BRADLEY *and* DAROFF'S

# NEUROLOGY
## IN CLINICAL PRACTICE

*We dedicate this book to our families in acknowledgement of their understanding and support.*

EIGHTH EDITION

BRADLEY *and* DAROFF'S

# NEUROLOGY IN CLINICAL PRACTICE

**Volume I**

**Joseph Jankovic, MD**
Professor of Neurology
Distinguished Chair in Movement Disorders
Director of Parkinson's Disease Center and Movement Disorders Clinic
Department of Neurology
Baylor College of Medicine
Houston, TX, United States

**John C. Mazziotta, MD, PhD**
Vice Chancellor of UCLA Health Sciences
Dean, David Geffen School of Medicine
CEO UCLA Health
University of California, Los Angeles
Los Angeles, CA, United States

**Scott L. Pomeroy, MD, PhD**
Bronson Crothers Professor of Neurology
Director, Intellectual and Developmental Disabilities Research Center
Harvard Medical School
Chair, Department of Neurology
Neurologist-in-Chief
Boston Children's Hospital
Boston, MA, United States

**Nancy J. Newman, MD**
LeoDelle Jolley Professor of Ophthalmology
Professor of Ophthalmology and Neurology
Instructor in Neurological Surgery, Emory University School of Medicine
Director, Section of Neuro-Ophthalmology
Emory Eye Center
Emory University
Atlanta, GA, United States

For additional online content visit ExpertConsult.com

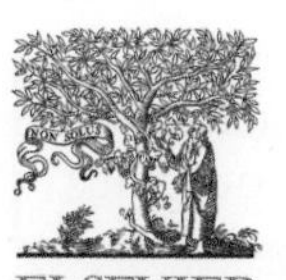

ELSEVIER Edinburgh London New York Oxford Philadelphia St Louis Sydney 2022

First edition 1991
Second edition 1996
Third edition 2000
Fourth edition 2004
Fifth edition 2008
Sixth edition 2012
Seventh edition 2016



**Notices**

Practitioners and researchers must always rely on their own experience and knowledge in evaluating and using any information, methods, compounds or experiments described herein. Because of rapid advances in the medical sciences, in particular, independent verification of diagnoses and drug dosages should be made. To the fullest extent of the law, no responsibility is assumed by Elsevier, authors, editors or contributors for any injury and/or damage to persons or property as a matter of products liability, negligence or otherwise, or from any use or operation of any methods, products, instructions, or ideas contained in the material herein.

**ISBN: 978-0-323-64261-3**

*Content Strategist:* Melanie Tucker
*Content Development Specialist:* Joanne Scott
*Project Manager:* Andrew Riley
*Design:* Margaret Reid
*Illustration Manager:* Paula Catalano
*Illustrator:* Joe Chovan
*Marketing Manager:* Claire McKenzie

Printed in India

Last digit is the print number: 9 8 7 6 5 4 3

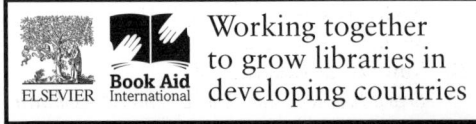

# CONTENTS

# PREFACE

From the very beginning, *Neurology in Clinical Practice* has served as a textbook of neurology that comprehensively covers the clinical neurosciences and provides, not only a description of neurological diseases and their pathophysiology, but also a practical approach to their diagnosis and management. Following the publication of the last edition our colleague, Dr. Robert Daroff, decided to step down. In recognition of his distinguished contributions from the inception, the book has been renamed as *"Bradley and Daroff's Neurology in Clinical Practice"*. We are delighted that Dr. Nancy Newman has joined the current team of editors. With her many scientific contributions to the field of neuro-ophthalmology and her long-standing commitment to excellence in neurologic education she is eminently qualified to continue Dr. Daroff's legacy.

In the preface to the 1991 first edition of this book, we forecast that major technological and research advances would soon reveal the underlying cause and potential treatment of an ever-increasing number of neurological diseases. This prediction has been realized. The three decades since that initial prediction have been marked with the excitement of new discoveries resulting from the blossoming of neurosciences. Advances in genetics, molecular biology, pharmacology, imaging, and surgery have revolutionized our approach to neurological disorders. Pathogenesis-targeted therapies, coupled with improved symptomatic management, have improved outcomes and changed the course of patients with many neurological diseases. Therapies are now available that slow the course of diseases such as multiple sclerosis and other neuroimmune disorders, neurologic and systemic neoplasms, and spinal muscular atrophy which until the past several years were relentlessly progressive. Advances in neuroimaging now enable the precise identification of functional regions and fine neuroanatomy of the human brain in health and disease. The important and challenging problems of neuroprotection are being addressed in both neurodegenerative disorders and acute injuries to the nervous system, such as stroke, hypoxic brain injury, and trauma. In line with this effort, basic science progress in areas of neuroplasticity and neural repair is yielding important results that should translate into disease-modifying therapies in the near future. New advances in immunology and the study of gut flora have important implications in the understanding of gut-brain interaction of many neurological disorders including Parkinson's disease.

When the first edition of this textbook was published, there was essentially no effective means of treating acute ischemic stroke. Today we have numerous opportunities to help such patients, and campaigns continue to educate the general public about the urgency of seeking treatment when stroke symptoms occur. These and other advances have changed neurology to a field in which interventions are increasingly improving the outcomes for patients with disorders that were previously considered to be untreatable.

The advent of teleneurology and wearables are increasingly used to assess neurologic symptoms and signs and to enhance access to medical providers. Teleneurology is now used by nearly all subspecialties, with a particular emphasis on patients who need intraoperative monitoring, critical care neurology, and stroke interventions.

To the benefit of patients, clinical neuroscience has partnered with engineering. Neuromodulation has become an important part of clinical therapy for patients with Parkinson's disease and other movement disorders, and has applications in pain management and seizure control. Along these same lines, brain-controlled devices are already helping to provide assistance to individuals whose mobility or communication skills are compromised. Recent advances in optogenetics have led to development of techniques that allow exploration and manipulation of neural circuitry, which likely have therapeutic applications in a variety of neurologic disorders.

Age-related neurodegenerative diseases, such as Alzheimer disease and Parkinson disease, are increasingly prevalent and represent a growing health and socioeconomic burden. A search for biomarkers that reliably identify a preclinical state and track progression of disease is an important goal for many neurodegenerative disorders. The costs in terms of suffering and hardship for patients and their families are too immense to quantify. As such, there is an urgent need for basic and clinical neuroscience to make progress in finding ways to delay the onset and slow progression of neurodegenerative disorders and, ultimately, prevent them.

There are startling new advances changing the neurosciences. The engineering of nanotechnologies into strategies to treat patients with neurological disorders is just beginning. Advances in genetics, including whole exome and whole genome sequencing, allow for not only discoveries of new genes, but also new disease mechanisms. Novel imaging techniques provide insights into connectivity deficits in sensory and motor networks that are associated with several neurological disorders. Innovative neurosurgical techniques and robotics are increasingly being utilized in enhancing function and optimizing quality of life of patients with neurological disorders.

We still have a long way to go to reach the ultimate goal of being able to understand and treat all neurological diseases. Neurology remains an intellectually exciting discipline, both because of the complexity of the nervous system and because of the insight that the pathophysiology of neurological disease provides into the workings of the brain and mind. Accordingly, we offer the eighth edition of *Neurology in Clinical Practice* as the updated comprehensive and most authoritative presentation of both the art and the science of neurology.

For this edition, the text has been rewritten and updated, and over 60 new authors have been added to the cadre of contributors. New chapters have been added covering ocular functional and structural investigations, cerebral palsy and palliative and end of life care, and chapters have been reorganized and consolidated. The eighth edition includes an interactive online version housed on *www.expertconsult.com*, which can be also downloaded for offline use on phones or tablets. The electronic version of the text contains even more video and audio material, as well as additional illustrations and references.

This new and expanded volume would not have been possible without the contributions of many colleagues throughout the world. We are deeply grateful to them for their selfless devotion to neurological education. We are also grateful to our Elsevier partners, Lucia Gunzel, Senior Content Development Manager, Joanne Scott, Deputy Content Development Manager and Melanie Tucker, Senior Acquisitions Editor, Neuroscience and Neurology who were key in drawing this project together. Additionally, we thank Andrew Riley, Senior Project Manager, without whose energy and efficiency we would not have achieved the high quality of production and rapidity of publication of this work. We also gratefully acknowledge the contributions of our readers, whose feedback regarding the print and online components of *Bradley and Daroff's Neurology in Clinical Practice* has been invaluable in refining and enhancing our educational goals. Finally, we wish to express our deep appreciation to our families for their support throughout this project and over the many decades of our shared lives.

**Joseph Jankovic, MD**
**John C. Mazziotta, MD, PhD**
**Scott L. Pomeroy, MD, PhD**
**Nancy J. Newman, MD**

# LIST OF CONTRIBUTORS

The editor(s) acknowledge and offer grateful thanks for the input of all previous editions' contributors, without whom this new edition would not have been possible.

**Bassel W. Abou-Khalil, MD**
Professor of Neurology
Director of Epilepsy Division, Neurology
Vanderbilt University Medical Center
Nashville, TN, USA

**Peter Adamczyk, MD**
Neurosciences Department Chair
Eden Medical Center
Castro Valley, CA, USA

**Bela Ajtai, MD, PhD**
Attending Neurologist
DENT Neurologic Institute
Amherst, NY, USA

**Jeffrey C. Allen, MD**
Director, Pediatric Neuro-oncology and Neurofibromatosis Programs
Department of Pediatrics, Division of Pediatric Hematology-Oncology
NYU Langone Medical Center
New York, NY, USA

**Brandon Ally, PhD**
Assistant Professor
Department of Neurology
Vanderbilt University
Nashville, TN, USA

**Andrea A. Almeida, MD**
BA Sports Neurology Fellow
Clinical Lecturer, Neurology
University of Michigan
Ann Arbor, MI, USA

**Anthony A. Amato, MD**
Vice-Chairman Neurology
Brigham and Women's Hospital;
Professor of Neurology
Harvard Medical School
Boston, MA, USA

**Michael J. Aminoff, MD, DSc, FRCP**
Distinguished Professor
Department of Neurology
School of Medicine
University of California
San Francisco, CA, USA

**Nicolaas C. Anderson, DO, MS**
Assistant Professor
Department of Neurology
Baylor College of Medicine
Houston, TX, USA

**Tetsuo Ashizawa, MD**
Professor
Department of Neurology
Houston Methodist Research Institute
Houston, TX, USA

**Hatim Attar, MD**
Assistant Professor of Neurology
Department of Neurology
Medical College of Wisconsin and Zablocki VA Medical Center, Milwaukee, WI
Milwaukee, WI, USA

**Alon Y. Avidan, MD, MPH**
Director, UCLA Sleep Disorders Center
Director, UCLA Neurology Clinic
University of California at Los Angeles
David Geffen School of Medicine at UCLA
Los Angeles, CA, USA

**Joachim M. Baehring, MD, DSc**
Associate Professor
Departments of Neurology, Neurosurgery and Medicine
Chief
Section of Neuro-Oncology
Yale Cancer Center
Yale School of Medicine
New Haven, CT, USA

**Asim K. Bag, MD**
Associate Member
Department of Diagnostic Imaging,
St. Jude Children's Research Hospital
Memphis, TN, USA

**Laura J. Balcer, MD, MSCE**
Professor of Neurology and Population Health
Vice Chair, Department of Neurology
NYU Langone Medical Center
New York, NY, USA

**Leomar Y. Ballester, MD, PhD**
Assistant Professor
Co-Director, Molecular Diagnostics Laboratory
Department of Pathology and Laboratory Medicine
Department of Neurosurgery
University of Texas Health Science Center at Houston, TX, USA

**Robert W. Baloh, MD**
Professor, Department of Neurology
Division of Head and Neck Surgery
University of California School of Medicine
Los Angeles, CA, USA

**Elizabeth Barkoudah, MD**
Program Director, Neurodevelopmental Disabilities Residency
Program Director, Children with Disabilities HMS Student Clerkship
Co-Director Cerebral Palsy and Spasticity Center
Department of Neurology
Boston, MA, USA

**Roger A. Barker, BA, MBBS, MRCP PhD**
Professor of Clinical Neuroscience
Honorary Consultant Neurologist
Department of Clinical Neurosciences
University of Cambridge
Addenbrooke's Hospital
Cambridge, UK

**Ryan Barmore, MD**
Adjunct Clinical Postdoctoral Associate
Neurology
University of Florida
Gainesville, FL, USA

**J.D. Bartleson, MD, FAAN**
Emeritus Professor of Neurology
Mayo Clinic
College of Medicine and Science
Rochester, MN, USA

**Amit Batla, MBBS MD DM (Neurology) FRCP**
Honorary Consultant Neurologist
National Hospital for Neurology and Neurosurgery and Royal Free London Hospital
UCL Queen Square Institute of Neurology, London, UK

**John David Beckham, MD**
Associate Professor
Departments of Medicine, Neurology, and Immunology and Microbiology
University of Colorado Anschutz Medical Campus
Aurora, CO, USA

**Leigh Beglinger, PhD**
Neuropsychologist
Elks Rehab System
Boise, ID, USA

**David H. Benninger, PD Dr**
Senior Consultant and Lecturer in Neurology
Department of Clinical Neurosciences
University Hospital of Lausanne (CHUV)
Lausanne, Switzerland

**Joseph R. Berger, MD, FACP, FAAN, FANA**
Professor of Neurology and Associate Chief of the Multiple Sclerosis Division
Perelman School of Medicine
University of Pennsylvania
Philadelphia, PA, USA

**José Biller, MD, FACP, FAAN, FAHA, FANA**
Professor and Chairman
Department of Neurology
Loyola University Chicago Stritch School of Medicine
Maywood, IL, USA

**David F. Black, MD**
Assistant Professor of Neurology and Radiology
Mayo Clinic
Rochester, MN, USA

**Nicholas Boulis, MD**
Associate Professor
Department of Neurosurgery, Emory University
Atlanta, GA, USA

**Michael P. Bowley, MD, PhD**
Staff Neurologist
Massachusetts General Hospital
Instructor
Harvard Medical School
Boston, MA, USA

**Sherri A. Braksick, MD**
Assistant Professor
Department of Neurology
Senior Associate Consultant
Neurosciences ICU
Mayo Clinic
Rochester, MN, USA

**Helen M. Bramlett, PhD**
Professor, Neurological Surgery
University of Miami Miller School of Medicine
Research Health Scientist, Research Service
Bruce W. Carter Department of Veterans Affairs Medical Center
Miami, FL, USA

**Steven M. Bromley, MD**
Director
Bromley Neurology
Audubon, NJ, USA

**Joseph Bruni, MD, FRCPC**
Consultant Neurologist
St. Michael's Hospital;
Associate Professor of Medicine
University of Toronto
Toronto, ON, Canada

**John C.M. Brust, AB, MD**
Professor of Neurology
Columbia University College of Physicians and Surgeons
New York, NY, USA

**W. Bryan Burnette, MD, MS**
Associate Professor
Pediatrics and Neurology
Vanderbilt University School of Medicine,
Nashville, TN, USA

**Carol Camfield, MD**
Professor Emeritus
Pediatrics
Dalhousie University
Halifax, NS, Canada

**Peter Camfield, MD**
Professor Emeritus
Pediatrics
Dalhousie University
Halifax, NS, Canada

**Alan Carson, MB, ChB, MD, FRCPsych, FRCP, MPhil**
Consultant Neuropsychiatrist
Senior Lecturer in Psychological Medicine
Department of Clinical Neurosciences
University of Edinburgh
Edinburgh, United Kingdom

**Dimitri Cassimatis, MD**
Associate Professor of Medicine
Emory University School of Medicine
Atlanta, GA, USA

**Robert Cavaliere, MD**
Assistant Professor
The Ohio State University
Columbus, OH, USA

**David A. Chad, MD**
Staff Neurologist
Reliant Medical Group
Saint Vincent Hospital
Worcester, MA, USA

**Vijay Chandran, MBBS, DM**
Clinical Fellow
Pacific Parkinson's Research Centre
University of British Columbia
Vancouver, BC, Canada

**Gisela Chelimsky, MD**
Professor of Paediatrics
The Medical College of Wisconsin
Milwaukee, WI, USA

**Thomas Chelimsky, MD**
Professor of Neurology
The Medical College of Wisconsin
Milwaukee, WI, USA

**Tanuja Chitnis, MD**
Professor of Neurology
Harvard Medical School
Boston, MA, USA

**Sudhansu Chokroverty, MD, FRCP**
Professor and Co-Chair
Program Director of Clinical Neurophysiology and Sleep Medicine
NJ Neuroscience Institute at JFK
Clinical Professor, Robert Wood Johnson Medical School
New Brunswick, NJ, USA

**Ugonma N. Chukwueke, MD**
Center for Neuro-Oncology
Dana-Farber Cancer Institute
Boston, MA, USA

**Paul E. Cooper, MD, FRCPC, FAAN**
Professor of Neurology,
Schulich School of Medicine and Dentistry and
University Hospital, London Health Sciences Centre,
London, ON, Canada

**Dany Cordeau, RN, PhD(c)**
Registered Nurse
Department of Sexology
Université du Québec à Montréal
Montreal, QC, Canada

**Frédérique Courtois, PhD**
Chair, Full Professor
Department of Sexology
Université du Quéébec à Montréal
Montreal, QC, Canada

**Claire J. Creutzfeldt, MD**
Harborview Comprehensive Stroke Center
University of Washington
Seattle, WA, USA

**Josep Dalmau, MD, PhD**
ICREA Research Professor
Hospital Clinic, IDIBAPS/University of Barcelona
Barcelona, Spain, Adjunct Professor
Neurology
University of Pennsylvania
Philadelphia, PA, USA

**Robert B. Daroff, MD**
Professor and Chair Emeritus
Department of Neurology
Case Western Reserve School of Medicine
University Hospitals Case Medical Center
Cleveland, OH, USA

**Ranan DasGupta, MBBChir, MA, MD, FRCS(Urol)**
Consultant Urological Surgeon
Department of Urology
Imperial College Healthcare NHS Trust
London, UK

**Mariel B. Deutsch, MD**
Behavioral Neurology and Neuropsychiatry Fellow
V.A. Greater Los Angeles Healthcare System
David Geffen School of Medicine at UCLA
Los Angeles, CA, USA

**Michael W. Devereaux, MD**
Professor of Neurology
University Hospitals Case Medical Center
Case Western Reserve University
Cleveland, OH, USA

**Melissa DiBacco, MD**
Postdoctoral Clinical Research Fellow
Department of Neurology – Epilepsy Division
Boston Children's Hospital
Boston, MA, USA

**W. Dalton Dietrich, PhD**
Scientific Director
The Miami Project to Cure Paralysis
Professor of Neurological Surgery, Neurology, Cell Biology and Biomedical Engineering
University of Miami
Leonard M. Miller School of Medicine
Center
Miami, FL, USA

**Pradeep Dinakar, MD, MS, MBA, FAAP**
Director, Interventional Pain Program
Boston Children's Hospital
Pain Management Center
Mass General Brigham
Assistant Professor of Anesthesiology
Harvard Medical School Boston, MA, USA

**Bruce H. Dobkin, MD**
Professor of Neurology
University of California Los Angeles
Los Angeles, CA, USA

**Richard L. Doty, BS, MA, PhD**
Director, Smell and Taste Center
Hospital of the University of Pennsylvania
Professor, Otorhinolaryngology: Head and Neck Surgery
University of Pennsylvania, Perelman School of Medicine
Philadelphia, PA, USA

**Gary R. Duckwiler, MD**
Professor and Director Interventional Neuroradiology
Director, INR Fellowship Program
Co-Director UCLA HHT Center of Excellence
David Geffen School of Medicine at UCLA
Los Angeles, CA, USA

**Ronald G. Emerson, MD**
Attending Neurologist and Director Intraoperative Monitoring Program
Hospital for Special Surgery
New York, NY, USA

**Michelle T. Fabian, MD**
Assistant Professor
Icahn School of Medicine at Mount Sinai
New York, NY, USA

**Alireza Faridar, MD**
Assistant professor
Neurology
Houston Methodist
Houston, TX, USA

**Conor Fearon, BE, MB, BCh, BAO**
Clinical Fellow
Department of Neurology
University of Toronto
Toronto, ON, Canada

**Marcia V. Felker, MD**
Clinical Assistant Professor of Pediatric Neurology
Indiana University School of Medicine
Riley Hospital for Children
Indianapolis, IN, USA

**Richard D. Fessler, MD, PhD**
Neurosurgery Resident
Rush University Medical Center
Chicago, IL, USA

**Richard G. Fessler, MD, PhD**
Professor, Neurosurgery
Rush University Medical Center,
Chicago, IL, USA

**Kathryn C. Fitzgerald, ScD**
Assistant Professor of Neurology and Epidemiology, Johns Hopkins University, Baltimore, MD, USA

**Laura Flores-Sarnat, MD**
Adjunct Research Professor of Clinical Neurosciences and Paediatrics
University of Calgary and Alberta Children's Hospital Research Institute
Calgary, AB, Canada

**Brent L. Fogel, MD, PhD**
Associate Professor of Neurology and Human Genetics
David Geffen School of Medicine
University of California, Los Angeles
Los Angeles, CA, USA

**Brent P. Forester, MD, MSc**
Associate Professor of Psychiatry
Chief, Division of Geriatric Psychiatry
McLean Hospital, Harvard Medical School, Belmont, MA, USA

**Jennifer E. Fugate, DO**
Assistant Professor of Neurology
Divisions of Critical Care and Cerebrovascular Neurology
Mayo Clinic
Rochester, MN, USA

**Martin J. Gallagher, MD, PhD**
Associate Professor of Neurology
Vanderbilt University School of Medicine
Nashville, TN, USA

**Sharon L. Gardner, MD**
Associate Professor, Pediatrics
Stephen D Hassenfeld Childrens Center For Cancer and Blood Disorders
New York University Langone Medical Center
New York, NY, USA

**Jarred Garfinkle, MDCM, MSc, FRCPC**
Neonatologist, Department of Pediatrics
McGill University/Montreal Children's Hospital Montreal, QC, Canada

**Ivan Garza, MD**
Assistant Professor of Neurology
Department of Neurology
Mayo Clinic
Rochester, MN, USA

**Claudio Melo de Gusmao, MD**
Clinical Director, Movement Disorders Program
Neurology
Boston Children's Hospital
Boston, MA, USA

**Carissa Gehl, PhD**
Clinical Associate Professor
Department of Psychiatry
University of Iowa
Iowa City, IA, USA

**Christopher D. Geiger, DO**
Assistant Professor
Department of Neurology
Case Western Reserve School of Medicine
University Hospitals Cleveland Medical Center
Cleveland, OH, USA

**David S. Geldmacher, MD**
Professor
Department of Neurology
University of Alabama at Birmingham
Birmingham, AL, USA

**Carter Gerard, MD**
Neurosurgery Resident
Rush University Medical Center
Chicago, IL, USA

**Daniel H. Geschwind, MD, PhD**
David Geffen School of Medicine
University of California, Los Angeles
Los Angeles, CA, USA

**Michael D. Geschwind, MD, PhD, FAAN, FANA**
Professor, Michael J. Homer Family Chair in Neurology
Department of Neurology, Memory and Aging Center
University of California, San Francisco
San Francisco, CA, USA

**Katherine A. Gifford, PhD**
Assistant Professor of Neurology
Vanderbilt University Medical Center
Nashville, TN, USA

**K. Michael Gibson, PhD**
Professor of Pharmacotherapy
College of Pharmacy and Pharmaceutical Sciences
Washington State University
Spokane, WA, USA

**Meredith R. Golomb, MD, MSc**
Associate Professor
Division of Child Neurology
Department of Neurology
Indiana University School of Medicine
Indianapolis, IN, USA

**Rachel Goode, MD**
Assistant Professor of Pediatrics
Department of Pediatrics
Vanderbilt University Medical Center
Nashville, TN, USA

**Jonathan Graff-Radford, MD**
Assistant Professor of Neurology
Mayo Clinic College of Medicine
Rochester, MN, USA

**Olivia Groover, MD**
Assistant Professor of Neurology
Emory University
Atlanta, GA, USA

**Jeffrey T. Guptill, MD, MA, MHS**
Professor of Neurology
Director, Duke University School of Medicine, Faculty
Duke Clinical Research Unit
Durham, NC, USA

**Cecil D. Hahn, MD, MPH**
Associate Professor
Paediatrics (Neurology)
University of Toronto
Director
Critical Care EEG Monitoring Program
The Hospital for Sick Children
Toronto, ON, Canada

**Christine Hall, PhD**
Adjunct Professor
Department of Psychology
Emory University
Atlanta, GA, USA

**Mark Hallett, MD**
Chief, Human Motor Control Section
National Institute of Neurological Disorders and Stroke
National Institutes of Health
Bethesda, MD, USA

**Aline I. Hamati, MD**
Clinical Assistant Professor of Pediatric Neurology
Indiana University School of Medicine
Riley Hospital for Children
Indianapolis, IN, USA

**David Hart, MD**
Director, Neurosurgery Spine
The Neurological Institute
University Hospitals Case Medical Center
Associate Professor of Neurological Surgery
Department of Neurological Surgery
Case Western Reserve University
Cleveland, OH, USA

**Sabine Hellwig, MD**
Neurologist
Assistant in Psychiatry
Department of Psychiatry and Psychotherapy
University Hospital Freiburg
Freiburg, Germany

**Karl Herholz, MD**
Professor in Clinical Neuroscience
Division of Neuroscience and Experimental Psychology
University of Manchester
Manchester, UK

**Alan Hill, MD, PhD**
Professor, Pediatrics
University of British Columbia
Child Neurologist
British Columbia's Children's Hospital
Vancouver, BC, Canada

**Benjamin D. Hill, PhD**
Assistant Professor
Psychology Department/CCP
University of South Alabama
Mobile, AL, USA

**Fred H. Hochberg, MD**
Visiting Scientist, Neurosurgery
University of California at San Diego
San Diego, CA, USA

**Kristin Huntoon, PhD, DO**
University of Texas
MD Anderson Cancer Center
Houston, TX, USA

**Jason T. Huse, MD, PhD**
Associate Professor
Departments of Pathology and Translational Molecular Pathology
University of Texas MD Anderson Cancer Center
Houston, TX, USA

**Monica P. Islam, MD, FAES, FACNS**
Associate Professor of Clinical Pediatrics
Section of Child Neurology
Nationwide Children's Hospital
The Ohio State University College of Medicine
Columbus, OH, USA

**Michael Iv, MD**
Clinical Associate Professor, Radiology
Stanford University
Stanford, CA, USA

**Reza Jehan, MD**
Professor
Department of Radiological Sciences
David Geffen School of Medicine at UCLA
Los Angeles, CA, USA

**Joseph Jankovic, MD**
Professor of Neurology
Distinguished Chair in Movement Disorders
Director of Parkinson's Disease Center and Movement Disorders Clinic
Department of Neurology
Baylor College of Medicine
Houston, TX, USA

**S. Andrew Josephson, MD**
Carmen Castro Franceschi and Gladyne K. Mitchell
Neurohospitalist Distinguished Professor and Chair
Department of Neurology
University of California, San Francisco
San Francisco, CA, USA

**Tudor G. Jovin, MD**
Neurology
Cooper University Hospital
Camden, NJ, USA

**Min K. Kang, MD**
Assistant Clinical Professor
Department of Neurology
University of California, San Francisco
San Francisco, CA, USA

**Matthias A. Karajannis, MD, MS**
Chief, Pediatric Neuro-Oncology Service
Attending Physician
Department of Pediatrics
Memorial Sloan Kettering Cancer Center
New York, NY, USA

**Carlos S. Kase, MD**
Professor of Neurology
Emory University School of Medicine
Atlanta, GA, USA

**Bashar Katirji, MD**
Director, Neuromuscular Center and EMG Laboratory
University Hospitals Cleveland Medical Center
Professor
Department Neurology
Case Western Reserve University School of Medicine
Cleveland, OH, USA

**Kevin A. Kerber, MD**
Professor
University of Michigan Health System
Ann Arbor, MI, USA

**Geoffrey A. Kerchner, MD, PhD**
Global Development Leader
Product Development Neuroscience
F. Hoffman-La Roche, Ltd.
Basel, Switzerland

**Ryan Khanna, MD**
Neurosurgery Resident
Rush University Medical Center
Chicago, IL, USA

**Samia J. Khoury, MD**
Director of Abou-Haider Neuroscience Institute
Professor of Neurology
American University of Beirut Medical Center
Beirut, lebanon;
Visiting Professor of Neurology
Harvard Medical School
Boston, MA, USA

**Howard S. Kirshner, BA, MD**
Professor and Vice Chairman
Department of Neurology
Vanderbilt University Medical Center
Nashville, TN, USA

**Stefan Klöppel, MD**
Head of Memory Clinic
Department of Psychiatry and Psychotherapy
University Medical Center Freiburg
Freiburg, Germany

**Anita A. Koshy, MD**
Assistant Professor
Department of Neurology
Department of Immunobiology
University of Arizona, College of Medicine
Tucson, AZ, USA

**Stephen C. Krieger, MD**
Associate Professor of Neurology
Corinne Goldsmith Dickinson Center for MS
Icahn School of Medicine at Mount Sinai
New York, NY, USA

**Abhay Kumar, MD**
Assistant Professor
Neurology
Saint Louis University
Saint Louis, MO, USA

**John F. Kurtzke, MD, FACP, FAAN**
Professor Emeritus, Neurology
Georgetown University;
Consultant, Neurology
Veterans Affairs Medical Center
Washington, DC, USA

**Jeffrey S. Kutcher, MD, FAAN**
Director, Kutcher Clinic for Sports Neurology
Brighton, Michigan
Park City, UT, USA

**Sheng-Han Kuo, MD**
Assistant Professor
Department of Neurology
College of Physicians and Surgeons
Columbia University
New York, NY, USA

**Anthony E. Lang, MD, FRCPC**
Professor
Department of Medicine, Neurology
University of Toronto
Director of Movement Disorders Center and the Edmond J. Safra Program in Parkinson's Disease
Toronto Western Hospital
Toronto, ON, Canada

**Patrick J.M. Lavin, MB, BCh, BAO, MRCPI**
Professor, Neurology and Ophthalmology
Department of Neurology
Vanderbilt University Medical School
Nashville, TN, USA

**Alice Lawrence, PT, MD**
Assistant Professor of Pediatrics
Department of Pediatrics
Vanderbilt University Medical Center
Nashville, TN, USA

**Marc A. Lazzaro, MD**
Assistant Professor of Neurology and Neurosurgery
Director, Neurointerventional Fellowship Training Program
Medical Director, Telestroke Program
Medical College of Wisconsin and Froedtert Hospital
Milwaukee, WI, USA

**Sönke Langner**
Department of Diagnostic Radiology and Neuroradiology, University Medicine, Greifswald, Germany

**David S. Liebeskind, MD, FAAN, FAHA**
Professor of Neurology
Neurology Director, Stroke Imaging
Co-Director, UCLA Cerebral Blood Flow Laboratory
Director, UCLA Vascular Neurology Residency Program;
Associate Neurology Director, UCLA Stroke Center
UCLA Department of Neurology
Los Angeles, CA, USA

**Chih-Chun Lin, MD, PhD**
Movement Disorders fellow
Department of Neurology
College of Physicians and Surgeons
Columbia University
New York, NY, USA

**Eric Lindzen, MD, PhD**
Jacobs Neurological Institute School of Medicine and Biomedical Sciences
State University of New York at Buffalo
Buffalo, NY, USA

**Alan H. Lockwood, MD, FAAN, FANA**
Emeritus Professor
Neurology and Nuclear Medicine
University at Buffalo
Buffalo, NY, USA

**Glenn Lopate, MD**
Professor of Neurology
Department of Neurology
Washington University School of Medicine
Saint Louis, MO, USA

**Fred D. Lublin, MD**
Saunders Family Professor of Neurology;
Director, The Corinne Goldsmith Dickinson Center for MS
Icahn School of Medicine at Mount Sinai
New York, NY, USA

**Michael J. Lyerly, MD**
Associate Professor
Director, Birmingham VA Medical Center Stroke Center
Department of Neurology
University of Alabama at Birmingham
Birmingham, AL, USA

**Robert L. Macdonald, MD, PhD**
Professor of Neurology
Vanderbilt University Medical Center
Nashville, TN, USA

**Devin D. Mackay, MD**
Associate Professor of Neurology, Ophthalmology and Neurosurgery
Director of Neuro-Ophthalmology
Indiana University School of Medicine
Indianapolis, IN, USA

**Robert Mallery, MD**
Assistant Professor
Neurology
Brigham and Women's Hospital
Boston, MA, USA

**Joseph C. Masdeu, MD, PhD**
Graham Family Distinguished Chair in Neurological Sciences
Director, Nantz National Alzheimer Center and Neuroimaging
Houston Methodist Neurological Institute
Houston Methodist Hospital
Houston, TX, USA

**John C. Mazziotta, MD, PhD**
Vice Chancellor of UCLA Health Sciences
Dean, David Geffen School of Medicine
CEO UCLA Health
University of California, Los Angeles
Los Angeles, CA, USA

**Mario F. Mendez, MD, PhD**
Director, Behavioral Neurology Program, and Professor Neurology and Psychiatry
David Geffen School of Medicine at UCLA
Director, Neurobehavior
V.A. Greater Los Angeles Healthcare System
Los Angeles, CA, USA

**Philipp T. Meyer, MD, PhD**
Medical Director and Professor
Department of Nuclear Medicine
Medical Center - University of Freiburg
Faculty of Medicine, University of Freiburg
Freiburg, Germany

**Dominique S. Michaud, ScD**
Professor, Department of Public Health and Community Medicine
Tufts University School of Medicine
Boston, MA, USA

**Amanda Miller, LMSW**
Social Worker
University of Iowa Huntington's Disease Society of America Center of Excellence
University of Iowa Carver College of Medicine
Iowa City, IA, USA

**Karl E. Misulis, MD, PhD**
Professor of Clinical Neurology and Clinical Biomedical Informatics
Director of Neurology Hospitalist Service
Vanderbilt University School of Medicine
Nashville, TN, USA

**Hiroshi Mitsumoto, MD, DSc**
Director
Eleanor and Lou Gehrig MDA/ALS Research Center
The Neurological Institute
New York, NY, USA

**Brian Murray, MB, BCh, BAO, MSc**
Consultant Neurologist
Hermitage Medical Clinic
Old Lucan Road
Dublin, Ireland

**E. Lee Murray, MD, FACP**
Clinical Assistant Professor of Neurology
University of Tennessee Health Science Center
Memphis, TN, USA
Attending Neurologist
West Tennessee Neuroscience
Jackson, TN, USA

**Evan D. Murray, MD**
Assistant in Neurology/ Instructor in Neurology
Department of Neurology
McLean Hospital/ Massachusetts General Hospital/ Harvard Medical School
Belmont, MA, USA;
Director, Traumatic Brain Injury Service
Manchester VA Medical Center
Manchester, NH, USA

**Fadi Nahab, MD**
Associate Professor of Neurology and Pediatrics
Emory University
Atlanta, GA, USA

**Ruth Nass, MD**
Professor of Child Neurology, Child and Adolescent Psychiatry, and Pediatrics
New York University Langone Medical Center
New York, NY, USA

**Lakshmi Nayak, MD**
Assistant Professor of Neurology, Harvard Medical School
Center for Neuro-Oncology, Dana-Farber/ Brigham and Women's Cancer Center
Boston, MA, USA

**Nancy J. Newman, MD**
LeoDelle Jolley Professor of Ophthalmology
Professor of Ophthalmology and Neurology
Instructor in Neurological Surgery, Emory University School of Medicine
Director, Section of Neuro-Ophthalmology
Emory Eye Center
Emory University
Atlanta, GA, USA

**Thanh N. Nguyen, MD**
Neurology, Radiology
Boston Medical Center
Boston University School of Medicine
Boston, MA, USA

**Raul G. Nogueira, MD**
Neurology
Marcus Stroke and Neuroscience Center
Grady Memorial Hospital
Emory University School of Medicine
Atlanta, GA, USA

**John G. Nutt, MD**
Professor of Neurology
Oregon Health & Science University
Portland, OR, USA

**Marc R. Nuwer, MD, PhD**
Department Head, Clinical Neurophysiology
Ronald Reagan UCLA Medical Center;
Professor, Neurology
David Geffen School of Medicine at UCLA
Los Angeles, CA, USA

**D. David O'Banion, MD FAAP**
Assistant Professor of Pediatrics, Developmental and Behavioral Pediatrics, Neurology
Emory University School of Medicine
Children's Healthcare of Atlanta Pediatrics Institute
Atlanta, GA, USA

**Michael S. Okun, MD**
Adelaide Lackner Professor of Neurology and Neurosurgery
UF Center for Movement Disorders and Neurorestoration
Gainesville, FL, USA

**Justin J.F. O'Rourke, PhD**
Clinical Neuropsychologist
South Texas Veterans Healthcare System
San Antonio, TX, USA

**Claudia R. Padilla, MD**
Behavioral Neurology and Neuropsychiatry Fellow
David Geffen School of Medicine
University of California at Los Angeles
Neurobehavior Unit
VA Greater Los Angeles Healthcare System
Los Angeles, CA, USA

**Jalesh N. Panicker, MD, DM, MRCP(UK)**
Consultant and Honorary Senior Lecturer
Department of Uroneurology
The National Hospital for Neurology and Neurosurgery and UCL Institute of Neurology
London, UK

**Leila Parand, MD**
Behavioral Neurology Fellow
David Geffen School of Medicine
University of California at Los Angeles
V.A. Greater Los Angeles Healthcare System
Los Angeles, CA, USA

**Jane S. Paulsen, PhD**
Professor
Department of Neurology
University of Wisconsin-Madison
Madison, WI, USA

**Phillip L. Pearl, MD**
Director of Epilepsy and Clinical Neurophysiology
William G. Lennox Chair, Department of Neurology
Boston Children's Hospital
Professor of Neurology, Harvard Medical School
Boston, MA, USA

**Zhongxing Peng-Chen, MD**
Neurologist
Movement Disorder Specialist
Neurología
Universidad del Desarrollo, Hospital Padre Hurtado
Facultad de Medicina Clínica Alemana
Santiago, Chile

**David L. Perez, MD, MMSc**
Assistant Professor of Neurology
Departments of Neurology and Psychiatry
Massachusetts General Hospital
Harvard Medical School
Boston, MA, USA

**Ronald C. Petersen, PhD, MD**
Professor of Neurology
Cora Kanow Professor of Alzheimer Disease Research
Department of Neurology
Mayo Clinic College of Medicine
Rochester, MN, USA

**Ronald F. Pfeiffer, MD**
Professor
Department of Neurology
Oregon Health & Science University
Portland, OR, USA

**Robert D.S. Pitceathly, MBChB, PhD**
MRC Clinician Scientist and Honorary Consultant Neurologist
Department of Neuromuscular Diseases
University College London Queen Square Institute of Neurology and
The National Hospital for Neurology and Neurosurgery
London, UK

**Scott L. Pomeroy, MD, PhD**
Bronson Crothers Professor of Neurology
Director, Intellectual and Developmental Disabilities
Research Center
Harvard Medical School
Chair, Department of Neurology
Neurologist-in-Chief
Boston Children's Hospital
Boston, MA, USA

**Sashank Prasad, MD**
Associate Professor of Neurology
Harvard Medical School
Chief, Division of Neuro-Ophthalmology
Brigham and Women's Hospital
Director, Harvard-Brigham and Women's-Massachusetts
General Hospital Neurology Residence Program
Boston, MA, USA

**Bruce H. Price, MD**
Chief, Department of Neurology
McLean Hospital
Associate Neurologist
Massachusetts General Hospital
Associate Professor of Neurology
Harvard Medical School
Boston, MA, USA

**Raymond S. Price, MD**
Associate Professor of Clinical Neurology and Neurology Residency Program Director
Perelman School of Medicine
University of Pennsylvania
Philadelphia, PA, USA

**Louis J. Ptáček, MD**
Distinguished Professor
Department of Neurology
University of California, San Francisco
San Francisco, CA, USA

**Alejandro A. Rabinstein, MD**
Professor
Department of Neurology
Consultant
Neurosciences ICU
Mayo Clinica
Rochester, MN, USA

**Vijay Ramaswamy, MD, PhD, FRCPC**
Assistant Professor and Staff Neuro-Oncologist
Division of Haematology/Oncology
Departments of Medical Biophysics and Paediatrics
Hospital for Sick Children and University of Toronto
Toronto, ON, Canada

**Tyler Reimschisel, MD, MHPE**
Founding Associate Provost for Interprofessional Education
Research and Collaborative Practice
Case Western Reserve University and Cleveland Clinic
Cleveland, OH, USA

**Bernd F. Remler, MD**
Professor of Neurology and Ophthalmology
Departments of Neurology and Ophthalmology
Medical College of Wisconsin
Chief, Section of Neurology, Zablocki VA Medical Center, Milwaukee, WI
Milwaukee, WI, USA

**Michel Rijntjes, MD**
Department of Neurology and Neuroscience
University Medical Center Freiburg
Freiburg, Germany

**E. Steve Roach, MD**
Professor of Neurology
University of Texas Dell Medical School
Austin, TX, USA

**Carrie E. Robertson, MD**
Assistant Professor
Department of Neurology
Mayo Clinic
Rochester, MN, USA

**Maisha T. Robinson, MD, MS**
Departments of Neurology and Family Medicine
Mayo Clinic
Jacksonville, FL, USA

**Michael Ronthal, MbBCh, FRCP, FRCPE, FCP(SA)**
Professor of Neurology Emeritus
Department of Neurology
Beth Israel Deaconess Medical Center
Harvard Medical School
Boston, MA, USA

**Karen L. Roos, MD**
John and Nancy Nelson Professor of Neurology
Department of Neurology
Indiana University School of Medicine
Indianapolis, IN, USA

**Ashley M. Roque, MD**
Assistant Professor
Department of Neuro-Oncology
Mount Sinai Hospital
New York, NY, USA

**Gary A. Rosenberg, MD**
Professor of Neurology
Director, UNM Center for Memory and Aging
University of New Mexico Health Sciences Center
Albuquerque, NM, USA

**Myrna R. Rosenfeld, MD, PhD**
Senior Investigator
Neuroimmunology Program
Hospital Clinical/IDIBAPS
Barcelona, Spain
Adjunct Professor, Neurology
University of Pennsylvania
Philadelphia, PA, USA

**Janet C. Rucker, MD**
Bernard A. and Charlotte Marden Professor
Departments of Neurology and Ophthalmology
New York University School of Medicine
New York, NY, USA

**Sean D. Ruland, DO**
Professor
Department of Neurology
Loyola University Chicago Stritch School of Medicine
Maywood, IL, USA

**Delaram Safarpour, MD, MSCE**
Assistant Professor of Neurology
Department of Neurology
Oregon Health and Science University
Portland, OR, USA

**Donald B. Sanders, MD**
Professor of Neurology
Duke University Medical School
Durham, NC, USA

**Harvey B. Sarnat, MS, MD, FRCPC**
Professor
Departments of Paediatrics, Pathology (Neuropathology)
and Clinical Neurosciences
University of Calgary, Cumming School of Medicine
Calgary, AB, Canada

**Jeffrey L. Saver, MD, FAHA, FAAN, FANA**
Professor of Neurology
Senior Associate Vice Chair for Clinical Research
Department of Neurology
Director, UCLA Comprehensive Stroke and Vascular Neurology Program
David Geffen School of Medicine at UCLA
Los Angeles, CA, USA

**Komal T. Sawlani, MD**
Assistant Professor
Department of Neurology
Case Western Reserve University School of Medicine
Cleveland, OH, USA

**Anthony H.V. Schapira, MD, DSc, FRCP, FMedSci**
Chairman and Professor of Clinical Neurosciences
Department of Clinical and Movement Neurosciences
University College London Queen Square Institute of Neurology
London, UK

**David Schiff, MD**
Harrison Distinguished Teaching Professor
Departments of Neurology, Neurological Surgery, and Medicine
University of Virginia School of Medicine
Charlottesville, VA, USA

**Michael J. Schneck, MD, FACP, FAAN, FAHA, FANA**
Professor Department of Neurology Loyola University Chicago
Stritch School of Medicine
Maywood, IL, USA

**Kirsten M. Scott, MRCP, PhD**
Neurology Registrar
Department of Neurology
Addenbrooke's hospital
Cambridge, UK

**Meagan D. Seay, DO**
Assistant Professor
Department of Ophthalmology and Visual Sciences
Assistant Professor
Department of Neurology
University of Utah
Moran Eye Center
UT, USA

**D. Malcolm Shaner, MD, FAAN**
Clinical Professor of Neurology
Department of Neurology
David Geffen School of Medicine, UCLA
Kaiser Permanente West Los Angeles Medical Center
Los Angeles, CA, USA

**Kaveh Sharzehi, MD, MS**
Assistant Professor of Medicine
Department of Medicine
Division of Gastroenterology and Hepatology
Oregon Health & Science University
Portland, OR, USA

**Ashkan Shoamanesh, MD, FRCPC**
Assistant Professor of Medicine (Neurology)
Director, Hemorrhagic Stroke Research Program
Marta and Owen Boris Chair in Stroke Research and Care
McMaster University / Population Health Research Institute
Hamilton, ON, Canada

**Reet Sidhu, MD**
Director, Developmental Neurology Program
Assistant Professor of Pediatrics, Neurology
Emory University School of Medicine
Children's Healthcare of Atlanta Pediatrics Institute
Atlanta, GA, USA

**Jonathan H. Smith, MD, FAHS**
Associate Professor of Neurology
Department of Neurology
Mayo Clinic
Scottsdale, AZ, USA

**Laura A. Snyder, MD, FAANS**
Attending Neurosurgeon
Barrow Neurological Institute
Phoenix, AZ, USA

**Yuen T. So, MD, PhD**
Professor of Neurology
School of Medicine
Stanford University
Palo Alto, CA, USA

**Marylou V. Solbrig, MD**
Formerly Professor
Departments of Medicine (Neurology) and Medical Microbiology
University of Manitoba
Winnipeg, MB, Canada

**Siddharth Srivastava, MD**
Instructor of Neurology
Department of Neurology
Boston Children's Hospital
Harvard Medical School
Boston, MA, USA

**Martina Stippler, MD, AANS, FACS**
Director of Neurotrauma
Department of Neurosurgery Harvard Medical School
Beth Israel Deaconess Medical Center
Boston, MA, USA

**Jon Stone, MB ChB FRCP PhD**
Honorary Professor (University of Edinburgh)
Department Clinical Neurosciences
Western General Hospital
Edinburgh, UK

**Jerry W. Swanson, MD, MHPE**
Professor of Neurology
Department of Neurology
Mayo Clinic College of Medicine and Science
Rochester, MN, USA

**Viktor Szeder, MD, PhD, MSc**
Associate Clinical Professor
Department of Radiological Sciences
David Geffen School of Medicine at UCLA
Los Angeles, CA, USA

**Lee A. Tan, MD**
Assistant Professor
Department of Neurosurgery
UCSF Medical Center
San Francisco, CA, USA

**Satoshi Tateshima, MD, DMSc**
Professor
Division of Interventional Neuroradiology
Department of Radiological Sciences
Ronald Reagan UCLA Medical Center
David Geffen School of Medicine at UCLA
Los Angeles, CA, USA

**Boon Lead Tee, MD, MSc**
Assistant Professor
Department of Neurology
Memory and Aging Center
University of California, San Francisco
San Francisco, CA, USA

**Stefan J. Teipel, MD**
Head of Section for Gerontopsychosomatic and Dementia Diseases
Deputy DZNE Site Speaker Rostock
Greifswald and Head of the Section for Clinical Research
Clinic for Psychosomatic and Psychotherapeutical Medicine
Section of Gerontopsychosomatic
Universitiy Medicine Rostock
German Center for Neurodegenerative Diseases, Site Rostock/Greifswald
Rostock, Germany

**Reena P. Thomas, MD PhD**
Clinical Assistant Professor
Division of Neuro-Oncology
Department of Neurology
Stanford University
Stanford, CA, USA

**Philip D. Thompson, MBBS PhD FRACP**
Emeritus Professor of Neurology
Department of Medicine
University of Adelaide
Adelaide, SA, Australia

**Matthew J. Thurtell, MBBS, MSc, FRACP**
Associate Professor, Ophthalmology and Neurology
Director, Neuro-Ophthalmology Service
Department of Ophthalmology and Visual Sciences
Department of Neurology
University of Iowa
Iowa City, IA, USA

**Robert L. Tomsak, MD, PhD**
Professor of Ophthalmology and Neurology
Wayne State University School of Medicine
Specialist in Neuro-ophthalmology
Kresge Eye Institute
Detroit, MI, USA

**Bryan Tsao, MD, MBA, FAAN, FANA**
Professor and Chair
Department of Neurology
Loma Linda University Health
School of Medicine
Loma Linda, CA, USA

**Chris Turner, FRCP PhD**
Consultant Neurologist
Queen Square Centre for Neuromuscular Diseases
The National Hospital for Neurology and Neurosurgery
Queen Square
London, UK

**Kenneth L. Tyler, MD**
Louise Baum Endowed Chair
Chairman of the Department of Neurology
University of Colorado School of Medicine
Aurora, CO, USA

**Stan H.M. Van Uum, MD, PhD, FRCPC**
Professor of Medicine,
Schulich School of Medicine and Dentistry,
St. Joseph's Health Care
London, ON, Canada

**Ashok Verma, MD, DM, MBA, FAAN, FANA**
Professor of Neurology
Staff Neurologist, Miami VA Medical Center
Director, Neuromuscular Medicine Fellowship Training Program
Medical Director, Bruce W. Carter VAMC ALS Program
Department of Neurology
University of of Miami Miller School of Medicine
Miami, FL, USA

**Michael Wall, MD**
Professor of Ophthalmology and Neurology
University of Iowa, College of Medicine
Iowa City, IA, USA

**Mitchell T. Wallin, MD, MPH**
Associate Professor of Neurology, Department of Neurology,
George Washington University & University of Maryland
Washington, DC, USA

**Leo H. Wang, MD, PhD**
Associate Professor of Neurology
Department of Neurology
University of Washington School of Medicine
Seattle, WA, USA

**Karin Weissenborn, MD, FRCP**
Associate Professor
Clinic for Neurology
Hannover Medical School
Hannover, Germany

**Cornelius Weiller, MD**
Director and Chair
Department of Neurology and Clinical Neuroscience Medical Faculty
University Hospital Freiberg
Freiberg, Germany

**Patrick Y. Wen, MD**
Center for Neuro-Oncology
Dana-Farber Cancer Institute
Boston, MA, USA

**Mark A. Whealy, MD**
Assistant Professor of Neurology
Department of Neurology
Mayo Clinic Rochester
Rochester, MN, USA

**Eelco F.M. Wijdicks, MD PhD**
Professor of Neurology
Consultant Neurosciences intensive Care Unit
Division of Neurocritical Care and Hospital Neurology
Mayo Clinic
Rochester, MN, USA

**Stephen M. Wilson, PhD**
Associate Professor
Department of Hearing and Speech Sciences
Vanderbilt University Medical Center
Nashville, TN, USA

**Daniel Winkel, MD**
Assistant Professor of Neurology
Department of Neurology
Emory University School of Medicine
Atlanta, GA, USA

**Oleg Y. Yerstein, MD**
Director
Center for Memory and Cognitive Disorders
Lahey Hospital and Medical Center
Los Angeles, CA, USA

**Osama O. Zaidat, MD, MS**
Neuroscience Institute
Bon Secours Mercy Health System
St Vincent Hospital
Toledo, OH, USA

# VIDEO TABLE OF CONTENTS

**Chapter 101 Video 5** Middle-Aged Woman with Restless Legs Syndrome

*(From Kryger, M. H. Gallery of Patient Interview Chapters. Atlas of Clinical Sleep Medicine,Second Edition. Copyright © 2014, 2010 by Saunders, an imprint of Elsevier Inc., Chapter 20, 478-482.)*

**Chapter 101 Video 6** Restless Legs Syndrome with Periodic Limb Movements During Sleep (x25)

*(From Kryger, M. H. Gallery of Sleep Laboratory Chapter Findings. Atlas of Clinical Sleep Medicine,Second Edition. Copyright © 2014, 2010 by Saunders, an imprint of Elsevier Inc., Chapter 21, 483-495.)*

**Chapter 101 Video 7** Periodic Limb Movements in Sleep

*(From Sleep Medicine Pearls, 3rd Edition, 3rd edn, Berry, Richard B., MD; Wagner, Mary H., MD. Copyright © 2015, 2003, 1999 by Saunders, an imprint of Elsevier Inc.)*

**Chapter 101 Video 8** Parasomnias and Nocturnal Frontal Lobe Epilepsy (NFLE): Lights and Shadows – Controversial points in the differential diagnosis

*(From Bisulli, F. et al, Sleep Medicine Volume 12. Copyright © 2011 Elsevier B.V.)*

**Chapter 101 Video 9** Fatal Familial Insomnia

*(From Chokroverty, S., Thomas, R. J. (eds). Atlas of Sleep Medicine, Copyright © 2014 by Saunders, an imprint of Elsevier Inc.)*

**Chapter 101 Video 10** Bruxism

*(From Berry, R. B., Wagner, M. H . Sleep Medicine Pearls, 3rd Edition. © 2015 Elsevier. All Rights Reserved.)*

**Chapter 101 Video 11** NREM Parasomnia (Confusional Arousal)

*(From Pincherle, A. et al. Epilepsy and NREM-parasomnia: A complex and reciprocal relationship. Sleep Medicine. 13(4), 2012. Pages 442–444. © Elsevier. doi:10.1016/S1389-9457(12)00144-X.)*

**Chapter 101 Video 12** NREM Parasomnia (Confusional Arousal)

*(From Pincherle, A. et al. Epilepsy and NREM-parasomnia: A complex and reciprocal relationship. Sleep Medicine. 13(4), 2012. Pages 442–444. © Elsevier. doi:10.1016/S1389-9457(12)00144-X)*

**Chapter 101 Video 13** REM Sleep Behavior Disorder 1

*(From Berry, R. B., Wagner, M. H . Sleep Medicine Pearls, 3rd Edition. © 2015 Elsevier. All Rights Reserved.)*

**Chapter 101 Video 14** REM Sleep Behavior Disorder 2

*(From Berry, R. B., Wagner, M. H . Sleep Medicine Pearls, 3rd Edition. © 2015 Elsevier. All Rights Reserved.)*

**Chapter 101 Video 15** Willis-Ekbom Disease Foundation Revised Consensus Statement on the Management of Restless Legs Syndrome

*(From Silber, M. H., et al. Mayo Clinic Proceedings, 2013-09-01, Volume 88, Issue 9, Pages 977-986, Copyright © 2013 Mayo Foundation for Medical Education and Research.)*

**Chapter 101 Video 16** Explaining the Results

*(From Kryger, M. H. Gallery of Patient Interview Chapters. Atlas of Clinical Sleep Medicine,Second Edition. Copyright © 2014, 2010 by Saunders, an imprint of Elsevier Inc., Chapter 20, 478-482.)*

**Chapter 101 Video 17** A 58-Year-Old Man With Position-Dependent Nocturnal Dyspnea

*From Schertel, A. et al. Chest, Volume 152, Issue 2 Copyright © 2017 American College of Chest Physicians.*

**Chapter 101 Video 18** A 12-Year-Old Boy with Sleep Apnea and Restless Sleep

*(From Kryger, M. H. Gallery of Sleep Laboratory Chapter Findings. Atlas of Clinical Sleep Medicine,Second Edition. Copyright © 2014, 2010 by Saunders, an imprint of Elsevier Inc., Chapter 21, 483-495.)*

**Chapter 101 Video 19** Pediatric Sleep Surgery

*(From Resnick, C. M. Atlas of the Oral and Maxillofacial Surgery. Clinics of North America. Published March 1, 2019. Vol. 27, Issue 1. Pages 67-75. Copyright © 2018 Elsevier Inc.)*

**Chapter 101 Video 20** 70-Year-Old Male Patient With a 15-Year History of Parkinson's Disease, Severe Depression and Longstanding RBD Displaying Marked Episodes of Laughter During REM Sleep

*(From Siclari, F. et al. Parkinsonism and Related Disorders, Vol. 17, Issue 5. Copyright © 2011 Elsevier Ltd.)*

**Chapter 101 Video 21** Ictal Bruxism Treated with Temporal Lobectomy

*(From Guaita, M.et al. Sleep Medicine, Volume 16, Issue 11, Copyright © 2015 Elsevier B.V.)*

**Chapter 101 Video 22** Familial Idiopathic Rapid Eye Movement Sleep Behavior Disorder

*(From Aurélie, P-J., Lannuzel, A., Arnulf, I. Sleep Medicine, 2017-02-01, Volume 30, Pages 29-30, Copyright © 2016 Elsevier.)*

**Chapter 103 Video 1** Large Left Hypertropia Secondary to Right Oculomotor Nerve Palsy

**Chapter 103 Video 2** Left Appendicular Ataxia

**Chapter 103 Video 3** Prominent Left Ptosis

**Chapter 103 Video 4** Cranial Neuropathies/Impaired Adduction, Elevation, and Depression with Intact Abduction of the Left Nerve

**Chapter 103 Video 5** Bilateral Abduction Deficits Secondary to Demyelinating Bilateral Abducens Palsies

**Chapter 103 Video 6** Esotropia

**Chapter 103 Video 7** Facial Nerve Function in a Patient with a History of Right Facial Palsy Two Years Ago and Current Left Facial Palsy

**Chapter 103 Video 8** Other Babinski Sign

*(Clips 103.1–2 from Leigh R. J., Zee, D. S. The Neurology of Eye Movements, 5th Edition, 2015. © Oxford University Press; Clips 103.2 - 103.7 © Janet C. Rucker, All rights reserved; Clip 103.8 Courtesy of Joseph Jankovic, MD)*

*(Clip 113.6 From Stone J, Hoeritzauer I, Brown K, Carson A. Therapeutic Sedation for Functional (Psychogenic) Neurological Symptoms. J Psychosom Res 2014; 76:165–8.)*

1

# Diagnosis of Neurological Disease

*Joseph Jankovic, John C. Mazziotta, Nancy J. Newman, Scott L. Pomeroy*

## OUTLINE



Neurological diagnosis is sometimes easy, sometimes quite challenging, and specialized skills are required. If a patient shuffles into the physician's office, demonstrating a pill-rolling tremor of the hands and loss of facial expression, Parkinson disease comes readily to mind. Although making such a "spot diagnosis" can be very satisfying, it is important to consider that this clinical presentation may have another cause entirely—such as neuroleptic-induced parkinsonism—or that the patient may be seeking help for a totally different neurological problem. Therefore an evaluation of the whole problem is always necessary.

In all disciplines of medicine, the history of symptoms and clinical examination of the patient are key to achieving an accurate diagnosis. This is particularly true in neurology. Standard practice in neurology is to record the patient's chief complaint and the history of symptom development, followed by the history of illnesses and previous surgical procedures, the family history, personal and social history, and a review of any clinical features involving the main body systems. From these data, one formulates a hypothesis to explain the patient's illness. The neurologist then performs a neurological examination, which should support the hypothesis generated from the patient's history. Based on a combination of the history and physical findings, one proceeds with the differential diagnosis to generate a list of possible causes of the patient's clinical features.

What is unique to neurology is the emphasis on *localization* and *phenomenology*. When a patient presents to an internist or surgeon with abdominal or chest symptoms, the localization is practically established by the symptoms, and the etiology then becomes the primary concern. However, in clinical neurological practice, a patient with a weak hand may have a lesion localized to muscles, neuromuscular junctions, nerves in the upper limb, brachial plexus, spinal cord, or brain. The formal neurological examination allows localization of the offending lesion and then a focused list of potential causes of problems in that specific location can be generated. Similarly, a neurologist skilled in recognizing phenomenology should be able to differentiate between tremor and stereotypy, both rhythmical movements; among tics, myoclonus, and chorea, all jerklike movements; and among other rhythmical and jerklike movement disorders, such as seen in dystonia. In general, the history provides the best clues to localization, disease mechanisms and etiology, and the examination is essential for localization confirmation and appropriate disease categorization—all critical for proper diagnosis and treatment.

This diagnostic process consists of a series of steps, as depicted in Fig. 1.1. Although standard teaching is that the patient should be allowed to provide the history in his or her own words, the process also involves active questioning of the patient to elicit pertinent information and systematic review of previous pertinent medical records. At each step, the neurologist should consider the possible anatomical localizations, the potential pathophysiological mechanisms of disease, and the possible etiologies of the symptoms, especially for the most likely localizations (see Fig. 1.1). From the patient's chief complaint and a detailed history, an astute neurologist can derive clues that lead first to a hypothesis about the location and then to a hypothesis about the etiology of the neurological lesion. From these hypotheses, the experienced neurologist can predict what neurological abnormalities

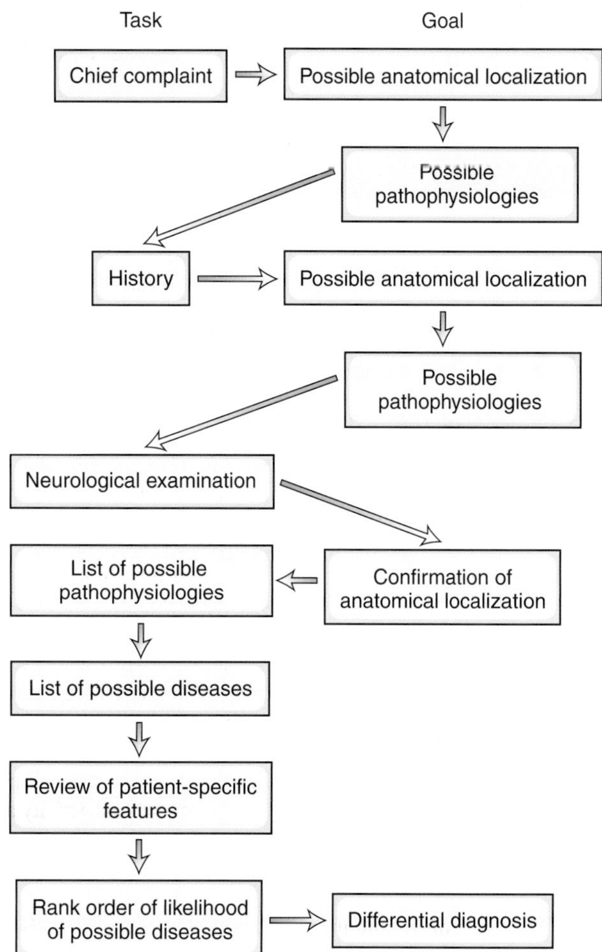


**Fig. 1.1** The diagnostic path is illustrated as a series of steps in which the neurologist collects data (Task) with the objective of providing information on the anatomical localization and nature of the disease process (Goal).

*should be present* and what *should be absent*, thereby allowing confirmation of the site of the dysfunction during the neurological examination. Alternatively, analysis of the history may suggest two or more possible anatomical locations and disease mechanisms and etiologies, each with a different predicted constellation of neurological signs. The findings on neurological examination can be used to determine which of these various possibilities is the most likely. To achieve a diagnosis, the neurologist needs to have a good knowledge not only of the anatomy and physiology of the nervous system but also of the clinical features and pathology of neurological diseases.

## NEUROLOGICAL INTERVIEW

The neurologist may be an intimidating figure for some patients. To add to the stress of the neurological interview and examination, the patient may already have a preconceived notion that the disease causing the symptoms may be progressively disabling and possibly life threatening. Because of this background, the neurologist should present an empathetic demeanor and do everything possible to put the patient at ease. It is important for the physician to introduce himself or herself to the patient and exchange social pleasantries before leaping into the interview. A few opening questions can break the ice: "Who is your doctor, and who would you like me to write to?" "What type of work have you done most of your life?" "How old are you?" "Are you right or left handed?" For children, questions like "Where do you go to school?" or "What sports or other activities do you like?" After this, it is easier to ask, "How can I be of service?" "What brings you to see me?" or "What is bothering you the most?" Such questions establish the physician's role in the relationship and encourage the patient to volunteer an initial history. At a follow-up visit, it often is helpful to start with more personalized questions: "How have you been?" "Have there been any changes in your condition since your last visit?"

Another technique is to begin by asking, "How can I help you?" This establishes that the doctor is there to provide a service and allows patients to express their expectations for the consultation. It is important for the physician to get a sense of the patient's expectations from the visit. Usually the patient wants the doctor to find or confirm the diagnosis and cure the disease. Sometimes the patient comes hoping that something is *not* present ("Please tell me my headaches are *not* caused by a brain tumor!"). Sometimes the patient claims that other doctors "never told me anything" (which may sometimes be true, although in some cases the patient did not hear, did not understand, or did not like what was said).

## CHIEF COMPLAINT

The chief complaint (or the several main complaints) is the usual starting point of the diagnostic process. The complaints serve to focus attention on the questions to be addressed in taking the history and provide the first clue to the anatomy and etiology of the underlying disease. The chief complaint also provides insight into the patient's level of understanding of his or her symptoms. For example, the patient may present with the triad of complaints of headache, clumsiness, and double vision. In this case, the neurologist would be concerned that the patient may have a tumor in the posterior fossa affecting the cerebellum and brainstem. The mode of onset is critically important in investigating the etiology. For example, in this case, a sudden onset usually would indicate a stroke in the vertebrobasilar arterial system. A course characterized by exacerbations and remissions may suggest multiple sclerosis, whereas a slowly progressive course points to a neoplasm. Paroxysmal episodes suggest the possibility of seizures, migraines, or some form of paroxysmal dyskinesia, ataxia, or periodic paralysis.

## HISTORY OF THE PRESENT ILLNESS

As one continues interviewing the patient, localization, figuring out from where the problem originates, remains paramount. In addition, a critical aspect of the information obtained from this portion of the interview has to do with establishing the temporal-severity profile of each symptom reported by the patient. Such information allows the neurologist to categorize the patient's problems based on the profile. For example, a patient who reports the gradual onset of headache and slowly progressive weakness of one side of the body over weeks to months could be describing the growth of a space-occupying lesion in a cerebral hemisphere. The same symptoms occurring rapidly, in minutes or seconds, with maximal severity from the onset, might be the result of a hemorrhage in a cerebral hemisphere. The symptoms and their severity may be equal at the time of the interview, but the temporal-severity profile leads to totally different hypotheses about the mechanism and etiology.

Often the patient will give a very clear history of the temporal development of the complaints and will specify the location and severity of the symptoms and the current level of disability. However, in other instances, the patient, particularly if elderly, will provide a tangential account and insist on telling what other doctors did or said, rather than relating specific signs and symptoms. Direct questioning often is needed to clarify the symptoms, but it is important not to "lead" the patient. Patients frequently are all too ready to give a positive response to an authority figure, even if it is incorrect. It is important to consider whether the patient is reliable. Reliability depends on the patient's intelligence, memory, language function, and educational and social status and on the presence of secondary gain issues, such as a disability claim or pending lawsuit.

The clinician should suspect a *somatoform* or *psychogenic* disorder in any patient who claims to have symptoms that started suddenly, particularly after a traumatic event, manifested by clinical features that are incongruous with an organic disorder, or with involvement of multiple organ systems. The diagnosis of a psychogenic disorder is based not only on the exclusion of organic causes but also on positive criteria. Getting information from an observer other than the patient is important for characterizing many neurological conditions such as seizures and dementia. Taking a history from a child is complicated by shyness with strangers, a different sense of time, and a limited vocabulary. In children, the history is always the composite perceptions of the child and the parent.

Patients and physicians may use the same word to mean very different things. If the physician accepts a given word at face value without ensuring that the patient's use of the word matches the physician's, misinterpretation may lead to misdiagnosis. For instance, patients often describe a limb as being "numb" when it is actually paralyzed. Patients often use the term "dizziness" to refer to lightheadedness, confusion, or weakness, rather than vertigo as the physician would expect. Although a patient may describe vision as being "blurred," further questioning may reveal diplopia. "Blackouts" may indicate loss of consciousness, loss of vision, or simply confusion. "Pounding" or "throbbing" headaches are not necessarily pulsating.

The neurologist must understand fully the nature, onset, duration, and progression of each sign or symptom and the temporal relationship of one finding to another. Are the symptoms getting better, staying the same, or getting worse? What relieves them, what has no effect, and what makes them worse? In infants and young children, the temporal sequence also includes the timing of developmental milestones.

An example may clarify how the history leads to diagnosis: A 28-year-old woman presents with a 10-year history of recurrent headaches associated with her menses. The unilateral quality of pain in some attacks and the association of flashing lights, nausea, and vomiting together point to a diagnosis of migraine. On the other hand, in the same patient, a progressively worsening headache on wakening, new-onset seizures, and a developing hemiparesis suggest an intracranial space-occupying lesion. Both the absence of expected features and the presence of unexpected features may assist in the diagnosis. A patient with numbness of the feet may have a peripheral neuropathy, but the presence of backache combined with loss of sphincter control suggests that a spinal cord or cauda equina lesion is more likely. Patients may arrive for a neurological consultation with a folder of results of previous laboratory tests and neuroimaging studies. They often dwell on these test results and their interpretation by other physicians. However, the opinions of other doctors should never be accepted without question, because they may have been wrong! The careful neurologist takes a new history and makes a new assessment of the problem. However, integration of objective data such as dates and test results into the patient's subjective narrative is essential.

The history of how the patient or caregiver responded to the signs and symptoms may be important. A pattern of overreaction may be of help in evaluating the significance of the complaints. Nevertheless, a night visit to the emergency department for a new-onset headache should not be dismissed without investigation. Conversely, the child who was *not* brought to the hospital despite hours of seizures may be the victim of child abuse or at least of neglect.

## REVIEW OF PATIENT-SPECIFIC INFORMATION

Information about the patient's background often greatly helps the neurologist to make a diagnosis of the cause of the signs and symptoms. This information includes the history of medical and surgical illnesses; current medications and allergies; a review of symptoms in non-neurological systems of the body; the personal history in terms of occupation, social situation, and alcohol, tobacco, and illicit drug use; and the medical history of the parents, grandparents, siblings, and children, looking for evidence of familial diseases. The order in which these items are considered is not important, but consistency avoids the possibility that something will be forgotten.

In the outpatient office, the patient can be asked to complete a form with a series of questions on all these matters before starting the consultation with the physician. This expedites the interview, although more details often are needed. What chemicals is the patient exposed to at home and at work? Did the patient *ever* use alcohol, tobacco, or prescription or illegal drugs? Is there excessive stress at home, in school, or in the workplace, such as divorce, death of a loved one, or loss of employment? Are there hints of abuse or neglect of children or spouse? A careful sexual history is also important information. The doctor should question children and adolescents away from their parents if obtaining more accurate information about sexual activity and substance abuse seems indicated.

### Review of Systems

The review of systems should include the elements of nervous system function that did not surface in taking the history, as well as at least, a general review of all systemic organ systems. Regarding the former, the neurologist should query the following: cognition, personality, and mood change; hallucinations; seizures and other impairments of consciousness; orthostatic faintness; headaches; special senses, including vision and hearing; speech and language function; swallowing; limb coordination; slowness of movement; involuntary movements or vocalizations; strength and sensation; pain; gait and balance; and sphincter, bowel, and sexual function. A positive response may help to clarify a diagnosis. For instance, if a patient complaining of ataxia and hemiparesis admits to unilateral deafness, an acoustic neuroma should be considered. Headaches in a patient with paraparesis suggest a parasagittal meningioma rather than a spinal cord lesion. The developmental history must be assessed in children and also may be of value in adults whose illness started during childhood.

The review of systems must also include all organ systems. Neurological function is adversely affected by dysfunction of many systems, including the liver, kidney, gastrointestinal tract, heart, and blood vessels. Multiorgan involvement characterizes several neurological disorders such as vasculitis, sarcoidosis, mitochondrial disorders, and storage diseases.

### History of Previous Illnesses

Specific findings in the patient's medical and surgical history may help to explain the present complaint. For instance, seizures and worsening headaches in a patient who previously had surgery for lung cancer suggest a brain metastasis. Chronic low back pain in a patient complaining of numbness and weakness in the legs on walking half a mile suggests neurogenic claudication from lumbar canal stenosis. The record of the history should include dates and details of all surgical procedures, significant injuries including head trauma and fractures, hospitalizations, and conditions requiring medical consultation and medications. For pediatric patients, obtain information on the pregnancy and state of the infant at birth.

Certain features in the patient's history should always alert the physician to the possibility that they may be responsible for the neurological complaints. Gastric surgery may lead to vitamin $B_{12}$ deficiency. Sarcoidosis may cause Bell palsy, diabetes insipidus, vision loss, and peripheral neuropathy. Disorders of the liver, kidney, and small bowel can be associated with a wide variety of neurological disorders. Systemic malignancy can cause direct and indirect (paraneoplastic) neurological problems. The physician should not be surprised if the patient fails to remember previous medical or surgical problems. It is common to observe abdominal scars in a patient who described no surgical procedures until questioned about the scars.

Medications often are the cause of neurological disturbances, particularly chemotherapy drugs. In addition, isoniazid may cause peripheral neuropathy and ethambutol a bilateral optic neuropathy. Lithium carbonate may produce tremor, ataxia, and nystagmus. Neuroleptic agents can produce a Parkinson-like syndrome or dyskinesias. Most patients do not think of vitamins, oral contraceptives, nonprescription analgesics, and herbal compounds as "medications," and specific questions about these agents are necessary.

### Family History

Some neurological disorders are hereditary. Accordingly, a history of similar disease in family members or of consanguinity may be of diagnostic importance. However, the expression of a gene mutation may be quite different from one family member to another with respect not only to the severity of neurological dysfunction but also to the organ systems involved. For instance, the mutations of the gene for Machado-Joseph disease *(SCA3)* can cause several phenotypes. A patient with Charcot-Marie-Tooth disease (hereditary motor-sensory neuropathy) may have a severe peripheral neuropathy, whereas relatives may demonstrate only pes cavus.

Reported diagnoses may be inaccurate. In families with dominant muscular dystrophy, affected individuals in earlier generations are often said to have had "arthritis" that put them into a wheelchair. Some conditions, such as epilepsy or Huntington disease, may be "family secrets." Therefore the physician should be cautious in accepting a patient's assertion that a family history of a similar disorder is lacking. If the possibility exists that the disease is inherited, it is helpful to obtain information from parents and grandparents and to examine relatives at risk. Some patients wrongly attribute symptoms in family members to a normal consequence of aging or to other conditions such as alcoholism. This is particularly true in patients with essential tremor. At a minimum, historical data for all first- and second-degree relatives should include age (current or at death), cause of death, and any significant neurological or systemic diseases.

### Social History

It is important to discuss the social setting in which neurological disease is manifest. Family status and changes in such can provide important information about interpersonal relationships and emotional stability. Employment history is often quite important. Has an elderly patient lost his or her job because of cognitive dysfunction? Do patients' daily activities put them or others at risk if their vision, balance, or coordination is impaired or if they have alterations in consciousness? Does the patient's job expose him or her to potential injury or toxin exposure? Are they in professions where the diagnosis of a neurological disorder would require reporting them to a regulatory agency (e.g., airline pilot, professional driver)? For children, asking whether they have successfully established friendships or other meaningful social connections, or whether they might be the victim of bullying is very important. A travel history is important, particularly if infectious diseases are a consideration. Hobbies can be a source of toxin exposure (e.g., welding sculpture). Level and type of exercise provide useful clues to overall fitness and can also suggest potential exposures to toxins and infectious agents (e.g., hiking and Lyme disease).

## EXAMINATION

### Neurological Examination

Neurological examination starts during the interview. A patient's lack of facial expression (hypomimia) may suggest parkinsonism or depression, whereas a worried or astonished expression may suggest progressive supranuclear palsy. Ptosis may suggest myasthenia gravis or a brainstem lesion. The pattern of speech may suggest dysarthria, aphasia, or spasmodic dysphonia. The presence of abnormal involuntary movements may indicate an underlying movement disorder. Neurologist trainees must be able to perform and understand the complete neurological examination, in which every central nervous system region, peripheral nerve, muscle, sensory modality, and reflex are tested. However, the full neurological examination is too lengthy to perform in practice. Instead, the experienced neurologist uses a *focused neurological examination* to examine in detail the neurological functions relevant to the history in addition to performing a *screening neurological examination* to check the remaining parts of the nervous system. This approach should confirm, refute, or modify the initial hypotheses of disease location and causation derived from the history (see Fig. 1.1).

Both the presence and absence of abnormalities may be of diagnostic importance. If a patient's symptoms suggest a left hemiparesis, the neurologist should search carefully for a left homonymous hemianopia and for evidence that the blink or smile is slowed on the left side of the face. Relevant additional findings would be that rapid, repetitive movements are impaired in the left limbs, that the tendon reflexes are more brisk on the left than the right, that the left abdominal reflexes are absent, and that the left plantar response is extensor. Along with testing the primary modalities of sensation on the left side, the neurologist may examine the higher integrative aspects of sensation, including graphesthesia, stereognosis, and sensory extinction with double simultaneous stimuli. The presence or absence of some of these features can separate a left hemiparesis arising from a lesion in the right cerebral cortex or from one in the left cervical spinal cord.

The screening neurological examination (Table 1.1) is designed for quick evaluation of the mental status, cranial nerves, motor system (strength, muscle tone, presence of involuntary movements, and postures), coordination, gait and balance, tendon reflexes, and sensation. More complex functions are tested first; if these are performed well, then it may not be necessary to test the component functions. For example, the patient who can walk heel to toe (tandem gait) does not have a significant disturbance of the cerebellum or of joint position sensation. Similarly, the patient who can do a pushup, rise from the floor without using the hands, and walk on toes and heels will have normal limb strength when each muscle group is individually tested. Asking the patient to hold the arms extended in supination in front of the body with the eyes open allows evaluation of strength and posture. It also may reveal involuntary movements such as tremor, dystonia, myoclonus, or chorea. A weak arm is expected to show a downward or pronator drift. Repeating the maneuver with the eyes closed allows assessment of joint position sensation.

**TABLE 1.1 Outline of the Screening Neurological Examination**

| Examination Component | Description/Observation/ Maneuver |
|---|---|
| **Mental Status** | Assessed while recording the history |
| **Cranial Nerves (CNs):** | |
| CN I | Should be tested in all persons who experience spontaneous loss of smell, in patients suspected to have Parkinson disease, and in patients who have suffered head injury |
| CN II | *Each eye:*<br>Visual acuity with glasses/contacts<br>Visual fields by confrontation<br>Swinging flashlight to detect relative afferent pupillary defect<br>Fundoscopy |
| CN III, IV, VI | Horizontal and vertical eye movements (saccades, pursuit, vestibulo-ocular reflex)<br>Pupillary symmetry and reactivity<br>Presence of nystagmus or other ocular oscillations |
| CN V | Pinprick and touch sensation on face, corneal reflex<br>Jaw strength |
| CN VII | Close eyes, show teeth |
| CN VIII | Perception of whispered voice in each ear or rubbing of fingers; if hearing is impaired, look in external auditory canals, and use tuning fork for lateralization and bone-versus-air sound conduction |
| CN IX, X | Palate lifts in midline, gag reflex present |
| CN XI | Shrug shoulders |
| CN XII | Protrude tongue |
| **Limbs** | *Separate testing of each limb:*<br>Presence of involuntary movements<br>Muscle mass (atrophy, hypertrophy) and look for fasciculations<br>Muscle tone in response to passive flexion and extension<br>Power of main muscle groups<br>Coordination<br>Finger-to-nose and heel-to-shin testing<br>Performance of rapid alternating movements<br>Tendon reflexes<br>Plantar responses<br>Pinprick and light touch on hands and feet<br>Double simultaneous stimuli on hands and feet<br>Joint position sense in hallux and index finger<br>Vibration sense at ankle and index finger |
| **Gait and Balance** | Spontaneous gait should be observed; stance, base, cadence, arm swing, tandem gait should be noted<br>Postural stability should be assessed by the pull test |
| **Romberg Test** | Stand with eyes open and then closed |

Of importance, the screening neurological examination may miss important neurological abnormalities. For instance, a bitemporal visual field defect may not be detected when the fields of both eyes are tested simultaneously; it will be found only when each eye is tested separately. Similarly, a parietal lobe syndrome may go undiscovered unless visuospatial function is specifically assessed.

It is sometimes difficult to decide whether something observed in the neurological examination is normal or abnormal, and only experience prevents the neurologist from misinterpreting as a sign of disease something that is a normal variation. Every person has some degree of asymmetry. Moreover, what is abnormal in young adults may be normal in the elderly. Loss of the ankle reflex and loss of vibration sense at the big toe are common findings in patients older than 70 years. The experienced neurologist appreciates the normal range of neurological variation, whereas the beginner frequently records mild impairment of a number of different functions. Such impairments include isolated deviation of the tongue or uvula to one side and minor asymmetries of reflexes or sensation. Such *soft signs* may be incorporated into the overall synthesis of the disorder if they are consistent with other parts of the history and examination; otherwise, they should be disregarded. If an abnormality is identified, seek other features that usually are associated. For instance, ataxia of a limb may result from a corticospinal tract lesion, sensory defect, or cerebellar lesion. If the limb incoordination is due to a cerebellar lesion, other findings will include ataxia on finger-to-nose and heel-to-shin testing, abnormal rapid alternating movements of the hands (dysdiadochokinesia), and often nystagmus and ocular dysmetria. If some of these signs of cerebellar dysfunction are missing, examination of joint position sense, limb strength, and reflexes may demonstrate that this incoordination is due to something other than a cerebellar lesion. At the end of the neurological examination, the abnormal physical signs should be classified as definitely abnormal *(hard signs)* or equivocally abnormal *(soft signs)*. The hard signs, when combined with symptoms from the history, allow the neurologist to develop a hypothesis about the anatomical site of the lesion or at least about the neurological pathways involved. The soft signs can then be reviewed to determine whether they conflict with or support the initial conclusion. An important point is that the primary purpose of the neurological examination is to reveal functional disturbances that localize abnormalities. The standard neurological examination is less effective when used to monitor the course of a disease or its temporal response to treatment. Measuring changes in neurological function over time requires special quantitative functional tests and rating scales.

### General Physical Examination

The nervous system is damaged in so many general medical diseases that a general physical examination is an integral part of the examination of patients with neurological disorders. Atrial fibrillation, valvular heart disease, or an atrial septal defect may cause embolic strokes in the central nervous system. Hypertension increases the risk for all types of stroke. Signs of malignancy raise the possibility of metastatic lesions of the nervous system or paraneoplastic neurological syndromes such as a subacute cerebellar degeneration or sensory peripheral neuropathy. In addition, some diseases such as vasculitis and sarcoidosis affect both the brain and other organs.

## ASSESSMENT OF THE CAUSE OF THE PATIENT'S SYMPTOMS

### Anatomical Localization

Hypotheses about lesion localization, neurological systems involved, and pathology of the disorder can be formed once the history is complete (see Fig. 1.1). The neurologist then uses the examination findings to confirm the localization of the lesion before trying to determine its cause. The initial question is whether the disease is in the brain, spinal cord, peripheral nerves, neuromuscular junctions, or muscles. Then it must be established whether the disorder is focal, multifocal, or systemic. A *system disorder* is a disease that causes degeneration of one part of the nervous system while sparing other parts of the nervous system. For instance, degeneration of the corticospinal tracts and spinal motor neurons with sparing of the sensory pathways of the central and peripheral nervous systems is the hallmark of the system degeneration termed *motor neuron disease*, or *amyotrophic lateral sclerosis*. Multiple system atrophy is another example of a system degeneration characterized by slowness of movement (parkinsonism), ataxia, and dysautonomia.

The first step in localization is to translate the patient's symptoms and signs into abnormalities of a nucleus, tract, or part of the nervous system. Loss of pain and temperature sensation on one half of the body, excluding the face, indicates a lesion of the contralateral spinothalamic tract in the high cervical spinal cord. A left sixth nerve palsy, with weakness of left face and right limbs, points to a left pontine lesion. A left homonymous hemianopia indicates a lesion in the right optic tract, optic radiations, or occipital cortex. The neurological examination plays a crucial role in localizing the lesion. A patient complaining of tingling and numbness in the feet initially may be thought to have a peripheral neuropathy. If examination shows hyperreflexia in the arms and legs and no vibration sensation below the clavicles, the lesion is likely to be in the spinal cord, and the many causes of peripheral neuropathy can be dropped from consideration. A patient with a history of weakness of the left arm and leg who is found on examination to have a left homonymous hemianopia has a right cerebral lesion, not a cervical cord problem.

The neurologist must decide whether the symptoms and signs could all arise from one focal lesion or whether several anatomical sites must be involved. The *principle of parsimony*, or *Occam's razor*, requires that the clinician strive to hypothesize only one lesion. The differential diagnosis for a single focal lesion is significantly different from that for multiple lesions. Thus a patient complaining of left-sided vision loss in both eyes and left-sided weakness is likely to have a lesion in the right cerebral hemisphere, possibly caused by stroke or tumor. On the other hand, if the visual difficulty is due to a central scotoma in the left eye only, and if the upper motor neuron weakness affects the left limbs but spares the lower cranial nerves, two lesions must be present: one in the left optic nerve and one in the left corticospinal tract below the medulla—as seen, for example, in multiple sclerosis. If a patient with slowly progressive slurring of speech and difficulty walking is found to have ataxia of the arms and legs, bilateral extensor plantar responses, and optic atrophy, the lesion must be either multifocal (affecting brainstem and optic nerves, and therefore probably multiple sclerosis) or a system disorder, such as a spinocerebellar degeneration. The complex vascular anatomy of the brain can sometimes cause multifocal neurological deficits to result from one vascular abnormality. For instance, a patient with occlusion of one vertebral artery may suffer coincident strokes from artery to artery emboli that result in a midbrain syndrome, a hemianopia, and an amnestic syndrome.

Synthesis of symptoms and signs for anatomical localization of a lesion requires a good knowledge of neuroanatomy, including the location of all major pathways in the nervous system and their interrelationships at different levels. In making this synthesis, the neurologist trainee will find it helpful to refer to diagrams that show transverse sections of the spinal cord, medulla, pons, and midbrain; the brachial and lumbosacral plexuses; and the dermatomes and myotomes. Knowledge of the functional anatomy of the cerebral cortex and the blood supply of the brain and spinal cord also is essential.

**TABLE 1.2 Pathophysiological Mechanisms of Neurological Disease**

| |
|---|
| Inflammatory |
| Infectious |
| Noninfectious (autoimmune) |
| Vascular |
| Arterial |
| Venous |
| Compressive/infiltrative |
| Neoplastic |
| Non-neoplastic |
| Degenerative/hereditary |
| Toxic/metabolic/nutritional |
| Mechanical |
| Trauma |
| Disorders of intracranial pressure |

Symptoms and signs may arise not only from disturbances caused at the focus of an abnormality—*focal localizing signs*—but also at a distance. One example is the damage that results from the shift of intracranial contents and alterations in intracranial pressure produced by an expansive supratentorial tumor. This may cause a palsy of the sixth cranial nerve, even though the tumor is located far from the cranial nerves. Clinical features caused by damage far from the primary site of abnormality sometimes are called *false localizing signs*. This term derives from the era before neuroimaging studies when clinical examination was the major means of lesion localization. In fact, these are not false signs but rather signs that the intracranial shifts are marked or the intracranial pressure is abnormal.

## Pathophysiological Mechanisms and Generating a Differential Diagnosis

Once the likely site of the lesion is identified, the next step is to consider all the possible pathophysiological mechanisms that can cause disease, especially in the nervous system and especially in the lesion location postulated (Table 1.2). Reviewing this "medical student" list is an extremely important next step in the process because it allows the clinician to systematically consider all the possible mechanisms of disease and hone down on those most likely to fit the anatomical location and the patient's symptoms and signs. Once the most likely pathophysiologies are selected, a focused list of diseases or conditions that may be responsible for the patient's symptoms and signs—the differential diagnosis—can be generated (see Fig. 1.1).

The experienced neurologist automatically first considers the most likely pathophysiology and causes, followed by less common causes. The beginner is happy to generate a list of the main causes of the signs and symptoms in whatever order they come to mind. Experience indicates the most likely causes based on specific patient characteristics, the portions of the nervous system affected, and the relative frequency of each disease. An important point is that *rare presentations of common diseases are more common than common presentations of rare diseases*. Equally important, the neurologist must be vigilant in including in the differential diagnosis less likely disorders that if overlooked can cause significant morbidity and/or mortality. A proper differential diagnosis list should include the most likely causes of the patient's signs and symptoms as well as the most ominous.

Keeping in mind the entire list of pathophysiological mechanisms will ensure that an important entity in the differential diagnosis will not be missed. Sometimes only a single disease is immediately incriminated, but usually several candidate diseases can be identified. The list of possibilities should take into account both the temporal features of the patient's symptoms and the pathological processes known to affect the relevant area of the nervous system. For example, in a patient with signs indicating a lesion of the internal capsule, the cause is likely to be stroke if the hemiplegia was of sudden onset. With progression over weeks or months, a more likely cause is an expanding tumor. As another example, in a patient with signs of multifocal lesions whose symptoms have relapsed and remitted over several years, the diagnosis is likely to be multiple sclerosis or multiple strokes (depending on the patient's age, sex, and risk factors). If symptoms appeared only recently and have gradually progressed, multiple metastases should be considered.

Again, the principle of parsimony or Occam's razor should be applied in constructing the differential diagnostic list. An example is that of a patient with a 3-week history of a progressive spinal cord lesion who suddenly experiences aphasia. Perhaps the patient had a tumor compressing the spinal cord and has incidentally incurred a small stroke. However, the principle of parsimony would suggest a single disease, probably cancer with multiple metastases. Another example is that of a patient with progressive atrophy of the small muscles of the hands for 6 months before the appearance of a pseudobulbar palsy. This patient could have bilateral ulnar nerve lesions and recent bilateral strokes, but amyotrophic lateral sclerosis is more likely. However, nature does not always obey the rules of parsimony, as Hickam's dictum—that a patient can have multiple coincident unrelated disorders—asserts.

As noted earlier, the differential diagnosis generally starts with a list of pathological processes (see Table 1.2) such as a stroke, a tumor, or an abscess. Each pathological process may result from any of several different diseases. Thus a clinical diagnosis of an intracranial mass lesion generates a list of the different types of tumors likely to be responsible for the clinical manifestations in the affected patient, as well as non-neoplastic causes of masses such as abscesses. Similarly, in a patient with a stroke, the clinical history may help to discriminate among hemorrhage, embolism, thrombosis, vascular spasm, and vasculitis. The skilled diagnostician is justly proud of placing the correct diagnosis at the top of the list, but it is more important to ensure that all possible diseases are considered. If a disease is not even considered, it is unlikely to be diagnosed. Treatable disorders should always be kept in mind, even if they have a very low probability. This is especially true if they may mimic more common incurable neurological disorders such as Alzheimer disease or amyotrophic lateral sclerosis.

### Investigations

Sometimes the neurological diagnosis can be made without any laboratory or imaging investigations. This is true for a clear-cut case of Parkinson disease, myasthenia gravis, or multiple sclerosis. Nevertheless, even in these situations, appropriate ancillary testing is important documentation for other physicians who will see the patient in the future. In other instances, the cause of the disease will be elucidated only by the use of ancillary tests. These tests may in individual cases include hematological and biochemical blood studies; neurophysiological testing (Chapters 35–39); neuroimaging (Chapters 40–42); organ biopsy; bacteriological and virological studies; and genetic testing. The use of ancillary tests in the diagnosis of neurological diseases is considered more fully in Chapter 34.

## MANAGEMENT OF NEUROLOGICAL DISORDERS

Not all diseases are curable. However, even if a disease is incurable, the physician should be able to reduce the patient's discomfort and assist the patient and family in managing the disease. Understanding a neurological disease is a science. Diagnosing a neurological disease is a combination of science and experience. Managing a neurological disease is an art, as illustrated in the chapters that comprise Part III of this book.

## THE EXPERIENCED NEUROLOGIST'S APPROACH TO THE DIAGNOSIS OF COMMON NEUROLOGICAL PROBLEMS

The skills of a neurologist are learned. Seeing many cases of a disease teaches us which symptoms and signs *should* be present and—just as important—which *should not* be present in a given neurological disease. Although there is no substitute for experience and pattern recognition, the trainee can learn the clues used by the seasoned practitioner to reach a correct diagnosis. Part I of this book covers the main symptoms and signs of neurological disease. These chapters describe how an experienced neurologist approaches common presenting problems such as a movement disorder, a speech disturbance, vision loss, or diplopia to arrive at the diagnosis. Part II of this book comprises the major fields of investigation and management of neurological disease. Part III provides a compendium of the neurological diseases themselves with their appropriate diagnoses and management.

2

# Episodic Impairment of Consciousness

*Daniel Winkel, Dimitri Cassimatis*

## OUTLINE



Temporary loss of consciousness may be caused by transient impaired cerebral perfusion (the presumed mechanism for syncope), cerebral ischemia, migraine, epileptic seizures, metabolic disturbances, sudden increases in intracranial pressure (ICP), or sleep disorders. These conditions may be difficult to distinguish from anxiety attacks, psychogenic nonepilcptic spells (PNESs), panic disorder, and malingering, which should always be considered.

Syncope is defined as an abrupt, transient, complete loss of consciousness, associated with inability to maintain postural tone, with rapid and spontaneous recovery (Shen et al., 2017). Syncope may result from both cardiac and noncardiac causes. Specific causes of a transient impairment in cerebral perfusion include vasovagal episodes (typically a surge in parasympathetic autonomic tone), decreased cardiac output secondary to cardiac arrhythmias, outflow obstruction, hypovolemia, orthostatic hypotension, and decreased venous return. Cerebrovascular disturbances from transient ischemic attacks of the posterior cerebral circulation perfusing the brainstem, or cerebral vasospasm from migraine, subarachnoid hemorrhage, or hypertensive encephalopathy may result in temporary loss of consciousness. Situational syncope may occur in association with cough, micturition, defecation, swallowing, Valsalva maneuver, or diving. These spells are often mediated via a decrease in venous return to the thorax and/or an increase in sympathetic tone. Metabolic disturbances due to hypoxia, drugs, anemia, and hypoglycemia may result in frank syncope or, more frequently, the sensation of an impending faint (presyncope).

Absence seizures, generalized tonic-clonic seizures, and complex partial seizures are associated with alterations of consciousness and are usually easily distinguished from syncope by careful questioning. Seizures may be difficult to distinguish from PNESs, panic attacks, and malingering. In children, breath-holding spells, a form of syncope (discussed later under "Miscellaneous Causes of Altered Consciousness"), can cause a transitory alteration of consciousness that may mimic epileptic seizures in this population. Although rapid increases in ICP (which may result from intermittent hydrocephalus, severe head trauma, brain tumors, intracerebral hemorrhage, certain severe metabolic derangements or Reye syndrome) may produce sudden loss of consciousness, affected patients frequently have other neurological manifestations that lead to this diagnosis.

In patients with episodic impairment of consciousness, diagnosis relies heavily on the clinical history described by the patient, and obtaining a detailed history from unaffected observers is often essential to clarifying the diagnosis. Laboratory investigations may also provide useful information. In a minority of patients, a cause for the loss of consciousness may not be established, and these patients may require longer periods of observation. Table 2.1 compares the clinical features of syncope and seizures.

## SYNCOPE

The pathophysiological basis of syncope is the temporary failure of cerebral perfusion, with a reduction in cerebral oxygen availability. *Syncope* refers to a symptom complex characterized by lightheadedness, generalized muscle weakness, giddiness, visual blurring, tinnitus, and gastrointestinal (GI) symptoms. The patient may appear pale and feel cold and "sweaty." The onset of loss of consciousness generally is gradual but may be rapid if related to certain conditions such as a cardiac arrhythmia or in the elderly. The gradual onset may allow patients to protect themselves from falling and injury. Factors precipitating a vasovagal syncopal episode (also known sometimes as a simple faint) include emotional stress, unpleasant visual stimuli, prolonged standing, venipuncture, and pain. Although the duration of unconsciousness is brief, it may range from seconds to minutes. During the faint, the patient may be motionless or display myoclonic jerks but never tonic-clonic movements. Urinary incontinence is uncommon. The pulse is weak and often slow because patients may be briefly bradycardic (from parasympathetic tone) and vasodilated. Breathing may be shallow and the blood pressure barely obtainable. As the fainting episode corrects itself by the patient becoming horizontal, normal color returns, breathing becomes more regular, and the pulse and blood pressure return to normal. After the faint, the patient experiences some residual weakness, but unlike the postictal state, confusion, headaches, and drowsiness are uncommon. Nausea may be noted before the episode and may still be present when the patient regains consciousness. The causes of syncope, which may often overlap, are classified by their pathophysiological mechanism (Box 2.1), but cerebral hypoperfusion is always the common final pathway. Rarely, vasovagal syncope may

**TABLE 2.1 Comparison of Clinical Features of Syncope and Seizures**

| Features | Syncope | Seizure |
|---|---|---|
| Relation to posture | Common | No |
| Time of day | Diurnal | Diurnal or nocturnal |
| Precipitating factors | Emotion, injury, pain, crowds, heat, exercise, fear, dehydration, coughing, micturition, venipuncture, prolonged standing | Sleep deprivation, drug/alcohol withdrawal, illness, medication nonadherence |
| Skin color | Pallor | Cyanosis or normal |
| Diaphoresis | Common | Rare |
| Aura or premonitory symptoms | Often minutes or longer, but can be very brief | Brief |
| Convulsion | Rare | Common |
| Other abnormal movements | Minor irregular twitching | Rhythmic jerks |
| Injury | Rare | Common (with convulsive seizures) |
| Urinary incontinence | Rare | Common |
| Tongue biting | No | Common with convulsive seizures |
| Postictal confusion | Rare | Common |
| Postictal headache | No | Common |
| Focal neurological signs | No | Occasional |
| Cardiovascular signs | Common to have low blood pressure and heart rate during event; cardiovascular exam may be completely normal after event unless there is an underlying cardiac disorder | Rare |
| Abnormal findings on EEG | Rare (generalized slowing may occur during the event) | Common |

*EEG*, Electroencephalogram.

**BOX 2.1 Classification and Etiology of Syncope**

- Arrhythmias:
  - Bradyarrhythmias
  - Tachyarrhythmias
  - Reflex arrhythmias (temporary sinus pause or bradycardia)
- Decreased cardiac output:
  - Outflow obstruction
  - Inflow obstruction
  - Cardiomyopathy
  - Hypovolemic
- Hypotensive:
  - Vasovagal attack
  - Drugs
  - Dysautonomia
- Cerebrovascular:
  - Carotid disease
  - Vertebrobasilar disease
  - Vasospasm
  - Takayasu disease
- Metabolic:
  - Hypoglycemia
  - Anemia
  - Anoxia
- Hyperventilation
- Multifactorial:
  - Vasovagal (vasodepressor) attack
  - Cardiac syncope
  - Situational: cough, micturition, defecation, swallowing, diving, Valsalva maneuver

have a genetic component suggestive of autosomal dominant inheritance (Klein et al., 2013). Wieling et al. (2009) reviewed the clinical features of the successive phases of syncope, as discussed earlier.

### History and Physical Examination

The history and physical examination are the most important components of the initial evaluation of syncope. Significant age and sex differences exist in the frequency of the various types of syncope. Syncope occurring in children and young adults is most frequently due to hyperventilation or vasovagal (vasodepressor) attacks and less frequently due to congenital heart disease (Lewis and Dhala, 1999). Fainting associated with benign tachycardias without underlying organic heart disease also may occur in children. Syncope due to basilar migraine is more common in young females. Although vasovagal syncope can occur in older patients (Tan and Perry, 2008), when repeated syncope begins in later life, organic disease of the cerebral circulation or cardiovascular system usually is responsible and requires exhaustive investigation.

A thorough history is the most important step in establishing the cause of syncope. The patient's description usually establishes the diagnosis. The neurologist should always obtain as full a description as possible of the first faint. The clinical features should be established, with emphasis on precipitating factors, posture, type of onset of the faint (including whether it was abrupt or gradual), position of head and neck, the presence and duration of preceding and associated symptoms, duration of loss of consciousness, rate of recovery, and sequelae. If possible, question an observer about clonic movements, color changes, diaphoresis, pulse, respiration, urinary incontinence, and the nature of recovery. Be certain to ask about any prior events, and gather these same details for each event that the patient recalls.

Cardiac syncope is defined as syncope caused by bradycardia, tachycardia, or hypotension due to low cardiac index, blood flow obstruction, vasodilation, or acute vascular dissection (Shen et al., 2017). Cardiac syncope should be suspected in patients with known cardiac disease. Clues in the history that suggest cardiac syncope include a history of palpitations or a fluttering sensation in the chest before loss of consciousness. These symptoms are common in arrhythmias but do not definitively establish that diagnosis as the cause for the syncope. In vasodepressor syncope and orthostatic hypotension, preceding symptoms of lightheadedness are common. Episodes of cardiac syncope generally are briefer than vasodepressor syncope, and the onset usually is rapid. Episodes due to cardiac arrhythmias occur independently of position, whereas in vasodepressor syncope and syncope due to orthostatic hypotension the patient usually is standing.

Attacks of syncope precipitated by exertion suggest a cardiac etiology. Exercise may induce arrhythmic syncope or syncope due to decreased cardiac output secondary to blood flow obstruction, such as may occur with hypertrophic cardiomyopathy with dynamic outflow obstruction, or with aortic or subaortic stenosis. Exercise syncope also may be due to cerebrovascular disease, aortic arch disease, congenital heart disease, severe stenosis of any of the cardiac valves, pulseless disease (Takayasu disease, a type of vasculitis), pulmonary hypertension, anemia, hypoxia, and hypoglycemia. A family history of sudden cardiac death, especially in females, suggests the long QT syndrome. Postexercise syncope may be secondary to orthostasis in the setting of dilated vascular beds in the large muscles (cardiac output may normalize faster than systemic vascular resistance), vasovagal syncope brought on by relative hypovolemia (in a setting of dilated vasculature), or autonomic dysfunction. A careful and complete medical and medication history is mandatory to determine whether prescribed drugs have induced either orthostatic hypotension or cardiac arrhythmias. To avoid missing a significant cardiac disorder, one should always consider a comprehensive cardiac evaluation in patients with exercise-related syncope. Particularly in the elderly, cardiac syncope must be distinguished from more benign causes because of increased risk of sudden cardiac death (Anderson and O'Callaghan, 2012).

The neurologist should inquire about the frequency of attacks of loss of consciousness and the presence of cerebrovascular or cardiovascular symptoms between episodes. Question the patient whether all episodes are similar, because some patients experience more than one type of attack. In the elderly, syncope may cause unexplained falls lacking prodromal symptoms. With an accurate description of the attacks and familiarity with clinical features of various types of syncope, the physician will correctly diagnose most patients (Brignole et al., 2006; Shen et al., 2004), but confirmatory testing to rule in, or to exclude, some high-risk diagnoses may be required. Features that distinguish syncope from seizures and other alterations of consciousness are discussed later in the chapter.

After a complete history, the physical examination is of next importance. Examination during the episode is very informative but frequently impossible unless syncope is reproducible by a Valsalva maneuver or by recreating the circumstances of the attack, such as by position change. In the patient with suspected cardiac syncope, pay particular attention to the vital signs and determination of supine and erect blood pressure. Normally, with standing, the systolic blood pressure is stable or *rises* and the pulse rate may *increase*. An orthostatic drop in blood pressure greater than 15 mm Hg may suggest autonomic dysfunction. Assess blood pressure in both arms when suspecting cerebrovascular disease, subclavian steal, or Takayasu arteritis.

During syncope due to a cardiac arrhythmia, a heart rate faster than 140 beats/ min often indicates that the rhythm is not sinus tachycardia (may be a supraventricular tachycardia, an ectopic atrial or ventricular tachycardia, or atrial fibrillation or flutter), whereas a bradycardia with heart rate of less than 40 beats/min suggests complete atrioventricular (AV) block or a prolonged sinus pause. An irregular pulse indicates possible atrial fibrillation but may also be seen with frequent premature atrial or ventricular contractions, and with intermittent AV block. Vagal maneuvers, which include Valsalva and cold water to the face, sometimes terminate a supraventricular tachycardia. Carotid sinus massage may also be effective, but this maneuver is not advisable in the acute setting because of the risk of cerebral embolism from potential atheroma in the carotid artery wall. In contrast, an ectopic atrial or ventricular tachycardia will usually not be terminated by vagal maneuvers. It is recommended that all patients with syncope undergo a resting electrocardiogram as part of their initial evaluation (Shen et al., 2017).

All patients with syncope should also undergo cardiac auscultation for the presence of cardiac murmurs and abnormalities of the heart sounds. Possible murmurs of concern include aortic stenosis, hypertrophic cardiomyopathy with outflow tract obstruction, and mitral valve stenosis. An intermittent posture-related murmur may be associated with an atrial myxoma. A systolic click and late systolic murmur of mitral regurgitation in a young person suggests mitral valve prolapse. A pericardial rub suggests pericarditis. The finding of a murmur, rub, or abnormal click in a patient with syncope should prompt the physician to order an echocardiogram.

All patients should undergo observation of the carotid and jugular venous pulses and auscultation of the neck. The degree of aortic stenosis may be reflected at times in a delayed or weakened carotid upstroke. Carotid, ophthalmic, and supraclavicular bruits suggest underlying cerebrovascular disease. Jugular venous distention suggests congestive heart failure or other abnormal filling of the right heart, whereas a very low jugular venous pressure suggests hypovolemia. Carotid sinus massage should be avoided in patients with carotid bruits but may be useful in patients suspected of having carotid sinus syncope. It is important to keep in mind that up to 25% of asymptomatic persons may have some degree of carotid sinus hypersensitivity. Carotid massage should be avoided in patients with suspected cerebrovascular disease, even if they have no carotid bruit, and when performed should be under properly controlled conditions with electrocardiographic (ECG) and blood pressure monitoring. The response to carotid massage may be vasodepressor, cardioinhibitory, mixed, or minimal.

## Causes of Syncope

### Cardiac Arrhythmias

Both bradyarrhythmias and tachyarrhythmias may result in syncope, and abnormalities of cardiac rhythm due to dysfunction from the sinoatrial (SA) node to the Purkinje network may be involved. Always consider arrhythmias in all cases in which an obvious alternative mechanism is not established. Syncope due to cardiac arrhythmias generally occurs more quickly than syncope from other causes. Cardiac syncope may occur in any position, is occasionally exercise induced, and may occur in both congenital and acquired forms of heart disease.

Although palpitations sometimes occur during arrhythmias, others are unaware of any cardiac symptoms. Syncopal episodes secondary to cardiac arrhythmias may be more prolonged than benign syncope and often occur with less warning. Patients may injure themselves significantly during their fall. The most common arrhythmias causing syncope are AV block, SA block, and paroxysmal supraventricular and ventricular tachyarrhythmias. *AV block* describes disturbances of conduction occurring in the AV conducting system, which include the AV node to the bundle of His and the Purkinje network. *SA block* describes a failure of consistent pacemaker function of the SA node. *Paroxysmal tachycardia* refers to a rapid heart rate that comes on intermittently. It may be secondary to an ectopic focus or reentrant loop outside the SA node but above the ventricle (supraventricular), or it may be from a source below the AV node (ventricular). In patients with implanted pacemakers, syncope can occur because of pacemaker malfunction.

#### Atrioventricular Block

AV block is probably the most common cause of arrhythmic cardiac syncope. The term *Stokes-Adams attack* describes disturbances of consciousness occurring in association with a complete AV block. Complete AV block occurs primarily in elderly patients and is often also seen in patients with a history of aortic valve disease. The onset of a Stokes-Adams attack generally is sudden, although a number of visual, sensory, and perceptual premonitory symptoms may be experienced. During the syncopal attack, the pulse disappears and no heart sounds are audible. The patient is pale and, if standing, falls down, often with resultant injury. If the attack is sufficiently prolonged, respiration may become labored, and urinary incontinence and clonic muscle jerks may occur. Prolonged confusion and neurological signs of cerebral ischemia may be present. Regaining of consciousness generally is rapid.

The clinical features of complete AV block include a slow pulse and elevation of the jugular venous pressure, sometimes with cannon waves. The first heart sound is of variable intensity, and heart sounds related to atrial contractions may be audible. An ECG confirming the diagnosis demonstrates independence of atrial P waves and ventricular QRS complexes. During Stokes-Adams attacks, the ECG generally shows ventricular standstill or a very slow ventricular escape rhythm, but ventricular fibrillation or tachycardia also may occur.

### Sinoatrial Block

SA block may result in dizziness, lightheadedness, and syncope. It is most frequent in the elderly. Palpitations are common, and the patient appears pale. Patients with SA node dysfunction frequently have other conduction disturbances, and certain drugs (e.g., verapamil, digoxin, beta-blockers) may further impair SA node function. On examination, the patient's pulse may be regular between attacks. During an attack, the pulse may be slow or irregular, and any of a number of rhythm disturbances may be present.

### Paroxysmal Tachycardia

Supraventricular tachycardias include atrial fibrillation with a rapid ventricular response, atrial flutter, AV nodal reentry, and the Wolff-Parkinson-White syndrome (AV reentry involving an accessory pathway). These arrhythmias may suddenly reduce cardiac output enough to cause syncope. Ventricular tachycardia may result in syncope if the heart rate is sufficiently fast, and ventricular fibrillation will almost always result in nearly immediate syncope. Ventricular arrhythmias are more likely in the elderly and in patients with cardiac disease. Ventricular fibrillation may be part of the long QT syndrome, which has a cardiac-only phenotype or may be associated with congenital sensorineural deafness in children. In most patients with this syndrome, episodes begin in the first decade of life, but onset may be much later. Exercise may precipitate an episode of cardiac syncope. Long QT syndrome may be congenital or acquired and sometimes is misdiagnosed in adults as epilepsy. Acquired causes include cardiac ischemia, mitral valve prolapse, myocarditis, and electrolyte disturbances; there are also many drugs that can prolong the QT. In the short QT syndrome, signs and symptoms are highly variable, ranging from complete absence of clinical manifestations to recurrent syncope to sudden death. The age at onset often is young, and affected persons frequently are otherwise healthy. A family history of sudden death in a patient with a short QT may indicate a familial short QT syndrome inherited as an autosomal dominant mutation. The ECG demonstrates a short QT interval and a tall and peaked T wave, and electrophysiological studies may induce ventricular fibrillation. Brugada syndrome may produce syncope as a result of ventricular tachycardia or ventricular fibrillation (Brugada et al., 2000). The ECG in Brugada syndrome may or may not show a typical Brugada pattern at rest (i.e., an incomplete right bundle-branch block in leads $V_1$ and $V_2$ and significant downsloping ST elevation leading to inverted T waves in those two leads).

### Reflex Cardiac Arrhythmias

A hypersensitive carotid sinus may be a cause of syncope in the elderly, most frequently men. Syncope may result from a reflex sinus bradycardia, sinus arrest, or AV block; peripheral vasodilatation with a fall in arterial pressure; or a combination of both. Although 10% of the population older than 60 years of age may have a hypersensitive carotid sinus, not all such patients experience syncope. Accordingly, consider this diagnosis only when the clinical history is compatible. Carotid sinus syncope may be initiated by wearing a tight collar, by rapidly turning the head (including when patients do so on their own), or by carotid sinus massage on clinical examination. When syncope occurs, the patient usually is upright, and the duration of the loss of consciousness generally is a few minutes. On regaining consciousness, the patient is mentally clear. Unfortunately, no accepted diagnostic criteria exist for carotid sinus syncope, and the condition is likely overdiagnosed.

Syncope in certain patients can be induced by unilateral carotid massage or compression; however, in those with atherosclerotic carotid disease, this can sometimes cause partial or complete occlusion of the ipsilateral carotid artery or release of atheromatous emboli and subsequent stroke. Because of these risks, carotid artery massage is contraindicated in those with known or suspected carotid atherosclerotic disease.

The rare syndrome of glossopharyngeal neuralgia is characterized by intense paroxysmal pain in the throat and neck accompanied by bradycardia or asystole, severe hypotension, and, if prolonged, seizures. Episodes of pain may be initiated by swallowing but also by chewing, speaking, laughing, coughing, shouting, sneezing, yawning, or talking. The episodes of pain always precede the loss of consciousness (see Chapter 20). Rarely, cardiac syncope may be due to bradyarrhythmias consequent to vagus nerve irritation caused by esophageal diverticula, tumors, or aneurysms in the region of the carotid sinus or by mediastinal masses or gallbladder disease.

### Decreased Cardiac Output

Syncope may occur as a result of a sudden and marked decrease in cardiac output. Causes are both congenital and acquired. Tetralogy of Fallot, the most common congenital malformation causing syncope, does so by producing hypoxia due to right-to-left shunting. Other congenital conditions associated with cyanotic heart disease also may cause syncope. Ischemic heart disease and myocardial infarction (MI), aortic stenosis, hypertrophic cardiomyopathy with outflow tract obstruction, pulmonary hypertension, pulmonic valve stenosis, acute massive pulmonary embolism, atrial myxoma, and cardiac tamponade may sufficiently impair cardiac output to cause syncope. Exercise-induced or effort syncope may occur in aortic or subaortic stenosis and other states in which there is limited cardiac output and associated peripheral vasodilatation induced by the exercise. Exercise-induced cardiac syncope and exercise-induced cardiac arrhythmias may be related.

In patients with valvular heart disease, the cause of syncope may be related to flow through the valve or to arrhythmias. Syncope in valvular disease may also be due to reduced cardiac output secondary to myocardial failure, to mechanical prosthetic valve malfunction, or to thrombus formation at a valve. Mitral valve prolapse generally is a benign condition, but, rarely, cardiac arrhythmias can occur. The most significant arrhythmias are ventricular. In atrial myxoma or with massive pulmonary embolism, a sudden drop in left ventricular output may occur. In atrial myxoma, syncope frequently is positional and occurs when the tumor falls into the AV valve opening during a change in position of the patient, thereby causing obstruction of the ventricular inflow.

Decreased cardiac output also may be secondary to conditions causing an inflow obstruction or reduced venous return. Such conditions include superior and inferior vena cava obstruction, tension pneumothorax, constrictive cardiomyopathies, constrictive pericarditis, and cardiac tamponade. Patients may also inadvertently cause reduced venous return and hypotension during a prolonged coughing fit or breath hold. Syncope associated with aortic dissection may be due to cardiac tamponade but also may be secondary to hypotension, obstruction of cerebral circulation, or a cardiac arrhythmia.

### Hypovolemia

Acute blood loss, usually due to GI tract bleeding, may cause weakness, faintness, and syncope if sufficient blood is lost. Blood volume depletion by dehydration may cause faintness and weakness, but true syncope is uncommon except when combining dehydration and exercise. Both anemia and hypovolemia may predispose a patient to vasovagal symptoms and vasovagal syncope when standing upright.

### Hypotension

Several conditions cause syncope by producing a fall in arterial pressure. Cardiac causes were discussed earlier. The common faint (synonymous with *vasovagal* or *vasodepressor syncope*) is the most frequent cause of a transitory fall in blood pressure resulting in syncope. It often is recurrent, tends to occur in relation to emotional stimuli, and may affect 20%–25% of young people. Less commonly, it occurs in older patients with cardiovascular disease.

The common faint may or may not be associated with bradycardia. The patient experiences impairment of consciousness, with loss of postural tone. Acutely, signs of autonomic hyperactivity are common, including pallor, diaphoresis, nausea, and dilated pupils. After recovery, patients may have persistent pallor, sweating, and nausea; if they get up too quickly, they may black out again. Presyncopal symptoms of lethargy and fatigue, nausea, weakness, a sensation of an impending faint, yawning, ringing in the ears, and blurred or tunnel vision may occur. It is more likely to occur in certain circumstances such as in a hot crowded room, especially if the affected person is volume-depleted and standing for a prolonged period, although it may still occur when sitting upright. Venipuncture, the sight of blood, or a sudden painful or traumatic experience may precipitate syncope. When the patient regains consciousness, there usually is no confusion or headache, although weakness is frequent. As in other causes of syncope, if the period of cerebral hypoperfusion is prolonged, urinary incontinence and a few clonic movements may occur (convulsive syncope).

Orthostatic syncope occurs when autonomic factors that compensate for the upright posture are inadequate. This can result from a variety of clinical disorders. Blood volume depletion or venous pooling may cause syncope when the affected person assumes an upright posture. Orthostatic hypotension resulting in syncope also may occur with drugs that impair sympathetic nervous system function. Diuretics, antihypertensive medications, nitrates, arterial vasodilators, sildenafil, calcium channel blockers, monoamine oxidase inhibitors, phenothiazines, opiates, L-dopa, alcohol, and tricyclic antidepressants all may cause orthostatic hypotension. Patients with postural orthostatic tachycardia syndrome (POTS) frequently experience orthostatic symptoms without orthostatic hypotension, but syncope can occur occasionally. Data suggest that there is sympathetic activation in this syndrome (Garland et al., 2007). Autonomic nervous system dysfunction resulting in syncope due to orthostatic hypotension may be a result of primary autonomic failure due to Shy-Drager syndrome (multiple system atrophy) or Riley-Day syndrome. Neuropathies that affect the autonomic nervous system include those of diabetes mellitus, amyloidosis, Guillain-Barré syndrome, acquired immunodeficiency syndrome (AIDS), chronic alcoholism, hepatic porphyria, beriberi, autoimmune subacute autonomic neuropathy, and small fiber neuropathies. Rarely, subacute combined degeneration, syringomyelia, and other spinal cord lesions may damage the descending sympathetic pathways, producing orthostatic hypotension. Accordingly, conditions that affect both the central and peripheral baroreceptor mechanisms may cause orthostatic hypotension (Benafroch, 2008).

### Cerebrovascular Ischemia

Syncope occasionally may result from reduction of cerebral blood flow in either the carotid or vertebrobasilar system in patients with extensive occlusive disease. Most frequently, the underlying condition is atherosclerosis of the cerebral vessels, but reduction of cerebral blood flow due to cerebral embolism, mechanical factors in the neck (e.g., severe osteoarthritis), and arteritis (e.g., Takayasu disease or cranial arteritis) may be responsible. In the subclavian steal syndrome, a very rare impairment of consciousness is associated with upper extremity exercise and resultant diversion of cerebral blood flow to the peripheral circulation. In elderly patients with cervical skeletal deformities, certain head movements such as hyperextension or lateral rotation can result in syncope secondary to vertebrobasilar arterial ischemia. In these patients, associated vestibular symptoms are common. Occasionally, cerebral vasospasm secondary to basilar artery migraine or subarachnoid hemorrhage may be responsible. Insufficiency of the cerebral circulation frequently causes other neurological symptoms, depending on the circulation involved.

Reduction in blood flow in the carotid circulation may lead to loss of consciousness, lightheadedness, giddiness, and a sensation of an impending faint. Reduction in blood flow in the vertebrobasilar system also may lead to loss of consciousness, but dizziness, lightheadedness, drop attacks without loss of consciousness, and bilateral motor and sensory symptoms are more common. However, dizziness and lightheadedness alone are not symptoms of vertebrobasilar insufficiency. Syncope due to compression of the vertebral artery during certain head and neck movements may be associated with episodes of vertigo, disequilibrium, or drop attacks. Patients may describe blackouts on looking upward suddenly or on turning the head quickly to one side. In general, symptoms persist for several seconds after the movement stops.

In Takayasu disease, major occlusion of blood flow in the carotid and vertebrobasilar systems may occur; in addition to fainting, other neurological manifestations are frequent. Pulsations in the neck and arm vessels usually are absent, and blood pressure in the arms is unobtainable. The syncopal episodes characteristically occur with mild or moderate exercise and with certain head movements. Cerebral vasospasm may result in syncope, particularly if the posterior circulation is involved. In basilar artery migraine, usually seen in young women and children, a variety of brainstem symptoms also may be experienced, and it is associated with a pulsating headache. The loss of consciousness usually is gradual, but a confusional state may last for hours.

### Metabolic Disorders

A number of metabolic disturbances, including hypoglycemia, anoxia, and hyperventilation-induced alkalosis, may predispose affected persons to syncope, but usually only lightheadedness and dizziness are experienced. The abruptness of onset of loss of consciousness depends on the acuteness and reversibility of the metabolic disturbances. Syncope due to hypoglycemia usually develops gradually. The patient has a sensation of hunger; there may be a relationship to fasting, a history of diabetes mellitus, and a prompt response to ingestion of food. Symptoms are unrelated to posture but may increase with exercise. During the syncopal attack, no significant change in blood pressure or pulse occurs. Hypoadrenalism may give rise to syncope by causing orthostatic hypotension. Disturbances of calcium, magnesium, and potassium metabolism are other rare causes of syncope. Anoxia may produce syncope because of the lack of oxygen or through the production of a vasodepressor type of syncope. A feeling of lightheadedness is common, but true syncope is less common. Patients with underlying cardiac or pulmonary disease are susceptible. In patients with chronic anemia or certain hemoglobinopathies that impair oxygen transport, similar symptoms may occur. Syncopal symptoms may be more prominent with exercise or physical activity.

Hyperventilation-induced syncope usually has a psychogenic origin. During hyperventilation, the patient may experience paresthesia of the face, hands, and feet, a buzzing sensation in the head, lightheadedness, giddiness, blurring of vision, mouth dryness, and occasionally tetany. Patients often complain of tightness in the chest and a sense of panic. Symptoms can occur in the supine or erect position and are gradual in onset. Rebreathing into a paper bag relieves the symptoms. During hyperventilation, a tachycardia may be present, but blood pressure generally remains normal.

### Miscellaneous Causes of Syncope

More than one mechanism may be responsible in certain types of syncope. Both vasodepressor and cardioinhibitory factors may be operational in common presentations of vasovagal syncope. In cardiac syncope, a reduction of cardiac output may be due to a single cause such as obstruction to inflow or outflow or a cardiac arrhythmia, but multiple factors are frequent.

Situational syncope, such as is associated with cough (tussive syncope) and micturition, are special cases of reflex syncope. In cough syncope, loss of consciousness occurs after a paroxysm of severe coughing. This is most likely to occur in obese men, usually smokers or patients with chronic bronchitis. The syncopal episodes occur suddenly, generally after repeated coughing but occasionally after a single cough. Before losing consciousness, the patient may feel lightheaded. The face often becomes flushed secondary to congestion, and then pale. Diaphoresis may be present, and loss of muscle tone may occur. Syncope generally is brief, lasting only seconds, and recovery is rapid. Several factors probably are operational in causing cough syncope. The most significant is blockage of venous return by raised intrathoracic pressure. In weight-lifting syncope, a similar mechanism is operational.

Micturition syncope most commonly occurs in men during or after micturition, usually after arising from bed in the middle of the night to urinate in the erect position. There may be a history of drinking alcohol before going to bed. The syncope may result from sudden reflex peripheral vasodilatation caused by the release of intravesicular pressure and bradycardia. The relative peripheral vasodilatation from recent alcohol use and a supine sleeping position is contributory because blood pressure is lowest in the middle of the night. The syncopal propensity may increase with fever. Rarely, micturition syncope with headache may result from a pheochromocytoma in the bladder wall. Defecation syncope is uncommon, but it probably shares the underlying pathophysiological mechanisms responsible for micturition syncope. Convulsive syncope is an episode of syncope of any cause that is sufficiently prolonged to result in a few clonic jerks; the other features typically are syncopal and should not be confused with epileptic seizures. Other causes of situational syncope include diving and the postprandial state. Syncope during sexual activity may be due to neurocardiogenic syncope, coronary artery disease, or the use of erectile dysfunction medications. Rare intracranial causes of syncope include intermittent obstruction to cerebrospinal fluid (CSF) flow such as with a third ventricular mass. Rarely, syncope can occur with Arnold-Chiari malformations, but these patients usually have other symptoms of brainstem dysfunction.

### Investigations of Patients with Syncope

In the investigation of the patient with episodic impairment of consciousness, the diagnostic tests performed depend on the initial differential diagnosis. It is best to individualize investigations, but some measurements such as hematocrit, blood glucose, and ECG are always appropriate. A resting ECG may reveal an abnormality of cardiac rhythm or conduction or suggest the presence of underlying ischemic or congenital heart disease. In the patient suspected of cardiac syncope, a chest radiograph may show evidence of cardiac hypertrophy, valvular heart disease, or pulmonary hypertension. Other noninvasive investigations that may be helpful include echocardiography, exercise stress testing, radionuclide cardiac scanning, prolonged Holter monitoring for the detection of cardiac arrhythmias, and cardiac magnetic resonance imaging (MRI). Echocardiography is useful in the diagnosis of valvular heart disease, cardiomyopathy, atrial myxoma, prosthetic valve dysfunction, pericardial effusion, aortic dissection, and congenital heart disease. Holter monitoring detects twice as many ECG abnormalities as those discovered on a routine ECG and may disclose an arrhythmia at the time of a syncopal episode. Holter monitoring typically for a 24-hour period is usual, although longer periods of recording may be required, typically up to 30 days. Implantable loop recorders can provide long-term rhythm monitoring in patients suspected of having a seldom but highly symptomatic cardiac arrhythmia (Krahn et al., 2004).

Exercise testing and electrophysiological studies are useful in selected patients. Exercise testing may be useful in detecting coronary artery disease, and exercise-related syncopal recordings may help to localize the site of conduction disturbances. Exercise testing should be considered in anyone with a history of exertional symptoms. Consider tilt-table testing in patients with unexplained syncope in high-risk settings or with recurrent faints in the absence of heart disease (Kapoor, 1999). Falsepositives occur, and 10% of healthy persons may faint during the test. Tilt testing frequently uses pharmacological agents such as nitroglycerin or isoproterenol, which increase sensitivity but decrease specificity. The specificity of tilt-table testing is approximately 90%, but the sensitivity differs in different patient populations. In patients suspected to have syncope due to cerebrovascular causes, noninvasive diagnostic studies including Doppler flow studies of the cerebral vessels and MRI or magnetic resonance angiography may provide useful information. The American Academy of Neurology recommends that carotid imaging not be performed unless there are other focal neurological symptoms (Langer-Gould et al., 2013). Cerebral angiography is sometimes useful. Electroencephalography (EEG) is useful in differentiating syncope from epileptic seizure disorders. EEG should be obtained only when a seizure disorder is suspected and generally has a low diagnostic yield (Poliquin-Lasnier and Moore, 2009).

A systematic evaluation can establish a definitive diagnosis in 98% of patients (Brignole et al., 2006). Neurally mediated (vasovagal or vasodepressor) syncope was found in 66% of patients, orthostatic hypotension in 10%, primary arrhythmias in 11%, and structural cardiopulmonary disease in 5%. Initial history, physical examination, and a standard ECG established a diagnosis in 50% of patients. A risk score such as the San Francisco Syncope Rule (SFSR) can help to identify patients who need urgent referral. The presence of cardiac failure, anemia, abnormal ECG, or systolic hypotension helps to identify these patients (Parry and Tan, 2010). A systematic review of the SFSR accuracy (Saccilotto et al., 2011) found that the rule cannot be applied safely to all patients and should only be applied to patients for whom no cause of syncope is identified. The rule should be used only in conjunction with clinical evaluation, particularly in elderly patients. The Risk Stratification of Syncope in the Emergency Department (ROSE) study is another risk stratification evaluation of patients who present to the emergency department (Reed et al., 2010). Independent predictors of 1-month serious outcome were elevated brain natriuretic peptide concentration, positive fecal occult blood, hemoglobin of 90 g/L or less, oxygen saturation of 94% or less, and Q wave on the ECG.

Although these risk scores can be used, there has been limited external validation, and there is no evidence to support that their use leads to better clinical outcomes than with unstructured clinical judgment (Shen et al., 2017).

In summary, the initial and most important parts of the evaluation of a patient with syncope are a detailed history from the patient and any witnesses of the syncopal event, followed by a thorough physical examination with a focus on the neurological and cardiovascular findings. It is recommended that all patients receive an ECG as part of an initial syncope evaluation. It is reasonable for most patients to undergo at least limited laboratory testing in the acute setting to rule out anemia and hypoglycemia. Beyond this, imaging and laboratory testing should be individualized and may not be necessary if the history and physical are highly suggestive of vasovagal syncope and if the exam and ECG show no concerning findings. In 2017 the American College of Cardiology, American Heart Association, and the Heart Rhythm Society released a joint guideline on the evaluation and management of patients with syncope that may further guide the clinician in the care of these patients (Shen et al., 2017).

## SEIZURES

Seizures can cause sudden, unexplained loss of consciousness in a child or an adult (see Chapter 100). Seizures and syncope are distinguishable clinically, and one should be familiar with the pathophysiology and clinical features for both.

### Pathophysiology

Epilepsy is the syndrome of recurrent unprovoked seizures. It is broadly dichotomized into generalized and partial (also known as focal). Generalized epilepsies are characterized by seizures that involve both hemispheres at onset rather than by electrographic spread. They are typically genetically predisposed and tend to manifest in childhood and adolescence in the form of discrete epilepsy syndromes (e.g., childhood absence epilepsy, juvenile myoclonic epilepsy). In contrast, partial or focal epilepsies are characterized by focal-onset seizures that may or may not secondarily generalize (i.e., propagate to various parts of the brain). These are often termed "localization related" or symptomatic due to the known local pathology (e.g., tumor, gliosis, abscess) that serves as an epileptogenic focus. If the pathology is suspected but not visualized, the term cryptogenic is instead used.

### History and Physical Examination

The most definitive way to diagnose epilepsy and the seizure type is clinical observation of the seizure, although this often is not possible, except when seizures are frequent. The history of an episode, as obtained from the patient and an observer, is of paramount importance. The neurologist should obtain a family history and should inquire about birth complications, central nervous system (CNS) infection, head trauma, and previous febrile seizures because they all may have relevance.

The neurologist should obtain a complete description of the episode and inquire about any warning before the event, possible precipitating factors, and other neurological symptoms that may suggest an underlying structural cause. Important considerations are the age at onset, frequency, and diurnal variation of the events. Seizures generally are brief and have stereotypical patterns, as described previously. With complex partial seizures and tonic-clonic seizures, a period of postictal confusion is highly characteristic and is much slower to resolve than the typical postsyncopal confusion. Unlike some types of syncope, seizures are unrelated to posture and generally last longer. In a tonic-clonic seizure, cyanosis frequently is present, pallor is uncommon, and breathing may be stertorous. In children with autonomic seizures (Panayiotopoulos syndrome) syncope-like epileptic seizures can occur, although usually accompanied by other features that help to clarify the diagnosis (Koutroumanidis et al., 2012).

Tonic-clonic and complex partial seizures may begin at any age, although young infants may not demonstrate the typical features because of incomplete development of the nervous system; specifically, the lack of CNS myelination in infants leads to more migratory jerking rather than the synchronous jerking seen with tonic-clonic seizures in children and adults.

The neurological examination may reveal an underlying structural disturbance responsible for the seizure disorder. Perinatal trauma may result in asymmetries of physical development, cranial bruits may indicate an arteriovenous malformation, and space-occupying lesions may result in papilledema or in focal motor, sensory, or reflex signs. In the pediatric age group, mental retardation occurs in association with birth injury or metabolic defects. The skin should be examined for abnormal pigment changes and other dysmorphic features characteristic of some of the neurodegenerative disorders.

If examination occurs immediately after a suspected tonic-clonic seizure, the neurologist should search for abnormal signs such as focal motor weakness ("Todd paralysis") and reflex asymmetry and for pathological reflexes such as a Babinski sign. Such findings may help to confirm that the attack was a seizure and suggest a possible lateralization or location of the seizure focus.

## SEIZURE CLASSIFICATION

Seizure classification is based on their functional distribution and on the structural neuroanatomy of the brain (see Chapter 100). The location and extent of a seizure's involvement is reflected in its clinical manifestation, termed its *semiology*.

### Absence Seizures

The onset of absence seizures is usually between the ages of 5 and 15 years, and a family history of seizures is present in 20%–40% of patients. The absence seizure is a well-defined clinical and electrographic event. The essential feature is an abrupt, brief episode of decreased awareness without any warning, aura, or postictal symptoms. At the onset of the absence seizure, there is an abrupt interruption of activity, or behavioral arrest. A simple absence seizure is characterized clinically only by an alteration of consciousness. Characteristic of a complex absence seizure is an alteration of consciousness and other signs such as minor motor automatisms (repetitive purposeless movements), most often fluttering of the eyelids. During a simple absence seizure, the patient remains immobile, breathing is normal, skin color remains unchanged, postural tone is not lost, and no motor manifestations occur. After the seizure, the patient immediately resumes the previous activities and may be unaware of the attack. An absence seizure generally lasts 10–15 seconds, but it may be shorter or as long as 40 seconds.

Complex absence seizures have additional manifestations such as diminution of postural tone that may cause the patient to fall, an increase in postural tone, minor clonic movements of the facial musculature or extremities, minor face or extremity automatisms, or autonomic phenomena such as pallor, flushing, tachycardia, piloerection, mydriasis, or urinary incontinence.

If absence seizures are suspected, office diagnosis is frequently possible by having the patient hyperventilate for 3–4 minutes, which often, although not always, induces an absence seizure.

### Tonic-Clonic Seizures

The tonic-clonic seizure is the most dramatic manifestation of epilepsy and is characterized by motor activity and loss of consciousness. Tonic-clonic seizures may be the only manifestation of epilepsy or may be associated with other seizure types. In a primary generalized tonic-clonic seizure, the affected person generally experiences no warning or aura, although a few myoclonic jerks may occur in some patients. The seizure begins with a tonic phase, during which there is sustained muscle contraction lasting 10–20 seconds. Following this phase is a clonic phase characterized by recurrent synchronous muscle contractions or rhythmic jerking. During a tonic-clonic seizure, a number of autonomic changes may be present, including an increase in blood pressure and heart rate, apnea, mydriasis, urinary or fecal incontinence, piloerection, cyanosis, and diaphoresis. Injury may result from a fall, shoulder dislocation, or tongue biting. In the postictal period, consciousness returns quite slowly, and the patient may remain lethargic and confused for a variable period. The patient may remain somnolent and wish to sleep for many hours. Pathologically brisk reflexes may be elicitable.

Some generalized motor seizures with transitory alteration of consciousness may have only tonic or only clonic components. Tonic seizures consist of an increase in muscle tone, and the alteration of consciousness generally is brief. Clonic seizures have a brief impairment of consciousness and bilateral clonic movements. Recovery may be rapid, but if the seizure is more prolonged, a postictal period of confusion may be noted.

## Complex Partial Seizures

In a complex partial seizure, the first seizure manifestation may be an alteration of consciousness, but the patient frequently experiences an aura or warning symptom. The seizure may have a simple partial onset that may include motor, sensory, visceral, or psychic symptoms. The patient initially may experience hallucinations or illusions, affective symptoms such as fear or depression, cognitive symptoms such as a sense of depersonalization or unreality, or aphasia. The particular symptoms are tightly correlated to the neuroanatomy of the seizure onset zone and eventually the extent of propagation.

The complex partial seizure generally lasts 1–2 minutes but may be shorter or longer. If it propagates widely, it may become secondarily generalized and evolve into a tonic-clonic convulsion. During a complex partial seizure, automatisms, generally more complex than those in absence seizures, may occur. The automatisms may involve continuation of the patient's activity before the onset of the seizure, or they may be new motor acts. Such automatisms are variable but frequently consist of oral automatisms (chewing or swallowing movements, lip smacking) or automatisms of the extremities, including fumbling with objects, walking, or trying to stand up. The duration of the postictal period after a complex partial seizure is variable, with a gradual return to normal consciousness and normal response to external stimuli. Table 2.2 provides a comparison of absence seizures and complex partial seizures.

**TABLE 2.2 Comparison of Absence and Complex Partial Seizures**

| Feature | Absence Seizure | Complex Partial Seizure |
|---|---|---|
| Neurological status | Normal | May have positive history or examination |
| Age at onset | Childhood or adolescence | Any age |
| Aura or warning | No | Common |
| Onset | Abrupt | Gradual |
| Duration | Seconds | Typically 1–2 minutes |
| Automatisms | Simple | More complex |
| Provocation by hyperventilation | Common | Uncommon |
| Termination | Abrupt | Gradual |
| Postictal phase | No | Confusion, fatigue |
| Frequency | Possibly multiple seizures per day | Occasional |
| Electroencephalogram | 3 Hz generalized spike-and-wave | Focal epileptic discharges or focal slowing |
| Neuroimaging | Usually normal findings | May demonstrate focal lesions |

## Investigations of Seizures

In the initial investigations of the patient with tonic-clonic or complex partial seizures, one should perform a complete blood cell count, urinalysis, biochemical screening, and determinations of blood glucose level and serum calcium concentration. Laboratory investigations generally are not helpful in establishing a diagnosis of absence seizures. In infants and children, consider biochemical screening for amino acid disorders. CSF examination is not necessary in every patient with a seizure disorder and should be reserved for those in whom a recent seizure may relate to an acute CNS infection.

MRI is the imaging modality of choice for the investigation of patients with suspected seizures. It is superior to computed tomography and increases the yield of focal structural disturbances.

EEG provides laboratory support for a clinical impression and helps to classify the type of seizure. Epilepsy is a clinical diagnosis; therefore an EEG cannot confirm the diagnosis with certainty unless the patient has a clinical event during the recording. Normal findings on the EEG do not exclude epilepsy, and minor nonspecific abnormalities do not confirm epilepsy. Some patients with clinically documented seizures show no abnormality even after serial or prolonged EEG recordings, including with special activation techniques. The EEG is most frequently helpful in the diagnosis of absence seizures. EEG supplemented with simultaneous video monitoring may document events of loss or alteration of consciousness, allowing for a strict correlation between EEG changes and the clinical manifestations in question. Video EEG is also is useful in distinguishing epileptic seizures from nonepileptic phenomena.

In most patients, an accurate diagnosis requires only a carefully taken clinical history, physical examination, and the aforementioned investigations. Others present a diagnostic dilemma and may require more extensive and invasive testing.

## Psychogenic Nonepileptic Spells

Nonepileptic spells are paroxysmal episodes of altered behavior that superficially resemble epileptic seizures but lack the expected EEG epileptic changes (Ettinger et al., 1999). However, 10%–20% of patients with nonepileptic spells also experience epileptic seizures and vice versa. In such cases, carefully determining semiological differences among the spell types is important when the spells are ongoing despite seemingly appropriate interventions.

A diagnosis often is difficult to establish based on the initial history alone. Establishing the correct diagnosis often requires observation of the patient's clinical episodes, but complex partial seizures of frontal lobe origin may be difficult to distinguish from nonepileptic spells. Most frequently, they superficially resemble tonic-clonic seizures, with whole-body shaking and unresponsiveness. They generally are abrupt in onset, typically occur in the presence of other people, and do not occur during sleep. Motor activity is uncoordinated, but urinary incontinence and physical injury are uncommon. Nonepileptic spells tend to be more prolonged than tonic-clonic seizures. Pelvic thrusting and back arching are common. Eye closure is common in nonepileptic spells, whereas the eyes tend to be open in epileptic seizures (Chung et al., 2006). During and immediately after the spell, the patient may not respond to verbal or painful stimuli. Cyanosis does not occur, and focal neurological signs and pathological reflexes are absent.

PNES syncope without prominent motor activity can resemble. These spells are not uncommon and are often referred to as psychogenic pseudosyncope (Tannemaat et al., 2013). The apparent loss of consciousness in these patients may be longer than in syncope. The diagnosis can be distinguished from syncope if tilt-table testing fails to document a decrease in heart rate or blood pressure.

In the patient with known epilepsy, consider the diagnosis of nonepileptic spells when previously controlled seizures become medically refractory. The patient should undergo psychological assessments because most affected persons are found to have specific psychiatric disturbances. In this patient group, a high frequency of hysteria, depression, anxiety, somatoform disorders, dissociative disorders, and personality disturbances is recognized. A history of physical or sexual abuse is also more prevalent in patients with PNESs. At times, a secondary gain is identifiable, although the absence of an identified gain or trigger should not preclude the diagnosis. In some patients with PNESs, the clinical episodes frequently precipitate by suggestion, by certain clinical tests such as hyperventilation and photic stimulation, and by placebo procedures such as intravenous saline infusion, tactile (vibration) stimulation, or pinching the nose to induce apnea. Hyperventilation and photic stimulation also may induce epileptic seizures, but their clinical features usually are distinctive. Some physicians avoid the use of placebo procedures because of the potential for an adverse effect on the doctor-patient relationship (Parra et al., 1998).

Findings on the EEG in patients with PNESs are normal during the clinical episode, demonstrating no evidence of an ictal process. However, it is important to note that a number of organic conditions may present with similar behavioral and motor symptoms and a nonepileptiform EEG (Caplan et al., 2011). These may include conditions such as frontal lobe seizures, limb-shaking transient ischemic attacks, and paroxysmal dyskinesias, and a careful clinical history and adjunct testing are paramount. With the introduction of long-term ambulatory EEG monitoring, correlating the episodic behavior of a patient with the EEG tracing is possible, and PNESs are distinguishable from epileptic seizures. Table 2.3 compares the features of PNES with those of epileptic seizures.

Although several procedures are used to help distinguish epileptic seizures from PNESs, none of these procedures have both high sensitivity and high specificity. No procedure attains the reliability of EEG-video monitoring, which remains the standard diagnostic method for distinguishing between the two (Cuthill and Espire, 2005).

**TABLE 2.3 Comparison of Psychogenic and Epileptic Seizures**

| Attack Feature | Psychogenic Seizure | Epileptic Seizure |
|---|---|---|
| Stereotypy of attack | Often variable | Stereotypical |
| Onset or progression | Gradual | More rapid |
| Duration | May be prolonged | Typically 1–2 minutes |
| Diurnal variation | Daytime | Nocturnal or daytime |
| Injury | Rare | Can occur with tonic-clonic seizures |
| Tongue biting | Rare (typically tip of tongue) | Can occur with tonic-clonic seizures (lateral tongue or inside of cheek) |
| Ictal eye closure | Common | Rare (eyes typically open) |
| Urinary incontinence | Rare | Frequent |
| Vocalization | May occur; variable (often crying, moaning) | Tonic-clonic seizures may have ictal cry at onset |
| Motor activity | Prolonged, uncoordinated; pelvic thrusting, back arching | Typically unilateral rhythmic jerking, dystonic posturing of a limb, or synchronous tonic-clonic activity |
| Prolonged loss of muscle tone | Common | Rare |
| Postictal confusion | Rare | Common (several minutes, often fatigued for hours desiring sleep) |
| Postictal headache | Rare | Common |
| Postictal crying | Common | Rare |
| Relation to medication changes | Unrelated | Usually related |
| Relation to menses in women | Uncommon | Occasionally increased |
| Triggers | Emotional disturbances | Sleep deprivation, illness, medication nonadherence |
| Frequency of attacks | More frequent, up to daily | Less frequent |
| Interictal EEG findings | Normal | Frequently abnormal |
| Reproduction of attack by suggestion | Sometimes | No |
| Ictal EEG findings | Normal | Abnormal |
| Presence of secondary gain | Common | Uncommon |
| Presence of others | Frequently | Variable |
| Psychiatric disturbances | Very common (though not always apparent) | Variable |

*EEG*, Electroencephalogram.

## MISCELLANEOUS CAUSES OF ALTERED CONSCIOUSNESS

In children, alteration of consciousness may accompany breath-holding spells and metabolic disturbances. Breath-holding spells and seizures are easily distinguished. Most spells start at 6–28 months of age, but they may occur as early as the first month of life; they usually disappear by 5 or 6 years of age. Breath-holding spells may occur several times per day and appear as either cyanosis or pallor.

The trigger for cyanotic breath-holding spells is usually a sudden injury or fright, anger, or frustration. The child initially is provoked, cries vigorously for a few breaths, and stops breathing in expiration, whereupon cyanosis rapidly develops. Consciousness is lost because of hypoxia. Although stiffening, a few clonic movements, and urinary incontinence occasionally are observed, these episodes can be clearly distinguished from epileptic seizures by the history of provocation and by noting that the apnea and cyanosis occur before any alteration of consciousness. In these children, findings on the neurological examination and the EEG are normal.

The provocation for pallid breath-holding is often a mild painful injury or a startle. The infant cries initially and then becomes pale and loses consciousness. As in the cyanotic type, stiffening, clonic movements, and urinary incontinence may rarely occur. In the pallid infant syndrome, loss of consciousness is secondary to excessive vagal tone, resulting in bradycardia and subsequent cerebral ischemia, as in a vasovagal attack.

Breath-holding spells do not require treatment, but when intervention is required, levetiracetam (Keppra) is effective for prophylaxis at ordinary anticonvulsant doses.

Several pediatric metabolic disorders may have clinical manifestations of alterations of consciousness, lethargy, or seizures (see Chapter 90).

*The complete reference list is available online at https://expertconsult.inkling.com/.* 

# 3

# Falls and Drop Attacks

Bernd F. Remler, Hatim Attar

## OUTLINE



## FALLS AND DROP ATTACKS—INTRODUCTION

Falling in childhood is part of growing up and usually medically insignificant, unless a serious childhood illness contributes. With advancing age, the potential for injury and other complications increases, and falling eventually develops into a dangerous burden for the elderly and the neurologically impaired. Quality of life can be severely affected by associated morbidity, immobilization, fear of falling (FOF), and growing dependency. Despite improved understanding of falls and their prevention, they remain a leading public health problem. The 2014 Behavioral Risk Factor Surveillance System (BRFSS) estimated that more than a fourth of adults older than 65 years have fallen, resulting in 29 million annual falls, more than 7 million injuries, and 800,000 hospital admissions in the United States. The corresponding cost to Medicare alone exceeded $31 billion and $50 billion for all medical care (Centers for Disease Control and Prevention, 2017, August 17). Fall-related injuries belong to the 20 most costly medical conditions.

Clinically, a large number of etiologies of falls have to be considered. A useful initial approach is to determine whether a patient has suffered a drop attack or an accidental fall. In this discussion the term drop attack describes a sudden fall occurring without a prodrome that may or may not be associated with loss of consciousness and cannot be prevented by assistive devices. In contrast, falls reflect an inability to remain upright during a postural challenge. Potential etiologies of drop attacks include cardiac, epileptic, vascular, sleep, and vestibular disorders, as well as congenital brain abnormalities and intracranial masses. In neurological practice, falling is most commonly associated with chronic disorders such as neuropathies, stroke, multiple sclerosis (MS), parkinsonism, and dementia. Affected patients have impaired control of stability and gait due to functional declines in neuromuscular, sensory, vestibulocerebellar, and cognitive systems. Finally, the elderly, with their inevitable infirmities and accumulating functional deficits, frequently fall. These associations permit a classification of falls and drop attacks, as presented in Box 3.1.

As is true for most neurological presentations, the medical history is essential in establishing the likely etiology of a patient's fall. Aside from gender, age, medications, and neurological conditions, which all affect fall risk, answers to the following questions should be sought:

What were the circumstances of the fall and has the patient fallen before?
Did the patient lose consciousness? If so, for how long?
Did lightheadedness, vertiginous sensations, or palpitations precede the event?
Is there a history of a seizure disorder, startle sensitivity, excessive daytime sleepiness, or falls precipitated by strong emotions?
Does the patient have headaches or migraine attacks associated with weakness?
Does the patient have vascular risk factors, and were there previous symptoms suggestive of transient ischemic attacks (TIAs)?
Are there symptoms of sensory loss, limb weakness, or stiffness?
Is there a history of visual impairment, hearing loss, vertigo, or tinnitus?

The neurological examination identifies predisposing functional deficits. However, in the case of drop attacks, the examination is often normal, posing a diagnostic challenge. In such patients, neuroimaging is necessary. Further workup is tailored to the clinical circumstance and may include vascular imaging, cardiac and autonomic studies, electroencephalogram (EEG), nocturnal polysomnography, and, rarely, genetic and metabolic testing when related conditions are suspected. Psychogenic disorders of station and gait need to be considered in patients who frequently experience near falls without injuries.

## DROP ATTACKS WITH LOSS OF CONSCIOUSNESS

### Syncope

The manifestations and causes of syncope are described in Chapter 2. Severe ventricular arrhythmias and hypotension lead to cephalic ischemia and falling. With sudden-onset third-degree heart block (Stokes-Adams attack), the patient loses consciousness and falls without warning. Other causes of decreased cardiac output, such as bradyarrythmias or tachyarrhythmias, are believed to be associated with prodromal faintness. However, reliance on history to determine a cardiac etiology of a fall may be inadequate because elderly patients with sick sinus syndrome can be amnestic for presyncopal symptoms. When occurring in young athletes, exertional drop attacks indicate the presence of potentially life-threatening structural heart disease, including

## BOX 3.1 Causes and Types of Falls and Drops

**Drop Attacks**

With loss of consciousness:
- Syncope
- Seizures

Without loss of consciousness:
- Transient ischemic attacks:
  - Vertebrobasilar insufficiency
  - Anterior cerebral artery ischemia
- Third ventricular and posterior fossa tumors
- Chiari malformation
- Otolithic crisis
  - Cataplexy

**Falls**

Neuromuscular disorders (neuropathy, radiculopathy, and myopathy)
Cerebral or cerebellar disorders
Cryptogenic falls in the middle-aged
Aging, neurodegeneration, and the neural substrate of gait and balance:
- Fear of falling
- Basal ganglia disorders:
  - Parkinson disease
  - Progressive supranuclear palsy and other parkinsonian syndromes
- The aged state

aortic stenosis or right ventricular dysplasia, among others. A large atrial myxoma can present in the same manner.

Cerebral hypoperfusion due to peripheral loss of vascular tone (orthostasis) is usually identifiable by a presyncopal syndrome of progressive lightheadedness, faintness, dimming of vision, and "rubbery"-feeling legs, but even in the context of positive tilt-table testing, up to 37% of patients report a clinically misleading symptom of true, "cardiogenic" vertigo (Newman-Toker et al., 2008). Vertigo and downbeat nystagmus may also occur with asystole (Choi et al., 2010).

### Seizures

Epileptic drop attacks are caused by several mechanisms, including asymmetrical tonic contractions of limb and axial muscles, loss of tone of postural muscles (atonic seizures), and seizure-related cardiac arrhythmias. Video-EEG monitoring of epileptic patients with a history of falls permits characterization of the various motor phenomena that cause loss of posture. Pediatric epileptic encephalopathy syndromes (e.g., Lennox-Gastaut syndrome and Dravet syndrome, as well as the myoclonic epilepsies) frequently present as drop attacks. A tilt-table test should be considered in children and adolescents to avoid overdiagnosing epilepsy (Sabri, Mahmodian, and Sadri, 2006). Epileptic drops in young patients with epileptic encephalopathy syndromes can be reduced with vagal nerve stimulation in some, as well as with clobazam, rufinamide (VanStraten and Ng, 2012) and cannabidiol oil (Thiele et al., 2018). Medically refractory cases may show improved control of epileptic drops, as well as developmental gains after callosotomy (Ueda, Sood, Asano, Kumar, and Luat, 2017). Falling as a consequence of the tonic axial component of startle-induced seizures may be controllable with lamotrigine. Paradoxically, some antiseizure drugs can precipitate epileptic drop attacks, such as carbamazepine in Rolandic epilepsy. In patients with a history of stroke, falling may be falsely attributed to motor weakness rather than to new-onset seizures. Destabilizing extensor spasms of spasticity can also be difficult to distinguish from focal seizures.

## DROP ATTACKS WITHOUT LOSS OF CONSCIOUSNESS

### Transient Ischemic Attacks

Drop attacks secondary to TIAs are sudden falls occurring without warning or obvious explanation such as tripping. Loss of consciousness either does not occur or is only momentary; the sensorium and lower limb strength are intact immediately or shortly after the patient hits the ground. Between episodes the neurological examination should not reveal lower limb motor or sensory dysfunction. The vascular distributions for drop attacks from TIAs are the posterior circulation and the anterior cerebral arteries.

#### Vertebrobasilar Insufficiency

Drop attacks caused by posterior circulation insufficiency result from transient ischemia to the corticospinal tracts or the paramedian reticular formation. They are rarely an isolated manifestation of vertebrobasilar insufficiency, because most patients have a history of TIAs that include the more common signs and symptoms of vertigo, diplopia, ataxia, weakness, and hemisensory loss. Occasionally, however, a drop attack is the ominous precursor of severe neurological deficits due to progressive thrombosis of the basilar artery and may precede permanent ischemic damage only by hours. Aside from embolism and focal stenosis in the posterior circulation, vertebrobasilar insufficiency can also be caused by the subclavian steal syndrome (Osiro S 2012).

#### Anterior Cerebral Artery Ischemia

Anterior cerebral artery (ACA) ischemia causes drop attacks by impairing perfusion of the parasagittal premotor and motor cortex controlling the lower extremities. Origination of both ACAs from the same root occurs in approximately 20% of the population and predisposes to ischemic drop attacks from a single embolus. Paraparesis and even tetraparesis can result from simultaneous infarctions in bilateral anterior cerebral artery (ACA) territories (Kang and Kim, 2008). Limb-shaking TIAs can be associated with drop attacks and occur in the context of the same vascular variant described earlier (Gerstner, Liberato, and Wright, 2005). Rare cases of drop attacks arising in the context of carotid dissection (Casana et al., 2011) and frontal arteriovenous (AV) fistulas (Oh, Yoon, Kim, and Shim, 2011) have been described.

### Third Ventricular and Posterior Fossa Abnormalities

Drop attacks can be a manifestation of colloid cysts of the third ventricle, Chiari malformation ("Chiari drop attack"), or mass lesions within the posterior fossa. With colloid cysts, unprovoked falling is the second most common symptom, after position-induced headaches. This history may be the only clinical clue to the diagnosis because the neurological examination can be entirely normal. Pineal cysts are also an occasional cause of drop attacks by producing a sudden rise in cerebrospinal fluid (CSF) pressure with position-dependent obstruction ("ball valve effect") of the ventricular system (Fernandez-Miranda, 2018). Drop attacks occur in 2%–3% of patients with Chiari malformation and can be associated with loss of consciousness. They often resolve after decompression surgery (Straus, Foster, Zimmerman, and Frim, 2009). Posterior fossa arachnoid cysts are common but only occasionally associated with tonsillar ectopia. This combination of anomalies has also been reported to cause drop attacks (Killeen, Tromop, Alexander, and Wickremesekera, 2013). Drops induced by rapid head turning were considered pathognomonic of cysticercosis of the fourth ventricle in the early twentieth century (Brun sign). The contemporary maneuver of cervical spine manipulation is rarely associated with a drop attack (Sweeney and Doody, 2010). Patients who experience sudden drop attacks in the context of intracranial mass lesions such as parasagittal meningiomas, posterior fossa and foramen magnum tumors, and subdural hematomas usually have baseline abnormalities of gait and strength. Falling may occur consequent to these impairments rather than to acute loss of muscle tone.

### Otolith Crisis

During attacks of vertigo, patients often lose balance and fall. Approximately one in five patients with peripheral vestibular disorders experience drop attacks (Tomanovic and Bergenius, 2010). Meniere disease (see Chapter 22) may be complicated by "vestibular drop attacks"—Tumarkin otolithic crisis (Tumarkin, 1936)—in approximately 6% of patients. Presumably, stimulation of otolith receptors in the saccule triggers inappropriate postural reflex adjustments via vestibulospinal pathways, resulting in falls without accompanying vertigo. Affected patients report feeling as if, without warning, they are being thrown to the ground. They may fall straight down or be propelled in any direction (Chen, Zhang, Zhang, and Tumarkin, 2020). One patient reported suddenly seeing and feeling her legs moving forward in front of her as she did a spontaneous backflip (personal communication Dr. R.B. Daroff). Vestibular drop attacks may also occur in elderly patients with unilateral vestibulopathies who do not satisfy diagnostic criteria for Meniere disease (H. Lee, Yi, Lee, Ahn, and Park, 2005).

#### Cataplexy

Cataplexy, the sudden loss of lower limb tone, is part of the tetrad of narcolepsy that also includes excessive daytime sleepiness, hypnagogic hallucinations, and sleep paralysis (see Chapter 101). Consciousness is preserved during a cataplectic attack, and the attack may vary in severity from slight lower limb weakness to generalized and complete flaccid paralysis with abrupt falling. Once on the ground, the patient is unable to move but continues to breathe. The attacks usually last less than 1 minute, only rarely exceeding several minutes in duration. Cataplectic attacks are provoked by strong emotion and associated with laughter, anger, surprise, or startle. Occasionally they interrupt or follow sexual orgasm. Cataplexy is rarely diagnosed in children, but a characteristic "cataplectic facies" with repetitive mouth opening, partial ptosis, and tongue protrusion has been described (Pillen, Pizza, Dhondt, Scammell, and Overeem, 2017). During the cataplectic attack, electromyographic silence in antigravity muscles is seen, and deep tendon reflexes and the H-reflex cannot be elicited. Cataplexy occurs in the absence of narcolepsy when associated with cerebral disease (symptomatic cataplexy), as in Niemann-Pick disease, Norrie disease, brainstem lesions, or as a paraneoplastic disorder (Farid et al., 2009). It can rarely occur as an isolated problem in normal individuals who have a family history of narcolepsy.

## FALLS

### Neuromuscular Disorders and Myelopathy

All conditions causing sensory and motor impairment in the lower limbs predispose to falls. Leg weakness, especially of the proximal type, and delayed sensory signals from the lower limbs lead to characteristic gait abnormalities in neuropathies (Wuehr et al., 2014). In diabetics, coexisting retinopathy and vestibulopathy further enhance the fall risk (Gioacchini et al., 2018). The multiple causes of neuropathy and myopathy are discussed in Chapters 106 and 109. Additional disorders increasing fall risk include lumbosacral radiculopathies, myelopathies, channelopathies associated with intermittent weakness, and neuromuscular transmission disorders. Falling may herald the onset of acute polyneuropathies such as Guillain-Barré syndrome. Patients with spinal cord disease (see Chapter 27) are at particularly high risk of falling because all descending motor and cerebellar tracts and ascending sensory tracts traverse the cord. This is particularly true for multiple sclerosis patients with gait and balance dysfunction, of whom at least half fall once or more a year (Cameron and Nilsagard, 2018). Multiple sclerosis patients older than 55 years have a high rate of injurious falls (Peterson, Cho, von Koch, and Finlayson, 2008), and FOF is common in this group (Kalron and Achiron, 2014). However, even elderly multiple sclerosis patients can attain marked reductions in fall risk with home-based balance and strength training (Sosnoff, Finlayson, McAuley, Morrison, and Motl, 2014).

#### Stroke

Strokes present with any combination of neurological deficits that predispose to falls in the acute and chronic state: weakness, ataxia, sensory deafferentation, hemianopsia, diplopia, anosognosia, hemineglect, vestibular tilting, and acquired gait abnormalities (Chen, Novak, and Manor, 2014) are obvious risk enhancing factors. Poststroke depression and immobilization further aggravate this risk, which is at least twice as high in stroke patients compared with age-matched controls. The majority of falls occur within the home environment and come with a high risk (>70%) of injuries (Schmid et al., 2013). The poststroke risk of a hip fracture is doubled and is particularly high in women within 3 months of the ischemic event (Pouwels et al., 2009). Concerns for such injuries have increased prevention efforts but have also provoked restrictions on patient mobility in acute care and rehabilitation facilities (Inouye, Brown, and Tinetti, 2009), because falls typically occur when patients attempt to get out of bed, stand up, or walk. Fortunately, concerted efforts have yielded significant reductions of fall and injury incidence in such institutions (Services, 2014, May 7).

### Other Cerebral or Cerebellar Disorders

Metabolic encephalopathies may cause a characteristic transient loss of postural tone (asterixis). If this is extensive and involves the axial musculature, episodic loss of the upright posture can mimic drop attacks in patients with chronic uremia. Cerebellar disease causes truncal instability and represents a prime cause of falling. Patients with degenerative cerebellar ataxias (see Chapter 23) have a 50% incidence of falls in any 3-month period of observation, which correlates with increased gait variability (Schniepp et al., 2014). Episodic ataxia syndromes and familial hemiplegic migraine are also associated with recurrent falls (Black, 2006). Severe attacks of hyperekplexia, a familial disorder of increased startle sensitivity, manifest with generalized hypertonia that can lead to uncontrollable falls. Effective prevention with clonazepam or valproate is available. Beneficial treatment can also be offered to properly diagnosed patients with normal-pressure hydrocephalus (see Chapter 88); ventriculoperitoneal shunting leads to dramatic improvement of gait and decreased risk of falls, albeit in a temporally limited manner.

### Cryptogenic Falls in the Middle-Aged

A diagnostic enigma is the occurrence of falls of unknown etiology among a subset of women older than 40 years of age. The fall usually is forward and occurs without warning during walking. The knees are often bruised (Thijs, Bloem, and van Dijk, 2009). Affected women report no loss of consciousness, dizziness, or even a sense of imbalance. They are convinced that they have not tripped but that their legs suddenly gave way. Gait is normal after the fall. This condition is estimated to affect 3% of women and develops after the age of 40 in the majority of patients. Originally described as a disorder of unknown causality, more recent inquiry into the frequency of falls in middle-aged and older women in the general population has elicited fall frequencies from 8% in women in their 40s to 47% in their 70s. Age and number of comorbidities such as diabetes and neuropathies are most predictive of falling (Nitz and Choy, 2008). Vestibular dysfunction of variable severity is also unexpectedly common and can be seen in 35% of individuals older than 40 years. Symptomatic (dizzy) patients have a 12-fold increase in the odds of falling (Agrawal, Carey, Della Santina, Schubert, and Minor, 2009). Fibromyalgia is associated with vestibular symptoms and an increased fall frequency (Jones, Horak, Winters-Stone, Irvine, and Bennett, 2009), as are migraine (Carvalho et al., 2018), poor sleep (Cauley et al., 2018), lower limb joint and foot problems (Afrin et al., 2018), and obesity (Ylitalo and Karvonen-Gutierrez, 2016). Indeed, obesity is associated with impaired dynamic balance functions already at a young age (do Nascimento, Silva, Dos Santos, de Almeida Ferreira, and de Andrade, 2017). When combined with sarcopenia, a clinically significant loss of muscle bulk and strength that can arise at any age throughout adulthood, the negative impact of obesity on mobility and associated FOF is magnified. Although beneficial in many regards, bariatric surgery has, unfortunately, been shown to increase the risk of fall-related, serious injuries (Carlsson et al., 2018). These observations indicate that risk factors for falls are prevalent already in middle age and correlate with falling later in life.

## Aging, Neurodegeneration, and the Neural Substrate of Gait and Balance

Significant alterations in quantitative gait characteristics (Chong, Chastan, Welter, and Do, 2009) evolve with advancing age, even in healthy individuals. It is estimated that by the age of 65, only 1 in 10 persons show gait abnormalities, but by the age of 85, only 1 in 10 have a normal gait. In the future, standardized measurement of gait speed could be included in the routine clinical assessment of the elderly, akin to a "vital sign" because slow speed (≤0.6 m/sec) has strong predictive power for all-cause mortality (Cummings, Studenski, and Ferrucci, 2014). Modern imaging methods are beginning to reveal the cerebral circuitry and brain centers supporting gait and balance. The midbrain contains a locomotor region within its reticular formation that includes the cholinergic pedunculopontine nucleus (PPN) and the cuneiform nucleus (CN). They are poorly delineated anatomically, but mesencephalic gray matter shows atrophy on magnetic resonance imaging (MRI) morphometry in non–dopa-responsive parkinsonism associated with gait and balance deficits (Sebille et al., 2019). The noradrenergic locus coeruleus is coactivated with the PPN (Benarroch, 2013) along with extensive pyramidal, extrapyramidal, and transcallosal networks. Cognitive circuitry in the frontal lobe and in the temporoparietal cortex (Takakusaki, 2017) is also involved in gait and balance functions, explaining the link between declining stability and cognition in the elderly, sometimes described as "brain failure." As expected, this is accelerated by subcortical white matter ischemic changes and neurodegenerative disorders (Montero-Odasso and Hachinski, 2014; Srikanth et al., 2010). For instance, patients with mild cognitive impairment (MCI) have a nearly threefold prevalence of gait abnormalities compared with healthy older adults (Allali and Verghese, 2017), and specific spatiotemporal gait features correlate with an increased risk of falls in dementia (Modarresi, Divine, Grahn, Overend, and Hunter, 2018). A clinically useful correlate of the parallel involvement of cognitive and locomotor pathways in the elderly is the failure of dual task execution when walking. Reduction of step length or stoppage when talking ("stops walking while talking") is a reliable indicator of an increased fall risk in the elderly (Ayers, Tow, Holtzer, and Verghese, 2014).

### Fear of Falling

FOF is a common and serious complication in patients with a history of falls and can also affect those at increased risk for falling. By itself, FOF increases the likelihood of such events, subsequent immobilization, and progression toward endstage disability. It is not limited to the elderly who have suffered injuries. FOF is prevalent among diabetics (Hewston and Deshpande, 2018), migraineurs (Carvalho et al., 2018), obese patients (Neri et al., 2017), and those with depression and sarcopenia (Gadelha et al., 2018). It tends to affect female patients more severely. Older adults should be queried about possible fear of outdoor falling, because their perceptions about the neighborhood environment can lead to self-imposed mobility restrictions (S. Lee et al., 2018).

FOF and its advancing severity in patients with recurrent falls is reliably assessed with the Falls Efficacy Scale-I (Gazibara et al., 2019). Brain mechanisms underlying FOF may relate to hypometabolism in the L supplementary motor area, a brain region involved in motor planning (Sakurai et al., 2017). FOF is augmented by underlying anxiety and may evolve into a specific phobia (basiphobia) in some patients (Grenier et al., 2019). Intervention in the form of structured exercise and cognitive behavioral therapy can alleviate the adverse effects of FOF (Wetherell et al., 2018; Liu, Ng, Chung, and Ng, 2018).

### Basal Ganglia Disorders

***Parkinson disease.*** Nearly all patients with Parkinson disease (PD) fall over the course of their illness and suffer twice as many fractures as age-matched controls. The fall risk increases with multiple factors, including disease duration, depression, cognitive impairment, treatment-related motor fluctuation, sedating drug use, coexisting rapid eye movement (REM) sleep behavior disorder (RBD) and, especially, cardiovascular autonomic dysfunction with orthostatic hypotension (Romagnolo et al., 2019). In addition, some patients may, without warning, drop directly to the ground. This is most commonly related to dopamine-induced motor fluctuations, particularly peak-dose dyskinesias and off periods (see Chapter 96). Freezing of gait (FOG), another fall-promoting feature of PD, shares a pathophysiological link with RBD because both conditions are associated with changes in the mesencephalic locomotor and balance centers (PPN and locus coeruleus) (Videnovic et al., 2013). FOG further correlates with dysfunction in cholinergic striatal pathways (Bohnen et al., 2019), while cholinergic dysinnervation of cortex relates to slowing of gait in PD (Bohnen et al., 2013). Dopamine substitution and deep brain stimulation (DBS) in PD patients improve gait characteristics but have less effect on axial locomotive components (Chastan et al., 2009), such as vertical breaking, which corresponds with an individual's ability to control falling. This appears to depend on nondopaminergic pathways, because PD patients who fall demonstrate cholinergic hypofunction, whereas nigrostriatal dopaminergic activity is the same as in nonfallers. Degeneration of the cholinergic PPN appears to be a key factor for impaired postural control in PD. These findings offer an explanation why standard DBS targeting the subthalamic nucleus does not diminish fall risk (Hausdorff, Gruendlinger, Scollins, O'Herron, and Tarsy, 2009) and may actually contribute to an increased fall incidence (Parashos, Wielinski, Giladi, Gurevich, and National Parkinson Foundation Quality Improvement Initiative, 2013). DBS of the PPN has yielded variable results with regard to improvement of gait and postural instability (Thevathasan et al., 2012). Although central mechanisms of gait and balance dysfunction predominate in falling PD patients, there is evidence that proprioceptive functions in the lower extremities also may be impaired, augmenting the fall risk (Teasdale, Preston, and Waddington, 2017). Consensus recommendations for fall assessment and prevention in PD patients have been published (van der Marck et al., 2014). However, falling still remains intractable in many PD patients, and prevention programs have demonstrated only limited and transient benefit.

***Progressive supranuclear palsy and other parkinsonian syndromes.*** Progressive supranuclear palsy (PSP) (see Chapter 96) manifests with parkinsonian features, axial rigidity, spasticity, and ophthalmoparesis. Falling affects all patients early in the course of the illness (Williams, Watt, and Lees, 2006) and is more likely in the backward direction than in those with PD, even with equivalent functional impairment. MRI tractography demonstrates overlapping but also differential involvement of brain circuitry in PD, in parkinsonism, and in normal elderly (Chan et al., 2014). RBD (see Chapter 101) is a precursor of PSP and an underrecognized cause of nocturnal falls. Clonazepam is commonly effective in the treatment of this parasomnia. Mechanisms similar to those described with PD and PSP contribute to falls in other parkinsonian syndromes, including multiple system atrophy, corticobasal ganglionic degeneration, and Lewy body disease (see Chapter 96). Falls are highly prevalent in the latter disorder because of the added cognitive dimension of neurological disability.

## Aged State

Most patients presenting to neurologists with a complaint of falling are elderly and chronically impaired. Approximately one-third of persons older than 65 years fall at least once every year (Centers for Disease and Prevention, 2008). As the likelihood of falling increases with age, so does the severity of injury. Next to fractures, falls are the single most disabling condition leading to admission to long-term care facilities. The increased risk of injuries and fractures with falling is explained by a declining ability to absorb fall energy with the upper extremities (Sran, Stotz, Normandin, and Robinovitch, 2010), the diminishing size of soft-tissue pads around joints (in particular the hips), and osteoporosis. As would be expected, elderly in sheltered accommodations have the highest frequency of falls, affecting up to 50% every year. Many of these patients fall repeatedly, with women bearing a higher risk than men. Women also experience more FOF and fractures after falling, whereas men are more likely to suffer traumatic brain injury (TBI) and die as a result. Additional gender differences exist in regards to fall circumstances. Men in long-term care facilities are more prone to fall from loss of support from an object and while rising from the seated position. Women are more likely to fall when walking (Yang et al., 2018). The high prevalence of anticoagulant and antiplatelet use in the elderly raises concern about the risk of intracranial bleeding in fall-related TBI. Paradoxically, low-dose aspirin may be protective (Gangavati et al., 2009) but can also cause delayed intracranial bleeding within 12–24 hours after head trauma (Tauber, Koller, Moroder, Hitzl, and Resch, 2009). The presence of an intracranial hemorrhage in conjunction with warfarin use indicates an increased risk for further clinical deterioration, even if the patient is awake upon admission (Howard et al., 2009). Recurrent falls while on anticoagulation do not appear to be associated with an increased bleeding risk, but there is a much greater risk of death if an intracranial hemorrhage or another bleeding injury in a solid organ has occurred (Chiu, Jean, Fleming, and Pei, 2018). In very old patients, falls constitute the leading cause of injury-related deaths, with TBI causing at least one-third of 15,000+ fall-related fatalities every year. Complications of hip fractures cause most of the other fatalities (Deprey, 2009).

The normal aging process is associated with a decline in multiple physiological functions that diminish the ability to compensate for challenges to the upright posture. Decreased proprioception (Suetterlin and Sayer, 2014), sarcopenia (Schaap, van Schoor, Lips, and Visser, 2018), orthopedic conditions, obesity (Follis et al., 2018), cardiovascular disturbances, deteriorating visual and vestibular functions (Liston et al., 2014), cognitive impairment, and failing postural reflexes (presbyastasis) (P. Y. Lee, Gadareh, and Bronstein, 2014) accrue to increase the risk of falling. Table 3.1 contains a steadily growing list of medical conditions that have been shown to increase falling risk in the elderly. Neurological conditions are not listed because all impairments of motor, cerebellar, sensory, and cognitive functions augment a patient's susceptibility to fall.

**TABLE 3.1 Medical Conditions Associated with an Increased Risk of Falls**

| | |
|---|---|
| History of falls | Orthostatic hypotension |
| Diabetes and other metabolic disorders | Carotid sinus hypersensitivity |
| Ischemic heart disease/heart failure | Low testosterone* |
| Persistent atrial fibrillation | Hearing and vision impairment |
| Cancer and chemotherapy | New spectacle lens prescription |
| Obesity | Smoking† |
| Low level of physical activity, apathy | UTI/ incontinence |
| Sarcopenia | Polypharmacy‡ |
| COPD | Depression |
| Frailty | Fear of falling |
| Migraine | Stressful life events* |
| Musculoskeletal pain/rheumatological disease | Elder abuse |
| Orthopedic/foot problems | Schizophrenia |
| Sleep apnea and other sleep disorders | Vestibular dysfunction |
| Delirium | |

*COPD,* Chronic Obstructive Pulmonary Disease; *UTI,* Urinary Tract Infection.
*Associated with falling in men.
†Associated with falling in women.
‡Benzodiazepines, psychotropic (antidepressants), and other centrally acting drugs (opioids, antiseizure agents, opioid analgesics, hypnotics). Antiarrhythmics; antihypertensives, especially after the onset of treatment.

The clinical evaluation aims to determine the fall mechanism and to identify predisposing medical conditions and correctable risk factors. In the absence of an overt explanation for falls, a syncopal event for which the patient may be amnestic becomes more likely. Orthostatic hypotension (Shaw and Claydon, 2014) and blood pressure drops associated with head turning (Schoon et al., 2013) are important contributors to falls but require a detailed evaluation of autonomic functions for adequate diagnosis. However, definitions of orthostasis vary significantly and diminish the relevance of an incidental measurement (Saedon, Tan, and Frith, 2018). A greater than 25% diastolic blood pressure drop is strongly correlated with previous falls, whereas a greater than 25% systolic drop correlates with orthostatic symptoms (Hartog et al., 2017). The implications of severe orthostatic blood pressure dysregulation are dire: failure of recovery of systolic blood pressure to at least 80% after 1 minute of standing is a strong predictor of mortality in elderly who fall (Lagro et al., 2014).

The immense burden of falling to patients and society necessitates recognition of an increased risk of future falls. Detailed practice parameters and guidelines have been published (Society, 2010; Thurman, Stevens, Rao, and Quality Standards Subcommittee of the American Academy of, 2008).

Intervention for falling elders requires a multifaceted approach (Society, 2010; Tinetti and Kumar, 2010). Depending on the clinical situation, this may include provision of assistive devices (orthotics, canes, and walkers), treatment of orthostasis or cardiac dysrhythmias, and modification of environmental hazards identified during home visits. All unnecessary medications that increase the risk of falls, especially sedatives, antihypertensives, and hypnotics, should be discontinued. High-risk behavior such as the use of ladders and moving about at low levels of illumination is discouraged, and women are advised to wear sturdy low-heeled shoes. Balance training such as tai chi and exercises aimed at improving strength and endurance diminish fall rates. Behavioral intervention for the development of FOF after such events can be effective and is strongly encouraged. Further useful interventions in the long term include vitamin D substitution (>800 international units (IU)/day), improvement of vision with cataract surgery (Foss et al., 2006), and statin treatment for prevention of osteoporotic fractures. However, none of these measures abolish the risk of falling, and even well-intended interventions may be associated with an increased fall risk. Unexpectedly, this was shown in patients who received new prescription eyeglasses (Campbell, Sanderson, and Robertson, 2010) and for the convenient annual dosing of 500,000 IU of vitamin D, which not only enhanced the risk of falls but also fractures (Sanders et al., 2010). Use of walkers is associated with the highest fall risk, raising the question whether these ubiquitous devices have inherent design flaws that are contributory (Stevens, Thomas, Teh, and Greenspan, 2009).

Currently, falls in the elderly remain an intractable problem. Exercise programs have been evaluated extensively, with variably beneficial results in terms of fall rates and cost-effectiveness (Hektoen, Aas, and Luras, 2009; Tinetti and Kumar, 2010). Elderly patients with high fall risk and dementia may not benefit at all (Peek et al., 2018), and, unexpectedly, a tendency toward greater rates of hospitalization and death were reported with long-term (>1 year) exercise programs. However, a meta-analysis indicated modest benefits and safety of long-term, moderate-intensity exercise participation, not exceeding 3 sessions per week (de Souto Barreto, Rolland, Vellas, and Maltais, 2018). Biomedical engineers are developing devices that aim to diminish falls and their adverse consequences, including sensors on the body, in beds, or in flooring that detect and announce falling. Low-stiffness walking surfaces, and soft, protective shells for major joints may reduce the risk of serious injuries. Advances like these, along with screening of elderly persons for fall risk and preventive program enrollment, may eventually diminish the burden of this epidemic.

*The complete reference list is available online at https://expertconsult.inkling.com.* 

# Delirium

*Mario F. Mendez, Oleg Yerstein*

## OUTLINE



Delirium is an acute mental status change characterized by abnormal and fluctuating attention. There is a disturbance in level of awareness and reduced ability to direct, focus, sustain, and shift attention (American Psychiatric Association [APA], 2013). These difficulties additionally impair other areas of cognition. The syndrome of delirium can be a physiological consequence of a medical condition or stem from a primary neurological cause.

Delirium is by far the most common behavioral disorder in a medical-surgical setting. Most physicians across medical and surgical specialties are faced with delirious patients at some point in their careers. In general hospitals, the prevalence of delirium ranges from 15% to 24% on admission. The incidence ranges between 6% and 56% of hospitalized patients, 11%–51% postoperatively in elderly patients, and 80% or more of intensive care unit (ICU) patients (Alce et al., 2013; Inouye et al., 2014). The consequences of delirium are serious: they include prolonged hospitalizations, increased mortality, high rates of discharges to other institutions, severe impact on caregivers and spouses, and approximately $150 billion annually in direct healthcare costs in the United States (Kerr et al., 2013; Leslie and Inouye, 2011). The 30-day cumulative cost of ICU delirium per patient is more than $17,000 and would be even higher if not for the high mortality associated with ICU care (Vasilevskis et al., 2018).

Knowledge of delirium dates to antiquity. Hippocrates referred to it as *phrenitis*, the origin of our word *frenzy*. In the first century AD, Celsus introduced the term *delirium*, from the Latin for "out of furrow," meaning derailment of the mind, and Galen observed that delirium was often due to physical diseases that affected the mind "sympathetically." In the nineteenth century, Gowers recognized that these patients could be either lethargic or hyperactive. Bonhoeffer, in his classification of organic behavioral disorders, established that delirium is associated with clouding of consciousness. Finally, Engel and Romano (1959) described alpha slowing with delta and theta intrusions on electroencephalograms (EEGs) and correlated these changes with clinical severity. They noted that treating the medical cause resulted in reversal of both the clinical and EEG changes of delirium.

In sharp contrast with this long history, physicians, nurses, and other clinicians often fail to diagnose delirium (Wong et al., 2010), and up to two-thirds of delirium cases go undetected or misdiagnosed (O'Hanlon et al., 2014). Healthcare providers miss this syndrome more from lack of recognition than from misdiagnosis. The elderly in particular may have a "quieter," more subtle presentation of delirium that may evade detection. Adding to the confusion about delirium are the many terms used to describe this disorder: acute confusional state, altered mental status, acute organic syndrome, acute brain failure, acute brain syndrome, acute cerebral insufficiency, exogenous psychosis, metabolic encephalopathy, organic psychosis, ICU psychosis, toxic encephalopathy, toxic psychosis, and others.

One of the most important clinical distinctions is that between delirium and dementia, the other common disorder impairing multiple cognitive domains. Delirium is acute in onset (usually hours to a few days), whereas dementia is chronic (usually insidious in onset and progressive). The definition of delirium must emphasize an acute behavioral decompensation with fluctuating attention, regardless of etiology or the presence of baseline cognitive deficits or preexisting dementia. Complicating this distinction is the fact that underlying dementia is a major risk factor for delirium.

Clinicians must also take care to define the terms used with delirium. *Attention* is the ability to focus on specific stimuli to the exclusion of others. *Awareness* is the ability to perceive or be conscious of events or experiences. *Arousal*, a basic prerequisite for attention, indicates responsiveness or excitability into action. *Coma*, *stupor*, *wakefulness*, and *alertness* are states of arousal. *Consciousness*, a product of arousal, means clarity of awareness of the environment. *Confusion* is the inability for clear and coherent thought and speech.

## CLINICAL CHARACTERISTICS

The essential elements of delirium are summarized in Boxes 4.1 and 4.2. Proposed criteria for this disorder are a neurocognitive disturbance that develops over a short period of time; tends to

**BOX 4.1 Clinical Characteristics of Delirium**

Acute onset of mental status change with fluctuating course
Attentional deficits
Confusion or disorganized thinking
Altered level of consciousness
Perceptual disturbances
Disturbed sleep/wake cycle
Altered psychomotor activity
Disorientation and memory impairment
Other cognitive deficits
Behavioral and emotional abnormalities

fluctuate; and impairs awareness, attention, and other areas of cognition (APA, 2013). In general, awareness, attention, and cognition fluctuate over the course of a day. Furthermore, delirious patients have disorganized thinking and an altered level of consciousness, perceptual disturbances, disturbance of the sleep/wake cycle, increased or decreased psychomotor activity, disorientation, and memory impairment. Other cognitive, behavioral, and emotional disturbances may also occur as part of the spectrum of delirium. Delirium can be summarized into the 10 clinical characteristics that follow.

### Acute Onset with Fluctuating Course

Delirium develops rapidly over hours or days but rarely over more than a week, and fluctuations in the course occur throughout the day. There are lucid intervals interspersed with the daily fluctuations. Gross swings in attention and awareness, arousal, or both occur unpredictably and irregularly and become worse at night. Because of potential lucid intervals, medical personnel may be misled by patients who exhibit improved attention and awareness unless these patients are evaluated over time.

### Cognitive and Related Abnormalities

#### Attentional Deficits

A disturbance of attention and consequent altered awareness is the cardinal symptom of delirium. Patients are distractible, and stimuli may gain attention indiscriminately, trivial ones often getting more attention than important ones. All components of attention are disturbed, including selectivity, sustainability, processing capacity, ease of mobilization, monitoring of the environment, and the ability to shift attention when necessary. Although many of the same illnesses result in a spectrum of disturbances from mild inattention to coma, delirium is not the same as a primary disorder of arousal.

#### Confusion or Disorganized Thinking

Delirious patients are unable to maintain the stream of thought with accustomed clarity, coherence, and speed. There are multiple intrusions of competing thoughts and sensations, and patients are unable to order symbols, carry out sequenced activity, and organize goal-directed behavior.

The patient's speech reflects this jumbled thinking. Speech shifts from subject to subject and is rambling, tangential, and circumlocutory, with hesitations, repetitions, and perseverations. Decreased relevance of the speech content and decreased reading comprehension are characteristic of delirium. Confused speech is further characterized by an abnormal rate, frequent dysarthria, and nonaphasic misnaming, particularly of words related to stress or illness, such as those referable to hospitalization.

#### Altered Level of Consciousness

Consciousness, or clarity of awareness, may be disturbed. Most patients have lethargy and decreased arousal. Others, such as those with delirium tremens, are hyperalert and easily aroused. In hyperalert patients, the extreme arousal does not preclude attentional deficits because patients are indiscriminate in their alertness, are easily distracted by irrelevant stimuli, and cannot sustain attention. The two extremes of consciousness may overlap or alternate in the same patient or may occur from the same causative factor.

#### Perceptual Disturbances

The most common perceptual disturbance is decreased perceptions per unit of time; patients miss things that are going on around them. Patients may experience visual distortions, such as illusions, misperceptions, and even pareidolias, or the recognition of familiar objects or patterns superimposed on random stimuli. These perceptual abnormalities may be multiple, changing, or abnormal in size or location. Hallucinations are particularly common among younger patients with the hyperactive subtype. They usually occur in the visual sphere and are often vivid, three dimensional, and in full color. Patients may see lilliputian animals or people that appear to move about. Hallucinations are generally unpleasant, and some patients attempt to fight them or run away with fear. Some hallucinatory experiences may reflect intrusions of dreams or visual imagery into wakefulness. Psychotic auditory hallucinations with voices commenting on the patient's behavior are unusual.

#### Disturbed Sleep/Wake Cycle

Disruption of the day/night cycle causes excessive daytime drowsiness and reversal of the normal diurnal rhythm. "Sundowning"—with restlessness and confusion during the night—is common, and, in some patients, delirium may be manifest only at night. Nocturnal peregrinations can result in a serious problem when the delirious patient, partially clothed in a hospital gown, has to be retrieved from the hospital lobby or from the street in the middle of the night. This is one of the least specific symptoms and also occurs in dementia, depression, and other behavioral conditions. However, in delirium, disruption of circadian sleep cycles may result in rapid eye movement (REM) or dream-state overflow into waking.

#### Altered Psychomotor Activity

There are three subtypes of delirium, based on changes in psychomotor activity. The hypoactive subtype is characterized by psychomotor retardation. These are the patients with lethargy and decreased arousal. The hyperactive subtype is usually hyperalert and agitated and has prominent overactivity of the autonomic nervous system. Moreover, the hyperactive type is more likely to have delusions and perceptual disorders such as hallucinations. Approximately half of patients with delirium manifest elements of both subtypes, called mixed subtype, alternating between hyperactive and hypoactive. Only approximately 15% are strictly hyperactive. In addition to the patients being younger, the hyperactive subtype has more drug-related causes, a shorter hospital stay, and a better prognosis. Many patients who present with an initial hyperactive phase evolve to a predominant hypoactive delirium.

#### Disorientation and Memory Impairment

Disturbances in orientation and memory are related. Patients are disoriented first to time of day, followed by other aspects of time, and then to place. They may perceive abnormal juxtapositions of events or places. Disorientation to person—in the sense of loss of personal identity—is rare. Disorientation is one of the most common findings in delirium but is not specific for delirium; it occurs in dementia and amnesia as well. Among patients with delirium, recent memory is disrupted in large part by the decreased registration caused by attentional problems.

## BOX 4.2 DSM-5 Diagnostic Criteria: Delirium*

A. A disturbance in attention (i.e., reduced ability to direct, focus, sustain, and shift attention) and awareness (reduced orientation to the environment).

B. The disturbance develops over a short period of time (usually hours to a few days), represents a change from baseline attention and awareness, and tends to fluctuate in severity during the course of a day.

C. An additional disturbance in cognition (e.g., memory deficit, disorientation, language, visuospatial ability, or perception).

D. The disturbances in Criteria A and C are not better explained by another preexisting, established, or evolving neurocognitive disorder and do not occur in the context of a severely reduced level of arousal, such as coma.

E. There is evidence from the history, physical examination, or laboratory findings that the disturbance is a direct physiological consequence of another medical condition, substance intoxication or withdrawal (i.e., due to a drug of abuse or to a medication), or exposure to a toxin, or is due to multiple etiologies.

*Specify* whether:

**Substance intoxication delirium:** This diagnosis should be made instead of substance intoxication when the symptoms in Criteria A and C predominate in the clinical picture and when they are sufficiently severe to warrant clinical attention.

- **Coding note:** The ICD-9-CM code for [specific medication]-induced delirium is **292.81.** The ICD-10-CM code depends on the type of medication. If the medication is an opioid taken as prescribed, the code is **F11.921.** If the medication is a sedative, hypnotic, or anxiolytic taken as prescribed, the code is **F13.921.** If the medication is an amphetamine-type or other stimulant taken as prescribed, the code is **F15.921.** For medications that do not fit into any of the classes (e.g., dexamethasone) and in cases in which a substance is judged to be an etiological factor but the specific class of substance is unknown, the code is **F19.921.**

**293.0 (F05) Delirium due to another medical condition:** There is evidence from the history, physical examination, or laboratory findings that the disturbance is attributable to the physiological consequences of another medical condition.

- **Coding note:** Use multiple spate codes reflecting specific delirium etiologies (e.g., 572.2 [K72.90] hepatic encephalopathy, 293.0 [F05] delirium due to hepatic encephalopathy). The other medical condition should also be coded and listed separately immediately before the delirium due to another medical condition (e.g., 572.2 [K72.90] hepatic encephalopathy; 293.0 [F05] delirium due to hepatic encephalopathy).

| | ICD-9-CM | ICD-10-CM | | |
|---|---|---|---|---|
| | | **With use disorder, mild** | **With use disorder, moderate or severe** | **Without use disorder** |
| Alcohol | 291.0 | F10.121 | F10.221 | F10.921 |
| Cannabis | 292.81 | F12.121 | F12.221 | F12.921 |
| Phencyclidine | 292.81 | F16.121 | F16.221 | F16.921 |
| Other hallucinogen | 292.81 | F16.121 | F16.221 | F16.921 |
| Inhalent | 292.81 | F18.221 | F18.221 | F18.921 |
| Opioid | 292.81 | F11.121 | F11.221 | F11.921 |
| Sedative, hypnotic, or anxiolytic | 292.81 | F13.121 | F13.221 | F13.921 |
| Amphetamine (or other stimulant) | 292.81 | F15.121 | F15.221 | F15.921 |
| Cocaine | 292.81 | F14.121 | F14.221 | F14.921 |
| Other (or unknown) substance | 292.81 | F19.221 | F19.221 | F19.921 |

- **Coding note**: The ICD-9-CM and ICD-10CM codes for the [specific substance] intoxication delirium are indicated in the table below. Note that the ICD-10-CM code depends on whether or not there is a comorbid substance use disorder present for the same class of substance. If a mild substance use disorder is comorbid with the substance intoxication delirium, the 4th position character is "1," and the clinician should record "mild [substance] use disorder," before the substance intoxication delirium (e.g., "mild cocaine use disorder is comorbid with the substance intoxication delirium"). If a moderate or severe substance use disorder is comorbid with the substance intoxication delirium, the 4th position character is "2,"and the clinician should record "moderate [substance] use disorder" or "severe [substance] use disorder," depending on the severity of the comorbid substance use disorder. If there is no comorbid substance use disorder (e.g., after a one-time heavy use of the substance), then the 4th position character is "9,"and the clinician should record only the substance intoxication delirium.

**Substance withdrawal delirium:** This diagnosis should be made instead of substance withdrawal when the symptoms in Criteria A and C predominate in the clinical picture and when they are sufficiently severe to warrant clinical attention.

- **Code** [specific substance] withdrawal delirium: **291.0 (F10.231)** alcohol; **292.0 (F11.23)** opioid; 292.0 (F13.231) sedative, hypnotic, or anxiolytic; **292.0 (F19.231)** other (or unknown) substance/medication.

**Medication-induced delirium:** This diagnosis applies when the symptoms in Criteria A and C arise as a side effect of a medication taken as prescribed.

**293.0 (F05) Delirium due to multiple etiologies:** There is evidence from the history physical examination, or laboratory findings that the delirium has more than one etiology (e.g., more than one etiological medical condition; another medical condition plus substance intoxication or medication side effect).

- **Coding note:** Use multiple separate codes reflecting specific delirium etiologies (e.g., 572.2 [K72.90] hepatic encephalopathy, 293.0 [F05] delirium due to hepatic failure; 291/0 [F10.231] alcohol withdrawal delirium). Note that the etiological medical condition both appears as a separate code that precedes the delirium code and is substituted into the delirium due to another medical condition rubric.

*Specify* if:

**Acute:** Lasting a few hours or days.

**Persistent:** Lasting weeks or months.

*Specify* if:

**Hyperactive:** The individual has a hyperactive level of psychomotor activity that may be accompanied by mood lability, agitation, and/or refusal to cooperate with medical care.

**Hypoactive:** The individual has a hypoactive level of psychomotor activity that may be accompanied by sluggishness and lethargy that approaches stupor.

**Mixed level of activity:** The individual has a normal level of psychomotor activity even though attention and awareness are disturbed. Also includes individuals whose activity level rapidly fluctuates.

* Previously referred to in DSM IV as "dementia, delirium, amnestic, and other cognitive disorders."



Note: The following supportive features are commonly present in delirium but are not key diagnostic features: sleep/wake cycle disturbance, psychomotor disturbance, perceptual disturbances (e.g., hallucinations, illusions), emotional disturbances, delusions, labile affect, dysarthria, and EEG abnormalities (generalized slowing of background activity).

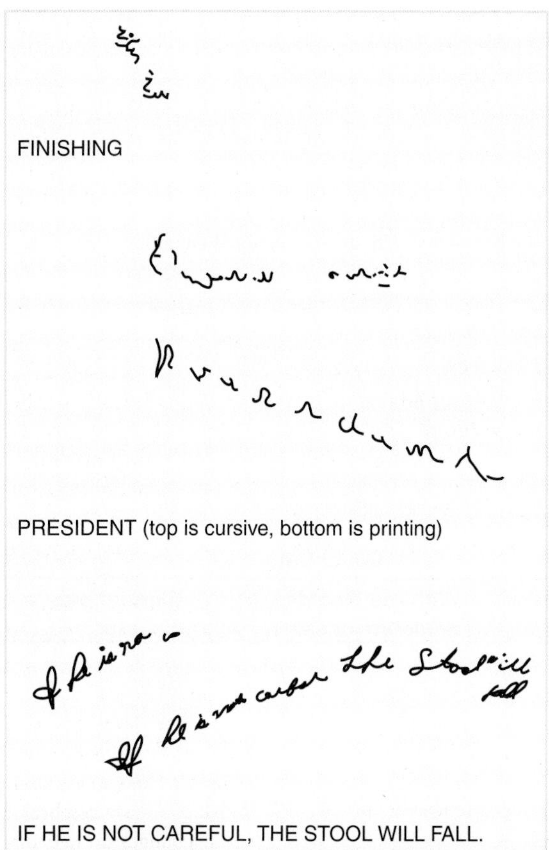

FINISHING
PRESIDENT (top is cursive, bottom is printing)
IF HE IS NOT CAREFUL, THE STOOL WILL FALL.


**Fig. 4.1 Writing Disturbances in Delirium.** Patients were asked to write indicated words to dictation. (Reprinted with permission from Chédru, J., Geschwind, N. (1972). Writing disturbances in acute confusional states. *Neuropsychologia 10,* 343–353.)

In delirium, reduplicative paramnesia, a specific memory-related disorder, results from decreased integration of recent observations with past memories. Persons or places are "replaced" in this condition. In general, delirious patients tend to mistake the unfamiliar for the familiar. For example, they tend to relocate the hospital closer to their homes. In a form of reduplicative paramnesia known as *Capgras syndrome*, a familiar person is mistakenly thought to be an unfamiliar impostor.

### Other Cognitive Deficits

Disturbances occur in visuospatial abilities and in writing. Higher visual-processing deficits include difficulties in visual object recognition, environmental orientation, and organization of drawings and other constructions.

Writing is easily disrupted in these disorders, possibly because it depends on multiple components. The most salient characteristics are abnormalities in the mechanics of writing. The formation of letters and words is indistinct, and words and sentences sprawl in different directions (Fig. 4.1). There is a reluctance to write, and there are motor impairments (e.g., tremors, micrographia) and spatial disorders (e.g., misalignment, leaving insufficient space for the writing sample). Sometimes the writing shows perseverations of loops in aspects of the writing. Spelling and syntax are also disturbed, with spelling errors particularly involving consonants, small grammatical words (prepositions and conjunctions), and the last letters of words.

### Behavioral and Emotional Abnormalities

Behavioral changes include poorly systematized delusions, often with persecutory and other paranoid ideation, and personality alterations. Delusions, like hallucinations, are generally fleeting, changing, and readily affected by sensory input. These delusions are most often persecutory. Some patients exhibit facetious humor and playful behavior, lack of concern about their illness, poor insight, impaired judgment, and confabulation.

There can be marked emotional lability. Patients can be agitated and fearful or depressed and apathetic. Dysphoric (unpleasant) emotional states are the more common. Up to half of elderly delirious patients display symptoms of depression with low mood, loss of interests, fatigue, decreased appetite and sleep, and other feelings related to depression. There may be mood-congruent delusions and hallucinations. The mood changes of delirium are probably due to direct effects of the confusional state on the limbic system and its regulation of emotions.

Finally, more elementary behavioral changes may be the principal symptoms of delirium. This is the case especially in the elderly, in whom decreased activities of daily living, urinary incontinence, and frequent falls are among the major manifestations of this disorder.

## PATHOPHYSIOLOGY

The pathophysiology of delirium is not entirely understood, but it depends on widely distributed neurological dysfunction. Delirium is the final common pathway of many pathophysiological disturbances that reduce or alter cerebral oxidative metabolism. These metabolic changes result in diffuse impairment in multiple neuronal pathways and systems.

Several brain areas involved in attention are particularly disturbed in delirium. Dysfunction of the anterior cingulate cortex is involved in disturbances of the management of attention (Reischies et al., 2005). Other areas include the bilateral or right prefrontal cortex in attentional maintenance and executive control, the temporoparietal junction region in disengaging and shifting attention, the thalamus in engaging attention, and the upper brainstem structures in moving the focus of attention. The thalamic nuclei are uniquely positioned to screen incoming sensory information, and small lesions in the thalamus may cause delirium. In addition, there is evidence that the right hemisphere is dominant for attention. Cortical blood flow studies suggest that right hemisphere cortical areas and their limbic connections are the "attentional gate" for sensory input through feedback to the reticular nucleus of the thalamus.

Another explanation for delirium is alterations in neurotransmitters, particularly a cholinergic-dopaminergic imbalance. There is extensive evidence for a cholinergic deficit in delirium (Alce et al., 2013). Anticholinergic agents can induce the clinical and EEG changes of delirium, which are reversible with the administration of cholinergic medications such as physostigmine. The beneficial effects of donepezil, rivastigmine, and galantamine—acetylcholinesterase-inhibitor medications used for Alzheimer disease—may be partly due to an activating or attention-enhancing role. Moreover, cholinergic neurons project from the pons and the basal forebrain to the cortex and make cortical neurons more responsive to other inputs. A decrease in acetylcholine results in decreased perfusion in the frontal cortex. Hypoglycemia, hypoxia, and other metabolic changes may differentially affect acetylcholine-mediated functions. Other neurotransmitters may be involved in delirium, including dopamine, serotonin, norepinephrine, γ-aminobutyric acid (GABA), glutamine, opiates, and histamine. Dopamine has an inhibitory effect on the release of acetylcholine, thereby contributing to the delirium-producing effects of L-dopa and other antiparkinsonism medications (Martins and Fernandes, 2012; Trzepacz and van der Mast, 2002). Opiates may induce the effects by increasing dopamine and glutamate activity. Polymorphisms in genes coding for a dopamine transporter and two dopamine receptors have been associated with the development of delirium (van Munster et al., 2010).

**BOX 4.3 Predisposing and Precipitating Factors for Delirium**

- Elderly, especially 80 years or older
- Dementia, cognitive impairment, or other brain disorder
- Fluid and electrolyte disturbances and dehydration
- Other metabolic disturbance, especially elevated BUN level or hepatic insufficiency
- Number and severity of medical illnesses, including cancer
- Infections, especially urinary tract, pulmonary, and AIDS
- Malnutrition, low serum albumin level
- Cardiorespiratory failure or hypoxemia
- Prior stroke or other nondementia brain disorder
- Polypharmacy and use of analgesics, psychoactive drugs, or anticholinergics
- Drug abuse, alcohol or sedative dependency
- Sensory impairment, especially visual
- Sensory overstimulation and "ICU psychosis"
- Sensory deprivation
- Sleep disturbance
- Functional impairment
- Fever, hypothermia
- Physical trauma or severe burns
- Fractures
- Male gender
- Depression
- Specific surgeries:
  - Cardiac, especially open heart surgery
  - Orthopedic, especially femoral neck and hip fractures, bilateral knee replacements
  - Ophthalmological, especially cataract surgery
  - Noncardiac thoracic surgery and aortic aneurysmal repairs
  - Transurethral resection of the prostate

*AIDS*, Acquired immunodeficiency syndrome; *BUN*, blood urea nitrogen; *ICU*, intensive care unit.

Inflammatory cytokines such as interleukins, interferon, and tumor necrosis factor alpha (TNF-$\alpha$) may contribute to delirium by altering blood-brain barrier permeability, by affecting neurotransmission (Cole, 2004; Fong et al., 2009; Inouye, 2006; Martins and Fernandes, 2012), and even by altering gut immune function (McCoy et al., 2018). The combination of inflammatory mediators and dysregulation of the limbic–hypothalamic–pituitary axis may lead to exacerbation or prolongation of delirium (MacLullich et al., 2008; Martins and Fernandes, 2012). Finally, secretion of melatonin, a hormone integral to circadian rhythm and the sleep/wake cycle, may be abnormal in delirious patients compared to those without delirium (Fitzgerald et al., 2013).

## DIAGNOSIS

Diagnosis is a two-step process. The first step is the recognition of delirium, which requires a thorough history, a bedside mental status examination focusing on attention, and a review of established diagnostic scales or criteria for delirium. The second step is to identify the cause from a large number of potential diagnoses. Because the clinical manifestations offer few clues to the cause, crucial to the differential diagnosis are the general history, physical examination, and laboratory assessments.

The general history assesses several elements. An abrupt decline in mentation, particularly in the hospital, should be presumed to be delirium. Although patients may state that they cannot think straight or concentrate, family members or other good historians should also be available to describe the patient's behavior and medical history. The observer may have noted early symptoms of delirium such as inability to perform at a usual level, decreased awareness of complex details, insomnia, and frightening or vivid dreams. It is crucial to obtain accurate information about systemic illnesses, drug use, recent trauma, occupational and environmental exposures, malnutrition, allergies, and any preceding symptoms leading to delirium. Furthermore, the clinician should thoroughly review the patient's medication list.

### Predisposing and Precipitating Factors

The greater the number of predisposing factors, the milder in severity the precipitating factors need be in order to result in delirium (Anderson, 2005; Box 4.3). Four factors independently predispose to delirium: vision impairments (<20/70 binocular), severity of illness, cognitive impairment, and dehydration (high ratio of blood urea to creatinine) (Inouye, 2006). Among these, cognitive impairment or dementia is worth emphasizing. Elderly patients with dementia are two to five times more likely to develop delirium than those without dementia, with increased admission to institutions and mortality (Fong et al., 2015; Inouye et al., 2014). Patients with dementia may develop delirium after minor medication changes or other relatively insignificant precipitating factors (Inouye et al., 2014). Moreover, premorbid impairment in executive functions may be independently associated with greater risk of developing delirium (Rudolph et al., 2006). Other important predisposing factors for delirium are advanced age, especially older than 80 years, and the presence of chronic medical illnesses (Johnson, 2001). Many of these elderly patients predisposed to delirium have cerebral atrophy or white matter and basal ganglia ischemic changes on neuroimaging. Additional predisposing factors are the degree of physical impairment, hip and other bone fractures, serum sodium changes, infections and fevers, and the use of multiple drugs, particularly those with narcotic, anticholinergic, or psychoactive properties. The predisposing factors for delirium are additive, each new factor increasing the risk considerably. Moreover, frail elderly patients often have multiple predisposing factors, the most common being functional dependency, multiple medical comorbidities, depression, and polypharmacy (Laurila et al., 2008).

In many cases the cause of delirium is multifactorial, resulting from the interaction between patient-specific predisposing factors and multiple precipitating factors (Inouye and Charpentier, 1996; Inouye et al., 2014; Laurila et al., 2008). Five specific factors that can independently precipitate delirium are use of physical restraints, malnutrition or weight loss (albumin levels <30 g/L), use of indwelling bladder catheters, adding more than three medications within a 24-hour period, and an iatrogenic medical complication (Inouye and Charpentier, 1996). Other precipitating factors for incident delirium, which is the term used to describe a delirium that newly occurs during the course of a stay in a clinical setting, include electrolyte disturbances (hyponatremia, hypercalcemia, etc.), major organ system disease, occult respiratory failure, occult infection, pain, specific medications such as sedative-hypnotics or histamine-2 blockers, sleep disturbances, and alterations in the environment. Novel situations and unfamiliar surroundings contribute to sensory overstimulation in the elderly, and sensory overload may be a factor in producing "ICU psychosis." Ultimately, delirium occurs in patients from a synergistic interaction of predisposing factors with precipitating factors.

In addition to the risk factors already discussed, heritability of delirium is an area of investigation. The presence of dopamine receptor genes *DRD2* and *DRD3*, and the dopamine transporter gene, *SLC6A3*, are possible pathophysiological vulnerabilities for delirium. Polymorphisms in *SLC6A3* and *DRD2* have occurred in association with delirium from alcohol and in elderly delirious patients with hip fractures (van Munster et al., 2009, 2010).

A locus on chromosome 2 spanning multiple genes including two for sodium/hydrogen exchange pumps and three interleukin-related genes correlate with an increased risk for delirium (McCoy et al., 2018). Finally, despite earlier conflicting data, a meta-analysis showed no association between apolipoprotein E (APOE) and delirium (Adamis et al., 2016).

## Mental Status Examination

Initial general behavioral observations are an important part of the neurological mental status examination. The most important are observations of attentiveness and arousability. Attention may wander so much that it must constantly be brought back to the subject at hand. General behavior may range from falling asleep during the interview to agitation and combativeness. Slow and loosely connected thinking and speech may be present, with irrelevancies, perseverations, repetitions, and intrusions. Patients may propagate their errors in thinking and perception by elaboration or confabulation. The examiner should evaluate the patient's general appearance and grooming, motor activity and spontaneity, mood and affect, propriety and witticisms, and the presence of any special preoccupations or inaccurate perceptions.

Bedside tests of attention can be divided into serial recitation tasks, continuous performance tasks, and alternate response tasks. The digit span test is a serial recitation task in which a series of digits is presented, one digit per second, and the patient is asked to repeat the entire sequence immediately after presentation. Perceptual clumping is avoided by the use of random digits and a regular rhythm of presentation. Correct recitation of seven (plus or minus two) digits is considered normal. The serial reversal test is a form of recitation task in which the patient recites a digit span backwards, the spelling of a word such as *world*, or the results of counting by ones, threes, or sevens from a predetermined number. Continuous performance tasks include the *A* vigilance test, in which the patient must indicate whenever the letter *A* is heard among random letters presented one per second. This can also be done visually by asking the patient to cross out every instance of a particular letter in a magazine or newspaper paragraph. Alternate response tasks are exemplified by the repetition of a three-step motor sequence (palm-side-fist), which is also a test of frontal functions. These attentional tests are not overly sensitive or specific, and they can be affected by the patient's educational background, degree of effort, or presence of other cognitive deficits. In sum, the best assessment of attention may be general behavioral observations and an appraisal of how "interviewable" the patient is and how much he stays on track with the interview.

Attentional or arousal deficits may preclude the opportunity to pursue the mental status examination much further, but the examiner should attempt to assess orientation and other areas of cognition. Patients who are off 3 days on the date, 2 days on the day of the week, or 4 hours on the time of day may be significantly disoriented to time. The examiner should inquire whether the patient knows where he or she is, what kind of place it is, and in what circumstances he or she is there. Disturbed recent memory is demonstrated by asking the patient to retain the examiner's name or three words for 5 minutes. A language examination should distinguish between the language of confusion and that of a primary aphasia (see "Special Problems in Differential Diagnosis," later in this chapter). Attempts at simple constructions such as copying a cube may be unsuccessful. Hallucinations can sometimes be brought out by holding a white piece of paper or an imaginary string between the fingers and asking the patient to describe what he or she sees.

## Diagnostic Scales and Criteria

The usual mental status scales and tests may not help in differentiating delirium from dementia and other cognitive disturbances. Specific criteria and scales are available for the diagnosis of delirium. Foremost among these are the *Diagnostic and Statistical Manual of Mental Disorders*, fifth edition DSM-5; APA, 2013), criteria for delirium (see Box 4.2).

### BOX 4.4 Diagnosis of Delirium by the Confusion Assessment Method

The diagnosis of delirium by the confusion assessment method requires the presence of features 1, 2, and either 3 or 4 (Inouye et al., 1990).

Feature 1: Acute onset and fluctuating course

Was there an acute change from the patient's baseline? Did the (abnormal) behavior fluctuate in severity?

Feature 2: Inattention

Did the patient have difficulty keeping track of what was being said?

Feature 3: Disorganized thinking

Was the patient's thinking disorganized or incoherent (rambling conversation, unclear or illogical flow of ideas)?

Feature 4: Altered level of consciousness

Overall, would you rate this patient's level of consciousness as alert (normal), vigilant (hyperalert), lethargic (drowsy, easily aroused), stupor (difficulty to arouse), or coma (unarousable)?

The confusion assessment method (CAM) is perhaps the most widely used instrument for screening for and diagnosing delirium (Ely et al., 2001) (Box 4.4). A brief version of the CAM, the 3-Minute Diagnostic Assessment (3D-CAM), which is aimed at healthcare staff with minimal additional training, shows high sensitivity and specificity for detecting delirium (Marcantonio et al., 2014). The Delirium Rating Scale-Revised-98 (DRS-R-98), a revision of the earlier DRS, is a 16-item scale with 13 severity items and 3 diagnostic items that reliably distinguish delirium from dementia, depression, and schizophrenia (Trzepacz et al., 2001). Both the CAM and the DRS-R-98 are best supplemented with other cognitive measures (Adamis et al., 2010). The 4 As Test (4AT) is a third brief screening tool for delirium, which has been validated in multiple clinical situations and suggests degree of cognitive impairment and the need for further testing (Bellelli et al., 2014).

There are additional scales used for specific situations. The Memorial Delirium Assessment Scale (MDAS) is a 10-item scale designed to quantify the severity of delirium in medically ill patients (Breitbart et al., 1997). Although it may also be useful as a diagnostic tool, it is best used after the initial delirium diagnosis is made (Adamis et al., 2010). The delirium symptom interview is also a valuable instrument but may not distinguish delirium from dementia. The Neelon and Champagne (NEECHAM) Confusion Scale (Neelon et al., 1996) is an easily administered screening tool widely used in the nursing community. It combines behavioral and physiological signs of delirium (Adamis et al., 2010). The Nursing Delirium Symptom Checklist (Nu-DESC) is a more recently validated screening tool that assesses inappropriate behavior and communication, disorientation, and hallucinations but may be more sensitive for hyperactive symptoms and may miss hypoactive delirium (Neufeld et al., 2013). The confusion assessment method for ICU (CAM-ICU) and the Intensive Care Delirium Screening Checklist (ICDSC) are two validated critical care assessment tools used to easily and relatively quickly screen for delirium in the ICU (Alce et al., 2013). Although highly specific, neither the CAM-ICU nor the NuDESC have shown high sensitivity for the identification of postoperative delirium (Neufeld et al., 2013).

The diagnosis of delirium is facilitated by the use of the CAM, DRS-R-98, 4AT, and the other instruments described earlier, along with the history from collateral sources such as family and nursing notes, a mental status examination focusing on attention, and specific tests such as a writing sample.

## Physical Examination

The physical examination should elicit any signs of systemic illness, focal neurological abnormalities, meningismus, increased intracranial pressure (ICP), extracranial cerebrovascular disease, or head trauma. In delirium, less specific findings include an action or postural tremor of high frequency (8–10 Hz), asterixis or brief lapses in tonic posture (especially at the wrist), multifocal myoclonus or shocklike jerks from diverse sites, choreiform movements, dysarthria, and gait instability. Patients may manifest agitation or psychomotor retardation, apathy, waxy flexibility, catatonia, or carphologia ("lint-picking" behavior). On physical examination, the presence of hyperactivity of the autonomic nervous system may be life threatening because of possible dehydration, electrolyte disturbances, or tachyarrhythmias.

### Laboratory Tests

Despite false-positive and false-negative rates on single tracings (Inouye, 2006), EEG changes virtually always accompany delirium when several EEGs are obtained over time (see Chapter 35). Disorganization of the usual cerebral rhythms and generalized slowing are the most common changes, as illustrated in Engel and Romano's classic paper (1959). The mean EEG frequency or degree of slowing correlates with the degree of delirium. Both hypoactive and hyperactive subtypes of delirium have similar EEG slowing; however, predominant low-voltage fast activity is also present on withdrawal from sedative drugs or alcohol. Additional EEG patterns from intracranial causes of delirium include focal slowing, asymmetric delta activity, and paroxysmal discharges (spikes, sharp waves, and spike-wave complexes). Periodic complexes such as triphasic waves and periodic lateralizing epileptiform discharges may help in the differential diagnosis (see Chapter 35). Investigators have considered bispectral EEG monitoring for adjustment of anesthetic depth and prevention of postoperative delirium (Wildes et al., 2019). In sum, EEGs are of value in deciding whether confusional behavior may be due to an intracranial cause, in making the diagnosis of delirium in patients with unclear behavior, in evaluating demented patients who might have a superimposed delirium, in differentiating delirium from schizophrenia and other primary psychiatric states, and in following the course of delirium over time.

Other essential laboratory tests include a complete blood cell count; measurements of glucose, electrolytes, blood urea nitrogen, creatinine, transaminase, and ammonia levels; thyroid function tests; arterial blood gas studies; chest radiographs; electrocardiogram; urinalysis; and urine drug screening. Less routine tests, such as antibody tests against Hu or *N*-methyl-D-aspartate receptors, should be considered when routine labs are unrevealing and there is a suspicion for malignancy. Although they are nonspecific, evoked potential studies often show prolonged latencies.

Because most cases of delirium are due to medical conditions, lumbar puncture and neuroimaging are needed in only a minority of delirious patients (Inouye, 2006). However, the need for a lumbar puncture deserves special comment. This valuable test, which is often neglected in the evaluation of delirious patients, should be performed as part of the workup when the cause is uncertain, especially in the presence of unexplained fever or meningismus. The lumbar puncture should be preceded by a computed tomographic (CT) or magnetic resonance imaging (MRI) scan of the brain, especially if there are focal neurological findings or suspicions of increased ICP, a space-occupying lesion, or head trauma. The yield of functional imaging is variable, showing global increased metabolism in patients with delirium tremens and global decreased metabolism or focal frontal hypoactivity in many other delirious patients.

**TABLE 4.1 Major Causes of Delirium**

| | |
|---|---|
| **Metabolic** | Electrolytes: hypo/hypernatremia, hypo/hypercalcemia, hypo/hypermagnesemia, hypo/hyperphosphatemia |
| | Endocrine: hypo/hyperthyroidism, hypo/hypercortisolism, hypo/hyperglycemia |
| | Cardiac encephalopathy, hepatic encephalopathy, uremic encephalopathy |
| | Hypoxia and hypercarbia |
| | Vitamin deficiencies: vitamin $B_{12}$, nicotinic acid, folic acid. Most notably Wernicke encephalopathy from thiamine deficiency |
| | Toxic and industrial exposures: carbon monoxide, organic solvent, lead, manganese, mercury, carbon disulfide, heavy metals |
| | Porphyria |
| **Toxic** | Intoxication and overdose |
| | Serotonin syndrome |
| | Malignant neuroleptic syndrome |
| | Withdrawal: alcohol, benzodiazepines, barbiturates, amphetamines, cocaine, coffee, phencyclidine, hallucinogens, inhalants, meperidine, and other narcotics |
| | Drugs: anticholinergic, benzodiazepines, opiates, antihistamines, antiepileptics, muscle relaxants, dopamine agonists, monoamine oxidase inhibitors, levodopa, corticosteroids, fluoroquinolone and cephalosporin antibiotics, beta-blockers, digitalis, lithium, clozapine, tricyclic antidepressants, calcineurin inhibitors |
| **Infectious** | Urinary tract infection, pneumonia, sepsis, meningitis, encephalitis, Creutzfeldt-Jakob and other prion diseases |
| **Neurological** | Vascular: ischemic stroke, intracerebral or subarachnoid hemorrhage, vasculitis |
| | Autoimmune and paraneoplastic encephalitides |
| | Neoplastic: brain tumors, carcinomatous meningitis |
| | Seizure related: postictal state, nonconvulsive status epilepticus |
| | Trauma: concussion, subdural hematoma |
| **Perioperative** | Surgery: thoracic (cardiac and noncardiac), vascular, and hip replacement, anesthetic and drug effects, hypoxia and anemia, hyperventilation, fluid and electrolyte disturbances, hypotension, embolism, infection or sepsis, untreated pain, fragmented sleep, sensory deprivation or overload |
| **Miscellaneous** | Hyperviscosity syndromes |

## DIFFERENTIAL DIAGNOSIS

### Common Causes of Delirium

The following discussion is a selective commentary that illustrates some basic principles and helps to organize the approach to working through the large differential diagnosis. Almost any sufficiently severe medical or surgical illness can cause delirium, and the best advice is to follow all available diagnostic leads (Table 4.1). (For further discussion of individual entities, the reader should refer to corresponding chapters in this book.) The confusion-inducing effects of these disturbances are additive, and there may be more than one causal factor, the individual contribution of which cannot be elucidated. Nearly half of elderly patients with delirium have more than one cause of their disorder, and clinicians should not stop looking for causes when a single one is found. Of the causes for delirium, the most common among the elderly are metabolic disturbances, infection, stroke, and drugs, particularly anticholinergic and narcotic medications. The most common causes among the young are drug abuse and alcohol withdrawal.

### Metabolic Disturbances

Metabolic disturbances are the most common causes of delirium (see Chapters 57 and 82). Fortunately, the examination and routine laboratory tests screen for most acquired metabolic disturbances that might be encountered. Because of the potential for life-threatening or permanent damage, some of these conditions—particularly hypoxia and hypoglycemia—must be considered immediately. Also consider dehydration, fluid and electrolyte disorders, and disturbances of calcium and magnesium. The rapidity of change in an electrolyte level may be as important a factor as its absolute value for the development of delirium. For example, some people tolerate chronic sodium levels of 115 mEq/L or less, but a rapid fall to this level can precipitate delirium, seizures, or even central pontine myelinolysis, particularly if the correction of hyponatremia is too rapid. Hypoxia from low cardiac output, respiratory insufficiency, or other causes is another common source of delirium. A cardiac encephalopathy may ensue from heart failure, increased venous pressure transmitted to the dural venous sinuses and veins, and increased ICP (Caplan, 2006). Also consider other major organ failures such as liver and kidney failure, including the possibility of unusual causes such as undetected portocaval shunting or acute pancreatitis with the release of lipases. Delirium due to endocrine dysfunction often has prominent affective symptoms such as hyperthyroidism and Cushing syndrome. Delirium occasionally results from toxins, including industrial agents, pollutants, and heavy metals such as arsenic, bismuth, gold, lead, mercury, thallium, and zinc. Other considerations are inborn errors of metabolism such as acute intermittent porphyria. Finally, it is particularly important to consider thiamine deficiency. In alcoholics and others at risk, thiamine must be given immediately to avoid precipitating Wernicke encephalopathy with the administration of glucose.

## Drugs

Drug intoxication and drug withdrawal are among the most common causes of delirium. Approximately 50% of patients older than 65 years take five or more chronic medications daily, and medications contribute to delirium in up to 39% of these patients (Inouye and Charpentier, 1996). Drug effects are additive, and drugs that are especially likely to cause delirium are those with anticholinergic properties, including many over-the-counter cold preparations, antihistamines, antidepressants, and neuroleptics.

Patients with anticholinergic intoxication present "hot as a hare, blind as a bat, dry as a bone, red as a beet, and mad as a hatter," reflecting fever, dilated pupils, dry mouth, flushing, and delirium. Both serotonin syndrome, due to excess serotonin from selective serotonin reuptake inhibitors (SSRIs; especially in combination with opioids and antiemetics) and neuroleptic malignant syndrome, due to an idiosynchratic and potentially life-threatening reaction to neuroleptics, may present with fever, dysautonomia, muscle rigidity, and mental disturbances manifested mostly as delirium (Oruch et al., 2017; van Ewijk et al., 2016).

Other important groups of drugs associated with delirium, especially in the elderly, are sedative hypnotics such as long-acting benzodiazepines, narcotic analgesics and meperidine, and histamine-2 receptor blockers. Antiparkinsonism drugs result in confusion with prominent hallucinations and delusions in patients with Parkinson disease who are particularly susceptible. Corticosteroid psychosis may develop in patients taking the equivalent of 40 mg/day or more of prednisone. The behavioral effects of corticosteroids often begin with euphoria and hypomania and proceed to a hyperactive delirium. Any drug administered intrathecally, such as metrizamide, is prone to induce confusional behavior.

Drug withdrawal syndromes can be caused by many agents, including barbiturates and other minor tranquilizers, sedative hypnotics, amphetamines, cocaine or "crack," and alcohol. Delirium tremens begins 72–96 hours after alcohol withdrawal, with profound agitation, tremulousness, diaphoresis, tachycardia, fever, and frightening visual hallucinations.

Excited delirium syndrome, also known as agitated delirium, is a drug-related alteration in mental status with combativeness or aggressiveness (Vilke et al., 2012). Similar to delirium tremens, these patients can develop severe psychomotor agitation, anxiety, hallucinations, elevated body temperature, tachycardia, diaphoresis, tolerance to significant pain, violent and bizarre behavior, and "superhuman strength." Excited delirium patients are commonly found to have acute drug intoxication or history of drug abuse. Most patients with excited delirium syndrome will survive, although there still is a high fatality rate estimated at 8.3%–16.5% (Gonin et al., 2017). Awareness among medical personnel regarding this syndrome is crucial for intervention and proactive treatment to prevent deaths.

## Infections

Infections and fevers often produce delirium. The main offenders are urinary tract infections, pneumonia, and septicemia. In a sporadic encephalitis or meningoencephalitis, important causal considerations are herpes simplex virus, Lyme disease, and acquired immunodeficiency syndrome (AIDS) (see Chapters 77–79). Patients with AIDS may be delirious because of the human immunodeficiency virus (HIV) itself or because of an opportunistic infection. Immunocompromised patients are at greater risk of infection, and any suspicion of infection should prompt culture of urine, sputum, blood, and cerebrospinal fluid (CSF). Prion disease can initially resemble delirium, but the former should be considered if there is prominent myoclonus and cerebellar symptoms in the setting of rapidly progressive cognitive decline.

## Strokes

Delirium can be the nonspecific consequence of any acute stroke, but most postinfarct confusion usually resolves in 24–48 hours (see Chapters 65 and 66). Sustained delirium can result from specific strokes, including right middle cerebral artery infarcts affecting prefrontal and posterior parietal areas, and posterior cerebral artery infarcts resulting in either bilateral or left-sided occipitotemporal lesions (fusiform gyrus). The latter lesions can lead to agitation, visual field changes, and even Anton syndrome (see Chapter 16). Delirium may follow occlusion of the anterior cerebral artery or rupture of an anterior communicating artery aneurysm with involvement of the anterior cingulate gyrus and septal region. Thalamic or posterior parietal cortex strokes may present with severe delirium, even with small lesions.

Other cerebrovascular conditions that can produce delirium include high-grade bilateral carotid stenosis, hypertensive encephalopathy, subarachnoid hemorrhage, and central nervous system (CNS) vasculitides such as systemic lupus erythematosus, temporal arteritis, and Behçet syndrome. Migraine can present with delirium, particularly in children. In contrast, the frequency of delirium in transient ischemic attacks, even in vertebrobasilar insufficiency, is low. Transient ischemic attacks should not be considered the cause of delirium unless there are other neurological signs and an appropriate time course.

## Epilepsy

Abnormal brain electrical activity is associated with delirium in four conditions: (1) ictally, with absence status, complex partial status, tonic status without convulsions, or periodic lateralizing epileptiform discharges; (2) postictally, after complex partial or generalized tonic-clonic seizures; (3) interictally manifested as increasing irritability, agitation, and affective symptoms associated with the prodrome of impending seizures; and (4) from the cognitive effects of anticonvulsant medications.

## Postoperative Causes

The cause of delirium in postoperative patients is often multifactorial (Robinson et al., 2009; Winawer, 2001). Predisposing factors to postoperative delirium include age older than 70 years, preexisting CNS disorders such as dementia and Parkinson disease, severe underlying medical conditions, a history of alcohol abuse, impaired functional status, and hypoalbuminemia. Precipitating factors include residual anesthetic and drug effects (especially after premedication with anticholinergic drugs), postoperative hypoxia, perioperative hypotension, electrolyte imbalances, infections, psychological stress, and multiple awakenings with fragmented sleep. There is no clear correlation of delirium with specific anesthetic route. Upon the cessation of general anesthesia, clinicians may observe the emergence of excitation, or an "emergence delirium" (Silverstein and Deiner, 2013). Otherwise, postoperative delirium may start at any time but often becomes evident about the third day and abates by the seventh, although it may last considerably longer. Clinicians may refer to a postoperative delirium that occurs 24–72 hours after the completion of a surgical procedure as an "interval delirium."

A number of surgeries are associated with a high rate of postoperative delirium. Between 30% and 40% of patients experience delirium after open heart or coronary artery bypass surgery. Patients older than 60 years are at special risk for postoperative delirium after cardiac surgery. Additional factors are decreased postoperative cardiac output and length of time on cardiopulmonary bypass machine, with its added risk for microemboli. In addition to an already high rate of delirium following fractures (up to 35.6% after hip fracture), orthopedic surgeries, particularly femoral neck fractures and bilateral knee replacements, further increase the frequency of delirium by approximately 18%. Emergency hip fracture repair is associated with a higher risk of delirium than elective hip surgery (Bruce et al., 2007). Elective noncardiac thoracic surgery is also associated with a 9%–14% frequency of delirium in the elderly. Cataract surgery is associated with a 7% frequency of delirium, possibly because of sensory deprivation. Patients who have undergone prostate surgery may develop delirium associated with water intoxication as a result of absorption of irrigation water from the bladder.

### Other Neurological Causes

Other CNS disturbances predispose to delirium. In general, patients with dementia, Lewy body disease, Parkinson disease, and atrophy or subcortical ischemic changes on neuroimaging are particularly susceptible. Autoimmune or paraneoplastic processes produce limbic and other encephalitides that may initially present with delirium. Autonomic instability, respiratory distress, and focal or generalized neurological symptoms such as seizures are key clinical findings that suggest the need for urgent further workup, including MRI and lumbar puncture, with prompt treatment if clinical suspicion is high. Electroconvulsive therapy often produces a delirium of 1 week or more. Head trauma can result in delirium as a consequence of brain concussion, brain contusion, intracranial hematoma, or subarachnoid hemorrhage (see Chapters 66 and 67). Moreover, subdural hematomas can occur in the elderly with little or no history of head injury. Rapidly growing tumors in the supratentorial region are especially likely to cause delirium with increased ICP.

Delirium can result from acute demyelinating diseases and other diffuse multifocal lesions and from obstructive forms of hydrocephalus. Patients with transient global amnesia have ongoing disorientation and appear confused but are not otherwise inattentive or manifest other signs of delirium. Transient global amnesia patients have prominent antegrade amnesia, limited retrograde amnesia for the preceding hours, and improve within 24 hours. In Wernicke encephalopathy, delirium accompanies ocular motor paresis, nystagmus, ataxia, and frequently residual amnesia (Korsakoff amnestic syndrome).

### Miscellaneous Causes

Various other disturbances can produce delirium. Bone fractures are associated with delirium in the elderly, and approximately 50% of those admitted with a hip fracture have delirium. Time from admission to operation in these patients is an additional risk factor for development of preoperative delirium (Juliebo et al., 2009). In orthopedic cases the possibility of fat emboli requires evaluation of urine, sputum, or CSF for fat. ICU psychosis is associated with sleep deprivation, immobilization, unfamiliarity, fear, frightening sensory overstimulation or sensory deprivation, isolation, transfer from another hospital ward, mechanical ventilation, psychoactive medications, and use of drains, tubes, and catheters (Van Rompaey et al., 2009). Delirium results from blood dyscrasias, including anemia, thrombocytopenia, and disseminated intravascular coagulopathy. Finally, physical factors such as heatstroke, electrocution, and hypothermia may be causal.

## Special Problems in Differential Diagnosis

Delirium must be distinguished from dementia, Wernicke aphasia, and psychiatric conditions (see Chapters 7, 9, 10, and 13). The main differentiating features of dementia are the longer time course and the absence of prominent fluctuating attentional and perceptual deficits. Chronic confusion states lasting 6 months or more are a form of dementia. Patients with delirium that becomes chronic tend to settle into a lethargic state without the prominent fluctuations throughout the day, and they have fewer perceptual problems and less disruption of the day/night cycle. In addition, delirium and dementia often overlap because demented patients have increased susceptibility for developing a superimposed delirium. The prevalence of delirium superimposed on dementia in community and hospital setting ranges from 22% to 89% (Morandi et al., 2012). Demented patients who suddenly get worse should always be evaluated for delirium. Patients with vascular dementia may have an acute onset or sharp decline in cognition similar to delirium.

Distinguishing delirium from dementia with Lewy bodies may be particularly difficult; both delirium and Lewy body dementia may present with prominent fluctuations in attention and alertness, visuospatial deficits and visual hallucinations. Key distinguishing features that suggest Lewy body dementia include a prior history of autonomic dysfunction, rapid eye movement (REM) behavior disorder and anosmia, followed by increasing frequency of falls and parkinsonism, and severe neuroleptic sensitivity, the constellation of which is not typical for delirium. On the other hand, acute onset, auditory hallucinations, and sleep/wake cycle disturbance without REM behavior disorder are consistent with delirium and not typically seen in Lewy body dementia. Further complicating the picture is that delirium may present superimposed on dementia and the aforementioned symptoms may be present concurrently. In such cases, collateral history is crucial to establish a timeline of progression and an accurate differential diagnosis may not be possible until after a diagnostic workup is completed (Morandi et al., 2017).

The language examination should distinguish Wernicke aphasia from the language of delirium. Aphasics have prominent paraphasias of all types, including neologisms, and they have relatively preserved response to axial or whole-body commands. Their agraphia is also empty of content and is paragraphic compared with the mechanical and other writing disturbances previously described in patients with delirium.

Psychiatric conditions that may be mistaken for delirium include schizophrenia, depression, mania, attention-deficit disorder, autism, dissociative states, and Ganser syndrome, which is characterized by ludicrous or approximate responses (see Chapters 9 and 10). In general, patients with psychiatric conditions lack the fluctuating attentional and related deficits associated with delirium. Schizophrenic patients may have a very disturbed verbal output, but their speech often has an underlying bizarre theme. Schizophrenic hallucinations are more

**TABLE 4.2 Special Problems in the Differential Diagnosis of Delirium***

| Clinical Feature | Delirium | Dementias | Stroke with Wernicke Aphasia | Schizophrenia | Depression |
|---|---|---|---|---|---|
| Course | Acute onset; hours, days, or more | Insidious onset†; months or years; progressive | Sudden onset; chronic, stable deficit | Insidious onset, 6 months or more; acute psychotic phases | Insidious onset, at least 2 weeks, often months |
| Attention | Markedly impaired attention and arousal | Normal early; impairment later | Normal | Normal to mild impairment | Mild impairment |
| Fluctuation | Prominent in attention arousal; disturbed day/night cycle | Prominent fluctuations absent; lesser disturbances in day/night cycle | Absent | Absent | Absent |
| Perception | Misperceptions; illusions and pareidolias; hallucinations, usually visual, fleeting; paramnesia | Perceptual abnormalities much less prominent‡; paramnesia | Normal | Hallucinations, auditory with personal reference | May have mood-congruent hallucinations |
| Speech and language | Abnormal clarity, speed, and coherence; disjointed and dysarthric; misnaming; characteristic dysgraphia | Early anomia; empty speech; abnormal comprehension | Prominent paraphasias and neologisms; empty speech; abnormal comprehension | Disorganized, with a bizarre theme | Decreased amount of speech |
| Other cognition | Disorientation to time, place; recent memory and visuospatial abnormalities | Disorientation to time, place; multiple other higher cognitive deficits | No other necessary deficits | Disorientation to person; concrete interpretations | Mental slowing; indecisiveness; memory retrieval difficulty |
| Behavior | Lethargy or delirium; nonsystematized delusions; emotional lability | Disinterested; disengaged; disinhibited; delusions and other psychiatric symptoms | Paranoia possibly ensuing | Systematized delusions; paranoia; bizarre behavior | Depressed mood; anhedonia; lack of energy; sleep and appetite disturbances |
| Electroencephalogram | Diffuse slowing; low-voltage fast activity; specific patterns | Normal early; mild slowing later | Normal | Normal | Normal |

*The characteristics listed are the usual ones and are not exclusive.
†Patients with vascular dementia may have an abrupt decline in cognition.
‡Patients with dementia with diffuse cortical Lewy bodies often have a fluctuating mental status and hallucinations.

often consistent persecutory voices rather than fleeting visual images, and their delusions are more systematized and have personal reference. Conversely, delirious hallucinations are usually visual, and the delusions are more transitory and fragmented. Mood disorders may also be mistaken for delirium, particularly if there is an acute agitated depression or a predominantly irritable mania. Often patients in a manic episode are inattentive, distractible, and hyperkinetic and look as if they are in a hyperactive delirium. A general rule is that psychiatric behaviors such as psychosis or mania may be due to delirium, called delirious mania, especially if they occur in someone who is 40 years or older without a prior psychiatric history. They should be regarded as delirium until proven otherwise. Table 4.2 outlines the special problems that must be considered in the differential diagnosis of delirium.

## PREVENTION AND MANAGEMENT

As many as 30%–40% of cases of delirium may be prevented with provision of high-quality care (Inouye et al., 2014). Misdiagnosis of delirium results in inadequate management in up to 80% of patients (Michaud et al., 2007), and approximately half of elderly patients affected by delirium actually develop symptoms *after* admission to the hospital. Early identification of patients with predisposing risk factors is important, especially in a frail geriatric population (Laurila et al., 2008). In addition, early intervention by geriatricians and others can reduce the rates of delirium (Deschodt et al., 2012). Multifactorial intervention programs can reduce the duration of delirium, length of hospital stay, need for institutionalization, and mortality (Hshieh et al., 2015). These programs, such as the Hospital Elder Life Program (HELP), focus on managing risk factors through interventions that include reorientation, therapeutic activities, reduced use and dose of psychoactive drugs, early mobilization, promotion of sleep, maintenance of adequate hydration and nutrition, and provision of vision and hearing adaptations (Inouye et al., 2014). They also focus on educational programs for physicians and nurses in the detection and management of delirium. Nurses, in particular, spend more time with patients than physicians do, and they may be in a better position to recognize delirium.

There are several steps in the management of delirium. First, attention is aimed at finding the cause and eliminating it, from removing the offending drug to treating the infection to administering high-dose thiamine for Wernicke encephalopathy. Second, the delirium is managed with symptomatic measures involving attention to fluid and electrolyte balance, nutritional status, and early treatment of infections. Third, management focuses on environmental interventions. Reduce unfamiliarity by providing a calendar, a clock, family pictures, and personal objects. Maintain a moderate sensory balance in the patient by avoiding sensory overstimulation or deprivation. Minimize staff changes, limit ambient noise and the number of visits from strangers, and provide a radio or a television set, a nightlight, and, where necessary, eyeglasses and hearing aids. Other environmental measures include providing soft music and warm baths and allowing the patient to take walks when possible. Physical restraints should be avoided if possible and a sitter used instead. Fourth, proper communication and support are critical with these patients. As much as possible, everything should be explained. Delusions and hallucinations should be neither endorsed nor challenged. Patients should receive emotional support, including frequent family visits. They also benefit from frequent reorientation to place, time, and situation. Finally, it is important to address safety for the patient, family, and caregivers to minimize the risks for suicidality, violence, falls, wandering, or inadvertent self-harm (Irwin et al., 2013).

In general, it is best to avoid the use of drugs in confused patients, because they further cloud the picture and may worsen delirium. All the patient's medications should be reviewed, and any unnecessary drugs should be discontinued. When medication is needed, the goal is to make the patient manageable, not to decrease loud or annoying behavior or to sedate them (Inouye, 2006). These patients should receive the lowest possible dose and should not get drugs such as phenobarbital or long-acting benzodiazepines. In particular, use of benzodiazepines can have a paradoxical effect in the elderly, causing agitation and confusion. Medication may be necessary if the patient's behavior is potentially dangerous, interferes with medical care, or causes the patient profound distress. Clinicians most often use haloperidol (starting at 0.25 mg daily) for these symptoms because of its higher dopamine receptor potency, lower anticholinergic effects, and the availability of various routes of use (Bledowski and Trutia, 2012). Haloperidol may be repeated every 30 minutes, orally (PO) or intramuscularly (IM), up to a maximum of 5 mg/day. After the first 24 hours; 50% of the loading dose may be given in divided doses over the next 24 hours; then the dose should be tapered off over the next few days (Inouye, 2004). There is mixed evidence to support the preventive use of haloperidol prior to the development of delirium, although it may reduce severity and duration postoperatively, as well as duration of hospital stay (Gosch and Nicholas, 2014; Kalisvaart et al., 2005). One multicenter study found no benefit of either haloperidol or ziprasidone compared with placebo specifically in the management of hypoactive or hyperactive ICU delirium (Girard et al., 2018). The atypical antipsychotics, including risperidone, olanzapine, quetiapine, and aripiprazole, may be used at low doses (Attard et al., 2008); however, safety and efficacy of the atypical and typical antipsychotics are similar (Toor et al., 2013). Results in favor of acetylcholinesterase inhibitors for delirium management have not been borne out in controlled trials, although in some cases, such as in patients with Lewy body dementia, they can be helpful (Attard et al., 2008; Martins and Fernandes, 2012; Tabet and Howard, 2009). In addition, the existing evidence does not support the use of acetylcholinesterase inhibitors after surgery for prevention of postoperative delirium (Alce et al., 2013; Attard et al., 2008; Tabet and Howard, 2009).

Other medications such as valproate, ondansetron, or melatonin may be effective and safe in selected cases. However, melatonin receptor agonists (melatonin, ramelteon, L-tryptophan) have shown inconsistent outcomes for delirium prevention (Choy et al., 2018; Walker et al., 2016).

There is growing evidence that the sedatives and hypnotics commonly used in the ICU can produce delirium (Hipp and Ely, 2012). Dexmedetomidine, an $\alpha_2$-agonist, has gained popularity in the ICU due to decreased respiratory suppression and evidence from recent trials demonstrating reduced delirium prevalence as compared with opioids and GABA-ergic drugs such as benzodiazepines (Hipp et al., 2012; Pavone et al., 2018). Dexmedetomidine has also been shown to reduce the incidence of postoperative delirium, especially after cardiac surgical procedures (Pavone et al., 2018).

## PROGNOSIS

The prognosis for recovery from delirium is variable. If the causative factor is rapidly corrected, recovery can be complete, with an average duration of delirium of approximately 8 days (2 days to 2 weeks). Delirium present at discharge is associated with a 2.6-fold increased risk of death or nursing home placement (McAvay et al., 2006), and delirium persisting after hospital discharge is associated with a 2.9-fold risk of death within the following year. This risk appears to be reversible with the resolution of delirium (Kiely et al., 2009). The link between delirium and subsequent long-term cognitive impairment is also firmly established (MacLullich et al., 2009; Morandi et al., 2012).

In the elderly, delirium may not be a transient disorder. For them, the duration of delirium is often longer than that of their underlying medical problem. Moreover, after hospital discharge, older patients who are delirious may not recover back to baseline (Inouye et al., 2014). In one study, 14.8% still met criteria for delirium 12 months after discharge, sometimes referred to as a "persistent delirium" (McCusker et al., 2004; Morandi et al., 2012). A partial nonprogressive delirium with some but not all criteria for delirium may persist in many elderly patients, sometimes referred to as a "subsyndromal delirium" (Martins and Fernendes, 2012).

Delirium is an independent predictor of adverse outcomes in older hospitalized patients; particularly in the presence of baseline cognitive impairment or dementia, it is associated with an increased mortality rate and may accelerate cognitive decline (Adamis et al., 2006; Inouye et al., 2014; MacLullich et al., 2009; McCusker et al., 2002). Delirium in the elderly predicts sustained poor cognitive and functional status and increased likelihood of nursing home placement after a medical admission. Hypoactive delirious patients appear to be at particular risk because of complications from aspiration and inadequate oral nutrition as well as falls and pressure sores. In general, however, clinicians can greatly improve prognosis with increased awareness of delirium, more rapid diagnosis of the causative factor(s), and better overall management.

*The complete reference list is available online at https://expertconsult.inkling.com/.* 

5

# Stupor and Coma

*Joseph R. Berger, Raymond Price*

## OUTLINE



## DEFINITIONS

*Consciousness* may be defined as a state of awareness of self and surroundings. Alterations in consciousness are conceptualized into two types. The first type affects arousal and is the subject of this chapter. Sleep, the only normal form of altered consciousness, is discussed in Chapter 101. The second type involves cognitive and affective mental function, sometimes referred to as the "content" of mental function. Examples of the latter type of alteration in consciousness are dementia (see Chapter 7), delusions, confusion, and inattention (see Chapter 9). These altered states of consciousness, with the exception of advanced dementia, do not affect the level of arousal.

Delirium is defined by American Psychiatric Association's *Diagnostic and Statistical Manual of Mental Disorders,* fifth edition (DSM-V), as a disturbance in attention and awareness (European Delirium Association). Delirium can occur without a reduced level of consciousness, such as a hyperactive delirium, and in this context would be classified as a disorder of the content or mental function. Alternatively, delirium can occur in conjunction with a mildly or moderately reduced level of consciousness, such as hypoactive delirium, and would be classified as a disorder of arousal. Delirium is a good example of a confusional state in which it may be clinically difficult to separate decreased arousal from a change in cognitive or affective mental function. In clinical practice, the exact boundary between different forms of altered consciousness may be vague. Diagnostic criteria for delirium from the American Psychiatric Association's DSM-V in addition to a disturbance in attention and awareness include an additional disturbance in cognition (memory, language, visuospatial ability, perception) that developed over hours to days as a change from the patient's baseline and is not better explained by a neurocognitive disorder. Patients with severely reduced levels of arousal such as coma cannot also be classified as delirious.

Alterations in arousal, although often referred to as altered levels of consciousness, do not actually form discrete levels but rather are made up of a continuum of subtly changing behavioral states that range from alert to comatose. These states are dynamic and thus may change with time. Four points on the continuum of arousal are often used in describing the clinical state of a patient: alert, lethargic, stuporous, and comatose. *Alert* refers to a perfectly normal state of arousal. *Lethargy* lies between alertness and stupor. *Stupor* is a state of baseline unresponsiveness that requires repeated application of vigorous stimuli to achieve arousal. *Coma* is a state of complete unresponsiveness to arousal. The terms *lethargy* and *stupor* cover a broad area on the continuum of behavioral states and thus are subject to misinterpretation by subsequent observers of a patient when used without further qualification. In clinical practice, in which relatively slight changes in arousal may be significant, only the terms *alert* and *comatose* (the endpoints of the continuum) have enough precision to be used without further qualification.

## CONDITIONS THAT MAY MIMIC COMA

Several different states of impaired cognition or consciousness may appear similar to coma or may be confused with it (Table 5.1). Moreover, patients who survive the initial coma may progress to certain of these syndromes after varying lengths of time. Once sleep/wake cycles become established, true coma is no longer present. Differentiation of these states from true coma is important to allow administration of appropriate therapy and to help determine prognosis.

In the *locked-in syndrome (de-efferented state)*, patients are alert and aware of their environment but are quadriplegic, with lower cranial nerve palsies resulting from bilateral ventral pontine lesions that involve the corticospinal, corticopontine, and corticobulbar tracts. The patients are awake and alert but are voluntarily able only to move

**TABLE 5.1 Behavioral States Confused with Coma**

| Behavioral State | Definition | Lesion | Comments |
|---|---|---|---|
| Locked-in syndrome | Alert and aware, quadriplegic with lower cranial nerve palsy | Bilateral ventral pontine | A similar state may be seen with severe polyneuropathies, myasthenia gravis, and neuromuscular blocking agents |
| Persistent vegetative state | Absent cognitive function but retained "vegetative" components | Extensive cortical gray or subcortical white matter with relative preservation of brainstem | Synonyms include apallic syndrome, coma vigile, cerebral cortical death |
| Abulia | Severe apathy, patient neither speaks nor moves spontaneously | Bilateral frontal medial | Severe cases resemble akinetic mutism, but patient is alert and aware |
| Catatonia | Mute, with marked decrease in motor activity | Usually psychiatric | May be mimicked by frontal lobe dysfunction or drugs |
| Pseudocoma | Feigned coma | | |

their eyes vertically or blink. The locked-in syndrome most often is observed as a consequence of pontine infarction due to basilar artery thrombosis. Other causes include central pontine myelinolysis and brainstem mass lesions. A state similar to the locked-in syndrome also may be seen with severe polyneuropathy—in particular, acute inflammatory demyelinating polyradiculoneuropathy, myasthenia gravis, and poisoning with neuromuscular blocking agents.

In the *persistent vegetative state* (PVS), patients do not demonstrate clinically the ability to engage in any of the following behaviors: awareness of self and environment, interaction with others, sustained, reproducible, or purposeful voluntary behavioral response to visual, auditory, tactile or noxious stimuli, language comprehension or expression, or blink to visual threat. However, these patients do retain vegetative functions such as cardiac action, respiration, maintenance of blood pressure, and a sleep/wake cycle. Spontaneous movements may occur and the eyes may open in response to external stimuli, but the patient does not speak or obey commands. Functional magnetic resonance imaging (MRI) and electroencephalogram (EEG) studies of patients who meet the aforementioned clinical criteria of PVS have shown that approximately 14% of these patients will activate brain regions similar to healthy subjects when following commands despite not being able to demonstrate clinically these behaviors. Diagnostic criteria for PVS are provided in Table 5.2. The diagnosis of this condition should be made cautiously and only after extended periods of observation. A number of poorly defined syndromes have been used synonymously with PVS, including *apallic syndrome* or *state*, *akinetic mutism*, *coma vigil*, *alpha coma*, *neocortical death*, and *permanent unconsciousness*. These terms, used variously by different authors, probably are best avoided because of their lack of precision.

A condition that has been estimated to be 10 times more common than PVS is the *minimally conscious state*, in which severe disability accompanies minimal awareness. A set of diagnostic criteria for the minimally conscious state have proposed (Table 5.3). In two separate studies in Europe, more than 40% of patients in a minimally conscious state were misdiagnosed as PVS, most commonly due to lack of appreciation of eye tracking. Some authors subdivide minimally conscious state into minimally conscious state plus for patients who demonstrated higher-level function such as command following or intelligible speech and minimally conscious state minus for patients who only rely to environmental stimuli or visually track objects. Similar to PVS patients, functional MRI and EEG studies of patients who meet the clinical criteria minimally conscious state have shown that approximately 32% of these patients will activate brain regions similar to healthy subjects when following commands despite not being able to demonstrate clinically these behaviors. Emergence from minimally conscious state occurs when there is recovery of appropriate yes or no answers to questions or when able to use two familiar objects correctly. *Abulia* is a severe apathy in which patients have blunting of feeling, drive, mentation, and behavior such that they neither speak nor move spontaneously. *Catatonia* may result in a state of muteness, with dramatically decreased motor activity. The maintenance of body posture, with preserved ability to sit or stand, distinguishes it from organic pathological stupor. It generally is a psychiatric manifestation but may

**TABLE 5.2 Criteria for the Diagnosis of a Persistent Vegetative State**

1. No evidence of awareness of themselves or their environment; they are incapable of interacting with others
2. No evidence of sustained, reproducible, purposeful, or voluntary behavioral responses to visual, auditory, tactile, or noxious stimuli
3. No evidence of language comprehension or expression
4. Intermittent wakefulness manifested by the presence of sleep/wake cycles
5. Sufficiently preserved hypothalamic and brainstem autonomic functions to survive if given medical and nursing care
6. Bowel and bladder incontinence
7. Variably preserved cranial nerve (pupillary, oculocephalic, corneal, vestibulo-ocular, and gag) and spinal reflexe

*Data from The Multi-Society Task Force on PVS. Medical aspects of the persistent vegetative state. N Engl J Med 1994;3330, 1499–1508, 1572–1579.*

**TABLE 5.3 Criteria for the Minimally Conscious State**

To diagnose a minimally conscious state, limited but clearly discernible evidence of self- or environmental awareness must be demonstrated on a reproducible or sustained basis by one or more of the following behaviors:

1. Follows simple commands
2. Gestural or verbal yes/no responses (regardless of accuracy)
3. Intelligible verbalization
4. Purposeful behavior, including movements or affective behaviors that occur in contingent relationship to relevant environmental stimuli and are not due to reflexive activity.

*Data from Giacino, J.T., Ashwal, S., Childs, N., et al., 2002. The minimally conscious state: definition and diagnostic criteria. Neurology 58, 349–353.*

be mimicked by frontal lobe dysfunction or drug effect. *Pseudocoma* is the term for a condition in which the patient appears comatose (i.e., unresponsive, unarousable, or both) but has no structural, metabolic, or toxic disorder.

## APPROACH TO THE PATIENT IN COMA

The initial clinical approach to the patient in a state of stupor or coma is based on the principle that *all* alterations in arousal constitute acute, life-threatening emergencies until vital functions such as blood pressure and oxygenation are stabilized, potentially reversible causes of coma are treated, and the underlying cause of the alteration in arousal is understood. Urgent steps may be necessary to avoid or minimize permanent brain damage from reversible causes. In view of the urgency of this situation, every physician should develop a diagnostic and therapeutic routine to use with a patient with an alteration in consciousness. A basic understanding of the mechanisms that lead to impairment in arousal is necessary to develop this routine. The anatomical and physiological bases for alterations in arousal are discussed in Chapter 101.

Although it is essential to keep in mind the concept of a spectrum of arousal, for the sake of simplicity and brevity only the term *coma* is used in the rest of this chapter. Table 5.4 lists many of the common causes of coma. More than half of all cases of coma are due to diffuse and metabolic brain dysfunction. In Plum and Posner's landmark study (1980, see 2007 revision) of 500 patients initially diagnosed as having coma of unknown cause (in whom the diagnosis was ultimately established), 326 patients had diffuse and metabolic brain dysfunction. Almost half of these had drug poisonings. Of the remaining patients, 101 had supratentorial mass lesions, including 77 hemorrhagic lesions and 9 infarctions; 65 had subtentorial lesions, mainly brainstem infarctions; and 8 had psychiatric coma. A logical decision tree often used in searching for the cause of coma divides the categories of diseases that cause coma into three groups: structural lesions, which may be above or below the tentorium; metabolic and toxic causes; and psychiatric causes. The history and physical examination usually provide sufficient evidence to determine the presence or absence of a structural lesion and quickly differentiate the general categories to decide what further diagnostic tests are needed or to allow for immediate intervention if necessary. Serial examinations are needed, with precise description of the behavioral state at different points in time, to determine if the patient is improving or—a more ominous finding—worsening, and to decide if a change in therapy or further diagnostic tests is necessary. Subtle declines in the intermediate states of arousal may herald precipitous changes in brainstem function, which may affect regulation of vital functions such as respiration or blood pressure. The dynamic quality of alterations of consciousness and the need for accurate documentation at different points in time cannot be overemphasized.

### Rapid Initial Examination and Emergency Therapy

A relatively quick initial assessment is conducted to ensure that the comatose patient is medically and neurologically stable before a more detailed investigation is undertaken. This rapid initial examination is essential to rule out the need for immediate medical or surgical intervention. In addition, various supportive or preventive measures may be indicated. Urgent and sometimes empirical therapy is given to prevent further brain damage. Potential immediate metabolic needs of the brain are supplied by empirical use of supplemental oxygen, intravenous thiamine (at least 100 mg), and intravenous 50% dextrose in water (25 g). A baseline serum glucose level should be obtained before glucose administration. The use of intravenous glucose in patients with ischemic or anoxic brain damage is controversial. Extra glucose may augment local lactic acid production by anaerobic glycolysis and may worsen ischemic or anoxic damage. However, clinically, empirical glucose administration is recommended when the cause of coma is unknown. There are two reasons for this approach: the frequent occurrence of alterations in arousal due to hypoglycemia and the relatively good prognosis for coma due to hypoglycemia when it is treated expeditiously; and the potentially permanent consequences if it is not treated. By comparison, the prognosis for anoxic or ischemic coma generally is poor and probably will remain poor regardless of glucose supplementation. Thiamine must always be given in conjunction with glucose to prevent precipitation of Wernicke encephalopathy. Naloxone hydrochloride may be given parenterally, preferably intravenously, in doses of 0.4–2.0 mg if opiate overdose is the suspected cause of coma. An abrupt and complete reversal of narcotic effect may precipitate an acute abstinence syndrome in persons who are physically dependent on opiates.

An initial examination should include a check of general appearance, blood pressure, pulse, temperature, respiratory rate and breath sounds, best response to stimulation, pupil size and responsiveness, and posturing or adventitious movements. The neck should be stabilized in all instances of trauma until cervical spine fracture or subluxation can be ruled out. The airway should be protected in all comatose patients and an intravenous line placed. However, in coma, the classic sign of an acute condition in the abdomen—namely, abdominal rigidity—may be subtle in degree or absent. In addition, the diagnosis of blunt abdominal trauma is difficult in patients with a change in mental status. Therefore, in unconscious patients with a history of trauma, a computed tomography (CT) scan of the abdomen or peritoneal lavage by an experienced surgeon may be warranted. Hypotension, marked hypertension, bradycardia, arrhythmias causing depression of blood pressure, marked hyperthermia, and signs of cerebral herniation mandate immediate therapeutic intervention. Hyperthermia or meningismus prompts consideration of urgent lumbar puncture. Examination of the fundus of the eye for papilledema and a CT scan of the brain should be performed before lumbar puncture in any comatose patient. Infection at the site of the lumbar puncture, papilledema, decerebrate posturing, and thrombocytopenia and other bleeding diathesis are contraindications to lumbar puncture and, even in their absence, medicolegal considerations may render a CT scan of the head preferable before proceeding to lumbar puncture. To avoid a delay in therapy when acute bacterial meningitis is strongly suspected, antibiotics and adjunctive corticosteroids should be administered within 1 hour of hospital admission (Brouwer et al., 2010) even if cerebrospinal fluid (CSF) collection cannot be obtained in a timely fashion. Corticosteroid administration should be avoided in the presence of septic shock. Blood cultures and throat swabs should be obtained on these patients prior to antibiotic administration. The risk of herniation from a lumbar puncture in patients with evidence of increased intracerebral pressure is difficult to ascertain from the literature; estimates range from 1% to 12%, depending on the series (Posner et al., 2007). It is important to recognize that both central and tonsillar herniation may increase neck tone. Despite an elevated intracranial pressure (ICP), sufficient CSF should always be obtained to perform the necessary studies. The performance of bacterial culture and cell count, essential in cases of suspected bacterial meningitis, requires but a few milliliters of fluid. Multiplex nucleic acid amplification tests may be helpful in diagnosing a central nervous system (CNS) infection, especially, when caused by fastidious or noncultivable microorganisms. Intravenous access and intravenous mannitol or hypertonic saline should be ready in the event that unexpected herniation begins after the lumbar puncture. When the CSF pressure is greater than 500 mm $H_2O$, some authorities recommend leaving the needle in place to monitor the pressure and administering

**TABLE 5.4 Causes of Coma**

**I. Symmetrical—Nonstructural**

***Toxins***

Lead
Thallium
Mushrooms
Cyanide
Methanol
Ethylene glycol
Carbon monoxide

**Drugs**

Sedatives
Barbiturates*
Other hypnotics
Tranquilizers
Bromides
Alcohol
Opiates
Paraldehyde
Salicylate
Psychotropics
Anticholinergics
Amphetamines
Lithium
Phencyclidine
Monoamine oxidase inhibitors

**II. Symmetrical—Structural**

***Supratentorial***

Bilateral internal carotid occlusion
Bilateral anterior cerebral artery occlusion

**III. Asymmetrical—Structural**

***Supratentorial***

Thrombotic thrombocytopenic purpura†
Disseminated intravascular coagulation
Nonbacterial thrombotic endocarditis (marantic endocarditis)
Subacute bacterial endocarditis
Fat emboli
Unilateral hemispheric mass (tumor, bleed) with herniation

***Metabolic***

Hypoxia
Hypercapnia
Hypernatremia
Hyponatremia*
Hypoglycemia*
Hyperglycemic nonketotic coma
Diabetic ketoacidosis
Lactic acidosis
Hypercalcemia
Hypocalcemia
Hypermagnesemia
Hyperthermia
Hypothermia
Reye encephalopathy
Aminoacidemia
Wernicke encephalopathy
Porphyria
Hepatic encephalopathy*
Uremia
Dialysis encephalopathy
Addisonian crisis

***Subarachnoid Hemorrhage***

Thalamic hemorrhage*
Trauma—contusion, concussion*
Hydrocephalus

***Subdural Hemorrhage, Bilateral***

Intracerebral bleed
Pituitary apoplexy†
Massive or bilateral supratentorial infarction
Multifocal leukoencephalopathy
Creutzfeldt-Jakob disease
Adrenal leukodystrophy
Cerebral vasculitis
Cerebral abscess

***Infections***

Bacterial meningitis
Viral encephalitis
Postinfectious encephalomyelitis
Syphilis
Sepsis
Typhoid fever
Malaria
Waterhouse-Friderichsen syndrome

***Psychiatric***

Catatonia

***Other***

Postictal
Diffuse ischemia (myocardial infarction, congestive heart failure, arrhythmia)
Hypotension
Fat embolism
Hypertensive encephalopathy
Hypothyroidism

***Infratentorial***

Basilar occlusion*
Midline brainstem tumor
Pontine hemorrhage*

***Subdural Empyema***

Thrombophlebitis†
Multiple sclerosis
Leukoencephalopathy associated with hemotherapy
Acute disseminated encephalomyelitis
Infratentorial
Brainstem infarction
Brainstem hemorrhage

*Relatively common asymmetrical presentation.
†Relatively symmetrical.
*Data from Plum, F., & Posner, J.B., 1980. The Diagnosis of Stupor and Coma, third ed. F. A. Davis, Philadelphia; and Fisher, C.M., 1969. The neurological evaluation of the comatose patient. Acta Neurologica Scandinavica 45 (Suppl 36), 5–56.*

intravenous mannitol or hypertonic saline to lower the pressure. If focal signs develop during or after the lumbar puncture, immediate intubation and hyperventilation also may be necessary to reduce intracerebral pressure urgently until more definitive therapy is available.

Ecchymosis, petechiae, or evidence of ready bleeding on general examination may indicate coagulation abnormality or thrombocytopenia. This increases the risk of epidural hematoma after a lumbar puncture, which may cause devastating spinal cord compression.

Measurements of prothrombin time, partial thromboplastin time, and platelet count should precede lumbar puncture in these cases, and the coagulation abnormality or thrombocytopenia should be corrected before proceeding to lumbar puncture.

## Common Presentations

Coma usually manifests in one of three ways. First, and most commonly, it occurs as an expected or predictable progression of an underlying illness. Examples are focal brainstem infarction with extension; chronic obstructive pulmonary disease in a patient who is given too high a concentration of oxygen, thereby decreasing respiratory drive and resulting in carbon dioxide narcosis; and known barbiturate overdose when the ingested drug cannot be fully removed and begins to cause unresponsiveness. Second, coma occurs as an unpredictable event in a patient whose prior medical conditions are known to the physician. The coma may be a complication of an underlying medical illness, such as in a patient with arrhythmia who suffers anoxia after a cardiac arrest. Alternatively, an unrelated event may occur, such as sepsis from an intravenous line in a cardiac patient or a stroke in a hypothyroid patient. Third, coma can occur in a patient whose medical history is totally unknown to the physician. Sometimes this type of presentation is associated with a known probable cause, such as head trauma incurred in a motor vehicle accident, but often the comatose patient presents to the physician without an obvious associated cause. Thorough objective systematic assessment must be applied in every comatose patient. Special care must be taken not to be lulled or misled by an apparently predictable progression of an underlying illness or other obvious cause of coma.

## History

Once the patient is relatively stable, clues to the cause of the coma should be sought by briefly interviewing relatives, friends, bystanders, or medical personnel who may have observed the patient before or during the decrease in consciousness. Telephone calls to family members may be helpful. The patient's wallet or purse should be examined for lists of medications, a physician's card, or other information. Attempts should be made to ascertain the patient's social background and prior medical history and the circumstances in which the patient was found. The presence of drug paraphernalia or empty medicine bottles suggests a drug overdose. Newer recreational drugs, such as γ-hydroxybutyrate and bath salts, must be considered in the differential diagnosis. An oral hypoglycemic agent or insulin in the medicine cabinet or refrigerator implies possible hypoglycemia. Antiarrhythmic agents such as procainamide or quinidine suggest existing coronary artery disease with possible myocardial infarction or warn that an unwitnessed arrhythmia may have caused cerebral hypoperfusion, with resulting anoxic encephalopathy. Oral anticoagulants, including direct thrombin inhibitors, factor Xa inhibitors, and warfarin, typically prescribed for patients with deep venous thrombosis or pulmonary embolism, atrial fibrillation or mechanical heart valve, may be responsible for massive intracerebral bleeding. In patients found to be unresponsive at the scene of an accident, the unresponsive state may be due to trauma incurred in the accident, or sudden loss of consciousness may have precipitated the accident.

The neurologist often is called when patients do not awaken after surgery or when coma supervenes following a surgical procedure. Postoperative causes of coma include many of those mentioned in Table 5.4. In addition, the physician also must have a high index of suspicion for certain neurological conditions that occur in this setting, including fat embolism, Addisonian crisis, and hypothyroid coma (precipitated by acute illness or surgical stress); Wernicke encephalopathy from carbohydrate loading without adequate thiamine stores; and iatrogenic overdose of a narcotic analgesic. Attempts should be made to ascertain if the patient complained of symptoms before onset of coma. Common signs and symptoms include headache preceding subarachnoid hemorrhage, chest pain with aortic dissection or myocardial infarction, shortness of breath from hypoxia, stiff neck in meningoencephalitis, and vertigo in brainstem stroke. Nausea and vomiting are common in poisonings. Coma also may be secondary to increased ICP. Observers may have noted head trauma, drug abuse, seizures, or hemiparesis. Descriptions of falling to one side, dysarthria or aphasia, ptosis, pupillary dilatation, or disconjugate gaze may help to localize structural lesions. The time course of the disease, as noted by family or friends, may help to differentiate the often relatively slow, progressive course of toxic-metabolic or infectious causes from abrupt, catastrophic changes that are seen most commonly with vascular events. Finally, family members or friends may be invaluable in identifying psychiatric causes of unresponsiveness. The family may describe a long history of psychiatric disease, previous similar episodes from which the patient recovered, current social stresses on the patient, or the patient's unusual, idiosyncratic response to stress. Special care must be taken with psychiatric patients because of the often-biased approach to these patients, which may lead to incomplete evaluation. Psychiatric patients are subject to all of the causes of coma listed in Table 5.4.

## General Examination

A systematic, detailed general examination is especially helpful in the approach to the comatose patient, who is unable to describe prior or current medical problems. This examination begins in the initial rapid examination with evaluation of blood pressure, pulse, respiratory rate, and temperature.

### Blood Pressure Evaluation

*Hypotension.* Cerebral hypoperfusion secondary to hypotension may result in coma if the mean arterial pressure decreases to less than the value for which the brain is able to autoregulate (normally 60 mm Hg). This value is substantially higher in chronically hypertensive persons, in whom the cerebral blood flow–mean arterial pressure curve is shifted to the right. Among the causes of hypotension are hypovolemia, massive external or internal hemorrhage, myocardial infarction, cardiac tamponade, dissecting aortic aneurysm, intoxication with alcohol or other drugs (especially barbiturates), toxins, Wernicke encephalopathy, Addison disease, and sepsis. Although most patients with hypotension are cold because of peripheral vasoconstriction, patients with Addison disease or sepsis may have warm shock due to peripheral vasodilation. Medullary damage also may result in hypotension because of damage to the pressor center.

*Hypertension.* Hypertension is the cause of alterations in arousal in hypertensive crisis and is seen secondarily as a response to cerebral infarction, in subarachnoid hemorrhage, with certain brainstem infarctions, and with increased intracerebral pressure. The Kocher-Cushing (or Claude Bernard) reflex is the development of hypertension associated with bradycardia and respiratory irregularity due to increased ICP. This response occurs more commonly in the setting of a posterior fossa lesion and in children. It results from compression or ischemia of the pressor area lying beneath the floor of the fourth ventricle. Hypertension is a common condition and thus may be present but unrelated to the cause of coma.

### Heart Rate

In addition to the Kocher-Cushing reflex, bradycardia can result from myocardial conduction blocks, with certain poisonings, and from effects of drugs such as the beta-blockers. Tachycardia is a result of hypovolemia, hyperthyroidism, fever, anemia, and certain toxins and drugs, including cocaine, atropine, and other anticholinergic medications.

### Respiration

The most common causes of decreased respiratory rate are metabolic or toxic, such as carbon dioxide narcosis or drug overdose with

CNS depressants. Increased respiratory rate can result from hypoxia, hypercapnia, acidosis, hyperthermia, hepatic disease, toxins or drugs (especially those that produce a metabolic acidosis, such as methanol, ethylene glycol, paraldehyde, and salicylates), sepsis, and pulmonary embolism (including fat embolism), and sometimes is seen in psychogenic unresponsiveness. Brainstem lesions causing hypopnea or hyperpnea are discussed later in the chapter. Changes in respiratory rate or rhythm in a comatose patient may be deceiving, because a metabolic disorder may coexist with a CNS lesion.

### Temperature

Core temperature is best measured with a rectal probe in a comatose patient because oral or axillary temperatures are unreliable. Pyrexia most often is a sign of infection. Accordingly, any evidence of fever in a comatose patient warrants strong consideration of lumbar puncture. Absence of an elevated temperature does not rule out infection. Immunosuppressed patients, elderly patients, and patients with metabolic or endocrine abnormalities such as uremia or hypothyroidism may not experience an increase in temperature in response to overwhelming infection. Pure neurogenic hyperthermia is rare and usually is due to subarachnoid hemorrhage or diencephalic (hypothalamus) lesions. A clue to brainstem origin is shivering without sweating. Shivering in the absence of sweating, particularly when unilateral in nature, also may be observed with a deep intracerebral hemorrhage. Other causes of increased temperature associated with coma are heatstroke, thyrotoxic crisis, and drug toxicity. (Atropine and other anticholinergics elevate core temperature but decrease diaphoresis, resulting in a warm, dry patient with dilated pupils and diminished bowel sounds.)

Except in heatstroke and malignant hyperthermia, fever does not result in stupor or coma by itself. Conversely, hypothermia, regardless of cause, is anticipated to lead to altered consciousness. Hypothermia causes diminished cerebral metabolism and, if the temperature is sufficiently low, may result in an isoelectric EEG. Hypothermia usually is metabolic or environmental in cause; however, it also is seen with hypotension accompanied by vasoconstriction and may occur with sepsis. Other causes of hypothermia associated with coma are hypothyroid coma, hypopituitarism, Wernicke encephalopathy, cold exposure, drugs (barbiturates), and other poisonings. Central lesions causing hypothermia are found in the posterior hypothalamus. The absence of shivering or vasoconstriction, or the presence of sweating, is a clue to the central origin of these lesions.

### General Appearance

The general appearance of the patient may provide further clues to the diagnosis. Torn or disheveled clothing may indicate prior assault. Vomiting may be a sign of increased ICP, drug overdose, or metabolic or other toxic cause. Urinary or fecal incontinence suggests an epileptic seizure or may result from a generalized autonomic discharge resulting from the same cause as for the coma. Examination of body habitus may reveal cushingoid patients at risk for an acute Addisonian crisis with abrupt withdrawal of their medications or additional stress from intercurrent illness. Cachexia suggests cancer, chronic inflammatory disorders, Addison disease, hypothyroid coma, or hyperthyroid crisis. The cachectic patient also is subject to Wernicke encephalopathy in association with carbohydrate loading. Gynecomastia, spider nevi, testicular atrophy, and decreased axillary and pubic hair are common in the alcoholic with cirrhosis.

### Head and Neck Examination

The head and neck must be carefully examined for signs of trauma. Palpation for depressed skull fractures and edema should be attempted, although this means of evaluation is not very sensitive. Laceration or edema of the scalp is indicative of head trauma. The term *raccoon eyes* refers to orbital ecchymosis due to anterior basal skull fracture. *Battle sign* is a hematoma overlying the mastoid, originating from basilar skull fracture extending into the mastoid portion of the temporal bone. The ecchymotic lesions typically are not apparent until 2–3 days after the traumatic event.

Meningismus, or neck stiffness, may be a sign of infectious or carcinomatous meningitis, subarachnoid hemorrhage, or central or tonsillar herniation. However, neck stiffness may be absent in coma from any cause but is likely to be present in less severe alterations in arousal. Scars on the neck may be from endarterectomy, implying vascular disease, or from thyroidectomy or parathyroidectomy, suggesting concomitant hypothyroidism, hypoparathyroidism, or both. Goiter may be found with hypothyroidism or hyperthyroidism.

### Eye Examination

Examination of the eyes includes observation of the cornea, conjunctiva, sclera, iris, lens, and eyelids. Edema of the conjunctiva and eyelids may occur in congestive heart failure and nephrotic syndrome. Congestion and inflammation of the conjunctiva may occur in the comatose patient from exposure. Enophthalmos indicates dehydration. Scleral icterus is seen with liver disease, and yellowish discoloration of the skin without scleral involvement may be due to drugs such as rifampin. Band keratopathy is caused by hypercalcemia, whereas hypocalcemia is associated with cataracts. Kayser-Fleischer rings are seen in progressive lenticular degeneration (Wilson disease). Arcus senilis is seen in normal aging but also in hyperlipidemia. Fat embolism may cause petechiae not only in skin of the upper body and oral mucosa but also in conjunctiva and eye grounds.

Funduscopic examination may demonstrate evidence of hypertension or diabetes. Grayish deposits surrounding the optic disk have been reported in lead poisoning. The retina is congested and edematous in methyl alcohol poisoning, and the disk margin may be blurred. Subhyaloid hemorrhage appears occasionally as a consequence of a rapid increase in ICP due to subarachnoid hemorrhage (Terson syndrome). Papilledema results from increased ICP and may be indicative of an intracranial mass lesion or hypertensive encephalopathy.

### Otoscopic Examination

Otoscopic examination should rule out hemotympanum or CSF otorrhea from a basilar skull fracture involving the petrous ridge, as well as infection of the middle ear. Infections of the middle ear, mastoid, and paranasal sinuses constitute the most common source of underlying infection in brain abscess. CSF rhinorrhea, which appears as clear fluid from the nose, may depend on head position. The presence of glucose in the watery discharge is virtually diagnostic, although false-positive results are possible.

### Oral Examination

Alcohol intoxication, diabetic ketoacidosis (acetone odor), uremia, and hepatic encephalopathy (musty odor of cholemia or *fetor hepaticus*) may be suspected from the odor of the breath. Arsenic poisoning produces the odor of garlic. Poor oral hygiene or oral abscesses may be a source of sepsis or severe pulmonary infection with associated hypoxemia. Pustules on the nose or upper lip may seed the cavernous sinus with bacteria by way of the angular vein. Lacerations on the tongue, whether old or new, suggest seizure disorder. Thin, blue-black pigmentation along the gingival margin may be seen in certain heavy metal poisonings (bismuth, mercury, and lead).

### Integument Examination

Systematic examination of the integument includes inspection of the skin, nails, and mucous membranes. A great deal of information can be gained by a brief examination of the skin (Table 5.5). Hot, dry skin is a feature of heat stroke. Sweaty skin is seen with hypotension or hypoglycemia. Drugs may cause macular-papular, vesicular, or petechial-purpuric rashes or bullous skin lesions. Bullous skin lesions most often are a result of barbiturates but also may be caused by imipramine, meprobamate, glutethimide, phenothiazine, and carbon monoxide. Kaposi sarcoma, anogenital herpetic lesions, or oral candidiasis should suggest the acquired immunodeficiency syndrome (AIDS), with its plethora of CNS abnormalities.

### Examination of Lymph Nodes

Generalized lymphadenopathy is nonspecific, because it may be seen with neoplasm, infection (including AIDS), collagen vascular disease, sarcoid, hyperthyroidism, Addison disease, and drug reaction (especially that due to phenytoin). However, local lymph node enlargement or inflammation may provide clues to a primary tumor site or source of infection.

**TABLE 5.5 Skin Lesions and Rashes in Coma**

| Lesion or Rash | Possible Cause |
|---|---|
| Antecubital needle marks | Opiate drug abuse |
| Pale skin | Anemia or hemorrhage |
| Sallow, puffy appearance | Hypopituitarism |
| Hypermelanosis (increased pigment) | Porphyria, Addison disease, chronic nutritional deficiency, disseminated malignant melanoma, chemotherapy |
| Generalized cyanosis | Hypoxemia or carbon dioxide poisoning |
| Grayish-blue cyanosis | Methemoglobin (aniline or nitrobenzene) intoxication |
| Localized cyanosis | Arterial emboli or vasculitis |
| Cherry-red skin | Carbon monoxide poisoning |
| Icterus | Hepatic dysfunction or hemolytic anemia |
| Petechiae | Disseminated intravascular coagulation, thrombotic thrombocytopenic purpura, drugs |
| Ecchymosis | Trauma, corticosteroid use, abnormal coagulation from liver disease or anticoagulants |
| Telangiectasia | Chronic alcoholism, occasionally vascular malformations of the brain |
| Vesicular rash | Herpes simplex |
| | Varicella |
| | Behçet disease |
| | Drugs |
| Petechial-purpuric rash | Meningococcemia |
| | Other bacterial sepsis (rarely) |
| | Gonococcemia |
| | Staphylococcemia |
| | ***Pseudomonas*** |
| | subacute bacterial endocarditis |
| | Allergic vasculitis |
| | Purpura fulminans |
| | Rocky Mountain spotted fever |
| | Typhus |
| | Fat emboli |
| Macular-papular rash | Typhus |
| | ***Candida*** |
| | ***Cryptococcus*** |
| | Toxoplasmosis |
| | Subacute bacterial endocarditis |
| | Staphylococcal toxic shock |
| | Typhoid |
| | Leptospirosis |
| | ***Pseudomonas*** sepsis |
| | Immunological disorders |
| | Systemic lupus erythematosus |
| | Dermatomyositis |
| | Serum sickness |
| **Other Skin Lesions** | |
| Ecthyma gangrenosu | Necrotic eschar often seen in the anogenital or axillary area *Pseudomonas* sepsis |
| Splinter hemorrhages | Linear hemorrhages under the nail, seen in subacute bacterial endocarditis, anemia, leukemia, and sepsis |
| Osler nodes | Purplish or erythematous painful, tender nodules on palms and soles, seen in subacute bacterial endocarditis |
| Gangrene of digits' extremities | Emboli to larger peripheral or arteries |

*Data on diseases associated with rashes from Corey, L., Kirby, P., 1987. Rash and fever. In: Braunwald, E., Isselbacher, K.J., Petersdorf, R.G. (Eds.), Harrison's Principles of Internal Medicine, eleventh ed. McGraw-Hill, New York, pp. 240–244.*

### Cardiac Examination

Cardiac auscultation will confirm the presence of arrhythmias such as atrial fibrillation, with its inherent increased risk of emboli. Changing mitral murmurs are heard with atrial myxomas and papillary muscle ischemia, which is seen with current or impending myocardial infarction. Constant murmurs indicate valvular heart disease and may be heard with the valvular vegetation of bacterial endocarditis.

### Abdominal Examination

Possibly helpful findings on abdominal examination include abnormal bowel sounds, organomegaly, masses, and ascites. Bowel sounds are absent in an acute abdominal condition, as well as with anticholinergic poisoning. Hyperactive bowel sounds may be a consequence of increased gastrointestinal motility from exposure to an acetylcholinesterase inhibitor (a common pesticide ingredient). The liver may be enlarged as a result of right heart failure or tumor infiltration. Nodules or a rock-hard liver may be due to hepatoma or metastatic disease. The liver may be small and hard in cirrhosis. Splenomegaly is caused by portal hypertension, hematological malignancies, infection, and collagen vascular diseases. Intraabdominal masses may indicate carcinoma. Ascites occurs with liver disease, right heart failure, neoplasms with metastasis to the liver, or ovarian cancer.

### Miscellaneous Examinations

A positive result on tests for blood in stool obtained at rectal examination is consistent with gastrointestinal bleeding and, possibly, bowel carcinoma. Large amounts of blood in the gastrointestinal tract may be sufficient to precipitate hepatic encephalopathy in the patient with cirrhosis.

## Neurological Examination

Neurological signs may vary depending on the cause of the impaired consciousness and its severity, and they may be partial or incomplete. For example, the patient may have a partial third nerve palsy with pupillary dilation, rather than a complete absence of all third nerve function, or muscle tone may be decreased but not absent. This concept is especially important in the examination of the stuporous or comatose patient because the level of arousal may also influence the expression of neurological signs. In the stuporous or comatose patient, even slight deviations from normal should not be dismissed as unimportant. Such findings should be carefully considered to discover their pattern or meaning.

The neurological examination of a comatose patient serves three purposes: (1) to aid in determining the cause of coma, (2) to provide a baseline, and (3) to help determine the prognosis. For prognosis and localization of a structural lesion, the following components of the examination have been found to be most helpful: state of consciousness, respiratory pattern, pupillary size and response to light, spontaneous and reflex eye movements, and skeletal muscle motor response.

### State of Consciousness

The importance of a detailed description of the state of consciousness is worth reemphasizing. It is imperative that the exact stimulus and the patient's specific response be recorded. Several modes of stimulation should be used, including auditory, visual, and noxious. Stimuli of progressively increasing intensity should be applied, with the maximal state of arousal noted and the stimuli, the site of stimulation, and the patient's exact response described. The examiner should start with verbal stimuli, softly and then more loudly calling the patient's name or giving simple instructions to open the eyes. If there is no significant response, more threatening stimuli, such as taking the patient's hand and advancing it toward the patient's face, are applied. However, a blink response to visual threat need not indicate consciousness. Finally, painful stimuli may be needed to arouse the patient. All patients in apparent coma should be asked to open or close the eyes and to look up and down; these voluntary movements are preserved in the locked-in syndrome but cannot be elicited in coma—an important distinction.

**TABLE 5.6 Glasgow Coma Scale**

| Best Motor Response | M |
|---|---|
| Obeys | 6 |
| Localizes | 5 |
| Withdraws | 4 |
| Abnormal flexion | 3 |
| Extensor response | 2 |
| Nil | 1 |
| **Verbal Response** | **V** |
| Oriented | 5 |
| Confused conversation | 4 |
| Inappropriate words | 3 |
| Incomprehensible sounds | 2 |
| Nil | 1 |
| **Eye Opening** | **E** |
| Spontaneous | 4 |
| To speech | 3 |
| To pain | 2 |
| Nil | 1 |

Supraorbital pressure evokes a response even in patients who may have lost afferent pain pathways as a result of peripheral neuropathy or spinal cord or some brainstem lesions. Nail bed pressure or pinching the chest or extremities may help to localize a lesion when it evokes asymmetrical withdrawal responses. Care must be taken to avoid soft-tissue damage. Purposeful movements indicate a milder alteration in consciousness. Vocalization to pain in the early hours of a coma, even if only a grunt, indicates relatively light alteration in consciousness. Later, primitive vocalization may be a feature of the vegetative state.

The Glasgow Coma Scale (Table 5.6) is used widely to assess the initial severity of traumatic brain injury. This battery assesses three separate aspects of a patient's behavior: the stimulus required to induce eye opening, the best motor response, and the best verbal response. Degrees of increasing dysfunction are scored. Its reproducibility and simplicity make the Glasgow Coma Scale an ideal method of assessment for non-neurologists involved in the care of comatose patients. However, its failure to assess other essential neurological parameters limits its utility. In addition, in patients who are intubated or who have suffered facial trauma, assessment of certain components of the Glasgow Coma Scale, such as eye opening and speech, may be difficult or impossible. An alternative scale referred to as the Full Outline of UnResponsiveness (FOUR) score has been proposed (Wijdicks et al., 2005a) and is based on eye response, motor response, brainstem reflexes (pupillary reaction, corneal reflex, and cough reflex), and respirations.

### Respiration

Normal breathing is quiet and unlabored. The presence of any respiratory noise implies airway obstruction, which must be dealt with immediately to prevent hypoxia. Normal respiration depends on (1) a brainstem mechanism, located between the midpons and cervical

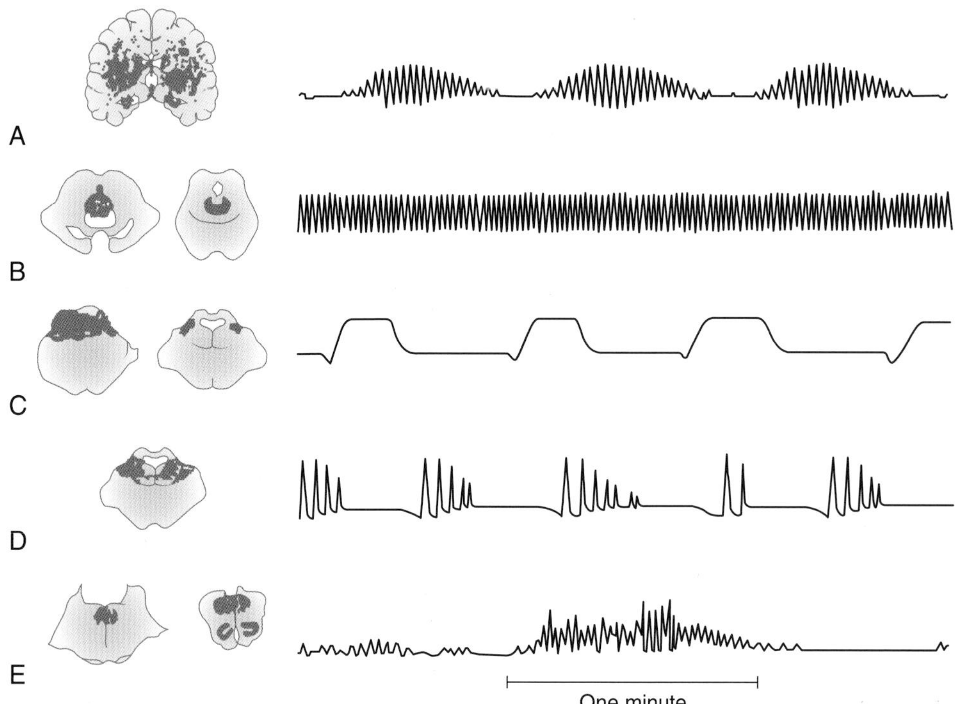


**Fig. 5.1** Abnormal respiratory patterns associated with pathological lesions *(shaded areas)* at various levels of the brain. The tracings were obtained by chest-abdomen pneumograph; inspiration reads up. **A**, Cheyne-Stokes respiration—diffuse forebrain damage. **B**, Central neurogenic hyperventilation—lesions of low midbrain ventral to aqueduct of Sylvius and of upper pons ventral to the fourth ventricle. **C**, Apneusis—dorsolateral tegmental lesion of middle and caudal pons. **D**, Cluster breathing—lower pontine tegmental lesion. **E**, Ataxic breathing—lesion of the reticular formation of the dorsomedial part of the medulla. *(Reprinted from Plum, F., Posner, J.B., 1995. The Diagnosis of Stupor and Coma, third ed. Oxford University Press, New York. Copyright 1966, 1972, 1980, 1996, Oxford University Press, Inc. Used by permission of Oxford University Press, Inc.)*

medullary junction, that regulates metabolic needs; and (2) forebrain influences that subserve behavioral needs such as speech production. The organization and function of brainstem mechanisms responsible for respiratory rhythm generation, as well as forebrain influences, are complex and beyond the scope of this chapter. Neuropathological correlates of respiration are presented in Fig. 5.1.

Respiratory patterns that are helpful in localizing levels of involvement include Cheyne-Stokes respiration, central neurogenic hyperventilation, apneustic breathing, cluster breathing, and ataxic respiration. *Cheyne-Stokes respiration* is a respiratory pattern that slowly oscillates between hyperventilation and hypoventilation. In 1818, Cheyne described his patient as follows: "For several days his breathing was irregular; it would entirely cease for a quarter of a minute, then it would become perceptible, though very low, then by degrees it became heaving and quick and then it would gradually cease again. This revolution in the state of his breathing occupied about a minute during which there were about 30 acts of respiration." Cheyne-Stokes respiration is associated with bilateral hemispheric or diencephalic insults, but it may occur as a result of bilateral damage anywhere along the descending pathway between the forebrain and upper pons. It also is seen with cardiac disorders that prolong circulation time. Alertness, pupillary size, and heart rhythm may vary during Cheyne-Stokes respiration (Posner et al., 2007). Patients are more alert during the waxing portion of breathing. A continuous pattern of Cheyne-Stokes respiration is a relatively good prognostic sign, usually implying that permanent brainstem damage has not occurred. However, the emergence of Cheyne-Stokes respiration in a patient with a unilateral mass lesion may be an early sign of herniation. A change in pattern from Cheyne-Stokes respiration to certain other respiratory patterns, described next, is ominous.

Two breathing patterns similar to Cheyne-Stokes respiration should not be confused with it. *Short-cycle periodic breathing* is a respiratory pattern with a shorter cycle (faster rhythm) than Cheyne-Stokes respiration, with one or two waxing breaths, followed by two to four rapid breaths, then one or two waning breaths. It is seen with increased ICP, lower pontine lesions, or expanding lesions in the posterior fossa (Posner et al., 2007). A similar type of respiration, in which there are short bursts of seven to ten rapid breaths, then apnea without a waning and waxing prodrome, has been erroneously referred to as Biot breathing. Biot, in fact, described an ataxic respiratory pattern, which is described later.

*Central neurogenic hyperventilation* refers to rapid breathing, from 40 to 70 breaths/min, usually due to central tegmental pontine lesions just ventral to the aqueduct or fourth ventricle (Posner et al., 2007). This type of breathing is rare and must be differentiated from reactive hyperventilation due to metabolic abnormalities of hypoxemia secondary to pulmonary involvement. Large CNS lesions may cause neurogenic pulmonary edema, with associated hypoxemia and increased respiratory rate. Increased intracerebral pressure causes spontaneous hyperpnea. Hyperpnea cannot be ascribed to a CNS lesion when arterial oxygen partial pressure is less than 70–80 mm Hg or carbon dioxide partial pressure is greater than 40 mm Hg.

*Kussmaul breathing* is a deep, regular respiration observed with metabolic acidosis. *Apneustic breathing* is a prolonged inspiratory gasp with a pause at full inspiration. It is caused by lesions of the dorsolateral lower half of the pons (Posner et al., 2007). *Cluster breathing,*

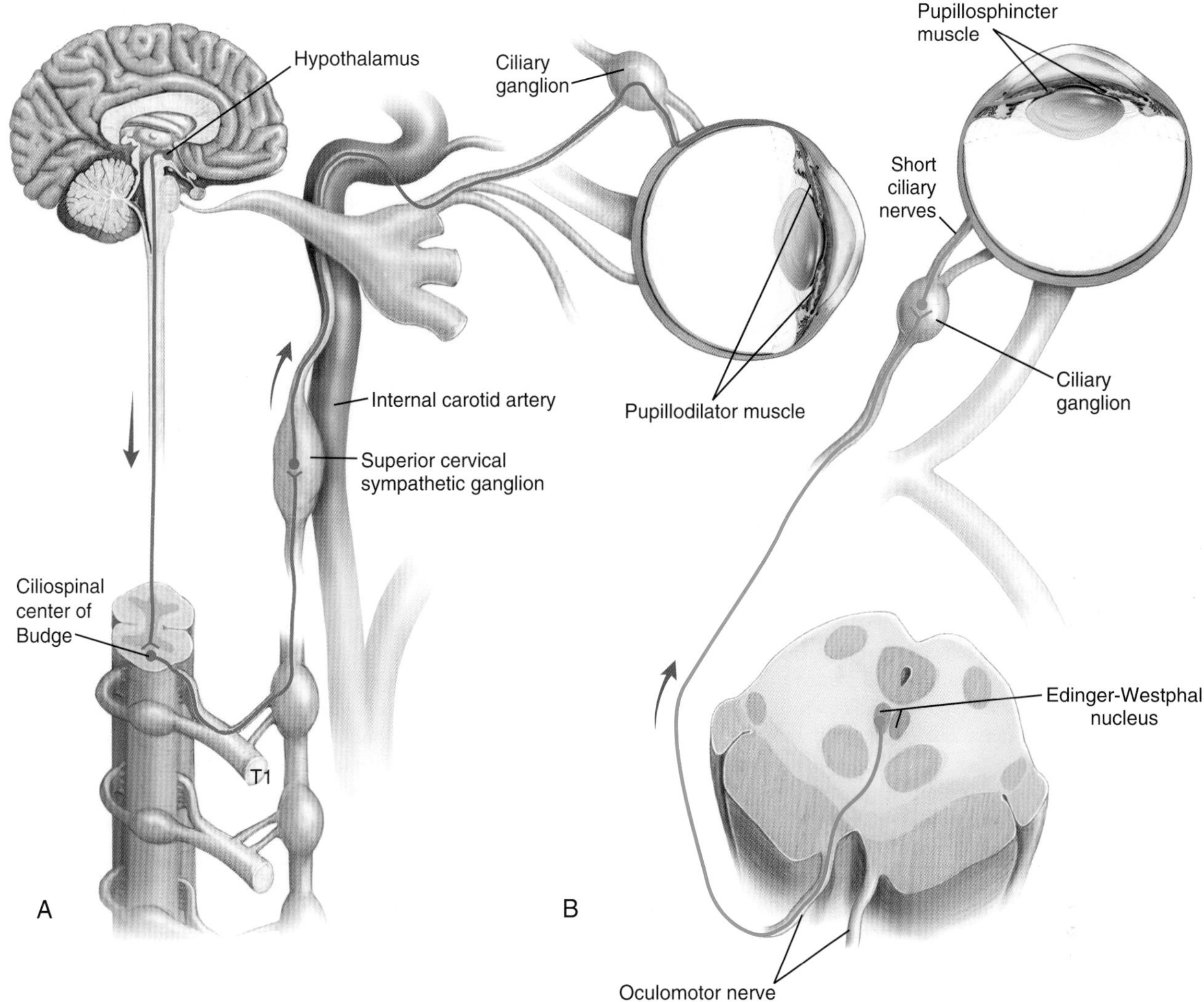


**Fig. 5.2** A, The sympathetic pupillodilator pathway. B, The parasympathetic pupilloconstrictor pathway. *(Reprinted from Plum, F., Posner, J.B., 1995. The Diagnosis of Stupor and Coma, third ed. Oxford University Press, New York.* Copyright 1966, 1972, 1980, 1996, *Oxford University Press, Inc. Used by permission of Oxford University Press, Inc.)*

which results from high medullary damage, involves periodic respirations that are irregular in frequency and amplitude, with variable pauses between clusters of breaths.

*Ataxic breathing* is irregular in rate and rhythm and usually is due to medullary lesions. The combination of ataxic respiration and bilateral sixth nerve palsy may be a warning sign of brainstem compression from an expanding lesion in the posterior fossa. This is an important sign because brainstem compression due to tonsillar herniation (or other causes) may result in abrupt loss of respiration or blood pressure. Ataxic and gasping respirations are signs of lower brainstem damage and often are preterminal respiratory patterns.

## Pupil Size and Reactivity

Normal pupil size in the comatose patient depends on the level of illumination and the state of autonomic innervation. The sympathetic efferent innervation consists of a three-neuron arc. The first-order neuron arises in the hypothalamus and travels ipsilaterally through the posterolateral tegmentum to the ciliospinal center of Budge at the T1 level of the spinal cord. The second-order neuron leaves this center and synapses in the superior cervical sympathetic ganglion. The third-order neuron travels along the internal carotid artery and then through the ciliary ganglion to the pupillodilator muscles. The parasympathetic efferent innervation of the pupil arises in the Edinger-Westphal nucleus and travels in the oculomotor nerve to the ciliary ganglion, from which it innervates the pupillosphincter muscle (Fig. 5.2).

Afferent input to the pupillary reflex depends on the integrity of the optic nerve, optic chiasm, optic tract, and projections into the midbrain tectum and efferent fibers through the Edinger-Westphal nucleus and oculomotor nerve. Abnormalities in pupil size and reactivity help to delineate structural damage between the thalamus and pons (Fig. 5.3), act as a warning sign heralding brainstem herniation, and help to differentiate structural causes of coma from metabolic causes.

Thalamic lesions cause small, reactive pupils, which often are referred to as *diencephalic pupils.* Similar pupillary findings are noted in many toxic-metabolic conditions resulting in coma. Hypothalamic lesions or lesions elsewhere along the sympathetic pathway result in *Horner syndrome.* Midbrain lesions produce three types of pupillary abnormality, depending on where the lesion occurs. (1) Dorsal tectal lesions interrupt the pupillary light reflex, resulting in *midposition*

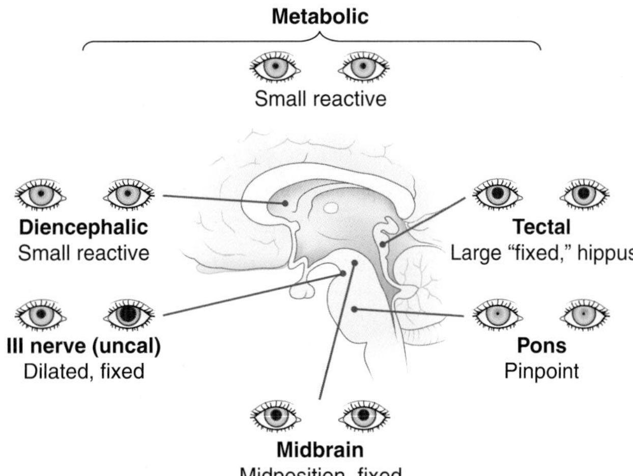


**Fig. 5.3** Pupils in Comatose Patients. *(Reprinted from Plum, F., Posner, J.B., 1995. The Diagnosis of Stupor and Coma, third ed. Oxford University Press, New York.* Copyright 1966, 1972, 1980, 1996, *Oxford University Press, Inc. Used by permission of Oxford University Press, Inc.)*

*pupils*, which are fixed to light but react to near vision; the latter is impossible to test in the comatose patient. Spontaneous fluctuations in size occur, and the ciliospinal reflex is preserved. (2) Nuclear midbrain lesions usually affect both sympathetic and parasympathetic pathways, resulting in *fixed, irregular midposition pupils*, which may be unequal. (3) Lesions of the third nerve fascicle in the brainstem, or after the nerve has exited the brainstem, cause *wide pupillary dilation*, unresponsive to light. Pontine lesions interrupt sympathetic pathways and cause small, so-called pinpoint pupils, which remain reactive, although magnification may be needed to observe this feature. Lesions above the thalamus and below the pons should leave pupillary function intact, except for Horner syndrome in medullary or cervical spinal cord lesions. The pathophysiology of pupillary response is discussed further in Chapter 17.

Asymmetry in pupillary size or reactivity, even of minor degree, is important. Asymmetry of pupil size may be due to dilation (mydriasis) of one pupil, such as with third nerve palsy, or contraction (miosis) of the other, as in Horner syndrome. This may be differentiated by the pupillary reactivity to light and associated neurological signs. A dilated pupil due to a partial third nerve palsy is less reactive and usually is associated with extraocular muscle involvement. The pupil in Horner syndrome is reactive; if the syndrome results from a lesion in the CNS, it may be associated with anhidrosis of the entire ipsilateral body. Cervical sympathetic chain lesions produce anhidrosis of only face, neck, and arm. A partial or complete third nerve palsy causing a dilated pupil may result from an intramedullary lesion, most commonly in the midbrain, such as an intramedullary glioma or infarction; uncal herniation compressing the third nerve; or a posterior communicating artery aneurysm. A sluggishly reactive pupil may be one of the first signs of uncal herniation, followed soon thereafter by dilation of that pupil and, later, complete third nerve paralysis.

Several caveats are important in examining the pupil or assessing pupillary reflexes. A common mistake is the use of insufficient illumination. The ophthalmoscope may be useful in this regard because it provides both adequate illumination and magnification. Rarely, preexisting ocular or neurological injury may fix the pupils or result in pupillary asymmetry. Seizures may cause transient anisocoria. Local and systemic medications may affect pupillary function. Topical ophthalmological preparations containing an acetylcholinesterase inhibitor, used in the treatment of glaucoma, produce miosis. The effect of a mydriatic agent placed by the patient or a prior observer may wear off unevenly, resulting in pupillary asymmetry. Some common misleading causes of a unilateral dilated pupil include prior mydriatic administration, old ocular trauma or ophthalmic surgery, and, more rarely, carotid artery insufficiency.

## Ocular Motility

Normal ocular motility (see Chapters 18 and 21) depends on the integrity of a large portion of the cerebrum, cerebellum, and brainstem. Preservation of normal ocular motility implies that a large portion of the brainstem from the vestibular nuclei at the pontomedullary junction to the oculomotor nucleus in the midbrain is intact. Voluntary ocular motility cannot be judged in the comatose patient, so the examiner must rely on reflex eye movements that allow for assessment of the ocular motor system. The eye movements normally are conjugate, and eyes are in the midposition in the alert person. Sleep or obtundation alone may unmask a latent vertical or horizontal strabismus, resulting in dysconjugacy; therefore patients must be examined when maximally aroused. The eyes return to the midposition in brain-dead patients. Evaluation of ocular motility consists of (1) observation of the resting position of the eyes, including eye deviation; (2) notation of spontaneous eye movements; and (3) testing of reflex ocular movements.

***Abnormalities in resting position.*** Careful attention must be paid to the resting position of the eyes. Even a small discrepancy in eye position may represent a partial extraocular nerve palsy. Partial nerve palsies or combined nerve palsies predictably result in a more complex picture on examination. Unilateral third nerve palsy from either an intramedullary midbrain lesion or extramedullary compression causes the affected eye to be displaced downward and laterally. A sixth nerve palsy produces inward deviation. However, isolated sixth nerve palsy is a poor localizer because of the extensive course of the nerve and because this palsy may be caused by nonspecific increases in ICP, presumably from stretching of the extramedullary portion of the nerve. A fourth nerve palsy is difficult to assess in the comatose patient because of the subtle nature of the deficit in ocular motility. Extraocular nerve palsies often become more apparent with the "doll's eye maneuver" or cold caloric testing in the comatose patient.

***Eye deviation.*** Spontaneous eye deviation may be conjugate or dysconjugate. Conjugate lateral eye deviation usually is due to an ipsilateral lesion in the frontal eye fields but may be due to a lesion anywhere in the pathway from the ipsilateral eye fields to the contralateral parapontine reticular formation (see Chapters 18 and 21). Dysconjugate lateral eye movement may result from a sixth nerve palsy in the abducting eye, a third nerve palsy in the adducting eye, or an internuclear ophthalmoplegia. An internuclear ophthalmoplegia may be differentiated from a third nerve palsy by the preservation of vertical eye movements. Downward deviation of the eyes below the horizontal meridian usually is due to brainstem lesions (most often from tectal compression); however, it also may be seen in metabolic disorders such as hepatic coma. Thalamic and subthalamic lesions produce downward and inward deviation of the eyes. Patients with these lesions appear to be looking at the tip of the nose. Sleep, seizure, syncope, apnea of Cheyne-Stokes respiration, hemorrhage into the vermis, and brainstem ischemia or encephalitis cause upward eye deviation, making this a poor localizing sign. Skew deviation is a maintained deviation of one eye above the other (hypertropia) that is not due to a peripheral neuromuscular lesion or a local extracranial problem in the orbit. It usually indicates a posterior fossa lesion (brainstem or cerebellar). Dysconjugate vertical eye position sometimes may occur in the absence of a brainstem lesion in the obtunded patient.

***Spontaneous eye movements.*** Spontaneous eye movements (see Chapter 18) are of many types. Purposeful-appearing eye movements in a patient who otherwise seems unresponsive should lead to consideration of the locked-in syndrome, catatonia, pseudocoma, or PVS. *Roving eye movements* are slow, conjugate, lateral to-and-fro movements. For roving eye movements to be present, the ocular motor nuclei and their connections must be intact. In general, when roving eye movements are present, the brainstem is relatively intact and coma is due to a metabolic or toxic cause or bilateral lesions above the brainstem. Detection of roving eye movements may be complicated by ocular palsies or internuclear ophthalmoplegia. These superimposed lesions produce relatively predictable patterns but often obscure the essential roving nature of the movement for the inexperienced observer.

*Nystagmus* occurring in comatose patients suggests an irritative or epileptogenic supratentorial focus. An epileptogenic focus in one frontal eye field causes contralateral conjugate eye deviation. Nystagmus due to an irritative focus may rarely occur alone, without other motor manifestations of seizures. In addition, inconspicuous movements of the eye, eyelid, face, jaw, or tongue may be associated with electroencephalographic status epilepticus. An EEG is required to ascertain the presence of this condition.

Spontaneous conjugate vertical eye movements are separated into different types according to the relative velocities of their downward and upward phases. In *ocular bobbing*, rapid downward, jerks of both eyes are observed, followed by a brief pause in downgaze, followed by the slow return to the midposition. In the typical form, there is associated paralysis of both reflex and spontaneous horizontal eye movements. *Monocular* or *paretic bobbing* occurs when a coexisting ocular motor palsy alters the appearance of typical bobbing. The term *atypical bobbing* refers to all other variations of bobbing that cannot be explained by an ocular palsy superimposed on typical bobbing. Most commonly, this term is used to describe ocular bobbing when lateral eye movements are preserved. *Typical ocular bobbing* is specific but not pathognomonic for acute pontine lesions. Atypical ocular bobbing occurs with anoxia and is nonlocalizing. In *reverse ocular bobbing,* there is a slow initial downward phase, followed by a rapid return that carries the eyes past the midposition into full upward gaze. Then the eyes slowly return to the midposition. Reverse ocular bobbing is nonlocalizing. *Ocular dipping,* also known as *inverse ocular bobbing,* refers to spontaneous eye movements in which an initial slow downward phase is followed by a relatively rapid return. Reflex horizontal eye movements are preserved. It usually is associated with diffuse cerebral damage.

*Vertical nystagmus,* due to an abnormal pursuit or vestibular system, is slow deviation of the eyes from the primary position, with a rapid (saccadic), immediate return to the primary position. It is differentiated from bobbing by the absence of latency between the corrective saccade and the next slow deviation. *Ocular-palatal myoclonus* (the palatal movement also is called *palatal tremor*) occurs after damage to the lower brainstem involving the Guillain-Mollaret triangle, which extends between the cerebellar dentate nucleus, red nucleus, and inferior olive. It consists of a pendular vertical nystagmus, in synchrony with the palatal movements. Ocular flutter is back-to-back saccades in the horizontal plane and usually is a manifestation of cerebellar disease.

***Reflex ocular movements.*** Examination of ocular movement is not complete in the comatose patient without assessment of reflex ocular movements, including the oculocephalic reflex ("doll's eye phenomenon") and, if necessary, the caloric (thermal) testing. In practice, the terms *doll's eye phenomenon* and *doll's eye maneuver* are used synonymously to refer to the *oculocephalic reflex,* which is the preferred term for the description of the response. This reflex is tested by observation of the motion of the eyes during sudden rotation of the head, by the examiner, in both directions laterally and then with flexion and extension of the neck, also performed by the examiner. When supranuclear influences on the ocular motor nerves are removed, the eyes move in the orbit opposite to the direction of the head turn, and maintain their position in space. *This maneuver should not be performed on any patient until the stability of the neck has been adequately assessed.* If there is any question of neck stability, a neck brace should be applied and caloric testing substituted. In the normal oculocephalic reflex (normal or positive doll's eye phenomenon), the eyes move conjugately in a direction opposite to the direction of movement of the head. Cranial nerve palsies predictably alter the response to this maneuver (Table 5.7).

Clinical caloric testing (as distinct from quantitative calorics, used to assess vestibular end-organ disorders; see Chapter 22) is commonly done by applying cold water to the tympanic membrane. With the patient supine, the head should be tilted forward 30 degrees to allow maximal stimulation of the lateral semicircular canal, which is most responsible for reflex lateral eye movements. After the ear canal is carefully checked to ensure that it is patent and the tympanic membrane is free of defect, 10 mL of ice-cold water is slowly instilled into one ear canal. For purposes of the neurological examination, irrigation of each ear with 10 mL of ice water generally is sufficient.

Cold water applied to the tympanic membrane causes currents of endolymph flow in the semicircular canal, simulating a contralateral

**TABLE 5.7 Oculocephalic Reflex***

| Method | Response | Interpretation |
|---|---|---|
| Lateral head rotation | Eyes remain conjugate, move in direction opposite to head movement, and maintain position in space | Normal |
| | No movement in either eye on rotating head to left or right | Bilateral pontine gaze palsy, bilateral labyrinthine dysfunction, drug intoxication, anesthesia |
| | Eyes move appropriately when head is rotated in one direction but do not move when head is rotated in opposite direction | Unilateral pontine gaze palsy |
| | One eye abducts, the other eye does not adduct | Third nerve palsy<br>Internuclear ophthalmoplegia |
| Vertical head flexion and extension | Eyes remain conjugate, move in direction opposite to head movement, and maintain position in space | Normal |
| | No movement in either eye | Bilateral midbrain lesions |
| | Only one eye moves | Third nerve palsy |
| | Bilateral symmetrical limitation of upgaze | Aging |

*To be performed only after neck stability has been ascertained.

head turn. This results in a change in the baseline firing of the vestibular nerve and slow (tonic) conjugate deviation of the eyes toward the stimulated ear. In an awake person or a patient in pseudocoma, the eye deviation is corrected with a resulting nystagmoid jerking of the eye toward the midline (fast phase). Warm-water irrigation produces reversal of flow of the endolymph, simulating an ipsilateral head turn, which causes conjugate eye deviation with a slow phase away from the stimulated ear. In an awake person or a patient in pseudocoma, the eye deviation is corrected with a saccadic fast phase toward the ear. By tradition, the nystagmus is named by the direction of the fast phase. The mnemonic COWS (cold *o*pposite, *w*arm *s*ame) refers to the fast phases. Simultaneous bilateral cold water application results in slow downward deviation, whereas simultaneous bilateral warm water application causes upward deviation.

Oculocephalic or caloric testing may elicit subtle or unsuspected ocular palsies. Abnormal dysconjugate responses occur with cranial nerve palsies, internuclear ophthalmoplegia, or restrictive eye disease. Movements may be sluggish or absent. Sometimes reinforcement of cold caloric testing with superimposed passive head turning after injection of cold water into the ear may reveal eye movement when either test alone shows none.

False-negative or misleading responses on caloric testing occur with preexisting inner ear disease, vestibulopathy such as that due to ototoxic drugs such as streptomycin, vestibular paresis caused by illnesses such as Wernicke encephalopathy, and drug effects. Subtotal labyrinthine lesions decrease the response; there is no response when the labyrinth is destroyed. Lesions of the vestibular nerve cause a decreased or absent response. Drugs that suppress either vestibular or ocular motor function, or both, include sedatives, anticholinergics, anticonvulsants, tricyclic antidepressants, and neuromuscular blocking agents. If the response from one ear is indeterminate, both cold- and warm-water stimuli should be applied to the other ear. If the test remains equivocal, superimposition of the doll's eye maneuver is recommended. The interpretation of abnormal cold caloric responses is summarized in Table 5.8.

An unusual ocular reflex that has been observed in the setting of PVS is reflex opening of both eyes triggered by flexion of an arm at the elbow. This reflex is distinct from reflex eye opening in the comatose patient induced by raising the head or turning it from side to side.

### Motor System

Examination of the motor system of a stuporous or comatose patient begins with a description of the resting posture and adventitious movements. Purposeful and nonpurposeful movements are noted and the two sides of the body compared. Head and eye deviation to one side, with contralateral hemiparesis, suggests a supratentorial lesion, whereas ipsilateral paralysis indicates a probable brainstem lesion. External rotation of the lower limb is a sign of hemiplegia or hip fracture.

*Decerebrate posturing* is bilateral extensor posture, with extension of the lower extremities and adduction and internal rotation of the shoulders and extension at the elbows and wrist. Bilateral midbrain or pontine lesions usually are responsible for decerebrate posturing. Less commonly, deep metabolic encephalopathies or bilateral supratentorial lesions involving the motor pathways may produce a similar pattern.

*Decorticate posturing* is bilateral flexion at the elbows and wrists, with shoulder adduction and extension of the lower extremities. It is a much poorer localizing posture, because it may result from lesions in many locations, although usually above the brainstem. Decorticate posture is not as ominous a sign as decerebrate posture because the former occurs with many relatively reversible lesions.

Unilateral decerebrate or decorticate postures also are less ominous. Lesions causing unilateral posturing may be anywhere in the motor system from cortex to brainstem. Unilateral extensor posturing is common immediately after a cerebrovascular accident, followed in time by a flexor response.

Posturing may occur spontaneously or in response to external stimuli such as pain or may even be set off by such minimal events as the patient's own breathing. These postures, although common, may also be variable in their expression because of other associated brainstem or more rostral brain damage. Special attention should be given to posturing because it often signals a brainstem herniation syndrome. Emergency room personnel and inexperienced physicians may mistake these abnormal postures for convulsions (seizures) and institute anticonvulsant therapy, resulting in an unfortunate delay of appropriate therapy for the patient.

Adventitious movements in the comatose patient may be helpful in separating metabolic from structural lesions. Tonic-clonic or other stereotyped movements signal seizure as the probable cause of decreased alertness. *Myoclonic jerking*, consisting of nonrhythmic jerking movements in single or multiple muscle groups, is seen with anoxic encephalopathy or other metabolic comas, such as hepatic encephalopathy. *Rhythmic myoclonus*, which must be differentiated from epileptic movements, usually is a sign of brainstem injury. Tetany occurs with hypocalcemia. *Cerebellar fits* result from intermittent tonsillar herniation and are characterized by deterioration of level of arousal, opisthotonos, respiratory rate slowing and irregularity, and pupillary dilatation.

The motor response to painful stimuli should be tested, but the pattern of response may vary depending on the site stimulated. Purposeful responses may be difficult to discriminate from more primitive

**TABLE 5.8 Caloric Testing**

| Method | Response | Interpretation |
|---|---|---|
| Cold water instilled in right ear | Slow phase to right, fast (corrective) phase to the left | Normal |
| | No response (make sure canal is patent, apply warm water stimulus to opposite ear | Obstructed ear canal, "dead" labyrinth, eighth nerve or nuclear dysfunction, false-negative result (see text) |
| | Slow phase to right, no fast phase | Toxic-metabolic disorder, drugs, structural lesion above brainstem |
| | Downbeating nystagmus | Horizontal gaze palsy |
| Cold water instilled in left ear | Responses should be opposite those for right ear | Peripheral eighth nerve or labyrinth disorder n right (provided that right canal is patent) |
| Warm water instilled in left ear after no response from cold water in right ear | Slow phase to right, fast phase to left | |

reflexes. Flexion, extension, and adduction may be either voluntary or reflex in nature. In general, abduction is most reliably voluntary, with shoulder abduction stated to be the only definite nonreflex reaction. This is tested in the comatose patient with noxious stimuli, such as pinching the medial aspect of the upper arm. Reflex flexor response to pain in the upper extremity consists of adduction of the shoulder, flexion of the elbow, and pronation of the arm. The *triple flexion response* in the lower extremities refers to reflex withdrawal, with flexion at the hip and knee and dorsiflexion at the ankle, in response to painful stimulation on the foot or lower extremity. Such reflexes seldom are helpful in localizing a lesion

*Spinal reflexes* are reflexes mediated at the level of the spinal cord and do not depend on the functional integrity of the brain or brainstem. Most patients with absent cortical or brainstem function have some form of spinal reflex. The *plantar reflex* may be extensor in coma from any cause, including drug overdoses and postictal states. It becomes flexor on recovery of consciousness if there is no underlying structural damage. Muscle tone and asymmetry in muscle tone are helpful in localizing a focal structural lesion and may help to differentiate metabolic from structural coma. Acute structural damage above the brainstem usually results in decreased or flaccid tone. In older lesions, tone usually is increased. Metabolic insults generally cause a symmetrical decrease in tone. Finally, generalized flaccidity is ultimately seen after brain death.

### Coma and Brain Herniation

Herniation syndromes are explained in Chapter 53. Knowledge of some of the clinical signs of herniation is especially important in the clinical approach to coma. Traditional signs of herniation due to supratentorial masses usually are variations of either an uncal or a central pattern. Classically, the uncal pattern includes early signs of third nerve and midbrain compression. The pupil initially dilates as a result of third nerve compression but later returns to the midposition with midbrain compression that involves the sympathetic and parasympathetic tracts. In the central pattern, the earliest signs are mild impairment of consciousness, with poor concentration, drowsiness, or unexpected agitation; small but reactive pupils; loss of the fast component of cold caloric testing; poor or absent reflex vertical gaze; and bilateral corticospinal tract signs, including increased tone of the body ipsilateral to the hemispheric mass lesion responsible for herniation (Posner et al., 2007).

Signs of herniation tend to progress generally in a rostrocaudal manner. An exception occurs when intraventricular bleeding extends to the fourth ventricle and produces a pressure wave compressing the area around the fourth ventricle. In addition, when a lumbar puncture reduces CSF pressure suddenly, in the face of a mass lesion that produced increased ICP, sudden herniation of the cerebellar tonsils through the foramen magnum may result (Posner et al., 2007). Both of these clinical scenarios may be associated with sudden, unexpected failure of medullary functions that support respiration or blood pressure. In patients with herniation syndromes, the clinical picture may be confusing because of changing signs or the expression of scattered, isolated signs of dysfunction in separate parts of the brain. In addition, certain signs may be more prominent than others.

Increased ICP invariably accompanies brainstem herniation and may be associated with increased systolic blood pressure, bradycardia, and sixth nerve palsies. However, these signs, as well as many of the traditional signs of herniation as described, actually occur relatively late. Earlier signs of potential herniation are decreasing level of arousal, slight change in depth or rate of respiration, and the appearance of a Babinski sign. Tonsillar herniation may be suggested by an altered level of consciousness, opisthotonic posturing, dilated pupils, and irregular breathing. These manifestations may occur in a paroxysmal fashion consequent to increases in ICP and have been referred to as the cerebellar fits of Hughlings Jackson. It is important to suspect herniation early because, once advanced changes develop, structural injury is likely to have occurred; subsequently, there is less chance of reversal.

## DIFFERENTIAL DIAGNOSIS

### Differentiating Toxic-Metabolic Coma from Structural Coma

Many features of the history and physical examination help to differentiate structural from metabolic and toxic causes of coma. Some features have already been mentioned. When the history is available, the patient's underlying illnesses and medications, or the setting in which they are found, often help to guide the physician to the appropriate cause. The time course of the illness resulting in coma can be helpful. In general, structural lesions have a more abrupt onset, whereas metabolic or toxic causes are more slowly progressive. Multifocal structural diseases such as vasculitis or leukoencephalopathy are an exception to this rule because they may exhibit slow progression, usually in a stepwise manner. Supratentorial or infratentorial tumors characterized by slow growth and surrounding edema may also mimic metabolic processes.

The response to initial emergency therapy may help to differentiate metabolic or toxic causes of coma. The hypoglycemic patient usually awakens after administration of glucose, the hypoxic patient responds to oxygen, and the patient experiencing an opiate drug overdose responds to naloxone. In general, structural lesions have focal features or at least notable asymmetry on neurological examination. Toxic, metabolic, and psychiatric diseases are characterized by their symmetry. Bilateral and often multilevel involvement frequently is seen with metabolic causes. Asymmetries may be observed but generally are of small degree and tend to fluctuate over time.

Many features of the neurological examination differentiate metabolic or toxic causes from structural lesions:

*State of consciousness.* Patients with metabolic problems often have milder alterations in arousal, typically with waxing and waning of the behavioral state. Patients with acute structural lesions tend to stay at the same level of arousal or progressively deteriorate. Toxins may also cause progressive decline in level of arousal.

*Respiration.* Deep, frequent respiration most commonly is due to metabolic abnormalities, although rarely it is caused by pontine lesions or by neurogenic pulmonary edema secondary to acute structural lesions.

*Funduscopic examination.* Subhyaloid hemorrhage or papilledema are almost pathognomonic of structural lesions. Papilledema due to increased ICP may be indicative of an intracranial mass lesion or hypertensive encephalopathy. Papilledema does not occur in metabolic diseases except hypoparathyroidism and lead intoxication.

*Pupil size.* The pupils usually are symmetrical in coma from toxic-metabolic causes. Patients with metabolic or toxic encephalopathies often have small pupils with preserved reactivity. Exceptions occur with methyl alcohol poisoning, which may produce dilated and unreactive pupils, or late in the course of toxic or metabolic coma if hypoxia or other permanent brain damage has occurred. In terminal asphyxia the pupils dilate initially and then become fixed at midposition within 30 minutes. The initial dilation is attributed to massive sympathetic discharge.

*Pupil reactivity.* Assessment of the pupillary reflex is one of the most useful means of differentiating metabolic from structural causes of coma. Pupillary reactivity is relatively resistant to metabolic insult and usually is spared in coma from drug intoxication or metabolic causes, even when other brainstem reflexes are absent. Hypothermia may fix pupils, as does severe barbiturate intoxication; neuromuscular blocking agents produce midposition or small pupils, and glutethimide and atropine dilate them.

*Ocular motility.* Asymmetry in oculomotor function typically is a feature of structural lesions.

*Spontaneous eye movements.* Roving eye movements with full excursion are most often indicative of metabolic or toxic abnormalities.

*Reflex eye movements.* Reflex eye movements normally are intact in toxic-metabolic coma, except rarely in phenobarbital or phenytoin intoxication or deep metabolic coma from other causes.

*Adventitious movement.* Periods of motor restlessness, tremors, or spasm punctuating coma often are due to drugs or toxins such as chlorpromazine or lithium. Brainstem herniation or intermittent CNS ischemia also may produce unusual posturing movements. Myoclonic jerking generally is metabolic and often anoxic in origin.

*Muscle tone.* Muscle tone usually is symmetrical and normal or decreased in metabolic coma. Structural lesions cause asymmetrical muscle tone. Tone may be increased, normal, or decreased by structural lesions.

The examiner should be aware of common structural lesions that mimic toxic-metabolic causes and, conversely, toxic or metabolic causes of coma that may be associated with focal abnormalities on examination. Structural lesions that may mimic toxic-metabolic causes include subarachnoid hemorrhage, sinus vein thrombosis, chronic or bilateral subdural hemorrhage, and other diffuse or multifocal disorders, such as vasculitis, demyelinating diseases, or meningitis. Any toxic-metabolic cause of coma may be associated with focal features; however, such features most often are observed with barbiturate or lead poisoning, hypoglycemia, hepatic encephalopathy, and hyponatremia. Old structural lesions such as prior stroke may be the origin of residual abnormalities found on neurological examination in a patient who is comatose from toxic or metabolic causes. Moreover, metabolic abnormalities such as hypoglycemia may unmask relatively silent structural abnormalities. Detailed descriptions of the toxic and metabolic encephalopathies are provided in Chapter 53.

## Differentiating Psychiatric Coma and Pseudocoma from Metabolic or Structural Coma

The patient who appears unarousable as a result of psychiatric disease and the patient who is feigning unconsciousness for other reasons may be difficult to differentiate from each other. In such instances, the history, when available, and findings on the physical examination may suggest to the physician that a nonphysiological mechanism is at work. Multiple inconsistencies are present on examination, and abnormalities that are found do not fit the pattern of usual neurological syndromes. Examinations of the eyelid, pupil, adventitious eye movements, and vestibulo-oculogyric reflex by cold caloric testing are especially useful to confirm the suspicion of pseudocoma.

Eyelid tone is difficult to alter voluntarily. In the patient with true stupor or coma, passive eyelid opening is easily performed and is followed by slow, gradual eyelid closure. The malingering or somatiform patient often gives active resistance to passive eye opening and may even hold the eyes tightly closed. It is nearly impossible for the psychiatric or malingering patient to mimic the slow, gradual eyelid closure. Blinking also increases in psychiatric and malingering patients but decreases in patients in true stupor. The pupils normally constrict in sleep or (eyes-closed-type) coma but dilate with the eyes closed in the awake state. Passive eye opening in a sleeping person or a truly comatose patient (if pupillary reflexes are spared) results in pupillary dilation. Opening the eyes of an awake person produces constriction. This principle may help to differentiate coma from pseudocoma. Roving eye movements cannot be mimicked and thus also are a good sign of true coma. Finally, if during cold caloric testing, the eyes do not tonically deviate to the side of the caloric instillation, and the fast phases are preserved, stupor or true coma is essentially ruled out. Moreover, cold caloric testing with the resultant vertigo usually "awakens" psychiatric and malingering patients.

## Helpful Laboratory Studies

Laboratory tests that are extremely helpful in evaluating the comatose patient are listed in Table 5.9. Arterial blood gas determinations rule out hypoxemia and carbon dioxide narcosis and help to differentiate primary CNS problems from secondary respiratory problems. Liver disease, myopathy, and rhabdomyolysis all elevate alanine aminotransferase and aspartate aminotransferase levels. Liver function test results may be misleading in end-stage liver disease because values may be normal or only mildly elevated with markedly abnormal liver function. Although the blood ammonia level does not correlate well with the level of hepatic encephalopathy, it often may be markedly elevated and thus helpful in cases of suspected liver disease with relatively normal liver function studies. Hepatic encephalopathy may continue for up to 3 weeks after liver function values return to normal.

Thyroid function studies are necessary to document hypothyroidism or hyperthyroidism. When addisonian crisis is suspected, a morning serum cortisol level should be obtained. A low or normal level in the stressful state of coma or illness strongly suggests adrenal insufficiency. Further testing of adrenal function should be performed as appropriate.

When the cause of coma is not absolutely certain or in possible medicolegal cases, a blood alcohol level and a drug and toxin screen are mandatory. The results of these tests usually are not available immediately but may be invaluable later. Serum osmolality can usually be measured rapidly by the laboratory and may be used to estimate alcohol level because alcohol is an osmotically active particle and increases the osmolar gap in proportion to its blood level. Serum osmolality can be calculated using the following:

$$\begin{aligned}\textbf{Serum osmolality} &= \textbf{2 Na}^{+}\textbf{(mEq/L) + blood urea nitrogen (mg/dL)/2.8}\\ &= \textbf{glucose (mg/dL)/18}\end{aligned}$$

The osmolar gap, which is the difference between the measured serum osmolality and the calculated serum osmolality, represents unmeasured osmotically active particles. Creatine kinase levels should routinely be measured in comatose patients initially and then at least daily for the first several days because of the great risk of rhabdomyolysis and subsequent preventable acute tubular necrosis in these patients. Measuring creatine kinase myocardial band (MB) isoenzyme levels every 8 hours for the first 24 hours helps to rule out a myocardial infarction.

## Other Useful Studies

### Electrocardiography

The electrocardiogram is useful to show myocardial infarction, arrhythmia, conduction blocks, bradycardia, or evidence of underlying hypertension or atherosclerotic coronary vascular disease. Hypocalcemia causes QT prolongation. Hypercalcemia shortens the QT interval. The heart rate is slow in hypothyroid patients with low-voltage QRS, flat or inverted T waves, and flattened ST segments. Hyperthyroid patients are generally tachycardic.

**TABLE 5.9 Laboratory Tests Helpful in Differential Diagnosis for Coma**

| Laboratory Study | Result | Associated Disorders |
|---|---|---|
| Electrolytes (Na, K, Cl, $CO_2$) | | See Chapters 58, 59 and 84 for discussion of disorders associated with abnormalities of electrolytes, glucose, BUN, calcium, and magnesium |
| Glucose | | |
| BUN | | |
| Creatinine | | |
| Calcium | | |
| Magnesium | | |
| Complete blood count with differential | **Hematocrit:** | |
| | Increased | Volume depletion, underlying lung disorder, myeloproliferative disorder, cerebellar hemangioblastoma; may be associated with vascular sludging (hypoperfusion) |
| | Decreased | Anemia, hemorrhage |
| | **White blood cell count:** | |
| | Increased | Infection, acute stress reaction, steroid therapy, after epileptic fit, myeloproliferative disorder |
| | Decreased | Chemotherapy, immunotherapy, viral infection, sepsis |
| | **Lymphocyte count:** | |
| | Decreased | Viral infection, malnutrition, acquired immunodeficiency syndrome |
| Platelet count | Decreased | Sepsis, disseminated intravascular coagulation, thrombotic thrombocytopenic purpura, idiopathic thrombocytopenic purpura, drugs; may be associated with intracranial hemorrhage |
| Prothrombin time | Increased | Coagulation factor deficiency, liver disease, anticoagulants, disseminated intravascular coagulation |
| Partial thromboplastin time | Increased | Heparin therapy, lupus anticoagulant |
| Arterial blood gases | | See text |
| Creatine phosphokinase | | See text |
| Liver function studies | | See text |
| Thyroid function studies | | See text |
| Plasma cortisol level | | See text |
| Drug and toxin screen | | See text |
| Serum osmolality | | See text |

*BUN,* Blood urea nitrogen.

## Neuroradiological Imaging

Once the patient is stabilized, necessary treatment is given, the initial examination is complete, and appropriate laboratory studies are ordered, the next test of choice is a CT scan of the brain, without contrast but with 5-mm cuts of the posterior fossa. Alternatively, MRI may be performed, depending on the clinical setting, the stability of the patient's condition, and availability. MRI provides superb visualization of the posterior fossa and its contents, an extremely useful feature when structural disease of the brainstem is suspected. However, MRI is not as specific as CT scanning for visualizing early intracranial hemorrhage, and it is limited at present by the length of time required to perform the imaging, image degradation by even a slight movement of the patient, and the relative inaccessibility of the patient during the imaging process. The CT scan, when performed as described, is currently the most expedient imaging technique, giving the physician the most information about possible structural lesions with the least risk to the patient. Repeating the scan with intravenous dye may be necessary later to better define lesions seen on the initial scan.

The value of the CT scan in demonstrating mass lesions and hemorrhage is undeniable. Furthermore, it may demonstrate features of brain herniation. Uncal herniation is characterized on CT scan by (1) displacement of the brainstem toward the contralateral side, with increase in width of subarachnoid space between the mass and ipsilateral free edge; (2) medial stretching of the posterior cerebral and posterior communicating arteries; (3) obliteration of the interpeduncular cistern; (4) occipital lobe infarction; and (5) distortion and elongation of the U-shaped tentorial incisura. The clinician should be aware that the CT scan may miss early infarction, encephalitis, and isodense subdural hemorrhage. Special caution must be taken in evaluating CT scans in comatose patients, especially before lumbar puncture, to rule out isodense subdural or bilateral subdural hemorrhage. Interpretation of CT scans is discussed in Chapter 40. In severe head injury, studies of cerebral metabolism employing single-photon emission computed tomography (SPECT) may be of prognostic value. Although cerebral blood flow in the first 48 hours after trauma does not appear to correlate with severity or prognosis, the cerebral metabolic rate of oxygen ($CMRO_2$), like the Glasgow Coma Scale, may be useful in predicting prognosis.

## Electroencephalography

The EEG is helpful in many situations and disorders, including confirming underlying cortical structural damage in patients too unstable to travel to the CT scanner; postictal states in patients slow to wake after a presumed seizure; partial complex seizures; electroencephalographic or nonconvulsive status epilepticus, as is seen in comatose patients after anoxic ischemic damage; and toxic-metabolic disturbances. With metabolic disorders, the earliest EEG changes are typically a decrease in the frequency of background rhythms and the appearance of diffuse theta activity that progresses to more advanced slowing in association with a decrease in the level of consciousness.

In hepatic encephalopathy, bilaterally synchronous and symmetrical, medium- to high-amplitude, broad triphasic waves, often with a frontal predominance, may be observed. Herpes simplex encephalitis may be suggested by the presence of unilateral or bilateral periodic sharp waves with a temporal preponderance. The EEG also can help to confirm a clinical impression of catatonia, pseudocoma, the locked-in syndrome, PVS, and brain death. EEGs are discussed further in Chapter 35.

### Evoked Potentials

Evoked potentials may help in evaluating brainstem integrity and in assessing prognosis for comatose patients. A study of 50 hemodynamically stable patients remaining in coma 4 hours after resuscitation from cardiopulmonary arrest who were not treated with hypothermia with short-latency somatosensory evoked potentials within 8 hours after arrest found that none of the 30 patients without cortical potentials recovered cognition. Five of the 20 patients with cortical potentials recovered. Forty percent of the patients who did not recover had preserved brainstem reflexes, allowing some evaluation of prognosis in a group of patients in whom prognosis is difficult to assess by other means. There have been reports of patients with bilateral absent N20 responses treated with targeted hypothermia after cardiopulmonary arrest who made a meaningful recovery, with an estimated false-positive rate of 2.2%. Event-related potentials may prove particularly useful as an objective assessment of cognitive function in patients with the locked-in syndrome. The N100 component of the auditory evoked potential and cognitive evoked potentials (mismatch negativity obtained after novel stimuli) appear to have predictive value for awakening from coma, but the pupillary reflex remains the strongest prognostic variable. Absence of evoked potentials in response to somatosensory stimuli also is highly predictive of nonawakening from coma.

### Intracranial Pressure Monitoring

ICP measurements provide an index of the degree of brain swelling and are particularly useful in the management of patients who have suffered severe head injury. Postmortem studies of fatal head injuries demonstrate a direct correlation between very elevated ICP and death due to tentorial herniation. The use of ICP monitoring in treating intracranial hypertension following traumatic brain injury significantly lowers mortality (Farahvar et al., 2012). However, in the absence of intracranial hematomas, comatose patients with normal findings on brain imaging studies have a low frequency of increased ICP and almost never develop uncontrolled intracranial hypertension.

## PROGNOSIS

In view of the current state of knowledge, outcome in any comatose patient cannot be predicted with 100% certainty unless that patient meets the criteria for brain death, as described later in the chapter. The available evidence is not sufficient to permit a definitive statement that a particular non–brain-dead patient will *not* recover from coma, nor does it allow prognostication regarding how much recovery may occur in specific cases. However, general statistics on the outcome of coma, based on serial examinations at various times after the onset of coma, have been compiled and give the examiner a general idea of how patients may do. Although a variety of neuroimaging techniques, such as diffusion tensor imaging, positron emission tomography, functional MRI, and transcranial magnetic stimulation, have been proposed as tools to determine the conscious state and assist in prognostication, large-scale randomized trials will be required before they are widely used for these reasons (Bodart et al., 2013).

The natural history of coma can be considered in terms of three subcategories: drug-induced, nontraumatic, and traumatic coma. Drug-induced coma usually is reversible unless the patient has not had appropriate systemic support while comatose and has sustained secondary injury from hypoperfusion, hypoxia, or lack of other necessary metabolic substrates.

### Nontraumatic Coma

Only approximately 15% of patients in nontraumatic coma make a satisfactory recovery. Functional recovery is related to the cause of coma. Diseases causing structural damage, such as cerebrovascular disease including subarachnoid hemorrhage, carry the worst prognosis; coma from hypoxia-ischemia due to such causes as cardiac arrest has an intermediate prognosis; coma due to hepatic encephalopathy and other metabolic causes has the best ultimate outcome. Age does not appear to be predictive of recovery. The longer a coma lasts, the less likely the patient is to regain independent functioning. Factors that adversely impact brain injury following cardiac arrest include cerebral edema, pyrexia, hyperglycemia, and seizures.

In the early days after the onset of nontraumatic coma, it is not possible to predict with certainty which patients will ultimately enter or remain in a vegetative state. In individuals who have suffered an out-of-hospital cardiac arrest, the combination of no prehospital return of spontaneous circulation, an unshockable initial rhythm, and unwitnessed onset by bystanders carries a very poor outcome in greater than 99% of the patients. An end-tidal $CO_2$ value of less than 1.9 kPa (14.3 mm Hg) after 20 minutes of cardiopulmonary respiration (CPR) also indicates an unfavorable outcome (Haenggi et al., 2014). Although rare cases have been reported of patients awakening after prolonged vegetative states, patients with nontraumatic coma who have not regained awareness by the end of 1 month are unlikely to do so. Even if they do regain consciousness, they have practically no chance of achieving an independent existence. A large multiinstitutional study determined that within 3 days of cardiac arrest, evaluation in the intensive care unit is sufficiently predictive of neurological outcome to allow for informed decisions regarding life support. Absence of pupillary light or corneal reflexes at least 24 hours after insult and no motor response to noxious stimuli no greater than limb extension after 3 days of observation suggest a poor prognosis for recovery. Other poor prognostic signs are myoclonic status epilepticus, bilateral absence of the N20 response from the somatosensory cortex, and several neuroimaging signs (Young, 2009). MRI of the brain has also provided assistance in predicting prognosis. Apparent diffusion coefficient (ADC) values less than $665 \times 10^{-6}$ mm$^2$/sec correlated with poor outcome regardless of the time to MRI, with a specificity of 100% but low sensitivity of 21% (wu et al., 2009). More recently, functional MRI has been applied to evaluating the patient with altered level of consciousness but continues to remain investigational.

### Traumatic Coma

The prognosis for traumatic coma differs from that for nontraumatic coma in many ways. First, many patients with head trauma are young. Second, prolonged coma of up to several months does not preclude a satisfactory outcome in traumatic coma. Third, in relationship to their initial degree of neurological abnormality, traumatic coma patients do better than nontraumatic coma patients.

The prognosis for coma from head trauma may be considered in terms of survival; however, because many more patients survive traumatic coma than nontraumatic coma, it is equally important to consider the ultimate disabilities of the survivors because many who survive are left with profound disabilities. The Glasgow Outcome Scale is a practical system for describing outcome in traumatic coma. As originally proposed, this scale includes five categories: (1) death,

(2) PVS, (3) severe disability (conscious but disabled and dependent on others for activities of daily living), (4) moderate disability (disabled but independent), and (5) good recovery (resumption of normal life even though there may be minor neurological and psychiatric deficits). In their landmark 1979 report, Jennett and colleagues studied 1000 patients in coma longer than 6 hours from severe head trauma: 49% of these patients died, 3% remained vegetative, 10% survived with severe disability, 17% survived with moderate disability, and 22% had good recovery. The most reliable predictors of outcome 6 months later were depth of coma as evaluated by the Glasgow Coma Scale; pupil reaction, eye movements, and motor response in the first week after injury; and patient age. Evidence of damage to the internal capsule, corpus callosum, cerebral peduncle, and white matter tracts on MRI in patients with traumatic coma carry an unfavorable prognosis.

In summary, early predictors of the outcome of posttraumatic coma include patient's age, motor response, pupillary reactivity, eye movements, and depth and duration of coma. The prognosis worsens with increasing age. Cause of injury, skull fracture, lateralization of damage to one hemisphere, and extracranial injury appear to have little influence on the outcome.

### Persistent Vegetative State

As a rule, chronic PVS can be reliably diagnosed 12 months after a traumatic brain injury and 3 months after other cerebral insults. Recovery after 3 years for patients in PVS has not been reported (Wijdicks et al., 2005b). Those patients who have been reported to "improve" remain severely disabled, bed or wheelchair bound, and fully dependent on care. At 5 years, the mortality rate for PVS is in excess of 80%. Prolonged survival is rare and requires exquisite medical attention. Death typically results from untreated infection or overwhelming sepsis. "Miracle awakenings," such as with the sudden appearance of communicative speech, have been observed rarely in patients in the minimally conscious state but not in those in PVS (Wijdicks, 2005).

## BRAIN DEATH

### Clinical Approach to Brain Death

A thorough knowledge of the criteria for brain death is essential for the physician whose responsibilities include evaluation of comatose patients. Despite differences in state laws, the criteria for the establishment of brain death are fairly standard within the medical community. These criteria include the following:

*Absence of any potentially reversible causes of marked CNS depression.* Such causes include hypothermia (temperature 32°C [89.6°F] or less), drug intoxication (particularly barbiturate overdose), and severe metabolic disturbance. Patients must be evaluated in the absence of sedatives and paralytics, allowing adequate time, which is typically five half-lives in the setting of normal hepatic and renal function for these medications to be metabolized and excreted. The absence of paralytic medications can be confirmed with peripheral nerve electrical stimulation, such as a train of four.

*Coma.* The patient should exhibit an unarousable unresponsiveness. There should be no meaningful response to noxious, externally applied stimuli. The patient should not obey commands or demonstrate any verbal response, either reflexively or spontaneously. However, spinal reflexes may be retained.

*No spontaneous respirations.* The patient should be removed from ventilatory assistance, and carbon dioxide should be allowed to build up because of the respiratory drive that hypercapnia produces. The diagnosis of absolute apnea requires the absence of spontaneous respiration at a carbon dioxide tension of at least 60 mm Hg. A safe means of obtaining this degree of carbon dioxide retention involves the technique of apneic oxygenation, in which 100% oxygen is delivered endotracheally through a thin sterile catheter for 10 minutes. Arterial blood gas levels should be obtained to confirm the arterial carbon dioxide pressure.

*Absence of brainstem reflexes.* Pupillary, oculocephalic, corneal, and gag reflexes all must be absent, and there should not be any vestibulo-ocular responses to cold calorics. The use of an automated infrared pupillometer that assesses pupil reactivity independent of the examiner is becoming increasingly more common in clinical practice.

In cases of diagnostic uncertainty after the aforementioned clinical examination or based on individual hospital policies, ancillary testing to confirm brain death can be performed. These ancillary tests assess for:

*Electrocerebral silence.* An isoelectric EEG should denote the absence of cerebrocortical function. Some authorities do not regard the performance of an EEG as mandatory in assessing brain death, and instances of preserved cortical function, despite irreversible and complete brainstem disruption, have been reported.

*Absence of cerebral blood flow.* Cerebral contrast angiography or radionuclide angiography can substantiate the absence of cerebral blood flow, which is expected in brain death. These tests are considered confirmatory rather than mandatory. On rare occasions, in the presence of supratentorial lesions with preserved blood flow to the brainstem and cerebellum, findings on cerebral radionuclide angiography may be misleading.

Despite aggressive therapeutic measures, *maintenance of cardiopulmonary function* of "brain-dead" persons for more than 1 week has been considered unlikely. In a series of 175 "brain-dead" persons with maintenance of cardiopulmonary function longer than 1 week after diagnosis, the potential to maintain cardiopulmonary function decreased exponentially with an initial half-life of 2–3 months followed at 1 year by a slow decline (Shewmon, 1998). One patient maintained cardiopulmonary function for more than 14 years. Survival was found to correlate inversely with age, and prolonged survival was more common with primary brain pathology. The tendency to cardiovascular collapse in brain death may be transient and is more likely to be attributable to systemic than to brain pathology.

*The complete reference list is available online at https://expertconsult.inkling.com/.*

6

# Prolonged Comatose States and Brain Death

Eelco F.M. Wijdicks

## OUTLINE



Consciousness refers to normal wakefulness with awareness of self and the external environment, interactions, and decisions. Explanations and descriptions of consciousness are complex and cross the disciplines of neuroscience, psychology, and philosophy. In medicine, the assessment of consciousness is a clinical assessment done by observing a patient's alertness, willful interaction to stimuli, and thought content as expressed by language. Consciousness implies there is the possibility of expressing a considered thought and not just a reflexive response. Consciousness can decline through a continuum from full wakefulness and awareness, to drowsiness, disorientation, loss of meaningful communication, and coma. Terms such as "stupor," "semicoma," "somnolence," "altered mental status," "encephalopathy," and "quiet delirium" are unfortunately often vaguely applied. A precise description of neurological findings is required and more useful in localizing the lesion. The first course of action is to determine whether the comatose patient is comatose from a lesion in one hemisphere causing mass effect, in both hemispheres or in the posterior fossa. Next is to determine whether structural brain injury, seizures, a toxin, or acute metabolic or endocrine derangement is responsible for its presentation.

## CONCEPTS OF ABNORMAL CONSCIOUSNESS

Consciousness is traditionally dichotomized into two components in a conceptually useful approach. The *content* of consciousness includes all cognitive functions, emotions, and intuitions of the brain. The *level* of consciousness refers to global alertness and behavioral responsivity. Several key anatomical structures control the conscious state: the ascending reticular activating system (ARAS) in the midbrain and upper pons, the diencephalon (thalamus and hypothalamus), anterior cingulate cortex, association cortices (precuneus and cuneus), and the cortex proper (Fig. 6.1). The neurochemistry driving this complex system consists of several important neurotransmitters: norepinephrine (originating from the locus ceruleus and pontine lateral tegmentum), dopamine (ventral tegmentum), serotonin (raphe nuclei), acetylcholine (basal forebrain), histamine (posterior hypothalamus), and orexin-hypocretin (lateral hypothalamus) (McClenathan et al., 2013). As the target of all incoming signals, the thalamus is central in governing consciousness and relays and gates information diffusely to brain networks.

Major mechanisms of coma involve destructive lesions of the thalamus or diffuse connections to the cortex or ARAS. These structures can be directly damaged or injured by compression or shifts, and the changes often alter consciousness permanently. More selective lesions involving a unilateral hemisphere or thalamus will not substantially impair long-term consciousness.

## PROLONGED DISORDERS OF CONSCIOUSNESS

### Vegetative State

The advent of intensive care units and mechanical ventilation has allowed patients with devastating brain injuries to survive. While deeply comatose during the acute phase, some of these patients transition to a different clinical state in which they regain awake and sleep cycles, but remain unaware of their surroundings. This clinical syndrome—named persistent vegetative state (PVS) in the early 1970s—described patients with no evidence of a functioning mind (Jennett and Plum, 1972). This state has also been referred to as "unresponsiveness wakefulness syndrome" because of the alleged negative connotation of the word "vegetative" (Laureys et al., 2010). After prolonged coma, patients begin to have periods of spontaneous eye-opening but do not visually fixate or track objects with their eyes. The key feature is that patients show "no evidence of sustained, reproducible, purposeful, or voluntary behavioral responses" to external stimuli (Multi-Society Task Force, 1994a). A patient's eyes may open wide, but consistently demonstrated visual pursuit and fixation are absent. A large mirror held in front of the patient—to track his or her own face—is a useful test and probably the best stimulus to assess whether visual fixation and pursuit occur. A startle response is often present and may manifest as myoclonus, head flexion, or a decorticate response (Wijdicks and Cranford, 2005). Primitive reflexes such as snout, glabella, and palmomental reflexes may be easily elicited. Random movements of the limbs and trunk, occasional grunts, and even occasional tears or smiles are all signs consistent with PVS but may provoke uncertainty for family members or inexperienced clinicians. Autonomic and brainstem functions are preserved so that patients generally can maintain adequate circulation and breathe spontaneously without difficulty. The clinical picture fits with what is seen pathologically, with the majority of brains

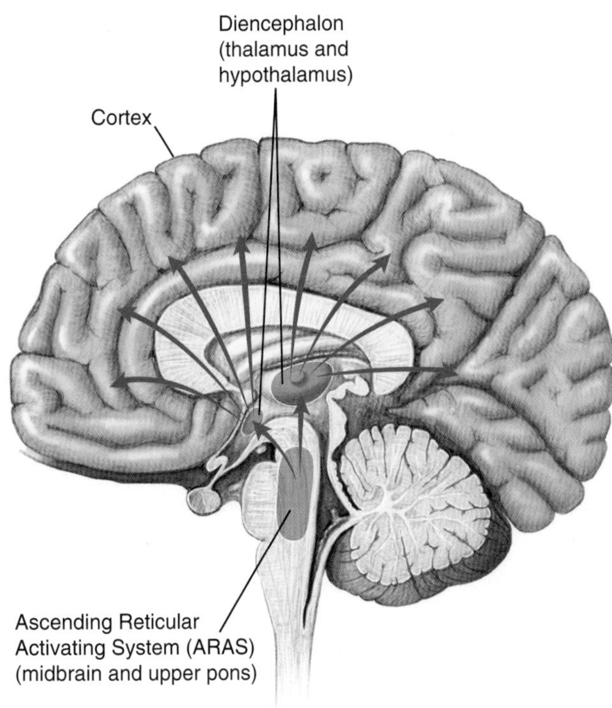


**Fig. 6.1** Key structures in maintaining an awake state and awareness. *(From Wijdicks, E.F., 2014. The Comatose Patient, second ed. Oxford University Press, New York.)*

at autopsy showing extensive damage to the subcortical white matter or thalamus, with sparing of the brainstem (Adams et al., 2000).

At what point can a vegetative state (VS) be considered permanent? When is there a high degree of clinical certainty that the clinical state is irreversible and the chance of regaining consciousness is exceedingly unlikely? The clinical course of PVS depends in large part on the underlying etiology and the duration of unconsciousness. The most common causes are traumatic brain injury (TBI) and hypoxic-ischemic brain injury. The traditional approach to prognostication has been that patients in posttraumatic VS are unlikely to regain consciousness after 12 months, whereas those with anoxic brain injury have even less potential for improvement and very rarely recover consciousness after 3 months (Multi-Society Task Force, 1994b). Although this is true for the majority of patients, a minority of patients may recover from PVS beyond these cutoffs (Matsuda et al., 2003). A small prospective study of patients with anoxic VS found that 7 of 43 patients (16%) recovered responsiveness and were living at 2 years, 12 (28%) remained vegetative, and 24 (56%) died (Estraneo et al., 2013). All responsive survivors had preserved pupillary light reflexes and present cortical responses with somatosensory-evoked potentials during the acute phase of injury. Notably, those who do become aware again often find themselves severely disabled. Age also plays a key role, particularly in TBI, with younger patients showing better recovery rates. The American Academy of Neurology, in collaboration with the American Congress of Rehabilitation Medicine and the National Institute on Disability, Independent Living, and Rehabilitation Research, formed a committee to develop a guideline on prolonged disorders of consciousness (DOC) (Giacino et al., 2018). The committee advocated more caution in prognostication and warned against clear time cutoff points beyond where no recovery occurs. The guideline suggests late (after 1 year) improvements primarily occurring in younger patients and approximately 20% of patients initially meeting PVS criteria.

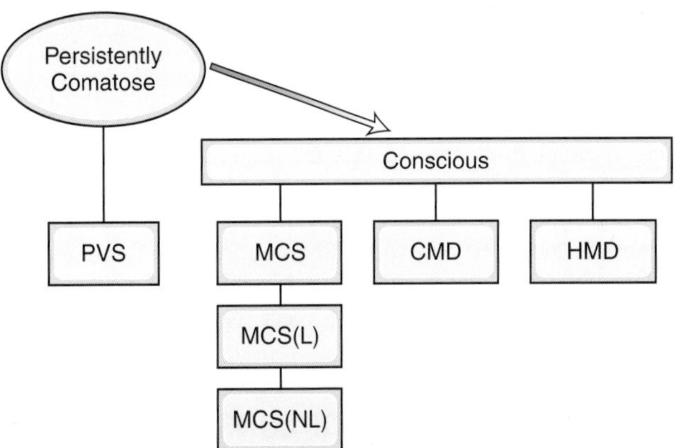


**Fig. 6.2** A concept of categories of persistent disorders of consciousness. (See text for explanation.) *CMD,* Cognitive motor dissociation; *HMD,* higher-order cortex-motor dissociation; *MCS,* minimally conscious state; *PVS,* persistent vegetative state.

The clinical assessment of a patient who is unconscious can be very challenging (Fig. 6.2). The examination may need to be repeated at different times of the day because of fluctuations in awareness and circadian oscillations affecting arousal. Some studies suggest a misdiagnosis in a substantial minority of patients in PVS and a reclassification of 13%–28% of supposedly vegetative patients using formal scales such as the Full Outline of UnReponsiveness (FOUR) score or the Coma Recovery Scale-Revised (CRS-R) (Giacino et al., 2004; Schnakers et al., 2009; Wijdicks et al., 2005). Diagnostic error rates of 40% have been cited, but this frequency might be falsely high because the evidence is based on poor reporting standards and insufficient follow-up (Wade, 2018).

## Minimally Conscious State

In the 1990s, clinicians involved in the care of brain-injured patients began to recognize that some patients previously diagnosed as vegetative showed subtle and partial awareness of their environment. This emerging clinical state was characterized and defined as the minimally conscious state (MCS) by expert consensus of members of a multidisciplinary work group in 2002 (Giacino et al., 2002). The distinguishing feature of MCS from PVS is the presence, albeit partial, of conscious awareness. A patient must demonstrate one or more specific reproducible behaviors to meet criteria for a diagnosis of MCS. These include following simple commands, responding with verbal or gestural yes/no answers, understandable verbalization, and purposeful behavior. The boundaries of chronic DOC are arbitrarily defined on a broad continuum. When patients reliably demonstrate functional interactive communication or can functionally use two different objects, they are generally considered no longer in MCS and then more appropriately characterized as severely disabled. Coma is typically a transient state, and one of several distinct clinical states emerges within days to weeks. This may be in response to rehabilitation physicians, who often reject the PVS diagnoses of patients referred to them, changing them to a MCS or better. MCS has some awareness and interaction and, of course, is more common than PVS. Some rehabilitation physicians have subclassified MCS into MCS with (MCS+) or without (MCS−) language. In addition, functional magnetic resonance imaging (MRI) scan-based categorization, including cognitive motor dissociation (CMD), has revealed a patient subset fulfilling all PVS criteria but showing command-following response on functional MRI. Another patient subset, higher-order cortex-motor dissociation (HMD), exhibits cortical response to auditory stimuli, again without evident awareness (see Fig. 6.2).

The clinical course of patients with MCS is still being defined. One of the reasons that it is important to differentiate PVS from MCS is that the prognosis for recovery appears to be different, with MCS patients recovering at better rates than those in PVS (Giacino and Kalmar, 2005). A small study showed that the majority of patients in MCS eventually "emerge" and that duration of MCS and age are the best predictors of outcome as measured by the disability rating scale (DRS) (Katz et al., 2009). Patients with TBI are more likely to progress than patients with nontraumatic disorders. For those with traumatic injuries, recovery can continue for 2–5 years (Nakase-Richardson et al., 2012).

## IMAGING IN DISORDERS OF CONSCIOUSNESS

Although the diagnosis of VS or MCS has always been a purely clinical determination, there has been interest in defining imaging correlates and predictors of these states. Structural injury on conventional MRI sequences within the corpus callosum and dorsal brainstem in subacute posttraumatic vegetative patients predicts a lack of recovery (Kampfl et al., 1998). Diffusion tensor imaging (DTI), which evaluates the structural integrity of white matter pathways, can detect structural abnormalities not visualized on conventional MRI sequences and may be a useful adjunct. Patients with more extensive white matter abnormalities on DTI MRI tend to score lower on the CRS-R (Newcombe et al., 2010).

Some investigators have pioneered the use of functional neuroimaging to complement the examination to determine whether a patient has any evidence of cerebral activity, which is often extrapolated to imply the presence of consciousness. Functional MRI involves T2-weighted images with gradient echo pulse sequence changes of deoxyhemoglobin in the perfused area, which is thought to imply neuronal activation. In a typical paradigm, the patient is instructed to perform basic cognitive tasks while in the scanner. In a pivotal case report, a patient classified clinically as vegetative 5 months after TBI had cortical activation on functional MRI with two different mental imagery tasks (Owen et al., 2006). Cortical activation was seen in the supplementary motor region after the patient was instructed to imagine playing tennis. The frequency of this finding—which is of uncertain clinical significance—appears to be rare. In one study, 5 of 54 patients with chronic DOC had cortical activation on functional MRI when asked to perform imagery tasks (play tennis or navigate their home) (Monti et al., 2010). However, activation of cortex does not necessarily prove consciousness and instead might be automatic. The use of functional MRI in patients with chronic DOC is further limited by low sensitivity and practical difficulties (e.g., patient movement requiring sedation), which preclude at least half of patients from being studied (Stender et al., 2014).

Neuronal activity has also been assessed by $^{18}$F-fluorodeoxyglucose (FDG) positron emission tomography (PET), which demonstrates brain glucose metabolism. Diminished metabolism is seen in the frontoparietal cortices of patients with DOC. Some studies have shown that in MCS, partial metabolism is maintained, whereas in PVS, the frontoparietal dysfunction is broader and more extensive (Thibaut et al., 2012). Predicting the absence of recovery of consciousness using $^{18}$F-FDG PET may be more reliable than predicting the presence of recovery (Stender et al., 2014). However, both false positives and false negatives occur, and the practical value of these imaging studies is not clear. They remain areas of research to further our understanding of conscious states but cannot be considered part of routine clinical practice at this time. A recent study using machine learning applied to electroencephalograms (EEGs) found that 15% of 104 "unresponsive" patients had brain activation detected by EEGs at a median of 4 days after injury (Claassen et al., 2019). However, approximately half of the small subset of patients with brain activation and approximately one in four patients without brain activation followed commands before discharge. At 12 months, patients showing early brain activation had three times more often independent function than patients without brain activation. This technology is not widely available, interpretation parameters are not firmly established, and false negatives are substantial.

**BOX 6.1 Suggested Interventions to Facilitate Recovery in Persistent Vegetative State or Minimally Conscious State (Many Unproven)**

**Pharmaceutical**
Amantadine*
Levodopa
Methylphenidate
Bromocriptine
Zolpidem
Dopamine agonists
Tricyclic antidepressants
Intrathecal baclofen

**Nonpharmaceutical**
Deep brain stimulation
Dorsal column stimulation
Transcortical magnetic stimulation
Transcortical direct cortical stimulation
Multisensory environmental stimulation
Music therapy

*Only drug tested in a randomized trial.

## TREATMENT OPTIONS

guidelines regarding treatment of patients with chronic DOC, but interventions to accelerate recovery in patients with chronic DOC is a topic of ongoing research, particularly in the rehabilitation community. A randomized trial of 184 patients with chronic DOC due to TBI showed that recovery (rated by the DRS) was faster in patients who were treated with amantadine for 4 weeks than in patients receiving placebo (Giacino et al., 2012). Both groups had significant improvements in the DRS score over 4 weeks, but the amantadine group improved faster. The dose of amantadine was 100 mg twice daily for 2 days, titrated up to 200 mg twice daily if no effect was seen. Overall outcomes were still discouraging, with 74% of patients in the amantadine group remaining with severe-to-extremely-severe disability or VS (compared with 83% in the placebo group) (Giacino et al., 2012). Many other drug therapies have been proposed and are shown in Box 6.1 (Lemaire et al., 2014; Martin and Whyte, 2007; Matsuda et al., 2005; Thonnard et al., 2013, Thibaut, 2019). Most agents have not been proven to be effective, but results have been mixed and the literature is limited by small numbers and publication bias.

In addition to medications, nonpharmaceutical interventions using electrical stimulation are also under investigation as therapy to spur recovery of consciousness in brain-injured patients. A study randomized 55 patients with chronic DOC to transcranial direct current stimulation over the left dorsolateral prefrontal cortex compared with sham stimulation. There was no observed effect in vegetative patients, but 13 patients in MCS showed a transient improvement in consciousness (assessed by the CRS-R) following stimulation. However,

12-month functional outcomes in this heterogeneous sample did not differ between responders and nonresponders. Only one clinical assessment was performed prestimulation and poststimulation, and further research is needed to confirm the findings and exclude the possibility that these were spontaneous fluctuations. The role of thalamic deep brain stimulation (DBS) for patients in VS or MCS is another area of investigation (Lemaire et al., 2014; Schiff et al., 2007). The most common targets for DBS in this population are the central intralaminar nuclei of the thalamus with the intent of activating the cortex through the reticular-thalamic complex. Several reports suggest that DBS has the potential to promote recovery in patients with prolonged DOC, but the series typically involved small numbers of patients and was limited by their observational nature. In most, it is difficult to parse out direct DBS effects from spontaneous or postrehabilitation recovery.

## BRAIN DEATH

Deeply comatose patients who lose *all* clinical signs of brain and brainstem function due to a major destructive lesion are dead and should be clearly distinguished from other comatose states. Death by these neurological criteria is a medically and legally accepted way of determining a person's death (Wijdicks, 2011). Before proceeding with a brain death evaluation, it is crucial that the irreversible cause of coma is established and there are no potential factors confounding the neurological examination. In most cases the patient should have been treated aggressively with measures such as administration of hyperosmolar agents, surgical evacuation of space-occupying lesions producing brainstem displacement, ventriculostomy, or other intracranial pressure (ICP)-lowering therapies. Once an untreatable catastrophic neurological structural injury has been proven while in this supported state, recovery does not occur and there is no known effective medical or surgical intervention. Irreversibility is determined by absent motor responses, loss of all brainstem reflexes, and the apnea test (described later). Brain death is relatively uncommon because the brainstem is very resilient to injury. When it does occur, the most common causes are severe TBI, aneurysmal subarachnoid hemorrhage (aSAH), massive intraparenchymal hemorrhage, or on rare occasion anoxic-ischemic brain injury. Neurological criteria for determining death first took shape in the 1950s and have been refined and developed throughout the world. The American Academy of Neurology has issued adult guidelines for brain death determination based on a thorough review of existing evidence (Wijdicks et al., 2010, Wijdicks, 2019). Brain death is based on a detailed and thorough clinical evaluation and in most countries (including the United States) confirmatory tests are not required if the clinical examination—including a formal apnea test—can be completed.

It is essential that certain prerequisites be met prior to the clinical examination. The main confounding factors that need to be excluded are hypothermia (core body temperature should be ≥36°C); drug intoxication or poisoning; lingering effects of sedatives, analgesics, and neuromuscular blockers; and severe electrolyte or acid-base disturbances (Fig. 6.3). Once the cause of coma has been established by the history and neuroimaging and all prerequisites are met, the clinical examination is performed. A period of time, usually hours, should have passed after the onset of brain injury to exclude the possibility of recovery. Because the history early in the course is often fragmentary and the use of sedative and analgesic medications is often unknown, brain death should not be determined within hours of emergency department evaluation or transfer from an outside facility.

A detailed examination of brainstem reflexes is the crux of the clinical assessment. Most pupils in brain death have a 4- to 6-mm diameter, and the pupillary response to bright light should be absent in both eyes. Constricted pupils should not be seen and should raise the concern of medication effect (often opioids). Corneal reflexes should be absent bilaterally. Caloric testing of the oculovestibular reflexes is performed with the head elevated to 30 degrees so that the horizontal semicircular canal becomes vertical. A small suction catheter is connected to a 50-mL syringe filled with ice water. In brain death, the reflex is absent, and after irrigation of the tympanum on each side, there are no eye movements. In a comatose, non–brain-dead patient with intact oculovestibular reflexes, the eyes slowly deviate toward the side of the cold stimulus. The eyes should be observed for at least 1 full minute after injection, and the time between stimulation of each side should be at least 5 minutes. The gag reflex in response to stimulation of the posterior oropharynx should be absent and can be tested by inserting a finger deep into the oral cavity and actually feeling the absence of contraction. The lack of a cough response is demonstrated by passing a suction catheter through the endotracheal tube and providing suctioning pressure all the way to the level of the carina.

The application of deep pressure on both condyles at the temporomandibular joint, supraorbital notch, fingernail beds, or sternal rubbing should elicit no grimacing and no motor response in the extremities. Decerebrate and decorticate posturing are motor responses that are not compatible with brain death, but some limb movements may be produced by spinally mediated reflexes. Clinical findings not consistent with a diagnosis of brain death are shown in Box 6.2.

Following the confirmation of absent motor responses, lack of respiratory drive is documented by an apnea test. This is most commonly performed using the apneic oxygenation-diffusion technique and involves preoxygenation with 100% oxygenation. A systolic blood pressure of 90–100 mm Hg is needed prior to the apnea test and most often vasopressors are already required to meet that goal (Fugate et al., 2011). Doses of vasopressors might need to be increased if persistent hypotension is problematic. A baseline arterial blood gas should show adequate oxygenation ($Pao_2 \geq 200$ mm Hg) and normal $Paco_2$ (35–45 mm Hg). Artificial ventilation is then removed for a period of 8–10 minutes, allowing buildup of arterial tension of carbon dioxide and the pH to be lowered, which under normal circumstances would stimulate respiratory centers. After disconnection from the ventilator, the patient is observed for breathing efforts (chest expansion, abdominal excursion, or gasping). The lack of respiratory drive is demonstrated when there have been no breathing efforts despite a rise in $Paco_2$ to 60 mm Hg or an increase of 20 mm Hg or greater from a normal baseline $Paco_2$. The apnea test using oxygen diffusion with oxygen insufflation at the level of the carina is very safe (Daneshmand et al., 2019), but the acidosis may reduce myocardial contractility, causing transient hypotension and there may be a need for a temporary increase in vasopressors.

Brain death is a clinical determination, and in the United States does not require additional ancillary tests in most cases. Occasionally, there are times when these are needed if certain parts of the examination cannot be properly conducted (e.g., major facial trauma that precludes a reliable assessment). When required, electrophysiological tests include EEG, auditory evoked potentials, and somatosensory evoked potentials. The EEG (with minimum of eight scalp electrodes and an interelectrode distance of at least 10 cm) should show electrocerebral silence, which necessitates no electrical potentials of more than 2 mV during a 30-minute recording. Artifacts created by the ventilator, pulse, or surrounding electrical devices are often seen and may lead to uncertainty in the interpretation. The clinical examination and the excluding of confounders remains the foundation of brain death determination. It should be noted that unresponsive patients could have "flat" EEGs despite intact brainstem reflexes (Heckmann et al., 2003),

**25 Assessments to Declare a Patient Brain Dead**

Prerequisites (ALL MUST BE CHECKED)

1. ☐ Coma, irreversible and cause known
2. ☐ Neuroimaging explains coma
3. ☐ Sedative drug effect absent *(if indicated, order a toxicology screen)*
4. ☐ No residual effect of paralytic drug *(if indicated, use peripheral nerve stimulator)*
5. ☐ Absence of severe acid-base, electrolyte, or endocrine abnormality
6. ☐ Normal or near normal temperature *(core temperature ≥ 36°C)*
7. ☐ Systolic blood pressure ≥ 100 mm Hg
8. ☐ No spontaneous respirations

Examination (ALL MUST BE CHECKED)

9. ☐ Pupils non-reactive to bright light *(typically mid-position at 5–7 mm)*
10. ☐ Corneal reflexes absent *(use both saline jet and tissue touch)*
11. ☐ Eyes immobile, oculocephalic reflexes absent *(tested only if C-spine integrity ensured)*
12. ☐ Oculovestibular reflexes absent *(50 mL of ice water in each ear sequentially)*
13. ☐ No facial movement to noxious stimuli at supraorbital nerve or temporomandibular joint compression. *(absent snout and rooting reflexes in neonates)*
14. ☐ Gag reflex absent *(gloved index finger to posterior pharynx)*
15. ☐ Cough reflex absent to tracheal suctioning *(at least 2 passes)*
16. ☐ No motor response to noxious stimuli in all 4 limbs *(triple flexion response is most common spinal-mediated reflex)*

Apnea Testing (ALL MUST BE CHECKED)

17. ☐ Patient is hemodynamically stable *(systolic blood pressure ≥ 100 mm Hg)*
18. ☐ Ventilator adjusted to normocapnia *($Paco_2$ 35–45 mm Hg)*
19. ☐ Patient pre-oxygenated with 100% oxygen for 10 minutes *($Pao_2$ ≥ 200 mm Hg)*
20. ☐ Patient maintains oxygenation with a PEEP of 5 cm $H_2O$ *(if not, consider recruitment maneuver )*
21. ☐ Disconnect ventilator
22. ☐ Provide oxygen via an insufflation catheter to the level of the carina at 6 liters/min or attach T-piece with CPAP valve @ 10–20 cm $H_2O$ and resuscitation bag
23. ☐ Spontaneous respirations absent
24. ☐ Arterial blood gas drawn at 8–10 minutes, patient reconnected to ventilator
25. ☐ *$Paco_2$* ≥ 60 mm Hg, or 20 mm Hg rise from normal baseline value
    or
    Apnea test aborted and confirmatory ancillary test *(EEG or cerebral blood flow study)*

Repeat Examinations

- Newborn (≥ 37 weeks gestational age) to 30 days: 2 examinations, 2 separate physicians, 24 hours apart
- 30 days to 18 years: 2 examinations, 2 separate physicians, 12 hours apart
- ≥18 years: 1 examination *(a second examination is needed in some* US *states: AL, CA, FL, IA, KY, LA)*

Documentation

- Time of death *(use time of final blood gas result or use time of completion of ancillary test)*

**Fig. 6.3** A clinical determination of brain death requires 25 tests. *CPAP,* Continuous positive airway pressure; *EEG,* electroencephalogram; *PEEP,* positive end-expiratory pressure.

**BOX 6.2 Clinical Findings Not Compatible with Brain Death**

Nystagmus or other spontaneous eye movements
Conjugate eye deviation
Pinpoint pupils
Grimacing to noxious stimulation
Decerebrate or decorticate motor posturing

or in profound hypothermia or drug overdose. Cerebral angiography, cerebral perfusion scintigraphy, or transcranial Doppler have been used to demonstrate the cessation of cerebral blood flow as ancillary tests, but there are technical pitfalls with these methods and they have not been validated (Wijdicks, 2010).

When the determination of brain death is made clinically, and the apnea test is the last component of the examination, the time of brain death is the time that the arterial $Pco_2$ reached the target value in the absence of respiratory effort. The family is told that their loved one has died. After adequate time has passed, the family should then be approached regarding the possibility of organ transplantation. Federal laws require the physician to contact an organ procurement organization, and in the United States and other countries, members of this organization will approach the family separately from the medical team.

The announcement of brain death should not come as a surprise to the family, and with ongoing contact, they should become aware of the patient's prognosis following a catastrophic brain injury. Brain-death examinations should be undertaken only under near certainty that the patient is brain dead. Then the family should be told that the patient has died but remains supported by artificial means. A discussion on organ donation follows.

## DECISION MAKING AND BIOETHICS

Statistics and probabilities of survival or recovery of consciousness do not always easily translate to decisions for individual patients with differing values. In large part, surrogates make decisions based on how information is communicated to them. Seeing relatives in a VS or an MCS is distressing and might be a source of dissension within families, and between families and physicians. The already complex situation could be further complicated by research studies suggesting that the detection of cortical activation or regionally increased metabolism on imaging scans implies "consciousness" in patients who appear clinically unconscious. These findings are subject to sensationalism, and families of patients in persistent coma may believe that functional MRI or $^{18}$F-FDG PET scans may be better than a clinical examination. False positives, false negatives, or inconclusive tests could lead to even further ambiguity and confusion (Wijdicks, 2012).

Should patients with prolonged DOC be kept alive? If so, for how long, and how is that determination best made? Ambiguity abounds. In a survey of 199 lay people in the United States, approximately 40% were uncertain about withdrawing life-sustaining treatments for either vegetative patients or patients in MCS (Gipson et al., 2014). Forty percent agreed that stopping treatment was morally acceptable for patients in VS, whereas 21% agreed for MCS. The most important factors in the decision about withdrawing treatments were the presence of consciousness, autonomy, and the ability to interact with others. Individuals were more likely to want treatment withdrawn from themselves than to endorse it more generally (Gipson et al., 2014). Although justice is one of the main components of medical ethics, it appears to be much less of a factor in lay person attitudes—despite unsustainable healthcare spending—which suggests that many reject a utilitarian approach in life-death circumstances.

This topic has received considerable attention from ethicists, legal experts, and the media, but only rare, exceptional situations are in the spotlight. Many cases in daily clinical practice are appreciably more straightforward. In some cases the poor neurological prognosis is very clear, and surrogates decide that even the "best case scenario" is not a situation thought to be acceptable to the patient. These decisions are obviously easier when the patient has previously and explicitly expressed wishes about type or level of disability they would find acceptable. In many young unfortunate patients, this is unknown. It is important to seek out prior advanced directives or living wills because all decisions should be made with one underlying principle: what is most important is what the patient wanted. Any physician would want to be more cautious in younger individuals—whatever the cause—and certainly if the MRI does not show overwhelming extensive injury. There are also possible ethical tensions when families protest and intervene with brain death testing—either full examination or the apnea test. Brain death determination is a neurological examination, and medical decisions are based on these findings. This examination does not require informed consent. If families object to organ donation or object to withdrawal of the mechanical ventilator and other intensive care measures, support is continued until legal issues have been resolved. In many instances, cardiac arrest will occur from terminal fatal arrhythmias.

## CONCLUSIONS

Catastrophic injury to the brain may cause permanent coma which often transitions to different states of impaired consciousness. New imaging and computer-assisted technology has suggested that some elements of awareness (not the same as consciousness) may exist in some patients who, on the surface, appear severely affected and unaware of the surroundings. Recovery may occur in some, but prediction is far from accurate. Loss of all brainstem function in a massive hemispheric lesion does not lead to recovery, and this state is accepted as death of the person.

*The complete reference list is available online at https://expertconsult.inkling.com/.* 

7

# Intellectual and Memory Impairments

*Howard S. Kirshner, Katherine A. Gifford*

## OUTLINE



The term *intellect* designates the totality of the mental or cognitive operations that compose human thought—the higher cortical functions that make up the conscious mind. The intellect and its faculties, the subject matter of human psychology, are the qualities that most separate human beings from other animals. Memory is a specific cognitive function: the storage and retrieval of information. As such, it is the prerequisite for learning, the building block of all human knowledge. Other "higher" functions such as language, calculations, spatial topography and reasoning, executive function, music, and creativity all represent functions of specific brain systems. The relationship of the mind and brain has long been of philosophical interest. Recent advances in cognitive neuroscience have made mind-brain questions the subject of practical scientific and clinical study. It is now possible to study how the metabolic activation of brain regions and the firing patterns of neurons give rise to the phenomenon of consciousness, the sense of self, the ability to process information, and the development of decisions and attitudes. The pattern of an individual's habitual decisions and attitudes becomes one's personality.

Francis Crick (1994), who with James Watson won the Nobel Prize for the discovery of the structure of DNA, expressed the "astonishing hypothesis" that "you, your joys and your sorrows, your sense of personal identity and free will, are in fact no more than the behavior of a vast assembly of nerve cells and their associated molecules" (p. 3). This chapter considers our knowledge of intellect and memory, mind and brain, from the perspective of the clinical neurologist who must assess disorders of the higher functions.

## NEURAL BASIS OF COGNITION

### Cerebral Cortex

The cognitive operations discussed in this chapter take place among a large network of cortical cells and connections, the neural switchboard that gives rise to conscious thinking. The cortical mantle of the human brain is very large compared with animal brains, containing more than 14 billion neurons. The information stored in the human cerebral cortex rivals that found in large libraries. Within the cortical mantle, the areas that have expanded the most from animal to human are the association cortices, cortical zones that do not carry out primary motor or sensory functions but rather interrelate the functions of the primary motor and sensory areas. According to Nauta and Feirtag's (1986) text, 70% of neurons in the human central nervous system reside in the cerebral cortex, and 75% of those are in the association cortex. Higher cortical functions, with few exceptions, take place in the association cortex.

The neuroanatomy of the cerebral cortex has been known in considerable detail since the 1800s. Primary cortical sensory areas include the visual cortex in the occipital lobe, the auditory cortex in the temporal lobe, the somatosensory cortex in the parietal lobe, and probably gustatory and olfactory cortices in the frontal and temporal lobes. Each of these primary cortices receives signals in only one modality (vision, hearing, or sensation) and has cortical-cortical connections only to adjacent portions of the association cortex also dedicated to this modality, called *unimodal association cortex*. Sensory information is sequentially processed in an increasingly complex fashion, leading from raw sensory data to a unified percept. Within each cortical area are columns of cells with similar function, called *modules*.

The organization of the primary sensory cortex and unimodal association cortex has been especially well worked out in the visual system through the Nobel Prize–winning research of Hubel and Wiesel and others. Retinal ganglion cells are activated by light within a bright center, with inhibition in the surround. These cells project through the optic nerve to the lateral geniculate body of the thalamus, then via the optic radiations to the primary visual cortex in the occipital lobes. In the primary visual cortex, a vertical band of neurons may be dedicated to the detection of a specific bright area, but in the cortex this is usually a bar or edge of light rather than a spot. These "simple" cells of the visual cortex respond to bright central bars with dark surroundings. Several such cells project to complex cells, which may detect an edge or line with a specific orientation, or a specific direction of movement, but with less specificity about the exact location within the visual field. Visual shapes are perceived by the operation of these cells. Complex cells in turn project to cells in the visual unimodal association cortex (the Brodmann areas 18 and 19), where cells may detect movement or patterns. Complex cells also respond to movement anywhere in the visual field, an important characteristic because of the organism's need to maintain visual attention for possible hazards in the environment. In the visual association cortex, columns may respond to specific shapes, colors, or qualities such as novelty. In this fashion, the functions of cell columns or modules become more sophisticated from the primary cortex to the association cortex. In Fodor's model, the modules of primary visual perception project to central systems. Cognitive science has made tremendous strides in the understanding of the neurobiology of specific functions such as vision, but it has yet to fathom the higher perceptual functions such as the concept of beauty in a starry sky or in a painting or the cross-modality processes that underlie, for example, the adaptation of a ballet to a specific musical accompaniment.

Unimodal association cortices communicate with each other via still more complex connections to the heteromodal association cortex, of which there are two principal sites. The posterior heteromodal association cortex involves the posterior inferior parietal lobe, especially the angular gyrus. The posterior heteromodal cortex makes it possible to perceive an analogy between an association in one modality (e.g., a picture of a boat and the printed word *boat* in the visual modality) with a percept in a different modality (e.g., the sound of the spoken word *boat*). These intermodality associations are difficult for animals, even chimpanzees, but easy for human beings. Cross-sensory associations involve the functioning of *cortical networks* of multitudes of neurons; the analogy drawn by neuroscientists is to the vast arrays of circuits active in computer networks. The product of such associations is a concept.

The second heteromodal association cortex involves the lateral prefrontal region (Goldman-Rakic, 1996). This region is thought to be involved with attention or "working memory" and with sequential processes such as storage of temporally ordered stimuli and the planning of motor activities. This temporal sequencing of information and motor planning is referred to by neuropsychologists as the *executive function* of the brain—the decisions we make every instant regarding which of the myriad of sensory stimuli reaching the sensory cortices merit attention, which require a motor response, and in what sequence and timing these motor responses will occur.

Another frontal cortical area, the orbitofrontal portion of the prefrontal cortex, is thought to be involved in emotional states, appetites, and drives, or in the integration of internal bodily states with sensations from the external world. The orbitofrontal cortex is known as the *supramodal cortex* (Benson, 1996) because it relates the functions of the heteromodal cortex regarding attention and sequencing of responses with interoceptive inputs from the internal milieu of the body. The orbitofrontal area has close connections with the limbic system and autonomic, visceral, and emotional processes. In studying brain evolution from primitive reptiles to humans, the neurobiologist Paul MacLean hypothesized that the internal and emotional parts of the brain, the limbic system, must be tied into the newer neocortical areas responsible for intellectual function, and that the linking of these two systems must underlie the phenomenon of consciousness. In a review of neuronal mechanisms of consciousness, Ortinski and Meador (2004) defined *conscious awareness* as "the state in which external and internal stimuli are perceived and can be intentionally acted on" (p. 1017). Benson and Ardila (1996), in reviewing clinical data from individuals with frontal lobe damage, state that the supramodal cortex is the brain system that "anticipates, conjectures, ruminates, plans for the future, and fantasizes." In other words, this part of the brain brings specific cognitive processes to conscious awareness and may be responsible for the phenomena of consciousness and self-awareness themselves.

## Consciousness

All human beings have a subjective understanding of what it means to be conscious and to have a concept of self, yet the neural basis for conscious awareness and the sense of self remains poorly understood. Until recently, many neuroscientists left the study of consciousness to the realm of religion and philosophy. Even Hippocrates knew that consciousness emanated from the brain, "to consciousness the brain is messenger." Francis Crick devoted the last part of his career to the understanding of consciousness. For Crick, the best model for the study of consciousness is visual awareness because the anatomy and physiology of the visual system are well understood. Crick argued that neurons in the primary visual cortex likely do not have access to conscious awareness. Stated another way, we do not pay attention to much of what our eyes see and our visual cortex analyzes. However, a perceived object excites neurons in several areas of the visual association cortex, each with associations that enter consciousness or are stored in short-term memory.

Activation of the frontal cortex is necessary for visual percepts to enter consciousness (Crick and Koch, 1995; Gelbard-Sagiv et al., 2018), although subconscious awareness in the form of blindsight may exist within the occipital cortex and subcortical structures (Celeghin et al., 2018). Conscious visual perception involves interactions between the visual parts of the brain and the prefrontal systems for attention and working memory (Ungerleider et al., 1998). The orbitofrontal cortex contains neurons that integrate interoceptive stimuli related to changes in the internal milieu with exteroceptive sensory inputs such as vision. Ortinski and Meader (2004) also point out the varying latencies of perception of specific sensory stimuli, such as color versus identification of a visual object. A synchronization of inputs through the thalamus to the cortex may be necessary before the perception becomes conscious. As stated earlier, the interaction between attention to external stimuli and internal stimuli underlies conscious awareness.

In the visual system, Goodale and Milner, (1992); Milner and Goodale, (2008); and also McIntosh and Schenk, (2009) have divided the visual system, after processing in the occipital cortex, into a ventral and a dorsal stream. The ventral stream, involved in perception of objects, is usually subject to conscious awareness and involves an occipital-temporal pathway, whereas the dorsal stream, involved in spatial localization of perceived objects to plan action, is usually less conscious.

There are many clinical examples of "unconscious" mental processing, and a number of these involve vision. Patients with cortical blindness sometimes show knowledge of items they cannot see, a phenomenon called *blindsight.* Patients with right hemisphere lesions who extinguish objects in the left visual field when presented with bilateral stimuli nonetheless show activation of the right visual cortex by functional magnetic resonance imaging (MRI), indicating that the objects are perceived, although not with conscious awareness (Rees et al., 2000). Libet (1999) demonstrated experimentally that visual and other sensory stimuli have to persist at least 500 msec to reach conscious awareness, yet stimuli of shorter duration can elicit reactions. An experimental example of unconscious visual processing comes from Gur and Snodderly (1997), who tested color vision in monkeys. When two colors were projected at a frequency of greater than 10 Hz, the monkey perceived a fused color, yet cellular recordings clearly demonstrated coding of information about the two separate colors in the monkey's visual cortex. Motor responses to sensory stimuli can occur before conscious awareness, as in the ability to pull one's hand away from a hot stove before feeling the heat. Racers begin running before they are aware of having heard the starting gun (Crick and Koch, 1998). A familiar example of unconscious visual processing is the drive home from work; most individuals can remember very little they see on the trip, yet they avoid oncoming vehicles and obstacles, stop for red lights, and drive without accidents. Crick and Koch (1998) refer to the unconscious visual processing as an "online" visual system. We shall discuss unconscious or "implicit" memories later in this chapter.

In language syndromes, patients can match spoken to written words without knowledge of their meaning, suggesting that there are unconscious rules of language. Brust (2000) has called all of these unconscious mental processes the "non-Freudian unconscious."

Research has linked the right frontal cortex to the sense of self. Keenan and colleagues (2001) studied patients undergoing the Wada test, in which a barbiturate is injected into the carotid artery to determine cortical language dominance. They presented subjects with a self-photograph and a photograph of a famous person, followed by a "morphed" photograph of a famous person and the patient. When the left hemisphere was anesthetized, the subjects said that the morphed photograph represented the subject himself, whereas with right hemisphere anesthesia, the subject selected the famous face. Patients with frontotemporal dementia also indicate a relationship between the right frontal lobe and self-concept. In the series by Miller and colleagues (2001), six of the seven patients who developed a major change in self-concept during their illness had predominant atrophy in the nondominant frontal lobe. A last example of the sense of self is the so-called Theory of Mind, which alludes to the understanding of another person as a conscious human being. Keenan and colleagues (2005) cite evidence that the right hemisphere frontotemporal cortex is dominant for both the sense of self and the recognition of other people.

The frontal lobes, as the executive center of the brain and the determining agent for attention and motor planning, are the origin of several critical networks for cognition and action. Cummings (1993) described five frontal networks for consciousness and behavior. These networks function as a circuit between the frontal lobe and subcortical regions: the frontal cortex projects to the basal ganglia, then to thalamic nuclei, and back to the cortex.

Clinical neurology provides important information about how lesions in the brain impair consciousness. The functioning of the awake mind requires the ascending inputs referred to as the *reticular activating system*, with its way stations in the brainstem and thalamus, as well as an intact cerebral cortex. Bilateral lesions of the brainstem or thalamus produce coma. Very diffuse lesions of the hemispheres produce an "awake" patient who shows no responsiveness to the environment, a state sometimes called *coma vigil* or *persistent vegetative state*, as in the well-known Terri Schiavo case (Bernat, 2006; Perry et al., 2005). Patients with very slight responses to environmental stimuli are said to be in a *minimally conscious state* (Wijdicks and Cranford, 2005). Recently, functional brain imaging studies have suggested that at least in a few patients labeled as having persistent vegetative state or minimally conscious state after traumatic brain injury, patients can think of playing tennis or standing in their home and seeing the other rooms, and the brain areas activated are similar to those of normal subjects. These same subjects, a small minority of patients with chronically impaired consciousness secondary to traumatic brain injury, showed evidence of conscious modulation of brain activity to indicate "yes" or "no" responses (Monti et al., 2010). This report has engendered controversy over our ability to determine when a patient truly lacks consciousness. In an accompanying editorial, Ropper noted that activation on brain imaging studies does not equal conscious awareness, and the concept that "I have brain activation, therefore I am … would seriously put Descartes before the horse" (Ropper, 2010).

Still less severe diffuse abnormalities of the association cortex produce encephalopathy, delirium, or dementia. These topics involve very common syndromes of clinical neurology. Stupor and coma are discussed in Chapter 5, and encephalopathy, or delirium, is covered in Chapter 4.

Focal lesions of the cerebral cortex generally produce deficits in specific cognitive systems. A detailed listing of such disorders would include much of the subject matter of behavioral neurology. Examples include Broca aphasia from a left frontal lesion, Wernicke aphasia from a left temporal lesion, Gerstmann syndrome (acalculia, left-right confusion, finger agnosia, and agraphia) from a left parietal lesion, visual agnosia or failure to recognize visual objects (usually from bilateral posterior lesions), apraxia from a left parietal lesion, and constructional impairment from a right parietal lesion. Multiple focal lesions can affect cognitive function in a more global fashion, as in the dementias (Chapter 66). Some authorities separate "cortical" dementias such as Alzheimer disease, in which combinations of cortical deficits are common, from "subcortical" dementias, in which mental slowing is the most prominent feature.

The frontal lobes are heavily involved in integration of the functions provided by other areas of cortex, and lesions there may affect personality and behavior in the absence of easily discernible deficits of specific cognitive, language, or memory function. In severe form, extensive lesions of the orbitofrontal cortex may leave the individual awake but staring, unable to respond to the environment, a state called *akinetic mutism*. With lesser lesions, patients with frontal lobe lesions may lose their ability to form mature judgments, reacting impulsively to incoming stimuli in a manner reminiscent of animal behavior. Such patients may be inappropriately frank or disinhibited. A familiar example is the famous case of Phineas Gage, a worker who sustained a severe injury to the frontal lobes. Gage became irritable, impulsive, and so changed in personality that coworkers said he was "no longer Gage." Bedside neurological testing and even standard neuropsychological tests of patients with frontal lobe damage may reveal normal intelligence except for concrete or idiosyncratic interpretation of proverbs and similarities. Experimentally, subjects with frontal lobe lesions can be shown to have difficulty with sequential processes or shifting of cognitive sets, as tested by the Wisconsin Card Sorting Test or the Category Test of the Halstead-Reitan battery. Luria introduced a simple bedside test of sequential shapes (Fig. 7.1) to assess for deficits indicative of frontal lesions. In contrast to the subtlety of these deficits to the examiner, the patient's family may state that there is a dramatic change in the patient's personality.

Another clinical window into the phenomena of consciousness comes from surgery to separate the hemispheres by cutting the corpus callosum. In split-brain or commissurotomized patients, each hemisphere seems to have a separate consciousness. The left hemisphere, which has the capacity for speech and language, can express this consciousness in words. For example, a split-brain patient can report words or pictures that appear in the right visual field. The right hemisphere cannot produce verbal accounts of items seen in the left visual field, but the subject can choose the correct item by pointing with the left hand; at the same time, the subject claims to have no conscious knowledge of the item. In terms of the speaking left hemisphere, the right hemisphere has "unconscious" visual knowledge, or *blindsight.* At times, the left hand of the patient may seem to operate under a different agenda from the right hand. A split-brain patient may select a dress from a rack with the right hand while the left hand puts it back or selects a more daring fashion. This rivalry of the left hand with the right is called the *alien hand syndrome*, a striking example of the

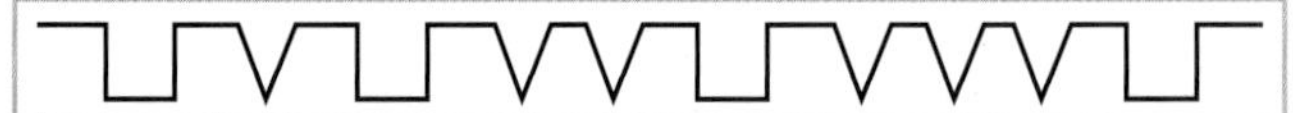

**Fig. 7.1 Luria's Test of Alternating Sequences.** (*Adapted from Luria, A.R., 1969. Frontal lobe syndromes. In: Vynken, P., Bruyn, G.W. (Eds.), Handbook of Clinical Neurology, vol. 2, Elsevier, New York. Reprinted with permission from Kirshner, H.S., 2002. Behavioral Neurology: Practical Science of Mind and Brain, second ed. Butterworth-Heinemann, Boston.*)

separate consciousnesses of the two divided hemispheres (Gazzaniga, 1998). Callosal syndromes, including the alien hand syndrome, have also been described in patients with strokes involving the corpus callosum (Chan and Ross, 1997) or the medial frontal lobe (Scepkowski and Cronin-Golomb, 2003).

## MEMORY

### Forms and Stages of Declarative Memory

Generally defined, *memory* refers to the ability of the brain to store and retrieve information, the necessary prerequisite for all learning. Some memories are so vivid they seem like a reliving of a prior experience, as in Marcel Proust's sudden recollections of his youth on biting into a madeleine pastry. Other memories are more vague or bring up a series of facts rather than a perceptual experience. Memory has been divided into several types and stages, leading to a confusing set of terms and concepts. Clinical neurologists have historically divided memory into three temporal stages. These stages can be helpful when conceptualizing diagnosis and difficulties in independent living and have a general correspondence to the stages and concepts of memory proposed by cognitive neuroscientists. The first stage, referred to as *immediate memory* by clinicians, corresponds to Baddeley's concept of *working memory* (Baddeley, 2010). *Immediate or working memory* refers to the system that actively holds pieces of transitory information in conscious awareness, where it can be subsequently manipulated or used to perform a task. There has been recent debate over the true capacity of working memory (Cowan, 2001), but the general consensus is that the normal adult human being can retain 5–9 meaningful items in working memory (Miller, 1956). This information can generally reside in conscious awareness indefinitely with attention and rehearsal. However, without rehearsal, this information is lost in approximately 18–20 seconds (Brown, 1958; Peterson and Peterson, 1959). As an example, most people can hear or see a telephone number, walk across the room, and dial the number without difficulty. Once the number is dialed and conversation is started, the number fades from working memory. Relying primarily on prefrontal brain regions, working memory declines with normal aging. Furthermore, disorders of attention, focal lesions of the superior frontal neocortex affecting Brodmann areas 8 and 9, and patients with aphasia secondary to left frontal lesions can show profound impairment in working memory (Goldman-Rakic, 1996).

The second stage of memory, referred to by clinicians as *short-term* or *recent memory*, involves the ability to encode and retrieve specific items, such as words or events, after a delay of minutes or hours. Some of the aforementioned confusion over terminology comes from the fact that cognitive psychologists posit that working memory underlies short-term memory and consider it distinct from episodic learning and memory. In clinical parlance, short-term memory is synonymous with recent episodic memory, whereas some cognitive psychologists use "short-term" to mean immediate memory. Short-term or recent episodic memory requires the function of the hippocampus and parahippocampal areas of the medial temporal lobe for both encoding and storage. The amygdala, a structure adjacent to the medial temporal cortex, is not essential for episodic memory but seems crucial for the encoding of emotional or social contexts of specific events (Markowitsch and Staniloiu, 2011). In contrast, the retrieval of recent episodic memories tends to rely on a delicate interaction between prefrontal regions and medial temporal regions. Budson and Price (2005) provide a simple analogy for remembering the anatomical organization of recent episodic memory. In this analogy, the frontal lobes are considered the "filing clerk" of the memory system, deciding what memories to retrieve and from where to retrieve them. The medial temporal lobes are the "recent memory filing cabinet," where recent memories are stored. Patients with medial temporal lobe damage (e.g., Alzheimer disease) have a damaged file cabinet, in which memories are unable to be stored. In contrast, patients with frontal lobe damage (e.g., stroke, tumor) have difficulty in properly organizing the files in the cabinet or difficulty locating them during retrieval. Finally, in patients with subcortical white matter pathology (e.g., ischemic disease, multiple sclerosis), the file clerk has difficulty gaining access to the file cabinet, which makes retrieval difficult. However, once given an option between multiple files—through a recognition or multiple-choice test—the file clerk can correctly identify the needed file. Commonly used bedside tests assess recent episodic memory. The patient is asked to recall three to five unrelated items at 5 minutes (testing the file cabinet). For any unrecalled words, the patient is given a hint or cue (testing the file clerk). Questions about this morning's breakfast are also effective. It is relatively easy to test for impairment in recent episodic memory by including general questions about recent events in one's life or the news in rapport building and interview.

The third stage, referred to as *remote* or *long-term* episodic memory, refers to the ability to retrieve specific items, such as words or events, after a delay of weeks, months, or years. An example of this would be asking patients about the last movie they have seen or what they did on their last birthday. Retrieval of remote episodic memories tends to require less hippocampal and medial temporal lobe involvement (Dudai, 2004). Consolidation of long-term memories can occur at the synaptic and systems levels. Synaptically, consolidation occurs through long-term potentiation and protein synthesis in the hippocampus during the first few hours of learning (Roediger et al., 2007). In contrast, on a systems level, consolidation occurs over long periods of time where hippocampal-dependent memory representations are stored in the neocortex. Hippocampal activation appears to decline linearly as time passes (Frankland and Bontempi, 2005; Squire et al., 2015. In other words, the older the memory, the less the hippocampus and medial temporal regions are needed for retrieval. This was previously demonstrated through patient H.M. and patients with Alzheimer disease who cannot retrieve recent information or events, but can easily recall events from many years ago. Similarly to short-term episodic memory, the frontal lobes are required to retrieve memories, but rather than the hippocampus, the file clerk must access memories in cortical regions.

Remaining within the realm of long-term declarative memory, there appears to be overlap in the type of information retrieved for remote memories. In addition to episodic memory, which according to Tulving (1985) requires some type of "mental time travel" to revisit the original experience, *semantic memories* can be retrieved. Semantic memory is referred to as factual knowledge that includes memory of meanings, understandings, and other concept-based knowledge as well as general knowledge about the world. Recall of famous figures or events, such as presidents or wars, and knowledge of semantic information, such as the definitions of words and the differences between words, are examples of semantic memory. Semantic memory differs from personal long-term memory in that the subject can continuously replenish such knowledge by reading and conversation.

Semantic memory is thought to reside in multiple cortical regions such as the visual association cortex for visual memories and the temporal cortex for auditory memories. This concept of multiple localizations of semantic memory is supported by functional brain imaging research (Cappa, 2008). Specific semantic knowledge of word meanings is thought to reside in the left lateral temporal cortex. Remote memory, as we shall see later, resists the effects of medial temporal damage; once memory is well stored in the neocortex, it can be retrieved without use of the hippocampal system.

TABLE 7.1 **Memory Stages**

| Traditional Term | Cognitive Neuroscience Term | Awareness Level | Anatomy |
|---|---|---|---|
| Immediate memory | Working memory | Explicit | Prefrontal cortex |
| Short-term memory | Episodic memory | Explicit | Medial temporal lobe |
| Long-term memory | Semantic memory | Explicit | Lateral temporal and other cortices |
| Motor memory | Procedural memory | Implicit | Basal ganglia, cerebellum |

Other nondeclarative categories of memory, such as motor and procedural memories, will be discussed later in this chapter. Table 7.1 is a classification of memory stages.

## Formation and Retrieval of Episodic Memories

Recently, the use of functional brain imaging in healthy human subjects and computational modeling has contributed to knowledge of the anatomy of episodic memory function. A network of structures has been identified in the encoding or formation of episodic memory. Although the hippocampus and all of its subregions are critical to the encoding of information, it is highly connected (both structurally and functionally) to the amygdala, entorhinal cortex, perirhinal cortex, temporal pole, insula, ventromedial prefrontal cortex, anterior and posterior cingulate, precuneus, and inferior parietal cortex (Kier et al., 2004; Poppenk and Moscovitch, 2011), which have all been implicated in the role of episodic memory. When sensory information is processed by specific sensory cortices (e.g., the occipital lobe for visual information), prefrontal regions attend and select important information to be encoded into memory. To-be-remembered information passes through the entorhinal cortex and into the hippocampus through the dentate gyrus (Rolls, 2007). The dentate gyrus acts as a "pattern separator" creating unique memory representations as it passes information to hippocampal subregion CA3 (Yassa and Stark, 2011). Subregion CA3 acts as its own autoassociation network whereby recurrent projections onto itself work to store a memory representation temporarily for later recall (Hunsaker and Kesner, 2013; for review see Rebola et al., 2017).

According to early positron emission tomography (PET) work, several brain regions show consistent activation in healthy subjects during memory retrieval. These brain regions include (1) the prefrontal cortex, especially on the right; (2) the hippocampus and adjacent medial temporal regions; (3) the anterior cingulate cortex; (4) the posterior midline regions of the cingulate, precuneate, and cuneate gyri; (5) the inferior parietal cortex, especially on the right; and (6) the cerebellum, particularly on the left (Cabeza et al., 1997). A model for the functions of these areas in memory is as follows: the prefrontal cortex appears to relate to attention, retrieval activation, and memory search; the hippocampi, particularly subregions CA3 and CA1, to conscious recollection of recently learned information; the cingulate cortex to the activation of memory and selection of a specific response; the posterior midline regions to visual imagery; the parietal cortex to spatial and memory awareness; and the cerebellum to voluntary self-initiated retrieval (Cabeza et al., 1997; Dickerson and Eichenbaum, 2010; Wagner et al., 1998). In subjects asked to recognize previously presented pairs of associated words, the right prefrontal cortex, anterior cingulate cortex, and inferior parietal region were the most activated. When the subject had to recall the words, the basal ganglia and left cerebellum also became active. In similar studies using functional MRI, Wagner and colleagues (1998) found that the left prefrontal region was predominantly involved when words were semantically encoded in memory; the right frontal activations seen in the previous study reflected nonverbal memory stimuli. Even in the hippocampus, words elicited activation of the left hippocampus, objects evoked activation in both hippocampi, and faces mainly activated the right hippocampus (Fliessbach et al., 2010; Rosazza et al., 2009). In studies of the recognition of visual designs, Petersson and colleagues (1997) found that the medial temporal cortex activates more during new learning tasks than during previously trained and practiced memory tasks. Other areas activated during the new learning task included the prefrontal and anterior cingulate areas, more on the right side, and the parieto-occipital lobes bilaterally. Trained tasks activated the hippocampi much less but did activate the right infero-occipitotemporal region. This finding correlates with human studies indicating that overlearned memories gradually become less dependent on the hippocampus. Rugg and colleagues (1997) also found greater activation of the left medial temporal cortex in tasks in which the subject remembered words by "deep encoding" of their meaning compared with simpler "shallow" encoding of the specific word. Other studies have shown that the deeper the encoding of a word's meaning, the better the subject remembers it (Schacter, 1996). Finally, the amygdala appears necessary for affective aspects of memory items, such as recall of fear associated with a specific stimulus (Knight et al., 2009).

Basic research on animals has begun to unravel the fundamental biochemical processes involved in memory. Bailey et al. (1996) have studied memory formation in the giant snail, *Aplysia*. Development of long-term facilitation, a primitive form of memory, requires activation of a gene called *CREB* (cyclic adenosine monophosphate response element-binding protein) in sensory neurons. This work formed the basis of the Nobel Prize awarded to Eric Kandel, who has remained prolific in the field of memory (for review see Kandel, 2012). In this system and also in similar studies on the fruit fly, *Drosophila*, gene activation and protein synthesis are necessary for memory formation. Injection of protein-synthesis inhibitors into the hippocampus can prevent consolidation of memories (McGaugh, 2000). Although similar studies have not been performed in humans, it is likely that similar gene activation and protein synthesis, perhaps beginning in the hippocampi but proceeding through its neocortical connections, are necessary for the transition from immediate working memory to longer-term storage of memory (Bear, 1997). This field of research may hold promise for the development of drugs to enhance memory storage.

## Amnestic Syndrome

*The amnestic syndrome* (Box 7.1) refers to profound loss of recent or short-term episodic memory. These patients, most of whom have bilateral hippocampal damage, have normal immediate and working memory span and largely normal ability to recall remote and semantic memories such as their childhood upbringing and education. Other cognitive or higher cortical functions may be completely intact (e.g., attention, executive functioning, language), which distinguishes these patients from those with dementias such as Alzheimer disease. Procedural or motor memory (see "Other Types of Memory," later in this chapter) tends to remain preserved in patients with amnestic syndrome, who may be taught to perform a new motor skill such as mirror writing. When asked to perform the newly learned skill again, the patient will typically not recall knowing how to do it, but the motor skill remains active, and the patient can easily demonstrate the

## BOX 7.1 Amnestic Syndrome Features

Impaired recent memory (anterograde, retrograde)
Global amnesia
Spared procedural memory
Preserved immediate memory
Preserved remote memory
Intact general cognitive function
Disorientation to time or place
Confabulation

skill. Other more variable features of the amnestic syndrome include potential disorientation to time and place. Furthermore, the amnestic syndrome can include *confabulation*, or making up information the memory system does not supply. Amnestic patients live in an eternal present in which they can interact, speak intelligently, and reason appropriately, but they do not remember anything about the interaction a few minutes after it ends. An amnestic patient may complete an IQ test within the normal or even above-normal range but not recall taking the examination minutes later. These patients are condemned to repeat the same experiences without learning from them. Memory research owes a great debt to the patient H.M., who underwent bilateral medial temporal resection for intractable epilepsy and lost all short-term memory, surviving for more than 50 years in this amnestic state (Corkin, 2002, Dittrich and Patient, 2016; Squire, 2009; ). He was the experimental subject from whom much of our knowledge of the amnestic syndrome derives.

The registration of short-term episodic memory involves a consolidation period during which a blow to the head, as in a football injury, can prevent memories from being stored or recalled. The recognition or recall of newly learned information appears to require the hippocampus. The site of storage of memories, as noted earlier, likely involves large areas of the neocortex specialized for specific cognitive functions such as auditory or visual analysis. Once processed in the neocortex and stored for a long period of time, items can be recalled even in the presence of hippocampal damage, as in the case of remote or semantic memories. After an injury producing hippocampal damage, a retrograde period of memory loss may extend back from minutes to years, and the subject cannot form new anterograde memories. As the ability to form new memories returns, the period of retrograde amnesia shortens or "shrinks" ("shrinking retrograde amnesia"). After a minor head injury, the permanent amnestic period may involve a few minutes of retrograde amnesia and a few hours or days of anterograde amnesia. In experimental studies in which amnestic subjects are shown famous people from past decades, a temporal gradient has been found in which subjects have excellent memory for remote personages but recall progressively less from periods dating up to the recent past.

The neuroanatomy of the amnestic syndrome is one of the best-studied areas of cognitive neuropsychology. In animal models, bilateral lesions of the hippocampus, parahippocampal gyrus, and entorhinal cortex produce profound amnesia (Squire and Zola, 1996). Human patients undergoing temporal lobectomy for epilepsy have shown very similar syndromes. In the early period of this surgery, a few patients were deliberately subjected to bilateral medial temporal ablations, with disastrous results for memory, as seen in H.M. (Corkin, 2002; Squire, 2009). In other cases, unilateral temporal lobectomy caused severe amnesia. In one such case, published by the neurosurgeon Wilder Penfield late in his life, an autopsy many years after the surgery showed preexisting damage to the contralateral hippocampus. Patients currently receive extensive evaluation (e.g., the Wada intracarotid barbiturate infusion test) to ensure that

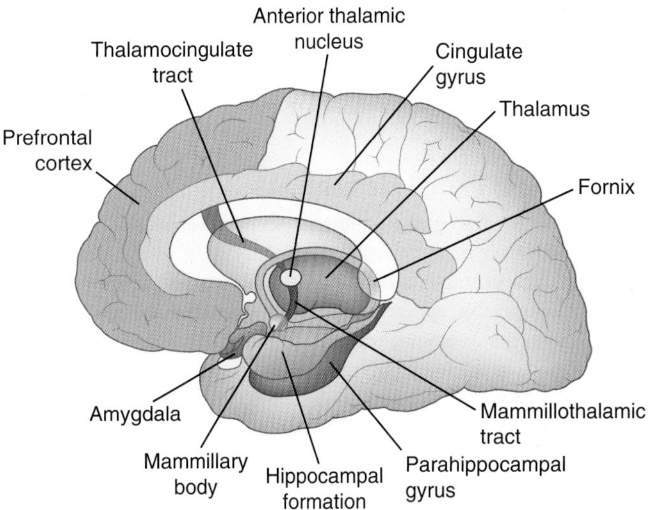


**Fig. 7.2 Episodic Memory.** The medial temporal lobes, including the hippocampus and parahippocampus, form the core of the episodic memory system. Other brain regions are also necessary for episodic memory to function correctly. (*Adapted from Budson, A.E., Price, B.H., 2005. Memory dysfunction. N Engl J Med 352, 692–699.*)

ablation of one hippocampus will not result in an amnestic syndrome, although partial memory deficits still occur. Other common causes of the amnestic syndrome involving bilateral medial temporal lesions include bilateral strokes in the posterior cerebral artery territory, involving the hippocampus, and herpes simplex encephalitis, which has a predilection for the orbitofrontal and medial temporal cortices. Gold and Squire (2006) described three new cases of the amnestic syndrome with detailed neurobehavioral testing in life and neuropathology at autopsy. One had bilateral hippocampal damage, one had Wernicke-Korsakoff syndrome with damage in the mammillary bodies and dorsomedial thalamus, and one had bilateral thalamic infarctions. We will return to these other anatomical substrates of memory later.

Although the neuroanatomy of memory storage and retrieval has been known for many years, numerous recent refinements have been made. Fig. 7.2 shows a simplified diagram of the memory system in the human brain. The hippocampus on each side projects via the fornix to the septal areas, then to the mammillary bodies, which in turn project to the anterior nucleus of the thalamus and on to the cingulate gyrus of the frontal lobe, which projects back to the hippocampus. This circuit (Papez circuit) is critical for short-term memory registration and retrieval. Disease processes that affect extrahippocampal parts of this circuit also cause amnesia. One well-studied example is the Wernicke-Korsakoff syndrome induced by thiamine deficiency, usually in the setting of alcoholism, with damage to the mammillary bodies and dorsomedial thalamic nuclei (Gold and Squire, 2006). A second clinical example is that of patients with ruptured aneurysms of the anterior communicating artery, which are associated with damage to the deep medial frontal areas such as the septal nuclei. These two amnestic syndromes are commonly associated with confabulation. The anterior communicating artery aneurysm syndrome also involves frontal executive dysfunction (Diamond et al., 1997). Traumatic brain injuries commonly produce memory loss, probably because the most common sites of damage are in the frontal and temporal lobes, but other deficits besides memory frequently occur. Of course, memory loss can be seen in several other neurological conditions, including brain tumors of the thalamus or temporal lobes, white matter diseases such as multiple sclerosis, and dementing diseases such as Alzheimer disease, which has a predilection for the entorhinal cortex, perirhinal cortex, hippocampus, basal frontal nuclei, and neocortex (Braak and Braak, 1991). In these other disorders, memory loss is usually not as isolated a deficit as in the amnestic syndrome.

### Syndromes of Partial Memory Loss

In contrast to the global amnesia seen in amnestic syndrome, patients who have memory loss for selected classes of items have been described. For example, patients who undergo left temporal lobectomy for intractable epilepsy usually have detectable impairment of short-term verbal memory, whereas those undergoing right temporal resection have impairment only of nonverbal memory. Isolated sensory-specific memory loss syndromes have also been described, such as pure visual or tactile memory loss. Ross (1980) described two patients with bilateral occipital lesions that disconnected the visual cortex from the memory structures. These patients could draw a diagram of their homes but could not learn new spatial layouts. Ross postulated that diagnosis of a selective visual recent memory deficit requires documentation of normal visual perception, absence of aphasia sufficient to impair testing, intact immediate visual memory, intact remote visual memory, and normal recent memory in other modalities. A similar syndrome of isolated tactile memory loss has also been described.

### Transient Amnesia

Transient amnesia is a temporary version of the amnestic syndrome. The most striking example of transient amnesia is the syndrome of transient global amnesia, lasting from several to 24 hours (Kirshner, 2011, 2017). In this syndrome, an otherwise cognitively intact individual suddenly loses memory for recent events, asks repetitive questions about his or her environment, and sometimes confabulates. During the episode, the patient has both anterograde and retrograde amnesia, as in the permanent amnestic syndrome. However, as recovery occurs, the retrograde portion "shrinks" to a short period, leaving a permanent gap in memory of the brief retrograde amnesia before the episode and the period of no learning during the episode. The syndrome is of unknown cause but can be closely imitated by disorders of known etiology such as partial complex seizures, migraine, and possibly transient ischemia of the hippocampus on one or both sides. Strupp and colleagues (1998) reported that 7 of 10 patients imaged during episodes of transient global amnesia showed abnormal diffusion MRI signal in the left hippocampus; 3 of these had bilateral hippocampal abnormalities. Permanent infarctions were not found. More specifically, the CA1 region within the hippocampus has been strongly implicated in transient global amnesia (for review see Bartsch & Deuschl, 2010) with many studies showing lesions using diffusion-weighted MRI in the CA1 region in cases of transient global amnesia (TGA) (Bartsch et al., 2006; Lee et al., 2007; Yang et al., 2008). Other investigators have found frontal lobe abnormalities by diffusion-weighted MRI or PET. Gonzalez-Martinez and colleagues (2010) reported a case in which a small left thalamic infarction found by diffusion-weighted MRI was associated with hypometabolism in the left thalamic region, seen on fluorodeoxyglucose (FDG) PET. These studies do not prove an ischemic etiology for transient global amnesia; rather, they indicate transient dysfunction in the hippocampus or its connections. The last several patients with transient global amnesia observed at our hospital have had normal diffusion-weighted MRI studies, except for two patients who had incomplete recovery; these patients both had left medial temporal infarctions. Confusional migraine, partial epilepsy (Bilo et al., 2009), drug intoxication, alcoholic "blackouts," and minor head injuries can also produce transient amnesia.

**TABLE 7.2 Types of Memory and Their Localization**

| Types of Recent Memory | Localization |
|---|---|
| **Declarative (Explicit)** | |
| Facts, events | Medial temporal lobe |
| **Nondeclarative (Implicit)** | |
| Procedural skills | Basal ganglia, frontal lobes |
| Classical conditioning | Cerebellum (+ amygdala) |
| Probabilistic classification learning | Basal ganglia |
| Priming | Neocortex |

## OTHER TYPES OF MEMORY (NONDECLARATIVE OR IMPLICIT MEMORY)

A confusing array of memory classifications and terminology has arisen, as shown in Table 7.2. Several aspects of memory do not involve the conscious recall involved in the three temporal memory stages. A simple example is motor memory, such as the ability to ride a bicycle, which is remarkably resistant to hippocampal damage. Such motor memories probably reside in the basal ganglia and cerebellum. In Squire and Zola's (1996) classification, motor memories of this type are called *procedural* or *implicit nondeclarative memories*; note that all three of the temporal stages of memory—working (immediate) memory, episodic (short-term) memory, and semantic (long-term) memory—are *declarative, explicit.*

Another term for the class of memories for which subjects have no conscious awareness is *implicit* or *nondeclarative memory* (in contrast to the explicit, declarative memory of episodic events). Implicit memories have in common storage and retrieval mechanisms that do not involve the hippocampal system; perhaps for this reason, the subject has no conscious knowledge of them. These procedural memories involve "knowing how" rather than "knowing that." Amnestic patients can learn new motor memories such as mirror drawing, which they can perform once started, although they have no recollection of knowing the task. Motor learning likely involves the supplementary motor cortex, basal ganglia, and cerebellum. Strokes in the territory of the recurrent artery of Heubner (affecting the caudate nucleus) can affect procedural memory (Mizuta and Motomura, 2006). Another type of memory localized to the cerebellum is *classical conditioning*, in which an unconditioned stimulus becomes associated with a reward or punishment given when the conditioned stimulus is presented (Clark et al., 2002; Thompson and Kim, 1996). The conditioning itself clearly involves the cerebellum, but the emotional aspect of the reward or punishment stimulus may reside in the amygdala. Classical conditioning can continue to function after bilateral hippocampal damage. Squire and Zola (1996) outlined other types of nondeclarative memory that take place independent of the hippocampal system. Probabilistic classification learning (e.g., predicting the weather from a combination of cues that are regularly associated with sunny or rainy weather) is unaffected by hippocampal damage but impaired in diseases of the basal ganglia such as Huntington and Parkinson diseases (Gluck et al., 2002; Thompson and Kim, 1996). Learning artificial grammar can also take place in the presence of amnestic syndrome, with functional imaging showing activation in the left parietal and occipital lobes (Skosnik et al., 2002). In all these memory experiments, the subject has no awareness of how he or she is able to answer the questions. The last form of nondeclarative memory is called *priming*, the presentation of a stimulus associated with the word or idea to be remembered, which then aids in retrieval of the item (e.g., recalling the word *doctor* when *nurse* appears on a priming list). Priming appears to involve the neocortex (Levy et al., 2004; Thompson and Kim, 1996). Schacter and Buckner (1998) have shown that deliberate use of priming can help amnestic patients to compensate for their memory loss in everyday life.

## BEDSIDE TESTS OF MEMORY AND COGNITIVE FUNCTION

The most important point to be made about bedside evaluations of cognition and memory is that they are an integral part of the neurological examination and a tool by which the neurologist localizes lesions affecting the higher cortical functions, just as the motor or cerebellar examinations localize neurological deficits. The most common error made by neurologists is to omit a systematic evaluation of mental function in patients who seem "alert and oriented." Deficits of memory, deficits in fund of knowledge, or focal deficits such as alexia, apraxia, agnosia, acalculia, or constructional impairment can be missed. Some patients have a "cocktail party" conversational pattern that belies such deficits; others become expert at deferring questions to a spouse or family member. Every neurologist has the task of deciding which patients need formal cognitive testing and whether to make up an individual test routine or to rely on one of the standard tests. Again, it is more important to make the assessment than to follow a specific format.

The formal mental status examination should always include explicit testing of orientation including the date, place, and situation. Memory testing should include an immediate attention test, of which the most popular are forward digit span, serial-7 subtractions from 100, or "spell world backward." Short-term memory should include recall of three to five unrelated words at 5 minutes followed by a recognition paradigm to elicit recall of unremembered words. Importantly, the patient must say all the words after presentation to make sure the items have been properly registered. At times, nonverbal short-term memory, such as recalling the locations of three hidden coins or reproducing drawings, can be useful to test, especially in the case of profound aphasia or verbal impairments. Remote memory can be tested by having the patient name children or siblings. Fund of information can be tested with recall of recent presidents or other political figures. For patients who do not pay attention to politics, use of athletic stars or television celebrities may be more appropriate. Language testing should include spontaneous speech, naming, repetition, auditory comprehension, reading, and writing (the bedside language test is described in more detail in Chapter13) . In our practice, we show patients more difficult naming items such as the drawings from the National Institutes of Health (NIH) Stroke Scale or body parts such as the thumb or the palm of the hand. Praxis testing should include the use of both imaginary and real (e.g., saw, hammer, pencil) objects. Both hands should be tested separately. Calculation tasks include the serial-7 subtraction test and simple change-making problems. Visual-spatial-constructional tasks can include line bisection, copying a cube or intersecting pentagons or another design, or drawing a clock or a house (Fig. 7.3). Many neurologists supplement assessment of this domain with the clock-drawing test. Insight and judgment are generally best tested by assessing the patient's understanding of his own illness. Formal assessment includes interpretation of proverbs (e.g., "Those who live in glass houses should not throw stones") or abstraction (stating how an apple and an orange are similar). Another bedside tool used to test frontal lobe processing, or executive function, is the copying and continuation of Luria's test of alternating sequences (sequential squares and triangles; see Fig. 7.1). A similar measure, also attributed to Luria, is the "fist/side/palm" repetitive movement. With these tests, preliminary localization can be made in the deep memory structures of the medial temporal lobes, the left hemisphere language cortex in the frontal and temporal lobes, the left parietal region (calculations, apraxia), and the right parietal lobe (visual-constructional tasks), or the frontal lobes (insight and judgment, proverbs, similarities, Luria's sequence test).

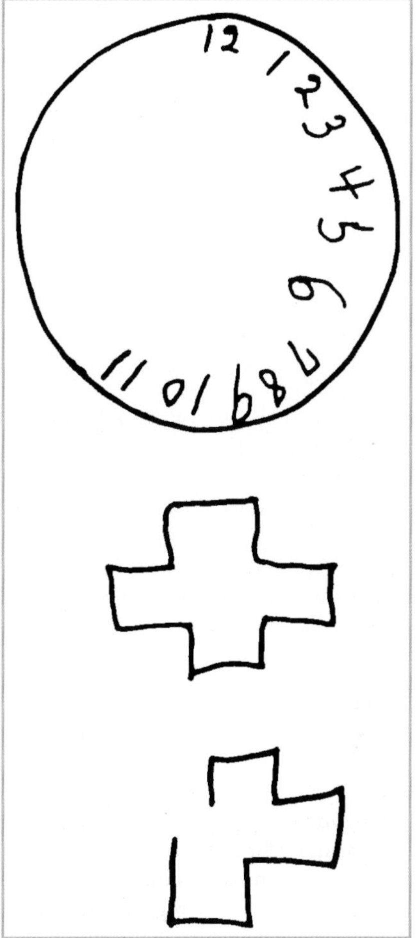

**Fig. 7.3** Spontaneous clock drawing and copying of a cross by a patient with a right parietal infarction. The patient had only mild hemiparesis but dense left hemianopia and neglect of the left side of the body. The neglect of the left side of space is evident in both drawings. (*Reprinted with permission from Kirshner, H.S., 2002. Behavioral Neurology: Practical Science of Mind and Brain, second ed. Butterworth-Heinemann, Boston.*)

Several versions of formal bedside mental status testing have been published, including Folstein's Mini-Mental State Examination (MMSE), the Montreal Cognitive Assessment (MoCA) tool, Kokmen Short Test of Mental Status, Saint Louis University Mental Status (SLUMS), and the Mini Cog (3-word recall and Clock Drawing Test). Perhaps the most widely used is the MMSE, consisting of 30 points: 5 for orientation to time (year, season, month, date, and day), 5 for orientation to place (state, county, town, hospital, and floor), 5 for attention (either serial 7s with 1 point for each of the first five subtractions or "spell *world* backward"), 3 for registration of three items, 3 for recall of three items after 5 minutes, 2 for naming a pencil and a watch, 1 for repeating "no ifs, ands, or buts," 3 for following a three-stage command, 1 for following a printed command ("close your eyes"), 1 for writing a sentence, and 1 for copying a diagram of two intersecting pentagons.

The advantages of the MMSE are short time of administration and quantitation, useful in documentation for insurance benefits, such as rehabilitative therapies or drug therapy, and for disability assessment.

Several disadvantages of the MMSE have been identified. First, the normal range of scores depends on education. The low-normal cutoff is estimated by Crum and colleagues (1993) to be 19 for uneducated people, 23 for graduates of elementary or junior high school, 27 for high school graduates, and 29 for college graduates. Second, age is also a factor. Third, even an abnormal score does not distinguish a focal lesion from a more diffuse disorder such as an encephalopathy or dementia. Fourth, the test is weighted toward orientation and language, and results can be normal in patients with right hemisphere or frontal lobe damage. Finally, the test is less sensitive to very early or subtle cognitive decline, such as within the mild cognitive impairment or prodromal phase of Alzheimer disease. To address these latter limitations, the MoCA was developed to assess more comprehensively multiple cognitive domains and provide more sensitivity to the identification of mild cognitive impairment. Like the MMSE, the MoCA is a 30-point test assessing executive functioning and abstraction, visuospatial skills, language, attention, verbal recall, and orientation. The SLUMS and Kokmen have similar designs.

One answer to the dilemma of mental status testing is to use one of the aforementioned assessment tools as a screening test and then supplement it with more focused tests. Box 7.2 lists the key elements of a mental status examination, whether the examiner chooses to adopt the MMSE or one of the other bedside cognitive instruments, or to create an individual test battery. Several texts provide further detail on such a battery. Although the mental status examination is the most neglected area of the neurological examination, it generally requires only a few minutes, and its cost-effectiveness compares well with brain imaging studies such as MRI or PET.

In addition to formal examination, an experienced clinician can learn much about the patient's mental status by careful observation during the history. Considerable insight can be gained into the patient's recent memory, orientation, language function, affect or mood, insight, and judgment. Affect and mood are best assessed in this fashion; if there is doubt, the clinician should consider how the patient makes the clinician feel: a depressed patient often elicits sadness or depressed mood, whereas a manic patient makes the clinician feel happy and amused.

In conclusion, this chapter considers the areas of neurology that most physicians find the most abstruse—namely, the higher cortical functions, intellect, and memory. As stated at the outset, this area of neurology can be treated as a series of specific functions to be analyzed at the bedside and localized, just like other functions of the nervous system. In fact, the rapidly increasing knowledge of cognitive neuroscience and our vastly improved ability to image the brain both at rest and during functional activities promise a new era of practical diagnosis of higher cognitive disorders.

### BOX 7.2 Bedside Mental Status Examination

Orientation (time, place, person, situation)
Memory (immediate, short term, long term)
Fund of information
Speech and language
Praxis
Calculations
Visual-constructional abilities
Abstract reasoning, sequential processes

*The complete reference list is available online at https://expertconsult.inkling.com/.* 

# 8

# Global Developmental Delay and Regression

*Rachel Goode, Alice Lawrence, Tyler Reimschisel*

## OUTLINE



Developmental delay occurs in approximately 1%–3% of children. Since developmental delay is common, monitoring a child's development is an essential component of well-child care. Ongoing assessment of the child's development at each well-child visit creates a pattern of development that is more useful than measuring the discrete milestone achievements at a single visit; therefore, developmental screening should be completed at each well-child visit (Council on Children with Disabilities, 2006). Identification of a child with developmental delays should be accomplished as early as possible, because the earlier a child is identified, the sooner the child can receive a thorough evaluation and begin therapeutic interventions that can improve the child's outcome. Developmental delay is common and one of the most frequent presenting complaints to a pediatric neurology clinic; therefore, neurologists should have a systematic approach to the child with developmental delay.

This chapter begins with a brief discussion of child development concepts related to typical and atypical development. Next, the clinical evaluation and management of developmental delay is reviewed. The chapter closes with a discussion of neurological regression.

## TYPICAL AND ATYPICAL DEVELOPMENT

### Child Development Concepts

A child's development is a continuous process of acquiring new and advanced skills. This development depends on maturation of the nervous system. Although typical child development follows a relatively consistent sequence, it is not linear. Instead, there are spurts and lags. For example, motor development in the first year of life proceeds relatively rapidly. Babies typically mature from being completely immobile to walking in just over 12 months, but then motor development progresses less dramatically during the second year of life. Conversely, language development in the first year of life occurs slowly, but there is an explosion of language acquisition between a child's first and second birthdays.

On average, most children achieve each developmental milestone within a defined and narrow age range (Table 8.1). Since each developmental skill can be acquired within an age range, it is imperative that professionals know what is typical to better determine when a child's development falls outside this range. These so-called red flags are important because they can be used to identify when a child has developmental delay for specific skills. For example, although the average age of walking is approximately 13 months, a child may walk as late as 17 months and still be within the typical developmental range. In this example, the red flag for independent walking is 18 months, and a child who is not walking by 18 months of age is delayed.

## GLOBAL DEVELOPMENTAL DELAY

### Developmental History

Child development is classically divided into five interdependent domains or streams: motor (gross and fine), problem-solving/cognitive, language (receptive and expressive), socialization, and adaptive. The approach to a child with possible developmental delays is based on a working knowledge of these domains and the typical age ranges for acquiring specific milestones within each domain. Therefore, the clinician should begin the evaluation of a child with developmental concerns by obtaining a developmental history, and emphasis should be placed on the pattern of milestone acquisition as well as the child's current developmental skills. Clinicians working in a busy clinical setting may need to base this history primarily on the caregiver's report of the child's developmental abilities. Clinicians may also use standardized tools to aid in this portion of the history, including the Ireton Child Development Inventory (CDI), the Ages and Stages Questionnaire (ASQ), the Parents' Evaluation of Developmental Status (PEDS), and/or the Modified Checklist for Autism in Toddlers (MCHAT) (Council on Children with Disabilities, 2006, 2007). However, if the clinician's history confirms a developmental disability, standardized testing by a developmental specialist or clinical psychologist should be strongly considered; this formal evaluation will provide a much better assessment of the child's developmental abilities.

When there is concern about developmental delay in a child, a developmental quotient should be calculated. The *developmental quotient* is the ratio of the child's developmental age over the chronological age. The developmental quotient should be calculated for each developmental stream. Typical development is a developmental quotient greater than 70%, and atypical development is a developmental

**TABLE 8.1 Typical Developmental Milestones by Age (50th–75th Percentile)**

| Age | Language | Socialization | Motor | Cognitive | Adaptive |
|---|---|---|---|---|---|
| 2 months | Coos (ooh, ah) Video 8.1c | Smiles with social contact (Video 8.1a) | Holds head up 45 degrees (Video 8.1b) | Focus on face, follows large contrasting object | |
| 3–4 months | Laughs and squeals Video 8.2a, "ah-goo" sound | Sustains social contact, soothes to parent voice | Grasps objects, rolls front to back (4 months), stands with support (Video 8.2c), no head lag (Video 8.2b) | Mouths objects, inspects own hands, shakes rattle | |
| 5–6 months | Razzes, reciprocal vocalizations | Prefers mother, smile/ vocalize to mirror, stranger anxiety | Transfers objects between hands (Video 8.3f), uses a raking grasp (Video 8.3e), rolls back to front (5 months) (Video 8.2d), sits with support (Video 8.3a), hands to feet in supine (Video 8.3b), pivots in prone (Video 8.3c) | Turns head to look for dropped object, removes cloth from face, bangs/ shakes toys | Places hand on breast/ bottle, opens mouth for spoon |
| 8–9 months | Nonspecific "mama/dada," inflection with babbling, looks for family member "where's mama?," orients to name | Uses sound to get attention, separation anxiety, follows a point | Sits alone (Video 8.4c), creeps or crawls (Video 8.4d), pulls to stand (Video 8.4b), radial-digital grasp (Video 8.4e) | Object permanence (Video 8.4a) | Holds bottle, finger feeds diced foods |
| 10–12 months | Says "dada/mama" specifically plus one other word, understands "no," follows one-step command with gestures | Plays simple ball games, plays peek-a-boo, looks preferentially when name is called (Video 8.5c) | Stands alone, cruises (10 months), beginner walking (12 months) (Video 8.5b), inferior pincer grasp | Looks at pictures in book, purposeful release | Adjusts body to dressing, finger feeds well |
| 12–1 months | Immature jargon (13 months), says 2–4 words and/or signs (13 months) (Video 8.6e), follows one-step command without gesture, understands 50–100 words | Indicates desires by pointing (12 months), points to indicate items of interest (14 months), functional play with toys | Walks alone (Video 8.6d), stoops and recovers, transitions floor sit to stand (12–13 months) (Video 8.6c), mature pincer grasp (Video 8.6a) | Dumps pellet from bottle, turns pages in book (Video 8.6b), places circle in single shape puzzle | Cooperates in dressing, removes shoes/ socks, spoon to mouth (flips the spoon) |
| 15–18 months | Says 4–6 words (15 months), says 10–15 words (18 months), uses giant words, animal sounds, points to self | Emerging pretend play, shows empathy | Walks up steps with a hand held, imitates scribbling, stacks two blocks | Points to one body part (15 months), points to three body parts (18 months) | Uses spoon, drinks from cup, removes garment |
| 18–24 months | Emerging 2 word phrases, 25–50 words, points to 2–4 pictures | Reciprocal pretend play, kisses with pucker | Walks with reciprocal arm swing and heel strike (Video 8.8c), kicks a ball (Video 8.8a), goes up stairs holding rail one step at a time (Video 8.8b), tower of 5–6 cubes, imitates vertical line | Points to 5–6 body parts (22 months), matches pairs of objects | Feeds self with spoon for entire meal, drinks from open cup, unzips zipper |
| 24–30 months | Uses at least 50 words and 2-word sentences (Video 8.9g), understands 250 words, follows two-step command, 50% intelligible | Parallel play, imitates adult activity | Runs well (Video 8.9e), goes down stairs holding rail one step at a time, jumps clearing floor (Video 8.9d), imitates circle, copies a horizontal line (Video 8.9b) | Sorts objects, matches object to picture, matches shapes, matches colors (Video 8.9c) | Takes off clothing without buttons, washes hands, verbalizes toileting needs |
| 30–36 months | Uses pronouns, knows first and last name, counts to 3, asks questions | Reciprocally pretends in play, helps put things away | Climbs stairs with alternate feet, walks on tip-toe ×4 steps (Video 8.10b), copies a vertical and horizontal line, imitates cross | 8–10 cube tower (Video 8.10a), 4-cube train (Video 8.9a), points to body part by function, understands concept of one (Video 11c) | Toilet trained, puts on coat unassisted, brushes teeth without assistance |
| 3 years | Counts 3 objects, 200+ words, three-word sentences, 75% intelligible, understands negatives | Emerging fears, imaginary play, begins to share | Rides a tricycle (Video 8.11d), goes up stairs alternating feet without rail (Video 8.11b), stands on one foot briefly, copies a circle, strings small beads | Copies 3 cube bridge (Video 8.11a), knows age and gender, understands big versus little (Video 8.11e), sorts by shape(Video 8.11f), draws two-part person | Independent eating, unbuttons, toilet trained |

TABLE 8.1 Typical Developmental Milestones by Age (50th–75th Percentile)—cont'd

| Age | Language | Socialization | Motor | Cognitive | Adaptive |
|---|---|---|---|---|---|
| 4 years | Counts 4 objects, 300–1000+ words, tells a story, 100% intelligible, follows three-step instruction | Labels emotions with words, has a preferred friend, engages in group play, understands deception | Hops on one foot, one-leg balance (Video 8.12b), standing broad jump (Video 8.12a), uses scissors to cut out pictures (Video 8.12c), copies a square and a cross | Draws 4–6 part person (Video 8.12d), counts to 4, points to 4 colors | Independent toileting, washes own hands, uses fork well |
| 5 years | Counts 10 objects (Video 8.13a), 2000+ words, speaks in complete sentences, tells stories with beginning, middle, and end, responds to "why" questions | Makes friendships and has a preferred group of friends, apologizes for mistakes | Skips (Video 8.13d), copies a triangle, uses dynamic tripod/quadruped grasp (Video 8.13b), in-hand manipulation (Video 8.13e), rotates pencil (Video 8.13f), puts penny in bank | Draws 8–10 part person, names 8–10 colors (Video 8.13c), identifies coins | Participates in domestic chores, spreads with knife well, dresses and bathes independently |

quotient less than 70%. Toddlers and young children with atypical development are at risk for lifelong developmental problems. The term *global development delay* is used if a child younger than 5–6 years of age has a developmental quotient less than 70% in two or more domains. Children with global developmental delay should receive a thorough medical evaluation to try to determine the cause of the delay and begin management for their developmental disabilities.

## Neurological and Other Medical History

For children with global developmental delay, the clinician should obtain a thorough medical history, including a detailed neurological history. Pertinent aspects of the history include the presence of any other neurological condition such as epilepsy, vision or hearing impairments, ataxia or a movement disorder, sleep impairment, and behavioral problems. The clinician should also inquire about prenatal, perinatal, and postnatal factors that can impact a child's development (Tables 8.2 and 8.3). The social history should probe for environmental factors that can affect development, including physical or other forms of abuse, neglect, psychosocial deprivation, family illness, impaired personalities in family members, sociocultural stressors, and the economic status of the family.

Though families now typically have fewer children, and the caregivers' knowledge of family history is frequently quite limited, the clinician should still make an effort to obtain a three-generation pedigree. The pertinent aspects of the family history include neurodevelopmental disabilities, special education services or failure to graduate from school, neurodegenerative disorders, multiple miscarriages or early postnatal death, ethnicity, and consanguinity. If a specific genetic syndrome is suspected, the clinician should inquire about the presence in other family members of medical problems associated with that syndrome. For example, if the child has the features of fragile X syndrome, the family history should include questions about maternal premature ovarian failure, parkinsonism or ataxia of unknown etiology in the maternal grandfather, and intellectual disability or learning problems in an X-linked pattern.

## Physical Examination

The growth parameters of the child should be measured, and the growth charts should be reviewed to determine the child's rate of growth. This is pertinent because many chromosomal anomalies and other genetic disorders that cause global developmental delay and intellectual disability are associated with failure to thrive or short stature, large stature, microcephaly, and macrocephaly.

TABLE 8.2 Etiology of Developmental Delay by Time of Onset

| Prenatal/Perinatal | Examples |
|---|---|
| Congenital malformations of the CNS | Lissencephaly, holoprosencephaly |
| Chromosomal abnormalities | Down syndrome, Turner syndrome |
| Endogenous toxins | Maternal hepatic or renal failure |
| Exogenous toxins from maternal use | Anticonvulsants, anticoagulants, alcohol, drugs of abuse |
| Fetal infection | Congenital infections |
| Prematurity and/or fetal malnutrition | Periventricular leukomalacia |
| Perinatal trauma | Intracranial hemorrhage, spinal cord injury |
| Perinatal asphyxia | Hypoxic-ischemic encephalopathy |
| **Postnatal** | **Examples** |
| Inborn errors of metabolism | Aminoacidopathies, mitochondrial diseases |
| Abnormal storage of metabolites | Lysosomal storage diseases, glycogen storage diseases |
| Abnormal postnatal nutrition | Vitamin or calorie deficiency |
| Endogenous toxins | Hepatic failure, kernicterus |
| Exogenous toxins | Prescription drugs, illicit substances, heavy metals |
| Endocrine organ failure | Hypothyroidism, Addison disease |
| CNS infection | Meningitis, encephalitis |
| CNS trauma | Diffuse axonal injury, intracranial hemorrhage |
| Neoplasia | Tumor infiltration, radiation necrosis |
| Neurocutaneous syndromes | Neurofibromatosis, tuberous sclerosis complex |
| Neuromuscular disorders | Muscular dystrophy, myotonic dystrophy |
| Vascular conditions | Vasculitis, ischemic stroke, sinovenous thrombosis |
| Other | Epilepsy, mood disorders, schizophrenia |

*CNS*, Central nervous system.

**TABLE 8.3 Perinatal Risk Factors for Neurological Injury**

| Maternal/Prenatal | Natal | Postnatal |
|---|---|---|
| Age <16 years or >35 years | Intrauterine hypoxia: prolapsed umbilical cord, abruptio placentae, circumvallate placenta | Abnormal feeding: poor sucking, weight gain, malnutrition, vomiting |
| Cervical or pelvic abnormalities | Midforceps delivery or breech presentation | Abnormal crying |
| Maternal illnesses: infection, shock, diabetes, nephritis, phlebitis, proteinuria, renal hypertension, thyroid disease, drug addiction, malnutrition | Poor Apgar scores: cyanosis, poor respiratory effort, bradycardia, poor reflexes, hypotonia | Abnormal examination: asymmetrical face, asymmetrical extremities, dysmorphic features, hypotonia, birth injuries, seizures |
| Maternal features: unmarried, uneducated, nonwhite, low-income, thin, short | Need for resuscitation: respiratory distress, bradycardia, hypotension | Abnormal findings: hyperbilirubinemia, fever, hypothermia, hypoxia |
| Consanguinity | Gestational age <30 weeks | |
| Prior abnormal pregnancy, miscarriages, stillbirths, abortions, neonatal deaths, infants less than 1500 g, abnormal placenta | Vaginal bleeding in the second or third trimester | |
| | Hypoxic-ischemic encephalopathy | |
| | Polyhydramnios or oligohydramnios | |

*From Sherr, E.H., Shevell, M.I., 2006. Mental retardation and global developmental delay. In: Swaiman, K.F., Ashwal, S., Ferriero, D.I. (Eds.), Pediatric Neurology, Principles and Practice, fifth edn. Mosby, Philadelphia.*

**TABLE 8.4 Ocular Findings Associated With Selected Syndromic Developmental Disorders**

| Finding | Examples |
|---|---|
| Cataracts | Cerebrotendinous xanthomatosis, galactosemia, Lowe syndrome, LSD, Wilson disease |
| Chorioretinitis | Congenital infections |
| Corneal opacity | Cockayne syndrome, Lowe syndrome, LSD, xeroderma pigmentosa, Zellweger syndrome |
| Glaucoma | Lowe syndrome, mucopolysaccharidoses, Sturge-Weber syndrome, Zellweger syndrome |
| Lens dislocation | Homocystinuria, sulfite oxidase deficiency |
| Macular cherry-red spot | LSD, multiple sulfatase deficiency |
| Nystagmus | Aminoacidopathies, AT, CDG, Chédiak-Higashi syndrome, Friedreich ataxia, Leigh syndrome, Marinesco-Sjögren syndrome, metachromatic leukodystrophy, neuroaxonal dystrophy, Pelizaeus-Merzbacher disease, SCD |
| Ophthalmoplegia | AT, Bassen-Kornzweig syndrome, LSDs, mitochondrial diseases |
| Optic atrophy | Alpers disease, Leber optic atrophy, leukodystrophies, LSDs, neuroaxonal dystrophy, SCD |
| Photophobia | Cockayne syndrome, Hartnup disease, homocystinuria |
| Retinitis pigmentosa or macular degeneration | AT, Bassen-Kornzweig syndrome, Cockayne syndrome, CDG, pantothenate kinase-associated neurodegeneration syndrome, Laurence-Moon-Biedl syndrome, LSD, mitochondrial diseases, Refsum disease, Sjögren-Larsson syndrome, SCD |

*AT,* Ataxia-telangiectasia; *CDG,* congenital disorders of glycosylation; *LSD,* lysosomal storage disease; *SCD,* spinocerebellar degeneration.
*From Sherr, E.H., Shevell, M.I., 2006. Mental retardation and global developmental delay. In: Swaiman, K.F., Ashwal, S., Ferriero, D.I. (Eds.), Pediatric Neurology, Principles and Practice, fifth edn. Mosby, Philadelphia.*

In the mental status portion of the examination, the clinician should note the interactions the child has with his or her caregivers and the clinician. Abnormal behaviors such as impaired eye contact, limited or absent social reciprocity, restricted or repetitive behaviors, and communication impairment may indicate that the child has an autism spectrum disorder, and the child should be referred to a psychologist or developmental pediatrician for assessment or confirmation of this condition. Other abnormal behaviors such as hyperactivity, impulsivity, and inattention, as well as suboptimal parenting skills, may also be noted during these observations. However, the clinician should use caution when raising concerns about a behavior problem based solely on the child's behavior in clinic, since this stressful situation may lead the child to manifest uncharacteristic behaviors.

A complete general physical and neurological examination should be performed to the extent the child will allow. The general examination should include but not be limited to an evaluation for dysmorphic features: abnormalities of the eyes (Table 8.4), skin, and hair; and organomegaly (Table 8.5). The neurological examination should include signs of impairment in extraocular movements; hypertonia or hypotonia; focal or generalized weakness; abnormal posture or movements; abnormal or asymmetrical tendon reflexes; ataxia, incoordination or other signs of cerebellar dysfunction; and gait abnormalities (see Table 8.5).

## Diagnostic Testing

Diagnostic testing in an individual with global developmental delay should be offered to the family, because the testing may provide an etiology for the developmental delays, could alert the physician and family to comorbid conditions the child is at risk for developing, can help provide recurrence information to the family, and may rarely lead to specific medical treatments or therapeutic interventions.

TABLE 8.5 **Other Findings Associated With Selected Syndromic Developmental Disorders**

| Finding | Examples |
|---|---|
| Cerebellar dysfunction | Aminoacidopathies, AT, Bassen-Kornzweig syndrome, CDG, cerebrotendinous xanthomatosis, Chédiak-Higashi syndrome, Cockayne syndrome, Friedreich ataxia, Lafora disease, LSD, Marinesco-Sjögren syndrome, mitochondrial disease, neuroaxonal dystrophy, Pelizaeus-Merzbacher disease, Ramsay Hunt syndrome, SCD, Wilson disease |
| **Hair Abnormalities** | |
| Synophrys | Cornelia de Lange syndrome |
| Fine hair | Homocystinuria, hypothyroidism |
| Kinky hair | Argininosuccinic aciduria, Menkes disease |
| Hirsutism | LSD |
| Balding | Leigh syndrome, progeria |
| Gray hair | AT, Chédiak-Higashi syndrome, Cockayne syndrome, progeria |
| **Hearing Abnormalities** | |
| Hyperacusis | LSD, SSPE, sulfite oxidase deficiency |
| Conductive loss | Mucopolysaccharidoses |
| Sensorineural loss | Adrenoleukodystrophy, CHARGE, Cockayne syndrome, mitochondrial diseases, SCD, Refsum disease |
| Infantile hypotonia | Canavan disease, myopathies, LSD, Leigh syndrome, Menkes disease, neuroaxonal dystrophy, spinal muscular atrophy, Zellweger disease |
| **Limb Abnormalities** | |
| Micromelia | Cornelia de Lange syndrome |
| Broad thumbs | Rubinstein-Taybi syndrome |
| Macrocephaly | Alexander disease, Canavan histiocytosis X, LSD |
| Microcephaly | Alpers disease, CDG, Cockayne syndrome, incontinentia, pigmenti, neuronal ceroid lipofuscinoses, Krabbe disease, neuroaxonal dystrophy, Rett syndrome |
| Movement disorders | AT, LSD, dystonia musculorum deformans, pantothenate kinase-associated neurodegeneration syndrome, juvenile Huntington disease, juvenile Parkinson disease, Lesch-Nyhan disease, phenylketonuria, Wilson disease, xeroderma pigmentosa |
| **Odors** | |
| Cat urine | β-Methyl-crotonyl-CoA carboxylase deficiency |
| Maple | Maple syrup urine disease |
| Musty | Phenylketonuria |
| Rancid butter | Methionine malabsorption syndrome |
| Sweaty feet | Isovaleric academia |
| Organomegaly | Aminoacidopathies, CDG, galactosemia, glycogen storage diseases, LSD, Zellweger syndrome |
| Peripheral neuropathy | AT, Bassen-Kornzweig syndrome, cerebrotendinous xanthomatosis, Cockayne syndrome, LSD, Refsum disease |
| Short stature | Cockayne syndrome, Cornelia de Lange syndrome, hypothyroidism, leprechaunism, LSD, Prader-Willi syndrome, Rubinstein-Taybi syndrome, Seckel bird-headed dwarfism |
| Seizures | Aminoacidopathies, CDG, glycogen synthetase deficiency, HIE, LSD, Menkes disease, mitochondrial diseases, neuroaxonal dystrophy |
| **Skin Abnormalities** | |
| Hyperpigmentation<br>Hypopigmentation | Adrenoleukodystrophy, AT, Farber disease, neurofibromatosis, Niemann-Pick disease, tuberous sclerosis complex, xeroderma pigmentosa |
| Nodules | Chédiak-Higashi syndrome, incontinentia pigmenti, Menkes disease, tuberous sclerosis complex |
| Thick skin | Cerebrotendinous xanthomatosis, Farber disease, neurofibromatosis, LSD, Refsum disease |
| Thin skin | Sjögren-Larsson syndrome, AT, Cockayne syndrome, progeria, xeroderma pigmentosa |

*AT*, Ataxia-telangiectasia; *CDG*, congenital disorders of glycosylation; *CHARGE*, coloboma, heart disease, choanal atresia, retardation, genital anomalies, ear anomalies; *HIE*, hypoxic-ischemic encephalopathy; *LSD*, lysosomal storage diseases; *SCD*, spinocerebellar degeneration; *SSPE*, subacute sclerosing panencephalitis.

*From Sherr, E.H., Shevell, M.I., 2006. Mental retardation and global developmental delay. In: Swaiman, K.F., Ashwal, S., Ferriero, D.I. (Eds.), Pediatric Neurology, Principles and Practice, fifth edn. Mosby, Philadelphia.*

### Genetic Testing

Based on the developmental history obtained, a diagnosis of global developmental delay can be made. In addition, the clinician should attempt to identify an underlying etiology for the delay. Occasionally, the history and examination suggest a specific recognizable genetic condition or other cause. In these situations, confirmatory testing should be performed if possible. For example, a girl with a history of global developmental delay who has acquired microcephaly, epilepsy, and midline hand wringing should be tested for Rett syndrome.

Frequently, however, the underlying cause is unknown despite the acquisition of a comprehensive history and physical examination. In these situations, a chromosomal microarray analysis (CMA) should be offered to the family, since it has the highest diagnostic yield of any single assay for children with global developmental delay: approximately 8%–12%. A clinical CMA tests for submicroscopic deletions or duplications that can be associated with a variety of neurodevelopmental delays, including global developmental delay. This is also the first-line test for individuals with nonspecific intellectual disability, an autism spectrum disorder, and multiple congenital anomalies (Miller et al., 2010). Though this test has a relatively high diagnostic yield, it will typically not detect inversions and other balanced rearrangements. Consequently, if the microarray is within normal limits, a follow-up high-resolution karyotype can be considered.

The CMA is also unable to detect trinucleotide repeat expansions, point mutations, and imprinting abnormalities. Therefore, every child with nonspecific global developmental delay **regardless of gender** should also have fragile-X testing performed. Based on the phenotype, the clinician should also consider performing methylation testing for Angelman and Prader-Willi syndrome, since the microarray analysis will miss the uniparental disomy or imprinting center abnormalities associated with these syndromes. Based on the patient's constellation of clinical features, molecular testing for UBE3A (Angelman syndrome), MeCP2 (Rett syndrome), and other genetic disorders may be considered if the microarray analysis is within normal limits.

In children with global developmental delay, it is important to confirm that the universal newborn screening test was normal at birth. Nonetheless, the diagnostic yield of biochemical testing in a child with nonspecific global developmental delay is quite low (<1%) (Moeschler and Shevell, 2006). The yield may be slightly higher if there is a history of (1) metabolic decompensation, hyperammonemia, hypoglycemia, protein aversion, acidosis, or other evidence of an inborn metabolic disease; (2) neonatal seizures, stroke, movement disorder, or other neurological diagnosis; (3) a family history of unexplained death or neurological disease in a first-degree relative; (4) parental consanguinity; or (5) prenatal history of acute fatty liver of pregnancy (AFLP) or toxemia with hemolysis, elevated liver enzymes, and low platelets (HELLP). Physical examination findings that should increase the suspicion of a metabolic disease include microcephaly, macrocephaly, growth failure, unusual odor, coarse facial features, unusual birthmarks, abnormal hair, hypotonia, dystonia, and focal weakness.

Biochemical tests from the blood to consider in the evaluation of a child with global developmental delay include complete blood count, comprehensive metabolic panel, serum lactate (and possibly serum pyruvate if the result is reliable at the clinician's institution), plasma amino acids, serum creatinine kinase level, uric acid level, and creatine metabolites (in girls). Urine studies to consider include organic acid analysis, purine and pyrimidine metabolites, and creatine metabolites (in boys). Selective metabolic testing may be warranted in specific clinical cases, such as serum 7-dehydrocholesterol level for Smith-Lemli-Opitz syndrome, screening for congenital disorders of glycosylation, biotinidase activity in the blood, cerebrospinal fluid (CSF) neurotransmitter metabolites for neurotransmitter deficiencies, and white blood cell enzyme analysis and urine glycosaminoglycans and oligosaccharides for lysosomal storage diseases.

If the clinical presentation is strongly suggestive of an underlying genetic condition, the microarray analysis is normal, and the other testing discussed earlier is normal or unwarranted based on the phenotype, disability-specific panels (autism panel, intellectual disability panel, etc.) or whole-exome sequencing (WES) using massively parallel next-generation sequencing technologies can be considered (Yang et al., 2013). It is important to note that this testing requires careful pretest and post-test counseling from a geneticist, genetic counselor, or other healthcare professional capable of interpreting and following up on the various results that can be provided through this new technology.

### Neuroimaging

Magnetic resonance imaging (MRI) of the brain has a yield of 65% in children with developmental delay (Shevell et al., 2003). The abnormalities most frequently identified include cerebral malformations, cerebral atrophy, delayed myelination, other white matter changes, postischemic changes, widened Virchow-Robin spaces, and phakomatoses. However, many of these changes are nonspecific and do not lead to the diagnosis of a specific etiology for the developmental delay. The yield of a brain MRI is higher if the child has neurological abnormalities on physical examination such as microcephaly, macrocephaly, focal neurological deficits, epilepsy, strokes, or a movement disorder. Given the non-negligible risk of sedation in a child with global developmental delay, neuroimaging with an MRI should be recommended as a first-line study in children with focal neurological findings and may be offered as a second-line study if genetic testing is nondiagnostic.

Because the diagnostic yield of head computed tomography (CT) is much lower than brain MRI, head CT is primarily indicated in children with global developmental delay who are suspected of having calcifications.

### Other Tests

Electroencephalography (EEG) should be performed in children with global developmental delay who are suspected of having seizures. An EEG should also be obtained in children with regression, even in the absence of spells, to rule out treatable causes of regression, including Landau-Kleffner syndrome, severe absence epilepsy, and electrical status epilepticus during slow-wave sleep. If the child has no history of spells or regression, an EEG is not indicated for routine evaluation of all children with global developmental delay.

Additional diagnostic tests are rarely warranted in children with nonspecific global developmental delay. Specifically, with the advent of massively parallel next-generation sequencing technology, invasive tests such as CSF analysis, muscle and/or nerve biopsies, and cell culture for enzyme analysis or other biochemical testing have been supplanted. However, these studies may be warranted in order to provide better phenotyping in situations when molecular testing has identified variants of unknown significance or when the patient has a classic presentation of a specific genetic condition and the molecular testing has been negative.

## MANAGEMENT

Medical management of global developmental delay begins with a disclosure to the family of the clinician's concern for the diagnosis. As with any situation in which the physician discloses difficult news, this must be done gently but clearly. The clinician should be prepared to respond to a full range of emotions including doubt, denial, sorrow, and anger. Furthermore, the family will usually need time to process the information that their child has or is at risk for having lifelong developmental problems. Therefore, a follow-up appointment should be scheduled to review the diagnosis and address additional questions or concerns the family may have.

In addition, any comorbid conditions should be treated, or the clinician should refer the patient to the appropriate subspecialist who can provide treatment for the comorbid condition. The clinician can also help facilitate social, community, or educational supports for the family. These may include family support groups, national parent organizations, and other resources in the community for families of children with developmental disabilities.

One of the most important aspects of the management of a child with global developmental delay is ensuring that the child receives early and appropriate therapeutic and educational interventions. Children younger than 3 years of age with developmental delays can be enrolled in early intervention programs. Each state's program includes a multidisciplinary team of therapists who complete a comprehensive assessment and provide appropriate interventions. Their assessment is summarized in a report called the *Individualized Family Service Plan*; this plan serves as the basis for provision of therapeutic services.

Children who are older than 3 years of age receive services through the special education program within the local school district. These services are usually provided by a multidisciplinary team of therapists and educators as well as a psychologist. They also complete an assessment and summarize their findings in a report called the Individualized Education Plan (IEP). The IEP serves as the basis for the services that will be provided to the child within the school system. Federal law mandates that children receive the special services they need in the least restrictive environment (LRE) possible. Therefore, many children with developmental disabilities are now educated in the regular ("mainstream") education classroom with an aide or co-teacher instead of being placed in a separate classroom. However, some children with more significant intellectual or behavioral problems may require placement in a special education classroom for part or all of the day.

## PROGNOSIS

Once a child is diagnosed with global developmental delay, the family will inquire about the child's ultimate developmental outcome, including cognitive and motor abilities, future level of independence, and life expectancy. In young children with mild developmental delay, it is not prudent to predict a developmental outcome with certainty. Instead, the potential range of outcomes should be discussed. Depending on the severity of the delays and associated medical problems, this range may include typical development once the child is school-aged. In an otherwise healthy individual with developmental delay, the life expectancy is normal. Children with significantly impaired mobility or other neurological impairments may have a shortened life expectancy.

Though some toddlers and young children with developmental delay may "catch up" and ultimately have typical development, global developmental delay is associated with an increased risk for having a *developmental disability*—a lifelong and chronic condition due to mental and/or physical impairments that impacts major life activities such as language function, learning, mobility, self-help, and independent living. Several types of developmental disabilities exist, including cerebral palsy, learning disabilities like dyslexia, intellectual disability, autism spectrum disorders, attention deficit-hyperactivity disorder, hearing impairment, and vision impairment.

These developmental disabilities are predominantly impairments in a specific subset of the developmental domains. For example, cerebral palsy is primarily an impairment of gross and fine motor skills; intellectual disability is primarily an impairment of language, problem-solving, and social-adaptive abilities; and autism spectrum disorders are primarily disorders of social-adaptive behaviors with or without language and communication impairments.

Developmental disabilities are common. Approximately 16%–18% of children have a developmental disability that includes behavior problems, and 1%–3% of the population has an intellectual disability. Approximately 1%–2% of children have an autism spectrum disorder.

Toddlers or preschool children who are diagnosed with global developmental delay are at highest risk for being diagnosed with intellectual disability at an older age, especially as the developmental quotient worsens. *Intellectual disability* is defined as significantly subaverage general intellectual functioning (IQ $< 70$) with limitations in adaptive functioning in at least two of the following skill areas: communication, self-help, social skills, academic skills, work, leisure, and health and/or safety. The incidence of intellectual disability is 1%–3% in the general population. Males are more likely to be affected than females; occurrence rates are 1:4000 males and only 1:6000 females.

In general, the diagnosis of intellectual disability is not made in a toddler or preschool child unless they have been diagnosed with a specific genetic condition associated with intellectual disability. In the absence of a specific genetic diagnosis, the diagnosis of intellectual disability in most children is made once they are able to complete formal psychology testing at approximately 5–7 years of age.

In our practice, when the developmental delays of a child younger than four are very severe, we will occasionally tell the family that the child will likely have intellectual disability. In these situations, we may share this concern even if the child does not have a formal diagnosis of a genetic syndrome or before the child is able to complete formal psychology testing. Children with severe developmental delays may in fact be too impaired to perform formal psychology testing.

## RECURRENCE RISK

Many couples are interested in knowing what their risk is for having another child with similar developmental concerns. A recurrence risk can only be provided with certainty if a specific etiology has been confirmed. Despite extensive genetic testing and other evaluations, the majority of children with developmental delays will not be diagnosed with a specific named genetic condition or other etiology for the delays. Consequently, the clinician can only provide an empirical recurrence risk based on population data and family history information. Though each case is unique, the most prudent approach is to remind the family that 1%–3% of the population has intellectual disability, and their risk for having another child with global developmental delay and subsequent intellectual disability is greater than the population risk. It is helpful to double-frame the risk by also stating that it is more likely that they would have an *unaffected* child than an *affected* child.

## REGRESSION

A regressive or neurodegenerative disease should be suspected when a child has ongoing and relentless loss of developmental skills. In addition, a regressive disease may begin to manifest itself as the development of a new neurological problem, such as a new-onset seizure disorder or movement disorder, development of a different type of seizure in a child with epilepsy, vision impairment, behavior problems, and dementia or cognitive decline.

In a child with neurological regression, a thorough neurological history and examination is warranted. The history should focus on any modifiable factors that could contribute to neurological decline, including worsening of another medical problem, recent modification to an existing medication regimen or initiation of a new medication, recovery from a prolonged acute illness or surgery, or a psychosocial stressor. All children with neurological decline should receive an extensive physical examination, with attention to those aspects of the examination that could provide clues to an underlying neurodegenerative disease (see Table 8.5). A pediatric ophthalmologist should also examine the patient for ocular stigmata of a neurodegenerative disease (see Table 8.4). A brain MRI should be performed to assess for changes that can be seen in many regressive diseases—atrophy, ventriculomegaly, white matter changes, and infarcts. Additional studies should be considered based on the patient's clinical presentation: comprehensive metabolic panel, lipid panel, creatine kinase, EEG, electromyography EMG, and nerve conduction studies, echocardiogram, and hearing test.

The need for genetic testing is based on the patient's presentation and results of the recommended studies. Categories of genetic diseases that should be considered include aminoacidopathies, organic acidurias, fatty acid oxidation defects, glycogen storage diseases, mitochondrial cytopathies, lysosomal storage diseases, neuronal ceroid lipofuscinoses, peroxisomal disorders, neurotransmitter synthesis disorders, spinal muscular atrophy syndromes, creatine synthesis disorders, congenital disorders of glycosylation, metal metabolism disorders (Menkes, Wilson, pantothenate kinase-associated neurodegeneration), and purine and pyrimidine disorders. Testing for most conditions can be done on blood, urine, and/or CSF samples. Alternatively, if the presentation is nonspecific and not pathognomonic for one of the above conditions, it may be most prudent and productive to perform WES as a first-line test. It is now very rare that more invasive procedures are warranted, including biopsies of the skin, muscle, liver, nerve, bone marrow, or conjunctiva.

Many reasons exist for aggressively pursuing a diagnosis of an underlying neurodegenerative disease. Most regressive disorders are irreversible, and the treatment is symptomatic. However, early diagnosis can reverse the neurological impairment or prevent future morbidity in some conditions such as Wilson disease, homocystinuria, and glutaric aciduria type I. Occasionally, pharmaceutical trials may be available to patients. Furthermore, a correct diagnosis can help the clinician provide better information about prognosis and life expectancy. Recurrence risk information and prenatal diagnosis may also be offered to families. For those conditions that are progressive and life limiting, the clinician should collaborate with a pediatric palliative care team to discuss end-of-life goals of care with the family.

*The complete reference list is available online at https://expertconsult.inkling.com/.* 

9

# Behavior and Personality Disturbances

*Carissa Gehl, Jane S. Paulsen*

## OUTLINE



Mental health has become a public health crisis (Hedegaard et al., 2018). In the past decade, suicide rates have increased 33%, mental illness has become the group of disorders with the highest years lost to disability (Global Health Data Exchange; http://ghdx.healthdata.org), and depression surpassed all other chronic illnesses as a source of global disability (World Health Organization [WHO]; https://apps.who.int/iris/bitstream/handle/10665/254610/WHO-MSD-MER-2017.2-eng.pdf;jsessionid=87FBBD04685D824264F8EF206FF39FC7?sequence=1). It has been suggested that every medical healthcare provider become familiar with the detection of mental illness; indeed, epidemiological studies find more than half of the population with mental illness is not receiving health care (Wang, 2005). Healthy aging across the life span is also a topic of importance for evaluation of behavior and personality changes in persons with neurological disorders or diseases. A primary domain to consider when working with persons with acquired brain disorders or degenerative brain diseases is the changing ability of the individual's communication. Fig. 9.1 shows the areas of the brain involved in pain sensation and gating. A brief evaluation of the figure shows the vast regions of the brain that can be interrupted by brain disease and numerous behavior challenges can arise when pain circuitry is interrupted. Behavior evaluation should always include a general evaluation of potential needs that a neurological patient may be unable to communicate such as pain, pressure, discomfort (from constipation), or other basic sensory disruptions such as temperature, hunger, or overstimulation. Common changes that occur over time in the brain can also impact behavioral changes associated with brain disease. For instance, data have suggested that brain processing shows a shift away from cognitive control toward greater activation of dorsolateral prefrontal cortex, which involves processing of affective stimuli, such as emotion. Behavioral assessment can benefit from using environmental efforts to engage cognitive appraisals that may decrease with brain disease or impairment. Fig. 9.2 shows the typical cognitive and emotional processing changes that occur over the life span.

Behavioral and personality disturbances commonly occur in individuals with neurological disease or injury (Table 9.1). Identification and treatment of behavioral disturbances are critical to neurology health care because they are frequently associated with reduced functional capacity, decreased quality of life, greater economic cost, more caregiver burden, placement in facilities, and morbidity. Common behavioral and personality disturbances in individuals with neurological disease or injury include depression (see Chapter 10 for additional information), anxiety, agitation, disinhibition, apathy, obsessional thinking, psychosis (i.e., hallucinations and delusions), and unawareness, among others. Etiology of behavioral and personality change is likely multifactorial, including physiological disruption of various brain circuits, most notably the frontosubcortical circuits, neurochemical disruption within the brain, and/or psychological and cognitive factors, including impact of disability and memory. Although these symptoms can be challenging to fully realize in a clinical examination room, clear identification and appropriate management is of utmost importance. The aim of this chapter is fourfold. First, factors contributing to behavioral and personality change in neurological illness and injury are discussed. Second, assessment methods for behavior and personality in persons with cerebral dysfunction are detailed. Third, information regarding the prevalence, phenomenology, and treatment of behavior and personality disturbances in dementia, movement disorders, epilepsy, stroke, and traumatic brain injury (TBI) is presented. Finally, discussion regarding the treatment and management of behavioral and personality dysfunction is outlined.

The current chapter focuses on behavioral and personality changes in neurological disease and injury. Please see Chapter 44 for detailed information on assessment and description of common cognitive changes observed in neurological disease and injury.

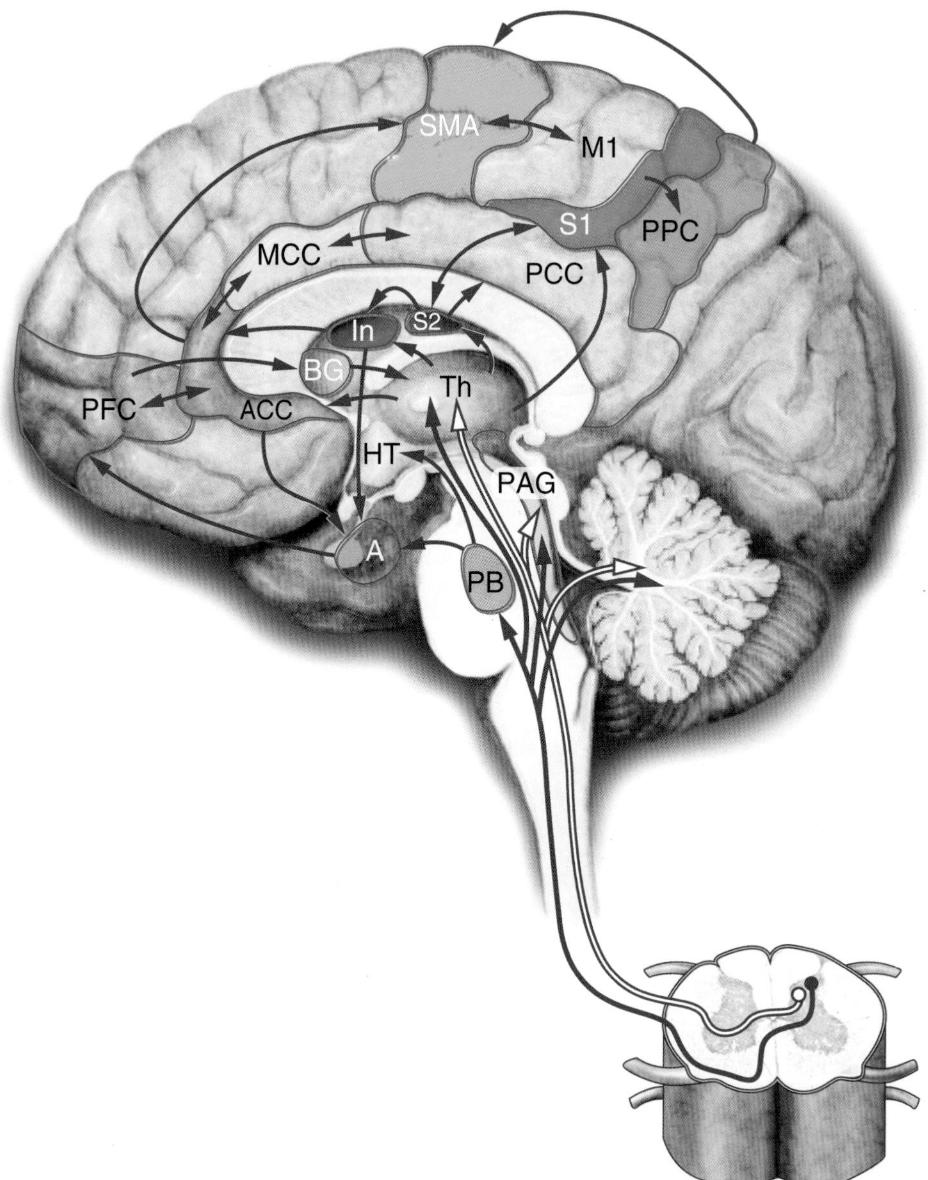


**Fig. 9.1 Schematic Representation of Brain Connectome and the Pain Matrix.** Cortical and subcortical pain networks and pathways involved in pain perception. Locations of brain regions involved in pain perception are shown in a schematic drawing showing the regions, their interconnectivity, and afferent pathways. There are 15 areas in this matrix: anterior cingulate *(ACC)*, medial cingulate *(MCC)*, insula *(In)*, thalamus *(Th)*, prefrontal cortex *(PFC)*, primary and secondary somatosensory cortices *(S1, S2)*, primary and supplementary motor cortices (*M1* and *SMA*), posterior parietal cortex *(PPC)*, posterior cingulate *(PCC)*, basal ganglia *(BG)*, hypothalamus *(HT)*, amygdala *(A)*, parabrachial nuclei *(PB)*, and periaqueductal gray *(PAG)*. (*From Duque, L., Fricchione, G., 2019. Fibromyalgia and its new lessons for neuropsychiatry. © Med. Sci. Monit. Basic Res. 25, 169–178.*)

## ETIOLOGY OF BEHAVIOR AND PERSONALITY CHANGE IN NEUROLOGICAL ILLNESS AND INJURY

### Frontosubcortical Circuitry

The frontosubcortical circuits provide a unifying framework for understanding the behavioral changes that accompany cortical and subcortical brain dysfunction. Alexander and colleagues described five discrete parallel circuits linking regions of the frontal cortex to the striatum, the globus pallidus and substantia nigra, and the thalamus (Alexander, DeLong and Strick, 1996). Five frontosubcortical circuits were initially described as motor, oculomotor, dorsolateral prefrontal, lateral orbitofrontal, and anterior cingulate gyrus. Disruption of dorsolateral prefrontal, lateral orbitofrontal, and anterior cingulate gyrus circuits have been associated with behavioral and personality disruptions. Specific behavioral syndromes have been attributed to dysfunction in these circuits (Box 9.1) (Mega and Cummings, 2001). Disruptions at any point in the circuit (e.g., the frontal cortex, corpus striatum, globus pallidus) may result in alterations of behavior. Disruption of the dorsolateral circuit (Fig. 9.3) is associated with executive dysfunction, which results in problematic behavior secondary to poor planning, organization, and decision making. Moreover, stimulus-bound behavior sometimes seen in late dementia may be attributable to disruptions in this circuit. Disruption of the orbitofrontal circuit (Fig. 9.4) is believed to be associated with increased irritability, impulsivity, mood lability,

Aging Paradox

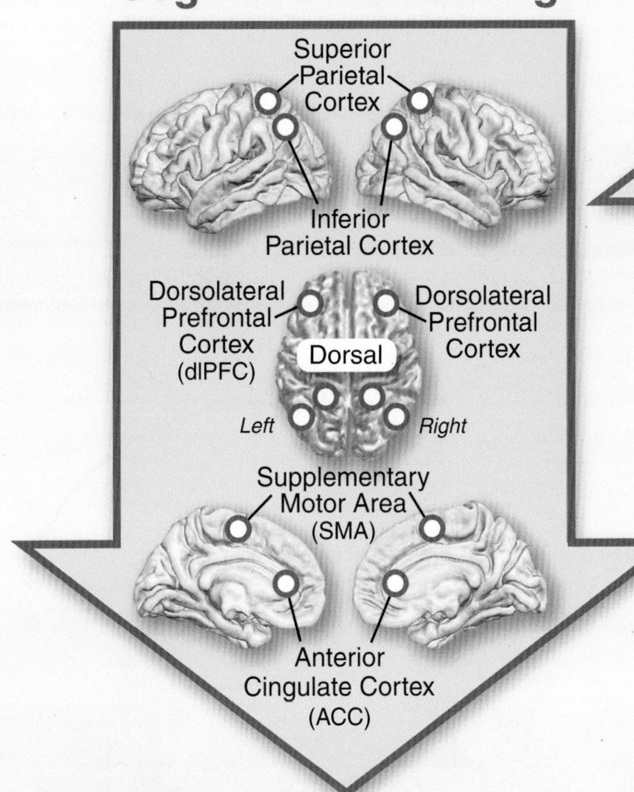


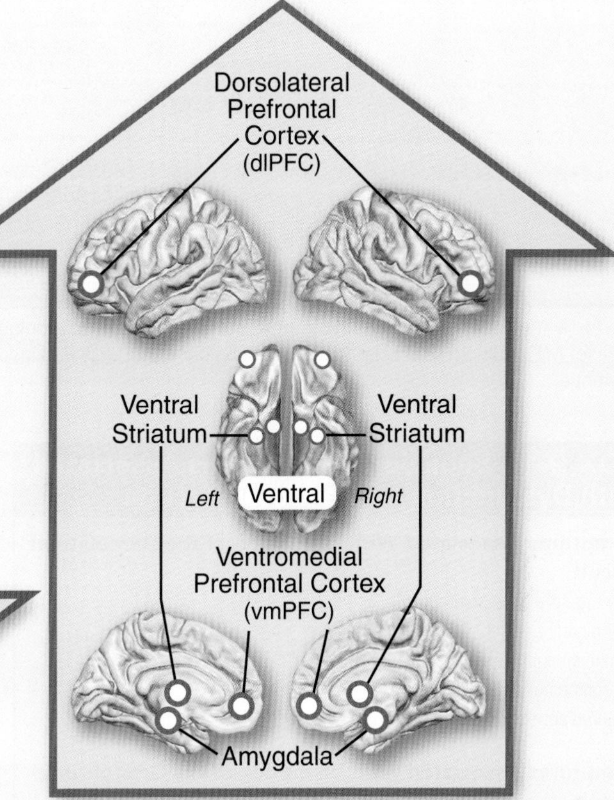


- Older adults exhibit over activation of the CNN during tasks of cognitive control (Cabeza et al., 2004)
- Older adults show reduced recruitment of posterior processing regions during cognitive control tasks (Davis et al., 2008)
- Older adults display reduced modulation of the CNN in response to varying task load (Prakash et al., 2012)
- Older adults exhibit a temporally lagged, late-onset CCN activation pattern during controlled cognitive processing (Velanova et al., 2011)
- Goal maintenance failure, utilizing the dlPFC, is at the crux of cognitive control decline (Braver & Barch, 2002)

- Older adults display greater activation of the dlPFC while processing affective stimuli (Leclerc & Kensinger, 2011)
- Older adults exhibit up-regulation of the dlPFC and vmPFC in response to negatively valenced stimuli, compared to positive (Leclerc & Kensinger, 2011)
- Older adults show greater amygdala activation in response to positive stimuli (Mather et al., 2004)
- Older adults engage in spontaneous emotion regulation during the perception of negative emotional stimuli, reflected by reduced amygdala activation, coupled with increased recruitment of the medial and lateral regions of the PFC (Mather et al., 2004)

**Fig. 9.2** Schematic Representation of the Aging Paradox. Older adults show a decline in incognitive processing, including impaired performance on tasks of cognitive control and alterations in the neural correlates of cognitive control. However, emotional processing, and, at times, emotional regulation is well maintained and even enhanced in older adults. (*From Prakash, R.S., De Leon, A.A., Patterson, B., Schirda, B.L., Janssen, A.L., 2014. Mindfulness and the aging brain: a proposed paradigm shift. Front. Aging Neurosci. 6, Article 120.*)

**TABLE 9.1 Prevalence of Behavioral and Psychiatric Disturbances in Neurological Disorders**

| | Depression | Apathy | Anxiety | Psychosis | Aggression | PBA |
|---|---|---|---|---|---|---|
| AD | 0%–86% | Up to 92% | — | 10%–73% | 33%–67% | — |
| ALS | 40%–50% | — | — | — | — | 10%–49% |
| FTD | — | 95% | — | 20% del., 7% hall. | — | — |
| VaD | 32% | — | 19%–70% | 33% del., 13%–25% hall. | — | — |
| PD | 40%–50% | 16.5%–40.0% | — | 16% del., 30% hall. | — | 4%–6% |
| HD | Up to 63% | 59% | — | 3%–12% | 19%–59% | — |
| TS | 73% | — | — | — | — | — |
| MS | 37%–54% | — | 9.2%–25.0% | — | — | 10% |
| Epilepsy | 8%–63% | — | 19%–50% | 0.6%–7.0% | 4.8%–50.0% | — |
| Stroke | 30%–40% | — | Up to 27% | — | Up to 32% | 11%–34% |
| TBI | 6%–77% | 10%–60% | 11%–70% | 2%–20% | 11%–98% | 5%–11% |

*AD*, Alzheimer disease; *ALS*, amyotrophic lateral sclerosis; *del.*, delusions; *FTD*, frontotemporal dementia; *hall.*, hallucinations; *HD*, Huntington disease; *MS*, multiple sclerosis; *PBA*, pseudobulbar affect; *PD*, Parkinson disease; *TBI*, traumatic brain injury; *TS*, Tourette syndrome; *VaD*, vascular dementia.

**BOX 9.1 Behavioral Syndromes Associated With Dysfunction of the Motor Circuits**

**Symptoms Associated With Disruption of the Dorsolateral Circuit**

Poor organizational strategies
Poor memory search strategies
Stimulus-bound behavior
Environmental dependency
Impaired set-shifting and maintenance

**Symptoms Associated With Disruption of the Orbitofrontal Circuit**

Emotional incontinence
Tactlessness
Irritability
Undue familiarity
Antisocial behavior
Environmental dependency
Mood disorders (depression, lability, mania)
Obsessive-compulsive disorder

**Symptoms Associated With Disruption of the Anterior Cingulate Circuit**

Impaired motivation
Akinetic mutism
Apathy
Poverty of speech
Psychic emptiness
Poor response inhibition

tactlessness, and socially inappropriate behavior. Finally, disruption of the anterior cingulate gyrus circuit is believed to be associated with decreased motivation, apathy, decreased speech, and akinesia.

## Behavioral Factors

In addition, nonneural factors likely contribute to behavioral and personality change in neurological illness and injury. Kales et al., (2015) provide a model of these factors in dementia. This model lends itself well to other neurological syndromes and injuries. They describe the contribution of patient, caregiver, and environmental factors (Fig. 9.5).

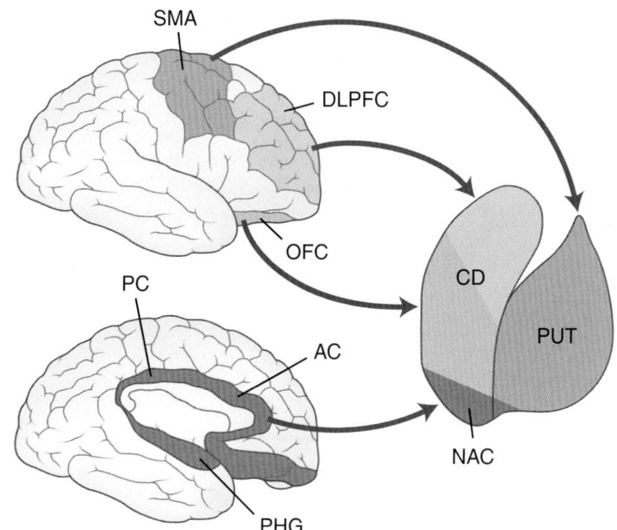


**Fig. 9.3 Frontostriatal Projections.** *AC*, Anterior cingulate gyrus; *CD*, caudate nucleus; *DLPFC*, dorsolateral prefrontal cortex; *NAC*, nucleus accumbens; *OFC*, orbital frontal cortex; *PC*, posterior cingulate gyrus; *PHG*, parahippocampal gyrus; *PUT*, putamen; *SMA*, supplementary motor area. (*Reprinted with permission from Brody, A.L., Saxena, S., 1996. Brain imaging in obsessive-compulsive disorder: evidence for the involvement of frontal-subcortical circuitry in the mediation of symptomatology. CNS Spectr. 1, 27–41. Copyright 1996 by MBL Communications. Reproduced with permission.*)

Patient factors include an individual's premorbid personality and psychiatric disorders. For example, disinhibition that starts secondary to disruption of frontal subcortical circuits may result in exacerbation of preexisting traits, such as irritability. Other factors related to the injury/illness can also contribute to behavioral and personality change. Cognitive factors such as memory impairment may additionally impact behavior and personality change, such as delusional thinking. In many situations, behavioral disturbances may reflect an individual with impaired cognitive and language abilities attempting to communicate information to their care providers (Sutor et al., 2006). Other aspects of illness and injury such as disability (which has been linked with depression) or anosognosia additionally impact behavior and personality. Unmet needs that may or may not be related to the primary neurological diagnosis may impact behavior and personality. For example, pain, hunger, or sleep

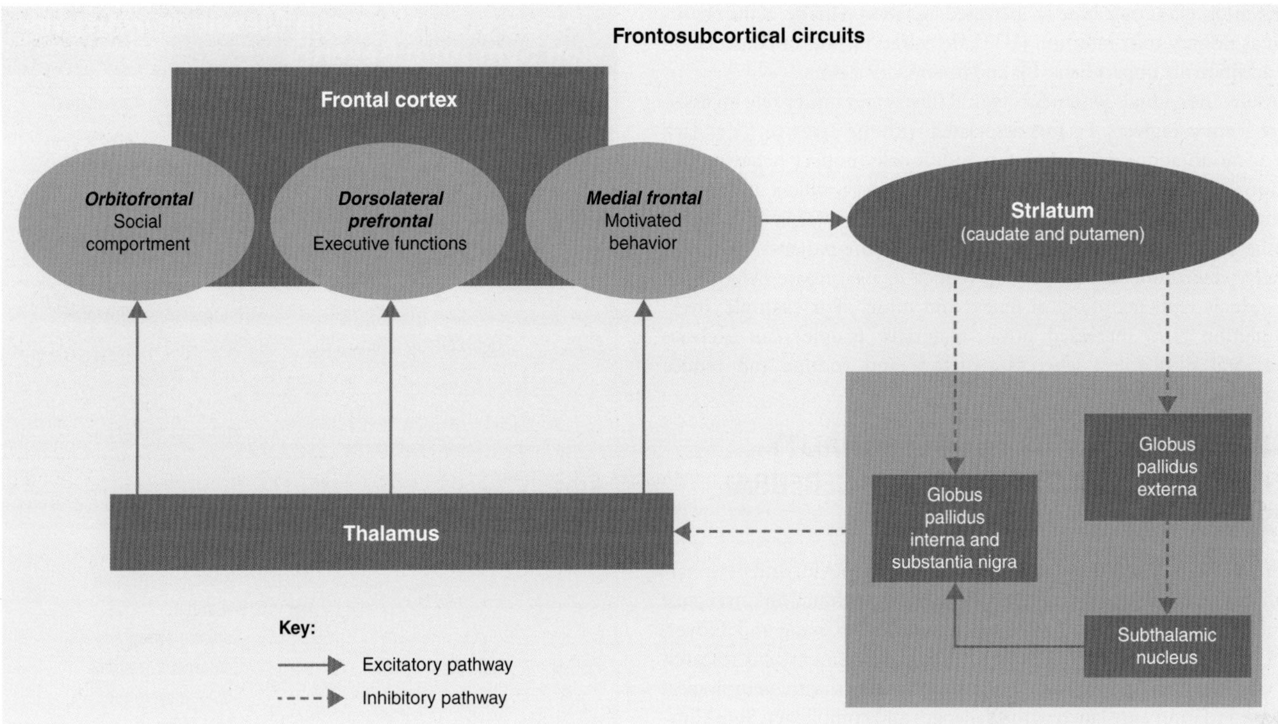


**Fig. 9.4** Outline of frontal subcortical circuits relevant to common neurobehavioral sequelae of traumatic brain injury. (*Adapted from Arciniegas, D.B., Beresford, T.P., 2001. Neuropsychiatry: An Introductory Approach. Cambridge University Press, Cambridge, UK, p. 58. Copyright © Cambridge University Press, 2001.*)

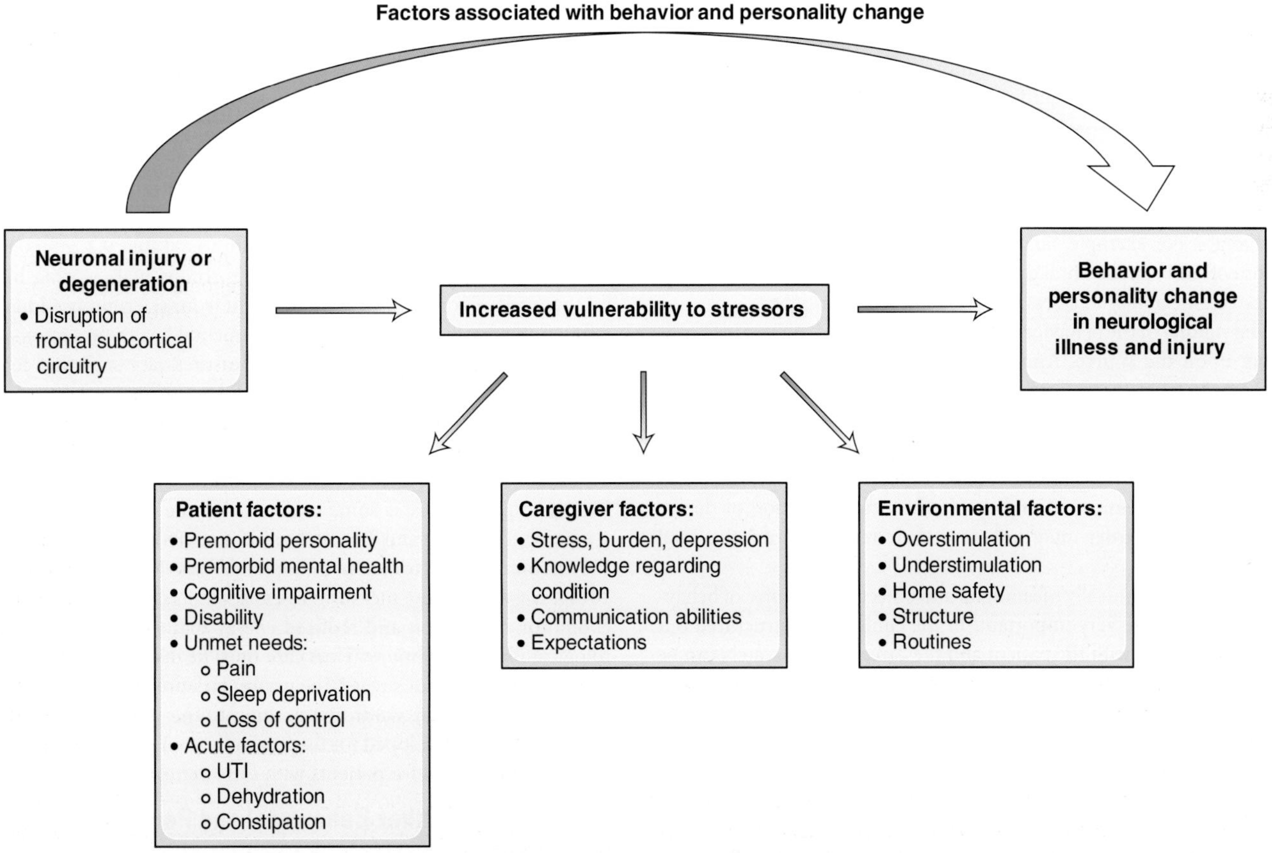


**Fig. 9.5** Factors Associated With Behavior and Personality Change. *UTI*, Urinary tract infection. (*From Kales, J.C., Gitlin, L.N., Lyketsos, C.G., 2015. Assessment and management of behavioral and psychological symptoms of dementia. BMJ 350:h369.*)

deprivation may contribute to increased agitation. Finally, acute factors such as urinary tract infection (UTI), dehydration, and/or constipation can additionally impact behavior and personality factors.

Many individuals with neurological illness and injury rely on assistance from caregivers. Factors associated with the caregiver (e.g., lack of education about dementia) can additionally impact behavior and personality change among those with neurological illness and injury. Strain in relationships either due to preexisting patterns of behavior or due to caregiver stress or burden impacts the patient's behavior. Finally, environmental factors can reduce or exacerbate behavior in individuals with neurological illness and injury. For example, overstimulation (i.e., increased noise, materials, people) can increase behavioral difficulties, whereas structure and routine can reduce behavioral symptoms.

## ASSESSING BEHAVIOR AND PERSONALITY DISTURBANCES IN PATIENTS WITH CEREBRAL DYSFUNCTION

There is evidence that appropriate treatment of behavior and personality disturbances in patients with acquired brain dysfunction can reduce required care levels and prevent hospitalizations (Chang and Troyer, 2011; Davydow et al., 2013, 2014). Clinical assessment and research of behavior and personality change in individuals with neurological disease and injury are laden with challenges and complexity. Some limitations of the available research are as follows:

1. Treatment of other symptoms (such as a movement disorder) may mask psychiatric and behavioral symptoms.
2. Most available neuropsychiatric assessment tools use conventional psychiatric terminology based on idiopathic psychiatric illness, which sometimes fails to distinctly reflect the symptoms associated with acquired disease and/or trauma.
3. There is overlap between symptoms of cerebral dysfunction and symptoms of behavior and personality disturbances; for example, psychomotor retardation or reduced energy, libido, or appetite might reflect an underlying syndrome (Parkinson disease [PD]), an acquired injury (e.g., TBI), or a major depressive episode.
4. Cognitive impairments may confound the detection of behavioral changes. For example, language and memory deficits occurring in individuals with cerebral dysfunction can limit self-reports and can restrict the ability to assess changes in mood or insight.
5. The validity of the behavioral dysfunction assessed can vary depending upon the source. Ample research shows that clinical ratings acquired from the patient, a collateral or spouse, and a healthcare worker can vary widely (see, e.g., Hoth et al., 2007). Patients with cerebral dysfunction may have impaired insight; thus they may underreport behavioral difficulties. Similarly, caregivers may also provide biased information because their current mood or degree of caregiver burden may influence their reporting of behavioral symptoms.

Nevertheless, clinically meaningful and objective measures of behavioral symptoms are very important. In the clinic, an unstructured but targeted interview with the patient and the caregivers separately can be useful. Inventories and scales based on semistructured interviews give valuable insight when used with appropriate training.

### Assessment of Depression

Neurological illness or injury may manifest as depression. In fact, depression is frequently a very early symptom or precedes onset of illness in many neurodegenerative disorders (Green et al., 2003; Ishihara and Brayne, 2006). There are several scales available for the assessment of mood disorders that might be useful in patients with acquired cerebral dysfunction. When clinicians think time is limited, self-report scales can be helpful in determining which symptoms are present and how bothersome or severe each symptom is. Table 9.2 offers additional information regarding these scales. Individuals scoring highly on these self-report measures may benefit from referral for additional evaluation and possible intervention by mental health professionals.

**TABLE 9.2 Common Measures of Depression Symptom Severity**

| Scale | Method | Items | Domains Assessed |
|---|---|---|---|
| BDI-II | Self-administered | 21 | Cognitive symptoms<br>Performance impairments<br>Somatic symptoms |
| CES-D | Self-administered | 20 | Somatic symptoms<br>Depressed affect<br>Positive affect<br>Interpersonal problems |
| GDS | Self-administered | 30 | Sad mood<br>Lack of energy<br>Positive mood<br>Agitation/anxiety<br>Social withdrawal |
| HADS | Self-administered | 14 | General depression<br>Anxiety |
| HDRS | Interview | 21 | Anxiety<br>General depression<br>Insomnia<br>Somatic symptoms |
| PHQ-9 | Self-administered | 9 | Cognitive symptoms<br>Somatic symptoms<br>Level of functional impairment |
| ZDS | Self-administered | 20 | Positive affect<br>Negative symptoms<br>Somatic symptoms |

*BDI-II*, Beck Depression Inventory, second edn. (Beck et al., 1996); *CES-D*, Center for Epidemiologic Studies Depression Scale (Radloff, 1997); *GDS*, Geriatric Depression Scale (Brink et al., 1982); *HADS*, Hospital Anxiety and Depression Scale (Zigmond and Smith, 1983); *HDRS*, Hamilton Depression Rating Scale (Hamilton, 1960); *PHQ-9*, Patient Health Questionnaire (Kroenke et al., 2001); *ZDS*, Zung Depression Scale (Zung, 1965).

Domains assessed by the different measures vary such that certain scales may not detect some symptoms of depression. Two of the most commonly used measures are the Beck Depression Inventory (BDI) and the Patient Health Questionnaire-9 (PHQ-9). Although research assessing the appropriateness of these measures in neurological populations is sparse, there is some evidence that the BDI may be a useful screening tool in PD and Tourette syndrome (TS), and the PHQ-9 has shown some support for use in multiple sclerosis (MS) (Amtmann et al., 2014). However, these measures assess several symptoms such as psychomotor retardation and reduced energy that are common in neurological illness and injury. Thus care must be taken to be certain that these measures do not suggest the person is depressed based on symptoms of neurological syndrome or injury. The Geriatric Depression Scale (GDS) was developed for use in elderly populations and may be a useful screening tool for patients with early dementia and PD.

### Assessment of Other Behavioral and Personality Disturbances

Several measures have been created to assess other behavioral and personality disturbances that occur in patients with cerebral dysfunction

**TABLE 9.3 Common Measures for Assessing Behavior and Personality in Patients With Cerebral Dysfunction**

| | ADMINISTRATION | | BEHAVIORS ASSESSED | | | | |
|---|---|---|---|---|---|---|---|
| Scale | Source | Time (Minutes) | Depression | Apathy | Anxiety | Psychosis | Aggression |
| ADAS | Patient and caregiver<br>Trained examiner | 45 | Yes | No | No | Yes | No |
| BEHAVE-AD | Caregiver interview | 20 | Yes | No | Yes | Yes | Yes |
| C-BRSD | Caregiver interview | 20–30 | Yes | Yes | No | Yes | Yes |
| FBI | Caregiver interview | 10–15 | No | Yes | No | No | Yes |
| FrSBe | Patient questionnaire<br>Caregiver questionnaire | 10 | No | Yes | No | No | No |
| NPI | Caregiver interview | 10 | Yes | Yes | Yes | Yes | Yes |
| NPI-Q | Caregiver | 5 | Yes | Yes | Yes | Yes | Yes |
| NRS-R | Patient/caregiver interview | 15–20 | Yes | No | Yes | No | Yes |

*ADAS*, Alzheimer Disease Assessment Scale; *BEHAVE-AD*, Behavioral Pathology in Alzheimer Disease Rating Scale; *C-BRSD*, CERAD (Consortium to Establish a Registry for Alzheimer Disease) Behavior Rating Scale for Dementia; *FBI*, Frontal Behavior Inventory; *FrSBe*, Frontal Systems Behavior Scale; *NPI*, Neuropsychiatric Inventory; *NPI-Q*, Neuropsychiatric Inventory-Questionnaire; *NRS-R*, Neurobehavioral Rating Scale-Revised.

(Table 9.3). These measures were specifically designed to assess behavioral symptoms in specific diagnoses, such as Alzheimer disease (AD): Alzheimer Disease Assessment Scale (ADAS); Behavioral Pathology in Alzheimer Disease Rating Scale (BEHAVE-AD); Consortium to Establish a Registry for Alzheimer Disease (CERAD) Behavior Rating Scale for Dementia (C-BRSD); general dementia: Neuropsychiatric Inventory (NPI); frontal lobe dementia: Frontal Behavior Inventory (FBI); TBI: Neurobehavioral Rating Scale-Revised (NRS-R); and damage to frontal regions: Frontal Systems Behavior Scale (FrSBe). Some measures such as the NPI and the FrSBe have been implemented in diverse conditions, including AD, PD, Huntington disease (HD), and MS. In addition, the NPI, which is available in an interview and a questionnaire format, has been frequently used as an outcome measure in clinical trials. More recently, efforts to better assess apathy have emerged (Agüera-Ortiz et al., 2013; Radakovic and Abrahams, 2014). Many of these measures might be useful ways to screen for a wide variety of potential behavioral disruptions among patients with neurological illness or injury. For individuals with limited insight and awareness, collateral reports of these difficulties may be of particular importance.

## BEHAVIOR AND PERSONALITY DISTURBANCES ASSOCIATED WITH CEREBRAL DYSFUNCTION

### Alzheimer Disease

Behavioral and psychological symptoms of dementia (BPSD) is reported to occur in at least 90% of individuals diagnosed with AD and related disorders (Chakrabortya et al., 2019). Patients with AD experience a wide range of behavioral disturbances, including affective symptoms, agitation, aggression, disinhibition, anxiety, apathy, and psychosis. Behavioral disturbances in AD are associated with increased caregiver burden, patient and caregiver abuse, greater use of psychotropic medications, more rapid cognitive decline, and earlier institutionalization. Unfortunately, there are no US Food and Drug Administration (FDA)-approved drugs to treat BPSD and off-label pharmacological approaches perform poorly in AD (Zdanys et al., 2016). New approaches must be considered to address the multiple consequences of these symptoms for independence and care programs. Current research involves review of the serotonergic system for cognition and BPSD in AD (Chakrabortya et al., 2019), identification of methylation differences for specific genes involved in mood, stress, and hippo signaling (Bhak et al., 2019), and efforts to group behavior irregularities into conceptual/biological domains (Keszycki et al., 2019). These newer research efforts require replication; however, translation to clinical care is expected within the next decade for biological markers of BPSD as well as more formal treatment strategies (Kales et al., 2019). For instance, one group reported that anhedonia is more highly associated with cognitive decline, whereas dysphoria was more associated with anxiety and mood disturbances (Lee et al., 2019).

Use of atypical antipsychotic medications has historically been the preferred method of treatment for behavioral disturbances in AD, including irritability, aggression, and psychosis. However, use of atypical antipsychotic medications in elderly adults may be associated with a nearly twofold increase in risk for mortality (Kuehn, 2005). In addition, a multisite study of atypical antipsychotics (olanzapine, quetiapine, and risperidone) showed no significant difference in Clinical Global Impression Scale scores for any antipsychotic medication over a placebo group (Schneider et al., 2006). Moreover, more participants found the side effects of the atypical antipsychotic medications to be intolerable compared with the placebo group (Schneider et al., 2006). In a retrospective observational study, behavioral symptoms were reduced in more than 20% of patients following treatment with antipsychotics, while a full half of participants exhibited worsening of symptoms (Kleijer et al., 2009). However, other retrospective observational studies have reported improvements in 33%–43% of individuals with AD and behavioral disturbances treated with atypical antipsychotics (Rocca et al., 2007). In addition, a retrospective cohort study showed that men display higher risk than women of developing a serious adverse event when started on an oral atypical antipsychotic (Rochon et al., 2013). The FDA have issued a black-box warning on the use of antipsychotics in elderly persons with dementia. Antipsychotics may be beneficial in a small subgroup of individuals, but care must be taken in prescribing such medications, owing to the potential side effects in the context of questionable effectiveness. A review of the clinical trial literature for cholinesterase inhibitors and memantine suggests that individuals treated with these pharmaceuticals typically do experience a reduction in behavioral symptoms, including improved mood and abatement of apathy (Cummings et al., 2008).

#### Depression

The true prevalence of depression in AD is controversial, with estimates up to 86%. One reason for the mixed findings lies in the

**TABLE 9.4 Clinical Aspects Differentiating Dementia From Depression**

| Major Depression | Dementia |
|---|---|
| Acute, nonprogressive | Insidious and progressive |
| Affective before cognitive | Cognitive before affective |
| Attention impaired | Memory impaired |
| Orientation intact | Orientation impaired |
| Complains of memory | Minimizes/normalizes memory |
| Gives up on testing | Obvious effort on testing |
| Language intact | Aphasic errors |
| Better at night | Sundowning |
| Self-referred | Referred by others |

different methods used to assess depression in AD, such as family interviews and patient self-report. Some symptoms of depression are confounded with components of AD (e.g., concentration, energy, interest). The probability of depression in AD appears to be greater if there is a history of depression either in the patient or in the family. Table 9.4 suggests differences between the signs of depression and confounding signs of dementia. Interestingly, there does not appear to be a clear relationship between depressive symptoms and severity of AD (Verkaik et al., 2007). Depression is associated with greater social and functional impairments in patients with AD (Starkstein et al., 2005), although others have not observed a correlation between depression and functional impairment (Landes et al., 2005).

Selective serotonin reuptake inhibitors (SSRIs) remain the preferred mode of treatment for depression in AD, and, although sertraline and citalopram have been shown to be effective (Lyketsos et al., 2000), findings are mixed. Although discontinuation of current antidepressant treatment shows worsening (Bergh et al., 2012), one review (Banerjee et al., 2011) suggests that secondary to the absence of benefit compared with placebo and the increased risk of adverse events (Rosenberg et al., 2010), the use of antidepressants for first-line treatment of depression in AD should be reconsidered. One recent paper formulated recommendations for future work:

1. It remains both ethical and essential for trials of new medication for depression in dementia to have a placebo arm.
2. Further research is required to evaluate the impact that treatments for depression in dementia have on carers in terms of quality of life and the time they spend caregiving.
3. Alternative biological and psychological therapies for depression in dementia should be considered, including new classes of antidepressants (such as venlafaxine) or antidementia medication (e.g., cholinesterase inhibitors).
4. Research is needed to investigate the natural history of depression in dementia in the community when patients are not referred to secondary care services.
5. Further work is needed to investigate the costs of depression in dementia, including caregiver burden and moderators to the treatment effects (Banerjee et al., 2013). A recent publication suggests that antidementia medication and nonpharmacological interventions can be potential choices (Chi et al., 2014).

## Apathy

*Apathy*, defined as diminished motivation not attributable to decreased level of consciousness, cognitive impairment, or emotional distress, is among the most common behavioral changes noted in AD. Assessment of apathy in AD may be difficult because it may be unclear whether decreased activity is due to apathy or inability to perform activities. Consistent with expectations based on frontal subcortical circuitry,

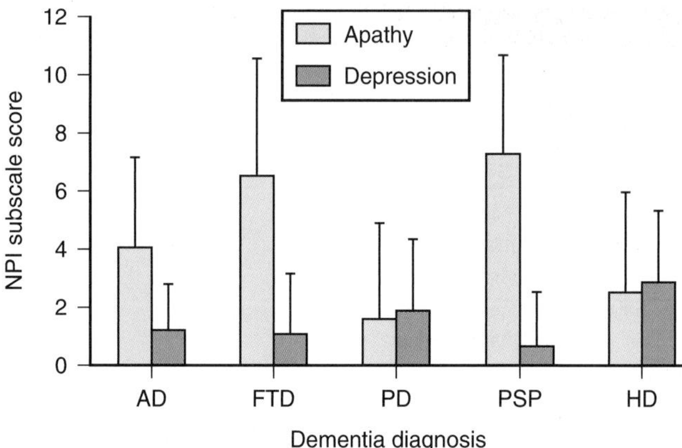


**Fig. 9.6** Incidence of Psychosis in Patients With Alzheimer Disease *(AD). FTD,* Frontotemporal dementia; *HD,* Huntington disease; *NPI,* neuropsychiatric inventory; *PD,* Parkinson disease; *PSP,* progressive supranuclear palsy. (*Reprinted with permission from Paulsen, J.S., Salmon, D.P., Thal, L.J., et al., 2000. Incidence of and risk factors for hallucinations and delusions in patients with probable AD. Neurology 54, 1965–1971.*)

apathy in AD has been shown to be associated with bilateral reductions in gray matter volume in the anterior cingulate cortex, orbitofrontal cortex, dorsolateral prefrontal cortex, and putamen (Bruen et al., 2008). Apathy in AD is associated with greater functional and cognitive impairment (Landes et al., 2005) and lower quality of life (Hurt et al., 2008).

## Aggression

Aggressive verbalizations and acts are common in AD. Reported prevalence rates range from 25% to 67%; studies have indicated that verbal aggression is more common in men and in individuals with delusions or agitation (Eustace et al., 2001) and is associated with increased placement in skilled nursing facilities. Sertraline has been associated with a 38% response rate for the treatment of aggression and irritability in AD (Lanctot et al., 2002).

## Psychosis

Prevalence rates of psychotic symptoms in AD range from 10% to 73%, with rates in clinical populations exceeding community-based samples. Interestingly, hallucinations and delusions are significantly less common among individuals with early-onset AD (Toyota et al., 2007). Once present, delusions recur or persist for several years in most patients with AD (Fig. 9.6). The presence of hallucinations is associated with increased placement in skilled nursing centers.

The delusions reported in AD are typically paranoid type, nonbizarre, and simple. Complex or bizarre delusions seen in patients with schizophrenia are conspicuously absent in patients with AD. However, misidentification phenomena are common in AD. Hallucinations in AD are more often visual than auditory, whereas the reverse is true for schizophrenia (Table 9.5).

Previously it was believed that individuals with AD experienced delusions secondary to significant cognitive difficulties. Evidence from neuropsychological investigations suggests more executive and frontal dysfunction in AD with psychotic symptoms than AD without these symptoms. The presence of delusions in AD is associated with poorer performance on the Frontal Assessment Battery (FAB) but was not related to global measures of cognitive impairment (i.e., Mini Mental Status Examination [MMSE]) (Nagata et al., 2009). However, more recent research has identified additional correlates and biological markers of psychosis. For example, delusions have been associated with reduced gray matter volume in the inferior right frontal gyrus and

**TABLE 9.5 Psychotic Symptoms in Alzheimer Disease Versus Schizophrenia in Elderly Patients**

| | Psychosis in Alzheimer Disease | Schizophrenia in the Elderly |
|---|---|---|
| Incidence | 30%–50% | <1% |
| Bizarre or complex delusions | Rare | Common |
| Misidentification of caregivers | Common | Rare |
| Common form of hallucinations | Visual | Auditory |
| Schneiderian first-rank symptoms | Rare | Common |
| Active suicidal ideation | Rare | Common |
| History of psychosis | Rare | Very common |
| Eventual remission of psychosis | Common | Uncommon |
| Need for many years of maintenance on antipsychotics | Uncommon | Very common |
| Average optimal daily dose of an antipsychotic | 15%–25% of that in young adult with schizophrenia | 40%–60% of that in a young adult with schizophrenia |

*Reprinted with permission from Jeste, D.V., Finkel, S.I., 2000. Psychosis of Alzheimer's disease and related dementias. Am. J. Geriatr. Psychiatry 8, 29–34.*

the inferior parietal lobule (Bruen et al., 2008). Persons with AD and hallucinations (but not delusions) are at significantly increased risk for mortality (Wilson et al., 2005).

## Frontotemporal Dementia

Frontotemporal dementia (FTD) is a heterogeneous group of syndromes, including primary progressive aphasia (PPA) and behavioral variant frontotemporal dementia (bvFTD). Consensus criteria for diagnosis of FTD have been described, with presence of behavioral change an important feature, especially in bvFTD. Behavioral changes may also be present in PPA, particularly later in the course. Caregiver distress is greater among individuals with FTD and behavioral changes, particularly apathy and disinhibition, versus those with primarily aphasic difficulties (Massimo et al., 2009).

### Behavioral Disruption

Atrophy within the frontal lobes leads to disruption of thc frontosubcortical circuits and the characteristic behavioral syndromes in FTD. Two classic behavioral syndromes have been described among individuals with FTD: an apathetic and a disinhibited subtype. Apathy is a very common symptom in individuals with FTD. Individuals may show little concern for personal hygiene and may appear unkempt. Moreover, symptoms of orbitofrontal syndrome, such as disinhibition, poor impulse control, tactlessness, and poor judgment are common. Loss of empathy, mental inflexibility, and stereotyped behaviors are also common. Symptoms similar to those observed in Klüver-Bucy syndrome, such as hyperorality and hypersexuality, may occur in late stages. Frequently the family members and caregivers are the ones who report these behavioral disturbances, because many patients with FTD experience reduced insight into their current difficulties. Behavioral change to varying degrees has been described in all FTD syndromes, including PPA (Grossman, 2012; Kertesz et al., 2010), although they frequently are less severe and/or occur later in the progression of the illness.

From a pathological perspective, individuals with FTD vary with regard to the degree to which the frontal versus temporal lobes and right versus left hemispheres are affected. Significant research has looked at the relationship between patterns of behavioral syndromes and underlying neuropathology (see Josephs, 2007, for a review). Individuals with bvFTD typically exhibit greater frontal versus temporal atrophy, which is typically symmetrical. Evidence shows that individuals with bvFTD and primarily apathetic behavioral changes show greater frontal involvement, particularly from/in the right dorsolateral prefrontal cortex (Massimo et al., 2009; Zamboni et al., 2008). Individuals with primarily disinhibited behavioral change show greater involvement of the right mediotemporal limbic and temporal lobe (Zamboni et al., 2008), although others have described increased atrophy within the left dorsolateral prefrontal cortex (Massimo et al., 2009). Individuals with semantic dementia (SD), a variant of PPA, most typically exhibit atrophy and dysfunction within the left anterior temporal lobe, whereas individuals with SD and behavioral changes are more likely to also exhibit changes in the ventromedial and superior frontal lobes. Individuals with progressive nonfluent aphasia (PNFA), another PPA variant, are more likely to show changes in left frontal and perisylvian areas.

No curative treatments exist for FTD. However, there has been some success with pharmacological intervention for behavioral dyscontrol. Although few large-scale studies have been completed, evidence suggests that behavioral disturbances such as disinhibition, overeating, and compulsions may show some response to treatment with SSRIs (Huey et al., 2006).

### Anosognosia

As noted in the consensus criteria, individuals with FTD frequently exhibit anosognosia. This loss of insight may manifest as an inability to perceive symptoms or a lack of concern for their current difficulties. Among individuals with frontotemporal lobar degeneration (FTLD), individuals with bvFTD exhibit greater anosognosia than individuals with the aphasic subtypes of FTLD (Zamboni et al., 2010). Patients with FTD frequently describe significantly fewer problems with cognition and behavior than what their caregivers describe. Moreover, this observed discrepancy between patient and caregiver report is greater among individuals with FTD than in individuals with AD, particularly for language, behavior, and functioning difficulties (Salmon et al., 2008). Severity of anosognosia is not typically associated with severity of dementia (Zamboni et al., 2010). The relationship between impaired awareness and specific neuropathology is somewhat unclear. Some studies have shown an association between impaired awareness and right frontal disruptions (Mendez and Shapira, 2005), whereas others have shown a link between anosognosia and involvement of the right temporoparietal cortex (Zamboni et al., 2010).

## Vascular Dementia

Dementia secondary to vascular changes is among the most common causes of dementia in older adults. National Institute of Neurological Disorders and Stroke and Association Internationale pour la Recherche et l'Enseignement en Neurosciences (NINDS-AIREN) diagnostic

**TABLE 9.6 Neuropsychiatric Features and Treatment in Parkinson Disease**

| Syndrome | Subtype | Key Feature | Treatment |
|---|---|---|---|
| Depression | Major depression | Low mood or loss of interest/pleasure | No large controlled trials published to date. Nonpharmacological (counseling), dopamine agonists (pramipexole, ropinirole), antidepressants (tricyclics, trazodone, SSRIs, SSNRI, SNRI, mirtazapine) |
| | Minor depression | Low mood and/or loss of interest/pleasure | No available evidence |
| | Dysthymia | Low mood ≥2 years | No available evidence |
| Anxiety | Panic attacks | Episodic panic attacks | Poor evidence for benzodiazepines, clomipramine, nonpharmacological |
| | GAD | Excessive, often irrational anxiety or worry | Same as above |
| Psychosis | Hallucinations | Seeing imaginary people or animals | Clozapine: two randomized trials showing improvement |
| | Delusions | False, fixed idiosyncratic beliefs, maintained despite contrary evidence | Same as above |
| Apathy | | Lack of initiative, motivation | Limited evidence: dopamine agonists, stimulants, modafinil |

*Modified with permission from Aarsland, D., Marsh, L., Schrag, A., 2009. Neuropsychiatric symptoms in Parkinson's disease. Mov. Disord. 24, 2175–2186. GAD, Generalized Anxiety Disorder.*

criteria for vascular dementia (VaD) include the presence of dementia and cerebrovascular disease, including evidence of such disease on imaging, with a documented relationship between these two criteria (see Sachdev et al., 2014, for a recent review). Pathologically, VaD frequently involves small-vessel disease involving white matter hyperintensities and/or lacunar strokes, most commonly affecting subcortical regions; therefore frontosubcortical circuits are frequently disrupted, and behavioral disturbances are common. Apathy, depression, and behavioral changes are common in VaD. The presence of significant cerebrovascular changes is observed among individuals with AD, suggesting that both pathologies may be present among a large subgroup of individuals with dementia.

### Depression

The mean reported prevalence of depression in VaD is 32%, although rates vary widely between studies (Ballard and O'Brien, 2002). Sample source likely influences the reported prevalence rates, with community samples endorsing lower rates of depression than clinic samples. Individuals with VaD and depression are less likely to have had a stroke and are more likely to have a prior history of depression and impairments in memory or attention than patients with VaD without depression. The relationship between age and depression in VaD is unclear, with increased rates of depression being reported in both younger and older samples.

### Additional Behavioral and Psychiatric Disorders

Apathy in VaD is associated with increased impairment in both basic and instrumental activities of daily living (Zawacki et al., 2002). This relationship is particularly apparent in patients with VaD who have also experienced a stroke. Rates of psychotic symptoms are similar in AD and VaD. Delusions (33%) and visual hallucinations (13%–25%) are reported in VaD and are associated with impaired cognitive functioning (Ballard and O'Brien, 2002). Care must be taken in the assessment of delusions in VaD and in dementia in general. It is important to differentiate delusions from confabulation or thought processes based on impaired cognitive functioning.

## Parkinson Disease

Behavioral changes are common in PD, and, although research has adequately characterized these difficulties, little controlled research has assessed the effectiveness of various interventions. The majority of neuropsychiatric symptoms in PD are more common in patients with mild cognitive decline or dementia, possibly related to shared underlying pathologies (Aarsland et al., 2014). Accurate diagnosis of neuropsychiatric syndromes in PD is important but can be difficult, due to overlapping of motor signs of parkinsonism: cognitive impairment, mood disorders, and apathy. Table 9.6 offers more detailed information regarding characteristics of behavioral change observed in PD as well as recent reviews of neurotherapeutic methods (Connolly and Fox, 2014; Tan, 2012). See a recent review of the neuropsychiatry of PD whose authors report that these symptoms remain underrecognized and undertreated (Weintraub and Mamikonyan, 2019).

### Depression

Depression is the most common psychiatric disturbance in persons with PD. Depending on the threshold for diagnosis and sample assessed, reported rates vary. Depression may predate the onset of motor symptoms in PD (Ishihara and Brayne, 2006). Risk factors for depression in PD include greater cognitive impairment, earlier disease onset, and family history of depression. Depression is *not* associated with increased motor symptom severity (Holroyd et al., 2005). The correlation between depression and disability is equivocal. Although the precise etiology is unknown, it is believed that depression in PD results from disruptions in dopamine (D2), noradrenaline, and serotonin pathways (Veazey et al., 2005).

Very few well-controlled studies have assessed antidepressant therapy in PD. Available research suggests that SSRIs are well tolerated and likely effective in the treatment of depression in PD (see McDonald et al., 2003, for a review). SSRIs are frequently implemented as a first-line therapy for depression in patients with PD, although SSRIs may worsen motor symptoms. In such cases, tricyclic antidepressants may be an effective alternative. Successful treatment of depressive symptoms with an SSRI may also result in reductions in anxiety and decreased disability.

### Psychosis

Hallucinations, typically visual, occur in up to 40% of patients with PD, with 16% reporting delusions (Fenelon et al., 2000). Psychotic symptoms are very uncommon early in the course of PD. Other diagnoses

**TABLE 9.7 Differentiating Psychosis in Parkinson Disease and Dementia With Lewy Bodies**

| Psychosis in Parkinson Disease | Psychosis in Dementia With Lewy Bodies |
|---|---|
| • Psychosis occurs in many but not all patients.<br>• Visual hallucinations are more common than delusions.<br>• Psychosis is generally medication induced.<br>• Hallucinations are usually fleeting and nocturnal.<br>• Fluctuating level of consciousness represents onset of delirium.<br>• Dementia may or may not accompany psychosis.<br>• Motor impairment virtually always precedes psychosis.<br>• Neuroleptics worsen motor function, but "neuroleptic sensitivity" associated with DLB is not a feature of PD.<br>• Disordered dopaminergic (and possibly serotonergic) transmissions are the most frequently hypothesized underlying mechanisms. | • Psychosis is a core feature for diagnosis.<br>• Visual hallucinations and delusions occur at similar frequencies.<br>• Psychosis occurs in the absence of antiparkinsonian medications.<br>• Hallucinations are generally persistent/recurrent.<br>• Fluctuating level of consciousness can be a core feature.<br>• Presence of dementia is required for a diagnosis of DLB.<br>• Motor impairment may occur after psychosis.<br>• Neuroleptic sensitivity characterized by dramatic motor and cognitive worsening and associated with increased morbidity and mortality has been reported.<br>• Disordered cholinergic transmission may be the most important underlying mechanism. |

*DLB*, Dementia with Lewy bodies; *PD*, Parkinson disease.
*From Ismail, M.S., Richard, I.H., 2004. A reality test: how well do we understand psychosis in Parkinson's disease? J. Neuropsychiatry Clin. Neurosci. 16, 8–18. Copyright 2004 by American Psychiatric Press Inc. Reproduced with permission.*

such as dementia with Lewy bodies (DLB) should be considered in patients exhibiting hallucinations early in the course of the disease. Table 9.7 summarizes important distinctions between psychosis in PD and DLB. Psychotic symptoms are more common in PD patients with greater cognitive impairment, longer duration of illness, greater daytime somnolence, and older age and in those who are institutionalized. Psychotic symptoms are strong predictors of nursing home placement and mortality in PD (Fenelon et al., 2000).

Historical accounts of PD rarely described psychotic symptoms, and it has been postulated that psychosis occurred secondary to dopamine agonist use. Although dopamine agonists may contribute to the development of psychosis, additional factors are also important. For example, individuals with psychosis are more likely to exhibit cholinergic deficits and have Lewy bodies in the temporal lobe observed at autopsy (Aarsland et al., 2009).

Intervention for remediation of psychotic symptoms in PD can involve several processes. Discontinuation of anticholinergics, selegiline, and amantadine before reducing L-dopa is recommended. Following these discontinuations, reduction and simplification of dopamine agonists may be beneficial. Atypical antipsychotics are added only when a reduction of other medications has not resulted in improvement, because even atypical antipsychotics have been associated with worsening of PD motor symptoms (Goetz et al., 2000).

### Apathy

Individuals with PD often experience increased rates of apathy. Estimates of apathy in PD have ranged from 16.5% to 40.0%. Individuals with apathy exhibit greater cognitive impairment (Dujardin et al., 2007). Controlled clinical trials for apathy in PD are very limited. Environmental and other behavioral interventions including establishment of a routine, structured schedule, and cuing from others can be helpful in some settings. Dopamine agonists, psychostimulants, modafinil, dopamine agonists, and testosterone have been reported to be helpful in decreasing apathy (see Aarsland et al., 2009, for more detailed information).

### Impulse Control Disorders

Among the most difficult-to-treat patients with PD are those with impulse control disorders (ICDs) or dopamine dysregulation syndrome (DSS). ICDs include compulsive gambling as well as compulsive sexual, spending, and eating behaviors, and DDS includes compulsive PD medication use, particularly short-acting agents. Patients are often unaware of the severity and impact of these behaviors and can be reluctant to try recommended treatments (Okun and Weintraub, 2013). Although evidence in support of pharmacological treatments and behavioral therapy for management of these symptoms is accruing, some have suggested deep brain stimulation (DBS) and intestinal L-dopa. Research is needed to compare and document the efficacy of suggested treatments for ICDs in PD (Weintraub et al., 2010).

Suicide rates have been increasing, and suicide rates in PD are no exception. Recent efforts have been made to better understand the combination of depressed mood, impulse control, and suicidality in PD. Because depression and impulsivity can independently be considered risk factors for suicide, these symptoms in PD require careful assessment. Some data suggest that an increase in suicide and suicide attempts in patients with PD might be secondary to DBS surgery, although findings are mixed secondary to differences in population characteristics and study design (Buhmann, C. et al., 2017). Giannini and colleagues (2019) retrospectively examined 534 PD patients who underwent bilateral subthalamic nucleus stimulation DBS surgery between 1993 and 2016 and reported that suicide rates were higher than national averages adjusted for age and sex. Findings suggest that PD patients with history of depression, psychosis, family psychiatric history, greater impulsivity, and depression were at increased risk for both attempting and completing suicide.

### Neuropsychiatric Effects of Deep Brain Stimulation

DBS is a well-recognized treatment for motor complications of L-dopa therapy in patients with PD. Although patient selection, surgical procedure, mechanisms of DBS, postoperative management, and motor outcomes have been extensively reviewed, details regarding nonmotor aspects of DBS are still emerging. A recent review evaluated five randomized clinical trials comparing DBS with the best available medical treatment (Castrioto et al., 2014). Although nonmotor symptoms were not systematically assessed, eTable 9.8  summarizes changes in depression, suicidal ideation, fatigue, apathy, anxiety, lability, impulse control, and psychosis. Although firm conclusions are not possible due to nonstandard methodology, the following summary might suffice: (1) anxiety was improved, (2) outcomes for impulse control were mixed, (3) weight gain secondary to increased eating behaviors was consistent, (4) depressive episodes were more frequent although less severe, (5) apathy worsened, and (6) no conclusion could be reached from suicidal ideation assessment. Given the lack of standard methodology used across studies, interpretations are difficult to make and further research is warranted to better characterize behavioral and personality changes following DBS. Authors provided prevention and management recommendations for clinicians to use to provide the best clinical care for PD  patients undergoing DBS (eBox 9.3).

## Dementia With Lewy Bodies

DLB is increasingly being recognized as a common cause of dementia in older adults. DLB is associated with fluctuating cognitive difficulties, parkinsonism, and hallucinations. Clinical presentation overlap occurs between the presentation of DLB with AD and PD. Research has observed greater overall behavioral symptoms among individuals with DLB than in individuals with AD, particularly with regard to hallucinations and apathy (Ricci et al., 2009). Recent imaging research suggests that depressive symptoms in mild AD and DLB are associated with cortical thinning in prefrontal and temporal areas, suggesting a need to reevaluate antidepressants in these patients (Lebedev et al., 2014; Lebedeva et al., 2014).

### Psychosis

Psychotic symptoms, particularly hallucinations, are a hallmark feature of DLB. Insight is typically poor. Unlike patients with AD or PD, patients with DLB exhibit hallucinations early in the course of the illness. Delusions are also common in DLB. The neuropathological correlates of hallucinations in DLB are somewhat unclear. It has been suggested that hallucinations are likely due to decreased acetylcholine as well as to changes in the basal forebrain and the ventral temporal lobe (Ferman and Boeve, 2007).

Hallucinations are correlated with poorer functioning with regard to instrumental activities of daily living (Ricci et al., 2009). Typical neuroleptics are avoided in DLB, because patients exhibit high sensitivity to these drugs and may experience severe parkinsonian symptoms and other side effects. In contrast, atypical neuroleptics such as clozapine and quetiapine, as well as cholinesterase inhibitors, are associated with improved cognition and decreased psychotic symptoms (McKeith, 2002).

## Huntington Disease

Up to 79% of individuals with HD report psychiatric and behavioral symptoms as the presenting manifestation of the disease. Symptom presentation varies across stage of illness in HD (Table 9.9). Behavioral symptoms are commonly observed among institutionalized patients with HD (Table 9.10). The behavioral difficulties can lead to placement difficulties in these patients.

### Depression

Depression is one of the most common concerns for individuals and families with HD, occurring in up to 69% of patients (van Duijn et al., 2008). Depression in HD is associated with worse cognitive performance (Smith et al., 2012) and contributes to significant morbidity (Beglinger et al., 2010) as well as early mortality due to suicide (Fiedorowicz et al., 2011). Depression may precede the onset of neurological symptoms in HD by 2–20 years, although large-scale empirical research has been minimal. Depression is common immediately before diagnosis, when neurological soft signs and other subtle abnormalities become evident (Epping et al., 2013). However, following a definite diagnosis of HD, depression is most prevalent in the middle stages of the disease (i.e., Shoulson-Fahn stages 2 and 3) and may diminish in the later stages (Paulsen et al., 2005b). Positron emission tomography (PET) studies indicate that patients with HD with depression have hypermetabolism in the inferior frontal cortex and thalamus relative to nondepressed patients with HD or normal age-matched controls. Efforts to understand the cellular and molecular mechanisms underlying behavioral disorders in patients with HD have suggested that dysfunctional huntingtin (HTT) affects cellular pathways that are involved in mood disorders or in the response to antidepressants, including BDNF/TrkB and serotonergic signaling. Thus the pathogenic polyQ expansion in HTT could lead to mood disorders not only by the gain of a new toxic function but also by the perturbation of its normal function (Pla et al., 2014).

### Suicide

Suicide is more common in HD than in other neurological disorders with high rates of depression such as stroke and PD. Most studies have found a fourfold to sixfold increase of suicide in HD, with reports as high as 8–20 times greater than the general population. Two "critical periods" during which suicidal ideation in HD increases dramatically have been identified. First, frequency of suicidal ideation doubles from 10.4% in at-risk persons with a normal neurological examination to 20.5% in at-risk persons with soft neurological signs. Second, in persons with a diagnosis of HD, 16% had suicidal ideation in stage 1, whereas nearly 21% had suicidal ideation in stage 2. Although the underlying mechanisms for suicidal risk in HD are poorly understood, it may be beneficial for healthcare providers to be aware of periods during which patients may be at an increased risk of suicide (Paulsen et al., 2005a). A history of suicide attempts and the presence of depression were strongly predictive of suicidal behavior in a large sample of prodromal HD ($n = 735$; Fiedorowicz et al., 2011).

### Psychosis

Psychosis occurs with increased frequency in HD, with estimates ranging from 3% to 12%. Psychosis is more common among early adulthood-onset cases than among those whose disease begins in middle or late adulthood. Psychosis in HD is more resistant to treatment than psychosis in schizophrenia. Huntington Study Group data suggest that psychosis may increase as the disease progresses (see Table 9.9), although psychosis can become difficult to measure in the later stages of disease.

### Obsessive-Compulsive Traits

Although true obsessive-compulsive disorder (OCD) is rare in HD, obsessive and compulsive behaviors are prevalent (13%–30%). Obsessive thinking often increases with proximity to disease onset and then remains stable throughout the illness. Obsessive thinking associated with HD is reminiscent of perseveration, such that individuals get "stuck" on a previous occurrence or need and are unable to shift.

### Aggression

Aggressive behaviors ranging from irritability to intermittent explosive disorders (IEDs) occur in 19%–59% of patients with HD. Although aggressive outbursts are often the principal reason for admission to a psychiatric facility, research on the prevalence and incidence of irritability and aggressive outbursts in HD is sparse. The primary limitation in summarizing these symptoms in HD is the varied terminology used to describe this continuum of behaviors. Clinicians and HD family members report that difficulty with placement attributable to the patient's aggression was among the principal obstacles to providing placement, although recent research demonstrates that problematic behaviors are evident in a minority of HD patients in nursing homes (Zarowitz et al., 2014).

### Apathy

Early signs of HD may include withdrawal from activities and friends, decline in personal appearance, lack of behavioral initiation, decreased spontaneous speech, and constriction of emotional expression. Frequently, these symptoms are considered reflective of depression.

**TABLE 9.9 Percentage of Patients With Huntington Disease Endorsing Psychiatric Symptoms by Total Functional Capacity (TFC) Stage**

| Symptom | Stage 1 (*n* = 432) | Stage 2 (*n* = 660) | Stage 3 (*n* = 520) | Stage 4 (*n* = 221) | Stage 5 (*n* = 84) |
|---|---|---|---|---|---|
| Depression | 57.5% | 62.9% | 59.3% | 52.1% | 42.2% |
| Suicide | 6.0% | 9.7% | 10.3% | 9.9% | 5.5% |
| Aggression | 39.5% | 47.7% | 51.8% | 54.1% | 54.4% |
| Obsessions | 13.3% | 16.9% | 25.5% | 28.9% | 13.3% |
| Delusions | 2.4% | 3.5% | 6.1% | 9.9% | 2.2% |
| Hallucinations | 2.3% | 4.2% | 6.3% | 11.2% | 3.3% |

*Data provided by the Huntington Study Group.*

**TABLE 9.10 Ratings by Nursing Home Staff of Problematic Behaviors in Patients With Huntington Disease**

| Behavior Problem | Percentage | Rank |
|---|---|---|
| Agitation | 76 | 2.0 |
| Irritability | 72 | 2.9 |
| Disinhibition | 59 | 3.3 |
| Depression | 51 | 4.2 |
| Anxiety | 50 | 4.4 |
| Appetite | 54 | 5.1 |
| Delusions | 43 | 5.5 |
| Sleep disorders | 50 | 5.5 |
| Apathy | 32 | 6.8 |
| Euphoria | 40 | 6.9 |

*From Paulsen and Hamilton, unpublished data.*

Although difficult to distinguish, apathy is defined as diminished motivation not attributable to cognitive impairment, emotional distress, or decreased level of consciousness. Depression involves considerable emotional distress evidenced by tearfulness, sadness, anxiety, agitation, insomnia, anorexia, feelings of worthlessness and hopelessness, and recurrent thoughts of death. Both apathy (59%) and depression (70%) are common in HD. However, 53% of individuals experienced only one of these symptoms rather than the two combined. Furthermore, depression and apathy were not correlated. Recent reports suggest that apathy is one of the most common symptoms reported in HD (van Duijn et al., 2014) and severity of apathy may progress with disease duration.

## Tourette Syndrome

TS is associated with disinhibition of frontosubcortical circuitry; as a result, it is not surprising that increased rates of psychiatric and behavioral symptoms are observed. These behavioral difficulties are more strongly associated with psychosocial functioning than the presence of tics (Zinner and Coffey, 2009). Rates of psychiatric disorders vary widely; significantly higher rates of psychiatric disorders are reported when samples are drawn from psychiatric clinics than from movement disorder clinics. Given the correlation between psychiatric symptoms and changes in psychosocial functioning, treatments in TS that consider psychiatric and behavioral symptoms are encouraged (Shprecher et al., 2014).

Approximately 20%–40% of individuals with TS meet criteria for OCD, whereas up to 90% of individuals in a clinic-referred sample may exhibit subthreshold levels of obsessive-compulsive symptoms (Zinner and Coffey, 2009). The frequency and severity of tics often decrease as individuals enter adulthood, but the comorbid obsessive-compulsive symptoms are more likely to continue into adulthood and are associated with difficulties in psychosocial functioning (Cheung et al., 2007). Mood and anxiety symptoms are common in TS. The relationship between severity of depression and presence/prevalence of tics is unclear. The comorbid presence of obsessive-compulsive symptoms is associated with increased risk for depressive symptoms (Zinner and Coffey, 2009).

## Multiple Sclerosis

The assessment of behavioral symptoms in MS is complicated because one of the hallmark symptoms of MS is variability of symptoms across time. In addition, there is significant heterogeneity within patients with MS. Finally, a disconnection between the experience of emotion and the expression of emotion has historically been observed in individuals with MS.

### Depression

Depression is the most common behavioral symptom in MS, occurring at rates of 37%–54%. Patients with MS may report symptoms of depression even with outward signs of euphoria. Although depression is frequently associated with reduced quality of life, the correlation between depressive symptoms and disability in MS is equivocal. Depression in MS is *not* consistently associated with increased rates of stressful events, disease duration, sex, age, or socioeconomic status. Among the subtypes of MS, depression may be most common in those with relapsing-remitting MS (Beiske et al., 2008). Fatigue is a strong predictor of depression among individuals with MS (Beiske et al., 2008). Depression in MS is largely chronic and may require intervention at various times throughout the course of disease (Koch et al., 2014).

Increased rates of suicidal ideation, suicide attempts, and completed suicides have been observed in individuals with MS. Suicide rates in MS are between two and seven times higher than in the general population (Bronnum-Hansen et al., 2005). Risk factors for suicidal ideation in MS include social isolation, current depression, and lifetime diagnosis of alcohol abuse disorder. Although suicide attempts occur throughout the progression of the disease, some have suggested that increased risk may be particularly high in the year following diagnosis (Bronnum-Hansen et al., 2005).

Biological factors likely contribute to depressive symptoms in MS. It has been hypothesized that the inflammatory process associated with MS may directly lead to depressive symptoms. Similarly, demyelination lesions in MS may directly contribute to the etiology of depression. However, imaging studies in MS have failed to show clear neuropathological correlates of depression. Disruptions have been observed in right parietal, right temporal, and right frontal areas (Zorzon et al., 2001) as well as the limbic cortex, implying disruption of frontosubcortical circuitry. It is likely that depression in MS results from a combination of psychosocial and biological factors.

Although controversial, depression may be a side effect for some individuals treated with interferon beta-1b (IFN-β-1b) (Feinstein, 2000). Patients with severe depression should be closely monitored while receiving IFN-β-1b. The relationship between depression and

## BOX 9.2 Strategies to Minimize Anxiety in Patients With Multiple Sclerosis

- Respect adaptive denial as a useful coping mechanism.
- Provide referrals to the National Multiple Sclerosis Society (1-800-Fight-MS) early in disease.
- Help patients to live "one day at a time," and restrict predictions regarding the future.
- Help patients to manage stress with relaxation techniques.
- Involve occupational therapists for energy conservation techniques.
- Focus on the patient's abilities, not disabilities.
- Consider patient's educational and financial background when giving explanations and referrals.
- Realize that patients have access to the Internet, self-help groups, and medical journals and may ask "difficult" questions.
- Expect grief reactions to losses.
- Deal with losses one at a time.
- Attend to the mental health needs of patients' families and caregivers.
- Respect the patient's symptoms as real.
- Avoid overmedicating.
- Focus supportive psychotherapy on concrete, reality-based cognitive and educational issues related to multiple sclerosis.
- Provide targeted pharmacotherapy.
- Refer appropriate patients for cognitive remediation training.
- Ask about sexual problems, as well as bowel and bladder dysfunction.
- Keep an open dialogue with the patient about suicidal thoughts.

*Modified with permission from Riether, A.M., 1999. Anxiety in patients with multiple sclerosis. Semin, Neuropsychiatry 4, 103–113.*

## TABLE 9.11 Neuroanatomical Structures and Pseudobulbar Affect

| Structure | Neuroanatomical Significance |
|---|---|
| Prefrontal cortex and anterior cingulate | A major component of the limbic lobe, with motor efferents to the brainstem structures involved in emotional expression |
| Internal capsule | A white matter structure consisting of pathways descending from the brain to the brainstem and spinal cord. Some of these pathways are related to the brainstem nuclei, some to the cerebellum (via basis pontis), and some reach the spinal cord |
| Thalamus | A node in the pathways to the cortex originated from the brainstem, cerebellum, and basal ganglia |
| Subthalamic nucleus | A crucial node in the indirect pathways that carry signals from the striatum to the frontal lobe via the thalamus |
| Basis pontis | Relay center for pathways entering the cerebellum |
| Cerebellar white and gray matter | Receives inputs from many parts of the nervous system and sends its signals to the spinal cord, brainstem, and cerebral cortex (mostly frontal lobe and some to somatomotor parietal cortical areas) through the thalamus |

*Modified with permission from Parvizi, J., Coburn, K.L., Shillcutt, S.D., et al., 2009. Neuroanatomy of pathological laughing and crying: a report of the American Neuropsychiatric Association Committee on Research. J. Neuropsychiatry Clin. Neurosci. 21, 75–87. Copyright 2009, American Psychiatric Association.*

IFN-β-1a and interferon alpha (IFN-α) is equivocal, because conflicting results have been reported. In contrast, glatiramer acetate has not been associated with increased depressive symptoms (Feinstein, 2000). Because of the potential relationship between depression and treatment for MS, as well as the high rates of depression in MS, it is critical that physicians take care to thoroughly assess a patient's current and past history of depression. This may be particularly important prior to beginning IFN interventions, as patients with histories of depression may be more likely to experience symptoms of depression following IFN treatment.

Few randomly assigned clinical trials have been conducted for the treatment of depression in MS. Several open-label trials of SSRIs have been conducted, which suggest that SSRIs may be effective in the treatment of depression in MS (Siegert and Abernethy, 2005). In addition, psychotherapy, particularly that focusing on coping skills, is efficacious in the reduction of depressive symptoms.

### Anxiety

Although common, anxiety is often overlooked because anxiety symptoms may be viewed as a result of poor coping skills. Some strategies to minimize anxiety in individuals with MS are described in Box 9.2. Comorbid anxiety and depression are associated with greater somatic complaints, social difficulties, and suicidal ideation than either anxiety or depression alone. Predictors of anxiety in individuals with MS include fatigue, pain, and younger age of onset (Beiske et al., 2008).

### Euphoria

Increased rates of cheerfulness, optimism, and denial of disability may occur in MS. Early studies suggested that more than 70% of individuals with MS experienced periods of euphoria. However, more recent studies suggest that prevalence rates of euphoria are between 10% and 25%. Euphoria frequently co-occurs with disinhibition, impulsivity, and emotional lability. Individuals with euphoria are more likely to have cerebral involvement, enlarged ventricles, poorer cognitive and neurological function, and increased social disability.

### Pseudobulbar Affect

Pseudobulbar affect (PBA) occurs when there is disparity between an individual's emotional *experience* and his or her emotional *expression*; affected individuals are unable to control laughter or crying. Approximately 10% of individuals with MS exhibit periods of PBA (Parvizi et al., 2009). PBA is more common in MS patients who have entered the chronic-progressive disease course, have high levels of disability, and have cognitive dysfunction. The neuropathological substrate for PBA is believed to involve several aspects of the frontosubcortical circuits as well as the cerebellum (Parvizi et al., 2009). Table 9.11 gives more detailed information. Dextromethorphan/quinidine may be effective in treating such symptoms (Panitch et al., 2006; Pioro et al., 2010) and is FDA approved. In addition, tricyclic and SSRI antidepressant medications may be helpful in reducing PBA symptoms (Parvizi et al., 2009).

## Amyotrophic Lateral Sclerosis

Historically, amyotrophic lateral sclerosis (ALS) has been largely viewed as a pure motor neuron disease. Increased awareness of cognitive and behavioral changes in individuals with ALS has burgeoned over the past few years. Mutations in the gene *C9orf72*, which causes TDP-43 positive inclusions, have been implicated in a large number of cases of both conditions. In fact, the two can coexist in the same family or in the same individual with a single mutation (Bennion Callister and Pickering-Brown, 2014; Seelaar et al., 2007). Patients with ALS and the C9orf72 repeat expansion seem to present a recognizable phenotype characterized by earlier disease onset, the presence of cognitive and behavioral impairment, specific neuroimaging changes, a family history of autosomal dominant neurodegeneration, and reduced survival (Byrne et al., 2012). It is currently well understood that behavioral and cognitive disturbances occur in a substantial proportion of patients, a subgroup of whom present with frontotemporal dementia. Deficits are characterized by executive and working memory impairments extending to changes in language and social cognition. Behavior and social cognition deficits closely resemble those reported in the behavioral variant of frontotemporal dementia, and consensus criteria for diagnosis of cognitive and behavioral syndromes related to ALS are reprinted in Table 9.12.

### Depression

Depressive symptoms occur in 40%–50% of individuals with ALS (Kubler et al., 2005), although most individuals exhibit subsyndromal depression. Depression in ALS has historically been thought to be associated with increased physical impairment, although these results are increasingly overturned (Kubler et al., 2005; Lule et al., 2008). Individuals with low psychological well-being were at increased risk of mortality (Fig. 9.7). Mortality risk was more strongly associated with psychological distress than age and was similar to the association of risk associated with severity of illness. Depression is correlated with duration of illness; however, depression is not associated with ventilator use or tube feeding (Kubler et al., 2005). Quality of life is highly impacted by presence of depressive symptoms, more so than the presence of physical limitations, indicating that physicians should be aware of available treatments for depressive symptoms (Lule et al., 2008).

### Pseudobulbar Affect

Up to 50% of individuals with ALS, most often those with pseudobulbar syndrome, report PBA (Parvizi et al., 2009). Individuals with PBA may be more likely to exhibit behavioral changes similar to those observed among individuals with FTD (Gibbons et al., 2008). Little research has assessed treatment of PBA. Potential pharmacological interventions include use of tricyclic and SSRI antidepressant medications (Parvizi et al., 2009). Dextromethorphan/quinidine may also be an effective treatment for PBA (Parvizi et al., 2009) and is currently FDA approved. Reduction in PBA symptoms was associated with improved quality of life and quality of relationships.

### Personality Change

With recognition of the correlation between ALS and FTD, increased interest has been placed on assessing for potential behavioral changes in ALS. Minimal research has fully explored this question. Gibbons and colleagues (2008) assessed behavioral changes among a small group of individuals with ALS by using a structured interview of close family members of those with ALS. In this small study, 14 of 16 individuals with ALS exhibited behavioral changes. Of those with behavioral changes, 69% exhibited reduced concern for others, 63% exhibited increased irritability, and 38% exhibited increased apathy. A questionnaire to assess behavioral change has been developed specifically for ALS to minimize exaggerations of behavior related to motor dysfunction (Raaphorst et al., 2012). Additional screening instruments for the detection and tracking of these syndromes in ALS are provided in Table 9.13.

## Epilepsy

Behavioral and personality disturbances occur in up to 50% of individuals with epilepsy. Identification and treatment of these behavioral disturbances remain inadequate, with less than half of individuals with epilepsy and major depressive disorder (MDD) being treated for depression. Presence of a psychiatric disorder is an independent predictor of quality of life in individuals with epilepsy (Kanner et al., 2010). In epilepsy, psychiatric disturbances are classified based on their chronological relationship to seizures. Ictal disturbances occur during the seizure. Periictal disturbances occur immediately before (preictal) or after (postictal) a seizure. Finally, interictal disturbances are those that occur independently of seizure states (Table 9.14). To facilitate patient understanding and provide accurate treatment of psychiatric symptoms, it is important to recognize that behavioral and personality disturbances can occur during the ictal state. Individuals in the ictal period may experience episodes of anxiety, depression, psychosis, and aggression. In addition, some seizures can cause uncontrollable but mirthless laughter, so-called gelastic epilepsy, which is classically seen with hypothalamic hamartomas (Parvizi et al., 2011). However, because much of the research regarding psychiatric disturbances in epilepsy has focused on interictal behavioral and personality disturbances, these disturbances will be the focus of this section.

### Depression

Depression is the most common psychiatric disorder in epilepsy. Rates of depression vary as a function of the sample assessed (clinical samples report higher rates of depression than population samples) and the measures used to diagnose depression. Depression often goes undiagnosed in patients with epilepsy, because symptoms of depression may be viewed as a normal reaction to illness. However, accurate diagnosis of depression is critical because depression is associated with poorer quality of life, underemployment, and family dysfunction (Ettinger et al., 2004). Interestingly, presurgical depression is associated with poorer postsurgical seizure outcomes (Metternich et al., 2009).

Attempted and completed suicides are common in epilepsy. The suicide rate in epilepsy is two or more times greater than in the general population (Stefanello et al., 2010). Rates of suicide are even higher in temporal lobe epilepsy. Risk factors for suicide include history of self-harm, family history of suicide, stressful life situations, poor morale, stigma, and psychiatric disorders. Individuals with comorbid anxiety and depression are at greater risk for suicidal ideation than individuals with only one syndrome (Stefanello et al., 2010). People with drug-resistant epilepsy have a particularly high rate of suicide, and efforts to better predict risk factors in this cohort are underway (Kwon and Park, 2019).

The cause of depression in epilepsy is unclear. Psychosocial stressors, genetic disposition, and neuropathology may play contributing roles. Although psychosocial stressors have been suggested as important in the cause of depression in epilepsy, observed rates of depression in epilepsy are higher than those in other chronically ill patient populations, lending support to theories of biological causes. Perception of seizure control is an important psychosocial variable to consider because a lower perception of seizure control is associated with increased depressive symptoms. Although results are somewhat mixed, there appears to be no relationship between age of onset or duration of epilepsy and depression. Depression appears to be more common in individuals with focal epilepsy than in those with primarily generalized epilepsy. Lateralization of seizure foci may be related to depression, with left-sided foci being more commonly associated with depression.

Pharmacological treatment of epilepsy may contribute to depression and psychiatric symptoms in general. Table 9.15 notes commonly used antiepileptic drugs (AEDs) and their psychotropic effects. Medications associated with sedation (e.g., barbiturates, benzodiazepines) may lead to depression, fatigue, and mental sluggishness.

Although the phenomenology of depression in epilepsy may prove dissimilar from that in patients with general depression, similar treatments are efficacious in the treatment of depression. Supportive psychotherapy may prove beneficial, particularly after initial diagnosis as

**TABLE 9.12 Consensus Criteria (Strong et al., 2009) for Diagnosis of Cognitive and Behavioral Syndromes Related to Amyotrophic Lateral Sclerosis and Their Potential Limitations**

| | Features Listed by Strong et al. (2009) | Comments |
|---|---|---|
| Relevant background characteristics for assessment of cognitive impairment | Premorbid intellectual ability; bulbar dysfunction; motor weakness; neurological comorbidities; systemic disorders (e.g., diabetes, hypothyroidism); drug effects (e.g., substance use, narcotic analgesics, psychotropics); psychiatric disorders (e.g., severe anxiety or depression, psychosis); respiratory dysfunction (measured by forced vital capacity, maximum inspiratory force, nocturnal oximetry or carbon dioxide readings); disrupted sleep; delirium; pain; fatigue; low motivation to undertake tests | A comprehensive list of potential confounds that might underlie or affect the presentation of cognitive impairment and behavioral change and that should be considered on a case-by-case basis |
| Background characteristics to be taken into account in diagnosis of behavioral impairment | Psychiatric disorders; psychological reaction to diagnosis of amyotrophic lateral sclerosis; premorbid diagnosis of personality disorder; pseudobulbar affect/emotional lability/pathological laughing and crying should be differentiated from depression | A comprehensive list of potential confounds that might underlie or affect the presentation of cognitive impairment and behavioral change and that should be considered on a case-by-case basis |
| Amyotrophic lateral sclerosis–cognitive impairment | Patient should have impaired scores (i.e., ≤5th percentile) on standardized neuropsychological tests compared with age-matched and education-matched norms, on two or more separate neuropsychological tests that are sensitive to executive dysfunction; domains other than executive functions should be assessed | Full assessments should control adequately for motor dysfunction and speech difficulties or use of assistive communication; examination of executive dysfunction only might underestimate prevalence of cognitive impairment; (Taylor et al., 2012) no data yet as to whether inclusion of measures of social cognition or theory of mind would affect detection; should ensure that impairments cannot be better explained by the potential confounds |
| Amyotrophic lateral sclerosis–behavioral impairment | Patient should meet two or more nonoverlapping supportive diagnostic features from established criteria for behavioral variant frontotemporal dementia (Neary et al., 1998; Rascovsky et al., 2007) (presence of only one feature might lead to overdiagnosis); presence of two behavioral abnormalities necessitates support obtained from two or more sources selected from interview or observation of the patient, report from a carer, or structured interview or questionnaire; reports from family or friends are essential; need to clarify that changes in behavior should be new, disabling, and not better accounted for by physical limitations that result from the disease | Tests of social cognition or the theory of mind might corroborate informants' reports; questionnaires specific to amyotrophic lateral sclerosis might improve correct identification of behavioral change (most available tests do not take into account the physical and resulting functional restrictions imposed by the disease); should ensure that impairments cannot be better explained by the potential confounds |
| Amyotrophic lateral sclerosis–frontotemporal dementia | Three categories are commonly recognized—behavioral variant frontotemporal dementia (progressive behavioral change characterized by insidious onset, changed social behavior, impaired self-control of interpersonal behavior, emotional blunting, and loss of insight); progressive nonfluent aphasia (progressively nonfluent speech accompanied by agrammatism, paraphasias, or anomia); and semantic dementia (fluent speech but impaired comprehension of word meaning or object identity, or both) | Criteria for frontotemporal lobar degeneration syndromes (of which behavioral variant frontotemporal dementia, progressive nonfluent aphasia, and semantic dementia are subtypes) were not originally defined for amyotrophic lateral sclerosis; should ensure that impairments cannot be better explained by the potential confounds<br>For behavioral variant frontotemporal dementia, diagnosis is mainly based on behavioral symptoms—thus the illness will not be diagnosed in patients without behavioral change but with primary executive dysfunction; diagnosis does not place main emphasis on evidence of executive dysfunction as measured with cognitive tests (although such evidences does contribute) |
| Amyotrophic lateral sclerosis–comorbid dementia | Association with a dementia not typical of frontotemporal dementia (e.g., Alzheimer disease, vascular dementia, mixed dementias) | Alzheimer pathological changes might be noted in patients presenting with behavioral variant frontotemporal dementia (Snowden et al., 2011), so this possible classification should not be discounted in amyotrophic lateral sclerosis |

*With permission from Goldstein, L.H., Abrahams, S., 2013. Changes in cognition and behaviour in amyotrophic lateral sclerosis: nature of impairment and implications for assessment. Lancet Neurol. 12, 368–380.*

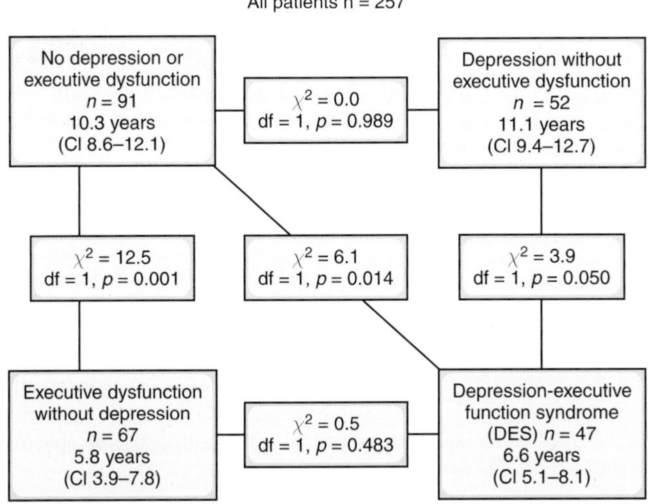


**Fig. 9.7** Poststroke survival by presence or absence of depression and executive dysfunction (endpoint, all causes of death). NOTE: determined by Kaplan-Meier Logistic-Rank Analysis. *(Reprinted with permission from Melkas, S., Vataja R., Oksala, N.K., et al., 2010. Depression-executive dysfunction syndrome relates to poor poststroke survival. Am. J. Geriatr. Psychiatry 18, 1007–1016.)*

patients begin to adapt to their illness. Few clinical trials have assessed the efficacy of antidepressant medications in patients with epilepsy. Older antidepressants and the antidepressant bupropion have been associated with increased seizures and should be avoided. Prueter and Norra (2005) suggest that citalopram and sertraline be considered first-line antidepressant medications in epilepsy because of their limited interactions with antiepileptic medication.

## Anxiety

Increased rates of anxiety disorders occur in patients with epilepsy. Between 19% and 50% of individuals with epilepsy meet criteria for one or more Diagnostic and Statistical Manual of Mental Disorders Fifth Editions (DSM-V) anxiety disorders (Beyenburg et al., 2005). Individuals with comorbid anxiety and depressive disorders report lower quality of life than individuals with either disorder alone (Kanner et al., 2010). Common anxiety disorders include agoraphobia, generalized anxiety disorder, and social phobia. Fear of having a seizure and anticipatory anxiety are quite common. Care must be taken to distinguish between panic attacks and fear occurring in the context of a seizure ("ictal fear"). Fear is the most common psychiatric symptom to manifest during a seizure.

The relationship between AEDs and anxiety is complex. Some AEDs appear to exacerbate anxiety symptoms, whereas others are associated with reductions in anxiety symptoms. Antidepressant

**TABLE 9.13 Screening Instruments for Cognitive Impairment and Behavioral Change in Amyotrophic Lateral Sclerosis**

| | Description | Strengths | Weaknesses |
|---|---|---|---|
| Penn State screen exam (Flaherty-Craig et al., 2006, 2009) | Neurobehavioral cognitive status examination, letter and category fluency, and the American National Adult Reading Test | Multidomain assessment; includes premorbid functions | Developed for other neurological disorders; not designed or modified for physical disability (Wicks et al., 2007); not formally validated |
| Screening assessment for cognitive impairment in amyotrophic lateral sclerosis (Gordon et al., 2007) | Verbal fluency and frontal behavior inventory | Brief; verbal fluency is particularly sensitive to cognitive impairment | Only one cognitive subtest (fluency); not adapted for physical disability; not formally validated |
| Amyotrophic Lateral Sclerosis Cognitive Behaviour Screen (Woolley et al., 2010) | Eight short cognitive tasks (executive functions) and carer behavior questionnaire | Brief; validated against neuropsychological battery in patients with amyotrophic lateral sclerosis | Assesses executive functions only; no language or memory assessment |
| Written verbal fluency (Abrahams et al., 2000) | Verbal fluency with motor control condition producing verbal fluency index | Designed to accommodate motor slowing; sensitive to frontal lobe dysfunction; validated with brain imaging | Only one cognitive test; needs further validation and normative data |
| Frontal Assessment Battery (Dubois et al., 2000) | Brief six-item screen | Brief; sensitive in patients with severe cognitive impairment | Investigated in a small sample of patients; not designed for patients with physical disability; assesses only one cognitive domain |
| Amyotrophic lateral sclerosis–frontotemporal dementia questionnaire (Raaphorst et al., 2012) | Behavioral screen, informant based | Developed for amyotrophic lateral sclerosis; good construct and clinical validity | Further validation data not yet available |
| Frontal Systems Behavior Scale (Grace and Malloy, 2002; Grossman et al., 2007) | Behavioral screen (patient and carer); three subscales (apathy, disinhibition, executive dysfunction) | Determines change in behavior from before illness to after onset | Not designed for amyotrophic lateral sclerosis; overlapping with physical symptoms particularly for apathy scale; potentially exaggerates behavioral change |
| Frontal Behavior Inventory (Kertesz et al., 1997) | Carer interviewed about patients' behavior and personality change; two subscales—negative behavior and disinhibition; modified version (Heidler-Gary and Hillis, 2007) is a self-complete measure* | Sensitive to subtypes of frontotemporal dementia and amyotrophic lateral sclerosis–frontotemporal dementia | Not designed for amyotrophic lateral sclerosis (items overlap with physical symptoms) |
| Neuropsychiatric Inventory (Cummings et al., 1994) | Carer-completed questionnaire with 12 neuropsychiatric domains | Used widely in other neurological groups; sensitive to moderate and severe dementia | Not designed for amyotrophic lateral sclerosis (items overlap with physical symptoms) |

*Frontal Behaviour Inventory—modified as described by Heidler-Gary and Hillis (2007). For a comprehensive list, including further recommendations on depression and pseudobulbar affect, see NINDS Common Data Elements.

*With permission from Goldstein, L.H., Abrahams, S., 2013, Changes in cognition and behaviour in amyotrophic lateral sclerosis: nature of impairment and implications for assessment. Lancet Neurol. 12, 368–380.*

medication, particularly the SSRIs, is the most common pharmacological treatment for anxiety in epilepsy. See the review by Beyenburg and colleagues (2005) for a more detailed discussion of treatment of anxiety in epilepsy.

### Psychosis

The association between epilepsy and psychosis has been debated throughout the past century. Individuals with epilepsy onset before age 20 years, duration of illness greater than 10 years, history of complex partial seizures, and temporal lobe epilepsy are at increased risk of psychotic disturbances. Postictal and interictal psychosis are most commonly reported. Postictal psychosis most commonly develops after many years of epilepsy (Devinsky, 2003). Episodes of postictal psychosis are short in duration, lasting from a few hours to a few months. Postictal psychosis is more common with limbic lesions (Devinsky, 2003). In interictal psychosis, episodes of psychosis are not temporally tied to seizure onset and typically last for more than 6 months.

**TABLE 9.14 Psychiatric Disturbances in Ictal, Postictal, and Interictal States**

| Ictal | Postictal | Interictal |
|---|---|---|
| Anxiety | Agitation | Panic disorder |
| Intense feelings of horror | | Generalized anxiety disorder |
| Panic attacks | | Phobias |
| Depressed mood | Depression | Major depressive disorder |
| Tearfulness | | Dysthymic disorder |
| | | Atypical depressive syndromes |
| | | Medication-induced mood changes |
| | | Adjustment disorder |
| Paranoia | Paranoia | Psychotic syndromes |
| Hallucinations | Hallucinations | |
| Illusions | | |
| Forced thoughts resembling obsessions | | Obsessive-compulsive disorder |
| Obsessions | | |
| Aggression/violence | Aggression/violence | Aggression/violence |
| Confusion | Confusion | |
| Sexual excitement | | |
| Laughter | Mania | |
| Déjà vu and other memory experiences | | |
| | | Conversion disorder |
| | | Medication-induced conditions |

*Reprinted with permission from Marsh, L., Rao, V., 2002. Psychiatric complications in patients with epilepsy: a review. Epilepsy Res. 49, 11–33.*

### Aggression

The relationship between epilepsy and aggression remains controversial. Early research suggested that the prevalence of aggression in epilepsy ranged from 4.8% to 50.0%. Aggression occurring in the context of a seizure is quite rare (Devinsky, 2003). Rates of aggression are believed to be higher in individuals with temporal lobe epilepsy. Results vary owing to the definition of aggression used and the method of group selection. Interictal aggression may be described as episodic dyscontrol or, as in the DSM nosology, IED, which is characterized by periods of largely unprovoked anger, rage, severe aggression, and violent behavior. Hippocampal sclerosis is less common in individuals with epilepsy and aggression (Tebartz van Elst et al., 2000). A subgroup of individuals with epilepsy and aggression has significant amygdala atrophy (Tebartz van Elst, 2002).

## Stroke

Neuropsychiatric disorders after stroke are common and distressing to patients and their families but often go undertreated. The most common neuropsychiatric outcomes of stroke are depression, anxiety, fatigue, and apathy, which each occur in at least 30% of patients and have substantial overlap. Emotional lability, personality changes, psychosis, and mania are less common. Neuropsychiatric complications of stroke are challenging to manage and require more research (Hackett et al., 2014).

### Depression

Within the first year following a stroke, 30%–40% of patients experience depression, with most developing depression within the first month (Ballard and O'Brien, 2002). Interestingly, rates appear to be similar for individuals in early, middle, and late stages following stroke.

**TABLE 9.15 Psychotropic Effects of Antiepileptic Drugs**

| Drug | Positive Effects | Negative Effects | Complications |
|---|---|---|---|
| Barbiturates | — | Aggression, depression, withdrawal syndromes | ADHD in children |
| Benzodiazepines | Anxiolytic, sedative | Withdrawal syndromes | Disinhibition |
| Ethosuximide | — | Insomnia | Alternative psychoses |
| Phenytoin | — | — | Toxic schizophreniform psychoses, encephalopathy |
| Carbamazepine | Mood stabilizing/impulse control | Rarely, mania and depression | — |
| Valproate | Mood stabilizing, antimanic | — | Acute and chronic encephalopathy |
| Vigabatrin | — | Aggression, depression, psychosis, withdrawal syndromes | ADHD, encephalopathy, alternative psychoses |
| Lamotrigine | Mood stabilizing, antidepressive | Insomnia | Rarely psychoses |
| Felbamate | Stimulating? | Agitation | Psychoses possible |
| Gabapentin | Anxiolytic, antidepressive? | Rarely aggression in children | — |
| Tiagabine | — | Depression | Nonconvulsive status epilepticus |
| Topiramate | Mood stabilizing? | Depression | Psychoses |
| Levetiracetam | — | — | — |

*ADHD*, Attention-deficit/hyperactivity disorder; *?*, Minimal data; *—*, not applicable.

*Reprinted with permission from Schmitz, B., 2002. Effects of antiepileptic drugs on behavior, in: Trimble, M., Schmitz, B. (Eds.), The Neuropsychiatry of Epilepsy. Cambridge University Press, Cambridge, UK.*

Depression after a stroke is associated with age, time since stroke, cognitive impairment, and social support. Significantly higher rates (five to six times more likely) of poststroke depression have been reported among individuals with a premorbid diagnosis of depression (Ried et al., 2010).

Depression is associated with longer hospital stays, suggesting that it affects rehabilitation efforts. Depression is associated with poorer recovery of activities of daily living and increased morbidity. Depression and executive dysfunction commonly co-occur following a stroke. The presence of executive dysfunction with or without co-occurring depressive symptoms may be the strongest predictor of morbidity following stroke (Melkas et al., 2010) (see Fig. 9.7). Studies assessing the relationship between disability and depression in stroke patients have been equivocal. Depression is associated with poorer quality of life in individuals who have had a stroke, even when neurological symptoms and disability are held constant.

The relationship between depression and lesion location has been the focus of significant research and controversy. Early research by Robinson and Price showed that left anterior lesions were associated with increased rates and severity of depression. Lesions nearer the left frontal pole or left caudate nucleus were associated with increased rates of depression. Some researchers have replicated these findings, but others have failed to do so. More recent review articles have not supported a relationship between lesion location and depression in poststroke patients (Bhogal et al., 2004). Of note, there is significant heterogeneity in previous studies, particularly between different sample sources.

If more homogeneous groups of patients are considered, some relationships emerge. Depression is associated with left-sided lesions in studies using hospital samples, whereas depression is associated with right-sided lesions in community samples (Bhogal et al., 2004). Time since stroke is an additional important variable to consider. Poststroke depression is associated with left-sided lesions in individuals in the first month following stroke (Bhogal et al., 2004). However, poststroke depression is associated with right-sided lesions in individuals more than 6 months after the stroke (Bhogal et al., 2004). Other differences in previous research, such as method of depression diagnosis, may contribute to the mixed results.

Few studies have assessed the effectiveness of various treatments for depression in these patients. A recent review suggests that there is no clear evidence that standard antidepressant medications are effective in the treatment of poststroke depression (Hackett et al., 2005). Although such interventions may not lead to effective cessation of depressive disorders, they may result in overall reductions in depressive severity. One study suggests that nortriptyline was more effective in the treatment of depression than either placebo or fluoxetine (Robinson et al., 2000). In this study, response to treatment with nortriptyline was associated with improvement in cognitive and functional abilities. This improvement in cognition and functional abilities following reduction in depressive symptoms has not always been replicated (Hackett et al., 2005).

### Pseudobulbar Affect

A portion of individuals experience PBA after a stroke. Between 11% and 35% of individuals experience emotional incontinence after stroke (Parvizi et al., 2009). Emotional incontinence is associated with lesions of the brainstem and cerebellar region (see Parvizi et al., 2009 for a review). Dextromethorphan with quinidine is currently FDA approved for PBA. Preliminary evidence suggests that tricyclic and SSRI antidepressants may be helpful in alleviating symptoms of PBA (Parvizi et al., 2009).

**TABLE 9.16 Lifetime Prevalence of Major Psychiatric Disorders by Head Injury Status From the New Haven Epidemiologic Catchment Area Study ($n$ = 5034)**

| | Head Injury (%) | No Head Injury (%) |
|---|---|---|
| Major depression ($n$ = 242) | 11.1 | 5.2 |
| Dysthymia ($n$ = 172) | 5.5 | 2.9 |
| Bipolar disorder ($n$ = 45) | 1.6 | 1.1 |
| Panic disorder ($n$ = 60) | 3.2 | 1.3 |
| Obsessive-compulsive disorder ($n$ = 102) | 4.7 | 2.3 |
| Phobic disorder ($n$ = 361) | 11.2 | 7.4 |
| Alcohol abuse/dependence ($n$ = 412) | 24.5 | 10.1 |
| Drug abuse/dependence ($n$ = 175) | 10.9 | 5.2 |
| Schizophrenia ($n$ = 73) | 3.4 | 1.9 |

Note: Adjusted for age, sex, marital status, socioeconomic status, alcohol abuse, and quality of life.

*Reprinted with permission from Silver, J.M., Kramer, R., Greenwald, S., et al., 2001. The association between head injuries and psychiatric disorders: findings from the New Haven NIMH epidemiologic catchment area study. Brain Inj. 15, 935–945.*

### Aggression

Reports have suggested that individuals have difficulty controlling aggression and anger following a stroke. Inability to control anger or aggression was associated with increased motor dysfunction and dysarthria. Aggression following stroke is associated with increased rates of MDD and generalized anxiety disorder. There is some evidence that lesions in the area supplied by the subcortical middle cerebral artery are associated with inability to control anger. Poststroke irritability and aggression are associated with lesions nearer to the frontal pole. Fluoxetine has been shown to successfully reduce levels of poststroke anger (Choi-Kwon et al., 2006). Similarly, reductions in irritability and aggression have been associated with reductions in depression following pharmacological intervention (Chan et al., 2006).

### Psychosis

Psychosis appears to be a rare sequela of stroke but has been reported to happen in the setting of large strokes in the right hemisphere. Preexisting atrophy (Rabins et al., 1991), preexisting untreated psychiatric disorders, and right inferior frontal gyrus involvement appear to be risk factors (Devine et al., 2014) for poststroke psychosis.

## Traumatic Brain Injury

TBI is a significant public health concern, affecting approximately 1.7 million individuals annually, with 275,000 individuals hospitalized each year in the United States. Public interest in TBI has increased secondary to recent military conflicts resulting in frequent blast injuries, as well as growing recognition of sports-related head injury. Significant behavioral and psychiatric disturbances are common following TBI, are typically chronic and a major cause of disability, and remain one of the most consistent risk factors for dementia in later life (Table 9.16) (Kim et al., 2007; Mortimer et al., 1991). Behavioral or mood disturbances are associated with decreased quality of life, increased caregiver burden, and more challenges to the treating physician and can significantly affect daily functioning, including management of close relationships and employment. Psychiatric diagnoses following TBI

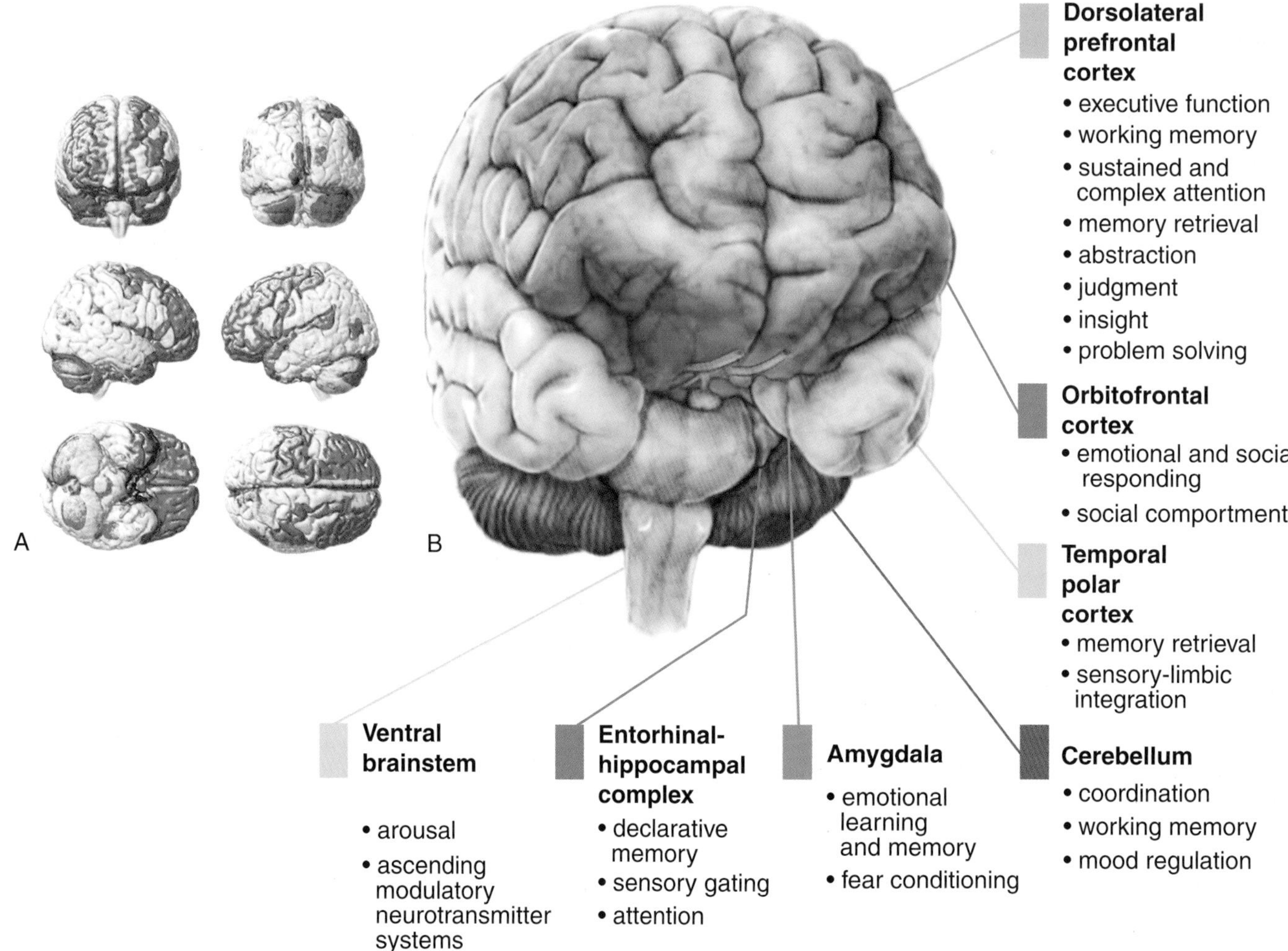


**Fig. 9.8** (A) Brain regions vulnerable to damage in a typical traumatic brain injury *(TBI)*; (B) Relationship of vulnerable brain regions to common neurobehavioral sequelae associated with TBI. *(A, Adapted from Bigler, E., 2005. Structural imaging. In: Silver, J., McAllister, T., Yudofsky, S. (Eds.), Textbook of Traumatic Brain Injury. American Psychiatric Press, Washington, DC, p. 87. Copyright © American Psychiatric Press, 2005. B, Adapted from Arciniegas, D.B., Beresford, T.P., 2001. Neuropsychiatry: An Introductory Approach. Cambridge University Press, Cambridge, UK, p. 58. Copyright © Cambridge University Press, 2001.)*

are more common in individuals with a history of psychiatric illness, poor social functioning, alcoholism, arteriosclerosis, lower MMSE score, and fewer years of education. Many behavioral changes such as increased disinhibition are associated with dysfunction within the frontal cortex. Fig. 9.8 (McAllister, 2011) depicts brain regions vulnerable to TBI and the associated relationships to neurobehavioral sequelae.

## Anosognosia

Although TBI is often associated with changes in motor, cognitive, and behavioral functioning, individuals with TBI frequently do not accurately assess these changes. Impairments in awareness have been associated with functional outcomes. Although it is most commonly reported that individuals with TBI underreport their difficulties, a subgroup of individuals appears to overreport their difficulties. It has been reported that individuals with mild to moderate TBI report greater impairments than their family members do of them, whereas those with more severe TBI report fewer impairments than their family members. Overreporting may be associated with depressive symptoms or litigation. Although symptoms of TBI frequently lead to difficulties in independent living and in the workplace, accurate assessment of these difficulties serves to mitigate this relationship. Thus it is possible that improved levels of awareness may lead to reductions in disability.

## Depression

Depression following TBI is common. Diagnosis of depression in TBI is complicated because symptoms of depression (e.g., fatigue, concentration difficulties, sleep disturbances) are common following TBI. For further discussion regarding the diagnosis of depression in TBI, see Seel et al. (2010). MDD occurs in up to 60% of individuals who have suffered TBI (Kim et al., 2007). Rates of depression in TBI vary as a function of severity of TBI assessed, method of depression diagnosis, and sample source. The best predictor of depression after TBI is the presence of premorbid depression; however, some have failed to replicate this finding. Other factors associated with post-TBI depression

TABLE 9.17 **Core Features of Behavioral Symptoms in Traumatic Brain Injury**

| Core Features | Depression | Apathy | Anxiety | Dysregulation |
|---|---|---|---|---|
| Mood (Intensity, scope) | Sad, irritable, frustrated (constant, global) | Flat, unexcited (constant, global) | Worried, distressed (frequent, situational) | Angry, tense (frequent, global) |
| Activity level | Low activity | Lack of initiative, behavior | Restless, "keyed up" | Impulsive, physically aggressive, argumentative |
| Attitude | Loss of interest, pleasure | Lack of concern | Overconcern | Argumentative |
| Awareness | Overestimates problems | Does not notice problems | Overestimates problems | Underestimates problems |
| Cognitions | Rumination on loss, failures | Unresponsive to events | Rumination on harm, danger | Rumination on tension, arousal |
| Physiological | Underaroused or hyperaroused | Underaroused | Hyperaroused | Underaroused or agitated |
| Coping style | Avoidance, social withdrawal | Compliant, dependent | Avoidance, checking behaviors | Uncontrolled outbursts |

*Modified from Seel, R.T., Macciocchi, S., Kreutzer, J.S., 2010. Clinical considerations for the diagnosis of major depression after moderate to severe TBI. J. Head Trauma Rehabil. 25, 99–112.*

include poor coping styles, social isolation, and increased stress (Kim et al., 2007). Depression in TBI is associated with increased suicidality, increased cognitive problems, greater disability, and aggression. See Table 9.17 for additional information regarding differentiating features associated with depression in TBI.

Suicidal ideation (65%) and attempts (8.1%) are common following TBI (Silver et al., 2001). In contrast to sex differences reported in the general population, women with TBI are more likely to commit suicide than men with TBI. Furthermore, suicide was more common in individuals with more severe injury and those younger than 21 years or older than 60 years at the time of injury.

No large class I studies of use of antidepressant medications, particularly SSRIs, in TBI have been completed, but small studies provide preliminary support for their use to treat depressive symptoms following TBI. Care must be taken in certain situations, because some antidepressants (i.e., bupropion) are associated with increased risk of seizures. Close monitoring following the beginning of a trial of antidepressant medication is encouraged; in some settings, such medications can increase agitation or anxiety in individuals with TBI. Please see Alderfer and colleagues (2005) for more details regarding recommendations for treatment of depression following TBI.

### Anxiety

Less research has assessed the prevalence of anxiety disorders in TBI; however, studies suggest that 11%–70% of individuals meet criteria for an anxiety disorder. A meta-analysis suggested that the mean prevalence of anxiety disorders following TBI is 29%. Panic disorder occurs in 3.2%–9.0% of individuals with a TBI (Silver et al., 2001).

### Apathy

Symptoms of apathy are reported in 10%–60% of individuals with a TBI. Among individuals with TBI referred to a behavioral management program, lack of initiation was among the most commonly reported problems, occurring in approximately 60% of the sample (Kelly et al., 2008). Apathy in TBI is often associated with depressive symptoms, although a significant number of individuals (28%) report experiencing apathy but not depression. Lesions affecting the right hemisphere and subcortical regions are more strongly associated with apathy than lesions affecting the left hemisphere.

### Personality Change

Personality change following TBI is common secondary to frequent injury to the frontal lobe and disruption of the frontosubcortical circuitry. Common changes include increased irritability, aggression, disinhibition, and inappropriate behavior. Although these difficulties can be among the most disabling for individuals with TBI, research in these areas is limited, and no uniform, agreed-upon diagnostic criteria for these behavioral changes exist.

Aggression within 6 months of TBI has been reported in up to 60% of individuals with TBI (Baguley et al., 2006). Among individuals referred to a TBI behavior management service, verbal aggression and inappropriate social behavior were among the most commonly reported behavioral difficulties and occurred in more than 80% of individuals (Kelly et al., 2008). Aggression following TBI is associated with depression, poorer psychosocial functioning, and greater disability (Rao et al., 2009).

A number of pharmacological interventions have been used to reduce and remediate behavioral changes following brain injury. See Nicholl and LaFrance (2009) for a review. One class of medication used in these settings is AEDs, currently routinely used to treat aggression, disinhibition, and mania following TBI. Again, few large-scale studies have assessed the effectiveness of AEDs in the treatment of behavioral change following TBI. Historically, neuroleptic drugs were used in high doses to treat behavioral dyscontrol in individuals with cognitive impairment. More recently, there has been increased interest in the use of atypical neuroleptics to treat both psychosis and behavioral changes following TBI.

In addition to pharmacological interventions, behavioral and environmental interventions have been shown to be effective at remediating behavioral dyscontrol following TBI. The discussion of behavioral and environmental techniques aimed at decreasing behavioral dyscontrol, including aggression and irritability, is beyond the scope of this chapter (see Sohlberg and Mateer, 2001, for more information). Providers may find referrals for such interventions within rehabilitation programs. Briefly, interventions may seek to reduce stimulation in the environment, increase structure and predictability, reinforce good behavior with limited response to undesired behavior, and use structured problem-solving strategies.

## Nonpharmacological Management of Behavior and Personality Change

Although there have been increasing improvements to pharmacological strategies used to treat behavior and personality change in those with neurological illness and injury, often some degree of these symptoms persists following pharmacological intervention. In addition, side effects of pharmacological interventions may make pharmacological interventions nontenable. In these situations, nonpharmacological interventions can be of benefit. Consideration of referral to geriatric psychiatry, neuropsychology, psychology, or other specialized providers is encouraged.

**TABLE 9.18 Nonpharmacological Intervention for Behavior and Personality Change**

**Modification of Patient Variables**
- Psychotherapy for individuals with less severe cognitive impairment
- Reinforce desired behaviors
- Distraction
- Provide with two appropriate choices (i.e., walk with walker or my arm)
- Acknowledge emotions even if rationale for emotions is faulty/unclear
- Assess for unmet or acute needs (i.e., pain, urinary tract infection (UTI), constipation)

**Modification of Caregiver Variables**
- Psychoeducation
- Psychotherapy for caregiver
- Support groups
- Working to change their expectations of patient
- Respite

**Modification of Environmental Variables**
- Limit access to safety concerns (i.e., car keys, guns)
- Increase supervision in the home setting
- Reduce degree of stimulation (i.e., noise, number of people, number of requests)
- Bed or door alarms

*UTI,* Urinary tract infection.

One might use the model by Kales and colleagues discussed before (see Fig. 9.5). Briefly, interventions might focus on behavioral strategies, caregiver education and intervention, and environmental changes (see Kales et al., 2015, for example). Behavioral interventions focus on use of strategies to directly change an individual's behavior. For example, it is not uncommon for undesired behaviors (e.g., aggression) to receive significant attention while preferred behaviors (e.g., working on quiet activity) receive no reinforcement. To successfully reduce undesired activities, individuals need to increase desired activities through reinforcing preferred behavior, offering desired activities, and reducing reinforcement of undesired behavior. Furthermore, redirection is frequently attempted in individuals with impaired cognition who are engaging in undesired behavior. Redirection is likely to be most successful if done in a multistep process involving validation of emotion, joining of behavior, distraction, and only then followed by redirection (Sutor et al., 2006). Caregiver interventions aim to assist caregivers in making internal changes that improve the quality of life for families touched by neurological illness and disease by improving psychoeducation, increasing coping strategies, and facilitating acceptance and/or changing expectations. Finally, environmental strategies focus on changing an individual's environment to reduce and ameliorate behavioral difficulties (i.e., limiting access to car, reducing environmental stimulation, and use of familiar and personal belongings the environment to reduce confusion and agitation). Unfortunately, there has been limited research to assess the success of these interventions. See Table 9.18 for additional information.

*The complete reference list is available online at https://expertconsult.inkling.com/.* 

# 10

# Depression and Psychosis in Neurological Practice

David L. Perez, Evan D. Murray, Brent P. Forester, Bruce H. Price

## OUTLINE



The disciplines of behavioral neurology, neuropsychiatry, and geriatric psychiatry are undergoing a scientific renaissance on a global scale (Perez et al., 2018; Price et al., 2000). The distinctions between traditional neurological and idiopathic psychiatric conditions are eroding, and the time is ripe to deconstruct the implicit Cartesian dualism that divides the clinical neurosciences—neurology, psychiatry, and neurosurgery. Brain–behavior relationships are bidirectional and should be considered within social and environmental contexts. Patients with neurological disorders presenting with prominent mood, perceptual, or thought disturbances, the focus of this chapter, exemplify the need to integrate neurological and psychiatric perspectives to assess and manage neuropsychiatrically complex patient populations in a comprehensive manner.

The most widely recognized nomenclature used for discussion of mental disorders derives from the classification system developed for the *Diagnostic and Statistical Manual of Mental Disorders* (DSM). The American Psychiatric Association introduced the DSM in 1952 to facilitate psychiatric diagnosis through improved standardization of nomenclature. There have been consecutive revisions of this highly useful and relied-upon document since its inception, with the last revision being in 2013. Discussion about the potential secondary causes of depression and psychosis requires a familiarity with the most salient features of the primary (idiopathic) psychiatric conditions. A brief outline of selected conditions is included in eBoxes 10.1 and 10.2, along with other content in this chapter marked "online only."

## PRINCIPLES OF DIFFERENTIAL DIAGNOSIS

Emotional and cognitive processes are based on brain structure and physiology. Abnormal behavior can be attributable to the complex interplay of neural physiology, social influences, and physical environment (Andreasen, 1997). Psychosis, mania, depression, disinhibition, obsessive compulsive behaviors, and anxiety all can occur as a result of neurological disease and can be virtually indistinguishable from the idiopathic forms (Rickards, 2005; Robinson and Travella, 1996). Neurological conditions should be considered in the differential diagnosis of any disorder with psychiatric symptoms.

Neuropsychiatric abnormalities can be associated with altered functioning in anatomical regions. Any disease, toxin, drug, or process that affects a particular region can be expected to show changes in behavior mediated by the distributed network encompassing that region. The limbic system and the frontosubcortical circuits are most commonly implicated in neuropsychiatric symptoms. This neuroanatomical conceptual framework can provide useful information for localization and thus differential diagnosis. For example, the Klüver-Bucy syndrome—which consists of placidity, apathy, visual and auditory agnosia, hyperorality, and hypersexuality—occurs in processes that cause injury to the bilateral medial temporoamygdalar regions. A few of the most common causes of this syndrome include herpes encephalitis, traumatic brain injury (TBI), frontotemporal dementias (FTDs), and late-onset or severe Alzheimer disease (AD). Disinhibition, a particularly common neuropsychiatric symptom, may be observed in patients with brain trauma, cerebrovascular ischemia, demyelination, abscesses, or tumors as well as neurodegenerative disorders. Damage to any portion of the cortical and subcortical portions of the orbitofrontal-striatal-pallidal-thalamic circuit can result in disinhibition (Bonelli and Cummings, 2007).

Mood disorders, paranoia, disinhibition, and apathy derive in part from dysfunction in the limbic system and basal ganglia, which are phylogenetically more primitive (Mesulam, 2000). In some cases, the behavioral changes represent a psychological response to the underlying disability; in others, neuropsychiatric abnormalities manifest as a result of intrinsic alterations of the neural network caused by the disease itself. For example, studies have shown that apathy in Parkinson disease (PD) is probably related to the underlying disease process rather than being a psychological reaction to disability or to depression and is closely associated with cognitive impairment (Kirsch-Darrow et al., 2006). Positron emission tomography (PET), single-photon emission computed tomography (SPECT), and functional magnetic resonance imaging (fMRI) studies suggest the involvement of similar regions of abnormality in acquired (secondary) forms of depression, mania, obsessive-compulsive disorder (OCD), and psychosis as in their primary psychiatric presentations (Lee et al., 2019; Milad and Rauch, 2012; Rubinsztein et al., 2001). Table 10.1 summarizes neuropsychiatric symptoms and their anatomical correlates. Additionally, the developmental phase during which a neurological illness occurs influences the frequency with which some neuropsychiatric syndromes are manifested. Adults with post-TBI sequelae tend to exhibit a higher rate of depression and anxiety. In contrast, post-TBI sequelae in children often involve attention deficits, hyperactivity, irritability, aggressiveness, and oppositional behavior (Max, 2014). When temporal lobe epilepsy or Huntington disease (HD) begins in adolescence, a higher incidence of psychosis is noted than when their onset occurs later in life. Earlier onset of multiple sclerosis (MS) and stroke are associated with a higher incidence of depression (Rickards, 2005).

Patients with AD, PD, HD, and FTDs can develop multiple coexisting symptoms such as irritability, agitation, impulse-control disorders, apathy, depression, delusions, and psychosis, many of which may be exacerbated by medications used to treat the underlying disorder (Table 10.2). For example, in patients with PD, dopamine (DA) agonists such as pramipexole and ropinirole have been found to increase the risk of pathological gambling, compulsive shopping, hypersexuality, and other impulse-control disorders, sometimes referred to as *dopamine dysregulation* (Voon et al., 2006; Weintraub et al., 2006). Management outcome can be influenced by multiple factors. For instance, the complex relationship between behavioral changes and the caregiver's ability to cope play a role in illness management and nursing home placement (de Vugt et al., 2005). For example, behavioral disturbances in patients with neurological illnesses are well described to be associated with caregiver distress and fatigue (Adams and Dahdah, 2016).

**TABLE 10.1 Neuropsychiatric Symptoms and Corresponding Neuroanatomy**

| Symptom | Neuroanatomical Region |
|---|---|
| Depression | Prefrontal cortex (particularly left anterior regions, anterior cingulate gyrus, subgenu of the corpus callosum, orbitofrontal cortex), basal ganglia, left caudate |
| Mania | Inferomedial and ventromedial frontal cortex, right inferomedial frontal cortex, anterior cingulate, caudate nucleus, thalamus, and temporothalamic projections |
| Apathy | Anterior cingulate cortex, nucleus accumbens, globus pallidus, thalamus |
| OCD | Orbital or medial frontal cortex, caudate nucleus, globus pallidus |
| Disinhibition | Orbitofrontal cortex, hypothalamus, septum |
| Paraphilia | Mediotemporal cortex, hypothalamus, septum, rostral brainstem |
| Hallucinations | Unimodal association cortex, orbitofrontal cortex, paralimbic cortex, limbic cortex, striatum, thalamus, midbrain |
| Delusions | Orbitofrontal cortex, amygdala, striatum, thalamus |

*OCD*, Obsessive-compulsive disorder.

**TABLE 10.2 Neurological Disorders and Associated Prominent Behavioral Features**

| Neurological Disorder | Associated Behavioral Disturbances |
|---|---|
| Alzheimer disease | Depression, irritability, anxiety, apathy, delusions, paranoia, psychosis |
| Lewy body dementia | Fluctuating confusion, hallucinations, delusions, depression, RBD |
| Vascular dementia | Depression, apathy, psychosis |
| Parkinson disease | Depression, anxiety, drug-associated hallucinations and psychosis, RBD |
| FTD | Early impaired judgment, disinhibition, apathy, loss of empathy, depression, delusions, psychosis |
| PSP | Disinhibition, apathy |
| TBI | Depression, disinhibition, apathy, irritability, psychosis (uncommon) |
| HD | Depression, irritability, delusions, mania, apathy, obsessive-compulsive tendencies, psychosis |
| Corticobasal degeneration | Depression, irritability, RBD, alien hand syndrome |
| Epilepsy | Depression, psychosis |
| HIV infection | Apathy, depression, mania, psychosis |
| MS | Depression, irritability, anxiety, euphoria, psychosis, pseudobulbar affect |
| ALS | Depression, disinhibition, apathy, impaired judgment; can coexist with FTD |

*ALS*, Amyotrophic lateral sclerosis; *FTD*, frontotemporal dementia; *HD*, Huntington disease; *HIV*, human immunodeficiency virus; *MS*, multiple sclerosis; *PSP*, progressive supranuclear palsy; *RBD*, rapid-eye-movement behavior disorder; *TBI*, traumatic brain injury.

## PRINCIPLES OF NEUROPSYCHIATRIC EVALUATION

A number of important principles must be considered when patients are being evaluated and treated for behavioral disturbances.

1. The clinical history may offer clues to the index of suspicion for a secondary (neuropsychiatric) etiology versus an idiopathic presentation. For example, late-life initial onset of mania or depression is more commonly associated with central nervous system (CNS) pathology (van Agtmaal et al., 2017).
2. A normal neurological examination does not exclude neurological conditions. Lesions in the limbic, paralimbic, and prefrontal regions may manifest with cognitive-affective-behavioral changes in the absence of elemental neurological abnormalities.
3. Normal routine laboratory testing, brain imaging, electroencephalography, and cerebrospinal fluid (CSF) analysis do not necessarily exclude diseases of neurological origin.
4. New neurological complaints or behavioral changes that are atypical for a coexisting primary psychiatric disorder should not be dismissed as being of psychiatric origin in a person with a preexisting psychiatric history.
5. The possibility of iatrogenically induced symptoms—such as lethargy with benzodiazepines, parkinsonism with neuroleptics, or hallucinations with dopaminergic medications—must be taken into account. Medication side effects can significantly complicate the clinical history and physical examination in both the acute and long-term setting. Medication side effects can also potentially be harbingers of underlying pathology or progression of illness. For example, marked parkinsonism occurring after neuroleptic exposure can be a feature of PD and dementia with Lewy bodies (DLB)

(Aarsland et al., 2005) before the underlying neurodegenerative condition becomes clinically apparent. PD patients may develop hallucinations as a side effect of dopaminergic medications (Starkstein et al., 2012).

6. Treatments of primary psychiatric and neurological behavioral disturbances share common principles. A response to therapy does not constitute evidence for a primary psychiatric condition.

The medical evaluation of affective and psychotic symptoms must be individualized based on the patient's family history, social environment (including social network), habits, risk factors, age, gender, clinical history, and examination findings. A careful review of the patient's medical history and a general physical examination as well as a neurological examination (Murray and Price, 2008; Ovsiew et al, 2008) should be performed to assess for possible neurological and medical causes. The most basic evaluation should include vital signs (blood pressure, pulse, respirations, and temperature) and a laboratory evaluation that minimally includes a complete blood cell count (CBC), electrolyte panel, serum glucose, blood urea nitrogen (BUN), creatinine, calcium, total protein and albumin as well as assessments of liver and thyroid function. Additional laboratory testing may be considered according to the clinical history and risk factors. These studies might include a toxicology screen, cobalamin (vitamin $B_{12}$), homocysteine, methylmalonic acid, folate, vitamin D, human immunodeficiency virus (HIV) serology, rapid plasma reagin (RPR), antinuclear antibodies (ANAs), erythrocyte sedimentation rate (ESR), C-reactive protein (CRP), ceruloplasmin, heavy metal screen, ammonia, serum and CSF paraneoplastic panel, urine porphobilinogen, number of cytosine-adenine-guanine (CAG) repeats for HD, and other specialized rheumatologic, metabolic, and genetic tests. Consideration should also be given to checking (especially in the elderly) the patient's oxygen saturation on room air. Neurological abnormalities suggested by the clinical history or identified on examination, especially those attributable to the CNS, should prompt further evaluation for neurological and medical causes of psychiatric illness. A clear consensus has not been reached as to when neuroimaging is indicated as part of the evaluation of new-onset depression in patients without focal neurological complaints and a normal neurological examination. This must be individualized based on clinical judgment. Treatment-resistant depression should prompt reassessment of the diagnosis and evaluation to rule out secondary causes of depressive illness, including cerebrovascular (small vessel) disease. A careful history to rule out a primary sleep disorder such as obstructive sleep apnea should be considered in the evaluation of refractory depressive symptoms (Haba-Rubio, 2005) or cognitive complaints. When new-onset atypical psychosis presents in the absence of identifiable infectious/inflammatory, metabolic, toxic, or other causes, we recommend that magnetic resonance imaging (MRI) of the brain be incorporated into the evaluation. In our experience, 5%–10% of such patients have MRI abnormalities that identify potential neurological contributions (particularly in those 65 years of age and older). The MRI will help to exclude lesions (e.g., demyelination, ischemic disease, neoplasm, congenital structural abnormalities, evidence of metabolic storage diseases) in limbic, paralimbic, and frontal regions that may not be clearly associated with neurological abnormalities on elemental examination (Walterfang et al., 2005). An electroencephalogram (EEG) should be considered to evaluate for complex partial seizures if there is a history of intermittent, discrete, or abrupt episodes of psychiatric dysfunction (e.g., confusion, spells of lost time, psychotic symptoms), stereotypy of hallucinations, automatisms (e.g., lip smacking, repetitive movements) associated with episodes of psychiatric dysfunction (or confusion), or a suspicion of encephalopathy (or delirium). Sensitivity of the EEG for detecting seizure activity is highest when the patient has experienced the specific symptoms while undergoing the study. Selected cases may require 24-hour or prolonged EEG monitoring to capture a clinical event and thus to clarify whether a seizure disorder is present.

## COGNITIVE-AFFECTIVE-BEHAVIORAL BRAIN–BEHAVIOR RELATIONSHIPS

We begin with a brief overview of cortical functional anatomy related to perceptual, cognitive, affective, and behavioral processing. Thereafter a synopsis of frontal network functional anatomy will follow, describing the distinct prefrontosubcortical circuits subserving important cognitive-affective-behavioral domains.

The cerebral cortex can be subdivided into five major functional subtypes: primary sensorimotor, unimodal association, heteromodal association, paralimbic, and limbic (Fig. 10.1). The primary sensory areas are the points of entry for sensory information into the cortical circuitry. The primary motor cortex conveys complex motor programs to motor neurons in the brainstem and spinal cord. Processing of sensory information occurs as information moves from primary sensory areas to adjacent unimodal association areas. The unimodal and heteromodal cortices are involved in perceptual processing and motor planning. The complexity of processing increases as information is then transmitted to heteromodal association areas, which receive input from more than one sensory modality. Examples of heteromodal association cortices include the prefrontal cortex, posterior parietal cortex, parts of the lateral temporal cortex, and portions of the parahippocampal gyrus. These cortical regions have a six-layered cytoarchitecture. Further cortical processing occurs in areas designated as *paralimbic*. These regions demonstrate a gradual transition of cortical architecture from the six-layered areas to the more primitive and simplified allocortex of limbic structures. The paralimbic regions, implicated in idiopathic and secondary neuropsychiatric symptoms, consist of the orbitofrontal cortex (OFC), cingulate gyrus, insula, temporal pole, and parahippocampal cortex. Cognitive, emotional, and visceral inputs merge in these regions. The limbic subdivision is composed of the hippocampus, amygdala, substantia innominata, prepiriform olfactory cortex, and septal area (Fig. 10.2). Limbic structures are to a great extent reciprocally interconnected with the hypothalamus. Limbic regions are intimately involved with processing and regulation of emotion, memory, motivation, and autonomic and endocrine function. The highest level of cognitive processing occurs in regions referred to as *transmodal areas*. These are composed of heteromodal, paralimbic, and limbic regions, which are collectively linked, in parallel, to other transmodal regions. Interconnections among transmodal areas (e.g., Wernicke area, posterior parietal cortex, hippocampal-enterorhinal complex) enable the integration of distributed perceptual processing systems, resulting in perceptual recognition (i.e., of phenomena such as scenes and events becoming experiences and words taking on meaning) (Mesulam, 2000).

### Cortical Networks

Classically, five distinct cortical networks have been conceptualized as governing various aspects of cognitive functioning:

1. The language network, which includes transmodal regions or "epicenters" in the Broca and Wernicke areas located in the pars opercularis/triangular portions of the inferior frontal gyrus and posterior aspect of the superior temporal gyrus, respectively
2. Spatial awareness, based in transmodal regions in the frontal eye fields and posterior parietal cortex

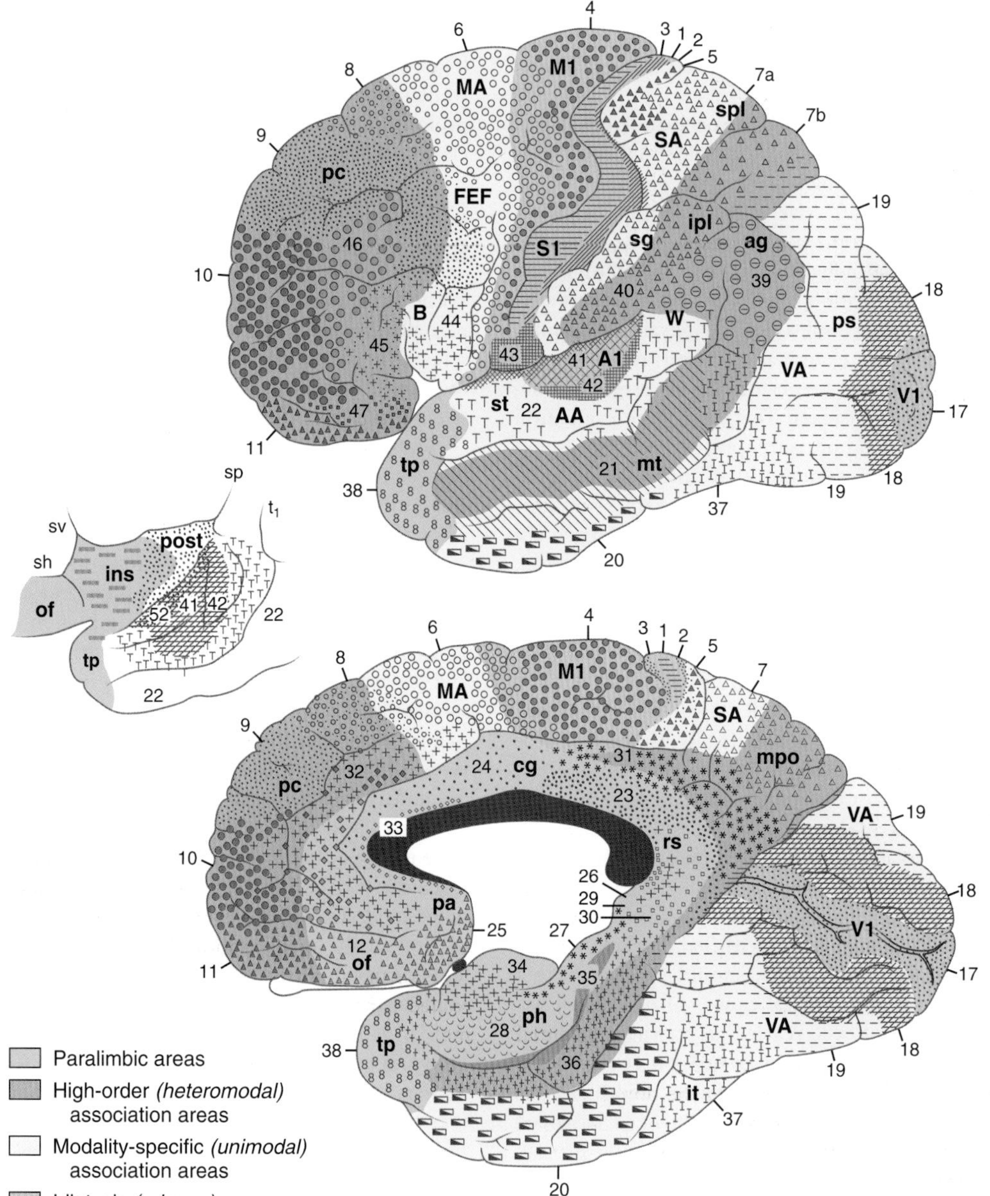


**Fig. 10.1** Cortical anatomy and functional subtypes (areas) described by Brodmann's map of the human brain. The boundaries are not intended to be precise. Much of this information is based on experimental evidence obtained from laboratory animals and remains to be confirmed in the human brain. *AA*, Auditory association cortex; *ag*, angular gyrus; *A1*, primary auditory cortex; *B*, Broca area; *cg*, cingulate gyrus; *f*, fusiform gyrus; *FEF*, frontal eye fields; *ins*, insula; *ipl*, inferior parietal lobule; *it*, inferior temporal gyrus; *MA*, motor association cortex; *mpo*, medial parieto-occipital area; *mt*, middle temporal gyrus; *M1*, primary motor area; *of*, orbitofrontal region; *pc*, prefrontal cortex; *ph*, parahippocampal region; *po*, parolfactory area; *ps*, peristriate cortex; *rs*, retrosplenial area; *SA*, somatosensory association cortex; *sg*, supramarginal gyrus; *spl*, superior parietal lobule; *st*, superior temporal gyrus; *S1*, primary somatosensory area; *tp*, temporopolar cortex; *VA*, visual association cortex; *V1*, primary visual cortex; *W*, Wernicke area. *(From Mesulam, M.M., 2000. Behavioral neuroanatomy. Large-scale networks, association cortex, frontal syndromes, the limbic system and hemisphere specializations. In: Mesulam, M.M. [Ed.], Principles of Behavioral and Cognitive Neurology. Oxford University Press, New York, p. 13.)*

3. The memory and emotional network, located in the hippocampal-enterorhinal region and amygdala
4. The executive function–working memory network, based in transmodal regions in the lateral prefrontal cortex and possibly the inferior parietal cortices
5. The face-object recognition network, based in the temporopolar and middle/ventral temporal cortices (Mesulam, 1998)

Lesions of transmodal cortical areas result in global impairments such as hemineglect, anosognosia, amnesia, and multimodal anomia. Disconnection of transmodal regions from a specific unimodal input will result in selective perceptual impairments such as category-specific anomias, prosopagnosia, pure word deafness, or pure word blindness.

The emergence of functional neuroimaging technologies—including task-based (Pan et al., 2011) and resting-state functional

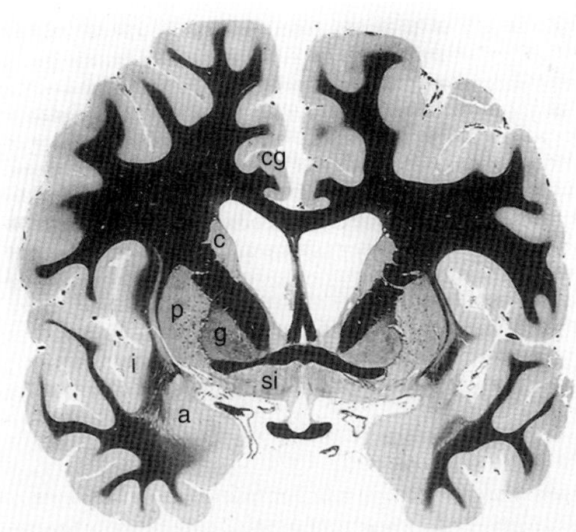


**Fig. 10.2** Coronal section through the basal forebrain of a 25-year-old human brain stained for myelin. The substantia innominata *(si)* and the amygdaloid complex *(a)* are located on the undersurface of the brain. *c,* Head of caudate nucleus; *cg,* cingulate gyrus; *g,* globus pallidus; *i,* insula. *(From Mesulam, M.M., 2000. Behavioral neuroanatomy. Large-scale networks, association cortex, frontal syndromes, the limbic system and hemisphere specializations. In: Mesulam, M.M. (Ed.), Principles of Behavioral and Cognitive Neurology. Oxford University Press, New York, p. 4.)*

connectivity analyses (Zhang and Raichle, 2010)—has over the past several decades allowed for the in vivo inspection of brain networks. Apart from the five networks already described, several additional networks have emerged as particularly important to the understanding of brain–behavior relationships in behavioral neurology and neuropsychiatry:

1. The default mode network (DMN)—which includes areas along the anterior and posterior cortical midline (medial prefrontal cortex, posterior cingulate cortex, precuneus), posterior inferior parietal lobules, and medial temporal lobe—is linked to self-referential processing (Buckner et al., 2008, Raichle, 2010).
2. The salience network—which is anchored in the dorsal anterior cingulate cortex (ACC) and insular cortex—has strong subcortical and limbic connections and is linked with reactions to the external world and homeostasis (Seeley et al., 2007).
3. The parietofrontal mirror neuron system—which includes the parietal lobe and the premotor cortex plus the caudal part of the inferior frontal gyrus—is involved in the recognition of voluntary behavior in other people (Cattaneo and Rizzolatti, 2009).

The limbic mirror system, formed by the insula and the anterior mesial frontal cortex, is devoted to the recognition of affective behavior. DMN and parietofrontal mirror neuron system abnormalities have been linked to mentalization deficits including impairments of theory of mind, while the right anterior insula and ACC have been implicated in emotional and self-awareness (Craig, 2009).

## Frontosubcortical Networks

Five frontosubcortical circuits subserve cognition, emotion, behavior, and movement. Disruption of these networks at the cortical or subcortical level can be associated with similar neuropsychiatric symptoms (Perez et al., 2015). Each of these circuits shares similar nonoverlapping components: (1) frontal cortex; (2) striatum (caudate, putamen, ventral striatum); (3) globus pallidus and substantia nigra; and (4) thalamus (which then projects back to frontal cortex) (Alexander et al., 1986, Bonelli and Cummings, 2007) (Fig. 10.3). Integrative connections also occur to and from other subcortical and distant cortical regions related to each circuit. Neurotransmitters such as DA, glutamate, γ-aminobutyric acid (GABA), acetylcholine, norepinephrine, and serotonin are involved in various aspects of neural transmission and modulation in these circuits. The frontosubcortical networks are named according to their site of origin or function. Somatic motor function is mediated by the motor circuit originating in the supplementary motor area. Oculomotor function is governed by the oculomotor circuit originating in the frontal eye fields. Three of the five circuits are intimately involved in cognitive, emotional, and behavioral functions: the dorsolateral prefrontal, the orbitofrontal, and the anterior cingulate circuits. Each circuit has both efferent and afferent connections with adjacent and distant cortical regions.

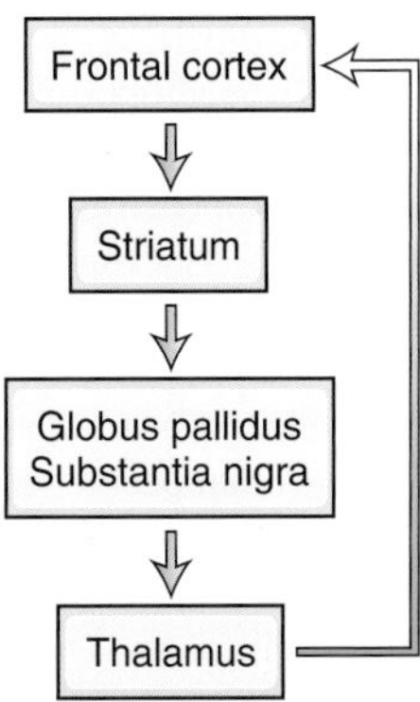


**Fig. 10.3** General Structure of Frontal Subcortical Circuits.

The dorsolateral prefrontal cortex (DLPFC)–subcortical circuit is principally involved in attentional and higher-order cognitive executive functions. These functions include the ability to shift sets, organize, and solve problems, as well as the abilities of cognitive control and working memory. Shifting sets is related to mental flexibility and consists of the ability to move between different concepts or motor plans or the ability to shift between different aspects of the same or related concept. Working memory is the online maintenance and manipulation of information. The DLPFC–subcortical circuit includes the dorsolateral head of the caudate, the lateral mediodorsal globus pallidus interna, and the parvocellular aspects of the mediodorsal and ventral anterior thalamic nuclei. Dysfunction in this circuit has been linked with environmental dependency syndromes (including utilization and imitation behavior), poor organization and planning, mental inflexibility, and working memory deficits. Executive dysfunction is also a principal component of subcortical dementias. Deficits identified in subcortical dementias include slowed information processing, memory retrieval deficits, mood and behavioral changes, gait disturbance, dysarthria, and other motor impairments. Vascular dementias, PD, and HD are a few examples of conditions that affect this circuit.

The OFC–subcortical circuit is implicated in socially appropriate and empathic behavior, value-based decision making, mental flexibility, response inhibition, and emotion regulation. It pairs thoughts, memories, and experiences with corresponding visceral and emotional states. The OFC has functional specificity along its anteroposterior and mediolateral axes. The medial OFC has been linked to reward processing and behavioral responses in the context of viscerosomatic evaluations, whereas more lateral regions mediate more external, sensory evaluations including decoding punishment. Anterior subregions process the reward value for more abstract and complex secondary reinforcing factors such as money, whereas more concrete factors such as touch and taste are encoded in the posterior areas. The posteromedial OFC is particularly implicated in evaluating the emotional significance of stimuli (Barbas and Zikopoulos, 2007). The OFC–subcortical connections include the ventromedial caudate, mediodorsal aspects of the globus pallidus interna, and the medial ventral anterior and inferomedial aspects of the magnocellular mediodorsal thalamus. OFC dysfunction, depicted in the classic personality change experienced by Phineas Gage following injury of his left medial prefrontal cortex by a metal rod in a construction accident, is associated with impulsivity, disinhibition, irritability, aggressive outbursts, socially inappropriate behavior, and mental inflexibility. Persons with bilateral OFC lesions may manifest "theory of mind" deficits. *Theory of mind* is a model of how a person understands and infers other people's intentions, desires, mental states, and emotions (Bodden et al., 2010). Conditions that exhibit OFC and related neurocircuit impairment include schizophrenia (Bora et al., 2009), depression (Price and Drevets, 2010), OCD (Milad and Rauch, 2012), FTD (Adenzato et al., 2010), and HD. Other conditions that may affect this circuit include closed head trauma, rupture of anterior communicating aneurysms, and subfrontal meningiomas.

The ACC and its subcortical connections are implicated in motivated behavior, conflict monitoring, cognitive control, and emotion regulation. Regions of the ACC located subgenually and rostral to the genu of the corpus callosum have reciprocal amygdalar connections and are implicated in the regulation of emotion. Dorsal ACC regions are interconnected to lateral and mediodorsal prefrontal regions and are involved in cognitive functions and the behavioral expression of emotional states (Devinsky et al., 1995, Etkin et al., 2011). An important function of the dorsal ACC is the ability to engage in aspects of *cognitive control*—the ability to pursue and regulate goal-oriented behavior. ACC–subcortical connections include the nucleus accumbens/ventromedial caudate, ventral globus pallidus, and ventral aspects of the magnocellular mediodorsal and ventral anterior thalamic nuclei. Deficit syndromes linked to the ACC–subcortical circuit include the spectrum of amotivational syndromes (apathy, abulia, akinetic mutism) and cognitive impairments including poor response inhibition, error detection, and goal-directed behavior. Some conditions that may affect this circuit include AD, FTD, PD, HD, head trauma, brain tumors, cerebral infarcts, and obstructive hydrocephalus.

### Cerebrocerebellar Networks

The cerebellum is engaged in the regulation of cognition and emotion through a feed-forward and feedback loop. The cortex projects to pontine nuclei, which in turn project to the cerebellum. The cerebellum projects to the thalamus, which then projects back to the cortex. Cognitive processing tasks such as language, working memory, and spatial and executive tasks appear to activate the posterior cerebellar lobe. The posterior cerebellar vermis may function as a putative limbic cerebellum, modulating emotional processing (Stoodley and Schmahmann, 2010). Distractibility, executive and working memory problems, impaired judgment, reduced verbal fluency, disinhibition, irritability, anxiety, emotional lability or blunting, obsessive-compulsive behaviors, depression, and psychosis have been reported in association with cerebellar pathology in the context of the cognitive-affective cerebellar syndrome (Schmahmann, 2004).

## BIOLOGY OF PSYCHOSIS

Schizophrenia is a chronic disintegrative thought disorder where patients frequently experience auditory hallucinations and bizarre or paranoid delusions. Among several etiological hypotheses for schizophrenia, the neurodevelopmental model is one of the most prominent. This model generally posits that schizophrenia results from processes that begin long before clinical symptom onset and is caused by a combination of environmental and genetic factors (Murray and Lewis, 1987; Weinberger, 1987). Several postmortem and neuroimaging studies support this hypothesis with findings of brain developmental alterations such as agenesis of the corpus callosum, arachnoid cysts, and other abnormalities in a significant number of schizophrenic patients (Hallak et al., 2007; Kuloglu et al., 2008). Environmental factors are associated with an increased risk for schizophrenia. These factors include being a first-generation immigrant or the child of a first-generation immigrant, urban living, drug use, head injury, prenatal infection, maternal malnutrition, obstetrical complications during delivery, and winter birth (Tandon et al., 2008). Genetic risks are clearly present but not well understood (Smoller 2014). The majority of patients with schizophrenia lack a family history of the disorder. The population lifetime risk for schizophrenia is 1%; it is 10% for first-degree relatives and 4% for second-degree relatives. There is an approximately 50% concordance rate for monozygotic twins as compared with approximately 15% for dizygotic twins. Advancing paternal age increases risk in a linear fashion, which is consistent with the hypothesis that de novo mutations contribute to the genetic risk for schizophrenia. It is most likely that many different genes make small but important contributions to susceptibility. The disease typically manifests only when these genes are combined or certain adverse environmental factors are present. A number of susceptibility genes show an association with schizophrenia: catechol-*O*-methyl-transferase, neuroregulin 1, dysbindin, disrupted in schizophrenia 1 (DISC1), metabotropic glutamate receptor type 3 gene, and G27/G30 gene complex (Nothen et al., 2010; Tandon et al., 2008). Research in twins and first-degree relatives of patients has shown that genes predisposing to schizophrenia and related disorders affect heritable traits related to the illness. Such traits include neurocognitive functioning, structural MRI brain volume measures, neurophysiological informational processing traits, and sensitivity to stress (van Os and Kapur, 2009). A small proportion of schizophrenia incidence may be explained by genomic structural variations known as *copy number variants* (CNVs). CNVs consist of inherited or de novo small duplications, deletions, or inversions in genes or regulatory regions. CNV deletions generally show higher penetrance (more severe phenotype) than duplications, and larger CNVs often have higher penetrance and/or more clinical features than smaller CNVs. These genomic structural variations contribute to normal variability, disease risk, and developmental anomalies; they also act as a major mutational mechanism in evolution. The most common CNV disorder, 22q11.2 deletion syndrome (velocardiofacial syndrome), has an established association with schizophrenia. Individuals with 22q11.2 deletions have a 20-fold increased risk for schizophrenia and constitute about 0.9%–1% of schizophrenia patients. When this syndrome is present, genetic counseling is helpful (Bassett and Chow, 2008). Studies are also identifying shared genetic risk for schizophrenia and autism spectrum disorders (McCarroll and Hyman, 2013).

A wide variety of neurological conditions, medications, and toxins are associated with psychosis. No consensus is available in the literature regarding the precise anatomical localization of various psychotic syndromes. Evidence from neurochemistry, cellular neuropathology, and neuroimaging studies supports that schizophrenia is a brain disease that affects multiple interacting neural circuits. The two best-known neurotransmitter models offered to explain the various manifestations of schizophrenia are the "dopamine hypothesis" (Howes and Kapur, 2009) and the "glutamate hypothesis." Schizophrenia has been associated with frontal lobe dysfunction and abnormal regulation of subcortical DA and glutamate systems (Keshavan et al., 2008).

Advances in structural and functional neuroimaging techniques over the past 30 years have greatly aided our understanding of neurocircuit alterations in schizophrenia. Structural studies have commonly identified diminished whole brain volume, increased ventricular size, and regional atrophy in hippocampal, prefrontal, superior temporal, and inferior parietal cortices in schizophrenic patients compared with control groups (Keshavan et al., 2008; Pearlson and Marsh, 1999; Shenton et al., 2001). A reversal of or diminished hemispheric asymmetry has also been characterized. Functional neuroimaging studies have commonly identified decreased cerebral blood flow (CBF) and blood oxygen level–dependent (BOLD) hypoactivation of the prefrontal cortex (including the DLPFC) during cognitive task performance and temporal lobe dysfunction (Brunet-Gouet and Decety, 2006; Keshavan et al., 2008). Schizophrenic patients with prominent negative symptoms have displayed reduced glucose utilization in the frontal lobes. A clinical and neurobiological overlap across schizophrenia, schizoaffective disorder, and bipolar disorder is also increasingly recognized (Clementz et al., 2016). Overall, functional imaging studies suggest that the DLPFC, OFC, ACC, ventral striatum, thalamus, temporal lobe subregions, and cerebellum are sites of prominent functional alterations. Several neurological conditions that may manifest psychosis (e.g., HD, PD, frontotemporal degenerations, stroke) are commonly also associated with frontal and subcortical dysfunction. For example, dorsolateral and mediofrontal hypoperfusion on functional imaging has been demonstrated in a subset of AD patients with delusions (Ismail et al., 2012).

## BIOLOGY OF DEPRESSION

The intersection of neurology and psychiatry is nowhere more evident than the remarkable comorbidity of psychiatric illness, especially depression, in many neurological disorders, with a 20%–60% prevalence rate of depression in patients with stroke, neurodegenerative diseases, MS, headache, HIV, TBI, epilepsy, chronic pain, obstructive sleep apnea, intracranial neoplasms, and motor neuron disease. Depression amplifies the physiological response to pain (Perez et al., 2015), whereas pain-related symptoms and limitations frequently lead to the emergence of depressive symptoms. In a community-based study, almost 50% of adolescents with chronic daily headaches had at least one psychiatric disorder, most commonly major depression and panic. Women with migraine who have major depression are twice as likely as those with migraine alone to report having been sexually abused when they were children. If the abuse continued past age 12, women with migraine were five times more likely to report depression (Tietjen et al., 2007). Despite the proliferation of antidepressant therapeutics, major depression is often a chronic and/or recurrent condition that remains difficult to treat. Up to 70% of patients taking antidepressants in a primary care setting may be poorly adherent, most often due to adverse side effects during both short- and long-term therapy.

Although the heritability of idiopathic depression based on twin studies is estimated to be between 40% and 50% (Levinson, 2006), the genetics of depression have thus far proven difficult to fully elucidate (Fabbri et al., 2018). Depression is a polygenetic condition that does not adhere to simple Mendelian genetics, and genetic mechanisms implicated in depression suggest complex gene–environment interactions. An individual's genetic makeup may lead to increased susceptibility for the development of depression in the context of adverse environmental (psychosocial) influences. Behavioral genetics research based on stress-diathesis models of depression demonstrates that the risk of depression after a stressful event is enhanced in populations carrying genetic risk factors and is diminished in populations lacking such risk factors. A gene's contribution to depression may be missed in studies that do not account for environmental interactions and may be revealed only when studied within the context of environmental stressors specifically mediated by that gene (Uher, 2008). Genotype–environment interactions are ubiquitous because genes not only affect the risk for depression by creating susceptibility to specific environmental stressors but may also predispose individuals to persistently place themselves in highly stressful environments. Approaches to the study of genetic influences in depression include association studies of candidate genes, genetic linkage studies of pedigrees with a strong family history of depression, and genome-wide association studies.

Association studies in depression have focused on monoaminergic candidate genes (Levinson, 2006). An intriguing interaction between polymorphisms in the promoter region of the serotonin transporter (5-HTT) gene and depression as well as an association between 5-HTT promoter region polymorphisms and depression-related neurocircuit activation patterns has emerged. The promoter activity of the 5-HTT gene is modified by sequence elements proximal to the 5′ regulatory region, termed the 5-HTT gene-linked polymorphic region (5-HTTLPR). The short "s" allele of the 5-HTTLPR is associated with lower transcription output of 5-HTT mRNA compared with the long "l" allele. A prospective longitudinal study has demonstrated that individuals with one or two copies of the short allele exhibited more depressive symptoms and suicidality following stressful life events in their early 20s compared with individuals homozygous for the long allele (Caspi et al., 2003; Karg et al., 2011). Genome-wide association studies in depression, including treatment-refractory depression (TRD), have largely failed to identify robust, reproducible findings (Fabbri et al., 2018, Lewis et al., 2010, Wray et al., 2012). This suggests that genome-wide association studies in depression have been underpowered to date.

Studies of epigenetic mechanisms in depression, though in their early stages, appear to hold promise in elucidating the mechanisms by which environmental factors affect gene expression. Epigenetics is the study of changes in gene activity caused by factors other than changes in the underlying nucleotide sequence. Whereas the genomic sequence defines the potential genetic repertoire of a given individual, the epigenome delineates which genes in the repertoire are expressed (along with the degree of expression) (Booij et al., 2013). As an example, DNA methylation is one of several epigenetic modifications that influence gene expression. In a pioneering animal study probing the impact of early life experiences on subsequent epigenetic programming, rat pups who experienced high rates of licking and grooming behaviors (positive influences) exhibited decreased methylation at the glucocorticoid receptor transcription factor binding site (Weaver et al., 2004). A postmortem human study examining epigenetic glucocorticoid receptor regulation revealed increased methylation in the neuron-specific glucocorticoid receptor and decreased glucocorticoid receptor mRNA in suicide victims with a history of childhood abuse compared with nonabused suicide victims and nonsuicide controls (McGowan et al., 2009).

At the cellular neurobiological level, the potential clinical relevance of neurogenesis in the adult mammalian brain represents a recent major breakthrough in depression studies. Imaging studies have demonstrated a 10%–20% decrease in the hippocampal volume of patients with chronic depression (Colle et al., 2018). Cell proliferation studies using 5-bromo-2′-deoxyuridine injection to label dividing cells show that antidepressants also lead to increased cell numbers in the mammalian hippocampus. This effect is seen with chronic but not acute treatment; the time course of the effect mirrors the known time course of the therapeutic action of antidepressants in humans (approximately 2 weeks for initial effect, upward of 4–8 weeks for maximal benefit) (Czeh et al., 2001; Samuels and Hen, 2011). Although a role for neurogenesis in the pathophysiology of depression appears to be a promising avenue of research, the relevance of animal studies described here with respect to humans remains controversial (Reif et al., 2006).

From a systems-level perspective, amygdalar-hippocampal, ACC, OFC, DLPFC, and subcortical regions are implicated in the neurobiology of primary and acquired depression (Perez et al., 2016). Increased basal and stimuli-driven amygdalar activity has been extensively characterized in depression (Drevets, 2003). In an early PET imaging study, depressed patients with a family history of depression demonstrated increased activation of the left amygdala; this pattern of amygdalar hyperactivation was also observed in remitted subjects with a family history of depression (Drevets et al., 1992). This suggests that enhanced amygdalar activity potentially represents a trait vulnerability biomarker for depressive illness. A number of studies have specifically linked enhanced amygdalar activity to the negative attentional bias of information processing in depression. Increased amygdalar metabolic activity has also been positively correlated with plasma cortisol levels (Drevets et al., 2002), suggesting a link between elevated amygdalar activity and dysfunction of the hypothalamic–pituitary–adrenal axis.

Dysfunction of the prefrontal cortex also plays an important role in the pathophysiology of depression. The subgenual ACC has been implicated in the modulation of negative mood states (Hamani et al., 2011). Several neuroimaging studies characterized elevated baseline subgenual activation in depression (Dougherty et al., 2003; Gotlib et al., 2005; Konarski et al., 2009; Mayberg et al., 2005), whereas other investigations have described reduced subgenual activations (Drevets et al., 1997). Mayberg and colleagues have suggested that depression can be potentially defined phenomenologically as "the tendency to enter into, and inability to disengage from, a negative mood state" (Holtzheimer and Mayberg, 2011). Subgenual ACC dysfunction may play a critical role in the inability to effectively modulate mood states. In addition to the ACC, the OFC and DLPFC exhibit abnormalities in depression. Consistent with OFC lesions linked to increased depression risk, depression severity is inversely correlated with medial and posterolateral OFC activity in neuroimaging studies (Drevets, 2007; Price and Drevets, 2010). Reduced OFC activations may lead to amygdalar disinhibition in depression. Meanwhile, the DLPFC potentially exhibits a lateralized dysfunctional pattern in depression. Though not consistently identified, depressed patients have shown left DLPFC hypoactivity and right DLPFC hyperactivity (Grimm et al., 2008); left DLPFC hypoactivity was linked to negative emotional judgments whereas right DLPFC hyperactivity was associated with attentional deficits. Subcortically, decreased ventral striatum/nucleus accumbens activation has been linked with anhedonia (Epstein et al., 2006; Keedwell et al., 2005; Pizzagalli et al., 2009). In neurological disorders, damage to the prefrontal cortex from stroke or tumor or to the striatum from degenerative diseases such as PD and HD is associated with depression (Charney and Manji, 2004). Functional imaging studies of subcortical disorders such as these reveal that hypometabolism in paralimbic regions, including the anterotemporal cortex and anterior cingulate, correlates with depression (Bonelli and Cummings, 2007). Depression in PD, HD, and epilepsy has been associated with reduced metabolic activity in the OFC and caudate nucleus.

Functional imaging studies of untreated depression have been extended to evaluate responses to pharmacological, cognitive-behavioral, and surgical treatments. Clinical improvement after treatment with selective serotonin reuptake inhibitors (SSRIs) such as fluoxetine correlates with increased activity on PET in brainstem and dorsal cortical regions including the prefrontal, parietal, anterior, and posterior cingulate areas and with decreased activity in limbic and striatal regions including the subgenual cingulate (Hamani et al., 2011), hippocampus, insula, and pallidum. These findings are consistent with the prevailing model for the involvement of a limbic-cortical-striatal-pallidal-thalamic circuit in major depression. The same group has shown that imaging can be used to identify patterns of metabolic activity predictive of treatment response. Hypometabolism of the rostral anterior cingulate characterized patients who failed to respond to antidepressants, whereas hypermetabolism characterized responders. Dougherty and coworkers (2003) used PET to search for neuroimaging profiles that might predict clinical response to anterior cingulotomy in patients with TRD. Responders displayed elevated preoperative metabolism in the left prefrontal cortex and the left thalamus. A combination of functional imaging and pharmacogenomic technologies might allow subsets of treatment responders to be classified and outcomes to be predicted more precisely than with either technology alone. Goldapple and coinvestigators (2004) used PET to study the clinical response of cognitive-behavioral therapy (CBT) in patients with unipolar depression; they found increases in the hippocampus and dorsal cingulate and decreases in the dorsal, ventral, and medial frontal cortex activity (Goldapple et al., 2004). The authors speculate that the same limbic-cortical-striatal-pallidal-thalamic circuit is involved but that differences in the direction of metabolic changes may reflect different underlying mechanisms of action of CBT and SSRIs. Resting-state metabolism of the right anterior insula as determined by PET has also been identified as a potential treatment-selective biomarker in depression for CBT and SSRI treatment response (McGrath et al., 2013), although reliable neuroimaging biomarkers of treatment response in major depression remain ill defined (Fonseka et al., 2018).

## CLINICAL SYMPTOMS AND SIGNS SUGGESTING NEUROLOGICAL DISEASE

Many neurological conditions have associated psychiatric symptoms. Psychiatrists and neurologists must be intimately acquainted with features of the clinical history and examination that point to the need for further investigation. Box 10.3 outlines some key features that have historically suggested an underlying neurological condition. eBox 10.4 reviews some key areas of the review of systems that can be helpful when a patient is being assessed for neurological and medical causes of psychiatric symptoms. eTable 10.3 reviews abnormalities in the elemental neurological examination associated with diseases that can exhibit significant neuropsychiatric features.

## PSYCHIATRIC MANIFESTATIONS OF NEUROLOGICAL DISEASE

Virtually any process that affects the neurocircuits described earlier can result in behavioral changes and psychiatric symptoms at some point. Psychiatric symptoms may be striking and can precede any neurological manifestation by years. eTable 10.4 lists conditions that can be associated with psychosis or depression. Box 10.5 summarizes some key points from the preceding discussion. A general overview and discussion of a number of major categories of neurological and systemic conditions with prominent neuropsychiatric features follows. More detailed information regarding the evaluation, natural history, pathology, and specific treatment recommendations for these conditions is beyond the scope of this chapter.

### Stroke and Cerebral Vascular Disease

Stroke is the leading cause of neurological disability in the United States and one of the most common causes of acquired behavioral changes in adults. The neuropsychiatric consequences of stroke depend on the location and size of the stroke, preexisting brain pathology, baseline intellectual capacity and functioning, age, and premorbid psychiatric history. Neuropsychiatric symptoms may occur in the setting of first strokes and multi-infarct dementia. In general, interruption of bilateral frontotemporal lobe function is associated with an increased risk of depressive and psychotic symptoms. Specific stroke-related syndromes such as aphasia and visuospatial dysfunction are beyond the

**BOX 10.3 Historical Features Suggesting Neurological Disease in Patients With Psychiatric Symptoms**

**Presence of Atypical Psychiatric Features**
Late or very early age of onset
Acute or subacute onset
Lack of significant psychosocial stressors
Catatonia
Diminished comportment
Cognitive decline
Intractability despite adequate therapy
Progressive symptoms

**History of Present Illness Includes**
New or worsening headache
Inattention
Somnolence
Incontinence
Focal neurological complaints such as weakness, sensory changes, incoordination, or gait difficulty
Neuroendocrine changes
Anorexia/weight loss

**Patient History**
Risk factors for cerebrovascular disease or central nervous system infections
Malignancy
Immunocompromise
Significant head trauma
Seizures
Movement disorder
Hepatobiliary disorders
Abdominal crises of unknown cause
Biological relatives with similar diseases or complaints

**Unexplained Diagnostic Abnormalities**
Screening laboratories
Neuroimaging studies or possibly imaging of other systems
Electroencephalography
Cerebrospinal fluid

**BOX 10.5 Key Points**

1. Affective and psychotic disorders may occur as a result of neurological disease and be indistinguishable from the idiopathic forms.
2. Neuropsychiatric and cognitive dysfunction can be correlated with altered functioning in anatomical regions.
3. Cortical processing of sensory information proceeds from its point of entry through association areas with progressively more complex interconnections with other regions having sensory, memory, cognitive, emotional, and autonomic information, resulting ultimately in perceptual recognition and emotional meaning for experiences.
4. Frontosubcortical circuits are heavily involved in cognitive, affective, and behavioral functioning. Disruption of frontal circuits at the cortical or subcortical level by various processes can be associated with similar neuropsychiatric symptoms.
5. Features of the patient's clinical history and examination can be suggestive of a medical or neurological cause of psychiatric symptoms.

Many medical and neurological conditions are associated with neuropsychiatric symptoms. Each condition may carry unique implications for prognosis, treatment, and long-term management.

scope of this chapter; therefore only the abnormalities in mood and emotion after stroke are discussed. A common misconception is that depressive symptoms can be explained as a response to the associated neurological deficits and impairment in function. Evidence supports a higher incidence of depression in stroke survivors than occurs in persons with other equally debilitating diseases. Minor depression is more closely related to the patient's elemental deficits. Emotional and cognitive disorders may occur independently of or in association with sensorimotor dysfunction in stroke. Poststroke depression (PSD) is the most common neuropsychiatric syndrome, occurring in 30%–50% of survivors at 1 year, with irritability, agitation, and apathy often present as well (Robinson and Jorge, 2016). About 50% of patients with depressive symptoms will meet criteria for a major depressive episode. Although somewhat controversial, onset of depression within the first few weeks after a stroke is most commonly associated with lesions affecting the frontal lobes, especially the prefrontal cortex and head of the caudate (Starkstein et al., 1987). The frequency and severity of depression increase with closer proximity to the frontal poles. Left prefrontal lesions are more commonly associated with acute depression and may be complicated by aphasia, resulting in the patient's inability to express the symptoms. Mania is much less common but usually occurs in relation to lesions of the right hemisphere, particularly with involvement of the OFC–subcortical circuit and medial temporal structures (Lee et al., 2019, Perez et al., 2011). Single manic events as well as recurrent manic and depressive episodes have been reported. Nondominant hemispheric strokes may also result in aprosody without associated depression. Currently the standard treatment of PSD is CBT and pharmacotherapy (Wang et al., 2018).

Apart from the association between large-territory strokes and depression, the "vascular depression" hypothesis denotes the potential of increased association between cerebrovascular disease and late-life depression (Alexopoulos, 2005; Alexopoulos et al., 1997). Clinically, vascular or late-life depression is characterized by executive deficits, slowed processing speed, psychomotor retardation, lack of insight, and disability out of proportion to depressive symptoms. Cerebrovascular white matter T2 MRI hyperintensities from diabetes, hyperlipidemia, cardiac disease, and hypertension have been linked with this condition. Some studies have localized white matter lesions to the prefrontal cortex and temporal lobe, including particular fiber tracts (e.g., cingulum bundle, uncinate fasciculus [Sheline et al., 2008]). Vascular depression has been associated with poor antidepressant response and higher relapse rates (Alexopoulos et al., 2000). Frontolimbic disconnection and cerebrovascular hypoperfusion are some of the theorized mechanisms linking cerebrovascular disease to late-life depression.

Psychosis or psychotic features may present as a rare complication of a single stroke, but the prevalence of these features is not well established. Manifestations may include paranoia, delusions, ideas of reference, hallucinations, or psychosis. Paranoia and psychosis have been reported in association with left temporal strokes resulting in Wernicke aphasia. Other regions producing similar neuropsychiatric symptoms include the right temporoparietal region and the caudate nuclei. Right hemispheric lesions may also be more associated with visual hallucinations and delusions. Reduplicative paramnesia and misidentification syndromes such as Capgras and Fregoli syndromes have also been reported. Reduplicative paramnesia is a syndrome in which patients claim that they are simultaneously in two or more locations. It has been observed to occur in patients with combined lesions of frontal and right temporal lobes but has also been described as due to temporal-limbic-frontal dysfunction (Politis and Loane, 2012). Capgras syndrome is the false belief that someone familiar, usually a family member or close friend, has been replaced by an identical-appearing imposter. It has been proposed that this results from right temporal-limbic-frontal disconnection resulting in a disturbance in the ability to recognize familiar people and places (Feinberg et al., 1999). A role for the left hemisphere in generating a fixed false narrative in the context of right lateralized perceptual deficits has also been postulated (Devinsky, 2009). In Fregoli syndrome, the patient believes that a persecutor is able to take on a variety of faces, like an actor. Psychotic episodes can also be a manifestation of complex partial seizures secondary to stroke. Patients with poststroke psychosis are more prone to have comorbid epilepsy than poststroke patients without associated psychosis. Lesions or infarcts of the ventral midbrain can result in a syndrome characterized by well-formed and complex visual hallucinations referred to as *peduncular hallucinosis,* and novel lesion mapping techniques suggest that subcortical lesions associated with peduncular hallucinosis are all functionally coupled with the extrastriate visual cortex (Boes et al. 2015). Obsessive-compulsive features have also been reported with strokes. These symptoms have been postulated to be due to dysfunction in the orbitofrontal-subcortical circuitry.

Consensus criteria for accurately diagnosing vascular cognitive impairments and dementia are lacking (Skrobot et al., 2017). The vascular cognitive impairments can be conceptualized as being made up of three groups: vascular dementia, mixed vascular dementia and AD pathology, and vascular cognitive impairment not meeting the criteria for dementia. These conditions may have variable contributions from mixed forms of small-vessel disease, large-vessel disease, and cardioembolic disease, which accounts for the clinical phenotypic heterogeneity. AD pathology is commonly found in association with cerebrovascular disease pathology, leading to uncertainty with respect to the relative contributions of each in some cases. A temporal relationship between a stroke and the onset of dementia or a stepwise progression of cognitive decline with evidence of cerebrovascular disease on examination and neuroimaging are considered most helpful. No specific neuroimaging profile exists that is diagnostic for pure cerebrovascular disease–related dementia. Vascular dementia may present with prominent cortical, subcortical, or mixed features. Cortical vascular dementia may manifest as unilateral sensorimotor dysfunction; abrupt onset of cognitive dysfunction and aphasia; and difficulties with planning, goal formation, organization, and abstraction. Subcortical vascular dementia often affects frontosubcortical circuitry, resulting in executive dysfunction, cognitive and psychomotor slowing, difficulties with abstraction, apathy, memory problems (recognition and cued recognition relatively intact), impairment of working memory, and decreased ability to perform activities of daily living. Memory difficulties tend to be less severe than in AD. Limited data suggest that cholinesterase inhibitors are beneficial for the treatment of vascular dementia as demonstrated by improvements in cognition, global functioning, and performance of activities of daily living (Chen et al., 2016).

## Infectious

An expansive list of infections that result in behavioral changes during the early, middle, or late phases of illness or as a result of treatments or subsequent opportunistic infections could be generated. This portion of the present chapter focuses on only a few salient examples with contemporary relevance and illustrative complexity.

### Human Immunodeficiency Virus

Individuals infected with HIV can be affected by a variety of neuropsychiatric and neurological problems independent of opportunistic infections and neoplasms. These include cognitive impairment, behavioral changes, and sensorimotor disturbances. Neurologists and psychiatrists must anticipate a spectrum of psychiatric phenomena that can include depression, paranoia, delusions, hallucinations, psychosis, mania, irritability, and apathy. *HIV-associated dementia* (HAD) is the term given to the syndrome that presents with bradyphrenia, memory decline, executive dysfunction, impaired concentration, and apathy. These features are compatible with a subcortical dementia with prominent dysfunction in the ganglia of the frontobasal ganglia (Woods et al., 2004). *Minor cognitive motor disorder* (MCMD) refers to a milder form of this syndrome that has become more common since the advent of highly active antiretroviral therapy (HAART). HAD may be the acquired immunodeficiency virus syndrome (AIDS)–defining illness in up to 10% of patients. It has been estimated to occur in 20%–30% of untreated adults with AIDS. HAART has reduced its frequency by approximately 50%, but the frequency of pathologically proven HIV encephalitis remains high.

Lifetime prevalence of depression in HIV-infected individuals is 22%–45%, with depressed individuals demonstrating reduced compliance with antiretroviral therapy and increased HIV-related morbidity. Antidepressants have been efficacious in treating HAD (Himelhoch and Medoff, 2005). Psychostimulants may also be a helpful adjunct in treating HAD. Evidence suggests that HIV-infected patients with new-onset psychosis usually respond well to typical neuroleptic medications, but they are more sensitive to the side effects of these medications, particularly extrapyramidal symptoms (EPS) and tardive dyskinesias. This sensitivity is thought to be due to HIV's effect on the basal ganglia, resulting in a loss of dopaminergic neurons. When typical neuroleptics are being prescribed, caution is warranted owing to this sensitivity and the additional possible pharmacological interactions with antiretroviral medications. Atypical neuroleptics are favored.

HAART and other medications used in HIV patients can have neuropsychiatric side effects. For example, the nucleoside reverse transcriptase inhibitor zidovudine (AZT) may lead to mania, delirium, or depression. Moreover, many medications used in the treatment of HIV inhibit or induce the cytochrome P450 system, thereby altering psychotropic drug levels. Therefore drug interactions in HIV patients with psychiatric disorders are common and require close monitoring.

### Creutzfeldt-Jakob Disease

Prion diseases are a group of fatal degenerative disorders of the nervous system caused by a conformational change in the prion protein, a normal constituent of cell membranes. These conditions are characterized by long incubation periods followed by a relatively rapid neurological decline and death (Johnson, 2005). Creutzfeldt-Jakob disease (CJD) is the most common human prion disease but is rare, with an incidence of between 0.5 and 1.5 cases per million people per year. The sporadic form of the disease accounts for about 85% of cases; it typically occurs later in life (mean age, 60 years), and manifests with a rapidly progressive course characterized by cerebellar ataxia, dementia, myoclonus, exaggerated startle reflex, seizures, and psychiatric symptoms progressing to akinetic mutism and complete disability within months after disease onset. Analysis of CSF may prove positive for 14-3-3 protein, which has been shown to have a sensitivity of 92% and a specificity of 80% (Muayqil et al., 2012). Diffusion-weighted imaging may show posterior cortical ribbon or striatal hyperintensities, whereas middle- to late-stage sporadic CJD may show periodic sharp-wave complexes on the EEG (Geschwind et al., 2008). Psychiatric symptoms such as personality changes, anxiety, depression, paranoia, obsessive-compulsive features, and psychosis occur in about 80% of patients during the first 100 days of illness (Wall et al., 2005). About 60% present with symptoms compatible with a rapidly progressive dementia. The mean duration of the illness is 6–7 months.

The autosomal dominant familial form of CJD accounts for 10%–15% of cases; iatrogenically caused cases account for about 1%.

New-variant CJD is a new form of acquired spongiform encephalopathy that emerged in 1994 in the United Kingdom. This form has been linked with consumption of infected animal products. Patients with the new variant have a different course characterized by younger age at onset (mean age, 29 years), prominent psychiatric and sensory symptoms, and a longer disease course. Spencer and colleagues reported that 63% demonstrated purely psychiatric symptoms at onset (dysphoria, anxiety, anhedonia), 15% had purely neurological symptoms, and 22% had features of both (Spencer et al., 2002). New-variant CJD may be distinguished from sporadic CJD by hyperintensities in the pulvinar on MRI. Median duration of illness was 13 months; by the time of death, prominent neurological and psychiatric manifestations were universal.

### Neurosyphilis

A resurgence of neurosyphilis has accompanied the AIDS epidemic in the industrialized world. Neurosyphilis may occur in any stage of syphilis. Early neurosyphilis, seen in the first weeks to years of infection, is primarily a meningitic process in which the parenchyma is not typically involved. It can coexist with primary or secondary syphilis and be asymptomatic. Inadequate treatment of early syphilis and coinfection with HIV predispose to early neurosyphilis. Epidemiological studies in HIV-infected patients have documented increased HIV shedding associated with genital ulcers, suggesting that syphilis increases the susceptibility of infected persons to the acquisition and transmission of HIV (Lynn and Lightman, 2004). Symptomatic early neurosyphilis may present with meningitis with or without cranial nerve involvement or ocular changes, meningovascular disease, or stroke. Late neurosyphilis affects the meninges, brain, or spinal cord parenchyma and usually occurs years to decades after primary infection. Manifestations of late neurosyphilis include tabes dorsalis, a rapidly progressive dementia with psychotic features, general paresis (also known as general paralysis of the insane), or both. Pupillary abnormalities are common, the most classic being Argyll Robertson pupils: miotic, irregular pupils showing light-near dissociation (Berger and Dean, 2014). Dementia as a symptom of neurosyphilis is unlikely to improve significantly with treatment, yet the course of the illness can be arrested. The presenting psychiatric symptoms of neurosyphilis can include personality changes, hostility, confusion, hallucinations, expansiveness, delusions, and dysphoria. Symptoms also reported in association with neurosyphilis include explosive temper, emotional lability, anhedonia, social withdrawal, decreased attention to personal affairs, unusual giddiness, histrionicity, hypersexuality, and mania. A significant incidence of depression has been associated with general paresis.

There is no uniform consensus for the best approach to diagnosing neurosyphilis. Diagnosis usually depends on various combinations of reactive serological tests, CSF cell count or protein, Venereal Disease Research Laboratories (VDRL) testing of the CSF, and clinical manifestations. Some authorities argue that all patients with syphilis should have CSF examination, since asymptomatic neurosyphilis can be identified only by changes in the CSF. The CSF VDRL is the standard serological test for CSF and is highly specific but insensitive. When reactive in the absence of substantial contamination of CSF with blood, it is usually considered diagnostic. Its titer may be used to assess the activity of the disease and response to treatment. Two tests of CSF may be used to confirm a diagnosis of neurosyphilis: the *Treponema pallidum* hemagglutination assay (TPHA) and fluorescent treponemal antibody absorption (FTA-ABS) assay. No single serology screen is perfect for diagnosing neurosyphilis. Other indicators of disease activity include CSF abnormalities such as elevated white blood cell count, elevated protein, and increased γ-globulin (IgG) levels. Treatment of neurosyphilis consists of a regimen of aqueous penicillin G, 18–24 million units per day administered as 3–4 million units intravenously every 4 hours or continuous infusion for 10–14 days. An alternative treatment is procaine penicillin G, 2–4 million units intramuscularly daily, with probenecid 500 mg orally, both daily for 10–14 days. A common recommendation to ensure an adequate response and cure is to repeat CSF studies 6 months after treatment.

## Metabolic and Toxic

Essentially any metabolic derangement, if severe enough or combined with other conditions, can adversely affect behavior and cognition (eTable 10.5 ). Metabolic disorders should remain within the differential diagnosis when patients with psychiatric symptoms are being evaluated.

### Thyroid Disease

Hypothyroidism results from a deficiency in circulating thyroxine ($T_4$). It can be due to impaired function at the level of the hypothalamus (tertiary hypothyroidism), the anterior pituitary (secondary hypothyroidism), or the thyroid gland (primary hypothyroidism, the most common cause of hypothyroidism). Neurological symptoms and signs can include headache, fatigue, apathy, inattention, slowness of speech and thought, sensorineural hearing loss, sleep apnea, and seizures. Some of these symptoms may mimic depression. Hypothyroidism can worsen or complicate the course of depression, resulting in a seemingly refractory depression. More rare findings include polyneuropathy, cranial neuropathy, muscle weakness, psychosis (referred to as *myxedema madness*), dementia, coma, and death. Psychosis typically presents with paranoid delusions and auditory hallucinations.

Hyperthyroidism may be due to a number of causes that produce increased serum $T_4$. With mild hyperthyroidism, patients are typically anxious, irritable, emotionally labile, tachycardic, and tremulous. Other symptoms can include apathy, depression, panic attacks, feelings of exhaustion, inability to concentrate, and memory problems. When apathy and depression are present, the term *apathetic hyperthyroidism* is often used. Thyroid storm results from an abrupt elevation in $T_4$, often provoked by significant stress such as that due to surgery. It can be associated with fever, tachycardia, seizures, and coma; if untreated, it is often fatal. Psychosis and paranoia frequently occur during thyroid storm but are rare with milder hyperthyroidism, as is mania. Many patients will experience complete remission of symptoms 1–2 months after a euthyroid state is obtained, with a marked reduction in anxiety, sense of exhaustion, irritability, and depression. Some authors, however, report an increased rate of anxiety in patients, as well as persistence of affective and cognitive symptoms for several months up to 10 years after a euthyroid state has been established.

Steroid-responsive encephalopathy associated with autoimmune thyroiditis (STREAT), also known as Hashimoto encephalopathy, is a rare disorder involving thyroid autoimmunity (Castillo et al., 2006). Antibodies associated with this condition include antithyroid peroxidase antibodies (previously known as *antithyroid microsomal antibodies*) and antithyroglobulin antibodies. The clinical syndrome may manifest with a progressive or relapsing and remitting course consisting of tremor, myoclonus, transient aphasia, stroke-like episodes, psychosis, seizures, encephalopathy, hypersomnolence, stupor, or coma. Encephalopathy usually develops over 1–7 days. The underlying mechanism of Hashimoto encephalopathy remains under investigation; importantly, levels of thyroid-stimulating hormone can be normal in this disorder. CSF most often shows an elevated protein level with almost no nucleated cells, whereas oligoclonal bands are often present. The EEG is abnormal in almost all cases, showing generalized slowing or frontal intermittent rhythmic δ activity. Triphasic waves, focal slowing, and epileptiform abnormalities may also be seen. MRI of the brain is often normal but may reveal hyperintensities on T2-weighted or fluid-attenuated inversion recovery (FLAIR) imaging in the subcortical white matter or at the gray/white matter junction. SPECT may show regions of hypoperfusion. The neurological and psychiatric symptoms respond well to treatment, which generally involves high-dose steroids. The associated abnormal findings on EEG, and often the MRI abnormalities, resolve with effective treatment.

## Wilson Disease

Wilson disease (WD), also known as *hepatolenticular degeneration*, is an autosomal recessive disorder produced by a mutation on chromosome 13. The gene encodes a transport protein, the mutation of which causes abnormal deposition of copper in the liver, brain (especially the basal ganglia), and the corneas of the eyes. WD typically begins in childhood but in some cases has its onset as late as the fifth or sixth decade. About one-third of patients present with psychiatric symptoms, one-third present with neurological features, and one-third present with hepatic disease. Neurological manifestations are largely extrapyramidal, including chorea, tremor (infrequently including wing beating–like characteristics), and dystonia. Other symptoms include dysphagia, dysarthria, ataxia, gait disturbance, and a fixed (sardonic) smile. Seizures may also occur in a minority of patients. Potential neuropsychiatric symptoms are numerous, with at least half of patients manifesting symptoms early in the disease course. Personality and mood changes are the most common neuropsychiatric features, with depression occurring in approximately 30% of patients. Bipolar spectrum symptoms occur in about 20% of patients. Suicidal ideation is recognized in about 5%–15%. WD patients can present with increased sensitivity to neuroleptics. Other symptoms include irritability, aggression, and psychosis. Cognitively, the profile is consistent with disturbance of the frontosubcortical networks. Despite long-term treatment, about 70% of WD patients develop psychiatric symptoms (Srinivas et al., 2008; Svetel et al., 2009).

Diagnosis is suggested by the identification of Kayser-Fleischer (KF) rings in patients with the appropriate clinical picture. The KF ring is a yellow-brown discoloration of the Descemet membrane in the limbic area of the cornea, best visualized with slit-lamp examination. A KF ring is present in 98% of patients with neurological disease and in 80% of all cases of WD. Reduced serum ceruloplasmin levels and elevated 24-hour urine copper excretion are consistent with this disorder. A liver biopsy is sometimes necessary to make the diagnosis. MRI studies may show abnormal T2 signal in the putamen, midbrain, pons, thalamus, cerebellum, and other structures. Atrophy is commonly present. The initial treatment for symptomatic patients is chelation therapy with either penicillamine or trientine. An estimated 20%–50% of patients with neurological manifestations treated with penicillamine experience an acute worsening of their symptoms, and some of these patients do not recover to their pretreatment neurological baseline. Alternatives that may lead to a lower incidence of neurological worsening include trientine or tetrathiomolybdate. Both may be used in combination with zinc therapy. Treatment of presymptomatic patients or maintenance therapy of successfully treated symptomatic patients can be accomplished with a chelating agent or zinc. Early treatment may result in partial improvement of the MRI changes as well as most of the neurological and psychiatric symptoms.

## Vitamin $B_{12}$ and Folic Acid Deficiency

The true prevalence of vitamin $B_{12}$ deficiency in the general population is unknown. The Framingham study demonstrated a prevalence of 12% among elderly persons living in the community. Other studies have suggested that the incidence may be as high as 30%–40% among the sick and institutionalized elderly. The most common sign of vitamin $B_{12}$ deficiency is macrocytic anemia. However, signs and symptoms attributed to the nervous system are diverse and can occur in the absence of anemia or macrocytosis. Furthermore, a normal serum cobalamin level does not exclude the possibility of a clinical deficiency. Serum homocysteine levels, which are elevated in more than 90% of deficiency states, and serum methylmalonic acid levels can be used to verify deficiency states in the appropriate settings.

*Subacute combined degeneration* (SCD) refers to the combination of spinal cord and peripheral nerve pathology associated with vitamin $B_{12}$ deficiency. Patients often complain of unsteady gait and distal paresthesias. The examination may demonstrate evidence of posterior column, pyramidal tract, and peripheral nerve involvement. Cognitive, behavioral, and psychiatric manifestations can occur in isolation or together with the elemental signs and symptoms. Personality change, cognitive dysfunction, mania, depression, and psychosis have been reported. Prominent psychotic features include paranoid or religious delusions and auditory and visual hallucinations. Dementia is often comorbid with cobalamin deficiency; however, the causative association is unclear. There are few research data to support the existence of reversible dementia due to vitamin $B_{12}$ deficiency. Cobalamin deficiency–associated cognitive impairment is more likely to improve when it is mild and of short duration. Folate deficiency can produce a clinical picture similar to cobalamin deficiency, although some investigators report that folate deficiency tends to produce more depression, whereas vitamin $B_{12}$ deficiency tends to produce more psychosis. Elevated serum homocysteine is also seen with a functional folate deficiency state wherein folate utilization is impaired. Repletion of folate if comorbid vitamin $B_{12}$ deficiency is not first corrected can result in an acute exacerbation of the neuropsychiatric symptoms.

## Porphyrias

The porphyrias are caused by enzymatic defects in the heme biosynthetic pathway. Porphyrias with neuropsychiatric symptoms include acute intermittent porphyria (AIP), variegated porphyria (VP), hereditary mixed coproporphyria (HMP), and plumboporphyria (extremely rare and autosomal recessive), which may give rise to acute episodes of potentially fatal symptoms such as neurovisceral crisis, abdominal pain, delirium, psychosis, neuropathy, and autonomic instability. AIP, the most common type reported in the United States, follows an autosomal dominant pattern of inheritance and is due to a mutation in the gene for porphobilinogen deaminase. The disease is characterized by attacks that may last days to weeks, with relatively normal function between attacks. Infrequently, the clinical course may exhibit persisting clinical abnormalities with superimposed episodes of exacerbation. The episodic nature, clinical variability, and unusual features of this condition may cause symptoms to be misattributed to somatoform, functional (psychogenic), or other psychiatric disorders. Attacks may be spontaneous but are typically precipitated by a variety of factors such as infection, alcohol use, pregnancy, anesthesia, and numerous medications including antidepressants, anticonvulsants, and oral contraceptives.

Porphyric attacks usually manifest with a triad consisting of abdominal pain, peripheral neuropathy, and neuropsychiatric symptoms. Seizures may also occur. Abdominal pain is the most common symptom, which can result in surgical exploration if the diagnosis is unknown. A variety of cognitive and behavioral changes can occur, including anxiety, restlessness, insomnia, depression, mania, hallucinations, delusions, confusion, catatonia, and psychosis. The diagnosis can be confirmed during an acute attack of AIP, HMP, or VP by measuring urine porphobilinogens. Acute attacks are treated with avoidance of precipitating factors (e.g., medications), intravenous hemin, intravenous glucose, and pain control.

### Drug Abuse

Common neurological manifestations are broad and include the direct effects of intoxication, side effects, and withdrawal syndromes as well as indirect effects. Direct effects can range from somnolence with sedatives to psychosis from hallucinogens and stimulants. Side effects may be as severe as stroke or vasculitis from stimulant abuse. Withdrawal may be lethal, as in the case of alcohol withdrawal and delirium tremens. Indirect effects can occur as a result of trauma, such as head injury, suffered while under the influence. Substance abuse has a high comorbidity with a variety of psychiatric conditions. Neuropsychiatric manifestations occur with abuse of all classes of drugs and are summarized in eBox 10.6. The behavioral and cognitive manifestations of substance abuse may be transient; in a vulnerable subset of individuals, however, they may be chronic. Growing evidence suggests that drug use (e.g., 3,4-methylenedioxymethamphetamine [MDMA, "ecstasy"]) may promote the development of chronic neuropsychiatric states such as depression and impaired cognition due to changes in structural and functional neuroanatomy (Parrott, 2013). Although the use of *Cannabis sativa* seems to be neither a sufficient nor a necessary cause of psychosis, it does confer an increased relative risk for developing psychosis in dose-dependent fashion (Marconi et al., 2016).

### Systemic Lupus Erythematosus

Systemic lupus erythematosus (SLE, lupus) is a multisystem inflammatory disorder that affects all ages, although young females are at a significantly elevated risk. CNS involvement is common, with clinical manifestations seen at some point during the disease course in up to 90% of patients. Primary neurological and psychiatric manifestations of SLE are likely due to a mixture of pathogenic mechanisms that include vascular abnormalities, autoantibodies, and the local production of inflammatory mediators. Secondary neurological and psychiatric manifestations occur as a result of various therapies (e.g., immunosuppression with steroids) or complications of the disease.

Neuropsychiatric symptoms are common, often episodic, and may occur in association with steroid treatment, which creates significant dilemmas in management. Depression and anxiety each occur in approximately 25% of SLE patients. Reports of the prevalence of overall mood disturbances range between 16% and 75%, and reports of anxiety disorders occur in 7%–70%. Psychosis is rarer and tends to occur in the context of confusional states. Its overall prevalence has been reported to range from 5% to 8%. The incidence of psychotic symptoms in patients receiving prednisone in doses between 60 and 100 mg/day is approximately 30%. These symptoms are reported to respond favorably to reduction in steroid dose and psychotropic management. Focal or generalized seizures may occur in the setting of active generalized SLE or as an isolated event. The prevalence of seizures ranges from 3% to 51%. Cognitive manifestations of SLE—including temporary, fluctuating, or relatively stable characteristics—eventually occur in up to 75% of patients; these manifestations range from mild attentional difficulties to dementia. In some patients, cognitive performance improves with resolution of any concurrent psychiatric disturbances. Cerebrovascular disease may underlie nonreversible cognitive dysfunction; when progressive, it may cause atrophy and multi-infarct dementia. Many patients with cognitive impairment have no demonstrable vascular lesions on neuroimaging. Cognitive impairment may manifest as subcortical features with deficits in processing speed, attention, learning and memory, conceptual reasoning, and cognitive flexibility. Reports of the prevalence of subclinical cognitive impairment range from 11% to 54% of patients. A number of brain-specific antibodies have been studied as potential diagnostic markers of psychosis associated with neuropsychiatric SLE (NPSLE), but none appear to be specific (Kimura et al., 2010). SLE patients identified as having a persistently positive immunoglobulin (Ig)G anticardiolipin antibody over a 5-year period have been demonstrated to have a greater reduction in psychomotor speed than antibody-negative SLE patients. Patients with a persistently elevated immunoglobulin A (IgA) anticardiolipin antibody level have been demonstrated to have poorer performance on tests of conceptual reasoning and executive function than antibody-negative SLE patients. Elevated IgG and IgA anticardiolipin antibody levels may be causative or a marker of long-term subtle deterioration in cognitive function in SLE patients. However, their role in routine evaluation and management remains controversial. Cerebrovascular disease is a well-known cause of neuropsychiatric dysfunction and is reported to occur in 5%–18% of SLE patients.

The criteria set most widely used for diagnosing SLE is that developed by the American College of Rheumatology (ACR). An antinuclear antibody (ANA) titer to 1:40 or higher is the most sensitive of the ACR criteria and is present in up to 99% of persons with SLE at some point in their illness. The ANA titer, however, is not specific. It can be positive in several other rheumatological conditions, in nonclinical populations, and in relation to some medication exposures. Anti–double-stranded DNA and anti-Smith antibodies, particularly in high titers, have high specificity for SLE, although their sensitivity is low. The rapid plasma reagin (RPR) test, a syphilis serology, may be falsely positive.

Treatment of NPSLE includes corticosteroids and immunosuppressive therapy, including pulse intravenous cyclophosphamide or plasmapheresis when NPSLE is thought to occur secondary to an inflammatory process. Anticoagulation is used in patients with thrombotic disease in the setting of antiphospholipid antibody syndrome.

### Multiple Sclerosis

MS is an inflammatory demyelinating disease that manifests the pathological hallmark findings of multifocal demyelinated plaques in the brain and spinal cord. MS lesions are typically disseminated throughout the CNS, with a predilection for the optic nerves, brainstem, spinal cord, cerebellum, and periventricular white matter. Its cause remains unknown, but it is thought to be an immune-mediated disorder affecting individuals with a genetic predisposition. The heterogeneity of clinical, pathological, and MRI findings suggest involvement of more than one pathological mechanism. It is the leading cause of nontraumatic disability among young adults. Socioepidemiological studies indicate that MS leads to unemployment within a 10-year disease course in as many as 50%–80% of patients. Females are more affected than males at a 2:1 ratio. It is characterized either by attacks of neurological deficits with variable remittance or by a steadily progressive course of neurological decline. Neuropsychiatric manifestations of MS are common, occurring in up to 60% of patients at some point in their disease. The lifetime prevalence of major depression in MS is approximately 50%. The lifetime prevalence of bipolar disorder is twice the prevalence in the general population. Euphoria may be present in more advanced MS, usually in association with cognitive deficits. *Pseudobulbar affect*—defined as outbursts of involuntary, uncontrollable, stereotypical episodes of laughing or crying—occurs in varying degrees of severity in approximately 10% of patients. Other symptoms include anxiety, sleep disorder, emotional lability/irritability, apathy, mania, suicidality, and rarely psychosis. Occasionally psychiatric symptoms may present as the major manifestation of an episode of demyelination. The presence of psychiatric symptomatology does not preclude the use of steroids to abbreviate clinical attacks of MS. There is ongoing debate about whether interferon therapy is associated with a higher incidence of depression in MS patients. Clinically, pharmacological and behavioral treatment mirrors the management of depression and psychosis in patients without MS. Recently published guidelines for management of the psychiatric symptoms of MS suggest that there is insufficient evidence to refute or support the use of antidepressants for depression or anxiety disorders in this population, although a combination of dextromethorphan and quinidine may be considered for the treatment of pseudobulbar affect (Minden et al., 2014).

Cognitive impairment is found in approximately 40% of patients. Deficits have been described in working, semantic, and episodic memory as well as in the person's ability to accurately assess his or her own memory function. Patients may also suffer from impaired attention, cognitive slowing, reduced verbal fluency, and difficulties with abstract reasoning and concept formation. Correlations between cognitive impairment and the MRI location of lesions and indices of total lesion area are actively under investigation (Charil et al., 2003; Reuter et al., 2011). There are few data on the treatment of cognitive dysfunction in MS (Amato et al., 2013). The disease-modifying agent interferon β-1a was noted to be associated with improvements in information-processing and problem-solving abilities over a 2-year longitudinal study. A small trial demonstrated an improvement in complex attention, concentration, and visual memory in a group of patients treated for 1 year with interferon β-1b compared with controls (Barak and Achiron, 2002). Donepezil, 10 mg daily, has been reported to improve verbal learning and memory in some MS patients.

## Neoplastic

A variety of neoplasms cause cognitive and behavioral disorders. Of particular relevance are mass lesions and paraneoplastic syndromes. Mass lesions can be single or multiple and can be primary to the CNS or metastatic. The most common intracranial primary tumors are astrocytomas (e.g., glioblastoma multiforme), meningiomas, pituitary tumors, vestibular schwannomas, and oligodendrogliomas. Common metastatic tumors include primary lung and breast tumors, melanoma, and renal and colon cancers. The number of patients presenting with a primary psychiatric diagnosis secondary to an unidentified brain tumor is likely to be less than 5%. However, 15%–20% of patients with intracranial tumors may present with neuropsychiatric manifestations before the development of primary neurological problems such as motor or sensory deficits. The behavioral manifestations of mass lesions are diverse and related to a number of factors including direct disruption of local structures or circuits, rate of growth, seizures, and increased intracranial pressure. A relationship between tumor location and specific psychiatric symptoms has not been established. Meningiomas, given their slow growth over years, are classic examples of tumors that can present solely with behavioral manifestations. Common locations include the olfactory groove and sphenoid wings, which can disrupt adjacent limbic structures such as the orbital frontal gyri and medial temporal lobes.

Paraneoplastic syndromes represent remote nonmetastatic manifestations of malignancy. Neurological paraneoplastic syndromes are primarily immune-mediated disorders that may develop as a result of antigens shared between the nervous system and tumor cells (Berzero and Psimaras, 2018). The most common primary malignancies that promote neurological paraneoplastic syndromes are ovarian and small-cell lung cancer (SCLC). These syndromes generally develop subacutely, often before the primary malignancy is identified, and may preferentially involve selected regions of the CNS. Typical sites of involvement include muscle, neuromuscular junction, peripheral nerve, cerebellum, and limbic structures. Limbic encephalitis—associated with SCLC, testicular cancer, and ovarian teratomas among other pathologies—produces a significant amnestic syndrome and neuropsychiatric symptoms including agitation, depression, personality changes, apathy, delusions, hallucinations, psychosis, and complex partial and generalized seizures. Anti *N*-methyl-D-aspartate (NMDA) receptor encephalitis associated with antibodies against the NR1-NR2 heterodimer of the receptor has been increasingly recognized as presenting commonly in young women with ovarian teratomas and psychiatric symptoms including anxiety, agitation, bizarre behavior, paranoid delusions, visual or auditory hallucinations, and/or memory loss. Additional frequently encountered symptoms include seizures, decreased consciousness, dyskinesias, autonomic instability, and hypoventilation (Dalmau and Rosenfeld, 2014). Elevated markers in paraneoplastic syndromes may include (1) intracellular paraneoplastic antigens, such as Hu, associated with SCLC, and Ta and Ma-2 (Hoffmann et al., 2008), associated with testicular cancer; and (2) cell membrane antigens such as the NMDA receptor and voltage-gated potassium channels. Paraneoplastic disorders are often progressive and refractory to therapy, although in some cases significant improvement follows tumor resection and early initiated immunotherapy interventions. Significant neuropsychiatric sequelae can arise from the various chemotherapeutic and radiation therapies used for cancer treatment.

## Degenerative

Neuropsychiatric symptoms are common in most degenerative disorders that produce significant dementia. In this chapter, the term *dementia* is used synonymously with the DSM-5 diagnostic category of major neurocognitive disorder; mild cognitive impairment (MCI) is synonymous with mild neurocognitive disorder. The individual presentations of such symptoms are related to a number of factors specific to the disease: location of lesion burden, rate of progression of disease, and factors specific to the individual (e.g., premorbid personality, education level, psychiatric history, social support system, and coping skills). Neurodegenerative diseases are increasingly recognized as involving abnormalities of protein metabolism. About 70% of dementias in the elderly and more than 90% of neurodegenerative dementias can be linked to abnormalities of three proteins: β-amyloid, α-synuclein, and tau. Disorders of protein metabolism have associated neuroanatomical regions of vulnerable cell populations that are related to the clinical manifestations. AD, for example, has associated disorders of β-amyloid and tau. PD, DLB, and multisystem atrophies are synucleinopathies. α-Synuclein is the main component of Lewy bodies, which are a major histological marker seen in PD and DLB. In these disorders, Lewy bodies may be found in the substantia nigra, locus coeruleus, nucleus basalis, limbic system, and transitional and neocortex. FTD, progressive supranuclear palsy (PSP), and corticobasal ganglionic degeneration implicate abnormal tau metabolism in their pathogenesis. Tauopathies are associated with selective involvement of the frontal and temporal cortex and frontosubcortical circuitry.

### Alzheimer Disease and Mild Cognitive Impairment

Neuropsychiatric symptoms of AD may include agitation, aggression, delusions including paranoia, hallucinations, anxiety, apathy, social withdrawal, reduced speech output, reduction or alteration of long-standing family relationships, and loss of sense of humor. With disease progression, patients often lose awareness (insight) into the nature and severity of their deficits. A review of 100 cases of autopsy-proven AD demonstrated that 74% of patients had behavioral symptoms detected at the time of the initial evaluation. Symptoms included apathy (51%), hallucinations (25%), delusions (20%), depressed mood (6.6%), verbal aggression (36.8%), and physical aggression (17%). The presence of behavioral symptoms at the initial evaluation was associated with greater functional impairment not directly related to the cognitive impairments. Depressive symptoms, dysphoria, or major depression eventually occur in approximately 50% of patients. Psychosis has been reported to occur in 30% to 50% of patients at some time during the course of the illness, more commonly in the later stages. Mania occurs in less than 5%. Behavioral changes have been shown to be problematic and to precipitate earlier nursing home placement. Social comportment has been viewed as being relatively spared in AD, but subtle personality changes occur in nearly every individual over time. Significant impairment in the ability to recognize facial expressions of emotion and an inability to repeat, comprehend, and discriminate affective elements of language have been reported. It has been hypothesized that 15% of AD patients may have a frontal variant wherein they present with difficulties attributable to frontal lobe circuitry rather than an amnestic syndrome. Impairments in driving ability (Dawson et al., 2009) and decision-making abilities such as medical decision making (Okonkwo et al., 2008) and financial management (Marson et al., 2009) may be present even in early AD.

Atypical antipsychotic drugs are widely used to treat psychosis, aggression, and agitation in patients with AD. Efficacy is modest and concerns about safety have emerged, including increased risk of mortality, cerebrovascular events, metabolic derangements, EPS, falls, cognitive worsening, cardiac arrhythmia, and pneumonia, among other symptoms (Steinberg and Lyketsos, 2012). Adverse effects may offset advantages in the efficacy of atypical antipsychotic drugs for the treatment of psychosis, aggression, or agitation in AD patients, particularly if used chronically. Limited evidence suggests that electroconvulsive therapy (ECT) may be effective for the management of severe agitation (Acharya et al., 2015). Early evidence also suggests that dronabinol may be helpful in the management of aggressive behavior in severely demented patients (Woodward et al., 2014).

The concept of MCI was developed to characterize a population of individuals exhibiting symptoms that are between normal age-related cognitive decline and dementia. These patients have minimal decline from their prior level of functioning and remain independent. MCI (*amnestic single domain*) was initially defined as a condition of memory impairment beyond what was expected for age in the absence of impairments in other domains of cognitive functioning such as working memory, executive function, language, and visuospatial ability. This concept has since evolved and now includes four subtypes of impairment that are not of sufficient severity to warrant the diagnosis of dementia. The second type of MCI, called *amnestic multiple domain*, is associated with memory impairment plus impairment in one or more other cognitive domains. The third subtype is called *nonamnestic single domain*, and the fourth is known as *nonamnestic multiple domain* MCI. In many cases the natural history of these subtypes leads to different endpoint conditions. Combining the clinical syndrome with the presumed cause may allow for reliable prediction of outcome of the MCI syndrome. When associated with only memory impairment, MCI may represent normal aging, depression, or progress to AD. Amnestic MCI involving multiple domains has a higher association with depression or progression to AD or vascular dementia. Nonamnestic single-domain MCI may have a higher likelihood of progression to FTD. Nonamnestic multiple-domain MCI may have a higher likelihood of progression to Lewy body dementia or vascular dementia (Petersen and Negash, 2008).

In 2008, it was estimated that more than 5 million people in the United States above 71 years of age had MCI. The prevalence of MCI among persons younger than 75 years has been estimated to be 19% and 29% for those older than 85 years. Almost one-third of these individuals have amnestic MCI, which may progress to AD at a rate of 10%–15% per year. The conversion rate of amnestic MCI to dementia over a 6-year period may be as high as 80%. Neuropsychiatric symptoms (also known as mild behavioral impairment) are common in persons with MCI. Depression occurs in 20%, apathy in 15%, and irritability in 15%. Increased levels of agitation and aggression are also present. Almost half of MCI patients demonstrate one of these neuropsychiatric symptoms coincident with the onset of cognitive impairment. Impaired awareness of memory dysfunction may also be present to a degree comparable with that found in persons with early AD. Evidence suggests that persons with MCI have an increased risk of motor vehicle accidents when risk factors such as having a history of driving citations, crashes, reduced driving mileage, situational avoidance, or aggression or impulsivity are present. Difficulties with medical decision making have also been identified in some individuals with MCI (Okonkwo et al., 2008).

### Frontotemporal Dementia

FTD, the most common progressive focal cortical syndrome, is characterized by atrophy of the frontal and anterotemporal lobes. Age at presentation is usually between 45 and 65 years (almost invariably before age 65), and reports of its incidence range from being equal in males and females to (more recently) predominating in males by a ratio of 14:3. The prevalence of FTD is equal to that of AD for early-onset (age <65) dementia. Features of behavioral variant FTD may include apathy, social withdrawal, loss of empathy or sympathy, disinhibition, impulsivity, poor insight, anosognosia, ritualistic or obsessive tendencies, and inappropriate sexual behavior; infrequently, particularly in the early stages of the disease, agitation, delusions, hallucinations, and psychosis may also occur (Rascovsky et al., 2011). Elements of the Klüver-Bucy syndrome may be present. Memory and language are usually spared during the early disease course. Depressive symptoms occur in 30%–40% of patients. SSRIs are somewhat effective in treating behavioral symptoms, including disinhibition, but are less effective in treating cognitive symptoms. About 30% of patients with FTD have a positive family history, and first-degree relatives of patients have a 3.5 times higher risk of developing dementia. Genes known to be mutated in this disorder include those encoding microtubule-associated protein tau and progranulin; the gene *C9ORF72* is a common genetic cause of both FTD and amyotrophic lateral sclerosis; it is also linked to the development of psychosis (Snowden et al., 2012). Semantic dementia, also known as primary progressive aphasia–semantic variant, is also associated with a neuropsychiatric syndrome that partially overlaps with behavioral variant FTD (Elahi and Miller, 2017).

### Idiopathic Parkinson Disease

Neuropsychiatric manifestations of PD are common. Depression is the most common psychiatric symptom, with a reported prevalence of 25%–50%. Establishing the diagnosis of depression is complicated by the presence of comorbid confounding symptoms that include dementia, facial masking, bradykinesia, apathy, and hypophonia. Menza et al. (2009) conducted a placebo-controlled trial in PD patients with depression and found that nortriptyline was efficacious in treating them but paroxetine was not. Psychosis is also particularly prevalent and generally related to dopaminergic agents (Menza et al., 2009). The onset of motor impairment almost always precedes that of psychosis. Hallucinations, usually fleeting and nocturnal, are typically visual and occur in 30% of treated patients. Auditory and olfactory hallucinations, however, are rare. Visual hallucinations are associated with impaired cognition, use of anticholinergic medications, and impaired vision. In contrast to the hallucinations associated with DLB, patients with PD generally have at least partial insight into the nature of their hallucinations. Delusions occur less commonly and are often persecutory in nature. Management is complicated by neuroleptic sensitivity to both typical and atypical agents. Typical neuroleptics should be avoided. Novel atypical neuroleptics with potentially more favorable pharmacological properties, such as quetiapine and clozapine, may have theoretical advantages over other agents for treating PD. Evidence suggests that clozapine is effective, quetiapine may be effective, and olanzapine is not effective. Impulse-control disorders—including pathological gambling, binge-eating, and compulsive sexual behavior and buying—are associated with DA agonist treatment in PD (Weintraub et al., 2010).

Many PD patients will develop dementia 10 years or more after the onset of motor symptoms. Up to 80% of PD patients will eventually develop frank dementia, a majority of whom will show comorbid AD pathology. Initial deficits may include cognitive slowing, memory retrieval deficits, attentional difficulties, visuospatial deficits, and mild executive impairments. In advanced disease, memory encoding and storage can become impaired. Primary language difficulties are not involved until the disease has significantly progressed. Some evidence suggests that patients with an akinetic-dominant form of PD with hallucinations are at higher risk of developing dementia than those with a tremor-dominant form who have no hallucinations. Dementia is a major prognostic factor for progressive disability and nursing home placement. In a placebo-controlled trial, cholinesterase inhibitors have been shown to produce moderate but significant improvements in global ratings of dementia, cognition, and behavioral symptoms in patients with mild to moderate PD (Wang et al., 2015).

### Dementia With Lewy Bodies

By some accounts, DLB is the second most common cause of dementia. The revised consensus criteria for the clinical diagnosis of DLB reiterate dementia as an essential feature for the diagnosis of DLB occurring before or concurrently with parkinsonism. Criteria developed for research purposes to distinguish DLB from PD with dementia use an arbitrary period of 1 year within which the occurrence of dementia and EPS suggests the diagnosis of possible DLB. If the clinical history of parkinsonism is longer than 1 year before dementia occurs, a diagnosis of PD with dementia is more accurate. Deficits of attention, executive function, and visuospatial ability may be prominent. These deficits may be worse in DLB than in patients with AD. Prominent or persistent memory impairment may not necessarily occur in the early stages but is usually evident with progression. Memory impairment is a less prominent feature than in AD. According to the revised consensus criteria, two core features are sufficient for the diagnosis of probable DLB and one feature for the diagnosis of possible DLB. Core features include fluctuating cognition, recurrent visual hallucinations, and spontaneous features of parkinsonism. Other suggestive and supportive features associated with DLB include delusions, hallucinations in other modalities, rapid-eye-movement (REM) sleep behavior disorder, depression, severe neuroleptic sensitivity, autonomic dysfunction, repeated falls/syncope, and episodes of unexplained transient loss of consciousness.

Hallucinations are characteristically seen early in the disease course and are persistent and recurrent. Visual hallucinations tend to occur early in the illness, are typically well formed and complex, and occur in 50%–80% of patients. Auditory hallucinations occur in approximately 30% of patients and olfactory hallucinations in 5%–10%. Delusions may be systematized and are present in 50% of patients over the course of the disease. Depression is estimated to be nearly as common as that in AD. Treatment is complicated by hypersensitivity to the adverse effects of antidopaminergic neuroleptic agents (both typical and atypical). Typical agents should be avoided. Atypical neuroleptics with potentially more favorable pharmacological properties (e.g., quetiapine and clozapine) may have theoretical advantages over other agents in treating DLB as with PD. Cholinesterase inhibitors are helpful for managing neuropsychiatric symptoms and may be beneficial for treating fluctuating cognitive impairment and visual hallucinations; they may also improve global functioning and activities of daily living.

### Huntington Disease

HD is a degenerative disorder of autosomal dominant inheritance resulting from an expanded trinucleotide (CAG) repeat on chromosome 4. Symptoms typically develop during the fourth or fifth decade, initially manifesting with neurological features, psychiatric features, or both. Neurologically, patients often demonstrate generalized chorea, motor impersistence, and oculomotor dysfunction. In the juvenile form, the Westphal variant, early parkinsonian features are prominent, as are seizures, ataxia, and myoclonus. Significant cognitive impairment is inevitable and is often present early in the disease. Features of a subcortical dementia are present with involvement of frontosubcortical circuits. Common features include cognitive slowing, memory retrieval deficits, attentional difficulties, and executive dysfunction. Patients often lack awareness of their chorea and their cognitive and emotional deficits. Psychiatric features such as personality changes, apathy, irritability, and depression are common. Depression may be exacerbated by tetrabenazine used for the treatment of chorea, since this drug is a DA-depleting agent. Psychosis may occur in up to 25% of patients with HD. Anxiety and obsessive tendencies also occur (Phillips et al., 2008).

### Epilepsy

Behavioral and cognitive dysfunction is frequently observed in patients with epilepsy and represents an important challenge in treating these patients. A complex array of factors influences the neuropsychiatric effect of epilepsy: cause, location of epileptogenic focus, age at onset, duration of epilepsy, nature of the epilepsy syndrome, seizure type, frequency, medications used for treatment, and psychosocial factors. Epilepsies that develop subsequent to brain trauma and stroke may be associated with cognitive and behavioral changes due to brain injury quite apart from those associated with the secondary seizures. The localization of an epileptogenic focus is also an important determinant of cognitive deficits. For example, temporal lobe epilepsy may be associated with memory defects, and frontal lobe epilepsy may be associated with performance deficits in executive functioning. Behavioral disturbances are most common with complex partial seizures and seizures involving foci in the temporolimbic structures. The age of onset can affect cognitive and behavioral functioning; onset of epilepsy before 5 years of age appears to be a risk factor for a lower intelligence quotient (IQ). Attention-deficit hyperactivity disorder, inattentive type, has been observed to be 2.5 times more common in children younger than 16 years with newly diagnosed unprovoked seizures than in controls. Behavioral symptoms may be more prominent in later-onset seizures. Duration of epilepsy and seizure type and frequency are other factors that affect cognition and behavior. Individuals with generalized tonic-clonic seizures may have greater associated cognitive impairment than that observed in persons with partial seizures; compared with patients experiencing fewer seizures, those who experience repeated generalized tonic-clonic seizures generally have increased cognitive impairment. A single seizure can be associated with postictal attentional deficits lasting 24 hours or longer. Antiepileptic medications add another level of complexity to management by introducing their associated side effects, which may include impairment of working memory, slowed cognitive processing, language disturbances, and behavioral changes. Anticonvulsants have been reported to be associated with a host of effects on sleep, such as insomnia, alterations of sleep architecture, and in some cases worsening of sleep-disordered breathing (barbiturates and benzodiazepines). These may all adversely affect cognition. On the other hand, anticonvulsants may reduce seizure activity, interictal activity, and arousals from sleep, thereby contributing to improved cognitive function.

Cognitive adverse side effects are more prominent in patients receiving polytherapy and have been noted to improve with a switch to monotherapy. It is estimated that more than 60% of patients with epilepsy meet diagnostic criteria for at least one psychiatric disorder over the course of their lives. Depression is the most common symptom, occurring with an estimated prevalence of 11%–44%. The prevalence of psychosis is estimated at between 2% and 8%. Other prominent psychiatric symptoms associated with epilepsy include anxiety, aggression, personality disorders, and panic disorders. Mania is considered rare. When symptoms of mood disorder or psychosis are being evaluated in a patient with epilepsy, it is important to take into account the chronological relationship of the seizures with the symptoms. Conceptually these symptoms can be classified into peri-ictal or preictal, ictal, postictal, and interictal. Paradoxically, depression or psychosis can follow remission of epilepsy, either after epilepsy surgery or the initiation of effective antiepileptic drug therapy, as part of the phenomenon of forced normalization. Peri-ictal or preictal dysphoric or depressive syndromes frequently precede a seizure. They may last hours to days and resolve with the occurrence of the seizure or persist for hours to days afterward. Peri-ictal depressive symptoms are more common in focal seizures than in generalized seizures. Ictal depressive symptoms occur in approximately 10% of temporal lobe epilepsy patients. Ictal depression is most often characterized by a sudden onset of symptoms independent of external stressors. No associated hemispheric lateralization of the epileptic focus has been clearly demonstrated. Anxiety is the most common ictal psychiatric symptom, with ictal panic being a mimic for idiopathic panic disorder. Treatment of preictal and ictal depressive symptoms does not usually require antidepressant therapy. Treatment should be directed at reducing the frequency of seizures.

The prevalence of postictal depressed mood has not been established. Patients with poorly controlled simple focal seizures have been reported to have postictal depressive symptoms averaging approximately 37 hours. After a seizure, depressive symptoms have been known to last up to 2 weeks, with some reports suggesting increased suicide risk. Investigation of patients with postictal depression has revealed unilateral frontal or temporal foci without hemispheric predominance. Interictal depression is considered the most common type of depression in epileptic patients. Its estimated prevalence ranges from 20% to 70%, depending on the patient group characteristics. Episodic major depression and dysthymia are common, whereas bipolar affective symptoms are rare. Interictal depressive symptoms are often chronic and less prominent than those with a frank major depressive disorder (MDD), resulting in patients not reporting their symptoms and healthcare providers not recognizing them. Treatment may be required for postictal depressive symptoms and usually is required for interictal depressive symptoms. Treatment should consist of an antidepressant medication and optimized seizure control. SSRIs have a lower risk of associated seizures and should be considered as first-line pharmacotherapy. ECT is not contraindicated in patients with epilepsy and should be considered for severe or TRD. The incidence of seizures in epilepsy patients after ECT is not increased compared with that in patients without epilepsy.

Psychosis is a rare primary manifestation of a seizure focus. When present, it is best treated by controlling the ictus and thus by administering antiepileptic medications. Psychosis may commonly manifest as a postictal phenomenon (representing approximately 25% of all psychosis associated with epilepsy). Diagnostic criteria for postictal psychosis (PIP) include (1) an episode of psychosis emerging within 1 week after the return of normal mental function following a seizure; (2) an episode length between 24 hours and 3 months; and (3) no evidence of EEG-supported nonconvulsive status epilepticus, anticonvulsant toxicity, previous history of interictal psychosis, recent head injury, or alcohol or drug intoxication. PIP may manifest with affect-laden symptomatology. Commonly there is a prompt response to low-dose antipsychotics or benzodiazepines. The annual incidence of PIP among patients who undergo inpatient video EEG monitoring was estimated to be approximately 6%. The prevalence of having experienced PIP among treatment-resistant partial epilepsy outpatients has been reported to be 7%. PIP is most commonly associated with temporal lobe epilepsy. Psychotic symptoms may include auditory, visual, or olfactory hallucinations. Abnormalities of thought content or form may include ideas of reference, paranoia, delusions, grandiosity, religious delusions, thought blocking, tangentiality, or loose associations. Manic symptoms may briefly occur in a minority of patients but are usually not of sufficient duration to meet criteria for a manic episode. In patients with temporal lobe epilepsy and PIP, studies have shown a higher incidence of bilateral cerebral injury or dysfunction, bilateral independent temporal region EEG discharges, and bifrontal and bitemporal hyperperfusion patterns on SPECT. These data suggest that bilateral cerebral abnormalities may be an important feature of PIP.

There has been speculation that PIP may sometimes be caused by complex partial (limbic) status (Elliott et al., 2009). When this is thought to be the case, acute therapy with antiepileptic medications would be advised, possibly in conjunction with antipsychotic medication. Risk factors for PIP include a cluster of seizures, insomnia within 1 week of onset of PIP (particularly within 1–3 days), epilepsy of more than 10 years' duration, generalized tonic-clonic seizures or secondarily generalized complex partial seizures, prior episodes of PIP, prior psychiatric hospitalizations or a history of psychosis, bilateral independent seizure foci (particularly temporal), history of TBI or encephalitis, and low intellectual function. PIP is usually short lived, lasting several days to weeks, but chronic psychosis may develop after recurrent episodes or even after a single episode. Research data are lacking for treatment of PIP, and recommendations are based on expert opinion. Recommendations include vigilant monitoring of patients with risk factors for PIP after a cluster of seizures, ensuring that there is no ongoing seizure activity, early implementation of antipsychotic medications (preferably atypical agents) after the emergence of symptoms, consideration of treatment after a cluster of seizures in patients with a history of PIP, and consideration of treatment with the emergence of sleeplessness, which can be a harbinger of PIP. PIP can respond to ECT, but it is rarely necessary to utilize this resource.

Interictal psychosis manifesting similar positive psychopathological phenomena as schizophrenia has been felt to be more common in patients with temporolimbic foci. This idea has been challenged by a population-based study using a cohort comprising 2.27 million people derived from the Danish longitudinal registers. These data support the premise that all types of epilepsy increase the risk of developing a schizophrenia-like psychosis. Furthermore, compared with the general population, persons with epilepsy have nearly 2.5 times the risk of developing schizophrenia and almost 3 times the risk of developing a schizophrenia-like psychosis. The risk for psychosis also increases with an increasing number of hospital admissions for epilepsy and with people first admitted for epilepsy at later ages. Some experts have suggested that interictal psychosis differs from primary psychosis insofar as the former tends to be associated with preserved affect, fewer negative symptoms, and arguably greater insight. The greatest similarities can be seen in the presence of positive symptoms such as delusions and hallucinations. The underlying causal mechanism for the association of epilepsy with schizophrenia or schizophrenia-like psychosis is unknown, but it may have features in common with PIP and likely involves bilateral cerebral dysfunction within frontal subcortical circuits and probably temporal subcortical circuits as well. Treatment for PIP is based primarily on the use of antipsychotic medications once status epilepticus has been diagnostically eliminated from consideration.

Treatment of epilepsy-related psychosis is complicated by the propensity of antipsychotics to cause paroxysmal EEG abnormalities (Centorrino et al., 2002; Kanner, 2008) and to lower the seizure threshold. EEG changes occur in the nonepileptic population treated with antipsychotics but in most circumstances are of little consequence. Studies defining the effects of neuroleptics on the EEG of persons with epilepsy are lacking. The potential for increasing seizures has led to some anxiety about the use of antipsychotics in individuals with epilepsy. In most circumstances, the risk of increasing seizures is considered low, but formal studies investigating the efficacy of antipsychotic medications for treating epilepsy-related psychosis and the risks for precipitating seizures are lacking. The specific causes and characteristics of a given epilepsy must be considered carefully, as these may increase risk. Seizure potential is generally dose related, so high-dose therapy should be avoided. Careful monitoring of anticonvulsants is advised. The lowest possible effective dose should be used, medications selected carefully, and psychiatric polypharmacy avoided if possible, since this may increase the risk of seizures. Seizure risk is particularly increased with use of clozapine and chlorpromazine. Potential problems with antipsychotic treatment in persons with epilepsy include pharmacokinetic interactions due to common metabolism with P450 isoenzymes, as well as side effects (sedation, weight gain, hyperlipidemia, decreased glycemic control, hematotoxicity, and hepatotoxicity).

## Traumatic Brain Injury

Each year approximately 1.7 million people in the United States sustain a TBI. It is estimated that 80% of these are of mild severity, and the remaining 20% are about evenly split between moderate and severe injuries. The leading causes of TBI in the United States are motor vehicle accidents, falls, assaults, and recreational accidents. The wars in Iraq and Afghanistan have increased the numbers of injuries suffered by US military personnel; 15%–20% of military and civilian personnel serving in these theaters have experienced mild TBI during their deployments.

The pathological correlates of moderate to severe TBI are numerous and particular to the types and mechanisms of injuries suffered. Various types of pathology, which are often found in combination, include penetrating wounds, depressed skull fractures, diffuse axonal injury (DAI), petechial hemorrhages, contusions, lacerations, hematomas (epidural, subdural, and intraparenchymal), subarachnoid hemorrhage, edema, herniation, and focal or diffuse hypoxic ischemic injury. Many of these specific types of injuries have their own prognosis and time course of recovery. Concussion or mild TBI occurs most frequently in young adults. There is ongoing debate about what clinical findings constitute mild TBI, with many practitioners advocating that loss of consciousness is not an absolute requirement. Others differ on the required duration of loss of consciousness, with ranges from 20 minutes to any event lasting less than 1 hour. Any traumatic process associated with a generalized alteration in cerebral function, including amnesia (retrograde or anterograde) or alteration in consciousness at the time of the accident, may be associated with brain injury. Persons who sustain a mild TBI often complain of a number of emotional/behavioral, cognitive, and physical symptoms, which can persist for months to years after the injury and rarely may be permanent. Such symptoms can include anxiety, depression, irritability, mood lability, cognitive slowing, judgment problems, difficulty concentrating, memory problems, fatigue, sensitivity to noise, dizziness, and headaches. Postconcussive symptoms occur after moderate and severe TBI as well. It is estimated that 80%–90% of persons sustaining a mild TBI make a favorable recovery. When symptoms persist, the patient is said to suffer from a *postconcussive syndrome*. The overall prevalence for postconcussive symptoms, self-limited and persistent at 3 months after injury, ranges from approximately 25% to 85%. Well-controlled research data are not available on optimal pharmacological management or rehabilitation strategies for post-TBI neuropsychiatric and cognitive difficulties. Limited evidence supports the effectiveness of methylphenidate for enhancing attention, processing speed, and memory function. Other medications—such as D-amphetamine, amantadine, donepezil, levodopa, and bromocriptine—may also have some benefit for treating symptoms that include attentional difficulties, cognitive slowing, poor initiation, aspects of poor memory, fatigue, or motor deficits. Cognitive rehabilitation may be helpful for management of attention and executive difficulties as well as improving communication skills (Cicerone et al., 2009). Evidence-based reviews generally support holistic rehabilitation programs that support community reintegration, awareness of deficits, regulation of behavior and affect, improved physical and social function, and effective communication (Cernich et al., 2010). Psychiatric disorders occur at high rates in TBI patients, with criteria for axis I disorders (as defined by the DSM-IV-TR) being met in 50%–80% of patients in a community sample of patients with a mixed level of severity. The experience of a concussion or mild TBI event has also been connected with a twofold increased risk of suicide (Fralick et al., 2019). Personality disorders were identified in 25%–65% of patients (Price, 2004; Warriner and Velikonja, 2006). Major psychiatric disorders included mood and anxiety disorders, schizophrenia, and other psychoses; personality disorders included major personality disorders and other maladaptive personality traits. Psychiatric symptoms have been observed to occur immediately after injury up to decades later. It is likely that a complex interplay of factors results in the particular cognitive and psychiatric manifestations in a given individual. These factors include the nature and severity of the neurological injury, premorbid personality and cognition, preexisting psychiatric illness, substance abuse history, family psychiatric history, educational level, occupational status, coping strategies, age at injury, stressors, support systems, and the possibility of psychological or financial gains.

Post-TBI depression occurs in up to 60% of patients, with comorbid anxiety and aggressive behavior being common. Both right and left hemispheric lesions have been implicated. SSRIs are most commonly prescribed and may be helpful for management of depression, irritability, agitation, and aggression. CBT may decrease depression, anxiety, and anger and improve problem-solving skills (Silver et al., 2009). TBI-associated hypomania and mania have also been observed, although at much lower frequencies. Psychosis in association with TBI has a reported incidence ranging from 0.7% to 20%. Reliable incidence and prevalence information is unavailable. An increased risk of developing chronic psychosis has been observed in individuals suffering severe diffuse brain injury involving the temporal and frontal lobes. Patients undergoing evaluation for potential TBI-related psychosis must be carefully distinguished from those with preexisting psychotic symptoms and schizophrenia. The mean delay to the onset of psychotic symptoms after injury has been reported to be about 4 years (Guerreiro et al., 2009). The latency of the injury to the onset of symptoms has been reported to range from 2 days to 48 years. Delusions occur in more than 75%, and hallucinations occur in almost 50% of patients. Approximately 70% of affected individuals were noted to have abnormal findings on EEG. Neuropsychological testing demonstrated abnormalities in almost 90%. Psychosis in the majority of patients eventually improves with antipsychotics.

## Depression-Related Cognitive Impairment

*Depression-related cognitive impairment* (DRCI) refers to the complex pattern of cognitive impairment seen in association with affective disorders such as major depression. Notably the DLPFC, ACC, related subcortical connections, and the hippocampus have been implicated in both cognitive and mood functions. Several factors are thought to be helpful in distinguishing DRCI from dementia. Patients with DRCI tend to complain of memory and concentration problems, whereas demented patients often deny (or underreport) that problems exist despite impairment that is obvious to their family members. The distinction between dementia and DRCI is often difficult to achieve because of the increased comorbidity of affective disorders in MCI and dementias. More recent research has added considerable complexity to the considerations involved in evaluating persons with DRCI. It is widely accepted that during an episode of MDD, patients can show deficits on neuropsychological testing in several domains including selective and sustained attention, alertness as assessed by reaction time tasks, memory, verbal and nonverbal learning, problem solving, planning, and monitoring. Recent data suggest that some deficits, particularly attentional and executive dysfunctions, do not remit in a subset of patients and may increase with recurrent episodes of depression or as the MDD proceeds.

The neuropsychology of late-life depression is poorly understood and may have some different considerations than its counterpart earlier in life. Impairments on measures of word generation, visuoconstruction, short-term memory, visual memory, executive functioning, and psychomotor and information-processing speed have been reported. Successful treatment of depression results in improvement of cognitive performance yet not necessarily to premorbid levels, particularly in memory and executive domains. A growing body of evidence suggests that late-life depression associated with cognitive dysfunction is due to deficits in frontosubcortical networks. Neuroimaging findings suggest a relationship among late-onset depression, executive dysfunction, and white matter hyperintensities, particularly in the frontal lobe deep white matter and caudate nucleus. Neuropsychological impairments in patients with major depressive symptoms predict a less favorable outcome with antidepressant therapy and CBT. Furthermore, late-life depression refractory to initial treatments should prompt an additional workup for cerebrovascular or neurodegenerative conditions as potential underlying mechanisms of treatment-resistant depression.

Converging evidence suggests that late-onset depressive symptoms may be both a prodrome of and an independent risk factor for cognitive decline as seen in AD and vascular dementia (Saczynski et al., 2010). Late-onset depression is also a risk factor for MCI (Dotson et al., 2010). Four possible mechanisms may underlie the association between depression and dementia/MCI. First, depression may cause cognitive impairment. For example, depression produces excessive release of glucocorticoids, which may lead to hippocampal damage. Second, depression may be an emotional reaction on the part of the patient to the onset of dementia. Third, an underlying neurodegenerative process may cause both the depression and the dementia. Fourth, there may be a synergistic interaction between depression and a neurodegenerative process that produces dementia, given that depression is a risk factor for the later-life development of dementia (Byers et al., 2011). Although a causal relationship between depression and dementia is speculative at this time, future studies may distinguish between these four possible mechanisms (Geda, 2010).

## Delirium

Delirium, acute confusional state, or encephalopathy is considered to be a subacute- to acute-onset disorder of attentional mechanisms that subsequently affects all other aspects of cognition. Three primary features include disturbance of vigilance, inability to maintain a coherent stream of thought, and difficulty or inability to carry out goal-directed movements. Disturbances in vigilance and behavior may manifest as hyperalertness, agitation, lethargy, or fluctuations in arousal. An impaired sleep/wake cycle is often seen and may be a presenting symptom. Other manifestations may include mild anomia, slurred speech, dysgraphia, dyscalculia, constructional deficits, perceptual distortions leading to illusions and hallucinations (which may be florid and frequently visual), tremor, myoclonus, asterixis, or gait imbalance. Delirium represents one of the most common causes of acute neuropsychiatric disturbances in the hospital setting and is often multifactorial in nature. Advanced age is an independent risk factor for its development, as are metabolic derangements, infections, medications, withdrawal syndromes, toxic exposures, major surgeries, head trauma, other CNS disease, and sensory deprivation (especially impaired eyesight). Focal damage to the following regions may also be associated with a confusional state: unilateral or bilateral fusiform gyri and lingual gyri, nondominant posteroparietal regions, and inferior prefrontal regions. A common comorbidity of delirium is underlying dementia that may or may not have been diagnosed previously. In these patients, return to their predelirium cognitive state may be prolonged or incomplete despite elimination of the offending factor or factors. The EEG findings are almost always abnormal, with changes paralleling the degree of behavioral impairment. Early EEG changes show slowing of α rhythms, which may be succeeded by further slowing described as medium- to high-voltage generalized activity in the theta-δ range. Triphasic waves may be seen in a number of conditions that commonly include hepatic and renal encephalopathy. Fast rhythms superimposed on slow activity are characteristic of sedative-hypnotic drug ingestion. The EEG is an indispensable tool for diagnosing nonconvulsive status epilepticus causing acute confusional states. Resolution of delirium is reflected by a reversal of these changes, although resolution may lag behind recovery, particularly in the elderly.

## Catatonia

Catatonia, once felt to be rare, has been reported to occur among psychiatric inpatients with a prevalence ranging from 7% to 30%. Up to 20% of catatonia in psychiatric inpatients is associated with mania, and 5%–15% is associated with schizophrenia. In general, catatonia is characterized by motor abnormalities that occur in association with changes in thought, mood, and vigilance. The specific manifestations vary and commonly include mutism, stupor, stereotypies, mannerisms, diminished motor function (including waxy flexibility or rigidity), staring, negativism, automatic obedience, echopraxia, and echolalia. *Stereotypies* are purposeless repetitions of sounds, words, phrases, or movements. Unexplained foreign accents, whispered or robotic speech, and tiptoe walking have also been observed. There are two principal forms of catatonia: a hypokinetic retarded-stuporous variety and a hyperkinetic excited-delirious variety. Patients with the excited form can present with impulsive or combative behavior that may be difficult to distinguish from mania. If untreated, catatonia may progress to a malignant state marked by fever, hyperexcitability, and autonomic instability, which after several days can be followed by exhaustion, dehydration, coma, cardiac arrest, and death. An overlap between malignant catatonia and the neuroleptic malignant syndrome has also been also described. Although many patients with catatonia have an underlying affective (most often mania) or psychotic disorder, some 10%–20% have significant medical or neurological conditions that contribute to their catatonic state. Stroke, demyelinating disease, encephalitis, head trauma, medications, and CNS malignancy are individually associated with catatonia. Medical disorders that can result in catatonia include heat stroke, autoimmune disease, uremia, hyperthyroidism, diabetic ketoacidosis, porphyria, and Cushing disease, among other conditions. Catatonia has been reported in association with the use of illicit recreational drugs, antipsychotics, and opiates as well as withdrawal from benzodiazepines and dopaminergic drugs. Important considerations in the differential diagnosis include neuroleptic malignant syndrome, serotonin syndrome, and nonconvulsive status epilepticus. Treatment with intravenous benzodiazepines, intravenous sodium amobarbital, or ECT can result in dramatic improvement. Bilateral ECT is more effective than unilateral in patients who are febrile or delirious or who do not respond to benzodiazepines (Fink and Taylor, 2009).

## TREATMENT MODALITIES

Persons with mild to moderate major depression may benefit equally from psychotherapy or medication. Severely depressed patients benefit more from antidepressant medication, alone or in combination with psychotherapy, than from psychotherapy alone. Three types of psychotherapeutic options have proven to be effective for the treatment of depression: CBT, interpersonal therapy (IPT), and problem-solving therapy (PST). The aim of CBT is to modify distorted thoughts and problematic reinforcing behaviors to yield more positive emotions. It may help to prevent relapse in patients with a history of recurrent depression. IPT requires the capacity for insight and targets conflicts and role transitions that may be contributing to depression. In PST, patients learn to cope better with specific everyday problems.

Clinicians face a wide array of antidepressant drug options (Table 10.6). The most commonly prescribed drugs are the second-generation antidepressants: SSRIs, serotonin and norepinephrine reuptake inhibitors (SNRIs), and bupropion. First-generation antidepressants (tricyclic antidepressants [TCAs] and monoamine oxidase inhibitors [MAOIs]) offer similar effectiveness but with more toxicity. Generally, TCAs are avoided because of considerable degrees of dry mouth, constipation, and dizziness; they are relatively contraindicated in patients with coronary artery disease, congestive heart failure, and arrhythmias. TCAs are also potentially fatal in overdose. MAOIs are also used infrequently, even by psychiatrists, because of the many associated dietary restrictions and the potential for hypertensive crisis. The selegiline patch (20-mg formulation) is a MAOI approved by the US Food and Drug Administration (FDA) that does not require dietary tyramine restrictions. Antidepressant selection is based on tolerability, safety, evidence of effectiveness in the patient or a first-degree relative, and cost. The goal of treatment is complete remission of symptoms and return to normal functioning. About 50% of patients achieve full remission with antidepressant therapy, whereas the other half achieve partial remission or are nonresponders. For the first episode, antidepressant treatment may take 1 to several months until remission is achieved, and medication should be continued for another 4–9 months. Some clinicians advocate treatment for at least 1 year to maintain remission for a full annual cycle of holidays and anniversaries. For patients older than 70 years who respond to an SSRI, treatment for 2 years may be considered in order to prevent recurrence. Increasing the dose of the current medication or changing medications is often necessary. For a partial response, the dose of the initial agent should be maximized as tolerated before switching to another medication or adding a second drug. When a partial response continues, the clinician can refer for psychotherapy, change antidepressants, or augment treatment with bupropion, mirtazapine, or a nontraditional agent. Compared with withdrawing one drug and initiating another, combination therapy offers faster effects and avoids withdrawal symptoms when stopping the first agent. Combinations of MAOIs and either SSRIs or TCAs are not recommended because of an increased risk for serotonin syndrome (with confusion, nausea, autonomic instability, and hyperreflexia). Although more research is needed, adding adjunctive atypical antipsychotics, psychostimulants, and thyroid hormone are other potential therapeutic options. Antipsychotics added to SSRIs for treatment-resistant depression show some benefit but also carry significant risks, so they should be used with caution and prescribed in collaboration with a psychiatrist (Shelton and Papakostas, 2008). A Cochrane review of monotherapy treatment with psychostimulants (dexamphetamine, methylphenidate, methyl amphetamine, and pemoline) for moderate to severe depression found short-term improvement in depression symptoms and fatigue (Candy et al., 2008). A second review of 19 controlled trials in adults older than 65 years supported this recommendation for methylphenidate (Hardy, 2009).

Studies are conflicting about the effectiveness of adding thyroid hormone (triiodothyronine [$T_3$] and levothyroxine [$T_4$]) to antidepressants. More research is needed before these therapies can be recommended. Augmentation with other nontraditional agents has also shown mixed results: ω-3 fatty acids added to sertraline in patients with coronary heart disease did not improve depressive outcomes (Carney et al., 2009). For seasonal depression, light therapy (6000–10,000 lux for 30–90 minutes each morning) may be helpful (Golden et al., 2005). Yoga, exercise (Cooney et al., 2013), self-help books, and relaxation therapy (Morgan and Jorm, 2008) may also be useful. Specific types of side effects are more common with particular drugs and should guide the choice of medications (see Table 10.6). Sexual side effects of SSRIs include decreased libido or interest, anorgasmia, and delayed ejaculation. To address these side effects, consider pretreatment counseling, switching to a drug with a different mechanism of action (e.g., bupropion, mirtazapine), use of planned 1-day drug holidays, or, if there are no contraindications, use of sildenafil for SSRI-associated erectile dysfunction. Switching to bupropion can reduce undesired weight gain. Agitation or excessive activation may occur with fluoxetine and warrants a switch to a different SSRI. In addition, ketamine is emerging as a rapidly effective pharmacotherapy for treatment-refractory major depression, although its study in neurologically complex patient populations has been limited to date (Bobo et al., 2016).

Treatment for schizophrenia is most successful when antipsychotic medications are combined with psychological and social supports. These supports may include CBT, vocational interventions, and the use of multidisciplinary mental health professional teams who work with the patient and caregivers inside and outside the hospital to ensure the patient's health and social care (van Os and Kapur, 2009). CBT may improve coping and reduce distress and affective symptoms associated with psychotic symptoms. Despite these interventions, about one-third of these individuals may remain symptomatic. Most antipsychotics share varying degrees of striatal $D_2$ receptor blockade. The first-generation antipsychotics (e.g., haloperidol, perphenazine, chlorpromazine) possess equivalent efficacy but differ in potency and side effects. All potentially produce hyperprolactinemia and EPS, including tardive dyskinesia (Waln and Jankovic, 2013). The second-generation antipsychotics, which also antagonize serotonin-2A receptors (e.g., clozapine, risperidone, olanzapine, quetiapine), are also known as *atypical antipsychotics*. They generally produce fewer EPS, less risk of tardive dyskinesia, and less hyperprolactinemia. eTable 10.7 lists selected antipsychotic side effects. Some atypical antipsychotics such as clozapine and olanzapine have been associated with weight gain, impairment of glucose metabolism, and dyslipidemia. Clozapine has greater efficacy than first-generation drugs but requires regular blood test monitoring throughout the course of treatment owing to

**TABLE 10.6 Medication Treatment for Depression**

| Agent, Daily Dose* | Benefits/Selected Side Effects |
|---|---|
| First-generation antidepressants | As a class: dry mouth, dizziness, nausea, sedation, anticholinergic effects, orthostatic hypotension. Contraindicated with MAOIs. Do not use with prolonged QT interval. Use with caution in patients with cardiovascular disease or predisposition to urinary retention or narrow-angle glaucoma. Follow ECGs and orthostatic blood pressure changes |
| Amitriptyline, 25–300 mg | May aid with sleep and treat neuropathic pain and migraines. Highly sedating and anticholinergic |
| Clomipramine, 25–250 mg | Possibly useful in comorbid anxiety, panic disorders, and OCD. |
| Desipramine, 25–300 mg | |
| Imipramine, 25–300 mg | |
| Nortriptyline, 25–150 | Less anticholinergic and antihistaminergic than amitriptyline and imipramine. Less prone to causing orthostatic hypotension |
| Protriptyline, 15–60 mg | |
| MAOIs | As a class: hypertensive crisis, orthostatic hypotension, insomnia, agitation, sedation, weight change, dry mouth, urinary hesitancy, and sexual dysfunction. Special dietary restrictions except for selegiline patch. Potential severe drug-drug interactions |
| Phenelzine, 45–60 mg | |
| Tranylcypromine, 30–50 mg | |
| Selegiline transdermal patch, 6–12 mg/day | |
| Second-generation antidepressants | Nausea, diarrhea, decreased appetite, nervousness, insomnia, somnolence, sweating, impaired sexual function; hyponatremia in the elderly.[†] Contraindicated with MAOIs. Potential for drug interactions with drugs metabolized in liver. Risk/benefit analysis needed in pregnancy |
| Bupropion, 100–450 mg | Norepinephrine/dopamine reuptake inhibitor. Less weight gain and fewer sexual side effects than other agents. Lowers seizure threshold. Relatively contraindicated in patients with history of seizures, family history of seizures, or head trauma |
| Citalopram, 10–40 mg | SSRI |
| Escitalopram, 5–20 mg | SSRI; similar to citalopram |
| Fluoxetine, 20–60 mg | SSRI; long half-life mitigates effects of missed doses. Withdrawal symptoms rare. Potent 2D6 inhibitor, raising concern for drug-drug interactions |
| Paroxetine, 5–40 mg (5–40 mg) | SSRI; more weight gain and sexual adverse events. Withdrawal syndrome not uncommon. High anticholinergic side-effect profile. Potent 2D6 inhibitor, raising concern for drug-drug interactions |
| Sertraline, 50–200 mg | SSRI |
| Trazodone, 50–400 mg | SRA/A; less effective as antidepressant in doses <300 mg. Somnolence, rare priapism in young men. Useful in low doses (50–100 mg) as a sleeping aid |
| Duloxetine, 30–120 mg | SNRI; may be effective in major depression, generalized anxiety disorder, chronic pain disorders[‡] |
| Venlafaxine, 37.5–225 mg | SNRI; higher incidence of nausea, vomiting, dry mouth, sexual side effects, and hypertension. Occasional hypertensive urgencies |
| Desvenlafaxine, 50–400 mg | SNRI |
| Mirtazapine, 7.5–45 mg | ARA; In addition to depression/anxiety efficacy, may be useful in older adults to increase appetite and improve sleep. Use caution with renal impairment. Avoid concomitant benzodiazepines and alcohol |
| Vilazodone, 10–40 mg | Selective serotonin reuptake inhibitor/5-$HT_{1A}$ receptor partial agonist |
| Vortioxetine, 10–20 mg | SSRI; serotonin 5-$HT_{1A}$ receptor agonist; serotonin 5-$HT_3$ receptor antagonist |
| Levomilnacipran, 20–120 mg | Serotonin/norepinephrine reuptake inhibitor |

*Dose range for geriatric patients is in parentheses.

*ARA*, $\alpha_2$-receptor antagonist; *ECG*, electrocardiogram; *MAOI*, monoamine oxidase inhibitor; *OCD*, obsessive-compulsive disorder; *SNRI*, serotonin and norepinephrine reuptake inhibitor; *SRA/A*, serotonin receptor antagonists/agonists; *SSRI*, selective serotonin reuptake inhibitor.

[†]*Wright, S.K., Schroeter, S., 2008. Hyponatremia as a complication of selective serotonin reuptake inhibitors. Journal of the American Association of Nurse Practitioners 20, 47–51.*

[‡]*Kroenke, K., Krebs, E.E., Bair, M.J., 2009. Pharmacotherapy of chronic pain: a synthesis of recommendations from systematic reviews. General Hospital Psychiatry 31, 206–19.*

an increased risk for agranulocytosis (1%–4%). Risperidone is known for its association with hyperprolactinemia. The primary symptom targets for antipsychotics are positive psychotic symptoms, agitation, and negative symptoms (e.g., apathy, social withdrawal, diminished affect). Response times for psychotic symptoms may range from responding within hours of administration to several weeks of administration. Maximal response may require months. Some patients are nonresponders. Agitation responds well to most antipsychotics, but negative symptoms generally respond only modestly.

## Electroconvulsive Therapy

MDD is the most common indication for ECT. The mechanisms by which this procedure alleviates depressive symptoms are not fully understood. Remission rates of 70%–90% have been reported in clinical trials of ECT for MDD (Popeo, 2009). It is also an effective treatment for bipolar disorder but may uncommonly precipitate hypomania or mania. Suicidal thoughts respond favorably to ECT and are an indication for early transition from drug therapy. ECT is not routinely used for the treatment of schizophrenia. When combined with antipsychotic medications, however, it may result in improvement in 80% of patients with drug-resistant chronic schizophrenia. Patients with mania also respond favorably to ECT. There are few absolute contraindications to ECT, but cardiac conditions may worsen and should be addressed. Conditions such as vascular aneurysms and aortic stenosis should preferably be repaired prior to ECT, but persons with such conditions have been reported to tolerate the procedure. Those with properly functioning cardiac pacemakers generally tolerate ECT well. Case reports of ECT performed on individuals with a recent cerebral infarction suggest a low complication rate and a favorable response to treatment. ECT has been successfully used in persons with mental retardation, MS, HD, arteriovenous malformations, and hydrocephalus (Ducharme et al., 2015). Patients with depression and PD may experience improvement of mood and motor symptoms with ECT. Some research supports the effectiveness of ECT for treatment of the core motor symptoms of PD (Popeo and Kellner, 2009). There is no evidence of structural brain damage due to ECT. Posttreatment memory difficulty (anterograde amnesia) is usually experienced during the course of ECT treatments but normally resolves within 1 month after the last treatment. Retrograde amnesia is more prominent for the events closer to the time of ECT treatment. Posttreatment confusion is variable and may be associated with bilateral electrode placement, high stimulus intensity, prolonged seizure activity, and inadequate oxygenation. There is controversy about whether unilateral electrode placement for ECT is as effective as bilateral placement. Several studies have shown equal efficacy as long as unilateral ECT is performed with a stimulus intensity well above seizure threshold (Lisanby, 2007). Studies also indicate a lower incidence of cognitive side effects with right unilateral electrode placement and electrical brief pulse waveform stimulus. There is uncertainty about the efficacy of ultrabrief pulse stimulus, but preliminary evidence suggests that it is associated with a significant reduction in memory-related side effects (Peterchev et al., 2010).

## Vagus Nerve Stimulation

The FDA approved vagus nerve stimulation (VNS) for TRD in July 2005 (Rush et al., 2000; Wani et al., 2013). Consensus criteria are unavailable for what constitutes TRD. Interest in VNS as a treatment for depression arose when it was noticed that persons being treated with VNS for treatment-resistant epilepsy (which is associated with an increased prevalence of depression) experienced improvements in their mood. Long-term studies of VNS for use as an adjunct to medications and therapy showed that it was well tolerated and resulted in a successful response in half of the patients and complete remission in one-third (Andrade et al., 2010). The mechanism of VNS's effects is not completely understood. It is believed that input information from the vagus nerve projects to the solitary tract nucleus and follows an ascending pathway to modulate various structures such as the amygdala, dorsal raphe, locus coeruleus, and the ventromedial prefrontal cortex that produce its effects on mood. The solitary tract nucleus also communicates with the parabrachial nucleus (PBN), cerebellum, and periaquaductal gray matter. The PBN communicates with other regions implicated in the pathophysiology of depression such as the hypothalamus, thalamus, amygdala, and nucleus of the stria terminalis. Only the left vagus nerve is used for VNS, because the right vagus nerve has parasympathetic branches to the heart. Aside from standard surgical risks, the most common side effects are voice alteration (54%–60% of patients), cough, neck pain, paresthesia, and dyspnea. These side effects typically decrease over time. It is recommended that VNS be used as an adjunctive treatment to medications and psychotherapy. Right unilateral ECT has been well tolerated by persons with VNS (Sharma et al., 2009).

## Repetitive Transcranial Magnetic Stimulation

Repetitive transcranial magnetic stimulation (rTMS) is an emerging, FDA-approved, noninvasive, well-tolerated treatment modality for MDD in adults (Perera et al., 2016). It is being studied for potential therapeutic applications in OCD, posttraumatic stress disorder, and auditory hallucinations in schizophrenia. The rTMS procedure uses a pulsed magnetic field introduced on the scalp surface to generate focal electrical stimulation of the cortical surface; it does not require anesthesia, does not produce a seizure, and can be administered in the office setting. The rTMS field can be pulsed at different frequencies to produce excitatory or inhibitory effects on cortical neurons. Frequencies of less than or equal to 1 Hz (slow rTMS) are believed to have mostly inhibitory neuronal effects by means of preferentially activating GABA-ergic interneurons in the cortex; this may result in transsynaptic depression. Use of rTMS frequencies greater than 1 Hz (fast rTMS) is believed to have mostly glutamatergic or excitatory neuronal effects (Kim et al., 2009). In depression, the target area is the left DLPFC. Left DLPFC high-frequency rTMS has shown effectiveness in almost one-third of pharmacotherapy-resistant MDD patients (Andrade et al., 2010). Although the mechanism of action for rTMS treatment of depression is not fully understood, emerging evidence suggests that one may be transsynaptic modulation of subgenual ACC activity through DLPFC stimulation (Fox et al., 2012; Weigand et al., 2018). Headaches and site application pain are the most common side effects; the risk for seizure is estimated at less than 1 per 10,000 rTMS sessions. Monotherapy with rTMS is associated with few adverse effects but significant antidepressant effects for patients with unipolar depression who do not respond to medications or cannot tolerate them (George et al., 2010).

## Psychiatric Neurosurgery or Psychosurgery

Neurosurgical procedures are not commonly used for treatment of neuropsychiatric symptoms but should be considered for selected conditions when patients have failed combined multiple, adequate trials of pharmacotherapy and psychotherapy (Ducharme et al., 2018). Psychosurgery, both ablative and by deep brain stimulation, is still experimental and should be performed at institutions that support psychosurgery research and also have multidisciplinary involvement and appropriate follow-up. In the middle of the twentieth century, procedures such as frontal lobotomy were performed without defined indications or an understanding of the limbic system. This resulted in severe adverse events, even death. During the latter half of the twentieth century, smaller stereotactically targeted lesions were used, resulting in benefits for patients, useful research data, and a precipitous decline in adverse events. Currently used ablative procedures include anterior cingulotomy, subcaudate tractotomy, limbic leucotomy (combined anterior cingulotomy and subcaudate tractotomy), and anterior capsulotomy. Carefully selected patients with intractable mood and anxiety disorders have experienced response rates ranging from 30% to 70%. Postoperative side effects are mostly transient and include headache, nausea, and edema. More serious adverse events include infection, urinary dysfunction, seizures, cognitive deficits, and cerebral infarct or hemorrhage (Andrade et al., 2010).

*Deep brain stimulation* involves the placement of electrodes into targeted deep brain regions so that electrical stimulation can be delivered. Its advantages over ablative procedures are its adjustability (by manipulation of stimulation parameters) and reversibility. Published brain targets include the subcallosal cingulate gyrus (Hamani et al., 2009; Holtzheimer et al., 2012), nucleus accumbens, ventral internal capsule/ventral striatum, inferior thalamic peduncle, and lateral habenula. Early-phase deep brain stimulation response rates for MDD ranged from 40% to 70% (Morishita et al., 2014); however, results of a multicenter clinical trial were modest and FDA approval for deep brain stimulation in treatment-refractory major depression has not yet been secured (Bari et al., 2018). Targets for OCD include the anterior limb of the internal capsule, ventral striatum, nucleus accumbens, or subthalamic nucleus (Denys et al., 2010). Transient hypomania may occur with deep brain stimulation for OCD. Response rates for OCD range from 20% to 75% (Haynes and Mallet, 2010). Upward of nine brain regions have been targeted for treatment of Gilles de la Tourette syndrome, which in most cases results in some diminution of tics (Hariz and Robertson, 2010; Porta et al., 2009). The effects on other neuropsychiatric comorbidities are uncertain.

## TREATMENT PRINCIPLES

The unique features of each condition discussed should be carefully taken into account when a treatment plan is being developed. Transient, progressive, or static impairments in abilities such as driving, medical decision making, and management of finances may be present. Increased vigilance when patients are being monitored for these impairments may improve care and allow for earlier interventions to protect the welfare of the patients, their families, and society. Patients with underlying neurological conditions tend to be more likely to react adversely to psychotropic medications, particularly with regard to extrapyramidal and cognitive side effects. These adverse reactions tend to be minimized with initiation of medications at low doses and the use of gentle titration. When clinically indicated, atypical antipsychotics are often preferred over typical agents because of their fewer adverse side effects, but longitudinal studies are needed to better confirm this impression (Lieberman et al., 2005; Tarsy et al., 2011). Further options to consider for treatment of refractory primary depression and other carefully selected psychiatric conditions include ECT, VNS, transcranial magnetic stimulation, deep brain stimulation, or stereotactic ablative surgery (Cook et al., 2014; Dougherty and Rauch, 2007; Wani et al., 2013). There is currently little evidence to guide the optimal treatment approach for patients with neurological disease and comorbid psychiatric symptoms.

In conclusion, advances in clinical neuroscience have improved our understanding of the neural substrates of cognition, perception, and emotional behavior. The traditional boundaries between neurology and psychiatry have become obsolete, and there is a continued need to bridge the divide across the clinical neurosciences (Fig. 10.4). The future of neurological and psychiatric care, training, and research will inevitably require effective collaboration between both disciplines (Cunningham et al., 2006; Perez et al., 2018; Price et al., 2000).

*The complete reference list is available online at https://expertconsult.inkling.com/.* 

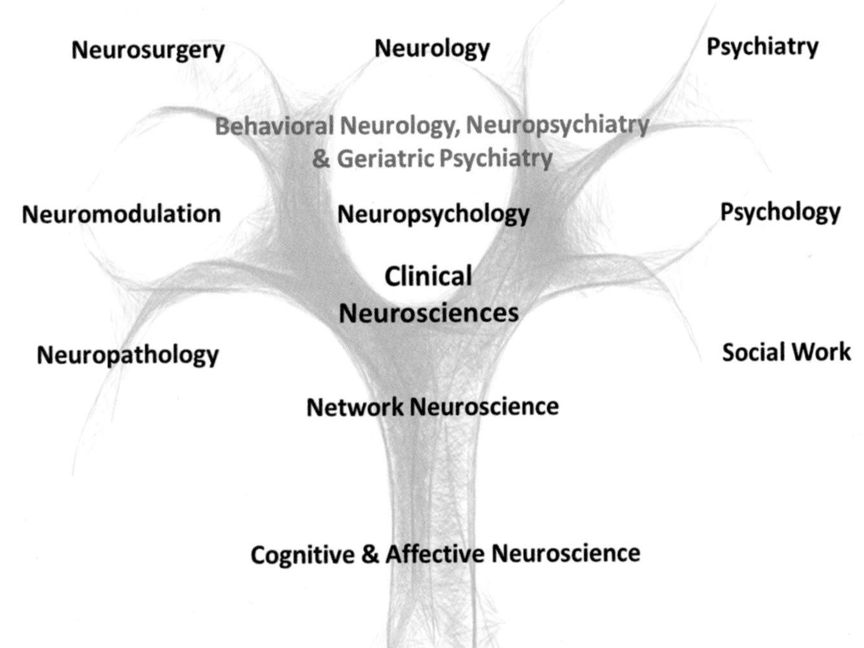


**Fig. 10.4** An integrated clinical neuroscience approach for the assessment, management, and investigation of patients with neuropsychiatrically complex brain disorders. Adapted from Perez et al., (2018).

# 11

# Limb Apraxias and Related Disorders

*Mario F. Mendez, Leila Parand*

## OUTLINE



*Apraxia* is an inability to correctly perform learned skilled movements. In limb apraxias, there is an inability to correctly execute these movements in an arm or hand owing to neurological dysfunction. Apraxia is essentially a cognitive deficit in motor programming and results in errors either of the spatiotemporal processing of the movements or in the content of the actions. During the course of an apraxia examination, these errors can help distinguish the major types of limb apraxias.

A first step in recognizing the limb apraxias is distinguishing them from other causes of impaired movement. First, apraxia is distinct from elementary motor deficits such as weakness, hemiparesis, spasticity, ataxia, or extrapyramidal disturbances. Second, apraxia is distinguishable from impaired movements due to primary sensory deficits, hemispatial neglect, spatial or object agnosia, or other sensory or spatial disorders. Third, apraxia is distinct from abnormal movements or postures such as tremor, myoclonus, choreoathetosis, or dystonic posturing. Finally, it is not apraxia if the impaired movements result from other cognitive disorders involving attention, memory, language comprehension, or executive functions (Leiguarda and Marsden, 2000).

Limb apraxia is not rare or insignificant. Apraxia occurs in about 50%–80% of patients with left hemisphere lesions and can persist as a chronic deficit in 40%–50% of these. It occurs in a variety of disorders, including stroke (Donkervoort et al., 2000), multiple sclerosis (Kamm et al., 2012, Rapaić et al., 2014), tumors such as parietal gliomas (Liouta et al., 2018), corticobasal syndrome (Armstrong et al., 2013), Alzheimer disease (Stamenova et al., 2014), some forms of primary progressive aphasia (Adeli et al., 2013), Parkinson disease, dementia with Lewy bodies (Nagahama et al., 2015), Huntington disease (Zadikoff and Lang, 2005), Creutzfeldt-Jakob disease (Gonzales and Soble, 2017), and even some patients with schizophrenia (Dutschke et al., 2018, Stegmayer et al., 2016). A careful examination for limb apraxia can lead to the differentiation of diseases such as Alzheimer disease from frontotemporal dementia, or dementia with Lewy bodies from other disorders (Ahmed et al., 2016; Nagahama et al., 2015).

Limb apraxia often results in major functional impairment, even when subtle, as it affects critical movements of the arms, hands, and fingers. Limb apraxia correlates with greater caregiver dependence and need for help with activities of daily living (ADLs) (Smania et al., 2006), and it can also interfere with rehabilitation therapy and the use of gestural communication.

Despite its importance, clinicians often fail to recognize limb apraxia. In many left hemisphere strokes, right hemiparesis masks the presence of right limb apraxia, and the assumption of normal clumsiness of the nondominant hand may mask the presence of left limb apraxia. Patients with limb apraxia from left hemisphere strokes can have a reduced awareness of limb apraxia (Kusch et al., 2018), making recovery more difficult. Even when there are no masking factors, the presence of limb apraxia may still go undetected. Many examiners do not evaluate patients for limb apraxia, do not know how to test for apraxia, or cannot recognize the spatiotemporal or content errors produced by this condition.

This chapter is about the limb apraxias. The term *apraxia* occurs broadly in neurology and is usually interchangeable with *dyspraxia*. Clinicians use apraxia to describe nonlearned motor dysfunctions including oculomotor movements, gait initiation (magnetic apraxia), and eyelid opening. They also use *apraxia* to describe skilled motor tasks that are dependent on visuospatial processing, including optic, constructional, and dressing apraxia. *Apraxia* correctly applies to conditions that are more clearly consistent with the definition of disturbances in learned skilled movements but involve body parts other than the limbs, including oro-buccal-facial and speech apraxias. These clinical entities are not included in this chapter, because they are either not limb apraxias or not true disorders of "praxis" in the sense of disturbances in learned skilled movements (Zadikoff and Lang, 2005). The focus of this chapter is on the seven major limb apraxias of the upper extremities. They include ideomotor apraxia, parietal variant; ideomotor apraxia, disconnection variant; dissociation apraxia; ideational apraxia; and conceptual apraxia. Also included is limb-kinetic apraxia, a disorder that some argue is not a true apraxia, but instead a more basic disturbance in fine motor movements. Callosal apraxias comprise a separate category because of their unique unilateral and varied manifestations.

## HISTORICAL PERSPECTIVE

Many clinicians and investigators helped develop the current concept of limb apraxia. In 1866, John Hughlings Jackson probably recognized limb apraxia when he observed that the patient had "power in his muscles and in the centres for coordination of muscular groups, but he—the whole man, or the 'will'—cannot set them agoing" (Pearce, 2009). In 1870, Carl Maria Finkelnburg used "asymbolia" to describe the clumsy and incomprehensible communicative gestures in aphasics, and in 1890, Meynert distinguished motor asymbolia from decreased motor "images" for movement. In 1899, D. De Buck used "parakinesia" to describe a patient who "though retaining the concepts for her actions, did not succeed in awakening the corresponding kinetic image." By this time, the stage was set for Hugo Karl Liepmann's seminal model of the limb apraxias.

In the early 1900s, Liepmann published a series of papers that led to the contemporary concept of limb apraxias. He proposed that the execution of purposeful movements could be divided into three steps (Goldenberg, 2003). First is the retrieval of the spatial and temporal representation or "movement formulas" of the intended action from the left hemisphere. Second is the transfer and association of these movement formulas via cortical connections with the "innervatory patterns" or motor programs located in the left "sensomotorium" (which includes premotor and supplementary motor areas [SMAs]). Third is the transmission of the information to the left primary motor cortex for performance of the intended actions in the right limb. Finally, in order for the left limb to perform the movements, the information traverses the corpus callosum to the right sensomotorium to activate the right primary motor cortex. Using Heymann Steinthal's term of "apraxia," Liepmann classified disturbances in these connections as "ideational, ideo-kinetic (melokinetic), and limb-kinetic apraxia." Over the years, this classification nomenclature has evolved and the application of these terms has shifted, but Liepmann's basic formulation of apraxia has persisted to the present day.

## A MODEL FOR PRAXIS

Models of apraxia emerge from this historical perspective. Most models of praxis include a left parietal hub with connections to anterior motor areas with a central role of learning and converting mental images of intended action into motor execution (Heilman and Rothi, 2012) (Fig. 11.1). These spatiotemporal movement formulas, also known as praxicons or visuokinesthetic motor engrams, are necessary for learned skilled movements. Multiple input modalities including visual, verbal-auditory, and tactile can activate these movement formulas. Cells in the inferior parietal lobule fire selectively in response to hand movements, visually presented information about object size and shape, or the actual manipulation of objects, and functional neuroimaging studies show activity of this region in response to recognition of actions associated with object or tool use (transitive actions) (Damasio et al., 2001). Functional neuroimaging studies have also shown activity in left parietal sub-regions with privileged connectivity to premotor and sensory areas (Garcea and Mahon, 2014). In addition to movement formulas, the left parietal region appears to contain action semantics and conceptual systems such as tool action, tool–object association

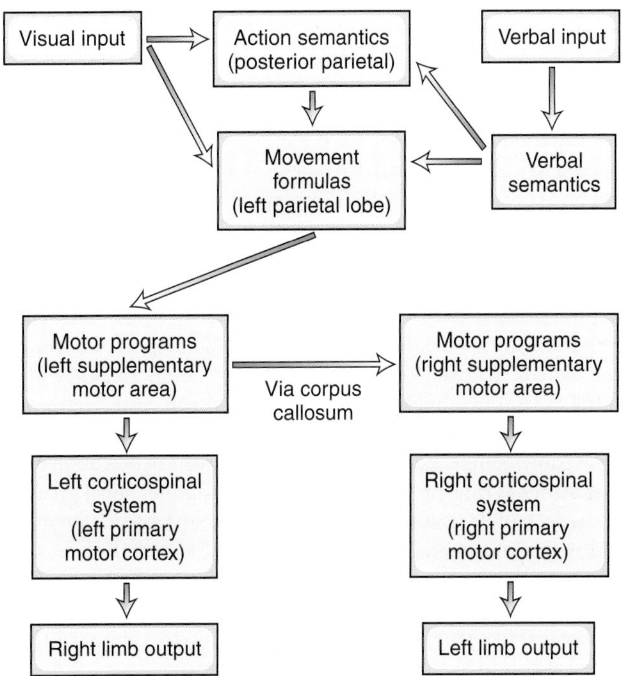


**Fig. 11.1** A Model of Praxis.

information, and general principles of tool use (Goldenberg and Spatt, 2009; Ochipa et al., 1992).

If a movement involves the use of a tool or object, action semantics specify knowledge of tool action (turning, pounding, etc.) and the knowledge of which tool or object to use for a task (Leiguarda and Marsden, 2000).

Beyond movement formulas and action semantics, a third important element of models of praxis is the motor programs themselves. In the premotor region, the SMA translates the movement formulas into motor programs before sending them on to primary motor cortex (Roy and Square, 1985). The SMA, which is involved in sequential movements and bimanual coordination of the upper extremities, receives projections from parietal neurons and in turn projects axons to motor neurons in the primary motor cortex. The SMA translates the parietal time-space movement formulas to specific motor programs that activate the motor neurons such that the contralateral extremity moves in the proscribed spatial trajectory and timing. For movements in the ipsilateral extremity, the brain further conveys these programs across the corpus callosum to the opposite premotor cortex.

Beyond this traditional model for praxis, apraxia may result from damage in other regions including the prefrontal cortex, right hemisphere, basal ganglia (putamen and globus pallidus), thalamus, and their white-matter connections.

The prefrontal region participates in sequencing multiple arm, hand, and finger movements. Functional magnetic resonance imaging studies suggest that proximal limb control representations are associated with bilateral inferior frontal gyri for both limbs, while distal limb control areas generally left lateralized for both limbs (Mäki-Marttunen et al., 2014). Both parietal regions participate in the integration of visual information and upper-extremity movement, and in performing nonpurposeful movements—a necessary aspect for learning new purposeful movements. Although the left inferior parietal lobule is more active than the right during action imagery and actual discrimination of nonpurposeful gestures, the right parietal region is more active during imitation and when these gestures consist of finger postures (Buccino et al., 2001; Hermsdorfer et al., 2001).

The role of basal ganglia and thalamus is less clear, but they function as part of cortical–subcortical motor loops. Apraxia could, theoretically, result from damage to any of these areas outside the traditional model of praxis.

Newer models of praxis have focused on network activation as opposed to isolated regional activation. The posterior left parietal and temporal cortices as well as the dorsolateral prefrontal cortex are activated when hand gestures are planned and executed. This left parieto-fronto-temporal network, or "praxis representation network" (Króliczak and Frey, 2009; Roy et al., 2014), includes two main streams: a ventral stream that processes semantic knowledge (the "what" pathway) and a dorsal stream that processes spatiotemporal information (the "where" pathway) (Brandi et al., 2014). Abnormalities of the ventral stream may impair action semantics such as the retrieval of tool-action concepts (Hoeren et al., 2014), and abnormalities of the dorsal pathway may result in spatiotemporal errors in executing movement formulas (Martin et al., 2017). The left supramarginal gyrus and left caudal middle temporal gyrus contribute to the integration of concepts with motor representations into actions (Króliczak et al., 2016). Consistent with a left parieto-fronto-temporal network, damage in the inferior frontal cortex reaching to the temporal pole is associated with an increased frequency of Body-Part-as-Object errors on praxis testing (Finkel et al., 2018).

This left parieto-fronto-temporal praxis network significantly overlaps with the mirror neuron network for understanding the intentional actions of others (Cattaneo, 2009). Left hemisphere stroke patients with apraxia with deficits in gesture comprehension have had lesions in more anterior parts of the mirror neuron system, whereas those with gesture imitation deficits have had lesions in more posterior parts (Binder et al., 2017).

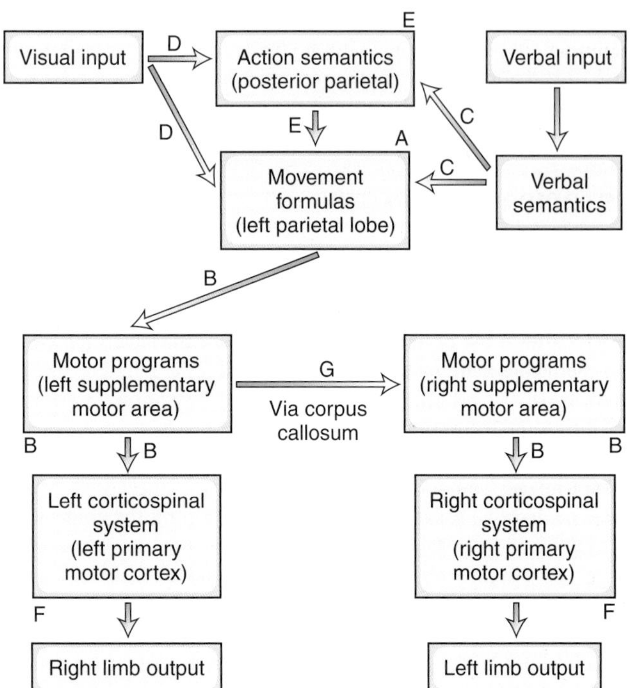


**Fig. 11.2 Lesions in Limb Apraxias.** Praxis disturbances can result from various brain localizations as illustrated here. **A**, Ideomotor apraxia, parietal variant. **B**, Ideomotor apraxia, disconnection variant. **C**, Verbal dissociation apraxia. **D**, Visual dissociation apraxia. **E**, Conceptual apraxia. **F**, Limb-kinetic apraxia. **G**, Callosal apraxia.

## CLASSIFICATION OF LIMB APRAXIAS

Beginning with Liepmann, there have been multiple attempts to classify and define the limb apraxias (Hanna-Pladdy and Rothi, 2001). The classification presented here is based on the seminal work of Heilman and associates, who have significantly contributed to the understanding of the limb apraxias (Heilman and Rothi, 2012). Depending on the location of the lesion, the patient has different patterns of ability to imitate and recognize gestures, perform sequential movements, and do fine motor activities (Fig. 11.2). The presence of production and content errors further characterizes the subtypes of limb apraxia.

### Ideomotor Apraxia, Parietal Variant

The parietal variant of ideomotor apraxia may be the most common and prototypical limb apraxia. Disruption of the movement formulas in the inferior parietal lobule impairs skilled movements on command and to imitation, as well as the recognition of gestures (see Fig. 11.2, A). Patients make spatial and temporal errors while producing movements. There is a failure to adopt the correct posture or orientation of the arm and hand or to move the limb correctly in space and at the correct speeds. Spatial errors involve the configuration of the hand and fingers, the proper orientation of the limb to the tool or object, and the spatial trajectory of the motion. A major distinguishing feature of the parietal variant of ideomotor apraxia is difficulty recognizing or identifying gestures, implicating damage to the praxicons, visuokinesthetic motor engrams, or movement formulas themselves.

### Ideomotor Apraxia, Disconnection Variant

This form of ideomotor apraxia is a disconnection of an intact parietal region from the pathways to primary motor cortices. The disconnection variant of ideomotor apraxia results from disruptions of motor programs in the SMA or in their intra- and interhemispheric connections (Heilman and Watson, 2008). These lesions result in impaired pantomime to verbal commands, impaired imitation of gestures, and the presence of spatiotemporal production errors. The movement formulas themselves are preserved and, in contrast to the parietal variant of ideomotor apraxia, these patients can recognize and identify gestures. The lesions lie along the route from the left inferior parietal cortex to primary motor cortices (see Fig. 11.2, B). Although SMA lesions tend to affect both upper extremities, if the SMA lesion is limited to the right, apraxia may be limited to the left upper extremity.

### Dissociation Apraxia

Patients with dissociation apraxia only exhibit errors when the movement is evoked by stimuli in one specific modality, usually the verbal or language modality. Dissociation apraxia is usually a specific disconnection between language areas and movement formulas in the inferior parietal lobule. However, information can reach the inferior parietal lobe via input modalities other than language. Patients with dissociation apraxia may be impaired when attempting to perform skilled movements in response to verbal commands, but they are able to imitate gestures and to indicate or use actual objects correctly. An important distinguishing feature of dissociation apraxia is errors that are often unrecognizable movements, rather than the spatiotemporal or content errors of other apraxia syndromes. In addition to verbal dissociation apraxia (see Fig. 11.2, C), there can be visual (see Fig. 11.2, D) and tactile dissociation apraxias as well.

### Ideational Apraxia

Ideational apraxia is the inability to correctly order or sequence a series of movements to achieve a goal. It is a disturbance in an overall ideational action plan. When these patients are given components necessary to complete a multistep task, they have trouble carrying out the steps in the proper order, such as preparing, addressing, and then mailing a letter. However, the individual steps are performed accurately. The lesions responsible for ideational apraxias are not clear; the deficits usually occur in patients with diffuse cerebral processes such as dementia, delirium, or extensive lesions in the left hemisphere that involve the frontal lobe and SMA. Unfortunately, use of the term *ideational apraxia* has been confusing, with the term erroneously applied to conceptual apraxia and other disorders. Ideational apraxia is not a conceptual problem in the proper application or use of tools or objects, but rather a problem in sequencing of actions in multistep behaviors.

### Conceptual Apraxia

Conceptual apraxia results in errors in action semantics, specifically involving the content of the action, such as in tool-selection errors or in tool–object knowledge. Whereas dysfunction of praxis production results in ideomotor apraxia, defects in the conceptual knowledge needed to successfully select tools and objects results in conceptual apraxia. Although conceptual apraxia often co-occurs with ideomotor apraxia, it can occur by itself, indicating that praxis production and praxis conceptual systems are independent. Patients with conceptual apraxia are unable to name or point to a tool when its function is discussed, or recall the type of actions associated with specific tools, utensils, or objects. They make content errors in which they substitute the action associated with the wrong tool for the requested tool. For example, when asked to demonstrate the use of a hammer or a saw either by pantomiming or using the tool, the patient with the loss of tool–object action knowledge may pantomime a screwing twisting movement as if using a screwdriver. Other terms used to describe these errors include *disturbances in mechanical knowledge* or *in action semantics* (see Fig. 11.2, E). Conceptual apraxia is most common in Alzheimer disease, in other dementias (Ochipa et al., 1992), and in patients with diffuse posterior cerebral lesions, particularly involving the left hemisphere.

### Limb-Kinetic Apraxia

Limb-kinetic apraxia results from disturbed motor programs. These patients have an inability to make finely graded, precise, coordinated individual finger movements. Limb-kinetic apraxia is not an apraxia in the traditional definition, but it is prominently considered in the differential diagnosis of the limb apraxias, and, therefore, discussed here. Patients with limb-kinetic apraxia complain of a loss of dexterity or deftness that makes fine motor movements such as buttoning or tying shoes difficult. Weakness or changes in muscle tone do not account for this "clumsiness," and limb-kinetic apraxia may be intermediate between paresis and other limb apraxias. Limb-kinetic apraxia is usually confined to the limb contralateral to a hemispheric lesion; however, when limb-kinetic apraxia occurs in the preferred hand, it may also be present in the nonpreferred hand (Hanna-Pladdy et al., 2002). Clinicians need to distinguish limb-kinetic apraxia from right parietal functions such as nonsymbolic gestures (e.g., copying meaningless fine finger movements) and from optic ataxia, or decreased coordination of the hands under visual guidance. Limb-kinetic apraxia results from lesions in the left SMA, the primary motor cortex, or even in the corticospinal system (see Fig. 11.2, F) (Kubel et al., 2018). Liepmann (1920) also thought that limb-kinetic apraxia could result from lesions in the sensory motor cortex, and Kleist (1931) attributed it to damage in the premotor areas.

### Callosal Apraxia

Several limb apraxia syndromes can result from callosal lesions (see Fig. 11.2, G). What distinguishes these patients is that their apraxia is confined to the nondominant limb, usually the left arm or hand in right-handed individuals. The right limb may be affected in left-handed individuals, or they may have a similar lateralization as right-handers. Liepmann and others described left-sided disconnection-variant ideomotor apraxia due to callosal lesions and strokes (Heilman and Watson, 2008). These patients cannot pantomime with their left hand to verbal command or imitate but can recognize and identify gestures. Others described left-sided dissociative apraxia due to callosal lesions (Gazzaniga et al., 1967; Geschwind and Kaplan, 1962). Patients who have had surgical disconnection of the corpus callosum could not gesture normally to command with their left arm and hand but performed well with imitation and actual tools. Some patients have had a combination of both disconnection-variant ideomotor and dissociative apraxia of their left arm and hand manifested by unrecognizable movements on verbal command and spatiotemporal errors on imitation. There is also the possibility of developing both limb-kinetic apraxia and ideomotor apraxia in the left hand with focal mesial lesions of the corpus callosum (Acosta et al., 2014).

Other patients have a callosal "alien limb" with independent movements of the nondominant limb, sometimes with "diagonistic apraxia," or the intermanual conflict of the hands acting in opposition to each other. The classic example of this is the split-brain patient who has undergone a corpus callosotomy and finds that his or her left hand is unbuttoning his shirt or blouse while the right one is trying to button it. Finally, there is a rare description of callosal lesions resulting in conceptual apraxia, indicating that conceptual knowledge as well as movement formulas have lateralized representations, and that such representations are contralateral to the preferred hand (Heilman et al., 1997).

## TESTING FOR LIMB APRAXIAS

Apraxia testing requires a systematic approach (Box 11.1). Prior to testing of praxis, a neurological examination excludes the presence of significant motor, sensory, or cognitive disorders that could explain the inability to perform learned skilled movements. First, the testing of praxis itself begins with asking the patient to pantomime to command. The movements are transitive (associated with tool or instrument use) and intransitive (associated with communicative gestures such as waving goodbye). For transitive movements, the examiner asks patients to demonstrate how to comb their hair, brush their teeth, or use a pair of scissors. For intransitive movements, the examiner asks patients to demonstrate how to wave goodbye, beckon somebody to come, or hitchhike. The testing involves the right and left limbs independently. The examiner observes the patients' responses for the presence of temporal-spatial or content errors. Second, if patients have difficulty pantomiming movements, the examiner tests their ability to imitate gestures. For gesture imitation, the examiner performs both transitive and intransitive movements and asks the patient to copy the movements. Gesture imitation should also include meaningless, or nonrepresentational, gestures such as linking pinkies or interlocking circles made with the thumb and index finger on each hand. Disturbed meaningless gestures can signify a number of conditions including an inability to apprehend spatial relationships involving the hands and arms in parietal-variant ideomotor apraxia, a basic disturbance in idiokinetic movements, or abnormalities in spatial processing from the right parietal lobe (Goldenberg, 2013). Imitating meaningless gestures bimanually may be particularly disturbed if there is biparietal disease, such as with Alzheimer disease (Sanin and Benke, 2017).

Third, for gesture knowledge, the examiner performs the same transitive and intransitive gestures and asks the patient to identify the gesture. The patient must identify the gesture and discriminate between those that are well and those that are poorly performed.

**BOX 11.1 The Examination for Limb Apraxia**

I. DOMINANT UPPER EXTREMITY
  1. PANTOMIME TO VERBAL COMMAND
    a. Transitive actions:
      Comb hair
      Brush teeth
      Flip a coin
      Use scissors
      Use a hammer
      Use a key
      Use a screwdriver
    b. Intransitive actions:
      Wave goodbye
      Beckon someone to come
      Indicate someone to stop
      Salute
      Show how to hitchhike
      Give the peace sign
      Give the OK sign
  2. IMITATION OF GESTURES
    The examiner demonstrates the same actions without naming them and asks the patient to copy them.
    The examiner also tests the imitation of meaningless gestures such as linking pinkies or interlocking circles made with the thumb and index finger on each hand.
  3. GESTURE KNOWLEDGE
    The examiner demonstrates different actions and asks the patient to identify their function/purpose and how well they were performed.
  4. SEQUENTIAL ACTIONS
    The examiner asks the patient to show how to prepare a letter for mailing, a sandwich for eating, a bowl of cereal with milk. The examiner instructs the patient that the imaginary elements needed for the task are laid out in front of them.
  5. CONCEPTUAL KNOWLEDGE
    The examiner shows the patient either pictures or the actual tools or objects and asks the patient to pantomime or demonstrate their use or function. The examiner may also show a task, such as holding a nail, and ask the patient to pantomime the correct tool use and action.
  6. LIMB-KINETIC MOVEMENTS
    Finger tapping
    Alternate touching each fingertip with thumb
    Pick up a coin without sliding
    Twirl coin between thumb, index, and middle fingers
  7. REAL OBJECT USE
    If limb apraxia is present, test with real object use. Most limb apraxias improve when using real objects for transitive actions and when gesturing spontaneously with intransitive actions.

II. NONDOMINANT UPPER EXTREMITY
  The examiner repeats the same procedures as for the dominant upper extremity.

Fourth, the patient must perform tasks that require several motor acts in sequence, such as making a sandwich or preparing a letter for mailing. Fifth, the examiner shows the patient pictures of tools or objects or the actual tools or objects themselves. The examiner then requests that the patient pantomime the action associated with the tool or object. Finally, the examiner checks for fine finger movements by asking the patient to do repetitive tapping, picking up a coin with a pincer grasp, and twirling the coin. Additional impairment in the patient's ability to use real objects usually indicates a marked severity of the limb apraxia. The pattern of deficits will determine the types of apraxia (Table 11.1). Specialists in occupational therapy, physical therapy, speech pathology, and neuropsychology can further assess and quantify the deficits in limb apraxia using instruments like the Apraxia Battery for Adults-2, the Florida Apraxia Battery, the Cologne Apraxia Screening, the Test of Upper Limb Apraxia, Short screening Test for Ideomotor Apraxia (STIMA), Diagnostic Instrument of Limb Apraxia (DILA) and its short version (DILA-S), and others (Buchmann and Randerath, 2017; Dovern et al., 2012; Power et al., 2010; Tessari et al., 2015; Vanbellingen et al., 2010).

## Testing for Ideomotor Apraxia, Parietal and Disconnection Variants

Patients with the ideomotor apraxias cannot pantomime to command or imitate the examiner's gestures. These patients improve only partially with intransitive acts, imitation, and real object use. Ideomotor apraxia results in spatiotemporal errors in the positioning and orientation of the arm, hand, and fingers to the target and in the timing of the movements, but the goal of the action is still recognizable. In addition to poor positioning of the limb in relation to an imagined object, patients with ideomotor apraxia have an incorrect trajectory of their limb through space owing to poor coordination of multiple joint movements. Patients with ideomotor apraxia also have hesitant, stuttered movements rather than smooth, effortless ones. The difference between parietal variant and disconnection types of ideomotor apraxia is that patients with the disconnection variant can comprehend gestures and pantomimes and discriminate between correctly and incorrectly performed pantomimes.

On attempting to pantomime, patients with ideomotor apraxia may substitute a body part for the tool or object ("Body-Part-as-Object" error) (Raymer et al., 1997). For example, when attempting to pantomime combing their hair or brushing their teeth, they substitute their fingers for the comb or toothbrush. Normal subjects may make the same errors, so the examiner should ask patients not to substitute their fingers or other body parts but to pantomime using a "pretend tool." Patients with ideomotor apraxia may not improve with these instructions and continue to make Body-Part-as-Object errors. The persistent substitution of a body part for a tool or object may indicate a left frontal disturbance. In addition, this type of error activates the right inferior parietal lobe; hence, patients with ideomotor apraxia with left parietal injury may be using their normal right parietal lobe in order to pantomime gestures (Ohgami et al., 2004).

## Testing for Dissociation Apraxia

The testing for dissociation apraxia is the same as for ideomotor apraxia. An important feature of dissociation apraxia when attempting to pantomime is the absence of recognizable movements. When asked to pantomime to verbal command, these patients may look at their hands but fail to perform any pertinent actions. However, unlike patients with ideomotor apraxia, they can imitate the examiner's actions. Given the language–motor disconnection, it is important to evaluate the patient for language disorders and to exclude aphasia. Similar defects in other modalities are possible as well. For example, some patients who are asked to pantomime in response to visual or tactile stimuli may be unable to do so but can correctly pantomime to verbal command.

## Testing for Ideational Apraxia

The test for ideational apraxia involves pantomiming multistep sequential tasks to verbal command. Examples are asking the patient

**TABLE 11.1 Testing in Limb Apraxias**

| | Ideomotor, parietal | Ideomotor, disconnection* | Dissociation* | Ideational* | Conceptual* | Limb-kinetic |
|---|---|---|---|---|---|---|
| Pantomime to verbal command | **Abnormal**† | **Abnormal**† | **Abnormal**‡ | Normal§ | **Abnormal**ǁ | Normal |
| Imitation of gestures | **Abnormal**† | **Abnormal**† | Normal | Normal§ | Normal | Normal¶ |
| Gesture knowledge | **Abnormal** | Normal | Normal | Normal | Normal | Normal |
| Sequential actions | Normal† | Normal | **Abnormal** | **Abnormal** | **Abnormal** | Normal |
| Conceptual knowledge of tool use | Normal | Normal | Normal | **Abnormal**/normal§ | **Abnormal** | Normal |
| Limb-kinetic movement | Normal | Normal | Normal | Normal | Normal | **Abnormal** |
| Real object use | Normal/**abnormal**# | Normal/**abnormal**# | Normal | Normal/**abnormal**# | **Abnormal**ǁ | Normal/**abnormal**# |

*Callosal apraxia, which is limited to the nondominant limb, can present as disconnection-variant ideomotor apraxia, a dissociative apraxia, or (rarely) a conceptual apraxia.
†Spatiotemporal production errors on single, individual ideomotor tasks.
‡Unrecognizable movements or attempts.
§Errors on performing sequential actions only (i.e., individual actions and their conceptual knowledge are normal).
ǁContent and tool use errors on individual ideomotor tasks.
¶Decreased dexterity in fine finger movements.
#Errors depend on severity. In general, errors are worse with verbal commands>imitation>real spontaneous object use and worse for transitive rather than intransitive actions.

to demonstrate how to prepare a letter for mailing or a sandwich for eating. The examiner instructs the patient that the imaginary elements needed for the task are laid out in front of them; the patient is then observed to see whether the correct sequence of events is performed. Ideational apraxia manifests as a failure to perform each step in the correct order. If disturbed, the examiner can repeat this testing with a real object, such as providing the patient with a letter and stamp.

### Testing for Conceptual Apraxia

Patients with conceptual apraxia make content errors and demonstrate the actions of tools or objects other than the one they were asked to pantomime. For example, the examiner shows the patient either pictures or the actual tools or objects and asks the patient to pantomime or demonstrate their use or function. Patients with conceptual apraxia pantomime the wrong use or function, but they are able to imitate gestures without spatiotemporal errors (see Table 11.1).

### Testing for Limb-Kinetic Apraxia

For limb-kinetic apraxia testing, the examiner asks the patient to perform fine finger movements and looks for evidence of incoordination. For example, the examiner asks the patient to pick up a small coin such as a dime from the table with the thumb and the index finger only. Normally, people use the pincer grasp to pick up a dime by putting a forefinger on one edge of the coin and the thumb on the opposite edge. Patients with limb-kinetic apraxia will have trouble doing this without sliding the coin to the edge of the table or using multiple fingers. Another test involves the patient rotating a nickel between the thumb, index, and middle fingers 10 times as rapidly as they can. Patients with limb-kinetic apraxia are slow and clumsy at these tasks (Hanna-Pladdy et al., 2002). In addition, they may also have disproportionate problems with meaningless gestures. These tasks, particularly the simple coin rotation test, provide valuable information about dexterity skills for ADLs (Foki et al., 2016).

### Testing for Callosal Apraxia

The examination for callosal apraxias is the same as for the other limb apraxias except that the abnormalities are limited to the nondominant hand. The testing for callosal apraxia may reveal a disconnection-variant ideomotor apraxia, a dissociative apraxia, or even a conceptual apraxia in the nondominant limb (Heilman et al., 1997).

## PATHOPHYSIOLOGY OF LIMB APRAXIAS

Ideomotor apraxia is associated with left hemispheric lesions in a variety of structures including the inferior parietal lobe, the frontal lobe, and the premotor areas, particularly the SMA. There are reports of ideomotor apraxia due to subcortical lesions in the basal ganglia (caudate-putamen), thalamus (pulvinar), and associated white-matter tracts including the corpus callosum. Limb apraxias can be caused by any central nervous system disorder that affects these regions. The different forms of limb apraxia result from cerebrovascular lesions, especially left middle cerebral artery strokes with right hemiparesis and apraxia evident in the left upper extremity. Right anterior cerebral artery strokes and paramedian lesions could produce ideomotor apraxia, disconnection variant. Ideomotor apraxia and limb-kinetic apraxia can be the initial or presenting manifestation of disorders such as corticobasal syndrome, primary progressive aphasia, parietal-variant Alzheimer disease, and other disorders (Rohrer et al., 2010).

There are important considerations of hemispheric specialization and handedness on praxis. Early investigators proposed that handedness was related to the hemispheric laterality of the movement formulas. Studies using functional imaging have provided converging evidence that in people who are right-handed, it is the left inferior parietal lobe that appears to store the movement formulas needed for learned skilled movements (Muhlau et al., 2005). However, left-handed people may demonstrate an ideomotor apraxia from a right hemisphere lesion, because their movement formulas can be stored in their right hemisphere. It is not unusual to see right-handed patients with large left hemisphere lesions who are not apraxic, and there are rare reports of right-handed patients with right hemisphere lesions and limb apraxia (Schell et al., 2014). These findings suggest that hand preference is not entirely determined by the laterality of the movement formulas, and praxis and handedness can be dissociated.

## REHABILITATION FOR LIMB APRAXIAS

Because many instrumental and routine ADLs depend on learned skilled movements, patients with limb apraxia usually have impaired functional abilities. The presence of limb apraxia, more than any other neuropsychological disorder, correlates with the level of caregiver assistance required 6 months after a stroke, whereas the absence of apraxia is a significant predictor of return to work after a stroke (Saeki et al., 1995). The treatment of limb apraxia is therefore important for improving the quality of life of the patient.

Even though many apraxia treatments have been studied, none has emerged as the standard. There are no effective pharmacotherapies for limb apraxia, and treatments primarily involve rehabilitation strategies. Buxbaum and associates (2008) surveyed the literature on the rehabilitation of limb apraxia and identified 10 studies with 10 treatment strategies: multiple cues, error type reduction, six-stage task hierarchy, conductive education, strategy training, transitive/intransitive gesture training, rehabilitative treatment, error completion, exploration training, and combined error completion and exploration training. Most of these approaches emphasize cueing with multiple modalities, with verbal, visual, and tactile inputs, repetitive learning, and feedback and correction of errors. If possible, rehabilitation techniques should involve activities that are akin to a natural setting (Baak et al., 2015). The timing of rehabilitation may be an important factor as well. Apraxia patients with acute lesions, such as left hemisphere strokes, appear to respond better if the therapy is initiated early (Mutha et al., 2017). Patients with post-stroke apraxia have had generalization of cognitive strategy training to other ADLs (Geusgens et al., 2006), but, unfortunately, many others have not (Bickerton et al., 2006; Shimizu and Tanemura, 2017). Newer technologies such as transcranial stimulation of left parietal cortex or primary motor cortex, can temporarily improve praxis in some patients (Bianchi et al., 2015; Bolognini et al., 2015; Park 2018). Other novel techniques for apraxia rehabilitation include embedding sensors in household tools in order to guide rehabilitation (Hughes et al., 2013), using a videogame-based feedback system to improve pinch and grasp forces (Fusco et al., 2018), and evaluating apraxia with a virtual partner (Candidi et al., 2017).

In summary, patients can learn and produce new gestures, and new technologies, including transcranial stimulation, may play a role in rehabilitation, but the re-learned specific movements may not persist or generalize well to contexts outside the rehabilitation setting.

Nevertheless, some patients with ideomotor apraxia have improved with gesture-production exercises (Smania et al., 2000), with positive effects lasting 2 months after completion of gesture training (Smania et al., 2006). Patients with apraxia would benefit from referral to a rehabilitation specialist with experience in treating apraxias (Cantagallo et al., 2012; Dovern et al., 2012).

Additional practical interventions for the management of limb apraxias involve making environmental changes. This includes removing unsafe tools or implements, providing a limited number of tools to select from, replacing complex tasks with simpler ones that require few or no tools and fewer steps, as well as similar modifications.

## RELATED DISORDERS

Other movement disturbances may be related to or confused with the limb apraxias. The *alien limb phenomenon*, a potential result of callosal lesions, is the experience that a limb feels foreign and has involuntary semipurposeful movements, such as spontaneous limb levitation. This disorder can occur from neurodegenerative conditions, most notably corticobasal syndrome. *Akinesia* is the inability to initiate a movement in the absence of motor deficits, and *hypokinesia* is a delay in initiating a response. Akinesia and hypokinesia can be directional, with decreased initiation of movement in a specific spatial direction or hemifield. Akinesia and hypokinesia result from a failure to activate the corticospinal system due to Parkinson disease and diseases that affect the frontal lobe cortex, basal ganglia, or thalamus.

Several other movement disturbances are associated with frontal lobe dysfunction. *Motor impersistence* is the inability to sustain a movement or posture and occurs with dorsolateral frontal lesions. *Magnetic grasp and grope reflexes* with automatic reaching for environmental stimuli are primitive release signs. In *echopraxia*, some patients automatically imitate observed movements. Along with utilization behavior, echopraxia may be part of the environmental dependency syndrome of some patients with frontal lesions. *Catalepsy* is the maintenance of a body position into which patients are placed (waxy flexibility). Two related terms are *mitgehen* ("going with"), where patients allow a body part to move in response to light pressure, and *mitmachen* ("doing with"), where patients allow a body part to be put into any position in response to slight pressure, then return the body part to the original resting position after the examiner releases it. *Motor perseveration* is the inability to stop a movement or a series of movements after the task is complete. In recurrent motor perseveration, the patient keeps returning to a prior completed motor program, and in afferent or continuous motor perseveration, the patient cannot end a motor program that has just been completed.

## SUMMARY

Limb apraxia, or the disturbance of learned skilled movements, is an important but often missed or unrecognized impairment. Clinicians may misattribute limb apraxia to weakness, hemiparesis, clumsiness, or other motor, sensory, spatial, or cognitive disturbance. Apraxia may only be evident on fine, sequential, or specific movements of the upper extremities and requires a systematic praxis examination (Zadikoff and Lang, 2005). Apraxia is an important cognitive disturbance and a salient sign in patients with strokes, Alzheimer disease, corticobasal syndrome, and other conditions. The model of left parietal movement formulas and disconnection syndromes introduced by Liepmann over 100 years ago continues to be compelling today. This model, in the context of a dedicated apraxia examination and analysis for spatiotemporal or content errors, clarifies and classifies the limb apraxias. Although more effective treatments need to be developed, rehabilitation strategies can be helpful interventions for these disturbances. Fortunately, recent advances in technology and rehabilitation continue to enhance our understanding and management of limb apraxias.

*The complete reference list is available online at https://expertconsult.inkling.com/.* 

12

# Agnosias

*Howard S. Kirshner*

## OUTLINE



Agnosias are disorders of recognition. The general public is familiar with agnosia from Oliver Sacks' patient, who not only failed to recognize his wife's face but also mistook it for a hat. Sigmund Freud originally introduced the term *agnosia* in 1891 to denote disturbances in the ability to recognize and name objects, usually in one sensory modality, in the presence of intact primary sensation. Another definition, that of Milner and Teuber in 1968, referred to agnosia as a "normal percept stripped of its meaning." The agnosic patient can perceive and describe sensory features of an object yet cannot recognize or identify the object.

Criteria for the diagnosis of agnosia include: (1) failure to recognize an object; (2) normal perception of the object, excluding an elementary sensory disorder; (3) ability to name the object once it is recognized, excluding anomia as the principal deficit; and (4) absence of a generalized dementia. In addition, agnosias usually affect only one sensory modality, and the patient can identify the same object when presented in a different sensory modality. For example, a patient with visual agnosia may fail to identify a bell by sight but readily identifies it by touch or by the sound of its ring.

Agnosias are defined in terms of the specific sensory modality affected—usually visual, auditory, or tactile—or they may be selective for one class of items within a sensory modality, such as color agnosia or prosopagnosia (agnosia for faces). To diagnose agnosia, the examiner must establish that the deficit is not a primary sensory disorder, as documented by tests of visual acuity, visual fields, auditory function, and somatosensory functions, and not part of a more general cognitive disorder, such as aphasia or dementia, as established by the bedside mental status examination. Naming deficits in aphasia or dementia are, with rare exceptions, not restricted to a single sensory modality.

Clinically, agnosias seem complex and arcane, yet they are important in understanding the behavior of neurological patients, and they provide fascinating insights into brain mechanisms related to perception and recognition. Part of their complexity derives from the underlying neuropathology; agnosias frequently result from bilateral or diffuse lesions such as hypoxic encephalopathy, multiple strokes, and major head injuries, and agnosic phenomena also play a role in neurodegenerative disorders and dementias, despite the earlier definitions.

Agnosias have aroused controversies since their earliest descriptions. Some authorities have attributed agnosic deficits to primary perceptual loss in the setting of general cognitive dysfunction or dementia. However, abundant case studies argue in favor of true agnosic deficits. In each sensory modality, a spectrum of disorders can be traced from primary sensory dysfunction to agnosia. We approach agnosias by sensory modality, with progression from primary sensory deficits to disorders of recognition.

## VISUAL AGNOSIAS

### Cortical Visual Disturbances

Patients with bilateral occipital lobe damage may have complete "cortical" blindness. Some patients with cortical blindness are unaware that they cannot see, and some even confabulate visual descriptions or blame their poor vision on dim lighting or not having their glasses (Anton syndrome, originally described in 1899). Patients with Anton syndrome may describe objects they "see" in the room around them but walk immediately into a wall. The phenomena of this syndrome suggest that the thinking and speaking areas of the brain are not consciously aware of the lack of input from visual centers. Anton syndrome can still be thought of as a perceptual deficit rather than a visual agnosia, but one in which there is unawareness or neglect of the sensory deficit. Such visual unawareness is also frequently seen with hemianopic visual field defects (e.g., in patients with R hemisphere strokes), and it even has a correlate in normal people; we are not conscious of a visual field defect behind our heads, yet we know to turn when we hear a noise from behind. In contrast to Anton syndrome, some cortically blind patients actually have preserved ability to react to visual stimuli, despite the lack of any conscious visual perception—a phenomenon termed *blindsight* or *inverse Anton syndrome* (Leopold, 2012; Ro and Rafal, 2006). Blindsight may be considered an agnosic deficit, because the patient fails to recognize what he or she sees. Residual vision is usually absent in blindness caused by disorders of the eyes, optic nerves, or optic tracts. Patients with cortical vision loss may react to more elementary visual stimuli such as brightness, size, and movement, whereas they cannot perceive finer attributes such as shape, color, and depth. Subjects sometimes look toward objects they cannot consciously see. One study reported a woman with postanoxic cortical blindness who could catch a ball without awareness of seeing it. Blindsight may be mediated by subcortical connections such as those from the optic tracts to the midbrain.

Lesions causing cortical blindness may also be accompanied by visual hallucinations. Irritative lesions of the visual cortex produce unformed hallucinations of lines or spots, whereas those of the temporal lobes produce formed visual images. Visual hallucinations in blindness are referred to as *Bonnet syndrome* (Teunisse et al., 1996). Although Bonnet originally described this phenomenon in his grandfather, who had ocular blindness, complex visual hallucinations occur more typically with cortical visual loss (Manford and Andermann, 1998). Visual hallucinations can occur during recovery from cortical blindness; positron emission tomography (PET) has shown metabolic activation in the parieto-occipital cortex associated with hallucinations, suggesting hyperexcitability of the recovering visual cortex (Wunderlich et al., 2000). The late Oliver Sacks reported numerous examples of visual hallucinations in his 2012 book, *Hallucinations* (Sacks, 2012).

In practice, we diagnose cortical blindness by the absence of ocular pathology, the preservation of the pupillary light reflexes, and the presence of associated neurological symptoms and signs. In addition to blindness, patients with bilateral posterior hemisphere lesions are often confused and agitated, and have short-term memory loss. Amnesia is especially common in patients with bilateral strokes within the posterior cerebral artery territory, which involves not only the occipital lobe but also the hippocampi and related structures of the medial temporal region. Cortical blindness occurs as a transient phenomenon after traumatic brain injury, in migraine, in epileptic seizures, and as a complication of iodinated contrast procedures such as arteriography. Cortical blindness can develop in the setting of hypoxic-ischemic encephalopathy (Wunderlich et al., 2000), posterior reversible encephalopathy syndrome (PRES), meningitis, systemic lupus erythematosus, dementing conditions such as the Heidenhain variant of Creutzfeldt–Jakob disease, or the posterior cortical atrophy syndrome described in Alzheimer disease and other dementias (Kirshner and Lavin, 2006).

## Cortical Visual Distortions

Positive visual phenomena frequently develop in patients with visual field defects and even in migraine: distortions of shape called *metamorphopsia*, scintillating scotomas, irregular shapes (teichopsia, or fortification spectra), macropsia and micropsia, peculiar changes of shape and size known as the *Alice in Wonderland syndrome* (described by Golden in 1979), achromatopsia (loss of color vision), akinetopsia (loss of perception of motion), palinopsia (perseveration of visual images), visual allesthesia (spread of a visual image from a normal to a hemianopic field), and even polyopia (duplication of objects). All these phenomena are disturbances of higher visual perception rather than agnosias.

Two types of color vision deficit are associated with occipital lesions. First, a complete loss of color vision, or achromatopsia, may occur either bilaterally or in one visual hemifield with lesions that involve portions of the visual association cortex (Brodmann areas 18 and 19). Second, patients with pure alexia and lesions of the left occipital lobe fail to name colors, although their color matching and other aspects of color perception are normal. Patients often confabulate an incorrect color name when asked what color an object is. This deficit can be called *color agnosia*, in the sense that a normally perceived color cannot be properly recognized. Although this deficit has been termed *color anomia*, these patients can usually name the colors of familiar objects such as a school bus or the inside of a watermelon.

## Balint Syndrome and Simultanagnosia

In 1909, Balint described a syndrome in which patients act blind, yet can describe small details of objects in central vision (Rizzo and Vecera, 2002). The disorder is usually associated with bilateral hemisphere lesions, often involving the parietal and frontal lobes. Balint syndrome involves a triad of deficits: (1) psychic paralysis of gaze, also called *ocular motor apraxia*, or difficulty directing the eyes away from central fixation; (2) optic ataxia, or incoordination of extremity movement under visual control (with normal coordination under proprioceptive control); and (3) impaired visual attention. These deficits result in the perception of only small details of a visual scene, with loss of the ability to scan and perceive the "big picture." Patients with Balint syndrome literally cannot see the forest for the trees. Some, but not all, patients have bilateral visual field deficits. In bedside neurological examination, helpful tests include asking the patient to interpret a complex drawing or photograph, such as the "Cookie Theft" picture from the Boston Diagnostic Aphasia Examination and the National Institutes of Health Stroke Scale.

Partial deficits related to Balint syndrome, including isolated optic ataxia, or impaired visually guided reaching toward an object, have also been described. Optic ataxia likely results from disruption of the transmission of visual information for visual direction of motor acts from the occipital cortex to the premotor areas. This function involves portions of the dorsal occipital and parietal areas as part of the "dorsal visual stream" (Himmelbach et al., 2009). A second partial Balint syndrome deficit is simultanagnosia, or loss of ability to perceive more than one item at a time, first described by Wolpert in 1924. The patient sees details of pictures, but not the whole. Many such patients have left occipital lesions and associated pure alexia without agraphia; these patients can often read "letter-by-letter," or one letter at a time, but they cannot recognize a word at a glance (see Chapter 13). Robertson and colleagues (1997) emphasized deficient spatial organization as a contributing factor to the perceptual difficulties of a patient with Balint syndrome secondary to bilateral parieto-occipital strokes. Balint syndrome has also been reported in patients with posterior cortical atrophy and related neurodegenerative conditions involving the posterior parts of both hemispheres (Kirshner and Lavin, 2006; McMonagle et al., 2006).

## Visual Object Agnosia

Visual object agnosia is the quintessential visual agnosia: the patient fails to recognize objects by sight, with preserved ability to recognize them through touch or hearing, in the absence of impaired primary visual perception or dementia (Biran and Coslett, 2003). In 1890, Lissauer distinguished two subtypes of visual object agnosia: *apperceptive visual object agnosia*, referring to the synthesis of elementary perceptual elements into a unified image, and *associative visual object agnosia*, in which the meaning of a perceived stimulus is appreciated by recall of previous visual experiences.

### Apperceptive Visual Agnosia

The first type, apperceptive visual agnosia, is difficult to separate from impaired perception or partial cortical blindness. Patients with apperceptive visual agnosia can pick out features of an object correctly (e.g., lines, angles, colors, movement), but they fail to appreciate the whole object (Grossman et al., 1997). Warrington and Rudge (1995) pointed to the right parietal cortex for its importance in visual processing of objects, and they found this area critical to apperceptive visual agnosia. A patient described by Luria misnamed eyeglasses as a bicycle, pointing to the two circles and a crossbar. Apperceptive visual agnosia can be related to damage to the primary visual cortex by bilateral occipital lesions (Serino et al., 2014). Recent evidence of the functions of specific cortical areas has included the specialization of the medial occipital cortex for appreciation of color and texture, whereas the lateral occipital cortex is more involved with shape perception. Deficits in these specific visual functions can be seen in patients with visual object agnosia (Cavina-Pratesi et al., 2010). On the other hand, a patient reported by Karnath et al. (2009) had visual form agnosia with bilateral medial occipitotemporal lesions.

Another way of analyzing apperceptive visual agnosia is by the focusing of visual attention. Theiss and DeBleser in 1992 distinguished two features of visual attention: a wide-angle attentional lens that sees the figure generally but perceives only gross features (the forest), and a narrow-angle spotlight that focuses on the fine visual details (the trees). They described a patient with a faulty wide-angle attentional beam; she could identify small objects within a drawing but missed what the drawing represented. Fink and colleagues (1996), in PET studies of visual perception in normal subjects, found that right hemisphere sites, particularly the lingual gyrus, activated during global processing of figures, whereas left hemisphere sites, particularly the left inferior occipital cortex, activated during more local processing. The ability of patients with apperceptive visual agnosia to perceive fine details but not the whole picture (missing the forest for the trees) is closely related to Balint syndrome and simultanagnosia.

As with most cortical visual syndromes, apperceptive visual agnosia usually occurs in patients with bilateral occipital lesions. It may represent a stage in recovery from complete cortical blindness. Deficits in recognition of visual objects may be especially apparent with recognition of degraded images, such as drawings rather than actual objects. Apperceptive visual agnosia can also be part of dementing syndromes (Kirshner and Lavin, 2006; McMonagle et al., 2006) (Fig. 12.1).

## Associative Visual Agnosia

Associative visual agnosia—Lissauer's second type—has to do with recognition of appropriately perceived objects. Some patients can copy or match drawings of objects they cannot name, thus excluding a primary defect of visual perception. Aphasia is excluded because the patient can identify the same object presented in the tactile or auditory modality. Patients with associative visual agnosia often have other related recognition deficits such as color agnosia, prosopagnosia, and alexia. Associative visual agnosia is usually associated with bilateral posterior hemisphere lesions, often involving the fusiform or occipitotemporal gyri, sometimes the lingual gyri and adjacent white matter. Jankowiak and colleagues described a patient with bilateral parieto-occipital damage from gunshot injuries. Visual acuity was nearly normal except for bilateral upper "altitudinal" visual field defects. He had difficulty recognizing and naming colors, faces, objects, and pictures. He could copy drawings he could not recognize, and he could draw images from memory or after tachistoscopic presentation. The crux of this patient's deficit was an inability to match an internal visual percept with representations of visual objects; in other words, he could perceive visual stimuli normally but failed to assign meaning or identity to them.

Geschwind postulated in 1965 that visual agnosia results from a disconnection syndrome in which bilateral lesions prevent visual information from the occipital lobes from reaching the left hemisphere language areas. Most but not all cases of associative visual agnosia have involved the fusiform or occipitotemporal gyri bilaterally, presumably interrupting connections between the visual cortex and the language areas for naming, or the medial temporal region for identification from memory. The disconnection hypothesis of visual agnosia is likely an oversimplification of the complexities of visual perception and recognition, but it provides a useful way to remember the syndrome.

A recent review divided visual agnosias into those affecting the ventral (or "what") visual network or stream, including visual object agnosia, cerebral achromatopsia, prosopagnosia (see below), topographagnosia, and pure alexia, versus those affecting the dorsal (or "where") stream, including akinetopsia (agnosia for movement), simultanagnosia, and optic ataxia (Haque et al., 2018). However, another recent review placed prosopagnosia and topographagnosia (agnosia for landmarks) in the ventral pathway. Orientation agnosia (agnosia for the placement of objects in space) belongs with the dorsal

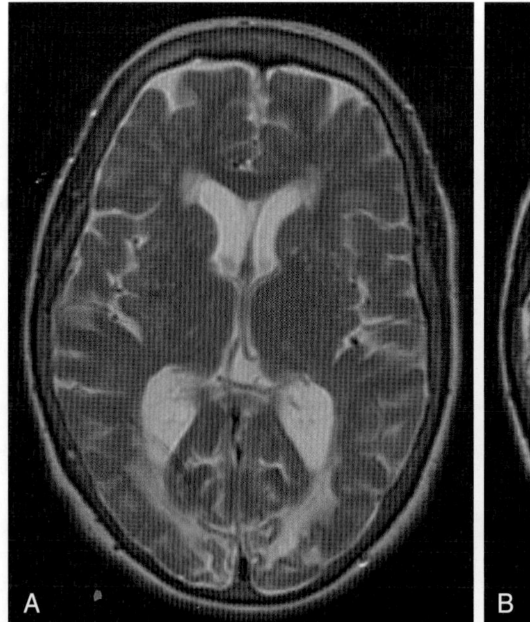

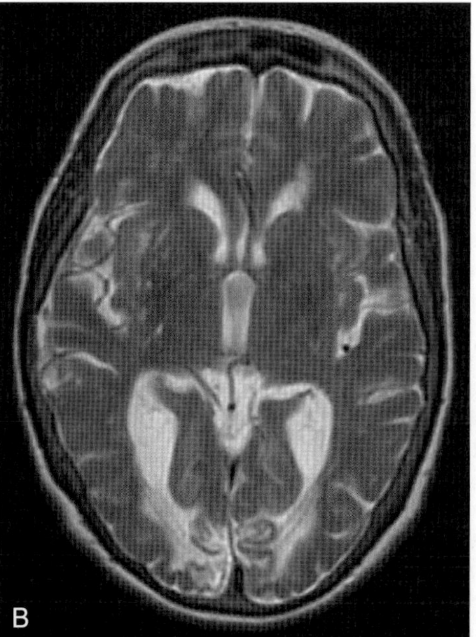


**Fig. 12.1** T2-weighted magnetic resonance images from a patient with progressive loss of vision, misidentification of objects, and the inability to describe the whole of a picture, mentioning only small details. The clinical diagnosis was posterior cortical atrophy, a neurodegenerative condition. Both A and B show atrophy of the occipital cortex bilaterally, with T2 hyperintensity in the occipital white matter.

pathway, along with akinetopsia (Martinaud, 2017). Landmark agnosia can be specific for recently learned landmarks or for all landmarks. The disorder can be distinguished from knowledge of routes. Lesions involve the right temporal lobe and right hippocampus (van der Ham et al., 2017). The ventral stream is thought to be conscious, the dorsal stream unconscious. Yet another recent paper points to greater interaction between the ventral and dorsal streams, from a detailed study of a patient with visual agnosia (Milner, 2017).

Rehabilitation of patients with visual agnosia and Balint syndrome has been studied to a limited extent. A recent review suggests that compensatory measures are more effective than restorative attempts in making these patients function better (Heutink et al., 2018).

## Optic Aphasia

The syndrome of optic aphasia, or optic anomia, is intermediate between agnosias and aphasias. The patient with optic aphasia cannot name objects presented visually but can demonstrate recognition of the objects by pantomiming or describing their use. The preserved recognition of the objects distinguishes optic aphasia from associative visual agnosia. Like visual agnosics, patients with optic aphasia can name objects presented in the auditory or tactile modalities, distinguishing them from anomic aphasics. In optic aphasia, information about the object must reach parts of the cortex involved in recognition, perhaps in the right hemisphere, but the information is not available to the language cortex for naming. This explanation also fits Geschwind's disconnection hypothesis. Patients with optic aphasia may confabulate incorrect names when asked to name an object they clearly recognize, just as the patient with color agnosia confabulates incorrect color names. The language cortex appears to supply a name from the class of items when specific information is not forthcoming, without the conscious awareness that the information is not correct. Patients with optic aphasia frequently manifest associated deficits of alexia without agraphia and color agnosia, suggesting a left occipital lesion. Optic aphasia bears great similarity to pure alexia without agraphia; just as optic aphasics may recognize objects they cannot name, pure alexics sometimes recognize words they cannot read.

## Prosopagnosia

*Prosopagnosia* refers to the inability to recognize faces. Patients fail to recognize close friends and relatives or pictures of famous people, except by memorizing details of shape or hairstyle, but they learn to compensate by identifying a person by voice, mannerisms, gait patterns, and apparel. Prosopagnosia is restricted not only to the visual modality but also to the class of faces.

Facial recognition is a complex function. First, patients who cannot match pictures of faces must have defective face processing, or apperceptive prosopagnosia, whereas those who can match faces but simply fail to recognize familiar examples (either friends and relatives or famous personages) have associative prosopagnosia (Barton et al., 2004). There has been some opinion that faces are not a unique perceptual entity but just representative of complex stimuli; however, a study by Busigny and colleagues (2010) found that their patient performed normally in perceptual tasks involving cars, objects, and geometric shapes, while being deficient with faces. Transient prosopagnosia has been reported after focal electrical stimulation of the right inferior occipital gyrus (Jonas et al., 2012). Another aspect of facial recognition is the perception of emotion in facial expressions, a function that appears localized to the right hemisphere. A recent study suggested that white-matter lesions disconnecting the occipital cortex from "emotion-related regions" might be responsible for agnosia for emotional facial expression (Philippi et al., 2009).

In clinical studies, prosopagnosia may occur either as an isolated deficit or as part of a more general visual agnosia for objects and colors. Faces are likely the most complex and individualized visual displays to recognize, but some patients with visual object agnosia can recognize faces, suggesting that there are specific brain areas devoted to facial recognition. Humphreys (1996) reviewed evidence that living things may be recognized in a different part of the occipital cortex from nonliving things.

The anatomical localization of prosopagnosia is similar to that of the other visual agnosias, but we have better knowledge of the anatomy and physiology of face recognition. Most studies have reported bilateral temporo-occipital lesions, often involving the fusiform or occipitotemporal gyri, but cases with unilateral posterior right hemisphere lesions have also been described. There is an occipital face area, presumably involved in facial perception, a fusiform gyrus face area, involved in recognition of faces, and most recently an anterior temporal center that appears to be involved in details of perception that may not be limited strictly to faces (Barton, 2003; Gainotti, 2013). In short, there is a right hemisphere network for facial recognition. A recent study involving both functional magnetic resonance imaging (fMRI) and neuropsychological testing found the inferior occipital ("occipital face area") lobe critical for the identification of specific individual faces, whereas the "fusiform face area" in the middle fusiform gyrus was involved in other aspects of face perception (Steeves et al., 2009). The disconnection hypothesis has been invoked in prosopagnosia, reflecting interruption of fibers passing from the occipital cortices to the centers where memories of faces are stored. Prosopagnosia also occurs in dementing illnesses such as frontotemporal dementia (Joubert et al., 2004) and posterior cortical atrophy (Kirshner and Lavin, 2006), and impaired facial recognition has also been reported in amnestic mild cognitive impairment (Lim et al., 2011). Two recent reviews discussed the rehabilitation of prosopagnosia (Corrow et al., 2016; Davies-Thompson et al., 2017).

## Klüver-Bucy Syndrome

Another form of visual agnosia is the psychic blindness syndrome described by Klüver and Bucy in 1939. They reported the syndrome originally in monkeys with bilateral temporal lobectomies, but similar symptoms develop in humans with bilateral temporal lesions (Trimble et al., 1997). An animal may inappropriately try to eat or mate with objects or fail to show customary fear when confronted with a natural enemy. Human Klüver-Bucy patients manifest visual agnosia and prosopagnosia as well as memory loss, language deficits, and changes in behavior such as placidity, altered sexual orientation, and excessive eating. Cases of the human Klüver-Bucy syndrome have been reported with bitemporal damage from surgical ablation, herpes simplex encephalitis, and dementing conditions such as Pick disease. Patients with Klüver-Bucy syndrome appear to have no major deficits of primary visual perception, but connections appear to be disrupted between vision and memory and limbic structures, so visual percepts do not arouse their ordinary associations.

A recent review of the Klüver-Bucy syndrome discussed more specific anatomical considerations in both animals and man. Bilateral ventral temporal lobe resections or lobectomies resulted in impaired visual discrimination, which was not seen following lateral temporal resections or unilateral resections. The temporal portion of limbic networks are disrupted in this syndrome, interfering with cortical and subcortical circuits involved in emotional behavior and mood. Bilateral resections of the lateral amygdala resulted in not only the loss of fear that is part of the Klüver-Bucy syndrome but also a "hypersexed state." Humans usually have partial syndromes, as compared with animals subjected to complete bilateral temporal lobectomy, but this syndrome also involves related deficits such as aphasia and memory loss. The author states that the treatment of these patients is "difficult and often unsatisfactory" (Lanska, 2018).

## AUDITORY AGNOSIAS

Like cortical visual syndromes, cortical auditory disorders range from primary auditory syndromes of cortical deafness to partial deficits of recognition of specific types of sound. As with the visual agnosias, most cortical auditory deficits require bilateral cerebral lesions, usually involving the temporal lobes, especially the primary auditory cortices in the Heschl gyri.

### Cortical Deafness

Profound hearing deficits are seen in patients with acquired bilateral lesions of the primary auditory cortex (Heschl gyrus, Brodmann areas 41 and 42) or of the auditory radiations projecting to the Heschl gyri. In general, unilateral lesions of the auditory cortex have little effect on hearing. Only rarely are patients with bilateral auditory cortex lesions completely deaf, even to loud noises; most retain some pure tone hearing but have deficits in higher-level acoustic processing such as identification of meaningful sounds, temporal sequencing, and sound localization. As in visual agnosia, the cortical hearing deficits blend imperceptibly into the auditory agnosias (Brody et al., 2013).

A patient with auditory agnosia can hear noises but not appreciate their meanings, as in identifying animal cries or sounds associated with specific objects, such as the ringing of a bell. Most such patients also cannot understand speech or appreciate music. Auditory agnosias can be divided into (1) pure word deafness, (2) pure auditory nonverbal agnosia, (3) phonagnosia, or the inability to identify persons by their voices (Gainotti, 2011; Hailstone et al., 2010; Polster and Rose, 1998), and (4) pure amusia. Patients may have one or a mixture of these deficits.

### Pure Word Deafness

The syndrome of pure word deafness involves an inability to comprehend spoken words, with an ability to hear and recognize nonverbal sounds. Pure word deafness often evolves out of an initial deficit of cortical deafness or severe cortical auditory disorder. Pure word deafness has traditionally been explained as a disconnection of both primary auditory cortices from the left hemisphere Wernicke area. Engelien and colleagues (2000) showed activation on PET scanning during auditory stimulation in a patient with extensive bilateral temporal lesions, a phenomenon they referred to as *deaf hearing* (analogous to blindsight). Unilateral left hemisphere lesions have also been associated with pure word deafness; by Geschwind's disconnection theory, such a lesion might be strategically placed so as to disconnect both primary auditory cortices from the Wernicke area. Occasionally patients with Wernicke aphasia have more severe involvement of auditory comprehension than reading comprehension, also resembling pure word deafness. In fact, most cases of pure word deafness also have paraphasic speech, further linking the syndrome to Wernicke aphasia (Fig. 12.2).

### Auditory Nonverbal Agnosia

*Auditory nonverbal agnosia* refers to patients who have lost the ability to identify meaningful nonverbal sounds but have preserved pure tone hearing and language comprehension. These cases also tend to have bilateral temporal lobe lesions. A reported case had a unilateral

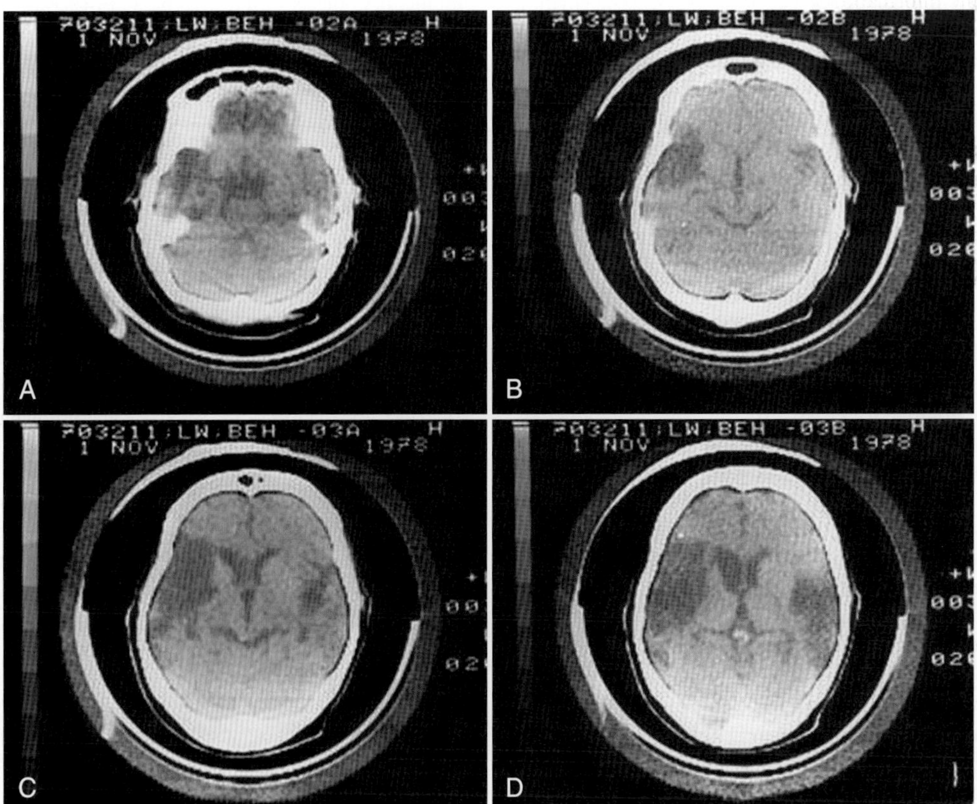


**Fig. 12.2** A computed tomography scan from a patient with extensive bilateral infarctions involving the temporal lobes. The patient could hear pure tones and nonverbal sounds, but she was completely unable to comprehend speech. These 4 slices of a computerized axial tomogram (CT scan) show old strokes affecting the temporal lobes bilaterally, in a patient with cortical deafness. (*From Kirshner, H.S., Webb, W.G., 1981. Selective involvement of the auditory-verbal modality in an acquired communication disorder: benefit from sign language therapy, Brain and Language, 13, 161–170.*)

left temporal lesion with evidence of reorganization of auditory word perception involving the adjacent left and contralateral right temporal cortex (Saygin et al., 2010).

### Phonagnosia

Phonagnosia is analogous to prosopagnosia in the visual modality; it is a failure to recognize familiar people by their voices. Again, apperceptive deficits can occur in the matching of unfamiliar voices, usually reflecting unilateral or bilateral temporal damage, but failure to recognize a familiar voice may involve a right parietal locus corresponding to the specific area for recognition of voices. Gainotti (2011) reviewed evidence that voice recognition deficits correlated with right anterior temporal lesions, but in many cases this is "multimodal," affecting recognition of familiar persons not only by voice but also by facial appearance. A related deficit is auditory affective agnosia, or failure to recognize the emotional intonation of speech, usually associated with right hemisphere lesions (Polster and Rose, 1998). Two cases of progressive phonagnosia have been reported in frontotemporal dementia (Hailstone et al., 2010).

A recently published case report of a bird enthusiast with semantic dementia described very specific impairments of bird call recognition, whereas the patient could recognize human faces and voices. There were also very focal deficits in bird knowledge referable to bird names and habitats (Muhammed, et al., 2018).

### Amusia

The loss of musical abilities after focal brain lesions is another complex topic, reflecting the complexity of musical appreciation and analysis (Alossa and Castelli, 2009). Traditional lesion-deficit analysis has suggested that recognition of melodies and musical tones is a right temporal function, whereas analysis of learned or skilled aspects of pitch, rhythm, and tempo involves the left temporal lobe. In a study of patients with temporal lobe lesions and epilepsy, those with left hemisphere lesions were more impaired in temporal sequencing of music as well as speech (Samson et al., 2001). The left hemisphere is likely more activated when a trained musician listens to music, as compared with an untrained listener. In a study of PET brain imaging during musical performance in 10 professional pianists, sight-reading of music activated both visual association cortices and the superior parietal lobes, areas distinct from those utilized in reading words. Listening to music activated both secondary auditory cortices, and playing music activated frontal and cerebellar areas. The authors commented that widespread as these areas were, the study did not examine the whole musical experience, let alone the pleasure afforded by music.

The composer, Maurice Ravel, whose case was originally described in 1948 by Alajouanine, suffered a progressive fluent aphasia that gradually took his ability to read or write music but spared his capacity to listen to and appreciate it. Another study also reported progressive musical dysfunction in two professional musicians with dementing illness. A recently described patient with resection of a right temporoparietal tumor had a loss of sad or happy music perception but preserved meter and beat (Baird et al., 2014).

## TACTILE AGNOSIAS

As we have seen with the syndromes of cortical loss of visual and auditory perception, a range of somatosensory deficits is seen with cortical lesions. Patients with lesions of the parietal cortex may have preserved ability to feel pinprick, temperature, vibration, and proprioception, yet they fail to identify objects palpated by the contralateral hand or to recognize numbers or letters written on the opposite side of the body. These deficits, called *astereognosis* and *agraphesthesia*, represent deficits of cortical sensory loss rather than agnosias. Alternatively, they could be considered as apperceptive tactile agnosias. Rarely, patients who can describe the shape and features of a palpated object, yet cannot identify the object, have been reported. The patient can readily identify the object by sound or sight, thereby fulfilling the criteria for associative tactile agnosia (Bottini et al., 1995).

Caselli (1991a) investigated 84 patients with unilateral hemisphere lesions for deficits in tactile perception. Seven patients had tactile agnosia for objects palpated by the contralateral hand. These deficits occurred in the absence of primary somatosensory loss. Some patients had severe hemiparesis or hemianopia yet performed well in tactile object recognition, but patients with neglect secondary to right hemisphere lesions tended to have more severe deficits. A second study reported that only patients with neglect had bilateral tactile object recognition deficits, whereas patients with left parietal lesions had tactile agnosia only for items in the right hand (Caselli, 1991b). However, the study did not include patients with bilateral lesions, and agnosia in the visual and auditory modalities is clearly more profound when bilateral lesions are present.

The mechanisms of tactile agnosia may vary. First, appreciation of shape may be a property of the sensory cortex. In the studies of Bottini and colleagues (1995), matching of shapes (an apperceptive task) was more sensitive to right hemisphere damage, whereas matching of meaningful shapes (the associative task) was more sensitive to left hemisphere lesions. Second, the right parietal cortex is also involved in spatial and topographical functions, and spatial disorders may account for some of the tactile recognition deficits of patients with right parietal lesions. Third, attentional deficits and neglect seen with right hemisphere lesions may increase the lack of tactile recognition. Fourth, disconnection syndromes may be involved in tactile agnosia. The famous 1962 patient of Geschwind and Kaplan with a lesion of the corpus callosum could not identify objects with the left hand, by speech, but could point to the correct object in a group. Patients with surgical section of the corpus callosum have similar deficits; these patients can feel the object with the left hand but cannot name it, presumably because the callosal lesion disconnects the right parietal cortex from left hemisphere language centers.

### Tactile Aphasia

*Tactile aphasia* is an inability to name a palpated object despite intact recognition of the object and intact naming when the object is presented in another sensory modality. This syndrome is closely analogous to optic aphasia and has been recognized only rarely.

## SUMMARY

Agnosias are disorders of sensory perception and recognition. The cortical mechanisms of the agnosias span a spectrum from primary sensory cortical deficits to disorders of the association cortex, or disconnection syndromes between cortical areas. Recognition of objects requires not only primary sensation but also association of the perceived item with previous sensory experiences and associative memories. The agnosias open a window into the brain's ability to perceive and recognize aspects of the world around us.

*The complete reference list is available online at https://expertconsult.inkling.com/.*

### Acknowledgment

Portions of this chapter appeared in Kirshner, H.S., 2002. Agnosias, in: *Behavioral neurology: Practical science of mind and brain.* Butterworth-Heinemann, Boston, pp. 137–158.

13

# Aphasia and Aphasic Syndromes

*Howard S. Kirshner, Stephen M. Wilson*

## OUTLINE



The study of language disorders involves the analysis of that most human of attributes, the ability to communicate through common symbols. Language has provided the foundation of human civilization and learning, and its study has been the province of philosophers as well as physicians. When language is disturbed by neurological disorders, analysis of the patterns of abnormality has practical usefulness in neurological diagnosis. Historically, language was the first higher cortical function to be correlated with specific sites of brain damage. It continues to serve as a model for the practical use of a cognitive function in the localization of brain lesions and for the understanding of human cortical processes in general.

*Aphasia* is defined as a disorder of language that is acquired secondary to brain damage. This definition, adapted from Alexander and Benson (1997), separates aphasia from several related disorders. First, aphasia is distinguished from congenital or developmental language disorders. Second, aphasia is a disorder of language rather than speech. *Speech* is the articulation and phonation of language sounds; *language* is a complex system of communicative symbols and rules for their use. Aphasia is distinguished from motor speech disorders, which include dysarthria, dysphonia (voice disorders), stuttering, and apraxia of speech. *Dysarthrias* are disorders of muscular control of speech. Dysarthria may result from mechanical disturbance of the tongue or larynx or from neurological disorders, including dysfunction of the muscles, neuromuscular junction, cranial nerves, bulbar anterior horn cells, corticobulbar tracts, cerebellar connections, or basal ganglia. Dysarthrias are discussed in Chapter 14.

Apraxia of speech is a syndrome of misarticulation of phonemes, especially consonant sounds. Unlike dysarthria, in which certain phonemes are consistently distorted, apraxia of speech contains inconsistent distortions and substitutions of phonemes. The disorder is called an *apraxia* because there is no primary motor deficit in articulation of individual phonemes. Clinically, speech-apraxic patients produce inconsistent articulatory errors, usually worse on the initial phonemes of a word and with polysyllabic utterances. Apraxia of speech, so defined, is commonly involved in speech production difficulty in the aphasias.

Third, aphasia is distinguished from disorders of thought. Thought involves the mental processing of images, memories, and perceptions, usually but not necessarily involving language symbols. Psychiatric disorders derange thought and alter the content of speech without affecting its linguistic structure. Schizophrenic patients, for example, may manifest bizarre and individualistic word choices, with loose associations and a loss of organization in discourse, together with vague or unclear references and communication failures (Docherty et al., 1996). Elementary language and articulation, however, are intact. Abnormal language content in psychiatric disorders is therefore not considered aphasia because the disorder is one of thought rather than one of language. Language disorders associated with diffuse brain diseases, such as encephalopathies and dementias, do qualify as aphasias, but the involvement of other cognitive functions distinguishes them from aphasia secondary to focal brain lesions.

An understanding of language disorders requires an elementary review of linguistic components. *Phonemes* are the smallest distinctive sound units; *morphology* is the use of appropriate word endings and connector words for grammatical categories such as tenses, possessives, and singular versus plural; *semantics* refers to word meanings; the *lexicon* is the internal dictionary; and *syntax* is the grammatical construction of phrases and sentences. *Discourse* refers to the use of these elements to create organized and logical expression of thoughts. *Pragmatics* refers to the proper use of speech and language in a conversational setting, including pausing while others are speaking, taking turns properly, and responding to questions. Specific language disorders affect one or more of these elements.

Language processes have a clear neuroanatomical basis. In simplest terms, the reception and processing of spoken language take place in the auditory system, beginning with the cochlea and proceeding through a series of way stations to the auditory cortex, Heschl gyrus, in each superior temporal gyrus. The decoding of sounds into linguistic information involves the left superior temporal gyrus and sulcus. The recognition of the role of the left temporal cortex in linking sound to meaning dates back to Wernicke (1874) and has been refined over the

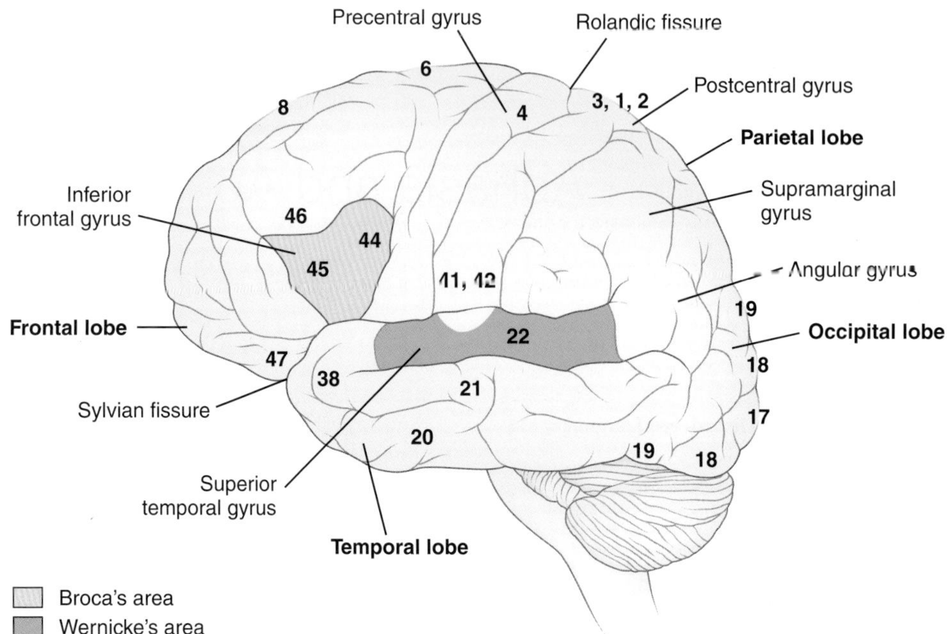


Fig. 13.1 The lateral surface of the left hemisphere, showing a simplified gyral anatomy and the relationships between Wernicke area and Broca area. Not shown is the arcuate fasciculus, which connects the two cortical speech centers via the deep, subcortical white matter.

last few decades based on numerous studies using the diverse methodologies of cognitive neuroscience.

For both repetition and spontaneous speech, auditory information is transmitted via direct and indirect dorsal pathways to Broca area in the posterior inferior frontal gyrus. This area of cortex "programs" the neurons in the adjacent motor cortex, subserving the mouth and larynx, from which descending axons travel to the brainstem cranial nerve nuclei. The inferior parietal lobule, especially the supramarginal gyrus, may also be involved in encoding of speech sounds for production. These anatomical relationships are shown in Figs. 13.1 and 13.2. Reading requires the perception of visual language stimuli by the occipital cortex, followed by processing into auditory language information. Writing involves the activation of motor neurons projecting to the arm and hand. A French study of 107 stroke patients, investigated with aphasia testing and magnetic resonance imaging (MRI) scans, confirmed the general themes of nearly 150 years of clinical aphasia research: frontal lesions caused nonfluent aphasia, whereas posterior temporal lesions affected comprehension (Kreisler et al., 2000).

These pathways, and doubtless others, constitute the cortical circuitry for language comprehension and expression. In addition, other cortical centers involved in cognitive processes project into the primary language cortex, influencing the content of language. Finally, subcortical structures play increasingly recognized roles in language functions. The thalamus, a relay for the reticular activating system, appears to alert the language cortex, and lesions of the dominant thalamus frequently produce fluent aphasia. Nuclei of the basal ganglia involved in motor functions, especially the caudate nucleus and putamen, participate in expressive speech. No wonder, then, that language disorders are seen with a wide variety of brain lesions and are important in practical neurological diagnosis and localization.

In almost all right-handed people, and in a majority of left-handers as well, clinical syndromes of aphasia result from left hemisphere lesions. Rarely, aphasia may result from a right hemisphere lesion in a right-handed patient, a phenomenon called *crossed aphasia* (Bakar et al., 1996).

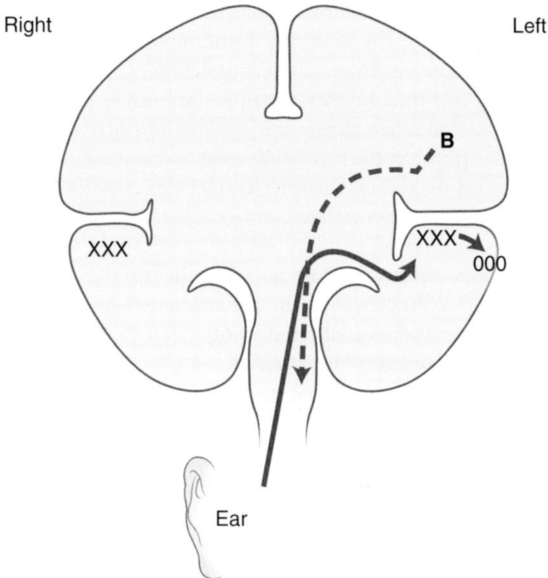


Fig. 13.2 Coronal plane diagram of the brain, indicating the inflow of auditory information from the ears to the primary auditory cortex in both superior temporal regions *(xxx)* and then to the Wernicke area *(ooo)* in the left superior temporal gyrus. The motor outflow of speech descends from the Broca area *(B)* to the cranial nerve nuclei of the brainstem via the corticobulbar tract *(dashed arrow)*. In actuality, the Broca area is anterior to the Wernicke area, and the two areas would not appear in the same coronal section.

## SYMPTOMS AND DIFFERENTIAL DIAGNOSIS OF DISORDERED LANGUAGE

*Muteness*, a total loss of speech, may represent severe aphasia (see the section Aphemia, a rare syndrome, later in this chapter). Muteness can also be a sign of dysarthria; frontal lobe dysfunction with akinetic mutism; severe extrapyramidal system dysfunction, as in Parkinson disease; non-neurological disorders of the larynx and pharynx; or even psychogenic syndromes, such as catatonia. Caution must therefore be taken in diagnosing the mute patient as aphasic. A good rule of thumb is that if the patient can write or type and the language form and content are normal, the disorder is probably not aphasic in origin. If the patient cannot speak or write but makes apparent effort to vocalize, and if there is also evidence of deficient comprehension, aphasic muteness is likely. Associated signs of a left hemisphere injury, such as right hemiparesis, also aid in diagnosis. Finally, if the patient gradually begins to make sounds containing paraphasic errors, aphasia can be identified with confidence.

Halting and effortful speech is a symptom of aphasia, but also of motor speech disorders, such as dysarthria or stuttering, and it may be a manifestation of a psychogenic disorder (see under Differential Diagnosis of Causes of Aphasia, later in this chapter; Binder et al., 2012). A second rule of thumb is that if one can transcribe the utterances of an effortful speaker into normal language, the patient is not aphasic. Effortful speech occurs in many aphasia syndromes for varying reasons, including difficulty in speech initiation, imprecise articulation of phonemes, deficient syntax, or word-finding difficulty.

*Anomia*, or inability to produce a specific name, is generally a reliable indicator of language disorder, although it may also reflect memory loss. Anomia is manifest in aphasic speech by word-finding pauses and circumlocutions or use of a phrase where a single word would suffice.

*Paraphasic speech* refers to the presence of errors in the patient's speech output. Paraphasic errors are divided into literal or phonemic errors, involving substitution of an incorrect sound (e.g., shoon for spoon), and verbal or semantic errors, involving substitution of an incorrect word (e.g., fork for spoon). A related language symptom is *perseveration*, the inappropriate repetition of a previous response. Occasionally, aphasic utterances involve nonexistent word forms called *neologisms*. A pattern of paraphasic errors and neologisms that so contaminate speech that the meaning cannot be discerned is called *jargon*.

Another cardinal symptom of aphasia is the failure to comprehend the speech of others. Most aphasic patients also have difficulty with comprehension and production of written language (reading and writing).

Fluent, paraphasic speech usually makes an aphasic disorder obvious. The chief differential diagnosis here involves aphasia, psychosis, acute encephalopathy or delirium, and dementia. Aphasic patients are usually not confused or inappropriate in behavior; they do not appear agitated or misuse objects, with occasional exceptions in acute syndromes of Wernicke or global aphasia. By contrast, most psychotic patients speak in an easily understood, grammatically appropriate manner, but their behavior and speech content are abnormal. Only rarely do schizophrenics speak in "clang association" or "word salad" speech. Sudden onset of fluent, paraphasic speech in a middle-aged or elderly patient should always be suspected of representing a left hemisphere lesion with aphasia.

Patients with acute encephalopathy or delirium may manifest paraphasic speech and "higher" language disorders, such as inability to write, but the grammatical expression of language is less disturbed than is its content. These language symptoms, moreover, are less prominent than accompanying behavioral disturbances, such as agitation, hallucinations, drowsiness, or excitement, and cognitive difficulties, such as disorientation, memory loss, and delusional thinking.

Chronic encephalopathies, or dementias, pose a more difficult diagnostic problem because involvement of the language cortex produces readily detectable language deficits, especially involving naming, reading, and writing. These language disorders (see Language in Dementing Diseases, later in this chapter) differ from aphasia secondary to focal lesions mainly by the involvement of other cognitive functions, such as memory and visuospatial processes.

**BOX 13.1 Bedside Language Examination**

1. Spontaneous speech
   a. Informal interview
   b. Structured task
   c. Automatic sequences
2. Naming
3. Auditory comprehension
4. Repetition
5. Reading
   a. Reading aloud
   b. Reading comprehension
6. Writing
   a. Spontaneous sentences
   b. Writing to dictation
   c. Copying

## BEDSIDE LANGUAGE EXAMINATION

The first part of any bedside examination of language is the observation of the patient's speech and comprehension during the clinical interview. A wealth of information about language function can be obtained if the examiner pays deliberate attention to the patient's speech patterns and responses to questions. In particular, minor word-finding difficulty, occasional paraphasic errors, and higher-level deficits in discourse planning and in the pragmatics of communication, such as turn-taking in conversation and the use of humor and irony, can be detected principally during the informal interview.

D. Frank Benson and Norman Geschwind popularized a bedside language examination of six parts, updated by Alexander and Benson (1997) (Box 13.1). This examination provides useful localizing information about brain dysfunction and is well worth the few minutes it takes.

The first part of the examination is an analysis of spontaneous speech. A speech sample may be elicited by asking the patient to describe the weather or the reason for coming to the doctor. If speech is sparse or absent, recitation of lists, such as counting or listing days of the week, may be helpful. The most important variable in spontaneous speech is fluency: fluent speech flows rapidly and effortlessly; nonfluent speech is uttered in single words or short phrases, with frequent pauses and hesitations. Attention should first be paid to such elementary characteristics as initiation difficulty, articulation, phonation or voice volume, rate of speech, prosody or melodic intonation of speech, and phrase length. Second, the content of speech utterances should be analyzed in terms of the presence of word-finding pauses, circumlocutions, and errors such as literal and verbal paraphasias and neologisms.

Naming, the second part of the bedside examination, is tested by asking the patient to name objects, object parts, pictures, colors, or body parts. A few items from each category should be tested because anomia can be specific to word classes. Proper names of persons are often affected severely. The examiner should ask questions to be sure that the patient recognizes the items or people that he or she cannot name.

Auditory comprehension is tested first by asking the patient to follow a series of commands of one, two, and three steps. An example of a one-step command is "stick out your tongue"; a two-step command is "hold up your left thumb and close your eyes." Successful following of commands ensures adequate comprehension, at least at this simple level, but failure to follow commands does not automatically establish a loss of comprehension. The patient must hear the command, understand the language the examiner speaks, and possess the motor ability to execute it, including the absence of apraxia. *Apraxia* (see Chapter 11 for full discussion) is defined operationally as the inability to carry out a motor command despite normal comprehension and normal ability to carry out the motor act in another context, such as to imitation or with use of a real object. Because apraxia is difficult to exclude with confidence, it is advisable to test comprehension by tasks that do not require a motor act, such as yes–no questions, or by commands that require only a pointing response. The responses to nonsense questions (e.g., "Do you vomit every day?") quickly establish whether the patient comprehends. Nonsense questions often produce surprising results, given the tendency of some aphasics to cover up comprehension difficulty with social chatter.

Repetition of words and phrases should be deliberately tested. Dysarthric patients have difficulty with rapid and variable sequences of consonants, such as "Methodist Episcopal," whereas people with aphasia have particular difficulty with grammatically complex sentences. The phrase "no ifs, ands, or buts" is especially challenging for individuals with aphasia. Often, they can repeat familiar or "high-probability" phrases much better than unfamiliar ones.

Reading should be tested both aloud and for comprehension. The examiner should carry a few printed commands to facilitate a rapid comparison of auditory with reading comprehension. Of course, the examiner must have some idea of the patient's premorbid reading ability.

Writing, the element of the bedside examination most often omitted, not only provides a further sample of expressive language but also allows an analysis of spelling, which is not possible with spoken language. A writing specimen may be the most sensitive indicator of mild aphasia, and it provides a permanent record for future comparison. Spontaneous writing, such as a sentence describing why the patient has come for examination, is especially sensitive for the detection of language difficulty. When spontaneous writing fails, writing to dictation and copying should be tested as well.

Finally, the neurologist combines the results of the bedside language examination with those of the rest of the mental status examination and of the neurological examination in general. These "associated signs" help to classify the type of aphasia and to localize the responsible brain lesion.

## DIFFERENTIAL DIAGNOSIS OF APHASIC SYNDROMES

### Broca Aphasia

In 1861, the French physician Paul Broca described a nonfluent speech disorder in two patients, one of whom could say only "tan.. tan". He proposed the term aphemia, but aphasia was adopted. In Broca aphasia, the speech pattern is nonfluent; on bedside examination, the patient speaks hesitantly, often producing the principal, meaning-containing nouns and verbs but omitting small grammatical words and morphemes. This pattern is called *agrammatism* or telegraphic speech. An example is "wife come hospital." Patients with acute Broca aphasia may be mute or may produce only single words, often with dysarthria and apraxia of speech. They make many phonemic errors, inconsistent from utterance to utterance, with substitution of phonemes usually differing only slightly from the correct target (e.g., p for b). Naming is deficient, but the patient often manifests a "tip of the tongue" phenomenon, getting out the first letter or phoneme of the correct name. Paraphasic errors in naming are more frequently of literal than verbal type. Auditory comprehension seems intact, but detailed testing usually reveals some deficiency, particularly in the comprehension of complex syntax. For example, sentences with embedded clauses involving prepositional relationships cause difficulty for patients with Broca aphasia in comprehension as well as in expression ("The rug that Bill gave to Betty tripped the visitor"). This may reflect the demands that these types of sentences make on working memory and other functions that depend on the frontal lobe. A study of grammatical comprehension in normal subjects with positron emission tomography (PET) scanning did show activation of the left frontal, Broca area during this function (Caplan et al., 1998). Repetition is hesitant in these patients, resembling their spontaneous speech. Reading is often impaired, despite relatively preserved auditory comprehension. Patients with Broca aphasia may have difficulty with syntax in reading, just as in auditory comprehension and speech. Writing is virtually always deficient in Broca aphasia. Most patients have a right hemiparesis, necessitating use of the nondominant, left hand for writing, but this left-handed writing is far more abnormal than the awkward renditions of a normal right-handed subject. Many patients can scrawl only a few letters.

**TABLE 13.1 Bedside Features of Broca Aphasia**

| Feature | Syndrome |
|---|---|
| Spontaneous speech | Nonfluent, mute, or telegraphic, sometimes dysarthric |
| Naming | Impaired |
| Comprehension | Intact (mild difficulty with complex grammatical phrases) |
| Repetition | Impaired |
| Reading | Often impaired ("third alexia") |
| Writing | Impaired (dysmorphic, dysgrammatical) |
| Associated signs | Right hemiparesis<br>Right hemisensory loss<br>± Apraxia of left limbs |

Associated neurological deficits of Broca aphasia include right hemiparesis, hemisensory loss, and apraxia of the oral apparatus and the nonparalyzed (typically left) limbs. Apraxia in response to motor commands is important to recognize because it may be mistaken for comprehension disturbance. Comprehension should be tested by responses to yes-no questions or commands to point to an object. The common features of Broca aphasia are listed in Table 13.1.

An important clinical feature of Broca aphasia is its frequent association with depression (Robinson 1997). Patients with Broca aphasia are typically aware of and frustrated by their deficits. At times, they become withdrawn and refuse help or therapy. Usually, the depression lifts as the deficit recovers, but it may be a limiting factor in rehabilitation.

The lesions responsible for Broca aphasia usually include the traditional Broca area in the posterior part of the inferior frontal gyrus, along with damage to adjacent cortex and subcortical white matter. Most patients with lasting Broca aphasia, including Broca original cases, have much larger left frontoparietal lesions, including most of the territory of the upper division of the left middle cerebral artery. Such patients typically evolve from global to Broca aphasia over weeks to months. Patients who manifest Broca aphasia immediately after their strokes, by contrast, have smaller lesions of the inferior frontal region, and their deficits generally resolve quickly.

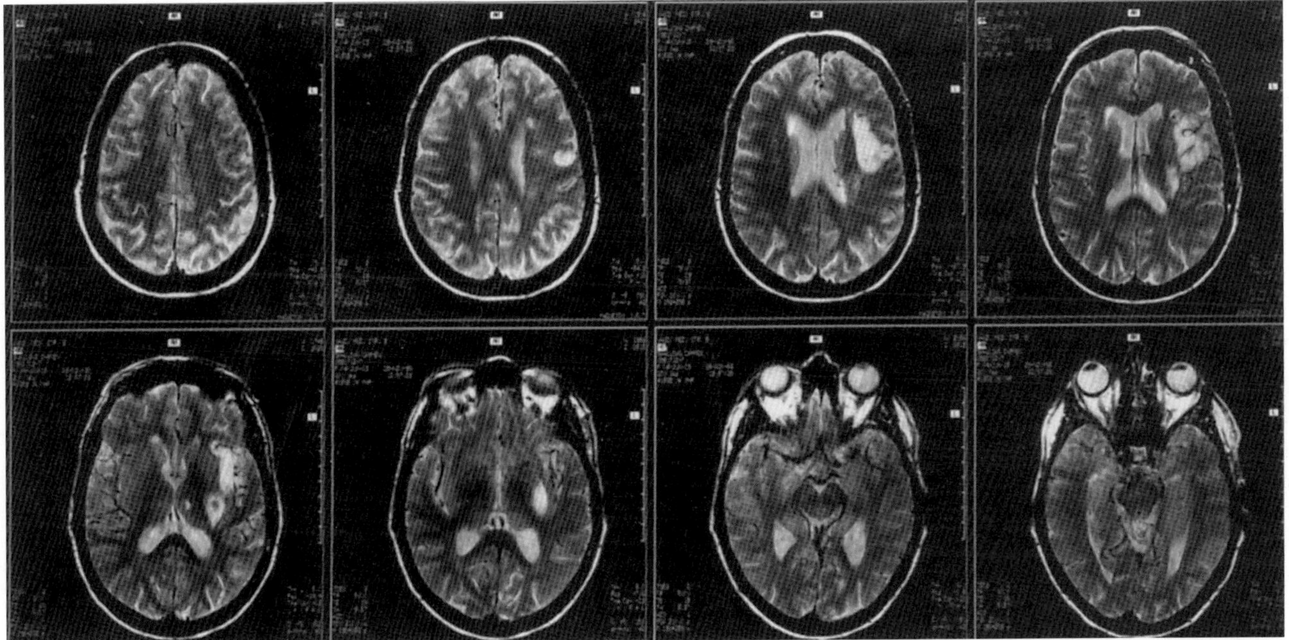

**Fig. 13.3** Magnetic resonance imaging scans from a patient with Broca aphasia. In this patient, the cortical Broca area, subcortical white matter, and the insula were all involved in the infarction. The patient made a good recovery.

In computed tomography (CT) scan analyses at the Boston Veterans Administration Medical Center, lesions restricted to the lower precentral gyrus produced only dysarthria and mild expressive disturbance. Lesions involving the traditional Broca area (Brodmann areas 44 and 45) resulted in difficulty initiating speech, and lesions combining Broca area, the lower precentral gyrus, and subcortical white matter yielded the full syndrome of Broca aphasia (Alexander et al., 1990). In studies by the same group, damage to two subcortical white matter sites—the rostral subcallosal fasciculus deep to the Broca area and the periventricular white matter adjacent to the body of the left lateral ventricle—was required to cause permanent nonfluency. Fig. 13.3 shows an MRI scan from a case of Broca aphasia.

## Aphemia

This rare syndrome, not much discussed currently, involves transient muteness in patients with isolated lesions centered on the left frontal Broca area, its subcortical white matter, or the inferior precentral gyrus. Aphemia may not classify as a language disorder if writing is normal.

## Wernicke Aphasia

Wernicke aphasia may be considered a syndrome opposite to Broca aphasia, in that expressive speech is fluent, but comprehension is impaired. The speech pattern is effortless and sometimes even excessively fluent (logorrhea). A speaker of a foreign language might notice nothing amiss, but a listener who shares the patient's language detects speech empty of meaning, containing verbal paraphasias, neologisms, and jargon productions. In milder cases, the intended meaning of an utterance may be discerned, but the sentence goes awry with paraphasic substitutions. Naming in Wernicke aphasia is deficient, often with bizarre, paraphasic substitutions for the correct name. Auditory comprehension is impaired, sometimes even for simple nonsense questions. Repetition is impaired; whispering a phrase in the patient's ear, as in a hearing test, may help cue the patient to attempt repetition. Reading comprehension is usually affected similarly to auditory comprehension, but occasional patients show greater deficits in one modality versus the other. The discovery of relatively spared reading ability in Wernicke aphasics is important in allowing these patients to communicate. Writing is also impaired, but in a manner quite different from that of Broca aphasia. The patient usually has no hemiparesis and can grasp the pen and write easily. Written productions are even more abnormal than oral ones, however, in that spelling errors are also evident. Writing samples are especially useful in the detection of mild Wernicke aphasia.

**TABLE 13.2 Bedside Features of Wernicke Aphasia**

| Feature | Syndrome |
|---|---|
| Spontaneous speech | Fluent, with paraphasic errors<br>Usually not dysarthric<br>Sometimes logorrheic |
| Naming | Impaired (often bizarre paraphasic misnaming) |
| Comprehension | Impaired |
| Repetition | Impaired |
| Reading | Impaired for comprehension, reading aloud |
| Writing | Well-formed, paragraphic |
| Associated signs | ± Right hemianopia<br>Motor, sensory signs usually absent |

Associated signs are limited in Wernicke aphasia; most patients have no elementary motor or sensory deficits, although a partial or complete right homonymous hemianopia may be present. The characteristic bedside examination findings in Wernicke aphasia are summarized in Table 13.2.

The psychiatric manifestations of Wernicke aphasia are quite different from those of Broca aphasia. Depression is less common; many Wernicke aphasics seem unaware of or unconcerned about their communicative deficits. With time, some patients become angry or

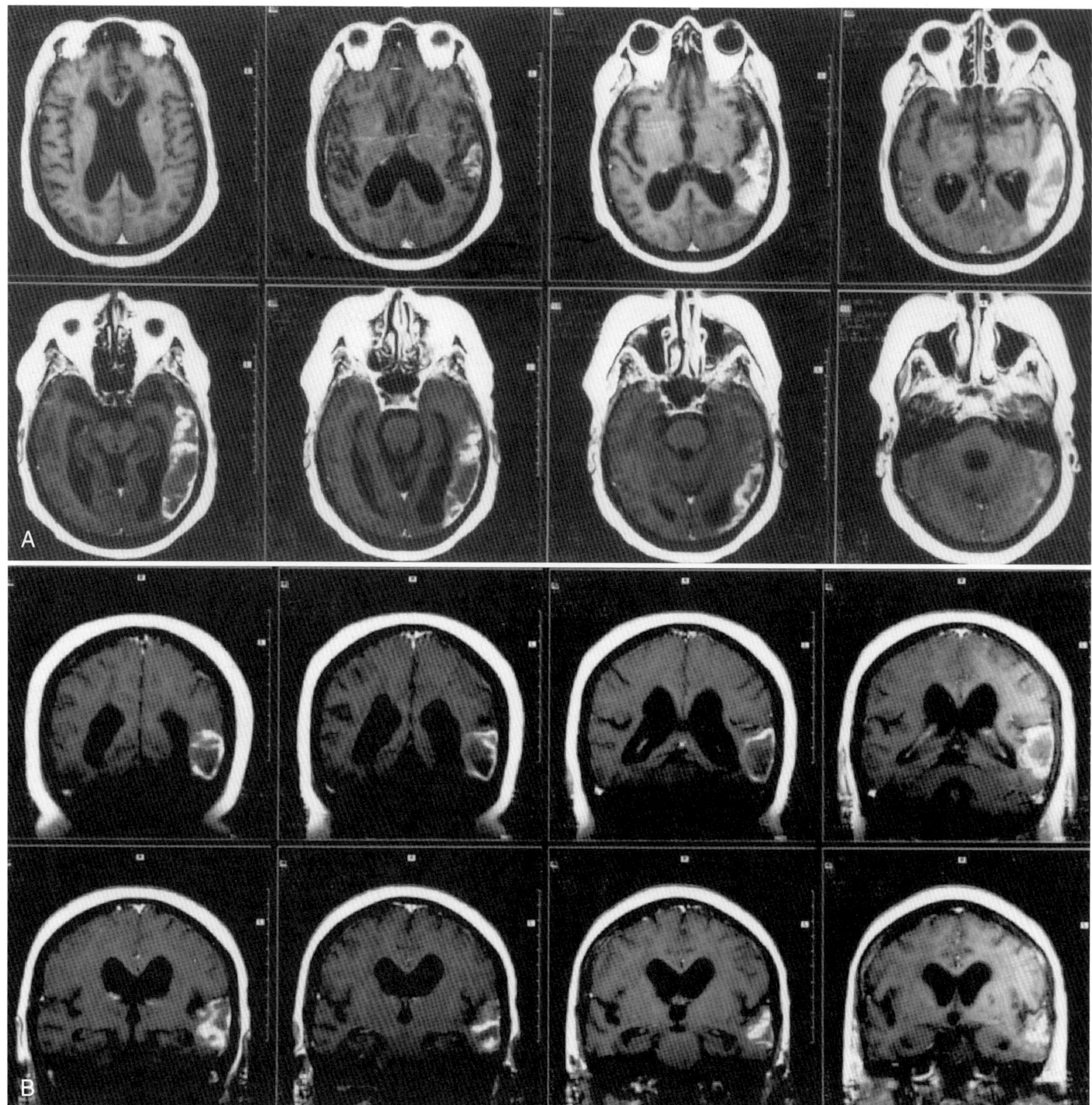

**Fig. 13.4** Axial and coronal magnetic resonance imaging slices (**A** and **B**), and an axial positron emission tomographic (PET) scan view (**C**) of an elderly woman with Wernicke aphasia. There is a large left superior temporal lobe lesion. The onset of the deficit was not clear, and the PET scan was useful in showing that the lesion had reduced metabolism, favoring a stroke over a tumor.

paranoid about the inability of family members and medical staff to understand them. This behavior, similarly to depression, may hinder rehabilitative efforts.

The lesions of patients with Wernicke aphasia are usually centered on the posterior portion of the superior temporal gyrus, extending into the inferior parietal lobule and middle temporal gyrus Kertesz et al., 1993). Fig. 13.4 shows a typical example. In the acute phase, the ability to match a spoken word to a picture is quantitatively related to decreased perfusion of the Wernicke area on perfusion-weighted MRI, indicating less variability during the acute phase than after recovery has taken place (Hillis et al., 2001). Recent literature (see Binder, 2015; Bonilha et al., 2017) has suggested that auditory comprehension is subserved by wider regions of the left temporal lobe. Electrical stimulation of the Wernicke area produces consistent interruption of auditory comprehension, supporting the importance of this region for decoding auditory language (Boatman et al., 1995). A receptive speech area in the left inferior temporal gyrus has also been suggested by electrical stimulation studies and by a few descriptions of patients with seizures involving this area (Kirshner et al., 1995). In terms of vascular anatomy, Wernicke aphasia is generally associated with the inferior division of the left middle cerebral artery.

## Pure Word Deafness

Pure word deafness is a rare but striking syndrome of isolated loss of auditory comprehension and repetition, without any abnormality of speech, naming, reading, or writing. Hearing for pure tones and for

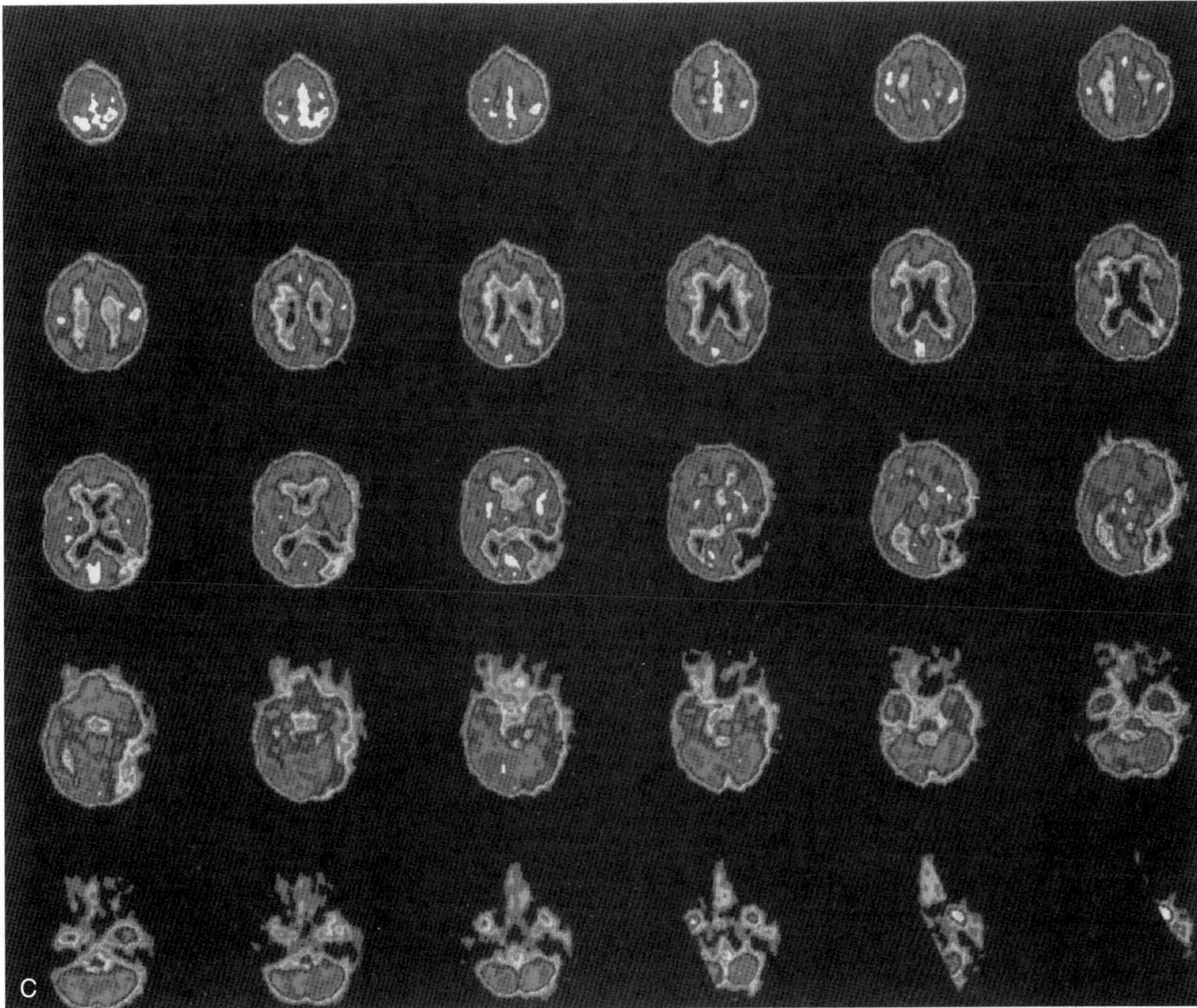


Fig. 13.4–Cont'd

nonverbal noises, such as animal cries, is intact. Most cases have mild aphasic deficits, especially paraphasic speech. Classically, the anatomical substrate is a bilateral lesion, isolating Wernicke area from input from the primary auditory cortex, in the bilateral Heschl gyri. Pure word deafness is thus an example of a "disconnection syndrome," in which the deficit results from loss of white matter connections rather than of gray matter language centers. Some cases of pure word deafness, however, have unilateral, left temporal lesions, if the lesion is placed such as to disconnect Wernicke area from primary auditory cortex of both hemispheres.

## Global Aphasia

Global aphasia may be thought of as a summation of the deficits of Broca aphasia and Wernicke aphasia. Speech is nonfluent or mute, but comprehension is also poor, as are naming, repetition, reading, and writing. Most patients have dense right hemiparesis, hemisensory loss, and often hemianopia, although occasional patients have little hemiparesis. Milder aphasic syndromes in which all modalities of language are affected are often called *mixed aphasias*. The lesions of patients with global aphasia are usually large, involving both the inferior frontal and the superior temporal regions and often much of the parietal lobe in between. This lesion represents most of the territory of the left middle cerebral artery. Patients in whom the superior temporal gyrus is spared tend to recover their auditory comprehension and to evolve toward the syndrome of Broca aphasia. Recovery in global aphasia may be prolonged; global aphasics may recover more during the second 6 months than during the first 6 months after a stroke (Sarno and Levita, 1979). Characteristics of global aphasia are presented in Table 13.3.

## Conduction Aphasia

Conduction aphasia is a theoretically important syndrome that can be remembered by its striking deficit of repetition. Most patients have relatively fluent spontaneous speech but make literal paraphasic errors and hesitate frequently for self-correction. Naming may be impaired, but auditory comprehension is preserved. Repetition may be disturbed to seemingly ridiculous extremes, such that a patient who can express himself or herself at a sentence level and comprehend conversation may be unable to repeat even single words. One such patient could not repeat the word "boy" but said "I like girls better." Reading and writing are somewhat variable, but reading aloud may share some of the same difficulty as repeating. Associated deficits include hemianopia in some patients; right-sided sensory loss may be present, but right hemiparesis is usually mild or absent. Some patients have limb apraxia, creating a

**TABLE 13.3 Bedside Features of Global Aphasia**

| Feature | Syndrome |
|---|---|
| Spontaneous speech | Mute or nonfluent |
| Naming | Impaired |
| Comprehension | Impaired |
| Repetition | Impaired |
| Reading | Impaired |
| Writing | Impaired |
| Associated signs | Right hemiparesis<br>Right hemisensory loss<br>Right hemianopia |

**TABLE 13.4 Bedside Features of Conduction Aphasia**

| Feature | Syndrome |
|---|---|
| Spontaneous speech | Fluent, hesitancy, literal paraphasic errors |
| Naming | Moderately impaired |
| Comprehension | Intact |
| Repetition | Impaired |
| Reading | + Reading aloud moderately impaired; reading comprehension largely intact |
| Writing | Variable deficits |
| Associated signs | + Apraxia of left limbs<br>+ Right hemiparesis, usually mild<br>+ Right hemisensory loss<br>+ Right hemianopia |

misimpression that comprehension is impaired. Bedside examination findings in conduction aphasia are summarized in Table 13.4.

The lesions of conduction aphasia usually involve either the superior temporal or the inferior parietal regions. Benson and associates suggested that patients with limb apraxia have parietal lesions, whereas those without apraxia have temporal lesions (Benson et al., 1973). Conduction aphasia may represent a stage of recovery in patients with Wernicke aphasia in whom the damage to the superior temporal gyrus is not complete.

Conduction aphasia has been advanced as a classical disconnection syndrome. Wernicke originally postulated that a lesion disconnecting the Wernicke and Broca areas would produce this syndrome; Geschwind later pointed to the arcuate fasciculus, a white matter tract traveling from the deep temporal lobe, around the sylvian fissure to the frontal lobe, as the site of disconnection. Anatomical involvement of the arcuate fasciculus is present in most, if not all, cases of conduction aphasia, but some doubt has been raised about the importance of the arcuate fasciculus to conduction aphasia or even to repetition (Bernal and Ardila, 2009). In cases of conduction aphasia, there is usually also cortical involvement of the supramarginal gyrus or temporal lobe. The supramarginal gyrus appears to be involved in auditory immediate memory and in phoneme perception related to word meaning, as well as phoneme generation (Hickok and Poeppel, 2000). Lesions in this area are associated with conduction aphasia and phonemic paraphasic errors. Others have pointed out that lesions of the arcuate fasciculus do not always produce conduction aphasia. Another theory of conduction aphasia has involved a defect in auditory verbal short-term (or what most neurologists would call immediate) memory.

**TABLE 13.5 Bedside Features of Anomic Aphasia**

| Feature | Syndrome |
|---|---|
| Spontaneous speech | Fluent, some word-finding pauses, circumlocution |
| Naming | Impaired |
| Comprehension | Intact |
| Repetition | Intact |
| Reading | Intact |
| Writing | Intact, except for anomia |
| Associated signs | Variable or none |

## Anomic Aphasia

*Anomic aphasia* refers to aphasic syndromes in which naming, or access to the internal lexicon, is the principal deficit. Spontaneous speech is normal except for the pauses and circumlocutions produced by the inability to name. Comprehension, repetition, reading, and writing are intact, except for the same word-finding difficulty in written productions. Anomic aphasia is common but less specific in localization than other aphasic syndromes. Isolated, severe anomia may indicate focal left hemisphere pathology. Alexander and Benson (1997) refer to the angular gyrus as the site of lesions producing anomic aphasia, but lesions there usually produce other deficits as well, including alexia and the four elements of Gerstmann syndrome: agraphia, right-left disorientation, acalculia, and finger agnosia, or the inability to identify fingers. Isolated lesions of the temporal lobe can produce pure anomia. Inability to produce nouns is characteristic of temporal lobe lesions, whereas inability to produce verbs occurs more with frontal lesions (Damasio, 1992). Even specific classes of nouns may be selectively affected in some cases of anomic aphasia. Anomia is also seen with mass lesions elsewhere in the brain, and in diffuse degenerative disorders, such as Alzheimer disease (AD). Anomic aphasia is also a common stage in the recovery of many aphasic syndromes. Anomic aphasia thus serves as an indicator of left hemisphere or diffuse brain disease, but it has only limited localizing value. The typical features of anomic aphasia are presented in Table 13.5.

## Transcortical Aphasias

The transcortical aphasias are syndromes in which repetition is normal, presumably because the causative lesions do not disrupt the perisylvian language circuit from the Wernicke area through the arcuate fasciculus to the Broca area. Instead, these lesions disrupt connections from other cortical centers into the language circuit (hence the name "transcortical"). The transcortical syndromes are easiest to think of as analogues of the syndromes of global, Broca, and Wernicke aphasias, with intact repetition. In addition, because transcortical aphasias spare the perisylvian language circuit, they are often associated with watershed lesions, in the anterior frontal region between the anterior cerebral artery (ACA) and middle cerebral artery (MCA) distribution, or in the parietal region, between the MCA and posterior cerebral artery (PCA) distributions.

Mixed transcortical aphasia, or the syndrome of the isolation of the speech area, is a global aphasia in which the patient repeats, often echolalically, but has no propositional speech or comprehension. This syndrome is rare, occurring predominantly in large, watershed infarctions of the left hemisphere or both hemispheres that spare the perisylvian cortex, or in advanced dementias.

Transcortical motor aphasia is an analogue of Broca aphasia in which speech is hesitant or telegraphic, comprehension is relatively spared, but repetition is fluent. This syndrome occurs with lesions in

**TABLE 13.6 Bedside Features of Transcortical Aphasias**

| Feature | Isolation Syndrome | Transcortical Motor | Transcortical Sensory |
|---|---|---|---|
| Speech | Nonfluent, echo-lalic | Nonfluent | Fluent, echolalic |
| Naming | Impaired | Impaired | Impaired |
| Comprehension | Impaired | Intact | Impaired |
| Repetition | Intact | Intact | Intact |
| Reading | Impaired | ± Intact | Impaired |
| Writing | Impaired | ± Intact | Impaired |

the frontal lobe, anterior to the Broca area, in the deep frontal white matter, or in the medial frontal region, in the vicinity of the supplementary motor area. All of these lesion sites are within the territory of the anterior cerebral artery, separating this syndrome from the aphasia syndromes of the middle cerebral artery (Broca, Wernicke, global, and conduction).

The third transcortical syndrome, transcortical sensory aphasia, is an analogue of Wernicke aphasia in which fluent, paraphasic speech, paraphasic naming, impaired auditory and reading comprehension, and abnormal writing coexist with normal repetition. This syndrome is relatively uncommon, occurring in strokes of the left temporo-occipital area and in dementias. Bedside examination findings in the transcortical aphasias are summarized in Table 13.6.

## Subcortical Aphasias

A current area of interest in aphasia research involves the "subcortical" aphasias. Although all the syndromes discussed so far are defined by behavioral characteristics that can be diagnosed on the bedside examination, the subcortical aphasias are defined by lesion localization in the basal ganglia, thalamus, or deep cerebral white matter. As knowledge about subcortical aphasia has accumulated, two major groups of aphasic symptomatology have been described: aphasia with thalamic lesions and aphasia with lesions of the subcortical white matter and basal ganglia.

Left thalamic hemorrhages frequently produce a Wernicke-like fluent aphasia, with better comprehension than cortical Wernicke aphasia. A fluctuating or "dichotomous" state has been described, alternating between an alert state with nearly normal language and a drowsy state in which the patient mumbles paraphasically and comprehends poorly. Luria has called this a quasi-aphasic abnormality of vigilance, in that the thalamus plays a role in alerting the language cortex. Whereas some skeptics have attributed thalamic aphasia to pressure on adjacent structures and secondary effects on the cortex, cases of thalamic aphasia have been described with small ischemic lesions, especially those involving the paramedian or anterior nuclei of the thalamus, in the territory of the tuberothalamic artery. Because these lesions produce little or no mass effect, such cases indicate that the thalamus and its connections play a definite role in language function (Carrerra and Bogousslavsky, 2006). A case report found fluent aphasia in a left-handed patient with a right thalamic hemorrhage, raising the possibility that language dominance extends to the level of the thalamus (Kirshner & Kistler, 1982).

Lesions of the left basal ganglia and deep white matter also cause aphasia. As in thalamic aphasia, the first syndromes described were in basal ganglia hemorrhages, especially those involving the putamen, the most common site of hypertensive intracerebral hemorrhage. Here, the aphasic syndromes are more variable but most commonly involve global or Wernicke-like aphasia. As in thalamic lesions, ischemic strokes have provided better localizing information. The most common lesion is an infarct involving the anterior putamen, caudate nucleus, and anterior limb of the internal capsule. Patients with this lesion have an "anterior subcortical aphasia syndrome" involving dysarthria, decreased fluency, mildly impaired repetition, and mild comprehension disturbance (Mega and Alexander, 1994). This syndrome most closely resembles Broca aphasia, but with greater dysarthria and less language dysfunction. Fig. 13.5 shows an example of this syndrome. More restricted lesions of the anterior putamen, head of caudate, and periventricular white matter produce hesitancy or slow initiation of speech but little true language disturbance. More posterior lesions involving the putamen and deep temporal white matter, referred to as the *temporal isthmus*, are associated with fluent, paraphasic speech and impaired comprehension resembling Wernicke aphasia (Naeser et al., 1990). Small lesions in the posterior limb of the internal capsule and adjacent putamen cause mainly dysarthria, but mild aphasic deficits may occasionally occur. Finally, larger subcortical lesions involving both the anterior and the posterior lesion sites produce global aphasia. A wide variety of aphasia syndromes can thus be seen with subcortical lesion sites. Nadeau and Crosson (1997) presented an anatomical model of basal ganglia and deep white matter involvement in speech and language, based on the known motor functions and fiber connections of these structures.

Controversy has followed the identification of the insula as a source of speech production; Dronkers (1996) suggested this based on a lesion overlap analysis of cases of apraxia of speech. Hillis and colleagues (2004), however, showed that in acute aphasia, the left frontal cortex, and not the insula, is related to apraxia of speech.

In clinical terms, subcortical lesions do produce aphasia, although less commonly than cortical lesions do, and the language characteristics of subcortical aphasias are often atypical. The presentation of a difficult-to-classify aphasic syndrome, in the presence of dysarthria and right hemiparesis, should lead to suspicion of a subcortical lesion.

## Pure Alexia Without Agraphia

*Alexia*, or acquired inability to read, is a form of aphasia, according to the definition given at the beginning of this chapter. The classic syndrome of alexia, pure alexia without agraphia, was described by the French neurologist Dejerine in 1892. This syndrome may be thought of as a linguistic blindfolding: patients can write but cannot read their own writing. On bedside examination, speech, auditory comprehension, and repetition are normal. Naming may be deficient, especially for colors.

Patients initially cannot read at all; as they recover, they learn to read letter by letter, spelling out words laboriously. They cannot read words at a glance, as normal readers do. By contrast, they quickly understand words spelled orally to them, and they can spell normally. Some patients can match words to pictures, indicating that some subconscious awareness of the word is present, perhaps in the right hemisphere. Associated deficits include a right hemianopia or right upper quadrant defect in nearly all patients and, frequently, a deficit of short-term memory. There is usually no hemiparesis or sensory loss.

The causative lesion in pure alexia is nearly always a stroke in the territory of the left posterior cerebral artery, with infarction of the medial occipital lobe, often the splenium of the corpus callosum, and often the medial temporal lobe. Dejerine postulated a disconnection between the intact right visual cortex and left hemisphere language centers, particularly the angular gyrus. (Fig. 13.6 is an adaptation of Dejerine's original diagram.) Geschwind later rediscovered this disconnection hypothesis. Although Damasio and Damasio (1983) found splenial involvement in only 2 of 16 cases, they postulated a disconnection within the deep

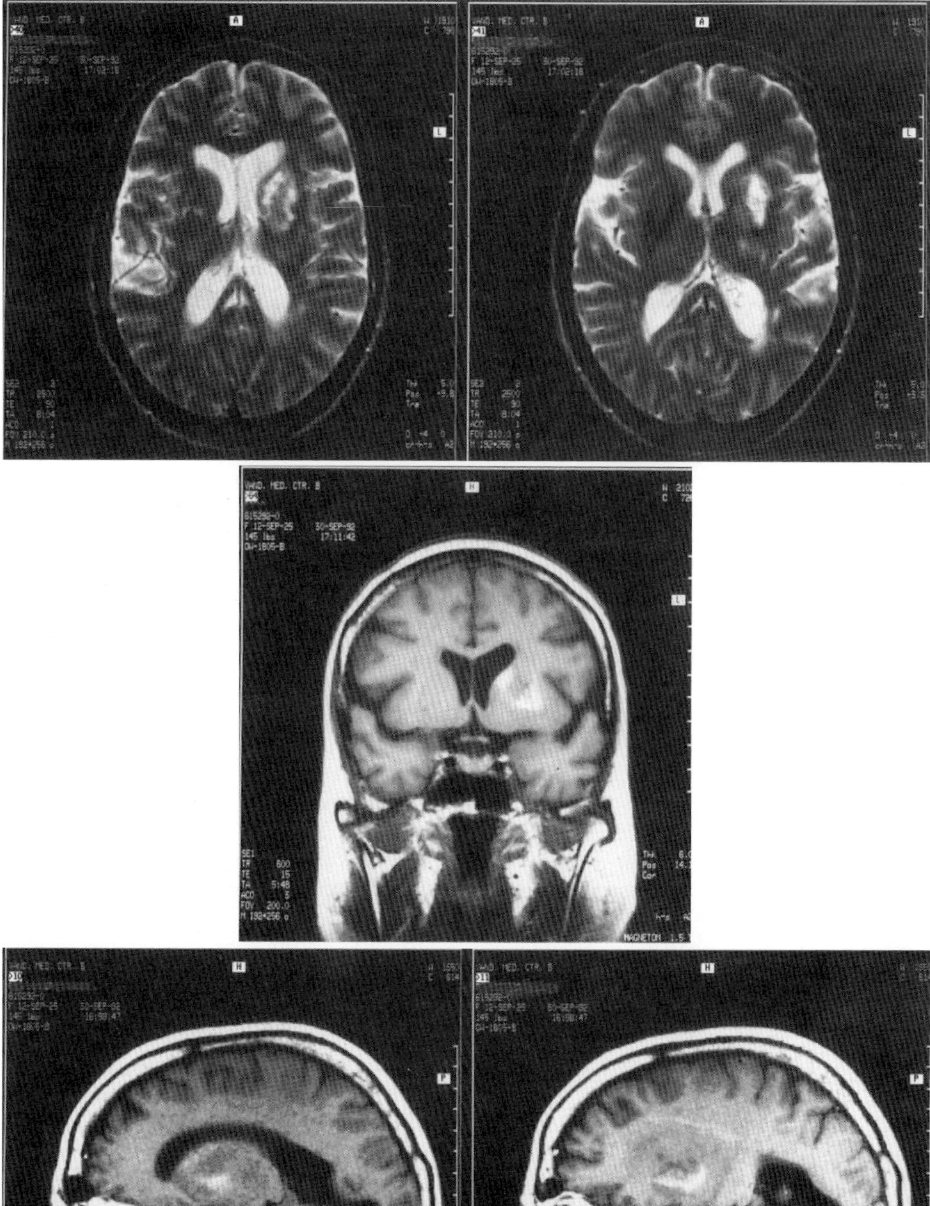

**Fig. 13.5** Magnetic resonance imaging (MRI) scan slices in the axial, coronal, and sagittal planes from a patient with subcortical aphasia. The lesion is an infarction involving the anterior caudate, putamen, and anterior limb of the left internal capsule. The patient presented with dysarthria and mild, nonfluent aphasia with anomia, with good comprehension. The advantage of MRI in permitting visualization of the lesion in all three planes is apparent.

white matter of the left occipital lobe. As in the disconnection hypothesis for conduction aphasia, the theory fails to explain all the behavioral phenomena, such as the sparing of single letters. A deficit in short-term memory for visual language elements, or an inability to perceive multiple letters at once (simultanagnosia), can also explain many features of the syndrome. Typical findings of pure alexia without agraphia are presented in Table 13.7 (Fig. 13.7).

## Alexia With Agraphia

The second classic alexia syndrome, alexia with agraphia, described by Dejerine in 1891, may be thought of as an acquired illiteracy, in which a previously educated patient is rendered unable to read or write. The oral language modalities of speech, naming, auditory comprehension, and repetition are largely intact, but many cases manifest a fluent, paraphasic speech pattern with impaired naming. This syndrome thus

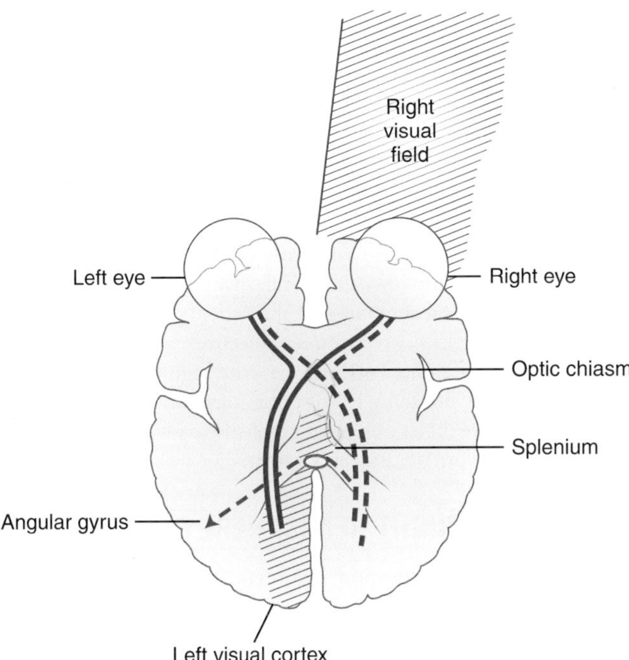


**Fig. 13.6** Horizontal brain diagram of pure alexia without agraphia, adapted from that of Dejerine in 1892. Visual information from the left visual field reaches the right occipital cortex but is "disconnected" from the left hemisphere language centers by the lesion in the splenium of the corpus callosum.

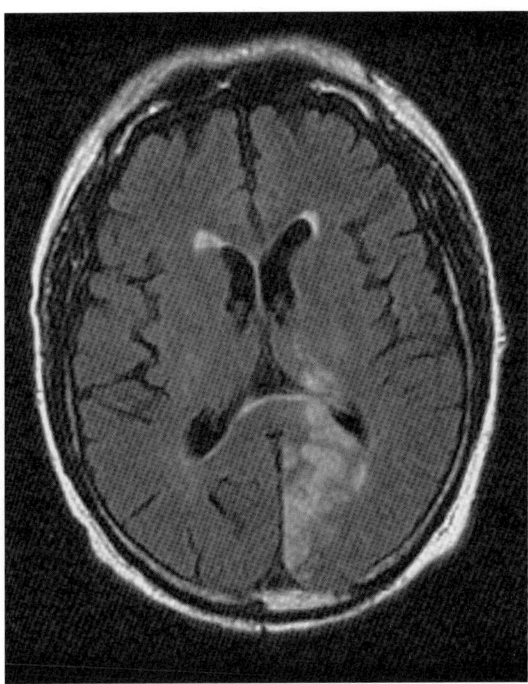

**Fig. 13.7** Fluid attenuated inversion recovery (FLAIR) magnetic resonance image of an 82-year-old male patient with alexia without agraphia. The infarction involves the medial occipital lobe and the splenium of the corpus callosum, within the territory of the left posterior cerebral artery.

**TABLE 13.7 Bedside Features of Pure Alexia Without Agraphia**

| Feature | Syndrome |
|---|---|
| Spontaneous speech | Intact |
| Naming | ± Impaired, especially colors |
| Comprehension | Intact |
| Repetition | Intact |
| Reading | Impaired (some sparing of single letters) |
| Writing | Intact |
| Associated signs | Right hemianopia or superior quadrantanopia<br>Short-term memory loss<br>Motor, sensory signs usually absent |

**TABLE 13.8 Bedside Features of Alexia With Agraphia**

| Feature | Syndrome |
|---|---|
| Spontaneous speech | Fluent, often some paraphasia |
| Naming | + Impaired |
| Comprehension | Intact, or less impaired than reading |
| Repetition | Intact |
| Reading | Severely impaired |
| Writing | Severely impaired |
| Associated signs | Right hemianopia<br>Motor, sensory signs often absent |

overlaps Wernicke aphasia, especially in cases in which reading is more impaired than auditory comprehension. Associated deficits include right hemianopia and elements of Gerstmann syndrome: agraphia, acalculia, right–left disorientation, and finger agnosia. The lesions typically involve the inferior parietal lobule, especially the angular gyrus. Etiologies include strokes in the territory of the angular branch of the left middle cerebral artery or mass lesions in the same region. Characteristic features of the syndrome of alexia with agraphia are summarized in Table 13.8.

## Aphasic Alexia

In addition to the two classic alexia syndromes, many patients with aphasia have associated reading disturbance. Neurolinguists and cognitive psychologists have divided alexias according to breakdowns in specific stages of the reading process. The linguistic concepts of surface structure versus the deep meanings of words have been instrumental in these new classifications. Four patterns of alexia (or dyslexia) have been recognized: letter-by-letter reading, deep, phonological, and surface dyslexia. Fig. 13.8 diagrams the steps in the reading process and the points of breakdown in the four syndromes. Letter-by-letter reading is equivalent to pure alexia without agraphia. Deep dyslexia is a severe reading disorder in which patients recognize and read aloud only familiar words, especially concrete, imageable nouns and verbs. They make semantic or visual errors in reading and fail completely in reading nonsense syllables or nonwords. Word reading is not affected by word length or by regularity of spelling; one patient, for example, could read "ambulance" but not "am." Most cases have severe aphasia, with extensive left frontoparietal damage.

Phonological dyslexia is similar to deep dyslexia, with poor reading of nonwords, but single nouns and verbs are read in a nearly normal fashion, and semantic errors are rare. The fourth type, surface dyslexia, involves spared ability to read by grapheme-phoneme conversion but inability to recognize long words, at a glance, or irregular words. These patients can read nonsense syllables but not words of irregular spelling, such as "colonel" or "yacht." Their errors tend to be phonological rather than semantic or visual (e.g., pronouncing rough and though alike).

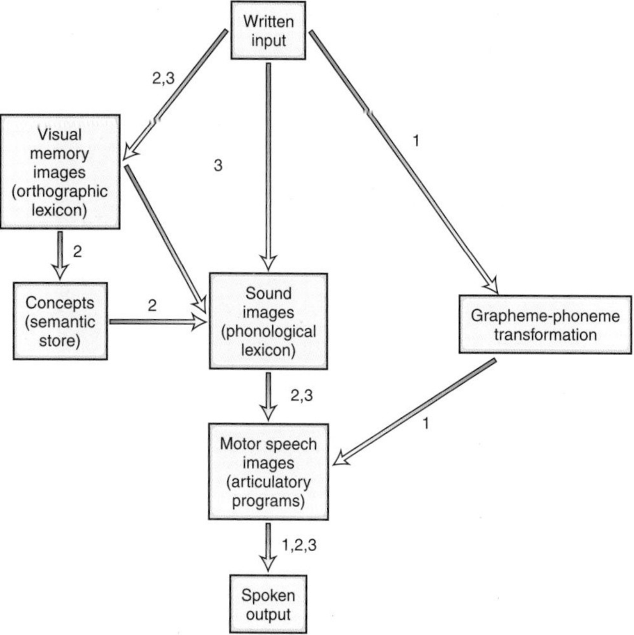


**Fig. 13.8 Neurolinguistic Model of the Reading Process.** According to evidence from the alexias, there are three separate routes to reading: 1 is the phonological (or grapheme-phoneme conversion) route; 2 is the semantic (or lexical-semantic-phonological) route; and 3 is the nonlexical phonological route. In deep dyslexia, only route 2 can operate; in phonological dyslexia, 3 is the principal pathway; in surface dyslexia, only 1 is functional. (*Adapted with permission from Margolin, D.I., 1991. Cognitive neuropsychology. Resolving enigmas about Wernicke aphasia and other higher cortical disorders. Arch. Neurol. 48, 751–765.*)

## Agraphia

Similarly to reading, writing may be affected either in isolation (pure agraphia) or in association with aphasia (aphasic agraphia). In addition, writing can be impaired by motor disorders, by apraxia, and by visuospatial deficits. Isolated agraphia has been described with left frontal or parietal lesions.

Agraphias can be analyzed in the same way as the alexias (Fig. 13.9). Thus, phonological agraphia involves the inability to convert phonemes into graphemes or to write pronounceable nonsense syllables, in the presence of ability to write familiar words. Deep dysgraphia is similar to phonological agraphia, but the patient can write nouns and verbs better than articles, prepositions, adjectives, and adverbs. In lexical or surface dysgraphia, patients can write regularly spelled words and pronounceable nonsense words but not irregularly spelled words. These patients have intact phoneme-grapheme conversion but cannot write by a whole-word or "lexical" strategy.

# LANGUAGE IN RIGHT HEMISPHERE DISORDERS

Language and communication disorders are important even in patients with right hemisphere disease. First, some patients, especially left-handed patients, may have right hemisphere language dominance and may develop aphasic syndromes from right hemisphere lesions. Second, rare right-handed patients develop aphasia after right hemisphere strokes, a phenomenon called "crossed aphasia" (Bakar et al., 1996). Third, even right-handed persons with typical left hemisphere dominance for language have subtly altered language function after right hemisphere damage. Such patients are not aphasic, in that the fundamental mechanisms of speech production, repetition, and comprehension are undisturbed. Affective aspects of language are impaired, however, such that the speech sounds flat and unemotional; the normal prosody, or emotional intonation, of speech is lost. Syndromes of loss of emotional aspects of speech are termed aprosodias. Motor aprosodia involves loss of expressive emotion with preservation of emotional comprehension; sensory aprosodia involves loss of comprehension of affective language, also called *affective agnosia*. More than

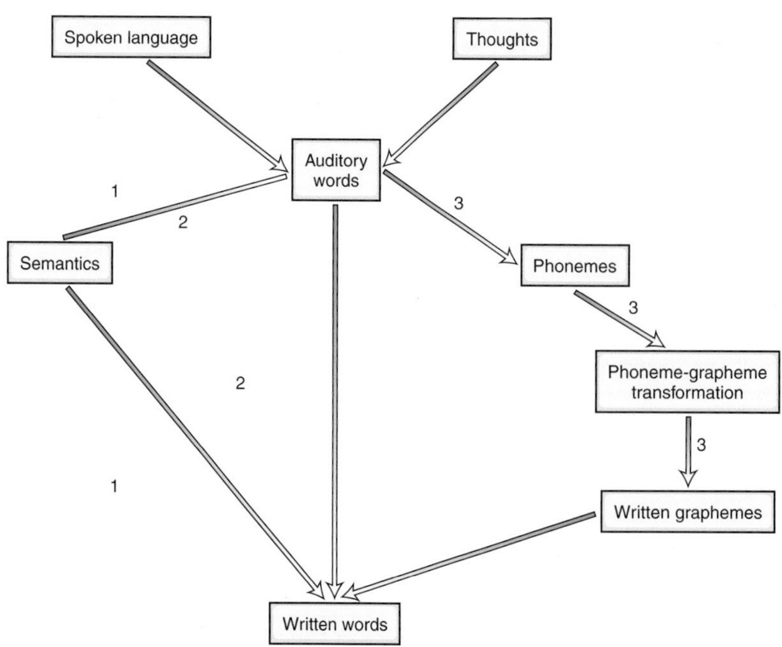


**Fig. 13.9 Neurolinguistic Model of Writing and the Agraphias.** In deep agraphia, only the semantic (phonological-semantic-lexical) route *(1)* is operative; in phonological agraphia, route *(2)*, the nonlexical phonological route produces written words directly from spoken words; in surface agraphia, only route *(3)*, the phoneme-grapheme pathway, can be used to generate writing.

just emotion, stress and emphasis within a sentence are also affected by right hemisphere dysfunction. More importantly, such vital aspects of human communication as metaphor, humor, sarcasm, irony, and related constituents of language that transcend the literal meaning of words are especially sensitive to right hemisphere dysfunction. These deficits significantly impair patients in the pragmatics of communication. In other words, right hemisphere–damaged patients understand what is said, but not how it is said. They may have difficulty following a complex story (Rehak et al., 1992). Such higher-level language deficits are related to the right hemisphere disorders of inattention and neglect, discussed in Chapters 4 and 45.

## LANGUAGE IN DEMENTING DISEASES

Language impairment is commonly seen in patients with dementia. Despite considerable variability from patient to patient, two patterns of language dissolution can be described. The first, the common presentation of AD, involves early loss of memory and general cognitive deterioration. In these patients, mental status examinations are most remarkable for deficits in short-term memory, insight, and judgment, but language impairments can be found in naming and in discourse, with impoverished language content and loss of abstraction and metaphor. The mechanics of language—grammatical construction of sentences, receptive vocabulary, auditory comprehension, repetition, and oral reading—tend to remain preserved until later stages. By aphasia testing, patients with early AD have anomic aphasia. In later stages, language functions become more obviously impaired. In terms of the components of language mentioned earlier in this chapter, the semantic aspects of language tend to deteriorate first, then syntax, and finally phonology. Reading and writing—the last-learned language functions—are among the first to decline. Auditory comprehension later becomes deficient, whereas repetition and articulation remain normal. The language profile may then resemble that of transcortical sensory or Wernicke aphasia. In terminal stages, speech is reduced to the expression of simple biological wants; eventually, even muteness can develop. By this time, most patients are institutionalized or bedridden.

The second pattern of language dissolution in dementia, less common than the first, involves the gradual onset of a progressive aphasia, often without other cognitive deterioration. Auditory comprehension is involved early in the illness, and specific aphasic symptoms are evident, such as paraphasic or nonfluent speech, misnaming, and errors of repetition. These deficits worsen gradually, mimicking the course of a brain tumor or mass lesion rather than a typical dementia (Grossman et al., 1996; Mesulam, 2001, 2003; Mesulam et al., 2014). The syndrome is referred to as "primary progressive aphasia (PPA)." MRI or CT scans may show focal atrophy in the left perisylvian region, while EEG studies may show focal slowing. PET has shown prominent areas of decreased metabolism in the left hemisphere regions.

Three variants of PPA are commonly recognized (Gorno-Tempini et al., 2011). Progressive nonfluent aphasia involves deficits in speech production and grammar, resembling Broca aphasia. Semantic dementia (Hodges and Patterson, 2007; Snowden et al., 1989) is a progressive fluent aphasia with impaired naming and loss of understanding of even single words. In reading, these patients may have a surface alexia pattern. The third variant of PPA, logopenic progressive aphasia, involves anomia and some repetition difficulty, with intact single-word comprehension (Gorno-Tempini et al., 2008). These three patterns of PPA are associated with different patterns of atrophy on MRI and hypometabolism on PET: progressive nonfluent aphasia is associated with left frontal and insular atrophy; semantic dementia is associated with bilateral anterior temporal atrophy; logopenic progressive aphasia is associated with left posterior temporal and inferior parietal atrophy (Diehl et al., 2004; Josephs et al., 2010). Progressive nonfluent aphasia and semantic dementia usually reflect different forms of frontotemporal lobar degeneration (FTLD), whereas logopenic progressive aphasia is most commonly due to Alzheimer pathology with an atypical anatomical distribution. Progressive nonfluent aphasias are often tauopathies, in familial cases related to mutations on chromosome 17 (Heutink et al., 1997), while semantic dementia may be related to ubiquitin deposition and mutations in the progranulin gene, with production of TDP-43 (Baker et al., 2006; Cruts et al., 2006). Another neurodegenerative diseases that can present with language abnormalities or PPA is corticobasal degeneration (Kertesz et al., 2000, Litvan et al., 1998). Creutzfeldt–Jakob disease can present with a rapidly progressive aphasia.

## INVESTIGATION OF THE APHASIC PATIENT

### Clinical Tests

The bedside language examination is useful in forming a preliminary impression of the type of aphasia and the localization of the causative lesion. Follow-up examinations are also helpful; as in all neurological diagnosis, the evolution of a neurological deficit over time is the most important clue to the specific disease process. For example, an embolic stroke and a brain tumor might both produce Wernicke aphasia, but strokes occur suddenly, with improvement thereafter, whereas tumors produce gradually worsening aphasia.

In addition to the bedside examination, a large number of standardized aphasia test batteries have been published. The physician should think of these tests as more detailed extensions of the bedside examination. They have the advantage of quantitation and standardization, permitting comparison over time and, in some cases, even a diagnosis of the specific aphasia syndrome. Research on aphasia depends on these standardized tests.

For neurologists, the most helpful battery is the Boston Diagnostic Aphasia Examination, or its Canadian adaptation, the Western Aphasia Battery. Both tests provide subtest information analogous to the bedside examination, and are therefore meaningful to neurologists, as well as aphasia syndrome classification. The Porch Index of Communicative Ability quantifies performance in many specific functions, allowing comparison over time. Other aphasia tests are designed to evaluate specific language areas. For example, the Boston Naming Test provides a large graded set of naming stimuli, while the Token Test evaluates higher-level comprehension deficits. Further information on neuropsychological tests can be found in Chapter 43.

Further diagnosis of the aphasic patient rests on the confirmation of a brain lesion by neuroimaging (Fig. 13.10). The advent of CT and MRI (discussed in Chapter 40) revolutionized the localization of aphasia by permitting "real-time" delineation of a focal lesion in a living patient; previously, the physician had to outlive the patient to obtain a clinical–pathological correlation at autopsy. MRI scanning provides better resolution of areas difficult to see on CT, such as the temporal cortex adjacent to the petrous bones, and more sensitive detection of tissue pathology, such as early changes of infarction. The anatomical distinction of cortical from subcortical aphasia is best made by MRI. Acute strokes are visualized early on diffusion-weighted MRI.

The EEG is helpful in aphasia in localizing seizure discharges, interictal spikes, and slowing seen after destructive lesions, such as traumatic contusions and infarctions. The EEG can provide evidence that aphasia is an ictal or postictal phenomenon and can furnish early clues to aphasia secondary to mass lesions or to herpes simplex encephalitis. In research applications, electrophysiological testing via subdural grid and depth electrodes, or stimulation mapping of epileptic foci in preparation for epilepsy surgery, has aided in the identification of cortical areas involved in language.

Cerebral arteriography is useful in the diagnosis of aneurysms, arteriovenous malformations (AVMs), arterial occlusions, vasculitis,

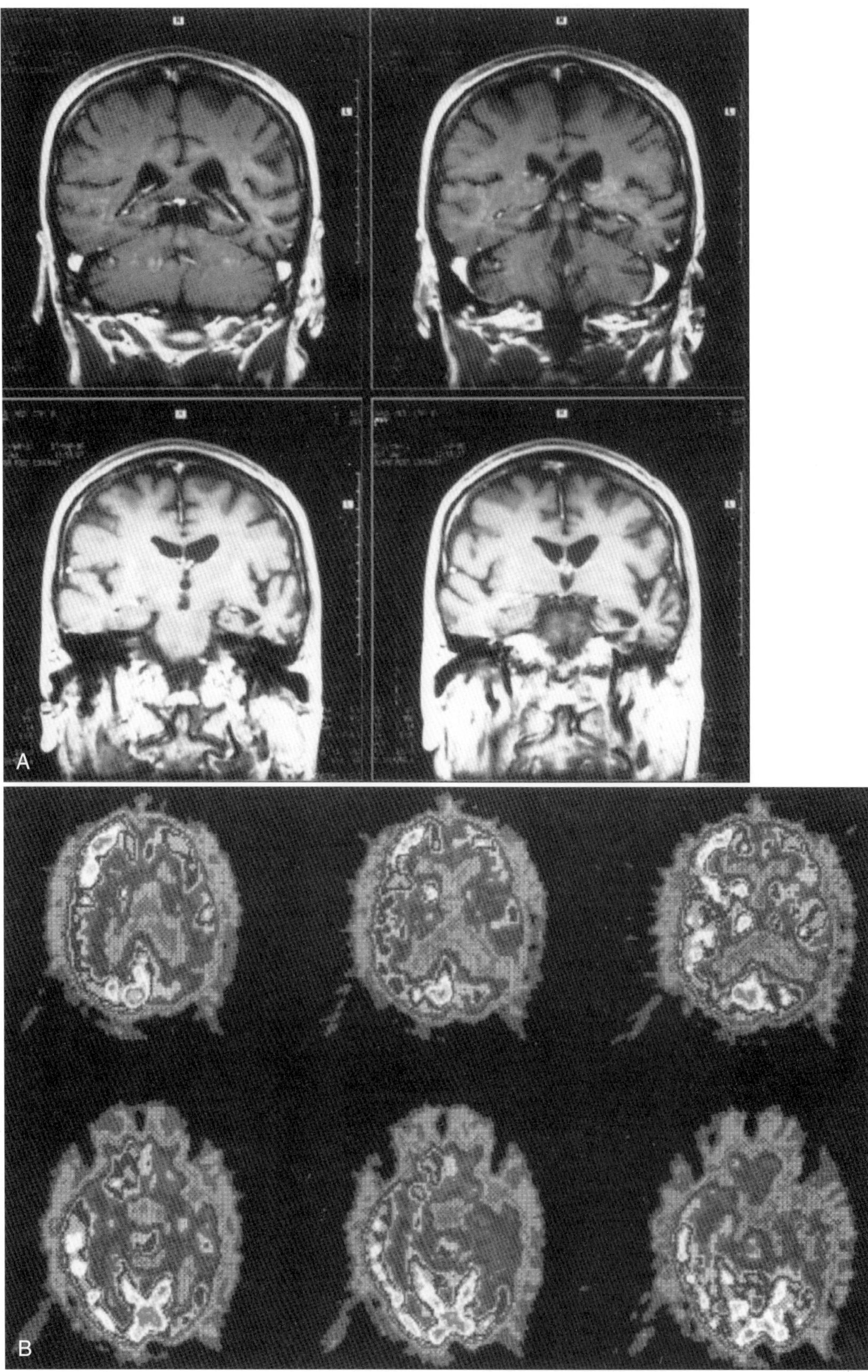

**Fig. 13.10** Coronal T1-weighted magnetic resonance imaging scans of a patient with primary progressive aphasia. Note the marked atrophy of the left temporal lobe. **A,** Axial fluoro-2-deoxyglucose positron emission tomography (FDG PET). **B,** Tomographic scan showing extensive hypometabolism in the left cerebral hemisphere, especially marked in the left temporal lobe.

and venous outflow obstructions. In preparation for epilepsy surgery, the Wada test, or infusion of amobarbital through an arterial catheter, is useful in the determination of language dominance. Other, related studies by language activation with functional MRI (fMRI) or PET now rival the Wada test for the study of language dominance (Abou-Khalil and Schlaggar, 2002).

Single-photon emission CT (SPECT), PET, and functional MRI (see Chapter 40) are contributing greatly to the study of language. Patterns of brain activation in response to language stimuli have been recorded in neurologically normal research participants as well as individuals with aphasia, and these studies have broadly confirmed the localizations based on pathology such as stroke over the past 140 years (Posner et al., 1988). In addition, these techniques can be used to map areas of the brain that activate during language functions after insults such as strokes, and the pattern of recovery can be studied. Some such studies have indicated right hemisphere activation in patients recovering from aphasia, whereas others have concluded that return to function of left hemisphere language regions is necessary for full recovery. An fMRI study (Saur et al., 2006) has suggested dysfunction in the language cortex shortly after an ischemic insult, followed by increased activation of right frontal cortex, and then a shift back to the more normal pattern of left hemisphere activation. These techniques provide the best correlation between brain structure and function currently available and should help advance our understanding of language disorders and their recovery.

## DIFFERENTIAL DIAGNOSIS

Vascular lesions, especially ischemic strokes, are the most common causes of aphasia. Historically, most research studies in aphasia have used stroke patients because stroke is an "experiment" of nature in which one area of the brain is damaged, while the rest remains theoretically intact. Strokes are characterized by the abrupt onset of a neurological deficit in a patient with vascular risk factors. The precise temporal profile is important: most embolic strokes are sudden and maximal at onset, whereas thrombotic strokes typically wax and wane or increase in steps. The bedside aphasia examination is helpful in delineating the vascular territory affected. For example, the sudden onset of Wernicke aphasia nearly always indicates an embolus to the inferior division of the left middle cerebral artery. Global aphasia may be caused by an embolus to the middle cerebral artery stem, thrombosis of the internal carotid artery, or even a hemorrhage into the deep basal ganglia. Whereas most aphasic syndromes involve the territory of the left middle cerebral artery, transcortical motor aphasia is specific to the anterior cerebral territory, and pure alexia without agraphia is specific to the posterior cerebral artery territory. The clinical features of the aphasia are thus of crucial importance to the vascular diagnosis.

Hemorrhagic strokes are also an important cause of aphasia, most commonly the basal ganglionic hemorrhages associated with hypertension. The deficits tend to worsen gradually over minutes to hours, in contrast to the sudden or stepwise onset of ischemic strokes. Headache, vomiting, and obtundation are more common with hemorrhages. Because hemorrhages compress cerebral tissue without necessarily destroying it, the ultimate recovery from aphasia is often better in hemorrhages than in ischemic strokes, although hemorrhages are more often fatal. Other etiologies of intracerebral hemorrhage include anticoagulants, head injury, blood dyscrasias, thrombocytopenia, and bleeding into structural lesions, such as infarctions, tumors, AVMs, and aneurysms. Hemorrhages from AVMs mimic strokes, with abrupt onset of focal neurological deficit. Ruptured aneurysms, on the other hand, present with severe headache and stiff neck or with coma; most patients have no focal deficits, but delayed deficits (e.g., aphasia) may develop secondary to vasospasm. Lobar hemorrhages may occur in elderly patients without hypertension. These hemorrhages occur near the cortical surface, sometimes extending into the subarachnoid space, and they may be recurrent. Pathological studies have shown amyloid deposition in small arterioles, or cerebral amyloid angiopathy. A final vascular cause of aphasia is cerebral vasculitis (see Chapter 70).

Traumatic brain injury is a common cause of aphasia. Cerebral contusions, depressed skull fractures, and hematomas of the intracerebral, subdural, and epidural spaces all cause aphasia when they disrupt or compress left hemisphere language structures. Trauma tends to be less localized than ischemic stroke, and thus, aphasia is often admixed with the general effects of the head injury, such as depressed consciousness, encephalopathy or delirium, amnesia, and other deficits. Head injuries in young people may be associated with severe deficits but excellent long-term recovery. Language deficits, especially those involving discourse organization, can be found in most cases of significant closed head injury (Chapman et al., 1992). Gunshot wounds produce focal aphasic syndromes, which rival stroke as a source of clinical-anatomical correlation. Subdural hematomas are infamous for mimicking other neurological syndromes. Aphasia is occasionally associated with subdural hematomas overlying the left hemisphere, but it may be mild and may be overlooked because of the patient's more severe complaints of headache, memory loss, and drowsiness.

Tumors of the left hemisphere frequently present with aphasia. The onset of the aphasia is gradual, and other cognitive deficits may be associated because of edema and mass effect. Aphasia secondary to an enlarging tumor may thus be difficult to distinguish from a diffuse encephalopathy or early dementia. Any syndrome of abnormal language function should therefore be investigated for a focal, dominant hemisphere lesion.

Infections of the nervous system may cause aphasia. Brain abscesses can mimic tumors in every respect, and those in the left hemisphere can present with progressive aphasia. Chronic infections, such as tuberculosis or syphilis, can result in focal abnormalities that run the entire gamut of central nervous system symptoms and signs. Herpes simplex encephalitis has a predilection for the temporal lobe and orbital frontal cortex, and aphasia can be an early symptom, along with headache, confusion, fever, and seizures. Aphasia is often a permanent sequela in survivors of herpes encephalitis. Acquired immunodeficiency syndrome (AIDS) can cause language disorders. Opportunistic infections can cause focal lesions anywhere in the brain, and the neurotropic human immunodeficiency virus agent itself produces a dementia (AIDS dementia complex), in which language deficits play a part.

Aphasia is frequently caused by degenerative central nervous system diseases. Reference has already been made to the focal, progressive aphasia in patients with FTLD and progressive nonfluent aphasia or atypical AD with logopenic primary progressive aphasia as compared with the more diffuse cognitive deterioration characteristic of AD.

Language dysfunction in AD may be more common in familial cases and may predict poor prognosis. Cognitive deterioration in patients with Parkinson disease may also include language deterioration similar to that of AD, although Parkinson disease tends to involve more fluctuation in orientation and greater tendency to active visual hallucinations and acting out of dreams (Rapid Eye Movement [REM] sleep behavior disorder). Corticobasal degeneration is also associated with PPA and FTD, as noted earlier. A striking abnormality of speech (i.e., initial stuttering followed by true aphasia and dementia) has been described in the dialysis dementia syndrome. This disorder may be associated with spongiform degeneration of the frontotemporal cortex, similar to Creutzfeldt–Jakob disease. Paraphasic substitutions and nonsense speech are also occasionally encountered in acute encephalopathies, such as hyponatremia or lithium toxicity.

Another cause of aphasia is seizures. Seizures can be associated with aphasia in children as part of the Landau-Kleffner syndrome or in adults as either an ictal or postictal Todd phenomenon. Epileptic aphasia is important to recognize, in that anticonvulsant drug therapy can prevent the episodes, and unnecessary investigation or treatment for a new lesion, such as a stroke, can be avoided. As mentioned earlier, localization of language areas in epileptic patients has contributed greatly to the knowledge of language organization in the brain. A new language area, the basal temporal language area (BTLA), was discovered through epilepsy stimulation studies, and only later confirmed in patients with spontaneous seizures (Kirshner et al., 1995).

Another transitory cause of aphasia is migraine. Wernicke aphasia may be seen in a migraine attack, usually with complete recovery over a few hours. Occasional patients may have recurrent episodes of aphasia associated with migraine (Mishra et al., 2009).

Finally, aphasia can be psychogenic, often associated with stuttering or stammering. A recent report (Binder et al., 2012) concerned three patients with stuttering or stammering, letter reversals (e.g. "low the mawn" instead of "mow the lawn"), and naming difficulty after minor head injuries. In all three, language productions were inconsistent; for example, when a subject became angry, the speech productions were much more normal. All three failed neuropsychological tests designed to detect a lack of effort (such as a digit span of only two). Patients failed to improve on easier speech production tasks such as speaking in unison, shouting, or speaking while finger-tapping. In addition, whereas developmental stutterers generally have difficulty only with the initial phoneme of a phrase, psychogenic stutterers, but also some acquired cases of stuttering, may hesitate on any word of a phrase.

## RECOVERY AND REHABILITATION OF APHASIA

Patients with aphasia from acute disorders, such as stroke, generally show spontaneous improvement over days, weeks, and months. In general, the greatest recovery occurs during the first few weeks and months with a decelerating time course. While a commonly stated dogma is that patients reach a plateau after 6 months to a year, several recent studies have clearly demonstrated that many patients continue to make gains years after a stroke. The aphasia type often changes during recovery: global aphasia evolves into Broca aphasia, and Wernicke aphasia into conduction or anomic aphasia (Pashek and Holland, 1988). Language recovery may be mediated by shifting of functions to the right hemisphere or to adjacent left hemisphere regions. As mentioned earlier, studies of language activation using fMRI and PET are advancing our understanding of the neuroanatomy of language recovery (Heiss et al., 1999; Thompson and den Ouden, 2008). These studies suggest that aphasia recovers best when left hemisphere areas, either in the direct language cortex or in adjacent areas, recover function. Right hemisphere activation seems to be a "second best" type of recovery.

In addition, a study of patients in the very acute phase of aphasia, with techniques of diffusion and perfusion-weighted MRI, has suggested less variability in the correlation of comprehension impairment with left temporal ischemia than has been suggested from testing of chronic aphasia, after recovery and compensation have commenced (Hillis et al., 2001).

Speech-language therapy, provided by speech-language pathologists, attempts to facilitate language recovery by a variety of techniques and to help the patient compensate for lost functions (see Chapter 57). Some of the main approaches that are commonly used include script training, response elaboration training, constraint-induced aphasia therapy, speech entrainment, and melodic intonation therapy. In script training, individuals rehearse personally relevant scripts for commonly encountered situations (e.g., visiting a coffee shop) in order to increase independence in communication. Response elaboration training involves clinicians using a cueing hierarchy to support patients in producing increasingly longer utterances by building on prior successful responses. Constraint-induced aphasia therapy involves minimizing the use of gesture or other alternative forms of communication in order to encourage practice with producing language. Speech entrainment depends on the surprisingly preserved ability of some patients with aphasia to speak along with an audiovisual model (i.e., hearing and watching the lips of another talker). This facilitation can be leveraged in support of script training and in the hope of promoting generalization to unsupported situations. Melodic intonation therapy is based on the premise of the right hemisphere's involvement in prosodic aspects of language, which can provide a substrate for recovery when the left hemisphere is damaged. There is robust evidence for the efficacy of speech-language therapy in randomized controlled trials. Some patients may also benefit from using an Augmentative and Alternative Communication (AAC) device to communicate. The recent explosion of mobile computing technology has led to a proliferation of high-quality applications that allow nonverbal patients to communicate common and personally relevant concepts.

A new approach to language rehabilitation is the use of pharmacological agents to improve speech. Albert and colleagues (1988) first reported that the dopaminergic drug bromocriptine promotes spontaneous speech output in transcortical motor aphasia. Several other studies have supported the drug in nonfluent aphasias, although a recent controlled study showed no benefit (Ashtary et al., 2006). Stimulant drugs are also being tested in aphasia rehabilitation. In a double-blind, placebo-controlled, parallel-group study, Berthier et al. (2009) observed the effect of memantine and constraint-induced aphasia therapy (CIAT) on chronic poststroke aphasia. Memantine and CIAT alone improved aphasia compared with placebo, but the best and most durable outcomes were observed when memantine and CIAT were combined. As new information accumulates on the neurochemistry of cognitive functions, other pharmacological therapies may be forthcoming.

Finally, stimulation techniques such as transcranial magnetic stimulation (Martin et al., 2009; Wong and Tsang, 2013) and direct cortical stimulation (Monti et al., 2013) are being applied to patients with aphasia, and several early trials indicate benefit from these techniques (Fridriksson et al., 2018; Saxena and Hillis, 2017; Tippett et al., 2014).

### Acknowledgment

The authors would like to thank Sarah Schneck, MS, CCC-SLP, in the Department of Hearing and Speech Sciences, Vanderbilt University Medical Center, for assistance, especially with the discussion about speech and language therapy.

*The complete reference list is available online at https://expertconsult.inkling.com/.* 

14

# Dysarthria and Apraxia of Speech

Howard S. Kirshner

## OUTLINE



## MOTOR SPEECH DISORDERS

Motor speech disorders are syndromes of abnormal articulation, the motor production of speech, without abnormalities of language. A patient with a motor speech disorder should be able to produce normal expressive language in writing and to comprehend both spoken and written language. If a listener transcribes into print or type the speech of a patient with a motor speech disorder, the text should read as normal language. Motor speech disorders include dysarthrias, disorders of speech articulation, apraxia of speech, a motor programing disorder for speech, and four rarer syndromes: aphemia, foreign accent syndrome, acquired stuttering, and the opercular syndrome. Duffy (1995), in an analysis of speech and language disorders at the Mayo Clinic, reported that 46.3% of the patients had dysarthria, 27.1% aphasia, 4.6% apraxia of speech, 9% other speech disorders (such as stuttering), and 13% other cognitive or linguistic disorders.

### Dysarthrias

*Dysarthrias* involve the abnormal articulation of sounds or phonemes, or more precisely, abnormal neuromuscular activation of the speech muscles, affecting the speed, strength, timing, range, or accuracy of movements involving speech (Duffy, 1995). The most consistent finding in dysarthria is the distortion of consonant sounds. Dysarthria is neurogenic, related to dysfunction of the central nervous system, nerves, neuromuscular junction, or muscle, with a contribution of sensory deficits in some cases. Speech abnormalities secondary to local, structural problems of the palate, tongue, or larynx do not qualify as dysarthrias. Dysarthria can affect not only articulation but also phonation, breathing, or prosody (emotional tone) of speech. Total loss of ability to articulate is called *anarthria.*

Like the aphasias, dysarthrias can be analyzed in terms of the specific brain lesion sites associated with specific patterns of speech impairment. Analysis of dysarthria at the bedside is useful for the localization of neurological lesions and the diagnosis of neurological disorders. An experienced examiner should be able to recognize the major types of dysarthria, rather than referring to "dysarthria" as a single disorder.

The examination of speech at the bedside should include repeating syllables, words, and sentences. Repeating consonant sounds (such as /p/, /p/, /p/) or shifting consonant sounds (/p/, /t/, /k/) can help to identify which consonants consistently cause trouble.

The Mayo Clinic classification of dysarthria (Duffy, 1995), widely used in the United States, includes six categories: (1) flaccid, (2) spastic and "unilateral upper motor neuron," (3) ataxic, (4) hypokinetic, (5) hyperkinetic, and (6) mixed dysarthria. These types of dysarthria are summarized in Table 14.1.

*Flaccid* dysarthria is associated with disorders involving lower motor neuron weakness of the bulbar muscles, such as polymyositis, myasthenia gravis, and bulbar poliomyelitis. The speech pattern is breathy and nasal, with indistinctly pronounced consonants. In the case of myasthenia gravis, the patient may begin reading a paragraph with normal enunciation, but by the end of the paragraph the articulation is soft, breathy, and frequently interrupted by labored respirations.

*Spastic* dysarthria occurs in patients with bilateral lesions of the motor cortex or corticobulbar tracts, such as bilateral strokes. The speech is harsh or "strain-strangle" in vocal quality, with reduced rate, low pitch, and consonant errors. Patients often have the features of "pseudobulbar palsy," including dysphagia, exaggerated jaw jerk and gag reflexes, and easy laughter and crying (emotional incontinence, pseudobulbar affect, or pathological laughter and crying). Another variant is the "opercular syndrome," described later in this chapter.

A milder variant of spastic dysarthria, "unilateral upper motor neuron" dysarthria, is associated with unilateral upper motor neuron lesions (Duffy, 1995). This type of dysarthria has features similar to those of spastic dysarthria, only in a less severe form. Unilateral upper motor neuron dysarthria is one of the commonest types of dysarthria, occurring in patients with unilateral strokes. Strokes, depending on their location, can also cause mixed patterns of dysarthria (see later). There is considerable evidence for the efficacy of speech therapy for poststroke dysarthria (Mackenzie, 2011).

*Ataxic* dysarthria or "scanning speech," associated with cerebellar disorders, is characterized by one of two patterns: irregular breakdowns of speech with explosions of syllables interrupted by pauses, or a slow cadence of speech, with excessively equal stress on every syllable. The second pattern of ataxic dysarthria is referred to as "scanning speech." A patient with ataxic dysarthria, attempting to repeat the phoneme /p/ as rapidly as possible, produces either an irregular rhythm, resembling popcorn popping, or a very slow rhythm. Causes of ataxic dysarthria include cerebellar strokes, tumors, multiple sclerosis, and cerebellar degenerations.

*Hypokinetic* dysarthria, the typical speech pattern in Parkinson disease, is notable for decreased and monotonous loudness and pitch, rapid rate, and occasional consonant errors. In a study of brain activation by positron emission tomography (PET) methodology (Liotti et al., 2003), premotor and supplementary motor area activations were seen in untreated patients with Parkinson disease and hypokinetic dysarthria but not in normal subjects. Following a voice treatment protocol, these premotor and motor activations diminished, whereas right-sided basal ganglia activations increased. Hypokinetic dysarthria

**TABLE 14.1 Classification of the Dysarthrias**

| Type | Localization | Auditory Signs | Diseases |
|---|---|---|---|
| Flaccid | Lower motor neuron | Breathy, nasal voice, imprecise consonants | Stroke, myasthenia gravis |
| Spastic | Bilateral upper motor neuron | Strain-strangle, harsh voice, slow rate, imprecise consonants | Bilateral strokes, tumors, primary lateral sclerosis |
| | Unilateral upper motor neuron | Consonant imprecision, slow rate, harsh voice quality | Stroke, tumor |
| Ataxic | Cerebellum | Irregular articulatory breakdowns, excessive and equal stress | Stroke, degenerative disease |
| Hypokinetic | Extrapyramidal | Rapid rate, reduced loudness, monopitch and monoloudness | Parkinson disease |
| Hyperkinetic | Extrapyramidal | Prolonged phonemes, variable rate, inappropriate silences, voice stoppages | Dystonia, Huntington disease |
| Spastic and flaccid | Hypernasality, lower motor neuron | Amyotrophic strain-strangle, harsh voice, slow rate, imprecise consonants | Upper lateral sclerosis, multiple strokes |

Adapted from Duffy, J.R., 1995. Motor Speech Disorders: Substrates, Differential Diagnosis, and Management. Mosby, St. Louis; and from Kirshner, H.S., 2002. Behavioral Neurology: Practical Science of Mind and Brain. Butterworth-Heinemann, Boston.

responds both to behavioral therapies and to pharmacological treatment of Parkinson disease, although the efficacy of speech therapy in Parkinson disease has not been proved (Herd et al., 2012).

*Hyperkinetic* dysarthria, a pattern in some ways opposite to hypokinetic dysarthria, is characterized by marked variation in rate, loudness, and timing, with distortion of vowels, harsh voice quality, and occasional, sudden stoppages of speech. This speech pattern is seen in hyperkinetic movement disorders such as Huntington disease and dystonia musculorum deformans.

The final category, *mixed* dysarthria, involves combinations of the other five types. One common mixed dysarthria is a spastic-flaccid dysarthria seen in amyotrophic lateral sclerosis (ALS). The ALS patient has the harsh, strain-strangle voice quality of spastic dysarthria, combined with the breathy and hypernasal quality of flaccid dysarthria. Multiple sclerosis may feature a spastic-flaccid-ataxic or spastic-ataxic mixed dysarthria, in which slow rate or irregular breakdowns are added to the other characteristics seen in spastic and flaccid dysarthria. A recent publication found that tongue movements were particularly affected by multiple sclerosis (Mefford et al., 2019). Wilson disease can involve hypokinetic, spastic, and ataxic features.

The management of dysarthria includes speech therapy techniques for strengthening muscles, training more precise articulations, slowing the rate of speech to increase intelligibility, or teaching the patient to stress specific phonemes. Devices such as pacing boards to slow articulation, palatal lifts to reduce hypernasality, amplifiers to increase voice volume, communication boards for subjects to point to pictures, and augmentative communication devices and computer techniques can be used when the patient is unable to communicate in speech. Surgical procedures such as a pharyngeal flap to reduce hypernasality or vocal fold Teflon injection or transposition surgery to increase loudness may help the patient to speak more intelligibly. In Parkinson disease, most patients have elements of dysarthria and dysphonia, and treatment can include speech therapy, drug treatment, deep brain stimulation, and even surgical options (Baumann et al., 2018; Dashtipour et al., 2018;). Deep brain stimulation may improve motor speech, although with variations depending on location and frequency of stimulation (Morello et al., 2020).

## Apraxia of Speech

Apraxia of speech is a disorder of the programing of articulation of sequences of phonemes, especially consonants (Ziegler et al., 2012). The motor speech system makes errors in selection of consonant phonemes, in the absence of any "weakness, slowness or incoordination" of the muscles of speech articulation (Wertz et al., 1991). The term "apraxia of speech" implies that the disorder is one of a skilled, sequential motor activity (as in other apraxias), rather than a primary motor disorder. Hillis and colleagues (2004) gave a more informal definition of apraxia of speech, in terms of a patient who "knows what he or she wants to say and how it should sound" yet cannot articulate it properly. Consonants are frequently substituted rather than distorted, as in dysarthria. Patients have special difficulty with polysyllabic words and consonant shifts, as well as in initiating articulation of a word. Errors are inconsistent from one attempt to the next, in contrast to the consistent distortion of phonemes in dysarthria. This inconsistency can be documented by asking the patient to repeat a difficult word such as "catastrophe" five times.

The four cardinal features of apraxia of speech are: (1) effortful, groping, or "trial-and error" attempts at speech, with efforts at self-correction; (2) dysprosody; (3) inconsistencies in articulation errors; and (4) difficulty with initiating utterances. Usually the patient has the most difficulty with the first phoneme of a polysyllabic utterance. The patient may make an error in attempting to produce a word on one trial, a different error the next time, and a normal utterance the third time.

Apraxia of speech is rare in isolated form, but it frequently contributes to the speech and language deficit of Broca aphasia. A patient with apraxia of speech, in addition to aphasia, will often write better than he or she can speak, and comprehension is relatively preserved. Dronkers (1996) and colleagues have presented evidence from computed tomography (CT) and magnetic resonance imaging (MRI) scans indicating that, although the anatomical lesions vary, patients with apraxia of speech virtually always have damage in the left hemisphere insula, whereas patients without apraxia of speech do not. However, this "overlapping lesion" approach to brain localization can be misleading. Moreover, recent MRI correlations of apraxia of speech in acute stroke patients by Hillis and colleagues (2004) have pointed to the traditional Broca area in the left frontal cortex as the site of apraxia of speech and as the site where programing of articulation takes place. Recent publications have drawn attention to primary progressive apraxia of speech as a progressive disorder, related to primary progressive aphasia and frontotemporal dementia (Croot et al., 2012; Duffy and Josephs, 2012; Utianski et al., 2018). See Chapter 13 for a discussion of primary progressive aphasia and frontotemporal dementia.

Testing of patients for speech apraxia includes the repetition of sequences of phonemes (pa/ta/ka), as discussed previously under testing for dysarthria. Repetition of a polysyllabic word (e.g., "catastrophe" or "television") is especially likely to elicit apraxic errors, and having the subject repeat the same word five times will bring out the inconsistency in the apraxic utterances.

## Oral or Buccolingual Apraxia

Apraxia of speech is not the same as oral-buccal-lingual apraxia or ideomotor apraxia for learned movements of the tongue, lips, and larynx. Oral apraxia can be elicited by asking a subject to lick his or her upper lip, smile, or stick out the tongue. Oral apraxia is discussed in Chapter 13, Aphasia and Aphasic Syndromes. Both oral apraxia and apraxia of speech can coexist with Broca aphasia.

## Aphemia

Another differential diagnosis with both apraxia of speech and dysarthria is the syndrome of *aphemia.* Broca first used the term "aphemie" to designate the syndrome later called "Broca aphasia," but in recent years the term has been reserved for a syndrome of near muteness, with normal comprehension, reading, and writing. Aphemia is clearly a motor speech disorder rather than an aphasia, if written language and comprehension are indeed intact. Patients are often anarthric, with no speech whatever, and then effortful, nonfluent speech emerges. Some patients have persisting dysarthria, with dysphonia and sometimes distortions of articulation that sound similar to foreign accents (see next section). Alexander et al. (1990) associated pure anarthria with lesions of the face area of motor cortex. Functional imaging studies also suggest that articulation is mediated at the level of the primary motor face area (Riecker et al., 2000), and disruption of speech articulation can be produced by transcranial magnetic stimulation over the motor face area (Epstein et al., 1999). Controversy remains as to whether aphemia is equivalent to apraxia of speech, as suggested by Alexander et al. (1989). In general, aphemia is likely to involve lesions in the vicinity of the primary motor cortex and perhaps Broca area.

## "Foreign Accent Syndrome"

The "foreign accent syndrome" is an acquired form of motor speech disorder, related to the dysarthrias, in which the patient acquires a dysfluency resembling a foreign accent, usually after a unilateral stroke (Kurowski et al., 1996; Marien et al., 2019; Takayama et al., 1993). Lesions may involve the motor cortex of the left hemisphere. The disorder can also be mixed with aphasia.

## Acquired Stuttering

Another uncommon motor speech disorder following acquired brain lesions is a pattern resembling developmental stuttering, referred to as "acquired" or "cortical stuttering." Acquired stuttering involves hesitancy in producing initial phonemes, with an associated dysrhythmia of speech. Acquired stuttering clearly overlaps with apraxia of speech but may lack the other features of apraxia of speech discussed earlier. Acquired stuttering has been described most often in patients with left hemisphere cortical strokes (Franco et al., 2000; Turgut et al., 2002), but the syndrome has also been reported with subcortical lesions including infarctions of the pons, basal ganglia, and subcortical white matter (Ciabarra et al., 2000). Stuttering-like dysfluencies can also occur in acquired apraxia of speech (Bailey et al., 2017). Acquired stuttering can also be psychogenic; Binder and colleagues (2012) discuss ways of detecting psychogenic acquired stuttering. A more general review of psychogenic speech and language abnormalities was recently published by Barnett and colleagues (2019). They believed that no uniform set of criteria exists for the reliable diagnosis of functional speech disorder.

## Opercular Syndrome

The opercular syndrome, also called Foix-Chavany-Marie syndrome or cheiro-oral syndrome (Bakar et al., 1998; Bogousslavsky et al., 1991), is a severe form of pseudobulbar palsy in which patients with bilateral lesions of the perisylvian cortex or subcortical connections become completely mute. These patients can follow commands involving the extremities but not the cranial nerves; for example, they may be unable to open or close their eyes or mouth or smile voluntarily, yet they smile when amused, yawn spontaneously, and even utter cries in response to emotional stimuli. The ability to follow limb commands shows that the disorder is not an aphasic disorder of comprehension. The discrepancy between automatic activation of the cranial musculature and inability to perform the same actions voluntarily has been called an "automatic-voluntary dissociation."

*The complete reference list is available online at https://expertconsult.inkling.com/.*

15

# Neurogenic Dysphagia

*Delaram Safarpour, Kaveh Sharzehi, Ronald F. Pfeiffer*

## OUTLINE



The mechanics of swallowing are like those of an elegant wristwatch. On the surface, this appears to be a simple, perhaps even pedestrian process, but it is actually both tremendously complex and remarkably fascinating. Humans swallow approximately 500 times daily (Shaw and Martino, 2013). Normally, swallowing occurs unobtrusively and is afforded scant attention. Malfunction can go completely unnoticed for a time; but when it finally becomes manifest, serious—sometimes catastrophic—consequences can ensue.

Impaired swallowing, or *dysphagia*, can originate from disturbances in the mouth, pharynx, or esophagus that may be generated by mechanical, musculoskeletal, or neurogenic mechanisms. Although mechanical dysphagia is an important topic, this chapter primarily focuses on neuromuscular and neurogenic causes of dysphagia, because processes in these categories are most likely to be encountered by the neurologist.

Dysphagia is surprisingly common and has been reported to be present in 3% of the general population and in 10% of individuals over age 65. Dysphagia occurs quite frequently in neurological patients and can occur in a broad array of neurological or neuromuscular conditions. It has been estimated that neurogenic dysphagia develops in approximately 400,000 to 800,000 people per year, and that dysphagia is present in roughly 50% of inhabitants of long-term care units. Moreover, dysphagia can lead to superimposed problems such as inadequate nutrition, dehydration, recurrent upper respiratory infections, and frank aspiration with consequent pneumonia and even asphyxia. It thus constitutes a formidable and frequent problem confronting the neurologist in everyday practice.

## NORMAL SWALLOWING

Swallowing is a surprisingly complicated and intricate phenomenon. It comprises a mixture of voluntary and reflex, or automatic, actions engineered and carried out by some of the more than 30 pairs of muscles within the oropharyngeal, laryngeal, and esophageal regions along with five cranial nerves and two cervical nerve roots that, in turn, receive directions from centers within the central nervous system (Sasegbon and Hamdy, 2017; Shaw and Martino, 2013). Reflex swallowing is coordinated and carried out at a brainstem level, where centers act directly on information received from sensory structures within the oropharynx and esophagus. A differentiation can be made between voluntary swallowing, which occurs when a person desires to eat or drink during the awake and aware state, and spontaneous swallowing in response to accumulated saliva in the mouth (Ertekin, 2011). Volitional swallowing is, not surprisingly, accompanied by additional activity that originates not only in motor and sensory cortices but also in other cerebral structures (Hamdy et al., 1999; Sasegbon and Hamdy, 2017; Zald and Pardo, 1999).

The process of swallowing can conveniently be broken down into three or four distinct stages or phases: oral (which some subdivide into oral preparatory and oral propulsive), pharyngeal, and esophageal. These components have also been distilled into what have been designated the *horizontal* and *vertical subsystems*, reflecting the direction of bolus flow in each component (when the individual is upright while swallowing). The horizontal subsystem comprises the *oral phase* of swallowing and is largely volitional in character; the vertical subsystem comprises the *pharyngeal* and *esophageal phases*, which are primarily under reflex control.

In the oral preparatory phase, food is taken into the mouth and, if needed, chewed. Saliva is secreted to provide both lubrication and the initial “dose” of digestive enzymes; the food bolus is then formed and shaped by the tongue. In the oral propulsive phase, the tongue propels the bolus backward to the pharyngeal inlet where, in a piston-like action, it delivers the bolus into the pharynx. This initiates the pharyngeal phase, in which a cascade of intricate, extremely rapid, and exquisitely coordinated movements sealoff the nasal passages and protects the trachea while the cricopharyngeal muscle, which functions as the primary component of the upper esophageal sphincter (UES), relaxes and allows the bolus to enter the esophagus. As an example of the intricacy of movements during this phase of swallowing, the UES, prompted in part by traction produced by elevation of the larynx, actually relaxes just prior to arrival of the food bolus, creating suction that assists in guiding the bolus into the esophagus. The bolus then enters the esophagus, where peristaltic contractions usher it distally and, on relaxation of the lower esophageal sphincter, into the stomach. Swallowing is synchronized with respiration, such that expiration rather than inspiration immediately follows a swallow, thus reducing the risk of aspiration—another example of the finely tuned coordination involved in the swallowing mechanism (Mehanna and Jankovic, 2010).

## NEUROPHYSIOLOGY OF SWALLOWING

Central control of swallowing has traditionally been ascribed to brainstem structures, with cortical supervision and modulation emanating from the inferior precentral gyrus. However, positron emission tomography (PET), transcranial magnetic stimulation (TMS), and functional magnetic resonance imaging (fMRI) studies of volitional swallowing reveal a considerably more complex picture in which a broad network of brain regions is active in the control and execution of swallowing.

It is perhaps not surprising that in PET studies, the strongest activation of volitional swallowing occurs in the lateral motor cortex within the inferior precentral gyrus, wherein lie the cortical representations of tongue and face. There is disagreement among investigators, however, in that some have noted bilaterally symmetrical activation of the lateral motor cortex (Zald and Pardo, 1999) whereas others have noted a distinctly asymmetrical activation, at least in some of the subjects tested (Hamdy et al., 1999).

Additional and perhaps somewhat surprising brain areas also are activated during volitional swallowing (Hamdy et al., 1999; Sasegbon and Hamdy, 2017; Schaller et al., 2006; Zald and Pardo, 1999). The supplementary motor area may play a role in preparing for volitional swallowing, and the anterior cingulate cortex may be involved with monitoring autonomic and vegetative functions. Another area of activation during volitional swallowing is the anterior insula, particularly on the right. It has been suggested that this activation may provide the substrate that allows gustatory and other intraoral sensations to modulate swallowing. Lesions in the insula may also increase the swallowing threshold and delay the pharyngeal phase of swallowing (Schaller et al., 2006). PET studies also consistently demonstrate distinctly asymmetrical left-sided activation of the cerebellum during swallowing. This activation may reflect cerebellar input concerning the coordination, timing, and sequencing of swallowing. Activation of putamen has also been noted during volitional swallowing, but it has not been possible to differentiate this activation from that seen with tongue movement alone.

Within the brainstem, swallowing appears to be regulated by central pattern generators that contain the programs directing the sequential movements of the various muscles involved (Steuer and Guertin, 2019). The *dorsomedial pattern generator* resides in the medial reticular formation of the rostral medulla and the reticulum adjacent to the nucleus tractus solitarius and is involved with the initiation and organization of the swallowing sequence (Schaller et al., 2006). A second central pattern generator, the *ventrolateral pattern generator*, lies near the nucleus ambiguus and its surrounding reticular formation (Schaller et al., 2006). It serves primarily as a connecting pathway to motor nuclei such as the nucleus ambiguus and the dorsal motor nucleus of the vagus, which directly control motor output to the pharyngeal musculature and proximal esophagus. The enteric nervous system also plays a role in controlling esophageal function, apparently involving both motor and sensory components (Woodland et al., 2013).

It has become evident that a large network of structures participates in the act of swallowing, especially volitional swallowing. The presence of this network presumably accounts for the broad array of neurological disease processes that can produce dysphagia as a part of the clinical picture.

## MECHANICAL DYSPHAGIA

Structural abnormalities—both within and adjacent to the mouth, pharynx, and esophagus—can interfere with swallowing on a strictly mechanical basis despite fully intact and functioning nervous and musculoskeletal systems (Box 15.1). Within the mouth, macroglossia, temporomandibular joint dislocation, certain congenital anomalies, and intraoral tumors can impede effective swallowing and produce mechanical dysphagia. Pharyngeal function can be compromised by processes such as retropharyngeal tumor or abscess, cervical anterior

### BOX 15.1 Mechanical Dysphagia

**Oral**
- Amyloidosis
- Congenital abnormalities
- Intraoral tumors
- Lip injuries:
  - Burns
  - Trauma
- Macroglossia
- Scleroderma
- Temporomandibular joint dysfunction
- Xerostomia:
  - Sjögren syndrome

**Pharyngeal**
- Cervical anterior osteophytes
- Infection:
  - Diphtheria
- Thyromegaly
- Retropharyngeal abscess
- Retropharyngeal tumor
- Zenker diverticulum

**Esophageal**
- Aberrant origin of right subclavian artery
- Caustic injury
- Esophageal carcinoma
- Esophageal diverticulum
- Esophageal infection:
  - *Candida albicans*
  - Cytomegalovirus
  - Herpes simplex virus
  - Varicella zoster virus
- Esophageal intramural pseudodiverticula
- Esophageal stricture
- Esophageal ulceration
- Esophageal webs or rings
- Gastroesophageal reflux disease
- Hiatal hernia
- Metastatic carcinoma
- Posterior mediastinal mass
- Thoracic aortic aneurysm

osteophyte formation, Zenker diverticulum, or thyroid gland enlargement. An even broader array of structural lesions can interfere with esophageal function, including malignant or benign esophageal tumors, metastatic carcinoma, esophageal stricture from numerous causes, vascular abnormalities such as aortic aneurysm or aberrant origin of the subclavian artery, or even primary gastric abnormalities such as hiatal hernia or complications from gastric banding procedures. Gastroesophageal reflux can also produce dysphagia. However, individuals with these problems are more likely to be seen by the gastroenterologist than the neurologist.

## NEUROMUSCULAR DYSPHAGIA

A variety of neuromuscular disease processes of diverse etiology can involve the oropharyngeal and esophageal musculature and produce dysphagia as part of their broader neuromuscular clinical picture (Box 15.2). Certain muscular dystrophies, inflammatory myopathies, and mitochondrial myopathies can all display dysphagia, as can disease processes affecting the myoneural junction, such as myasthenia gravis (MG).

### Oculopharyngeal Muscular Dystrophy

Oculopharyngeal muscular dystrophy (OPMD) is a rare disorder that has a worldwide distribution. It was initially described and is most frequently encountered in individuals with a French-Canadian ethnic background, although its highest reported prevalence is among the Bukhara Jews in Israel (Abu-Baker and Rouleau, 2007). OPMD is the consequence of a GCG trinucleotide repeat expansion in the polyadenylate-binding protein nuclear 1 gene (*PABPN1*; also known as poly[A]-binding protein 2 [PABP2]) on chromosome 14. The inheritance pattern of OPMD is primarily autosomal dominant, although a rare autosomal recessive form has been described. OPMD is unique among the muscular dystrophies because of its appearance in older individuals, with symptoms typically first appearing between ages 40 and 60. It is characterized by slowly progressive ptosis, dysphagia, and proximal limb weakness. Facial weakness, changes in voice quality, and excessive fatigue may develop; impaired cognitive function also has been described (Waito et al., 2018). Because of the ptosis, patients with OPMD may assume an unusual posture characterized by raised eyebrows and extended neck.

Dysphagia in OPMD is due to impaired function of the oropharyngeal musculature. Impaired swallow efficiency due to reduced pharyngeal constriction, speed of hyoid movement, and degree of airway closure may lead to oral and nasal regurgitation, aspiration, postswallow pharyngeal residue, and esophageal retention (Waito et al., 2018). Although it evolves slowly over many years, OPMD may eventually result not only in difficulty or discomfort with swallowing but also in weight loss, malnutrition, and aspiration.

No specific treatment for the muscular dystrophy itself is available, but both cricopharyngeal myotomy and botulinum toxin injection into the cricopharyngeal muscle are effective in diminishing dysphagia in the setting of OPMD. However, both worsened dysphagia and dysphonia may be complications of botulinum toxin injections (Youssof et al., 2014).

### BOX 15.2 Neuromuscular Dysphagia

**Oropharyngeal**

- Inflammatory myopathies:
  - Dermatomyositis
  - Inclusion body myositis
  - Polymyositis
- Mitochondrial myopathies:
  - Kearns-Sayre syndrome
  - MNGIE
- Muscular dystrophies:
  - Duchenne
  - Facioscapulohumeral
  - Limb girdle
  - Myotonic
  - Oculopharyngeal
- Neuromuscular junction disorders:
  - Botulism
  - Lambert-Eaton syndrome
  - Myasthenia gravis
  - Tetanus
- Scleroderma
- Stiff man syndrome

**Esophageal**

- Amyloidosis
- Inflammatory myopathies:
  - Dermatomyositis
  - Polymyositis
- Scleroderma

*MNGIE*, Myoneurogastrointestinal encephalomyopathy.

### Myotonic Dystrophy

Myotonic dystrophy is an autosomal dominant disorder whose phenotypic picture includes not only skeletal muscle but also cardiac, ophthalmological, endocrinological, and even central nervous system involvement. It is the most common form of adult-onset muscular dystrophy. Mutations at two distinct locations are associated with the clinical picture of myotonic dystrophy. Type 1 myotonic dystrophy is due to a CTG expansion in the myotonic dystrophy protein kinase (*DMPK*) gene on chromosome 19; type 2 is the consequence of a CCTG repeat expansion in the zinc finger protein 9 (*ZNF9*) gene on chromosome 3.

Gastrointestinal (GI) symptoms develop in more than 50% of individuals with the clinical phenotype of myotonic dystrophy. These may be the most disabling component of the disorder in 25% of individuals with type 1 myotonic dystrophy, and GI symptoms may actually antedate the appearance of other neuromuscular features. Subjective dysphagia is one of the most prevalent GI features and has been reported in 37%–56% of patients (Ertekin et al., 2001b). Coughing when eating, suggestive of aspiration, may occur in 33%. Objective measures paint a picture of even more pervasive impairment, demonstrating disturbances in swallowing in 70%–80% of persons with myotonic dystrophy (Ertekin et al., 2001b). In one study, 75% of patients asymptomatic for dysphagia were still noted to have abnormalities on objective testing (Marcon et al., 1998).

A variety of abnormalities in objective measures of swallowing have been documented in myotonic dystrophy. Abnormal cricopharyngeal muscle activity is present in 40% of patients during electromyographic (EMG) testing (Ertekin et al., 2001b). Impaired esophageal peristalsis has also been noted in affected individuals studied with esophageal manometry. On videofluoroscopic testing, incomplete relaxation of the UES and esophageal hypotonia were the most frequently noted abnormalities (Marcon et al., 1998). Both muscle weakness and myotonia are felt to play a role in the development of dysphagia in persons with myotonic dystrophy (Ertekin et al., 2001b); in at least one study, a correlation was noted between the size of the CTG repeat expansion and the number of radiological abnormalities in myotonic patients

(Marcon et al., 1998). In a systematic review of oropharyngeal dysphagia in type 1 myotonic dystrophy, Pilz and colleagues identified pharyngeal pooling, decreased pharyngeal contraction amplitude, and reduced UES resting pressure as the primary findings responsible for dysphagia (Pilz et al., 2014). Cognitive dysfunction also may predispose individuals with myotonic dystrophy to be less aware of dysphagia and less likely to employ measures such as proper diet and eating methods to minimize it (Umemoto et al., 2012).

## Other Muscular Dystrophies

Although less well characterized, dysphagia also occurs in other types of muscular dystrophy. Difficulty swallowing and choking while eating occur with increased frequency in children with Duchenne muscular dystrophy. Dysphagia has also been documented in patients with limb-girdle dystrophy and facioscapulohumeral dystrophy (FSHD). Dysphagia associated with reduced cheek compression strength and reduced endurance of cheek compression and anterior tongue elevation is evident in 25% of patients with FSHD (Mul et al., 2019).

## Inflammatory Myopathies

Dermatomyositis and polymyositis are the most frequently occurring of the inflammatory myopathic disorders. Both are characterized by progressive, usually symmetrical weakness affecting proximal muscles more prominently than distal. Fatigue and myalgia also may occur. Malignant disease is associated with the disorder in 10%–15% of patients with dermatomyositis and 5%–10% of those with polymyositis. Among individuals older than age 65 with these inflammatory myopathies, more than 50% are found to have cancer.

Although dysphagia can develop in both conditions, it more frequently is present in dermatomyositis; when present, it is more severe. Dysphagia is present in 20%–55% of individuals with dermatomyositis but in only 18% with polymyositis (Parodi et al., 2002). The risk of dysphagia in dermatomyositis is associated with the presence of internal malignancy and anti–transcription intermediary factor 1$\gamma$ (TIF-1$\gamma$) antibody (Mugii et al., 2016). It is the consequence of involvement of striated muscle in the pharynx and proximal esophagus. Involvement of pharyngeal and esophageal musculature in polymyositis and dermatomyositis is an indicator of poor prognosis and can be the source of significant morbidity. A 1-year mortality rate of 31% has been reported in individuals with inflammatory myopathy and dysphagia (Williams et al., 2003), although other investigators have reported a 1-year survival rate of 89% (Oh et al., 2007).

Dysphagia in persons with inflammatory myopathy may be due to restrictive pharyngoesophageal abnormalities such as cricopharyngeal bar, Zenker diverticulum, and stenosis. In fact, in one study of 13 patients with inflammatory myopathy, radiographic constrictions were noted in 9 (69%) individuals, compared with 1 of 17 controls with dysphagia of neurogenic origin (Williams et al., 2003). Aspiration was also more common in the patients with myositis (61% vs. 41%). The resulting dysphagia can be severe enough to require enteral feeding. Acute total obstruction by the cricopharyngeal muscle has been reported in dermatomyositis, necessitating cricopharyngeal myotomy. Other investigators have reported improvement in 50% of individuals 1 month following cricopharyngeal bar disruption; improvement was still present in 25% at 6 months (Williams et al., 2003). The reason for the formation of restrictive abnormalities in inflammatory myopathy is uncertain, but it may be that long-standing inflammation of the cricopharyngeus muscle impedes its compliance and ability to open fully (Williams et al., 2003).

Dysphagia also may develop in inclusion body myositis and may even be the presenting symptom. In the late stages of the disorder, the frequency of dysphagia may actually exceed that seen in dermatomyositis and polymyositis. In a group of individuals in whom inclusion-body myositis mimicked and was confused with motor neuron disease, dysphagia was present in 44% (Dabby et al., 2001). In another study, dysphagia was documented in 37 of 57 (65%) patients with inclusion-body myositis (Cox et al., 2009). Abnormal function of the UES, probably due to inflammatory involvement of the cricopharyngeal muscle with consequent reduced compliance, was documented in 37%. A focal inflammatory myopathy involving the pharyngeal muscles and producing isolated pharyngeal dysphagia also has been described in individuals older than age 69. It has been suggested that this is a distinct clinical entity characterized by cricopharyngeal hypertrophy, although polymyositis localized to the pharyngeal musculature has been reported.

Dysphagia in both dermatomyositis and polymyositis may respond to corticosteroids and other immunosuppressive drugs, and these remain the mainstay of treatment. Intravenous immunoglobulin (IVIG) therapy has produced dramatic improvement in dysphagia in individuals who were unresponsive to steroids. Although inclusion-body myositis usually responds poorly to these agents, there are reports of long-lasting stabilization of dysphagia with either intravenous or subcutaneous immunoglobulin therapy (Pars et al., 2013). More often, cricopharyngeal myotomy is necessary (Oh et al., 2007).

## Mitochondrial Disorders

The mitochondrial disorders are a family of diseases that develop as a consequence of dysfunction in the mitochondrial respiratory chain. Most are the result of mutations in mitochondrial deoxyribonucleic acid (DNA) genes, but nuclear DNA mutations may be responsible in some. Mitochondrial disorders are by nature multisystemic, but myopathic and neurological features often predominate, and symptoms may vary widely even between individuals within the same family.

In addition to the classic constellation of symptoms—including progressive external ophthalmoplegia, retinitis pigmentosa, cardiac conduction defects, and ataxia—individuals with Kearns-Sayre syndrome also may develop dysphagia. Severe abnormalities of pharyngeal and upper esophageal peristalsis have been documented in this disorder. Cricopharyngeal dysfunction is common and impaired deglutitive coordination may develop.

Dysphagia has also been described in other mitochondrial disorders, but these descriptions are only anecdotal and formal study has not been undertaken.

## Myasthenia Gravis

MG is an autoimmune disorder characterized by the production of autoantibodies directed against the $\alpha_1$ subunit of the nicotinic postsynaptic acetylcholine receptors at the neuromuscular junction, causing destruction of the receptors and a reduction in their number. The clinical consequence of this process is the development of fatigable muscle weakness that progressively increases with repetitive muscle action and improves with rest. MG occurs more frequently in women than in men. Although symptoms can develop at any age, the reported mean age of onset in women is between 28 and 35 years and in men between 42 and 49 years. Although myasthenic symptoms remain confined to the extraocular muscles in approximately 20% of patients, more widespread muscle weakness becomes evident in most individuals.

Initial involvement of the bulbar musculature, sometimes labeled laryngeal MG and characterized by dysphagia or dysarthria, is surprisingly common in MG (Yang et al., 2019). Bulbar involvement is evident from the beginning in approximately 6%–30% of MG patients (Koopman et al., 2004); with disease progression, most eventually develop bulbar symptoms such as dysphagia and dysarthria. It is important to recognize, however, that swallowing function may be abnormal even without the presence of symptomatic dysphagia in individuals with MG (Umay et al., 2018). Dysphagia in MG can be due to dysfunction at the oral, pharyngeal, or even esophageal levels, and many patients experience it at multiple levels. In a study of 20 myasthenic patients experiencing dysphagia, abnormalities in the oral preparatory phase were evident in 13 individuals (65%), oral phase dysphagia in 18 (90%), and pharyngeal phase involvement in all 20 (100%; Koopman et al., 2004). Oral phase involvement can be due to fatigue and weakness of the tongue or masticatory muscles. In MG patients with bulbar symptoms, repetitive nerve stimulation studies of the hypoglossal nerve have demonstrated abnormalities, as have studies utilizing EMG of the masticatory muscles recorded while chewing. Pharyngeal dysfunction is also common in MG patients who have dysphagia, as demonstrated by videofluoroscopy (VFS). Aspiration, often silent, may be present in 35% or more of these individuals; in elderly patients the frequency of aspiration may be considerably higher. Bedside speech pathology assessment is not a reliable predictor of aspiration (Koopman et al., 2004). Motor dysfunction involving the striated muscle of the proximal esophagus also has been documented in MG. In one study that used testing with esophageal manometry, 96% of patients with MG demonstrated abnormalities such as decreased amplitude and prolongation of the peristaltic wave in this region. Cricopharyngeal sphincter pressure was also noted to be reduced.

It is important to remember that dysphagia can also precipitate myasthenic crisis in individuals with MG. In fact, in one study, dysphagia was considered to be a major precipitant of myasthenic crisis in 56% of patients (Koopman et al., 2004).

## NEUROGENIC DYSPHAGIA

A variety of disease processes originating in the central and peripheral nervous systems can disrupt swallowing mechanisms and produce dysphagia. Processes affecting cerebral cortex, subcortical white matter, subcortical gray matter, brainstem, spinal cord, and peripheral nerves can all elicit dysphagia as a component of the clinical picture (Box 15.3). In addition, oropharyngeal dysphagia is reported in 23% of independently living elderly (Serra-Prat et al., 2011). The term *presbyphagia* describes multifactorial changes of swallowing physiology associated with aging. These changes are more likely to be related to stroke and neurodegenerative disorders in older individuals; in patients younger than age 60, oncological or other neurological pathologies are more probable (Baijens et al., 2016).

In individuals with neurogenic dysphagia, prolonged swallow response, delayed laryngeal closure, and weak bolus propulsion combine to increase the risk of aspiration and the likelihood of malnutrition.

### Stroke

Stroke is the fifth leading cause of death, claiming 133,000 lives annually; it is the number one cause of adult disability in the United States. Each year, close to 800,000 people experience a new or recurrent stroke. On average, every 40 seconds, someone in the United States has a stroke. The mechanism of stroke is ischemic in 87% of cases; of the remaining cases, 10% are due to intracerebral hemorrhage and 3% the result of subarachnoid hemorrhage. Although stroke can occur at any age, its prevalence increases with advancing age in both males and females, and 75% of strokes occur in individuals older than 75 years.

Dysphagia develops in 28%–65% of individuals following acute stroke, and its presence is associated with increased likelihood of severe disability or death (Falsetti et al., 2009; Runions et al., 2004; Schaller et al., 2006). This wide range reflects differences in the manner of assessment of dysphagia, the setting, and the timing of the test used. Although many stroke patients recover swallowing spontaneously in the early days after stroke, 11%–50% will continue to have dysphagia at 6 months (Mann et al., 2000; Martino et al., 2005). Aspiration and pneumonia are the most widely recognized complications of dysphagia

**BOX 15.3 Neurogenic Dysphagia**

**Oropharyngeal**

- Arnold-Chiari malformation
- Basal ganglia disease:
  - Biotin responsive
  - Corticobasal degeneration
  - DLB
  - HD
  - Multiple system atrophy
  - Neuroacanthocytosis
  - PD
  - PSP
  - WD
- Central pontine myelinolysis
- Cerebral palsy
- Drug related:
  - Cyclosporine
  - Tardive dyskinesia
  - Vincristine
- Infectious:
  - Brainstem encephalitis
  - Diphtheria
  - Epstein-Barr virus
  - *Listeria*
  - Poliomyelitis
  - Progressive multifocal leukoencephalopathy
  - Rabies
- Mass lesions:
  - Abscess
  - Hemorrhage
  - Metastatic tumor
  - Primary tumor
- Motor neuron diseases:
  - ALS
  - MS
- Peripheral neuropathic processes:
  - Charcot-Marie-Tooth disease
  - Guillain-Barré syndrome (Miller Fisher variant)
- Spinocerebellar ataxias
- Stroke
- Syringobulbia

**Esophageal**

- Achalasia
- Autonomic neuropathies:
  - Diabetes mellitus
  - Familial dysautonomia
  - Paraneoplastic syndromes
- Basal ganglia disorders:
  - PD
- Chagas disease
- Esophageal motility disorders
- Scleroderma

*ALS*, Amyotrophic lateral sclerosis; *DLB*, dementia with Lewy bodies; *HD*, Huntington disease; *MS*, multiple sclerosis; *PD*, Parkinson disease; *PSP*, progressive supranuclear palsy; *WD*, Wilson disease.

following stroke, but undernourishment and even malnutrition also occur with surprising frequency (Finestone and Greene-Finestone, 2003). Using screening assessment tools, there is evidence that 12%–41% of stroke survivors are at risk of malnutrition at 6 months (Brynningsen et al., 2007) and 11% at 16–18 months (Jönsson et al., 2008). Poststroke dysphagia is an independent predictor of poor outcome, institutionalization, and significant costs (Kumar et al., 2012). The risk of developing pneumonia is three times higher in stroke patients with dysphagia; in patients with confirmed aspiration, the risk is elevated 11-fold (Smithard et al., 2007). The individual cost of pneumonia and associated mortality in a large retrospective US study of stroke patients was quantified as $27,633 (Wilson, 2012).

Finestone and Greene-Finestone (2003) have delineated a number of warning signs that can alert physicians to the presence of poststroke dysphagia. Some are obvious and others more subtle. They include drooling, excessive tongue movement or spitting food out of the mouth, poor tongue control, pocketing of food in the mouth, facial weakness, slurred speech, coughing or choking while eating, regurgitation of food through the nose, wet or "gurgly" voice after eating, hoarse or breathy voice, complaints of food sticking in the throat, absence or delay of laryngeal elevation, prolonged chewing, prolonged time to eat or reluctance to eat, and recurrent pneumonia.

Although it is commonly perceived that the presence of dysphagia following stroke indicates a brainstem localization for the stroke, this is not necessarily so. Impaired swallowing has been documented in a significant proportion of strokes involving cortical and subcortical structures. The pharyngeal phase of swallowing is primarily impaired in brainstem infarction; in hemispheric strokes, the most striking abnormality is often a delay in initiation of voluntary swallowing. Strokes involving the right hemisphere tend to produce more impairment of pharyngeal motility, whereas left hemispheric lesions have a greater effect on oral stage function (Ickenstein et al., 2005). Dysphagia has been reported as the sole manifestation of infarction in both medulla and cerebrum.

Approximately 50%–55% of patients with lesions in the posterior inferior cerebellar artery distribution with consequent lateral medullary infarction (Wallenberg syndrome) develop dysphagia (Teasell et al., 2002). The fact that unilateral medullary infarction can produce bilateral disruption of the brainstem's swallowing centers suggests that they function as one integrated center. Infarction in the distribution of the anteroinferior cerebellar artery can also result in dysphagia.

Following stroke within the cerebral hemispheres, dysphagia can develop by virtue of damage to either cortical or subcortical structures involved with volitional swallowing. Cortical reorganization then plays a key role in swallowing recovery. The mechanism of swallowing recovery after stroke was studied in 28 hemispheric stroke patients using VFS and TMS. After hemispheric stroke, nondysphagic subjects displayed greater pharyngeal cortical representation in the contralesional hemisphere compared with dysphagic subjects. TMS follow-up data at 1 and 3 months indicated that subjects who recovered swallowing function had significantly greater pharyngeal representation in the unaffected hemisphere compared with baseline. These findings highlight the importance of the contralesional hemisphere in swallowing recovery and suggest that bilateral hemispheric damage is more likely to produce dysphagia (Cohen et al., 2016). Bilateral infarction of the frontoparietal operculum may result in the anterior operculum syndrome (Foix-Chavany-Marie syndrome), which is characterized by inability to perform voluntary movements of the face, jaw, tongue, and pharynx but with fully preserved involuntary movements of the same muscles. Impairment of volitional swallowing may be a component of this syndrome. Although tongue deviation is classically associated with medullary lesions damaging the hypoglossal nucleus, it has also been documented in almost 30% of persons with hemispheric infarctions. When present in hemispheric stroke, tongue deviation is always associated with facial weakness and dysphagia is present in 43% of affected patients.

Individuals with subcortical strokes have a higher incidence of dysphagia and aspiration than those with cortical damage. In one study, more than 85% of individuals with unilateral subcortical strokes demonstrated videofluoroscopic evidence of delayed initiation of the pharyngeal stage of swallowing; in 75%, some radiographic aspiration was noted. Using magnetoencephalography (MEG), Teismann and colleagues compared swallowing activation in subacute stroke patients with and without dysphagia with healthy controls. Increased contralesional activity was predictive of no dysphagia in this study, suggesting that neuroplasticity plays an important role in the recovery of swallowing function (Teismann et al., 2011).

Aspiration is a potentially life-threatening complication of stroke. Studies have documented its occurrence in 30%–55% of stroke patients. In one study, videofluoroscopic evidence of aspiration was observed in 36% of patients with unilateral cerebral stroke, 46% with bilateral cerebral stroke, 60% with unilateral brainstem stroke, and 50% with bilateral brainstem lesions. Other studies have suggested that the incidence of aspiration in brainstem strokes may be considerably higher—more than 80%—and that subcortical strokes may result in aspiration in 75% of cases. Kemmling and colleagues (2013) have reported that individuals with right peri-insular strokes have an increased risk of developing hospital-acquired pneumonia and suggest that this may be related to impairment in host immunity due to autonomically induced immunosuppression rather than being a direct consequence of aspiration secondary to dysphagia. Additionally, two symptom mapping studies showed a strong association between dysphagia and right hemispheric opercular and primary sensorimotor cortex strokes (Galovic et al., 2013; Suntrup et al., 2015). In individuals with left hemispheric middle cerebral artery stroke, the presence of aphasia or buccofacial apraxia is a highly significant predictor of dysphagia (Somasundaram et al., 2014).

Individuals with signs of aspiration within the first 72 hours following acute stroke have a 12-fold higher risk of being dependent on a feeding tube 3 months later (Ickenstein et al., 2012). On the other hand, aspiration in dysphagic patients may not be associated with obvious signs such as a cough response or overt swallowing difficulty. In fact, silent aspiration (aspiration with absence of any outward signs of distress) occurs in over 2%–25% of patients (Ramsey et al., 2005). Furthermore, an absent gag reflex does not help to differentiate those aspirating from those who are not (Finestone and Greene-Finestone, 2003). In one study, only 44% of patients with suspected oropharyngeal dysphagia following stroke had an impaired gag reflex, and only 47% coughed during oral feeding (Terré and Mearin, 2006). Therefore the employment of objective testing measures to detect the presence and predict the risk of aspiration has been advocated. Dysphagia after stroke can be diagnosed by clinical bedside assessments or instrumentally. Instrumental assessment utilizing modified barium swallow testing with VFS is considered the gold standard in the diagnosis of dysphagia but requires specialist staff and equipment and may not be possible within the first few hours after stroke; clinical bedside assessment is the only option in these cases (Cohen et al., 2016). Simple bedside techniques such as a water-swallowing test have been advocated as practical though somewhat less sensitive alternatives.

Ickenstein and colleagues (2010) emphasize the value of a stepwise assessment of swallowing in patients admitted to the hospital with stroke, with the assessment beginning on the first day of admission. The first step is a modified swallowing assessment performed by the nursing staff on the day of admission; the second step is a clinical swallowing examination performed within 72 hours of admission by a swallowing therapist; the third step is performance of flexible transnasal swallowing endoscopy performed by a physician within 5 days of admission. Appropriate diet and treatment are then determined after each step. Employment of such a stepwise assessment of dysphagia resulted in a significant reduction in the rate of pneumonia and in antibiotic consumption in a stroke unit (Ickenstein et al., 2010). Instrumental methods of assessment of dysphagia include the videofluoroscopic swallowing study (VFS) and fiberoptic endoscopic evaluation of swallowing (FEES). VFS involves swallowing a radiological contrast agent. It is an expensive test, requires travel to a radiology suite, and it involves radiation. Hence it is impractical to perform VFS in every case. In FEES, a laryngoscope is passed transnasally to the hypopharynx to view the larynx and pharynx. The FEES study enables assessment of anatomy, secretions, and of food and drink management. The equipment is portable, sitting is not essential, and the procedure can be performed at the bedside. However, FEES and VFS are not routinely available in many hospitals worldwide. When available, these two instrumental assessments are consistent and interchangeable. They are the only two assessments that can diagnose aspiration reliably.

Swallowing often improves spontaneously in the days and weeks after stroke. Improvement is more likely to occur after cortical strokes compared with those of brainstem origin; the improvement is probably the result of compensatory reorganization of undamaged brain areas (Schaller et al., 2006). Given this natural ability of the brain to reorganize, there has been increased interest in the therapeutic potential of neuromodulation to treat oropharyngeal dysphagia. One of these methods is transcranial direct current stimulation (tDCS), which promotes brain plasticity by tonic stimulation. A recent double-blind randomized study in 60 patients with acute dysphagic stroke showed that those who received tDCS over the contralesional swallowing motor cortex had more rapid rehabilitation of acute poststroke dysphagia. Early intervention seemed to be beneficial in this study. Nasogastric tube feeding can temporarily provide adequate nutrition and buy time until swallowing improves sufficiently to allow oral feeding, but it entails some risks itself, such as increasing the possibility of reflux with consequent aspiration. For individuals in whom significant dysphagia persists after stroke, placement of a percutaneous endoscopic gastrostomy (PEG) tube may become necessary. Ickenstein and colleagues (2005) documented this necessity in 77 of 664 (11.6%) stroke patients admitted to their rehabilitation hospital. Continued need for a PEG tube after discharge from the unit carried with it a somber prognosis.

Various methods of behavioral swallowing therapy have traditionally been used in managing persistent poststroke dysphagia. However, the treatment landscape may be changing. Early application of neuromuscular electrical stimulation therapy in conjunction with traditional dysphagia therapy appears to be more effective in improving swallowing function than traditional therapy by itself (Lee et al., 2014). The combination of bilateral repetitive TMS and traditional therapy may also be more effective than traditional therapy alone (Momosaki et al., 2014). In individuals who experience dysfunction of the UES poststroke, a single botulinum toxin injection into the cricopharyngeal muscle may afford an improvement in swallowing that may last for up to 12 months, although care must be taken in choosing appropriate patients (Terré et al., 2013). In a small percentage of individuals, however, placement of a PEG tube will be necessary.

In an individual patient data meta-analysis of three randomized controlled trials of pharyngeal electrical stimulation (PES) for poststroke dysphagia, reduced radiological aspiration, reduced dysphagia, and reduced length of hospital stay were documented (Scutt et al., 2015). However, a subsequent large randomized controlled trial involving 162 patients did not demonstrate benefit for the procedure, although possible undertreatment was suggested as a potential explanation for the absence of benefit (Bath et al., 2016). Reduction in salivary substance P has been associated with reduced swallowing frequency poststroke (Niimi et al., 2018). In another study in which PES (which increases salivary substance P levels) was performed on 23 tracheotomized stroke patients who could not be decannulated due to severe dysphagia, 61% were decannulated after the first treatment cycle and success in achieving decannulation was closely correlated with increased salivary substance P levels (Muhle et al., 2017).

Dysphagia can also develop in the setting of other cerebrovascular processes. Within the anterior circulation, dysphagia has been reported with carotid artery aneurysms. Within the posterior circulation, processes such as elongation and dilatation of the basilar artery, posterior inferior cerebellar artery aneurysm, intracranial vertebral artery dissections, giant dissecting vertebrobasilar aneurysms, and cavernous malformations within the medulla may produce dysphagia in addition to other symptoms.

Dysphagia is also a potential complication of carotid endarterectomy, not on the basis of stroke but due to laryngeal or cranial nerve injury. In one study, careful otolaryngologic examination demonstrated such deficits in almost 60% of patients postoperatively (Monini et al., 2005). Most deficits were mild and transient, but some persistent impairment was noted in 17.5% of those studied, and 9% required some rehabilitative procedures. Some investigators recommend careful evaluation and early rehabilitation to improve swallowing function at 1 and 3 months after the procedure (Masiero et al., 2007).

## Multiple Sclerosis

MS is an inflammatory demyelinating disease of the central nervous system that primarily though not exclusively affects young adults. The mean age of onset is approximately age 30. In its most common guise, MS is characterized by exacerbations and remissions, although some individuals may follow a chronic progressive course right from the start. The etiology of MS is uncertain but an autoimmune process is presumed.

Dysphagia is a frequent problem that presents challenges for the management of MS patients. Survey studies report subjective difficulty swallowing in approximately 38% of adults with MS (Alali et al., 2018; Levinthal et al., 2013), but studies utilizing objective measures, such as swallowing videoendoscopy, demonstrate abnormalities in approximately 90% of patients (Fernandes et al., 2013). The prevalence of dysphagia in MS rises with increasing disability; about 17% of individuals with mild disability may develop neurogenic dysphagia, with the percentage escalating to 65% in the most severely affected. Dysphagia in MS is caused by a combination of impairments in several structures including the corticobulbar tracts, cerebellum, brainstem, and lower cranial nerves (Alali et al., 2016). On the other hand, cognitive and affective impairments may also influence the type and severity of symptoms observed. Adults with MS-related dysphagia report reduced scores across all domains of swallowing-related quality of life, including burden of dysphagia, eating duration, food selection, fear related to eating, and social concerns related to swallowing problems (Alali et al., 2018).

Abnormalities in the oral, pharyngeal, and even esophageal phases of swallowing have been documented. Rare instances of the anterior operculum syndrome with buccolinguofacial apraxia have been reported in MS. Abnormalities in the oral phase of swallowing are common in MS patients with mild disability, but additional pharyngeal phase abnormalities develop in those with more severe disability. Disturbances in both the sequencing of laryngeal events and function of the pharyngeal constrictor muscles are typically present in persons experiencing dysphagia. Pharyngeal sensory impairment may play a role in the development of dysphagia in some patients.

If untreated, dysphagia may lead to reduced quality of life, increased risk of weight loss and dehydration, and aspiration pneumonia; therefore dysphagia should be identified and treated at the early stages of the disease (Poorjavad et al., 2010). Steps in the diagnosis of dysphagia in MS include bedside evaluation, questionnaires, and FEES (Giusti and Giambuzzi, 2008). Although treatment approaches are limited, intraluminal PES has been demonstrated to provide sustained benefit in a blinded pilot study of a small number of patients (Restivo et al., 2013a).

## Parkinson Disease

PD is a neurodegenerative disorder in which symptoms typically emerge between 55 and 65 years of age. The most prominent neuropathology in PD involves the pigmented dopaminergic neurons in the substantia nigra, but neuronal loss in other areas of the nervous system, including the enteric nervous system, has also been documented.

Dysphagia was first described in PD by none other than James Parkinson himself in his original description of the illness in 1817. It now is recognized as a frequent component of PD. Results of a meta-analysis indicated that subjective dysphagia is acknowledged by 35% of individuals with PD; studies utilizing objective measures show a much higher prevalence estimate of 82% (Kalf et al., 2012; Takizawa et al., 2016). Sex, age, disease duration, and dementia all seem to contribute to the occurrence of swallowing disturbances (Cereda et al., 2014).

Dysphagia in PD may be due to oral, pharyngeal, or esophageal dysfunction. Within the oral phase, difficulty with bolus formation, delayed initiation of swallowing, repeated tongue pumping, and other abnormalities have been demonstrated with modified barium swallow testing. Pharyngeal dysmotility, retention of tablets in the epiglottic vallecula, and impaired relaxation of the cricopharyngeal muscle constitute examples of abnormalities noted in the pharyngeal phase. All of these abnormalities can delay the onset of symptom relief after PD medications are taken and may easily be overlooked because they cannot be assessed visually; diagnosis requires laryngoscopy or videofluorographic examination of swallowing (Sato et al., 2018). Individuals with PD are more likely to swallow during inspiration and also to inhale post swallow, both of which increase the risk of aspiration (Gross et al., 2008). The esophageal phase is the most automatic stage of swallowing and esophageal dysfunction also can trigger dysphagia in PD. Impairment of UES movement is common in PD and can result in esophageal dysphagia (Van Hooren et.al., 2014). Esophageal manometry has demonstrated abnormalities in 61%–73% of PD patients studied; videofluoroscopic studies show a broader range, with some abnormality reported in 5%–86% of individuals (Pfeiffer, 2018). A wide variety of abnormalities of esophageal function have been described, including slowed esophageal transit, both segmental and diffuse esophageal spasm, ineffective or tertiary contractions, and even aperistalsis. Dysfunction of the lower esophageal sphincter may also be present in PD and can produce not only symptoms of reflux but also dysphagia.

Aspiration has been noted to be present in 15%–56% of patients with PD and completely silent aspiration in 15%–33% (Pfeiffer, 2003). Even more striking is a study in which vallecular residue, believed to indicate an increased risk of aspiration, was found to be present in 88% of PD patients without clinical dysphagia. Silent aspiration and laryngeal penetration of saliva have been noted to occur in a significant percentage (10.7% and 28.6%, respectively) of individuals with PD who exhibit daily drooling (Rodrigues et al., 2011). In another study by the same group of investigators, a 9.75-fold increased risk of respiratory infection was documented in PD patients with daily drooling and silent aspiration or silent laryngeal penetration of food who were followed for 1 year (Nóbrega et al., 2008). However, a cross-sectional study of 119 patients with PD and 32 controls did not support drooling as a hallmark symptom for critical dysphagia in that 39% of patients with critical aspiration had no drooling and 41% of patients with severe drooling had no clinically relevant dysphagia on FEES (Nienstedt et al., 2018). The increased risk of aspiration in individuals with PD is associated with a prolonged swallowing time (Lin et al., 2012).

Dysphagia in PD has traditionally been attributed to rigidity and bradykinesia of the involved musculature secondary to basal ganglia dysfunction. However, alpha-synuclein deposition and axonal degeneration have been documented in peripheral motor nerves innervating the pharynx, along with evidence of denervation in pharyngeal muscles (Mu et al., 2013). Hypesthesia of laryngeal structures has also been noted in PD patients, possibly contributing to the risk of aspiration (Rodrigues et al., 2011). Utilizing MEG, diminished cortical activation also has been documented in individuals with PD experiencing dysphagia (Suntrup et al., 2013).

Whether dysphagia responds to levodopa or dopamine agonist therapy is controversial. Objective improvement in swallowing, documented by modified barium swallow testing, has been observed in 33%–50% of patients in some but not all studies. It has also been suggested that improvement in motor function with levodopa may make possible the adoption of compensatory swallowing postures (Nóbrega et al., 2014).

The effect of deep brain stimulation (DBS) on swallowing is also disputed. Studies assessing the effect of DBS on swallowing using subthalamic nucleus (STN) or globus pallidus internus (GPi) targeting did not identify clinically significant improvement or deterioration. Despite patient reports of improvement in swallowing function, no clinically relevant changes in deglutition were found using FEES or VFS (Silbergleit et al., 2012; Troche et al., 2013).

In patients with cricopharyngeal muscle dysfunction, both cricopharyngeal myotomy and botulinum toxin injections have been used successfully. Traditional behavioral swallowing therapy approaches are of benefit to some individuals. Newer techniques—such as expiratory muscle strength training (EMST) and video-assisted swallowing therapy (VAST)—show promise, but surface electrical stimulation (SES) of the neck does not appear to be effective (van Hooren et al., 2014). On rare occasions, PEG tube placement may be necessary.

## Other Basal Ganglia Disorders

In the PD-plus syndromes—such as progressive supranuclear palsy (PSP), multiple system atrophy, corticobasal degeneration, and dementia with Lewy bodies (DLB)—dysphagia is a frequent problem; in contrast to PD, it often develops relatively early in the course of the illness. The median latency to the development of dysphagia in PD is more than 130 months, whereas it is 67 months in multiple system atrophy, 64 months in corticobasal degeneration, 43 months in DLB, and 42 months in PSP (Muller et al., 2001). In fact, the appearance of dysphagia within 1 year of symptom onset virtually eliminates PD as a diagnostic possibility, although it does not help to distinguish between the various PD-plus syndromes (Muller et al., 2001). In persons with PSP, the presence and severity of dysphagia does not correlate well with the presence and severity of dysarthria, so the decision to evaluate swallowing function should not be based on the presence or absence of speech impairment.

Dysphagia can be a prominent problem in patients with Wilson disease and is frequently a component of the clinical picture in chorea-acanthocytosis. Dysphagia in chorea-acanthocytosis is primarily the result of prominent orolingual dyskinesia, which pushes food out of the mouth and is pathognomonic of this disorder. A unique basal ganglia process characterized by the presence of subacute encephalopathy, seizures, dysarthria, dysphagia, rigidity, dystonia, and eventual quadriparesis—now labeled biotin thiamine-responsive basal ganglia disease—has been shown to improve promptly and dramatically after biotin and thiamine administration (Algahtani, et al., 2017). Dysphagia may also develop in the setting of spinocerebellar ataxia.

Dysphagia is also a well-documented complication of botulinum toxin injections for cervical dystonia, presumably as a consequence of diffusion of the toxin. It should be noted, however, that 11% of patients with cervical dystonia experience dysphagia as part of the disease process itself, and 22% may display abnormalities on objective testing. Whether the dysphagia in individuals with cervical dystonia is mechanical or neurogenic has been the topic of debate. In a study of 25 patients with cervical dystonia, clinical assessment suggested the presence of dysphagia in 36% and electrophysiological evaluation demonstrated abnormalities in 72% (Ertekin et al., 2002). The electrophysiological abnormalities strongly suggested a neurogenic basis for the dysfunction.

## Amyotrophic Lateral Sclerosis

Amyotrophic lateral sclerosis (ALS) is the most common form of motor neuron disease. It is characterized by progressive loss of motor neurons in the cortex, brainstem, and spinal cord, which results in a clinical picture of progressive weakness that combines features of both upper motor neuron dysfunction with spasticity and hyperreflexia and lower motor neuron dysfunction with atrophy, fasciculations, and hyporeflexia. The mean age of symptom onset is between ages 54 and 58 years. ALS is categorized into two forms. The most common form is sporadic (90%–95%); the remaining 5%–10% are familial ALS (FALS). There is no obvious genetic inheritance in the former group, whereas there is a dominant inheritance pattern in the latter group (Valdmanis and Rouleau, 2018).

Although dysphagia eventually develops in most individuals with ALS, bulbar symptoms can be the presenting feature in approximately 25% of patients. Individuals with bulbar onset of symptoms have a fivefold greater risk of developing dysphagia than those with spinal onset (Ruoppolo et al., 2013). A sensation of solid food sticking in the esophagus may provide the initial clue to emerging dysphagia, but abnormalities in the oral phase of swallowing are most often evident in patients with early ALS. Impaired function of the lips and tongue (particularly the posterior portion of the tongue) due to evolving muscle weakness typically appears first, followed next by involvement of jaw and suprahyoid musculature, and finally by weakness of pharyngeal and laryngeal muscles. Lip weakness can result in spillage of food from the mouth; tongue weakness leads to impaired food bolus formation and transfer. Inadequate mastication due to jaw muscle weakness adds to the difficulty with bolus formation, and the eventual development of pharyngeal and laryngeal weakness opens the door for aspiration. Neurophysiological testing in patients with ALS who have dysphagia demonstrates delay in the triggering of the swallowing reflex for voluntarily initiated swallows and its eventual abolishment with relative preservation of spontaneous reflexive swallows until the terminal stages of the disease. Videofluoroscopic studies have demonstrated that reduced pharyngeal constriction is associated with impaired swallowing efficiency in individuals with ALS (Waito et al., 2018b). Although VFS is the most precise means of evaluating dysphagia in individuals with ALS, scales such as the Norris ALS Scale provide an adequate method for deciding on the need for dysphagia treatment. The development of oropharyngeal dysphagia in individuals with ALS has a discernible effect on quality of life and is associated with increased depression and social withdrawal (Paris et al., 2013).

Spasm of the UES, with hyperreflexia and hypertonicity of the cricopharyngeal muscle, has been reported in ALS patients with bulbar dysfunction, presumably as a consequence of upper motor neuron involvement, and has been considered to be an important cause of aspiration (Ertekin et al., 2001a). This has prompted the employment of cricopharyngeal myotomy and more recently botulinum toxin injection (Restivo et al., 2013b) as a treatment measure in such patients, but these approaches should be limited to those with objectively demonstrated UES spasm.

Control of oral secretions can be a difficult problem for patients with ALS. Peripherally acting anticholinergic drugs such as glycopyrrolate are the first line of treatment for this problem. Because beta-adrenergic stimulation increases production of protein and mucus-rich secretions that may thicken saliva and make it especially difficult for patients to handle, administration of beta-blockers such as metoprolol has been proposed to reduce thickness of oral, nasal, and pulmonary secretions. Surgical procedures to reduce the production of saliva (e.g., tympanic neurectomy, submandibular gland resection) have also been employed but have not been extensively studied.

Behavioral therapy approaches can be useful in treating mild to moderate dysphagia in ALS. Alterations in food consistency (e.g., thickening liquids), swallowing compensation techniques, and voluntary airway protection maneuvers all provide benefit and can be taught by speech/swallowing therapists. Eventually, however, enteral feeding becomes necessary in many individuals with advanced ALS. Placement of a PEG tube can stabilize weight loss, relieve nutritional deficiency, and improve quality of life for individuals with advanced ALS and severe dysphagia. A radiologically inserted gastrostomy (RIG) has been advocated in patients with respiratory compromise. However, with appropriate precautions, PEG may be equally safe in carefully selected high-risk patients (Talbot et al., 2018). A recent large prospective study of gastrostomy insertion in ALS—comparing RIG, PEG, and per oral radiologically inserted gastrostomy (PIG)—showed no difference in mortality between PEG and RIG, including patients with forced vital capacity (FVC) below 50% (ProGas Study Group, 2015).

## Cranial Neuropathies

Pathological processes involving the lower cranial nerves can produce dysphagia, usually as a part of a broader clinical picture. Dysphagia can be prominent in the Miller Fisher variant of acute inflammatory demyelinating polyneuropathy (Guillain-Barré syndrome). Response to plasmapheresis is expected in this situation. The pharyngo-cervical-brachial variant of Guillain-Barré syndrome manifests with dysphagia; including weakness of facial muscles, neck flexors, and proximal upper limb muscles; ophthalmoplegia; ataxia; and autonomic dysfunction (heart rate, bladder). Laboratory and electrophysiological investigations are similar to those in evaluating typical Guillain-Barré syndrome.

Dysphagia also may be present in herpes zoster infection, where it has been attributed to cranial ganglionic involvement. Examples of other processes in which cranial nerve involvement can result in dysphagia include Charcot-Marie-Tooth disease and primary or metastatic tumors involving the skull base. Severe but reversible dysphagia with significantly prolonged esophageal transit time has been attributed to vincristine therapy.

Facial onset sensory and motor neuronopathy (FOSMN) syndrome is a rare, slowly progressive neurodegenerative disorder characterized initially by sensory symptoms involving the face with subsequent development of motor weakness involving bulbar, neck, and upper limb muscles, with resultant dysphagia, dysarthria, and arm weakness. It has been proposed that FOSMN syndrome should be considered to be a variant of ALS (Dalla Bella et al., 2014).

## Brainstem Processes

Any process damaging the brainstem's swallowing centers or lower cranial nerve nuclei can lead to dysphagia. Therefore, in addition to stroke and MS, a number of other processes affecting brainstem function may display dysphagia as part of their clinical picture. Brainstem tumors, both primary and metastatic, may be responsible for dysphagia, as can central pontine myelinolysis, progressive multifocal leukoencephalopathy, and leukoencephalopathy due to cyclosporine toxicity. Brainstem encephalitis produced by organisms such as *Listeria* and Epstein-Barr virus may also result in dysphagia.

## Cervical Spinal Cord Injury

Dysphagia may develop in individuals with cervical spinal cord injury, especially if the injury is associated with respiratory insufficiency. In a study of 51 persons with cervical spinal cord injury and respiratory insufficiency, 21 (41%) suffered from severe dysphagia with aspiration and another 20 (39%) had mild dysphagia (Wolf and Meiners, 2003). Previous studies have reported the incidence of dysphagia following spinal cord injury to range from 16.6% to 60% (Shem et al., 2012). Individuals with higher spinal cord injury were statistically more likely to experience more prominent dysphagia after undergoing therapy, although this difference was not evident on admission. In a retrospective consecutive case series involving 298 patients following acute cervical spinal cord injury, old age, severe paralysis, and the presence of tracheostomy were risk factors for dysphagia (Hayashi et al., 2017). Iruthayarajah and colleagues performed a systematic review and meta-analysis that documented age, injury severity, level of injury, presence of tracheostomy, coughing, voice quality, bronchoscopy need, pneumonia, mechanical ventilation, nasogastric tubes, comorbid injury, and cervical surgery as significant risk factors for dysphagia following spinal cord injury (Iruthayarajah et al., 2018). With treatment and time, most patients demonstrate improvement in their dysphagia. The characteristics of dysphagia in traumatic spinal cord injury suggest an underlying mechanism of neurologic injury to structures and nerves necessary for swallowing.

Dysphagia may also develop in the setting of nontraumatic cervical spinal column disease. For example, dysphagia is one of the most frequent symptoms experienced by individuals with diffuse idiopathic skeletal hyperostosis (DISH, Forestier disease).

## Other Processes

Although rare in developed countries, rabies is encountered more frequently in developing nations. In endemic areas, approximately 10% of affected individuals do not report any prior exposure to animal bite. Dysphagia, typically accompanying phobic spasms in the classic "furious" form of rabies, is a well-recognized feature of the human disease. A hyperactive gag reflex is usually also present in this situation. However, dysphagia may also develop in the "paralytic" form of rabies, which can be more difficult to diagnose because the classically recognized features are often absent.

Neurogenic oropharyngeal dysphagia has also been reported as a consequence of severe hypothyroid coma.

## Evaluation of Dysphagia

Various diagnostic tests ranging from simple bedside analysis to sophisticated radiological, endoscopic, and neurophysiological procedures have been developed to evaluate dysphagia (Box 15.4). Although most are performed by primary care providers or gastroenterologists, it is important for neurologists to be aware of them so that diagnostic tests can be employed when clinical circumstances are appropriate (Box 15.5).

History and examination can provide useful clues to localization and diagnosis (Table 15.1). In fact, it has been reported that a good history will accurately identify the location and cause of dysphagia in 80% of cases (Cook, 2008). Odynophagia, or pain on swallowing, is suggestive of an inflammatory process of the esophageal mucosa and should be distinguished from the usually painless dysphagia. Difficulty initiating swallowing, the need for repeated attempts to succeed at swallowing, the presence of nasal regurgitation during swallowing, and coughing or choking immediately after attempted swallowing all suggest an oropharyngeal source for the dysphagia. A sensation

### BOX 15.4 Diagnostic Tests

**Oropharyngeal**
Clinical examination
Cervical auscultation
Timed swallowing tests
3-oz water swallow test
Modified barium swallow test
Pharyngeal videoendoscopy
Pharyngeal manometry
Videomanofluorometry
Electromyographic recording
Dysphagia limit

**Esophageal**
Endoscopy
Esophageal manometry
Videofluoroscopy

### BOX 15.5 Dysphagia Testing

**If Oral Phase Dysfunction Is Suspected**
Screening tests:
- Clinical examination
- Cervical auscultation
- 3-oz water swallow

Primary test:
- Modified barium swallow

**If Pharyngeal Phase Dysfunction Is Suspected**
Screening tests:
- Clinical examination
- 3-oz water swallow
- Timed swallowing

Primary test:
- Modified barium swallow

Complementary tests:
- Pharyngeal videoendoscopy
- Pharyngeal manometry
- Electromyography
- Videomanofluorometry

**If Esophageal Dysfunction Is Suspected**
Primary tests:
- Videofluoroscopy
- Endoscopy

Complementary test:
- Esophageal manometry

of food "hanging up" in the area of the xiphoid process implicates esophageal dysfunction, whereas a perception of the bolus "sticking" in the sternal notch may occur as a result of an oropharyngeal process or a lesion anywhere along the course of the esophagus (Fig. 15.1). Therefore the patient's localization of the site of dysphagia is not always reliable in determining the site of the pathology (Trate et al., 1996). Differentiation between obstructive disease and motor disease can be assessed based on the type of food bolus being held up and the progression of dysphagia. In individuals with motor disorders, dysphagia to solid and liquid occur simultaneously, whereas in patients with mechanical obstruction, dysphagia initially involves solids and later progresses to include liquids (Abdel Jalil et al., 2015).

Physical examination may reveal evidence suggesting a cause for dysphagia. Lip and tongue function can easily be assessed during routine neurological examination, and both palatal and gag reflexes can be evaluated. Signs of residual cerebrovascular disease, gait changes of PD, and wasting typical of muscular dystrophies can be elicited during a thorough examination. Hyporeflexia of hypothyroidism; cervical lymphadenopathy of esophageal cancer; and thickened, sclerotic skin lesions of scleroderma are other useful findings that may be evident during general physical examination (Trate et al., 1996).

Cervical auscultation is not widely used to evaluate swallowing, but it may be useful to assess coordination between respiration and swallowing. In the normal situation, swallowing occurs during exhalation, which reduces the risk of aspiration. Conversely, discoordinated swallowing in the midst of inhalation increases the possibility that food might be drawn into the respiratory tract.

**TABLE 15.1 Clues to Dysphagia**

| Clue | Cause of Dysphagia |
|---|---|
| Difficulty initiating swallowing | Oropharyngeal dysfunction |
| Repetitive swallowing | Oropharyngeal dysfunction |
| Retrosternal "hanging-up" sensation | Esophageal dysfunction |
| Difficulty with solids but not liquids | Mechanical obstruction |
| Difficulty with both solids and liquids | Esophageal dysmotility |
| Regurgitation of undigested food | Zenker diverticulum |
| Halitosis | Zenker diverticulum |

One of the easiest and potentially most important parts of the physical examination is watching the patient swallow in the office. A standardized 3-oz water swallow test has been advocated as a simple bedside evaluation for oropharyngeal dysphagia. The presence of cough on swallowing during this test has been reported to provide a positive predictive value of 84% with regard to the presence of aspiration and a negative predictive value of 78%. However, the test does not provide any information regarding the specific mechanism of dysphagia.

Timed swallowing tests that require repetitive swallowing of specific amounts of water have also been employed to evaluate dysphagia. Individuals with swallowing impairment may display a number of abnormalities including slower swallowing speed (<10 mL/sec) and coughing, which may indicate the presence of dysphagia or aspiration. However, some concern has been voiced that the relatively large amounts of fluid used in these timed tests could present a significant risk for pulmonary complications due to aspiration even if only water is used.

The modified barium swallow test has become a standard method for assessing oropharyngeal dysphagia. Patients are observed via VFS swallowing barium-impregnated food of differing consistencies (thin liquid, pudding, cookie). Both oral and pharyngeal function can be characterized and the four categories of oropharyngeal swallowing dysfunction can be assessed: (1) inability or excessive delay in initiation of pharyngeal swallowing, (2) aspiration of ingestate, (3) nasopharyngeal regurgitation, and (4) residue of ingestate within the pharyngeal cavity after swallowing (Kahrilas, 1999). Furthermore, VFS can assess the response to corrective measures such as positioning techniques and dietary modifications. Increasing bolus viscosity typically improves swallowing function in individuals with neurogenic dysphagia.

Videoendoscopy of the pharynx via the nasal passageway allows direct visualization of the pharyngeal component of swallowing before

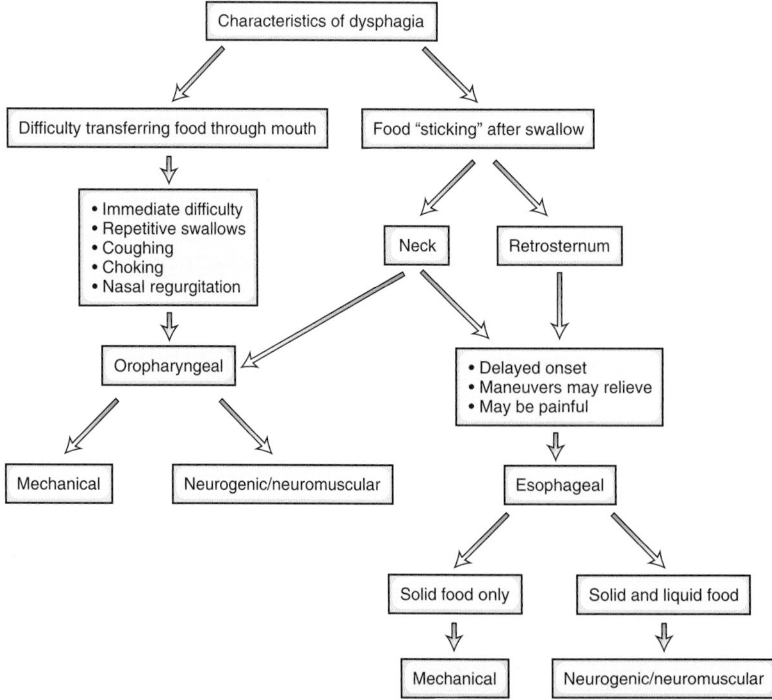


**Fig. 15.1** Assessment of Dysphagia.

and after passage of the food bolus. Its primary value is to demonstrate the presence of residual material in the pharynx after a swallow, indicative of increased risk of aspiration.

Pharyngeal manometry provides physiological information regarding function of both the pharynx and the UES; the information derived is complementary to that obtained by VFS. A combined procedure, termed *videomanofluorometry*, in which VFS and manometry are performed simultaneously, can also be utilized. Although useful, this procedure is not always readily available.

Esophageal function can be assessed by endoscopy, barium swallow, and esophageal manometry. Endoscopy and barium swallow are often complementary and not duplicative. Endoscopy can provide accurate information on esophageal anatomy and mucosal integrity and allows biopsy and tissue diagnosis. Endoscopy also serves as a potential therapeutic tool if a maneuver such as dilation is needed. Barium esophagography can also provide anatomical information but provides far greater information for motility disorders. Transnasal high-resolution esophageal manometry provides detailed information on peristaltic and sphincter function (both upper and lower esophageal sphincters) with little anatomical information (ASGE Standards of Practice Committee et al., 2014; Ott, 1990). Scintigraphic procedures can be employed to evaluate oral, pharyngeal, and esophageal function but are not widely utilized. It has been suggested that scintigraphic examination with documentation of piecemeal deglutition and determination of the dysphagia limit may be particularly useful in centers where more sophisticated electrophysiological techniques are not available (Argon et al., 2004).

More sophisticated electrodiagnostic procedures have been developed to study dysphagia. EMG recording of cricopharyngeal function and integrated submental activity has been useful in a research setting to characterize aspects of swallowing. Ertekin and colleagues (2002) have used EMG recordings to define an indicator of dysphagia they term the *dysphagia limit*. Normal subjects can swallow a 20-mL bolus of water in a single attempt, but persons with dysphagia must divide the bolus into two or more parts in order to complete the swallow. If individuals are given stepwise increases in bolus volume, the volume of fluid at which the division of the bolus first occurs is labeled the dysphagia limit. The investigators consider a dysphagia limit of less than 20 mL as abnormal and indicative of dysphagia.

In conclusion, because of the broad network of structures involved in the control and execution of swallowing, dysphagia can be an important component of the clinical picture in patients with a wide variety of neurological diseases. In both the diagnosis and treatment of dysphagia, it can be of great value to determine the specific mechanism responsible for this condition in individual patients.

*The complete reference list is available online at https://expertconsult.inkling.com/.* 

16

# Neuro-Ophthalmology: Afferent Visual System

Matthew J. Thurtell, Sashank Prasad, Robert L. Tomsak

## OUTLINE



## AFFERENT VISUAL SYSTEM ANATOMY AND PHYSIOLOGY

From a conceptual standpoint, it is useful to consider vision as having two components: *central* or *macular* vision (high acuity, color perception, and light-adapted) and *peripheral* or *ambulatory* vision (low acuity, poor color perception, and dark-adapted). Light, refracted by the cornea and lens, is focused on the retina. For the best possible vision, the image of the object of regard must fall onto the *fovea*, which is the most sensitive part of the macula. The cone photoreceptors, which mediate central and color vision, are the greatest in density at the fovea. The cone system functions optimally in conditions of light adaptation. Visual acuity and cone density fall off rapidly as eccentricity from the fovea increases. For example, the retina 20 degrees eccentric to the fovea can only resolve objects equivalent to Snellen 20/200 (6/60 metric) optotypes or larger. Rod photoreceptors are present in the highest numbers approximately 20 degrees from the fovea and are more abundant than cones in the more peripheral retina; rods function best in dim illumination. The total extent of the normal peripheral visual field in each eye is approximately 60 degrees superior, 60 degrees nasal, 70–75 degrees inferior, and 100 degrees temporal to fixation (Fig. 16.1). Because of the optical properties of the eye, the nasal retina receives visual information from the temporal visual field, while the temporal retina receives visual information from the nasal visual field (see Fig. 16.1). Similarly, the superior retina receives visual information from the inferior visual field and vice versa. These points are clinically important when evaluating visual loss.

The signal from cone and rod photoreceptors reaches a ganglion cell after being modulated by bipolar, horizontal, and amacrine cells (Fig. 16.2). Two main types of retinal ganglion cell exist: *parasol cells* (M retinal ganglion cells, which project to the magnocellular pathway) and *midget cells* (P retinal ganglion cells, which project to the parvocellular pathway). Retinal nerve fibers form arcuate bundles respecting the midline horizontal raphe and enter the optic disc superiorly and inferiorly (Fig. 16.3). Nerve fibers exit the globe via the scleral canal, where they receive physical support from the lamina cribrosa and metabolic support from intertwining astrocytes. Once nerve fibers pass through the lamina cribrosa, they are supported by oligodendrocytes and become myelinated. Nerve fibers that arise from the ganglion cells of the nasal retina of each eye decussate in the optic chiasm to the contralateral optic tract, while those from the temporal retina do not decussate. The percentages of crossed and uncrossed fibers in the human optic chiasm are approximately 53% and 47%, respectively.

Visual information stratifies further in the lateral geniculate nucleus (LGN), which is the only way station between the retinal ganglion cells and the primary visual cortex. The LGN, a portion of the thalamus, has six layers. Axons from ipsilateral retinal ganglion cells synapse in layers 2, 3, and 5; contralateral axons synapse in layers 1, 4, and 6. Layers 1 and 2 of the LGN are the *magnocellular layers*, and these receive input from M retinal ganglion cells. The magnocellular pathway is concerned mainly with movement detection, detection of low contrast, and dynamic form perception. After projecting to the primary visual cortex (visual area 1, V1, or Brodmann area 17), information from the M pathway is distributed

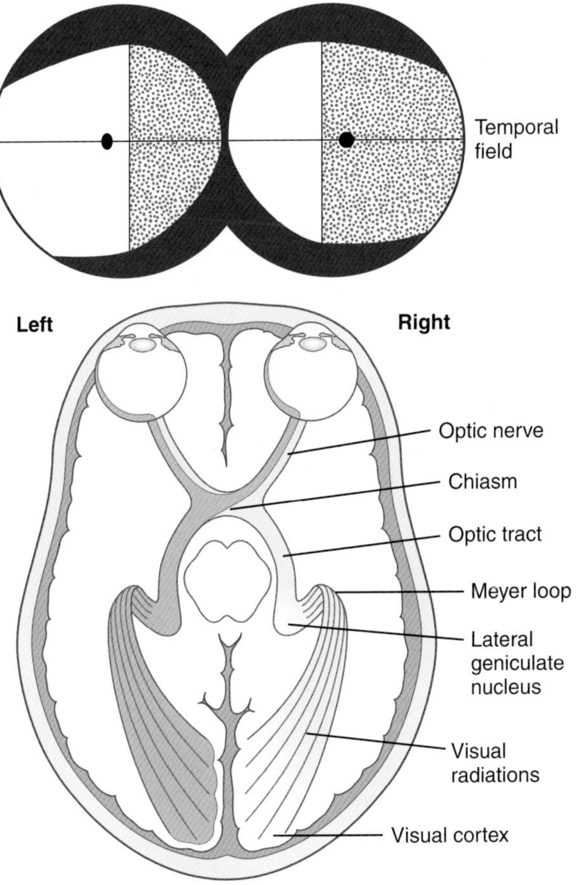


**Fig. 16.1** Visual Pathways.

to V2 (part of area 18) and V5 (junction of areas 19 and 37). Layers 3–6 of the LGN are the *parvocellular layers* and receive input from P retinal ganglion cells, which are color selective and responsive to high contrast. Information from the P pathway is distributed to V2 and V4 (fusiform gyrus). Superior fibers that leave the LGN go straight back to the primary visual cortex, while inferior fibers loop anteriorly around the temporal horn of the lateral ventricle *(Meyer loop)*. Because these fibers pass close to the tip of the temporal lobe, temporal lobectomy sometimes damages these fibers, causing a "pie-in-the-sky" homonymous visual field defect.

The primary visual cortex (striate cortex, V1, or Brodmann area 17) is in the occipital lobe. Fibers from the macula project to the portion of the visual cortex closest to the occipital poles, while fibers from the peripheral retina project to the visual cortex lying more anteriorly. The nonoverlapping part of the most peripheral temporal visual field (*monocular temporal crescent*) arises from unpaired crossed axons from the nasal retina that project to the most anterior portion of the visual cortex. The primary visual cortex has interconnections with visual association areas concerned with color, motion, and object recognition.

## NEURO-OPHTHALMOLOGICAL EXAMINATION OF THE AFFERENT VISUAL SYSTEM

The neuro-ophthalmological examination makes use of ophthalmic tools and techniques but aims at neurological diagnosis. Because many neurologists are not familiar with ophthalmic examination techniques, and ophthalmologists are often not experienced with neurological localization, the neuro-ophthalmological subspecialty provides a bridge between the two disciplines.

### Examination of Visual Acuity

*Visual acuity* is the spatial resolution of vision. Visual acuity should always be measured in each eye individually and with the best possible optical correction (i.e., with the patient's glasses); other optical means such as a pinhole device or refraction may be needed if optical correction is not available. The resulting measure, called *best-corrected visual acuity*, is the only universally interpretable measurement of central visual function. Ideally, visual acuity should be measured both at distance (usually 20 feet or 6 m) and near (usually 14 inches or 0.33 m). The notation 20/20 (6/6) indicates that the patient (numerator) is able to see the optotypes seen by a normal person at 20 feet (denominator). A visual acuity of 20/60 (6/18) indicates that the patient sees an optotype at 20 feet that a normal person would see at 60 feet.

A disparity between the distance and near visual acuities is often indicative of a specific problem. For example, the most common cause of better distance than near acuity is uncorrected presbyopia. Common causes of better near than distance acuity include myopia and congenital nystagmus. In the latter disorder, convergence needed for near vision dampens the nystagmus.

When measuring near vision, the reading card should be held at the specified distance of 14 inches (or 0.33 m) to control for variation in image size on the retina. The medical record should clearly specify if a nonstandard distance is used. Two types of near cards are readily available; one has numbers, and the other has written text (Fig. 16.4). In neurological practice, a near card with text measures visual acuity as well as reading ability to some degree. A disparity between the measurements from the two types of near card might suggest a disturbance of some other cortical function, such as language function (see Chapter 13).

### Contrast Vision Testing

*Contrast vision*, the ability to distinguish adjacent areas of differing luminance, can be evaluated by assessing the perception of lines or optotypes of different sizes (spatial frequencies) with varying degrees of contrast. Contrast vision can be impaired in numerous diseases of the eye (e.g., cataract) and retrobulbar visual pathways (e.g., optic neuropathies). Special charts—the Pelli–Robson chart (sensitivity) and Sloan chart (acuity)—are required to assess contrast vision.

### Light-Stress Test

In some disorders of the macula, abnormalities are not apparent with the ophthalmoscope. The light-stress (or photo-stress) test is a useful method for determining whether reduced central vision is a consequence of macular dysfunction. Prior to the test, the best-corrected visual acuity is measured in each eye. Then, with the eye with decreased vision occluded, the other eye is exposed to a bright light for 10 seconds. Immediately thereafter, the patient is instructed to read the next largest line on the eye chart, and the recovery period is timed. The same procedure is followed for the eye with decreased vision, and the results are compared. Fifty seconds is the upper limit of normal for visual recovery, although most normal subjects recover within several seconds. In patients with macular disease, the recovery period often takes several minutes.

### Color Vision Testing

Dyschromatopsia, especially if asymmetrical between the eyes, is an indication of optic nerve dysfunction but can also occur with retinal disease (Almog and Nemet, 2010). Symmetrical acquired dyschromatopsia might indicate a retinal degeneration, such as a cone–rod dystrophy. Congenital dyschromatopsia occurs in about 8% of men and 0.5% of women.

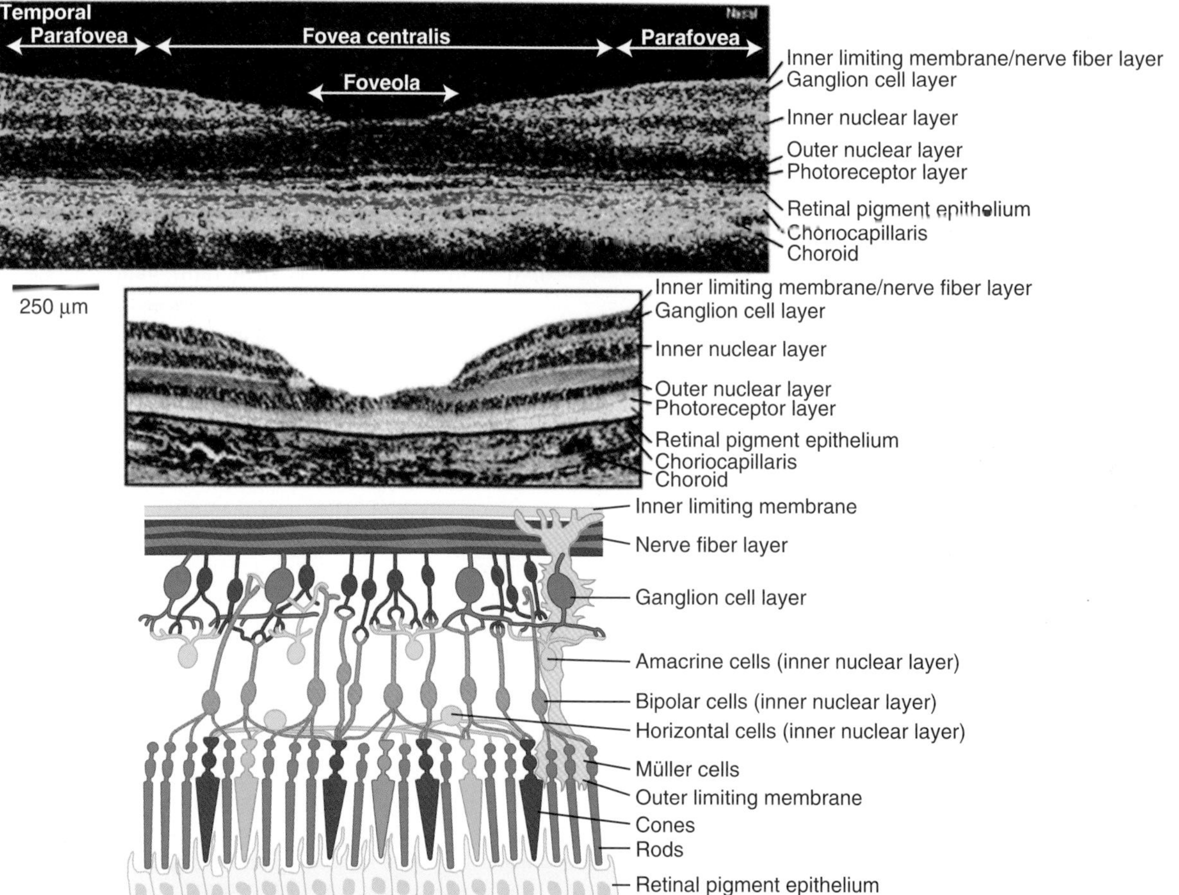


**Fig. 16.2** Structures of the Neurosensory Retina. *Top*, high-resolution optical coherence tomography. *Middle*, histological section. *Bottom*, schematic depiction of retinal layers. *(Adapted and reprinted with permission from Jaffe, G., Caprioli, J., 2004. Optical coherence tomography to detect and manage retinal disease and glaucoma. Am J Ophthalmol 137[1], 156–169 and* http://www.webvision.med.utah.edu.*)*

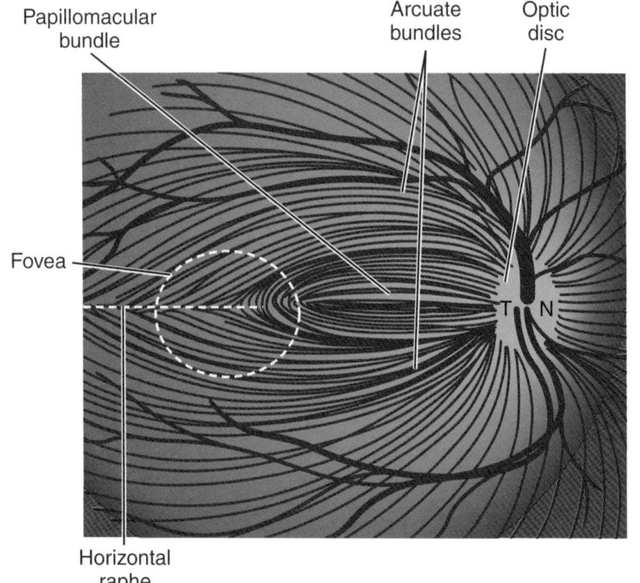


**Fig. 16.3** Arrangement of Retinal Nerve Fiber Layer, Composed of Ganglion Cell Axons. The papillomacular bundle conveys axons from the fovea directly to the temporal margin *(T)* of the optic disc. The remainder of temporal ganglion cell axons is arranged in arcuate bundles above and below the fovea, arriving at the superior and inferior disc margins. Finally, axons originating nasal to the disc arrive at its nasal border *(N)*.

Techniques for assessing color vision range from the simple to the sophisticated. A gross color vision defect is identifiable at the bedside by assessing for red desaturation. The clinician holds a bright red object in front of each of the patient's eyes individually and asks for a comparison of both brightness and color intensity. Asking for a comparison of red saturation on each side of fixation sometimes detects a subtle hemianopia. Formal measurements of color vision can be obtained with pseudoisochromatic color plates (e.g., Ishihara or Hardy–Rand–Rittler plates) or with sorting tests (e.g., Farnsworth–Munsell test).

## Examination of the Pupils

Examination of the pupils involves assessing pupil size and shape, the direct and consensual reactions to light, and the near response. The examination should also include an assessment for a relative afferent pupillary defect (RAPD). If a difference in pupil size *(anisocoria)* is noted, look for ptosis and ocular motility deficits, keeping in mind the possibility of Horner syndrome or third cranial nerve palsy. Record findings in an easily understood format (Table 16.1).

Measurements of pupil size and light reaction are made in dim illumination with the patient fixating on an immobile distant target. If there is anisocoria, it is useful to measure pupil size in both darkness and bright light. Anisocoria due to oculosympathetic paresis (Horner syndrome) is greater in the dark because the affected pupil does not dilate well. Conversely, anisocoria due to parasympathetic denervation (e.g., Adie tonic pupil) is more evident in bright light because the affected pupil does not constrict well (see Chapter 17).

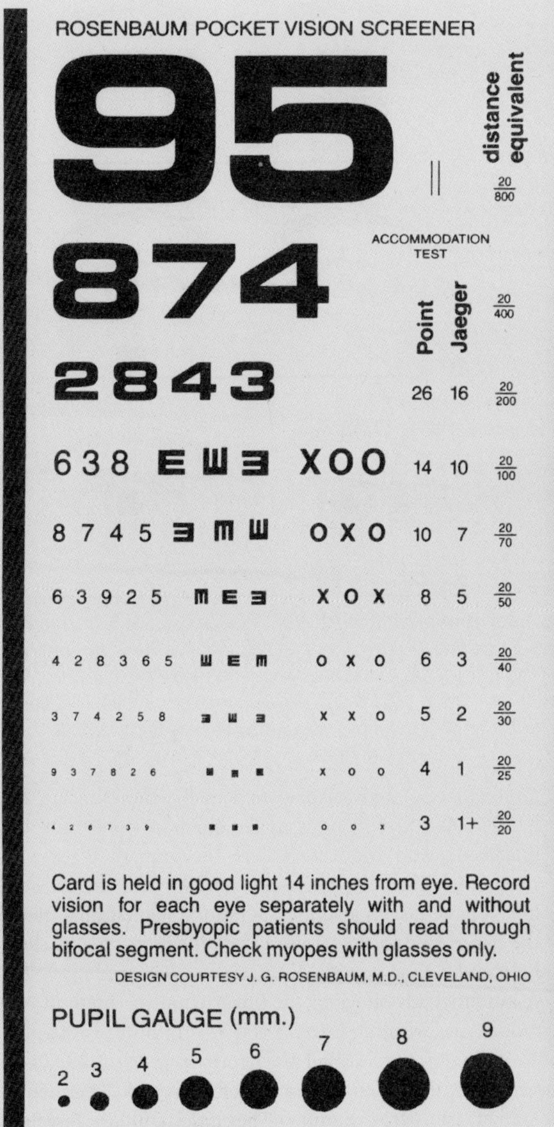


V = .50 D.

The fourteenth of August was the day fixed upon for the sailing of the brig Pilgrim, on her voyage from Boston round Cape Horn, to the western coast of North America. As she was to get under way early in the after noon I made my appearance on board at twelve o'clock in full sea rig, and with my chest, containing an outfit for a two or three years voyage, which I had undertaken from a determination to cure, if possible, by an entire change of life, and by a long absence from books and study, a weakness of the eyes which had obliged me to give up my pursuits, and which no medical aid seemed likely to cure. The change from the tight dress coat, silk cap and kid gloves of an undergraduate at Cambridge to the

V = .75 D.

loose duck trousers, checked shirt and tarpaulin hat of a sailor, though somewhat of a transformation, was soon made, and I supposed that I should pass very well for a Jack tar. But it is impossible to deceive the practiced eye in these matters; and while I supposed myself to be looking as salt as Neptune himself, I was, no doubt, known for a landsman by every one on board, as soon as I hove in sight. A sailor has a peculiar cut to his clothes, and a way of wear-

V = 1. D.

ing them which a green hand can never get. The trousers, tight around the hips, and thence hanging long and loose around the feet, a superabundance of checked shirt, a low-crowned, well-varnished black hat, worn on the back of the head, with half a fathom of black ribbon hanging over the left eye, and a peculiar tie to the black silk neckerchief, with sundry other *details*, are signs the want of which betray the beginner at once.

V = 1.25 D.

Beside the points in my dress which were out of the way, doubtless my complexion and hands would distinguish me from the regular *salt*, who, with a sun-browned cheek, wide step and rolling gait, swings his bronzed and toughened hands athwart-ships half open, as though just ready to grasp a rope. "With all my imperfections

V = 1.50 D.

on my head," I joined the crew, and we hauled out into the stream and came to anchor for the night. The next day we were employed in preparation for sea, reeving and studding-sail gear, crossing royal yards, putting on chafing gear, and taking on board our powder. On the

V = 1.75 D.

following night I stood my first watch. I remained awake nearly all the first part of the night, from fear that I might not hear when I was called; and when I went on deck, so great were my ideas of the importance of my trust, that I

V = 2. D.

walked regularly fore and aft the whole length of the vessel, looking out over the bows and taffrail at each turn, and was not a little surprised at the unconcerned manner in which the billows turned up their

Your glasses are of value to you only as they accurately interpret your prescription and this only as they are fitted and serviced in accordance with these needs. They are a therapeutic device.

A B

**Fig. 16.4** A, Rosenbaum-style near vision card. B, Near vision card with written text.

**TABLE 16.1 Simple Method of Recording Pupillary Examination**

| | Size (mm) | Direct Light Reaction | Consensual Light Reaction | Near Reaction |
|---|---|---|---|---|
| Right eye | 4.0 | 4+ | 2+ | 4+ |
| Left eye | 4.0 | 2+ | 4+ | 4+ |

When measuring light reactions or assessing for an RAPD, the brightest light available should be used. The near reaction can be elicited by having the patient look at his or her thumb, positioned at a distance of 15–30 cm. With this method, a near reaction can be elicited even in a completely blind patient, owing to proprioceptive influences. The pupil shows *light-near dissociation* when the direct light reaction is less prominent than the near reaction. Light-near dissociation can be seen with parasympathetic denervation of the pupil (e.g., Adie tonic pupil), with dorsal midbrain lesions (e.g., as part of the dorsal midbrain syndrome), and in patients with severe bilateral optic neuropathies.

The presence of an RAPD (formerly called a *Marcus Gunn pupil*) is an invaluable sign of a unilateral or asymmetric optic neuropathy. An RAPD is best detected by alternately illuminating the pupils by swinging a flashlight between them at a frequency of about once per second—hence the name, *swinging flashlight test.* The swinging flashlight test compares the direct and consensual light reactions in the same eye. Normally, these reactions are equal. However, in patients with a unilateral or asymmetric optic neuropathy, because of reduction in the direct reaction as compared with the consensual reaction, the pupil of the eye with decreased vision dilates when reilluminated (both pupils are actually "dilating" in that they are both resetting at the size commensurate with the amount of light transmitted back to the brain by the damaged optic nerve). Box 16.1 and Fig. 16.5 describe the method for detecting an RAPD. Two caveats exist. The test brings out an asymmetry of optic nerve conduction, so an RAPD is not present when both optic nerves are injured to the same extent. In addition, severe inner retinal pathology can produce an RAPD, but the abnormality is usually obvious on funduscopic examination. In contrast, an optic neuropathy with minimal loss of visual acuity often gives an obvious RAPD. The magnitude

**BOX 16.1 Testing for a Relative Afferent Pupillary Defect**

1. The patient should fixate on an immobile distant target to minimize fluctuations in pupillary size and accommodative miosis.
2. A light bright enough to cause maximum pupillary constriction should be used.
3. Each pupil should be checked individually for its direct light response, which can be graded on a scale of 1–4 (see Table 16.1).
4. The light should be moved quickly to illuminate each eye alternately every 1 second (the swinging flashlight test).
5. The pupil should be observed for initial constriction or dilation.
6. Only three or four swings of the light should be made, to minimize bleaching of the retina, and subsequent slowing of the pupillary reactions.

of an RAPD can be quantified using neutral density filters. See Chapter 17 for further discussion of pupillary abnormalities.

## Light Brightness Comparison

Light brightness comparison is a subjective swinging flashlight test. The subjective appreciation of light intensity is often impaired in patients with optic neuropathies, but not in macular disease. The clinician shines a bright light into both eyes in succession and asks the patient to estimate the difference in brightness. For example, the clinician could ask, "If this light (normal eye illuminated) were worth $1 in terms of light brightness or intensity, what would this one be worth (abnormal eye illuminated)?"

## Visual Field Testing

Evaluation of the visual fields is vital in patients with visual loss. Several techniques can be used for visual field examination, ranging from simple confrontation testing to sophisticated threshold static perimetry. Confrontation testing should be part of the routine neurological examination, although it is insensitive for detection of mild visual field loss (Kerr et al., 2010). For the purposes of this discussion, the emphasis is on simple and practical techniques, while more sophisticated methods are briefly summarized.

In the first assessment, the patient is asked to observe the clinician's face with each eye in turn and to report if any part of the clinician's face is missing, blurred, or distorted when the patient's line of sight is directed to the nose. For example, a patient with a central scotoma may report that the eyes and nose are missing, a patient with an inferior altitudinal visual field defect may report that the lower half of the face is missing, while a patient with homonymous hemianopia may report that one side of the face is missing.

Confrontation testing should follow. Although many methods are available, a simple, thorough examination can be done by finger counting in all four quadrants, coupled with hand comparison. The steps are as follows:

1. The clinician has the patient occlude one eye and maintain fixation on the clinician's nose.
2. *Finger counting in the quadrants:* The clinician holds up fingers sequentially in each of the four quadrants of the visual field and asks the patient to count the number seen.
3. *Simultaneous finger counting using both hands:* If step 2 is completed normally, the clinician asks the patient to count the number of fingers displayed with both hands, first in both of the upper quadrants of the patient's visual field and then in the lower quadrants. Then, the patient is asked to add the total number of fingers shown with both hands. Visual inattention is often identifiable during this step of confrontation testing.

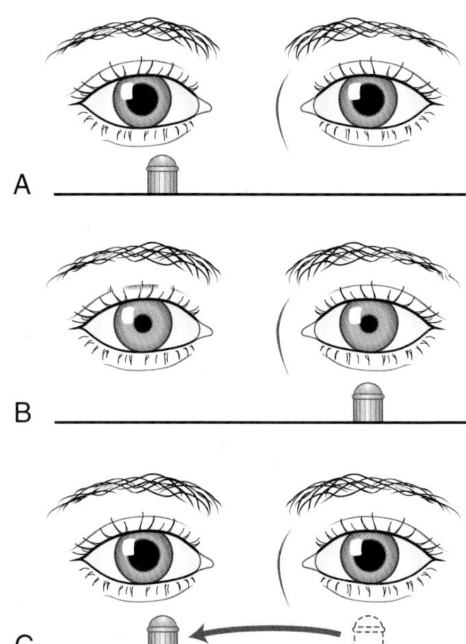


**Fig. 16.5 Right Relative Afferent Pupillary Defect from a Right Optic Nerve Lesion. A,** Poor direct and consensual reaction with illumination of the right eye. **B,** Excellent direct and consensual reaction with illumination of the left eye. **C,** Poor direct and consensual reaction, manifest as redilation of both pupils when the light is swung back to the right eye.

4. *Simultaneous hand comparison:* Finally, the clinician holds both hands open, first in both upper quadrants and then both lower quadrants, and asks the patient to compare the quality of the images. For example, when shown hands on either side of the midline, a patient with a subtle bitemporal hemianopia may state that the hands held in the temporal hemifields are not as clear as those held in the nasal hemifields.

A potential advantage of the finger counting method over kinetic methods (e.g., wiggling fingers) is that it minimizes the potential for confounding by the *Riddoch phenomenon*, which refers to a dissociation between the visual perception of form and movement such that the patient can perceive moving but not stationary targets in half of the visual field (Zeki and Ffytche, 1998). The Riddoch phenomenon can occur when homonymous hemianopia results from visual cortex lesions. Accordingly, the clinician may miss a hemianopia when using only a moving target, such as wiggling fingers, in the far periphery.

Confrontation methods using colored (e.g., red) objects can be effective in detecting subtle visual field defects (Kerr et al., 2010). Confrontation testing is also useful for assessing patients with constricted visual fields. As the distance between the clinician and the patient increases, the visual field should expand, producing a *funnel*. However, with nonorganic (functional) visual field constriction, the visual field often does not expand as the distance between the clinician and the patient increases, thereby producing a *tunnel* (Fig. 16.6).

The central 20 degrees of the visual field can be assessed in each eye separately using the Amsler grid (Fig. 16.7). With the grid held in good light at a distance of 30 cm from the eye and the patient wearing his or her reading glasses, if needed, the following questions are asked:

1. Can you see the spot in the center of the grid?
2. While looking at the center spot, can you see the entire grid or are any sides or corners missing?
3. While you are looking at the center spot, are any of the lines in the grid missing, blurred, or distorted?

If the patient indicates an abnormality, the clinician should ask the patient to draw the abnormal areas on the grid. The grid can then be kept

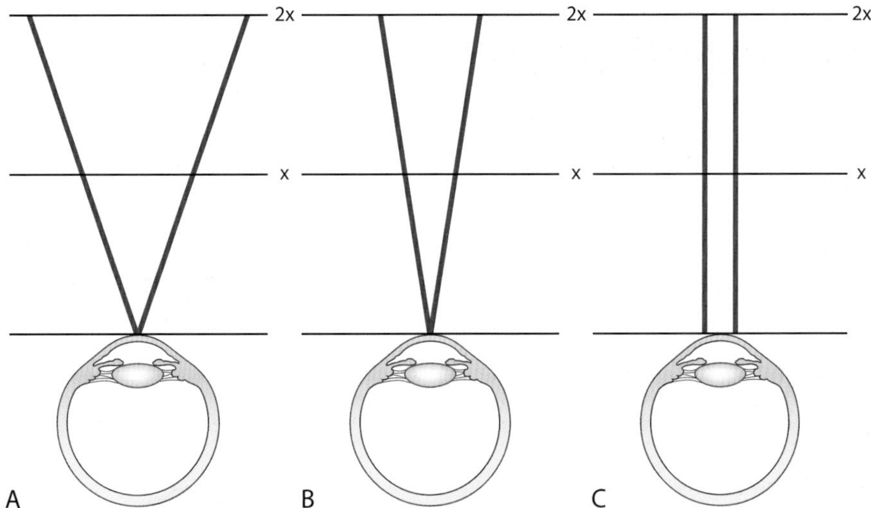


**Fig. 16.6** **A,** The normal visual field enlarges with an increase in testing distance; it "funnels." **B,** The constricted visual field from organic disease also proportionally enlarges. **C,** The constricted visual field from nonorganic disease does not usually enlarge as testing distance increases; rather, it "tunnels." *(Adapted from Trobe, J.D., Glaser, J.S., 1983. The Visual Fields Manual: a Practical Guide to Testing and Interpretation. Gainesville, Triad, p. 135.)*

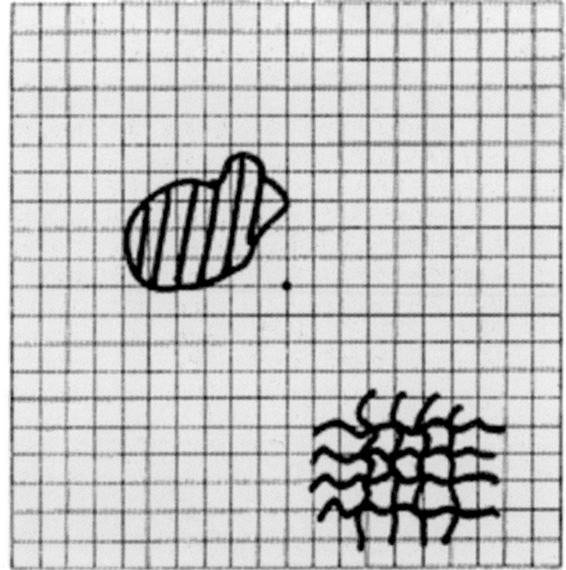

**Fig. 16.7** **Amsler Grid.** *Upper left,* Paracentral scotoma. *Lower right,* Metamorphopsia (straight lines appear wavy).

in the patient's medical record. Patients with a central scotoma may report that the center of the grid is missing, those with a hemianopic defect may report that half of the grid is missing, and those with macular disease may report that the lines are wavy or distorted (i.e., metamorphopsia).

## Interpretation of Visual Field Defects

Eight general rules for visual field interpretation are summarized in Box 16.2. Comments relating to six of these general rules are presented here.

### Rule 1

Optic nerve lesions can produce prechiasmal visual field abnormalities that are characteristic. Nonarteritic anterior ischemic optic neuropathy (NAION) often produces an inferior altitudinal defect, optic neuritis often produces a central or cecocentral scotoma, and compressive optic neuropathy often produces abnormalities in both the peripheral and the central portions of the visual field (Fig. 16.8).

A lesion at the junction of the optic nerve and chiasm produces a junctional scotoma (i.e., ipsilateral cecocentral scotoma and contralateral temporal defect) due to involvement of both ipsilateral fibers and crossing fibers from the contralateral nasal retina. Binasal field defects (Fig. 16.9) can result from papilledema, anterior ischemic optic neuropathy, glaucoma, optic nerve head drusen, optic nerve pits, optic nerve hypoplasia, and sectoral retinitis pigmentosa (RP). Binasal field defects that are organic in etiology do not respect the vertical meridian, whereas nonorganic binasal defects may.

### Rule 2

True bitemporal hemianopias are the hallmark of chiasmal disease. Bitemporal field defects that do not respect the vertical meridian (pseudobitemporal hemianopias) are almost always due to congenital rotation or tilting of the optic discs (Fig. 16.10). Bilateral cecocentral scotomas can masquerade as bitemporal field defects, and the distinguishing feature is whether the defect respects the vertical meridian of the visual field.

### Rule 3

A homonymous visual field defect is present in the same hemifield (i.e., right or left) or visual quadrant (i.e., upper or lower) of each eye. The only exception to this rule is with the monocular temporal crescent syndrome, in which only unpaired visual fibers residing in the contralateral anteromedial occipital lobe are affected.

### Rule 4

Incongruent hemianopias tend to result from more anterior retrochiasmal lesions (e.g., those affecting the optic tract or temporal lobe; Fig. 16.11; Kedar et al., 2007). Optic tract lesions often produce a contralateral RAPD (i.e., in the eye with the temporal visual field defect), which is helpful for clinical localization.

### Rule 5

Congruent homonymous hemianopias have patterns that are very similar or identical in the two eyes. Highly congruent hemianopias usually result from occipital lobe infarcts (Fig. 16.12) but can sometimes occur with more anterior retrochiasmal lesions (Kedar et al., 2007).

**BOX 16.2 General Rules of Visual Field Interpretation**

1. Lesions of the retina and optic nerve produce visual field defects in the ipsilateral eye only, unless the lesions are bilateral.
2. Only a lesion of the optic chiasm causes true bitemporal hemianopia.
3. Retrochiasmal lesions produce homonymous visual field defects.
4. Anterior retrochiasmal lesions produce incongruent homonymous visual field defects.
5. Posterior retrochiasmal lesions produce congruent homonymous visual field defects.
6. Temporal lobe lesions give slightly incongruent homonymous hemianopias involving the upper quadrant.
7. No localizing value can be assigned to a complete homonymous hemianopia, except that the lesion is retrochiasmal and contralateral to the visual field defect.
8. A unilateral homonymous hemianopia does not reduce visual acuity.

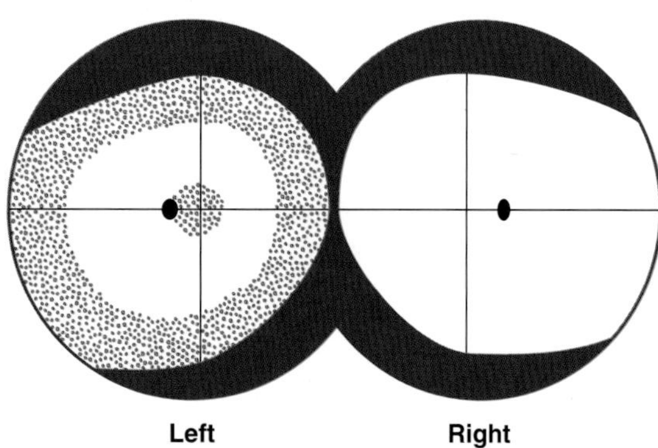


**Fig. 16.8** Constriction of the left visual field with a cecocentral scotoma due to compressive optic neuropathy, with a normal right visual field.

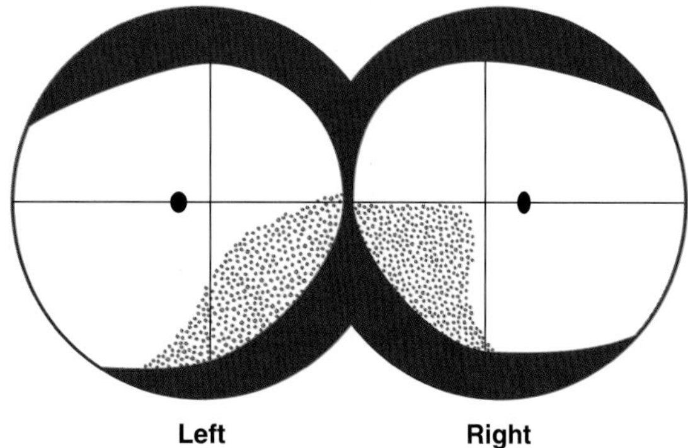


**Fig. 16.9** Binasal visual field defects (e.g., due to glaucoma). Note that the vertical meridian is not respected.

### Rule 8

Even a complete unilateral homonymous hemianopia does not decrease visual acuity because the macular cortex in the opposite hemisphere is intact. If the input to both macular cortices is impaired, central acuity is often diminished *(cortical blindness)*, but the visual acuities should be equally diminished. If the visual acuities are not similar, the clinician should search for another (or additional) explanation for the asymmetry.

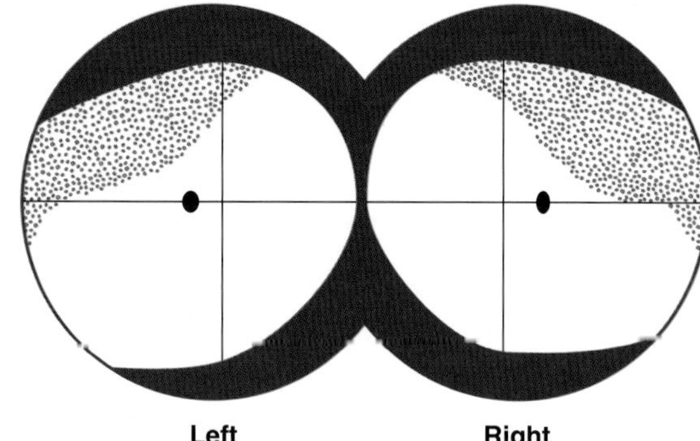


**Fig. 16.10** Pseudobitemporal hemianopia (e.g., due to tilted optic discs). Note that the vertical meridian is not respected.

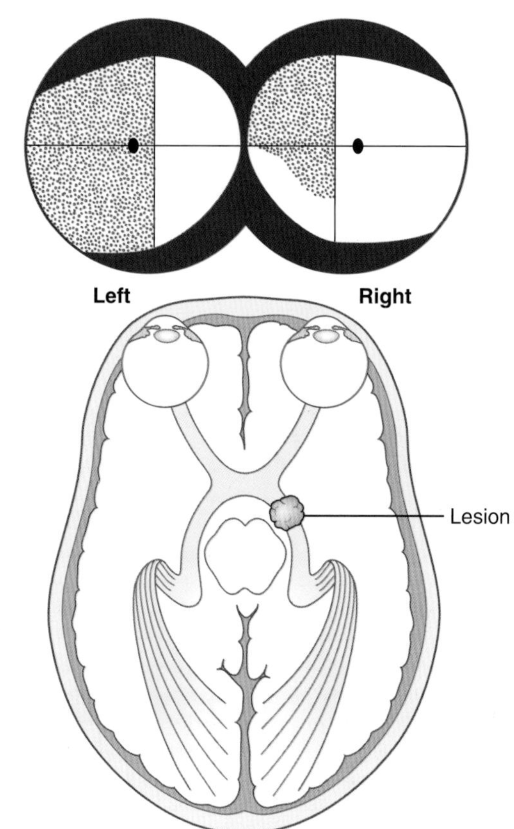


**Fig. 16.11** Incongruent left homonymous hemianopia from a right optic tract lesion.

## Examination of the Ocular Fundus

Examination of the ocular fundus, to evaluate for abnormalities in the appearance of the optic disc, retinal vasculature, and macula, is mandatory in patients with visual loss. The steps, when using the direct ophthalmoscope, are as follows:

1. The room lights are dimmed.
2. The clinician has the patient maintain fixation on a distant target to minimize miosis due to accommodation.
3. The clinician holds the ophthalmoscope with their right hand and looks through their right eye when evaluating the patient's right eye, and vice versa when evaluating the left eye.
4. The clinician begins the examination positioned temporally to the patient at arm's length.

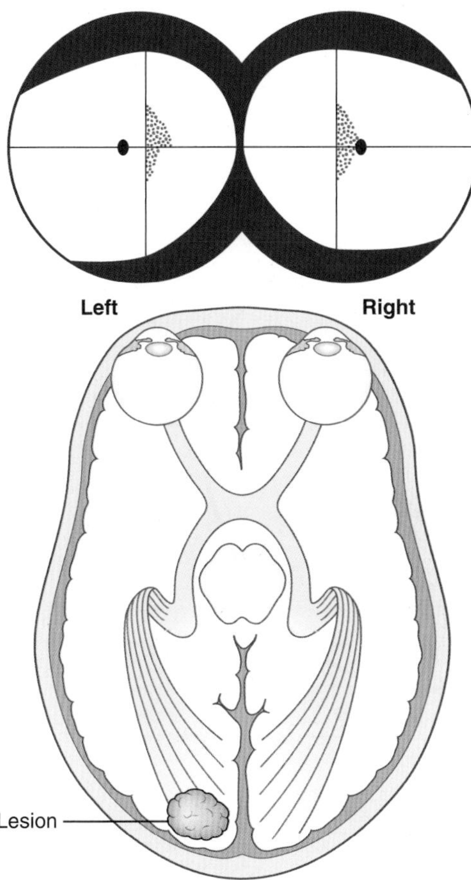


**Fig. 16.12** Congruent paracentral right homonymous hemianopia from a left occipital pole lesion.

5. The clinician evaluates for the red reflex, which may be absent when there is a media opacity (e.g., dense cataract or vitreous hemorrhage).
6. The clinician moves closer to the patient while adjusting the focus of the ophthalmoscope.
7. When the clinician is close to the patient and the retina is in focus, a retinal vessel is followed until the optic disc is found.
8. The clinician evaluates the appearance of the optic disc for edema, pallor, and cupping, and then the peripapillary region for the presence of hemorrhages, cotton-wool spots, exudates, and retinal folds.
9. The clinician evaluates the appearance of the retinal vasculature arising from the optic disc.
10. Lastly, the clinician evaluates the appearance of the macula, which is located temporal to the optic disc.

Examination with the direct ophthalmoscope can be difficult in patients who have small pupils. In such patients, pharmacological dilation of the pupils should be considered; there is minimal risk of inducing angle-closure glaucoma in patients with normal anterior chamber anatomy (Patel et al., 1995).

## ANCILLARY DIAGNOSTIC TECHNIQUES

Ancillary diagnostic tests may be obtained to further characterize and determine the cause of visual loss (see Chapter 43). Formal visual field testing (perimetry) allows for characterization and quantification of visual field defects. Ophthalmic imaging techniques may not only be used to image the ocular fundus and blood vessels but also now allow for measurement of the thickness of individual retinal layers and detection of subtle architectural abnormalities. Electrophysiological techniques may be used to evaluate objectively the function of the retina and optic nerves. Imaging techniques for evaluating the afferent visual pathways and cortical areas involved in visual processing are discussed in Chapter 40.

### Perimetry

Numerous techniques for examining the visual fields are available (Sample et al., 2011), but a detailed discussion of these is beyond the scope of this chapter. Examination of the entire visual field requires a perimeter; the tangent screen measures only the central 30 degrees of the visual field at a distance of 1 m. Perimeters can be divided into those that use a moving (kinetic) stimulus and those that use a static stimulus. Most static perimeters are automated and driven by computer. Static perimeters can determine the visual threshold at defined points in the visual field (threshold static perimetry) or may evaluate these points using stimuli of set luminance (suprathreshold static perimetry). The Goldmann perimeter is the most commonly used kinetic perimeter (see Fig. 16.13, *A* for a normal visual field obtained using the Goldmann perimeter), although kinetic perimetry can also be performed with the Humphrey and Octopus perimeters. The Humphrey and Octopus perimeters are the most commonly used static perimeters (see Fig. 16.13, *B* for a normal visual field obtained using the Humphrey perimeter). Threshold static perimeters are the most sensitive and quantitative, allowing for a comparison of the patient's responses with those of age-matched normal controls, but testing can be time consuming and tiring for the patient. To gain useful information from static perimetry, the patient must be alert, cooperative, and able to maintain steady central fixation. Many patients with neurological disorders are unable to concentrate for an examination that can take as long as 15 minutes per eye, and, thus, static perimetry findings may be unreliable in such patients. Recent refinements in testing strategy have made it possible to reduce testing time and thereby increase reliability, but many neuro-ophthalmologists continue to use Goldmann perimetry to assess the visual fields in selected patients.

### Ophthalmic Imaging

Photographs of the ocular fundus may be obtained to identify and document ophthalmoscopic findings. Retinal vascular abnormalities, such as occlusions (e.g., central retinal artery occlusion [CRAO]) and microvascular disease (e.g., diabetic retinopathy), may be evaluated when red-free fundus photographs are taken following intravenous (IV) injection of fluorescein *(fluorescein angiography). Fundus autofluorescence* photography allows for topographical mapping of lipofuscin in the retinal pigment epithelium layer. Lipofuscin is a fluorescent pigment that accumulates in retinal pigment epithelial cells following photoreceptor degradation, and, thus, autofluorescence may be used to detect subtle abnormalities in patients with retinal diseases (Schmitz-Valckenberg et al., 2008). Because optic nerve head drusen exhibit autofluorescence, they may be detected on fundus autofluorescence even when they are not visible on ophthalmoscopy (Kurz-Levin and Landau, 1999).

*Optical coherence tomography* (OCT) uses light waves to generate high-resolution cross-sectional images of the optic nerve and retina. As the retinal layers have differing optical reflectivity, they can be distinguished using OCT. The thickness of the layers can be determined from OCT and compared with age-matched normal controls. Measurement of the peripapillary retinal nerve fiber layer and macular ganglion cell layer thicknesses with OCT may help with the detection of mild optic neuropathy (Fig. 16.14). Measurement of the thickness of retinal layers or identification of architectural changes on OCT can aid the diagnosis and management of retinal disease.

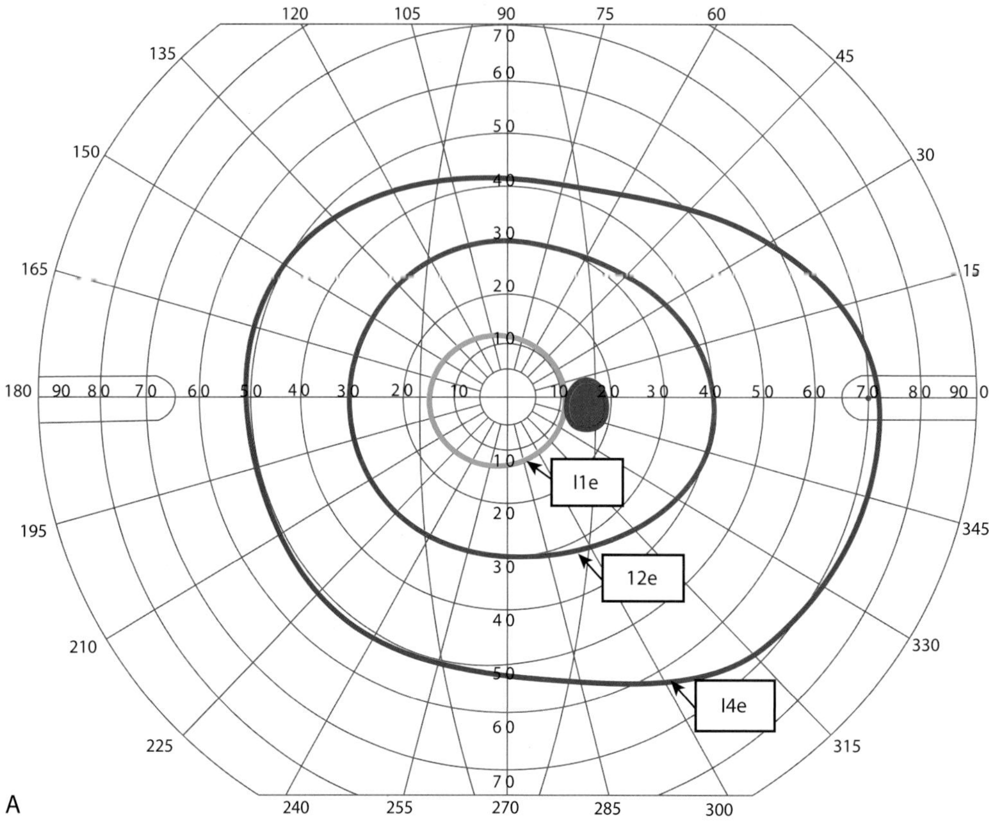


**Fig. 16.13 Kinetic and Automated Static Perimetry. A,** Kinetic perimetry of the right visual field using the Goldmann perimeter demonstrates an intact visual field. The isopters (*I1e*, *I2e*, and *I4e*) indicate the locations in the visual field where the subject perceived each stimulus. The scotoma 10–20 degrees right of center is the physiological blind spot.

### Electrophysiology

Electrophysiology may help in the investigation of unexplained visual loss or in identification of subclinical optic nerve dysfunction. Measurement of *visual-evoked potentials* (VEPs) has long been used for the evaluation of demyelinating optic neuropathies, which produce a delayed P-100. However, VEP findings can be misleading; a low-amplitude VEP could be misinterpreted as indicating optic neuropathy in a patient with retinal disease. *Electroretinography* (ERG) is useful for the evaluation of suspected retinal dysfunction, especially when ophthalmoscopic findings are subtle or absent. *Full-field ERG* evaluates the response of the entire retina to flashes of light. A variety of stimuli are presented in differing states of light adaptation, allowing for evaluation of different retinal elements, including the rod and cone photoreceptors. Because full-field ERG evaluates the response of the entire retina, it may not be abnormal in patients with focal retinal dysfunction (e.g., macular dysfunction). *Multifocal ERG* allows for the topographic evaluation of macula ERG responses and is more sensitive for detecting macular dysfunction (Sutter and Tran, 1992); multifocal ERG findings can be grossly abnormal even when ophthalmoscopic changes are absent or subtle.

## APPROACH TO THE PATIENT WITH VISUAL LOSS

Visual loss commonly accompanies neurological disease and is one of the most disturbing symptoms a patient may experience. While visual loss is often due to a benign or treatable process, it can be the first sign of a blinding or life-threatening disease. Common causes of visual loss include uncorrected refractive error, corneal disease, cataract, glaucoma, retinal disease (e.g., age-related macular degeneration), and amblyopia. Ophthalmic causes of visual loss are often not readily apparent to the neurologist, whereas neurological causes of visual loss often confuse ophthalmologists. Thus, the approach to evaluating visual loss must be systematic, so that sinister causes are not missed, and simple causes are not overinvestigated. The localization and cause of visual loss can often be inferred from the pattern and temporal profile of visual loss. Here, we briefly discuss the differential diagnosis of visual loss based on its pattern and temporal profile, as well as nonorganic (functional) visual disturbances. A comprehensive description of optic nerve and retinal disorders is presented in the final section of the chapter.

## PATTERN OF VISUAL LOSS

### Central Visual Loss

A defect in the visual field surrounded by normal vision is called a *scotoma*, from the Greek word meaning "darkness." Loss of central vision, resulting in a central or cecocentral scotoma, is usually quickly noticed, while peripheral visual field defects, such as homonymous hemianopia, can be asymptomatic. However, when noticed, they are frequently referred to the eye with the greater extent of field loss (i.e., the eye with temporal field loss; Fig. 16.15). Central and cecocentral scotomas are usually due to lesions of the optic nerve or macula. A lesion at the junction of the optic nerve and chiasm produces a *junctional scotoma* with an ipsilateral central scotoma, due to optic nerve involvement, and a contralateral temporal field defect, due to chiasmal involvement (Fig. 16.16). Patients with junctional scotomas are often unaware of the contralateral temporal field defect, emphasizing the importance of assessing each eye separately during visual field evaluation.

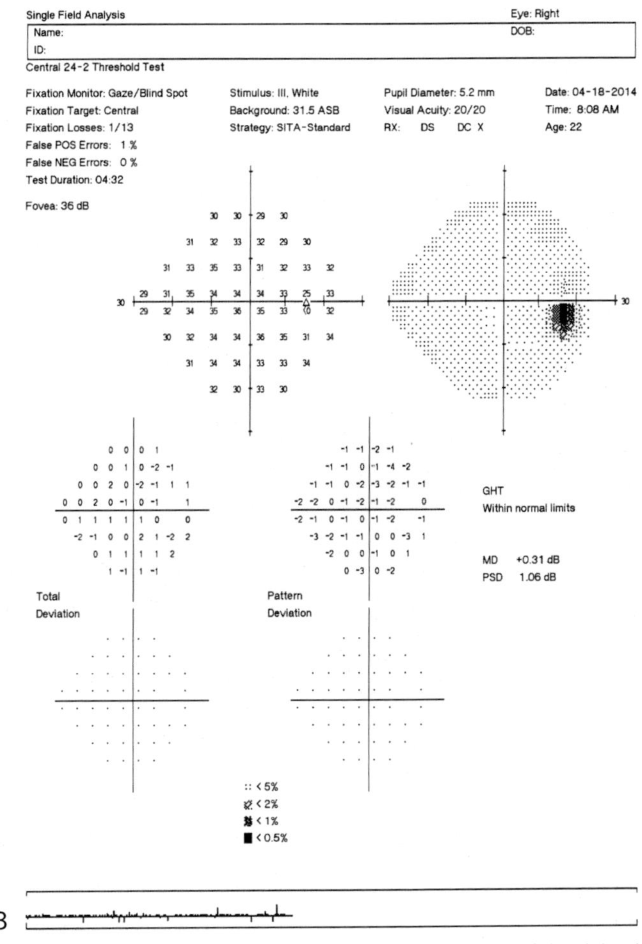


B

**Fig. 16.13, cont'd** B, Automated static perimetry of the central 24 degrees of the right visual field using the Humphrey perimeter (24-2 *SITA*-standard program) demonstrates an intact visual field. *Upper,* The testing strategy, stimulus size, and stimulus color are indicated. *Upper left,* The reliability indices (number of fixation losses, false-positive rate, and false-negative rate) and the foveal visual threshold (in decibels) are displayed. The decibel *(dB)* is a logarithmic relative scale to quantify differential light sensitivity (1 dB = 0.1 log-unit of stimulus intensity). *Upper center and right,* Threshold sensitivity plot (displays raw threshold data for each test location) and grayscale plot (displays interpolated data; darker areas indicate areas of visual field loss). The physiological blind spot is 10–20 degrees right of center. *Lower left and center,* The total deviation plots indicate deviations from age-adjusted normal values at each test location (in dB and as a probability of being abnormal). The pattern deviation plots indicate the deviations with adjustment for generalized depression of the visual field (e.g., due to refractive error, media opacity, or pupillary miosis). *Lower right,* The mean deviation (*MD,* mean of all total deviation values) is a global indicator of the severity of visual field loss. Negative values indicate greater visual field loss. The pattern standard deviation *(PSD)* provides a measure of the uniformity of the visual field loss, such that diseases causing highly focal defects (e.g., glaucoma) will have a high PSD, whereas those causing diffuse visual field loss will have a low PSD.

In general, scotomas caused by retinal disease are so-called positive scotomas because they are perceived as a black or gray spot in the visual field. Patients with macular pathology can also have metamorphopsia; metamorphopsia is almost always caused by retinal disease (e.g., age-related macular degeneration, macular edema, and epiretinal membrane). In contrast, optic nerve lesions characteristically produce negative scotomas, areas of absent vision that are otherwise not perceivable, in conjunction with decreased color vision, contrast vision, and light brightness perception. On occasion, paradoxical photophobia, especially with fluorescent lighting, can occur with optic nerve lesions. Photopsias (light flashes) can occur with vitreoretinal traction (e.g., posterior vitreous detachment), retinal disease (e.g., cancer-associated retinopathy [CAR]), toxicity from certain drugs (e.g., digitalis), or optic nerve disease (e.g., in the healing phase of optic neuritis, in which case they may be evoked by sound). Photopsias can also occur as part of migraine visual aura. Aside from ocular diseases, bilateral central visual loss can result from lesions involving both optic nerves, the optic chiasm, or the visual cortex concerned with central vision. The possibility of nonorganic (functional) visual loss must be considered, but it remains a diagnosis of exclusion.

## Peripheral Visual Loss

For simplicity, visual field defects can be classified into one of three groups: prechiasmal, chiasmal, or retrochiasmal. Unilateral prechiasmal lesions affect the visual field of one eye only, chiasmal lesions affect the visual fields of both eyes in a nonhomonymous bitemporal fashion, and retrochiasmal lesions cause homonymous visual field defects with varying degrees of congruity depending on their location (Fig. 16.17).

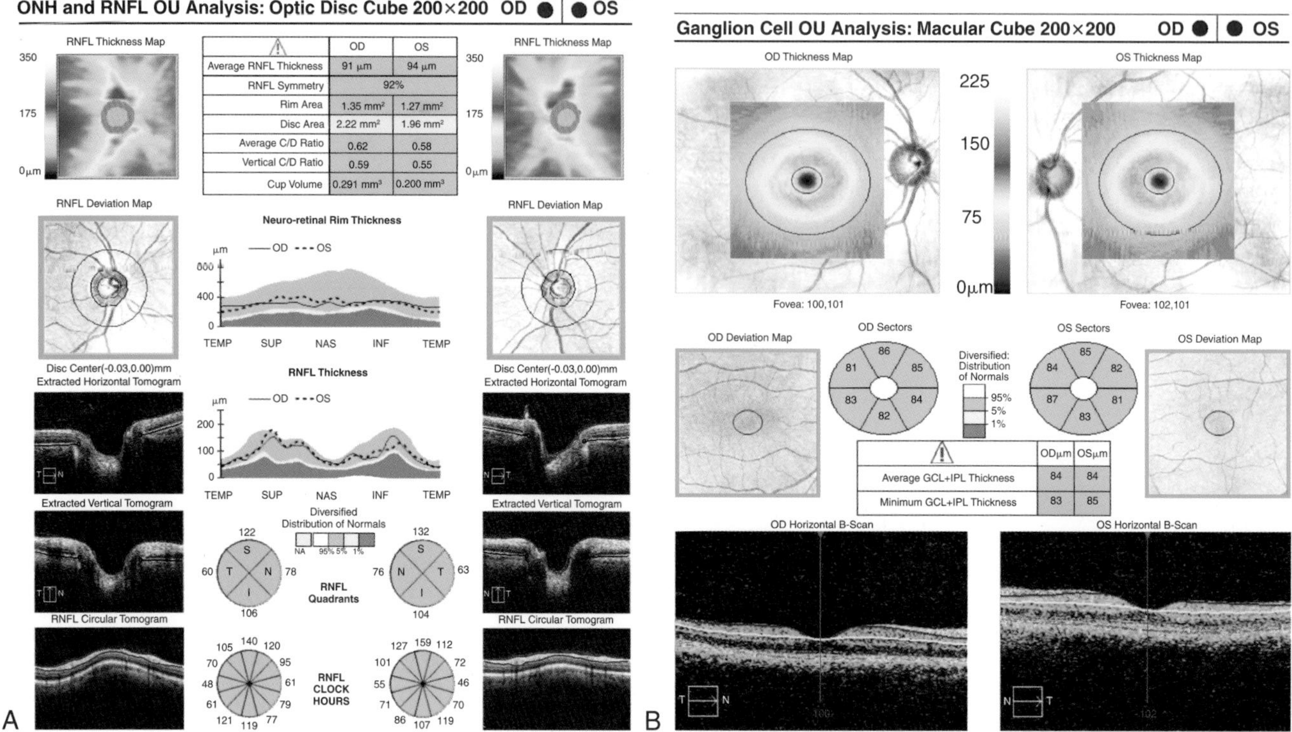


**Fig. 16.14 Optical Coherence Tomography of the Optic Nerves and Macula. A,** Optical coherence tomography of the optic nerve head *(OHN)* and retinal nerve fiber layer *(RNFL)* from the right eye *(OD)* and left eye *(OS)*, obtained using the Cirrus optic disc cube protocol. The top panel shows the RNFL thickness map, with the average RNFL thickness (in micrometers), optic disc area, and the cup-to-disc *(C/D)* ratio for each eye. Neuro-retinal rim and RNFL thicknesses are plotted below for quadrants of the optic nerves (*S*, superior; *N*, nasal; *I*, inferior; *T*, temporal) compared with the distribution from age-matched normal controls. The RNFL thicknesses fall within the normal range in both eyes. **B,** Optical coherence tomography showing the macular ganglion cell analysis from the right eye and left eye, obtained using the Cirrus macular cube protocol. The top panel shows the ganglion cell thickness map for each eye. The ganglion cell layer thicknesses are plotted below for the six sectors of the macula compared with the distribution from age-matched normal controls. The ganglion cell layer thicknesses fall within the normal range for both eyes *(OU)*.

## TEMPORAL PROFILE OF VISUAL LOSS

### Sudden-Onset Visual Loss

Visual loss of sudden onset can be divided into three temporal patterns: transient (Box 16.3; Thurtell and Rucker, 2009), nonprogressive, and progressive.

#### Transient Monocular Visual Loss

***Amaurosis fugax*** The term *amaurosis fugax* is often used to describe the transient monocular visual loss (TMVL) caused by emboli from the carotid arteries, aorta, or heart to the retinal circulation. Typically, these attacks are sudden in onset, last for several minutes, and are characterized by altitudinal visual field loss that is often described as being similar to a curtain descending over the eye (Donders, 2001). Patients may also describe having separate attacks with hemispheric symptoms, such as weakness and aphasia, rather than visual loss.

***Retinal artery vasospasm*** TMVL can be caused by retinal artery vasospasm and is called *retinal migraine* when accompanied by migraine headache (Hill et al., 2007). Vasospastic TMVL is usually benign and often responds to calcium channel blockers (Winterkorn et al., 1993).

***Angle-closure glaucoma*** Attacks of angle-closure glaucoma should also be considered in the differential diagnosis of TMVL, especially if the patient reports seeing halos around lights or has associated eye pain, injection, or vomiting. Urgent ophthalmic consultation should be obtained to prevent irreversible visual loss.

***Visual loss in bright light*** Some patients with reduced blood supply to the eye due to a high-grade stenosis or occlusion of the internal carotid artery report TMVL in bright light, which is thought to be due to impaired regeneration of photopigments secondary to ocular ischemia (Kaiboriboon et al., 2001). The TMVL can also occur following meals or with postural changes. A variety of ophthalmic abnormalities can be present and collectively comprise the *ocular ischemic syndrome* (Chen and Miller, 2007). Other retinal diseases, such as cone dystrophies and age-related macular degeneration, can cause evanescent visual loss in bright light, also known as *hemeralopia* or *day blindness*. The visual loss in these diseases is usually bilateral, whereas it is unilateral in patients with unilateral carotid disease.

***Uhthoff phenomenon*** TMVL with increases in body temperature is known as the *Uhthoff phenomenon* and most commonly occurs in patients with a history of optic neuritis, but it can also occur in patients with other optic neuropathies. The phenomenon is thought to arise as a result of transient conduction block within the optic nerve. Vision returns to baseline when the body temperature returns to normal.

***Transient visual obscurations*** Transient visual obscurations are brief episodes of monocular or binocular visual loss in patients with optic disc edema due to increased intracranial pressure (ICP). The visual loss is often precipitated by postural changes or Valsalva-like maneuvers (e.g., coughing and straining) and probably occurs secondary to transient hypoperfusion of the edematous optic nerve head. The visual loss lasts for only a few seconds, with vision rapidly

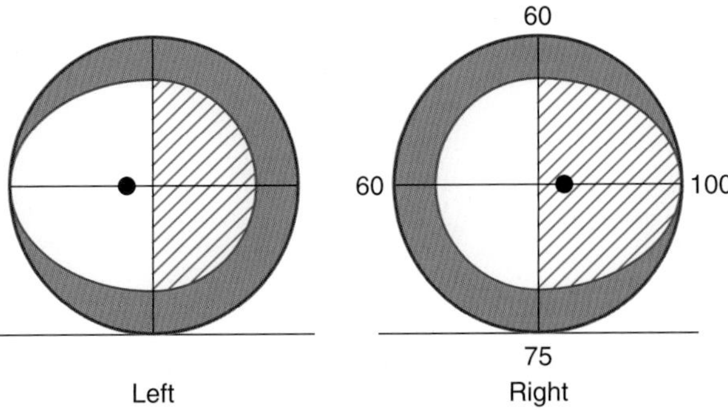


Fig. 16.15 Right Homonymous Hemianopia. The visual loss is often referred to the right eye because the right temporal visual field is larger than the left nasal visual field. *Numbers* refer to the normal extent of the visual field in degrees.

returning to baseline thereafter. Similar episodes of visual loss can occur with systemic hypotension, giant cell arteritis (GCA), or retinal venous stasis. Gaze-evoked transient visual loss has been reported with orbital tumors but can occasionally occur with optic disc edema.

***Other causes of transient visual loss*** Transient visual loss can also occur as a result of transient optic nerve compression by cystic lesions, such as paranasal sinus mucoceles and craniopharyngiomas. Other ophthalmic causes of TMVL include impending central retinal vein occlusion and recurrent hyphema, although it is important to note that some causes (e.g., corneal basement membrane dystrophy and tear film dysfunction) produce visual blurring rather than actual visual loss.

### Transient Binocular Visual Loss

Other than transient visual obscurations occurring in patients with bilateral optic disc edema, simultaneous complete or incomplete transient binocular visual loss is almost always due to transient dysfunction of the visual cortex. Visual migraine aura is probably the most common cause of transient binocular visual loss (see Chapter 102). Transient binocular visual loss can also result from cerebral hypoperfusion due to vasospasm, thromboembolism, systemic hypotension, hyperviscosity, or vascular compression (Box 16.4; Thurtell and Rucker, 2009). Transient binocular visual loss can occur in association with seizures, although they more commonly cause visual hallucinations, which can be elementary or complex, depending on the location of the seizure focus (Bien et al., 2000). Transient cortical blindness can occur in association with headache, altered mental status, and seizures in the posterior reversible encephalopathy syndrome (PRES; Hinchey et al., 1996). Transient cortical blindness can sometimes occur after head trauma, especially in children. Lastly, transient bilateral visual loss can occasionally be nonorganic in etiology, but this should remain a diagnosis of exclusion.

### Sudden Monocular Visual Loss Without Progression

Visual loss due to optic nerve or retinal ischemia is characteristically sudden in onset (Box 16.5) and is usually nonprogressive, although a stepwise decline in vision may occur over several weeks in some patients with anterior ischemic optic neuropathy. *Anterior ischemic optic neuropathy* is a common cause of optic neuropathy and occurs due to loss of blood supply to the optic nerve head, resulting in optic disc edema (Rucker et al., 2004). In affected patients younger than 50 years, it is usually nonarteritic in etiology, being caused by a combination of factors that impair blood supply to the optic nerve head. In patients older than 50 years, giant cell (temporal or cranial) arteritis must be considered. *Posterior ischemic optic neuropathy*

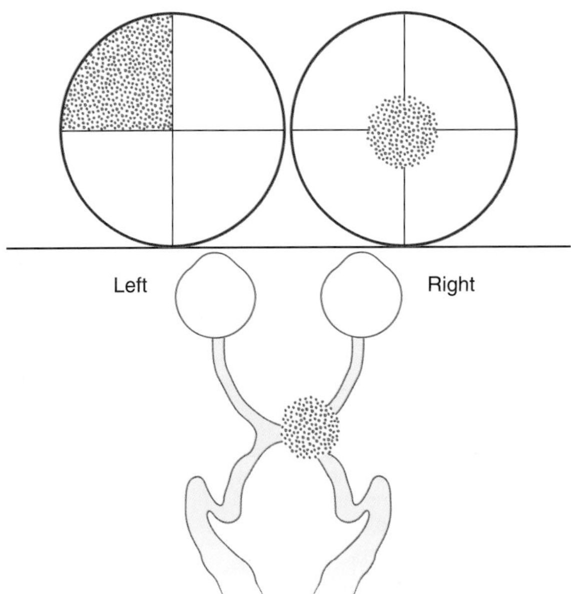


Fig. 16.16 Junctional Scotoma from a Lesion at the Junction of the Optic Nerve and Chiasm. The lesion affects both the right optic nerve, producing a cecocentral scotoma in the right eye, and crossing fibers in the optic chiasm, producing a temporal visual field defect in the left eye. The temporal visual field defect of a junctional scotoma often goes unnoticed by the patient and may only be detected with visual field testing.

(PION), occurring due to loss of blood supply to the retrobulbar portion of the optic nerve, is far less common but can occur in the perioperative period (e.g., during prolonged prone spine surgery or cardiac bypass surgery) or with hemodynamic shock (Rucker et al., 2004). GCA should be specifically considered in elderly patients with PION.

Optic nerve ischemia almost never results from embolism. In contrast, central or branch retinal artery occlusions (BRAOs) are caused mostly by embolic or thrombotic events. Opacification of the retinal nerve fiber layer with a cherry-red spot at the macula is the classic funduscopic appearance of acute CRAO. Retinal arterial occlusions can produce altitudinal, quadrantic, or complete monocular visual loss. The triad of BRAOs, hearing loss, and encephalopathy results from a rare microangiopathy known as *Susac syndrome* (Susac et al., 2007).

Occlusion of the central retinal vein can result in sudden visual loss and an unmistakable hemorrhagic retinopathy. It usually occurs in patients with risk factors for atherosclerosis and results from venous thrombosis at the level of the lamina cribrosa of the sclera. When ischemic, it causes a dense central scotoma with sparing of peripheral vision.

Idiopathic central serous retinopathy can manifest as a positive central scotoma of sudden onset, often with metamorphopsia or micropsia and a positive light-stress test result. It results from leakage of fluid into the subretinal space and most often occurs in young adult men with type A personalities. The diagnosis can be difficult to make without the aid of fluorescein angiography or OCT, as the retinal findings are subtle. Spontaneous recovery usually occurs within weeks to months, but occasionally laser photocoagulation is required to seal leaking vessels.

Traumatic optic neuropathy (TON) usually results in sudden permanent optic nerve dysfunction. The trauma can be severe or deceptively minor, causing a contusion or laceration of the optic nerve or a shearing of its nutrient vessels with subsequent infarction.

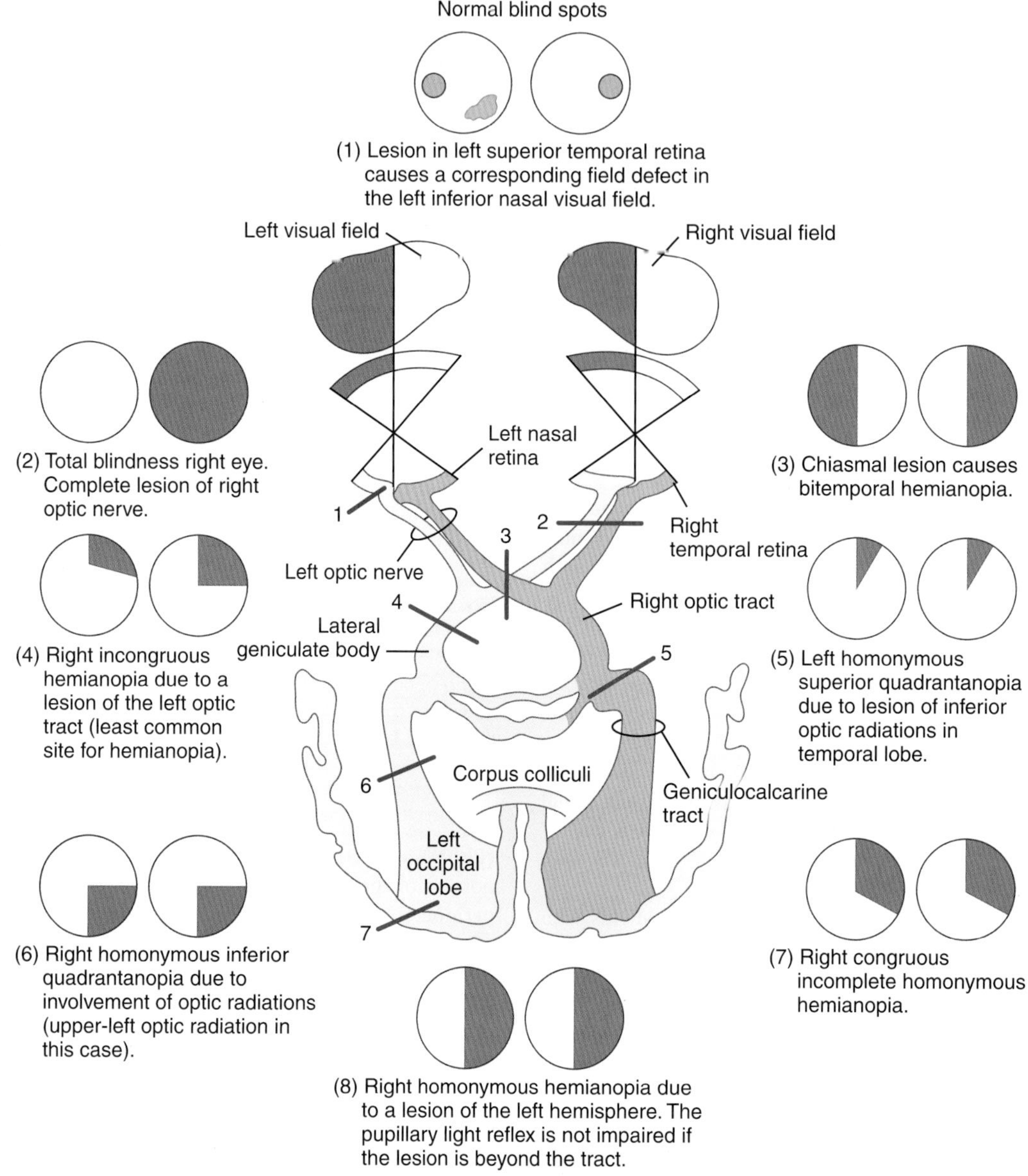
Normal blind spots
(1) Lesion in left superior temporal retina causes a corresponding field defect in the left inferior nasal visual field.
Left visual field
Right visual field
(2) Total blindness right eye. Complete lesion of right optic nerve.
Left nasal retina
(3) Chiasmal lesion causes bitemporal hemianopia.
1
2
3
Right temporal retina
Left optic nerve
4
Right optic tract
Lateral geniculate body
(4) Right incongruous hemianopia due to a lesion of the left optic tract (least common site for hemianopia).
5
(5) Left homonymous superior quadrantanopia due to lesion of inferior optic radiations in temporal lobe.
6
Corpus colliculi
Geniculocalcarine tract
Left occipital lobe
7
(6) Right homonymous inferior quadrantanopia due to involvement of optic radiations (upper-left optic radiation in this case).
(7) Right congruous incomplete homonymous hemianopia.
(8) Right homonymous hemianopia due to a lesion of the left hemisphere. The pupillary light reflex is not impaired if the lesion is beyond the tract.

**Fig. 16.17** Topographical Diagnosis of Visual Field Defects. *(Reprinted with permission from Vaughn, C., Asbury, T., Tabbara, K.F., 1989. General Ophthalmology, twelfth ed. Appleton & Lange, Norwalk, CT, p. 244.)*

## Sudden Binocular Visual Loss Without Progression

Sudden, permanent, binocular visual loss most commonly results from strokes involving the retrochiasmal visual pathways and causes homonymous visual field defects (Box 16.6; Rizzo and Barton, 2005). In patients who have no other neurological symptoms or signs, the lesion is usually in the occipital lobe. Bilateral occipital lobe infarcts can result in tubular visual field defects, checkerboard visual field defects, or complete loss of vision in both eyes, a condition called *cortical* or *cerebral blindness*. Cortical blindness, especially from infarction, can be accompanied by a denial of the visual loss and confabulation, a condition known as *Anton syndrome*.

Sudden binocular visual loss can occasionally result from simultaneous bilateral ischemic optic neuropathies (especially in the perioperative period) or from chiasmal compression due to *pituitary apoplexy*. Pituitary apoplexy can also cause headache, diplopia, ptosis, altered mental status, and hemodynamic shock (Sibal et al., 2004), but the presentation can be subtle such that the diagnosis is missed.

## Sudden Visual Loss with Progression

Sudden-onset, painful monocular visual loss that subsequently worsens is commonly due to optic neuritis. The visual loss typically progresses over days before stabilizing and then improving. Optic neuritis is well known to be associated with multiple sclerosis (MS) and may be the first sign of the disease. The prognosis for visual recovery without treatment is excellent in most patients, although there is a poor recovery in some, such as those with optic neuritis occurring in association with neuromyelitis optica (NMO; Wingerchuk et al., 2007).

Leber hereditary optic neuropathy (LHON), a maternally transmitted disease resulting from mutations in the mitochondrial deoxyribonucleic acid (DNA) genes encoding subunits of respiratory chain complex I, can also cause sudden painless central visual loss with subsequent progression. The visual loss initially may be monocular or binocular, but the fellow eye is almost always affected within a few weeks to months and certainly by 1 year. Visual recovery is variable and infrequent and depends on the mitochondrial DNA mutation.

**BOX 16.3 Causes of Transient Monocular Visual Loss**

Retinal circulation emboli
Migraine/vasospasm
Hypoperfusion (hypotension, hyperviscosity, hypercoagulability)
Ocular (optic disc edema, intermittent angle-closure glaucoma, hyphema, impending central retinal vein occlusion)
Vasculitis (e.g., giant cell arteritis)
Other (Uhthoff phenomenon, idiopathic, nonorganic)

**BOX 16.4 Causes of Transient Binocular Visual Loss**

Migraine
Cerebral hypoperfusion:
- Thromboembolism
- Systemic hypotension
- Hyperviscosity

Seizures
Posterior reversible encephalopathy syndrome
Head trauma
Optic disc edema (transient visual obscurations)

**BOX 16.5 Causes of Sudden Monocular Visual Loss Without Progression**

Central or branch retinal artery occlusion
Anterior ischemic optic neuropathy, arteritic or nonarteritic
Posterior ischemic optic neuropathy
Branch or central retinal vein occlusion
Traumatic optic neuropathy
Central serous retinopathy
Retinal detachment
Vitreous hemorrhage
Nonorganic (functional) visual loss

Careful questioning of the patient with "sudden" visual loss may reveal a long-standing deficit that has suddenly been noticed (e.g., when covering the fellow eye) or that has worsened over time. In such cases, the clinician should evaluate for a slow-growing compressive lesion (Box 16.7).

## Progressive Visual Loss

Progressive visual loss is the hallmark of a lesion compressing the afferent visual pathways. Common compressive lesions include pituitary tumors, aneurysms, craniopharyngiomas, and meningiomas (see Box 16.7; Gittinger, 2005; Glaser, 1999). Granulomatous disease of the optic nerve from sarcoidosis or tuberculosis can cause chronic progressive visual loss. Optic nerve compression at the orbital apex from thyroid eye disease can occur with minimal orbital signs or ocular motility disturbance. In each of these cases, the visual loss can be so insidious as to go unnoticed until it is fortuitously discovered during a routine examination.

Hereditary or degenerative diseases of the optic nerves or retina must be included in the differential diagnosis of gradual-onset visual loss. The hereditary optic neuropathies are bilateral and are usually diagnosed during the first two decades of life (Yu-Wai-Man et al., 2009). The most common inherited optic neuropathy is the autosomal dominant variety, known as *dominant optic atrophy*. Characteristically,

**BOX 16.6 Causes of Sudden Binocular Visual Loss Without Progression**

Occipital lobe stroke
Bilateral ischemic optic neuropathies
Pituitary apoplexy
Head trauma
Nonorganic (functional) visual loss

**BOX 16.7 Causes of Progressive Visual Loss**

Anterior visual pathway inflammation:
- Optic neuritis
- Sarcoidosis
- Meningitis

Anterior visual pathway compression:
- Tumors
- Aneurysms
- Thyroid eye disease

Hereditary optic neuropathies:
- Leber hereditary optic neuropathy
- Dominant optic atrophy

Optic nerve head drusen
Glaucoma and normal-tension glaucoma
Chronic papilledema
Toxic (e.g., ethambutol) and nutritional optic neuropathies
Radiation damage to anterior visual pathways
Paraneoplastic (cancer-associated) retinopathy or optic neuropathy

there are central or cecocentral scotomas with sparing of the peripheral visual field and temporal pallor and cupping of the optic discs. Color vision is usually abnormal. Other ophthalmic and neurological abnormalities may be present (Yu-Wai-Man et al., 2009).

Optic disc drusen are a common cause of pseudopapilledema and can produce visual field defects including enlargement of the physiological blind spot, arcuate defects, and generalized constriction (Lee and Zimmerman, 2005). Loss of visual acuity is atypical but can result from development of a secondary choroidal neovascular membrane, with subsequent hemorrhage into the macula, or anterior ischemic optic neuropathy.

Glaucoma is a common cause of progressive visual field loss. The visual field defects are arcuate, and central vision is spared until late. Glaucoma is usually bilateral and symmetric, with associated increased intraocular pressure and optic disc cupping. In normal-tension glaucoma, glaucomatous optic disc and visual field changes develop despite normal intraocular pressure (Anderson et al., 2001).

Chronic papilledema from any cause of intracranial hypertension can produce progressive optic neuropathy (see Chapter 88). The visual fields become constricted, with nasal defects occurring initially, followed by gradual constriction, with central vision being spared until late.

Toxic and nutritional optic neuropathies are bilateral and usually progressive (Phillips, 2005; Tomsak, 1997). The nutritional variety is characterized by gradual onset of painless visual loss over weeks to months, prominent dyschromatopsia, cecocentral scotomas, and development of optic atrophy late in the disease. Medications that are toxic to the optic nerves, including ethambutol, amiodarone, and linezolid, can cause a gradual onset of painless visual loss (Phillips, 2005). Retinal toxins, such as vigabatrin, digitalis, chloroquine, hydroxychloroquine, and phenothiazines, can also cause painless progressive binocular visual loss.

**BOX 16.8 Some Forms of Nonorganic Visual Disturbance**

Visual acuity loss (one or both eyes)
Visual field loss (unilateral or bilateral)
Color perception abnormalities
Convergence/accommodative insufficiency
Spasm of the near triad
Loss of depth perception
Diplopia
Night blindness
Photophobia
Pharmacological pupils
Voluntary nystagmus

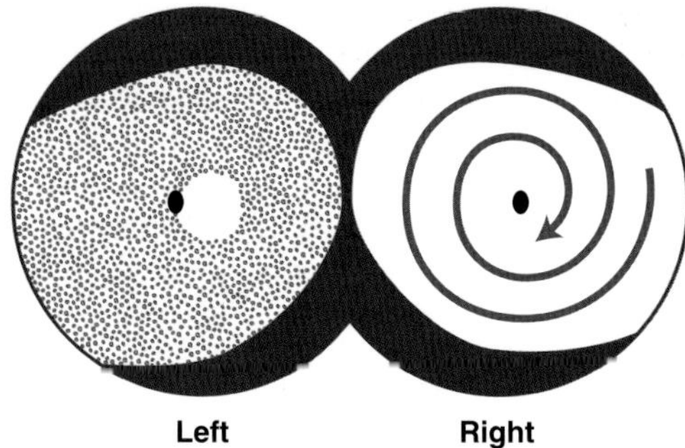


**Fig. 16.18** Two common visual field abnormalities with nonorganic visual loss. *Left,* Concentric (tubular) constriction. *Right,* Spiraling of an isopter (seen only with kinetic visual field testing).

Slowly progressive visual loss from radiation damage to the anterior visual pathways or retina can result from direct radiation therapy to the eye or periocular irradiation. It can also occur after whole-brain irradiation or parasellar irradiation (Lessell, 2004). Its incidence relates to fraction size and total radiation dose. Radiation-induced capillary endothelial cell damage is the initial event that triggers the damage. Radiation retinopathy may be indistinguishable from diabetic retinopathy.

Rapidly progressive bilateral visual loss can be caused by paraneoplastic processes that affect the retina or, less commonly, optic nerves (Ko et al., 2008). Small-cell carcinoma of the lung is the most commonly associated tumor, but gynecological, endocrine, and breast tumors have been implicated. With CAR, features include photopsias, night blindness or *nyctalopia*, constricted visual fields, and an extinguished electroretinogram. Combined treatment with chemotherapy and immunosuppression may be effective in occasional cases.

## NONORGANIC (FUNCTIONAL) VISUAL DISTURBANCES

Nonorganic (functional) visual disturbances can have a variety of manifestations (Box 16.8). Similarly to other nonorganic conditions, they can be a challenge to diagnose and manage (Friedman and LaFrance, 2010).

### Diagnostic Techniques

A careful social and family history must be obtained when evaluating a patient with suspected nonorganic visual disturbance, especially regarding abuse, peer pressure, and visually impaired friends and family members. Different examination approaches are needed, depending on the type of nonorganic visual disturbance. For example, if a patient reports total blindness, the clinician should examine the pupils, check for the optokinetic response using an optokinetic drum, and oscillate a large mirror in front of the patient to try inducing pursuit eye movements. If the patient claims visual loss in one eye, the clinician should examine the pupils to assess for an RAPD and test stereopsis. In this situation, normal visual acuity can sometimes be demonstrated using the vertical prism dissociation test (Golnik et al., 2004). In this test, a vertical prism is placed over the eye with intact vision, such that the images from the two eyes become vertically separated. If the patient is able to read the optotypes on the two vertically separated 20/20 (6/6) lines, normal visual acuity can be confirmed for both eyes. Specialized ophthalmic techniques such as a "fogging" refraction can also be helpful in this situation but require the assistance of an ophthalmologist or, ideally, a neuro-ophthalmologist.

Testing of visual fields in patients with suspected nonorganic visual loss may reveal one of several patterns, including tubular constriction, cloverleaf constriction, spiraling of an isopter, crossing isopters, or inverted isopters (Fig. 16.18). Confrontation or tangent screen testing done at different distances can be useful in evaluating a patient with visual field constriction, as the visual field area should increase as the distance between the patient and the clinician increases. Lack of expansion of visual field area with increasing distance from the clinician suggests nonorganic visual field constriction (see Fig. 16.6). Cloverleaf constriction is best detected using automated static perimetry and cannot be produced by organic disease. Spiraling, crossing, and inversion of isopters can be detected using kinetic perimetry and cannot be produced by organic disease. Kinetic perimetry with both eyes opened in a patient with suspected nonorganic monocular visual loss may demonstrate nonphysiological visual field constriction on the side of the reported visual loss.

The use of VEPs to diagnose nonorganic visual loss can be unreliable. If the VEP is normal, useful information is gained, but factitious abnormalities in the VEP can be induced if patients defocus their vision during the test. Therefore, an abnormal VEP is not always diagnostic of organic visual disturbance.

### Prognosis

About half of patients with nonorganic visual disturbance improve with time and reassurance. Factors that indicate a good prognosis include youth and the presence of anxiety, whereas older age and depression are usually associated with a poor prognosis.

## OPTIC NERVE AND RETINAL DISORDERS

Disorders of the optic nerve and retina are common causes of afferent visual loss in clinical neurology. The diagnosis of optic neuropathy should be considered when visual loss (affecting visual acuity, color vision, or visual field) is accompanied by an abnormal optic disc appearance or an RAPD. The specific cause for an optic neuropathy often can be established on the basis of clinical history (i.e., character and progression of vision loss) and examination (i.e., pattern of visual field loss and optic disc appearance). Furthermore, optic neuropathies are classifiable by appearance of the optic disc: normal, swollen, or pale. This section discusses the differential diagnosis for optic neuropathies, based on optic disc appearance, and retinal disorders of particular interest in neurology.

## OPTIC DISC EDEMA

In assessing an elevated optic disc, the examiner must first make the important distinction between true disc swelling and pseudopapilledema. Disc swelling caused by increased ICP is referred to as *papilledema* and may be accompanied by headache, transient visual obscurations, nausea, vomiting, and pulse-synchronous tinnitus. In addition, papilledema usually is bilateral and symmetric, in contrast with other optic neuropathies including optic neuritis or NAION. Causes of pseudopapilledema include congenital anomalies and optic disc drusen.

## Unilateral Optic Disc Edema

The most common causes of unilateral optic disc edema are NAION, optic neuritis, and orbital compressive lesions. Although characteristics of the optic disc appearance may overlap among these entities, certain features may suggest a specific diagnosis. These are described and illustrated in the following sections. Briefly, in NAION, the disc typically has an edematous appearance that is often sectoral, and disc hemorrhages are frequently present. On the other hand, only one-third of patients with optic neuritis will have optic disc swelling, and, when present, it is typically mild. Disc hemorrhages are uncommon with optic neuritis, and this finding should suggest an alternative diagnosis. Finally, compressive lesions may lead to chronic disc edema, optociliary collateral vessels, and glistening white bodies on the disc surface (pseudodrusen from extruded axoplasm).

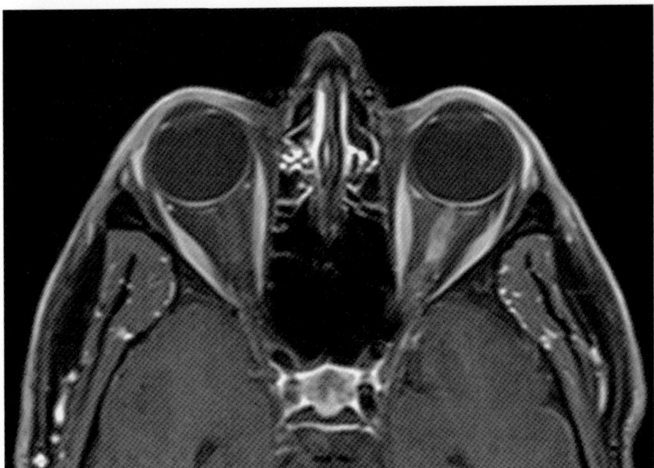

**Fig. 16.19** Axial T1-weighted postgadolinium magnetic resonance imaging with fat saturation in a patient with left optic neuritis. Note enhancement of the left optic nerve consistent with acute inflammation.

Despite suggestive patterns in the appearance of the optic nerve, it is often not possible to distinguish NAION, optic neuritis, and compressive optic neuropathies on this basis alone. Typically, these diagnoses also rely on the clinical history and the pattern of the visual field deficit. Vision loss generally is slowly progressive in patients with compressive lesions, it is rapidly progressive with subsequent improvement in those with optic neuritis, while it is most often maximal at onset with minimal improvement in patients with NAION. Both optic neuritis and compressive lesions generally produce central visual loss, whereas NAION typically produces a nerve fiber bundle-type field defect (originating from the physiological blind spot and respecting the horizontal meridian, owing to the arrangement of retinal ganglion cell axons traveling to the optic disc). However, considerable overlap exists in the patterns of visual field loss caused by the different forms of optic neuropathy.

### Optic Neuritis

Typical *optic neuritis* is an inflammatory optic neuropathy caused by demyelinating disease (Toosy et al., 2014; Fig. 16.19). Visual loss in the affected eye typically occurs rapidly over several hours to a few days. Decreased color vision and contrast sensitivity are characteristic (Baier et al., 2005; Trobe et al., 1996). In addition, pain with eye movements precedes the vision loss in approximately 90% of cases (Optic Neuritis Study Group, 1991). The pain typically lasts 3–5 days; if it persists for longer than 7 days, optic neuritis should be considered less likely, and further workup should be pursued. Visual field defects commonly are present; they can be either diffuse or discrete scotomas and are nonspecific. Fundus examination shows mild disc edema in approximately one-third of affected eyes, which is typically less prominent than the disc swelling associated with papilledema (Fig. 16.20). In the majority of patients, the fundus appearance is normal.

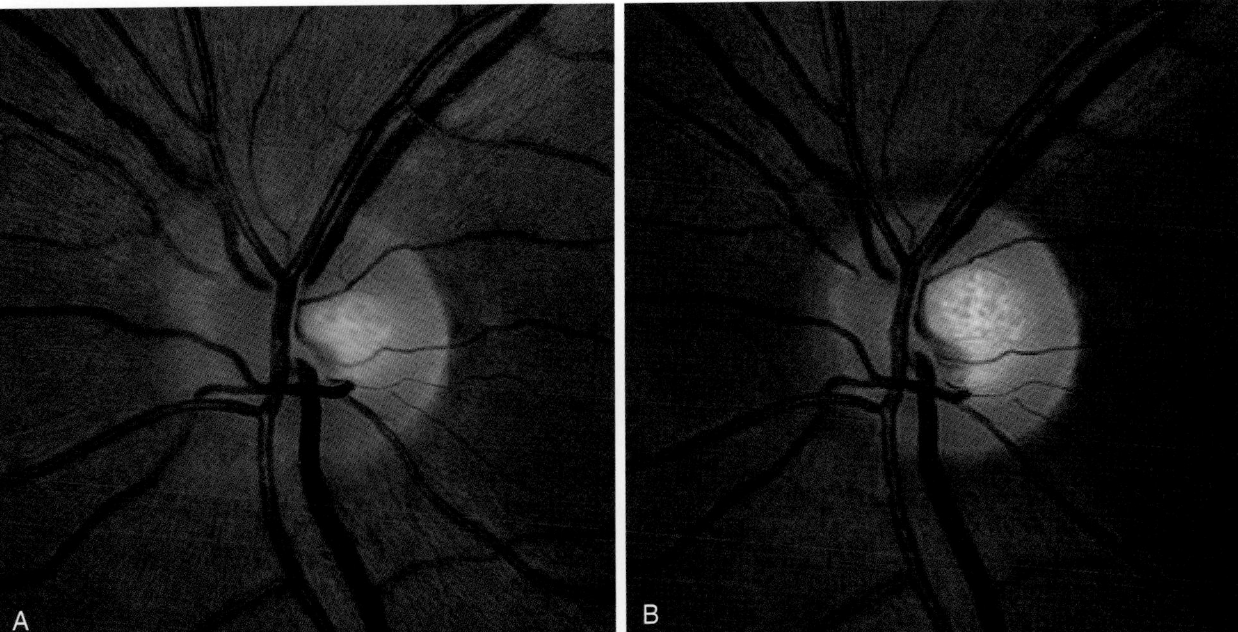


**Fig. 16.20** A, Fundus photograph of the left eye in a patient with acute left optic neuritis. Note mild nerve fiber layer edema, greatest at the nasal portion of the disc, without hemorrhages or cotton-wool spots. B, Fundus photograph of the left eye from the same patient taken 3 months after initial presentation. Note resolution of edema and presence of mild temporal pallor.

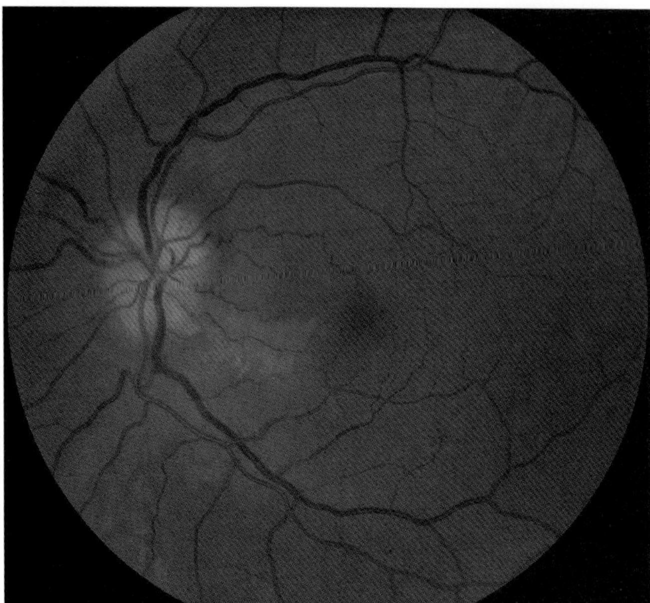

**Fig. 16.21** Fundus photograph of the left eye in a patient with anterior ischemic optic neuropathy from giant cell arteritis. Note pallor and edema of the nerve head. The patient also has inner retinal ischemia evidenced by cotton-wool spots in the macula.

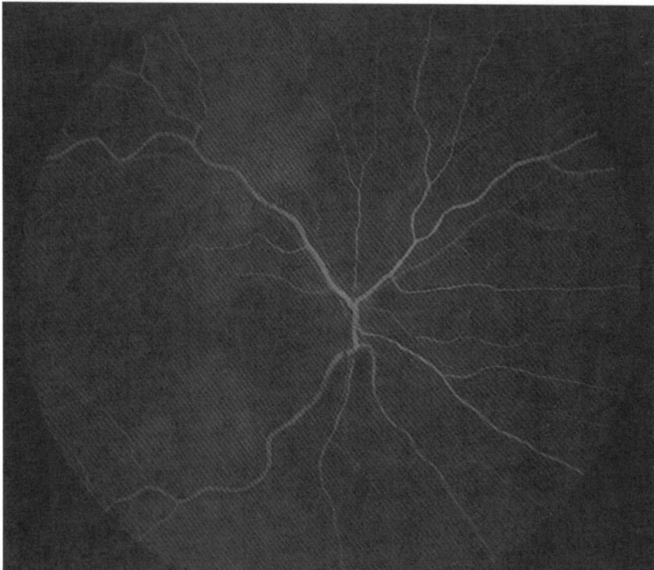

**Fig. 16.22** Fluorescein angiography of the right eye in a patient with giant cell arteritis, showing nonperfused choroid consistent with inflammatory occlusion of posterior ciliary arteries.

The prognosis for recovery of vision generally is good but is in relation to the severity of the initial deficit. Recovery typically begins within 1 month. The likelihood of progression of optic neuritis to MS is best predicted by brain magnetic resonance imaging (MRI) at the time of diagnosis. In the Optic Neuritis Treatment Trial, the risk of developing MS within 15 years was 72% among patients with one or more characteristic brain lesions, whereas it was 25% if the MRI was normal (Optic Neuritis Study Group, 2008). With features that are atypical for optic neuritis (e.g., painless visual loss, severe disc edema, disc or peripapillary hemorrhages, and macular exudate), the risk of developing MS is negligible (Beck et al., 1993).

Following an episode of optic neuritis, the optic nerve usually demonstrates pallor, suggesting that axonal loss has accompanied the episode of demyelination (see Fig. 16.20). OCT usually demonstrates atrophy of the retinal nerve fiber and ganglion cell layers (Frohman et al., 2008), providing a reliable structural marker that complements clinical assessments of visual function.

Treating optic neuritis with high-dose IV corticosteroids reduces the risk of developing MS over the following 2 years (Beck et al., 1993). In the long term, however, this acute treatment is unlikely to affect the likelihood of progression to MS (Optic Neuritis Study Group, 1997). In addition, IV corticosteroid treatment may hasten visual recovery but does not significantly affect long-term visual outcomes (Beck and Cleary, 1993). Because oral prednisone (1 mg/kg) may be associated with an increased risk of recurrence of optic neuritis when not used in conjunction with high-dose IV corticosteroids, this therapy should be avoided (Beck et al., 1992). In addition to IV corticosteroids, studies support the early use of immunomodulating treatments for high-risk patients to reduce the likelihood of progression to MS within 2–5 years (Toosy et al., 2014). Trials are ongoing to assess the efficacy of newer oral immunomodulatory agents to reduce the risk of relapse after an initial clinical presentation with optic neuritis.

NMO, or Devic disease, is characterized by necrotizing demyelinating lesions of the optic nerves and the spinal cord (Wingerchuk and Weinshenker, 2014). The spinal lesion characteristic of NMO often extends contiguously over three or more vertebral segments. NMO is a humorally mediated disease distinct from MS. The majority of patients with NMO have serum antibodies that target aquaporin 4 (NMO-IgG, which is a water channel that has a role in cell water homeostasis in the brain and spinal cord), while a minority have serum antibodies that target myelin oligodendrocyte glycoprotein (MOG-IgG, which is a cell membrane protein that has a role in myelin sheath construction and integrity; Probstel et al., 2015). Optimal treatment regimens for optic neuritis occurring in patients with underlying NMO have not been established. Plasmapheresis may be beneficial in the acute stage, and treatment with rituximab (a chemotherapeutic monoclonal antibody that depletes B cells) may be an effective disease-modifying agent (Wingerchuk and Weinshenker, 2014).

### Ischemic Optic Neuropathy

Arteritic anterior ischemic optic neuropathy (AAION) is usually related to GCA, also referred to as *temporal* or *cranial arteritis*. Its incidence increases with age, with most patients being older than 70 years.

GCA typically affects the extracranial medium- to large-caliber arteries because they possess elastic lamina, which is the initial site of inflammation in this disorder (Salvarani et al., 2012). The condition is associated with polymyalgia rheumatica, consisting of proximal muscle ache, arthralgia, and stiffness, as well as with jaw claudication, fever, malaise, and scalp tenderness. The diagnosis is suggested by an elevated erythrocyte sedimentation rate and C-reactive protein and is confirmed by evidence of giant cells and endovascular inflammation on temporal artery biopsy. Vision loss is the presenting symptom in up to 60% of cases and is generally more severe than in NAION. In approximately 25% of cases, vision is limited to hand motion perception or worse. In suspected cases, treatment with corticosteroids should not be delayed. IV corticosteroids may help delay the progression of visual loss and decrease the likelihood of fellow eye involvement. The prognosis for recovery in the affected eye, however, is poor despite treatment.

The optic disc in AAION typically has a chalky-white edematous appearance, and disc hemorrhages are likely to be present (Fig. 16.21). Coexisting retinal ischemia with cotton-wool spots is very suggestive of AAION. Fluorescein angiography reveals choroidal hypoperfusion (Fig. 16.22). Occasionally, the ischemic insult is to the retrobulbar portion of the optic nerve and causes visual loss without disc edema; this condition is termed *arteritic posterior ischemic optic neuropathy*.

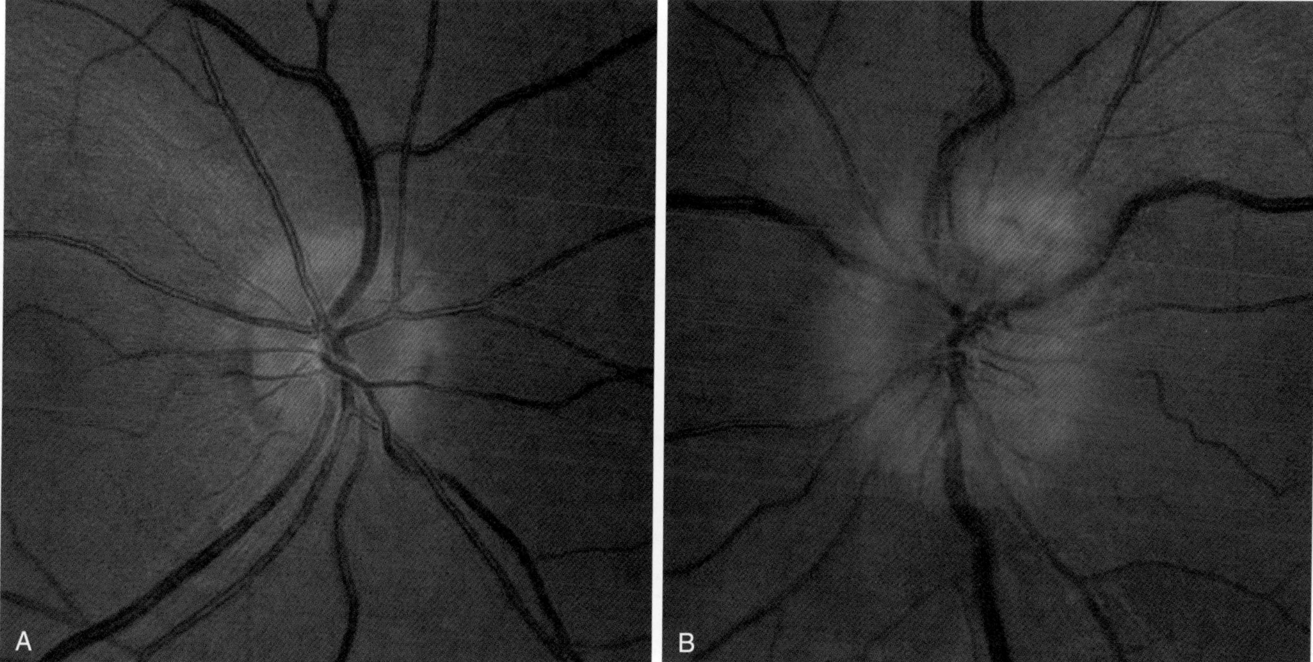


**Fig. 16.23** Fundus photographs in a patient with acute nonarteritic ischemic optic neuropathy in the left eye, demonstrating disc edema in the left eye with a small cup-to-disc ratio in the right eye, suggesting a "disc at risk."

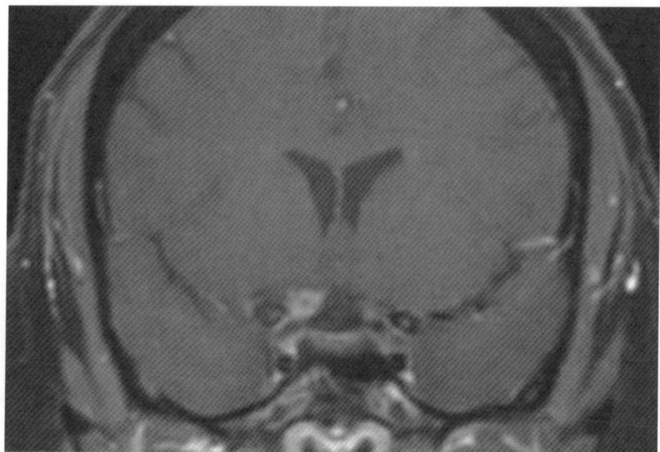

**Fig. 16.24** Coronal T1-weighted postgadolinium magnetic resonance imaging in a patient with right optic neuropathy from neurosarcoidosis. Note enlargement and enhancement of the right optic nerve.

NAION is the most common cause of unilateral optic nerve edema in adults older than 50 years and is commonly associated with vascular risk factors such as diabetes or hypertension (Fontal et al., 2007). Other risk factors include a congenitally crowded optic nerve head, obstructive sleep apnea, and nocturnal hypotension, possibly precipitated by antihypertensive therapy (Arnold, 2003). Swelling of a crowded optic nerve within the scleral canal may produce a compartment syndrome, provoking further vascular compression, ischemia, and swelling.

Although the clinical profile of NAION may occasionally overlap with the findings of optic neuritis (Rizzo and Lessell, 1991), typical features of NAION include nerve fiber hemorrhages, altitudinal visual field defects, moderate to severe disc edema, and the absence of pain (Fig. 16.23). Because the optic nerve head is supplied by an end-arterial system of short posterior ciliary arteries and the circle of Zinn-Haller, sectoral disc edema is common. NAION may follow ocular surgery because associated increases in intraocular pressure may compromise optic nerve head perfusion (Fontal et al., 2007).

Many patients with NAION will have a stable deficit, although a minority may experience stepwise visual loss progressing over 1 month. Spontaneous improvement may occur in the first 6 months, although in many patients, this reflects improved ability with eccentric fixation (Hayreh and Zimmerman, 2008). In 15%–20% of patients, subsequent involvement of the fellow eye occurs, and this rate is increased by the presence of vascular risk factors and younger age, especially if there are crowding optic disc anomalies such as optic disc drusen and congenitally small optic discs. When the second eye is affected in NAION, optic atrophy has already developed in the first eye, and acute disc edema is present in the fellow eye; this clinical presentation is called the *pseudo-Foster Kennedy syndrome.* (A true Foster Kennedy syndrome is characterized by optic atrophy due to compression, typically from an expanding tumor, and papilledema in the fellow eye secondary to increased ICP.) Occasionally, premonitory disc swelling in an asymptomatic eye will be noted, which may progress to frank visual loss or remit spontaneously (Hayreh and Zimmerman, 2007). Recurrence of NAION in an affected eye, however, is rare, possibly because optic nerve atrophy following the initial event decompresses the nerve. There does not appear to be a significantly higher rate of stroke in patients with NAION, suggesting that its pathophysiology may differ from atherosclerotic disease (Arnold and Levin, 2002).

### Other Causes

Inflammatory conditions can also cause a subacute optic neuropathy. Optic discs may appear edematous or normal, the latter indicating retrobulbar involvement. Optic nerve involvement is common in neurosarcoidosis, which can be accompanied by anterior uveitis or posterior segment vitritis (Prasad et al., 2008; Fig. 16.24). Visual loss in this condition is often steroid responsive. Optic neuropathy and retinal involvement may also occur with other inflammatory conditions, such as systemic lupus erythematosus and Sjögren disease. Occasionally, optic nerve infiltration produces optic disc edema without affecting

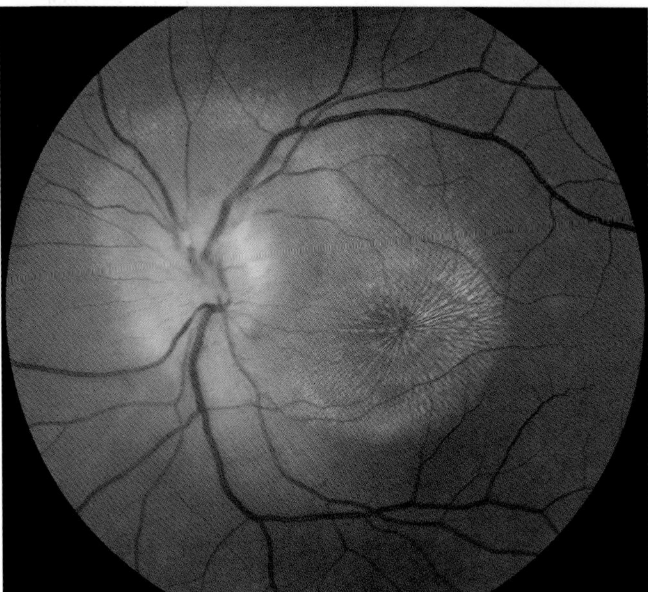

**Fig. 16.25 Ophthalmoscopic Appearance of *Bartonella* Neuroretinitis.** Fundus photograph of the patient's left eye taken 2 weeks after onset of visual loss shows optic disc edema and a macular star.

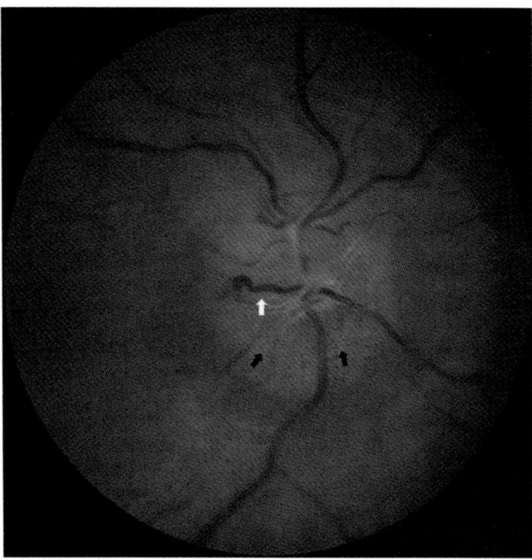

**Fig. 16.26** Fundus photograph of the right eye in a patient with chronic disc edema. Note the indistinct disc margins *(black arrows)* and an optociliary collateral vessel *(white arrow)*. *(Reprinted with permission from Prasad S., Volpe, N.J., Balcer, L.J., 2010. Approach to optic neuropathies: clinical update. Neurologist 16, 23–34.)*

visual function, but more often, there is a decrease in visual acuity and visual field loss. In some cases, inflammation of the optic nerve is not just steroid-responsive but steroid-dependent, indicating that long-term immunomodulatory treatment is necessary to prevent relapsing symptoms; this clinical entity has been called chronic relapsing inflammatory optic neuropathy (Petzold and Plant, 2014). A proportion of patients with this entity have NMO-IgG or MOG-IgG serum antibodies (Petzold et al., 2019).

Infectious conditions are another frequent cause of optic neuropathy (March and Lessell, 1996). Neuroretinitis, in which optic neuropathy coexists with characteristic peripapillary or macular exudates, should be distinguished from acute demyelinating optic neuritis (Fig. 16.25). The initial clinical presentation of these conditions may be similar, but the characteristic macular star of neuroretinitis will appear within 1–2 weeks, establishing the diagnosis. The distinction is critical because neuroretinitis has no association with an increased risk of MS and may be due to cat scratch disease (*Bartonella henselae*), syphilis (*Treponema pallidum*), Lyme disease (*Borrelia burgdorferi*), or sarcoidosis. In most cases, *Bartonella* infection is self-limited and does not require treatment, but in severe cases, doxycycline or azithromycin may be effective. Other infectious causes of optic neuropathy include human immunodeficiency virus (HIV) and opportunistic infections including toxoplasmosis, cytomegalovirus, and cryptococcosis.

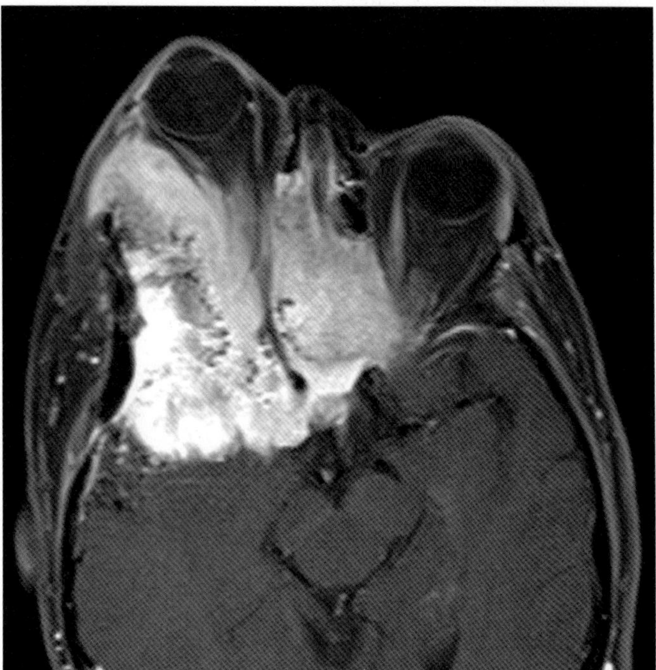

**Fig. 16.27** Axial T1-weighted postcontrast magnetic resonance imaging in a patient with a large sphenoid wing meningioma causing right optic nerve compression, cranial nerve palsies, and proptosis.

Paranasal sinus disease can cause a condition that mimics optic neuritis, with acute optic neuropathy and pain on eye movements, or can cause a progressive optic neuropathy resulting from compression (Rothstein et al., 1984). Optic neuropathy due to sinusitis and mucocele should be considered in patients who have clinical evidence of optic neuritis with seemingly atypical features, particularly in elderly patients with severe sinus disease, a history of fevers, ophthalmoplegia, or progression of vision loss beyond 2 weeks. Presentations after dental infection also occur.

Several compressive mass lesions cause a progressive optic neuropathy. The optic disc is edematous in cases of intraorbital compression, but in cases of retro-orbital compression, disc edema typically only occurs if ICP is elevated. Chronic disc edema due to compressive lesions may be accompanied by optociliary collateral vessels and glistening white bodies on the disc surface (pseudodrusen from extruded axoplasm; Fig. 16.26). Important causes of compressive optic neuropathy include neoplasm (including optic nerve sheath or skull base meningioma, pituitary adenoma, craniopharyngioma, dermoid and epidermoid tumors, and metastases), sinus lesions, bony processes (such as fibrous dysplasia), enlarged extraocular muscles (such as in thyroid eye disease), or aneurysms (Fig. 16.27). Meningiomas of the optic nerve sheath occur primarily in women and can cause visual loss associated with either disc swelling or atrophy.

Primary optic nerve neoplasms include benign juvenile pilocytic glioma in children and (rarely) malignant glioblastoma in adults

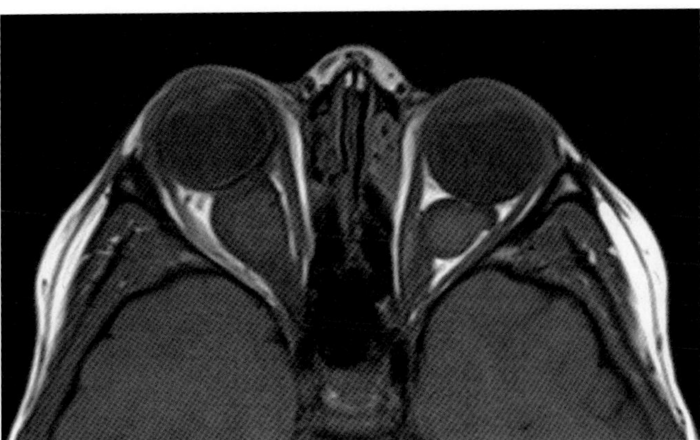

**Fig. 16.28** Axial T1-weighted magnetic resonance imaging in a patient with bilateral optic nerve gliomas (juvenile pilocytic astrocytomas). The patient had stigmata of type 1 neurofibromatosis.

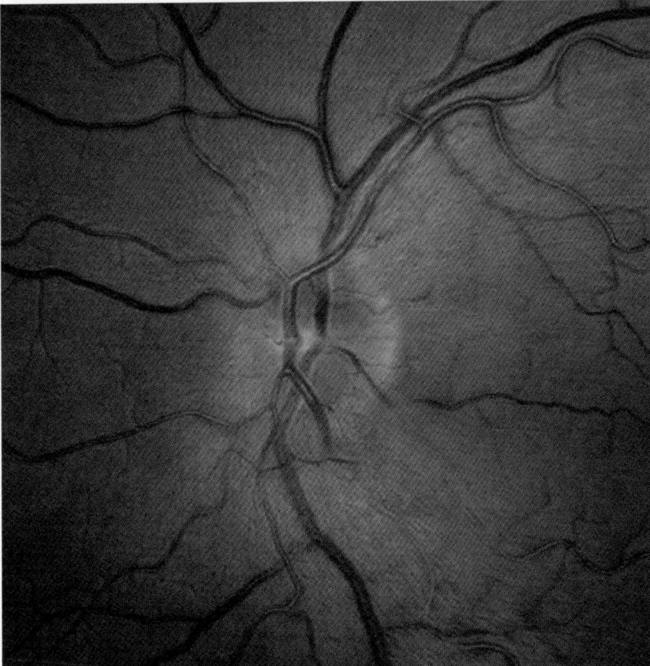

**Fig. 16.29** Fundus photograph of the left eye in a patient with Leber hereditary optic neuropathy. Note hyperemia with appearance of slight disc edema and peripapillary telangiectatic vessels.

(Fig. 16.28). Juvenile pilocytic astrocytoma is often associated with neurofibromatosis type 1 and may be managed conservatively with frequent ophthalmological examination through adolescence (Avery et al., 2011; Listernick et al., 2007). When clinical or radiographic progression is detected, chemotherapy should be first-line therapy, followed by radiation and, rarely, surgery. Malignant optic nerve glioblastoma is much rarer, affects adults, and has a poor prognosis (Spoor et al., 1980). Other neoplastic conditions include lymphoma, leukemia, carcinomatous meningitis, and optic nerve metastasis. Almost any form of carcinoma can metastasize to the optic nerve; breast and lung carcinomas are the most common.

Optic neuropathy may occur as a delayed effect of radiation therapy. It can occur with or without disc edema and can sometimes be difficult to distinguish from tumor recurrence (Danesh-Meyer, 2008). Radiation optic neuropathy is suggested by exposure (typically at least 50-Gy dosage), characteristic 6- to 24-month time lag to symptoms, and accompanying radiation changes in proximal tissues. Progression occurs over weeks to months,

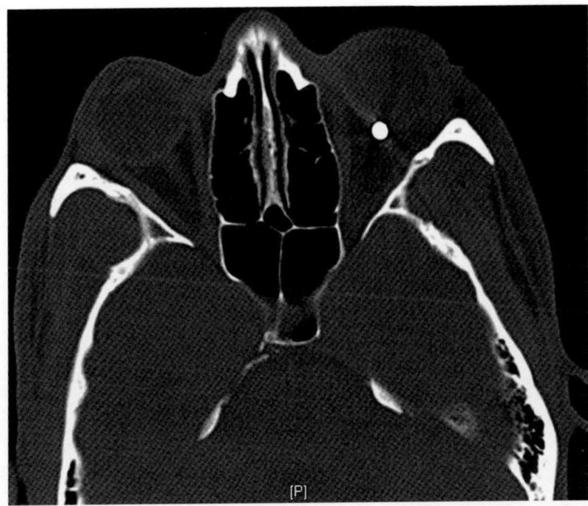



**Fig. 16.30** Axial computed tomography scan *(bone windows)* from a patient with direct left traumatic optic neuropathy due to avulsion by a BB pellet. *(Reprinted with permission from Prasad S., Volpe, N.J., Balcer, L.J., 2010. Approach to optic neuropathies: clinical update. Neurologist 16, 23–34.)*

and spontaneous recovery is rare. Several treatments, including corticosteroids, hyperbaric oxygen, and vascular endothelial growth factor inhibitors, have been reported in occasional cases to halt progression of visual loss.

Visual loss in a patient with known or suspected cancer raises the possibility of a paraneoplastic optic neuropathy or retinopathy (Damek, 2005). In paraneoplastic optic neuropathy, evidence of other neurological dysfunction is common, and the antibody most commonly identified is directed toward collapsin response mediator protein 5 (CRMP5). Paraneoplastic retinopathies, on the other hand, include CAR (with antibodies to recoverin protein) and melanoma-associated retinopathy (with antibodies to rod ganglion cells).

LHON is a subacute, sequential, maternally inherited optic nerve disorder in which 80%–90% of affected persons are males in the second or third decade of life (Newman, 2005; Yu-Wai-Man et al., 2009). The optic disc may appear hyperemic and mildly edematous in the acute phase, although fluorescein angiography does not demonstrate capillary leakage because true disc edema is not present. Circumpapillary telangiectatic vessels, present in the peripapillary nerve fiber layer, are an important clue to the diagnosis (Fig. 16.29). These early funduscopic changes may be noted in presymptomatic eyes. As the condition progresses, the discs become atrophic. Because fibers mediating the pupillary light reflex may be selectively spared, the light reflex may be preserved despite significant visual loss. Genetic diagnosis of LHON is based on the identification of mitochondrial DNA mutations (see Chapter 93). Most patients have permanent visual loss, although a minority will experience some recovery. The prognosis depends on the mutation harbored; patients with mtDNA mutation 14484 are more likely to have spontaneous recovery than patients with mutations 11778 or 3460 (Newman, 2005). At present, no effective treatment for this condition is available, although idebenone has been studied and might promote some improvement of vision (Chinnery and Griffiths, 2005; Klopstock et al., 2011).

Direct TON may include nerve avulsion or transection and is easily recognized by the history of injury (Sarkies, 2004; Fig. 16.30). Fundus examination may reveal extensive intraocular hemorrhages. On the other hand, posterior indirect TON will present with visual loss in the absence of fundus abnormalities; it may result from shearing forces and subsequent edema within the optic canal. Up to half of these patients may improve spontaneously (Sarkies, 2004). Treatments, including corticosteroids and surgical decompression, remain controversial and mostly ineffective (Yu-Wai-Man and Griffiths, 2005, 2013).

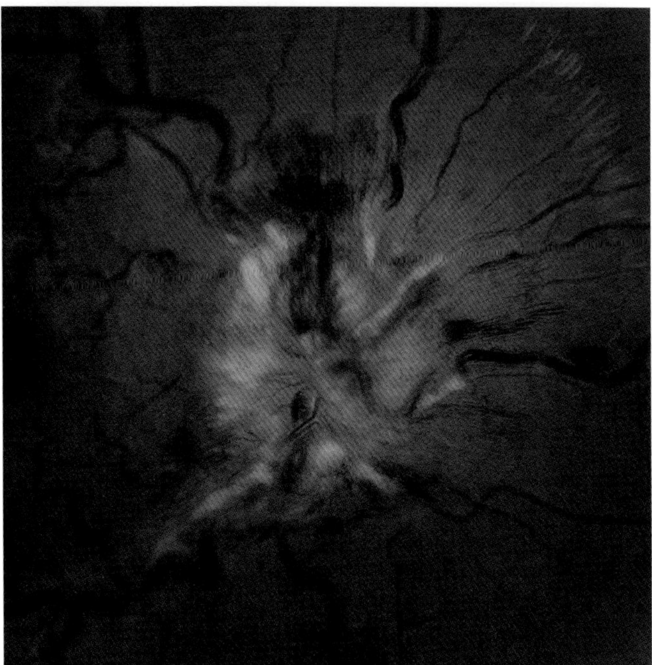

**Fig. 16.31** Fundus photograph of the right eye in a patient with acute papilledema. Note that swelling of the peripapillary nerve fiber layer causes an obscured view of underlying retinal vessels. Splinter hemorrhages and cotton-wool spots, which suggest true papilledema rather than pseudopapilledema, are seen.

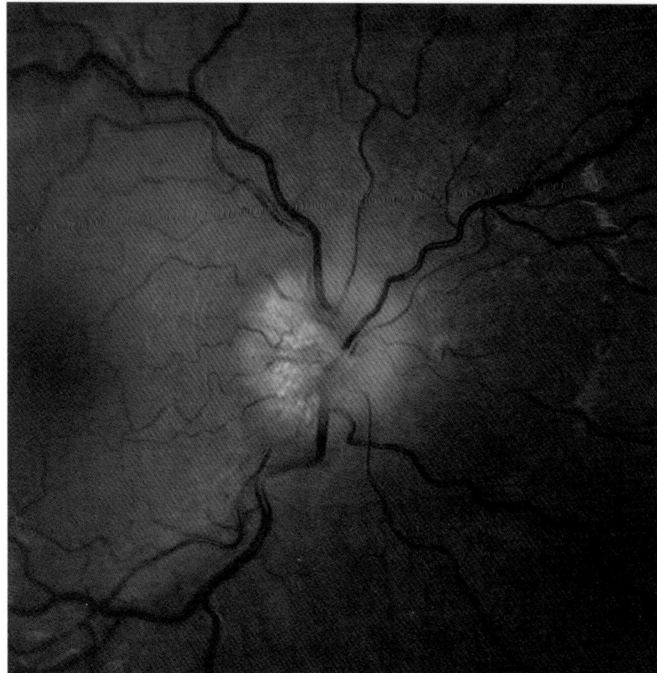

**Fig. 16.32** Fundus photograph of the right eye in a patient with chronic papilledema. Note pale, gliotic disc appearance with pseudodrusen overlying the temporal disc.

## Bilateral Optic Disc Edema

### Papilledema

The term *papilledema* refers specifically to optic disc edema secondary to increased ICP. Disc edema in papilledema results from blockage of axoplasmic flow in nerve fibers, increasing the volume of axoplasm in the optic disc (Hayreh, 1977). On the basis of the chronicity and fundus appearance, papilledema can be divided into four stages: early, fully developed (acute), chronic, and atrophic. The acute phase of papilledema is often suggested by a mismatch between optic disc edema and relatively spared optic nerve function, particularly central visual acuity. The most common visual field defects encountered in patients with early or acute papilledema are enlargement of the physiological blind spot, arcuate visual field defects (typically inferonasal), and concentric constriction. When acute papilledema is accompanied by decreased acuity (and often metamorphopsia), fluid typically extends from the peripapillary region to the macula itself (Chen et al., 2015).

In early papilledema, edema is most prominent at the superior and inferior poles of the optic disc where the nerve fiber layer is thickest. With further development of papilledema, edema encompasses the disc surface more uniformly, and the degree of disc elevation increases (Fig. 16.31). The retinal veins may distend slightly, and the disc may appear mildly hyperemic. These vascular changes result from nerve fiber edema causing compression of capillaries and venules, leading to venous stasis and dilation, formation of microaneurysms, and finally flame-shaped disc and peripapillary hemorrhages (see Fig. 16.31). Concentric retinal folds may be seen in the peripapillary region, and radial retinal folds may be seen extending into the macula (Sibony et al., 2015). Retinal cotton-wool spots may occur secondary to infarction of the nerve fiber layer that is normally transparent. Spontaneous venous pulsations (SVPs) usually are absent with increased ICP. Although papilledema typically is bilateral, it can be asymmetrical because of differences in the pressure transmitted to the retrolaminar portion of the optic nerve related to anatomical variation in the subarachnoid septations of the optic nerves (Killer et al., 2003).

Fluorescein angiography in the setting of acute papilledema may reveal absent fluorescence during the retinal arterial phase as a result of delayed circulation caused by disc swelling. Dilated capillaries and microaneurysms may appear in the arteriovenous phase. Fluorescein may leak from dilated capillaries in the venous phase.

The disc appearance changes as papilledema becomes chronic, usually after weeks to months. The nerve fiber layer may appear pale and take on a gliotic appearance as a result of optic atrophy and astrocytic proliferation (Fig. 16.32). Hemorrhages are less prominent (and often have resolved completely). The disc takes on a "champagne cork" appearance in which small, glistening white bodies (pseudodrusen) are present owing to extruded axoplasm after prolonged stasis (see Fig. 16.32). Collateral vessels due to dilation of preexisting communications between the retinal and ciliary circulation may appear.

If increased ICP and papilledema persist, optic nerve axons become damaged, and visual field loss develops; optic disc edema lessens, and pallor develops (atrophic papilledema). Finally, patients with end-stage papilledema exhibit optic nerve atrophy (disc pallor) without evidence of swelling. Chronic atrophic papilledema, unlike the acute phase, is often characterized by loss of visual acuity with severely constricted visual fields.

Papilledema can be the consequence of numerous disease processes that increase ICP. An expanding mass lesion such as a brain tumor, cerebral edema due to stroke, or intracranial hemorrhage will increase ICP, particularly in a younger patient without age-related brain atrophy. Compression of the ventricular system in the posterior fossa is particularly likely to cause papilledema. Venous sinus thrombosis is another common cause, especially in pregnancy and other states of hypercoagulability. Cryptococcal meningitis is the infectious disorder most commonly associated with significant papilledema.

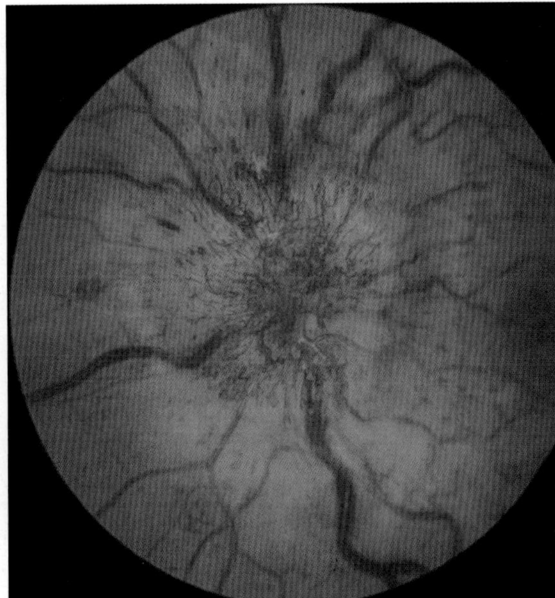

Fig. 16.33 Diabetic papillopathy (incipient nonarteritic anterior ischemic optic neuropathy) in a patient with type 1 diabetes. Note the telangiectatic vessels on the disc surface.

Idiopathic intracranial hypertension (which is also known as pseudotumor cerebri or benign intracranial hypertension) can lead to disc edema and progressive visual loss. The condition is most common in obese women, but modest weight gain (by 5%–15%) even in nonobese women is a risk factor for the disease. Additional risk factors are the use of tetracycline antibiotics or vitamin A derivatives, and if these agents are being taken, they should be discontinued. Weight loss should be imperative in the management of idiopathic intracranial hypertension. In patients with mild visual loss, treatment with acetazolamide can improve symptoms and reduce optic disc swelling (Wall et al., 2014). In patients with more severe visual loss or a fulminant presentation, surgical interventions, such as optic nerve sheath fenestration, cerebrospinal fluid (CSF) shunting, or transverse venous sinus stenting, may be indicated to reduce the possibility of permanent visual loss.

### Malignant Hypertension

A marked elevation in blood pressure may produce bilateral optic disc edema indistinguishable from papilledema (Hayreh, 1977). Peripapillary cotton-wool spots and retinal hemorrhages are other prominent features in patients with malignant hypertension. Encephalopathy and vision loss owing to PRES are common but not always present. The changes associated with malignant hypertension can occur at lower blood pressures in patients with renal failure.

### Diabetic Papillopathy

Diabetic papillopathy is a rare cause of bilateral (or sometimes unilateral) disc edema in patients with diabetes (Barbera et al., 1996). This entity is distinct from typical NAION in that there is often bilateral, simultaneous optic nerve involvement. Visual loss is typically minimal, with the exception of an enlarged physiological blind spot. Disc edema may be accompanied by marked capillary telangiectasias overlying the disc surface (Fig. 16.33). Neuroimaging and lumbar puncture may be necessary to distinguish this condition from papilledema. The pathogenesis is unclear but may relate to a mild impairment of blood flow causing disc edema without infarction of the optic nerve head, as in the case of premonitory NAION; consequently, this condition has also been called *incipient NAION* (Hayreh and Zimmerman, 2008). In many cases, the optic disc edema resolves without residual visual deficit.

**TABLE 16.2 Differentiation of Early Papilledema and Pseudopapilledema**

| Feature | Papilledema | Pseudopapilledema |
|---|---|---|
| Disc color | Hyperemic | Pink, yellowish pink |
| Disc margins | Indistinct early at superior and inferior poles, later entire margin | Usually distinct, may be lumpy |
| Vessels | Normal distribution, slight fullness; spontaneous venous pulsations absent | Emanate from center, frequent anomalous pattern, ± spontaneous venous pulsations |
| Nerve fiber layer | Dull as a result of edema, which may obscure blood vessels | No edema; may glisten with peripapillary halo of feathery light reflections |
| Hemorrhages | Splinter | Subretinal, retinal, vitreous |

*Reprinted with permission from Beck, R.W., Smith, C.H., 1988. Neuro-Ophthalmology: A Problem-Oriented Approach. Little, Brown, Boston.*

### Other Causes

LHON, as discussed earlier, frequently presents with simultaneous bilateral visual loss and the appearance of mild disc edema. Anemia, hyperviscosity states, pickwickian syndrome, hypotension, and severe blood loss are other uncommon causes of bilateral optic disc edema. The clinical setting generally provides clues to the diagnosis. In addition, any of the entities described under unilateral optic disc edema, particularly the infiltrative disorders, rarely can cause bilateral disc edema. In children, optic neuritis commonly is bilateral and is often associated with bilateral disc edema. Bilateral simultaneous ischemic optic neuropathies should prompt immediate evaluation for GCA in patients older than 55 years. Although most toxic optic neuropathies manifest with normal-appearing optic discs, disc edema is seen acutely with methanol poisoning.

## Pseudopapilledema

In patients with pseudopapilledema, visible optic disc drusen (hyaline bodies) may be present. Even when drusen are not visible (i.e., *buried*), the distinction between true disc edema and pseudopapilledema can frequently be made on the basis of examination findings (Table 16.2). The most important distinguishing feature is the clarity of the peripapillary nerve fiber layer. In patients with true disc edema, the nerve fiber layer is hazy, obscuring the underlying retinal vessels, while in pseudopapilledema, this layer can remain distinct. In addition, the presence of SVPs supports the diagnosis of pseudopapilledema, although SVP can be absent in pseudopapilledema as well. Although subretinal hemorrhages may be present in patients with pseudopapilledema (particularly in the setting of optic disc drusen), flame-shaped hemorrhages are characteristic of true papilledema. When drusen are buried, the clinical distinction between papilledema and pseudopapilledema can be challenging, and ocular ultrasonography can help demonstrate hyperechoic signals consistent with drusen.

### Optic Disc Drusen

*Optic disc drusen* constitute a common cause of pseudopapilledema. Although their etiology is unclear, drusen may result from altered axoplasmic flow, particularly in the setting of a small optic canal (Lam et al., 2008). In children, disc drusen tend to be buried, whereas in adults, they are often visible (i.e., *exposed*) on the disc surface (Figs. 16.34 and 16.35). The progression from buried to exposed drusen in individual patients has been well documented. Buried drusen can be diagnosed by identifying calcified deposits in the optic nerve head on ophthalmic ultrasound and by characteristic OCT findings. They can also be seen on computed tomography if they are large enough (see Fig. 16.34, B). The prevalence of optic

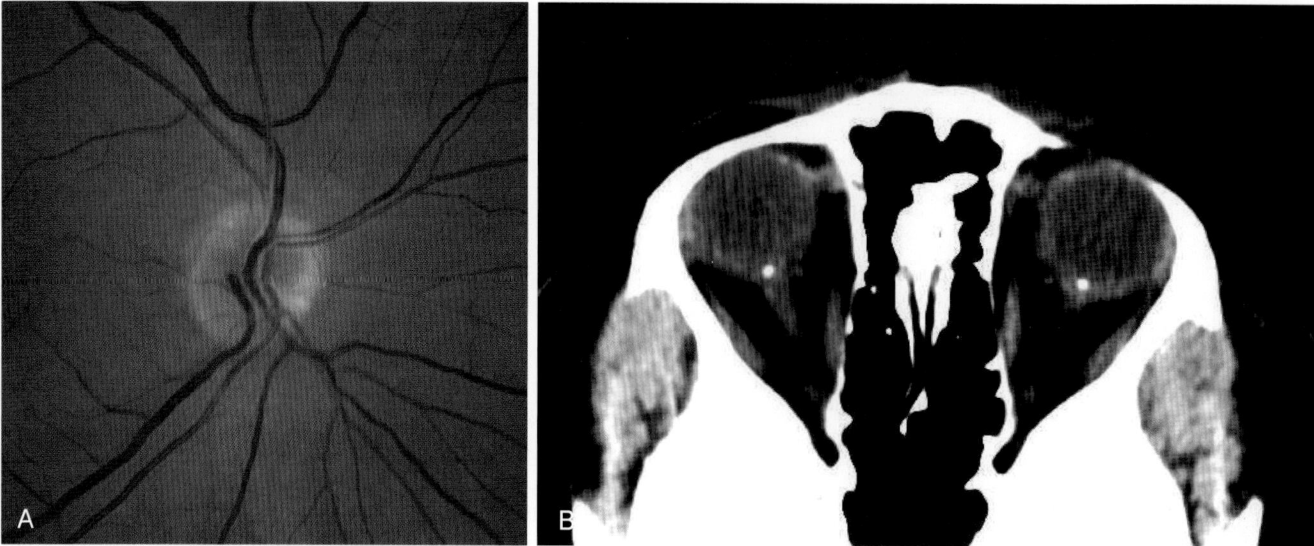


**Fig. 16.34** **A,** Fundus photograph of the right eye in a patient with pseudopapilledema. There is a "lumpy-bumpy" disc appearance and visible disc drusen at the nasal aspect of the disc. Note that retinal vessels are not obscured by nerve fiber layer edema. Spontaneous venous pulsations may also indicate pseudopapilledema. **B,** Axial computed tomography scan from the same patient shows calcified material at both optic nerve heads consistent with calcified optic disc drusen.

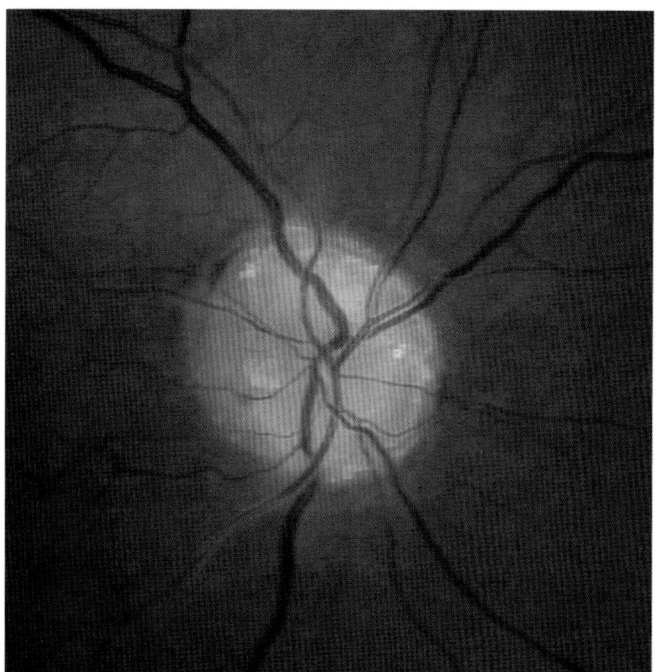

**Fig. 16.35** **Optic Disc Drusen.** Visible excrescences on the disc surface represent optic disc drusen, which are one example of pseudopapilledema.

disc drusen is approximately 2% within the general population, and they can be bilateral in two-thirds of cases. Optic disc drusen are much more common in Caucasian patients than in African Americans and may be inherited in an autosomal dominant pattern with incomplete penetrance.

Patients with optic disc drusen generally do not complain of visual symptoms, although rarely a patient may experience transient visual obscurations similar to those described by patients with true papilledema. Although patients may be unaware of a visual field defect, such deficits are common, occurring in approximately 70% of eyes with exposed disc drusen and in 35% of those with buried drusen (Lam et al., 2008). These deficits can slowly progress and probably result from nerve fiber layer thinning and axonal dysfunction caused by the drusen. The visual field defects, therefore, generally follow a nerve fiber bundle distribution, most commonly affecting the inferior nasal visual field. Enlargement of the blind spot and generalized field constriction may also occur. In addition, visual field loss in the setting of optic disc drusen can occur secondary to superimposed ischemic optic neuropathy or an associated retinal degeneration.

## OPTIC NEUROPATHIES WITH NORMAL-APPEARING OPTIC DISCS

Many optic neuropathies manifest initially with a normal disc appearance; these are classified as retrobulbar optic neuropathies. The disc appearance is normal because the pathological process is posterior to the lamina cribrosa. As with the edematous disc, the differential diagnosis depends on whether optic nerve involvement is unilateral or bilateral.

### Unilateral Presentations

The most common causes of unilateral retrobulbar optic neuropathy are optic neuritis and compressive lesions. The time course of vision loss usually is helpful in distinguishing between these two entities. No definite way exists to differentiate these disorders on examination, but the detection of a superior temporal field defect in the fellow eye (a junctional scotoma) is highly suggestive of a compressive lesion affecting the anterior optic chiasm and the posterior optic nerve, involving the decussating fibers (termed *Wilbrand knee* or *genu*; see Fig. 16.16). Posterior (retrobulbar) ischemic optic neuropathy (PION) may occur in patients with GCA, other vasculitides, or severe blood loss (Chang and Miller, 2005; Hayreh, 2004). It can also occur in the perioperative setting (e.g., during prolonged prone spine surgery or cardiac bypass surgery).

### Bilateral Presentations

Bilateral optic neuropathies in which the optic discs appear normal include nutritional optic neuropathy (including so-called tobacco–alcohol amblyopia), vitamin $B_{12}$ or folate deficiencies, toxic optic neuropathy (from heavy metals), drug-related optic neuropathy (due to ethambutol, amiodarone, linezolid, and others), and

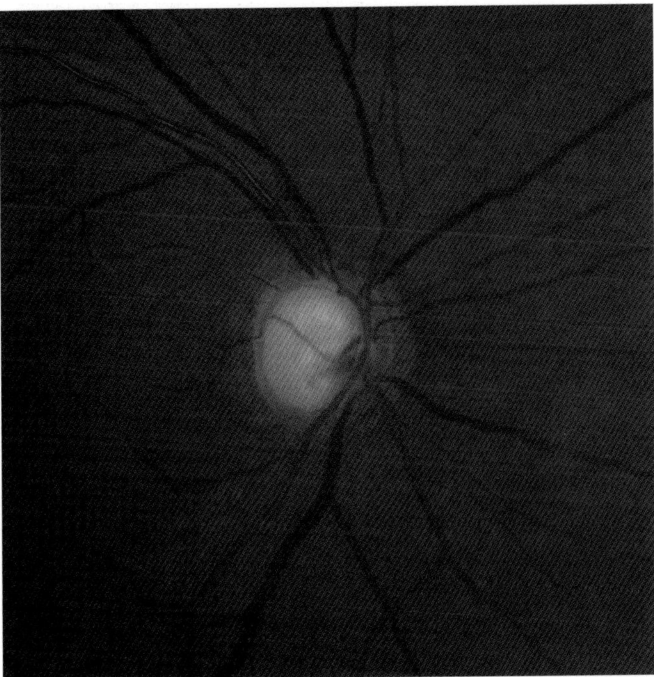

**Fig. 16.36** Fundus photograph of the right eye in a patient with glaucoma. There is severe disc cupping, but the remaining neuroretinal rim is normal in color.

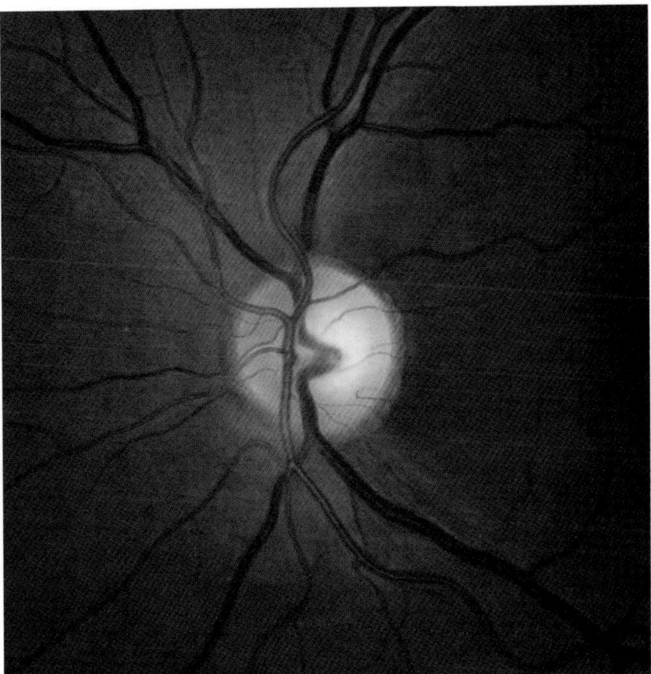

**Fig. 16.37** Fundus photograph of the left eye in a patient with dominant optic atrophy. Note temporal pallor and temporal cupping.

inherited optic neuropathies. When these conditions are chronic, optic atrophy may ensue. Other diagnostic considerations in this category include bilateral compressive lesions and bilateral retrobulbar optic neuritis. Finally, posterior indirect TON can result from shearing forces and subsequent edema within the optic canal.

## OPTIC NEUROPATHIES WITH OPTIC ATROPHY

Any optic neuropathy that produces damage to the optic nerve may result in optic atrophy. Compressive lesions characteristically will cause progressive visual loss and optic atrophy. The presence of gliotic changes over the disc suggests prior disc edema.

Glaucoma is the most common type of optic neuropathy, and it is typically identified by elevated intraocular pressure and disc cupping without disc pallor (Fig. 16.36; Jonas and Budde, 2000). However, angle-closure glaucoma may present with acute painful visual loss, resembling the features of optic neuritis. Distinguishing characteristics include the severity of pain (which can be excruciating), presence of visual halos, and an injected eye with an enlarged, nonreactive pupil. Normal-tension glaucoma is more difficult to recognize but will present with optic disc cupping and progressive field constriction, despite normal intraocular pressures (Anderson et al., 2001). Compressive optic neuropathy can occasionally produce disc cupping and, consequently, mimic glaucoma; the presence of central visual loss and disc pallor helps to distinguish patients with compressive optic neuropathy from those with glaucoma and should prompt neuroimaging.

Dominantly inherited optic atrophy typically presents with insidious visual loss in childhood (Newman, 2005). These patients often have a characteristic disc appearance, with pallor and excavation of the temporal portion of the disc (Fig. 16.37). The disorder is most often due to mutations of the *OPA1* gene, with autosomal inheritance and variable penetrance. The *OPA1* gene product is believed to target the mitochondria and support membrane stability. A mutation of the *OPA1* gene is present in approximately two-thirds of pedigrees with dominant optic atrophy, and, thus, the absence of a mutation does not exclude the diagnosis.

Optic atrophy also occurs as a consequence of disorders of the retina, optic chiasm, and optic tract. Patients with lesions of the optic chiasm or tract can demonstrate bow-tie atrophy, with pallor of the nasal and temporal portions of the disc in the setting of temporal visual field loss. Acquired postgeniculate lesions (i.e., posterior to the LGN) do not produce disc pallor, although congenital lesions may lead to pallor through transsynaptic degeneration.

## CONGENITAL OPTIC DISC ANOMALIES

Congenital optic nerve anomalies (in addition to optic disc drusen, as discussed earlier) include tilted optic discs and optic nerve dysplasia. Visual loss associated with congenital disc anomaly can range from total blindness to minimal dysfunction.

### Tilted Optic Disc

A tilted optic disc usually is easily recognizable on fundus examination. The disc may appear foreshortened on one side, and one portion may appear elevated, with the opposite end depressed (Fig. 16.38). Often, the retinal vessels run in an oblique direction. Tilted optic discs are of neurological importance in that they usually are bilateral and may be associated with temporal field loss, thus mimicking a chiasmal syndrome. However, differentiation from chiasmal disease usually is possible because the visual field defects in patients with tilted discs typically do not respect the vertical meridian (see Fig. 16.10).

### Optic Nerve Dysplasia

Of the several types of optic nerve dysplasia, optic nerve hypoplasia is the most common (Taylor, 2007). In this condition, the optic disc appears small and surrounded by choroid and retinal pigment changes that resemble a double ring (Fig. 16.39). The abnormality may be unilateral or bilateral. In most cases, no specific cause is identifiable. The frequency of optic nerve hypoplasia appears to be increased in children of mothers who had diabetes mellitus or ingested antiepileptic drugs, quinine, or lysergic acid diethylamide (LSD) during pregnancy. De Morsier syndrome (septo-optic dysplasia)

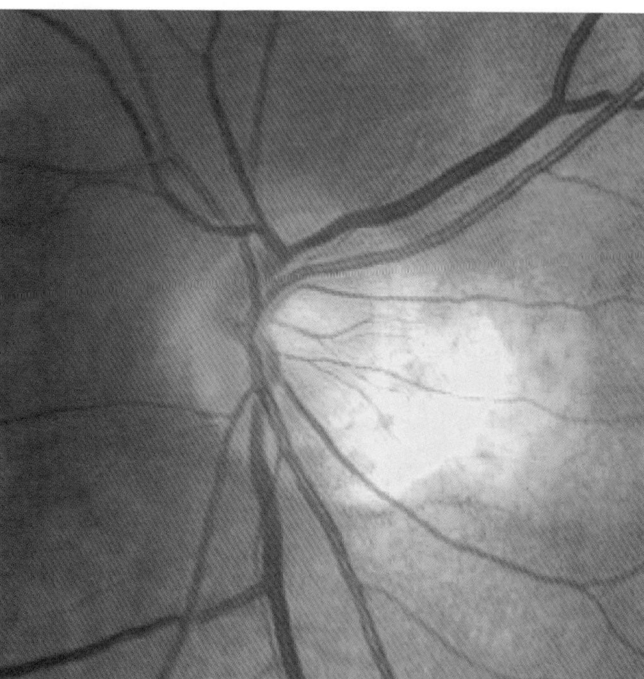

Fig. 16.38 Fundus photograph of the left eye in a patient with a tilted optic disc. The disc in the fellow eye had a similar appearance.

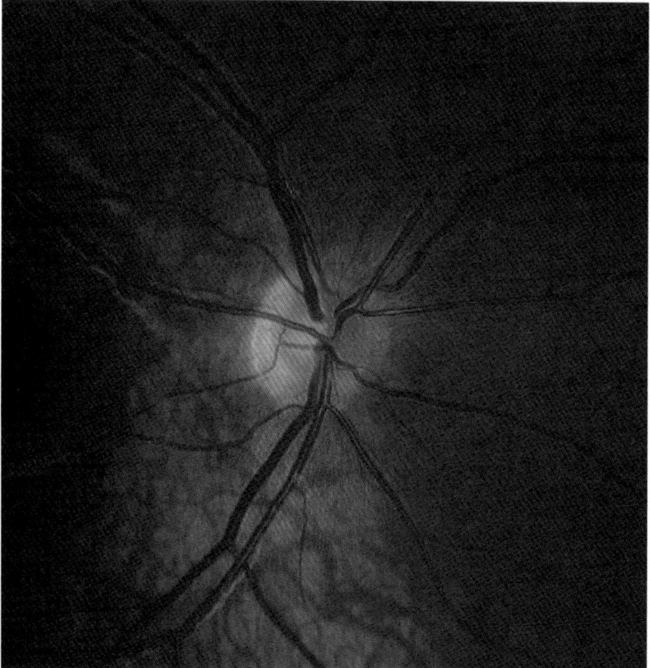

Fig. 16.39 Fundus photograph of the right eye in a patient with optic nerve hypoplasia (ONH). The disc is the inner circle of the two seen on the photograph: hence the term double-ring of ONH. Note the relatively large size of the blood vessels at the surface of the disc.

is characterized by developmental abnormalities of structures sharing an embryological forebrain derivation, including optic nerve hypoplasia, absent septum pellucidum, and pituitary gland dysfunction (Taylor, 2007). Optic nerve aplasia, or complete absence of the optic discs, is extremely rare.

Optic nerve coloboma is more common than optic nerve hypoplasia and results from incomplete closure of the fetal fissure (Fig. 16.40). It may occur as an isolated finding or as part of a congenital syndrome including Aicardi syndrome and trisomy 13. Another type

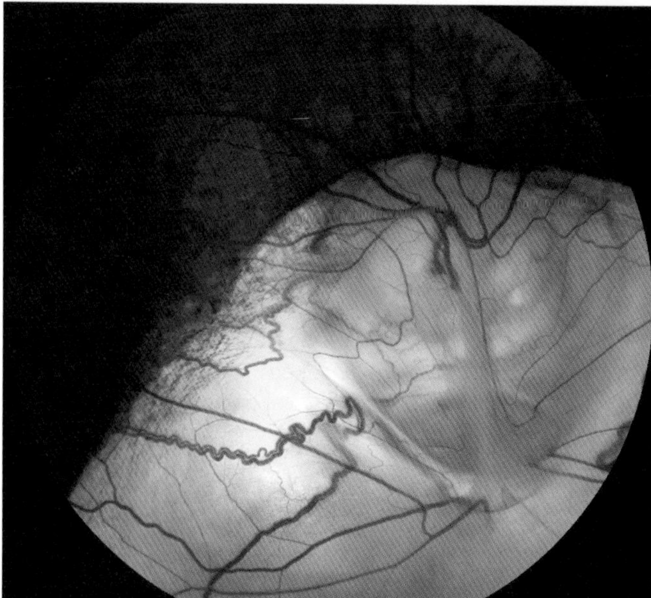

Fig. 16.40 Fundus photograph of the right eye in a patient with inferior optic disc and retinal colobomas.

of congenital anomaly, the optic pit, is manifested as a small grayish area, usually located in the inferior temporal portion of the optic disc. In some optic nerve dysplasias, the disc appears enlarged. This is true of the so-called morning glory disc in which a large whitish concavity is surrounded by pigmentation that resembles a morning glory flower. This appearance occurs because defective closure of the embryonic fissure is followed by growth of glial tissue and vascular remnants.

## RETINAL DISORDERS

### Retinal Arterial Disease

Retinal arterial disease can manifest as a CRAO/BRAO, or TMVL. Carotid artery atherosclerosis is the most common cause, but aortic atherosclerosis and cardiac valvular disease must also be considered. Evaluation and treatment for retinal arterial disease are similar to those for stroke and cerebrovascular disease in general because the annual risk of stroke or death in patients with visible retinal emboli can be increased 10-fold to 8.5% compared with controls. Acute retinal artery occlusion (CRAO/BRAO) is characterized by retinal whitening (edema) secondary to infarction. In CRAO, these findings usually are more prominent in the posterior pole than they are in the periphery (Fig. 16.41). A marked narrowing of the retinal arterioles is often noted. Because the fovea (the center of the macula) receives the majority of its blood supply from the choroid and there are no overlying retinal ganglion cells, this area retains its normal reddish-orange color, producing the characteristic cherry-red spot. The retinal edema usually subsides fairly rapidly over days to weeks. After resolution, the retinal appearance typically returns to normal, although the prognosis for visual recovery generally is poor.

When present, retinal emboli most often are located at arteriolar bifurcations. Visualization of retinal emboli is more common in BRAO than in CRAO. They may be located on or near the optic disc or in the retinal periphery (Fig. 16.42). The three major types of retinal emboli are (1) cholesterol (Hollenhorst plaques, most commonly from the carotid artery), (2) platelet-fibrin (most commonly from the cardiac valves), and (3) calcific (from either an arterial or a cardiac source). It is difficult to distinguish accurately among these on the basis of fundus examination alone. With impaired blood flow after a CRAO, a portion of a retinal arteriole may take on a whitish appearance. This represents not an embolus, but rather stagnant lipid in the blood or changes in the arteriole wall.

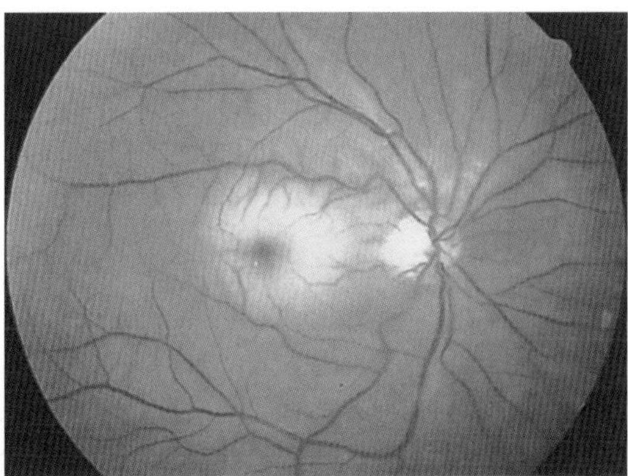

**Fig. 16.41** Fundus photograph of the right eye in a patient with a central retinal artery occlusion. Note the cherry-red spot in the center of the macula, with surrounding whitening of the retina.

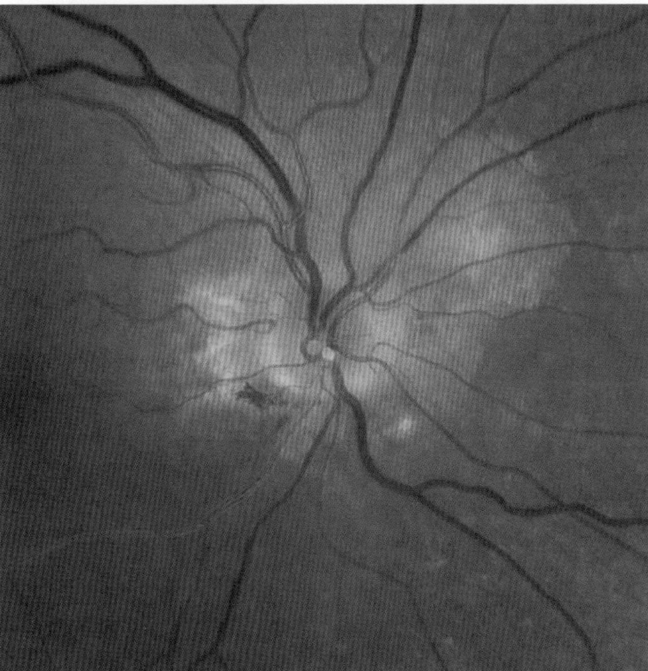

**Fig. 16.42** Fundus photograph of the right eye in a patient with a calcium embolus lodged at the disc. Note the accompanying attenuation of the inferior retinal arteries.

## Branch Retinal Artery Occlusions and Encephalopathy (Susac Syndrome)

Branch retinal artery occlusions and encephalopathy (Susac syndrome) is a rare disorder characterized by multiple branch retinal artery occlusions and neurological dysfunction (Susac et al., 2007). Susac syndrome most commonly affects women between the ages of 20 and 40 years. A viral syndrome may precede the development of ocular and neurological signs. The most prominent neurological manifestations are impaired mentation, sensorineural hearing loss, and visual deficits relating to BRAOs, although the full triad of these symptoms is rarely present initially. CSF in patients with Susac syndrome shows a mild lymphocytic pleocytosis and elevated protein. Antinuclear antibody (ANA) testing and cerebral arteriography are generally normal, but brain MRI most often demonstrates multiple areas of high signal intensity that resemble demyelinating plaques on T2-weighted images and characteristically involve the corpus callosum. Fluorescein angiography can be very helpful to demonstrate characteristic areas of vascular permeability and arteriolar blockage (Fig. 16.43).

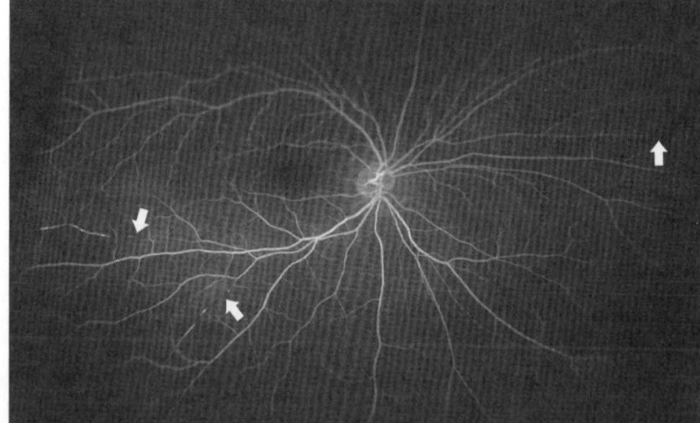

**Fig. 16.43** Fluorescein angiogram of the right eye in a patient with Susac syndrome showing multiple branch retinal arteriolar occlusions *(arrows)*.

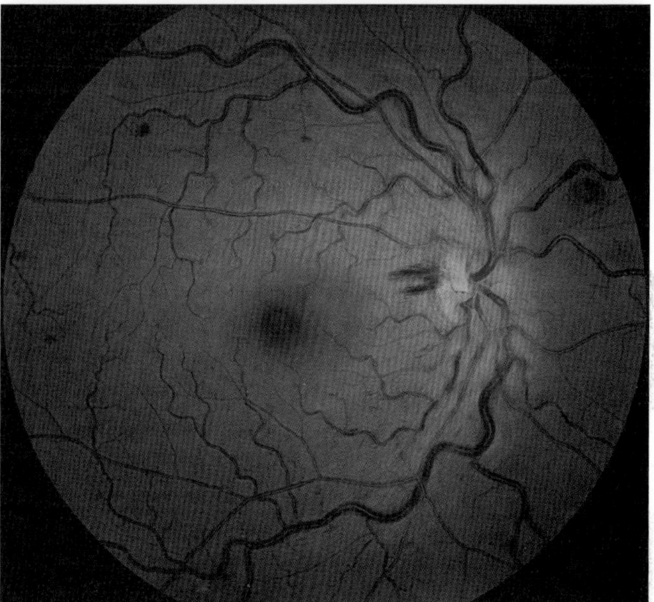

**Fig. 16.44** Fundus photograph of the right eye in a patient with central retinal vein occlusion. Note mild disc edema and hyperemia, engorgement of retinal veins, and scattered intraretinal hemorrhages.

## Ocular Ischemic Syndrome

Generalized ocular ischemia indicates involvement of both retinal and ciliary circulations in the eye. Signs of optic nerve and retinal ischemia may be present, as well as ophthalmoplegia and evidence of anterior segment ischemia (iris atrophy, loss of pupil reactivity, cataract formation, and neovascularization of the iris). Carotid artery occlusion or dissection and GCA are the primary considerations in patients with ocular ischemia (Chen and Miller, 2007).

## Retinal Vein Occlusion

Central or branch retinal vein occlusions rarely occur in patients younger than 50 years. The diagnosis is established clinically by the presence of characteristic retinal hemorrhages in the setting of acute vision loss. These occur diffusely in central retinal vein occlusion and focally in branch retinal vein occlusion (Fig. 16.44). Disc edema is often present and in some cases is the predominant fundus feature. No direct associations between retinal vein occlusion and carotid artery atherosclerotic disease are recognized. Patients require evaluation for vascular risk factors but generally do not require carotid imaging or ultrasound examination. In cases of bilateral retinal vein occlusion, patients should be evaluated for hyperviscosity syndromes or hypercoagulable states.

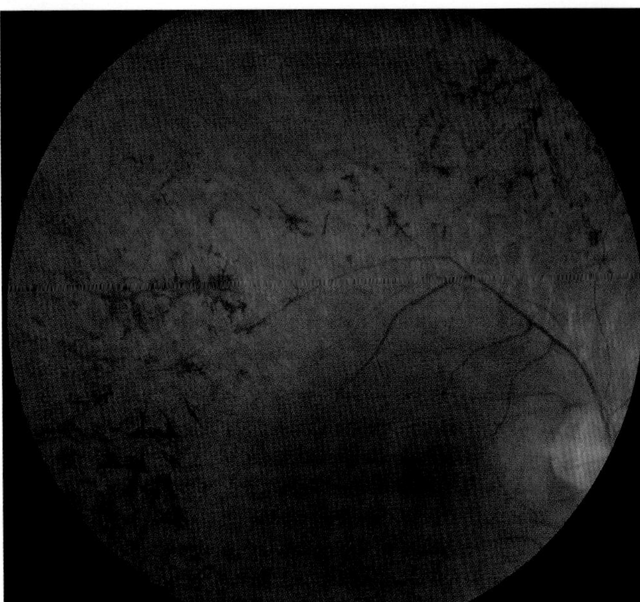

Fig. 16.45 Fundus photograph of the right eye in a patient with retinitis pigmentosa. Note retinal arteriolar attenuation and prominent bony spicule changes in the retinal midperiphery.

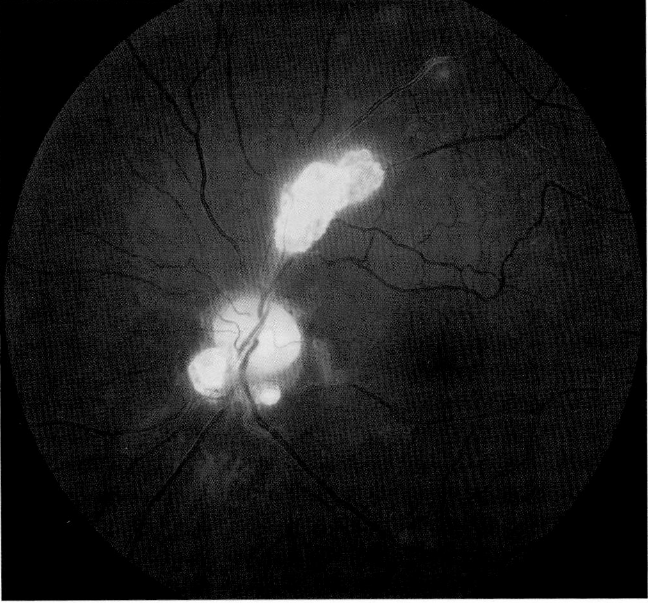

Fig. 16.46 Fundus photograph of the left eye in a patient with multiple astrocytic hamartomas in the setting of tuberous sclerosis. The patient also has optic atrophy secondary to papilledema from obstructive hydrocephalus.

## Retinal Degenerations

Among the many diseases of retinal degeneration, several are associated with neurological disease. The cause of RP is degeneration of the retinal rods and cones. Rods are predominantly affected early in the course of RP, impairing night vision. Visual field loss occurs first in the midperiphery and progresses to severe field constriction. Pigmentary retinal changes that look similar to bony spicules are the hallmark of RP (Fig. 16.45). In some cases, however, pigment changes are not prominent, and the visual field loss may be mistaken for a neurological disorder. Even without the characteristic bony spicule-type changes, the diagnosis of RP can be made on the basis of the retinal thinning, narrowing of retinal arterioles, and waxy optic disc pallor.

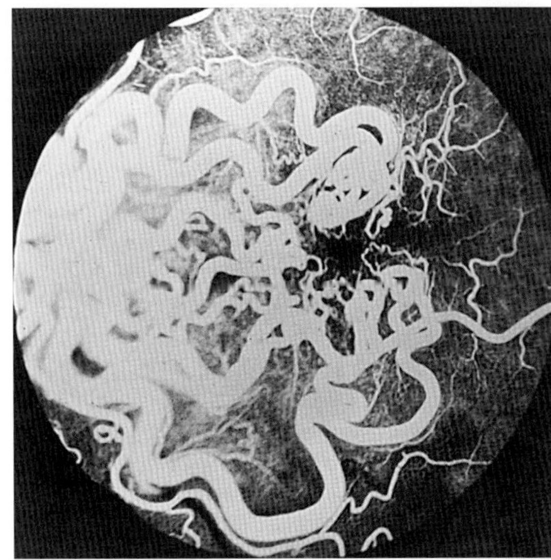

Fig. 16.47 Fluorescein angiogram of a racemose arteriovenous malformation in the retina in a patient with Wyburn-Mason disease.

RP may be associated with Kearns-Sayre syndrome, Cockayne syndrome, Refsum syndrome, and inherited vitamin E deficiency. Retinal degenerations with prominent involvement of the macula, sometimes producing a characteristic "bull's eye" appearance, can occur with Batten disease, spinocerebellar ataxia type 7, and toxic exposures (e.g., chloroquine).

Retinal photoreceptor degenerations can occur as a remote effect of cancer (the paraneoplastic retinopathies). These include CAR, which affects primarily rods and manifests with night blindness; cancer-associated cone dysfunction, which manifests as dyschromatopsia; and melanoma-associated retinopathy, which has a relatively better prognosis. Initial visual acuity in these conditions can range from normal to significantly impaired, typically with a rapid rate of deterioration. Arteriolar narrowing is a consistent finding, and pigmentary changes in the retina are variable. ERG is markedly abnormal. Antiphotoreceptor antibodies often can be identified in the serum, although the specificity of these tests remains imperfect. Treatment of the underlying malignancy rarely improves vision, but immunosuppression with steroids can be effective.

Progressive cone dystrophies are retinal degenerations that commonly demonstrate autosomal dominant inheritance. Typically, vision loss develops in both eyes, beginning in adolescence and worsening over several years. Early in the course, the fundus may appear normal; with time, however, pigmentary changes develop in the macula, and ERG demonstrates characteristic reductions of the photopic response.

## Phakomatoses

Retinal findings are common in phakomatoses that affect the nervous system, particularly tuberous sclerosis and von Hippel-Lindau disease. Neurological features of phakomatoses are described in Chapter 99. In tuberous sclerosis, retinal astrocytic hamartomas are characteristic (Fig. 16.46). These usually are multiple and may appear either as a fullness in the retinal nerve fiber layer or as a nodular refractile lesion resembling a mulberry. Von Hippel-Lindau disease is characterized by the presence of one or more retinal angiomas that appear as reddish masses with a feeding artery and draining vein. Treatment with photocoagulation or cryotherapy may be necessary. Lastly, Wyburn-Mason disease is characterized by racemose arteriovenous malformations in the retina (Fig. 16.47).

*The complete reference list is available online at https://expertconsult.inkling.com/.*

17

# Pupillary and Eyelid Abnormalities

*Matthew J. Thurtell, Janet C. Rucker*

## OUTLINE



## PUPILLARY ABNORMALITIES

### Pupil Anatomy and Neural Control

The size of the pupil is determined by the balance of action between two muscles embedded in the iris: the sphincter pupillae, under parasympathetic control, and the dilator pupillae, under sympathetic control. The sphincter is located circumferentially around the pupil and constricts the pupil. The dilator is situated radially and dilates the pupil. On exposure to light, the pupil constricts as a result of the pupillary light reflex (Fig. 17.1). The afferent limb of the light reflex originates in the retinal ganglion cells and travels via the optic nerve, chiasm, and optic tract to the dorsal midbrain pretectum, just rostral to the superior colliculus, from which neuronal signals are relayed bilaterally to the paired parasympathetic Edinger-Westphal nuclei (Nester et al., 2010; Papageorgiou et al., 2009). In primate studies, the pretectal olivary nucleus is identified as the primary relay between retinal ganglion cells and the Edinger-Westphal nuclei (see Fig. 17.1) (Warwick, 1954). The efferent limb of the light reflex consists of the preganglionic parasympathetic fibers traveling from the Edinger-Westphal nuclei in both oculomotor nerves to the ciliary ganglion and the postsynaptic, postganglionic short ciliary nerves carrying the parasympathetic innervation from the ciliary ganglion to the sphincter muscle (see Chapter 103 for a more extensive discussion of the oculomotor nucleus and nerve anatomy). The pupillary near reflex consists of pupillary constriction as a response to viewing of a near target. Thus miosis is a component of the near triad, along with lens accommodation and eye convergence. The anatomical substrate of the pupillary near reflex is less well defined than that of the light reflex, although a network of neurons including near-response cells has been identified in primates and may play a role in the near triad—especially the vergence and accommodation components (Zhang et al., 1992; Rucker et al., 2019).

The sympathetic innervation destined for the dilator muscle passes along a chain of three neurons: first-, second-, and third-order neurons (Fig. 17.2). First-order neurons originate in the posterolateral hypothalamus and descend in the dorsolateral brainstem and intermediolateral cell column of the spinal cord to the upper thoracic cord (T2). After the first-order neurons synapse in the spinal cord, second-order neurons exit to the paravertebral sympathetic chain via the ventral horns. They pass by the lung apex and then ascend with the common and internal carotid arteries to reach the superior cervical ganglion in the neck, at the angle of the jaw, where they synapse with the third-order neurons. At this point, sudomotor fibers related to facial sweating separate anatomically from those fibers serving pupillary dilation. From the superior cervical ganglion, third-order neurons continue their ascent with the internal carotid artery through the skull base and into the cavernous sinus, where they temporarily join the abducens nerve. They then join branches of the trigeminal nerve, with which they enter the orbit and reach the dilator muscle via the long ciliary nerves (see Fig. 17.2).

### Normal Pupil Phenomena

Hippus, or pupillary unrest, is a nonrhythmical, small-amplitude (<1 mm) variation in pupil size that occurs in normal eyes after light stimulation and is not triggered by accommodation (Hunter et al., 2000; Thompson et al., 1971). After a light stimulus, the pupil constricts, redilates, and then oscillates. The role (if any) of these oscillations in pupillary or visual function is unclear.

Physiological anisocoria (also termed *central*, *simple*, or *benign anisocoria*; unequal pupils) occurs in up to 20% of the population; the difference in pupil size ranges from approximately 0.4 to 1 mm. The amount of anisocoria is usually the same in light compared with darkness, although it is sometimes slightly greater in darkness. It should not be accompanied by abnormalities of the pupillary light or near responses, nor should it be accompanied by ptosis or ophthalmoplegia.

With age, the pupils become smaller and less reactive to light. Such pupils generally do not require diagnostic evaluation. Although not a normal condition, diabetes similarly affects the pupils sufficiently often as to make small and poorly reactive pupils common in that clinical setting in the absence of any other pathological pupil state. Both parasympathetic and sympathetic pupillary dysfunction can occur in diabetes, and pupillary abnormalities are correlated with a number of other disease processes, including the presence of cardiovascular autonomic dysfunction, peripheral neuropathy, and retinopathy (Bremner and Smith, 2006; Bremner, 2009).

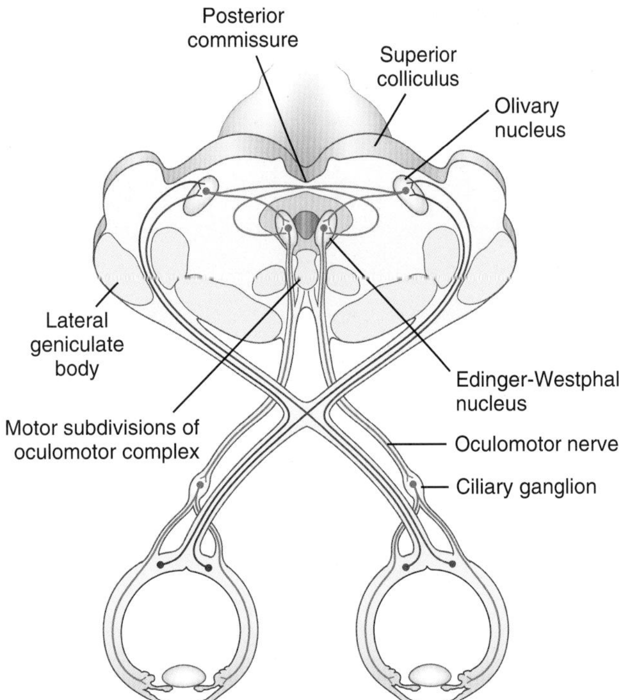


**Fig. 17.1** Schematic diagram of the pupillary light reflex in the macaque monkey, showing the afferent limb via the retina, optic nerve, chiasm, and optic tract; the midbrain connections between the pretectal olivary nuclei and Edinger-Westphal nuclei; and the efferent limb via the oculomotor nerve and ciliary ganglion. For simplicity, a single neuron in the olivary nucleus is shown projecting to both Edinger-Westphal nuclei, and inputs from both olivary nuclei converge on a single neuron in the Edinger-Westphal nucleus. (*Courtesy J.C. Horton; republished with permission from Kourouyan, H.D., Horton, J.C., 1997. Transneuronal retinal input to the primate Edinger–Westphal nucleus. J Comp Neurol 381, 78.*)

## Afferent Pathological Conditions of the Pupils

The relative afferent pupillary defect (RAPD), or Marcus Gunn pupil, is a hallmark of optic nerve disease. However, given that the initial synapse of the pupillary light reflex pathway occurs in the dorsal midbrain pretectal olivary nucleus, a unilateral lesion of the dorsal midbrain may also rarely produce an RAPD in the absence of vision loss (Kawasaki et al., 2010). It is a manifestation of unilateral or asymmetrical bilateral disruption of the afferent limb of the pupillary light reflex and occurs as a result of the consensual and bilateral nature of the light reflex. When a light stimulus is applied to one eye, both pupils constrict due to the bilateral connections between the pretectal olivary and Edinger-Westphal nuclei. When the swinging flashlight test is performed to evaluate for an RAPD, the light will be transmitted normally via an intact optic nerve and to a lesser extent by a diseased optic nerve. This results in the appearance of a brisk bilateral pupillary constriction when the light stimulus is applied to the normal eye and a lesser constriction with initial relative dilation when the light stimulus is transferred to the eye with the optic neuropathy, thus the RAPD. The greater the extent of retinal ganglion cell and optic nerve damage, the larger the relative dilation of the pupil will appear (Lagreze and Kardon, 1998; Tatham et al., 2014). See Chapter 16 for a more detailed description and a table with step-by-step instructions on how to evaluate for an RAPD and for a more extensive discussion of optic nerve disease.

## Efferent Pathological Conditions of the Pupils

### Clinical Presentation and Examination

The medical history of a patient rarely begins with the statement "I noticed that I have unequal pupils." Most patients have anisocoria brought to their attention by a doctor, friend, or relative. Those who notice anisocoria themselves may give a misleading account of the duration of the condition; magnification of old photographs of the patient may prove helpful in clarifying the duration of the anisocoria. Occasionally, a patient has visual symptoms caused solely by an abnormality in pupillary size. Photophobia can occur when a dilated pupil fails to protect the retina from increased illumination. Less often, a complaint of poor night vision (or dim daytime vision) may arise in patients with small, poorly reactive pupils; this occurs as a result of the pupils not dilating normally, thereby decreasing the light-gathering power of the eye under conditions of dim illumination.

The pupil examination of a patient being evaluated for a pupillary abnormality should begin with observation of the resting size of the pupils in ambient room light and of resting eyelid position. If anisocoria is present, the amount of anisocoria in light versus in darkness should be determined. Pupil size can be determined in the dark by having the patient look at a distant target in a dark room while the examiner shines just enough light indirectly from below to allow visualization of the pupils. Assessment in the light versus in darkness will help determine which pupil, if either, is the abnormal pupil. Anisocoria that is more pronounced in the light suggests that the large pupil is the abnormal pupil, because the small pupil will constrict normally to light, enhancing the difference in size between the small pupil and the large, nonconstricting pupil. The differential diagnosis for anisocoria greater in light includes parasympathetic outflow damage (tonic pupil, oculomotor palsy), iris sphincter injury or ischemia, pharmacological pupil dilation, and asymmetrical sympathetic activation. Anisocoria that is more pronounced in the dark suggests that the small pupil is the abnormal pupil, because the large pupil will dilate normally in the dark, enhancing the difference in size between the large pupil and the small, nondilating pupil. A caveat to the suggestion that the small pupil is abnormal in this situation is that physiological anisocoria will often be slightly greater in the dark (Lam et al., 1987). The differential diagnosis for pathological anisocoria greater in the dark includes sympathetic outflow damage (Horner syndrome), iris pathology such as trauma or inflammation, and asymmetrical parasympathetic stimulation (e.g., pharmacological stimulation).

The next step in the examination is evaluation of the direct and consensual pupillary light reflexes, followed by evaluation of the pupillary near response (Kasthurirangan and Glasser, 2006). The near response can be elicited by having the patient shift gaze from a distant target to their thumb, held several inches in front of their eyes. Under certain conditions, the pupils may have light-near dissociation with poor direct responses to light but relatively preserved constriction to near stimuli.

Once the abnormal pupil is identified, pharmacological testing with a number of topical eye drops can be used for confirmation of the diagnosis and assistance with localization (Table 17.1). The general method is application of 1–2 drops of the pharmacological agent into each eye, followed by reexamination of the pupils 30–45 minutes later. Sensitivity of accurate response detection is increased with before-and-after photographic documentation. Diagnostic use of topical pharmacological agents and additional helpful examination findings for each of the specific disorders are described in detail in the sections of this chapter covering these disorders and outlined in a systematic guideline in Fig. 17.3. The presence of mild ptosis on the side of the small pupil may indicate sympathetic dysfunction, whereas ptosis on the side of the large pupil may indicate oculomotor nerve dysfunction. Careful examination of vision, ocular motility, facial strength and sensation, and the ocular fundus should also be performed.

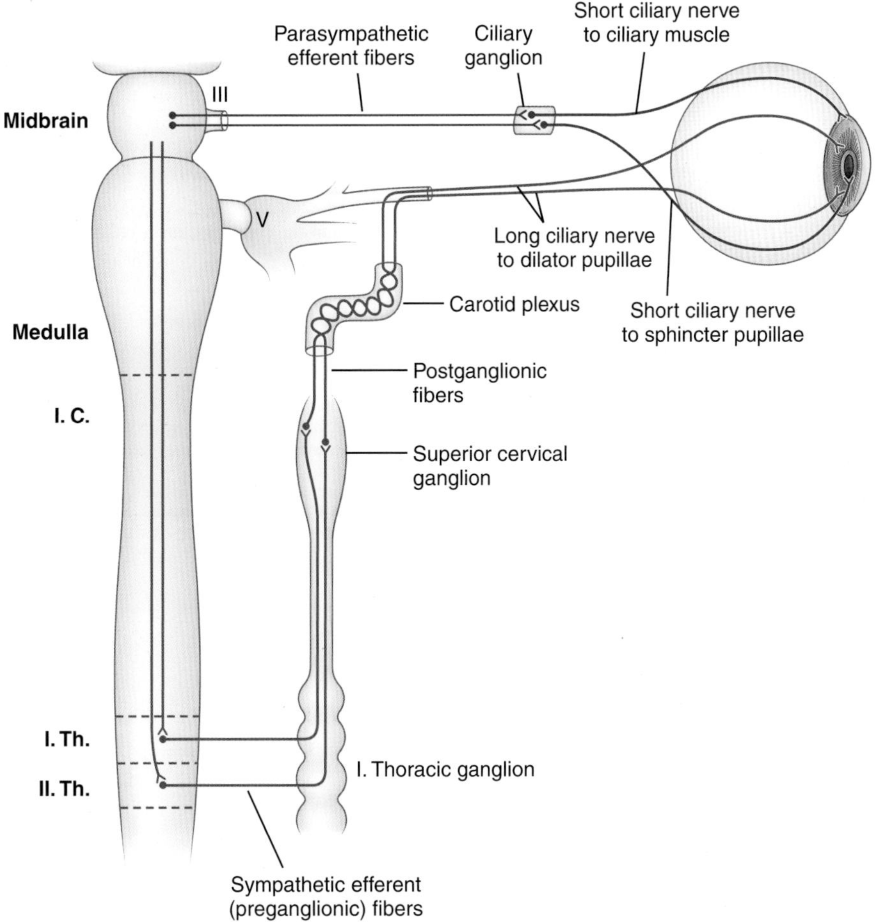


**Fig. 17.2** Parasympathetic and sympathetic pathways for innervation of the sphincter pupillae and dilator pupillae. *I. C.*, First cervical spinal cord segment; *I. Th.*, first thoracic segment; *II. Th.*, second thoracic segment; *III*, oculomotor nerve; *V*, trigeminal nerve. (*Adapted from Gray, H., 1918. Anatomy of the Human Body, plate 840.*)

## Anisocoria Greater in the Light

***Postganglionic parasympathetic dysfunction—tonic pupil.*** A tonic pupil is large and reacts poorly to light and slowly to near stimuli. After distance refixation, it exhibits a slow, tonic redilation (Fig. 17.4), which transiently reverses the anisocoria, making the tonic pupil smaller, because the normal pupil quickly redilates whereas the tonic pupil does not (see Fig. 17.4, D). In the ophthalmology office, evaluation of a tonic pupil at the slit lamp reveals segmental constriction of some portions of the pupil and absent constriction of other portions. Denervation supersensitivity can occur with parasympathetic denervation of the iris sphincter muscle. As a result, instillation of a dilute solution of pilocarpine, the cholinergic agent, can be used to confirm the diagnosis (Fig. 17.5; see Table 17.1). A 0.1% solution is often suggested, but false-positive results may be more frequent than with a more dilute solution (Leavitt et al., 2002). Dilute pilocarpine will constrict the tonic pupil but not a normal pupil or a dilated pupil from pharmacological stimulation. Dilute pilocarpine is not commercially available and must be prepared by dilution with preservative-free normal saline.

Tonic pupils result from damage to the intraorbital ciliary ganglion or short ciliary nerves from a variety of etiologies, including focal infectious (herpes zoster, syphilis) or noninfectious (giant cell arteritis) inflammation (Prasad et al., 2009), malignant infiltration, paraneoplastic processes (Horta et al., 2012), and trauma. Tonic pupils may also be seen as a component of a systemic autonomic neuropathy (see Chapter 107) (Bremner and Smith, 2006; Yamashita et al., 2010), Guillain-Barré syndrome or its Miller Fisher variant (Kaymakamzade et al., 2013), and botulism. Perhaps the most common and most easily recognizable tonic pupil is the benign Adie pupil, which often presents with acute painless enlargement of the pupil and may be accompanied by complaints of photophobia and blurred near vision due to involvement of fibers traveling to the ciliary body for lens accommodation. In 80% of patients, the condition is unilateral. It is most common in healthy young women and is thought to be due to a viral ciliary ganglionitis. Additional examination findings may include decreased corneal sensation and, in the Holmes-Adie syndrome, decreased deep tendon reflexes (Kelly-Sell and Liu, 2011). The affected pupil tends to become smaller with time and can sometimes become smaller than the unaffected pupil. Ross syndrome is the triad of tonic pupils, hyporeflexia, and segmental anhidrosis (Ross, 1958). It is unclear whether this syndrome is a variant of the Holmes-Adie syndrome or a mechanistically distinct disorder, but impaired sweating is the distinguishing feature (Nolano et al., 2006). Harlequin syndrome, in which there is asymmetrical impairment of facial flushing to thermal or emotional stress, may also occur in patients with tonic pupils and hyporeflexia, although Horner syndrome is more common (Bremner and Smith, 2008).

***Preganglionic parasympathetic dysfunction—oculomotor palsy.*** Pupillary enlargement from oculomotor palsy may be

**TABLE 17.1 Diagnostic Pupillary Eyedrop Testing**

| Testing | Mechanism of Action | Diagnostic Utility and Expected Response |
|---|---|---|
| **Anisocoria Greater in the Light (Abnormal Larger Pupil)** | | |
| Dilute pilocarpine (0.0625% or 0.1%) | Parasympathomimetic; direct sphincter stimulation | Tonic pupil will constrict and pupil affected by oculomotor palsy may constrict (denervation supersensitivity)<br>Normal pupil and pupil affected by pharmacological blockade will not respond |
| Pilocarpine (1%) | Parasympathomimetic; direct sphincter stimulation | Normal pupil and pupil affected by oculomotor palsy will constrict fully<br>Pupil affected by pharmacological blockade will not or only partially respond |
| **Anisocoria Greater in the Dark (Abnormal Smaller Pupil)** | | |
| Cocaine (2%–10%) | Inhibits norepinephrine reuptake at the sympathetic terminus | Horner pupil will not dilate<br>Normal pupil will dilate |
| Hydroxyamphetamine (1%) | Induces third-order sympathetic neuron to release any stored norepinephrine | Preganglionic (first- or second-order neuron) Horner pupil will dilate<br>Postganglionic (third-order neuron) Horner pupil will not dilate |
| Apraclonidine (0.5%) | Weak sympathetic agonist | Horner pupil will dilate (denervation supersensitivity)<br>Normal pupil will not change or will constrict slightly |

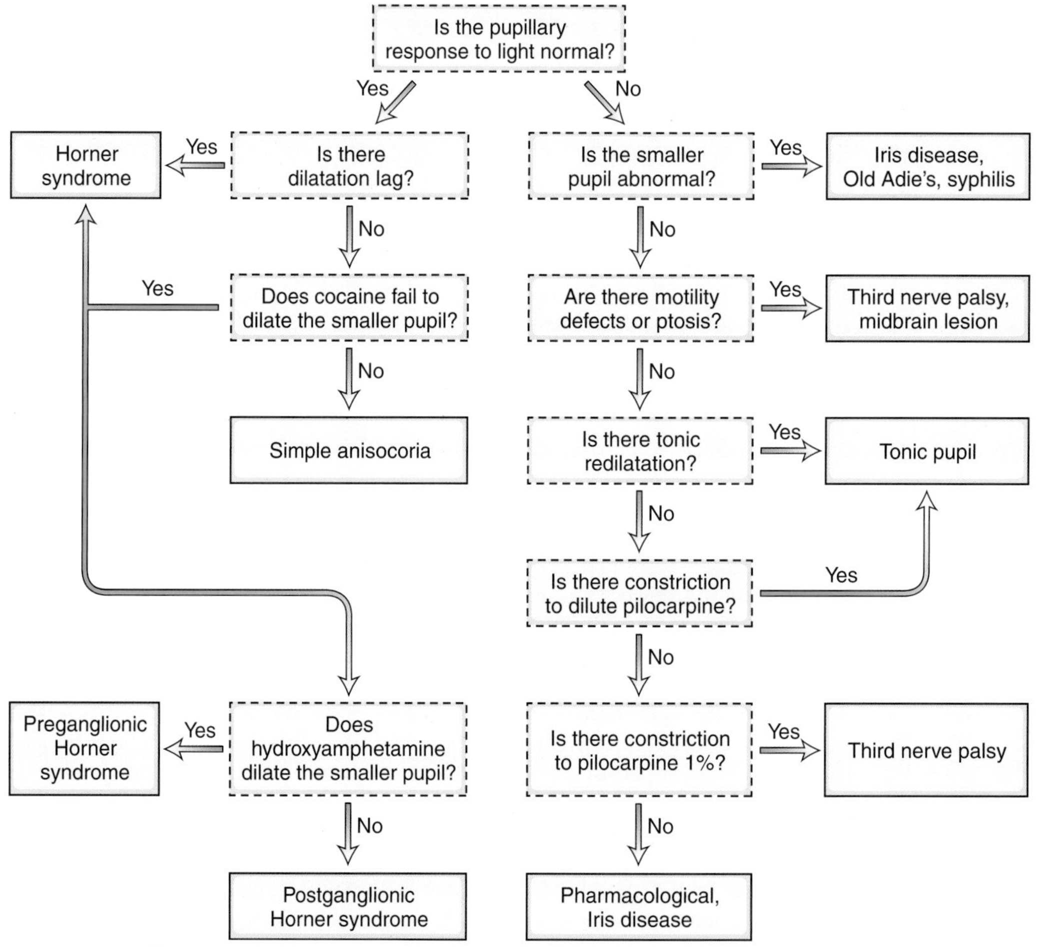


**Fig. 17.3** Flowchart with Systematic Guidelines for Evaluation of Anisocoria.

accompanied by ocular motor deficits due to weakness of the oculomotor-innervated medial, inferior, and superior rectus and inferior oblique muscles and by ptosis due to weakness of the levator palpebrae superioris muscle. Pupillary involvement may be an early sign of compression by a posterior communicating artery aneurysm because the pupillary fibers are located superficially on the superomedial surface of the nerve. It may also be a sign of herniation of the temporal lobe uncus from increased intracranial pressure. A fixed and dilated pupil at the initial presentation of head trauma, stroke, or an intracranial mass lesion is associated with 75% mortality (Clusmann et al., 2001). Although dilute pilocarpine has been reported to produce constriction of the pupil in this situation, the pupil should

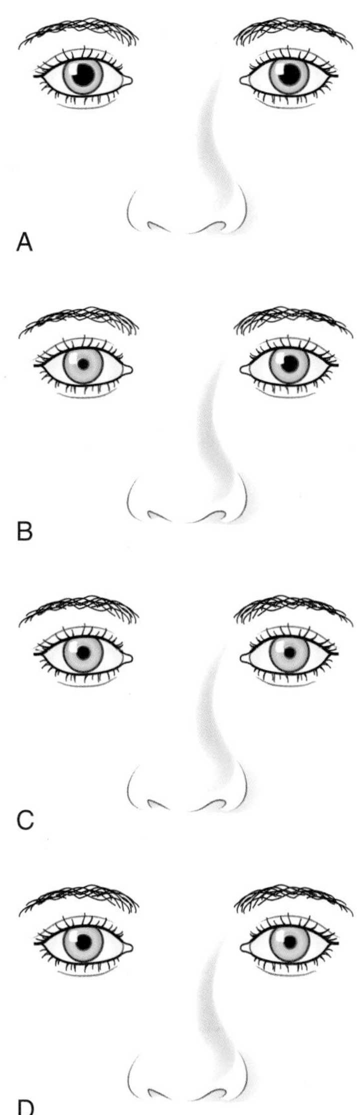


Fig. 17.4 Left Tonic Pupil. A, In darkness, anisocoria is minimal because the normal right pupil is dilated. B, In bright light, anisocoria is enhanced because the normal right pupil constricts, whereas the tonic pupil does not. C, A near stimulus results in constriction of the tonic pupil, giving light-near dissociation. D, A few seconds after return of gaze to a distant target, the normal right pupil has redilated, but the tonic pupil remains small.

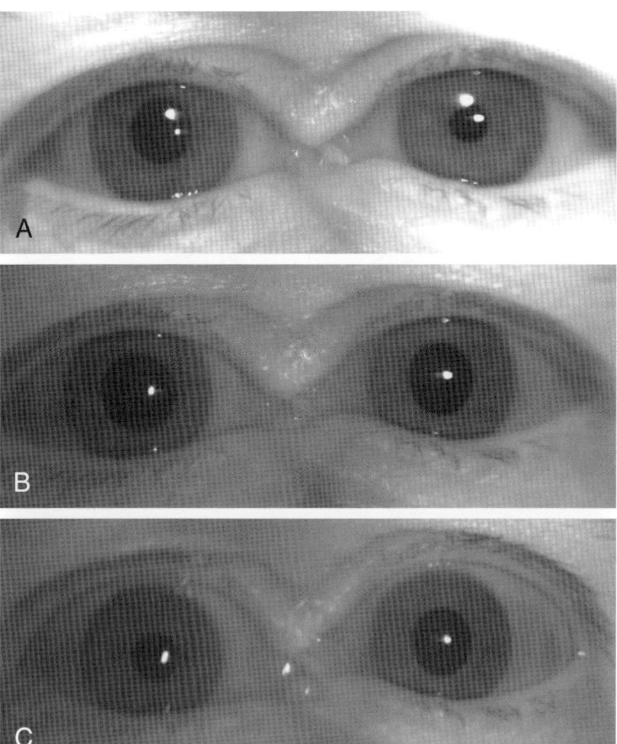


Fig. 17.5 Right Tonic Pupil. A, When viewed in bright light, there is anisocoria with a larger right pupil. B, When viewed in dim light, the anisocoria is less prominent due to dilation of the normal left pupil. C, Thirty minutes after instillation of dilute pilocarpine, the right pupil is constricted due to the presence of cholinergic supersensitivity.

definitely constrict after administration of 1% pilocarpine (see Table 17.1). This may help in differentiating isolated pupillary enlargement from oculomotor palsy from pharmacological pupillary enlargement, because a pharmacological pupil should not constrict with pilocarpine. See Chapter 103 for a complete discussion of oculomotor nerve anatomy and clinical lesions.

***Iris sphincter injury and ischemia.*** Blunt trauma to the eye can damage the iris sphincter, causing mydriasis (pupillary enlargement) with poor pupillary constriction to both light and near stimuli. Tears at the pupillary margin may be evident. The pupil may be smaller than normal (spastic miosis) immediately after the injury, but it becomes dilated and poorly reactive after a few minutes. This course of events may simulate those of uncal herniation. Iris ischemia may cause mydriasis, poor pupillary reactivity, and iris transillumination defects. Iris ischemia may occur with acute angle-closure glaucoma and ocular ischemic syndrome, both of which are usually accompanied by poor vision and pain. Additional signs of acute angle-closure glaucoma include corneal edema and ocular injection. The ocular ischemic syndrome can occur in patients with severe stenosis of an internal carotid artery or stenoses of the internal and external carotid arteries on one side. Associated eye findings include neovascularization of the retina, optic disc, or iris (rubeosis iridis), anterior uveitis (iritis), ocular hypotony, and midperipheral retinal hemorrhages. Some forms of iris degeneration, such as iris atrophy, may cause pupillary dilation, often with irregularity of the pupillary outline.

***Pharmacological mydriasis.*** Pharmacological mydriasis usually occurs after accidental or intentional instillation of anticholinergic agents such as atropine. Accidental mydriasis usually occurs with hand-to-eye contact in individuals who have contact with dilating agents; examples include following application of a scopolamine skin patch for motion sickness, administration of eye drops to a family member with eye disease, or exposure to plants with parasympathetic blocking activity such as angel's trumpet or jimson weed (Andreola et al., 2008; Spina and Taddei, 2007). Inadvertent administration of nebulized ipratropium into the eye via an ill-fitting face mask in a critically ill patient may result in unilateral mydriasis that mimics isolated pupillary involvement from oculomotor nerve compression due to intracranial hypertension with uncal herniation (Eustace et al., 2004). However, pharmacologically dilated pupils tend to be larger than the dilated pupil of oculomotor nerve palsy. Sympathomimetic agents, such as phenylephrine, give mydriasis that is less marked and prolonged than that caused by anticholinergic agents. Pharmacologically dilated pupils either do not constrict or only partially constrict after administration of 1% pilocarpine, whereas all preiris sphincter causes of pupillary dilation will fully constrict (see Table 17.1).

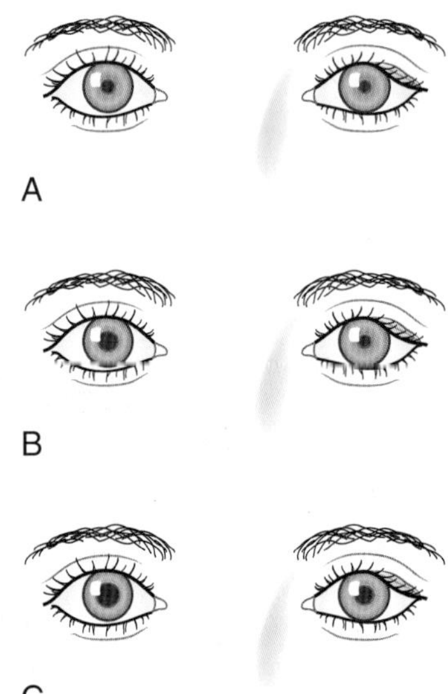

Fig. 17.6 Left Horner Syndrome. A, Mild upper lid ptosis and miosis in room light. B, Anisocoria is increased at 5 seconds after the lights are dimmed, due to dilation lag of left pupil. C, Fifteen seconds after the lights are dimmed, left pupil exhibits increased dilation compared to the image in B.

## Anisocoria Greater in the Dark

***Horner syndrome.*** The classic Horner syndrome triad of sympathetic dysfunction consists of ipsilateral ptosis, miosis, and facial anhidrosis. The lesion may be anywhere along the three-neuron sympathetic pathway (described in Pupil Anatomy and Neural Control). Anhidrosis is present only with lesions of the first- or second-order (preganglionic) neurons because the fibers serving facial sweating take a pathway distinct from those destined for the dilator muscle after synapsing in the superior cervical ganglion. The ptosis results from impaired innervation of the Müller muscle, which contributes only slightly to maintenance of lid opening. As a result, only mild ptosis will be evident with sympathetic dysfunction. Apparent enophthalmos (an illusion of a "sunken" eye) due to palpebral fissure narrowing from involvement of the Müller muscle in combination with subtle elevation of the lower lid ("reverse" or "upside down" ptosis) from involvement of lower lid smooth muscle may occur. An additional finding on examination is dilation lag, the delayed dilation of the Horner pupil in darkness (Pilley and Thompson, 1975) (Fig. 17.6).

The differential diagnosis for Horner syndrome varies for a preganglionic lesion (first- or second-order neuron) versus a postganglionic (third-order neuron) lesion; differentiation between the two will dictate the diagnostic approach. Localization of a preganglionic versus a postganglionic lesion can be made with topical eye drops (Mughal and Longmuir, 2009). Hydroxyamphetamine (1%) is used for this purpose. However, some prefer to confirm the presence of Horner syndrome using cocaine or apraclonidine eye drop testing rather than proceeding directly to localization testing. Administration of diagnostic and localizing drops cannot be done on the same day; at least 24 hours must separate the eye drop tests. From a practical standpoint, cocaine and hydroxyamphetamine are difficult to obtain. Cocaine is a controlled substance, must be kept under lock and key, and results in positive urine toxicology for 2 days after ocular administration (Jacobson et al., 2001). Hydroxyamphetamine eye drops can be obtained from compounding pharmacies. Cocaine inhibits reuptake of norepinephrine at the sympathetic terminus. The result is dilation of a normal pupil but impaired dilation of the sympathetically denervated pupil, with a resultant increase in the anisocoria. Lack of dilation after cocaine administration occurs with both preganglionic and postganglionic lesions. Hydroxyamphetamine induces the third-order neuron to release any stored norepinephrine. It will dilate a normal pupil and a pupil with an intact third-order sympathetic neuron. Therefore, if pupillary dilation occurs in a Horner pupil, the lesion is localized to the preganglionic first- or second-order neurons. If pupillary dilation fails to occur, a third-order neuron lesion is likely (Fig. 17.7, A, B).

Apraclonidine, in a 0.5% solution, is a recent addition to the diagnostic armamentarium for Horner syndrome (Koc et al., 2005). It is an α-adrenergic agonist approved for lowering of intraocular pressure. After bilateral instillation of apraclonidine in a patient with Horner syndrome, there is reversal of the anisocoria caused by dilation of the Horner pupil and either constriction of or no change in the normal pupil (Fig. 17.8). This occurs because apraclonidine is a weak $\alpha_1$-agonist; the Horner pupil dilates due to denervation supersensitivity. In addition, the Horner-induced ptosis resolves; however, this alone cannot be used to confirm diagnosis, because elevation of the eyelid may be seen in normal eyes. Apraclonidine as a replacement for cocaine in the diagnosis of Horner syndrome is promising, but further study is needed; it remains unclear how much time is needed for denervation supersensitivity to develop (Bremner, 2019; Kardon, 2005). A positive apraclonidine test has been reported within 3 hours of lesion onset; however, a false-negative result has been reported up to 16 days after carotid dissection (Cooper-Knock et al., 2011; Dewan et al., 2009; Lebas et al., 2010).

Any lesion along the course of the three-neuron sympathetic pathway may cause Horner syndrome. Two conditions deserve detailed description, owing to their clinical importance and potential ominous prognosis if left undetected; these are carotid dissection, with presentation as an isolated painful Horner syndrome, and Pancoast tumor. Acute onset of a painful Horner syndrome, especially after neck trauma or manipulation (e.g., chiropractic manipulation), should lead to suspicion for a carotid dissection. The intracranial precavernous portion of the carotid artery can be affected and it is not uncommon for a dissection in this portion to be missed on magnetic resonance angiography (MRA) and detected only by careful examination of non–contrast-enhanced fat-saturated axial T1-weighted magnetic resonance imaging (MRI) through the base of the skull, looking for a crescent of hyperintense T1 signal surrounding the carotid artery flow void (see Fig. 17.7, C, D). Treatment typically consists of antiplatelet therapy with aspirin to minimize the risk of emboli from the dissected artery (Kennedy et al., 2012). A preganglionic Horner syndrome, particularly in a patient with a history of tobacco use, should prompt a search for a pulmonary apical neoplasm or Pancoast tumor. Outside of these two settings, the work-up for Horner syndrome consists of neuroimaging of the affected portion of the sympathetic pathway: brain and spine (the entire cervical and first two thoracic segments) MRI with contrast for a preganglionic lesion, and brain MRI with contrast and head and neck MRA for a postganglionic lesion (Almog et al., 2010; Davagnanam et al., 2013). Despite the many potential causes of Horner syndrome, imaging of the entire three-neuron sympathetic pathway identifies a causative lesion in a minority (approximately 20%) of patients with isolated Horner syndrome (Beebe et al., 2017). In children, the majority of Horner syndromes are congenital; however, birth trauma, vascular malformations, carotid dissection, and neoplasm (neuroblastoma) are possible causes. The recommended evaluation in children includes neuroimaging and urinary catecholamine testing to screen for neuroblastoma (Smith et al., 2010).

***Anterior uveitis (iris inflammation).*** Acute inflammatory disease involving the iris (anterior uveitis or iritis) may cause pupillary constriction. If inflammation persists, adhesions between the iris

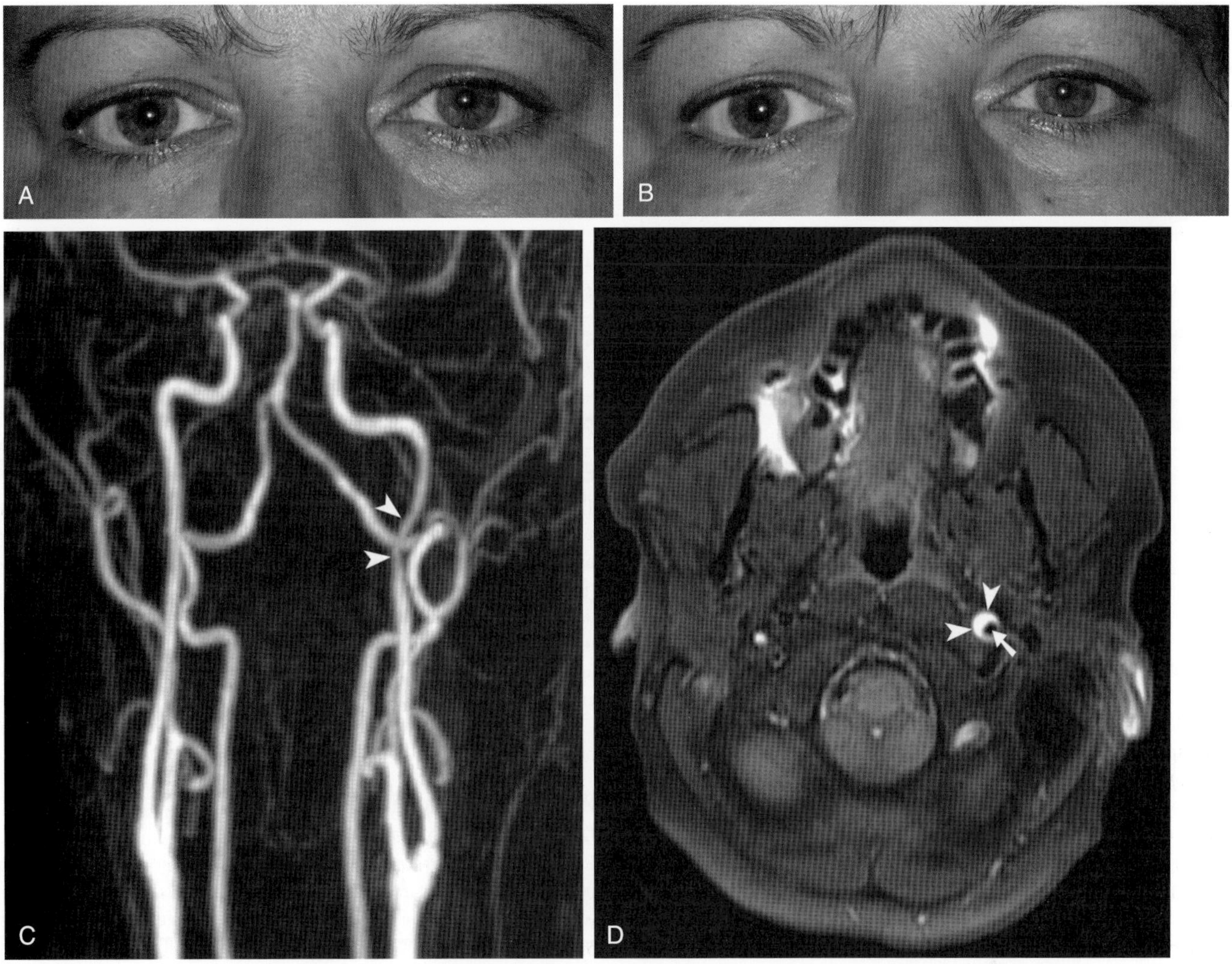

**Fig. 17.7** Acute, painful, left postganglionic (third-order neuron) Horner syndrome secondary to a left internal carotid artery dissection. **A,** Left miosis and slight ptosis. **B,** Failure of left pupil to dilate after 1% hydroxyamphetamine instillation, confirming the postganglionic location of the lesion. **C,** Magnetic resonance angiography, showing subtle focal narrowing of the left internal carotid artery *(arrowheads).* **D,** T1-weighted axial magnetic resonance image without contrast, showing a left internal carotid artery dissection with a crescent of hyperintense blood in the wall of the artery *(arrowheads)* causing narrowing of the artery lumen *(white arrow).*

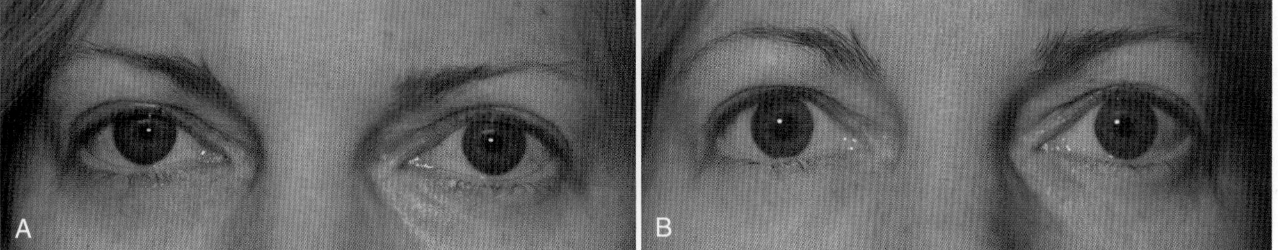


**Fig. 17.8** **A,** Right Horner syndrome with mild right ptosis and anisocoria with a small right pupil. **B,** Forty minutes after administration of 0.5% apraclonidine. Note reversal of anisocoria secondary to dilation of the Horner pupil and resolution of the ptosis.

and lens (posterior synechiae) may lead to pupillary irregularity and immobility. Usually the inflamed eye is red and the patient reports pain and photophobia. However, some chronic forms of anterior uveitis can cause iris adhesions without these manifestations. Syphilis most commonly causes Argyll Robertson pupils but may cause focal iris inflammation and degeneration. Infiltration of the iris by tumor or amyloid can also cause irregular pupils.

## Episodic Anisocoria

Anisocoria may be intermittent. Physiological anisocoria can vary from week to week and occasionally from hour to hour. A rare condition known as *tadpole pupil* results from intermittent spasms of segments of the dilator muscle; often, these patients have an underlying Horner syndrome (Thompson et al., 1983). A related phenomenon is oculosympathetic spasm associated with lesions of the cervical spinal cord.

**BOX 17.1 Clinical Examination of the Eyelids**

Observe for at least 1 minute, looking for the following:
- Palpebral fissure asymmetry
- The resting position of each upper and lower eyelid relative to the iris edge
- Upper or lower lid retraction and scleral show
- Ptosis
- Proptosis (protruding eye) or enophthalmos (inward or "sunken" eye)
- Eyelid edema or scarring
- Blink rate (normal is roughly 18 times/min)

Assess lid position in different gaze directions
If ptosis is present, assess for worsening with prolonged upgaze
Observe gentle and forced lid closure
Examine for pupillary abnormalities, ocular motor abnormalities, and facial weakness

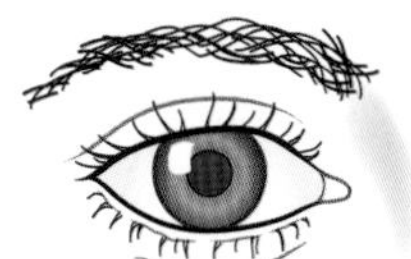
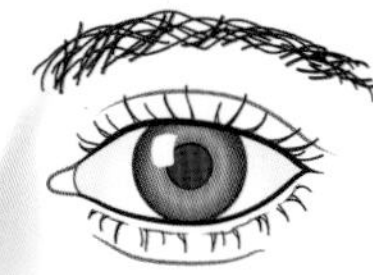

**Fig. 17.9** Normal Eyelid Position. Upper lid covers the upper 1–2 mm of the iris. Lower lid just touches the lower edge of the iris.

Benign episodic unilateral mydriasis is a diagnosis of exclusion in which episodes of pupillary dilation last from minutes to a few days (Jacobson, 1995). Some patients have migraine or a trigeminal autonomic cephalgia, but many patients have isolated monocular visual blurring or are asymptomatic during episodes (Antonaci et al., 2010). The frequency of episodes varies from several per week to one every few years. Some patients have asymmetrical parasympathetic insufficiency as a cause of the episodes, whereas others have asymmetrical sympathetic hyperactivity. Cyclical oculomotor palsy is a rare condition in which periodic oculomotor spasms occur in a patient with oculomotor nerve palsy. During the spasms, the eyelid rises, the exotropic eye moves to the midline, and the pupil constricts. In some cases the spasms involve only the pupil. Intermittent spasm of portions of the pupillary sphincter may occur in traumatic oculomotor nerve paralysis and with aberrant regeneration. Unilateral pupillary dilation and other pupillary signs can also occur during seizures, and rhythmic pupillary oscillations have been reported with Creutzfeldt-Jakob disease (Nagasaka et al., 2010).

### Pupillary Light-Near Dissociation

The term *light-near dissociation* refers to pupils that have marked diminution of constriction to light, with better constriction to near stimuli. The differential diagnosis includes tonic pupil, Argyll Robertson pupil, the dorsal midbrain syndrome, and severe bilateral optic neuropathy (Han et al., 2010). Tonic pupils were described earlier (Anisocoria Greater in the Light). Argyll Robertson pupils are small and irregular. In the past, this condition was most commonly seen in the setting of syphilis, but currently diabetes is thought to be the most common cause, although the pupils are not miotic. Localization of the underlying lesion is unclear, but possibilities include the ciliary ganglion and the dorsal midbrain (Thompson and Kardon, 2006). The dorsal midbrain or Parinaud syndrome (see Chapter 21) consists of impaired vertical gaze, convergence-retraction nystagmus, and lid retraction (Collier sign), in addition to pupillary light-near dissociation. It is often due to pineal gland lesions, hydrocephalus, or stroke. Light-near

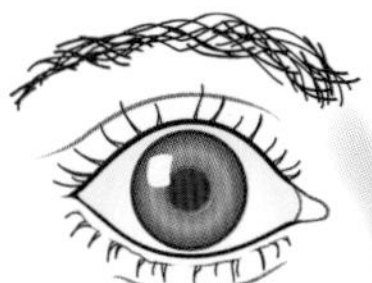
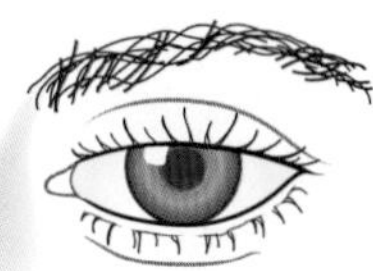

**Fig. 17.10** Mild lid retraction with superior scleral show on the right and ptosis on the left.

dissociation in this syndrome may be due to destruction of the dorsally located olivary pretectal nuclei involved in the pupillary light reflex (see Pupil Anatomy and Neural Control), with relative sparing of the fibers serving the pupillary near response, which arise from a more ventral pathway.

## EYELID ABNORMALITIES

### Eyelid Anatomy and Neural Control

The width of the palpebral fissure is determined by the balance of action of the orbicularis oculi muscle, the levator palpebrae superioris muscle, smooth Müller muscle, and the periorbital and eyelid connective tissues. The orbicularis oculi is innervated by the facial nerve, the levator palpebrae superioris by the oculomotor nerve, and the Müller muscle by the sympathetic nervous system. Activation of the orbicularis oculi results in eye closure. The levator palpebrae and, to a lesser extent, Müller muscle are responsible for maintaining eye opening. See Chapter 103 for a complete discussion of the anatomy of the facial and oculomotor nerves.

### Pathological Conditions of the Eyelids

#### Clinical Presentation and Examination

Patients with abnormal eyelids may present complaining of a change in the physical appearance of one or both eyelids, or they may complain of symptoms related to impaired eyelid function such as eye pain or blurred vision from exposure keratopathy due to excessive eyelid opening or incomplete eyelid closure. In contrast, patients may be unaware of a problem but have had an asymmetrical eye appearance brought to their attention by an acquaintance or family member. Patients will often indicate that they have a "droopy eye" even if the side with the smaller palpebral fissure is the normal side and the side with the widened palpebral fissure is abnormal. It is up to the examiner to determine which side is abnormal. Familiarity with the resting position of the eyelids is therefore essential for determining whether a pathological state exists.

Steps in the examination of the eyelids are summarized in Box 17.1. The normal palpebral fissure is between 12 and 15 mm wide. At rest, the upper eyelid normally covers the upper 1–2 mm of the iris, and the margin of the lower eyelid just touches the lower border of the iris (Fig. 17.9). In an eye with upper lid retraction, the lid touches the upper border of the iris or sclera is visible between the iris and the upper lid margin (superior scleral show) (Fig. 17.10). With lower lid retraction, sclera is visible between the iris and the lower lid margin (inferior scleral show). Patients with factitious (voluntary) ptosis display contraction of the orbicularis oculi with wrinkling of the skin near the lid margin and a lowered eyebrow. An example of true upper lid ptosis is shown in Fig. 17.10. In an effort to elevate the lids, patients with bilateral ptosis often have frontalis contraction with eyebrow elevation. Proptosis (exophthalmos, or eye protrusion) can be evaluated by inspecting the globe position with respect to the orbital rim by looking tangentially across the orbital margin from above, below, or laterally.

Assessment of lid position in different gaze positions may reveal lid retraction on downgaze, which suggests orbital disease such as thyroid

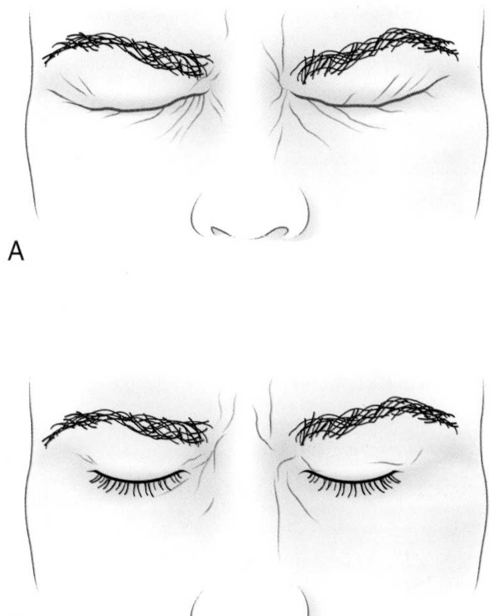


Fig. 17.11 Forced Eyelid Closure. A, Normal forced eyelid closure, with buried lashes. B, Weak forced eyelid closure. Note that lashes remain visible.

eye disease or aberrant regeneration of the oculomotor nerve. The latter condition may also cause lid retraction on adduction. There are many potential lid abnormalities with neuromuscular junction disease, such as myasthenia gravis, including increased ptosis or induction of ptosis with prolonged upgaze, a Cogan lid twitch, enhanced ptosis, and the peek sign. A Cogan lid twitch can be seen with rapid return of the eyes to primary position after sustained downgaze; the upper eyelid elevates excessively, twitches, and then returns to its ptotic position. Enhanced ptosis is increased ptosis in a less or nonptotic eyelid with manual elevation of the more ptotic lid. The peek sign is positive when prolonged eye closure increases orbicularis oculi weakness and causes lid separation with eye exposure despite initial complete eye closure. Incomplete gentle eye closure may also suggest facial weakness from causes other than myasthenia gravis, including facial nerve palsy or a myopathic process such as chronic progressive external ophthalmoplegia (CPEO). Subtle weakness of the orbicularis oculi muscles may be detected with forced eye closure (Fig. 17.1 and Box 17.1). Forced lid closure followed by rapid reopening can be used for evaluating hemifacial spasm, apraxia of lid opening, and blepharospasm, which are often worsened by this maneuver. Patients with apraxia of lid opening show frontalis contraction and brow elevation when asked to open their eyes, but their eyes remain closed. Patients with blepharospasm have persistent orbicularis oculi contraction after being asked to open their eyes.

The final steps in evaluation are to look for abnormalities of the pupil and ocular motility and to perform a full neurological examination. Ophthalmological consultation may be helpful if the etiology of the lid abnormality is not readily apparent; it will also help with evaluation of corneal health in patients with lid abnormalities. After completion of these examination steps (outlined in Table 17.2), it should be possible to determine which side is abnormal and to determine whether the dynamics of eyelid opening and closure are normal.

### Pathologically Widened Palpebral Fissures

When the palpebral fissure is too wide, the differential diagnosis includes lid retraction from orbital disease (e.g., thyroid eye disease) or facial nerve dysfunction with resultant orbicularis oculi weakness. Less common, but also to be considered in the differential diagnosis, are the stare and decreased blinking associated with parkinsonism; Summerskill sign, lid retraction associated with end-stage hepatic disease; and Collier sign, lid retraction seen as a component of the dorsal midbrain syndrome. These conditions may result in exposure keratopathy, causing the patient to complain of eye pain and blurred vision.

Patients with thyroid eye disease may be clinically and serologically hyperthyroid, hypothyroid, or euthyroid. In addition to lid lag (higher-than-normal lid position in downgaze), thyroid eye disease is often accompanied by periorbital edema, conjunctival injection and chemosis, proptosis, eyelid retraction, lagophthalmos (inability to close the eye completely), and the von Graefe sign (dynamic slowing of lid descent during eye movement from upgaze into downgaze) (Gaddipati and Meyer, 2008). Diagnosis is confirmed by demonstration of enlarged extraocular muscles on orbital computed tomography or MRI. There may be thyroid-stimulating antibodies.

Lower lid retraction deserves special mention because it may suggest a different differential when found in the absence of upper lid retraction. It may be congenital or mechanical due to lower lid laxity but most often is a sign of proptosis. As with upper lid retraction, thyroid eye disease is the most common cause, but the lower lid may appear to be spuriously retracted in three situations: (1) when the contralateral lower lid is elevated (as in Horner syndrome), (2) when the globe is elevated in conditions that cause hypertropia (e.g., trochlear nerve palsy), and (3) when the orbicularis oculi is weak from myasthenia gravis or facial nerve palsy.

**TABLE 17.2 Lid Abnormalities Associated with Cerebral Hemisphere Lesions**

| Lid Abnormality | Pathological Findings |
|---|---|
| Unilateral ptosis | Contralateral hemisphere lesions; contralateral and ipsilateral hemisphere lesions |
| Bilateral ptosis | Bilateral frontal lobe lesions; unilateral and bilateral hemisphere lesions |
| Impairment of voluntary lid opening and closure | Dominant hemisphere or bilateral hemisphere lesions or basal ganglia disease |
| Impairment of voluntary and reflex lid opening (apraxia of lid opening) | Basal ganglia disease; bilateral hemisphere lesions; nondominant cerebral lesion |
| Difficulty maintaining lid closure (motor impersistence) | Nondominant hemisphere or bilateral hemisphere lesions |
| Difficulty maintaining lid opening (reflex blepharospasm) | Nondominant hemisphere or bilateral hemisphere lesions |

*Modified with permission from Nutt, J.G., 1977. Lid abnormalities secondary to cerebral hemisphere lesions. Ann Neurol 1, 149–151; and from Johnston, J.C., Rosenbaum, D.M., Picone, C.M., et al., 1989. Apraxia of eyelid opening secondary to right hemisphere infarction. Ann Neurol 25, 622–624.*

### Pathologically Narrowed Palpebral Fissures

When the palpebral fissure is too narrow, the differential diagnosis includes pseudoptosis and true ptosis (Figueiredo, 2010). Pseudoptosis may result from dermatochalasis (redundancy of eyelid skin) or contralateral lid retraction. True ptosis may be congenital or acquired via mechanical, myopathic, or neurogenic factors. Congenital ptosis can be caused by abnormalities of the levator muscle or its innervation and can be unilateral or bilateral. Additional congenital anomalies resulting in ptosis include trigeminal-levator synkinesis (Marcus Gunn jaw-wink phenomenon), in which unilateral ptosis occurs with jaw movements;

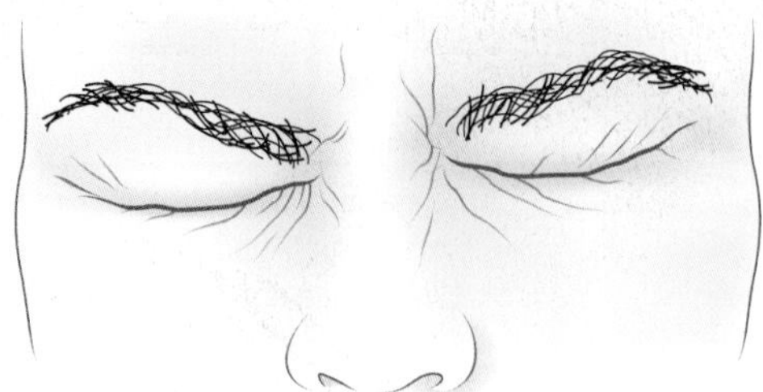

**Fig. 17.12 Blepharospasm, Involuntary Forced Eye Closure.**

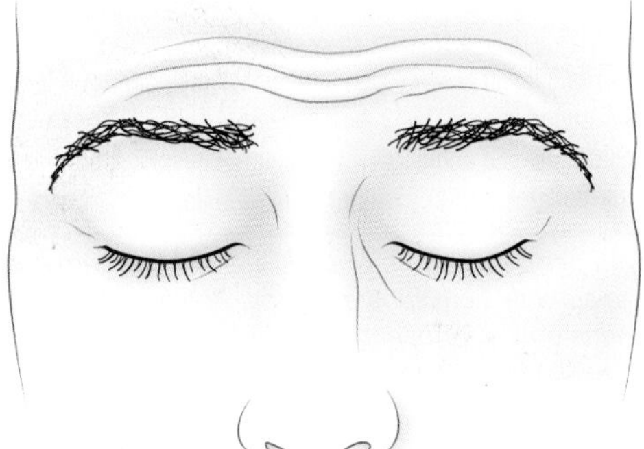

**Fig. 17.13 Apraxia of Lid Opening.** Note elevated eyebrows and frontalis contraction with persistent eye closure.

Duane syndrome with paresis of abduction, adduction, or both, associated with ptosis and globe retraction on attempted adduction; congenital oculomotor palsies; and congenital Horner syndrome (Demirci et al., 2010).

Acquired mechanical causes of ptosis include dehiscence of the levator aponeurosis secondary to aging (involutional blepharoptosis, or senile ptosis) or trauma and inflammation or infiltration of the lid. Dehiscence of the levator aponeurosis is the most common cause of ptosis in the elderly and is accompanied by an elevated superior eyelid crease. The most common myopathic cause of ptosis is CPEO, which is most frequently a manifestation of a mitochondrial myopathy (see Chapter 93). CPEO may occur in isolation or as a component of a wider mitochondrial defect such as Kearns-Sayre syndrome, with pigmentary retinopathy and cardiac conduction defects. Oculopharyngeal muscular dystrophy and myotonic dystrophy are additional myopathic causes of ptosis. Myasthenia gravis is a frequent cause of acquired ptosis—either in isolation or accompanied by ocular motor defects, bulbar weakness, or generalized weakness. The diagnosis is most reliably confirmed with acetylcholine receptor antibodies, a decremental response with repetitive nerve stimulation, or single-fiber electromyography. Neurogenic etiologies include Horner syndrome, oculomotor paresis, and, rarely, disease of the cerebral hemispheres (cerebral ptosis)—particularly right hemispheric lesions (Averbuch-Heller et al., 2002; Manconi et al., 2006) (see Table 17.2). Rightward gaze deviation and upgaze paresis often accompany cerebral ptosis. Horner syndrome and oculomotor paresis are described in detail earlier in this chapter. Lower lid elevation may accompany upper lid ptosis in Horner syndrome and may occur secondary to enophthalmos (e.g., from orbital blowout fractures), local lid edema, excessive lid closure, or factitious ptosis.

## Dynamic Eyelid Abnormalities

Dynamic lid abnormalities include blepharospasm, apraxia of lid opening, hemifacial spasm, myokymia, and myotonia. Blepharospasm consists of uncontrolled bilateral orbicularis oculi contraction causing eyelid closure (Fig. 17.12) (Peckham et al., 2011). Secondary

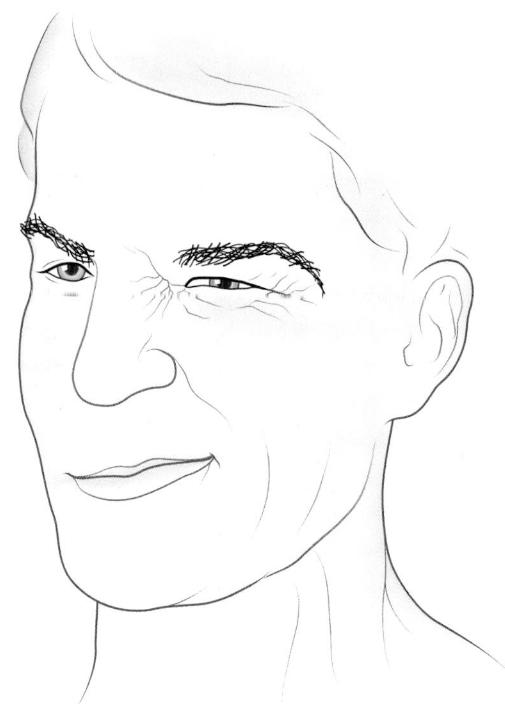

**Fig. 17.14 Hemifacial Spasm.** Synchronous contraction of muscles innervated by the left facial nerve.

blepharospasm may occur as a result of photophobia from ocular diseases such as dry eye, corneal disease (abrasion, keratitis), and ocular inflammation. When the condition is bilateral with no associated ocular or neurological abnormalities, the diagnosis is benign essential blepharospasm, which is a focal dystonia. When there are dystonic movements of the lower face, jaw, tongue, or neck, the designation is oromandibular dystonia with blepharospasm (Meige syndrome), a segmental dystonia. When orbicularis oculi contraction occurs only with lid manipulation or other stimulation, the term *reflex blepharospasm* is sometimes used. Most patients with parkinsonism have reflex blepharospasm, and all types of blepharospasm are made worse by lid manipulation and photophobia. Factitious (voluntary) blepharospasm is rare. The term *apraxia of lid opening* describes inappropriate inhibition of the levator palpebrae muscle that occurs in some patients with bilateral or nondominant cerebral hemisphere lesions or in association with benign essential blepharospasm (Fig. 17.13).

Hemifacial spasm is characterized by paroxysmal, involuntary, synchronous contraction of muscles innervated by the facial nerve on one side (Fig. 17.14) (see Chapter 103). Involuntary twitches of portions of the orbicularis oculi muscle (orbicularis myokymia) are common in normal individuals; these usually involve the lower eyelid. In facial myokymia, these muscular contractions involve other facial muscles. Occasionally, facial myokymia is associated with spastic paretic hemifacial contracture, a condition characterized by tonic contraction of facial muscles on one side with associated weakness of the same muscles. Facial myokymia may be unilateral or bilateral. This sign may indicate brainstem disease; the most common causes are multiple sclerosis and brainstem neoplasm (usually gliomas), but Guillain-Barré syndrome and extraaxial neoplasms may be causal. Myotonia of lid closure may occur in myotonic dystrophy, hypothyroidism, and hyperkalemic (and more rarely, hypokalemic) familial periodic paralysis.

*The complete reference list is available online at https://expertconsult.inkling.com/.*

18

# Neuro-Ophthalmology: Ocular Motor System

Janet C. Rucker, Patrick J.M. Lavin

## OUTLINE



## GENERAL PRINCIPLES OF OCULAR MOTOR CONTROL

*I do not know of any kind of work better fitted for correcting loose habits of observation and careless thinking than a study of the ocular motor nerves.*

***John Hughlings Jackson, 1877***

This chapter includes an outline of ocular motor anatomy and physiology pertaining to clinical disorders of eye movements and is divided into two broad categories: those disorders that result in insufficient eye movements and ocular misalignment, thereby causing disorders of gaze and binocular diplopia, and those that result in abnormal spontaneous eye movements, causing a subjective sense of visual motion called oscillopsia. Competence in accurate diagnosis in such disorders is dependent on the skills of attentive listening, probing questions, extensive knowledge of neuroanatomy and of disorders that affect the efferent visual pathways, and eye movement examination. Objective measurement of abnormal eye movements can increase the sensitivity of detecting subtle deficits to confirm clinical suspicions.

A reasonable understanding and interpretation of abnormal eye movements requires appreciation of the anatomy and physiology of eye movement control. Normal vision is accomplished by a continuous cycle of visual fixation and visual analysis, interrupted by rapid gaze-shifting eye movements called saccades. Subjects with intact afferent visual systems are capable of discerning small details comparable to a Snellen acuity of 20/13 provided that the target image is maintained within 0.5 degree of the fovea centralis. However, 10 degrees from fixation, the resolving power of the retina drops to 20/200. Although the peripheral retina has poor spatial resolution, it is exquisitely sensitive to movement (temporal resolution). The image of an object entering the peripheral visual field stimulates the retina to signal the ocular motor system to make a saccade to fixate the image on the fovea. Visual information concerning spatial resolution (fine detail) and color travels via retinal ganglion (P) cells to the parvocellular layers of the lateral geniculate nucleus (LGN), whereas information concerning temporal resolution (movement) travels via retinal ganglion (M) cells to the magnocellular layer of the LGN. In turn, LGN neurons project via the optic radiations to the primary visual area (V1), the striate cortex (area 17). From here, two processing streams project (Fig. 18.1): the ventral stream, responsible for form and object recognition dominated by foveal representation, projects to the temporal lobe; the dorsal stream, responsible for movement recognition and visuospatial processing dominated by peripheral visual field representation, projects to the prestriate cortex and then to the superior temporal sulcus region. This contains cortical middle temporal (MT) areas and middle superior temporal (MST) areas in monkeys, roughly equivalent to the parietotemporal-occipital (PTO) junction in humans. Both streams converge on the frontal eye fields (FEFs) and are involved in controlling saccades and other eye movements. Thus, with the exception of reflexive vestibular eye movements, cerebral structures determine *when* and *where* the eyes move, whereas brainstem mechanisms determine *how* they move. In other words, voluntary eye movements are generated in the brainstem but triggered by the cerebral cortex.

## EYE MOVEMENT ANATOMY

### Functional Classes of Eye Movements

The goal of visual fixation and all normal eye movements is to place and maintain an object of visual interest on each fovea simultaneously to allow visualization of a single, stable object. To meet this goal, several types, or functional classes, of eye movements exist, including saccades, smooth pursuit, vestibular reflexes, optokinetic nystagmus (OKN), and vergence. Anatomically and physiologically, separate supranuclear (i.e., prenuclear) neuronal networks coordinate their activity to initiate and modulate each type of eye movement.

#### Saccades

The saccadic system moves the eyes rapidly (up to 800 degrees/sec) and conjugately to fixate new targets (Fig. 18.2, *A*). Saccades may be generated voluntarily or in response to verbal commands in the absence of a visible target. Reflexive saccades occur in response to peripheral retinal stimuli such as visual threat or to sounds. Also, saccades create the fast components of nystagmus, including OKN. In general, voluntary saccades

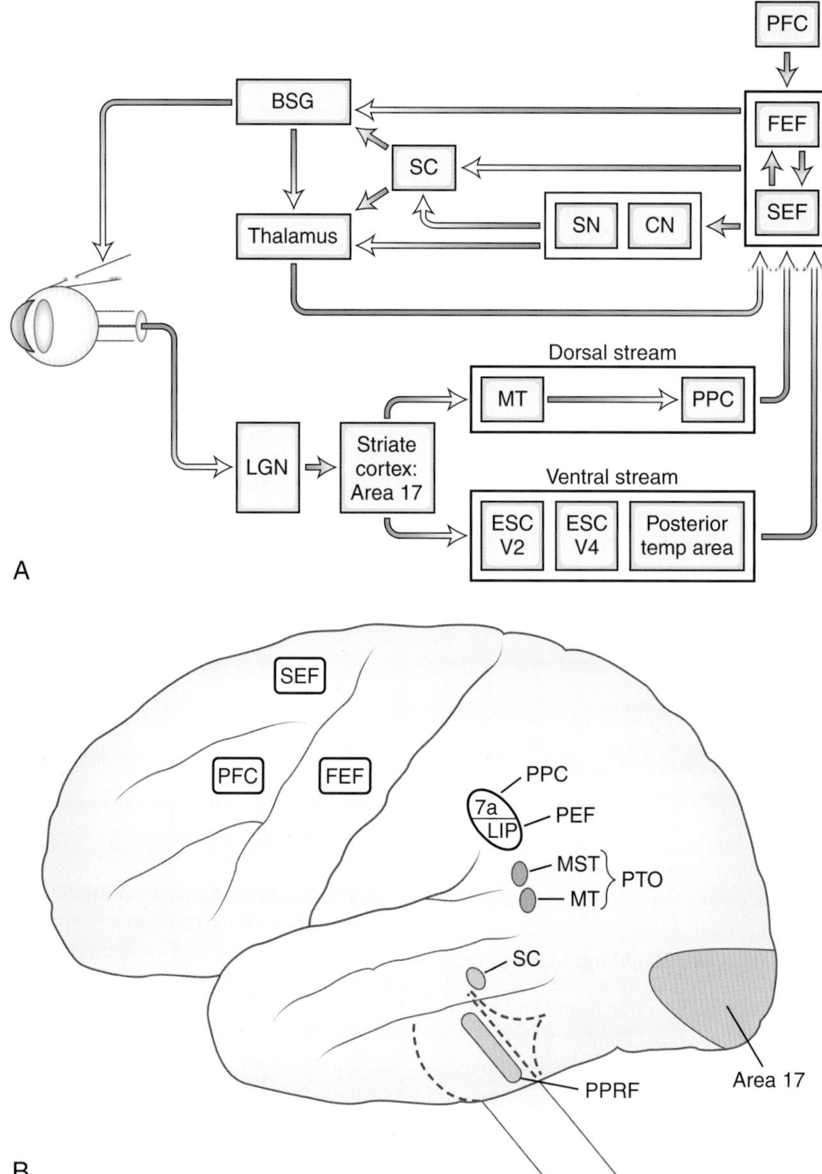


**Fig. 18.1** **A,** Overview of the combined afferent and efferent visual system. **B,** Areas in the human brain that are believed to be important in generating saccades and pursuit. *BSG,* Brainstem saccadic generator; *CN,* caudate nucleus; *ESC,* extrastriate cortex; *FEF,* frontal eye field; *LGN,* lateral geniculate nucleus; *LIP,* lateral intraparietal area; *MST,* medial superior temporovisual area; *MT,* middle temporovisual area; *PEF,* parietal eye field; *PFC,* prefrontal cortex; *PPC,* posterior parietal cortex area; *PPRF,* paramedian pontine reticular formation; *PTO,* parietotemporo-occipital junction; *SC,* superior colliculus; *SEF,* supplementary eye field in the supplementary motor area; *SN,* substantia nigra; *7a,* area 7a. ***(A,** Redrawn from Stuphorn, V., Schall, J.D., 2002. Neuronal control and monitoring of the initiation of movements. Muscle Nerve 26, 326–339.)*

are generated in the contralateral frontal cortex and reflexive saccades in the contralateral parietal cortex. More specifically, several specialized areas in the cortex—identified by pathological lesions, transcranial magnetic stimulation, and neurophysiological studies (particularly in monkeys)—play a major role in controlling saccades (see Fig. 18.1, *B*). These include the FEFs in the precentral gyrus and sulcus (Brodmann area 6 in humans); the supplementary eye fields (SEFs) on the dorsomedial aspect of the superior frontal gyrus anterior to the supplementary motor area; the parietal eye fields (PEFs) in the lateral intraparietal (LIP) area in monkeys which is equivalent to an area in the intraparietal sulcus near the angular gyrus region (Brodmann areas 39 and 40 in humans); the posterior parietal cortex (PPC) (Brodmann area 39 in the upper angular gyrus in humans); the dorsolateral prefrontal cortex (PFC) (Brodmann area 46); the vestibular cortex in the posterior superior temporal gyrus; and the hippocampus in the medial temporal lobe. Collectively, these cortical areas and the superior colliculus are parts of a network that determines when different types of saccades occur and where they go: that is, they calculate their direction and amplitude (accuracy).

To enable the small, strap-like extraocular muscles to move the relatively large globes and overcome inertia and elastic recoil of the viscous orbital contents, the yoked agonist muscles for a conjugate saccade require a *burst* of innervation (called the pulse) to occur simultaneously with reciprocal inhibition of yoked antagonist muscles (Robinson, 1970) (Fig. 18.3, *A*). The saccadic pulse is generated by excitatory burst neurons (EBNs) in the brainstem: for horizontal saccades, EBNs are located in the ipsilateral paramedian pontine reticular

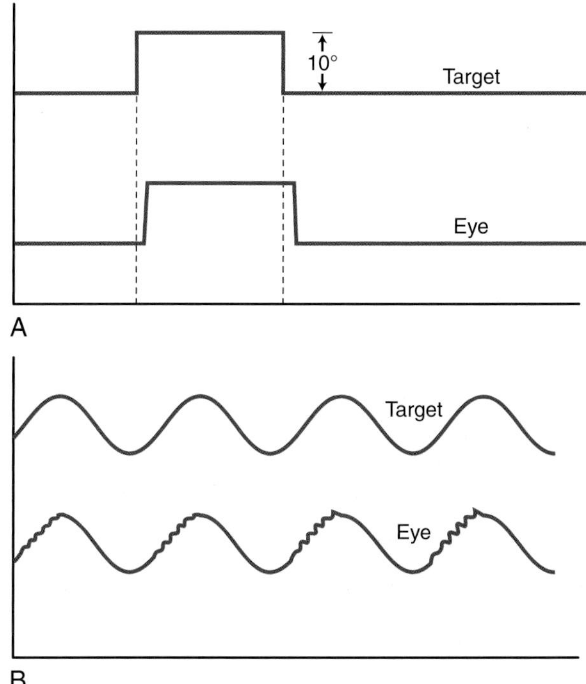


Fig. 18.2 **Simulated Eye Movement Recordings.** By convention for horizontal movements, upward deflections represent rightward eye movements and downward deflections represent leftward eye movements. **A,** Saccades. A target moves rapidly 10 degrees to the right. After a latency of about 200 msec, the eye follows with a fast saccade to target. When the target returns to the center, the sequence is repeated in the opposite direction. **B,** Pursuit. The target moves in a sinusoidal pattern in front of the patient. The eye follows the target after a latency of about 120 msec, but pursuit movements to the right are defective, resulting in the rightward "cogwheel" (saccadic) pursuit. Pursuit to the left is normal.

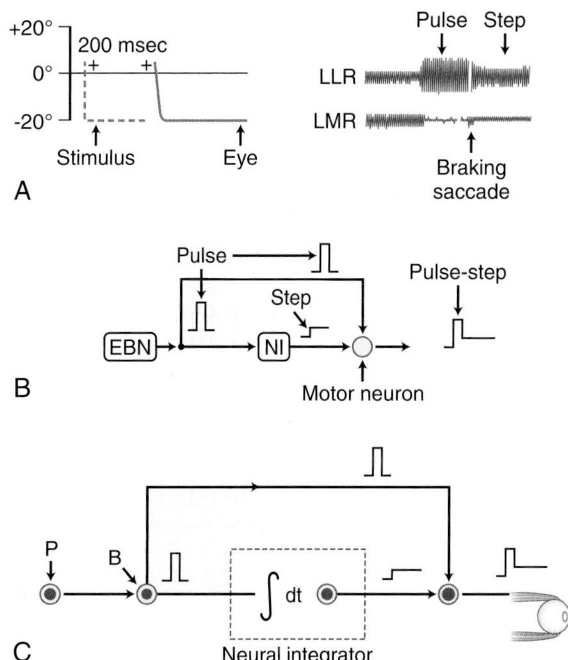


Fig. 18.3 **Ocular Motor Events for a Leftward Saccade. A,** After the appearance of a stimulus 20 degrees to the left of fixation (−20 degrees), the eyes move to the target with a saccade after a latency of 200 msec. Idealized electromyography of the left extraocular muscles shows the activity of the agonist (the left lateral rectus *[LLR]*) and the antagonist (the left medial rectus *[LMR]*) muscles. **B,** The pulse originates in the excitatory burst neurons *(EBNs)* and is mathematically integrated by the neural integrator *(NI)*; both signals are added to produce the pulse-step of the innervation to the ocular motor neurons. **C,** The pause cells *(P)* discharge continuously, suppressing the burst cells *(B)*, except during a saccade, when they "pause," allowing the burst cells to discharge and generate a pulse. *(Reprinted with permission from Lavin, P.J.M., 1985. Conjugate and disconjugate eye movements. In: Walsh, T.J. [Ed.], Neuro-ophthalmology: Clinical Signs and Symptoms. Lea & Febiger, Philadelphia.)*

formation (PPRF) just rostral to the abducens nucleus (Horn et al., 1995); for vertical and torsional saccades, EBNs are located in the rostral interstitial medial longitudinal fasciculus (RIMLF) in the midbrain (Horn and Büttner-Ennever, 1998). Whereas EBNs discharge to generate the pulse, inhibitory burst neurons (IBNs) discharge to inhibit the yoked antagonist muscles (Strassman et al.,1986; Scudder et al., 1988).

At saccade end, maintenance of the eyes on target in an eccentric position requires transition of the pulse command into a new lower-level tonic step command provided by neural integrators (NIs) (see Fig. 18.3, *B*). The NIs for horizontal eye movements include the medial vestibular nucleus and nucleus prepositus hypoglossi (Langer et al., 1986), whereas vertical integration occurs in the interstitial nucleus of Cajal (INC). The cerebellum and EBNs maintain the output of the NIs by controlling gain, via a positive feedback loop, to keep the eyes on target.

Just before and during saccades, EBNs are inhibited tonically by omnipause neurons (OPNs) located in the nucleus raphe interpositus (RIP) in the caudal pons (Büttner-Ennever et al., 1988). Thus, OPNs—which receive input from the cerebrum, cerebellum, and superior colliculus—allow a saccade when they cease discharging and permit EBNs to fire (see Figs. 18.3, *C* and 18.4). For example, for a leftward saccade, OPNs cease discharging, the left lateral rectus and the right medial rectus muscles receive a pulse of innervation to generate the saccade, and their antagonists, the left medial and right lateral rectus muscles, are reciprocally inhibited. Upon reaching the visual target, the pulse command, mediated by the NIs, transitions to tonic step command to hold the eyes in place. The saccade has ended and OPNs resume firing.

Typically, saccades are assessed clinically by asking the subject to make rapid eye movements between two stationary visual targets in the horizontal and then vertical planes. The examiner should observe for abnormalities of saccade onset, speed, conjugacy, accuracy, and trajectory.

## Smooth Pursuit

The pursuit system enables the eyes to track slowly moving targets (up to 70 degrees/sec) to maintain the image stable on the fovea. Specially trained subjects (e.g., baseball players) are capable of smooth-pursuit eye movements as fast as 100 degrees/sec. Control of smooth-pursuit eye movements is complex (see Fig. 18.1) but essentially consists of three components: sensory, motor, and attentional-spatial. The stimulus for pursuit is movement of an image across the fovea at velocities greater than 3 to 5 degrees/sec. The sensory component includes the striate cortex (area 17), which receives information from the retinal ganglion (M) cells via the magnocellular layer of the LGN and the optic radiations. The striate cortex projects to the prestriate cortex (parieto-occipital areas 18 and 19) and then to the superior temporal sulcus region, which contains cortical areas MT and MST in monkeys, equivalent to the PTO junction in humans. This sensory subsystem encodes for location, direction, and velocity of objects moving in the contralateral visual field and is the major afferent input driving smooth pursuit.

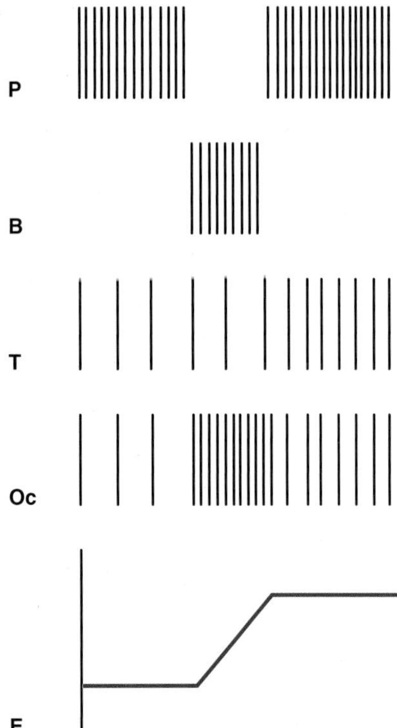


Fig. 18.4 Electrophysiological Events During a Saccade. *P* represents an intraneuronal recording from a pause cell and demonstrates a constant discharge, which ceases just before and during a saccade, allowing an excitatory burst neuron *(B)* to discharge during the saccade pulse. *T* represents the discharge in a tonic neuron, which increases after the pulse as a result of integration of the pulse to a step. Both the pulse (P) and the tonic output (T) of burst-tonic neurons innervate the ocular motor neurons *(Oc)*. The result is a rapid contraction of the extraocular muscle, which moves the eye from primary position and holds it in an eccentric position *(E)*.

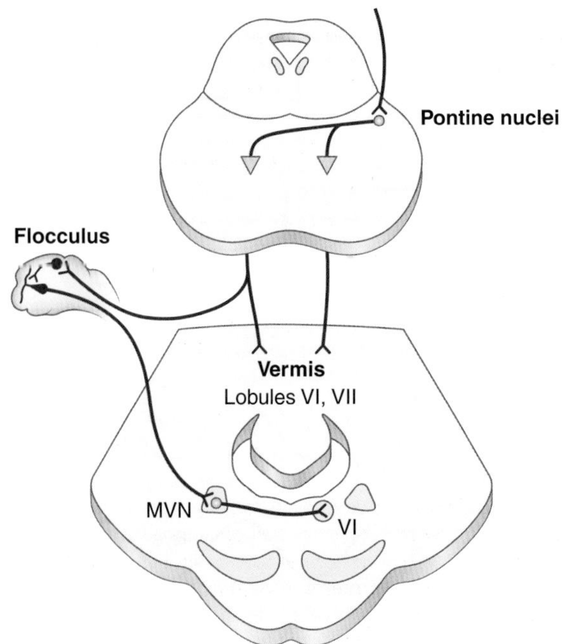


Fig. 18.5 Postulated double decussation of pursuit pathways in the brainstem and cerebellum. The first decussation consists of excitatory mossy fiber projections from the pontine nuclei to granule cells, which excite basket cells and stellate cells in the contralateral cerebellar flocculus. The basket and stellate cells inhibit Purkinje cells, which in turn inhibit neurons in the medial vestibular nucleus *(MVN)*. The second decussation consists of excitatory projections from the MVN to the opposite abducens nucleus *(VI)*. *(Reprinted with permission from Johnston, J.L., Sharpe, J.A., Morrow, M.J., 1992. Paresis of contralateral smooth pursuit and normal vestibular smooth eye movements after unilateral brainstem lesions. Ann Neurol 31, 495–502.)*

It projects to the pursuit motor subsystem bilaterally, also located in the PTO region, as well as to frontal and SEFs. This pursuit pathway is indirect and focuses attention on small moving targets. A direct pathway bypassing the attentional-spatial subsystem enables large moving objects, such as full-field optokinetic stimuli, to generate smooth pursuit contralaterally even when the subject is inattentive. The superior colliculus also contributes to pursuit drive. The PTO projects to the ipsilateral dorsolateral and lateral pontine nuclei. To control ipsilateral tracking, pursuit pathways undergo a double decussation from the pontine nuclei to the contralateral cerebellar flocculus and medial vestibular nucleus and then back to the ipsilateral abducens nucleus (Fig. 18.5).

Clinically, smooth pursuit is assessed by having the subject follow a very slowly moving visual target in the horizontal and then vertical planes while the examiner observes for any corrective saccades superimposed upon pursuit. If the target moves too quickly or changes direction abruptly, even in healthy individuals, or if the pursuit system is impaired, the eyes become unable to maintain pace with the target and fall behind. Consequently the image moves off the fovea, producing a retinal error signal that provokes a corrective (catch-up) saccade and again fixates the target. Then the cycle repeats itself, resulting in saccadic ("cogwheel") pursuit (see Fig. 18.2, *B*). Bidirectional defective pursuit eye movements, a normal finding in infants, are nonspecific and occur under conditions of stress or fatigue or with sedative medication. However, impaired tracking in one direction suggests a structural lesion of the ipsilateral pursuit system (see Fig. 18.2, *B*).

Pursuit defects fall into four categories:

1. Retinotopic defects: Lesions of the geniculostriate pathway cause impaired pursuit in both directions in the contralateral visual field defect. Defects also occur with lesions of areas MST or MT; these patients have apparently normal visual fields but selective "blindness" for movement.
2. Impaired pursuit, worse in the ipsilateral direction in both hemifields, occurs with lesions in the lateral aspect of area MST and the foveal representation of area MT in monkeys, similar to a focal PTO lesion in humans. Lesions in the FEF, posterior thalamus, midbrain, ipsilateral pons, contralateral cerebellum, contralateral pontomedullary junction, and ipsilateral abducens nucleus can also impair pursuit in both hemifields but more markedly in the ipsilateral direction.
3. Symmetrically impaired pursuit in both horizontal directions occurs with focal lesions in the parieto-occipital region (area 39), medication (e.g., anticonvulsants, sedatives, and psychotropic agents), alcohol, fatigue, inattention, schizophrenia, encephalopathy, a variety of neurodegenerative disorders, and age (infants and the elderly).
4. An acute nondominant (e.g., parietal, frontal) hemispheric lesion associated with a hemispatial neglect syndrome causes transient loss of pursuit beyond the midline into contralateral hemispace.

## Vestibular Eye Movements

The vestibular eye movement system maintains a stable image on the retina during head movements. The semicircular canals respond to rotational acceleration of the head by driving the vestibulo-ocular reflex

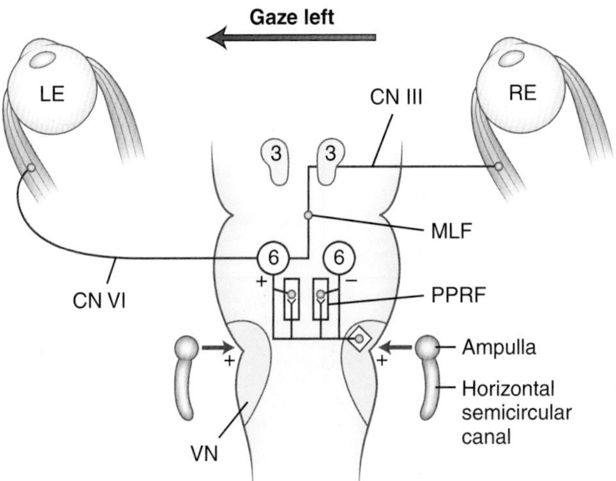


**Fig. 18.6** A lateral head turn (yaw, or side to side) induces movement of the endolymph in the ipsilateral horizontal semicircular canal toward the ampulla (as would warm water caloric stimulation of the external auditory meatus/tympanic membrane) and thus excites the contralateral abducens nucleus and inhibits the ipsilateral abducens nucleus via the vestibular nuclei *(VN)*. Each abducens nucleus innervates the ipsilateral lateral rectus muscle via the abducens nerve and the contralateral medial rectus muscle via the abducens nucleus interneurons, the medial longitudinal fasciculus *(MLF)*, and the neurons for the medial rectus (part of cranial nerve *[CN]* III nucleus). Neurons in each paramedian pontine reticular formation *(PPRF)* also have an excitatory input to the ipsilateral abducens nucleus and an inhibitory input to the contralateral abducens nucleus for saccades and quick phases of nystagmus. *LE,* Left eye; *RE,* right eye. *(Adapted from Lavin, P.J.M., 1985. Conjugate and disconjugate eye movements. In: Walsh, T.J. [Ed.], Neuro-ophthalmology: Clinical Signs and Symptoms. Lea & Febiger, Philadelphia.)*

(VOR) to maintain the eyes in the same direction in space during head movements. The otoliths (utricle and saccule) are gravity receptors that respond to linear acceleration and static head tilt (gravity)—that is, with ocular counter-rolling. The vestibular system stabilizes the direction of gaze during head movements by virtue of changes in its tonic input to the ocular motor nuclei. This is illustrated most clearly by the horizontal VOR (Fig. 18.6). Each horizontal semicircular canal innervates the ipsilateral medial vestibular nucleus to inhibit the ipsilateral abducens nucleus and excite the contralateral abducens nucleus. The ampulla of the right horizontal semicircular canal is stimulated by turning the head to the right (or by warm caloric stimulation). This mechanical information is transduced by the vestibular end organ to electrical signals and transmitted to the ipsilateral vestibular nucleus. Excitatory information is then relayed to the contralateral abducens nucleus and inhibitory information to the ipsilateral abducens nucleus, causing the eyes to deviate in the direction opposite to head rotation, thus maintaining the direction of gaze. The vestibular system is discussed further in Chapter 22.

Vestibular eye movements are assessed most readily on clinical examination by testing visually enhanced oculocephalic reflexes in horizontal and vertical directions. The subject is asked to maintain fixation on a visual target as the examiner actively rotates the head in the horizontal and vertical directions while noting the range of excursions of the eyes and the smoothness of the eye movement.

## Optokinetic Nystagmus

The optokinetic system uses visual reference points in the environment to maintain orientation. It complements the vestibulo-ocular system, which becomes less responsive during slow or sustained head movements, to stabilize images on the retina in situations such as large turns or spinning. When the eyes reach their limit of movement in the orbits, a reflexive saccade allows refixation to a point further forward in the direction of head rotation. The sequence repeats itself, resulting in OKN, comprising slow following pursuit-like movements and rapid saccadic resetting quick phases.

In humans, the optokinetic system predominantly responds to fixation and pursuit of a moving target (immediate component) and to a lesser extent velocity storage (delayed component), which involves neural circuitry in the vestibular system. *Velocity storage* is a mechanism by which the central nervous system (CNS), predominantly the vestibular system including the vestibulocerebellum, prolongs or causes perseveration of short signals generated by the vestibular end organ to enhance orientation in space. Velocity storage is largely involuntary. Probably, the optokinetic system evolved to supplement the vestibular system during sustained rotations.

True OKN is a rhythmic involuntary conjugate ocular oscillation provoked by a compelling full visual field stimulus, such as that produced by rotating an image of the environment around the patient or by turning the patient in a revolving chair. Elicitation of OKN using a pocket tape is a useful bedside test but evaluates only foveal pursuit and refixation saccades, which is helpful in several circumstances, as pointed out in respective sections further on. The subject is asked to directly look at the stimulus without following the motion. The examiner should note the presence or absence of slow and quick phases of eye movement in response to stimulus motion. OKN is a very reflexive eye movement that cannot actively be suppressed while attending to the stimulus.

## Vergence

In humans and other frontal-eyed animals capable of binocular fusional vision, disconjugate (vergence) eye movements are necessary to maintain ocular alignment on an approaching or retreating object (convergence and divergence, respectively). Vergence movements are essential for binocular single vision and stereoscopic depth perception. Electromyography demonstrates that divergence is an active movement (Tamler and Jampolsky, 1967), although it is not as dynamic or as much under voluntary control as convergence. The principal driving stimuli for vergence movements, relayed from the occipital cortex, are accommodative retinal blur (unfocused vision) and fusional disparity (diplopia). Each of these stimuli can operate independently. Convergence occurs predominantly via activation of the medial rectus muscles, though each eye also excyclotorts (more so in downgaze) to facilitate stereoscopic perception (Brodsky, 2002). In addition, the pupils change size as part of the near reflex to increase the depth of field and sharpen the focus of the optical system.

Although the source of adduction commands for versional horizontal eye movements originates in the abducens nucleus, signals for convergence-mediated adduction do not arise here (Gamlin et al., 1989; Gamlin and Mays, 1992). Although the precise locations of the convergence and divergence centers are unknown, important areas include the rostral superior colliculus, the mesencephalic reticular formation (MRF) dorsolateral to the oculomotor nucleus, and the supraoculomotor area above the oculomotor nucleus; further, separate pathways controlling fast (saccade-like) and slow convergence also exist (Bohlen et al., 2016, 2017; Cohen and Büttner-Ennever, 1984; May, et al., 2016, 2018; Rucker et al., 2019; Van Horn et al., 2013).

Clinically, vergence is tested by asking the subject to either follow a slowly moving target as it moves toward and away from him or her on a midline horizontal plane extending centrally toward the examiner between the subject's eyes (slow vergence) or to make rapid jumps of the eyes between near and distant midline visual targets (fast vergence).

**TABLE 18.1 Actions of Extraocular Muscles**

| Muscle | Primary | Secondary | Tertiary |
|---|---|---|---|
| Medial rectus | Adduction | | |
| Lateral rectus | Abduction | | |
| Superior rectus | Elevation | Intorsion | Adduction |
| Inferior rectus | Depression | Extorsion | Adduction |
| Superior oblique | Intorsion | Depression | Abduction |
| Inferior oblique | Extorsion | Elevation | Abduction |

**TABLE 18.2 Yoked Muscle Pairs**

| Ipsilateral | Contralateral |
|---|---|
| Medial rectus | Lateral rectus |
| Superior rectus | Inferior oblique |
| Inferior rectus | Superior oblique |

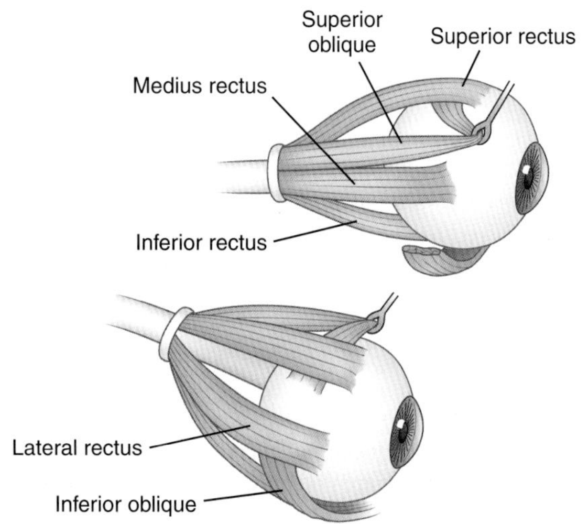


**Fig. 18.7** The Six Extraocular Muscles for Each Eye.

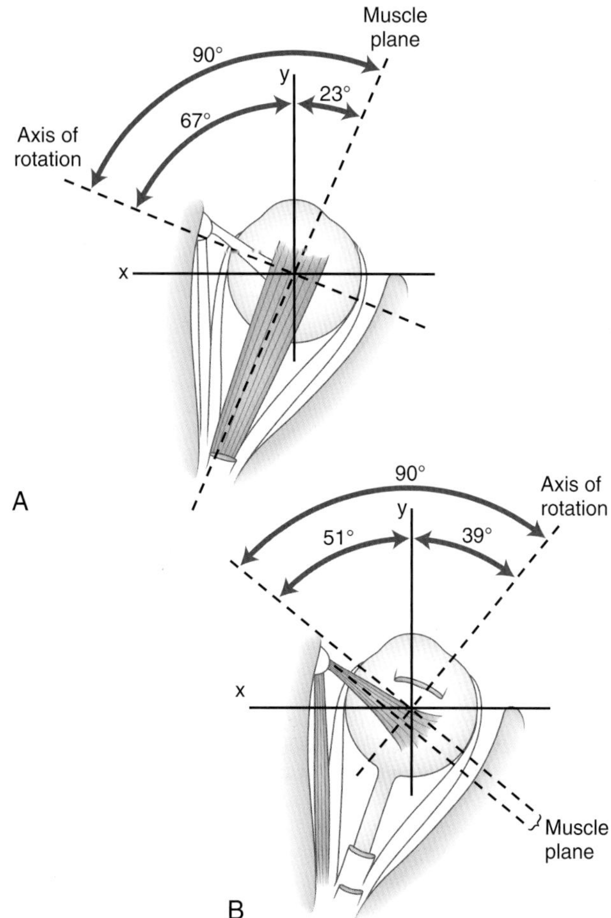


**Fig. 18.8 A,** Relationship of the muscle plane of the vertical rectus muscles to *x*- and *y*-axes. **B,** Relationship of the muscle plane of the oblique muscles to the *x*- and *y*-axes. *(Reprinted with permission from Von Noorden, G.K., 1985. Burian-Von Noorden's Binocular Vision and Ocular Motility, third ed. Mosby, St. Louis.)*

## The Final Common Pathway of Eye Movements

The supranuclear networks send command signals to a "final common pathway" that includes the ocular motoneuron, neuromuscular junction, and the final effector organ of eye movements—the extraocular muscle. For some time it was believed that all motoneurons and extraocular muscle fibers participate fully in all types of eye movements (Scott and Collins, 1973); however, more recently it was shown that specific neuronal and muscle fiber types may be more important for certain types of eye movements.

Each eye receives input from three ocular motor cranial nerves: oculomotor or cranial nerve III, trochlear or cranial nerve IV, and abducens or cranial nerve VI. (See Chapter 103 for a review of the anatomy of each ocular motor cranial nerve.) The six extraocular muscles (Table 18.1) of each eye are yoked in pairs (Table 18.2), so that the eyes move conjugately (versions) to maintain alignment of the visual axes (Fig. 18.7). The actions of the medial and lateral recti are confined to the horizontal plane. The actions of the superior and inferior recti are solely vertical when the eye is abducted 23 degrees. The oblique muscles, the main cyclotorters, also act as pure vertical movers when the eye is adducted 51 degrees (Fig. 18.8). For practical purposes, the vertical actions may be tested at 30 degrees of adduction and abduction. According to the Hering law of dual innervation, yoked muscles receive equal and simultaneous innervation while their antagonists are inhibited (the Sherrington law of reciprocal inhibition), thereby allowing the eyes to move conjugately and with great precision. The pulling actions of the extraocular muscles evolved to move the eyes in the planes of the semicircular canals, which are not strictly horizontal or vertical. These pulling actions are influenced by both the conventional insertions of the global layer of each extraocular muscle directly into the eyeball and by the insertion of the orbital layer into the fibromuscular connective tissue sheath that envelopes each rectus muscle (Fig. 18.9). This arrangement forms a pulley system that is innervated actively (Demer, 2002), stabilizes rotation of the globes in three-dimensional space during complex eye movements (e.g., when a horizontal muscle contracts during upgaze), and prevents excessive retraction of the globe within the orbit during extraocular muscle contraction. Techniques for examining the final common pathway are discussed further on.

# DISORDERS OF EYE MOVEMENTS—OPHTHALMOPLEGIA AND OCULAR MISALIGNMENT

## Approach to History and Examination

### History

The most common symptom with disorders of ocular misalignment, with or without ophthalmoplegia (i.e., reduced range of movement of

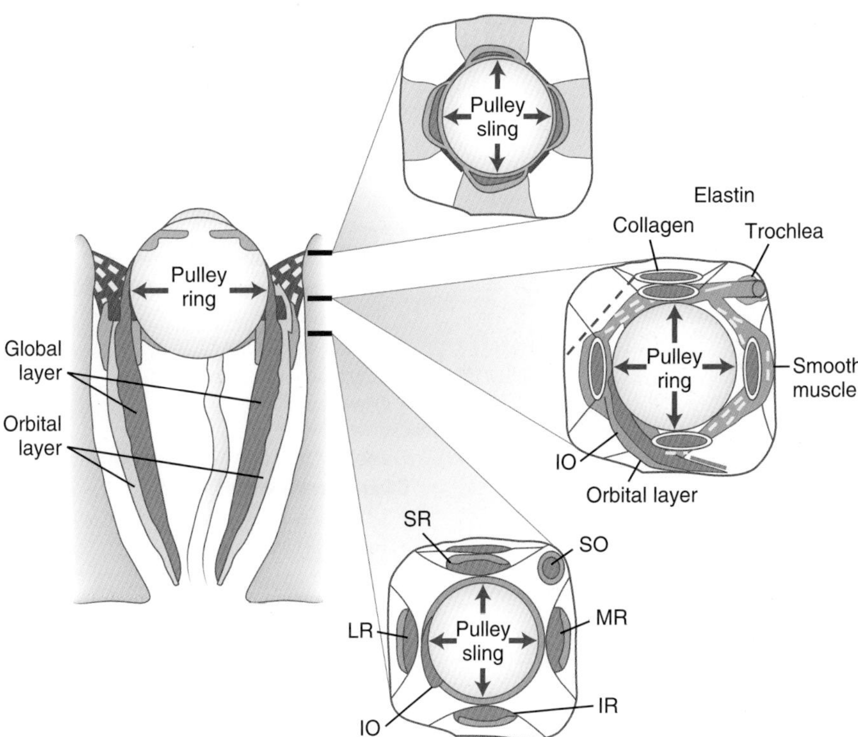


**Fig. 18.9** Diagrammatic representation of the structure of orbital connective tissues and their relationship to the fiber layers of the rectus extraocular muscles. Coronal views are represented at levels indicated by the arrows in horizontal section. *IO,* Inferior oblique; *IR,* inferior rectus; *LR,* lateral rectus; *MR,* medial rectus; *SO,* superior oblique; *SR,* superior rectus. *(Redrawn from Demer, J.L., 2002. The orbital pulley system: a revolution in concepts of orbital anatomy. Ann N Y Acad Sci 956, 17–32.)*

one or both eyes), is diplopia (double vision). Diplopia is encountered frequently in neurological practice and may reflect an emergency with high morbidity and mortality or a benign acquired or lifelong condition. Box 18.1 gives for a summary of the general approach to diplopia. The first question (and exam technique, if the patient is uncertain) is to assess if the diplopia is monocular (fails to resolve by covering each eye) or binocular (resolves with covering each eye). Most often monocular diplopia is due to refractive error or dry eye, which is confirmed if double revolves when the patient looks through a pinhole or some other ocular cause (Box 18.2). An exception to the "rule" that intraocular pathology causes monocular diplopia may occur if a retinal distortion such as an epiretinal membrane displaces the fovea to an extrafoveal location; thus, an intraocular process results in binocular diplopia (Verveka et al., 2017). This is the "dragged-foveal diplopia syndrome" and likely results from rivalry between central and peripheral fusional mechanisms (Guyton, 2018). Anisoconia (aniseikonia), defined as a difference of 20% or more between the image size from each eye and usually due to an optical aberration caused by anisometropia or cataract surgery, can cause diplopia, which may resolve with complex optical correction. Small differences in image size, even less than 3%, can cause visual discomfort or asthenopia without frank diplopia.

Images of the same object must fall on corresponding points of each retina to maintain binocular single vision (fusion) and stereopsis (Fig. 18.10). If the visual axes are not aligned, the object is seen by noncorresponding (disparate) points of each retina and diplopia results (Fig. 18.11). Also, it is helpful to remember that patients with poor vision in one eye may not experience diplopia and that binocular visual blurring (visual blur that resolves completely with each eye covered) or vague "eye strain" may represent ocular misalignment. Theoretically, the onset of double vision should be abrupt. However, in practice, the history of onset may be vague due to misinterpretation as blurring, intermittent occurrence, small amplitude, or compensation by head position. Occasionally visual confusion occurs because each fovea fixates a different object simultaneously, causing the perception of two objects in the same place at the same time (Fig. 18.12). Patients may misinterpret physiological diplopia, a normal phenomenon, as a pathological symptom. Physiological diplopia occurs when a subject fixates an object in the foreground and then becomes aware of another object farther away but in the direction of gaze. The nonfixated object is seen by noncorresponding parts of each retina and is perceived by the mind's (cyclopean) eye as double (Fig. 18.13).

Box 18.1 gives additional historical elements and examination techniques for diplopia. Horizontal diplopia is caused by impaired abduction or adduction of an eye and vertical, by impaired elevation or depression. Diplopia that is worse in one particular direction of gaze suggests that motility in that direction is impaired. Diplopia that is worse at distance usually accompanies impaired abduction or divergence, whereas worsening at near accompanies impaired adduction or convergence. For example, lateral rectus muscle weakness causes horizontal diplopia worse at distance and on looking to the side of the weak muscle. Medial rectus weakness causes horizontal diplopia that is worse at near and to the contralateral side. Care should be taken not to localize too early, as a suspected lateral rectus weakness by history could turn out to be due to myasthenia or a restrictive process in the orbit that affects the medial rectus (Box 18.3). Isolated vertical diplopia (Box 18.4) is commonly caused by superior oblique weakness. If acquired, one image is usually tilted—an infrequent finding when the condition is congenital.

## BOX 18.1 Assessment of the Patient with Diplopia

**History**

- Monocular or binocular?
- Horizontal, vertical, or oblique separation of the images?
- Effect of distance of target (worse at near or far)?
- Effect of fatigue? Worse in morning or evening?
- Transient or persistent? If transient, effect of gaze direction or truly transient (consider giant cell arteritis)?
- Tilting of one image?
- Is there is a history of head trauma, cancer, "lazy eye," eye surgery, or botulinum toxin?
- What other symptoms are present (i.e., headache, eye pain, dizziness, weakness)?

**Observation**

- Head tilt or turn? ("FAT* scan")
- Ptosis (fatigue)?
- Pupil size? Anisocoria?
- Proptosis?

**Eye Examination**

- Visual acuity (each eye separately, and binocularly if primary position nystagmus present)
- Versions (pursuit, saccades, and muscle overaction)
- Convergence (does miosis occur?)
- Ductions
- Ocular alignment (muscle balance) in the "forced primary position" and comitance pattern
- Pupils
- Lids (examine palpebral fissures, levator function, fatigue)
- Vestibulo-ocular reflexes (doll's eye reflex)
- Bell phenomenon
- Prism measurements
- Stereopsis (Titmus stereo test)
- Optokinetic nystagmus

**General Neurological Examination**

**Other Tests Where Indicated**

- Listen for bruits
- Forced ductions
- Edrophonium (Tensilon) test
- Lights on-off test for *the dragged-fovea diplopia syndrome*
- Ice-pack test for ptosis

* *FAT,* Family album tomography—review of old photographs for head tilt, pupil size, lids, ocular alignment, etc. For magnification, use an ophthalmoscope, magnifying glass, or slit lamp.

## BOX 18.2 Causes of Monocular Diplopia

- Uncorrected refractive error
- Equipment failure (defective contact lens, ill-fitting bifocals in patients with dementia)
- Corneal disease (e.g., astigmatism, dry eye, keratoconus)
- After surgery for long-standing tropia (eccentric fixation)
- Corrected long-standing tropia (eccentric fixation)
- Foreign body in aqueous or vitreous media
- Iris abnormalities (polycoria, trauma)
- Lens: multirefractile (combined cortical and nuclear) cataracts, subluxation
- Occipital cortex (bilateral monocular): migraine, epilepsy, stroke, tumor, trauma (palinopsia, polyopia)
- Psychogenic
- Retinal disease (rare)

### Examination

To evaluate disorders causing ocular misalignment with or without ophthalmoplegia, first note any abnormal resting head turn or tilt and then determine the range of versions (Fig. 18.14, *A*) (conjugate eye movements) and ductions. Ductions involve the range of motion monocularly (see Fig. 18.14, *B*). If ductions are not full, restrictive limitation should be assessed by moving the eye forcibly (see the section titled "Forced Ductions," further on). If a conjugate defect (i.e., gaze palsy of both eyes to movement in the same direction) is present, determine whether the eyes move reflexively (i.e., whether the range limitation can be overcome) by testing for the oculocephalic reflex and the Bell phenomenon (spontaneous deviation of the eyes, usually upward, with eye closure). Causes of gaze palsies and ophthalmoplegia are outlined in Table 18.3 and discussed in the following paragraphs.

***Heterophorias versus heterotropias.*** When no ocular misalignment of the eyes is present, the patient is said to have an "ortho" pattern of alignment. A "hetero" pattern indicates a misalignment. Two different terms are used, *heterotropia or heterophoria,* depending on whether binocular fusion must be disrupted for misalignment to be detected. With a tropia, there is a manifest deviation of one eye that can be readily seen. With a phoria, disruption of binocular fusion must occur to detect an ocular misalignment. Many individuals have a latent horizontal heterophoria, which may become manifest (heterotropia) under conditions of stress such as fatigue, exposure to bright sunlight, or ingestion of alcohol, anticonvulsants, or sedatives. Divergent eyes are said to be *exotropic* and convergent eyes *esotropic.* With vertical misalignment, when the nonfixating eye is higher, the patient is said to have a *hypertropia,* and when it is lower, a *hypotropia*—although by convention, *right* or *left hypertropia* is more often used than the term *hypotropia.*

***Techniques to assess ocular alignment.*** Examination of ocular alignment should be performed for binocular diplopia. The alignment pattern of the eyes in primary position should be assessed first. Horizontal diplopia is accompanied by either an eso- or exo- deviation. Vertical diplopia is accompanied by either a left or right hyperdeviation. With diplopia from paralytic strabismus, the image from the nonfixating paretic eye is the false image and is displaced in the direction of action of the weak muscle. Thus, a patient with esotropia has uncrossed diplopia (see Fig. 18.11, *A*) and a patient with exotropia has crossed diplopia (see Fig. 18.11, *B*). After a variable period, a patient may learn to ignore or suppress the false image. If suppression occurs before visual maturity (approximately 6 years of age) and persists, central connections in the afferent visual system fail to develop fully, leading to permanent visual impairment in the deviated nonfixating eye (developmental amblyopia). Amblyopia is more likely to develop with esotropia than with exotropia because exotropia is commonly intermittent. After visual maturity, suppression and amblyopia do not occur; instead, the patient may learn to avoid diplopia by ignoring the false image.

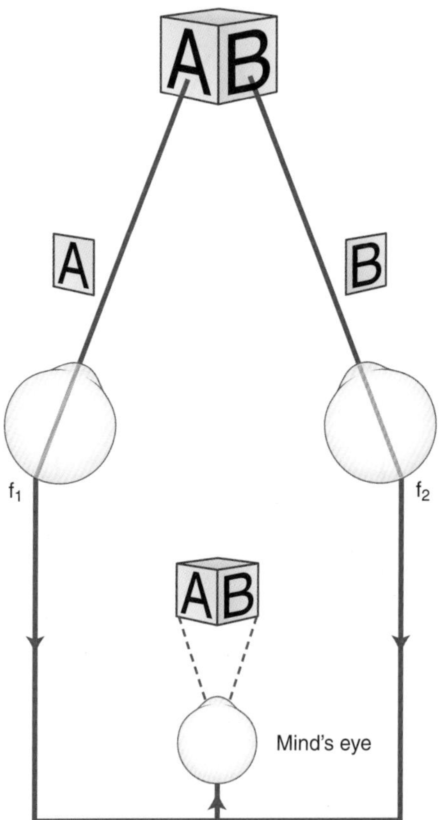


**Fig. 18.10** Each eye views the target, *AB*, from a different angle. The fovea of the left eye *($f_1$)* views the "A" side of the target and the fovea of the right eye *($f_2$)* views the "B" side of the target. The occipital cortex—the cyclopean (mind's) eye—integrates the disparate images so that a three-dimensional image (AB) of the target is perceived. This phenomenon is called *sensory fusion*.

Before determining ocular alignment, the examiner must neutralize a head tilt or turn by placing the head in the "controlled (forced) primary position"; otherwise, misalignment may go undetected because of the compensating head posture. Subjective tests of ocular alignment include the red glass, Maddox rod, Lancaster red-green, and Hess screen tests.

With the *red glass test*, the patient views a penlight while a red filter or glass is placed, by convention, over the right eye. This allows easier identification of the image seen by each eye; the right eye views a red light and the left a white light. The addition of a green filter over the left eye, using red-green glasses, further simplifies the test for younger or less reliable individuals. The target light is shown in the nine diagnostic positions of gaze (see Fig. 18.14, *A*). As the light moves into the field of action of a paretic muscle, the images separate. The individual is asked to signify where the images are most widely separated and to describe their relative positions. Interpretation of the results is summarized in Fig. 18.15.

The *Maddox rod test* uses the same principle as the red glass test, but the images are completely dissociated. A point of light seen through the rod, which is a series of half cylinders, is changed to a straight line that is seen perpendicular to the cylinders (Fig. 18.16). This dissociation of images (a point of light and a line) breaks fusion, enabling the detection of heterophorias as well as heterotropias. Cyclotorsion may be detected by asking if the image of the line is tilted (Fig. 18.17). The Maddox rod can be positioned to produce a horizontal, vertical, or oblique line.

Similar tests include the *Lancaster red-green test* and the *Hess screen test*, which use the same principles, although they are unlikely to be used by a neurologist. Each eye views a different target (a red light through the red filter and a green light through the green filter). The relative positions of the targets are plotted on a grid screen and analyzed to identify the paretic muscle. These haploscopic tests are used mainly by ophthalmologists to quantitatively follow patients with motility disorders.

The *Hirschberg test*, an objective method of determining ocular deviation in young or uncooperative patients, is performed by observing the point of reflection of a penlight held approximately 30 cm from the eyes (Fig. 18.18). The light should be centered on the cornea in

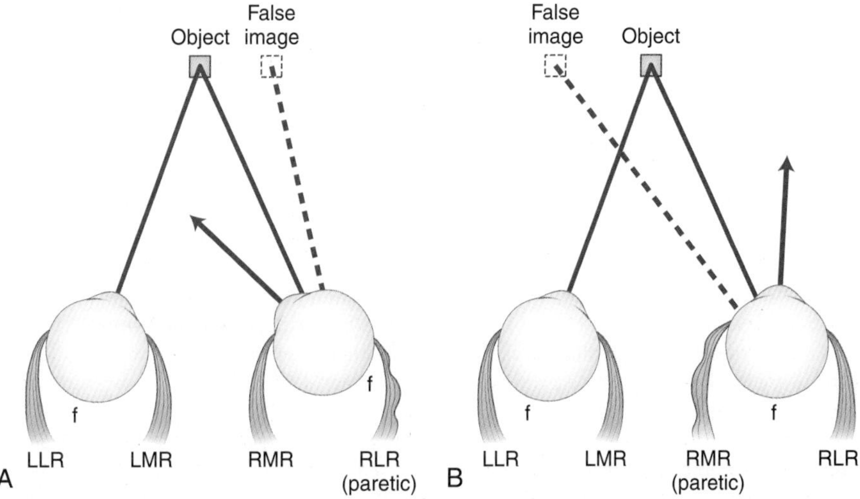


**Fig. 18.11 Misalignment of the Visual Axes. A,** Esotropia caused by a right lateral rectus *(RLR)* palsy results in the right eye turning inward so that the image falls on the retina, nasal to the fovea *(f)*, and is projected by the mind's eye to the temporal field. That is, the false image is projected in the direction of action of the paretic muscle, causing uncrossed (homonymous) diplopia. **B,** Exotropia caused by a paretic right medial rectus *(RMR)* muscle results in the image falling on the retina temporal to the fovea, with projection to the nasal field in the direction of the action of the paretic RMR, causing crossed (heteronymous) diplopia. *LLR,* Left lateral rectus; *LMR,* left medial rectus.

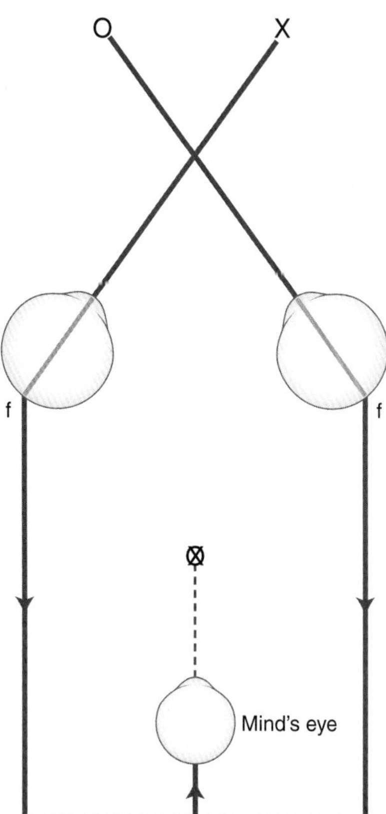


**Fig. 18.12 Visual Confusion (a rare occurrence).** Each fovea *(f)* views a different object, which is projected to the visual cortex by the cyclopean (mind's) eye and perceived in the same place at the same time.

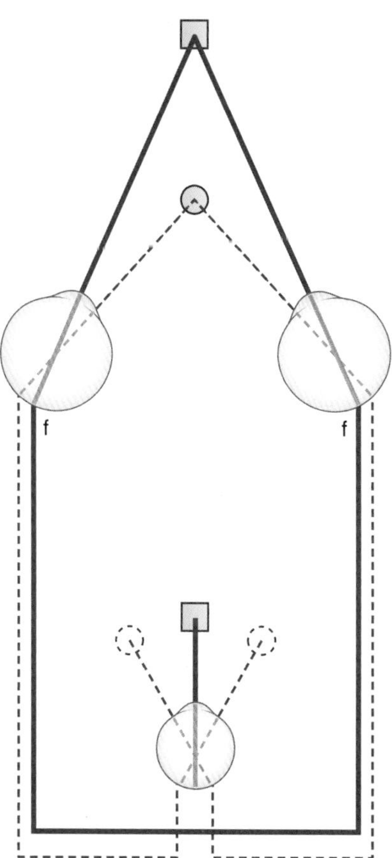


**Fig. 18.13 Physiological Diplopia.** The cyclopean eye views the object *(the square)* as a single object because each fovea *(f)* fixates it. The images of a nonfixated target *(the circle)* fall on noncorresponding points of each retina, so the object appears double.

one eye; if it is not also seen in the center of the other eye, an ocular misalignment is likely to be present. One millimeter of decentration is equal to 7 degrees of ocular deviation. One degree is equal to approximately 2 prism diopters. One prism diopter is the power required to deviate (diffract) a ray of light by 1 cm at a distance of 1 m (Fig. 18.19).

The *cover-uncover test* is determined for both distance (tested at 6 m) and near (tested at 33 cm) vision. The patient is asked to fixate an object at the appropriate distance. The left eye is covered while the patient maintains fixation on the object. If the right eye is fixating, it remains on target, but if the left eye alone is fixating, the right eye moves onto the object. If the uncovered right eye moves in (adducts), the patient has a right exotropia; if it moves out (abducts), the patient has an esotropia; if it moves down, a right hypertropia; if it moves up, a right hypotropia (otherwise called a left hypertropia). The physician should *always* observe the uncovered eye. The test should be repeated by covering the other eye. Prisms are used—mainly by neuro-ophthalmologists, ophthalmologists, orthoptists, and optometrists—to measure the degree of any ocular deviation (see Fig. 18.19). If diplopia is due to breakdown of a long-standing (congenital) deviation, prism measurement can also be used to detect supranormal fusional amplitudes (large fusional reserves) to help confirm the long-standing nature. If no manifest deviation of the visual axes is found using the cover-uncover test, the patient is orthotropic. Then the physician may perform the cross-cover test.

During the *cross-cover test* (alternate-cover test), the patient is asked to fixate an object, and then one eye is covered for at least 4 seconds before the second eye is covered. The examiner should observe the uncovered eye. If the patient is orthotropic, the uncovered eye does not move but the covered eye loses fixation and assumes its position of rest—latent deviation (heterophoria or phoria). In that case, when the covered eye is uncovered, it refixates by moving back; the uncovered eye is immediately covered and loses fixation. The cross-cover test prevents binocular viewing, and thus foveal fusion, by always keeping one eye covered. Many normal subjects without a history of diplopia are exophoric because of the natural alignment of the orbits.

*Fixation switch diplopia* occurs in patients with long-standing strabismus who partially lose visual acuity in the fixating eye, usually because of a cataract or refractive error (Pineles, 2016). Such patients avoid double vision usually by ignoring the false image from the nonfixating eye, but a significant decrease in acuity in the "good" eye forces them to fixate with the weak eye. This causes misalignment of the previously good eye and results in diplopia. Fixation switch diplopia can usually be treated successfully with appropriate optical management.

***Comitance versus incomitance.*** If a patient has an ocular misalignment (tropia or phoria), the physician must determine whether it is comitant or incomitant (i.e., noncomitant) by checking the degree of deviation in the nine diagnostic cardinal positions of gaze (see Fig. 18.14, *A*). When the pattern and degree of ocular misalignment—that is, the angle of deviation of the visual axes—is constant regardless of the direction of gaze, the patient has a comitant strabismus (heterotropia). For example, if a patient has an esotropia in primary position that does not change (and the degree of diplopia does not change) in right and left gaze compared with primary position, the misalignment is comitant. When the degree of misalignment varies with gaze direction, the patient has an incomitant (paralytic due to a weak eye muscle or restrictive due to a stiff eye muscle in the orbit) strabismus.

### BOX 18.3 Causes of Esotropia

- Abducens palsy (unilateral or bilateral)
- Abducens palsy with contracture of antagonist (ipsilateral medial rectus) during recovery
- Accommodative esotropia
- Acute thalamic esotropia
- Chiari malformation (via abducens palsy or increased convergence tone due to cerebellar dysfunction)
- Congenital esotropia (also acquired, cyclic)
- Cyclical oculomotor palsy (spastic phase)
- Divergence insufficiency or paralysis
- Duane syndrome
- Medial rectus entrapment (blowout fracture)
- Myasthenia gravis
- Nystagmus blockage syndrome (in congenital and latent nystagmus)
- Ocular neuromyotonia
- Orbital disorders (orbital varix, infiltrative lesions)
- Posterior internuclear ophthalmoplegia of Lutz (pseudo-sixth)
- Pseudo–sixth cranial nerve palsy of Fisher
- Rippling muscle disease
- Sagging eye syndrome (see section in chapter)
- Spasm of the near reflex (near triad) (accompanied by miosis)
- Stiff person syndrome (associated with abduction deficits, hypometric saccades)
- Thyroid eye disease (often involves medial rectus, leading to restrictive abduction defect)
- Tonic convergence spasm (part of dorsal midbrain syndrome)
- Wernicke encephalopathy (bilateral abducens palsies)

### BOX 18.4 Causes of Vertical Diplopia

**Common Causes**

- Superior oblique palsy
- Thyroid eye disease (muscle infiltration)
- Myasthenia gravis
- Skew deviation (brainstem, cerebellar, hydrocephalus)

**Less Common Causes**

- Orbital inflammation (myositis, idiopathic orbital inflammatory syndrome [previously designated "orbital pseudotumor"])
- Orbital infiltration (lymphoma, metastases, amyloid, IgG-4–related disease)
- Primary orbital tumor
- Entrapment of the inferior rectus (blowout fracture)
- Third nerve palsy with or without aberrant innervation
- Superior division third nerve palsy
- Partial third nuclear lesion (very rare)
- Brown syndrome (congenital, acquired)
- Congenital extraocular muscle fibrosis or muscle absence
- Double elevator palsy (monocular elevator deficiency); controversial in origin
- Sagging eye syndrome (see discussion in section on sixth nerve mimics)

**Other Causes**

- Chronic progressive external ophthalmoplegia
- Miller Fisher syndrome
- Botulism
- Monocular supranuclear gaze palsy
- Stiff person syndrome
- Superior oblique myokymia
- Dissociated vertical deviation (divergence)
- Wernicke encephalopathy
- Vertical one-and-a-half syndrome

When a patient with incomitant strabismus fixates on an object with the nonparetic eye, the angle of misalignment is referred to as the *primary deviation*. When the patient fixates with the paretic eye, the angle of misalignment is referred to as the *secondary deviation*. Secondary deviation is always greater than primary deviation in incomitant strabismus because of the Hering law of dual innervation; it may mislead the examiner to believe that the eye with the greater deviation is the weak one (Fig. 18.20).

Often, comitant strabismus is ophthalmological in origin. In contrast, incomitant strabismus is neurological (though a common exception to this generalization is skew deviation [discussed later]). As an example of incomitance, a right lateral rectus palsy will cause an esotropia that increases upon looking to the right, the side of the weak muscle, and decreases upon looking to the left, opposite side where the weak muscle is out of its plane of action (see Fig. 18.15, *A*). Similarly, with a right medial rectus weakness, an exotropia will be present that increases on looking left and decreases in right gaze (see Fig. 18.15, *B*). Of importance to accurate neurological localization and diagnosis is the concept of spread of comitance with a chronic lesion, which means that there is a tendency for a chronic ocular deviation to "spread" to all fields of gaze, thereby becoming comitant over time; thus, the usual localizing rules of comitance may not apply.

The Parks-Bielschowsky three-step test enables the examiner to assess the pattern of a vertical misalignment of the eyes to identify the paretic muscle. Eight muscles are involved in vertical eye movements: four elevators (two superior recti and two inferior obliques) and four depressors (two inferior recti and two superior obliques). The three-step test endeavors to determine whether a single paretic muscle is responsible for vertical diplopia (see Fig. 18.17). Using the cover-uncover test, which is objective, or one of the subjective tests such as the red glass test, the physician can perform the three-step test for vertical diplopia. When one of the subjective methods for test performance is used, it is important to remember that the hypertropic eye views the lower image. The examiner should also be aware of the pitfalls of the three-step test—namely, the conditions in which the rules break down. These include restrictive ocular myopathies (Box 18.5), long-standing strabismus, skew deviation, and disorders involving more than one muscle. The test is most helpful for confirming the pattern of a fourth nerve palsy.

- *Step 1* determines which eye is higher (hypertropic) in primary position. The patient's head may have to be repositioned (controlled primary position) to neutralize any compensatory tilt. If the right eye is higher, the weak muscle is either one of the two depressors of the right eye (inferior rectus or superior oblique) or one of the two elevators of the left eye (superior rectus or inferior oblique).
- *Step 2* determines whether the hypertropia increases on left or right gaze. If a right hypertropia increases on left gaze, the weak muscle is either the depressor in the right eye, which acts best in adduction (i.e., the superior oblique), or the elevator in the left eye, which acts best in abduction (i.e., the superior rectus).
- *Step 3* determines whether the hypertropia changes when the head tilts to the left or the right. If a right hypertropia increases on head tilt right, the weak muscle must be an intortor of the right eye (superior oblique); if it increases on head tilt left, the weak muscle must be an intortor of the left eye (superior rectus).

Three additional optional steps have been described:

- *Step 4* uses one of several techniques (e.g., double Maddox rod, visual field blind spots, indirect ophthalmoscopy, fundus photography)

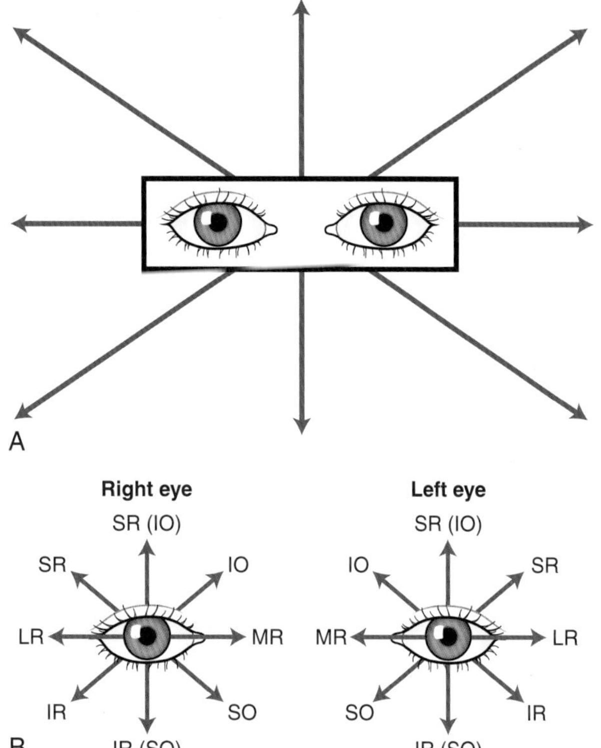


**Fig. 18.14** **A,** The nine diagnostic positions of gaze used for testing versions (saccades and pursuit). **B,** Ductions are used to test the isolated action of each of the six muscles of each eye (the other five muscles are assumed to be functioning normally). Pure elevation (supraduction) and depression (infraduction) of the eyes are predominantly functions of the superior *(SR)* and inferior *(IR)* rectus muscles, respectively, with some help from the oblique muscles. That is, the eyes are rotated directly upward primarily by the SR with some help from the inferior oblique *(IO)*. The eyes are rotated directly downward primarily by the IR with some help from the superior oblique *(SO)*. *LR,* Lateral rectus; *MR,* medial rectus.

to determine whether ocular torsion is present. Establishing the degree and direction of ocular torsion, if any, can differentiate a skew deviation from a superior oblique palsy. Because the primary action of the superior oblique muscle is incyclotorsion (see Table 18.1), typically an acute palsy results in approximately 5 degrees of excyclotorsion of the affected eye due to unopposed action of the ipsilateral inferior oblique muscle; greater than 10 degrees suggests bilateral involvement. If either eye is intorted, a superior oblique palsy is not responsible and the patient may have a skew deviation (Donahue et al., 1999).

- *Step 5* is helpful in the acute phase. If the deviation is greater on downgaze, the weak muscle is a depressor; if it is worse on upgaze, the weak muscle is likely to be an elevator. This fifth step is helpful only in the acute stage, because with time the deviation becomes more comitant.
- *Step 6* involves assessing the size of the vertical deviation in a supine position. If the deviation improves in a supine position, a skew deviation is more likely than a superior oblique palsy (Wong, 2015).

***Head position, eyelids, and other exam techniques*** (Video 18.1). Patients with diplopia may compensate by tilting or turning the head in the direction of action of the weak muscle to move the eyes into a position where the weak muscle is not needed (Fig. 18.21). For example, with right lateral rectus palsy, the head is turned slightly to the right; then, on attempted right gaze, the patient turns the head farther to the right (see Fig. 18.21, *A*). With a right superior oblique palsy, the head tilts forward and to the left (see Fig. 18.21, B). The rule is as follows: The head turns or tilts in the direction of action of the weak muscle.

Careful examination of the eyelids and external appearance of the eyes in the presence of diplopia can provide clues for accurate localization (Box 18.6). Visual acuity, stereopsis, color vision, and confrontation visual fields should be checked carefully and separately in each eye, along with a complete neurological examination.

Nonfatigable limitation of eye movements may suggest a restrictive process such as a tethered extraocular muscle (entrapment) or an infiltrative process such as with thyroid eye disease (TED), idiopathic orbital inflammatory syndrome (IOIS), lymphoma, and so on. Assessment for such restriction is performed with *forced duction testing* under topical anesthesia. The use of phenylephrine hydrochloride eye drops beforehand reduces the risk of subconjunctival hemorrhage. Although this test is in the realm of the ophthalmologist, it may be performed in the office using topical anesthesia and a cotton-tipped applicator, but great care must be taken to avoid injuring the cornea. The causes of restrictive myopathy are listed in Box 18.5; however, any cause of prolonged extraocular muscle paresis can result in contracture of its antagonist muscle.

## Localization and Diagnosis

### Comitant Congenital Strabismus

Comitant strabismus occurs early in life; the magnitude of misalignment (deviation) is similar in all directions of gaze, and each eye has a full range of movement (i.e., full ductions). Some form of comitant ocular misalignment is present in 2% to 3% of preschool children and some form of amblyopia in 3% to 4% (Hunter, 2005). Likely this occurs because of failure of central mechanisms in the brain that keep the eyes aligned. Infantile (congenital) esotropia may be associated with maldevelopment of the afferent visual system, including the visual cortex, and presents within the first 6 months of life; those with comitant esotropia of more than 40 prism diopters (20 degrees) do not "grow out of it" and require surgical correction (Donahue, 2007). Evidence using cortical motion visual evoked potentials indicates that early correction of strabismus (before 11 months of age) improves visual cortical development (Gerth et al., 2008). Esotropia after the age of 3 months is abnormal and, if constant, usually associated with development delay, cranial facial syndromes, or structural abnormalities of the eye. It should be corrected early unless contraindicated by one of the previously mentioned underlying conditions. Intermittent exotropia is common and can be treated with exercises, minus-lens spectacles to stimulate accommodation, or surgery.

Comitant esotropia that manifests between the ages of 6 months and 6 years (average 2½ years) is usually caused by hyperopia (farsightedness), resulting in *accommodative esotropia*: such children with excessive farsightedness must accommodate to have clear vision; the constant accommodation causes excessive convergence and leads to persistent esotropia. Accommodative esotropia responds well to spectacle correction alone. Evidence indicates that high-level stereopsis is restored in these children (unlike those with uncorrected infantile esotropia) if treatment is initiated within 3 months of the onset of constant esotropia (Fawcett et al., 2005).

New-onset strabismus at school age (after age 6 years) is unusual and warrants evaluation for a neurological disorder. Occasionally children with Chiari malformations or posterior fossa tumors present with isolated esotropia before other symptoms or signs develop. Features that suggest a structural cause for esotropia include presentation after age 6, complaints such as diplopia or headache, incomitance in horizontal gaze, esotropia greater at distance than near, and neurological

**TABLE 18.3 Causes of Ophthalmoplegia and Gaze Palsies**

| Site | Disorder |
|---|---|
| Muscle | Ocular myopathies: |
| | Congenital myopathies: |
| | Central core |
| | Centronuclear (myotubular) |
| | Fiber-type disproportion |
| | Multicore (ptosis, spares EOM) |
| | Nemaline |
| | Neurocristopathy (EOM fibrosis) |
| | Oculopharyngodistal myopathy (Satoyoshi myopathy) |
| | Autosomal dominant |
| | Autosomal recessive |
| | Reducing body myopathy (ptosis, spares EOM) |
| | Dystrophies: |
| | Myotonic dystrophy (ptosis, usually spares EOM) |
| | Oculopharyngeal dystrophy |
| | Inflammatory myopathies: |
| | Dermatomyositis |
| | Giant cell arteritis (typically by muscle ischemia) |
| | Idiopathic orbital inflammatory syndrome (orbital pseudotumor) |
| | Metabolic and toxic myopathies (act at multiple sites, e.g., anticonvulsants) |
| | Mitochondrial cytopathy: |
| | Chronic progressive external ophthalmoplegia (CPEO) |
| | CPEO-like syndrome: mitochondrial toxicity in long-standing AIDS and long exposure to HAART |
| | Kearns-Sayre syndrome |
| | Pearson syndrome |
| | POLIP syndrome (polyneuropathy, ophthalmoplegia, leukoencephalopathy, intestinal pseudo-obstruction) |
| | Infiltrative disorders (thyroid, amyloid, metastases, congenital familial fibrosis, cystinosis) |
| | High myopia (large globes cause mechanical restriction) Trauma (orbital entrapment) |
| Neuromuscular junction | Myasthenia gravis |
| | Toxins (e.g., botulism, cosmetic botulinum toxin, organophosphates) |
| | Lambert-Eaton syndrome (rarely affects EOM, mainly causes ptosis) |
| Ocular motor nerves | See Chapter 103 |
| Gaze palsies | Nuclear and paranuclear: |
| | Brainstem injury (vascular, multiple sclerosis, neuromyelitis optica, encephalitis, paraneoplastic, toxins, tumor) |
| | Familial congenital gaze palsy |
| | Glycine encephalopathy (nonketotic hyperglycinemia: hiccups, seizures, apneic spells) |
| | Internuclear ophthalmoplegia |
| | Leigh disease |
| | Machado-Joseph disease (SCA3) |
| | Maple syrup urine disease |
| | Möbius and Duane syndromes (agenesis of cranial nerve nuclei) |
| | One-and-a-half syndrome |
| | Progressive encephalitis with rigidity and myoclonus (PERM), a variant of the stiff person syndrome |
| | Spinocerebellar degeneration |
| | Tangier disease |
| | Vitamin E deficiency |
| | Prenuclear: |
| | Monocular "supranuclear" elevator palsy |
| | Ocular tilt reaction |
| | Skew deviation |
| | Vertical one-and-a-half syndrome |
| | Supranuclear (predominantly horizontal): |
| | Acutely, after hemispheric stroke: |
| | Congenital ocular motor apraxia or congenital saccadic palsy |
| | Ipsiversive or contraversive (wrong-way eyes) |
| | Gaucher disease (types 2 and 3) |
| | Ictal (transient, adversive) |
| | Juvenile-onset GM2 gangliosidosis (mimics juvenile SMA) |
| | Postictal (transient, ipsiversive) |
| | Paraneoplastic disorders |

Continued

**TABLE 18.3 Causes of Ophthalmoplegia and Gaze Palsies—cont'd**

| Site | Disorder |
|---|---|
| | Supranuclear (predominantly vertical): |
| | Adult-onset GM2 gangliosidosis (mimics multisystem atrophy or spinocerebellar degeneration) (V > H) |
| | Amyotrophic lateral sclerosis (rare, V > H) |
| | Autosomal dominant parkinsonian-dementia complex with pallidopontonigral degeneration (dementia, dystonia, frontal and pyramidal signs, urinary incontinence) |
| | Cerebral amyloid angiopathy with leukoencephalopathy |
| | Congenital vertical ocular motor apraxia (rare) |
| | Dentatorubral-pallidoluysian atrophy (autosomal dominant, dementia, ataxia, myoclonus, choreoathetosis) |
| | Diffuse Lewy body disease (ophthalmoplegia may be global) |
| | Dorsal midbrain syndrome |
| | Familial Creutzfeldt-Jakob disease (U > D) |
| | Familial paralysis of vertical gaze |
| | Gerstmann-Sträussler-Scheinker disease (U > D, dysmetria, nystagmus) |
| | Guamanian Parkinson disease-dementia complex (Lytico-Bodig disease) |
| | HARP syndrome (hypoprebetalipoproteinemia, acanthocytosis, retinitis pigmentosa, pallidal degeneration) |
| | Hydrocephalus (untreated, decompensated shunt) |
| | Joseph disease |
| | Kernicterus (U > D) |
| | Late-onset cerebellopontomesencephalic degeneration (D > U) |
| | Neurovisceral lipidosis; synonyms: DAF syndrome (downgaze palsy-ataxia-foamy macrophages); dystonic lipidosis; Niemann-Pick disease type C (initially loss of downgaze, which may become global, and be associated with ataxia, cognitive changes, sensory neuropathy, and pyramidal findings) |
| | Pallidoluysian atrophy (dysarthria, dystonia, bradykinesia) |
| | Paraneoplastic disorders |
| | Progressive supranuclear palsy (PSP) |
| | Stiff person syndrome |
| | Subcortical gliosis (U > D) |
| | Variant Creutzfeld-Jakob disease (U > D) |
| | Vitamin $B_{12}$ deficiency (U > D) |
| | Wilson disease (also slow horizontal saccades) (U > D) |
| | Supranuclear (global): |
| | Abetalipoproteinemia |
| | AIDS encephalopathy |
| | Alzheimer disease (pursuit) |
| | Cerebral adrenoleukodystrophy |
| | Corticobasal ganglionic degeneration |
| | Fahr disease (idiopathic striatopallidodentate calcification) |
| | Gaucher disease |
| | Hexosaminidase A deficiency |
| | Huntington disease |
| | Joubert syndrome |
| | Leigh disease (infantile striatonigral degeneration) |
| | Malignant neuroleptic syndrome (personal observation) |
| | Methylmalonohomocystinuria |
| | Neurosyphilis |
| | Opportunistic infections |
| | Paraneoplastic disorders |
| | Pelizaeus-Merzbacher disease (H > V) |
| | Pick disease (impaired saccades) |
| | Progressive multifocal leukoencephalopathy |
| | Pseudo-PSP, a selective saccadic palsy, associated with progressive ataxia, dysarthria, and dysphagia over several months following aortic/cardiac surgery under hypothermic circulatory arrest |
| | Stiff person syndrome-late |
| | Tay-Sachs disease (infantile GM2 gangliosidosis) (V > H) |
| | Wernicke encephalopathy |
| | Whipple disease (V > H) |
| | X-linked dystonia-parkinsonism (Lubag disease) |

*AIDS*, Acquired immunodeficiency syndrome; *D*, loss of downgaze; *EOM*, extraocular muscles; *global*, loss of horizontal and vertical gaze; *H*, loss of horizontal gaze; *HAART*, highly active antiretroviral therapy; *SMA*, spinal muscular atrophy; *U*, loss of upgaze; *V*, loss of vertical gaze.

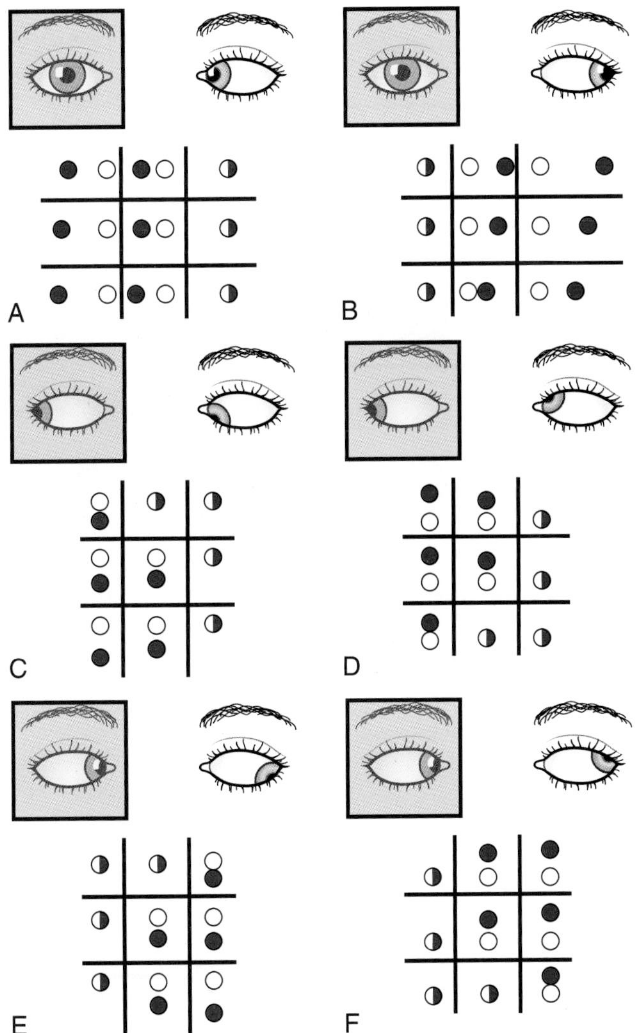


**Fig. 18.15 The Red Glass Test.** Diplopia fields for each type of muscle paralysis are shown. By convention, the red glass is placed over the right eye. The charts below each case are displayed as the subject, facing the examiner, indicates the position of the red *(red circle)* and the white *(white circle)* images in the nine diagnostic positions of gaze. **A,** Right lateral rectus palsy. **B,** Right medial rectus palsy. **C,** Right inferior rectus palsy. **D,** Right superior rectus palsy. **E,** Right superior oblique palsy. **F,** Right inferior oblique palsy. *(Reprinted with permission from Cogan, D.G., 1956. Neurology of the Ocular Muscles, second ed. Charles C Thomas, Springfield, IL. Courtesy Charles C Thomas, Publisher, 1956.)*

findings such as abduction deficits, ataxia, optic disc edema, pathological nystagmus, and saccadic pursuit. Adults who develop isolated esotropia, particularly when they become presbyopic in their early 40s, should have a cycloplegic refraction to detect *latent hyperopia,* although other acquired causes of adult-onset esotropia should be considered (see Box 18.3).

*Dissociated vertical deviation* (DVD), though not a comitant strabismus, is an asymptomatic congenital anomaly that is usually discovered during the cover test or pupil light reflex testing. While the patient fixates an object, one eye is covered, loses fixation, and rises; the uncovered eye maintains fixation. This congenital ocular motility phenomenon is usually bilateral but frequently asymmetric and often is associated with amblyopia, esotropia, and latent nystagmus (LN). Controversy remains as to whether the number of axons decussating in the chiasm is excessive, as suggested by evoked potential studies. DVD has no other clinical significance.

## Infranuclear Eye Movements

***Extraocular muscles and orbit.*** Proptosis, eyelid retraction, lid lag (i.e., delayed lowering of the upper lid margin with depression of an eye), conjunctival injection, and periorbital swelling suggest an orbital/extraocular muscle process, such as an orbital mass lesion, thyroid eye disease (TED), or idiopathic orbital inflammatory syndrome (IOIS, also called orbital pseudotumor). Inflammation, infiltration, or fibrosis of an extraocular muscle often restricts the range of eye movement in the direction opposite that muscle's field of action (for example, left medial rectus involvement leads to a left abduction defect) and occasionally may cause weakness and impair movement in the direction of action of the muscle.

The two most common conditions resulting in diplopia secondary to extraocular muscle disease are TED and IOIS. TED is typically painless except for a foreign body sensation (grittiness) and may present with unilateral or bilateral signs. IOIS is most often unilateral, with subacute painful onset. Classically, TED affects the inferior and medial rectus muscles early, leading to restriction of elevation and abduction of the eye. Both entities may cause vision loss from optic nerve involvement, by compression in TED, or inflammation with IOIS. Chronic progressive external ophthalmoplegia (CPEO) can also cause painless, slowly progressive loss of eye movements (usually without diplopia due to insidious progression and symmetry of the process). Unlike other causes of ophthalmoplegia, classic signs of orbital disease are not present; rather, unilateral or bilateral progressive ptosis is characteristic. Mitochondrial myopathy is the most common etiology of CPEO, either isolated or as part of a syndrome such as Kearns-Sayre.

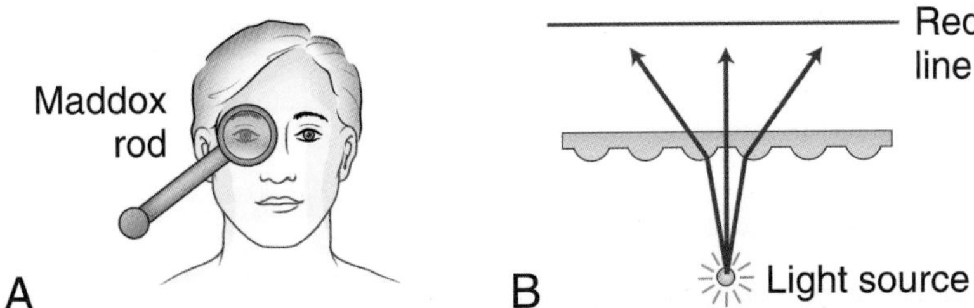


**Fig. 18.16 The Maddox Rod Test.** (Unlike in Fig. 18.15, the images are displayed from the patient's perspective as the patient perceives them.) **A,** By convention, the right eye is covered by the Maddox rod, which may be adjusted so that the patient sees a red line at right angles to the cylinders in the horizontal or vertical plane as desired (red image seen by the right eye; light source seen by the left eye). **B,** The Maddox rod is composed of a series of cylinders that diffract a point of light to form a line.

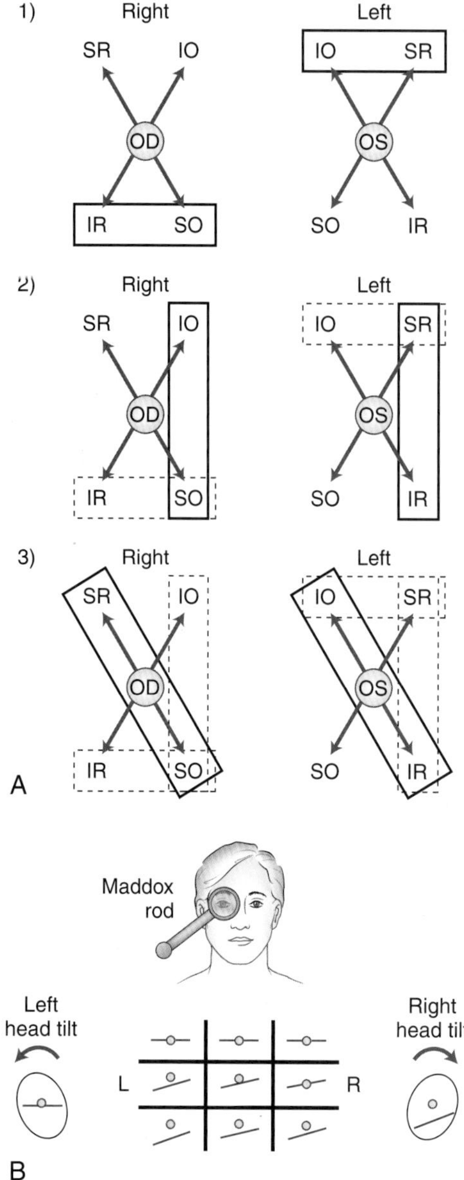


**Fig. 18.17** Example of the three-step test in a patient with an acute right superior oblique palsy. **A,** If a patient has a hypertropia, one of eight muscles may be responsible for the vertical ocular deviation. Identifying the higher eye eliminates four muscles. Step 1: With a right hypertropia, the weak muscle is either one of the two depressors of the right eye (IR or SO) or one of the two elevators of the left eye (IO or SR) *(enclosed by solid line)*. Step 2: If the deviation (or displacement of images) is greater on left gaze, one of the muscles acting in left gaze *(enclosed by solid line)* must be responsible; in this case either the depressor in the right eye (SO) or the elevator in the left eye (SR). Step 3: If the deviation is greater on right head tilt, the incyclotortors of the right eye (SR and SO) or the excyclotortors of the left eye (IR and IO) *(enclosed)* must be responsible, in this case, the right SO—that is, the muscle enclosed three times. If the deviation was greater on left head tilt, the left SR would be responsible. *IO,* Inferior oblique; *IR,* inferior rectus; *SO,* superior oblique; *SR,* superior rectus. **B,** The Maddox rod test (displayed as in Fig. 18.16, as the subject perceives the images) in a patient with a right SO palsy shows vertical separation of the images that is worse in the direction of action of the weak muscle and demonstrates subjective tilting of the image from the right eye. When the head is tilted toward the left shoulder, the separation disappears; but when the head is tilted to the right shoulder, to the side of the weak muscle, the separation is exacerbated (Bielschowsky third step).

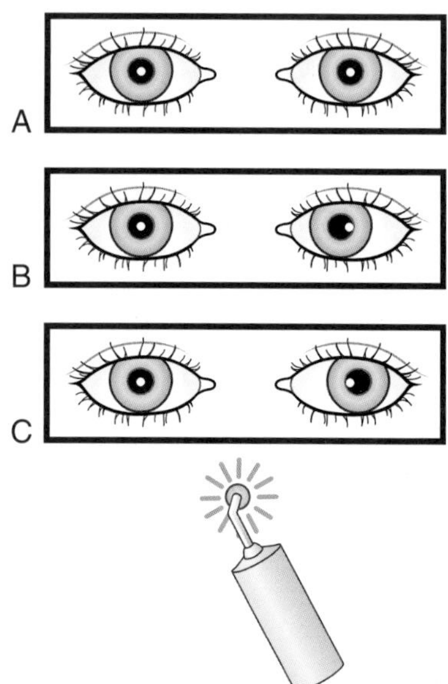


**Fig. 18.18** The Hirschberg method for estimating the amount of ocular deviation. Displacement of the corneal light reflex of the deviating eye varies with the amount of ocular misalignment. One millimeter is equivalent to approximately 7 degrees of ocular deviation, and 1 degree equals approximately 2 prism diopters. **A,** No deviation (orthotropic). **B,** Left esotropia. **C,** Left exotropia.

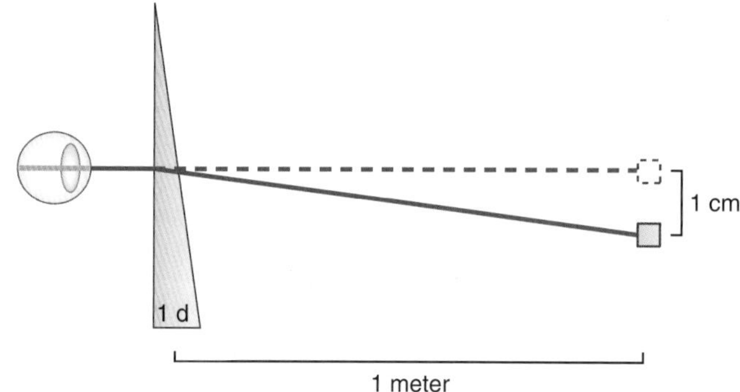


**Fig. 18.19** A prism with the power of 1 prism diopter *(d)* can diffract a ray of light 1 cm at 1 m.

An orbital CT scan may suffice to identify enlarged extraocular muscles (Fig. 18.22, *A*) in TED and IOIS; however, orbital magnetic resonance imaging (MRI) with contrast is preferred and should include both axial and coronal images to assess for optic nerve compression; muscle enlargement may be underestimated with axial images alone. Involvement of the tendon of the enlarged extraocular muscle distinguishes IOIS from TED (see Fig. 18.22, *B*).

Serological thyroid function studies, including thyroid-stimulating hormone (TSH), tri-iodothyronine (T3) and thyroxine (T4), and TSH-receptor antibodies should be assessed if TED is suspected. Patients with TED may be serologically hyper-, hypo-, or euthyroid. Antithyroglobulin and antimicrosomal antibodies may be elevated with TED, whereas serum IgG subtyping may be helpful in identifying those patients with IOIS who have IgG4 disease, which can affect up to 50% (Abad et al., 2019; Andrew et al., 2015).

***Neuromuscular junction.*** Myasthenia gravis (MG) is the most common disease of the neuromuscular junction. Ocular motor dysfunction can mimic virtually any pupil-sparing abnormal eye movement, from pupil-sparing third nerve palsies to fourth and sixth nerve palsies to brainstem supranuclear gaze palsies to internuclear

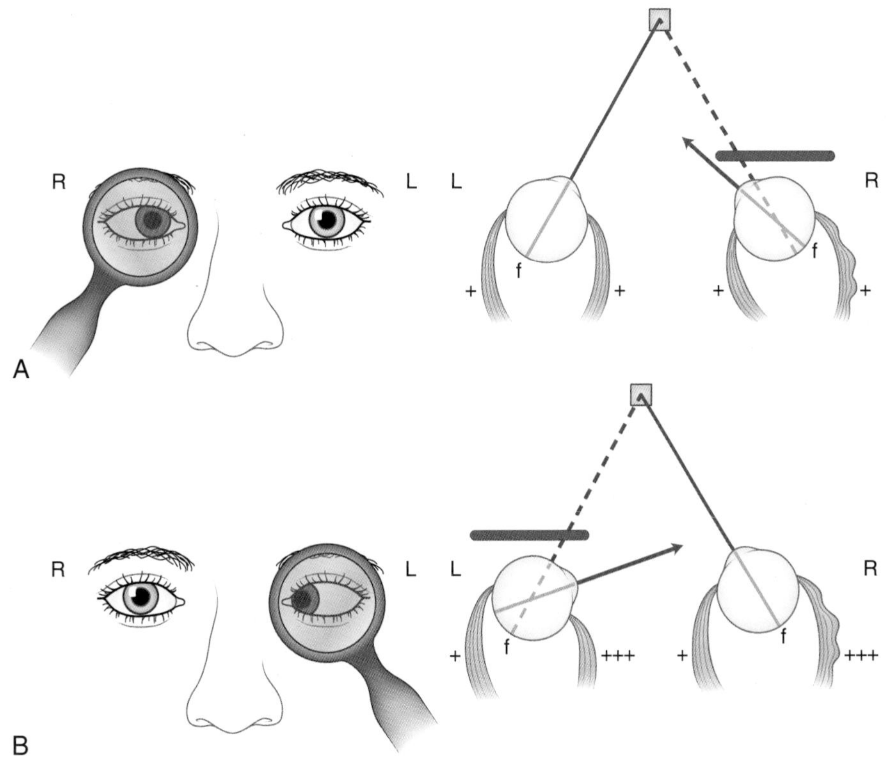


**Fig. 18.20 Primary and Secondary Deviation with Palsy of the Right Lateral Rectus Muscle. A,** The right eye is covered with an occluder while the left eye fixates on the object. A small right esotropia (primary deviation) is demonstrated. (The opaque occluder is shown here to be partly transparent so that the reader can observe the position of the covered eye but the patient cannot see through it.) **B,** The left eye is covered while the paretic right eye fixates on the object. The right eye can fixate on the object despite the weak right lateral rectus muscle because that muscle is overdriven by the central nervous system. The normal left medial rectus muscle is also overdriven (the Hering law of dual innervation), resulting in a large esotropia (secondary deviation). *f*, fovea.

## BOX 18.5 Causes of Positive (Restrictive) Findings on Testing Forced Ductions

- Acquired: superior oblique tendinitis, myositis, or injury
- Brown syndrome
- Carotid-cavernous or dural shunt fistula
- Congenital: superior oblique tendon sheath syndrome
- Duane syndrome
- Entrapment (blowout fracture)
- Extraocular muscle fibrosis (congenital, postoperative)
- Long-standing muscle weakness
- Orbital infiltration: myositis, lymphoma, metastasis, amyloidosis, cysticercosis, trichinosis
- Thyroid ophthalmopathy

ophthalmoplegia (INO). Diagnostic confusion often arises when the eye movements of MG mimic another disorder and ptosis is not present to raise suspicion of MG. It is always appropriate to keep MG in the differential diagnosis for any unexplained eye movement abnormality and to have a low threshold for pursuing diagnostic testing.

Botulism from *Clostridium botulinum* neurotoxin blockade also affects neuromuscular junction transmission. The eye movements are like those seen in MG, with variable patterns of ophthalmoplegia. However, unlike the lack of pupillary involvement in MG, tonic pupillary involvement (with slow tonic reaction and redilation to light and pupillary light-near dissociation manifested as better reaction to a near stimulus than to a light stimulus) is typical of botulism. A third disorder of the neuromuscular junction is the Lambert-Eaton myasthenic syndrome (LEMS), which is due to presynaptic neuromuscular junction failure (in contrast to MG, which is a postsynaptic disorder). The primary clinical manifestation is skeletal muscle weakness that may improve, rather than fatigue, with repetitive movement. Ptosis is common with LEMS; however, eye movements are affected less often (Young and Leavitt, 2016), and when affected are, rarely, the presenting clinical feature.

Historic features such as fatigability with diplopia more common toward the end of the day and/or variability in the pattern of diplopia among horizontal, vertical, and oblique patterns make MG more likely in a patient with diplopia. Signs of MG (Video 18.2) include  moment-to-moment or visit-to-visit variability in ocular misalignments, fatigability of eye movements or lids with prolonged upgaze, Cogan lid twitch, orbicularis oculi weakness, ptosis and curtaining or enhanced ptosis, and faster than normal "twitchy" saccades (i.e., lightning saccades). The finding of lid retraction should suggest coexisting TED, especially with proptosis. The incidence of thyroid dysfunction is higher in MG, particularly if seropositive (Lin et al., 2017; Toth et al., 2016). Cogan lid twitch is an excessive twitch of the upper lid upon return of the eyes to central position after 10 seconds of sustained downgaze. The basis for eyelid curtaining is the Hering law of equal (dual) neural innervation to each eyelid: Manually elevating the more ptotic lid results in increased ptosis in the less ptotic or nonptotic eyelid. These signs are not pathognomonic for

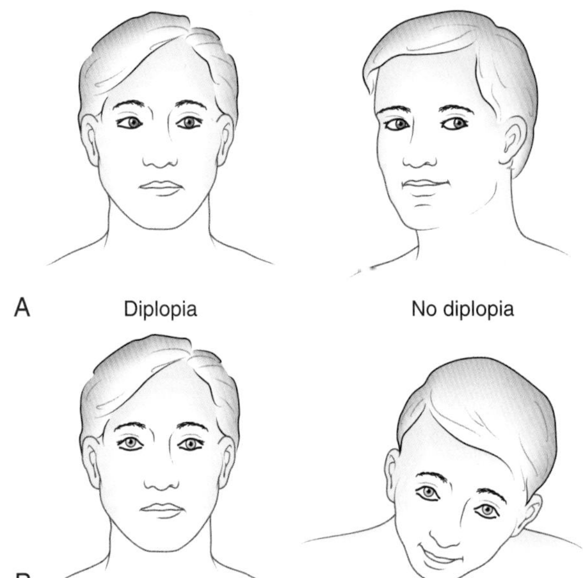


**Fig. 18.21 Compensatory Head Positions for Diplopia. A,** Right lateral rectus palsy. A right esotropia is present in primary gaze; however, by turning the head to the right (in the direction of action of the weak right lateral rectus muscle), the patient can move the eyes into left gaze and maintain both eyes on target (orthotropia), thereby achieving binocular single vision. **B,** Acute right superior oblique muscle palsy. The right eye extorts (excycloduction) because of the unopposed action of the right inferior oblique muscle. When the patient tilts the head to the left and forward (in the direction of action of the weak muscle), the right eye is passively intorted while the left eye actively intorts to compensate and maintain binocular single vision. The head also tilts forward to compensate for the weak depressor action of the weak right superior oblique.

### BOX 18.6 Signs Associated with Diplopia

- Extraocular muscle or lid fatigue, suggests myasthenia gravis (MG)
- Cogan lid twitch, suggests MG
- Weakness of other muscles (e.g., orbicularis oculi, other facial muscles, neck flexors, bulbar muscles), suggests MG or oculopharyngeal dystrophy
- Narrowing of the palpebral fissure and retraction of the globe on adduction, associated with an abduction deficit, suggests Duane retraction syndrome
- Paradoxical elevation of upper lid on attempted adduction or downgaze, and pupil constriction on attempted adduction or downgaze, occurs with aberrant reinnervation of the third cranial nerve, which is nearly always a result of trauma or compression caused by tumor or aneurysm
- Ptosis with elevation of deep upper lid creases, baggy eyelids, superior sulcal enlargement or deformity, and previous eyelid surgical repair, suggest sagging eye syndrome
- Miosis accompanying intermittent esotropia with a variable abduction deficit, occurs with spasm of the near reflex (also called convergence spasm)
- Horner syndrome, ophthalmoplegia, and impaired sensation in the distribution of the first division of the trigeminal nerve occur with superior orbital fissure and anterior cavernous sinus lesions; Horner syndrome with a contralateral superior oblique palsy occurs with a lower midbrain trochlear nucleus lesion
- Proptosis, suggests an orbital lesion such as thyroid eye disease, inflammatory or infiltrative orbital disease (tumor, orbital pseudotumor, or amyloidosis), or a carotid-cavernous sinus fistula (in which case it may be pulsatile)
- Ocular bruits, often heard by both patient and doctor, occur with carotid-cavernousor dural shunt fistulas
- Ophthalmoplegia, ataxia, nystagmus, and confusion, suggest Wernicke encephalopathy
- Facial pain, hearing loss, and ipsilateral lateral rectus weakness, indicate the Gradenigo syndrome
- Myotonia and retinal pathology in the setting of diplopia and ophthalmoplegia, suggest more widespread disorders such as mitochondrial disease

MG (Kao et al., 1999; Van Stavern et al., 2007); thus confirmatory laboratory testing is important.

Although diagnostic testing for MG is covered in more detail in Chapter 108, it is important to note here that the edrophonium test must have an objective endpoint (e.g., ptosis, a tropia, limited ductions), and that the physician must observe an objective change. When forced ductions are positive, indicating a restrictive myopathy, the edrophonium test will be negative and therefore is not indicated. Myasthenic ptosis may be reversed temporarily with application of an ice pack over the affected lid for 1 to 2 minutes (Marinos et al,., 2018; Yamamoto et al., 2017) or after having the patient rest with closed eyes for 30 to 60 minutes. Acetylcholine receptor antibodies are elevated (abnormal) in about 80% of patients with generalized MG but in only 38% to 71% of those with ocular MG (Benatar, 2006; Costa et al., 2004; Padua et al., 2000; Peeler et al., 2015). Anti-MuSK (anti–muscle specific receptor tyrosine kinase) antibodies are rarely associated with chronic ocular MG (Bennett et al., 2006; Hanisch et al., 2006), although ocular manifestations are a common presenting feature in disease that then generalizes (Evoli et al., 2017) and MuSK antibodies are more likely if there is significant bulbar involvement. A decremental response on repetitive electromyographic (EMG) stimulation is highly specific but has a low sensitivity in ocular MG (Benatar, 2006; Costa et al., 2004; Padua et al., 200); single-fiber EMG of the orbicularis oculi has a high sensitivity and specificity (Benatar, 2006; Costa et al., 2004; Padua et al., 2000). A decremental response of the inferior oblique muscle on ocular vestibular evoked myogenic potential (oVEMP) stimulation is a novel and evolving ocular MG diagnostic test (Wirth et al., 2019). Conversion to generalized myasthenia will occur in up to 55% of patients presenting with isolated ocular symptoms (Hendricks et al., 2019).

***Ocular motor cranial nerves.*** See Chapter 103 for full coverage of the anatomy and clinical lesions of the third (III, oculomotor), fourth (IV, trochlear), and sixth (VI, abducens) cranial nerves. Supplementary comments are included here.

**Single Versus Multiple Nerves.** Differential diagnosis varies substantially between a clinically isolated cranial mononeuropathy and a process involving multiple ocular motor nerves simultaneously. The former, in adults, is often due to microvascular ischemia, trauma, or a focal structural lesion on a single nerve. Unilateral involvement of multiple nerves suggests an orbital apex or cavernous sinus lesion. Bilateral involvement of multiple nerves suggests a leptomeningeal process or Miller Fisher syndrome (triad: ophthalmoplegia, ataxia, and areflexia, associated with GQ1b antibodies). The differential diagnosis of diffuse ophthalmoplegia is broad (Boxes 18.7 and 18.8).

**Mimics.** An examination consistent with weakness of a specific single cranial nerve will typically be due to a lesion of that nerve, although MG can present with weakness identical to a pupil-sparing third, fourth, or sixth nerve palsy. Other mimics of sixth nerve dysfunction include TED (see earlier), divergence insufficiency due to the sagging and heavy-eye syndromes, pseudo–sixth nerve palsy from a midbrain/thalamic lesion, convergence spasm as a component of the spasm of the near triad (see later), and the Duane syndrome.

Divergence insufficiency can mimic chronic sixth nerve dysfunction with spread of comitance. Divergence insufficiency presents as

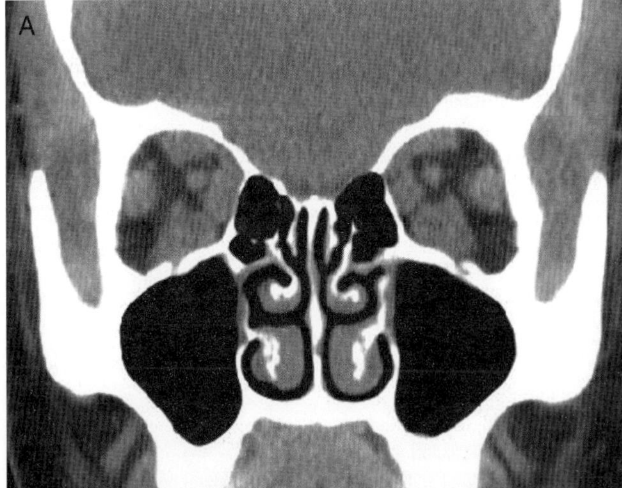


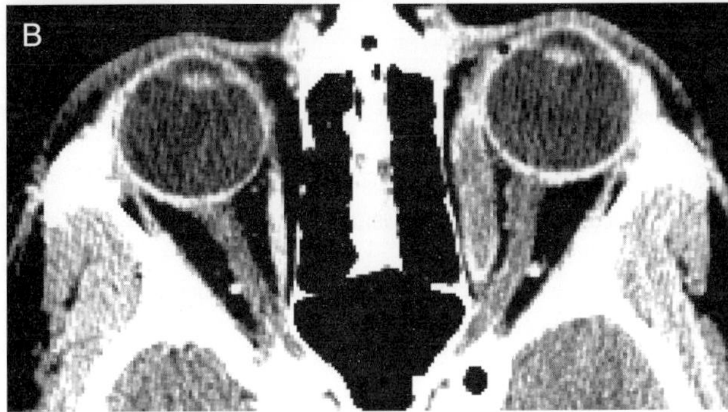


**Fig. 18.22** Extraocular Muscle Imaging in Orbital Conditions. **A**, Coronal orbital computed tomography (CT) showing enlargement of the extraocular muscles bilaterally, most notable in the bilateral inferior recti, in an individual with painless progressive diplopia from thyroid eye disease. **B**, Axial orbital CT showing enlargement of the left medial rectus muscle body and the muscle tendon insertion in an individual with painful horizontal diplopia in primary and left gaze from idiopathic orbital inflammation.

**BOX 18.7 Causes of Acute Bilateral Ophthalmoplegia***

- Basilar meningitis, hypertrophic cranial pachymeningitis, or neoplastic infiltration†
- Botulism
- Brainstem encephalitis†
- Brainstem stroke†
- Carotid-cavernous or dural shunt fistula†
- Cavernous sinus thrombosis (febrile, ill patient)†
- Central herniation syndrome
- Ciguatera poisoning
- Diphtheria
- Fisher syndrome (Miller Fisher syndrome) with or without ataxia
- Intoxication (sedatives, tricyclics, organophosphates, anticonvulsants—consciousness impaired)
- Leigh disease (subacute necrotizing encephalomyelitis)
- Multiple sclerosis
- Myasthenia
- Neuroleptic malignant syndrome (personal observation)
- Orbital pseudotumor†
- Paraneoplastic encephalomyelitis
- Pituitary apoplexy†
- Progressive encephalomyelitis with rigidity and myoclonus, a variant of stiff person syndrome
- Psychogenic
- Stiff person syndrome
- Thallium poisoning
- Tick paralysis
- Tolosa-Hunt syndrome†
- Trauma (impaired consciousness, signs of injury)†
- Wernicke encephalopathy

*All may be unilateral.
†Pain may be present.

binocular horizontal diplopia at distance with full ductions, and at distance greater than near either a comitant eso-deviation of the eyes or an eso-deviation in primary position that becomes smaller in right and left gaze. Though previously thought to have the same localizing value as sixth nerve dysfunction, it is recognized now as a common cause of diplopia, typically in patients over 70 years of age, due to the *sagging eye syndrome* (Chaudhuri and Demer, 2013). Age-related involution (atrophy) of orbital connective tissue can cause "sagging" of the orbital pulleys (see earlier) and extraocular muscles, particularly affecting the lateral recti. Symmetrical involvement of the orbits causes divergence insufficiency and impaired elevation of both eyes; when it occurs asymmetrically, it causes a small angle hypertropia with excylotorsion of the contralateral eye (opposite to the excyclotorsion seen in the hypertropic eye with superior oblique weakness) and vertical diplopia. A similar process, the *heavy-eye syndrome*, may occur due to high myopia (Tan and Demer, 2015). Lesions at the level of the thalamus, midbrain, and cerebellum can all cause eso-deviations of the eyes, likely from effects related to the convergence system. Midbrain lesions can cause a pseudo–sixth nerve palsy with limitation of abduction of one eye and a consequent eso-deviation. The Duane syndrome is a congenital disorder of maldevelopment of the sixth cranial nerve (Gunduz et al., 2019). The most common form, type 1, involves impaired abduction associated with retraction of the eye and a narrowed palpebral fissure upon attempted abduction. Typically, patients with type 1 Duane syndrome do not have diplopia.

### Nuclear

See Chapter 21 for a more detailed description of anatomy and clinical conditions of the third (III, oculomotor), fourth (IV, trochlear), and sixth (VI, abducens) cranial nerve nuclei. The abducens nucleus contains two populations of motoneurons: those that innervate the ipsilateral lateral rectus for abduction and those that decussate in the pons and ascend in the contralateral medial longitudinal fasciculus (MLF) to the medial rectus for adduction to allow conjugate horizontal eye movements.

A lesion of the abducens nucleus produces paralysis of all ipsilateral versional eye movements. By example, a right abducens nucleus lesion results in right horizontal gaze palsy affecting all eye movements except convergence, as convergence signals do not travel in the MLF. Lesions of the bilateral abducens nucleus result in bilateral horizontal gaze palsies (i.e., loss of all horizontal eye movements, with spared ability to converge). With rare exceptions, lesions of the abducens nucleus that cause an acquired ipsilateral gaze palsy almost always involve the facial nerve fasciculus as it loops around the abducens nucleus and result in an associated facial nerve palsy.

**BOX 18.8 Causes of Chronic Ophthalmoplegia**

- Brainstem neoplasm
- Chronic ataxic neuropathy, ophthalmoplegia, monoclonal protein, cold agglutinins, and disialosyl antibodies (CANOMAD)
- Chronic basal meningitis (infection, sarcoid, or carcinoma)
- Chronic ophthalmoplegia with anti-GQ1b antibody
- Congenital extraocular muscle fibrosis
- Dysthyroidism
- Leigh disease
- Multiple sclerosis
- Myasthenia gravis
- Myopathies (e.g., mitochondrial, fiber-type disproportion (see Table 18.3)
- Nuclear, paranuclear, and supranuclear gaze palsies (see Table 18.3)

### Internuclear

***Internuclear ophthalmoplegia* (Video 18.3).** Damage to the medial longitudinal fasciculus (MLF) connecting the third and sixth cranial nerve nuclei impairs transmission of neural impulses from the abducens nucleus to the contralateral medial rectus muscle (see Fig. 18.6). This results in an *internuclear ophthalmoplegia* (INO) manifest as impaired adduction of the eye ipsilateral to the lesion, slowed adducting saccades in that eye, and abducting "nystagmus" upon abduction in the contralesional eye, which is an adaptive response (overshoot dysmetria) because the medial rectus muscle's weakness causes increased innervation to both itself and the yoked contralateral lateral rectus (the Hering law of dual innervation). Patching the eye with the abducting "nystagmus" can decrease the oscillation, supporting this hypothesis (Zee et al., 1987). Acutely, upward-beating nystagmus and torsional nystagmus (TN) may be present (Choi et al., 2012; Jeong et al., 2011). Convergence may be preserved with an INO, as signals for convergence of the medial rectus muscles are not carried in the MLF. Patients with bilateral INO may be exotropic, designated as the *wall-eyed bilateral INO* (WEBINO) *syndrome*, and have slow-abducting saccades because of impaired inhibition of tone in the medial recti. Other clinical features associated with unilateral INO include a partial contralateral ocular tilt reaction (OTR) (Choi et al., 2017 et al., 2017), manifest as a skew deviation with ipsilesional hypertropia (Zwergal et al., 2008), and defective vertical smooth pursuit, OKN, and vertical VORs.

A subtle INO is demonstrated by having the patient make repetitive horizontal saccades, which typically discloses slow adduction of the ipsilateral eye and may sometimes be the only sign of an INO. Alternatively, an optokinetic tape may be used to induce repetitive saccades in the direction of action of the suspected weak medial rectus muscle by moving the tape in the opposite direction and observing for slower and adducting saccades of smaller amplitude.

INO may occur with a variety of disorders (Box 18.9) affecting the brainstem, although demyelinating lesions in younger patients and ischemic lesions in older patients are most common. INO must be distinguished from the many (primarily peripheral infranuclear) causes of pseudo-INO (see Box 18.9).

Rarely, patients with small lesions in the rostral pons or midbrain, remote from the abducens nerve and nucleus, may have a Lutz posterior INO (also called INO of abduction [Kommerell, 1975]). In this condition, abduction is impaired, but the adducting eye has nystagmus. The mechanism is impaired inhibition of the antagonist medial rectus muscle secondary to damage to uncrossed fibers from the PPRF to the oculomotor nucleus, running close to but separate from the MLF. MG can mimic a Lutz posterior INO (Zheng and Lavin, 2018).

**BOX 18.9 Causes of Internuclear Ophthalmoplegia**

- Brainstem (pontine) stroke—unilateral
- Multiple sclerosis—unilateral or bilateral
- Intrinsic tumor—primary or metastatic
- Meningitis (especially tuberculosis, also acquired immunodeficiency syndrome, brucellosis, cystercosis, syphilis)
- Brainstem encephalitis (infective, inflammatory, lupus, paraneoplastic, sarcoid)
- Chemotherapy with radiation therapy
- Drug intoxication:
  - Comatose—anticonvulsants, phenothiazines, tricyclics
  - Awake—lithium
- Spinocerebellar degeneration
- Fabry disease (vascular)
- Herniation (epidural and acute and chronic subdural hemorrhage, cerebral hematoma)
- Vascular malformations
- Vasculitis
- Wernicke encephalopathy
- Progressive supranuclear palsy
- Syringobulbia associated with a Chiari malformation
- Trauma (closed head injury, neck/vertebral artery injury)
- Hexosaminidase A deficiency
- Kennedy disease (X-linked recessive progressive spinomuscular atrophy)
- Maple syrup urine disease
- Cerebral air embolism
- Vitamin $B_{12}$ deficiency
- Pseudointernuclear ophthalmoplegia
  - Long-standing exotropia
  - Myasthenia
  - Myotonic dystrophy
  - Neuromyotonia of the lateral rectus muscle
  - Partial palsy of cranial nerve III
  - Previous extraocular muscle surgery
  - Thyroid orbitopathy (lateral rectus restriction)
  - Orbital pseudotumor
  - Other infiltrative disorders of extraocular muscle (neoplasm, amyloid, etc.)
  - Miller Fisher syndrome (sometimes may be a true internuclear ophthalmoplegia)

### Supranuclear

#### *Brainstem*

**Saccadic gaze palsy** A number of congenital and acquired conditions—including degenerative, inflammatory, neoplastic and paraneoplastic, ischemic, metabolic, and hereditary conditions—can cause saccadic gaze palsies with slow saccades (see **Table 18.3**) (Lloyd-Smith Sequeira et al., 2017). Examination of the different functional classes of eye movements—specifically, saccades, smooth pursuit, and vestibular reflexes—helps to distinguish nuclear, paranuclear, and supranuclear gaze palsies. EBNs in the brainstem are located in the PPRF just rostral to the abducens nucleus (Horn, et al., 1995) for horizontal saccades and in the RIMLF in the midbrain (Horn and Büttner-Ennever, 1998) for vertical and torsional saccades. It follows that a lesion of the PPRF can cause a horizontal saccadic gaze palsy and a lesion in the RIMLF can cause a vertical and torsional saccadic gaze palsy. Thus the clinical hallmark of a supranuclear gaze palsy is disproportionate involvement of saccades, which classically is manifest as slow saccades with or without limitation of gaze. Eliciting OKN is helpful in identifying saccadic gaze palsies; also, as the quick phases of OKN are saccades and are lost in brainstem supranuclear gaze palsies. Smooth pursuit may be affected, but usually to a lesser extent than saccades. Vestibular eye movements are typically spared. In other words, any limitation in the range of eye movement seen with saccades or smooth pursuit should be overcome with vestibular stimulation. In contrast to supranuclear disorders, nuclear and infranuclear (extraocular muscle, neuromuscular junction, and cranial nerve) processes affect saccades, smooth pursuit, and vestibular reflexes equally. The caveat is that, with acute catastrophic lesions (ischemia or hemorrhage), supranuclear eye movement lesions may affect all classes of eye movements, but the deficits still tend to affect saccades most dramatically.

***Horizontal.*** A right PPRF lesion causes impaired conjugate gaze to the right (right eye abduction and left eye adduction). Acutely, gaze may be deviated contralaterally because of unopposed resting innervation from the intact left PPRF. Bilateral PPRF lesions result in absent horizontal gaze (or selective loss of saccades) (Video 18.4) and slowed vertical saccades (Hanson et al., 1986; Pierrot-Deseilligny et al., 1984; Slavin, 1986), as some vertical saccades are programmed in the PPRF and relayed to the midbrain via a juxta-MLF pathway, presumably to coordinate horizontal, vertical, and oblique trajectories as well as head movement.

***One-and-a-half syndrome.*** A lesion involving both the PPRF (or the abducens nucleus) and the crossed MLF (with decussated fibers that originated in the contralateral abducens nucleus) on one side of the pons causes the *one-and-a-half syndrome* (see Fig. 18.6 and Video 18.5). The PPRF lesion causes an ipsilateral horizontal gaze palsy and the MLF lesion causes an ipsilateral INO with impaired ipsilateral adduction (see earlier section on INO). The only horizontal eye movement that remains intact is abduction of the eye contralateral to the lesion; thus "one and a half" of the horizontal eye movements are impaired. Typically an exotropia (outward deviation of the eyes) is present. Also, some patients have a contralateral OTR (Zwergal et al., 2008); those with abducens nucleus, rather than PPRF involvement, have an accompanying facial nerve palsy and may develop oculopalatal myoclonus later, probably because of the proximity of the central tegmental tract to the facial nerve fascicle. MG can cause a pseudo–one-and-a-half syndrome.

***Vertical.*** Lesions of the RIMLF result in slowed or absent vertical saccades, especially when bilateral, with or without limitation in vertical gaze range. The RIMLF EBNs for upward saccades are likely caudal, ventral, and medial in the RIMLF and project to the elevator muscles (superior rectus and inferior oblique) bilaterally, with axons crossing within the oculomotor nucleus (Fig. 18.23) and not in the posterior commissure (PC), as previously thought (Bhidayasiri et al., 2000). The RIMLF EBNs for downward saccades are more rostral, dorsal, and lateral in the RIMLF and project only to the ipsilateral depressor muscles (inferior rectus and superior oblique) (see Fig. 18.23). Each RIMLF also projects only ipsilaterally for control of torsional saccades.

Given this anatomy, RIMLF lesions might be expected to have a more profound effect on downgaze. Bilateral RIMLF lesions cause either loss of downward saccades or of all vertical saccades. The effects of unilateral lesions are less well understood, as in theory they should cause only mild slowing of downward saccades and loss of torsional quick phases (saccade-like resetting movements seen with torsion VOR testing); however, a wide range of vertical gaze deficits are reported with unilateral RIMLF involvement. Deficits from RIMLF lesions tend to affect the eyes conjugately, as each RIMLF sends signals to vertical eye muscles for each eye. However, unilateral (or monocular) vertical gaze palsies are occasionally seen.

Two forms of the vertical one-and-a-half syndrome occur with discrete lesions in the upper midbrain. One, which consists of bilateral upgaze palsy associated with monocular paresis of downward movement, can occur with either ipsilateral or contralateral thalamomesencephalic infarction. The other consists of a downgaze palsy associated with monocular elevator paresis that can occur with bilateral mesodiencephalic lesions. A crossed vertical gaze paresis, with supranuclear weakness of elevation of the contralateral eye and weakness of depression of the ipsilateral eye, may occur with a lesion involving the mesodiencephalic junction and medial thalamus.

Monocular elevator deficiency, also termed *monocular elevator palsy* or *double elevator palsy*, is characterized by limitation of elevation of one eye. The limitation is the same in both adduction and abduction, unlike the Brown superior oblique tendon sheath syndrome, in which the limitation is predominantly in adduction. This can result from a lesion either in supranuclear or infranuclear structures (Gauntt et al., 1995; Jampel and Fells, 1968), such as paretic or restrictive disorders of the extraocular muscles, orbital floor fractures, myasthenia, and fascicular lesions of the oculomotor nerve. When monocular elevator deficiency is congenital or occurs early in life, it may be associated with abnormalities of convergence, amblyopia, a chin-up head position, and ptosis or pseudoptosis (pseudoptosis occurs when a patient with a hypotropic eye fixates with the other eye; the upper lid follows the hypotropic eye and appears ptotic. When the patient fixates with the hypotropic eye, the apparent ptosis disappears. Some patients may have both a true ptosis and a superimposed pseudoptosis). Some congenital cases are supranuclear because of congenital unilateral midbrain lesions; when they are of long standing, inferior rectus restriction and fibrosis prevent reflex elevation of the eye (the Bell phenomenon). In those cases, primary orbital disorders such as myositis, thyroid orbitopathy, orbital floor fractures, and infiltrative disease must be excluded. Corrective surgery is helpful. Acquired supranuclear monocular elevator palsy results in limitation of elevation of one eye on attempted upgaze despite intact downgaze and orthotropia in primary position (unlike patients with monocular elevator deficiency, who have an abnormal head posture). This rare condition occurs with unilateral vascular or neoplastic lesions involving either the ipsilateral or contralateral midbrain. Usually the affected eye can be elevated in response to vestibular stimulation, and ptosis is usually absent. When asymmetrical, the sagging eye syndrome (see earlier section titled "Mimics" [of cranial nerve disorders]) can cause impaired elevation of one eye that cannot be overcome by vestibular stimulation.

Acute-onset vertical gaze palsy is due most often to midbrain infarction. The RIMLF is supplied by the thalamic-subthalamic paramedian artery, which originates from the posterior cerebral artery (PCA) at the bifurcation of the basilar artery and the PCAs. A single thalamic-subthalamic paramedian (the artery of Percheron) artery supplies both RIMLF in roughly 20% of people (Lasjaunias et al., 2000), making bilateral RIMLF lesions possible from a single vessel infarct (Matheus and Castillo, 2003). Disorders of vertical gaze, particularly downgaze and combined upgaze and downgaze paresis, may be overlooked in patients with brainstem vascular disease because of impaired consciousness due to concomitant damage to the reticular activating system.

The classic cause of chronic progressive vertical saccadic slowing is progressive supranuclear palsy (PSP), a neurodegenerative tauopathy causing rapid deterioration with early falls, akinetic-rigid parkinsonism, and swallowing difficulty. The hallmark feature is slowing of

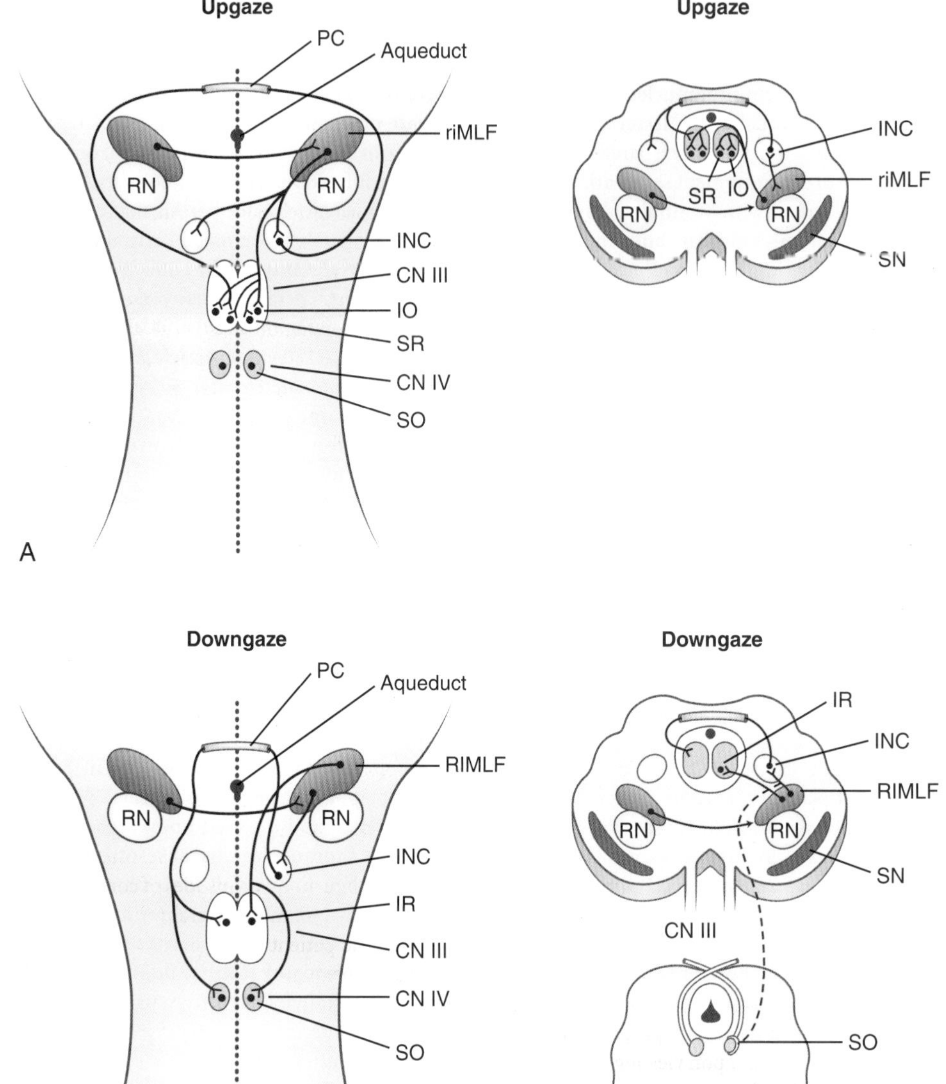


**Fig. 18.23 Hypothetical Pathways Involved in Controlling Vertical Eye Movements. A,** Upward eye movements. Burst neurons for upward saccades are shown projecting from the medial rostral interstitial nucleus of the medial longitudinal fasciculus *(RIMLF)* to the elevator muscles, superior recti, and inferior obliques bilaterally, with axons crossing within the oculomotor nucleus. **B,** Burst neurons for downward saccades are shown projecting only to the ipsilateral depressor muscles, the inferior rectus, and the superior oblique. The axons of the burst neurons for upward saccades also project to the interstitial nucleus of Cajal *(INC)*, which plays a role in neural integration for vertical and torsional gaze. From the INC, the axons project dorsally and laterally to cross in the posterior commissure before turning ventrally to the oculomotor and trochlear nerve nuclei. *CN III,* Third nerve nuclear complex; *CN IV,* fourth nerve nucleus; *IO,* inferior oblique subnucleus; *IR,* inferior rectus subnucleus; *PC,* posterior commissure; *RN,* red nucleus; *SN,* substantia nigra; *SO,* superior oblique nucleus; *SR,* superior rectus subnucleus *(Redrawn from Bhidayasiri, R., Plant, G.T., Leigh, R.J., 2000. A hypothetical scheme for the brainstem control of vertical gaze. Neurology 54, 1985–1993.)*

vertical saccades early in the disease. A common clinical misconception is that downward saccades are impaired more than upward saccades early in the disease (Chen et al., 2010); however, slowing of both downward and upward saccades is common and limitation of upward gaze is more common than that of downward gaze (Chen et al., 2010). Early in the disease course, horizontal saccades are slowed also, but much less than vertical. Late in the disease course, saccades and smooth pursuit may be lost both vertically and horizontally, although VOR still tends to overcome the range limitations. In end-stage disease, even the VOR is lost.

*A pseudo-PSP syndrome*, characterized by a selective saccadic palsy (sometimes associated with ataxia, dysarthria, and dysphagia) that progresses over several months can follow aortic or cardiac surgery under hypothermic circulatory arrest, usually with a normal MRI (Bernat and Lukovits, 2004; Solomon et al., 2008). Injury to the EBNs or their supporting perineural net structures in the PPRF is likely

**BOX 18.10 Features of Spasm of the Near Reflex (Psychogenic)**

- Near tetrad:
  - Convergence
  - Miosis
  - Accommodation (blur at distance, myopia by retinoscopy)
  - Excyclotorsion (extorsion)
- Neurasthenic symptoms
- Blepharoclonus (frequent blink rate)
- Poor cooperation in other motor tasks
- Obstructive behavior (e.g., closing eyes, or not responding to commands such as "look to the right" despite being observed to do so during the interview)
- Other behavioral changes (e.g., tunnel vision)
- May disappear with rapid saccades
- Full range of eye movement:
  - With pursuit of own hand
  - With one eye covered
  - Doll's eyes with fixation
- Ice-cold calorics:
  - Normal response
  - Bizarre behavioral response
- Normal optokinetic nystagmus if patient encouraged or distracted (e.g., count stripes)
- Demeanor:
  - Affective disorder
  - Tinted glasses or sunglasses

(Eggers et al., 2015). The delayed progression of this syndrome remains unexplained but may represent a form of decelerated apoptosis.

***Dorsal midbrain syndrome.*** The features of the dorsal midbrain syndrome (the Parinaud syndrome) (Video 18.6) include a supranuclear saccadic upgaze palsy, convergence-retraction "nystagmus" (often elicited by attempted upgaze), lid retraction (Collier sign), and pupillary light-near dissociation (pupillary constriction upon viewing a near target but not with direct light testing). Pineal region tumors, ischemic stroke, hemorrhage, and decompensated hydrocephalus are common etiologies.

The EBNs for vertical saccades also project to the INC, which plays a major role in neural integration for vertical and torsional gaze (Bhidayasiri et al., 2000). From the INC, the pathways project dorsally and laterally to cross in the PC before turning ventrally to the oculomotor and trochlear nerve nuclei (see Fig. 18.23). The axons to the elevator muscles travel more dorsally and thus are more susceptible to extrinsic compression, as often occurs with the dorsal midbrain syndrome. Convergence-retraction nystagmus is not a true nystagmus as it lacks slow phases or drifts (see section titled "Nystagmus," later), but a rapid dysmetric horizontal eye movement induced by attempted upward saccades. This is assessed clinically by having the patient look at an OKN tape moving downward in an attempt to induce upward saccades. Rapid convergence with synchronous retraction of both globes caused by simultaneous cocontraction of the extraocular muscles is followed by a slow divergent movement. Less commonly, if lateral rectus innervation is dominant, a rapid divergent movement occurs initially. The pupillary light-near dissociation occurs because the light reflex pathways are more superficial. In contrast, intrinsic midbrain lesions cause impairment of convergence and accommodation (the near reflex) while sparing the light reflex.

**Vergence deficits** Disorders of vergence include convergence insufficiency, convergence spasm, and divergence insufficiency. *Convergence insufficiency* is most commonly seen clinically as a benign, often self-limited condition in children or as an acquired deficit after traumatic head injury or with parkinsonian disorders. Occasionally it is seen as an isolated phenomenon in adults without neurological illness. Convergence is very dependent on effort, so repeated examination to ensure maximum effort is important. Symptoms include words running together when reading; frank binocular horizontal diplopia at near; and vague symptoms such as eyestrain, headache, and burning eyes that are often associated with asthenopia. Examination signs of convergence insufficiency include a reduced near point of convergence (inability to convergence the eyes to within a few centimeters of the nose), an exophoria with near fixation larger than any exophoria with distance fixation, and low convergence amplitudes (inability to fuse an image at near with base-out prisms placed in front of one eye). Orthoptic exercises (pencil push-ups) (Rucker and Phillips, 2018), reading glasses with base-in prisms, and myopic correction are useful in management.

Central disruption of fusion, or posttraumatic fusion deficiency, can occur after moderate head injury and causes intractable diplopia despite the patient's ability to fuse intermittently and, even briefly, achieve stereopsis. The diplopia fluctuates and varies between crossed, uncrossed, and vertical. Versions and ductions may be full, but vergence amplitudes are greatly reduced. Prism therapy or surgery is ineffective, but an eye patch or centrally frosted lens may provide symptomatic relief. The location of injury is presumed to be in the midbrain. Also, central disruption of fusion is reported with brainstem tumors, stroke, following removal of long-standing cataracts, uncorrected aphakia, and neurosurgical procedures. This condition must be distinguished from bilateral fourth cranial nerve palsies, when diplopia is constant and associated with cyclodiplopia and excyclotropia (>10 degrees) and also from psychogenic disorders of vergence.

*Convergence spasm*, or spasm of the near reflex, is a disorder characterized by intermittent episodes of convergence, miosis, and accommodation. It may mimic bilateral (and occasionally unilateral) abducens paresis. The patient may complain of double or blurred vision and is esotropic, particularly at distance; however, prominent miosis is the clue, as is variability in the exam over time (i.e., one moment there appears to be an abduction defect and the next moment it is gone). Spasm of the near reflex is reported in patients with organic disorders but is more commonly psychogenic, either in patients with conversion reactions or in anxious patients in whom the "spasm" is a manifestation of misdirected effort. The differential diagnosis is that of esotropia (see Box 18.3). Miosis on gaze testing generally establishes the diagnosis but can be difficult to discern. Accommodative esotropia and latent hyperopia must be excluded by obtaining a cycloplegic refraction. Patients with psychogenic spasm of the near reflex often have associated somatic complaints and obstructionist behavior such as blepharoclonus on lateral gaze and poor cooperation in performing motor tasks such as smiling, opening the mouth, and protruding the tongue (features of neurasthenia and asthenopia) (Box 18.10). Management should focus on identifying the source of the psychopathology and may require psychiatric evaluation. Strategies such as the use of cycloplegia (homatropine eye drops) to prevent accommodative spasm, thus inhibiting the near triad, may be helpful.

*Divergence insufficiency* is characterized by esotropia that is either comitant or reduced in lateral gaze and uncrossed horizontal diplopia at distance in the absence of other neurological symptoms or signs. The esotropia may be intermittent or constant, but the patients can fuse at near. Versions and ductions are full, and saccadic velocities, if measured quantitatively, appear normal. The origin of divergence insufficiency is unclear, but it may result from a break in fusion in an individual with a congenital esophoria usually coming on later in life; it also occurs in patients with midline cerebellar disease. The condition is easily treated with base-out prisms for the distance correction

**Eye position during head tilt**

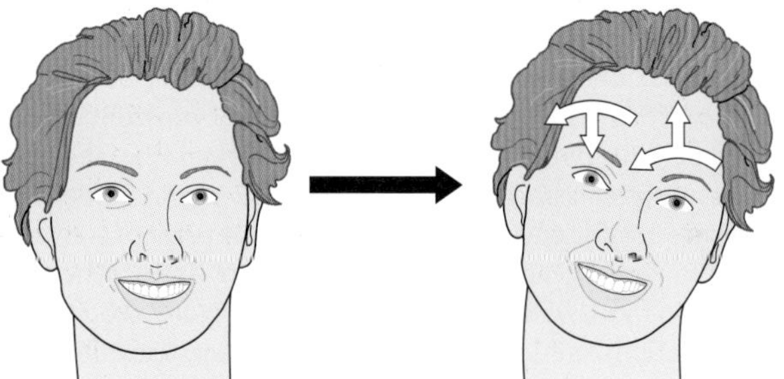

Normal ocular counter-rolling reflex

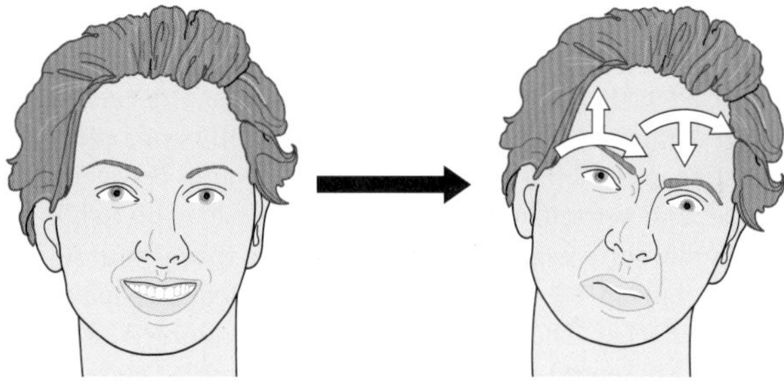

Ocular tilt reaction

**Fig. 18.24** **A,** Normal ocular counter-rolling phenomenon during head tilt. **B,** Ocular tilt reaction consists of spontaneous skew deviation, cyclotorsion of both eyes (upper poles rotated toward lower eye), paradoxical head tilting, and displacement of the subjective visual vertical toward the side of the lower eye. *(From Lavin, P.J.M., Donahue, S.P., 2013. Disorders of supranuclear control of ocular motility. In: Yanoff, M., Duker, J.S. [Eds.], Ophthalmology, fourth ed. Elsevier.)*

and rarely requires extraocular muscle surgery. Divergence insufficiency in the elderly occurs with the sagging eye syndrome (see earlier); it is recognized by the associated signs of involutional changes such as ptosis and/or elevated upper lid creases, superior sulcus enlargement, deformity, or baggy eyelids; it is differentiated from divergence insufficiency of neurogenic origin by the absence of nystagmus, saccadic dysmetria, and ataxia.

Divergence paralysis, a controversial entity that may be difficult to distinguish from divergence insufficiency, usually occurs in the context of a severe head injury or other cause of raised intracranial pressure. Such patients have horizontal diplopia at distance; however, quantitatively, in contrast to divergence insufficiency, abducting saccades are slow. Patients with bilateral palsies of the sixth cranial nerve who recover gradually may go through a phase in which the esotropia becomes comitant with full ductions, mimicking divergence paralysis. Divergence paralysis can also occur with Miller Fisher syndrome, Chiari malformations, pontine tumors, and excessive sedation from drugs.

**Ocular tilt reaction and skew deviation** In normal circumstances, a synkinetic movement, ocular counter-rolling, allows people to maintain horizontal orientation of the environment while tilting the head to either side (**Fig.** 18.24, *A*). When the head is tilted to the left, the left eye rises and intorts as the right eye falls and extorts within the range of the ocular tilt reflex (approximately 10 degrees from the vertical). The initial transient dynamic (phasic) counter-rolling response results from stimulation of the semicircular canals, whereas the sustained (tonic) response is mediated by the otolith organs and holds the eyes in their new position. Lesions of these pathways result in an inappropriate OTR and skew deviation.

The OTR consists of spontaneous skew deviation, cyclotorsion of both eyes (the upper poles rotated toward the lower eye), paradoxical head tilting (see Fig. 18.24, *B*), and displacement of the subjective visual vertical, all toward the side of the lower eye. A tonic (sustained) OTR occurs with a prenuclear (i.e., supranuclear) lesion causing imbalance in the otolithic (gravireceptive) pathways to the ocular motor system anywhere along the pathway from the ipsilateral utricle, vestibular nerve, nuclei, or the contralateral MLF, contralateral INC, to the medial thalamus. A phasic (paroxysmal) OTR occurs with a lesion, such as a cavernoma, in the region of the INC, and may respond to baclofen or carbamazepine (Rodriguez et al., 2009). An OTR can be induced by sound in patients with perilymph fistulas of the vestibular end organ (the Tullio phenomenon). A partial OTR in which there is no head tilt or there is merely ocular torsion, can occur with lesions of the cerebellar nodulus and uvula. This is attributed to an increase in the tonic resting activity of secondary otolithic neurons in the ipsilesional vestibular nucleus because of loss of inhibition from the injured nodulus. A contralateral OTR occurs in individuals with INO and those with the one-and-a-half syndrome (Zwergal et al., 2008).

A variant of the OTR, characterized by the alternating tonic conjugate ocular torsion that accompanies congenital ocular motor apraxia (COMA), occurs in Joubert syndrome. The eyes rotate, cycling every 10 to 15 seconds, with torsional amplitudes of 30 to 45 degrees in each direction. Affected individuals may have an intermittent skew deviation with intermittent head tilting. Neuroimaging demonstrates superior cerebellar hypoplasia, with elongation of the superior cerebellar peduncles producing a *molar tooth sign* (Papanagnu et al., 2014).

*Skew deviation* is a vertical divergence of the ocular axes caused by a prenuclear asymmetry of ascending utricular input to the cranial nerve nuclei serving vertical eye movements. Lesions causing skew are typically in the brainstem or cerebellum, involving the vertical vestibulo-ocular pathways; occasionally they occur peripherally in the vestibular nerve or end organ. Skew deviation is particularly common with vascular lesions of the pons or lateral medulla (Wallenberg syndrome). A skew deviation is usually but not always comitant; when incomitant, it may mimic a partial third cranial nerve or a fourth cranial nerve palsy. Dieterich and Brandt demonstrated ocular torsion of one or both eyes associated with subjective tilting of the visual vertical toward the lower eye in most patients with skew deviations (Dieterich and Brandt, 1993). With lesions caudal to the lower pons, the ipsilateral eye is lower (ipsiversive skew); but with lesions rostral to the midpontine level, the contralateral eye is lower (contraversive skew). Ocular torsion may be present without a vertical deviation and, in either situation, can be detected by blind spot mapping, indirect ophthalmoscopy, fundus photography, double Maddox rod test, or settings of the visual vertical.

**Lateropulsion** Saccadic lateropulsion is characterized by hypermetric (overshoot) saccades (**Fig.** 18.25, *B*) to the side of the lesion (ipsipulsion) and hypometric (undershoot) saccades (see Fig. 18.25, *C*) to the opposite side. In darkness or with the eyelids closed, the patient may have conjugate deviation toward the side of the lesion (ipsipulsion). Saccadic lateropulsion occurs with lesions of the lateral medulla (most commonly ischemic) involving cerebellar inflow (inferior cerebellar peduncle). Saccadic lateropulsion with a bias away from the side of the lesion (contrapulsion) may occur with lesions involving the region of the superior cerebellar peduncle (outflow tract) and adjacent cerebellum (superior cerebellar artery territory). Pulsion of vertical saccades with a parabolic trajectory occurs in patients with lateral medullary injury: both upward and downward saccades deviate toward the side of the lesion with corrective oblique saccades; whereas

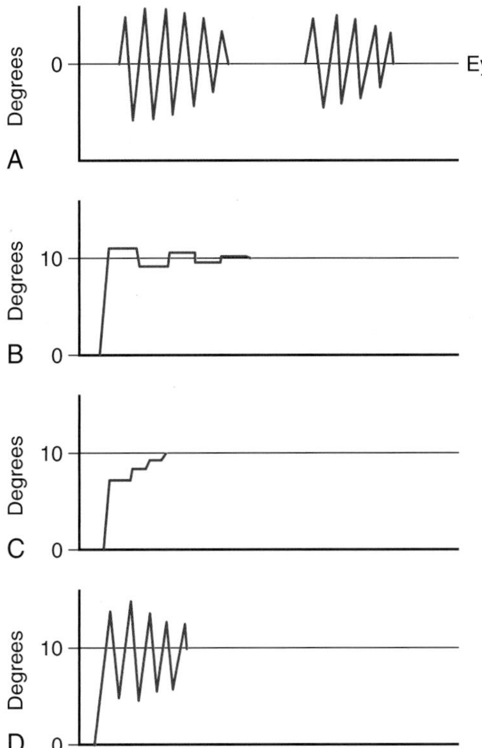


**Fig. 18.25 Oculographic Diagrams of Waveforms in Various Non-nystagmus Oscillations. A,** Spontaneous ocular flutter in primary position. **B,** Overshoot dysmetria (hypermetria). **C,** Undershoot dysmetria (hypometria). **D,** Flutter dysmetria exacerbated by refixation of 1–10 degrees.

in those with lesions involving cerebellar outflow, vertical saccades deviate away from the side of the injury.

***Cerebellum.*** Several eye movement abnormalities or combinations thereof strongly suggest a cerebellar localization. Some of these are mentioned in the earlier discussion, such as impaired smooth pursuit, eso-deviations and divergence weakness, and skew deviations. Cerebellar forms of nystagmus are covered later, in the section titled "Nystagmus."

The cerebellum coordinates the ocular motor system to drive the eyes smoothly and accurately and is supplied richly by afferent fibers conveying ocular information (e.g., velocity, position, neural integration) from the vestibular system, the afferent visual system, the PPRF, and the MRF. The dorsal vermis and fastigial nuclei determine the accuracy of saccades by modulating saccadic amplitude; also, they adjust the innervation to each eye selectively to ensure precise conjugate movements. Lesions of the dorsal vermis and fastigial nuclei result in saccadic dysmetria (often, overshoot dysmetria that is greater centripetally), macrosaccadic oscillations (MSO) (see the section titled "Saccadic Intrusions," further on), and disorders of vergence (see the section titled "Vergence deficits").

Selective cerebellar lesions have differential effects on eye movements. Bilateral lesions of the fastigial and globose (interpositus) nuclei cause hypermetria of externally triggered saccades but do not affect internally triggered saccades. Bilateral lesions of the posterior vermis (lobules VI and VII) cause hypometric horizontal and vertical saccades and impaired pursuit. Unilateral lesions of the posterior vermis cause hypometric ipsilateral and hypermetric contralateral saccades, whereas unilateral lesions of the caudal fastigial nucleus cause hypermetric ipsilateral and hypometric contralateral saccades.

The flocculus, part of the vestibulocerebellum, is responsible for matching the saccadic pulse and step appropriately and for stabilizing images on the fovea. It adjusts the output of the NI and participates in long-term adaptive processing to ensure that eye movements remain appropriate to the stimulus. For example, the amplitude (gain) and even the direction of the slow phases of the VOR are adjusted by the flocculus. Lesions of the flocculus result in gaze-holding deficits such as gaze-evoked, rebound, and downbeat nystagmus (see the section titled "Nystagmus," later). Floccular lesions also impair smooth pursuit, cancelation (suppression) of the VOR by the pursuit system during combined head and eye tracking, and the ability to suppress nystagmus (and vertigo) by fixation. The nodulus, also part of the vestibulocerebellum, influences vestibular eye movements and vestibular optokinetic interaction. Lesions of the nodulus in monkeys and humans produce periodic alternating nystagmus (PAN) (see the section titled "Nystagmus," later).

A specific form of skew deviation, called *alternating skew deviation on lateral gaze,* in which the hypertropia changes sides (i.e., right hyper on right gaze, left hyper on left gaze), often results from lesions affecting the cerebellar pathways or cervicomedullary junction. This is probably the result of asymmetrical vestibular input to the yoked superior oblique and contralateral inferior rectus muscles (see Table 18.2) because of increased central otolithic tone for downgaze. Skew deviation that alternates between up- and downgaze can occur with spinocerebellar degeneration. Congenital superior oblique overaction causes an A-pattern exotropia (eyes diverge on downgaze) and an abducting hypertropia on lateral gaze; often it is associated with disorders of the posterior fossa, such as hydrocephalus, meningomyelocele, and Chiari II malformations. Congenital inferior oblique overaction causes a V-pattern esotropia (eyes converge or cross on downgaze) and is otherwise benign. Bilateral fourth cranial nerve palsies may mimic gaze-dependent alternating skew, in which the adducting eye is hypertropic; however, diplopia is worse on downgaze, with significant excyclotorsion and a V-pattern esotropia.

Cerebellar lesions can impact torsional eye movements. Pathological rapid torsional eye deviation during voluntary saccades may occur with large lesions involving the midline cerebellum, deep cerebellar nuclei, and dorsolateral medulla. The amplitudes of these torsional saccades ("blips") are larger for ipsilesional (hypermetric) than for contralesional (hypometric) horizontal saccades. Eye movement recordings using a scleral search coil (see the section titled "Recording of Eye Movements," further on) demonstrated that the blips are followed by an exponentially slow torsional drift toward the initial torsional eye position. These blips may be a form of torsional saccadic dysmetria.

### Cortex

**Horizontal gaze deviations** Transient gaze deviation, usually of the head and eyes, occurs in about 20% of patients with acute hemisphere stroke and other insults. Because of gaze paresis to the hemiplegic side (i.e., paralyses of gaze and limbs are on the same side), the eyes are deviated toward the side of the lesion (ipsiversive gaze deviation), which may be seen on imaging studies performed at presentation. With stroke, right-sided lesions are more common but smaller; consequently, patients with left-sided lesions (gaze deviation to the left) have a worse prognosis. Ipsiversive gaze deviation occurs more often when the inferior parietal lobule (IPL) or circuits between the FEF and the IPL or their projections to the brainstem (superior colliculus or PPRF) are involved; the FEF usually are spared. After about 5 days, the intact hemisphere, which contains neurons for bilateral gaze, takes over. Thereafter, subtle abnormalities such as prolonged saccadic latencies and impaired saccadic suppression can be detected only by quantitative oculography. Bilateral lesions of the frontomesencephalic pathways cause loss of horizontal saccades in both directions and impair vertical saccades (particularly upward) but spare pursuit, VORs, and the slow phases of OKN.

Conjugate eye deviation to the "wrong" side—that is, away from the lesion and toward the hemiplegia (contraversive gaze deviation)—may occur with supratentorial lesions, particularly thalamic lesions, such as hemorrhage, and (rarely) large perisylvian or lobar hemorrhage. The mechanism is unclear, but possibilities include the following:

1. An irritative or seizure focus causing "contraversive ocular deviation" is unlikely, because neither clinical nor electrical seizure activity is reported in these patients.
2. Because eye movements are represented bilaterally in each frontal lobe, it is conceivable that the center for ipsilateral gaze alone may be damaged, resulting in contraversive ocular deviation.
3. An irritative lesion of the intralaminar thalamic neurons, which discharge for contralateral saccades, could theoretically cause contraversive ocular deviation.
4. Damage to the contralateral inhibitory center could be responsible also.

Postictal "paralytic" conjugate ocular deviation occurs after adversive seizures as part of a Todd paresis. Spasticity of conjugate gaze (lateral deviation of both eyes away from the lesion) during forced eyelid closure can occur in patients with large, deep parietotemporal lesions; eye movements are otherwise normal except for ipsilateral saccadic pursuit. Psychogenic ocular deviation can occur in patients feigning unconsciousness; the eyes are directed toward the ground irrespective of which way the patient is turned.

**Ocular motor apraxia** *Ocular motor apraxia (OMA)* is the inability to perform voluntary eye movements, including saccades and smooth pursuit, while spontaneous saccades and reflexive eye movements (vestibular and OKN fast and slow phases) are preserved. Individuals with OMA often utilize head thrusting or blinking behaviors to initiate eye movements. OMA represents a type of supranuclear gaze palsy that can be congenital or acquired and that is distinct etiologically, mechanistically, and on examination from brainstem supranuclear saccadic gaze palsies. Acquired forms generally localize to either bifrontal or biparietal lesions and occur with illness such as posterior cortical atrophy, corticobasal degeneration, and others (see Table 18.3). OMA is a component of the triad of the Balint syndrome, which also includes simultanagnosia (ability to see components of a visual scene but not the cohesive scene) and optic ataxia (impaired visually guided limb movements).

*Spasm of fixation*, a term introduced by Gordon Holmes in 1930, describes patients who have difficulty shifting visual attention because of impaired initiation of voluntary saccades when looking at a fixation target but are capable of normal initiation of saccades in the absence of such a target or when it is removed. Their saccades have a prolonged latency and may be hypometric in the presence of a central visual target; however, blinks or combined eye and head movements may sometimes facilitate normal saccades. Holmes stressed that fixation was an active process and attributed spasm of fixation to "exaggerated" fixation; evidence from other studies supports this concept. The lesions that cause spasm of fixation may be bihemispheric and interrupt indirect FEF projections via the caudate nucleus and substantia nigra reticularis to the superior colliculus. Normally, during saccades to auditory, visual, and remembered targets, neurons in the FEFs discharge via these pathways and disinhibit the superior colliculus to allow the saccades and disengage fixation. Interruption of these and perhaps other pathways might contribute to spasm of fixation by maintaining tonic inhibitory suppression of saccades by the SC (Leigh and Zee, 2015).

*Congenital ocular motor apraxia* is more common in boys than in girls and is characterized by impaired voluntary horizontal pursuit and saccadic movements but preservation of vertical eye movements; reflex saccades may be retained partly. Because random eye movements also are absent in many of these children, the term *apraxia* is strictly incorrect; *congenital saccadic palsy* or *congenital gaze palsy* is more accurate, but the term *COMA* is now established in the literature. By 4 to 8 months of age, the child develops a thrusting head movement strategy, often with prominent blinking, to overcome the eye movement deficit. Because the VOR prevents a change in direction of gaze on head turning, the child closes the eyes to reduce the degree of reflex eye movement (the gain of the VOR falls with the eyes closed) while thrusting the head beyond the range of the VOR arc to bring the eyes in line with the target. Then, with the eyes open, the child slowly straightens the head while the contralateral VOR maintains fixation. Some patients may use dynamic head thrusts to facilitate saccadic eye movements or reflexively to induce fast phases of vestibular nystagmus.

Because children with COMA cannot easily refixate or pursue new targets, particularly in the first 6 months of life, before they develop the head-thrusting strategy, they are sometimes misdiagnosed as being blind. After 6 months of age, children with COMA present because of the head thrusts. The diagnosis of COMA can be confirmed by demonstrating the inability to make saccades; this is most easily done by spinning the infant. In normal infants, the eyes tonically deviate in the same direction as head movement; persistent absence of reflex saccades (fast phases in the opposite direction) after 2 to 3 weeks of age is abnormal and indicates saccadic palsy. As children with COMA reach school age, pursuit and voluntary saccades improve variably. However, the condition does not resolve completely and can be detected in adulthood. COMA may be associated with structural abnormalities (Box 18.11) and occasionally strabismus, psychomotor developmental delay (particularly reading and expressive language ability), clumsiness, and gait disturbances. COMA may be familial.

Congenital vertical ocular motor apraxia is rare and must be differentiated from metabolic and degenerative disorders that cause progressive neurological dysfunction (e.g., neurovisceral lipidosis) and from stable disorders such as birth injury, perinatal hypoxia, and Leber congenital amaurosis.

*Early-onset ataxia with ocular motor apraxia and hypoalbuminemia (EAOH)*, an autosomal recessive disorder described in Japanese families, presents in childhood and is associated with progressive ataxia with marked cerebellar atrophy on imaging, horizontal and vertical OMA, a peripheral neuropathy with early areflexia and late distal wasting and weakness, and hypoalbuminemia. Some patients have foot deformities, kyphoscoliosis, choreiform movements, facial grimacing, and exaggerated blinking (perhaps to initiate saccades). When the condition is advanced, external ophthalmoplegia can mask the saccadic failure. This disorder is associated with hypercholesterolemia and mimics Friedreich ataxia; patients with EAOH have OMA, chorea, and intention tremor but not extensor plantar responses or cardiomyopathy. Leg edema correlates with the degree of albumen; the *pseudo*hypercholesterolemia resolves with replacement of albumen. EAOH is likely a variant of autosomal recessive ataxia with ocular motor apraxia (AOA), described next. Both disorders have missense mutations in the aprataxin *(APTX)* gene.

*Ataxia with ocular motor apraxia*, an autosomal recessive disorder described in Portuguese families, presents in early childhood and is associated with cerebellar ataxia, horizontal and vertical OMA, and very early areflexia that later progresses to a full-blown axonal neuropathy. Some patients have pes cavus, scoliosis, dystonia, and optic atrophy. In advanced cases, external ophthalmoplegia can mask the saccadic failure, as in EAOH. AOA resembles ataxia telangiectasia but without the telangiectasia, developmental delay, and immune dysfunction. It is very similar to ataxia with ocular motor apraxia type 1 (AOA1) syndrome.

**BOX 18.11 Disorders Associated with Ocular Motor Apraxia**

- Aicardi syndrome
- Aplasia or hypoplasia of the corpus callosum
- Aplasia or hypoplasia of the cerebellar vermis (up to 53% of patients)
- Ataxia with "ocular motor" apraxia type I syndrome
- Ataxia telangiectasia
- Autosomal recessive AOA associated with axonal peripheral neuropathy, areflexia, and pes cavus (may be the same as EOAH)
- Bardet-Biedl syndrome
- Bilateral cerebral cortical lesions
- Birth injuries (see perinatal/postnatal disorders)
- Carbohydrate-deficient glycoprotein syndrome type Ia
- Carotid fibromuscular hypoplasia
- Cockayne syndrome
- COMA (occasionally may be familial)
- Congenital vertical ocular motor apraxia (rare)
- Cornelia de Lange syndrome
- Dandy-Walker malformation
- EOAH (may be the same disorder as AOA)
- GM1 gangliosidosis
- Hydrocephalus
- Infantile Gaucher disease
- Infantile Refsum disease
- Joubert syndrome
- Krabbe leukodystrophy
- Leber congenital amaurosis
- Megalocephaly
- Microcephaly
- Microphthalmos
- Neurovisceral lipidosis (e.g., Niemann-Pick type C)
- Occipital porencephalic cysts
- Pelizaeus-Merzbacher disease
- Perinatal and postnatal disorders (hypoxia, meningitis, PV leukomalacia, athetoid cerebral palsy, perinatal septicemia and anemia, herpes encephalitis, epilepsy)
- Propionic acidemia
- Succinic semialdehyde dehydrogenase deficiency
- Wieacker syndrome

*AOA*, Ataxia with ocular motor apraxia; *COMA*, congenital ocular motor apraxia; *EOAH*, early-onset ataxia with ocular motor apraxia and hypoalbuminemia; *PV*, periventricular.

*Ataxia with ocular motor apraxia type 1*, a late-onset autosomal recessive neurodegenerative form with progressive ataxia and peripheral neuropathy, can mimic ataxia telangiectasia but without the extraneurological features (Criscuolo et al., 2004). It is associated with mutations of the *APTX* gene. *Ataxia with ocular apraxia type 2 (AOA2)*, a juvenile-onset autosomal recessive disorder, is a slowly progressive cerebellar ataxia characterized by cerebellar atrophy and a sensorimotor neuropathy. Almost all patients have elevated serum alpha-fetoprotein levels, but OMA is observed in only 47% of patients (Asaka et al., 2006). Thus the disease name, AOA2, could be misleading. The responsible gene (*SETX*) maps to chromosome 9q34.

## Treatment of Diplopia

Patching (occlusive) therapy is used to eliminate one image, mainly during the acute phase of diplopia. In children younger than age 6, each eye should be patched alternately to prevent developmental amblyopia. Such young patients should be under the care of an experienced ophthalmologist, with regular follow-up evaluations. Adults may wear the patch over whichever eye is more comfortable, although some clinicians feel that alternating the patch reduces the incidence of contractures. An excellent method of patching utilizes spectacles. If the patient does not wear glasses, an inexpensive pair of plano (nonprescription plain lenses) glasses or sunglasses can be used. Options include clip-on occluders that can be switched from lens to lens or placement of frosted plastic tape on one lens. The use of tape also allows the option of partial occlusion, which can be very useful in selected cases. For example, if fusion can be obtained at distance but diplopia occurs with reading, occlusion of the lower portion of a bifocal lens often works well.

Prisms are helpful in eliminating double vision if the deviation is not too great. A reasonable range of binocular single vision may be achieved with prisms provided that the individual's expectations are not too high and there is no significant cyclodeviation.

Botulinum toxin injections into selected eye muscles is used with mixed success in patients with both comitant and incomitant strabismus. It may be helpful in patients with acute abducens palsies, particularly if they are bilateral and traumatic in origin. This treatment should be performed only by an ophthalmologist experienced in orbital injections. The main drawbacks are the variability and transience of effect and complications. The most common untoward effects are ptosis, dry-eye problems, and worsening diplopia. As a rule, the beneficial effects wear off in 3 to 4 months.

Extraocular muscle surgery can correct long-standing strabismus (comitant or noncomitant). Generally a period of at least 6 months of stable ocular alignment measures is required for consideration of surgery.

Finally, orthoptic exercises are of use in patients with convergence insufficiency.

# DISORDERS OF EYE MOVEMENTS—ABNORMAL SPONTANEOUS MOVEMENTS AND OSCILLATIONS

## Approach to History and Examination

The main forms of abnormal spontaneous eye movements include nystagmus, which may be congenital or acquired, and saccadic intrusions. Often, congenital nystagmus is asymptomatic and rarely causes oscillopsia (a subjective sense of visual motion). The physician should determine whether the nystagmus was present since birth or is acquired and whether there is a family history or a history of amblyopia or lazy eye. A list of current medications should be reviewed. For any spontaneous abnormal eye movement, the presence or absence of visual impairment (i.e., reduced visual quality, blurred vision, oscillopsia) should be queried and symptoms such as headache, diplopia, vertigo, or other neurological abnormalities must be taken into account. Examination should include assessment of visual acuity, confrontation visual fields, ocular motility, pupillary reflexes, observation for ocular albinism, and ophthalmoscopy. Ophthalmoscopy may be used to detect subtle nystagmus not apparent to the naked eye. Clinical features that must be determined are listed in Box 18.12.

### Examine All Classes of Eye Movements

Fixation and stability of gaze holding should be checked. This is done by having the individual look at a target and observing for spontaneous eye movements such as drift, microtremor, nystagmus, opsoclonus, ocular myokymia, ocular myoclonus, or saccadic intrusions. If spontaneous primary-position nystagmus is present, the effects of changes in the direction of gaze and convergence on the nystagmus should be determined. Pursuit movements provide an opportunity to

## BOX 18.12 Clinical Features to Look for in Patients with Nystagmus

- Are there signs of ocular albinism?
- Is there a spontaneous head tilt or turn?
- Is the nystagmus present in primary position or only with eccentric gaze (gaze-evoked nystagmus)?
- Is the nystagmus binocular and conjugate or is it dissociated?
- Is the waveform pendular or jerk? If jerk, what is the direction of the fast phase?
- Is there a latent component (i.e., an increase in nystagmus intensity when one eye is covered)?
- Is there a torsional component?
- Is there spontaneous alteration of direction, as with periodic alternating nystagmus? This entity, for which recognition requires observation over time, must be distinguished from rebound nystagmus.
- Is there a null zone (a direction of gaze in which the nystagmus is minimal or absent)?
- Determine whether convergence damps the nystagmus or changes its direction.
- Is the nystagmus altered (accentuated or suppressed) by head positioning or posture or by head shaking (as in spasmus nutans)?
- Do the following provocative maneuvers—elimination of visual fixation, supine positioning, head shaking, hyperventilation, mastoid vibration—unmask or modify the appearance of nystagmus?
- What is the effect of optokinetic stimulation? In infantile nystagmus syndrome, the response is paradoxical—that is, the fast phase is in the direction of the slow-moving target.
- Are there associated rhythmic movements of other muscle groups (e.g., face, tongue, ears, neck, palate [as in oculopalatal myoclonus/tremor], limbs)?

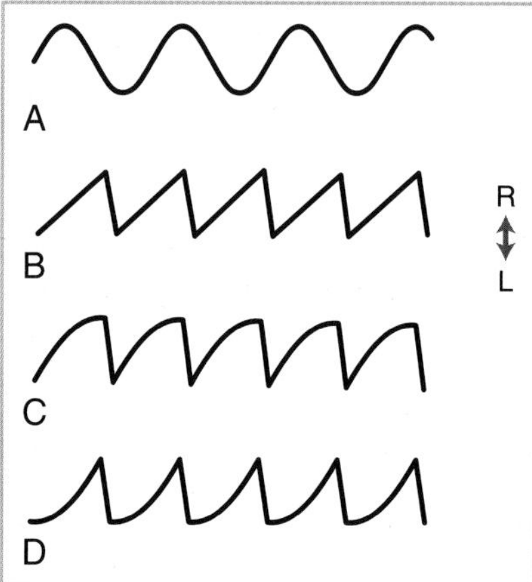


**Fig. 18.26** Oculographic Diagrams of Nystagmus Waveforms. By convention, a downward deflection in the horizontal position trace of the eye movement is a leftward eye movement. **A,** Pendular (sinusoidal) nystagmus. **B,** Left-beating jerk nystagmus with a constant (linear) velocity slow phase. **C,** Left-beating jerk nystagmus with a decreasing (exponential) velocity slow phase. **D,** Left-beating jerk nystagmus with an increasing (exponential) velocity slow phase.

observe for gaze-evoked nystagmus (GEN). Gaze shifts with saccades offer an opportunity to determine if saccadic intrusions are provoked by these movements. Changes in the amplitude, frequency, or even direction of nystagmus may be elicited by convergence and may have diagnostic and therapeutic implications. OKN testing is particularly helpful with congenital nystagmus, wherein the fast phase may be absent or the direction paradoxical—that is, in the direction of the slowly moving tape or drum.

## BOX 18.13 Causes of Monocular Oscillopsia and/or Nystagmus

- Acquired monocular blindness (nystagmus in blind eye)
- Alternating hemiplegia of childhood
- Amblyopia
- Brainstem infarction (thalamus and upper midbrain)
- Ictal nystagmus
- Internuclear and pseudointernuclear ophthalmoplegia
- Multiple sclerosis
- Nystagmus with monocular ophthalmoplegia
- Nystagmus with one eye absent
- Pseudonystagmus (lid fasciculations)
- Spasmus nutans
- Superior oblique myokymia

## Clinical Disorders

### Nystagmus

Nystagmus is an involuntary biphasic rhythmic ocular oscillation in which one or both phases are slow (Fig. 18.26). The slow phase of nystagmus is the pathological component responsible for the initiation and generation of the nystagmus. With pendular nystagmus, only back-to-back slow phases are present, whereas with jerk forms of nystagmus, the fast (saccadic) phase is a corrective movement bringing the fovea back toward the target. Often, nystagmus interferes with vision by blurring the object of regard (poor foveation), or making the environment appear to oscillate (oscillopsia), or both.

For clinical purposes, nystagmus may be divided into pendular and jerk forms. Nystagmus may result from dysfunction of the vestibular end organ, vestibular nerve, brainstem, cerebellum, or cerebral centers for ocular pursuit. *Pendular nystagmus* (see Fig. 18.26, *A*) is central (brainstem or cerebellum) in origin, whereas *jerk nystagmus* may be either central or peripheral. Either form may have horizontal, vertical, or torsional components. Disconjugate (dissociated) nystagmus occurs when the ocular oscillations are out of phase (in different directions) in each eye. It is seen with brainstem lesions (see following discussion of pendular vergence nystagmus), and spasmus nutans. Monocular nystagmus is also disconjugate and may be associated with amblyopia and other forms of vision loss (Box 18.13).

Jerk nystagmus is named conventionally by the direction of the fast phase and is divided into three types (increasing, decreasing, or linear velocity) on the basis of the shape of the slow-phase tracing on oculographic recordings (see Fig. 18.26). Jerk nystagmus with a linear (constant velocity) slow phase (see Fig. 18.26, *B*) is caused by vestibular dysfunction, either peripheral or central, resulting in an imbalance in vestibular input to the brainstem gaze centers. When the slow phase has a decreasing velocity exponential (see Fig. 18.26, *C*), the brainstem NI that holds the eyes in eccentric gaze positions is at fault and is said to be "leaky." The integrator is unable to maintain a constant output to the gaze center to hold the eyes in an eccentric position, resulting in gaze-paretic nystagmus. An increasing velocity exponential slow phase (see Fig. 18.26, *D*) is central in origin and is the usual form of congenital nystagmus (now termed *infantile nystagmus syndrome* [INS]), although it is not pathognomonic, as it is also reported in forms of acquired nystagmus (Bakaeva et al., 2018; Zee et al., 1980).

**TABLE 18.4 Localizing Value of Nystagmus Syndromes and Nonnystagmus Ocular Oscillations**

| Nystagmus Syndrome | Localization |
|---|---|
| Downbeat nystagmus | Bilateral cervicomedullary junction (flocculus) |
| | Floor of the fourth ventricle |
| Periodic alternating nystagmus (PAN) | Cervicomedullary junction (nodulus) |
| Alternating windmill nystagmus (a variant of PAN) | Bilateral pontomesencephalic junction |
| Upbeat nystagmus | Bilateral pontomedullary junction |
| Bow-tie nystagmus (a variant of upbeat nystagmus) | Cerebellar vermis |
| | Medial medulla, syringomyelia, syringobulbia, tobacco inhalation |
| Pendular nystagmus | Paramedian pons |
| | Deep cerebellar (fastigial) nuclei |
| Seesaw nystagmus (SSN): | Mesodiencephalic junction, chiasm, disorders that disrupt central vision |
| Hemi-jerk SSN | Unilateral mesodiencephalic lesions: upper poles of the eyes jerk toward side of the lesion, and vertical component is always disjunctive (eyes oscillate in opposite directions, with the intorting eye rising and the extorting eye falling) |
| | Lateral medullary lesions: upper poles of the eyes jerk away from the side of lesion; but the vertical component may be either conjugate, usually upward, or disjunctive |
| Alternating hemi-SSN with direction of vertical pursuit | Middle cerebellar peduncle |
| Rebound nystagmus | Cerebellum |
| Bruns nystagmus | Cerebellopontine angle, AICA territory stroke |
| Torsional nystagmus, jerk | Central vestibular system |
| Torsional nystagmus, pendular | Medulla |
| Atypical infantile nystagmus syndrome: | |
| Asymmetric horizontal | Ocular albinism |
| Vertical (pendular, downbeat, or upbeat) | Retina: congenital cone dysfunction, congenital stationary night blindness |
| **Nonnystagmus Ocular Oscillations** | **Localization** |
| Convergence-retraction "nystagmus" | Dorsal midbrain |
| Opsoclonus | Cerebellar fastigial nuclei or brainstem |
| Ocular flutter | Deep cerebellum nuclei or brainstem |
| Ocular dysmetria | Cerebellum (dorsal vermis and fastigial nuclei) |
| Ocular myoclonus (oculopalatal) | Guillain-Mollaret triangle (central tegmental tract in the pons) |
| Ocular bobbing | Pons |
| Square-wave jerks | Superior colliculus or its inputs, cerebellum |
| Square-wave pulses | Cerebellar outflow tracts (may be associated with rubral tremor) |

*AICA,* Anteroinferior cerebellar artery.

A helpful approach in understanding the various mechanisms of nystagmus is to consider the mechanisms by which a visual target is maintained on the fovea: (1) stabilization of fixation, including via visual feedback mechanisms by which the visual system suppresses unwanted saccades and detects retinal drifts followed by programming of corrective eye movements; (2) VORs, by which eye position is maintained despite small head and body movements; and (3) NIs, which largely serve to maintain the eyes in a desired eccentric gaze position by counteracting the elastic pull of orbital tissues that draws the eyes back toward the center (Leigh and Zee, 2015). Table 18.4 summarizes the localizing value of nystagmus syndromes and nonnystagmus ocular oscillations.

### *Acquired Nystagmus.*

#### Impaired fixational mechanisms.

***Nystagmus in blindness.*** Large-amplitude ("searching") pendular nystagmus is usually associated with poor vision because of afferent disorders such as optic neuropathy, which can be unilateral, and retinal disorders. Pendular waveforms are common with optic nerve causes of vision loss, whereas jerk nystagmus is more often seen with retinal causes of vision loss. The *Heimann-Bielschowsky phenomenon* is a rare form of monocular vertical or occasionally oblique pendular oscillation, with a frequency of 1 to 5 Hz, that occurs in an amblyopic eye or after acquired monocular vision loss, as with cataract (Nguyen and Borruat, 2019). In the latter situation, it may be reversible after successful treatment of the underlying condition or with gabapentin (Rahman et al., 2006).

Monocular nystagmus may be pendular or jerk and may be horizontal, vertical, or oblique. Oculographic recordings may reveal small-amplitude oscillations in the fellow eye. Monocular nystagmus may occur with amblyopia, blindness, and in several other conditions (see Box 18.13). Superior oblique myokymia (SOM) may be mistaken for a monocular torsional or vertical nystagmus.

***Acquired pendular nystagmus.*** Acquired pendular nystagmus (APN) may have horizontal, vertical, and torsional components, although one is usually dominant. The most common cause of APN is multiple sclerosis (MS), followed by brainstem vascular disease. Other disorders of myelin—including Cockayne syndrome, Pelizaeus-Merzbacher disease, peroxisomal disorders, disorders associated with toluene abuse, as well as spinocerebellar disease, hypoxic encephalopathy, and Whipple disease—can cause pendular nystagmus.

Pendular nystagmus likely results from disruption of normal feedback from cerebellar nuclei to the NIs (Das et al., 2000). This is in keeping with the predominance of paramedian pontine lesions on MRI in patients with horizontal pendular nystagmus and with the predominance of medullary lesions in those with torsional pendular nystagmus (Lopez et al., 1996). The rhythmic pendular oscillations may be the result of deafferentation of the inferior olive by lesions involving the central tegmental tracts, medial vestibular nuclei, or paramedian tracts, causing instability in the system. Disruption of prenuclear ocular motor pathways necessary for orthotropia (and conjugacy) may be a factor as well. A similar mechanism may be responsible for oculopalatal myoclonus (discussed later in this section).

In demyelinating diseases, APN most often is horizontal and/or elliptical in trajectory, with a frequency of 3 to 5 Hz (Gresty et al., 1982). MS patients frequently have optic neuropathy that usually is worse in the eye with the larger oscillations. The oscillations of each eye may be so different that the nystagmus may appear monocular clinically (Leigh and Zee, 2015). Elliptical APN with a larger vertical component and superimposed or interposed upbeat nystagmus is characteristic of Pelizaeus-Merzbacher disease. This nystagmus can be difficult to discern with the naked eye. It is seen more easily with an ophthalmoscope, but oculography using scleral search coils may be necessary to detect it.

*Oculopalatal myoclonus* (Video 18.7), also called oculopalatal tremor, is a pure vertical or vertical-torsional pendular oscillation with a frequency of 1 to 3 Hz, usually associated with similar oscillations of the soft palate (palatal tremor) and sometimes other muscles of branchial origin. The classic presentation is delayed development of the nystagmus and palatal tremor, often with one beginning prior to the other, that occurs weeks or months after brainstem infarction or hemorrhage of a brainstem cavernoma. Typically the location of the original insult is the pons, involving the central tegmental tract. Following a latency of months, hypertrophic degeneration of the inferior olives, which can be seen on MRI as increased T2 signal, ensues and the oculopalatal tremor begins. Dissociated nystagmus is predictive of unilateral inferior olivary changes on MRI, with the MRI changes being on the side of the eye with larger-amplitude oscillations (Kim, et al., 2007). The association of a facial nerve palsy with the one-and-a-half syndrome may predict the development of oculopalatal myoclonus, probably because of the proximity of the central tegmental tract to the facial nerve. Also, oculopalatal myoclonus can have an insidious onset in the absence of an original vascular insult in association with progressive ataxia, a condition called progressive ataxia with palatal tremor (PAPT) (Samuel et al., 2004). *Cyclovergent nystagmus* (i.e., disconjugate TN in which the upper poles of the eyes oscillate in opposite directions) was detected by scleral search coil oculography in a patient with progressive ataxia and palatal myoclonus. On rare occasions, cyclovergent nystagmus may be observed clinically. PAPT is attributed to superficial siderosis, adult-onset Alexander disease, and mitochondrial disease (Nicastro et al., 2016).

Dysfunction of the cerebellar nuclei or their connections (Guillain-Mollaret triangle) and disruption of retinal error signals relayed to the inferior olive may be responsible for oculopalatal myoclonus, which is confined to the muscles of branchial origin. The current hypothesis relates to the development of new soma-to-soma electrical coupling via gap junctions (connexins) in inferior olivary neurons that in a healthy normal state fire only dysychronously via dendrite-to-dendrite connections (Shaikh et al., 2010, 2017).

*Pendular vergence nystagmus*, previously called *convergent-divergent nystagmus*, a very rare variant of APN, is disconjugate and occurs in patients with MS, brainstem stroke, Chiari malformations, cerebral Whipple disease as oculomasticatory myorhythmia (OMM), occasionally oculopalatal myoclonus, and pseudo-Whipple disease (anti-Ma2–associated encephalitis). OMM, to date, is pathognomonic of Whipple disease. It consists of continuous rhythmic jaw contractions synchronous with dissociated pendular vergence oscillations present in primary position. It may be associated with supranuclear vertical gaze palsy, altered mentation, somnolence, mild uveitis, or retinopathy. With pendular vergence nystagmus, the eyes oscillate, mainly horizontally, in opposite directions simultaneously, although they sometimes form circular, elliptical, or oblique trajectories, depending on the phase relationship of the horizontal, vertical, and torsional vectors responsible for the oscillations.

*Convergence-evoked nystagmus* is an unusual ocular oscillation that is usually pendular and is induced by voluntary convergence. The movements may be conjugate or dissociated. This condition may be congenital or acquired, as in patients with MS. A jerk form occurs with Chiari type I malformations. Convergence-evoked vertical nystagmus (upbeat more common than downbeat) also occurs. Convergence-evoked nystagmus should be distinguished from voluntary nystagmus and from convergence retraction nystagmus (see later section titled "Saccadic Intrusions" for the former and, earlier, "Dorsal midbrain syndrome" for the latter).

*See-saw nystagmus* (SSN) is a spectacular ocular oscillation in which one eye rises and intorts as the other eye falls and extorts. The waveform is pendular (see later section titled "Vestibular nystagmus" for discussion of a jerk form of see-saw). The oscillations usually become faster and smaller on upgaze but slower and larger on downgaze; they may cease in darkness. Disordered control of the normal ocular counter-rolling reflex may be responsible.

Bitemporal hemianopia, caused by acquired chiasmal defects or impaired central vision, plays a significant role in generating SSN. Disruption of retinal error signals necessary for VOR adaptation, normally conveyed to the inferior olive by the chiasmal crossing fibers, results in an unstable visuovestibular environment. Fixation and pursuit feedback accentuate this instability, causing synchronous oscillations of floccular Purkinje cells, which relay to the nodulus, resulting in SSN. This mechanism also may be the basis for the ocular oscillations of oculopalatal myoclonus. The observations of SSN and INS in achiasmatic humans and achiasmatic Belgian sheepdogs support this hypothesis (Dell'Osso and Daroff, 1998). Significantly, the onset of both SSN and oculopalatal myoclonus may be delayed after CNS lesions.

SSN occurs with lesions in the region of the mesodiencephalic junction, particularly the zona incerta and the INC. Congenital SSN may be associated with a superimposed horizontal pendular nystagmus; some patients with congenital SSN may be achiasmatic or have septo-optic dysplasia. Reverse congenital SSN is a rare condition in which the rising eye extorts as the falling eye intorts. Acquired SSN may be associated with suprasellar tumors, Joubert syndrome, and Leigh disease (particularly the jerk form described further on in the section "Vestibular nystagmus"). Acquired pendular SSN may be accompanied by a bitemporal hemianopia from trauma, an expanding lesion in the third ventricular region, or severe loss of central vision due to disorders such as choroiditis, cone-rod dystrophy, whole-brain radiation, intrathecal methotrexate, and vitreous hemorrhage. Transient (latent) SSN may occur for a few seconds after a blink, perhaps because of loss of fixation, in patients with chiasmal region lesions. If SSN damps with convergence, base-out prisms may be helpful. Baclofen also may be beneficial in SSN.

APN is severely disabling due to the incessant to-and-fro foveal drift it creates, which is typically accompanied by constant oscillopsia. APN in demyelinating disease tends to respond fairly well to treatment with gabapentin or memantine (Thurtell et al., 2010) (Table 18.5), though APN with oculopalatal myoclonus often is refractory to treatment. Clonazepam and valproic acid may also be helpful, as can chronically patching the eye with larger oscillations if they are dissociated. Palatal

**TABLE 18.5 Treatment of Nystagmus and Nonnystagmus Oscillations***

| Nystagmus Syndrome | Treatment |
|---|---|
| Infantile nystagmus syndrome | Prisms |
| | Contact lenses |
| | Extraocular muscle surgery |
| | Kestenbaum-Anderson procedure |
| | Tenotomy and reattachment procedure (experimental) |
| | Acetazolamide 250–1000 mg bid (Thurtell et al., 2010a) |
| | Brinzolamide 1% eye drops, 1 drop OU bid (Aygit et al., 2018; Dell'osso et al., 2011; Hertle et al., 2015) |
| | Memantine (Sherry et al., 2006) |
| | Gabapentin 300–600 mg qid (Sherry et al., 2006) |
| | Gene therapy (experimental) when the nystagmus is associated with retinal disorders (Leigh and Zee, 2015) |
| Acquired pendular nystagmus | Trihexyphenidyl 5–20 mg tid, benztropine, clonazepam 0.5–1 mg bid, gabapentin 300 mg qid, isoniazid, memantine 10 mg qid† (Starck et al., 2010; Thurtell et al., 2010b), valproate, diethylpropion hydrochloride, tenotomy followed by memantine, hand held muscle massager (vibrator) held to the head (Beh et al., 2014) |
| Convergence-evoked horizontal | Base-in prisms |
| Downbeat nystagmus | Base-out prisms (if nystagmus damps with convergence) |
| | Base-down prisms over both eyes if intensity of nystagmus diminishes in upgaze |
| | Contact lenses (personal observation) |
| | Extraocular muscle surgery realignment (Donahue, personal communication, and observation) |
| | Baclofen 5 mg tid, chlorzoxazone 500 mg tid (Feil et al., 2013), betahistine, clonazepam 0.5–1 mg bid, gabapentin, scopolamine, 4-AMP 5–10 mg tid (dalfampridine, the sustained-release form of 4-AMP at 10 mg bid may be more effective than 4-AMP [Claassen et al., 2013]), 3,4-diaminopyridine 10–20 mg bid |
| | Brinzolamide 1% eye drops, 1 drop OU bid (personal observation) |
| Periodic alternating nystagmus: | |
| Congenital | Dextroamphetamine, baclofen 5–10 mg tid (occasionally), 5-HT |
| Acquired | Baclofen 5–10 mg tid, phenytoin, memantine 5–10 mg qid |
| Upbeat nystagmus | Base-up prisms over both eyes if intensity of nystagmus diminishes in downgaze |
| | Baclofen 5–10 mg tid, gabapentin, 4-AMP 5–10 mg tid-qid, memantine 10 mg qid (Thurtell et al., 2010b), thiamine |
| Oculopalatal myoclonus | Chronically patch one eye |
| | Baclofen, carbamazepine, cerulein, clonazepam, gabapentin 300 mg qid, memantine 10 mg qid, scopolamine, trihexyphenidyl 5–20 mg tid, valproate |
| Seesaw nystagmus (SSN) | Baclofen, clonazepam 0.5–1 mg bid, gabapentin, memantine 10 mg qid (Huppert et al., 2011), base-out prisms |
| Hemi-SSN | Memantine (Thurtell et al., 2010b) |
| Ictal nystagmus | AEDs |
| Episodic nystagmus: | |
| Episodic ataxia-1 | Acetazolamide 125–1000 mg bid |
| Episodic ataxia-2 | Acetazolamide 125–1000 mg bid, 4-AMP 5–10 mg tid, dalfampridine 10 mg bid |
| Oculomasticatory myorhythmia | Antibiotics for Whipple disease; consider gabapentin or memantine |
| Torsional nystagmus | Gabapentin 300 mg qid, memantine (Thurtell et al., 2010b) |
| **Nonnystagmus Ocular Oscillations** | **Treatment** |
| Opsoclonus | Treat underlying condition when possible, ACTH, thiamine, clonazepam, gabapentin, ondansetron, steroids; if paraneoplastic, protein A immunoabsorption |
| Superior oblique myokymia | Carbamazepine, gabapentin, oxcarbazepine, other AEDs, topical beta-blockers, memantine, base-down prism over the affected eye, muscle/tendon surgery, microvascular decompression |
| Ocular neuromyotonia | Carbamazepine, oxcarbazepine (Whitted and Lavin, personal observation) |
| Microflutter | Propranolol, verapamil |
| Square-wave jerks and square-wave oscillations | Valproate, amphetamines, barbiturates, diazepam, clonazepam, memantine (Rosini et al., 2013; Serra et al., 2008) |

*Treat underlying cause when possible.
†Memantine is reported to exacerbate multiple sclerosis (Villoslada et al., 2009).
*ACTH,* Adrenocorticotropic hormone; *AEDs,* antiepileptic drugs; *4-AMP,* 4-aminopyridine; *5-HT,* 5-hydroxytryptamine.

tremor may respond to botulinum injections. Palatal tremor should be distinguished from pulsations of the uvula that are synchronous with the systolic pulse (Muller sign) in patients with aortic regurgitation (Williams and Steinberg, 2006).

**Vestibular nystagmus.** Vestibular nystagmus results from damage to the labyrinth, vestibular nerve, vestibular nuclei, or their connections in the brainstem or cerebellum. Vestibular nystagmus may be divided into central and peripheral forms based on the associated features outlined in Chapter 22.

Vestibular nystagmus is jerk nystagmus that tends to follow Alexander's law, with increasing amplitude and frequency in the direction of the fast phases of the nystagmus.

**BOX 18.14 Causes of Downbeat Nystagmus**

- Congenital (rare)
- Transiently in normal neonates
- Idiopathic (common)
- Craniocervical junction abnormalities:
  - Basilar invagination (e.g., Paget disease)
  - Chiari malformations
  - Dolichoectasia of the vertebrobasilar arterial system
  - Foramen magnum tumors
  - Syringobulbia
- Cerebellar disorders:
  - Alcoholic cerebellar degeneration (chronic usage)
  - Anoxic cerebellar degeneration
  - Anti–glutamic acid decarboxylase antibodies (anti-GAD65 antibodies)
  - Cerebellar degeneration following human T-lymphotropic virus types I and II
  - Episodic ataxia
  - Familial spinocerebellar degeneration, particularly SCA-6, and with multiple system atrophy
  - Heat stroke–induced cerebellar degeneration
  - Paraneoplastic cerebellar degeneration
- Metabolic disorders (drugs, toxins, and deficiencies):
  - Alcohol intoxication
  - Amiodarone
  - Anticonvulsants
  - Lithium
  - Magnesium depletion
  - Opioids
  - Toluene abuse
  - Vitamin $B_{12}$ deficiency
  - Wernicke encephalopathy (as a chronic, persistent late-stage finding)
- Other:
  - Benign paroxysmal positional vertigo: positional downbeat nystagmus with an anterior canal lesion
  - Brainstem encephalitis
  - Cardiogenic vertigo
  - Cephalic tetanus
  - Finger extensor weakness and downbeat nystagmus motor neuron disease (FEWDON-MND)
  - Hydrocephalus
  - Leukodystrophy
  - Multiple sclerosis
  - Small-amplitude downbeat nystagmus in carriers of blue-cone monochromatism
  - Syncope
  - Vertebrobasilar ischemia

***Peripheral vestibular nystagmus.*** Peripheral vestibular nystagmus (see Chapter 22), caused by dysfunction of the vestibular end organ or nerve, has a linear slow phase (see Fig. 18.26, *B*), whereas with central lesions, the slow phase may be variable. Nystagmus in specific patterns induced by provocative maneuvers such as elimination of visual fixation, head shaking, hyperventilation, or supine positioning, often is the key to establishing a peripheral localization. Peripheral vestibular nystagmus is usually associated with vertigo, nausea, vomiting, perspiration, diarrhea, hearing loss, and tinnitus. These symptoms, as opposed to oscillopsia, are typically the reason the individual seeks medical attention. With central vestibular nystagmus, symptoms such as nausea are less severe, but other neurological features may be present, such as headache, ataxia, diplopia, and pyramidal tract signs.

***Downbeat nystagmus*** **(Video 18.8).** Downbeat nystagmus is the most common form of acquired primary positional nystagmus; it is a spontaneous downward-beating jerk nystagmus (i.e., slow drifts of the eyes upward, followed by fast-resetting downward movements) present in primary position and is attributed to either (1) interruption of the posterior semicircular canal projections, which are responsible for the downward VOR, causing upward drift of the eyes with corrective downward saccades; (2) impaired cerebellar inhibition of the vestibular circuits for upward eye movements, resulting in uninhibited upward drifting of the eyes, with corrective downward saccades; or (3) dysfunction of pursuit pathways. The amplitude of the oscillations increases significantly when the eyes are deviated laterally and slightly downward (Daroff sign, "side-pocket" nystagmus), particularly when the oscillations are subtle in primary gaze.

Downbeat nystagmus may be precipitated or worsened by horizontal or vertical head shaking or with changes in posture (positional downbeat nystagmus), particularly the head-hanging position (Choi et al., 2015), although the latter may also signify benign paroxysmal positional vertigo (Oh et al., 2019). Development of downbeat nystagmus after horizontal head shaking, called perverted nystagmus, is a definite sign of CNS disease and is suggested to be due to enhanced activity in central anterior semicircular canal pathways (Choi et al., 2016).

Downbeat nystagmus results from either damage to the commissural fibers between the vestibular nuclei in the floor of the fourth ventricle or bilateral damage to the vestibulocerebellum (flocculus, paraflocculus, nodulus, and uvula) that disinhibits the VOR in pitch. Rarely it is due to a brainstem lesion, typically involving a group of neurons called the paramedian tracts (Nakamagoe et al., 2013). It frequently occurs with structural lesions at the craniocervical junction; MRI of the foramen magnum region (in the sagittal plane) is the imaging investigation of choice. A wide variety of other pathologies can also cause downbeat nystagmus, and a large percentage of cases are idiopathic (Box 18.14). In some cases of unexplained downbeat nystagmus, the cause is a radiographically occult infarction; however, lesions that cause downbeat nystagmus are bilateral. The treatment of downbeat nystagmus involves correction of the underlying cause when possible. When downbeat nystagmus damps on convergence, it may be treated successfully with base-out prisms, reducing the oscillopsia and improving visual acuity. Medications including clonazepam, chlorzoxazone, and 4-aminopyridine may help as well (see Table 18.5); 4-aminopyridine is more effective in downbeat nystagmus associated with cerebellar atrophy rather than structural lesions (Huppert et al., 2011), and the sustained-release form (dalfampyridine) may be more effective (Claassen et al., 2013).

***Upbeat nystagmus.*** Upbeat nystagmus is a spontaneous jerk nystagmus with the fast phase upward while the eyes are in primary position (Video 18.9). It is attributed to interruption of the anterior semicircular canal projections, which are responsible for the upward VOR, resulting in downward drift of the eyes with corrective upward saccades. The amplitude and intensity of the nystagmus usually increase on upgaze. This finding strongly suggests bilateral paramedian lesions of the brainstem, usually at the pontomedullary (or, less often pontomesencephalic) junction, affecting perihypoglossal nuclei in the lower medulla that project to the cerebellum. Upbeat nystagmus is most common with Wernicke encephalopathy (WE) and MS. Upbeat nystagmus that converts to downbeat nystagmus on examination may specifically suggest WE; conversion to a chronic persistent downbeat nystagmus may occur over time after resolution of the acute phase

of WE (Kattah et al., 2018). Upbeat nystagmus may also be seen with intoxication from anticonvulsants, organophosphates, lithium, nicotine, or thallium (author's personal observation, PL). Rarely, upbeat nystagmus may be congenital. In infants, upbeat nystagmus may be a sign of anterior visual pathway disease, such as Leber congenital amaurosis, optic nerve hypoplasia, aniridia, or cataracts. Small-amplitude upbeat nystagmus may be seen in individuals who are carriers of blue-cone monochromatism, whereas affected individuals may have intermittent pendular oblique nystagmus. If the intensity of upbeat nystagmus diminishes in downgaze, base-up prisms over both eyes may improve the oscillopsia. Medications such as memantine may also be helpful (see Table 18.5). A comprehensive list of causes of upbeat nystagmus can be found elsewhere (Leigh and Zee, 2015).

A variant of upbeat nystagmus, so-called bow-tie nystagmus, is reported with posterior fossa medial medullary stroke (Choi et al., 2004) and is characterized by oblique upward fast phases alternating to the left or right because of the changing direction of each horizontal component (Leigh and Zee, 2015).

***Torsional and jerk see-saw nystagmus.*** In torsional nystagmus (TN), the eye oscillates in a pure rotary plane. TN may be present in primary position or with either head positioning or gaze deviation. It usually results from lesions in the central vestibular pathways. Pure TN occurs with central vestibular dysfunction only, whereas mixed torsional-horizontal nystagmus is common with peripheral vestibular disease. In patients with lesions of the middle cerebellar peduncle, TN with a jerk waveform—like jerk see-saw nystagmus—may be evoked by vertical pursuit eye movement and during fixation suppression of the vertical VOR. The direction of the fast phase changes with pursuit direction; it usually is toward the side of the lesion on downward pursuit and away from the side of the lesion on upward pursuit (FitzGibbon et al., 1996). When the waveform of TN is pendular (i.e., torsional pendular nystagmus), the lesion is usually in the medulla. Skew deviation frequently coexists with TN. Gabapentin may help (see Table 18.5).

A jerk waveform hemi-SSN (see earlier section titled "Acquired pendular nystagmus" for pendular forms of SSN) occurs with unilateral mesodiencephalic lesions, presumably because of selective unilateral inactivation of the torsional eye-velocity integrator in the INC; during the fast (jerk) phases, the upper poles of the eyes rotate toward the side of the lesion. In hemi-jerk SSN caused by lateral medullary lesions, the fast phases jerk away from the side of the lesion. In both situations, the torsional component is always conjugate. With mesodiencephalic lesions, the vertical component is always disjunctive (the eyes oscillate in opposite directions, with the intorting eye rising and the extorting eye falling), but with medullary lesions it may be either conjugate (usually upward) or disjunctive. Other features of brainstem dysfunction may be necessary to localize the lesion.

***Periodic alternating nystagmus.*** PAN is a horizontal jerk nystagmus in which the fast phase beats in one direction and then damps or stops for a few seconds before changing direction to the opposite side; the cycle repeats every 30 to 180 seconds. During the short transition period, vertical nystagmus or square-wave jerks (SWJs) may occur. PAN localizes to the cerebellar nodulus and uvula. PAN may occur with any lesion affecting this location, including Chiari malformations, infarction, encephalitis, and Creutzfeldt-Jacob disease. When PAN is congenital, it may be associated with albinism. In one series of patients with congenital PAN, none had pure vertical oscillations, even during the transition period (Gradstein et al., 1997). Although not all patients with acquired PAN have vertical nystagmus during the transition period, its presence may distinguish acquired from congenital PAN (personal observation); this finding does not obviate further evaluation when appropriate. Transient episodes of PAN were provoked by attacks of Meniere disease in a patient with a hypoplastic cerebellum and an enlarged cisterna magna (Chiu and Hain, 2002). Episodic PAN can be a manifestation of a seizure (see later discussion of eye movements in seizure and coma). A variant of PAN called "alternating windmill nystagmus," consisting of oscillations in both the horizontal and vertical planes, 90 degrees out of phase, occurred in a blind patient (Leigh and Zee, 2015).

Lesions of the cerebellar nodulus cause loss of γ-aminobutyric acid (GABA)–mediated inhibition from the Purkinje cells to the vestibular nuclei, impairing the velocity storage mechanism. It is likely that overcompensation in feedback loops causes cyclical firing between reciprocally connected inhibitory neurons and generates the unusual oscillations of acquired PAN. Affected patients have hyperactive vestibular responses and poor vestibular fixation suppression, attributed to involvement of the nodulus and uvula (Leigh and Zee, 2015).

Treatment of PAN should be directed at correcting the cause, such as a Chiari malformation, when possible. Baclofen, a $GABA_B$ agonist, replaces the missing inhibition and is usually effective in stopping the nystagmus completely in the acquired form and occasionally in the congenital form. Dextroamphetamine is a second option (see Table 18.5).

### Nystagmus in eccentric gaze

***Gaze-evoked nystagmus.*** GEN may also be called direction-changing nystagmus or gaze-paretic nystagmus. GEN is an appropriate term to use when there is uncertainty as to whether the nystagmus is physiological or pathological. The term gaze-paretic nystagmus implies pathology.

Gaze-paretic nystagmus, the most common type of nystagmus, is usually symmetrical and evoked by eccentric gaze to either side but is absent in the primary position (Video 18.10). Frequently it is present  on eccentric vertical gaze, especially upward with upward-beating nystagmus on upgaze. It may be asymmetric with asymmetric CNS disease. With myasthenia, fatigue of gaze maintenance with drifts of the eyes toward primary position and resetting saccades may mimic the appearance of gaze-paretic nystagmus. The latter has a jerk waveform, with the fast phase in the direction of gaze (i.e., right beating in right gaze). Oculographic recordings show a decreasing exponential slow phase (see Fig. 18.26, *C*). Gaze-paretic nystagmus results from dysfunction of the NIs and is commonly caused by alcohol or drug intoxication as from anticonvulsants or tranquilizers. When it is caused by structural disease, it tends to be asymmetric.

*Bruns nystagmus* occurs in patients with large cerebellopontine angle tumors. The nystagmus is bilateral but asymmetrical, with a jerk waveform. It is characterized by large-amplitude low-frequency fast phases on gaze toward the side of the lesion but small-amplitude high-frequency fast phases on gaze to the opposite side. The ipsilateral large-amplitude (coarse) nystagmus has an exponentially decreasing velocity slow phase attributed to compression of the brainstem NI, which includes the ipsilateral medial vestibular nucleus. The contralateral small-amplitude high-frequency nystagmus has a linear slow phase attributed to ipsilateral vestibular dysfunction (see Fig. 18.26). Occasionally a stroke in the territory of the anteroinferior cerebellar artery can cause Bruns nystagmus (personal observation).

*Physiological (endpoint) nystagmus* is a jerk nystagmus observed on extreme lateral or, rarely, upward gaze. If the bridge of the nose obstructs the view of the adducting eye, it may be disconjugate because the amplitude is greater in the abducting eye. A torsional component is sometimes seen. Physiological nystagmus is distinguished from pathological nystagmus by its symmetry on right and left gaze and by the absence of other neurological features. It is not present when the angle of gaze is less than 30 degrees from primary position. Oculographic recordings demonstrate a linear slow phase (see Fig. 18.26, *B*) and may detect transient small-amplitude rebound nystagmus.

*Rebound nystagmus* is a horizontal GEN in which the direction of the fast phase reverses with sustained lateral gaze or beats transiently in the opposite direction when the eyes return to primary position. The latter is occasionally a physiological finding. Rebound nystagmus is caused by dysfunction of the cerebellum or the perihypoglossal nuclei in the medulla. Occasionally rebound nystagmus may be torsional.

Cerebellar dysfunction can cause a form of GEN in which the fast phase beats toward primary position (i.e., centripetally) and the slow phase drifts peripherally toward an eccentric target. Centripetal nystagmus is like rebound nystagmus and may result from overcompensation by the cerebellar nodulus and uvula to adjust for a directional bias by temporarily moving the null zone during eccentric gaze. Centripetal nystagmus in both the horizontal and vertical planes may be associated with Creutzfeldt-Jakob disease.

***Congenital Nystagmus.*** The three distinct nystagmus syndromes seen in infancy and childhood were renamed by the Classification of Eye Movement Abnormalities and Strabismus (CEMAS) Working Group, sponsored by the National Eye Institute (Hertle, National Eye Institute Sponsored Classification of Eye Movement Abnormalities and Strabismus Working Group, 2002). The first of these syndromes, previously known as *congenital nystagmus*, is now called *infantile nystagmus syndrome*; the second, *fusion maldevelopment nystagmus syndrome* (FMNS), includes the latent form and manifest latent nystagmus (MLN); and the third, *spasmus nutans syndrome* (SNS), remains unchanged.

**Infantile nystagmus syndrome (congenital).** INS is usually present from birth but may not be noticed for the first few weeks or occasionally even years of life. It may be accompanied by severe visual impairment but is not the result of poor vision. Disorders that, through genetic association, are responsible for poor vision in patients with INS include those designated by the mnemonic of A's—*a*chiasma, *a*chromatopsia, *a*lbinism (both ocular and oculocutaneous forms), *a*maurotic idiocy of Leber (Leber congenital amaurosis), *a*niridia, *a*plasia (usually hypoplasia) of the fovea, and *a*plasia (usually hypoplasia) of the optic nerve—and congenital cataracts and congenital stationary night blindness. Paradoxical pupil constriction in darkness, particularly in patients with poor vision, suggests an associated retinal or optic nerve disorder. High myopia (uncommon early in life) in infants with INS suggests congenital stationary night blindness, and high hyperopia suggests Leber congenital amaurosis; such retinal disorders can be confirmed by electroretinography. INS may be familial and is inherited in an autosomal recessive X-linked dominant or recessive pattern. Genetic defects identified in some families include a dominant form of INS linked to chromosomal region 6p12, an X-linked form of INS with incomplete penetrance among female carriers associated with a defect on the long arm of the X chromosome, a deletion in the *OA1* gene (ocular albinism) in a family with X-linked INS associated with macular hypoplasia and ocular albinism, and three mutations in the *OA1* gene in families with hereditary nystagmus and ocular albinism (Faugere et al., 2003). For a review of the molecular genetics of INS see Self and Lotery (2007).

INS appears horizontal in most patients and may be either pendular or jerk in primary position. Pendular nystagmus often becomes jerk on lateral gaze. The horizontal oscillations may be accentuated during vertical tracking. Oculography with three-dimensional scleral search coils demonstrates that many patients with INS have a torsional component phase locked with the horizontal component. Individuals with INS often have good vision unless an associated afferent defect is present (see earlier discussion). In INS, the nystagmus damps with convergence; latent superimposition (an increase in nystagmus amplitude occurring when one eye is covered) may be present. A null zone wherein the nystagmus intensity is minimal may be found; if this zone is to one side, the affected individual turns the head to improve vision. Often the head "oscillates" as well. Both features—damping of nystagmus with convergence and a null zone—can be used in therapy by changing the direction of gaze with prisms or extraocular muscle surgery to improve head posture and visual acuity. Oculographic recordings usually demonstrate either a sinusoidal (see Fig. 18.26, *A*) or a slow phase with an increasing exponential waveform (see Fig. 18.26, *D*). However, in the first few months of life, the waveform of INS may be more variable, evolving into the more classic pattern as the child grows older. Outside the null zone, the nystagmus follows Alexander's law and increases in intensity (amplitude × frequency) on lateral gaze. Thus patients with INS or FMNS may induce an esotropia intentionally to suppress the nystagmus in the adducting eye. This strategy is called the *nystagmus blockage syndrome*.

Patients with INS do not experience oscillopsia (an illusory oscillation of the environment) unless a head injury, decompensated strabismus, or retinal degeneration causes a decline in vision, ocular motor function, or both. Prisms or strabismus surgery may correct such late-onset oscillopsia. Up to 50% of patients with INS have strabismus (Brodsky and Fray, 1997).

Rarely in INS, the nystagmus is in the vertical plane, or circumductory where the eyes move conjugately in a circular or cycloid pattern. In patients with retinal disorders such as achromatopsia, albinism, congenital cone dysfunction, or congenital stationary night blindness, INS can have an asymmetrical horizontal or vertical waveform that varies among pendular, downbeat, and upbeat. Occasionally INS may be unilateral, occur later in the teens or adult life, or become symptomatic if changes in the internal or external environment alter foveation stability and duration, causing oscillopsia. Less common patterns of INS such as periodic alternating, upbeat, downbeat, and SSN are discussed later.

**Fusional maldevelopment syndrome (FMNS) (latent).** FMNS includes both LN and MLN. LN occurs with monocular fixation: that is, when one eye is covered. The slow phase is directed toward the covered eye. The amplitude of the oscillations increases on abduction of the fixating eye. With MLN, the oscillations are present with both eyes open, but only one eye is fixating; vision in the other is ignored or suppressed because of strabismus or amblyopia. The nystagmus waveform has a linear (decreasing velocity) slow phase (see Fig. 18.26, *B*), which differs from that of true INS. Some patients with LN can suppress it at will.

The pathogenesis of LN may be related to impaired development of binocular vision mechanisms. Under monocular viewing conditions, rhesus monkeys deprived of binocular vision early in life have poor nasal-to-temporal optokinetic responses. The pretectal nucleus of the optic tract (NOT) is necessary for generation of slow-phase eye movements in response to horizontal full-field visual motion. In normal monkeys, the NOT on each side is driven binocularly and responds well to visual stimuli presented to either eye. In monkeys with LN, each NOT is driven mainly by the contralateral eye. Thus, in the altered monkeys, when only one eye is viewing, one optic tract nucleus is stimulated, causing an imbalance between each NOT. This imbalance is believed to be responsible for LN. Of interest, under monocular viewing conditions, patients with congenital esotropia have poor temporal-to-nasal pursuit, and some have LN or MLN. Indeed, in esotropic patients, LN may be unmasked in dim light or by shining a bright light at the dominant eye, as when pupil reflexes are being tested.

**Spasmus nutans syndrome.** SNS is a transient high-frequency, low-amplitude pendular nystagmus with onset between the ages of 6 and 12 months that lasts approximately 2 years but occasionally can continue for as long as 5 years. The direction of the oscillations may be

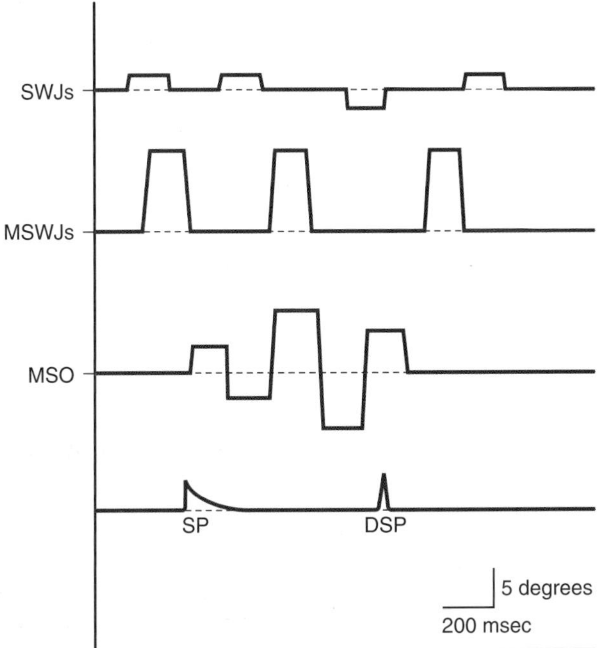


**Fig. 18.27** Simulated eye movement recordings of square-wave jerks *(SWJs)*, macro–square wave jerks or square-wave pulses *(MSWJs)*, macrosaccadic oscillations *(MSOs)*, a saccadic pulse *(SP)*, and a double saccadic pulse *(DSP)*.

**BOX 18.15 Saccadic Intrusions and Oscillations**

- Square-wave jerks and square-wave oscillations
- Flutter (voluntary, involuntary)
- Flutter dysmetria
- Microsaccadic flutter (variant of voluntary flutter?)
- Opsoclonus
- Macro–square wave jerks (now designated *square-wave pulses*)
- Ocular bobbing, reverse and inverse bobbing, dipping, and reverse dipping
- Superior oblique myokymia
- Convergence-retraction nystagmus
- Abduction nystagmus with internuclear ophthalmoplegia
- Tic-like ocular myoclonic jerks (eye tics)

horizontal, vertical, or torsional; the oscillations are often disconjugate, asymmetrical (usually greater in the abducting eye if seen in lateral gaze), even monocular, and variable. SNS may be associated with torticollis and head titubation; these three features constitute the *spasmus nutans triad*. The titubation has a lower frequency than that of the nystagmus and thus is not compensatory. Patients can improve their vision by vigorously shaking the head, presumably to stimulate the VOR and suppress or override the ocular oscillations. Some patients may have esotropia. Clinically, spasmus nutans is distinguished from INS and FMNS by its intermittency, high frequency, vertical component, and dysconjugacy (Leigh and Zee, 2015).

Although spasmus nutans is a benign and transient disorder, it must be distinguished from acquired nystagmus caused by structural lesions involving the anterior visual pathways in approximately 2% of patients. In the latter situation, a careful ophthalmological examination reveals abnormalities such as impaired vision, a relative afferent pupillary defect, or optic atrophy. Also, retinal disorders may masquerade as spasmus nutans; paradoxical pupil constriction in darkness

**BOX 18.16 Square-Wave Jerks**

- Normal subjects (<2 degrees)
- Aging
- AIDS-dementia complex (HIV encephalitis)
- Carriers of blue-cone monochromatism
- Catecholamine depletion in normals
- Cerebral hemisphere tumors and stroke
- Congenital nystagmus
- Dyslexia (suppressed by methylphenidate)
- Excitement in normals
- Friedreich ataxia
- Gerstmann-Sträussler-Scheinker disease
- Joseph disease
- Latent nystagmus
- Lewy body disease
- Lithium
- MS (cerebellar dysfunction)
- MSA
- OPCA
- PD; small SWJs may develop or increase after pallidotomy
- PSP
- Schizophrenia
- Square-wave pulses (macro–SWJs)
- Strabismus
- Tobacco
- Wernicke encephalopathy

*AIDS*, Acquired immunodeficiency syndrome; *HIV*, human immunodeficiency virus; *MS*, multiple sclerosis; *MSA*, multiple system atrophy; *OPCA*, olivopontocerebellar atrophy; *PD*, Parkinson disease; *PSP*, progressive supranuclear palsy; *SWJs*, square-wave jerks.

is suggestive, but an electroretinogram is confirmatory. Spasmus nutans can be associated in a patient with COMA and cerebellar vermian hypoplasia.

### Saccadic Intrusions

Saccadic intrusions are brief, unwanted saccadic interruptions of fixation (see Figs. 18.25 and 18.27 and Box 18.15). Other intrusions are saccadic pulses (stepless saccades) that interrupt fixation and are followed by a slow drift back on target (glissade), double saccadic pulses (fragment of flutter with two back-to-back saccades), and dynamic overshoots (see Fig. 18.27). Saccadic intrusions tend to be precipitated by gaze shifts. They are divided into two broad categories depending on whether they have an intersaccadic interval (or pause) between the back-to-back saccades. With the exception of SWJs, saccadic intrusions tend to result in the symptom of oscillopsia and may require treatment.

#### *With Intersaccadic Interval*

**Square-wave jerks.** SWJs (Box 18.16 Video 18.11) are spontaneous  small-amplitude paired saccades with an intersaccadic interval of 150 to 200 msec that briefly interrupt fixation (see Fig. 18.27). They may occur physiologically in normal subjects (particularly without fixation and in darkness) and are usually about 2 degrees in amplitude. They are more common in the elderly and in carriers of blue-cone monochromatism. SWJs are prominent in PSP, multiple system atrophy (MSA), and cerebellar disease; the increased frequency of SWJs in these less dopamine-responsive parkinsonian syndromes such as olivopontocerebellar atrophy (autosomal dominant cerebellar atrophy), PSP, Lewy body disease, and MSA may distinguish them from idiopathic Parkinson disease (PD), although they may also occur in PD at any disease stage (Shaikh et al., 2011). Because of the intersaccadic interval, SWJs are thought to be triggered supratentorially, whereas other saccadic intrusions (e.g., saccadic pulses) and oscillations (e.g., flutter and opsoclonus) are caused by dysfunction in the brainstem and cerebellum. However, square-wave oscillations (runs of otherwise typical SWJs that may clinically be mistaken for ocular flutter) are most often reported in the context of cerebellar injury (Brokalaki et al., 2015; Optikan and Pretegiani, 2017; Pretegiani et al., 2017; Rosini et al., 2013), in which case they may be responsive to memantine.

Square-wave pulses (SWPs), previously termed *macrosquare-wave jerks*, also interrupt fixation but differ from SWJs, having larger amplitudes (10–40 degrees) and shorter latencies (about 80 msec) before the eyes return to the target; they occur in patients with MS and olivopontocerebellar degeneration and may accompany rubral tremor. SWJs and SWPs should be distinguished from MSOs, which wax and wane across fixation (see Fig. 18.27), are not present in darkness, and occur with midline cerebellar lesions.

**Macrosaccadic oscillations.** MSOs (see Fig. 18.27) are runs of horizontal saccades with intersaccadic intervals that are larger than those of SWJs and that oscillate about the midline of fixation with a crescendo-decrescendo pattern depending on their size. They represent cerebellar disease, specifically of the caudal fastigial nucleus, and can be considered as an extreme along the spectrum of cerebellar saccadic hypermetria. Ocular dysmetria occurs with refixation saccades that overshoot the target (see Fig. 18.25, *B*) and often oscillate with an intersaccadic interval of approximately 200 msec before coming to rest.

#### *Without Intersaccadic Interval*

**Ocular flutter and opsoclonus** (Videos 18.12 and 18.13). Ocular flutter (see Fig. 18.25, *A*) and opsoclonus occur with brainstem or cerebellar disease and consist of conjugate back-to-back saccades without an intervening intersaccadic interval; they occur spontaneously in intermittent bursts. Ocular flutter, by definition, occurs only in the horizontal plane, whereas opsoclonus has horizontal, vertical, and torsional trajectories. Flutter and opsoclonus are often are precipitated by gaze shifts (see Fig. 18.25, *D*). Rarely, they are triggered by a change in posture (Martins et al., 2019) or occur only in eccentric gaze (Rizzo et al., 2019). Usually these oscillations are large enough to be seen on clinical examination; however, ocular microflutter, previously called *microsaccadic ocular flutter*, is a rare symptomatic ocular oscillation requiring magnification for detection (Ashe et al., 1991). Patients complain of episodes of "shimmering" vision. It is reported with cerebellar degeneration and MS and as a benign phenomenon in some individuals. When it is persistent, patients should be evaluated for occult neoplasms and have long-term follow-up.

These oscillations result from pathology that disinhibits saccadic EBNs, which have an inherent tendency to oscillate due to membrane properties of postinhibitory rebound firing and reciprocal synaptic feedback loops (Shaikh et al., 2008). Increased sensitivity of the $GABA_A$ receptor in a circuit involving the cerebellum, inferior olives, and EBNs provides a link between the various brainstem and cerebellar dysfunctions that can result in flutter and opsoclonus (Optican and Pretegiani, 2017).

The most common causes (Box 18.17 and Table 18.6) of flutter and opsoclonus include viral or postviral encephalitis and toxic, metabolic, and paraneoplastic disorders. Parainfectious states are typically accompanied by emotional lability, myoclonus, and ataxia. Several paraneoplastic antibodies are associated with flutter and opsoclonus in adults; however, antibodies are often not detected. In children, the opsoclonus-myoclonus-cerebellar syndrome is often a manifestation of neuroblastoma and may be responsive to adrenocorticotropic hormone. The efficacy of immunotherapy in adults with paraneoplastic syndromes is difficult to assess. However, in addition to treatment of the underlying neoplasm, early and aggressive immunotherapy, including the use of immunoadsorption therapy with plasma exchange, may be effective. Responsiveness probably depends on the degree of the inflammatory component rather than on neuronal loss. Flutter and opsoclonus occasionally may respond to thiamine, clonazepam, and antiepileptic agents.

**Voluntary "nystagmus."** Voluntary nystagmus is not true nystagmus as it consists of voluntarily produced back-to-back saccades and has no slow phases. It is more accurately called voluntary flutter. The oscillations are horizontal and thus consistent with the term *flutter*;

### BOX 18.17 Causes of Opsoclonus

- Acquired immunodeficiency syndrome-related brainstem encephalitis or lymphoma
- Adults: carcinoma (thiamine-responsive)
- Biotin-responsive multiple carboxylase deficiency
- Celiac disease
- Children: neuroblastoma (corticotropin responsive)
- Drugs (amitriptyline, chlordecone, cocaine, dichlorodiphenyltrichloroethane, haloperidol, phencyclidine, phenytoin, diazepam, thallium, toluene, strychnine, vidarabine)
- Encephalitis (viral, pyogenic)
- Hashimoto encephalopathy
- Hydrocephalus
- Hyperosmolar coma
- Lipidoses
- Multiple sclerosis
- Paraneoplastic
- Pontine hemorrhage
- Postencephalitic
- Sarcoid
- Thalamic glioma
- Thalamic hemorrhage
- Transient phenomenon in healthy neonates
- Viral hepatitis
- Wernicke encephalopathy

### TABLE 18.6 Age-Related Likely Causes and Features of Opsoclonus

| | |
|---|---|
| **Neonates** | Parainfectious<br>Paraneoplastic (neuroblastoma in chest or abdomen) |
| **Older infants:** | |
| **8 months to 3 years** | Neural crest tumor or regressed neural crest tumor |
| **Older than 3 years** | Regressed neural crest tumor |
| **Children with opsoclonus** | Good prognosis for tumor<br>Poor prognosis for ocular movements (Respond to ACTH) |
| **Adults** | Parainfectious: enterovirus, West Nile, Lyme, mumps, HIV, malaria, dengue, Zika<br>Paraneoplastic (breast, ovary, lung)/autoimmune: reported with the following antibodies: Hu, Yo, Ma, amphiphysin, P/Q calcium channel, NMDAR, GAD, GQ1b; may respond to protein A immunoabsorption |

*ACTH*, Adrenocorticotropic hormone; *HIV*, human immunodeficiency virus.

however, some individuals can evoke oscillations in other planes, including vertical, torsional, or (rarely) cycloid—a phenomenon reported as "volitional opsoclonus." The ability to induce flutter voluntarily can be familial; however, some individuals are able to learn to do this eye movement. It may be confused with pathological ocular flutter, but clues include the fact that individuals with this ability typically must converge their eyes to initiate the oscillation and are unable to sustain it for longer than 30 seconds or so. Occasionally, subjects use this ability to feign illness, but the phenomenon should easily be recognized.

### Eye Movements in Seizures and Coma

***Ictal nystagmus.*** Often ictal nystagmus accompanies adversive seizures and beats to the side opposite the focus. Ictal nystagmus may be associated with transient pupillary dilation of either the abducting or adducting eye. Pupillary oscillations synchronous with the nystagmus may occur rarely. Ictal nystagmus associated with unformed visual hallucinations, homonymous hemianopia, and unusual MRI findings occurs in patients with nonketotic hyperglycemia (Lavin, 2005; Stayman et al., 2013). Nystagmus as the only motor manifestation of a seizure is rare; however, there are reports of isolated ictal nystagmus, as occurs with vivid ictal visual hallucinations. Monocular nystagmus associated with ipsilateral hemianopic visual hallucinations in a binocular patient can occur as the only manifestation of a partial seizure caused by a focal discharge in the contralateral medial occipital lobe. It is difficult to draw any clinical conclusion regarding the location of the seizure discharge in these patients because seizure foci have been found in occipital, parietal, temporal, and frontal areas. Usually the nystagmus is horizontal, but vertical nystagmus, mainly in comatose patients, occurs on occasion. In comatose patients, periodic eye movements should alert the physician to the possibility of status epilepticus; indeed, PAN associated with periodic alternating gaze deviation (PAGD) and periodic alternating head rotation may be a manifestation of seizure. The monocular abducting nystagmus seen in alternating hemiplegia of childhood is likely ictal in origin.

***Ping-Pong Gaze and Periodic Alternating Gaze Deviation.*** *Ping-pong gaze* is characterized by slow, conjugate, horizontal rhythmic oscillations that cycle every 4–8 seconds (short-cycle PAGD) and occurs in comatose patients because of bilateral cerebral or upper brainstem lesions or metabolic dysfunction; one patient had a vermian hemorrhage. The oscillations can be saccadic. Ping-pong gaze implies that the horizontal gaze centers in the pons are intact. The prognosis for recovery is generally poor except in patients with a toxic or metabolic cause; occasionally patients with structural lesions recover (Diesing and Wijdicks, 2004).

*Periodic alternating gaze deviation* is a rare cyclical ocular motor disorder in which the direction of gaze alternates every few minutes. Lateral deviation can be sustained for up to 15 minutes; gaze then returns to the midline for 10–20 seconds before changing to the other side. Occasionally PAGD is associated with structural lesions such as pontine vascular disorders; Chiari malformations; congenital absence or abnormalities of the inferior cerebellar vermis, the uvula, and nodulus; Creutzfeldt-Jakob disease involving the flocculonodular lobe; spinocerebellar degeneration; occipital encephaloceles; and paraneoplastic brainstem encephalitis. A reversible form of PAGD occurs with hepatic encephalopathy and is attributed to derangement of GABA metabolism. PAN has a similar time cycle to PAGD and results from lesions of the uvular and nodular regions. Indeed, PAGD may be PAN with loss of corrective saccades because of concomitant saccadic palsy or immaturity of the saccadic system in infants.

***Ocular Bobbing.*** *Ocular bobbing* is a rapid downward movement of both eyes followed by a slow drift back to primary position. The movement recurs between 2 and 15 times/min and is found in patients who are usually comatose, with severe central pontine destruction and horizontal gaze palsies (Table 18.7). In typical bobbing, horizontal eye movements are spared. Other forms of bobbing are described and are listed in Table 18.7.

### Miscellaneous Abnormal Spontaneous Eye Movements

*Superior oblique myokymia* is a paroxysmal, rapid, small-amplitude monocular torsional-vertical oscillation caused by contraction of the superior oblique muscle. Patients may complain of monocular blurring, torsional or vertical oscillopsia, torsional or vertical diplopia, or twitching of the eye. Oculography using magnetic search coils demonstrates both phasic and tonic contractions of intorsion, depression, and—to a much lesser extent—abduction of the superior oblique muscle (Leigh and Zee, 2015). MRI may show a smaller superior oblique muscle on the affected side, suggesting antecedent injury to the fourth nerve; this hypothesis is supported by an MRI finding of neurovascular compression of the fourth nerve at its root exit zone. SOM may be difficult to detect with the unaided eye and is more easily detected with a direct ophthalmoscope. It may be precipitated by activating the superior oblique muscle when the patient looks down in the direction of action of that muscle or tilts the head toward the affected eye. SOM has a relapsing-remitting course in otherwise healthy adults. It is reported with adrenoleukodystrophy, lead poisoning, cerebellar astrocytoma, dural arteriovenous fistula, and microvascular

**TABLE 18.7 Ocular Bobbing**

| Type | Movement | Cause |
|---|---|---|
| Ocular bobbing (atypical bobbing, horizontal eye movements preserved) | Fast down, slow upward return to primary position | Severe central pontine destruction, central pontine myelinolysis, encephalitis, extra-axial pontine compression (usually a cerebellar hematoma), organophosphate poisoning |
| Reverse bobbing | Fast up, slow downward return to primary position | Usually nonlocalizing encephalopathy: anoxia, metabolic encephalopathy, head injury, post–status epilepticus |
| Dipping (inverse bobbing) | Slow down, fast upward return to primary position | Anoxic, metabolic, and toxic position encephalopathies, post status epilepticus |
| Reverse dipping | Slow up, fast downward return to primary position | Cryptococcal meningitis or obtundation (in a patient with acquired immunodeficiency syndrome), pontine stroke |
| V-pattern pretectal pseudobobbing | Fast downward convergent movements at higher frequency and slower return to primary position than with typical bobbing | Acute obstructive hydrocephalus |

compression. It may respond dramatically to medication such as carbamazepine or gabapentin, propranolol in low dosage, amitriptyline, baclofen, phenytoin, benzodiazepines, or topical beta-blockers used for glaucoma (see Table 18.5). A base-down prism in front of the affected eye may alleviate the patient's symptoms, avoid potential side effects of long-term medication, and obviate the superior oblique muscle or tendon surgery that is occasionally used in resistant cases. Disabling SOM may respond to microvascular decompression of the trochlear nerve at its root exit.

*Episodic nystagmus* is associated with disorders in which the patient has paroxysmal episodes of vertigo, ataxia, and nystagmus lasting up to 24 hours. The nystagmus may be torsional, vertical, or dissociated. The frequency of attacks varies, ranging from once a day to only a few times per year. Such periodic ataxias occur in patients with hereditary inborn errors of metabolism in an autosomal dominant form without any detectable metabolic defect (channelopathy), in some forms of spinocerebellar degeneration, and in basilar migraine. Acetazolamide or 4-aminopyridine may alleviate or prevent attacks in the familial form.

*Oculogyric crises* are spasmodic conjugate ocular deviations, usually in an upward direction. They occurred in the late stages of postencephalitic PD after the 1918 influenza epidemic, but now most often are caused by neuroleptic medication, particularly haloperidol. Also, they may occur with head injury, neurosyphilis, herpetic brainstem encephalitis, bilateral paramedian midbrain inflammation, NMDA-receptor encephalitis, and carbamazepine or lithium carbonate toxicity. Oculogyric crises can occur in the early stages of autosomal dominant "rapid-onset dystonia-parkinsonism." A typical attack or crisis lasts about 2 hours, during which the eyes are tonically deviated upward, repetitively, for periods of seconds to minutes. The spasms may be preceded or accompanied by disturbing emotional symptoms, including anxiety, restlessness, compulsive thinking, and sensations of increased brightness or distortions of visual background (resembling occipital lobe seizures). The patient may be able to force the eyes back to the primary position temporarily by using voluntary saccades, optokinetic tracking, head rotation, or blinking. Electroencephalographic recordings during the attacks show no epileptiform activity. The eyelids are usually open, although they may jerk rhythmically at times from twitching of the orbicularis oculi, and the pupils are usually not involved. Attacks may be precipitated by excitement. They should be differentiated from benign paroxysmal tonic upward (PTU) gaze (see later). Treatment for oculogyric crises includes diphenhydramine, L-dopa, and high-dose trihexyphenidyl; anticholinergic agents terminate the thought disorders as well.

*Tonic upward deviation of gaze* (forced upgaze), a rare sign, is seen in unconscious patients and must be distinguished from oculogyric crises, petit mal seizures, and psychogenic coma. Comatose patients with sustained upgaze after diffuse brain injury (e.g., hypotension, cardiac arrest, heatstroke) usually have cerebral and cerebellar hypoxic damage with relative sparing of the brainstem; it generally appears within the first few hours of the insult (Johkura et al., 2004). Those patients who develop myoclonic jerks and large-amplitude downbeat nystagmus later have a very poor prognosis. Rarely, tonic upward gaze deviation may be psychogenic but can be overcome, indeed cured, by cold caloric stimulation of the eardrums.

*"Benign" paroxysmal tonic upward gaze* may occur in association with ataxia in young children who have downbeat nystagmus on attempted downgaze. The duration of the deviation is variable (seconds to hours), but it is usually short and occurs frequently throughout the day. PTU gaze usually starts in the first year of life and lasts about 2 years; the onset may be during or shortly after an infection or vaccination. PTU gaze may be exacerbated by fatigue, relieved by sleep, and sometimes provoked by car travel; there is no evidence that the episodes are seizures or oculogyric crises. The cause of PTU gaze is unknown, but at follow-up a significant number of patients have developmental delay, intellectual disability, language delay, or ocular motility disorders; these findings imply that PTU gaze is a marker for underlying neurological or developmental abnormalities. The condition is reminiscent of the intermittent or periodic ataxias, which may respond to drugs such as acetazolamide.

*Tonic downward deviation of gaze* (forced downgaze) is associated with impaired consciousness in patients with medial thalamic hemorrhage, acute obstructive hydrocephalus, severe metabolic or hypoxic encephalopathy, or massive subarachnoid hemorrhage (SAH). Also, the eyes may converge, as if looking at the nose. When tonic downward gaze deviation is the result of hypoxic encephalopathy, it appears later (1–7 days) than upward tonic gaze deviation (hours) and almost always predicts a persistent vegetative state (Johkura et al., 2004). Tonic downward gaze deviation may also occur in psychogenic illness, especially feigned coma, but can also be overcome by caloric stimulation. In young children with acute hydrocephalus, tonic downward deviation may be associated with upper lid retraction; because of its appearance, this is called the *setting sun sign*.

In otherwise healthy neonates, downward deviation of the eyes or tonic upgaze while awake may occur as a transient phenomenon caused by uneven delayed development in the vertical otolithic-ocular pathways. Tonic vertical deviation due to ictal activity is rare. A form of paroxysmal ocular downward deviation that lasts seconds and occurs in neurologically impaired infants with poor vision may also be seen in preterm infants with bronchopulmonary dysplasia but subsequent normal development.

Cyclical esotropia, also called *circadian*, *alternate-day*, or *clock-mechanism esotropia*, usually begins in childhood, although it can occur at any age and can also follow surgery for intermittent esotropia. The cycles of orthotropia and esotropia may run 24–96 hours, similar to many other cyclical or periodic biological phenomena with obscure mechanisms. Patients with cyclical esotropia can decompensate into a constant esotropia that can be corrected surgically.

*Ocular neuromyotonia* is a brief episodic myotonic contraction of one or more muscles supplied by the ocular motor nerves, most commonly the oculomotor nerve. It may occur spontaneously or be provoked by prolonged gaze in a particular direction. It usually results in esotropia of the affected eye accompanied by failure of elevation and depression of the globe. When the oculomotor nerve is affected, there may be associated signs of aberrant reinnervation (see Chapter 103). The pupil may be fixed to both light and near stimuli or become myotonic. Ocular neuromyotonia occurs most often after radiation therapy for sellar region tumors. Less often it is associated with compressive lesions such as pituitary adenomas, cavernous sinus meningiomas or aneurysms, thyroid orbitopathy, radiation of a frontal lobe lesion, following myelography with thorium dioxide, with Paget disease of the skull base, or with neurovascular compression by a dolichoectatic basilar artery. Demyelinating lesions in the region of the third cranial nerve fascicle also can cause "paroxysmal spasm" of the muscles innervated by the oculomotor nerve but are usually accompanied by other findings such as eyelid retraction or paroxysmal limb dystonia. Occasionally no cause can be found. Ocular neuromyotonia may respond to carbamazepine or other antiepileptic drugs. It should be distinguished from SOM and the spasms of cyclical oculomotor palsy.

*Cyclical oculomotor palsy* is characterized by paresis alternating with "cyclic" spasms of both the extra- and intraocular muscles supplied by the oculomotor nerve. It is a rare condition usually noted in the first 2 years of life, although most cases are believed to

**BOX 18.18 Gaze-Evoked Phenomena**

**Physiological Phenomena**
- Blinks
- Endpoint nystagmus
- Flaring of the nostrils during vertical saccades
- Mentalis contraction during horizontal saccades (personal observation)
- Oculoauricular phenomenon: retraction of ear during lateral gaze (or convergence)
- Orbicularis oculi myokymia
- Phosphenes (more intense in patients with optic neuritis, retinal/vitreous detachment: Moore lightning streaks)

**Pathological Sensory Phenomena**
- Gaze-evoked amaurosis in the eye ipsilateral to an orbital apex tumor
- Gaze-evoked tinnitus with cerebellopontine angle tumors or following posterior fossa surgery
- Reverse-Tullio phenomenon (gaze-evoked swooshing sound) caused by end-organ damage in a patient with Tullio phenomenon (sound-evoked nystagmus and vertigo) (personal observation)
- SUNCT (sudden unilateral conjunctival injection and tearing) syndrome with saccades
- Tinnitus with periodic saccadic oscillations
- Vertigo

**Pathological Motor Phenomena**
- Convergence retraction nystagmus on attempted upgaze (dorsal midbrain syndrome)
- Facial twitching, clonic limb movements, blepharoclonus, lid nystagmus, involuntary laughter and seizures
- Gaze-evoked nystagmus
- Neuromyotonia
- Retraction of the globe in Duane syndrome
- Superior oblique myokymia
- Synkinetic movements with cyclical oculomotor palsy and with aberrant reinnervation of the oculomotor nerve (see Chapter 103)

be congenital and are often associated with other features of birth trauma. During the spasms, which last for 10–30 seconds, the upper eyelid elevates, the globe adducts, and the pupil and ciliary muscle constrict, causing miosis and increased accommodation; the paretic phase usually lasts longer. Signs of aberrant oculomotor reinnervation (see Chapter 103) are usually present. Spasms, often heralded by twitching of the upper lid, may be precipitated by intentional accommodation or adduction. Cycles occur irregularly, vary from 1.5–3 minutes in duration, persist during sleep, may be suppressed by topical cholinergic agents (eserine, pilocarpine), and are abolished by topical anticholinergic agents (atropine, homatropine) or general anesthesia. The cycles usually persist throughout life, but the spasms of the extraocular muscles may abate, leaving only intermittent miosis. Symptomatic cyclical oculomotor palsy may occur in later life in patients with underlying lesions involving the third cranial nerve, but the features and cycles are atypical.

*Gaze-evoked phenomena* such as endpoint nystagmus, the oculoauricular phenomenon, and orbicularis oculi myokymia are physiological or benign. Others, such as GEN or tinnitus, are pathological (Box 18.18) and may be the result of damage to the horizontal NI.

### Treatment of Oscillations

Treatments used for the different types of nystagmus are summarized in Table 18.5. Underlying causes should be rectified where possible, and visual acuity should be maximized. Prisms, surgery, and contact lenses are the mainstays of treatment for INS, although memantine has been shown to also be effective. Medications are the mainstays of therapy for acquired forms of nystagmus, although prisms may also be helpful.

## DEVELOPMENT OF THE OCULAR MOTOR SYSTEM

At birth, the vestibular system is the most developed of the ocular motor subsystems and is easily tested by rotating the infant, held at arm's length, with the head tilted 30 degrees forward. In normal neonates, the eyes deviate tonically in the same direction as head movement; reflex saccades develop by 2–3 weeks after birth. Smooth-pursuit movements may be detected in neonates but only with large targets (such as a human face) at low velocities. These findings, although not well quantified, are consistent with histological maturation of the fovea after at least 8 weeks of age. Also, neonates can generate the smooth-pursuit component of OKN with full-field stimulation.

Fixation is not well developed until about 2 months of age, although some infants younger than 1 month of age can fixate targets provided that the stimuli are engaging and the infant is alert. By 9 weeks, 90% of full-term infants can fixate and follow the human face. Full-field OKN and larger targets stimulate the parafoveal retina, which matures earlier than the fovea. Stimulation of the saccadic system, also immature in the neonate, is influenced by the infant's attention as well as by the size and appropriateness of the target. Vertical saccades mature more slowly than horizontal saccades and may not be detected for the first month after birth. Also, vergence movements are slow to mature but are seen after about the first month.

Ocular alignment in the newborn is usually poor, with transient shifts from esotropia to exotropia during the first few weeks. Ocular alignment depends on both visual input and the maturity of the vergence system. In most infants, ocular alignment is established by 3–4 weeks of age but may be delayed until as late as 5 months. Small-angle esotropia and intermittent esotropia may spontaneously resolve in infants younger than 20 weeks of age; constant esotropia greater than 40 prism diopters is unlikely to resolve spontaneously. Esotropia after 3 months and exotropia after 5 months are considered abnormal and require appropriate evaluation. Large-angle exotropia may be associated with craniofacial, genetic, or other neurological abnormalities.

Paroxysmal phenomena are common in infancy and may occur in as many as one in four. Ocular motor anomalies may occur in the neonate without any pathological significance. About 2% of newborns have a tendency for tonic downward deviation of the eyes in the waking state; during sleep, however, the eyes assume the normal position, and the VORs are intact. Other uncommon abnormalities seen in newborns include opsoclonus, which may regress through a phase of ocular flutter, skew deviation, apparent bilateral INO, transient downbeat nystagmus, and tonic upward deviation. These findings likely represent delayed maturity of the ocular motor system in neonates.

## RECORDING OF EYE MOVEMENTS

### How Can They Help?

Oculographic techniques provide clinicians and researchers with objective and quantitative means of analysis that have led to a better understanding of eye movement neurophysiology and ocular motility disorders. Quantitative oculography can measure saccadic latency, velocity, accuracy, pursuit and VOR gain as well as nystagmus slow phase velocity; it can detect unsuspected oscillations and intrusions and identify different nystagmus waveforms. Oculography is used to record both spontaneous and induced eye movements to a target, such as a projected light in front of the subject, or to vestibular and optokinetic stimuli.

### Methods of Recording

Electro-oculography, also known as *electronystagmography* is a popular method of quantitative oculography but has a limited range and is unreliable for vertical eye movements because of eyelid artifact. Infrared oculography is more accurate but challenged by the need for patient cooperation with calibration and lid artifacts. The most quantitatively accurate technique involves use of the scleral search coil.

*The complete reference list is available online at https://expertconsult.inkling.com/.*

19

# Disturbances of Smell and Taste

*Richard L. Doty, Steven M. Bromley*

## OUTLINE



Disorders of smell and taste can jeopardize human safety and produce loss of appetite, unintended weight loss, malnutrition, occupational disability, and reduced quality of life. In a study of 750 patients with chemosensory disturbances, 68% reported altered quality of life, 46% changes in appetite or body weight, and 56% adverse influences on daily living or psychological well-being (Deems et al., 1991a). In another study of 445 such patients, at least one hazardous event, such as food poisoning or failure to detect fire or leaking natural gas, was reported by 45.2% of those with anosmia, as compared with 19.0% of those with normal function (Santos et al., 2004). Importantly, older persons with smell loss are three times more likely to die over the course of 4 or 5 years (Devanand et al., 2015; Pinto et al., 2014). Of particular relevance to the neurologist is the fact that smell dysfunction is among the earliest "preclinical" or "presymptomatic" signs of neurodegenerative diseases such as Alzheimer disease (AD) and Parkinson disease (PD) (Doty, 2012). Indeed, olfactory tests are as effective in detecting PD as single-photon emission computed tomography (SPECT) imaging of the dopamine transporter (Deeb et al., 2010).

Both smell and taste disorders have been documented in a wide range of diseases, although meaningful smell disturbances are much more common than taste disorders. The vast majority of patients complaining of "taste" disturbances actually have decreased smell, not taste, function (Deems et al., 1991a). Flavor sensations such as cola, coffee, chocolate, strawberry, pizza, licorice, steak sauce, and vanilla depend upon stimulation of the olfactory receptors by molecules that enter the nasal pharynx during deglutition (Burdach and Doty 1987). Such "taste" sensations disappear when the olfactory epithelium is severely damaged, leaving intact only tactile and the taste bud–mediated sensations of sweet, sour, salty, bitter, and savory.

In this chapter, olfactory and gustatory system anatomy and physiology are reviewed, with an emphasis on pathophysiology. Chemosensory disturbances in diseases commonly encountered by the neurologist are described, along with means for patient assessment and symptom management.

## ANATOMY AND PHYSIOLOGY

### Olfaction

The approximately 6 million olfactory receptor cells are located within a pseudostratified columnar neuroepithelium lining the cribriform plate and sectors of the superior septum, the middle turbinate, and the superior turbinate. This epithelium also contains sustentacular, microvillar, and basal cells (the precursors of other cell types within the epithelium) and is supported by a highly vascularized lamina propria containing Bowman glands, the major source of the olfactory mucus. The bipolar receptor cells, which project 3–30 receptor-bearing cilia into the mucus, serve as both a receptor cell and a first-order neuron and can regenerate, to some degree, from basal cells after being damaged. Such cells exhibit the most diverse molecular phenotype of any neuron, expressing a wide range of receptor protein types and cell surface antigens. A photomicrograph of the surface of the olfactory epithelium is shown in Fig. 19.1.

Each olfactory receptor cell expresses only 1 of nearly 400 functional types of receptor proteins. Odor receptor genes are found in approximately 100 locations on all chromosomes except 20 and Y. Remarkably, the olfactory subgenome spans 1%–2% of the total genomic DNA. Most single-chemical odorants stimulate more than one type of receptor and overlap typically exists among the sets of receptors stimulated by various chemicals, implying complex across-fiber sensory coding.

After coalescing into bundles (fila) within the lamina propria, the olfactory receptor axons traverse the foramina of the cribriform plate and enter sphere-like glomeruli located within an outer layer of the olfactory bulb, an ovid structure composed of afferent and efferent nerve fibers, multiple interneurons, microglia, astrocytes, and blood vessels (Fig. 19.2). Those receptor cells expressing the same odorant protein converge onto the same glomerulus. The bulb's primary output neurons—the mitral and tufted cells—are modulated by input from olfactory receptor cells and local interneurons, including the γ-aminobutyric acid (GABA) ergic granule cells, the most numerous cells of the bulb. Granule cells receive numerous inputs from central brain regions and, unlike nearly all other central nervous system (CNS) neurons, undergo periodic replacement from neuroblasts that migrate from the anterior subventricular zone of the brain. Some of these differentiating neuroblasts further migrate within the bulb to repopulate periglomerular cells (Rousselot et al., 1995).

The axons of the mitral and tufted cells project centrally, via the lateral olfactory tract, to the anterior olfactory nucleus, the piriform cortex, the anterior cortical nucleus of the amygdala, the periamygdaloid complex, and the rostral entorhinal cortex. Pyramidal cells from the anterior olfactory nucleus project to numerous ipsilateral and contralateral brain structures, the latter via the anterior commissure. Although most bulbar output neurons project ipsilaterally to cortical structures without synapsing in the thalamus, connections via the thalamus do exist between primary (e.g., entorhinal) cortex and secondary (i.e., orbitofrontal) olfactory cortices.

The relative roles of central brain structures in odor perception are poorly understood. The piriform cortex encodes higher-order representations of odor quality, identity, and familiarity, and is involved in odor learning and memory (Gottfried et al., 2002). The entorhinal cortex preprocesses information entering the hippocampus, whereas the amygdala seems to respond to the intensity of emotionally significant odors. The orbitofrontal cortex combines input from taste, texture, and smell and plays a vital role in flavor perception and hedonics (Rolls and Grabenhorst, 2008).

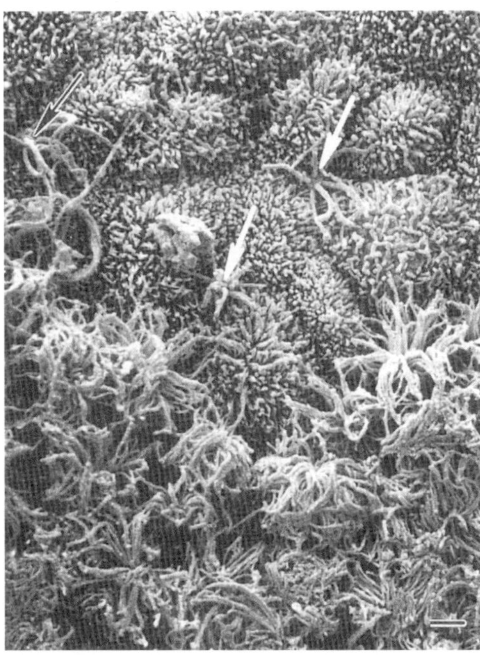

**Fig. 19.1 A Surface Transition Region Between the Olfactory and Respiratory Epithelia.** The bottom half displays olfactory epithelium, the top half respiratory epithelium. *Arrows* identify olfactory receptor cell dendritic endings with cilia. Bar = 5 μm. *(From Menco, B.P.M., Morrison, E.E., 2003. Morphology of the mammalian olfactory epithelium: form, fine structure, function, and pathology. In: Doty, R.L. (Ed.), Handbook of Olfaction and Gustation, second ed. Marcel Dekker, New York, pp. 17–49, with permission.)*

## Gustation

Taste is critical for identifying substances in foods and beverages, such as sugars and poisonous alkaloids, that promote or disrupt homeostasis. In addition to being located within the oral cavity, bitter and sweet taste–related receptors are found in the alimentary and respiratory tracts, where they are involved in metabolism and bacterial defense. In the oral cavity, the taste receptor cells are located within taste buds, small flask-like structures on the surface of the oral epithelium, mostly on protuberances called papillae (Figs. 19.3 and 19.4). Like olfactory receptor cells, taste receptor cells periodically die and become replaced.

Humans possess approximately 7500 oral taste buds. Those on the fungiform papillae are innervated by the chorda tympani division of the facial nerve (cranial nerve [CN] VII). The palatine branch of the greater superficial petrosal division of CN VII innervates the taste buds on the soft palate, whereas taste buds on the anterior *foliate papillae* are innervated by CN VII. The buds on the posterior foliate papillae are innervated by CN IX, as are those located on the *circumvallate papillae.* Taste buds within the oral pharynx are supplied by the vagus (CN X) nerve.

A small family of three G protein–coupled receptors (GPCRs), termed T1R1, T1R2, and T1R3, encode sweet and umami (monosodium glutamate–like) sensations. Bitter is mediated by the T2R receptors, a family of approximately 30 GPCRs expressed on cells different from those that express sweet and umami receptors. Salty sensations arise from the entrance of $Na^+$ ions into the cells via specialized membrane channels, such as the amiloride-sensitive $Na^+$ channel. Although sour taste has been suggested to depend upon a range of receptors, PKD2L1 is likely the primary sour taste receptor. The nerves innervating the taste buds converge centrally into the nucleus of the solitary tract of the brainstem. From there, fibers project to centers within the upper regions of the ventral posterior nuclei of the thalamus via the

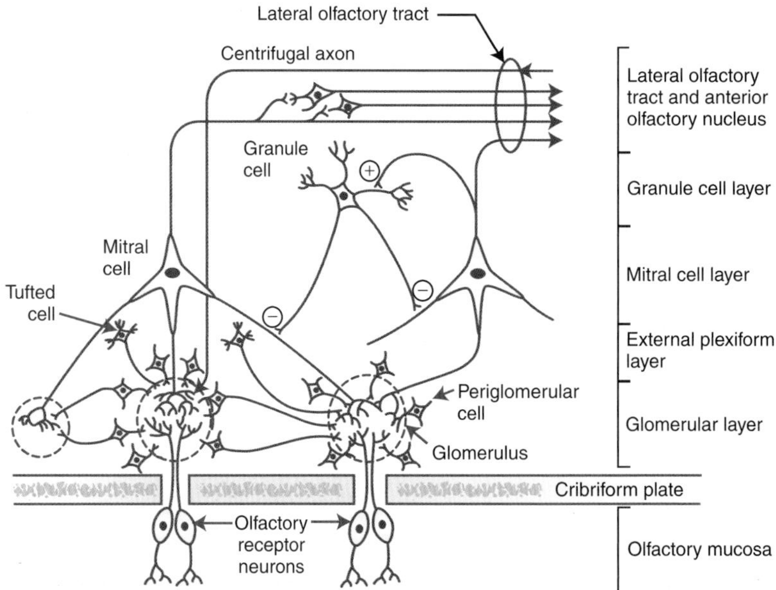


**Fig. 19.2 Schematic of Olfactory Bulb Structures, Neurons, and Layers.** *(From Alloway, K.D., Pritchard, T.C., 2007. Medical Neuroscience, second ed. Hayes Barton, Raleigh, NC, with permission.)*

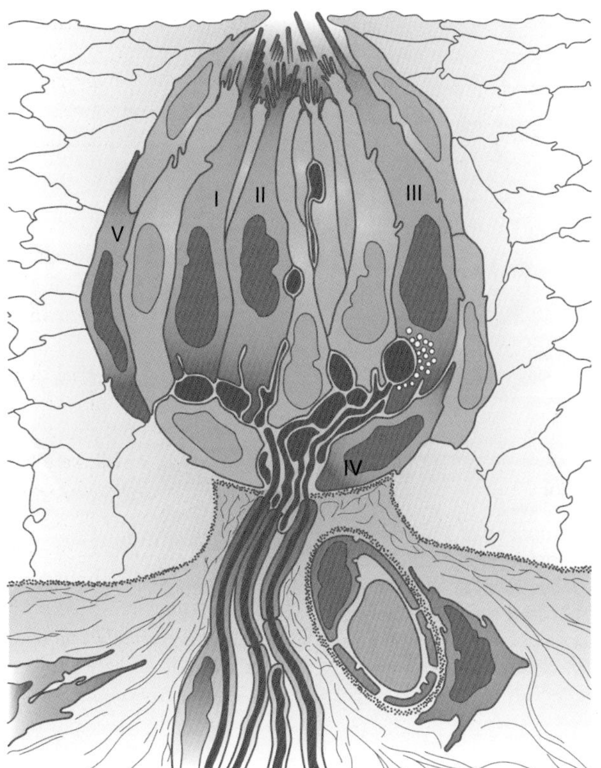


Fig. 19.3 **Idealized Drawing of Longitudinal Section of Mammalian Taste Bud.** Cells of type I, II, and III are elongated and form the sensory epithelium of the bud. These cells have different types of microvillae within the taste pit and may reach the taste pore. Type IV are basal cells, and type V are marginal cells. Synapses are most apparent at the bases of type III cells. The connecting taste nerves have myelin sheaths. *(From Witt, M., Reutter, K., Miller, I.J., Jr., 2003. Morphology of the peripheral taste system. In: Doty, R.L., (Ed.), Handbook of Olfaction and Gustation, second ed. Marcel Dekker, New York, pp. 651–677. Copyright © 2003 Marcel Dekker, Inc.)*

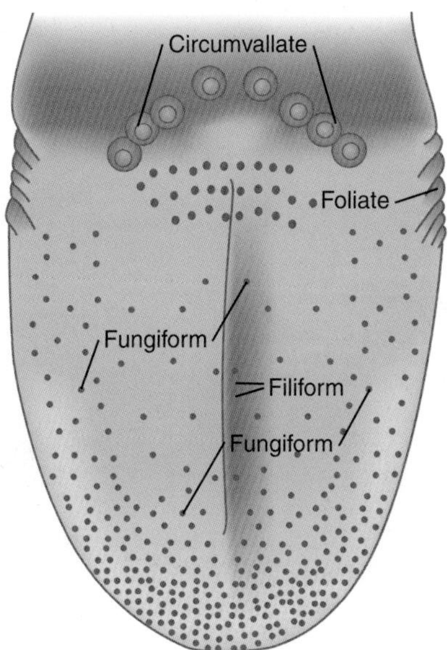


Fig. 19.4 **Schematic Representation of the Tongue Demonstrating the Relative Distribution of the Four Main Classes of Taste Papillae.** Note that the fungiform papillae can vary considerable in size and that they are more dense on the anterior and lateral regions of the tongue. *(Copyright © 2006 Richard L. Doty.)*

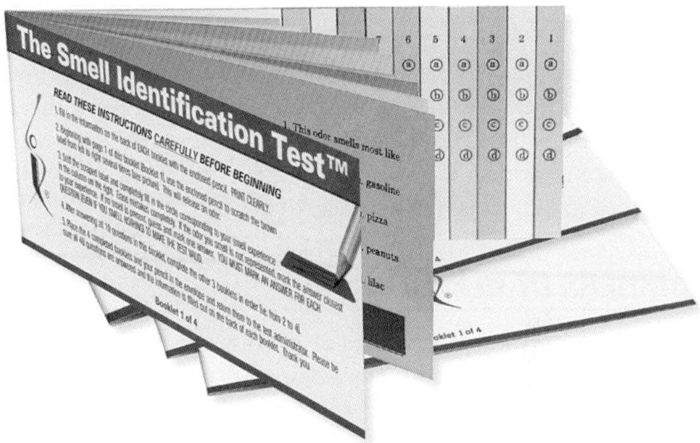


Fig. 19.5 **Booklets of the University of Pennsylvania Smell Identification Test (UPSIT).** The test is composed of four booklets, each containing 10 microencapsulated scratch and sniff odorants that are released by a pencil tip. Associated with each odorant is a multiple-choice question about which of four possibilities is correct. Forced-choice answers are recorded on the last page of each booklet and assessed with a simple scoring key. *(Copyright © 2004 Sensonics, Inc., Haddon Heights, NJ. Reprinted with permission.)*

medial lemniscus. Information is then sent to the amygdala and several cortical regions, including the primary somatosensory cortex and the anterior insular cortex. Neurons within these regions respond to taste, touch, and in some cases odors.

The "taste code" interpreted by the brain depends on the specific neurons that are activated and the patterns of firing that occur both within and between these neurons. As with odors, the brain must remember what a particular tastant tastes like (e.g., sweet) and a matching or comparison of information coming from the taste pathways must be made at some point in the CNS. Much of the "integration" of gustatory information with other sensory input occurs at the level of the orbitofrontal cortex. Secondary connections through anterior limbic structures are involved in emotion, reward valuation, and reward-related decision making (Rolls, 2013).

## CHEMOSENSORY TESTING

The most widely used olfactory tests are psychophysical tests of odor identification and detection (Doty, 2007; Doty and Laing, 2015). Psychophysical tests require that a patient signifies some aspect of conscious perception in relation to a stimulus. In identification tests, a subject is typically asked to identify, usually from a list of alternatives, the quality of the sensation experienced when sniffing or tasting a stimulus. A response is required even if no sensation is perceived, a procedure called forced-choice responding. For example, the most popular odor identification test—the 40-item "scratch and sniff" University of Pennsylvania Smell Identification Test (UPSIT)—requires a subject to identify the name of each odor from a list of four alternatives (Fig. 19.5) (Doty et al., 1984b). The number of correct answers determines the degree of deficit and allows for both an overall absolute classification of function (i.e., normosmia, mild microsmia, moderate microsmia, severe microsmia, anosmia) and a relative classification based upon percentiles from age- and sex-related norms. Malingering can be discerned from improbable responses in the forced-choice situation.

Odor detection threshold tests—tests akin to pure-tone hearing threshold tests—are also commonly used clinically to assess olfactory function. The goal of such tests is to establish the lowest concentration of an odorant that can be reliably discerned from a blank stimulus. The odorant phenyl ethyl alcohol is commonly employed in such testing

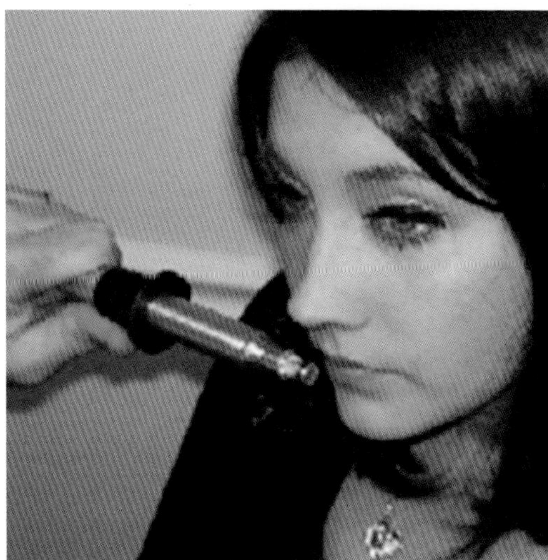
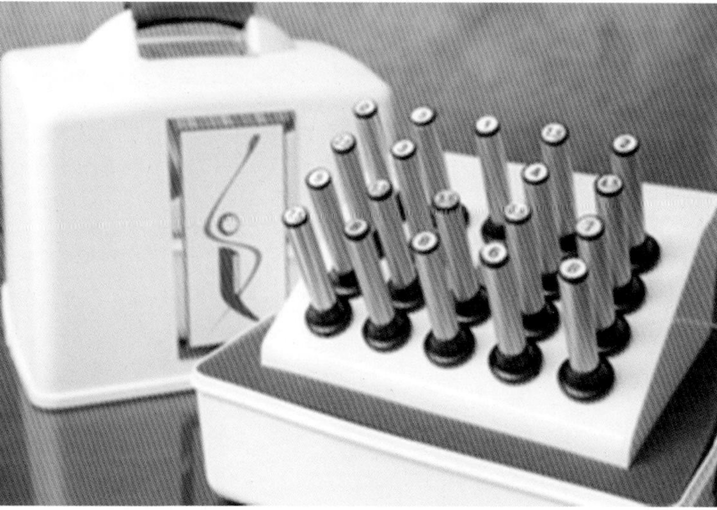

**Fig. 19.6 The Snap & Sniff threshold test.** The test kit is composed of 20 smell "wands." Five contain no odor and the others contain, in the case of the standard odorant phenyl ethyl alcohol, half-log stimulus dilutions ranging from $10^{-2}$ (strongest) to $10^{-9}$ (weakest) concentrations. When the thumb of the operator pushes the black ring forward, an odorized tip is presented to the subject. Releasing the ring retracts the tip back into the wand's housing. This test makes it impossible to touch the nose to the odor source, unlike other similar tests. Other tests, including odor identification tests, use Snap & Sniff technology. *(Photographs courtesy Sensonics International, Haddon Heights, New Jersey. Copyright © 2017, Sensonics International.)*

given its relatively low propensity to stimulate intranasal trigeminal afferents and its pleasant smell at higher concentrations. Some threshold tests, like those based upon Snap & Sniff "smell wands" (Fig. 19.6), use staircase procedures to establish a reliable threshold and can be administered in many cases in less than 10 minutes.

## DISORDERS OF OLFACTION

Olfactory loss can be total (anosmia) or less than total (hyposmia or microsmia). Strange and distorted smells, sometimes described as "chemical-like or garbage-like," can occur either in the absence of a stimulus (phantosmia) or when an odorant or warm air is smelled (dysomia or parosmia). When a fecal-like character is present, this is often termed cacosmia. Usually dysosmia or phantosmia is due to peripheral neurological causes, such as altered firing of the receptor cells during degeneration or regeneration, although central lesions, as in epilepsy, can be involved in some cases. In rare instances, bacterial infections within the nose, sinuses, or oral cavity can be the source of foul smells. Olfactory agnosia—the inability to recognize odors by an otherwise intact olfactory system—may occur secondary to some brain lesions. Distinguishing this problem from other forms of dysfunction is challenging. Hypersensitivity to odorants (hyperosmia) has been reported, although many persons claiming hypersensitivity are experiencing dysosmias and show decrements in function upon testing.

Many factors influence the ability to smell, including age, sex, smoking behavior, reproductive state, nutrition, toxic exposures, head trauma, and numerous diseases (Table 19.1). Men generally perform less well than women on olfactory tests. Age is a major correlate of smell dysfunction, with significant decrements occurring in more than 50% of those between 65 and 80 years of age and in 75% of those 80 years of age and older (Fig. 19.7) (Doty et al., 1984a). Such losses help to explain why many of the elderly find food distasteful and succumb to nutritional deficiencies and, in rare instances, natural gas poisoning. Among the causes of age-related changes are: (a) cumulative damage to olfactory epithelium from viral and other environmental xenobiotics; (b) loss of mucosal metabolizing enzymes; (c) ossification of the cribriform plate foramina; (d) loss of selectivity of receptor cells to odorants; (e) alterations in nasal engorgement; (f) increased susceptibility to nasal disease; (g) changes in neurotransmitter systems; and (h) neuronal deposition of aberrant proteins associated with neurodegenerative diseases (Doty and Kamath, 2014). Aside from age, the three most common causes of long-lasting or permanent smell loss are, in order of frequency, upper respiratory infections, head trauma, and chronic rhinosinusitis (Deems et al., 1991a). Congenital, iatrogenic, and toxic chemical exposures are the next most common causes.

Although the symptoms of the common cold and influenza are readily apparent to the patient, it is important to remember that most viral infections are either entirely asymptomatic or so mild that they go unrecognized. Thus, during seasonal epidemics, the number of serologically documented influenza or arboviral encephalitis infections exceeds the number of acute cases by several hundred-fold (Stroop, 1995). For these and other reasons, many idiopathic cases of smell dysfunction likely reflect unrecognized viral infections. Under certain circumstances, some viruses can enter the brain after incorporation into the olfactory receptor cells, possibly catalyzing neurodegenerative disease (Doty, 2008). Such viruses as herpes simplex types 1 and 2, polio, the Indiana strain of wild-type vesicular stomatitis, rabies, mouse hepatitis, Borna disease, and canine distemper viruses are neurotropic for peripheral olfactory structures.

A large number of systemic medical conditions are accompanied by some degree of smell or taste loss, including such common disorders as diabetes, hypertension, hypothyroidism, kidney disease, and liver disease, as reviewed in detail elsewhere (Doty, 2019a). It is remarkable that most immune-related diseases are accompanied by demonstrable loss of olfactory function, including allergic rhinitis, asthma, autoimmune pancreatitis, Behçet disease, Churg-Strauss syndrome, Crohn disease, fibromyalgia, giant cell arteritis, lupus, Mikulicz disease, multiple sclerosis, myasthenia gravis, neuromyelitis optica, pemphigus vulgaris, psoriasis vulgaris, rheumatoid arthritis, sclerodermia, and Sjögren syndrome (DeLuca et al., 2014).

**TABLE 19.1 Disorders and Conditions Associated with Compromised Olfactory Function, as Measured by Olfactory Testing**

| | |
|---|---|
| 22q11 deletion syndrome | Medications |
| AIDS/HIV infection | Migraine |
| Adenoid hypertrophy | Multiple sclerosis |
| Adrenal cortical insufficiency | Multiple system atrophy |
| Age | Multiinfarct dementia |
| Alcoholism | Narcolepsy with cataplexy |
| Allergies | Neoplasms, cranial/nasal |
| Alzheimer disease | Nutritional deficiencies |
| Amyotrophic lateral sclerosis | Obesity |
| Anorexia nervosa | Obsessive compulsive disorder |
| Asperger syndrome | Obstructive pulmonary disease |
| Ataxias | Orthostatic tremor |
| Attention-deficit/hyperactivity disorder | Panic disorder |
| Bardet-Biedl syndrome | Parkinson dementia complex of Guam |
| Chemical exposure | Parkinson disease |
| Chronic obstructive pulmonary disease | Pick disease |
| Congenital | Posttraumatic stress disorder |
| Creutzfeldt-Jakob disease | Pregnancy |
| Cushing syndrome | Pseudohypoparathyroidism |
| Cystic fibrosis | Psychopathy |
| Degenerative ataxias | Radiation (therapeutic, cranial) |
| Diabetes | REM behavior disorder |
| Down syndrome | Refsum disease |
| Epilepsy | Renal failure/end-stage kidney disease |
| Facial paralysis | Restless leg syndrome |
| Frontotemporal lobe degeneration | Rhinosinusitis/polyposis |
| Gonadal dysgenesis (Turner syndrome) | Schizophrenia |
| Guamanian ALS/PD/dementia syndrome | Seasonal affective disorder |
| Head trauma | Sjögren syndrome |
| Herpes simplex encephalitis | Stroke |
| Hypothyroidism | Tobacco smoking |
| Huntington disease | Toxic chemical exposure |
| Iatrogenesis | Upper respiratory infections |
| Kallmann syndrome | Usher syndrome |
| Korsakoff psychosis | Vascular disorders (e.g., aneurysms, hemorrhages) |
| Leprosy | Vitamin $B_{12}$ deficiency |
| Liver disease | |
| Lubag | |

*AIDS*, Acquired immunodeficiency syndrome; *ALS*, advanced life support; *HIV*, human immunodeficiency virus; *PD*, Parkinson disease; *REM*, rapid eye movement.

Traumatic brain injury (TBI) resulting in olfactory impairment is common and should be considered in even mild TBI (Schofield and Doty, 2019). In one study of boxers, many of whom are currently active in the sport and as many as one-third suffering a "knock-out" at one point, 28% were found to be hyposmic relative to matched controls (Vent et al., 2010). As one might expect, the more severe the trauma—measured by Glasgow Coma Rating Scale on presentation and the length of posttraumatic amnesia—the higher risk of olfactory impairment. Approximately 10% of posttraumatic anosmic patients will recover age-related normal function over time. This increases to nearly 25% of those with less-than-total loss (London et al., 2008). Loss of smell function from head trauma usually reflects coup-contrecoup movement of the brain that abnormally stretches the olfactory bulbs and tracts and, in some cases, shears off the olfactory fila at the level of the cribriform plate (Doty et al., 1997).

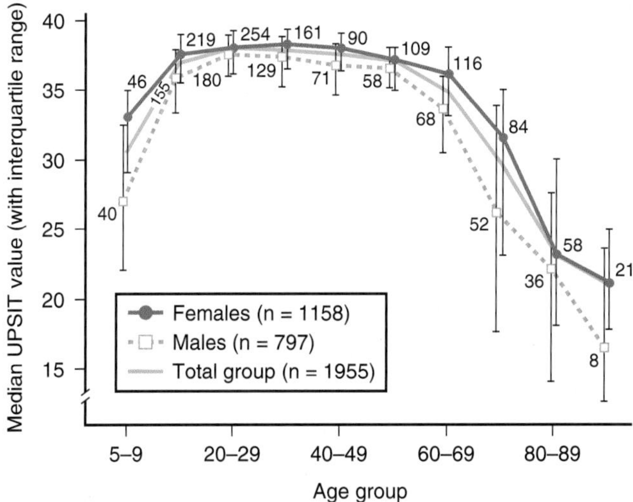


**Fig. 19.7 Scores on the University of Pennsylvania Smell Identification Test (UPSIT) as a function of subject age and sex.** Numbers by each data point indicate sample sizes. Note that women identify odorants better than men at all ages. *(From Doty, R.L., Shaman, P., Applebaum, S.L., et al., 1984a. Smell identification ability: changes with age. Science 226, 1441–1443. Copyright © 1984 American Association for the Advancement of Science.)*

A major development in neurology is the discovery that a number of neurodegenerative diseases are associated with smell loss early in their course, most notably AD and PD. In most cases the loss precedes the classic clinical phenotype by several years. Interestingly, a number of disorders often confused with these two diseases are unaccompanied by meaningful olfactory dysfunction, making smell testing potentially useful as an aid in differential diagnosis. For AD, major affective disorder is an example (McCaffrey et al., 2000). For PD, such examples include progressive supranuclear palsy (PSP) (Doty et al., 1993), essential tremor (Busenbark et al., 1992), 1-methyl-4-phenyl-1,2,3,6-tetrahydropyridine (MPTP)-induced parkinsonism (Doty et al., 1992), and vascular parkinsonism (Katzenschlager et al., 2004). The relative severity of olfactory dysfunction in a range of neurodegenerative diseases and in schizophrenia is shown in Table 19.2.

It is noteworthy that the olfactory loss is present in idiopathic rapid eye movement (REM) sleep behavior disorder (iRBD), because individuals with iRBD frequently develop PD. The fact that REM behavior disorder is seen not only in its idiopathic form but also in association with narcolepsy has led to findings that narcolepsy—independent of REM behavior disorder—is associated with a significant impairment in olfactory function (Stiasny-Kolster et al., 2007). Orexin A (hypocretin-1) is decreased or undetectable in the cerebrospinal fluid (CSF) of patients with narcolepsy and cataplexy. Because orexin-containing hypothalamic neurons project throughout the entire olfactory system (Caillol et al., 2003), damage to these projections may impair olfactory function in narcoleptic patients. Intranasal administration of orexin A to narcoleptic patients with cataplexy improves their olfactory function, implying that mild olfactory impairment is not only a primary feature of this disorder but also that CNS orexin deficiency could cause this loss (Baier et al., 2008).

In the headache world, the search for potential cranial neuropathies in association with idiopathic intracranial hypertension (IIH) has led to the discovery that IIH patients have impairment in olfactory sensitivity (Bershad et al., 2014). Migraines are also of interest considering frequent reports of osmophobia during attacks or even olfactory auras. Migraneurs with episodic migraine appear to have similar olfactory function to age- and sex-matched controls, but some exhibit microsmia or hyposmia during acute attacks (Marmura et al., 2014).

**TABLE 19.2 Relative Degree of Olfactory Dysfunction in Various Neurological Diseases on an Arbitrary Scale**

| Disease | Relative Severity of Smell Loss |
|---|---|
| Idiopathic Parkinson disease, Alzheimer disease, dementia with Lewy bodies, Guam PD-dementia complex. Idiopathic rapid eye movement sleep behavior disorder | ++++ |
| Huntington disease, Down syndrome, PARK8 PD | +++ |
| Multiple system atrophy (type-P), PARK1 PD, pallidopontonigral degeneration, drug-induced PD?, schizophrenia. Semantic dementia?, X-linked dystonia-parkinsonism (Lubag), narcolepsy | ++ |
| Motor neuron disease, SCA2 PD, Friedreich ataxia, PARK3, corticobasal degeneration, frontotemporal dementia | + |
| Major affective disorder, essential tremor, vascular parkinsonism, MPTP-induced parkinsonism, idiopathic dystonia, SCA3 PD, progressive supranuclear palsy; PARK2 | 0 |

Key: ++++ marked damage; + mild damage; 0 normal. Note that most of the values are based on relatively small patient numbers except for idiopathic Parkinson disease. *SCA*, Spinocerebellar atrophy.
*Modified and updated from Hawkes, C.H., Doty, R.L., 2009. The Neurology of Olfaction. Cambridge University Press, Cambridge, with permission.*

## DISORDERS OF TASTE

Impairment of whole mouth gustatory function is rare outside of generalized metabolic disturbances, such as diabetes, chronic renal failure, end-stage liver disease, thyroid disease, hypothyroidism, medications, and vitamin and mineral deficiencies. Nonetheless, taste perception can be altered by (a) viral invasion of one or more taste nerves, (b) the release of foul-tasting materials from the nasal and oral cavities secondary to medical conditions and oral appliances (e.g., rhinosinusitis, gingivitis, purulent sialadenitis), (c) transport problems of tastants to the taste buds (e.g., scaring of the lingual surface, mucosal drying, inflammatory conditions, infections), (d) damage to the taste buds (e.g., invasive carcinomas, local trauma), (e) damage to the taste nerves (e.g., chorda tympani damage from Bell palsy, middle ear infections, or operations), and (f) damage to taste-related CNS structures from disorders such as multiple sclerosis, tumors, epilepsy, and stroke. Lesions caudal to the pons produce ipsilateral deficits, whereas lesions within the pons proper can produce ipsilateral, contralateral, or bilateral deficits. Both ipsilateral and contralateral taste deficits have been noted in patients with lesions of the insular cortex, reflecting the bilateral representation of taste function at this level (Pritchard et al., 1999). Unlike CN VII, CN IX is relatively protected along its path, although iatrogenic interventions can result in CN IX injury (e.g., from tonsillectomy, bronchoscopy, laryngoscopy, and radiation therapy), and this nerve is not immune to damage from tumors, vascular lesions, and infection. On rare occasion, epilepsy or migraine is associated with a gustatory prodrome or aura, and some tastes may actually trigger seizures or migraine attacks.

A number of medications have been implicated in taste dysfunction, including antineoplastic agents, antirheumatic drugs, antibiotics, and blood pressure medications (Doty et al., 2008; Schiffman, 2018). Terbinafine, a popular antifungal, can produce long-lasting loss of sweet, sour, bitter, and salty taste perception (Doty and Haxel, 2005). A double-blind study found that eszopiclone, a widely used sleep medication, induces a bitter dysgeusia in approximately two-thirds of individuals tested (Doty et al., 2009). This sensation was related to the time since drug administration, was stronger for women than for men, and correlated with both saliva and blood levels of the drug.

Alterations in chemosensory function are well established as a consequence of radiation and chemotherapy for cancer patients. Taste thresholds can increase during chemotherapy and qualitative changes, such as the development of a metallic taste, are frequently reported (Gamper et al., 2012). In one study of nasopharyngeal cancer patients receiving radiotherapy who developed impairment in olfactory function, decreased olfactory bulb volume was noted (Veyseller et al., 2014).

## CLINICAL EVALUATION OF TASTE AND SMELL

Etiology can usually be established from a clinical history that explores symptom nature, onset, duration, pattern of fluctuations, and potential precipitating events, such as upper respiratory infections that occurred prior to symptom onset. Information regarding head trauma, smoking habits, drug and alcohol abuse (e.g., intranasal cocaine, chronic alcoholism in the context of Wernicke and Korsakoff syndromes), exposures to pesticides and other toxic agents, and medical interventions are informative. The possibility of multiple or cumulative effects cannot be discounted. A determination of all the medications that the patient was taking before and at the time of symptom onset is important, as are comorbid medical conditions potentially associated with taste and smell impairment, such as renal failure, liver disease, hypothyroidism, diabetes, and dementia. Delayed puberty in association with anosmia (with or without midline craniofacial abnormalities, deafness, and renal anomalies) suggests the possibility of Kallmann syndrome. Recollection of epistaxis, discharge (clear, purulent or bloody), nasal obstruction, allergies, and somatic symptoms, including headache or irritation, have potential localizing value. Questions related to memory, parkinsonian signs, and seizure activity (e.g., automatisms, occurrence of black-outs, auras, and déjà vu) should be posed. The possibility of malingering should be considered, particularly if litigation is involved. Intermittent smell loss usually implies an obstructive disorder, such as from rhinosinusitis or other inflammatory problem. Sudden smell loss alerts the practitioner to head trauma, ischemia, infection, or a psychiatric condition. Gradual smell loss can be a marker for the development of a progressive obstructive lesion, cumulative drug effects, or simply presbyosmia or presbygeusia. Although losses secondary to head trauma are most commonly abrupt, in some cases the loss appears over time or becomes apparent to the patient only after a long interval. In addition to quantitative sensory evaluation, which is key in defining the dysfunction, neurological and otorhinolaryngological (ORL) examinations, along with appropriate brain and nasosinus imaging, aid in the evaluation of patients with olfactory or gustatory complaints. Blood serum tests may be helpful to identify such conditions as diabetes, infection, heavy metal exposure, nutritional deficiency (e.g., vitamins $B_6$ and $B_{12}$), allergy, and thyroid, liver, and kidney disease.

## TREATMENT AND MANAGEMENT

Management of chemosensory disorders is condition specific. Many chemosensory disorders, if present for a long period of time, cannot be reversed, whereas others spontaneously remit without any therapeutic intervention (Deems et al., 1996; London et al., 2008). The literature is replete with multiple claims of therapeutic successes, although when critically evaluated, few are convincing and properly controlled studies are rare. In a recent review, nearly 30 claims of treatments for olfaction or taste disorders were noted (Doty, 2019b). Putative therapies included acupuncture, continuous positive airway pressure (CPAP), corticosteroids, exercise, sodium citrate, theophylline, vitamins (A, $B_{12}$, D, and E) and such antioxidants as caroverine and α-lipoic acid. The use of artificial saliva, changing metallic dental appliances, medication adjustments or discontinuances, mouthwashes, improved oral hygiene, and zinc or iron repletion were noted for a range of taste disorders. As noted in that review, double-blind studies were rare and the quality of most of these studies was poor.

That being said, bona fide medical or surgical interventions for patients with obstructive or inflammatory disorders (e.g., allergic rhinitis, glossitis, polyposis, intranasal or intraoral neoplasms) are available. In cases of chronic rhinosinusitis, an oral taper of prednisone can initially be used to quell general inflammation followed by topical administration of the nasal spray or drops in the inverted head position, such as the Moffett position (Canciani and Mastella, 1988). Although several well-designed studies found no influence of either azithromycin or minocycline on the olfactory function of patients with chronic rhinosinusitis (Reden et al., 2011; Videler et al., 2011), a retrospective study of 280 patients with smell dysfunction due to rhinosinusitis or upper respiratory infections found a positive association between olfactory thresholds and the reported use of bactericidal antibiotics (Wang et al., 2018). Moreover, thresholds were significantly lower for bactericidal antibiotic users than for bacteriostatic antibiotic users with either etiology. However, like many other studies, such findings need confirmation in double-blind interventional studies.

It is well established that candidiasis or other oral infections can be quelled with topical antifungal and antibiotic treatments. Some salty or bitter dysgeusias respond to chlorohexidine mouthwash, possibly as a result of its strong positive charge (Wang et al., 2009). Patients with excessive oral dryness, including dryness due to medications, often benefit from the use of mints, lozenges, or sugarless gum, as well as oral pilocarpine or artificial saliva.

Many medications induce taste distortions and their discontinuance can eliminate the problem, although reversal of the dysfunction may take months (Doty et al., 2008). Despite being widely mentioned in the medical literature, zinc and vitamin A therapies are unlikely to benefit olfactory disturbances except when frank deficiencies are present, although both of these agents may improve taste dysfunction secondary to hepatic deficiencies (Deems et al., 1991b). Studies reporting positive effects of theophylline, acupuncture, and transcranial magnetic stimulation are not convincing and generally lack appropriate control groups. There are reports that some antiepileptics and antidepressants (e.g., amitriptyline) may be value in treating some chemosensory disturbances, particularly following head trauma. Donepezil (an acetylcholinesterase inhibitor) has been reported to improve both cognitive and odor identification scores in patients with AD (Velayudhan and Lovestone, 2009).

It is of interest that repeated exposure to odorants may, in fact, increase sensitivity to them in both animals and humans, providing a rationale for therapies in which multiple odors are smelled before and after going to bed (Hummel et al., 2009). In one study, patients with postinfectious and posttraumatic olfactory impairment were put through 16 weeks of "training" of smelling four separate odorants, which resulted in an increase in function for both groups (Konstantinidis et al., 2013). Importantly, spontaneous recovery over time occurs in some instances, providing hope to at least some patients. In a longitudinal study of 542 patients with smell loss from a variety of causes, modest improvement occurred over an average time period of 4 years in approximately half of the participants (London et al., 2008). Nonetheless, normal age-related function returned in only 11% of the anosmic and 23% of the hyposmic patients. The amount of dysfunction present at the time of presentation, not etiology, was the best predictor of prognosis.

An important but overlooked element of therapy comes from chemosensory testing itself. Confirmation or lack of conformation of loss is beneficial to patients, particularly ones who come to believe they may be "crazy" as a result of unsupportive medical providers or family members. Quantitative testing places the patient's problem into overall perspective and if considerable function is present, patients can be informed of a more positive prognosis. It is extremely therapeutic for an older person to become aware that, although his or her smell function is not what it used to be, it still is greater than the average percentile of his or her peer group. It is unfortunate that many such patients are simply told by their physician they are getting old and nothing can be done for them, often exacerbating or leading to depression and decreased self-esteem.

*The complete reference list is available online at https://expertconsult.inkling.com/.* 

# 20

# Cranial and Facial Pain

*Jerry W. Swanson, J.D. Bartleson*

## OUTLINE



Headache is an exceedingly common symptom that affects virtually everyone at some time in life. It is estimated that nearly half of the world's adults have an active headache disorder (Robbins and Lipton, 2010). Headache is one of the most common reasons for outpatient healthcare visits in the United States. Patients with head and/or face pain typically present for medical attention because the discomfort is severe, interferes with work and/or leisure activities, or raises the patient's or family's concern about a serious underlying cause.

Headache disorders are classified as primary or secondary (Box 20.1; IHS, 2018). The primary headache disorders do not have an underlying structural or exogenous cause, but all of them can be simulated by secondary conditions. The diagnosis of head and face pain depends on three elements: the history, neurological and general examinations, and other appropriate investigations if needed. The treatment of headaches is discussed in Chapter 102.

## HISTORY

The gold standard for the diagnosis and management of headache is a careful interview and neurological and general medical examinations (De Luca and Bartleson, 2010). In the vast majority of patients with headache, the neurological and general examinations will be normal; in such cases the diagnosis is based entirely on the history and the absence of objective abnormalities on examination. A minority of patients will require testing to help establish a diagnosis. Therefore clinicians are well advised to spend most of their time interviewing the patient.

History taking for head and face pain is similar to that for other presenting complaints, but several specific aspects should be addressed. The questions listed in Box 20.2 are useful, and the discussion that follows illustrates some responses and their implications. Usually one begins by asking the patient to describe the symptoms or, alternatively, simply by asking how he or she can be helped. This approach allows patients to relax and say what they had planned to say. Usually, if not interrupted, they will speak for less than 2 minutes. Once the patient has had an opportunity to speak, directed but open-ended questions (see Box 20.2) can be asked.

### Types of Headaches

Many individuals have more than one type of headache. It is valuable to establish this information at the beginning of the interview so that each type of pain can be carefully delineated. For example, both migraine headaches and tension-type headaches often occur in the same individual. Additionally, change in an established headache pattern can indicate a new condition.

### Onset of Headaches

A stable headache disorder of many years' duration is almost always of benign origin. Migraine headaches often begin in childhood, adolescence, or early adulthood. A headache of recent onset obviously has many possible causes, including the new onset of either a benign or serious condition. "Recent onset" has been defined differently by various authors; the typical range is from 1 to 12 months. In general, the more recent the onset of headache, the greater the risk of a possible secondary cause. The "worst ever" headache, an increasingly severe headache, or change for the worse in an existing headache pattern all raise the possibility of an intracranial lesion. Headaches of rapid (over seconds to minutes) onset suggest an intracranial hemorrhage, usually in the subarachnoid space, but they also can be caused by intracerebral hemorrhage, cerebral venous thrombosis, intra- and extracranial arterial dissection, pituitary apoplexy, spontaneous intracranial hypotension, reversible cerebral vasoconstriction syndrome (RCVS), acute hypertensive crisis, and other conditions that must be excluded with the first occurrence of "thunderclap headache" (Schwedt, 2015). If no underlying cause is discovered despite an expedited and thorough investigation, a diagnosis of primary thunderclap headache can be considered. Onset of a new headache in patients older than 50 years raises suspicion of an

**BOX 20.1 Classification of Headaches**

**The Primary Headaches**
Migraine and its subtypes
Tension-type headache and its subtypes
Trigeminal autonomic cephalalgias:
Cluster headache
Paroxysmal hemicrania
Short-lasting unilateral neuralgiform headache attacks
Hemicrania continua
Other primary headache disorders:
Primary cough headache
Primary exercise headache
Primary headache associated with sexual activity
Primary thunderclap headache
Cold-stimulus headache
External-pressure headache
Primary stabbing headache
Nummular headache
Hypnic headache
New daily persistent headache

**The Secondary Headaches**
Headache attributed to trauma or injury to the head and/or neck
Headache attributed to cranial and/or cervical vascular disorder
Headache attributed to nonvascular intracranial disorder
Headache attributed to a substance or its withdrawal
Headache attributed to infection
Headache attributed to disorder of homeostasis
Headache or facial pain attributed to disorder of the cranium, neck, eyes, ears, nose, sinuses, teeth, mouth, or other facial or cervical structure
Headache attributed to psychiatric disorder

**Painful Cranial Neuropathies, Other Facial Pains, and Other Headaches**
Painful cranial neuropathies and other facial pains
Other headache disorders

*From The International Classification of Headache Disorders, 3rd edition, 2018.*

**BOX 20.2 Useful Questions to Ask the Patient with Headache**

- How many types of headache do you have?
- When and how did each type begin?
- If the headaches are episodic, what is the frequency and duration?
- How long does it take for your headaches to reach maximal intensity?
- How long do your headaches last?
- When do the headaches tend to occur, and what factors trigger your headaches?
- Where does your pain start, and how does it evolve?
- What is the quality of your pain?
- How severe is your pain?
- Is the pain steady or pulsating (throbbing), or both?
- Are there symptoms that herald the onset of your headache?
- What are they, when do they begin, and how long do they last?
- Are there symptoms that accompany your headaches?
- Do you get nauseated with your headaches?
- Does light and/or noise bother you a lot more when you have a headache than when you don't?
- Do your headaches limit your ability to work, study, or participate in other activities?
- Does anything aggravate your pain (e.g., exertion)?
- Are your headaches getting better or worse or are they about the same?
- What treatments have been used to treat the headaches, both acutely and preventively?
- What helps your pain?
- Is there a family history of headaches?
- What previous testing have you had?
- Do you have other medical or neurological problems?
- What do you think might be causing your headaches?
- How disabling are your headaches?
- Why are you seeking help now?

intracranial lesion (e.g., subdural hematoma) or giant cell (temporal or cranial) arteritis (GCA). A history of antecedent head or neck injury should be sought; even a relatively minor injury can be associated with subsequent development of subdural hemorrhage (especially in the elderly) and posttraumatic dissection of the carotid or vertebral arteries (Debette and Leys, 2009). However, posttraumatic headaches can occur following head injury in the absence of any demonstrable pathology.

## Frequency and Periodicity of Episodic Headaches

Migraine may be episodic or chronic. Chronic migraine is defined as headache occurring on more than 15 days per month for 3 or more months that has the features of migraine headache on 8 or more days per month. Chronic migraine usually develops in individuals with a history of episodic migraine headaches. Chronic migraine may occur with or without medication overuse. Some patients with medication overuse do not improve after drug withdrawal.

Episodic cluster headaches typically occur daily for several weeks or months and are followed by a lengthy headache-free interval. Chronic cluster headaches occur at least every other day for more than 1 year or with remissions lasting less than 3 months. If there is no regular periodicity, it is useful to inquire about the longest and shortest periods of freedom between headaches. Having the patient monitor headache frequency, duration, intensity, headache triggers, and medication use on a headache calendar or in a diary is helpful in diagnosis and measuring response to treatment. Tension-type headaches can be episodic (infrequent, <12 days per year) or frequent (≥12 and <180 days per year) or chronic (≥15 days per month on average for more than 3 months).

Thunderclap headache recurring over a few days or weeks raises the possibility of RCVS, a diagnosis that requires the exclusion of aneurysmal subarachnoid hemorrhage (Ducros, 2012; IHS, 2018).

## Temporal Profile

A chronic daily headache without migrainous or autonomic features is likely to be a chronic tension-type headache. Untreated migraine pain usually peaks within 1–2 hours of onset and lasts 4–72 hours. Cluster headache is typically maximal immediately (if the patient awakens with the headache in progress) or peaks within minutes (if it begins while the patient is awake). Cluster headaches are more common in men and are infrequently inherited. They last from 15 to 180 minutes (usually 45–120 minutes). Headaches similar to cluster but lasting only 2–30 minutes and occurring several or many times a day are typical of episodic or chronic paroxysmal hemicrania, both of which are more common in women and are prevented by indomethacin (Goadsby, 2012). Primary stabbing headaches ("ice-pick pains") are momentary, typically lasting seconds. Stabbing headaches are more common in patients with migraine, tend to vary in location, and do not have identifiable triggers. Tension-type headaches commonly build up over hours and last hours to days to years. Headache that is daily and unremitting from onset, usually in patients without prior headaches, is classified as new daily persistent headache and may have features suggestive of migraine or tension-type headache. A chronic, continuous, unilateral headache of moderate severity with superimposed attacks of more intense pain associated with autonomic features suggests the diagnosis of hemicrania continua, an indomethacin-responsive syndrome. Occipital neuralgia and trigeminal neuralgia manifest as brief shock-like pains, often triggered by stimulation in the territory served by the affected nerve. Occasionally a dull pain in the same nerve distribution persists longer, often after a series of brief, sharp pains. *S*hort-lasting *u*nilateral *n*euralgiform headache with *c*onjunctival injection and *t*earing (SUNCT) is a rare syndrome consisting of paroxysms of first-division trigeminal nerve pain lasting 5–240 seconds but occurring 3–200 times per day with the associated autonomic symptoms for which it is named (Goadsby, 2012). SUNA (short-lasting neuralgiform headache attacks with autonomic symptoms) is a related disorder and differs from SUNCT only in that not more than one of the following occurs ipsilateral to the pain: (1) conjunctival injection or (2) lacrimation (tearing).

## Time of Day and Precipitating Factors

Cluster headaches often awaken patients from a sound sleep and may occur at the same time each day in an individual person. Hypnic headaches usually begin after age 50 years and regularly awaken the patient at a particular time of night. Unlike cluster headaches, they are usually bilateral and not associated with autonomic phenomena (Lanteri-Minet, 2014). Migraine headaches can occur at any time but often begin in the morning. A headache of recent onset that disturbs sleep or is worse on waking may be caused by increased intracranial pressure. Tension-type headaches can be present during much of the day and are often more severe later in the day. Obstructive sleep apnea may be accompanied by the frequent occurrence of headache on awakening, as might medication overuse headache ("rebound headache") and headache due to caffeine withdrawal. If headache begins while the patient is asleep, it is impossible to tell whether the onset was gradual or abrupt.

Patients with chronic recurrent headaches often recognize factors that trigger an attack. Migraine headaches may be precipitated by bright light, menstruation, weather changes, caffeine withdrawal, fasting, alcohol, sleeping more or less than usual, stress and release from stress, certain foods and food additives, perfume and smoke, and others. Alcohol can trigger a cluster headache within minutes of ingestion. If bending, lifting, coughing, or Valsalva maneuver brings on a headache, an intracranial lesion, especially one involving the posterior fossa, must be considered. Exertional headache and headache associated with sexual activity are both worrisome. Although either can occur as a primary headache disorder unassociated with structural disease or can be associated with migraine, both types can also be due to subarachnoid hemorrhage, arterial dissection, and RCVS, which must be excluded with the first occurrence of such headaches. Intermittent headaches that are worsened by sitting or standing and improved by lying down are characteristic of a cerebrospinal fluid (CSF) leak, although other headache patterns may occur. If there is no history of lumbar puncture, head trauma, or neurosurgical intervention, a spontaneous CSF leak may be the cause (Mokri, 2013). Lancinating face pain triggered by facial or intraoral stimuli occurs with trigeminal neuralgia. Glossopharyngeal neuralgia typically causes throat or ear pain that is triggered by chewing, swallowing, or talking, although cutaneous trigger zones in and about the ear are occasionally present.

## Location

Asking the patient to outline the location of the pain with his or her finger can be very helpful. Trigeminal neuralgia is confined to one or more branches of the trigeminal nerve. The patient may be able to localize one or more trigger points on the face or in the mouth and then show how the pain spreads. Pain in the throat may be due to a local process or to glossopharyngeal neuralgia. Carotid artery dissection commonly presents with unilateral neck, face, and head pain; is frequently associated with an ipsilateral Horner syndrome; and often follows head or neck trauma.

Migraine is commonly unilateral, can be confined to the front or back of the head, and can affect the neck. Migraine pain can start on one side and spread to the other or be bilateral from onset. Cluster headaches are unilateral during an attack and typically are centered in, behind, or around one eye. Some patients' cluster headaches switch sides with different cluster periods, and a smaller number of patients experience side shifts within a cluster period. The typical tension-type headache is generalized, although it may begin in the neck muscles and affect chiefly the occipital region or predominate frontally. When pain is localized to the eye, mouth, or ear, local processes involving these structures must be considered. Otalgia may be caused by a process involving the tonsil and posterior tongue. With chronic unilateral facial pain, an underlying lesion often cannot be identified. Occasionally facial pain may be a symptom of nonmetastatic lung cancer (Pembroke et al., 2013).

## Quality and Severity

The character and quality of the patient's pain can have significance. In most cases, the type of pain can be designated as sharp, aching, or burning. Headaches may be steady or throbbing (pulsating) in character. It may be helpful to ask the patient to grade the severity of pain on a scale of 1–10. Patients who report that their pain is at level 20 are hurting but may be prone to exaggerate. Another useful approach is to ask the patient to indicate the severity of their headache pain as follows: mild = no impact on function, moderate = able to function with difficulty, severe = unable to function. Migraine pain often has a pulsating quality that may be superimposed on a more continuous pain. The pain of cluster headache is characteristically severe, boring, and steady and often described as a "hot poker." SUNCT produces moderately severe pain in the orbital or temporal region and may be described as sharp and stabbing or (rarely) pulsatile. Tension-type headaches are often described as a steady feeling of fullness, tightness, or pressure or like a cap, band, or vise. Headaches caused by meningeal irritation, whether related to infectious meningitis or blood, are typically severe. Trigeminal neuralgia pain is severe, brief, sharp, electric shock–like, or stabbing; pains can occur up to several times per minute, and a milder ache may persist between paroxysms of pain. Glossopharyngeal neuralgia pain is similar in character to that of trigeminal neuralgia.

## Premonitory Symptoms, Aura, and Accompanying Symptoms

Some patients have premonitory symptoms that precede a migraine headache by hours. These can include psychological changes (e.g., depression, euphoria, irritability) or somatic symptoms (e.g., constipation, diarrhea, abnormal hunger, fluid retention, increased urination). The term *aura* refers to focal cerebral symptoms associated with a migraine attack. These symptoms can last 5–60 minutes but usually last 10–30 minutes. Aura symptoms typically precede the headache but can continue into the headache phase or begin during the headache. Visual symptoms are most common and may consist of either positive (scintillating lights, spots, or zig-zag lines) or negative (scotomas or visual field loss) phenomena or both. The visual symptoms characteristically affect both eyes simultaneously but can rarely affect one eye alone. Less common hemispheric symptoms, such as unilateral somatosensory disturbances (tingling and/or numbness) or dysphasic language disturbance, may occur with or without visual symptoms. Aura symptoms usually have a gradual onset and offset; they typically increase and decrease over minutes. If more than one symptom occurs (e.g., visual plus somatosensory), the onsets usually are staggered and not simultaneous. Patients can experience migraine aura without an associated headache. Positive symptoms, the slow spread of symptoms, and staggered onsets help differentiate migraine aura from focal symptoms caused by cerebrovascular disease.

Symptoms originating from the brainstem or both cerebral hemispheres simultaneously—such as vertigo, dysarthria, ataxia, auditory symptoms, diplopia, bilateral visual symptoms in both eyes, bilateral numbness and/or paresthesias, and decreased level of consciousness—may accompany migraine with brainstem aura (formerly called basilar-type migraine) (IHS, 2018). Vertigo without other brainstem signs can also accompany migraine headaches. Migraine with aura that includes motor weakness can be due to familial hemiplegic migraine if there is a family history in at least one first- or second-degree relative or due to sporadic hemiplegic migraine if there is no family history. It can be difficult for the patient to differentiate sensory loss from true weakness, but this must be carefully delineated. Nausea, vomiting, photophobia, phonophobia, and osmophobia characteristically accompany migraine attacks. In addition, lacrimation, rhinorrhea, and nasal congestion can accompany migraine headache and mimic headache of sinus origin (Cady et al., 2005). Ipsilateral miosis, ptosis, lacrimation, conjunctival injection, and nasal stuffiness commonly accompany cluster headache; sweating and facial flushing on the side of the pain are much less common. Similar autonomic features also accompany episodic and chronic paroxysmal hemicrania and hemicrania continua. Very short attacks (5–240 seconds) with ipsilateral conjunctival injection and tearing suggest SUNCT (Goadsby, 2012). Horner syndrome is common in carotid artery dissection. In the setting of acute transient or persistent monocular visual loss, GCA and carotid dissection and stenosis should be considered. Temporomandibular joint dysfunction includes jaw pain precipitated or aggravated by movement of the jaw or clenching of the teeth and is associated with reduced range of jaw movement, joint clicking, and tenderness over the joint. Headache accompanied by fever suggests an infection. Headache associated with persistent or progressive diffuse or focal central nervous system (CNS) symptoms, including seizures, implies a structural cause. Purulent or bloody nasal discharge suggests an acute sinus cause for the headache. Likewise, a red eye raises the possibility of an ocular process such as infection or acute glaucoma. A history of polymyalgia rheumatica, jaw claudication, or tenderness of the scalp arteries in an older person strongly suggests GCA. Transient visual obscurations upon standing, usually pulsatile tinnitus, diplopia (especially for objects in the distance), and papilledema may be associated with increased intracranial pressure from any cause, including idiopathic intracranial hypertension (pseudotumor cerebri).

### Aggravating and Mitigating Factors

Worsening of headache as a result of a cough or physical jolt suggests an intracranial component to the pain. Sufferers of cluster headache tend to endure their pain in an agitated state, pacing and moving about, whereas patients with migraine typically prefer to lie still. *Precipitation* or marked worsening of headache in the upright position and/or relief with recumbency suggests intracranial hypotension. Routine physical activity, light, sound, and smells typically aggravate migraine headaches. Rest, especially sleep, and avoidance of light and noise as well as the application of cold tend to benefit the migraineur. Massage, ice, or heat may reduce the pain associated with tension-type headache. Local application of pressure over the affected eye or ipsilateral temporal artery, local application of heat or cold, and (rarely) brief intense physical activity may alleviate the pain of cluster headache.

### Family History of Headaches

Migraine is often an inherited disorder, and a family history of migraines (sometimes referred to as "sick headaches") is present in about two-thirds of patients. Tension-type headaches can also be familial. In individuals with cluster headaches, studies have shown a family history of cluster headaches in 5%–20%. Familial hemiplegic migraine is a rare autosomal dominant variant of migraine with aura, wherein the aura includes hemiparesis lasting from minutes to 24 hours.

### Prior Evaluation

The patient should be asked about prior consultations and testing. If appropriate, those records and imaging studies can be obtained for review.

### Prior Treatment

Response to treatment should be sought, including agents used to treat individual headache attacks acutely and those used prophylactically. The dose, frequency, and duration of each treatment should be reviewed. This information provides an opportunity to determine whether acute medications have been overused or underused and whether prophylactic medications were optimized. A history of the use of caffeine-containing substances should also be elicited because they may cause or aggravate headaches through rebound withdrawal.

### Disability

Baseline and follow-up assessment of headache-related disability is helpful in judging the effects of treatment and guiding headache therapy. The Migraine Disability Assessment Scale (MIDAS) is a useful and validated clinical tool (Andrasik et al., 2005).

### Patient Concerns and Reasons for Seeking Help

Headache pain can produce significant fear and anxiety regarding serious disease. The patient should be encouraged to express any concerns so that each can be appropriately addressed.

The question of why the patient is seeking help may be obvious if the problem is of recent onset. If the problem is chronic, however, it can be useful to inquire why the patient has come for aid at this time. Red and yellow flags (Box 20.3) help identify which patients are more likely to have a secondary cause of their pain.

### Other Medical or Neurological Problems

A history of past and current medical and neurological conditions, injuries, operations, and medication allergies should be obtained. A list of all current medications and dietary supplements should be recorded. A number of medications can cause headache, including hormonal, cardiovascular, and gastrointestinal agents (De Luca and Bartleson, 2010).

## EXAMINATION

The examination begins the moment the physician encounters the patient. Careful observation helps determine whether the patient appears ill, anxious, or depressed and whether the history is reliable. The patient who is unable to give a reasonably coherent history should be suspected of having an abnormal mental status. Although, typically, the physical examination of the headache patient shows no abnormalities, findings on examination may yield important clues about the underlying cause.

Vital signs, especially blood pressure and pulse, should be assessed. Extremely high blood pressure can cause headache. If there is a question of fever, temperature can be measured. The body habitus should be noted. Patients with idiopathic intracranial hypertension, typically young women, are usually obese. The general examination can include auscultation of the heart and lungs, palpation of the abdomen, and examination of the skin. A neurologic examination—including assessment of the mental status, gait, cranial nerves, reflexes, and motor and sensory systems—is essential. The skull and cervical spine should be examined. The area over an infected sinus may be tender. Thickened, tender, irregular temporal arteries with a reduced pulse suggest GCA. In both migraine and tension-type headaches, the scalp may be tender. A short neck or low hairline suggests basilar invagination or a Chiari malformation. In an infant, bulging of the fontanelles suggests increased intracranial pressure, most commonly caused by hydrocephalus. It is important to measure head circumference in a child. The cervical spine also should be tested for tenderness and mobility. Nuchal rigidity on passive neck flexion and a Kernig sign indicate meningeal irritation.

**BOX 20.3 Headache Warning Flags**

**Red Flags for Worrisome Headaches**

- Head or neck injury
- New onset or new type or worsening pattern of existing headache
- New level of pain (e.g., worst ever)
- Abrupt or split-second onset
- Triggered by Valsalva maneuver or cough
- Triggered by exertion
- Triggered by sexual activity
- Headache during pregnancy or puerperium
- Age >50 years
- Neurological signs or symptoms
  - Seizures
  - Confusion
  - Impaired alertness
  - Weakness
  - Papilledema
- Systemic illness
  - Fever
  - Nuchal rigidity
  - Weight loss
  - Scalp artery tenderness
- Secondary risk factors
  - Cancer
  - Immunocompromised host
  - Human immunodeficiency virus (HIV)
  - On immunosuppressants
- Recent travel
  - Domestic
  - Foreign

**Yellow Flags for Worrisome Headaches**

- Wakes patient from sleep at night
- New onset side-locked headaches
- Postural headaches

*From De Luca, G.C., Bartleson, J.D., 2010. When and how to investigate the patient with headache. Semin Neurol 30, 133–134. Used with permission.*

## DIAGNOSTIC TESTING

In most cases the history, together with the neurological and physical examinations, is all that is needed to make a diagnosis, especially in the patient with long-standing headaches. Migraine, tension-type headaches, and cluster headaches can usually be diagnosed with a high degree of certainty, and it is often possible to proceed directly to management.

In some situations the diagnosis is uncertain and additional diagnostic testing should be considered. The worrisome headache "warning flags" that increase the likelihood of a serious underlying intracranial process and often lead to additional testing are listed in Box 20.3. Red flags are more worrisome than yellow flags. Investigation of the patient with headache includes almost all tests used in neurology and neurosurgery as well as various medical studies. Selection of appropriate tests depends on the diagnostic formulation after the history and examination; indiscriminate use of batteries of tests is unwarranted.

### Neuroimaging and Other Imaging Studies

#### Computed Tomography and Magnetic Resonance Imaging

Computed tomography (CT) and magnetic resonance imaging (MRI) are extremely useful tests in evaluating patients with headache. CT is best utilized when investigating for acute intracranial hemorrhage, assessing bony anatomy, or evaluating for sinusitis. Althugh CT can detect intracranial processes such as tumors, hematomas, cerebral infarctions, abscesses, hydrocephalus, and meningeal processes, MRI provides higher sensitivity and specificity, and is therefore the preferred diagnostic study for these entities. Advantages of CT over MRI include lower cost, a faster scan for those patients who either cannot remain still or are claustrophobic, compatibility with pacemakers and other retained metal objects, and widespread availability. The iodinated contrast used in CT has been associated with allergic reactions and contrast-induced nephropathy. The contrast agent used in MRI is less likely to produce allergic reactions or renal damage, but it has been associated with nephrogenic systemic fibrosis, typically in patients with preexisting renal impairment. The imaging modality of choice to investigate various causes of headache is shown in Box 20.4.

CT can detect acute subarachnoid hemorrhage in at least 95% of patients if sufficient bleeding has occurred and the patient is scanned promptly. If findings on the CT scan are normal and the history is suggestive of recent subarachnoid hemorrhage, a lumbar puncture should be performed to assess for red blood cells and xanthochromia. Evidence of bleeding (i.e., red blood cells and xanthochromia) can last for up to 1–2 weeks after a subarachnoid hemorrhage.

CT can be helpful for evaluating abnormalities of the skull, orbit, sinuses, facial bones, and the bony cervical spine. Changes associated with intracranial hypotension are best shown with MRI and include enhancement of the pachymeninges, sagging of the brain, engorged veins, and subdural fluid collections (Mokri, 2013). The cervical spinal cord and exiting nerve roots are much better shown with MRI than with plain CT. Myelography with CT can be used to image the spine as an alternative to MRI. MR angiography is a noninvasive method that can demonstrate intracranial and extracranial vascular occlusive disease including large-vessel dissection, intracranial arteriovenous malformations, and aneurysms. CT angiography can also show arterial disease, although arterial calcifications may confound accurate luminal diameter measurements. Intracranial venous sinus thrombosis is best shown with gadolinium-enhanced MR venography, but CT venography is an alternative when MRI is unavailable or contraindicated. For headache that is acute in onset or that follows trauma, CT is the preferred imaging study to look for subarachnoid and other intracranial bleeding. For the evaluation of patients with subacute and chronic headache, MRI is recommended (Sandrini et al., 2004). MRI can reveal more than CT, but many of the abnormalities will be incidental, including asymptomatic cerebral infarctions, small aneurysms, and benign brain tumors (Vernooij et al., 2007).

#### Plain Radiographs and Other Imaging of the Skull, Sinuses, and Cervical Spine

Plain radiographs of the skull are unnecessary in the routine evaluation of patients with headache, but they can infrequently be useful in patients with an unusual bony abnormality found on physical examination. Although plain radiographs of the sinuses can show infection, hemorrhage, fracture, or tumor, CT provides much greater definition and has become the test of choice for these conditions. Occipitonuchal pain may result from degenerative disk and joint disease of the upper cervical spine. Rheumatoid arthritis and ankylosing spondylitis can lead to craniocervical junction instability and pain. Fat-saturated postgadolinium T1-weighted MR images as well as inversion recovery sequences can be very helpful in demonstrating marrow edema and joint fluid abnormalities seen in many spondyloarthropathies (Lacout et al., 2008). Tomographic images or CT may be needed to show bony changes in the upper cervical spine and craniocervical junction. Flexion and extension, odontoid, and pillar views of the cervical spine can help to exclude ligamentous damage and fractures in patients with a history of head and neck injury. MRI is the imaging study of choice for spinal cord and nerve root pathology.

**BOX 20.4 Imaging Modality of Choice to Investigate Causes of Headache**

**MRI Preferred**

***Vascular Disease***
Cerebral infarction
Venous infarction

***Neoplastic Disease***
Primary and secondary brain tumors (especially in posterior fossa)
Skull base tumors
Meningeal carcinomatosis and lymphomatosis
Pituitary tumors

***Infections***
Cerebritis and brain abscess
Meningitis
Encephalitis

***Other***
Chiari malformation
Cerebrospinal fluid hypotension with pachymeningeal enhancement and brain sag
Foramen magnum and upper cervical spine lesions
Pituitary apoplexy
Rare encephalopathies with headache (CADASIL,* MELAS,† SMART‡)

**CT Preferred**

***Fractures (Calvarium)***
Acute hemorrhage (subarachnoid, intracerebral)
Paranasal sinus and mastoid air cell disease

**MRI and CT Equal**

***MR Angiography/CT Angiography***
Vasculitis (large and medium-sized vessels)
Intracranial aneurysms
Carotid and vertebral artery dissections
Reversible cerebral vasoconstriction syndrome

***MR Venography/CT Venography***
Cerebral venous thrombosis
Increased intracranial pressure in absence of structural lesion on MRI

* CADASIL—cerebral autosomal dominant arteriopathy with subcortical infarcts and leukoencephalopathy.
† MELAS—mitochondrial encephalomyopathy, lactic acidosis, and stroke-like episodes.
‡ SMART—stroke-like migraine attacks after radiation therapy.
*CT*, Computed tomography; *MRI*, magnetic resonance imaging.
*Copyrighted and used with permission of Mayo Foundation for Medical Education and Research.*

### Temporomandibular Joint/Dental Imaging Studies

Panoramic x-ray examination, MRI, or CT of the temporomandibular joints may be helpful in selected patients. The presence of temporomandibular joint disease should not be taken as proof that the patient's headaches are related. Dental radiographs are useful if a dental origin for the pain is suspected.

### Cerebral Angiography

Cerebral angiography is rarely needed in the initial investigation of headache. It can be helpful in confirming vascular disease, including arterial dissections, arteriovenous malformations, intracranial aneurysms, RCVS, and CNS vasculitis.

### Myelography with Computed Tomography and Radioisotope Studies for the Detection of Cerebrospinal Fluid Leaks

In addition to MRI of the brain and spine, radioisotope cisternography (typically with indium-111) can be helpful in determining the presence and location of a spontaneous or posttraumatic CSF leak. Myelography with CT or MR myelography is often necessary to determine the site of a leak.

## Cerebrospinal Fluid Tests

CSF examination can diagnose or exclude meningitis, encephalitis, subarachnoid hemorrhage, and leptomeningeal cancer and lymphoma. It can also document increased or decreased intracranial pressure and confirm the diagnosis of *h*eada*c*he and *n*eurological *d*eficits with CSF *l*ymphocytosis (HaNDL) (Gomez-Aranda et al., 1997). The opening CSF pressure should always be measured.

## Electrophysiological Testing

Electroencephalography is not useful in the investigation of headache unless the patient also has a history of seizures, syncope, or episodes of altered awareness, and there is no indication for use of evoked potentials (Sandrini et al., 2004).

## General Medical Tests

A few blood tests are important in the investigation of headache. Elevation of the erythrocyte sedimentation rate (ESR), often to 100 mm per hour or higher, is frequently seen in GCA. A normal ESR does not exclude the condition because 4% of patients with positive findings on temporal artery biopsy have a normal ESR (Smetana and Shmerling, 2002). C-reactive protein and platelet count are also often elevated in patients with GCA. Rarely, episodic headaches associated with unusual behavior or impairment of consciousness can suggest an insulinoma, which is supported by elevated serum insulin and C-peptide levels in the face of a low or relatively low fasting glucose level. Levels of carboxyhemoglobin can be measured in patients complaining of early morning headaches during the home heating season, especially when several members of the same household are affected. Drug and alcohol screening may be helpful in certain patients. Thyroid function should be checked in patients with chronic headache because hypothyroidism can present with headaches. Plasma and urine levels of catecholamines and metanephrines should be measured if a pheochromocytoma is suspected.

Rarely, cigarette smokers can present with face pain that frequently includes the ear and is due to an underlying ipsilateral lung tumor without CNS involvement. Chest radiograph or CT of the chest can confirm the diagnosis (Pembroke et al., 2013).

## Special Examinations and Consultations

In patients who wake from sleep with headache, overnight pulse oximetry and/or polysomnography can be performed to look for a treatable sleep disorder such as sleep apnea.

Formal visual field testing can be useful (e.g., may show enlarged blind spots and constricted fields from increased intracranial pressure, or characteristic field loss due to glaucoma). Tonometry can document elevated intraocular pressure in glaucoma, but unless the eye is red or the cornea is cloudy, glaucoma is an uncommon cause of head or even eye pain. These tests are routinely done by ophthalmologists, who also have the equipment and expertise to perform slit-lamp and other specialized examinations. If pain of dental or temporomandibular joint origin is suspected, an oral surgeon or dentist skilled in the detection and treatment of these disorders should be consulted. Diagnosis of tumors of the sinuses, nasopharynx, and neck, as well as inflammation of the sinuses, is aided by consultation with

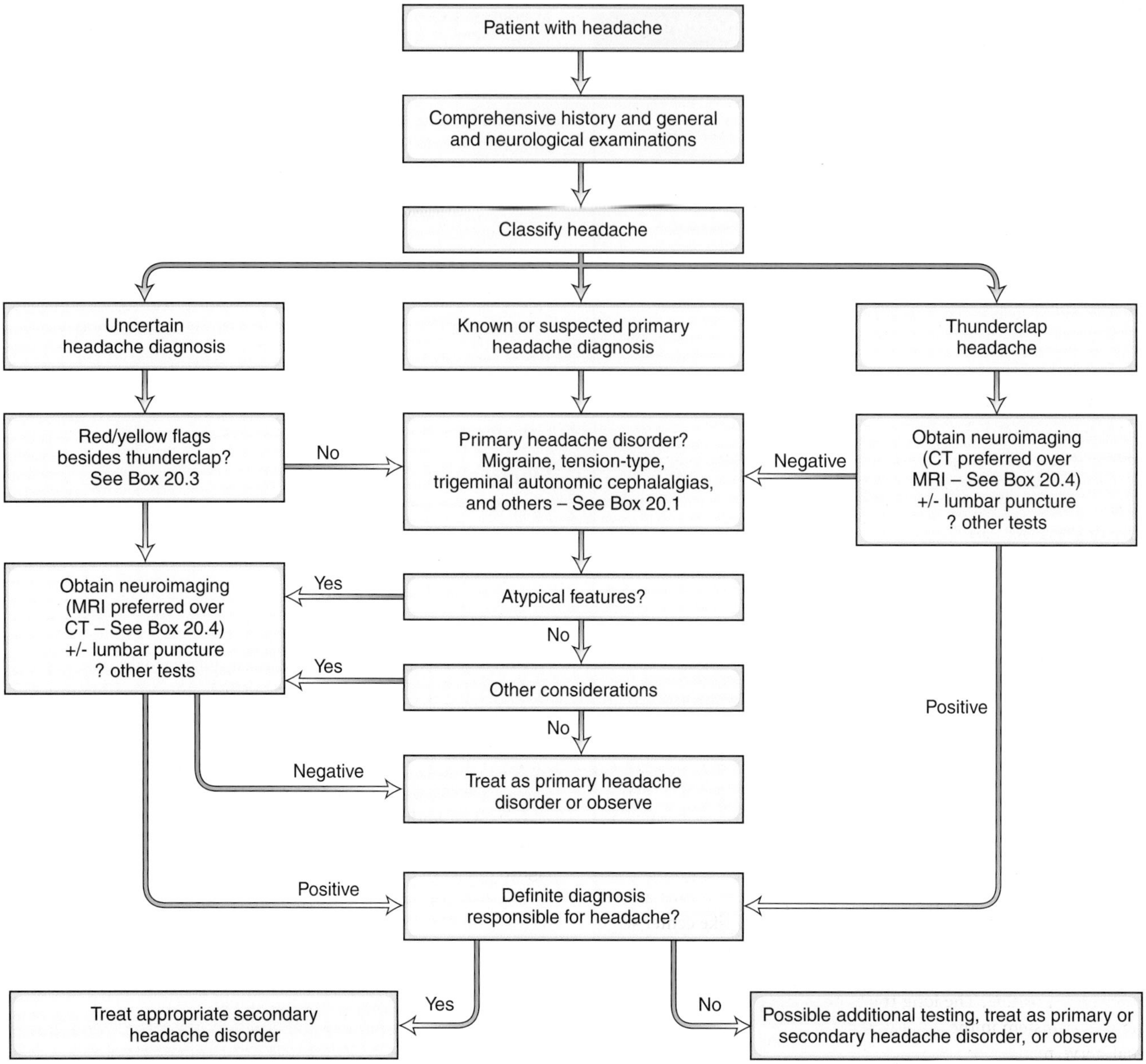

Patient with headache

Comprehensive history and general and neurological examinations

Classify headache

Uncertain headache diagnosis

Known or suspected primary headache diagnosis

Thunderclap headache

Red/yellow flags besides thunderclap? See Box 20.3

No

Primary headache disorder? Migraine, tension-type, trigeminal autonomic cephalalgias, and others – See Box 20.1

Negative

Obtain neuroimaging (CT preferred over MRI – See Box 20.4) +/- lumbar puncture ? other tests

Obtain neuroimaging (MRI preferred over CT – See Box 20.4) +/- lumbar puncture ? other tests

Yes

Atypical features?

No

Yes

Other considerations

Positive

No

Negative

Treat as primary headache disorder or observe

Positive

Definite diagnosis responsible for headache?

Treat appropriate secondary headache disorder

Yes

No

Possible additional testing, treat as primary or secondary headache disorder, or observe

**Fig. 20.1** Algorithm for the Evaluation of Headache Disorders. *(Copyrighted and used with permission of Mayo Foundation for Medical Education and Research.)*

an otorhinolaryngologist. Temporal artery biopsy is performed to confirm or exclude GCA. In some selected cases (e.g., headaches as a manifestation of a chronic pain disorder or a history of drug abuse), psychiatric consultation may be helpful in diagnosis and management.

## FURTHER OBSERVATION

Sometimes a definitive diagnosis cannot be reached despite a careful history, thorough examination, and appropriate investigations. In such cases, further observation, with or without a trial of therapy, often reveals the diagnosis. An algorithm showing one approach to diagnosis of the patient who presents with headache is shown in Fig. 20.1.

*The complete reference list is available online at https://expertconsult.inkling.com/.*

# 21

# Brainstem Syndromes

*Devin D. Mackay, Michael Wall*

## OUTLINE



Other chapters in this book that deal with symptoms emphasize history as the starting point for generating possibilities for the differential diagnosis. This list of diagnostic considerations is then refined during the examination. This chapter calls for a different approach. When the neurologist evaluates a patient with a brainstem disorder, often the most effective method of diagnosis is to organize the differential diagnosis around the objective physical findings, particularly in patients with an altered mental status such as coma. The symptoms are still integrated in the approach, but the physical findings take center stage.

Organization around the physical findings is efficient because very specific neurological localization, which limits the diagnostic alternatives, often is possible. The long tracts of the nervous system traverse the entire brainstem in the longitudinal (rostrocaudal) plane, whereas cranial nerve nuclei and their respective cranial nerves originate and exit at distinct levels of the brainstem. This arrangement allows for exquisite localization of function based on the findings of the neurological examination.

The chapter begins with a discussion of the brainstem ocular motor syndromes, followed by descriptions of miscellaneous brainstem, brainstem stroke, and thalamic syndromes.

## OCULAR MOTOR SYNDROMES

### Combined Vertical Gaze Ophthalmoplegia

*Combined vertical gaze ophthalmoplegia* is defined as paresis of both upward and downward gaze. Vertical gaze ophthalmoplegia is an example of a brainstem syndrome in which the objective physical findings dictate the diagnostic approach to the problem. Symptoms of vertical gaze ophthalmoplegia, when present, are relatively nonspecific and usually occur in patients who have difficulty looking down, as required for reading, eating from a table, and walking down a flight of stairs. In addition, the patient's report of symptoms may be unobtainable because of mental status changes caused by dysfunction of the reticular formation that lies adjacent to the vertical gaze generator in the rostral midbrain (see Chapter 18).

The neurological examination discloses associated signs of the disorders listed in the differential diagnosis (Box 21.1) (Graff-Redford et al., 1985). Coma may occur due to reticular system involvement. Long-tract signs and loss of the pupillary reflexes are commonly associated. The syndrome of combined vertical gaze ophthalmoplegia is diagnosed when the ocular findings occur in isolation from long-tract signs.

With combined vertical gaze ophthalmoplegia, vertical saccades and pursuit are lost. This gaze limitation may be overcome by the oculocephalic (doll's head or doll's eye) maneuver, which tests the vestibuloocular reflex (VOR) (see Chapter 18); a conjugate eye movement in the direction opposite to that of head movement is the expected response with this maneuver. The Bell phenomenon (reflex movement of the eyes up and out in response to forced eye closure) often is absent and skew deviation (vertical misalignment of the eyes) may occur. Absence of convergence and loss of the pupillary reactions to light are common.

The location of the lesion for combined vertical gaze ophthalmoplegia is the rostral interstitial nucleus of the medial longitudinal fasciculus (riMLF) (Leigh and Zee, 2006). Box 21.1 lists the disorders involving the rostral mesodiencephalic region (for the differential diagnosis) that cause combined vertical gaze ophthalmoplegia (see Chapter 18). The most common causes of isolated combined vertical gaze ophthalmoplegia are stroke and progressive supranuclear palsy (PSP). In cortical-basal ganglionic degeneration, ocular motility findings can be similar to those in PSP but are less severe. Although the supranuclear vertical gaze ophthalmoplegia may be prominent early in the course of PSP, obvious vertical and horizontal gaze limitation usually is a late finding in cortical-basal ganglionic degeneration (Rottach et al., 1996).

The diagnostic formulation varies with the age of the patient. Isolated combined vertical gaze ophthalmoplegia usually is due to infarction of the rostral dorsal midbrain. When onset is gradual instead of abrupt or if the patient is young, other disorders should be considered (see Box 21.1). In the elderly, PSP (see Chapter 96) is likely if the onset is gradual. PSP can be mimicked by several disorders, including the treatable Whipple

**BOX 21.1 Differential Diagnosis for Combined Vertical Gaze Ophthalmoplegia**

Stroke
Progressive supranuclear palsy
Cortical-basal ganglionic degeneration
Arteriovenous malformation
Multiple sclerosis
Tumor (thalamic, mesencephalic, pineal)
Hydrocephalus
Whipple disease
Syphilis
Metabolic disorders:
- Lipid and lysosomal storage diseases (e.g., Niemann-Pick type C)
- Wilson disease
- Kernicterus

Wernicke encephalopathy
Bulbar-onset amyotrophic lateral sclerosis (associated with TDP-43–positive inclusions)
Paraneoplastic brainstem encephalitis (e.g., with Ma-2 antibodies)
Creutzfeldt-Jakob disease

**BOX 21.2 Differential Diagnosis for Dorsal Midbrain Syndrome**

Pineal and other tumors
Stroke
Trauma (including iatrogenic from surgery)
Hydrocephalus and shunt malfunction
Multiple sclerosis
Transtentorial herniation
Congenital aqueductal stenosis
Infections:
- Encephalitis
- Cysticercosis

Midbrain arteriovenous malformation
Metabolic disorders:
- Lipid storage disease
- Wilson disease
- Kernicterus

Wernicke encephalopathy

disease (Averbuch-Heller et al., 1999). For Whipple disease, oculomasticatory myorhythmia, which consists of pendular converging and diverging eye oscillations with synchronous jaw oscillations, is pathognomonic. Laboratory investigations used to evaluate combined vertical gaze ophthalmoplegia include computed tomography (CT) or, preferably, magnetic resonance imaging (MRI). Care should be taken not to overlook lesions inferior to the floor of the third ventricle. Lumbar puncture (LP), syphilis serology, erythrocyte sedimentation rate, and antinuclear antibody assay complete the evaluation when the cause is not obvious. Small-bowel biopsy should be considered if Whipple disease is a possible diagnosis. A polymerase chain reaction (PCR) assay performed on the small-bowel biopsy, cerebrospinal fluid (CSF), or other tissues for the 16S ribosomal ribonucleic acid (RNA) gene of *Tropheryma whipplei* appears to have both sensitivity and specificity for the diagnosis of Whipple disease (Lee, 2002).

## Upgaze Paresis (Dorsal Midbrain or Parinaud Syndrome)

Another brainstem syndrome that can occur without symptoms is the dorsal midbrain syndrome. When symptoms do occur, the patient reports difficulty looking up and may have blurred distant vision caused by accommodative spasm.

The tetrad of findings in the dorsal midbrain syndrome are (1) loss of upgaze, which usually is supranuclear (loss of pursuit and saccades with preservation of the VOR); (2) normal to large pupils with light-near dissociation (loss of the pupillary light reaction with preservation of the response to a near stimulus) or pupillary areflexia; (3) convergence-retraction nystagmus, in which the eyes make converging and retracting movements during attempted upward saccades; and (4) lid retraction (Collier sign).

The location of the lesion causing the upgaze paresis of the dorsal midbrain syndrome is the posterior commissure and its interstitial nucleus (Leigh and Zee, 2006). The presence of the full syndrome implies a lesion of the dorsal midbrain (including the posterior commissure), bilateral lesions of the pretectal region, or a large unilateral tegmental lesion. The differential diagnosis is presented in Box 21.2. Other than the mild upgaze limitation that can occur with aging, which is caused by involutional changes in the orbital connective tissues (Chaudhuri and Demer, 2013), the most common cause of isolated loss of upgaze is a tumor in the pineal region. The next most common causes are stroke and trauma. The upgaze palsy portion of the syndrome can be mimicked by any of several conditions: double elevator palsy, PSP, orbital causes such as thyroid eye disease, the bilateral Brown superior oblique tendon sheath syndrome, pseudodorsal midbrain syndrome secondary to myasthenia gravis (MG), Guillain-Barré syndrome, Miller Fisher syndrome, and congenital upgaze limitation. Forced ductions (see Chapter 18) may be performed by grasping anesthetized conjunctiva with forceps and moving the globe through its range of motion; the presence of restriction of movement with forced ductions implies a lesion within the orbit.

The diagnostic formulation for the dorsal midbrain syndrome varies with age. In children and adolescents, pineal region tumors or obstructive hydrocephalus are usually the cause. In young and middle-aged adults, the disorder is uncommon, and the cause may be trauma, multiple sclerosis (MS), or arteriovenous malformation (AVM). In the elderly, stroke and PSP are the most common causes.

The investigation needed to evaluate dorsal midbrain syndrome is MRI. If no structural lesion is present and an infectious or inflammatory cause is suspected, an LP should be performed.

## Downgaze Paresis

Isolated downgaze paresis is uncommon. Symptoms, when they occur, are related to difficulty in reading, eating, and walking down stairs.

Neurological examination reveals loss of downward pursuit and saccades, although pursuit may sometimes be spared. The vertical oculocephalic maneuver may be normal or may disclose gaze limitation. Convergence may be lost, and gaze-evoked upbeat nystagmus may be present on upward gaze. In young patients, forced ductions should be performed to assess for congenital restrictive downgaze limitation.

The site of the lesion for isolated downgaze paresis is bilateral involvement of the lateral portions of the riMLF. The main considerations in the differential diagnosis are ischemic stroke, PSP, and Whipple disease. Investigations to support the clinical diagnosis include CT or MRI. Lesions may be detected in the rostral mesodiencephalic junction inferior to the floor of the third ventricle.

The diagnostic formulation for isolated downgaze limitation is uncomplicated. When acute in onset, this disorder usually is due to stroke. In an elderly patient with a progressive course, PSP should be considered.

## Internuclear Ophthalmoplegia

Internuclear ophthalmoplegia (INO) is characterized by paresis or slowing of adduction of one eye, with horizontal nystagmus in the contralateral eye when it is abducted (Video 21.1). It is due to a lesion of the MLF ipsilateral to the side of the adduction weakness.

Surprisingly, most patients with INO do not have symptoms. The symptoms that may be associated with INO are diplopia, oscillopsia of one of the two images, and blurred vision. When diplopia is present, it can be due to medial rectus paresis (horizontal diplopia) or skew deviation (vertical diplopia).

The MLF carries information for vertical pursuit and the vertical VOR. Consequently, other associated findings with MLF lesions are abnormal vertical smooth pursuit and impaired reflex vertical eye movements (VOR, Bell phenomenon). Vertical saccadic eye movements are unaffected. Gaze-evoked vertical nystagmus (usually on upgaze) and skew deviation may be present with the higher eye on the side of the lesion. Skew deviation is a pure vertical ocular misalignment that is not due to a cranial nerve palsy, orbital lesion, or strabismus but is caused by unilateral or asymmetrical damage to the otolith-ocular pathways (Zwergal et al., 2008).

INO, discussed further in Chapter 18, may be a false localizing sign. Brainstem compression due to subdural hematoma with transtentorial herniation and cerebellar masses may cause INO. MG, Guillain-Barré syndrome, and Miller Fisher syndrome also may simulate INO.

The diagnostic considerations are many and varied. Examination can differentiate a lesion of the MLF from a partial third cranial nerve palsy, MG, strabismus, or thyroid eye disease. For example, intact convergence eye movements would be expected in an isolated MLF lesion but not in conditions affecting the third cranial nerve, medial rectus muscles, or neuromuscular junction. The common causes of INO are stroke (including vertebral artery dissection) in older age groups and MS in the young. One series reported that approximately one-third of INO cases are caused by stroke, one-third by MS, and one-third by other causes (Keane, 2005). Less common causes include trauma, herniation, infections, tumor, vasculitis, and surgical procedures.

Investigations that are performed to elucidate the cause include MRI. Thin cuts are often needed to find the lesion when INO is isolated. Investigations should be performed to evaluate for MG unless there are associated signs of obligatory brainstem dysfunction.

The diagnostic formulation for INO first necessitates accurate localization of the lesion. Limitation or slowing of adduction initially is formulated simply as an adduction deficit. It may also be due to (1) a lesion of the midbrain or third cranial nerve disrupting innervation; (2) a disorder of the neuromuscular junction (MG); or (3) a lesion involving the medial rectus muscle.

## Horizontal Gaze Paresis

Although there are no common symptoms of horizontal gaze paresis, this condition seldom occurs in isolation. Patients may complain of inability to see or to look to the side. Because supranuclear gaze pareses are conjugate by definition, diplopia does not occur.

On examination, with unilateral isolated involvement of the paramedian pontine reticular formation (PPRF), loss of ipsilateral saccades and pursuit is evident. However, full horizontal eye movements can be demonstrated with the oculocephalic maneuver (VOR).

Lesions of the sixth cranial nerve nucleus cause horizontal gaze paresis with inability of the oculocephalic maneuver (VOR) to overcome the limitation. Although an associated ipsilateral peripheral facial palsy is usually seen due to involvement of the fascicle of the seventh cranial nerve coursing over the sixth cranial nerve nucleus, cases of isolated horizontal gaze paresis caused by sixth nerve nuclear lesions have been reported (Miller et al., 2002). With bilateral lesions, loss or limitation of horizontal saccades and (usually) pursuit in both directions is characteristic. Gaze-paretic nystagmus may be present. In the acute phase, transient vertical gaze paresis and vertical nystagmus or upgaze paresis can also be seen. In the chronic phase, vertical eye movements are full, although nystagmus may be noted on upgaze.

The location of the lesion for horizontal gaze paresis is the frontopontine tract, mesencephalic reticular formation, PPRF, and sixth cranial nerve nucleus. The explanation for gaze palsy occurring with a nuclear lesion is given later in the chapter (see Syndromes Involving Ocular Motor Nuclei).

The diagnostic possibilities are varied. As with other ocular motility disorders, MG may cause gaze limitation that simulates a central nervous system (CNS) lesion. The diagnostic formulation varies with age, rapidity of onset, and associated clinical findings. For patients with an acute onset who are older than 50 years of age, stroke is a likely cause. With a subacute onset before the age of 50 years, a diagnosis of MS should be considered. Congenital cases usually are due to Möbius syndrome (Rucker et al., 2014). Systemic lupus erythematosus (SLE), syphilis, and Wernicke encephalopathy should be considered for any acquired cases.

Investigations for horizontal gaze paresis should include MRI. If there are no obligatory signs of CNS dysfunction, MG must be considered.

### BOX 21.3 Differential Diagnosis for Total Ophthalmoplegia

Acute:
- Miller Fisher syndrome
- Guillain-Barré syndrome
- Bilateral pontine or midbrain-thalamic stroke
- Myasthenia gravis
- Pituitary apoplexy
- Botulism
- Anticonvulsant intoxication
- Multiple cranial neuropathies from infection or neoplasm
- Wernicke encephalopathy

Chronic/Progressive:
- Chronic progressive external ophthalmoplegia syndromes
- Oculopharyngeal muscular dystrophy
- Myotonic dystrophy and other congenital myopathies
- Congenital cranial dysinnervation syndromes
- Neurodegenerative diseases (e.g., progressive supranuclear palsy, late spinocerebellar ataxia type 2)
- Myasthenia gravis
- Thyroid eye disease (especially in combination with myasthenia gravis)

## Global Paralysis of Gaze

The characteristic symptom of global paralysis of gaze is an inability to look voluntarily in any direction. However, global paralysis of gaze rarely occurs in isolation, and signs and symptoms of involvement of other local structures usually are present.

The location of the lesion is the frontopontine tract for saccades, and the parietooccipitopontine tract for pursuit, where they converge at the subthalamic and upper midbrain level (Thurtell and Halmagyi, 2008). The differential diagnosis for total ophthalmoplegia is given in Box 21.3. The common causes for this presentation are diseases that do not involve the CNS, such as Miller Fisher syndrome, Guillain-Barré syndrome, MG, and chronic progressive external ophthalmoplegia (CPEO); for intraaxial lesions, considerations include stroke, Wernicke encephalopathy, PSP, and other neurodegenerative disorders (e.g., spinocerebellar ataxias).

The diagnostic formulation usually is focused on extraaxial (cranial nerve, neuromuscular junction, or muscle) pathology, because a brainstem lesion rarely causes isolated complete ophthalmoplegia. Miller Fisher syndrome, Guillain-Barré syndrome, bilateral cavernous sinus lesions (e.g., metastases, pituitary apoplexy), meningitis, and MG (sometimes in combination with thyroid eye disease) are likely possibilities if the onset is subacute (Keane, 2007). If the presentation is long-standing, slowly progressive, and accompanied by ptosis, CPEO syndromes, such as Kearns-Sayre, and other myopathic processes, such as oculopharyngeal muscular dystrophy (particularly in patients of French-Canadian descent), should be considered. In these extraaxial disorders, the gaze limitation cannot be overcome with the oculocephalic maneuver (VOR). PSP is a diagnostic possibility in the elderly, whereas Wernicke encephalopathy should be considered in alcoholics and nutritionally deprived patients. Whipple disease also can cause this rare clinical presentation.

Investigations for patients with global paralysis of gaze should include MRI. Investigations for MG should be considered. When botulism is suspected, electromyography with repetitive nerve stimulation and serum or stool assay for botulinum toxin should be performed.

### One-and-a-Half Syndrome

The one-and-a-half syndrome is characterized by an ipsilesional horizontal gaze palsy, together with an ipsilesional INO (impaired adduction of the ipsilesional eye). The common symptoms are diplopia, oscillopsia (the illusion that objects or scenes are oscillating), and blurred vision. Associated findings include skew deviation and gaze-evoked nystagmus on upgaze or lateral gaze. Acutely, there may be an exotropia (one eye deviated outward) in primary position. Other features may include limitation of upgaze, impaired vertical pursuit, and loss of convergence.

The location of the lesion is the PPRF or sixth cranial nerve nucleus, with extension to involve the internuclear fibers crossing from the contralateral sixth cranial nerve nucleus, which causes the INO. Entities to consider in the differential diagnosis include MS, stroke, AVM, and tumor of the lower pons. A pseudo-one-and-a-half syndrome may occur with MG, Miller Fisher syndrome, or Guillain-Barré syndrome. The diagnostic formulation for the one-and-a-half syndrome is similar to that for INO. Before the age of 50 years, the cause usually is MS; after age 50 years, it usually is stroke.

Variations of the one-and-a-half syndrome have been described, including the eight-and-a-half syndrome, which consists of a one-and-a-half syndrome with an ipsilateral facial palsy, and eight syndrome, which consists of a lateral gaze palsy (without INO) and a facial palsy (Eggenberger, 1998; Green et al., 2018).

Appropriate investigations for the one-and-a-half syndrome and its variants are MRI and, if indicated, LP.

## SYNDROMES INVOLVING OCULAR MOTOR NUCLEI

Patients with lesions involving the third or sixth cranial nerve nucleus present not only with accompanying long-tract signs but also show different ocular motility disturbances than seen with lesions involving the third or sixth fascicle or cranial nerve.

### Third Cranial Nerve Nucleus

The common manifestations of third cranial nerve nucleus lesions are diplopia and ptosis. The signs present on the side of the lesion are weakness of the inferior and medial recti and the inferior oblique muscles. Upgaze limitation is present in both eyes because the superior rectus subnucleus is contralateral, and the axons from this subnucleus cross within the nuclear complex. In addition, ptosis and dilated unreactive pupils may be present on both sides because the levator subnucleus (also known as the central caudal nucleus) and Edinger-Westphal nuclei are bilaterally represented.

The main considerations in the differential diagnosis are stroke (either ischemic or hemorrhagic), metastatic tumor, and MS. Of these diagnoses, only ischemic stroke is common. Disorders that simulate nuclear third cranial nerve palsy include MG, CPEO, thyroid eye disease, Miller Fisher syndrome, and Guillain-Barré syndrome.

The pertinent investigation for this syndrome is MRI, which usually demonstrates an ischemic stroke. Once the proper localization has been made, the diagnostic formulation is straightforward.

### Sixth Cranial Nerve Nucleus

The sixth cranial nerve nucleus has two populations of neurons. The abducens motor neurons innervate the ipsilateral lateral rectus muscle. Internuclear neurons decussate at the level of the sixth cranial nerve nucleus, travel up the MLF, and terminate on the medial rectus subnucleus of the contralateral third cranial nerve. Accordingly, a lesion of the sixth cranial nerve nucleus causes ipsilateral horizontal gaze palsy.

Patients with an isolated horizontal gaze palsy are often asymptomatic. If they do have symptoms, they report difficulty looking to one side. On examination, a conjugate horizontal gaze paresis is present, which cannot be overcome by the oculocephalic maneuver or caloric stimulation. A peripheral seventh cranial nerve palsy usually accompanies a lesion of the sixth cranial nerve nucleus. Considerations in the differential diagnosis include stroke (Miller et al., 2002), Wernicke encephalopathy, MS, and a tumor of the pontomedullary junction.

Evaluation of a lesion of the sixth cranial nerve nucleus includes MRI, possibly LP, and investigations (e.g., edrophonium or prostigmine test) for MG if there are no long-tract signs to indicate intraaxial disease.

## OTHER BRAINSTEM AND ASSOCIATED SYNDROMES

### Diencephalic Syndrome (Russell Syndrome)

Common symptoms of the diencephalic syndrome include emaciation with increased appetite, euphoria, vomiting, and excessive sweating (Fleischman et al., 2005). Patients also may have an alert appearance with motor hyperactivity. Most cases occur in children younger than 3 years.

The differential diagnosis should include hyperthyroidism, diabetes mellitus, a tumor in the region of the fourth ventricle, vein of Galen malformation, and a hypothalamic tumor. Most patients appear pale despite lack of anemia. Ophthalmological findings include optic atrophy and, less commonly, nystagmus.

Investigations for diencephalic syndrome may show an elevated serum growth hormone level that is incompletely suppressed by hyperglycemia. MRI often demonstrates a hypothalamic mass lesion. Malignant cells may be present in the CSF and are diagnostic. The CSF also may contain human chorionic gonadotropin in patients with germinomas. An LP should not be performed if neuroimaging studies demonstrate a mass effect.

### Thalamic Syndrome

The common symptoms of thalamic syndrome include pain (thalamic pain), numbness, and hemisensory loss. The pain may be spontaneous or evoked by any form of stimulation. It often has a disagreeable and lasting quality. Patients also may complain of a distorted sense of taste. Right thalamic lesions appear to predominate.

On examination, a marked hemianesthesia is present which may be dissociated: that is, pain and temperature or light touch and vibration sense may be separately lost. Proprioceptive loss, often with astereognosis, is a common feature. A transitory hemiparesis sometimes occurs.

The usual location of the lesion for this type of pain is the ventroposterolateral nucleus of the thalamus. In addition to the thalamus, thalamic-type pain can occur with lesions of the parietal lobe, medial lemniscus, and dorsolateral medulla (MacGowan et al., 1997). The differential diagnosis includes stroke and tumor. The diagnostic formulation depends on the rate of onset of symptoms, associated signs, and findings on neuroimaging studies. The apoplectic onset of symptoms implicates stroke. Gradual onset is characteristic of tumor. Neuroimaging studies, preferably MRI, should confirm the clinical impression.

## Tectal Deafness

The symptoms associated with tectal deafness are bilateral deafness associated with other related CNS symptoms such as poor coordination, weakness, or vertigo. The main considerations in the differential diagnosis for the deafness are conductive hearing loss, cochlear disorders, bilateral eighth cranial nerve lesions, tectal deafness, and pure word deafness.

On examination, deafness that usually spares pure tones is confirmed. Pure word deafness with lesions of the inferior colliculi has been reported (Vitte et al., 2002). Other brainstem signs, including the dorsal midbrain syndrome, often are associated. The location of the lesion is the inferior colliculi; the most common causes are trauma, stroke, or a tumor of the brainstem, cerebellum, or pineal region. The diagnostic formulation for hearing loss caused by lesions rostral to the cochlear nuclei is the presence of hearing loss characterized by sparing of pure tone, with marked deterioration when background noise distortion or other aural stimuli are added. Signs of damage to adjacent nervous system structures are often present.

The pertinent investigations include MRI and an audiogram. Tests that reveal CNS auditory loss are distorted speech audiometry, dichotic auditory testing, and auditory brainstem evoked responses, although findings on evoked responses may be normal (Vitte et al., 2002).

## Foramen Magnum Syndrome

Foramen magnum syndrome is characterized by upper motor neuron–type weakness and sensory loss in any modality below the head. Detecting this syndrome is important because it often is caused by benign tumors such as meningiomas or fibromas, which may be removed completely when detected early in their course. Its only manifestations may be identical to those of a high spinal cord syndrome (see Chapter 27).

The common initial symptoms include neck stiffness and pain, which may radiate into the shoulder. Occipital headache also may be an early symptom. Other common symptoms are weakness of the upper or lower extremities, numbness (most commonly of hands or arms), clumsiness, and gait disturbance.

Considerations in the differential diagnosis include cervical spondylosis, syringomyelia, MS, transverse myelitis, atlantoaxial subluxation (e.g., in rheumatoid arthritis), Chiari malformation, and foramen magnum or upper cervical cord tumor.

On examination, hemiparesis or quadriparesis and sensory loss are common. The loss of sensation may involve all modalities. It may be dissociated and capelike or may occur in a C2 distribution. Some patients have hemisensory loss below the cranium or involvement of only the lower extremities.

Pseudoathetosis resulting from loss of joint position sense may be an early sign. Atrophy of muscles of the upper extremities may occur at levels well below that of the lesion. Electric shock–like sensations radiating down the spine, which may be transmitted into the extremities, may occur with neck flexion (Lhermitte sign). This phenomenon may occur with lesions of the posterior columns, most commonly from MS. Lower cranial nerve palsies are less common. The presence of downbeat nystagmus in primary position or lateral gaze strongly suggests a lesion involving the craniocervical junction; this may be missed unless the nystagmus is sought when the patient gazes laterally and downward.

The differential diagnosis includes a foramen magnum or upper cervical cord tumor. The tumor is often a meningioma, neurofibroma, glioma, or metastasis. Cervical spondylosis, MS, syringobulbia, and the Chiari malformation (often accompanied by a syrinx) are other diagnostic considerations. The definitive investigation for evaluation of this syndrome is MRI.

Patients with foramen magnum tumors may have a relapsing-remitting clinical course with features that simulate those of MS. Because many of the tumors are meningiomas, the clinician should be alert for patients at risk. Meningiomas occur with increased frequency in women in their childbearing years and increase in size during pregnancy. Cervical spondylosis usually is associated with a related radiculopathy and is not accompanied by downbeat nystagmus or lower cranial nerve abnormalities. Diagnosis requires a high index of suspicion; foramen magnum tumors are often difficult to diagnose early because signs may be minimal despite a large tumor.

## Syringobulbia

Syringobulbia is a disorder of the lower brainstem caused by progressive enlargement of a fluid-filled cavity that involves the medulla and almost invariably the spinal cord (syringomyelia). The symptoms and signs are caused by dysfunction of the central spinal cord.

The common symptoms of syringobulbia and syringomyelia are lack of pain with accidental burns, hand numbness, neck and arm pain, leg stiffness, and headache, together with oscillopsia, diplopia, or vertigo. On examination, signs of lower brainstem dysfunction are evident. Lower motor neuron signs of the ninth through twelfth cranial nerves may be present. Nystagmus, if present, can be horizontal, vertical, or torsional. Signs of a spinal cord lesion characteristically coexist. In the upper extremities, dissociated anesthesia of an upper limb or forequarter (i.e., loss of pain and temperature sensation with sparing of other modalities) may be noted. The sensory loss also may be in a hemisensory distribution and deep tendon reflexes in the upper extremities are often absent or decreased.

Spastic paraparesis, usually asymmetrical, may occur. Loss of facial sensation can occur in an onion-skin pattern emanating from the corner of the mouth. Charcot (neuropathic) joints and trophic skin disorders may be present in long-standing cases. Horner syndrome and sphincter disturbances are other occasional findings.

The lesion is located in a rostrocaudal longitudinal cavity from the medulla into the spinal cord. The cavity usually is located near the fourth ventricle or central canal of the spinal cord. The most reliable and sensitive investigation for syringobulbia is MRI.

The main considerations in the differential diagnosis are an intrinsic central cord and lower brainstem lesion (syrinx, tumor, or trauma) and compressive foramen magnum syndrome caused by a tumor or a Chiari type I malformation. Less likely causes are MS and spinal arachnoiditis.

The diagnostic formulation for syringobulbia is based on data from the history, examination, and investigations. It most often is a disease of young adults, with a peak incidence in the third and fourth decades of life. Painless burns and dissociated segmental anesthesia of the upper extremities are highly suggestive of the diagnosis. A diagnosis of MS requires the presence of other noncontiguous lesions, oligoclonal bands in the CSF, and characteristic MRI findings. Tumors usually produce a more rapid course.

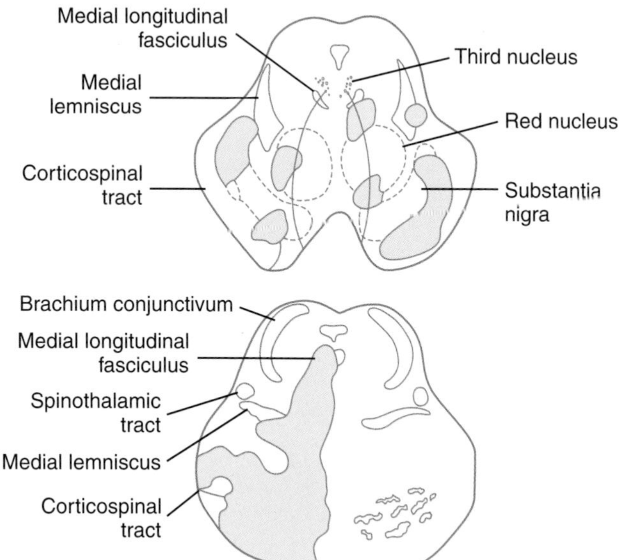


**Fig. 21.1 Distribution of Brainstem Infarction in a Patient with Basilar Artery Embolism.** Note the rostrocaudal extension of the infarction, along with its patchy nature. (*Reprinted with permission from Kubik, C.S., Adams, R.D., 1946. Occlusion of the basilar artery: a clinical and pathological study. Brain 59, 73–121.*)

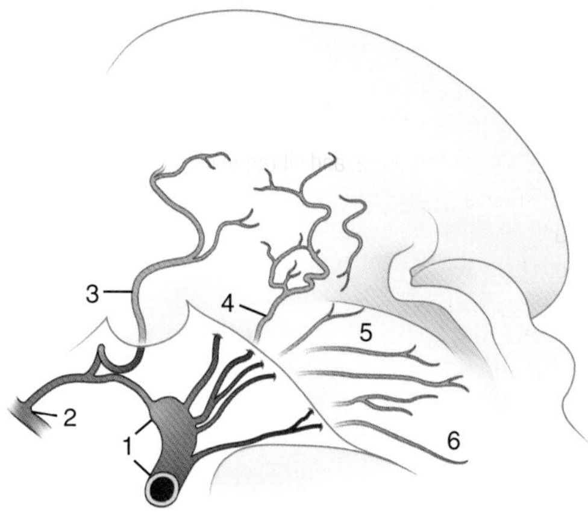


**Fig. 21.2** Branches of the basilar communicating artery (P1 segment of posterior cerebral artery), as seen in a sagittal section of the brainstem: thalamic polar *(1)*, posterior communicating *(2)*, posterior thalamosubthalamic paramedian *(3)*, superior paramedian *(4)*, inferior paramedian *(5)*, and mesencephalic paramedian *(6)*. (*Reprinted with permission from Percheron, G., 1976. Les artères et territoires du thalamus humain: II. Artères et territoires thalamiques paramédians de l'artère basilare communicante. Rev. Neurol. 132, 309–324.*)

## BRAINSTEM ISCHEMIC STROKE SYNDROMES

Vertebrobasilar ischemic lesions often have a rostrocaudal or patchy distribution (Fig. 21.1), rather than a simplified transverse distribution (Kubik and Adams, 1946). Thus a single lesion may not explain all of the clinical features.

The cardinal manifestations of brainstem stroke are involvement of the long tracts of the brainstem in combination with cranial nerve deficits. Crossed cranial nerve and motor or sensory long-tract deficits are characteristic. The cranial nerve palsy is ipsilateral to the lesion, whereas the long-tract signs are contralateral—hence the term *crossed*. Coma, ataxia, and vertigo, which are common with vertebrobasilar (posterior circulation) stroke, are uncommon with carotid (anterior circulation) stroke. INO, unreactive pupils, lower motor neuron cranial nerve impairment, and skew deviation, when caused by stroke, occur only with posterior circulation lesions. The same is usually true for nystagmus and most other ocular oscillations.

Another characteristic of vertebrobasilar ischemia is bilateral involvement of the long tracts. This can result in locked-in syndrome, which is usually caused by a lesion of the basis pontis and characterized by quadriplegia, corticobulbar tract involvement, and loss of the ability to produce speech. The reticular activating system is spared, so consciousness is preserved. Eye movements and blinking may be all that is left under voluntary control.

Another feature of bilateral lesions of the long tracts is pseudobulbar palsy. The symptoms resemble those that occur with medullary lesions. However, the cranial nerve nuclei have lost their cortical input, which results in dysarthria, dysphagia, bilateral facial weakness, extremity weakness, and emotional lability. A more appropriate term for this syndrome is *supranuclear bulbar palsy*.

Cortical blindness occurs with bilateral posterior cerebral artery occlusion and concomitant occipital lobe infarction.

Ischemic stroke syndromes are outlined next. These syndromes can occur in isolation, as presented here, or in combination. The combinations can be medial with lateral involvement or often rostrocaudal extension. Several classic stroke syndromes, such as the Wallenberg lateral medullary syndrome and Weber cerebral peduncle syndrome, exist. However, an investigation that looked prospectively at 304 cases of brainstem stroke found one of 24 eponymous syndromes in only 20 cases; approximately 20% of cases showed different unnamed crossed brainstem syndromes (Marx and Thömke, 2009).

### Thalamic Stroke Syndromes

The blood supply of the thalamus arises from the posterior cerebral, posterior communicating, basilar communicating (P1 segment of the posterior communicating artery) (Fig. 21.2), and anterior and posterior choroidal arteries. Thalamic stroke syndromes are listed in Box 21.4. Fig. 21.3 illustrates the arterial territories of the thalamus.

### Midbrain Stroke Syndromes

Midbrain stroke is characterized by long-tract signs combined with involvement of the third and fourth cranial nerves (Bogousslavsky et al., 1994). Anterior circulation stroke may also produce midbrain signs when there is transtentorial herniation. Classifications of the blood supply to the brainstem are numerous, and this variability is nowhere more apparent than in the midbrain.

Blood flows to the upper midbrain via perforating branches of the posterior cerebral artery. The P1 segment of the posterior cerebral artery (basilar communicating artery or mesencephalic artery) arises from the basilar artery. A simplified scheme divides the vascular territories into medial and lateral transverse regions.

The medial midbrain syndromes are characterized by an ipsilateral third cranial nerve palsy associated with a contralateral hemiparesis. Involvement of the medial lemniscus may result in loss of the discriminative sensations (proprioception, vibration, and stereognosis). The lateral syndromes are characterized by contralateral loss of pain and temperature sensation, ipsilateral Horner syndrome, and loss of facial sensation. Ataxia may occur on either side. Ischemic stroke syndromes of the midbrain are outlined in Box 21.5. Figs. 21.4 and 21.5 show the territories involved with occlusive and ischemic stroke syndromes in this area. A caudal paramedian midbrain stroke can produce bilateral cerebellar (truncal and gait) ataxia, eye motility disorders (nuclear third nerve palsy, INO), and palatal myoclonus (Mossuto-Agatiello, 2006). A variation of a caudal midbrain stroke that involves the fourth nerve nucleus and adjacent oculosympathetic pathways can cause an ipsilateral Horner syndrome and

## BOX 21.4 Ischemic Stroke Syndromes of the Thalamus

**Anterolateral**

***Common Symptoms***

Contralateral weakness, vision loss
Confusion
Disorientation
Language disturbance

***Signs***

Contralateral:
- Hemiparesis
- Hemiataxia
- Hemisensory loss
- Homonymous hemianopia

Right-sided lesion: visuospatial abnormalities, hemineglect, nonverbal intellect affected
Left-sided lesion: disorientation, aphasia

***Arterial Territory Involved***

Thalamic polar (tuberothalamic) artery (see Figs. 21.2 and 21.3)

**Medial**

***Common Symptoms***

Disorientation and confusion
Coma with occlusion of mainstem variant
Visual blurring

***Signs***

Vertical gaze ophthalmoplegia
Loss of pupillary reflexes
Loss of convergence
Disorientation and confusion, stupor, coma, and various neuropsychiatric disturbances

***Arterial Territory Involved***

Posterior thalamosubthalamic paramedian artery (thalamic paramedian or deep interpeduncular profundus artery; see Figs. 21.2 and 21.3)

**Lateral and Posterior Internal Capsule**

***Common Symptoms***

Contralateral:
- Weakness
- Numbness
- Confusion

***Signs***

Contralateral:
- Hemiparesis
- Diminished pain and temperature
- Dysarthria
- Homonymous hemianopia; usually with a tongue of sparing along the horizontal meridian

Memory impairment
With right-sided lesions: visuoperceptual abnormalities

***Arterial Territory Involved***

Anterior choroidal artery (see Fig. 21.3)

**Posterolateral**

***Common Symptoms***

Contralateral:
- Weakness
- Numbness
- Vision loss
- Neglect
- Confusion

***Signs***

Contralateral:
- Loss of touch, pain, temperature, and vibration sense (common)
- Hemiparesis in some
- Hemiataxia
- Homonymous hemianopia

Left hemispatial neglect
Poor attention span

***Arterial Territory Involved***

Geniculothalamic artery (see Fig. 21.3)

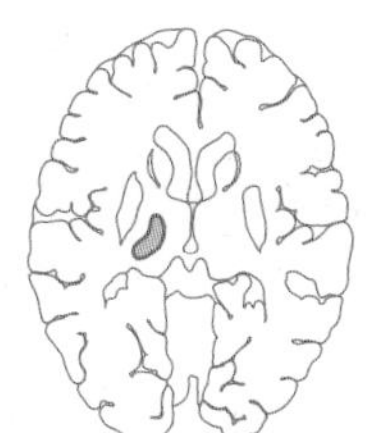
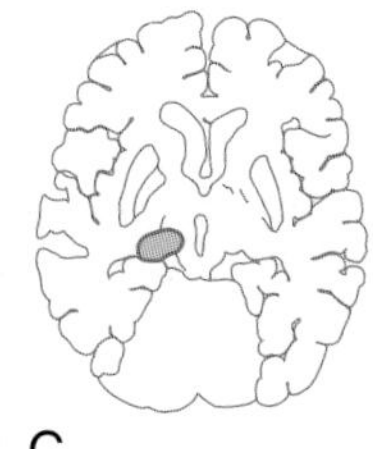
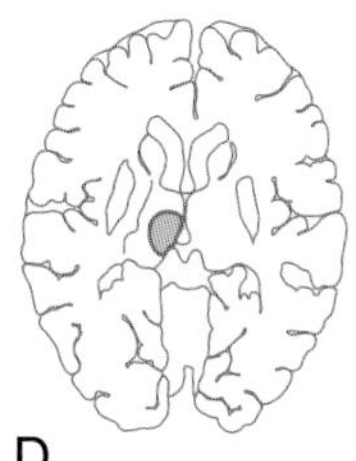
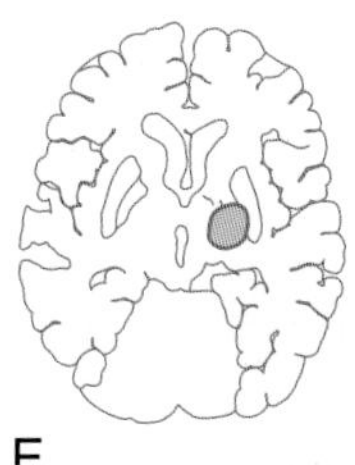
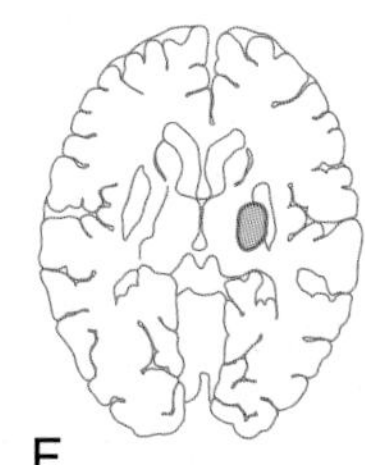

A B C D E F

**Fig. 21.3 Schematic Axial Sections Showing the Five Arterial Territories of the Thalamus.** **A,** Geniculothalamic (inferolateral) artery territory. **B,** Anterior thalamosubthalamic paramedian (tuberothalamic) territory. **C,** Posterior choroidal territory. **D,** Posterior thalamosubthalamic paramedian territory. **E** and **F,** Anterior choroidal territory. (*Modified with permission from Bogousslavsky, J., Regli, F., Uske, A., 1988. Thalamic infarcts: clinical syndromes, etiology and prognosis. Neurology 38, 837–848.*)

**BOX 21.5 Ischemic Stroke Syndromes of the Midbrain**

**Middle Median Midbrain Syndrome**

***Common Symptoms***

Contralateral:
- Weakness
- Ataxia
- Tremor
- Numbness

Ipsilateral:
- Eyelid ptosis
- Ataxia
- Diplopia

***Signs***

Contralateral:
- Weakness
- Ataxia
- Tremor
- Pseudoabducens palsy

Ipsilateral:
- Third cranial nerve palsy (nuclear or fascicular)

Internuclear ophthalmoplegia

***Arterial Territory Involved***

Median and paramedian perforating branches of the basilar or posterior cerebral (mesencephalic) arteries

**Middle Lateral Midbrain Syndrome (see Fig. 21.4)**

***Common Symptoms***

Numbness: contralateral
Clumsiness: ipsilateral

***Signs***

Contralateral:
- Hemianesthesia
- Ataxia

Ipsilateral:
- Facial hemianesthesia (or contralateral)
- Horner syndrome
- Ataxia (if lesion is ventral to brachium conjunctivum)

***Arterial Territory Involved***

Superior cerebellar artery

**Inferior Medial Midbrain Syndrome (see Fig. 21.5)**

***Common Symptoms***

Diplopia
Contralateral weakness
Clumsiness

***Signs***

Contralateral:
- Fourth cranial nerve palsy
- Ataxia (may be ipsilateral, depending on whether the lesion is before or after the decussation of the brachium conjunctivum)
- Hemiparesis
- Supranuclear horizontal gaze paresis (ipsilateral if below decussation in lower midbrain)

Ipsilateral:
- Internuclear ophthalmoplegia

***Arterial Territory Involved***

Median branches of the basilar artery

**Inferior Lateral Midbrain Syndrome (see Fig. 21.5)**

***Common Symptom***

Contralateral numbness

***Signs***

Contralateral:
- Hemianesthesia

Ipsilateral:
- Hemianesthesia of face
- Horner syndrome

***Arterial Territory Involved***

Superior cerebellar artery

contralateral fourth nerve palsy; the fourth nerve fibers decussate in the superior (anterior) medullary velum before exiting the brainstem.

## Pontine Stroke Syndromes

The pons is supplied by numerous penetrating branches of the basilar artery. These arteries have little collateral supply; consequently, lacunar syndromes (see Chapter 65) can occur (Box 21.6). These syndromes (Figs. 21.6–21.8) may be clinically indistinguishable from lacunar syndromes from stroke of the internal capsule. More extensive paramedian syndromes are accompanied by characteristic pontine findings. The findings may initially fluctuate (pontine warning syndrome).

Contralateral hemiparesis, ipsilateral ataxia, INO, and conjugate horizontal gaze paresis characterize the medial syndromes. The lateral syndromes are distinguished by contralateral hemianesthesia and loss of discriminative sensation with ipsilateral Horner syndrome, facial hemianesthesia, and ataxia. Ipsilateral lower motor neuron–type facial paresis, sixth cranial nerve paresis, deafness, and vertigo occur with inferior pontine stroke.

## Medullary Stroke Syndromes

Medial medullary ischemia (Fig. 21.9) can cause crossed hypoglossal hemiparesis syndrome. In addition, patients may have loss of discriminative sensation (position sense, graphesthesia, and stereognosis) when there is associated medial lemniscus involvement. Four patterns of medial medullary stroke have been described: (1) the most frequent, classic crossed hypoglossal hemiparesis syndrome; (2) sensorimotor stroke without lingual palsy; (3) pure hemiparesis; and (4) bilateral medial medullary stroke (Kumral et al., 2002). Ocular motor findings often are prominent and can include ocular contrapulsion, ocular tilt reaction, and nystagmus (gaze-evoked, upbeat, and hemiseesaw) (Kim et al., 2005).

Lateral medullary syndrome (Wallenberg syndrome; see Fig. 21.9) is one of the most dramatic clinical presentations in neurology (Box 21.7). Long-tract signs (i.e., contralateral loss of pain and temperature sensation over half of the body, ipsilateral ataxia, ipsilateral axial lateropulsion [Eggers et al., 2009], Horner syndrome) are accompanied by involvement of the nuclei and fasciculi of cranial nerves V, VIII, IX,

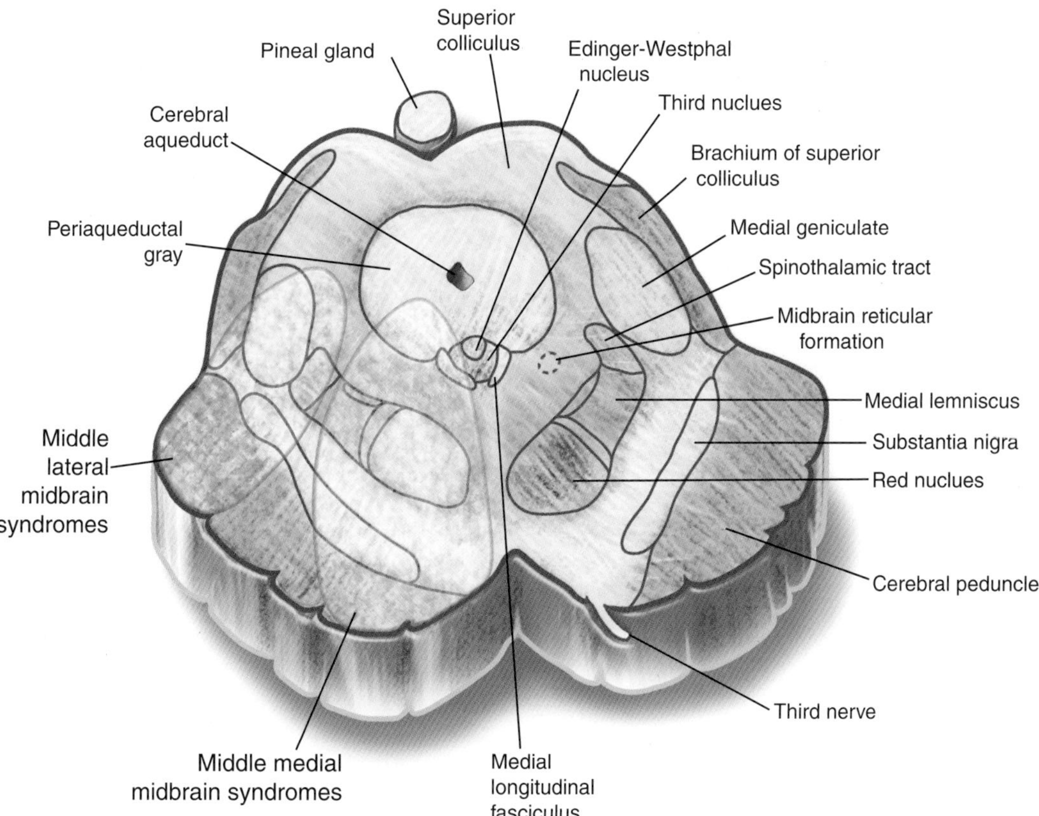


**Fig. 21.4** Midbrain at the level of the superior colliculus, showing the medial and lateral territories involved with ischemic stroke syndromes in this area.

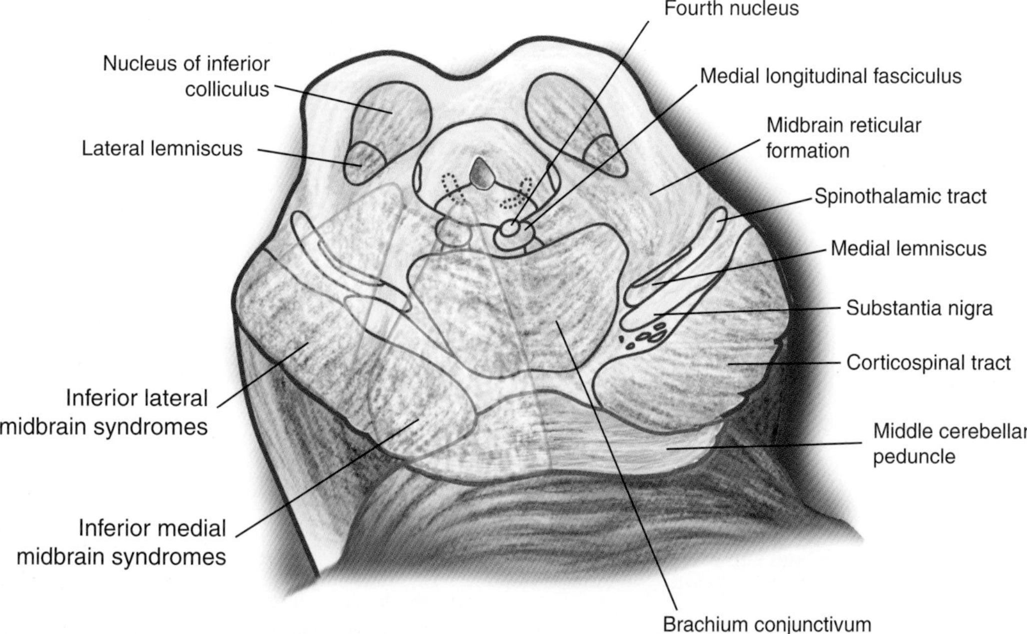


**Fig. 21.5** Midbrain at the level of the inferior colliculus, showing the medial and lateral territories involved with ischemic stroke syndromes in this area.

## BOX 21.6 Ischemic Stroke Syndromes of the Pons

### Superior Medial Pontine Syndrome (See Fig. 21.6)

***Common Symptoms***

Contralateral weakness
Clumsiness

***Signs***

Ipsilateral:
- Ataxia
- Internuclear ophthalmoplegia
- Oscillations of palate, pharynx, vocal cords with nystagmus (oculopalatal tremor, occurs after weeks to months rather than acutely)

Contralateral:
- Paralysis of face, arm, and leg

***Arterial Territory Involved***

Median branches of the basilar artery

### Superior Lateral Pontine Syndrome (see Fig. 21.6)

***Common Symptoms***

Ipsilateral clumsiness
Contralateral numbness
Dizziness, nausea, vomiting

***Signs***

Ipsilateral:
- Ataxia of limbs and gait, falling to side of lesion
- Horner syndrome
- Facial hemianesthesia
- Paresis of muscles of mastication

Contralateral:
- Hemianesthesia (trigeminothalamic tract)
- Impaired touch, vibration, and position sense

***Arterial Territory Involved***

Superior cerebellar artery

### Middle Medial Pontine Syndrome (see Fig. 21.7)

***Common Symptoms***

Contralateral hemiparesis
Ipsilateral clumsiness

***Signs***

Ipsilateral:
- Ataxia of limbs
- Conjugate gaze paresis toward the side of the lesion
- Internuclear ophthalmoplegia

Contralateral:
- Paresis of face, arm, and leg
- With bilateral lesions, locked-in syndrome may occur

***Arterial Territory Involved***

Median branches of the basilar artery

### Middle Lateral Pontine Syndrome (see Fig. 21.7)

***Common Symptoms***

Numbness
Clumsiness
Chewing difficulty

***Signs***

Contralateral:
- Hemisensory loss

Ipsilateral:
- Ataxia of limbs
- Paralysis of muscles of mastication
- Impaired pain sensation over side of face
- Horner syndrome

***Arterial Territory Involved***

Long lateral branches of basilar artery

### Inferior Medial Pontine Syndrome (Foville Syndrome) (see Fig. 21.8)

***Common Symptoms***

Contralateral weakness and numbness
Ipsilateral facial weakness
Diplopia

***Signs***

Contralateral:
- Paralysis of arm and leg
- Impaired tactile and proprioceptive sense over half the body

Ipsilateral:
- Paresis of conjugate gaze to side of lesion; to oculocephalic maneuver also if the sixth cranial nerve nucleus is involved
- Internuclear ophthalmoplegia or one-and-a-half syndrome
- Lower motor neuron–type facial palsy

Other:
- Nystagmus

***Arterial Territory Involved***

Median branches of the basilar artery

### Inferior Lateral Pontine Syndrome (Anterior Inferior Cerebellar Artery Syndrome) (see Fig. 21.8)

***Common Symptoms***

Vertigo, nausea, vomiting
Oscillopsia
Deafness, tinnitus
Facial numbness
Incoordination

***Signs***

Contralateral:
- Impaired pain and thermal sense over half the body (may include the face)

Ipsilateral:
- Deafness
- Facial paralysis
- Ataxia
- Impaired sensation over face

Other:
- Nystagmus

***Arterial Territory Involved***

Anterior inferior cerebellar artery

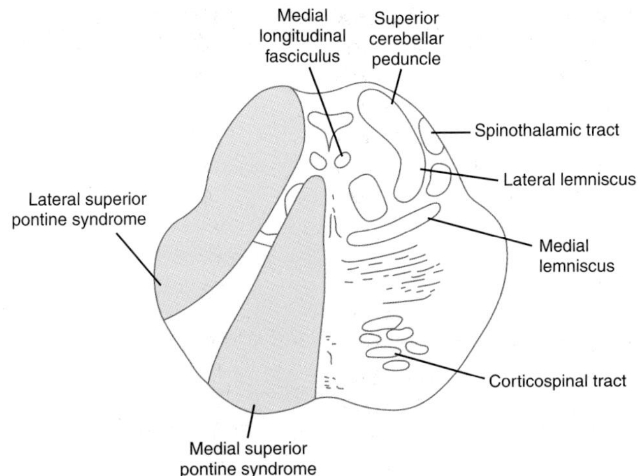


**Fig. 21.6** Superior pontine level, showing the medial and lateral territories involved with ischemic stroke syndromes in this area. (*Reprinted with permission from Adams, R.D., Victor, M., 1993. Principles of Neurology, fifth ed. McGraw-Hill, New York.*)

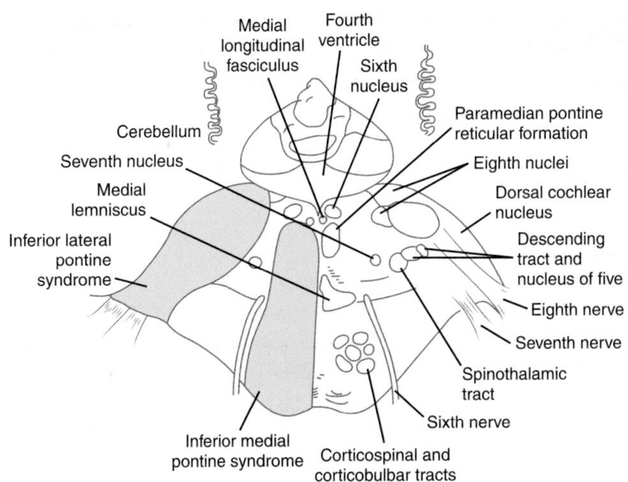


**Fig. 21.8** Inferior pons at the level of the sixth cranial nerve nucleus, showing the medial and lateral territories involved with ischemic stroke syndromes in this area. (*Reprinted with permission from Adams, R.D., Victor, M., 1993. Principles of Neurology, fifth ed. McGraw-Hill, New York.*)

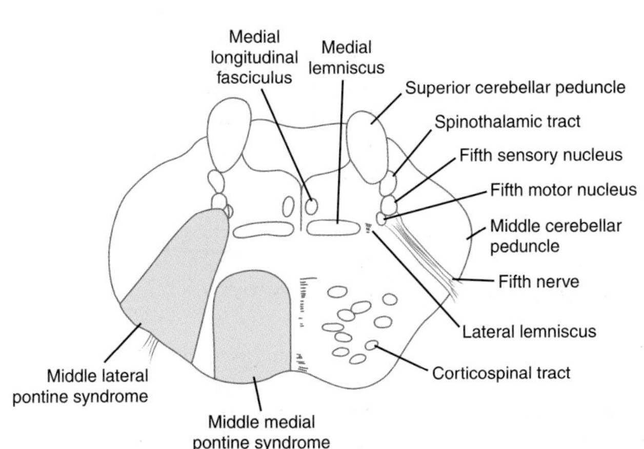


**Fig. 21.7** Middle pontine level, showing the medial and lateral territories involved with ischemic stroke syndromes in this area. (*Reprinted with permission from Adams, R.D., Victor, M., 1993. Principles of Neurology, fifth ed. McGraw-Hill, New York.*)

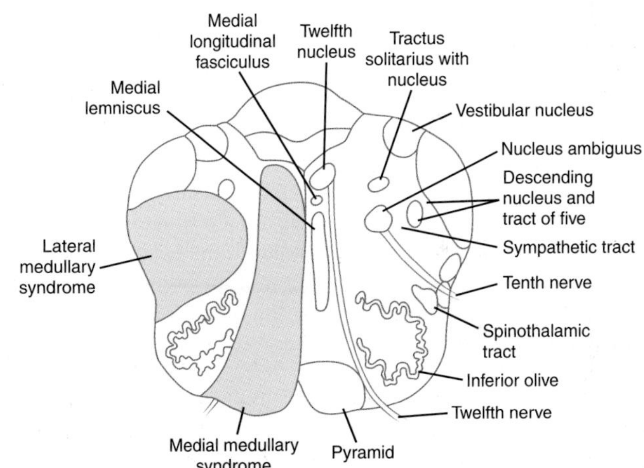


**Fig. 21.9** Medulla at the level of the inferior olivary complex, showing the medial and the more common lateral territory involved with ischemic stroke in this brainstem area. (*Reprinted with permission from Adams, R.D., Victor, M., 1993. Principles of Neurology, fifth ed. McGraw-Hill, New York.*)

## BOX 21.7 Ischemic Stroke Syndromes of the Medulla

**Medial Medullary Syndrome (see Fig. 21.9)**

***Common Symptoms***

Contralateral weakness
Dysarthria

***Signs***

Contralateral:
- Paralysis of arm and leg, sparing face
- Impaired tactile, vibratory, and proprioceptive sense over half the body

Ipsilateral:
- Paralysis with atrophy (late) of half the tongue

Other:
- Primary-position upbeat nystagmus

***Arterial Territory Involved***

Occlusion of vertebral artery or branch of vertebral or lower basilar artery or anterior spinal artery

**Lateral Medullary Syndrome (Wallenberg Syndrome) (see Fig. 21.9)**

***Common Symptoms***

Ipsilateral facial pain and numbness
Vertigo, nausea, and vomiting
Ipsilateral clumsiness
Diplopia, oscillopsia
Contralateral numbness
Dysphagia, hoarseness

***Signs***

Contralateral:
- Impaired pain sensation over half the body, sometimes including the face

Ipsilateral:
- Impaired sensation over half the face
- Ataxia of limbs, falling to side of lesion (lateropulsion)
- Horner syndrome
- Dysphagia, hoarseness, paralysis of vocal cords
- Diminished gag reflex
- Loss of taste

Other:
- Nystagmus (torsional, horizontal, gaze-evoked horizontal, or downbeat on lateral gaze)
- Skew deviation
- Hiccup

***Arterial Territory Involved***

Occlusion of any of five vessels may be responsible: vertebral; posterior inferior cerebellar; or superior, middle, or inferior lateral medullary artery

and X. Torsional nystagmus often is present, and affected patients may have singultus (hiccups). The critical sign that distinguishes this from a lateral pontine syndrome is involvement of the nucleus ambiguous or its fasciculus and consequent weakness of the ipsilateral palate and vocal cord. It is increasingly found in the setting of vertebral artery dissection. (See Chapter 65 for a more detailed discussion of stroke.)

Eponymous name designations for all the cranial nerve syndromes are provided in Chapter 103.

*The complete reference list is available online at https://expertconsult.inkling.com/.*

22

# Neuro-Otology: Diagnosis and Management of Neuro-Otological Disorders

*Kevin A. Kerber, Robert W. Baloh*

## OUTLINE



*Dizziness* is a term patients use to describe a variety of symptoms including spinning or movement of the environment (vertigo), lightheadedness, presyncope, or imbalance. Patients may also use the term for other sensations such as visual distortion, internal spinning, nonspecific disorientation, and anxiety.

Patients may experience dizziness in isolation or with other symptoms. Neurological causes should be considered when other neurological signs and symptoms are present and also whenever specific peripheral vestibular or general medical disorders have not been identified. It is critical to ask the patient about associated symptoms, since they may be the key to diagnosis. *Vertigo*, a sensation of spinning of the environment, suggests a lesion within the vestibular pathways, either peripheral or central. Associated ear symptoms such as hearing loss and tinnitus can suggest a peripheral localization (i.e., inner ear, eighth nerve). Many different types of hearing loss occur with or without dizziness, and an understanding of common auditory disorders is important to the practicing neurologist. With an understanding of the neuro-otological bedside examination, specific findings can often be identified.

In this chapter, we provide background information regarding dizziness, vertigo, and hearing loss and the clinical information necessary for making specific diagnoses. We also include details on testing and management of these patients.

## HISTORICAL BACKGROUND

In 1861, Prosper Meniere was the first to recognize the association of vertigo with hearing loss and thus to localize the symptom to the inner ear (Baloh, 2001). Caloric testing, the most widely used test of the vestibulo-ocular reflex (VOR), was introduced by Robert Barany in 1906. He was later awarded the Nobel Prize for proposing the mechanism of caloric stimulation. Barany also provided the first clinical description of benign paroxysmal positional vertigo (BPPV) in 1921. Endolymphatic hydrops was identified in postmortem specimens of patients with Meniere disease in 1938. A method for measuring eye movements in response to caloric and rotational stimuli (electronystagmography [ENG]) was introduced in the 1930s, and in the 1970s digital computers began to be used to quantify eye movement responses.

Neuroimaging in the late 1970s and 1980s greatly expanded our understanding of causes of dizziness and vertigo. Prior to this time, stroke was considered an exceedingly rare cause of vertigo (Fisher, 1967). However, we now know that cerebellar and brainstem infarctions are identified in about 10%–15% of acute dizziness presentations that do not have obvious other central findings (Kerber, 2015). Imaging studies continue to lead to new discoveries of causes of vertigo, as demonstrated by the recently described disorder of superior canal dehiscence (SCD). But the most common causes of vertigo—Meniere disease, BPPV, and vestibular neuritis—still have no identifiable imaging characteristics.

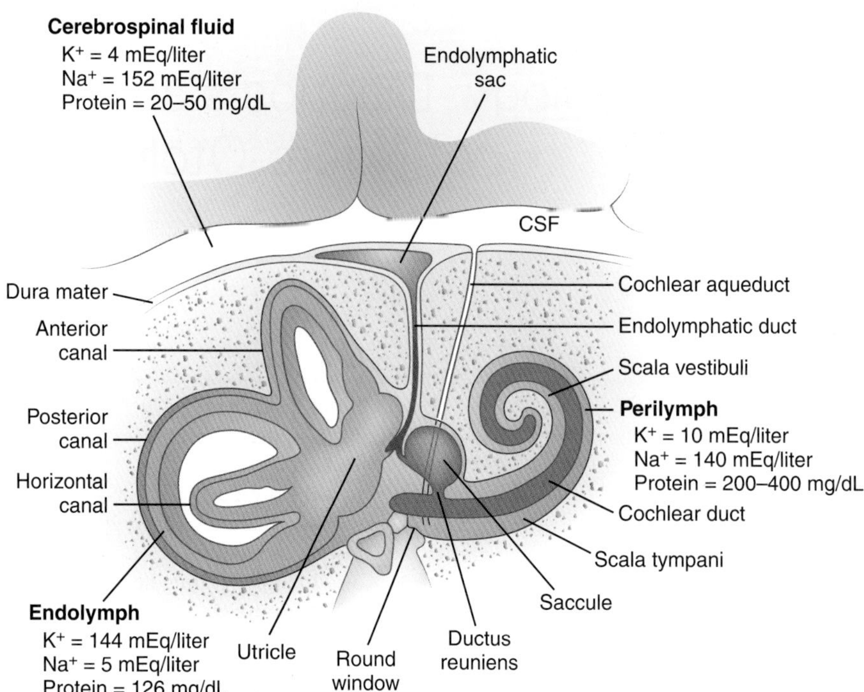


**Fig. 22.1** Anatomy of the Inner Ear. *CSF*, Cerebrospinal fluid. *(From Baloh, R.W., 1998. Dizziness, Hearing Loss, and Tinnitus. F.A. Davis Company, Philadelphia, Figure 6, p. 16.)*

Over the past 25 years, our understanding of the mechanisms for the common neuro-otological disorders has been greatly enhanced. BPPV can now be readily identified and cured at the bedside with a simple positional maneuver, and variants have also been described (Bhattacharyya, 2017). The head-thrust test can be used at the bedside to identify a vestibular nerve lesion, and because of this it has particular utility in helping distinguish vestibular neuritis from a posterior fossa stroke (Halmagyi and Curthoys, 1988; Kerber, 2015; Newman-Toker et al., 2008). Controversies regarding Meniere disease have been clarified, and medical and surgical treatments have improved (Minor et al., 2004). It is now clear that patients with recurrent episodes of vertigo without hearing loss, a condition once called *vestibular Meniere disease*, do not actually have Meniere disease.

Migraine is now recognized as an important cause of dizziness, even in patients without simultaneous headaches (Lempert, 2012). In fact, benign recurrent vertigo (BRV; patients with recurrent episodes of vertigo without accompanying auditory symptoms or other neurological features) is usually a migraine equivalent (Oh et al., 2001b). A more detailed description of the rotational vertebral artery syndrome has led to appreciation of the high metabolic demands of the inner ear and its susceptibility to ischemia (Choi et al., 2005). Genetic research has identified ion channel dysfunction in disorders such as episodic ataxia (EA) and familial hemiplegic migraine, and patients with these disorders also commonly report vertigo (Jen et al., 2004a). It is hoped that identifying specific genes causing vertigo syndromes will lead to a better understanding of the mechanisms and also create the opportunity to develop specific treatments in the future.

## EPIDEMIOLOGY OF VERTIGO, DIZZINESS, AND HEARING LOSS

Dizziness is a very common symptom. About 15%–20% of the adult US population reports problems with dizziness within a 12-month period (Kerber, 2017). Though most people report nonspecific types of dizziness, more than one-third report vertigo. Dizziness is more common among females and older people and has important healthcare utilization implications because up to 80% of patients with dizziness seek medical care at some point. In the United States, the National Centers for Health Statistics report 7.5 million annual ambulatory visits to physician offices, hospital outpatient departments, and emergency departments (EDs) for dizziness, making it one of the most common principal complaints (Burt and Schappert, 2004).

Hearing loss affects approximately 16% of adults (age >18 years) in the United States (Lethbridge-Cejku et al., 2006). Men are more commonly affected than women, and the prevalence of hearing loss increases dramatically with age, so that by age 75, nearly 50% of the population reports hearing loss, which is a common cause of disability. The most common type of hearing loss is sensorineural, and both idiopathic presbycusis and noise-induced forms are common etiologies. Bothersome tinnitus is less frequent in the US population, with about 3% reporting it, although this increases to about 9% for subjects older than 65 (Adams et al., 1999). The most common type of tinnitus is a high-pitched ringing in both ears.

## NORMAL ANATOMY AND PHYSIOLOGY

The inner ear is composed of a fluid-filled sac enclosed by a bony capsule with an anterior cochlear part, central chamber (vestibule), and a posterior vestibular part (Fig. 22.1). Endolymph fills up the fluid-filled sac and is separated by a membrane from the perilymph. These fluids primarily differ in their composition of potassium and sodium, with the endolymph resembling intracellular fluid with a high potassium and low sodium content, and perilymph resembling extracellular fluids with a low potassium and high sodium content. Perilymph communicates with the cerebrospinal fluid (CSF) through the cochlear aqueduct.

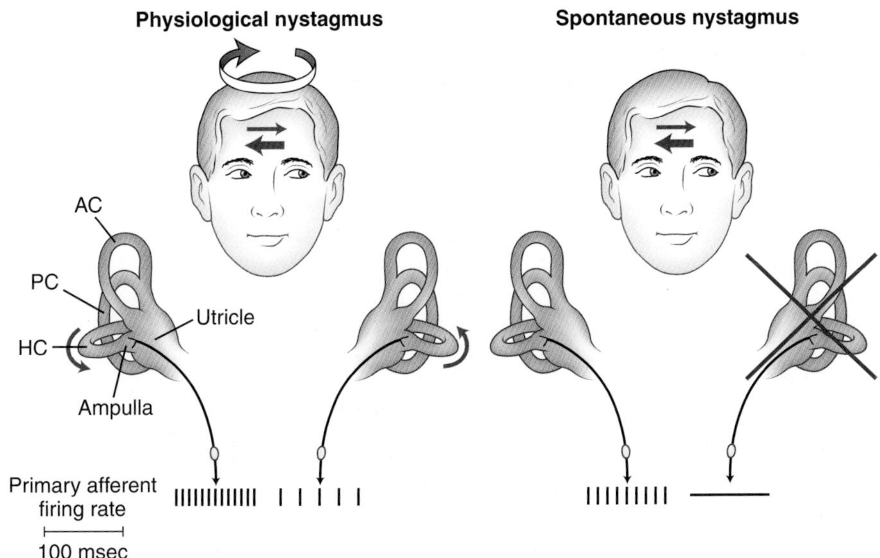


**Fig. 22.2** Primary afferent nerve activity associated with rotation-induced physiological nystagmus and spontaneous nystagmus resulting from a lesion of one labyrinth. *Thin straight arrows* indicate the direction of slow components; *thick straight arrows* indicate the direction of fast components; *curved arrows* show the direction of endolymph flow in the horizontal semicircular canals. *AC,* Anterior canal; *HC,* horizontal canal; *PC,* posterior canal. *(From Baloh, R.W., 1998. Dizziness, Hearing Loss, and Tinnitus. F.A. Davis Company, Philadelphia, Figure 16, p. 36.)*

The cochlea senses sound waves after they travel through the external auditory canal and are amplified by the tympanic membrane and ossicles of the middle ear (Baloh and Kerber, 2011). The stapes, the last of three ossicles in the middle ear, contacts the oval window, which directs the forces associated with sound waves along the basilar membrane of the cochlea. These forces stimulate the hair cells, which in turn generate neural signals in the auditory nerve. The auditory nerve enters the lateral brainstem at the pontomedullary junction and synapses in the cochlear nucleus. The trapezoid body is the major decussation of the auditory pathway, but many fibers do not cross to the contralateral side. Signals then travel to the superior olivary complex. Some projections travel from the superior olivary complex to the inferior colliculus through the lateral lemnisci, and others terminate in one of the nuclei of the lateral lemniscus. Next, fibers travel to the ipsilateral medial geniculate body, and then auditory radiations pass through the posterior limb of the internal capsule to reach the auditory cortex of the temporal lobe.

The peripheral vestibular system is composed of three semicircular canals, the utricle and saccule, and the vestibular component of the eighth cranial nerve (Baloh and Kerber, 2011). Each semicircular canal has a sensory epithelium called the *crista*; the sensory epithelium of the utricle and saccule is called the *macule*. The semicircular canals sense angular movements, and the utricle and saccule sense linear movements. Two of the semicircular canals (anterior and posterior) are oriented in the vertical plane nearly orthogonal to each other; the third canal is oriented in the horizontal plane (horizontal canal). The crista of each canal is activated by movement occurring in the plane of that canal. When the hair cells of these organs are stimulated, the signal is transferred to the vestibular nuclei via the vestibular portion of cranial nerve VIII. Signals originating from the horizontal semicircular canal then pass via the medial longitudinal fasciculus along the floor of the fourth ventricle to the abducens nuclei in the middle brainstem and the ocular motor complex in the rostral brainstem. The anterior (also referred to as the *superior*) and posterior canal impulses pass from the vestibular nuclei to the ocular motor nucleus and trochlear nucleus, triggering eye movements roughly in the plane of each canal. A key feature is that once vestibular signals leave the vestibular nuclei they divide into vertical, horizontal, and torsional components. As a result, a lesion of central vestibular pathways can cause a pure vertical, pure torsional, or pure horizontal nystagmus.

The primary vestibular afferent nerve fibers maintain a constant baseline firing rate of action potentials (APs). When the baseline rate from each ear is symmetrical (or an asymmetry has been centrally compensated), the eyes remain stationary. With an uncompensated asymmetry in the firing rate, resulting from either increased or decreased activity on one side, slow ocular deviation results. By turning the head to the right, the baseline firing rate of the horizontal canal is physiologically altered, causing an increased firing rate on the right side and a decreased firing rate on the left side (Fig. 22.2). The result is a slow deviation of the eyes to the left. In an alert subject, this slow deviation is regularly interrupted by quick movements in the opposite direction (nystagmus), so the eyes do not become pinned to one side. In a comatose patient, only the slow component is seen because the brain cannot generate the corrective fast components ("doll's eyes").

The plane in which the eyes deviate as a result of vestibular stimulation depends on the combination of canals that are stimulated (Table 22.1). If only the posterior semicircular canal on one side is stimulated (as occurs with BPPV), a vertical-torsional deviation of the eyes can be observed, which is followed by a fast corrective response generated by the conscious brain in the opposite direction. However, if the horizontal canal is the source of stimulation (as occurs with the horizontal canal variant of BPPV [HC-BPPV]), a horizontal deviation with a slight torsional component (because this canal is slightly off the horizontal plane) results. If the vestibular nerve is lesioned (vestibular neuritis) or stimulated (vestibular paroxysmia), a horizontal greater than torsional nystagmus is seen that is the vector sum of all three canals—the two vertical canals on one side cancel each other out.

Over time, either an asymmetry in the baseline firing rates resolves (the stimulation has been removed) or the central nervous system (CNS) compensates for it. This explains why an entire unilateral peripheral vestibular system can be surgically destroyed and patients only experience vertigo for several days to weeks. It also explains why patients with slow-growing tumors affecting the vestibular nerve, such as an acoustic neuroma, generally do not experience vertigo or nystagmus.

**TABLE 22.1 Physiological Properties and Clinical Features of the Components of the Peripheral Vestibular System**

| Localization | Component(s) | Triggered Eye Movements | Common Clinical Conditions | Localizing Features |
|---|---|---|---|---|
| **Semicircular Canals** | | | | |
| Posterior canal | PC | Vertical, torsional | BPPV-PC | Nystagmus |
| Anterior canal | AC | Vertical, torsional | BPPV-AC, SCD | Nystagmus, fistula test |
| Horizontal canal | HC | Horizontal ≫ torsional | BPPV-HC, fistula | Nystagmus |
| **Vestibular Nerve** | | | | |
| Superior division | AC, HC, utricle | Horizontal > torsional | VN, ischemia | Nystagmus, head-thrust test |
| Inferior division | PC, saccule | Vertical, torsional | VN, ischemia | Nystagmus |
| Common trunk (cranial nerve 8) | AC, HC, PC, utricle, saccule | Horizontal > torsional | VN, VP, ischemia | Nystagmus, head-thrust test, auditory findings |
| Labyrinth | AC, HC, PC, utricle, saccule | Horizontal > torsional | EH, labyrinthitis | Nystagmus, auditory findings |

*AC*, Anterior canal; *BPPV*, benign paroxysmal positional vertigo; *EH*, endolymphatic hydrops; *HC*, horizontal canal; *PC*, posterior canal; *SCD*, superior canal dehiscence; *VN*, vestibular neuritis; *VP*, vestibular paroxysmia.

## HISTORY OF PRESENT ILLNESS

The history and physical examination provide the most important information when evaluating patients complaining of dizziness (Colledge et al., 1996; Lawson et al., 1999). Often, patients have difficulty describing the exact symptom experienced (Kerber, 2017), so the onus is on the clinician to elicit pertinent information. The first step is to define the symptom. No clinician should ever be satisfied to record the complaint simply as "dizziness." For patients unable to provide a more detailed description of the symptom, the physician can ask the patient to place their symptom into one of the following categories: movement of the environment (vertigo), lightheadedness, or strictly imbalance without an abnormal head sensation. However, caution must be taken in placing too much emphasis on the type of dizziness because patient descriptions about dizziness can be unreliable, inconsistent, and overlap (Newman-Toker et al., 2007; Kerber, 2017). Most dizziness patients report more than one type of dizziness, and specific types of dizziness symptoms have a stronger correlation with each other than they do with disease-based constructs (Kerber, 2017). Therefore other details about the symptom (e.g., timing, triggers) need to be considered as well. Table 22.2 displays the key distinguishing features of common causes of dizziness. One key point is that any type of dizziness may worsen with position changes, but some disorders such as BPPV only occur after position change.

## PHYSICAL EXAMINATION

### General Medical Examination

A brief general medical examination is important. Identifying orthostatic drops in blood pressure can be diagnostic in the correct clinical setting. Orthostatic hypotension is probably the most common general medical cause of dizziness among patients referred to neurologists. Identifying an irregular heart rhythm may also be pertinent. Other general examination measures to consider in individual patients include a visual assessment (adequate vision is important for balance) and a musculoskeletal inspection (significant arthritis can impair gait).

### General Neurological Examination

The general neurological examination is very important in patients complaining of dizziness, because dizziness can be the earliest symptom of a neurodegenerative disorder (de Lau et al., 2006) and can also be an important symptom of stroke, tumor, demyelination, or other pathologies of the nervous system. One should ensure that the patient has full ocular ductions. A posterior fossa mass can impair facial sensation and the corneal reflex on one side. Assessing facial strength and symmetry is important because of the close anatomical relationship between the seventh and eighth cranial nerves. The lower cranial nerves should also be closely inspected by observing palatal elevation, tongue protrusion, and trapezius and sternocleidomastoid strength.

The general motor examination determines strength in each muscle group and also assesses bulk and tone. Increased tone or cogwheel rigidity could be the main finding in a patient with an early neurodegenerative disorder. The peripheral sensory examination is important because a peripheral neuropathy can cause a nonspecific dizziness or imbalance. Temperature, pain, vibration, and proprioception should be assessed. Reflexes should be tested for their presence and symmetry. One must take into consideration the normal decrease in vibratory sensation and absence of ankle jerks that can occur in elderly patients. Coordination is an important part of the neurological examination in patients with dizziness because disorders characterized by ataxia can present with the principal symptom of dizziness. Observing the patient's ability to perform the finger-nose-finger test, the heel-knee-shin test, and rapid alternating movements adequately assesses extremity coordination (Schmitz-Hubsch et al., 2006).

### Neuro-Otological Examination

When the general neurological examination is not revealing, the neuro-otological exam can be the critical element. The neuro-otological examination is a specialty examination expanding upon certain aspects of the general neurological examination and also includes an audio-vestibular assessment.

#### Ocular Motor

The first step in assessing ocular motor function is to search for spontaneous involuntary movements of the eyes. The examiner asks the patient to look straight ahead while observing for nystagmus or saccadic intrusions. Nystagmus is characterized by a slow- and fast-phase component and is classified as spontaneous, gaze-evoked, or positional. The direction of nystagmus is conventionally described by the direction of the fast phase, which is the direction it appears to be "beating" toward. Recording whether the nystagmus is vertical, horizontal, torsional, or a mixture of these provides important localizing information. Spontaneous nystagmus can have either a peripheral or central pattern. Although central lesions can mimic a "peripheral" pattern of nystagmus (Lee and Cho, 2004; Newman-Toker et al., 2008), unusual circumstances are required for peripheral

**TABLE 22.2 Distinguishing Among Common Peripheral and Central Vertigo Syndromes**

| Cause | History of Vertigo | Duration of Vertigo | Associated Symptoms | Physical Examination |
|---|---|---|---|---|
| **Peripheral** | | | | |
| Vestibular neuritis | Single prolonged episode | Days to weeks | Nausea, imbalance | "Peripheral" nystagmus, positive head-thrust test, imbalance |
| BPPV | Positionally triggered episodes | <1 min | Nausea | Characteristic positionally triggered burst of nystagmus |
| Meniere disease | May be triggered by salty foods | Hours | Unilateral ear fullness, tinnitus, hearing loss, nausea | Unilateral low-frequency hearing loss |
| Vestibular paroxysmia | Abrupt onset; spontaneous or positionally triggered | Seconds | Tinnitus, hearing loss | Usually normal |
| Perilymph fistula | Triggered by sound or pressure changes | Seconds | Hearing loss, hyperacusis | Nystagmus triggered by loud sounds or pressure changes |
| **Central** | | | | |
| Stroke/TIA | Abrupt onset; spontaneous | Stroke, >24 h; TIA, < 24 h | Brainstem, cerebellar | Spontaneous "central" nystagmus; gaze-evoked nystagmus; focal neurological signs; negative head-thrust test; skew deviation |
| MS | Subacute onset | Minutes to weeks | Unilateral visual loss, diplopia, incoordination, ataxia | "Central" types or rarely "peripheral" types of spontaneous or positional nystagmus; usually other focal neurological signs |
| Neurodegenerative disorders | May be spontaneous or positionally triggered | Minutes to hours | Ataxia | "Central" types of spontaneous or positional nystagmus; gaze-evoked nystagmus; impaired smooth pursuit; cerebellar, extrapyramidal and frontal signs |
| Migraine | Onset usually associated with typical migraine triggers | Seconds to days | Headache, visual aura, photo-/phonophobia | Normal interictal examination; ictal examination may show "peripheral" or "central" types of spontaneous or positional nystagmus |
| Familial ataxia syndromes | Acute-subacute onset; usually triggered by stress, exercise, or excitement | Hours | Ataxia | "Central" types of spontaneous or positional nystagmus Ictal, or even interictal, gaze-evoked nystagmus; ataxia; gait disorders |

*BPPV*, Benign paroxysmal positional vertigo; *MS*, multiple sclerosis; *TIA*, transient ischemic attack.

lesions to cause "central" patterns of nystagmus. The peripheral pattern of spontaneous nystagmus is unidirectional: that is, the eyes beat only to one side (Video 22.1). Peripheral spontaneous nystagmus never changes direction. It is usually a horizontal greater than torsional pattern because of the physiology of the asymmetry in firing rates within the peripheral vestibular system whereby the vertical canals cancel each other out. The prominent horizontal component results from the unopposed horizontal canal asymmetry. Other characteristics of peripheral spontaneous nystagmus are suppression with visual fixation, increase in velocity with gaze in the direction of the fast phase, and decrease with gaze in the direction opposite of the fast phase. Some patients are able to suppress this nystagmus so well at the bedside, or have partially recovered from the initiating event, that spontaneous nystagmus may only appear by removing visual fixation. Several simple bedside techniques can be used to remove the patient's ability to fixate. Frenzel glasses are designed to remove visual fixation by using +30 diopter lenses. An ophthalmoscope can be used to block fixation. While the fundus of one eye is being viewed, the patient is asked to cover the other eye. Probably the simplest technique involves holding a blank sheet of paper close to the patient's face (so as to block visual fixation) and observing for spontaneous nystagmus from the side.

*Saccadic intrusions* are spontaneous, involuntary saccadic movements of the eyes, without the rhythmic fast and slow phases characteristic of nystagmus. *Saccades* are fast movements of the eyes normally under voluntary control and used to shift gaze from one object to another. Square-wave jerks and saccadic oscillations are the most common types of saccadic intrusions. *Square-wave jerks* refer to small-amplitude, involuntary saccades that take the eyes off a target, followed after a normal intersaccadic delay (around 200 msec) by a corrective saccade to bring the eyes back to the target. Square-wave jerks can be seen in neurological disorders such as cerebellar ataxia, Huntington disease (HD), or progressive supranuclear palsy (PSP), but they also occur in normal individuals. If the square-wave jerks are persistent or of large amplitude (macro-square wave jerks), pathology is more likely.

*Saccadic oscillations* refer to back-to-back saccadic movements without the intersaccadic interval characteristic of square-wave jerks, so their appearance is that of an oscillation. When a burst occurs only in the horizontal plane, the term *ocular flutter* is used (Video 22.2). When vertical and/or torsional components are present, the term *opsoclonus* (or so-called dancing eyes) is used. The eyes make constant random conjugate saccades of unequal amplitude in all directions. Ocular flutter and opsoclonus are pathological findings typically seen in several different types of CNS diseases involving brainstem–cerebellar pathways. Paraneoplastic disorders should be considered in patients presenting with ocular flutter or opsoclonus.

### Gaze Testing

The patient should be asked to look to the left, right, up, and down; the examiner looks for gaze-evoked nystagmus in each position (Video 22.3). A few beats of unsustained nystagmus with gaze greater than 30 degrees is called *end-gaze nystagmus* and variably occurs in normal subjects. Gaze-evoked downbeating nystagmus (Video 22.4), vertical nystagmus that increases on lateral gaze, localizes to the craniocervical junction and midline cerebellum. Gaze testing may also trigger saccadic oscillations (see Videos 22.3 and 22.4).

### Smooth Pursuit

*Smooth pursuit* refers to the voluntary movement of the eyes used to track a target moving at a low velocity. It functions to keep the moving object on the fovea to maximize vision. Though characteristically a very smooth movement at low frequency and velocity testing, smooth pursuit inevitably breaks down when tested at high frequencies and velocities. Though smooth pursuit often becomes impaired with advanced age, a longitudinal study of healthy elderly individuals found no significant decline in smooth pursuit over 9 years of evaluation (Kerber et al., 2006). Patients with impaired smooth pursuit require frequent small saccades to keep up with the target; thus the term *saccadic pursuit* is used to describe this finding. Abnormalities of smooth pursuit occur as the result of disorders throughout the CNS and with tranquilizing medicines, alcohol, inadequate concentration or vision, and fatigue. However, in a cognitively intact individual presenting with dizziness or imbalance symptoms, bilaterally impaired smooth pursuit is highly localizing to the cerebellum. Patients with early or mild cerebellar degenerative disorders may have markedly impaired smooth pursuit with mild or minimal truncal ataxia as the only findings.

### Saccades

Saccades are fast eye movements (velocity of this eye movement can be as high as 600 degrees per second) used to quickly bring an object onto the fovea. Saccades are generated by the burst neurons of the pons (horizontal movements) and midbrain (vertical movements). Lesions or degeneration of these regions leads to slowing of saccades, which can also occur with lesions of the ocular motor neurons or extraocular muscles. Severe slowing can be readily appreciated at the bedside by instructing the patient to look back and forth from one object to another. The examiner observes both the velocity of the saccade and the accuracy. Overshooting saccades (missing the target and then needing to correct) indicates a lesion of the cerebellum (Video 22.5). Undershooting saccades are less specific and often occur in normal subjects.

### Optokinetic Nystagmus and Fixation Suppression of the Vestibulo-Ocular Reflex

Optokinetic nystagmus (OKN) and fixation suppression of the VOR suppression can also be tested at the bedside. OKN is a combination of fast (saccadic) and slow (smooth pursuit) movements of eyes and can be observed in normal individuals when, for example, watching a moving train. OKN is maximally stimulated with both foveal and parafoveal stimulation, so the proper laboratory technique for measuring OKN uses a full-field stimulus by having the patient sit stationary while a large rotating pattern moves around them. This test can be approximated at the bedside by moving a striped cloth in front of the patient, though this technique only stimulates the fovea. Patients with disorders causing severe slowing of saccades will not be able to generate OKN, so their eyes will become pinned to one side. VOR suppression can be tested at the bedside using a swivel chair. The patient sits in the chair and extends his or her arm in the "thumbs-up" position out in front. The patient is instructed to focus on the thumb and to allow the extended arm to move with the body so the visual target of the thumb remains directly in front of the patient. The chair is then rotated from side to side. The patient's eyes should remain locked on the thumb, demonstrating the ability to suppress the VOR stimulated by rotation of the chair. Nystagmus will be observed during the rotation movements in patients with impairment of VOR suppression, which is analogous to impairment of smooth pursuit. Both OKN and VOR suppression can also be helpful when examining patients having difficulty following the instructions for smooth pursuit or saccade testing.

### Vestibular Nerve Examination

Often omitted as part of the cranial nerve examination in general neurology texts, important localizing information can be obtained about the functioning of the vestibular nerve at the bedside. A unilateral or bilateral vestibulopathy can be identified using the *head-thrust test* (Halmagyi et al., 2008) (Fig. 22.3 and Video 22.6). To perform the head-thrust test, the physician stands directly in front of the patient, who is seated on the examination table. The patient's head is held in the examiner's hands, and the patient is instructed to focus on the examiner's nose. The head is then quickly moved about 5–10 degrees to one side. In patients with normal vestibular function, the VOR results in movement of the eyes in the direction opposite the head movement. Therefore the patient's eyes remain on the examiner's nose after the sudden movement. The test is repeated in the opposite direction. If the examiner observes a corrective saccade bringing the patient's eyes back to the examiner's nose after the head thrust, impairment of the VOR in the direction of the head movement is identified. Rotating the head slowly back and forth (the doll's eye test) also induces compensatory eye movements, but both the visual and vestibular systems are activated by this low-velocity test, so a patient with complete vestibular function loss and normal visual pursuit will have normal-appearing compensatory eye movements on the doll's eye test. This slow rotation of the head, however, is helpful in a comatose patient who is not able to generate voluntary visual tracking eye movements. Slowly rotating the head can also be a helpful test in patients with impairment of the smooth-pursuit system, because smooth movements of the eyes during slow rotation of the head indicates an intact VOR, whereas continued saccadic movements during slow rotation indicates an accompanying deficit of the VOR (Migliaccio et al., 2004).

### Positional Testing

Positional testing can help identify peripheral or central causes of vertigo. The most common positional vertigo, BPPV, is caused by free-floating calcium carbonate debris, usually in the posterior semicircular canal, occasionally in the horizontal canal, or rarely in the anterior canal. The characteristic burst of upbeat torsional nystagmus is triggered in patients with BPPV by a rapid change from the sitting-up position to supine head-hanging left or head-hanging right (the Dix–Hallpike test; Video 22.7). When present, the nystagmus is usually only triggered in one of these positions. A burst of nystagmus in the opposite direction (downbeat torsional) occurs when the patient resumes the sitting position since the debris moves in the opposite direction. A repositioning maneuver can be used to move the debris out of the canal. The modified Epley maneuver (Fig. 22.4 and Video 22.8) is more than 80% effective in treating patients with posterior canal BPPV, compared with 10% effectiveness of a sham procedure (Hilton, 2014). The key feature of this maneuver is the roll across in the plane of the posterior canal so that the debris rotates around the posterior canal and out into the utricle. Once the debris enters the utricle, it no longer disrupts semicircular canal function. Recurrences are common, however (see Videos 22.7 and 22.8).

If the debris is in the horizontal canal, direction-changing horizontal nystagmus is seen. Patients are tested for HC-BPPV by turning the head to each side while lying in the supine position. The nystagmus can be either paroxysmal geotropic (beating toward the ground) or persistent apogeotropic nystagmus (beating away from the ground). In the case of geotropic nystagmus, the debris is in the posterior segment (or "long arm") of the horizontal canal, whereas the debris is in

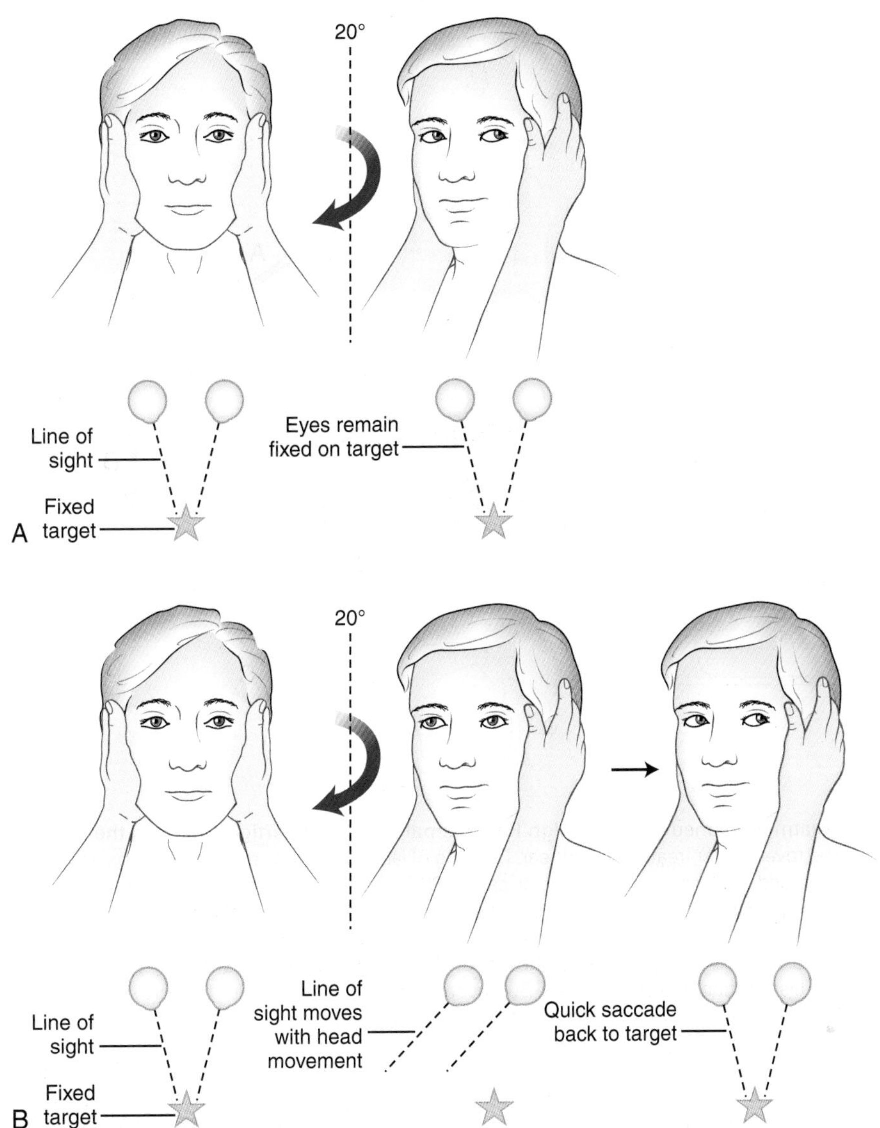


**Fig. 22.3 Head-Thrust Test.** The head-thrust test is a test of vestibular function that can be easily done during the bedside examination. This maneuver tests the vestibulo-ocular reflex (VOR). The patient sits in front of the examiner and the examiner holds the patient's head steady in the midline. The patient is instructed to maintain gaze on the nose of the examiner. The examiner then quickly turns the patient's head about 10–15 degrees to one side and observes the ability of the patient to keep the eyes locked on the examiner's nose. If the patient's eyes stay locked on the examiner's nose (i.e., no corrective saccade) **(A)**, then the peripheral vestibular system is assumed to be intact. If, however, the patient's eyes move with the head **(B)** and then the patient makes a voluntary eye movement back to the examiner's nose (i.e., corrective saccade), then this indicates a lesion of the peripheral vestibular system and not the central nervous system (CNS). Thus, when a patient presents with the acute vestibular syndrome, the test result shown in A would suggest a CNS lesion (because the VOR is intact), whereas the test result in B suggests a peripheral vestibular lesion on the right side (because the VOR is not intact). *(From Edlow, J.A., Newman-Toker, D.E., Savitz, S.I., 2008. Diagnosis and initial management of cerebellar infarction. Lancet Neurology 7, 951–964.)*

the anterior segment (or "short arm") when apogeotropic nystagmus is triggered. When geotropic nystagmus is triggered, the side with the stronger nystagmus is the involved side. However, when apogeotropic nystagmus is observed, the involved side is generally opposite the side of the stronger nystagmus. With the geotropic variant, class I evidence supports treatment with the barbecue maneuver or the Gufoni maneuver (Kim et al., 2012a). Another maneuver for HC-BPPV is the "forced prolonged position" (Vannucchi et al., 1997). In cases of the apogeotropic variant of HC-BPPV, a variation of the Gufoni maneuver or a head-shaking maneuver can effectively treat the condition, though patients may require a second maneuver to clear the debris from the long arm of the horizontal canal (the same maneuver to treat geotropic HC-BPPV; Kim et al., 2012b).

Positional testing can also trigger central types of nystagmus (usually persistent downbeating), which may be the most prominent examination finding in patients with disorders like Chiari malformation or cerebellar ataxia (Kattah and Gujrati, 2005; Kerber et al., 2005a). Central positional nystagmus can also mimic the nystagmus of HC-BPPV. Positional nystagmus may also be prominent in patients with migraine-associated dizziness (von Brevern et al., 2005).

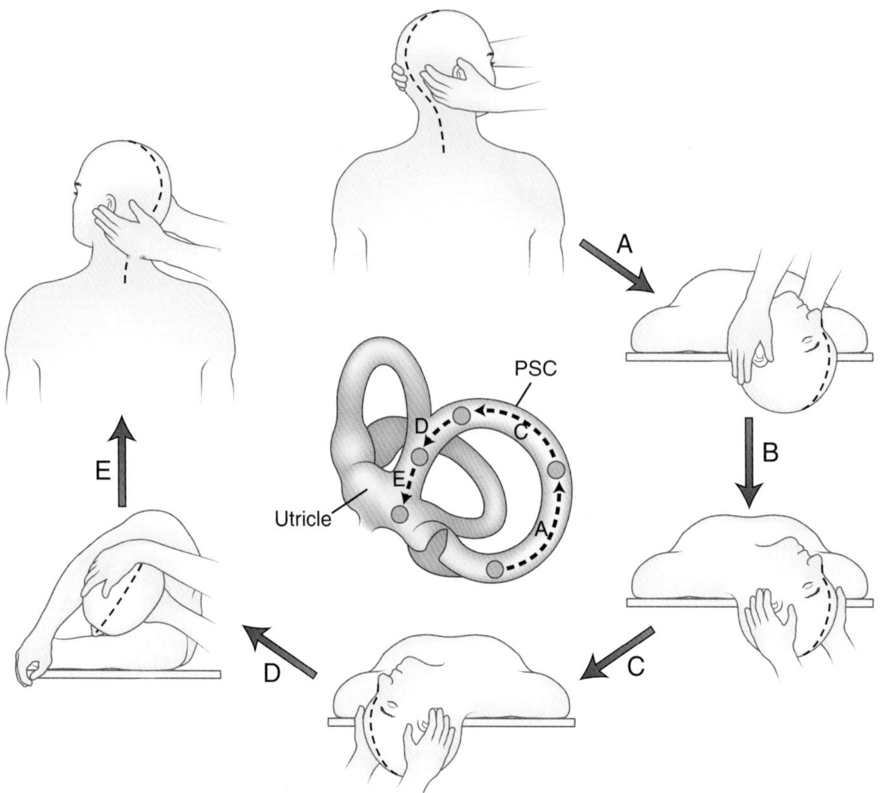


**Fig. 22.4 Treatment Maneuver For Benign Paroxysmal Positional Vertigo Affecting the Right Ear.** Procedure can be reversed for treating the left ear. Drawing of labyrinth in the center shows position of the debris as it moves around the posterior semicircular canal *(PSC)* and into the utricle. **A,** Patient is seated upright with head facing examiner, who is standing on the right. **B,** Patient is then rapidly moved to head-hanging right position (Dix–Hallpike test). This position is maintained until nystagmus ceases. Examiner moves to the head of the table, repositioning hands as shown. **C,** Patient's head is rotated quickly to the left, with right ear upward. This position is maintained for 30 seconds. **D,** Patient rolls onto the left side while examiner rapidly rotates the head leftward until the nose is directed toward the floor. This position is then held for 30 seconds. **E,** Patient is then rapidly lifted into the sitting position, now facing left. The entire sequence should be repeated until no nystagmus can be elicited. Following the maneuver, the patient is instructed to avoid head-hanging positions to prevent the debris from re-entering the posterior canal. *(From Baloh, R.W., 1998. Dizziness, Hearing Loss, and Tinnitus. F.A. Davis Company, Philadelphia, Figure 69, p. 166.)*

## Fistula Testing

In patients reporting sound- or pressure-induced dizziness, a defect of the bony capsule of the labyrinth can be tested for by pressing and releasing the tragus (small flap of cartilage that can be used to occlude the external ear canal) and observing the eyes for brief associated deviations. Pneumatoscopy (introducing air into the external auditory canal through an otoscope) or Valsalva against pitched nostrils or closed glottis can also trigger associated eye movements. The direction of the triggered nystagmus helps identify the location of the fistula.

## Gait

Casual gait is examined for initiation, heel strike, stride length, and base width. Patients are then observed during tandem walking and while standing in the Romberg position (with eyes open and closed). A decreased heel strike, stride length, flexed posture, and decreased arm swing suggest Parkinson disease. A wide-based gait with inability to tandem walk is characteristic of truncal ataxia. Patients with acute vestibular loss will veer toward the side of the affected ear for several days after the event. Patients with peripheral neuropathy or bilateral vestibulopathy may be unable to stand in the Romberg position with eyes closed.

## Auditory Examination

The bedside examination of the auditory system begins with otoscopy. The tympanic membrane is normally translucent; changes in color indicate middle ear disease or tympanosclerosis, a semicircular crescent or horseshoe-shaped white plaque within the tympanic membrane. Tympanosclerosis is rarely associated with hearing loss but is an important clue to past infections. The area just superior to the lateral process of the malleus should be carefully inspected for evidence of a retraction pocket or cholesteatoma. Findings on otoscopy are usually not associated with causes of dizziness because the visualized abnormalities typically do not involve the inner ear.

Finger rubs at different intensities and distances from the ear are a rapid, reliable, and valid screening test for hearing loss in the frequency range of speech (Torres-Russotto et al., 2009). If a patient can hear a faint finger rub stimulus at a distance of 70 cm (approximately one arm's length) from one ear, then a hearing loss on that side—defined by a gold-standard audiogram threshold of greater than 25 dB at 1000, 2000, and 4000 Hz—is highly unlikely. On the other hand, if a patient cannot hear a strong finger rub stimulus at 70 cm, hearing loss on that side is highly likely. The whisper test can also be used to assess hearing at the bedside (Bagai et al., 2006). For this test, the examiner stands behind the patient to prevent lip reading and occludes and masks the nontest ear, using a finger to rub and close the external auditory canal. The examiner then whispers a set of three to six random numbers and letters. Overall, the patient is considered to have passed the screening test if they repeat at least 50% of the letters and numbers correctly. The Weber and Rinne tests are commonly used bedside tuning fork tests. To perform these, a tuning fork (256 Hz or 512 Hz) is gently struck on a hard rubber pad, the elbow, or the knee about two-thirds of the way along the tine. To conduct the Weber test, the base of the vibrating fork is placed on the vertex (top or crown of the head), bridge of the nose, upper incisors, or forehead. The patient is asked if the sound is heard and whether it is heard in the middle of the head or in both ears equally, toward the left, or toward the right. In a patient with normal hearing, the tone is heard centrally. In asymmetrical or a unilateral hearing impairment, the tone lateralizes to one side. Lateralization indicates an element of conductive impairment in the ear in which the sound localizes, a sensorineural impairment in the contralateral ear, or both. The Rinne test compares the patient's hearing by air conduction with that by bone conduction. The fork is first held against the mastoid process until the sound fades. It is then placed 1 inch from the ear. Normal subjects can hear the fork about twice as long by air as by bone conduction. If bone is greater than air conduction, a conductive hearing loss is suggested.

## SPECIFIC DISORDERS CAUSING VERTIGO

### Peripheral Vestibular Disorders

Peripheral vestibular disorders are important for neurologists to understand because they are common, readily identified at the bedside, and often missed by frontline physicians (see Table 22.2).

#### Acute Unilateral Vestibulopathy (Vestibular Neuritis)

A common presentation to the ED or outpatient clinic is the rapid onset of severe vertigo, nausea, vomiting, and imbalance. The symptoms gradually resolve over days to weeks, but about 20% of patients report some dizziness even 12 months later (Shupak, 2008). The typical etiology of this disorder is vestibular neuritis, which is presumed to be viral because the course is generally benign and self-limited, similar to Bell palsy. Small histopathological studies support the etiology of a viral cause. However, ischemia or demyelination can also cause an acute unilateral vestibulopathy. The key to identifying an acute unilateral vestibulopathy is recognizing the peripheral vestibular pattern of nystagmus and identifying a positive head-thrust test in the setting of a rapid onset of vertigo without other neurological symptoms. The course of vestibular neuritis is self-limited, and the mainstay of treatment is symptomatic. A course of corticosteroids might improve recovery of the caloric response but symptomatic and functional outcomes were not clinically different (Fishman et al., 2011). Vestibular physical therapy—delivered with in person sessions or even home training—can help patients compensate for the vestibular lesion (Hillier et al., 2011).

#### Benign Paroxysmal Positional Vertigo

BPPV has a lifetime cumulative incidence of nearly 10% (von Brevern, 2005). Patients typically experience brief episodes of vertigo when getting in and out of bed, turning in bed, bending down and straightening up, or extending the head back to look up. As noted earlier, the condition is caused when calcium carbonate debris dislodged from the otoconial membrane inadvertently enters a semicircular canal. The debris can be free-floating within the affected canal (canalithiasis) or stuck against the cupula (cupulolithiasis). Though the positional attacks are the hallmark feature, some BPPV patients also report constant mild unsteadiness (Von Brevern, 2015). The gold standard test is the Dix-Hallpike test with the positive finding being the hallmark triggered and transient upbeat-torsional nystagmus. Repositioning maneuvers are highly effective in removing the debris from the canal, though recurrence is common (see Fig. 22.4; Fife et al., 2008). Once the debris is out of the canal, patients are instructed to avoid extreme head positions to prevent the debris from re-entering the canal. Patients can also be taught to perform a repositioning maneuver, should they have a recurrence of the positional vertigo.

#### Meniere Disease

Meniere disease is characterized by recurrent attacks of vertigo associated with auditory symptoms (hearing loss, tinnitus, aural fullness) during attacks. Over time, progressive hearing loss develops. Attacks are variable in duration, most lasting longer than 20 minutes, and are associated with severe nausea and vomiting. The course of the disorder is also highly variable. For some patients, the attacks are infrequent and decrease over time, but for others they can become debilitating. Occasionally, auditory symptoms are not appreciated by the patients or identified by interictal audiograms early in the disorder, but inevitably patients with Meniere disease develop these features, usually within the first year. Thus the term *vestibular Meniere disease*, previously used for patients with recurrent episodes of vertigo but no hearing loss, is no longer used. Though usually a disorder involving only one ear, Meniere disease becomes bilateral in about one-third of patients.

Endolymphatic hydrops, or expansion of the endolymph relative to the perilymph, is regarded as the etiology, though the underlying cause is unclear. In addition, the characteristic histopathological changes of endolymphatic hydrops have been identified in temporal bone specimens of patients with no clinical history of Meniere disease (Merchant et al., 2005). Some patients with well-documented Meniere disease experience abrupt episodes of falling to the ground, without loss of consciousness or associated neurological symptoms. Patients often report the sensation of being pushed or thrown to the ground. The falls are hard and often result in fractures or other injuries. These episodes have been called *otolithic catastrophes of Tumarkin* because of the suspicion that they represent acute stimulation of the otoliths. The bedside interictal examination of patients with Meniere disease may identify asymmetrical hearing, but the head-thrust test is usually normal. Treatment is initially directed toward an aggressive low-salt diet and diuretics, though the evidence for these treatments is poor. Intratympanic gentamicin injections can be effective and are minimally invasive. Sectioning of the vestibular nerve and destruction of the labyrinth are other procedures (Minor et al., 2004). Autoimmune inner-ear disease presents as a fulminate variant of Meniere disease. Another variant is so-called delayed endolymphatic hydrops. Patients with this disorder report recurrent episodes of severe vertigo without auditory symptoms developing years after a severe unilateral hearing loss caused by a viral or bacterial infection.

#### Vestibular Paroxysmia

Vestibular paroxysmia is characterized by brief (seconds to minutes) episodes of vertigo, occurring suddenly without any apparent trigger (Strupp, 2016). The disorder may be analogous to hemifacial spasm and trigeminal neuralgia, which are felt to be due to spontaneous discharges from a partially damaged nerve. In patients with vestibular paroxysmia, unilateral dysfunction can sometimes be identified on vestibular or auditory testing. Like the analogous disorders, it is conceivable that a normal vessel could be compressing the cranial nerve, and surgical removal of the vessel might seem to be a treatment option. However, many asymptomatic subjects have a normal vessel lying on the eighth nerve (usually the anterior inferior cerebellar artery), and most vestibular paroxysmia patients have a favorable course with conservative or medication management (Strupp, 2016), so the decision to operate in this delicate region is rarely indicated. Medications associated with a reduction in episodes include carbamazepine, oxcarbazepine, and gabapentin (Strupp, 2016).

### Vestibular Fistulae

*Superior canal dehiscence* was first described in 1998 (Minor et al., 1998). As the name implies, dehiscence of the bone overlying the superior canal results in a fistula between the superior canal and the middle cranial fossa. Normally the semicircular canals are enclosed by the rigid bony capsule, so these vestibular structures are unaffected by sound pressure changes. The oval and round windows direct the forces associated with sound waves into the cochlea and along the spiral basilar membrane. A break in the bony capsule of the semicircular canals can redirect some of the sound or pressure to the semicircular canals, causing vestibular activation, a phenomenon known as *Tullio phenomenon*. Prior to the discovery of SCD, fistulas were known to occur with rupture of the oval or round window or erosion into the horizontal semicircular canal from chronic infection. Pressure changes generated by increasing intracranial pressure (ICP; Valsalva against closed glottis) or increasing middle ear pressure (Valsalva against pinched nostrils or compression of the tragus) triggers brief nystagmus in the plane of the affected canal. Surgically repairing the defect can be attempted if the patient is debilitated by the symptoms, but most patients do well with conservative management (Ward, 2017). A study looking at long-term outcome after SCD surgical treatment had a low follow-up rate (43%; 93/218) but reported trends in improved audio-vestibular symptoms that were greatest for autophony, pulsatile tinnitus, audible body sounds, and sensitivity to loud sounds, and least for dizziness (Alkhafaii, 2017). Patients with SCD may have hypersensitivity to bone-conducted sound and bone-conduction thresholds on the audiogram lower than the normal 0 dB hearing levels, even though air conduction thresholds remain normal (Minor, 2005).

### Other Peripheral Disorders

There are many other peripheral vestibular causes of vertigo, but most are uncommon. Vertigo often follows a blow to the head, even without a corresponding temporal bone fracture. This so-called labyrinthine concussion results from the susceptibility of the delicate structures of the inner ear to blunt trauma. Vestibular ototoxicity, usually from gentamicin, can cause a vestibulopathy that is usually bilateral but rarely can be unilateral (Waterston and Halmagyi, 1998). A bilateral vestibulopathy can also occur from an immune-mediated disorder (e.g., autoimmune inner-ear disease, Cogan syndrome), infectious process (e.g., meningitis, syphilitic labyrinthitis), structural lesion (bilateral acoustic neuroma), or a genetic disorder (e.g., neurodegenerative or isolated vestibular). The bilateral vestibular loss often goes unrecognized because the vestibular symptoms can be overshadowed by auditory or other symptoms. Although the most prominent vestibular symptoms of bilateral vestibulopathy are oscillopsia and imbalance, some nonspecific dizziness and vertigo attacks may occur as well. Vestibular schwannomas typically present with slowly progressive unilateral hearing loss, but rarely vertigo can occur. Because the tumor growth is slow, the vestibulopathy is compensated by the CNS. Finally, any disorder affecting the skull base, such as sarcoidosis, lymphoma, bacterial and fungal infections, or carcinomatous meningitis, can cause either unilateral or bilateral peripheral vestibular symptoms.

## Central Nervous System Disorders

The key to the diagnosis of CNS disorders in patients presenting with dizziness is the presence of other focal neurological symptoms or identifying central ocular motor abnormalities or ataxia. Because central disorders can mimic peripheral vestibular disorders, the most effective approach in patients with isolated dizziness is first to rule out common peripheral causes.

### Brainstem or Cerebellar Ischemia/Infarction

Ischemia affecting vestibular pathways within the brainstem or cerebellum often causes vertigo. Brainstem ischemia is normally accompanied by other neurological signs and symptoms, because motor and sensory pathways are in close proximity to vestibular pathways. Vertigo is the most common symptom with Wallenberg syndrome, infarction in the lateral medulla in the territory of the posterior inferior cerebellar artery (PICA), but other neurological symptoms and signs (e.g., diplopia, facial numbness, Horner syndrome) are typically present. Ischemia of the cerebellum can cause vertigo as the most prominent or only symptom, and a common dilemma is whether the patient with acute-onset vertigo needs a magnetic resonance imaging (MRA) scan to rule out cerebellar infarction. Computed tomography (CT) scans of the posterior fossa are not a sensitive test for acute ischemic stroke (Chalela et al., 2007). Abnormal ocular motor findings in patients with brainstem or cerebellar strokes include (1) spontaneous nystagmus that is purely vertical or torsional, (2) direction-changing gaze-evoked nystagmus (patient looks to the left and has left-beating nystagmus, looks to the right, and has right-beating nystagmus), (3) impairment of smooth pursuit, and (4) overshooting saccades. Central causes of nystagmus can sometimes closely mimic the peripheral vestibular pattern of spontaneous nystagmus (Lee et al., 2006b; Kerber, 2015; Newman-Toker et al., 2008). In these cases, a negative head-thrust test (i.e., no corrective saccade) or a skew deviation could be the key indicators of a central rather than a peripheral vestibular lesion (Newman-Toker et al., 2013a, 2013b). Cardiovascular risk factors are also independent predictors of stroke in dizziness patients (Kerber, 2015) and therefore should be considered in evaluation and management plans.

### Multiple Sclerosis

Dizziness is a common symptom in patients with multiple sclerosis (MS). Vertigo is the initial symptom in about 5% of patients with MS. A typical MS attack has a gradual onset, reaching its peak within a few days. Milder spontaneous episodes of vertigo, not characteristic of a new attack, and positional vertigo lasting seconds are also common in MS patients. Nearly all varieties of central spontaneous and positional nystagmus occur with MS, and occasionally patients show typical peripheral vestibular nystagmus when the lesion affects the root entry zone of the vestibular nerve. MRI of the brain identifies white matter lesions in about 95% of MS patients, although similar lesions are sometimes seen in patients without the clinical criteria for the diagnosis of MS.

### Posterior Fossa Structural Abnormalities

Any structural lesion of the posterior fossa can cause dizziness. With the Chiari malformation, the brainstem and cerebellum are elongated downward into the cervical canal, causing pressure on both the caudal midline cerebellum and the cervicomedullary junction. The most common neurological symptom is a slowly progressive unsteadiness of gait, which patients often describe as dizziness. Vertigo and hearing loss are uncommon, occurring in about 10% of patients. Ocular motor abnormalities (e.g., spontaneous or positional downbeat nystagmus, impaired smooth pursuit) are particularly common with Chiari malformations. Dysphagia, hoarseness, and dysarthria can result from stretching of the lower cranial nerves, and obstructive hydrocephalus can result from occlusion of the basilar cisterns. MRI is the procedure of choice for identifying Chiari malformations; midline sagittal sections clearly show the level of the cerebellar tonsils. The most common

CNS tumors in the posterior fossa are gliomas in adults and medulloblastoma in children. Ocular motor dysfunction (impaired smooth pursuit, overshooting saccades), impaired coordination, or other central findings occur in these patients. An early finding of patients with cerebellar tumors can be central positional nystagmus. Vascular malformations (arteriovenous malformations [AVMs], cavernous hemangiomas) can similarly cause dizziness but generally are asymptomatic until bleeding occurs.

### Neurodegenerative Disorders

Patients with neurodegenerative disorders (e.g., Parkinson disease, other parkinsonian syndromes, or progressive ataxia) can present with the main complaint of dizziness (de Lau et al., 2006). However, dizziness in these patients is usually better clarified as imbalance. Positional downbeat nystagmus occurs in patients with spinocerebellar ataxia type 6 (SCA6) and other progressive ataxia disorders (Kattah and Gujrati, 2005; Kerber et al., 2005a).

### Epilepsy

Vestibular symptoms are common with focal seizures, particularly those originating from the temporal and parietal lobes. The key to differentiating vertigo with seizures from other causes of vertigo is that seizures are almost invariably associated with an altered level of consciousness. Episodic vertigo as an isolated manifestation of a focal seizure is a rarity if it occurs at all.

## Vertigo in Inherited Disorders

The clinical evaluation of patients presenting with dizziness has traditionally hinged on the history of present illness and examination. However, with the recent rapid advances in molecular biology, it has become apparent that many causes of vertigo have a strong genetic component. Because of this, obtaining a complete family history is very important, particularly in patients without a specific diagnosis for their dizziness. Since the symptoms of these familial disorders are often not debilitating and can be highly variable, simply asking the patient about a family history at the time of the appointment may not be adequate. The patient should be instructed to specifically interview other family members regarding the occurrence of these symptoms.

### Migraine

Migraine is a heterogeneous genetic disorder characterized by headaches in addition to many other neurological symptoms. Several rare monogenetic subtypes have been identified. Linkage analysis has identified a number of chromosomal loci in common forms of migraine, but no specific genes have been found. Dizziness has long been known to occur among patients with migraine headaches, and BRV is usually a migraine equivalent because no other signs or symptoms develop over time, the neurological examination remains normal, and a family or personal history of migraine headaches is common, as are typical migraine triggers. Interestingly, some patients with BRV also report auditory symptoms similar to patients with Meniere disease, and a mild hearing loss may also be seen on the audiogram (Battista, 2004). The key distinguishing factor between migraine and Meniere disease is the lack of progressive unilateral hearing loss in patients with migraine. Other types of dizziness are common in patients with migraine as well, including nonspecific dizziness and positional vertigo (von Brevern et al., 2005). The cause of vertigo in migraine patients is not yet known, but the diagnosis of migraine should be entertained in any patient with chronic recurrent attacks of dizziness of unknown cause. Long-standing motion sensitivity including carsickness, sensitivities to other types of stimuli, and a clear family history of migraine help support the diagnosis. Also, some patients have a typical migraine visual aura or other focal neurological symptoms associated with headache. Though the diagnosis of migraine-associated dizziness remains one of exclusion, little else can cause recurrent episodes without any other symptoms over a long period of time. In a genome-wide linkage scan of BRV patients (20 families), linkage to chromosome 22q12 was found, but genetic heterogeneity was evident (Lee et al., 2006a). Testing linkage using a broader phenotype of BRV and migraine headaches weakened the linkage signal. Thus no evidence exists at this time that migraine is allelic with BRV, even though migraine has a high prevalence in BRV patients.

### Familial Bilateral Vestibulopathy

Familial bilateral vestibulopathy (FBV) patients typically have brief attacks of vertigo followed by progressive loss of peripheral vestibular function leading to imbalance and oscillopsia, usually by the fifth decade. The recurrent attacks of vertigo may somehow cause damage to vestibular structures, leading to progressive vestibular loss. Quantitative rotational testing shows gains greater than 2 standard deviations below the normal mean for both sinusoidal and step changes in angular velocity. Caloric testing is insensitive for identifying bilateral vestibulopathy because of the wide range of normal caloric responses. The bedside head-thrust test may show bilateral corrective saccades when vestibulopathy is severe. As the vestibulopathy becomes more severe, attacks of vertigo become less frequent and eventually cease. Despite the high prevalence of familial hearing loss and enormous progress in identifying the genetic basis of deafness, to date no gene mutations that lead to isolated bilateral vestibulopathy in humans have been identified (Jen, 2011; Strupp, 2017). Only a few FBV families have been described (Brantberg, 2003; Jen et al., 2004b). Given the high prevalence and genetic diversity of familial hearing loss, it seems reasonable to suspect that bilateral vestibulopathy would have a similar prevalence and genetic diversity. The huge disparity in knowledge about genetic deafness and genetic vestibulopathy might stem from our inadequacy to identify vestibulopathy rather than the rareness of the disorder. It is much more straightforward for healthcare providers to identify the symptoms of hearing loss than the symptoms of vestibular loss. Adequate laboratory testing for hearing loss is also much more readily available than it is for vestibular loss. Increased knowledge and use of the bedside head-thrust test, however, has the potential to substantially enhance the identification of bilateral vestibular loss.

## Familial Hearing Loss and Vertigo

Familial progressive vestibular-cochlear dysfunction was first identified in 1988. Linkage to chromosome 14q12–13 was later found, and the disorder was designated DFNA9 (DFNA = deafness, familial, nonsyndromic, type A [autosomal dominant]; Manolis et al., 1996). Using an organ-specific approach, mutations within *COCH* were found to cause DFNA9 (Robertson et al., 1998). This disorder of progressive hearing loss is unique because no other autosomal dominant genetic hearing loss syndromes have vertigo as a common symptom. Progressive hearing loss is the most prominent symptom of DFNA9. Vertigo occurs in about 50% of DFNA9 patients. When present, vertigo may be spontaneous in onset or positionally triggered (Lemaire et al., 2003). Age of onset is variable, with some patients developing symptoms in the second to third decade and others developing symptoms later. Vertigo attacks last minutes to hours and can be accompanied by worsening of hearing, aural fullness, or tinnitus, thus closely mimicking Meniere syndrome. Vertigo episodes can precede or accompany onset of hearing loss. In addition to severe progressive hearing loss, eventually DFNA9 patients develop progressive loss of vestibular function and corresponding symptoms of imbalance and oscillopsia. Because some patients have attacks closely resembling Meniere syndrome, the

*COCH* gene was screened for mutations in idiopathic Meniere disease patients, but none were found. No studies report the use of effective treatments for vertigo attacks, but like FBV patients, these attacks generally only last a few years and then become less frequent, presumably due to loss of vestibular function. Of the many autosomal dominant genes that cause hearing loss, *DFNA11* is the only other one associated with vestibulopathy.

Enlarged vestibular aqueduct (EVA) syndrome, designated DFNB4 (DFNB = deafness, familial, nonsyndromic, type B [autosomal recessive]), is characterized by early-onset hearing loss with enlargement of the vestibular aqueduct best seen on temporal bone CT. Normally, the vestibular aqueduct is less than 1.5 mm in diameter, but in EVA it is much larger. The mechanism leading to hearing loss and vertigo is unclear. The vestibular aqueduct contains the endolymphatic duct, which connects the medial wall of the vestibule to the endolymphatic sac and is an important structure in the exchange of endolymph. Enlargement may cause increased transmission of ICPs to the inner-ear structures. However, the Valsalva maneuver—which increases ICP—does not trigger symptoms in EVA patients. Vertigo attacks last 15 minutes to 3 hours and are not associated with changes in hearing. Vertigo attacks may begin at the onset of hearing loss (early childhood) or years later and can be triggered by blows to the head or vigorous spinning (Oh et al., 2001a). Quantitative vestibular testing may be normal in EVA patients or reveal mild to moderate loss of vestibular function. Enlargement of the vestibular aqueduct has also been observed in Pendred syndrome (PS), branchio-oto-renal syndrome, CHARGE (*c*oloboma of the eye, *h*eart defects, *a*tresia choanae, *r*etardation of growth or development, *g*enitourinary anomalies, and *e*ar abnormalities or hearing impairment), Waardenburg syndrome, and distal renal tubular acidosis with deafness. EVA syndrome is allelic to PS, which is characterized by developmental abnormalities of the cochlea in combination with thyroid dysfunction and goiter.

### Familial Ataxia Syndromes

Vestibular symptoms and signs are common with several of the hereditary ataxia syndromes including SCA types 1, 2, 3, 6, and 7, Friedreich ataxia, Refsum disease, and EA types 2, 3, 4, and 5. In most of these disorders, the symptoms are slowly progressive, with the cerebellar ataxia and incoordination overshadowing the vestibular symptoms. Head movement-induced oscillopsia commonly occurs because the patient is unable to suppress the VOR with fixation. Attacks of vertigo may occur in up to half of patients with SCA6 (Takahashi et al., 2004), many of which are positionally triggered (Jen et al., 1998). Persistent downbeating nystagmus is often seen with the Dix-Hallpike test; the positional vertigo and nystagmus can even be the initial symptom in these patients. Most of the EA syndromes have onset before the age of 20 (Jen et al., 2004a). The attacks are characterized by extreme incoordination, leading to severe difficulty walking during attacks. Vertigo can occur as part of these attacks, and migraine headaches are common in these patients as well. In fact EA2, SCA6, and familial hemiplegic migraine type 1 are all caused by mutations with the same gene, *CACNA1A*. An additional feature of EA2 and EA4 is the eventual development of interictal nystagmus and progressive ataxia. Patients with EA2 may experience reduced attacks with acetazolamide or 4-aminopyridine (Zesiewicz, 2018).

## COMMON CAUSES OF NONSPECIFIC DIZZINESS

Patients with nonspecific dizziness are probably referred to neurologists more frequently than patients with true vertigo. These patients are usually bothered by lightheadedness (wooziness), presyncope, imbalance, motion sensitivity, or anxiety. Side effects or toxicity from medications are common causes of nonspecific dizziness. Bothersome lightheadedness can be a direct effect of the medication itself or the result of lowering of the patient's blood pressure. Ataxia can be caused by antiepileptic medications and is usually reversible once the medication is decreased or stopped. Patients with peripheral neuropathy causing dizziness report significant worsening of their balance in poor lighting and also the sensation that they are walking on cushions. Drops in blood pressure can be caused by dehydration, vasovagal attacks, or as part of an autonomic neuropathy. Patients with panic attacks can present with nonspecific dizziness, but their spells are invariably accompanied by other symptoms such as sense of fear or doom, palpitations, sweating, shortness of breath, or paresthesias. Persistent postural perceptual dizziness (PPPD) is a new label for a form of chronic dizziness manifested by sensations of postural instability and sensitivity to self and surround motion that is often associated with migraine, panic attacks, and generalized anxiety (Popkirov, 2018). Other medical conditions such as cardiac arrhythmias or metabolic disturbances can also cause nonspecific dizziness. In the elderly, confluent white matter hyperintensities have a strong association with dizziness and balance problems. Presumably the result of small vessel arteriosclerosis, decreased cerebral perfusion (Marstrand et al., 2002) has been identified in these patients even when blood pressure taken at the arm is normal. Patients with dizziness related to white matter hyperintensities on MRI usually feel better sitting or lying down and typically have impairment of tandem gait. Since many elderly patients are taking blood pressure medications, at least a trial of lowering or discontinuing these medications is warranted.

## COMMON PRESENTATIONS OF VERTIGO

Patients present with symptoms rather than specific diagnoses. The most common presentations of vertigo are the following.

### Acute Severe Vertigo

The patient presenting with new-onset severe vertigo probably has an acute unilateral vestibulopathy caused by vestibular neuritis; however, stroke should also be a concern. In the absence of focal neurological symptoms or signs on the general evaluation, attention should focus on the neuro-otological evaluation. If no spontaneous nystagmus or gaze nystagmus is observed, a technique to block visual fixation should be applied. The direction of the nystagmus should be noted and the effect of gaze assessed. If a peripheral vestibular pattern of nystagmus is identified, a positive head-thrust test in the direction opposite the fast phase of nystagmus suggests a lesion of the vestibular nerve. Vestibular neuritis is presumed to be the most common cause of this presentation but there is no mechanism to confirm a viral/postviral etiology. A central vestibular lesion (e.g., ischemic stroke) becomes a serious concern if there are "red flags" such as other central signs or symptoms, direction-changing nystagmus, vertical nystagmus, a negative head-thrust test (i.e., no corrective saccade after the head-thrust test to the direction opposite the fast phase of spontaneous nystagmus), a skew deviation, or substantial stroke risk factors (Kerber, 2015; Newman-Toker, 2013a; Newman-Toker, 2013b). Vertebral artery dissection can lead to an acute vertigo presentation, but the most common symptom is severe, sudden-onset occipital or neck pain, with additional neurological signs and symptoms (Arnold et al., 2006). If hearing loss accompanies the episode, either labyrinthitis or an ischemic lesion via the anterior inferior cerebellar artery are possible. When hearing loss and facial weakness accompany the acute onset of vertigo, one should closely inspect the outer ear for vesicles characteristic of herpes zoster (Ramsay Hunt syndrome). An acoustic neuroma is a slow-growing tumor, so only rarely is it associated with acute-onset vertigo. Migraine can mimic vestibular neuritis, though the diagnosis of migraine-associated vertigo hinges on recurrent episodes and lack of progressive auditory symptoms.

### Recurrent Attacks of Vertigo

In patients with recurrent attacks of vertigo, the key diagnostic information lies in the details of the attacks. Meniere disease is the likely cause in patients with recurrent vertigo lasting longer than 20 minutes and associated with unilateral auditory symptoms. If the Meniere-like attacks present in a fulminate fashion, the diagnosis of autoimmune inner-ear disease should be considered. Transient ischemic attacks (TIAs) should be suspected in patients having brief episodes of vertigo, particularly when vascular risk factors are present and other neurological symptoms are reported (Josephson et al., 2008). Case series of patients with rotational vertebral artery syndrome demonstrate that the inner ear and possibly central vestibular pathways have high energy requirements and are therefore susceptible to levels of ischemia tolerated by other parts of the brain (Choi et al., 2005). Crescendo TIAs can be the harbinger of impending stroke or basilar artery occlusion. As with acute severe vertigo, accompanying auditory symptoms do not exclude the possibility of an ischemic disorder. Migraine and the migraine equivalent, BRV, are characterized by a history of similar symptoms, a normal examination, family or personal history of migraine headaches and/or BRV, other migraine characteristics, and typical triggers. Attacks are otherwise highly variable, lasting anywhere from seconds to days. If the attacks are consistently seconds in duration, the diagnosis of vestibular paroxysmia should be considered (Strupp, 2016). MS may be the cause when patients have recurrent episodes of vertigo and a history of other attacks of neurological symptoms, particularly when fixed deficits such as an afferent pupillary defect or internuclear ophthalmoplegia are identified on the examination.

### Recurrent Positional Vertigo

Positional vertigo is defined by the symptom being *triggered*, not simply worsened, by certain positional changes. Physicians often confuse vestibular neuritis with BPPV because vestibular neuritis patients can often settle into a relatively comfortable position and then experience dramatic worsening with movement. The patient complaining of recurrent episodes of vertigo triggered by certain head movements likely has BPPV, but this is not the only possibility. BPPV can be identified and treated at the bedside, so positional testing should be performed in any patient with this complaint. Positional testing can also uncover the other causes of positionally triggered dizziness (Bertholon et al., 2002). The history strongly suggests the diagnosis of BPPV when the positional vertigo is brief (<1 minute), has typical triggers, and is unaccompanied by other neurological symptoms. A burst of triggered and transient vertical torsional nystagmus is specific for BPPV of the posterior canal (Aw et al., 2005). If the Dix–Hallpike test does not trigger the characteristic nystagmus, the examiner should search for the HC-BPPV with supine positional testing. Central positional nystagmus occurs as the result of disorders affecting the posterior fossa, including tumors, cerebellar degeneration, Chiari malformation, or MS. The nystagmus of these disorders is typically downbeating and persistent, though a pure torsional nystagmus may occur as well. Patients with loss of one vertebral artery may develop vertigo or significant dizziness after head turns to the direction opposite the intact artery because the bony structures of the spinal column can pinch off the remaining vertebral artery (Choi et al., 2005). Central types of nystagmus develop as a result, and vertigo can be the most prominent symptom. Finally, migraine can also closely mimic BPPV and central positional nystagmus (von Brevern et al., 2005). Patients with migraine as the cause typically report a longer duration of symptoms once the positional vertigo is triggered, and the nystagmus may be of a central or peripheral type. The mechanisms are not clear, but the disorder is usually self-limited and not progressive. Associations between migraine and typical BPPV have also been made, but the link between these disorders is unclear.

## HEARING LOSS

Neurologists generally do not encounter patients principally bothered by auditory symptoms such as hearing loss or tinnitus, as opposed to patients with dizziness, who are frequently referred for evaluation. Nevertheless, an understanding of the auditory system, certain disorders causing auditory symptoms, and audiograms can enhance the diagnostic abilities of the neurologist.

### Conductive Hearing Loss

Conductive hearing loss results from lesions involving the external or the middle ear. The tympanic membrane and ossicles act as a transformer, amplifying the airborne sound and effectively transferring it to the inner-ear fluid. If this normal pathway is obstructed, transmission can occur across the skin and through the bones of the skull (bone conduction) but at the cost of significant energy loss. Patients with a conductive hearing loss can hear speech in a noisy background better than a quiet background, since they can understand loud speech as well as anyone. The most common cause of conductive hearing loss is impacted cerumen in the external canal. The most common serious cause of conductive hearing loss is otitis media, which can result from either infected fluid (suppurative otitis) or noninfected fluid (serous otitis) accumulating in the middle ear and impairing conduction of airborne sound. With chronic otitis media, a cholesteatoma may erode the ossicles. Otosclerosis produces progressive conductive hearing loss by immobilizing the stapes with new bone growth in front of and below the oval window. Other common causes of conductive hearing loss are trauma, congenital malformations of the external and middle ear, and glomus body tumors.

### Sensorineural Hearing Loss

Sensorineural hearing loss results from lesions of the cochlea, the auditory division of the acoustic nerve, or both and results in inability to normally perceive both bone- and air-conducted sound. The spiral cochlea mechanically analyzes the frequency content of sound. For high-frequency tones, only sensory cells in the basilar turn are activated, but for low-frequency tones, all sensory cells are activated. Therefore, with lesions of the cochlea and its afferent nerve, the hearing levels for different frequencies are usually unequal, and the phase relationship between different frequencies may be altered. Patients with sensorineural hearing loss often have difficulty hearing speech that is mixed with background noise, and they may be annoyed by loud speech. Distortion of sounds is common with sensorineural hearing loss. A pure tone may be heard as noisy, rough, or buzzing, or it may be distorted so that it sounds like a complex mixture of tones.

### Central Hearing Loss

Central hearing loss results from lesions of the central auditory pathways. These lesions involve the cochlear and dorsal olivary nuclear complexes, inferior colliculi, medial geniculate bodies, auditory cortex in the temporal lobes, and interconnecting afferent and efferent fiber tracks. As a rule, patients with central lesions do not have impaired hearing levels for pure tones, and they understand speech so long as it is clearly spoken in a quiet environment. If the listener's task is made more difficult with the introduction of background or competing messages, performance deteriorates more markedly in patients with central lesions than it does in normal subjects. Lesions involving the eighth nerve root entry zone or cochlear nucleus (demyelination or infarction in the lateral pontomedullary region), however, can cause unilateral hearing loss for pure tones. Because about half of afferent nerve fibers cross central to the cochlear nucleus, this is the most central structure in which a lesion can result in a unilateral hearing loss.

## SPECIFIC DISORDERS CAUSING HEARING LOSS

### Meniere Disease

Auditory symptoms in Meniere disease consist of a fluctuating sense of fullness and pressure along with tinnitus and decreased hearing in one ear. In the early stages, the hearing loss is completely reversible, but in later stages a residual hearing loss remains. Tinnitus may persist between episodes but usually increases in intensity immediately before or during the acute episode. It is typically described as a roaring sound like the sound of the ocean or a hollow seashell. The hearing loss on the audiogram appears in the early stages as a low-frequency loss. However, as the disorder progresses, a more complete hearing loss occurs. In about one-third of patients, the disorder becomes bilateral. Eventually, severe permanent hearing loss develops and the episodic nature spontaneously disappears. When the progression of hearing loss (particularly when bilateral) is fulminant and rapidly progressive, the diagnosis of autoimmune inner-ear disease should be considered. Also see the section on Meniere disease under Specific Disorders Causing Vertigo.

### Cerebellopontine Angle Tumors

Acoustic neuromas (vestibular schwannoma) account for about 5% of intracranial tumors and more than 90% of cerebellopontine angle tumors. These tumors usually begin in the internal auditory canal, producing symptoms by compressing the nerve in its narrow confines. As the tumor grows, it protrudes through the internal auditory meatus, stretches adjacent nerves over the surface of the mass, and deforms the cerebellum and brainstem. By far the most common symptoms associated with acoustic neuromas are slowly progressive unilateral hearing loss and tinnitus from compression of the cochlear nerve. Rarely, acute hearing loss occurs, possibly from compression of the labyrinthine vasculature. Vertigo occurs infrequently, but approximately half of patients with an acoustic neuroma complain of mild imbalance or disequilibrium. An epidermoid tumor, meningioma, facial nerve schwannoma, or metastatic disease can also cause mass lesions within the cerebellopontine angle. The audiometric pattern is variable; however, patients with cerebellopontine angle tumors causing hearing loss usually have poor speech discrimination, acoustic reflex decay, and pure tone decay rather than a marked asymmetry of pure tones.

### Superior Canal Dehiscence

Patients with SCD may experience conductive hyperacusis (hearing their eye move or the impact of their feet during walking or running) and autophony (hearing their own breath and voice sounds) in the affected ear. An air/bone gap, with preserved acoustic reflexes, may be identified on standard audiograms. The Weber tuning fork test typically lateralizes to the affected ear, and the Rinne turning fork test may show bone conduction greater than air conduction (see Specific Disorders Causing Vertigo).

### Otosclerosis

Otosclerosis is a metabolic disease of the bony labyrinth that usually manifests by immobilizing the stapes, thereby producing a conductive hearing loss. A positive family history for otosclerosis is reported in 50% to 70% of cases. Bilateral involvement is usual, but about one-fourth of cases are unilateral. Although conductive hearing loss is the hallmark of otosclerosis, a combined conductive-sensorineural hearing loss pattern is frequent. Although otosclerosis is primarily a disorder of the auditory system, vestibular symptoms and signs are more common than generally appreciated.

### Noise-Induced Hearing Loss

Noise-induced hearing loss is extremely common. About one-third of individuals with hearing loss can attribute at least part of the loss to noise exposure. The loss almost always begins at 4000 Hz, creating the typical notched appearance on the audiogram, and does not affect speech discrimination until late in the disease process. Typically, levels of noise exposure greater than 85 dB are required to cause the changes in the ear induced by loud noise. Examples of noise greater than 85 dB that are common sources of exposure include motorcycles, firecrackers, factory machinery, and music concerts.

### Genetic Disorders

Many genetic causes of hearing loss have been identified, including syndromic and nonsyndromic phenotypes and inheritance types that are autosomal dominant, autosomal recessive, and mitochondrial. Typically these disorders start early in life and cause profound hearing loss. Vestibular symptoms are not common but may not be thoroughly assessed in affected individuals.

### Ototoxicity

The most common medications causing hearing loss are aminoglycoside antibiotics, loop diuretics, and cisplatin. Impaired elimination of these drugs, such as occurs in patients with renal insufficiency, predisposes to ototoxicity. Patients receiving high-dose salicylate therapy frequently complain of hearing loss, tinnitus, and dizziness. These symptoms and signs are rapidly reversible after cessation of the salicylate ingestion.

## COMMON PRESENTATIONS OF HEARING LOSS

### Asymmetrical Sensorineural Hearing Loss

Evaluation of patients identified as having an asymmetrical sensorineural hearing loss is primarily the search for a tumor in the area of the internal auditory canal or cerebellopontine angle, or more rarely other lesions of the temporal bone or brain. With an asymmetry of hearing defined as 15 dB or greater in two or more frequencies or a 15% or more asymmetry in speech discrimination scores, approximately 10% of patients will have lesions identified on MRI (Cueva, 2004). A simple management guide that has been proposed is to order an MRI if there is a ≥15 dB asymmetry at 3000 Hz, or instead a follow-up audiogram if the asymmetry is less than 15 dB at 3000 Hz (Saliba et al., 2011). Acoustic neuromas are by far the most common abnormality found. Other causative lesions may include glomus jugulare tumors, ectatic basilar artery with brainstem compression, or petrous apex cholesterol granuloma. Auditory brainstem response (ABR) testing shows a sensitivity and specificity around 70%, with a false-positive rate of 77%, but a false-negative rate of 29% (Cueva, 2004).

### Sudden Sensorineural Hearing Loss

The etiology of sudden sensorineural hearing loss is similar to both Bell palsy and vestibular neuritis in that a viral cause is presumed in the majority of cases, but proof of a viral pathophysiology in a given case is difficult to obtain. The hearing loss can abruptly develop or evolve over several hours. Acoustic neuromas may be found in around 5% of patients with this presentation (Aarnisalo et al., 2004), but one should also be aware of false-positive MRIs, particularly for lesions smaller than 6 mm (Arriaga et al., 1995). Focal ischemia to the cochlea, cochlear nerve, or the root entry zone can also cause an abrupt loss of hearing over several minutes. In the setting of a patient at risk for stroke, this cause should be considered early, because it can be the harbinger of basilar artery occlusion (Toyoda et al., 2002). Sudden-onset bilateral hearing loss can rarely result from bilateral lesions of the primary auditory cortex in the transverse temporal gyri of

Heschl. Deficits can range from auditory agnosia for speech or nonspeech sounds, with relatively normal hearing thresholds, to rare cases of cortical deafness characterized by markedly elevated pure-tone thresholds.

### Hearing Loss with Age

The bilateral hearing loss commonly associated with advancing age is called *presbycusis*. It is not a distinct entity but rather represents multiple effects of aging on the auditory system. It may include conductive and central dysfunction, but the most consistent effect of aging is on the sensory cells and the neurons of the cochlea. The typical audiogram appearance in patients with presbycusis is that of symmetrical hearing loss, with the tracing gradually sloping downward with increasing frequency. The most consistent pathology associated with presbycusis is a degeneration of sensory cells and nerve fibers at the base of the cochlea.

## TINNITUS

Tinnitus is a noise in the ear that is usually audible only to the patient, although occasionally the sound can be heard by the examining physician. It is a symptom that can be associated with a variety of disorders that may affect the ear or the brain. The most important piece of information is whether the patient localizes it to one or both ears or if it is nonlocalizable. Tinnitus localized to one ear is probably more likely to have an identifiable cause than when localized to both ears or nonlocalizable. The characteristics of the tinnitus should be described by the patient, as this can provide helpful information. For an example, the typical tinnitus associated with Meniere disease is described as a roaring sound like listening to a seashell. The tinnitus associated with an acoustic neuroma is typically a high-pitched ringing or like the sound of steam blowing from a tea kettle. If the tinnitus is rhythmic, the patient should be asked whether it is synchronous with the pulse or with respiration. Recurrent rhythmic or even nonrhythmic clicking sounds in one ear can indicate stapedial palatal myoclonus. However, the most common form of tinnitus is a bilateral high-pitched sound that is usually worse at night when it is quiet and there is less background noise to mask it. Tinnitus can be worse when the patient is under stress or with the use of caffeine.

## LABORATORY INVESTIGATIONS IN DIAGNOSIS AND MANAGEMENT

### Dizziness and Vertigo

The history and physical examination should determine what diagnostic tests if any are necessary in patients presenting with dizziness or vertigo. Studies have repeatedly shown that MRI, audiogram, and vestibular tests are not more likely to be abnormal in unselected patients complaining of dizziness when compared with age-matched controls (Colledge et al., 1996, 2002; Hajioff et al., 2002; Lawson et al., 1999; Yardley et al., 1998). Many disorders causing dizziness can be diagnosed and even treated at the bedside, with no further diagnostic tests indicated.

#### General Tests

General tests such as blood work, chest x-ray, or electrocardiograms are only indicated when searching for a specific abnormality. If a patient has otherwise unexplained nonspecific dizziness, ruling out metabolic causes is indicated.

#### Imaging

Brain imaging is commonly ordered in patients complaining of dizziness. Though a CT scan can rule out a large mass, smaller lesions cannot be excluded because of artifact and poor resolution in the posterior fossa (Chalela et al., 2007). MRI is the imaging modality of choice but is expensive and generally a much less practical test than CT. Determining which patients should have an MRI can be difficult, which is why an understanding of the common peripheral vestibular disorders is important. Patients identified as having BPPV, vestibular neuritis, or Meniere disease do not require an imaging study. In addition, patients with normal neurological and neuro-otological examinations reporting episodes of dizziness dating back more than several months are highly unlikely to have a relevant abnormality on MRI. Though studies suggest improved hearing preservation after surgery in patients with acoustic neuromas when diagnosed early, this does not mean that every patient complaining of dizziness requires an MRI to exclude this cause. Acoustic neuromas are rare, whereas dizziness and vertigo are extremely common. On the other hand, for any patient experiencing focal neurological symptoms or having unexplained neurological deficits or an otherwise rapid, unexplained progression of symptoms, an MRI should be strongly considered to rule out a mass lesion, stroke, structural abnormality, or MS. In dizzy patients with gradually progressive hearing loss, MRI may also be helpful.

#### Vestibular Testing

***Eye movement recording.***

**Methods of recording eye movements.** Eye movement recordings can be made with *electronystagmography* or videonystagmography (VNG). ENG equipment is less expensive to purchase, and the test provides reliable clinical information (Furman et al., 1996). Artifacts from lid movements or muscle APs are common; thus the "noise" is greater in ENG than in VNG. Probably the main clinical advantage of video-oculography (VOG) is the ability to go back and observe the actual video recording of the eye movements. Measuring torsional eye movements is also possible with VNG, although systems for doing so are still being developed. Disadvantages of VNG are the inability to measure eye movements with the eyes closed and difficulties stabilizing the head gear.

***Eye movement subtests.*** A standard test battery includes a search for pathological nystagmus or saccadic intrusions with fixation and with eyes open in the darkness, tests of visual ocular control (saccades, smooth pursuit, OKN), and the bithermal caloric test (Baloh and Kerber, 2011).

***Recording pathological spontaneous eye movements.*** Once the equipment has been set up and calibrated, the patient is asked to look straight ahead, both when fixating on a target and in darkness with eyes open (removing fixation). In this manner, spontaneous nystagmus or saccadic intrusions can be recorded. Patients are then instructed to look about 30 degrees from the midline in each direction, maintaining gaze for about 10–20 seconds in each direction. Gaze-evoked nystagmus is demonstrated when nystagmus not seen in the primary position appears with gaze. The most common type of gaze-evoked nystagmus has approximately equal amplitude in all directions and results from either medication toxicity or cerebellar dysfunction. In patients with a partially compensated peripheral vestibular lesion, nystagmus in one direction may be present. Small-amplitude nystagmus with gaze more than 30 degrees is typically a physiological nystagmus appearing in normal individuals and is referred to as *end-gaze nystagmus*. Positional testing using both the head-hanging positions and supine positions is used to search for positional nystagmus. A characteristic burst of nystagmus is seen in patients with BPPV. Persistent positional nystagmus (i.e., no burst) is a common finding when recordings are made with eyes open in darkness. When the average slow-phase velocity exceeds 4 degrees per second, it is outside the normal range but nonlocalizing. When patients are able to suppress this nystagmus when presented with a visual target, a peripheral cause is suggested.

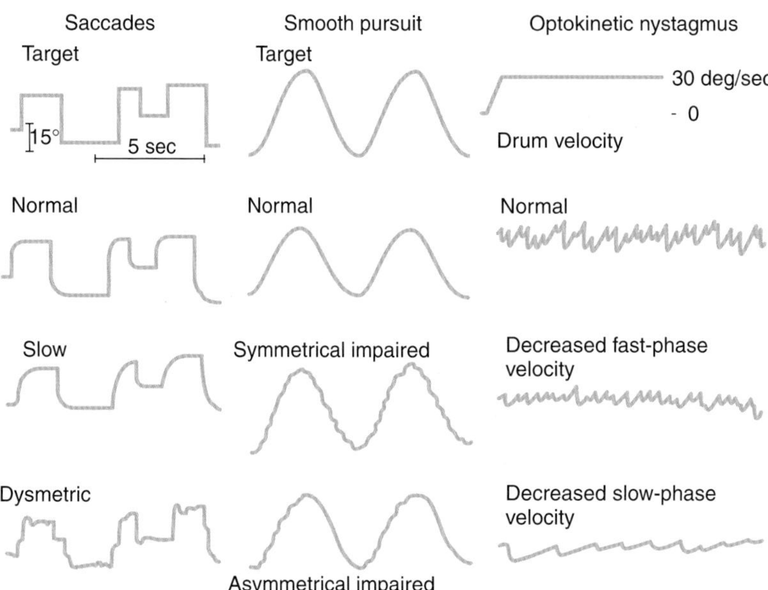


**Fig. 22.5** Electronystagmographic recordings of normal and abnormal saccades, smooth pursuit, and optokinetic nystagmus. *(From Baloh, R.W., 1998. Dizziness, Hearing Loss, and Tinnitus. F.A. Davis Company, Philadelphia, Figure 37, p. 84.)*

***Visual ocular motor control.***

**Saccades.** By presenting the patient with visual targets that move 10–30 degrees in the horizontal and vertical planes, measurements of saccade onset, velocity, and accuracy can be made. Patients are instructed to "jump" from target to target. Normal subjects, elderly and young alike, achieve a highly reproducible pattern of saccadic velocity that has a nonlinear relationship between peak velocity and amplitude of the eye movement. Velocities initially increase from about 5-degree to 30-degree movements, and then a maximum velocity is achieved. Saccade velocity remains intact through late age in individuals without focal neurological disease. Slowing of saccades can occur with lesions anywhere in the diffuse central pathways involved in generating saccades, but the most pronounced slowing occurs with lesions affecting the brainstem (pretectal and paramedian pontine gaze centers or ocular motor neurons) and the extraocular muscles. Typical disorders with slowing of saccades are PSP and HD. Slowing can also result if the patient has taken tranquilizing drugs. A lesion of medial longitudinal fasciculus results in slowing of the adducting eye, often more easily appreciated with quantitative measures than bedside testing. Normal subjects consistently undershoot target jumps larger than 20 degrees and will require a small corrective saccade to achieve the final position. Overshooting saccades, however, are rare and do not consistently occur in normal patients. Overshooting saccades typically are seen in patients with cerebellar dysfunction.

**Smooth pursuit.** Recordings of smooth pursuit are made by having the patient follow a target back and forth. The slope of this eye/target velocity relationship represents the gain of the smooth pursuit system, which depends on the velocity and frequency of the target movements. Higher velocity and frequency testing results in lower gains. Though each laboratory must establish normal values, typically normal subjects have very high mean gains (0.92 ± 0.05 at 0.2 Hz, 22.6 degrees per second). Though a patient's age is typically considered when interpreting results, a recent study shows smooth-pursuit gains can be well maintained in subjects well into their ninth decade (Kerber et al., 2006).

**Optokinetic nystagmus.** Laboratory testing of OKN uses a full-field visual stimulus (typically a patterned drum) that moves at a constant velocity and frequency around the subject, who is either instructed to follow the target (resulting in large-amplitude nystagmus) or stare through it (resulting in small-amplitude nystagmus). This stimulus also causes a sensation of self-rotation called *circular vection*, even though the peripheral vestibular system is not being stimulated. The OKN gain is measured by comparing the slow-component velocity of the eye movement to the target velocity. As with smooth-pursuit testing, gain drops off with increasing frequency and velocity of the target in normal subjects. The normal and abnormal ENG appearance of saccades, smooth pursuit, and OKN are demonstrated in Fig. 22.5.

***Bithermal caloric testing.*** With the bithermal caloric test, each ear is irrigated alternately for a fixed duration (30–40 seconds) with a constant flow of water that is either 7°C above or below body temperature. The external auditory canal should first be inspected to make sure that cerumen does not occlude it and that the tympanic membrane is intact. The different temperatures of the water induce a movement of the endolymph mainly within the horizontal semicircular canal, because this canal is anatomically closest to the tympanic membrane. The resulting temperature gradient from one side of the canal to the other causes flow of the endolymph that triggers a very low-frequency stimulus of the horizontal canal. The advantages of this test method are that the endolymph can be triggered to flow in both directions (ampullopetal and ampullofugal), each ear can be stimulated separately, and the test is tolerated by most patients. Limitations include the need for constant temperature baths and plumbing to maintain continuous circulation of the water through the infusion hose, the interindividual variability of caloric vestibular responses, and only being able to apply a single frequency stimulus.

The conventional method for measuring caloric stimulation is to compare the maximum slow-phase velocities achieved on one side to that of the other side, using the vestibular paresis formula

$$\frac{(R30° + R44°) - (L30° + L44°)}{(R30° + R44° + L30° + L44°)} \times 100.$$

Directional preponderance is also calculated using the formula

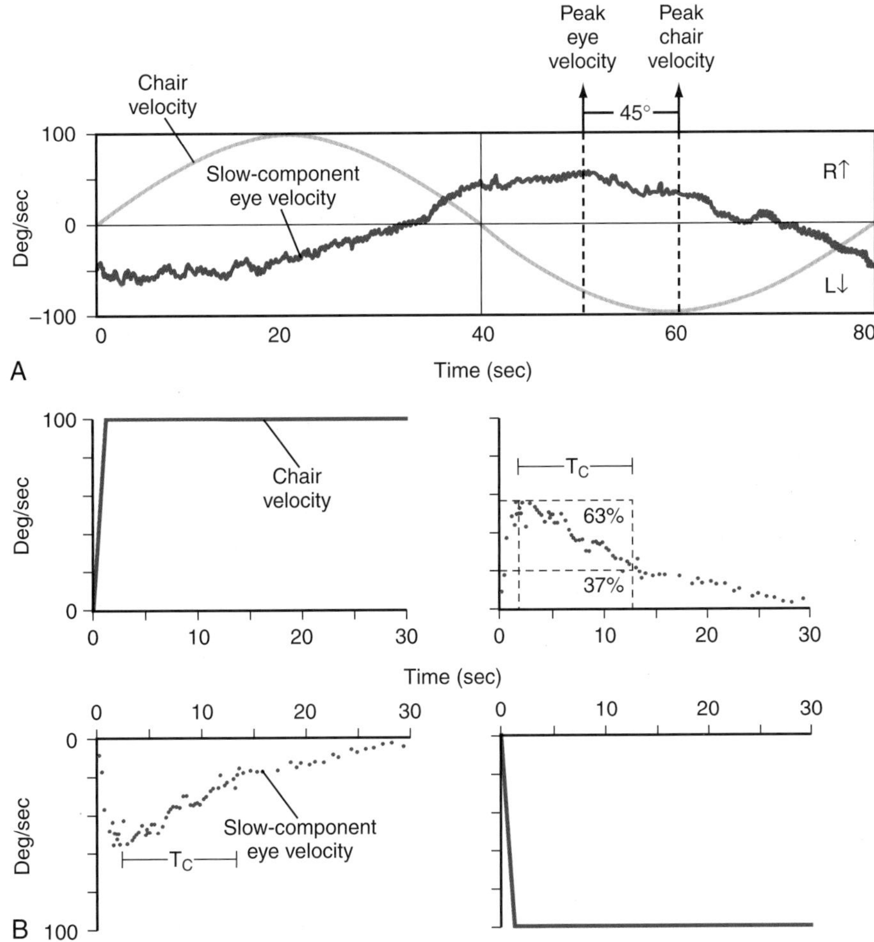


**Fig. 22.6** Plots of slow-component eye velocity versus time for nystagmus induced by sinusoidal angular rotation in the horizontal plane at 0.0125 Hz and a peak velocity of 100 deg/sec **(A)** and by step changes in angular velocity of 100 deg/sec occurring with an acceleration of approximately 140 deg/sec$^2$ **(B)**. Subject is seated on a motorized rotating chair with eyes open in darkness. Eye movements are recorded with electronystagmography. Fast components are identified and removed, and slow-component eye velocity is measured every 20 msec. The gain of the response (peak slow-component eye velocity/peak chair velocity) is about 0.6 for both types of stimulation. The phase lead with sinusoidal stimulation is the difference in timing between the peak eye velocity and peak chair velocity (in this case 45 degrees). The time constant ($T_C$) is the time required for the response to decay to 37% of its initial value (about 10 seconds in B). *(From Baloh, R.W., 1998. Dizziness, Hearing Loss, and Tinnitus. F.A. Davis Company, Philadelphia, Figure 36, p. 81.)*

$$\frac{(L30° + R44°) - (L44° + R30°)}{(L30° + R44° + L44° + R30°)} \times 100.$$

Dividing by the total response normalizes the measurements to remove the large variability in absolute magnitude of normal caloric responses. Typically, the finding of significant vestibular paresis of 25% to 30% with bithermal caloric stimulation suggests a lesion in the vestibular system that is located anywhere from the end organ to the vestibular nerve root entry zone in the brainstem. This finding is a strong indicator of a unilateral peripheral lesion, but it must be placed in the context of the patient's clinical history and bedside examination; a caloric paresis can also occur in central vestibular disorders. High rates of significant vestibular paresis as measured by the caloric test have been reported in patients with acute vertigo presentations caused by stroke (Newman-Toker et al., 2008). It is also common to find a caloric asymmetry in control subjects without dizziness (particularly those with migraine or diabetes) who undergo this test. A significant directional preponderance on caloric testing (>30%) indicates an imbalance in the vestibular system but is nonlocalizing, occurring with both peripheral and central lesions.

***Rotational testing.*** For rotational testing, the patient sits in a motorized chair that rotates under the control of a computer, and the patient's head and body move in unison with the chair. The chair is in a dark room, so visual fixation is removed. Eye movements induced by the vestibular system stimulating movements of the patient's head and body within the chair are recorded using ENG or VNG. The computer precisely controls the velocity and frequency of rotations so that the VOR can be measured at multiple frequencies in a single session. Sinusoidal and step (impulse) changes in angular velocity are routinely used (Fig. 22.6). In clinical testing, generally only rotations about the vertical axis are used, which maximally stimulates the horizontal canals. Off-vertical rotation can be used to measure the function of the vertical semicircular canals and otoliths, but typically this is only done in research studies. For sinusoidal rotations, results are reported as gain (peak slow-component eye velocity divided by peak chair velocity) and phase (timing between the peak velocity of eye and head) at different frequencies.

Because both inner ears are stimulated at the typically low velocities and frequencies used, rotational testing is most effective at determining a bilateral peripheral vestibular hypofunction that leads to a decreased gain and increased phase. Unilateral vestibular hypofunction can be suggested by a normal gain with increased phase on standard testing or a decreased unilateral gain with shortened time constant on impulse (rapid movement) testing. Normal rotational testing results in gains around 0.5 at low-frequency rotation (0.05 Hz), with gains approaching 1.0 at higher-frequency rotations (>1 Hz). Even patients with partial loss of bilateral vestibular function may have gains in the normal range at the higher-frequency rotations, probably owing to the contribution of additional sensory systems (Jen et al., 2005; Wiest et al., 2001). The main disadvantage of rotational chair testing is the expense associated with setting it up. As a result, this vestibular test is typically only available at large academic centers. Because of this, portable devices using either passive (examiner-generated) head rotations or active (patient-generated) head turns have been developed, but the quality of evidence to support the use of these tests is low (Fife et al., 2000).

Rotational chair testing can also be used to measure the patient's ability to suppress the VOR and a combined measure of both OKN and rotational testing (visual VOR).

***Quantitative head-thrust testing.*** New devices that enable quantitative measurement of the vestibular-ocular reflex as elicited by the head-thrust test have been developed (Halmagyi, 2017). The devices consist of goggles that contain a video camera to measure eye movement velocity and an accelerometer to measure head movement velocity. Because of its ability to determine eye and head velocity, the device-based head-thrust test is mainly focused on measuring the VOR gain to each side rather than on the presence or absence of corrective saccades, which are the focus of the non—device-based head-thrust test. The quantitative measure of the head-thrust test is an advantage of the device because corrective saccades can be imperceptible, so-called covert saccades. The head-thrust test uses much higher acceleration than caloric testing to elicit eye movements via the vestibular system so that a direct comparison of the results of these tests is not entirely appropriate. However, one comparison found that a clinically significant abnormal device-based head-thrust test result is unlikely to occur in subjects with only a mild caloric asymmetry (Mahringer and Rambold, 2014). For acute peripheral lesions, the VOR gain is typically substantially reduced on the affected side (side opposite the fast phase of nystagmus; gain ~0.2–0.4) and normal to mildly reduced to the unaffected side (Choi, 2018). Acute lesions of the central vestibular system are typically normal to mildly reduced bilaterally when the lesion is in the distribution of the PICA. However, the VOR gains can closely mimic peripheral disorders when the lesion is in the distribution of the anterior inferior cerebellar artery.

***Posturography.*** Posturography is a method for quantifying balance. This testing consists of measuring sway while standing on a stable platform and also with tilt or linear displacement of the platform, both with eyes open and eyes closed, and also with movement of the visual surround. Posturography is not a diagnostic test and is of little use for localizing a lesion. It can be helpful for following the course of a patient and may serve as a quantitative measure of the response to therapy or in research studies. Posturography may be useful for identifying people at risk for falling, though whether it is better at this than a careful clinical assessment is unclear (Piirtola and Era, 2006). Posturography may be helpful in identifying patients with factitious balance disorders (Gianoli et al., 2000).

***Vestibular evoked myogenic potentials.*** It has long been known that the sacculus, which during the course of its evolution functioned as an organ of hearing and still does in primitive vertebrates, can be stimulated by loud sounds. As a result of this stimulation, a signal travels via the inferior trunk of the vestibular nerve to cranial nerve VIII and into the brainstem. From there, inhibitory postsynaptic potentials travel to the ipsilateral sternocleidomastoid muscle (SCM), essentially allowing the individual to reflexively turn toward the sound. To generate this vestibular evoked myogenic potential (VEMP) response, intense clicks of about 95–100 dB above normal hearing level (NHL) are required (Fife, 2017). The response is measured from an activated ipsilateral SCM. Tonic contraction of the muscle is required to demonstrate the inhibitory response. The amplitude of the response and also the threshold needed to generate it are measured. Because the absolute amplitudes vary greatly from patient to patient, the more reliable abnormality is detecting a side-to-side difference in an individual. In addition, responses are unreliable in subjects older than 60 years and in patients with middle ear abnormalities. Abnormal VEMP responses can be detected in most disorders affecting the peripheral vestibular system, but this test may help identify disorders that selectively affect the inferior vestibular nerve or SCD (Fife, 2017). Because caloric and rotational testing mainly stimulate the horizontal semicircular canal (which sends afferent responses via the superior vestibular nerve), the rare disorder affecting only the inferior vestibular nerve will not be identified with these tests. In patients with SCD, VEMP testing leads to increased amplitudes and lowered thresholds due to the low-impedance pathway created by the third window.

## Hearing Loss and Tinnitus

### Auditory Testing

Audiological assessment is the basis for quantifying auditory impairment. Most neurologists rely on bedside assessments of hearing. In defining an auditory abnormality, tuning forks are no substitute for a complete audiological battery. Audiological testing is most reliable in defining peripheral or cochlear auditory disturbances and often may provide useful information, based on subtests, to diagnose retrocochlear disorders such as an acoustic neuroma. Tests for central auditory dysfunction are more difficult and poorly understood. Detailed descriptions of audiological tests, both peripheral and central, are provided in standard texts (Katz et al., 2009).

The basic audiological evaluation establishes the degree and configuration of hearing loss, assesses ability to discriminate a speech signal, and provides some insight into the type of loss and possible cause. The test battery consists of pure-tone air- and bone-conduction thresholds, speech thresholds, speech discrimination testing, and immittance measures.

***Pure-tone testing.*** Pure-tone air-conduction thresholds provide a measure of hearing sensitivity as a function of frequency and intensity. When a hearing loss is present, the pure-tone air-conduction test indicates reduced hearing sensitivity. Pure tones are defined by their frequency (pitch) and intensity (loudness). NHLs for pure tones are defined by international standards. Brief-duration pure tones at selected frequencies are presented through earphones (air conduction) or a bone-conduction oscillator on the mastoid bone (bone conduction). The audiogram indicates the lowest intensity at which a person can hear at a given frequency and displays the degree (in decibels) and configuration (sensitivity loss as a function of frequency) of a hearing loss. Thresholds in audiology are usually defined as the lowest-intensity signal a person can detect approximately 50% of the time during a given number of presentations. Bone-conduction tests are intended to be a direct measure of inner-ear sensitivity. Pure-tone

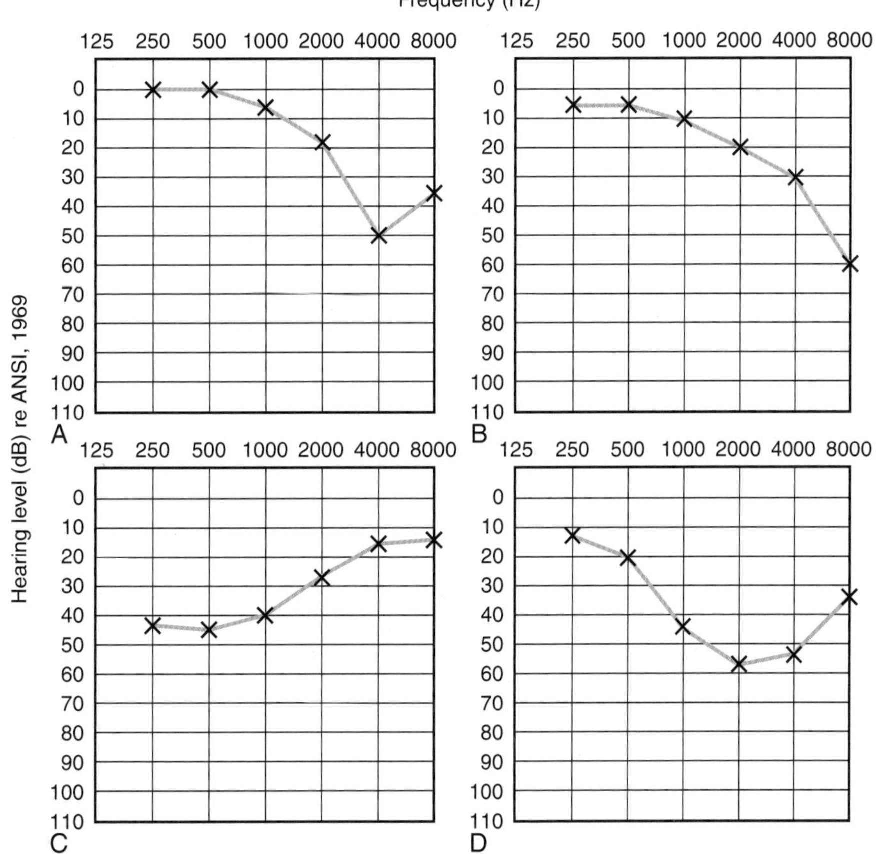


**Fig. 22.7 Audiograms Illustrating Four Characteristic Patterns of Sensorineural Hearing Loss.** A, Notched pattern of noise-induced hearing loss. B, Downward-sloping pattern of presbycusis. C, Low-frequency trough of the Meniere syndrome. D, Pattern of congenital hearing loss. *(From Baloh, R.W., 1998. Dizziness, Hearing Loss, and Tinnitus. F.A. Davis Company, Philadelphia, Figure 39, p. 95.)*

bone-conduction thresholds are obtained when a stimulus is presented by bone conduction.

Comparison of air- and bone-conduction thresholds establishes the type of hearing loss. Conductive loss results from disorders in the outer or middle ear. The audiogram of patients with SCD may also have an air/bone gap, even though there is no abnormality of the outer or middle ear. This exception results from the third window created by the dehiscence, which increases bone conduction. Sensorineural loss is associated with disorders of the cochlear and eighth cranial nerves. Mixed loss is a conductive and sensorineural loss coexisting in the same ear. Typical audiogram pure-tone patterns seen in patients with four common causes of sensorineural hearing loss are shown in Fig. 22.7.

***Speech testing.*** The speech reception threshold (SRT) is the lowest-intensity level at which the listener can identify or understand two-syllable spoken words 50% of the time. This test provides a check on the validity of the pure-tone test, as it should agree (±5 dB) with an average of the two best pure-tone thresholds in the speech range (500–2000 Hz). Once the SRT is determined, the audiologist measures speech discrimination ability by presenting a standardized list of 50 phonetically balanced monosyllabic words at volume levels approximately 35–40 dB above SRT. The speech discrimination score is reported as the percentage of words the subject can correctly repeat back to the audiologist.

Pure tone, SRT, and speech discrimination testing comprise the major routine measures of hearing. Considering these tests together can also provide localizing information. In patients with retrocochlear lesions, speech discrimination can be severely reduced even when pure-tone levels are normal or near normal, whereas in patients with cochlear lesions, discrimination tends to be proportional to the magnitude of hearing loss.

***Middle ear testing.*** Immittance measures assess the status of the middle ear and confirm information obtained in other tests of the battery. The basic immittance battery consists of tympanometry, static immittance, and acoustic reflex thresholds. Data from the tympanogram permit determination of the static compliance of the middle ear system. A result of "type A tympanogram" means that mobility of the tympanic membrane and middle ear structures is within normal limits.

***Acoustic reflex testing.*** Acoustic reflex measures the contraction of the stapedius muscle (innervated by the seventh cranial nerve) in response to a loud sound. The afferent limb of the reflex arch is through the auditory portion of the eighth cranial nerve, and the efferent portion of the reflex arch is through the seventh cranial nerve. The stapedius muscle normally contracts on both sides when an adequate sound is presented in one ear. As a result of contraction of the stapedius muscle, the tympanic membrane tightens or stiffens, thereby increasing the impedance or resistance of the eardrum to acoustic energy and resulting in a slight attenuation of sound transmitted through the middle ear system. In a normal subject, the acoustic reflex occurs in response to a pure tone between 70 and 100 dB above hearing level or when a white noise stimulus is presented at 65 dB above hearing level. Patients with conductive hearing loss due to middle ear pathology do not have reflexes because the lesion prevents a change in compliance with stapedius muscle contraction. With cochlear lesions, the acoustic reflex may be present at sensation levels less than 60 dB above the auditory pure-tone threshold, which is a form of abnormal loudness growth or recruitment. Cochlear hearing losses must be moderate or severe before the acoustic reflex is lost. In contrast, patients with retrocochlear or eighth cranial nerve lesions often have abnormal acoustic reflexes with normal hearing. The reflex may be absent or exhibit an elevated threshold or abnormal decay. Reflex decay is present if the amplitude of the reflex decreases to half its original size within 10 seconds of stimulation at 1000 Hz, 10 dB above reflex threshold. Observation of the pattern of acoustic reflex testing, along with hearing evaluation, permits inferences to support the presence of a cochlear, conductive, or retrocochlear lesion of the seventh or eighth cranial nerves.

**Evoked potentials.** Brainstem auditory evoked potentials are also known as *brainstem auditory evoked responses* or *auditory brainstem responses*. These physiological measures can be used to evaluate the auditory pathways from the ear to the upper brainstem. In addition, ABR threshold testing, although not a test of hearing sensitivity, may be used to determine behavioral threshold sensitivity in infants or uncooperative patients. The most consistent and reproducible potentials are a series of five submicrovolt waves that occur within 10 msec of an auditory stimulus. These potentials are recorded by averaging 1000–2000 responses from click stimuli by use of a computer system and amplifying the response. The anatomical correlates of the five reliable potentials have been only roughly approximated. Wave I of the brainstem auditory evoked potential is a manifestation of the APs of the eighth cranial nerve and is generated in the distal portion of the nerve adjacent to the cochlea. Wave II may be generated by the eighth cranial nerve or cochlear nuclei. Wave III is thought to be generated at the level of the superior olive, and waves IV and V are generated in the rostral pons or in the midbrain near the inferior colliculus. The complex anatomy of the central auditory pathway, with multiple crossing of fibers from the level of the cochlear nuclei to the inferior colliculus, makes the interpretation of central disturbances in the evoked responses difficult.

Abnormal interwave latencies (I–III or I–V) are seen with retrocochlear lesions (cerebellopontine angle tumors) and can even be seen when only mild or no hearing loss is detected on pure-tone audiometry. However, compared with brain MRI with gadolinium, the sensitivity of the ABR test is low, particularly with small tumors (Cueva, 2004). The least specific finding is the absence of all waves. This occurs in some patients with acoustic neuroma and in some with cerebellopontine angle meningiomas. Such patients often have marked hearing deficits with poor discrimination, suggesting retrocochlear disease. The absence of all waves should not occur unless a severe hearing loss exists.

**Other tests.** Electrocochleography is a method of recording the stimulus-related electrical potentials associated with the inner ear and auditory nerve, including the cochlear microphonic, summating potential (SP), and compound AP of the auditory nerve. The amplitude of the SP and compound AP is measured; an increased SP/AP ratio suggests increased endolymphatic pressure. This test is sometimes used in an attempt to distinguish Meniere disease from other causes of dizziness and hearing loss but lacks a rigorous analysis of its usefulness when there is clinical uncertainty.

## MANAGEMENT OF PATIENTS WITH VERTIGO

### Treatments of Specific Disorders

BPPV can be diagnosed and treated at the bedside, requiring no further treatment. Once repositioning is confirmed to be successful (see Fig. 22.4), patients are instructed to avoid head-hanging positions such as those used by dentists and hairdressers. These positions can cause the particles to reaccumulate in the posterior semicircular canals. For patients with HC-BPPV, the "barbeque" rotation, Gufoni maneuver, or forced prolonged position can be used (Fife et al., 2008; Kim et al., 2012a; Tirelli and Russolo, 2004; Vannucchi et al., 1997). The management of patients with vestibular neuritis is primarily symptomatic. Prolonged use of sedating medications to treat symptoms is not recommended, because it can slow down the vestibular compensation process. Randomized controlled trials have found that vestibular physical therapy improves outcomes in patients with unilateral vestibulopathy, though very few of these studies were specifically performed in a vestibular neuritis population (Hillier and McDonnell, 2011). A course of corticosteroids may improve recovery of the caloric response, but studies have not revealed evidence of symptomatic and functional improvements compared with placebo (Fishman et al., 2011; Ismail, 2019). The early treatment of Meniere disease continues to be a low-salt diet and diuretics, though the evidence to support these interventions is weak (Minor et al., 2004). Minimally invasive intratympanic gentamicin injections can be used for patients with debilitating symptoms. Surgical ablation of the labyrinth and sectioning of the vestibular nerve are other options. Patients with vestibular paroxysmia may benefit from carbamazepine, oxcarbamazepine, or gabapentin (Strupp, 2017). The third window in patients with SCD can be surgically repaired but is only recommended in patients debilitated by the symptoms (Ward, 2017).

Patients identified as having an infarction in the posterior fossa should be closely monitored, as herniation or recurrent stroke can occur. Patients with acute infarction presentations should be considered for tissue plasminogen activator (tPA) eligibility. Stenting of a symptomatic (i.e., TIA or nonsevere stroke) stenosis of the basilar artery or an intracranial vertebral artery has been shown to be substantially inferior to medical management (Chimowitz et al., 2011). Patients identified with demyelinating lesions may be candidates for disease-modifying treatments even after presenting with a clinically isolated syndrome. Patients with EA are typically highly responsive to treatment with acetazolamide or 4-aminopyridine, and there is anecdotal evidence of benefit of the use of acetazolamide in patients with BRV, a migraine equivalent. Patients with migraine-associated dizziness should first attempt to identify and eliminate triggers of their symptoms and also obtain adequate sleep and cardiovascular exercise. If these general measures are not adequate in controlling symptoms, a migraine prophylactic medication could be tried but clinical trials are lacking. Small trials of triptan medications in patients with migrainous vertigo suggest safety of these medicines but no significant benefit (Neuhauser et al., 2003). A phase II/III trial of rizatriptan for acute vestibular migraine has an estimated completion date of June 2019 (NCT02447991).

### Symptomatic Treatment of Vertigo

The commonly used antivertiginous drugs and their dosages are listed in Table 22.3 (Huppert et al., 2011). It is often difficult to predict which drugs or combinations of drugs will be most effective in individual patients, and large trials are lacking. In addition, the mechanisms of these medications are not specific to the vestibular system, so side effects are common. Anticholinergic or antihistamine drugs are usually effective in treating patients with mild to moderate vertigo, and sedation is minimal. If the patient is particularly bothered by nausea, the antiemetics prochlorperazine and metoclopramide can be effective and combined with other antivertiginous medications. For severe vertigo, sedation is often desirable, and drugs such as promethazine and diazepam are particularly useful, though prolonged use is not recommended.

**TABLE 22.3 Medical Therapy for Symptomatic Vertigo***

| Class | Dosage† |
|---|---|
| **Antihistamines** | |
| Meclizine | 25 mg PO q 4–6 h |
| Dimenhydrinate | 50 mg PO or IM q 4–6 h, or 100 mg suppository q 8 h |
| Promethazine | 25–50 mg PO or IM or as a suppository q 4–6 h |
| **Anticholinergic Agent** | |
| Scopolamine | 0.2 mg PO q 4–6 h, or 0.5 mg transdermally q 3 days |
| **Benzodiazepines** | |
| Diazepam | 5 or 10 mg PO, IM, IV q 4–6 h |
| Lorazepam | 0.5–2 mg PO, IM, IV q 6–8 h |
| **Phenothiazine** | |
| Prochlorperazine | 5 or 10 mg PO or IM q 6 h, or 25 mg suppository q 12 h |
| **Benzamide** | |
| Metoclopramide | 5 or 10 mg PO, IM, or IV q 4–6 h |

*IM*, Intramuscular; *IV*, intravenous; *PO*, oral.
**Huppert, D., Strupp, M., Muckter, H., et al., 2011. Which medication do I need to manage dizzy patients? Acta Otolaryngol 131, 228–241.*
†Usual adult starting dosage; maintenance dosage can be increased by a factor of 2–3. The most common side effect is drowsiness.

## MANAGEMENT OF PATIENTS WITH HEARING LOSS AND TINNITUS

Hearing aids continue to become more effective and better designed for patient comfort and acceptance, although cost remains the major limiting factor in their more widespread use. Cochlear implants have revolutionized the approach to treatment of profound sensorineural loss. The management of tinnitus remains difficult, and specific treatments are often ineffective. Patients with a specific cause for the problem usually have the most potential for improvement. Idiopathic high-pitched tinnitus may diminish with avoidance of caffeine, other stimulants, and alcohol. A masking device used in quiet environments may also provide some relief. For patients with intolerable idiopathic tinnitus, a trial of a tricyclic amine antidepressant may be of benefit.

*The complete reference list is available online at https://expertconsult.inkling.com/.* 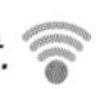

# 23

# Cerebellar Ataxia

*Sheng-Han Kuo, Chih-Chun Lin, Tetsuo Ashizawa*

## OUTLINE



The cerebellum, a unique brain structure with distinctly organized neuronal circuits, is critical for motor and cognitive functions. The cerebellum has dense neuronal connections with almost all regions of the cerebral cortex and brainstem, and can serve as a "hub" to regulate the many brain functions. While cerebellar dysfunction has been implicated in tremor, dystonia, and autism, the prototypical disorder of the cerebellum is cerebellar ataxia, a clinical sign that can have a variety of causes, including nutritional deficiency, immunological dysfunction, vascular and degenerative etiologies, and genetic mutations. Searching for genetic causes for ataxia is particularly relevant because the genetic mutations for ataxia often have very high penetrance; therefore, genetic identification for cerebellar ataxia is often diagnostic. In addition, there are many genetic mutations associated with cerebellar ataxia, which indicates that these genetic mutations converge at the dysfunction of the cerebellar circuitry, highlighting the complex biological processes required to maintain the integrity of this brain structure. The diagnosis of cerebellar ataxia is often regarded as very complicated by neurologists. To simplify and streamline the search for the causes of cerebellar ataxia, this chapter aims to provide a step-by-step approach. In brief, the first step is to recognize the signs and symptoms for ataxia and associated neurological features. The second step is to search for the structural, nutritional, and immunological causes of ataxia. If genetic ataxias are considered, repeat expansions needed to be determined before genetic sequencing for mutations because repeat expansion–associated ataxias are much more common, and more difficult to detect using conventional sequencing technologies. Finally, degenerative etiologies are likely the causes for ataxia onset at an old age. Of note, a significant portion of ataxia patients might eventually have no identifiable causes during life; these patients usually follow a slowly progressive clinical course. Complex environmental and genetic interactions, epigenetic alterations, or regional genetic somatic mosaicism might explain some of these cases; these remain underexplored areas in cerebellar ataxia.

This chapter describes clinical features, imaging findings, and genetics for the differential diagnoses of cerebellar ataxia, providing a guide for clinicians. However, the detailed genetic diagnosis of cerebellar ataxia can be very extensive, and is beyond the scope of this chapter. Instead, this chapter only includes the common causes of genetic ataxia.

## FUNCTION OF THE CEREBELLUM

The motor part of the cerebellum receives sensory inputs from the outside environment to calculate the proper movements in response. These sensory inputs could be either from tactile sensory nerves or from the vestibular system; therefore, the dysfunction of these systems is sometimes difficult to distinguish from the primary problems of the cerebellum. The current understanding of how the cerebellum integrates sensorimotor information is based on Marr-Albus-Ito theory, in which the cerebellum can function as a neuronal learning machine (Boyden et al., 2004). This theory is based on the physiological recording and anatomical connections of the cerebellar circuitry that are capable of altering synaptic strength in responses to motor learning. Dysfunction of the cerebellar circuitry thus results in erroneous motor

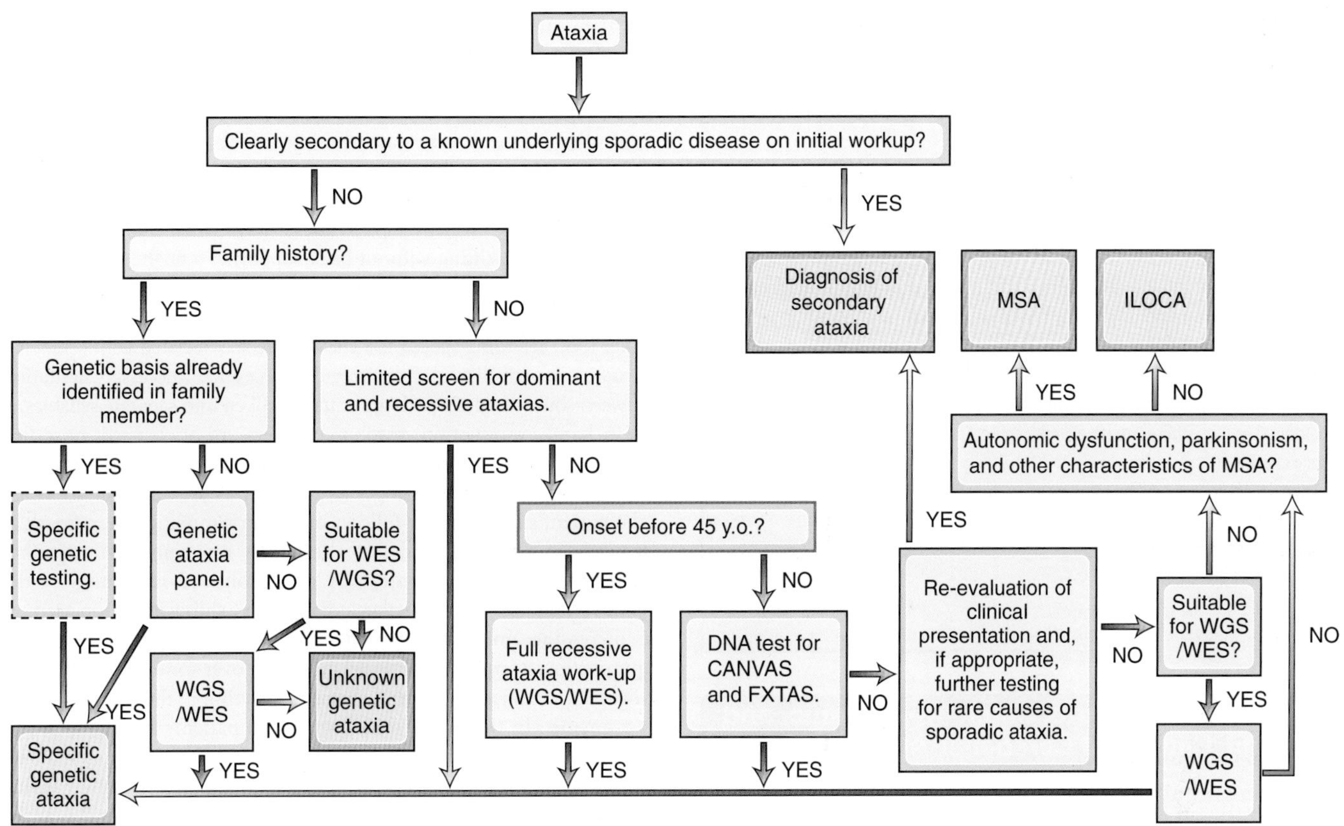


**Fig. 23.1 The Diagnostic Workflow for Cerebellar Ataxia.** *AD,* Autosomal dominant; *AR,* autosomal recessive; *CANVAS,* cerebellar ataxia, neuropathy, vestibular areflexia syndrome; *Cbl,* cerebellum; *FA,* Friedreich ataxia; *FXTAS,* fragile X-associated tremor and ataxia syndrome; *GAD,* glutamate decarboxylase; *ILOCA,* idiopathic late-onset cerebellar ataxia; *MSA,* multiple system atrophy; *RBD,* rapid eye movement behavior disorder; *SCA,* spinocerebellar ataxia; *WES,* whole exome sequencing; *WGS,* whole genome sequencing. (*Modified from* Continuum, 2019.)

learning and improper motor predictions and commands, leading to symptoms of ataxia and/or tremor.

The same principles that hold for the motor cerebellum can be applied to nonmotor regions of the cerebellum, which have many connections to frontal, parietal, and temporal areas of the cerebral cortex. Therefore, dysfunction of the nonmotor cerebellum has been postulated to cause inappropriate prediction of emotional and cognitive responses; this is known as cerebellar cognitive affective syndrome (Schmahmann and Sherman, 1998). Further studies in physiology and anatomy of the cerebellum will provide a more comprehensive understanding of cerebellar function and will accelerate therapy development for cerebellar ataxia.

## SIGNS AND SYMPTOMS FOR CEREBELLAR ATAXIA

Recognizing the early symptoms of cerebellar ataxia is an important first step in establishing the symptom onset and the chronicity of the disease. Table 23.1 lists the common early symptoms of cerebellar ataxia. The first symptom is usually gait difficulty (Luo et al., 2017), which can manifest as "walking as if one is drunk," difficulty in running, turning, walking on high heels, and walking up or down stairs without holding on to the railings. These symptoms could be intermittent in the very early stage and patients might experience these symptoms only after ingestion of small amount of alcohol. Later on, these symptoms could become constant. Beyond abnormal gait, slurred speech, from occasional word pronunciation difficulty to persistent speech problems, is often encountered.

Tremor of the hands is also commonly experienced by patients with ataxia (Gan et al., 2017). Clumsiness and bad handwriting are sometimes described by patients. Dizziness (vertiginous or nonvertiginous) is another symptom associated with cerebellar ataxia. Double vision, particularly when patients turn their heads quickly, is also another common symptom.

In the later stages of cerebellar ataxia, patients might experience falls, swallowing difficulty, blurry vision, and loss of hand dexterity in performing daily activities such as dressing and using utensils.

After establishing the symptoms of cerebellar ataxia, the next step is to determine the chronicity of these symptoms (acute vs. subacute vs. chronic) and the rate of progression, which will be important for the differential diagnosis (Table 23.2). In acute-onset cerebellar ataxia, infectious, vascular, and toxic causes need to be considered. For subacute-onset cerebellar ataxia, immune-mediated etiology would be on top of the differential diagnoses. Genetic and degenerative cerebellar ataxias usually have insidious onset with progressive clinical courses. Another category is episodic cerebellar ataxia, which encompasses various causes (see Table 23.2).

Besides recognizing the symptoms of cerebellar ataxia, identification of associated neurological signs is equally important, because these additional symptoms can often provide diagnostic clues. The commonly associated symptoms are peripheral neuropathy, parkinsonism, dystonia, tremor, sleep dysfunction, autonomic symptoms, seizures, and hearing loss.

## NEUROLOGICAL EXAMINATION OF CEREBELLAR ATAXIA

The neurological examination of cerebellar ataxia constitutes five domains: eyes, speech, hands, legs, and gait. Scale for Assessment and Rating of Ataxia (SARA) is a commonly used clinical scale to assess different domains of cerebellar ataxia, except for the eye movements (Schmitz-Hubsch et al., 2006). The SARA scale encompasses the

**TABLE 23.1 Signs and Symptoms for Cerebellar Ataxia**

| Early Signs and Symptoms |
|---|
| Difficulty in running |
| Difficulty in walking |
| Difficulty in turning |
| Difficulty in walking in high heels |
| Difficulty in walking up and down stairs without holding on to the railings |
| Sensitive to alcohol; balance become worse after a small amount of alcohol |
| Slurred speech; occasionally difficult to be understood |
| Clumsiness in handwriting |
| Dizziness |
| Double vision, particularly when turning head quickly |
| Incidental finding of cerebellar atrophy on neuroimaging studies |
| Hand tremor |
| **Late Signs and Symptoms** |
| Falls |
| Swallowing difficulty |
| Blurry vision |
| Clumsiness in hands, difficulty in dressing and using utensils |

**TABLE 23.2 Acute, Subacute, Chronic, and Episodic Causes of Cerebellar Ataxia**

| Acute Causes of Cerebellar Ataxia (Minutes to Few Days) |
|---|
| Vascular causes: ischemic or hemorrhagic cerebellar strokes |
| Alcohol intoxication |
| Toxins (mercury, thallium, toluene, solvents) |
| Medication-related (phenytoin, carbamazepine, phenobarbital, lithium) |
| Multiple sclerosis |
| Meningitis, particularly basilar meningitis |
| Viral cerebellitis |
| Cerebellar abscess |
| Wernicke encephalopathy/thiamine deficiency |
| **Subacute Causes of Cerebellar Ataxia (Weeks to Months)** |
| Paraneoplastic cerebellar degeneration |
| Brain tumors |
| Creutzfeldt-Jakob disease |
| Superficial siderosis |
| Anti-GAD ataxia* |
| Tuberculosis meningitis |
| **Chronic Causes of Cerebellar Ataxia (Months to Years)** |
| Ataxia associated with gluten sensitivity |
| Genetic ataxia |
| Mitochondrial disease |
| Multiple system atrophy |
| Idiopathic late-onset cerebellar ataxia |
| **Episodic Causes of Cerebellar Ataxia** |
| Genetic episodic ataxia |
| Psychogenic ataxia |
| Mitochondrial disease |
| Multiple sclerosis |

**GAD*, Glutamate decarboxylase.

following: (1) gait, (2) stance, (3) sitting, (4) speech, (5) finger chase, (6) nose-finger, (7) fast alternating hand movements, and (8) heel-shin slide. Video 23.1 demonstrates a complete examination of the SARA scale. For the gait examination, ataxia patients are asked to walk normally. Variable stride length and/or veering toward one side are common gait patterns in the early stage of cerebellar ataxia. A wide-based gait usually develops as a compensatory mechanism in the moderate and severe stage of cerebellar ataxia (Video 23.2). In other words, depending on the disease stage and individual compensatory strategy, the ataxic gait might differ. To detect subtle difficulty in gait, observing patients running or walking up or down stairs can be useful.

Ataxia patients usually have truncal sways while standing still and sometimes when sitting without back support. To further identify subtle ataxia in the stance examination, patients are asked to stand with feet together, to stand on tandem stance, to stand on either foot, or to hop on either foot. Scanning speech is a classic speech associated with cerebellar ataxia, slow, with characteristic irregular force and unnecessary hesitation between some words. Words are usually broken into separate syllables.

In hand examination, three maneuvers are often used: nose-finger tests (the patient points repeatedly with his index finger from his nose to examiner's index finger as precisely as possible), finger chase (the patient's index finger follows examiner's moving index finger as precisely as possible), and fast alternating movements (the patient performs repetitive alternation of pronation and supination of the hand). Patients with cerebellar ataxia often exhibit intention tremor, as increasing amplitude of oscillatory movements when voluntarily approaching a target, in the finger-nose test; over- or undershoot in the finger chase test; and slow and abnormal rhythm in the fast alternating movements. In the leg examination, ataxia patients are instructed to lift one leg, point with the heel to the opposite knee, and slide down along the shin to the ankle. Ataxia patients often have the heel falling off the shin during the slide. Functionally, one can consider this as the leg equivalent of the nose-finger test.

In patients with cerebellar ataxia, abnormal eye movements are common and sometimes can be diagnostic (Video 23.3). Neurologists should assess eyes in the fixation position, during smooth pursuit, and in saccadic movements. Certain eye movement abnormalities might be associated with specific types of ataxias: for example (1) square-wave jerks (saccadic intrusion in the fixed gaze) in Friedreich ataxia, (2) end-gaze nystagmus in many types of ataxia, (3) hypo- or hypermetric saccades, also in many types of ataxia, (4) breakdown of smooth pursuit (saccadic pursuit) in spinocerebellar ataxia type 3 (SCA3), (5) slow saccades in SCA2 (Video 23.4), (6) ophthalmoplegia/ophthalmoparesis in sensory axonal neuropathy with dysarthria and ophthalmoplegia (SANDO) syndrome with DNA polymerase gamma-1 (*POLG*) mutations, (7) ptosis in SANDO syndrome and mitochondrial ataxia, and (8) impaired vertical saccades in Niemann-Pick type C.

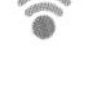

Many mimickers resemble cerebellar ataxia or present with overlapping symptoms (Table 23.3). As such, neurological examinations should also assess the associated signs, such as tremor, dystonia, myoclonus, parkinsonism, sensory neuropathy, muscle weakness, and pyramidal signs. Note that sensory neuropathy could be a predominant feature in certain ataxia syndromes in the early stage of the disease, such as Friedreich ataxia and *POLG*-ataxia. Detailed physical examination sometimes can yield additional information for the diagnosis, such as telangiectasia for ataxia telangiectasia, splenomegaly for Niemann-Pick type C, scoliosis and pes cavus for Friedreich ataxia.

## LABORATORY TESTS FOR CEREBELLAR ATAXIA

Serum and cerebrospinal fluid (CSF) biomarkers can be useful in diagnosing nutritional, immune-mediated, and autosomal recessive ataxia with metabolic dysfunction (certain forms of the latter). Serum levels of vitamin $B_1$, $B_{12}$, and E should be tested for deficiency. Vitamin $B_1$ deficiency causes Wernicke encephalopathy and can occur in a variety of clinical settings, such as cancer and malnutrition, besides alcoholism (Kuo et al., 2009). Vitamin E deficiency is relatively rare and can occur

**TABLE 23.3 Differential Diagnosis and Conditions That Might Mimic Cerebellar Ataxia**

| |
|---|
| Sensory neuropathy |
| Parkinsonism |
| Magnetic gait/normal-pressure hydrocephalus |
| Vestibular problems |
| Upper motor neuron symptoms/spasticity |
| Muscle weakness |
| Orthopedic issues |
| Pain-related gait disturbance |

in two forms of recessive ataxia: ataxia with vitamin E deficiency and abetalipoproteinemia.

Serum autoantibodies can indicate specific immune-mediated causes of ataxia, such as ataxia associated with anti-glutamate acid decarboxylase (GAD) antibodies, anti-thyroperoxidase (TPO) antibodies (for steroid-responsive encephalopathy), paraneoplastic antibodies, anti-gliadin and anti-tissue transglutaminase antibodies (for gluten ataxia). Serum antibody levels are often diagnostic, especially when high levels of antibodies are present; occasionally, these autoantibodies can be only be detected in the CSF. Therefore, a lumbar puncture is warranted when immune-mediated ataxia is suspected, especially in cases with subacute onset of ataxia without marked cerebellar atrophy in the imaging studies. Infectious and inflammatory etiologies should also be examined in the CSF.

CSF analysis can provide additional information; for instance, a high protein 14-3-3 level can be seen in Creutzfeldt-Jakob disease (CJD), whereas a low CSF glucose level might point toward ataxia with glucose transporter type 1 deficiency.

Serum metabolic biomarkers sometimes can be helpful in identifying several forms of autosomal recessive ataxia. Ataxia telangectasia and ataxia with oculomotor apraxia type 2 both have elevated serum alpha fetoprotein levels, and cerebrotendinous xanthomatosis can have elevated blood cholestanol levels.

## NEUROIMAGING FOR CEREBELLAR ATAXIA

Brain magnetic resonance imaging (MRI) should be obtained in ataxia patients. This enables visualization of demyelinating, vascular, and structural causes for ataxia, such as multiple sclerosis, brain tumors, abscess, and ischemic or hemorrhagic strokes. Cerebellar cortical atrophy is the most common finding, and clinicians should assess the degree of the cerebellar atrophy in different cerebellar lobules and in vermis, paravermis, and hemisphere (Fig. 23.2, *A–C*). Prominent CSF space between cerebellar folia indicates the underlying degeneration. An enlarged fourth ventricle is often associated with cerebellar atrophy (see Fig. 23.2, *D*). The cerebellum is divided into motor (predominantly anterior) and nonmotor (predominantly posterior) regions (Stoodley and Schmahmann, 2010). Therefore, clinicians should pay special attention to patients with prominent atrophy in the posterior lobules of the cerebellum and assess their cognitive dysfunction and emotional liability. In addition, speech and gait ataxia is associated with vermal atrophy, whereas appendicular ataxia is associated with paravermal atrophy. As mentioned above, certain forms of ataxia have predominant sensory neuropathy in the early stage (e.g., Friedreich ataxia, ataxia with vitamin E deficiency and *POLG*-ataxia); therefore, there might be no obvious cerebellar atrophy on the brain MRI.

Clinicians should also look for specific changes associated with certain forms of cerebellar ataxia. Fragile X–associated tremor and ataxia syndrome has T2-hyperintensity in the bilateral middle cerebellar peduncles (see Fig. 23.2, *E*). Wernicke encephalopathy has T2 hyperintensity in the mamillary bodies, periaqueductal gray, and paraventricular thalamus (Kuo et al., 2009). and adult-onset Alexander disease can have prominent subcortical white matter changes. *POLG*-ataxia, adult-onset Alexander disease, and ataxia with gluten sensitivity can have T2 hyperintensity in the bilateral inferior olivary nucleus (see Fig. 23.2, *F*). Multiple system atrophy can have either a hot-cross-bun sign (a T2 hyperintense cross sign in the pons, associated with the cerebellar type, Fig. 23.2, *G*) or linear T2 hyperintensity along the outer rim of the striatum (associated with the parkinsonism type, Fig. 23.2, *H*). Superficial siderosis has hypointensity along the surface of the cerebellum and brainstem in the gradient echo sequence (GRE; see Fig. 23.2, *I*). CJD has cortical ribboning on the diffusion-weighted imaging (DWI). While the presence of these features can help with the diagnosis, the absence of these features does not exclude these causes of cerebellar ataxia.

In addition to brain MRI, a dopamine transporter scan can be used to test the involvement of the dopamine system, which can be seen in multiple system atrophy.

## OTHER DIAGNOSTIC TESTS FOR ATAXIA

In addition to brain imaging studies, physiological measures can help to identify the involvement of additional systems. Autonomic nervous tests for orthostatic hypotension and/or urinary disturbance together with a sleep study to demonstrate rapid eye movement behavior disorder suggest the diagnosis of MSA. Electromyography and conduction studies can assess the associated motor-sensory neuropathy. In patients with ataxia and sensory neuropathy, the diagnosis of *POLG*-ataxia can be supported by muscle biopsy, demonstrating increased succinate dehydrogenase (SDH) expression as the result of mitochondrial proliferation (Fig. 23.3, *A*). In patients with CJD, an electroencephalogram may show typical periodic sharp-wave complexes, and brain biopsy may demonstrate spongiform changes (see Fig. 23.3, *B*).

## ACQUIRED CAUSES FOR ATAXIA

Before one starts searching for genetic causes of cerebellar ataxia in a patient, it is important to identify acquired causes of ataxias, as some of them are potentially treatable or partially reversible, in contrast to genetic cerebellar ataxias. Common acquired causes of ataxias include metabolic (nutrition, toxins), vascular insults (ischemic stroke, bleed), neoplasms, infections, and autoimmune reactions (Table 23.4).

### Nutritional

#### Vitamin $B_1$/Thiamine

Thiamine deficiency can lead to Wernicke encephalopathy, which may present with altered mental status, ophthalmoplegia, and ataxia (Zubaran et al., 1997). While thiamine deficiency is frequently associated with chronic alcohol use, there is evidence that thiamine deficiency can cause cerebellar dysfunction independent of alcohol toxicity (Collins and Converse, 1970). Proposed mechanisms of thiamine-deficiency-induced ataxia include tissue edema, altered blood-brain barrier integrity, impaired energy metabolism, reduced thiamine-utilizing enzymes in cerebellum and subsequent loss of amino acids, lactic acidosis, excitotoxicity, mitochondrial uncoupling, oxidative stress, reactive microglia, apoptosis, and microvascular damage (Mulholland, 2006).

#### Vitamin E ($\alpha$-Tocopherol)

Acquired vitamin E ($\alpha$-tocopherol) deficiency can occur in patients with insufficient intake or poor absorption. Vitamin E deficiency can also be hereditary, stemming from mutations in the gene for $\alpha$-tocopherol

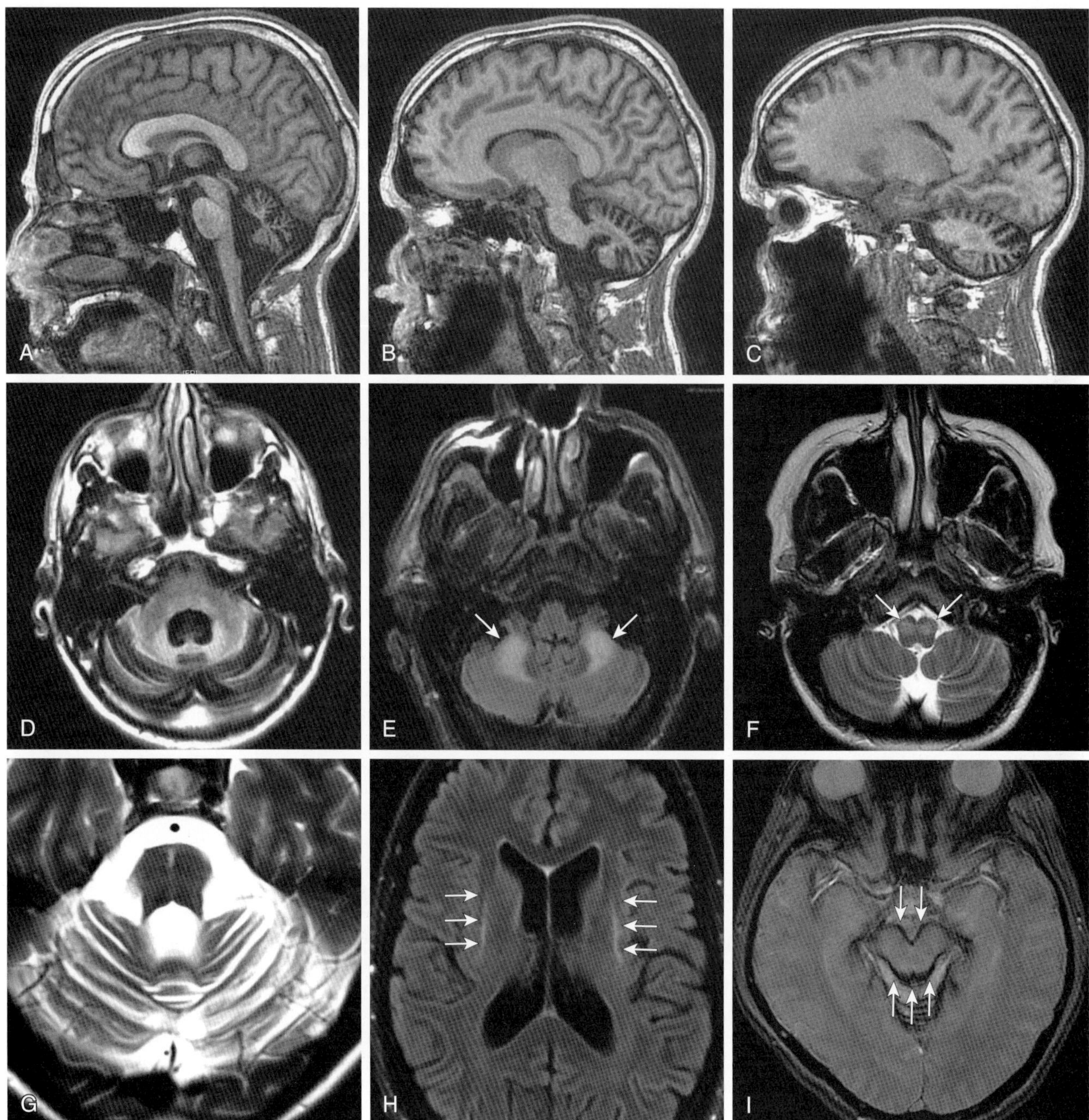


**Fig. 23.2** Sagittal T1 brain magnetic resonance imaging (MRI) demonstrates cerebellar atrophy in a patient with idiopathic late onset cerebellar ataxia. There is prominent cerebellar foliation and sulci in the vermis (**A**), paravermis (**B**), and hemisphere (**C**). Prominent sulci also noted in the axial fluid-attenuated inversion recovery (FLAIR) sequence in the same individual (**D**). T2 sequence of the axial brain MRI demonstrates hyperintensity in the bilateral cerebellar peduncles in a patient with fragile X–associated tremor and ataxia syndrome (*arrows*, **E**). T2 sequence of the axial brain MRI demonstrates hyperintensity in the bilateral inferior olivary nuclei in a patient with *POLG*-ataxia (*arrows*, **F**). T2 sequence of the axial brain MRI shows the hyperintensity of a cross sign in the pons (hot-cross-bun sign) in a patient with multiple system atrophy (**G**). Another patient with multiple system atrophy has bilateral linear hyperintensity in the outer rim of the striatum in the FLAIR sequence (*arrows*, **H**). Gradient echo sequence (GRE) of the axial brain MRI demonstrates linear hypointensity surrounding the brainstem in a patient with superficial siderosis (*arrows*, **I**).

transfer protein in ataxia with vitamin E deficiency or mutations in the *MTTP* gene in abetalipoproteinemia (Harding et al., 1985; Ouahchi et al., 1995). Patients typically present with progressive cerebellar ataxia with limb and gait changes, titubation of the head, and evidence of peripheral neuropathy. Ataxia with vitamin E deficiency and abetalipoproteinemia are further discussed under genetic ataxias (see below).

## Autoimmune

### Paraneoplastic Cerebellar Degenerations

Paraneoplastic cerebellar degenerations (PCDs) are the most frequently encountered paraneoplastic neurological syndrome (around 24.3%; Giometto et al., 2010). Patients with PCDs usually present with a subacute-onset cerebellar syndrome over several months (Shams'ili

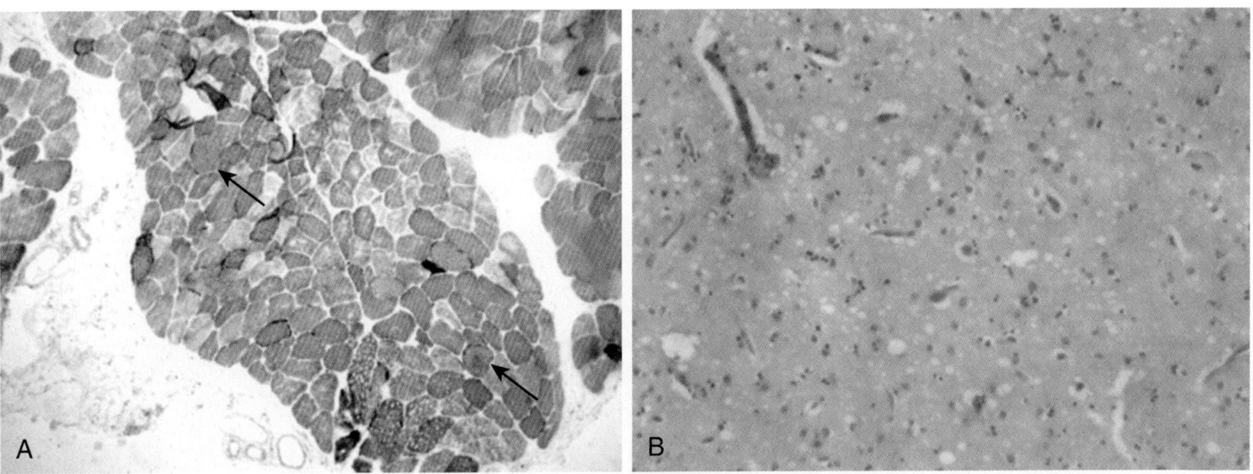


**Fig. 23.3** Muscle biopsy demonstrates mitochondrial dysfunction in a patient with *POLG*-ataxia. Combined succinate dehydrogenase (SDH) *(blue)* and cytochrome *c* oxidase (COX) *(brown)* stain shows COX-negative fibers with strong SDH expression, indicating that these muscle fibers have respiratory chain defects with corresponding mitochondrial proliferation as a compensatory response (*arrows*, **A**). *(Modified from Kuo et al., 2017. Neurology 89, e1–e5.)* Postmortem examination of the basal ganglia in a case of Creutzfeldt-Jakob disease demonstrates spongiform changes (**B**).

**TABLE 23.4 Acquired Causes of Ataxia**

| Entity | Diagnostic Process |
|---|---|
| **Vascular Disease** | History of strokes, imaging |
| Hypoxic encephalopathy | History of hypoxic episodes |
| Demyelinating disease | Remitting and relapsing episodes, imaging, CSF analysis |
| Tumors in the posterior fossa | Imaging |
| Cranio-vertebral junction anomalies | Imaging |
| **Toxic Disorders** | History |
| Alcohol | |
| Chemotherapy (5-fluorouracil, ara-C, methotrexate) | |
| Metals (mercury, bismuth, lithium, lead) | |
| Solvents (toluene) | |
| Anticonvulsants (phenytoin) | |
| **Infectious/Inflammatory Disease** | History, imaging, serology, CSF analysis |
| Acute cerebellar ataxia of childhood, acute cerebellitis | History, imaging, CSF analysis |
| Post-infectious | Imaging, CSF analysis |
| Bickerstaff encephalitis | Serology |
| Human immunodeficiency virus (HIV) | CSF 14-3-3, imaging, electroencephalogram, biopsy |
| Creutzfeldt-Jakob disease (CJD) | Small intestine biopsy |
| Whipple disease | |
| **Autoimmune:** | Serology |
| Paraneoplastic | Anti-Hu, anti-Yo, anti-Ri, others |
| Gluten sensitivity | Anti-gliadin, anti-tissue transglutaminase |
| Anti-GAD ataxia | Anti-GAD |
| Anti-GluRδ2 ataxia | Anti-GluRδ2 |
| Superficial siderosis | Imaging |
| **Nutritional:** | Blood |
| Vitamin $B_1$ deficiency | Vitamin $B_1$ level |
| Vitamin $B_{12}$ deficiency | Vitamin $B_{12}$ level |
| Vitamin E deficiency | Vitamin E level |

*CSF*, Cerebrospinal fluid; *GAD*, glutamate decarboxylase.

et al., 2003). Neurological symptoms may precede the diagnosis of the neoplasm (Ducray et al., 2014; Shams'ili et al., 2003). Brain MRI typically demonstrates cerebellar atrophy, although it may be normal at an early stage (de Andres et al., 2006; Mitoma et al., 2017). Onconeural antibodies associated with PCDs include anti-Yo, anti-Hu, anti-Ma, anti-Ri, anti-VGCC, anti-CV2/CRMP5, anti-Tr/DNER, and anti-mGluR1 (Ducray et al., 2014; Shams'ili et al., 2003). The most common cancers associated with PCDs are small-cell lung cancer, ovarian

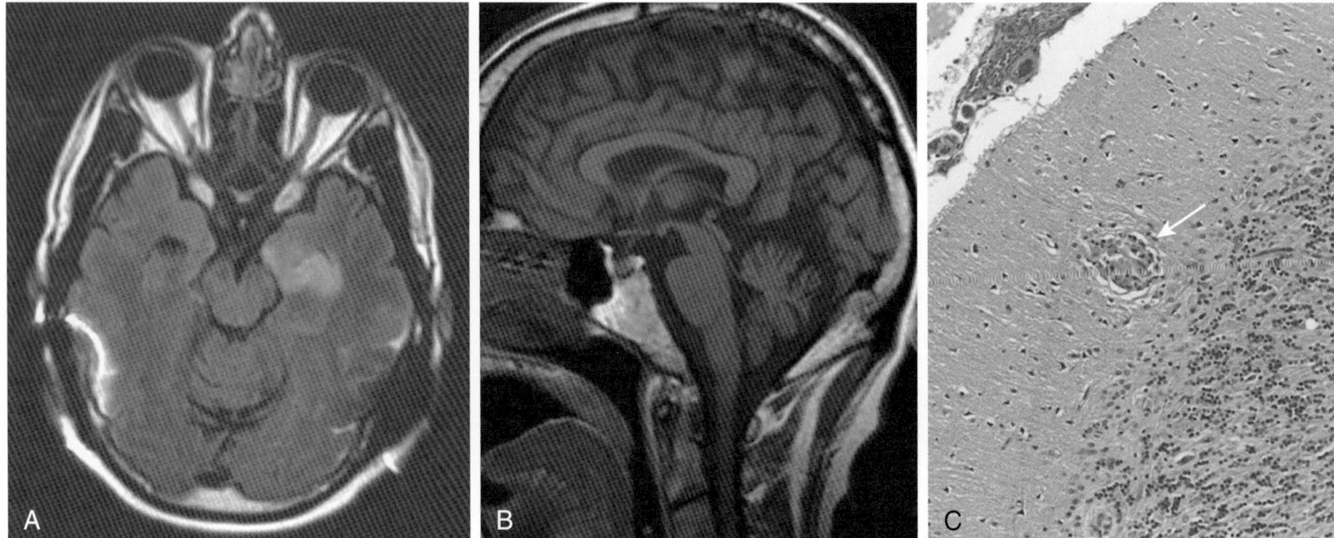


**Fig. 23.4** A 51-year-old man with bilateral hearing loss and progressive ataxia. Brain magnetic resonance imaging (MRI) demonstrates hyperintensity in the left medial temporal region on an axial fluid-attenuated inversion recovery (FLAIR) sequence (**A**) and cerebellar atrophy on a sagittal T1 sequence (**B**). Postmortem examination shows the granuloma in the cerebellar cortex (**C**), confirming the diagnosis of neurosarcoidosis.

tumor, breast cancer, and Hodgkin lymphoma (Ducray et al., 2014; Shams'ili et al., 2003). The role of onconeural antibodies is still unclear as most of the targets are intracellular antigens, which limits antibody accessibility (Mitoma et al., 2017). The mainstream treatment is to identify and treat underlying cancer. However, the response to either immunotherapy or to the tumor itself has been poor (Hoffmann et al., 2008; Shams'ili et al., 2003).

### Neurosarcoidosis

Sarcoidosis is a chronic inflammatory disease with formation of non-caseating granulomas. About 3%–10% of patients with sarcoid have involvement of the central nervous system (CNS; Ungprasert and Matteson, 2017). Cerebellar symptoms arise when the cerebellum or its in- or outflow tracts are affected by neurosarcoid. The brain MRI typically shows hyperintensity changes on fluid-attenuated inversion recovery (FLAIR) images (Fig. 23.4, *A*). In chronic cases, cerebellar atrophy may be seen (see Fig. 23.4, *B*). Confirmation of diagnosis requires biopsy demonstrating non-caseating granulomas (see Fig. 23.4, *C*).

### Gluten-Sensitive Ataxia

Gluten-sensitive ataxia was initially categorized as part of the extra-intestinal manifestation of celiac disease (gluten-sensitive enteropathy), but increasing evidence suggests that these and gluten-sensitivity with skin involvement (dermatitis herpetiformis) may all belong to the spectrum of "gluten sensitivity" (Hadjivassiliou et al., 2003). Patients with gluten-sensitive ataxia manifest with progressive ataxia, with limb, truncal, and ocular involvement that worsens slowly over the years (Hadjivassiliou et al., 2003). Thirteen percent of the patients have gastrointestinal symptoms, suggesting an overlapping syndrome with gluten-sensitive enteropathy. Similar to celiac disease, adopting a gluten-free diet may improve the symptoms of gluten-sensitive ataxia (Hadjivassiliou et al., 2003a, 2003b, 2013). In addition to anti-gliadin antibodies found in patients with gluten sensitivity, antibodies against transglutaminase 6 (anti-TG6) are recently found to be associated with gluten-sensitive ataxia (Hadjivassiliou et al., 2008). Injection of antibodies with reactivity to TG2 and TG6 to mice can cause ataxia, suggesting that anti-TG6 may have a pathogenic role (Boscolo et al., 2010).

### Anti-Glutamic Acid Decarboxylase Ataxia

Antibodies against GAD, the rate-limiting enzyme for γ-aminobutyric acid (GABA) synthesis, are associated with neurological conditions including stiff person syndrome, limbic encephalitis, epilepsy, and cerebellar ataxia (Saiz et al., 2008). Most of the patients with cerebellar ataxia with anti-GAD antibodies present with an insidious-onset gait and limb ataxia, dysarthria, and nystagmus. Peripheral neuropathy or rigidity in the leg may also be seen (Honnorat et al., 2001). It is more commonly seen in women (80%–90%; Mitoma et al., 2017). MRI may show cerebellar atrophy (Honnorat et al., 2001). The pathogenic role of anti-GAD antibody is still unclear, although rats infused with anti-GAD antibodies seem to have more irregular gait (Manto et al., 2015). In patients with subacute-onset anti-GAD ataxia treated with intravenous immunoglobulin (IVIG) with corticosteroid or other immunosuppressors, 35% showed improvement (Arino et al., 2014).

### Steroid-Responsive Encephalopathy Associated with Autoimmune Thyroiditis

Steroid-responsive encephalopathy associated with autoimmune thyroiditis (SREAT) is also called Hashimoto encephalopathy. It is an encephalopathy associated with antithyroid antibodies (e.g., antithyroperoxidase and antithyroglobulin antibodies; Castillo et al., 2006). The role of antithyroid antibodies is still unclear, and there is still debate whether its presence is coincidental. Another antibody associated with SREAT is anti-NAE, an antibody against the N-terminus of α-enolase, and its pathogenic role is again undetermined (Yoneda et al., 2007). Patients may present with a wide range of neuropsychiatric symptoms, including altered mental status, psychosis, cognitive impairment, seizure, cerebellar ataxia, and other involuntary movements (Brain et al., 1966; Shaw et al., 1991).

### Acute Cerebellitis

Acute cerebellitis is an inflammatory process involving the cerebellum, affecting children more than adults. Clinical presentation includes ataxia, nausea, vomiting, headache, dysarthria, fever, nystagmus, vertigo, and altered mental status. The onset of symptoms is typically preceded by a viral infection or recent vaccination (Connolly et al., 1994; De Bruecker et al., 2004; van der Maas et al., 2009). The delayed onset of ataxia after a prodromal infection and the specific targeting of cerebellum suggest acute cerebellitis is more likely an immune-mediated inflammatory disorder rather than the result of a direct infection to the cerebellum. The infectious agent may be detected by polymerase chain reaction (PCR) or by elevated serum immunoglobulin M (IgM) titer against an organism, but in most cases, the etiology was never identified. Organisms associated with acute cerebellitis include varicella zoster virus, Epstein-Barr virus, mumps, influenza, herpes simplex virus 7, cytomegalovirus, Coxsackie virus, enterovirus, and *Mycoplasma pneumoniae* (Desai and Mitchell, 2012; Sawaishi and Takada, 2002; Van Samkar et al., 2017). The prognosis is usually self-limiting, but severe cases may sustain permanent neurological deficits.

### Bickerstaff Encephalitis

Bickerstaff encephalitis is characterized by progressive ophthalmoplegia, ataxia, and altered consciousness or hyperreflexia (Bickerstaff and Cloake, 1951). Bickerstaff encephalitis is similar to Fisher syndrome, which consists of ophthalmoplegia, ataxia, and areflexia (Fisher, 1956). Both are associated with elevated serum anti-GQ1b antibodies (Chiba et al., 1992; Yuki et al., 1993), and now the two are considered entities that are in the same spectrum. Patients with Bickerstaff encephalitis may have hyperintensity on the T2-weighted images, involving brainstem, cerebellum, thalamus, or subcortical white matter (Odaka et al., 2003). The imaging findings of cerebellar and brainstem involvement as well as the few autopsy cases (Al-Din et al., 1982; Bickerstaff, 1957; Odaka et al., 2003) suggest that the ataxia in Bickerstaff encephalitis is more likely to be cerebellar. In contrast, the ataxia in Fisher syndrome is more likely the result of proprioception impairment: namely, sensory ataxia. However, patients with Fisher syndrome may also have abnormalities on MRI, making the debate unsettled (Ito et al., 2008).

### CLIPPERS

As the name indicates, chronic lymphocytic inflammation with pontine perivascular enhancement responsive to steroids (CLIPPERS) is a chronic inflammatory process of the pontine region that responds to steroids, and pathological findings showed predominant perivascular lymphocytic inflammation (Tobin et al., 2017). Patients present with subacute-onset gait ataxia and diplopia along with dysarthria, tingling of the face, dizziness, nystagmus, and paraparesis (Pittock et al., 2010). MRI shows small punctate of gadolinium enhancement (Tobin et al., 2017). Corticosteroid is the treatment of choice, but maintenance immunosuppressant is required. Most patients experienced improvement with treatment, and in a study 10 out of 23 patients had complete resolution of MRI findings (Tobin et al., 2017).

## Infections

### Creutzfeldt-Jakob Disease

CJD can present with mainly cerebellar ataxia before developing other cognitive symptoms (Jellinger et al., 1974). CJD is a form of rapidly progressive dementia caused by misfolded prion protein, PrP, encoded by the gene *PRNP* (Goldgaber et al., 1989; Prusiner, 1998). Polymorphism of the *PRNP* gene affects the clinical phenotype (Parchi et al., 1999). In patients expressing a 21 kDa PrP with homozygous methionine at codon 129 (MM1), 33% presented with cerebellar ataxia at symptoms onset, whereas in patients carrying heterozygous methionine/valine at codon 129 (MV1), 75% presented with cerebellar ataxia at onset (Parchi et al., 1999). Diagnostic tools include MRI DWI sequence showing cortical ribbon sign and double hockey stick sign, elevated CSF 14-3-3 protein, CSF RT-QuIC and protein misfolding cyclic amplification (PMCA) test, electroencephalogram with periodic sharp wave complex, and spongiform pathology on brain biopsy (see Fig. 23.3, *B*).

### Whipple Disease

Whipple disease is a chronic multisystemic infectious disease caused by *Tropheryma whipplei*. The incidence is about 1 per 1,000,000 (Sieracki, 1958). It predominantly affects the gastrointestinal tract, leading to abdominal pain, diarrhea, and weight loss. Involvement of the CNS can occur in 6%–43% of the patients (Louis et al., 1996). Among the patients with CNS Whipple disease, 11%–45% have cerebellar ataxia. Other neurological symptoms include cognitive impairment, seizure, psychiatric symptoms, supranuclear gaze palsy, cranial nerve involvement, upper motor neuron signs, and myoclonus. The pathognomonic symptoms for CNS Whipple disease, oculomasticatory myorhythmia, and oculo-facial-skeletal myorhythmia, occur in about 20% of patients (Compain et al., 2013; Louis et al., 1996; Matthews et al., 2005). PCR can detect *T. whipplei* in CSF in 92% of patients with CNS Whipple disease (Compain et al., 2013).

### *Listeria* Encephalitis

Infection caused by *Listeria monocytogenes* typically presents as self-limited gastroenteritis. However, *L. monocytogenes* can also cause meningitis, encephalitis, and brain abscess owing to its CNS tropism (Lorber, 2007; Moragas et al., 2011; Streharova et al., 2007). Interestingly, *Listeria* encephalitis tends to involve just the brainstem: hence the term "rhombencephalitis". Clinical symptoms may include cranial nerve palsy (single or multiple), altered mental status, and cerebellar ataxia. Arrhythmia or respiratory compromise may occur, depending on the extent of the brainstem involvement. Although less frequent, basal ganglia, thalami, cerebral cortex, and spinal cord may also be affected (Arslan et al., 2018).

### Human Immunodeficiency Virus

In patients with human immunodeficiency virus (HIV) infection, neurological symptoms may arise from direct toxicity of HIV to the nervous system, opportunistic infection, side effects of antiretroviral agents, and increased risk of developing CNS lymphoma (Gerstner and Batchelor, 2010). Cerebellar ataxia can be the result of lymphoma or a localized opportunistic infection in the posterior fossa (e.g., progressive multifocal leukoencephalopathy [PML] or toxoplasmosis). PML is caused by the death of the oligodendrocytes and loss of myelination as the result of JC virus reactivation in immunocompromised patients. Initiation of antiretroviral agents may unmask or worsen PML because of immune reconstitution inflammatory syndrome (PML-IRIS; Sidhu and McCutchan, 2010). A study reviewed literature between 1998 and 2016, finding that 28% of patients with PML-IRIS have cerebellar ataxia (Fournier et al., 2017). In rare cases, HIV patients may develop a pure cerebellar syndrome not associated with cognitive impairment, opportunistic infection, or CNS lymphoma (Elsheikh et al., 2010; Pedroso et al., 2018; Tagliati et al., 1998).

## Toxins

### Ethanol

Cerebellar symptoms can occur in both acute and chronic alcohol intoxication, in addition to other neurological symptoms including cognitive impairment, seizure, slurred speech, and peripheral neuropathy. Ethanol has a direct effect on ion channels such as receptors for *N*-methyl-D-aspartate (NMDA), GABA, and glycine as well as neuronal nicotinic receptors and potassium channels (Harris et al., 2008). Ethanol can cause secondary thiamine deficiency from malnutrition and direct impairment of thiamine metabolism (Laforenza et al., 1990), leading to Wernicke encephalopathy, characterized by the triad of altered mental status, ophthalmoplegia, and ataxia (Zubaran et al., 1997).

#### Anticonvulsants

Multiple anticonvulsants can cause ataxia, including phenytoin, valproic acid, carbamazepine, oxcarbazepine, lamotrigine, zonisamide, lacosamide, vigabatrin, and gabapentin (van Gaalen et al., 2014). The majority of cases are reversible with discontinuation or reduction of the offending medication. Chronic phenytoin use can cause cerebellar atrophy, but cerebellar symptoms may not always be present, and most seemed to correlate with supratherapeutic serum level of phenytoin (Koller et al., 1981; Luef et al., 1994; McLain et al., 1980). Valproic acid can itself cause ataxia, but more often it acts through lowering the metabolism of other medications. Benzodiazepine-related ataxia occurs more often in children, and symptoms are usually milder and reversible (van Gaalen et al., 2014).

#### Chemotherapy Agents

Several chemotherapy agents can cause cerebellar ataxia among other neurological symptoms, including 5-fluorouracil (5-FU), capecitabine (prodrug of 5-FU), cytarabine, and methotrexate (Boesen et al., 1988; Dworkin et al., 1985; Gonzalez-Suarez et al., 2014; Lam et al., 2008; Pazdur et al., 1992).

#### Metronidazole

Metronidazole is associated with cerebellar toxicity and reversible hyperintensity signal on T2 FLAIR, DWI, and apparent diffusion coefficient map (Heaney et al., 2003).

#### Heavy Metals

Lithium overdose may result in action tremor, cerebellar ataxia, and altered mental status. Methylmercury can cause cerebellar ataxia, tunnel vision, hearing deficits, and peripheral neuropathy. Lead poisoning can result in cognitive impairment, attention deficits, motor-predominant neuropathy, and cerebellar edema. Excessive intake of bismuth subsalicylate has been associated with ataxia, confusion, and myoclonus (Gordon et al., 1995).

#### Toluene

Toluene exposure can result in cognitive impairment, seizure, encephalopathy, postural tremor, and cerebellar ataxia (King, 1982; Saito and Wada, 1993). Sources of exposure are typically organic solvent in paint spray, paint thinner, or glues.

### Vascular Disease

Blood supply to the cerebellum consists of three arteries of the vertebral-basilar system: the posterior inferior cerebellar artery (PICA), anterior inferior cerebellar artery (AICA), and superior cerebellar artery (Fig. 23.5). Clinical presentation of a stroke depends on which of the three arteries is involved, although symptoms of more than vascular territory may be seen if the site of an arterial occlusion is a vertebral or basilar artery. PICA (Wallenberg) syndrome involves the lateral medulla, inferior cerebellar peduncle, inferior vermis, cerebellar tonsils, and inferior cerebellar hemisphere. Patients may present with acute-onset vertigo, unsteady gait, limb ataxia, hemifacial sensory loss to pain and temperature, and hoarseness. In addition to cerebellar signs, a neurological examination may reveal asymmetric elevation of the soft palate, nystagmus, and Horner syndrome (because of the involvement of the descending sympathetic tract). Infarct of the AICA affects the inferior lateral pons part of the middle cerebral peduncle, the anterior cerebellum, and the flocculus. Clinical symptoms are very similar to PICA infarct, including vertigo, cerebellar ataxia, nystagmus, hemifacial sensory loss, as well as Horner syndrome. Patients may have acute-onset hearing loss, owing to the labyrinth artery arising from AICA, distinguishing itself from a PICA syndrome. Sometimes AICA infarct is indistinguishable from PICA infarct, requiring neuroimaging for accurate assessment. The superior cerebellar artery is responsible for the superior aspect of the cerebellar hemisphere, and part of the midbrain tectum. In addition to cerebellar ataxia and gaze-evoked nystagmus, the oculomotor or trochlear nucleus may be involved.

Ataxia-hemiparesis can be caused by a lacunar stroke located at the corona radiata, posterior limb of internal capsule, or ventral pons contralateral to the side of symptoms.

### Superficial Siderosis

Superficial siderosis is the result of iron and/or hemosiderin deposition at the pial and subpial regions. Involvement of cerebellum can lead to cerebellar ataxia. Superficial siderosis can be the result of subarachnoid hemorrhage or from arteriovenous malformation. More recently it is linked to cerebral amyloid angiopathy (Linn et al., 2008, 2010). The actual mechanism of how deposition of iron and/or hemosiderin can cause ataxia is still unclear.

### Neoplastic

Among all primary CNS tumors, 2% are located in the cerebellum (Ostrom et al., 2016). Neoplasms in the posterior fossa are more common in children between 4 to 10 years old and relatively rare in adults. For adults, metastases account for the majority of cerebellar neoplasms (Pfiffner et al., 2014). The common origins of the metastatic tumors include lung, breast, and gastrointestinal tract (Yoshida and Takahashi, 2009). Primary CNS tumors include medulloblastoma, ependymoma, hemangioblastoma, low-grade glioma, dysplastic gangliocytoma, atypical teratoid/rhabdoid tumors, and embryonal tumors with abundant neuropil and true rosettes (ETANTR, also known as embryonal tumors with multilayered rosettes, ETMR. These were formerly known as primitive neuroectodermal tumors, PNETs). Diagnosis largely depends on neuroimaging studies and biopsy.

## GENETIC CAUSES FOR ATAXIA

Genetic diagnostic approaches for common cerebellar ataxias involve screening for repeat expansions, then sequencing (see Fig. 23.1).

Genetic mutations are a major cause of ataxia. These should be looked for when the patient has one or more affected family members. However, family history is frequently lacking in autosomal recessive cerebellar ataxias (ARCAs). The absence of family history may also be attributable to early death of the affected parent or separation from them, adoption, non-paternity, or germline mutation, in autosomal dominant ataxias. Furthermore, a recent study suggests an unexpectedly high prevalence of premutation alleles which could serve as a reservoir for de novo mutations in some SCAs caused by repeat expansions (Gardiner et al., 2019).

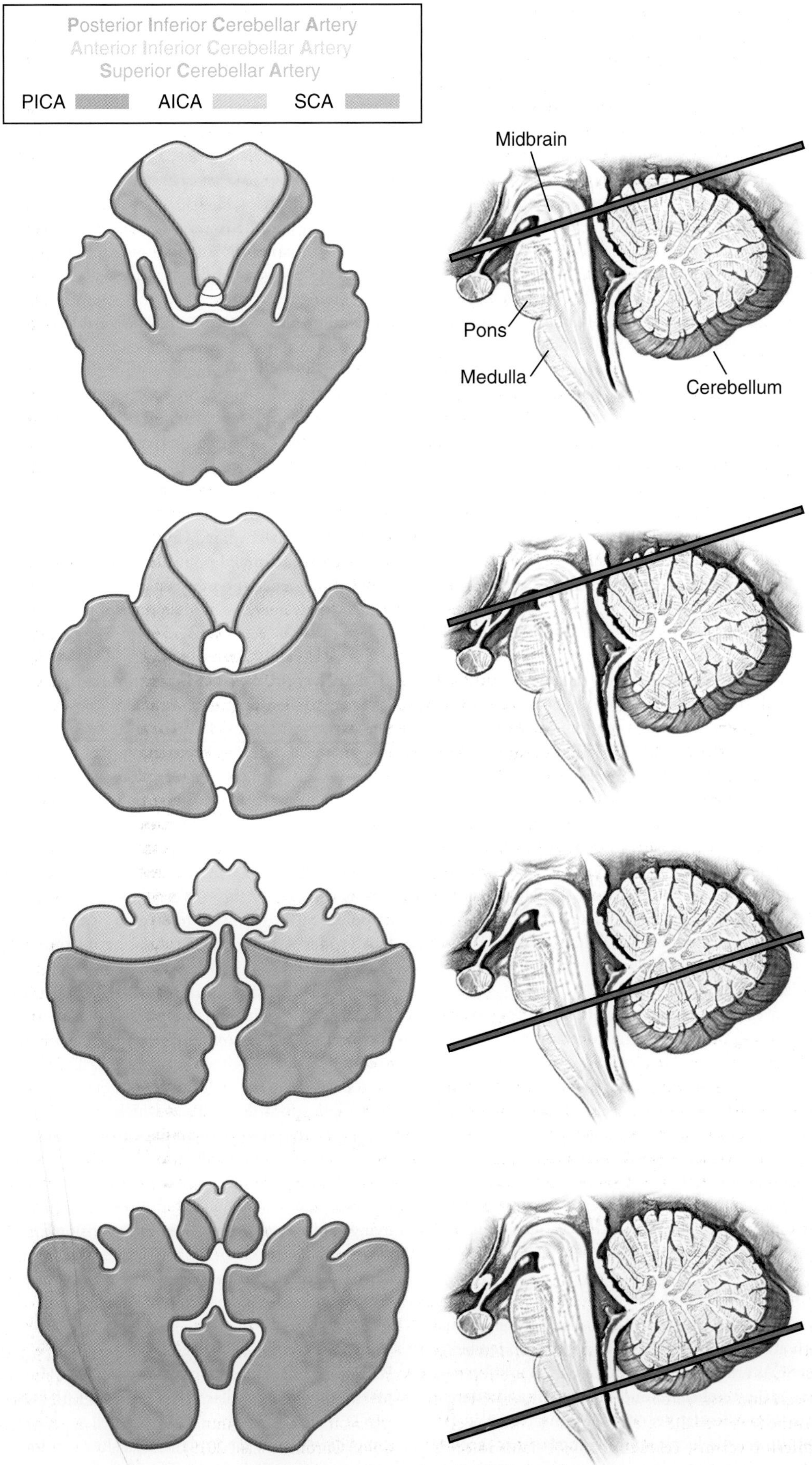

**Fig. 23.5** Vascular Supply for Cerebellum.

ARCAs are usually, but not always, early onset. Patients are usually under the care of pediatric neurologists, geneticists, or pediatricians. However, when these patients reach adulthood, they may come to visit neurologists who work with adults. For example, patients with Friedreich ataxia, the most common inherited ataxia in regions where people speak Indo-European and Afro-Asiatic languages (Bidichandani and Delatycki, 1993; Labuda et al., 2000), typically develop symptoms in childhood, and usually survive into adulthood. The transition to adult care can be challenging and disruptive without appropriate expertise of adult neurologists. The prevalence of autosomal recessive cerebellar ataxias may have been underestimated in late-onset ataxic disorders. A recent study showed that an autosomal recessive mutation with intronic pentanucleotide repeat expansions causing cerebellar ataxia, neuropathy, vestibular areflexia syndrome (CANVAS) and related disorders may account for up to 20% of unexplained ataxias (Cortese et al., 2019). Thus, recessive ataxias are commonly overlooked but must be taken into the differential diagnoses of ataxic disorders in adult clinics.

For a patient with familial ataxias, one should attempt to obtain available results of genetic testing of any relative who may have the same disease. If no such relative is available, genetic testing of common ataxias should be done. For dominantly inherited ataxia, common SCAs are caused by an expansion of a short tandem repeat, and for ARCA autosomal cerebellar, Friedreich ataxia and several other common recessive ataxias should be tested. Expanded repeats are not readily detectable by whole exome sequencing (WES) or whole genome sequencing (WGS) based on next-generation sequencing (NGS) technology. Thus, unless the phenotype of the test subject points to a specific diagnosis, a panel of repeat expansion mutations should be done first (see Fig. 23.1). If these diagnoses are excluded, then WES is considered. If the WES result includes only variations of unknown significance (VUS), pedigree analysis for co-segregation of the VUS and the disease and biological functional testing in experimental systems may be needed in determining the pathogenicity. Synonymous mutations (that do not change the amino acid coding) are unlikely to be, but cannot be dismissed as, the pathogenic mutation. Similar genetic testing approaches should be considered for apparently sporadic disorders if secondary causes (especially those that are treatable) of ataxia are excluded. The remaining sporadic ataxias may be classified into two major types by clinical manifestations: (1) idiopathic late-onset cerebellar ataxia (ILOCA), and (2) multiple system atrophy—cerebellar type (MSA-C; Ashizawa et al., 2018; see Fig. 23.1).

Among the secondary causes of progressive ataxia, immune-mediated ataxias may present with neurodegenerative features, which may respond to timely immunotherapy. However, the presence of autoantibodies does not necessarily mean they are pathogenic, and consequently immune-mediated ataxias may be overdiagnosed. In genetic ataxias, on the other hand, pathogenic mutations may be frequently labeled as VUS, and structural genomic mutations such as large deletions, inversions, duplications, and translocations, and repeat expansions are not readily captured by the WES. Therefore, limitations in detecting the mutation and interpreting genetic test results may lead to underdiagnosing many genetic disorders.

## Autosomal Dominant Cerebellar Ataxias

Spinocerebellar ataxias (SCAs) are a group of autosomal dominant disorders presented with ataxia variably accompanied by extracerebellar manifestations. Most SCAs are progressive adult-onset neurodegenerative disorders affecting the cerebellum and its afferent and efferent pathways. In the genetic nomenclature, SCAs are numbered in the order of discovery of the genetic locus, and the number has recently reached 48.

### Frequency of Spinocerebellar Ataxia

The collective prevalence of all known types of SCAs has been estimated as 1.0–5.6 in 100,000 (Leone et al., 1995; Ruano et al., 2014; van de Warrenburg et al., 2002). Thus, all SCAs are rare diseases by the United States government's definition (Mulberg et al., 2019). A recent study of expanded polyglutamine (polyQ) alleles of known disease loci in five large population-based European cohorts showed that 10.7% had at least one CAG repeat expansion allele within the intermediate range, while up to 1.3% had a CAG repeat number within the disease range, mostly in the lower pathological range associated with elderly onset (Gardiner et al., 2019). Although intermediate alleles potentially mutable to become the disease-range allele may be overestimated due to including interrupted alleles (e.g., SCA1 repeat), the size of reservoir populations for polyQ SCA may be alarmingly high.

### Regional and Ethnic Distributions of Spinocerebellar Ataxia

SCAs 1, 2, 3, 6, 7, and 8 are most common in the United States and Europe, while geographic predilection of specific SCAs and distinctive founder effects exist in various parts of the world (Fig. 23.6). For example, a high prevalence has been found for SCA1 in Poland; SCA2 in Cuba, Mexico, and Italy; SCA6 in UK, Germany, and Japan; SCA7 in South Africa, Mexico, and Venezuela; SCA10 in Latin America; SCA12 in India and Italy; while SCA3 is the most common SCA worldwide. However, only limited population-based data (Coutinho et al., 2013) exist for incidence and prevalence of SCAs, and estimated frequency of SCAs in a given region is often reflecting founder effects.

### Genetic Mutations in Spinocerebellar Ataxia

SCA 1, 2, 3, 6, 7, 17 and (Dentatorubral-pallidoluysian atrophy) are all caused by an expansion of a CAG repeat encoding a polyQ peptide in respective genes (Ashizawa et al., 2018; Klockgether et al., 2019; Paulson et al., 2017). The mutation of SCA8 is an expanded CTG repeat in the 3′ untranslated region (3′UTR) of the *ATXN8OS* gene, while the same repeat on the opposite strand encodes polyQ in the *ATXN8* gene. SCA10, SCA31, and SCA37 are autosomal dominant ataxias caused by a large expanded intronic pentanucleotide repeat. SCA36 is the only SCA caused by an hexanucleotide repeat expansion (Fig. 23.7) (Ashizawa et al., 2018). The pathogenic mechanism of polyQ SCAs points to toxic gain of function by the mutant protein products, while SCAs caused by intronic repeat expansions are thought to be caused by toxic untranslated RNAs that contain large repeats (Table 23.5) (Ashizawa et al., 2018; Paulson et al., 2017). Most other mutations in remaining SCAs are missense mutations, which may lead to either toxic gain of function of the mutant protein or dominant negative effect (Table 23.6). There are a handful of SCAs caused by deletions (SCA15/16 and SCA14), translocation (SCA27), and duplications (SCA20), of which SCA15/16 and SCA27 show loss of function of the gene (haploinsufficiency) (Iwaki et al., 2008; Misceo et al., 2009). Haploinsufficiency may also play a pathogenic role in SCA47 (Gennarino et al., 2018). These mechanisms have important implications in the ongoing and future development of disease-modifying molecular therapy. Repeat expansion and missense mutations are generally good targets of RNA silencing therapy, while haploinsufficiency would be addressed by gene replacement therapy or transcription enhancers to increase the lacking protein.

### Genotype-Phenotype Correlation

Phenotypically, Harding has classified SCAs into three types: autosomal dominant cerebellar ataxia (ADCA) I, II, and III (Harding, 1982). ADCA I is a phenotype with cerebellar ataxia plus variable extracerebellar (mainly CNS) signs, e.g., slow saccades in SCA2 (see Video 23.4) and dystonia in SCA3 (Fig. 23.8, *A*). Patients with ADCA II show 

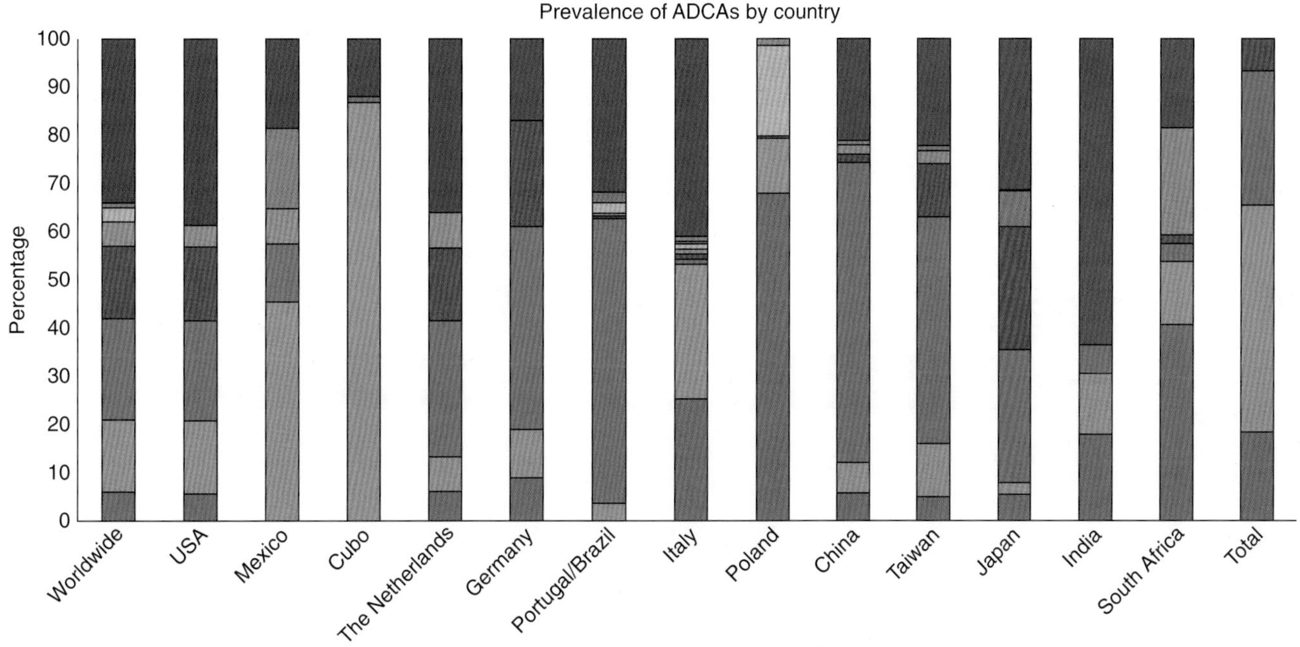


**Fig. 23.6** **The Prevalence of Spinocerebellar Ataxia *(SCA)* by Country.** The category "Rare" includes other spinocerebellar ataxias (SCAs), e.g., SCA10, SCA12, SCA17, etc. Note that in Mexico, SCA10 represents 13.9% of all SCA patients. *ADCA*, Autosomal dominant cerebellar ataxia. (Worldwide: *Bird, T.D., 1993. Hereditary ataxia overview. In: Adam, M.P., Ardinger, H.H., Pagon, R.A., et al. (Eds.), GeneReviews((R)). Seattle, WA.*

USA: *Moseley, M.L., Benzow, K.A., Schut, L.J., et al., 1998. Incidence of dominant spinocerebellar and Friedreich triplet repeats among 361 ataxia families. Neurology. 51(6), 1666–1671.* https://doi.org/10.1212/wnl.51.6.1666.

Mexico: *Velazquez Perez, L., Cruz, G.S., Santos Falcon, N., et al., 2009. Molecular epidemiology of spinocerebellar ataxias in Cuba: insights into SCA2 founder effect in Holguin. Neurosci. Lett. 454(2), 157–160.* https://doi.org/10.1016/j.neulet.2009.03.015.

Cuba: *Velazquez Perez, L., Cruz, G.S., Santos Falcon, N., et al., 2009. Molecular epidemiology of spinocerebellar ataxias in Cuba: insights into SCA2 founder effect in Holguin. Neurosci. Lett. 454(2), 157–160.* https://doi.org/10.1016/j.neulet.2009.03.015.

The Netherlands: *van de Warrenburg, B.P., Sinke, R.J., Verschuuren-Bemelmans, C.C., et al., 2002. Spinocerebellar ataxias in the Netherlands: prevalence and age at onset variance analysis. Neurology. 58(5), 702–708.* https://doi.org/10.1212/wnl.58.5.702.

Germany: *Schols, L., Amoiridis, G., Buttner, T., et al., 1997. Autosomal dominant cerebellar ataxia: phenotypic differences in genetically defined subtypes? Ann. Neurol. 42(6), 924–932.* https://doi.org/10.1002/ana.*410420615.*

Portugal/Brazil: *Silveira, I., Miranda, C., Guimaraes, L., et al., 2002. Trinucleotide repeats in 202 families with ataxia: a small expanded (CAG)n allele at the SCA17 locus. Arch. Neurol. 59(4), 623–629.* https://doi.org/10.1001/archneur.59.4.623.

Italy: *Brusco, A., Gellera, C., Cagnoli, C., et al., 2004. Molecular genetics of hereditary spinocerebellar ataxia: mutation analysis of spinocerebellar ataxia genes and CAG/CTG repeat expansion detection in 225 Italian families. Arch. Neurol. 61(5), 727–733.* https://doi.org/10.1001/archneur.61.5.*727.*

Poland: *Krysa, W., Sulek, A., Rakowicz, M., et al., 2016. High relative frequency of SCA1 in Poland reflecting a potential founder effect. Neurol. Sci. 37(8), 1319–1325. doi:10.1007/s10072-016-2594-x.*

China: *Wang, J., Shen, L., Lei, L., et al., 2011. Spinocerebellar ataxias in mainland China: an updated genetic analysis among a large cohort of familial and sporadic cases. Zhong Nan Da Xue Xue Bao Yi Xue Ban 36(6), 482–489.* https://doi.org/10.3969/j.issn.1672-7347.2011.06.*003.*

Taiwan: *Soong, B.W., Lu, Y.C., Choo, K.B., et al., 2001. Frequency analysis of autosomal dominant cerebellar ataxias in Taiwanese patients and clinical and molecular characterization of spinocerebellar ataxia type 6. Arch. Neurol. 58(7), 1105–1109.* https://doi.org/10.1001/archneur.58.7.*1105.*

Japan: *Maruyama, H., Izumi, Y., Morino, H., et al., 2002. Difference in disease-free survival curve and regional distribution according to subtype of spinocerebellar ataxia: a study of 1,286 Japanese patients. Am. J. Med. Genet. 114(5), 578–583.* https://doi.org/10.1002/ajmg.10514.

India: *Krishna, N., Mohan, S., Yashavantha, B. S., et al., 2007. SCA 1, SCA 2 and SCA 3/MJD mutations in ataxia syndromes in southern India. Indian J. Med. Res. 126(5), 465–470.*

South Africa: *Bryer, A., Krause, A., Bill, P., et al., 2003. The hereditary adult-onset ataxias in South Africa. J. Neurol. Sci. 216(1), 47–54. doi:10.1016/s0022-510x(03)00209-0.*)

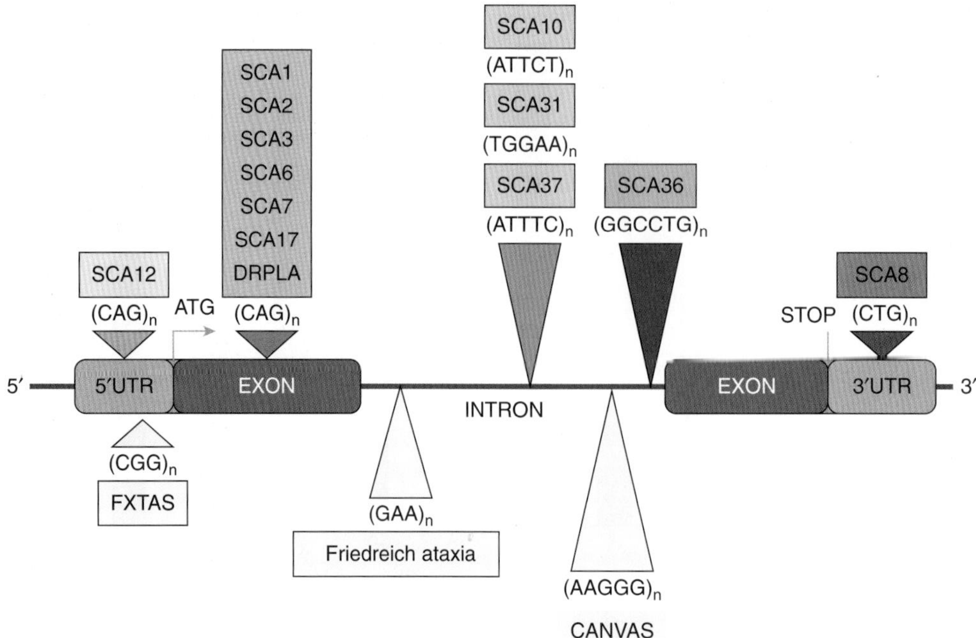


**Fig. 23.7 Ataxias Caused by Repeat Expansions.** *3′UTR*, 3′ Untranslated region; *5′UTR*, 5′ untranslated region; *CANVAS*, cerebellar ataxia, neuropathy, vestibular areflexia syndrome; *FXTAS*, fragile X associated tremor ataxia syndrome.

pigmentary macular degeneration, and SCA7 is the only known ADCA  II among SCAs (see Fig. 23.8, *B* and Video 23.5). Patients with ADCA III present almost pure cerebellar signs throughout the course of disease, and SCA6 could be considered in this category.

Cerebellar cognitive affective syndrome (CCAS or Schmahmann syndrome) (Schmahmann, 2004), which consists of underrecognized cognitive impairments may be present in patients with SCAs. The onset of most SCAs is typically with balance loss and gait ataxia, although oculomotor abnormalities may be present early on examination. Besides SCA7, different SCAs may show some distinct clinical features. These features, combined with information about ethnicity and anticipation, may provide a useful guidance for efficient genetic testing in some families (see Tables 23.5 and 23.6).

## Anticipation

Progressively earlier onset of the disease in successive generations with increasing severity within a family, known as genetic anticipation, is a hallmark of most polyQ SCAs (McInnis, 1996). Anticipation is attributed to intergenerational increase of the number of CAGs. It is the mechanism underlying the juvenile-onset disease and de novo cases of polyQ SCAs. The small size of CAG repeat expansion in SCA6 and CAA interruptions within the expanded CAG repeat of SCA17 make the mutant expanded allele stable, leading to the lack of anticipation in these SCAs. Anticipation has also been reported in SCA5, SCA10, and SCA31. The instability of repeat size would explain anticipation in SCA10 and SCA31. However, the case of SCA5 is puzzling because the SCA5 is not a repeat expansion disorder and caused by point mutations in the *SPNBII* gene. Additional mechanisms of observed anticipation other than repeat size changes, such as ascertainment bias and epigenetics, may need to be explored (Petronis et al., 1997).

## Genetic Testing

The National Ataxia Foundation posts its guidelines for genetic testing (https://ataxia.org/wp-content/uploads/2017/07/SCA-Making_an_Informed_Choice_About_Genetic_Testing.pdf), which are similar to those established for Huntington disease. While genetic testing of subjects who are exhibiting clinical ataxia is straightforward, presymptomatic testing involves the issue of "to know or not to know" (Robins Wahlin, 2007), and this issue is further complicated in testing at-risk subjects before adulthood (Quarrell et al., 2018). When efficacious treatments become available, the guidelines for presymptomatic genetic diagnosis would be changed to enable early diagnosis and treatment. Although preimplantation genetic diagnosis (PGD) of SCAs is technically feasible, no report of PGD has emerged in the literature for SCAs. Genetic counseling is always recommended before and after the genetic testing.

## Pathogenic Mechanism

***PolyQ Spinocerebellar Ataxias.*** The pathogenic mechanism of polyQ SCAs is a toxic gain of function by the protein that the mutant gene encodes (Coarelli et al., 2018). The toxic effect differs from one SCA to another depending on the structural and functional context of the mutant protein(s), including the splice variants and posttranslational modifications (Ashizawa et al., 2018; Carroll et al., 2018; Du et al., 2013, 2019, Friedrich et al., 2018; Karam and Trottier, 2018; Klockgether et al., 2019; Paulson et al., 2017; Perez Ortiz and Orr, 2018; Scoles and Pulst, 2018; Ward et al., 2019; Yang et al., 2016). Interruption(s) of the SCA1 CAG repeat by histidine-coding CAT units decreases the pathogenicity (Opal and Ashizawa, 1993). Although interruptions of CAG repeats by synonymous CAA units would not change the PolyQ repeat in the protein product, it may change the stability of the repeat length and might affect the age at onset and the severity of the disease (Menon et al., 2013; Wright et al., 2019). Patients with SCA2 expansions may present with L-dopa responsive parkinsonism or amyotrophic lateral sclerosis, and long normal *ATXN2* alleles are risk factors for amyotrophic lateral sclerosis (Antenora et al., 2017).

Existing data suggest that pathogenic pathways involved in the toxic gain of function in different SCAs may interact with each other in the ataxia interactome (Fernandez-Funez et al., 2000; Vazquez et al., 2019). The interaction of polyQ tract of ATXN3 and beclin 1 can be affected by polyQ tracts of other SCAs, individually leading

**TABLE 23.5 Spinocerebellar Ataxias Caused by Expanded Microsatellite Repeats**

| Disease | Gene and Protein (Repeat Location) | REPEATS, PRINCIPAL REPEAT UNIT | | | Notable Characteristic Clinical Signs | Anticipation |
|---|---|---|---|---|---|---|
| | | Normal | Intermediate | Disease | | |
| **SCAs Caused by Polyglutamine-Coding CAG Repeat Expansions** | | | | | | |
| SCA1 | *ATXN1* | 6–39* | 40 | 41–83 | Hypermetric saccades, pyramidal signs | + |
| SCA2 | *ATXN2* | <31 | 31–33 | 34–200 | Slow saccades, areflexia | +[†] |
| SCA3 | *ATXN3* | 12–44 | 45–55 | 56–86 | Bulged eyes, motor neuron signs | + |
| SCA6 | *CACNA1A* | <18 | 19 | 20–33 | Downbeat nystagmus | – |
| SCA7 | *ATXN7* | 4–19 | 28–33 | 34–>460 | Visual loss | + |
| SCA17 | *TBP* | 25–40 | – | 4 | Huntington disease-like | –[†] |
| DRPLA | *ATN1* | 6–35 | 36–48 | 49–88 | Huntington disease-like | + |
| **SCAs Caused by Noncoding Microsatellite Repeat Expansions** | | | | | | |
| SCA8[‡] | *OSATXN8* (3′UTR) | 15–34, CTG or CAG | 34–89, CTG or CAG | 89–250, CTG or CAG | Reduced penetrance | – |
| SCA10 | *ATXN10* (intron) | 8–32, ATTCT[§] | 33–799 ATTCT[‖] | 800–4500, ATTCT[¶] | Some families with epilepsy | ± |
| SCA12 | PPP2R2B (5′ UTR) | 7–28, CAG | 29–66, CAG | 67–78, CAG | Tremor | – |
| SCA31[#] | *BEAN* (intron) | <400, ATTTT | Unknown | 500–760 TGGAA | Pure cerebellar ataxia | + |
| SCA36 | *NOP56* (intron) | 3–14, GGCCTG | Unknown | 650–2500 | Motor neuron disease | – |
| SCA37** | *DAB1* (5′UTR; intron) | <400, ATTTT | Unknown | 31–75, ATTTC | Pure cerebellar ataxia | – |

*SCA*, Spinocerebellar ataxias.
*CAT interruptions are present in many normal CAG repeat alleles. The length of the uninterrupted stretch CAG repeat seems to determine whether they are pathogenic (Opal and Ashizawa, 2017).
†CAA interruptions affect repeat stability in SCA2 and SCA17, and affect toxicity and, potentially, phenotype in SCA2.
‡Expanded SCA8 repeats can contain one or more CCG, CTA, CTC, CCA, or CTT interruptions, which affect the stability of the repeat and, potentially, the penetrance.
§In SCA10, long normal alleles may contain TTTTC units or ATTGT-TTTTC units.
‖Some intermediate alleles may be interrupted by ATGCT, ATATTCT, and ATTTCT units.
¶Fully expanded alleles may be interrupted by a stretch of ATCCT repeat or a segment of an ATTCC repeat followed by an ATCCC repeat may be inserted within the expanded ATTCT repeat. The presence of the $(ATCCT)_n$–$(ATCCC)_n$ insertion is associated with epilepsy and alters the pattern of repeat instability and anticipation.
#In SCA31, the presence of TGGAA repeats is essential for pathogenicity.
**In SCA37, the presence of ATTTC repeats is pathogenic.
Data were extracted from OMIM and GeneReviews of corresponding SCAs.

to alterations of autophagy (Ashkenazi et al., 2017). Interactions between polyQ-containing proteins are also important in transcription-coupled DNA repair (TCR) in SCA3 (Chatterjee et al., 2015; Gao et al., 2019). The TCR complex is a multiprotein assembly that consists of POLR2A, PNKP, LIG3, TBP, CREB, CBP, TAFII130, HAP1, Huntingtin and ATXN3. PNKP plays the key role in repair of single-strand break in nuclear and mitochondrial DNA in SCA3 and HD (Gao et al., 2019).

## Somatic Instability of Expanded Repeats

A genome-wide association study (GWAS) identified three significant loci associated with the age at onset in Huntington disease (Genetic Modifiers of Huntington's Disease, 2015). An additional study of polyQ SCAs and HD suggested single nucleotide polymorphisms (SNPs) of DNA repair genes, *FAN1* and *PMS2*, are significant modifiers of the age at onset (Bettencourt et al., 2016). An SNP in *ERCC6*, another DNA repair gene, was also identified as a significance modifier of an expansion bias of the expanded SCA3 CAG repeat (Martins et al., 2014). DNA repair genes regulate germline and somatic instability of CAG repeats and have been postulated to play a role in further expansion of CAG repeats related to anticipation, disease progression, and tissue-specific pathology (Larson et al., 2015). While the CAG repeat size has been shown to be smaller in the cerebellum than other parts of brain, the repeat size was not studied specifically for Purkinje cells or deep cerebellar nuclei, where degeneration primarily occurs. Since these neurons are the minority among other cerebellar cells, the repeat size in Purkinje cells and deep cerebellar nuclei needs to be determined to assess the pathogenic impact of the instability of expanded CAG repeats in SCAs.

## Noncoding Repeat Spinocerebellar Ataxias

In SCA8 expanded noncoding CUG repeat is transcribed from the 3′UTR of the *ATXN8OS* gene. There is another gene, *ATXN8*, on the opposite strand encoding a polyQ-coding CAG repeat. The pathogenic mechanism of SCA8 is further confounded by frequent incomplete penetrance of the disease (Moseley et al., 2006). In SCA10, SCA31, and SCA37 the expanded repeat consists of AT-rich

**TABLE 23.6 Spinocerebellar Ataxias Caused by Expanded Microsatellite Repeats**

| Disease | Gene and Protein | Mutation | Notable Characteristic Clinical Signs |
|---|---|---|---|
| SCA5 | *SPTBN2* | Missense | Downbeat nystagmus and some patients with spasticity, anticipation |
| SCA11 | *TTBK2* | Missense | Some patients with pyramidal signs |
| SCA13 | *KCNC3* | Missense | Variable between families |
| SCA14 | *PRKCG* | Missense | Tremor or myoclonus, facial myokymia |
| SCA15 and 16 | *ITPR1* | Deletion | Pure cerebellar ataxia with tremor |
| SCA18 | *IFRD1* | Missense | Sensorimotor neuropathy |
| SCA19 and 22 | *KCND3* | Missense, in-frame 3 bp deletion | Extracerebellar features variable between families |
| SCA20 | *Multiple (DAGLA)** | 260 kb duplication | Pure cerebellar ataxia with spasmodic dysphonia, palatal tremor |
| SCA21 | *TMEM240* | Missense | Cognitive impairment, extrapyramidal signs |
| SCA23 | *PDYN* | Missense | Extracerebellar features variable between families |
| SCA26 | *EEF2* | Missense | Pure cerebellar ataxia |
| SCA27 | *FGF14* | Missense | Mental retardation, tremor |
| SCA28 | *AFG3L2* | Missense | Spastic ataxia |
| SCA29 | *ITPR1* | Missense | Pure cerebellar ataxia, congenital nonprogressive |
| SCA34 | *ELOVL4* | Missense | Hyperkeratosis, MSA-C like |
| SCA35 | *TGM6* | Missense | Hyperreflexia and variable other extracerebellar features |
| SCA38 | *ELOVL5* | Missense | Pure cerebellar ataxia, some patients have sensory neuropathy |
| SCA40 | *CCDC88C* | Missense | Spastic ataxia |
| SCA41 | *TRPC3* | Missense | Pure cerebellar ataxia |
| SCA42 | *CACNA1G* | Missense | Dementia |
| SCA43 | *MME* | Missense | Peripheral neuropathy |
| SCA44 | *GRM1* | Missense, +1 bp frame shift | Spasticity |
| SCA45 | *FAT2* | Missense | Pure cerebellar ataxia (single family) |
| SCA46 | *PLD3* | Missense | Sensory neuropathy |
| SCA47 | *PUM1* | Missense | Pure cerebellar ataxia in adults. Juvenile forms have developmental complex phenotype. |
| SCA48 | *STUB1* | Frame shift | Cerebellar ataxia or cognitive/affective disorder |

Data were extracted from OMIM and GeneReviews of corresponding SCAs.
MSA-C, Multiple system atrophy—cerebellar type; *SCA*, spinocerebellar ataxias.
*The duplicated region in direct orientation contains 12 or more genes, including the *DAGLA* gene.
*Ashizawa, T., Oz, G., Paulson, H. L., 2018. Spinocerebellar ataxias: prospects and challenges for therapy development. Nat. Rev. Neurol. 14(10), 590–605. https://doi.org/10.1038/s41582-018-0051-6.*

pentanucleotide units, ATTCT in *ATXN10*, GGAAT in *BEAN*, and ATTTT in *DAB1*, respectively (Matsuura et al., 2000; Sato et al., 2009; Seixas et al., 2017). In SCA36 an intronic hexanucleotide GGCCTG repeat is expanded in *NOP56* (Kobayashi et al., 2011). Existing evidence points to toxic gain of function by the respective expanded RNA repeat playing major roles in their pathogenic mechanisms. In SCA12 an expanded CAG repeat in 5′UTR of *PPP2R2B* has been thought to cause the disease by misregulating the host gene expression (Cohen and Margolis, 2016; Holmes et al., 1999). *PPP2R2B* appears to produce at least eight transcript isoforms, each with a different N-terminal region. The repeat is included in several splice variants (Cohen and Margolis, 2016).

### Repeat Associated Non-AUG Translation

Many but not all expanded repeats that cause SCAs are translated in different frames by a mechanism(s) that is not dependent on the start codon (AUG). This RAN translation may also occur with the antisense transcript from the opposite strand (Cleary et al., 2018). The mechanism of this RAN translation is not fully understood. Evidence for pathogenic contributions of RAN translation in SCAs is becoming increasingly compelling. RAN translation products accumulate in cells as toxic aggregates (Lee et al., 2017) and disrupt functions of nuclear pores and integrity of membraneless organelles (Lee et al., 2016). However, the magnitude of pathogenic contribution of RAN translation relative to other gain-of-function mechanisms remains to be investigated.

### Transcripts from the Opposite Strand

In SCA8 bidirectional expression of a CAG•CUG repeat potentially causes dual pathogenesis (Ikeda et al., 2006; Nemes et al., 2000). Similar bidirectional expression of expanded repeats occurs in SCA2 (Li et al., 2016), SCA7 (Sopher et al., 2011), and fragile X-tremor and ataxia syndrome (FXTAS) (Ladd et al., 2007; Vittal et al., 2018), as well as myotonic dystrophy type 2 (Zu et al., 2017), and C9ORF2 amyotrophic lateral sclerosis/ frontotemporal dementia (Cleary et al., 2018). The bidirectional transcription and RAN translation together express multiple mutant proteins depending on the context of the expanded repeat within the gene as well as the length and motif of the repeat unit.

### Other Mutations Causing Spinocerebellar Ataxias

The application of WES and WGS to genetic diagnosis of ataxia has led to discovery of a rapidly increasing number of genetic variations that include both disease-causing mutations and VUS. Most known disease-causing mutations are missense mutations in SCAs. Considering the dominant inheritance, the mutation is likely to exert toxic effects or dominant negative effect. However, haploinsufficiency (i.e., 50% reduction of the gene product) may be sufficient to cause the disease, as in SCA15/16 and SCA27 (Obayashi et al., 2012; Shimojima et al.,

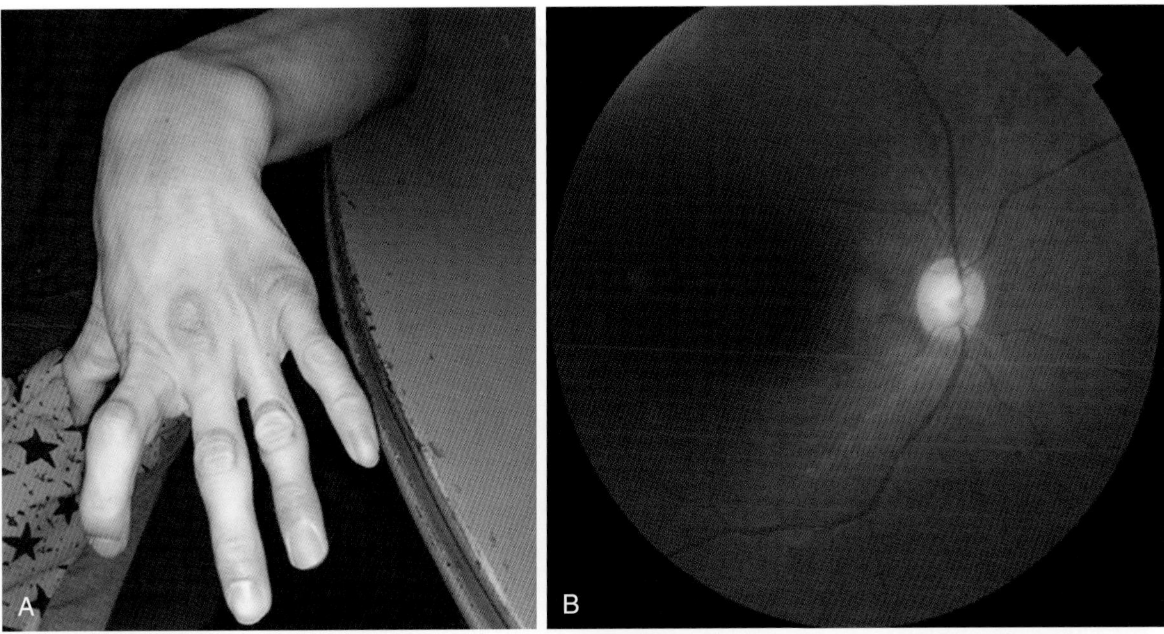


**Fig. 23.8** Prominent hand dystonia in a patient with SCA3 (**A**). Retinal degeneration in a patient with SCA7 (**B**).

2012). In SCA20 the mutation is heterozygous duplication of a 260-kb segment at 11q12.2-11q12.3, harboring 10 known genes including *DAGLA* and 2 unknown genes (Knight et al., 2008).

## Autosomal Recessive Cerebellar Ataxias

ARCAs comprise a group of disorders with cerebellar and spinal cord degeneration typically presenting in childhood, adolescence, or early adulthood, often accompanied by other neurological and systemic manifestations (Anheim et al., 2012; Crockett et al., 1987; Fogel, 2018; Renaud et al., 2017; Synofzik and Nemeth, 2018; Synofzik et al., 2019). ARCAs often affect siblings, but parents are usually asymptomatic heterozygous carriers. The common forms of genetically defined ARCAs are shown in Table 23.7. With the increasing availability of WES, the number of ARCAs now exceeds 90, and an equivalent number of additional autosomal recessive disorders show ataxia as a part of the phenotypic spectrum. Friedreich ataxia is the most common and well-recognized ARCA in the United States and Europe, although there have been no reports of genetically confirmed Friedreich ataxia among sub-Saharan Africans, Amerindians, and people from Central, East, and Southeast Asia [7,8,16,17]. In adults, a recent report described a new late-onset ARCA that shows complete or incomplete presentations of CANVAS caused by a biallelic intronic AAGGG repeat expansion in the replication factor C subunit 1 *(RFC1)* gene (Cortese et al., 2019). This new ARCA may be common in European and US populations. The next common ARCAs are spastic paraplegia 7 (SPG7), autosomal recessive spastic ataxia of Charlevoix-Saguenay (ARSACS), ataxia with oculomotor apraxia 2 (AOA2), spectrin repeat-containing nuclear envelope protein type 1 (SYNE1) ataxia, ataxia telangiectasia, ataxia with oculomotor apraxia 1 (AOA1) and *POLG*-ataxia, each accounting for 2% or more of all ARCAs (Synofzik and Schule, 2017; see Table 23.7).

### Autosomal Recessive Cerebellar Ataxias Caused by Expansion of Intronic Repeats

***Friedreich ataxia.*** Patients with Friedreich ataxia show an afferent/sensory ataxia as a prominent feature (Fig. 23.9), although neuropathological and imaging studies often show cerebellar pathology, in addition to spinal cord, pathology (see Fig. 23.9, *B* and *C*; Marty et al., 2019; Pandolfo, 2008; Pandolfo and Manto, 2013). Additional key features are abnormal eye movements (90.5%), scoliosis (73.5%), deformities of the feet (58.8%), urinary dysfunction (42.8%), cardiomyopathy and cardiac hypertrophy (40.3%), and decreased visual acuity (36.8%; Reetz et al., 2018). Optic neuropathy and sensorineural hearing loss may occur. Hypertrophic cardiomyopathy with conduction defects, arrhythmias and late congestive heart failure shorten the life expectancy to 40–50 years of age. Approximately 95% of patients with Friedreich ataxia carry two copies of large GAA repeat expansion alleles in intron 1 of the *FXN* gene. The discovery of the GAA expansion mutations in Friedreich ataxia led to identification of atypical Friedreich ataxia patients who would not meet the earlier diagnostic criteria (Harding, 1981b; Parkinson et al., 2013), including late-onset Friedreich ataxia (LOFA; Bhidayasiri et al., 2005; Martinez et al., 2017), Friedreich ataxia with retained reflexes (FARR; Geschwind et al., 1997; Harding, 1981a), and various movement disorders that accompany small GAA expansions (Galimanis et al., 2008; Wali, 2000). Some patients are compound-heterozygous with a GAA expansion in one allele of the *FXN* gene and a point mutation in the other. *FXN* encodes frataxin, the key mitochondrial iron transporter, and loss of function of frataxin leads to impaired mitochondrial iron transport and iron-sulfur (Fe-S) cluster metabolism. There are excellent reviews on recent progress in understanding pathogenic mechanisms and therapeutic development in FA (Bidichandani and Delatycki, 1993; Burk, 2017; Strawser et al., 2017; Tai, et al., 2018).

***Cerebellar ataxia neuropathy vestibular areflexia syndrome (CANVAS) and related late-onset ataxias.*** Cortese and colleagues (2019) identified homozygous intronic AAGGG repeat expansion in the *replication factor C subunit 1 (RFC1)* gene at chromosome 4p14 as a common cause of late-onset ataxia (the mean age at onset 54 ± 9 years). Some patients showed typical CANVAS syndrome while others often lacked either sensory neuropathy or vestibulopathy; some patients lacked both and were presented as ILOCA (i.e., isolated cerebellar ataxia). Sensory ataxia and vestibulopathy appear to result from large-fiber neuropathy and ganglionopathy. Chronic cough and autonomic dysfunctions may be seen in 25%–35% of patients. Cognitive and motor functions are generally spared, Bilateral

**TABLE 23.7 Common Autosomal Recessive Cerebellar Ataxias (ARCAs)**

| ARCAs | Gene | Protein (Function) | Diagnostic Biomarker | Pathogenic Pathway | Clinical Features |
|---|---|---|---|---|---|
| FA | *FXN* | Frataxin (Fe-S biogenesis) | | Mitochondrial dysfunction | Sensory and cerebellar ataxia, square-wave jerks, areflexia, Babinski sign, scoliosis, pes caves, cardiomyopathy, diabetes |
| CANVAS | *RFC1* | Replication factor C subunit 1 | | Unknown | Cerebellar ataxia, sensory polyneuropathy, vestibular areflexia |
| SPG7 | *SPG7* | Paraplegin (mitochondrial protease) | | Mitochondrial dysfunction | Cerebellar ataxia, spastic paraparesis, optic neuropathy |
| AVED | *TTPA* | α-Tocopherol transfer protein | Low serum vitamin E | | Sensory ataxia, cerebellar ataxia, areflexia, Friedreich ataxia-like |
| ARSACS | *SACS* | Sacsin (mitochondrial fission and localization) | | Mitochondrial dysfunction | Spastic ataxia, axonal sensorimotor polyneuropathy |
| A-T | *ATM* | Ataxia telangiectasia mutated (serine protein kinase) | Elevated AFP | DNA repair (DSB) | Cerebellar ataxia, telangiectasia, oculomotor apraxia, choreoathetosis, myoclonus, dystonia, polyneuropathy, sensitivity to ionizing radiation, immune deficiency, cancers, frequent infections |
| ATLD | *MRE11* | Meiotic recombination 11 | | DNA repair (DSB) | A-T like phenotype |
| AOA1 | *APTX* | Aprataxin | Low serum albumin, elevated serum cholesterol | DNA repair | Cerebellar ataxia, oculomotor apraxia, polyneuropathy |
| AOA2 | *SETX* | Senataxin | Elevated AFP | DNA repair | Cerebellar ataxia, oculomotor apraxia, polyneuropathy |
| ANS | *POLG1* | DNA polymerase subunit g-1 | | Mitochondrial dysfunction | Sensory ataxia, neuropathy, dysarthria, external ophthalmoparesis, epilepsy |
| ARCA1 | *SYNE1* | Nesprin-1 (structural protein) | | Cytoskeletal alterations | Cerebellar ataxia with the onset in childhood to middle age, extracerebellar disorders including motor neuron disease. |
| Nieman-Pick C (NPC) | *NPC1, NPC2* | Sterol lipid | Plasma oxysterols, bile acids, and sphingolipids | Lipid metabolism abnormalities | Ataxia with other neurological, psychiatric, and visceral signs |
| CTX | | Mitochondrial cytochrome P450 enzyme sterol 27-hydroxylase | Plasma cholestanol | Lipid metabolism abnormalities | Cerebellar ataxia, xanthoma of tendons |

*ANS*, Ataxia neuropathy spectrum; *AOA1*, ataxia with oculomotor apraxia type 1; *AOA2*, ataxia with oculomotor apraxia type 2; *ARCA1*, autosomal recessive cerebellar ataxia type 1; *ARCA2*, autosomal recessive cerebellar ataxia type 2, with coenzyme Q10 deficiency; *ARCA3*, autosomal recessive cerebellar ataxia type 3 caused by mutations in *ANO10; CANVAS*, cerebellar ataxia, neuropathy, vestibular areflexia syndrome; *ARSACS*, autosomal recessive spastic cerebellar ataxia of Charlevoix-Saguenay; *A-T*, ataxia telangiectasia; *ATLD*, ataxia telangiectasia-like disorder; *AVED*, ataxia with vitamin E deficiency; *CTX*, cerebrotendinous xanthomatosis; *FA*, Friedreich ataxia.

vestibular areflexia may be detected as diminished vestibulo-ocular reflex gain on the head impulse test, abnormal dynamic visual acuity, and abnormal occlusive fundoscopy (Zee test; Szmulewicz et al., 2016). Nerve conduction studies readily detect sensory neuropathy, and brain MRI shows cerebellar atrophy in most cases. Core histopathological findings are widespread depletion of Purkinje cells with prominent Bergmann gliosis.

After genetic mapping of the disease locus to 4p14, a region of reduced read depth (number of unique reads that include a given nucleotide) on WGS was identified in a *RFC1* intron 2 region, where expanded tandemly repeated AAGGG units were detected by repeat-primed PCR and Southern blot analyses. Analysis of DNA from 16 sporadic cases showed two AAGGG expansion alleles. Normal alleles are polymorphic and consisted of either $(AAAAG)_{11}$ (75%), expanded AAAAG (13%), or AAAGG (8%) repeats, but did not include AAGGG repeats. The allelic carrier frequency of the expanded AAGGG repeat was 0.7%, and 22% of patients with sporadic late-onset ataxia showed the homozygous AAGGG expansions, indicating that this is the second most common recessive ataxia after Friedreich ataxia in the European population. There was no correlation between age at onset and the number of AAGGG repeat units. The pathogenic mechanism remains to be determined. There are no changes in levels of *RFC1* mRNA or protein. RNAseq data showed a profile similar to that found in controls. Dosage effects of toxic gain of function by the AAGGG repeat RNA may be a plausible explanation worth investigating. While it is premature to exclude the possibility of spliceopathy as the disease mechanism, the mutant RNA-mediated toxic function, as well as RAN translation, may be involved in activation of other cell death pathways in Purkinje cells.

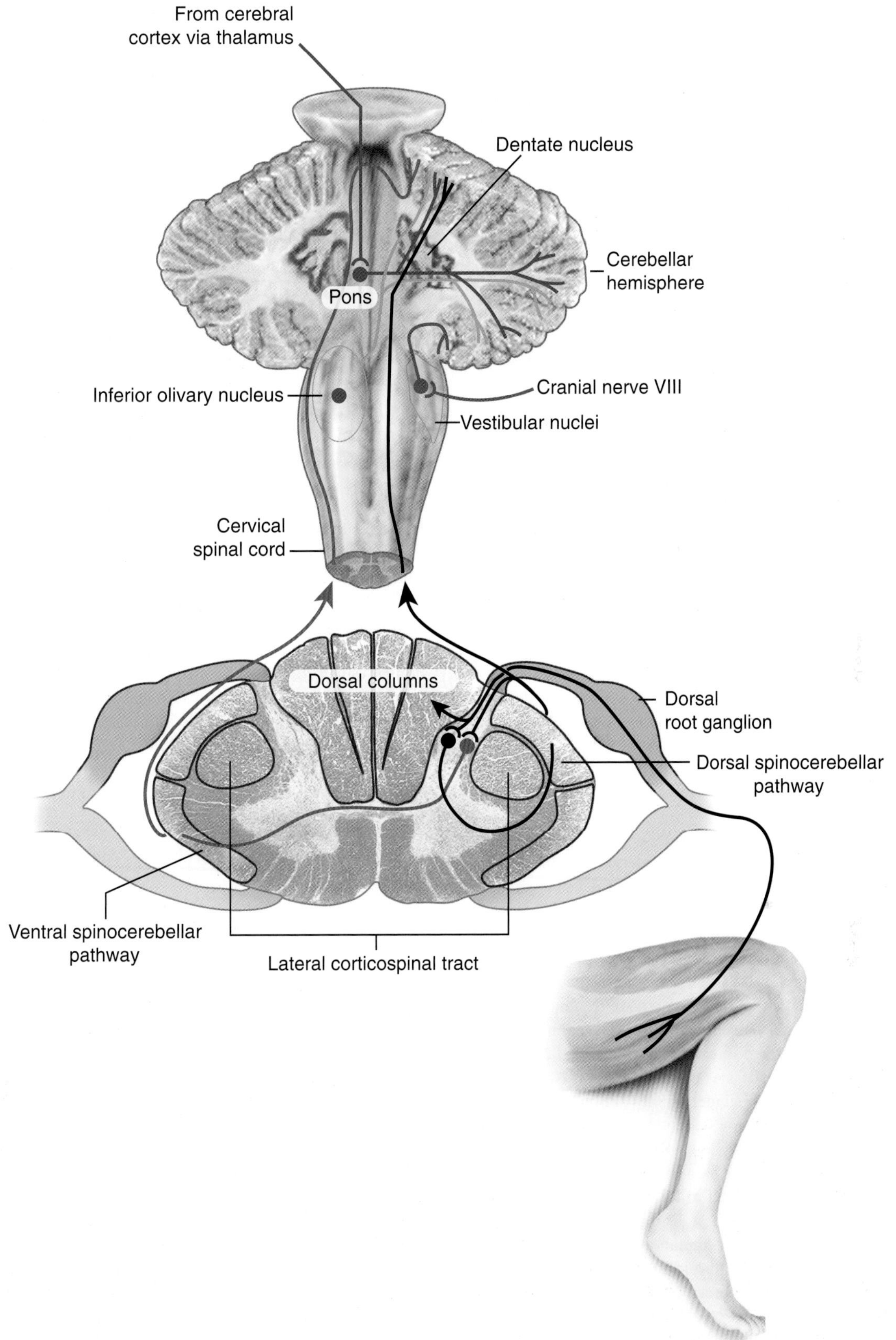


**Fig. 23.9 Friedreich Ataxia.** Structures involved in Friedreich ataxia pathology. Neurons in the dorsal root ganglia and dentate nuclei are primarily affected. The dorsal spinocerebellar tracts and dorsal columns show degeneration. There is also atrophy in Gracilis, cuneatus, and Clarke's nuclei.

### Autosomal Recessive Cerebellar Ataxias Caused by Conventional (Non-Repeat Expansion) Mutations

ARCAs show correlations between key features of the clinical phenotype and the function of mutated genes. Synofzik and colleagues recently classified mutated genes in ARCAs in groups involved in mitochondrial functions, DNA repair, and complex lipid metabolism, to delineate pathogenic pathways that may be targeted by future therapeutics (see Table 23.7 column of Pathogenic pathway). Below, we describe common ARCAs that belong to each of these groups.

## Autosomal Recessive Cerebellar Ataxias with Abnormal Mitochondrial Function

While any neurodegenerative disease can involve mitochondrial dysfunction in the final common pathway, here we will describe ARCAs that are caused by mutations in genes whose protein products play essential roles in mitochondrial functions. Since we have already described Friedreich ataxia, which is one of the prime examples of mitochondrial ARCAs, we describe here the rest of the mitochondrial ARCAs.

### Autosomal Recessive Spastic Ataxia of Charlevoix–Saguenay

Sucsin is a large 520 kDa multidomain protein which facilitates mitochondrial fission and controls intracellular localization of mitochondria. Patients with ARSACS have mutations in the *SACS* gene that encodes sacsin. While the founder effect of ARSACS is striking in Quebec, this disease exists in many other regions of the world (Baets et al., 2010; Kuchay et al., 2019; Vermeer et al., 2008). The triad of cerebellar ataxia, lower extremity spasticity, and axonal-demyelinating sensorimotor neuropathy characterizes clinical features of ARSACS. About 70% of ARSACS patients have mild learning disability, and 15% develop epilepsy (Duquette et al., 2013). The disease starts at 30 years of age, and the age of death widely varies, averaging at 41 years. Atrophy of the vermis accompanies T2-hypointense stripes in the central pons, diffuse T2-hyperintensity in the lateral pons, and thickened middle cerebellar peduncles on brain MRI of greater than 90% of ARSACS patients (Synofzik et al., 2013).

### Spastic Paraplegia Type 7

Although SPG7 also belongs to a group of disorders designated "familial spastic paraparesis", patients with SPG7 frequently develop cerebellar ataxia, which can be the presenting symptom and the most conspicuous clinical sign particularly in those with the p.Ala510Val missense mutation (Parodi et al., 2018). Some patients with SPG7 also show ophthalmoparesis, optic neuropathy, vertical gaze palsy, or blepharoptosis. The onset is usually in mid-30s with a slow progression leading to a loss of independent ambulation (van Gassen et al., 2012). The paraplegin from the mutated SPG7 shows altered interactions with AFG3L2, a protein involved in SCA28 and spastic ataxia 5, in an m-AAA metalloprotease complex at the inner mitochondrial membrane (Patron et al., 2018).

### POLG Ataxia

Mutations in the *POLG* gene cause a continuum of overlapping phenotypes, and ataxia is a prominent feature in the ataxia neuropathy spectrum of *POLG*-related neurological disorders (Cohen et al., 1993; Rahman and Copeland, 2019). *POLG* mutations are the most common cause of hereditary mitochondrial disorders. The ataxia neuropathy spectrum includes the phenotypes previously referred to as mitochondrial recessive ataxia syndrome (MIRAS) and sensory ataxia neuropathy dysarthria and ophthalmoplegia (SANDO). Ataxia and neuropathy are core features. Approximately two-thirds of patients with POLG ataxia develop seizures and almost one-half develop ophthalmoplegia, while clinical myopathy is rare. In patients with myopathy, muscle biopsy demonstrates increased SDH expression, indicating mitochondrial proliferation (see Fig. 23.3, *A*). Myoclonus, blindness, and liver dysfunction of various severity may occur (Tzoulis et al., 2006; Wong et al., 2008).

***ARCAs with impaired DNA repair.*** In 14 or more ARCAs, mutations have been found in genes involved in repair of single-strand break, double-strand break, or base excision repair (see Table 23.7). Some of the non-neurological clinical features of ataxia-telangiectasia, such as immune deficiency, sensitivity to ionizing radiation, oculomotor apraxia, malignancy, and polyneuropathy, are also associated with these diseases, depending on the involved DNA repair mechanism.

### Ataxia Telangiectasia

Ataxia-telangiectasia typically affects young children. The prevalence of ataxia-telangiectasia is ~1 in 40,000 live births in the United States. Ataxia-telangiectasia in children almost always accompanies oculomotor apraxia, choreoathetosis, and telangiectasia (especially in ocular conjunctivae). Myoclonus and dystonia are also frequently seen. Sensitivity to ionic radiation, immune deficiency with frequent infections, and increased incidence of lymphoma, leukemia, and other malignancies are important issues in management of ataxia-telangiectasia patients. The life span of these patients is significantly shortened to, usually, less than 50 years. However, atypical clinical presentations of ataxia-telangiectasia have been increasingly recognized, with adolescent- and adult-onset milder disease with isolated ataxia or dystonia. Elevated serum alpha-fetoprotein (AFP) levels serve as an important diagnostic biomarker, especially when greater than 20 ng/mL. Brain MRI shows cerebellar atrophy. Ataxia-telangiectasia is caused by mutations in the *ATM* gene, which encodes a serine/threonine kinase that is recruited and activated by DNA double-strand breaks and phosphorylates key proteins to initiate activation of the DNA damage checkpoint. *ATM* also regulates nuclear localization, gene transcription, oxidative stress response, apoptosis, and nonsense-mediated decay (Ambrose and Gatti, 2013). Several reports, including one randomized controlled trial (Zannolli et al., 2012), suggested beneficial effect of glucocorticoids, including dexamethasone encapsulated in autologous erythrocytes which alleviate chronic side effects (Chessa et al., 2014). Glucocorticoids may induce splicing of ATM transcript to a short but active ATM variant. For treatment of immunodeficiency, IVIG replacement is useful.

### Autosomal Recessive Cerebellar Ataxias with Oculomotor Apraxia

Oculomotor apraxia is defined as the inability to initiate horizontal saccades in the head-fixed condition. Head rotation is usually necessary to initiate gaze shifts. Oculomotor apraxia is largely attributable to defective saccadic initiation and hypometria (Salman, 2015). Ataxia with oculomotor apraxia type 1 (AOA1), AOA2, and AOA4, as well as ataxia-telangiectasia, exhibit oculomotor apraxia, ataxia, and neuropathy with variably elevated serum level of alpha fetal protein while AOA3, which has been described in a single Arabic family with homozygous missense mutation in the *PIK3R5* gene, showed infantile onset of ataxia with no elevation of serum alpha fetal protein (Bohlega et al., 2011). While patients with these AOAs have neurological features very similar to those of ataxia-telangiectasia, they show neither telangiectasia nor immunological deficiency. AOA1 and AOA2 may be clinically difficult to distinguish from ataxia-telangiectasia when ataxia-telangiectasia does not accompany non-neurological features, especially in late-onset patients. However, the presence of hypoalbuminemia and hypercholesterolemia indicates the diagnosis of AOA1. AOA4 is a rapidly progressive disease, and most patients became wheelchair-bound in the second or third decade due to severe muscle weakness and atrophy. Genetic mutations of AOAs are in genes involved in repair of single-strand breaks (*APTX* in AOA1 [Moreira et al., 2001] and *PNKP* in AOA4 [Bras et al., 2015]) and double-strand breaks (*SETX* in AOA2 [Moreira et al., 2004]). Several allelic variants of *SETX* gene have been associated with autosomal recessive spinocerebellar ataxia with axonal neuropathy 2 (SCAN2) (Airoldi et al., 2010; Anheim et al., 2008;

Asaka et al., 2006; Bassuk et al., 2007; Duquette et al., 2005; Fogel and Perlman, 2006; Moreira et al., 2004), while other *SETX* variants cause autosomal dominant juvenile amotrophic lateral sclerosis (ALS4) (Chen et al., 2004). The protein product senataxin is required for resolving RNA-DNA hybrids in R-loops (Zhao et al., 2016).

Other ARCAs with impaired DNA repair also have some of characteristic manifestations of ataxia-telangiectasia. For example, RIDDLE (radiosensitivity, immunodeficiency dysmorphic features and learning difficulties; Stewart et al., 2007) and Nijmegen breakage syndrome (NBS; Antoccia et al., 2006), which are caused by mutations in genes involved in double-strand breaks repair, show immune deficiency and radiosensitivity. Although neuropathy is often associated with inherited ataxias, it is a cardinal feature of patients with mutations in SSB repair genes, including *APTX (AOA1)* (Moreira et al., 2001) , *PNKP (AOA4)* (Bras et al., 2015), *TDP1 (SCAN1)* (Takashima et al., 2002), and *XRCC1 (SCAR26)* (Takashima et al., 2002), as well as in some double strand breaks repair genes, including *ATM (ataxia-telangiectasia)* and *SETX (AOA2)* (Takashima et al., 2002).

***Autosomal recessive cerebellar ataxias with complex lipid metabolism abnormalities.*** ARCAs are also caused by mutations of genes regulating metabolism of lipids, including sterols, sphingolipids, glycerophospholipids, glucosylceramides, fatty acyls, and prenol lipids (Synofzik et al., 2019). These ARCAs show disorders of various intracellular organelles, such as lysosomes, peroxisomes, and endoplasmic reticula. The list of genetic mutations of ARCAs involved in lipid metabolism has become long, as the WES becomes common in genetic testing. Here we will focus on Niemann-Pick type C and cerebrotendinous xanthomatosis.

### Niemann-Pick C

Niemann-Pick C accounts for about 1%–2% of all ARCAs (Synofzik et al., 2015). Niemann-Pick C is caused by mutations in the *NPC1*, or rarely *NPC2*, gene and primarily affects the cholesterol trafficking in the brain and peripheral organs. In a late stage of the disease cerebellar Purkinje cells are primarily affected. Clinical phenotype is predominantly ataxia across age groups while hypotonia and delayed developmental milestones are seen in infantile patients and visceral signs precede neurological signs in patients with juvenile-onset Niemann-Pick C. In adult patients, a range of neurological, psychiatric, and visceral signs appear years before diagnosis. Miglustat treatment significantly delays the disease progression and death (Pineda et al., 2019).

### Cerebrotendinous Xanthomatosis

Cerebrotendinous xanthomatosis is an ARCA caused by mutations in the *CYP27A1* gene (Nie et al., 2014). Clinically, patients with cerebrotendinous xanthomatosis show adult-onset progressive cerebellar ataxia, dystonia, dementia, epilepsy psychiatric disorders, polyneuropathy, and myopathy, accompanied by tendon xanthoma, and other premature systemic manifestations, including childhood cataracts, atherosclerosis, osteoporosis, and respiratory insufficiency. An elevated plasma cholestanol level provides the diagnostic confirmation before genetic diagnosis (Stelten et al., 2019).

### Ataxia with Vitamin E Deficiency

Vitamin E deficiency caused by hereditary disorders such as α-tocopherol transferase deficiency and abetalipoproteinemia leads to ataxia. Ataxia with vitamin E deficiency typically has juvenile onset with progressive ataxia, loss of proprioception, areflexia, decreased visual acuity and Babinski sign, which resembles the phenotype of Friedreich ataxia. Reduced plasma vitamin E (α-tocopherol) level with normal lipoproteins and the presence of biallelic *TTPA* pathogenic variants on genetic testing establish the diagnosis (Schuelke, 1993). Vitamin E deficiency is also seen in infants with abetalipoproteinemia (Hentati et al., 2012). These diseases are treatable by timely dietary supplements.

***Autosomal recessive cerebellar ataxias with cytoskeleton protein.*** SYNE1 ataxia accounts for about 5% of recessive ataxias (Synofzik et al., 2016). Although initial reports portrayed pure cerebellar ataxia in patients with this disease (Dupre et al., 2007; Gros-Louis et al., 2007), subsequent cases indicated that the majority of patients show various extracerebellar signs, including motor neuron disease (Mademan et al., 2016; Synofzik et al., 2016). The onset of ataxia varies from childhood to middle age, generally with slow progression of the disease. *SYNE1* encodes a large synaptic nuclear envelope protein of the spectrin family, Nesprin 1 (Gros-Louis et al., 2007). The *SYNE1* mutations include intronic mutations and truncating mutations.

Remaining ARCAs can be searched in OMIM (https://www.omim.org/).

### X-linked Ataxia

There are only a handful of X-linked ataxias, among which FXTAS is the most well recognized because of the mutation related to fragile X syndrome (Hagerman and Hagerman, 2016). FXTAS is associated with CGG triplets in the premutation range (55–200 CGG repetitions) in the *FMR1* gene on X chromosome. FXTAS, a late-onset neurodegenerative disorder, typically affects male premutation carriers with a constellation of neurological manifestations, including tremor (essential tremor–like tremor, resting tremor, and intention tremor) and cerebellar ataxia, often associated with parkinsonism, and cognitive impairments (Fay-Karmon and Hassin-Baer, 2019). Women with premutation alleles of *FMR1* less frequently have FXTAS but may show fragile X–associated primary ovarian insufficiency, which is a chronic disorder characterized by oligo/amenorrhea and hypergonadotropic hypogonadism before 40 years of age (Fink et al., 2018). MRI of the brain of FXTAS and female premutation carriers shows white matter intensity characteristically with T2 intensities in middle cerebellar peduncles (Fig. 23.2 E) (Apartis et al., 2012; Shelton et al., 2017). The premutation shows further pleiotropic phenotype, including a wide variety of somewhat elusive neuropsychiatric disorders (Hagerman et al., 2018).

The premutation expansion of the CGG repeat increases the level of FMR1 mRNA with the equivalent or slightly decreased level of FMR1 protein. The pathogenic mechanism is, thus, not a loss of function of the FMR1 protein. The RNA with the premutation CGG repeat (and CCG repeat from the opposite strand) may gain a toxic function through interactions with RNA-binding proteins and the RAN translation (Glineburg et al., 2018). Furthermore, the toxic RNA and translated proteins are shown to influence liquid-liquid phase separation, membraneless organelle dynamics, and nucleocytoplasmic transport (Rodriguez and Todd, 2019). Although the pathogenic contribution of each mechanism in FXTAS needs further investigation, the disease mechanism of FXTAS is clearly different from that of fragile X syndrome, which is caused by a loss of FMR1 protein function.

## DEGENERATIVE CAUSE

### Idiopathic Late-Onset Cerebellar Ataxia

ILOCA was first used by Harding for all nonhereditary progressive cerebellar ataxias with no identifiable secondary causes (Harding, 1981). MSA-C was included at the time and later separated from ILOCA. Unlike MSA-C, which has a distinct pathology feature of glial cytoplasmic inclusion (Gilman et al., 2008; Quinn, 1989), ILOCA does not have a signature pathology finding.

The prevalence of ILOAC may range from 2.2 to 12.4 cases in every 100,000 people (Leone et al., 1995; Muzaimi et al., 2004; Polo et al., 1991; Tsuji et al., 2008).

Patients with ILOCA have cerebellar ataxia as the core clinical feature, including wide-based gait and stance, appendicular ataxia, such as dysmetria on finger-to-nose or heel-to-shin tests, as well as dysdiadochokinesia with rapid alternating movements. Scanning speech is also common. Ocular findings on examination may include saccadic pursuit, saccade hyper- or hypometria, gaze-evoked nystagmus, and impaired optokinetic nystagmus. In addition, patients may have signs of pyramidal tract involvement, such as hyper- or hyporeflexia, positive Babinski signs, or spasticity (Abele et al., 2002, 2007; Burk et al., 2005). Bladder dysfunction may be seen in about 30% of ILOCA patients, making it more difficult to distinguish ILOCA and MSC-C. Image findings of patients with ILOCA include isolated cerebellar atrophy or possibly concomitant brainstem or spinal cord atrophy (Abele et al., 2007).

The etiology of ILOCA is still unclear. Whether it is a uniform group of patients is still under debate. It can be caused by a combination of genetic and environmental factors, similar to other neurodegenerative diseases such as sporadic amyotrophic lateral sclerosis.

### Multiple System Atrophy—Cerebellar Type

MSA-C is a late-onset, idiopathic degenerative disorder that presents with autonomic symptoms and cerebellar ataxia with or without parkinsonian features (Video 23.6). It was initially termed olivopontocerebellar atrophy (OPCA) and was included in ILOCA by Harding (1981). However, it is defined by its pathological hallmark, α-synuclein-positive glial cytoplasmic inclusions, setting itself apart from ILOCA (Gilman et al., 2008). The incidence of MSA is about 0.6–0.7 cases per 100,000 person-years (Bower et al., 1997; Schrag et al., 1888; Tison et al., 2000). Among MSA patients, MSA parkinsonian-type (MSA-P) is 2–4 times more prevalent than MSC-C (Gilman et al., 2005; Kollensperger et al., 2011).

Patients with MSA-C have autonomic symptoms such as urinary incontinence, dizziness, and syncopal episodes as the consequences of orthostatic hypotension, constipation, and sweating abnormalities. Motor symptoms are predominantly cerebellar ataxia (wide-based gait, truncal ataxia, limb dysmetria, and change in speech), while there may be a combination of parkinsonian symptoms (rigidity, tremor, and bradykinesia) and pyramidal tract involvement. Neurological examination may reveal square-wave jerks, saccadic pursuit, nystagmus, and scanning speech. The progression is much faster than idiopathic Parkinson disease. Patients require walking aids in about 3–5 years after the onset of symptoms and become bedridden in about 6–7 years. The average life expectancy after diagnosis is about 7–9 years, and patients commonly succumb to pneumonia or urosepsis (Klockgether, 2010; Watanabe et al., 2002; Wenning et al., 2013).

The definitive diagnosis mandates the finding of widespread cerebral α-synuclein-positive glial cytoplasmic inclusions on postmortem pathology (Gilman et al., 2008). Clinically, it is a diagnosis of exclusion. The diagnostic challenge frequently is to distinguish MSA-C from ILOCA. Age of onset for MSA-C and ILOCA are both in the mid-50s. Patients with ILOCA progress more slowly and about 50% of the patients can still walk without walking aids 11 years after symptom onset. Patients with ILOCA may have normal life span (Abele et al., 2002).

MRI of MSA-C patients have profound cerebellar atrophy but may also have atrophy of the pons and putamen. Two findings are consistent with the diagnosis of MSA-C, the putaminal hyperintense rim and the "hot-cross-bun" sign; both are seen on T2-weighted or FLAIR imaging. (Fig. 23.2, G and H) The former is a slit-like hyperintense rim at the lateral aspect of the putamen. The latter is a hyperintense cruciform appearance of the pons (Lee et al., 2005). However, these are nonspecific findings. The putaminal hyperintense rim may be seen in normal subjects and "hot-cross-bun" sign can occur in any patients with pontocerebellar degeneration and gliosis (Burk et al., 2001).

Despite extensive efforts to distinguish ILOCA from MSA-C, about 30% of patients who were initially diagnosed as ILOCA eventually develop into MSA-C, demonstrating the difficulty of making the diagnosis (Abele et al., 2002; Gilman et al., 2000).

Unlike SCAs, no single-gene mutation leads to MSA-C. Functionally impaired coenzyme CoQ2 (CoQ2) variants are associated with the development of MSA-C in two families (Multiple-System Atrophy Research, 2013). The CoQ2 model is particularly of interest because the synthesis of coenzyme CoQ10 (CoQ10) relies on CoQ2, and CoQ10 levels in the cerebellum were decreased (Barca et al., 2016; Schottlaender et al., 2016). However, a large scale of GWAS was unable to associate MSA-C with CoQ2 (Sailer et al., 2016).

## FUNCTIONAL (PSYCHOGENIC) ATAXIA

Functional ataxia can present with ataxic limb movements, but more commonly with gait imbalance. They are more commonly categorized under functional movement disorder or functional gait disorders. Clues in clinical history consistent with functional ataxia include abrupt onset, fluctuation of symptoms with spontaneous remissions, and multiple somatizations. Sometimes one may identify a secondary gain or pending litigation. Upon neurological examination, it is important to pay attention to inconsistencies. Patients may demonstrate fluctuation of impairment (51%), excessive slowness of movements (35%), hesitation (16%), assume uneconomical postures (30%), "walking on ice" gait pattern (30%), and frequent buckling without actual falls (22%) (Lempert et al., 1991). Romberg test may demonstrate building up of amplitudes of swaying after a delay or shaking the upper torso during the test, but the legs are completely steady. Many of the symptoms or signs may be ameliorated with distraction: dysmetric movements on one side got better or were interrupted when patients were asked to perform tasks on the contralateral side. Patients may have dysmetria or erratic trajectory with centrifugal limb movements while centripetal movements were perfectly fine (Lempert et al., 1991; Manto, 2001; Miyasaki et al., 2003). It is not uncommon to see functional movement disorders present together with a true movement disorder. It is therefore important for the clinician to exclude other causes or concomitant true ataxia before making the diagnosis of a functional movement disorder, even if the neurological examination is highly consistent with functional movement disorders.

## MANAGEMENT

### Pharmacological Treatments

Treatment for cerebellar ataxia has been a challenge. Ataxias of secondary causes require treatment of the underlying disorders: for example, autoimmune, vitamin deficiency, toxic agents, or overdosed medications. However, for symptomatic treatments of genetic or degenerative ataxias, few pharmacological agents have shown benefits. Many medications targeting polyQ have been tested in animal models with a wide range of mechanisms, including histone deacetylation inhibitor, adenosine receptor antagonist, autophagy inducer, serotonin reuptake inhibitor, and modulators of chaperone functions. (Ashizawa et al., 2018; Buijsen et al., 2019). However, most agents have no proven benefit clinically. The 2018 American Academy of Neurology guideline reviewed the literature extensively and deemed that only 4-aminopyridine, riluzole, valproic acid, and thyrotropin-releasing hormone may improve symptoms of ataxia in selected populations of patients (Zesiewicz et al., 2018).

### 4-Aminopyridine

Evidence suggests that 4-aminopyridine acts through blocking potassium channels to prolong the duration of the action potential and increase the action potential after hyperpolarization, therefore restoring the pacemaking precision of Purkinje cells in an episodic ataxia type 2 mouse model (Alvina and Khodakhah, 2010). The median monthly attack frequency in patients with episodic ataxia type 2 was significantly reduced when the patients were treated with 4-aminopyridine over the course of 3 months (Strupp et al., 2011).

### Valproic Acid

Valproic acid is widely used as an anticonvulsant, believed to act through inhibiting sodium channels. Interestingly, it is also a histone deacetylase inhibitor, and in animal models of SCA3, it can reduce polyQ-mediated cytotoxicity (Yi et al., 2013). A recent clinical trial showed valproic acid improved stance in patients with SCA3 at 12 weeks (Lei et al., 2016).

### Thyrotropin-Releasing Hormone

A clinical trial conducted before cerebellar ataxia was routinely genetically diagnosed showed that thyrotrophin-releasing hormone possibly improves speech, gait, and standing in patients with cerebellar ataxia in 10–14 days (Sobue et al., 1983). However, given that the genetic or molecular identity of these cerebellar ataxia patients was unclear, the significance or the applicability of these results remains to be determined or verified.

### Riluzole and Its Precursor

Riluzole, a medication approved for treatment of amyotrophic lateral sclerosis, had been shown to improve ataxia symptoms for several SCAs at 8 weeks and 12 months (Ristori et al., 2010; Romano et al., 2015). The rationale is supported by normalization of firing patterns of Purkinje cells in brain slices of SCA3 mice. It is believed that riluzole acts through modulating SK channel activities to correct burst firing of Purkinje cells in transgenic mice to tonic firing seen in wild-type animals (Shakkottai et al., 2011; Walter et al., 2006). However, the preliminary results of a recent open pilot trial with a precursor of riluzole, trigriluzole/troriluzole, which supposedly has better CNS penetrance, showed the trigriluzole is safe for patients, although no significant benefit was found in mixed SCAs (SCA1, 2, 3, 6, 7, 8 10) in a short term. Another phase III randomized controlled trial, again aiming at the same SCAs, is at the initiation phase (www.clinicaltrials.gov) to test long-term effects.

### Varenicline

Varenicline (Chantix), a ligand of nicotinic acetylcholine receptors (Mihalak et al., 2006), has been reported to improve SCA3 and SCA14 (Zesiewicz et al., 2012; Zesiewicz and Sullivan, 2008). However, other investigators have yet to repeat the results (Connolly et al., 2012).

## Nonpharmacological Treatments

### Noninvasive Brain Stimulators

Transcranial magnetic stimulation and transcranial direct current stimulation are believed to modulate the excitability of different areas of the nervous system and may have effects on motor, cognitive, and affective functions (van Dun et al., 2017). Transcranial magnetic stimulation targeting the cerebellum has been shown to improve ataxic gait and truncal ataxia in patients with SCA after 21 days of treatment (Shiga et al., 2002; Shimizu et al., 1999).

It has been demonstrated that a single session of transcranial direct current stimulation stimulating the cerebellar region has at least transient benefits in patients including mixed SCAs, Friedreich ataxia, MSA-C, FXTAS, and AOA (Benussi et al., 2015). A 2-week treatment course can have benefit that lasts up to 3 months (Benussi et al., 2017). A more recent study applied anodal cerebellum and cathodal spinal transcranial direct current stimulation to patients, including 9 SCAs, 5 MSA-C, and 6 other ataxias, and demonstrated that after 2 weeks of treatment, there was an improvement in ataxia symptoms (Benussi et al., 2018).

### Physical and Occupational Therapy

Intensive physical and occupational therapy for 4 weeks has shown benefit in ataxia, gait speed, and activity of daily living in patients with SCA6, SCA31, and patients with pure cerebellar ataxia of unknown causes. The effect may last for as long as 24 weeks in about 50% of the patients (Miyai et al., 2012). On the other hand, pressure splints in addition to neuromuscular rehabilitation have no benefit on ataxia resulting from multiple sclerosis (Armutlu et al., 2001). Stochastic vibration therapy has been shown to improve walking and speech in patients with SCA1, 2, 3, and 6 in one study (Kaut et al., 2014). However, the SARA scores, the primary outcome, did not show a significant difference between control and sham groups. There is not sufficient evidence to determine whether this mode of intervention is beneficial to SCAs.

## Targeted Molecular Therapy

### Antisense Oligonucleotides

Antisense oligonucleotides (ASOs) are short segments of single-strand oligonucleotides that are designed to have sequences complementary to specific targets in RNAs or genomic DNA, leading to mRNA degradation or interference of transcription, splicing, or translation. Recent success with ASOs in spinal muscular atrophy showed that ASOs can be promising and safe therapeutic agents to treat neurodegenerative diseases (Mousa et al., 2018). Ongoing clinical trials of ASOs include amyotrophic lateral sclerosis (targeting ...) (SOD1 and C9ORF72), HD (targeting HTT), and Alzheimer disease (targeting APP). In two mouse models of SCA2, intraventricularly administered ASOs targeting ATXN2 were able to reduce ATXN2 expression in the cerebellum and improve motor function, compared with control mice injected with saline (Scoles et al., 2017). Similarly, ASOs administered to SCA3 mice lowered the expression of ATXN3 with expanded polyQ (McLoughlin et al., 2018). These preclinical data provide scientific rationale to develop ASO therapies for SCAs.

### Gene Therapy

Gene therapy is a molecular method aiming to replace defective or absent genes, or to counteract the ones undergoing overexpression. Virally-mediated knockdown of gene expression can be promising to treat PolyQ SCAs, whereas virally-mediated gene over-expression is useful for ARCAs, such as Friedreich ataxia. Various viral vectors have been developed and tested in preclinical models with success. Among the different approaches, gene editing with CRISPR/Cas9 has received attention because of its precision and easy personalization. CRISPR/Cas9 is capable of specific genomic editing through the combination of a guide RNA that is complementary to the target sequence and a Cas9 (or Cpf1) with endonuclease activity to cleave the target DNA. CRISPR/Cas9 has been adopted widely in the biomedical field. However, technical difficulties such as delivery and off-target effects set the limit. A recent study deleted the CAG repeat expansion region in induced pleural potent cells (iPSCs) from SCA3 patients, setting evidence for the technical feasibility for clinical application (Ouyang et al., 2018).

*The complete reference list is available online at https://expertconsult.inkling.com/.*

24

# Diagnosis and Assessment of Parkinson Disease and Other Movement Disorders

*Joseph Jankovic, Anthony E. Lang*

## OUTLINE



The term *movement disorders* is often used synonymously with *basal ganglia* or *extrapyramidal diseases.* However, neither of the two latter terms adequately encompasses all the disorders included under the broad umbrella of movement disorders. Movement disorders are neurological motor disorders manifested by slowness or poverty of movement (bradykinesia or hypokinesia, such as that seen in parkinsonian disorders) at one end of the spectrum and abnormal involuntary movements (hyperkinesias) such as tremor, dystonia, chorea, stereotypy, athetosis, ballism, tics, myoclonus, stereotypies, akathisias, and other dyskinesias at the other. Although motor dysfunctions resulting from upper and lower motor neuron, spinal cord, peripheral nerve, and muscle diseases usually are not classified as movement disorders, abnormalities in muscle tone (e.g., rigidity, spasticity), incoordination (cerebellar ataxia; see Chapters 23 and 94), and complex disorders of execution of movement denoted by the term *apraxia* (see Chapter 11) are generally included among movement disorders.

The term *movement disorder* refers to a clinical condition for which there are many possible causes. In most fields of neurology, the recommended initial clinical approach is to determine where in the nervous system the disease process is located and what that process could be. When dealing with movement disorders, however, rather than localizing the lesion the first step is to classify the movement disorder based on knowledge and recognition of phenomenology. Some abnormal movements may appear to be bizarre and therefore difficult to categorize. Despite attempts at uniformity in definition, classification errors are common. Inaccurate categorization occasionally has resulted in clinical, genetic, and epidemiological misinformation embedded in the literature. This is even more evident in complex conditions that have a combination of a variety of hypokinetic and hyperkinetic movement disorders such as tardive dyskinesia and N-methyl-D-aspartate receptor (NMDAR) antibody-mediated encephalitis (Varley et al., 2019). Video documentation is very useful in clarifying the phenomenology, thereby minimizing the risk of misdiagnosis.

Many movement disorders have no known or established cause. These disorders, sometimes called *essential* or *idiopathic movement disorders*, are now best classifiable as *primary movement disorders* and distinguished from those that are secondary to identifiable diseases. In the following sections, the emphasis is on historical and clinical features that help the clinician make this distinction. Family history, including parental consanguinity (suggestive of autosomal recessive disorder) and ethnic origin (e.g., Ashkenazi Jewish) (Inzelberg et al., 2014), often is helpful in arriving at a diagnosis. It is crucial to recognize that the symptoms in other family members may be different from those in the patient because of variability of gene expression and penetrance or because they may have an entirely different disorder. For example, some family members of patients with primary dystonia may have dystonic features, whereas others may have predominantly a tremor. Additional problems that may hamper the acquisition of an adequate family history include adoption, uncertain paternity, and even the deliberate withholding of important family information. Denial of positive family history is particularly common in patients with Huntington disease (HD) and the genetic ataxias. An adult-onset disorder may not have been evident in a family member who died at an early age. It is particularly important to exclude Wilson disease (WD) because of the specific therapy available and the universally fatal outcome of the disease if left untreated (Lin et al., 2014).

Obtaining a birth history (e.g., Apgar score, history of anoxia, jaundice, or traumatic birth) and early developmental abnormalities (e.g., delayed milestones) is essential, especially when considering the possibility of cerebral palsy or kernicterus (Monbaliu et al., 2017). Also, a history of perinatal infection or childhood encephalitis or meningitis is important. Certain drugs and toxins have a strong potential for causing movement disorders, particularly drugs that block dopamine receptors. These include antipsychotic drugs (e.g., all the typical and atypical neuroleptics), certain antiemetic drugs, and other drugs used for various gastrointestinal (GI) disorders (e.g., metoclopramide, prochlorperazine, promethazine), calcium channel blockers (e.g., cinnarizine, flunarizine), central nervous system (CNS) stimulants (e.g., methylphenidate, cocaine), and dopaminergic drugs (e.g., levodopa).

Besides documenting the movement disorder, neurological examination should search for additional findings that would help indicate the secondary nature of the problem. General physical examination must be thorough. An extremely important component of the examination in individuals suspected of WD is a corneal evaluation, including slit-lamp examination, to exclude the presence of a Kayser-Fleischer ring, a characteristic finding in this autosomal recessive disorder that may be manifested by a broad variety of movement disorders (Fig. 24.1). The phenomenology of the movement disorder should be described in detail while the patient is at rest and during various positions and activities. Whenever possible, particularly if there are some unusual or atypical features, the movement disorder should be video recorded (after patient's written permission). The nature and extent of laboratory investigations depend on clinical suspicions, based on the history and physical examination.

## PARKINSONISM

The initial feature of many basal ganglia diseases is slowness of movement (bradykinesia) and paucity or absence of movement (akinesias), often associated with rigidity and tremor (Jankovic, 2008). Some authors have used the term *hypokinesia* to describe a reduction in amplitude of movement. The combination of slowness and poverty of movement and increase in muscle tone is characteristic of many parkinsonian disorders. The term *parkinsonism* is used to describe a syndrome manifested by a combination of the following six cardinal features: (1) tremor at rest, (2) bradykinesia, (3) rigidity, (4) loss of postural reflexes, (5) flexed posture, and (6) freezing (motor blocks). The four major characteristics of parkinsonism account for most of the described clinical abnormalities: tremor, rigidity, akinesia, and postural disturbances (forming the acronym *TRAP*).

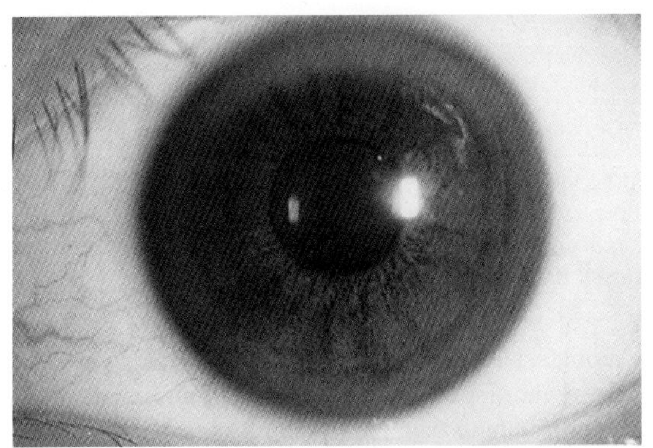

**Fig. 24.1 Kayser-Fleischer Ring.** Note the golden-brown full-circumference ring, thickest and most readily seen between the 11 o'clock and 1 o'clock positions of the cornea.

The most common cause of idiopathic parkinsonism (akinetic-rigid syndrome) is Parkinson disease (PD) (Obeso et al., 2017). As a result of advances in genetics, many forms of idiopathic parkinsonism have been found to result from mutations in specific genes, such as those coding for α-synuclein (*SNCA* gene), parkin (*PARK2* gene), leucine-rich repeat kinase 2 (*LRRK2* gene), PTEN-induced putative kinase 1 (*PINK1* gene) protein, and a growing number of other gene mutations (Table 24.1) (Deng et al., 2018). Whereas some of the gene mutations (e.g., *SNCA*) are very rare causes of parkinsonism, *PARK2* mutations account for up to 50% of all patients with early-onset parkinsonism, and *LRRK2* mutations may account for a large proportion of cases in selected populations (e.g., North Africans, Ashkenazi Jews) (Inzelberg et al., 2014). Although less than 10% of all patients with PD have a causative genetic mutation, clinicians must learn about these genetic forms of parkinsonism not only to understand the pathogenic mechanisms but also to learn how to interpret and use the increasingly available gene tests, including whole-exome and whole-genome sequencing, for genetic counseling (MacArthur et al., 2014). There is growing appreciation for different subtypes of PD and the need to develop diagnostic criteria based on clinical, genetic, and pathological features (Thenganatt and Jankovic, 2015). Besides genetic causes, there are many other causes of parkinsonism and of parkinsonism combined with other neurological deficits (atypical parkinsonism or parkinsonism-plus syndromes) (Box 24.1).

### Motor Abnormalities

Early in the course of the disease, many patients with parkinsonism are unaware of any motor deficit. Often the patient's spouse comments on a reduction in facial expression (often misinterpreted as

**TABLE 24.1 Genetic Causes of Parkinsonism (Excludes Unconfirmed Genes and Genes Thought to Serve as Risk Factors)**

| Disease Classification with Gene (Marras et al., 2016) | Inheritance | Gene Locus | Protein |
|---|---|---|---|
| PARK-*SNCA* (PARK1)—typical PD | AD | 4q21-23 includes missense mutations and duplications and triplications | α-Synuclein |
| PARK-*Parkin* (PARK2)—juvenile parkinsonism, dystonia | AR | 6q25.2-27 | Parkin |
| PARK-*PINK1* (PARK6)—early onset | AR | 1p36 | (PTEN-induced kinase 1) |
| PARK-*DJ-1* (PARK7)—early onset | AR | 1p36 | DJ-1 |
| PARK-*LRRK2* (PARK8)—PD | AD | 12p11.23-q13.11 | LRRK2 (dardarin) |
| PARK-*ATP13A2* (PARK9) (Kufor-Rakeb syndrome)—early onset, spasticity, dementia, ophthalmoparesis, pallidal atrophy | AR | 1p36 | Lysosomal type 5 P-type ATPase |
| NBIA/DYT/PARK-*PLA2G6* (PARK14)—adult-onset dystonia-parkinsonism, subtype of NBIA | AR | 22q13.1 | Phospholipase $A_2$ |
| PARK-*FBXO7* (PARK15)—early-onset parkinsonian-pyramidal syndrome | AR | 22q12-q13 | F-box Protein7 |
| PARK-*VPS35* (PARK17) | AD | 16q11.2 | VPS35 |
| PARK- *DNAJC6* (PARK19) | AR | 1p31.3 | Auxilin |
| PARK-*SYNJ1* (PARK20) | AR | 21q22.11 | Synaptojanin 1 |
| PARK-*CHCHD2* (PARK22) | AD | 7p11.2 | CHCHD2 |
| PARK-*VPS13C* (PARK23) | AD | 15q22.2 | Vacuolar Protein Sorting 13 |

*AD*, Autosomal dominant; *AR*, autosomal recessive; *ATP*, adenosine triphosphate; *GCI*, glial cytoplasmic inclusions; *LB*, Lewy bodies; *NBIA*, neurodegeneration with brain iron accumulation; *PD*, Parkinson disease.

## BOX 24.1 Classification of Parkinsonism

I. Parkinson disease
  Parkinson disease—sporadic
  Parkinson disease—hereditary (see Table 24.1)
II. Multisystem degenerations ("parkinsonism plus")
  Progressive supranuclear palsy
  Multiple system atrophy (Shy-Drager syndrome):
    MSA-P (striatonigral degeneration)
    MSA-C (olivopontocerebellar atrophy)
  Lytico-bodig disease, or amyotrophic lateral sclerosis and parkinsonism-dementia complex of Guam
  Corticobasal degeneration
  Progressive pallidal atrophy
III. Heredodegenerative parkinsonism
  Dopa-responsive dystonia
  Huntington disease
  Wilson disease
  Neurodegenerations with brain iron accumulation (including pantothenate kinase-associated neurodegeneration and aceruloplasminemia)
  Spinocerebellar atrophies, including Machado-Joseph disease
  Frontotemporal dementia with parkinsonism (FTDP)
  Gerstmann-Sträussler-Scheinker syndrome
  Familial progressive subcortical gliosis
  Lubag (X-linked dystonia-parkinsonism)
  Primary familial brain calcification
  Mitochondrial cytopathies with striatal necrosis
  Ceroid lipofuscinosis
  Familial parkinsonism with peripheral neuropathy
  Parkinsonian-pyramidal syndrome
  Neuroacanthocytosis
  Neuroferritinopathy
IV. Secondary (acquired, symptomatic) parkinsonism
  Infectious: postencephalitic, acquired immunodeficiency syndrome, subacute sclerosing panencephalitis, Creutzfeldt-Jakob disease, prion diseases
  Drugs: dopamine receptor blocking drugs (antipsychotic, antiemetic drugs), reserpine, tetrabenazine, methyldopa, lithium, flunarizine, cinnarizine
  Toxins: MPTP, carbon monoxide, manganese, mercury, carbon disulfide, cyanide, methanol, ethanol
  Vascular: multi-infarct disease
  Trauma: pugilistic encephalopathy disease
  Other: parathyroid abnormalities, hypothyroidism, hepatocerebral degeneration, brain tumor, paraneoplastic, normal-pressure hydrocephalus, noncommunicating hydrocephalus, syringomesencephalia, hemiatrophy-hemiparkinsonism, peripherally induced tremor and parkinsonism, psychogenic

*MSA-C*, Multiple system atrophy, cerebellar type; *MSA-P*, multiple system atrophy, parkinsonian type; *MPTP*, 1-methyl-4-phenyl-1,2,3,6-tetrahydropyridine.

depression), a reduction in arm swing while walking, and a slowing of activities of daily living, most notably dressing, feeding, and walking. The patient may then become aware of a reduction in manual dexterity, with slowness and clumsiness interfering with activities. PD is typically asymmetrical, especially early in the course. A painful or even frozen shoulder is one of the most common early symptoms of PD, possibly related to decreased arm swing and secondary joint changes or shoulder muscle rigidity, often misdiagnosed as bursitis, arthritis, or a rotator cuff disorder. Indeed, many PD patients have a variety of joint (e.g., striatal hand or foot) and skeletal deformities (e.g., scoliosis, Pisa sign, camptocormia) which are often wrongly attributed to arthritis or orthopedic problems (Wijemanne and Jankovic, 2019).

## TABLE 24.2 Parkinsonian Syndromes: Differential Diagnosis

| | PD | PSP | MSA-P | MSA-C | CBS | DLB |
|---|---|---|---|---|---|---|
| *Bradykinesia* | + | + | + | ± | + | ± |
| *Rigidity* | + | + | + | + | + | ± |
| *Gait disturbance* | + | + | + | + | + | ± |
| *Tremor* | + | – | ± | ± | ± | ± |
| *Ataxia* | – | – | – | + | – | – |
| *Dysautonomia* | ± | ± | + | + | – | ± |
| *Dementia* | ± | + | ± | – | ± | + |
| *Dysarthria or dysphagia* | ± | + | + | + | + | ± |
| *Dystonia* | ± | ± | ± | – | + | – |
| *Eyelid apraxia* | ± | + | ± | – | ± | – |
| *Limb apraxia* | – | ± | – | – | + | ± |
| *Motor neuron disease* | – | – | ± | – | – | – |
| *Myoclonus* | ± | – | ± | ± | + | ± |
| *Neuropathy* | – | – | – | ± | – | – |
| *Oculomotor deficit* | – | + | – | + | + | ± |
| *Sleep impairment* | ± | ± | ± | ± | – | ± |
| *Asymmetrical findings* | + | ± | ± | – | + | ± |
| *L-dopa response* | + | ± | ± | ± | – | ± |
| *L-dopa dyskinesia* | + | – | ± | – | – | – |
| *Family history* | ± | – | – | – | – | – |
| *Putaminal T2 hypointensity* | – | ± | + | + | – | – |

*CBS*, Corticobasal syndrome; *DLB*, dementia with Lewy bodies; *MSA-C*, multiple system atrophy, cerebellar type; *MSA-P*, multiple system atrophy, parkinsonian type; *PD*, Parkinson disease; *PSP*, progressive supranuclear palsy; +, present; –, absent.

Besides shoulder pain as one example of a sensory symptom related to underlying motor abnormality, painful dystonia and other etiologies can contribute to pain and discomfort associated with PD (Ha and Jankovic, 2012). Handwriting often becomes slower and smaller (micrographia), with speed and size decreasing as the task continues. Eventually the writing may become illegible. Dressing tasks such as fastening small buttons or getting arms into sleeves are often slow and difficult. Hygiene, including taking a shower or bath, becomes impaired. As with most other tasks, disability is greater if the dominant arm is more affected; shaving, brushing teeth, and other repetitive movements usually are affected the most. Use of eating utensils becomes difficult, chewing is laborious, and choking while swallowing may occur. If the latter is an early and prominent complaint, one must consider bulbar involvement in one of the parkinsonism-plus syndromes, such as progressive supranuclear palsy (PSP) and multiple system atrophy (MSA) (Jellinger, 2014; Low et al., 2015) (Table 24.2).

Speech becomes slurred and loses its volume (hypophonia), and as a result, patients often must repeat themselves. Like gait, speech may be *festinating*; that is, it gets faster and faster (tachyphemia). A large number of additional speech disturbances may occur, including stuttering and *palilalia*, an involuntary repetition of a phrase with increasing rapidity. When hypophonia and speech problems occur as presenting symptoms or in early stage of the disease one should consider a diagnosis other than PD (e.g., hypophonia and palilalia are more common features of PSP and MSA, particularly when present early in the course, than of PD). A monotone, nasal quality of the voice, which is quite distinctive from the hypokinetic dysarthria of PD, also suggests the diagnosis of PSP. A higher-pitched quivering, "whiny" voice may suggest MSA, especially if it is associated with frequent sighing, respiratory gasps, laryngeal stridor, and other respiratory problems (Mehanna and Jankovic, 2010).

Another problem related to impairment of bulbar function is excessive salivation and drooling. Initially this may occur only at night, but later it can be also present throughout the day, at times necessitating the constant use of a tissue or handkerchief.

Getting in and out of a chair or car, and climbing in and out of the bathtub, may cause problems and most patients switch to showering instead of bathing. Many patients misinterpret these difficulties as resulting from "weakness," but there is usually no evidence of weakness in PD until patients develop frailty related to physical inactivity. Generalized loss of energy and fatigability are among the most common complaints by patients with PD (Siciliano et al., 2018). Walking becomes slowed and shuffling, with flexion of the knees and a narrow base. When involvement is asymmetrical, one leg may drag behind the other. Stride then shortens, and turns include multiple steps (turning en bloc). Later, patients may note a tendency to advance more and more rapidly with shorter and shorter steps (festination), at times seemingly propelled forward with a secondary inadequate attempt to maintain the center of gravity over the legs. When this occurs, a nearby wall or an unobstructed fall may be the only method of stopping. Alternatively, the feet may seem glued to the floor, the so-called freezing phenomenon, or motor block. Early on, this is appreciated when the patient initiates walking (start hesitation), especially when turning (particularly in an enclosed space), or attempts to walk through an enclosed area or a narrow passage such as a doorway or walking in or out of an elevator. When combined with poor postural stability, prominent freezing results in the tendency to fall forward or to the side while turning. Later, impaired postural reflexes may cause falls without a propulsive or freezing precipitant. The early occurrence of falls suggests a diagnosis of PSP or other parkinsonian disorder rather than PD. Turning over in bed and adjusting the bedclothes often become difficult. Patients may have to sit up first and then turn, and later the spouse may have to help roll the person over or adjust position for comfort.

## Non-Motor Abnormalities

The complaints of patients with parkinsonism are not limited to the motor system, and a large variety of non-motor symptoms, many of which are probably not directly related to dopaminergic deficiency, often emerge as the disease progresses. In many cases, they become more disabling than the classic motor problems (Lim et al., 2009; Marinus et al., 2018; see Table 24.2). Non-motor features can precede the motor abnormalities and these are increasingly recognized as important features during the prodromal (pre-motor) phase of PD (Postuma and Berg, 2019).

Cognitive decline and dementia occur in a variety of parkinsonian syndromes that are discussed elsewhere (see Chapter 96). Depression is also a common problem, and patients often lose their assertiveness and become withdrawn, more passive, and less motivated to socialize. The term *bradyphrenia* describes the slowness of thought processes and inattentiveness often seen.

Complaints related to autonomic dysfunction are also common in PD, even in the prodromal phase. In all parkinsonian syndromes, constipation is a common complaint and may become severe. However, fecal incontinence does not occur in PD unless the motor disability is such that the patient cannot maneuver to the bathroom, dementia is superimposed, or impaction has led to overflow incontinence. Bladder complaints such as frequency, nocturia, and the sensation of incomplete bladder emptying are also common. Urinary incontinence and bladder retention are especially suggestive of MSA. A mild to moderate degree of orthostatic hypotension is common in parkinsonian disorders, and antiparkinsonian drugs often aggravate the problem. If the autonomic features, particularly erectile dysfunction, sphincter problems, and orthostatic lightheadedness, occur early or become the dominant feature, one must consider the possibility of MSA. Impotence with early loss of nocturnal or morning erections and inability to maintain erection during intercourse is suggestive of MSA (see Chapter 46). The other symptom that may precede the onset of motor problems associated with several parkinsonian disorders, particularly PD, MSA, or dementia with Lewy bodies, is rapid eye movement (REM) sleep behavior disorder (see Chapter 101). One characteristic non-motor feature of PD is excessive greasiness of the skin and seborrheic dermatitis, characteristically seen over the forehead, eyebrows, and malar area.

In addition to pain, there are many other sensory symptoms associated with PD (Patel et al., 2014). Visual complaints are usually not a prominent feature, with the following specific exceptions. In PD (and many other parkinsonian disorders), diplopia may occur during reading secondary to impaired convergence (Waln and Jankovic, 2018). Visual complaints sometimes occur in other parkinsonian disorders, particularly PSP. Oculogyric crises, which are sudden episodes of involuntary ocular deviation (most often up and to the side) in the absence of neuroleptic drug exposure, are virtually pathognomonic of parkinsonism after encephalitis lethargica, although they may occur in rare neurometabolic disorders as well (Slow and Lang, 2017). Sensory loss is not part of parkinsonism, although patients with PD may have poorly explained positive sensory complaints such as numbness and tingling, aching, and painful sensations that are sometimes quite disabling (Patel et al., 2014). Peripheral neuropathy suggests another disorder or an unrelated problem (e.g., diabetes mellitus), although a higher-than-expected incidence of peripheral neuropathy, possibly related to levodopa treatment and elevated methylmalonic acid levels, has been suggested (Toth et al., 2010).

Although a variety of neurophysiological and computer-based methods for quantitating the severity of the various parkinsonian symptoms and signs have been proposed, most studies rely on clinical rating scales. Non-demented patients can reliably self-administer and complete the *Movement Disorder Society (MDS)-UPDRS* (http://www.movementdisorders.org). The revision clarifies some ambiguities and more adequately assesses the non-motor features of PD (Goetz et al., 2010). Some clinical research studies also use more objective timed test such as the Purdue Pegboard Test, movement and reaction times, and a variety of wearable devices are increasingly used in clinical trials to provide another, more quantitative, assessment of motor function. Many scales, such as the Parkinson's Disease Questionnaire-39 (PDQ-39) and the Parkinson's Disease Quality of Life Questionnaire (PDQL), attempt to assess the overall quality of life (Jankovic, 2008).

## Onset and Course

As in other movement disorders, the age at onset of a parkinsonian syndrome is clearly important in considering a differential diagnosis. Although the majority of patients are adults, parkinsonism may have onset in childhood or adolescence (juvenile parkinsonism) and between 21 and 40 years (young-onset parkinsonism; see Box 24.1). The younger the age at onset the more likely it is that the etiology of the parkinsonism is genetic. Besides categorizing patients with PD according to age at onset, there are other subtypes of PD. For example, the "tremor-dominant" subtype typically has a slow progression and more favorable long-term prognosis than the "postural instability gait difficulty" (PIGD) subtype which is more rapidly progressive and is more likely associated with non-motor problems including cognitive decline (Thenganatt and Jankovic, 2014a). Other parkinsonian disorders (e.g., those due to toxins, vascular causes) may present abruptly or progress more rapidly or may even improve spontaneously (e.g., those due to drugs, certain forms of encephalitis).

## Examination and Clinical Signs

The diagnosis of parkinsonism often is immediately apparent on first contact with the patient. The facial expression, low-volume voice, tremor, slowness and poverty of movement, shuffling gait, and stooped posture provide an immediate and irrevocable first impression of parkinsonism. However, the physician must perform a detailed assessment, searching for any atypical features to distinguish between PD and other parkinsonian disorders (Morris and Jankovic, 2012). Loss of facial expression *(hypomimia)* often is an early sign of PD. But occasional patients have a wide-eyed, anxious, worried expression due to furrowing of the brow ("procerus sign") and deep facial folds, which strongly suggests PSP. Blink frequency usually is reduced, although *blepharoclonus* (repetitive spasms of the lids on gentle eye closure) and reflex blepharospasm (e.g., precipitated by shining a light into the eyes or manipulating the lids) also may be seen. Spontaneous blepharospasm and apraxia of lid opening occur less often (Waln and Jankovic, 2018). Patients with apraxia of lid opening (not a true apraxia) are not able to open their eyes after spontaneous or voluntary closure and often must use their fingers to forcefully open their eyes, and once the eyes are fixated on an object, the eyelids remain open. Primitive reflexes, including the inability to inhibit blinking in response to tapping over the glabella (Myerson sign) and palmomental reflexes, are nonspecific and are commonly present in many parkinsonian disorders (Brodsky et al., 2004).

Various types of tremor, most notably rest and postural varieties, often accompany parkinsonian disorders. Patients should be observed with hands resting on their laps or thighs, and they should be instructed to hold their arms in an outstretched position or in a horizontal position with shoulders abducted, elbows flexed, and hands palms-down in front of their faces in the so-called "wing-beating position." Rest tremor often re-emerges after a period of quiescence in a new position (*re-emergent tremor*; Jankovic, 2016). This re-emergent tremor, which is often the most troublesome parkinsonian tremor because it interferes with holding objects steadily against gravity, may be wrongly attributed to postural tremor and lead to misdiagnosis as essential tremor. A true kinetic (intention) tremor, elicited by the finger-to-nose maneuver, is much less common in patients with PD and other parkinsonian disorders and usually indicates involvement of cerebellar connections. A jerky (myoclonic) postural tremor is suggestive of a diagnosis of MSA rather than PD. Head tremor *(titubation)* suggests a diagnosis other than PD, such as essential tremor, dystonic neck tremor, or a cerebellar tremor associated with the cerebellar form of MSA (MSA-C), spinocerebellar atrophy, or multiple sclerosis (MS).

*Rigidity,* an increase in muscle tone, is usually equal in flexors and extensors and present throughout the passive range of movement. This contrasts with the distribution and velocity-dependent nature of spasticity (the clasp-knife phenomenon). Paratonia (or Gegenhalten), on the other hand, increases with repetitive passive movement and attempts to get the patient to relax. It may be difficult to distinguish between milder forms of paratonia and rigidity, especially in the legs. Characteristically, the performance of voluntary movements in the opposite limb (e.g., opening and closing the fist or abduction-adduction of the shoulder) brings out rigidity, a phenomenon known as *activated rigidity* (Froment sign). Superimposed on the rigidity may be a tremor or cogwheel phenomenon. This, like the milder forms of rigidity, is better appreciated by placing one hand over the muscles being tested (e.g., placing the left thumb over the biceps and the remaining fingers over the triceps while flexing and extending the elbow with the right hand). The distribution of the rigidity sometimes is helpful in differential diagnosis. For example, pronounced nuchal rigidity with much less hypertonicity in the limbs suggests the diagnosis of PSP, whereas an extreme degree of unilateral arm rigidity or paratonia suggests *corticobasal syndrome* (CBS), diagnosed clinically, or *corticobasal degeneration* (CBD), diagnosed by autopsy (Ling et al., 2014).

Bradykinesia (slow movement) or akinesia (absence of movement) are appreciable on examination in several ways. Automatic movements normally expressed in conversation, such as gesturing with hands while speaking, crossing and uncrossing the legs, and repositioning the body in the chair diminish or are absent. The performance of rapid, repetitive, and alternating movements such as finger tapping, opening and closing the fist, pronation-supination of the forearm, and foot tapping is slow, with a gradual reduction in amplitude and eventual cessation of movement *(freezing)*. The decrement in amplitude of repetitive movements is characteristic of the bradykinesia of PD and is often considered mandatory for the diagnosis. In contrast, bradykinesia in PSP may not be associated with decrementing amplitude on repetitive movements (Ling et al., 2012). Watching the patient write is an important part of the examination. Observation of writing in a patient with PD may reveal great slowness and effort, even in someone with minimal change in the size of the script. In contrast, patients with PSP may have "fast micrographia" with a rapid production of an illegible script. In addition to micrographia, writing and drawing show a tendency to fatigue, with a further reduction in size as the task proceeds and a concomitant action tremor. This is in contrast to handwriting in patients with essential tremor (ET), which tends to be larger and tremulous.

Postural disturbances are common in parkinsonian disorders. The head usually tilts forward and the body becomes stooped, often with pronounced kyphosis and varying degrees of scoliosis, typically away from the side of the onset of parkinsonian signs, such as rest tremor. The arms become flexed at the elbows and wrists, with varying postural deformities in the hands, the most common being flexion at the metacarpophalangeal joints and extension at the interphalangeal joints, with adduction of all the fingers and opposition of the thumb to the index finger (*striatal hand*; Fig. 24.2, *A*; Wijemanne and Jankovic, 2019). Flexion with contracture may also occur in the joints of the legs, particularly the knees, contributing to the typical flexed posture. Variable foot deformities occur, the most common being hammer toe-like disturbances in most of the toes, occasionally with extension of the great toe (*striatal foot*; see Fig. 24.2, *B*), which may be misinterpreted as an extensor plantar response. Initially, abnormal foot posturing may be induced by action, occurring only during walking or weight bearing. The flexed or simian posture sometimes is extreme, with severe flexion at the waist (*camptocormia*; Jankovic, 2010; see Fig. 24.2, *C*). Some patients, particularly those with MSA, exhibit scoliosis or tilted posture (*Pisa sign*; see Fig. 24.2, *D*). Despite the truncal flexion, the position of the hands in patients with PD often remains above the beltline because of flexion of the elbows. Occasional patients remain upright or even demonstrate a hyperextended posture. Hyperextension of the neck is particularly suggestive of PSP, whereas extreme flexion of the neck (head drop or bent spine) suggests MSA (see Fig. 24.2, *D*) but also PD.

Postural instability is characteristic of all parkinsonian disorders, particularly the postural instability and gait difficulty forms of PD, PSP, and MSA. As patients rise from a sitting position, poor postural stability, slowness, rigidity, narrow base, and not repositioning the feet often combine to cause them to fall back into the chair "in a lump"; this is especially prominent in patients with PSP. These patients also may "rocket" out of the chair inappropriately quickly, failing to recognize their inability to maintain stability on their feet. The PD patient may require several attempts, push off the arms of the chair, or need to be pulled up by an assistant. Gait disturbances in typical parkinsonism include lack of arm swing, shortened and later shuffling stride, narrow base, flexed knees, freezing in the course of walking (especially when initiating gait and when approaching a door frame or a potential obstruction or a chair). Patients with PD turn en bloc, whereas patients

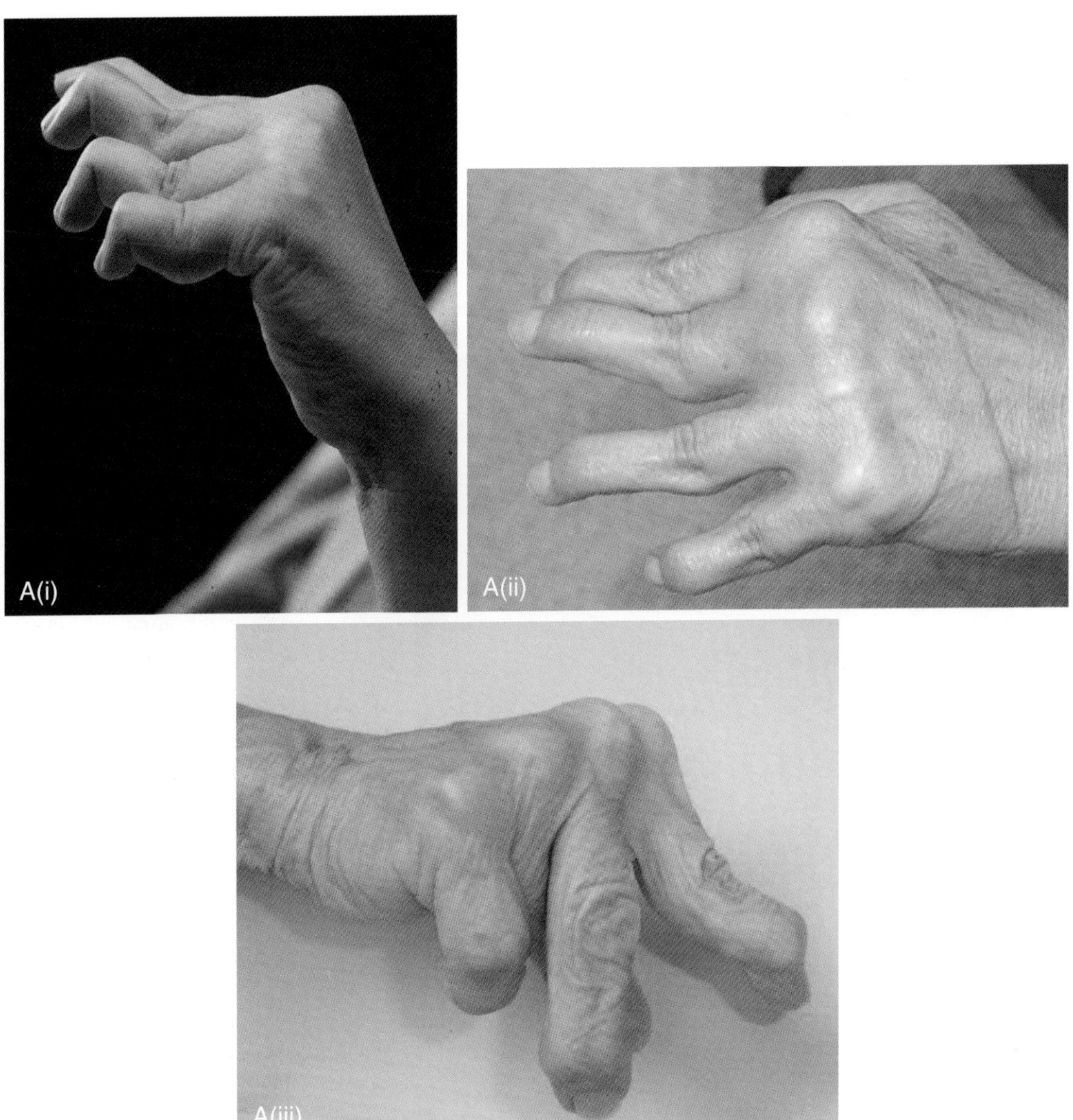


**Fig. 24.2** Parkinsonian Deformities. A, Striatal hand deformities.

with PSP tend to pivot when they turn. In more severe cases of PD or PSP, propulsion and retropulsion may occur spontaneously, resulting in falls (Jankovic, 2008). In addition, walking often brings out or exacerbates a hand tremor in patients with PD. To assess postural instability, the physician performs the pull test. Standing behind the patient, the examiner pulls the patient backward by the shoulders, carefully remaining close behind to prevent a fall (Morris and Jankovic, 2012). Once postural reflexes are impaired, there may be retropulsion or multiple backward steps in response to the postural perturbation. Later there is a tendency to fall en bloc without retropulsion or even normal attempts to recover or to cushion the fall.

In PD, the base of the gait is usually narrow but when the gait is wide-based, atypical parkinsonism should be considered (see Chapter 96; Mirelman et al., 2019). Toe walking *(cock-walk)* is seen in some parkinsonian disorders (e.g., due to manganese poisoning), and a peculiar loping gait may indicate the rare patient with akinesia in the absence of rigidity, which may be one phenotype of PSP. The so-called magnetic foot, or marche à petits pas, is typically seen in vascular parkinsonism, Binswanger disease, and normal pressure hydrocephalus. Lower-body parkinsonism in which the gait is slightly broad-based and shuffling (with possible freezing) but normal arm swing and minimal or no impairment in upper limbs is typically associated with a history or stroke risk factors and evidence of cerebrovascular disorders such as lacunar strokes, although some patients may have microinfarcts not necessarily appreciated on brain imaging (Mehanna and Jankovic, 2013). A striking discrepancy of involvement between the lower body and the upper limbs, with normal or even excessive arm swing, is an important clue to the diagnosis of vascular parkinsonism or normal pressure hydrocephalus.

## Differential Diagnosis

Although dementia commonly occurs in PD, this feature, particularly when present relatively early in the course, must alert the physician to other possible diagnoses (see Chapter 96), including dementia with Lewy bodies, particularly if the cognitive deficit is accompanied by visual hallucinations and the course is fluctuating, or the coincidental association with other common causes of cognitive decline, such as Alzheimer disease (Svenningsson et al., 2012). Prominent eye movement disturbances are found in a number of conditions, including

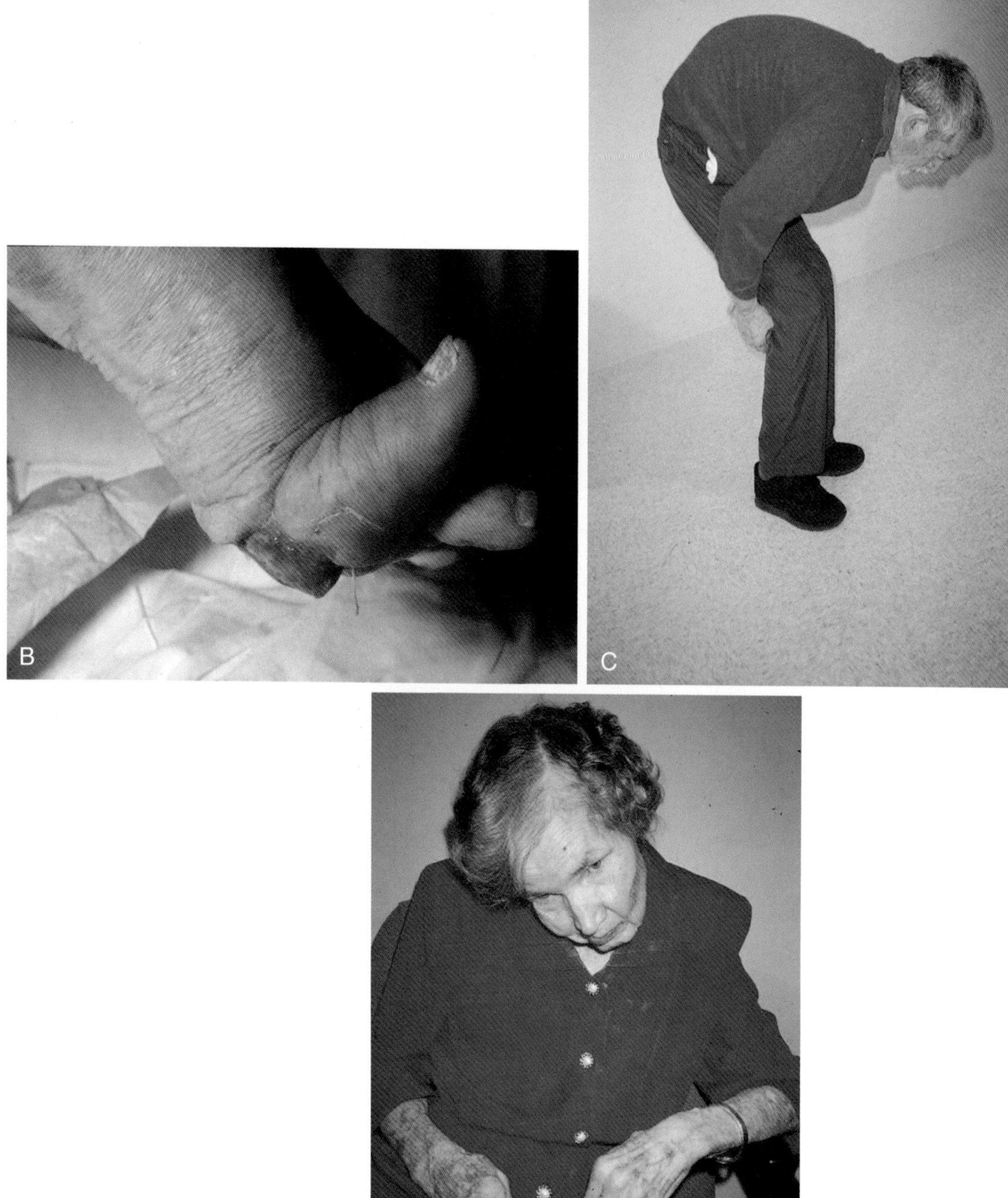

**Fig. 24.2—cont'd, B,** Striatal foot deformity. **C,** Camptocormia in a patient with Parkinson disease. **D,** Pisa sign and anterior neck flexion in a patient with multiple system atrophy.

PSP, MSA-C, postencephalitic parkinsonism, CBD, and Machado-Joseph disease (SCA3). It is important to assess both horizontal and vertical pursuit and saccadic eye movements. Slowing of vertical saccades is characteristic of PSP and is particularly noticeable when evaluating vertical optokinetic nystagmus and the optokinetic tape moves in upward direction during which there is slowing or impairment of downward saccades (Waln and Jankovic, 2018). The oculocephalic (doll's eye) maneuver must be performed when ocular excursions are limited, seeking supportive evidence of supranuclear gaze palsy. Patients with PSP typically have trouble making eye contact because of disturbed visual refixation. As a result of persistence of visual fixation when PSP patients turn, their head turn lags behind their body turn.

Obvious pyramidal tract dysfunction usually suggests diagnoses other than PD. An exaggerated grasp response indicates disturbance of the frontal lobes and the possibility of a concomitant dementing process. Occasionally a pronounced flexed posture in the hand may be confused with a grasp reflex, and the examiner must be convinced that there is active contraction in response to stroking of the palm. The abnormalities of rapid, repetitive, and alternating movements described earlier can be confused with the clumsy awkward performance of limb-kinetic apraxia (Zadikoff and Lang, 2005). More importantly, the abnormalities in performance of repetitive movement must not be confused with the disruption of rate, rhythm, and force typical of the dysdiadochokinesia of cerebellar disease. A helpful maneuver in testing for the presence of associated cerebellar dysfunction is to have the patient tap with the index finger on a hard surface. Watching and, in particular, listening to the tapping often allows a distinction to be made between the slowness and decrementing response of parkinsonism and the irregular rate and force of cerebellar ataxia (dysdiadochokinesia). Testing for ideomotor apraxia, as seen in CBS, also should be performed by asking the patient to mimic certain hand gestures (intransitive tasks) such as the "victory sign" or the University of Texas "hook 'em horns sign" (extension of the second and fifth finger and flexion of the third and fourth finger) or to simulate certain activities (transitive tasks [using a tool or utensil]) such as brushing teeth and combing hair. However, in the later stages of many parkinsonian disorders, rigidity and other motor disturbances may make results of these tests difficult to interpret. In PD or MSA, the less affected limb may show mirror movements as the patient attempts to perform rapid repetitive or alternating movements with the most affected limb (Espay et al., 2005). On the other hand, in CBS, the most affected limb may mirror movements performed in the less affected limb. Some patients with parkinsonism and frontal lobe involvement exhibit signs of perseveration such as the applause sign, manifested by persistence of clapping after instructing the patient to clap consecutively three times as quickly as possible. Although initially thought to be characteristic of PSP, it is also present in some patients with other parkinsonian disorders (Wu et al., 2008).

The presence of other abnormal movements in an untreated patient may indicate a diagnosis other than PD. Seek evidence of stimulus-sensitive myoclonus by producing a sudden loud noise or using a light touch or pinprick in the digits and the proximal palm or the sole of the foot. Easily elicited and nonfatiguing myoclonic jerks in response to these stimuli may be seen not only in patients with CBS and MSA but also in some patients with PD and dementia.

Despite a variety of sensory complaints, patients with PD do not show prominent abnormalities on the sensory examination, aside from the normal increase in vibration threshold that occurs with age (Patel et al., 2014). Cortical sensory disturbances suggest a diagnosis of CBS. Wasting and muscle weakness are not characteristic of PD, although later in the course of the disease, severely disabled patients show disuse atrophy and severe problems in initiating and maintaining muscle activation that are often difficult to separate from true weakness. Combinations of upper and lower motor neuron weakness occur in several other parkinsonian disorders (see Table 24.2).

Assessing autonomic function is important not only in patients suspected of having MSA but also in patients with PD, many of whom have dysautonomia. At the bedside, this includes an evaluation of orthostatic changes in blood pressure and pulse (in supine position and at least 3 minutes after standing) and, in appropriate circumstances, the patient's response to the Valsalva maneuver, mental arithmetic, and the cold pressor test, among others. Finally, perform sequential examinations over time, carefully searching for the development of additional findings that may provide a clue to the diagnosis. Several parkinsonian syndromes present initially as pure parkinsonism; only later with disease progression do other signs develop.

## TREMOR

*Tremor* is rhythmic oscillation of a body part, produced by either alternating or synchronous contractions of reciprocally innervated antagonistic muscles. The International Parkinson and Movement Disorder Society (IPMDS) has provided a "consensus" statement on classification of tremors according to Axis 1 (clinical characteristics) and Axis 2 (etiology) (Bhatia et al., 2018). While tremors may vary in amplitude, they typically have a fixed frequency. The basis of further categorization is the position, posture, and motor performance necessary to elicit it. A *rest tremor* occurs with the body part in complete repose, although when a patient totally relaxes or sleeps this tremor usually disappears. Maintenance of a posture, such as extending the arms parallel to the floor, reveals a *postural tremor*; moving the body part to and from a target brings out an *intention tremor*. The use of other descriptive categories has caused some confusion in tremor terminology. *Action tremor* has been used for both postural and kinetic (also known as *intention*) tremors. Whereas a *kinetic tremor* is present throughout goal-directed movement, the term *terminal* tremor applies to the component of kinetic tremor that exaggerates when approaching the target. *Dystonic tremor* is a relatively slow, irregular, and sometimes jerky movement occurring in the body part affected by dystonia (discussed below), even though the dystonia may not be obvious. Ataxic tremor refers to a combination of kinetic tremor plus limb ataxia. Box 24.2 provides a list of differential diagnoses for the three major categories of tremor and other rhythmic movements that occasionally are confused with tremor.

A description of symptoms occurs under the various categories of tremor. All people have a normal or physiological tremor demonstrable with sensitive recording devices. Two common pathological tremor disorders that are often confused are parkinsonian rest tremor and essential tremor. Although Chapter 96 discusses both conditions in detail, we discuss helpful distinguishing points here in view of the frequency of misdiagnosis.

### Rest Tremor

A rest tremor occurs with the body part in complete repose and often dampens or subsides entirely with action. For this reason, patients with pure rest tremor experience greater social embarrassment than functional disability, unless, as noted earlier, the rest tremor re-emerges during postural holding. Indeed, in some cases it is a family member or friend who first observes the tremor, which is noticeable to the patient only later. Alternatively, some patients complain of the sensation of trembling inside long before a rest tremor becomes overt. Early on, rest tremor may be intermittent and often precipitated only by anxiety or stress. The onset of most types of tremor is in the arms, often beginning asymmetrically. In the face, rest tremor usually affects the tongue, lips and jaw, and the patient may note a rhythmic clicking of the teeth. In the limbs, the tremor usually is most distally in the fingers (pill rolling) or may manifest by flexion-extension or a supination-pronation, oscillatory movement of the wrist and forearm, and flexion-extension movement of the ankle. In severe forms, it may be present more proximally, causing the entire body to shake. The presence of head tremor (titubation) should raise the possibility of essential tremor or of dystonic tremor associated with cervical dystonia or cerebellar outflow tremor, as is seen in patients with MS or posterior fossa disorders rather than PD. Tremor in the legs, and especially in the feet while sitting, is usually caused by parkinsonian rest tremor. A history of progression from unilateral arm tremor to additional involvement of the ipsilateral leg suggests parkinsonism rather than essential tremor. Once the tremor has become noticeable to the patient, a variety of methods are used to conceal the movement, such as holding one hand with the other, sitting on the affected hand, or crossing the legs to dampen a tremulous lower limb. Many patients find that they can briefly abort the tremor by conscious effort.

## BOX 24.2 Classification and Differential Diagnosis of Tremor

**Resting Tremors**

PD
Other parkinsonian syndromes (less common)
Midbrain (rubral) tremor (Holmes tremor): rest < postural < intention
WD (also acquired hepatocerebral degeneration)
Essential tremor

**Postural Tremors**

Physiological tremor
Exaggerated physiological tremor; these factors can also aggravate other forms of tremor:
- Stress, fatigue, anxiety, emotion
- Endocrine: hypoglycemia, thyrotoxicosis, pheochromocytoma
- Drugs and toxins: adrenocorticosteroids, β-agonists, dopamine agonists, amphetamines, lithium, tricyclic antidepressants, neuroleptics, theophylline, caffeine, valproic acid, alcohol withdrawal, mercury ("hatter's shakes"), lead, arsenic, others

Essential tremor (familial or sporadic)
Primary writing tremor and other task-specific tremors
Orthostatic tremor
With other CNS disorders:
- PD (postural tremor, re-emergent tremor, associated essential tremor)
- Other akinetic-rigid syndromes
- Idiopathic dystonia, including focal dystonias

With peripheral neuropathy:
- Charcot-Marie-Tooth disease (called the *Roussy-Lévy syndrome*)
- Other peripheral neuropathies

Cerebellar tremor

**Intention Tremors**

Diseases of cerebellar outflow (dentate nuclei, interpositus nuclei, or both, and superior cerebellar peduncle):
- MS, trauma, tumor, vascular disease, WD, acquired hepatocerebral degeneration, drugs, toxins (e.g., mercury), others

**Miscellaneous Rhythmic Movement Disorders**

Functional/Psychogenic tremor
Rhythmic movements in dystonia (dystonic tremor, myorhythmia)
Rhythmic myoclonus (segmental myoclonus, e.g., palatal or branchial myoclonus, spinal myoclonus), myorhythmia
Oscillatory myoclonus
Asterixis
Clonus
Epilepsia partialis continua
Hereditary chin quivering
Spasmus nutans
Head bobbing with third ventricular cysts
Nystagmus

*CNS*, Central nervous system; *MS*, multiple sclerosis; *PD*, Parkinson disease; *WD*, Wilson disease.

## Postural and Action Tremor

In contrast to a pure rest tremor, postural tremors, especially with pronounced terminal accentuation, can result in significant disability. Many such patients are mistaken as having "bad nerves." People who perform delicate work with their hands (e.g., jewelers, surgeons) become aware of this form of tremor earlier than most. The average person usually first appreciates tremor in the acts of feeding and writing. Carrying a cup of liquid, pouring, or eating with a spoon often brings out the tremor. Writing is tremulous and sloppy, sometimes causing a bank to question the patient's signature on a check. The voice may be involved in essential tremor. Again, anxiety and stress worsen the tremor, and patients often notice that their symptoms are especially bad in public. The most common cause of postural tremor seen in movement disorders clinics is essential tremor (Jankovic, 2009) or accentuated physiological tremor, sometimes as a result of various drugs.

Patients often adopt compensatory mechanisms to lessen the disability caused by tremor. Many give up certain tasks such as serving drinks and eating specific foods (e.g., soup), especially in public. When the tremor is very asymmetrical, patients often switch to using the less-affected hand for many tasks, including writing. Bringing a cup to the mouth becomes difficult; later, a straw is required. When writing, patients may use the other hand to steady the paper or the writing hand itself. Patients often switch from cursive to print, and the use of heavier or thicker writing instruments sometimes makes the script more legible. In some patients with parkinsonian disorders and severe rest tremor, the tremor may also be present while the patient holds an outstretched or wing-beating posture. This tremor usually occurs after a latency of several seconds: hence the term *re-emergent tremor* (Dirks et al., 2018; Jankovic, 2016); in contrast, in essential tremor the tremor is evident immediately on taking up a new posture. Some patients with essential tremor also have rest tremor and develop other parkinsonian features. There is also evidence that some patients with a past history of long-standing postural and action tremor diagnosed as "essential tremor" have an increased risk for developing PD (Tarakad and Jankovic, 2019).

## Other Types of Tremor

Various types of writing disturbances may combine with tremor. Primary writing tremor is one form of task-specific tremor that affects the writing act in isolation, with little or no associated postural or terminal tremor interfering with other acts. Dystonic writer's cramp can involve additional tremulousness on writing. Distinction is required from the voluntary excessive squeezing of the pen or pressing onto the page often seen in patients with essential tremor or primary writing tremor, which is attributable to their attempts to lessen the effect of tremor on writing. In addition, patients with postural tremor may consciously slow their writing to improve accuracy, but this is a voluntary compensatory mechanism not associated with the micrographia and fatigue that accompany parkinsonism.

Tremor in the head and neck, or titubation, occurs in isolation or combined with a postural tremor elsewhere, especially in the arms, as is seen in patients with essential tremor. When the head tremor is irregular and is associated with abnormal head posture and uneven contractions or hypertrophy of the neck muscles, the possibility of cervical dystonia and dystonic tremor of the head should be considered. Head tremor at disease onset may be a form of cervical dystonia, typically affecting older women (Merola et al., 2019). Head tremor is rarely a source of physical disability but may create social embarrassment. Patients occasionally complain of a similar tremor of the voice. This is particularly noticeable to others who are listening to the patient on the telephone, and many ask the patient whether they are sad or have been crying.

Less often, patients with postural tremors note a similar tremor in the legs and trunk. The awareness of this form of tremor clearly depends on the activity performed. One form of postural tremor, orthostatic tremor, characteristically presents not as tremor but rather as difficulty and insecurity on standing. It is associated with a 14- to 16-Hz tremor in the legs and trunk (Yaltho and Ondo, 2014). This tremor typically subsides if the patient walks about, leans against something, or sits down.

Although patients with several different types of tremor may indicate that alcohol transiently reduces their shaking, a striking response to small amounts of alcohol is particularly characteristic of essential tremor (Mostile and Jankovic, 2010). Clues to the possible presence of factors aggravating the normal physiological tremor (see Box 24.2) require further inquiry.

In addition to clinical examination, various physiological, accelerometric, and other computer-based techniques can be employed to assess tremor, but a clinical rating scale usually is most practical, particularly in clinical trials. The Tremor Research Group (TRG) has developed a rating scale that can be used to quantitatively assess all types of tremor, particularly essential tremor, the most common type encountered in clinical practice. The TRG Essential Tremor Rating Scale (TETRAS) has been found to correlate well with the Fahn-Tolosa-Marin tremor scale (Ondo et al., 2017) and quantitative computer-based systems (Mostile et al., 2010). Besides rest tremor, postural tremor, and kinetic limb tremor, examine patients for tremor of the head. With the patient seated or standing, head tremor may be evident as vertical ("yes-yes") nodding *(tremblement affirmatif)* or side-to-side ("no-no") horizontal or lateral shaking *(tremblement negatif)*. There may be combinations of the two, with rotatory movements. Subtle head tremors may only be appreciated when the examiner holds the patient's cranium while testing with the other hand for extreme lateral eye movements. Head tremors usually range from 1.5 Hz to 5 Hz and are most commonly associated with essential tremor or cervical dystonia and with diseases of the cerebellum and its outflow pathways. A parkinsonian rest tremor may involve the tongue, jaw, and lips, but almost never involves the head. A similar tremor of the perioral and nasal muscles, the *rabbit syndrome*, has been associated with antipsychotic drug therapy but may also occur in PD. In many disorders, voluntary contraction of the facial muscles induces an action tremor. In addition, a postural tremor of the tongue often is present on tongue protrusion. It is important to observe the palate at rest for the slower rhythmic movements of palatal myoclonus (also called *palatal tremor*). Occasionally, tremor spares the palate, with similar movements affecting other branchial structures. Demonstration of a voice tremor requires asking the patient to hold a note as an "ah" or "eh" sound as long as possible. Superimposed on the vocal tremulousness may be a harsh, strained quality or abrupt cessation of airflow during the course of maintaining the note (voiceless pause), which suggests a superimposed dystonia of the larynx *(spasmodic dysphonia)*.

A parkinsonian rest tremor characteristically has a frequency in the range 4–6 Hz. The frequency of postural arm tremors varies, depending on cause and severity; essential tremor usually is in the range of 5–10 Hz, with the greater-amplitude tremors tending to be slower. Exaggerated physiological tremor has a frequency of 8–12 Hz. Many patients with parkinsonism demonstrate a combination of slower resting and faster postural tremors. Some patients with slower, larger-amplitude forms of essential tremor have a definite resting component.

A rest tremor in the limbs occurs even with the muscles in complete repose. Even a small amount of muscle activity, as may occur if the patient is somewhat anxious or the limb is not completely at rest, may bring out a higher-frequency action postural tremor. It is sometimes impossible to abate this postural tremor during a stressful office interview. Stress and concentration may bring out an occult rest tremor, such as the performance of serial sevens. Although a rest tremor characteristically subsides when the patient maintains a posture (e.g., holding the arms outstretched parallel to the floor), it may recur after a few seconds. As noted earlier, the re-emergent tremor that occurs after a latency of a few seconds (and sometimes as long as 1 minute) suggests an underlying parkinsonian disorder (Dirks et al., 2018; Jankovic, 2016). Carrying out goal-directed movements, such as finger-to-nose testing, usually causes the tremor to dampen further or subside completely. On the other hand, a typical postural tremor associated with essential tremor usually occurs without latency after the initiation of a posture and may worsen further at the endpoints of goal-directed movement *(terminal tremor)*. The slower kinetic tremor of cerebellar disease occurs throughout the movement but also worsens upon reaching the target. Occasionally, pronounced bursts of muscle activity in a patient with terminal tremor cause individual separate jerks, which give the impression of superimposed myoclonus. *Essential myoclonus* (an older term) is an autosomal dominant disorder, and affected patients and their relatives have both jerk-like myoclonus and sometimes postural tremor phenomenologically similar to essential tremor.

Having the patient point the index fingers at each other under the nose (without touching the fingers together or touching the face) with the arms abducted at the sides and the elbows flexed can demonstrate both distal tremor in the hands and proximal tremors. An example of proximal tremor is the slower wing-beating tremor of cerebellar outflow pathway disease, as may be seen in WD. Tremor during the course of slowly pronating and supinating the forearms with the arms outstretched or with forceful abduction of the fingers can occur in patients with primary writing tremor. Holding a full cup of water with the arm outstretched often amplifies a postural tremor, and picking up the full cup, bringing it to the mouth, and tipping it to drink enhances the terminal tremor, often causing spillage. Pouring water between two cups, monitoring the amount of spillage, is a common evaluation tool for tremors. In addition to writing, one should have the patient draw with both hands separately. Useful drawing tasks include an Archimedes spiral, a wavy line from one side of the page to the other (Fig. 24.3), and an attempt to carefully draw a line or spiral between two well-defined, closely opposed borders. Another useful test designed to bring out position-specific tremor is the dot approximation test, in which the

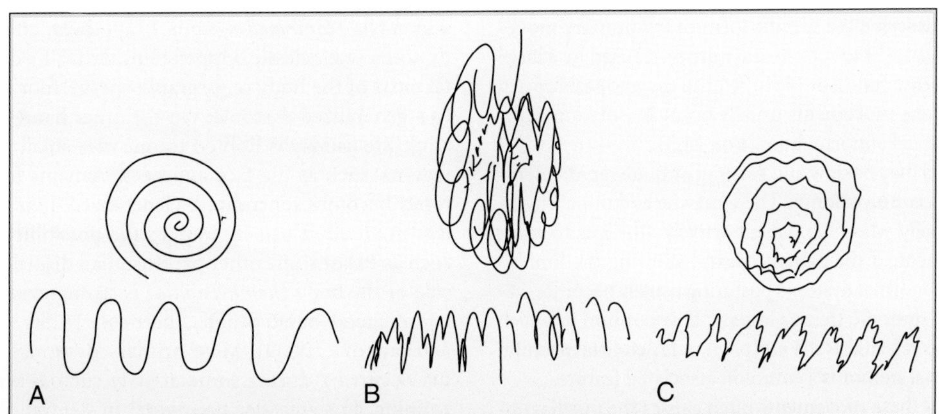


**Fig. 24.3** Archimedes spiral and wavy-line drawings by the examiner (A) and by a patient with essential tremor (B, C), in whom the tremor is asymmetrical and more evident in the right hand (B) than in the left hand (C).

patient is instructed to be seated at the desk with elbow elevated and to hold the tip of the pen or pencil (for at least 10 seconds) as close as possible to a dot drawn on a sheet of paper without touching it. Many patients with action tremors note marked exacerbation of their tremor during this specific task. Most patients with action tremor also have "isometric" tremor noted while the patient squeezes the examiner's fingers or maintains a flexed position of hips against gravity while seated.

In the legs, in addition to the standard heel-to-shin testing which brings out kinetic and terminal tremors, it may be possible to demonstrate a postural tremor by having the patient hold the leg off the bed and attempt to touch the examiner's finger with the great toe. Patients with orthostatic tremor develop rapid (14–16 Hz), rhythmic contractions of leg muscles after standing for a few seconds or minutes, which they may perceive as a cramp or unsteadiness and insecurity on standing rather than tremor. This dampens or subsides on walking, sitting, or lying down. Because of the rapidity of the tremor, the oscillatory movement of the legs may not be obvious to a casual observer but palpation, auscultation of electrophysiological recordings from the leg muscles can confirm the presence of the tremor. If the patient has similar symptoms on standing that are not significantly improved by walking, electrophysiological studies may confirm a diagnosis of orthostatic myoclonic rather than orthostatic tremor. Diseases or lesions involving the midbrain or the superior cerebellar peduncle result in the so-called midbrain, or rubral, tremor *(Holmes tremor)*. Characteristically, this form of tremor combines features of the three tremor classes. It is often present at rest, increases with postural maintenance, and increases still further, sometimes to extreme degrees, with goal-directed movement. Another form of rest tremor is *myorhythmia*, defined as repetitive, rhythmic, slow (1–4 Hz) tremor affecting chiefly cranial and limb muscles (Baizabal-Carvallo et al., 2015). It is typically associated with lesions involving the brainstem, thalamus, or other diencephalic structures, some with potentially treatable etiologies.

Tremor or shaking also may be a feature of a functional (psychogenic) movement disorder or psychiatric disease, representing a conversion reaction or even malingering (Baizabal-Carvallo et al., 2019). This functional (psychogenic) tremor differs from most organic tremors in that the frequency is often quite variable, concentration and distraction often abate the tremor or profoundly change its frequency instead of increasing it, and the phenomenology is atypical or incongruous with any organic tremor (Thenganatt and Jankovic, 2014b).

## DYSTONIA

Dystonia is a disorder dominated by sustained muscle contractions, which often cause twisting and repetitive movements or abnormal postures (Albanese et al., 2013). The term *dystonia* is used in three major contexts: (1) to describe the specific form of involuntary movement (i.e., a physical sign), (2) to refer to a syndrome caused by a large number of different disease states, or (3) to refer to the idiopathic form of dystonia, in which these movements usually occur in isolation without additional neurological abnormalities (Box 24.3).

Dystonic movements may be slow and twisting or quite rapid, resembling the shock-like jerks of myoclonus. There may be additional rhythmic movements, especially when the patient actively attempts to resist the involuntary movement. If the patient relaxes, allowing the limb to move as it pleases, the abnormal dystonic posturing usually becomes evident, and the rhythmic dystonic tremor lessens. This position in which dystonic tremor ceases is referred as the *null point*. A faster distal postural tremor similar to essential tremor is a common associated feature.

The varied nature of these movements often causes the misdiagnosis of dystonia as some other type of movement disorder. One common error in diagnosis is the mislabeling of dystonia as hysteria or a functional (psychogenic) disorder. This misperception is often fueled by the observation that stress and anxiety aggravate the movements, and rest and even hypnosis alleviate the movements. Furthermore, patients with dystonia often discover a variety of peculiar maneuvers (sensory tricks or alleviating maneuvers) that they can use to lessen or even completely abate the dystonic movements and postures (Patel et al., 2014). The abnormal movements and postures may occur only during the performance of certain acts and not others that use the same muscles. An example of this action, *task-specific dystonia*, is involvement of the hand only in writing (writer's cramp or graphospasm) or playing a musical instrument, but not with other manual tasks such as using utensils. Dystonia of the oromandibular region only on speaking or eating is another example of task-specific dystonia, as is dystonia in legs and trunk that occurs only on walking forward but not on walking backward, climbing stairs, or running. On the other hand, some dystonias occur only during running (Wu and Jankovic, 2006). A final source of possible confusion with hysteria is the occurrence of dystonia after injury to the affected limb or after prolonged immobilization such as casting. Such peripherally induced dystonia, which is usually fixed rather than mobile, may be associated with a complex regional pain syndrome (previously referred to as *reflex sympathetic dystrophy*), depression, and personality changes and may occur on a background of secondary gain or litigation and other features of psychogenic dystonia (Thenganatt and Jankovic, 2014c; van Rooijen et al., 2011).

Dystonia can affect almost all striated, skeletal muscle groups. Common symptoms include forced eyelid closure *(blepharospasm)*; jaw clenching, forced jaw opening, or involuntary tongue protrusion (oromandibular or lingual dystonia); a harsh, strained, or breathy voice (laryngeal dystonia or spasmodic dysphonia); and involuntary deviation of the neck in any plane or combination of planes (cervical dystonia or spasmodic torticollis) (Albanese et al., 2013; Balint et al., 2018). Other symptoms are spasms of the trunk in any direction, which variably interfere with lying, sitting, standing, or walking (axial dystonia); interference with manual tasks (often only specific tasks in isolation—the occupational cramps); and involvement of the leg, usually with inversion and plantar flexion of the foot, causing the patient to walk on the toes. All these disorders may slowly progress to the point of complete loss of voluntary function of the affected part. On the other hand, only certain actions may be impaired, and the disorder may remain focal in distribution.

The age at onset and distribution of dystonia often are helpful in determining the possible cause. Box 24.3 details the many causes of inherited and acquired dystonias (dystonia due to a known specific cause; Albanese et al., 2013). Whereas some patients with dystonia have "pure dystonia" without any other neurological deficit *(isolated dystonia)*, others have additional clinical features such as parkinsonism, spasticity, weakness, myoclonus, dementia, seizures, and ataxia *(combined dystonia)*. Typically, childhood-onset primary dystonia (e.g., classic, Oppenheim, or DYT1 dystonia) begins in distal parts of the body (e.g., graphospasm, foot inversion) and spreads to a generalized dystonia. On the other hand, dystonia beginning in adult life usually is limited to one or a small number of contiguous regions, such as the face and neck, remains focal or segmental, and rarely becomes generalized. Generalized involvement or onset in the legs in an adult usually implies the possibility of a secondary cause such as PD or some other parkinsonian disorder. Involvement of one side of the body *(hemidystonia)* is strong evidence of a lesion in the contralateral basal ganglia, particularly the putamen (Wijemanne and Jankovic, 2009). Most primary dystonias start as action dystonia occurring during some activity such as writing and walking or running, but consider peripheral or central trauma and functional (psychogenic) dystonia when the dystonia occurs at rest and consists of a fixed posture (Thenganatt and Jankovic, 2014c). A fixed posture

## BOX 24.3 Etiological Classification of Dystonia

I. Inherited (see Tables 24.6A and 24.6B)
   A. Inherited (isolated)
   B. Inherited (combined)
II. Acquired dystonia (dystonia due to a known specific cause)
   Parkinson disease
   Progressive supranuclear palsy
   Multiple system atrophy
   Corticobasal degeneration
   Alternating hemiplegia of childhood
   Pelizaeus-Merzbacher disease
   Dystonia deafness
   Huntington disease
   Spinocerebellar degenerations
   Dentatorubral-pallidoluysian atrophy
   Hereditary spastic paraplegia with dystonia
   Thalamo-olivary degeneration with encephalopathy
   Wilson disease
   Neurodegeneration with brain iron accumulation
   Hypoprebetalipoproteinemia, acanthocytosis, retinitis pigmentosa, and pallidal degeneration
   Ataxia-telangiectasia
   Ataxia oculomotor apraxia
   Neuroacanthocytosis
   Rett syndrome
   Intraneuronal inclusion disease
   Infantile bilateral striatal necrosis
   Familial basal ganglia calcifications
   Hereditary spastic paraplegia with dystonia
   Associated with metabolic disorders:
   1. Amino acid disorders
      Glutaricacidemia
      Methylmalonicacidemia
      Homocystinuria
      Hartnup disease
      Tyrosinemia
      Glucose transporter-1 (GLUT-1) deficiency
   2. Lipid disorders
      Metachromatic leukodystrophy
      Ceroid lipofuscinosis
      Niemann-Pick disease type C (dystonic lipidosis, histiocytosis); defect in cholesterol esterification; caused by mutation in *NPC1* gene (18q11) and *HE1* gene (14q24.3)
      Gangliosidoses (GM1, GM2 variants)
      Hexosaminidase A and B deficiency
   3. Other metabolic disorders
      Bioamine metabolism disorders (dopamine responsive dystonia)
      Deficiencies in GTP-cyclohydrolase 1, sepiapterin reductase, aromatic amino acid decaraboxylase, tyrosine hydroxylase
      Biopterin-deficient diseases
      Lesch-Nyhan syndrome
      Triosephosphate isomerase deficiency
      Biotin-responsive basal ganglia disease
      Leigh disease
      Leigh disease
   Perinatal cerebral injury and kernicterus: athetoid cerebral palsy,, delayed-onset dystonia
   Infection: viral encephalitis, encephalitis lethargica, Reye syndrome, subacute sclerosing panencephalitis, Creutzfeldt-Jakob disease, human immunodeficiency virus
   Other: tuberculosis, syphilis, acute infectious torticollis
   Drugs: L-dopa and dopamine agonists, dopamine receptor-blocking drugs, fenfluramine, anticonvulsants, flecainide, ergots, certain calcium channel blockers
   Toxins: magnesium, carbon monoxide, carbon disulfide, cyanide, methanol, disulfiram, 3-nitroproprionic acid, wasp sting
   Metabolic: hypoparathyroidism
   Paraneoplastic brainstem encephalitis
   Vitamin E deficiency
   Primary antiphospholipid syndrome
   Cerebrovascular or ischemic injury, Sjögren syndrome
   Multiple sclerosis
   Central pontine (and extrapontine) myelinolysis
   Brainstem lesions
   Spinal cord lesions
   Syringomyelia
   Brain tumor
   Arteriovenous malformation
   Head trauma and brain surgery (thalamotomy)
   Lumbar stenosis
   Peripheral trauma (with causalgia)
   Electrical injury
III. Functional/Psychogenic
IV. Pseudodystonia
   Atlanto-axial subluxation
   Syringomyelia
   Arnold-Chiari malformation
   Trochlear nerve palsy
   Vestibular torticollis
   Posterior fossa mass
   Soft-tissue neck mass
   Congenital postural torticollis
   Congenital Klippel-Feil syndrome
   Isaacs syndrome
   Satoyoshi syndrome
   Stiff person syndrome
   Dupuytren contractures
   Trigger digits
   Ventral hernia

maintained during sleep or anesthesia implies superimposed contractures or a musculoskeletal disturbance mimicking the postures of dystonia. Although rest and sleep lessen dystonia in many, some note a striking diurnal variation. The diurnal variation manifests with little or no dystonia on rising in the morning, followed by the progressive development of problems as the day goes on, sometimes to the point of becoming unable to walk late in the day. This diurnal variability strongly suggests a diagnosis of dopa-responsive dystonia, although this feature is present in only about half of these patients (Wijemanne and Jankovic, 2015). Important clues to the cause of dystonia are (1) the nature of symptom onset (sudden versus slow), and (2) its course, whether rapid or slow progression or episodes of spontaneous remission.

The family history must be reviewed in detail with the awareness that affected relatives may have limited or distinctly different involvement from that of the patient. The categorization of genetic dystonias according to loci is somewhat arbitrary (Balint et al., 2018; Moghimi et al., 2014; Lohmann and Klein, 2013). Obtaining a birth and developmental history is critical in view of the frequency of dystonia after birth trauma, birth anoxia, and kernicterus.

Action dystonia is commonly the earliest manifestation of primary (idiopathic) dystonia. It is important to observe patients performing the acts that are most affected. Later, other tasks precipitate similar problems, the use of other parts of the body causes the dystonia to become evident in the originally affected site, and the dystonia may overflow to other sites including the opposite side of the body ("mirror dystonia") (Sitburana et al., 2009). Still later, dystonia is periodically evident at rest, and even later the posturing may be persistent and difficult to correct passively, especially when secondary joint contractures develop. A significant deviation from this progression, particularly with the early appearance of dystonia at rest, should encourage the physician to search carefully for a secondary cause (see Box 24.3).

It is important to recognize the natural variability of dystonia, which may be influenced by stress and anxiety. This is exemplified by blepharospasm, in which sunlight or stress often exacerbate the eyelid closure but increased concentration associated with singing or talking such as occurs during a conversation or a visit to the doctor often reduces the severity of the problem. If only placing reliance on the degree of disability seen in the office, the physician may underestimate the severity of the blepharospasm and may misdiagnose the problem as hysterical.

Depending on the cause of the dystonia, several other neurological abnormalities may be associated. Consider WD in any patient with onset of dystonia before age 60 (Mak and Lam, 2008). Many secondary dystonic disorders (listed in Box 24.3 and discussed in Chapter 96) result in additional psychiatric or cognitive disturbances, seizures, or pyramidal tract or cerebellar dysfunction. Ocular motor abnormalities suggest a diagnosis of Leigh disease, Niemann-Pick type C, ataxia-telangiectasia, ataxia-oculomotor apraxia syndrome, HD, Machado-Joseph disease (SCA3), or other spinocerebellar atrophies. Optic nerve or retinal disease raises the possibility of Leigh disease, other mitochondrial cytopathies, GM2 gangliosidosis, ceroid lipofuscinosis, and neurodegeneration with brain iron accumulation (NBIA) (McNeill et al., 2008; Schneider et al., 2013). One of the most common causes of NBIA is pantothenate kinase–associated neurodegeneration (PKAN), previously called Hallervorden-Spatz disease (Schneider et al., 2013). Other causes include neuroferritinopathy, infantile neuroaxonal dystrophy, aceruloplasminemia, and PLA2G6-associated neurodegeneration. Lower motor neuron and peripheral nerve dysfunction occur with neuroacanthocytosis, ataxia-telangiectasia, ataxia-oculomotor apraxia syndrome, metachromatic leukodystrophy, Machado-Joseph disease (SCA3), and other multisystem degenerations. Occasionally, prominent dystonic postures or pseudoathetosis occurs secondary to profound proprioceptive loss due to peripheral nerve, spinal cord, or brain (e.g., thalamic) lesions. The dystonia itself may cause additional neurological problems such as spinal cord or cervical root compression from long-standing torticollis, and peripheral nerve entrapment from limb dystonia. Also, independent of the cause, long-standing dystonic muscle spasms often result in hypertrophy of affected muscles (e.g., the sternocleidomastoid muscle in cervical dystonia).

Although the general medical examination must be thorough, the diagnosis is largely based on the history and observed phenomenology of the movement disorder (Morris and Jankovic, 2012). As always, carefully seek the ophthalmological and systemic signs of WD. Abdominal organomegaly also may indicate a storage disease. Tongue and lip mutilation are seen in neuroacanthocytosis or PKAN, in which orolingual action dystonia may be prominent (Walker et al., 2006). Oculocutaneous telangiectasia and evidence of recurrent sinopulmonary infections suggest ataxia-telangiectasia (Levy and Lang, 2018). Musculoskeletal abnormalities may simulate dystonia; rarely, dysmorphic features may serve as a clue to a mucopolysaccharidosis.

## CHOREA/ATHETOSIS

The term *chorea* derives from the Greek *choreia*, meaning "a dance." This hyperkinetic movement disorder consists of irregular, unpredictable, brief, jerky movements that flow randomly from one part of the body to another (Jankovic and Roos, 2014). The term *athetosis* describes slow chorea, typically seen in patients with cerebral palsy. Besides these disorders, there are numerous other causes of chorea, especially HD (Jankovic, 2009; Testa and Jankovic, 2019), most of which are listed in Box 24.4.

Initially, patients, particularly those with HD, often are unaware of the presence of involuntary movements, and the family may simply interpret the chorea as normal fidgetiness (Jankovic and Roos, 2014). The earliest patient complaints usually are those of clumsiness and incoordination, such as dropping objects or bumping into things. The limbs occasionally strike closely placed objects. In moderate to severe cases, patients may complain of abnormal involuntary jumping or jerking of the limbs and trunk. However, even when movements are overt, many patients deny their presence or only admit to being minimally aware of them.

Other features often associated with chorea, particularly HD, include motor impersistence manifested by inability to maintain tongue protrusion *(trombone tongue)* and pendular reflexes, probably caused by motor hypotonia (Jankovic and Roos, 2014). Speech may be slurred, halting, and periodically interrupted, especially in HD, in which speech disturbances are severe and often do not correlate with the severity of chorea. Here, in addition to dysarthria, there is usually a reduction in the spontaneity and quantity of speech output. Problems with feeding result from a combination of limb chorea, which causes sloppiness, and swallowing difficulties, which can result in choking and aspiration. Eating is particularly difficult for patients with *neuroacanthocytosis* (previously termed *chorea-acanthocytosis*), in which severe orolingual dystonia (eating dystonia) can cause the tongue to push the food out of the mouth almost as quickly as the patient puts it in. Patients with this dystonia often place food at the back of the tongue and throw the head back to initiate swallowing. One form of choreic movement in patients with neuroacanthocytosis is continuous truncal bending and extending movements, giving the appearance of a "rubber man," most apparent while the patient is standing or walking. Disturbances of stance and gait can be an early complaint in patients with chorea. The patient may note a tendency to sway and jerk while standing and an unsteady, uneven gait often likened to a drunken stagger. Later still, added postural instability in HD results in falls. Respiratory dyskinesias may cause the patient to feel short of breath or unable to obtain enough air (Mehanna and Jankovic, 2010). Patients with involvement of the pelvic region may complain bitterly of thrusting and rocking movements in the lower trunk and pelvis. Respiratory and pelvic involvements are sources of complaint more often in tardive dyskinesia than in other choreic movement disorders.

It is obvious from a review of Box 24.4 that it is impractical to discuss additional historical clues for every cause of chorea. We therefore limit discussion here to a few practical and important points.

Age at onset and manner of progression vary depending on the cause. A helpful distinction made here is between benign hereditary chorea, associated with *NKX2-1* (formerly called *TITF1*) gene (14q13.1–q21.1) mutation, and HD (Patel and Jankovic, 2014). In the *NKX2-1* syndrome chorea typically begins in childhood with a slow progression and little cognitive change, although a more disabling and progressive forms have been described: hence the term "benign hereditary chorea" should be abandoned (Parnes et al., 2018). In contrast, HD presenting in childhood is more often of the akinetic-rigid variety, with severe mental changes and rapid progression.

## BOX 24.4 Etiological Classification of Chorea

Developmental and aging choreas:
- Physiological chorea of infancy
- Cerebral palsy (anoxic), kernicterus
- Buccal-oral-lingual dyskinesia and edentulous orodyskinesia
- In older adults, senile chorea (probably several causes)

Hereditary choreas:
- Huntington disease
- Benign hereditary chorea (*TITF1* gene mutations)
- Neuroacanthocytosis
- Other central nervous system degenerations: "Huntington disease–like" disorders (e.g., PRNP, junctophilin or *JPH3* mutations, neuroferritinopathy, SCA17, c9orf72) dentratorubropallidoluysian atrophy (DRPLA), some spinocerebellar atrophies, ataxia-telangiectasia, ataxia oculomotor apraxia types 1 and 2, tuberous sclerosis of basal ganglia, neurodegeneration with brain iron accumulation (e.g., pantothenate kinase-associated neurodegeneration ),
- Neurometabolic disorders: Wilson disease, Lesch-Nyhan syndrome, lysosomal storage disorders, amino acid disorders, Leigh disease, porphyria

Drugs: neuroleptics (tardive dyskinesia), antiparkinsonian drugs, amphetamines, cocaine, tricyclic antidepressants, oral contraceptives

Toxins: alcohol intoxication and withdrawal, anoxia, carbon monoxide, manganese, mercury, thallium, toluene

Metabolic:
- Hyperthyroidism
- Hypoparathyroidism (various types)
- Pregnancy (chorea gravidarum)
- Hypernatremia and hyponatremia, hypomagnesemia, hypocalcemia
- Hypoglycemia and hyperglycemia (the latter may cause hemichorea, hemiballism)
- Acquired hepatocerebral degeneration
- Nutritional (e.g., beriberi, pellagra, vitamin $B_{12}$ deficiency in infants)

Infectious and postinfectious:
- Sydenham chorea
- Encephalitis lethargica
- Various other infectious and postinfectious encephalitis, Creutzfeldt–Jakob disease

Immunological:
- Systemic lupus erythematosus
- Henoch-Schönlein purpura
- Others (rarely): sarcoidosis, multiple sclerosis, Behçet disease, polyarteritis nodosa

Vascular (often hemichorea):
- Infarction or hemorrhage
- Arteriovenous malformation, moyamoya disease
- Polycythemia rubra vera
- Migraine
- Following cardiac surgery with hypothermia and extracorporeal circulation in children

Tumors (direct brain involvement; paraneoplastic)

Trauma, including subdural and epidural hematoma

Miscellaneous, including paroxysmal choreoathetosis

*PRNP*, prion protein.

In most cases of HD, the onset of chorea occurs in mid to late or adult life and is slow and insidious (Testa and Jankovic, 2019). An abrupt or subacute onset is more typical of many of the symptomatic causes of chorea, such as Sydenham chorea, hyperthyroidism, cerebral infarcts, and neuroleptic drug withdrawal (withdrawal emergent syndrome; Mejia and Jankovic, 2010), systemic lupus erythematosus (SLE), and other autoimmune choreas (Baizabal-Carvallo et al., 2013a; Baizabal-Carvallo and Jankovic, 2018). A pattern of remissions and exacerbations suggests the possibility of drugs, SLE, and rheumatic fever, whereas brief (minutes to hours) bouts of involuntary movement indicate a paroxysmal dyskinesia (Waln and Jankovic, 2015).

A recent history of streptococcal throat infection and musculoskeletal or cardiovascular problems in a child suggests a diagnosis of rheumatic (Sydenham) chorea. One may obtain a previous history of rheumatic fever, particularly in women who develop chorea during pregnancy or while taking birth control pills. Chorea gravidarum may be more common in women with prior history of rheumatic chorea. The individual contractions in Sydenham disease are slightly longer (>100 msec) than those in HD (50–100 msec), and there are often associated features such as dysarthria, oculogyric deviations, "milkmaid's grip," obsessive-compulsive behavior, and other features, including the prior history of streptococcal infection, that support the diagnosis of Sydenham disease.

In women, chorea during pregnancy or a history of previous fetal loss suggests the possibility of SLE with anticardiolipin antibodies, even in the absence of other features of collagen vascular disease. Symptoms isolated to one side of the body suggest a structural lesion in the contralateral basal ganglia. Some patients with Sydenham chorea have unilateral involvement. However, many patients who complain of unilateral involvement have abnormalities of both sides on examination.

A careful family history is crucial. The most common cause of inherited chorea is HD, which has fully penetrant autosomal dominant transmission (Testa and Jankovic, 2019). However, the family history can be misleading because the clinical features of the disease in other family members may have been mainly behavioral (including a history of suicides), and psychiatric disturbances and the chorea hardly noticed.

The range of choreiform movements in HD is quite broad, including eyebrow lifting or depression, lid winking, lip pouting or pursing, cheek puffing, lateral or forward jaw movements, tongue rolling or protruding, head jerking in any plane (a common pattern is a sudden backward jerk followed by a rotatory sweep forward), shoulder shrugging, trunk jerking or arching, pelvic rocking, and flitting movements of the fingers, wrists, toes, and ankles. Patients incorporate choreic jerks into voluntary movements, perhaps in part to mask the presence of the dyskinesia (so-called parakinesis).

Chorea often alters the performance of various tasks such as finger-to-nose testing and rapid alternating movements, causing a jerky, interrupted performance. Standing and walking often aggravate the chorea. The gait in HD may be particularly difficult to characterize under a single movement disorder rubric; it is irregular and lurching and has bizarre characteristics, not simply explained by increased chorea. This usually is wide based, despite the absence of typical ataxia. Patients may deviate from side to side in a zigzag fashion with lateral swaying and additional spontaneous flexion. In addition, the stride may be irregularly longer or shorter and the speed slowed, with some features similar to those of a parkinsonian gait, such as loss of arm swing, festination, propulsion, and retropulsion. Finally, one or both arms may be flexed at the elbow as if holding a purse over the forearm.

Respiratory irregularities, possibly related to chorea of the chest muscles, are common in HD, tardive dyskinesia, and a variety of other movement disorders (Mehanna and Jankovic, 2010). Periodic grunting, respiratory gulps, humming, and sniffing may be present in this and other choreic disorders, including HD. Other movement disorders often combine with chorea. Dystonic features probably are the most common and are seen in many conditions. Less common but well

**TABLE 24.3 Neuroleptic-Induced Movement Disorders**

| Acute, Transient | Chronic, Persistent |
|---|---|
| *Dystonic reaction* | *Tardive dyskinesia/stereotypy* |
| *Parkinsonism* | *Tardive chorea* |
| *Akathisia* | *Tardive dystonia* |
| *Withdrawal emergent syndrome* | *Tardive akathisia* |
| *Neuroleptic malignant syndrome* | *Tardive tics* |
| | *Tardive tremor* |
| | *Tardive gait disorder* |
| | *Persistent parkinsonism* |
| | *Tardive sensory syndrome* |

recognized are parkinsonism (e.g., with juvenile HD, neuroacanthocytosis, and WD), tics (e.g., in neuroacanthocytosis), myoclonus (e.g., in juvenile HD), tremor (e.g., in WD and HD), and ataxia (e.g., in juvenile HD and some spinocerebellar ataxias such as SCA17). Tone usually is normal to low. Muscle bulk is typically preserved, although weight loss and generalized wasting are common in HD. When distal weakness and amyotrophy are present, one must consider accompanying anterior horn cell or peripheral nerve disease, as in neuroacanthocytosis including McLeod's syndrome, ataxia-telangiectasia, Machado-Joseph disease, and spinocerebellar ataxias (see Chapter 96). Reduced tendon reflexes occur. On the other hand, chorea often results in hung-up and pendular reflexes, probably caused by the occurrence of a choreic jerk after the usual reflex muscle contraction.

Depending on the cause (see Box 24.4), several other neurological disturbances may be associated with chorea. In HD, for example, cognitive changes, motor impersistence (e.g., difficulty maintaining eyelid closure, tongue protrusion, constant handgrip), apraxias (especially orolingual), and oculomotor dysfunction are all quite common (see Chapter 96). *Milkmaid's grip*, appreciated as an alternating squeeze and release when the patient is asked to maintain a constant, firm grip of the examiner's fingers, probably is caused by a combination of chorea and motor impersistence.

## STEREOTYPY

Stereotypy is a continuous, repetitive, coordinated movement that may be associated with a variety of disorders and rarely occurs as an isolated, idiopathic movement disorder (Edwards et al., 2012; Frei et al., 2018; Savitt and Jankovic, 2018). Stereotypy is often confused with chorea, which, in contrast to stereotypy, is a random movement. One of the most common causes of stereotypy is tardive dyskinesia, associated with the use of dopamine receptor blockers (Table 24.3) (discussed in more detail in Chapter 96). In contrast to chorea associated with HD, which often predominantly involves the upper face (Jankovic and Roos, 2014), patients with tardive dyskinesia have repetitive, coordinated (stereotypic) movement of their tongue and mouth. Although the involuntary movements associated with tardive dyskinesia may superficially seem choreic, the muscle contractions are more predictable and repetitive, and the movements are more coordinated, often resembling seemingly purposeful motor acts such as chewing. Patients with orofacial stereotypy often have difficulties keeping their dentures in place and they may grind their teeth (bruxism) or cause biting of the tongue or inner cheek. These include chewing and smacking of the mouth and lips, rolling of the tongue in the mouth or pushing against the inside of the cheek *(bon-bon sign)*, and periodic protrusion or fly-catcher movements of the tongue. The speed and amplitude of these movements can increase markedly when the patient is concentrating on performing rapid alternating movements in the hands. Patients often have a striking degree of voluntary control over the movements and may be able to suppress them for a prolonged period when asked to do so. However, on distraction, the movements return immediately. Despite severe facial movements, voluntary protrusion of the tongue is rarely limited, and this act often dampens or completely inhibits the ongoing facial movements. This contrasts with the pronounced impersistence of volitional tongue protrusion seen in HD, which is far out of proportion to the degree of choreic involvement of the tongue. Despite the rocking movements of the pelvis, tapping of the feet, and shifting of the weight from side to side while standing (some of which may be caused by akathisia), the gait often is normal in patients with tardive dyskinesia, although a bizarre duck-like gait can be seen.

Other causes of stereotypies, besides tardive dyskinesia, include autistic disorders, schizophrenia, and restless legs syndrome, but perhaps the most common stereotypy is the leg stereotypy syndrome (Lotia et al., 2018). This condition is typically manifested by repetitive, continuous movement present almost exclusively in the legs while the patient is seated but may also occur while standing during which time it involves not only the legs but also may be manifested by swaying of the trunk. While some individuals describe these movements as soothing, there is no evidence that they are associated with or driven by anxiety or an irresistible urge to move, as is typically seen with akathisia or restless legs syndrome. Frequently familial, the epidemiology, pathophysiology, or treatment of leg stereotypy syndrome has not been studied.

Other causes of stereotypy include multiple infarctions in the basal ganglia, and possibly lesions in the cerebellar vermis result in similar movements. Older adults, especially the edentulous, often have a form of stereotypic orofacial movement, usually with minimal lingual involvement. Here, as in tardive dyskinesia, inserting dentures in the mouth may dampen the movements, and placing a finger to the lips can also suppress them. Another important diagnostic consideration and source of clinical confusion is idiopathic oromandibular dystonia. The abnormal movements tend to interfere more with the eating or speaking than those of classical tardive dyskinesia, and when these problems occur in patients with a tardive syndrome the movements are typically more dystonic (i.e., tardive dystonia). Orofacial and limb stereotypies, often preceded by psychiatric symptoms, may also be seen in children and adults as part of anti-NMDAR encephalitis (Baizabal-Carvallo et al., 2013b; Balu et al., 2019).

## BALLISM

Ballism, or ballismus, from the Greek word for "to throw," refers to flinging or flailing movements that are non-patterned, usually involving proximal muscles of the limbs. Lower-amplitude distal choreic movements also may be seen, and occasionally there is even intermittent prolonged dystonic posturing. Although considered unique hyperkinetic movement disorders, it is more likely that ballism and chorea represent a continuum rather than distinct entities. The coexistence of distal choreic movements, the discontinuous nature in less-severe cases, and the common evolution of ballism to typical chorea during the natural course of the disorder or with treatment all support this theory (Jankovic 2009). Ballism is usually confined to one side of the body, called *hemiballismus*. Occasionally, only one limb is involved *(monoballism)*; rarely, both sides are affected *(biballism)* or both legs *(paraballism)*. Box 24.5 lists the various causes of hemiballism.

The flinging movements of ballism often are extremely disabling to patients, who drop things from their hands or damage closely placed objects. Self-injury is common, and examination often reveals multiple bruises and abrasions. Additional signs and symptoms depend on the cause, location, and extent of the lesion, which is usually in the contralateral subthalamic nucleus or striatum (see Chapter 96).

**BOX 24.5 Causes of Ballism**

Infarction or ischemia, including transient ischemic attacks; usually lacunar disease, hypertension, diabetes, atherosclerosis, vasculitis, polycythemia, thrombocytosis, other causes
Hemorrhage
Tumor:
Metastatic
Primary
Other focal lesions (e.g., abscess, arteriovenous malformation, tuberculoma, toxoplasmosis, multiple sclerosis plaque, encephalitis, subdural hematoma)
Hyperglycemia (nonketotic hyperosmolar state)
Drugs (phenytoin, dopamine agonists in Parkinson disease)

**BOX 24.6 Phenomenological Classification of Tics**

**Simple Motor Tics**
Eye blinking; eyebrow raising; nose flaring; grimacing; mouth opening; tongue protrusion; platysma contractions; head jerking; shoulder shrugging, abduction, or rotation; neck stretching; arm jerks; fist clenching; abdominal tensing; pelvic thrusting; buttock or sphincter tightening; hip flexion or abduction; kicking; knee and foot extension; toe curling

**Simple Phonic Tics**
Sniffing, grunting, throat clearing, shrieking, yelping, barking, growling, squealing, snorting, coughing, clicking, hissing, humming, moaning

**Complex Motor Tics**
Head shaking, teeth gnashing, hand shaking, finger cracking, touching, hitting, jumping, skipping, stamping, squatting, kicking, smelling hands or objects, rubbing, finger twiddling, echopraxia, copropraxia, spitting, exaggerated startle

**Complex Phonic Tics**
Coprolalia (wide variety, including shortened words), unintelligible words, whistling, panting, belching, hiccupping, stuttering, stammering, echolalia, palilalia (also mental coprolalia and palilalia)

## TICS

Tics are the most varied of all movement disorders. Patients with Tourette syndrome, the most common cause of tics, manifest motor or phonic tics and a wide variety of associated symptoms (Jankovic and Kurlan, 2011; Robertson et al., 2017). Tics are brief and intermittent movements (motor tics) or sounds (phonic tics). Motor tics typically consist of sudden, abrupt, transitory, often repetitive, and coordinated (stereotypical) movements that may resemble gestures and mimic fragments of normal behavior, vary in intensity, and are repeated at irregular intervals. The movements are most often brief and jerky (clonic); however, slower, more prolonged movements (tonic or dystonic tics) also occur. Several other characteristic features are helpful in distinguishing this movement disorder from other dyskinesias. Patients usually experience an inner urge or local premonitory sensations before making the movement, which is temporarily relieved by its performance. Tics are voluntarily suppressible for variable periods, but this occurs at the expense of mounting inner tension and the need to allow the tic to occur. Indeed, a large proportion of people with tics, when questioned carefully, admit that they intentionally produce the movements or sounds that comprise their tics (in contrast to most other dyskinesias) in response to the uncontrollable inner urge or a premonitory sensation. Box 24.6 provides examples of the various types of tics. Motor and phonic tics are divisible further as simple or complex. Simple motor tics are random, brief, irregular muscle twitches of isolated body segments, particularly the eyelids and other facial muscles, the neck, and the shoulders. In contrast, complex motor tics are coordinated, patterned movements involving a number of muscles in their normal synergistic relationships. Some Tourette syndrome patients also manifest sudden and transitory cessation of all motor activity *(blocking tics)*, including speech, without alteration of consciousness.

**BOX 24.7 DSM-5 Diagnostic Criteria: Tourette's Disorder (307.23 [F95.2])**

1. Both multiple motor and one or more vocal tics have been present at some time during the illness, although not necessarily concurrently.
2. The tics may wax and wane in frequency but have persisted for more than 1 year since first tic onset.
3. Onset is before age 18 years.
4. The disturbance is not attributable to the physiological effects of a substance (e.g., cocaine) or another medical condition (e.g., Huntington disease, postviral encephalitis).

Reprinted with permission from the American Psychiatric Association, DSM-5 Task Force. Diagnostic and Statistical Manual of Mental Disorders: DSM-5™, 5th ed. Arlington: American Psychiatric Publishing; 2013.

Simple and complex phonic tics comprise a wide variety of sounds, noises, or formed words (see Box 24.6). The term *vocal tic* usually applies to these noises. However, because many of these sounds do not use the vocal cords, we prefer the term *phonic tic*. Although the presence of phonic tics is required for the diagnosis of definite Tourette syndrome, this criterion is artificial because phonic tics are essentially motor tics that result in abnormal sounds. Possibly the best-known (although not the most common) example of complex phonic tic is *coprolalia*, the utterance of obscenities or profanities. These are often slurred or shortened or may intrude into the patient's thoughts but not become verbalized (mental coprolalia; Freeman et al., 2009). In addition, patients with Tourette syndrome often exhibit copropraxia (obscene gestures) and echopraxia (mimicked gestures).

A wide variety of other behavioral disturbances may be associated with tic disorders, and it is sometimes difficult to separate complex tics from some of these comorbid disorders. These comorbid disturbances include attention deficit with or without hyperactivity, obsessive-compulsive behavior, impulsive behavior, and externally directed and self-destructive behavior, including self-mutilation (Jankovic and Kurlan, 2011). In some cases, the self-injurious behavior can be quite serious and even life threatening ("malignant Tourette").

Like most dyskinesias, tics usually increase with stress. However, in contrast to other dyskinesias, relaxation (e.g., watching television at home) often results in an increase in the tics, probably because the patient does not feel the need to suppress them voluntarily. Distraction or concentration usually diminishes tics, which also differs from most other types of dyskinesia. Many patients with idiopathic tics note spontaneous waxing and waning in their nature and severity over weeks to months, and periods of complete remission are possible. Many people with tics are only mildly affected, and many are even unaware that they demonstrate clinical features. This must be kept in mind when reviewing the family history and planning treatment. Finally, tics are one of the few movement disorders that can persist during all stages of sleep, although they usually subside in sleep.

There is no diagnostic test for Tourette syndrome; the diagnosis is based on clinical criteria according to the DSM-5 (American Psychiatric Association, 2013), which appears in Box 24.7.

**BOX 24.8 Etiological Classification of Tics**

I. Physiological tics
  A. Mannerisms
II. Pathological tics
  A. Primary
    Sporadic:
      1. Transient motor or phonic tics (<1 year)
      2. Chronic motor or phonic tics (>1 year)
      3. Adult-onset (recurrent) tics
      4. Tourette syndrome
    Inherited:
      1. Tourette syndrome
      2. Huntington disease
      3. Neuroacanthocytosis
  B. Secondary ("tourettism")
      1. Infections: encephalitis, Creutzfeldt-Jakob disease, Sydenham chorea
      2. Drugs: stimulants, L-dopa, carbamazepine, phenytoin, phenobarbital, antipsychotics
      3. Toxins: carbon monoxide
      4. Developmental: static encephalopathy, chromosomal abnormalities
      5. Other: head trauma, stroke, neurocutaneous syndromes, chromosomal abnormalities, schizophrenia, neuroacanthocytosis, degenerative disorders
III. Related disorders
  A. Stereotypies
  B. Self-injurious behaviors
  C. Hyperactivity syndrome
  D. Compulsions
  E. Excessive startle
  F. Jumping disease, latah, myriachit

*Modified from Jankovic, J., 2001. Tourette's syndrome. N. Engl. J. Med. 345, 1184–1192.*

Box 24.8 lists causes of tic disorders. Most are primary or idiopathic, and within this group, the onset almost always occurs in childhood or adolescence (Tourette syndrome). The male-to-female ratio in patients with Tourette syndrome is approximately 3:1. Idiopathic tics occur on a spectrum from a mild, transitory, single, simple motor tic to chronic, multiple, simple, and complex motor and phonic tics.

Patients and their families complain of a wide variety of symptoms (see Box 24.7). They may have seen numerous other specialists (e.g., allergists for repetitive sniffing, otolaryngologists for throat clearing, ophthalmologists for excessive eye blinking or eye rolling, and psychologists and psychiatrists for various neurobehavioral abnormalities). Often, someone close to the patient or a teacher suggests the diagnosis of Tourette syndrome to the family after learning about it in the media. Children may verbalize few complaints or feel reluctant to speak of the problem, especially if they have been subject to ridicule by others. Even young children, when questioned carefully, can provide the history of urge to perform the movement that gradually culminates in the release of a tic and the ability to control the tic voluntarily at the expense of mounting inner tension. Children may be able to control the tics for prolonged periods but often complain of difficulty concentrating on other tasks while doing so. Some give a history of requesting to leave the schoolroom and then releasing the tics in private (e.g., in the washroom). Peers and siblings often chastise or ridicule the patient, and parents or teachers, not recognizing the nature of the disorder, may scold or punish the child for what are thought to be voluntary bad habits (indeed, an older term for tics is *habit spasms*).

The history may include an exposure to stimulants for hyperactivity. Review the family history for the wide range of associated symptoms such as obsessive-compulsive behavior and attention deficit disorder. Additional neurological complaints, including other dyskinesias, suggest the possibility of a secondary cause of the tics. Although tics may sometimes appear as highly unusual and bizarre movements and sounds, tics are rarely of psychogenic origin (Baizabal-Carvallo and Jankovic, 2014).

In most patients with tics, the neurological examination is entirely normal except for the motor or phonic tics, or both. In patients with primary tic disorders, the presence of other neurological, cognitive, behavioral, and neuropsychological disturbances may simply relate to extension of the underlying cerebral dysfunction beyond the core that accounts for pure tic phenomena. Patients with secondary forms of tics (e.g., neuroacanthocytosis, tardive tics) may demonstrate other involuntary movements such as chorea, dystonia, and other neurological deficits (see Box 24.6). Careful interview stressing the subjective features that precede or accompany tics usually allows the distinction between true dystonia or myoclonus, and dystonic or clonic tics.

Despite bitter complaints by the family, it is common for patients to show little or no evidence of a movement disorder during an office appointment. Aware of this, the physician must attempt to observe the patient at a time when he or she is less likely to be exerting voluntary control, such as in the waiting room. If no movements have been witnessed during the interview, the physician should seemingly direct attention elsewhere (e.g., to the parents) while observing the patient out of the corner of the eye. The patient often releases the tics while changing in the examining room, particularly after suppressing tics during the interview. The physician should attempt to view the patient at this time or at least listen for the occurrence of phonic tics. If all else fails, ask the patient voluntarily to mimic the movements. This, in combination with associated symptoms such as urge, voluntary release, control, and the often varied and complex nature of the movements, usually is enough to provide the diagnosis, even if the physician never witnesses spontaneous tics in the office. Finally, ask the parents to provide home videos of the patient. Although tics usually start in childhood, some adults may present with tics and other features of Tourette syndrome. In most of these adults with tics one can find evidence of childhood onset of tics which spontaneously remitted after adolescence and recurred later during adulthood (Jankovic and Kurlan, 2011; Robertson et al., 2017).

## MYOCLONUS

Myoclonus is a sudden, brief, shock-like involuntary movement possibly caused by active muscle contraction *(positive myoclonus)* or inhibition of ongoing muscle activity *(negative myoclonus)*. The differential diagnosis of myoclonus is broader than that of any other movement disorder (Box 24.9). To exclude muscle twitches, such as fasciculations caused by lower motor neuron lesions, some authors have insisted that an origin in the CNS be a component of the definition. Although the majority of cases of myoclonus originate in the CNS, occasional cases of brief shock-like movements clinically indistinguishable from CNS myoclonus occur with spinal cord or peripheral nerve or root disorders.

The clinical patterns of myoclonus vary widely. The frequency varies from single, rare jerks to constant, repetitive contractions. The amplitude may range from a small contraction that does not move a joint to a very large jerk that moves the entire body. The distribution ranges from focal involvement of one body part, to segmental (involving two or more contiguous regions), to multifocal, to generalized. When the jerks occur bilaterally, they may be symmetrical or asymmetrical. When they occur

**BOX 24.9 Etiological Classification of Myoclonus**

**Physiological Myoclonus (Normal Subjects)**
Sleep jerks (hypnagogic jerks)
Anxiety-induced
Exercise-induced
Hiccup (singultus)
Benign infantile myoclonus with feeding

**Essential Myoclonus (No Known Cause and No Other Gross Neurological Deficit)**
Hereditary (phenotype may be pure myoclonus or myoclonus-dystonia)
Sporadic

**Epileptic Myoclonus (Seizures Dominate and no Encephalopathy, at Least Initially)**
Fragments of epilepsy
Isolated epileptic myoclonic jerks
Epilepsia partialis continua
Idiopathic stimulus-sensitive myoclonus
Photosensitive myoclonus
Myoclonic absences in petit mal
Childhood myoclonic epilepsies
Infantile spasms
Myoclonic astatic epilepsy (Lennox-Gastaut syndrome)
Cryptogenic myoclonus epilepsy
Myoclonic epilepsy of Janz
Benign familial myoclonic epilepsy (Rabot syndrome)
Progressive myoclonic epilepsy: Baltic myoclonus (Unverricht-Lundborg syndrome)

**Symptomatic Myoclonus (Progressive or Static Encephalopathy Dominates)**
Storage diseases
Lafora body disease
Lipidoses, such as GM2 gangliosidosis, Tay-Sachs disease, Krabbe disease
Ceroid lipofuscinosis (Batten disease, Kufs disease)
Sialidosis (cherry-red spot)
Spinocerebellar degeneration
Ramsay Hunt syndrome (many causes)
Friedreich ataxia
Ataxia-telangiectasia
Basal ganglia degenerations:
- Wilson disease
- Neurodegeneration with brain iron accumulations
- Progressive supranuclear palsy
- Huntington disease
- Parkinson disease
- Corticobasal degeneration
- Pallidal degenerations
- Multiple system atrophy
- Mitochondrial encephalopathies, including myoclonic epilepsy and ragged-red fibers

Dementias:
- Creutzfeldt-Jakob disease
- Alzheimer disease
- Viral encephalopathies
- Subacute sclerosing panencephalitis
- Encephalitis lethargica
- Arbovirus encephalitis
- Herpes simplex encephalitis
- Postinfectious encephalitis

Inflammatory/autoimmune:
- Autoimmune encephalitis including anti-NMDA-receptor antibody encephalitis, etc. Paraneoplastic
- Celiac disease

Metabolic:
- Hepatic failure
- Renal failure
- Dialysis syndrome
- Hyponatremia
- Hypoglycemia
- Infantile myoclonic encephalopathy (polymyoclonus, with or without neuroblastoma)
- Nonketotic hyperglycemia
- Multiple carboxylase deficiency

Toxic encephalopathies:
- Bismuth
- Heavy metal poisons
- Methyl bromide, dichlorodiphenyltrichloroethane
- Drugs, including L-dopa, tricyclic antidepressants

Other encephalopathies

Post hypoxia (Lance-Adams syndrome):
- Post-traumatic
- Heat stroke
- Electric shock
- Decompression injury

Focal central nervous system damage:
- Post stroke
- Post thalamotomy
- Tumor
- Trauma
- Olivodentate lesions (palatal myoclonus)
- Spinal cord lesions (segmental or spinal myoclonus) disease

*NMDA*, N-methyl-D-aspartate.

in more than one region, they may be synchronous in two body parts (within milliseconds) or asynchronous. Myoclonus usually is arrhythmic and irregular, but in some patients it is very regular (rhythmic), and in others there may be jerky oscillations that last for a few seconds and then fade away (oscillatory). Myoclonic jerks may occur spontaneously without a clear precipitant or in response to a wide variety of stimuli, including sudden noise, light, visual threat, pinprick, touch, and muscle stretch. Attempted movement (or even the intention to move) may initiate the muscle jerks (action or intention myoclonus). *Palatal myoclonus* is a form of segmental myoclonus manifested by rhythmic contractions of the soft palate. The rhythmicity has led to the alternative designation of *palatal tremor*, but the latter is an oscillatory movement produced by synchronous or alternating contractions of antagonist muscle. In contrast, segmental myoclonus, such as palatal myoclonus, is produced by rhythmical contractions of agonists only. Symptomatic palatal myoclonus is usually manifested by contractions of the levator veli palatini, whereas essential palatal myoclonus consists of rhythmic contractions of the tensor veli palatini, which is often associated with a clicking sound in the ear, and disappears with sleep. Symptomatic but not essential palatal myoclonus often is associated with hypertrophy of the inferior olive evident on magnetic resonance imaging (MRI). There is a growing body of evidence that palatal myoclonus can be produced volitionally, which has been increasingly reported as a manifestation of functional/psychogenic movement disorder (Dijk and Tijssen, 2010; Zadikoff et al., 2006).

As may be seen from the foregoing description and the long list of possible causes of myoclonus, the symptoms in these patients are quite varied. For simplification, we briefly review the possible symptoms with respect to four major etiological subcategories in Box 24.9.

*Physiological forms of myoclonus* occurring in normal subjects vary depending on the precipitant. Probably the most common form is the jerking most of us have experienced on falling asleep (*hypnagogic myoclonus*, or *jactitation*). This very familiar phenomenon is rarely a source of concern. Occasionally, anxiety- or exercise-induced myoclonus causes concern. The history usually is clear, and there is little to find (including abnormal movements) when the patient is seen.

In the *essential myoclonus* group, patients usually complain of isolated muscle jerking in the absence of other neurological deficits (with the possible exception of tremor and dystonia). The movements may begin at any time from early childhood to late adult life and may remain static or progress slowly over many years. The family history may be positive, and some patients note a striking beneficial effect of alcohol (Mostile and Jankovic, 2010). Associated dystonia, present in some patients, also may respond to ethanol.

Myoclonus occurring as one component of a wide range of seizure types is *epileptic myoclonus*. Many of these patients give a clear history of seizures as the dominant feature. Myoclonic jerks may be infrequent and barely noticeable to the patient or may occur frequently and cause pronounced disability. Myoclonus on waking in the morning or an increasing frequency of the myoclonic jerks may forewarn of a seizure soon to come. The clinical pattern of myoclonus in this instance also varies widely. Sensitivity to photic stimuli and other sensory input may be prominent. Occasional patients demonstrate isolated myoclonic jerks in the absence of additional seizure activity. In these cases, the family history may be positive for seizures, and the electroencephalogram (EEG) often demonstrates a typical centrencephalic seizure pattern that is otherwise asymptomatic (such as a 3-Hz spike-and-wave pattern). In others, myoclonus and seizures are equally prominent (the myoclonic epilepsies). These may or may not be associated with an apparent progressive encephalopathy (most often with cognitive dysfunction and ataxia) in the absence of a definable, underlying, symptomatic cause.

In the *disorders classified as causing symptomatic myoclonus*, seizures may occur, but the encephalopathy (either static or progressive) is the feature that predominates. Many different myoclonic patterns occur in this broad category. As can be appreciated from a review of Box 24.9, a plethora of other neurological and systemic symptoms may accompany the encephalopathy. Two clinical subcategories of this larger grouping are distinguishable to assist in differential diagnosis. In progressive myoclonic epilepsy, myoclonus, seizures, and encephalopathy predominate, whereas in progressive myoclonic ataxia (often called *Ramsay Hunt syndrome*), myoclonus and ataxia dominate the clinical picture, with less frequent or severe seizures and mental changes. Myoclonus may also originate in the brainstem and spinal cord. Spinal segmental myoclonus often is rhythmic and limited to muscles innervated by one or a few contiguous spinal segments. Propriospinal myoclonus is another type of spinal myoclonus that usually results in flexion jerks of the trunk. This type of myoclonus is often of psychogenic origin.

Considering the varied causes, the possible range of neurological findings is wide. Alternatively, despite the complaint of abnormal movements, some patients with myoclonus (e.g., those with tics and certain paroxysmal dyskinesias) have little to reveal on examination. This is particularly the case for the physiological forms of myoclonus and for those associated with epilepsy and some symptomatic causes. When myoclonus is clearly present on examination, the physician should try to characterize the movement, as outlined in this chapter. When the jerks are single or repetitive but arrhythmic, one must differentiate these movements from tics. Myoclonus usually is briefer and less coordinated or patterned. Furthermore, myoclonus is not associated with a premonitory urge or sensation. Rhythmic forms of myoclonus may be confused with tremors. Here, the pattern of movement is more one of repetitive, abrupt-onset, square-wave movements caused by contractions of the agonists, in contrast to the smoother sinusoidal activity of tremor produced by alternating or synchronous contractions of antagonist muscles. Rhythmic myoclonus usually is in the range 1–4 Hz, in contrast to the faster frequencies seen in most types of tremor. The oscillations of so-called oscillatory myoclonus may be faster. These are distinguishable by their bursting or shuddering nature, usually precipitated by sudden stimulus or movement, lasting for a few seconds and then fading away.

The distribution of the myoclonus is helpful in classifying the myoclonus and considering possible etiologies. Focal myoclonus may be more common in disturbances of an isolated region of the cerebral cortex. Segmental involvement, particularly when rhythmic, may occur with brainstem lesions (e.g., branchial or palatal myoclonus) or spinal lesions (spinal myoclonus) (Esposito et al., 2009). Multifocal or generalized myoclonus suggests a more diffuse disorder, particularly involving the reticular substance of the brainstem. When multiple regions of the body are involved, it is helpful to attempt to estimate whether movements are occurring in synchrony. It is sometimes difficult to do this clinically, and multichannel electromyographic (EMG) monitoring is needed.

Throughout the examination, it is important to define whether the movements occur spontaneously or with various precipitants such as sudden loud noise, visual threat, perturbation, or a pinprick. Test several special-sense and somesthetic sensory inputs. In addition, it is important to evaluate the effects of passive and active movement. In the case of action or intention myoclonus, jerking occurs during voluntary motor activity, especially when the patient attempts to perform a fine motor task such as reaching for a target. This disturbance is often confused with severe ataxia. Action myoclonus may be evident in such activities as voluntary eyelid closure, pursing of lips or speaking, holding the arms out, finger-to-nose testing, writing, bringing a cup to the mouth, holding the legs out against gravity, heel-to-shin testing, and walking. In addition to the positive myoclonus that results from a brief active muscle contraction, negative myoclonus may occur. Although clinically these appear as brief jerks, causation is periodic inhibition of ongoing muscle activity and sudden loss of muscle tone.

The most common example of negative myoclonus is *asterixis*, which may be seen in liver failure (liver flap) and, to a lesser extent, in other metabolic encephalopathies and occasionally with focal brain lesions. The best-recognized location of asterixis is the forearm muscles, where it causes a flapping, irregular tremor-like movement with wrist extension. When mild and of low amplitude, this may be confused with 5- to 6-Hz postural tremor. A similar form of negative myoclonus accounts for the periodic loss of postural tone in axial and leg muscles in some patients with action myoclonus syndromes such as postanoxic action myoclonus. This results in a bobbing movement of the trunk while standing and may culminate in falls.

## MISCELLANEOUS MOVEMENT DISORDERS

*Hemifacial spasm* is a relatively common disorder in which irregular tonic and clonic movements involve the muscles of one side of the face innervated by the ipsilateral seventh cranial nerve. Unilateral eyelid twitching usually is the first symptom, followed at variable intervals by lower-facial muscle involvement. Rarely, the spasm affects both sides of the face, in which case the spasms are asynchronous on the two sides, in contrast to other pure facial dyskinesias such as cranial dystonia (Yaltho and Jankovic, 2011).

The term *akathisia* refers to a sense of restlessness and the feeling of a need to move (Frei et al., 2018; Waln and Jankovic, 2013). This was first used to describe what was thought to be a hysterical condition, and later the term was applied to the restlessness with inability to sit or stand still (motor impatience) seen in patients with idiopathic and postencephalitic parkinsonism. The most common cause of the syndrome is as a side effect of major tranquilizing or antiemetic drugs (neuroleptics) that act by blocking dopamine receptors, often accompanied by other features of tardive dyskinesia. A classic example of "sensory" movement disorder (Patel et al., 2014), akathisic movements occur in response to the subjective inner feeling of restlessness and need to move. The movements of akathisia are varied and complex. They include repetitive rubbing; crossing and uncrossing the arms; stroking the head and face; repeatedly picking at clothing; abducting and adducting, crossing and uncrossing, swinging, or up-and-down pumping of the legs; and shifting weight, rocking, marching in place, or pacing while sitting and standing. Occasionally, patients demonstrate a variety of vocalizations such as moans, grunts, and shouts. Akathisia can be an acute or delayed complication of antipsychotic drug therapy (acute akathisia and tardive akathisia, respectively). It also occurs in PD, secondary to selective serotonin reuptake inhibitors, and in certain confusional states or dementing processes.

Another disorder in which most movements are secondary to the subjective need to move is the *restless legs syndrome*, perhaps the most common of all movement disorders, occurring in approximately 14% of women and 7% of men older than 50 years of age (Trenkwalder and Paulus, 2010). Unlike in akathisia, the patient with restless legs syndrome typically complains of a variety of sensory disturbances in the legs, including pins and needles, creeping or crawling, aching, itching, stabbing, heaviness, tension, burning, and coldness. Occasionally, similar symptoms occur in the arms. These complaints usually are experienced during prolonged immobility such as during car trips, on an airplane, or during recumbency in the evening just before falling asleep. This condition commonly is associated with another movement disorder, periodic leg movements of sleep, sometimes inappropriately called *nocturnal myoclonus*. These periodic slow, sustained (1- to 2-second) movements range from synchronous or asynchronous dorsiflexion of the big toes and feet to triple flexion of one or both legs. More rapid myoclonic movements or slower, prolonged, dystonic-like movements of the feet and legs also may be present in these patients while awake, and these too may have a natural periodicity. Leg myoclonus or foot dystonia may also be the presenting feature of the stiff person syndrome (Baizabal-Carvallo and Jankovic, 2015).

Another uncommon but well-defined movement disorder of the lower limbs is painful legs and moving toes. Here, the patient typically complains of a deep pulling or searing pain in the lower limb and foot (a small proportion of patients have a painless variant) associated with continuous wriggling or writhing of the toes, occasionally the ankle, and less commonly more proximal muscles of the leg. Rarely, a similar problem is seen in the upper limb as well. In some cases, there is a history of root or nerve injury, and the examination may demonstrate evidence of peripheral nerve dysfunction.

Some dyskinesias occur intermittently rather than persistently. This is typical of tics and certain forms of myoclonus. Dystonia often occurs only with specific actions, but this is usually a consistent response to the action rather than a periodic and unpredictable occurrence. Some patients with dystonia have a diurnal variation (dopa-responsive dystonia) characterized by more normal motor function in the morning with the emergence or worsening of dystonia as the day progresses, so that by the end of the day the patients may be unable to ambulate because of severe generalized dystonia (Wijemanne and Jankovic, 2015). A small group of patients with chorea or dystonia have bouts of sudden-onset, short-lived, involuntary movements known as *paroxysmal choreoathetosis* or, more appropriately, *paroxysmal dyskinesia* (Waln and Jankovic, 2015) (Table 24.4). Certain features such as precipitants, duration, frequency, age of onset, and family history (see Chapter 96) characterize these disorders and sometimes help to separate them into diagnostic categories. Thus, paroxysmal dyskinesias may be categorized as kinesigenic (precipitated by voluntary movement such as arising from a chair or starting to run),

**TABLE 24.4 Classification of Paroxysmal Dyskinesias**

| | Paroxysmal Kinesigenic Dyskinesia | PNKD | PED | PHD |
|---|---|---|---|---|
| Inheritance | AD | AD | AD | Usually sporadic |
| Gender M:F | 4:1 | 2:1 | 2:3 | 7:3 |
| Age at onset, years | <1–20 | <1–20 s | 2–30 | 4–20 s |
| Phenomenology of abnormal movements | Dystonia with or without chorea/ballism, uni- or bilateral | Dystonia with or without choreoathetosis, uni- or bilateral, rarely spasticity | Dystonia, sometimes in combination with choreoathetosis, uni- or bilateral | Dystonia, chorea, ballism<br>May be a form of frontal epilepsy |
| Triggers | Sudden movement, change in direction, acceleration, startle | Alcohol, caffeine, emotions, fatigue | Prolonged exercise, muscle vibration | Sleep |
| Duration of paroxysms | Seconds up to 5 min | 2 min to 4 h | 5 min to 2 h | 30 min up to 50 min |
| Frequency of paroxysms | 1 per month to 100 per day | Few per week to few in a lifetime | Few per month | Few per year to few per night |
| Genetics | 1. EKD1: 16p11.2-q12.1 (DYT10) with *PRRT2* gene within this region<br>2. EKD2: 16q13-q22.1 (DYT19)<br>3. EKD3: no mutation on chromosome 16 | 1. *PNKD*: 2q35 (DYT8)<br>2. *SCL2A1*: chromosome 1 (DYT9)<br>3. *KCNMA1*: 10q22<br>4. locus on 2q31 (DYT20) | 1. *SCL2A1*: 1p35-p31.3 (DYT18) | 1. *CHRNA4*: 20q13.2-q13.3<br>2. *CHRNB2*: chromosome 1q21<br>3. locus on chromosome 15q24<br>4. locus on chromosome 8p21 |
| Treatment | Anticonvulsants (carbamazepine, phenytoin, others) | Avoiding triggers, benzodiazepines (clonazepam) | Avoiding triggers, ketogenic diet (in GLUT1 deficiency) | Anticonvulsants |

*AD*, Autosomal dominant; *PED*, paroxysmal exercise-induced dyskinesia; *PHD*, paroxysmal hypnogenic dyskinesia; *PNKD*, paroxysmal nonkinesigenic dyskinesia.

**BOX 24.10 Clues to the Presence of a Functional (Psychogenic) Movement Disorder**

**Physical Factors**

***Movement Disorder***

Abrupt onset
Incongruous movements
Inconsistent movements
Response to placebo or suggestion
Selective disability
Dramatic resolution
Maximum early disability
Deliberate slowing
Rhythmic shaking
Bizarre gait

***Other Neurological Findings***

Giveway weakness
Non-anatomical sensory loss
Dizziness and fainting
"Seizures"
Convergence spasm
Bursts of verbal gibberish
Visual disturbances
Headache
Chronic pain
Amnesia
Insomnia
Exhaustion/Fatigue

***Multiple Somatizations***

Self-inflicted injuries
Unwitnessed paroxysmal disorders

***Psychiatric Problems***

Depression
Anxiety disorder
Somatization disorder
Predisposing event
Trauma
Surgery
Major life event

**Social Factors**

Work-related injuries
Litigation
Relationship problems (spouse or children)
Physical abuse
Sexual abuse
Substance abuse
Secondary gain
Factitious disorder/malingering

nonkinesigenic, exertional, or nocturnal. In many cases, the movements are so infrequent that the physician never sees them, so a careful history is needed to determine the nature of the disorder, and having the patient provide a videotape of the events is often invaluable. On the other hand, typical paroxysmal kinesigenic dyskinesia (PKD) can occur many times per day, each event usually lasting seconds to a few minutes, and often can be triggered on examination in the office (e.g., sudden initiation of movement such as running on the spot from a resting state). There may be a family history of seizures or migraines. Am increasing number of paroxysmal dyskinesias are being recognized as genetic channelopathies or mitochondrial disorders (Waln and Jankovic, 2015). The glucose transporter-1 (GLUT-1) deficiency syndrome often results in paroxysmal exercise-induced dyskinesia as well as other clinical features (Pons et al., 2010). Periodic ataxias often are included in the group of paroxysmal movement disorders.

Also, there are disorders in which an abnormal or excessive response to startle occurs. In some patients, one simply finds an exaggerated startle response, which habituates poorly after repeated stimuli. In others, there is an abnormal response to the stimuli that normally evoke startle. Hyperekplexia, also known as *startle syndrome*, may be more akin to certain forms of myoclonus than to a normal startle response. Several other unusual disorders, first described in the nineteenth century together with Tourette syndrome, manifest excessive startle. Jumping disease (Jumping Frenchmen of Maine), latah, and myriachit also involve sudden striking out, echo phenomena, automatic obedience, and several other less common features. These disorders are quite distinct from Tourette syndrome and possibly represent culturally related operant-conditioned behavior rather than true neurological disease, although this point remains controversial.

Finally, functional (psychogenic) movement disorders characterized by abnormal slowness or excessive movements or postures that cannot be directly attributed to a lesion or an organic dysfunction in the nervous system are emerging as one of the most common groups of disorders encountered in movement disorder clinics (Thenganatt and Jankovic, 2014; Baizabal-Carvallo et al., 2019). Derived primarily from psychiatric or psychological disorders, because of their rich spectrum of phenomenology and variable severity, functional (psychogenic) movement disorders present a major diagnostic and therapeutic challenge. Facilitating the diagnosis of functional (psychogenic) movement disorders are various clues that include somatic and psychiatric complaints (especially chronic fatigue and pain syndromes) and movement disorders whose phenomenology is incongruous with typical movement disorders. These include sudden onset (often related to some emotional or minor physical trauma), secondary gain, variable frequency of tremor, distractibility, and exaggeration of symptoms (Box 24.10). Functional movement disorders must be differentiated from catatonia, a complex neuropsychiatric syndrome characterized by a broad range of motor, speech, and behavioral abnormalities, including "waxy flexibility," "posturing," and a variety of other motor and behavioral abnormalities (Wijemanne and Jankovic, 2015).

## INVESTIGATION OF MOVEMENT DISORDERS

The nature and extent of the investigation of a patient presenting with a movement disorder vary depending on the clinical circumstances. When the historical and clinical features are typical of certain primary (idiopathic) disorders, further investigations may be unnecessary. Examples of these include normal physiological tremor and myoclonus, essential tremor (especially if familial), adult-onset focal dystonias, childhood tic disorders, and even PD. However, one must always be mindful of the possibility of additional occult aggravating factors superimposed on a known pre-existing movement disorder. The reverse is also possible, in which the presumed cause is actually an aggravating factor or simply a coincidental association, particularly in the case of patients thought to have drug-induced disturbances. For example, chorea apparently caused by the birth control pill (or chorea gravidarum) may be a manifestation of underlying SLE. When dealing with presumed neuroleptic-induced movement disorders, it is important to

**TABLE 24.5 Investigation of Movement Disorders**

| Movement Disorder Investigation | A | C | B | D | T | M |
|---|---|---|---|---|---|---|
| *Routine hematology (including sedimentation rate)* | + | + | + | + | − | + |
| *Routine biochemistry (including $Ca^{2+}$, uric acid, liver function tests)* | + | + | + | + | + | + |
| *Serum copper, ceruloplasmin (with or without 24-h urine Cu, liver biopsy, radiolabeled Cu studies)* | ++ | ++ | − | ++ | + | + |
| *Slit-lamp examination* | ++ | ++ | − | ++ | + | + |
| *Thyroid function* | + | ++ | − | + | − | + |
| *Antistreptolysin O test, anti-DNase B, antihyaluronidase* | − | + | − | + | + | − |
| *Antinuclear factor, LE cells, other immunological studies, anticardiolipin antibodies, Venereal Disease Research Laboratories test* | + | ++ | + | + | − | + |
| *Blood acanthocytes* | + | + | − | + | + | + |
| *Lysosomal enzymes* | + | + | − | + | + | + |
| *Urine organic and amino acids* | + | + | − | + | − | + |
| *Urine oligosaccharides and mucopolysaccharides* | + | + | − | + | − | + |
| *Serum lactate and pyruvate* | + | + | − | + | − | + |
| *DNA tests for gene mutations* | + | + | − | + | − | + |
| *Bone marrow for storage cells (including electron microscopy)* | + | + | − | + | − | + |
| *Electron microscopy of leukocytes; biopsy of liver, skin, and conjunctiva* | + | + | − | + | − | + |
| *Nerve or muscle biopsy* | + | + | − | + | − | + |
| *Oligoclonal bands* | ± | + | ± | ± | − | + |
| *Computed tomography or magnetic resonance imaging* | ++ | ++ | ++ | ++ | + | ++ |
| *Electroencephalography* | + | + | − | + | + | ++ |
| *Electromyography and nerve conduction studies* | + | + | − | + | + | + |
| *Evoked potentials* | ± | ± | − | ± | − | ++ |
| *Electroretinogram* | + | + | − | + | − | + |
| *Neuropsychological testing* | + | + | − | − | + | − |

Note: The extent of investigation depends on factors such as age of onset, nature of progression, and presence of historical or clinical atypical features suggesting a secondary cause of the movement disorder in question.

++, Very important or often useful; +, sometimes helpful; ±, questionably helpful; − rarely or never helpful. *A*, Akinetic rigid syndrome; *B*, hemiballism; *C*, chorea; *D*, dystonia; *LE*, Lupus erythematosus; *M*, myoclonus; *T*, tics.

consider the possibility that the antipsychotic drug was given for initial psychiatric manifestations of an unrecognized/undiagnosed underlying brain disease that is now *causing* the movement disorder in question. HD and WD are two disorders in which this may occur.

The importance of excluding WD cannot be overemphasized. This includes slit-lamp examination, measurement of serum ceruloplasmin and copper, liver function tests, measurement of 24-hour urinary copper excretion, and, if necessary, liver biopsy and genetic testing. Children, adolescents, and young adults presenting with parkinsonism, chorea, or a dystonic or myoclonic syndrome need additional careful hematological and biochemical assessment, as indicated in Table 24.5.

Although in the majority of movement disorders, the diagnosis depends on recognizing typical clinical phenomena, certain movement disorders require specific investigations. For example, when neuroacanthocytosis is suspected, demonstrating blood acanthocytes, elevated serum creatine kinase, and altered nerve conduction studies are needed to support the diagnosis (Walker et al., 2006). Biochemical screening may also reveal evidence of hypoparathyroidism, which can cause calcification of the basal ganglia, resulting in several movement disorders (Deng et al., 2015). Hyperthyroidism, polycythemia rubra vera, SLE, and antiphospholipid syndrome should be considered in the differential diagnosis of chorea. Early clues are a history of recurrent fetal loss, a prolonged partial thromboplastin time, a false-positive Venereal Disease Research Laboratories (VDRL) test, and thrombocytopenia, which indicates the presence of antiphospholipid immunoglobulins such as the lupus anticoagulant and anticardiolipin antibodies (Baizabal-Carvallo et al., 2013a). In addition to the classic autoimmune conditions including celiac disease (antigliadin antibodies), and stiff person syndrome (anti-GAD and other antibodies), paraneoplastic movement disorders should be considered in any patient with subacute onset of hyperkinetic movement disorder or ataxia. Consider Sydenham chorea in a child presenting with chorea of unknown origin, and obtain antistreptolysin O titer, antihyaluronidase, and electrocardiogram. In a patient with hemiballism, one should search for potential risk factors for vascular disease by measuring levels of blood sugar (often very high in patients with hyperglycemic nonketotic states which first can present with hemiballism [see below]), hemoglobin, platelets, erythrocyte sedimentation rate, cholesterol, and triglycerides.

Genetic DNA tests are increasingly being used in the evaluation of patients with familial and even sporadic PD and other movement disorders, but such testing should only be done with proper counseling, given the existing uncertainties, including incomplete penetrance and other difficulties interpreting such tests (MacArthur et al., 2014). Genetic panels are now widely available for most movement disorder phenotypes (parkinsonism, dystonia, HD and other choreas, NBIAs, myoclonic encephalopathies, etc. (Tables 24.6, A and B). Whole-exome or whole-genome sequencing is increasingly utilized in evaluation of disorders without obvious diagnosis.

**TABLE 24.6A Etiological Classification of Dystonia-Inherited (Isolated)**

| Classification | Chromosome Gene Mutation Gene Product | Pattern of Inheritance | Onset | Distribution, Additional Features | Origin/Comment |
|---|---|---|---|---|---|
| DYT-*TOR1A* (DYT1) | 9q34, GAG deletion, *TOR1A*/TorsinA | AD | C | Distal limbs, generalized | Penetrance: 30% AJ, 70% NJ |
| DYT-*THAP1* (DYT6) | 8q21-22 *THAP1* | AD | A, C | Cervical, cranial, brachial | German-American Mennonite-Amish |
| DYT-*ANO3* (DYT24) | 3, *ANO3* | AD | A | Cranial-cervical-laryngeal, tremor, myoclonus | European |
| DYT-*GNAL* (DYT25) | 18p, *GNAL* | AD | A | Cervical > cranial > arm | European |

*A*, adult onset; *AD*, Autosomal dominant *C*, childhood onset; *AJ*, Ashkenazi Jewish; *NJ*, Non-Ashkenazi Jewish; *OCD*, obsessive compulsive disorder; *XR*, X-linked recessive.

**TABLE 24.6B Etiological Classification of Dystonia-Inherited (Combined)**

| Classification | Chromosome Gene Mutation Gene Product | Pattern of Inheritance | Onset | Distribution, Additional Features |
|---|---|---|---|---|
| DYT/PARK-*TAF1* (DYT3) | Xq<br>*TAF1* | XR | A | Parkinsonism |
| DYT-*TUBB4* (DYT4) | 19p13.3-p13.2<br>*TUBB4* (β-tubulin 4a) | AD | C, A | Whispering dysphonia, cranial, cervical, limb, gait disorder, facial atrophy, ptosis, edentulous |
| DYT/PARK-*GCH1* (DYT5a) | 14q22.1<br>*GCH1*/GTP cyclohydrolase I | AD | C | Dopa-responsive dystonia, diurnal fluctuation<br>Gait disorder, parkinsonism, myoclonus, spasticity |
| DYT/PARK-*TH* (DYT5b) | 11p15.5<br>tyrosine hydroxylase | AR | C | Dopa-responsive dystonia<br>Gait disorder, parkinsonism, myoclonus, spasticity |
| DYT-*SGCE* (DYT11) | 7q21.3<br>*SGCE*<br>Epsilon-sarcoglycan | AD | C | Myoclonus-dystonia<br>Alcohol-responsive, OCD, drug addiction |
| DYT/PARK-*ATP1A3* (DYT12) | 19q13.2<br>*ATP1A3*<br>$Na^+/K^+$-ATPase alpha3 | AD | C | Rapid-onset-dystonia- parkinsonism<br>Alternating hemiplegia of childhood, cerebellar ataxia, areflexia, pes cavus, optic atrophy, and sensorineural hearing loss (CAPOS) syndrome |
| DYT-*PRKRA* (DYT16) | 2q31.2<br>*PRKRA* | AD | C | Predominantly lower limb, axial, oromandibular, and laryngeal dystonia, parkinsonism, unresponsive to levodopa |
| DYT-*KCTD17* (DYT26) | 22q12, *KCTD17* | AD | C, A | Myoclonus-dystonia<br>Cranial-cervical |

*AD*, Autosomal dominant; *AR*, autosomal recessive.

Imaging studies such as computed tomography (CT) and particularly MRI are useful in certain disorders. Most patients with hemidystonia have a definable lesion in the contralateral basal ganglia (most often the putamen). The cause of hemiballism or hemichorea is usually a structural lesion in the contralateral subthalamic nucleus or striatum. The cause is commonly a small lacunar infarction, so MRI typically is more successful than CT in localizing the lesion. A pattern of high signal in the striatum (especially the putamen) on T1 imaging is characteristic of hemiballism due to hyperosmolar nonketotic hyperglycemia. In patients with parkinsonism, imaging must assess the possibility of hydrocephalus (either obstructive or communicating), midbrain atrophy (as in PSP), and cerebellar and pontine atrophy (as in MSA). MRI clearly is much more effective in demonstrating these posterior fossa abnormalities than is CT. Atrophy of the head of the caudate nucleus occurs in HD, but it is not specific for this disorder and does not correlate with the presence or severity of chorea. Multiple infarctions, intracerebral calcification (better seen on CT), mass lesions (e.g., tumors, arteriovenous malformations), and basal ganglia lucencies (as seen in various disorders) may be found in patients with several movement disorders such as parkinsonism, chorea, and dystonia. In patients with striatonigral degeneration (one subcategory of MSA with prominent parkinsonism), T2-weighted and proton-density MRI scans often demonstrate a combination of striatal atrophy and hypointensity, with linear hyperintensity in the posterolateral putamen. T2-weighted gradient echo MRI often demonstrates hypointense putaminal changes (Brooks et al., 2009). The "hot cross bun" sign in the pons and hyperintensity in the middle cerebellar peduncles on fluid-attenuated inversion recovery (FLAIR) imaging also suggest MSA-C. The latter feature as well as additional supratentorial white-matter changes, especially in the splenium of the corpus callosum, and atrophy also occur in the fragile X tremor ataxia syndrome (FXTAS). Sagittal-view MRI in patients with PSP can show atrophy of the rostral midbrain tegmentum; the most rostral midbrain, the midbrain tegmentum, the pontine base, and the cerebellum appear to correspond to the bill, head, body, and wing, respectively, to form a "hummingbird" or "penguin" sign (although this is a rather late imaging feature). Further developments in MRI promise to improve our ability to differentiate between various degenerative disorders, especially if they are associated with characteristic pathological features. Examples are deposition of pigments or heavy metals. T1-weighted hyperintensity in the basal ganglia occurs in hyperglycemia, manganese toxicity, hepatocerebral disease, WD, abnormal calcium metabolism, neurofibromatosis, hypoxia, and hemorrhage. Striatal T1-weighted hypointensity and T2-weighted hyperintensity suggest mitochondrial disorders. Striatal T2-weighted hypointensity, with hyperintensity of the mesencephalon sparing the red nucleus and the lateral aspect of the substantia nigra, gives the appearance of "face of the giant panda" sign, the typical MRI appearance of WD. T2-weighted MRI in PKAN typically shows hypointensity in the globus pallidus surrounding an area of hyperintensity, the "eye of the tiger" sign (McNeill et al., 2008; Schneider et al., 2013).

Magnetic resonance spectroscopy also holds promise for differentiating disorders with various neurodegenerative patterns or neurometabolic disturbances. Positron emission tomography (PET) using fluorodeoxyglucose, fluorodopa, and other radiolabeled compounds (e.g., demonstrating labeling of dopamine receptors) has shown reproducible changes in such conditions as HD and parkinsonian disorders. For example, F-dopa PET scans show reduced uptake in both the putamen and caudate in patients with atypical parkinsonism (e.g., PSP, MSA), whereas the caudate uptake is relatively preserved in patients with PD. The patterns of abnormalities seen may predict the underlying pathological changes and thus may be useful in differential diagnosis. Developments in single-photon emission computed tomography (SPECT) suggest that this will probably become a useful diagnostic tool in evaluating and diagnosing certain movement disorders. For example, SPECT study of the dopamine active transporter (DAT) helps differentiate PD (and other parkinsonian disorders with degeneration of the substantia nigra) from other tremor disorders such as essential tremor. Finally, recent studies suggest that transcranial ultrasound demonstrating hyperechogenicity in the region of the substantia nigra compacta in PD may be a useful diagnostic tool.

Routine electrophysiological testing including EEG, somatosensory evoked potentials, EMG, and nerve conduction studies may provide supportive evidence of disease involving structures outside the basal ganglia. Although these and other electrophysiological procedures have contributed to our understanding of the pathophysiology of movement disorders, they have been most crucial to the study of myoclonus. Here, EEG shows a variety of disturbances such as spikes, spike-and-wave patterns, and periodic discharges. Occasionally, spikes precede EMG myoclonic discharges, particularly if the myoclonus is associated with epilepsy. However, in the majority of cases, it is impossible to determine a correlation between spike discharges and myoclonic jerks by simple visual inspection. Special electrophysiological techniques averaging cortical activity that occurs before a myoclonic jerk (triggered back-averaging) may show focal contralateral central negativity lasting 15–40 µsec, preceding the muscle jerk by 10–25 µsec in the upper limbs and 30–35 µsec in the legs. This is evidence of so-called cortical myoclonus, indicating that cortical activity results in the muscle jerks (although the primary pathology may not be in the cerebral cortex). In other forms of myoclonus that originate in subcortical areas, cortical discharges may be seen but are not time-locked in the same fashion to the jerks. In these cases, there may be generalized 25- to 40-µsec negativity before, during, or after the muscle jerking. The muscle bursts seen on EMG typically are synchronous in antagonistic muscles and usually are less than 50 µsec in duration. In one form of essential myoclonus, ballistic reflex myoclonus, the EMG bursts show alternating activity in antagonists that lasts 50–150 µsec. With multichannel EMG recording, it may be possible to demonstrate the activation order of muscles. In cortical myoclonus, muscles activate in a rostrocaudal direction, with cranial nerve muscles firing in descending order before the limbs. In myoclonus originating from subcortical or reticular sources, it may be possible to show that the myoclonus propagates in both directions from a point source, up the brainstem, usually starting in muscles innervated by cranial nerve XI, and down the spinal cord. In propriospinal myoclonus, the spread up and down the spinal cord occurs at a speed that suggests the involvement of a slowly conducting polysynaptic pathway. However, this pattern also can be mimicked voluntarily and may be present in psychogenic myoclonus.

Somatosensory evoked potentials and late EMG responses (C reflexes) often are enhanced in patients with myoclonus. Giant sensory evoked potentials occur in the hemisphere contralateral to the jerking limb in patients with cortical myoclonus. This is especially true in patients with focal myoclonus that is sensitive to a variety of sensory stimuli applied to the affected part (cortical reflex myoclonus). The cortical components of the sensory evoked potentials usually are not enhanced in subcortical or spinal myoclonus, but the latencies may be prolonged, depending on the location of the disease process. Electrophysiological studies are also useful in differentiating functional (psychogenic) from organic movement disorders, particularly in the case of myoclonus and tremor (Thenganatt and Jankovic, 2015).

In addition to blood and cerebrospinal fluid proteins, there are genetic, imaging, neurophysiological, and other biomarkers currently being investigated in attempts to diagnose presymptomatic or early disease (Espay et al., 2017; Saeed et al., 2017; Wu et al., 2011). In caring for a patient with a movement disorder, the clinician must always keep an open mind to the possibility of finding a secondary cause. This should be the case even when the onset, progression, and clinical features of the movement disorder in question are typical of an idiopathic condition and the preliminary laboratory testing has not revealed another cause. Repeated thorough neurological examinations should be undertaken periodically in the search for clues that might indicate the need to pursue the investigation further.

*The complete reference list is available online at https://expertconsult.inkling.com/.* 

25

# Gait Disorders

*Philip D. Thompson, John G. Nutt*

## OUTLINE



The maintenance of an upright posture and the act of walking are among the first and ultimately most complex motor skills humans acquire. From an early age, walking skills are modified and refined. In later years, the interplay between voluntary and automatic control of posture and gait provides a rich and complex repertoire of motion that ranges from walking and running to complex sports and dancing. An individual's pattern of walking may be so distinctive that he or she can be recognized by the characteristics of the gait or even the sound of the steps. Many diseases of the nervous system are identified by the disturbances of gait and posture they produce.

## PHYSIOLOGICAL AND BIOMECHANICAL ASPECTS OF GAIT

Humans assume a stable upright posture before beginning to walk. Stability when standing is based on mechanical musculoskeletal linkages between the trunk and legs and neurological control detecting and correcting body sway. Coordinated synergies of axial and proximal limb muscle contraction and a hierarchy of postural responses maintain standing or static postural control. Postural responses encompass automatic righting reflexes keeping the head upright on the trunk, supporting reactions controlling antigravity muscle tone, anticipatory (feedforward) postural reflexes occurring before limb movement, and reactive (feedback) postural adjustments counteracting body perturbations during movement. Postural responses are also modified by voluntary control according to the circumstances in which balance is threatened. For example, rescue reactions such as a step or windmill arm movements preserve the upright posture and protective reactions, such as an outstretched arm breaks a fall to prevent injury. Postural reflexes and responses are generated by the integration of visual, vestibular, and proprioceptive inputs in the context of voluntary intent and the environment in which the subject is moving.

Once the trunk is upright and stable, locomotion can begin. The initiation of gait is heralded by a series of shifts in the center of pressure beneath the feet during the course of an anticipatory postural adjustment—first posteriorly, then laterally toward the stepping foot, and finally toward the stance foot to allow the stepping foot to swing forward. This sequence is then followed by the stereotyped stance, swing, and step phases of the gait cycle. Dynamic equilibrium—during walking, turning, and the avoidance of obstacles—poses even more challenges to the postural system. Moreover, the effects of disease or aging on postural control commonly first appear when walking (Earhart, 2013).

## ANATOMICAL ASPECTS OF GAIT

The neuroanatomical structures responsible for equilibrium and locomotion in humans, inferred from studies in lower species, indicate two basic systems (Takakusaki, 2013). First, brainstem (subthalamic, midbrain) and cerebellar locomotor regions project through descending reticulospinal pathways from the pontomedullary reticular formation into the ventromedial spinal cord. Stimulation of brainstem locomotor centers leads to an increase in axial and limb muscle tone followed by the adoption and maintenance of an upright posture before stepping begins. Second, descending pontomedullary reticular projections activate assemblies of spinal interneurons (central pattern generators or spinal locomotor centers) that drive motoneurons of limb and trunk muscles in a patterned and repetitive manner to produce stepping movements. Propriospinal networks link motoneurons of the trunk and limbs, facilitating synergistic coordinated limb and trunk movements during locomotion. In quadrupeds, spinal locomotor centers are capable of maintaining and coordinating rhythmic stepping movements after spinal transection. The cerebral cortex and corticospinal tract are not necessary for experimentally induced locomotion in quadrupeds but are required for precision stepping. In monkeys, descending ventromedial brainstem and ventrolateral spinal motor pathways are necessary for stepping and balance. Lesions of the medial brainstem in monkeys that interrupt descending reticulospinal, vestibulospinal, and tectospinal systems produce marked postural dysequilibrium. Control of posture and locomotion in humans appears to be mediated by similar networks. The isolated spinal cord in humans with spinal cord transection can produce spontaneous movements but cannot generate rhythmic stepping, indicating that brainstem and higher cortical connections are necessary for bipedal walking in humans. Neuroimaging of imagined gait suggests that the prefrontal cortex via corticobulbar and indirectly via corticostriatal tracts modulates midbrain and cerebellar locomotor regions (Zwergal, et al., 2012). Frontal motor projections to the pontomedullary reticular formation that innervate axial muscles modulate postural responses associated with stepping and spinal motoneurons, enabling precision foot movements. The parietal cortex integrates sensory inputs that convey position and orientation in space, the relationship to gravitational forces, the speed and direction of movement, and the characteristics of the terrain and environment. The cerebellum modulates the rate, rhythm, amplitude, and force of stepping and also contributes to the medial brainstem efferent system controlling truncal posture and equilibrium through projections from the flocculonodular and anterior lobes. Although neuroimaging reveals locomotor circuitry, the means by which these control the automatic and voluntary movements of walking remain unknown.

## HISTORY: COMMON SYMPTOMS AND ASSOCIATIONS

A detailed history of the walking difficulty provides the first clues to diagnosis. It is helpful to note the circumstances in which walking difficulty occurs, the leg movements most affected, and any associated symptoms, especially falls (which may be the presenting feature). Walking over uneven ground exacerbates most walking difficulties, leading to tripping, stumbling, and falls. Fear of falling may lead to a variety of voluntary protective measures to minimize the risk of injury. In some patients, particularly the elderly, compensatory strategies and a fear of falling lead to a "cautious" gait pattern that dominates the clinical picture. Often individuals are unaware of their gait abnormality but family or friends note altered cadence, shuffling, veering, or slowness. Because disorders at many levels of the musculoskeletal, peripheral, and central nervous systems give rise to difficulty walking, it is necessary to consider whether orthopedic problems, muscle weakness, a neurological defect of motor control, or sensory disturbance is contributing to the gait problem.

### Weakness

Many patients attribute any gait or balance problem to leg weakness even though none is detected on examination. However, weakness of certain muscle groups produces characteristic difficulties during particular movements of the gait cycle. Catching or scraping a toe on the ground and a tendency to trip may be the presenting symptom of hemiplegia (causing a spastic equinovarus foot posture) or foot drop caused by weakness of ankle dorsiflexion. Weakness of knee extension presents with a sensation that the legs will give way while standing or walking down stairs. Weakness of ankle plantarflexion interferes with the ability to stride forward, resulting in a shallow stepped gait. Difficulty in climbing stairs or rising from a seated position is suggestive of proximal muscle weakness. Axial muscle weakness due to peripheral neuromuscular disease may also interfere with truncal mobility. Fatigue during walking accompanies muscular weakness of any cause and is a frequent symptom of the extra effort required to walk in the presence of upper motor neuron syndromes and basal ganglia disease.

### Slowness and Stiffness

Slowness of walking is encountered in the elderly and in most gait disorders. Walking slowly is a normal reaction to unstable or slippery surfaces that cause postural insecurity and threaten balance. Similarly, those who feel that their balance is less secure because of any musculoskeletal or neurological disorder walk slowly. In Parkinson disease (PD) and other basal ganglia diseases, slowness of walking is due to shuffling with short, shallow steps. Difficulty initiating stepping when starting to walk (start hesitation), when an obstacle is encountered, or turning (freezing) are common in advanced stages of parkinsonian syndromes.

Difficulty rising from a chair or turning in bed and a general decline in agility may be clues to loss of truncal mobility in diffuse cerebrovascular disease, hydrocephalus, and basal ganglia diseases. Complaints of stiffness, heaviness, or "legs that do not do what they are told" may be the presenting symptoms of a spastic paraparesis or hemiparesis. Patients with spastic paraparesis frequently report that they drag their legs, catch the toes of their shoes on any surface irregularity, and that their legs may suddenly give way, causing stumbling and falls. The circumstances in which leg stiffness occurs while walking may be revealing. It is important to remember that leg muscle tone in some upper motor neuron syndromes and dystonia may be normal when the patient is examined in the supine position but is increased during walking. In childhood, an action dystonia of the foot is a common initial symptom of primary dystonia with stiffness, inversion, plantarflexion of the foot, and walking on the toes becoming evident only after walking or running. In adults, exercise-induced foot dystonia when running may be the presenting symptom of PD. Patients with dopa-responsive dystonia typically develop symptoms in the afternoon ("diurnal fluctuation").

### Imbalance

Complaints of poor balance and unsteadiness are cardinal features of cerebellar and sensory ataxia (due to proprioceptive sensory loss) but they may also occur in other neurological disorders and are particularly common in the elderly. The patient with a cerebellar gait ataxia complains of unsteadiness, staggering, inability to walk in a straight line, and near falls. Turning and suddenly changing direction results in veering to one side or staggering as if intoxicated. Symptoms are exacerbated by an uneven support surface. A sensory ataxia presents with unsteadiness when walking in the dark because visual compensation for the proprioceptive loss is not possible. Patients with impaired proprioception and sensory ataxia complain of being uncertain of the exact position of their feet when walking. They are unable to appreciate the texture of the ground beneath their feet and may describe abnormal sensations in the feet that give the impression of walking on a spongy surface or cotton wool. Acute vestibulopathy is associated with vertigo and severe imbalance. Chronic vestibular dysfunction often causes veering and a sense of imbalance when walking in environments with many moving objects, as in shopping malls or streets crowded with pedestrians and vehicles. Chronic vestibular lesions may be well compensated and revealed only when visual or proprioceptive input is compromised. Acute disturbances of balance and loss of truncal equilibrium also occur in vascular lesions of the cerebellum, thalamus, and basal ganglia. A wide-based unsteady gait is also a feature of frontal lobe diseases such as normal pressure hydrocephalus, diffuse small vessel ischemia of frontal subcortical white matter, and—as discussed further on—higher-level gait disorders. Imbalance in subcortical cerebrovascular disease and basal ganglia disorders commonly manifests when turning while walking, stepping backward, bending over to pick up something, or performing several tasks simultaneously, such as walking and carrying an object.

### Falls

Falls may be classified according to whether muscle tone is retained ("falling like a tree trunk," or toppling) or tone is lost (collapsing falls). Collapsing falls associated with sudden loss of muscle tone imply a loss of consciousness characteristic of orthostatic hypotension, cardiovascular syncope, or seizures. Toppling falls with retained muscle tone are due to impaired static and dynamic postural responses that control body equilibrium during standing and walking. Accordingly it is important to establish the circumstances in which falls occur, whether consciousness was retained, and any clear precipitants or associated symptoms.

Since many people attribute falls to tripping when in fact tripping did not occur, details of how tripping occurred are important. Tripping may be due to foot drop or shallow steps, and this tendency is exaggerated when walking on uneven ground. Tripping may also be a consequence of poor vision or carelessness secondary to inattention, cognitive impairment, or delirium. Proximal muscle weakness may cause the legs to give way and thus lead to falls. Unsteadiness and poor balance in an ataxic syndrome can also lead to falls. More commonly, apparently spontaneous falls, falls associated with postural adjustments, or falls occurring when an individual is performing multiple tasks suggest an impairment of postural responses. In the early stages of an akinetic-rigid syndrome, spontaneous falls, especially backward, are an important clue to diagnoses such as multiple system atrophy and progressive supranuclear palsy (Steele-Richardson-Olszewski syndrome) rather than PD. Falls do occur in PD but are a late feature, and a number of causes must be considered. These include festinating steps that are too small to restore balance, tripping or stumbling over rough surfaces because shuffling shallow steps fail to clear small obstacles, and failure to step because of start hesitation or freezing. In each of these examples, falling stems from locomotor hypokinesia and a lack of normal-sized, rapid, compensatory voluntary movements. The direction of these falls is usually forward onto knees and outstretched arms (indicating preservation of rescue reactions). Other falls, in any direction, when changing posture or turning in small spaces generally result from loss of postural and righting responses, either spontaneously when multitasking or after minor perturbations. It is also important to consider collapsing falls related to orthostatic hypotension, a common finding in PD. Falls are often multifactorial; contributing factors may include structural obstacles in a cluttered environment, uneven walking surfaces, stairs, improper use of walking aids, muscle weakness, neurological disturbances of vision, vestibular or sensory function, and polypharmacy.

### Sensory Symptoms and Pain

The distribution of any accompanying sensory complaints provides a clue to the site of the lesion producing walking difficulties. A common example is cervical spondylotic myelopathy and a spastic paraparesis with cervical radicular pain or paresthesias, sensations of tight bands around the trunk (due to spinal sensory tract compression). Distal symmetrical paresthesias of the limbs suggest peripheral neuropathy. It is important to determine whether leg pain and weakness during walking are caused by focal neural pathology (a radiculopathy or neurogenic claudication of the cauda equina) or whether the pain is of musculoskeletal origin and is exacerbated by walking. Neurogenic intermittent claudication of the cauda equina should be distinguished from vascular intermittent claudication, in which ischemic leg muscle pain typically affects the calves and interrupts walking. Neurogenic claudication is exacerbated by extension of the spine and relieved by leaning forward or sitting down. Skeletal pain due to degenerative joint disease is aggravated by movement of the affected joints and often persists at rest (in contrast to claudication). The normal pattern of walking is frequently modified by joint disease (especially of the hip). Voluntary strategies to minimize pain by avoiding full weight bearing on the affected limb or by limiting its range of movement are a common cause of antalgic gait patterns (i.e., limping).

### Urinary Incontinence

Urinary urgency and incontinence often accompany neurological gait disorders. A spastic paraparesis with loss of voluntary control of sphincter function suggests a spinal cord lesion. Parasagittal cerebral lesions such as frontal lobe tumors (parasagittal meningioma), frontal lobe infarction caused by anterior cerebral artery occlusion, and hydrocephalus should also be considered. Impairment of higher mental function and incontinence may be important clues to a cerebral cause of paraparesis. Urinary urgency and urge incontinence are also common in parkinsonism and subcortical white matter ischemia.

### Cognitive Changes

Cognitive deterioration is associated with slowing of gait speed. Slowing of gait may be a marker of impending cognitive impairment and dementia (Mielke et al., 2013). Conversely, cognitive impairment characterized by executive dysfunction, inattention, impaired multitasking, and set switching may predict later development of falls in older adults without dementia or impaired mobility (Mirelman et al., 2012). Dementia with disinhibition and impulsivity is associated with reckless gait patterns and falls.

## EXAMINATION OF POSTURE AND WALKING

A scheme for the examination of posture and walking is summarized in Box 25.1. A convenient starting point is to observe the overall pattern of limb and body movement during walking. Normal walking progresses in a smooth and effortless manner. The truncal posture is upright, and the legs swing in a fluid motion with a regular stride length. Synergistic head, trunk, and upper limb movement flow with each step. Observation of the pattern of body and limb movement during walking also helps the examiner decide whether the gait problem is caused by a focal abnormality (e.g., leg shortening, hip disease, muscle weakness) or a generalized disorder of movement and whether the problem is unilateral or bilateral. After the overall walking pattern has been observed, the specific aspects of posture and gait should be examined (see Box 25.1).

### Arising From Sitting

Watching the patient rise from a chair without using the arms informs the examiner about the patient's pelvic girdle strength, control of truncal movement, coordination, and balance. Inability to rise when the feet are appropriately placed under the body while sitting and the trunk is leaning forward may indicate proximal weakness. An abnormally wide stance base when rising to stand from a seated position often signals incoordination or imbalance. Inappropriate strategies in which the feet are not positioned directly under the body or the trunk leans backward while a person is trying to stand are seen in frontal lobe disease and higher-level gait disorders.

**BOX 25.1 Examination of Gait and Balance**

**Arising to Stand From Seated Position**
Proximal muscle strength
Organization of truncal and limb movements
Stability
Stance base

**Standing**
Posture
Stance base
Body sway
Romberg test
Reactive postural responses (pull test)

**Walking**
Initiation of stepping
Speed of walking
Stance base width
Step length
Cadence, rhythm, and tempo of stepping
Step trajectory (shallow, shuffling, or high stepping)
Associated trunk and arm movements
Trunk posture

**Turning While Walking**
Number of steps to turn
Stabilizing steps
En bloc (truncal and limb movement)
Freezing

**Other Maneuvers**
Tandem walking
Walking backward
Running
Walking on toes, heels

**TABLE 25.1 Summary of Clinical Features Distinguishing Different Types of Gait Ataxia**

| Feature | Cerebellar | Sensory | Frontal Lobe |
|---|---|---|---|
| Trunk posture | Leans forward | Stooped | Upright |
| Stance | Wide-based | Wide-based | Wide-based |
| Postural responses | Variable | Intact | Impaired |
| Initiation of gait | Normal | Normal | Start hesitation |
| Steps | Staggering, lurching | High-stepping | Short, shuffling |
| Speed | Normal, slow | Normal, slow | Very slow |
| Heel-to-toe | Unable | Variable | Unable |
| Turning corners | Veers away | Minimal effect | Freezing, shuffling |
| Romberg test | Variable | Positive; increased unsteadiness | Variable |
| Heel-to-shin test | Usually abnormal | Variable | Normal |
| Falls | Uncommon | Yes | Very common |

## Stance

The width of the stance base (the distance between the feet) when rising from sitting, standing, and walking gives an indication of balance. Wide-based gaits are typical of cerebellar or sensory ataxia but may also be seen in diffuse cerebrovascular disease and frontal lobe lesions (Table 25.1). In mild ataxia, a widened base may be evident only during turning and may disappear when walking in a straight line. Widening the stance base is an efficient method of reducing body sway in the lateral and anteroposterior planes. Persons whose balance is insecure for any reason tend to adopt a wider stance, assume a posture of mild generalized flexion, and take shorter steps. Those who have attempted to walk on ice or other slippery surfaces will recognize these strategies to avoid falls. Eversion of the feet is a strategy to increase stability and is particularly common in patients with diffuse cerebrovascular disease. Spontaneous sway, drift of the body in any direction, actively pushing the body out of balance to one side or backward, and the ability to stay upright without seeking the support of furniture or assistance of another person are important clues to imbalance. Tandem (heel-to-toe) walking is a good objective measure of walking stability.

## Trunk Posture

The trunk is normally upright during standing and walking. Flexion of the trunk and a stooped posture are characteristic features in PD. Slight flexion at the hips to lower the trunk and shift the center of gravity forward is intended to minimize posterior body sway and reduce the risk of falling backward; it is common in many unsteady or cautious gait syndromes. In contrast, an upright posture with neck and trunk extension is typical of progressive supranuclear palsy. A posture of neck flexion occurs with weakness of the neck extensors in motor neuron disease, myasthenia gravis, and some myopathies. It is also a dystonic manifestation (antecollis) in multiple system atrophy and PD. Dystonia and parkinsonism may also alter truncal posture, leading to camptocormia or lateral truncal flexion (Pisa syndrome). Tilt of the trunk to one side in dystonia is accompanied by muscle spasms, the most common being an exaggerated flexion movement of the trunk and hip with each step. Paraspinal muscle spasm and rigidity also produce an exaggerated lumbar lordosis in the stiff person syndrome.

An exaggerated lumbar lordosis, caused by hip girdle weakness, is typical of proximal myopathies. Truncal tilt away from the side of the lesion is observed in some acute vascular lesions of the thalamus and basal ganglia. Misperception of the vertical posture and truncal tilt in posterolateral thalamic vascular lesions results in inappropriate movements to correct the perceived tilt in the "pusher syndrome" (Karnath et al., 2005). Acute vestibular imbalance in the lateral medullary syndrome leads to tilt toward the side of the lesion (lateropulsion).

Truncal flexion (camptocormia) may occur in paraspinal myopathies that produce weakness of trunk extension. Abnormal thoracolumbar postures also result from spinal ankylosis and spondylitis. A restricted range of spinal movement and persistence of the abnormal spinal posture when supine or during sleep are useful pointers toward a bony spinal deformity as the cause of an abnormal truncal posture. Truncal postures, particularly in the lumbar region, can be compensatory for shortening of one lower limb; lumbar or leg pain; or disease of the hip, knee, or ankle.

## Postural Responses

Reactive postural responses are examined by "the pull test," or sharply pulling the upper trunk backward or forward while the patient is standing (Hunt and Sethi, 2006). The pull should be sufficient to require the patient to step to recover balance. The examiner must be prepared to prevent the patient from falling. A few short shuffling steps backward (retropulsion) or an impending fall backward or forward (propulsion) suggests impairment of righting reactions. Falls after postural changes such as arising from a chair or turning while walking suggest impaired anticipatory postural responses. Falls without rescue arm movements or stepping movements to break or arrest the fall indicate loss of protective postural responses and result in head injuries or a fractured neck of femur. Accordingly, the nature of the injuries sustained during falls provide a clue to the loss of these postural responses. A tendency to fall backward spontaneously is a sign of impaired postural reflexes in progressive supranuclear palsy and gait disorders associated with frontal lobe diseases.

## Walking

### Initiation of Gait

Difficulty initiating the first step (start hesitation) ranges in severity from a few short shuffling steps, to repeated small shallow steps on the spot without forward progress ("slipping clutch" phenomenon) to complete immobility with the feet seemingly glued to the floor ("magnetic feet" phenomenon). Patients may use exaggerated upper body movements or alter the step pattern, such as stepping sideways or lifting the feet very high in an effort to engage their legs in motion. The magnetic feet phenomenon suggests frontal lobe disease, diffuse cerebrovascular disease, or hydrocephalus. Start hesitation is a feature of the "freezing gait" of PD. Isolated start hesitation is seen in the syndrome of gait ignition failure and discussed further in the later section titled "Higher-Level Gait Disorders."

### Stepping

Once walking is under way, the length and trajectory of each step and the rhythm and tempo of stepping should be noted. Short, regular, shallow steps or shuffling and a slow gait are characteristic of the akinetic-rigid syndromes. Shuffling is most evident when starting to walk, stopping, or turning corners; specific examination of these maneuvers may reveal a subtle tendency to shuffle and freeze. Once under way, freezing may interrupt walking, with further shuffling and start hesitation. Freezing typically occurs during turning, when walking in confined spaces, after encountering an obstacle, with visual distraction such as walking through a doorway, or if attention is diverted for any reason. The small shuffling steps of freezing are often accompanied by trembling of the knees, standing on the toes, and forward tilt of the trunk. Festination (increasingly rapid small steps) is common in PD but rare in other akinetic-rigid syndromes, which are frequently associated with poor balance and falls rather than festination. A slow gait is also seen in ataxia (sensory and cerebellar), spasticity, and cautious gait syndromes, but the stepping patterns differ. Jerky steps of irregular variable rhythm, length, and direction suggest ataxic or choreic syndromes. Subtle degrees of cerebellar ataxia may be unmasked by asking the patient to walk heel to toe in a straight line (tandem gait), to stand on one leg, or to walk and turn quickly. When vision is important in helping to maintain balance, as in sensory ataxia caused by proprioceptive loss, the removal of vision greatly exaggerates the ataxia. This is the basis of the Romberg test, in which eye closure leads to a dramatic increase in unsteadiness and even falls in the patient with sensory ataxia. In conducting the Romberg test, it is important for the patient to be standing comfortably before eye closure and for the examiner to remember that a modest increase in body sway is a normal response to eye closure. Distinctive leg postures and foot trajectories occur during stepping in sensory ataxia, foot drop, spasticity, and dystonia. It may be necessary to examine the patient while he or she is running so as to identify an action dystonia of the legs in the early stages of primary torsion dystonia.

### Turning

Turning while walking stresses balance more than walking in a straight line and is often where gait abnormalities first appear. Slowing on turns may be the first abnormality in walking in a patient with PD. Multiple steps on turning are common in PD and diffuse cerebrovascular disease. An extra step or mild widening of the base on turning may herald the onset of ataxia.

**BOX 25.2 Causes of Foot Drop and an Equinovarus Foot Posture When Walking**

Peripheral nerve:
- L5 radiculopathy
- Lumbar plexopathy
- Sciatic nerve palsy
- Peroneal neuropathy (compression)
- Peripheral neuropathy (bilateral)
- Anterior horn cell disease (motor neuron disease)

Myopathy
Scapuloperoneal syndromes
Spasticity
Dystonia
Sensory ataxia

### More Challenging Tests of Walking

Walking on the toes and heels may bring out abnormal movements and also reveal subtle weakness of dorsiflexion and plantarflexion of the ankle. In action dystonia of the foot, walking backward will sometimes reduce or abolish the dystonic foot posturing that is observed when walking forward.

### Associated Synergistic Limb Movements While Walking

Unilateral loss of associated synergistic arm swing while walking is a valuable sign of early PD but may also be seen in acute unilateral cerebellar lesions and hemiparesis. Exaggerated arm swing is observed in the "military two step" gait of a *marche à petit pas*. Involuntary movements are often superimposed on synergistic arm swing during walking. Dystonic posturing of an arm or leg may be indicative of dystonia, parkinsonism, and old hemiparesis. Choreiform limb movements are more prominent in walking than at rest in most chorea syndromes, levodopa-induced dyskinesia, and tardive dyskinesia. Parkinsonian tremor of the dependent upper limb is often observed during walking.

## MOTOR AND SENSORY EXAMINATION

After observing the patient walk, motor and sensory function in the limbs is examined with the patient sitting or supine. The size and length of the limbs should be measured in any child presenting with a limp. Asymmetry in leg size suggests a congenital malformation of the spinal cord or brain or (rarely) local overgrowth of tissue. The spinal column should be inspected for scoliosis and the lumbar region for skin defects or hairy patches indicative of spinal dysraphism.

Muscle bulk, tone, tendon reflexes and plantar responses are examined. Changes in muscle tone—such as spasticity, lead-pipe or cogwheel rigidity, or paratonic rigidity (gegenhalten)—point to diseases of the upper motor neuron, basal ganglia, and frontal lobes, respectively. In the patient who complains of symptoms in only one leg, a detailed examination of the other leg is important. If signs of an upper motor neuron syndrome are present in both legs, a disorder of the spinal cord or parasagittal region is likely. The presence and distribution of muscle wasting and muscle weakness should be noted. Examination reveals whether the abnormal leg and foot posture in a patient with foot drop (Box 25.2) is caused by spasticity or weakness of ankle dorsiflexors due to anterior horn cell disease, a peripheral neuropathy, a peroneal compression neuropathy, or an L5 root lesion. Joint position sense should be examined for defects of proprioception in the ataxic patient or for awkward posturing of the foot. Examination of various voluntary leg movements, such as the heel shin test, may reveal lower limb ataxia; the inability to perform rapid regular foot tapping is a sign of bradykinesia; and difficulty drawing a circle with the foot or making alternating bicycling leg movements may indicate dyspraxia, as seen in corticobasal syndromes. Other signs, such as a supranuclear gaze palsy and frontal lobe release signs, should be sought where relevant.

## DISCREPANCIES ON EXAMINATION OF GAIT

Several conditions are notable for producing minimal abnormal signs on examination of the recumbent patient, in contrast to the observed difficulty when walking. A patient with cerebellar gait ataxia caused by a vermis lesion may perform the heel-to-shin test normally when supine but be ataxic when walking. The finding of normal muscle strength, muscle tone, and tendon reflexes is common in dystonic syndromes in which an action dystonia causes abnormal posturing of the feet only when walking. A dystonic gait may be evident only when running or walking forward but not when walking backward. Gegenhalten (paratonia), with or without brisk tendon reflexes, may be the only abnormal sign in the recumbent patient with a frontal lobe lesion, hydrocephalus, or diffuse cerebrovascular disease who is totally unable to walk when standing. Such patients perform the heel-to-shin test and make bicycling movements of their legs normally when lying on a bed. In spastic paraplegia caused by hereditary spastic paraplegia, cerebral palsy (Little disease), or cervical spondylotic myelopathy, only minor changes in muscle tone, strength, and tendon reflexes may be evident during the supine examination, in contrast to profound leg spasticity when standing and attempting to walk. The leg tremor of orthostatic tremor appears only during weight bearing, especially when standing still. Incongruous signs and "give way" weakness, along with bizarre sensory disturbances that do not correlate with the gait pattern, often signal psychogenic or functional disorders.

## CLASSIFICATION OF GAIT PATTERNS

The goal of classifying gait patterns is to develop a scheme reflecting the physiological basis of human gait and thereby to recognize the level at which the nervous system derangement is occurring. A scheme based on Hughlings Jackson's three levels of neurological function—lower (simplest), middle, and higher (complex, integrative)—enables a classification according to function. Each level contributes sensory and motor function, but the function of higher centers is more complex and dispersed within the nervous system.

### Lower-Level Gait Disorders

Lower-level disorders manifest physical signs such as weakness or sensory loss. Lower-level motor gait disorders are due to diseases of the muscle and peripheral nerves that produce muscle weakness. Lower-level sensory gait disorders follow loss of one of the three basic senses important for gait and balance: proprioception, vision, and vestibular sensation.

#### Myopathic Weakness and Gait

Weakness of proximal leg and hip girdle muscles interferes with stabilizing the pelvis and trunk on the legs during all phases of the gait cycle. Failure to stabilize the pelvis produces exaggerated rotation of the pelvis with each step and a waddling gait. The hips are slightly flexed as a result of weakness of hip extension, leading to an exaggerated lumbar lordosis. Weakness of hip extension interferes with standing from a squatting or lying position and patients push themselves up with their arms (Gower sign). A myopathy is the most common cause of proximal muscle weakness, but neurogenic weakness of proximal muscles can also produce this clinical picture.

#### Neurogenic Weakness and Gait

Muscle weakness of peripheral nerve origin, as in a neuropathy, typically affects distal leg muscles and results in a steppage gait. The patient lifts the leg and foot high above the ground with each step because of weakness of ankle dorsiflexion and foot drop. When this clinical picture is confined to one leg (unilateral foot drop), a common peroneal or sciatic nerve palsy or an L5 radiculopathy is the usual cause (see Box 25.2). Weakness of ankle plantarflexion produces a shallow stepped gait. A femoral neuropathy, as in diabetes mellitus, produces weakness of knee extension and buckling of the knee when walking or standing. This may first be evident when walking down stairs. Progressive muscular atrophy in motor neuron disease or a quadriceps myopathy caused by inclusion body myositis may result in similar focal weakness.

#### Sensory Ataxia

Loss of proprioceptive input and joint position sense from the lower limbs deprives the patient of knowledge of the position of the legs and feet in space, the progress of ongoing movement, the state of muscle contraction, and finer details of the texture of the surface on which the patient is walking. Walking on uneven surfaces is particularly difficult. Patients with sensory ataxia adopt a wide base and advance cautiously, taking slow steps under visual guidance. During walking, the feet are thrust forward with variable direction and height. The sole of the foot strikes the floor forcibly with a slapping sound (slapping gait). The absence of visual information when walking at night or during the Romberg test leads to imbalance and falls. Sensory ataxia is the result of deafferentation due to interruption of large-diameter proprioceptive afferent fibers in peripheral neuropathies, posterior root or dorsal root ganglionopathies, and dorsal column lesions.

#### Vestibular Imbalance, Vertigo, and Gait

Acute peripheral vestibular disorders result in leaning and unsteady veering to the side of the lesion (depending on the position of the head). Paradoxically, unsteadiness and veering may be less evident when running than when walking in acute vestibulopathy. In general, patients with an acute vestibulopathy prefer to lie still to minimize the symptoms of acute vestibular imbalance. In chronic vestibular failure, gait may be normal, although unsteadiness can be unmasked during eye closure and rotation of the head from side to side while walking. Acute vestibular imbalance in the lateral medullary syndrome leads to tilt and veering toward the side of the lesion (lateropulsion).

### Middle-Level Gait Disorders

Gait disorders related to abnormalities of the middle-level motor disorders include (1) spasticity from corticospinal tract lesions; (2) ataxia arising from disturbances of the cerebellum and its connections; (3) hypokinetic gaits associated with parkinsonism; and (4) hyperkinetic gaits associated with chorea, dystonia, and other movement disorders.

#### Spastic Gait

Spasticity of the arm and leg on one side produces the characteristic clinical picture of a spastic hemiparesis, in which the arm is adducted, internally rotated at the shoulder, and flexed at the elbow, with pronation of the forearm and flexion of the wrist and fingers. The leg is slightly flexed at the hip and extended at the knee, with plantarflexion and inversion of the foot. The swing phase of each step is accomplished by slight lateral flexion of the trunk toward the unaffected side and hyperextension of the hip on that side to allow slow circumduction of the extended paretic leg as it swings forward from the hip, dragging the foot or catching the toe on the ground beneath. Minimal associated arm swing occurs on the affected side. The stance may be slightly widened, and the speed of walking is slow. Balance may be poor because the hemiparesis interferes with corrective postural adjustments on the affected side. Muscle tone in the affected limbs is increased, clonus may be present, and tendon reflexes are abnormally brisk, with an extensor plantar response. Examination of the sole of the shoe may reveal wear of the toe and outer borders of the shoe, suggesting that the spastic gait is of long standing. After a spastic hemiparesis is identified, the site of the corticospinal tract lesion is determined by magnetic resonance imaging (MRI) of the brain (and, where indicated, the spinal cord).

Spasticity of both legs gives rise to a spastic paraparesis. The legs are stiffly extended at the knees, plantarflexed at the ankles, and slightly flexed at the hips. Both legs circumduct, and the toes of the plantarflexed feet catch on the floor with each step. The gait is slow and labored as the legs are dragged forward with each step. There is a tendency to adduct the legs, particularly when the disorder begins in childhood, an appearance described as "scissors gait." The causes of a spastic paraparesis include hereditary spastic paraplegia, in which the arms and sphincters are unaffected and there may be little or no leg weakness, and other myelopathies. An indication of the extent and level of the spinal cord lesion can be obtained from the presence or absence of weakness or sensory loss in the arms, a spinothalamic sensory level or posterior column sensory loss, and alterations in sphincter function. Patients with paraparesis of recent onset should be investigated with MRI of the spinal cord to exclude potentially treatable causes such as spinal cord compression.

Occasionally bilateral leg dystonia (dystonic paraparesis) mimics a spastic paraparesis. This typically occurs in dopa-responsive dystonia in childhood and may be misdiagnosed as hereditary spastic paraplegia or cerebral diplegia. Clinical differentiation between these conditions can be difficult. Brisk tendon reflexes occur in both, and isolated spontaneous extension of the great toe in patients with striatal disorders (a "striatal" toe) may be misinterpreted as a Babinski response. A "true" Babinski sign comprises extension of the great toe accompanied by fanning of the other toes and knee flexion in response to lateral plantar stimulation along with other features of spasticity and an upper motor neuron (corticospinal) lesion. In young children, the distinction is important because a proportion of such patients can be treated successfully with levodopa (discussed in the following sections).

### Cerebellar Ataxia

Disease of the midline cerebellar structures, the vermis, and anterior lobe produces loss of truncal balance, increased body sway, dysequilibrium, and gait ataxia. When standing, the patient adopts a wide-based stance; the legs are stiffly extended and the hips slightly flexed to crouch forward and minimize truncal sway. The truncal gait ataxia of midline cerebellar pathology has a lurching and staggering quality that is more pronounced when walking on a narrow base or during heel-to-toe walking. A pure truncal ataxia may be the sole feature of a midline (vermis) cerebellar syndrome and may escape notice if the patient is not examined when standing because leg coordination during the heel-to-shin test may be relatively normal when the patient is examined supine. Midline cerebellar pathologies include structural lesions (masses, hemorrhage), paraneoplastic syndromes, and malnutrition in alcoholism. Patients with anterior lobe atrophy develop a 3-Hz anteroposterior sway of the trunk and a rhythmic truncal and head tremor (titubation) that is superimposed on the gait ataxia. This combination of truncal gait ataxia and truncal tremor is characteristic of some late-onset anterior lobe cerebellar degenerations.

Lesions of the cerebellar flocculonodular lobe (the vestibulocerebellum) exhibit multidirectional body sway, dysequilibrium, and severe impairment of body and truncal motion. Standing and even sitting can be impossible, although the heel-shin test may appear normal when the patient is lying down, and upper limb function may be relatively preserved.

Limb ataxia due to involvement of the cerebellar hemispheres is characterized by a decomposition of normal leg movement. Steps are irregular and variable in timing (dyssynergia), length, and direction (dysmetria). Steps are taken slowly and carefully so as to reduce the tendency to lurch and stagger. These defects are accentuated when the patient is attempting to walk heel to toe in a straight line. With lesions confined to one cerebellar hemisphere, ataxia is limited to the ipsilateral limbs, and there is little postural instability or truncal imbalance if the vermis is not involved. Vascular disease and mass lesions are generally responsible for unilateral hemispheric lesions.

Cerebellar gait ataxia is exacerbated by the rapid postural adjustments needed to change direction, turn a corner, or avoid obstacles, and when stopping or starting to walk. Minor support, such as holding the patient's arm during walking, and visual compensation, reduce body sway in cerebellar ataxia. Eye closure may heighten anxiety about falling and increase body sway, but not to the extent observed in a sensory ataxia. Episodic ataxias produce periods of impaired gait that typically last seconds to hours. Alcohol and drug use must be considered in the differential of episodic ataxia.

### Spastic Ataxia

A combination of spasticity and ataxia produces a distinctive "bouncing" gait (Box 25.3). Such gaits are seen in multiple sclerosis, the Arnold-Chiari malformation, and hydrocephalus in young people. Gait is wide based and clonus is precipitated by standing or walking, creating a bouncing motion. Compensatory movements, made in an effort to regain balance, set up a vicious cycle of ataxic movements, clonus, and increasing unsteadiness, rendering the patient unable to stand or walk. Bouncing gaits must be distinguished from action myoclonus of the legs and cerebellar truncal tremors.

### Hypokinetic (Parkinsonian) Gait

The most common hypokinetic-bradykinetic gait disturbance is that encountered in PD. In early PD, an asymmetrical reduction of arm swing and slight slowing in gait, particularly when turning, is characteristic. In more advanced PD, the posture is stooped, with flexion of the shoulders, neck, trunk, and knees. During walking, there is little associated or synergistic limb and body movement, and the arms are held immobile at the sides or slightly forward of the trunk. During walking, parkinsonian tremor of the upper limbs is often apparent but leg tremor is rare. A characteristic feature of a parkinsonian gait is the tendency to begin walking with a few rapid, short, shuffling steps (start hesitation) before breaking into a more normal stepping pattern with small, shallow steps on a narrow base. Once under way, walking may be interrupted by shuffling or even cessation of movement (freezing) if an obstacle is encountered, when walking through doorways or other confined spaces, or when attempting to undertake multiple tasks at once. These signs may be alleviated by levodopa treatment. In the long term, levodopa therapy may induce dyskinesias, resulting in choreic and dystonic gaits as described later.

**BOX 25.3 Differential Diagnosis of Involuntary Movements of the Legs When Standing**

- Action myoclonus and asterixis of legs
- Benign essential tremor
- Orthostatic tremor
- Cerebellar truncal tremor
- Clonus in spasticity
- Spastic ataxia
- Parkinson disease

The posture of generalized flexion of the patient with PD exaggerates the normal tendency to lean forward when walking. To maintain balance when walking and avoid falling forward, the patient may advance with a series of rapid small steps (festination). Retropulsion and propulsion are similar manifestations of a flurry of small shuffling steps made in an effort to preserve equilibrium. Instead of a single large step, a series of small steps are taken to maintain balance. Freezing becomes increasingly troublesome in the later stages of PD, at which time auditory or visual sensory cues may be more useful in triggering a step than medication. The shuffling gait of PD that is responsive to levodopa characterizes the middle-level gait pattern. As the disease progresses, dysequilibrium and falls emerge as features of a higher-level gait disorder (discussed later).

### Choreic Gait

The random movements of chorea are accentuated and often most noticeable during walking. The superimposition of chorea on the trunk and limb movements of the walking cycle gives the gait a dancing quality owing to the exaggerated leg motion and arm swing. Chorea can also interrupt the walking pattern, leading to a hesitant gait. Additional voluntary compensatory movements appear in response to perturbations imposed by chorea. Chorea in Sydenham chorea or chorea gravidarum may be sufficiently violent to throw patients off their feet. Severe chorea of the trunk may render walking impossible. The chorea of Huntington disease causes a lurching, stumbling, stuttering gait with steps forward, backward, or to one side. Walking is slow, the stance varies step to step, but it is generally wide based and the trunk sways excessively with the variable length and timing of steps. These characteristics may be misinterpreted as ataxia. Dystonic posturing such as hip or knee flexion and leg-raising movements commonly punctuate the stepping motion. Balance and equilibrium are usually maintained until the terminal stages of Huntington disease, when an akinetic-rigid syndrome may supervene. Neuroleptics such as haloperidol reduce chorea but do not improve gait in Huntington disease. Other causes of chorea can produce similar changes in gait and balance; a differential for chorea is covered in Chapters 24 and 96.

### Dystonic Gait

Of all gait disturbances, dystonic syndromes produce the more bizarre and difficult diagnostic problems. The classic presentation of childhood-onset primary torsion dystonia is an action dystonia of a leg, with sustained abnormal posturing of the foot (typically plantarflexion and inversion) on attempting to run. In contrast, walking forward or backward or even running backward may be normal at an early stage. An easily overlooked sign in the early stages is tonic extension of the great toe (the striatal toe) when walking. This may be a subtle finding but occasionally it is so pronounced that a hole is worn in the toe of the shoe. With the passage of time, dystonia may progress to involve the whole leg and then become generalized.

More difficult to recognize are those dystonic syndromes that present with bizarre, seemingly inexplicable postures of the legs and trunk when walking. A characteristic feature common to dystonic gaits is excessive flexion of the hip when walking. Patients may hop or walk sideways in a crab-like fashion. Hyperflexion of the hips and knee produces an attitude of general body flexion in a simian posture or excessive flexion of the hip and knee and plantarflexion of the foot in a bird-like (peacock) gait during the swing phase of each step. Many patients have been thought to be hysterical because of these unusual gait disturbances, particularly when formal neurological examination with the patient supine is normal. Each of these gait patterns is well described in primary and secondary dystonic syndromes. Tardive dystonia following neuroleptic drug exposure may produce similar bizarre abnormalities of gait.

It is important to look for asymmetry in the assessment of childhood-onset dystonia. Hemidystonia and isolated leg dystonia in an adult suggest symptomatic or secondary dystonia, particularly when accompanied by falls due to early loss of postural responses and righting reflexes.

Dopa-responsive dystonia characteristically presents in childhood with walking difficulties and diurnal fluctuations in the severity of dystonia. The child typically walks normally in the early morning but develops increasing rigidity and dystonic posturing of the legs as the day progresses or after exercise. Symptoms may be relieved by a nap ("sleep benefit"). Examination reveals dystonic plantarflexion and inversion of the foot, with brisk tendon reflexes. Some of these patients respond dramatically to levodopa. Indeed, all children presenting with a dystonic foot or leg should have a therapeutic trial of levodopa before other therapies such as anticholinergic drugs are commenced.

Paroxysmal dyskinesias may also present with difficulty walking. Paroxysmal kinesigenic choreoathetosis may present with the sudden onset of difficulty walking as the result of dystonic postures and involuntary movements of the legs, often appearing after standing from a seated position. These attacks are typically brief, lasting for only seconds.

### Mixed Movement Disorders and Gait

Many conditions, notably athetoid cerebral palsy, produce motor signs reflecting abnormalities at many levels of the nervous system, all of which disrupt normal patterns of walking. These include spasticity of the legs, truncal and gait ataxia, dystonia, and dystonic trunk and limb spasms. Difficulties arise in distinguishing this clinical picture from that of primary torsion dystonia, which may begin at a similar age in childhood. The patient with cerebral palsy usually has a history of hypotonia and delayed achievement of developmental motor milestones, especially truncal control (sitting up) and walking. Often there is a history of perinatal injury or birth asphyxia. In a substantial proportion of patients, however, such an event cannot be identified. A major distinguishing feature is poor balance at an early age, which may be a contributing factor to the delay in sitting and later walking. As the child begins to walk, the first signs of dystonia and athetosis appear. The presence of spasticity and ataxia also helps to distinguish this condition from primary dystonia. Childhood neurodegenerative diseases may first manifest as difficulty walking, stemming from a combination of motor syndromes. A progressive course raises the possibility of a symptomatic or secondary movement disorder.

### Tremor of the Trunk and Legs

Leg tremor in benign essential tremor is occasionally symptomatic but is generally overshadowed by upper limb tremor. Trunk and leg tremor may contribute to unsteadiness in cerebellar disease (see the earlier discussion on cerebellar gait ataxia). Orthostatic tremor has a unique frequency (16 Hz) and distribution, affecting trunk and leg muscles while standing. This rapid tremor produces an intense sensation of unsteadiness, often with little obvious shaking of the legs or body, which is relieved by walking or sitting down. Patients avoid standing still (e.g., in a queue) and may shuffle on the spot or pace about in an effort to relieve the unsteadiness experienced when standing still. Falls are rare. Examination reveals a rippling of the quadriceps muscles during standing, and the tremor is often only appreciated by palpation of leg muscles. Recording leg muscle electromyographic activity assists the differential diagnosis of involuntary movements of the legs when standing (see Box 25.3).

### Action Myoclonus

Postanoxic action myoclonus of the legs is often accompanied by negative myoclonus (asterixis) that disrupts standing and walking (see Box 25.3). Repetitive action myoclonus produces jerky movements of the legs, throwing the patient off balance. Lapses of muscle activity (negative myoclonus) between the jerks cause the patient to sag toward the ground. This sequence of events gives the stance an exaggerated bouncing appearance, which is

**BOX 25.4 Differential Diagnosis of an Akinetic-Rigid Syndrome and Gait Disturbance**

Parkinson disease
Drug-induced parkinsonism
Multiple system atrophy:
- Striatonigral degeneration
- Shy-Drager syndrome (idiopathic orthostatic hypotension)
- Olivopontocerebellar atrophy

Progressive supranuclear palsy (Steele-Richardson-Olszewski syndrome)
Corticobasal degeneration
Frontotemporal dementia
Creutzfeldt-Jakob disease
Cerebrovascular disease (Binswanger disease)
Hydrocephalus
Frontal lobe tumor
Juvenile Huntington disease
Wilson disease
Cerebral anoxia, carbon monoxide poisoning
Manganese toxicity
Neurosyphilis

sustainable for only a few seconds before the patient falls or seeks relief by sitting down. Difficulty walking is one of the major residual disabilities of postanoxic myoclonus. Many patients remain wheelchair bound as a result. The stance is wide based, and there is often an element of cerebellar ataxia, although this may be difficult to distinguish from severe action myoclonus. Stimulus-sensitive cortical reflex myoclonus also produces a similar disorder of stance and gait, with reflex myoclonus of the quadriceps resulting in a bouncing posture. Negative myoclonus of the legs interfering with stance has been described as an acute phenomenon after vascular lesions in many parts of the brain, particularly of the thalamus and frontal lobes.

## Higher-Level Gait Disorders

Higher level gait disorders are characterized by varying combinations of dysequilibrium (unsteadiness due to inappropriate or absent postural responses), falls, wide stance base, short shuffling steps, and freezing. In contrast to lower- and middle-level gait patterns, formal neurological examination fails to reveal signs that adequately explain the gait disturbance, although brisk tendon reflexes and extensor plantar responses or depressed reflexes and minor distal sensory loss may be encountered. Slowness of sequential leg movement and poor truncal control are often present. Stepping patterns are influenced by environmental cues that induce freezing of gait. Freezing or falling while performing multiple simultaneous tasks is common; such reactions are important clues to the diagnosis of higher-level gait disorders (Nutt, 2013; Thompson, 2007).

There are many descriptions of similar gait patterns in the literature, often focusing on one element of the gait disturbance. This has generated a variety of terms for higher-level gait disorders, such as *apraxia of gait, magnetic gait, lower-half parkinsonism, frontal gait*, and *marche à petit pas*. Because of uncertainty about the pathophysiology of these clinical manifestations, there has been no agreement on the terminology used to describe them.

### Hypokinetic Higher-Level and Freezing Gait Patterns

With progression of PD, freezing of gait, dysequilibrium, loss of postural, and righting responses and falls become increasingly troublesome and, unlike the hypokinetic steps and flexed truncal posture, do not respond to increasing doses of levodopa. There is some evidence from clinical, imaging, and pathological studies to suggest that dysequilibrium in the late stages of PD is mediated via mechanisms other than dopaminergic deficiency, and subcortical cholinergic projections from the pedunculopontine nucleus have been implicated. Deep brain stimulation (DBS) of the subthalamic nucleus (STN) or globus pallidus interna (GPi) can improve gait (Katz et al., 2015; Schlenstedt et al., 2017). DBS in the region of the pedunculopontine nucleus remains a subject of investigation for freezing of gait, postural instability, and falls (Thevathasan et al., 2018).

**TABLE 25.2 Summary of Clinical Features Differentiating Parkinson Disease From Symptomatic Parkinsonism in Patients With an Akinetic-Rigid Gait Syndrome**

| Feature | Parkinson Disease | Symptomatic Parkinsonism |
|---|---|---|
| Posture | Stooped (trunk flexion) | Stooped or upright (trunk flexion/extension) |
| Stance | Narrow | Often wide-based |
| Initiation of walking | Start hesitation | Start hesitation, magnetic feet |
| Steps | Small, shuffling | Small, shuffling |
| Stride length | Short | Short |
| Freezing | Common | Common |
| Leg movement | Stiff, rigid | Stiff, rigid |
| Speed | Slow | Slow |
| Festination | Common | Rare |
| Arm swing | Minimal or absent | Reduced or excessive |
| Heel-to-toe walking | Normal | Poor (truncal ataxia) |
| Reactive postural responses | Preserved in early stages | Absent at early stage |
| Falls | Late (forward, tripping) | Early and severe (backward, tripping, or without apparent reason) |

Slowness of leg movement and shuffling occur in a variety of akinetic-rigid syndromes other than PD (Box 25.4); the most common of these are multiple system atrophy, corticobasal degeneration, and progressive supranuclear palsy (Jankovic, 2015). A number of clinical signs can help distinguish between these conditions (Table 25.2). In progressive supranuclear palsy, the typical neck posture is one of extension, with axial and nuchal rigidity rather than neck and trunk flexion as in PD. A stooped posture with exaggerated neck flexion is sometimes a feature of multiple system atrophy. A distinguishing feature of progressive supranuclear palsy and multiple system atrophy is the early appearance of falls due to loss of postural and righting responses. By comparison, these reactions are preserved in PD until later stages of the illness. There also may be an element of ataxia in these akinetic-rigid syndromes that is not evident in PD. The disturbance of postural control and dysequilibrium in progressive supranuclear palsy is coupled with impulsivity due to frontal executive dysfunction, leading to reckless lurching movements during postural changes when sitting or rising as well as to toppling falls. Falls occur in 80% of patients with progressive supranuclear palsy and can be dramatic, leading to injury. Accordingly, the patient who presents with falls and an akinetic-rigid syndrome is more likely to have one of these conditions rather than PD. Finally, the dramatic response to levodopa that is typical of PD does not occur in these other akinetic-rigid syndromes, although some cases of multiple system atrophy respond partially for a short period.

In addition to the hypokinetic disorders discussed previously, diseases of the frontal lobe—including tumors (glioma or meningioma), anterior cerebral artery infarction, obstructive or communicating hydrocephalus (especially normal-pressure hydrocephalus), and diffuse small vessel cerebrovascular disease (multiple lacunar infarcts and Binswanger disease)—also disturb gait and balance. These pathologies interrupt connections between the frontal lobes, other cortical areas, and subcortical structures, especially the striatum. The clinical appearance of the gait in frontal lobe lesions varies from a predominantly wide-based unsteady ataxic gait to an akinetic-rigid gait with slow short steps and a tendency to shuffle. It is common for a patient to present with a combination of these features. In the early stages, the stance base is wide, with an upright posture of the trunk and shuffling when starting to walk or turning corners. There may be episodes of freezing. Arm swing is normal or even exaggerated, giving the appearance of a "military two-step" gait. The normal fluidity of trunk and limb motion is lost. In contrast, voluntary upper limb and hand movements are normal and there is a lively facial expression. This "lower half parkinsonism" is commonly seen in diffuse small vessel cerebrovascular disease. The *marche à petit pas* of Dejerine and Critchley's atherosclerotic parkinsonism refers to a similar clinical picture. Patients with this clinical syndrome are commonly misdiagnosed as having PD. The normal motor function of the upper limbs, retained arm swing during walking, upright truncal posture, wide-based stance, upper motor neuron signs including pseudobulbar palsy, and the absence of a resting tremor distinguish this syndrome from PD. In addition, the lower-half parkinsonism of diffuse cerebrovascular disease generally does not respond to levodopa treatment (see Box 25.4). Walking speed in subcortical arteriosclerotic encephalopathy is slower than in cerebellar gait ataxia or PD (Ebersbach et al., 1999). Slowness of movement and the lack of lower limb (heel-to-shin) ataxia distinguish the wide-based stance of this syndrome from that of cerebellar gait ataxia (see Table 25.1).

As the underlying condition progresses, the unsteadiness and slowness of movement become more pronounced. There may be great difficulty initiating a step (start hesitation, "slipping clutch") as if the feet were glued to the floor ("magnetic feet"). Attempts to take a step require assistance and the patient seeks support from nearby objects or persons. There may be excessive upper body movement as the patient tries to free the feet to initiate walking. Once walking is under way, steps may be better, but small, shuffling, ineffective steps (freezing) reemerge when attempting to turn. Such patients rarely exhibit the festination of PD, but a few steps of propulsion or retropulsion may be taken. Postural and righting reactions are impaired and eventually lost. Falls are common and follow the slightest perturbation. In contrast, these patients are often able to make stepping, walking, or bicycling leg movements with the legs when seated or lying supine, but they cannot step or walk when standing. This discrepancy may reflect poor control of truncal motion and dysequilibrium when standing, making stepping impossible without falling (Thompson, 2007). The inability to stand from sitting or lying and difficulty turning over in bed are other signs of impaired truncal movement in the higher-level gait disorder of frontal lobe gait disease. Frontal signs such as paratonic rigidity (gegenhalten) of the arms and legs, grasp reflexes in the fingers and toes, and brisk tendon reflexes with extensor plantar responses are common. Urinary incontinence and dementia frequently occur. Brain imaging with MRI reveals the majority of conditions causing this syndrome, such as diffuse cerebrovascular disease, cortical atrophy, or hydrocephalus.

Some patients display fragments of this clinical picture. Those with the syndrome of gait ignition failure or gait initiation failure exhibit profound start hesitation and freezing, but step size and rhythm are normal once walking is under way. Sensory cues may facilitate stepping. Balance while standing or walking is normal. These findings are similar to those seen with walking in PD, but speech and upper limb function are normal and there is no response to levodopa. Brain imaging results are normal. This syndrome has also been described as "pure akinesia" and "primary progressive freezing of gait." Some cases develop stuttering speech and hypokinetic handwriting. The slowly progressive evolution of symptoms suggests a degenerative condition. Follow-up studies indicate that this may be one expression of progressive supranuclear palsy (Riley et al., 1994) or another form of neurodegeneration (Factor et al., 2006). Occasionally isolated episodic festination with truncal flexion is encountered. Others complain of a loss of the normal fluency of stepping when walking and say that a conscious effort is required to maintain a normal stepping rhythm and step size. These symptoms may be associated with subtle dysequilibrium, manifesting as a few brief staggering steps to one side or a few steps of retropulsion after standing up, turning quickly, or making other rapid changes in body position. Finally, some elderly patients experience severe walking difficulties that resemble those described in frontal lobe disease. The history in these syndromes is one of gradual onset, without stroke-like episodes or identifiable structural or vascular lesions of the frontal lobes or cerebral white matter on imaging. The criteria for normal pressure hydrocephalus are not fulfilled, there are no signs of parkinsonism, and levodopa is ineffective. There is no evidence of more generalized cerebral dysfunction, as occurs in Alzheimer disease. Indeed, it is rare for patients with Alzheimer disease to develop difficulty walking until the later stages. The cause of these syndromes is unknown, although it is increasingly recognized that subcortical white matter pathology may exist without apparent MRI lesions (Jokinen et al., 2013).

## ELDERLY GAIT PATTERNS, CAUTIOUS GAITS, AND FEAR OF FALLING

Healthy, neurologically normal elderly people tend to walk at slower speeds than their younger counterparts. The slower speed of walking is related to shorter and shallower steps with reduced excursion at lower limb joints. In addition, stance width may be slightly wider than normal, and synergistic associated arm swing and trunk movements are less vigorous. The rhythmicity of stepping is preserved. These changes give the normal elderly gait a cautious or guarded appearance and provide a more secure base to compensate for a subtle age-related deterioration in balance. Factors contributing to a general decline in mobility of the elderly include degenerative joint disease, which reduces the range of limb movement and decreased cardiovascular fitness, thus limiting exercise capacity.

In unselected elderly populations including those who fall, a more pronounced deterioration in gait and postural control with dysequilibrium is evident. Walking speed is slower, steps are shorter, stride length is reduced, the stance phase of walking is increased, and variability in stride time is increased.

Elderly patients with an insecure gait characterized by slow short steps, en bloc turns, and falls often have signs of multiple neurological deficits, such as (1) mild proximal weakness of neuromuscular origin, (2) subtle sensory loss (mild distal light touch and proprioceptive loss, blunted vestibular or visual function), (3) mild spastic paraparesis due to cervical myelopathy, and (4) impaired truncal control—as discussed earlier—without any one lesion being severe enough to explain the walking difficulty. The cumulative effect of these multiple deficits may account for perceived instability and dysequilibrium. Musculoskeletal disorders, postural hypotension, and loss of confidence (especially after falls) are further factors contributing to a cautious gait pattern. In this situation, brain imaging is valuable to look for frontal and periventricular white matter ischemic lesions that correlate with imbalance, increased body sway, falls, and cognitive decline (Baezner et al., 2008) and also to exclude treatable causes of gait disorders such as a frontal meningioma.

Falls lead to a marked loss of confidence when walking and a cautious or protected gait. A cautious gait is a normal response to the perception of impaired or threatened balance and a fear of falling. Such patients adopt a crouched posture and take short shallow steps. They may be unable to walk without support, holding onto furniture, leaning on walls, and avoiding crowded or open spaces because of a fear of falling. The gait improves dramatically when support is provided. Accordingly, a cautious gait should be interpreted as compensatory and not specific for any level of the gait classification. A formal program of gait retraining may help to restore confidence and improve the ability to walk.

## PERCEPTIONS OF INSTABILITY AND ILLUSIONS OF MOVEMENT

A number of syndromes have been described in which middle-aged individuals complain of unsteadiness and imbalance associated with "dizziness," sensations or illusions of semicontinuous body motion, sudden brief body displacements, or body tilt. These symptoms develop in open spaces where there are no visible supports (space phobia) or in particular situations such as on bridges, stairs, and escalators or in crowded rooms. Such symptoms are associated with the development of phobic avoidance behavior and the syndrome of phobic postural vertigo (Brandt, 1996). Prolonged illusory swaying and unsteadiness after sea or air travel is referred to as the *mal de débarquement* syndrome. Past episodes of a vestibulopathy may suggest a subtle semicircular canal or otolith disturbance, but a disorder of vestibular function is rarely confirmed in these syndromes. Fear of falling and anxiety are common accompaniments. These symptoms must be distinguished from the physiological "vertigo" and unsteadiness accompanying visual-vestibular mismatch or conflict when observing moving objects, focusing on distant objects in a large panorama, or looking upward at a moving object.

## RECKLESS GAIT PATTERNS

Reckless gaits are seen in patients with impaired postural responses and poor truncal control who do not recognize their instability and take risks that result in falls and injuries. Such patients make inappropriate movements of the feet and trunk when sitting or standing without due caution or monitoring of body posture and position. The most striking examples occur in frontal dementias such as progressive supranuclear palsy and frontotemporal dementias, in which impulsivity and a failure to adapt to the precarious balance are part of the cognitive decline.

## HYSTERICAL AND PSYCHOGENIC GAIT DISORDERS

A gait disorder is one of the commoner manifestations of a psychogenic, functional, or hysterical movement disorder. The typical gait patterns encountered are listed in Box 25.5.

The more acrobatic hysterical disorders of gait indicate the extent to which the nervous system is functioning normally and capable of high-level coordinated motor skills and postural control to perform complex maneuvers. Suggestibility, variability, improvement with distraction, and a history of sudden onset or a rapid, dramatic, and complete recovery are common features of functional or psychogenic gait (and movement) disorders in general. For example, a suggestible patient with an exaggerated positive Romberg sign may paradoxically improve when instructed to perform a distracting task. Another classical discrepancy is illustrated by the Hoover sign in the patient with an apparently paralyzed leg when examined supine. As the patient lifts the normal leg, the examiner places a hand under the "paralyzed" leg and feels the presence (and strength) of synergistic hip extension. The general neurological examination often reveals a variety of other signs suggestive of psychogenic origin such as "giveway weakness" and nonphysiological sensory disturbances. Other functional movement disorders are often present and a long history of vague medical conditions is common. One must be cautious in accepting a diagnosis of hysteria, however, because a bizarre gait may be the presenting feature of primary torsion dystonia. Unusual truncal and leg postures may be encountered in truncal and leg tremors, and higher-level gait disorders are often not adequately explained by the standard neurological examination.

**BOX 25.5 Characteristic Psychogenic or Functional Gait Patterns**

Transient fluctuations in posture while walking
Knee buckling without falls
Excessive slowness and hesitancy
A crouched, stooped, or other abnormal posture of the trunk
Complex postural adjustments with each step
Exaggerated body sway or excessive body motion, especially when tandem walking
Trembling or "weak" legs

*From Hayes, M.W., Graham, S., Heldorf, P., et al., 1999. A video review of the diagnosis of psychogenic gait: appendix and commentary. Mov Disord 14, 914–921.*

## MUSCULOSKELETAL DISORDERS AND ANTALGIC GAIT

### Skeletal Deformity and Joint Disease

Degenerative osteoarthritis of the hip may produce leg shortening in addition to mechanical limitation of leg movement at the hip, giving rise to a waddling gait or a limp. Leg shortening with limping in childhood may be the presenting feature of hemiatrophy due to a cerebral or spinal lesion or spinal dysraphism. Examination of the legs may reveal lower motor neuron signs, sensory loss with trophic ulcers of the feet, and occasionally upper motor neuron signs such as a brisk knee reflex. Lumbosacral vertebral abnormalities (spina bifida), bony foot deformities, and a cutaneous hairy patch over the lumbosacral region are clues to the diagnosis. In adult life, spinal dysraphism (diastematomyelia with a tethered cord) may first become symptomatic after a back injury, with the development of walking difficulties, leg and lower back pain, neurogenic bladder disturbances, and sensory loss in a leg. Imaging of the spinal canal reveals the abnormality.

### Painful (Antalgic) Gaits

Most people at one time or another experience a limp caused by a painful or an injured leg. Limps and gait difficulties due to joint disease, bone injury, or soft-tissue injury are not usually accompanied by muscle weakness, reflex change, or sensory loss. Limitation of the range of joint movement at the hip, knee, or ankle to reduce pain leads to short steps with a fixed leg posture. Hip disease causes a variety of gait adjustments; it is important to examine the range of hip movements (while supine) and any associated pain during passive movements of the hip in a patient with a gait disorder. Pain due to intermittent claudication of the cauda equina is most commonly caused by lumbar spondylosis and, rarely, by a spinal tumor. Diagnosis is confirmed by spinal imaging. It may be difficult to distinguish this syndrome from calf muscle claudication secondary to peripheral vascular disease. Examination after exercise may resolve the issue by revealing a depressed ankle jerk or radicular sensory loss with preservation of arterial pulses in the leg. Other painful conditions affecting the spine, lower limbs, and soft tissue, such as plantar fasciitis, can affect gait.

*The complete reference list is available online at https://expertconsult.inkling.com/.*

26

# Hemiplegia and Monoplegia

E. Lee Murray, Karl E. Misulis

## OUTLINE



Hemiplegia and monoplegia are more likely to be due to discrete focal lesions than diffuse lesions, so these presentations are especially suited to clinical-anatomical localization. Similarly, imaging studies are likely to be revealing with hemiplegia or monoplegia, but the focus of imaging must be directed by clinical suspicion.

Hemiplegia and monoplegia are motor symptoms and signs; however, associated sensory abnormalities are essential to localization, so these are discussed when appropriate. Sensory deficit syndromes are discussed in more depth in Chapter 31. Motor power begins with volition, the conscious effort to initiate movement. Lack of volition does not produce weakness but rather results in akinesia. Projections from the premotor regions of the frontal lobes to the motor strip result in activation of corticospinal tract (CST) neurons, which then have a descending pathway, which is detailed later.

Localization begins with identification of weakness. Differentiation is made among the following distributions:

- Generalized weakness
- Monoplegia
- Hemiplegia
- Paraplegia

Only hemiplegia and monoplegia are discussed in this chapter.

## ANATOMY AND PHYSIOLOGY

### Motor System Anatomy

Anatomical localization begins with a good understanding of anatomy and physiology. Focal deficits such as hemiplegia and monoplegia are more likely to be due to a focal structural lesion than diffuse disorders, so anatomy is of prime importance.

The neuroanatomical locus of motor initiative is unknown and likely diffuse, but motor planning probably begins in the premotor cortex. Integrating sensory information into the planning stage, neurons of the premotor cortex project widely to targets including the motor cortex, prefrontal cortex, parietal cortex, supplementary motor cortex area, basal ganglia, thalamus, and spinal cord. Output from the primary motor cortex descends through the internal capsule to the brainstem and spinal cord as the pyramidal tract.

#### Pyramidal Tract

Pyramidal tract axons become the corticobulbar and corticospinal tracts. Most of the descending axons cross in the brainstem to activate contralateral cranial nerve nuclei or descend into the spinal cord in the lateral corticospinal tract. These neurons generally supply limb muscles. A minority of the motor axons descend in the spinal cord uncrossed in the anterior corticospinal tract, where some of these axons cross before they supply contralateral motoneurons. Some of the descending neurons that are uncrossed supply ipsilateral axial muscles.

The premotor cortex is divided into divisions that have cytoarchitectural foundations and some functional implications, but real topographic organization develops in the primary motor cortex, where mapping of the body areas served by regions of the cortex produces a distorted representation of the body—the homunculus (Fig. 26.1).

Descending corticospinal pathways through the internal capsule are topographically organized, though not as precisely as in the motor cortex. Within the internal capsule, the corticospinal tracts are generally in the posterior limb, with the face and arm axons anteriorly and the leg axons posteriorly.

As the corticospinal axons descend through the spinal cord, the presence of crossed and uncrossed axons makes for complex effects of lesions on motor function. In addition, whereas there is some topographic organization to the corticospinal tracts, this is not as precise or clinically relevant as in the motor cortex or even internal capsule (Morecraft et al., 2002).

#### Basal Ganglia

The basal ganglia likely modulate motor activity rather than directly activating it. They seem to play a role in control of initiation of movement by the premotor and motor cortical regions. In addition to the

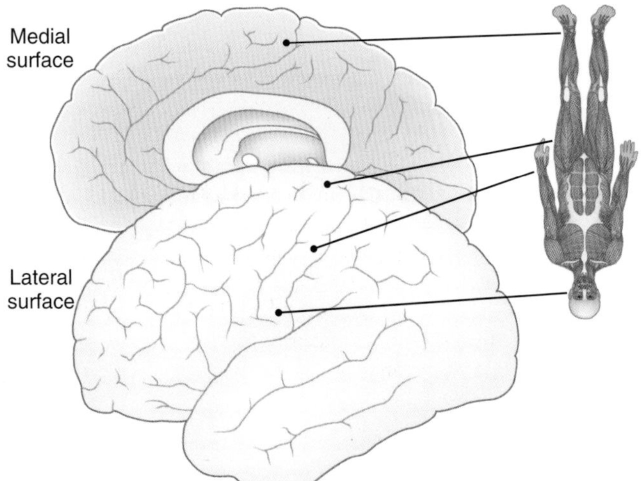


Fig. 26.1 Representation of the body on the Motor Cortex. Face and arms are represented laterally, and legs are represented medially, with cortical representation of the distal legs bordering on the central sulcus.

**TABLE 26.1 Cerebral Lesions**

| Lesion Location | Symptoms | Signs |
|---|---|---|
| Motor cortex | Weakness and poor control of the affected extremity, which may involve face, arm, and leg to different degrees | Incoordination and weakness that depends on the location of the lesion within the cortical homunculus; often associated with neglect, apraxia, aphasia, or other signs of cortical dysfunction |
| Internal capsule | Weakness that usually affects the face, arm, and leg almost equally | Often associated with sensory impairment in same distribution |
| Basal ganglia | Weakness and incoordination on the contralateral side | Weakness, often without sensory loss; no neglect or aphasia |
| Thalamus | Sensory loss | Sensory loss with little or no weakness |

role of the basal ganglia in motor function, they are implicated in other functions, including memory and particularly the initiation, execution, and termination of learned motor tasks (Packard et al., 2002). There is also evidence of involvement of the basal ganglia in nonmotor cognitive tasks (Calabresi et al., 2016).

Afferents to the basal ganglia are from the cerebral cortex and thalamus to the striatum. Efferents from the striatum are largely to the globus pallidus and substantia nigra. The globus pallidus, in turn, projects to the thalamus.

### Cerebellum

The cerebellum monitors and modulates motor activities, responding to motor commands and inputs from sensory receptors of the joints, muscles, and vestibular system. The cerebellum is somewhat topographically organized, with gait and axial musculature represented at and near the midline and limb motor activity served laterally in the cerebellar hemispheres.

### Localization of Motor Deficits

The topographic organization of the cerebral cortex dictates that lesions produce weakness depending on location and size. The homunculus roughly predicts which muscles are affected. If the lesion is small and localized to the motor cortex, the deficit can be purely or solely motor. If the lesion is larger and involves sensory regions, a sensory deficit is expected.

Lesions of the internal capsule can potentially involve only motor axons; but because of the proximity of adjacent structures, some sensory involvement is more common. Lesions producing limited motor involvement of one limb are not commonly associated with the internal capsule.

Lesions of the descending corticospinal tracts in the brainstem produce hemiplegia, typically with other brainstem signs, such as crossed sensory symptoms, cranial nerve deficits, or ataxia not explained by weakness.

Lesions of the corticospinal tract in the spinal cord usually produce upper motoneuron (UMN) deficits below the level of the lesions but also often lower motoneuron (LMN) deficits at the level of the lesion. Lesions so restricted in the cord as to produce hemiparesis or the Brown-Séquard syndrome are rare.

Lesions and disorders of the basal ganglia commonly produce contralateral motor dysfunction, although they are more likely to manifest as difficulty with motor control rather than hemiplegia or monoplegia. Disorders with focal motor symptoms from basal ganglia dysfunction include Parkinson disease, dystonia, hemiballismus, and Huntington disease.

Lesions of the cerebellum do not produce hemiplegia or monoplegia. Instead, a lateral lesion will produce ipsilateral limb ataxia and a midline lesion gait ataxia.

## HEMIPLEGIA

### Cerebral Lesions

Cerebral lesions constitute the most common cause of hemiplegia. Lesions in either cortical or subcortical structures may be responsible for the weakness (Table 26.1). Some lesions are both cortical and subcortical, and some these can include mass lesions, infarctions, and hemorrhages.

### Cortical Lesions

Cortical lesions produce weakness that is more focal than the weakness seen with subcortical lesions. Fig 26.1 is a diagrammatic representation of the surface of the brain, showing how the body is mapped onto the surface of the sensorimotor cortex: the homunculus. The face and arm are laterally represented on the hemisphere, whereas the leg is draped over the top of the hemisphere and into the interhemispheric fissure.

Small lesions of the cortex can produce prominent focal weakness of one area, such as the leg or the face and hand; but hemiplegia—paralysis of both the leg and arm on the same side of the body—is not expected from a cortical lesion unless the damage is extensive. The most likely cause of cortical hemiplegia would be a stroke involving the entire territory of the internal carotid artery.

***Seizure-related weakness.*** Seizures can present with hemiparesis due either to ictal paralysis or postictal (Todd) paralysis. The latter is much more common than the former.

**Todd paralysis.** Postictal (Todd) paralysis is a transient weakness that develops contralateral to the seizure focus. The preceding motor activity is followed by weakness lasting from minutes to hours, as long as 36 hours, with a median duration of about 15 hours (Rolak et al., 1992). Depending on the anatomy of the distribution of the seizure activity, nonmotor manifestations such as aphasia may occur, although aphasia can be ictal as well as postictal (Loesch et al., 2017).

There is no specific diagnostic test, but with prolonged hemiparesis after a seizure, electroencephalography (EEG) is often indicated to rule out nonconvulsive status epilepticus. If the patient has no history of seizures, particularly focal seizures, emergent evaluation for acute stroke is warranted because both ischemic and hemorrhagic stroke can present with seizure activity (Brosinski, 2014).

**Ictal paralysis.** Ictal paralysis is weakness due to the discharge rather than the after effects of the discharge, as with Todd paralysis (Dale and Cross, 1999). This is much less common. It can be confused with stroke, and some patients with ictal paralysis may be treated with reperfusion therapy for acute ischemic stroke (Sanghvi et al., 2016). Luckily, the risk of these treatments is relatively low in patients without an acute stroke (Chernyshev et al., 2010). Ictal paralysis is seen mainly in children, making confusion with stroke less likely.

Diagnosis of ictal paralysis depends on obtaining an EEG during the episode. EEG often shows slow-wave activity. Periodic lateralized epileptiform discharges (PLEDs) have also been described (Calarese et al., 2008; Tseng et al., 2006).

***Alternating hemiplegia of childhood.*** Alternating hemiplegia of childhood is a rare condition characterized by attacks of unilateral weakness, often with signs of other motor deficits (e.g., dyskinesias, stiffness) and oculomotor abnormalities (e.g., nystagmus) (Zhang et al., 2003). Attacks begin in early childhood, usually before age 18 months; they last hours and deficits accumulate over years. Initially patients exhibit normal neurological function between attacks, but with time persistent neurological deficits become obvious. A benign form can occur on awakening in patients who are otherwise normal and do not develop progressive deficits; this entity is related to migraine. Diagnostic studies are often performed, including magnetic resonance imaging (MRI), EEG, and angiography, but these usually show no abnormalities. Alternating hemiplegia is suggested when a young child presents with episodes of hemiparesis, especially on awakening, not associated with headache.

***Hemiconvulsion-hemiplegia-epilepsy syndrome.*** In young children with the rare condition called hemiconvulsion-hemiplegia-epilepsy syndrome, unilateral weakness develops after the sudden onset of focal seizures. The seizures are often incompletely controlled. Neurological deficits are not confined to the motor system and may include cognitive, language, and visual deficits. Unlike alternating hemiplegia, the seizures and motor deficits are initially consistently unilateral, although eventually the unilateral seizures may become generalized. Imaging findings may be normal initially but eventually atrophy of the affected hemisphere is seen (Freeman et al., 2002). Cerebrospinal fluid (CSF) analysis is not specific, but a mild mononuclear pleocytosis may develop because of central nervous system (CNS) damage and seizures. Rasmussen encephalitis is a cause of this syndrome.

### Subcortical Lesions

Subcortical lesions are more likely than cortical lesions to produce equal weakness of the contralateral face, arm, and leg because of the convergence of the descending axons in the internal capsule. The internal capsule is a particularly common location for lacunar infarctions and can also be affected by hemorrhage in the adjacent basal ganglia or thalamus. Weakness of sudden onset is most likely to be the result of infarction, with hemorrhage in a minority of cases. Demyelinating disease is characterized by a subacute onset. Tumors are associated with a slower onset of deficit and can grow quite large in subcortical regions before the patient presents for medical attention.

***Infarction.*** Infarction is usually a clinical diagnosis but can be confirmed by computed tomography (CT) or MRI, as discussed earlier (see "Cortical Lesions"). Infarction manifests with an acute onset of deficit, although the course may be one of steady progression or stuttering. Lacunar infarctions are more likely than cortical infarctions to be associated with a stuttering course.

**Lenticulostriate arteries.** Lenticulostriate arteries are small penetrating vessels that arise from the proximal middle cerebral artery (MCA) and supply the basal ganglia and internal capsule. Infarction commonly produces contralateral hemiparesis with little or no sensory involvement. This is one cause of the syndrome of pure motor stroke, which can also be due to a brainstem lacunar infarction (Lastilla, 2006).

**Thalamoperforate arteries.** These are small penetrating vessels that arise from the posterior cerebral artery (PCA) and supply mainly the thalamus. Infarction in this distribution produces contralateral sensory disturbance but can also cause movement disorders such as choreoathetosis or hemiballismus; hemiparesis is not expected.

***Leukoencephalopathies***

**Multiple sclerosis.** MS manifests with any combination of deficits due to white matter dysfunction. Hemiparesis can develop, especially if large plaques affect the CST fibers in the hemispheres. Hemiparesis is even more likely with brainstem or spinal demyelinating lesions because small lesions in these areas can produce more profound deficits. The diagnosis is suggested by progression over days plus a prior history of episodes of relapsing and remitting neurological deficits. Episodes of weakness that last for only minutes are unlikely to be due to demyelinating disease but rather to a transient ischemic attack (TIA), migraine equivalent, or seizure.

Diagnosis is based on clinical grounds for most patients, but the finding of areas of increased signal intensity on MRI T2-weighted images is suggestive of MS. Active demyelinating lesions often show enhancement on gadolinium-enhanced T1-weighted images. CSF examination is usually performed and can show normal findings or elevated protein, a mild lymphocytic pleocytosis, or oligoclonal bands of immunoglobulin G (IgG).

**Progressive multifocal leukoencephalopathy.** Progressive multifocal leukoencephalopathy (PML) is a demyelinating disease caused by reactivation of the JC virus, usually seen in immunodeficient patients. Predisposed patients include those with acquired immunodeficiency syndrome (AIDS), leukemia, lymphoma, tuberculosis, or sarcoidosis. Patients receiving immunosuppressive therapies—such as natalizumab, rituximab, cyclophosphamide, or cyclosporine for various autoimmune diseases—are also at risk. Visual loss is the most common presenting symptom, and weakness is the second. MRI shows multiple white matter lesions. CSF either reveals no abnormality or shows a lymphocytic pleocytosis or elevated protein, or both. Brain biopsy is required for specific diagnosis, although JC virus deoxyribonucleic acid (DNA) can be detected in the CSF by polymerase chain reaction (PCR) assay in most patients. PML is suggested when a patient with immunodeficiency presents with subacute to chronic onset of neurological deficits and multifocal white matter lesions on MRI.

Although there are no proven treatments, general principles can be applied—namely, improving immunological status by the treatment of underlying disease and the removal of immunosuppressive therapies. Caution should be taken when discontinuing immunosuppressants, since recovery of the immune system can lead to immune reconstitution inflammatory syndrome (IRIS) and consequently to worsening neurological status. IRIS can be managed with a short course of high-dose intravenous corticosteroids. Natalizumab-induced PML can be managed by plasma exchange.

### Both cortical and subcortical

***Infections.*** Infections can present as hemiplegia, usually with a subacute onset. Bacterial abscess of the brain can present with subacute progressive hemiparesis. This can occur in isolation, from dental or other sources, or in the bed of an infarction, as in a patient with bacterial endocarditis (Mori et al., 2003; Okubo et al., 1998). With acute onset of weakness and then progressive worsening, embolic infarction and then abscess in the region of the infarction has to be considered.

Viral infections such as encephalitis can present with hemiplegia but usually are associated with other symptoms. Hemiparesis from herpes simplex virus (HSV) encephalitis would be expected to be associated with fever, mental status changes, headache, and/or seizures (Ahmed et al., 2013).

**Migraine.** Migraine has many subdivisions, and the classification scheme is evolving. Among the subdivisions in the 2013 scheme (Headache Classification Committee of the International Headache Society, 2013) are the following:

- Migraine without aura
- Migraine with aura, including typical aura, hemiplegic migraine, brainstem aura, and retinal migraine
- Chronic migraine
- Complications of migraine, including migrainous infarction, persistent aura without infarction, and aura-triggered seizure
- Probable migraine
- Episodic syndromes that may be associated with migraine

Many of these can cause hemiplegia (Black, 2006). *Migraine without aura* is episodic headache without aura; by definition, there should be no deficit. *Migraine with aura* is episodic headache with aura, most commonly visual. The subtypes of hemiplegic migraine, brainstem aura, and retinal migraine all have associated neurological deficit, but hemiplegia is typical of only the first subtype. *Hemiplegic migraine*, as its name suggests, is characterized by paralysis of one side of the body, typically with onset before the headache; this variant is often familial. *Migraine with brainstem aura* is episodic headache with brainstem signs including vertigo and ataxia; this variant is a disorder mainly of childhood. *Migrainous infarction* features sustained deficit plus MRI evidence of infarction that had developed from the migraine. Definitive diagnosis is problematic because patients with migraine have a higher incidence of stroke not associated with a migraine attack. *Persistent aura without infarction* is persistence of the aura for a week or longer without evidence of infarction on MRI.

The diagnosis of migraine is suggested by the combination of young age of the patient with few vascular risk factors and a marching deficit that can be conceptualized as migration of spreading electrical depression across the cerebral cortex. Imaging is often necessary to rule out hemorrhage, infarction, and demyelinating disease.

**Mass lesion.** Although infarction presents with deficits with localization dependent on vascular anatomy, mass lesions are not so constrained. Lesions may affect motor and sensory systems with complex symptomatology. The etiology of these nonvascular cortical lesions is usually trauma, tumor, or infection. Diagnosis of acute trauma is typically easy but identification of the remote effects of trauma may be difficult, especially when limited history is available.

Hemiplegia from mass lesion can be produced by a large lesion of the cerebral hemisphere, at which point nonmotor symptoms would be evident, including cortical signs, sensory abnormalities, and/or visual field abnormalities. Subcortical mass lesions are seldom as restricted to internal capsule/basal ganglia as infarction.

**Infarction.** Both cortical and subcortical infarctions can produce weakness, but cortical infarctions are more likely than subcortical infarctions to be associated with sensory deficits. Also, many cortical infarctions are associated with cortical signs—neglect with nondominant hemisphere lesions and aphasia with dominant hemisphere lesions. Unfortunately this distinction is not absolute because subcortical lesions can also occasionally produce these signs.

Initial diagnosis of infarction is usually made on clinical grounds. An abrupt onset of the deficit is typical. Weakness that progresses over several days is unlikely to be caused by infarction, although some infarcts can show worsening for a few days after onset. Progression over days suggests demyelinating disease or infection. Progression over weeks suggests a mass lesion such as tumor. Progression over seconds to minutes in a marching fashion suggests either epilepsy or migraine; not all migraine-associated deficits are associated with concurrent or subsequent Headache.

Head CTs often do not show infarction for up to 3 days after the event but are performed emergently to rule out mass lesion or hemorrhage. Small infarctions may never be seen on CT. MRI is superior in showing both old and new infarctions; diffusion-weighted imaging (DWI) in conjunction with apparent diffusion coefficient (ADC) on MRI distinguishes recent infarction from old lesions.

**Middle cerebral artery.** The MCA supplies the lateral aspect of the motor sensory cortex, which controls the face and arm. On the dominant side, speech centers are also supplied—the Broca area (expression) in the posterior frontal region and the Wernicke area (reception) on the superior aspect of the temporal lobe.

Cortical infarction in the territory of the MCA produces contralateral hemiparesis, which is usually associated with other signs of cortical dysfunction such as aphasia with left hemispheric lesions or neglect with right hemispheric lesions. Weakness is much more prominent in the arm, hand, and face than in the leg. Hemianopia is sometimes seen, especially with large MCA infarctions, as a result of infarction of the optic radiations. MCA infarction is suspected with hemiparesis plus cortical signs of aphasia or neglect. Confirmation is with imaging.

**Anterior cerebral artery.** The ACA supplies the inferior frontal and parasagittal regions of the frontal and anterior parietal lobes. This region is responsible for leg movement and is important for bowel and bladder control. Infarction in the ACA distribution produces contralateral leg weakness. The arm may be slightly affected, especially the proximal arm, with sparing of hand and face. In some patients, both ACAs arise from the same trunk, so infarction produces bilateral leg weakness; this deficit can be mistaken clinically for myelopathy and is in the differential diagnosis for suspected cord infarction or other acute myelopathy.

ACA infarction is suggested by a clinical presentation of unilateral or bilateral leg weakness and CST signs. Confirmation is with MRI.

**Posterior cerebral artery.** The PCAs are the terminal branches of the basilar artery. They supply most of the occipital lobes and the medial aspect of the temporal lobes. PCA infarction is not expected to produce weakness but produces contralateral hemianopia, often with memory deficits due to bilateral hippocampal infarction.

The clinical diagnosis of PCA infarction may be missed because an examiner may not look for hemianopia in a patient who otherwise presents only with confusion. Visual complaints may be vague or nonexistent.

PCA infarction is suggested by a clinical presentation of acute confusion, visual disturbance, or both. A finding of hemianopia is supportive evidence. Imaging can show not only the area of infarction but also the location of the vascular defect—unilateral or bilateral PCA or basilar artery.

**Hemorrhages.** A wide range of intracranial hemorrhages (ICHs) can produce hemiparesis. The development of ICH, as opposed to infarction, is suggested especially by drowsiness, seizures, and progression of the deficit. CT of the brain promptly makes the diagnosis in most circumstances. Occasionally small subdural hematomas (SDHs) may not be seen on CT but are seen on MRI and may produce hemiparesis.

Hemorrhages are of the multiple types: intraparenchymal hemorrhage (IPH), subdural hemorrhage (SDH), epidural hemorrhage (EDH), intraventricular hemorrhage (IVH), and subarachnoid hemorrhage (SAH).

**Intraparenchymal hemorrhage.** IPH is often hypertensive and may be predisposed by a vascular malformation. Trauma can produce IPH, but there are usually other associated ICHs with this. Associated IVH, SDH, and SAH are common. Hemiparesis can be produced especially by IPH and SDH.

**Subarachnoid hemorrhage.** Nontraumatic SAH predisposes to the development of vasospasm and infarction, resulting in hemiplegia. This is discussed in detail in Chapter 67. Traumatic brain injury is associated with an increased risk of subsequent stroke and resultant hemiparesis, but traumatic SAH does not seem to enhance this risk (Morris et al., 2017).

**Subdural hematoma.** Subdural hematoma is often associated with hemiparesis, and the presence of this deficit is one indicator of whether surgical intervention is needed (Motiei-Langroudi et al., 2019). The exact mechanism of hemiparesis under a subdural hematoma is not known, but recent data suggest that mechanical tension on the cortex is a strong correlate and likely a larger determinant than actual SDH size (Tomita et al., 2018).

**Epidural hematoma.** Epidural hematoma (EDH) commonly presents with alteration of consciousness after an inciting trauma. If consciousness recovers, hemiparesis may be evident. Sometimes a history is provided of transient improvement in mental status with hemiparesis noted and then a lapse into unconsciousness, so that the focality cannot be clearly demonstrated. This pattern is of strong concern for EDH. Not only cerebral but also spinal EDH can present with hemiparesis (Nakanishi et al., 2011; Patel et al., 2018 ).

**Intraventricular hemorrhage.** IVH without any associated IPH is uncommon and usually due to vascular malformations and intraventricular tumors. These isolated IVHs are seldom associated with focal signs but rather present with headache and altered mental status. IVH due to breakthrough from IPH from either hypertension, vascular malformation, or trauma is associated with focal signs including hemiparesis but due to the parenchymal damage, not the IVH itself.

***Tumors.*** Tumors affecting the cerebral hemispheres commonly present with progressive deficits including hemiparesis. Coordination deficit usually develops before the weakness. Cortical dysfunction, such as aphasia with dominant hemispheric lesions and neglect, is commonly present. Other signs of expanding tumors may include headache, seizures, confusion, and visual field defects.

Tumor should be suspected in a patient with progressive motor deficit over weeks, especially with coexistent seizures or headache. MRI with contrast enhancement is more sensitive than CT for identification of tumors. Although there are many exceptions, generally, benign tumors tend to present with seizures and malignant tumors with progressive deficit including hemiparesis.

Abrupt onset of hemiparesis can develop with tumors, especially if there is hemorrhage into the tumor or the tumor affects the vasculature, producing infarction.

Hemiparesis from infarction in patients with primary brain tumors is often related to treatments (radiation vasculopathy and surgical manipulation), but a substantial proportion are embolic and of uncertain relation to the tumor (Parikh et al., 2017). Infarction in patients with brain metastases is usually linked with cancer-related hypercoagulability (Nam et al., 2017).

***Autoimmune.***

**Demyelinating disease.** Demyelinating disease comprises a group of conditions whose pathophysiology implicates the immune system.

**Acute disseminated encephalomyelitis.** Acute disseminated encephalomyelitis (ADEM) is a demyelinating illness that is monophasic but in other respects manifests like a first attack of MS (Wingerchuk, 2006). This entity is sometimes called *parainfectious encephalomyelitis*, although the association with infection is not always certain. Symptoms and signs at all levels of the CNS are common, including hemiparesis, paraplegia, ataxia, and brainstem signs. Diagnosis is based on clinical grounds because MRI may not definitively distinguish between MS and ADEM. CSF examination may show a mononuclear pleocytosis and elevation in protein, but these findings are neither always present nor specific. Even the presence or absence of oligoclonal IgG in the CSF cannot differentiate between ADEM and MS. Patients who present clinically with ADEM should be warned of the possibility of having recurrent events indicative of MS.

**Sarcoid.** Sarcoid can affect almost any part of the nervous system. Neurosarcoidosis can manifest as cranial neuropathies, radiculopathy, myelopathy, meningitis, hydrocephalus, and neuropathy of various types. Hemiparesis is uncommon, but hemiparesis due to intraparenchymal lesions has been described (Galdys et al., 2016). Hemiparesis in the absence of any other manifestations of neurosarcoid would be unusual.

Neurosarcoid is suspected with almost any neurological symptoms in a patient with known sarcoid. When the patient has not been diagnosed with sarcoid, neurosarcoid may be suspected when a patient has neurological deficits of no known etiology and is found to have any of the following: aseptic meningitis, enhancement on MRI of lesions in the brain or spinal parenchyma, meninges, on nerve roots, or multiple mononeuropathies. Diagnosis is usually confirmed by biopsy of lymph node or lung lesion, since biopsy of neural tissue is more difficult and destructive.

## Brainstem Lesions

Brainstem lesions producing hemiplegia are among the easiest to localize because associated signs of cranial nerve and brainstem dysfunction are almost always present.

### Brainstem Motor Organization

Fig 26.2 shows the anatomical organization of the brainstem's motor systems. Motor pathways descend through the CST to the pyramidal decussation in the medulla, where they cross to innervate the contralateral body. Lesions of the pons and midbrain above this level produce contralateral hemiparesis, which may involve the contralateral face. Rostral lesions of the medulla produce contralateral weakness, whereas more caudal medullary lesions produce ipsilateral cranial nerve signs with a contralateral hemiparesis and sensory deficit.

Sensory pathways from the nucleus gracilis and nucleus cuneatus cross at about the same level as the motor fibers of the CST, so deficits in light touch and position sense tend to parallel the distribution of the motor deficit. By contrast, the spinothalamic tracts have already crossed in the spinal cord and ascend laterally in the brainstem. Accordingly, lesions of the lower medulla may produce contralateral loss of pain and temperature sensation and ipsilateral loss of touch and position sense. Lesions above the mid-medulla produce a contralateral sensory defect of all modalities similar to that from cerebral lesions, yet the clues to brainstem localization can include the following:

- Ipsilateral facial sensory deficit from a trigeminal lesion
- Ipsilateral hemiataxia from damage to the cerebellar hemispheres or nuclei
- Ocular motor weakness from any of multiple lesion locations
- Ipsilateral Horner syndrome from damage of the descending sympathetic tracts

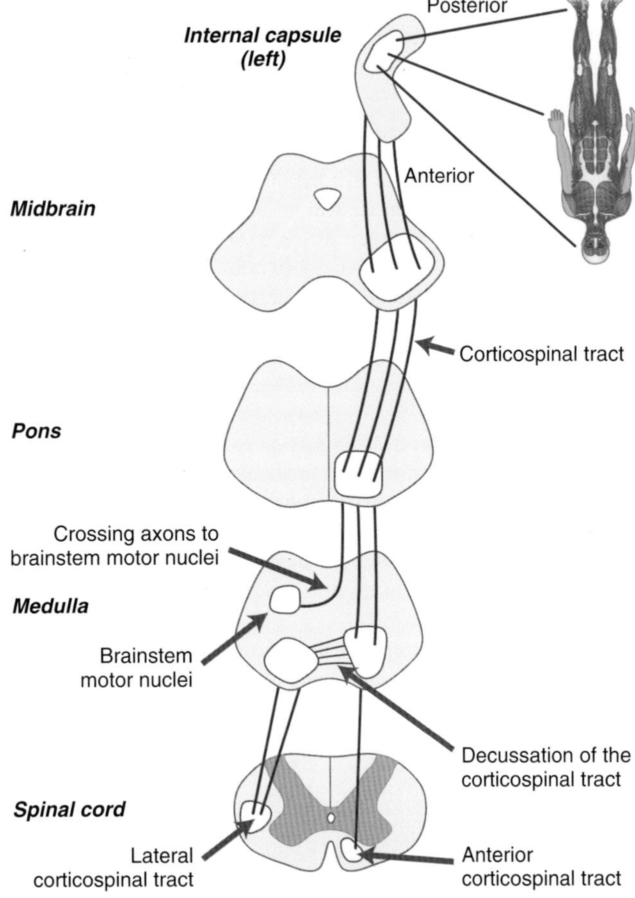


**Fig. 26.2 Brainstem motor organization, beginning with Internal Capsule.** Corticospinal tract remains topographically organized throughout brainstem and spinal cord, although isolated lesions below cerebral cortex are unlikely to produce topographically specific damage.

## Common Lesions

Table 26.2 shows some of the important lesions of the brainstem and their associated motor deficits. Brainstem lesions are usually due to damage to the penetrating branches of the basilar artery. Patients present with contralateral weakness along with other deficits that help to localize the lesion. Hemiataxia often develops and can be mistaken for hemiparesis, so careful examination is essential.

## Spinal Lesions

Spinal lesions can produce hemiplegia sparing the face, although they mostly will cause bilateral deficits typical of myelopathy. A spinal cord lesion should be suspected in a patient with bilateral weakness, bowel or bladder control deficits, and back pain.

### Spinal Hemisection (Brown-Séquard Syndrome)

Spinal hemisection is seldom seen in clinical practice. This entity is usually associated with intradural tumors, trauma, inflammatory conditions such as demyelinating disease, and occasionally spinal infarction. Spondylotic myelopathy, disc disease, and most extradural tumors typically produce symmetrical deficits. Patients with the spinal hemisection syndrome present with weakness ipsilateral to and below the lesion. In addition, segmental motor loss may be seen with involvement of the motoneurons at the level of the lesion. Sensory abnormalities include loss of pain and temperature contralateral to and below the lesion. Position sense may be affected ipsilateral to the lesion.

### Transverse Myelitis

Transverse myelitis is an acute myelopathic process that is presumed to be autoimmune in origin. Patients present with motor and sensory deficits below the lesion, usually in the form of a paraplegia. The abnormalities are typically bilateral but may be asymmetrical. MRI may show increased signal on T2 images, enlargement of the cord, and/or enhancement in the spinal cord, which has an appearance that differs subtly from that in involvement in MS.

**TABLE 26.2 Brainstem Syndromes**

| Named Disorder | Lesion Location | Signs |
|---|---|---|
| **Midbrain** | | |
| Weber syndrome | CN III, ventral midbrain, CST | Contralateral hemiparesis, CN III palsy |
| Benedikt syndrome | CN III, ventral midbrain, CST, red nucleus | Contralateral hemiparesis, third nerve palsy, intention tremor, cerebellar ataxia |
| Top-of-the-basilar syndrome | Occipital lobes, midbrain oculomotor nuclei, cerebral peduncle, medial and temporal lobe, thalamus | Contralateral hemiparesis, cortical blindness, oculomotor deficits, memory difficulty, contralateral sensory deficit |
| **Pons** | | |
| Millard-Gubler syndrome | CN VI, CN VII, ventral pons | Contralateral hemiparesis, CN VI and CN VII palsies |
| Clumsy hand syndrome | CST | Contralateral hemiparesis, dysarthria, often with facial weakness |
| Pure motor hemiparesis (due to pons lesion) | Ventral pons | Contralateral hemiparesis with corticospinal tract signs |
| Ataxic hemiparesis (due to pons lesion) | CST, cerebellar tracts | Contralateral hemiparesis with impaired coordination |
| Foville syndrome | CN VII, ventral pons, paramedian pontine reticular formation | Ipsilateral CN VII palsy, contralateral hemiparesis, gaze palsy to the side of the lesion |
| **Medulla** | | |
| Medial medullary syndrome | CST, medial lemniscus, hypoglossal nerve | Contralateral hemiparesis, loss of position and vibratory sensation, ipsilateral tongue paresis |
| Lateral medullary syndrome | Spinothalamic tract, trigeminal nucleus, cerebellum and inferior cerebellar peduncle, vestibular nuclei, nucleus ambiguus | No hemiparesis usually produced, but hemiataxia may be mistaken for hemiparesis; dysphagia, hemisensory loss, face weakness, Horner syndrome are common |

*CN*, Cranial nerve; *CST*, corticospinal tract.

Transverse myelitis is a clinical diagnosis. The primary differential diagnosis is between MS and neuromyelitis optica (NMO).

### Spinal Cord Compression

Spinal cord compression is usually due to disk protrusion, spondylosis, or acute trauma, but neoplastic and infectious causes should always be considered (Shedid and Benzel, 2007). Disc disease and spondylosis are typically in the midline, so bilateral findings are expected. Extradural tumors also usually produce bilateral findings. Intradural tumors may produce unilateral deficits and can occasionally manifest as Brown-Séquard syndrome.

Lesions below the cervical spinal cord would produce not hemiplegia but rather monoplegia of a lower limb or paraplegia. Spondylosis with cord compression produces LMN weakness at the level of the lesion and CST signs below the level of the lesion. Spinal cord compression resulting in paralysis should be evaluated as quickly as possible with MRI. Myelography should be considered if MRI is not urgently available.

### Spinal Cord Infarction

Anterior spinal artery infarction usually causes paraparesis and spinothalamic sensory loss below the level of the lesion; dorsal column function is preserved. Rarely, one segmental branch of the anterior spinal artery can be involved with unilateral spinal cord damage and monoparesis or hemiparesis. Spinal cord infarction is suggested when a patient presents with paraparesis or paraplegia of acute onset and MRI of the spine does not show cord compression and MRI of the brain does not show bilateral ACA infarction.

### Spinal Cord Tumor

*Peripheral lesions.* Peripheral lesions are not expected to produce hemiplegia. A pair of peripheral lesions affecting an arm and leg on the same side, however, may occasionally masquerade as hemiplegia. Differentiation depends on identification of the individual lesions as being within the distribution of one nerve, nerve root, or plexus division. The tendon reflexes are likely to be depressed in patients with peripheral lesions, rather than increased as with CST lesions.

*Amyotrophic lateral sclerosis* can produce weakness of one limb, followed by weakness of the other limb on the same side, with progression over months or even years. Usually the combined presence of UMN and LMN involvement without sensory changes and lack of bowel/bladder involvement supports the diagnosis. If the predominant involvement is UMN in type, the picture can look like that of a progressive hemiparesis.

*Mononeuropathy multiplex* can manifest as separate lesions affecting individual limbs; involvement of an arm and leg on the same side can give the impression of hemiparesis. Diabetes is the most common cause, but other causes include leprosy, vasculitis, and predisposition to pressure palsies. Diagnosis is by electromyography (EMG), which can differentiate mononeuropathies from polyneuropathy (Misulis, 2003).

## Psychogenic Hemiplegia

*Psychogenic* or *functional* weakness includes both conversion reaction and malingering. In conversion reaction, the patient is not conscious of the nonorganic nature of the deficit, whereas in malingering, the patient makes a conscious effort to fool the examiner. Some secondary gain for the patient, either psychological or economic, is a factor with both types. In malingering, the secondary gain is usually more obvious and may involve disability payments, litigation, family attention, or avoidance of stressors or tasks. Clues to functional weakness include the following:

- Improvement in strength with coaching
- Give-way weakness
- Inconsistencies in examination—for example, inability to extend the foot but ability to walk on the toes
- Hoover sign (The patient lies supine on the bed and lifts one leg at a time. If the tested leg is truly paralyzed, the examiner should feel an effort to press down with the opposite heel. Failure to do so constitutes the Hoover sign)
- Paralysis in the absence of other signs of motor system dysfunction, including tone and reflex changes

Diagnosis of functional weakness is based on inconsistencies on examination and elimination of the possibility of organic disease. Functional weakness should be diagnosed with caution. It is easy to dismiss the patient's complaints after an inconsistent feature is seen, especially if some secondary gain is obvious. Unfortunately a patient with organic problems may have a functional overlay, which may exaggerate otherwise subtle clinical findings.

If functional weakness is suspected, some diagnostic testing is often required to rule out neurological disease, although such investigations should be kept to a minimum.

# MONOPLEGIA

## Cerebral Lesions

Cerebral lesions more commonly produce hemiplegia than monoplegia, but isolated limb involvement can occasionally occur, especially with cortical involvement. The arm segment of the sensorimotor cortex lies on the lateral aspect of the hemisphere adjacent to the sylvian fissure. Subcortical lesions are less likely than cortical lesions to produce monoplegia because of the dense packing of the fibers of the CST in the internal capsule.

### Infarction

The arm region of the motor cortex is supplied by the MCA. Infarction of a branch of the MCA can produce isolated arm weakness, although facial involvement and cortical signs are expected (Paciaroni et al., 2005). With more extensive lesions, visual fields can be abnormal because of infarction of the optic radiations. Mild leg weakness can also occur with medial cortical involvement of the infarct. The leg segment of the cortex lies in the parasagittal region and is supplied by the ACA. ACA infarction produces weakness of the contralateral leg.

### Transient Ischemic Attack

Episodic paralysis of one limb sometimes is due to a TIA. The main considerations in the differential diagnosis are migraine and seizure. Abrupt onset and absence of positive (muscle activating) motor symptoms argue in favor of TIA.

### Migraine

Migraine can a produce a sensation that marches along one limb, usually the arm. This marching pattern differs from the abrupt onset of stroke. Involvement of only the leg is unusual. The headache phase typically begins as the neurological deficit is resolving. Weakness can develop as part of the migraine aura, but this is much less likely than sensory disturbance. Not all migrainous weakness is followed by headache.

### Seizure

Seizure classically produces positive motor symptoms with jerking or stiffness. Focal seizures can rarely produce negative motor symptoms, including paralysis. In such cases, the seizure can be impossible to diagnose without EEG, so EEG may be indicated in selected patients with unexplained focal weakness. Ictal paralysis can have abrupt onset and offset and can even resemble negative myoclonus.

Focal seizure activity may be suggested by subtle twitching or disturbance of consciousness associated with the episodes. In comparison with TIAs, seizures are usually more frequent and have a shorter duration. Postictal weakness of only one limb can occur.

### Multiple Sclerosis

MS can produce monoplegia secondary to a discrete white matter plaque in the cerebral hemisphere, but because MS is a subcortical disease, hemiparesis is more common. The corticospinal tracts are somatotopically organized, so monoparesis is theoretically possible but uncommon. Onset of symptoms is subacute.

### Tumors

Tumors deep to the cortex rarely produce monoplegia because the involvement is not sufficiently discrete to affect only one limb. Cortical involvement makes single-limb involvement more likely. Parasagittal lesions often produce leg involvement, which initially can be unilateral. Meningiomas often arise from one side of the falx, so they predominantly affect the opposite leg, initially with weakness, incoordination, and CST signs. With progression, bilateral symptoms develop.

Bilateral leg weakness with CST signs can be due to either cerebral or spinal lesions, although a single leg deficit is only rarely due to a spinal cause. Metastatic tumors often are found at the gray/white junction; in this location, they can produce focal cortical damage. Early on, the lesion may be too small to produce other neurological symptoms, but with increasing growth, it is more likely to produce focal seizures. Tumor is suspected with insidious progression of focal deficit, especially if combined with headache or seizures.

### Infections

Infections are an uncommon cause of monoplegia, but this presentation is possible. Brain abscess in the region of the motor strip can produce weakness largely confined to one extremity, arm more than leg. Viral encephalitis produces different patterns of involvement depending on whether it is HSV. Non-HSV encephalitis commonly produces an encephalopathy, with focal motor deficit being unlikely. HSV encephalitis, often with temporal lobe involvement, can produce arm and face weakness; but hemiparesis, seizures, and language deficits are more common (Mekan et al., 2005). Involvement of the brain outside of the temporal lobes is seen in a small but important group of patients and can produce symptoms appropriate to the lesion (e.g., frontal or occipital). The brainstem can rarely be affected with no evident hemispheric involvement (Jereb et al., 2005).

## Brainstem Lesions

Brainstem lesions seldom produce monoplegia because of the tight packing of the fibers of the CSTs in the brainstem. Unilateral cerebellar hemispheric lesions may produce appendicular ataxia, which is most obvious in the arm, although this should be distinguished from monoparesis by the absence of weakness or CST signs.

## Spinal Lesions

Spinal lesions can produce weakness from segmental damage to nerve roots or CSTs. Weakness at the level of the lesion is in a radicular distribution and may be associated with muscle atrophy and loss of segmental reflexes. Weakness below the lesion can be unilateral or bilateral and is associated with CST signs.

With a spinal cord lesion, monoplegia of a lower extremity is more common than that of an upper extremity unless only the nerve roots are affected. Leg monoplegia can occur from a variety of spinal cord lesions including tumors, other mass lesions causing compression, immune and inflammatory disorders, and stroke (Nelson et al., 2016; Waters et al., 2012).

## Peripheral Lesions

Peripheral lesions usually produce monoparetic weakness in the distribution of a single nerve, nerve root, or plexus. A few conditions, such as amyotrophic lateral sclerosis and focal spinal muscular atrophy, may produce weakness in a monomelic (monoplegic) distribution.

### Pressure Palsies

Intermittent compression of a peripheral nerve can produce transient paresis of part of a limb. The patient may think that the entire limb is paralyzed, but detailed examination shows that the paresis is limited to a nerve distribution. Recovery from the weakness usually occurs so rapidly that examination is often not possible before the improvement. Predisposition to pressure palsies can be seen in two main circumstances: on a hereditary basis and in the presence of peripheral polyneuropathy.

***Hereditary neuropathy with predisposition to pressure palsies.*** Hereditary neuropathy with a predisposition to pressure palsies is associated with episodic weakness and sensory loss associated with compression of isolated nerves. This disorder is inherited as an autosomal dominant condition with a deletion or mutation in the gene for peripheral myelin protein 22 (*PMP-22*). Nerve conduction studies (NCS) will show slowing, commonly across the compression area (carpal tunnel, cubital tunnel, and femoral head) (Robert-Varvat et al., 2018). Nerve conduction velocities (NCVs) may also be reduced in asymptomatic gene carriers (Chance, 2006).

***Pressure palsies in polyneuropathy.*** Patients with polyneuropathy may have an increased susceptibility to pressure palsies. Areas of demyelination are more likely to have a depolarizing block produced by even mild pressure.

### Mononeuropathies

Table 26.3 shows some important peripheral nerve lesions of the arm. Table 26.4 shows some important peripheral nerve lesions of the leg.

***Median nerve.*** The most common median neuropathy is carpal tunnel syndrome, but other important anatomical lesions, including anterior interosseus syndrome and pronator teres syndrome, have been described.

**Carpal tunnel syndrome.** Carpal tunnel syndrome is the most common mononeuropathy. The median nerve is compressed as it passes under the flexor retinaculum at the wrist. Patients present with numbness on the palmar aspect of the first through the third digits. Forced flexion or extension of the wrist commonly exacerbates the sensory symptoms. Weakness of the abductor pollicis brevis may develop in advanced cases.

This condition would not normally be considered in the differential diagnosis for monoparesis, but because the patient can complain of weakness that is more extensive than the actual deficit, it is considered here. Clinical diagnosis can be confirmed by EMG.

**Anterior interosseus syndrome.** The anterior interosseous nerve is a branch of the median nerve in the forearm that supplies some of the forearm muscles. Damage can occur distal to the elbow, producing a syndrome that is essentially purely motor. Weakness of finger flexion is prominent. Affected muscles include the flexor digitorum profundus to the second and third digits (the portion to the fourth and fifth digits is innervated by the ulnar nerve). The distal median nerve entering the hand is unaffected because the anterior interosseous nerve arises from the main trunk of the median nerve.

Diagnosis is suspected by weakness of the median nerve–innervated finger flexors with sparing of the abductor pollicis brevis and ulnar nerve–innervated flexors. EMG can confirm the diagnosis.

**TABLE 26.3 Peripheral Nerve Lesions of the Arm**

| Lesion | Clinical Findings | Electromyography Findings |
|---|---|---|
| **Median Neuropathy** | | |
| Carpal tunnel syndrome | Weakness and wasting of abductor pollicis brevis if severe; sensory loss on palmar aspect of first through third digits | Slow median motor and sensory NCV through the carpal tunnel; denervation of abductor pollicis brevis if severe |
| Anterior interosseous syndrome | Weakness of flexor digitorum profundus, pronator quadratus, flexor pollicis longus | Denervation in flexor digitorum profundus, flexor pollicis longus, pronator quadratus |
| Pronator teres syndrome | Weakness of distal median-innervated muscles; tenderness of pronator teres | Slow median motor NCV through proximal forearm denervation of distal median-innervated muscles |
| Compression at the ligament of Struthers | Weakness of distal median-innervated muscles | As for pronator teres syndrome, with the addition of denervation of pronator teres |
| **Ulnar Neuropathy** | | |
| Palmar branch damage | Weakness of dorsal interossei; no sensory loss | Normal ulnar NCV; denervation of first dorsal interosseus but not abductor digiti minimi |
| Entrapment at Guyon canal | Weakness of ulnar intrinsic muscles; numbness over fourth and fifth digits | Slow ulnar motor and sensory NCV through wrist |
| Entrapment at or near the elbow | Weakness of ulnar intrinsic muscles; numbness over fourth and fifth digits | Slow ulnar motor NCV across elbow, denervation in first dorsal interosseus, abductor digiti minimi, and ulnar half of flexor digitorum profundus |
| **Radial Neuropathy** | | |
| Posterior interosseus syndrome | Weakness of finger and wrist extensors; no sensory loss | Denervation in wrist and finger extensors; sparing of the supinator and extensor carpi radialis |
| Compression at the spiral groove | Weakness of finger and wrist extensors; triceps usually spared; sensory loss on dorsal aspects of first digit | Slow radial motor NCV across spiral groove; denervation in distal radial-innervated muscles; triceps may be affected with proximal lesions |

*NCV*, Nerve conduction velocity.

**TABLE 26.4 Peripheral Nerve Lesions of the Leg**

| Lesion | Clinical Findings | Electromyography Findings |
|---|---|---|
| Sciatic neuropathy | Weakness of tibial- and peroneal-innervated muscles, with sensory loss on posterior leg and foot | Denervation distally in tibial- and peroneal-innervated muscles |
| Peroneal neuropathy | Weakness of foot extension and eversion and toe extension | Denervation in tibialis anterior; NCV across fibular neck may be slowed |
| Tibial neuropathy | Weakness of foot plantar flexion | Denervation of gastrocnemius |
| Femoral neuropathy | Weakness of knee extension; weakness of hip flexion if psoas involved | Denervation in quadriceps, sometimes psoas |

*NCV*, Nerve conduction velocity.

**Pronator teres syndrome.** The median nerve distal to the elbow can be damaged as it passes through the pronator teres muscle. All median-innervated muscles of the arm are affected except for the pronator teres itself. The clinical picture is that of an anterior interosseous syndrome plus distal median neuropathy. The pronator teres may be tender, and palpation may exacerbate some of the distal pain.

***Ulnar nerve.*** Ulnar entrapment is most common near the elbow and at the wrist. Entrapment at the elbow produces weakness of the ulnar-innervated intrinsic muscles. Weakness of long flexors of the fourth and fifth digits also can develop. When the entrapment is at the wrist, the weakness is isolated to the intrinsic muscles of the hand, and more proximal muscles are unaffected. Although most of the intrinsic muscles of the hand are ulnar innervated, a few are median innervated and are unaffected in ulnar neuropathy.

The diagnosis of ulnar neuropathy is suggested when a patient complains of pain or numbness on the ulnar aspect of the hand. Additional findings that support this diagnosis include weakness and wasting of the intrinsic muscles of the hand, which is especially easy to see in the first dorsal interosseous.

***Radial nerve palsy.*** Radial neuropathy is most commonly seen above the elbow, such that wrist and finger extensors are mainly affected. The triceps also can be affected. Radial nerve palsy is most commonly due to a pressure palsy in alcoholic intoxication. Peripheral neuropathy makes the development of pressure neuropathy of the radial nerve more likely.

***Femoral neuropathy.*** Femoral neuropathy can occur at the level of the lumbar plexus secondary to compression by intraabdominal contents (fetus or neoplasm), but we have also seen it from damage incurred during angiography or surgery. Patients present with pain in the thigh and weakness of knee extension. They usually report that the leg "gives out" during walking or that they cannot get out of a chair without using their arms. Examination may show quadriceps weakness, but this muscle group is so strong that the examiner may not be able to detect the deficit. Lower leg muscles must be examined to ensure that muscles in the sciatic distribution are normal. Diagnosis is confirmed by EMG showing denervation confined to the femoral nerve distribution. Unfortunately electrical signs of denervation may not be obvious for up to 4 weeks after the injury. CT of the abdomen and pelvis should be considered to evaluate for possible mass compression of the femoral nerve.

**TABLE 26.5 Radiculopathies**

| Level | Motor Deficit | Sensory Deficit |
|---|---|---|
| **Cervical Radiculopathy** | | |
| C5 | Deltoid, biceps | Lateral upper arm |
| C6 | Biceps, brachioradialis | Radial forearm and first and second digits |
| C7 | Wrist extensors, triceps | Third and fourth digits |
| C8 | Intrinsic hand muscles | Fifth digit and ulnar forearm |
| T1 | Intrinsic muscles of the hand, especially APB | Axilla |
| **Lumbar Radiculopathy** | | |
| L2 | Psoas, quadriceps | Lateral and anterior thigh |
| L3 | Psoas, quadriceps | Lower medial thigh |
| L4 | Tibialis anterior, quadriceps | Medial lower leg |
| L5 | Peroneus longus, gluteus medius, tibialis anterior, extensor hallucis longus | Lateral lower leg |
| S1 | Gastrocnemius, gluteus maximus | Lateral foot and fourth and fifth digits |

*APB*, Abductor pollicis brevis.

***Sciatic neuropathy.*** Sciatic neuropathy can have multiple causes, including acute trauma and chronic compressive lesions. The term *sciatica* describes pain in the distribution of the sciatic nerve in the back of the leg. It is usually due to radiculopathy (see "Radiculopathies," later). An intramuscular injection into the sciatic nerve rather than the gluteus muscle is an occasional cause of sciatic neuropathy, which is characterized by initial severe pain followed by a lesser degree of pain and weakness.

*Piriformis syndrome* is a condition in which the sciatic nerve is compressed by the piriformis muscle. This is a difficult diagnosis to make, requiring demonstration of increased pain on tensing the piriformis muscle by flexing and adducting the hip. Piriformis syndrome should be considered in patients presenting with symptoms and signs referable to the sciatic nerve but with no evident cause seen on imaging of the lumbar spine and plexus.

Diagnosis of sciatic neuropathy is considered when a patient presents with pain or weakness of the lower leg muscles. EMG can confirm the distribution of denervation. Nerve Conduction Study (NCS) are usually normal.

***Peroneal (Fibular) neuropathy.*** The *peroneal nerve* is appropriately designated as the *fibular nerve* in many modern scientific publications and texts because of its proximity to the fibula and to distinguish it from *perineal nerves*. Although this may become standard, we continue to use the term *peroneal* for this discussion. Peroneal neuropathy can develop from a lesion at the fibular neck, the popliteal fossa, or even the sciatic nerve in the thigh. The peroneal division of the sciatic nerve is more susceptible to injury than the tibial division, so incomplete sciatic injury affects predominantly the peroneal innervated muscles—tibialis anterior, extensor digitorum brevis, and peroneus. In addition, the peroneal division innervates the short head of the biceps femoris. This is an important muscle to remember because distal peroneal neuropathy spares it, whereas a proximal sciatic neuropathy, a peroneal division lesion, or a radiculopathy is expected to cause denervation not only in the tibialis anterior but also the short head of the biceps femoris (Marciniak et al., 2005).

## Radiculopathies

Radiculopathy produces weakness of one portion of a limb. Common radiculopathies are summarized in Table 26.5. Complete paralysis of all of the muscles of an arm or leg is not caused by radiculopathy other than in traumatic avulsion of multiple nerve roots. Roots serving arm power include chiefly C5 to T1. Roots serving leg power are chiefly L2 to S1. A lesion at the L5 level often elicits a complaint of weakness of the entire limb because of the foot drop, which interferes with gait. Reflex abnormalities are often present early in a radiculopathy and are a manifestation of the sensory component. Motor deficits develop with increasingly severe radiculopathy.

Radiculopathy should be suspected when a patient presents with pain radiating down one arm or leg, especially if neck or low back pain corresponding to the level of the deficit is a feature as well. Motor and sensory symptoms and signs should conform to one nerve root distribution.

Diagnosis of radiculopathy can be confirmed by MRI for structural evidence and EMG for signs of denervation.

## Plexopathies

***Brachial and lumbar plexitis (or plexopathy).*** Brachial plexitis, is an acute neuropathic syndrome of possible autoimmune etiology (Van Eijk et al., 2016). Other terms include brachial neuritis and neuralgic amyotrophy. Patients present with shoulder and arm pain followed by weakness as the pain abates. Eventual functional recovery is the rule, although this takes months and is occasionally incomplete. Brachial plexitis is somewhat more common than lumbosacral plexitis. The upper plexus, C5 and C6, is most commonly affected, although the lower plexus can be involved.

A diagnosis of plexitis is considered when a patient presents with single limb pain and weakness that does not follow a single root or nerve distribution. MRI appearance of the region is normal unless neoplastic infiltration has occurred.

NCS are usually normal except for slow or absent F waves. EMG may be normal initially but eventually shows denervation in the distribution of the affected portion of the plexus.

Differentiation of plexitis from radiculopathy is accomplished on the basis of not only the more extensive deficits in patients with plexitis but also the time course of pain followed by weakness as the pain abates; this pattern is not expected in patients with radiculopathy. EMG of paraspinal muscles at the level of involvement will show denervation changes in a radiculopathy but not a plexopathy. Sensory nerve action potentials may be lost distally in a plexopathy but not in a radiculopathy because of its preganglionic location, leaving the distal branches of the sensory neurons intact.

***Neoplastic plexus infiltration.*** The brachial and lumbar plexuses are in proximity to the areas that can be infiltrated by tumors, including those involving the lymph nodes, lungs, kidneys, and other abdominal organs. The first symptom of tumor infiltration is usually pain. Weakness and sensory loss are less common symptoms. Neoplastic plexus compression or infiltration manifests as a progressive painful monoparesis. Limb movements that stretch the plexus elicit pain, and the patient tends to hold the limb immobile to avoid exacerbating the pain.

Neoplastic infiltration of the brachial plexus usually involves the lower plexus, C8 to T1. Lung cancer and lymphoma are the most common tumors to cause this. Horner syndrome can develop with lower brachial plexus involvement. The main consideration in the differential diagnosis is radiation plexopathy. The diagnosis is suspected on the basis of the severe pain and weakness. EMG often shows denervation that spans single nerve and root distributions. Detailed knowledge of the plexus anatomy is essential during examination and EMG. MRI usually shows infiltration or compression of the plexus.

***Radiation plexopathy.*** Radiation therapy in the region of the plexus can produce progressive dysfunction. The upper brachial plexus is especially susceptible because of the lesser amount of surrounding tissues to attenuate the radiation. Symptoms are dysesthesias and weakness. The dysesthesias may be associated with discomfort but are seldom described as painful. This absence of pain is one key to differentiation from neoplastic plexus infiltration, which is typically quite painful.

Diagnosis is suspected in the clinical setting of progressive painless weakness in a patient with cancer who has received radiation to the region. MRI is essential for ruling out tumor infiltration. EMG shows denervation, which is not a differentiating feature, but myokymia is more commonly seen in patients with radiation plexopathy than in those with neoplastic infiltration.

***Plexopathy from hematomas.*** Hematomas can develop adjacent to the brachial and lumbosacral plexuses and compress them, producing motor and sensory findings. Brachial plexus hematomas are usually from bleeding disorders or instrumentation such as central line placement. Lumbosacral plexus hematomas can also develop from coagulopathies, including coagulopathy associated with anticoagulant treatment, and after procedures such as abdominal surgery or femoral artery catheterization.

The prognosis is generally good as long as the plexus or nerve has not been directly injured, because the condition is usually neurapraxia rather than neurotmesis, and conduction is usually restored when the blood is resorbed. Large hematomas should be considered for evacuation if severe plexus damage is present.

***Plexus trauma.*** A history of trauma makes the etiology of the plexopathy quite obvious. The main difficulty is in differentiating traumatic plexopathy from radiculopathy (nerve root avulsion) or peripheral nerve damage. Also, spinal cord damage must be considered because cord contusion and hematomyelia may manifest with weakness that is most prominent in one extremity. Motor vehicle accidents, childbirth, and occupational injuries are the most common causes of traumatic plexopathy. Forced extension of the arm over the head damages the lower plexus, with the intrinsic muscles of the hand being especially affected (Klumpke palsy). Forced depression of the shoulder produces damage to the upper plexus, producing prominent weakness of the deltoid, biceps, and other proximal muscles (Erb palsy).

Trauma includes not only stretch injury but also penetrating injury such as knife and bullet wounds. Knife wounds can easily damage the brachial plexus but are much less likely to involve the lumbosacral plexus. Gunshot wounds may directly affect either the brachial or lumbosacral plexus, and the shock waves of high-velocity bullets may damage the plexus without direct contact. Unfortunately the speed and extent of recovery from these types of injuries are poor.

Diagnostic studies should include imaging not only of the plexus but also of the adjacent spinal cord, looking for disc herniation, spondylosis, subluxation, or other anatomical deformity. Plain radiographs should be obtained to ensure skeletal integrity. MRI or CT of the region will visualize the soft tissues.

***Thoracic outlet syndrome.*** Thoracic outlet syndrome is an overdiagnosed condition characterized by weakness of muscles innervated by the lower trunk of the brachial plexus (Ferrante and Ferrante, 2017). The motor axons in the lower trunk supply both the median- and ulnar-innervated intrinsic muscles of the hand. Finger and wrist flexors occasionally may be affected, causing marked impairments in use of the hand, which is not restricted to a single nerve distribution. Sensory loss is mainly in an ulnar distribution, because the sensory fibers of the median nerve ascend through the middle trunk rather than the lower trunk.

Diagnosis of thoracic outlet syndrome depends on demonstration of low-amplitude median and ulnar nerve compound motor action potentials and ulnar sensory nerve action potentials. Median sensory nerve action potentials are normal. CT or MRI of the plexus may be necessary to rule out infiltration by nearby tumor. Imaging of the neck and cervical spine occasionally reveals cervical ribs. These are usually asymptomatic, so their presence does not confirm the diagnosis of thoracic outlet syndrome.

***Diabetic amyotrophy.*** Diabetic amyotrophy is a lumbar plexopathy affecting axons mainly forming the femoral nerve. Patients present with weakness and pain in a femoral nerve distribution. Although a length-dependent diabetic peripheral neuropathy may be an accompanying feature, the femoral distribution symptoms and signs overshadow the other findings. Patients eventually improve, although the recovery is often prolonged and incomplete. It is difficult to study the conduction of the femoral nerve, so this test is diagnostically helpful only if results are normal. EMG usually shows denervation, although up to 4 weeks may pass before electrical signs of axonal dysfunction are seen.

### Neuronopathies

Neuronal degenerations usually affect multiple individual nerve distributions and usually involve more than one limb. A few focal motor neuropathies, however, can produce single limb defects.

***Monomelic amyotrophy.*** Monomelic amyotrophy is a condition in which motoneurons of one limb degenerate; often the distribution suggests involvement of specific motoneuron columns in the spinal cord. The arm is more often affected than the leg. The opposite limb can be affected to a much lesser extent. Pain and sensory loss are not expected. Progressive weakness develops over months to years and may eventually plateau without further worsening. Onset usually is in young adulthood, at the age of approximately 20 years, and men are predominantly affected. Diagnosis is confirmed by clinical presentation and EMG findings.

***Poliomyelitis.*** Poliomyelitis is now uncommon but still occurs in some parts of the world. A poliomyelitis-like syndrome can result from viruses other than the poliovirus itself, including West Nile virus. The illness usually manifests with acute asymmetrical weakness after an initial phase of encephalitic symptoms including headache, meningeal signs, and possibly confusion or seizures. The paralysis may involve only one limb but is more commonly generalized. After recovery, only one limb may remain weak (monoparesis).

***Multifocal motor neuropathy.*** Multifocal motor neuropathy is a progressive autoimmune muscle disease commonly associated with anti-GM1 antibodies. A common presentation is predominant unilateral weakness, cramping, and fasciculations and wasting in the hand and arm, but the legs can also be affected. NCS show conduction block in noncompressible areas (Gilhus et al., 2010). Presentation is often confused with ALS but lacks UMN and bulbar involvement.

## PITFALLS IN THE DIFFERENTIAL DIAGNOSIS OF HEMIPLEGIA AND MONOPLEGIA

*Additional text available at http://expertconsult.inkling.com.*

*The complete reference list is available online at https://expertconsult.inkling.com/.*

27

# Paraplegia and Spinal Cord Syndromes

*Bruce H. Dobkin*

## OUTLINE



Paraplegia and quadriplegia may result from a variety of systemic and primary central nervous system medical conditions as well as trauma at all segmental levels of the spinal cord (Box 27.1). A spinal cord syndrome may develop from extramedullary and intramedullary pathological processes. Initial symptoms may be gradual in onset and progressive, including pain, dysesthesia, or subtle upper or lower extremity weakness. In other cases, such as an inflammatory myelitis, acute onset of severe motor, sensory, and autonomic deficits may develop without premonitory symptoms. Trauma from a cervical flexion-extension injury, for example, may produce a central cord injury of the lower cervical spinal cord with incomplete quadriparesis, whereas a complete transection injury at the lower thoracic spinal cord from a fall may result in complete paraplegia. Thus both the rostrocaudal segmental level of disease involvement or trauma and completeness of the lesion in the transverse plane anticipate the person's impairments and disability. Details about the relationships between specific spinal cord segments and sensory dermatomes are reviewed in Chapter 31, and the segmental innervations of specific muscle groups are reviewed in Chapters 32 and 33. The sensorimotor clinical examination enables localization of the lesion (Fig. 27.1).

When a patient who presents with paraparesis or paraplegia is being examined, a careful neurological examination is critical for planning additional diagnostic workup and care. Identifying distinct spinal cord syndromes and determining the likely location of the underlying pathological process will guide subsequent imaging and electrodiagnostic studies. As in most upper motor neuron or motor unit diseases, fatigability of strength occurs with repetitive movements against light resistance. For example, even when the initial manual muscle exam does not detect iliopsoas weakness, 10 leg raises from the supine position against light downward hand compression may reveal mild paresis upon immediately retesting hip flexion. Structural information about the integrity of the spine may be obtained from radiographic plain films and computed tomography (CT) for bone pathology. Myelography is indicated when extrinsic cord compression is suspected, especially when magnetic resonance imaging (MRI) is contraindicated. MRI with contrast best reveals intrinsic and extrinsic cord pathology. Spinal angiography identifies vascular pathology. A review of imaging of the spine is provided in Chapters 40 and 41.

Acute and long-term patient care is influenced by the clinical presentation, severity of neurological deficits, underlying pathology, and prognosis for gains over time. Patients presenting with an acute spinal cord syndrome after trauma show both early (days to 3 months) and late (up to 2 years) changes in their motor and sensory deficits (Fawcett et al., 2007). Both neurological improvements and clinical worsening may occur. When some sparing of sensation and movement is present in the first 72 hours after trauma, the prognosis for walking is rather good. Indeed, up to 90% of patients with a cervical central cord injury who have any spared sensation and movement below the level of injury by 4 weeks after trauma will become functional ambulators (Dobkin et al., 2006). Thus serial and careful neurological examinations are important for monitoring the injury-related deficits, especially in the first weeks after onset. Rehabilitation of patients with paraplegia follows after the acute medical needs have been addressed. The aim is to promote as much functional independence as possible with and without assistive devices, decrease the risk of complications, and reintegrate the patient into home and community. Neurological rehabilitation for paraparesis after spinal cord syndromes is reviewed in Chapter 55.

## COMMON SPINAL CORD SYNDROMES

The clinical presentation of a spinal cord injury depends on whether the injury is complete or spares selected fiber tracts. A number of clinically characterized spinal cord syndromes may develop as a result of the involvement of different portions of the spinal cord's gray and white matter.

### Spinal Shock

*Spinal shock* refers to the period of depressed spinal reflexes caudal to an acute spinal cord injury; it is followed by the emergence of pathological reflexes and return of cutaneous and muscle stretch reflexes (see Chapter 63). The bulbocavernosus and cremasteric reflexes commonly return before the ankle jerk, Babinski sign, and knee jerk.

**BOX 27.1 Differential Diagnosis of Diseases Affecting the Spinal Cord**

**Compressive Lesions**

***Nonneoplastic***

Trauma:
- Vertebral body fracture/dislocation
- Hyperextension injury
- Direct puncture, stab, or missile

Spondylosis:
- Cervical stenosis
- Lumbar stenosis

Intervertebral disc herniation
Infectious disorders (e.g., abscess, tuberculosis)
Inflammatory (e.g., rheumatoid arthritis, ankylosing spondylitis, sarcoid)
Hemorrhage:
- Epidural hematoma

Congenital disorders
Arachnoid cysts
Paget disease
Osteoporosis

***Neoplastic***

Epidural metastasis
Intradural extramedullary (e.g., meningioma, neurofibroma, leptomeningeal metastasis)
Intramedullary

***Noncompressive Myelopathies***

Demyelinating (e.g., MS, ADEM)
Hereditary (e.g., spastic paraplegia)
Viral myelitis (e.g., varicella-zoster, AIDS–related myelopathy, human T-lymphotropic virus type I infection)
Syringomyelia
Vitamin $B_{12}$ deficiency and other nutritional deficiencies
Infarction
Ischemia and hemorrhage from vascular malformations or cavernoma
Spirochetal diseases (syphilis and Lyme disease)
Toxic myelopathies (e.g., radiation-induced)
Autoimmune diseases (e.g., lupus, Sjögren syndrome)
Paraneoplastic
Neuronal degenerations
Tethered cord at the cauda equina
Acute and subacute transverse myelitis of unknown cause

*ADEM*, Acute disseminated encephalomyelitis; *AIDS*, acquired immunodeficiency syndrome; *MS*, multiple sclerosis.

## Incomplete Lesions of the Spinal Cord

### Unilateral Transverse Lesion

A hemisection lesion of the spinal cord causes a Brown-Séquard syndrome. A pure hemisection is unusual, but patients may show features of a unilateral lesion or hemisection. A Brown-Séquard lesion is characterized by ipsilateral weakness and loss of both vibration and position sense below the level of the injury. In addition, there is a loss of temperature and pain sensation below the level of the lesion on the contralateral side. As pain and temperature fibers extend rostrally a few segments before crossing the midline to enter the lateral spinothalamic tract, the loss of pain and temperature sensory modalities extends rostrally on the contralateral side to a segmental level that is a few segments below the level of the lesion. In addition, at the segmental level of the hemisection injury, a limited patch of ipsilateral loss of pain and temperature in combination with a lower motor neuron weakness is often detected. Brown-Séquard syndrome may be caused by a variety of etiologies but is commonly encountered after traumatic injuries, including bullet and stab wounds.

### Central Cord Syndrome

Traumatic cervical central cord syndrome is commonly characterized by the triad of (1) motor impairment disproportionately more severe in the upper than the lower extremities, (2) bladder dysfunction usually including urinary retention, and (3) sensory dysfunction of varying degrees. An international consensus group suggested that an upper and lower extremity difference of at least 10 motor score points, based on the Medical Research Council scale, can be considered as a quantitative addition to the commonly used qualitative criteria for making the diagnosis (van Middendorp et al., 2010). An additional clinical feature of the traumatic central cord syndrome is a dissociated sensory loss for pain and temperature, whereas vibration and position sense remain preserved. This sensory presentation may be explained by a direct injury to intramedullary decussating fibers, which normally would ascend contralaterally as part of the spinothalamic tract. As a result, a cape-like sensory deficit may be encountered in patients with a cervical level injury, but sensation within more caudal dermatomes would generally be spared (Fig. 27.2).

A traumatic central cord syndrome is mostly encountered in elderly patients who have suffered a relatively minor trauma in the form of a cervical hyperextension injury, commonly in the setting of an underlying cervical spondylosis. Falls and motor vehicle injuries are common etiologies. Syringomyelia or tumors may also produce a central cord syndrome.

### Anterior Spinal Artery Syndrome

An anterior cord syndrome involves the anterior two-thirds of the spinal cord, sparing the posterior columns. The corticospinal and spinothalamic tracts are both affected. The syndrome is clinically characterized by paralysis and sensory impairments below the level of the lesion, with impaired sensation of pain and temperature; vibration sense and proprioception are preserved. Fiber tracts for autonomic control are also typically compromised, resulting in bladder, bowel, and sexual dysfunction. In the acute phase after injury, a spinal shock phase with decreased muscle tone and areflexia may present, followed by a gradual return of reflexes and hypertonicity and perhaps spasms.

An anterior cord syndrome may be caused by trauma from central disc compression or a bone fragment as well as a myelitis. Vascular occlusive causes are perhaps the most common etiology. For instance, the anterior cord syndrome may present as a spinal cord stroke from atherothrombotic or embolic occlusion of the anterior spinal cord artery. Invasive vascular and thoracoabdominal surgical procedures may be complicated by impaired blood flow to the spinal cord, especially due to obstruction or hypoperfusion of the artery of Adamkiewicz near the T6 level. This may also follow surgery at the distal aorta and proximal iliac arteries with the use of aortic counterpulsation devices and, occasionally, from retroperitoneal hematomas or abscesses. Similarly, survivors of cardiac arrest and significant hypotensive episodes may demonstrate a midthoracic anterior cord ischemic syndrome, as the vascular supply near the T6 segment is particularly susceptible to distal field ischemia.

### Anterior Horn and Pyramidal Tract Syndromes

Paralysis may be encountered in the setting of motor impairments in combination with relative sparing of sensory and autonomic functions, as seen in motor neuron disease including amyotrophic lateral sclerosis (ALS). Lower motor neuron weakness with atrophy and loss

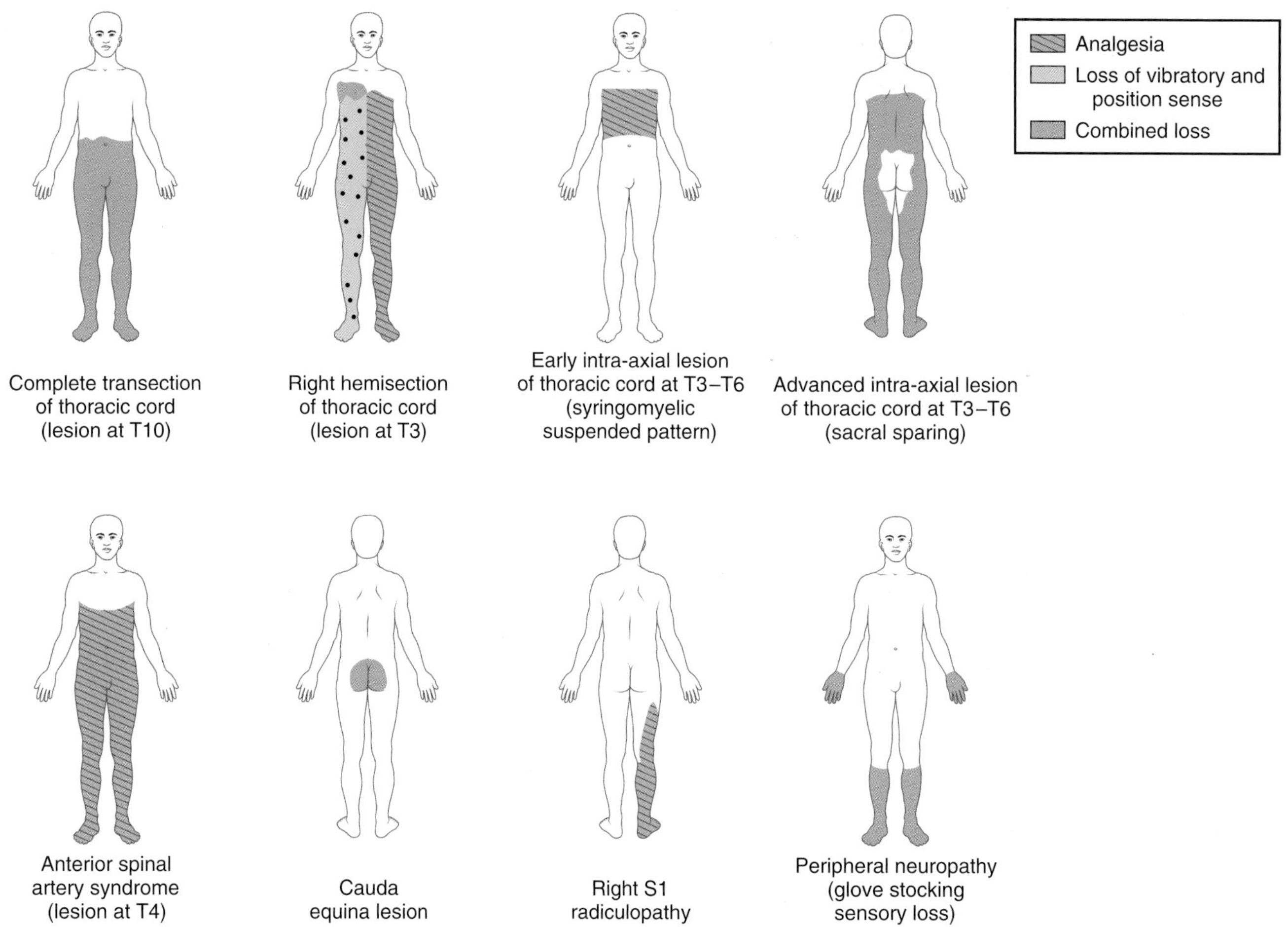


**Fig. 27.1** Characteristic sensory disturbances found in various spinal cord lesions in comparison with peripheral neuropathy.

of reflexes is typically seen in combination with upper motor neuron weakness, signs of spasticity, and hyperreflexia. Different limbs may be affected to various degrees, but symptoms are progressive over the course of the disease. However, innervation of the external anal and urethral sphincters is normally preserved in ALS, with sparing of bladder and bowel function.

### Combined Posterior and Lateral Column Disease

A clinical syndrome characterized by the development of a spastic ataxic gait pattern may be caused by lesions affecting the posterior and lateral white matter tracts. Friedreich ataxia represents a genetic etiology, and vitamin $B_{12}$ deficiency may result in subacute combined degeneration with spastic paretic gait and sensory ataxia. Dorsal horn and column injury alone may result from tabes dorsalis.

## CHARACTERISTIC CLINICAL FEATURES OF LESIONS AT DIFFERENT LEVELS

Paralysis may be caused by lesions at any segmental level of the spinal cord from both intramedullary and extramedullary disease. The characteristic symptoms and signs affecting motor and sensory functions typically depend on the segmental level of injury.

### Foramen Magnum and Upper Cervical Spine

When structural lesions are located in or adjacent to the foramen magnum, several different neurological patterns are possible. For example, brainstem signs may occur together with symptoms from a spinal cord injury. Involvement of the lower portion of the brainstem is suggested by speech impairments, including dysarthria and dysphonia, as well as by dysphagia. In addition, facial numbness and nystagmus may be detected in association with tumors or other structural lesions in the foramen magnum. When compression of the spinal cord occurs, long-tract signs may present from injury to the corticospinal tract with, for instance, a spastic hemiparesis or quadriparesis. A lower motor neuron injury component may also be detectable from lesions at the craniocervical junction and the foramen magnum, with upper extremity weakness, muscular atrophy, and decreased muscle stretch reflexes.

Several pathological processes and lesions may be present at the level of the foramen magnum and its immediate vicinity. These conditions include Arnold-Chiari malformations; traumatic injuries; rheumatoid arthritis; syringomyelia; vascular lesions such as vertebral artery thrombosis, dissection, or an arteriovenous malformation; and a variety of tumors including meningiomas. Multiple sclerosis may also cause intramedullary lesions of the brainstem and the upper cervical spinal cord and selectively affect long white matter tracts. Imaging studies, especially MRI, help determine the nature and precise anatomical location for pathological processes in the foramen magnum and upper cervical spine region.

Lesions affecting the uppermost portion of the cervical spine may be challenging to diagnose owing to a nonlocalizing symptom complex upon initial presentation. Pain is a common early symptom and may be localized to the neck or occipital region. Sometimes the pain may be aggravated by neck movement. When upper cervical nerve roots are compressed, a radicular pain may present in the corresponding

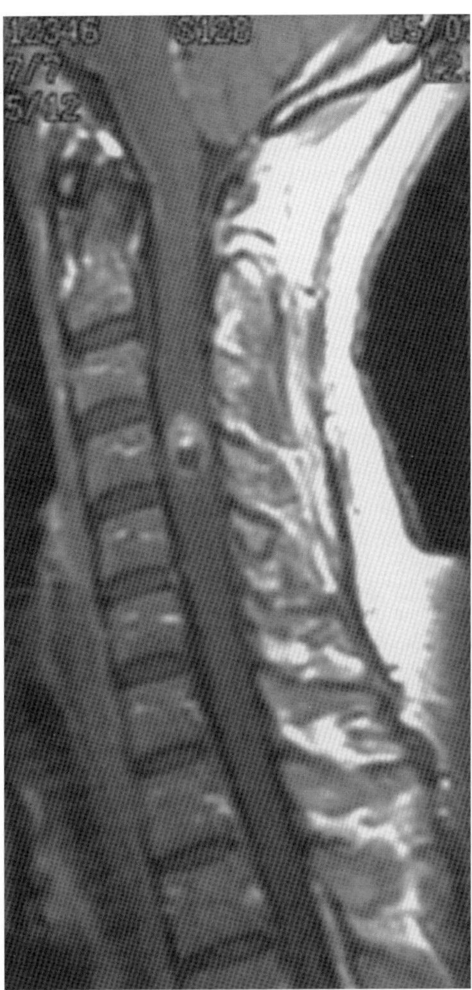

Fig. 27.2 Magnetic resonance image of the cervical spine showing a contrast-enhancing mass. Patient presented with a cape-like sensory loss for pain and temperature. Resection of the mass revealed a glioma.

dermatome. Irritation of the second cervical nerve root, for example, may present with a pain localized within the posterior aspect of the scalp, whereas an injury to the third and fourth nerve roots may induce pain projected to the neck or shoulder. A lower motoneuron injury presentation with upper extremity muscular weakness and atrophy may also be part of the clinical presentation. When the spinal cord is compressed by epidural or subdural space-occupying lesions, spastic weakness of upper and lower extremities typically follows.

An injury or disease process affecting the upper cervical spinal cord may also compromise breathing. Normal respiration requires functional use of the diaphragm muscle, which is innervated by the phrenic nerve. Motoneurons contributing to the phrenic nerve are located within the cervical spinal cord and contribute efferent axons to the C3–C5 ventral roots. Therefore complete injuries affecting the spinal cord above the C3 segment will compromise the function of the diaphragm, and respiratory failure may follow.

## Lower Cervical and Upper Thoracic Spine

Injuries to the lower part of the cervical spine and upper thoracic spine may be caused by extramedullary compression of nerve roots and the spinal cord or by an intramedullary disease process. The correlation between presenting symptoms and localization of the underlying lesion is most precise for the extramedullary pathological processes (e.g., tumors, herniated discs) that compress individual segmental nerve roots or spinal nerves. Intramedullary lesions may also present with pain, but the segmental localization is commonly less precise.

Extramedullary lesions typically first irritate segmental nerve roots and the spinal nerve, with radicular pain and sensory deficits typically following the corresponding dermatomal distribution. Similarly, motor deficits involve each myotome affected by the lesion. Muscle stretch reflexes may also provide helpful information with regard to the primary level of injury, as the affected segmental reflex is typically depressed or absent and caudal reflexes are hyperactive. For instance, when a lesion is at the C4–C6 level, a radicular pattern of pain and sensory symptoms may typically involve the radial side of the arm, forearm, and hand. Motor deficits include weakness in elbow flexion. In addition, the biceps and brachioradialis muscle stretch reflexes may be depressed or absent, especially when the C5–C6 levels are involved.

In contrast, lesions at the C7–T1 level usually present with pain and sensory impairments over the ulnar side of the upper extremity, including the arm, forearm, and hand. Motor deficits related to affected myotomes commonly involve elbow extension, the intrinsic hand muscles, and the triceps reflex.

Lower and upper motoneuron signs may also be present in adjacent segments. If segmental nerve roots and the spinal cord are compressed by a herniated disc or space-occupying lesion at the C5–C6 level, for example, a decreased brachioradialis reflex may reflect a C6 radiculopathy, whereas a brisk and hyperactive finger flexor reflex reflects an upper motoneuron syndrome.

## Thoracic Levels

Traumatic spinal cord injury at the thoracic level usually produces a complete lesion. The segmental level of injury is best determined by a careful sensory examination of dermatomes. Useful clinical landmarks are the nipple line for the T4 dermatome and the umbilicus for the T10 dermatome. Pain may follow a radicular pattern around the chest or abdomen corresponding to the segmental levels of injury. Sensory testing of pin, temperature, pressure, and light touch appreciation may determine the most caudal dermatome of normal sensation as well as a zone of partial preservation. The sensory testing should include evaluation of dermatomes of the left and right side of the body, with comparisons of homologous levels. In addition to a combination of at-level pain, sensory deficits, and muscular weakness, autonomic dysfunction may develop from long-tract involvement and include urinary retention, bladder sphincter dyssynergia, and bladder hyperreflexia.

## Conus Medullaris and Cauda Equina

The conus medullaris of the spinal cord terminates approximately at the level of the L1 vertebra, although the precise location of the tip of the conus may show marked variability between subjects. This anatomical aspect of the spinal cord is important because spinal trauma commonly takes place at the thoracolumbar junction, and the extent of such injuries is highly variable (Kingwell et al., 2008). Traumatic injuries to the conus medullaris usually result in weakness or paralysis of the lower extremities, absence of lower extremity reflexes, and saddle anesthesia (Fig. 27.3). However, some patients with conus medullaris injuries exhibit a mixed upper and lower motoneuron syndrome. In contrast, a cauda equina injury that lesions lumbosacral roots below the level of the conus medullaris is a pure lower motoneuron syndrome. Cauda equina injuries present with lower extremity weakness, areflexia, decreased muscle tone, and variable sensory deficits. At least one-third of these patients suffer considerable central pain. Affected limb and pelvic floor muscles develop flaccid weakness, and electromyography shows denervation after either a conus medullaris or cauda equina injury, especially following anatomically complete lesions.

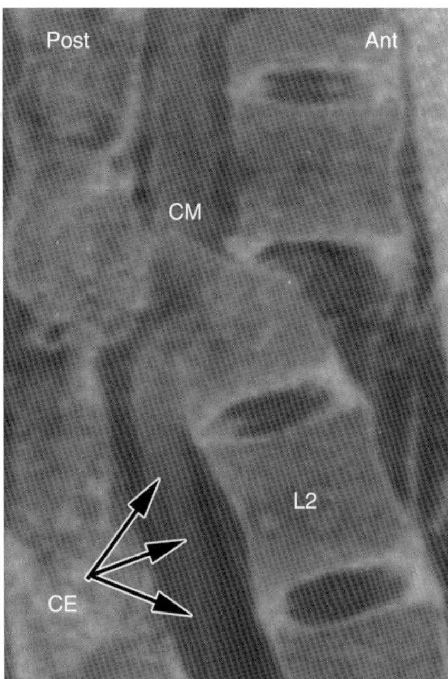


**Fig. 27.3** Magnetic resonance imaging demonstrating the effects of trauma to the thoracolumbar portion of the spine with a crush injury of the cauda equina (CE) and conus medullaris (CM) portion of the spinal cord. Note T12–L1-level spine fracture and dislocation.

Both conus medullaris and cauda equina injuries are associated with bladder, bowel, and sexual dysfunction. Urodynamic evaluations typically demonstrate detrusor areflexia, and a rectal exam identifies a flaccid anal sphincter. In addition, the bulbocavernosus reflex is typically absent or diminished, and reflexogenic erection in males is commonly lost.

Imaging studies (e.g., plain radiographs, CT, MRI) identify structural pathology. Burst fractures and fracture dislocations are common injuries to the spinal column that result in neurological deficits, suggesting a conus medullaris or cauda equina involvement. Following trauma to the thoracolumbar spine, imaging studies can be used to assess spinal stability and identify detailed aspects of spinal fractures, including the presence and location of bone fragments, spinal canal encroachment, epidural hematomas, and herniated discs. A variety of treatment options exist (e.g., surgical stabilization of the spine, decompression of the conus medullaris and nerve roots).

A lumbar spinal stenosis due to a congenitally small-diameter spinal canal or central disc and spondylotic narrowing one or more levels below L1 may present with a subtle course. Over months to years, lower extremity numbness or pain, usually in an L3–S1 single or multiradicular pattern, accompanies standing and walking, often gradually progressing to limit walking distance. Pain is commonly accompanied by weakness, but patients may not be aware of their deficit. Clinical insight into this diagnosis and the upper level of cauda compression is gained by a manual muscle examination after a few minutes of being supine, followed by having the subject walk for about 500 ft and then immediately retesting strength. Transient paresis or greater paresis in the affected root distribution is often found immediately after the walk and resolves within a minute or two.

## PAIN AND AUTONOMIC DYSFUNCTION

In addition to motor and sensory impairments, pain and dysfunction in the autonomic nervous system can aid in the localization of spinal cord syndromes. Pain is frequently associated with spinal cord injuries, along with autonomic impairments that may affect blood pressure and heart rate, bladder, bowel, sexual, and cardiorespiratory function. The type and severity of autonomic dysfunction depends on the location of pathology and severity of the spinal cord injury. International spinal cord injury societies recommend a systematic approach to the documentation of remaining autonomic function after a spinal cord injury (Alexander et al., 2009).

### Pain Syndromes

Distinct pain syndromes may develop as a result of compression, inflammation, or injury to the vertebral column, ligaments, dura mater, nerve roots, dorsal horn, and ascending spinal cord sensory tracts. Neuropathic pain may take the form of *paresthesia* (abnormal but not unpleasant sensation that is either spontaneous or evoked), *dysesthesia* (an abnormal unpleasant sensation that is spontaneous or evoked), *allodynia* (pain evoked by ordinary stimuli such as touch or rubbing), and *hyperalgesia* (an augmented response to a stimulus that is usually painful).

### Local Pain

Localized neck or back pain may result from irritation or injury to innervated spine structures including ligaments, periosteum, and dura. The pain is typically deep and aching, may vary with a change in position, and often becomes worse from increased load or weight bearing on affected structures. Percussion or palpation over the spine may in some patients worsen the local pain. When the injured or diseased spinal structures are irritated, secondary symptoms may develop, including muscle spasm and a more diffusely located pain. Musculoligamentous sources of pain often persist for more than a week after spinal surgery and develop with compensatory overuse of joints and muscles. Such pain must be distinguished from central neurogenic pain but can also amplify it.

### Projected Pain

A pathological process involving the facet joints may be experienced as focal or radiating pain in an upper or lower extremity. When a nerve root is irritated or injured, the projected pain is radicular.

Radicular pain commonly has a sharp, stabbing quality or causes dysesthesia. It may be exacerbated by activities that stretch the affected nerve root (e.g., straight leg raising or flexion of the neck). Straining or coughing may also increase the intensity and severity of radicular pain. Nerve root irritation may also result in sensory and motor deficits following the same dermatome and myotome distribution as the affected nerve root. This helps localize the level of spinal cord injury that is causing paraplegia.

### Central Neurogenic Pain

*Paresthesia*, *dysesthesia*, *allodynia*, and *hyperalgesia* accompany injury to the spinal cord in at least half of patients and also occur after thalamocortical stroke. Regardless of segmental level or completeness of injury, most patients with a traumatic spinal cord injury develop a clinically significant pain syndrome at some time after sustaining the lesion (Waxman and Hains, 2006). Neuropathic pain after spinal cord injury may affect different locations. At-level pain is primarily derived from local cellular and neuroplastic changes in the dorsal horn and sensory roots at the segments of injury. Below-level pain is located in body segments receiving innervation from the spinal cord caudal to the lesioned segments. Above-level neurogenic pain is less common.

Pain developing after a spinal cord injury is commonly described as burning, pricking, or aching in quality. It can be experienced as deep or superficial. Some patients develop a severe and excruciating pain syndrome after cord or cauda trauma that is at-level and below-level even in the absence of any cutaneous or proprioceptive sensation, which requires centrally acting medications to control. The medication most recently approved by the US Food and Drug Administration for spinal pain is pregabalin. The mechanisms for such painful phantom phenomena are not well understood but include structural and molecular dorsal horn, thalamic, and cortical adaptations to ordinary and noxious inputs.

## Autonomic Dysreflexia

Injuries to the spinal cord that result in paraplegia from a lesion above T6 may also impair autonomic control and result in episodes of severe hypertension or hypotension. Autonomic dysreflexia represents an acute syndrome characterized by excessive and uncontrolled sympathetic output from the spinal cord. As a result, the blood pressure is suddenly and markedly elevated. Associated symptoms include headache; malaise; blurring of vision; flushed, sweaty skin above the level of injury; and pale, cool skin below it. An episode of autonomic dysreflexia can be triggered by any noxious stimulus below the segmental level of injury. Common triggers include bladder distention, constipation, rectal fissures, joint injury, and urinary tract infection. Autonomic dysreflexia may present soon after the initial injury but more commonly becomes symptomatic several months after the spinal cord injury. Prevention is the best approach. Treatment of acute symptoms targets removal of noxious stimuli and cautious lowering of the blood pressure (see Chapter 63).

## Bowel and Bladder Dysfunction

Normal bladder and bowel control depend on segmental reflexes involving both autonomic and somatic motor neurons as well as descending and ascending tracts of the spinal cord (Fowler et al., 2008). As a result, bladder and bowel function may be impaired after an injury to any segmental level of the spinal cord. Different clinical syndromes develop depending on whether the injury or disease process affects the sacral spinal cord directly or higher segmental levels. Traumatic spinal cord injuries with paraplegia taking place above the T12 vertebra will interrupt spinal cord long-tract connections between supraspinal micturition centers in the brainstem and cerebral cortex and the sacral spinal cord. An upper motoneuron syndrome follows, with detrusor-sphincter dyssynergia caused by impaired coordination of autonomic and somatic motor control of the bladder detrusor and external urethral sphincter, respectively. Incomplete bladder emptying results. In addition, the upper motoneuron syndrome also includes detrusor hyperreflexia with increased pressure within the bladder. In contrast, injury to the T12 vertebra and below results in a direct lesion to the sacral spinal cord and associated nerve roots. A direct lesion to preganglionic parasympathetic neurons and somatic motoneurons of the Onuf nucleus located within the S2–S4 spinal cord segments results in the denervation of pelvic targets. Injuries to both the conus medullaris and cauda equina present as a lower motoneuron syndrome characterized by weak or flaccid detrusor function. Urinary retention follows, with risk of overflow incontinence. The goal of all bladder care is to avoid retrograde urine flow, urinary tract infections, and renal failure. Management of both upper and lower motoneuron bladder impairment commonly includes clean intermittent bladder catheterizations. Chapter 45 discusses evaluation and treatment.

*The complete reference list is available online at https://expertconsult.inkling.com/.*

28

# Proximal, Distal, and Generalized Weakness

*Komal T. Sawlani, Christopher D. Geiger*

## OUTLINE



Muscle weakness may be due to disorders of the central nervous system (CNS) or peripheral nervous system (PNS). The PNS includes the primary sensory neurons in the dorsal root ganglia, nerve roots, peripheral nerves, neuromuscular junctions, and muscles. Although not strictly peripheral, the primary motor neurons (anterior horn cells) in the brainstem and spinal cord are also conventionally included as part of the PNS. The neurological examination allows separation of the causes of weakness arising at these different locations. If the pattern of weakness is characteristic of upper motor neuron (UMN) dysfunction (i.e., weakness of upper-limb extensors and lower-limb flexors) together with hyperreflexia and extensor plantar responses, the weakness clearly is of CNS origin. Weakness with sensory loss may occur in both CNS disorders and disorders of the nerve roots and peripheral nerves. Weakness without sensory loss may also occur from CNS disorders, but in the PNS, this pattern of weakness occurs in disorders of the anterior horn cell, neuromuscular junction, or muscle. Rarely in the PNS are peripheral motor fibers the site of pathology (i.e., multifocal motor neuropathy with conduction block [MMNCB]). Although fatigue often accompanies most disorders of weakness, marked fatigue, especially when involving the extraocular, bulbar, and proximal upper limb muscles, often indicates a disorder of the neuromuscular junction.

The motor unit is the primary building block of the PNS and includes the anterior horn cell, its motor nerve, terminal nerve fibers, and all their accompanying neuromuscular junctions and muscle fibers. This chapter concentrates on disorders of the motor unit and disorders that may also involve the peripheral sensory nerves. The pattern of weakness often localizes the pathological process to the primary neurons, nerve roots, peripheral nerves, neuromuscular junctions, or muscles. Muscle weakness changes functional abilities that are more or less specific to the muscle groups affected. Recognizable patterns of symptoms and signs often allow a reasonable estimation of the anatomical involvement. Identifying these patterns is the first step in the differential diagnosis of weakness, as certain disorders affect specific muscle groups. This chapter begins with a review of the symptoms and signs of muscular weakness with respect to the muscle groups affected. A discussion follows of the bedside examinations, functional examinations, and laboratory tests often used in evaluating patients with muscle weakness. The chapter concludes with an approach to the differential diagnosis of muscle weakness based on which muscle groups are weak, whether the muscle weakness is constant or fluctuating, and whether the disorder is genetic or acquired.

## CLINICAL PRESENTATION BY AFFECTED REGION

### General Considerations

As muscles begin to weaken, the associated clinical features depend more on which muscles are involved than on the cause of involvement. A complicating factor in evaluating weakness is the patient's interpretation of the term *weak*. Although physicians use this term to denote a loss of muscle power, patients tend to apply it more loosely in describing their symptoms. Even more confusing, many people use the words *numb* and *weak* interchangeably, so the clinician should not accept a complaint of weakness at face value; the patient should be questioned further until it is clear that weakness means loss of muscle strength.

If the patient has no objective weakness when examined, the clinician must rely on the history. In patients with weak muscles, a fairly stereotypical set of symptoms emerges according to which muscle groups are weak (discussed later in this section). The patient whose weakness is caused by depression or malingering has vague symptoms, avoids answering leading questions, and the stereotypical symptoms of weakness are seldom volunteered. Instead, these patients make such statements as "I just can't do (the task)," or "I can't climb the stairs because I get so tired and have to rest." When pressed regarding these symptoms, it becomes apparent that specific details are lacking. Patients who cannot get out of a low chair because of real weakness explain exactly how they have to maneuver themselves into an upright position (e.g., pushing on the chair arms, leaning forward in the seat, and bracing their hands against the furniture). The examiner should avoid providing patients with clinical details they appear to be searching for. Asking whether pushing on the arms of the chair is required to stand up provides the patient with key information that may later be used in response to the questions of baffled successive examiners. In addition, it often is difficult to differentiate true muscle weakness from apparent weakness that accompanies tendon or joint contractures or is secondary to pain. For example, patients with primary orthopedic conditions often complain of weakness. In these patients, however, pain with passive or active motion often is a prominent part of the symptoms.

In evaluating weakness, the first key task is to discern which muscle groups are affected. In this regard, it is helpful to consider the involvement of specific body regions: ocular; facial and bulbar; neck, diaphragm, and axial; proximal upper extremity; distal upper extremity; proximal lower extremity; and distal lower extremity.

### Ocular Muscles

Extraocular muscle weakness results in ptosis or diplopia. When looking in the mirror, the patient may notice drooping of the eyelids, or family and friends may point it out. It is important to keep in mind that ptosis occasionally develops in older patients as a consequence of aging (i.e., partial dehiscence of the levator muscles) or a sequela of ocular surgery (i.e., lens implantation for cataracts). To differentiate between acute and chronic ptosis, it helps to look at prior photographs. Because the ocular myopathies often are familial, examination of family members is useful. Bilateral ptosis may result in compensatory backward tilting of the neck to look ahead or upward. Rarely, this postural adaptation may lead to neck pain and fatigue as the prominent symptoms. In addition, true ptosis often results in compensatory contraction of the frontalis muscles to lessen the ptosis, resulting in a characteristic pattern of a droopy eyelid with prominent forehead furrowing produced by contraction of the frontalis muscle. Weakness of extraocular muscles may result in diplopia. Mild diplopia, however, may cause only blurring of vision, sending the patient to the ophthalmologist for new eyeglasses. It is also worth asking the patient whether closing one eye corrects the diplopia because neuromuscular weakness is not among the causes of monocular diplopia.

### Facial and Bulbar Muscles

Patients experience facial weakness as a feeling of stiffness or sometimes as a twisting or altered perception in the face (note that patients often use the word *numbness* in describing facial weakness). Drinking through a straw, whistling, and blowing up balloons are all particularly difficult tasks for these patients and may be sensitive tests for facial weakness, particularly when such weakness dates from childhood. Acquaintances may notice that the patient's expression is somehow changed. A pleasant smile may turn into a snarl because of weakness of the levator anguli oris muscles. In lower facial weakness, patients may notice drooling and difficulty retaining their saliva, often requiring them to carry a tissue in the hand—the so-called napkin sign—which often accompanies bulbar involvement in amyotrophic lateral sclerosis (ALS). A common observation in mild, long-standing facial weakness, as in patients with facioscapulohumeral (FSH) muscular dystrophy, is a tendency for the patient to sleep with the eyes open from weakness of the orbicularis oculi. Weakness of masticatory muscles may result in difficulty chewing, sometimes with a sensation of fatigue and discomfort, as may occur with myasthenia gravis (MG). Pharyngeal, palatal, and tongue weakness disturbs speech and swallowing. A flaccid palate is associated with nasal regurgitation, choking spells, and aspiration of liquids. Speech may become slurred or acquire a nasal or hoarse quality. In contrast with central lesions, no problem with fluency or language function is observed.

### Neck, Diaphragm, and Axial Muscles

Neck muscle weakness becomes apparent when the patient must stabilize the head. Riding as a passenger in a car that brakes or accelerates, particularly in emergencies, may be disconcerting for the patient with neck weakness because the head rocks forward or backward. Similarly, when the patient is stooping or bending forward, weakness of the posterior neck muscles may cause the chin to fall on the chest. A patient with neck-flexion weakness often notices difficulty lifting the head off the pillow in the morning. As neck weakness progresses, patients may develop the *dropped head syndrome*, in which they no longer can extend the neck, and the chin rests against the chest (Fig. 28.1). This posture leads to several secondary difficulties, especially with vision and swallowing.

Shortness of breath often develops when diaphragm muscles weaken, especially when individuals lie flat or must exert themselves. These symptoms can be mistakenly attributed to lung or heart disease. Severe diaphragmatic weakness leads to hypoventilation and carbon dioxide retention. This may first be manifested as morning headaches or vivid nightmares. Later, hypercapnia results in sedation and a depressed

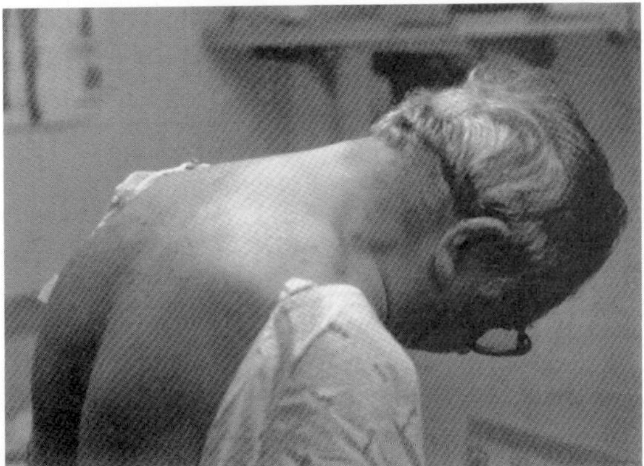

**Fig. 28.1 Dropped Head Syndrome.** With severe weakness of the neck extensor muscles, the patient no longer can extend the neck, and the chin rests against the chest.

mental state. Rarely, axial and trunk muscles can be involved early in the course of a neuromuscular disorder. Weakness of the abdominal muscles may make sit-ups impossible. Focal weakness of the lower abdominal muscles results in an obvious protuberance that superficially mimics an abdominal hernia. Patients with weakness of the paraspinal muscles are unable to maintain a straight posture when sitting or standing, although they can do so when lying on the bed (so-called *bent spine syndrome*).

### Proximal Upper Extremity

A feeling of tiredness often is the first expression of shoulder weakness. The weight of the arms is sufficient to cause fatigue. Early on, the patient experiences fatigue while performing sustained tasks with the hands held up, especially over the head. The most problematic activities include painting the ceiling, shampooing or combing the hair, shaving, and simply trying to lift an object off a high shelf.

### Distal Upper Extremity

Hand and forearm weakness interferes with many common activities of daily living. Difficulty with activities that require dexterity, such as buttoning and using a zipper, is an early sign. With further decreased hand strength, other activities affected include opening a jar, turning on a faucet or the car ignition, using a key, holding silverware, writing, and opening a car door.

### Proximal Lower Extremity

Weakness of the proximal lower extremities often is responsible for the earliest symptoms experienced by patients who develop weakness. Patients notice that they have difficulty arising from the floor or from a low chair and have to use the support of the hands or knees. Getting out of a bath or getting up from a toilet without handrails is particularly difficult. Older patients may attribute this limitation to arthritis or some similar minor problem. Walking becomes clumsy, and the patient may stumble. In descending stairs, people with quadriceps weakness tend to keep the knee locked and stiff. If the knee bends slightly as the weight of the body transfers to the lower stair, the knee may collapse. Greater problems with coming down stairs than with going up suggest quadriceps weakness, whereas the reverse is true for hip extensor weakness. Once patients with hip-girdle weakness are up and on level ground, they feel more secure. Family and friends, however, often will notice an obvious change in the affected person's gait. In patients with hip-girdle weakness, a waddling gait often develops because weakness of the hip abductors of the weight-bearing leg results in the hip's falling as the patient walks (*Trendelenburg gait*).

### Distal Lower Extremity

Symptoms localized to deficits in the anterior compartment (i.e., peroneal muscle weakness) often constitute the first sign of weakness of the distal lower extremity. Weakness of the anterior tibial and ankle evertor muscles often results in tripping, even over small obstacles, and an increased tendency to repeatedly sprain the ankle. If the weakness becomes severe, a foot drop develops, and the gait incorporates a slapping component. To compensate for the foot drop, patients must raise the knee higher when they walk so that the sagging foot and toes clear the floor *(steppage gait)*. Weakness of both anterior and posterior muscles of the lower leg often makes the stance unstable, which causes the patient to complain of poor balance. Isolated weakness of the posterior calf muscles makes standing on tiptoes impossible.

## BEDSIDE EXAMINATION OF THE WEAK PATIENT

The neurological examination of patients with muscle weakness is the same as that used for patients with other neurological problems. Special attention to the observational and functional components of the evaluation, however, is particularly rewarding in the patient with weakness.

### Observation

It is useful to spend a few moments observing the patient and noting natural posture and motion. When patients, particularly children, are aware of the examination, they often concentrate on performing as normally as possible. When unaware of scrutiny, their posture and movements may be more natural. At one time or another, we have heard the parent's exasperated cry, "He never does it that way at home." For example, ptosis may be obvious on inspection of the head and neck. The more severe the ptosis, the greater the patient's tendency to throw the head backward. The eyebrows are elevated and the forehead wrinkled in an attempt to raise the upper lids. This sometimes is so successful that ptosis is apparent only when the examiner smooths out the wrinkled forehead and allows the eyebrows to assume a more normal position. Psychogenic ptosis is easy to detect: the lower lid elevates with contraction of both parts of the orbicularis oculi muscles (i.e., blepharospasm) to accompany the lowered upper lid.

Weakness of the facial muscles present since childhood may give a smooth, unlined appearance to the adult face. In addition, facial expression diminishes or changes. A smile may become a grimace or a snarl, with eversion of the upper lip. The normal blink may slow, or eyelid closure may be incomplete so that the sclera is always visible. The normal preservation of the arch of the upper lip may be lost, and the mouth may assume either a tented or a straight-line configuration. Actual wasting of the facial muscles is difficult to see, but temporalis and masseter atrophy produce a characteristic scalloped appearance above and below the cheekbone. Because rearranging the hair style may cover the muscle wasting, the examiner should make a conscious effort to check the upper portion of the patient's face. The tongue is inspected for atrophy and fasciculations. Inspecting the tongue at rest with the mouth open, looking for the random irregular twitching movements of fasciculations, is the best method. When the tongue is fully protruded, many patients have some normal quivering movements that can easily be mistaken for fasciculations. It is wise to diagnose fasciculations of the tongue only when there is associated atrophy.

Facial weakness causes the normal labial sounds (that of *p* and *b*) to be softened. The examiner with a practiced ear can detect other alterations of speech. Lower motor neuron (LMN) involvement of the palate and tongue gives speech a hollow, nasal, echoing timbre, whereas UMN dysfunction causes the speech to be monotonous, forced, and strained. Laryngeal weakness may also be noticed in speech when the voice becomes harsh or brassy, often associated with loss of the glottal stop (the small sound made by the larynx closing, as at the start of a cough).

Weakness of the shoulder muscles causes a characteristic change in posture. Normally, the shoulders brace back by means of the tone of the muscles, so the hands are positioned with the thumbs forward when the arms are by the side. As the shoulder muscles lose their tone, the point of the shoulder rotates forward. This forward rotation of the shoulder is associated with a rotation of the arm so that the backs of the hands now are forward facing. In addition, the loss of tone causes a rather loose swinging movement of the arms in normal walking. When shoulder weakness is severe, the patient may fling the arms by using a movement of the trunk, rather than lifting the arms in the normal fashion. In the most extreme example, the only way the patient can get the hand above the head on a wall is to use a truncal movement to throw the whole arm upward and forward so the hand rests on the wall and then to creep the hand up the wall using finger movements. Atrophy of the pectoral muscles leads to the development of a horizontal or upward sloping of the anterior axillary fold. This is especially the case in FSH muscular dystrophy. The examiner may observe *winging of the scapula*, a characteristic finding in weakness of muscles that normally fix the scapula to the thorax (e.g., the serratus anterior, rhomboid, or trapezius). As these muscles become weak, any attempted movement of the arm causes the scapula to rise off the back of the rib cage and protrude similarly to a small wing. The arm and shoulder act as a crane—the boom of the crane is the arm, and the base is the scapula. Obviously, if the base is not fixed, any attempt to use the crane results in the whole structure's falling over. This is the operative mechanism with attempts to elevate the arm; the scapula simply pops off the back of the chest wall in a characteristic fashion. In the most common type of winging, the entire medial border of the scapula protrudes backward. In some diseases, particularly FSH muscular dystrophy, the inferomedial angle juts out first, and the entire scapula rotates and rides up over the back. This often is associated with a *trapezius hump*, in which the middle part of the trapezius muscle in the web of the neck mounds over the upper border of the scapula. Note that when examining a slender person or a child, in whom prominent shoulder blades are common, the shoulder configuration returns to normal with forcible use of the arm, as in a pushup.

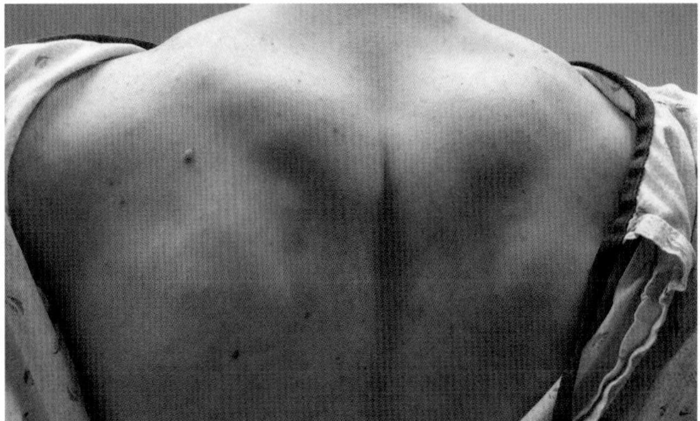

**Fig. 28.2** Hypertrophy of shoulder and posterior neck muscles in a 20-year-old male with myotonia since childhood.

## Muscle Bulk and Deformities

Assessment of muscle bulk looking for atrophy and hypertrophy is an important part of the neuromuscular examination. Prominent muscle wasting usually accompanies neurogenic disorders associated with axonal loss. However, severe wasting also occurs under chronic myopathic conditions. Wasting is best appreciated in the distal hand and foot muscles and around bony prominences. In the arm, wasting of the intrinsic hand muscles produces a characteristic hand posture in which the thumb rotates outward so that it lies in the same plane as that of the fingers (the *simian hand*), and the interphalangeal joints flex slightly with slight extension of metacarpophalangeal joints (the *claw hand*). Wasting of the small muscles leaves the bones easily visible through the skin, resulting in the characteristic guttered appearance of the back of the hand. In the foot, one of the easier muscles to inspect is the extensor digitorum brevis, a small muscle on the lateral dorsum of the foot that helps dorsiflex the toes. It often wastes early in neuropathies and anterior horn cell disorders. Under myopathic conditions in which proximal muscles are affected more than distal muscles, the extensor digitorum brevis may actually hypertrophy to try to compensate for weakness of the long toe dorsiflexors above it.

Muscle mass of the leg is so variable among individuals that it is sometimes difficult to decide whether wasting of the muscles has occurred. Any marked asymmetry indicates an abnormality, but distinguishing a slender thigh from quadriceps muscle atrophy often is difficult. One way to try to distinguish these conditions is to ask the patient to tighten the knee as firmly as possible. The firm medial and lateral bellies of the normal quadriceps that bunch up in the distal part of the thigh just above the knee fail to appear in the wasted muscle. The same technique can be used to evaluate anterior tibial wasting. In a severely wasted muscle, a groove on the lateral side of the tibia (which normally is filled by the anterior tibial muscles) is apparent. A moderate degree of wasting is difficult to distinguish from thinness of the leg, but if the patient dorsiflexes the foot, the wasted muscle fails to develop the prominent belly seen in a normal muscle.

Abnormal muscle hypertrophy is uncommon but may be a key finding when present. Beyond the expected increase in muscle bulk that accompanies exercise, generalized muscle hypertrophy is a feature of *myotonia congenita* and *paramyotonia congenita*, giving the appearance of the extreme development typically seen in weight lifters (Fig. 28.2). Hypertrophy is a common finding in the rare syndrome of *acquired neuromyotonia,* in which the continuous discharge of motor axons results in the muscle effectively exercising itself. Rarely, hypertrophy occurs in some chronic denervating disorders, especially in the posterior calf muscle in S1 radiculopathies. Electromyography (EMG) in affected patients often reveals spontaneous discharges in these muscles (usually complex

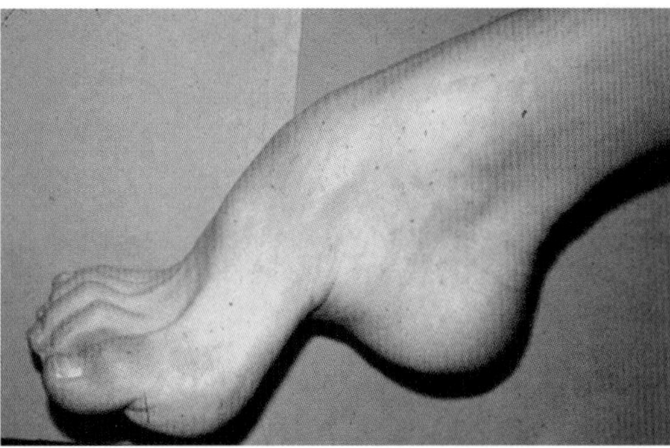

**Fig. 28.3** *Pes cavus* is caused by intrinsic foot muscle weakness during early growth and development. This condition is recognized as a high arch, foreshortened foot, and hammer toes. It often is a sign that weakness has been present since early childhood and implies an inherited disorder in most patients. (*From Krause, F.G., Guyton, G.P. Mann's surgery of the foot and ankle, In: Coughlin, M.J., Saltzmanand, C.L., Anderson, R.B. (Eds.), Mann's Surgery of the Foot and Ankle, ninth ed. pp. 1361–1382. Copyright © 2014 by Saunders, an imprint of Elsevier Inc.*)

repetitive discharges) consequent to chronic denervation. By contrast, conditions exist in which muscle hypertrophy is not from true muscle enlargement but from infiltration of fat, connective tissue, and other material (i.e., pseudohypertrophy). *Pseudohypertrophy* occurs in calf muscles of patients with Duchenne and Becker muscular dystrophy, as well as in patients with limb-girdle muscular dystrophy, spinal muscular atrophy (SMA), and some glycogen storage disorders. Similarly, pseudohypertrophy occurs rarely in sarcoidosis, cysticercosis, amyloidosis, hypothyroid myopathy, and focal myositis. Palpable masses in muscles occur with muscle tumors, ruptured tendons, or muscle hernias.

Several bony deformities often provide important clues to the presence of neuromuscular conditions. Proximal and axial muscle weakness often leads to scoliosis. Intrinsic foot muscle weakness present from childhood often leads to the characteristic foot deformity of *pes cavus*, in which the foot is foreshortened with high arches and hammer toes (Fig. 28.3). Pes cavus is a sign that weakness has been present at least since early childhood and implies a genetic disorder in most patients. Likewise, a high-arched palate often develops from chronic neuromuscular weakness present from childhood.

## Muscle Palpation, Percussion, and Range of Motion

Palpation and percussion of muscle provide additional information. Fibrotic muscle may feel rubbery and hard, whereas denervated muscle may separate into discrete strands that roll under the fingers. Muscle in inflammatory myopathies or rheumatological conditions may be tender to palpation, but severe muscle pain on palpation is unusual. An exception to this rule occurs with a patient experiencing an acute phase of viral myositis or rhabdomyolysis, whose muscles may be very sensitive to either movement or touch. Percussion of muscle may produce the phenomenon of *myotonia*, in which a localized contraction of the muscle persists for several seconds after percussion (Video 28.1). Percussing the thenar eminence and watching for a delayed relaxation of the thumb abductors will best show this phenomenon. Gripping the hands and opening them may also demonstrate delayed relaxation, known as grip myotonia (Video 28.2). This defining characteristic of myotonic dystrophy and myotonia congenita is distinguishable from myoedema, which occasionally occurs in patients with thyroid disorders and other metabolic conditions. In *myoedema*, the development of a dimple in the muscle, which then mounds to form a small hillock, follows the percussion.

In addition to its diagnostic value, the presence of a muscle contracture across a joint may cause disability, even in the absence of weakness. Thus, an evaluation of range of motion at major joints is an important part of the clinical examination. A standard examination includes evaluation for contractures at the fingers, elbows, wrists, hips, knees, and ankles. At the hips, both flexion and iliotibial band contractures should be looked for.

## Muscle Tone

The physiological origin of muscle tone is complex and outside the scope of this chapter. In examining the weak patient, however, muscle tone offers valuable information regarding the origins of the weakness. Variations from a normal muscle tone result in increased tone *(hypertonicity)* or decreased tone *(hypotonicity)*. Increased tone results from the loss of CNS influences on the tonic contraction of muscle. Decreased tone usually implicates a problem with the proprioceptive or peripheral motor innervation of a muscle but may also result from an acute spinal cord or cerebral lesions. Patients usually do not complain directly of increased or decreased tone; for example, the spastic patient may complain of heaviness, stiffness, or slowness of movement.

Several methods are used to examine tone. First is the spontaneous posture of the extremities. With spasticity, the upper limbs often are in a fixed flexed posture, and affected muscles are firm to palpation. The examiner should attempt to relax the patient to allow free passive movement; helpful instructions may include statements such as "Don't try to help me do the work," or "just let your arm or leg go floppy." Normally, resistance is the same throughout the range of motion and does not change with changes in the velocity of the movement. In a patient with spasticity, rapid passive displacement of the extremity results in increased resistance followed by relaxation *(clasp-knife phenomenon)*. Resistance varies with the speed and direction of passive motion. Examination of tone in the legs should include supine examination because with the patient in this position, the examiner easily accomplishes hip and knee flexion by grasping the back of the knee and lifting briskly. In spasticity, the heel elevates off the examination table, while normally the heel remains in contact with the table. Hypotonia is the loss of normal tone and is felt as increased ease of passive movements during these maneuvers, or floppiness. In patients with severe hypotonia, the joints may be passively hyperextended.

## Strength

Evaluation of individual muscle strength is an important part of the clinical examination. Many methods are available. Fixed myometry has become popular within the research community. This method uses a strain gauge attached to a rigid supporting structure, often integrated into the examining couch on which the patient lies. The patient then uses maximum voluntary contraction, quantitated in newtons (N). The merits of this method are debatable, and, for the average clinician, the equipment expense is prohibitive.

In an office situation and in many clinical drug trials, manual muscle testing gives perfectly adequate results and is preferable to fixed myometry in young children. The basis is the Medical Research Council grading system, with some modification (Table 28.1). This method is adequate for use in an office situation, particularly if supplemented by the functional evaluation. A scale of 0–5 is used, in which 5 indicates normal strength. A grade of 5 indicates that the examiner is certain a muscle is normal and never used to compensate for slightly weak muscles. Muscles that can move the joint against resistance may vary quite widely in strength; grades of 4+, 4, and 4− often are used to indicate differences, particularly between one side of the body and the other. Grade 4 represents a wide range of strength, from slight weakness to moderate weakness, which is a disadvantage. For this reason, the scale has been more useful in following the average strength of many muscles during the course of a disease, rather than the course of a single muscle. Averaging many muscle scores smooths out the stepwise progression noted in a single muscle. This may demonstrate a steadily progressive decline. A grade of 3+ is assigned when the muscle can move the joint against gravity and can exert a tiny amount of resistance but then collapses under the pressure of the examiner's hand. It does not denote the phenomenon of *sudden give-way*, which occurs in conversion disorders and in patients limited by pain. Grade 3 indicates that the muscle can move the joint throughout its full range against gravity but not against any added resistance. Sometimes, particularly in muscles acting across large joints such as the knee, the muscle is capable of moving the limb partially against gravity but not through the full range of movement. A muscle that cannot extend the knee horizontally when the patient is in a sitting position but can extend the knee to within 30–40 degrees of horizontal is graded 3−. Grades 2, 1, and 0 are as defined in Table 28.1.

Although it is commendable and sometimes essential to examine each muscle separately, most clinicians test muscle groups rather than individual muscles. In our clinic, we test neck flexion, neck extension, shoulder abduction, internal rotation, external rotation, elbow flexion and extension, wrist flexion and extension, finger abduction and adduction, thumb abduction, hip flexion and extension, thigh abduction and adduction, knee flexion and extension, ankle dorsiflexion and plantar flexion, and dorsiflexion of the great toe.

## Fatigue

Fatigue is a common symptom in many neuromuscular disorders and many medical conditions. Anemia, heart disease, lung disease, cancer, poor nutrition, deconditioning, and depression are among the many disorders that can result in fatigue. Under certain neuromuscular conditions, however, strength is normal at rest but progressively decays

**TABLE 28.1 The Medical Research Council Scale for Grading Muscle Strength**

| Grade | Description |
|---|---|
| 0 | No contraction |
| 1 | Flicker or trace of contraction |
| 2 | Active movement with gravity eliminated |
| 3 | Active movement against gravity |
| 4 | Active movement against gravity and resistance |
| 5 | Normal power |

with muscle use. This clinical scenario most often characterizes the postsynaptic neuromuscular transmission disorders, especially MG. Repetitive or sustained muscle testing brings out true muscle fatigue. Always test fatigue in patients with a suspected neuromuscular transmission disorder. Ptosis is provoked by sustained upgaze for 2–3 minutes. Counting out loud from 1 to 100 may result in slurred, nasal, or hoarse speech. Repetitive testing of the strength of shoulder abduction or hip flexion may result in progressive weakness in patients with MG.

### Reflexes

In motor unit disorders, reflexes are normal, reduced, or absent. ALS is the exception because both UMN and LMN dysfunctions coexist, so hyperreflexia and spasticity often accompany signs of LMN loss. In neurogenic disorders with demyelination, reflexes are lost early in the disease, as occurs in Guillain-Barré syndrome, from blocking and desynchronization of muscle-spindle afferents and motor efferents. With disorders resulting in axonal loss, reflexes are depressed in proportion to the amount of loss. Because most axonal neuropathies predominantly affect distal axons, the distal reflexes (ankle reflexes) are depressed or lost early, and the more proximal ones remain normal. In myopathies, reflexes tend to diminish in proportion to the amount of muscle weakness. The same is true for postsynaptic neuromuscular transmission disorders. With presynaptic neuromuscular transmission disorders (e.g., Lambert-Eaton myasthenic syndrome), reflexes tend to be depressed or absent at rest but return to normal or at least improve after brief (10-second) periods of exercise.

### Sensory Disturbances

Disorders of the motor unit generally are not associated with disturbances of sensation unless a second condition is superimposed. Motor neuron disorders, neuromuscular transmission disorders, and myopathies generally follow this rule. Among the few exceptions is the minor sensory loss in patients with X-linked spinobulbar muscular atrophy (Kennedy disease) and inclusion-body myositis, both of which may have coexistent degeneration of the peripheral nerves and dorsal root ganglion cells. In the paraneoplastic Lambert-Eaton myasthenic syndrome, patients often have minor sensory signs reflecting a more widespread paraneoplastic process.

Sensory deficits often accompany peripheral neuropathies that are predominantly motor and usually thought of as motor neuropathies. Such disorders include Guillain-Barré syndrome, Charcot-Marie-Tooth disease, and some toxic neuropathies (e.g., lead). Under these conditions, sensory abnormalities on examination or electrophysiological testing help identify the disorder as a neuropathy, thereby narrowing the differential diagnosis.

### Peripheral Nerve Enlargement

Palpation of peripheral nerves may yield important information in several neuromuscular conditions. Diffusely enlarged nerves occur in some patients with chronic demyelinating peripheral neuropathies, especially Charcot-Marie-Tooth disease type 1, Dejerine-Sottas syndrome, and Refsum disease. In addition, focal enlargement occurs in nerve sheath tumors (neurofibromatosis) or with infiltrative lesions (e.g., amyloidosis and leprosy). Easily palpated nerves are the greater auricular nerve in the neck, the ulnar nerve at the elbow, the superficial radial sensory nerve as it crosses the extensors to the thumb distal to the wrist, and the peroneal nerve at the fibular head at the knee.

### Fasciculations, Cramps, and Other Abnormal Muscle Movements

All limbs are examined to determine the presence or absence of fasciculations. A *fasciculation* is a brief twitch caused by the spontaneous firing of one motor unit. Fasciculations may be difficult or impossible to see in infants or obese patients. They can be present in normal people, so their presence in the absence of wasting or weakness is of no significance *(benign fasciculations)*. Fasciculations that are widespread and seen on every examination may indicate denervating disease, particularly anterior horn cell disease. Mental or physical fatigue, caffeine, cigarette smoking, or drugs such as amphetamines exacerbate fasciculations.

In some patients who have been careful to avoid exposure to exacerbating factors, disease-related fasciculations may be absent or appear benign. This should be kept in mind during the evaluation. Abundant fasciculations may be difficult to differentiate from *myokymia,* which is a more writhing, bag of worms–like motion of muscle (Video 28.3). Myokymia results from repetitive bursting of a motor unit (i.e., grouped fasciculations) and characteristically is associated with certain neuromuscular conditions (e.g., radiation injury and Guillain-Barré syndrome).

Similar to fasciculations, cramps may be benign or accompany several neuropathic conditions. A *cramp* is a painful involuntary muscle contraction. Cramps occur when a muscle is contracting in a shortened position. During a cramp, the muscle becomes hard and well defined. Stretching the muscle relieves the cramp. Superficially, a muscle contracture that occurs in a metabolic myopathy may resemble a cramp, although these two entities are completely different on electrophysiological testing. During a contracture, electrical silence is characteristic, whereas numerous motor units fire at high frequencies during a cramp.

## FUNCTIONAL EVALUATION OF THE WEAK PATIENT

### Walking

Alteration of gait may occur with weakness of the muscles of the hip and back, leg, and shoulder. In normal walking, when the heel hits the ground, the action of the hip abductors, which stabilize the pelvis, serves to counteract the shock. Weakness of these muscles on one side leads to the pelvis to dip to the other side; bilateral weakness produces a waddle. In addition, weakness of the hip extensors and back extensors makes it difficult for the patient to maintain a normal posture. Ordinarily, the body is carried so that the center of gravity is slightly forward of the hip joint. If these muscles become weak, the patient often throws the shoulders back so that the weight of the body falls behind the hip joints. This postural adjustment accentuates the lumbar lordosis. Alternatively, with pronounced weakness of the quadriceps muscles, the patient stabilizes the knee by throwing it backward. When the knee is hyperextended, it locks, deriving its stability from the anatomy of the joint rather than from muscular support. Finally, weakness of the muscles of the lower leg may result in a *steppage gait,* in which a short throw at the ankle midswing affects dorsiflexion of the foot. The foot then rapidly comes to the ground before the toes fall back into plantar flexion. Shoulder weakness may be observed as the patient walks; the arms hang loosely by the sides and tend to swing in a pendular fashion rather than with a normal controlled swing.

### Arising from the Floor

The normal method for arising from the floor depends on the age of the patient. The young child can spring rapidly to the feet without the average observer being able to dissect the movements. The elderly patient may turn to one side, place a hand on the floor, and rise to a standing position with a deliberate slowness. The patient with hip muscle weakness will turn to one side or the other to put the hand on the floor for support. The degree of turning is proportional to the severity of the weakness. Most people arise to a standing position from a squatting position, but the patient with hip extensor and quadriceps muscle weakness finds it easier to keep the hands on the floor and raise the hips high in the air. This has been termed the *butt-first maneuver*; the patient forms a triangle with the hips at the apex and the base of support provided by both hands and feet on the floor and then laboriously rises from this position, usually by pushing on the thighs with both hands to brace the body upward. The progress of recovery or progression of weakness can be documented by noting whether the initial turn is greater than 90 degrees, whether unilateral or bilateral hand support is used on the floor and thighs, whether this support is sustained or transitory, and whether a butt-first maneuver is used. The entire process is known as the *Gower maneuver,* but it is useful to break it up into its component parts (Fig. 28.4).

### Psychogenic Weakness

An experienced examiner should be able to differentiate real weakness from psychogenic weakness. The primary characteristic of psychogenic weakness is that it is unpredictable and fluctuating. Muscle strength may suddenly give out when a limb is being evaluated. The patient has difficulty knowing the exact muscle strength expected and cannot adequately counter the examiner's resistance. This gives rise to a wavering, collapsing force. Tricks are useful to bring out the discrepancy in muscle performance. For example, if the weak thigh cannot lift off the chair in a seated position, then the legs should not swing up onto the mattress when being seated on the examining table. When the examiner suspects that weakness of shoulder abduction is feigned, the patient's arm is placed in abduction. With the examiner's hand on the elbows, the examiner can instruct the patient to push toward the ceiling. At first, the downward pressure is very light, and the patient is unable to move the examiner's hand toward the ceiling. However, the arm does not fall down either, and as the downward pressure is gradually increased, continued exhortation to push the examiner's hand upward results in increasing resistance to the downward pressure. The examiner ends up putting maximum weight on the outstretched arm, which remains in abduction. The logical conclusion is that the strength is normal. Patients do not realize this because they believe that because they did not move the examiner's hand upward, they must be weak.

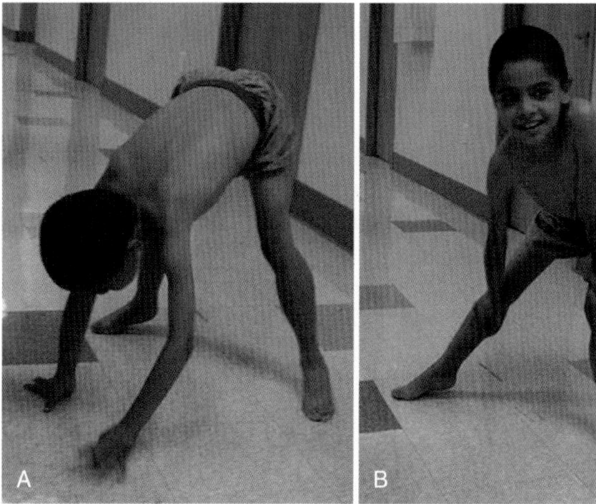


**Fig. 28.4 Gower Sign in a 7-Year-Old Boy With Duchenne Muscular Dystrophy. A,** Butt-first maneuver as hips are hoisted in the air. **B,** Hand support on the thighs. *(From McDonald, C.M., 2012. Clinical approach to the diagnostic evaluation of hereditary and acquired neuromuscular diseases. Phys. Med. Rehabil. Clin. N. Am. 23(3), 495–563. Copyright © 2012 Elsevier Inc.)*

## CLINICAL INVESTIGATIONS IN MUSCULAR WEAKNESS

As is so often the case, the most critical components to evaluating a patient with weakness are a thorough history and physical examination. Key elements of the interview should focus on the distribution of weakness, duration of symptoms, and their persistence. It is also useful to determine if there were any delays in the patient's motor or cognitive development or if there is any family history of similar symptomatology. It should be determined if there were any potential toxic exposures (e.g., statins, colchicine, alcohol, steroids, and amiodarone) or if there are any general medical conditions that may be related (e.g., mixed connective tissue disorder, hypothyroidism, sarcoidosis, and malignancy). It is important to query about difficulties swallowing, chewing, or breathing. Any symptoms that may suggest underlying heart failure or cardiac arrhythmia should be elicited. The presence of dysphagia, diaphragmatic weakness, or cardiac dysfunction is not only important to identify for the patient's safety but also significantly narrows the potential differential diagnosis.

Although a complete motor examination as previously outlined is paramount, special attention should be given to certain distinctive features. These include the presence of ptosis, ophthalmoparesis, facial weakness, scapular winging, joint contractures, and skin changes. These findings are often pathognomonic and essential to the diagnosis. That said, there are cases in which even the most seasoned clinician cannot localize the origin of weakness or identify the underlying disease process. In this situation, there are a number of investigations at the physician's disposal. Initial considerations include serum creatine kinase (CK) levels, electrodiagnostic testing, and muscle biopsy. Recently, neuromuscular imaging has proven an invaluable adjunct to traditional electrodiagnosis. If an inflammatory myopathy is considered, there are serological tests for myositis-specific antibodies (MSAs). Finally, commercial genetic testing is becoming increasing available and affordable for a number of hereditary neurological conditions.

### Creatine Kinase

CK is an enzyme specific to muscle, and therefore, the degree of its presence in the serum can be used as a surrogate marker of muscle membrane integrity. However, hyperCKemia (as it is sometimes dubbed) is not always due to an underlying myopathy. Serum CK elevations can be seen in response to exercise or trauma. In these situations, elevations are often transient. Sustained increases in these levels can be a sensitive indicator of underlying muscle damage. Notable exceptions exist. CK concentrations may rarely be elevated as high as *10 times normal in patients with SMA* and occasionally in those with ALS (see Chapter 97).

Measurements of serial CK concentrations generally follow the progression of the disease. However, problems have been recognized with both of these uses. Foremost is the determination of the normal level. Race, gender, age, and activity level are important in determining normal values. All studies on CK concentration show that gender and race affect values. In a survey of 1500 hospital employees, using carefully standardized methods, it was possible to detect three populations, each with characteristic CK values (Wong et al., 1983). The upper limits of normal (97.5th percentile) were as follows:

- Black men only: 520 U/L
- Black women, nonblack men: 345 U/L
- Nonblack women: 145 U/L

The nonblack population included Hispanics, Asians, and Caucasians. Because expression of the upper limit is as a percentile of the mean, by definition, 2.5% of the normal population will have levels above the upper limit of normal. Although this does not seem like a large proportion, in a town of 100,000, a total of 2500 people would have abnormal levels. The point is that the upper limit of normal CK concentration is not rigid and requires intelligent interpretation. Although the serum CK concentration can be useful in determining the course of an illness, judgment is required because changes in CK values do not always mirror the clinical condition. In treating inflammatory myopathies with immunosuppressive drugs or corticosteroids, a steadily declining CK concentration is reassuring, whereas concentrations that are creeping back up when the patient is presumably in remission may be concerning.

Serum CK concentrations are also useful for determining whether an illness is monophasic. A bout of myoglobinuria is usually associated with very high concentrations of CK. The concentration then declines steadily by approximately 50% every 2 days. This pattern indicates that a single episode of muscle damage has occurred. Patients with CK concentrations that do not decline in this fashion or that vary from high to low on random days have an ongoing illness.

It is important to note that patients with very chronic muscle weakness or very focal involvement may have a normal or mildly elevated CK level. Classically, these conditions include FSH muscular dystrophy, metabolic myopathies, inclusion body myositis, myotonic dystrophy, or oculopharyngeal muscular dystrophy (OPMD). On the other end of the spectrum, conditions with a rapid clinical course or diffuse muscle involvement may have more impressive CK elevations. These include the dystrophinopathies, polymyositis, toxic myopathies, and rhabdomyolysis.

Finally, there are other muscle enzymes to be aware of. Most notably, these include aldolase, lactate dehydrogenase, and aminotransferases. In general, none of these markers is as specific for muscle disease as CK. For example, elevated transaminases can be seen in diseases of bone, liver, and muscle. With that said, there are rare instances where these markers may be elevated in patients with myositis and normal CK levels (Bohlmeyer et al., 1994). It is well advised to avoid sending these laboratory tests routinely in a "shotgun approach" to the workup of weakness. At best, they increase the cost of care without significantly impacting the diagnostic yield. At worst, an elevated alanine aminotransferase (AST) may lead to an unnecessary liver biopsy. A judicious, evidence-based use of these tests on a case-by-case basis is best practice.

## Antibody Testing

Serum antibody testing can be helpful in establishing and further narrowing the differential diagnosis of weakness from the motor unit. The most notable example is acetylcholine receptor (AChR) antibodies being present in 80%–85% of patients with generalized MG, a postsynaptic neuromuscular junction disorder (Ruff et al., 2018). Alongside history, physical examination, and electrodiagnosis, a positive AChR antibody result in a patient with a history suggestive of MG will aid in securing the diagnosis. Muscle-specific kinase (MuSK) autoantibody is present in 4%–6% of individuals with MG (Ruff et al., 2018). There is a growing literature regarding other antibodies in MG including lipoprotein receptor-related protein 4 (LRP4). In all likelihood, those patients currently deemed "seronegative" may have autoimmunity aimed at a postsynaptic membrane protein or enzyme yet to be established. Identification of these antibodies is helpful in aiding diagnosis and also in understanding pathophysiology of neuromuscular junction dysfunction. This can advance the development of different therapies for MG.

There are many other conditions of the motor unit associated with particular antibodies as well. For example, certain antiganglioside (GM1) antibodies have been found in individuals with an acquired demyelinating neuropathy known as MMNCB.

In addition, sending for myositis-associated antibody panels in certain inflammatory myopathies can help in determining a particular association with extraskeletal muscle manifestations (i.e., interstitial lung disease), involvement of connective tissue disease, as well as the disease severity and possible association with an underlying malignancy. This is by no means a complete list, and other chapters will review individual diseases in detail and the relevant workup including known antibody associations.

## Electrodiagnostic Testing

Electrodiagnostic testing consists of nerve conduction studies and needle EMG. This is an operator-dependent study, and an experienced electromyographer is essential to perform and interpret an EMG correctly. Chapter 36 discusses the principles of EMG. The EMG study may provide much useful information. An initial step in the assessment of the weak patient is to localize the abnormality within the motor unit: neuropathic, myopathic, or neuromuscular junction. Nerve conduction studies and the needle electrode examination are particularly useful for identifying neuropathic disorders and localizing the abnormality to anterior horn cells, roots, plexus, or peripheral nerve territories (see Chapters 97, 105, and 106). Repetitive nerve stimulation and single-fiber EMG can aid in elucidating disorders of the neuromuscular junction. Short and long exercise testing are specialized nerve conduction studies that are used in the evaluation of periodic paralysis and nondystrophic myotonic disorders (Tan et al., 2011). The needle electrode examination may help distinguish between the presence of abnormal muscle versus nerve activity, depending on the presence of acute and chronic denervation, myotonia, neuromyotonia, fasciculations, cramps, and myokymia (Videos 36.4–36.6, 36.8, 36.9, 36.12, 36.13).

## Muscle Biopsy

The use of muscle biopsy is important for establishing the diagnosis in most disorders of the motor unit, although for some diseases, definitive genetic tests have made biopsy unnecessary. Histochemical evaluation is available at most hospitals and is particularly useful, and electron microscopy may provide a specific diagnosis. An important aspect of the muscle biopsy study is the analysis of the muscle proteins. Individual muscle proteins, including dystrophin, sarcoglycans, and other structural proteins, may be missing or deficient in specific illnesses, and the diagnosis is often definitive with these analyses. Some laboratories perform specialized studies on fresh and frozen muscle to assess mitochondrial function, including oxidative phosphorylation assays to assess respiratory chain function and electron transport chain analysis. With the growing availability of genetic testing, extensive immunohistochemical stains may be unnecessary.

Chapter 109 reviews the details of muscle biopsy, but a word about the selection of the muscle to be biopsied is appropriate here. All biopsy procedures carry a risk of sampling error. Not all muscles are equally involved in any given disease, and it is important to select a muscle that is likely to give the most useful information. The gastrocnemius muscle, often chosen for muscle biopsy, is not ideal because it demonstrates a predominance of type 1 fibers in the normal person and often shows denervation changes caused by minor lumbosacral radiculopathy. In addition, it has more than its fair share of random pathological changes, such as fiber necrosis and small inflammatory infiltrates, even when no clinical suspicion of a muscle disease exists. For this reason, it is preferable to select either the quadriceps femoris or the biceps brachii if either of these muscles is weak. A biopsy should never be performed on a muscle that is the site of a recent EMG or intramuscular injection because these procedures produce focal muscle damage. If such a muscle has to be biopsied, at least 2–3 months should elapse after the procedure before the biopsy is performed. In the patient with a relatively acute (duration of weeks) disease, it is wise to select a muscle that is obviously clinically weak. In patients with long-standing disease, it may be better to select a muscle that is almost normal to avoid an "end-stage" muscle. Sometimes, an apparently normal muscle is biopsied. For example, in a patient who is suspected of having motor neuron disease and has wasting and weakness of the arms, with EMG changes of denervation in the arms but no apparent denervation of the legs, biopsy of the biceps muscle would show the expected denervation and would add no useful information. Biopsy evidence of denervation in a quadriceps muscle, however, would be consistent with widespread involvement, supporting the diagnosis of motor neuron disease. On the other hand, if biopsy of the quadriceps muscle yielded normal results, this would make the diagnosis of motor neuron disease less likely because even strong muscles in patients with motor neuron disease usually show some denervation. Motor neuron disease is not usually an indication for biopsy unless the diagnosis is in question.

## Imaging

An adjunct in the workup of conditions of the motor unit is neuromuscular ultrasound. This test has the advantage of being noninvasive, painless, and inexpensive. As with EMG, this is operator dependent, and a firm knowledge of neuroanatomy and sonography is needed to perform quality studies. Neuromuscular ultrasound allows for the direct visualization of nerves and muscles and can give additive, important information to EMG, history, and the physical examination. For example, an individual who presents with numbness and tingling in digits 4 and 5 with weakness of intrinsic hand muscles may be sent for an EMG to evaluate for ulnar neuropathy. Although an ulnar nerve injury may be identified by EMG, the exact location at which the nerve is injured may not be concluded by the data of the EMG study alone (Alrajeh and Preston, 2018). A neuromuscular ultrasound tracing the pathway of the ulnar nerve from wrist to the upper arm can help in determining if there is an area of focal enlargement as the point of injury or if there are any external compressing structures. Tumors, aneurysms, and ganglion cysts are examples of mass lesions that may result in nerve compression (Fig. 28.5). This information is useful in determining the appropriate treatment plan—especially when decompressive surgery is being considered.

Another area where ultrasound shines is in the evaluation of acquired demyelinating polyneuropathies. For example, a patient may present with progressive weakness and sensory symptoms over months to years. Suspecting a severe peripheral neuropathy, electrodiagnostic testing would be an appropriate first step. However, in some cases, all nerve conduction responses may be absent. This leaves the physician unable to comment on the underlying pathophysiology of the neuropathy—whether there is primary axonal loss or demyelinating features. This is a particularly important question when considering the diagnosis of chronic inflammatory demyelinating polyneuropathy (CIDP), which may be amenable to immunotherapy. Normative data for nerve cross-sectional area have been well established (Cartwright et al., 2008), and neuromuscular ultrasound may reveal focal nerve hypertrophy at nonentrapment sites in an acquired demyelinating neuropathy (Fig. 28.6). This is a marker of the chronic denervation and subsequent reinnervation seen in CIDP and is analogous to the classic "onion bulb" formation seen on nerve biopsy.

The information from ultrasound can help in muscle conditions as well. In general, myopathic processes will result in homogenously increased muscle echogenicity (brightness). Neurogenic conditions result is a more heterogeneous or "moth-eaten" pattern. In addition to the quality of the echogenic changes, the pattern of involved muscles can be equally useful. It may identify an appropriate muscle for biopsy or be a clue to the underlying diagnosis itself. In certain muscle conditions, such as inclusion body myositis, the typical pattern of weakness involves forearm flexor and knee extensors (sparing the rectus femoris) muscles. Thus, an ultrasound revealing changes in this particular pattern may be helpful in further supporting a diagnosis of inclusion body myositis, even if these muscles were not noticeably weak on clinical examination (Karvelas et al., 2019).

Diaphragmatic ultrasound is another area that has seen an increase in utilization over recent years. Traditionally, diaphragm function has been evaluated with phrenic nerve conduction studies, but these can be technically challenging—especially in patients with a large body habitus. In the intensive care unit (ICU), the presence of a central venous catheter (e.g., internal jugular and subclavian) is a contraindication for these studies, which can be problematic when evaluating a patient with failure to wean from the ventilator. Likewise, needle EMG of the diaphragm is difficult to perform and carries a risk of significant complications such as pneumothorax. Ultrasound, however, is a noninvasive alternative to electrodiagnostic testing for evaluation of both the structure and the dynamic function of the diaphragm (Sarwal et al., 2013).

While not as cost-effective as sonography, MRI can have similar utility in determining the pattern of muscle involvement and in some cases may be superior. While ultrasound performs well with superficial anatomy, MRI can better characterize deep musculature and give a more "global" assessment. In fact, MRI patterns have been at the center of proposed diagnostic algorithms for evaluation of distal myopathies (Udd, 2012). Narrowing the differential diagnosis by way of clinical

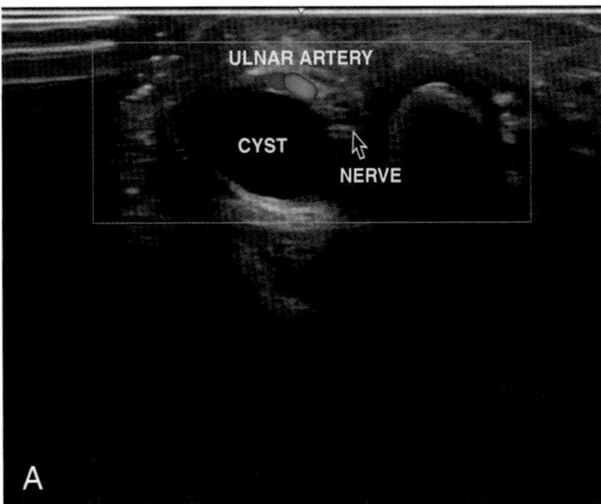


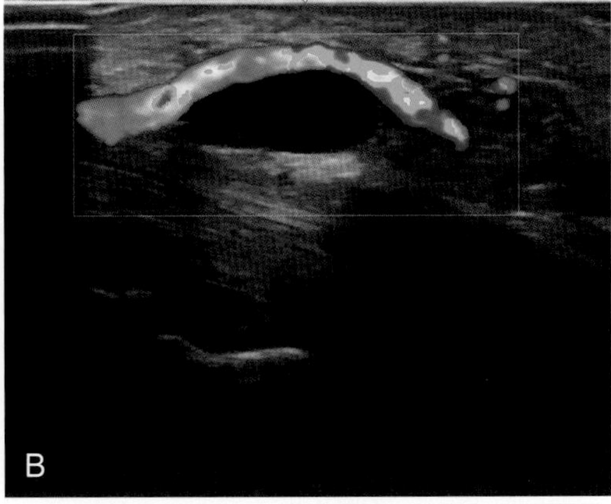


**Fig. 28.5 Sonograms of Focal Ulnar Nerve Entrapment at Guyon Canal. A,** Short-axis view of the distal, volar wrist revealing the ulnar nerve impinged between the pisiform bone and a ganglion cyst arising from the wrist joint. **B,** Long-axis view demonstrates the mass effect of this cyst as it displaces the ulnar artery superficially.

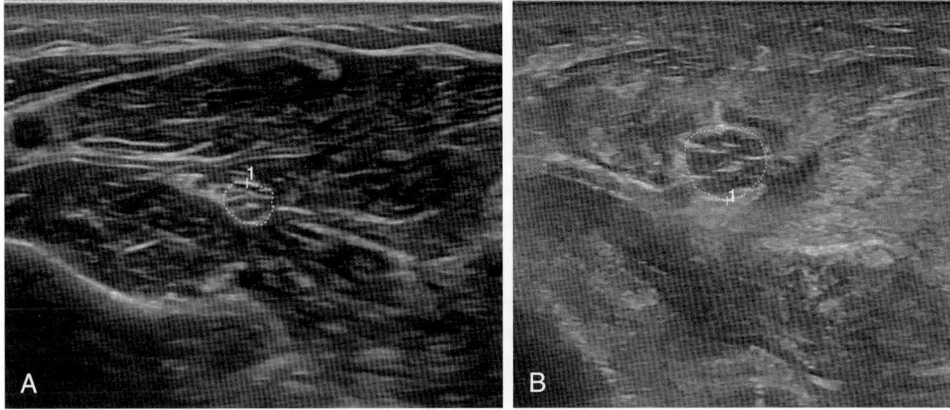

**Fig. 28.6 Focal Nerve Hypertrophy at Nonentrapment Sites. A**, Short-axis sonogram of the midforearm reveals the median nerve with a normal echogenicity, architecture, and size. This nerve measures 7.6 $mm^2$ in cross-sectional area (NL < 10 $mm^2$). **B**, The same location in a patient with chronic inflammatory demyelinating polyneuropathy. Note enlarged nerve fascicles within the nerve as well as the overall increased cross-sectional area (24.5 $mm^2$). In addition, the surrounding muscle reveals increased echogenicity (brightness) characteristic of denervation.

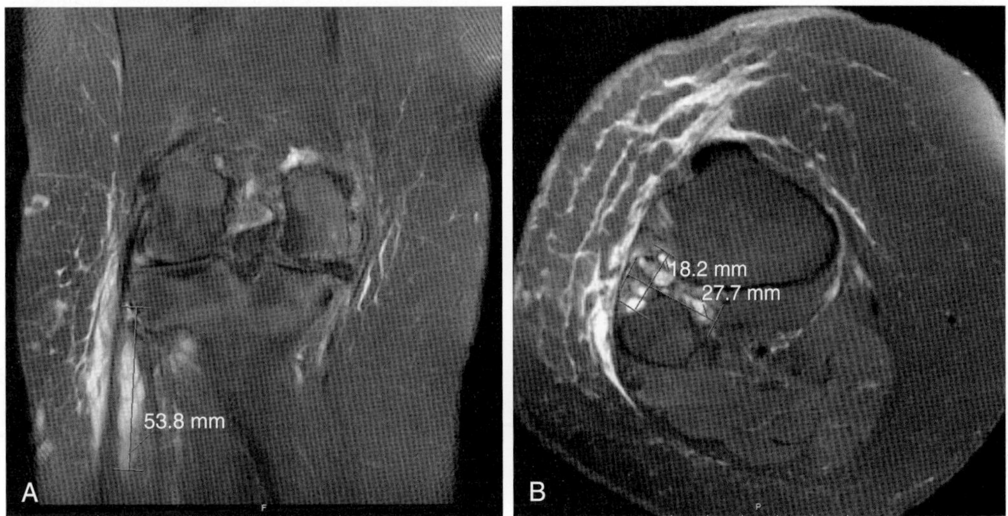


**Fig. 28.7 MRI of an Intraneural Ganglion Cyst. A**, Coronal view of the knee reveals a cystic structure within the peroneus longus muscle. **B**, Axial view of the knee demonstrates a complex, multilobulated, cystic mass between the tibia and head of the fibula.

evaluation and imaging phenotype may be an effective way to perform more targeted genetic investigations.

Finally, MRI can be the key diagnostic modality in peripheral nerve injury. Take, for example, a patient presenting with an acute-onset, painful foot drop. Electrodiagnostic testing demonstrated electrophysiological evidence of a severe, axonal, nonlocalizable peroneal neuropathy. A neuromuscular ultrasound of the common peroneal nerve was underwhelming, but the peroneus longus muscle revealed a well-circumscribed, hypoechoic structure within the muscle belly. A follow-up MRI showed a multilobulated intraneural cyst dissecting down the articular branch of the peroneal nerve into the peroneus longus muscle (Fig. 28.7). This finding allowed for appropriate referral to neurosurgery for ligation and decompression.

## Genetic Testing

Chapter 48 covers the details of genetic testing and counseling. Genetic analysis has become a routine part of the clinical investigation of neuromuscular disease and in many situations has supplanted muscle biopsy and other diagnostic tests. Furthermore, genetic testing is becoming increasingly important in certain conditions of the motor unit where treatment is now available. The use of genetic testing for diagnosis in a specific patient implies that the genetic cause of a specific disease is established and that intragenic probes that allow the determination of whether the gene in question is abnormal are available. Examples of such abnormalities are deletions in the dystrophin gene, seen in many cases of Duchenne muscular dystrophy (DMD), mutations or deletions of *SMN1* in SMA, and the expansion of the triplet repeat in the myotonic dystrophy gene. In 2016, the US Federal Drug and Administration (FDA) approved an antisense oligonucleotide called eteplirsen for individuals with DMD with deletions located in exon 51, about 14% of patients with DMD (Goyal and Narayanaswami, 2018). Also in 2016, the FDA approved nusinersen, an antisense oligonucleotide, for patients with SMA. Individuals with SMA have homozygous mutations or deletions in the *SMN1* gene and thus do not make a necessary amount of functional protein that is important for alpha-motor neuron survival; thus, this is a progressive condition of alpha-motor neuron loss, leading to weakness. There is a second gene called *SMN2*, which can be present as 0–8 copies in all individuals. This gene leads to an SMN protein product, although only results in 10% of full-length protein when spliced normally. Nusinersen targets the *SMN2* gene product with the goal of increasing the number of full-length functional SMN protein, thereby helping the alpha-motor neurons survive (Goyal et al., 2018). There has been ongoing research for other genetic conditions of the motor unit, and likely in the future, more treatment options will become available. Thus, genetic testing will become even more important in helping to more definitively diagnose conditions in which there will exist treatments. It is difficult to keep up with the mushrooming list of genes known to be associated with neuromuscular diseases, yet maintaining current knowledge is imperative if patients are to be provided with suitable advice. Useful references can be found in the journal *Neuromuscular Disorders*, which carries a list of all known neuromuscular genetic abnormalities each month, and on the websites Online Mendelian Inheritance in Man (http://www.ncbi.nlm.nih.gov/omim/) and GeneTests-GeneClinics (http://www.ncbi.nlm.nih.gov/sites/GeneTests/).

### Exercise Testing

Exercise testing may be an important part of the investigation of muscle disease, particularly in metabolic disorders. The two types of exercise tests used are forearm exercise testing and bicycle exercise ergometry. Forearm (grip) exercise protocols are designed to provide a test of glycolytic pathways, particularly those involved in power exercise. Incremental bicycle ergometry gives additional information regarding the relative use of carbohydrates, fats, and oxygen.

Several types of forearm exercise testing are used. Hogrel et al., 2001 The traditional method has been to have the patient grip a dynamometer repetitively, with a blood pressure cuff on the upper arm raised above systolic pressure. The necessity of the blood pressure cuff is now questionable. If the work performed by the patient is sufficiently strenuous, the cuff is unnecessary because the muscle is working at a level that surpasses the ability of blood-borne substances to sustain it. In addition, ischemic exercise may result in rhabdomyolysis in patients with defects in the glycolytic enzyme pathway and is best avoided.

After an adequate level of forceful exercise is maintained for 1 minute, samples of venous blood can be obtained at intervals after exercise to monitor changes in metabolites. In normal persons, the energy for such short-duration work derives from intramuscular glycogen. Thus, lactate forms when exercise is relatively anaerobic, as with strenuous activity. In addition, serum concentrations of hypoxanthine and ammonia, as well as lactate, are elevated with short-duration strenuous activity. Patients with certain defects in the glycolytic pathways produce normal to excessive amounts of ammonia and hypoxanthine, but no lactate. Patients with adenylate deaminase deficiency show the reverse: neither ammonia nor hypoxanthine appears, but lactate production is normal. Patients who cannot cooperate with the testing and show poor effort produce neither high lactate nor ammonia concentrations.

In mitochondrial disorders and other instances of metabolic stress, the production of both lactate and hypoxanthine is excessive. A modified ischemic forearm test has been used as a sensitive and specific screen for mitochondrial disorders. During exercise in normal persons, mitochondrial oxidative phosphorylation increases 100-fold from that measured during rest. In mitochondrial disorders, the disturbed oxidative phosphorylation results in an impaired systemic oxygen extraction. In one study comparing 12 patients with mitochondrial myopathy, 10 patients with muscular dystrophy, and 12 healthy subjects, measurement was made of cubital venous oxygen saturation after 3 minutes at 40% of maximal voluntary contraction of the exercised arm (Jensen et al., 2002). Oxygen desaturation in venous blood from exercising muscle was markedly lower in patients with mitochondrial myopathy than in patients with other muscle diseases and healthy subjects. Random measurement of serum lactate was not reliable at differentiating patients with mitochondrial myopathy from normal subjects.

## DIFFERENTIAL DIAGNOSIS BY AFFECTED REGION AND OTHER MANIFESTATIONS OF WEAKNESS

Once the presence of weakness has been established by means of either the history or the physical examination, the clinical features may be so characteristic that the diagnosis is obvious. At other times, the cause of the weakness may be less certain. Fig. 28.8 displays an outline of diagnostic considerations based on the characteristics of the weakness, such as whether it is fluctuating or constant. This approach can be used in the differential diagnosis of weakness affecting specific body regions and with other manifestations of weakness, as described in the following sections.

### Disorders With Prominent Ocular Weakness

*OPMD* involves slowly progressive weakness of the eye muscles, causing ptosis and external ophthalmoplegia, and is associated with difficulty in swallowing. This disorder is inherited as an autosomal dominant condition, with symptom onset usually after the age of 50 years. Many patients also have facial weakness and hip and shoulder weakness. Swallowing difficulty may become severe enough to necessitate cricopharyngeal myotomy or gastrostomy tube placement; however, life span in this condition appears to be normal.

*Kearns-Sayre syndrome* is a distinctive collection of features including ptosis, external ophthalmoplegia, cardiac conduction defects, pigmentary degeneration of the retina, cerebellar ataxia, pyramidal tract signs, short stature, and mental retardation, with symptom onset before the age of 20 years. These findings accompany an abnormality of the mitochondria in muscle and other tissues. Kearns-Sayre syndrome usually is sporadic. It may be slowly progressive or nonprogressive. Other mitochondrial disorders may also include chronic progressive external ophthalmoplegia (CPEO) as a feature of a more widespread syndrome.

In addition, several other disorders may display prominent extraocular muscle involvement. Among these is *centronuclear myopathy*, one of the congenital myopathies. This condition is not restricted to the eye muscles and has prominent involvement of the limbs as well. External ophthalmoplegia of subacute progressive onset, with or without other bulbar and limb muscle involvement, may occur in variant forms of Guillain-Barré syndrome (i.e., Miller Fisher syndrome) and in botulism. Finally, isolated ptosis or extraocular muscle weakness often is a presenting feature of MG and occasionally of Lambert-Eaton myasthenic syndrome.

### Disorders With Distinctive Facial or Bulbar Weakness

The diagnosis of *FSH muscular dystrophy* may be delayed until early adult life. Weakness of the face may lead to difficulty with whistling or blowing up balloons and may be severe enough to give the face a smooth, unlined appearance with an abnormal pout to the lips (Fig. 28.9, *A*). Weakness of the muscles around the shoulders is constant, although the deltoid muscle is surprisingly well preserved and may even be pseudohypertrophic in its lower portion. When the patient attempts to hold the arms extended in front, winging of the scapula occurs that is quite characteristic. The whole scapula may slide upward on the back of the thorax. The inferomedial border always juts backward, producing the appearance of a triangle at right angles to the back, with the base of the triangle still attached to the thorax. In addition, a discrepancy in power often occurs between the wrist flexors, which are strong, and the wrist extensors, which are weak. Similarly,

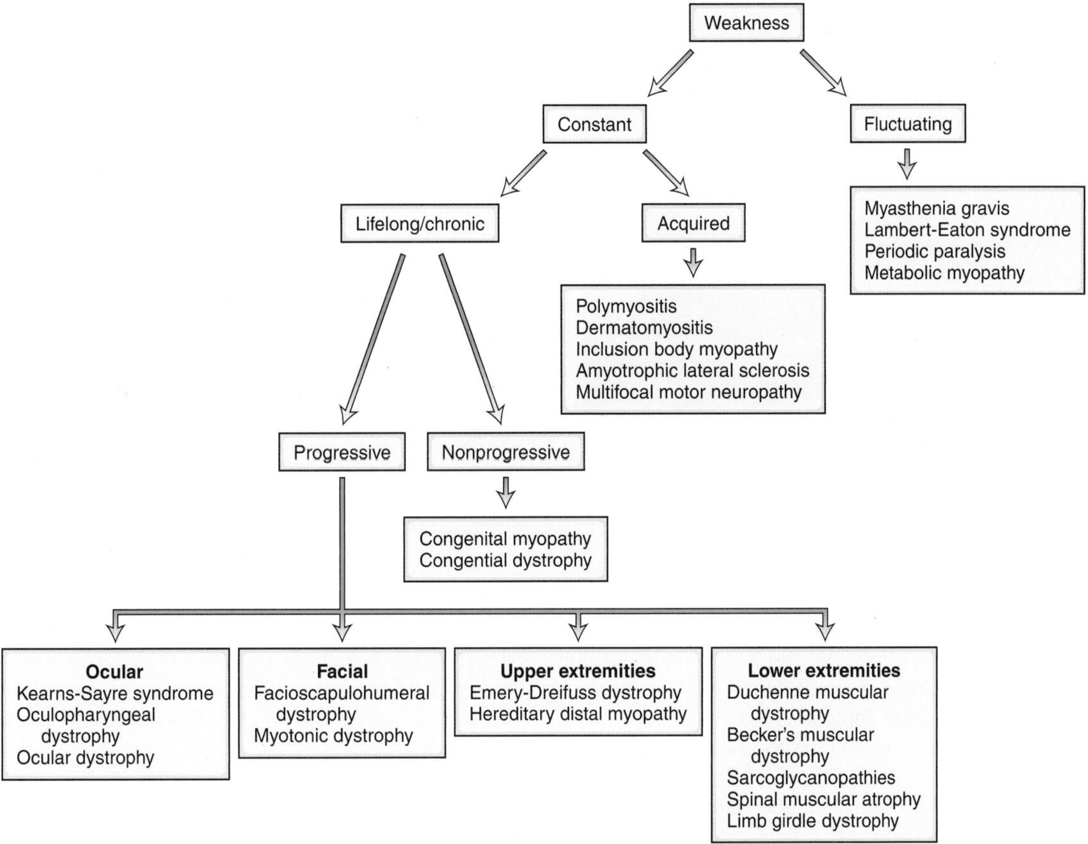


**Fig. 28.8** Algorithm for the Diagnostic Approach to the Patient With Weakness.

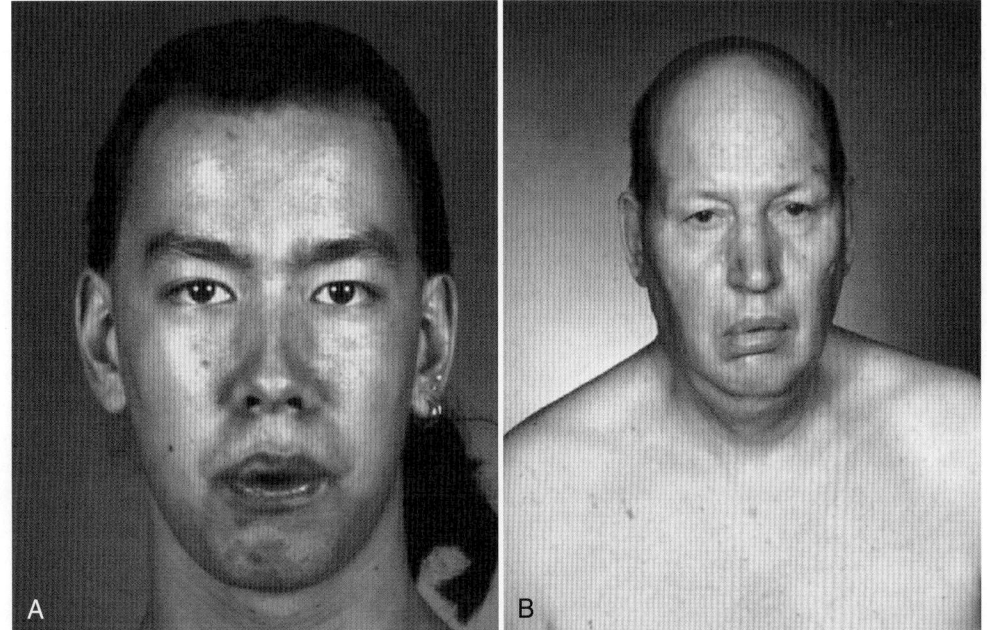


**Fig. 28.9** Facial weakness is a prominent feature of both facioscapulohumeral (FSH) dystrophy and myotonic dystrophy, but characteristic features of each are so distinctive that the conditions are readily recognizable and not easily confused. **A,** Patient with FSH dystrophy is unable to purse the lips when attempting to whistle. **B,** Typical appearance of a patient with myotonic dystrophy is marked by frontal balding, temporalis muscle wasting, ptosis, and facial weakness. Related to FSH dystrophy is scapuloperoneal dystrophy, which has similar features but lacks the facial weakness.

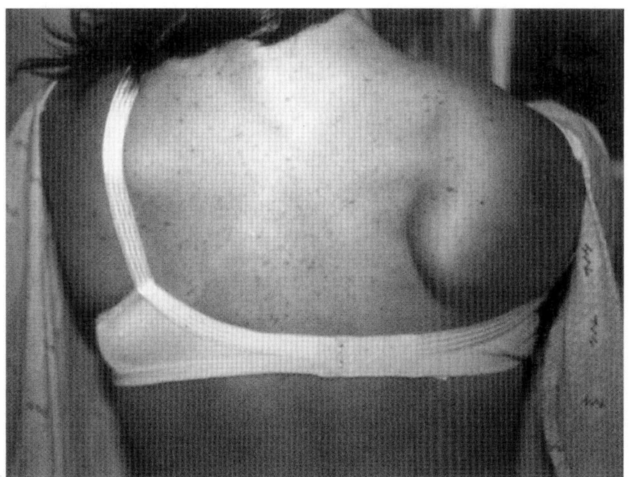

**Fig. 28.10** Asymmetrical Scapular Winging in Facioscapulohumeral Muscular Dystrophy.

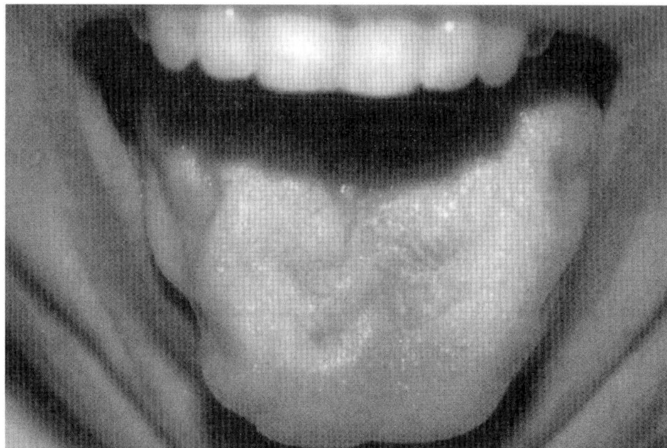

**Fig. 28.11** Tongue Atrophy in a Patient with Amyotrophic Lateral Sclerosis. *(Reprinted with permission from Katirji, B., Kaminski, H.J., Preston, D.C., et al. (Eds), 2002. Neuromuscular Disorders in Clinical Practice. Butterworth-Heinemann, Boston.)*

the ankle plantar flexors may be strong, whereas the ankle dorsiflexors are weak. It is common for the weakness to be asymmetrical, with one side much less involved than the other (Fig. 28.10). Inheritance of the disorder is as an autosomal dominant trait. FSH muscular dystrophy is associated with a contraction of the D4Z4 microsatellite repeat in the subtelomeric region of chromosome 4q35. Mild forms of the illness may be asymptomatic.

*Myotonic dystrophy type I* is a common illness with distinctive features including distal predominance of weakness. Inheritance is as an autosomal dominant trait, caused by a heterozygous trinucleotide (CTG) repeat expansion in the 3′ untranslated region of the dystrophia myotonica protein kinase (*DMPK*) gene on chromosome 19q13. The family history is often negative because patients may be unaware that other family members have the illness. This is due to the phenomenon of *anticipation,* whereby more severe syndromes appear in successive generations because of the expansion of the trinucleotide repeat. This diagnosis is suggested in any patient with muscular dystrophy and predominantly distal weakness. The neck flexors and temporalis and masseter muscles often are wasted. More characteristic than the distribution of the weakness is the long, thin face with hollowed temples, ptosis, and frontal balding (see Fig. 28.9, *B*). Percussion myotonia and grip myotonia occur in most patients after the age of 13 years. An EMG study can be diagnostic, showing myotonic discharges predominantly in distal limb muscles. Muscle biopsy usually is not necessary but may show characteristic changes.

A subset of patients with ALS presents with isolated bulbar weakness of LMN type (i.e., progressive bulbar palsy) or UMN type (i.e., progressive pseudobulbar palsy). Frequently, the condition shows a combination of UMN and LMN involvement. In these patients, dysarthria, dysphagia, and difficulty with secretions are the prominent symptoms. On examination, the tongue often is atrophic and fasciculating (Fig. 28.11), and the jaw and facial reflexes are exaggerated. The voice often is harsh and strained as well as slurred, reflecting the coexistent UMN and LMN dysfunction. In patients with X-linked spinobulbar muscular atrophy (Kennedy disease), bulbofacial muscles are also prominently affected. Patients often have a characteristic finding of chin fasciculations.

## Disorders With Prominent Respiratory Weakness

Disorders with prominent respiratory muscle weakness include inherited and acquired myopathies, disorders of the neuromuscular junction or peripheral nerves, motor neuron diseases, and CNS processes involving the brainstem or high cervical spinal cord. Adult-onset acid maltase deficiency (i.e., adult-onset Pompe disease), a glycogen storage disorder, frequently manifests with respiratory system–related symptoms of dyspnea or excessive daytime sleepiness, although proximal muscle weakness is present in most patients. Chronic progressive respiratory weakness occurs in DMD late in the course as well as in some other dystrophies including Becker and Emery-Dreifuss. Certain inflammatory myopathies such as polymyositis and dermatomyositis can result in dyspnea. In the ICU setting, critical illness myopathy may result in difficulty weaning from a ventilator, although limb muscles are also weak in this condition. MG occasionally manifests with respiratory failure, although usually myasthenic crisis occurs in patients already known to have myasthenia. Botulism results in respiratory compromise when severe, but the onset usually is stereotypical, with oculobulbar weakness followed by descending weakness, which aids in diagnosis. Guillain-Barré syndrome is a frequent cause of neuromuscular respiratory failure, with subacute onset of ascending weakness and numbness as the most common presentation. ALS leads to respiratory muscle weakness, usually late in the course of the disease. The occasional patient with weakness in the ICU setting, however, is found to have ALS after evaluation for failure to wean from a ventilator. In a patient with limb and respiratory muscle weakness, but normal bulbar muscle strength, the possibility of a high cervical cord lesion should be considered.

## Disorders With Distinctive Shoulder-Girdle or Arm Weakness

In *Emery-Dreifuss muscular dystrophy*, clinical features include prominent early contractures of the elbows, posterior neck, and Achilles tendons, with atrophy and weakness of muscles around the shoulders, upper arms, and lower part of the legs. Cardiac conduction abnormalities are common, and acute heart block is a frequent cause of death. Shoulder-girdle and arm weakness are also prominent features of FSH muscular dystrophy, discussed earlier.

Distal muscular weakness and atrophy are most common in neurogenic disorders. Benign focal amyotrophy, also known as *Sobue disease* or *monomelic amyotrophy*, manifests with the insidious onset of weakness and atrophy of the hand and forearm muscles, predominantly in men between the ages of 18 and 22 years. ALS often begins as weakness and wasting in one distal limb. More important to identify because it is treatable is MMNCB, a rare demyelinating polyneuropathy that may be confused clinically with ALS with LMN dysfunction. The initial features often are weakness, hyporeflexia, and fasciculations, especially of the hands. Clues to the diagnosis are a slow indolent course, weakness out of proportion to the amount of atrophy, and asymmetrical involvement of muscles of the same myotome but with a different peripheral nerve supply (e.g., weakness of ulnar nerve-innervated C8 muscles out of proportion to weakness of median nerve-innervated C8 muscles—the so-called "split hand" sign). Charcot-Marie-Tooth disease usually manifests with distal weakness and wasting that starts in the distal lower limbs before involving the hands, although, eventually, the hand and arm muscles are involved.

Distal muscular disorders that may manifest with upper-extremity complaints include myotonic dystrophy, and *Welander myopathy*, a hereditary distal myopathy caused by heterozygous mutation in the *TIA1* gene on chromosome 2p13. Welander myopathy, transmitted as an autosomal dominant trait, has a predilection for the finger and wrist extensor muscles. Other hereditary distal myopathies typically present first in the lower extremities.

Insidious onset of weakness of the finger flexors with relative preservation of finger extensor strength is common in *inclusion-body myositis*, a condition that generally manifests after the age of 50 years. In patients with this disorder, however, weakness is also prominent in the lower extremities, especially the quadriceps.

## Disorders With Prominent Hip-Girdle or Leg Weakness

Although patients with these disorders often have diffuse weakness, including arm and shoulder-girdle weakness, it is usually their hip and leg weakness that brings them to medical attention.

The SMAs are hereditary neuronopathies manifesting with prominent proximal weakness. The atrophy results from the death of anterior horn cells in the spinal cord. This condition spares extraocular muscles, and reflexes are absent. The natural history classification of the SMAs is by age at onset and severity; most forms share a defect in the *survival motor neuron* (*SMN1*) gene on chromosome 5q and are of autosomal recessive inheritance. Acute infantile SMA (*Werdnig-Hoffmann disease*) is a severe and usually fatal illness characterized by marked weakness of the limbs and respiratory muscles. Children with the intermediate form of SMA (chronic Werdnig-Hoffmann disease or SMA type 2) also have severe weakness, rarely maintaining the ability to walk for more than a few years. However, with the use of antisense oligonucleotide therapy for SMA discussed in the genetics section of this chapter, the clinical phenotype of patients with SMA, especially those treated early in life, is changing; the strength and ability to reach motor milestones are improved compared with the natural history of the disease. The chronic juvenile form of SMA (*Kugelberg-Welander syndrome*) begins sometime during the first decade of life, and patients walk well into the second decade or even into early adult life. Scoliosis is less common than in SMA type 2. This condition is consistent with a normal life span. Finally, adult-onset SMA leads to slowly progressive proximal muscle weakness after the age of 20 years.

The inherited muscular dystrophies cause progressive, nonfluctuating weakness. Aside from the inherited distal muscular dystrophies discussed earlier in the chapter, other muscular dystrophies manifest with proximal muscle weakness. *DMD*, inherited as an X-linked recessive trait caused by mutations in the *DMD* gene, is associated with an absence of dystrophin. Clinically, the combination of proximal weakness in a male child with hypertrophic calf muscles and contractures of the Achilles tendons gives the clue to the diagnosis. The serum CK concentration is markedly elevated. Although muscle biopsy is diagnostic, genetic testing is now preferred to confirm the diagnosis (see Chapter 48). The clinical features of *Becker muscular dystrophy* are identical except for later onset and slower progression. Cardiomyopathy is also a feature. Female carriers of the gene usually are free of symptoms but may present with limb-girdle distribution weakness or cardiomyopathy.

The limb-girdle dystrophies constitute a well-accepted diagnostic classification despite their clinical and genetic heterogeneity. Weakness begins in the hips, shoulders, or both and spreads gradually to involve the rest of the limbs and the trunk. The genetics of these disorders is constantly expanding (see Chapter 48), and genetic testing is now available for many limb-girdle dystrophies.

Severe early-onset limb-girdle dystrophy similar in phenotype to DMD, including calf hypertrophy, occurs in the *sarcoglycanopathies*. The cause is a deficiency in one of the dystrophin-associated glycoproteins (sarcoglycans α, β, γ, and δ). The inheritance pattern in these disorders is autosomal recessive, not X-linked, and the sarcoglycanopathies affect both genders equally. Cardiac involvement is rare, and mental retardation is not part of the phenotype. Another cause of a severe Duchenne-like phenotype is mutation of the *FKRP* gene, also inherited in an autosomal recessive manner.

With less severe limb-girdle phenotypes, several genetic causes have been recognized, and inheritance is both autosomal recessive and autosomal dominant. In general, the phenotype in the autosomal recessive group is clinically more severe, with earlier onset of weakness and more rapid progression.

Diagnostic evaluation of limb-girdle muscular dystrophies is rapidly evolving and covered in greater depth in Chapter 109. Genetic testing for dystrophin, sarcoglycans, and other genes may be appropriate before performance of muscle biopsy. If the appropriate genetic tests are uninformative, then muscle biopsy is indicated. The biopsy specimen will show dystrophic changes, separating limb-girdle dystrophy from other (inflammatory) myopathies and from denervating diseases such as SMA. Immunohistochemical analysis of dystrophic muscle may provide a specific diagnosis, but not in all cases. Unfortunately, many patients with limb-girdle muscular dystrophies do not receive a specific diagnosis.

With the exception of Welander myopathy, predominantly lower-extremity weakness is the usual presentation of hereditary distal myopathies. Among these disorders are the Markesbery-Griggs-Udd, Nonaka, and Laing myopathies, which affect anterior compartment muscles in the leg, and Miyoshi myopathy, which affects predominantly the posterior calf muscles.

In patients with inclusion-body myositis, the quadriceps and forearm finger flexor muscles often are preferentially involved. In some patients, this involvement may be asymmetrical at the onset. The other inflammatory myopathies—polymyositis and dermatomyositis—affect proximal, predominantly hip-girdle muscles in a symmetrical fashion. Although rare, the Lambert–Eaton myasthenic syndrome manifests with proximal lower-extremity weakness in more than half of patients, similar to a myopathy. Hyporeflexia and autonomic and sensory symptoms may suggest the diagnosis. EMG often is diagnostic.

Ascending weakness of subacute onset with hyporeflexia, usually with numbness, is the hallmark of Guillain-Barré syndrome. The examiner should take care to look for a spinal sensory level and UMN signs because a spinal cord lesion can mimic this presentation. When present, bulbar weakness is helpful in the diagnosis. Respiratory weakness may result. As discussed earlier, multiple neuromuscular causes of weakness of subacute onset with respiratory failure are recognized.

Distal muscle weakness and atrophy are the hallmarks of neurogenic disorders. In both the demyelinating and axonal forms of Charcot-Marie-Tooth disease, the problem in the legs antedates that in the hands. In ALS, the weakness often is asymmetrical and may combine with UMN signs.

## Disorders With Fluctuating Weakness

An important consideration in the differential diagnosis is whether the weakness is constant or fluctuating. Even constant weakness may vary somewhat in degree, depending on how the patient feels. It is well recognized that an individual's physical performance is better on days when they feel energetic and cheerful and is less optimal on days when they feel depressed or are sick. Such factors can also be expected to affect the patient with neuromuscular weakness. The examiner should make specific inquiries to determine how much variability exists. Does the strength fluctuation relate to exercise or time of day? Pathological fatigue is the hallmark of neuromuscular junction abnormalities.

Factors other than exercise may result in worsening or improvement of the disease. Some patients notice that fasting, carbohydrate loading, or other dietary manipulations make a difference in their symptoms. Such details may provide a clue to underlying metabolic problems. Patients with a defect in lipid-based energy metabolism are weaker in the fasting state and may carry a candy bar or sugar with them. The patient with hypokalemic periodic paralysis may notice that inactivity after a high-carbohydrate meal precipitates an attack.

The usual cause of weakness that fluctuates markedly on a day-to-day basis or within a space of several hours is a defect in neuromuscular transmission, metabolic abnormality, or channel disorder (e.g., periodic paralysis), rather than one of the muscular dystrophies. Most neurologists recognize that the cardinal features of MG are ptosis, ophthalmoparesis, dysarthria, dysphagia, and proximal weakness (see Chapter 108). On clinical examination, the hallmark of MG is pathological muscle fatigue. Normal muscles fatigue if exercised sufficiently, but in MG, fatigue occurs with little effort. Failure of neuromuscular transmission may prevent holding the arms in an outstretched position for more than a few seconds or maintenance of sustained upgaze. Frequently, the patient is relatively normal in the office, making the diagnosis of myasthenia more difficult; the history and ancillary studies (assay for AChR antibodies, anti-MuSK antibodies, and EMG with repetitive stimulation or single-fiber EMG) must be relied on to establish the diagnosis.

In the Lambert-Eaton myasthenic syndrome, fluctuating weakness may also occur, but the fluctuating character is less marked than in MG. Weakness of the shoulder and especially the hip girdle predominates, with the bulbar, ocular, and respiratory muscles relatively spared. Exceptions to this latter rule are recognized, and some presentations of Lambert-Eaton myasthenic syndrome mimic MG. Typically, reflexes are reduced or absent at rest. After a brief period of exercise, weakness and reflexes often are improved (facilitation), which is the opposite of the situation in MG. The electrophysiological correlate of this phenomenon is the demonstration of a marked incremental response to rapid, repetitive nerve stimulation or brief exercise. The underlying pathophysiology of Lambert-Eaton myasthenic syndrome is an autoimmune or paraneoplastic process mediated by anti–voltage-gated calcium channel antibodies; commercial testing for these antibodies is available.

Patients with periodic paralysis note attacks of weakness, typically provoked by rest after exercise. Inheritance of the primary periodic paralyses is as an autosomal dominant trait secondary to a sodium or calcium channel defect (see Chapter 98). In the hyperkalemic (sodium channel) form, patients experience weakness that may last from minutes to days; beginning in infancy to early childhood, the provocation is by rest after exercise or potassium ingestion. Potassium levels generally are high during an attack. In the hypokalemic (calcium channel) form, weakness may last hours to days, is quite severe beginning in the early teens, manifests more in male than in female individuals, and the provocation is by rest after exercise or carbohydrate ingestion. Potassium levels generally are low during an attack.

Secondary hypokalemic periodic paralysis occurs in a subset of patients with thyrotoxicosis. The syndrome is clinically identical to primary hypokalemic periodic paralysis, except for the age at presentation, which usually is in adulthood. In both types of primary periodic paralysis, paralysis may be total, but with sparing of bulbofacial muscles. Respiratory muscle paralysis is rare in hypokalemic periodic paralysis. Patients with paramyotonia congenita may also experience attacks of weakness, especially in the cold. EMG with special protocols for exercise and cooling may be diagnostic; genetic testing is also available for these disorders.

## Disorders Exacerbated by Exercise

Fatigue and muscle pain provoked by exercise, the most common complaints in patients presenting to the muscle clinic, often are unexplained. Diagnoses such as fibromyalgia (see Chapter 104) may confound the examination. Biochemical defects are being detected in an increasing number of patients with exercise-induced fatigue and myalgia. The metabolic abnormalities that impede exercise are disorders of carbohydrate metabolism, lipid metabolism, and mitochondrial function (see Chapter 109). The patient's history may give some clue to the type of defect.

Fatty acids provide the main source of energy for resting muscle. Initiation of vigorous exercise requires the use of intracellular stores of energy because blood-borne metabolites initially are inadequate. It takes time for the cardiac output to increase, for capillaries to dilate, and for the blood supply to muscle to be increased, and an even longer time to mobilize fat stores in the body in order to increase the level of fatty acids in the blood. Because muscle must use its glycogen stores for energy in this initial phase of heavy exercise, defects of glycogen metabolism cause fatigue and muscle pain in the first few minutes of exercise. As exercise continues, the blood supply increases, resulting in an increased supply of oxygen, glucose, and fatty acids. After 10–15 minutes, the muscle begins to use a mixture of fat and carbohydrate. The use of carbohydrate is not tolerated for long periods, however, because it would deplete the body's glycogen stores, potentially resulting in hypoglycemia. After 30–40 minutes of continued endurance exercise, the muscle is using chiefly fatty acids as an energy source. Patients with defective fatty acid metabolism easily tolerate the initial phase of exercise. With endurance exercise lasting 30–60 minutes, however, they may become incapacitated. Similarly, in the fasting state, the body is more dependent on fatty acids, which it uses to conserve glucose. Thus, the patient with a disorder of fatty acid metabolism may complain of increased symptoms when exercising in the fasting state. Ingestion of a candy bar may give some relief because this quickly boosts the blood glucose level. Patients with fatty acid metabolism defects often have well-developed muscles because they prefer relatively intense, brief, power exercise such as weightlifting.

Disorders of mitochondrial metabolism vary in presentation. In some types, recurrent encephalopathic episodes occur, often noted in early childhood and resembling Reye disease (see Chapter 92). In other types, particular weakness of the extraocular and skeletal muscles is a presenting feature. In still other types, usually affecting young adults, the symptoms are predominantly of exercise intolerance. Defects occur in the electron transport system or cytochrome chain that uncouples oxygen consumption from the useful production of adenosine triphosphate (ATP). The resulting limit on available ATP causes metabolic pathways to operate at their maximum with even a light exercise load. Resting tachycardia, high lactic acid levels in the blood, excessive sweating, and other indications of hypermetabolism may be noted. This clinical picture may lead to an erroneous diagnosis of hyperthyroidism. It is essential always to measure the serum lactic acid concentration when a mitochondrial myopathy is suspected, although the level is normal in some patients. In addition to lactate, ammonia and hypoxanthine concentrations may also be elevated.

Patients with suspected metabolic defects should undergo forearm exercise testing. A blood pressure cuff should not be used for the ischemic portion of the test because this may be hazardous in patients with defects in the glycolytic pathway.

## Disorders With Constant Weakness

With disorders characterized by constant weakness, the course is one of stability or steady deterioration. Without treatment, periods of sustained objective improvement or major differences in strength on a day-to-day basis are lacking. The division of this group of disorders into subacute and chronic also needs clarification. *Subacute* means that weakness appeared over weeks to months in a previously healthy person. In contrast, *chronic* implies a much less definite onset and prolonged course. Although the patient may say that the weakness came on suddenly, a careful history elicits symptoms that go back many years. This division is not absolute. Patients with polymyositis, usually a subacute disease, may have a slow course mimicking a muscular dystrophy. Patients with a muscular dystrophy may have a slow decrease in strength but suddenly lose a specific function such as standing from a chair or climbing stairs and believe their deterioration to be acute in onset.

## Acquired Disorders Causing Weakness

The usual acquired disorders that produce weakness are motor neuron diseases; inflammatory, toxic, or endocrine disorders of muscle; neuromuscular transmission disorders; and peripheral neuropathies with predominantly motor involvement. The first task is to determine whether the weakness is neuropathic, myopathic, or secondary to a neuromuscular transmission defect. In some instances, this is straightforward, and in others, it is very difficult. For instance, some cases of motor neuron disease with predominantly LMN dysfunction may mimic inclusion-body myositis, and Lambert-Eaton myasthenic syndrome may mimic polymyositis. If fasciculations are present, the disorder must be neuropathic. If reflexes are absent and muscle bulk is preserved, suspect a demyelinating neuropathy, although presynaptic neuromuscular junction disorders (e.g., Lambert-Eaton myasthenic syndrome) also show hyporeflexia with normal muscle bulk. The presence of sensory signs or symptoms, even if mild, may indicate a peripheral neuropathy or involvement of the CNS. Often, separating these conditions requires serum CK testing, EMG, and muscle biopsy.

ALS is the most common acquired motor neuron disease. Although peak age at onset is from 65 to 70 years, the disorder can occur at any adult age. It often follows a relatively rapid course preceded by cramps and fasciculations. Examination shows muscle atrophy and often widely distributed fasciculations. If the bulbar muscles are involved, difficulties with swallowing and speaking are also present. The diagnosis is relatively simple if unequivocal evidence of UMN dysfunction accompanies muscle atrophy and fasciculations. UMN signs include slowness of movement, hyperreflexia, Babinski sign, and spasticity. A weak, atrophic muscle associated with an abnormally brisk reflex is almost pathognomonic for ALS. The finding of widespread denervation on needle electrode examination in the absence of any sensory abnormalities or demyelinating features on nerve conduction testing supports the diagnosis. In all patients without bulbar involvement, it is important to rule out spinal pathology, because the combination of cervical and lumbar stenosis occasionally may mimic ALS with respect to clinical and electrophysiological findings.

In patients with only LMN dysfunction, it is essential to exclude the rare diagnosis of *MMNCB*, a condition usually treatable with intravenous gamma globulin. Patients with MMNCB usually have no bulbar features or UMN signs, and a characteristic finding includes demyelination (i.e., conduction block) on motor nerve conduction testing. Because the underlying pathophysiological process is conduction block, weakness usually is more severe than expected for the observed degree of atrophy. However, atrophy occurs, especially when the condition is of long duration.

Although most adults with motor neuron disease have ALS or one of its variants, sporadic forms of adult-onset SMA and especially X-linked spinobulbar muscular atrophy (Kennedy disease) can occur as well. In these cases, the progression of weakness is much slower, and UMN involvement is absent. Of importance, these latter cases, especially Kennedy disease, often have elevated CK levels in the range of 500–1500 U/L.

If the patient has a myopathy, acquired and inherited causes should be considered. A discussion of the presentation of inherited myopathic disorders appears earlier in the chapter. Causes of acquired myopathies include inflammatory conditions and a large number of toxic, drug-induced, and endocrine disorders. Inflammatory myopathies include polymyositis, dermatomyositis, and inclusion-body myositis and often run a steadily progressive course, although some fluctuations occur, particularly in children. Onset of weakness in polymyositis and dermatomyositis is subacute, weakness is proximal, and serum CK levels usually are increased. If an associated rash is present, little doubt exists about the diagnosis of dermatomyositis. If a rash is absent, polyomyositis may be difficult to differentiate clinically from any of the other causes of proximal weakness. Sometimes, the illness occurs as part of an overlap syndrome in which fragments of other autoimmune diseases (e.g., scleroderma, lupus, and rheumatoid arthritis) are involved. Polymyositis sometimes is difficult to differentiate from a muscular dystrophy, even after muscle biopsy; some inflammatory changes occur in muscular dystrophies, most notably in FSH muscular dystrophy. Other signs of systemic involvement such as malaise, transitory aching pains, mood changes, and loss of appetite are more common in polymyositis than in limb-girdle dystrophy.

Inclusion-body myopathy typically has a chronic, insidious onset. It occasionally mimics polymyositis but more often mimics ALS associated with LMN dysfunction. Clues to the diagnosis are male gender, onset after the age of 50 years in most patients, slower progression, and characteristic involvement of the quadriceps and long finger flexors. Some patients may have proximal muscle weakness, as in polymyositis, whereas others may have predominantly distal weakness mimicking that of ALS and other neuropathic conditions. Serum CK generally is elevated but occasionally may be normal. As with other chronic inflammatory myopathies, interpreting the EMG study may be difficult and requires an experienced examiner because inclusion-body myopathy often shows a combination of myopathic and neuropathic features. Inclusion-body myopathy, unlike polymyositis, often is unresponsive to immunosuppressive therapy. Pathological features include rimmed vacuoles and intracytoplasmic and intranuclear filamentous inclusions.

Toxic, drug-induced, and endocrine disorders are always considerations in the differential diagnosis of acquired myopathies. Among toxins, alcohol is still one of the most common and may produce both an acute and a chronic myopathic syndrome. Several prescription medicines are associated with myopathies. Most prominent are corticosteroids, cholesterol-lowering agents (i.e., statins), and colchicine.

Although neuromuscular transmission disorders are always diagnostic considerations in patients with fluctuating symptoms, the Lambert-Eaton myasthenic syndrome may be an exception. It often manifests with progressive proximal lower-extremity weakness without fluctuations. Clues to the diagnosis include a history of cancer, especially small-cell lung cancer (although in many patients the myasthenic syndrome may predate the discovery of the cancer), hyporeflexia, facilitation of strength and reflexes after brief exercise, and coexistent autonomic symptoms, especially urinary and sexual dysfunction in men.

Sensory features separate peripheral neuropathies from disorders of the motor unit. The notable exception is MMNCB, discussed earlier. Other neuropathies may also manifest with predominantly motor symptoms. Among these are toxic neuropathies (from dapsone, vincristine, lead, or an acute alcohol-related neuropathy) and some variants of Guillain-Barré syndrome (especially the acute motor axonal neuropathy syndrome).

## Lifelong Disorders

Most patients presenting to the neuromuscular clinic will have lifelong or at least very chronic, presumably inherited, disorders. These include inherited disorders of muscle (e.g., dystrophies and congenital myopathies), anterior horn cell (e.g., Kennedy disease), peripheral nerves (e.g., Charcot-Marie-Tooth polyneuropathy), or very rarely, neuromuscular transmission (e.g., congenital myasthenic syndromes). In some of these disorders, the responsible genetic abnormality has been identified. An important point in the differential diagnosis is to determine whether the weakness is truly progressive. The examiner should ask questions until the progressive or nonprogressive nature of the disease is ascertained. The severity of the disease is not proof of progression. It is difficult to imagine that a 16-year-old girl confined to her wheelchair with SMA and scoliosis and having difficulty breathing has a relatively nonprogressive disorder, but careful questioning may reveal no loss of function for several years. Furthermore, it is not sufficient to ask the patient in vague and general terms whether the illness is progressive. Questioning should be specific; for example, "Are there tasks you cannot perform now that you could perform last week (month, year)?" The examiner must also be alert for denial, which is common in young patients with increasing weakness. The 18-year-old boy with limb-girdle dystrophy may claim to be the same now as in years gone by, but questioning may reveal that he was able to climb stairs well when he was in high school, whereas he now needs assistance in college.

### Lifelong Nonprogressive Disorders

Some patients complain of lifelong weakness that has been relatively unchanged over many years. Almost by definition, such disorders have to start in early childhood. Nonprogression of weakness does not preclude severe weakness. Later-life progression of such weakness may occur as the normal aging process further weakens muscles that have little functional reserve. One major group of such illnesses is the congenital nonprogressive myopathies, including central core disease, nemaline myopathy, and congenital fiber-type disproportion. The typical clinical picture in these diseases is that of a slender dysmorphic patient with diffuse weakness. Other features may include skeletal abnormalities such as high-arched palate, pes cavus, and scoliosis, which are supportive of the presence of weakness in early life. Deep tendon reflexes are depressed or absent. Although unusual, severe respiratory involvement may occur in all these diseases. The less severe (non-X-linked) form of myotubular (centronuclear) myopathy is suggested by findings of ptosis, extraocular muscle weakness, and facial diplegia. Muscle biopsy usually provides a specific morphological diagnosis in the congenital myopathies; specific genetic testing is now available for many of the congenital myopathies. Several varieties of congenital muscular dystrophy (CMD) are recognized. The weakness in CMD manifests in the newborn period, with the affected child presenting as a floppy baby. Skeletal deformities and contractures may be present. CNS abnormalities, including cognitive impairment, seizures, and structural brain or eye abnormalities, may be present. The classification is based on the involved protein function and causative gene mutation. The main CMD subtypes, grouped by the involved protein function and gene in which causative mutations occur, include defects in structural proteins, glycosylation, proteins of the endoplasmic reticulum and nuclear envelope, and mitochondrial membrane proteins. The disorders with CNS structural abnormalities are very severe; for example, characteristics of Fukuyama CMD include microcephaly, mental retardation, and seizures with severe disability. The serum CK concentration may be markedly elevated in CMDs. The muscle biopsy specimen shows dystrophic changes, and immunohistochemistry often provides a specific diagnosis. Tests for some of the gene mutations are commercially available.

### Lifelong Disorders Characterized by Progressive Weakness

Most diseases in the category of lifelong disorders characterized by progressive weakness are inherited progressive disorders of anterior horn cells, peripheral motor nerve, or muscle. Among these are the spinal muscular atrophies, Charcot-Marie-Tooth polyneuropathies, and muscular dystrophies. Mild day-to-day fluctuations in strength may occur in these disorders, but the overall progression is steady (i.e., the disorder is slowly progressive from the start and remains that way); it will not suddenly change course and become rapidly progressive. As mentioned earlier, patients may experience long periods of stability when their disease is seemingly nonprogressive.

Traditional attempts to categorize disorders are based on whether the disorder is caused by anterior horn cell, peripheral motor nerve, or muscle disease, along with a specific pattern of muscle weakness. Certain characteristic patterns of weakness often suggest specific diagnoses. For example, the names of FSH and oculopharyngeal muscular dystrophies reflect their selective involvement of muscles. Today, all disorders are redefined and categorized in accordance with their specific genetic abnormality.

## Other Conditions

No scheme of analysis is perfect in clinical medicine, and many exceptions to the guidelines provided earlier exist. Most notable are disorders restricted to various parts of the body. The etiology for such localized illness is often unclear but may represent a forme fruste of a disorder with a specific gene defect. Examples include branchial myopathy and quadriceps myopathy, as well as the focal forms of motor neuron disease such as benign monomelic amyotrophy. These diseases often are "benign" in that they do not shorten life. The weakness may cause disability, although it is usually mild.

*The complete reference list is available online at https://expertconsult.inkling.com/.*

29

# Muscle Pain and Cramps

*Leo H. Wang, Glenn Lopate*

## OUTLINE



## GENERAL FEATURES OF PAIN

Pain is an uncomfortable sensation with sensory and emotional components. Short episodes of pain or discomfort localized to muscle are a near universal experience. Common causes of short-term muscle discomfort are unaccustomed exercise, trauma, cramps, and systemic infections. Pain localized to muscle may be due to noxious stimuli in muscle or referral from other structures including skin, nerves, connective tissue, joints, and bone. Common syndromes with pain localized to muscle but no histological muscle pathology include fibromyalgia and small-fiber neuropathies. The referral of pain from other structures to muscle may involve stimulation of central neural pathways or secondary noxious contraction of muscle.

The best categorization of pain in muscle and other tissues is by temporal and qualitative features. Cutaneous pain is thought to be subjectively experienced as two phases: the first phase perceived as sharp, well-localized, and lasting as long as the stimulus. A delayed second phase of pain is experienced as dull, aching or burning, and more diffuse. In contrast to cutaneous pain, visceral, muscular, or chronic pain is more likely experienced subjectively similar to the second phase of cutaneous pain, and has more sensory and affective components. Pain from stimulation of diseased tissue is often associated with *hyperalgesia*, in which a noxious stimulus produces an exaggerated pain sensation, or with *allodynia*, pain induced by a normally innocuous stimulus.

Sensitization is the reduction of the pain threshold and can be the result of changes in molecular composition, cellular interactions, and network connectivity throughout the pain system. Neuropathic pain, localized to muscle or other tissues, is associated with increased afferent axon activity and occurs spontaneously or after peripheral stimuli. It may be related to central or peripheral sensitization.

## MUSCLE PAIN: BASIC CONCEPTS

Generation of pain localized to muscle involves activation of afferent axons, conduction of pain signals through the peripheral and central nervous systems (PNS and CNS), and central processing of properties of the afferent signals.

### Nociceptor Terminal Stimulation and Sensitization

Stimuli of afferent axons can be mechanical or chemical (for review see Khan, 2019). Mechanosensory transduction is mediated by mechanosensitive ion channels such as piezo2, transient receptor potential cation channel, subfamily A, member 1 (TRPA1), transient receptor potential cation channel, subfamily V, member 4 (TRPV4), or members of the degenerin/epithelial sodium channel (DEG/ENaC) family.

Endogenous chemical stimuli of muscle nociceptors include protons ($H^+$) and adenosine triphosphate (ATP), which are increased in muscle with damage. In humans, injection of acidic buffered solution into muscle elicits pain, which activate the acid-sensing ion channels (ASICs), a subfamily of the DEG/ENaC superfamily. ASICs are expressed on sensory axons innervating skeletal and/or cardiac muscles. One member, ASIC3, may initiate the anginal pain associated with myocardial ischemia. The heat and capsaicin receptor TRPV1 can also be activated under strong acidic conditions.

The second important chemical cause of muscle pain is ATP. ATP is present in increased levels in muscle interstitium during ischemic muscle contraction. Injection of ATP also elicits pain. Many peripheral nociceptors express purinergic receptors, which include two subfamilies: the P2Y receptors (G-protein-coupled receptors) and P2X receptors (ATP-gated ion channels formed from a trimer of P2X receptors). In muscle, the release of ATP primarily activates the receptor complexes composed of a combination of $P2X_2$ and/or $P2X_3$ receptors. Pharmacological inhibition or genetic deletion of $P2X_2$ or $P2X_3$ receptor antagonists can reverse mouse models of hyperalgesia induced mechanically or by inflammation.

Other chemical substances (bradykinin, serotonin, prostaglandin E2 [PGE2] and nerve growth factor [NGF]) that most likely do not activate pain afferents at physiological levels can induce pain at supraphysiological levels, or can sensitize peripheral nociceptive afferents. Sensitization of nociceptive axon terminals is reduction of the threshold for their stimulation into the innocuous range. Sensitization of nociceptor terminals can have two effects on axons: (1) an increase in the frequency of action potentials in normally active nociceptors or (2) induction of new action potentials in a population of normally silent small axons.

Bradykinin, serotonin, and prostaglandins are normally sequestered in normal tissue and increase in damaged tissue. Bradykinin is the protease product of the plasma protein kallidin. In damaged tissue, kallidin is exposed to and cleaved by tissue kallikreins forming bradykinin. Serotonin is normally stored in platelets and is released when the platelets are in damaged tissue. Bradykinin and serotonin are only mildly painful when injected into human muscle. Bradykinin produces more pain after the injection of PGE2 or serotonin.

PGE2 is present in delayed-onset muscle soreness (DOMS). PGE2 is released from endothelial and other tissue cells. The depression of muscle nociceptor activity by aspirin may reflect inhibition of the effects of PGE2.

Endogenous substances proposed to play roles in activating or sensitizing peripheral nociceptive afferents include neurotransmitters (serotonin, histamine, glutamate, nitric oxide, adrenaline), neuropeptides (substance P [SP], tachykinins, bradykinin, NGF, calcitonin gene-related peptide [CGRP], endothelin 1), proteases (that activate proteinase-activated receptor 2 [PAR2]), and inflammatory mediators (prostaglandins, cytokines). In humans, intramuscular injection of glutamate, capsaicin, levoascorbic acid, hypertonic saline (sodium chloride 5%–6%), and potassium chloride causes pain. Glutamate is an important neurotransmitter in the CNS pain pathway, and, peripherally, is probably more important in sensitizing muscle afferents. Increased levels of glutamate in muscle correlate temporally with the appearance of pain after exercise or experimental injections of hypertonic saline. There are no specific membrane receptors for hypertonic saline (sodium chloride 5%–6%) and potassium chloride; they activate muscle nociceptors through changing membrane equilibrium potential.

Lactate, an anaerobic metabolite, probably does not play a primary role in directly stimulating muscle pain. Patients with myophosphorylase deficiency do not produce lactate under ischemia yet experience pain. Lactate may potentiate the effects of $H^+$ ions on ASIC3 channels in activating pain-related axons.

Many receptors that respond to chemical stimuli are also activated by changes in temperature: TRPA1, TRPM3, and TRPM8 receptors are activated by cold temperatures; TRPV1 and TRPV3 by warm temperatures. Gain-of-function TRPA1 mutations are associated with familial episodic pain syndromes (Kremeyer et al., 2010).

No matter what the stimuli, the propagation of generated pain signal is dependent on sodium channels. Important sodium channels expressed in muscle nociceptive afferents include the sodium channels ($Na_V$) 1.7, 1.8, and 1.9 (*SCN9A*, *SCN10A*, and *SCN11A*, respectively). $Na_V$ 1.7 and 1.9 act as threshold channels—causing an initial depolarization leading to additional sodium channels to open; $Na_V$ 1.8 acts to sustain depolarization in the setting of sustained noxious stimuli. Mutations in genes for these channels may cause loss or increase of pain (Dib-Hajj and Waxman, 2019).

## Nociceptive Axons

Many of the afferent axons that transmit painful stimuli from muscle (nociceptors) have free nerve endings (see review by Mense and Gerwin, 2010). These free nerve endings do not have corpuscular receptive structures such as pacinian or paciniform corpuscles. They appear as a "string of beads," thin stretches of axon (with diameters of 0.5–1.0 μm) with intervening varicosities. Most free nerve endings are ensheathed by a single layer of Schwann cells that leave bare some of the axon membranes, where only the basal membrane of the Schwann cell separates the axon membrane from the interstitial fluid. A single fiber has several branches that extend over a broad area. These terminal axons (nerve endings) end near the perimysium, adventitia of arterioles, venules, and lymphatic vessels, but do not contact muscle fibers (Fig. 29.1, *A*). It is not clear whether nociceptive afferents can have both cutaneous and muscle branches. The varicosities in the free terminals contain granular or dense core vesicles containing glutamate and neuropeptides such as SP, vasoactive intestinal peptide (VIP), CGRP, and somatostatin. When the afferents are activated, neuropeptides are released into the interstitial tissue and may activate other nearby muscle nociceptors.

Action potentials arising in nociceptor terminals induce or potentiate pain by two mechanisms: *centripetal conduction* to central branches of afferent axons brings nociceptive signals directly to the CNS. *Centrifugal conduction* of action potentials along peripheral axon branches causes indirect effects by activating other unstimulated nerve terminals of the same nerve and causing release of glutamate and neuropeptides into the extracellular medium. These chemical substances can stimulate or sensitize terminals on other nociceptive axons. This is the basis for the axon reflex and the wheal and flare around a cutaneous lesion.

Group III (class Aδ cutaneous afferent) thinly myelinated and group IV (class C cutaneous afferent) unmyelinated afferent axons conduct the pain-inducing stimuli from muscle to the CNS. Group III nociceptive axons are thinly myelinated and conduct impulses at moderately slow velocities (3–13 m/sec). Group III fibers can end in free nerve terminals (possibly for mediating a more spontaneous pain) or other receptors such as paciniform corpuscles. Group IV fibers are unmyelinated, conduct impulses at very slow velocities (0.6–1.2 m/sec), end as free nerve endings, and are the main mediators of the diffuse, dull, or burning muscle pain.

Group II axons are large and myelinated, and conduct impulses at rapid velocities, mainly from muscle spindles. They normally mediate innocuous stimuli, and stimulation may reduce the perception of pain (by acting on the nociceptive afferents in the spinal cord). Inflammation or repetitive stimulation can sensitize group II afferents (phenotypic switch), which then mediate mechanical allodynia in some tissues.

The cell bodies of all afferents are located in the dorsal root ganglion; the central process enters the CNS through the dorsal root (Fig. 29.2). Central terminals of nociceptive axons from muscle end in lamina I of the superficial dorsal horn and laminae IV–VI of the neck of the dorsal horn of the spinal cord. Cutaneous afferents end in the same areas, but in addition can also terminate in lamina II. Dorsal horn neurons have convergent inputs from afferents from both muscle and skin, and therefore activation of cutaneous afferents may be experienced as muscle pain.

The central terminals of the peripheral nociceptors express N-type ($Ca_V2.2$) channels, which control calcium entry and release of synaptic transmitter spinal dorsal horn neurons. One of its auxiliary (and not pore-forming) subunits is the α2-delta (α2δ) subunit; one of its subunit family member, α2δ-1, is the target of gabapentinoids.

Glutamate is the main neurotransmitter of pain in the CNS and binds N-methyl-D-aspartate (NMDA) and α-amino-3-hydroxy-5-methyl-4-isoxazolepropionic acid (AMPA) receptors. With short-lasting or low-frequency discharges, glutamate is only able to activate AMPA receptors, causing short-lasting and ineffective depolarization of the dorsal horn neuron. Additional inhibitory signals are also present to suppress the conductance of the pain signal: (1) inhibitory signal from the group II myelinated peripheral afferent; and (2) the inhibitory descending pain tracts which contact the central process of the peripheral afferent using glycine and γ-aminobutyric acid (GABA) as inhibitory neurotransmitters. With long-lasting and high-frequency discharges, persistent glutamate signal activates NMDA receptors, which have been shown to be critically important in the development of chronic nociceptive hypersensitivity. In addition, SP, when released, activates tachykinin receptor NK1 receptors, which lead to increased NMDA receptor conductivity and de novo expression

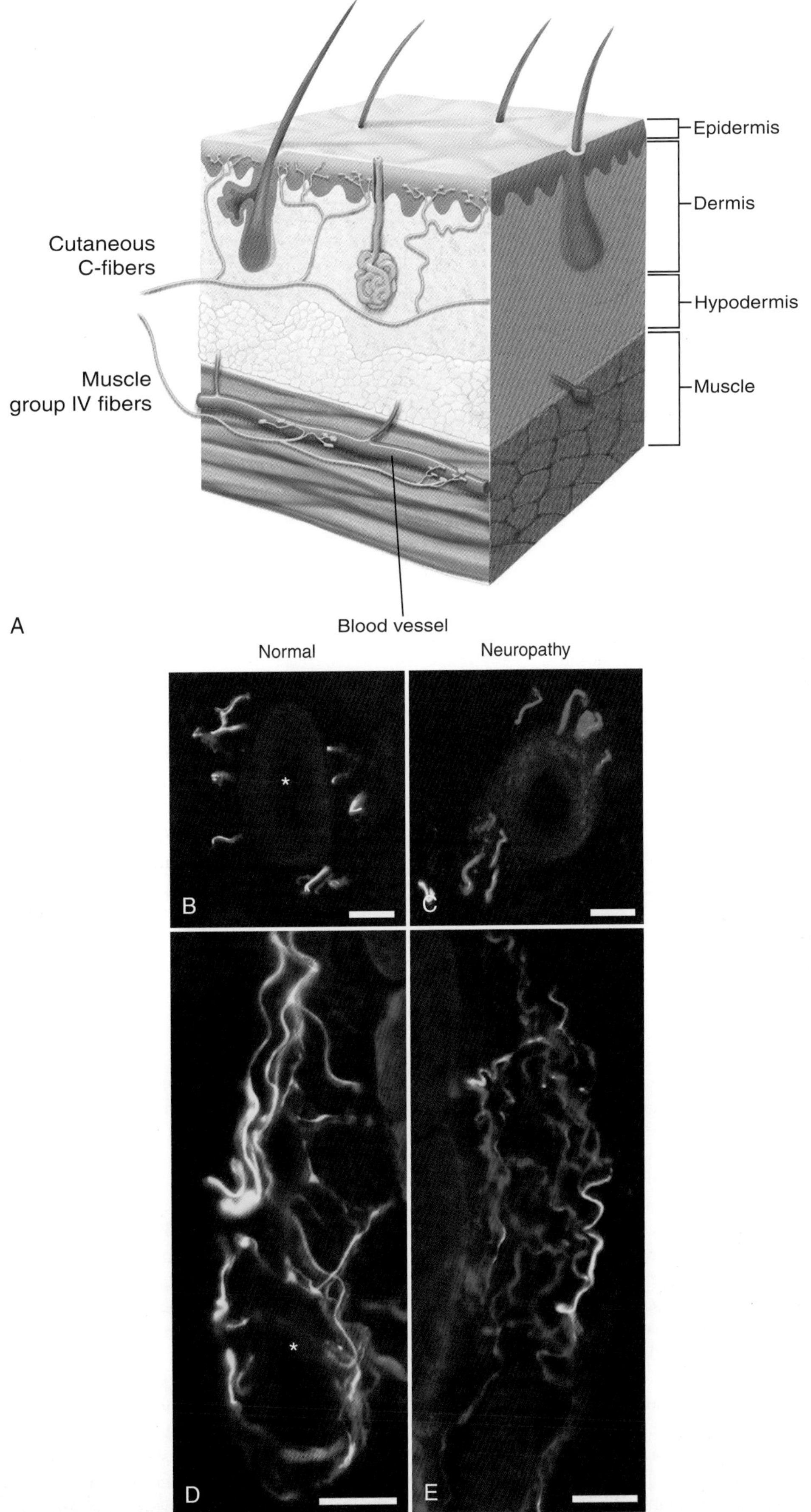


**Fig. 29.1 Sensory Innervation of the Skin and Muscle. A,** C-fiber and group IV fiber innervation of the skin and muscle. **B–E,** Double label staining (yellow) of nonmyelinating Schwann cell cytoplasm by neural cell adhesion molecule (NCAM) (red) and unmyelinated axons by peripherin (green) is much more abundant in the blood vessels (labeled with *) of normal muscle compared with muscle from a patient with -fiber neuropathy where the majority of Schwann cell processes are devoid of axons (bar = 20 μm). *(Courtesy Amir Dori, Glenn Lopate, and Alan Pestronk.)*

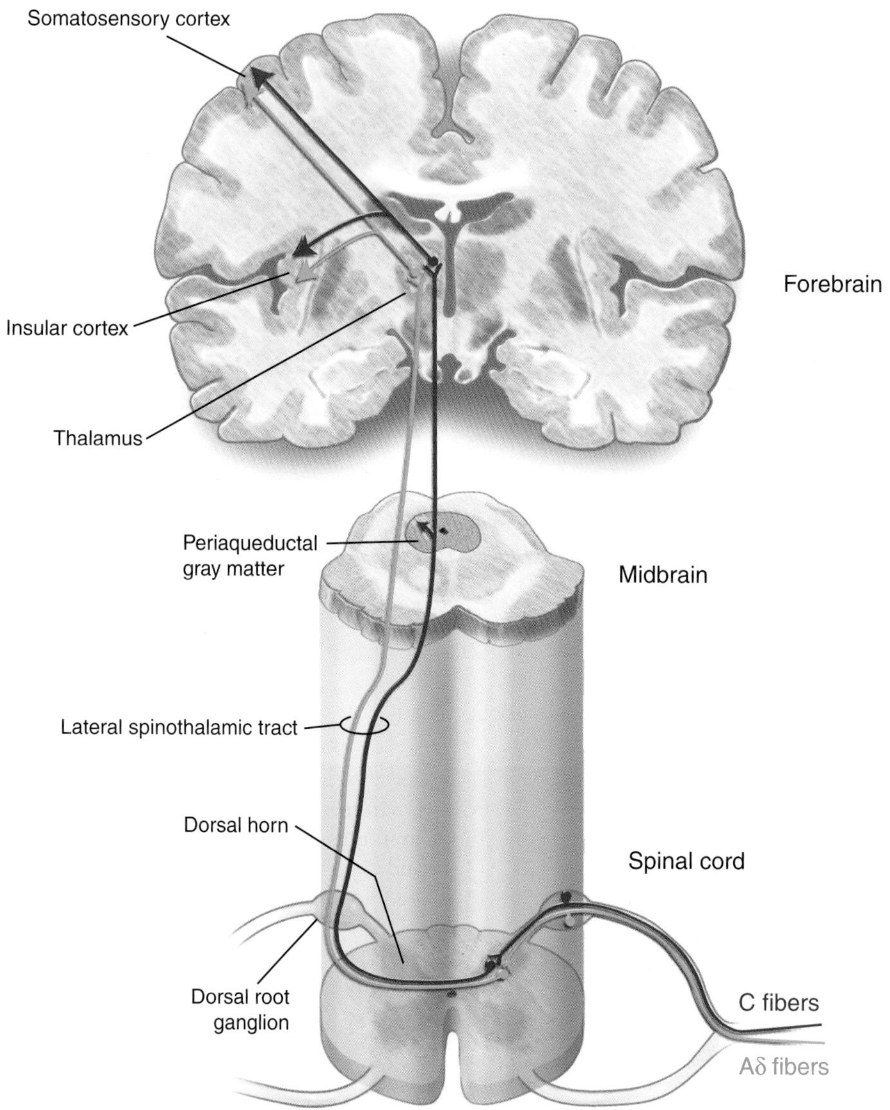


**Fig. 29.2** The Central Nervous System Pain Pathway.

of NMDA receptors. Functional changes in AMPA/NMDA receptor activity are one mechanism resulting in central sensitization. Other mechanisms include metabolic changes in neurons and surrounding glia, and changes in synaptic structure.

Dorsal horn neurons convey pain signals primarily through the contralateral lateral spinothalamic tract, with minor projections through the spinoreticular and spinomesencephalic tracts. The spinothalamic tract terminates in the lateral thalamic nuclei and then relays to the primary and secondary somatosensory cortex, prefrontal cortex (for cognitive and affective pain), anterior cingulate cortex, and insular cortex.

The spinoreticular tract relays information to the medial nuclei of the thalamus, and mediates the autonomic component of pain sensations. The spinomesencephalic tract projects to the amygdala (which processes the emotional and memory aspect of pain).

Afferents conveying muscle pain have different midbrain and thalamic relays than do cutaneous afferents and activate different cortical areas. In addition, interneurons and descending CNS pathways modulate muscle afferents differently than cutaneous afferents. For example, descending antinociceptive pathways that originate in the mesencephalon with connections in the medulla and spinal cord are an important modulator of pain and may be stronger for muscle afferents. These pathways utilize $\alpha_2$-adrenergic, cannabinoid, opioid, and serotonin (5-HT) receptors.

## CLINICAL FEATURES OF MUSCLE PAIN

### General Features of Muscle Pain

In the clinical setting, patients describe muscle discomfort using a variety of terms: pain, soreness, aching, fatigue, cramps, or spasms. Pain with muscle cramps has an acute onset and short duration. Cramp pain is associated with palpable muscle contraction, and stretching the muscle provides immediate relief. Pain originating from fascia and periosteum has relatively precise localization. Cutaneous pain differs from muscle pain by its distinct localization and sharp, pricking, stabbing, or burning nature. Pain with small-fiber neuropathies is often present outside length-dependent distributions and may be located in proximal as well as distal regions. In fibromyalgia syndromes, it is common for patients to complain that fatigue accompanies their muscle discomfort. Depression is more common in patients with chronic musculoskeletal pain than in a population without chronic pain.

**BOX 29.1 Myopathic Pain Syndromes***

**Inflammatory**

Inflammatory and immune myopathies:
- Systemic connective tissue disease
- Perimysial pathology: tRNA synthetase antibodies
- Fasciitis
- Childhood dermatomyositis

Muscle infections:
- Viral myositis (including hepatitis C [possibly], enterovirus, dengue virus)
- Pyomyositis
- Toxoplasmosis
- Trichinosis
- Spirochete (*Borrelia burgdorferi*/Lyme disease)

**Rhabdomyolysis ± Metabolic Disorder**

Glycogen storage disease type V (myophosphorylase deficiency): McArdle disease
Glycogen storage disease type VII (phosphofructokinase deficiency)
Carnitine palmitoyltransferase II
Mitochondrial myopathies
Malignant hyperthermia syndromes
Familial recurrent rhabdomyolysis (myoglobinuria) in childhood (*LPIN1* mutations)

**Other Myopathies With Pain or Discomfort**

Myopathy with tubular aggregates ± cylindrical spirals
Adult-onset nemaline rod myopathy
Multicore disease
Fiber-type disproportion myopathy
Myopathy with deficiency of iron-sulfur clusters
Myopathy with tubulin-reactive crystalline inclusions
Myopathy with hexagonally cross-linked crystalloid inclusions
Myoadenylate deaminase deficiency
Neuromyopathy with internalized capillaries
Myotonias: myotonic dystrophy 2; dominant myotonia congenita (occasional)
Muscular dystrophies (occasional): Duchenne, Becker, limb-girdle dystrophy types 1A, 1C, 2C, 2D, 2E, 2H, 2I, 2L; ANO5-deficient myopathy
Selenium deficiency
Vitamin D deficiency
Toxic myopathy: eosinophilia myalgia, rhabdomyolysis
Hypothyroid myopathy
Mitochondrial disorders (fatigue or myalgias with exercise)
Camurati-Engelmann syndrome (bone pain)

**Drugs and Toxins**

*Usual associated features: weakness, abnormal electromyogram.

## Evaluation of Muscle Discomfort

The basis for the classification of disorders underlying muscle discomfort can be anatomical, temporal in relation to exercise, muscle pathology, and the presence or absence of active muscle contraction during the discomfort (Pestronk, 2019). Evaluation of muscle discomfort typically begins with a history that includes the type, localization, inducing factors, and evolution of the pain; drug use; and mood disorders. The physical examination requires special attention to the localization of any tenderness or weakness. The pain may produce the appearance of weakness by preventing full effort. Typical of this type of "weakness" on examination is sudden reduction in the apparent level of effort, rather than smooth movement through the range of motion expected with true muscle weakness. The sensory examination is important because small-fiber neuropathies commonly cause discomfort with apparent localization in muscle. A general examination is needed to evaluate the possibility that pain may be arising from other tissues such as joints. Blood studies may include creatine kinase (CK), aldolase, complete blood cell count, sedimentation rate, potassium, magnesium, calcium, phosphate, lactate, thyroid functions, and evaluation for systemic immune disorders. CK values of African Americans are higher than those of other races (up to 3 times higher than Caucasian Americans) (Kenney et al., 2012). Evaluate urine myoglobin in patients with a high CK and severe myalgias, especially when they relate to exercise. Electromyography (EMG) may suggest myopathy or if normal may indicate that muscle pain is arising from anatomical loci other than muscle. Nerve conduction studies may detect an underlying neuropathy, but objective documentation of small-fiber neuropathies can require quantitative sensory testing or skin biopsy with staining of intraepidermal nerves. There is reduced innervation of blood vessels within muscle in patients with small-fiber neuropathy (see Fig. 29.1, *B–E*) (Dori et al., 2015).

Magnetic resonance imaging (MRI) could show increased muscle signal on short tau inversion recovery (STIR) sequences. Muscle ultrasound can be a useful and noninvasive method of localizing and defining types of muscle pathology. Muscle biopsy is most often useful in the presence of another abnormal test result such as a high serum CK, aldolase, lactate, or an abnormal EMG. However, important clues to treatable disorders such as fasciitis or systemic immune disorders (connective tissue pathology, perivascular inflammation, or granulomas) may be present in muscle in the absence of other positive testing. Examination of both muscle and connective tissue increases the yield of muscle biopsy in syndromes with muscle discomfort. There is increased diagnostic yield from muscle biopsies if in addition to routine morphological analysis and processing, histochemical analysis includes staining for acid phosphatase, alkaline phosphatase, esterase, mitochondrial enzymes, glycolytic enzymes, $C_{5b-9}$ complement, and major histocompatibility complex (MHC) class I. While disorders of glycogen and lipid metabolism often result in abnormal muscle histochemistry, deficiencies in some enzymes (e.g., phosphoglycerate kinase or carnitine palmitoyltransferase [CPT] II deficiencies) may not cause muscle pathology and diagnosis is best made by genetic testing. Ultrastructural examination of muscle rarely provides additional information in muscle pain syndromes.

# MUSCLE DISCOMFORT: SPECIFIC CAUSES

Muscle pain is broadly divisible into groups, depending on its origin and relation to the time of muscle contraction. Myopathies may be associated with muscle pain without associated muscle contraction (myalgias) (Boxes 29.1 and 29.2). Muscle pain during muscle activity (Box 29.3; also see Box 29.2) may occur with muscle injury, myopathy, cramps, or tonic (relatively long-term) contraction. Some pain syndromes perceived as arising from muscle originate in other tissues, such as connective tissue, nerve, or bone, or have no clear morphological explanation for the pain (Box 29.4).

## Myopathies with Muscle Pain

Myopathies that produce muscle pain (see Box 29.1) are usually associated with weakness, a high serum CK or aldolase, or an abnormal EMG (Pestronk, 2019). Immune-mediated or inflammatory myopathies may produce muscle pain or tenderness (including anti-HMG-CoA reductase [anti-HMGCR] myopathy), especially with an associated systemic connective tissue disease or pathological involvement of connective tissue (including myopathies with anti-tRNA synthetase antibodies). Pain is common in childhood dermatomyositis, immune myopathies associated with systemic disorders, eosinophilia-myalgia syndromes, focal myositis, and infections. Myopathies due

**BOX 29.2 Muscle Discomfort Associated with Drugs and Toxins**

**Inflammatory Myopathy**

Definite:

- Hydralazine
- Penicillamine
- Procainamide
- 1,1′- Ethylidenebis [tryptophan]
- Immune checkpoint inhibitors (ipilimumab, nivolumab, more so anti-PD-1 agents)
- Statin (HMG-CoA reductase antibody myopathy)
- Toxic oil syndrome

Possible:

- Cimetidine
- Imatinib mesylate
- Interferon-α
- Ipecac
- Lansoprazole
- Leuprolide
- Levodopa
- Penicillin
- Phenytoin
- Propylthiouracil
- Proton pump inhibitors
- Sulfonamide

**Rhabdomyolysis ± Chronic Myopathy**

Alcohol
ε-Amino caproic acid
Amphetamines
Cocaine
Cyclosporine
Daptomycin
Hypokalemia
Isoniazid
Lipid-lowering agents*:

- Bezafibrate
- Clofibrate
- Fenofibrate
- Gemfibrozil
- Lovastatin
- Simvastatin
- Pravastatin
- Fluvastatin
- Atorvastatin
- Cerivastatin
- Nicotinic acid
- Red yeast rice

Labetalol
Lithium
Organophosphates
Propofol
Snake venom
Tacrolimus
Zidovudine

**Painful Myopathy ± Rhabdomyolysis**

Colchicine
Emetine
Fenoverine
Germanium
Hypervitaminosis E
Taxenes
Zidovudine

**Myalgia ± Myopathy**

Amiodarone
Amphotericin
Aromatase inhibitors
Azathioprine
Beta-blockers (rare)
Bevacizumab
Bisphosphonates
Bortezomib
Brentuximab
Bumetanide
Calcium channel blockers
Cholesterol-lowering agents
Corticosteroid withdrawal
Danazol
Denosumab
Eculizumab
Estrogen
Evolocumab
Fluoroquinolones
HER2 antibodies (trastuzumab, pertuzumab)
Inotersen
Interferon-α: 2a and 2b
Ivosidenib
Lanadelumab (anti-kallikrein monoclonal antibody)
Mercury (organic)
Methotrexate†
Metolazone
Mushrooms (orellanine/*Psilocybe*)
Opioids
Oral contraceptives
Paclitaxel
Retinoids (all-*trans*-retinoic acid, isotretinoin)
Rifampin
Serotonin reuptake inhibitor treatment and withdrawal‡
Succinylcholine
Tyrosine kinase inhibitors (alectinib, acalabrutinib, dasatinib, imatinib, larotrectinib, lenvatinib, lorlatinib, nilotinib, pazopanib, sunitinib, trametinib, as well as BRAF inhibitors [dabrafenib, vemurafenib])
Vaccines
Vinca alkaloids

**Cramps**

Albuterol
Anticholinesterase
Bergamot (bergapten)
Caffeine
Clofibrate
Cyclosporine
Diuretics (chronic, excessive use)
Lithium
Nifedipine
Terbutaline
Tetanus
Theophylline
Vitamin A

*Especially with concurrent cyclosporine A, danazol, erythromycin, gemfibrozil, niacin, colchicine.
†With concurrent pantoprazole.
‡Especially withdrawal of medications with short half-life (paroxetine, venlafaxine).

## BOX 29.3 Cramps* and Other Involuntary Muscle Contraction Syndromes

**Cramp Syndromes**

Ordinary:
- Common in normal individuals, especially gastrocnemius muscle, older age
- Pregnancy

Systemic disorders:
- Dehydration: hidrosis, diuretics, hemodialysis
- Metabolic: low $Na^+$, $Mg^{2+}$, $Ca^{2+}$, glucose, uremia, cirrhosis, Gitelman syndrome
- Endocrine: thyroid (hyper- or hypothyroid), hypoadrenal, hyperparathyroid

Ischemia

Drug-induced

Denervation, partial: motor neuron disease, spinal stenosis, radiculopathy, neuropathy (including small-fiber neuropathy)

Syndromes: cramp-fasciculation, Satoyoshi syndrome

**Other Contraction Syndromes**

Central disorders: stiff person syndrome, spasticity, tetanus, dystonia

Peripheral nerve disorders: neuromyotonia, tetany, myokymia, partial denervation

Muscle: contractures, myotonia, myoedema

**Genetic Muscle Contraction Syndromes**

Muscular dystrophy: Becker; LGMD 1C

Myotonia: myotonia congenita, myotonia fluctuans, acetazolamide-responsive myotonia, myotonic dystrophy

Contractures:
- Brody syndrome: *ATP2A1*
- Glycogen storage disorders: deficiency of myophosphorylase; phosphorylase kinase regulatory subunit $\alpha 1$; phosphoglycerate mutase; phosphofructokinase, muscle
- Rippling muscle syndrome: Caveolin-3
- Hereditary angiopathy with nephropathy, aneurysms, and muscle cramps (HANAC): *COL4A1*
- Neuropathic

Cramps: autosomal dominant:
- Schwartz-Jampel: perlecan, *LIFR*
- Neuromyotonia and myokymia: *KCNQ2; KCNA1*
- Geniospasm
- Crisponi: *CRLF1*
- Myofibrillar myopathy

Cramps: autosomal recessive:
- Autosomal recessive axonal neuropathy with neuromyotonia *HINT1*

**Possible Treatments for Cramps and Other Muscle Spasms**

Normalize metabolic abnormalities

Quinine sulfate

Carbamazepine

Phenytoin

Gabapentin

Tocainide

Verapamil

Amitriptyline

Vitamin E

Riboflavin

Mexiletine

*Usual features: sudden involuntary painful muscle contractions (usually involve single muscles, especially gastrocnemius); local cramps in other muscles often associated with neuromuscular disease. Precipitants: muscle contraction, occasionally during sleep. Relief: passive muscle stretch, local massage.

## BOX 29.4 Pain Syndromes Without Chronic Myopathy*

**Pain of Uncertain Origin**

Polymyalgia rheumatica

Infections:
- Viral and postviral syndromes
- Brucellosis

Endocrine
- Thyroid: decreased (mainly) or increased
- Parathyroid: increased or decreased
- Adrenal insufficiency

Familial Mediterranean fever

**Pain with Defined Origin**

Connective tissue disorders:
- Systemic
- Fasciitis

Joint disease

Bone: osteomalacia, fracture, neoplasm

Vascular: ischemia, thrombophlebitis

Polyneuropathy:
- Small-fiber polyneuropathies
- Guillain-Barré syndrome

Radiculoneuropathy

Central nervous system: restless legs syndrome, dystonias (focal)

**Pain of Muscle from Central Sensitization**

Fibromyalgia

Chronic fatigue syndrome/systemic exertion intolerance disease

Myofascial pain syndrome

Joint hypermobility syndrome/Ehlers-Danlos syndrome

**Pain of Muscle Origin without Chronic Myopathy**

Muscle ischemia: atherosclerosis, calciphylaxis

Muscle overuse syndromes:
- Delayed-onset muscle soreness (DOMS)
- Cramps

Drugs, toxins

Muscle injury (strain)

*Usual features: muscle pain; may interfere with effort but no true weakness; present at rest, may increase with movement; muscle morphology and serum creatine kinase normal.

to direct infections (e.g., bacterial, viral, toxoplasmosis, trichinosis) are usually painful. Metabolic myopathies, including myophosphorylase and CPT II deficiencies, typically produce muscle discomfort or fatigue with exercise more so than rest. As a rule, disorders of carbohydrate utilization (e.g., myophosphorylase deficiency) produce pain and fatigue after short, intense exercise, whereas lipid disorders (e.g., CPT II deficiency) cause muscle discomfort with sustained exercise. Myophosphorylase deficiency causes exercise intolerance with myalgias, weakness, and painful contractures. The pain is proportional to the amount of exercise. Rhabdomyolysis is usually associated with muscle pain and tenderness that can persist for days after the initial event. It may occur with a defined metabolic or toxic myopathy or sporadically in the setting of unaccustomed exercise, especially in hot weather. Rhabdomyolysis may produce renal failure—a life-threatening complication and therefore the etiology and any precipitants should be aggressively pursued. Normal physiological responses to strenuous exercise (such as basic training) can result in CK up to 50 times the upper limit of normal (Kenney et al., 2012). These patients experience muscle soreness but not weakness or swelling. They have no myoglobinuria, renal failure, or electrolyte disturbances and the condition is probably benign. Medications, such as cholesterol-lowering agents, may produce a painful myopathy with prominent muscle fiber necrosis and a very high serum CK. Rhabdomyolysis can occur, especially at high doses. However, more commonly, cholesterol-lowering agents produce a myalgia syndrome with no defined muscle pathology.

Muscular dystrophy and mitochondrial disorders are usually painless. Patients with mild dystrophinopathies (such as Becker muscular dystrophy) or mitochondrial syndromes with minimal or no weakness may experience a sense of discomfort such as myalgias, fatigue, or cramps, especially after exercise. Hereditary myopathies with occasional reports of muscle discomfort or spasms in patients (or carriers) include certain limb–girdle muscular dystrophies, facioscapulohumeral dystrophy, myotonic dystrophy type 2, and some mild congenital myopathies. Pain in genetic myopathies is often due to musculoskeletal problems secondary to the weakness. Several myopathies defined by specific morphological changes in muscle but whose cause is unknown commonly have myalgias or exercise-related discomfort. These syndromes include tubular aggregates with or without cylindrical spirals, focal depletion of mitochondria, internalized capillaries, and adult-onset rod myopathies.

## Muscle Cramps

Muscle cramps (see Box 29.3) are localized, typically uncomfortable muscle contractions (Miller and Layzer, 2005). Characteristic features include a sudden involuntary onset in a single muscle or muscle group, with durations of seconds to minutes and a palpable region of contraction. Occasionally there is distortion of posture. Fasciculations often occur before and after the cramp. Muscle cramps are thought to originate in motor axons or nerve terminals. EMG during cramps demonstrates rapid, repetitive motor unit action potentials ("cramp discharges") at rates from 40 to 150 per second that increase and then decrease during the course of the cramp. CNS influences on cramps are minor and probably involve modulation of cramp thresholds. The EMG can distinguish cramps from other types of muscle contraction (e.g., contracture and myoedema are electrically silent).

Cramps usually arise during sleep or exercise and are more likely to occur when muscle contracts. Pain syndromes associated with cramps include discomfort during a muscle contraction and soreness after the contraction due to muscle injury. Cramps, especially those in the calf or foot muscles, are common in normal people of any age. They may be more common in the elderly (up to 50%), at the onset of exercise, at night, during pregnancy, and with fasciculations. These types of cramps are usually idiopathic and benign. In up to 60% of patients with cramps, small-fiber neuropathy may be the only underlying disease discovered after routine evaluation (Lopate et al., 2013).

Cramps that occur frequently in muscles other than the gastrocnemius often herald an underlying neuromuscular disorder. The presence of fasciculations with mild cramps but no weakness usually represents benign fasciculation syndrome. When the muscle cramps are more disabling, the condition is often called cramp-fasciculation syndrome. EMG is normal except for the presence of fasciculations. Repetitive nerve stimulation at 10 Hz provokes after-discharges of motor unit action potentials.

While neurogenic disorders that produce partial denervation of muscles (e.g., amyotrophic lateral sclerosis, radiculopathies, polyneuropathies) are a common cause of cramps, other etiologies (see Boxes 29.2 and 29.3) include drugs and metabolic, neuropathic, and genetic disorders.

When EMG shows neuropathy, myokymia, and/or neuromyotonia, the diagnosis is Isaacs syndrome. This is an autoimmune condition with antibodies to the voltage-gated potassium channel complex and has overlap with Morvan syndrome (which affects the CNS predominantly) and, rarely, cramp-fasciculation syndrome or neuropathic pain.

Treatment of cramp syndromes involves management of the underlying disorder and/or symptomatic trials of medications. Active stretching, by contracting the antagonist, may be helpful because it evokes reciprocal inhibition; however, there is no clear evidence that prophylactic stretching abates the frequency of cramps. Symptomatic treatment can reduce abnormal muscle contractions or the discomfort produced by the contractions. Mexiletine is helpful in treating cramps. Quinine, tonic water, and related drugs can be effective in treating nocturnal muscle cramps, but side effects may outweigh benefits. Increased salt intake and magnesium lactate or citrate may help treat leg cramps during pregnancy.

## Other Involuntary Muscle Contraction Syndromes

Diffuse muscle contraction syndromes, usually arising from the PNS or CNS (dystonias), often show widespread and continuous spontaneous motor unit fiber discharges. They may produce considerable discomfort. Causes are hereditary syndromes, CNS disorders, drugs, or toxins (see Boxes 29.2 and 29.3). Tetany, typically associated with hypocalcemia or alkalosis, causes spontaneous repetitive discharges often at very high rates. Myokymia can often be seen on the skin as vermicular or spontaneous rippling. EMG shows rhythmic or semi-rhythmic bursts of normal-appearing motor units at 30–80 Hz. Malignant hyperthermia and neuroleptic malignant syndrome both cause diffuse muscle rigidity and, if severe, rhabdomyolysis, as well as dysautonomia. They are usually triggered after drug exposure, immediately after halothane or depolarizing muscle relaxant in malignant hyperthermia, and days to weeks after exposure to a variety of dopamine antagonists for neuroleptic malignant syndrome.

Muscle contractions originating from muscle include electrically active forms due to myotonia and electrically silent contractures. *Myotonia* is repetitive firing of muscle fibers at rates of 20–80 Hz, with waxing and waning of the amplitude and frequency. Triggering the action potentials may be mechanical or electrical stimulation. Myotonic contractions are usually not painful, except for exercise-induced muscle cramps in myotonia fluctuans or acetazolamide-responsive myotonia (both a result of mutations in *SCN4A*). Mexiletine helps the stiffness and improves quality of life. Patients with recessive myotonia congenita often note fatigue. *Muscle contractures* are active, painful muscle contractions in the absence of electrical activity. (The term is also used to describe fixed resistance to stretch of a shortened muscle due to fibrous connective tissue changes or loss of sarcomeres in the muscle.) Contractures differ clinically from cramps, having a more prolonged time course, no resolution by muscle stretch, and occurrence only in an exercised muscle. Electrically silent muscle contractures occur in myopathies including myophosphorylase deficiency and other glycolytic disorders, Brody syndrome, rippling muscle disease, and hypothyroidism (myoedema).

## Myalgia Syndromes Without Chronic Myopathy

Pain originating from muscle, often acute, may occur in the absence of a chronic myopathy (see Box 29.4). Muscle ischemia causes a squeezing pain in the affected muscles during exercise. Ischemia produces pain that develops especially rapidly (within minutes) if muscle is forced to contract at the same time; the pain subsides quickly with rest. Cramps and overuse syndromes are associated with pain during or immediately after muscle use. DOMS occurs 12–48 hours after exercise and lasts for hours to days. Muscle contraction or palpation exacerbates discomfort. Serum CK is often increased and STIR MRI changes may be present. DOMS is most commonly precipitated by eccentric muscle contraction (contraction during muscle stretching) or unaccustomed exercise, and may be associated with repetitive overstretching of elastic noncontractile tissues. Disruption of the myofibril structure may be seen in muscle biopsy, as well as activation of secondary responses (protein degradation, autophagy, inflammation); see Hotfiel et al., (2018). Exercise training and gentle stretching typically protects against DOMS.

Polymyalgia syndromes have pain localized to muscle and other structures. Polymyalgia pain is often present at rest and variably affected by movement. Serum CK and EMG are normal. No major pathological change in muscle occurs unless the discomfort produces disuse and atrophy of type II muscle fibers. Muscle biopsies may also show changes associated with systemic immune disorders, including inflammation around blood vessels or in connective tissue. Polymyalgia syndromes can have identified causes, including systemic immune disease, drug toxicity, and small-fiber polyneuropathies.

A series of clinical criteria define some syndromes of uncertain pathophysiology associated with muscle discomfort (polymyalgia rheumatica, myalgic encephalomyelitis/chronic fatigue syndrome, fibromyalgia, myofascial pain syndrome, and joint hypermobility syndrome). *Polymyalgia rheumatica* usually occurs after age 50 years and manifests with pain and stiffness in joints and muscles, weight loss, and low-grade fever. The pain is symmetrical, involving the shoulder, neck, and hip girdle, and is greatest after inactivity and sleeping. Polymyalgia rheumatica can be associated with temporal arteritis and an elevated sedimentation rate (>40 mm/h). Pain improves within a few days after treatment with corticosteroids (prednisone, 20 mg/day).

Appreciation of the disability that occurs with *myalgic encephalomyelitis/chronic fatigue syndrome* has deepened. The National Academy of Medicine published a 2015 report (IOM, 2015) proposing that the name "systemic exertion intolerance disease" may better represent the characteristics that patients experience. The disease affects a patient's ability to perform at premorbid function and is accompanied by persistent and unexplained fatigue that is unremitting even with rest. The report proposed that the diagnosis require: (1) a substantial reduction or impairment in the ability to engage in premorbid levels of occupational, educational, social, or personal activities that persists for more than 6 months and is accompanied by fatigue, which is often profound, is of new or definite onset (not lifelong), is not the result of ongoing excessive exertion, and is not substantially alleviated by rest; (2) post-exertional malaise; and (3) unrefreshing sleep. Post-exertional malaise is described as exacerbations (including muscle pain) after (minor) physical, mental, or emotional effort. Other common symptoms include cognitive impairment and/or orthostatic intolerance. The orthostatic symptoms may overlap with vasovagal syncopes/neurallymediated hypotension or postural orthostatic tachycardia syndrome. The disease has a wide spectrum of presentations and severity with biological changes to multiple organ systems. The etiologies appear multifactorial, and can include infection, physical or emotional trauma, genetics, and/or environmental factors. Treatment is symptomatic and supportive. Exercise, once enthusiastically recommended because of evidence from clinical trials, is now recommended according to each patient's ability to tolerate exercise.

*Fibromyalgia* is diagnosed when there is a history of at least 3 months of widespread/multisite musculoskeletal pain. Examination findings can include excessive tenderness in predefined anatomical sites on the trunk and extremities. Patients may also note fatigue and disturbed sleep, headache, cognitive difficulty, and aggravation of symptoms by exercise, anxiety, or stress. The etiology of fibromyalgia can be a combination of CNS sensitization and/or peripheral nerve abnormalities. The loss of or dysfunction of cutaneous C-fibers (possibly muscle nociceptor) may underlie the pathophysiology of a subset of patients with fibromyalgia.

In contrast to the chronic widespread pain of fibromyalgia, patients with *myofascial pain syndrome* experience more localized pain arising from myofascial trigger points. These areas may be what some patients describe as "knots" in the muscle; they are taut, palpable, and painful. These trigger points are postulated to be at activated motor endplate region of muscles. The pain elicited upon palpation can be localized or in a stereotypical referred region. Sensory, motor, or autonomic symptoms may accompany trigger points. Interestingly, there appears to be an overlap between trigger points and acupuncture points; and mechanical interruptions of those points with (dry) needles, acupuncture needles, needles with local anesthetic, botulinum toxin, saline, or sterile water is a treatment.

*Joint hypermobility syndrome* is a large subset of clinically defined Ehlers-Danlos syndrome and is frequently characterized by musculoskeletal pain, albeit not the defining characteristics.

A commonality to fibromyalgia, myofascial pain syndrome, and muscle pain in joint hypermobility syndrome is central sensitization.

Decreasing the central sensitization to pain is the focus of the pharmacological treatment of these pain conditions. Medications include tricyclic antidepressants, selective serotonin and norepinephrine reuptake inhibitors, and gabapentinoids. No clear evidence exists for the superiority of any one medication. Opioids are most likely last-line treatments and only in situations where clear improvement of quality of life can be demonstrated. Low-impact aerobic exercise training improves/maintains mental and cardiovascular health, prevents deconditioning, and may reduce pain. It may be contraindicated in a subset of patients with chronic fatigue syndrome/systemic exertion intolerance disease but should be encouraged in all who can tolerate. Cognitive behavioral therapy may be useful.

Pain or discomfort localized to muscle may arise in other structures. For example, hip disease can suggest the misdiagnosis of a painful proximal myopathy with apparent leg weakness. In this situation, external or internal rotation of the thigh commonly evokes proximal pain. Radiological studies can confirm the diagnosis. Disorders of bone and joints, connective tissue, endocrine systems, vascular supply, peripheral nerves and roots, and the CNS may also present with discomfort localized to muscle.

Regardless of the etiology of the muscle pain, muscle pain is real to patients. There are probably fewer patients who complain of muscle pain for malingering purposes or secondary gain than there are patients who complain of muscle pain due to sensitization with no clear examination findings or objective test abnormalities. Treating these patients as true sufferers of complicated but sometimes undefined and many times unexplainable syndromes may be ultimately more helpful than outright dismissal as "psychological."

*The complete reference list is available online at https://expertconsult.inkling.com/.*

# 30

# Hypotonic (Floppy) Infant

W. Bryan Burnette

## OUTLINE



A floppy, or hypotonic, infant is a common scenario encountered in the clinical practice of child neurology. It can present significant challenges in terms of localization and is associated with an extensive differential diagnosis (Box 30.1). As with any clinical problem in neurology, attention to certain key aspects of the history and examination allows correct localization within the neuraxis and narrows the list of possible diagnoses. Further narrowing of the differential is achievable with selected testing based on the aforementioned findings. Understanding the anatomical and etiological aspects of hypotonia in infancy necessarily begins with an understanding of the concept of tone. *Tone* is the resistance of muscle to stretch. Categorization of tone differs among authors, but assessment is performed with the patient at rest and all parts of the body fully supported; examination involves tonic or phasic stretching of a muscle or the effect of gravity. Tone is an involuntary function and therefore separate and distinct from strength or power, which is the maximum force generated by voluntary contraction of a muscle. Function at every level of the neuraxis influences tone, and disease processes affecting any level of the neuraxis may reduce tone. Although a comprehensive review of conditions associated with hypotonia in infancy is beyond the scope of a single chapter, this chapter considers the basic approach to evaluating the floppy infant and considers several key disorders.

## APPROACH TO DIAGNOSIS

### History

Several features of the history may point to a specific diagnosis or category of diagnoses leading to hypotonia, or may permit distinguishing disorders present during fetal development from disorders acquired during the perinatal period. Thoroughly investigate a family history of disorders known to be associated with neonatal hypotonia, especially in the mother or in older siblings. Certain dominantly inherited genetic disorders (e.g., myotonic dystrophy) are associated with *anticipation* (earlier or more severe expression of a disease in successive generations). Such disorders may be milder and therefore undiagnosed in the mother. A maternal history of spontaneous abortion, fetal demise, or other offspring who died in infancy may also provide clues to possible diagnoses. A history of reduced fetal movement is a common feature of disorders associated with hypotonia, and may indicate a peripheral cause (Vasta et al., 2005). A history of maternal fever late in pregnancy suggests in utero infection, while a history of a long and difficult delivery followed by perinatal distress suggests hypoxic-ischemic encephalopathy with or without accompanying myelopathy. Among the many potential causes of neonatal hypotonia, acquired perinatal injury is far more common than inherited disorders and is rarely overlooked. However, also consider the possibility of a motor unit disorder leading to perinatal distress and hypoxic-ischemic encephalopathy.

### Physical Examination

#### General Features of Hypotonia

Assessing tone in an infant involves both observation of the patient at rest and application of certain examination maneuvers designed to evaluate both axial and appendicular musculature. Beginning with observation, a normal infant lying supine on an examination table will demonstrate flexion of the hips and knees so that the lower extremities are clear of the examination table, flexion of the upper extremities at the elbows, and internal rotation at the shoulders (Fig. 30.1). A hypotonic infant lies with the lower extremities in external rotation, the lateral aspects of the thighs and knees touching the examination table, and the upper extremities either extended down by the sides of the trunk or abducted with slight flexion at the elbows, also lying against the examination table. Evaluation of the *traction response* is done with the infant in supine position; the hands are grasped and the infant pulled toward a sitting position. A normal response includes flexion at the elbows, knees, and ankles, and movement of the head in line with the trunk after no more than a brief head lag. The head should then remain erect in the midline for at least a few seconds. An infant with axial hypotonia demonstrates excessive head lag with this maneuver (Fig. 30.2, *A*), and once upright, the head may continue to lag or may fall forward relatively quickly. Absence of flexion of the limbs may also be seen and indicates either appendicular hypotonia or weakness. The traction response is normally present after 33 weeks, postconceptional age. *Vertical suspension* is performed by placing hands under the infant's axillae and lifting the infant without grasping the thorax. A normal infant has enough power in the shoulder muscles to remain suspended without falling through, with the head upright in the midline and the

## BOX 30.1 Differential Diagnosis of the Floppy Infant

**Cerebral Hypotonia**

***Chromosomal Disorders***
Prader-Willi syndrome
Chronic nonprogressive encephalopathy
Chronic progressive encephalopathy
Benign congenital hypotonia

***Combined Cerebral and Motor Unit Disorders***
Acid maltase deficiency
Congenital myotonic dystrophy
Syndromic congenital muscular dystrophies
Congenital disorders of glycosylation
Lysosomal disorders
Infantile neuroaxonal dystrophy

***Spinal Cord Disorders***
Acquired spinal cord lesions
Spinal muscular atrophy
Infantile spinal muscular atrophy with respiratory distress
X-linked spinal muscular atrophy

***Peripheral Nerve Disorders***
Congenital hypomyelinating neuropathy/Dejerine-Sottas disease

***Neuromuscular Junction Disorders***
Juvenile myasthenia gravis
Neonatal myasthenia gravis
Congenital myasthenic syndromes
Infant botulism

***Muscle Disorders***
Congenital myopathies:
- Centronuclear myopathy
- Nemaline myopathy
- Central core disease

Nonsyndromic congenital muscular dystrophies:
- Merosin-deficient congenital muscular dystrophy
- Ullrich congenital muscular dystrophy

Other muscular dystrophies;
- Infantile facioscapulohumeral dystrophy

hips and knees flexed. In contrast, a hypotonic infant held in this manner slips through the examiner's hands (see Fig. 30.2, *B*), often with the head falling forward and the legs extended at the knees. Infants with axial hypotonia related to brain injury may also demonstrate crossing, or *scissoring*, of the legs in this position, which is an early manifestation of appendicular hypertonia. In *horizontal suspension*, the infant is held prone with the abdomen and chest against the palm of the examiner's hand (see Fig. 30.2, *C*). A normal infant maintains the head above horizontal with the limbs flexed, while a hypotonic infant drapes over the examiner's hand with the head and limbs hanging limply. Other examination findings in hypotonic infants include various deformities of the cranium, face, limbs, and thorax. Infants with reduced tone may develop occipital flattening, or *positional plagiocephaly*, as the result of prolonged periods of lying supine and motionless.

### Localization

Once the presence of hypotonia in an infant is established, the next step in determining causation is localization of the abnormality to the brain,

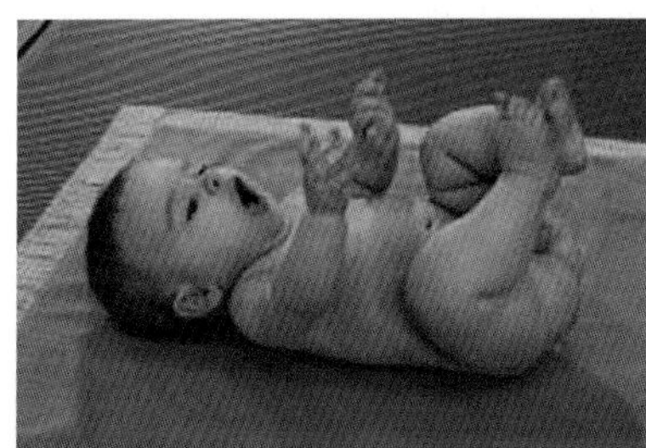

**Fig. 30.1** Normal Infant Lying Supine with Legs Flexed and Arms Adducted. (*With permission from Kobesova, A., Kolar, P., 2014, Developmental kinesiology: three levels of motor control in the assessment and treatment of the motor system. J Bodyw Mov Ther 18[1], 23–33, Elsevier.*)

spinal cord, motor unit, or multiple sites. A *motor unit* is a single spinal motor neuron and all the muscle fibers it innervates and includes the motor neuron with its cell body, axon, and myelin covering; the neuromuscular junction; and muscle. The major "branch point" at this stage of the assessment is whether the lesion is likely to be in the brain, at a more distal site, or at multiple sites. Review of the recent literature suggests that 60%–80% of cases of hypotonia in infancy are due to central causes, while 15%–30% are due to peripheral abnormalities (Peredo and Hannibal, 2009).

The key features of disorders of cerebral function, particularly the cerebral cortex, are encephalopathy and seizures. Encephalopathy manifesting as decreased level of consciousness may be difficult to ascertain, given the large proportion of time normal infants spend sleeping. However, full-term or near-term infants with normal brain function spend at least some portion of the day awake with eyes open, particularly with feeding. Encephalopathy also manifests with excessive irritability or poor feeding, although the latter problem is rarely the sole feature of cerebral hemispheric dysfunction and may occur with disorders at more distal sites. Infants with centrally mediated hypotonia of many different etiologies frequently have relatively normal power despite a hypotonic appearance. Power may not be observable under normal conditions because of a paucity of spontaneous movement, but it may be observable with application of a noxious stimulus such as a blood draw or placement of a peripheral intravenous catheter. Other indicators of central rather than peripheral dysfunction include *fisting* (trapping of the thumbs in closed hands), normal or brisk tendon reflexes, and normal or exaggerated primitive reflexes. Tendon reflexes should be tested with the infant's head in the midline and the limbs symmetrically positioned; deviations from this technique often result in spuriously asymmetrical reflexes. *Primitive reflexes* are involuntary responses to certain stimuli that normally appear in late fetal development and are supplanted within the first few months of life by voluntary movements. Abnormalities of these reflexes include absent or asymmetrical responses, obligatory responses (persistence of the reflex with continued application of the stimulus), or persistence of the reflexes beyond the normal age range. Two of the most sensitive primitive reflexes are the Moro and asymmetrical tonic neck. The *Moro reflex* is a startle response present from 28 weeks after conception to 6 months postnatal age (Gingold et al., 1998). Quickly dropping the infant's head below the level of the body while holding the infant supine with the head supported in one hand and the body supported in the other readily elicits this reflex. The normal response consists of initial abduction and extension of the arms with opening of the hands, followed quickly by adduction and flexion with closure of the hands. The *tonic neck reflex* is a vestibular response and is present from term until approximately 3 months of age. The response is elicited by rotating the head to one side while the infant is lying supine. The normal response is extension of the ipsilateral limbs while the contralateral

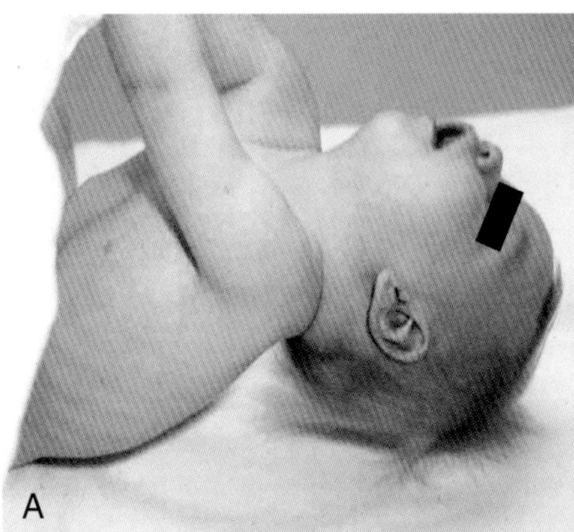


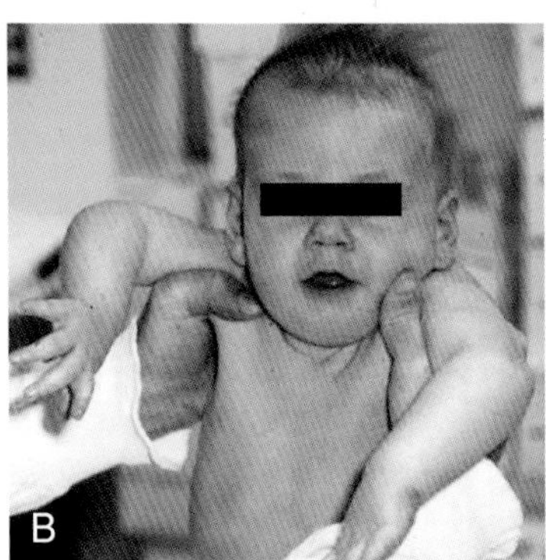


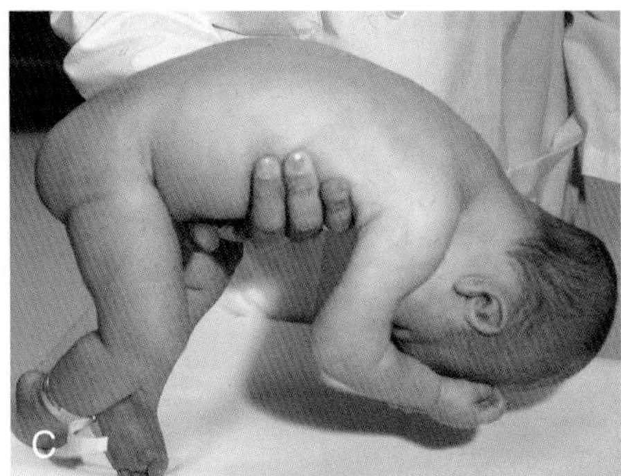


**Fig. 30.2** **A,** Hypotonic infant demonstrating abnormal traction response with excessive head lag. **B,** Vertical suspension in a hypotonic infant, with elevation of shoulders and arms (slip-through). **C,** Horizontal suspension with the head and limbs hanging limply. (*With permission from Bodensteiner, J. B., 2008, The evaluation of the hypotonic infant. Semin Pediatr Neurol 15[1], 10–20, Elsevier.*)

limbs remain flexed. Central disorders resulting in hypotonia also may be associated with dysmorphism of the face or limbs, or malformations of other organs. Various defects in *O*-linked glycosylation of α-dystroglycan, a protein associated with the dystrophin glycoprotein complex that stabilizes the sarcolemma, result in structural defects of the brain, eye, and skeletal muscle.

Disorders of the spinal cord leading to neonatal hypotonia are usually secondary to perinatal injury. Spinal cord injury may occur in the setting of a prolonged, difficult vaginal delivery with breech presentation, resulting in trauma to the spinal cord, or may result from hypoxic-ischemic injury to the cord concurrently with encephalopathy. In the latter case, hypotonia may initially be attributable to the encephalopathy. In cases of hypotonia resulting from spinal cord injury, diminished responsiveness to painful stimuli, sphincter dysfunction with continuous leakage of urine and abdominal distension, and priapism may provide clues to localization of the lesion.

The hallmark of disorders of the motor unit is weakness. Tendon reflexes are absent or reduced. Tendon reflexes reduced out of proportion to weakness usually indicate a neuropathy, often a demyelinating neuropathy, whereas tendon reflexes reduced in proportion to weakness are more likely to result from myopathy or axonal neuropathy. The motor unit is the final common pathway for all reflexes, and, for this reason, primitive reflexes are depressed or absent in motor unit disorders. This phenomenon may hinder detection of central nervous system (CNS) abnormalities when lesions at both levels coexist. Other abnormalities related to motor unit disorders in infants include underdevelopment of the jaw (micrognathia), a high-arched palate, and chest wall deformities, in particular pectus excavatum. Muscle atrophy may also occur but this also occurs in cerebral disorders. Sensory function is not assessable in detail in a neonate or young infant, particularly in the presence of encephalopathy, although reduced responsiveness to pinprick may provide clues to the presence of a polyneuropathy or spinal cord lesion in the setting of normal mental status. Some motor unit disorders may result in perinatal distress due to weakness and may result in a superimposed encephalopathy that confounds the localization of hypotonia.

Hypotonic infants may have reduced movement during fetal development, leading to fibrosis of muscles or of structures associated with joints, as well as foreshortening of ligaments. This results in restricted joint range of motion, or *contractures.* The term *arthrogryposis* refers to joint contractures that develop prenatally. The most common form of arthrogryposis is unilateral or bilateral clubfoot. The most severe end of this clinical spectrum is *arthrogryposis multiplex congenita,* or multiple joint contractures. The causes of this condition may be abnormalities of the intrauterine environment, motor unit disorders, or disorders of the CNS. Hypotonia in utero may also result in congenital hip dysplasia.

## Diagnostic Studies

Selective laboratory testing allows confirmation of the clinical localization of hypotonia, and in many cases leads to identification of a specific diagnosis. In all cases, ancillary testing guided by historical features and examination findings has the greatest chance of yielding a diagnosis. Available modalities include various forms of neuroimaging; electrophysiological techniques including electroencephalography (EEG), nerve conduction studies (NCS), electromyography (EMG), and repetitive nerve stimulation (RNS); muscle and nerve biopsy; and other laboratory studies such as serum creatine kinase (CK), metabolic studies, and genetic studies.

### Neuroimaging

Neuroimaging studies, in particular magnetic resonance imaging (MRI), are most useful when suspecting structural abnormalities of the CNS. T1-weighted images most readily detect congenital malformations of the brain and spinal cord, while T2-weighted images and various T2-based sequences reveal abnormalities of white matter and show evidence of ischemic injury. Specialized techniques, such as magnetic resonance spectroscopy, may show evidence of mitochondrial disease (Matthews et al., 1993) or disorders of cerebral creatine metabolism (Frahm et al., 1994). When performing neuroimaging studies that require sedation on hypotonic infants, give particular consideration to airway management and other safety issues.

### Electroencephalography

EEG may be informative when seizures are suspected as either a cause of unexplained encephalopathy or a result of a more global disturbance of brain function. EEG may also reveal evidence of underlying structural abnormalities and thus increase the pretest probability of a diagnostic finding on neuroimaging.

### Creatine Kinase

CK catalyzes the conversion of creatine to phosphocreatine, which serves as a reservoir for the buffering and regeneration of adenosine triphosphate (ATP). It expresses in many human tissues, in particular smooth muscle, cardiac muscle, and skeletal muscle. The concentration of CK detectable in serum increases in any condition in which tissues expressing high levels of the enzyme undergo breakdown. Serum CK concentration may be elevated in congenital myopathies, congenital muscular dystrophies, or spinal muscular atrophy (SMA), but levels may also be elevated transiently following normal vaginal deliveries or with perinatal distress. Conversely, serum CK is normal in some congenital myopathies and inherited neuropathies.

### Metabolic Studies

Removal of low-molecular-weight toxic metabolites across the placenta typically prevents inborn errors of metabolism (e.g., amino acidopathies, organic acidurias, urea cycle defects, fatty acid oxidation defects, mitochondrial disorders) from causing in utero injury. More commonly, these disorders manifest in a previously healthy newborn who develops hypotonia, encephalopathy, or seizures within the first 24–72 hours after birth, after oral feeding begins and toxic intermediates begin to accumulate in the blood. Although detection of many disorders is by state-mandated newborn screens, these results may not be available before an affected infant becomes symptomatic. For this reason, newborns who develop hypotonia and encephalopathy after an unremarkable first few days of life should have enteral feedings held until metabolic studies such as blood ammonia level, plasma amino acid, acylcarnitine profile, and urine organic acids have definitively excluded an inborn error of metabolism. Because neonatal sepsis has a similar presentation, undertake investigation for infection with cultures of blood, urine, and cerebrospinal fluid in such cases; empirical antimicrobial therapy should be initiated while diagnostic studies are pending.

### Nerve Conduction Studies and Electromyography

NCS and EMG are the studies of choice in a suspected motor unit disorder when other available clinical information does not suggest a specific diagnosis. The two techniques are complementary and always performed together. They allow distinction between primary disorders of muscle and peripheral nerve disorders when the two are indistinguishable on clinical grounds. RNS studies evaluate the integrity of the neuromuscular junction, abnormalities of which are not detectable with routine NCS or EMG. The most commonly observed abnormality on low-rate (2–3 Hz) RNS studies of patients with various forms of myasthenia is a significant decrement, usually defined as 10% or greater, in the amplitude of the compound motor action potential (CMAP) between the first and fourth or fifth stimuli of a series. Single-fiber EMG (SFEMG) is a highly specialized technique that evaluates the delay in depolarization between adjacent muscle fibers within a single motor unit, referred to as *jitter*. This modality is highly sensitive for neuromuscular junction abnormalities but has a low specificity and requires a cooperative patient. SFEMG with stimulation of the appropriate nerve has been described in pediatric patients (Tidwell and Pitt, 2007), but experience with this technique in infants is limited to a small number of centers. The utility of these neurophysiology studies is dependent on the skill and experience of the clinician performing the tests, as well as the precision of the question posed.

### Muscle Biopsy

Muscle biopsy is integral to the diagnosis of certain inherited muscle disorders, such as congenital myopathies, congenital muscular dystrophies, and metabolic myopathies, and may also aid in the distinction between myopathies and motor neuron disorders. Give careful consideration to the site chosen for biopsy. Ideally, a muscle should be chosen that is moderately but not severely weak and that has not undergone needle EMG. Another important consideration is the quantity of tissue obtained. Obtain a sufficient quantity of tissue to rapidly freeze a portion for routine histochemical stains, submit additional tissue for specialized studies such as biochemical assays, electron microscopy, or genetic studies, and have additional tissue available to be stored for possible future studies. In practical terms, this usually entails obtaining at least three separate specimens weighing 1–1.5 g each. Although needle biopsy may procure an adequate sample in some cases, open biopsy is more likely to yield an appropriate amount of tissue, thereby avoiding the need for a second surgical procedure and its attendant risks. The value of muscle biopsy, as with neurophysiology studies, depends on the experience of the interpreting laboratory and the focus of the question asked by the referring clinician. In addition to these factors, proper handling of the tissue between the operating room and the receiving laboratory is a critical link in the chain of custody. This step is often the most difficult to control, but it requires attention equal to the other steps in the process in order to maximize the probability of obtaining a diagnostic sample and to minimize the risk of subjecting the patient to a second procedure.

### Nerve Biopsy

Nerve biopsy plays a more limited role in the diagnosis of hypotonia in infancy. It is nevertheless appropriate when a peripheral neuropathy is suspected on clinical grounds, but available testing fails to yield a diagnosis. The sural nerve is usually chosen because of its accessibility and the relatively minor deficit produced by its removal. Sural nerve biopsy is most likely to be informative in the setting of an abnormal response on NCS. The limited choice of peripheral nerves available for biopsy confines the use of this procedure to centers with considerable experience. Submit portions of the nerve for routine histochemical stains, paraffin-embedded sections, and thin plastic sections, the latter processed for light microscopy or electron microscopy.

### Genetic Testing

In some cases of hypotonia in infancy, the combination of clinical history, examination, and ancillary testing points toward a specific genetic diagnosis. Genetic testing is commercially available for many conditions, and the number continues to expand rapidly. Consult one or more of the accessible resources such as the Internet-based Online Mendelian Inheritance in Man or GeneTests.org for the most current information on testing for specific disorders. When a chromosomal disorder is suspected, consider array comparative genomic hybridization (aCGH), a technique that has an increased diagnostic yield by 5%–17% over traditional karyotyping (Prasad and Prasad, 2011). The newer technique of whole exome sequencing will likely further increase the diagnostic yield of the genetic evaluation of hypotonia, but its application to this clinical problem has been limited to date.

### Serology

In cases of a suspected neuromuscular junction disorder such as myasthenia gravis, assays of antibodies directed against the sarcolemmal nicotinic acetylcholine receptor or muscle-specific kinase are commercially available. Autoimmune myasthenia gravis is rare in infancy, but absence of the antibodies is required for the diagnosis of a congenital myasthenic syndrome. Several forms of myasthenia gravis occur in infancy and are discussed in greater detail later in this chapter.

## SPECIFIC DISORDERS ASSOCIATED WITH HYPOTONIA IN INFANCY

### Cerebral Disorders

Regardless of etiology, hypotonia is a common feature of disturbed function of the cerebral hemispheres in neonates and infants and, as previously noted, is frequently characterized by diminished tone that is disproportionate to the degree of weakness. Disorders of cerebral function in infancy are also frequently associated with concurrent axial hypotonia and appendicular hypertonia. Overall, central disorders are a far more common cause of hypotonia than motor unit diseases. Although a comprehensive listing of all such disorders is beyond the scope of a single chapter, a number of important categories of cerebral causes of hypotonia are considered here.

### Chromosomal Disorders

Hypotonia is a prominent feature of many disorders associated with large- or small-scale chromosomal abnormalities. Such disorders also are frequently associated with a dysmorphic appearance of the face and hands. Among the most common of these disorders is *Prader-Willi syndrome* (PWS), which is caused by various abnormalities resulting in absence of paternally expressed genes within the PWS/Angelman syndrome (AS) region on chromosome 15 (Kim et al., 2012). Pathogenic defects in this region include paternal deletion, uniparental disomy, or an imprinting defect. Affected individuals often have profound hypotonia and poor feeding in infancy, suggesting a disorder of the motor unit or a combined cerebral and motor unit disorder. However, serum CK, EMG, muscle biopsy, and brain MRI are normal. The commonly recognized morphological features of almond-shaped eyes, narrow biparietal diameter, and relatively small hands and feet may not be readily apparent in early infancy. DNA methylation analysis is the only technique that will diagnose PWS in all three molecular classes and differentiate PWS from AS in deletion cases (Glenn et al., 1996, 1997; Kubota et al., 1996). A DNA methylation analysis consistent with PWS is sufficient for clinical diagnosis, though not for genetic counseling purposes. Parental DNA samples are not required to differentiate the maternal and paternal alleles. The most robust and widely used assay targets the 5′ CpG island of the SNURF-SNRPN (typically referred to as SNRPN) locus, and will correctly diagnose PWS in more than 99% of cases (Glenn et al., 1996; Kubota et al., 1997). The promoter, exon 1, and intron 1 regions of SNRPN are unmethylated on the paternally expressed allele and methylated on the maternally repressed allele. Normal individuals have both a methylated and an unmethylated SNRPN allele, while individuals with PWS have only the maternally methylated allele. Methylation-specific multiplex-ligation probe amplification (MS-MLPA) can also determine the parental origin in this region (Kim et al., 2012).

Failure to thrive in infancy gives way in early childhood to hyperphagia and a characteristic pattern of behavioral abnormalities, intellectual disability, and hypogonadism.

### Chronic Nonprogressive Encephalopathy

*Chronic nonprogressive encephalopathy* describes a clinical syndrome with many potential causes, including cerebral dysgenesis related to a genetic disorder, in utero infection, toxic exposure, inborn error of metabolism, or vascular insult. Perinatal brain injury resulting in a chronic encephalopathy is readily diagnosable and typically associated with a reduced level of consciousness and seizures. Hypoxic-ischemic brain injury in the newborn manifests with low Apgar scores, and lactic acidosis along with other indicators of injury to other vital organs, is often present. Hypotonia related to ischemic brain injury usually gives way to spasticity. In cases of remote in utero injury or cerebral dysgenesis, hypotonia may be the only manifestation of the problem in the perinatal period. Clues to the presence of cerebral dysgenesis include malformations of other organs and abnormalities of head size or shape. In such cases, obtain an MRI of the brain, and a chromosomal anomaly should be sought with karyotype and chromosomal microarray analysis. The onset of hypotonia in a previously healthy neonate or infant is almost always cerebral in origin and may also relate to infection, vascular injury, or an inborn error of metabolism.

### Chronic Progressive Encephalopathy

Chronic progressive encephalopathy more commonly presents with developmental regression than with hypotonia. Inborn errors of metabolism involving small molecules may cause this clinical presentation, but more frequently the cause is a disorder of lysosomal or peroxisomal metabolism leading to progressive accumulation of storage material in various tissues. These disorders frequently manifest with progressive facial dysmorphism, organomegaly, or skeletal dysplasia in addition to neurological decline. Among the disorders causing chronic progressive encephalopathy, various autosomal recessive defects of peroxisome biogenesis in the Zellweger syndrome spectrum (ZSS) are most commonly associated with profound hypotonia in infancy. The most severely affected individuals present with neonatal hypotonia, poor feeding, encephalopathy, seizures, and craniofacial dysmorphism (Steinberg et al., 2006). Stippling of the patellae and other long bones (chondrodysplasia punctata) may be seen on skeletal survey, and affected individuals may have evidence of hepatic dysfunction as well as hepatic cysts on abdominal imaging. Measurement of plasma very-long-chain fatty acid (VLCFA) concentrations identifies elevated levels of C26:0 and C26:1, and ratios of C24/C22 and C26/C22 indicate a defect in peroxisomal fatty acid metabolism. Abnormalities in 14 different *PEX* genes (Braverman et al., 2016), all of which encode peroxins (proteins required for peroxisome assembly), have been identified in ZSS, with a majority having pathogenic mutations in the *PEX1* gene (Collin and Gould, 1999; Maxwell et al., 2002; Walter et al., 2001). Management is supportive, and the most severely affected infants do not survive beyond the first year of life.

### Benign Congenital Hypotonia

*Benign congenital hypotonia* refers to infants with early hypotonia who later develop normal tone. It is a diagnosis made only in retrospect and has become less common in the era of high-resolution neuroimaging and genetic testing. Nevertheless, there remains a subset of children, often with a family history of a similarly affected parent or sibling who was undiagnosed. Intellectual disability of varying degrees frequently becomes apparent in later life.

## Combined Cerebral and Motor Unit Disorders

Several genetic diseases manifest with abnormalities of both the brain and the motor unit. These conditions can present considerable diagnostic challenges.

### Acid Maltase Deficiency

Acid maltase deficiency, an autosomal recessive deficiency of the lysosomal enzyme acid α-1,4-glucosidase, presents with a severe skeletal myopathy and cardiomyopathy and also may be associated with encephalopathy. Routine histochemical stains show accumulation of glycogen in lysosomal vacuoles and within the sarcoplasm. The diagnosis is confirmed with biochemical assay of enzyme activity in muscle or in cultured skin fibroblasts. Recombinant human enzyme is approved by the US Food and Drug Administration (FDA) for replacement therapy, which can prolong survival (Kishnani et al., 2006).

### Congenital Myotonic Dystrophy

Congenital myotonic dystrophy is an autosomal dominant disorder that typically presents in adolescence or early adulthood, but in some instances may be associated with profound hypotonia and weakness of the face, trunk, and limbs in infancy. Approximately 25% of infants born to mothers with myotonic dystrophy are affected in this way, although the diagnosis in the mother may be unrecognized (Rakocevic-Stojanovic et al., 2005). Survivors of perinatal distress often have global developmental delay, with both intellectual impairment and motor disability throughout childhood, then develop myotonia and other characteristic symptoms of the muscular dystrophy as they approach puberty. To date, only myotonic dystrophy type 1, caused by abnormal expansion of a trinucleotide repeat within the gene *DMPK*, has been associated with a congenital presentation. Genetic testing is commercially available.

### Infantile Facioscapulohumeral Dystrophy

Facioscapulohumeral dystrophy (FSHD) is another dominantly inherited muscular dystrophy presenting most frequently in early adulthood, but which may have a congenital presentation. The genetic abnormality is contraction of a 3.3-kb repeat array at the D4Z4 locus. Those with the smallest integral number of repeats may have diffuse hypotonia and weakness in infancy and account for less than 5% of cases (Klinge et al., 2006). Affected infants may have cognitive impairment, epilepsy, and progressive sensorineural hearing loss. Serum CK is normal or mildly elevated. Family history may include a mildly affected parent, although cases also result from de novo mutations. Genetic testing is commercially available.

### Syndromic Congenital Muscular Dystrophies

A group of congenital muscular dystrophies due to defects of *O*-linked glycosylation of dystroglycan, a component of the dystrophin–glycoprotein complex spanning the plasma membrane of skeletal myocytes, are associated with severe myopathy, a cerebral cortical malformation referred to as *cobblestone lissencephaly*, and ocular defects such as retinal dysplasia. In addition to profound hypotonia and weakness, affected infants often have intractable epilepsy. These diagnoses are suspected based on the characteristic constellation of abnormalities and have been clinically categorized as *Fukuyama congenital muscular dystrophy*, *Walker-Warburg syndrome*, and *muscle-eye-brain disease*. Thus far, 15 different causative genes have been identified (Schorling et al., 2017), and there appears to be a far greater degree of phenotypic overlap among the different genotypes than was previously appreciated.

### Congenital Disorders of Glycosylation

Congenital disorders of glycosylation are a group of recessively inherited defects in 21 different enzymes that modify *N*-linked oligosaccharides (Jaeken et al., 2009). Many forms present with hypotonia in infancy. The most common form, type Ia, results from a deficiency of the phosphomannomutase enzyme. In addition to hypotonia, affected infants may have hyporeflexia, global developmental delay, failure to thrive, seizures, and evidence of hepatic dysfunction, coagulopathy, and elevated thyroid-stimulating hormone (TSH). Characteristic examination findings include inverted nipples and an abnormal distribution of subcutaneous fat. Facial dysmorphism occurs but is not present in all cases. Brain MRI shows cerebellar hypoplasia. Analysis of transferrin isoforms in serum by isoelectric focusing reveals a characteristic pattern indicative of a defect in the early steps of the *N*-linked oligosaccharide synthetic pathway. Commercially available genetic testing identifies pathogenic sequence variants in 95% of affected individuals. Although cerebral dysfunction dominates the early clinical picture, some patients develop a demyelinating peripheral neuropathy in the first or second decade of life (Gruenwald, 2009).

### Lysosomal Disorders

Certain defects of lysosomal hydrolases, in particular *Krabbe disease* and *metachromatic leukodystrophy*, result in progressive degeneration of both central and peripheral myelin (Korn-Lubetzki et al., 2003), producing both an encephalopathy and motor unit dysfunction (Cameron et al., 2004). Both disorders are associated with characteristic white matter abnormalities on brain MRI, and biochemical assays on peripheral blood of β-galactocerebrosidase in the case of Krabbe, and of arylsulfatase A in the case of metachromatic leukodystrophy, confirm the diagnosis.

### Infantile Neuroaxonal Dystrophy

Neuroaxonal dystrophy is a rare autosomal recessive disorder caused by mutations in the *PLA2G6* gene, which encodes a calcium-independent phospholipase (Gregory et al., 2008). The classic form may present as early as 6 months of age with hypotonia, although psychomotor regression is more common, and progressive spastic tetraparesis and optic atrophy with visual impairment follow. Brain MRI shows bilateral T2 hypointensity of the globus pallidus, which is indicative of progressive iron accumulation, as well as thinning of the corpus callosum and cerebellar cortical hyperintensities. NCS show evidence of an axonal sensorimotor polyneuropathy with active denervation on EMG. The characteristic pathological finding is of enlarged and dystrophic-appearing axons on biopsy of skin, peripheral nerve, or other tissue-containing peripheral nerve. Commercially available genetic testing identifies abnormalities in approximately 95% of children with early symptom onset.

## Spinal Cord Disorders

Disorders of the spinal cord leading to generalized hypotonia in infancy usually involve the cervical spine at a minimum but may involve the entire cord. They include both acquired processes and genetic syndromes.

### Acquired Spinal Cord Lesions

Acquired spinal cord lesions relate to trauma sustained during delivery or occur as a part of the spectrum of hypoxic-ischemic encephalopathy. As previously noted, the highest risk of spinal cord injury occurs in vaginal deliveries with breech presentation, particularly when the head is hyperextended in utero. Herniation of the brainstem through the foramen magnum, as well as injury to the cerebellum, may also occur. Cervical spine injury may also occur in cephalic presentations with midforceps delivery, especially in cases of prolonged rupture of membranes. In both traction injury and hypoxic-ischemic injury, encephalopathy often dominates the early clinical picture and may obscure the extent of spinal cord dysfunction. Potential indicators in the acute phase include bladder distention with dribbling of urine and impaired sweating below the level of the lesion. Signs of spasticity gradually supplant early flaccid paraparesis. As mental status improves, the level and extent of motor impairment becomes apparent. MRI of the spine in the acute stage may show cord edema or hemorrhage, whereas imaging obtained later in the course may reveal cord atrophy.

### Spinal Muscular Atrophy

SMA is the most common inherited disorder of the spinal cord resulting in hypotonia in infancy, occurring with an incidence of approximately 1 in 10,000 live births per year (Sugarman et al., 2012). It is an autosomal recessive disorder in which the molecular defect leads to impaired regulation of programmed cell death in anterior horn cells and in motor nuclei of lower cranial nerves. Both populations of motor neurons are progressively lost, producing hypotonia and weakness of limb and truncal musculature, as well as bulbar dysfunction. In approximately 95% of cases, the genetic defect is homozygous deletion of the survival motor neuron 1 *(SMN1)* gene, which is located on the telomeric region of chromosome 5q13 (Ogino and Wilson, 2002). A virtually identical centromeric gene on 5q13, referred to as *SMN2*, encodes a similar but less biologically active product (Swoboda et al., 2005). While no more than two copies of *SMN1* are present in the human genome, variable numbers of *SMN2* copies are present. The protein product of *SMN2* appears to partially rescue the SMA phenotype such that a larger *SMN2* copy number generally results in a milder presentation and disease course.

Historically, SMA patients have been categorized into different phenotypes or syndromes based on age of presentation and maximum motor ability achieved. The disease results from a common genetic abnormality with a spectrum of phenotypic severity contingent upon modifying factors that include *SMN2* copy number and other loci not yet identified. The classification of the most severely affected patients, with weakness and hypotonia evident at birth, is SMA type 0. These infants may have arthrogryposis multiplex congenita in addition to diffuse weakness of limb and trunk muscles, but facial weakness is usually mild if present. Perinatal respiratory failure causes death in early infancy. SMA type 1, also referred to as *Werdnig-Hoffmann disease*, is a designation given to infants who develop weakness within the first 6 months of life. These infants may appear normal at birth or may appear hypotonic. Facial expression is usually normal, and arthrogryposis is usually absent. Weakness is worse in proximal than in distal muscles and worse in the lower extremities, which may lead to suspicion of a congenital myopathy or muscular dystrophy. Further confounding the diagnosis is the presence of an elevated serum CK in a substantial portion of patients (Rudnick-Schoneborn et al., 1998), although CK rarely rises above 1000 U/L. In addition to limb weakness, affected infants demonstrate abdominal breathing due to relative preservation of diaphragm function as compared with abdominal and chest wall musculature. Needle EMG shows evidence of both acute and chronic denervation in the limbs and serves to distinguish this disorder from myopathies with a similar presentation.

Genetic testing is commercially available for SMN-related SMA. Among the 5% of patients without homozygous deletion of *SMN1*, most are compound heterozygotes with the characteristic deletion on one allele and a point mutation on the other. Parents of affected children are heterozygotes for deletion of *SMN1* in a majority of cases, although a 2% rate of de novo mutations is reported in SMA patients (Wirth et al., 1997). The natural history of SMA is unique among anterior horn cell disorders in that the progression of weakness is most rapid early in the disease course and subsequently slows. Nevertheless, in the absence of supportive and therapeutic measures, median survival is 8 months, with death due to respiratory failure. Survivors have normal cognitive development. Nusinersen (Spinraza), an antisense oligonucleotide that alters *SMN2* messenger RNA splicing to increase the production of full-length transcript, was approved in the United States for the treatment of SMA in 2016. The drug is delivered intrathecally, and must be given in repeated doses. Clinical trials of the drug demonstrated improved survival and motor development, particularly in type 1 SMA patients treated in the early months of life (Finkel et al., 2017). Replacement of the missing *SMN1* gene by systemic delivery of human *SMN1* copy DNA in an adeno-associated virus (AAV) vector is the subject of active research (Mendell, et al., 2017).

### Infantile Spinal Muscular Atrophy With Respiratory Distress Type 1

Infantile spinal muscular atrophy with respiratory distress type 1 (SMARD1), previously classified as a variant of SMA type 1, is a rare and distinct autosomal recessive anterior horn cell disorder. Unlike SMN-related SMA, affected infants develop early diaphragmatic paralysis and distal limb weakness that progresses to complete paralysis. Many have intrauterine growth restriction and are born with ankle contractures. Approximately one-third are born prematurely. Similar to SMN-related SMA, EMG and muscle biopsy reveal evidence of chronic active denervation. The causative gene encodes the immunoglobulin μ-binding protein 2 (IGHMBP2), for which testing is commercially available (Grohmann et al., 2001).

### X-Linked Spinal Muscular Atrophy

This rare X-linked anterior horn cell degenerative disorder shares a considerable degree of phenotypic overlap with SMN-related SMA. Distinctive features include polyhydramnios secondary to impaired fetal swallowing, arthrogryposis, and axonal sensory and motor abnormalities on NCS (Dlamini et al., 2013). Consider the diagnosis in any simplex case of a male infant with an SMA phenotype and normal *SMN1* copy number. The only known causative gene encodes the ubiquitin-like modifier activating enzyme 1 (UBA1, formerly UBE1), for which commercial testing is available.

## Peripheral Nerve Disorders

Polyneuropathies, both inherited and acquired, are a rare cause of infantile hypotonia. The two most common clinical designations for infantile polyneuropathies are *congenital hypomyelinating neuropathy* (CHN) and *Dejerine-Sottas disease* (DSD). In recent years, mounting evidence reveals that neither entity is a monogenic disorder, nor are they clearly distinct from one another. Clinical features include hypotonia, distal or diffuse weakness, absent tendon reflexes, and evidence on NCS of a demyelinating polyneuropathy. Traditionally, DSD was classified as hereditary motor and sensory neuropathy (HMSN) type III, but at least four genes associated with various demyelinating HMSN subtypes have been linked to the DSD and CHN phenotypes: *PMP22, MPZ, EGR2,* and *PRX* (Plante-Bordenueve and Said, 2002). In general, patients with an infantile presentation are homozygotes or compound heterozygotes for mutations in the causative genes. The most common acquired autoimmune peripheral neuropathies, Guillain-Barré syndrome and chronic inflammatory demyelinating polyneuropathy (CIDP), occur rarely in the first year of life and typically present with weakness and hypotonia in a previously normal infant.

## Neuromuscular Junction Disorders

Disorders of neuromuscular transmission resulting in hypotonia in infancy also feature varying degrees of weakness or fatigability. Appreciation of the latter is by fluctuating ptosis, weak suck, or premature discontinuation of oral feedings. Neuromuscular junction disorders presenting with hypotonia in infancy include juvenile myasthenia gravis, neonatal myasthenia gravis resulting from placental transmission of maternal antibodies against the fetal postsynaptic acetylcholine receptor, congenital myasthenic syndromes (CMS), and infant botulism.

### Juvenile Myasthenia Gravis

Approximately 10%–15% of cases of autoimmune myasthenia gravis due to endogenous production of antibodies directed against sarcolemmal nicotinic acetylcholine receptors or muscle-specific kinase occur in individuals younger than 16 years of age. The disorder is particularly rare in the first year of life (Andrews, 2004). The small number of infantile cases reported in the literature limits the conclusions drawn with respect to the occurrence of measurable antibody titers, treatment, and outcomes in this age group.

### Neonatal Myasthenia

In approximately 15% of infants born to mothers with autoimmune myasthenia gravis, transitory symptoms of myasthenia occur in the neonatal period related to transfer of acetylcholine receptor antibodies across the placenta. Because the fetal nicotinic acetylcholine receptor is different from the adult form, the expression of myasthenic symptoms in newborns depends on the maternal production of antibodies against the fetal receptor (Gardnerova et al., 1997). These antibodies are not active against the adult form of the receptor and therefore do not contribute to maternal symptoms. Likewise, antibodies against the fetal receptor are not detectable by commercially available assays. For these reasons, neither maternal symptom severity nor the maternal antibody titer predicts the likelihood or severity of neonatal myasthenic symptoms. As with juvenile myasthenia gravis, the predominant symptoms are ocular or bulbar, although generalized hypotonia or weakness may occur. Rarely, affected infants have arthrogryposis due to prenatal exposure to fetal antibodies, leading to prolonged immobility in utero. Affected infants may require respiratory support temporarily or symptomatic therapy with subcutaneous neostigmine prior to oral feeds to prevent fatigue and premature discontinuation of feeding. In a majority of cases, the symptoms resolve within the first month of life (Papazian, 1992).

### Congenital Myasthenic Syndromes

Several genetic disorders of neuromuscular transmission have been identified as causing hypotonia; fluctuating or persistent weakness of ocular, bulbar, or limb muscles; or arthrogryposis in infancy. The basis of one widely used classification scheme of CMS is whether the abnormality occurs in the presynaptic motor nerve terminal, the synaptic cleft, or the postsynaptic sarcolemma. The cause of the presynaptic disorder is a defect in the enzyme choline acetyltransferase, which synthesizes the neurotransmitter, whereas the synaptic defect results from deficiency of the end-plate cholinesterase. The causes of the postsynaptic disorders are various abnormalities of the structure, localization, or kinetics of the acetylcholine receptor. Inheritance of most CMS is autosomal recessive, except for the slow-channel syndrome, which is autosomal dominant. The clinical presentation is similar to other forms of myasthenia occurring in infancy, although deficiencies of the presynaptic enzyme choline acetyltransferase and of the postsynaptic acetylcholine receptor-associated protein rapsyn are also associated with sudden episodes of apnea (Hantai et al., 2004). Infants with CMS have negative antibody studies and demonstrate a decremental response on RNS. Specialized electrophysiological testing on fresh muscle biopsy specimens has been useful as a diagnostic tool but is not widely available. Of the 29 different genes currently known to be associated with CMS (Farmakidis et al., 2018), testing is commercially available for 22, while testing of the others is available on a research basis only. Most forms of CMS are treated with cholinesterase inhibitors and/or the potassium channel inhibitor 3,4-diaminopyridine. However, cholinesterase inhibitors may exacerbate end-plate cholinesterase deficiency, defects in the postsynaptic DOK-7 protein, and slow-channel syndrome. The latter form of the disorder may respond to fluoxetine (Harper et al., 2003), while improvement with oral ephedrine (Lashley et al., 2010) or salbutamol (Lorenzoni et al., 2013) has been reported in patients with defects in the *DOK-7* gene. The natural history of CMS is highly variable, even among patients with the same genotype.

### Infant Botulism

Spores of the gram-positive anaerobe *Clostridium botulinum*, an organism found in soil and in some cases in contaminated foods, produce an exotoxin that prevents anchoring of acetylcholine-containing vesicles to the presynaptic nerve terminal of the neuromuscular junction, disrupting neuromuscular transmission and resulting in flaccid weakness. In adults, the cause of botulism is ingestion of the preformed toxin; the organism itself cannot survive in the acidic environment of the adult digestive tract. By contrast, infants who ingest spores may be colonized and develop botulism from in situ production of the toxin. Affected infants may present any time after 2 weeks of age and may have relatively greater involvement of bulbar than appendicular muscles. The characteristic finding on RNS is an increment in the CMAP with high-rate (50 Hz) stimulation (Cornblath et al., 1983). Diagnostic confirmation is obtained by testing a stool or enema specimen with a bioassay in mice inoculated against different strains of toxin. Aside from supportive measures, early administration of botulinum immune globulin shortens the course of the disease (Arnon et al., 2006). In most cases, treatment should be initiated based on the clinical suspicion and should not be delayed while awaiting results of the bioassay.

## Muscle Disorders

Subsets of disorders that cause hypotonia in infancy relate to developmental or structural defects of myocytes and do not affect cerebral function. The *congenital myopathies* are developmental muscle disorders with distinctive features on muscle histology. Most are autosomal recessive or X-linked, although some are allelic with dominantly inherited conditions with later symptom onset. Common features include diffuse weakness and hypotonia with normal or mildly elevated serum CK, nonspecific myopathic abnormalities on EMG, and predominance of type I fibers on muscle histology. The diagnosis is contingent upon biopsy findings and in some cases can be confirmed with commercially available genetic testing. A recommended diagnostic approach based upon clinical features and skeletal muscle pathology is outlined in a review by North et al. (2014). Cognition is usually normal, and there are no abnormalities of other organs. Weakness may be severe but is typically static or slowly progressive, and some affected infants show improved strength through the early childhood years. Treatment for these conditions is supportive. The nonsyndromic congenital muscular dystrophies also feature diffuse weakness and hypotonia and are often associated with significant elevations in serum CK. Although subcortical white matter abnormalities may be seen on brain MRI in affected patients (Mercuri et al., 1995), cognitive development is usually normal. Treatment of the disorders discussed in this section is largely supportive.

### Congenital Myopathies

***Centronuclear myopathy..*** Centronuclear myopathy has X-linked, recessive, and dominant forms due to defects in 10 different genes, although not all result in congenital weakness and hypotonia. X-linked centronuclear myopathy, caused by mutations in the *MTM1* gene, affects male infants. Clinical features include facial weakness, ptosis, and ophthalmoplegia, in addition to severe limb weakness. Affected infants may have macrocephaly, a thin face, and long digits. Serum CK is normal or mildly elevated, and EMG shows a nonspecific myopathic pattern. The characteristic findings on muscle pathology are the presence of large, single, centrally located nuclei in more than 5% of myofibers, and predominance of hypotrophic type I fibers (Pierson et al., 2007). Mutations in the *BIN1* gene result in a similar phenotype but with recessive inheritance (Nicot et al., 2007). A dominantly inherited form of centronuclear myopathy exists but presents beyond infancy. Evidence of impaired neuromuscular transmission and favorable clinical response to pyridostigmine has been reported in a small number of centronuclear myopathy patients (Robb et al., 2011).

***Nemaline myopathy..*** At least 11 different genes have been associated with this disorder, many of which encode different components of thin filaments within the sarcomere (Cassandrini et al., 2017; Miyatake et al., 2017). Inheritance may be recessive or dominant, and many cases are associated with de novo mutations. Characteristic of many forms is congenital weakness involving proximal limb muscles, the face, and extraocular muscles. Muscle biopsy reveals characteristic rod-shaped sarcoplasmic inclusions best visualized on Gomori trichrome staining of frozen muscle. The most common abnormality is in the gene encoding the skeletal muscle nebulin (NEB), accounting for approximately 50% of cases. Genetic testing is commercially available for all 11 genes associated with this disorder.

***Central core disease..*** The majority of individuals with central core disease have mild weakness, although congenital weakness with reduced fetal movement, arthrogryposis, and spinal deformities do occur. Sparing of the face and extraocular muscles is common. Histology of frozen muscle shows well-demarcated areas of absent staining by oxidative stains such as reduced nicotinamide adenine dinucleotide (NADH)-tetrazolium reductase. These areas tend to be centrally located within type I myofibers and run the entire length of the myofibers on longitudinal sections. The most common causative genetic abnormality affects the skeletal muscle ryanodine receptor 1 (RYR1), which mediates calcium release from the sarcoplasmic reticulum during excitation–contraction coupling. The disorder is allelic with susceptibility to malignant hyperthermia (Robinson et al., 2006). Some individuals have both phenotypes, others have only one of the two disorders. Both autosomal dominant and autosomal recessive inheritance of central core disease have been documented (Monnier et al., 2000). A pilot study of salbutamol treatment of a small cohort of children and adolescents with central core disease showed encouraging results, but has not been replicated (Messina et al., 2004).

### Nonsyndromic Congenital Muscular Dystrophies

***Merosin-deficient congenital muscular dystrophy..*** The etiology of the most common nonsyndromic congenital muscular dystrophy is a recessively inherited deficit of α-2 laminin (merosin), a component of the dystrophin-associated glycoprotein complex in skeletal muscle. Affected infants are hypotonic, with weakness of face and limb muscles and arthrogryposis. Extraocular and bulbar muscles are not usually affected. Serum CK is highly elevated, and hypomyelination of cerebral white matter is apparent on brain MRI by 6 months of age. EMG is myopathic, and some infants also have evidence of peripheral myelin dysfunction on NCS. Muscle biopsy shows evidence of a chronic necrotizing myopathy, and endomysial lymphocytic inflammation also occurs. Immunostaining demonstrates absence of skeletal muscle merosin. Sequencing of the *LAMA2* gene is commercially available. Weakness is usually static. Epilepsy occurs at a higher rate in affected infants than in the general population, although cognition is usually normal (Herrmann et al., 1996).

***Ullrich congenital muscular dystrophy..*** This autosomal recessive nonsyndromic congenital muscular dystrophy results from defects in the extracellular matrix protein collagen VI. The presence of proximal joint contractures with striking hyperlaxity of distal joints in early life distinguishes it from other disorders in this category (Muntoni et al., 2002). Serum CK ranges from normal to 10 times the upper limit of normal. Reduced immunostaining of frozen skeletal muscle for collagen VI and production of the protein in cultured fibroblasts are diagnostic. Both assays, as well as genetic testing for abnormalities in the three different *COL6A* genes, are commercially available.

## SUMMARY

The hypotonic infant remains a common yet challenging presenting problem in child neurology. Attention to details of the history, particularly regarding pregnancy, the perinatal period, and early infancy, as well as a focus on localization, which may require multiple examinations over time, aid with narrowing the differential diagnosis. The major branch point in the diagnostic evaluation is localization of the deficit to the CNS, peripheral nervous system, or multiple levels; CNS disorders are approximately twice as common as other etiologies. Recent literature on the evaluation of the hypotonic infant suggests that, through a systematic approach, a specific diagnosis can be achieved in up to 85% of cases (Jain and Jayawant, 2011; Peredo and Hannibal, 2009). Further advances in neuroimaging and in molecular genetic techniques will likely result in further increases in diagnostic success in this area, and may provide opportunities to develop more effective therapies.

*The complete reference list is available online at https://expertconsult.inkling.com/.* 

31

# Sensory Abnormalities of the Limbs, Trunk, and Face

*E. Lee Murray, Karl E. Misulis*

## OUTLINE



Clinical evaluation of sensory deficits is inherently more difficult than evaluation of motor deficits because of the subjective nature of the examination. Nevertheless, it is important to identify sensory deficits in order to localize lesions.

## ANATOMY AND PHYSIOLOGY

### Peripheral Pathways

Activation of sensory end organs produces a generator potential in the afferent neurons. If the generator potential reaches threshold, an action potential is produced that is conducted by the sensory axons to the spinal cord.

Sensory transducers are seldom directly affected by neuropathic conditions, although peripheral vascular disease can produce dysfunction of the skin's sensory axons, and systemic sclerosis can damage the skin sufficiently to produce a primary deficit of sensory transduction (eTable 31.1).

The rate of action potential propagation differs according to the diameter of the axons and depending on whether the fibers are myelinated or unmyelinated. In general, nociceptive afferents are small myelinated and unmyelinated axons. Nonnociceptive afferents are large-diameter myelinated axons. The characteristics of afferent fibers are shown in eTable 31.2.

### Spinal Cord Pathways

Sensory afferent information passes through the dorsal root ganglia to the dorsal horn of the spinal cord. Some of the axons pass through the dorsal horn without synapsing and ascend in the ipsilateral dorsal columns; these serve mainly joint position and touch sensations. Other axons synapse in the dorsal horns, and the second-order sensory neurons cross in the anterior white commissure of the spinal cord to ascend in the contralateral spinothalamic tract. Although this tract is best known for the conduction of pain and temperature information, some nonnociceptive tactile sensation is conducted as well.

The dorsal column tracts ascend to the cervicomedullary junction, where axons from the leg synapse in the nucleus gracilis and axons from the arms synapse in the nucleus cuneatus. Fig. 31.1 shows the ascending pathways through the spinal cord to the brain.

### Brain Pathways

#### Brainstem

Axons from the nucleus gracilis and nucleus cuneatus cross in the medulla and ascend in the medial lemniscus. The spinothalamic tracts in the brainstem are continuations of the same tracts in the spinal cord and ascend lateral to the medial lemniscus in the brainstem. Lesions of the brainstem can produce sensory deficits congruent with the anatomical localization, but these symptoms are usually eclipsed by motor and cranial nerve deficits.

#### Thalamus

Lesions of the thalamus rarely affect only a single region, but the functional organization of this structure may affect clinical findings. The ventroposterior complex is the main somesthetic receiving area and includes the ventroposterior lateral nucleus, which receives information from the body, and the ventroposterior medial nucleus, which receives sensory input from the head and face. Projections are to the primary somatosensory cortex on the postcentral gyrus. The posterior nuclear group receives nociceptive input from the spinothalamic tract and projects mainly to the secondary somesthetic region on the inner aspect of the postcentral gyrus, adjacent to the insula.

#### Cerebral Cortex

Classic neuroanatomical teaching presents a picture of the central sulcus bounded by the motor strip anteriorly and the sensory strip posteriorly. This division was derived largely from studying lower animals, in which the separation between these functions is marked. On ascending the evolutionary ladder, however, this division becomes less prominent, and many neurologists refer to the entire region as the motor-sensory strip. In general, sensory function is served prominently

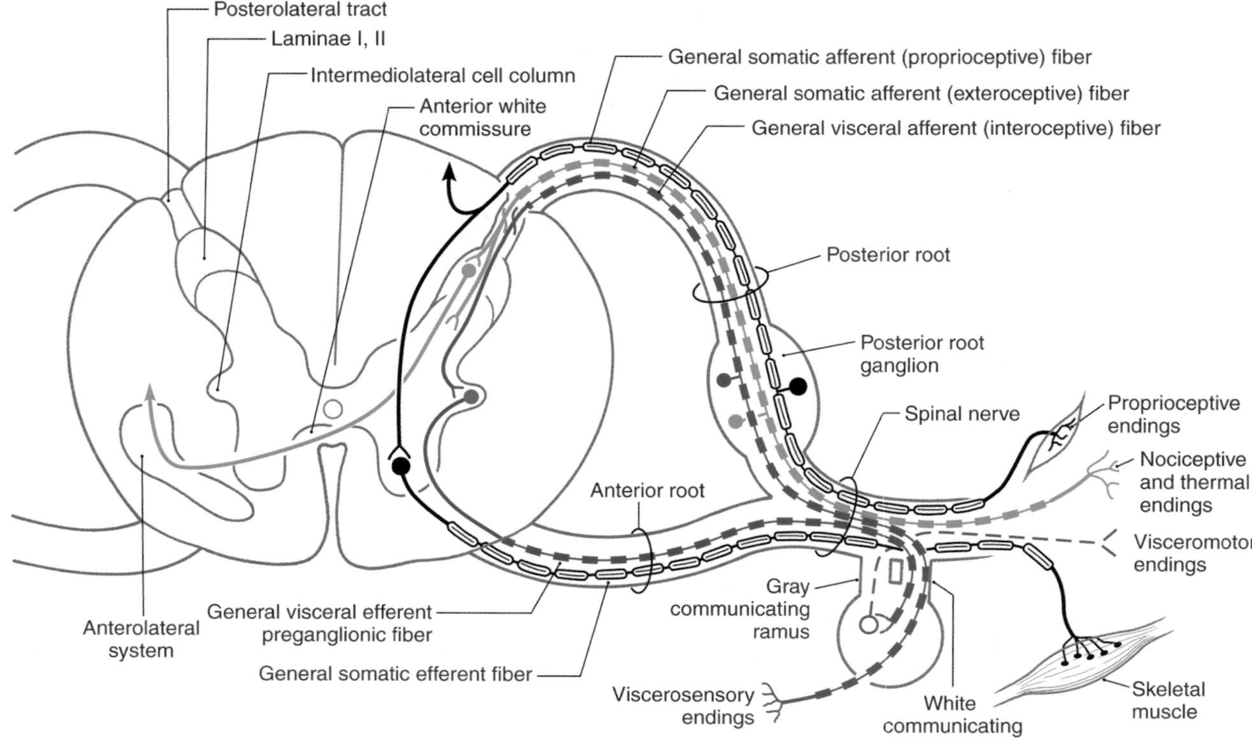


**Fig. 31.1** Axial Section of the Spinal Cord Showing Dorsal and Ventral Roots Forming a Spinal Nerve. Sensory afferents give rise to two major ascending pathways: the anterolateral system (nociceptive, serving thermal sensation primarily) and posterior columns (serving large-fiber modalities primarily, including touch, vibration, and proprioception). Inhibitory input derives from descending fibers as well as collaterals, via interneurons, from mechanoreceptive fibers. (*With permission from Haines, D.E., 2012. Fundamental Neuroscience for Basic and Clinical Applications, third ed. Elsevier, Saunders Philadelphia.*)

on the postcentral gyrus. The mapping of the cortex follows the same homunculus presented in Chapter 26 (see Fig. 26.1), with the head and arm portions located laterally on the hemisphere and the leg region located superiorly near the midline and wrapping onto the parasagittal cortex.

## Sensory Input Processing

Elementary sensory inputs of all modalities provide data to the brain; they are then processed at a higher cortical level. The locations of these areas for processing are not as discrete as the primary sensory cortical regions. However, disorders in higher-level function certainly exist. Just as presbyopia and presbycusis have central as well as peripheral components, there is evidence that higher-level cerebral processing of other sensory data can deteriorate with age as well as disease (Lee, 2013). Abnormalities in central sensory processing have been described in Alzheimer disease, autism, and stroke (Chang et al., 2014; de Tommaso et al., 2014; Puts et al., 2014; Sweetnam and Brown, 2013).

# APPROACH TO LOCALIZATION AND DIAGNOSIS

## Sensory Abnormalities

Abnormalities of sensory perception are varied, and the pattern of symptoms is often a clue to diagnosis:

- Loss of sensation (numbness)
- Dysesthesia and paresthesia
- Neuropathic pain
- Sensory ataxia

Patients often use the term *numbness* to mean any of a variety of symptoms. Strictly speaking, numbness is the loss of sensation and usually manifests as decreased sensory discrimination and elevated sensory threshold; these are negative symptoms. Some patients use the term *numbness* to mean weakness; others are referring to positive sensory symptoms such as dysesthesia and paresthesia.

*Dysesthesia* is an abnormal perception of a sensory stimulus, as when pressure produces a feeling of tingling or pain. If large-diameter axons are mainly involved, the perception is typically tingling; if small-diameter axons are involved, the perception is commonly pain. *Paresthesia* is an abnormal spontaneous sensation similar in quality to dysesthesia. Dysesthesias and paresthesias are usually seen in localized regions of the skin affected by peripheral neuropathic processes such as polyneuropathy or mononeuropathy. These perceptual abnormalities can also be seen in patients with central conditions such as myelopathy or cerebral sensory tract dysfunction.

*Neuropathic pain* can result from damage to the sensory nerves from any cause. Peripheral neuropathic conditions result in failure of conduction of the sensory fibers, giving decreased sensory function plus pain from electrical discharge of damaged nociceptive axons (Cohen and Mao, 2014). The pathophysiology of neuropathic pain partly involves lowering of the membrane potential of the axons so that minor deformation of the nerve can produce repetitive action potentials (Zimmermann, 2001). An additional feature with neuropathic conditions appears to be unstable membrane potential, so that the crests of fluctuations of membrane potential can produce action potentials. Finally, crosstalk between damaged axons allows an action potential in one nerve fiber to be abnormally transmitted

**TABLE 31.1 Sensory Localization**

| Level of Lesion | Features and Location of Sensory Loss |
|---|---|
| Cortical | Sensory loss in the contralateral body is restricted to the portion of the homunculus affected by the lesion. If the entire side is affected (with large lesions), either the face and arm or the leg will tend to be affected to a greater extent |
| Internal capsule | Sensory symptoms in the contralateral body that usually involve head, arm, and leg to an equal extent. Motor findings are common although not always present |
| Thalamus | Sensory symptoms in the contralateral body including the head. These may split at the midline. Sensory dysfunction without weakness is highly suggestive of a lesion of the thalamus |
| Spinal transection | Sensory loss at or below a segmental level, which may be slightly different for each side. Motor examination is also key to localization |
| Spinal hemisection | Sensory loss is ipsilateral for vibration and proprioception (dorsal columns) and contralateral for pain and temperature (spinothalamic tract) |
| Nerve root | Sensory symptoms follow a dermatomal distribution |
| Plexus | Sensory symptoms span two or more adjacent root distributions, corresponding to the anatomy of plexus divisions |
| Peripheral nerve | Distribution follows peripheral nerve anatomy or involves nerves symmetrically |

to an adjacent nerve fiber. These pathophysiological changes also produce exaggerated sensory symptoms, including hyperesthesia and hyperpathia. *Hyperesthesia* is increased sensory experience with a stimulus. *Hyperpathia* is augmented painful sensation.

Sensory ataxia is the difficulty in coordination of a limb that results from loss of sensory input, particularly proprioceptive input. The resulting deficit may resemble cerebellar ataxia, but other signs of cerebellar dysfunction are not seen on neurological examination.

## Localization of Sensory Abnormalities

A general guide to sensory localization is presented in Table 31.1. Guidelines for the diagnosis of sensory abnormalities are summarized in Table 31.2. Details of specific sensory levels of dysfunction are discussed next.

### Peripheral Sensory Lesions

Lesions of the peripheral nerves and the plexuses produce sensory loss that follows their peripheral anatomical distribution. Peripheral sensory loss produces a multitude of potential complaints. Clues to localization are as follows:

- Distal sensory loss and/or pain in more than one limb suggests peripheral neuropathy.
- Sensory loss in a restricted portion of one limb suggests a peripheral nerve or plexus lesion; mapping of the deficit should make the diagnosis.
- Sensory loss affecting an entire limb is seldom due to a peripheral lesion. A central lesion should be sought.

Unfortunately, especially with peripheral lesions, a discrepancy between the complaint and the examination findings is common.

**TABLE 31.2 Diagnosis of Sensory Abnormalities**

| Abnormality | Features | Lesion | Cause |
|---|---|---|---|
| Distal sensory deficit | Sensory loss with or without pain distal on the legs. Arms may also be affected | Peripheral nerve | Peripheral neuropathy |
| Proximal sensory deficit | Sensory loss on the trunk without limb symptoms | Neuropathy with predominantly proximal involvement | Porphyria, diabetes, other plexopathies |
| Dermatomal distribution of pain and/or sensory loss | Pain and/or sensory loss in the distribution of a single nerve root | Nerve root | Radiculopathy due to disk, osteophyte, tumor, herpes zoster |
| Single-limb sensory deficit | Loss of sensation on one entire limb that spans neural and dermatomal distributions | Plexus or multiple single nerves | Autoimmune plexitis, hematoma, tumor |
| Hemisensory deficit | Loss of sensation on one side of body. May be associated with pain. Face involved with brain lesions but not spinal lesions | Thalamus, cerebral cortex, or projections. Brainstem lesion, spinal cord lesion, and lower lesions do not involve the face | Infarction, hemorrhage, demyelinating disease, tumor, infection |
| Crossed sensory deficit: unilateral facial and contralateral body | Unilateral loss of pain and temperature sensation on contralateral body | Lesions of uncrossed trigeminal fibers and crossed spinothalamic fibers | Lateral medullary syndrome |
| Pain/temperature and vibration/proprioception deficits on opposite sides | Unilateral loss of sensation on face, unilateral loss of vibration and proprioception on the other side | Spinal cord lesion ipsilateral to vibration and proprioception deficit and contralateral to pain and temperature deficit | Disk protrusion, spinal stenosis, intraspinal tumor, transverse myelitis. Intraparenchymal lesions are more likely to produce dissociated sensory loss |
| Dissociated suspended sensory deficit | Loss of pain and temperature sensation on one or both sides with normal sensation above and below | Syringomyelia in the cervical or thoracic spinal cord | Chiari malformation, hydromyelia, central spinal cord tumor, or hemorrhage |
| Sacral sparing | Preservation of perianal sensation with impaired sensation in the legs and trunk | Lesion of the cord with mainly central involvement, sparing peripherally located sacral ascending fibers | Cord trauma, intrinsic tumors of the cord |

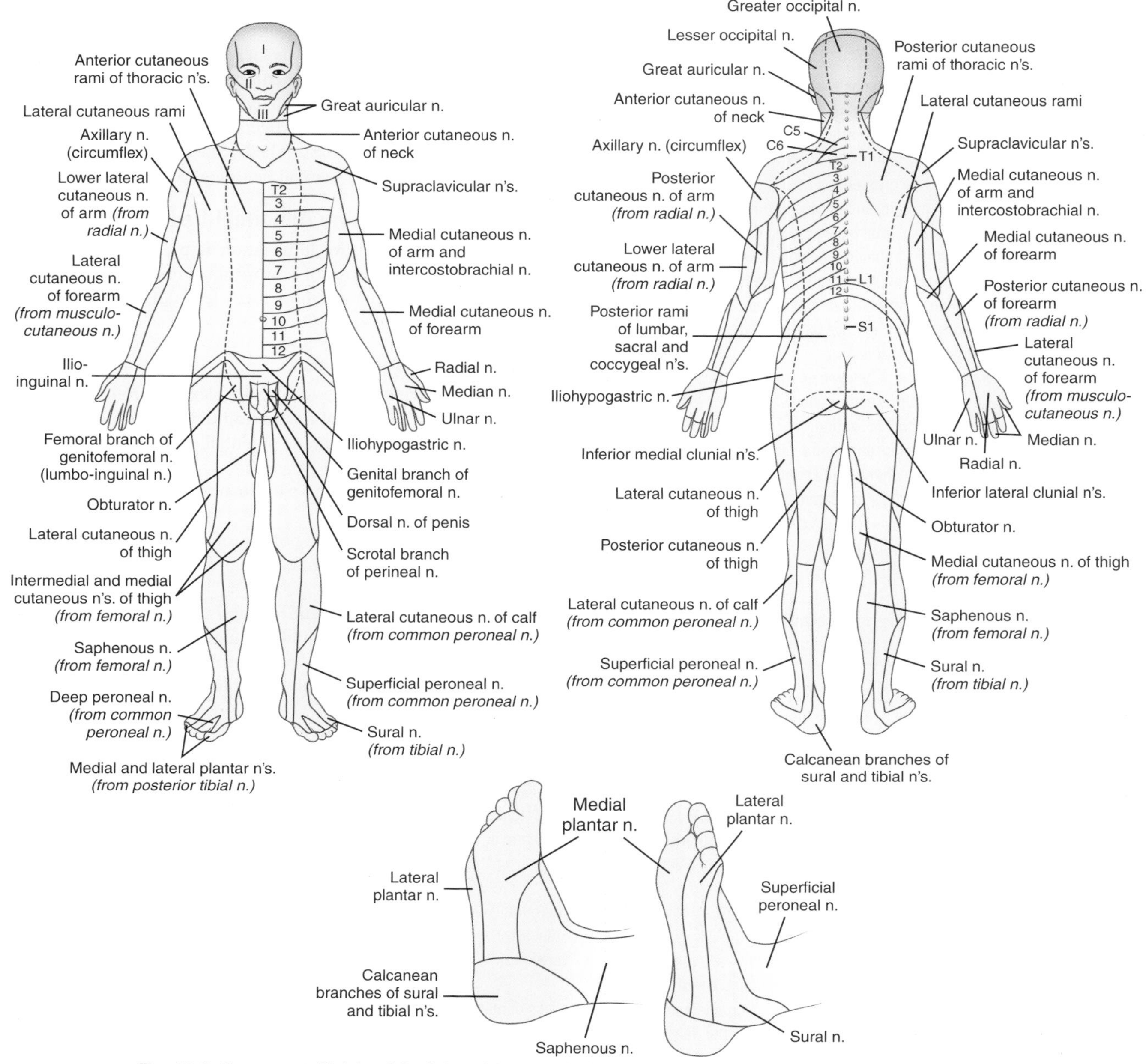


**Fig. 31.2** Cutaneous Fields of Peripheral Nerves *(n.)*. Note that thoracic dermatomes are innervated by primary anterior and posterior rami of spinal nerves from the respective level. Spinous processes of T1, L1, and S1 are indicated. *inf.*, Inferior; *lat.*, lateral; *med.*, median. (*Reprinted with permission from Haymaker, W., Woodall, B., 1953. Peripheral Nerve Injuries: Principles of Diagnosis. W.B. Saunders, Philadelphia.*)

The patient may complain of sensory loss affecting an entire limb when the examination shows a median or ulnar distribution of sensory loss. Alternatively, the patient may complain of sensory loss but examination fails to reveal a sensory deficit. This discrepancy is more likely to be due to limitations of the examination than to malingering. Also, patients may have significant sensory complaints as a result of pathophysiological dysfunction of the afferent axons while the integrity and conducting function of the axons are still intact, so that the examination will show no loss of sensory function.

Fig. 31.2 summarizes the peripheral nerve anatomy of the body and Fig. 31.3 shows the dermatomal distribution.

## Spinal Sensory Lesions

Certain sensory syndromes suggest a spinal lesion:

- Sensory level on the trunk
- Dissociated sensory loss on the trunk or limbs, sparing the face
- Suspended sensory loss
- Sacral sparing

*Sensory level* is a deficit below a certain level of the spinal cord segments. *Dissociated sensory loss* is disturbance of pain and temperature on one side of the body and of vibration and proprioception on the other. The term can also be used to describe loss of one sensory modality (e.g., pain and temperature) with normality of another—in this instance, vibration and proprioception. *Suspended sensory loss*

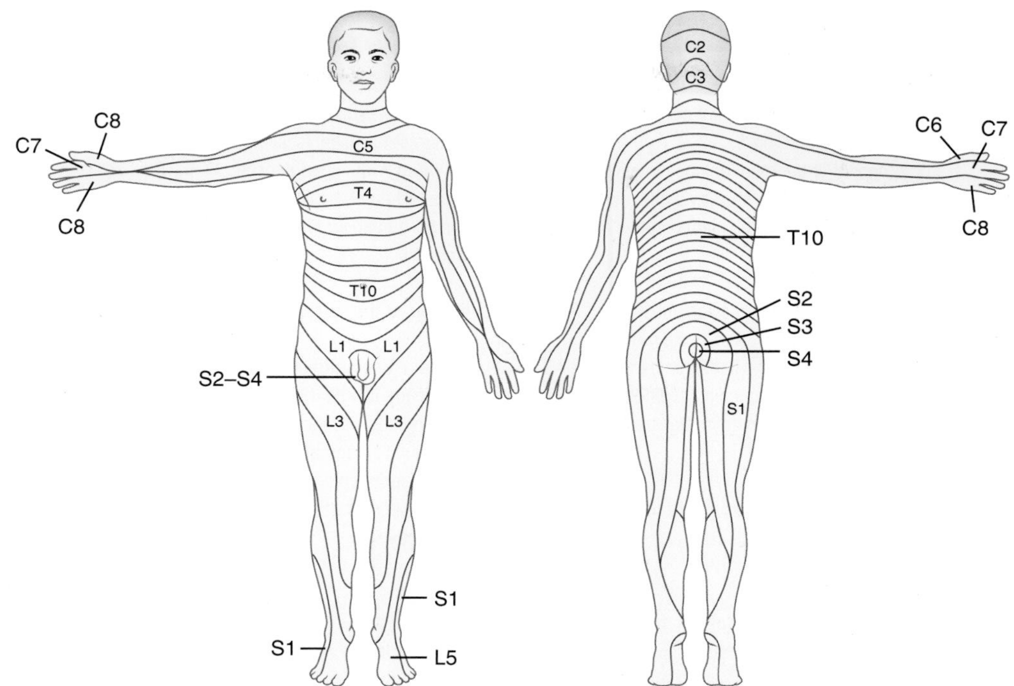


**Fig. 31.3** Dermatomes: Cervical *(C)*, Thoracic *(T)*, Lumbar *(L)*, and Sacral *(S)*. Boundaries are not quite as distinct as shown here because of overlapping innervation and variability among individuals. (*Reprinted with permission from Martin, J.H., Jessell, T.M., 1991. Anatomy of the somatic sensory system. In: Kandel, E.R. (Ed.), Principles of Neural Science. Appleton & Lange, Norwalk, CT.*)

describes the clinical situation in which sensory loss involves a number of dermatomes while those above and below are spared. *Sacral sparing* is a disturbance of sensory function in the legs with preservation of perianal sensation.

***Sensory level.*** With a sensory level, loss of sensation in a myelopathic distribution without weakness and reflex abnormalities would be very unusual. Sensory symptoms with incipient myelopathy are more often positive than negative; the Lhermitte sign (electric shock–like paresthesias radiating down the spine and often into the arms and legs produced by flexion of the cervical spine) is a common presentation of cervical myelopathy. Although the Lhermitte sign is commonly thought of as being associated with inflammatory conditions such as multiple sclerosis, it is more often seen with cervical spondylotic myelopathy and has been reported after radiation therapy affecting the cervical spinal cord as well as even after cervical injections.

Although a spinal cord localization is suspected with a sensory level, the level of the sensory loss may be slightly different between the two sides; this finding does not indicate a second lesion. Also, a basic tenet of neurology for the evaluation of spinal sensory levels is to look for a lesion not only at the upper level of the deficit but also higher. Magnetic resonance imaging (MRI) is the best noninvasive test for assessing sensory loss of spinal origin. Of note, demyelinating disease and other inflammatory conditions of the spinal cord may not be visualized on MRI; if an inflammatory lesion is suspected, however, a contrasted study on a high-field scanner will have greater diagnostic sensitivity (Runge et al., 2001).

***Dissociated sensory loss.*** Pain and temperature fibers cross shortly after entering the spinal cord and ascend contralaterally in the spinothalamic tract, whereas vibration and proprioception fibers ascend uncrossed in the dorsal columns. Therefore unilateral lesions of the spinal cord can produce loss of vibration and proprioception ipsilateral to the lesion and loss of pain and temperature sensation contralateral to it. This dissociation of sensory loss is most prominent in patients with intrinsic spinal cord lesions such as tumors, but it can also be seen with focal extrinsic compression. MRI usually shows the spinal lesion. The level of the deficits is often not congruent because of intersegmental projection of the pain and temperature axons in the posterolateral tract before synapsing on second-order neurons.

A second form of dissociated sensory loss can arise from selective lesions of the dorsal or ventral aspects of the cord. Anterior spinal artery syndrome produces infarction of the ventral aspect of the cord, sparing the dorsal columns; therefore a deficit of pain and temperature sensation is found below the level of the lesion but vibration and proprioception are spared. A selective lesion of the dorsal columns is less likely, but predominant dorsal column deficits can occur in patients with tabes dorsalis, multiple sclerosis, subacute combined degeneration, or Friedreich ataxia as well as occasionally in focal spinal cord mass lesions.

***Suspended sensory loss.*** A third form of dissociated sensory loss is seen in syringomyelia, with loss of pain and temperature sensation, sparing of touch and joint-position sensation (usually affecting the upper limbs), and normal sensation above and below the lesion (see "Syringomyelia," later).

***Sacral sparing.*** Ascending spinal afferents are topographically organized, with caudal fibers peripheral to more rostral fibers. Therefore central cord lesions can affect the higher fibers before the lower fibers, so that sensory loss throughout the legs with sparing of perianal sensation may be found. In some patients with severe cord lesions, this preserved sensation may be the only neurological function below the level of the lesion. The cause is usually trauma, but intrinsic mass lesions can also produce this clinical picture.

## Brainstem Sensory Lesions

Brainstem lesions uncommonly affect sensory function without affecting motor function. The notable exception is trigeminal neuralgia, characterized by lancinating pain without sensory loss in the distribution of a portion of the trigeminal nerve.

**TABLE 31.3 Common Sensory Syndromes**

| Syndrome | Localization | Sensory Features | Associated Findings |
|---|---|---|---|
| Acute inflammatory demyelinating poly radiculo neuropathy | Demyelinating lesion of peripheral nerves and roots | Dysesthesias and paresthesias that may be painful, along with sensory loss | Areflexia is common early in the course; motor findings predominate |
| Sensory neuropathy | Axonal or neuronal damage involving predominantly sensory axons | Burning pain, often with superimposed dysesthesias and paresthesias | Reflexes often suppressed distally early in the course |
| Carpal tunnel syndrome | Compression of the median nerve at the wrist | Numbness on the thumb and index and middle fingers | Weakness and wasting of the abductor pollicis brevis may occur in severe cases |
| Ulnar neuropathy | Ulnar nerve compression, most likely near the elbow and at the wrist | Loss of sensation on the fourth and fifth digits | Weakness of the interossei is often evident with advanced cases |
| Syringomyelia | Fluid-filled cavity that expands the spinal cord, damaging segmental neurons and white matter tracts | Loss of pain and temperature at the levels of the lesion (cape-like distribution; suspended sensory loss); dissociated sensory loss (i.e., affecting spinothalamic sensation and sparing posterior column sensation) | Weakness at the level of the lesion can develop with motoneuron damage; spasticity below the lesion can develop in severe cases |
| Thalamic infarction | Infarction of the territory of the thalamoperforate arteries | Sensory loss and sensory ataxia involving the contralateral body | Weakness may develop; aphasia or neglect suggesting cortical damage can rarely develop with involvement of thalamocortical connections |
| Thalamic pain syndrome | Previous sensory stroke in the thalamus produces neuropathic pain of central origin | Burning dysesthetic pain in the contralateral body, especially distally in the limbs | Other signs of the thalamic damage are typical, including sensory loss |
| Trigeminal neuralgia | Dysfunction of the trigeminal nerve root | Paroxysms of lancinating electric shock–like neuropathic pain but no other cranial nerve abnormality and no weakness | No sensory loss or motor findings |

Lateral medullary syndrome typically results from occlusion of the posteroinferior cerebellar artery and produces sensory loss on the ipsilateral face (from trigeminal involvement) plus loss of pain and temperature sensation on the contralateral body (from damage to the ascending spinothalamic tract). With this syndrome, however, the motor findings eclipse the sensory findings, which include ipsilateral cerebellar ataxia, bulbar weakness resulting in dysarthria and dysphagia, and Horner syndrome.

Medial medullary syndrome typically results from occlusion of a branch of the vertebral artery and is less common than lateral medullary syndrome. Patients have loss of contralateral position and vibration sensation, but again, the motor findings predominate, including contralateral hemiparesis and ipsilateral paresis of the tongue.

Ascending damage in the brainstem from vascular and other causes can also produce contralateral sensory loss. But as with the aforementioned syndromes, the sensory findings are trivial compared with the motor findings.

### Cerebral Sensory Lesions

***Thalamic lesions.*** Pure sensory deficit of cerebral origin usually arises from damage to the thalamus. The thalamus receives vascular supply from the thalamoperforate arteries—which are branches of the posterior cerebral arteries—often with some contribution from the posterior communicating arteries. In some patients, both thalami are supplied by one posterior cerebral artery, so bilateral thalamic infarction can develop from unilateral arterial occlusion. Thalamic pain syndrome is an occasional sequela of a thalamic sensory stroke and is characterized by spontaneous pain localized to the distal arm and leg and exacerbated by contact and stress.

***Cortical lesions.*** Lesions of the postcentral gyrus produce more sensory symptoms than motor symptoms. Infarction of this region involving a branch of the middle cerebral artery can produce sensory loss with little or no motor loss. More posterior lesions may spare the primary modalities of sensation (pain, temperature, touch, joint position) but instead impair higher sensory function, with manifestations such as graphesthesia, two-point discrimination, and the perception of double simultaneous stimuli.

## COMMON SENSORY SYNDROMES

Some common sensory syndromes are outlined in Table 31.3. Many of these are associated with motor deficits as well.

### Peripheral Syndromes

#### Sensory Polyneuropathy

The most common presenting complaint among patients with distal symmetrical peripheral polyneuropathy is sensory disturbance. The disturbance can be negative (decreased discrimination and increased threshold) or positive (neuropathic pain, paresthesias, dysesthesias) or both. Most neuropathies involve motor and sensory fibers, although the initial symptoms are usually sensory.

Nerve conduction studies can evaluate the status of the myelin sheath, thereby identifying patients with predominantly demyelinating polyneuropathies, including acute inflammatory demyelinating polyneuropathy (AIDP) and chronic inflammatory demyelinating polyneuropathy (CIDP). Electromyography (EMG) can demonstrate denervation and hence axonal damage, thereby identifying the motor involvement of many neuropathies with predominantly axonal features (Misulis and Head, 2002).

Cerebrospinal fluid (CSF) analysis can be helpful for identifying some immune-mediated and inflammatory neuropathies. Nerve biopsy can help with diagnosis of a variety of neuropathies.

#### Diabetic Neuropathies

Sensory involvement from diabetic neuropathy affects mainly small myelinated and unmyelinated axons, thereby producing disordered pain and temperature sensation. The findings often appear to be a paradox to the affected patient: loss of sensation yet with burning pain. Pathophysiologically, this makes perfect sense. The damaged axons cannot carry the patterns of action potentials, which accounts for the loss of sensation, yet spontaneous action potentials from damaged nerve endings plus increased susceptibility to discharge from mechanical stimuli cause the perceived neuropathic pain. Conventional neurodiagnostic testing often shows axonal neuropathy with sensory predominance (Perkins and Bril, 2014).

### Small-Fiber Neuropathy

Small-fiber neuropathies (SFNs) typically present as a progressive burning pain, commonly seen first in the feet. Lancinating pain, numbness, and paresthesias along with symptoms of autonomic dysfunction are commonly seen. Examination demonstrates abnormalities of pinprick and temperature sensation in most patients. Vibratory perception is often affected. Reflexes are commonly normal. Conventional electrodiagnostic studies are normal as they only access large fiber nerves. Since sweat glands are innervated by small fiber nerves, quantitative sudomotor axon reflex tests (QSARTs) are highly specific and sensitive. Improvements in pathology techniques have made skin biopsy an effective and safe method for diagnosing SFN.

Common etiologies include diabetes mellitus, autoimmune/paraneoplastic conditions, vitamin deficiencies/toxicities, toxic exposure to alcohol, heavy metals, and medications. Amyloidosis should also be considered, especially when it is accompanied by profound autonomic dysfunction.

### Acquired Immunodeficiency Syndrome–Associated Neuropathies

Human immunodeficiency virus type 1 (HIV-1) infection can produce a variety of neuropathic presentations. One of the most common is a painful, predominantly sensory polyneuropathy (Robinson-Papp and Simpson, 2009). The diagnosis can be confirmed by nerve conduction studies, EMG, and the appropriate clinical findings. CSF analysis and biopsy are usually not necessary unless an HIV-1–associated vasculitis or infection (such as cytomegalovirus) is present (Kaku and Simpson, 2014).

### Toxic Neuropathies

Some toxic neuropathies can be predominantly sensory. Such presentations are most commonly seen in patients with chemotherapy-induced peripheral neuropathy (Gutiérrez-Gutiérrez et al., 2010). Although motor abnormalities do occur, the sensory symptoms eclipse the motor symptoms for most patients. Development of dysesthesias, burning, and loss of sensation is the characteristic presentation. The neuropathy can be severe enough to be dose limiting for some patients and may continue to progress for months after the cessation of chemotherapy.

Patients with neuropathy that develops during chemotherapy can be presumed to have toxic neuropathy. If the association is not clear, however, other possibilities should be considered, including paraneoplastic and nutritional causes. Atypical features of chemotherapy-induced neuropathy include the appearance of symptoms after completion of the chemotherapy regimen and the development of prominent neuropathy with the administration of agents that are seldom neurotoxic.

Among the uncommon toxic neuropathies is that due to vitamin $B_{12}$/pyridoxine. Excess supplementation can cause a painful sensory neuropathy associated with degeneration of the dorsal root ganglia (Perry et al., 2004). With further excessive doses, motor involvement can occur, but this is far less common.

### Amyloid Neuropathy

Primary amyloidosis can produce a predominantly sensory neuropathy in approximately one-third of affected patients (Simmons and Specht, 2010). Familial amyloid polyneuropathy is a dominantly inherited condition. Patients present with painful dysesthesias plus loss of pain and temperature sensation. Weakness develops later. Autonomic dysfunction is typical. Eventually the sensory loss can be severe enough to make the affected extremities virtually anesthetic. The diagnosis can be suspected on clinical grounds, and confirmation requires positive results on either DNA genetic testing or nerve biopsy.

### Proximal Sensory Loss

Proximal sensory loss involving the trunk and upper aspects of the arms and legs is uncommon but can be seen in patients with porphyria or diabetes and in some with proximal plexopathies with a restricted distribution. Other rare causes of proximal sensory loss include Tangier disease, Sjögren syndrome, and paraneoplastic syndrome (Rudnicki and Dalmau, 2005). These neuropathic processes can be associated with pain in addition to the sensory loss. Motor deficit is also common, with weakness in a proximal distribution.

Patients with thoracic sensory loss should also be evaluated for thoracic spinal cord lesions, which may not always be associated with corticospinal tract signs.

### Temperature-Dependent Sensory Loss

Leprosy can produce sensory deficits that predominantly affect cooler regions of the skin, including the fingers, toes, nose, and ears (Wilder-Smith and Van Brakel, 2008). Temperature sensation is impaired initially, with subsequent involvement of pain and touch sensation in the cooler skin regions. The deficit gradually ascends to warmer areas, typically in a stocking-glove distribution, with frequent trigeminal and ulnar nerve involvement.

### Acute Inflammatory Demyelinating Polyradiculoneuropathy

Acute inflammatory demyelinating polyradiculoneuropathy (AIDP), or Guillain-Barré syndrome, is an autoimmune process characterized by rapid progression of inflammatory demyelination of the nerve roots and peripheral nerves. Patients present with generalized weakness that may spread from the legs upward or occasionally from cranial motor nerves downward. Sensory symptoms are generally are overshadowed by the motor loss. Tendon reflexes are lost as the weakness progresses (Hughes and Cornblath, 2005).

The diagnosis of AIDP is suspected in a patient who presents with progressive weakness with areflexia. Nerve conduction studies can confirm slowing, especially proximally (F-waves are particularly affected). CSF analysis shows an increased protein level without a prominent cellular response (albuminocytological dissociation).

### Mononeuropathy

Of the many recognized mononeuropathies, the most common is carpal tunnel syndrome, with ulnar neuropathy a close second. Although not classically considered a mononeuropathy, radiculopathy can be considered to fall into this category because one peripheral nerve unit is affected.

***Carpal tunnel syndrome.*** Compression of the median nerve at the wrist produces sensory loss on the palmar aspects of the first through the third digits. Motor symptoms and signs can develop with increasing severity of the mononeuropathy, but the sensory symptoms predominate, especially early in the course (Bland, 2005).

Nerve conduction studies usually show slowing of sensory and motor conduction of the median nerve through the carpal tunnel at the wrist. The slowing is present when conduction elsewhere is normal or at least

**TABLE 31.4 Radiculopathies**

| Nerve Root | Sensory Loss | Motor Loss | Reflex Abnormality |
|---|---|---|---|
| C5 | Radial forearm | Deltoid, biceps | None |
| C6 | Digits 1 and 2 | Biceps, brachioradialis | Biceps |
| C7 | Digits 3 and 4 | Wrist extensors, triceps | Triceps |
| C8 | Digit 5 | Intrinsic hand muscles | None |
| L2 | Lateral and anterior upper thigh | Psoas, quadriceps | None |
| L3 | Lower medial thigh | Psoas, quadriceps | Patellar (knee) |
| L4 | Medial lower leg | Tibialis anterior, quadriceps | Patellar (knee) |
| L5 | Lateral lower leg | Peronei, gluteus medius, tibialis anterior, toe extension | None |
| S1 | Lateral foot, digits 4 and 5, outside of sole | Gastrocnemii, gluteus maximus | Achilles tendon (ankle) |

when the distal slowing is far out of proportion to the slowing from neuropathy elsewhere. The EMG findings are usually normal, but denervation in the abductor pollicis brevis may develop with severe disease.

***Ulnar neuropathy.*** Ulnar neuropathy is commonly due to compression in the region of the ulnar groove. Patients present with numbness in the ulnar two fingers (fourth and fifth digits). Weakness of the interossei develops with advanced ulnar neuropathy in any location, but sensory symptoms predominate, especially early in the course (Cut, 2007).

Motor nerve conduction studies show slowing of conduction across the elbow or wrist—the two common sites for ulnar nerve entrapment. Findings on sensory nerve conduction studies will also be abnormal if the lesion is at the wrist. EMG can show denervation in the ulnar-innervated intrinsic muscles of the hand.

***Radial neuropathy.*** Radial neuropathy is often due to compression of the nerve in the spiral groove. Prototypically, this is seen in patients with alcohol intoxication, although cases are not confined to this association. Damage to the radial nerve in the spiral groove results in damage to muscles innervated distally to the triceps. Patients typically present with wrist drop, and sensory symptoms are minimal. Compression of the radial nerve distally in the forearm near the wrist can produce sensory loss and dysesthesias on the radial side of the dorsum of the hand; in this case there is no motor loss.

The diagnosis is suspected clinically from the wrist drop in the absence of weakness of muscles of the arm innervated by other nerves; examination of median and ulnar-innervated muscles can be difficult if the radial deficit is severe. Sensory findings, when present, are typical. Sensory findings in a radial nerve distribution without motor involvement suggest damage to the distal radial sensory nerve (e.g., from pressure, handcuffs, the insertion of an intravenous catheter, or other local trauma).

### Radiculopathy

Radiculopathy commonly produces pain, sensory loss, or both in the distribution of one or more nerve roots. Motor symptoms and signs develop with increasing severity, but sensory symptoms (usually pain) may be present for years without motor symptoms. Reflex abnormalities are common in radiculopathy.

Table 31.4 presents clinical features of common radiculopathies. Although cervical and lumbar radiculopathies are discussed here, any level can be affected. Diabetic radiculopathy and herpes zoster commonly affect thoracic dermatomes as well as cervical and thoracic dermatomes that are usually unaffected by spondylosis or disk disease.

Radiculopathy is best investigated using MRI. In patients below 45 years of age, the most common etiological disorder is disk disease. In older patients, spondylosis and osteophyte formation predominate. The latter is slower to progress and less likely to be associated with spontaneous remissions and exacerbations. EMG can be helpful to identify any axonal damage from radiculopathy, which may help determine the need, location, and timing of decompressive surgery.

## Spinal Syndromes

### Myelopathy

Myelopathy typically produces sensory loss, although the motor and reflex findings eclipse the sensory findings in most patients. Nevertheless, when a patient presents with back pain with or without leg weakness, a sensory level should be sought.

Some basic "pearls" regarding sensory testing in patients with suspected myelopathy follow:

- A defined line-like level is not expected.
- The sensory mapping is not as precise as that shown on dermatome charts.
- The sensory loss is seldom complete, which makes precise localization even more difficult.
- The sensory level may not be at the same level on the two sides of the body—a discrepancy of up to several levels can be seen.
- There may be dissociated sensory loss due to crossed projections of pain/temperature versus uncrossed touch/proprioception projections.
- Discrepancy in sensory level between posterior column and spinothalamic levels can occur because of intersegmental projections of the axons of the posterolateral (Lissauer) tract.
- The sensory level may be much higher than might be expected from motor examination or pain. This is because the lesion may be much higher than indicated by the levels of clinical findings, reinforcing the basic precept that the examiner must start from the level of the symptoms and consider higher levels.

The differential diagnosis of myelopathy is broad, with structural, ischemic, inflammatory, neoplastic, and metabolic disorders being the most common. Initial evaluation almost always involves imaging with MRI. If no structural cause is identified, then studies to consider are lumbar puncture (LP) for CSF indicators of infection, inflammation, cancer, vitamin $B_{12}$ and copper levels for metabolic etiologies of myelopathy, and additional questioning for a history of precipitants such as radiation therapy, recent infectious illness, trauma, or electrical injury. HIV-associated myelopathy is increasingly recognized and is not one disorder but a host of conditions that are predisposed by HIV, including infection, neoplasia, and immune-mediated myelitis (Levin and Lyons 2018).

### Syringomyelia

Syringomyelia is the presence of a syrinx, or fluid-filled space, in the spinal cord that extends over several to many segments. This is most commonly associated with a Chiari malformation (Koyanagi and Houkin, 2010). The mass effect of the syrinx produces damage to the fibers crossing in the anterior commissure that are destined for the spinothalamic tract, which conveys pain and temperature sensation. With more severe enlargement of the syrinx, damage to the surrounding ascending tracts may occur, affecting sensation below the level of the lesion. By the time this develops, segmental motoneuron and descending corticospinal tract damage are almost always present, and clinical signs of these changes can be seen.

### Spinal Hemisection

The spinal hemisection syndrome (Brown-Séquard syndrome) is classically described as the result of surgical or traumatic hemisection of the cord, but this presentation is rarely if ever encountered in clinical practice. Below the level of the lesion, ipsilateral deficits in vibration and proprioception from dysfunction of the dorsal columns as well as contralateral deficits in pain and temperature from damage to the spinothalamic tracts are the characteristic findings. Ipsilateral weakness also is seen from damage to the corticospinal tracts.

The diagnosis is suggested by the clinical presentation. This is a condition that can easily be missed unless the examiner assesses individual sensory modalities. MRI usually is performed to look for inflammatory or structural causes of the condition.

### Polyradiculopathies

A host of conditions can present with sensory symptoms due to involvement of multiple nerve roots. Many of these also have motor manifestations, but the focus here is on sensory presentations.

HIV can be associated with a rapidly progressive lumbosacral polyradiculopathy often with leg and/or saddle sensory deficits at the onset.

Neoplastic meningitis can present with sensory symptoms, with pain at multiple nerve roots. These are often associated with cranial neuropathies.

Neurosarcoid can produce granulomatous polyradiculopathy but can also produce parenchymal cord damage resulting in myelopathy (Reda et al, 2011; Uzawa et al, 2009).

Subacute sensory neuronopathy is a paraneoplastic condition, usually associated with anti-Hu antibodies. Symptoms can be related to sensory loss, including large and small-fiber involvement and/or pain. Loss of joint position and vibratory sense are common initial symptoms. Small cell lung cancer is the most common associated neoplasia, but others can produce this (Storstein et al, 2016). This often develops prior to the diagnosis of cancer.

### Tabes Dorsalis and Related Disorders

Tabes dorsalis is due to involvement of the dorsal roots by late neurosyphilis. Patients present with sensory ataxia, lightning pains, and often a slapping gait. Tendon reflexes are depressed (Marra, 2009).

Syphilitic myelitis is a rare complication of neurosyphilis, characterized by progressive weakness and spasticity. Motor symptoms dominate in this condition, with lesser sensory symptoms than with tabes dorsalis. MRI of the spine must be performed to look for other structural causes of myelopathy.

## Brain Syndromes

### Thalamic Infarction and Hemorrhage

Thalamic infarction typically produces contralateral hemisensory loss and is the main cause of a pure sensory stroke. All modalities are affected to variable degrees. The thalamus and its vascular supply are not organized so that specific portions of the sensory system are affected without dysfunction of other sensory systems and regions. MRI is most sensitive for visualization of acute thalamic lesions but computed tomography (CT) is performed when MRI is unavailable or contraindicated.

### Thalamic Pain Syndrome (Central Poststroke Pain)

Thalamic pain syndrome is an occasional sequela to thalamic infarction that usually affects the entire contralateral body, from face through arm, trunk, and leg. The pain, mainly distal in the limbs, is present at rest but is exacerbated by sensory stimulation. The distribution of the pain may shift so that the pain is poorly localized (Nicholson, 2004). Sensory detection thresholds are increased. Involvement of the posterior ventrobasal region is thought to be necessary for production of thalamic pain.

In a patient with a known history of thalamic infarction, additional study is usually not needed when thalamic pain occurs. If the pain develops long after the infarction, however, repeated scanning to look for a new pathological process—such as recurrent infarction, hemorrhage, or (less likely) tumor—is warranted.

The term *central poststroke pain syndrome* is increasingly used, since not all poststroke pain syndromes are due to primary thalamic damage, although the thalamus is still felt to be an important part of the pathophysiology (Klit et al., 2009).

Thalamic infarction and hemorrhage are often associated with nonsensory symptoms that can include deficits in memory, executive function, sleep cycle, and other functions (Chen et al., 2017).

### Trigeminal Neuralgia

Trigeminal neuralgia is a painful condition that produces lancinating pain in the distribution of part of the trigeminal nerve. This is prototypical neuropathic pain. Patients have paroxysms of pain that usually last for seconds. Sensory loss does not occur, so its presence encourages further search for other diagnoses. Imaging studies are commonly performed in the evaluation of trigeminal neuralgia but are seldom revealing.

### Mental Neuropathy (Numb Chin Syndrome)

Although the development of isolated numbness and/or pain in the chin region may seem insignificant, it is often an ominous finding suggestive of an underlying and possibly undiagnosed malignancy. The diagnosis of a mental neuropathy warrants an aggressive malignancy evaluation. Nonmalignant etiologies include trauma and other jaw pathologies, multiple sclerosis, infections, connective tissue diseases, vasculitis, and sickle cell crisis in both adult and pediatric patients (Hamdoun et al., 2012; Laurencet et al, 2000).

### Cortical Infarction

Infarction of the sensory cortex serving the face and arm is due to thromboembolism of branches of the middle cerebral artery. Infarction in the territory of the anterior cerebral artery produces sensory loss affecting the leg. Motor symptoms and signs are usually present, as are sensory abnormalities; however, if the region of infarction is limited, the sensory findings may be much more prominent than the motor findings.

### Deficits of Higher Sensory Perception

Multiple disorders have been described as producing defects in higher sensory processing. These include, in part, neonatal insult, autism, early developmental disorders, stroke, Alzheimer disease, head injury, and posttraumatic stress disorder. The total scope and features of these disorders are not completely understood, and since they are less able to be localized than more elemental sensory deficits, they are studied less often. Most of the clinical descriptions are anecdotal, with few control comparisons.

*Sensory processing disorder* is a term that has not yet been incorporated into standard diagnostic terminology, but there is increasing indication that this is likely a family of disorders with a variety of substrates and features (Koziol et al., 2011). The anatomical structures that serve higher sensory processing and integration are as broad as the brain itself and include cerebral cortex, basal ganglia, cerebellum, and the thalamus. The disorder can manifest as difficulty with processing sensory data into complex meaning and difficulty with attention to or interpretation of sensory stimuli and even electrophysiological responses from the brain. Sensory processing disorder crosses the border between sensory perception and attention—hence the multitude of studies examining sensory perception in autism spectrum disorder (Cygan et al., 2014).

The *sensory profile* is an assessment tool in the form of a long questionnaire that addresses, in part, some of the higher sensory processing without making a definitive diagnosis; it can be helpful for identifying patients who may have difficulty with sensory processing (Brown et al., 2001; Dunn, 1994). Although initially developed for use in children, an adult sensory profile assessment is now in use.

Infants with low birth weight and neonatal insult appear to be at increased risk for sensory processing disorder (Gill et al., 2013; Wickremasinghe et al., 2013). Not surprisingly, children with autism also exhibit increased risk for this (Puts et al., 2014). At present sensory processing is not routinely assessed in clinical practice, but the clinician should be aware of the concept and the potential manifestations of related disorders.

Clinical manifestations of sensory processing disorders can include misinterpretation of sensory data, resulting in poorly organized motor output and impaired incorporation of sensory stimuli in learning. This can affect not just responses to audio and visual stimuli but to almost any modality, cause deficiency or excess cognitive response to sensory stimulation, or even accentuate a drive to get sensory inputs. There is evidence for neurobehavioral consequences of sensory processing disorders, but some of this might be related to perinatal events rather than the sensory processing disorder per se (Ryckman et al., 2017).

### Functional (or Psychogenic) Sensory Loss

Functional sensory loss is less common than other positive functional neurological symptoms such as seizures or paralysis. In fact, it is easy to mistakenly ascribe a pattern of sensory loss to a nonanatomical cause when, in fact, true disease is present. Such misdiagnosis is particularly common with thalamic infarction and plexus dysfunction. Of note, embellished sensory or motor loss, although obvious to the examiner, may be superimposed on a real neurological deficit. The patient may be unintentionally helping the examiner yet essentially ruining the credibility of the report.

Cautionary notes should be borne in mind. In general, however, clinical presentations suggesting functional sensory loss include the following:

- Sensory loss exactly splitting the midline, with a minimal transition zone
- Circumferential sensory loss around the body or an extremity
- Failure to perceive vibration with a precise demarcation
- Loss of vision or hearing on the same side of the body as for the cutaneous sensory deficit
- Total anesthesia

The discrepancies in total anesthesia can be failure to perceive any sensory stimulus on an extremity that moves perfectly well. This degree of sensory loss would be expected to produce sensory ataxia. Another trap for a patient with psychogenic anesthesia of a limb involves tapping the limb while the patient's eyes are closed; consequent movement of the limb confirms the functional nature of the deficit. Third, if the anesthetic limb is an arm, examining for sensory abnormality while the arms are folded across the chest can be confusing for the malingering patient, especially if performed quickly.

## PITFALLS

Additional text available at http://expertconsult.inkling.com. 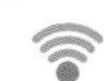

*The complete reference list is available online at https://expertconsult.inkling.com/.* 

32

# Arm and Neck Pain

Michael Ronthal

## OUTLINE



Evaluation of the patient with arm and/or neck pain is based on a meticulous history and clinical examination.

A useful approach is to consider the diagnosis in terms of pain-sensitive structures in the neck and upper limbs. These structures may be part of the nervous system or may involve joints, muscles, and tendons. Neurological causes of pain should be considered based on the innervation of the neck and arm; nonneurological causes are based on dysfunction of the other anatomical structures of the arm or neck. Because nerve root irritation generates neck muscle spasm, this type of pain is usually lumped into the "neurological" category. Some essentially nonneurological conditions have neurological complications and are grouped in this chapter as "in-between" disorders.

If the pain can be reproduced by joint movement at any level, the underlying cause is more likely to be rheumatological than neurological.

## CLINICAL ASSESSMENT

### History

#### Neurological Causes of Pain: Sites That Can Trigger Pain

***Muscle spasm.*** Posterior cervical muscles in spasm trigger local pain that is aggravated by neck movement, and the diagnosis is supported by the finding of palpable spasm and tenderness. The pain may radiate upward to the occipital region and over the top of the head to the bifrontal area. It is usually described as constant, aching, bursting, or as a tight band or pressure sensation on top of the head. Pain with similar characteristics can be triggered by pathology in the facet joints, cervical vertebrae, and even intervertebral disk pathology. These are often causative in the genesis of neck muscle spasm.

Neck mobility is best assessed by testing flexion and extension, lateral flexion to the right and left, and rotation to the right and left. Normally with flexion, the chin can touch the sternum; in rotation, the chin can approximate the point of the shoulder. Restriction of movement, particularly rotation, usually indicates the presence of cervical spondylosis.

***Central pain.*** Dysfunction affecting the ascending sensory tracts in the spinal cord may generate pain or paresthesias in the arms or down the trunk and lower limbs. An electric shock–like sensation provoked by neck flexion that spreads to the arms, down the spine, and even into the legs is thought to originate in the posterior columns of the cervical spinal cord (Lhermitte sign). Although this symptom is frequent in patients with multiple sclerosis (MS), it is nonspecific and simply indicates a pathological process in the cervical cord. Sharp superficial burning pain or itching points to dysfunction in the spinothalamic system, whereas deep aching boring pain with paresthesias of tightness, squeezing, or a feeling of swelling suggests dysfunction in the posterior column proprioceptive system. Sensory symptoms indicate which tract is dysfunctional, but they are poor segmental localizers.

***Nerve root pain.*** If the pathology involves a nerve root, it is referred to the upper limb in a dermatomal distribution. Brachialgia (arm pain) aggravated by neck movement, coughing, or sneezing suggests radiculopathy; when these trigger features are present, one can be fairly certain that the pain is radicular in origin. Nerve root pain is typically lancinating in character, but it can present as a dull ache in the arm.

Repetitive sudden shooting pains radiating from the occipital region to the temporal areas or vertex suggest the diagnosis of occipital neuralgia. There may be local tenderness over the greater or lesser occipital nerve, and a local injection of corticosteroid plus local anesthetic is both diagnostic and therapeutic. Failure to respond suggests that the area of the craniovertebral junction should be imaged.

***Ulnar nerve pain.*** Ulnar nerve entrapment triggers numbness or pain radiating down the medial aspect of the arm to the little and ring fingers. Symptoms are often worse at night when the patient sleeps with a flexed elbow, and they may interrupt sleep. Ulnar paresthesias are also triggered by pressure on the nerve when the patient is resting the elbow on the arm of a chair or desk. Tapping on the nerve in the ulnar groove at the elbow may evoke a tingly electrical sensation in the little and ring fingers (Tinel sign).

***Median nerve pain.*** Median nerve entrapment in the carpal tunnel classically awakens the patient from sleep with numbness and tingling in the thumb, index, and middle fingers, which is relieved by "shaking

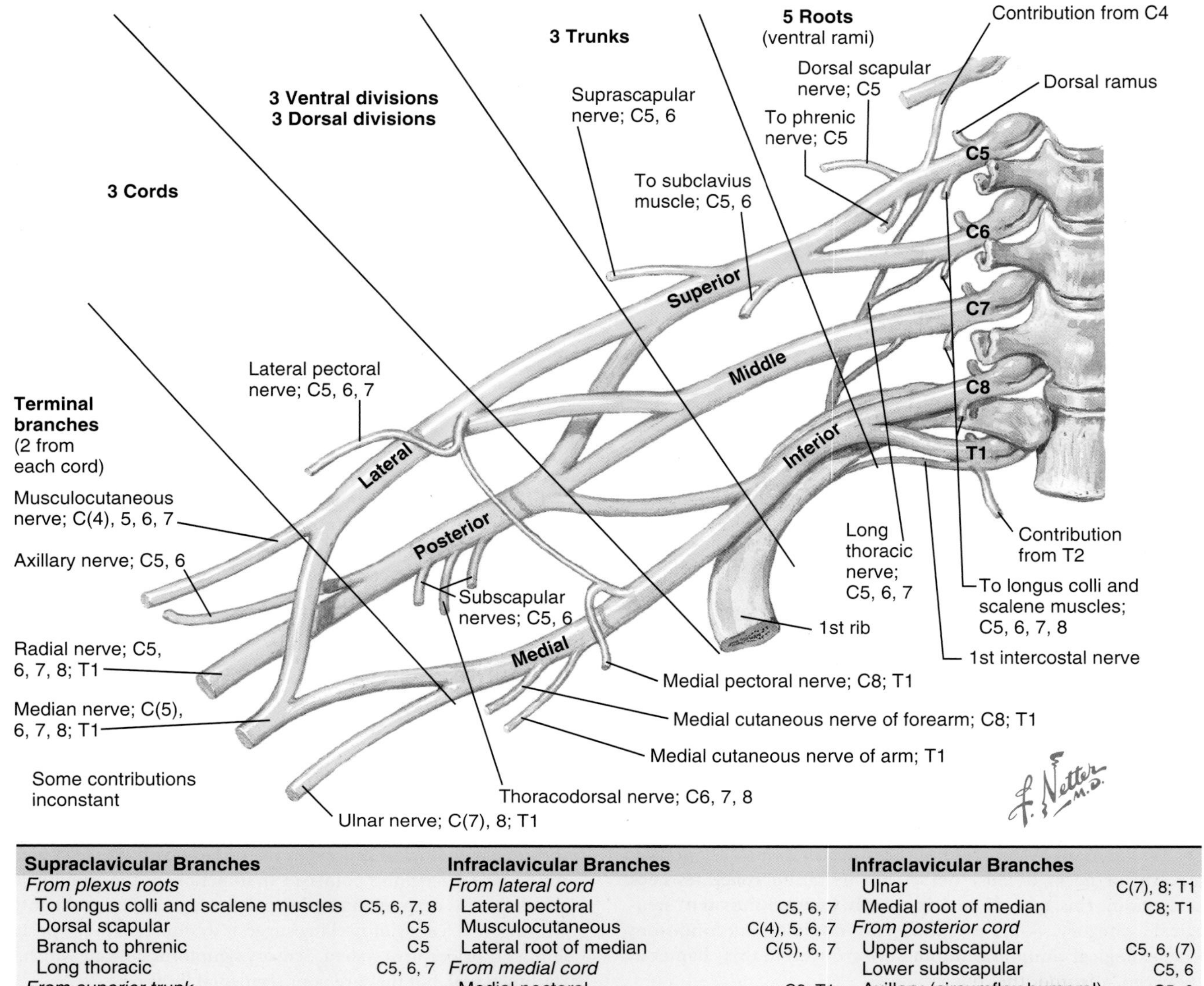


| Supraclavicular Branches | | Infraclavicular Branches | | Infraclavicular Branches | |
|---|---|---|---|---|---|
| *From plexus roots* | | *From lateral cord* | | Ulnar | C(7), 8; T1 |
| To longus colli and scalene muscles | C5, 6, 7, 8 | Lateral pectoral | C5, 6, 7 | Medial root of median | C8; T1 |
| Dorsal scapular | C5 | Musculocutaneous | C(4), 5, 6, 7 | *From posterior cord* | |
| Branch to phrenic | C5 | Lateral root of median | C(5), 6, 7 | Upper subscapular | C5, 6, (7) |
| Long thoracic | C5, 6, 7 | *From medial cord* | | Lower subscapular | C5, 6 |
| *From superior trunk* | | Medial pectoral | C8; T1 | Axillary (circumflex humeral) | C5, 6 |
| Suprascapular | C5, 6 | Medial cutaneous nerve of arm | T1 | Thoracodorsal | C5, 6 |
| To subclavius muscle | C5, 6 | Medial cutaneous nerve of forearm | C8; T1 | Radial | C5, 6, 7, 8 |

**Fig. 32.1** Brachial Plexus: Schema. *(Netter illustration from www.netterimages.com © Elsevier Inc. All rights reserved.)*

out" the hand. Pain generated in the median nerve can be sharp and lancinating and radiates to the thumb, index, and middle fingers. Although entrapment in the carpal tunnel is common, occasionally the site of entrapment is close to the elbow as the nerve passes under the pronator muscle.

***Plexus pain.*** Infiltrative or inflammatory lesions of the brachial plexus produce severe brachialgia radiating from the shoulder region and spreading down the arm. Radiation to the ulnar two fingers suggests that the origin is in the lower brachial plexus, and radiation to the upper arm, forearm, and thumb suggests an upper plexopathy. The thoracic outlet syndrome is an overdiagnosed condition but certainly exists. Patients with thoracic outlet syndrome complain of brachialgia and numbness or tingling in the upper limb or hand when they are working with objects above the head; thoracic outlet maneuvers are designed to test for compromise of the neurovascular structures passing through the thoracic outlet. The arm is extended at the elbow, abducted at the shoulder, and then rotated posteriorly. The examiner palpates the radial pulse while listening with a stethoscope over the brachial plexus in the supraclavicular fossa. The patient takes a deep inspiration and turns his or her head to one or the other side. Many normal individuals lose their radial pulse when doing this, but a bruit heard over the plexus does suggest, at the least, vascular entrapment (Adson test). The patient then exercises hands held above the head and extended elbows—numbness, pain, or paresthesias, often with pallor of the hand, support the diagnosis of thoracic outlet syndrome (Roos test) (Fig. 32.1).

## Nonneurological Causes of Neck Pain and Brachialgia

Muscle pain is deep, aching, and boring. In the cervical region, it is localized to the shoulders and sometimes radiates down the arm. If the patient with myalgia is over 50 years of age, a markedly elevated sedimentation rate would suggest the diagnosis of polymyalgia rheumatica. Patients with fibromyalgia may have pain in the neck, shoulders, and arms, with trigger spots or nodules that are exquisitely tender even to light pressure.

If pain is triggered or aggravated by joint movement of the upper limb, arthritis or tendonitis is the likely cause. Pain on shoulder abduction is usually related to Tendonitis, rotator cuff pathology, or pericapsulitis. The tendons anteriorly and at the lateral point of the shoulder may be tender to pressure. More diffuse tenderness anterior to the shoulder joint suggests bursitis. Tenderness over the medial or lateral epicondyle at the elbow indicates local inflammatory epicondylitis, and pain on active or passive wrist or finger joint movement suggests tendonitis or arthritis of the fingers. The pain of epicondylitis may radiate down the forearm in a pseudoneuralgic fashion, but precipitation by wrist extension or grip indicates a rheumatological cause.

## Examination

The physical examination is designed to define the neurological signs which localize the pathology to spinal cord, nerve roots, or peripheral nerves. Evaluation for nonneurological pathology is also necessary because rheumatological problems often complicate a primarily neurological problem. A detailed knowledge of motor and sensory neuroanatomy is required for accurate localization.

### Motor Signs—Atrophy and Weakness

The examination begins with inspection. Particular attention is paid to atrophy of muscles of the shoulders and arms and the small muscles of the hands. Fasciculations are associated with anterior horn cell disease, but they may be part of the neurology of cervical spondylosis and radiculopathy. Significant sensory signs would argue against anterior horn cell degeneration.

Muscles in the various myotomes are tested individually. When there is unilateral weakness, the contralateral side can act as a control, but some standard measure of strength is necessary for accurate evaluation when bilateral weakness is present. If one can overcome the action of a muscle by resisting or opposing its action close to the joint it moves, using an equivalent equipotent muscle of the examiner (fingers test fingers, whole arm tests biceps), then that muscle is by definition, weak. The degree of weakness can be graded, and the five-point (Medical Research Council [MRC]) grading scale is often used. Grade 5 represents normal strength. Grade 4 represents "weakness" somewhere between normal strength and the ability to move the limb only against gravity (grade 3). Grade 4 covers such a wide range of weakness that it is usually expanded. One simple expansion is into mild, moderate, or severe. When the muscle can move the joint only with the effect of gravity eliminated, it is graded at 2, and grade 1 is just a flicker of movement.

Hypertonia, weakness, sensory loss, increased tendon reflexes, and/or extensor plantar reflexes indicate cord dysfunction; when combined with radicular signs in the upper limbs, a spinal cord lesion in the neck at the level of the root signs is indicated. The distribution or pattern of weakness is all important in localizing the problem to root, plexus, peripheral nerve, muscle, or even upper motor neuron (central weakness). It is useful to use a simplified schema of radicular anatomical localization when one is evaluating nerve root weakness because overlap of segmental innervation of muscles can complicate the analysis (Table 32.1) If the pattern of weakness does not conform to a clearly defined anatomical distribution of cervical roots or a single peripheral nerve, a plexopathy is likely. Upper plexus lesions cause mainly shoulder abduction weakness, and lower plexus lesions cause weakness of the small muscles of the hand.

**TABLE 32.1 Segmental Innervation Scheme for Anatomical Localization of Nerve Root Lesions**

| Segment Level | Muscle(s) | Action |
|---|---|---|
| C4 | Supraspinatus | First 10 degrees of shoulder abduction |
| C5 | Deltoid | Shoulder abduction |
| | Biceps/brachialis/brachioradialis | Elbow flexion |
| C6 | Extensor carpi radialis longus | Radial wrist extension |
| C7 | Triceps | Elbow extension |
| C7 | Extensor digitorum | Finger extension |
| C8 | Flexor digitorum | Finger flexion |
| T1 | Interossei | Finger abduction and adduction |
| | Abductor digiti minimi | Abduction of the little finger |

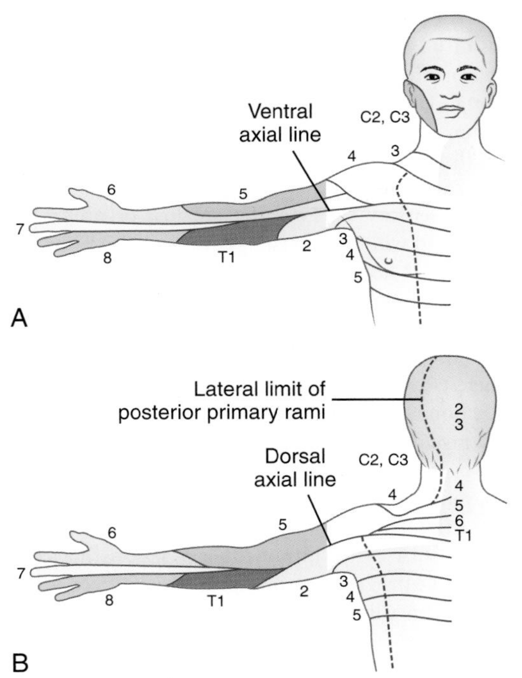


**Fig. 32.2 Diagram of the Dermatomes in the Upper Limbs. (A)** Anterior aspect. Although variability and overlap across the interrupted lines are evident, little or no overlap occurs across the continuous lines (i.e., dorsal and ventral axial lines). The examiner should routinely choose one spot in the "middle" of a dermatome and test at that point in all patients. C4 usually terminates at the point of the shoulder, T3 is almost always in the axilla, and T4 spreads across the chest so that C4 abuts T4 approximately at the nipple line. **(B)** Posterior aspect.

### Sensory Signs

Skin sensation is tested in a standardized manner, starting with pinprick appreciation at the back of the head (C2), followed by sequentially testing sensation in the cervical dermatomes, passing down the shoulder, over the deltoid, down the lateral aspect of the arm to the lateral fingers, and then proceeding to the medial fingers and up the medial aspect of the arm (Fig. 32.2). The procedure is repeated with a wisp of cotton to test light touch sensation; test tubes filled with cold and warm water are used to test temperature sensation. Position sense in the distal phalanx of a finger is tested by immobilizing the proximal joint and supporting the distal phalanx on its medial and lateral sides and then moving it up or down in small increments. The patient, with eyes closed, reports the sensation of movement and its direction. Loss of position sense in the fingers usually indicates a very high cervical cord lesion.

### Tendon Reflexes

An absent tendon reflex helps to localize segmental nerve root levels, but in cervical spondylosis, which is by far the most common underlying pathology, the reflexes are often preserved or even increased despite radiculopathy because of an associated myelopathy. An absent or decreased biceps reflex localizes the root level to C5, and an absent triceps reflex localizes the level to C6 or C7. An absent biceps reflex but with spread so that triceps or finger flexors contract is called an *inverted biceps jerk* and is strong evidence for C5 radiculopathy.

## PATHOLOGY AND CLINICAL SYNDROMES

### Spinal Cord Syndromes

#### Intramedullary Lesions

Primary intramedullary lesions may be neoplastic, inflammatory, or developmental. The most common presenting symptom of spinal cord tumor is pain, present in about two-thirds of patients, and usually radicular in distribution. It is often aggravated by coughing or straining and is worse at night.

Dissociated sensory signs (segmental loss of pinprick and temperature sensation with preserved light touch, vibration, and position sense) in the upper limbs indicates central cord dysfunction. In progressive acquired lesions, long tract signs will ultimately develop. If magnetic resonance imaging (MRI) reveals swelling of the spinal cord, the most common tumors are glioma, lymphoma, and ependymoma. A cavity suggests syringomyelia, but the most common cause of central cord dysfunction is cervical stenosis with extrinsic cord compression.

Cervical myelitis presents with the rapid onset of radicular and long-tract symptoms and signs and may be due to MS, postinfectious encephalomyelitis, or neuromyelitis optica, or it may be without an obvious cause (idiopathic).

Syringomyelia, a cystic intramedullary lesion of variable length and unpredictable progression, may present with deep aching or boring pain in the upper limb, often characteristically referred to the ear. Asymmetrical lower motor neuron (radiculopathic) signs in the upper limbs, with dissociated suspended sensory loss (i.e., an upper and lower border of the impairment of pinprick and temperature sensation), is suggestive of a syrinx.

### Extramedullary Lesions

***Cervical spondylosis.*** Extramedullary lesions, whatever the pathology, may result in any combination of root, central cord, and long-tract signs and symptoms. The most common cause of cervical nerve root and spinal cord compression is cervical spondylosis. This is a degenerative disorder of the cervical spine characterized by disk degeneration with disk space narrowing, bone overgrowth producing spurs and ridges, and hypertrophy of the facet joints, all of which can compress the cord and/or nerve roots. Hypertrophy of the spinal ligaments, with or without calcification, may contribute to compression. Hypertrophic osteophytes are present in approximately 30% of the population and therefore do not exclude other concomitant pathology. Furthermore, the degree of bony change does not always correlate with the severity of the signs and symptoms. This chronic degenerative process is sometimes referred to as a *hard disk* as opposed to an acute disk herniation or a *soft disk,* in which the onset is acute with severe neck pain and brachialgia. Patients with cervical spondylosis often wake up in the morning with a painful stiff neck and diffuse nonpulsatile headache that resolves in a few hours. The lesion is most commonly at C5/6 and/or C6/7 and the focal signs are likely to reflect root dysfunction at those levels. Wasting and weakness of the small muscles of the hands, but particularly weakness of abduction of the little finger, are often present. This sign localizes to lower segmental levels, but there may be no observable anatomical change at those levels and the sign is labeled a false localizer.

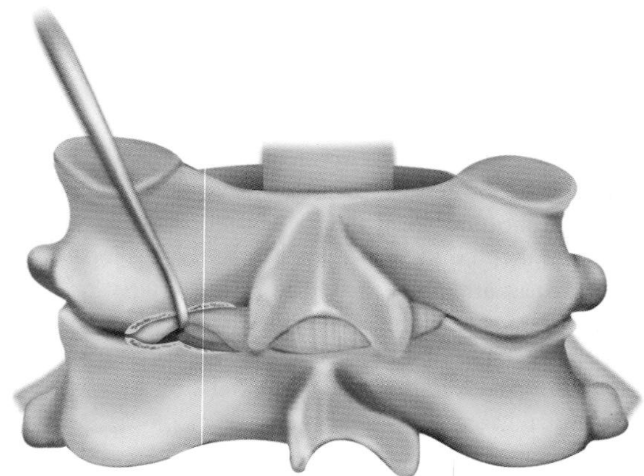

**Fig. 32.3 Cervical Disc Herniation.** The nerve root is gently mobilized and retracted upward to expose the herniated portion of the disk. (*From Ament, J.D., Kwon, H.D., Kim. K.D. Cervical microforaminotomy and decompressive laminectomy. In: Kim, D.H., et al. [Eds.], Surgical Anatomy and Techniques to the Spine, second ed. Copyright © 2006, 2013 by Saunders, an imprint of Elsevier Inc.*)

Restricted neck movement is always present with significant cervical spondylosis. Bladder dysfunction with frequency, urgency, and urgency incontinence or the finding of long-tract signs indicates the need for imaging of the cervical spine both to exclude pathology other than cervical spondylosis and also to define the severity of the spinal cord compression. Immobilization in a cervical collar, particularly in sleep, often helps with the symptoms and signs of cervical spondylosis. The role of surgery as treatment is discussed in Chapter 105 (Fig. 32.3).

### Other Cord Compression Syndromes

Extramedullary cord compression by pathology in the epidural space may be due to a primary or metastatic tumor. A schwannoma or nerve sheath tumor produces signs and symptoms related to the nerve root on which it arises; as it enlarges, progressive myelopathic dysfunction occurs. Plain radiographs of the cervical spine may demonstrate an enlarged intervertebral foramen; the MRI is diagnostic. A meningioma may present in a similar fashion and is more frequent in the thoracic region.

Over 90% of patients with metastatic malignancy present with pain. Malignant bone pain is usually localized to the vertebra involved and percussion tenderness over the vertebral spine is a good localizing sign. As the pathology spreads to the epidural space, radicular pain occurs. Plain radiographs of the cervical spine may show bony pathology with the preservation of disk spaces, but the imaging modality of choice is MRI. The whole spinal column should be scanned because metastases, some of which may be subclinical, often occur at multiple sites. Spinal cord compression due to metastatic disease is a neurological emergency requiring treatment with immediate high-dose steroids and either local irradiation or surgical decompression.

Epidural infection may be pyogenic and is often rapidly progressive; it may be chronic when the organism is likely to be mycobacterial or fungal. Pyogenic epidural abscess may present with fever, severe pain localized to a rigid neck, radicular pain, and rapidly progressive root and myelopathic signs; sometimes, however, the presentation is more subacute with less systemic evidence of infection. Imaging reveals early loss of the disk space, which enhances with contrast material. The infection then spreads into the epidural space and from there into the bone, resulting in vertebral collapse. Optimal therapy is surgical decompression and evacuation combined with 6–12 weeks of appropriate antimicrobial therapy for pyogenic infections and more prolonged treatment for tuberculosis.

A sudden onset of severe neck pain should raise the issue of spinal subarachnoid, subdural, or epidural hemorrhage. Bleeding is usually associated with some form of coagulopathy or anticoagulant therapy, but it also sometimes occurs with vascular anomalies.

## Radiculitis

Herpes zoster, which infects cervical sensory root ganglia, triggers radicular pain. The diagnosis becomes clear when, after 2–10 days, the typical vesicular rash appears. Motor involvement occasionally occurs, and, when it does, it has a predilection for the C5/6 segments. Myelitis with long-tract signs is seen in less than 1% of patients. If the pain lasts longer than 3 months after crusting of the skin lesions, postherpetic neuralgia has developed. The pain is described as constant, nagging, burning, aching, tearing, and itching, upon which are superimposed electric shocks and jabs. Treatment of postherpetic neuralgia pain is discussed in Chapters 102 and 105.

## Brachial Plexopathy

Brachialgia and physical signs not respecting a single nerve root that are associated with tenderness to palpation in the supraclavicular notch should arouse suspicion of a brachial plexopathy.

### Brachial Neuritis (Neuralgic Amyotrophy, Parsonage-Turner Syndrome)

Brachial neuritis is characterized by the abrupt onset of severe unilateral and constant unrelenting pain in the shoulder and arm, worse at night and rarely bilateral. The syndrome afflicts mainly young adult men. Within a week or so, muscle weakness, atrophy, and fasciculations develop, mainly in the shoulder girdle but occasionally more distally and distributed in more than one myotome. Despite the pain, there is usually little or no sensory loss. Pathogenesis is thought to be autoimmune/inflammatory, and antecedent inciting events include immunization, infections, heart pathology, and trauma. The syndrome is also associated with autoimmune diseases and Hodgkin disease. There is no proven specific treatment, but an initial short course of corticosteroids is usually prescribed. Treatment is supportive, and the pain mostly runs its course in 6–8 weeks. In some patients, recovery from paralysis can take up to a year, and occasionally there is some permanent mild weakness.

A subset of patients with a family history have recurrent attacks. Hereditary neuralgic amyotrophy is autosomal dominant, and many have deletions of the *PMP-22* gene in a portion of the distal long arm of chromosome 17.

### Brachial Plexopathy in Cancer Patients

Plexopathy in patients with a history of breast cancer or lymphoma who have been irradiated poses a problem: is this radiation plexopathy or malignant infiltration of the brachial plexus? Malignant infiltration is more likely to be extremely painful and to involve the lower plexus. There may be an associated Horner syndrome. Radiation plexitis is less likely to cause severe pain and often involves the upper plexus. Both syndromes are slowly progressive, but radiation plexitis is likely to be of longer duration. The electromyogram (EMG) can be helpful and myokymia and fasciculations support the diagnosis of radiation plexitis. Imaging with MRI to detect tumor infiltration has a sensitivity of 96%, specificity of 95%, and a positive predictive value of 95%. Occasionally locally malignant, relentless, and progressive, schwannoma occurs in a plexus that has been irradiated many years before.

## Thoracic Outlet Syndrome

Entrapment may involve the brachial plexus, subclavian artery, or both. Sagging musculature with postural abnormalities including droopy shoulders and a long neck contribute to the predisposition for thoracic outlet syndrome.

A supernumerary cervical rib or simply an elevated transverse process of the seventh cervical vertebra may be seen on plain radiographs. The extra rib may articulate with the superior aspect of the first rib, or a fibrous band may extend from its tip to the tip of the abnormal transverse process and connect to the first rib. The abnormal structure compresses the plexus, particularly when the upper limb is elevated above head level. Pain and paresthesias radiate to the ulnar side of the hand and fingers and there is weakness of the intrinsic muscles of the hand secondary to lower plexus compression. The thoracic outlet maneuvers (Adson and Roos tests) described previously are generally considered to be unreliable but do raise suspicion. The neurological examination may be normal or there may be weakness of the abductor digiti minimi with hypothenar sensory loss. Occasionally, the abductor pollicis brevis muscle is particularly atrophic and weak, mimicking carpal tunnel syndrome.

The diagnosis is usually one of exclusion: imaging of the cervical spine is normal, and nerve conduction studies below the clavicle are also normal. Venous and arterial anatomy can be studied by catheter angiography, Doppler, or MR angiography and venography. Electrophysiological studies that show partial denervation of the small muscles of the hand and a decreased sensory nerve action potential amplitude from the little finger are compatible with the diagnosis of thoracic outlet syndrome.

In all cases a conservative approach should be tried initially. Postural exercises and thoracic outlet muscle-strengthening exercises with instructions for ergodynamics at work and correction of unusual sleep posture provide relief in 50%–90% of patients, usually within 6 weeks. Failure of conservative treatment and ongoing symptoms prompts consideration of a surgical opinion (Fig. 32.4).

## Suprascapular Nerve Entrapment

The suprascapular nerve may be entrapped or injured as it passes through the suprascapular notch (see Chapter 106). It is occasionally cut in the process of lymph node biopsy. The branch to the infraspinatus muscle can be entrapped at the spinoglenoid notch by a hypertrophied inferior transverse scapular ligament. The patient complains of deep pain at the upper border of the scapula that is aggravated by shoulder movement, and there may be atrophy and weakness of the supra- and more commonly, the infraspinatus muscles. The supraspinatus muscle accounts for the first 10 degrees of shoulder abduction, and the infraspinatus muscle rotates the arm externally.

## Carpal Tunnel Syndrome

Carpal tunnel syndrome, the most common entrapment neuropathy, is more frequent in women and in pregnancy. It is now accepted as an occupational hazard secondary to repetitive stress as in, for example,

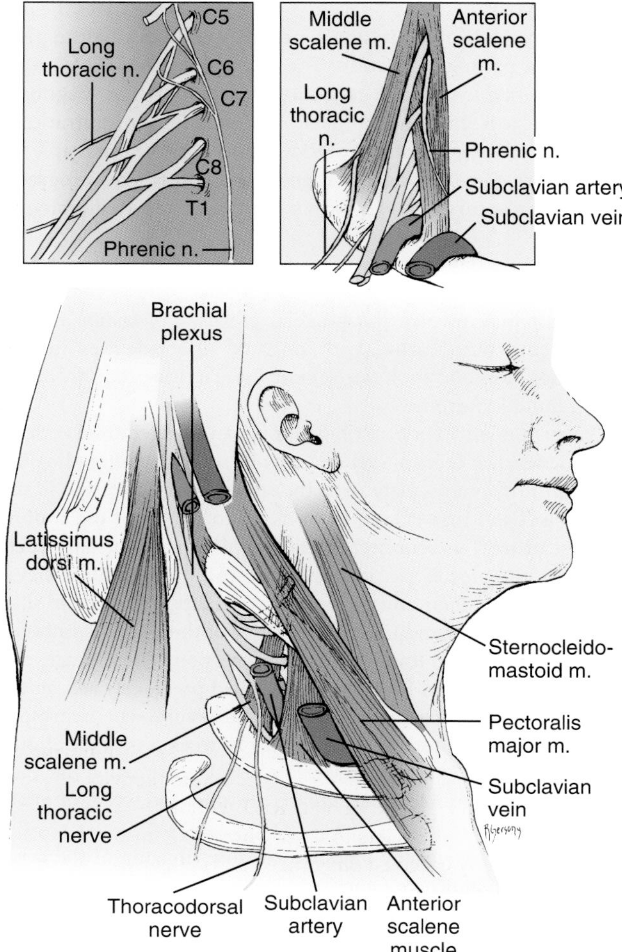


**Fig. 32.4 Anatomy of the Thoracic Outlet.** The surgical anatomy of the thoracic outlet is centered upon spinal nerve roots C5 through T1, which interdigitate to form the brachial plexus as they cross under the clavicle and over the first rib. The long thoracic and phrenic nerves also arise within the thoracic outlet region. The brachial plexus nerve roots pass through the scalene triangle, which is bordered by the anterior and middle scalene muscles on each side and the first rib at the base. The subclavian artery also courses through the scalene triangle in direct relation to the brachial plexus nerve roots. The subclavian vein crosses over the first rib immediately in front of the anterior scalene muscle before joining with the internal jugular vein to form the innominate vein. Symptoms of neurogenic thoracic outlet syndrome are often exacerbated by arm elevation, where greater strain is placed on the neurovascular structures passing through the scalene triangle. (*Modified from Thompson, R.W., Petrinec, D., 1997. Surgical treatment of thoracic outlet compression syndromes. I. Diagnostic considerations and transaxillary first rib resection. Ann. Vasc. Surg. 11, 315–323.*)

typing; occasionally it is the presenting symptom of underlying systemic disease. The nerve is entrapped in the bony confines of the carpal tunnel, which is roofed by the transverse carpal ligament.

Pregnancy, diabetes, rheumatoid arthritis, hypothyroidism, sarcoidosis, acromegaly, and amyloid infiltration of the ligament require appropriate screening blood studies, which should be checked in all patients with carpal tunnel syndrome.

Numbness or pain radiates to the thumb, index, and middle fingers and often wakes the patient at night. At times there is diffuse brachialgia. Atrophy and weakness of the abductor pollicis brevis muscle may be marked, but the motor deficit itself is rarely a cause of disability, although sensory loss in the distribution of the median nerve can be a handicap when the hand is being used out of sight.

Atrophy and weakness of the abductor pollicis brevis results in weakness of thumb abduction. There is also weakness of the opponens pollicis, but patients recruit the long flexor tendons when opposition is tested, so weakness is hard to identify. The palmar cutaneous nerve branch leaves the median nerve proximal to the flexor retinaculum and supplies the skin over the thenar eminence and proximal palm on the radial aspect of the hand. Hence sensory loss secondary to carpal tunnel syndrome involves the distal thumb, index, and middle fingers but not the thenar eminence itself, a useful diagnostic point.

The Phalen test is performed by holding the wrist in complete flexion for a few minutes. Precipitation of numbness or tingling in a median nerve distribution is supportive evidence. Sensitivity is about 74% and the false-positive rate is about 25%. The Tinel sign may be elicited by tapping the median nerve at the wrist.

Confirmation of the diagnosis is provided by nerve conduction studies and EMG: distal motor and sensory latencies are prolonged, and polyphasic reinnervation potentials are seen in the abductor pollicis brevis. More extensive and expensive investigations are usually not warranted, but sonography and MRI have been utilized in difficult cases.

Sleeping in wrist splints is sometimes helpful, but patients with unremitting pain or significant motor and sensory signs as well as confirmatory nerve conduction studies should be offered decompressive surgery. This is usually curative. The surgeon should send the excised flexor retinaculum for histopathological examination to exclude the deposition of amyloid.

Occasionally, carpal tunnel syndrome may be mimicked by entrapment of the median nerve more proximally at the elbow. Here it passes beneath the thick fascial band between the biceps tendon and the forearm fascia and then between the two heads of the pronator teres muscle. As the nerve passes between the heads of the pronator teres, it supplies that muscle as well as the flexor carpi radialis (which flexes and abducts the hand at the wrist) and the flexor digitorum superficialis (which flexes the fingers at the interphalangeal joints with the proximal phalanx fixed). After it passes between the two heads of the pronator teres muscle, it supplies the flexor pollicis longus (which flexes the distal phalanx of the thumb with the proximal phalanx fixed), the flexor digitorum profundus to the first and second digits (which flexes the distal phalanx with the middle phalanx fixed), and the pronator quadratus (which pronates the forearm with the elbow completely flexed). Nerve conduction studies may localize the site of pathology, and the EMG precisely defines which muscles are involved (Fig. 32.5).

## Ulnar Entrapment at the Elbow

The ulnar nerve can be entrapped proximal to the epicondylar notch or as it passes through the cubital tunnel at the elbow, where a fibro-osseous canal is formed by the medial condyle, ulnar collateral ligament, and the flexor carpi ulnaris. Structural narrowing of the canal aggravated by occupational stress and a sustained flexion posture, especially when sleeping, aggravates entrapment. Although numbness and tingling are more common than pain, both are referred to the hypothenar eminence and the little and ring fingers. A positive Tinel sign at the elbow over the ulnar nerve helps localize the site. There is wasting and weakness of the small muscles of the hand (excluding the abductor pollicis brevis and opponens, which are median innervated), and there is decreased sensation over the palmar aspect of the ring and little fingers. In severe chronic cases, clawing of the fourth and fifth digits results from weakness of the third and fourth lumbrical muscles. Nerve conduction studies localize the area of entrapment. If the symptoms do not resolve by avoiding prolonged elbow flexion and the physical signs are significant, surgical decompression should be considered (see Chapter 106) (Fig. 32.6).

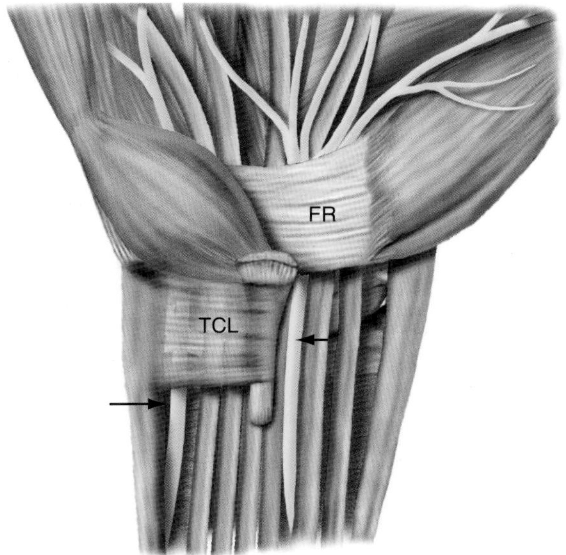


**Fig. 32.5 Anatomy of the Carpal Canal.** The median nerve gives off the palmar cutaneous branch before entering the canal *(short arrow)*. The median nerve then travels through the canal and gives off the motor branch. The *long arrow* indicates the ulnar nerve as it enters the Guyon canal. *FR*, Flexor retinaculum; *TCL*, transverse carpal ligament *(From Ma, C., Beltran, L.S., Bencardino, J.T., Beltran, J., 2015. Compressive and entrapment neuropathies of the upper extremities. In: Pope, T.L., Bloem, H.L., Beltran, J., et al. [Eds.], Musculoskeletal Imaging, second ed. Philadelphia, Elsevier, 2015.)*

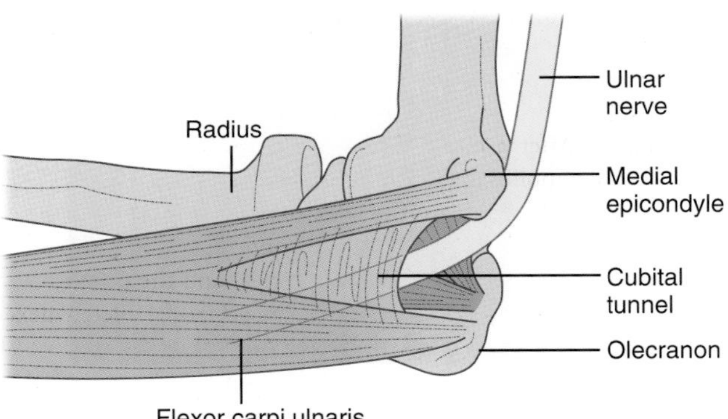


**Fig. 32.6 Detail of Ulnar Nerve Anatomy at the Elbow.** Entrapment of the ulnar nerve occurs both at the groove (between the medial epicondyle and the olecranon) or distally at the cubital tunnel. *(Reprinted with permission from Kincaid, J.C., 1988. AAEE minimonograph no. 31: the electrodiagnosis of ulnar neuropathy at the elbow. Muscle Nerve 11, 1005.)*

## Radial Nerve–Posterior Interosseus Nerve Syndrome

Having passed along the spiral groove of the humerus, the radial nerve pierces the lateral intermuscular septum to lie in front of the lateral condyle of the humerus between the brachialis and brachioradialis muscles. There it bifurcates to form the superficial branch, which provides sensory innervation to the lateral dorsal hand, and the deep branch, referred to as the *posterior interosseus nerve*. This branch supplies the finger and thumb extensors and the extensor carpi radialis brevis muscle, which is of lesser importance for radial wrist extension (extensor carpi radialis longus is dominant, and its nerve supply comes off slightly more proximally, so radial wrist extension is spared in lesions of the posterior interosseus nerve). The deep branch passes through the fibrous edge of the extensor carpi radialis muscle through a slit in the supinator muscle (arcade of Frohse). Entrapment of the posterior interosseous nerve here produces symptoms similar to those of lateral epicondylitis—lateral arm pain or a dull ache in the deep extensor muscle area, which radiates proximally and distally and is increased with resisted active supination of the forearm. Extension of the elbow, wrist, and middle fingers against resistance increases the lateral elbow pain. Tenderness may be elicited over the posterior interosseous nerve just distal and medial to the radial head. Posterior interosseous entrapment pain is typically seen in manual laborers and occasionally in typists. The site of pathology is easily localized by EMG and nerve conduction studies; surgical decompression is usually successful. Occasionally, a neoplasm of the nerve causes the same symptoms, and some surgeons prefer MRI prior to surgery (Fig. 32.7).

## Complex Regional Pain Syndrome

The complex regional pain syndrome (CRPS) encompasses syndromes previously called reflex sympathetic dystrophy (RSD), causalgia, shoulder-hand syndrome, Sudeck atrophy, transient osteoporosis, and acute atrophy of bone (see Chapters 52, 106, and 107). By consensus, the syndrome requires the presence of regional pain and sensory changes following a noxious event. The pain is of a severity greater than that expected from the inciting injury and is associated with abnormal skin color or temperature change, abnormal sudomotor activity, or edema. *Type I CRPS* refers to patients with RSD without a definable nerve lesion, and *type II CRPS* refers to cases where a definable nerve lesion is present (formerly called *causalgia*). A soft tissue injury is the inciting event in about 40% of patients, a fracture in 25%, and myocardial infarction in 12%.

The pathophysiology is unclear, but because many patients respond to sympathetic block and autonomic features are prominent, it has been suggested that there is an abnormal reflex arc that follows the route of the sympathetic nervous system and is modulated by cortical centers. There is decreased sympathetic outflow to the affected limb and autonomic manifestations previously ascribed to sympathetic overactivity are now thought to be due to catecholamine hypersensitivity. Significant emotional disturbance at the time of onset is present in many patients, and stress may be a precipitating factor.

Three stages of progression have been described:

- Stage I: sensations of diffuse burning, sometimes throbbing, aching, sensitivity to touch or cold, with localized edema. Vasomotor disturbances produce altered skin color and temperature.
- Stage II: progression of soft tissue edema, with thickening of skin and articular soft tissues and muscle wasting. This may last 3–6 months.
- Stage III: progression to limitation of movement, often with a frozen shoulder, contractures of the digits, waxy trophic skin changes, and brittle ridged nails. Plain radiographs show severe demineralization of adjacent bones.

Motor impairment is not necessary to make the diagnosis, but weakness, tremor, or dystonia is sometimes present.

The diagnosis is essentially clinical. Diffuse, severe, nonsegmental pain with cyanosis or mottling; increased sweating and shiny skin; swollen nonarticular tissue; and coldness to touch are characteristic. Hypersensitivity to pinprick may preclude precise sensory testing. There may be associated myofascial trigger points and tendonitis about the shoulder.

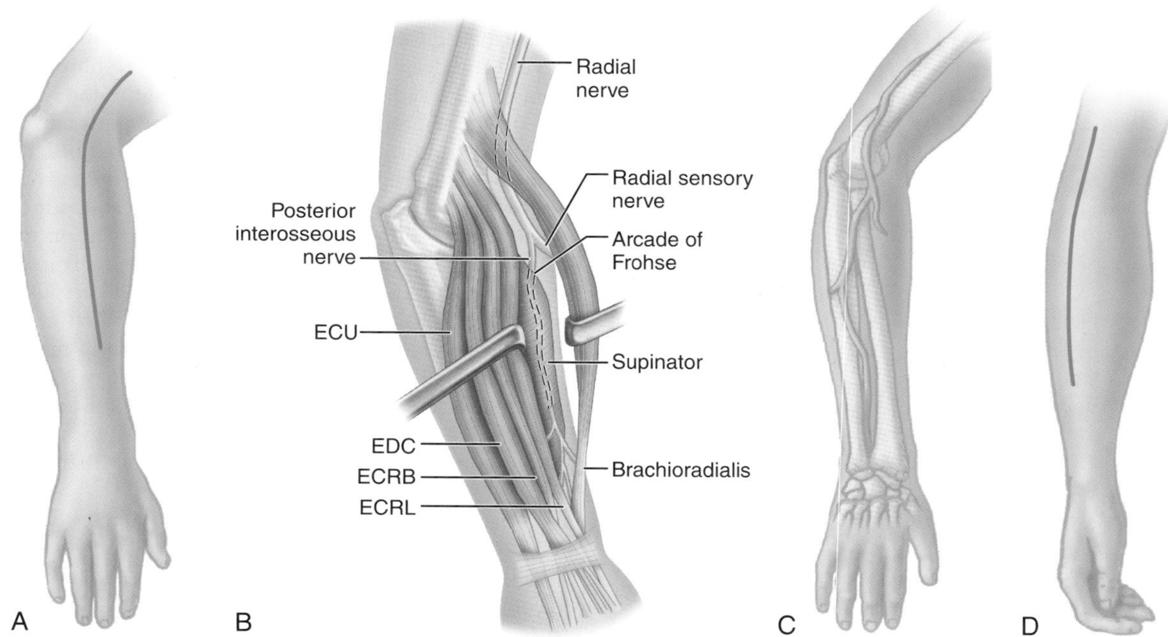


**Fig. 32.7 Radial Tunnel Syndrome.** Exposure of the posterior interosseous branch of the radial nerve for repair or decompression in radial tunnel syndrome. **(A)** Line of incision, forearm prone, elbow flexed. **(B)** Nerve exposed. **(C)** Diagram of course of nerve with arm in position A. **(D)** Line of incision, elbow extended. *(From Jobe, M.T., Martinez, S.F., 2017. Peripheral nerve injuries. In: Azar, F.M., et al. [Eds.], Campbell's Operative Orthopaedics, 13th ed. Copyright © 2017 by Elsevier, Inc. All rights reserved.)*

Autonomic testing may help with the diagnosis; the resting sweat output and quantitative sudomotor axon reflex test used together are 94% sensitive and 98% specific and are excellent predictors of a response to sympathetic block. Bony changes including osteoporosis and joint destruction may be seen. Bone scintigraphy is most sensitive in stage I and less useful in later stages. A stellate ganglion block may be useful both therapeutically and diagnostically (see Chapter 106).

These patients require a good deal of psychological support as well as trials of symptomatic medication. Drugs that sometimes work are prazosin, propranolol, nifedipine or verapamil, guanethidine or phenoxybenzamine, and antidepressants. Bisphosphonates may prevent bone resorption and are also helpful with pain control. A trial of stellate ganglion block, which can be repeated if successful, is worthwhile. Sympathectomy has been used for progressive disease in patients who have previously responded to sympathetic block (Fig. 32.8).

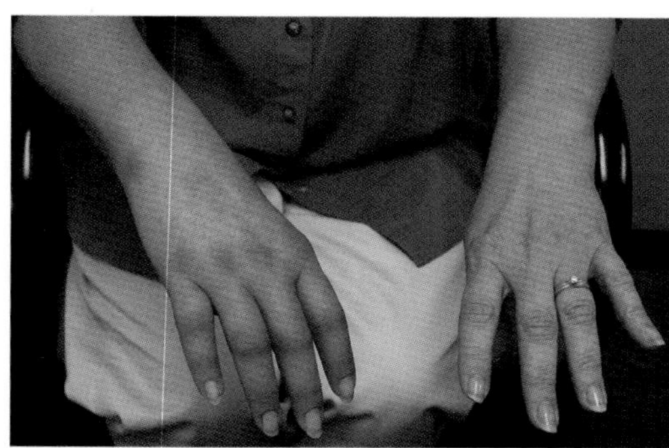

**Fig. 32.8 Skin Changes in Complex Regional Pain Syndrome.** Patient diagnosed with complex regional pain syndrome presenting with a shiny appearance of the right hand. *(From Mathews, A.L., Chung, K.C., 2015. Management of complications of distal radius fractures. Hand Clin. 31[2], 205–215. Copyright © 2015 Elsevier Inc.)*

## "In-Between" Neurogenic and Nonneurogenic Pain Syndrome—Whiplash Injury

> *Whiplash is an acceleration-deceleration mechanism of energy transfer to the neck. It may result from rear-end or side impact motor vehicle collisions but can also occur during diving or other mishaps. The impact may result in bony or soft tissue injuries (whiplash injury), which in turn may lead to a variety of clinical manifestations (whiplash-associated disorders).*
>
> ***Quebec Task Force on Whiplash-Associated Disorders (Spitzer, Skovron, Salmi, & et al, 1995a, 1995b)***

Rear-end motor vehicle collisions are responsible for 85% of whiplash injuries, and about 1 million such injuries occur in the United States every year. Severe injuries can cause rupture of ligaments, avulsion of vertebral endplates, fractures, and disk herniations, often associated with cervical nerve root or spinal cord damage. The severity of injury can be graded:

- Grade I injuries: pain, stiffness, and tenderness in the neck—no physical signs
- Grade II injuries: grade I symptoms together with physical signs of decreased range of movement and point tenderness
- Grade III injuries: neurological signs are present—weakness, sensory loss, absent reflex or long-tract signs.

The prognosis is related to the severity of injury:

- Neck pain lasting longer than 6 months after injury: grade I, 44%; grade II, 81%; grade III, up to 90%
- Headache lasting longer than 6 months after injury: grade I, 37%; grade II, 37%; grade III, 70%

- In general, about 40% of patients report complete recovery at 2 years, and about 45% continue to have major complaints 2 years after the injury.

The cause of persistent symptoms in patients with minor injuries is unknown, and little evidence exists for a structural basis for chronic whiplash pain in this group. The difference between a trivial injury and one of more significance should be based on the presence or absence of neurological signs.

About 20% of patients complain of cognitive symptoms after whiplash; cognitive dysfunction is likely to be functional or malingering.

The influence of compensation and legal action in whiplash-associated disorders remains controversial. Two studies from Lithuania, where only a minority of car drivers are insured for personal injury, demonstrated both retrospectively and prospectively significantly less symptomatology than for similar accidents in the United States; in Lithuania, at 1 year, no significant difference existed between collision and control groups. The Quebec Task Force emphasizes that whiplash is essentially a benign condition, with the majority of patients recovering, but it is the refractory minority that accounts for an inordinate proportion of the costs.

Support, physical therapy, muscle relaxants, and antidepressants are the main therapeutic options, but if neurological signs are present, imaging of the cervical spine with MRI is indicated. Persistence of pain for more than 6 weeks should indicate referral to a more specialized service; often a multidisciplinary team approach is best.

## Rheumatoid Arthritis of the Spine

Rheumatoid arthritis in the cervical spine involves all the synovial joints but it is particularly problematic when it involves the atlantoaxial articulation. Local inflammation and pannus formation cause pain on neck movement, and there may be rupture of the transverse ligament that holds the odontoid process in place, resulting in atlantoaxial subluxation. Pain is referred to the neck below the earlobe, and there may be a high myelopathy. Instability can cause sudden death. Spine radiographs show excessive space between the anterior arch of the atlas and the odontoid process.

## Nonneurological Neck/Arm Pain Syndromes

Patients with nonneurological causes for acute, subacute, or chronic neck and arm pain are frequently referred for neurological opinion. They may have no focal deficits or have minor nerve root or peripheral nerve signs that are incidental to their main complaint. Usually the clue to diagnosis is found in the history: a good history of movement aggravating or triggering the pain suggests the rheumatological cause.

### Fibromyalgia and Myofascial Syndrome

Within the group of rheumatological disorders, fibromyalgia is considered to be the most common cause of generalized musculoskeletal pain in women between the ages of 20 and 55 years; its prevalence is approximately 2%. The pain may initially be localized to the neck and shoulders but can spread diffusely over the body. It may follow an episode of physical or emotional trauma or a flu-like illness, and more than 90% of patients complain of depression and fatigue. Many patients may have a true sleep disorder. The only physical signs are muscle tenderness and the finding of "trigger spots," or multiple tender palpable nodules in the muscles. The diagnostic criteria require widespread musculoskeletal pain and excess tenderness in at least 11 of 18 predefined anatomical sites.

Myofascial pain is considered to be a localized form of fibromyalgia, with pain and tenderness in one anatomical region, such as the neck and shoulder. The cause and pathology of the condition are unknown and there is no specific treatment. Most patients are tried on muscle relaxants and antidepressants along with physical therapy and exercise. Failure to respond warrants a trial of trigger-point injections of corticosteroid in a local anesthetic.

### Polymyalgia Rheumatica

Polymyalgia rheumatica, more common in patients over the age of 50, presents with severe aching, pain, and tenderness in the neck and shoulder girdle muscles in association with a markedly elevated erythrocyte sedimentation rate. The condition responds dramatically to small doses of oral steroid. Some cases are associated with temporal arteritis. If there is weakness, one should consider the diagnosis of polymyositis, and the serum creatine kinase should be measured.

### Tendonitis, Bursitis, and Arthritis

***Shoulder.*** Pain triggered by shoulder joint movement suggests tendonitis, capsulitis, rotator cuff tear, or an internal derangement of the joint. Flexion and elevation of the shoulder that evokes pain is labeled the *impingement sign*. Patients with a painful arc syndrome often respond to local corticosteroid injections into the tender tendons. Tenderness anterior to the shoulder joint suggests bursitis, which also usually responds to local corticosteroid injection. Weakness of extreme shoulder abduction indicates a rotator cuff tear, but pain on movement makes clinical evaluation difficult, and MRI of the shoulder may be needed to establish the diagnosis. Acromioclavicular joint arthritis causes a more diffuse shoulder pain aggravated by arm elevation, and the diagnosis rests on radiographs of the shoulder joint. Nonsteroidal anti-inflammatory medications help.

Adhesive capsulitis or frozen shoulder presents with marked limitation of shoulder joint movement such that the scapula moves en bloc with the arm and is associated with movement-evoked pain. Treatment for adhesive capsulitis is not all that satisfactory. Analgesics and physical therapy help in a limited way; the course is likely to consist of many months of discomfort but, in the end, spontaneous resolution.

***Elbow***

**Epicondylitis.** Pain in the elbow region triggered by clenching the fist (which tenses the extensor muscles and irritates their points of origin), or pain that increases with resisted finger and/or wrist extension and flexion, suggests the diagnosis of epicondylitis. Local tenderness medially or laterally over the distal end of the humerus makes the diagnosis. Lateral epicondylitis is known as "tennis elbow" and medial epicondylitis as "golfer's elbow." Treatment with a Velcro rubber band over the tender area at the elbow supplemented by local corticosteroid injections is usually helpful. Occasionally, these patients require surgery.

**Olecranon bursitis.** Local tenderness and swelling at the point of the elbow ("Popeye joint") makes the diagnosis of olecranon bursitis. The condition may follow local irritation but can be a manifestation of gout and occasionally represents a pyogenic infection. The bursa should be aspirated for diagnosis.

***Wrist***

**Tendonitis.** Wrist tendonitis is diagnosed by finding local tendon tenderness to pressure or stretch over the tendons. In De Quervain tenosynovitis there is tenderness over the radial aspect of the wrist; pain is caused by ulnar flexion with the thumb held in the closed fist (Finkelstein test). Splinting or casting and topical steroids are of benefit.

***Hands.*** Digital arthritis causes pain on finger joint movement, and there may be swelling of the joints and joint inflammation, as indicated by rubor. Pain in the fingers—worse in the morning, aggravated by movement and not associated with numbness (as in carpal tunnel)—suggests rheumatoid arthritis. Fingers spindling or other joint deformity is seen in chronic arthritis.

Distal arthritis in the terminal interphalangeal joints suggests osteoarthritis or psoriatic arthropathy. Bony swelling of the terminal phalanges (Heberden nodes) supports the diagnosis of osteoarthritis. Red, hot, painful, hypersensitive extremities, especially when hypersensitive to heat, suggest the diagnosis of erythromelalgia. This may represent abnormal sensitization of thermal receptors or abnormal platelet function and is sometimes associated with blood dyscrasias. Erythromelalgia usually responds to medication with aspirin.

*The complete reference list is available at https://expertconsult.inkling.com/* 

33

# Lower Back and Lower Limb Pain

E. Lee Murray, Karl E. Misulis

## OUTLINE



Lower back pain is one of the most common reasons for neurological and neurosurgical consultation. In many of the patients who present with lower back pain, the pain either developed or was exacerbated as a result of occupational activity. Lower limb pain is a common accompaniment to lower back pain but can occur independently.

The list of considerations in the differential diagnosis of lower back and lower leg pain is extensive and includes neural, bone, and non-neurological disorders. Although lower back pain is usually thought of as either neuropathic (specifically, radiculopathy-associated) or mechanical in origin, other possible sources of pain, including urolithiasis, tumors, infections, vascular disease, and other intraabdominal processes, must be considered in the differential diagnosis.

## ANATOMY AND PHYSIOLOGY

The lumbosacral spinal cord terminates in the conus medullaris at the level of the body of the L1 vertebra (Fig. 33.1). The motor and sensory nerve roots from the lumbosacral cord form the cauda equina. From there, the motor and sensory nerve roots unite at the dorsal root ganglion to form the individual spinal nerves. These anastomose in the lumbosacral plexus (Fig. 33.2), from which run the major nerves supplying the leg (Table 33.1).

Pain in the lower back can have many origins. A good beginning for the differential diagnosis is determining whether the leg also has pain.

A complicating factor in this consideration is that local spine pain can be referred—that is, felt at a distance—because of the common nerve root innervation of the proximal spinal nerves and peripheral nerves supplying distal parts of the leg.

Causes of lower back pain without leg pain include:

- Ligamentous strain
- Muscle strain
- Facet pain
- Bony destruction
- Inflammation from many causes

Causes of lower back plus lower limb pain include:

- Radiculopathy
- Plexopathies
- Spinal stenosis

Important causes of leg pain without low back pain include:

- Peripheral mononeuropathies
- Polyneuropathies
- Plexopathies
- Select inflammatory conditions
- Vascular claudication

Individual peripheral nerve lesions are usually caused by local trauma, entrapment by connective tissue, or involvement with mass lesions.

Lower back pain occasionally is caused by non-neurological and non-skeletal lesions. Some of the most important causes are:

- Urolithiasis
- Ovarian cysts and carcinoma
- Endometriosis
- Bladder or kidney infection
- Abdominal aortic aneurysm
- Visceral ischemia or other aortic ischemic disease.

## APPROACH TO DIAGNOSIS OF LOW BACK AND LEG PAIN

The first step in diagnosis is localization of the causative lesion. History and examination usually allow differentiation among mechanical, neuropathic, and non-neurological pain.

### History and Examination

The history should focus first on features of the back and leg pain:

- Mode of onset
- Character
- Distribution
- Associated motor and sensory symptoms
- Bladder and bowel control
- Exacerbating and remitting factors
- History of predisposing factors (e.g., trauma, cancer, osteoporosis)

For example, the acute onset of lower back pain radiating down the leg suggests a lumbosacral radiculopathy. Onset with exertion suggests

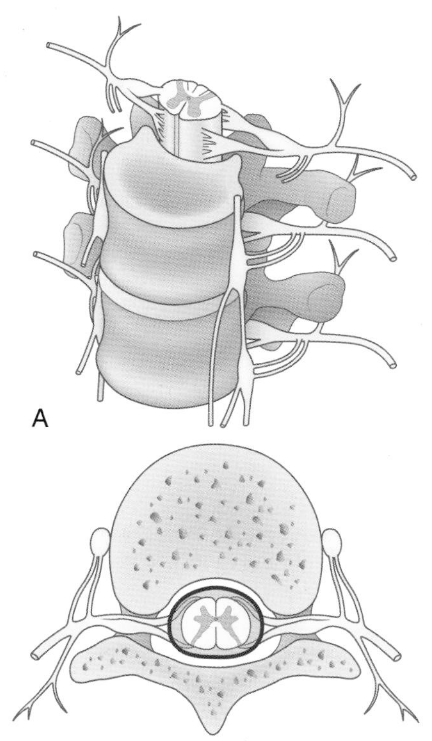

Fig. 33.1 Oblique (A) and axial (B) views of the spine showing anatomical relationships between neural and bone elements.

a herniated disk as a cause of the radiculopathy. Progressive symptom development can be from any expanding lesion, such as a tumor, infection, or disk extrusion.

Patients with lower back and leg pain usually have more symptoms than signs of neurological dysfunction. Therefore, if examination shows sensory and motor signs in a specific radicular or neural distribution, a detectable structural lesion is more likely.

The neurological examination is targeted to determine whether the symptoms are accompanied by abnormal neurological signs. General examination of the lower limb is important. Muscle groups that can be tested include:

- Hip–girdle muscles:
  - Hip flexors (psoas, sartorius)
  - Hip extensors (gluteus maximus, semitendinosus, semimembranosus, biceps femoris)
  - Hip adductors (adductor group: longus, brevis, magnus)
  - Hip abductors (gluteus medius, gluteus minimus, piriformis)
- Knee muscles:
  - Knee extension (quadriceps)
  - Knee flexion (semitendinosus, semimembranosus, biceps femoris)
- Ankle and foot muscles:
  - Foot plantar flexion (gastrocnemius)
  - Foot dorsiflexion (tibialis anterior)
  - Foot evertors (peronei)
  - Foot inverters (tibialis posterior)
  - Toe extension (extensor digitorum)
  - Great toe extension (extensor hallucis longus)

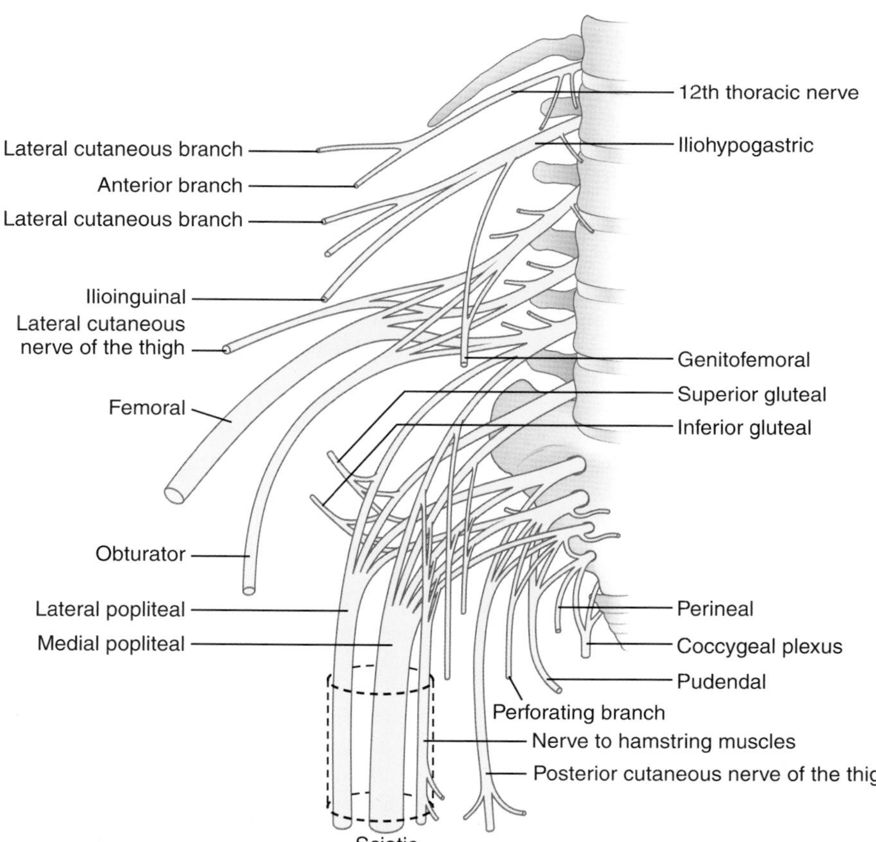

Fig. 33.2 Anatomy of the Lumbosacral Plexus. *(Reprinted with permission from Bradley, W.G., 1974. Disorders of the Peripheral Nerves. Blackwell, Oxford, p. 29.)*

**TABLE 33.1 Motor and Sensory Function of Lumbosacral Nerves**

| Nerve | Origin | Motor Function | Sensory Function |
|---|---|---|---|
| Femoral | Lumbar plexus, L2–L4 | Extension of knee, flexion of thigh | Anterior thigh |
| Saphenous | Distal sensory branch of femoral nerve | None | Inside aspect of lower leg |
| Lateral femoral cutaneous | Branch of lumbar plexus, L2–L3 | None | Lateral thigh |
| Obturator | Lumbar plexus, L2–L4 | Adduction of thigh | Medial aspect of upper thigh |
| Sciatic | Combined roots from lumbosacral plexus, partially separated into tibial and peroneal divisions | Foot plantar (tibial division) and dorsiflexion (peroneal division), foot inversion (tibial) and eversion (peroneal) | Lateral, anterior, and posterior aspects of lower leg and foot |
| Tibial | Lumbosacral plexus, L4–S3 | Plantar flexion and inversion of foot | Posterior lower leg and sole of foot |
| Peroneal | Lumbosacral plexus, L5–S2 | Dorsiflexion and eversion of foot | Dorsum of foot and lateral lower leg |
| Superficial peroneal | Distal sensory branch of peroneal nerve | None | Dorsum of foot |
| Sural | Cutaneous branches of peroneal and tibial nerves | None | Lateral foot to sole |

**TABLE 33.2 Classification of Lower Back and Lower Limb Pain**

| Type | Examples |
|---|---|
| Mechanical pain | Facet pain |
| | Bony destruction |
| | Sacroiliac joint inflammation |
| | Osteomyelitis |
| | Diskitis |
| | Lumbar spondylosis |
| Neuropathic pain | Polyneuropathy |
| | Radiculopathy from disk disease, zoster, and diabetes |
| | Mononeuropathy including sciatic, femoral, lateral femoral cutaneous, and peroneal neuropathies |
| | Plexopathy from cancer, abscess, hematoma, and autoimmune processes |
| Non-neurological pain | Urolithiasis |
| | Retroperitoneal mass |
| | Ovarian cyst or carcinoma |
| | Endometriosis |

- Toe plantar flexion (flexor digitorum longus)
- Great toe flexion (flexor hallucis longus)

Sensory examination should include the important nerve roots and peripheral nerve distributions: the femoral, peroneal, tibial, and lateral femoral cutaneous, lumbar roots L2–L5, and sacral root S1. Reflexes to be studied include the Achilles, patellar, and plantar reflexes.

Exacerbation of pain with some maneuvers also can be revealing. Stretch of damaged nerves results in increased pain by deforming the axon membrane, thereby increasing membrane conductance, depolarizing the nerve, and producing repetitive action potentials. Straight leg raising augments pain in a lumbosacral radiculopathy. Hip extension exacerbates pain of upper lumbar radiculopathy or that due to damage to the upper parts of the lumbar plexus, such as from carcinomatous infiltration or inflammation.

Armed with the abnormalities recognized from this history and examination, the neurologist may come to a conclusion about the localization of the lesion. This knowledge narrows the differential diagnosis substantially.

## Differential Diagnosis of Lower Back and Leg Pain

The differential diagnosis of lower back and leg pain can be addressed as shown in Tables 33.2 through 33.5. Classification into mechanical and neuropathic categories is useful for narrowing the scope of diagnostic considerations. The possibility of non-neurological causes should always be kept in mind.

Some basic guidelines for the differential diagnosis of lower back and leg pain are as follows:

- Pain confined to the lower back generally is caused by a low back disorder.
- Pain confined to the leg is usually caused by a leg disorder, although neuropathic pain from lumbar spine disease can radiate down the leg without back pain in a minority of patients.
- Pain in both the low back and the leg is usually caused by lumbar radiculopathy or, less commonly, lumbosacral plexopathy.
- Clinical abnormalities confined to one nerve root distribution are usually caused by intervertebral disk disease or lumbosacral spondylosis producing radiculopathy.
- Clinical abnormalities that involve several nerve distributions are usually caused by plexus lesions, with cauda equina lesions being the alternative diagnosis.
- Bilateral lesions suggest proximal damage in the spinal canal affecting the roots of the cauda equina.
- Impairment of bladder control indicates either a cauda equina lesion or, less commonly, a bilateral sacral plexopathy.
- Non-neurological causes of lower back pain are possible and particularly include urolithiasis, abdominal aortic aneurysm, ischemia, and other intraabdominal pathological processes.
- Multiple lesions can make the differential diagnosis more difficult. For example, radiculopathies at two or more levels may look like a plexopathy or peripheral neuropathic process.

Non-neurological causes of lower back pain include urolithiasis, ovarian cysts, endometriosis, pelvic carcinoma, bladder infection, and other retroperitoneal lesions including tumor, abscess, abdominal aortic aneurysm, visceral ischemia, and hematoma. These conditions produce pain that does not radiate unless neural structures are involved. Neural involvement in the abdomen and pelvis can produce radiating pain that can be clinically differentiated from radiculopathy only if multiple nerve roots are involved. Early involvement of bowel or bladder function together with abdominal pain suggests one of these non-neurological conditions.

## Evaluation

Diagnostic evaluation of lower back and lower leg pain begins with proper clinical localization and classification of the complaint. Diagnostic tests are summarized in Table 33.6 (Russo, 2006). The tests used depend on the clinical presentation, as discussed later (see the section Clinical Syndromes).

**TABLE 33.3 Differential Diagnosis of Lower Back and Leg Pain**

| Disorder | Clinical Features | Diagnostic Findings |
|---|---|---|
| Radiculopathy | Back pain radiating into leg in a dermatomal distribution. Sensory loss and motor loss are in a root distribution. Increased pain with coughing or straining. | Suspected when neuropathic pain radiates from back down into leg in a single root distribution. Disk or mass can be seen on MRI or CT. Zoster and diabetes can cause radiculopathy without abnormal studies. |
| Plexopathy | Back and leg pain with a neuropathic character, dysesthesias, burning, or electric sensation. Back pain can develop when cause is mass lesion in region of plexus. | Suspected when patient has leg pain in more than one peripheral nerve or root distribution. MRI of plexus or CT of abdomen and pelvis can show mass or hematoma. |
| Spinal stenosis | Pain in lower back, buttocks, and legs, especially with standing, walking, and lumbar spine extension. | MRI or CT shows obliteration of subarachnoid space. |

*CT*, Computed tomography; *MRI*, magnetic resonance imaging.

**TABLE 33.4 Differential Diagnosis of Isolated Lower Back Pain**

| Disorder | Clinical Features | Diagnostic Findings |
|---|---|---|
| Sacroiliac joint inflammation | Pain lateral to spine where sacrum inserts into top of iliac bone. Pain is exacerbated by movement and pressure but does not radiate down leg. | Clinical diagnosis. Radiographs can show degenerative changes in joint. Bone scan shows increased uptake in region. |
| Facet pain | Unilateral or bilateral paraspinal pain without radiation. Pain is increased by spine motion, especially extension. | Clinical diagnosis. Radiographs can show facet degeneration. |
| Ovarian cyst or cancer | Pain in hip and lower back, often but not always extending into lower quadrant. Bowel disturbance may develop with advanced disease. | Abdominal and pelvic CT shows mass lesion in ovary. |
| Endometriosis | Usually pelvic pain but occasionally pain in back and legs. Pain is often timed to menses. | Diagnosis suspected during pelvic examination. Vaginal ultrasound is supportive. Laparoscopy is diagnostic. |
| Retroperitoneal mass, abdominal aortic aneurysm, abscess, hematoma | Pain in back. May be bilateral to spine. May be associated with superimposed neuropathic pain in cases with plexus or proximal nerve involvement. | CT or MRI shows hematoma, aneurysm, eroding vertebral bodies, or abdominal mass. |
| Urolithiasis | Pain in upper to mid-back laterally that may radiate to groin. No radiation into leg. | Radiographs may show stones. Intravenous pyelography typically shows obstruction of flow.<br>Contrasted abdominal CT usually shows the stone and obstruction. |
| Diskitis | Pain in lower back exacerbated by movement. Some patients may have radiation of pain to abdomen, hip, or leg. | MRI shows characteristic changes in disk and surrounding tissues. |

*CT*, Computed tomography; *MRI*, magnetic resonance imaging.

### Magnetic Resonance Imaging

Magnetic resonance imaging (MRI) commonly is performed to assess the lumbosacral spine and lumbosacral plexus. It also can be used to evaluate the peripheral nerves in the pelvis and lower limbs.

MRI of the lumbosacral spine has the highest yield when the patient has back pain associated with radicular distribution of pain. Isolated back pain with no clinical symptoms or signs in the leg seldom is associated with significant findings on MRI. Intraspinal disorders that may not be revealed by MRI without contrast enhancement include neoplastic meningitis, epidural abscess, diskitis, and some chronic infectious meningitides (Tan et al., 2002).

Techniques for MRI of the lumbosacral plexus and peripheral nerves have greatly improved, so this modality can reveal masses, infiltration, and some inflammatory lesions, but MRI can miss disorders that are without a structural defect.

### Myelography and Postmyelographic Computed Tomography

With the advent of MRI, myelography has been performed less commonly. If adequate information is not obtained from noninvasive studies, myelography occasionally may be indicated. Modern uses of myelography are not only for patients who cannot have MRI due to size or implanted devices (Pomerantz, 2016).

For myelography, lumbar puncture is performed, and radiopaque dye is infused into the cerebrospinal fluid (CSF). Conventional radiographs are obtained as the dye is manipulated through the CSF pathways. Postmyelographic computed tomography (CT) is performed in most instances.

### Nerve Conduction Studies and Electromyography

Nerve conduction studies (NCS) and electromyography (EMG) are performed for four principal purposes:

- Assist localization of the lesion(s)
- Assist in evaluating the severity of the lesion(s)
- Determine whether the lesion is acute, subacute, or chronic
- Determine whether the lesion is neuropathic, axonal, or demyelinating

Axonal damage seen with radiculopathy or entrapment neuropathy suggests consideration of surgical decompression. Of note, signs of denervation may not appear on EMG until up to 4 weeks after onset of axonal damage.

**TABLE 33.5 Differential Diagnosis of Isolated Leg Pain**

| Disorder | Clinical Features | Diagnostic Findings |
|---|---|---|
| Peroneal neuropathy | Loss of sensation on dorsum of foot. Weakness of foot and toe dorsiflexion. | Slowed nerve conduction velocity across region of entrapment, usually at fibular neck. EMG may show denervation in peroneal-innervated muscles, especially tibialis anterior, without involvement of short head of biceps femoris. |
| Femoral neuropathy | Pain and sensory loss in anterior thigh, often with weakness of quadriceps and suppression of knee reflex. | NCS can sometimes be performed but may be technically difficult. EMG may show denervation in a distribution limited to femoral nerve. |
| Piriformis syndrome | Pain from back or buttock down posterior thigh. Pain is exacerbated by sitting or climbing stairs. Stretch of piriformis (flexion and adduction of the hip) worsens pain. | Clinical diagnosis. Pain radiating down leg in a sciatic nerve distribution. Exacerbation of pain by flexion and adduction of hip. EMG and NCS may show proximal sciatic nerve damage. |
| Meralgia paresthetica (lateral femoral cutaneous nerve dysfunction) | Pain and loss of sensation of lateral femoral cutaneous nerve on lateral aspect of thigh. | Clinical diagnosis. NCS is difficult to perform on this nerve. |
| Claudication | Pain in thigh and lower leg with exertion. Pain does not occur with lumbar spine extension. | Suspected with exertional leg pain without back pain. Ultrasonography or angiography confirms arterial insufficiency. |
| Plexopathy | Back and leg pain that has a neuropathic character. Dysesthesias, burning, or electric sensation. Plexitis has no associated back pain. | Suspected when a patient has leg pain in more than one peripheral nerve distribution. MRI of plexus or CT of abdomen can show a structural lesion in some patients. |
| Radiculopathy | Pain largely in one dermatomal distribution. May be motor and reflex loss. Most patients have back pain, but not all. | Suspected with pain radiating down one leg with or without back pain. Best imaged by MRI or postmyelographic CT. |

*CT*, Computed tomography; *EMG*, electromyography; *MRI*, magnetic resonance imaging; *NCS*, nerve conduction studies.

**TABLE 33.6 Diagnostic Studies for Lower Back and Lower Limb Pain**

| Diagnostic Test | Advantages | Disadvantages |
|---|---|---|
| Magnetic resonance imaging | Sensitive for identification of lumbar disk herniation, spinal stenosis, paravertebral mass in region of plexus, perineural tumors, and diskitis. | May overemphasize structural lesions. May miss vascular lesions of spinal cord. Paravertebral disorders may be overlooked if they are not the focus of interest. Cannot be performed on patients with some implanted metallic and electrical devices. |
| Noncontrast CT | Shows osteophytes and lateral disk herniations best. Can show bone fractures and extension of fragments into regions that may contain neural elements. | Cannot identify neural elements without intrathecal contrast. Disk herniations without bone involvement may be missed. |
| Myelography with postmyelographic CT | Many neurosurgeons consider this the definitive test for identification of lumbar disk herniation, osteophytes, and intervertebral foraminal stenosis. Postmyelographic CT should be routinely performed. | May miss far-lateral herniations. Is invasive with a small risk of serious adverse effects. |
| Nerve conduction studies and EMG | Sensitive for identification of specific nerve root or peripheral neuropathic involvement. | Patients may have clinically significant radiculopathy without EMG evidence of denervation (or vice versa if radiculopathy is old). |
| Diskogram | Can identify disk anatomy in comparison with bony and neural anatomy. May confirm disk level if it produces pain that reproduces patient's complaints. | Invasive test, but risk of serious complications is low. Seldom performed in routine practice. |

*CT*, Computed tomography; *EMG*, electromyography.

Entrapment neuropathy, or nerve root compression which can be responsible for lower limb pain, is likely to slow conduction velocity across the region of compression. Conduction velocities proximal and distal to the compression are usually normal, so conduction across the affected nerve segment must be studied.

Radiculopathy typically is associated with normal NCS findings in the peripheral branches of the nerves but with slowing of the F-wave. Asymmetry of tibial H-reflexes can suggest S1 radicular process on the side with the prolonged H-reflex Absence of abnormalities on NCSs and EMG does not rule out the presence of a radiculopathy.

Mechanical lower back pain is associated with no EMG or NCS alterations, so these studies are not usually indicated unless symptoms or signs of neural involvement are present.

### Radiography

Plain radiographs are obtained in patients with acute skeletal trauma and in almost all patients with isolated lower back pain. Among the potential findings are degenerative joint disease, vertebral body collapse, bony erosion, subluxation, and fracture. Radiographs of the pelvis and long bones also are obtained and may show fractures and destructive lesions.

### Bone Scan

Bone scan is especially important for examining multiple bone regions in cases of suspected neoplastic bone involvement. Multifocal involvement makes a neoplastic cause more likely than an infectious cause for the destruction.

## CLINICAL SYNDROMES

### Lower Back and Leg Pain

#### Lumbar Spine Stenosis

Lumbar spine stenosis is a disorder that affects mainly late middle-aged and older adults. The cause is multifactorial, with disk disease, bony hypertrophy, and thickening of the ligamentum flavum being the most important. Some of the symptoms are undoubtedly caused by direct pressure of these tissues on the cauda equina and exiting nerve roots, but a major contributor appears to be compression of the vascular supply of the nerve roots. Standing is associated with extension of the lumbar spine, which causes anterior bulging of the ligamentum flavum that lies posteriorly. Compression of the vascular supply creates nerve root ischemia, which can produce severe pain and weakness with exertion.

A diagnosis of lumbar spine stenosis should be suspected in patients with leg pain that is exacerbated by standing and walking and relieved promptly by sitting. Lying down, especially in the prone position, may exacerbate the low back pain, again through lumbar extension, a feature that helps differentiate lumbar spine stenosis from lumbar radiculopathy.

Confirmation of the diagnosis is by MRI or CT of the lumbar spine, which shows obliteration of the subarachnoid space at the level of the lesion. The hypertrophied ligamentum flavum and osteophyte formation are usually evident on these studies. If doubt about the diagnosis exists, myelography with postmyelographic CT scanning can be performed, but this is seldom needed.

Treatment can be conservative in the absence of neurological deficits. Physical therapy and medications can help, but surgical decompression may be required. Weakness of the legs or sphincter disturbance indicates a need for decompression. Although good evidence supports the benefit of surgical decompression at least in the short term, it is not clear that complex spine surgery with instrumentation produces substantial improvement in outcome especially when the etiology of the pain is not related to fracture or instability (Gibson and Waddell, 2005).

#### Cauda Equina Syndrome and Conus Medullaris Syndrome

Lesions of the lumbar spine can result in damage to the conus medullaris, cauda equina, or both. Cauda equina syndrome is compression of the nerve roots below the termination of the spinal cord. Nerve root dysfunction is due to direct compression by surrounding structures. Important causes include acute trauma; chronic degenerative bony disease with retropulsion of fragments into the spinal canal; lumbar disk disease; infections such as abscess; intraspinal and meningeal tumor; and intraspinal hematoma. This syndrome can be a rare complication of minor and major spinal procedures. Cauda equina syndrome usually develops as an insidious chronic process unless due to acute trauma. Symptoms can include back pain, leg pain, and weakness and cramps in the legs. Sensory symptoms can be sensory loss as well as neuropathic pain. Sphincter disturbance is common, especially with progression.

Conus medullaris syndrome is due to damage to the terminus of the spinal cord above most of the cauda equina and therefore at a higher spinal level. Etiology can be compression from all the conditions listed above plus occasional infiltrating lesions of the conus medullaris itself, especially by tumor. Conus medullaris syndrome is usually more rapidly progressive, is associated with earlier back pain and sphincter disturbance, and is more likely to be associated with preservation of some lower extremity reflexes, usually patellar.

MRI is the preferred diagnostic imaging method. If MRI cannot be performed, many causes of both syndromes can be identified on CT of the spine but contrast may be required.

**TABLE 33.7 Lumbosacral Radiculopathy**

| Root | Motor Deficits | Sensory Deficits | Reflex Deficits |
|---|---|---|---|
| L2 | Psoas, quadriceps | Lateral and anterior upper thigh | None |
| L3 | Psoas, quadriceps | Lower medial thigh | Patellar (knee) |
| L4 | Tibialis anterior, quadriceps | Medial lower leg | Patellar (knee) |
| L5 | Tibialis anterior, peroneus longus, gluteus maximus | Lateral lower leg | None |
| S1 | Gastrocnemii, gluteus maximus | Lateral foot, digits 4 and 5, outside of sole | Achilles (ankle) |

#### Lumbosacral Radiculopathy

Lumbosacral radiculopathy is usually caused by infringement on the neural foramen by either herniated disk material or osteophytes. Herniated disk is more common in young patients; osteophyte formation is more common in older patients.

Patients present with back pain radiating down the leg in a distribution appropriate to the involved nerve root. The most common lumbosacral radiculopathy is of the S1 nerve root, produced by a lesion at the L5–S1 interspace. Table 33.7 presents the typical motor, sensory, and reflex deficits associated with lumbosacral radiculopathy at individual levels.

The presence of lower back pain with radiating pain in a nerve root distribution points to a diagnosis of radiculopathy. Motor, sensory, and reflex deficits are not always present, so the diagnosis is suspected on the basis of symptoms without objective signs.

Confirmation of the diagnosis is by MRI, which can show disk protrusion or osteophyte encroachment with nerve root compression. MRI is the diagnostic procedure of choice for most surgeons, although postmyelographic CT is still occasionally used. Myelography with CT also may be used, especially in patients who cannot undergo MRI because of certain implanted electronic devices and metallic heart valves.

NCS findings are usually normal in patients with lumbosacral radiculopathy, although F-waves may be delayed in the affected root. EMG can reveal evidence of denervation in a nerve root distribution and can usually differentiate peripheral neuropathic processes from radiculopathy. This study also can determine whether denervation is present with radiculopathy.

Management of lumbosacral radiculopathy depends on the severity of symptoms, including pain and weakness. If the symptoms are mild, antiinflammatory agents may suffice. Muscle relaxants can produce short-term relief of muscle spasm and pain. Surgical options for lumbosacral radiculopathy are considered when the patient has intractable pain refractory to conservative care; when weakness is prominent, especially if it is unresponsive to conservative management; and when sphincter disturbance is present. Sphincter disturbance caused by lumbar disk disease or spondylosis necessitates consideration of urgent surgery. Patients with such deficits should not be given a trial of conservative therapy.

### Arachnoiditis

Arachnoiditis is inflammation of the arachnoid membranes surrounding the spinal cord. The inflammation can be caused by a number of processes including trauma to the spinal canal by injury or surgery, chronic compression of spinal nerves, chemicals such as intrathecal chemotherapy or contrast agents, blood products from subarachnoid hemorrhage, infections, or neoplasms. Some clinicians believe that arachnoiditis due to mechanical processes is overdiagnosed.

Common symptoms include pain in the back and legs which typically has a neuropathic character. Sensory symptoms can be loss of sensation or dysesthesias. Muscle symptoms can include twitching and cramps, and in severe cases, weakness or even paralysis can develop.

Diagnosis of arachnoiditis is suspected in patients with low back and leg pain who have radiological studies, which suggest the diagnosis; arachnoiditis is seldom a diagnosis of first consideration during initial evaluation. MRI shows thickened and clumped nerve roots. Careful examination of the imaging shows nerve roots adherent to each other and to the dura (Anderson et al., 2017). When MRI cannot be performed, myelography can show the same overall appearance. EMG can identify denervation spanning single root distributions and document motor dysfunction, but no EMG findings are specific for arachnoiditis. CSF analysis is performed if the differential diagnosis includes meningeal infection or tumor.

Treatment of arachnoiditis is usually symptomatic since the underlying cause is either remote or unknown. Preventing this disorder is the best approach and can be achieved by avoiding injury and sometimes by administering steroids with intrathecal medications.

### Plexopathy

***Plexus injury from retroperitoneal abscess.*** Retroperitoneal abscess is usually caused by peritonitis from gastrointestinal neoplasms or following surgery. Retroperitoneal abscess can affect the lumbosacral plexus. Patients present with abdominal and flank pain, often with overt signs of systemic infection, with fever, malaise, elevated white blood cell counts, and elevated C-reactive protein (CRP) concentration. The diagnosis is confirmed by CT of the abdomen. Management typically begins with surgical drainage followed by prolonged antibiotic treatment. Narcotics are usually needed for the pain of retroperitoneal abscess.

***Plexus injury from retroperitoneal hematoma.*** Retroperitoneal hematoma is usually caused by a bleeding disorder, a pelvic fracture, or abdominal surgery. Occasionally, bleeding from the site of arteriography puncture can result in tracking of blood into the region of the lumbosacral plexus, especially after thrombolytic therapy or anticoagulation. Hematoma also has been described in patients after lumbar plexus block and may be delayed (Aveline and Bonnet, 2004).

This diagnosis should be suspected in patients with leg motor and sensory symptoms who are at risk for intraabdominal hemorrhage; abdomen and leg pain are common. Confirmation of the diagnosis is by CT of the abdomen, which can show blood in the region of the plexus.

Treatment of plexus hematoma is supportive. Evacuation of the hematoma is seldom needed, and surgery commonly is reserved for patients with continued blood loss, which must be arrested.

***Neoplastic lumbosacral plexopathy.*** Neoplasms affecting the lumbosacral plexus can be solid or infiltrating. Both can produce severe neuropathic pain affecting one or both sides of the lumbosacral plexus. Diagnosis is suspected when a patient with known cancer presents with pain and often weakness of one or both legs. Diagnosis might be indirectly identified if there is no known cancer, with paravertebral tumor identified on lumbar spine MRI or other scan of the abdomen and pelvis.

The presence of back pain depends on the type of location of the lesion. About half of patients with neoplastic lumbosacral plexopathy have local pain in the back region (Jaeckle et al, 1985).

Diagnosis is usually established by MRI of the lumbar spine and plexus. Since the differential diagnosis might include radiation plexopathy, EMG can be helpful with that differentiation (Jaeckle, 2010).

Treatment depends on the tumor type and stage. If there is no known cancer diagnosis, then biopsy with or without excision is usually performed. Complete excision of some solid tumors is possible. Otherwise, radiation therapy is given initially. Pain often is relieved shortly after the radiation therapy has begun. During initial treatment, anticonvulsants can be used to relieve the neuropathic pain. Pure analgesics also may be used and sustained-release opiate formulations are effective in treating this condition.

### Acute Inflammatory Demyelinating Polyradiculoneuropathy

Acute inflammatory demyelinating polyradiculoneuropathy (AIDP) usually presents with motor and sensory deficits of the extremities but can be associated with back pain, usually in the lower back, but higher levels of pain can occur. The back pain may precede distal weakness, making the diagnosis not evident initially. The pain can be prominent and severe, and, in those cases, MRI may show enhancement of the lumbosacral nerve roots and cauda equina (Ding et al., 2018).

## Leg Pain Without Lower Back Pain

### Peripheral Nerve Syndromes

Peripheral nerve injury is commonly the result of sustained compression. Peroneal palsy is the most common lower extremity syndrome, usually caused by pressure at the fibular neck. Femoral neuropathy commonly results from intraabdominal causes and can be difficult to differentiate from upper lumbar plexopathy.

The diagnosis of peripheral nerve palsy is clinical, with symptoms and signs confined to one neural distribution. Patients usually present with neuropathic pain and sensory loss. Dysesthesias and paresthesias in the affected distribution are common. Reflex abnormalities depend on the individual nerves affected.

Definitive treatment of peripheral nerve entrapment is surgical release. Surgery is not always necessary, and conservative management may be successful. Tumor compression of peripheral nerves can be treated surgically, but radiation therapy can shrink the tumor, thereby relieving pain. Conservative management includes physical therapy to maximize comfort and improve function, antiinflammatory agents and anticonvulsants to alleviate pain, and counseling on methods to avoid subsequent damage. The counseling should address prevention of nerve compression and nerve stretch.

***Femoral neuropathy.*** The femoral nerve is usually injured in the pelvis as it passes beneath the inguinal ligament or in the leg. Intraabdominal disorders including mass lesions and hematoma are commonly implicated. Femoral artery puncture for angiography also may be a cause, either directly or via resultant hematoma.

Patients present with weakness that is most easily detected in the psoas, because the quadriceps are so strong. Sensory loss is over the anterior thigh and medial aspect of the calf and has a saphenous nerve distribution (the terminal sensory branch of the femoral nerve). This distribution of sensory loss is helpful to differentiate femoral neuropathy from lumbar radiculopathy. The patellar reflex is usually depressed.

The diagnosis can be supported by EMG evidence of denervation in the quadriceps but not in the lower leg or posterior thigh muscles. The adductors are especially important to test because they are innervated by the same nerve roots that supply the femoral nerve but instead are innervated by the obturator nerve. Normal EMG findings cannot rule out this diagnosis, because many patients do not have active or chronic denervation. NCS of the femoral nerve is difficult, especially in large patients, who are predisposed to the development of femoral neuropathy.

Treatment is seldom surgical, except for the removal of a massive psoas or iliacus hematoma or mass lesion. Weight loss and avoidance of marked hip flexion can reduce the chance of persistent damage. Physical therapy will aid recovery of motor power. Femoral neuropathy in the absence of marked damage usually resolves.

***Meralgia paresthetica.*** Dysfunction of the lateral femoral cutaneous nerve commonly is caused by compression as it passes beneath the inguinal ligament. Obesity and pregnancy predispose to this disorder, as does intraabdominal surgery of a variety of types. Recent reports have even described soldiers with body armor having meralgia paresthetica.

Meralgia paresthetica is the sensory syndrome of pain and sensory loss on the lateral thigh. Patients present with numbness and often pain on the lateral thigh. Motor deficits are not a feature. Meralgia paresthetica is differentiated from femoral neuropathy by the lateral distribution of the sensory findings and the absence of motor and reflex abnormalities.

Nerve conduction testing of the lateral femoral cutaneous nerve, although feasible, is technically difficult even in the best circumstances. It is even more difficult in obese patients, who are at particular risk for entrapment of the nerve.

Treatment is conservative. Weight loss is usually effective in preventing recurrence. Medications and blocks for neuropathic pain are sometimes helpful. The role of surgery is controversial and is rarely performed (Haim, et al., 2006; Harney and Patijn, 2007).

***Sciatic neuropathy.*** The sciatic nerve is most likely to be injured as it leaves the sciatic notch and descends into the upper leg. Compression can occur in patients in prolonged coma, especially those who are very thin. The sciatic nerve also is susceptible to injury from pelvic and sacral fractures, hip surgery or dislocation, needle injection injuries, and any penetrating injury.

Patients present with pain that is usually localized close to the level of the sciatic nerve lesion, although substantial radiation of the pain may be a feature. Loss of sensation is prominent below the knee, sparing the medial lower leg (the territory of the saphenous branch of the femoral nerve). Weakness can affect all muscles of the lower leg, but peroneal-innervated muscles are more likely to demonstrate weakness for two reasons. First, tibial-innervated foot extensors are so strong that substantial weakness would have to be present for weakness to be evident on examination. Second, the peroneal division of the sciatic nerve is more susceptible to compression injury than the tibial division, even high in the thigh.

Sciatic neuropathy is usually diagnosed clinically but can be supported by EMG evidence of denervation in sciatic-innervated muscles; signs of denervation may not be seen until 4 weeks after injury.

Treatment of sciatic compression is supportive, with avoidance of recurrent compression. Medications for neuropathic pain are often used. Surgical exploration and decompression are performed only in patients with clear evidence of a structural lesion.

***Piriformis syndrome.*** Piriformis syndrome is an uncommon condition in which the sciatic nerve is compressed by the piriformis muscle in the posterior gluteal area. Hypertrophy of the piriformis muscle and other anatomical variants predispose affected persons to development of the syndrome. This condition may affect not only the main sciatic trunk but also the superior gluteal nerve. The diagnosis and even existence of this as a singular condition is controversial (Halpin and Ganju, 2009).

Patients present with pain in the buttock that radiates down the leg and is exacerbated by adduction and flexion of the hip. Pain tends to be aggravated by prolonged sitting, climbing steps, and other maneuvers that irritate the piriformis muscle.

Piriformis syndrome is a clinical diagnosis. A patient with symptoms of sciatic neuropathy has no signs of radiculopathy or spinal stenosis on imaging. MRI neurography may show the lesion in many patients (Filler et al., 2005).

Piriformis syndrome is usually managed with antiinflammatory agents and sometimes local injections of steroids. Surgical treatment is rarely performed, and there is controversy about the indications and expected effectiveness of surgical treatment.

***Peroneal (fibular) neuropathy.*** Peroneal neuropathy is commonly caused by compression of the nerve as it passes from the popliteal fossa across the fibular neck into the anterior compartment of the lower leg. Patients often present with foot drop from weakness of the tibialis anterior muscle. The diagnosis is confirmed by NCS and EMG, with slowing of peroneal nerve conduction across the region of entrapment, usually across the fibular neck. The EMG shows evidence of active and chronic denervation in many patients, in keeping with the axonal damage indicated by the foot drop (Marciniak et al., 2005).

Peroneal neuropathy can develop in a variety of conditions which predispose to mechanical compression such as prolonged bed rest, hyperflexion of the knee, sitting with crossed legs, and lower leg cast. Peroneal neuropathy is of increased incidence in patients with peripheral neuropathy, those with a neurofibrous band attached to the peroneus longus, and ballet dancers (Dellon et al., 2002).

***Polyneuropathy.*** Peripheral neuropathy is a common cause of lower-extremity pain. The differential diagnosis for this condition is broad in scope, as would be expected. Among the most important causes are diabetes mellitus, familial neuropathy, metabolic neuropathies, and vasculitis. Pain is the presenting manifestation and differs in character according to the type of neuropathy. Small-fiber neuropathies manifest with burning pain that is often worse in the evening. Large-fiber neuropathies manifest with dysesthesias and paresthesias, often with electric shock-like pains.

Diagnosis is usually confirmed by NCS and EMG. Axonal neuropathy is more common than demyelinating neuropathy. Occasionally, patients with a predominantly small-fiber sensory neuropathy have normal NCS findings. Laboratory studies for peripheral neuropathy typically are performed as outlined in Chapter 34.

Treatment is with tricyclic antidepressants or anticonvulsants. Amitriptyline commonly is used for patients with small-fiber neuropathic pain. Anticonvulsants are used predominantly for patients with large-fiber neuropathic pain. When patients have symptoms of both, treatment with gabapentin, pregabalin, or oxcarbazepine can be helpful. Combination therapy with a tricyclic and anticonvulsant may be beneficial. Pure analgesics occasionally are used on a nightly basis to assist with sleep (Singleton, 2005).

### Plexopathy

***Diabetic lumbosacral plexopathy.*** Diabetic amyotrophy is a lumbosacral plexopathy that usually presents first with pain in the back, hip, lower back, or thigh and upper leg. In a minority of patients, pain develops in the lower leg. Diabetic amyotrophy can occur prior to the diagnosis of diabetes, although most have established disease.

The disorder is thought to be an inflammatory vasculopathy, with damage that probably is immune mediated. Patients present with pain in the hip and thigh associated with weakness of the quadriceps, psoas, and adductors. The plexopathy is more often unilateral than bilateral.

Pain develops prior to weakness in most patients. Weakness can be severe, and disabling. While this chapter focuses on lower back and leg pain, diabetic amyotrophy can affect the upper extremities.

Diagnosis is suspected by proximal pain and weakness of a leg in a patient with known diabetes. This disorder must be differentiated from lumbar radiculopathy and other structural lesions in the region of the plexus. NCS and EMG show coexistent peripheral polyneuropathy plus denervation in proximal muscles including quadriceps, psoas, and adductors. MRI and CT do not show a structural lesion.

Treatment is symptomatic. Immune-modulating treatments have been tried but are not standard. Most patients improve, although recovery is usually incomplete. The pain abates before recovery of muscle strength.

***Non-diabetic lumbosacral plexopathy.*** A condition similar to diabetic amyotrophy can develop in patients without diabetes. Presentation is similar. This is not necessarily associated with a prediabetic state (Ng et al. 2019).

Lumbosacral plexitis is similar to brachial plexitis, a presumed autoimmune process, but is less common. This entity is differentiated from radiculitis, which can be an inflammatory disorder of autoimmune or infectious origin (Tyler, 2008).

Management of idiopathic lumbosacral plexitis is supportive, with no medical intervention known to alter the course of the disease. Anticonvulsants are commonly used for pain management. Corticosteroids and high-dose intravenous immunoglobulin also are used occasionally, although it is not clear that their benefits outweigh the risks. The relatively short duration of the pain makes opiates appropriate for some patients if needed.

### Herpes Zoster

Reactivation of the varicella zoster virus first presents with hypersensitivity and pain in a single nerve root distribution. In most patients, a vesicular rash develops in the same cutaneous distribution usually several days after the onset of the pain. When the rash crusts over, there is commonly pigmentary changes of variable duration. The pain abates as the inflammation recedes, although the patient may be left with sensory or motor deficit. Weakness can be evident in muscles innervated predominantly by the single nerve root.

Diagnosis is clinical, and with a typical presentation including rash, structural imaging is usually not necessary. EMG and imaging are usually considered if the diagnosis is uncertain or with prolonged deficit. The differential diagnosis is broader in scope before development of the rash, and considerations include radiculopathy from other causes, including disk disease and osteophytes.

Treatment with antiviral agents such as acyclovir or famciclovir should begin within 72 hours of symptom onset. Early treatment may help hasten recovery and reduce the incidence of postherpetic neuralgia. Corticosteroids are often used in immunocompetent patients and especially for zoster ophthalmicus.

***Claudication of leg arteries.*** Arterial claudication is an important element in the differential diagnosis of spinal stenosis. Vascular disease of the iliac arteries and terminal branches results in marginal perfusion of lower limb muscles. Walking and other moderate activities exacerbate the ischemia, producing pain and weakness with exertion. The clinical picture may resemble that of spinal stenosis, but differentiating features include the lack of back pain, lack of exacerbation of leg pain with recumbent lumbar extension, and vascular changes in the leg.

Claudication is diagnosed by vascular imaging. Ultrasound examination can be a good screening test but angiography can provide a definitive diagnosis and, in some patients, can be the means for definitive treatment by angioplasty.

## Lower Back Pain Without Leg Pain

### Mechanical Lower Back Pain

Mechanical lower back pain is usually caused by strain of paraspinal muscles and ligaments with local inflammation. Muscle tears also may cause acute lower back pain. Therefore, mechanical lower back pain is usually a combination of bone, muscular, and connective tissue pain. Patients present with pain in the lower back without radicular symptoms and show no motor, sensory, or reflex abnormalities on examination. Any weakness or gait disturbance is due to pain and not neurological deficit.

Diagnosis is based on the clinical features and exclusion of other causes. In the absence of objective neurological deficits, imaging including spinal MRI is usually not needed initially. Depending on presentation and clinical course, radiography for bony changes may be needed. In the absence of signs of bony or neural destruction, conservative management may begin. If the patient does not respond to initial treatment, MRI may be indicated.

Mechanical lower back pain is usually treated by an initial period of rest of approximately 2 days, followed by an increase in activity including physical therapy. Muscle relaxants and antiinflammatories are often used. Surgery and repetitive nerve blocks are seldom indicated for mechanical back pain.

### Sacroiliac Joint Inflammation (Sacroiliitis)

Sacroiliitis is a term for sacroiliac (SI) joint inflammation, which presents with pain isolated to the back and just lateral to the spine in the region of the SI joint. This is often a component of more generalized arthritic conditions including ankylosing spondylitis but can also be seen in psoriatic and autoimmune arthritides (Miller et al., 2014).

Diagnosis is suspected with the local pain without radiation. MRI can show the inflammatory change (Boy et al., 2014). While a primary inflammatory or degenerative lesion is most common, in some cases infections and destructive processes can produce similar symptoms (Garg et al., 2014; Kim et al., 2013).

### Facet Joint Pain Syndrome

Pain from the facet joints of the lumbosacral spine is usually not an isolated entity but rather a component of mechanical back pain. Pain results from long-term degenerative changes in the facet joints, usually caused by strain. Repetitive strenuous activity, excessive weight, and abnormal posture may predispose affected persons to the development of facet pain. Acute trauma to the back may produce active joint inflammation that can be self-limited.

Diagnosis is suspected with pain usually lateral to the spine that is exacerbated by spine extension or bending toward the affected side. Facet pain often is bilateral. Pain can be exacerbated by prolonged sitting or walking up steps, as well as retaining one position for a prolonged time. Patients present with pain without motor, sensory, or reflex deficit unless radiculopathy or spinal stenosis is also present. Imaging may show chronic degenerative changes or be normal.

Facet pain is usually treated with antiinflammatory agents, physical therapy, and avoidance of precipitating activities. Facet blocks are usually not necessary, and effectiveness in terms of long-term relief is controversial (Varlotta et al., 2011).

### Lumbar Spine Osteomyelitis

Vertebral osteomyelitis is infection of the vertebrae, usually due to *Staphylococcus aureus*. This is most common in the lumbar region and may develop as a sequela of trauma or systemic infection. Adjacent structures are often affected with diskitis, often resulting from this, although the route of infection can be from infected disk to vertebra.

Diagnosis is suspected by lower back pain associated with systemic signs of infection—fever, elevated CRP, erythrocyte sedimentation rate (ESR), white blood cell (WBC) count (An and Seldomridge, 2006). Helpful clinical features include pain with percussion over the spine, marked limitation of motion of the spine, and tightness of paraspinal muscles that is more marked than usually seen with mechanical pain.

MRI shows changes in the vertebral body and often in the disk and the adjacent psoas muscle. Radiographs show degeneration of the disk margin of the vertebral body and disk space narrowing. Needle biopsy can reveal the causative organism in most cases. The diagnosis can easily be missed initially, since it can occur in patients with pre-existing lumbar spine pain, and inflammatory signs may not be marked early on (Mylona et al., 2009).

Treatment is with antibiotics and bed rest. Surgical debridement is needed in patients who do not respond to antibiotics.

### Lumbar Spine Compression

Compression of the lumbar vertebral bodies occurs in the setting of acute trauma, osteoporosis, infection, or tumor. Compression with minimal trauma is especially of concern for advanced osteoporosis or tumor. Patients present with severe lower back pain, usually without radicular symptoms. If the collapse results in impingement on nerve roots, radicular pain may develop. Compression of the cauda equina can result in weakness of the legs and sphincter disturbance.

The diagnosis of lumbar spine compression is suggested by a clinical presentation of lower back pain that is exacerbated by movement, jarring, or certain postures such as bending or twisting. Imaging of almost any type shows the bone deformation or destruction. MRI or a bone scan may be needed to help differentiate tumor or infection from degenerative causes.

Treatment consists of immobilization of the fracture site, which may include bracing. Pure analgesics often are needed, especially at night. Corticosteroids should be avoided if the cause is osteoporotic but can be very helpful for malignant vertebral collapse. Vertebroplasty can be very helpful. Surgery may be needed for unstable lesions or if there is spinal or neural compression. Radiation therapy is used for malignant collapse.

### Tumors Involving the Spinal Column

Tumors involving the spinal column can produce pain through destruction of the bone with subsequent collapse. Onset can be insidious or sudden. Sudden onset of severe local back pain can be a sign of vertebral body collapse, although the differential diagnosis is broader than this and includes nonmalignant mechanical pain. Insidiously progressive pain can be caused by tumor of the spine but the differential diagnosis includes epidural abscess, osteomyelitis, and other inflammatory conditions.

The cancers involved are of a broad range. Multiple myeloma is often characterized by involvement at multiple levels. Solid tumors with propensity for spinal involvement include lung, breast, thyroid, prostate, and renal cell cancers.

Benign tumors can involve the spine and some of these can present with back pain, although they often produce radicular pain. Some of these are meningiomas and neurofibromas. Osteomas produce bone inappropriately and present usually in childhood with pain in the femur and other long bones, but vertebrae can be involved. Osteoblastomas not only result in bony overgrowth but also predispose the patient to bone destruction and collapse, thereby producing local pain and radicular pain if neural elements are affected by impingement. In that case, pain would not be limited to the back and would involve the leg or other dermatomes.

### Lumbar Diskitis

Diskitis is an inflammatory process affecting the intervertebral disks of any level, often occurring in the lumbar spine. The responsible organism is dependent on the infectious source, with *S. aureus* and mycobacteria being among the most important causes. Diskitis associated with recent lumbar surgery is likely to be caused by resistant bacteria. In children, extraspinal manifestations of infection are less likely (Early et al., 2003).

Patients present with lower back pain, with marked restriction of flexion of the spine. Patients with postoperative diskitis usually have systemic inflammatory markers, but overt signs of infection with fever and chills may be absent.

A diagnosis of lumbar diskitis is suggested by the presence of severe lower back pain usually without a radicular component, often with tenderness and spasm of the paravertebral muscles associated with willingness of the patient to flex the hips but not the spine (Mikhael et al., 2009). ESR and CRP concentrations are usually increased. The diagnosis can be confirmed by MRI, and often shows changes in the endplates of the adjacent vertebrae. Bone scans show increased uptake in the region of the infected disk. Biopsy is often needed to identify an organism. The specific infectious agent may not be identified in as high as one-third of patients (Sheick et al., 2017).

Treatment begins with bed rest and antibiotics (Grados et al., 2007). Extensive surgery is not usually necessary; even tuberculous diskitis is successfully treated with antibiotics in more than 80% of cases (Bhojraj and Nene, 2002).

In some patients, diskectomy with fusion of the adjacent vertebral bodies may be required for relief of symptoms. Use of this management approach is usually restricted to adults; progression leading to surgery is less common in children.

### Spinal Epidural Abscess

Bacterial infection of the epidural space can develop into a spinal epidural abscess. The infectious organisms can spread from adjacent structures, the skin, or hematogenously. There is a triad of fever, back pain, and neurological deficits; however, the combination of all three is rarely seen. Most patients have limited symptomatology initially.

Diagnosis is confirmed by MRI, but contrast may be needed to reveal the infection. We have even seen cases where the lesion was not initially seen, but subsequently visualized on repeat scanning. Laboratory studies including elevated peripheral blood WBC, CRP, and ESR are frequently abnormal.

Treatment usually begins with identification of the organism from blood or surgery (Patel et al., 2014). An increasing proportion of patients are diagnosed by MRI when the epidural abscess is quite small. In this case, aspiration rather than open surgery or even empiric treatment may be appropriate. Close follow-up is needed in all patients.

## PITFALLS

Additional text available at http://expertconsult.inkling.com.

*The complete reference list is available online at https://expertconsult.inkling.com/.*

# 34

# Investigations in the Diagnosis and Management of Neurological Disease

*Joseph Jankovic, John C. Mazziotta, Nancy J. Newman, Scott L. Pomeroy*

## OUTLINE



The history and examination are key to making the diagnosis in a patient with neurological disease (see Chapter 1). However, ancillary testing is very important in diagnosis and management. Testing for specific disorders is addressed in detail in later chapters in Part III. This chapter provides a general overview of the principles that underlie obtaining investigations beyond the neurological examination.

Investigations beyond the history and examination should be directed to prove or disprove the hypothesis that a certain disease is responsible for the patient's condition. They should not be used as a "fishing expedition." Sometimes a physician who cannot formulate a differential diagnosis from the clinical history and examination is tempted to order a wide range of tests to see what might be abnormal. In addition to the high costs involved, this approach is likely only to add to the confusion, because "abnormalities" may be found that have no relevance to the patient's complaints. For instance, many patients are referred to neurologists to determine whether they have multiple sclerosis (MS) because their physicians requested magnetic resonance imaging (MRI) of the brain for some other purpose, such as the investigation of headaches. If the MRI shows small T2-weighted bright abnormalities in the centrum semiovale (changes that are seen in a proportion of normal older adults and in those with hypertension and diabetes), the neuroradiologist will report that the differential diagnosis includes MS, despite the fact that the patient has no MS symptoms and is unlikely to have MS.

There have been significant advances in laboratory technology; as a result, genetic, immunological, and other blood tests are expanding the ability of clinicians to confirm the diagnosis of an increasing number of neurological disorders, obviating more invasive studies. A test may be diagnostic (e.g., the finding of cryptococci in the cerebrospinal fluid [CSF] of a patient with a subacute meningitis, a low vitamin E level in a patient with ataxia and tremor, a low serum vitamin $B_{12}$ level in a patient with a combined myelopathy and neuropathy).One rapidly emerging area of diagnostic investigation is genetic testing. This can be targeted to a specific mutation when the level of suspicion for the genetic disorder is very high. However, there is an increasing utilization of new-generation diagnostic genetic testing such as whole-exome and whole-genome sequencing. The interpretation of these tests may require consultation with a geneticist and a genetic counselor. Another area of diagnostic testing that is rapidly expanding is immunology and testing for specific antibodies that may be involved in the pathogenesis of a variety of autoimmune and paraneoplastic disorders.

Results of laboratory tests can also be used to determine response to treatment. For instance, the high erythrocyte sedimentation rate (ESR) that is typically seen with giant cell arteritis falls with corticosteroid treatment and control of the condition. A rising ESR as the corticosteroid dosage is reduced indicates that the condition is no longer adequately controlled and that headaches and the risk of loss of vision may soon return.

Neuroimaging modalities have expanded remarkably, and the neurologist ordering these tests should be familiar with each one, so that appropriate sequences and methods are used to address the particular question presented by the patient's history. Also, because of the increasing use of pacemakers, deep brain stimulators, and other devices, the neurologist should be aware that certain precautions must be taken before MRI scans are ordered. MRI has replaced computed tomography for most conditions, and MR angiography and venography have largely replaced conventional catheter-based studies for the imaging of blood vessels.

It is important to use ancillary tests judiciously and to understand their sensitivity, specificity, risks, and costs. The physician must understand how to interpret hematological, biochemical, and bacteriological studies and specific neurodiagnostic investigations. These last studies include clinical neurophysiology, neuroimaging, and the pathological study of biopsy tissue. Knowledge of the various DNA tests available and their interpretation is critical before they are ordered; their results may have far-reaching implications not only for the patient but also for all of the patient's other family members.

The neurologist must know enough about each test to request it appropriately and interpret the results intelligently. As a rule, it is inappropriate to order a test if the result will not influence diagnosis or management. Tests should be used to diagnose and treat disease, not to protect against litigation. When used judiciously, investigations serve both purposes; when ordered indiscriminately, they serve neither. As we become more digitally advanced, functions in electronic medical record templates may suggest "best practices" as a guide to diagnostic investigations for given clinical presentations, but there is no substitute for physician-directed good clinical sense.

The neurologist must also have a working knowledge of several related disciplines that provide specific investigations to aid in a neurological diagnosis. These include neuropsychology, neuro-ophthalmology, neuro-otology, uroneurology, neuroepidemiology, clinical neurogenetics, neuroimmunology, neurovirology, and neuroendocrinology. Later chapters in Part II describe some of these disciplines and the investigations they offer.

## DIAGNOSTIC YIELD OF ANCILLARY TESTS

In choosing tests, the neurologist must decide what information will help to distinguish between the diseases on the differential diagnostic list. A test is justified if the result will confirm or rule out a certain disease or alter patient management provided that it is not too risky or painful. A lumbar puncture (LP) is justified if the clinical picture is that of meningitis, when the test may both confirm the diagnosis and reveal the responsible organism. However, culture and sensitivity testing should not be ordered on every sample of CSF sent to the laboratory if meningitis is not in the differential diagnosis. Because LP is invasive, with potential complications, it is not justified unless an abnormal finding will aid in the diagnosis. No test is justified unless the finding will influence the diagnostic process.

The physician should provide full clinical information and highlight the questions for which answers are being sought from the investigations. The electrophysiologist will look more carefully for evidence of denervation in a certain myotome if the patient has a syndrome suggesting herniation of that disk. The neuroradiologist will obtain additional views to search for evidence of a posterior communicating artery aneurysm if the neurologist reports a third nerve palsy in a patient with subarachnoid hemorrhage.

## INTERPRETATION OF RESULTS OF INVESTIGATIONS

Every biological measurement in a population varies over a normal range, which usually is defined as ±2 or 3 standard deviations (SDs) from the mean value; 2 SDs encompass 96%, and 3 SDs encompass 99% of the measurements from a normal population. Even with 3 SDs, 1 normal person in 100 has a value outside the normal range. Therefore an abnormal result may not indicate the presence of a disease. It is also important to know the characteristics of the normal population used to standardize a laboratory test. Ranges that were normalized using adults are almost never correct for newborns and children. Ranges normalized using a hospitalized population may not be accurate for ambulatory people.

An abnormal test result may not be caused by the disorder under investigation. For example, an elevated serum creatine kinase (CK) concentration can result from recent exercise, electromyography (EMG), intramuscular injection, liver disease, or myocardial infarction (MI) as well as from a primary muscle disease. A common problematic finding for pediatric neurologists is centrotemporal spikes on the electroencephalogram (EEG) of a child with headache or a learning disability who has never had a seizure. The EEG should not have been ordered in the first place, and to give such a patient antiepileptic drugs would compound poor judgment in diagnosis with worse judgment in management.

The neurologist should personally review the results of all tests that are ordered. In most instances, the actual imaging studies should be reviewed in addition to the report, and, when appropriate, the neuroradiologist should participate. Similarly, for neurologists experienced in pathology, biopsy findings may be reviewed with the neuropathologist. The neurologist who knows the patient may be of great help in interpreting imaging or pathological studies.

## RISK, COST, AND PRIORITIZATION OF INVESTIGATIONS

If two different tests provide equivalent information, the physician should choose the one that causes less pain and risk to the patient. The costs of the two tests should also be considered. The diagnostic capability of two tests may not be identical, and the more expensive test may not be better. The cost of a test must be considered in the context of the total cost of the illness. An expensive test that shortens a hospital stay may be cost-effective. Where only limited funding is available for health care, the money must be used to purchase the most cost-effective care for the greatest number of people. Clearly, physicians should acquaint themselves with the costs of the tests they order and practice cost-effective medicine.

The selection of ancillary tests and the sequence in which they are performed are important components of good medical practice. The order in which tests are requested depends on their diagnostic specificity, sensitivity, availability, cost, and invasiveness.

Sometimes a therapeutic trial is used as an investigation. Time may also be used as an investigation. For example, a patient on a statin medication who experiences gradual-onset muscle weakness and myalgias would be better served by stopping the drug and observing whether the muscle symptoms resolve rather than immediately performing a muscle biopsy.

## RELIABILITY OF INVESTIGATIONS

When a new test is developed, its sensitivity (the frequency with which the test is abnormal in patients with the particular disease) and specificity (the frequency with which the test is abnormal in people without the particular disease) must be determined. If a test is very sensitive but has poor specificity, it may not be useful for diagnosis. For instance, the ESR is very sensitive in giant cell arteritis, but it is elevated in so many other conditions that it cannot be used to diagnose the condition. Of more use is a test that is highly specific even if it has a lower sensitivity. An acetylcholine receptor antibody titer is abnormal in only about 50% of patients with ocular myasthenia gravis, for example, but it is very rarely abnormal in normal people or those with other conditions. The specificity and sensitivity can be useful to quantitate the extent to which a test result makes a diagnosis of the disease more or less likely.

## DECISION ANALYSIS

Diagnostic acumen and treatment success are the hallmarks of the experienced neurologist. This acumen can be taught and can be learned from years of practice. Decision analysis is a method developed to provide insight into the processes of diagnosis and management of a complex disease when sufficient data are unavailable. This method can help to identify areas of uncertainty in currently accepted diagnostic and management methods. Decision analysis forces the clinician to make quantitative estimates of each of the many factors entering into a clinical decision and to calculate the risk/benefit ratio of each management decision. Decision analysis is an excellent teaching tool. Because crucial quantitative data are often not easily available, this necessitates a search for such data, either from the literature or through new research.

## RESEARCH INVESTIGATIONS AND TEACHING HOSPITALS

Because many of our readers are neurologists in training, here we briefly mention the use of investigations in teaching and research centers. Clinical research is closely regulated in most parts of the world, and research investigations cannot be performed until the protocol is approved by an institutional review board or an ethics-in-research committee. The peer review process is designed to ensure that the risks of the research study are justified, taking into account the patient's particular disease and the likely benefits of the research. The institutional review board ensures that the patient receives the full information contained in an informed consent form and understands the risks of the study and what is likely to be learned from the research. Special policies and procedures also apply to minors, patients with cognitive dysfunction, those in emergency situations, or those with alterations in consciousness. No patient should be coerced, knowingly or unknowingly, into participating in a research procedure. Once the institutional review board has given permission for a research project, it continues to monitor the study to ensure that the research conforms to the protocol.

In a teaching hospital, the attending or consultant physician is legally and ethically responsible for the care provided to a patient by physicians in training. The attending neurologist must ensure that every investigation is justified for diagnostic and management purposes. All physicians are legally and ethically bound to make sure that the patient understands the reason for each investigation and gives informed consent. The neurologist in training must learn to use tests judiciously and not to perform tests simply for curiosity or education. The two-way discussion with more senior neurologists about the rationale, risk/benefit ratio, and cost/benefit ratio of each investigation is an important part of the learning process.

## PATIENT CONFIDENTIALITY

Some diagnostic tests, such as the DNA genetic test for Huntington disease, necessitate prior counseling about the implications of the tests for possibly affected persons and their families. Physicians and their staff in the United States must comply with the Health Insurance Portability and Accountability Act of 1996 (http://www.hhs.gov/ocr/privacy).

## THE ROLE OF ANCILLARY TESTS IN NEUROLOGICAL DISEASE MANAGEMENT

The standard neurological examination is designed more to detect abnormal function for diagnostic purposes than to quantify the neurological abnormalities. When possible, therefore, ancillary investigations are used to measure the disease's response to treatment. These investigations may be quantitative and therefore can be helpful in managing progression. Quantitative tools provide important information for measuring a patient's status objectively during the course of a disease. Generally, abnormal laboratory values return toward normal as a disease resolves or become increasingly abnormal as it worsens. Vital capacity in a patient with Guillain-Barré syndrome is an example of a measurement that improves as the disease improves. This is not always the case, however. In Duchenne muscular dystrophy, the serum CK concentration decreases as the disease worsens because fewer muscle fibers remain to release enzyme into the serum. In myasthenia gravis, the patient's condition can go from minimal weakness to total paralysis unrelated to the titers of acetylcholine receptor antibodies in the blood. Therefore laboratory values cannot always be used as indices of disease severity or response to treatment. Other limitations on the use of ancillary tests to monitor disease progression include sampling errors and test sensitivity and specificity. However, as compared with the routine neurological examination, quantitative measures of neurological function enable a much better assessment of a disease's response to treatment.

# 35

# Electroencephalography and Evoked Potentials

*Cecil D. Hahn, Ronald G. Emerson*

## OUTLINE



The techniques of applied electrophysiology are of practical importance in diagnosing and managing certain categories of neurological disease. Modern instrumentation permits the selective investigation of the functional aspects of the central and peripheral nervous systems. The electroencephalogram (EEG) and evoked potentials are measures of electrical activity generated by the central nervous system (CNS). Despite the introduction of positron emission tomography (PET), functional magnetic resonance imaging (fMRI), and magnetoencephalography (MEG), electroencephalography and evoked potential studies are currently the only readily available laboratory tests of brain physiology. As such, they are generally complementary to anatomical imaging techniques such as computed tomography (CT) or MRI, especially when it is desirable to document abnormalities that are not associated with detectable structural alterations in brain tissue. Furthermore, EEG provides the only continuous measure of cerebral function over time.

This chapter is not intended as a comprehensive account of all aspects of EEG and evoked potentials. Rather, the intent is to provide clinicians with an appreciation of the scope and limitations of these investigations as currently used.

## ELECTROENCEPHALOGRAPHY

### Physiological Principles of Electroencephalography

The cerebral cortex generates EEG signals. Spontaneous EEG activity reflects the flow of extracellular space currents generated by the summation of excitatory and inhibitory synaptic potentials occurring on thousands or even millions of cortical neurons. Individual action potentials do not contribute directly to EEG activity. A conventional EEG recording is a continuous graph, over time, of the spatial distribution of changing voltage fields at the scalp surface that result from ongoing synaptic activity in the underlying cortex.

EEG rhythms appear to be part of a complex hierarchy of cortical oscillations that are fundamental to the brain's information processing mechanisms, including input selection and transient "binding" of distributed neuronal assemblies (Buzsaki and Draguhn, 2004). In addition to reflecting the spontaneous intrinsic activities of cortical neurons, the EEG depends on important afferent inputs from subcortical structures including the thalamus and brainstem reticular formation. Thalamic afferents, for example, are probably responsible for entraining cortical neurons to produce the rhythmic oscillations that characterize normal patterns like alpha rhythm and sleep spindles. An EEG abnormality may occur directly from disruption of cortical neural networks or indirectly from modification of subcortical inputs onto cortical neurons.

A scalp-recorded EEG represents only a limited, low-resolution view of the electrical activity of the brain. This is due in part to the pronounced voltage attenuation and "blurring" that occurs from overlying cerebrospinal fluid (CSF) and tissue layers. Relatively large areas of cortex have to be involved in similar synchronized activity for a discharge to appear on the scalp EEG. For example, recordings obtained from arrays of microelectrodes penetrating into the cerebral cortex reveal a complex architecture of seizure initiation and propagation invisible to recordings from the scalp or even the cortical surface, with seizure-like discharges occurring in areas as small as a single cortical column (Schevon et al., 2008). Furthermore, potentials involving surfaces of gyri are more readily recorded than potentials arising in the walls and depths of sulci. Activity generated over the lateral convexities of the hemispheres records more accurately than does activity coming from interhemispherical, mesial, or basal areas. In the case of epileptiform activity, estimates are that 20%–70% of cortical spikes do not appear on the EEG, depending on the region of cortex involved. Additionally, although the scalp-recorded EEG consists almost entirely of signals slower than approximately 40 Hz, intracranial oscillations of several hundred hertz may be recorded and, of clinical importance, have been associated with both normal physiological processes and seizure initiation (Schevon et al., 2009).

Such considerations limit the usefulness of the EEG. First, surface recordings are not useful for unambiguously determining the nature of synaptic events contributing to a particular EEG wave. Second, the EEG is rarely specific as to cause because different diseases and conditions produce similar EEG changes. In this regard, the EEG is analogous to findings on the neurological examination—hemiplegia caused by a stroke cannot be distinguished from that caused by a brain tumor. Third, many potentials occurring at the brain surface involve such a small area or are of such low voltage that they cannot be detected at the scalp. The EEG results may then be normal despite clear indications from other data of focal brain dysfunction. Finally, abnormalities in brain areas inaccessible to EEG recording electrodes (some cortical areas and virtually all subcortical and brainstem regions) do not affect the EEG directly but may exert remote effects on patterns of cortical activity.

## Normal Electroencephalographic Activities

Spontaneous fluctuations of voltage potential at the cortical surface are in the range of 100–1000 mV, but at the scalp are only 10–100 mV. Different parts of the cortex generate relatively distinct potential fluctuations, which also differ in the waking and sleep states.

In most normal adults and children aged 3 years and older, the waking pattern of EEG activity consists mainly of sinusoidal oscillations occurring at 8–12 Hz, which are most prominent over the occipital area—the alpha rhythm (Fig. 35.1, *A*). Eye opening, mental activity, and drowsiness attenuate (block) the alpha rhythm. Activity faster than 12 Hz beta activity is normally present over the frontal areas and may be especially prominent in patients receiving barbiturate or benzodiazepine drugs. Activity slower than 8 Hz is divisible into delta activity (1–3 Hz) and theta activity (4–7 Hz). Adults may normally show a small amount of theta activity over the temporal regions; the percentage of intermixed theta frequencies increases after the age of 60 years. Delta activity is not normally present in adults when they are awake but appears when they fall asleep (see Fig. 35.1, *B*). The amount and amplitude of slow activity (theta and delta) correlate closely with the depth of sleep. Slow frequencies are abundant in the EEGs of newborns and young children, but these disappear progressively with maturation. A posterior dominant rhythm in the theta frequency range is apparent from about 3 months of age, which gradually increases in frequency to reach at least 8 Hz by 3 years.

An EEG undergoes characteristic changes during sleep. During stage I sleep, or drowsiness, the alpha rhythm becomes less regular, may slow slightly, and then disappears; theta activity becomes more prominent. During stage II sleep, sleep spindles, brief (1- to 2-second) runs of 12- to 14-Hz rhythmic waves, are seen synchronously over the central head regions. Vertex sharp waves are seen during stage II sleep and may also be present during stage I. With slow-wave sleep, diffuse delta activity dominates the EEG. During rapid-eye-movement (REM) sleep, which is associated with dreaming, the EEG demonstrates a low-voltage mixed-frequency pattern.

## Common Types of Electroencephalographic Abnormalities

### Focal Polymorphic Slow Activity

Polymorphic slow activity is irregular activity in the delta (1–4 Hz) or theta (4–7 Hz) range, which, when continuous, has a strong correlation with a localized cerebral lesion such as infarction, hemorrhage, tumor, or abscess. Intermittent focal slow activity may also indicate localized parenchymal dysfunction but is less predictive than continuous polymorphic slow activity.

### Generalized Polymorphic Slow Activity

Diffuse disturbances in background rhythms marked by excessive slow activity and disorganization of waking EEG patterns arise in encephalopathies of metabolic, toxic, or infectious origin and with brain damage caused by a static encephalopathy.

### Intermittent Monomorphic Slow Activity

Paroxysmal bursts of generalized bisynchronous rhythmic theta or delta waves usually indicate thalamocortical dysfunction and may be seen with metabolic or toxic disorders, obstructive hydrocephalus, deep midline or posterior fossa lesions, and also as a nonspecific functional disturbance in patients with generalized epilepsy. Focal bursts of rhythmic waves lateralized to one hemisphere usually indicate deep (typically thalamic or periventricular) abnormalities, often of a structural nature.

### Voltage Attenuation

Cortical disease causes voltage attenuation. Generalized voltage attenuation is usually associated with diffuse depression of function such as after anoxia or with certain degenerative diseases (e.g., Huntington disease). The most severe form of generalized voltage attenuation is electrocerebral inactivity, which is corroborative evidence of brain death in the appropriate clinical setting. Focal voltage attenuation reliably indicates localized cortical disease such as porencephaly, atrophy, or contusion, or an extra-axial lesion such as a meningioma or subdural hematoma.

### Epileptiform Discharges

Epileptiform discharges are spikes or sharp waves that occur interictally (between seizures) in patients with epilepsy and sometimes in persons who do not experience seizures but have a genetic predisposition to epilepsy. Epileptiform discharges may be focal or generalized, depending on the seizure type.

## Recording Techniques

The EEG recording methods in common use are summarized in the following discussion. Details can be found in guidelines of the American Clinical Neurophysiology Society, (2014).

A series of small gold, silver, or silver–silver chloride disks is symmetrically positioned over the scalp on both sides of the head in standard locations (the International 10–20 system). In practice, 20 or more channels of EEG activity are recorded simultaneously, each channel displaying the potential difference between two electrodes. Electrode pairs are interconnected in different arrangements called *montages* to permit a comprehensive survey of the brain's electrical activity. Typically, the design of montages is to compare symmetrical areas of the two hemispheres—anterior versus posterior regions or parasagittal versus temporal areas in the same hemisphere.

A typical study is about 30 to 45 minutes in duration and includes two types of "activating procedures": hyperventilation and photic stimulation. In some patients, these techniques provoke abnormal focal or generalized alterations in activity that are of diagnostic importance and would otherwise go undetected (Fig. 35.2). Recording during sleep and after sleep deprivation and placement of additional electrodes at other recording sites are useful in detecting specific kinds of epileptiform potentials. The use of other maneuvers depends on the clinical question posed. For example, epileptiform activity may occasionally activate only by movement or specific sensory stimuli. Vasovagal stimulation may be important in some types of syncope.

In the past, EEG recording instruments were simple analog devices with banks of amplifiers and pen writers. In contrast, modern EEG machines make use of digital processing and storage, and the electroencephalographer interprets the EEG from a computer display rather than from paper. Technological advances have not fundamentally changed the principles of EEG interpretation, but they have facilitated EEG reading. Early paper-based EEG systems

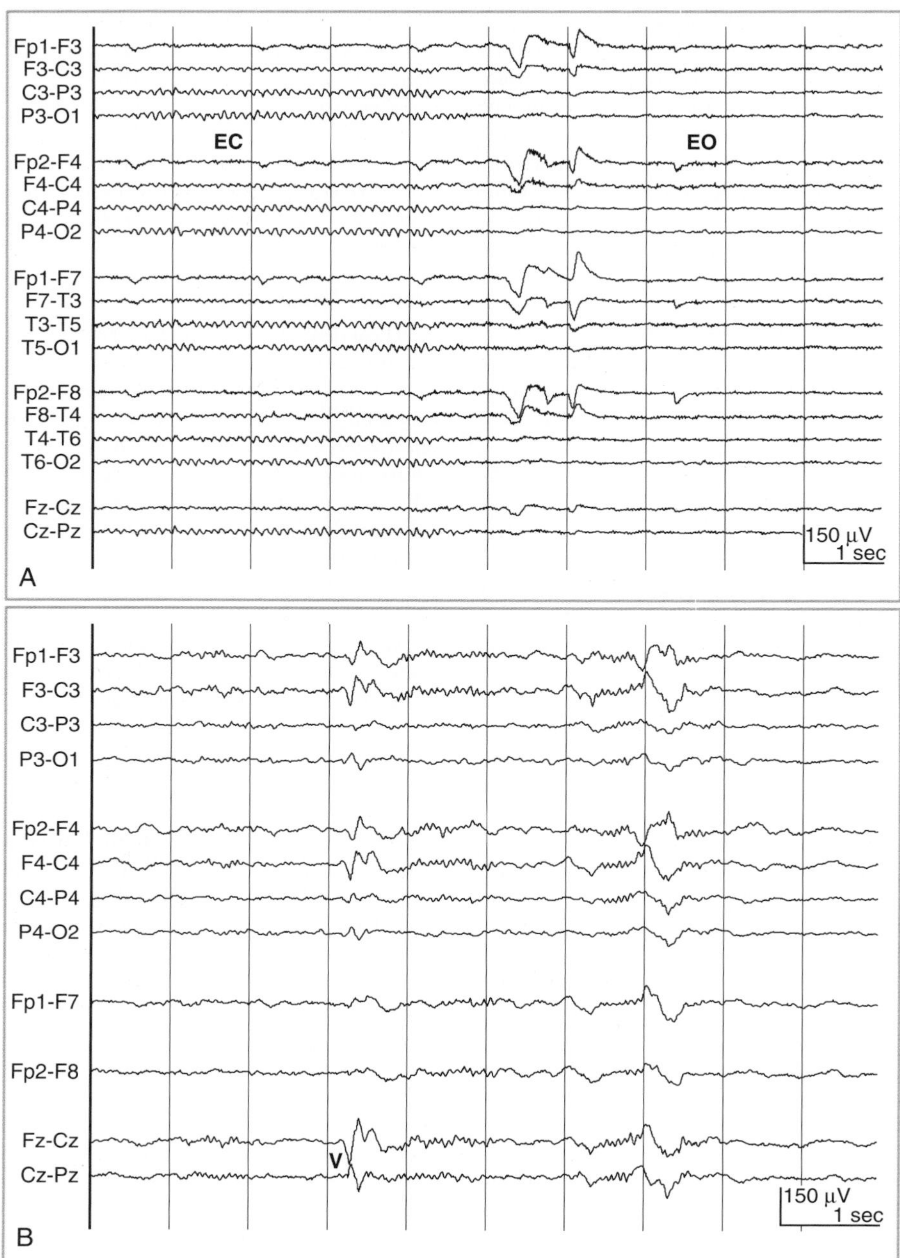


**Fig. 35.1 Samples of Normal Electroencephalographic Recordings from Two Patients. A,** Waking activity is characterized by a 9-Hz alpha rhythm that attenuates when the eyes are opened *(EO)* and resumes when the eyes are closed *(EC)*. **B,** Stage 2 sleep is characterized by 2- to 5-Hz background activity, on which are superimposed vertex *(V)* waves and sleep spindles.

required that all recording parameters—display gain, filter settings, and the manner in which scalp-recorded signals were combined and displayed (montages)—be fixed by the technologist at the time of recording. In contrast, digital EEG systems permit the electroencephalographer to adjust these settings at the time of interpretation. A given EEG waveform or pattern can be examined using a number of different instrument settings, including sophisticated montages (e.g., common average reference, Laplacian reference) that were unavailable using traditional analog recording systems. Although this flexibility does not change the interpretive strategies used to read an EEG, it does allow the electroencephalographer to apply them more effectively.

In addition to facilitating the standard interpretation of EEGs, mathematical techniques can also be used to reveal features that may not be apparent to visual inspection of raw EEG waveforms. For example, averaging techniques, useful in improving the signal-to-noise ratios of spikes and sharp waves, can reveal field distributions and timing relationships that are not otherwise appreciable. Dipole source localization methods have been used to characterize both interictal spikes and ictal discharges in patients with epilepsy and may contribute to localization of the seizure focus (Ebersole, 2000). Such methods are based on a number of critical assumptions that, if applied without recognition of their limitations, can result in anatomically and physiologically erroneous conclusions (Emerson et al., 1995). Therefore caution is warranted in their use.

For patients undergoing long-term EEG recordings as part of the diagnosis or management of epilepsy, a time-locked digital video image of the patient is recorded simultaneously with the EEG. EEG data are often processed by software that can automatically detect most seizure activity. Similar systems are finding increased use in intensive care units (ICUs), where EEG monitoring has become increasingly important in the management of patients with nonconvulsive seizure (NCS) activity, threatened or impending cerebral ischemia, severe head trauma, and metabolic coma (Drislane et al., 2008; Friedman et al., 2009).

## Clinical Uses of Electroencephalography

The EEG assesses physiological alterations in brain activity. Many changes are nonspecific, but some are highly suggestive of specific entities (epilepsy, herpes encephalitis, metabolic encephalopathy). The EEG is also useful in following the course of patients with altered states of consciousness and may, in certain circumstances, provide prognostic information. EEG can be used as an ancillary test in the determination of brain death.

EEG is not a screening test. It serves to answer a particular question posed by the patient's condition; therefore the provision of sufficient clinical information helps in designing an appropriate test with meaningful clinical correlation. The request for this study should specifically state the question addressed by the EEG.

EEG interpretation should be based on a systematic analysis using consistent parameters that permit comparisons with findings expected from the patient's age and circumstances of recording. Accurate interpretation requires high-quality recording. This depends on trained technologists who understand the importance of meticulous electrode application, proper use of instrument controls, recognition and (where possible) elimination of artifacts, and appropriate selection of recording montages to allow optimal display of cerebral electrical activity.

### Epilepsy

The EEG is usually the most helpful laboratory test when a diagnosis of epilepsy is being considered. Because the onset of seizures is unpredictable, and their occurrence is relatively infrequent in most patients, EEG recordings are usually obtained when the patient is not having a seizure (interictal recordings). Fortunately, electrical abnormalities in the EEG occur in most patients with epilepsy even between attacks.

The only EEG finding that has a strong correlation with epilepsy is *epileptiform activity*, a term used to describe spikes and sharp waves that are clearly distinct from ongoing background activity. Clinical and experimental evidence supports a specific association between epileptiform discharges and seizure susceptibility. Only about 2% of patients without epilepsy have epileptiform discharges on EEG, whereas as many as 90% of patients with epilepsy demonstrate epileptiform discharges, depending on the circumstances of the recording and the number of studies obtained.

Nonetheless, interpretation of interictal findings always requires caution. There is poor correlation between most epileptiform discharges and the frequency and likelihood of recurrence of epileptic seizures (Selvitelli et al., 2010). Furthermore, a substantial number of patients with unquestionable epilepsy have consistently normal interictal EEGs. The most convincing proof that a patient's episodic symptoms are epileptic is obtained by recording an electrographic seizure discharge during a typical behavioral attack.

Videos showing actual EEG recordings obtained during seizures (Videos 35.1–35.3) are available at http://www.expertconsult.com.

In addition to epileptiform patterns, EEGs in patients with epilepsy often show excessive focal or generalized slow-wave activity. Less often, asymmetries of frequency or voltage may be noted. These findings are not unique to epilepsy and are present in other conditions such as static encephalopathies, brain tumors, migraine, and trauma.

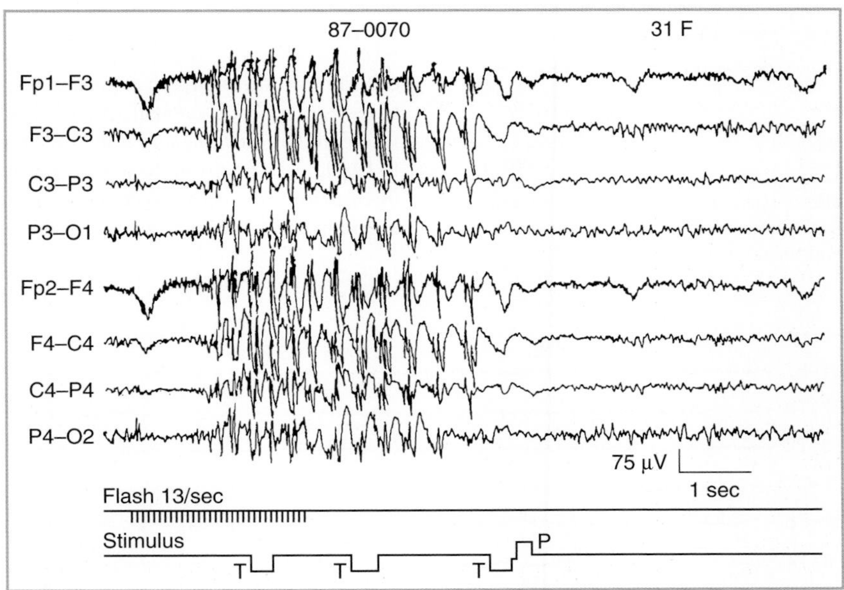


**Fig. 35.2** Intermittent stroboscopic light stimulation at 13 flashes per second elicited generalized bursts of 4- to 5-Hz spike-wave activity, termed a *photoparoxysmal* (photoconvulsive) *response*. The spike-wave paroxysm was associated with a brief absence, as documented by the patient's *(P)* inability to respond to a tone given by the technologist *(T)*. Normal responsiveness returned immediately on cessation of the spike-wave activity. The remainder of the electroencephalogram was normal.

In patients with unusual spells, nonspecific changes on EEG should be weighed cautiously and are not to be considered direct evidence for a diagnosis of epilepsy. On the other hand, when clinical data are unequivocal or when epileptiform discharges occur as well, the degree and extent of background EEG changes may provide information that is important for judging the likelihood of an underlying focal cerebral lesion, a more diffuse encephalopathy, or a progressive neurological syndrome. Additionally, EEG findings may help determine prognosis and aid in the decision to discontinue antiepileptic medication.

The type of epileptiform activity on EEG is helpful in classifying a patient's epilepsy correctly and sometimes in identifying a specific epilepsy syndrome (see Chapter 100). Clinically, generalized tonic-clonic seizures may be generalized from the onset (primary generalized seizures) or may begin focally and then spread to become generalized (secondary generalized seizures). Impairment of consciousness, with or without automatisms, may be a manifestation of either a generalized nonconvulsive epilepsy (e.g., absence seizures) or a focal epilepsy (e.g., temporal lobe epilepsy). The initial clinical features of a seizure may be uncertain because of postictal amnesia or nocturnal occurrence. In these and similar situations, the EEG can provide information crucial to the correct diagnosis and appropriate therapy.

In generalized seizures, the EEG typically shows bilateral synchronous diffuse bursts of spikes and spike-and-wave discharges (Fig. 35.3). All generalized EEG epileptiform patterns share certain common features, although the exact expression of the spike-wave activity varies depending on whether the patient has pure absence, tonic-clonic, myoclonic, or atonic-astatic seizures. The EEG also may help to distinguish between idiopathic and symptomatic generalized epilepsy. In idiopathic generalized epilepsy, no cerebral disease is demonstrable and EEG background rhythms are normal or near normal. In symptomatic generalized epilepsy, evidence can be found for diffuse brain damage and the EEG typically demonstrates some degree of generalized slow-wave activity.

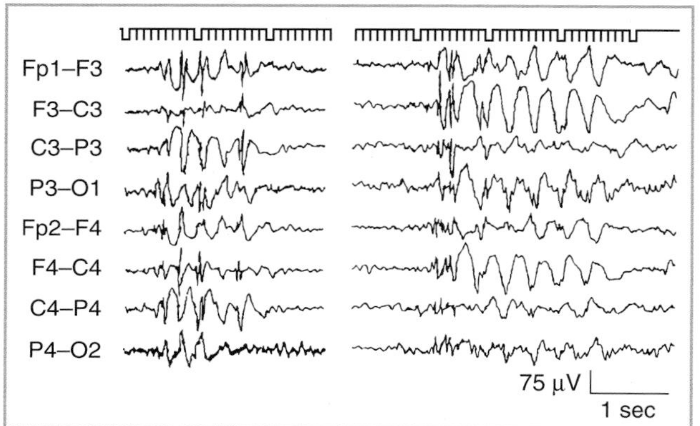


**Fig. 35.3** Example of generalized spike-wave patterns with primary generalized (idiopathic) epilepsy. The patient had mainly tonic-clonic seizures with occasional absence attacks.

Consistently focal epileptiform activity is the signature of focal-onset (partial) epilepsy (Fig. 35.4). With the exception of the benign focal epilepsies of childhood, focal epileptiform activity results from neuronal dysfunction caused by demonstrable brain disease. A reasonable correlation exists between spike location and the type of ictal behavior. Anterior temporal spikes are usually associated with complex partial seizures, rolandic spikes with simple motor or sensory seizures, and occipital spikes with primitive visual hallucinations or diminished visual function as an initial feature.

In addition to distinguishing epileptiform from nonepileptiform abnormalities, EEG analysis sometimes permits the identification of specific epilepsy syndromes. Such electroclinical syndromes include hypsarrhythmia associated with infantile spasms (West syndrome; Fig. 35.5); 3-Hz spike-and-wave activity associated with typical absence attacks (childhood or juvenile absence epilepsy; Fig. 35.6); generalized multiple spikes and waves (polyspike-wave pattern) associated with myoclonic epilepsy, including so-called juvenile myoclonic epilepsy of Janz (Fig. 35.7); generalized sharp and slow waves (slow spike-and-wave pattern) associated with Lennox-Gastaut syndrome (Fig. 35.8); and central-midtemporal spikes associated with benign rolandic epilepsy (Fig. 35.9).

The increased availability of special monitoring facilities for simultaneous video and EEG recording and of ambulatory EEG recorders has improved diagnostic accuracy and the reliability of seizure classification. Prolonged continuous recordings through one or more complete sleep/wake cycles constitute the best way to document ictal episodes and should be considered in patients whose interictal EEGs are normal or nondiagnostic and in clinical dilemmas that are resolvable only by recording actual behavioral events. Although EEG documentation of an ictal discharge establishes the epileptic nature of a corresponding behavioral change, the converse is not necessarily true. Sometimes muscle or movement artifacts so obscure the EEG recording that it is impossible to know whether any EEG change has occurred. In these circumstances, postictal slowing is usually indicative of an epileptic event if similar slow waves are not present elsewhere in the recording and if the EEG recording subsequently returns to baseline. In addition, focal seizures not accompanied by alteration in consciousness occasionally have no detectable scalp correlate. On the other hand, the persistence of alpha activity and absence of slowing

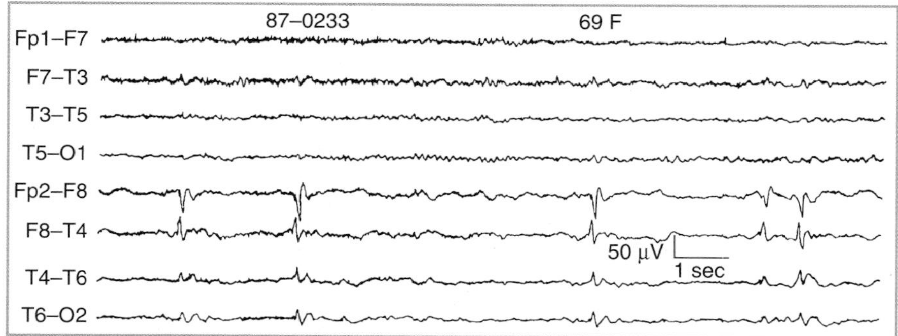


**Fig. 35.4** Focal right anterior temporal spikes occurring on the electroencephalogram of a 69-year-old woman with complex partial seizures after a stroke involving branches of the right middle cerebral artery.

during and after an apparent convulsive episode are inconsistent with an epileptic generalized tonic-clonic seizure.

## Focal Cerebral Lesions

The use of EEG to detect focal cerebral disturbances has declined because of the development and widespread availability of modern neuroimaging techniques. Nonetheless, the EEG has a role in documenting focal physiological dysfunction in the absence of discernible structural pathology and in evaluating the functional disturbance produced by known lesions.

Focal slow-wave activity (delta, theta) is the usual EEG sign of a focal disturbance. A structural lesion is likely if the slowing is (1) present continuously; (2) shows variability in waveform, amplitude, duration, and morphology (so-called arrhythmic or polymorphic activity); and (3) persists during changes in wake/sleep states (Fig. 35.10, *A* and *B*). The localizing value of focal slowing increases when it is topographically discrete or associated with depression or loss of superimposed faster background frequencies. The character and distribution of the EEG changes caused by a focal lesion depend on the lesion's size, its distance from the cortical surface, the specific structures involved, and its acuity. Superficial lesions tend to produce more focal EEG changes, whereas deep cerebral lesions produce hemispheric or even bilateral slowing. For example, a small stroke located in the thalamus may produce widespread hemispheric slowing and alteration in sleep spindles and alpha rhythm regulation, whereas a lesion of the same size located at the cortical surface may produce few if any EEG findings.

Bilateral paroxysmal bursts of rhythmic delta waves (Fig. 35.11) with frontal predominance—once attributed to subfrontal, deep midline, or posterior fossa lesions—are actually nonspecific and seen more often with diffuse encephalopathies. Focal or lateralized intermittent bursts of rhythmic delta waves as the prominent EEG abnormality suggest a deep supratentorial (periventricular or diencephalic) lesion.

Single lacunae usually produce little or no change in the EEG. Similarly, transient ischemic attacks not associated with chronic cerebral hypoperfusion or imminent occlusion of a major vessel do not significantly affect the EEG outside the symptomatic period. Superficial cortical or large, deep hemispheric infarctions are usually associated with localized EEG abnormalities.

EEG is generally not indicated for the diagnosis of headache. That being said, focal EEG changes (and other nonepileptiform abnormalities) may be seen during migraine. The likelihood of an abnormal EEG

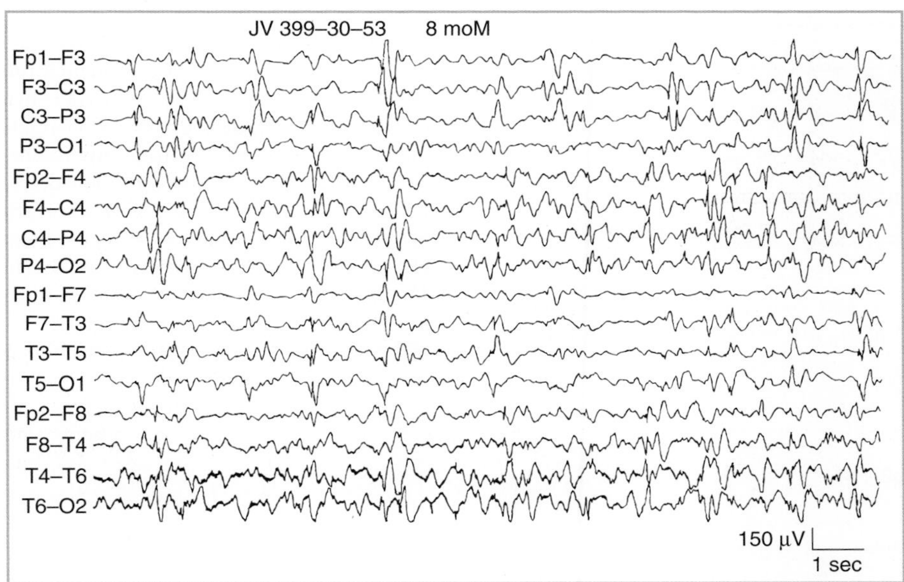


**Fig. 35.5** Electroencephalographic pattern, termed *hypsarrhythmia*, in a recording obtained in an 8-month-old boy with infantile spasms. Background activity is high-voltage and unorganized, with abundant multifocal spikes.

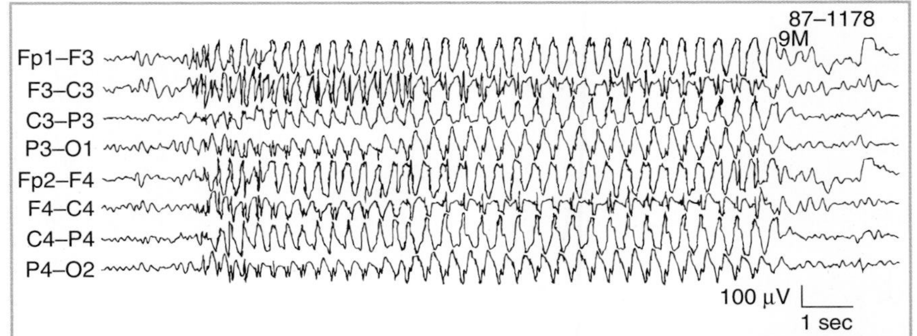


**Fig. 35.6** A 3-Hz spike-and-wave paroxysm on the electroencephalogram of a 9-year-old boy with absence seizures (petit mal epilepsy). During this 12-second discharge, the child was unresponsive and demonstrated rhythmic eye blinking.

and the severity of the abnormality relate to the timing and character of the migraine attack. EEGs are more likely to be focally abnormal with complicated rather than common migraine and during rather than between headaches.

EEG changes seen with brain tumors are caused by disturbances in bordering brain parenchyma, as most tumor tissue is electrically silent. Focal EEG changes are caused by interference with patterns of normal neuronal synaptic activity; by destruction or alteration of the cortical neurons; and by metabolic effects caused by changes in blood flow, cellular metabolism, or the neuronal environment. Diffuse EEG changes are the consequence of increased intracranial pressure, shift of midline structures, or hydrocephalus. EEG is especially helpful in following the extent of cerebral dysfunction over time; in distinguishing between direct effects of the neoplasm and superimposed metabolic or toxic encephalopathies; and in differentiating among epileptic, ischemic, and noncerebral causes for episodic symptoms.

The role of EEG in the management of patients with head injuries is limited. Transient generalized slowing is common after concussion. A persistent area of continuous localized slow-wave activity suggests cerebral contusion even in the absence of a focal clinical or CT abnormality, and unilateral voltage depression suggests subdural hematoma. EEG performed in the first 3 months after injury does not predict posttraumatic epilepsy.

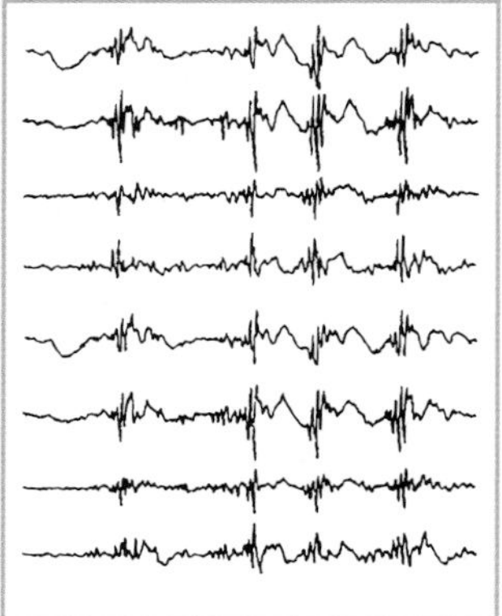

**Fig. 35.7** Example of generalized spike-wave patterns with primary generalized (idiopathic) epilepsy. The patient had juvenile myoclonic epilepsy.

### Altered States of Consciousness

The EEG has a major role in evaluating patients with altered levels of consciousness. Because EEG permits a reasonable assessment of supratentorial brain function, it complements the clinical examination in patients with significant depression of consciousness. Abnormalities are typically nonspecific with regard to etiology. In general, however, correlation with the clinical state is good. Some findings are more suggestive of particular causes than of others and are occasionally prognostically useful as well. Specific questions the EEG may help to answer (depending on the clinical presentation) are the following:

- Are psychogenic factors playing a major role?
- Is the process diffuse, focal, or multifocal?
- Is depressed consciousness due to unrecognized epileptic activity (nonconvulsive status epilepticus)?
- What evidence, if any, points to improvement, despite relatively little change in the clinical picture?
- What findings, if any, assist in assessing prognosis?

### Metabolic Encephalopathies

Metabolic derangements affecting the brain diffusely are among the most common causes of altered mental function in a general hospital. Generalized slow-wave activity is the main indication of decreased consciousness. The degree of EEG slowing closely parallels the patient's mental status and ranges from only minor slowing of alpha-rhythm frequency (slight inattentiveness and decreased alertness) to continuous delta activity (coma). Slow-wave activity sometimes becomes bisynchronous and assumes a high-voltage, sharply contoured triphasic morphology, especially over the frontal head regions (Fig. 35.12). These generalized periodic discharges (PDs) with triphasic morphology, originally considered diagnostic of hepatic failure, occur with equal frequency in other metabolic disorders, such as uremia,

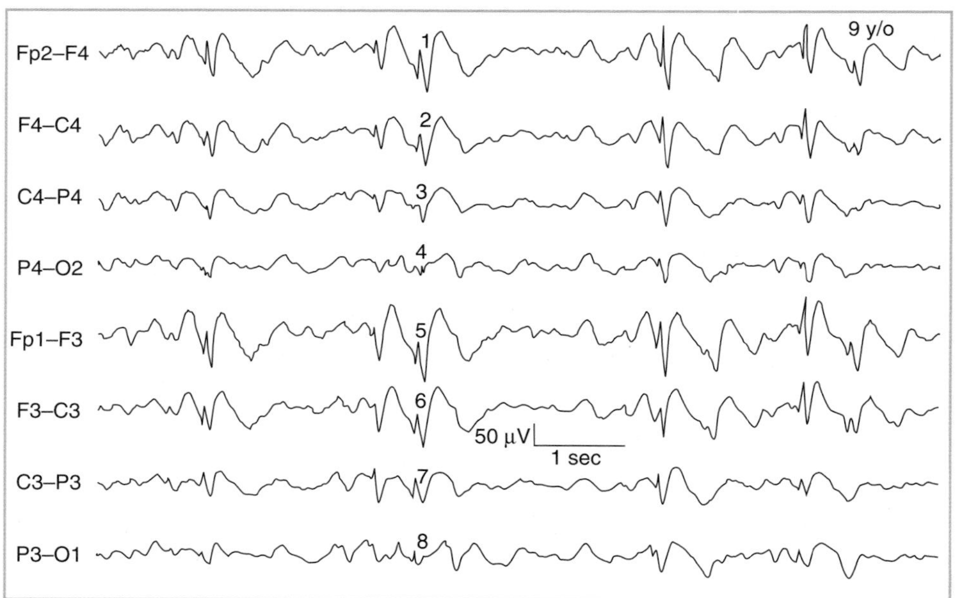


**Fig. 35.8** Generalized sharp- and slow-wave discharges on the electroencephalogram (EEG) of a 9-year-old child with intellectual disability and uncontrolled typical absence, tonic, and atonic generalized seizures. This constellation of clinical and EEG features constitutes the Lennox-Gastaut syndrome.

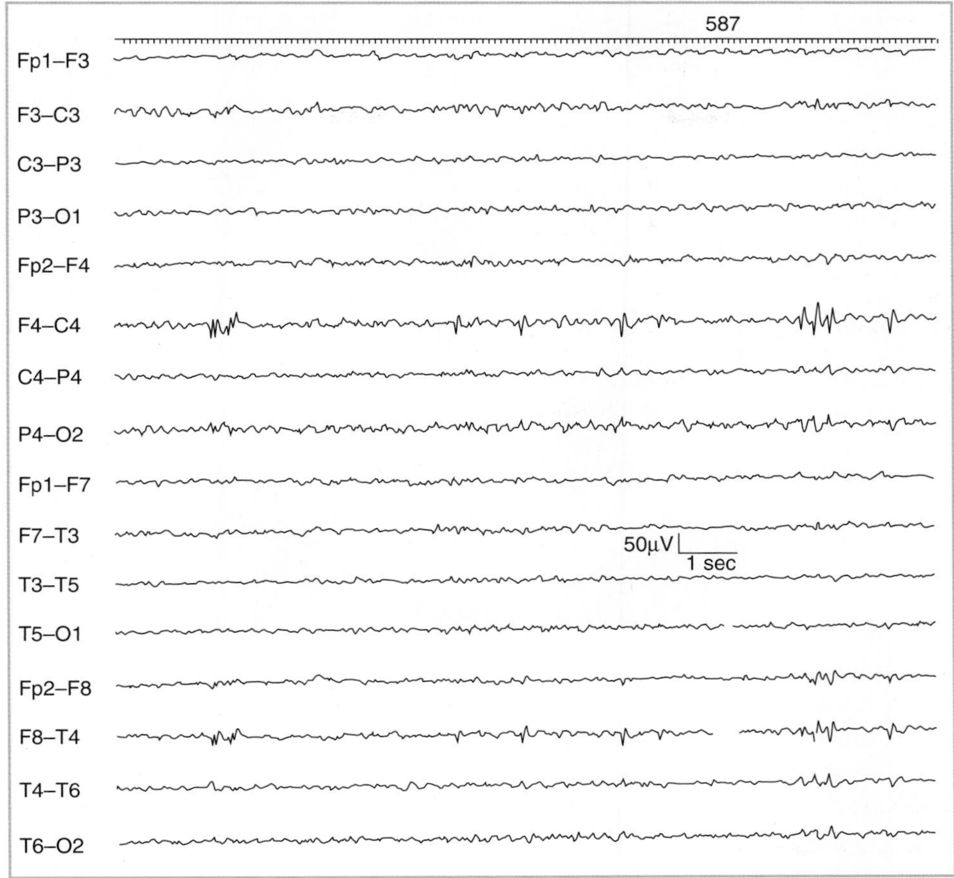


**Fig. 35.9** Electroencephalogram obtained during drowsiness in a 10-year-old boy with benign rolandic epilepsy. Stereotypical diphasic or triphasic sharp waves occur in the right central-parietal and midtemporal regions.

hyponatremia, hyperthyroidism, anoxia, and hyperosmolarity. The value of these so-called triphasic waves is that they suggest a metabolic cause in an unresponsive patient (Hirsch et al., 2013).

Some EEG features increase the likelihood of a specific metabolic disorder. Prominent generalized rhythmic beta activity raises the suspicion of drug intoxication in a comatose patient. Severe generalized voltage depression indicates impaired energy metabolism and suggests hypothyroidism if anoxia and hypothermia can be excluded. A photoconvulsive response is seen more often with uremia than with other causes of metabolic encephalopathy. Focal seizure activity is common in patients with hyperosmolar coma.

## Hypoxia

Hypoxia, with or without circulatory arrest, produces a wide range of EEG abnormalities depending on the severity and reversibility of the brain damage. EEGs obtained 6 hours or more after the hypoxic insult may show patterns that have prognostic value (see Chapter 5). Sequential EEGs strengthen the validity of such findings. EEG abnormalities associated with poor neurological outcome include alpha coma, burst suppression, and periodic patterns.

The term *alpha coma* refers to the apparent paradoxical appearance of monorhythmic alpha-frequency activity in the EEG of a comatose patient; the EEG recording may appear normal to the inexperienced observer (Fig. 35.13). In contrast to normal alpha activity, that seen with alpha coma is generalized, often maximal frontally, and unreactive to external stimuli.

The *burst suppression pattern* consists of occasional generalized bursts of medium- to high-voltage mixed-frequency slow-wave activity, sometimes with intermixed spikes, with intervening periods of severe voltage depression or cerebral inactivity (Fig. 35.14).

The *periodic pattern* consists of generalized spikes or sharp waves that recur with a relatively fixed interval, typically one or two per second (Fig. 35.15). Sometimes the periodic sharp waves occur independently over each hemisphere. Myoclonic jerks of the limbs or whole body usually accompany a postanoxic periodic pattern (Hirsch et al., 2013).

The prognostic value of these patterns relates exclusively to the cause. Similar features are recognized with potentially reversible causes of coma, including deep anesthesia, drug overdose, and severe liver or kidney failure.

## Infectious Diseases

Of all infectious diseases affecting the brain, herpes simplex encephalitis is the one for which EEG is most useful in initial assessment. Early and accurate diagnosis is important because the response to acyclovir is best when treatment is started early. Characteristic EEG changes in the clinical setting of encephalitis are helpful in selecting patients for early antiviral treatment, as the EEG is usually abnormal and suggestive of herpes infection before abnormalities are apparent on CT.

Viral encephalitis is expected to cause diffuse polymorphic slow-wave activity, and a normal EEG result raises doubt about the diagnosis. With herpes simplex encephalitis, a majority of patients show focal temporal or frontotemporal slowing that may be unilateral, or,

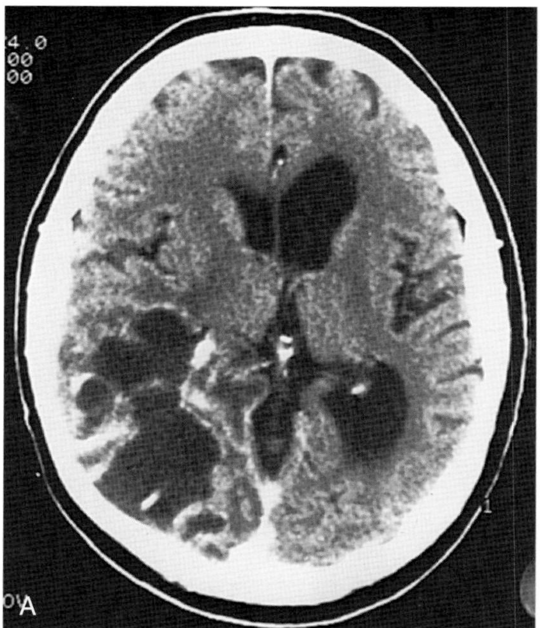

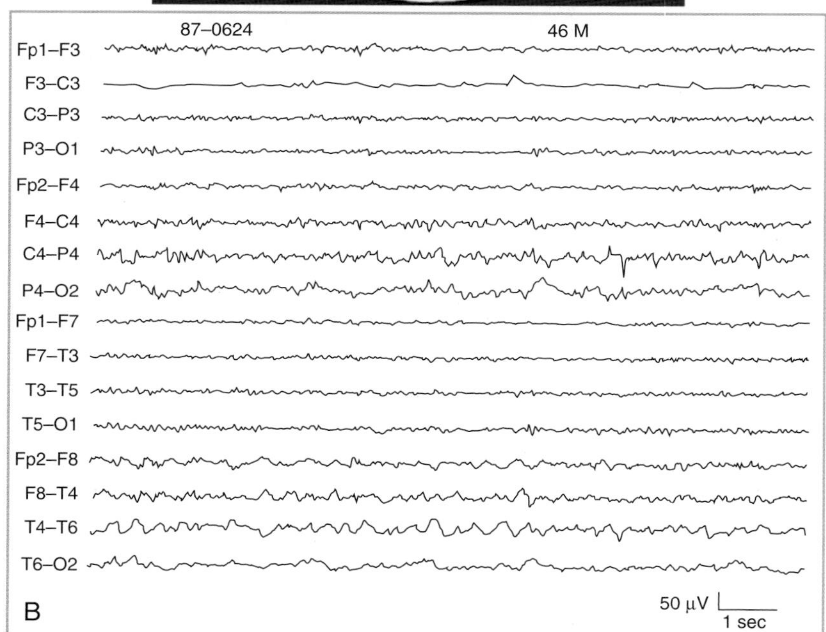


**Fig. 35.10** The patient was a 46-year-old man with a glioblastoma involving the right temporal and parietal lobes. **A,** Lesion is well demonstrated on this computed tomography scan of the brain. **B,** Electroencephalogram demonstrates continuous arrhythmic slowing over the right temporal and parieto-occipital areas. In addition, loss of the alpha rhythm and overriding faster frequencies are seen in corresponding areas of the left cerebral hemisphere.

if bilateral, asymmetrical. Lateralized PDs over one or both temporal regions (occasionally in other locations and sometimes generalized) add additional specificity to the EEG findings. These diagnostic features usually appear between days 2 and 15 of illness and are sometimes detectable only with serial tracings.

Bacterial meningitis causes severe and widespread EEG abnormalities, typically profound slowing and voltage depression, but viral meningitis produces little in the way of significant changes. Although CT and MRI have replaced EEG in evaluating patients with suspected brain abscess, focal EEG changes may occur in the early stage of cerebritis before an encapsulated lesion is demonstrable on CT or MRI.

EEG abnormalities usually resolve as the patient recovers, but the rate of resolution of clinical deficits and that of the electrographic findings may be different. It is not possible to predict either residual neurological morbidity or postencephalitic seizures by EEG criteria. An early return of normal EEG activity does not exclude the possibility of persistent neurological impairment.

## Brain Death

The diagnosis of brain death rests on strict clinical criteria that, when satisfied unambiguously, permit a conclusive determination of irreversible loss of brain function. In the United States, the usual

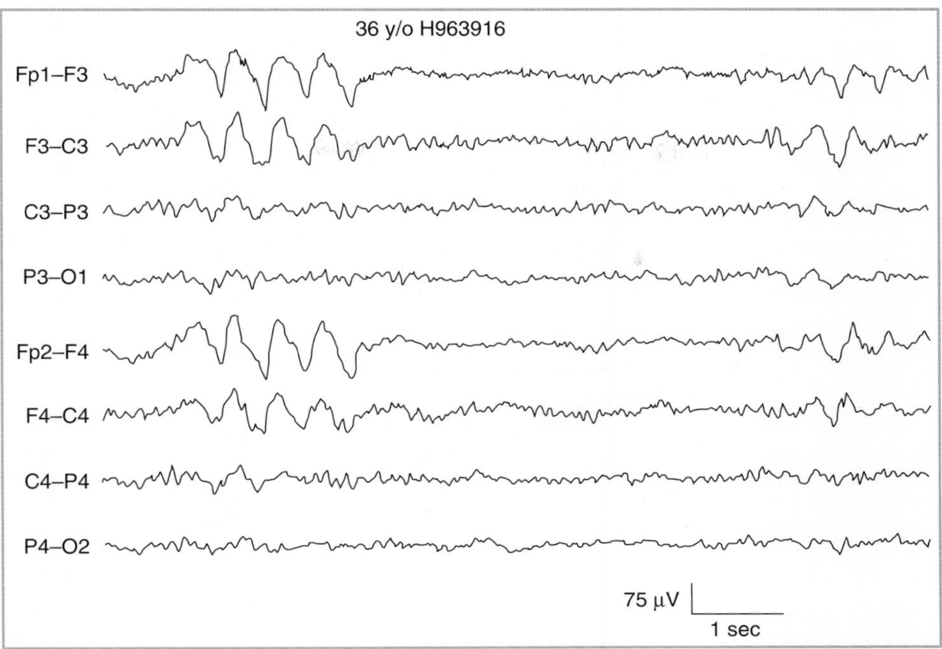


**Fig. 35.11** Bursts of intermittent rhythmic delta waves on the electroencephalogram (EEG) of a 36-year-old patient with primary generalized epilepsy and tonic-clonic seizures. Generalized spike-wave activity occurred elsewhere in the EEG. Intermittent rhythmic delta waves are a nonspecific manifestation of the patient's generalized epileptic disorder. (*Courtesy Dr. Bruce J. Fisch.*)

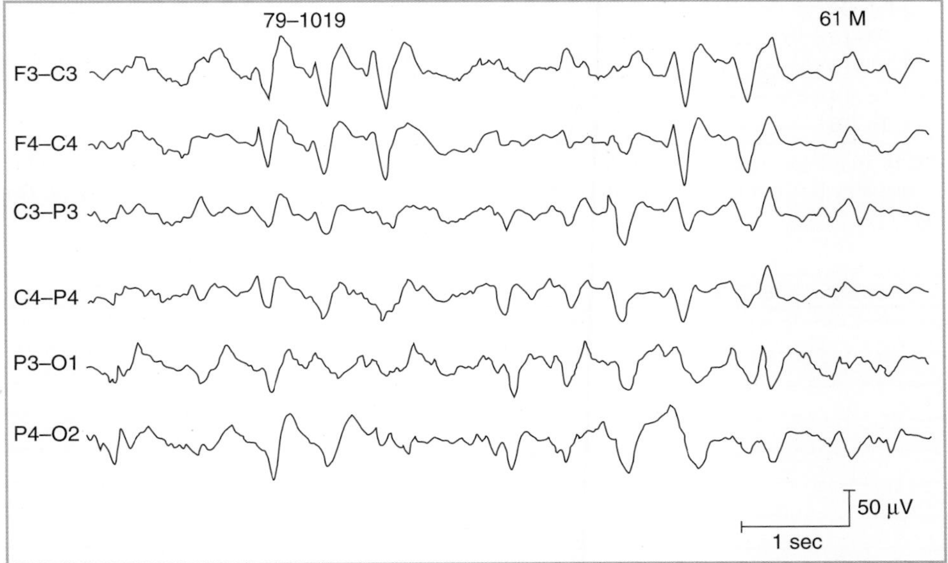


**Fig. 35.12** Triphasic waves on the electroencephalogram of a 61-year-old man with hepatic failure. *(Courtesy Dr. Bruce J. Fisch.)*

definition of brain death is irreversible cessation of all functions of the entire brain, including the brainstem. Because the EEG is a measure of cerebral—especially cortical—function, it has been widely used in association with clinical evaluation to provide objective evidence that brain function is lost. Several studies have demonstrated that enduring loss of cerebral electrical activity, termed *electrocerebral inactivity* or *electrocerebral silence*, accompanies clinical brain death and is never associated with recovery of neurological function. The determination of electrocerebral inactivity is technically demanding, requiring a special recording protocol. Minimum technical standards for EEG recording in suspected cerebral death have been established by the American Clinical Neurophysiology Society (American Clinical Neurophysiology Society, 2014).

Temporary and reversible loss of cerebral electrical activity is observable immediately after cardiorespiratory resuscitation, drug overdose from CNS depressants, and severe hypothermia. Therefore accurate interpretation of an EEG demonstrating electrocerebral inactivity must take into account these exceptional circumstances. Chapter 6 summarizes the clinical criteria for establishing the diagnosis of brain death.

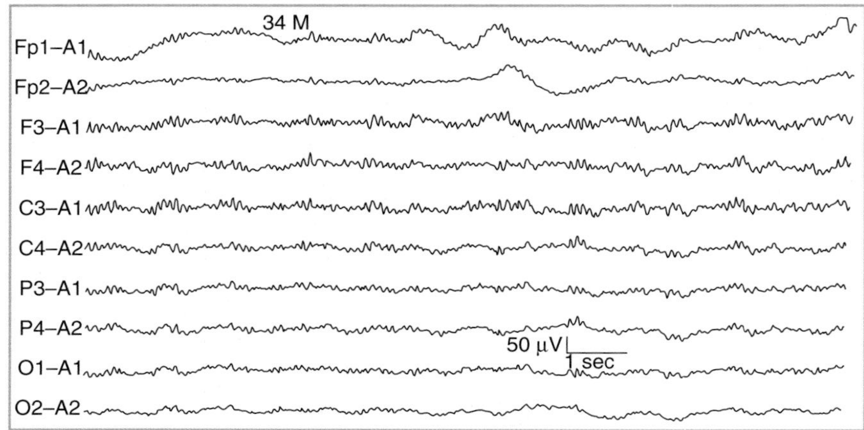


**Fig. 35.13** Alpha coma in a 34-year-old man with severe hypoxic-ischemic brain damage from a subarachnoid hemorrhage with diffuse prolonged cerebral vasospasm. Unlike the normal alpha rhythm, the alpha-range activity on the electroencephalogram of this comatose patient is widespread but maximal frontally, unreactive, and superimposed on low-voltage arrhythmic delta frequencies.

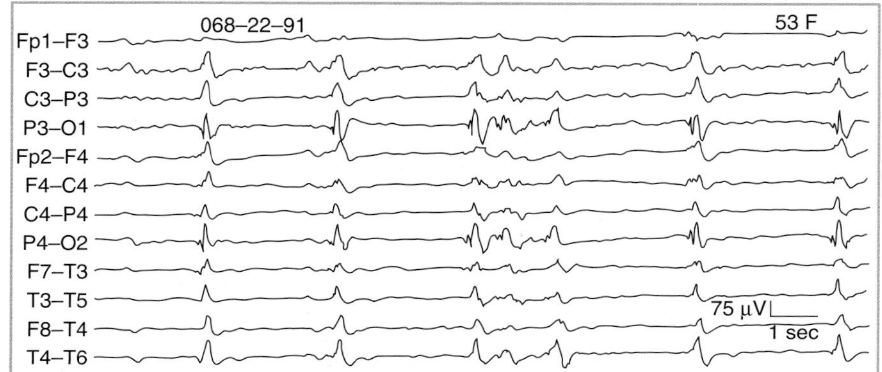


**Fig. 35.14** Burst suppression pattern on the electroencephalogram of a 53-year-old woman with anoxic encephalopathy following cardiorespiratory arrest. The patient died several days later. (*Courtesy Dr. Barbara S. Koppel.*)

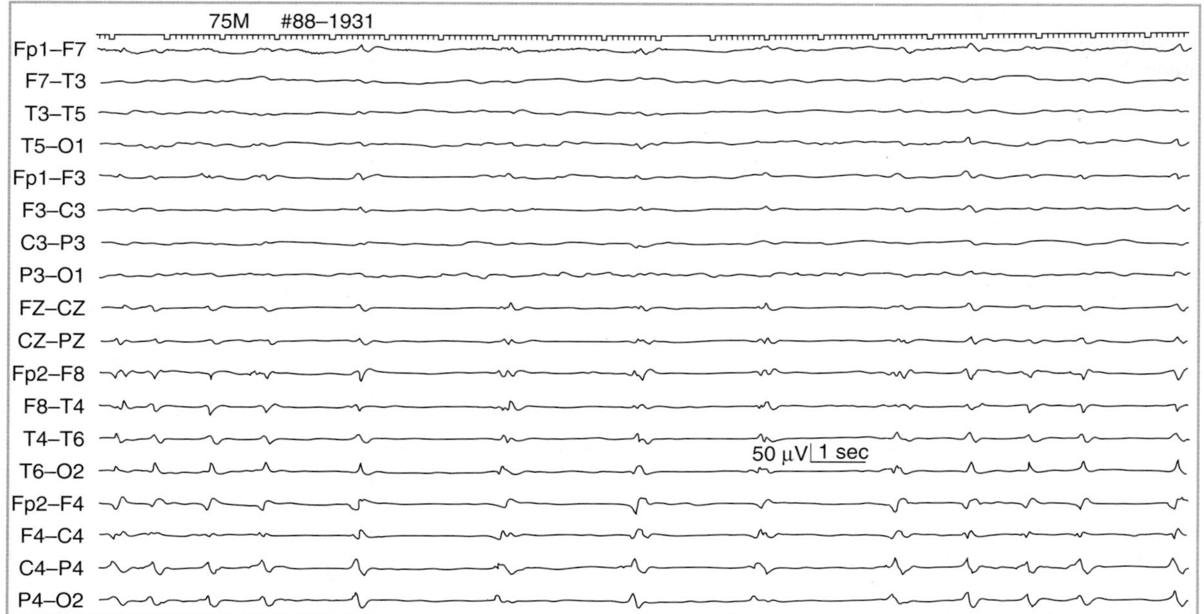


**Fig. 35.15** Periodic pattern on the electroencephalogram of a patient with anoxic encephalopathy following cardiorespiratory arrest. The patient was paralyzed with pancuronium because of bilateral myoclonus.

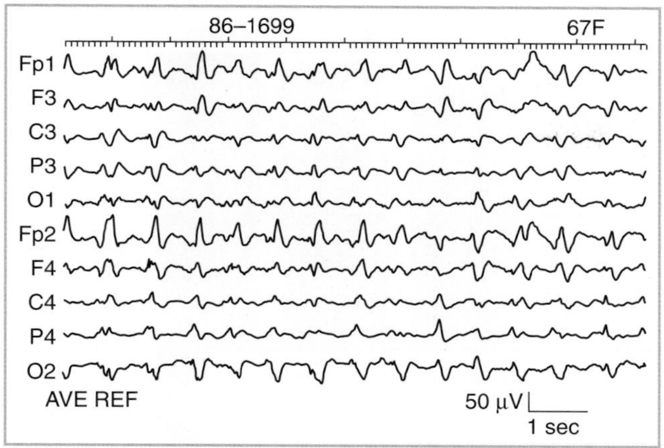


**Fig. 35.16** Periodic sharp-wave pattern on the electroencephalogram of a 67-year-old woman with Creutzfeldt-Jakob disease. Generalized bisynchronous diphasic sharp waves occur at approximately 1.5 to 2.0 per second. *AVE REF,* Average reference montage.

**BOX 35.1 Indications for Continuous Electroencephalography in the Intensive Care Unit**

Established seizures/status epilepticus, to guide titration of anticonvulsant therapy

Screen for nonconvulsive seizures among patients deemed to be at high risk:
- Hypoxic-ischemic encephalopathy (with or without hypothermia therapy)
- Stroke
- Meningitis
- Intraventricular hemorrhage
- Metabolic disturbance
- Sepsis

Screen for seizures in patients who are paralyzed and deemed to be at risk for seizures

Characterization of "spells" suspected to represent seizures

Detection of cerebral ischemia (i.e., delayed cerebral ischemia due to vasospasm following subarachnoid hemorrhage)

Prognostication by monitoring evolution of the electroencephalographic background

## Aging and Dementia

Because the EEG is a measure of cortical function, theoretically it should be useful in the diagnosis and classification of dementia. The utility of single EEG examinations in evaluating patients with known or suspected cognitive impairment, however, is often disappointing. Two important reasons for this limitation are (1) problems in distinguishing the effects on cerebral electrical activity of normal aging from those caused by disease processes and (2) the absence of generally accepted quantifiable methods of analysis and statistically valid comparison measures.

With increasing age beyond 65 years, a slight reduction in alpha-rhythm frequency and in the total amount of alpha activity is normal. Normal elderly persons also show slightly increased amounts of theta and delta activity, especially over the temporal and frontotemporal regions, as well as changes in sleep patterns. Early in the course of some dementing illnesses, no EEG abnormality may be apparent (this is the rule with Alzheimer disease), or the normal age-related changes may become exaggerated, differing more in degree than in kind.

In practice, the EEG can assist in the evaluation of suspected dementia by confirming abnormal cerebral function in patients with a possible psychogenic disorder and by delineating whether the process is focal or diffuse. Sequential EEGs usually are more helpful than a single tracing, and a test early in the course of the illness may provide more specific information than can be obtained later on. Overall, the degree of EEG abnormality shows good correlation with the degree of dementia.

EEG findings in Alzheimer disease are highly dependent on timing. The EEG is initially normal or shows an alpha rhythm at or just below the lower limits of normal. Generalized slowing ensues as the disease progresses. In patients with focal cognitive deficits, accentuation of slow-frequency activity over the corresponding brain area may be a feature. Continuous focal slowing is sufficiently unusual to suggest the possibility of another diagnosis. Prominent focal or bilateral independent slow-wave activity, especially if seen in company with a normal alpha rhythm, favors multifocal disease such as multiple cerebral infarcts. Sometimes a specific cause may be suggested. For example, an EEG showing generalized typical periodic sharp-wave complexes in a patient with dementia is virtually diagnostic of Creutzfeldt-Jakob disease (Fig. 35.16).

Event-related evoked potentials have application in the study of dementia. These long-latency events (i.e., potentials occurring more than 150 msec after the stimulus) are heavily dependent on psychic and cognitive factors. Ideally, they measure the brain's intrinsic mechanisms for processing certain types of information and are potentially valuable in the electrophysiological assessment of dementia. The best known of the event-related potentials is the P300, or P3, wave. The place of these long-latency evoked potentials in the evaluation of dementia is still under investigation, but the pattern of electrophysiological abnormality may be helpful in distinguishing among types of dementia (Comi and Leocani, 2000).

## Continuous Electroencephalographic Monitoring in the Intensive Care Unit

Recent technological advances have brought continuous EEG monitoring (cEEG) to the ICU bedside to assist in the evaluation of brain function in critically ill patients. As a real-time monitor of brain function, cEEG has the advantages that it is noninvasive and provides continuous high temporal resolution information about brain function. Perhaps most importantly, it is an extension of conventional EEG; as such, it remains the best tool for identifying electrographic seizures. Common indications for cEEG in the ICU are listed in Box 35.1.

Monitoring by cEEG has become common in specialized centers, and clinical practice has been guided by recent consensus statements published by the American Clinical Neurophysiology Society (Herman et al., 2015a, 2015b). Both the technology and clinical practice are evolving. Although recording is continuous, the review and interpretation are typically intermittent (e.g., they are performed two or three times daily, with more frequent review as necessary). Although this arrangement can result in delayed recognition of significant events (e.g., seizures, ischemia), it nonetheless represents an important improvement over the previous practice of intermittent, infrequent, standard EEG recording. Many centers employ remote networking to facilitate timely interpretation without requiring the physical presence of expert EEG readers in the ICU. Some institutions provide round-the-clock "neurotelemetry," with EEG technologists screening multiple cEEG recordings on a continuous basis.

### Continuous Electroencephalogram Monitoring for Nonconvulsive Seizures

Monitoring for the detection of NCSs is the most common indication for cEEG recording. The demand for cEEG monitoring has, in large

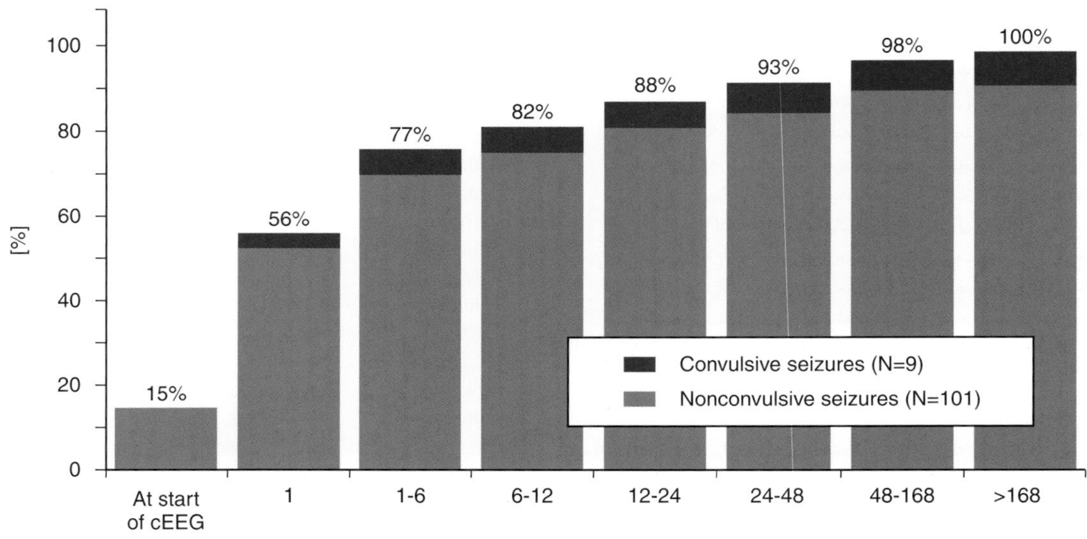


**Fig. 35.17 Time from Onset of Continuous Electroencephalographic** ***(cEEG)*** **Monitoring to the occurrence of the First Seizure.** *(Reprinted with permission from Claassen, J., Mayer, S.A., Kowalski, R.G., et al., 2004. Detection of electrographic seizures with continuous EEG monitoring in critically ill patients. Neurology 62[10], 1743–1748.)*

part, been driven by increased awareness of the prevalence of NCSs in certain groups of critically ill patients. The reported prevalence of NCSs in critically ill patients undergoing cEEG has varied considerably, depending on both the population studied and the study design (DeLorenzo et al., 1998; Towne et al., 2000; Treiman et al., 1998). Retrospective cohort studies in both adults and children undergoing EEG monitoring based on the clinical suspicion of NCSs report seizure detection rates between about 15% and 40% (Abend et al., 2013; Claassen et al., 2004; Jette et al., 2006). An important finding common to these studies is that the great majority (75%–92%) of critically ill adults and children who are found to have seizures had pure NCSs (Abend et al., 2013; Claassen et al., 2004). Risk factors for NCSs in the general ICU population include prior history of epilepsy, intracerebral and subarachnoid hemorrhage, CNS infection, brain tumors, severe traumatic brain injury, and sepsis. Patients with sepsis in the medical ICU setting are also at risk for NCSs (Oddo et al., 2009). In children, NCSs have most commonly been reported in the setting of coma following convulsive seizures as well as among patients with a past history of epilepsy, hypoxic brain injury, and traumatic brain injury (Abend et al., 2013; McCoy et al., 2011).

Fig. 35.17 illustrates that about 90% of critically ill patients who ultimately have seizures experience their first seizure within the first 24 hours of monitoring, and that half of these patients will have the first seizure within the first hour. Accordingly, many centers now monitor for 24 hours and then continue to record for 24 hours after the last electrographic seizure or for 24 hours after a change in therapy that might provoke seizures (such as tapering of anticonvulsant infusions or rewarming following hypothermia). The absence of epileptiform discharges during the first few hours of cEEG monitoring appears to predict a lower seizure risk (Shafi et al., 2012).

## Electrographic Identification of Nonconvulsive Seizures

Fig. 35.18 depicts an unequivocal NCS. The discharge lasts more than 10 seconds and has the classic electrographic features of a seizure, with clear evolution in frequency, amplitude, morphology, and spatial extent. However, not all NCSs are as clear cut, and the lack of concordant clinical signs can make some NCSs difficult to identify. Box 35.2 lists proposed criteria for NCS (Chong and Hirsch, 2005). Some cEEG patterns resemble electrographic seizures, but fail to meet all of these criteria. When the EEG pattern is equivocal, a therapeutic trial of benzodiazepines can be helpful. However, the interpretation of the benzodiazepine trial may itself be difficult, because clinical improvement may be delayed, and because electrographic and clinical improvement may require loading doses of other anticonvulsant medications.

## The "Ictal-Interictal Continuum"

In the ICU setting, the distinction between recurrent interictal epileptiform discharges and ictal discharges can be challenging. Electrographic patterns often wax and wane, evolving from patterns that are clearly ictal to those that are clearly interictal and vice versa. This can frustrate consistent EEG reporting; more importantly, it can present challenges to clinicians who must decide which EEG patterns warrant treatment and how aggressively they should be treated. Most experts recommend treating unequivocal NCSs and equivocal patterns with a clear clinical correlate. There is less consensus on treatment of equivocal patterns without clinical correlate. Chong and Hirsch have proposed a conceptual framework termed the "ictal-interictal continuum" (Chong and Hirsch, 2005; Fig. 35.19), in which various electrographic patterns are plotted according to their likelihood to represent an ictal phenomenon and their potential to cause secondary neuronal injury. Standardized terminology for rhythmic and periodic EEG patterns occurring during critical care EEG recordings has recently been developed by a committee of the American Clinical Neurophysiology Society (Hirsch et al., 2013).

## Periodic Discharges

PDs are characterized by spikes, sharp waves, or sharply contoured slow waves that recur periodically or pseudo-periodically, usually every 1 to 2 seconds. PDs may be generalized (GPDs: generalized PDs, formerly called GPEDs; Fig. 35.20), unilateral (LPDs: lateralized PDs, formerly called PLEDs), or bilaterally independent (BIPDs: bilateral independent PDs, formerly called BIPLEDs; Fig. 35.21). PDs are frequently associated with focal brain injury such as ischemia, hemorrhage, or

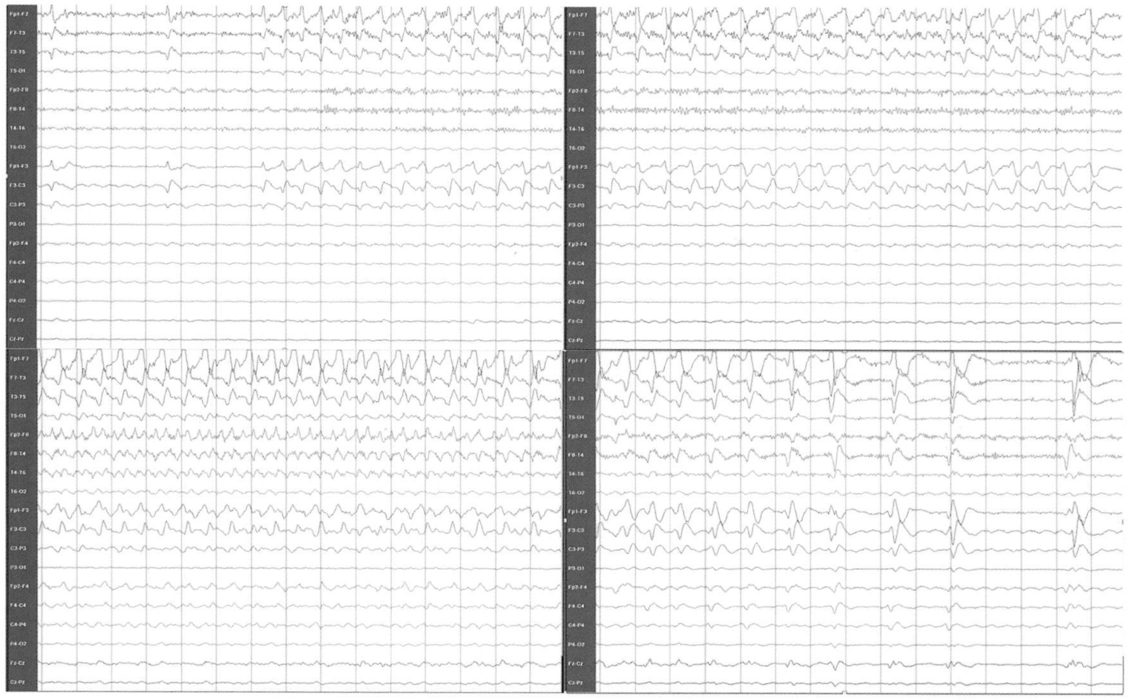

Fig. 35.18 Nonconvulsive Seizure (Arising From Left Hemisphere, Spreading to Right Hemisphere).

## BOX 35.2 Criteria for Nonconvulsive Seizures

Any pattern lasting at least 10 seconds satisfying any one of the following three primary criteria.

**Primary Criteria**

1. Repetitive generalized or focal spikes, sharp waves, spike-and-wave or sharp- and slow-wave complexes at three per second or greater.
2. Repetitive generalized or focal spikes, sharp waves, spike-and-wave, or sharp- and slow-wave complexes at three per second or less and the secondary criterion.
3. Sequential rhythmic, periodic, or quasi-periodic waves at one per second or greater and unequivocal evolution in frequency (gradually increasing or decreasing by at least one per second—for example, from two–three per second), morphology, or location (gradual spread into or out of a region involving at least two electrodes). Evolution in amplitude alone is not sufficient. Change in sharpness without any other change in morphology is not adequate to satisfy evolution in morphology.

**Secondary Criterion**

Significant improvement in clinical state or appearance of a previously absent normal electroencephalographic (EEG) pattern (such as a posterior dominant rhythm) temporally coupled to acute administration of a rapid-acting antiepileptic drug. Resolution of the "epileptiform" discharges, leaving diffuse slowing without clinical improvement and without appearance of previously absent normal EEG patterns, would not satisfy the secondary criterion.

*Reprinted with permission from Chong, D.J., Hirsch, L.J., 2005. Which EEG patterns warrant treatment in the critically ill? Reviewing the evidence for treatment of periodic epileptiform discharges and related patterns. J Clin Neurophysiol 22(2), 79–91.*

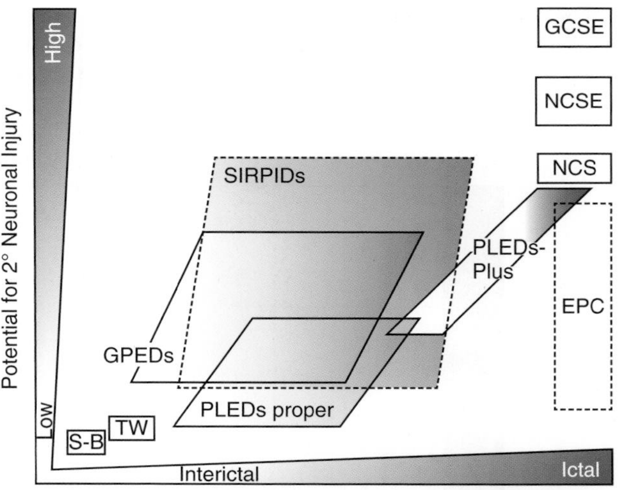


Fig. 35.19 The Ictal-Interictal Continuum. *EPC,* epilepsia partialis continua; *GCSE,* generalized convulsive status epilepticus; *GPEDs,* Generalized periodic discharges; *PLEDs,* lateralized periodic discharges; *NCS,* nonconvulsive seizures; *NCSE,* nonconvulsive status epilepticus; *SIRPIDs,* stimulus-induced rhythmic, periodic, or ictal discharges *TW,* triphasic waves. (*Reprinted with permission from Chong, D.J., Hirsch, L.J., 2005. Which EEG patterns warrant treatment in the critically ill? Reviewing the evidence for treatment of periodic epileptiform discharges and related patterns. J Clin Neurophysiol 22[2], 79–91.*)

infection. By definition, they do not meet the formal criteria for a seizure. However, they frequently occur following prolonged seizures. There is controversy about the meaning of PDs, their potential contribution to secondary brain injury, and consequently the need for their treatment. They may simply be markers of encephalopathy or focal brain injury rather than a pathological entity that requires treatment.

However, PDs have been associated with poor outcome following status epilepticus (Jaitly et al., 1997; Nei et al., 1999).

### Stimulus-Induced Rhythmic, Periodic, or Ictal Discharges

The periodic epileptiform discharges described earlier generally occur spontaneously and do not change in response to arousal or external stimulation. However, occasionally, electrographic patterns consistently occur following stimulation or arousal of a comatose patient (Fig. 35.22). These stimulus-sensitive EEG patterns have been termed stimulus-induced rhythmic, periodic, or ictal discharges, or SIRPIDs (Hirsch et al., 2004). It is often unclear whether SIRPIDs represent ictal phenomena such as reflex seizures or interictal phenomena such as an abnormal arousal pattern. There is debate about how aggressively these patterns should be treated. Most SIRPIDs are not accompanied by clinical signs, although occasionally they may correlate with focal motor seizures, in which case the case for treatment may be more compelling (Hirsch et al., 2008).

### Quantitative Electroencephalogram

Increasing awareness and concern about NCSs has led to a growing demand for continuous EEG monitoring in ICUs, generating large volumes of data that can be overwhelming to interpret using conventional reviewing techniques that display 10–20 seconds of raw EEG data per screen. To address this challenge and facilitate interpretation of prolonged EEG recordings, several quantitative EEG (QEEG) display tools have been developed to provide insight into trends in the EEG over time and to highlight significant electrographic events. However, it is important to emphasize that QEEG tools should not replace careful review of the underlying raw EEG. Table 35.1 lists QEEG display tools commonly available from various manufacturers and their primary clinical applications. One of the most appealing applications of QEEG displays is their potential use as a screening tool for seizures. Fig. 35.23, *A* and *B* illustrate the typical appearance of seizures on amplitude-integrated EEG (aEEG) and color density spectral array (CDSA) displays, respectively. aEEG is a technique that displays time-compressed and rectified EEG amplitude on a semilogarithmic scale. The top and bottom margins of the aEEG tracing reflect the maximum and minimum EEG amplitudes at a given time. CDSA is a technique that applies fast-Fourier transformation (FFT) to convert raw EEG signals into a time-compressed and color-coded display, also termed a color spectrogram. Frequency-specific EEG power is depicted on the *y*-axis, with varying degrees of EEG power (power = amplitude$^2$) depicted using a color-coded scale. The sensitivity of QEEG displays for seizure identification can reach as high as 80%; however, sensitivity varies by seizure type. Seizures of low amplitude or shorter duration are more challenging to identify by QEEG (Stewart et al., 2010). Many types of artifact may also resemble seizures on QEEG, leading to "false positives." Therefore QEEG trending displays should always be interpreted in conjunction with careful review of the accompanying raw EEG tracing.

### Magnetoencephalography

Additional text available at http://expertconsult.inkling.com.

## EVOKED POTENTIALS

Additional text available at http://expertconsult.inkling.com.

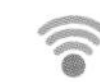

## INTRAOPERATIVE MONITORING

Additional text available at http://expertconsult.inkling.com.

*The complete reference list is available online at https://expertconsult.inkling.com/.*

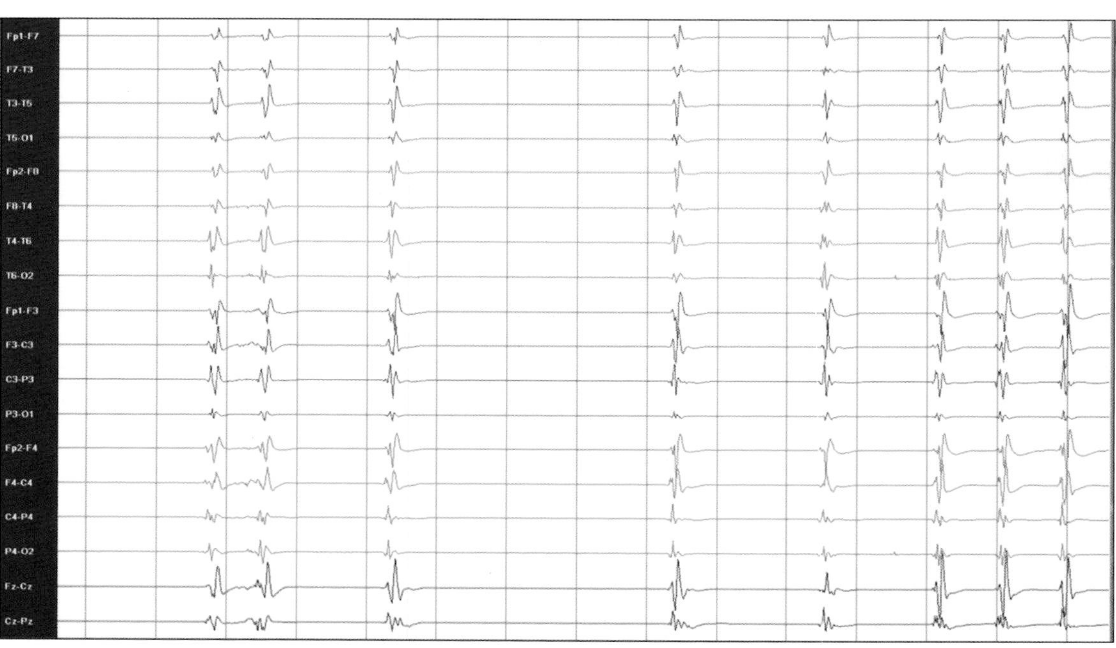


**Fig. 35.20** Generalized Periodic Discharges.

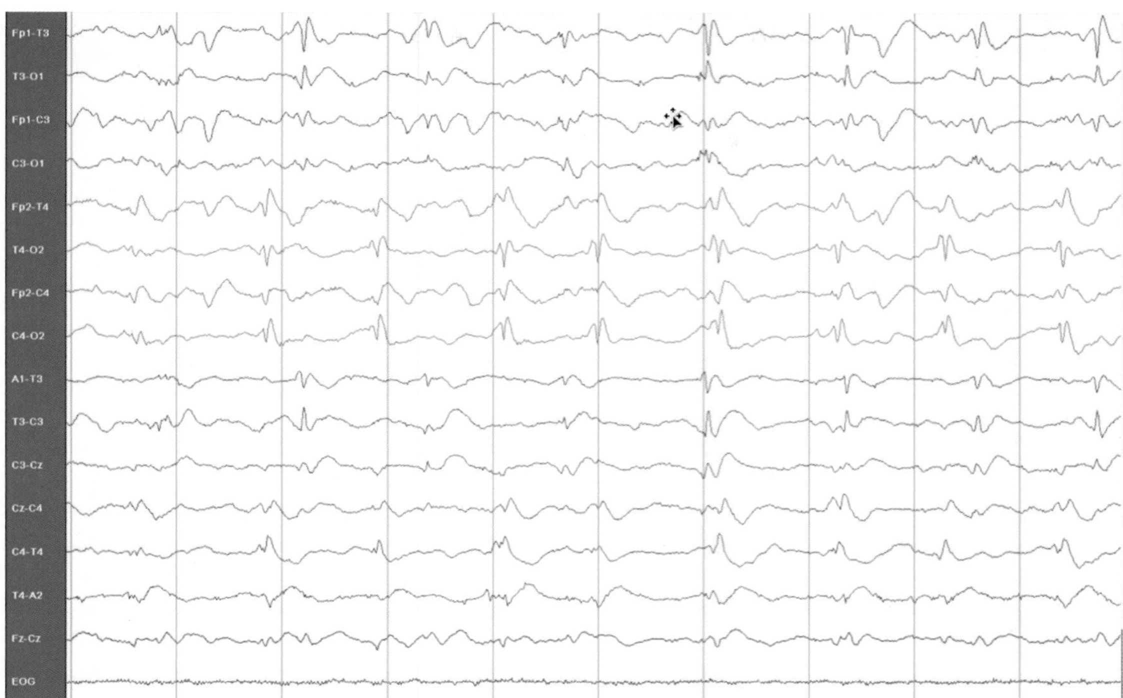


**Fig. 35.21** Bilateral Independent Periodic Discharges.

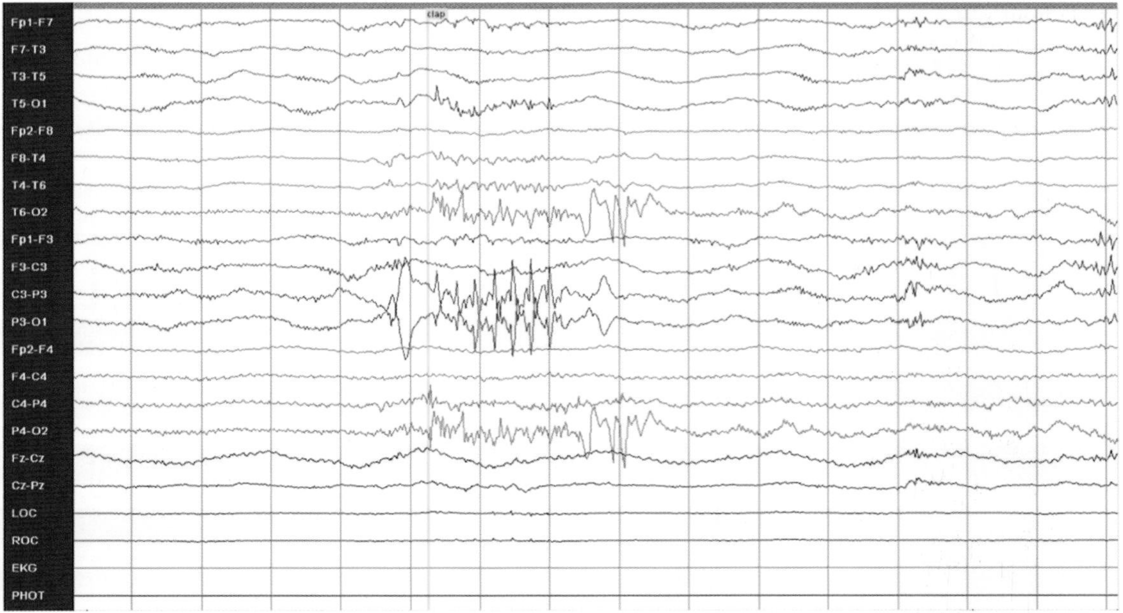


**Fig. 35.22** Stimulus-Induced Rhythmic, Periodic, or Ictal Discharges in Response to Noise.

**TABLE 35.1 Overview of Commonly Available Quantitative Electroencephalographic (EEG) Display Tools**

| Quantitative EEG Display Tool | Primary Clinical Applications |
|---|---|
| Amplitude-integrated EEG (aEEG) | Background assessment, seizure identification |
| Envelope trend | Seizure identification |
| Color spectrogram (CDSA, CSA, DSA) | Seizure identification |
| Total power | Seizure identification |
| Rhythmicity spectrogram | Seizure identification |
| Alpha-delta ratio | Background assessment, ischemia detection |
| Alpha variability | Background assessment, ischemia detection |
| Asymmetry indices | Background assessment, ischemia detection |
| Burst suppression index | Background assessment |

*CDSA*, color density spectral array; *CSA*, color spectral array; *DSA*, density spectral array

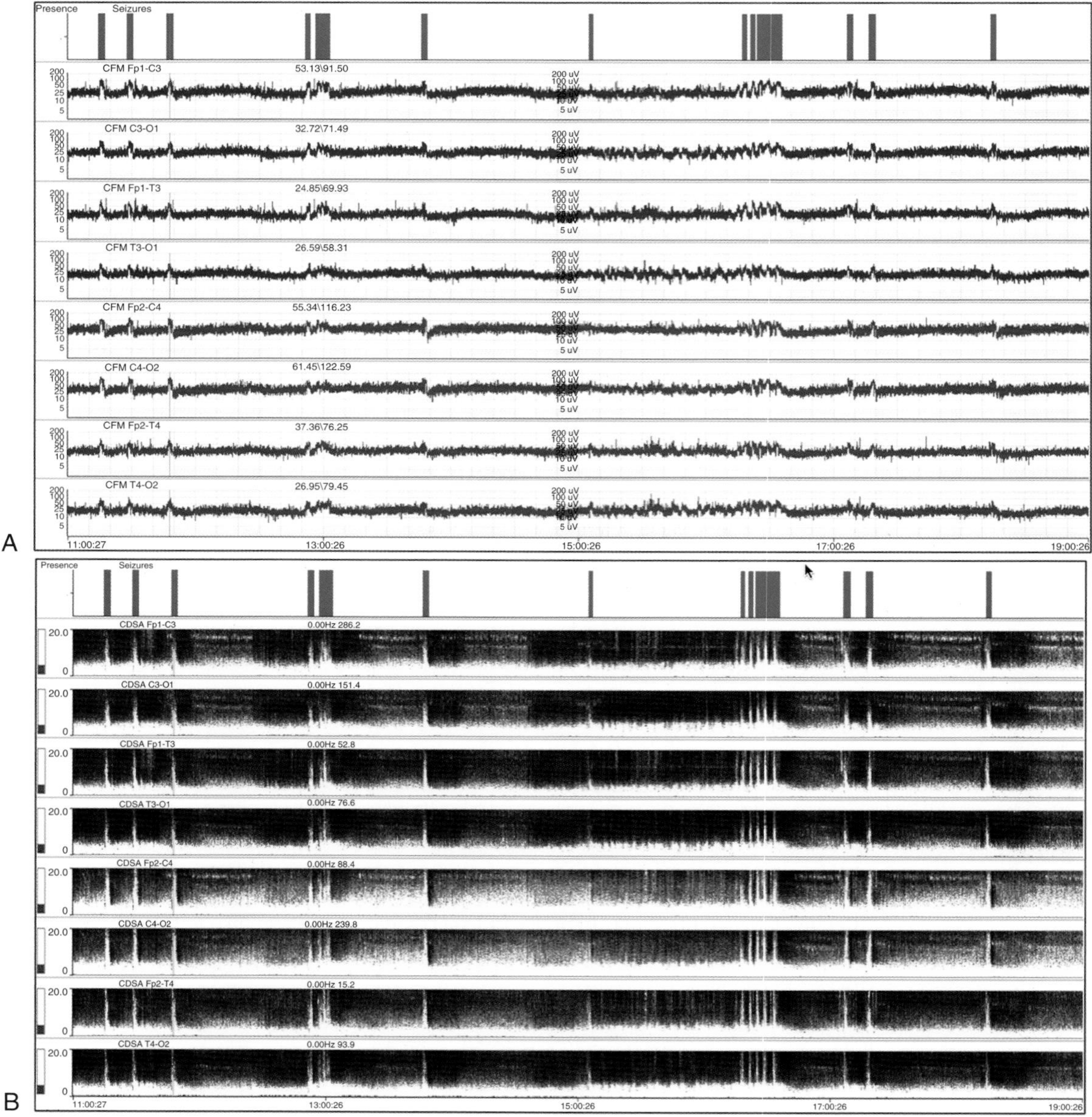


**Fig. 35.23 A,** Recurrent seizures depicted on an 8-hour amplitude-integrated electroencephalogram (aEEG) display. **B,** Recurrent seizures depicted on an 8-hour color density spectral array *(CDSA)* display. Electrographic seizures identified on the raw EEG are indicated by the blue bars at the top of each figure. An eight-channel double-distance longitudinal bipolar montage. On the aEEG display **(A)**, seizures are associated with a rise in both the bottom and top margin of the aEEG tracing. On the CDSA display **(B)**, seizures are associated with bright bands of color, indicating higher-power EEG activity across a wider range of frequencies.

36

# Clinical Electromyography

Bashar Katirji

## OUTLINE



Clinical electromyography is a distinct medical discipline that plays a pivotal role in the diagnosis of peripheral nerve and neuromuscular disorders (Katirji and Kaminsky, 2002). The designations *clinical electromyography (EMG)*, *electrodiagnostic (EDX) examination*, and *electroneuromyography (ENMG)* are used interchangeably to encompass the electrophysiological study of peripheral nerve, neuromuscular junction, and muscle; the terms *needle electromyography* and *needle electrode examination* are reserved for the specific testing that involves needle electrode evaluation of muscle. Although many still refer to all such testing as simply *electromyography*, use of the word without a descriptor is discouraged because it can be confusing, often implying only the needle electrode part of the evaluation. For clarity, the terms *clinical EMG* refers to the entire EDX study whereas *needle EMG* refers to the needle electrode component. These terms are used in this chapter.

The clinical EMG examination is an important diagnostic tool that helps localize a neuromuscular problem at the motor or sensory neuron cell body, nerve root, peripheral nerve, neuromuscular junction, muscle membrane, or muscle. It also helps to establish the underlying process in these disorders and assess their management and prognosis. EDX testing provides the most valuable diagnostic information when the clinical assessment suggests a short list of differential diagnoses. The clinician should perform a detailed or focused neurological examination before referring the patient for a clinical EMG, which in turn serves as an independent procedure to provide an objective assessment of the peripheral nervous system (PNS; Katirji, 2002). Patients with complex clinical pictures are best served by neurological consultations prior to performing EDX testing.

The clinical EMG examination is composed of two main tests: nerve conduction studies (NCSs) and needle EMG. These tests complement each other, and both are often necessary for a definite diagnosis. Additional EDX procedures include assessment of F waves, H reflexes, and blink reflexes; repetitive nerve stimulation (RNS); and single-fiber EMG (SFEMG). A focused history and examination will help the electromyographer design the most appropriate EDX study Katirji, 2018; (Preston and Shapiro, 2013). The electromyographer must be proficient in using modern EDX equipment and applying EDX techniques, know the normal values for commonly and uncommonly examined NCSs and for motor unit action potentials (MUAPs) in different muscles, and be familiar with the specific and nonspecific EDX findings in different neuromuscular disorders.

## NERVE CONDUCTION STUDIES

### Principles

Electrical stimulation of nerve fibers initiates impulses that travel along motor, sensory, or mixed nerves and evoke a compound action potential. The three types of NCSs are motor, sensory, and mixed. Analysis of the compound muscle action potential (CMAP), which is evoked by stimulating a nerve while recording from a muscle, indirectly assesses the conduction characteristics of motor fibers. Analysis of the sensory nerve action potential (SNAP) assesses the sensory fibers by stimulating a nerve and recording directly from a cutaneous nerve. Mixed NCSs directly assess the sensory and motor fibers simultaneously by stimulating and recording from a mixed nerve and analyzing the mixed nerve action potential (MNAP). Use of standard NCSs enables the precise localization of a lesion and accurate characterization of peripheral nerve function.

#### Stimulators

NCSs use two different kinds of surface (percutaneous) electrical stimulators. *Constant voltage stimulators* regulate voltage output so that current varies inversely with the impedance of the system, including the skin and subcutaneous tissues. *Constant current stimulators* change voltage according to impedance so that the amount of current that reaches the nerve is within the limits of skin resistance. As the current flows between the cathode (negative pole) and the anode (positive pole), negative charges accumulate under the cathode and positive charges under the anode, depolarizing and hyperpolarizing the nerve, respectively. In bipolar stimulation, both electrodes are over the nerve trunk, with the cathode closer to the recording site. Anodal conduction block of the propagated impulse may occur with inadvertent reversal of the cathode and anode of the stimulator. The cause of the block is hyperpolarization at the anode. This may prevent the nerve impulse evoked by the depolarization occurring under the cathode from proceeding past the anode.

Supramaximal stimulation of a nerve that results in depolarization of all available axons is a paramount prerequisite to accurate and reproducible NCS measurements. To achieve supramaximal stimulation, one slowly increases the current (or voltage) intensity until it reaches a level at which the recorded potential does not increase in size. Then, increasing the current an additional 20%–30% ensures that the potential does not change further.

### Recording Electrodes

Surface electrodes record the CMAP, SNAP, or MNAP. The advantages of surface recording are reproducible evoked responses that change only slightly with the position of the electrodes in relation to the recording muscle or nerve. In contrast, needle electrode recording registers only a small portion of the muscle or nerve action potentials; as a result, the evoked responses are variable and not reproducible, although they have less interference from neighboring discharges. Needle recordings improve the recording from small atrophic muscles or a proximal muscle that is not excitable in isolation. Most recording electrodes used in clinical practice are disk electrodes; ring electrodes are convenient for recording the antidromic sensory potentials from digital nerves over the proximal and distal interphalangeal joints.

### Recording Procedure

A prepulse preceding the stimulus triggers the sweep on a storage oscilloscope. The amplifier sensitivity determines the size (amplitude) of the potential. Overamplification truncates the response and underamplification prevents accurate measurements of the exact takeoff point from baseline. Digital averaging is very useful in recording low-amplitude SNAPs. Signals that are time locked to the stimulus summate with averaging at a constant latency and appear as an evoked potential distinct from the background noise. The signal-to-noise ratio increases in proportion to the square root of the trial number. For example, four trials give twice as big a response as a single stimulus, and nine trials give three times the amplitude. Most current instruments digitally indicate the latency and amplitude by cursors when the desired spot on the waveform is marked. The operator can override these cursors if needed.

## Motor Nerve Conduction Studies

The performance of motor NCSs requires stimulating a motor or mixed peripheral nerve while recording the CMAP from a muscle innervated by that nerve. Ideal muscles to record from are well isolated from neighboring muscles, which eliminates volume conduction. A pair of recording electrodes consists of an active lead, G1, placed on the belly of the muscle, and a reference (indifferent or inactive) lead, G2, placed on the tendon *(belly-tendon recording)*. The propagating muscle action potential, originating under G1 located near the motor point, gives rise to a simple biphasic waveform with an initial negativity. Initial positivity suggests incorrect positioning of the active electrode away from the motor end-plate zone or a volume-conducted potential from distant muscles activated by anomalous innervation or by accidental spread of stimulation to other neighboring nerves, thus generating potentials from distant muscles

The nerve is usually stimulated, whenever technically feasible, at two or more points along its course. Shorter nerves—such as the axillary, femoral, and facial nerves—are stimulated at only one point, because the more proximal portions of the nerves are inaccessible. Otherwise, the nerve is typically stimulated distally near the recording electrode and more proximally to evaluate one or more proximal segments. Motor NCSs evaluate several measurements (Fig. 36.1):

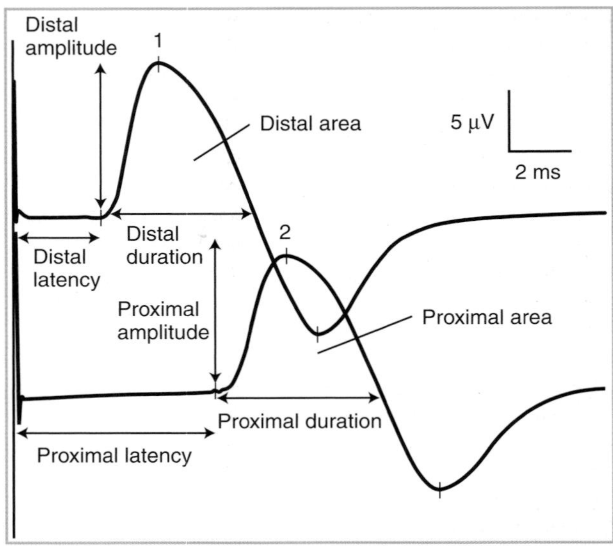


**Fig. 36.1** Motor nerve conduction study of the median nerve, revealing a typical compound muscle action potential (CMAP) with distal (wrist) and proximal (elbow) stimulations; it shows the distal and proximal latencies and CMAP amplitudes, durations, and areas. The proximal CMAP has a lower amplitude (12.6 mV vs. 11.3 mV) and area (37.3 mV/ms vs. 34.50 mV/ms) than the distal CMAP because of physiological temporal dispersion and phase cancellation. The proximal conduction velocity is calculated by measuring the distance of the elbow-to-wrist segment and using the formula:Thus, for the conduction velocity in this example, 210 mm/6.9 ms − 3.5 ms = 62 m/sec.

$$\text{Motor conduction velocity} = \frac{\text{Distance}}{\text{Proximal latency–Distal latency}}$$

- *CMAP amplitude:* The usual measure of amplitude is from baseline to negative peak and is expressed in millivolts. When recorded with surface electrodes, CMAP amplitude is a semiquantitative measure of the number of axons conducting between the stimulating and recording points. CMAP amplitude also depends on the relative conduction speed of the axons, the integrity of the neuromuscular junctions, and the number of muscle fibers that are able to generate action potentials.
- *CMAP duration:* This measurement is usually the duration of the negative phase of the evoked potential and is expressed in milliseconds. It is a function of the conduction rates of the various axons forming the examined nerve and the distance between the stimulation and recording electrodes. As a result of physiological temporal dispersion and phase cancellation, the CMAP generated from proximal stimulation is slightly longer in duration and lower in amplitude than that obtained from distal stimulation (see forthcoming section).
- *CMAP area:* This is usually limited to the negative phase area under the waveform and shows linear correlation with the product of amplitude and duration. Measurement is in millivolts per millisecond and requires electronic integration using computerized equipment. The ability to measure CMAP area has practically replaced the need to record its duration.
- *Latencies:* Latency is the time interval between nerve stimulation (shock artifact) and the CMAP onset. Expression of latency is in milliseconds and reflects the conduction rate of the fastest

conducting axon. Whenever technically possible, the nerve is stimulated at two points: a distal point near the recording site and a more proximal point. The measures obtained are the *distal latency* and *proximal latency*, respectively. Both latencies depend mostly on the length of the nerve segment and, to a much lesser extent, on neuromuscular transmission time and propagation time along the muscle membrane. When anatomically feasible, several proximal stimulation points may be done, generating several proximal latencies; in these situations the exact site of stimulation should be specified—for example, below elbow, above elbow, or axilla—referring to stimulation sites while the ulnar nerve is being tested.

- *Conduction velocity:* This is a computed measurement of the speed of conduction expressed in meters per second. Measurement of conduction velocity allows comparison of the speed of conduction of the fastest fibers between different nerves and subjects irrespective of the length of the nerve. The calculation requires measurement of the length of the nerve segment between distal and proximal stimulation sites. Measuring the surface distance along the course of the nerve estimates the nerve length; it should be more than 10 cm to improve the accuracy of surface measurement.

$$\text{Motor conduction velocity} = \frac{\text{Distance}}{\text{Proximal latency–Distal latency}}$$

As with latencies, motor conduction velocity measures the speed of conduction of the fastest axon. In contrast with motor latency, however, motor nerve conduction velocity is a pure nerve conduction time because neuromuscular transmission time and muscle fiber propagation time are common to both stimulation sites, and the latency difference between two points is the time required for the nerve impulse to travel from one stimulus point to the other. When the nerve is stimulated at multiple proximal sites, several proximal conduction velocity segments may be calculated, such as above-elbow to below-elbow segment and below-elbow to wrist segment when the ulnar nerve is being tested.

## Sensory Nerve Conduction Studies

Sensory axons are evaluated by stimulating a nerve while the transmitted potential from the same nerve is recorded at a different site. Therefore SNAPs are true nerve action potentials. The measurement of *antidromic* sensory NCSs requires recording potentials directed toward the sensory receptors, whereas obtaining *orthodromic* responses requires recording potentials directed away from these receptors. Sensory latencies and conduction velocities are identical with either method, but SNAP amplitudes are generally higher in antidromic studies. Orthodromic responses are sometimes low in amplitude, necessitating the use of averaging techniques. Action potentials from distal muscles may obscure antidromic responses because the thresholds of some motor axons are similar to those of large myelinated sensory axons. Fortunately, accurate measurement of SNAPs is still possible because the large-diameter sensory fibers conduct 5%–10% faster than motor fibers. This relationship may change in disease states that selectively affect different fibers.

SNAPs may be obtained by several methods: (1) stimulating and recording a pure sensory nerve (such as the sural and radial sensory nerves); (2) stimulating a mixed nerve while recording distally over a cutaneous branch (such as the antidromic median and ulnar sensory responses); or (3) stimulating a distal cutaneous branch while recording over a proximal mixed nerve (such as in orthodromic median and ulnar sensory studies). Similar to their motor counterparts, sensory NCSs record several measurements (Fig. 36.2):

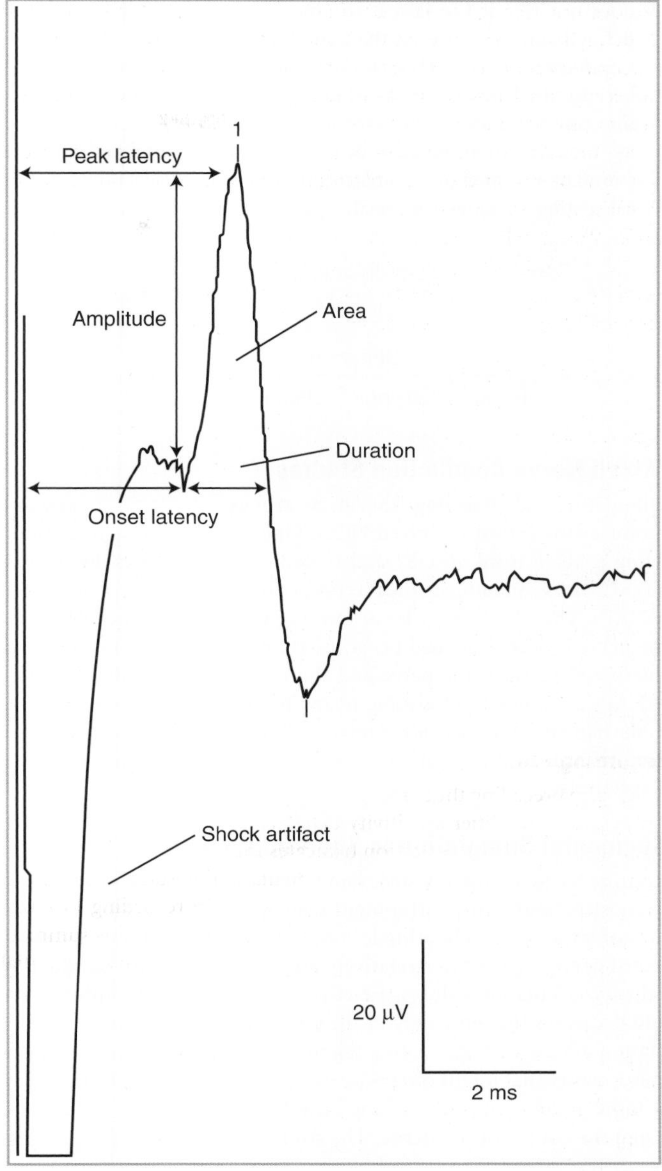


**Fig. 36.2** Antidromic median sensory nerve conduction study after stimulation at the wrist, revealing peak and onset latencies and sensory nerve action potential amplitude, duration, and area. The shock artifact interferes with accurate determination of onset latency, whereas peak latency is easily determined.

- *SNAP amplitude:* This semiquantitatively measures the number of sensory axons that conduct between the stimulation and recording sites. The calculation is from the baseline to negative peak or from positive peak to negative peak and is expressed in microvolts. SNAP duration and area may be measured, but such measurements are not useful because of significant temporal dispersion and phase cancellation (see later discussion).
- *Latencies:* Sensory distal latencies are measured (in milliseconds) from the stimulus artifact to the peak of the negative phase (peak latency) or from the stimulus artifact to the onset of the SNAP (onset latency). A large shock artifact, a noisy background, or a wavy baseline may obscure onset latency. Although peak latency

does not reflect the fastest conducting sensory fibers, it is easily defined and more precise than onset latency.

- *Conduction velocity:* This requires stimulation at a single site only because the latency consists of just the nerve conduction time from the stimulus point to the recording electrode. As with motor velocity, the calculation may also be done using both distal and proximal stimulations. Only onset latencies (not peak latencies) are useful for calculating velocities to assess the speed of the fastest conducting fibers.

$$\text{Sensory conduction velocity} = \frac{\text{Distance}}{\text{Onset latency}}$$

or

$$= \frac{\text{Distance}}{\text{Proximal latency} - \text{Distal latency}}$$

## Mixed Nerve Conduction Studies

Stimulating and recording from nerve trunks containing sensory and motor axons constitute mixed NCSs. Often these tests require stimulating a nerve trunk distally and recording more proximally because large CMAPs contaminate the reverse by obscuring the lower-amplitude MNAPs. The MNAP may be of low amplitude or not elicitable when the nerve is deeply situated (as at the elbow or knee) because of tissue interposed between the nerve and the recording electrode. Therefore MNAPs are limited to assessing mixed nerves in distal nerve segments in the hand or foot, such as the mixed palmar and mixed plantar studies used to evaluate carpal tunnel syndrome and tarsal tunnel syndrome, respectively.

## Segmental Stimulation in Short Increments

Routine NCSs are usually sufficient to localize the site of involvement in most patients with entrapment neuropathies. During the evaluation of a focal demyelinating lesion, however, inclusion of the unaffected nerve segment in a relatively long distal latency or conduction velocity calculation dilutes the effect of slowing at the injured site and decreases the sensitivity of the test. Therefore incremental stimulation across a shorter nerve segment is useful to help localize an abnormality that might otherwise escape detection. Localization that is more precise entails "inching" the stimulus in short increments along the course of the nerve. The study of short segments provides better resolution of restricted lesions. For example, a nerve impulse may be found to conduct at a rate of 0.2 ms per 1.0 cm (50 m/sec). For a 1-cm segment, then, demyelination would double the conduction time to 0.4 ms/cm. In a 10-cm segment, normally covered in 2.0 ms, a 0.2-ms increase would constitute a 10% change, or approximately 1 standard deviation, or well within the normal range of variability. However, the same 0.2-ms increase would represent a 100% change in latency if it were measured over a 1-cm segment. The large per-step increase in latency more than compensates for the inherent measurement error associated with stimulating multiple times in short increments.

The inching (or actually "centimetering") technique is particularly useful in assessing nerve conduction in patients with carpal tunnel syndrome or an ulnar neuropathy at the elbow or wrist (McIntosh et al., 1998). For example, stimulation of a normal median nerve in 1-cm increments across the wrist results in latency changes of approximately 0.16–0.21 ms/cm from midpalm to distal forearm (Fig. 36.3). A sharply localized latency increase across a 1-cm segment indicates a focal abnormality of the median nerve (Fig. 36.4). An abrupt change in waveform usually accompanies the latency increase across the site of compression.

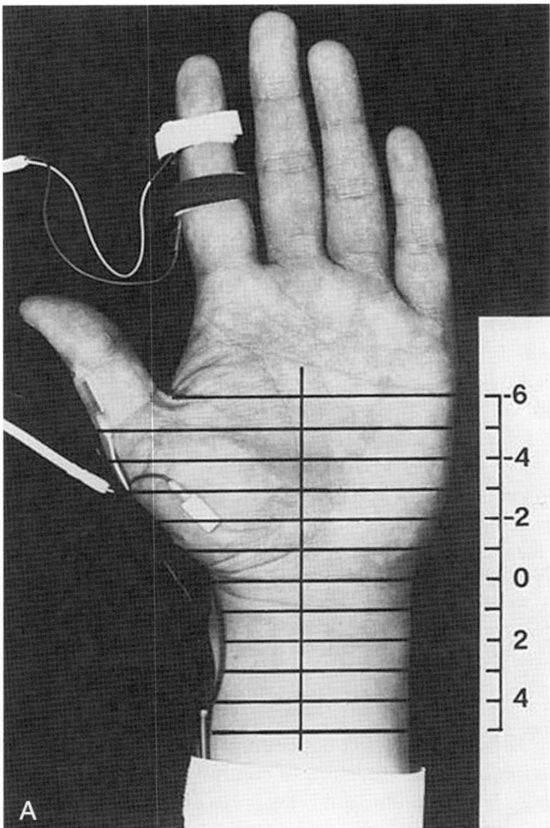


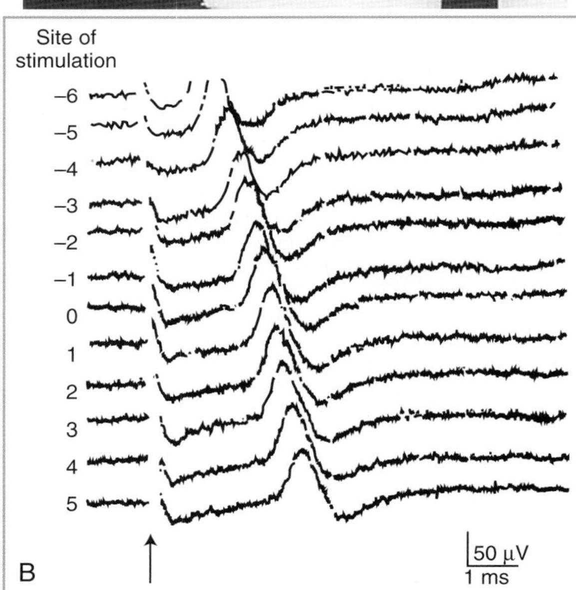


**Fig. 36.3** A, Twelve sites of stimulation in 1-cm increments along the length of the median nerve. The 0 level is at the distal crease of the wrist, corresponding to the origin of the transverse carpal ligament. Sensory nerve action potentials (SNAPs) and compound muscle action potentials are recorded from the second digit and abductor pollicis brevis, respectively. **B,** SNAPs in a normal subject recorded after stimulation of the median nerve at multiple points across the wrist. The site of each stimulus is indicated on the left. The latency changes increased linearly (approximately 0.16–0.21 ms) as the stimulus site was moved proximally in 1-cm increments. (*B, Reprinted with permission of the author and publisher from Kimura, J., 1979. The carpal tunnel syndrome: localization of conduction abnormalities within the distal segment of the median nerve. Brain 102, 619–635. By permission of Oxford University Press.*)

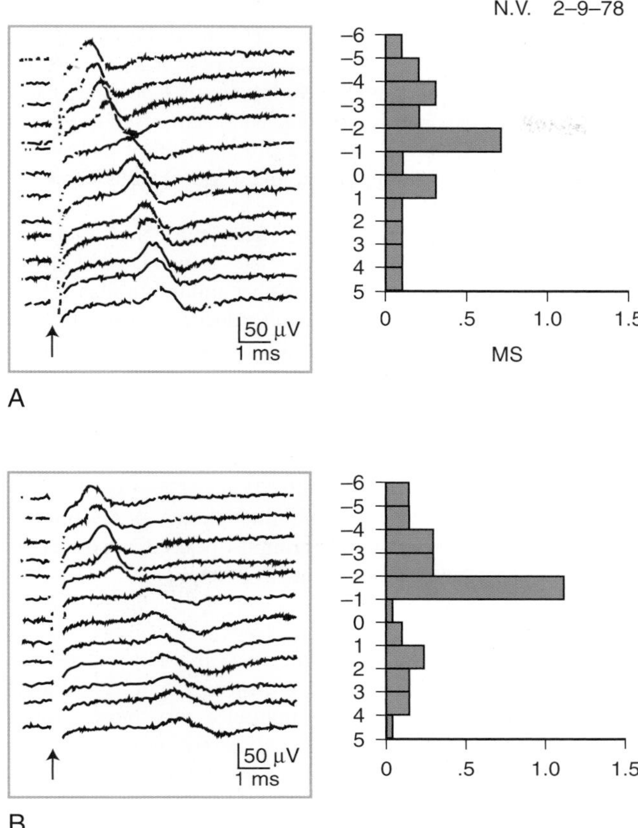


**Fig. 36.4** Sensory nerve action potentials in a patient with bilateral carpal tunnel syndrome (see also Fig. 36.3 for settings). A sharply localized slowing was found from point −2 to point −1 in both hands, with a latency change measuring 0.7 ms on the left (**A**) and 1.1 ms on the right (**B**), compared with the other segments with normal latency changes of approximately 0.16–0.21 ms. Note also a distinct change in waveform of the sensory potential at the point of localized conduction delay. (*Reprinted with permission of the author and publisher from Kimura, J., 1979. The carpal tunnel syndrome: localization of conduction abnormalities within the distal segment of the median nerve. Brain 102, 619–635. By permission of Oxford University Press.*)

## Physiological Variability and Common Sources of Error

The major pitfalls in NCS usually involve technical errors in the stimulating or recording system (Kimura, 1997). Common errors include large stimulus artifact, increased electrode noise, submaximal stimulation, costimulation of an adjacent nerve not under study, eliciting an unwanted potential from distant muscles, recording or reference electrode misplacement, and errors in measurement of nerve lengths and conduction times. Other errors are attributable to intertrial and physiological variability, including the effects of temperature, age, the length of the studied nerve, anomalous innervation, and temporal dispersion.

### Temperature

Nerve impulse propagation slows by 2.4 m/sec, or approximately 5%, per degree centigrade from 38°C to 29°C of body temperature. Also, cooling results in a higher CMAP and SNAP amplitude and longer response duration, probably because of accelerated and slowed sodium channel inactivation (Rutkove et al., 1997). Therefore a CMAP or SNAP with high amplitude and slow distal latency or conduction velocity should raise the suspicion of a cool limb. To reduce this type of variability, a plate thermistor is used to measure skin temperature. This measurement correlates linearly with the subcutaneous and intramuscular temperatures. If the skin temperature falls below 33°C, the limbs are warmed by immersion in warm water or by the application of warming packs or a hydrocollator. Adding 5% of the calculated conduction velocity for each degree below 33°C theoretically normalizes the result. The use of such conversion factors is based on evidence obtained in healthy persons; however, this may not be applicable in patients with abnormal nerves.

### Age

Because myelination is incomplete at birth, nerve conduction velocities are half the adult values in full-term newborns; in 23- to 24-week premature newborns, velocities are one-third the values for term newborns. They attain adult values at 3–5 years. Motor and sensory nerve conduction velocities tend to increase slightly in the arms and decrease in the legs during childhood up to the age of 19 years. Conduction velocities slowly decline after age 50, so the mean conduction velocity is reduced by approximately 10% at 60 years of age.

Aging also diminishes SNAP and CMAP amplitudes, which decline slowly after age 60. SNAP amplitudes are affected more prominently, so much so that normal upper limb SNAP amplitude drops to 50% by age 70 and lower limb SNAPs in many healthy persons older than 60 are low in amplitude or unevokable. Therefore the absence of lower extremity SNAPs in older adults must be interpreted with caution; the finding is not necessarily abnormal without other confirmatory data.

### Height and Nerve Segment Lengths

An inverse relationship between height and nerve conduction velocity suggests that longer nerves conduct more slowly than shorter nerves. For example, the nerve conduction velocities of the peroneal and tibial nerves in the lower extremities are 7–10 m/sec slower than those of the median and ulnar nerves in the upper extremities. The slightly lower temperature of the legs compared with the arms is not the entire explanation. Possible factors accounting for the length-related slowing include abrupt distal axonal tapering, progressive reduction in axonal diameter, and shorter internodal distances. For similar reasons, nerve impulses propagate faster in proximal than in distal nerve segments. Adjustments of normal values are necessary for patients of extreme height; this usually is no more than 2 m/sec below the lower limit of normal.

### Anomalies

Several anomalous peripheral innervations may influence interpretation of the EDX study. Two of these variants, the Martin-Gruber anastomosis and the accessory deep peroneal nerve, have a significant effect on NCSs.

***Martin-Gruber anastomosis.*** In the Martin-Gruber anastomosis, anomalous fibers cross from the median to the ulnar nerve in the forearm. The communicating branches usually consist of motor axons supplying the ulnar innervated intrinsic hand muscles, particularly the first dorsal interosseous muscle, the hypothenar muscles (abductor digiti minimi), and the thenar muscles (adductor pollicis, deep head of flexor pollicis brevis), or a combination of these muscles (Uchida and Sugioka, 1992). The Martin-Gruber anastomosis occurs in approximately 15%–20% of the population and is sometimes bilateral. This anomaly manifests as a drop in the ulnar CMAP amplitude between distal and proximal stimulation sites (simulating the appearance of conduction block on ulnar NCS recording from the abductor digiti minimi or first dorsal interosseous). With distal stimulation (at the wrist), the CMAP reflects all ulnar motor fibers, whereas proximal stimulation activates only the uncrossed fibers, which are fewer in number. This anomaly can be confirmed by median nerve stimulation at the elbow, which evokes a small CMAP from the abductor digiti minimi or first dorsal interosseous, which is not present on median nerve stimulation at the wrist. Although in the majority of subjects the abnormal decline in CMAP amplitude occurs across the forearm segment, this pseudo-conduction block may occasionally be encountered across the elbow segment, resembling partial conduction block in a patient with ulnar neuropathy at the elbow (Whitaker and Felice, 2004). When anomalous fibers innervate the thenar muscles, stimulation of the median nerve at the elbow activates the nerve and the crossing ulnar fibers, resulting in a large CMAP, often with an initial positivity caused by volume conduction of action potential from the ulnar thenar muscles to the median thenar muscles. By contrast, distal median nerve stimulation evokes a smaller thenar CMAP without the positive dip because the crossed fibers are not present at the wrist. In addition, the median nerve conduction velocity in the forearm is spuriously fast, particularly in the presence of carpal tunnel syndrome, because the CMAP onset represents a different population of fibers at the wrist than at the elbow. Collision studies obtain an accurate conduction velocity by using action potentials of the crossed fibers (Sander et al., 1997).

***Accessory deep peroneal nerve.*** About 20%–30% of subjects have an anomalous accessory deep peroneal nerve. It is a branch of the superficial peroneal nerve and usually arises as a continuation of the muscular branch that innervates the peroneus longus and brevis muscles. It passes behind the lateral malleolus and terminates in the extensor digitorum brevis (EDB) on the dorsum of the foot. During peroneal motor NCS recording from the EDB, the peroneal CMAP amplitude is larger-stimulating proximally than distally because the anomalous fibers are not present at the ankle. Stimulation behind the lateral malleolus confirms this anomaly, which yields a small CMAP that approximately equals the difference between the CMAP amplitudes evoked with distal and proximal peroneal nerve stimulations. Complete innervation of the EDB by the accessory deep peroneal nerve is rare but should be suspected if there is preservation of function in the EDB muscle (i.e., extension of lateral toes) in a patient with severe deep peroneal neuropathy (Kayal and Katirji, 2009).

***Pre- and postfixed brachial plexus.*** In most people, the brachial plexus arises from the C5 to T1 cervical roots. In some, the plexus origin shifts one level up (prefixed), arising from C4 to C8; in others, it shifts one level down (postfixed), originating from C6 to T2. These anomalies result in error in the precise localization of cervical root lesions based on myotomal and dermatomal representation. In a prefixed plexus, the location of the cervical lesion is one level higher than concluded from findings on the clinical examination and EDX studies. In contrast, with a postfixed plexus, the cervical root lesion is one level lower.

***Riche-Cannieu anastomosis.*** Riche-Cannieu anastomosis is a communication in the palm between the recurrent motor branch of the median nerve and the deep branch of the ulnar nerve. The result is dual innervation of some intrinsic hand muscles such as the first dorsal interosseous, adductor pollicis, and abductor pollicis brevis. Riche-Cannieu anastomosis is rather common but is often not clinically or electrophysiologically apparent. When this anomaly is prominent, denervation in ulnar muscles may follow a median nerve lesion, and vice versa. In addition, a complete median or ulnar nerve lesion may be associated with relative sparing of some median innervated muscles or ulnar innervated muscles in the hand.

### Temporal Dispersion and Phase Cancellation

The CMAP, evoked by supramaximal stimulation, represents the summation of all individual MUAPs directed to the muscle through the stimulated nerve. Typically, as the stimulus site moves proximally, the CMAP slightly drops in amplitude and area and increases in duration. This is caused by temporal dispersion in which the velocity of impulses in slow-conducting fibers lags increasingly behind those of fast-conducting fibers as conduction distance increases. With dispersion, a slight positive and negative phase overlap occurs, and phase cancellation of MUAP waveforms is seen (Fig. 36.5). The result of temporal dispersion and phase cancellation is a prolongation of CMAP duration, reduction of CMAP amplitude, and a less obvious decrease in CMAP area.

Physiological temporal dispersion affects the SNAP more than the CMAP (Fig. 36.6). This difference relates to two factors. The first relates to the disparity between sensory fiber and motor fiber conduction velocities. The range of conduction velocities between the fastest and slowest individual human myelinated sensory axons is almost twice that for the motor axons (25 m/sec and 12 m/sec, respectively). The second factor is the difference in duration of individual unit discharges between nerve and muscle. With short-duration biphasic or triphasic SNAPs, a slight latency difference could line up the positive peaks of the fast fibers with the negative peaks of the slow fibers and cancel both (Fig. 36.7). In longer-duration biphasic CMAPs, the same latency shift would only partially superimpose peaks of opposite polarity and phase cancellation would be less of a factor.

### Intertrial Variability

Principal factors contributing to an intertrial variability include errors in determining surface distance and measuring latencies and amplitudes of the recorded response. Amplitudes vary most, probably reflecting a shift in the recording site. NCSs are more reproducible when they are administered by the same examiner because there is a significant degree of interexaminer difference (Chaudhry et al., 1991).

## Electrodiagnosis by Nerve Conduction Studies

Although both NCSs and needle EMGs are required in most patients to confirm a neuromuscular diagnosis, certain peripheral nerve disorders are evident on NCSs alone.

### Focal Nerve Lesions

Peripheral nerve is composed of unmyelinated and myelinated axons surrounded by Schwann cells and a supporting tissue. Surrounding the unmyelinated axons are only the plasma membranes of Schwann cells. By contrast, wrapped around myelinated axons are multiple myelin layers that have a low capacitance and large resistance. Surrounding the myelinated axon is myelin, along with Schwann cells, except at certain gaps called the *nodes of Ranvier*, where sodium channels are highly concentrated and saltatory conduction occurs. Three supportive layers—the endoneurium, perineurium, and epineurium—surround nerves; they are highly elastic and protect the myelin and axon from external pressure and tension. Nerve fibers may be injured by a variety of mechanisms, including compression, ischemia, traction, and laceration.

The classification of peripheral nerve lesions is based on the extent of injury to the elements of peripheral nerve, including axon, myelin, and supportive layers. In *neurapraxia (first-degree injury)*, distortion of myelin occurs near the nodes of Ranvier, producing segmental conduction block without wallerian degeneration. In *axonotmesis (second-degree injury)*, the axon is interrupted but all the supporting nerve structures remain intact. In *neurotmesis*, the nerve injury is severe, resulting in complete disruption of the nerve with all the supporting structures (see Chapter 63). Often, the neurotmesis group is divisible into three degrees, as follows: *third-degree injury*, with disruption of the endoneurium and with intact perineurium and epineurium; *fourth-degree injury*, with disruption of all neural elements except the epineurium; and *fifth-degree nerve injury*, with complete nerve transection

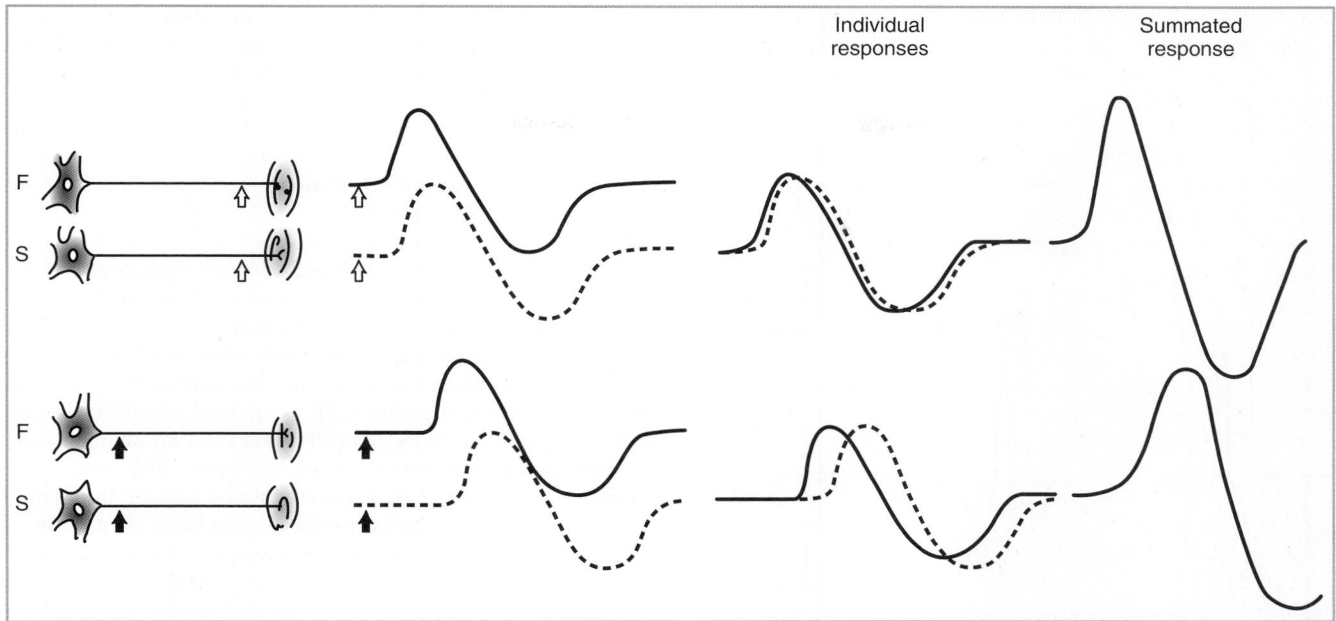


Fig. 36.5 Compound muscle action potentials showing the relationship between fast-conducting *(F)* and slow-conducting *(S)* motor fibers. With distal stimulation *(top)*, two unit discharges representing motor unit potentials sum to produce a muscle action potential twice as large. With proximal stimulation *(bottom)*, motor unit potentials of long duration still superimpose nearly in phase despite the same latency shift of the slow motor fiber. Thus, a physiological temporal dispersion alters the size of the muscle action potential only minimally if at all. Phase cancellation increases substantially when the latency difference between fast- and slow-conducting fibers is increased by a demyelinating neuropathy. This gives the false impression of motor conduction block. (*Reprinted with permission from Kimura, J., Machida, M., Ishida, T., et al., 1986. Relation between size of compound sensory or muscle action potentials and length of nerve segment. Neurology 36, 647–652.*)

resulting in complete discontinuity of the nerve. EDX studies alone cannot accurately distinguish between the five degrees of nerve injuries, but they can separate the first (neurapraxia) from the other axon-loss types (Wilbourn, 2002).

***Demyelinative mononeuropathy.*** When focal injury to myelin occurs, conduction along the affected nerve fibers may alter. This may result in conduction slowing or block along the nerve fibers. The cause of *conduction block* is interruption of action potential transmission across the nerve lesion; it is the electrophysiological correlate of neurapraxia and usually results from loss of more than one myelin segment *(segmental or internodal demyelination)*. Bracketing two stimulation points, one distal and one proximal to the site of injury, best localizes a nerve lesion with conduction block. With such lesions, stimulation distal to the lesion elicits a normal CMAP, whereas proximal stimulation evokes a response with reduced amplitude or fails to evoke any response; these are respectively defined as partial or complete conduction block (Fig. 36.8, *A*). There are several limitations to the diagnosis of demyelinative conduction block:

1. Phase cancellation between peaks of opposite polarity may reduce CMAP size because of abnormally increased temporal dispersion. Such excessive desynchronization often develops in acquired demyelinative neuropathies. If the distal and proximal responses have dissimilar waveforms, the discrepancy in amplitude or area between the two may be the result of phase cancellation rather than conduction block. Therefore, for a diagnosis of partial conduction block, findings should include a significantly lower CMAP amplitude as well as CMAP area with stimulation proximal to the injury site than with the CMAP distal to it, and without any significant prolongation of CMAP duration. More than 50% decay of both the CMAP amplitude and area across the lesion is usually the criterion for definite conduction block.
2. Distal demyelinating lesions causing conduction block of the nerve segment between the most distal stimulating point and the recording site manifest as unelicitable or low CMAP amplitudes at both distal and proximal stimulation sites. This finding mimics the NCSs seen with axonal degeneration. Repeated NCSs often show rapid improvement of CMAP within weeks, consistent with remyelination but not with axonal loss and reinnervation.
3. Conduction block may also follow axonal loss before the completion of wallerian degeneration. This is referred to as axon-loss conduction block, or axon-discontinuity conduction block. Repeated NCSs will show rapid decline of distal CMAP within a week, resulting in equal CMAPs at all points of stimulation (see "Axon-loss mononeuropathy," later).
4. The prominent temporal dispersion normally seen in evaluating SNAPs precludes the use of sensory potentials to diagnose conduction block.

*Focal slowing* of conduction is usually the result of widening of the nodes of Ranvier *(paranodal demyelination)*. Slowing, often synchronized, affects all large myelinated fibers equally. This results in prolongation of distal latency if the focal lesion is distal (see Fig. 36.8, *B, a*), or slowing in conduction velocity if the focal lesion is proximal (see Fig. 36.8, *B, b*). CMAP amplitude, duration, and area, however, are normal and do not change when the nerve is stimulated proximal to the lesion. Desynchronized slowing *(differential slowing)* occurs when conduction velocity reduces at the lesion site along a variable number of the medium-sized or small nerve fibers (average- or slower-conducting axons). Here the CMAP disperses with prolonged duration on stimulations proximal to the lesion. The

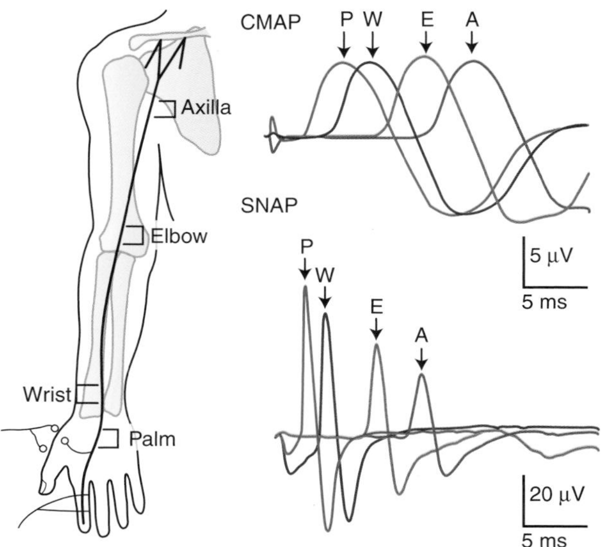


**Fig. 36.6** Simultaneous recordings of compound muscle action potentials *(CMAPs)* from the thenar eminence and sensory nerve action potentials *(SNAPs)* from index finger after stimulation of the median nerve at palm *(P)*, wrist *(W)*, elbow *(E)*, and axilla *(A)*. With progressively more proximal stimulation, CMAPs remained nearly the same; for SNAPs, however, both amplitude and the area under the waveform became much smaller.

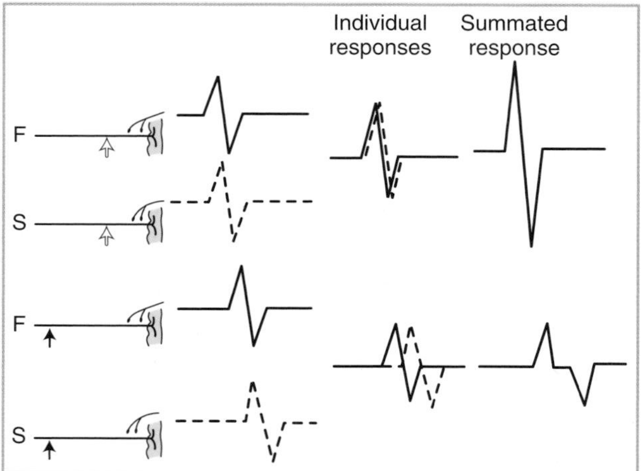


**Fig. 36.7 Sensory Nerve Action Potentials.** A model for phase cancellation between fast-conducting *(F)* and slow-conducting *(S)* sensory fibers. With distal stimulation *(top)*, two unit discharges sum in phase to produce a sensory action potential twice as large. With proximal stimulation *(bottom)*, a delay of the slow fiber causes phase cancellation between the negative peak of the fast fiber and positive peak of the slow fiber, resulting in a 50% reduction in size of the summated response. *(Reprinted with permission from Kimura, J., Machida, M., Ishida, T., et al., 1986. Relation between size of compound sensory or muscle action potentials and length of nerve segment. Neurology 36, 647–652.)*

speed of conduction along the injury site (latency or conduction velocity) is normal because of sparing of at least some of the fastest-conducting axons (see Fig. 36.8, *C*). When synchronized and desynchronized slowing coexist, slowing of distal latency or conduction velocity accompanies the dispersed CMAP with prolonged duration.

***Axon-loss mononeuropathy.*** After acute focal axonal damage, the distal nerve segment undergoes wallerian degeneration. Characteristically, unelicitable or low CMAP amplitudes with distal and proximal stimulations are signs of complete or partial lesions, respectively, involving motor axonal loss. The CMAP amplitudes provide a reliable estimate of the amount of axonal loss except in the chronic phase, in which effective reinnervation via collateral sprouting may increase the CMAP and give a misleadingly low estimate of the extent of original axonal loss.

In partial axon-loss lesions, distal latencies and conduction velocities are normal or borderline. Selective loss of fast-conducting fibers associated with more than a 50% reduction in mean CMAP amplitude may slow conduction velocity up to 80% of the normal value because the velocity represents the remaining slow-conducting fibers. Motor conduction velocity may slow to 70% of normal value with a reduction of CMAP amplitude to less than 10% of the lower limit of normal.

Soon after axonal transection (i.e., for the first 48 hours), the distal axon remains excitable. Therefore stimulation distal to the lesion elicits a normal CMAP, whereas proximal stimulation elicits a response with reduced amplitude and area, producing a conduction block pattern (see Fig. 36.8, *D, middle panel*). This pattern is axonal noncontinuity, early axon loss, or axon-discontinuity conduction block. Soon, however, the distal axons undergo wallerian degeneration, and the distal CMAP decreases in size to equal the proximal CMAP (see Fig. 36.8, *D, lower panel*). With wallerian degeneration, the distal CMAP decreases in amplitude and area starting 1 or 2 days after nerve injury and reaches its nadir in 5–6 days. In contrast, the distal SNAP lags slightly behind and reaches its nadir in 10 or 11 days (Fig. 36.9). The difference between the decline of the SNAP and CMAP amplitudes and areas after axon loss probably relates to neuromuscular transmission failure, which affects only the CMAP amplitude and area. Supporting this hypothesis is the fact that MNAPs recorded directly from nerve trunks follow the time course of SNAPs.

The study is repeated after 10 or 11 days, when degenerating axons have lost excitability, to distinguish between conduction block due to demyelination and that due to axonal loss. A reduction in amplitude and area of the evoked potential from stimulation above and below the lesion indicates axonal loss (see Fig. 36.8, *D*). By contrast, if the distally evoked CMAP still has preserved amplitude and area greater than that of the proximally elicited response, it indicates partial segmental demyelination.

Identification of conduction block in the early days of axonal loss is extremely helpful in localizing a peripheral nerve injury, particularly the closed type in which the exact site of lesion is not apparent. Awaiting the completion of wallerian degeneration leads to diffusely low or unevokable CMAPs (regardless of stimulation site), which does not allow accurate localization of the injury site. Needle EMG study is useful, but localization by this method is suboptimal (see later discussion).

***Preganglionic (intraspinal canal) lesions.*** Damage to the sensory axons in the nerve roots located proximal to the dorsal root ganglion does not affect the SNAP amplitude because the peripheral sensory axons originating from the unipolar dorsal root ganglion neurons remain intact. Because the dorsal root ganglia are usually located outside the spinal canal and within the intervertebral foramina, intraspinal canal lesions involving axonal loss (such as radiculopathies or root avulsions) have no effect on SNAP amplitudes. However, these nerve root lesions often result in the degeneration of motor axons, as reflected by abnormal needle EMG findings and, when severe, by CMAPs of low amplitude and area. In contrast to intraspinal canal lesions that are preganglionic, extraspinal lesions with axonal loss (such as plexopathies) are postganglionic and, when mixed nerves

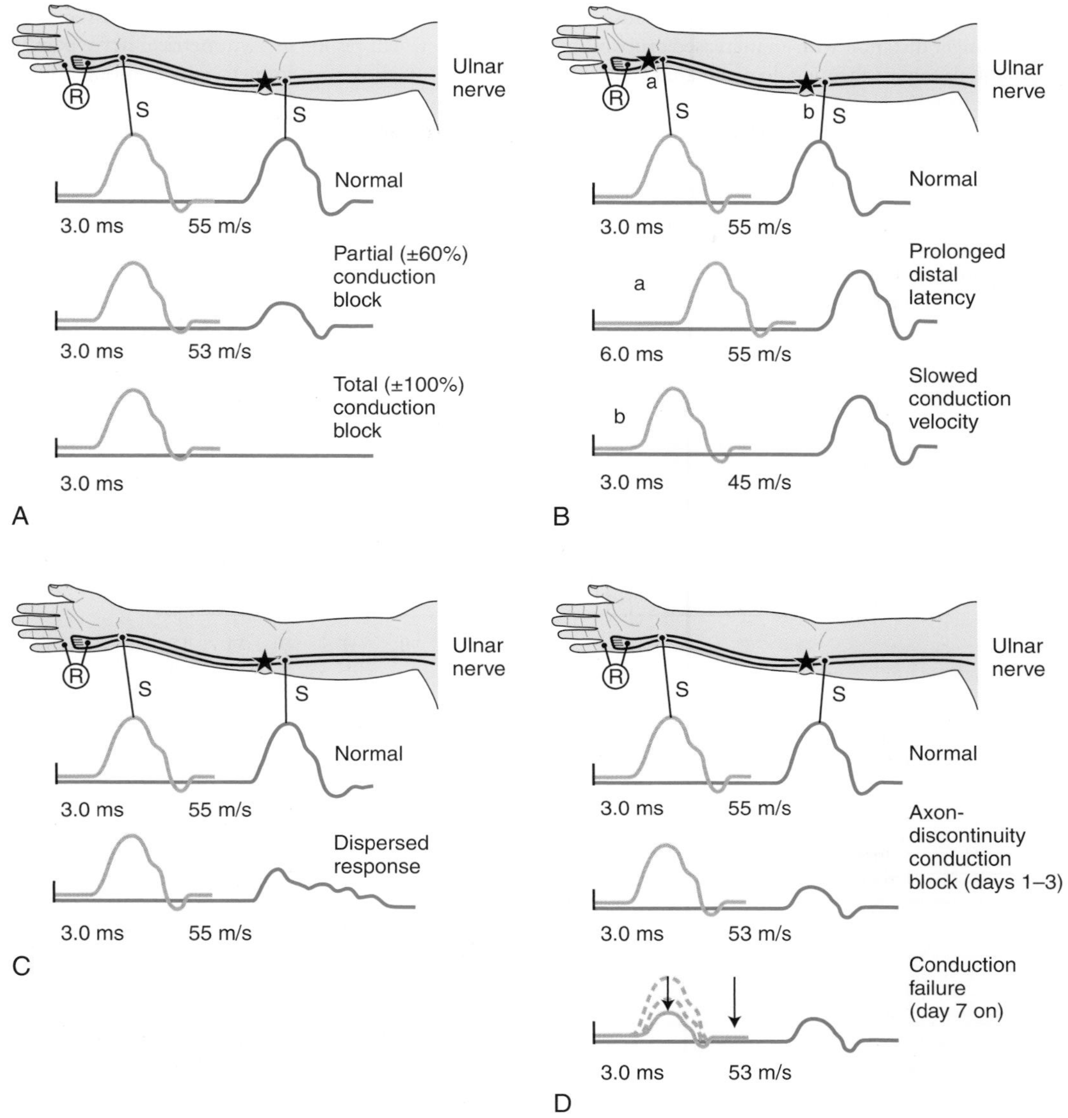


**Fig. 36.8 Findings on Nerve Conduction Studies. A,** Demyelinative conduction block. Note the proximal compound muscle action potential (CMAP) is either low in amplitude (partial block) or absent (complete block). **B,** Focal synchronized slowing of the distal nerve segment *(a)* or the proximal nerve segment *(b)*. **C,** Focal desynchronized slowing of the forearm nerve segment, resulting in significant dispersion of the proximal CMAP. **D,** Axon loss (partial), studied early and late after nerve trauma. *R,* Recording; *S,* stimulation. (*Reprinted with permission from Wilbourn, A.J., 2002. Nerve conduction studies. Types, components, abnormalities and value in localization. Neurol Clin 20, 305–338.*)

undergo wallerian degeneration, affect the CMAP as well as the SNAP amplitudes.

## Generalized Polyneuropathies

NCSs are essential in diagnosing peripheral polyneuropathies. They are very useful for endorsing the diagnosis or suggesting alternative diagnoses such as small-fiber sensory neuropathies or entrapment neuropathies. When confirmed, NCSs will also aid in establishing the types of fibers affected (large-fiber sensory, motor, or both). Of greatest importance, NCSs often identify the primary pathological process of the various polyneuropathies: axonopathy (axonal degeneration) versus myelinopathy (segmental demyelination). This helps greatly in identifying the cause of the polyneuropathy (Fig. 36.10, A, B & C).

***Axonal polyneuropathies.*** Axonal polyneuropathies produce length-dependent dying-back degeneration of axons. The major change on NCS is decrease of the CMAP and SNAP amplitudes and areas, more marked in the lower extremities. By contrast, conduction velocities and distal latencies are usually normal (Fig. 36.10, *B*). As with axonal loss mononeuropathies, selective loss of many fast-conducting fibers associated with more than a 50% reduction in CMAP amplitude may slow conduction velocity to more than 70%–80% of normal value.

***Demyelinating polyneuropathies.*** The hallmark of demyelinating polyneuropathies is a widespread increase in conduction time caused by impaired saltatory conduction. Therefore NCS findings are characterized by significant slowing of conduction velocities (<70% of the lower limit of normal) and distal latencies (>130% of the upper limit of normal). With distal stimulation, demyelination delays the distal latency and there is usually a moderate reduction of the CMAP amplitude because of abnormal temporal dispersion and phase cancellation. With proximal stimulation, the CMAP amplitude is lower and the proximal conduction velocity markedly slows because the action potentials travel a longer distance, with an increased probability for the nerve action potentials to pass through demyelinated segments (see Fig. 36.10, *C*). The proximal CMAP amplitude and/or area decay is the result of more prominent temporal dispersion and phase cancellation as well as possible conduction block along some fibers.

NCSs further separate chronic demyelinating polyneuropathies into inherited and acquired polyneuropathies. Characteristic of inherited demyelinating polyneuropathies, such as Charcot-Marie-Tooth disease type I, is uniform slowing, resulting in symmetrical abnormalities as well as the absence of conduction blocks. By contrast, acquired demyelinating polyneuropathies, such as chronic inflammatory demyelinating polyneuropathy, are often associated with nonuniform slowing, which results in asymmetrical nerve conductions even in the absence of clinical asymmetry. In addition, multifocal conduction blocks and excessive temporal dispersions at nonentrapment sites are characteristic of acquired demyelinating polyneuropathies.

In the most common form of Guillain-Barré syndrome, acute inflammatory demyelinating polyneuropathy, multifocal demyelination that fulfills the criteria for demyelination is evident in 35%–50% of patients during the first 2 weeks of illness, compared with 85% by the third week (Al-Shekhlee et al., 2005; Albers et al., 1985). Two other suggestive nerve conduction findings in this disorder are (1) abnormal upper extremity SNAPs with normal sural SNAPs (called *sural sparing pattern*), an unusual

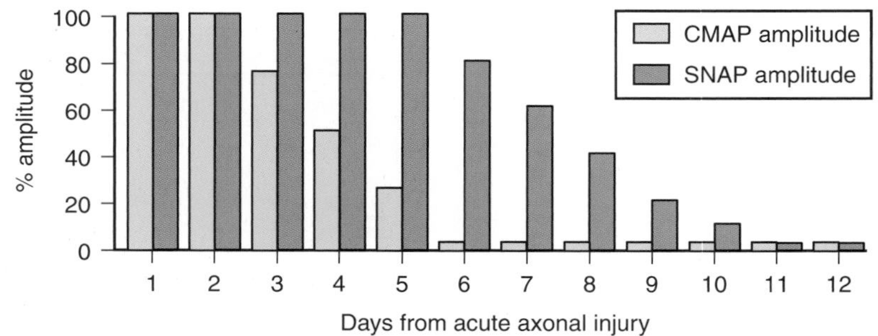


**Fig. 36.9** Distal compound muscle action potential *(CMAP)* and sensory nerve action potential *(SNAP)* amplitudes during wallerian degeneration after an acute axonal nerve injury. (*Reprinted with permission from Katirji, B., 2018. Electromyography in Clinical Practice: A Case Study Approach, third ed. Oxford University Press, New York.*)

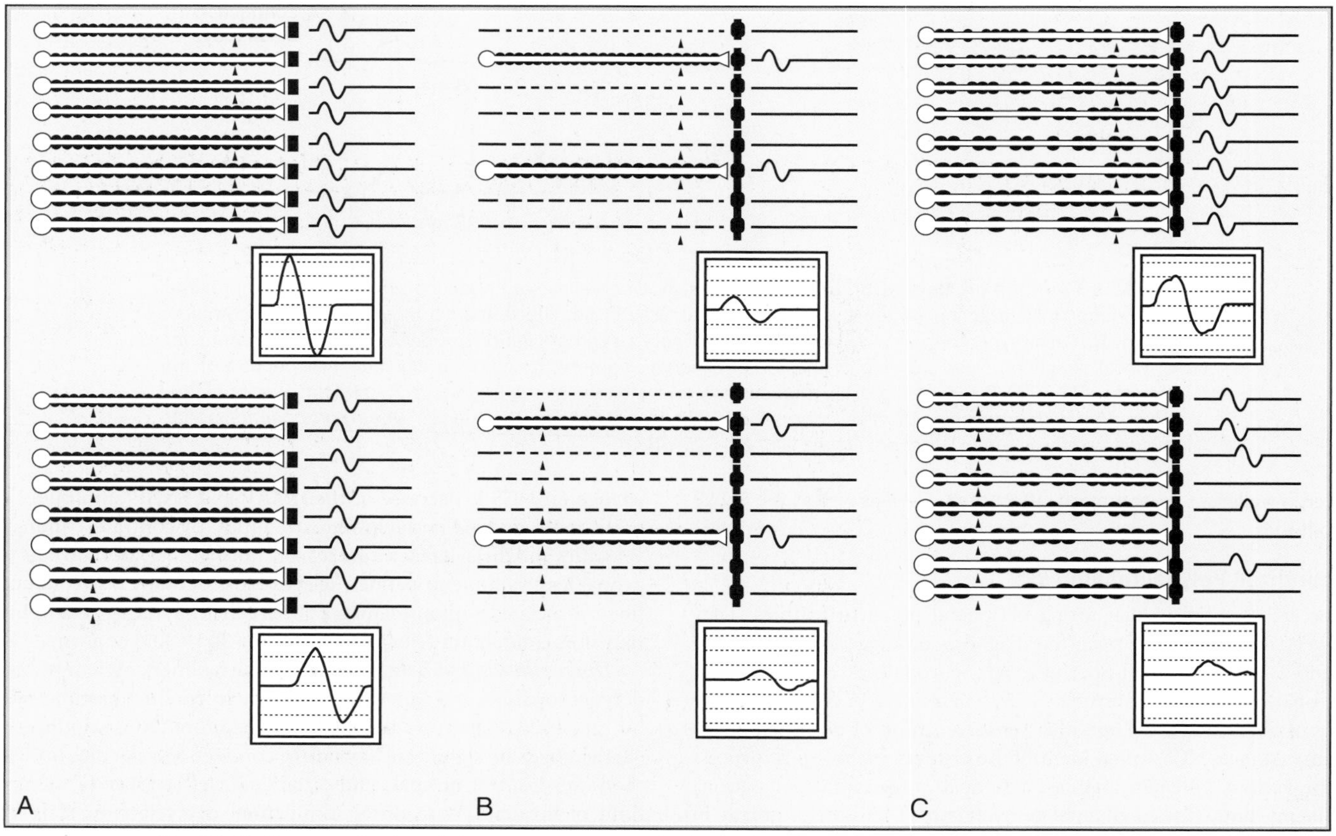

A B C

**Fig. 36.10** Computerized model of motor nerve conduction study of a peripheral nerve. **A,** Normal nerve. **B,** Nerve after axonal degeneration. **C,** Nerve with segmental demyelination. (*Reprinted with permission from Brown, W.F., Bolton, C.F. [Eds], 1989. Clinical Electromyography. Butterworth-Heinemann, Boston.*)

pattern in axonal length–dependent polyneuropathy, and (2) diffuse absence of F waves with normal results on motor conduction studies, findings consistent with proximal peripheral nerve or spinal root involvement.

## NEEDLE ELECTROMYOGRAPHIC EXAMINATION

### Principles and Techniques

The motor unit consists of a single motor neuron and all the muscle fibers it innervates. A single motor unit innervates either type I or type II muscle fibers but never both. All muscle fibers in one motor unit discharge simultaneously when stimulated by synaptic input to the lower motor neuron (LMN) or by electrical stimulation of the axon. The ratio of muscle fibers per motor neuron *(innervation ratio or motor unit size)* is variable and ranges from 3 to 1 for extrinsic eye muscles to several thousand to 1 for large limb muscles. The smaller ratio is generally characteristic of muscles that perform fine gradations of movement. The distribution of a single motor unit's muscle fibers in a muscle is wide, with significant overlap between different motor units.

The muscle fiber has a resting potential of 90 mV, with negativity inside the cell. The generation of an action potential reverses the transmembrane potential, which then becomes positive inside the cell. An extracellular electrode, as used in needle EMG, records the activity resulting from this switch of polarity as a predominantly negative potential (usually triphasic, positive-negative-positive waveforms). When they are recorded near a damaged region, however, action potentials consist of a large positivity followed by a small negativity.

Concentric and Teflon-coated monopolar needle electrodes are equally satisfactory in recording muscle potentials, with little appreciable difference. Although monopolar needles are less painful, they require an additional reference electrode placed nearby, which often results in greater electrical noise caused by electrode impedance mismatch between the intramuscular active electrode and the surface reference disk.

The electromyographer first identifies the needle insertion point by recognizing the proper anatomical landmark and the activation maneuver for the sampled muscle. Needle EMG evaluation requires appreciation of the following technical considerations:

1. Inserting or slightly moving the needle causes insertional activity that results from needle injury of muscle fibers.
2. Moving the needle a small distance and pausing a few seconds assesses spontaneous activity in relaxed muscle. From a single cutaneous insertion, relocating the needle in four quadrants of the muscle completes the evaluations.
3. Minimal contraction assesses the morphology of several MUAPs measured on the screen. The needle should be moved slightly (pulled back or moved deeper) if sharp MUAPs are not seen with minimal contraction.
4. Increasing the intensity of muscle contraction assesses the recruitment pattern of MUAPs. Maximal contraction normally fills the screen, producing the interference pattern.

An amplification of 50 μV per division best defines the insertional and spontaneous activity, whereas 200 μV per division is suited for voluntary activity. Most laboratories use a screen with sweep speeds of 10–20 ms per division for insertional, spontaneous, and voluntary activities.

### Insertional and Spontaneous Activity

#### Normal Insertional and Spontaneous Activity

Brief bursts of electrical discharges accompany insertion and repositioning of a needle electrode into the muscle, slightly outlasting the movement of the needle. On average, insertional activity lasts for a few hundred milliseconds. It appears as a cluster of positive or negative repetitive high-frequency spikes, which make a crisp static sound over the loudspeaker.

At rest, muscle is silent, with no spontaneous activity except in the motor end-plate region, the site of neuromuscular junctions, which are usually located along a line crossing the center of the muscle belly. Table 36.1 lists normal and abnormal insertional and spontaneous activities (Katirji et al., 2014). Two types of normal end-plate

**TABLE 36.1 Insertional and Spontaneous Activity on Needle Electromyography**

| Potential | Source Generator and Morphology | Sound on Loudspeaker | Stability | Firing Rate (Hz) | Firing Pattern |
|---|---|---|---|---|---|
| End-plate noise | Miniature end-plate potentials (monophasic negative) | Seashell | — | 20–40 | Irregular (hissing) |
| End-plate spike | Muscle fiber initiated by terminal axonal twig (brief spike, diphasic, initial negative) | Sputtering fat in a frying pan | — | 5–50 | Irregular (sputtering) |
| Fibrillation (brief spike) | Muscle fiber (brief spike, diphasic or triphasic, initial positive) | Rain on a tin roof or tick-tock of a clock | Stable | 0.5–10 (occasionally up to 30) | Regular |
| Positive sharp wave | Muscle fiber (diphasic, initial positive, slow negative) | Dull pops, rain on a tin roof, or tick-tock of a clock | Stable | 0.5–10 (occasionally up to 30) | Regular |
| Myotonia | Muscle fiber (brief spike, initial positive, or positive wave) | Revving engine or dive bomber | Waxing and waning amplitude | 20–150 | Waxing and waning |
| Complex repetitive discharge | Multiple muscle fibers time-linked together | Machine or motorcycle on highway | Usually stable, may change in discrete jumps | 5–100 | Perfectly regular |
| Fasciculation | Motor unit (motor neuron or axon) | Corn popping | | Low (0.1–10) | Irregular |
| Myokymia | Motor unit (motor neuron or axon) | Marching soldiers | | 1–5 (interburst), 5–60 (intraburst) | Bursting |
| Cramp | Motor unit (motor neuron or axon) | | — | High (20–150) | Interference pattern or several individual units |
| Neuromyotonia | Motor unit (motor neuron or axon) | Pinging | Decrementing amplitude | Very high (150–250) | Waning |

*Adapted with permission from Katirji, B., Kaminski, H.J., Ruff, R.L. (Eds), 2014. Neuromuscular Disorders in Clinical Practice. Springer, New York.*

spontaneous activity occur together or independently: end-plate noise and end-plate spikes (Fig. 36.11).

***End-plate noise (see Video 36.1).*** The tip of the needle approaching the end-plate region often registers recurring irregular negative potentials, 10–50 μV in amplitude and 1–2 ms in duration. These potentials are the extracellularly recorded miniature end-plate potentials, or nonpropagating depolarizations caused by spontaneous release of acetylcholine quanta. They produce a characteristic sound on the loudspeaker much like that of a seashell held to the ear.

***End-plate spikes (see Video 36.2).*** End-plate spikes are intermittent spikes, 100–200 μV in amplitude and 3–4 ms in duration, firing irregularly at 5–50 impulses per second. Their characteristic waveform (initial negative deflection) and irregular firing pattern distinguish them from the regular-firing fibrillation potentials. Furthermore, they are often associated with end-plate noise and sound on the loudspeaker like that of sputtering fat in a frying pan. The end-plate spikes are discharges of single muscle fibers generated by activation of intramuscular nerve terminals irritated by the needle. The similarity of the firing pattern of end-plate spikes to discharges of muscle spindle afferents suggests that they may originate in the intrafusal muscle fibers.

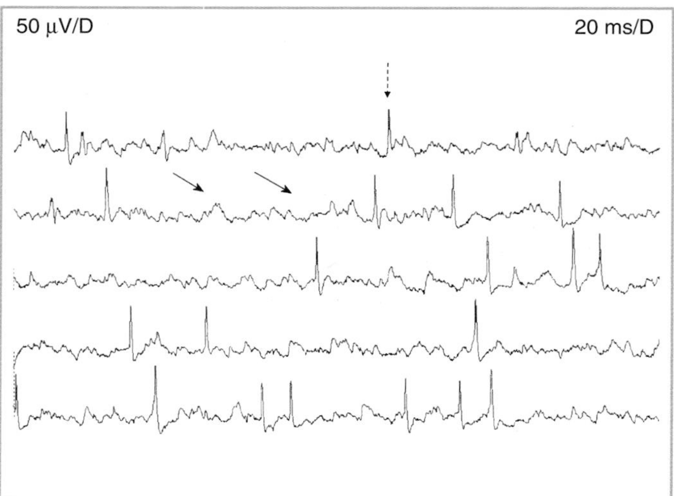


**Fig. 36.11** End-plate noise *(solid arrows)* and spikes *(dashed arrow)* representing normal spontaneous activities.

## Abnormal Insertional and Spontaneous Activity

***Prolonged versus decreased insertional activity.*** An abnormally prolonged (increased) insertional activity indicates instability of the muscle membrane, as is often seen in conjunction with denervation, myotonic disorders, or necrotizing myopathies such as inflammatory myopathies. Insertional positive waves, initiated by needle movements only and identical to the spontaneous discharges, may follow the increased insertional activity and last for a few seconds. This isolated activity usually signals early denervation of muscle fibers, such as occurs 1–2 weeks after acute loss of motor axons. A marked reduction or absence of insertional activity suggests either fibrotic or severely atrophied muscle or functionally inexcitable muscle, as during the paralytic attack of periodic paralysis.

A benign increased insertional activity, named by Wilbourn as "snap, crackle, pop" because of its characteristic sound, is a normal variant recorded from muscles of some healthy individuals (Daube and Rubin, 2009; Wilbourn 1982). This finding has no clinical significance when seen as an isolated finding but may be mistaken for abnormal types of increased insertional activity. It is much more common in men, particularly those who are well built and muscular. It is seen more often in the leg muscles than the arm muscles, most commonly in the gastrocnemius.

***Fibrillation potentials (see Video 36.3).*** Fibrillation potentials are spontaneous action potentials of denervated muscle fibers. They result from reduction of the resting membrane potential of the denervated muscle fiber to the level at which it can fire spontaneously. Fibrillation potentials, triggered by spontaneous oscillations in the muscle fiber membrane potential, typically fire in a regular pattern at a rate of 1–30 Hz. The sound they produce on the loudspeaker is crisp and clicking, reminiscent of rain on a tin roof or the tick-tock of a clock. Fibrillation potentials have two types of waveforms: brief spikes and positive waves. *Brief spikes* are usually triphasic with initial positivity (Fig. 36.12, *A*). They range from 1 to 5 ms in duration and 20–200 μV in amplitude when recorded with a concentric needle electrode. Brief-spike fibrillation potentials may be confused with physiological end-plate spikes but are distinguishable by their regular firing pattern and triphasic configuration with an initial positivity. Occasionally placement of the needle electrode near the end-plate zone of a denervated muscle results in brief spikes, morphologically resembling end-plate spikes with an initial negativity. *Positive waves* have an initial positivity and subsequent slow negativity with a characteristic saw tooth appearance (see Fig. 36.12, *B*). Recordings made near the damaged part of the muscle fiber (incapable of generating an action potential) account for the absence of a negative spike. Although usually seen together, positive sharp waves tend to precede brief spikes after nerve section, possibly because insertion of a needle in already irritable muscle membrane triggers the response.

Fibrillation potentials are the electrophysiological markers of muscle denervation. Based on their distribution, they are useful in localizing lesions to the anterior horn cells of the spinal cord, ventral root, plexus, or peripheral nerve. Insertional positive waves may appear within 2 weeks of acute denervation, but fibrillation potentials do not become full until approximately 3 weeks after axonal loss. Because of this latent period, their absence does not exclude recent acute denervation. In addition, late in the course of denervation, muscle fibers that are reinnervated, fibrotic, or severely atrophied show no fibrillation potentials. A numerical grading system (from 0 to 4) is the standard to semiquantitate fibrillation potentials. Their density is a rough estimate of the extent of denervated muscle fibers: 0, no fibrillations; +1, persistent single trains of potentials (<2 seconds) in at least two areas; +2, moderate number of potentials in three or more areas; +3, many potentials in all areas; +4, abundant spontaneous potentials nearly filling the screen.

Fibrillation potentials also occur in necrotizing myopathies such as the inflammatory myopathies and muscular dystrophies. The probable causes are (1) segmental necrosis of muscle fiber together with its central section (region of myoneural junction), leading to effective denervation of its distant muscle fiber segments as they become physically separated from the neuromuscular junction; (2) reduction of the resting membrane potential of partially damaged fibers to the level that allows spontaneous discharges to occur; and (3) damage to the terminal intramuscular motor axons, presumably by the inflammatory process, resulting in muscle fiber denervation. In disorders of the neuromuscular junction such as MG and botulism, fibrillation potentials are rare; when they are present, the explanation is a prolonged

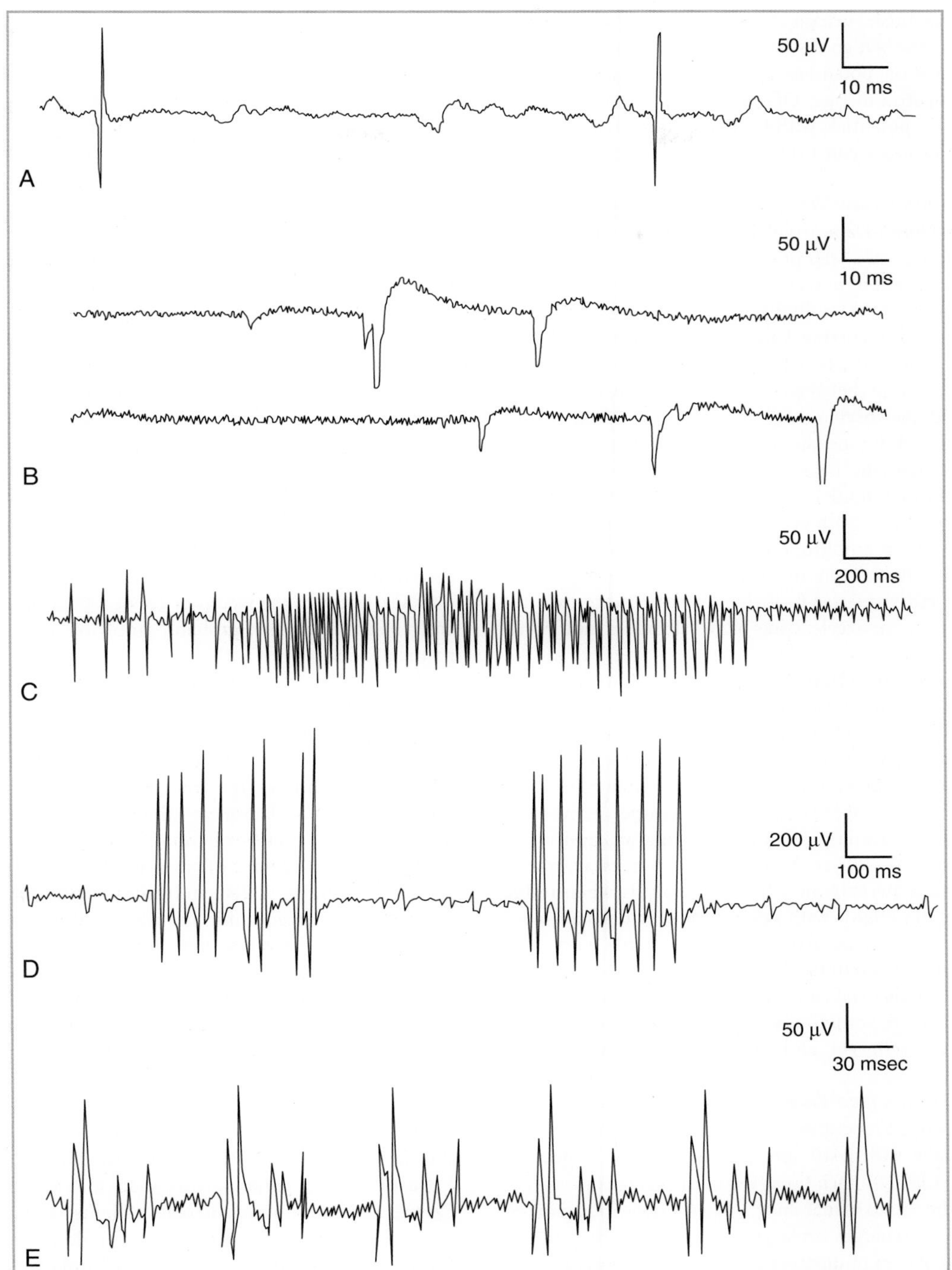


**Fig. 36.12 Abnormal Insertional Activities. A,** Brief spike fibrillation potentials. **B,** Positive waves. **C,** Myotonic discharge. **D,** Myokymic discharge. **E,** Complex repetitive discharge. (*Reprinted with permission from Preston, D.C., Shapiro, B.E., 2013. Electromyography and Neuromuscular Disorders, third ed., Elsevier/Saunders, Philadelphia..*)

neuromuscular transmission blockade resulting in effective denervation of muscle fibers.

***Fasciculation potentials (see Video 36.4).*** Fasciculation potentials are spontaneous discharges of a motor unit. They originate from the motor neuron or anywhere along its axon. Fasciculation potentials fire randomly and irregularly and undergo slight changes in amplitude and waveform from time to time, giving them a corn-popping sound on the loudspeaker. They have a much lower firing rate than that of voluntary MUAPs and are unaffected by slight voluntary contraction of agonist or antagonist muscles.

Fasciculation potentials are most common in diseases of anterior horn cells but also occur in radiculopathies, entrapment neuropathies, peripheral polyneuropathies, and the cramp fasciculation syndrome. Other causes are tetany, thyrotoxicosis, and overdose of anticholinesterase medication. In addition, they may occur in healthy people and are considered a normal variant when seen in isolation. No reliable method exists to distinguish "benign" from "malignant" fasciculation potentials except that the benign discharges tend to fire more quickly, and grouped fasciculation potentials from multiple units are more common in motor neuron disease. Of greatest importance, the association of fasciculation potentials with fibrillation potentials or other neurogenic MUAP changes constitutes strong evidence of a LMN disorder.

***Myotonic discharges (see Video 36.5, available at).*** Myotonic discharge, a special type of abnormal insertional activity, appears either as a sustained run of sharp positive waves, each followed by a slow negative component of longer duration, or as a sustained run of negative spikes with a small initial positivity (see Fig. 36.12, *C*). Myotonic discharges are recurring single-fiber potentials showing, as with fibrillation potentials, two types of waveforms depending on the spatial relationship between the recording surface of the needle electrode and the discharging muscle fibers. When muscle membranes are injured by needle insertion, positive waves are usually initiated, whereas the negative spikes, resembling the brief spike form of fibrillation potentials, tend to occur at the beginning of slight volitional contraction. Both positive waves and negative spikes typically wax and wane in amplitude over the range of 10 μV to 1 mV, varying inversely to the rate of firing. Their frequency ranges from 20 to 150 Hz and gives rise to a characteristic noise over the loudspeaker, simulating an accelerating or decelerating motorcycle or chainsaw.

Myotonic discharges are often abundant, with or without grip or percussion myotonia on clinical examination, in the myotonic dystrophies (types I and II), myotonia congenita, sodium channel myotonias, and paramyotonia congenita. They may also accompany other myopathies such as acid maltase deficiency (Pompe disease), myotubular myopathy, Schwartz-Jampel syndrome (chondrodystrophic myotonia), colchicine myopathy, and statin myopathy (Shapiro et al., 2014). Myotonic discharges are rarely seen in patients with hyperkalemic periodic paralysis when tested between attacks and in patients with polymyositis or dermatomyositis. They are reported in muscular dystrophy patients with caveolin-3 mutation (limb girdle muscular dystrophy type 1C; Milone et al., 2012). Rarely, single brief runs may be encountered in neurogenic disorders. These are sometimes referred to as myotonic-like or pseudomyotonic discharges and are never the predominant waveform.

***Myokymic discharges (see Video 36.6).*** Myokymia results from complex bursts of grouped repetitive discharges in which motor units fire repetitively, usually with 2–10 spikes discharging at a mean of 30–40 Hz (see Fig. 36.12, *D*). Each burst recurs at regular intervals of 1–5 seconds, giving the sound of marching soldiers on the loudspeaker. Clinically, myokymic discharges often give rise to sustained muscle contractions, which have an undulating ("*bag of worms*") appearance beneath the skin. The origin of myokymic discharges is probably ectopic in motor nerve fibers and amplified by increased axonal excitability, as after hyperventilation-induced hypocarbia.

Myokymic discharges in facial muscles are associated with brainstem glioma or multiple sclerosis (MS) or seen in the delayed phases of Bell palsy and Guillain-Barré syndrome. In limb muscles, myokymia may be focal, as with radiation plexopathies and carpal tunnel syndrome, or diffuse, as with Guillain-Barré syndrome, chronic inflammatory demyelinating polyneuropathy, gold intoxication, or thyrotoxicosis. Myokymic discharges often accompany neuromyotonic discharges in peripheral nerve hyperexcitability (PNH) syndromes, including Isaacs and Morgan syndromes (Jamieson and Katirji, 1994; Sawlani and Katirji, 2017).

***Complex repetitive discharges (see Video 36.7).*** A complex repetitive discharge results from the nearly synchronous firing of a group of muscle fibers. One fiber in the complex serves as a pacemaker, driving one or several other fibers ephaptically so that the individual spikes in the complex fire in the same order in which the discharge recurs. One of the late-activated fibers reexcites the principal pacemaker to repeat the cycle. The entire sequence recurs at a slow or fast rate, usually in the range of 5–100 Hz. The discharge ranges from 50 μV to 1 mV in amplitude and up to 50–1000 ms in duration. The complex waveform contains several distinct spikes and remains uniform from one discharge to another (see Fig. 36.12, *E*). These discharges typically begin abruptly, maintain a constant rate of firing for a short period, and cease as abruptly as they started when the chain reaction eventually blocks. They produce a noise on the loudspeaker that mimics the sound of a machine or a motorcycle.

Complex repetitive discharges are abnormal discharges but are less specific than other spontaneous discharges. They occur most often in myopathies but also occur in some neuropathic disorders such as radiculopathies. They most commonly accompany chronic conditions but are occasionally observed in subacute disorders. They may also occur in the iliacus or cervical paraspinal muscles of apparently healthy persons, probably implying a clinically silent neuropathic process.

***Neuromyotonic discharges (see Video 36.8).*** Neuromyotonic discharges are extremely rare discharges in which muscle fibers fire repetitively with a high intraburst frequency (40–350 Hz), either continuously or in recurring decrementing bursts, producing a pinging sound on the loudspeaker. The discharges are more prominent in distal than proximal muscles, probably implicating the terminal branches of motor axons as the site of generation (Maddison et al., 2006). Most cases of acquired neuromyotonia are associated with the PNH syndromes, including Isaacs and Morgan syndromes (Ahmed and Simmons, 2015; Sawlani and Katirji, 2017). In these disorders, neuromyotonia is often intermixed with diffuse myokymic discharges, fasciculation potentials, and cramp discharges. PNH syndromes are autoimmune antibody-mediated peripheral nerve voltage-gated potassium channelopathies that also include also limbic encephalitis and cramp-fasciculation syndrome, both sometimes exhibiting neuromyotonic discharges. It is now clear that the voltage-gated potassium channel antibodies are directed to the channel-associated proteins, mostly leucine-rich glioma inactivated 1 (LGI1) and contactin-associated protein-like 2 (Caspr2). Most patients with Isaacs and Morgan syndromes have Caspr2 autoimmunity, whereas patients with limbic encephalitis have LGI1 autoimmunity (Jammoul et al., 2016). Other conditions that may be associated with neuromyotonia include episodic ataxia type 1 and, rarely, chronic spinal muscular atrophies.

***Cramp discharges (see Video 36.9).*** A muscle cramp is a sustained involuntary muscle contraction. On needle EMG studies, cramp discharge consists of MUAPs usually firing at a rate of 40 to 60 Hz, with abrupt onset and cessation. Cramps most often occur in healthy people, but hyponatremia, hypocalcemia, hypomagnesemia, myxedema, pregnancy, postdialysis state, and the early stages of motor neuron disease exaggerate their frequency. Clinically, cramps may resemble muscle contractures accompanying several metabolic muscle diseases, but complete electrical silence on the needle EMG is characteristic of these contractures.

## Voluntary Motor Unit Action Potentials

### Morphology of Motor Unit Action Potentials (see Videos 36.10–36.13)

MUAP is the extracellular electrode recording of a small portion of a motor unit. The inherent properties of the motor unit and the spatial relationships between the needle tip and individual muscle fibers dictate the waveform. Slight repositioning of the electrode changes the electrical profile of the same motor unit. Therefore one motor unit can give rise to MUAPs of different morphology at different recording sites. Amplitude, duration, and number of phases characterize the MUAP waveform.

***Amplitude.*** MUAP amplitude is the maximum peak-to-peak amplitude. It ranges from several hundred microvolts to a few millivolts with a concentric needle and is substantially greater with a monopolar needle. The amplitude of an MUAP decreases to less than 50% at a distance of 200–300 μm from the source and to less than 1% a few millimeters away. Therefore the amplitude depends on the proximity of the tip of the needle electrode to the muscle fibers. Only a small number of individual muscle fibers located near the tip of the electrode determine the amplitude of an MUAP (probably less than 20 muscle fibers lying within a 1-mm radius of the electrode tip). In general, amplitude indicates muscle fiber density (FD), not the motor unit territory.

***Duration.*** MUAP duration reflects the activity from most muscle fibers belonging to a motor unit because potentials generated more than 1 mm away from the electrode contribute to the initial and terminal low-amplitude portions of the potential. The duration indicates the degree of synchrony among many individual muscle fibers that are variable in length, conduction velocity, and membrane excitability. A slight shift in needle position or rotation influences duration much less than amplitude. MUAP duration is a good index of the motor unit territory and is the parameter that best reflects the number of muscle fibers in a motor unit. The measure of duration is from the initial deflection away from baseline to the final return to baseline. It normally ranges from 5 to 15 ms, depending on the sampled muscle and the age of the subject (Daube and Rubin, 2009).

Long-duration MUAPs are often of high amplitude and are the best indicators of reinnervation, as seen with LMN disorders, peripheral polyneuropathies, mononeuropathies, and radiculopathies. They occur with increased number or density of muscle fibers or a loss of synchrony of fiber firing within a motor unit. Short-duration MUAPs are often of low amplitude. They occur in disorders associated with loss of muscle fibers, as in necrotizing myopathies (Fig. 36.13). These motor units may be seen with significant myoneural junction blockade in patients with neuromuscular junction disorders.

***Phases.*** A phase constitutes the portion of a waveform that departs from and returns to the baseline. The number of phases equals the number of negative and positive peaks extending to and from the baseline or the number of baseline crossings minus one. Normal MUAPs have four phases or less. However, approximately 5%–15% of MUAPs have five phases or more; this may increase up to 25% in proximal muscles such as the deltoid, gluteus maximus, and iliacus muscles. Increased polyphasia is an abnormal but nonspecific MUAP abnormality since it occurs in both myopathic and neurogenic disorders. An increased number of polyphasic MUAPs suggests desynchronized discharge, loss of individual fibers within a motor unit, or temporal dispersion of muscle fiber potentials within a motor unit. Excessive temporal dispersion, in

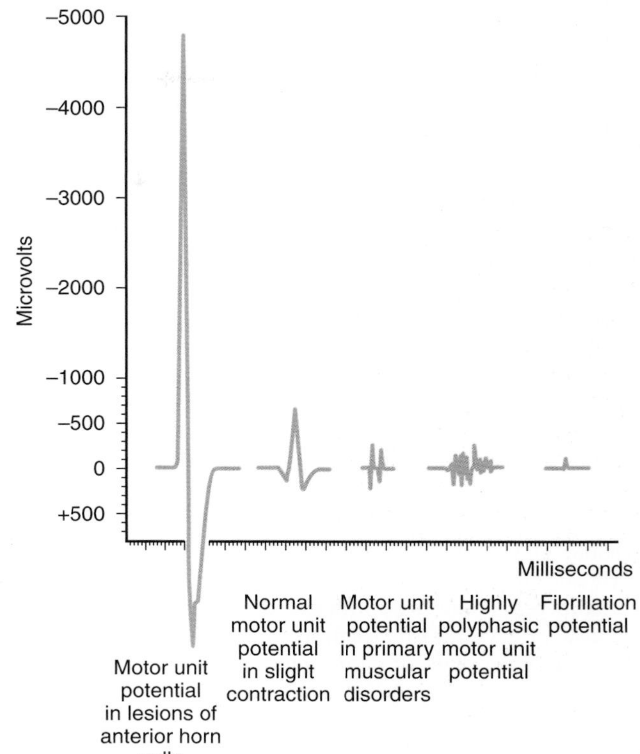


**Fig. 36.13** Motor unit action potentials (MUAPs) in health and disease. *(Reprinted with permission from Daube, J., 1991. Needle electromyography in clinical electromyography. Muscle Nerve 14, 685–700.)*

turn, results from differences in conduction time along the terminal branch of the nerve or over the muscle fiber membrane. In early reinnervation after severe denervation, the newly sprouting axons reinnervate only a few muscle fibers. Consequently, the MUAP may also be polyphasic, with short duration and low amplitude ("nascent" MUAP), which makes it difficult to distinguish from MUAPs seen in myopathies.

Some MUAPs have a serrated pattern characterized by several turns or directional changes without crossing the baseline. This also indicates desynchronization among discharging muscle fibers. Satellite potential (linked potential or parasite potential) is a late spike of MUAP, which is distinct but time locked with the main potential. It implicates early reinnervation of muscle fibers by newly formed collateral sprouts that are usually long, small, thinly myelinated, and slowly conducting. As the sprout matures, the thickness of its myelin increases and its conduction velocity increases. Hence the satellite potential fires more closely to the main potential and may ultimately become an additional phase or serration within the main complex.

### Stability of Motor Unit Action Potentials (see Video 36.14)

Motor units normally discharge semirhythmically, with successive MUAPs showing nearly identical configuration because all muscle fibers of the motor unit fire during every discharge. The morphology of a repetitively firing MUAP may fluctuate if individual muscle fibers forming the unit block intermittently. Moment-to-moment MUAP variability indicates deficient neuromuscular transmission as recurring discharges deplete the store of immediately available acetylcholine (Fig. 36.14). This instability occurs in neuromuscular junction disorders (such as MG, the Lambert-Eaton myasthenic syndrome, and botulism), in neurogenic disorders associated with recent reinnervation (such as motor neuron disease, subacute radiculopathy, and polyneuropathy), and during the early stages of reinnervation in acute peripheral nerve injuries.

### Firing Patterns of Motor Unit Action Potentials (see Videos 36.10, 36.13, 36.15, 36.16, )

During constant contraction in a healthy person, initially only one or two motor units activate semirhythmically. The motor units activated early are primarily those with small type I muscle fibers. Large type II units participate later during strong voluntary contraction. Greater muscle force brings about not only the recruitment of previously inactive units but also more rapid firing of already active units with both mechanisms operating simultaneously (Erim et al., 1996).

*Recruitment frequency* is a measure of motor unit discharge, defined as the firing frequency (rate) at the time of recruiting an additional unit. In normal muscles, mild contraction induces isolated discharges at a rate of 5–10 Hz. This rate depends on the sampled muscle and the types of motor units studied. The reported ranges for healthy people and those with neuromuscular disorders overlap. *Recruitment ratio* is the average firing rate divided by the number of active units. Normally this ratio should not exceed 5:1—for example, with three units each firing less than 15 Hz. Typically, when the firing frequency of the first MUAP reaches 10 Hz, a second MUAP should begin to fire; by 15 Hz, a third unit should fire, and so forth. A ratio of 10, with two units firing at 20 Hz each, indicates a loss of motor units. When such loss is severe, intact residual motor units can increase their firing rate to a maximum of 30–50 Hz in most human skeletal muscles.

*Activation* is the central control of motor units, which enables an increase in firing rate and force. Failure of descending impulses also limits recruitment, although here the excited motor units discharge more slowly than expected for normal maximal contraction. Thus a slow rate of discharge *(poor activation)* in an upper motor neuron (UMN) disorder (such as stroke or myelopathy) or in volitional lack of effort (as with pain, hysterical paralysis, or malingering) stands in sharp contrast to a fast rate of discharge in a LMN weakness *(decreased recruitment)*. With greater contraction, many motor units begin to fire rapidly, making recognition of individual MUAPs difficult; hence the name *interference pattern*. Several factors influence the spike density and average amplitude of the summated response. These include descending input from the cortex, number of motor neurons capable of discharging, firing frequency of each motor unit, waveform of individual potentials, and phase cancellation. The causes of an incomplete interference pattern are poor activation, reduced recruitment, or both. Methods for assessing recruitment during maximal contraction include examination of the interference pattern or, during moderate levels of contraction, estimation of the number of MUAPs firing for the level of activation. The evaluation of maximal contraction is most useful in excluding mild degrees of decreased recruitment. In the extreme case when only few motor units fire rapidly, a picket fence–like interference pattern results.

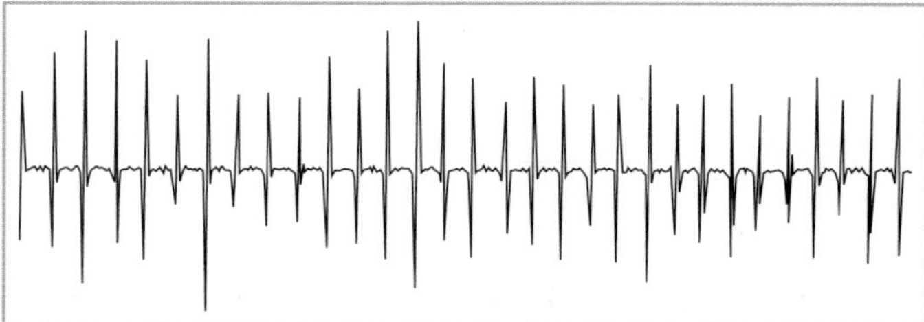

**Fig. 36.14** Unstable motor unit action potentials (moment-to-moment variation) in a patient with myasthenia gravis (recorded with a sweep speed of 100 ms per division and a sensitivity of 0.2 mV per division). Note the extreme amplitude variability of the activated single motor unit action potential. *(Reprinted with permission from Katirji, B., 2018. Electromyography in Clinical Practice: A Case Study Approach, third ed. Oxford University Press.)*

In myopathy, low-amplitude, short-duration MUAPs produce a smaller force per motor unit than normal MUAPs. The instantaneous recruitment of many units is required to support a slight voluntary effort in patients with moderate to severe weakness *(early or rapid recruitment)*. With early recruitment, a full interference pattern is attained at less than maximal contraction, but its amplitude is low because FD is below normal in individual motor units. In advanced myopathies with severe muscle weakness, loss of muscle fibers is so extensive that entire motor units effectively disappear, resulting in a decreased recruitment and an incomplete interference pattern mimicking the recruitment pattern of a neurogenic disorder.

## Electrodiagnosis by Needle Electromyography

### Lower Motor Neuron Disorders

The first needle EMG change occurring after an acute LMN insult is an abnormal recruitment pattern. Recruitment frequency and ratio increase in LMN lesions because fewer motor units fire for a given strength of contraction. Furthermore, the interference pattern with maximal contraction decreases.

Insertional activity increases after the first week, and insertional positive waves may appear within 2 weeks after acute denervation. However, spontaneous fibrillation potentials become apparent in all abnormal muscles after 3 weeks. Fasciculation potentials accompany electrical denervation changes in diseases of the anterior horn cells, roots, and peripheral nerves but do not have pathological significance when they are seen alone. Limb myokymic discharges occur, usually with entrapments, radiation plexopathy, or Guillain-Barré syndrome. Complex repetitive discharges denote a chronic myopathy or radiculopathy, although they may occur with other LMN disorders as well as in subacute disorders.

MUAPs are normal in morphology in the acute phase of denervation, but signs of reinnervation become apparent as early as 1 month later. Reinnervation causes first an increased number of MUAP turns and phases and later increased MUAP duration and amplitude. Amplitude generally reflects FD, whereas duration reflects motor unit territory. The expected MUAP from LMN lesions is a long-duration high-amplitude polyphasic unit (Fig. 36.15; see also Fig. 36.13). The exception is in early reinnervation, in which motor units acquire few muscle fibers, resulting in brief, small polyphasic MUAPs ("nascent" MUAPs), mimicking a myopathic process.

***Radiculopathies.*** Needle EMG is the most sensitive and specific EDX test for identifying cervical and lumbosacral radiculopathies, particularly those associated with axonal loss. Needle EMG is useful for accurate localization of the level of the root lesion. Finding signs of denervation (fibrillation potentials, decreased recruitment, and long-duration high-amplitude polyphasic MUAPs) in a segmental myotomal distribution (i.e., in muscles innervated by the same roots via more than one peripheral nerve), with or without denervation of the paraspinal muscles, localizes the LMN lesion to the root level (Wilbourn and Aminoff, 1998). In radiculopathies associated with axonal loss of proximal sensory fibers, the distal sensory axons do not degenerate, because the unipolar neurons of dorsal root ganglia and their distal axons usually escape injury. Hence a normal SNAP of the corresponding dermatome ensures that the root lesion is within the spinal canal (i.e., proximal to the dorsal root ganglia). For example, in an L5 radiculopathy, the tibialis anterior (peroneal nerve) and tibialis posterior (tibial nerve) muscles often are abnormal on needle EMG, as may be those from the lumbar paraspinal muscles, but the superficial peroneal SNAP is usually normal.

***Plexopathies.*** Plexopathies are extraspinal lesions that involve nerve plexus before the formation of the terminal peripheral nerves. The diagnosis of brachial or lumbosacral plexopathies requires a solid knowledge of peripheral nerve anatomy. Brachial plexus anatomy is particularly complex, so that multiple NCSs and muscle needle EMGs are needed for evaluation. An important task of the EDX evaluation is to differentiate between lesions affecting the brachial plexus (postganglionic lesions) and those involving the roots (preganglionic lesions). This distinction is particularly important in brachial plexus traction injuries, which may mimic root avulsions (Ferrante, 2014). In avulsions, the dorsal root ganglia remain intact and their peripheral axons do not undergo wallerian degeneration. Therefore root avulsions spare SNAPs, whereas SNAPs are low in amplitude or absent in brachial plexopathies when studied after the completion of wallerian degeneration (more than 10 days from injury).

***Mononeuropathies.*** Needle EMG is most useful in axonal mononeuropathies, particularly when they are examined after the completion of wallerian degeneration. These lesions are not localizable by NCSs because they are not associated with the slowing of focal conduction or with conduction block, as seen with demyelinating mononeuropathies. NCS in axon-loss peripheral nerve lesions often show low-amplitude or absent CMAPs and SNAPs following stimulations at distal and proximal sites, whereas distal latencies and conduction velocities are normal or slightly slowed.

The principle of localizing an axon-loss mononeuropathy by needle EMG is similar to manual muscle strength testing on clinical examination. Typically, the needle EMG reveals neurogenic changes (fibrillation potentials, reduced MUAP recruitment, and chronic neurogenic MUAP morphology changes) that are limited to muscles innervated by the involved nerve and located distal to the site of the lesion. Muscles innervated by branches arising proximal to the lesion are normal, however. Localization of axon-loss peripheral nerve lesions by needle EMG is suboptimal because some nerves have very long segments from which no motor branches arise, such as the median and ulnar nerves in the arm or the common peroneal nerve in the thigh. In addition, needle EMG may falsely localize a partial nerve lesion more distally along the affected nerve because of fascicular involvement of nerve fibers or effective reinnervation of proximally situated muscles (Wilbourn, 2002). An example is sparing of ulnar muscles in the forearm (flexor carpi ulnaris and ulnar part of flexor digitorum profundus) following an axon-loss ulnar nerve lesion at the elbow.

Needle EMG is particularly useful in assessing the progress of reinnervation occurring spontaneously or after nerve repair. MUAP recruitment and morphology help assess the process of muscle fiber reinnervation that occurs with proximal-distal regeneration of nerve fibers from the site of the injury or collateral sprouting. Early proximal-distal regeneration of nerve fibers in severe axon-loss lesions often manifests as brief, small, polyphasic (nascent) MUAPs. Collateral sprouting causes an increased number of MUAP turns and phases followed by an increased duration and amplitude of MUAPs (Katirji, 2006).

***Peripheral polyneuropathies.*** Widespread abnormalities on NCSs are characteristic of polyneuropathies. The needle EMG

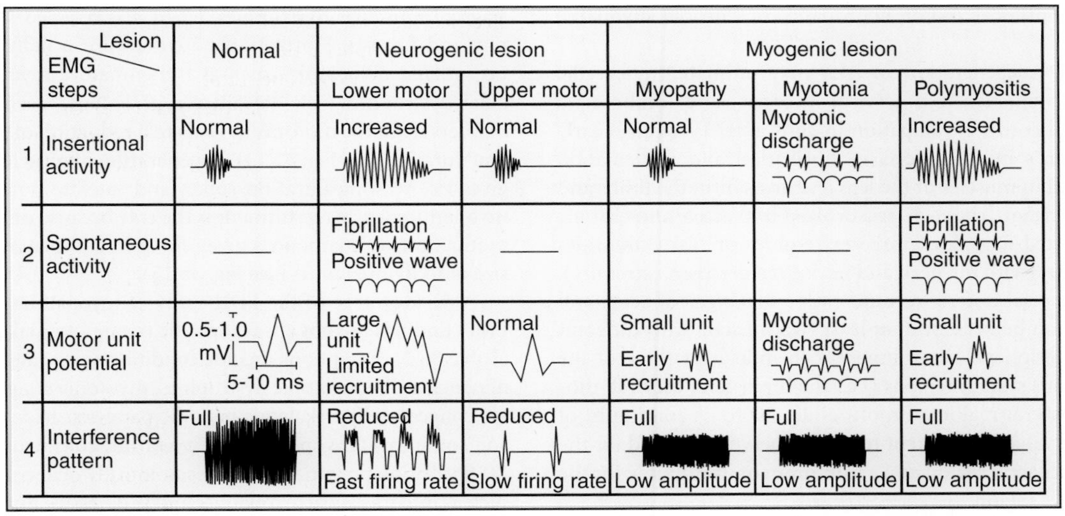

| | Lesion / EMG steps | Normal | Neurogenic lesion | | Myogenic lesion | | |
|---|---|---|---|---|---|---|---|
| | | | Lower motor | Upper motor | Myopathy | Myotonia | Polymyositis |
| 1 | Insertional activity | Normal | Increased | Normal | Normal | Myotonic discharge | Increased |
| 2 | Spontaneous activity | — | Fibrillation<br>Positive wave | — | — | — | Fibrillation<br>Positive wave |
| 3 | Motor unit potential | 0.5-1.0 mV<br>5-10 ms | Large unit<br>Limited recruitment | Normal | Small unit<br>Early recruitment | Myotonic discharge | Small unit<br>Early recruitment |
| 4 | Interference pattern | Full | Reduced<br>Fast firing rate | Reduced<br>Slow firing rate | Full<br>Low amplitude | Full<br>Low amplitude | Full<br>Low amplitude |

**Fig. 36.15** A summary of characteristic findings on needle electromyography *(EMG)* in normal subjects, patients with neurogenic lesions, and patients with myogenic lesions. Insertional activity is greater with lower motor neuron lesions and polymyositis and consists of myotonic discharges in myotonia. Spontaneous activity generally occurs with lower motor neuron disorders and inflammatory myopathy. Motor unit action potentials usually are large and polyphasic, with reduced recruitment in lower motor neuron conditions; in myopathies and polymyositis, motor units are small, with early recruitment. Interference pattern is reduced with both upper and lower motor neuron lesions, as well as in functional (nonorganic) weakness; however, firing rate is rapid in lower motor neuron lesions and slow with upper motor neuron lesions and functional (nonorganic) weakness (in which the rate may be irregular also). Interference pattern is full but of low amplitude in myopathic lesions. *(Reprinted from Kimura, J., 2013. Electrodiagnosis in Diseases of Nerve and Muscle: Principles and Practices, fourth ed. Oxford University Press. Copyright 2013. Used by permission of Oxford University Press.)*

depicts the temporal profile of the illness. In acute demyelinating polyneuropathies such as the Guillain-Barré syndrome, needle EMG during the acute phase of illness may show only reduced recruitment of MUAPs in weak muscles, with normal MUAP morphology and no spontaneous activity. In chronic demyelinating polyneuropathies such as chronic inflammatory demyelinating polyneuropathy, the needle EMG may show signs of mild axonal loss that is not always suspected on NCSs, with fibrillation potentials and reinnervated MUAPs. In acute axon-loss polyneuropathy, such as the axonal forms of Guillain-Barré syndrome or critical illness polyneuropathy, fibrillation potentials typically develop within 2–3 weeks and reinnervated MUAPs become apparent after 1–2 months. In progressive axon-loss polyneuropathies, fibrillation potentials denote active denervation, whereas long-duration high-amplitude polyphasic MUAPs confirm reinnervation. Both changes are usually symmetrical, follow a distal-to-proximal gradient, and are worse in the legs than in the arms. In chronic and very slowly progressive polyneuropathies, reinnervation may keep pace completely with denervation, yielding few or no fibrillation potentials but reduced recruitment of reinnervated long-duration and high-amplitude MUAPs.

***Anterior horn cell disorders.*** Needle EMG is the most important EDX study to provide evidence of diffuse LMN degeneration in patients with motor neuron disease. The needle EMG often shows signs of active denervation (fibrillation potentials), active reinnervation (long-duration high-amplitude polyphasic MUAPs and unstable MUAPs), and loss of motor units (reduced MUAP recruitment).

One disadvantage of needle EMG in motor neuron disease is that it evaluates only LMN degeneration; UMN degeneration requires clinical assessment. Therefore clinical evaluation is the basis for diagnosing amyotrophic lateral sclerosis (ALS), with the EDX studies playing a supporting role. The reasons to perform such studies in patients with suspected ALS are to (1) confirm LMN dysfunction in clinically affected regions, (2) detect evidence of LMN dysfunction in clinically uninvolved regions, and (3) exclude other pathophysiological processes such as multifocal motor neuropathy or chronic myopathy (Chad, 2002).

Although LMN degeneration in ALS may ultimately affect the entire neuraxis (brainstem and cervical, thoracic, and lumbosacral segments of spinal cord), participation in clinical trials requires early diagnosis. Lambert's initial criteria of fibrillation and fasciculation potentials detected in muscles of the legs and arms or in the limbs and the head were stringent. These criteria evolved into active and chronic denervation detected in at least three extremities or two extremities and cranial muscles (with the head and neck considered an extremity). The revised El Escorial criteria recommended that signs of acute and chronic denervation be present in at least two muscles with different spinal root and peripheral nerve innervation in at least three of the four central nervous system regions (i.e., the brainstem, cervical, thoracic, and lumbosacral regions; Brooks et al., 2000). A minimum of two muscles innervated by different roots and nerves is needed for the cervical and lumbosacral region and a minimum of one muscle for the bulbar and thoracic region.

Earlier criteria dismissed fasciculation potentials completely, since they may be benign. These criteria required active denervation in the form of fibrillation potentials as well as signs of chronic denervation and reinnervation. More recent criteria included fasciculation potentials and considered them equivalent in importance to the presence of fibrillation potentials as long as they are encountered in muscles showing chronic denervation and reinnervation. These revisions have had a significant clinical impact by allowing earlier diagnosis of ALS (Costa et al., 2012; de Carvalho et al., 2008).

In patients with suspected motor neuron disease, NCSs are useful mostly in excluding other neuromuscular diagnoses such as polyneuropathies. Sensory NCS findings usually are normal in anterior horn cell disorders, whereas motor NCSs show normal results or low CMAP amplitudes consistent with LMN loss. Motor nerve conduction velocities are normal or slightly slowed but never below 70% of the lower limits of normal, as often seen in demyelinating polyneuropathies. Furthermore, the NCSs do not show other demyelinating features such as conduction blocks; these are characteristic of multifocal motor neuropathy, a treatable disorder that may mimic LMN disease.

The most current diagnostic classification of ALS is as follows:

1. *Clinically definite ALS* is defined by clinical or electrophysiological evidence by the presence of LMN as well as UMN signs in the bulbar region and at least two spinal regions or in three spinal regions.
2. *Clinically probable ALS* is defined on clinical or electrophysiological evidence by LMN and UMN signs in at least two regions with some UMN signs necessarily rostral to (above) the LMN signs.
3. *Clinically possible ALS* is defined when clinical or electrophysiological signs of UMN and LMN dysfunction are found in only one region or UMN signs are found alone in two or more regions or LMN signs are found rostral to UMN signs.

### Upper Motor Neuron Lesions

In patients with UMN lesions, EDX studies show normal insertional activity, no spontaneous activity at rest, and normal MUAP morphology. The only abnormality is a reduced interference pattern due to poor activation with a slow rate of motor unit discharge (see Fig. 36.15). Recruitment measured by either recruitment frequency or ratio is normal. Nonorganic weakness or poor effort produces a similar pattern except that motor unit firing may be irregular.

### Myopathic Disorders

Insertional activity is usually normal or increased except in the late stage of muscular dystrophies, when it is reduced secondary to atrophy and fibrosis. Fibrillation potentials are usually absent except in necrotizing myopathies such as inflammatory myopathies and muscular dystrophies (see "Fibrillation potentials," earlier). Random loss of fibers from the motor unit leads to a reduction of MUAP amplitude and duration (see Fig. 36.13). Regeneration of muscle fibers sometimes gives rise to long-duration spikes and satellite potentials in chronic myopathies. Early recruitment is the rule because of the need for more motor units to maintain a given force in compensation for the small size of individual units (see Fig. 36.15).

A disadvantage of the EDX study of myopathies is that the needle EMG findings are not always specific enough to make a final diagnosis (Table 36.2). Exceptions include conditions associated with (1) myotonia, such as the myotonic dystrophies, myotonia congenita, paramyotonia congenita, hyperkalemic periodic paralysis, acid maltase deficiency, and some toxic myopathies (such as from colchicine and statins) and (2) fibrillation potentials, which occur mostly in necrotizing myopathies such as inflammatory myopathies and progressive muscular dystrophies (such as Becker and Duchenne muscular dystrophies). Another disadvantage of the needle EMG is that findings either are normal or include subtle abnormalities in some nonnecrotizing myopathies, such as the metabolic and endocrine myopathies (Lacomis, 2002). Therefore a normal needle EMG does not exclude a myopathy.

In polymyositis and dermatomyositis, it is essential to recognize the changing pattern on the needle EMG at diagnosis, after treatment, and during relapse. Fibrillation potentials appear first at diagnosis or relapse and disappear early during remission. Abnormal MUAP morphology becomes evident later and takes longer to resolve. The

**TABLE 36.2 Patterns of Needle Electromyographic Findings in Myopathies**

| Often Normal | Myopathic MUAPs with Fibrillation Potentials† | Myopathic MUAPs Only | Fibrillation Potentials Only | Myopathic MUAPs and Myotonia | Myotonia Only |
|---|---|---|---|---|---|
| Metabolic myopathies:<br>• McArdle disease<br>• Tarui disease<br>• Brancher deficiency<br>• Debrancher deficiency<br>• CPT deficiency<br>• Carnitine deficiency<br>• Adenylate deaminase deficiency<br>Mitochondrial myopathies:<br>• Kearns-Sayre syndrome<br>• MELAS<br>• MERRF endocrine myopathies:<br>Steroid (mild)<br>Hypothyroid<br>Hyperthyroid<br>Hyperparathyroid<br>Cushing<br>Others:<br>• Fiber type disproportion<br>• Acute rhabdomyolysis<br>• Periodic paralysis* | Inflammatory myopathies:<br>• Polymyositis<br>• Dermatomyositis<br>• Inclusion body myositis<br>• Sarcoid myopathy<br>• HIV-associated myopathy<br>Muscular dystrophies:<br>• Duchenne<br>• Becker<br>• Distal<br>Others:<br>• Critical illness myopathy<br>• Myotubular myopathy<br>• Parasitic infections (trichinosis) | Muscular dystrophies:<br>• FSH<br>• Limb girdle<br>• Oculopharyngeal<br>• Emery-Dreifus<br>Congenital myopathies<br>• Central core<br>• Nemaline rod<br>Endocrine myopathies:<br>• Steroid (severe)<br>• Hypothyroid<br>• Hyperthyroid<br>• Hyperparathyroid<br>Toxic myopathies:<br>• Alcohol<br>• Emetine | Inflammatory myopathies‡:<br>• Polymyositis<br>• Dermatomyositis<br>• Sarcoid myopathy<br>• HIV-associated myopathy<br>Others:<br>• Chloroquine | Myotonic dystrophies:<br>• DM1<br>DM2 muscle channelopathies:<br>• Paramyotonia congenita<br>• Hyperkalemic periodic paralysis*<br>Others:<br>• Acid maltase deficiency<br>• Myotubular myopathy<br>• Calpain-3 mutation (LGMD1C) Colchicine<br>• Statins | Myotonia congenita<br>• Thomsen disease<br>• Becker disease<br>Other myotonic disorders:<br>• Atypical painful myotonia<br>• Myotonia fluctuans |

*Between attacks.
†Mixed with large MUAPs in chronic myopathies.
‡Early or mild.
*CPT*, Carnitine palmitoyltransferase deficiency; *FSH*, facioscapulohumeral; *HIV*, human immunodeficiency virus; *McArdle disease*, myophosphorylase deficiency; *MELAS*, mitochondrial encephalomyopathy, lactic acidosis, and stroke-like episodes; *MERRF*, myoclonic epilepsy and ragged-red fibers; *MUAP*, motor unit action potential; *Tarui disease*, phosphofructokinase deficiency; *LGMD*, limb girdle muscular dystrophy.
*Adapted with permission and revisions from Katirji, B., Kaminski, H.J., Ruff, R.L. (Eds), 2014. Neuromuscular Disorders in Clinical Practice. Springer, New York.*

presence of fibrillation potentials also is helpful in distinguishing exacerbation of myositis from a corticosteroid-induced myopathy (Wilbourn, 1993).

## SPECIALIZED ELECTRODIAGNOSTIC STUDIES

### Late Responses

#### F Wave

A supramaximal stimulus applied at any point along the course of a motor nerve elicits a small and late motor response (F wave) after the CMAP (M response). The *F wave* derives its name from *foot*—the first recording was from the intrinsic foot muscles. The nerve action potential initiated during a motor NCS travels in two directions: distally (orthodromically) to depolarize the muscle and generate a CMAP, and proximally (antidromically) toward the spinal cord to trigger an F wave. The long-latency F wave is a very small CMAP that results from backfiring of antidromically activated anterior horn cells, averaging 5%–10% of the motor neuron pool. The F wave's afferent and efferent loops are the motor neuron, with no intervening synapse (Fisher, 2002). The F wave varies in latency, morphology, and amplitude with each stimulus because a different population of anterior horn cells backfires. Therefore an adequate study requires that about 10 F waves be clearly identified (Fig. 36.16, *A*). Moving the stimulator proximally decreases the F-wave latency because the action potential travels a shorter distance.

The *F-wave minimal latency*, measured from the stimulus artifact to the beginning of the evoked potential, is the most reliable and useful measurement and represents conduction of the largest and fastest motor fibers. The minimal F-wave latency depends on the length of the nerve studied (see Fig. 36.16, *B*). The most sensitive criterion of abnormality in a unilateral disorder affecting a single nerve is a minimum latency difference between the two sides or between two nerves in the same limb. Absolute latencies are useful only for sequential reassessment of the same nerve.

*F-wave persistence* is a measure of the number of F waves obtained for the number of supramaximal stimulations and is usually greater than 50% except with stimulation of the peroneal nerve during recording in the EDB. Although this measurement is very helpful in depicting the percentage of excitable motor axons, it is highly influenced by the level of patient relaxation and anxiety during testing. The *F-wave conduction velocity* provides a better comparison between proximal and distal (forearm or leg) segments. *F-wave chronodispersion* reflects the degree of scatter among consecutive F waves and can be determined by calculating the difference between the minimal and maximal F-wave latencies; this measure indicates the range of motor conduction velocities in the nerve.

Prolonged F-wave minimal latencies occur in most polyneuropathies, particularly the demyelinating type. In the early phases of Guillain-Barré syndrome, findings on routine motor nerve studies may be normal except for prolonged or absent F waves, which

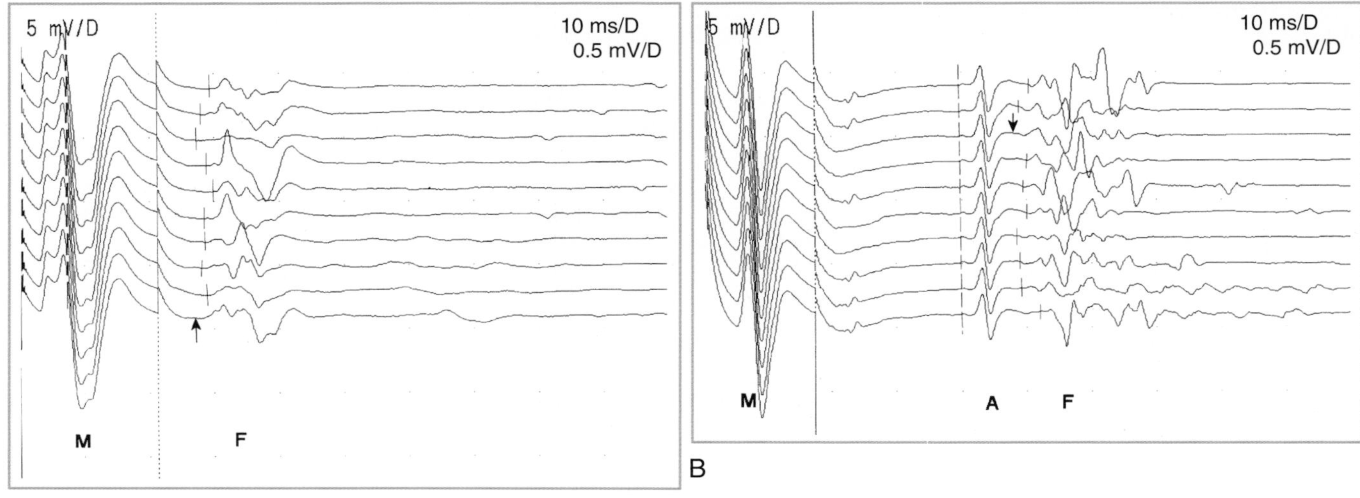


**Fig. 36.16** A, Normal *F* waves recorded from the hypothenar muscles after supramaximal stimulations of the ulnar nerve at the wrist. Ten consecutive traces are shown in a raster mode. Note the large *M* response and the significant variability of F-wave latencies (vertical cursors) and morphology. The minimum F-wave latency *(arrow)* is 28.5 ms. **B,** Normal F waves recorded from the abductor hallucis after supramaximal stimulations of the tibial nerve at the ankle. Ten consecutive traces are shown in a raster mode showing also the larger M response and the variability of F-wave latencies (vertical cursors) and morphology. Note that the minimum F-wave latency *(arrow)* is 48.5 ms owing to the greater length of the tibial nerve, compared with the ulnar nerve in *A*. Note also the presence of a simple A wave that precedes the F wave, with a constant morphology and latency *(dashed vertical line)*.

imply proximal demyelination (Al-Shekhlee et al., 2005; Gordon and Wilbourn, 2001). F-wave minimal latencies in radiculopathies have limited use. They may be normal despite partial motor axonal loss, since most muscles have multiple root innervations (Wilbourn and Aminoff, 1998).

## A Wave

The A wave (*a*xonal wave) is a potential seen occasionally during recording of F waves at supramaximal stimulation. The A wave follows the CMAP and often precedes but occasionally follows the F wave. The A wave may be seen in asymptomatic persons during studies of the tibial nerve. It may be mistaken for an F wave, but its constant latency and morphology differentiate it from the highly variable morphology and latency of the F wave (see Fig. 36.16, *B*). A waves are sometimes seen in axon-loss polyneuropathies, motor neuron disease, and radiculopathies, whereas multiple or complex A waves are often associated with acquired or inherited demyelinating polyneuropathies. The exact pathway of the A wave is unknown; the constant morphology and latency of the A wave are best explained by the fixed point of a collateral reinnervating sprout or an ephaptic transmission between two axons.

## H Reflex

The H reflex, named after Hoffmann for his original description, is an electrical counterpart of the stretch reflex elicited by a mechanical tap to the tendon. The group 1A sensory fibers and alpha motor neurons form the respective afferent and efferent arcs of this predominantly monosynaptic reflex. The H reflex and F wave can be distinguished by increasing stimulus intensity. The H reflex is best elicited by a long-duration stimulus, which is submaximal to produce an M response (Fig. 36.17). In contrast, the F wave requires supramaximal stimulus intensity. The H reflex from stimulating the tibial nerve while recording the soleus muscle (S1 arc reflex) is the most reproducible and commonly used in clinical practice. This is in contrast with the F wave, which can be elicited from any limb muscle.

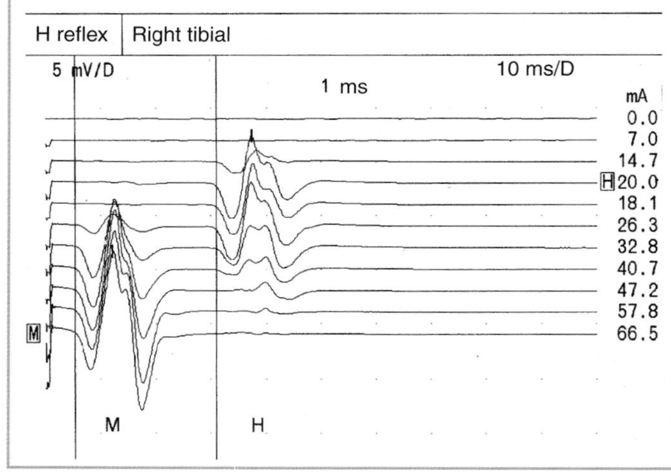


**Fig. 36.17** H reflex recorded from the soleus after stimulation of the tibial nerve at the knee. Shock intensity (in milliamperes) was gradually increased to supramaximal stimulation *(right panel)*. Note that the H reflex appeared with subthreshold level of stimulus (14.7 mA), followed by initial increase and subsequent decrease in amplitude with successive stimuli of progressively higher intensity. The H reflex disappeared with shocks of supramaximal intensity (66.5 mA), which elicited a maximal M response.

Absent H reflexes are seen in more than 90% of patients with Guillain-Barré syndrome. This includes the early phases of disease (Al-Shekhlee et al., 2005; Gordon and Wilbourn, 2001). However, this finding is not specific and is common in the majority of peripheral polyneuropathies. An asymmetrically absent or side-to-side latency difference greater than 1.5 ms or amplitude difference of more than 50% is common in S1 radiculopathy (Nishida et al., 1996).

### Blink Reflex

The blink reflex generally evaluates the trigeminal and facial nerves and their connections in the pons and medulla. It has an afferent limb mediated by sensory fibers of the supraorbital branch of the ophthalmic division of the trigeminal nerve and an efferent limb mediated by motor fibers of the facial nerve.

With two-channel recording, the blink reflex has two components: an early R1 and a late R2 response. The R1 response is present only ipsilateral to the stimulation and is usually a simple triphasic waveform with a dyssynaptic pathway between the main trigeminal sensory nucleus in the midpons and the ipsilateral facial nucleus in the lower pontine tegmentum. The R2 response is a complex waveform and is the electrical counterpart of the corneal reflex. It is typically present bilaterally, with an oligosynaptic pathway between the nucleus of the trigeminal spinal tract in the ipsilateral pons and medulla and interneurons forming connections to the ipsilateral and contralateral facial nuclei.

The blink reflex is most useful in evaluating unilateral lesions such as facial neuropathy, trigeminal neuropathy, or a pontine or medullary lesion. With a facial nerve lesion, the R1 and R2 potentials are absent or delayed with supraorbital stimulation ipsilateral to the lesion, whereas the R2 response on the contralateral side is normal. With a trigeminal nerve lesion, the ipsilateral R1 and R2 and contralateral R2 are absent or delayed, whereas all responses are normal with contralateral stimulation. With a midpontine lesion involving the main sensory trigeminal nucleus or the pontine interneurons to the ipsilateral facial nerve nucleus, supraorbital stimulation on the side of the lesion results in an absent or delayed R1 but an intact ipsilateral and contralateral R2. Finally, with a medullary lesion involving the spinal tract and trigeminal nucleus or the medullary interneurons to the ipsilateral facial nerve nucleus, supraorbital stimulation on the affected side results in a normal R1 and contralateral R2 but an absent or delayed ipsilateral R2. In demyelinating polyneuropathies such as Guillain-Barré syndrome or type 1 Charcot-Marie-Tooth disease, a marked delay of all blink responses may occur, reflecting slowing of motor fibers, sensory fibers, or both.

## Repetitive Nerve Stimulation

### Principles

Repetitive stimulation of motor or mixed nerves is performed to evaluate patients with suspected neuromuscular junction disorders, including MG, Lambert-Eaton myasthenic syndrome, botulism, and congenital myasthenic syndromes. The design and plans for RNS depend on physiological factors inherent in the neuromuscular junction that dictate the type and frequency of stimulations used in the diagnosis of neuromuscular junction disorders. The CMAP obtained during a routine NCS represents the summation of all muscle fiber action potentials generated in a muscle after supramaximal stimulation of all motor axons while recording via a surface electrode placed over the belly of a muscle.

- A *quantum* is the amount of acetylcholine in a single vesicle, which is approximately 5000–10,000 acetylcholine molecules. Each quantum (vesicle) released results in a 1-mV change of postsynaptic membrane potential. This occurs spontaneously during rest and forms the basis of the *miniature end-plate potential.*
- The number of quanta released after a nerve action potential depends on the number of quanta in the *immediately available* (i.e., *primary*) *store* and the probability of release: $m = p \times n$, where $m$ equals the number of quanta released during each stimulation, $p$ equals the probability of release (effectively proportional to the concentration of calcium and typically about 0.2, or 20%), and $n$ equals the number of quanta in the immediately available store. In normal conditions, a single nerve action potential triggers the release of 50–300 vesicles (quanta), with an average equivalent to about 60 quanta (60 vesicles). In addition to the immediately available store of acetylcholine located beneath the presynaptic nerve terminal membrane, a *secondary* (or *mobilization*) *store* starts to replenish the immediately available store after 1–2 seconds of repetitive nerve action potentials. A *large tertiary* (or *reserve*) *store* also is available in the axon and cell body.
- The *end-plate potential* is the potential generated at the postsynaptic membrane after a nerve action potential. Because each vesicle released causes a 1-mV change in the postsynaptic membrane potential, this results in an approximately 60-mV change in the amplitude of the membrane potential.
- Under normal conditions, the number of quanta (vesicles) released at the neuromuscular junction by the presynaptic terminal far exceeds the postsynaptic membrane potential change necessary to reach the threshold needed to generate a postsynaptic muscle action potential. This is the basis of the *safety factor*, which results in an end-plate potential that is always above threshold and able to generate a muscle fiber action potential. In addition to quantal release, other factors that contribute to the safety factor and the end-plate potential include acetylcholine receptor conduction properties, acetylcholine receptor density, and acetylcholinesterase activity (Boonyapisit et al., 1999).
- *Voltage-gated calcium channels* open after depolarization of the presynaptic terminal, leading to calcium influx. Through a calcium-dependent intracellular cascade, vesicles dock into active release zones, releasing acetylcholine molecules. Calcium then diffuses slowly out of the presynaptic terminal in 100–200 ms. The rate at which motor nerves are repetitively stimulated dictates whether or not calcium accumulation plays a role in enhancing the release of acetylcholine. At a slow rate of RNS (i.e., a stimulus every 200 ms or more; or a stimulation rate <5 Hz), the calcium role in acetylcholine release is not increased and subsequent nerve action potentials reach the nerve terminal long after calcium has dispersed. By contrast, with rapid RNS (i.e., a stimulus every 100 ms or less; a stimulation rate >10 Hz), calcium influx is greatly increased, and the probability of release of acetylcholine quanta increases.

### Slow Repetitive Nerve Stimulation

The application of three to five supramaximal stimuli to a mixed or motor nerve at a rate of 2–3 Hz is the technique of slow RNS. This rate is low enough to prevent calcium accumulation but high enough to deplete the quanta in the immediately available store before the mobilization store starts to replenish it. Three to five stimuli are adequate for the maximal release of acetylcholine.

Calculation of the decrement with slow RNS entails comparing the baseline CMAP amplitude with the lowest CMAP amplitude (usually the third or fourth). The CMAP decrement is expressed as a percentage and calculated as follows:

$$\%\ \text{Decrement} = \frac{\text{CMAP amplitude of 1st response} - \text{CMAP amplitude of 3rd or 4th response}}{\text{CMAP amplitude of 1st response}} \times 100$$

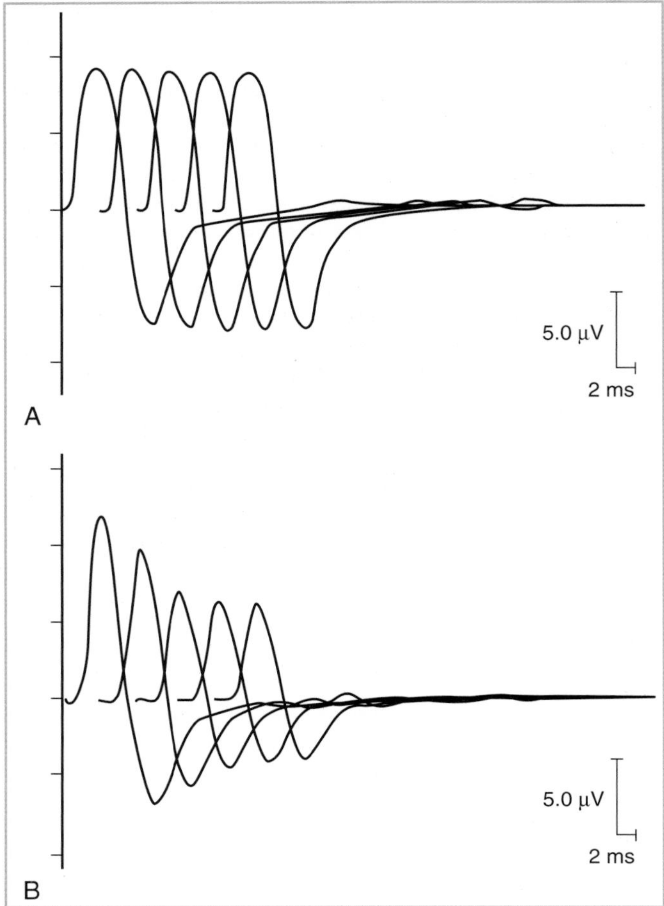


**Fig. 36.18** Slow (2-Hz) repetitive nerve stimulation in a healthy subject (**A**) and in a patient with generalized myasthenia gravis (**B**) showing compound muscle action potential decrement. *(Reprinted with permission from Katirji, B., 2018. Electromyography in Clinical Practice: A Case Study Approach, third ed. Oxford University Press, New York..)*

Under normal conditions, slow RNS does not cause a CMAP decrement. Although the second through fifth end-plate potentials fall in amplitude, they always remain above threshold (because of the normal safety factor) and ensure muscle fiber action potential generation after each stimulation. In addition, the secondary store begins to replace the depleted quanta after the first few seconds, with a subsequent rise in the end-plate potential. Therefore, all muscle fibers generate muscle fiber action potentials, and the CMAP does not change in size (Fig. 36.18 A). In *postsynaptic neuromuscular junction disorders* (such as MG), the safety factor is reduced because fewer acetylcholine receptors are available. Therefore the baseline end-plate potential reduces but is usually still above threshold. Slow RNS results in a decrease in end-plate potential amplitudes at many neuromuscular junctions. As end-plate potentials decline below the threshold, the number of muscle fiber action potentials produced declines, leading to a CMAP decrement (Fig. 36.18 B). In *presynaptic neuromuscular junction disorders* (such as Lambert-Eaton myasthenic syndrome), the baseline end-plate potential is low, with many end plates not reaching threshold. Therefore many muscle fibers do not fire, resulting in low baseline CMAP amplitude (Table 36.3). With slow RNS, further CMAP decrement occurs, caused by the further decline of acetylcholine release with the subsequent stimuli, resulting in further loss of many end-plate potentials and muscle fiber action potentials (Geiger and Katirji, 2018; Katirji and Kaminski, 2002).

**TABLE 36.3 Compound Muscle Action Potentials and Repetitive Nerve Stimulation in Neuromuscular Junction Disorders**

| Neuromuscular Junction Defect | Prototype Disorder | CMAP | Slow RNS | Rapid RNS* |
|---|---|---|---|---|
| Postsynaptic | Myasthenia gravis | Normal | Decrement | Normal or decrement |
| Presynaptic | Lambert-Eaton myasthenic syndrome | Low | Decrement | Increment |

*Or after brief exercise CMAP.
*CMAP*, compound muscle action potential; *RNS*, repetitive nerve stimulation.

In patients with suspected MG, the diagnostic yield of slow RNS increases if the following recommendations are applied:

- *Obtain slow RNS at rest and after exercise.* A reproducible decrement of more than 10% confirms a neuromuscular junction defect. Slow RNS should be repeated after the patient exercises for 10 seconds to demonstrate repair of the decrement *(posttetanic facilitation)*. The patient should then perform maximal voluntary exercise of the tested muscle for 1 minute. Then, repeat slow RNS every 30 seconds and for 3–5 minutes after exercise. This is most important when a reproducible but equivalent CMAP decrement (<10%) appears at rest. Because the amount of acetylcholine released with each stimulus is at its minimum 2–5 minutes after exercise, slow RNS after exercise increases the chance of detecting a defect of neuromuscular transmission at the neuromuscular junction by demonstrating a worsening and significant CMAP decrement *(postexercise exhaustion)*.
- *Record from clinically weakened muscles.* Most commonly used and technically feasible nerves for slow RNS are the median, ulnar, and spinal accessory nerves. The diagnostic sensitivity is clearly higher for slow RNS recording in proximal muscles than in distal muscles, whereas the distal ones are less technically demanding. Facial nerve repetitive stimulation is indicated in patients with oculobulbar weakness (Zinman et al., 2006), but this study is technically difficult and sometimes associated with a large stimulation artifact that renders waveform interpretation subject to error.
- *Warm the extremity studied* (skin temperature should be above 32°C). This precaution decreases false-negative results because cooling improves neuromuscular transmission and may mask the decrement.
- *Discontinue cholinesterase inhibitors* for 12–24 hours (if clinically possible). This measure also decreases the false-negative rate with slow RNS.

### Rapid Repetitive Nerve Stimulation

Rapid RNS is most useful in patients with suspected presynaptic neuromuscular junction disorders such as Lambert-Eaton myasthenic syndrome or botulism. The optimal frequency is 20–50 Hz for 2–10 seconds. A typical rapid RNS applies 200 stimuli at a rate of 50 Hz (i.e., 50 Hz for 4 seconds). Calculation of CMAP increment after rapid RNS is as follows:

$$\%\ \text{Increment} = \frac{\text{CMAP amplitude of the largest response} - \text{CMAP amplitude of 1st response}}{\text{CMAP amplitude of 1st response}} \times 100$$

A brief (10-second) period of maximal voluntary isometric exercise is much less painful and has the same effect as that of rapid RNS at 20–50 Hz. Application of a single supramaximal stimulus generates a baseline CMAP. Then the patient performs a 10-second maximal isometric voluntary contraction, followed by another stimulus that produces the postexercise CMAP.

With rapid RNS or postexercise CMAP evaluation, two competing forces act on the nerve terminal. First, stimulation tends to deplete the pool of readily available synaptic vesicles. This depletion reduces transmitter release by reducing the number of vesicles released in response to a nerve terminal action potential. Second, calcium accumulates in the nerve terminal, thereby increasing the probability of synaptic vesicle release. In a normal nerve terminal, the effect of depletion of readily available synaptic vesicles predominates, so that with rapid RNS, the number of vesicles released decreases. The end-plate potential does not fall below threshold, however, because of the safety factor. Therefore the supramaximal stimulus generates action potentials in all muscle fibers and no CMAP decrement occurs. In fact, rapid RNS or brief (10-second) exercise in normal subjects often leads to a slight physiological increment of the CMAP that does not exceed 40%–50% of the baseline CMAP. The probable cause is increased synchrony of muscle fiber action potentials after tetanic stimulation *(posttetanic pseudofacilitation).*

In a presynaptic disorder such as Lambert-Eaton myasthenic syndrome, very few vesicles release and many muscle fibers do not reach threshold, resulting in low baseline CMAP amplitude. With rapid RNS, the calcium concentrations in the nerve terminal rises high enough to enhance release of a sufficient number of synaptic vesicles to result in a larger end-plate potential that crosses threshold and is capable of generating action potentials. This results in many more muscle fibers firing and leads to a CMAP increment (see Table 36.3). The increment is often higher than 200% in Lambert-Eaton myasthenic syndrome (Fig. 36.19), with 10-second postexercise facilitation achieving the highest diagnostic sensitivity (Hatanaka and Oh, 2008). Patients with botulism have a less pronounced increment, ranging from 40% to 200%, due to the more severe neuromuscular blockade (Witoonpanich et al., 2009). In a postsynaptic disorder such as MG, rapid RNS causes no change of CMAP because the depleted stores are compensated by calcium influx. In severe postsynaptic blockade (as during myasthenic crisis), the increased quantal release cannot compensate for the marked

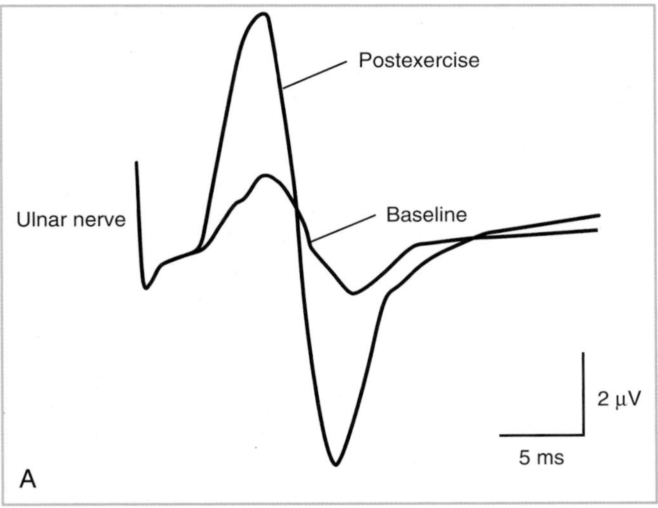


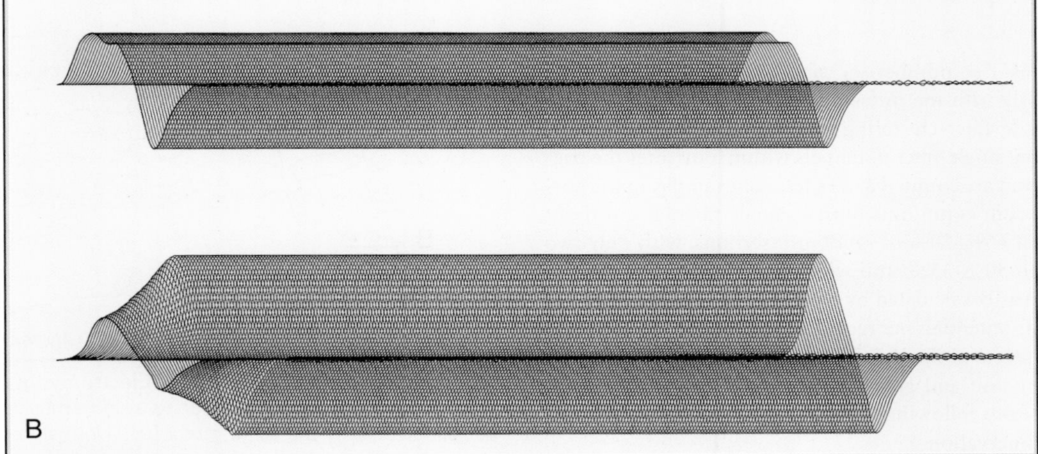


**Fig. 36.19** **A,** Baseline and compound muscle action potential (CMAP) after brief exercise (postexercise) in a patient with Lambert-Eaton myasthenic syndrome. Note the significant CMAP increment (294%) after brief (10 seconds) exercise. **B,** Rapid (50-Hz) repetitive nerve stimulation in a control subject *(top)* and in a patient with Lambert-Eaton myasthenic syndrome *(bottom)*. No CMAP increment is observed for the control subject, whereas a significant (250%) increment is apparent for the patient. (*Reprinted with permission from Katirji, B., 2018. Electromyography in Clinical Practice: A Case Study Approach, third ed. Oxford University Press, New York.*)

neuromuscular block, resulting in a drop in end-plate potential amplitude. Therefore fewer end plates reach threshold and fewer muscle fiber action potentials are generated, resulting in CMAP decrement.

## Single-Fiber Electromyography

### Principles

The technical requirements for performing SFEMG are as follows. First, a concentric single-fiber needle electrode allows the recording of single-muscle-fiber action potentials. The small side port on the cannula of the needle serves as the pickup area. A single-fiber needle electrode records from a circle of 300-µm radius, as compared with the 1-mm radius of a conventional concentric EMG needle. Recent studies, however, have shown no difference in sensitivity or specificity between the reusable single-fiber and disposable concentric-needle electrodes in healthy subjects and in patients with MG (Farrugia et al., 2009; Sarrigiannis et al., 2006; Stålberg and Sanders, 2009). Second, the amplifier must have an impedance of 100 megohms or greater to counter the high electrical impedance of the small leadoff surface, the gain is set higher for SFEMG recordings than for conventional EMG, the sweep speed is faster, and the filter should have a 500-Hz low frequency to attenuate signals from distant fibers. Third, an amplitude threshold trigger allows recording from a single muscle fiber, and a delay line permits viewing of the entire waveform even though the single-fiber potential triggers the sweep. Fourth, computerized equipment assists in data acquisition, analysis, and calculation.

*Voluntary (recruitment) SFEMG* is a common method for activating muscle fibers. A mild voluntary contraction produces a biphasic potential with duration of approximately 1 ms and amplitudes that vary with the recording site. Single-fiber potentials suitable for study must have peak-to-peak amplitude greater than 200 µV, rise time less than 300 µs, and a constant waveform. The electromyographer rotates, advances, and retracts the needle until a potential that meets these criteria is captured.

*Stimulation SFEMG* is performed by inserting another monopolar needle electrode near the intramuscular nerve twigs and stimulating through it at a low current and constant rate. Surface stimulation may be achieved, as with percutaneous stimulation of the temporal branch of the facial nerve recording the frontalis muscle (Kouyoumdjian and Stålberg, 2012). This method does not require patient participation and is therefore useful in children or in uncooperative or comatose patients. SFEMG is useful in assessing FD or in jitter analysis (see later discussion).

### Fiber Density

FD is calculated as the number of single-fiber potentials firing almost synchronously with the initially identified single-fiber potential. Increased muscle fiber clustering indicates collateral sprouting. Simultaneously firing single-fiber potentials within 5 ms after the triggering single-fiber unit are counted at 20 sites. For example, in the normal extensor digitorum communis muscle, single fibers fire without nearby discharges in 65%–70% of random insertions, with only two fibers discharging in 30%–35%, and with three fibers discharging in 5% or fewer. FD is easily calculated by hand by averaging the number of single fiber muscle potentials per recording site over 20 sites. The FD is useful to study the loss of the normal mosaic distribution of muscle fibers from a motor unit and grouping of muscle fibers of a motor unit within its territory following reinnervation. In neuropathy, FD increases due to reinnervation.

### Jitter

SFEMG measures *neuromuscular jitter*, which represents the variation in time intervals between pairs of single-fiber muscle action potentials obtained with voluntary activation or the variation in time measured between stimulus and individual single-fiber muscle action potentials with stimulation technique. Voluntary jitter is the variability of the time interval between two muscle fiber action potentials (a muscle pair) innervated by the same motor unit. It is the variability of the interpotential intervals between repetitively firing paired single-fiber potentials (Stålberg and Trontelj, 1997; Fig. 36.20). Neuromuscular jitter can be determined by using a commercially available computer program that calculates the mean value of consecutive interval differences over 50–100 discharges, as follows:

$$\mathrm{MCD} = \frac{[\mathrm{IPI}\ 1 - \mathrm{IPI}\ 2] + [\mathrm{IPI}\ 2 - \mathrm{IPI}\ 3] + \ldots + [\mathrm{IPI}\ (N-1) - \mathrm{IPI} N]}{N-1}$$

where MCD is the *mean consecutive difference*, IPI 1 is the interpotential interval of the first discharge, IPI 2 of the second discharge, and so on, and *N* is the number of discharges recorded.

Neuromuscular blocking is the intermittent failure of transmission of one of the two muscle fiber potentials. This reflects failure of one of the muscle fibers to transmit an action potential owing to failure of the end-plate potential to reach threshold. Blocking is the extreme abnormality of the jitter measured as the percentage of discharges of a motor unit in which a single-fiber potential does not fire. For example, in 100 discharges of the pair, if a single potential is missing 30 times, the blocking is 30%. In general, blocking occurs when the jitter values are significantly abnormal.

The results of SFEMG jitter studies are expressed by the mean jitter of all potential pairs, the percentage of pairs with blocking, and

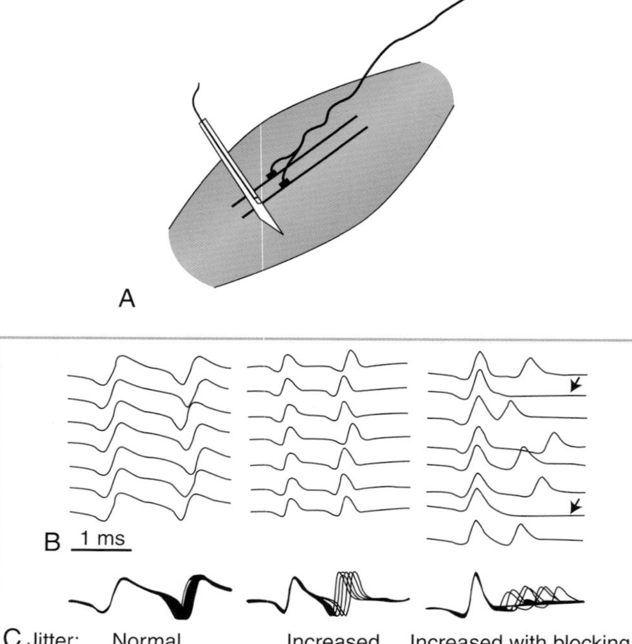


**Fig. 36.20** Voluntary Single-Fiber Electromyographic Jitter Study. **A,** The jitter is measured between two single muscle fiber action potentials innervated by the same motor unit. Normal, moderately increased jitter is seen in a patient with myasthenia gravis; greatly increased jitter with intermittent blocking *(arrows)* is evident in another patient with myasthenia gravis. The upper tracings (**B**) are shown in a raster mode, and the lower tracings (**C**) are superimposed. (*Reprinted from Stålberg, E., Trontelj, J.V., 1997. The study of normal and abnormal neuromuscular transmission with single fibre electromyography. J Neurosci Methods 74, 145–154, with permission from Elsevier Science.*)

the percentage of pairs with normal jitter (Fig. 36.21). Because jitter may be abnormal in 1 of 20 recorded potentials in healthy subjects, the study is considered to indicate defective neuromuscular transmission if the mean jitter value exceeds the upper limit of the normal jitter value for that muscle, if more than 10% of potential pairs (e.g., more than 2 of 20 pairs) exhibit jitter values above the upper limit of the normal jitter, or if any neuromuscular blocking is present.

Normal values for jitter may be affected by a number of different variables, including the specific muscle being examined, type of recording electrode used, mode of muscle fiber activation, and age of the subject. Reference values for jitter measurements with volitional muscle activation utilizing a traditional SFEMG needle or standard concentric EMG needles were different and published (Gilchrist 1992; Stålberg et al., 2016). As jitter values obtained by stimulation SFEMGs are calculated on the basis of one end plate, the normal values are lower than those obtained by volitional activation. To calculate the normal stimulation jitter value using a SFEMG needle, it is recommended that the reference data for volitional SFEMG be multiplied by 0.80.

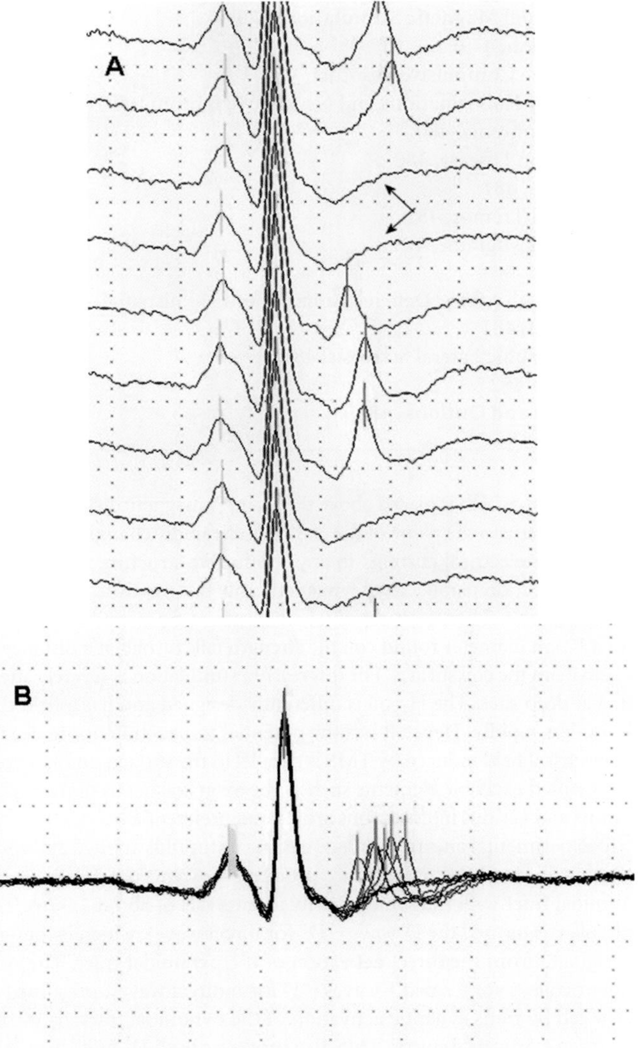


**Fig. 36.21** Single-fiber EMG jitter study (voluntary, using concentric needle electrode) from the frontalis muscle in a seronegative patient with ocular myasthenia gravis. **A**, Raster mode. **B**, Superimposed mode. Several discharges of three muscle fibers are shown, triggering on the second *(middle)* fiber. Note that the first potential *(on the left)* has a normal jitter value (MCD = 20 μs) while the third potential *(on the right)* has significant jitter (MCD = 116 μs) with frequent potential blocking *(arrows)*. *MCD,* Mean consecutive difference.

Jitter analysis is highly sensitive but not specific. Although jitter is often abnormal in MG and other disorders of the neuromuscular junction, it may also be abnormal in a variety of neuromuscular disorders, including motor neuron disease, peripheral neuropathies, and myopathies. Therefore the diagnostic value of jitter must be considered in light of the patient's clinical manifestations and other EDX findings.

SFEMG jitter studies have a high and equal sensitivity and specificity in acetylcholine receptor–seropositive and seronegative patients with MG. In clinical practice, it is most often used in patients who are seronegative to acetylcholine receptor and muscle-specific kinase (MuSK) antibodies. SFEMGs of limb muscles, such as the extensor digitorum, are often normal in MuSK-positive MG patients, whereas SFEMGs of facial muscles, such as the orbicularis oculi, have a similar sensitivity in MuSK-positive patients as in acetylcholine receptor–positive patients. SFEMG jitter study is useful as a prognostication tool in MG. Patients with higher mean jitter values, a greater percentage of fibers with increased jitter, and/or impulse blocking have a higher risk and frequency of a severe disease exacerbation (Abraham et al., 2017; Baruca et al., 2016). The degree of jitter change in patients with MG also predicts and correlates with the clinical change in MG patients, thus having a potential use as a biomarker of disease control when performed longitudinally (Sanders and Massey, 2017).

*The complete reference list is available online at https://expertconsult.inkling.com/.* 

37

# Extracranial Neuromodulation

*David H. Benninger, Zhen Ni, Mark Hallett*

## OUTLINE



At the beginning of the 1980s, Merton and Morton developed the first method of noninvasive brain stimulation, transcranial electrical stimulation (TES), and this had obvious clinical application. They used a single, brief, high-voltage electric shock and produced a relatively synchronous muscle response, the motor evoked potential (MEP). The latency of MEPs was compatible with activation of the fast-propagating corticospinal tract. It was immediately clear that this method would be useful for many purposes, but a problem with TES is that it is painful, because of simultaneous stimulation of pain fibers in the scalp. Five years later, Barker and colleagues demonstrated that it was possible to stimulate the brain (and nerve as well) using magnetic stimulation (transcranial magnetic stimulation [TMS]) with little or no pain. TMS is now commonly used in clinical neurology to study central motor conduction time. Depending on the stimulation techniques and parameters, TMS can excite or inhibit the brain activity, allowing functional mapping of cortical regions and creation of transient functional lesions. It is now widely used as a research tool to study aspects of human brain physiology including motor function and the pathophysiology of various brain disorders (Hallett, 2007). Because TMS can influence the brain, there have been attempts to use it as therapy, particularly when used repetitively (rTMS). Effects demonstrated so far are mild to moderate, and there are already therapeutic indications.

## METHODS AND THEIR NEUROPHYSIOLOGICAL BACKGROUND

For magnetic stimulation, a brief, high-current (usually several thousand amps within 200 μs) electrical pulse is produced in a coil of wire, called the magnetic coil, which is placed above the scalp. A magnetic field is induced perpendicularly to the plane of the coil. Such a rapidly changing magnetic field induces electrical currents in any conductive structure nearby, with the flow direction parallel to the magnetic coil, but opposite in direction. The magnetic field falls off rapidly with distance from traditional coils; with a 12 cm diameter round coil the strength falls by half at a distance of 4–5 cm from the coil surface. For this reason, stimulation is severely attenuated at deep sites. The H-coil is differently designed and has a field that falls off less rapidly. Hence it has the potential to penetrate more deeply. The electrical field induced by TMS is parallel to the surface, and horizontally oriented excitable elements such as the axon collaterals of pyramidal neurons and various interneurons are excited preferentially.

In experimental animals, a single electrical stimulus applied at threshold intensity to the motor cortex produces descending volleys in the pyramidal tract with the same velocity at intervals of about 1.5 ms. The first volley is termed the D-wave ("D" for direct wave), which is thought to originate from the direct activation of the pyramidal tract. The subsequent volleys are termed I-waves ("I" for indirect wave), presumed to be elicited by trans-synaptic activation of the pyramidal tract via intrinsic cortico-cortical circuitry. TMS also produces both D- and I-waves in descending pyramidal neurons. In contrast to electrical stimulation that preferentially evokes D-waves first, TMS at threshold intensity often produces a corticospinal volley with I-waves, but no early D-wave (Ziemann and Rothwell, 2000). This finding suggests that TMS activates pyramidal neurons indirectly through synaptic inputs, but does not activate them directly, presumably because of the direction of its current flow. Standards for the use of TMS and review of side effects have been published (Rossi et al., 2019; Rossini et al., 2015).

## STIMULATION PARAMETERS FOR DIAGNOSTIC USE OF TRANSCRANIAL MAGNETIC STIMULATION

### Central Motor Conduction Measurements

With TMS, it is possible to measure conduction in central motor pathways (central conduction time, or CCT). CCT can be estimated by subtracting the conduction time in the peripheral nerves and neuromuscular junction from the total latency of MEPs measured at the onset of the initial deflection. Peripheral motor conduction time is currently measured through two methods: (1) F-wave recordings for the measurement of spine-to-muscle conduction time and (2) direct stimulation of the efferent roots and nerves over the spine. Magnetic stimulation on the posterior neck or the dorsal spine activates spinal roots at the level of the intervertebral foramen. Since the cervical roots are excited about 3 cm away from the anterior horn cell, magnetic stimulation of the roots is not an accurate measurement of CCT and may miss a proximal partial or complete block of impulse propagation. F-waves are usually elicited in the relaxed state by delivering supramaximal stimulation to the peripheral motor nerve at a site near the muscle under examination. The stimulus evokes an orthodromic volley in the motor nerves, which produces a short latency response in the muscle (M wave). In addition, an antidromic volley travels back to the spinal cord, exciting the spinal motoneurons, and an efferent volley travels down to the motor nerve causing a late excitation of the muscle, known as the F-wave. Total peripheral motor conduction time can be estimated as: (F+M−1)/2 (1 is the time due to the central delay at the level of $\alpha$-motoneuron). Consequently, the CCT can be obtained as follows: MEP latency—−(F+M−1)/2. Using this method, the average CCT is about 6.4 ms for the thenar muscles and 13.2 ms for the tibialis anterior. The descending volley of action potentials from TMS desynchronize along their path, which causes phase cancellation. This explains why the amplitudes of conventional MEPs are usually small compared with motor responses from maximal peripheral nerve stimulation (compound muscle action potential [CMAP]) and of variable size. This phase cancellation limits the detection and the quantification of the central motor conduction and can be corrected by the triple stimulation technique (TST). The TST is a collision method and consists of a conventional TMS and two subsequent peripheral distal and proximal nerve stimulations, which "resynchronize" the descending action potentials. The TST allows better detection and quantification of corticospinal conduction deficits and offers an objective measure for clinical practice (Magistris et al., 1998, 1999). Combining the TST with paired-pulsed TMS paradigms of short-interval intracortical inhibition (SICI) and intracortical facilitation (ICF) improves their consistency, though the inter-individual variability alone precludes their clinical utility (Caranzano et al., 2017).

### Motor Excitability Measurements

#### Motor Thresholds

Motor threshold (MT) represents the minimal stimulation intensity producing MEPs in the target muscle. This can be measured in resting (resting motor threshold [RMT]) or contracting (active motor threshold [AMT]) muscles. RMT is determined to the nearest 1% of the maximum stimulator output and is commonly defined as the minimal stimulus intensity required to produce MEPs of greater than 50 μV in at least 5 out of 10 consecutive trials. Here the MEP amplitudes are usually measured peak to peak. AMT is determined in the moderately active muscle (usually between 5% and 10% of the maximal voluntary contraction) and is defined as the minimum intensity that produces either MEPs of greater than 100 μV or silent period (SP) or MEPs of greater than 200 μV in at least 5 out of 10 consecutive trials. Other methods are also used for MT and the adaptive method may be the most accurate (Groppa et al., 2012). MT in resting muscle reflects the excitability of a central core of neurons, depending on the excitability of individual neurons and their local density. Since MT can be influenced by drugs that affect voltage-gated sodium and calcium channels, it may represent membrane excitability.

#### Motor Evoked Potential Recruitment Curve (Stimulus Response Curve; Input-Output Curve)

The recruitment curve is the growth of MEP size as a function of stimulus intensity (Kukke et al., 2014). The underlying physiology is poorly understood, but appears to involve neurons in addition to the core region activated at threshold. The slope of the recruitment curve is related to the number of corticospinal neurons that can be activated at a given stimulus intensity, mainly indirectly through corticocortical connections. The neurons that can be activated at a lower threshold are highly excitable neurons located in core regions of corresponding motor cortex, while neurons recruited at a higher intensity may have a higher threshold for activation, either because they are intrinsically less excitable or because they are spatially further from the magnetic stimulus's center of activation. These neurons would be part of the "subliminal fringe." The changes in recruitment curve are usually more prominent with higher-intensity stimulations. This finding suggests that recruitment curve may represent the excitability of less excitable or peripherally located neurons, rather than highly excitable core neurons, or the connections between them. The slope of recruitment curve is increased by drugs that enhance adrenergic transmission, such as dextroamphetamine, and is decreased by sodium and calcium channel blockers and by gamma-aminobutyric acid (GABA) agonists.

#### Silent Period and Long-Interval Intracortical Inhibition

The SP is a pause in ongoing voluntary electromyography (EMG) activity produced by TMS (Fig. 37.1, *A*). The SP is usually measured with a suprathreshold stimulus in moderately active muscle (usually 5%–10% of maximal voluntary contraction). SP duration is usually defined as the interval between the magnetic stimulus and the first reoccurrence of rectified voluntary EMG activity (Chen et al., 1999; Curra et al., 2002). While the first part of the SP is due in part to spinal-cord refractoriness, the latter part is entirely due to cortical inhibition (cortical silent period [CSP]). If a second suprathreshold test stimulation (TS) is given during the SP following suprathreshold conditioning stimulus (CS; usually 50–200 ms after the first stimulus), its MEP is significantly suppressed (long intracortical inhibition [LICI]; Fig. 37.1, *B*; Chen et al., 1999; Curra et al., 2002). SP and LICI appear to assess $GABA_B$ function, although other drugs affecting membrane excitability or dopaminergic transmission also influence SP. Although LICI and SP share similar mechanisms, they may not be identical because they are affected differently in various diseases (Berardelli et al., 1996).

#### Short-Interval Intracortical Inhibition and Intracortical Facilitation

Various inhibitory and excitatory connections in the motor cortex can be evaluated by TMS using a paired-pulse technique. A subthreshold CS preferentially excites interneurons, by which MEPs from a following TS are suppressed at interstimulus intervals (ISIs) of 1–5 ms (intracortical inhibition; SICI for such inhibition at short intervals) or facilitated at ISIs of 8–20 ms (ICF; Fig. 37.2; Ilic et al., 2002; Ziemann, 1999). SICI and ICF reflect interneuronal activity in the cortex. SICI is likely largely a GABAergic effect, especially related to $GABA_A$ receptors. ICF is largely a glutamatergic effect. However, subcortical or even spinal activation may also be involved in ICF, as ICF is not related to changes in I-waves (Di Lazzaro et al., 2006b). SICI can be divided into two phases, with maximum inhibition at ISIs of 1 ms and 2.5 ms. SICI at 1 ms ISI is presumably caused either by neuronal refractoriness resulting in desynchronization of the corticospinal volley or by different inhibitory circuits, while SICI at ISI of 2 ms or longer is most likely a synaptic inhibition.

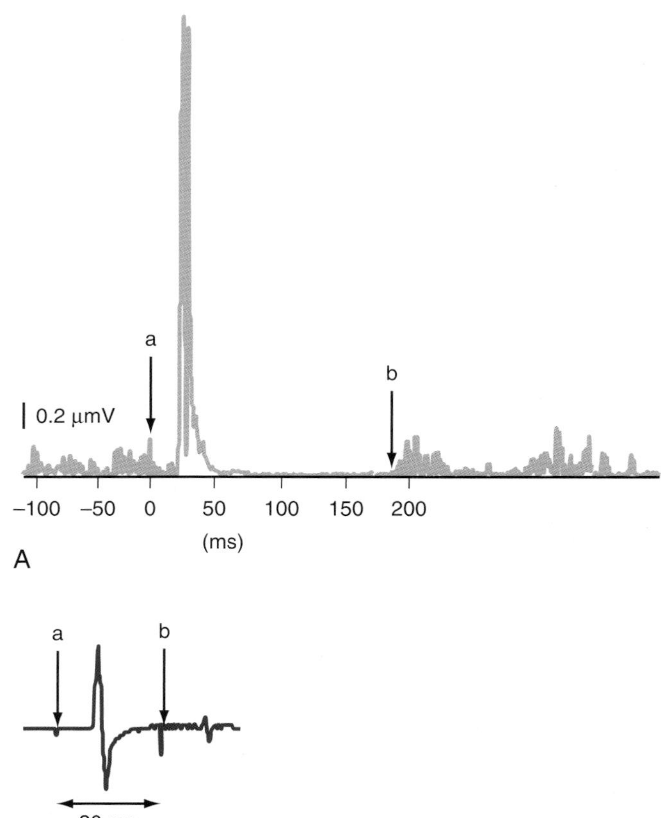


**Fig. 37.1** **A,** A rectified electromyography (EMG) recording of the first dorsal interosseus after single transcranial magnetic stimulation (TMS) under isometric contraction at 10% of maximal voluntary contraction. The silent period can be measured from TMS trigger *(a)* to reoccurrence of EMG activity *(b)*. **B,** Paired-pulse TMS with suprathreshold conditioning stimulation. Test stimulation *(b)* with the same stimulation intensity is applied at 80 ms after the conditioning stimulation *(a)*. Motor evoked potential of the test stimulation is significantly suppressed compared with that of the conditioning stimulation (long intracortical inhibition).

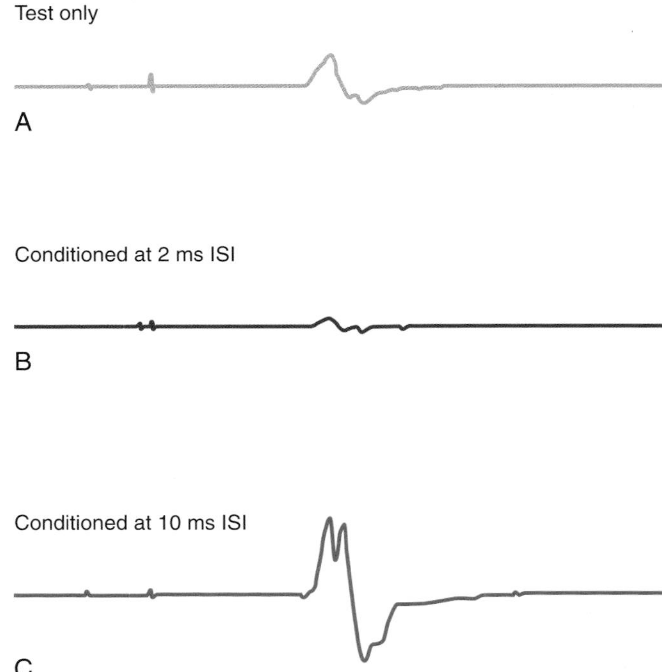


**Fig. 37.2** Paired-pulse transcranial magnetic stimulation with subthreshold conditioning stimulation. At 2 ms interstimulus interval *(ISI)* (**B**), motor evoked potential (MEP) amplitude is significantly suppressed compared with that in test stimulation alone (**A**) (short-interval intracortical inhibition). At 10 ms ISI, MEP amplitude is significantly increased (**C**) (intracortical facilitation).

The magnitude of SICI depends on the intensity of CS and TS. With a given CS, TS intensity variation results in a U-shaped variation of SICI magnitude with a maximum inhibition at TS producing MEPs with peak-to-peak amplitude of around 1 mV. Variation of CS intensity at a given TS intensity also leads to a U-shaped change in SICI magnitude, with maximum SICI occurring at CS intensity around 90% AMT or 70% RMT. The low end of CS intensity producing SICI represents SICI threshold. Increased magnitude of SICI with CS above SICI threshold may indicate increasing recruitment of inhibitory interneurons that contribute to SICI, while decreased magnitude of SICI with increased CS intensities above those producing maximum SICI may represent recruitment of facilitatory processes (presumably, those mediating short-interval intracortical facilitation [SICF]; see next section) that superimpose with SICI.

## Short-Interval Intracortical Facilitation

SICF is also known as facilitatory I-wave interactions; it is also measured in a paired-pulse TMS protocol. In contrast to SICI and ICF, however, SICF is elicited by a suprathreshold first stimulus and a subthreshold second stimulus, or two near-threshold stimuli. SICF is usually observed at discrete ISIs of 1.1–1.5 ms, 2.3–2.9 ms, and 4.1–4.4 ms. ISIs producing facilitatory response in SICF are about 1.5 ms apart, similar to the intervals of different I-waves, which suggests that SICF originates in those neural structures responsible for the generation of I-waves (Ziemann and Rothwell, 2000). The second pulse is thought to excite the initial axon segments of excitatory interneurons, which are depolarized by excitatory postsynaptic potentials from the first pulse without firing an action potential. In addition, it is important to mention that the final outcome measured as MEP induced by a paired-pulse TMS reflects a complex interplay between cortical inhibition and facilitation, because the stimulus parameters (stimulus intensities for the first and second stimuli and ISI between two stimuli) for testing SICI and SICF overlap (Peurala et al., 2008). Indeed, $GABA_A$ agonists reduce both SICI and SICF. Therefore, reduced SICI observed in various disease conditions may represent either a true reduction in SICI or enhanced facilitation, or both. Measuring the low and high ends of CS producing SICI is now considered to be a more sensitive and informative method to assess neurophysiological changes occurring in various conditions than simply measuring the magnitude of SICI.

## Short-Latency and Long-Latency Afferent Inhibition

Afferent inhibition can be measured by applying a conditioning sensory stimulus such as median nerve stimulation followed by a test stimulus over the contralateral motor cortex. MEP inhibition occurs usually at ISIs of approximately 20 ms (short-latency afferent inhibition [SAI]) and 200 ms (long-latency afferent inhibition [LAI]; Chen, 2004). SAI is thought to be of cortical origin because the recordings of corticospinal volleys demonstrate a strong suppression of later I-waves with unaffected earlier descending waves. SAI is reduced by the acetylcholine antagonist scopolamine, suggesting that SAI can be used to test the integrity of cholinergic neural circuits. Accordingly, SAI is reduced in patients with Alzheimer disease (AD), and is improved with a single dose of rivastigmine, an acetylcholinesterase inhibitor.

The mechanism mediating LAI is still unclear, but is thought to be different from that of SAI.

### Surround Inhibition

Surround inhibition (SI), suppression of excitability in an area surrounding an activated neural network, has been proposed to be an essential mechanism in the motor system where it could aid the selective execution of desired movements. Using a self-triggered TMS technique, in which TMS is set to be triggered by the EMG activity from the activated muscle (agonist), MEPs of the surround muscles (i.e., the muscles near to the agonist but unrelated to its movement) are suppressed during the movement (up to 80 ms after the EMG onset) despite enhanced spinal excitability (Jung et al., 2004). SI is reduced in patients with focal hand dystonia and may be altered in other disorders of human motor control, such as Parkinson disease (PD).

### Other Inhibitory Phenomena of the Motor Cortex

Interhemispheric inhibition (IHI) can also be assessed by TMS, by applying a CS to the motor cortex, which suppresses MEPs produced by a test stimulus over the contralateral motor cortex at ISIs of between 6 ms and 50 ms (Di Lazzaro et al., 1999; Ni et al., 2009). IHI is mediated by transcallosal fibers at the cortical level, although subcortical structures may also be involved (Wahl et al., 2007). Long-latency IHI at ISIs between 20 and 50 ms is likely mediated by $GABA_B$ receptors.

Magnetic stimulation of the cerebellum, which can be performed using a double-cone coil, inhibits the MEPs produced by stimulation of the contralateral motor cortex 5–7 ms later (cerebellar inhibition, CBI; Iwata and Ugawa, 2005). Cerebellar stimulation is thought to activate Purkinje cells in the cerebellar cortex, leading to inhibition of the deep cerebellar nuclei (such as the dentate nucleus) which have a dyssynaptic excitatory pathway to the motor cortex via the ventral thalamus. CBI is reduced or absent in patients with cerebellar degeneration or lesions in the cerebellothalamocortical pathway.

Table 37.1 summarizes the characteristics of different motor excitability measures using TMS.

### Interaction Between Different Cortical Circuits

The cortical circuits in the M1 are not independent of each other but are interconnected within a complex neural network. The interaction between two cortical circuits can be expressed as the changes in one circuit at the presence of the other and can be tested with a triple-pulse TMS paradigm (review see Ni et al., 2011a, 2011b). Notably, it was well demonstrated that SICI decreases when LICI is present (Ni et al., 2011a; Sanger et al., 2001), and the disinhibitory effect can be blocked by a $GABA_B$ antagonist (Florian et al., 2008), indicating that LICI inhibits SICI at a presynaptic level.

### Motor Cortical Plasticity Measurements—Paired Associative Stimulation

Paired associative stimulation (PAS) refers to a paradigm consisting of slow-rate repetitive low-frequency median or ulnar nerve stimulation combined with TMS over the contralateral motor cortex (usually, 0.1–0.25 Hz for 10–30 minutes). This protocol has been shown to induce plastic changes of excitability in the human motor cortex, similar to associative long-term potentiation in experimental animals (Classen et al., 2004). PAS-induced changes in MEP amplitudes depend on the interval between the afferent nerve stimulation and TMS (usually around 25 ms for enhanced excitability and around 10 ms for reduced excitability). PAS-induced plasticity measures may contribute to elucidating the pathogenesis of neurological disorders where abnormal neuroplasticity is thought to have a pathogenetic role, such as focal dystonia.

## CLINICAL APPLICATIONS FOR DIAGNOSTIC USE OF TRANSCRANIAL MAGNETIC STIMULATION

Since its introduction, TMS has increasingly been used to evaluate the underlying neurophysiological mechanisms in various neurological disorders (Table 37.2; (Badawy et al., 2012; R. Chen, 2004; Curra et al., 2002; Sohn and Hallett, 2004). In addition, many studies have been performed to investigate the effect of various

**TABLE 37.1 Summary of Motor Excitability Measurements Using Transcranial Magnetic Stimulation**

| | METHODS | | | |
|---|---|---|---|---|
| **Measurement** | **Conditioning** | **Test** | **ISIs (ms)** | **Proposed Mechanisms (Pharmacology)** |
| MT | | Near threshold | | Membrane excitability |
| RC | | Suprathreshold | | Recruitment of less excitable neurons |
| SP | | Suprathreshold | | $GABA_B$, $GABA_A$?, Dopamine? |
| LICI | Suprathreshold | Suprathreshold | 50–200 | $GABA_B$ |
| SICI | Subthreshold | Suprathreshold | 1–6 | $GABA_A$ |
| ICF | Subthreshold | Suprathreshold | 8–20 | Glutamate |
| SICF | Suprathreshold/near threshold | Subthreshold/near threshold | 1.1–1.5, 2.3–2.9, 4.1–5.0 | $GABA_A$* |
| SAI | Peripheral nerve | Suprathreshold | 20 | Acetylcholine |
| LAI | Peripheral nerve | Suprathreshold | 200 | |
| SI | Movement of unrelated muscle | Suprathreshold | –80 | $GABA_A$? |
| IHI | Opposite motor cortex | Suprathreshold | 8–50 | $GABA_B$? |
| CBI | Cerebellum | Suprathreshold | 5–7 | |

*Note: SICF is mediated by summation of different descending indirect waves. However, the activation of the GABAergic interneuron is responsible for the SICF troughs and contributes to the periodic facilitation of SICF.

*CBI*, Cerebellar inhibition; *GABA*, gamma-aminobutyric acid; *ICF*, intracortical facilitation; *IHI*, interhemispheric inhibition; *ISI*, interstimulus interval; *LAI*, long-latency afferent inhibition; *LICI*, long-interval intracortical inhibition; *MT*, motor threshold; *RC*, recruitment curve; *SAI*, short-latency afferent inhibition; *SI*, surround inhibition; *SICF*, short-interval intracortical facilitation; *SICI*, short-interval intracortical inhibition; *SP*, silent period.

**TABLE 37.2 Changes in Transcranial Magnetic Stimulation Measurements in Various Neurological Disorders**

| | MT | MEP/ RC | SP | LICI | SICI | ICF | SAI | SI | CBI |
|---|---|---|---|---|---|---|---|---|---|
| **Movement Disorders** | | | | | | | | | |
| Parkinson disease | — | | ↓ | ↑ | ↓ | — | — | ↓ | — |
| Dystonia | — | ↑ | ↓ | ↓/↑ | ↓ | — | — | ↓ | |
| Huntington | | | ↑ | | ↓ | ↑ | | | |
| PKD | — | — | — | ↓ | —/↓ | — | | | |
| **Other Degenerative Disorders** | | | | | | | | | |
| Alzheimer disease | ↓/— | ↑ | | | ↓ | — | ↓ | | |
| Cerebellar degeneration | ↑ | | ↑/— | ↑ | — | ↓ | | | ↓ |
| Amyotrophic lateral sclerosis | ↓/↑ | ↑ | ↓ | ↓ | ↓ | ↑ | | | — |
| Generalized epilepsy | ↓/— | | ↑/— | ↓/— | ↓ | — | | | |
| Migraine | ↑/— | | ↑/— | ↓ | —/↓ | ↑/— | | | |

*CBI*, Cerebellar inhibition; *ICF*, intracortical facilitation; *LICI*, long-interval intracortical inhibition; *MEP*, motor evoked potential; *MT*, motor threshold; *PKD*, paroxysmal kinesigenic dyskinesia; *RC*, recruitment curve; *SAI*, short-latency afferent inhibition; *SI*, surround inhibition; *SICI*, short-interval intracortical inhibition; *SP*, silent period; ↑, increased; ↓, reduced; —, unchanged.

**TABLE 37.3 Acute Effects of Neurological Drugs on Transcranial Magnetic Stimulation Measurements**

| Drugs | MT | MEP/ RC | CSP | LICI | SICI | ICF | SICF | SAI |
|---|---|---|---|---|---|---|---|---|
| Na$^+$ channel blockers | ⇈ | ═/↓ | ═ | | ═/↓ | ═/↓ | ═ | |
| GABA$_A$ agonists | ═ | ⇊ | —/↑ | | ⇊/— | ↓/— | ↓ | |
| GABA$_B$ agonists | — | | ↓ | ↓ | ↑ | ↓ | — | |
| Glutamate (*N*-methyl-D-aspartate) antagonists | ═ | ═ | ═ | | ↑ | ↓ | — | |
| Levodopa/ dopamine agonists | ═ | ═/↓ | ⇈/— | | ⇈/— | ═ | ↓ | |
| Dopamine antagonists | ═ | ↑ | ═ | | ═/↓ | —/↑ | | |
| Norepinephrine agonists | ═ | ↑ | — | | ═/↓ | ⇈ | | |
| Serotonin reuptake inhibitor | ═ | ↑ | — | | ↓ | ↔ | | |
| Anticholinergics | —/↓ | —/↑ | ═ | ↑ | —/↓ | —/↑ | | ↓ |
| **Other Drugs** | | | | | | | | |
| Ethanol | — | — | ↑ | | ↑ | ↓ | | |
| Gabapentin | ═ | | ⇈ | | ⇈ | ⇊ | | |
| Levetiracetam | —/↑ | ↓ | —/↑ | | ═ | ═ | | |
| Topiramate | — | | — | | ↑ | | | |
| Piracetam | | | | | | | ↓ | |

*CSP*, Cortical silent period; *ICF*, intracortical facilitation; *LICI*, long-interval intracortical inhibition; *MEP*, motor evoked potential; *MT*, motor threshold; *RC*, recruitment curve; *SAI*, short-latency afferent inhibition; *SICF*, short-interval intracortical facilitation; *SICI*, short-interval intracortical inhibition; *SP*, silent period; ↑, increased; ↓, reduced; —, unchanged; ⇈, ⇊, ═, indicate consistent observations in two or more studies.

neurologically acting drugs on TMS measurements (Table 37.3; Ziemann, 2004), and these provide useful information about the mechanisms mediating various TMS techniques as well as better understanding of the mechanism of these drugs. A report regarding the clinical diagnostic utility of TMS has been published by a committee of the International Federation of Clinical Neurophysiology (IFCN; Chen et al., 2008).

## Movement Disorders

### Parkinson Disease and Parkinson Plus Syndromes

CCT is normal in PD, but can be prolonged in patients with multisystem atrophy (MSA) and progressive supranuclear palsy (PSP), which suggest a possible role of CCT measurements in patients with Parkinson plus syndromes involving the pyramidal tracts. A reduction in SICI has been observed in various movement disorders, regardless of the nature of the disturbances (Berardelli, 1999). In PD, reduced SICI is only observed at high CS intensities (MacKinnon, et al., 2005). SICF is increased in PD and likely contributes to the reduced SICI at the same ISIs. Both the exaggerated SICF and reduced SICI at the ISIs when increased SICF is elicited can be normalized by dopaminergic medications. On the other hand, SICI measured with ISIs outside the range of SICF is also decreased in Parkinson's disease, and the impairment cannot be normalized by dopaminergic medications (Ni et al., 2013). In patients with corticobasal degeneration, SICI is often markedly reduced or turned into facilitation along with reduced IHI (Pal et al., 2008). SP is shortened in PD. Reduced LICI at both postsynaptic and presynaptic level has been reported in PD with the evidence from a triple-pulse TMS study showing that suppressed SICI in the presence of LICI seen in healthy controls disappeared in the patients (Chu et al., 2009). SAI is normal in patients with PD, but is reduced in patients with MSA. LAI is reduced in PD, which is not affected by dopaminergic medications. SI is reduced or absent in the asymptomatic side of patients with unilateral PD (Shin et al., 2007). Dopaminergic drugs enhance SICI and prolong SP, whereas dopamine-blocking agents reduce SICI and increase ICF. The effect of sensory inputs on the local M1 circuits may also be impaired in PD. LAI inhibited LICI in healthy controls with a triple-pulse paradigm, but the interaction was not observed in PD patients either with or without medication (Sailer et al., 2003). These observations suggest that motor cortex excitability depends on the balance between different inhibitory mechanisms, some of which are under the control of the basal ganglia. Several studies measured changes in TMS parameters after subthalamic nucleus deep brain stimulation (DBS). SP is lengthened and ICF is enhanced after DBS, but no SP change was observed in another study. Reduced SAI presumably associated with dopaminergic medications and reduced LAI were restored by DBS. Motor cortical plasticity tested with PAS decreases in patients with PD in an off-medication state. The impaired cortical plasticity can be restored by dopaminergic medication in patients without levodopa-induced dyskinesia, but not in patients with dyskinesia (Morgante et al., 2006). In advanced PD patients with levodopa-induced dyskinesia, cortical plasticity induced by PAS can be restored with both medication and subthalamic DBS, but not with either DBS or medication off (Kim et al., 2015).

### Dystonia

In patients with focal dystonia, reduced SICI is not site-specific and was also observed in unaffected sides in patients with upper limb dystonia, and in hand muscles in patients with cervical and facial dystonia. In patients with dystonia, shortening of SP is observed, but only in dystonic muscles. In writer's cramp, decrease in LICI was observed in the symptomatic hand during muscle activation. Both SICI and LICI were found to be abnormal in functional (psychogenic) dystonia, which limits the value of these measures in differentiating organic from functional disorders (Espay et al., 2006; Quartarone et al., 2009). SICI is normal in dopa-responsive dystonia (DYT5; Hanajima et al., 2017). Recruitment curve, SP, SICI, LICI, ICF, and SICF were all normal in patients with myoclonus-dystonia (DYT15; Li et al., 2008; van der Salm et al., 2009). In patients with focal dystonia, LAI is diminished or absent, but SAI is normal. SI is reduced or absent in patients with focal hand dystonia (Jung et al., 2004). On the other hand, SI in patients with paroxysmal kinesigenic dyskinesia may be prolonged and be present even after the self-initiated movement is terminated (Shin et al., 2010). In patients with focal dystonia, PAS-induced plasticity is abnormally enhanced with loss of topographic specificity, even in non-dystonic parts of the body (Quartarone et al., 2008; Weise et al., 2011). This abnormal enhancement is not observed in patients with psychogenic dystonia (Quartarone et al., 2009). Abnormally enhanced PAS-induced plasticity may also be helpful for distinguishing PD-like patients showing normal dopamine transporter scans (SWEDDs: Scans Without Evidence of Dopaminergic Deficit) from PD patients (Schwingenschuh et al., 2010).

### Huntington Disease

Although SP may be normal at the early or preclinical stage of Huntington disease (HD; Schippling et al., 2009), progressive shortening in SP with functional decline was found in symptomatic patients at 2-year follow-up (Lefaucheur et al., 2006b). This finding is consistent with the disease pathology with GABAergic neuronal loss in the brain and suggests that SP may be a potential biomarker of disease progression. SICI may be normal in symptomatic patients (Priori et al., 2000). However, the results may have been confounded by inclusion of patients with chorea due to various etiologies. The CS intensity for producing the same degree of SICI was found to be increased in early stages, and even in the preclinical stage, of the disease (Schippling et al., 2009). SAI was decreased in the same group of patients. These studies with paired-pulse measurements support the view that cortical functional impairments occur at an early stage in HD.

### Essential Tremor

Cortical inhibitory circuits including SICI, LICI, and CBI are normal in mild essential-tremor patients, indicating that the neural inputs to the M1 are preserved at the early disease stage (Pinto et al., 2003; Romeo et al., 1998). On the other hand, CBI was absent in more severe patients with DBS of the ventralis intermedius thalamus when the stimulation was turned off. DBS restored the lost inhibition in these advanced patients in the stimulation-on state, suggesting that thalamic DBS may functionally change the excitability of inhibitory neurons mediating CBI and normalize the activity along cerebello-thalamo-cortical pathways in the patients (Jung et al., 2004; Molnar et al., 2004, 2005).

### Mirror Movement

Mirror movement is characterized as an involuntary movement on one side of the body that occurs simultaneously as a mirror of a voluntary movement on the other side. TMS on one side of M1 produces bilateral MEPs in patients with congenital mirror movement, indicating that both contralateral (decussated) and ipsilateral (not decussated) motor pathways exist in the patients (Cohen et al., 1991; Gallea et al., 2013; Jung et al., 2004). In addition, IHI decreases in congenital mirror movement patients (Gallea et al., 2013), suggesting that mirror movements may be related to impairment in the transcallosal fibers. Similar results with ipsilateral MEP and decreased IHI were also reported in PD patients with mirror movements (Li et al., 2007).

## Other Neurodegenerative Disorders

### Dementia and Mild Cognitive Impairment

In AD, motor cortical hyperexcitability was demonstrated by TMS, which included reduced MT, enhanced MEP, and reduced SICI. However, motor cortical facilitatory circuits appeared normal, as measured by ICF and SICF. Reduced MT was significantly correlated with the severity of cognitive impairments. SAI, representing cholinergic system function, is reduced in patients with AD, and is reversed by the oral administration of cholinesterase inhibitors. Abnormal SAI in combination with a large increase in SAI after a single dose of anticholinesterase inhibitor may indicate a favorable response to these drugs. SAI was also found to be abnormal in patients with Lewy body dementia, but is usually normal in frontotemporal dementia (Di Lazzaro, et al., 2006a). SAI is usually normal in patients with MCI, but found to be reduced in amnestic MCI, with multiple domain impairments suggesting that this type of MCI might be a phenotype of incipient AD (Nardone et al., 2012). Cortical plasticity induced by PAS is lost in patients with mild to moderate AD (Battaglia et al., 2007).

### Amyotrophic Lateral Sclerosis

In amyotrophic lateral sclerosis (ALS), abnormalities in MT are inconsistent, presumably due to heterogeneity of the ALS phenotype and the stage of the disease at time of testing (Vucic et al., 2013). While some studies found an increased MT or even an absence of MEPs, others have reported either normal or reduced MT. Longitudinal studies have shown a reduction of MTs early in the disease course, increasing to the point of cortical inexcitability with disease progression (Vucic et al., 2013). Increases in MEP amplitudes along with reduced MT have been documented, particularly in early stage of ALS, suggesting that cortical hyperexcitability is an early feature of ALS (Vucic et al., 2013). Absence or reduction in CSP has been reported in ALS, most prominently in early stages of the disease; this appears to be specific for ALS among various neuromuscular disorders (Vucic et al., 2013). Decreased SICI has been demonstrated in ALS, but not observed in ALS mimic disorders (Vucic et al., 2011). It is important that reduction in SICI precedes the clinical development of familial ALS, which may help in establishing the diagnosis (Vucic et al., 2008), and indicates that this measure might be particularly sensitive. ICF is increased in ALS, suggesting that glutamate-mediated excitotoxicity may be involved in motoneuron hyperexcitablity (Vucic et al., 2008). The involvement of the glutamate circuit in ALS pathophysiology is further supported by the finding that riluzole (a glutamate antagonist) restores the decreased SICI in ALS patients (Stefan et al., 2001). CMCT is typically modestly prolonged in ALS, probably reflecting axonal degeneration of the upper motor neurons. Evaluation with these methods, particularly SICI, with a special TMS technique called threshold tracking, can be useful in differentiating ALS from look-alike lower motor neuron disorders (Geevasinga et al., 2019).

### Cerebellar Disorders

In patients with various types of cerebellar degeneration, MT, CSP, and LICI are often increased. ICF is reduced without change in SICI, and CBI is usually reduced or absent. However, these changes are different among the various types of cerebellar degeneration (Schwenkreis et al., 2002). In patients with inherited cerebellar ataxia, reduced ICF can be more specific for spinocerebellar ataxia (SCA) 2 and 3, while prolonged CCT was found in patients with Friedreich ataxia and SCA 1, 2, and 6.

### Epilepsy and Antiepileptic Drugs

There are several different mechanisms for the genesis of epileptic seizures and for the modes of action of antiepileptic drugs (AEDs). TMS can be used to give information about these mechanisms by measuring cortical excitability. For example, MT is decreased in untreated patients with idiopathic generalized epilepsy. On the other hand, in progressive myoclonic epilepsy, threshold is normal, but there is loss of cortical inhibition demonstrated with paired pulses at 100–150 ms and an increase in facilitation at 50 ms. Prolonged SP was found in idiopathic generalized epilepsy and also in partial motor seizure. Within 48 hours after a generalized tonic-clonic seizure, ICF is reduced while SICI is normal, presumably representing a protective mechanism against spreading or recurrence of seizures. Increased motor cortical excitability, including reduced MT, increased ICF, and reduced SICI and LICI, were observed in the 24 hours before a seizure, while the opposite changes in motor cortical excitability measures were seen in the 24 hours after a seizure (Badawy et al., 2009). SICI is reduced but ICF is normal in progressive or juvenile myoclonic epilepsy. LICI is also reduced in progressive myoclonic epilepsy and also in idiopathic generalized epilepsy. Weaker SICI and ICF in the hemisphere ipsilateral to seizure onset were found to have a predictive value for seizures in the subsequent 48 hours in temporal lobe epilepsy patients with acute drug withdrawal (Wright et al., 2006). A long-term follow-up study in drug-naïve patients with generalized or partial epilepsy demonstrated that a decrease in cortical excitability, such as increased MT and increased SICI and LICI after medication, predicted a high probability of being seizure-free after 1 year of treatment (Badawy et al., 2010).

Specific effects can be seen with various AEDs in normal subjects (Kimiskidis et al., 2014). AEDs which enhance the action of GABA, such as vigabatrin, gabapentin and lorazepam, increase SICI, but have no effect on MT. In contrast, the AEDs blocking voltage-gated sodium or calcium channels, phenytoin, carbamazepine, and lamotrigine, increase MT without significant effects on SICI (Ziemann et al., 1996). In addition to elucidating these mechanisms, TMS can potentially be used to quantify physiological effects in individual patients, and this may be more valuable in some circumstances than monitoring blood levels of AEDs.

### Stroke

Several studies have attempted to correlate clinical recovery from stroke to the characteristics of MEPs. MEPs are often absent in severely affected stroke patients. In mildly affected patients, MEPs are usually of longer latency, smaller amplitude, and higher MT. The presence of MEPs in the early stage of stroke is associated with a good functional recovery (Hendricks et al., 2002). Conversely, absence of MEPs in the paretic limb with concomitantly increased MEP amplitudes in the unaffected limb predicts poor recovery. In addition, the presence of ipsilateral MEPs in the paretic limb in response to the stimulation of the unaffected hemisphere is also associated with poor recovery. The recovery of MEP latency is highly correlated with return of hand function. Higher MT than normal is often associated with the signs of spasticity. Noninvasive mapping of the motor cortex can be carried out with TMS using the figure-of-eight-shaped coil. This technique has been used to evaluate cortical reorganization in various conditions. In stroke patients, it has been demonstrated that cortical reorganization of the motor output still occurs for several months after insult. There is progressive enlargement of the motor maps of the recovering affected part. SICI is reduced in the affected hemisphere in the acute phase of a motor cortical stroke and remains reduced regardless of functional recovery. SICI also tends to be reduced in the unaffected hemisphere, but returns to normal subsequently—or can be greater than that in the affected hemisphere in patients showing good recovery. Enhanced SICI may lead to reduced activity in the unaffected hemisphere, which enhances activity of the affected hemisphere and promotes recovery.

### Multiple Sclerosis

CCT measurement has been applied in the evaluation of patients with multiple sclerosis (MS), where there is frequent involvement of the corticospinal tract. Typically, there is either a unilateral or bilateral prolongation of CCT consistent with demyelinating lesions in the corticospinal tract (Schlaeger et al., 2013; Schmierer et al., 2002). Prolonged CCT is more pronounced in progressive MS than in relapsing-remitting MS. Similar to other evoked potential studies, MEPs vary considerably in latency, amplitude, and shape in patients with MS when they are measured consecutively. An increased MT is also frequently observed in patients with MS.

### Migraine

Several studies have shown an increased MT in patients with migraine, but some studies also showed normal MT. CSP is usually normal, but in some studies shortened CSP was found in the hand as well as facial muscles. SICI was normal in one study, but reduced in another study. ICF was normal in one study, but increased in another. Because of the high prevalence of visual symptoms, many studies have investigated the cortical excitability of the occipital cortex, and have found a reduced phosphene threshold for occipital TMS (similar to MT for motor cortical TMS) in patients with migraine with aura (Badawy et al., 2012).

### Cervical Myelopathy and Other Spinal Cord Lesions

TMS is a useful tool for detection of cervical myelopathy, along with somatosensory evoked potentials. In patients with cervical myelopathy, MEPs, as well as the ratio of MEP/CMAP compound muscle action potential (CMAP), are usually reduced. CCT is prolonged, and their interside difference is increased. Simultaneous recordings from muscles innervated by different myelomers can help define the spinal level where the lesion is involved. Prolonged CCT often correlates with the clinical severity and the degree of cord compression observed in MRI. In a study recruiting a large number of patients with cervical myelopathy (Lo et al., 2004), the sensitivity of TMS in differentiating the presence and absence of MRI cord abnormality was 100% and the specificity was around 85%. CCT measures of the muscles innervated by cranial nerves, such as the trapezius or the tongue, may help differentiate ALS from cervical myelopathy. Abnormal CCT to these muscles indicates high probability of ALS.

## RATIONALE FOR REPETITIVE TRANSCRANIAL MAGNETIC STIMULATION IN THERAPEUTIC APPLICATIONS

The rationale of repetitive TMS (rTMS) for the therapy of neurological and psychiatric disorders draws from the concept that stimulation can alter brain activity and physiology. The idea is to compensate or even to reverse functional abnormalities thought to cause clinical deficits, assuming that normal functioning can be restored. The rTMS modulates brain excitability, and possibly also plasticity itself (called metaplasticity), which could facilitate and promote training effects of a subsequent rehabilitative intervention (Rossini et al., 2015). Promising randomized controlled therapeutic studies may provide a proof of concept, and the clinical use of rTMS for the treatment of depression and obsessive-compulsive disorder (OCD) has been approved in the United States and in some European countries.

Currently the best evidence in support of the concept that brain stimulation can help patients comes from DBS, although with DBS the effect is contemporaneous with the stimulation, while with rTMS the desired effect is after the stimulation. The success of DBS raises hope that rTMS might also be effective. The motor cortex is of particular interest in relation to motor disorders, due to its accessibility for rTMS. Functional imaging demonstrates widespread activation of the motor circuit by rTMS targeting the primary motor cortex (M1; Okabe et al., 2003) and the dorsal pre-motor cortex (dPMC; Bestmann, et al., 2005), supporting this concept. Further support comes from rTMS of M1 and the prefrontal cortex, which release dopamine in the caudate and putamen, corresponding to their cortico-striatal projections (Strafella et al., 2001, 2003).

## BASIC PRINCIPLES OF REPETITIVE TRANSCRANIAL MAGNETIC STIMULATION

In addition to single and paired pulse stimulation, TMS can be applied repetitively (rTMS), inducing effects which persist beyond the stimulation. This persistence implies functional and structural changes in synaptic strength, which constitute the basic mechanisms of plasticity.

Plasticity is the ability of the brain to change. It underlies normal brain functions, such as motor learning or adaptation to an environmental change. Plasticity is also responsible for spontaneous recovery after brain injury, such as stroke. rTMS and other means of brain stimulation can induce plastic changes, and diverse patterns of stimulation will produce different effects and even metaplasticity.

Generally, early plastic changes are alterations in synaptic strength; later changes will include anatomical changes such as sprouting and alterations of dendritic spines. By analogy to basic synaptic physiology, increasing of synaptic strength is called long-term potentiation (LTP) and reducing synaptic strength is called long-term depression (LTD). Changes induced by rTMS are considered LTP-like or LTD-like, depending on whether excitability is increased or decreased (Quartarone and Hallett, 2013; Quatarone et al., 2006). Plastic changes at any one time can occur only within a certain range, which is referred to as homeostatic plasticity (Abraham and Tate, 1997; Bienenstock et al., 1982; Turrigiano and Nelson, 2004). The stimulation protocol defines the direction of effects, which can be excitatory or inhibitory. High-frequency, or rapid, rTMS, ≥5 Hz, generally increases excitability, whereas low-frequency or slow rTMS, usually 1 Hz, induces a decrease (inhibition). There are patterned stimulation protocols and some derive their rationale from studies in brain physiology. A promising stimulation protocol, Theta-Burst Stimulation (TBS), is thought to simulate normal firing patterns in the hippocampus by coupling gamma-frequency bursts (50 Hz) with theta-rhythm (5 Hz). TBS given continuously (cTBS) leads to depression, whereas, if the TBS is given in periodic short trains, there is an increase of excitability (Huang et al., 2005). Quadripulse TMS (QPS) is the delivery of clusters of four pulses at different intervals, given every 5 seconds. Short intervals in the cluster of about 5 ms will lead to facilitation, whereas longer intervals of about 50–100 ms will lead to depression (Hamada et al., 2008). These are all methods of homosynaptic plasticity where activity of a synapse will lead to its own change. Heterosynaptic plasticity involves two inputs into the same synapse; as described earlier, this can be done with the TMS technique called PAS which combines a peripheral nerve and subsequent motor cortex stimulation by TMS (Stefan et al., 2000) but this has not yet been applied in therapy. These stimulation effects have been explored principally in the motor cortex and are now being extended to nonmotor areas. The efficacy of intermittent rTMS is contingent on its ability to induce effects which persist minutes to hours beyond the stimulation period (Chen et al., 1997; Gangitano et al., 2002; Maeda et al., 2000). Plasticity has been probed in various brain disorders and appears preserved, for instance, in PD (Benninger, 2013).

There are safety concerns with rTMS and these have been summarized by an international committee (Rossi et al., 2009; Rossini et al., 2015). Seizures are the most serious acute adverse effect of rTMS, although this is extremely rare, and primarily results from excitatory stimulation protocols exceeding safety limits. Particular precaution is warranted in vulnerable patients with disease conditions or drugs that potentially lower the seizure threshold. There are no reports of irreversible stimulation effects.

## CURRENT CONCEPTS OF THERAPEUTIC APPLICATION OF REPETITIVE TRANSCRANIAL MAGNETIC STIMULATION

A rapidly growing number of randomized controlled studies have probed the therapeutic potential of rTMS in various brain disorders. Therapeutic applications include rTMS as an adjunct to conventional therapy, in treatment-refractory cases, and as a first-line therapy. rTMS promotes learning during repetitive practice (Ackerley et al., 2010), and combining rTMS with rehabilitative and other types of interventions may enhance the therapeutic benefit (Rossini et al., 2015). The rationale of rTMS is to induce plastic changes. It may offer an alternative to invasive procedures such as DBS and epidural cortex stimulation, and may simulate the condition after electrode implantation to determine the eligibility of candidates in a pre-surgical evaluation and contribute to validating a cortical target. rTMS also can assess the capability for plasticity and has advanced our knowledge of the pathophysiology of various brain disorders.

An extensive review of current concepts and guidelines for the potential therapeutic use of rTMS in various brain disorders has been published (Lefaucheur et al., 2014) and is currently being revised. This review focuses on approved applications and discusses other selected therapeutic approaches to illustrate the diversity of rationales and possibilities.

### Depression

Currently the strongest evidence for rTMS is found for the treatment of depression, and this indication is now clinically approved in the United States and in some countries in Europe (George et al., 2013). A large multicenter randomized controlled trial (RCT) found significant reduction in depression scores with high frequency (10 Hz) rTMS to the left dorsolateral prefrontal cortex (DLPFC) compared with placebo in the acute treatment of major depression (O'Reardon et al., 2007). This led to FDA approval, despite a negative multicenter RCT published in the same year (Herwig et al., 2007). There has been a discussion about this discrepancy, which some had attributed to the methodological differences between the studies. A subsequent RCT supported the antidepressant efficacy of rapid rTMS of the left DLPFC (George et al., 2010), and a current meta-analysis provides further support (Berlim et al., 2013b). Electroconvulsive therapy provided the initial rationale for rTMS, with the intent to modulate brain networks involved in the pathophysiology of depression. The targets had been derived from neurophysiological and imaging research in patients with depression, pointing to functionally opposite changes in the prefrontal cortices. This concept of disbalance has found support in therapeutic trials demonstrating similar efficacy of both the approved excitatory rapid rTMS of the left DLPFC and the inhibitory slow rTMS aimed at the hyperactivity of the right DLPFC (Chen et al., 2013). Interestingly, there are nonresponders to either protocol who have benefited from side switching, but no predictor of therapeutic success has been identified that could guide individual therapy. The few controlled studies found no superiority of bilateral over unilateral stimulation of either side (Berlim et al., 2013a).

Rapid rTMS of the left DLPFC offers a therapeutic option in medication-refractory major depression. The therapeutic effect increases with repeated interventions and may be stronger in younger patients and depression of recent onset (George and Post, 2011). Following the principles of evidence-based medicine (EBM), a consensus of European experts concluded in a review of RCT a definite efficacy (level A) of high-frequency (HF) rTMS of the left DLPFC for the treatment of medication-refractory major depression, while the issues of maintenance and prevention of relapses have not been resolved (Lefaucheur et al., 2014). Theta-burst TMS has now also been used and may produce much faster benefit (Blumberger et al., 2018).

### Obsessive Compulsive Disorder

OCD is a chronic anxiety disorder and the pathophysiology of OCD involves dysfunction of brain networks with abnormal activity in multiple frontal cortical areas (Abramowitz et al., 2009). rTMS enables modulation of neural activity in distinct target brain areas and may be a more suitable treatment for the OCD patients than the aspecific pharmacological therapy. As OCD is related to hyperactivity of the orbitofrontal-subcortical circuit, early study with high-frequency rTMS targeting DLPFC was designed to normalize the hyperactive circuit via activation of the inhibitory pathway between DLPFC and orbitofrontal cortex (Greenberg et al., 1997). Symptoms measured with the Yale-Brown Obsessive Compulsive Scale were improved in the patients. Further study showed that high-frequency (20 Hz) deep TMS delivered with an H coil over the medial prefrontal cortex and anterior cingulate cortex was effective in OCD patients (Carmi et al., 2018). The effect was demonstrated in the positive results of a multicenter phase 3 clinical trial with 6 weeks of treatment, which led to FDA approval for the treatment in OCD patients. On the other hand, low-frequency rTMS to the orbitofrontal cortex may also reduce obsessive-compulsive symptoms by inhibiting the orbitofrontal cortical hyperactivity directly (Ruffini et al., 2009). Similarly, low-frequency rTMS to the supplementary motor area (SMA) was tried and showed improved symptoms in patients as the reduced inhibition in motor areas may be related to OCD (Gomes et al., 2012). However, the effects of rTMS application to these and other new targets in the frontal cortex must be tested in clinical trials with large sample sizes.

### Auditory Hallucinations and Negative Symptoms in Schizophrenia

The increased pathological activity in the primary and associative auditory areas in the left temporo-parietal cortex (TPC) presumed to underlie auditory hallucinations provides the rationale for inhibitory rTMS protocols. The results are ambiguous, with both positive and negative studies (both of class II and III), though a few meta-analyses point to a possible therapeutic efficacy of inhibitory rTMS. Larger studies are needed.

Negative symptoms in schizophrenia may result from functional disturbance in the prefrontal cortex. Various stimulation protocols have targeted frontal areas, but only facilitatory rapid rTMS to the left DLPFC has been promising. A Cochrane review of 41 studies with 1473 participants found insufficient evidence to support or to refute clinical efficacy of rTMS for treating symptoms of schizophrenia and as an adjunctive therapy to antipsychotic medication, though considered temporo-parietal rTMS promising for auditory hallucinations and other positive symptoms (Dougall et al., 2015).

### Parkinson Disease

The success of DBS in PD has raised interest in rTMS as an alternative therapy. PD may offer a model to investigate whether rTMS can improve symptoms and reverse functional changes in the motor network. The motor system affected in PD lends itself ideally for cause-effect exploration.

The current disease model suggests that dysfunction of the cortico-striato-thalamo-cortical circuit results in a deficient thalamo-cortical drive and impaired facilitation of the motor cortex to cause motor symptoms (Mink, 1996; Wichmann, et al., 2011). Decreased cortical activation and excitability during planning and performance of voluntary activity may represent a neurophysiological correlate of bradykinesia (Chen et al., 2001). The rationale of rapid rTMS is to increase motor cortex activation and excitability. Though pilot studies were promising and meta-analyses concluded modest efficacy of rTMS in improving motor function (Chou et al., 2015; Elahi et al., 2009; Fregni et al., 2005; Jung et al., 2004), the results of recent class 1 therapeutic trials remain ambiguous regarding M1 stimulation (Benninger et al., 2012; Brys et al., 2016), while failing to confirm the efficacy of combined M1 and DLPFC stimulation (Benninger et al., 2011; Brys et al., 2016). Larger RCTs of different stimulation protocols are needed.

A promising therapeutic concept arises from the postulated role of oscillatory activity in normal brain physiology and in the pathogenesis of brain disorders (Benninger and Hallett, 2015). In PD, presumed pathological oscillatory $\beta$-activity in the motor cortex and basal ganglia characterizes bradykinesia and physiological $\gamma$ activity (>30 Hz) emerges along with clinical improvement (Brown, 2007). The rationale of rTMS in this regard is to entrain oscillatory activity into a physiological range (Thut and Miniussi, 2009) and to enhance "pro-kinetic" $\gamma$-activity while suppressing "akinetic" $\beta$-activity (Brown, 2007). An RCT of 50 Hz rTMS in PD modulated cortical excitability, but failed to improve motor function, which may require longer-lasting stimulation (Benninger et al., 2012).

Plasticity, while weakened, appears preserved in PD, but efficacy of rTMS may be contingent on prolonged stimulation, considering the sequential disappearance of tremor, rigidity, bradykinesia, and axial signs with continuing use of DBS over hours (Temperli et al., 2003). In dystonia, the clinical improvement with DBS takes months and goes along with a presumed restoration of normal physiology (Ruge et al., 2011). These observations highlight the role of plasticity in clinical improvement, which may depend on chronic stimulation. Plasticity may be maladaptive and contribute to the pathogenesis of dyskinesias (Morgante et al., 2006). Dyskinesias may respond to inhibitory stimulation of the cerebellum (Koch et al., 2009) and of the SMA (Sayin et al., 2014), while not of the M1 (Flamez et al., 2016), but larger studies are needed.

An interesting finding is that rTMS causes dopamine release in moderate PD (Strafella et al., 2005, 2006) which could contribute to the acute effects. A recent study combined rTMS with behavioral training to get an increased benefit (Yang et al., 2013), which is worth pursuing in this and other indications.

## Dystonia

Dystonia is a heterogeneous disorder characterized by involuntary muscle activity and impaired voluntary motor control. Neurophysiological investigations point to a deficiency of inhibitory circuits, sensory dysfunction, and maladaptive plasticity. Therapeutic options are scarce and rTMS is being investigated with the rationale to restore inhibition. There are a few controlled trials primarily in focal hand dystonia, cervical dystonia, and blepharospasm, and effects, if beneficial, have been modest and short-lived. The targets have included the primary motor and sensory cortices, the premotor cortex, and the cerebellum.

## Essential Tremor

Neurophysiology and functional imaging point to the key role of the cerebellum in the pathogenesis of essential tremor and of other types of tremor. The hyperactivity of both the deep cerebellar nuclei and cortex in essential tremor provides the rationale for inhibitory stimulation to restore normal excitability and suppress tremor (Kang and Cauraugh, 2017; Shih and Pascual-Leone, 2017). There are few controlled rTMS studies with promising results, but the evidence is insufficient to draw any conclusion about the efficacy of cerebellar stimulation for essential tremor (Badran et al., 2016; Bologna et al., 2015; Gironell et al., 2002; Hellriegel et al., 2012; Jung et al., 2004).

## Pain and Migraine

Chronic pain refractory to medical therapy is a challenge, and rTMS is being investigated as an alternative approach. Several therapeutic rTMS studies postulate efficacy in the treatment of chronic neuropathic and non-neuropathic pain. A Cochrane meta-analysis of 30 controlled studies with 528 patients did not find efficacy of rTMS in chronic pain, but the heterogeneity of causes, targets, and stimulation parameters may contribute to the negative conclusion. A subgroup analysis suggested efficacy of a single intervention of high-frequency (≥5 Hz) rTMS of the motor cortex, but the pain relief is minimal and of short duration (O'Connell et al., 2014). This intervention could be repeated, but longer-lasting efficacy still needs to be demonstrated.

Why stimulate the motor cortex for the modulation of nociception? Painful stimuli are reported to decrease the excitability of the motor cortex (Valeriani et al., 1999). In chronic pain, neurophysiological investigations and functional imaging demonstrate extensive changes in brain activity and cortical excitability, but their contribution to the pathogenesis of pain is not known. rTMS of the cortex changes the intracortical inhibition and may contribute to the reduction of chronic neuropathic pain (Lefaucheur et al., 2006a). In functional imaging, stimulation of the motor cortex modulates activity in the limbic circuits, brainstem, and spinal cord, which are the centers involved in affective-emotional integration of pain (Garcia-Larrea and Peyron, 2007). These studies suggest a functional interaction of the motor system and nociception, but the mechanisms are still under investigation.

A number of rTMS studies failed to reduce the frequency of migraine attacks. But, as an exception from the general therapeutic use of rTMS, single TMS pulses (sTMS) have been applied during the aura to prevent a migraine attack. The rationale is to interrupt cortical spreading depression, presumed to underlie the aura. In a controlled study, sTMS maintained pain freedom more than sham stimulation (Lipton et al., 2010). The clinical use has been approved, though it has fueled a critical discussion of the scientific evidence and lesser stringency in the evaluation of therapeutic devices by regulatory bodies. For this purpose, the FDA approved a portable TMS device.

Notwithstanding the heterogeneity of the RCTs, the consensus of European experts concluded a definite efficacy (level A) of HF rTMS of the contralateral (to the pain) primary motor cortex (M1) in reducing chronic neuropathic pain based on evidence from RCTs (Lefaucheur et al., 2014). The current IFCN guidelines consider it good clinical practice to select candidates for invasive cortical stimulation based on their response to HF rTMS of M1 (Rossini et al., 2015).

## Tinnitus

The rationale for rTMS derives from the hypothesis of hyperactivity in the auditory TPC as a potential cause of chronic tinnitus, which may result from the deafferentation process following a cochlear trauma or disease (Eggermont, 2007). The TPC has been the target of inhibitory slow rTMS studies with possible effects, but the evidence remains weak and recent RCTs have been negative (Langguth et al., 2014; Plewnia et al., 2012). In one of these studies (Langguth et al., 2014), stimulation of TPC (inhibition) was combined with facilitatory stimulation of the prefrontal cortex (facilitation) because of the increased frontotemporal connectivity in tinnitus (Sclee et al., 2008) and the role of the prefrontal cortex in higher-level auditory processing (Eggermont, 2007; Vanneste and De Ridder, 2011), but this did not provide any benefit.

## Stroke with Motor Deficits, Aphasia, and Hemispatial Neglect

The rationale for rTMS in subacute and chronic stroke has two principal aims: to enhance adaptive plasticity and to counteract compensatory mechanisms presumed to interfere with neuronal repair, considered maladaptive plasticity, which could impede functional recovery. For these purposes, facilitatory rTMS protocols have been applied to the perilesional area and inhibitory protocols principally to the unaffected hemisphere. The rationale draws from neurophysiological exploration pointing to an increased excitability of the contralateral hemisphere presumed to interfere with perilesional mechanisms of recovery, although it could also enhance functional recovery (Gerloff et al., 2006). The majority of studies have targeted motor deficits, aphasia, and hemispatial neglect in subacute and chronic stroke.

In stroke with motor deficits, despite promising results in a few controlled studies, a Cochrane review of 19 studies including 588 patients found no evidence of improvement of motor function nor in activities of daily living to support clinical use of rTMS in post-stroke rehabilitation (Hao et al., 2013).

In aphasia, the few class III/IV studies with either approach—enhancing perilesional mechanisms, or inhibition of the contralateral hemisphere, especially when combined with rehabilitative interventions—yielded promising results (Mylius et al., 2012), which need confirmation in larger controlled studies.

Most patients with hemispatial neglect recover spontaneously, but chronic forms may benefit from repeated inhibitory cTBS of the contralesional hemisphere, which improved performance in neuropsychological tests and activities of daily living for the follow-up period of 3 weeks in a controlled study (Cazzoli et al., 2012). A recent meta-analysis of 6 RCTs with a total of 163 patients found overall beneficial effects of rTMS on dysphagia after stroke, but the type of stimulation protocol and the target (unaffected versus affected, or both hemispheres) needs to be clarified in larger studies (Liao et al., 2017).

## Amyotrophic Lateral Sclerosis

The rationale for rTMS in the treatment of ALS is for reducing the cortical hyperexcitability and, thereby, counteracting the excitotoxicity by glutamate and other neurotransmitters presumed to be mechanisms of disease. A recent Cochrane meta-analysis of the few randomized studies found insufficient evidence for a conclusion conferring the efficacy and safety of rTMS (Fang et al., 2013).

### Epilepsy

The treatment-resistance of focal epilepsy is relatively prevalent and poses a challenge. The rationale for rTMS is to modulate the focal hyperexcitability presumed to be a central mechanism in seizure generation. Transcranial stimulation can also be used as an alternative approach to more invasive procedures to determine eligibility in a presurgical evaluation. Promising case series of focal and nonfocal, mainly inhibitory slow rTMS could not be confirmed by controlled trials (Chen et al., 2016; Nitsche and Paulus, 2009). There are reports of reduction of interictal EEG abnormalities after rTMS, but this does not translate into therapeutic efficacy. The small number and the heterogeneity of potentially underpowered studies preclude clinical recommendations. A recent Cochrane review of the few RCT found rTMS to be safe, and found reasons to support the efficacy of the technique in reducing epileptic activity, but could not draw any conclusion due to insufficient evidence (Chen et al., 2016).

## CONCLUSION AND OUTLOOK

The rationale for noninvasive brain stimulation in clinical practice is to provide benefit beyond conventional therapy, to offer an alternative approach for patients at risk or that are excluded from surgical interventions, and/or to treat refractory symptoms.

There is evidence for the therapeutic efficacy of rTMS in the treatments of medication-refractory major depression (rapid rTMS of left DLPFC) neuropathic pain (rapid rTMS of contralateral M1) and hand motor recovery in the post-acute stage of stroke (slow rTMS of contralesional M1). The evidence in these conditions was considered to indicate definite efficacy (level A recommendation) by a current consensus on therapeutic applications (Lefaucheur et al., 2014). This review concluded a probable efficacy (level B) for improving quality of life and pain in fibromyalgia, motor impairment and depression in PD, lower limb spasticity in MS, posttraumatic stress disorder and chronic post-stroke non-fluent aphasia. There is an official guidance for single-pulse TMS during aura to prevent migraine, though the evidence is still minimal.

The rapidly increasing number of trials reflects strong interest in pursuing the search for therapeutic applications of rTMS. Larger controlled studies will provide better evidence to specify and possibly extend the present recommendations. Despite the reports of therapeutic potential, clinical effects are often small and negligible regarding functional independence and quality of life. Looking to the future in regard to noninvasive brain stimulation for therapy, transcranial electrical stimulation is also promising and may well replace TMS for some indications.

*The complete reference list is available online at https://expertconsult.inkling.com/.*

38

# Intracranial Neuromodulation

*Ryan Barmore, Zhongxing Peng-Chen, Abhay Kumar, Michael S. Okun*

## OUTLINE



As early as the 1950s temporary deep brain stimulation (DBS) electrodes were implanted into the septal region. The procedure was performed for pain control and was reported to have beneficial effects (Hamani et al., 2006). There were various attempts at DBS, with most documented experiences revealing its usefulness in test stimulation prior to ablative brain lesions (Blomstedt and Hariz, 2010). In 1987, when Alim-Louis Benabid was operating on a chronic pain patient, he noticed that the patient's tremor improved during test stimulation and decided to chronically stimulate this patient. Over the ensuing decades, multiple DBS placements into several brain regions for a variety of clinical indications have been attempted (Awan, Lozano, and Hamani, 2009).

High-frequency stimulation (HFS) has been thought to affect the basal ganglia network and has been previously described to operate as an informational lesion, though this explanation continues to be modified and refined (Birdno and Grill, 2008; McIntyre, 2004a, 2004b and 2004c). HFS has been hypothesized to result in a decoupling of the cellular and the axonal output within a thalamocortical relay circuit. The firing rates and patterns of the cell body may be suppressed, while fibers of passage may be excited. DBS may, ultimately, affect a cortico-striatopallido-thalamo-cortical (CSPTC) network and result in upstream, as well as downstream, changes within this complex basal ganglia network (McIntyre and Hahn, 2010). The specific effects of an electrical field are thought to reflect changes relative to the position and orientation of the axon to the actual DBS lead and to exert trans-synaptic influences (McIntyre, 2004a, 2004b and 2004c).

The clinical benefits of DBS have been hypothesized to be due to more than just local neurotransmitter release (Stefani et al., 2005); however, several authors have argued that there is a collective effect and that transmitter release may be very important to the mechanism of action (Dostrovsky and Lozano, 2002; Lee Chang, Roberts, and Kim, 2004; Vitek, 2002). Animal models of DBS have revealed increased extracellular concentrations of glutamate, γ-aminobutyric acid (GABA), adenosine, and dopamine (Chang, Shon, Agnesi, and Lee, 2009; Shon et al., 2010; Windels et al., 2003). Depolarization blockade, synaptic inhibition, and synaptic depression (McIntyre, 2004b and 2004c) have also been proposed to play a role in the potential mechanisms of action of DBS. The mechanisms underpinning the therapeutic effects of DBS remain unknown; however, neurophysiological, neurochemical, neurovascular, neurogenic, and neuro-oscillations all play a role.

DBS technology involves placement of a lead with four to eight contacts into a specific and predetermined brain target (Fig. 38.1). Selective placement of the DBS leads within different anatomical regions. Somatotopies may affect the neuronal network and, in the best possible cases, lead to improvement in clinical symptoms. The lead is usually connected to a neurostimulator placed subcutaneously under the clavicle, although the battery can be placed in a multitude of regions. The neurostimulator can then be programmed or adjusted in order to tailor a setting to an individual patient. There are thousands of different combinations that may be chosen. The amplitude, frequency, pulse width, and electrode configuration may all be changed. The optimal settings are patient- and symptom-specific, and generally require that patients be reprogrammed frequently for the first 4–6 months. Additionally, medications as well as stimulation settings must be monitored (Ondo and Bronte-Stewart, 2005; Rodriguez, Fernandez, Haq, and Okun, 2007).

Each disorder or symptom considered for treatment with DBS should be carefully evaluated. Only a fraction of the patients with a given neurological or neuropsychiatric disorder may be eligible for this type of therapy. Most patients receiving DBS should be medication-resistant and should undergo a complete multidisciplinary screening by a neurologist, psychiatrist, neuropsychologist, neurosurgeon, and by physical, occupational, and speech/swallowing therapists. Following screening there should be a detailed interdisciplinary discussion about the goals of therapy including symptoms targeted, symptoms that will likely respond, symptoms that are not likely to respond, and an individual patient's expectations.

In cases of Parkinson disease (PD), patients should undergo an "off/on" levodopa medication challenge to determine which symptoms respond best to medication. The symptoms that respond best to medication usually are those that respond best to stimulation (with the

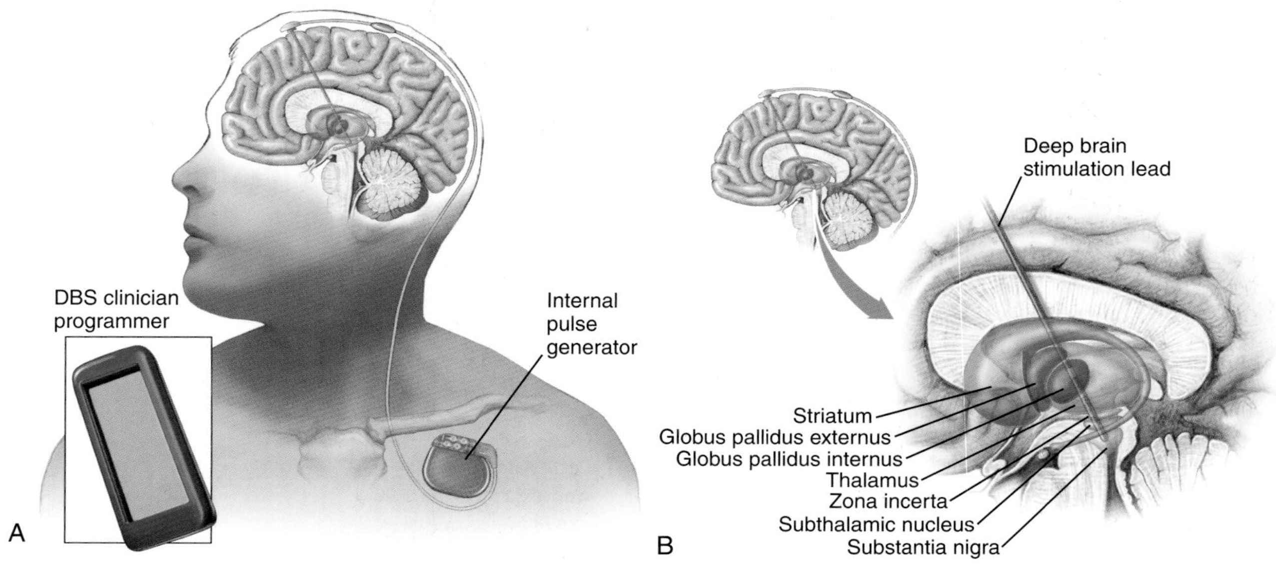


**Fig. 38.1** **A,** Deep brain stimulation *(DBS)* consists of a lead connected to an internal pulse generator placed subcutaneously, usually under the clavicle. **B,** This lead has four contacts that can be activated through a programmer. In this case, the lead is placed in the subthalamic nucleus.

exceptions of tremor and dyskinesia). Risks and benefits of a potential DBS surgery, as well as the potential brain target(s), and unilateral versus bilateral DBS should all be carefully addressed in preoperative conversations with patients and families (Alberts, Hass, Vitek, and Okun, 2008; Kluger, Klepitskaya, and Okun, 2009; Okun et al., 2004, 2007, 2009; Okun and Foote, 2004; Rodriguez et al., 2007; Skidmore et al., 2006; Ward, Hwynn, and Okun, 2010). There are many potential adverse events that may occur as a result of DBS, some of which may constitute emergencies (Morishita et al., 2010).

Depending on the region of the world and the preference of individual surgical teams, leads and batteries may be placed in a single setting or may be staged (separate operating room procedures). Additionally, one lead, two leads, or, in exceptional circumstances more than two leads, may be implanted in a single session. One review of DBS hardware-related complications cited lead migration, lead fracture, lead erosion/infection, and lead malfunctions as not uncommon occurrences (Lyons, Wilkinson, Overman, and Pahwa, 2004; Oh et al., 2002). Surgically related and stimulation-related complications can occur; they may include but are not limited to hemorrhage, infection, stroke, seizures, paresthesias, dysarthria, hypophonia, dystonia, mood worsening, suicide, apathy, and worsening of comorbidities. Difficulty with verbal fluency and anger seem to be common sequelae in PD patients (Blomstedt and Hariz, 2005; Blomstedt and Hariz, 2006; Hariz et al., 2008; Okun et al., 2008b; Saint-Cyr and Albanese, 2006). DBS teams must differentiate between lesion effects, stimulation-induced effects, and transient versus permanent neurological dysfunction.

## PARKINSON DISEASE

PD is a complex disorder thought to be the result of extensive loss of neurons and their projections within motor and nonmotor basal ganglia circuitry (Alexander, 1986). A rationale for neuromodulatory therapy has been developed as a result of models of basal ganglia physiology. Perhaps the most famous model reveals loss of dopaminergic neurons in the substantia nigra pars compacta with a resultant abnormal neuronal activity in both the direct and indirect basal ganglia circuitry. These changes are thought to result in the genesis of many of the motor symptoms of PD.

Initial treatment of PD is usually with dopaminergic therapy, although disease progression may lead to limitations in medical therapy including such symptoms as wearing "off" between doses, "on-off" fluctuations, and medication-related dyskinesia (Video 38.1). The subthalamic nucleus (STN) and the globus pallidus internus (GPi) DBS have been used to modulate basal ganglia pathways and to restore important functions in select patients, as can be seen in Video 38.2 (Pahwa, Wilkinson, Overman, and Lyons, 2005; Weaver et al., 2009). To date, STN and GPi DBS have shown similar motor outcomes and the potential benefits between these targets have been shown to manifest differences. STN DBS may have a slightly larger benefit in the medication off state, and may allow for larger dopaminergic medication reductions, though STN DBS may have an equal or higher risk of neuropsychiatric changes as compared with GPi DBS. GPi DBS may provide better dyskinesia suppression, better long-term flexibility, and a relatively safer risk–benefit profile (Anderson, Burchiel, Hogarth, Favre, and Hammerstad, 2005; Follett et al., 2010; Mikos, Zahodne, Okun, Foote, and Bowers, 2010; Moro et al., 2010; Odekerken et al., 2013; Odekerken et al., 2016; Okun et al., 2009; Weaver et al., 2012; Williams et al., 2010; Zahodne et al., 2009). GPi is also a better target for dyskinesia that tends to occur at very low medication doses, often referred to as "brittle" dyskinesia.

### Clinical Evidence: Randomized Controlled Trials

There have been multiple smaller studies to determine the efficacy of STN and/or GPi DBS in the treatment of PD symptoms. The best supporting evidence for the use of DBS in PD patients comes from several randomized clinical trials that compare these targets with the best medical treatment (Table 38.1).

In 2006, the German Parkinson Study Group published a comparison between bilateral STN stimulation and medication versus medical management alone (Deuschl et al., 2006). In this study, 156 patients with advanced PD younger than 75 years of age were enrolled and randomized into both groups. The primary outcome of the study was to assess changes in the quality of life per the Parkinson Disease Questionnaire

**TABLE 38.1 Deep Brain Stimulation—A Few Selected Deep Brain Stimulation Studies from the Literature**

| Author | Site/No. | Follow-up | Outcomes/Author Conclusions |
|---|---|---|---|
| **Parkinson Disease** | | | |
| (Timmermann et al., 2015) VANTAGE | STN (B/L): 40 | 12–52 weeks | Constant current, 8-contact DBS device was safe and effective. |
| (Odekerken et al., 2013) NSTAPS | GPi: 65<br>STN:63 | 1 year | STN stimulation showed greater improvement in UPDRS while off-medication and greater medication reduction, while there were no differences in cognition, mood, and behavior. |
| (Schuepbach et al., 2013) EARLYSTIM | STN (B/L) | 2 years | Early stimulation (*N* = 124) was superior to medical therapy alone (*N* = 127) in terms of motor disability, ADL, levodopa-induced complications, and time with good mobility. |
| (Okun et al., 2012) | STN (B/L): 136 | 1 year | Constant-current device DBS had better outcomes in terms of good quality on time and improved UPDRS motor score. |
| (Follett et al., 2010) | GPi (B/L): 152<br>STN (B/L):147 | 2 years | Similar improvement in motor function with stimulation of either target. STN group has lesser medication requirement and more decline in visuomotor skills and level of depression compared with GPi group. |
| (Okun et al., 2009) COMPARE | STN (U/L): 22<br>GPi (U/L): 23 | 7 months | UPDRS motor scores improved in STN and GPi; worsened mood with ventral DBS of both sites; worsened letter fluency more with STN; anger in both targets. |
| (Krack et al., 2003) | STN (B/L): 49 | 5 years | Improved motor function, dyskinesia, and ADLs off-medication. Worsened on medication akinesia, speech, postural instability, freezing, and cognitive problems. |
| **Tremor** | | | |
| (Wharen et al., 2017) | VIM (B/L): 47 (ET)<br>VIM (U/L): 80 | 6 months | Constant-current device showed improved upper extremity tremor, ADLs, quality of life and depression. |
| (Zhang et al., 2010) | VIM (B/L): 11 (ET)<br>VIM (U/L): 23 | 3–128 months | Overall 80.4% improvement in tremor with average follow-up of 56.9 months. |
| (Hariz et al., 2008) | VIM: 38 (PD) | 6 years | Tremor effectively controlled by DBS with stable appendicular rigidity and akinesia. Axial scores worsened. Improvement in ADLs disappeared despite tremor control. |
| (Blomstedt et al., 2007) | VIM: 19 (ET) | 7 years | Effective treatment for ET but improvement diminishes over time. |
| **Dystonia** | | | |
| (Ostrem et al., 2017) | STN (B/L): 20 | 3 years | BFMDRS motor scores improved 70.4%, TWSTRS scores improved 66.6%. Improvement at 36 months equivalent to 6 months. |
| (Volkmann et al., 2012) | GPi (B/L): 40 | 5 years | There is sustained improvement in dystonia and rating and disability at 5 years with B/L GPi in primary generalized or segmental dystonia. |
| **Pain** | | | |
| (Akram et al., 2016) | VTA: 21 (CH) | 4–60 months | Sixty percent improvement in headache frequency, 30% improvement in severity. Abortive medication usage dropped by 57%. QoL, disability and mood scales improved. |
| (Broggi 2007) | PH:<br>16 (CH)<br>1 (SUNCT)<br>3 (AFP) | 18 months | 10/16 CH patients completely pain-free, the SUNCT patient responded, no benefit in AFP. |
| **Epilepsy** | | | |
| (Geller et al., 2017) | RNS device at seizure focus: 111 | 2–6 years | Median seizure reduction of 70%. 29% of patients had at least one seizure-free period of ≥6 months, 15% with ≥1 year. |
| (Jobst et al., 2017) | RNS device at seizure focus: 126 | 2–6 years | Seventy percent median seizure reduction with frontal and parietal seizure onsets, 58% with temporal onsets, 51% with multilobar. No deficits seen in stim over eloquent cortex. |
| **Neuropsychiatry** | | | |
| (Kefalopoulou et al., 2015) | GPi: 15 | 8–36 months | 15.3% improvement in YGTSS scores at end of blinded stimulation period; 40.1% improvement in YGTSS after open-label phase. |
| (Ackermans et al., 2011) | CMN, substantia periventricularis, VO: 6 (TS) | 1 year | Stimulation effect persisted after a year with a 49% improvement in YGTSS. |

*Continued*

TABLE 38.1 **Deep Brain Stimulation—A Few Selected Deep Brain Stimulation Studies from the Literature—cont'd**

| Author | Site/No. | Follow-up | Outcomes/Author Conclusions |
|---|---|---|---|
| (Luyten et al., 2016) | ALIC/BNST area: 24 | 4–16 years | Significant improvement in obsessions, compulsions, anxiety, depression and function. |
| (Greenberg et al., 2010) | VC/VS: 26 (OCD) | 24–36 months | Two-thirds of patients improved; patients with more posterior target had more effective treatment. |
| (Goodman et al., 2010) | VC/VS: 6 (OCD) | 1 year | 4/6 patient responders, sham stimulation period for half the patients. |

This table is a summary of some of the major neuromodulatory studies, but for space considerations not all studies could be listed. We apologize to any authors who were excluded.

*ADLs,* Activities of daily living; *AFP,* atypical facial pain; *ALIC,* anterior limb of the internal capsule; *BFMDRS,* Burke-Fahn-Marsden Dystonia Rating Scale; *B/L,* bilateral; *BNST,* bed nucleus of the stria terminalis; *CH,* cluster headache; *CMN,* centromedian thalamic nucleus; *DBS,* deep brain stimulation; *ET,* essential tremor; *GPi,* globus pallidus internus; *OCD,* obsessive-compulsive disorder; *PD,* Parkinson's disease; *PH,* posterior hypothalamus; *QoL,* quality of life; *STN,* subthalamic nucleus; *SUNCT,* short-lasting unilateral neuralgiform headache attacks with conjunctival injection and tearing; *TS,* Tourette syndrome; *TWSTRS,* Toronto Western Spasmodic Torticollis Rating Scale; *U/L,* unilateral; *UPDRS,* United Parkinson Disease Rating Scale; *VC/VS,* ventral capsule/ventral striatum; *VIM,* ventral intermediate thalamic nucleus; *VO,* nucleus ventralis oralis of the thalamus; *VTA,* ventral tegmental area; *YGTSS,* Yale Global Tic Severity Scale.

(PDQ-39) and the severity of motor symptoms per the Unified Parkinson Disease Rating Scale motor score (UPDRS-III) between the stimulation-and-medication versus the medication-alone group. The stimulation group had a significant improvement in the PDQ-39 and UPDRS-III scores. One of the drawbacks of the German Parkinson Study Group trial was that the population studied was relatively young.

The Veterans Administration CSP 468 Study Group published a second randomized clinical trial 3 years later (Weaver et al., 2009). The objective of the study was to compare the outcomes of bilateral DBS implanted in either the STN ($N = 60$) or GPi ($N = 61$) versus best medical management ($N = 134$) stratified by site and age less than 70 years and more than 70 years. This trial demonstrated an improvement in quality of life and motor symptoms. The improvements persisted, despite the inclusion of an older population. However, the differences between targets were not analyzed. In 2012, the same group reported sustained benefits of stimulation of either the STN ($N = 70$) or the GPi ($N = 89$) on motor function after a 36-month follow-up (Weaver et al., 2012). The findings of the CSP 468 trial have been largely confirmed by a Dutch trial, the NSTAPS study, which also revealed similar outcomes for STN and GPi DBS (Odekerken et al., 2013). A 3-year follow-up, which included 90 of the 128 patients originally enrolled in the NSTAPS study, observed slightly more improvement in off-medication motor symptoms favoring STN and greater medication reduction, also favoring STN. There were similar risks of cognitive, mood, and behavioral outcomes though this study used some outcome variables that were not comparable to many other studies (Odekerken et al., 2016).

DBS plus best medical therapy versus best medical therapy alone for advanced PD, better known as the PD SURG trial, provided further evidence of the efficacy of DBS in the treatment of PD (Williams et al., 2010). In this study, 366 patients were randomized to surgical intervention with DBS and best medical treatment or best medical treatment alone. Again, the DBS group had better quality of life as assessed by the PDQ-39 a year after randomization. Long-term efficacy of DBS in PD has been excellent. Symptoms that respond to levodopa seem to continue to respond to DBS, with the exceptions of tremor and dyskinesia that may have persistent benefits despite waning levodopa responses (Krack et al., 2003; Schüpbach et al., 2005; Wider, Pollo, Bloch, Burkhard, and Vingerhoets, 2008). We know that as disease progresses, nonmotor complications emerge and these are often not responsive to levodopa or to DBS.

There has been much interest in delivering DBS earlier in the disease course. The EARLYSTIM trial studied 251 subjects between the ages of 18 and 60 years, disease duration of 4 years or more, with a severity rating below stage 3 on the Hoehn and Yahr scale, and presence of fluctuations or dyskinesia for 3 years or less (Schuepbach et al., 2013). Bilateral STN DBS devices were implanted on 124 subjects. When compared with the best medical treatment ($N = 127$), again the DBS group had better quality of life and motor scores per the PDQ-39 and UPDRS-III. All secondary outcome variables improved in this study. It has been suggested that the patient's expectation of a negative outcome (the patient was aware of randomization to the nonsurgical group) led to a placebo effect that may have positively biased the outcome. The behavioral effects of DBS were recently evaluated in a secondary analysis of the 251 patients in the EARLYSTIM trial with secondary behavioral outcomes of apathy, behavior, and depression evaluated at 2-year follow-up. This study reported a reduction in neuropsychiatric fluctuations and an improvement in the Ardouin Scale of Behavior (bilateral STN DBS plus medical therapy group alone). The scores of apathy and depression did not differ between treatment groups. A smaller number of antidepressant and antipsychotic medications were used in the DBS-plus-medical therapy group but the study was not powered to examine this relationship. Two suicides occurred in the DBS-plus-medical therapy group and one in the medical therapy-only group (Lhommée et al., 2018).

A pilot trial was completed comparing bilateral STN DBS plus optimal medical therapy to optimal medical therapy alone. It was conducted in 30 subjects who were between the ages of 50 and 75 years old, off-medication Hoehn and Yahr stage 2 (severity rating). Patients were treated for more than 6 months and for less than 4 years and without a history of motor fluctuations (Charles et al., 2014). There were 15 subjects who underwent bilateral STN DBS placement. Co-primary endpoints were: time to reach a 4-point worsening from baseline, the off-therapy UPDRS-III score, and the change in levodopa equivalent daily dose from baseline to 24 months. Total and part III UPDRS scores were not significantly different on or off therapy at 24 months. The DBS plus optimal medical therapy group required less medication at all time points, with the maximum difference reached at 18 months. Overall, the safety and feasibility study of DBS plus optimal medical therapy in early PD patients in whom motor complications *had not yet occurred*, found a 50%–80% reduction in the relative risk of worsening compared with optimal medical therapy alone when followed at 2 years (Hacker et al., 2015). A recent follow-up study suggested that DBS in early PD may possibly have an impact on the progression of rest tremor (Hacker et al., 2018).

Until recently, few fundamental technological advances in DBS have occurred in the era of modern usage. Traditional DBS has used a single-source voltage-driven system, which has the potential limitation of changes in the electrical field due to fluctuations in tissue impedance. Recently, constant-current devices have been developed and this technology has the theoretical advantage of improved field stability. The St. Jude Medical DBS Study Group investigated the impact of a constant-current DBS device implanted in bilateral STN on the change in "on" time without dyskinesia. The control group received the DBS with a delayed 3-month activation. The improvement of quality "on" time was observed in both groups, with greater benefit in the stimulated group. These findings confirmed the effect of lead implantation alone, in addition to the efficacy of constant-current devices.

Additional innovations in design have led to finer control over the electrical field's shape and direction of spread. A new development has been the use of multiple independent current sources, which facilitates the delivery of current to one or more DBS contacts. This approach has a goal of improved precision in electrical field shaping and a limitation of side effects. The VANTAGE study was a prospective, nonrandomized, unblinded, multicenter trial of unilateral and bilateral STN DBS in 40 PD patients in Europe, which evaluated the use of a new constant-current system and utilized eight circumferential contacts with independent current sources. This technology was manufactured by Boston Scientific (Timmermann et al., 2015). The primary endpoint was mean change in the UPDRS-III score at 26 weeks, and this was improved with a significant mean difference of 23.8 points, which was a 62% change. The use of anti-Parkinsonian medications was reduced; the amount of "on" time and also the quality of life was improved. This system was not formally compared with conventional DBS, but the frequency and severity of side effects were comparable to those reported in prior trials of STN DBS. This system was approved for use in Europe in 2012. The long-term results of the VANTAGE study at 5 years were recently presented, and it was shown that quality-of-life measures continued to improve from baseline (Timmermann et al., 2018). More recently, this system was evaluated in the INTREPID study, the results of which were recently presented. This was a multicenter, prospective, double-blind randomized controlled trial (RCT) of STN DBS that was conducted in the United States. The study met the primary outcome of change in mean hours per day of on time without troublesome dyskinesia (Vitek, Jain, and Starr, 2017). Based on this most recent study, the US Food and Drug Administration (FDA) approved the use of this device for PD in December 2017.

Traditional DBS leads utilize cylindrical contacts, which produce a circumferential field. Recently developed directional devices use radially segmented leads, which take advantage of independent current sources to activate one or more segments to create asymmetric field shapes. The therapy was designed so that the electrical current could be directed away from nontargeted structures and toward intended fiber bundles, thereby minimizing side effects. The PROGRESS trial is an ongoing nonrandomized, double-blind crossover trial comparing classic stimulation with directional stimulation of the STN in PD patients using a different constant-current device which incorporates radially segmented leads. The device was developed by Abbott. The primary outcome measure will be "the proportion of subjects for which at least one lead's therapeutic window (evaluated by a blinded evaluator) is greater using directional stimulation than omnidirectional stimulation; tested against a performance goal of 60%" (NCT02989610). This system was approved in the EU in 2015 and by the US FDA in 2016.

The DIRECT DBS trial is a multicenter study of STN DBS in PD utilizing a constant-current device with segmented leads and eight contacts with independent current sources. This device was developed by Boston Scientific. Preliminary results were presented showing the potential for directional stimulation–related differences in clinical responses (Steigerwald et al., 2018).

## DYSTONIA

Dystonia is characterized by sustained co-contraction of agonist and antagonist muscles. Sufferers may experience involuntary repetitive movements that result in twisted and sometimes painful postures. Dystonia may be focal, segmental, or generalized based on the body region affected. A 2013 consensus document revised the classification of dystonia into two axes (Albanese et al., 2013). Axis I categorizes dystonia by its clinical features and axis II by etiology. Lesion surgery (i.e., pallidotomy and thalamotomy) has been successfully employed for various primary and secondary dystonias (Lozano et al., 1995; Yoshor, Hamilton, Ondo, Jankovic, and Grossman, 2001), though most centers prefer DBS, as ablation is irreversible and bilateral lesions may result in speech or cognitive issues (Ondo et al., 1998), while stimulation parameters may be adjusted for benefit and to limit side effects.

DBS therapy is mainly performed in the GPi target, as stimulation in this region has provided a reasonable alternative to lesion therapy. Most DBS cases have responded best if the dystonia has been of primary origin, although select secondary dystonias as well as tardive dystonias have had meaningful improvements in small series (Capelle et al., 2010; Coubes et al., 1999; Gruber et al., 2009; Kumar, Dagher, Hutchison, Lang, and Lozano, 1999; Kupsch et al., 2003; Tronnier and Fogel, 2000; Vercueil et al., 2001). There have been multiple large randomized trials that address primary generalized dystonia, and each has demonstrated sustained improvement of dystonia rating scales up to 5 years after implantation (Coubes et al., 2004; Kupsch et al., 2006; Vidailhet et al., 2005, 2007; Volkmann et al., 2012). A recent longitudinal study including 61 patients with idiopathic inherited and also acquired dystonia who underwent GPi DBS observed overall sustained clinical improvements. Those with idiopathic and inherited isolated dystonia and acquired dystonia did best, while those with dystonia secondary to neurodegenerative disorders did poorly (Meoni et al., 2017). Additionally, the number of indications has been expanding within dystonia (e.g., cerebral palsy) and the number of brain targets continues to expand, with recent trials indicating the potential for STN DBS (Ostrem et al., 2011, 2017).

One interesting and unique aspect of DBS for dystonia has been the phenomenon that, in many cases, the effects seem to be delayed and appear gradually after stimulation initiation (weeks to months). It has been hypothesized that this phenomenon may be the result of neuroplasticity, with recent work suggesting the role of normalization of abnormal cortical plasticity by the electrical stimulation provided by DBS (Ni et al., 2018). The mechanisms underlying the benefit(s) of DBS in dystonia remain unknown. The other evolving story in dystonia DBS has been the utilization of lower stimulation frequencies for select cases (Alterman et al., 2007; Alterman, Shils, Miravite, and Tagliati, 2007; Goto, Mita, and Ushio, 2002; Kim, Chang, Park, and Chang, 2012; Limotai et al., 2011; Ostrem et al., 2014; Velez-Lago et al., 2012). Selecting which cases may respond to lower frequencies remains an area of investigation.

## TREMOR

Tremor has been broadly defined as an involuntary and rhythmic oscillation of a body part and has been classified according to its etiology and/or by its characteristics (e.g., phenomenology, physiology, etc.; Video 38.3). It has been hypothesized that physiological disturbances in the cerebellothalamic and pallidothalamic pathways may be the genesis of some tremor subtypes.

The ventralis intermedius (VIM) nucleus of the thalamus, which takes its input from the cerebellum, forms a vital piece of this regulatory network, and has been frequently targeted for HFS to address various medication-refractory tremors, with the most common being essential tremor (ET; Benabid et al., 1996). DBS therapy has been reported to have similar efficacy as thalamotomy (Schuurman et al., 2000) and fewer short-term side effects, but more long-term device-related adverse effects when compared to lesion therapy.

Typically, unilateral VIM DBS has been employed to control medication-refractory tremor in a contralateral extremity (Video 38.4). Unilateral DBS may result in side effects of ataxia and speech problems, and these issues may be more commonly encountered when bilateral DBS is utilized (Pahwa et al., 2006). Midline tremor, head tremor, and voice tremor seem to less consistently respond to DBS (Ondo, Almaguer, Jankovic, and Simpson, 2001). Longitudinal follow-up studies have revealed good long-term benefits, although there has been an emerging concern in the field about waning efficacy over time, with tolerance and disease progression among suspected causes (Blomstedt, Hariz, Hariz, and Koskinen, 2007; Pahwa et al., 2006; Rodríguez Cruz et al., 2016; Sydow, Thobois, Alesch, and Speelman, 2003; Zhang et al., 2010). A paper by Favilla et al. (2012) revealed that in ET, disease progression and not tolerance is the more common mechanism underpinning worsening tremor over time.

The largest prospective study in ET was recently published using the Abbott constant-current device for unilateral thalamic DBS. In this prospective, controlled, multicenter study, 127 patients were implanted with VIM DBS. The primary efficacy outcome at 180 days in 76 patients revealed a mean improvement of 1.25 ± 1.26 points in the target limb tremor rating scale (TRS). Improvements were also found in secondary outcome measures of quality of life, depression, and activities of daily living (ADLs). There were 47 patients who underwent placement of a second contralateral VIM DBS, with significant reduction in contralateral tremor at 180 days. The rate of adverse events was comparable with prior studies, with serious adverse events including three infections, three intracranial hemorrhages, and three device explants (Wharen et al., 2017).

While VIM DBS is preferred for pure ET and select cases of PD tremor, cerebellar/midbrain tremor, posttraumatic tremor, and MS tremor have had worse efficacy with this target when compared with ET. These more complex tremor disorders have been treated in small case series by either single or multiple leads in VIM, ventralis oralis posterior (VOP), or by zona incerta (ZI; Foote et al., 2006; Foote and Okun, 2005; Papavassiliou et al., 2008). The exact target(s) for these disorders remain to be investigated.

## DEMENTIA

Several reports of DBS implantation in Alzheimer disease (AD) over the last decade have suggested a possible role for DBS. The two primary targets studied have been the nucleus basalis of Meynert (NBM) and the fornix. The report of serendipitously evoked autobiographical memories in a case of bilateral hypothalamic DBS to treat obesity prompted the discovery that the fornix may be a potential DBS target. Early reports of DBS targeting the fornix revealed the possibility of improving symptoms and changes in temporal and/or parietal lobe hypometabolism (Fontaine et al., 2013; Laxton et al., 2010). Similar findings of increased functional connectivity and increased cortical metabolism were seen after 1 year in a study of five AD patients with stimulation of the fornix (Smith et al., 2012). A larger phase II RCT of DBS in the fornix of 42 patients with mild AD failed to meet its primary outcome. Patients in this trial older than 65 may have possibly benefited (Lozano et al., 2016).

A marked cholinergic deficit due to degeneration of the NBM, which is located in the basal forebrain, is thought to play a significant role in the cognitive and behavioral dysfunction in AD. Excitation of NBM output using low-frequency stimulation may be a method to improve cholinergic output to the cortex. This notion has been supported by work in animal models (Kurosawa, Sato, and Sato, 1989; Rasmusson, Clow, and Szerb, 1992). An early attempt of using NBM DBS in a patient with AD demonstrated no significant clinical benefit (Turnbull et al., 1985). Another pilot trial of NBM DBS in AD suggested stable or possibly improved cognition in four of six patients (Kuhn et al., 2015a). There was possible benefit in two younger AD patients with a higher level of baseline functioning (Kuhn et al., 2015b). A study of eight younger AD patients similarly suggested earlier-stage disease may respond better to NBM DBS.

A small study of two patients evaluated the effect of DBS on auditory processing, and supported the potential beneficial effects of NBM DBS on recognition of familiar stimuli (Dürschmid et al., 2020). Seeking to better define predictors of response, a recent study of NBM DBS utilized magnetic resonance imaging (MRI) to define preoperative cortical thickness and to identify networks modulated by stimulation. This study observed that preserved fronto-parieto-temporal cortical thickness and retained interplay were both associated with better outcomes (Baldermann et al., 2018). Expanding to a new target, there was a recently reported phase I open-label trial of ventral capsule/ventral striatum (VC/VS) in three AD patients. Two of three patients demonstrated meaningfully less decline in the primary outcome measure, with minimal to increased metabolism evident on 2-deoxy-2-[$^{18}$F]fluoro-D-glucose (FDG) positron emission tomography (PET) imaging of frontal cortical regions.

DBS for Parkinson disease dementia (PDD) is similarly an emerging area of exploration. The degeneration of the NBM in PDD typically leads to a cholinergic deficit that is greater than that observed in AD. The results of the first case of NBM DBS for PDD were potentially encouraging (Freund et al., 2009). This was followed by a pilot double-blind RCT of bilateral NBM DBS in six patients with PDD and, while it was found to be safe, no improvements were seen in the primary cognitive outcomes (Gratwicke et al., 2018). Future research directions may explore subregions of the NBM and the effects of different stimulation parameters.

## NEUROPSYCHIATRIC DISORDERS

### Tourette Syndrome

Tourette syndrome (TS) is a complex neuropsychiatric disorder with a usual onset in childhood. The disorder is characterized by changing motor and vocal tics that must be present for at least 1 year and be marked by fluctuations in number, frequency, and complexity (Robertson, 2000). Patients frequently have associated behavioral abnormalities including anxiety, attention deficit hyperactivity disorder, self-injurious behavior, and obsessive-compulsive behavior which may persist into their adult life, even when motor and phonic tics decline or disappear (Jankovic, 2001; Leckman et al., 1998). Only a small minority of patients diagnosed with TS progress to disabling refractory tic disorder or to malignant TS that is unresponsive to medical and behavioral therapy (Cheung, Shahed, and Jankovic, 2007). A very select group of TS patients may be candidates for DBS. The heterogeneity of the patient populations and the small size of studies have limited the interpretation of reported successes and failures. Because of the special risks in this population, the Tourette Association of America (TAA) and European Society for the Study of TS have published guidelines for selection of DBS candidates and for the preferred standardized outcome measures that should be employed if attempting these surgeries (Mink et al., 2006; Müller-Vahl et al., 2011). The TAA recommendations for patient selection, assessment, and management were updated recently, given the growing experience with DBS in these patients (Schrock et al., 2015).

Although the mechanisms which cause TS are unknown, abnormalities within the limbic and motor loops of the cortical-basal ganglia-thalamo-cortical circuitry that involve both dopaminergic and serotonergic neurotransmission are likely contributory to the motor and behavioral manifestations in mild and severe TS cases (Albin and Mink, 2006; Wichmann and DeLong, 2006). The centro-median-parafascicular complex (CM-Pf) of the thalamus (Ackermans et al., 2011; Houeto et al., 2005; Okun et al., 2013), the GPi (both motor and nonmotor territories; Cannon et al., 2012), and the anterior limb of internal capsule among several others have been utilized as targets for DBS therapy (ALIC; Flaherty et al., 2005).

While a number of brain targets have been used across studies and reports, the CM-Pf region has been the most commonly used. The pallidum is the second most widely used target. CM-Pf region and pallidum, to date, have better efficacy than the anterior limb target. More careful studies, including characterization of individual targets, will be needed to determine the optimal target (Burdick, et al., 2010; Flaherty et al., 2005; Maciunas et al., 2007; Porta et al., 2009; Servello et al., 2008; Shields et al., 2008; Visser-Vandewalle et al., 2003). There have been five double-blind RCTs of DBS in TS to date, and a number of open-label trials and case reports (Ackermans et al., 2011; Kefalopoulou et al., 2015; Maciunas et al., 2007; Schrock et al., 2015; Welter et al., 2008, 2017).

In 2012 the International Tourette Syndrome Database and Registry was launched in an effort to pool outcome data from around the world. Recently, the 1-year outcomes from this TS DBS cohort were published, with 171 of 185 patients analyzed. The authors found that 64.2% had symptoms of OCD, and 21.6% had a history of self-injurious behavior. One year after DBS implantation, the mean total Yale Global Tic Severity Scale score improved from baseline 75.01 (standard deviation [SD] 18.36) to 41.19 (SD 20.00; $P < .001$). The mean motor tic subscore improved from baseline 21.00 (SD 3.72) to 12.91 (SD 5.78; $P < .001$), and the mean phonic tic subscore improved from 16.82 (SD 6.56) at baseline to 9.63 (SD 6.99; $P < .001$) at 1 year. Adverse events occurred in 35.4% of patients. Intracranial hemorrhage occurred in two patients, infection in four patients with five events, and lead explantation in one patient (Martinez-Ramirez et al., 2018).

Given the fluctuations in the features of TS, alternative paradigms to classic, continuous stimulation are being explored. These include scheduled stimulation (Okun et al., 2013), as well as closed-loop, or adaptive, DBS, which responds dynamically to neurophysiological biomarkers in an effort to suppress tics. Few studies have investigated this to date (Bour et al., 2015; Jimenez-Shahed et al., 2016; Marceglia et al., 2010; Priori et al., 2013; Shute et al., 2016), with the most recent studies further suggesting the feasibility of this approach (Marceglia et al., 2017). Recently reported was a study in which a responsive neurostimulator (RNS; the NeuroPace RNS system) was chronically implanted in the CM-Pf region of the thalamus in a patient with TS (Molina et al., 2018). A spectral power increase in the 5–15 Hz band was found to have the highest sensitivity for tics and provided a control signal for responsive stimulation. There was a 64% improvement from baseline in the Modified Rush Tic Rating Scale and 48% improvement in the Yale Global Tic Severity Score at 12 months, a 63.3% improvement in the device's projected mean battery life and with the responsive stimulation found to be safe and well-tolerated in this patient. Larger studies will be needed to determine the effectiveness of this approach.

## Depression

The impact of treatment-resistant depression makes neuromodulation a potentially attractive alternative therapy for a select group of these patients (Ward et al., 2010). DBS for treatment-resistant depression remains investigational and should only be considered when medication, psychotherapy, and electrical convulsive therapy are not helpful and also when an institutional review board experimental protocol has been obtained.

Experts have hypothesized that there is an abnormality in the CSTC network in severely depressed humans and that by lesioning or neuromodulating at specific nodes clinical symptoms may be reduced. DBS targets have been rapidly emerging and may include subgenual cingulate cortex/outflow tract (SCC), VC/VS or the ventral aspect of the anterior limb of the internal capsule (vALIC), nucleus accumbens (NAc), medial forebrain bundle (MFB), lateral habenular complex (LHb), and the inferior thalamic peduncle (ITP; Dandekar et al., 2018; Greenberg et al., 2008; Mayberg et al., 2005; Ward et al., 2010). While the overall results from case reports and open-label trials have been promising (Morishita et al., 2014), data from blinded RCTs have been varied. Two RCTs were discontinued due to lack of efficacy, based on futility analyses (Morishita et al., 2014). Double-blind, sham-controlled RCTs have been mixed, with some negative results of DBS for resistant depression treatment (Dougherty et al., 2015), while others found positive or mixed results (Bergfeld et al., 2016; Holtzheimer et al., 2017; Merkl et al., 2013; Puigdemont et al., 2015; Ramasubbu et al., 2013). As the approach is refined, there is hope that continuous DBS and also closed-loop adaptive techniques may be utilized. There is also a notion that defining the subtypes of depression will lead to better patient selection and improved outcomes (Ramirez-Zamora et al. 2018).

## Obsessive-Compulsive Disorder

Another DBS indication that has received FDA approval, under a humanitarian device exemption, is OCD. OCD is characterized by recurrent intrusive thoughts or obsessions that may produce overwhelming anxiety and may be relieved in some cases by the indulgence in ritualistic, compulsive behaviors. Functional neuroimaging has revealed hyperactivity within the VS, medial thalamic region, and the orbitofrontal cortex as a potentially abnormal network in this disorder. A select group of patients who may be refractory to medical treatment or to behavioral approaches could be candidates for a neurosurgical intervention (Tye, Frye, and Lee, 2009).

Neurosurgical interventions have, in the recent past, involved lesioning of the ALIC, cingulotomies, leucotomies, as well as other approaches (Ward, Hwynn, and Okun, 2010). The idea underpinning early therapies was to create a disconnection between frontal lobe and basal ganglia circuitry to attempt to disrupt the abnormally firing neural network. Apathy and other irreversible complications resulted from early lesion approaches, and most were abandoned in favor of selective lesioning of the VS or DBS. It has been reported that HFS of the bilateral ALIC/NAc region may achieve remission in more than 50% of well-selected patients (Goodman et al., 2010; Greenberg et al., 2008; Nuttin et al., 2008). Other brain areas that have been successfully targeted include the STN, the VC/VS, the supero-lateral MFB, the ITP, as well as the internal capsule/bed nucleus of the stria terminalis (BNST; Coenen et al., 2017; Jiménez et al., 2013; Luyten et al., 2016; Mallet et al., 2008; Malone et al., 2009; Raymaekers et al., 2017; Ward et al., 2010). It should be stressed that expert interdisciplinary teams, including psychiatrists and psychologists, should be employed to carefully screen and follow patients who undergo DBS for OCD, depression, and other neuropsychiatric disorders (Okun et al., 2007, 2008a).

## Drug Addiction

Addiction is the behavior characterized by relentlessly seeking drugs despite knowledge of possible adverse consequences (Kreek, 2008).

Imaging studies in humans have revealed that addiction seems to involve sudden surges in extracellular dopamine in limbic areas including the NAc (shell and core) and the dorsal striatum. Prolonged drug abuse may result in reorganization of the reward and memory circuits and lead to increased sensitivity to various signals, which may trigger relapse (Koob and Volkow, 2010). As an alternative to medical therapy, stereotactic neurosurgery-leucotomy (Knight, 1969), hypothalamotomy (Dieckmann and Schneider, 1978), cingulotomy (Kanaka and Balasubramaniam, 1978), and ablation of the NAc (Gao et al., 2003) have been attempted and shown variable effectiveness. The irreversibility of lesions, the behavioral implications, and the trial designs of ablative procedures have led to uncertainty about their place in clinical practice (Stelten et al., 2008).

STN DBS in PD has been reported in some cases to help with dopamine dysregulation syndrome (Witjas et al., 2005), while there are reports of smoking cessation (Kuhn et al., 2009; Mantione et al., 2010) and treatment of alcohol dependency (Heldmann et al., 2012; Kuhn et al.. 2007, 2011, Müller et al., 2009, 2016; Voges et al., 2013) following DBS in the NAc. Improvement in drug-seeking behaviors following DBS of the NAc have also been reported in cases and an open-label pilot study for the treatment of heroin dependence (Chen et al., 2019; Kuhn et al., 2014; Valencia-Alfonso et al., 2012; Zhou, Xu, and Jiang, 2011), and cocaine dependence have recently been reported (Gonçalves-Ferreira et al., 2016).

### Anorexia Nervosa

Anorexia nervosa (AN) is a common, difficult-to-treat disorder and has one of the highest mortality rates of any psychiatric disorder. The marked compulsivity observed in AN along with frequent comorbidity with OCD has suggested there may be a common underlying pathophysiology (Altman and Shankman, 2009). It has been increasingly recognized that aberrant reward circuitry is involved in the genesis and perpetuation of AN, and that there are significant overlaps of these networks with circuitry involved in compulsive behaviors. These findings have supported the many clinical parallels between OCD, addiction, and eating disorders (Lee, Elias, and Lozano, 2017).

Several brain targets have been utilized for AN in cases and trials. These have included the NAc (Wang et al., 2013; Wu et al., 2013), SCC (Israël et al., 2010; Lipsman et al., 2013, 2017), the VC/VS (McLaughlin et al., 2013), the BNST (Barbier et al., 2011; Nuttin et al., 2003) and both the MFB and the BNST (Blomstedt, Naesström, and Bodlund. 2017). There have been promising results across most of these studies. A longitudinal feasibility and preliminary efficacy study of DBS directed to the NAc along with an integrated neuroethical substudy is ongoing (Park, Scaife, and Aziz 2018). The largest series to date, using DBS of the SCC, found an increase in average body mass index (BMI) in 14/16 patients at 12 months (with two having withdrawn for poorly defined reasons). This series also showed improvements in mood, anxiety, and affective regulation (Lipsman et al., 2017). Much remains to be learned about this potential adjunctive therapy, which remains experimental.

## PAIN

Neuromodulation has been specifically employed for pain due to phantom-limb, stroke, brachial plexus injury, and anesthesia dolorosa (Bittar et al., 2005). After it was appreciated by functional imaging that cluster headache (CH) and facial pain syndromes may be related to hypothalamic circuitry, neuromodulation of this region was attempted and has been reported successful in multiple cases (Akram et al., 2016, 2017; Bartsch et al., 2008; Broggi et al., 2007; Chabardès et al., 2016; Fontaine et al., 2010; Leone et al., 2006, 2013; Schoenen et al., 2005; Seijo et al., 2011; Starr et al., 2007; Vyas et al., 2019). Recently reported was DBS in a patient with CH, targeting the mamillotegmental fasciculus; there was significant improvement (Seijo-Fernandez et al., 2018). There was also a report of bilateral STN DBS for PD in a patient with comorbid CH with persistent resolution of headaches (Huotarinen et al., 2017).

## EPILEPSY

Despite active antiepileptic drug (AED) development, up to 20% of epileptic patients suffer from poor seizure control even with optimal medical therapy (Devinsky, 1999). First-line treatment for drug-resistant epilepsy has been resective surgery, most commonly anterior temporal lobectomy (ATL), which may result in 80%–90% seizure freedom (Yoon et al., 2003). For the remaining patients, alternative therapies such as vagal nerve stimulation (VNS) have proven to have variable efficacy, with one review of the literature finding approximately 50% of patients with a 50% reduction in seizure frequency (Connor et al., 2012).

Multiple targets have been evaluated for DBS in epilepsy with variable results (Li and Cook, 2018). One of many potential reasons that studies have reported variable results with the same DBS target may be that certain seizure types may respond differently to stimulation of a particular target.

Despite all the uncertainty, several trials have empirically demonstrated the efficacy of DBS for seizures, even in patients who have failed other therapies. These exciting results have fueled a number of studies designed to firmly establish DBS as an effective treatment for intractable epilepsy. In the largest controlled study of anterior nucleus DBS for epilepsy, those with diffuse, frontal, occipital, or parietal seizure foci failed to benefit, even though patients with a temporal lobe focus or foci had a significant reduction in seizure frequency (Fisher et al., 2010).

## CLOSED-LOOP STIMULATION—THE EPILEPSY EXPERIENCE

Closed-loop devices are devices programmed to respond to detection of ictal or epileptiform discharges that may abort impending seizures. An initial trial of closed-loop stimulation in eight patients with intractable epilepsy involved local closed-loop HFS directly to the epileptic focus in response to the abnormal electrocorticographic discharges detected by a seizure detection algorithm (Osorio et al., 2005). In four patients with multiple, remote seizure foci, closed-loop HFS was applied using the anterior nucleus of the thalamus. There was significant decrease (>50%) in seizures during experimental phase in both patient groups.

Four patients using an external RNS experienced clinical and electrographic suppression of seizures (Kossoff et al., 2004). These findings encouraged a multicenter trial of implantable RNS (NeuroPace, Inc. CA, US.) that continuously monitored electrographic activity through depth and/or strip leads. The RNS delivered electrical stimulation to the seizure focus when it detected the epileptic activity (Skarpaas and Morrell, 2009).

The SANTE study, involving 110 patients, found improvement at 25 months (Fisher et al., 2010). Long-term outcomes were reported in 2015, with 68% of patients having greater than 50% seizure frequency reduction at 5 years (Salanova et al., 2015). This approach recently received FDA approval.

Patients with pharmaco-resistant partial-onset epilepsy were recruited for a double-blinded, sham-controlled RCT (Morrell and RNS System in Epilepsy Study Group, 2011). Seizures were reduced in the treatment compared with the sham group, with a 53% median percent seizure reduction at 2 years (Heck et al., 2014), and the FDA granted approval for the Neuropace RNS device in 2014. There was a 48%–66% seizure reduction observed in the long-term, open-label study (Bergey et al., 2015). Recently, a long-term observational study of RNS in patients with intractable mesial temporal lobe epilepsy found a median 70% decrease in seizure frequency at mean follow-up of 6 years (Geller et al., 2017). A study of RNS in 126 patients with neocortical seizure foci found significant improvements without neurological deficits following stimulation in eloquent cortex (Jobst et al., 2017).

## CONCLUSIONS AND THE FUTURE OF DEEP BRAIN STIMULATION

In recent decades, chronic DBS has become routine for several diagnoses in neurological practice (e.g., PD, dystonia, and ET), and has been utilized experimentally for dementia and selected neuropsychiatric indications (e.g., OCD, depression, addiction, and TS). There are several other indications now under investigation for potential DBS therapies. Recently emerging indications are treatment-resistant PTSD, obesity, and AN.

Several companies have recently introduced novel lead designs and novel stimulation parameters to improve effectiveness and to reduce adverse events. It is likely that DBS therapy will continue to expand in indications and will become more personalized as the technology evolves and improves.

*The complete reference list is available online at https://expertconsult.inkling.com/.*

39

# Intraoperative Monitoring

*Marc R. Nuwer*

## OUTLINE



Neurophysiological intraoperative monitoring (IOM) uses electroencephalography (EEG), electromyography (EMG), and evoked potentials (EPs) during surgery to improve outcome. These techniques warn the surgeon of impending complications in time to intervene and correct problems before they become worse. IOM can also identify motor or language cortex to spare them from resection. A surgeon can rely on monitoring for reassurance about nervous system integrity, allowing the surgery to be more extensive than would have been safe without monitoring. Some patients are eligible for surgery with monitoring who may have been denied surgery without monitoring because of a high risk of nervous system complications. Patients and families can be reassured that certain feared complications are screened for during surgery. In these ways, monitoring extends the safety, range, and completeness of surgery.

Effective collaboration and communication are needed between surgeon, anesthesiologist, and neurophysiologist (Gertsch et al., 2019). The monitoring team maintains open communication throughout surgery. An experienced electrodiagnostic technologist applies electrodes and ensures technically accurate studies. The interpreting neurophysiologist is either in the operating room or monitors continuously online in real time.

## TECHNIQUES

Many IOM techniques are adapted from common outpatient testing: for example, EEG, brainstem auditory evoked potential (BAEP), and somatosensory evoked potential (SEP) tests. Box 39.1 lists various techniques used in the operating room. EEG is used when surgery risks cortical ischemia, such as aneurysm clipping or carotid endarterectomy. BAEP is used for procedures around the eighth nerve or when the brainstem is at risk in posterior fossa procedures: for example, Fig. 39.1. SEP is widely used for many procedures that risk impairment to the spinal cord, brainstem, or sensorimotor cortex.

Some IOM techniques are specific to the operating room. Transcranial electrical motor evoked potential (MEP) tests are evoked by several-hundred-volt electrical pulses delivered to motor cortex through the intact skull. Recordings are made from extremity muscles. MEP monitors corticospinal tracts during cerebral, brainstem, or spinal surgery. Electrocorticography (ECoG) measures EEG directly from the exposed cortex. ECoG guides the surgeon to resect physiologically dysfunctional or epileptogenic areas while sparing relatively normal cortex. Direct cortical stimulation applies very localized electrical pulses to cortex through a handheld wand. That electricity disrupts cortical function such as language, which can be tested in patients who are awake during a craniotomy. Direct cortical stimulation identifies language or motor regions so that they can be spared during resections. Similar direct nerve stimulation is used for cranial and peripheral nerves to locate them amid pathological tissue and to check whether a nerve is still intact. Electrical stimulation of the floor of the fourth ventricle during brainstem resection can identify tracts and nuclei of interest. The placement of spinal pedicle screws risks injury to nerve roots or spinal cord. To reduce that risk, EMG is monitored while electrical stimulation is delivered to the pedicle hole drilled in the spine or the screw. If the hole or screw has errantly broken through bone into the spinal canal or nerve foramen, the stimulation may elicit an EMG warning of misplacement. In-depth descriptions of each procedure are beyond the scope of this chapter. The reader is referred elsewhere for extensive coverage of intraoperative neurophysiological techniques (Nuwer, 2008).

### Spinal Cord Monitoring

SEP and MEP spinal cord monitoring is a good example of a common IOM technique. Electrical stimuli are delivered at a rate of several per second to the ulnar nerve at the wrist and the posterior tibial nerve at the ankle. Averaged SEP peaks are recorded at standardized surface locations over the spine and scalp. Small electrical potentials recorded during the 50 ms following stimulation indicate the transit and arrival of axonal volleys or synaptic events at peripheral, spinal, brainstem, and primary sensory cortical levels. SEP recordings are repeated every few minutes. MEP stimulating electrodes are located on the scalp over motor cortex. Electrical MEP pulses are strong enough to discharge the axon hillock of motor cortex pyramidal cells. The resulting action potentials travel down corticospinal tracts and discharge spinal anterior horn cells. MEP recordings are made from limb muscles at 25–45 ms after stimulation.

## BOX 39.1 Techniques Used for Intraoperative Monitoring and Testing

Electroencephalography
Electrocorticography
Direct cortical stimulation
Somatosensory evoked potentials
Transcranial electrical motor evoked potentials
Brainstem auditory evoked potentials
Deep brain and brainstem electrical stimulation
Electromyography
Nerve conduction studies
Direct spinal cord stimulation
Reflex testing
Pedicle screw stimulation testing

SEP and MEP peaks remain stable over time in uneventful spinal surgery. If values change beyond established limits, the monitoring team alerts the surgeon of increased risk of neurological impairment. Which peaks are preserved and which are changed can localize the side and level of impairment. In thoracolumbar surgery, SEP and MEP channels of the upper extremity serve as controls to separate systemic or anesthetic causes from thoracic or lumbar surgical reasons for change. The ulnar nerve is often used rather than the median nerve during cervical surgery for better coverage of the lower cervical cord. The peroneal nerve at the knee may substitute for the posterior tibial nerve at the ankle for elderly patients, those with diabetes, or others in whom a peripheral neuropathy may interfere with adequate distal peripheral conduction. Blockade of the neuromuscular junction is helpful in reducing muscle artifact in SEP but must be limited for use if MEP is monitored. Sometimes other incidental clinical problems are detected beyond the primary purpose of monitoring in the

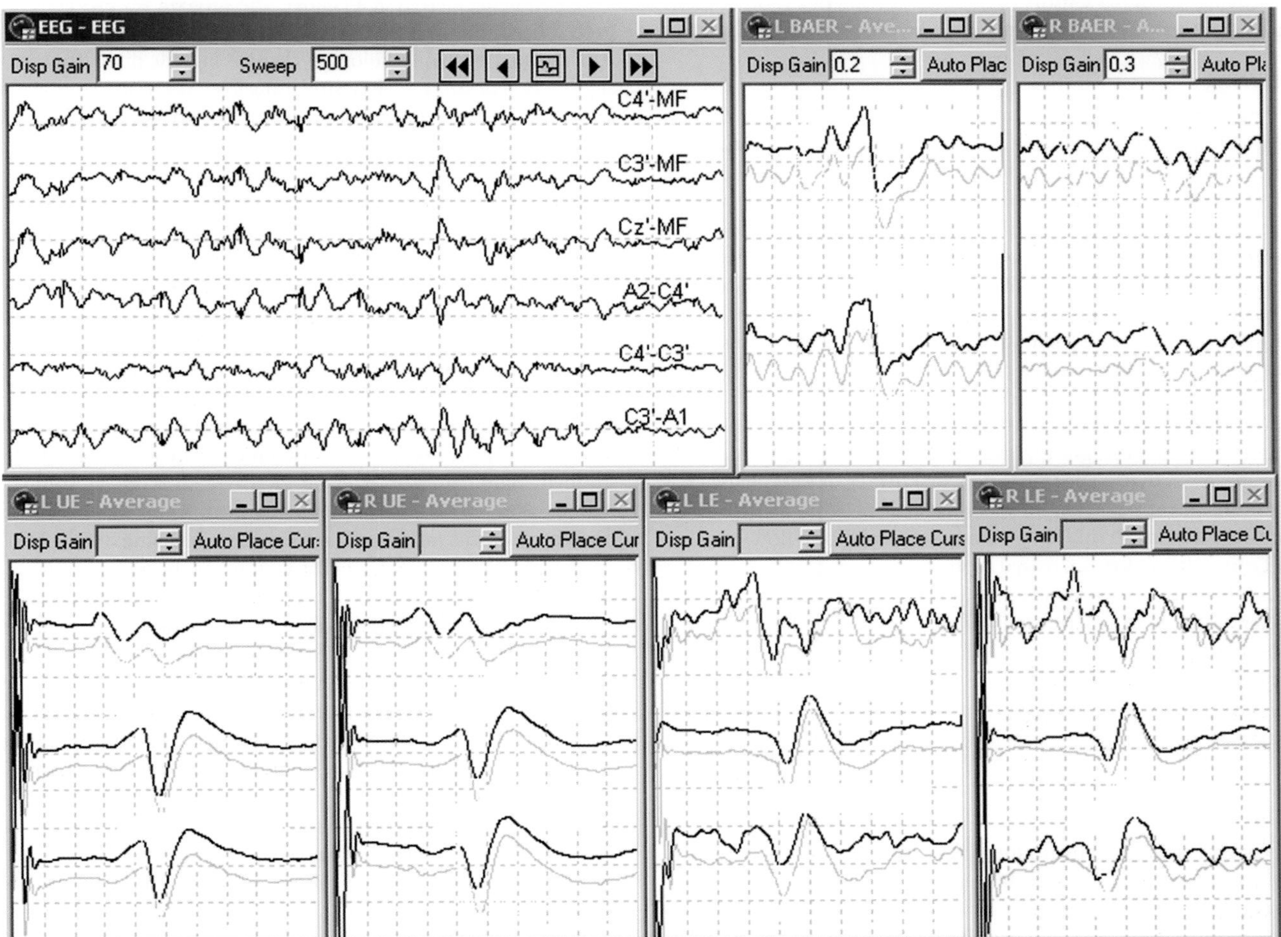


**Fig. 39.1** Typical Setup of Multimodal Intraoperative Monitoring. Several types of recordings are displayed simultaneously on one screen. *Top line*: electroencephalography *(EEG)*, six channels. Left *(L)* brainstem auditory evoked potential *(BAEP)*; right *(R)* BAEP. Each BAEP window shows ipsilateral ear and contralateral ear recordings in pairs. Each pair of tracings is the current tracing *(black)* compared with the baseline *(gray)* at the beginning of the procedure. *Bottom line*: Left median, right median, left posterior tibial, and right posterior tibial nerve somatosensory evoked potential (SEP). Each SEP window shows a subcortical and two cortical channel recordings in pairs. Each pair of tracings is the current tracing *(black)* compared with the baseline *(gray)* at the beginning of the procedure. Right BAEP wave V is of low amplitude because of the cerebellopontine angle tumor for which the surgery was undertaken. Other monitoring windows (not shown) assess muscle electromyography (EMG) for cranial nerve 5 and 7. Other monitoring pages available to the neurophysiologist (not shown) display a variety of other views and can be interrogated to interpret the signals online more accurately in real time.

spinal cord, brainstem, or cortical regions. For example, a developing plexopathy or peripheral nerve compression can be spotted by loss of the peripheral peak, which may be easily treated by repositioning an arm. Occasionally, IOM changes warn of a systemic problem such as hypoxia secondary to a ventilatory problem.

## INTERPRETATION

Interpretation of intraoperative neurophysiology includes two categories. One is *monitoring*, in which baseline findings are established and subsequent findings are compared with baseline. Alarm criteria are set in advance based on knowledge of how much change is acceptable without risk. The other category, *testing*, identifies structures and sets limits of resection. Testing is used in several ways. One is to identify a structure, such as finding the facial nerve buried within pathological tissue. Another is to identify motor or language cortex prior to a resection. A third example is identifying which cauda equina root is L5, or S1, or S2, identifying which is a sensory or a motor portion of a root, or identifying roots as opposed to filum terminale during tethered cord release.

### Monitoring

Interpretation relies on latency and amplitude criteria for raising a monitoring alarm. SEP and BAEP use a 50% decrease in amplitude or a 10% increase in latency as alarm criteria. The criteria must account for the effects of temperature and anesthesia—for example, from boluses or increased inhalation anesthetics. Technical problems can arise from the electrodes themselves (e.g., becoming dislodged). Equipment can malfunction. Systemic factors such as hypotension or hypoxia can also cause changes in IOM.

MEPs are judged more qualitatively. They either remain present or become absent. Some physicians raise an alarm if an MEP amplitude decreases by more than 80% (MacDonald et al., 2013).

A 50% loss of EEG fast activity is seen when cerebral blood flow drops below 20 mL/100 g/min. Still lower blood flow causes a 50% increase in slow activity. The third and worst degree of EEG change is a 50% or more loss of signal amplitude, which can progress all the way to an isoelectric state at 10 mL/100 g/min of cerebral blood flow.

EMG monitors for increased spontaneous activity. Excessive mechanical compression or ischemia can provoke a nerve to respond in a pattern referred to as a *neurotonic discharge* or *A-train*. Such a minute-long rapid firing is the same discharge as occurs when someone accidentally hits the ulnar nerve at the elbow and feels a minute-long painful sensation in the ulnar distribution. In the operating room, this warns of mechanical or ischemic nerve problems (Nichols and Manafov, 2012).

### Testing

Motor cortex is identified by finding the postcentral primary somatosensory gyrus by median nerve SEP testing. The N20 peak is located with good precision, thereby identifying the immediately anterior gyrus as motor cortex. For language localization, an awake surgical patient is tested repeatedly with various oral and visual verbal and nonverbal tasks. Language-active regions are identified as those where electrical stimulation disrupts the patient's ability to complete those tasks. Corticospinal tracts in hemispheric deep white matter are identified by electrical stimulation with muscle recording. When 5-mA stimulation produces no motor responses, the corticospinal tract is at least 5 mm from the site of stimulation; the general rule is 1-mm distance for each milliampere needed to elicit muscle responses. For cranial nerve nuclei, cranial nerves, or peripheral nerves, a direct or nearby stimulation produces responses in appropriate muscles. The pattern of muscle responses can separate root structures (i.e., L5, S1, and S2 roots). Motor roots and nerves respond with EMG to low stimulus intensity, whereas sensory nerves or roots require a 10-fold greater intensity to provoke an EMG response through reflex pathways. That enables the surgeon to identify which root or nerve is motor and which is sensory.

## RESPONSE TO CHANGE

When changes occur during monitoring, the team quickly assesses whether the change is likely due to a technical, systemic, or surgical problem. Occasional transient significant changes occur without significant risk for postoperative neurological problems. Transient changes for a few minutes can occur without substantial risk of postoperative problems, especially if the neurophysiological findings shortly return to baseline. Risk of neurological complications is higher when changes remain through the end of the procedure and when they are of a major degree. For example, a very high risk situation is the complete, permanent loss of EPs that previously had been normal and easily detected.

Upon being alerted of a change, the surgeon reviews actions of the preceding 15 minutes that may have caused the change. Surgical problems causing neurophysiological changes include direct trauma, excessive traction or compression, stretching from spinal distraction, vascular insufficiency from compression, clamping, embolus or thrombus, and other clinical circumstances. Clamping a carotid artery during an endarterectomy may produce EEG changes within 15 seconds. Many other changes are gradual or cumulative, so that monitoring alarms occur many minutes after the offending action. Two factors compound that delay: ischemia and compression can be tolerated for a short interval before nerves stop conducting. SEP and BAEP recordings take one to several minutes to average—sometimes longer when electrocautery or other electrical noise is ongoing—thereby delaying report of a change.

Many surgical or anesthetic actions can be taken in response to IOM alerts. Remedial measures depend on the recent surgical actions. The surgical maneuver under way can be paused, stopped, or reversed. Resection can be halted. An instrument can be removed or repositioned. Blood pressure can be increased. A vascular shunt can be placed, clamped vessels can be unclamped, a clip can be adjusted, or transected aortic intercostal arteries can be reimplanted. Retractors can be repositioned. Spinal distraction can be reduced. If no IOM recovery occurs in 20 minutes, the patient can be awakened on the operating table and ordered to move his or her legs ("wake-up test") to double check motor function. Steroids are sometimes given, although the literature about their usefulness is controversial. Causes can be sought through inspection and exploration for mechanical or hematoma nervous system impingement. Motor and language identified can be avoided during resection. Systemic or local hypothermia or barbiturate-induced coma can be implemented for nervous system protection. Lowering of cerebrospinal fluid pressure by free drainage can be used in some cases of spinal ischemia. Hemoglobin level can be increased by transfusion. Other interventions are also used.

## PREDICTION OF DEFICITS

IOM is effective at preventing many postoperative neurological complications (Ney et al., 2015; Nuwer et al., 2012). Risk depends on the severity and duration of IOM changes. Transient changes that revert to baseline within a few minutes are rarely followed by postoperative deficits. Many temporary changes represent clinically significant complications that are identified and then corrected promptly and completely; this is the goal of monitoring. In other cases, transient changes are false alarms. Both are combined in outcome studies as "false-positive" monitoring events since their causes cannot be directly separated. Outcomes studies show false positives in several percent of cases. New neurological postoperative impairment occurs in about half of cases, with persistent changes of moderate degree (Nuwer et al., 1995). Sometimes postoperative neurological impairment is less than might have occurred if monitoring had not initiated interventions that partially corrected the problem. Severe monitoring changes often predict postoperative neurological deficits. Some are due to intraoperative problems that were identified promptly but could not be adequately corrected.

## ANESTHESIA

Many inhalation anesthetics substantially affect cortical function (Sloan and Heyer, 2002). Commonly used agents attenuate or abolish cortical EP recordings. Limiting the dose of inhalation anesthesia often produces satisfactory anesthesia compatible with monitoring. Boluses of centrally active medication can cause transient IOM changes. Continuous-drip medication delivery is preferred. Much less susceptible to anesthetic effects are the nonsynaptic pathways such as peripheral nerve conduction. Subcortical monosynaptic pathways are less affected than cortical polysynaptic pathways. For example, in SEP monitoring, brainstem peaks remain relatively robust despite inhalation anesthesia levels that nearly eliminate cortical peaks in the same pathway. MEPs tolerate inhalation anesthesia poorly, so MEPs are often conducted with total intravenous anesthesia using propofol, a centrally excitatory anesthetic agent, along with little or no inhalation agent. Turning this effect around, anesthetic and drug effects can be monitored by the degree of EP or EEG changes. When a barbiturate-induced cortically protective burst suppression or isoelectric state is desired, EEG is the primary tool to identify that sufficient depth has been achieved.

A surgical patient's core temperature may drop by 1°C or more. Limb temperature may drop even more. Axonal conduction velocity depends on temperature, so peak latencies increase as temperature drops. Monitoring can help to identify therapeutic temperature effects. When a hypothermia-induced cortically protective isoelectric state is desired, EEG is the primary tool to identify that sufficient depth has been achieved.

## CLINICAL SETTINGS

Box 39.2 lists many clinical conditions and types of surgery for which IOM is used. Procedures involving the intracranial posterior fossa commonly use BAEP, SEP, and cranial nerve EMG monitoring. Typical applications include the resection of cerebellopontine angle and skull base tumors, brainstem vascular malformations and tumors, and microvascular decompressions (Møller, 1996). Intracranial supratentorial procedures include resections for epilepsy, tumors, and vascular malformations as well as aneurysm clipping. These use a combination of EEG and SEP monitoring, sometimes with functional cortical localization, direct cortical stimulation, and ECoG. Surgery of the carotid artery, aorta, or heart may use EEG to monitor hemispheric function or assess the need for shunting or testing the adequacy of protective hypothermia (Plestis et al., 1997). Some also use or prefer SEPs for these vascular procedures.

Spinal surgery is the most common setting for IOM (Nuwer et al., 2013). Disorders include cervical decompression and fusion for radiculopathy or myelopathy, deformity correction for scoliosis, resection of spinal column or cord tumors, and stabilization of fractures. Both SEP and MEP are often used in these cases to assess the posterior column and corticospinal tract functions. The use of MEP depends on the case, since it requires total intravenous anesthesia and incurs some movements during surgery. As a result, occasional spinal procedures still are done with SEP alone. In cases involving pedicle screw placement, EMG is monitored to detect screw misplacement (Shi et al., 2003). Spinal cord monitoring is also used for cardiothoracic procedures of the aorta that could jeopardize spinal perfusion (Jacobs et al., 2006). Peripheral nerve monitoring is carried out for cases risking injury to the nerves, plexus, or roots. Testing can also determine which segments of a nerve are damaged when a nerve graft is performed.

Outcomes for spinal cord surgery have been assessed (Nuwer et al., 1995, 2012). In one large multicenter study of SEP IOM involving 100,000 cases of spinal surgery, half with IOM, the rate of false-positive alarms was about 1%. The rate of false-negative alarms was about 0.1%, which involved those cases with postoperative neurological deficits without a monitoring alarm. Some were minor transient changes and others were neurological deficits that started during the hours or days postoperatively. The rate of major intraoperative changes missed by SEP monitoring was 0.06%. The risk of paraplegia was 60% less among the IOM-monitored cases than among those that were not monitored. That is equivalent to avoiding paraplegia or paraparesis at a rate of 1 case in every 200 when monitoring was used. To improve even further on these SEP IOM monitoring outcomes, MEPs are now used together with SEP for many spinal procedures. With MEP the expected rate of false-negative cases and postoperative neurological deficits should be reduced still further.

Comparative effectiveness studies and cost–benefit analysis favor IOM spinal cord monitoring (Ney and van der Goes, 2014). Ney and van der Goes suggest that IOM saves a hospital system between $64,075 and $102,193 in not having to deal with the effects of adverse outcomes (i.e., in having avoided such outcomes because of IOM monitoring) after accounting for the costs of IOM itself.

### BOX 39.2 Clinical Conditions Monitored During Surgery

Epilepsy surgery
Cerebral tumor and vascular malformation resection
Intracranial aneurysm clipping
Movement disorders electrode placement
Mapping of nerves, tracts, and nuclei during brainstem and cranial base surgery
Ear and parotid surgery near facial nerve
Thyroid and aortic arch surgery near the laryngeal nerve
Carotid endarterectomy
Carotid balloon occlusion
Endovascular spinal and cerebral procedures
Correction of spinal deformity
Stabilization of spinal fracture
Resection of spinal tumor
Decompression and fusion of cervical myelopathy
Decompression and fusion of cervical radiculopathy
Decompression and fusion of lumbar stenosis
Tethered cord and cauda equina procedures
Dorsal root entry zone surgery
Brachial and lumbosacral plexus surgery
Peripheral nerve surgery
Cardiac and aortic procedures

*The complete reference list is available online at www.expertconsult.com.*

40

# Structural Imaging Using Magnetic Resonance Imaging and Computed Tomography

*Joseph C. Masdeu, Bela Ajtai, Alireza Faridar*

## OUTLINE



## COMPUTED TOMOGRAPHY

Computed tomography (CT; other terms include *computer assisted tomography* [CAT]) has been commercially available since 1973. The term *tomography* (i.e., to slice or section) refers to a process for generating two-dimensional (2D) image slices of an examined organ of three dimensions (3D). CT imaging is based on the differential absorption of x-rays by various tissues. X-rays are electromagnetic waves with wavelengths falling in the range of 10–0.01 nm on the electromagnetic spectrum. X-rays can also be described as high-energy photons, with corresponding energies varying between 124 and 124,000 electron volts, respectively. X-rays in the higher range of energies, known as *hard x-rays*, are used in diagnostic imaging because of their ability to penetrate tissue, yet (to an extent), also be absorbed or scattered differentially by various tissues, allowing for the generation of image contrast.

Owing to their high energy, x-rays are also a form of ionizing radiation, and the health risks associated with their use, although minimal, should always be accounted for in diagnostic imaging. The x-rays generated by the x-ray source of the CT scanner are shaped into an x-ray beam by a *collimator*, a rectangular opening in a lead shield. The beam penetrates the slab of tissues to be imaged, which will absorb/deflect it to a varying degree depending on their atomic composition, structure, and density (*photoelectric effect* and *Compton scattering*). The remaining x-rays emerge from the imaged slab and are measured by detectors located opposite the collimator. In fourth-generation CT scanners, the detectors are in a fixed position and the x-ray source rotates around the patient. As the beam of x-rays is transmitted through the imaged body part, sweeping a 360-degree arc for each slice imaged, the emerging x-rays are collected; then a computer analyzes the output of the detectors and calculates the x-ray attenuation of each individual tissue volume (voxel).

The degree of x-ray absorption by the various tissues is expressed and displayed as shades of gray in the CT image. Darker shades correspond to less attenuation. The attenuation by each voxel of tissue is projected on the flat image of the scanned slice as a tiny quadrilateral, generally square, called a *pixel* or picture element. Depending on the reconstruction matrix, a slice will be represented by more or fewer pixels, corresponding to more or less resolution. The shade of gray in each pixel corresponds to a number on an arbitrary linear scale, expressed as Hounsfield units (HU). This number varies between approximately −1000 and 3000+, with values of greater magnitude corresponding to tissues or substances of greater radiodensity, which are depicted in lighter tones. The −1000 value is for air; 0 is for water. Bone is greater than several hundred units, but cranial bone can be 2000 or even more. Fresh blood (with a normal hematocrit) is about 80 units; fat is −50 to −80. Tissues or materials with higher degrees of x-ray absorption, shown in white or lighter shades of gray, are referred to as *hyperdense*, whereas those with lower x-ray absorption properties are *hypodense*; these are relative terms compared with other areas of any given image.

By changing the settings of the process of transforming the x-ray attenuation values to shades on the grayscale, it is possible to select which tissues to preferentially display in the image. This is referred to as *windowing*. Utilizing a bone window, for instance, is very useful for evaluating fractures in cases of craniofacial trauma (Fig. 40.1).

In CT imaging, contrast agents are frequently used for the purpose of detecting abnormalities that cause disruption of the blood–brain barrier (BBB; e.g., certain tumors, inflammation, etc.). The damaged BBB allows for the net diffusion of contrast material into the site of pathology, where it is detected; this is referred to as *contrast enhancement*. Contrast materials used in CT scanning contain iodine in an injectable water-soluble form. Iodine is a heavy atom; its inner electron shell absorbs x-rays through the process of *photoelectric capture*. Even a small amount of iodine effectively blocks the transmitted x-rays so they will not reach the detector. The high x-ray attenuation/absorption will result in hyperdense appearance in the image. Other CT techniques requiring contrast administration are CT angiography (CTA), CT myelography, and CT perfusion studies.

More than 20 years ago, a fast-imaging technique called *spiral* (or *helical*) *CT scanning* was introduced to clinical practice. With this technique, the x-ray tube in the gantry rotates continuously, but data acquisition is combined with continuous movement of the patient through the gantry. The circular rotating path of the x-rays, combined with the linear movement of the imaged body, results in a spiral or helix-shaped x-ray path—hence the name. These scanners can acquire data rapidly, and a large volume can be scanned in 20–60 seconds. This technique offers several advantages, including more rapid image acquisition. During the short scan time, patients can usually hold their breath, which reduces/minimizes motion artifacts. Timing of contrast bolus administration can be optimized, and less contrast material is sufficient. The short scan time, optimal contrast bolus timing, and better image quality are very useful in CTA, where cervical and intracranial blood vessels are visualized. These images can also be reformatted as 3D views of the vasculature, which are often displayed in color and can be depicted along with reformatted bone or other tissues in the region of interest (ROI; Fig. 40.2).

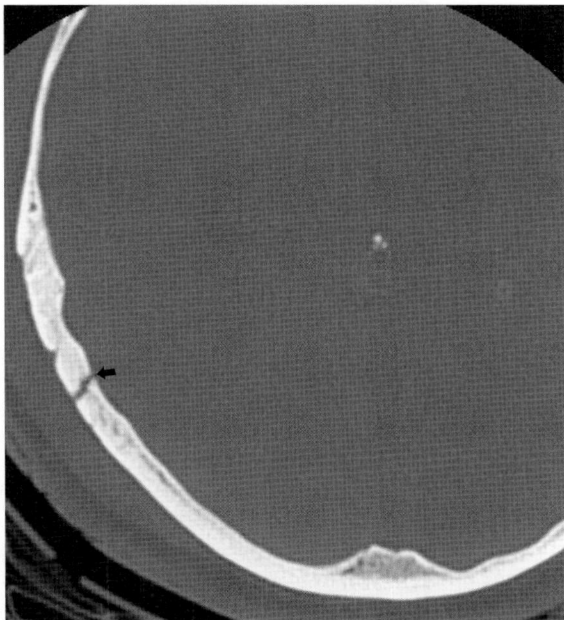

**Fig. 40.1 Computed Tomography Scan from a 32-Year-Old Patient After a Motor Vehicle Accident.** Axial bone window computed tomography image reveals a skull fracture *(arrow)*.

Superfast CT scanners have become available in the past 5 years. Multiplying the number of detectors by 4 can result in obtaining 64 slices of an organ in a fraction of a second. They are particularly useful in cardiology and also allow for the acquisition of perfusion images of the entire brain. One shortcoming is a greater exposure to ionizing radiation per scan.

## MAGNETIC RESONANCE IMAGING

### Basic Principles

Magnetic resonance imaging (MRI) is based on the magnetic characteristics of the imaged tissue. It involves creation of tissue magnetization (which can then be manipulated in several ways) and detection of tissue magnetization as revealed by signal intensity. The various degrees of detected signal intensity provide the image of a given tissue.

In clinical practice, MRI uses the magnetic characteristics inherent to the protons of hydrogen nuclei in the tissue, mostly in the form of water but to a significant extent in fat as well. The protons spin about their own axes, which creates a magnetic dipole moment for each proton (Fig. 40.3). In the absence of an external magnetic field, the axes of these dipoles are arranged randomly, and therefore the vectors depicting the dipole moments cancel each other out, resulting in a zero net magnetization vector and a zero net magnetic field for the tissue.

This situation changes when the body is placed in the strong magnetic field of a scanner (see Fig. 40.3, *A*). The magnetic field is generated by an electric current circulating in wire coils that surround the

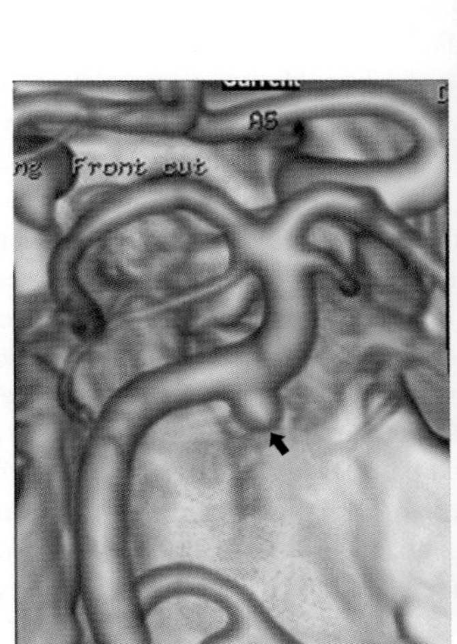



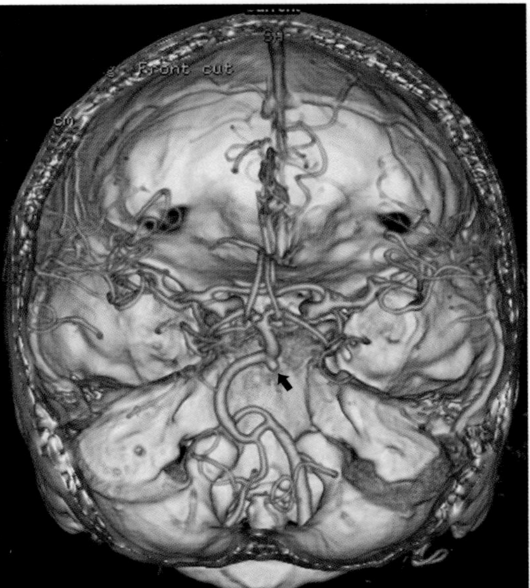



**Fig. 40.2 Computed Tomography Angiogram with 3D Reconstruction.** Reconstructed color images reveal a basilar artery aneurysm *(arrows)*.

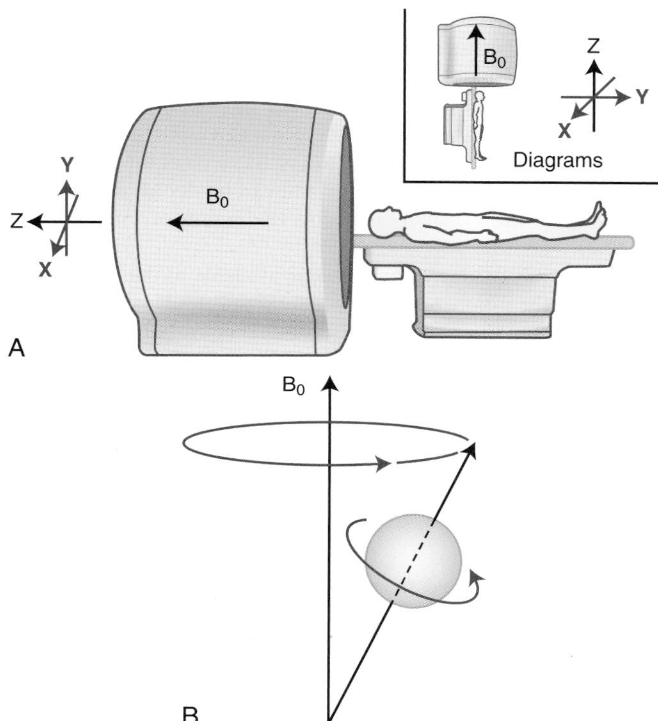


**Fig. 40.3** **A,** Magnetization in a magnetic resonance imaging scanner. Direction of external magnetic field is in the head–foot direction in the scanner. However, in diagrams that follow, the frame of reference is turned, so that the *z* direction is up *(inset)*. **B,** Precession. In an external magnetic field *($B_0$)*, protons spin around their own axis and "wobble" about the axis of the magnetic field. This phenomenon is called precession. (A, From *Higgins, D., 2010. ReviseMRI. Available from: http://www.revisemri.com/questions/basicphysics/precession,* B, Reprinted *with permission from Hashemi, R.H., Bradley, W.G., Lasanti, C.J., 2004. MRI—The Basics, second ed. Lippincott Williams & Wilkins, Philadelphia.*)

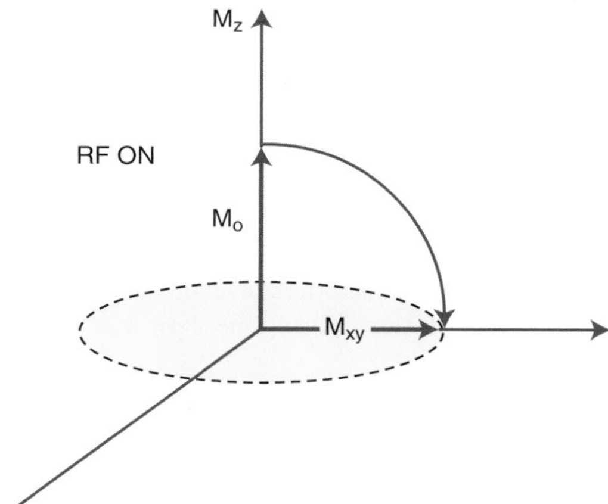


**Fig. 40.4 Flipping the Net Magnetization Vector.** When a 90-degree radiofrequency (RF) pulse is applied, the net magnetization vector of the protons *($M_0$)* is flipped from the vertical *(z)* plane to the horizontal *(xy)* plane. (*Reprinted with permission from Hashemi, R.H., Bradley, W.G., Lasanti, C.J., 2004. MRI—The Basics, second ed. Lippincott Williams & Wilkins, Philadelphia.*)

open bore of the scanner. Most MRI scanners used in clinical practice are superconducting magnets. Here the electrical coils are housed at near-absolute zero temperature, minimizing their resistance and allowing for the strong currents needed to generate the magnetic field without undue heating. The low temperature is achieved by cryogens (liquid nitrogen or helium). Most clinical scanners in commercial production today produce magnetic fields at strengths of 1.5 or 3.0 tesla (T).

When the patient is placed in the MRI scanner, the magnetic dipoles in the tissues line up relative to the external magnetic field. Some dipoles will point in the direction of the external field ("north"), some will point in the opposite direction ("south"), but the net magnetization vector of the dipoles (the sum of individual spins) will point in the direction of the external field ("north"), and this will be the tissue's acquired net magnetization. At this point, a small proportion of the protons (and therefore the net magnetization vector of the tissue) is aligned along the external field (longitudinal magnetization), and the protons precess with a certain frequency. The term *precession* describes a proton spinning about its own axis and its simultaneous wobbling about the axis of the external field (see Fig. 40.3, *B*). The frequency of precession is directly proportional to the strength of the applied external magnetic field.

As a next step, a radiofrequency pulse is applied to the part of the body being imaged. This is an electromagnetic wave, and if its frequency matches the precession frequency of the protons, *resonance* occurs. Resonance is a very efficient way to give or receive energy. In this process, the protons receive the energy of the applied radiofrequency pulse. As a result, the protons flip and the net magnetization vector of the tissue ceases transiently to be aligned with that of the external field but flips into another plane; thereby *transverse magnetization* is produced. One example of this is the 90-degree radiofrequency pulse that flips the entire net magnetization vector by 90 degrees to the transverse (horizontal) plane (Fig. 40.4). What we detect in MRI is this transverse magnetization, and its degree will determine the *signal intensity*. Through the process of electromagnetic induction, rotating transverse magnetization in the tissue induces electrical currents in *receiver coils*, thus accomplishing signal detection. Several cycles of excitation pulses by the scanner with detection of the resulting electromagnetic signal from the imaged subject are repeated per imaged slice. This occurs while varying two additional magnetic field gradients along the *x* and *y* axes for each cycle. Varying the magnetic field gradient along these two additional axes, known as *phase* and *frequency encoding*, is necessary to obtain sufficient information to decode the spatial coordinates of the signal emitted by each tissue voxel. This is accomplished using a mathematical algorithm known as a *Fourier transform*. The final image is produced by applying a gray scale to the intensity values calculated by the Fourier transform for each voxel within the imaging plane, corresponding to the *signal intensity* of individual tissue elements.

## T1 and T2 Relaxation Times

During the process of resonance, the applied 90-degree radiofrequency pulse flips the net magnetization vectors of the imaged tissues to the transverse (horizontal) plane by transmitting electromagnetic energy to the protons. The radiofrequency pulse is brief, and after it is turned off, the magnitude of the net magnetization vector starts to decrease along the transverse or horizontal plane and return ("recover or relax") toward its original position, in which it is aligned parallel to the external magnetic field. The relaxation process, therefore, changes the magnitude and orientation of the tissue's net magnetization vector. There is a decrease along the horizontal or transverse plane and an increase (recovery) along the longitudinal or vertical plane (Fig. 40.5).

To understand the meaning of T1 and T2 relaxation times, the decrease in the magnitude of the horizontal component of the net

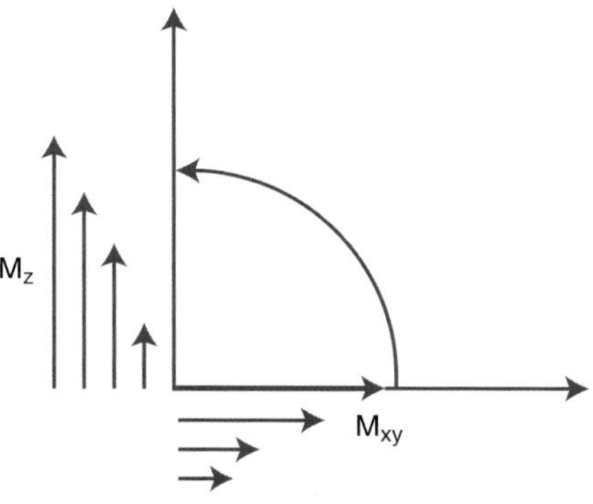


**Fig. 40.5 T1 and T2 Relaxation.** When the radiofrequency (RF) pulse is turned off, two processes begin simultaneously: gradual recovery of the longitudinal magnetization *($M_z$)* and gradual decay of the horizontal magnetization component *($M_{xy}$)*. These processes are referred to as T1 and T2 relaxation, respectively. (*Reprinted with permission from Hashemi, R.H., Bradley, W.G., Lasanti, C.J., 2004. MRI—The Basics, second ed. Lippincott Williams & Wilkins, Philadelphia.*)

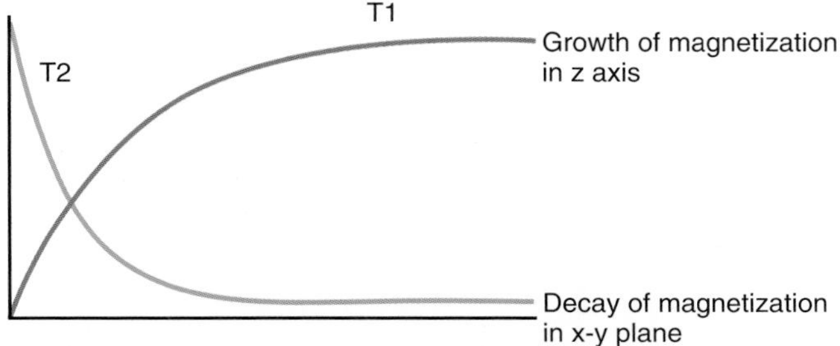


**Fig. 40.6** This diagram illustrates the simultaneous recovery of longitudinal magnetization (*T1* relaxation) and decay of horizontal magnetization (*T2* relaxation) after the radiofrequency pulse is turned off. (*Reprinted with permission from Hashemi, R.H., Bradley, W.G., Lasanti, C.J., 2004. MRI—The Basics, second ed. Lippincott Williams & Wilkins, Philadelphia.*)

magnetization vector and its simultaneous increase in magnitude along the vertical plane should be analyzed independently. These processes are in fact independent and occur at two different rates, with T2 relaxation always occurring more rapidly than T1 relaxation (Fig. 40.6). The *T1 relaxation time* refers to the time required by protons within a given tissue to recover 63% of their original net magnetization vector along the vertical or longitudinal plane immediately after completion of the 90-degree radiofrequency pulse. As an example, a T1 time of 2 seconds means that 2 seconds after the 90-degree pulse is turned off, the given tissue's net magnetization vector has recovered 63% of its original magnitude along the vertical (longitudinal) plane. Different tissues may have quite different T1 time values (T1 recovery or relaxation times). T1 relaxation is also known as *spin-lattice relaxation*.

While T1 relaxation relates to the longitudinal plane, *T2 relaxation* refers to the decrease of the transverse or horizontal magnetization vector. When the 90-degree pulse is applied, the entire net magnetization vector is flipped in the horizontal or transverse plane. When the pulse is turned off, the transverse magnetization vector starts to decrease. The T2 relaxation time is the time it takes for the tissue to lose 63% of its original transverse or horizontal magnetization. As an example, a T2 time of 200 ms means that 200 ms after the 90-degree pulse has been turned off, the tissue will have lost 63% of its transverse or horizontal magnetization. The decrease of the net

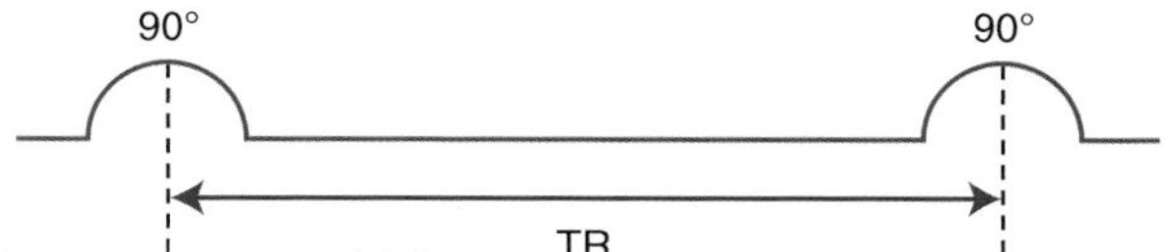


**Fig. 40.7 Repetition Time.** This pulse sequence diagram demonstrates the concept of repetition time *(TR)*, which is the time interval between two sequential radiofrequency pulses. (*Reprinted with permission from Hashemi, R.H., Bradley, W.G., Lasanti, C.J., 2004. MRI—The Basics, second ed. Lippincott Williams & Wilkins, Philadelphia.*)

magnetization vector in the horizontal plane is due to dephasing of the individual proton spins as they precess at slightly different rates owing to local inhomogeneities of the magnetic field. This dephasing of the individual proton magnetic dipole vectors causes a decrease of the transverse component of the net magnetization vector and loss of signal. T2 relaxation is also known as *spin-spin relaxation*. Just like the T1 values, the T2 time values of different tissues may also be quite different. Tissue abnormalities may alter a given tissue's T1 and T2 time values, ultimately resulting in the signal changes seen on the patient's MR images.

## Repetition Time and Time to Echo

As mentioned earlier, the amount of the signal detected by the receiver coils depends on the magnitude of the net magnetization vector along the transverse or horizontal plane. Using certain operator-dependent parameters, it is possible to influence how much net magnetization strength (in other words, vector length) will be present in the transverse plane for the imaged tissues at the time of signal acquisition. During the imaging process, the initial 90-degree pulse flips the entire vertical or longitudinal magnetization vector into the horizontal plane. When this initial pulse is turned off, recovery along the longitudinal plane begins (T1 relaxation). Subsequent application of a second radiofrequency pulse at a given time after the first pulse will flip the net magnetization vector that recovered so far along the longitudinal plane back to the transverse plane. As a result, we can measure the magnitude of the net longitudinal magnetization that had recovered within each voxel at the time of application of the second pulse, provided that signal acquisition is begun immediately afterward. The time between these radiofrequency pulses is referred to as *repetition time*, or TR (Fig. 40.7). It is important to realize that contrary to the T1 and T2 times, which are properties of the given tissue, the TR is a controllable parameter. By selecting a longer TR, for instance, we allow more time for the net magnetization vector to recover before we flip it back to the transverse plane for measurement. A longer TR, because it increases the amount of signal that can potentially be detected, will also result in a higher signal-to-noise ratio, with higher image quality.

As described earlier, the other process that begins after the initial radiofrequency pulse is turned off is the decrease of net horizontal or transverse magnetization, owing to dephasing of the proton spins (T2 relaxation). *Time to echo* (TE) refers to the time we wait until we measure the magnitude of the remaining transverse magnetization. TE, just like TR, is a parameter controlled by the operator. If we use a longer TE, tissues with significantly different T2 values (i.e., different rates of loss of transverse magnetization component) will show more difference in the measured signal intensity (transverse magnetization vector size) when the signals are collected. However, there is a tradeoff. If the TE is set too high, the signal-to-noise ratio of the resulting image will drop to a level that is too low, resulting in poor image quality.

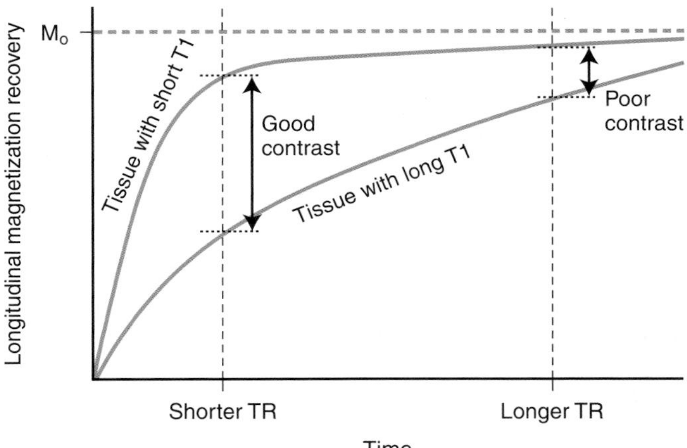


**Fig. 40.8 T1 Weighting.** When imaging tissues with different T1 relaxation times, selecting a short repetition time *(TR)* will increase T1 weighting, as the magnitudes of their recovered longitudinal magnetizations will be different. By selecting a longer TR, longitudinal magnetization of both tissues will recover significantly, and there will be a smaller difference between the magnitudes of their recovered magnetization vectors; therefore, the T1 weighting will be less.

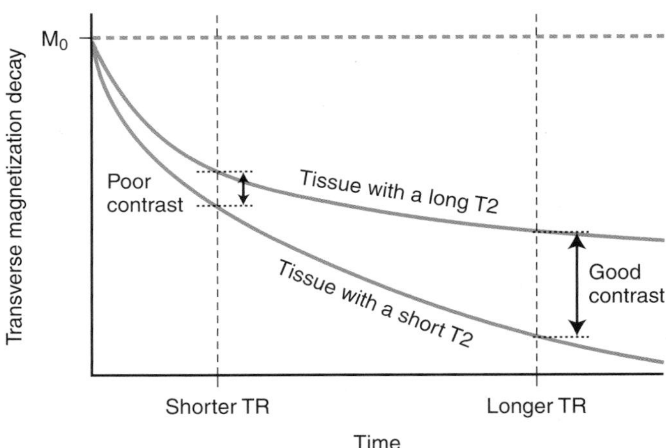


**Fig. 40.9 T2 Weighting.** In tissues with different T2 relaxation times, selecting a short time to echo (TE) will not result in much T2 weighting, because there is no major difference yet between the loss of their transverse magnetizations. However, by selecting a longer TE, we allow a significant difference to develop between the amount of transverse magnetization of the two tissues, so more T2 weighting is added to the image.

## Tissue Contrast (T1, T2, and Proton Density Weighting)

By using various TR and TE values, it is possible to increase (or decrease) the contrast between different tissues in an MR image. Achieving this contrast may be based on either the T1 or the T2 properties of the tissues in conjunction with their proton density (PD). Selecting a long TR value reduces the T1 contrast between tissues (Fig. 40.8). Thus, if we wait long enough before applying the second 90-degree pulse, we allow enough time for all tissues to recover most of their longitudinal or vertical magnetization. Because T1 is relatively short, even for tissues with the longest T1, this is possible without resulting in excessively long scan times. Since after a long TR the longitudinally oriented net magnetization vectors of separate tissue types are all of similar magnitudes prior to being flipped into the transverse plane by the second pulse, a long TR will result in little T1 tissue contrast. Conversely, by selecting a short TR value, there will be significant variation in the extent to which tissues with different T1 relaxation times will have recovered their longitudinal magnetization prior to being flipped by the second 90-degree pulse (see Fig. 40.8). Therefore, with a short TR, the second pulse will flip magnetization vectors of different magnitudes into the transverse plane for measurement, resulting in more T1 contrast between the tissues.

During T2 relaxation in the transverse plane, selecting a short TE will give higher measured signal intensities (as a short TE will not allow enough time for significant dephasing, i.e., transverse magnetization loss), but tissues with different T2 relaxation times will not show much contrast (Fig. 40.9). This is because by selecting a short time until measurement (short TE), we do not allow significant T2-related magnitude differences to develop. If we select longer TE values, tissues with different T2 relaxation times will have time to lose different amounts of transverse magnetization, and therefore by the time of signal measurement, different signal intensities will be measured from these different tissues (see Fig. 40.9). This is referred to as *T2 contrast*.

Based on the described considerations, selecting TR and TE values that are both short will increase the T1 contrast between tissues, referred to as *T1 weighting*. Selecting long TR and long TE values will cause increased T2 contrast between tissues, referred to as *T2 weighting*.

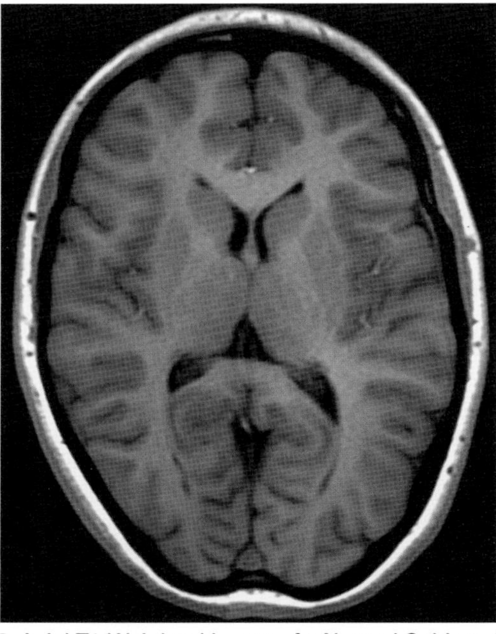

**Fig. 40.10** Axial T1-Weighted Image of a Normal Subject, Obtained With a 3-T Scanner.

On T1-weighted images, substances with a longer T1 relaxation time (such as water) will be darker. This is because the short TR does not allow as much longitudinal magnetization to recover, so the vector flipped to the transverse plane by the second 90-degree pulse will be smaller with a lower resulting signal strength. Conversely, tissues with shorter T1 relaxation times (such as fat or some mucinous materials) will be brighter on T1-weighted images, as they recover more longitudinal magnetization prior to their proton spins being flipped into the transverse plane by the second 90-degree pulse (Fig. 40.10). Among many other applications of T1-weighted images, they allow for evaluation of BBB breakdown: areas with abnormally permeable BBB show increased signal after the intravenous administration of

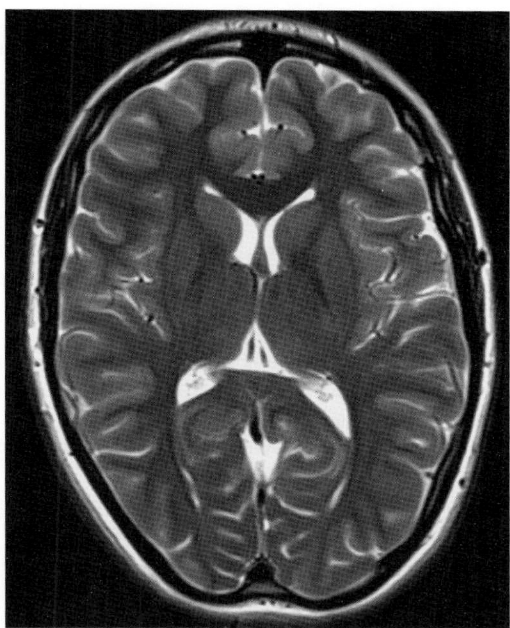

**Fig. 40.11** Axial T2-Weighted Image of a Normal Subject, Obtained With a 3-T Scanner.

**TABLE 40.1 Magnetic Resonance Imaging Signal Intensity of Some Substances Found in Neuroimaging**

| | T1-Weighted Image | T2-Weighted Image |
|---|---|---|
| Air | ↓↓↓↓ | ↓↓↓↓ |
| Free water/CSF | ↓↓↓ | ↑↑↑ |
| Fat | ↑↑↑ | ↑ |
| Cortical bone | ↓↓↓ | ↓↓↓ |
| Bone marrow (fat) | ↑↑ | ↑ |
| Edema | ↓ | ↑↑ |
| Calcification | ↓ (Heavy amounts of $Ca^{++}$)<br>↑ (Little $Ca^{++}$, some $Fe^{+++}$) | ↓ |
| Mucinous material | ↑ | ↓ |
| Gray matter | Lower than in T2-WI | |
| White matter | Higher than in T2-WI | |
| Muscle | Similar to gray matter | Similar to gray matter |
| Blood products: | | |
| • Oxyhemoglobin | Similar to background | ↑ |
| • Deoxyhemoglobin | ↓ | ↓ |
| • Intracellular met-hemoglobin | ↑↑ | ↓ |
| • Extracellular met-hemoglobin | ↑↑ | ↑↑ |
| • Hemosiderin | ↓ | ↓↓↓ |

*CSF,* Cerebrospinal fluid; *T2-WI,* T2-weighted image.

gadolinium. Gadolinium administration is contraindicated in pregnancy. Breastfeeding immediately after receiving gadolinium is generally regarded to be safe (Chen et al., 2008). Renally impaired patients are susceptible to an uncommon but serious adverse reaction to gadolinium, *nephrogenic systemic fibrosis* (Marckmann et al., 2006).

On T2-weighted images, substances with longer T2 relaxation times (e.g., water) will be brighter because they will not have lost as much transverse magnetization magnitude by the time the signal is measured (Fig. 40.11). The T1 and T2 signal characteristics of various tissues or substances found in neuroimaging are listed in Table 40.1.

What happens if we select long TR and short TE values? With the longer TR, the T1 differences between the tissues diminish, whereas the short TE does not allow much T2 contrast to develop. The signal intensity obtained from the various tissues, therefore, will mostly depend on their relative proton densities. Tissues having more PD, and thereby larger net magnetization vectors, will have greater signal intensity. This set of imaging parameters is referred to as *proton density weighting*.

## Magnetic Resonance Image Reconstruction

To construct an MR image, a slice of the imaged body part is selected; then the signal coming from each of the voxels making up the given slice is measured. Slice selection is achieved by setting the external magnetic field to vary linearly along one of the three principal axes perpendicular to the axial, sagittal, and coronal planes of the subject being imaged. As a result, protons within the slice to be imaged will precess at a Larmor frequency different from the Larmor frequency within all other imaging planes perpendicular to the axis along which the magnetic field gradient is applied. The *Larmor frequency* is the natural precession frequency of protons within a magnetic field of a given strength and is calculated simply as the product of the magnetic field, $B_0$, and the gyromagnetic ratio, $\gamma$. The precession frequency of a hydrogen proton is therefore directly proportional to the strength of the applied magnetic field. The gyromagnetic ratio for any given nucleus is a constant, with a value for hydrogen protons of 42.58 MHz/T. In slices at lower magnetic strengths of the gradient, the protons precess more slowly, whereas in slices at higher magnetic field strengths, the protons precess more quickly. Based on the property of nuclear magnetic resonance, the applied radiofrequency pulse (which flips the magnetization vector to the transverse plane) will stimulate only those protons with a precession frequency that matches the frequency of the applied radiofrequency pulse. By selecting the frequency of the stimulating radiofrequency pulse during the application of the slice selection gradient, we can choose which protons (those with a specific Larmor frequency) to stimulate ("make resonate"), and thereby we can select which slice of the body to image (Fig. 40.12).

After excitation of the slice to be imaged, using the slice selection gradient, the spatial coordinates of each voxel within the slice must be encoded to determine how much signal is coming from each voxel of that slice. This is achieved by means of two additional gradients that are orthogonal to each other within the imaging plane, known as the *frequency encoding gradient* and the *phase encoding gradient*. The phase encoding gradient briefly alters the precession frequency of the protons along the axis to which it is applied, thereby changing the relative phases of the precessing protons along this in-plane axis. The frequency encoding gradient, applied orthogonally to the phase encoding gradient within the imaging plane, alters the precession frequency of the protons along the axis to which it is applied, during the acquisition of the MRI signal. As a result of these encoding steps, each voxel will have its own unique frequency and its own unique phase shift, which upon repeating the acquisition with several incremental changes in the phase encoding gradient will allow for deduction of the spatial localization of different intensity values for each voxel using a mathematical algorithm known as a *Fourier transform*. Phase encoding takes time; it has to be performed for each row of voxels in the image along the

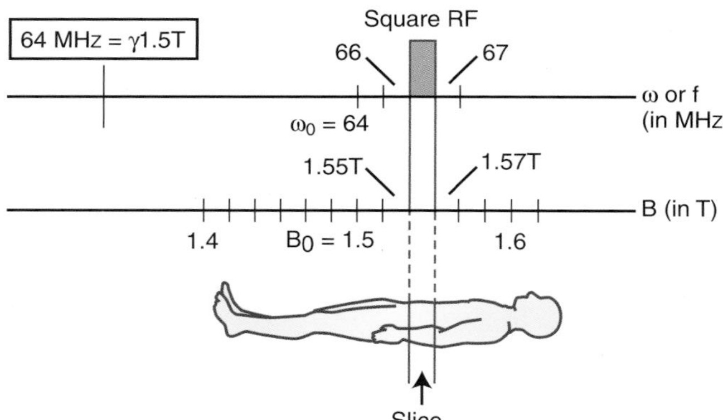


**Fig. 40.12 Slice Selection Gradient.** Using a gradient coil, a magnetic strength gradient is applied parallel to the long axis of the subject's body in the scanner. As a result, the magnetic field is weakest at the feet and gets gradually stronger toward the head. In this example, magnetic field strength is 1.4 T at the feet, 1.5 T at the mid-body, and 1.6 T at the head. Accordingly, protons in these regions will precess at different frequencies (ω): slowest in the feet and with gradually higher frequencies toward the head as the magnetic field gets gradually stronger. Since the radiofrequency *(RF)* pulse will resonate with those protons (and flip their magnetization vectors) that precess with the same frequency as that of the RF pulse, by selecting the frequency of the RF pulse, we can select which body region's protons to stimulate (i.e., which body slice to image). (*Reprinted with permission from Hashemi, R.H., Bradley, W.G., Lasanti, C.J., 2004. MRI—The Basics, second ed. Lippincott Williams & Wilkins, Philadelphia.*)

phase encoding axis. Therefore, the higher the resolution of the image along the phase encoding axis, the longer the time required to acquire the image for that slice of tissue.

In the online version of this chapter (available at http://www.expertconsult.com), there is a discussion of the nature and application of the following MRI sequences or techniques: spin echo and fast (turbo) spin echo; gradient-recalled echo (GRE) sequences, partial flip angle; inversion recovery sequences (FLAIR, STIR); fat saturation; echoplanar imaging; diffusion-weighted magnetic resonance imaging (DWI); perfusion-weighted magnetic resonance imaging (PWI); susceptibility-weighted imaging (SWI); diffusion tensor imaging (DTI); and magnetization transfer contrast imaging.

## STRUCTURAL NEUROIMAGING IN THE CLINICAL PRACTICE OF NEUROLOGY

For an expanded version of this section, go to http://www.expertconsult.com.

### Brain Diseases

Although a description of brain findings on CT and MRI with their differential diagnosis would be helpful (Masdeu et al., 2016), in this chapter we have chosen the traditional approach of listing the imaging findings caused by various brain diseases.

#### Brain Tumors

Epidemiology, pathology, etiology, and management of cancer in the nervous system are discussed in Chapters 71–76. From the standpoint of structural neuroimaging, a useful anatomical classification distinguishes two main groups: intra-axial and extra-axial tumors. Intra-axial tumors are within the brain parenchyma, extra-axial tumors are outside the brain parenchyma (involving the meninges or, less commonly, the ventricular system). Intra-axial tumors are usually infiltrative with poorly defined margins. Conversely, extra-axial tumors, even though they often compress or displace the adjacent brain, are usually demarcated by a cerebrospinal cleft or another tissue interface between tumor and brain parenchyma. For differential diagnostic purposes, intra-axial primary brain neoplasms can be further divided into the anatomical subgroups of supratentorial and infratentorial tumors (Table 40.2).

For evaluation of brain tumors, the structural imaging modality of choice is MRI. Due to their gradual expansion and often infiltrative nature, most brain tumors are already visible on MRI by the time patients become symptomatic. Exceptions to this rule are tumors that tend to involve the cortex or corticomedullary junction, such as small oligodendrogliomas or metastases, which may cause seizures early, even before being clearly visible on noncontrast MRI. Meningeal involvement is also often symptomatic, for instance by causing headaches and confusion, but may not be appreciated on noncontrast images. Higher magnetic field strength (e.g., a 3-T scanner) and contrast administration (in double or triple dose if necessary) can improve detection of small or clinically silent neoplastic lesions.

Neuroimaging is particularly useful in the assessment of brain tumors. Unlike destructive lesions such as ischemic strokes, brain tumors often cause clinical manifestations that are difficult to interpret. Sometimes the clinical presentation may provide clues to localization—for example, a seizure is suggestive of an intra-axial tumor, whereas cranial nerve involvement tends to signal an extra-axial pathology. But edema, mass effect, obstructive hydrocephalus, and elevated intracranial pressure (ICP) can give rise to nonspecific symptoms (e.g., headache, visual disturbance, altered mental status), and false localizing signs may also appear, such as oculomotor or abducens nerve compression due to an expanding intra-axial mass.

Neoplastic tissues most commonly prolong the T1 and T2 relaxation times, appearing hypointense on T1- and hyperintense on T2-weighted images, but different tumors differ in this property, facilitating tumor identification on MRI. MRI is also very sensitive for detection of other pathological changes that can be associated with tumors, such as calcification, hemorrhage, necrosis, and edema. The structural detail provided by MRI is useful for assessing involved structures and determining the number and macroscopic extent of the neoplasms, thereby guiding surgical planning or other treatment modalities.

#### Intra-axial Primary Brain Tumors

Certain brain tumor types are discussed in the online version of this chapter, available at http://www.expertconsult.com. 

***Ganglioglioma and gangliocytoma.*** *Gangliogliomas* (WHO grade I or II) are mixed tumors containing both neural and glial elements. *Gangliocytomas* (WHO grade I) are less common and contain well-differentiated neuronal cells without a glial component. Less commonly, gangliogliomas may exhibit anaplasia within the glial component and are classified as *anaplastic ganglioglioma* (WHO grade III). A rare type of gangliocytoma, dysplastic gangliocytoma of the cerebellum (also known as *Lhermitte-Duclos disease*) exhibits a characteristic "tiger-striped" appearance and is often present in association with Cowden disease, a phakomatosis.

The peak age of onset for gangliogliomas is the second decade. This tumor is usually supratentorial and is most commonly located in the temporal lobe. It is well demarcated, and a cystic component and mural nodule are often observed. Calcification is common.

TABLE 40.2 **Magnetic Resonance Imaging Characteristics of Brain Tumors**

| Tumor | Typical Location, Appearance | Typical T1 Signal Characteristics | Typical T2 Signal Characteristics | Typical Enhancement Pattern |
|---|---|---|---|---|
| **Ventricular Region** | | | | |
| Central neurocytoma | Intraventricular, at foramen of Monro | Isointense | Iso- to hyperintense | Variable, usually moderate and heterogeneous |
| Subependymal giant cell astrocytoma | Intraventricular, at foramen of Monro | Hypo- to isointense | Hyperintense with possible hypointense foci due to calcium | Intense |
| Choroid plexus papilloma | Intraventricular (lateral ventricle in children, fourth ventricle in adults)<br>Calcification and hemorrhage may be present | Iso- to hypointense | Iso- to hyperintense | Intense |
| Subependymoma | Mostly fourth ventricle but can be third and lateral ventricles | Iso- to hypointense | Hyperintense | Mild or absent |
| **Intra-axial, Mostly Supratentorial** | | | | |
| Ganglioglioma, gangliocytoma | Supratentorial, mostly temporal lobe.<br>Solid and cystic | Solid portion isointense, cyst hypointense | Solid portion hypo- to hyperintense, cyst hyperintense | From none to heterogeneous or rim |
| Pleomorphic xanthoastrocytoma | Cerebral cortex and adjacent meninges<br>Has cystic portions | Hypointense or mixed intensity | Hyperintense or mixed intensity | Solid portion and adjacent meninges enhance |
| Diffuse astrocytomas | Supratentorial in two-thirds of cases | Iso- to hypointense | Hyperintense | Grade II may enhance |
| Anaplastic astrocytoma | Frequently in frontal lobes | Iso- to hypointense | Hyperintense | Diffuse or ringlike |
| Oligodendroglioma | Supratentorial white matter and cortical mantle<br>May exhibit cyst or calcification | Hypo- to isointense | Hyperintense; also typically hyperintense on DWI | Variable, patchy |
| Glioblastoma | Frontal and temporal lobes, spreads along pathways such as corpus callosum | Mixed (edema, necrosis, hemorrhage) | Mixed (edema, necrosis, hemorrhage) | Intense, inhomogeneous, nodular or ringlike |
| Primary CNS lymphoma | Supratentorial or infratentorial<br>In immunocompetent host, usually solitary at ventricular border; in immunocompromised, multiple in white matter | Iso- to hypointense | Iso- to hyperintense | Intense<br>Typically ringlike in immunocompromised host |
| **Intra-axial, Posterior Fossa** | | | | |
| Pilocytic astrocytoma | Posterior fossa, sellar region<br>Usually large cyst with mural nodule | Iso- to hypointense | Iso- to hyperintense | Solid component enhances intensely |
| Ependymoma | Fourth ventricle<br>Cystic component | Iso- to hypointense | Iso- to hyperintense | Intense in solid portion, rim around cyst |
| Hemangioblastoma | Infratentorial<br>Vascular nodule and cystic cavity | Hypo- to isointense, but can be mixed due to hemorrhage | Hyperintense, but can be mixed due to hemorrhage | Solid component enhances |
| Medulloblastoma | Arises from roof of fourth ventricle | Iso- to hypointense | Iso-, hypo-, or hyperintense | Heterogeneous |
| **Extra-axial** | | | | |
| Esthesioneuroblastoma | Cribriform plate, anterior fossa | Isointense | Iso- to hyperintense | Heterogeneous |
| Meningioma | Falx, convexity, sphenoid wing, petrous ridge, olfactory groove, parasellar region, and the posterior fossa<br>Calcification may be present | Iso- to slightly hypointense | Can be hypo-, iso-, or hyperintense | Intense, homogeneous |
| Schwannoma | Cerebellopontine angle, vestibular portion of cranial nerve VIII<br>Cyst or calcification may be present | Iso- to hypointense | Iso- to hyperintense | Homogeneous |
| Neurofibroma | Arises from peripheral nerve sheath, any location | Iso- to hypointense | Hyperintense | Homogeneous |

*(Continued)*

**TABLE 40.2 Magnetic Resonance Imaging Characteristics of Brain Tumors—cont'd**

| Tumor | Typical Location, Appearance | Typical T1 Signal Characteristics | Typical T2 Signal Characteristics | Typical Enhancement Pattern |
|---|---|---|---|---|
| **Sella and Pineal Regions** | | | | |
| Pituitary adenoma | Sella, with potential supra- and parasellar extension | Hypo- or isointense | Hyperintense | Homogeneous, enhances in a delayed fashion (initially hypointense relative to the normally enhancing gland; on delayed images, hyperintense relative to the gland due to delayed contrast accumulation) |
| Craniopharyngioma | Suprasellar cistern, sometimes intrasellar<br>Solid and cystic components | Iso- to hypointense<br>Cyst has variable signal intensity | Solid and cystic component both hyperintense<br>Calcification may be hypointense | Solid component enhances homogeneously |
| Pineoblastoma | Tectal area | Isointense | Iso- to hypo- to hyperintense | Moderate heterogeneous |
| Pineocytoma | Tectal area<br>Well defined, noninvasive | Isointense | May be hypointense | Intense with variable pattern (central, nodular) |
| Germinoma | Tectal region | Variable, hypo- and hyperintense | Variable, hypo- and hyperintense | Intense |

*CNS*, Central nervous system; *DWI*, diffusion-weighted imaging.

On MRI (Provenzale et al., 2000), the solid component is usually isointense on T1 and hypo- to hyperintense on T2-weighted images. The cystic component, if present, exhibits CSF signal characteristics. The associated mass effect is variable. With contrast, various enhancement patterns are seen—homogeneous or rim pattern—but no enhancement is also possible.

***Pilocytic astrocytomas.*** Pilocytic astrocytomas have two major groups: juvenile and adult. These tumors are classified as WHO grade I. Juvenile pilocytic astrocytomas are the most common posterior fossa tumors in children. The most common locations are the cerebellum, at the fourth ventricle, third ventricle, temporal lobe, optic chiasm, and hypothalamus (Koeller and Rushing, 2004). The appearance is often lobulated, and the lesion appears well demarcated on MRI. Hemorrhage and necrosis are uncommon. Areas of calcification may be present. The tumor usually exhibits solid as well as cystic components, with or without a mural nodule. The adult form is usually well circumscribed, often calcified, and typically exhibits a large cyst with a mural nodule. On MRI, the solid portions of the tumor are iso- to hypointense on T1- and iso- to hyperintense on T2-weighted images (Arai et al., 2006). The cystic component usually exhibits CSF signal characteristics. The associated edema and mass effect is usually mild, sometimes moderate. With gadolinium, the solid components (including the mural nodule) enhance intensely, but not the cyst, which rarely may show rim enhancement.

***Pleomorphic xanthoastrocytoma.*** Pleomorphic xanthoastrocytoma is a rare variant of astrocytic tumors. It is thought to arise from the subpial astrocytes and typically affects the cerebral cortex and adjacent meninges and may cause erosion of the skull. The most common location is the temporal lobe. It is classified as WHO grade II. It usually occurs in the second and third decades of life, and patients often present with seizures. On MRI (Tien et al., 1992) usually a well-circumscribed cystic mass appears in a superficial cortical location. A solid portion or mural nodule is often seen, and the differential diagnosis includes pilocytic astrocytoma and ganglioglioma. The signal characteristics are hypointense or mixed on T1-, and hyperintense or mixed on T2-weighted images. With contrast, the solid portions and sometimes the adjacent meninges enhance. Calcification may be present. There is mild or no mass effect associated with this tumor.

***Diffuse astrocytomas.*** Diffuse astrocytomas are well-differentiated tumors (WHO grade II), usually arising from the fibrillary astrocytes of the white matter. Even though imaging may show a fairly well-defined boundary, these tumors are infiltrative and usually spread beyond their macroscopic border. In 2016 update to the WHO classification of central nervous system (CNS) tumors, astrocytoma is subdivided by the presence of isocitrate dehydrogenase (IDH) mutations, with IDH-mutant tumors carrying better prognoses. Although grade II astrocytoma is a relatively slow-growing tumor, they have a relatively high recurrence rate and an inherent malignant potential to transform into high-grade astrocytoma (Lind-Landström et al., 2012). Two-thirds of cases are supratentorial (Fig. 40.17). A subgroup of these astrocytomas involves specific regions such as the optic nerves/tracts or the brainstem (Fig. 40.18).

Diffuse astrocytomas are iso- or hypointense on T1-weighted images and hyperintense on T2-weighted images. Expansion of the adjacent cortex may be seen, and mass effect (if present) is generally modest. There is little to no surrounding edema. Diffuse astrocytoma usually do not enhance, however, small ill-defined areas of enhancement are not rare. The appearance of enhancement in a previously nonenhancing tumor is a worrisome sign of progression to higher grades.

***Anaplastic astrocytoma.*** Anaplastic astrocytoma is classified as grade III by the WHO grading system. It represents 25%–30% of gliomas, usually appears between 40 and 60 years of age, and is more common in men. Anaplastic astrocytoma is a diffuse infiltrating tumor that often evolves from a well-differentiated astrocytoma as a result of chromosomal and gene alterations. It is most frequently found in the frontal lobes. On MRI, anaplastic astrocytomas appear as poorly circumscribed heterogeneous tumors, which are iso- to hypointense on T1-weighted and hyperintense on T2-weighted images, with associated hyperintensity in the surrounding white matter representing vasogenic edema. Foci of hemorrhage may be present but not too commonly. There is moderate mass effect associated with the lesions, and, with contrast, a variable degree and pattern of enhancement is noted (diffuse or ringlike). This tumor is

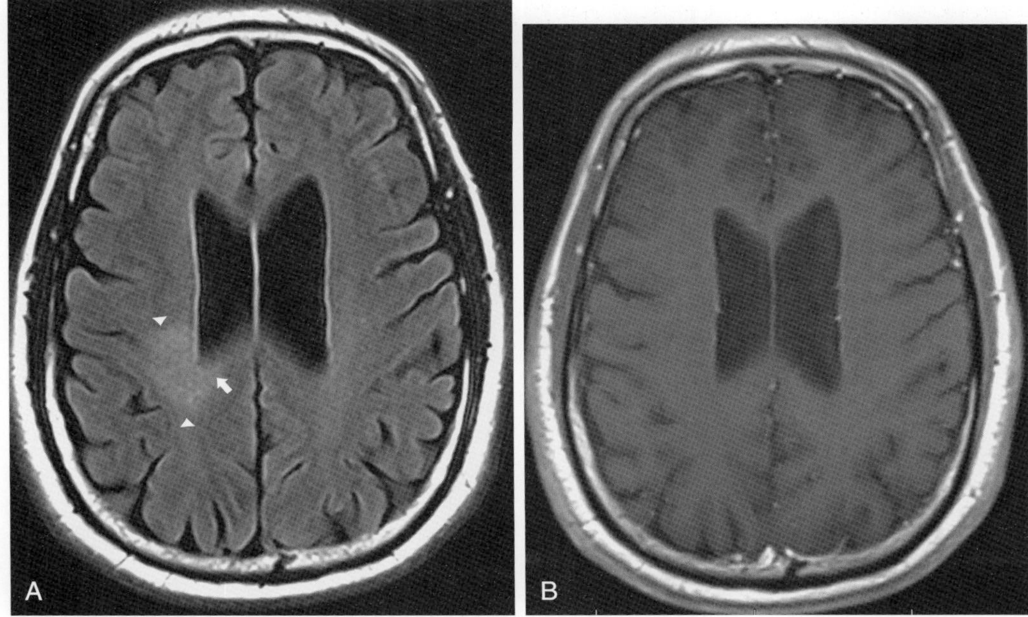


**Fig. 40.17 Low-Grade Glioma. A,** On FLAIR image, a faint hyperintense lesion is seen *(arrowheads)* with somewhat blurred margins in the right corona radiata at the border of the lateral ventricle, extending minimally toward the corpus callosum *(arrow)*. **B,** On T1-weighted postcontrast image, this lesion does not enhance.

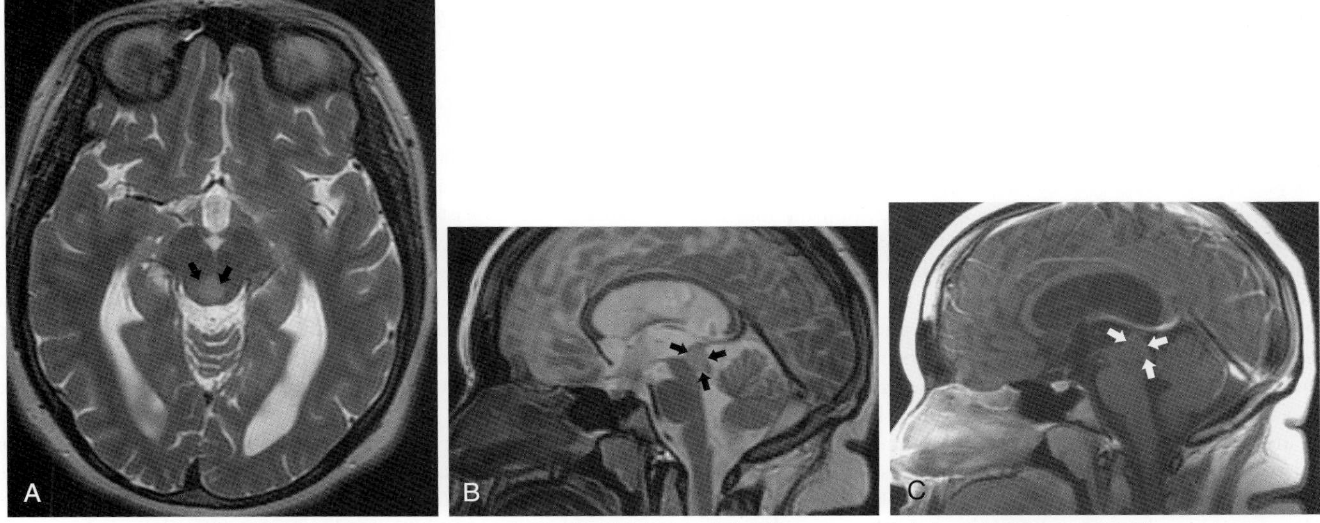


**Fig. 40.18 Tectal Glioma. A, B,** On axial and sagittal T2-weighted images, a faintly hyperintense mass lesion is seen involving the tectum of the midbrain *(arrows)*. There appears to be at least partial obstruction of the aqueduct, resulting in enlargement of the third and lateral ventricles. **C,** Following gadolinium administration, the tumor does not enhance *(arrows)*.

highly infiltrative, usually cannot be fully removed by surgery, and the median survival is 3–4 years.

***Gliomatosis cerebri*** was previously considered a distinct entity, but since the 2016 update to the WHO classification of CNS tumors, it is now being considered a growth pattern of many gliomas, most commonly, anaplastic astrocytoma. The glial tumor cells are disseminated throughout the parenchyma and infiltrate large portions of the neuraxis. Macroscopically it appears homogeneous and is seen as enlargement/expansion of the parenchyma; the gray/white matter interface may become blurred, but the architecture is otherwise not altered. Unilateral hemispheric white matter is generally involved first; then the pathology spreads to the contralateral hemisphere through the corpus callosum. Later, the deep gray matter (basal ganglia, thalamus, massa intermedia) may be affected as well. Diffuse tumor infiltration often extends into the brainstem, cerebellum, and even the spinal cord. Histologically, most cases of gliomatosis cerebri are WHO grade III.

The MRI appearance is iso- to hypointense on T1 and hyperintense on T2. Hemorrhage is uncommon, and enhancement is also rare, at least in the early stages (Fig. 40.19). Later, multiple foci of enhancement may appear, signaling more malignant transformation. The imaging appearance is similar to that of autoimmune or infectious encephalitis, including subacute sclerosing panencephalitis, but in these disorders, clinical findings are more pronounced.

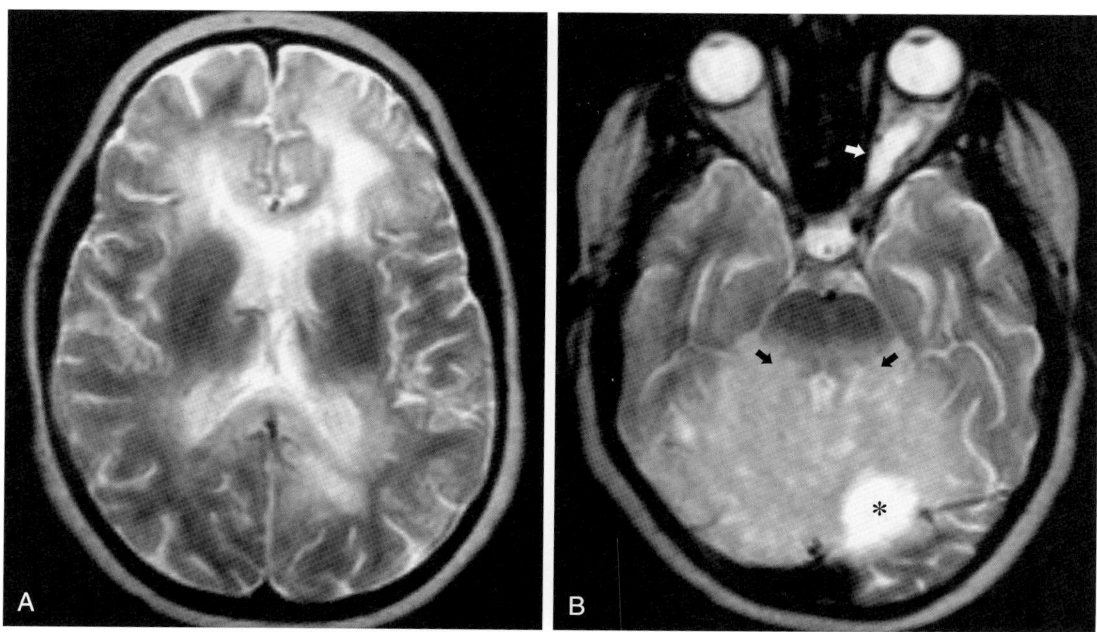


**Fig. 40.19** **Gliomatosis Cerebri. A,** Axial T2-weighted magnetic resonance (MR) image of the brain shows bilateral patchy areas of increased signal intensity in periventricular white matter. **B,** Axial T2-weighted MR image of brain obtained at the level of the upper pons shows diffuse thickening and hyperintensity of the left optic nerve *(white arrow)* and increased signal intensity in the posterior aspect of pons and in the cerebellum *(black arrows)*. A focus of very high signal intensity is present in posterior left cerebellar hemisphere *(asterisk)*. (*From Yip, M., Fisch, C., Lamarche, J.B., 2003. AFIP archives: gliomatosis cerebri affecting the entire neuraxis. Radiographics 23, 247–253.*)

***Oligodendroglioma.*** Oligodendroglioma, made up by IDH mutant and 1p/19q codeleted cells, accounts for 5%–10% of all gliomas. It arises from the oligodendroglia that form the myelin sheath of the CNS pathways. Oligodendroglioma occurs most commonly in young and middle-aged adults, with a median age of onset within the fourth to fifth decades and a male predominance of up to 2:1. Seizure is often the presenting symptom. The most common location is the supratentorial hemispheric white matter, and it also involves the cortical mantle. The tumor often has cystic components and at least, microscopically, in 90% of cases also shows calcification. Hemorrhage and necrosis are rare, and the mass effect is not impressive. On MRI (Koeller and Rushing, 2005) the appearance is heterogeneous, and the tumor is hypo- and isointense on T1 and hyperintense on T2. With gadolinium, the enhancement is variable, usually patchy, and the periphery of the lesion tends to enhance more intensely. Oligodendrogliomas are hypercellular and have been noted to appear hyperintense on diffusion-weighted images (Fig. 40.20).

***Glioblastoma.*** Glioblastoma (GBM), previously known as glioblastoma multiforme, is a highly malignant tumor classified as grade IV by the WHO. It is most common in older adults, usually appearing in the fifth and sixth decades and represents 40%–50% of all primary neoplasms and up to 20% of all intracranial tumors. It is subdivided into two types on the basis of the presence or absence of IDH mutation. It is likely that most of the previously recognized primary GBMs were IDH wild-type, and most of the secondary GBMs (from progression of a previous lower-grade tumor) were IDH mutant. Methylation of the promoter for O[6]-methylguanine-DNA methyltransferase (MGMT), the gene for methylguanine methyltransferase, is well recognized as a favorable prognostic factor in GBM (Binabaj et al., 2018).

Glioblastoma forms a heterogeneous mass exhibiting cystic and necrotic areas and often a hemorrhagic component as well. The most common locations are the frontal and temporal lobes. The tumor is highly infiltrative and has a tendency to spread along larger pathways such as the corpus callosum and invade the other hemisphere, resulting in a characteristic "butterfly" appearance. GBM has also been described to spread along the ventricular surface in the subarachnoid space and may also invade the meninges. There are reported cases of extracranial glioblastoma metastases.

Structural neuroimaging distinguishes between multifocal and multicentric glioblastomas. The term *multifocal glioblastoma* refers to multiple tumor islands in the brain that arose from a common source via continuous parenchymal spread or meningeal/CSF seeding; therefore, they are all connected, at least microscopically. *Multicentric glioblastoma* refers to multiple tumors that are present independently, and physical connection between them cannot be proven, implying they are separate de novo occurrences. This is less common, having been noted in 6% of cases.

On MRI (Fig. 40.21) glioblastomas usually exhibit mixed signal intensities on T1- and T2-weighted images. Cystic and necrotic areas are present, appearing as markedly decreased signal on T1-weighted and hyperintensity on T2-weighted images. Mixed hypo- and hyperintense signal changes due to hemorrhage are also seen. The hemorrhagic component can also be well demonstrated by gradient echo sequences or by SWI. The core of the lesion is surrounded by prominent edema, which appears hypointense on T1-weighted and hyperintense on T2-weighted images. Besides edema, the signal changes around the core of the tumor reflect the presence of infiltrating tumor cells and, in treated cases, postsurgical reactive gliosis and/or postirradiation changes. Following administration of gadolinium, intense enhancement is noted, which is inhomogeneous and often ringlike, also including multiple nodular areas of enhancement. The surrounding edema and ringlike enhancement at times makes it difficult to distinguish glioblastoma from cerebral abscess. DWI is helpful in these cases; glioblastomas are hypointense with this technique, whereas abscesses exhibit remarkable hyperintensity on diffusion-weighted images.

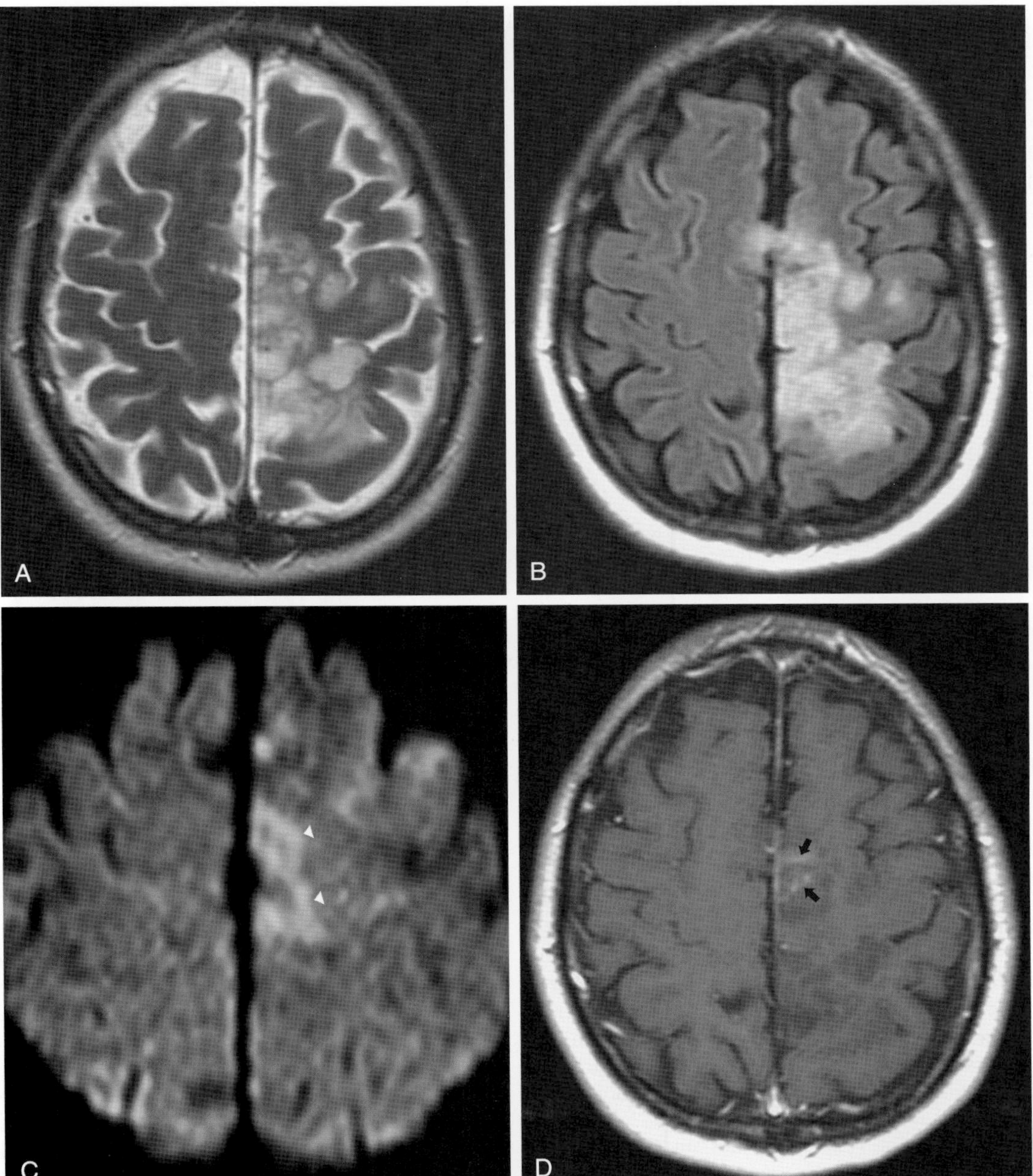


**Fig. 40.20 Oligodendroglioma.** A mass lesion is seen in the left medial frontal lobe, involving the cortical mantle and underlying white matter. **A, B,** On T2 and FLAIR images, the tumor is hyperintense. **C,** On diffusion-weighted image, faint hyperintensity due to the hypercellular nature of this tumor is noted *(arrowheads)*. **D,** With contrast, a few areas of enhancement are seen that tend to involve the periphery of the lesion *(arrows)*.

Owing to its aggressive growth (the tumor size may double every 10 days) and infiltrative nature, the prognosis for patients with glioblastoma is very poor. Despite surgery, irradiation, and chemotherapy the median survival is 1 year.

***Ependymoma.*** Although ependymomas are primarily extra-axial tumors (within the fourth ventricle), intraparenchymal ependymomas arising from ependymal cell remnants of the hemispheric parenchyma are also well known, so this tumor type is discussed here. Ependymomas comprise 5%–6% of all primary brain tumors; 70% of cases occur in childhood and the first and second decades, and ependymoma is the third most common posterior fossa tumor in children. Ependymomas arise from differentiated ependymal cells, and the most common location (70%) is the fourth ventricle. The tumor is usually well demarcated and is separated from the vermis by a CSF interface. The tumor may be cystic and may contain calcification and hemorrhage but these features are more common in supratentorial ependymomas. It may extrude from the cavity of the fourth ventricle through the foramina of Luschka and Magendie. Spreading via CSF to the spinal canal (drop-metastases) may occur, but on spine imaging ependymoma is more commonly noted to arise from the ependymal lining of the central canal, presenting as an intramedullary spinal cord tumor. A subtype, myxopapillary ependymoma, is almost always restricted to the filum terminale.

Ependymomas are hypo- to isointense on T1-weighted images and iso- to hyperintense on T2-weighted images. With gadolinium, intense enhancement is seen, mostly involving the solid components of the tumor, whereas the cystic components tend to exhibit rim enhancement.

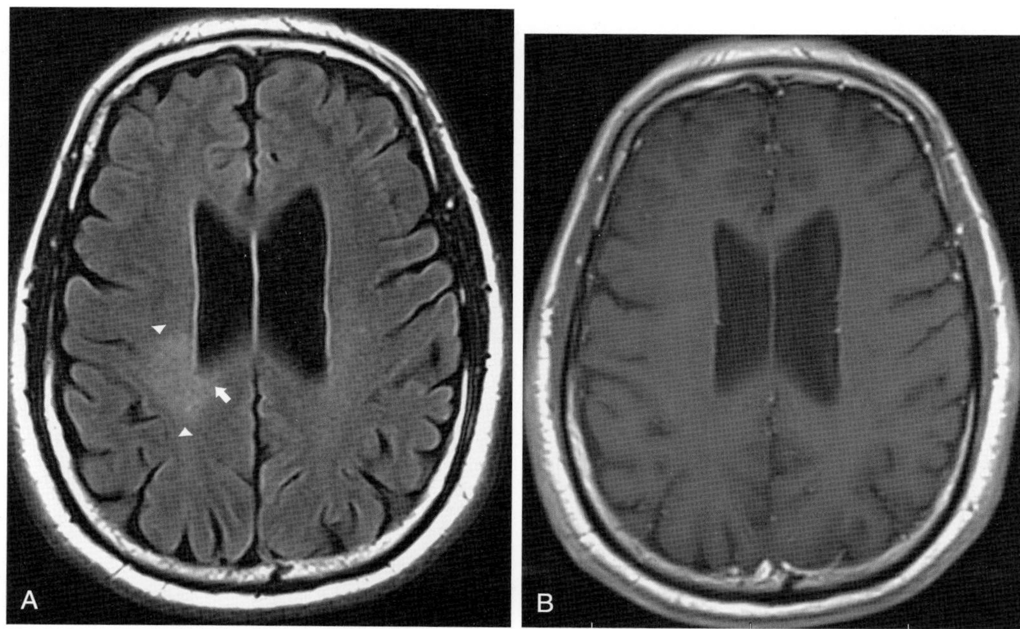


**Fig. 40.21** Glioblastoma Multiforme. **A,** Axial FLAIR image demonstrates a mass lesion spreading across the corpus callosum to involve both frontal lobes in a symmetrical fashion ("butterfly" appearance). The tumor is isointense, exerts mass effect on the sulci and the lateral ventricles, and is surrounded by vasogenic edema. **B,** On axial T1 postcontrast imaging, the tumor exhibits heterogeneous irregular enhancement, most marked at its periphery.

The differential diagnosis for infratentorial ependymoma includes medulloblastoma, pilocytic astrocytoma, and choroid plexus papilloma.

***Lymphoma.*** Primary CNS lymphoma (PCNSL) is a non-Hodgkin lymphoma, which in 98% of cases is a B-cell lymphoma. It once accounted for only 1%–2% of all primary brain tumors, but this percentage has been increasing, mostly because of the growing acquired immunodeficiency syndrome (AIDS) population. The peak age of onset is 60 in the immunocompetent population and age 30 in immunocompromised patients. Lesions may occur anywhere within the neuraxis, including the cerebral hemispheres, brainstem, cerebellum, and spinal cord, although the most common location (90% of cases) is supratentorial. PCNSL lesions are highly infiltrative and exhibit a predilection for sites that contact subarachnoid and ependymal surfaces as well as the deep gray nuclei.

The imaging appearance of PCNSL depends on the patient's immune status. The tumor is hypo- to isointense on T1-weighted and hypo- to slightly hyperintense on T2-weighted images. Contrast enhancement is usually intense. In immunocompetent patients (Zhang et al., 2010) the lesion is often single and tends to abut the ventricular border (Costa et al., 2006), and ring enhancement is uncommon (Fig. 40.22). In immunocompromised patients, usually multiple, often ring-enhancing lesions are seen, which are most commonly located in the PV white matter and the gray/white junction of the lobes of the hemispheres, but the deep central gray matter structures and the posterior fossa may be involved as well. Overall, the imaging appearance appears more malignant in the immunocompromised cases and may be difficult to differentiate from toxoplasmosis. Other components of the differential diagnosis in patients with multiple PCNSL lesions include demyelination, abscesses, neurosarcoidosis, and metastatic disease.

***Hemangioblastoma.*** Hemangioblastomas represent only 1%–2% of all primary brain tumors, but in adults they are the most common type of primary intra-axial tumor of the posterior fossa (cerebellum and medulla). These tumors are WHO grade I, well circumscribed, and exhibit a vascular nodule with a usually larger cystic cavity. On MRI the solid portion is hypo- to isointense on T1 and hyperintense on T2-weighted images. Sometimes hyperintense foci are noted on T1; this is due to occasional lipid deposition or hemorrhage within the tumor. The cystic component is usually hypointense on T1 (but may be hyperintense relative to CSF due to high protein content) and markedly hyperintense on T2. On FLAIR images, the cyst fluid is not completely nulled, resulting in a bright signal, and the nodule is also hyperintense. There is usually mild surrounding edema. With gadolinium, the solid component exhibits intense enhancement. Hemangioblastomas are seen in 50% of patients with von Hippel-Lindau disease, and approximately one-fourth of all hemangioblastomas occur in these patients (Neumann et al., 1989).

## Extra-axial Primary Brain Tumors

Descriptions of schwannomas and the more rare extra-axial primary brain tumor types—esthesioneuroblastoma, central neurocytoma, and subependymoma—are available in the online version of this chapter (http://www.expertconsult.com). 

***Meningiomas.*** Meningiomas are the most common primary brain tumors of nonglial origin and make up 15% of all intracranial tumors. The peak age of onset is the fifth decade, and there is a striking female predominance that may be related to the fact that some meningiomas contain estrogen and progesterone receptors. These tumors arise from meningothelial cells. In 1%–9% of cases, multiple tumors are seen. The most common locations are the falx (25%), convexity (20%), sphenoid wing, petrous ridge (15%–20%), olfactory groove (5%–10%), parasellar region (5%–10%), and the posterior fossa (10%). Rarely, an intraventricular location has been reported. Meningiomas often appear as smooth hemispherical or lobular dural-based masses (Fig. 40.23). Calcification is common, seen in at least 20% of these tumors. Meningiomas also often exhibit vascularity. The extra-axial location of the tumor is usually well appreciated owing to a visible CSF interface between tumor and adjacent brain parenchyma. Meningiomas may become malignant, invading the brain and eroding the skull. In such cases, prominent

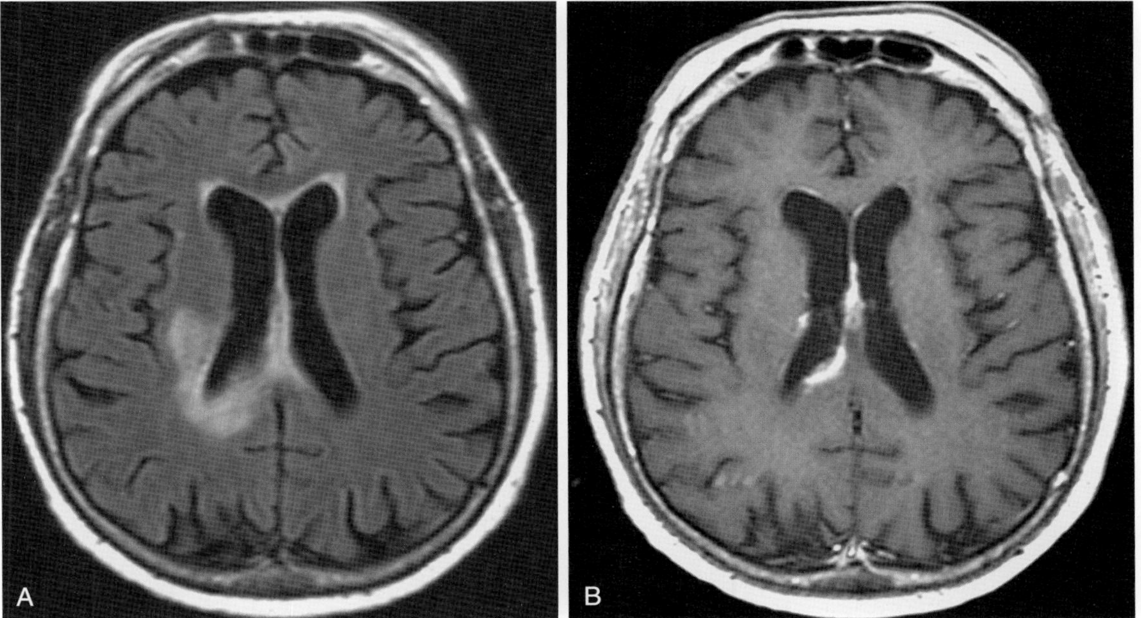


**Fig. 40.22 Central Nervous System Lymphoma in an Immunocompetent Individual. A,** FLAIR sequence depicts a single hyperintense lesion with spread along the ventricular border. **B,** After contrast administration, multiple areas of enhancement are seen within the lesion, without a ringlike enhancement pattern.

edema may be present in the brain parenchyma, to the extent that the extra-axial nature of the tumor is no longer obvious.

On T1-weighted images, meningiomas are usually iso- to slightly hypointense. The appearance on T2 can be iso-, hypo-, or hyperintense to the gray matter. Although MRI does not reveal the histological subtypes of meningiomas with absolute certainty, there have been observations according to which fibroblastic and transitional meningiomas tend to be iso- to hypointense on T2-weighted images, whereas the meningothelial or angioblastic type is iso- or more hyperintense. Not uncommonly, the skull adjacent to a meningioma will exhibit subtle thickening—a useful diagnostic clue in some cases.

After gadolinium administration, meningiomas typically exhibit intense homogeneous enhancement. A quite typical imaging finding on postcontrast images is the *dural tail sign*, which refers to the linear extension of enhancement along the dura, beyond the segment on which the tumor is based. Earlier this had been attributed to en plaque extension of the meningioma along these dural segments and was thought to be specific for this type of tumor. However, recently it has been recognized that this imaging appearance is not specific to this situation and may be seen in other tumors, secondary to increased vascularity/hyperperfusion or congestion of the dural vessels after irradiation and as a postsurgical change.

***Primitive neuroectodermal tumor.*** *Primitive neuroectodermal tumor* (PNET) is a collective term that includes several tumors arising from cells that are derived from the neuroectoderm and are in an undifferentiated state. The main tumors that belong to the PNET group are medulloblastomas, esthesioneuroblastomas, and pinealoblastomas. The tumors belonging to the PNET group are fast growing and highly malignant. The most common mode of metastatic spread for PNETs is via CSF pathways, an indication for imaging surveillance of the entire neuraxis when these tumors are suspected.

***Medulloblastoma.*** Medulloblastomas arise from the undifferentiated neuroectodermal cells of the roof of the fourth ventricle (superior or inferior medullary velum, vermis). They represent 25% of all cerebral tumors in children, usually presenting in the first and second decade. The tumor fills the fourth ventricle, extending rostrally toward the aqueduct and caudally to the cisterna magna, frequently resulting in obstructive hydrocephalus. Leptomeningeal and CSF spread may also occur, resulting in spinal drop metastases. Cystic components and necrosis may be present. Calcification is possible. On CT, medulloblastoma typically appears as a heterogeneous, generally hyperdense midline tumor occupying the fourth ventricle, with mass effect and variable contrast enhancement. The MRI signal (Koeller and Rushing, 2003) is heterogeneous; the tumor is iso- or hypointense on T1 and hypo-, iso-, or hyperintense on T2. Contrast administration induces heterogeneous enhancement (Fig. 40.24). Restricted diffusion may be seen on DWI/ADC (Gauvain et al., 2001). Consistent with its site of origin, indistinct borders between the tumor and the roof of the fourth ventricle may be observed, aiding in the differential diagnosis, which in children includes atypical, rhabdoid-teratoid tumor, brainstem glioma, pilocytic astrocytoma, choroid plexus papilloma, and ependymoma. The adult differential diagnosis includes the latter two entities in addition to metastasis and hemangioblastoma. Medulloblastoma does not tend to extrude via the foramina outside of the fourth ventricle, facilitating differentiation from ependymoma. In children, choroid plexus papilloma is more likely to occur within the lateral ventricle.

***Pineoblastoma.*** Pineoblastomas are highly cellular tumors that are similar in MRI appearance to pineocytomas. However, they tend to be larger (>3 cm), more heterogeneous, frequently cause hydrocephalus, and also may spread via the CSF. This tumor is isointense to gray matter on T1, with moderate heterogeneous enhancement following administration of gadolinium. Like other PNETs, the hypercellularity of pineoblastoma results in T2-weighted signal that tends to be iso- or hypointense relative to gray matter, and restricted diffusion may also be seen. Cysts within the tumor may appear markedly hyperintense on T2, peripheral edema less so. In cases accompanied by hydrocephalus, FLAIR imaging may reveal uniform hyperintensity in a planar distribution along the margins of the lateral ventricles due to transependymal flow of CSF. Peripheral calcifications or intratumoral hemorrhage will exhibit markedly hypointense signal with blooming artifact on T2* (pronounced *T2-star*) images. Differential diagnostic considerations include germ cell tumor, pineocytoma, and (uncommonly) metastases.

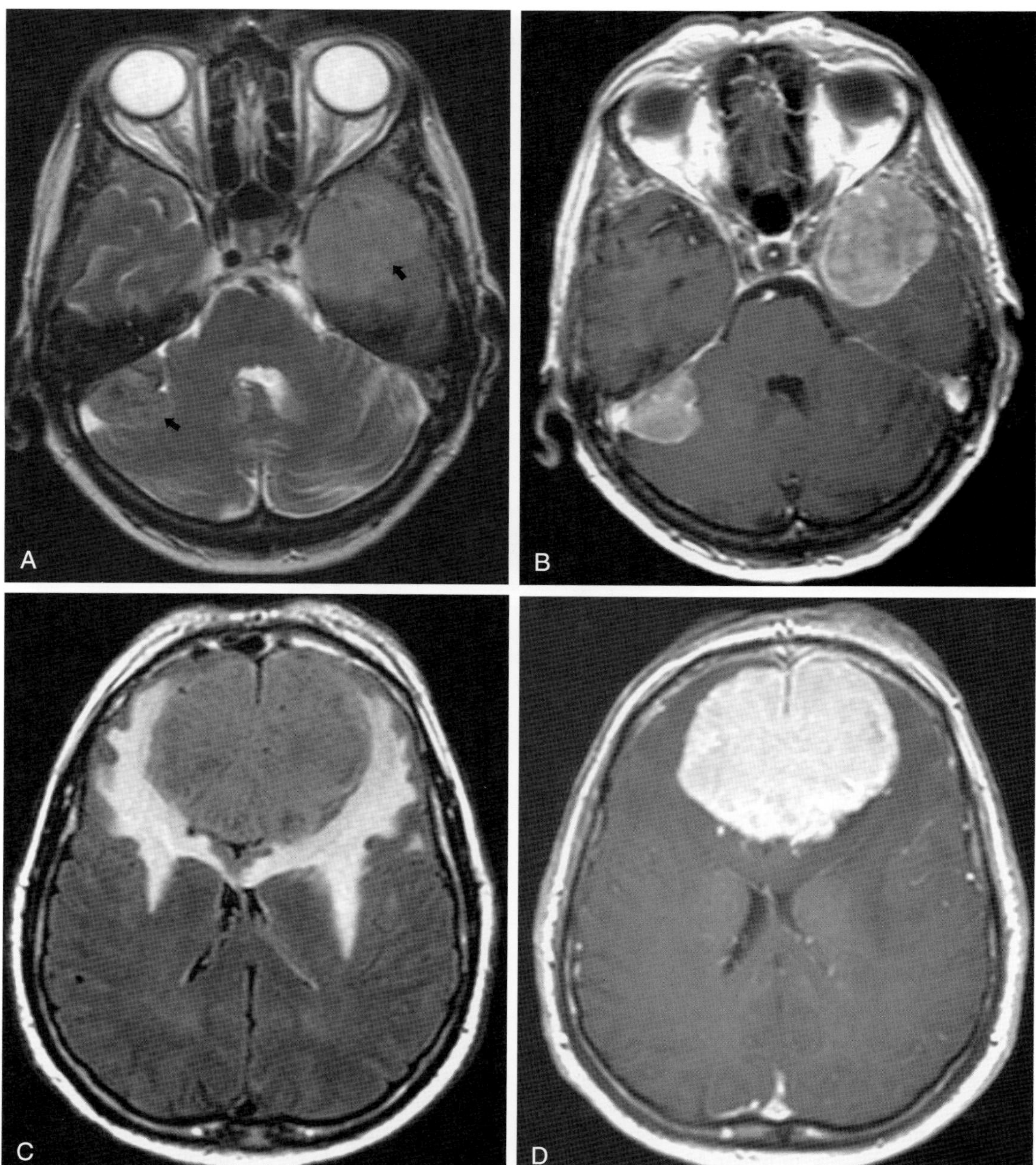

**Fig. 40.23 Two Cases of Meningioma.** In the first (**A, B**) two extra-axial mass lesions are seen, one arising from the tentorium and the other from the sphenoid wing in the left middle cranial fossa *(arrows)*. These compress the right cerebellar hemisphere and the left temporal lobe, respectively. **A,** On T2-weighted image, the masses are mostly isointense with foci of hypointensity. **B,** After gadolinium administration, the masses enhance homogeneously. Note the small dural tail along the tentorium. In the second case (**C, D**) a large olfactory groove meningioma that exerts significant mass effect on the frontal lobes, corpus callosum, and lateral ventricles is presented. **C,** On FLAIR image, hyperintense vasogenic edema is seen in the compressed brain parenchyma. **D,** Tumor enhances homogeneously with gadolinium.

***Other pineal region tumors.*** Besides pineoblastomas, which histologically belong to the group of PNETs, the pineal gland may also develop tumors of pinealocyte origin (pineocytoma) and germ cell tumors.

**Pineocytoma.** Pineocytomas are homogeneous masses containing more solid components, but cysts may also be present. These tumors have a round, well-defined, noninvasive appearance. Calcification is commonly seen, but hemorrhage is uncommon. These tumors may be hypointense on T2 and exhibit a variable (central, nodular) pattern of intense enhancement after gadolinium administration (Fakhran and Escott, 2008).

**Germ cell tumors (germinoma).** Masses in the pineal region are most often germ cell tumors, usually germinomas. Less common types include teratoma, choriocarcinoma, and embryonal carcinoma. Germinomas are well-circumscribed round or lobulated lesions. Hemorrhage and calcification are rare. Metastases may spread via CSF, so the entire neuraxis should be imaged if these tumors are suspected.

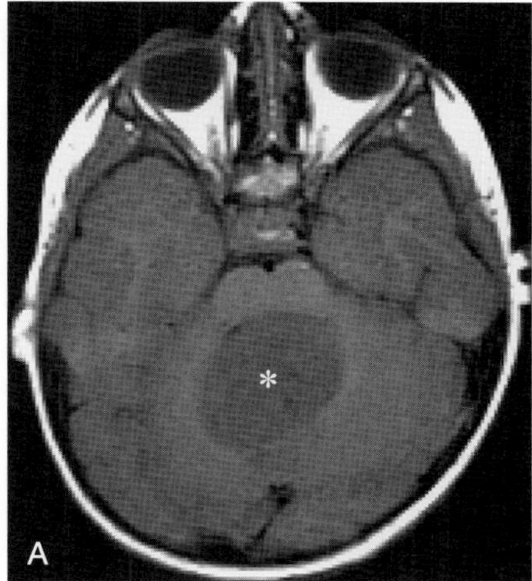

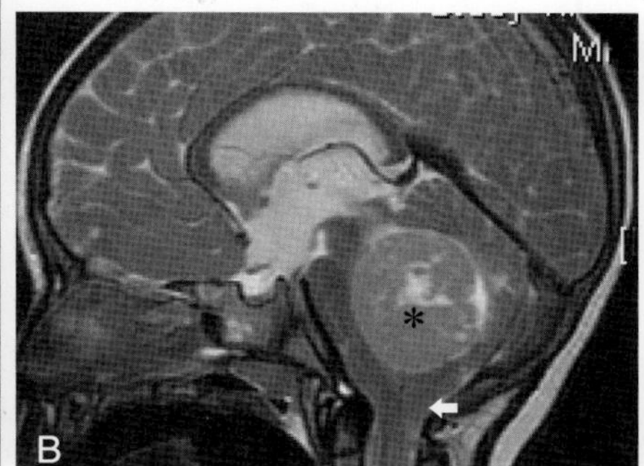

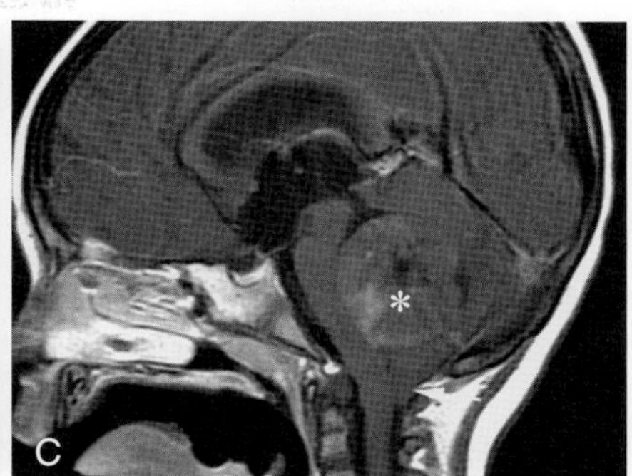


**Fig. 40.24 Medulloblastoma.** A large mass lesion is seen *(asterisk)* filling and expanding the fourth ventricle. **A,** On T1-weighted image, tumor is partially iso- but mostly hypointense. **B,** On T2-weighted image, tumor shows iso- and hyperintense signal change; it compresses/displaces the brainstem and cerebellum. On sagittal images, note the secondary Chiari malformation (caudal displacement of cerebellar tonsils) due to mass effect *(arrow)*. **C,** On T1 postcontrast image, there is a heterogeneous enhancement pattern.

MRI signal characteristics are variable, with iso- to hyperintense signal relative to gray matter on both T1 and T2. With gadolinium, intense contrast enhancement is seen.

**Subependymal giant cell astrocytoma.** Subependymal giant cell astrocytoma (SEGA), a WHO grade I tumor, arises from astrocytes in the subependymal zone of the lateral ventricles and develops into an intraventricular tumor in the region of the foramen of Monro. It is seen almost exclusively in patients with tuberous sclerosis. Just like central neurocytoma, this tumor is also prone to cause obstructive hydrocephalus. The tumor is heterogeneously hypo- to isointense on T1 and heterogeneously hyperintense on T2-weighted images, with possible foci of hypointensity due to calcification. On FLAIR, an isointense to hyperintense solid tumor background may be punctuated by hypointense cysts. FLAIR is also useful to assess for the possible presence of hyperintense cortical tubers, which if present aid in the differential diagnosis. With gadolinium, intense enhancement is seen.

**Choroid plexus papilloma.** Choroid plexus papilloma is a well-circumscribed, highly vascular, intraventricular WHO grade I tumor derived from choroid plexus epithelium. In children it is usually seen in the lateral ventricle, while in adults it tends to involve the fourth ventricle. General imaging characteristics include a villiform or bosselated "cauliflower-like" appearance. Hemorrhage and calcification are noted occasionally in the tumor bed. The tumor's location frequently causes obstructive hydrocephalus. On MRI, the appearance is hypo- or isointense to normal brain on T1 and iso- to hyperintense on T2-weighted images. The latter may also show punctate or linear/serpiginous signal flow voids within the tumor. Calcification (25%) or hemorrhage manifests as a markedly hypointense blooming artifact on T2* gradient echo images. With gadolinium, intense enhancement is seen. Choroid plexus carcinomas are malignant tumors that may invade the brain parenchyma and may also spread via CSF.

## Tumors in the Sellar and Parasellar Region

The sellar and parasellar group of extra-axial masses include pituitary micro- and macroadenomas and craniopharyngiomas. Meningiomas, arachnoid cysts, dermoid and epidermoid cysts, optic pathway gliomas, hamartomas, metastases, and aneurysms are also encountered in the para- and suprasellar region.

***Pituitary adenomas.*** The distinction between micro- and macroadenomas is based on their size: tumors less than 10 mm are microadenomas; the larger tumors are macroadenomas. These tumors may arise from hormone-producing cells, such as prolactinomas or growth hormone–producing adenomas, resulting in characteristic clinical syndromes. Pituitary adenomas are typically hypointense on T1-weighted and hyperintense on T2-weighted images, relative to the surrounding parenchyma. This signal change, however, is not always conspicuous, especially in the case of small microadenomas. Gadolinium administration helps in these cases, when the microadenoma is visualized as relative hypointensity against the background of the normally enhancing gland (Fig. 40.26). Following a delay, this difference in enhancement is often no longer apparent, and if the postcontrast images are obtained in a later phase, a reversal of contrast may be noted. The adenoma takes up contrast in a delayed fashion and is seen as hyperintense against the more hypointense gland from where the contrast has washed out. Sometimes when the signal characteristics are not conspicuous, only alteration of the size and shape of the pituitary gland or shifting of the infundibulum may indicate the presence of a microadenoma. Because of this, it is important to be familiar with the normal range of pituitary gland sizes, which depend on age and gender. In adults, a gland height of more than 9 mm is worrisome. In the younger population, however, different normal values have been established. Before puberty, the normal height is 3–5 mm. At puberty in girls, the gland height may be 10–11 mm and may exhibit an upward convex morphology. In boys at puberty, the height is 6–8 mm, and the upward convex morphology can be normal. The size and shape of the gland may also change during pregnancy: convex morphology may appear, and a gland height of 10 mm is considered normal.

While microadenomas are localized to the sellar region, macroadenomas may become invasive and extend to the suprasellar region and may displace/compress the optic chiasm or even the hypothalamus. Extension to the cavernous sinus is also possible (see eFig. 40.27).

***Craniopharyngioma.*** Craniopharyngiomas are believed to originate from the epithelial remnants of the Rathke pouch. This WHO grade I tumor may be encountered in children, and a second peak incidence is in the fifth decade (Eldevik et al., 1996). The most common location is the suprasellar cistern (Fig. 40.28), but intrasellar

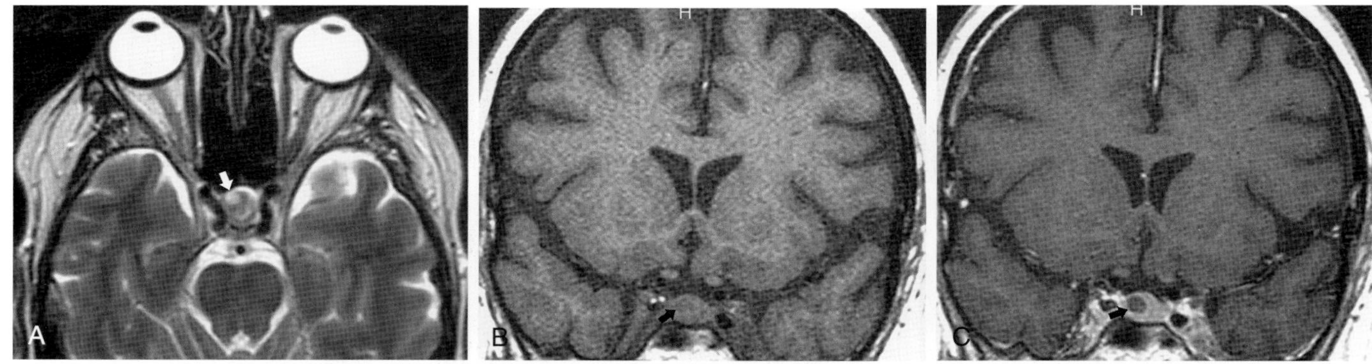


**Fig. 40.26 Pituitary Microadenoma. A,** Axial T2-weighted image demonstrates a round area of hyperintensity on right side of pituitary gland *(arrow)*. **B,** On coronal noncontrast T1-weighted image, the gland has an upward convex morphology, and there is a vague hypointensity in its right side *(arrow)*. **C,** On coronal T1-weighted postcontrast image, the microadenoma is well seen as an area of hypointensity *(arrow)* against the background of the normally enhancing gland parenchyma.

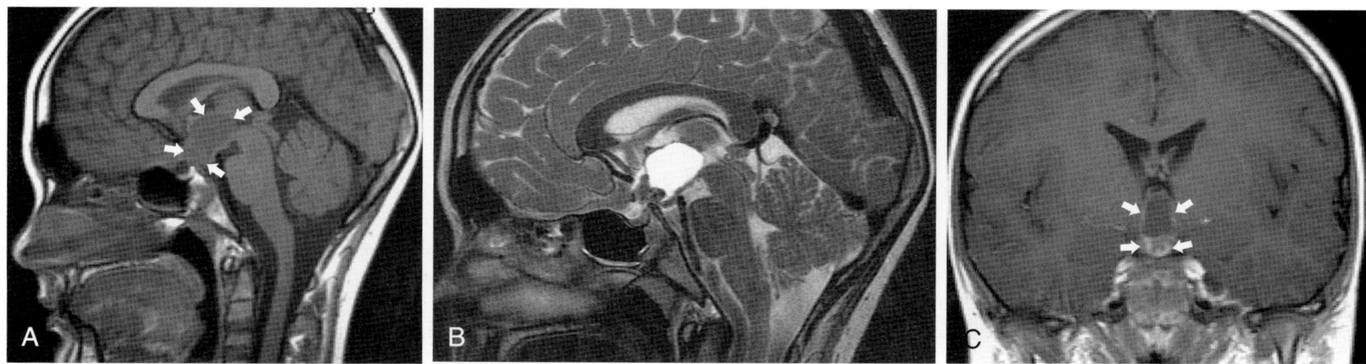


**Fig. 40.28 Craniopharyngioma. A,** On sagittal T1-weighted image, a suprasellar mass lesion has a prominent T1 hypointense cystic component *(arrows)*. **B,** On sagittal T2-weighted image, the cyst is hyperintense. **C,** With gadolinium, both the rim of the cyst and the solid portion of the mass exhibit enhancement *(arrows)*.

tumors are also possible. The tumor may cause expansion of the sella or erosion of the dorsum sellae. In the suprasellar region, displacement of the chiasm, the anterior cerebral arteries, or even the hypothalamus is possible. Craniopharyngiomas have both solid and cystic components. Histologically, the more common adamantinomatous and the less common papillary forms are distinguished. The adamantinomatous type frequently exhibits calcification. The MRI signal is heterogeneous. Solid portions are iso- or hypointense on T1, whereas cystic components exhibit variable signal characteristics depending on the amount of protein or the presence of blood products. On T2, the solid and cystic components are sometimes hard to distinguish, as they are both usually hyperintense. Areas of calcification may appear hypointense on T2. In contrast, the solid portions of the tumor exhibit intense enhancement.

## Metastatic Tumors

Intracranial metastases are detected in approximately 25% of patients who die of cancer. Cerebral metastases comprise over half of brain tumors (Vogelbaum and Suh, 2006) and are the most common type of brain tumor in adults (Klos and O'Neill, 2004). Most (80%) metastases involve the cerebral hemispheres, and 20% are seen in the posterior fossa. Pelvic and colon cancer have a tendency to involve the posterior fossa. Intracranial metastases, depending on the type of tumor, may involve the skull and the dura, the brain, and also the meninges in the form of meningeal carcinomatosis. Among all tumors that metastasize to the bone, breast and prostate cancer and multiple myeloma are especially prone to spread to the skull and dura. Most often, carcinomas involve the brain and get there by hematogenous spread. Systemic tumors with the greatest tendency to metastasize to brain are lung (as many as 30% of lung cancers give rise to brain metastases), breast (Fig. 40.29), and melanoma (Fig. 40.30). Cancers of the gastrointestinal tract (especially colon and rectum) and the kidney are the next most common sources. Other possibilities include gallbladder, liver, thyroid gland, pancreas, ovary, and testicles. Tumors of the prostate, esophagus, and skin (other than melanoma) hardly ever form brain parenchymal metastases.

It is important to highlight the potential imaging differences between primary and metastatic brain tumors, since a significant percentage of patients found to have brain metastasis have no prior diagnosis of cancer. Cerebral parenchymal metastases can be single (usually with kidney, breast, thyroid, and lung adenocarcinoma) or (more commonly) multiple (in small cell carcinomas and melanoma) and tend to involve the gray/white matter junction. Seeing multiple tumors at the corticomedullary junction favors the diagnosis of metastatic lesions over a primary brain tumor. The size of metastatic lesions is variable, and the mass effect and peritumoral edema is usually prominent and, contrary to that seen with primary brain tumors, frequently out of proportion to the size of the tumor itself. The edema is vasogenic, persistent, and involves the white matter, highlighting the intact cortical sulci as characteristic fingerlike projections. It is hypointense on T1 and hyperintense on T2 and FLAIR. The tumor itself exhibits variable, often heterogeneous signal intensity, especially if the metastasis is hemorrhagic (15% of brain metastases). Tumors that tend to cause hemorrhagic metastases include melanoma; choriocarcinoma; and lung, thyroid, and kidney cancer. The tumor signal characteristic can be unique in mucin-producing colon adenocarcinoma metastases, where the mucin and protein content cause a hyperintense signal on T1-weighted images.

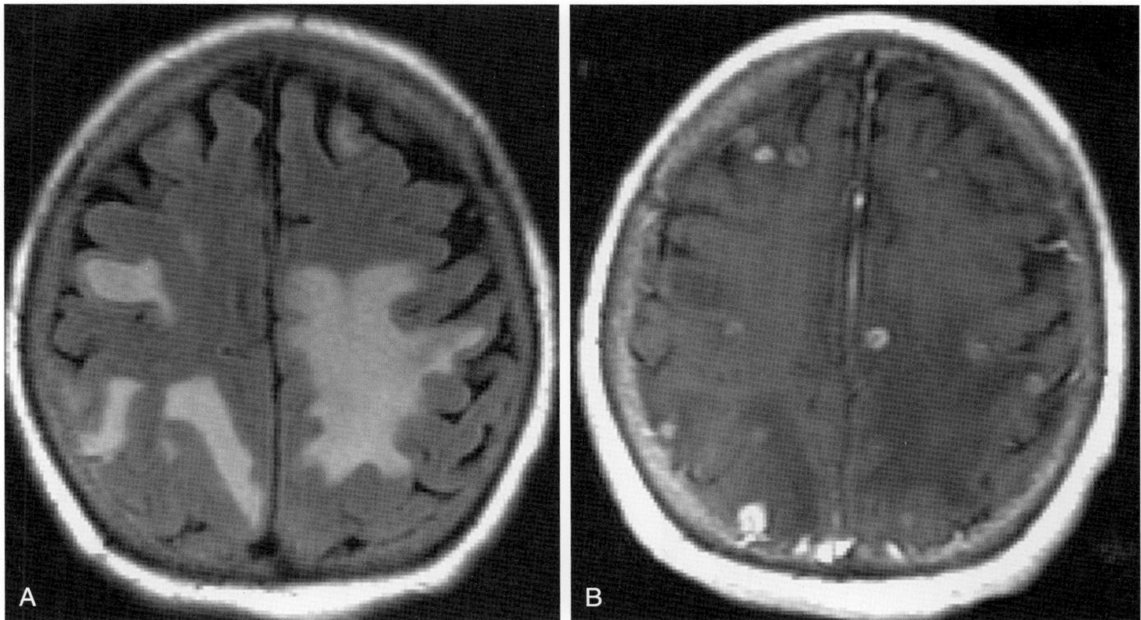


**Fig. 40.29 Brain Metastases from Breast Cancer. A,** On axial FLAIR image, multiple areas of vasogenic edema extend into subcortical white matter with fingerlike projections. **B,** On axial T1-weighted postcontrast image, numerous small enhancing mass lesions are scattered in both hemispheres at the gray/white junction. Both homogeneous and ringlike enhancement patterns are present.

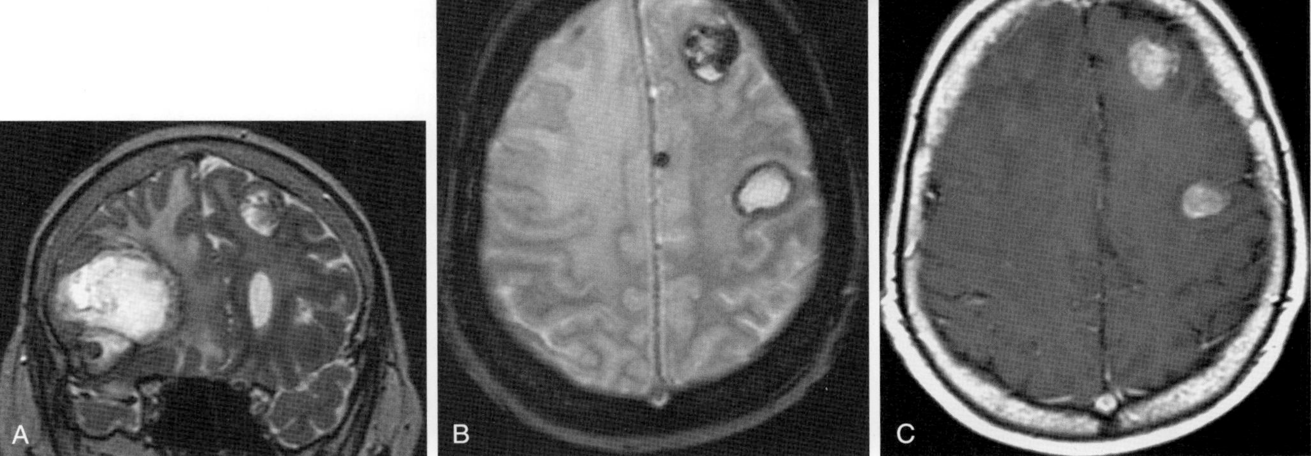


**Fig. 40.30 Hemorrhagic Melanoma Metastases. A,** Coronal T2-weighted image demonstrates a large hyperintense mass in the right frontal lobe, with associated hyperintense vasogenic edema and mass effect. A smaller mass lesion with similar signal characteristics is present at the gray/white junction in the left frontal lobe. Note surrounding rim of hypointensity, indicating hemosiderin deposition within these hemorrhagic metastases. **B,** On gradient echo, hypointense blood degradation products are well seen within the metastases. **C,** Following gadolinium administration, intense enhancement is noted.

Detection of intracerebral metastases is facilitated by administration of gadolinium, and every patient with neurological symptoms and a history of cancer needs to have a gadolinium-enhanced MRI study. The enhancement pattern of metastatic tumors can be solid or ringlike. To improve the diagnostic yield, triple-dose gadolinium or magnetization transfer techniques have been used, which improve detection of smaller metastases that are not so conspicuous with single-dose contrast administration. A triple dose of gadolinium improves metastasis detection by as much as 43% (van Dijk et al., 1997). Meningeal carcinomatosis can also be detected by contrast administration, which can reveal thickening of the meninges and/or meningeal deposits of the metastatic tumor.

For demonstration of the role of advanced structural neuroimaging in brain tumor surgery planning, see the online version of this chapter, available at http://www.expertconsult.com. 

## Ischemic Stroke

***Acute ischemic stroke.*** With the introduction of intravenous tissue plasminogen activator (IV tPA) and, later, mechanical thrombectomy in the treatment of acute ischemic stroke, timely diagnosis of an ischemic lesion, determining its location and extent, and demonstrating the amount of tissue at risk has become essential (see Chapters 65 and 68). CT imaging remains of great value in the evaluation of acute stroke; it is readily available, and newer CT modalities including CTA and CT perfusion imaging are coming into greater use. The applicability of CT to acute stroke continues to be enhanced by the ever-increasing rapidity with which scans can be acquired, allowing for greater coverage of tissues with thinner slices. The technological advances allowing for rapid acquisition of data have led to 4D imaging, where complete 3D data sets of the brain are serially obtained over very short time intervals, allowing for higher temporal and spatial resolutions in brain perfusion studies of acute ischemic stroke patients.

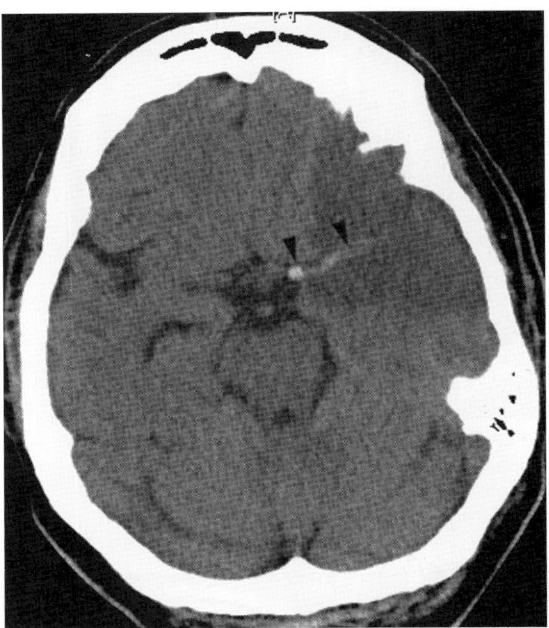

**Fig. 40.32 Evolving Ischemic Stroke in the Territory of the Left Middle Cerebral Artery.** On this noncontrast CT scan, a hyperdense signal is seen in the distal left internal carotid artery and in the M1 segment of the left middle cerebral artery, indicating the presence of a blood clot *(arrowheads)*. There is hypodensity in the corresponding area of the left hemisphere, demonstrating the evolving ischemic infarct.

CT is very useful in detecting hyperdense hemorrhagic lesions as the cause of stroke. Early ischemic stroke, however, may not cause any change on unenhanced CT, making it difficult to determine the extent of the ischemic lesion and the amount of tissue at risk. CT is especially limited in evaluating ischemia in the posterior fossa, owing to streak artifacts at the skull base. Despite these limitations, early signs of acute ischemia on unenhanced CT may be helpful in the first few hours after stroke. CT signs of acute ischemia include blurring of the gray/white junction and effacement of the sulci due to ischemic swelling of the tissues. Blurring of the contours of the deep gray matter structures is of similar significance. In cases of internal carotid artery occlusion, middle cerebral artery main segment (M1) occlusion, or more distal occlusions, intraluminal clot may be seen as a focal hyperdensity, sometimes referred to as a *hyperdense* middle cerebral artery (MCA), or *hyperdense dot sign* (Fig. 40.32).

Several MRI modalities, as well as CT perfusion studies, are capable of providing data regarding cerebral ischemia and perfusion to assist in the evaluation for possible thrombolytic therapy very early after symptom onset. DWI with ADC mapping is considered to be the most sensitive method for imaging acute ischemia (Figs. 40.33–40.36). In humans, the hyperintense signal indicating restriction of diffusion is detected within minutes after onset (Hossmann and Hoehn-Berlage, 1995).

***Temporal evolution of ischemic stroke on magnetic resonance imaging***

**Acute stroke.** Initially, the hyperintense signal on DWI is caused by decreased water diffusivity due to swelling of the ischemic nerve cells (for the first 5–7 days); then it increasingly results from the abnormal T2 properties of the infarcted tissue (T2 shine-through). For this reason, a reliable estimation of the age of the ischemic lesion is not possible by looking at DWI images alone. Imaging protocols for acute ischemic

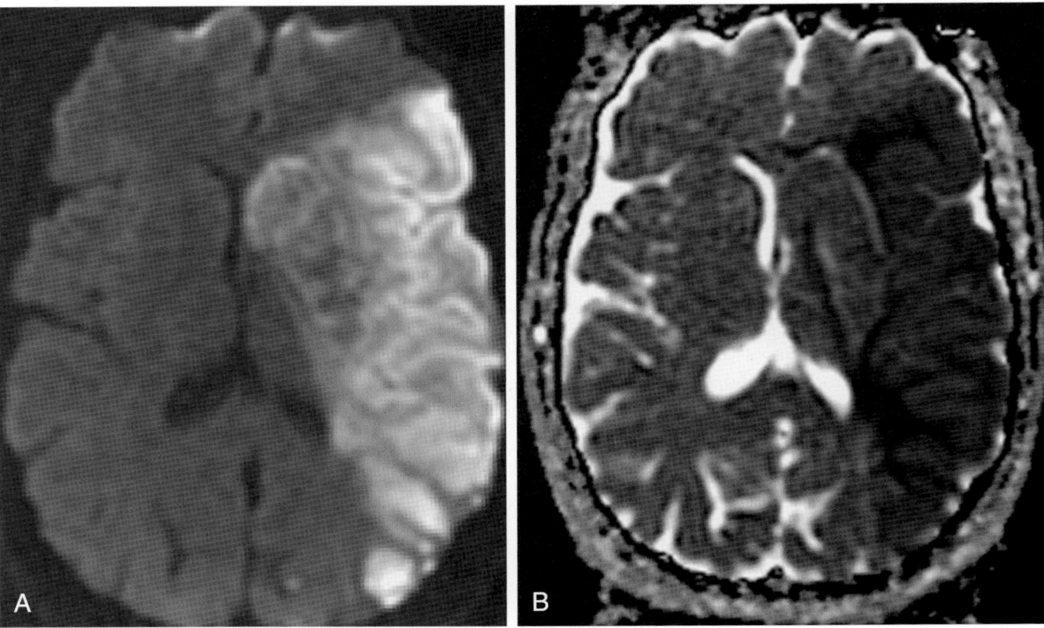


**Fig. 40.33 Acute Ischemic Stroke in the Territory of the Middle Cerebral Artery. A,** On diffusion-weighted imaging, a hyperintense area of restricted diffusion is seen in the territory of the left middle cerebral artery. Note evolving mass effect on the sulci and left lateral ventricle and the mild midline shift. **B,** On apparent diffusion coefficient map, corresponding hypointensity is seen in the same area.

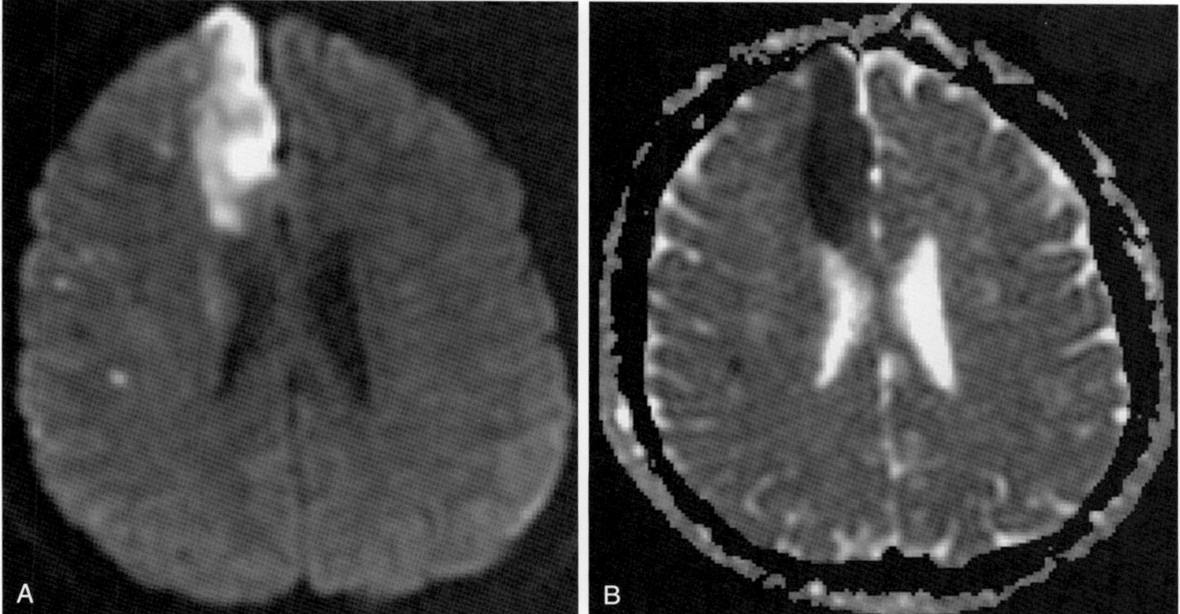


**Fig. 40.34 Acute Ischemic Stroke in the Territory of the Anterior Cerebral Artery. A,** On diffusion-weighted imaging, a hyperintense area of restricted diffusion is seen in the right medial frontal lobe, involving the territory of the anterior cerebral artery. **B,** On apparent diffusion coefficient map, corresponding hypointensity is seen in the same area.

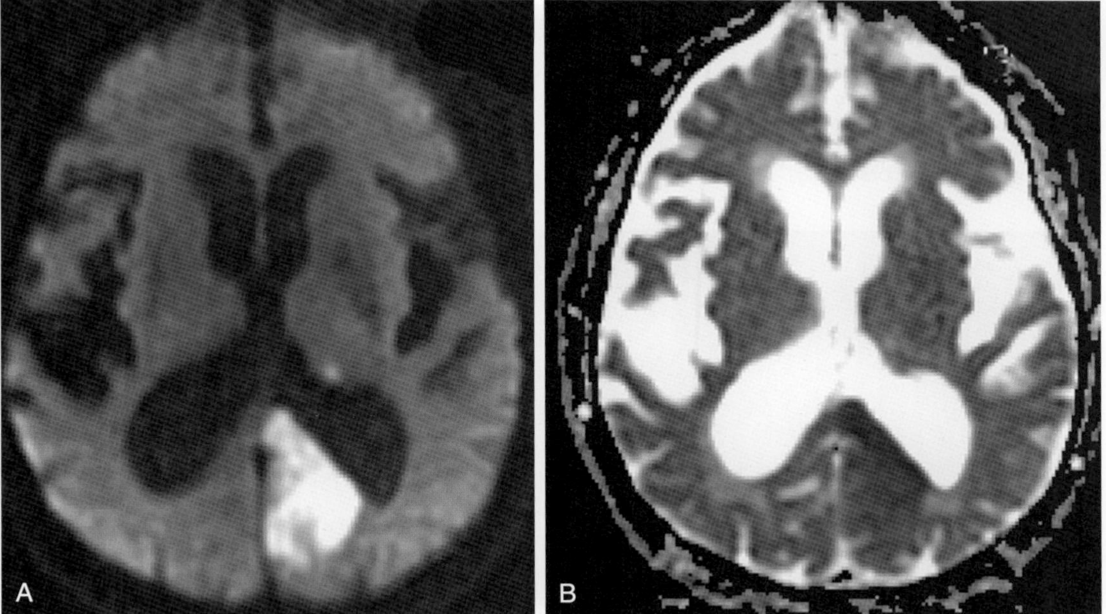


**Fig. 40.35 Acute Ischemic Stroke in the Territory of the Posterior Cerebral Artery. A,** On diffusion-weighted imaging, a hyperintense area of restricted diffusion is seen in the left medial occipital lobe, involving the territory of the posterior cerebral artery. **B,** On apparent diffusion coefficient map, corresponding hypointensity is seen in the same area.

stroke usually include T1- and T2-weighted fast spin echo images, FLAIR sequences, and DWI with ADC maps. These sequences together confirm the diagnosis of ischemia, determine its extent, and allow for an approximate estimation of the time of onset (Srinivasan et al., 2006). On ADC maps, the values decrease initially after the onset of ischemia (i.e., the signal from the affected area becomes progressively more hypointense). This reaches a nadir at 3–5 days but remains significantly low until the seventh day after onset. After this time, the values increase (the signal gets more and more hyperintense) and return to the baseline values in 1–4 weeks (usually in 7–10 days). Therefore, ADC maps are quite useful for the estimation of the age of the lesion: If the signal of the area is hypointense on an ADC map, the lesion is likely less than 7–10 days old. If the area is isointense or hyperintense on the ADC map, the onset was likely more than 7–10 days ago. As already noted, although these signal changes take place on ADC maps, the DWI images remain hyperintense, without noticeable changes of intensity by visual inspection.

On T2-weighted (including FLAIR) images, the signal intensity of the ischemic area is normal in the initial hyperacute stage, increases markedly over the first 4 days, then becomes stable. In a research setting, computing the numerical values of hyperintensity in infarcted tissue on serial T2-weighted scans can demonstrate a consistent sharp signal increase after 36 hours, distinguishing lesions younger or older than 36 hours. This is certainly not possible by visual inspection used in clinical practice.

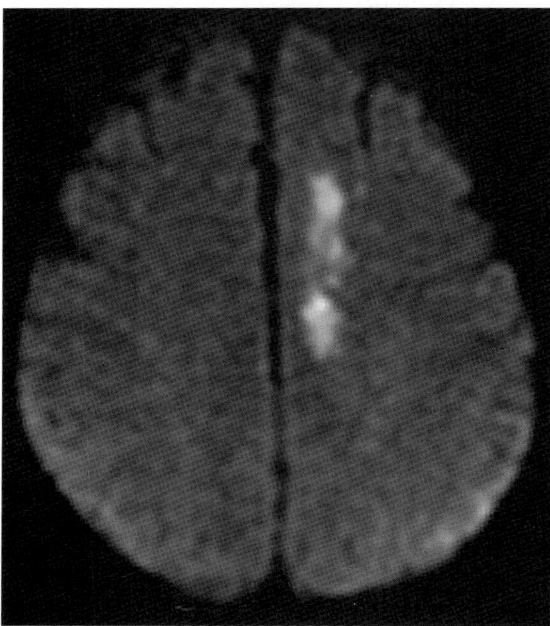

**Fig. 40.36 Acute Ischemic Stroke in the Left Anterior Watershed Area.** On diffusion-weighted imaging, a hyperintense area of restricted diffusion is seen in the left frontal lobe, involving the watershed zone between the anterior and middle cerebral artery.

One purpose of MRI in the evaluation of acute stroke is to determine the extent of irreversible tissue damage and to identify tissue that is at risk but potentially salvageable. The combination of DWI and PWI is frequently used for this purpose (Fig. 40.37). Evaluation is based on the premise that diffusion-weighted images delineate the tissue that suffered permanent damage (although in some cases, restricted diffusion is reversible, corresponding to ischemia without infarction), whereas areas without signal change on DWI but abnormal signal on perfusion-weighted images represent tissue at risk, the so-called ischemic penumbra. If there is a mismatch between the extent of DWI changes and perfusion deficits, the latter being larger, reperfusion treatment with mechanical thrombectomy is justified to salvage the brain tissue at risk up to 24 hours of last known normal (Powers et al., 2018). If the extent of diffusion and perfusion abnormalities is similar or the same, the tissue is thought to be irreversibly injured, with no penumbra, and therefore the potential benefit from reperfusion treatment may not be high enough to justify the risk of hemorrhage associated with thrombolytic treatment.

**Subacute ischemic stroke (1 day to 1 week after onset).** In this stage, there is an ongoing increase of cytotoxic edema due to swelling of the ischemic neurons. Parallel with this, the involved tissue becomes more and more hypointense on T1 and also gradually more hyperintense on T2 and FLAIR sequences. Cytotoxic edema is usually maximal 2–3 days after onset, but in the case of malignant middle cerebral artery strokes, it may keep increasing until day 5. Arterial wall enhancement is seen during this stage, whereas parenchymal enhancement usually begins at the end of the first week.

Reperfusion usually occurs at this stage and may be associated with petechial hemorrhages or even frank hemorrhage within the infarcted tissue. Petechial hemorrhages are very common; microbleeds (not always visible with CT or MRI) occur in as much as 65% of ischemic stroke patients (Werring, 2007). Frank hemorrhagic transformation, however, is much less common.

**Late subacute ischemic stroke (1–3 weeks after onset).** In this stage, gradual resolution of the edema is seen. As the infarcted

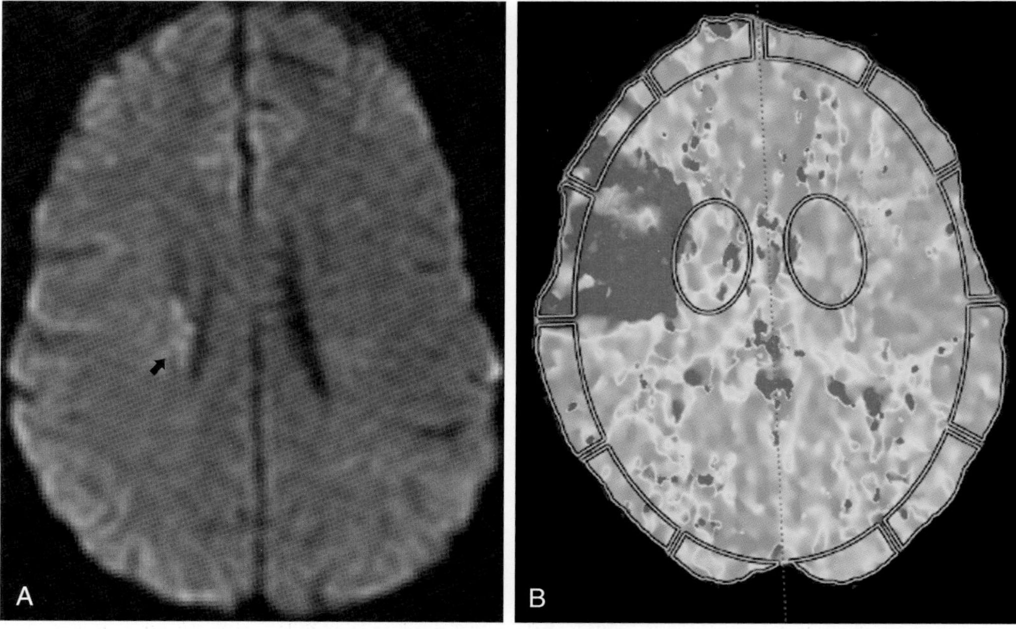


**Fig. 40.37 Ischemic Penumbra in Acute Right Middle Cerebral Artery Stroke. A,** Diffusion-weighted image reveals a small, circumscribed area of restricted diffusion in the paraventricular region of the right centrum semiovale *(arrow)*. **B,** Magnetic resonance perfusion-weighted image demonstrates a much larger perfusion deficit, as revealed by increased mean transit time, indicated in red. The perfusion deficit *(red)* outside the small area of restricted diffusion (*arrow,* **A**) represents the ischemic penumbra.

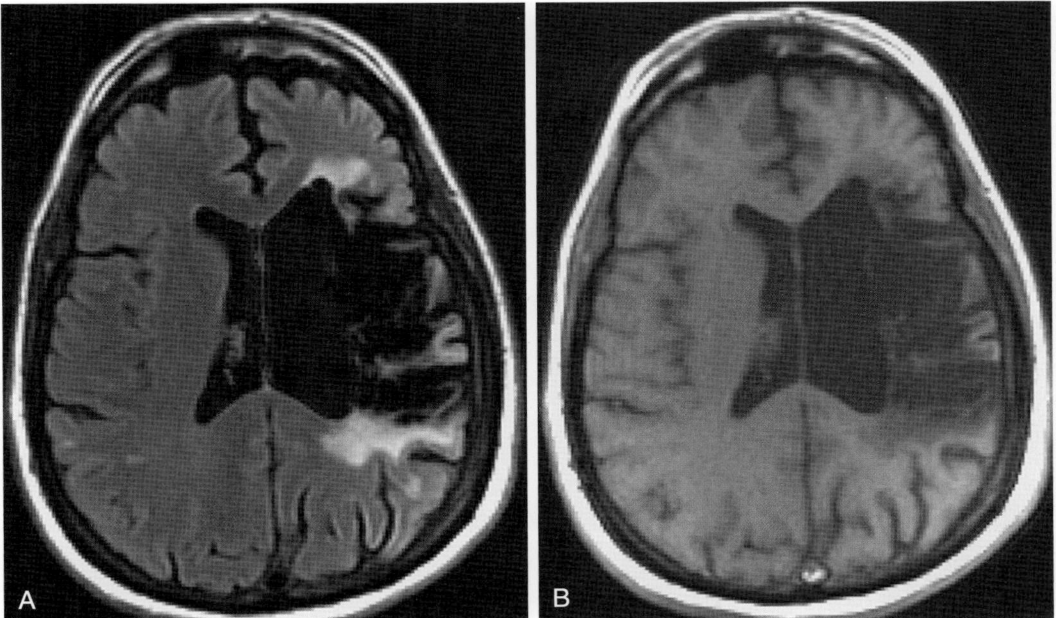


**Fig. 40.38 Chronic Ischemic Stroke. A,** On FLAIR image, a large area of encephalomalacia is seen in the territory of the left middle cerebral artery. Hypointense cerebrospinal fluid (CSF)-like cavity is surrounded by hyperintense signal change in adjacent parenchyma, indicating gliosis. Note ex vacuo enlargement of adjacent segment of left lateral ventricle. **B,** On noncontrast T1-weighted image, the cavity of encephalomalacia appears as CSF-like hypointensity. Areas of gliosis appear as faint zones of hypointensity.

tissue is disintegrating and resorbed, the T1 hypointensity and T2 hyperintensity of the lesion become more marked. Gray matter enhancement (which in the case of infarcted cortex has a gyriform pattern) is intense throughout this stage.

**Chronic ischemic stroke (3 weeks and older).** Areas of complete tissue destruction with death not only of neurons but of glia and necrosis of other supporting tissues as well, will eventually appear as cavitary lesions filled with fluid that have signal characteristics identical to CSF: hyperintensity on T2-weighted images and marked hypointensity on T1 images and FLAIR sequences. The region of encephalomalacia is bordered by a glial scar (reactive gliosis) that is hyperintense on T2 and FLAIR images (Fig. 40.38). Although the initial signal changes on DWI frequently predict the final extent of tissue destruction, changes on DWI can also disappear, and the final size of tissue cavitation can be best determined on T1-weighted images, which should be part of every stroke follow-up imaging protocol. Tissue in the margins of the cavitary lesion, and often in other areas of the brain as well, may have undergone extensive neuronal loss resulting only in atrophy but not in signal intensity changes, even on T2-weighted images (partial infarction).

Besides signal changes, chronic ischemic infarcts lead to secondary changes in the brain. Owing to the loss of tissue, ex vacuo enlargement of the adjacent CSF spaces (sulci and adjacent ventricular segments) occurs. Pathways that originate from or pass through the infarcted area undergo wallerian degeneration, which is seen as T2 hyperintense signal change along the course of these pathways (Fig. 40.39). Later, the hyperintensity may resolve, but the loss of pathways may result in volume loss of the structures they pass through (e.g., cerebral peduncle, pons, medullary pyramid), noted as decreased cross-sectional area.

## Stroke Etiology

Structural imaging provides data on the morphology and location of ischemic cerebral lesions, which can be very helpful to determine stroke etiology: lacunar, atherothrombotic, embolic, hypoperfusion-related, or venous. Diagnostic evaluation and treatment of a patient with stroke, as well as secondary stroke prevention, is often dependent upon structural imaging.

A discussion of the neuroimaging aspects of the various stroke etiologies is available at http://www.expertconsult.com. 

## Other Cerebrovascular Occlusive Disease

***Arteriolosclerosis (white matter hyperintensity of presumed vascular origin).*** Diffuse or patchy T2 hyperintense signal changes in the deep hemispheric and subcortical white matter are probably the most common abnormal findings on MRI in the adult and elderly patient population. The terms *microvascular ischemic changes, chronic small vessel disease, or leukoaraiosis* are alternatively used to describe these lesions on imaging studies. Their etiology and clinical significance have been debated extensively.

Certain hyperintense signal changes are considered normal incidental findings, with no clinical relevance. A uniformly thin, linear, T2 hyperintensity that has a smooth outer border along the border of the body of the lateral ventricles is often seen in the elderly population and likely represents fluid or gliotic changes in the subependymal zone. It tends to be more pronounced at the tips of the frontal horns *(ependymitis granularis).* This finding is thought potentially to be due to focal loss of the ependymal lining with gliosis and/or influx of interstitial fluid into these regions.

Patchy signal changes within the white matter of the cerebral hemispheres beyond a relatively low threshold (generally, one white matter hyperintensity per decade of life is felt to fall within the normal range) are pathological and are most commonly of ischemic origin. According to the most accepted hypothesis, these hyperintensities are the result of gradual narrowing or occlusion of the small vessels of the white matter, the diameters of which are less than 200 μm (hence the terms *microvascular lesions* or *small vessel disease*). Pathologically, these

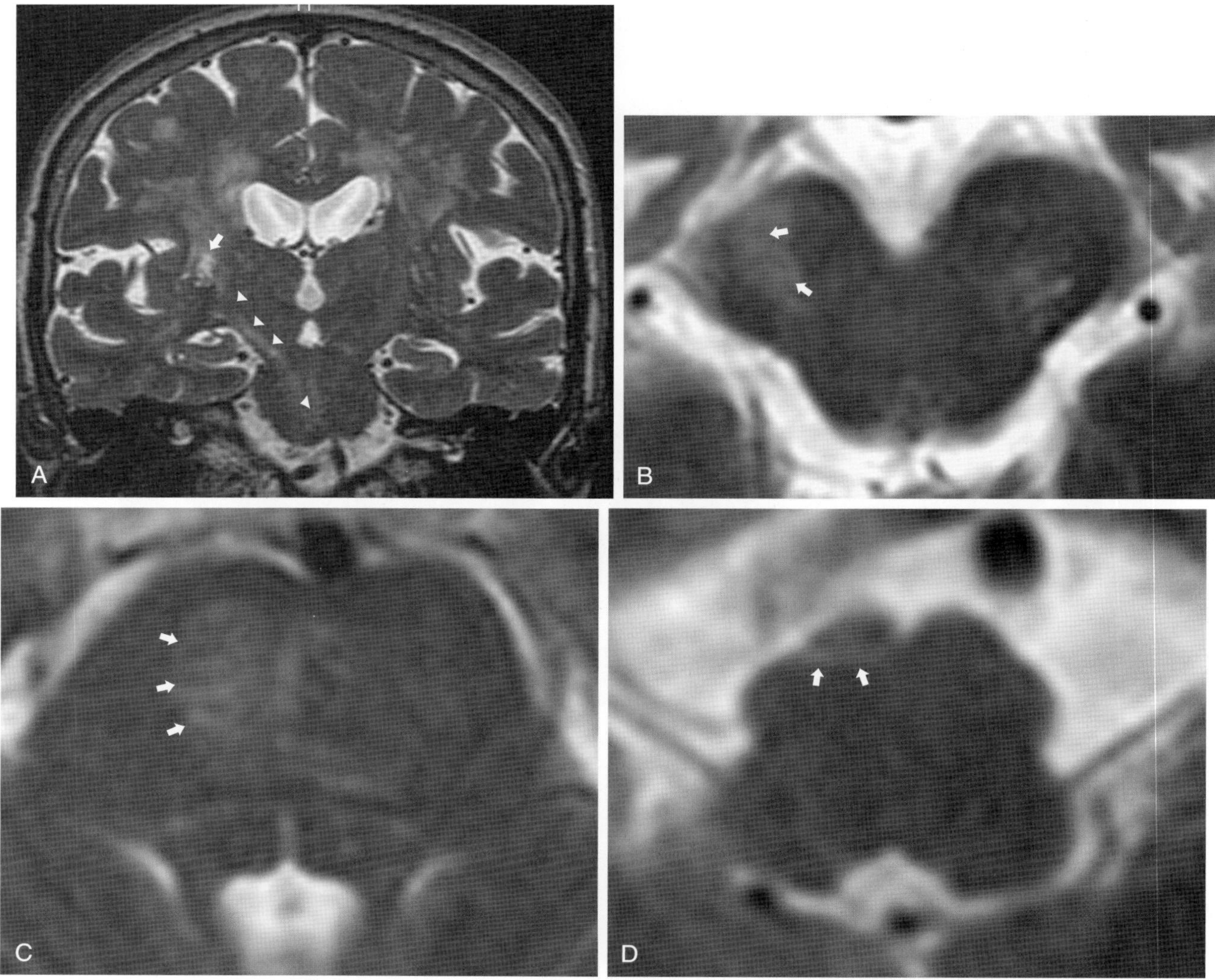

**Fig. 40.39 Wallerian Degeneration.** **A,** Coronal T2-weighted image demonstrates a chronic lacunar ischemic lesion in the right internal capsule *(arrow)*. From here, a linear hyperintense signal change is seen extending caudally along the course of the degenerating corticospinal tract fibers, through the right cerebral peduncle into the pons *(arrowheads)*. **B–D,** Serial T2-weighted axial images of the brainstem demonstrate the hyperintense signal of the degenerating fibers *(arrows)* in the right cerebral peduncle (**B**), right pontine tegmentum (**C**), and in the right medullary pyramid (**D**).

lesions are composed of focal demyelination and gliosis. The lumen of the involved vessels is narrow or occluded; their walls may exhibit arteriosclerotic changes and commonly amyloid deposits. On imaging studies, they have a chronic appearance, with diffuse borders and no surrounding edema or evidence of mass effect. They are generally associated with some degree of central atrophy, which tends to worsen with higher lesion loads. The distribution of these lesions changes only very gradually on serial scans, often showing minimal to no significant difference on studies spaced several years apart.

While age by itself can cause such changes, and the incidence of these lesions increases with age in people 40 years or older, there are several other risk factors that can make them more numerous. These include hypertension, diabetes, hypercholesterolemia, and smoking. Indeed, patients with these medical problems are more likely to have an elevated number of ischemic white matter lesions.

Chronic ischemic white matter lesions are hypodense on CT, but MRI is much more sensitive and reveals more extensive lesions (Fig. 40.41, *A*). On MRI, the lesions are hyperintense on T2 and FLAIR sequences. They may or may not be visible as T1 hypointensities. It is possible that only lesions visible on T1-weighted images may be clinically significant. Common locations are the PV and, more commonly, the deep white matter, but subcortical lesions are also common, with sparing of the U-fibers. The lesions can be isolated, scattered, or more confluent, especially in the PV zone. Morphologically, individual lesions generally exhibit indistinct borders with a diffuse "cotton-wool" appearance and range in size from punctate to small. Regions of confluent lesions may appear large and more commonly affect the deep white matter anterior and posterior to the bodies of the lateral ventricles, symmetrically within the parietal and frontal lobes. Deep white matter lesions also often occur in a distribution parallel to the bodies of the lateral ventricles on axial views, with an irregular band-like or "beads-on-string" appearance often separated from the PV lesions by an intervening band of relatively unaffected white matter. Involvement of the external capsules is also characteristic. These patterns of lesion

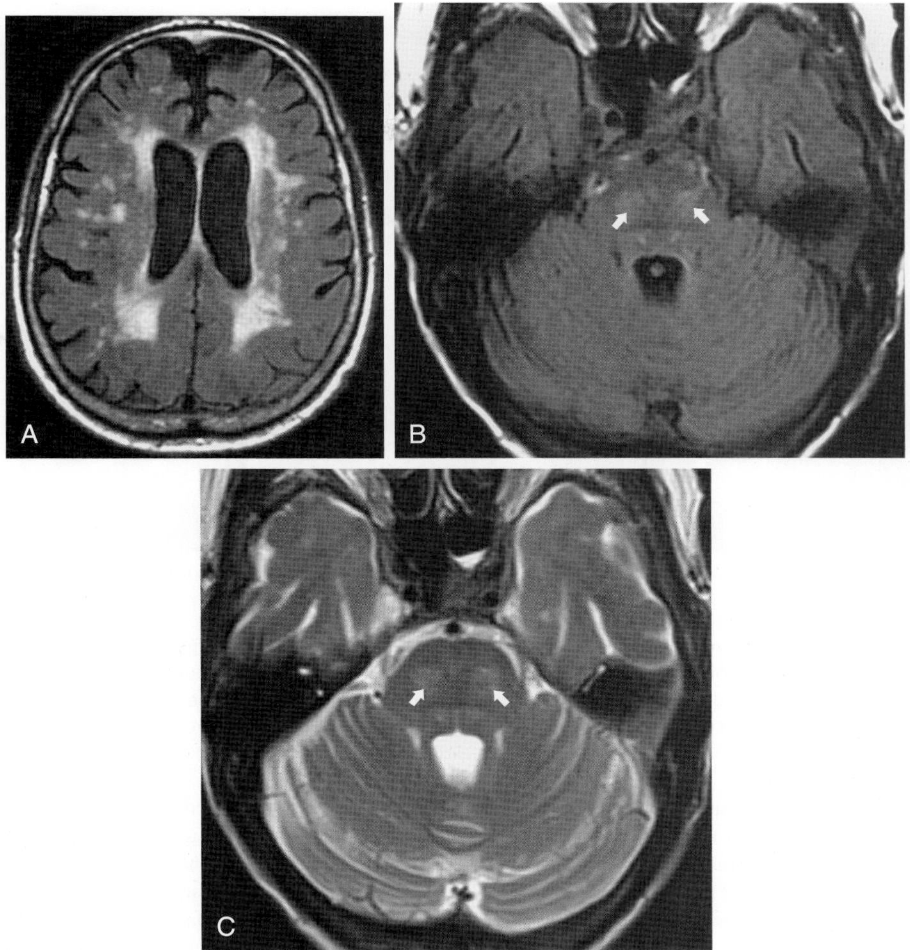


**Fig. 40.41 Microvascular Ischemic White Matter Changes. A,** Axial FLAIR image reveals extensive hyperintense areas in the hemispheric white matter bilaterally. Some are confluent at the borders of the ventricles, others are scattered in other regions. Note the "band" of hyperintensity in the left hemisphere parallel to the border of the lateral ventricle. **(B, C)** On axial FLAIR and T2-weighted images, faint hyperintense signal changes are seen in the pontine tegmentum bilaterally, exhibiting the typical imaging appearance of microvascular ischemia *(arrows)*.

distribution and morphology are often best seen on FLAIR. Contrary to the lesions of multiple sclerosis (MS), microvascular ischemia tends not to involve the temporal lobes or the corpus callosum. Besides the hemispheric white matter, microvascular ischemic lesions often also involve the basis pontis (see Fig. 40.41, *B* and *C*, available online).

The clinical significance of ischemic white matter lesions depends on their extent and location. The presence of a few small, scattered, ischemic white matter lesions on T2-weighted images is clinically meaningless, and these are usually considered a normal imaging manifestation of aging. Patients may feel more comfortable with descriptions such as "age spots of the brain" to convey their benign nature when verbally discussing results. More extensive lesions also visible on T1-weighted sequences, however, are more likely to be associated with neurological abnormalities such as abnormal gait, dementia, and incontinence. In ischemic arteriolar encephalopathy or Binswanger disease, there is pronounced, widely distributed, and confluent PV and deep white matter signal change. In more severe cases, the confluent hyperintensity also involves the internal and external capsules or subcortical white matter. Besides confluent lesions, coexisting multiple scattered T2 hyperintensities are also very common. Ischemic white matter lesions are often intermixed with lacunar ischemic strokes and generalized cerebral volume loss is also frequently noted.

eFig. 40.42 illustrates a case where the combination of various vascular pathologies, including large vessel stroke, and multiple lacunar infarcts led to vascular dementia.

Scattered small, nonspecific-appearing, seemingly microvascular white matter hyperintensities have a broader differential diagnosis in the younger patient population. Multiple small T2 hyperintense lesions in the hemispheric white matter can be caused by migraine, trauma, inborn errors of metabolism, vasculitis (including Sjögren syndrome, lupus, Behçet disease, and primary CNS vasculitis), Lyme disease, and MS. Since the MRI appearance of these is nonspecific, clinical correlation is always warranted. In many instances, these white matter lesions are idiopathic, and future serial imaging studies are needed for follow-up.

***Hippocampal sclerosis.*** Although ischemia may not be the only pathological mechanism underlying hippocampal sclerosis, this entity is discussed in conjunction with other ischemic lesions of the CNS, in the online version of this chapter available at http://www.expertconsult.com.

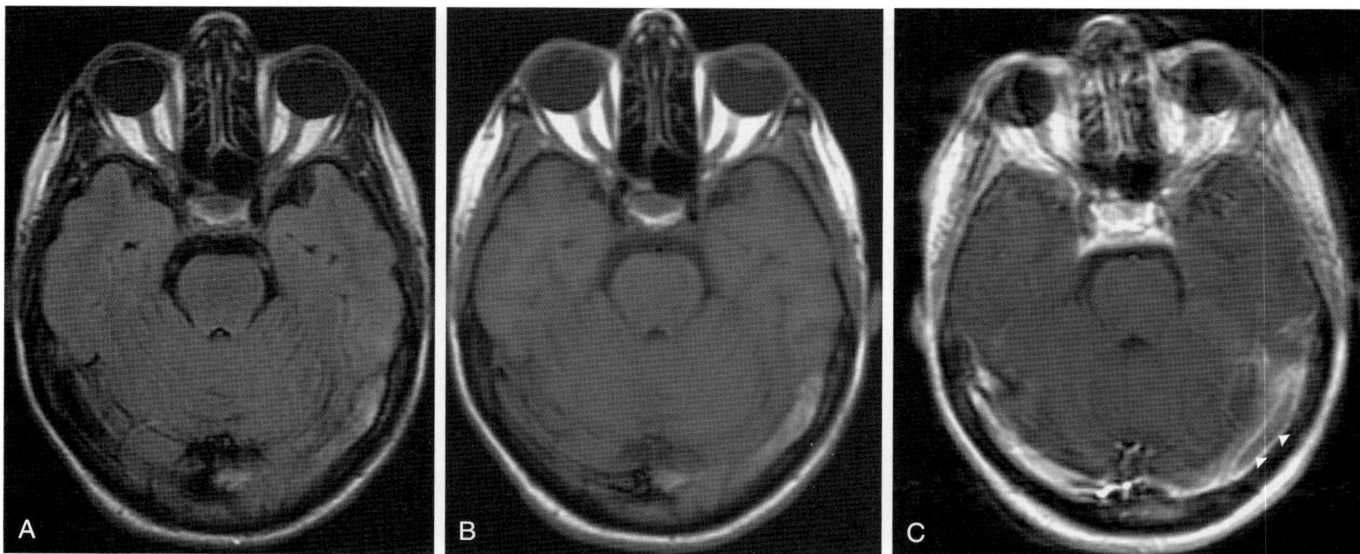


**Fig. 40.46 Left transverse and sigmoid sinus thrombosis with a small left temporal lobe area of venous ischemia.** This 48-year-old patient presented with a new-onset seizure and right visual field deficit that resolved later. **A,** Axial FLAIR image reveals abnormal hyperintense signal in the left transverse and sigmoid sinus, indicating thrombosis. Compare with the right transverse sinus, with the normal hypointense flow void. This FLAIR image also shows a small but noticeable area of hyperintensity due to venous ischemia in the left temporal lobe. **B,** Noncontrast T1-weighted image also reveals abnormal hyperintense signal in the involved venous sinuses. Again, compare with the contralateral sinus. **C,** Postcontrast T1-weighted image reveals normal filling in the sinus on the right, but there is no filling along the visualized segment of the left transverse sinus *(arrowheads)*.

***Cerebral venous sinus thrombosis.*** Acute cerebral venous sinus thrombosis results in diminished or absent flow in the involved sinuses. Cerebral venous sinus thrombosis usually causes typical signal changes on MRI (Fig. 40.46) and severely attenuated or absent flow signal on MRV. MRV techniques include flow-sensitive modalities such as 2D time-of-flight and phase contrast imaging, as well as postcontrast high-resolution three-dimensional spoiled gradient-recalled (3D SPGR), which offers excellent visualization of the sinuses with a very high spatial resolution and contrast-to-noise ratio.

In the appropriate clinical context, a useful sign of venous sinus thrombosis is the absence of a normal hypointense flow void in the involved sinuses on T1- and T2-weighted images and absent flow in the involved sinus on MRV. Nonflowing blood generally results in increased signal intensity on T1 and T2. In the early acute stage, however, the sinuses may still be hypointense. This is followed by signal that is isointense to the gray matter. The typical hyperintense signal on T1- and T2-weighted images appears when methemoglobin is present in the clot. At all stages, therefore, simultaneous review of the MRV or CT angiogram for lack of flow signal and lack of contrast filling in conjunction with conventional MRI may be particularly useful to increase the sensitivity and specificity of detection of sinus thrombosis while also adding information regarding the age of the clot.

Following administration of gadolinium, there may be enhancement of the dural wall of the sinus and along the periphery of the clot, but not within the clot itself, resulting in an "empty delta" appearance. This is classically a CT finding, but the same concept also applies to MRI in the context of the T1-weighted clot signal that varies with clot age. MR demonstrates lack of flow, appearing as absence of contrast-related signal in the involved sinuses. CT angiogram reveals no contrast filling in the thrombosed sinuses. The cortical veins that drain into the involved sinuses may appear engorged on MRV. However, if the thrombosis also involves these draining veins, they too may exhibit lack of signal on MRV, lack of filling on CT angiogram, and lack of flow voids in conjunction with iso- or hyperintense signal on T1- and T2-weighted images.

Variations in the speed of blood flow and anatomical variants of the venous sinuses may change their usual signal characteristics, leading to a false diagnosis of venous sinus thrombosis. Slow flow in a venous sinus may cause increased signal on T1- and T2-weighted images, potentially leading to a false assumption of thrombosis. Gadolinium-enhanced images help in these cases, demonstrating contrast filling/enhancement in the sinuses and confirming the absence of thrombosis. A normal variant of venous sinus hypoplasia/aplasia may result in decreased/absent flow signal on MRV, falsely interpreted as thrombosis. T1- and T2-weighted images, however, are usually able to demonstrate the absence of thrombus in the sinus. These examples highlight the importance of reviewing all necessary image modalities (MRV, T2-weighted images, T1-weighted images with and without contrast) to make or reject a diagnosis of venous sinus thrombosis.

## Hemorrhagic Cerebrovascular Disease

Structural neuroimaging is crucial in the evaluation of hemorrhagic cerebrovascular disease. Besides detection of the hematoma itself, its location can provide useful information regarding its etiology. Lobar hematomas, especially along with small, scattered, parenchymal microbleeds, raise the possibility of cerebral amyloid angiopathy, whereas putaminal, thalamic, or cerebellar hemorrhages are more likely to be of hypertensive origin. Other underlying lesions such as brain tumors causing hemorrhages can be detected by structural imaging. This section discusses hemorrhagic cerebrovascular disease and cerebral intraparenchymal hematoma, whereas other causes of hemorrhage such as trauma or malignancy are discussed in other sections. Refer to Chapters 66 and 67 for a clinical neurological review of intracerebral hemorrhages.

For decades, noncontrast CT scanning has been (and in most emergency settings still is) the essential tool for initial evaluation of intracerebral hemorrhage. In hyperacute (<12 hours after onset) and acute hemorrhage (12–48 hours), the patient's hematocrit largely determines the lesion's degree of density on CT. With a normal hematocrit, both retracted and unretracted clots exhibit hyperdensity that contrasts sufficiently with the isodense background of brain parenchyma to be easily detectable. In cases of anemia, however, small hemorrhagic lesions may potentially be overlooked owing to their lower CT density and may even be isodense to brain. The following sections describing the appearance of hemorrhage on CT and MRI studies all assume a normal hematocrit.

In the acute stage, the hematoma is seen as an area of hyperdensity on CT. The associated mass effect depends on the size and location. Effacement of the ventricles, cortical sulci, or basal cisterns is often seen. Various degrees of midline shift or subtypes of herniation (transtentorial, subfalcine, etc.) may occur. The surrounding edema is seen as hypodensity and tends to appear irregular with varying thickness depending on the degree of involvement of adjacent white matter tracts, which are preferentially affected. The initially distinct border of the hematoma changes within days to a few weeks after onset and becomes irregular and "moth-eaten" due to the phagocytic activity of macrophages. Small hematomas may disappear on CT within 1 week; in the case of larger hematomas, the process may take more than a month. Small hemorrhages may resolve without any residual change, while those that are larger are gradually replaced by an encephalomalacic cavity of decreased density and ex vacuo enlargement of the adjacent CSF spaces.

The appearance of hemorrhagic cerebrovascular disease on MRI is very complex regarding both signal heterogeneity on individual scans and subsequent changes in appearance over successive imaging studies. Signal characteristics of hemorrhage vary widely across different pulse sequences (T1, T2, T2* gradient echo), depending on the age of the hemorrhage; presence of oxyhemoglobin, deoxyhemoglobin, methemoglobin, and hemosiderin; changing water content within the clot; and integrity of erythrocyte membranes. Understanding the typical MRI appearance of each stage in the evolution of a hemorrhage allows one to estimate its age, because biochemical and structural changes characteristic of each stage (macroscopic and microscopic) occur along a predictable time line. In addition to conventional (T1- and T2-weighted) images, the gradient echo technique has been used to detect even small intracerebral hemorrhages, given its sensitivity to the paramagnetic properties (magnetic field distorting effects) of various blood products. More recently introduced into clinical practice, the technique of SWI offers the greatest sensitivity for chronic hemorrhage to date and is particularly useful in evaluating punctate hemorrhages in patients with diffuse shear injury secondary to prior head trauma.

A discussion of the MR imaging features of hemorrhage is best organized according to the stages of hemorrhage evolution as follows.

***Hyperacute hemorrhage (0–24 hours).*** In the early (hyperacute) phase of intraparenchymal hemorrhage (<24 hours) the red blood cells are intact, and a mixture of oxy- and deoxyhemoglobin is present (Bakshi et al., 1998). In this stage, the signal on T1-weighted images is isointense to the brain, so even larger hematomas may be missed on this pulse sequence. On T2-weighted images, the oxyhemoglobin portion is hyperintense and deoxyhemoglobin is hypointense, resulting in the gradual appearance of a hypointense rim and gradually increasing hypointense foci within the hematoma as the amount of deoxyhemoglobin increases from the periphery. Such hypointense foci are also seen on FLAIR. Between the clot and the deoxyhemoglobin-containing rim, thin intervening clefts of fluid-like T2 hyperintensity may be seen as an initial manifestation of clot retraction. On gradient echo images, hyperacute hemorrhage will exhibit heterogeneously isointense to markedly hypointense signals, the latter corresponding to deoxyhemoglobin content in more peripheral portions of the clot. The amount of edema is mild in this stage, usually seen as a thin rim that is hyperintense on T2 and FLAIR images and hypointense on T1-weighted images (Atlas and Thulborn, 1998).

***Acute hemorrhage (1–3 days).*** During this stage, hemoglobin is transformed to deoxyhemoglobin, but the membranes of the erythrocytes are still intact (Bakshi et al., 1998). The hematoma becomes slightly hypointense on T1 and strikingly hypointense on T2-weighted images (Fig. 40.47). On GRE, proton spins in the presence of paramagnetic deoxyhemoglobin dephase rapidly during TE, resulting in signal loss and, therefore, hypointensity of the hematoma on this pulse sequence. The surrounding edema, which is more extensive during this stage, is hypointense on T1 and hyperintense on T2.

***Early subacute hemorrhage (3 days to 1 week).*** As blood degradation evolves, deoxyhemoglobin is converted to methemoglobin. At this stage, the blood degradation products are still intracellular (Bakshi et al., 1998). Intracellular methemoglobin is hyperintense on T1 and hypointense on T2-weighted images. T1 shortening is primarily the result of dipole–dipole interactions between heme iron and adjacent water protons, facilitated by a conformational change that occurs when deoxyhemoglobin is converted to methemoglobin.

Signal changes on T2 occur via a different mechanism. Sequestration of methemoglobin within the intact red blood cell membrane results in a locally paramagnetic environment adjacent to the diamagnetic, methemoglobin-free extracellular compartment. These differences in the local magnetic fields, present at a microscopic level, cause rapid dephasing of proton spins and signal loss during TE as water molecules diffuse rapidly through this heterogeneous environment. Therefore, on T2-weighted images, the presence of intracellular methemoglobin results in hypointensity of the hemorrhage. These signal changes start from the periphery of the hematoma where the deoxyhemoglobin-to-methemoglobin transformation first occurs. During this stage, the amount of edema starts to decrease.

***Late subacute hemorrhage (1–4 weeks).*** In the late subacute phase, the membranes of the red blood cells disintegrate, and methemoglobin becomes extracellular (Bakshi et al., 1998). Extracellular methemoglobin contains $Fe^{3+}$, which has five unpaired electrons. This leads to a dipole–dipole interaction that, contrary to intracellular methemoglobin, causes hyperintense signal change on both T1- and T2-weighted images (Fig. 40.48).

During this stage (usually 2 weeks after the hemorrhage) hemosiderin deposition begins, typically at the periphery of the hematoma where macrophages reside. A dark peripheral rim appears on GRE and T2-weighted images, which is initially thin but then progressively thicker. The amount of edema around the hematoma continues to decrease gradually.

***Chronic hemorrhage (>4 weeks).*** In the chronic stage (Bakshi et al., 1998), the core of larger hematomas turns into a slitlike or linear cavity with CSF signal characteristics, being hypointense on T1 and FLAIR and hyperintense on T2-weighted images. At the periphery of the lesion, macrophages continue to remove iron from the extracellular methemoglobin; hemosiderin and ferritin are deposited in their lysosomes, resulting in a rim of hypointense signal on T2-weighted and GRE images. This hypointense rim becomes progressively more prominent during the transition from the late subacute to chronic stage (Fig. 40.49).

If the hemorrhage is small, eventually its entire area will be occupied by hemosiderin deposition. Smaller hemorrhages or microbleeds, such as those seen in amyloid angiopathy or after head trauma, are visualized as multiple uniformly hypointense foci on GRE images. Susceptibility-weighted images are even more sensitive to magnetic field distortion due to blood products and can reveal microbleeds that are missed even by conventional gradient echo images. It is important to keep in mind that because of magnetic field distortion, the area of hypointensity on GRE or susceptibility-weighted images is larger than the actual size of the bleed. GRE or, ideally, SWI should be part of every MRI protocol for brain trauma.

Hemorrhage, like many other lesions to the brain, provokes reactive gliosis. In the chronic stage, surrounding gliosis is seen as mildly hyperintense signal on T2 and FLAIR images.

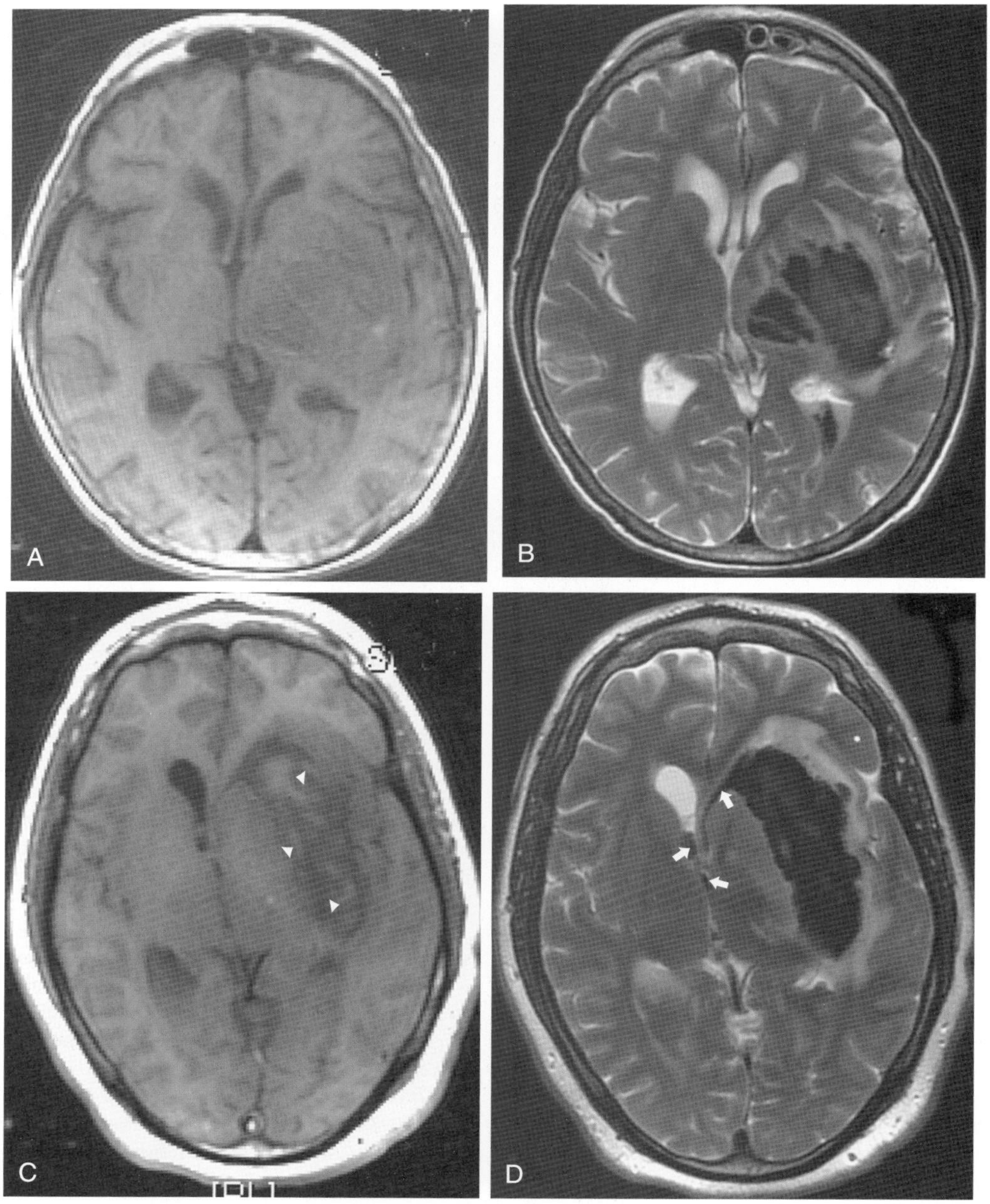

**Fig. 40.47** **Two Cases of Acute Parenchymal Hemorrhage.** **(A, B)** Large acute left basal ganglia hemorrhage. On noncontrast T1-weighted image **(A)** only faint hypointensity is noted. On axial T2-weighted image **(B)** the hematoma appears as a striking hypointensity with developing hyperintense edema in surrounding parenchyma. Note associated mass effect. **(C, D)** In this case, the basal ganglia hematoma is in a more advanced stage. On T1-weighted image **(C)** the area is still mostly hypointense, but its center is now turning hyperintense because of intracellular methemoglobin *(arrowheads)*. On corresponding T2-weighted image **(D)** the hematoma is still hypointense (as intracellular methemoglobin is also hypointense on T2), but the surrounding hyperintense edema is more prominent and the mass effect is increased as well. Note that hemorrhage is also present within the ventricle, making the prognosis worse *(arrows)*.

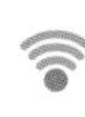

Superficial siderosis, a chronic sequela of bleeding into the subarachnoid space, and cerebral amyloid angiopathy, a hemorrhage-prone condition, are discussed in the online version of this chapter, available at http://www.expertconsult.com.

### Infection

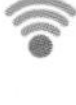

Structural neuroimaging can provide useful information for evaluating infectious diseases of the CNS. The imaging modality of choice is MRI, which is able to demonstrate even subtle parenchymal abnormalities and inflammatory involvement of the meninges. Visit http://www.expertconsult.com to view this section. For a review of the etiology, clinical presentation, and treatment of infections of the nervous system, see Chapters 77–79.

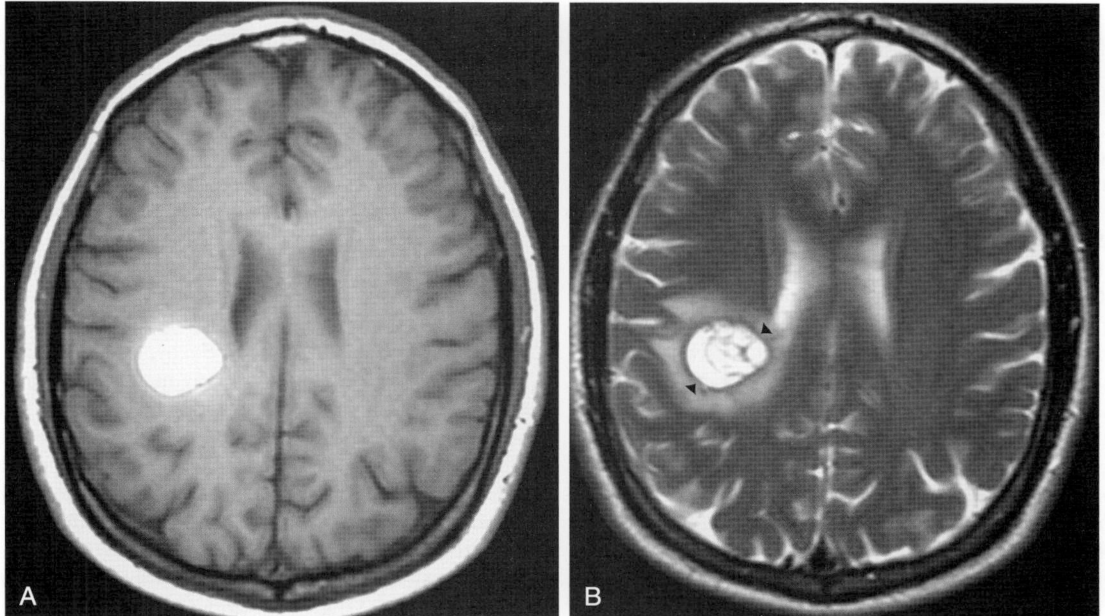


**Fig. 40.48 Late Subacute Parenchymal Hemorrhage. A,** On noncontrast T1-weighted image, there is a hematoma in the right corona radiata. This exhibits homogeneous hyperintense signal. **B,** On T2-weighted image, the hematoma also appears as homogeneous hyperintensity. Signal characteristics are typical for the presence of extracellular methemoglobin in a late subacute hematoma. Note beginning of hypointense hemosiderin deposition at the rim of the hematoma on T2-weighted image *(arrowheads)*.

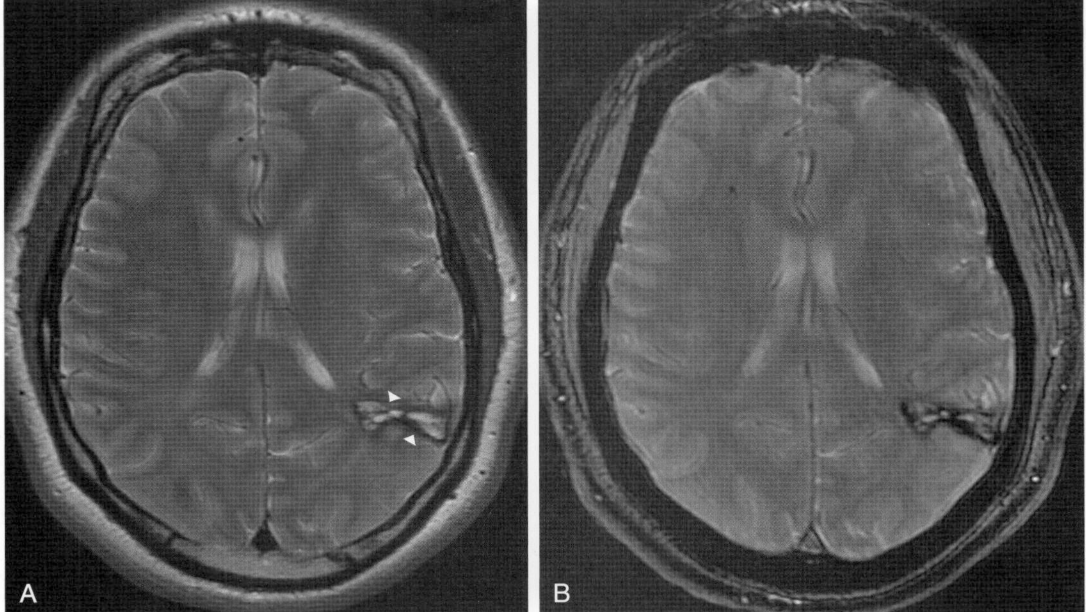


**Fig. 40.49 Chronic Parenchymal Hemorrhage. A,** Axial T2-weighted image reveals a slitlike cavitary lesion in the left parietal lobe. Its center has cerebrospinal fluid-like hyperintense signal, but there is a rim of hypointensity due to hemosiderin deposition along its border *(arrowheads)*. **B,** Axial gradient echo image reveals markedly hypointense hemosiderin deposition along the border of the chronic hemorrhage.

### Multiple Sclerosis and Other White Matter Diseases

Inflammatory and noninflammatory lesions of the corpus callosum, leukodystrophy (Krabbe disease, metachromatic leukodystrophy, adrenoleukodystrophy), radiation leukoencephalopathy, posterior reversible encephalopathy syndrome (PRES), and central pontine myelinolysis are discussed in the online version of this chapter, available at http://www.expertconsult.com.

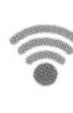

***Multiple sclerosis.*** MS is a demyelinating disease with autoimmune inflammatory reaction against the myelin sheath of CNS pathways (see Chapter 80). MRI is essential for the diagnosis of MS by demonstrating the typical inflammatory demyelinating lesions disseminated in time and space (Fig. 40.59). It is also used for disease monitoring and assessment of response to therapy.

MS white matter lesions may occur supratentorially or infratentorially, as well as within the spinal cord (imaging of spinal cord MS lesions is described later). Best evaluated on T2-weighted images, infratentorial lesions may be seen within the medulla, pons, midbrain, or cerebellum. Characteristic locations include the pontine tegmentum, periaqueductal region, cerebral peduncles, middle and superior cerebellar peduncles, and the white matter of the cerebellar hemispheres. Punctate or small lesions that are present directly adjacent to the fourth ventricle or cisterns are sometimes difficult to detect on T2-weighted images but are not uncommon. Infratentorial lesions are generally smaller than supratentorial lesions and are also less frequently hypointense on conventional T1-weighted images; they commonly appear hypointense on T1-weighted 3D spoiled gradient echo pulse sequences.

Supratentorial white matter lesions are usually best appreciated using the FLAIR pulse sequence, which nulls out CSF signal that may obscure PV abnormalities on conventional T2-weighted images. PV and subcortical white matter lesions typically are small in size and morphologically are generally ovoid or round on axial images. On sagittal views, PV lesions often exhibit a thin linear or fingerlike morphology (Dawson fingers), with the long axis of the lesion oriented perpendicularly to the wall of the lateral ventricle in a PV distribution. The PV distribution of many MS lesions is well demonstrated on SWI imaging, which reveals a single tiny, profoundly hypointense dot or thin linearity at the center of a significant proportion of demyelinating lesions. It represents a venule and is visible because of the magnetic susceptibility effects of deoxygenated venous blood, to which SWI is particularly sensitive.

Although the distribution of white matter lesions in MS has a somewhat random appearance, the hemispheres characteristically match each other in terms of lesion load, which typically is highest around the ventricles. On sagittal views, PV lesions are usually most numerous adjacent to the bodies and atria of the lateral ventricles, with less involvement of the white matter adjacent to the occipital and temporal horns. The deep white matter of the frontal and parietal lobes typically also tends to exhibit a greater number of lesions than either the occipital or temporal lobes. However, the presence of lesions adjacent to the temporal horns favors a diagnosis of MS. Juxtacortical demyelination is less commonly seen. Juxtacortical lesions, which involve the U-fibers, often exhibit a crescentic morphology and are usually seen only on FLAIR, PD, or T2-weighted images. Occasionally they are hypointense on T1 as well. When present, this type of lesion favors the diagnosis of MS. Corpus callosum lesions are also relatively specific for MS. They are best visualized on sagittal FLAIR images, typically as punctate hyperintensities along the septocallosal margin (undersurface of the corpus callosum). Thin hyperintense linearities that are contiguous with and perpendicular to the undersurface may also be present. These findings are often superimposed upon a thin irregular band of T2 hyperintensity running along the undersurface of the corpus callosum rostrocaudally. Isolated lesions within the central fibers of the corpus callosum that are noncontiguous with the septocallosal margin are less typical and should raise the level of suspicion for alternate differential diagnoses, discussed in the following section.

Although it is well known from histopathological studies that MS affects not only the hemispheric white matter but also the cortex and deep gray nuclei, cortical gray matter lesions are uncommonly seen on conventional MRI studies. They may be seen more often with the use of high-field scanners (3.0 T or higher). Of the conventional pulse sequences, high spatial resolution FLAIR images are the most sensitive for cortical gray matter lesions. Detection is limited because the subtle hyperintensity of cortical lesions on FLAIR is only slightly greater than the already relatively hyperintense background of the cortical gray matter. A cortical gray matter lesion may be verified by correlation of the finding on separate FLAIR image stacks acquired in orthogonal planes or by detection of a hypointense lesion of identical morphology and location on T1-weighted 3D spoiled gradient echo pulse sequences. Cortical gray matter lesions generally have a curvilinear contour that conforms to the topology of the cortex but may also overlap with the adjacent white matter. Like deep gray-matter lesions, cortical gray-matter hyperintensities visible on MRI are usually small, in the millimeter range. Deep gray-matter MS lesions tend to be round or oval and are most frequently seen in the thalami.

T1-weighted images are useful for the detection of "black holes," markedly hypointense lesions that have been shown histopathologically to exhibit more extensive demyelination and axonal loss than other lesions. They always exhibit a correlating hyperintensity on T2-weighted images but may appear centrally hypointense on FLAIR owing to their relatively high free water content. Conversely, not all T2-weighted lesions exhibit T1 hypointensity, and therefore the T1 lesion load is always less extensive than the T2 lesion load. Some MS cases, usually earlier in disease progression, exhibit no T1 hypointense lesions.

T1-weighted postcontrast images are useful for the detection of enhancing lesions in patients with clinical exacerbations. Enhancement may be solid or ringlike. Open-ring configurations are more typical for MS than other disease entities that also exhibit ring enhancement, such as tumors and infections (Masdeu et al., 2000). Five minutes between gadolinium injection and the acquisition of postcontrast images is the minimum acceptable delay for detecting acute demyelinating lesions. "Double or triple dose" and longer delays of up to 15 minutes for the postcontrast T-weighted imaging may detect more lesions but is not necessary for routine clinical practice (Traboulsee et al., 2016).

Chronic MS lesions do not exhibit restricted diffusion, appearing on DWI as either isointense to the surrounding brain parenchyma or, less commonly, hyperintense due to T2 shine-through artifact. On the corresponding ADC maps, chronic lesions exhibit normal or high ADCs. However, as recently described, acute enhancing demyelinating lesions may on rare occasions exhibit high signal on DWI, with corresponding low pixel values (hypointense) on the ADC map, consistent with restricted diffusion (Balashov et al., 2009). Rapid resolution of restricted diffusion in these acute lesions is the rule, and they often evolve to exhibit increased ADC values on follow-up studies.

Nonconventional MRI pulse sequences are commonly used to assess MS in the research environment. SWI is a newer technique that is exquisitely sensitive to the small venules as well as iron deposition, the latter thought to play a pathophysiological role in MS. Magnetization transfer imaging may be used to generate histograms of pixel values within the normal-appearing white matter; such histograms are typically shifted to the left, with lower peak values than in normal individuals. DTI is a more advanced application of DWI that is used to measure the directional diffusion of water molecules

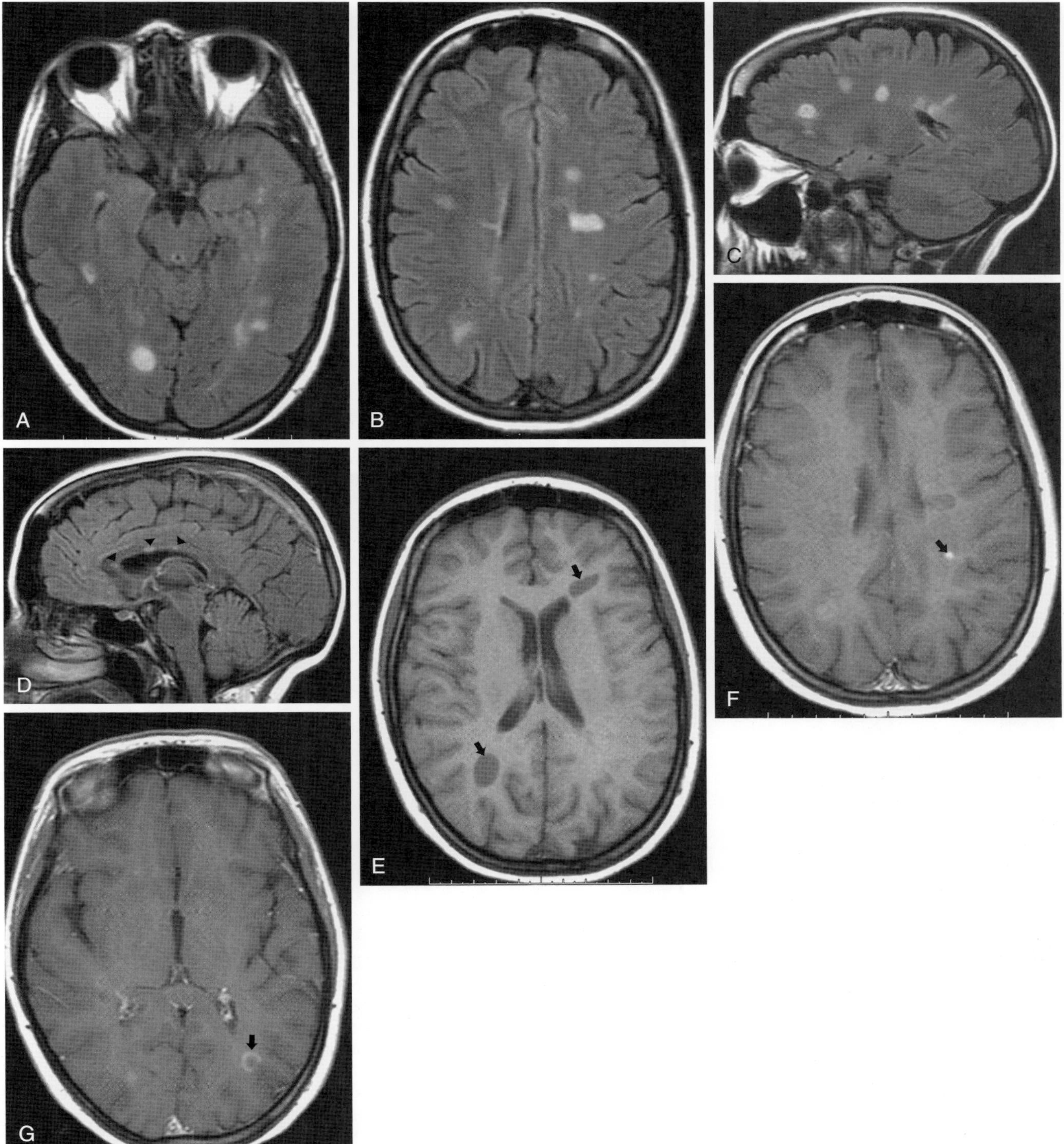


**Fig. 40.59 Multiple Sclerosis.** A–C, Axial and sagittal FLAIR images demonstrate multiple hyperintense lesions in the white matter. The majority of these abut the lateral ventricles, including the temporal horns bilaterally. Several lesions are linear and oriented perpendicular to ventricular borders. On sagittal FLAIR image (C) some lesions exhibit characteristic Dawson fingerlike appearance. D, On midsagittal FLAIR image, lesions are present in the corpus callosum *(arrowheads)*. E, On T1-weighted noncontrast image, two prominently hypointense lesions exhibit a "black hole" appearance *(arrows)*. (F, G) Axial T1 postcontrast images demonstrate two enhancing lesions. One is a small, homogeneously enhancing lesion in the left centrum semiovale *(arrow)*, the other is seen in the left parietal subcortical area *(arrow)*. This latter lesion exhibits an "open-ring" enhancement pattern which is very typical for active demyelinating lesions.

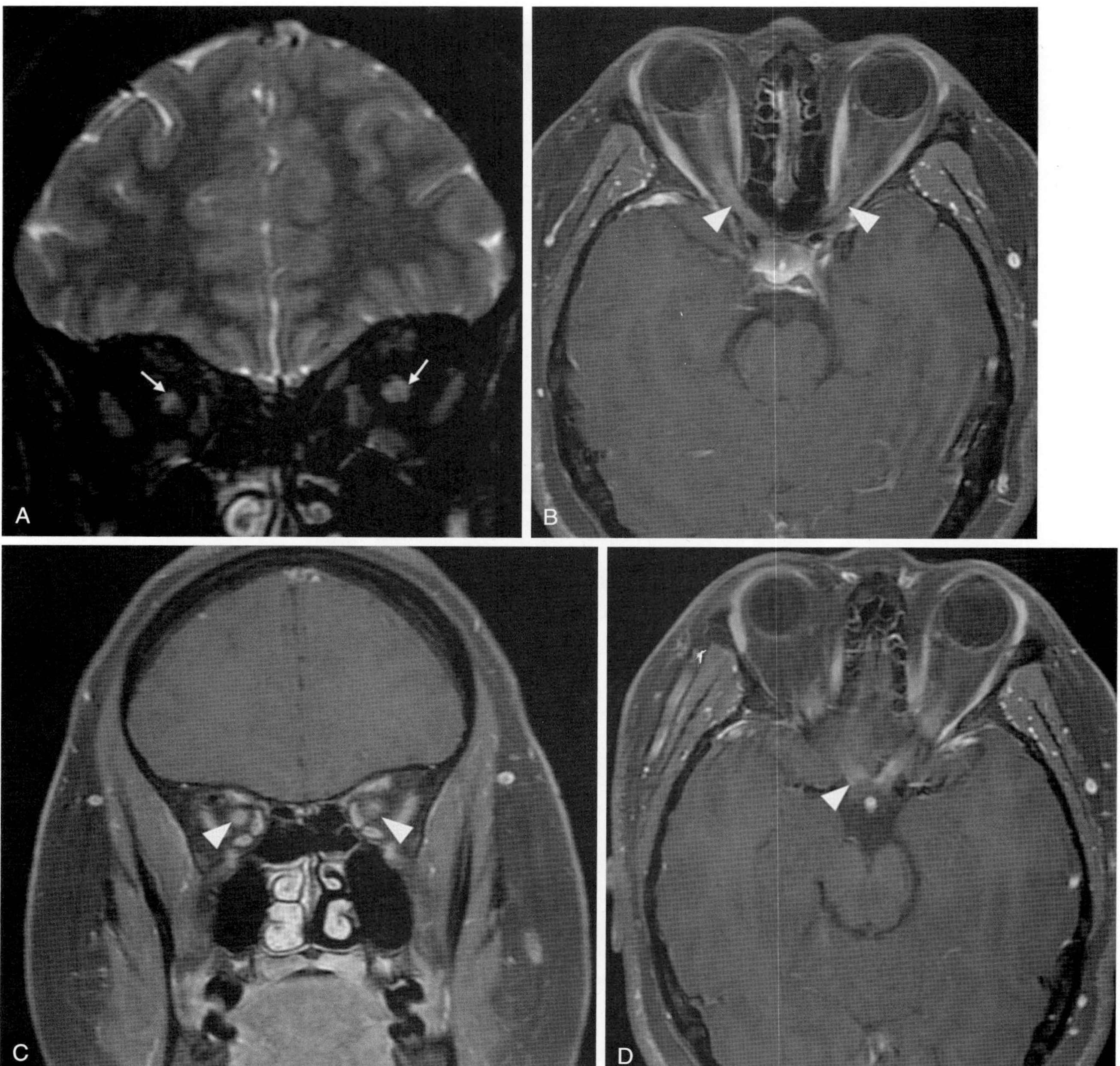


**Fig. 40.60 Neuromyelitis Optica.** MRI from a 26-year-old woman with serologically proven neuromyelitis optica. Both optic nerves appear hyperintense *(arrows)* on coronal T2-weighted images **(A)**. Axial and coronal T1-weighted postcontrast images **(B, C)**, demonstrate bilateral enhancement *(arrowheads)*, involving more than half of the length of the optic nerves and extending posteriorly to the optic chiasm **(D)**.

within white matter tracts. Like magnetization transfer imaging, DTI is useful for the quantification of pathology within normal-appearing white matter.

***Neuromyelitis optica spectrum disorder.*** Neuromyelitis optica (NMO) is a distinct severe demyelinating disorder with predilection for the optic nerves and spinal cord (spinal cord findings are discussed in the "Spinal Diseases" section), caused by an autoantibody to the aquaporin-4 (AQP4) water channel. In targeted imaging of the orbit, characteristics of optic neuritis will be visible, including swelling and signal changes on T2-weighted sequences (Fig. 40.60, *A*) and enhancement after contrast on T1-weighted images (see Fig. 40.60, *B*). Bilateral optic nerve involvement (see Fig. 40.60, *C*), those extending more than half of its lengths (see Fig. 40.60, *B*) and those involving the posterior aspects of the optic nerves or the chiasm (see Fig. 40.60, *D*), are more suggestive of neuromyelitis optica spectrum disorder (NMOSD) than of MS, which also causes optic neuritis. In chronic stages of the disease, atrophy of the optic nerves with associated hyperintensities on T2-weighted sequences may be seen (Wingerchuk et al., 2015). In addition to involvement of the orbit, 60% of patients develop brain MRI abnormalities including lesions localized in AQP4-rich circumventricular regions. One of the most specific brain MRI abnormalities in patients with NMOSD is a lesion in the dorsal brainstem adjacent to the fourth ventricle, including the area postrema and the nucleus tractus solitarius. Such lesions are highly associated with intractable hiccups, nausea, and vomiting. Diencephalic lesions surrounding the third ventricles and cerebral aqueduct, which include

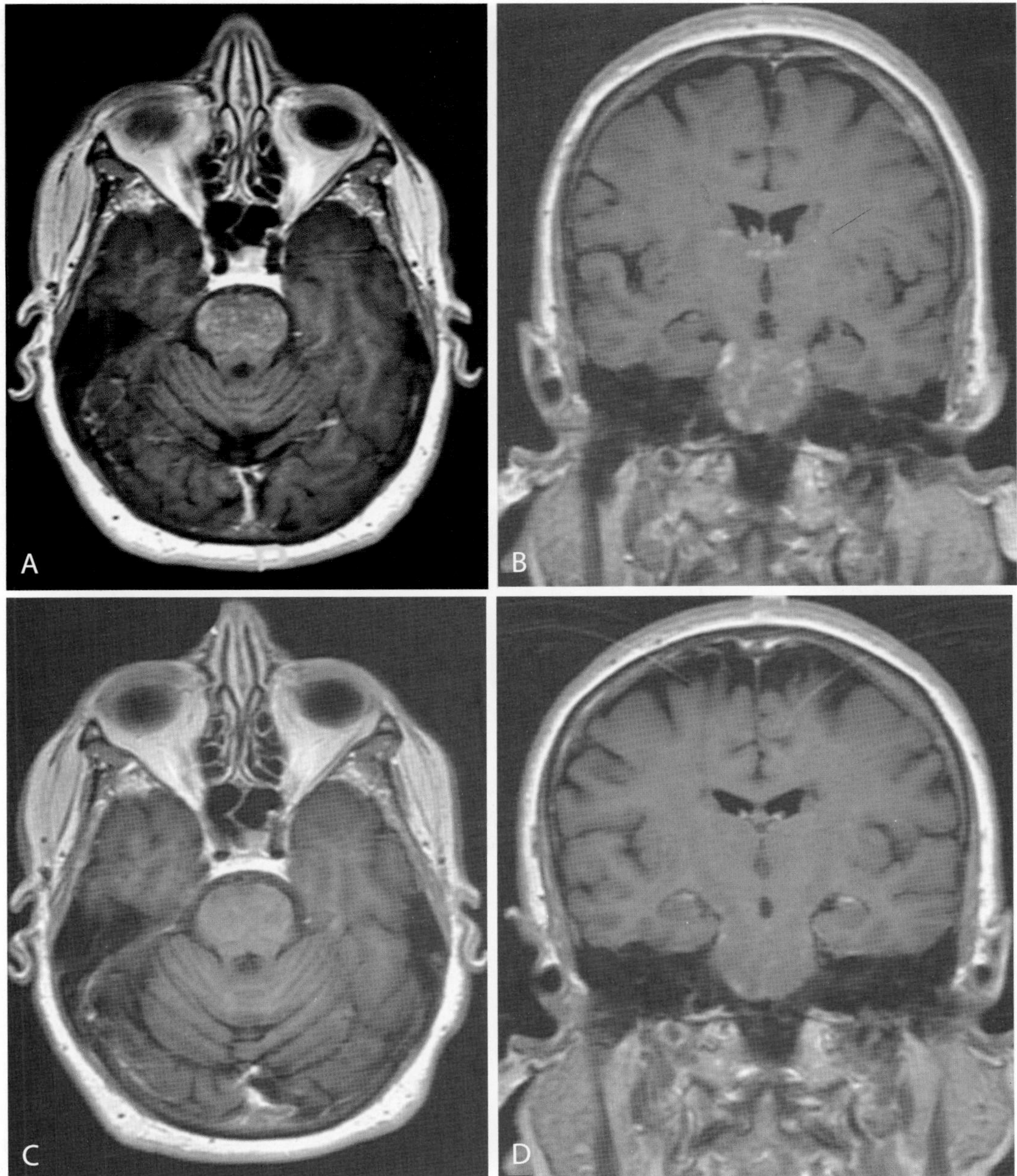


**Fig. 40.61 CLIPPERS.** MRI from a 69-year-old woman who presented with dysarthria and ataxia. Axial **(A)** and coronal **(B)** T1 postcontrast images show multiple punctate and curvilinear contrast-enhancing lesions in the pons. Almost complete resolution of contrast enhancement is noted following 5 days of steroid therapy **(C, D)**.

the thalamus, hypothalamus, and anterior border of the midbrain, have been reported in NMOSD (Kim et al., 2015, Wingerchuk et al., 2015). The most common pattern of gadolinium enhancement in brain lesions is cloud-like, characterized as patchy and inhomogeneous with poorly defined margins (Dutra et al., 2018).

***Acute disseminated encephalomyelitis.*** Acute disseminated encephalomyelitis (ADEM) is an acute demyelinating disease that, unlike MS, is typically monophasic. It may follow vaccination or a viral infection. On MRI, multiple hyperintense lesions are seen in the hemispheric white matter, cerebellum, and brainstem. The hemispheric lesions are often subcortical. Although MS may also involve the gray matter, this is much more common in ADEM, and basal ganglia or thalamic lesions are seen in 30%–40% of cases. The lesions may exhibit vasogenic edema, and hemorrhage may also be seen. Punctate, linear, ring, and incomplete ring patterns all occur; absence of enhancement does not exclude the diagnosis

***CLIPPERS.*** Chronic lymphocytic inflammation with pontine perivascular enhancement responsive to steroids (CLIPPERS) is a recently described brainstem encephalitis, characterized by white matter perivascular, predominantly T-lymphocytic, infiltrate without granulomas, infection, lymphoma, or vasculitis (Pittock et al., 2010). All CLIPPERS patients have the characteristic MRI pattern of symmetric curvilinear gadolinium enhancement peppering the pons (Fig. 40.61, *A–B*) and extending variably into the medulla, brachium

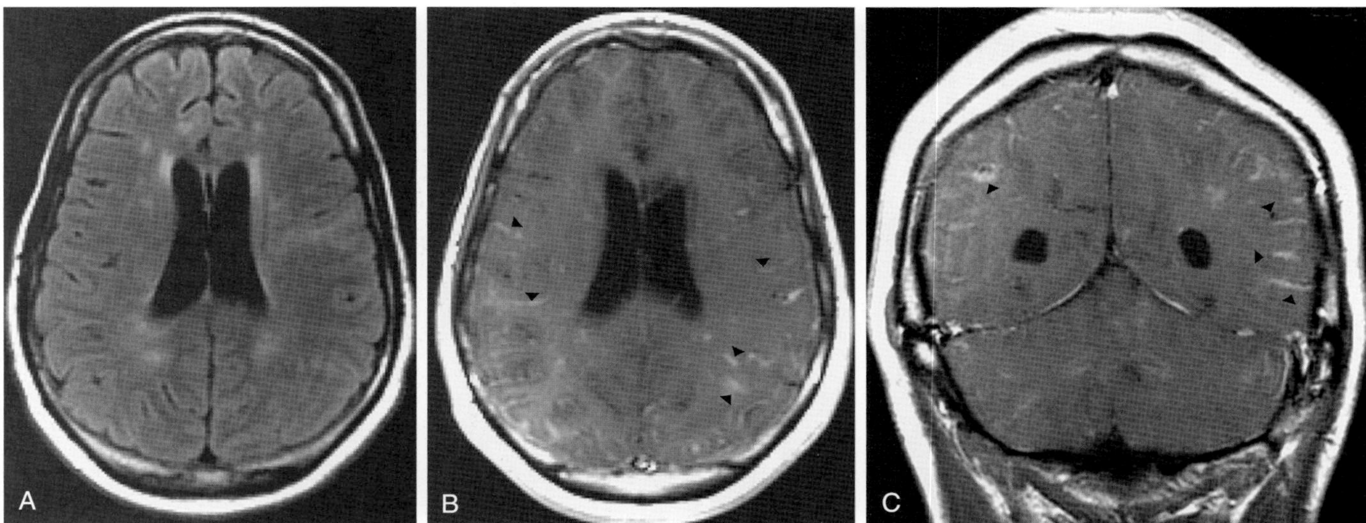


**Fig. 40.62 Neurosarcoidosis. A,** Axial FLAIR image reveals multiple hyperintense lesions in the deep and subcortical white matter bilaterally. **(B, C)** Axial and coronal T1 postcontrast images show multiple linear areas of enhancement in a leptomeningeal and perivascular distribution, a pattern characteristic of neurosarcoidosis *(arrowheads).*

pontis, cerebellum, midbrain, and occasionally, thalamus or spinal cord. In T2 sequences, the degree of signal abnormality does not significantly exceed the size of the area of postgadolinium enhancement. Corticosteroid therapy is typically associated with marked to complete resolution of postgadolinium T1 contrast enhancement (see Fig. 40. 61, *C–D*; Pittock et al., 2010).

***Neurosarcoidosis.*** The prevalence of nervous system involvement in sarcoidosis is approximately 5%. In the brain parenchyma, multiple PV T2 hyperintense lesions are frequently noted, which may be due to a vasculitic process and often cannot be distinguished from MS or ischemic microvascular changes. Sarcoidosis may also involve the pituitary infundibulum and hypothalamus (resulting in endocrine symptoms). The granulomatous inflammation may affect the cranial nerves and/or their meningeal coverings as well, resulting in enlargement, hyperintense signal change, and abnormal enhancement. Although sarcoidosis may involve the dura, following gadolinium administration, leptomeningeal enhancement is more commonly noted. It is typically seen along the penetrating blood vessels and the adjacent leptomeninges, and is due to perivascular spread of the granulomatous process (Fig. 40.62). Sometimes larger intraparenchymal or meningeal enhancing lesions are noted which may be mistaken for primary or metastatic tumors. When involved, the pituitary infundibulum and hypothalamus may also exhibit enhancement. Neurosarcoidosis may also lead to hydrocephalus, either by interfering with CSF absorption through the arachnoid granulations or by obstructing the ventricular system.

## Trauma

Both CT and MRI have a pivotal role in the evaluation of craniocerebral trauma (Chapters 60–62). In the emergency room setting, the first imaging modality is usually a noncontrast CT scan. CT bone windowing is the best tool for evaluating skull fractures (Fig. 40.66, *A*), whereas brain windowing is of great value for visualizing subarachnoid (see Fig. 40.66, *B*), epidural, subdural, intraventricular, or intraparenchymal hemorrhages. MRI is very useful in detecting traumatic lesions of the brain parenchyma, especially when more subtle changes are present, such as small contusions, parenchymal microbleeds, and the small or punctate lesions of diffuse axonal injury. The various consequences of trauma that we will review next seldom occur in isolation but tend to occur in various combinations (e.g., cortical contusion is frequently associated with subarachnoid hemorrhage).

***Traumatic subarachnoid hemorrhage.*** Traditionally, a noncontrast CT scan has been the first-line imaging study to demonstrate traumatic subarachnoid hemorrhage. Acute blood appears hyperdense in the subarachnoid space. The hemorrhage may be seen in the sylvian fissures, interhemispheric fissure, basal cisterns, or in the cortical sulci at the convexities, depending on the site of trauma. Subarachnoid hyperdensity tends to resolve within 5–7 days after the hemorrhage, but depending on the amount of subarachnoid blood, this may be a shorter or longer process.

Until FLAIR pulse sequences became available, MRI was inferior to CT in detecting subarachnoid blood, especially in the first few days. Conventional T1- and T2-weighted images may completely miss subarachnoid blood in these early stages. However, subarachnoid blood appears hyperintense on FLAIR images (see Fig. 40.66, *C*), and this pulse sequence is considered equal or superior to CT in detecting subarachnoid blood (Woodcock et al., 2001), especially in the posterior fossa and at the skull base, where CT images are often compromised by beam-hardening artifacts. The hyperintense signal change is due to the presence of blood, which changes the zero point of the TI of CSF, and therefore signal attenuation in subarachnoid regions containing hemorrhage will not be complete. An important caveat is that subarachnoid hyperintensity on FLAIR may also result from other causes. A common cause is magnetic susceptibility artifact, seen in patients who have braces or other metal devices that distort the magnetic field, which results in a lack of CSF signal suppression and the artifactually hyperintense appearance of CSF adjacent to the anterior frontal lobes.

Besides detection of blood in the acute phase, structural neuroimaging is also very useful to evaluate the potential later complications of subarachnoid hemorrhage. Subarachnoid blood may occlude the arachnoid granulations, leading to impaired CSF absorption, communicating hydrocephalus, and ventriculomegaly. Another late

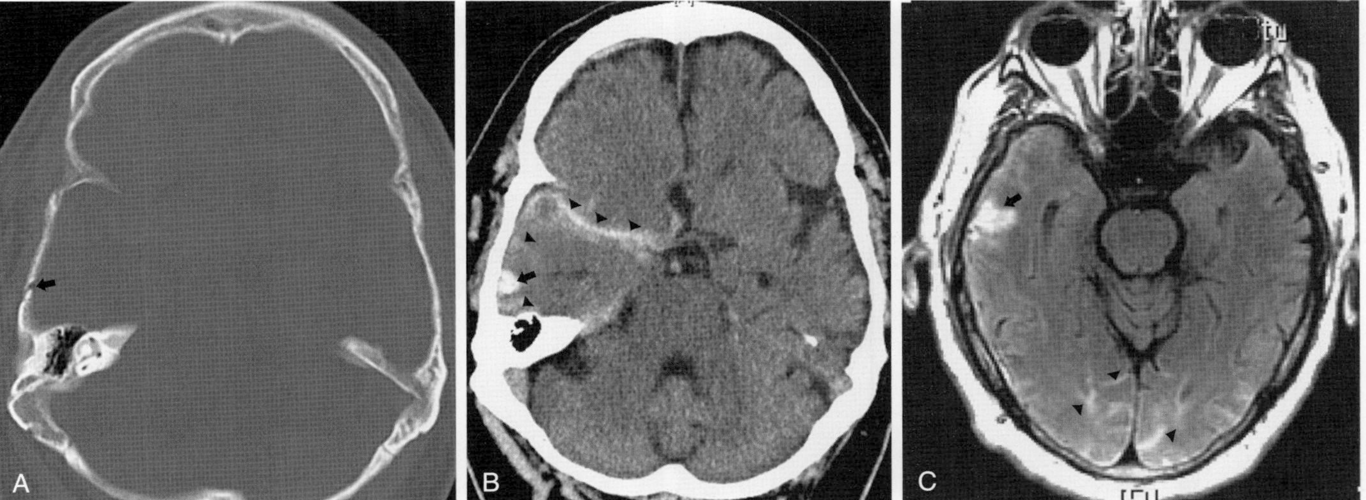


**Fig. 40.66 Skull Fracture and Contusion with Subarachnoid Hemorrhage.** **A,** Axial bone window computed tomography (CT) image demonstrates a right temporal bone fracture *(arrow)*. **B,** Axial brain window CT scan reveals a hyperdense area at the right temporal lobe surface, consistent with contusion and hemorrhage *(arrow)*. There is hyperdensity in the right temporal lobe sulci and even more so in the right middle cranial fossa of the brain, due to traumatic subarachnoid blood *(arrowheads)*. **C,** Axial FLAIR image demonstrates hyperintense signal change in the right temporal lobe, consistent with contusion *(arrow)*. There is also bilateral hyperintense signal due to the presence of subarachnoid blood in the sulci of the occipital lobes, which settled in these dependent regions because of the prolonged supine position of the patient *(arrowheads)*.

phenomenon that tends to follow repeated episodes of subarachnoid hemorrhage is superficial siderosis. In this condition, hemosiderin is deposited along the leptomeninges and appears as linear areas of hypointensity on T2-weighted images (see eFig. 40.50).

***Subdural hemorrhage.*** Subdural hematomas are common sequelae of head trauma and are thought to result from rupture of the bridging veins (veins that drain from the cerebral surface and pierce the dura to enter the adjacent venous sinus). Morphologically they follow the contour of the cerebral surface and can cross the cranial suture lines but not the midline at the falx cerebri and cerebelli. Depending on the size, there is a varying degree of mass effect on the adjacent brain; in the more severe cases, effacement of the adjacent ventricles, midline shift, and various herniation syndromes may occur.

As subdural hematomas age, their imaging appearance changes both on CT and MRI. On CT, acute subdural hematomas appear hyperdense. If the patient remains in a recumbent position, the cellular elements settle to the lower part of the hematoma, which will appear more hyperdense, whereas the "supernatant" is less so. With time, hemoglobin degradation occurs, and the density of the hematoma will decrease, eventually becoming hypodense. During this process there is a transitional stage when the density of the hematoma will be very similar or the same as that of the brain, rendering its detection more difficult. Just as with intraparenchymal hematomas, the density depends on the hematocrit, and in severely anemic patients, even acute subdural hematomas may appear iso- or hypodense, leading to erroneous dating.

On MRI, subdural hematomas exhibit a signal evolution similar to that seen with intraparenchymal hemorrhages, but the pace of evolution is different due to a slower decrease of the oxygen content within the hematoma. Acute subdural hematomas (Fig. 40.67) are initially isointense on T1 and hyperintense on T2, but as deoxyhemoglobin appears, the signal on T2-weighted images becomes hypointense. In the subacute phase, the signal is hyperintense on T1 and hypointense on T2, but in the late subacute stage, the signal will be hyperintense on both T1- and T2-weighted images because of extracellular methemoglobin (Fig. 40.68). It is important to remember that these stages are not separated sharply, and mixed patterns are often seen; this is due to the presence of oxy- and deoxyhemoglobin in the acute stage and intra- and extracellular methemoglobin in the chronic stage. Rebleeding into an existing subdural hematoma may also occur, resulting in the presence of clots of various ages.

Chronic subdural hematomas (Fig. 40.69) are hypointense relative to the brain but, having higher protein content, are mildly hyperintense relative to the CSF on T1-weighted images and hyperintense on T2-weighted images. Hemosiderin deposition is not as prominent as in parenchymal hemorrhages because macrophages tend to be cleared by the meningeal circulation. Chronic subdural hematomas may look similar to hyperacute ones on noncontrast images, but because of their vascular membrane, with gadolinium they exhibit enhancement along their periphery. On CT, chronic subdural hematomas appear as hypodense subdural collections. Mass effect is variable depending on the size of the hematoma and degree of cerebral atrophy. If repeated hemorrhage occurs into the subdural collection, the hyperdense fresh blood is seen within the chronic hypodense collection (Fig. 40.70).

***Epidural hemorrhage.*** Contrary to subdural hematoma, epidural hemorrhage is usually arterial in origin and due to laceration of a meningeal artery, most commonly the middle meningeal artery. Epidural hematomas are often lens shaped, respect cranial suture lines, and sometimes the dura itself is seen as a linear structure pushed toward the brain. The evolution of CT and MRI signal characteristics is similar to that of subdural hematomas.

***Cortical contusion.*** Cerebral contusions result from the brain hitting against the inner table of the skull or sliding against the bony ridges of the base of the skull. The most common locations include the poles and inferior surfaces of the frontal, temporal, and occipital lobes. The injured brain parenchyma exhibits foci of hemorrhage and varying degrees of edema, which may progress later to more confluent hematoma and more swelling. On CT, acute contusions appear as foci of hyperdense hemorrhage with or without swelling. The hematomas

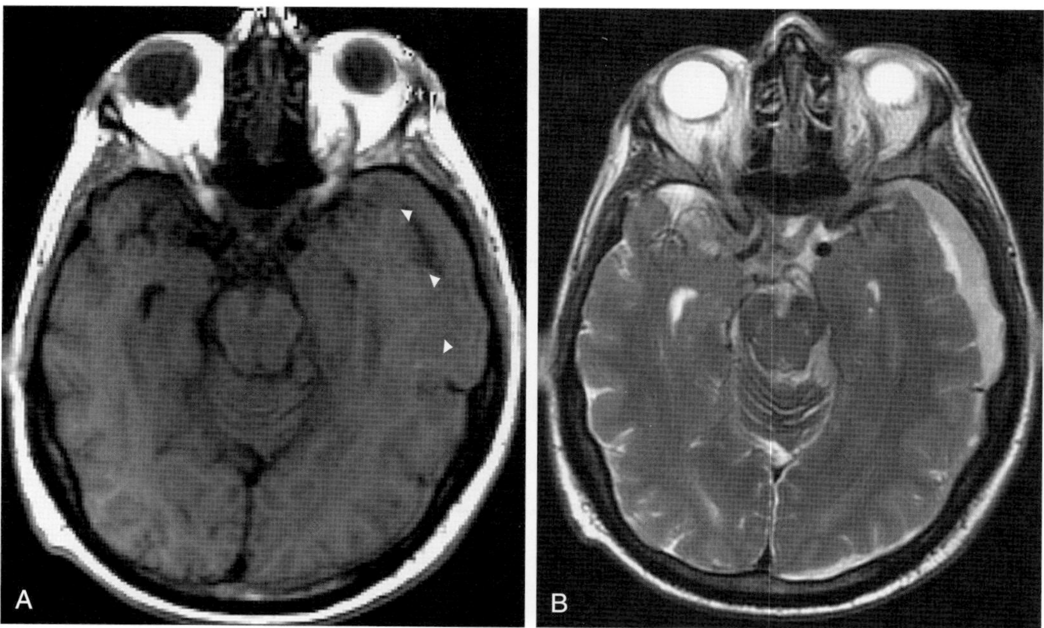

**Fig. 40.67 Acute Subdural Hematoma. A,** Axial noncontrast T1-weighted image shows a subdural collection over the left temporal lobe, which is isointense to the brain parenchyma and therefore somewhat difficult to notice *(arrowheads)*. **B,** Axial T2-weighted image helps by revealing a much more obvious hyperintense subdural collection in the same area.

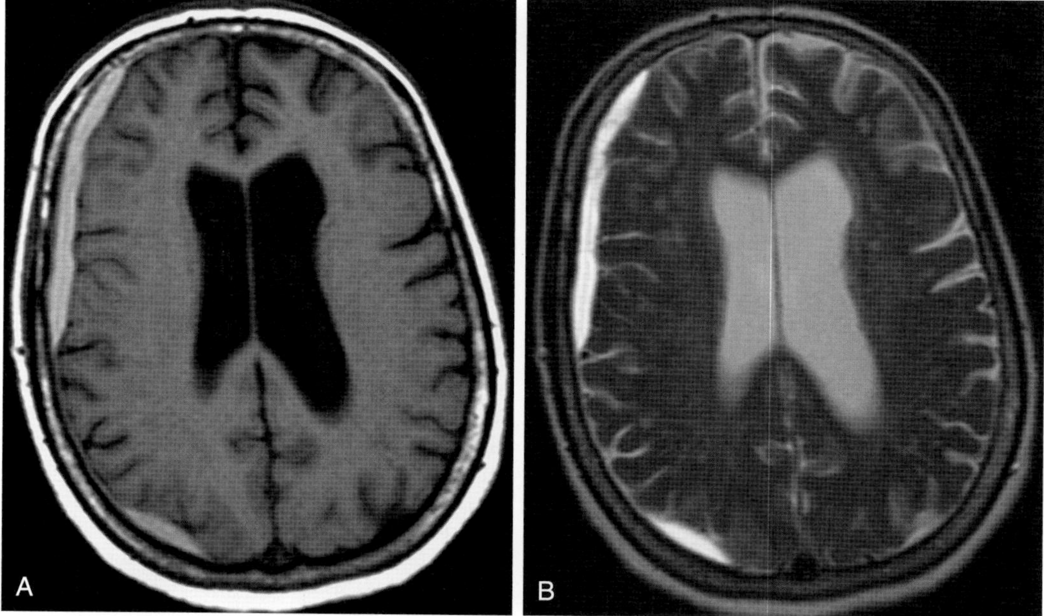

**Fig. 40.68 Subacute Subdural Hematoma. A,** On axial T1-weighted image, the subacute subdural hematoma over the right frontal and parietal lobes is hyperintense and easily noticeable. **B,** On axial T2-weighted image, the hematoma is also hyperintense.

get reabsorbed later, and the swelling decreases. In the chronic stage, no residual findings or varying degrees of encephalomalacia may be seen. On MRI, with the appearance of deoxyhemoglobin, a hypointense signal is seen on T2; the surrounding edema is hyperintense on T2 and FLAIR sequences (Fig. 40.71). Later, in the subacute stage, extracellular methemoglobin is hyperintense on T1- and T2-weighted images. Gradient echo and susceptibility-weighted images are very useful to show the hemorrhagic component of the lesion. Chronic contusions are associated with encephalomalacic cavities of various sizes, exhibiting CSF signal characteristics and surrounded by a hyperintense rim of reactive gliosis on T2 and FLAIR sequences. Variable degrees of hemosiderin deposition appear hypointense on FLAIR, gradient echo, and SWI.

***Diffuse axonal injury.*** The underlying pathomechanism of this entity is shearing injury of the white matter pathways. This may involve the corpus callosum or other fiber tracts of the corona radiata

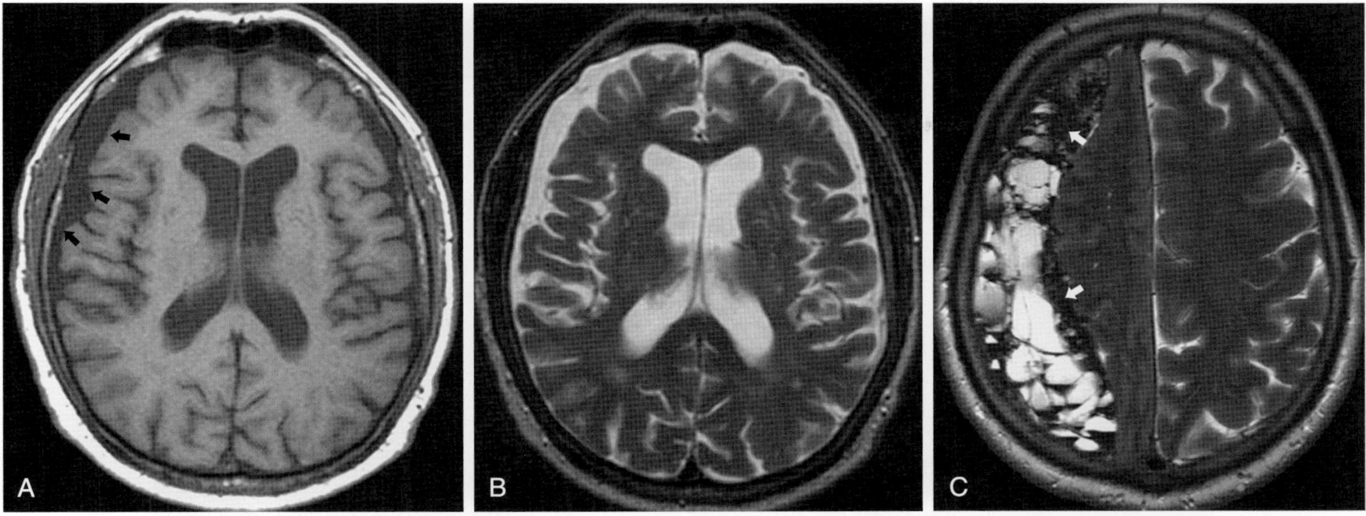


**Fig. 40.69 Chronic Subdural Hematoma. A,** Axial T1-weighted image reveals a right frontal chronic subdural hematoma with signal similar to cerebrospinal fluid *(arrows)*. **B,** On axial T2-weighted image, the chronic hematoma is hyperintense. **C,** Axial T2-weighted image of a different case. Within the hyperintense subdural collection, multiple hypointense zones are seen; these are due to hemosiderin deposition *(arrows)*. There is prominent mass effect on the hemisphere.

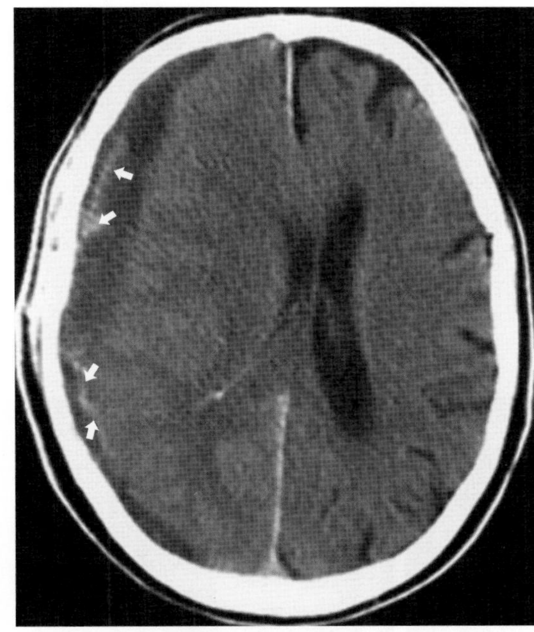

**Fig. 40.70 Chronic Subdural Hematoma on Computed Tomography (CT).** Axial noncontrast CT scan shows a hypodense subdural collection over the right frontal and parietal lobes. Right hemisphere is compressed, and midline shift is present. Note hyperdense areas within the subdural collection, suggestive of another more recent bleeding episode *(arrows)*.

and centrum semiovale, and may also involve the brainstem. The changes on structural neuroimaging can be very subtle, usually in the few-millimeter size range. Such lesions are usually not detected by CT. MRI is the study of choice. On MRI, the lesions appear as foci of hyperintensity seen on T2 and FLAIR sequences. Foci of hemorrhage (usually microbleeds) are also present. For detection of the microbleeds associated with axonal injury, gradient echo or susceptibility-weighted images (Fig. 40.72) are the most sensitive (Li and Feng, 2009).

***Cerebral parenchymal hematoma.*** The imaging appearance of cerebral hematomas is discussed in the section "Hemorrhagic Cerebrovascular Disease." As described there, for detection of smaller hemorrhagic lesions or microbleeds, gradient echo or SWI are the most sensitive techniques and should be part of every trauma imaging protocol.

### Metabolic and Toxic Disorders

This section is available at http://www.expertconsult.com. Refer to Chapters 84–87 for further discussions of these topics. 

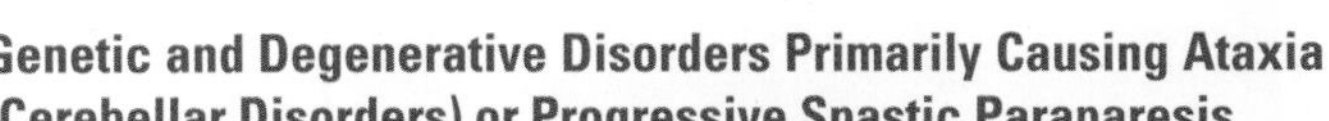

### Genetic and Degenerative Disorders Primarily Causing Ataxia (Cerebellar Disorders) or Progressive Spastic Paraparesis

Structural neuroimaging has a limited role in the evaluation of hereditary and degenerative spinocerebellar disorders. The neurological examination, family history, and genetic testing are most helpful in finding the specific diagnosis, whereas imaging usually has a supportive role—for instance, by defining the degree of involvement of the pontine nuclei in the differential diagnosis of olivopontocerebellar atrophy. Nevertheless, imaging is almost always obtained in patients who present with progressive ataxia or spastic paraparesis for the purpose of ruling out other potential causes, such as an enlarging posterior fossa neoplasm. In addition, certain spastic or ataxic disorders (hereditary spastic paraplegia with a thin corpus callosum, multiple system atrophy (MSA), spinocerebellar ataxias (SCA), Friedreich ataxia, ataxia-telangiectasia, fragile X premutation syndrome) may present with characteristic MRI changes.

These are discussed in the online version of this chapter, available at http://www.expertconsult.com. Refer to Chapter 23 for a review of ataxic disorders. 

### Genetic and Degenerative Disorders Primarily Causing Parkinsonism or Other Movement Disorders

Structural neuroimaging has a limited role in the evaluation of parkinsonian syndromes and other movement disorders. Diagnosis of these entities is still largely dependent on a detailed

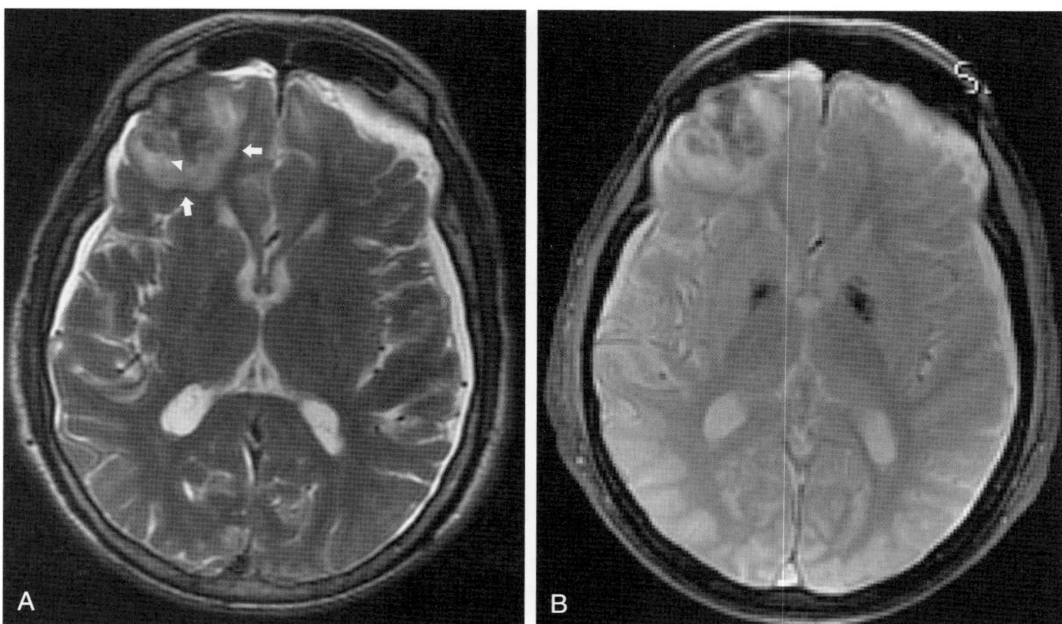


**Fig. 40.71 Contusion With Subdural Hematoma. A,** Axial T2-weighted image demonstrates an area of mixed signal change in the right frontal lobe *(arrows)*. Its center contains hypointense hemorrhagic changes *(arrowhead)* and is surrounded by hyperintense edema. Note coexisting bilateral traumatic subdural hematomas. **B,** Gradient echo image reveals more clearly a hypointense signal in the center of the contusion, owing to the presence of blood degradation products.

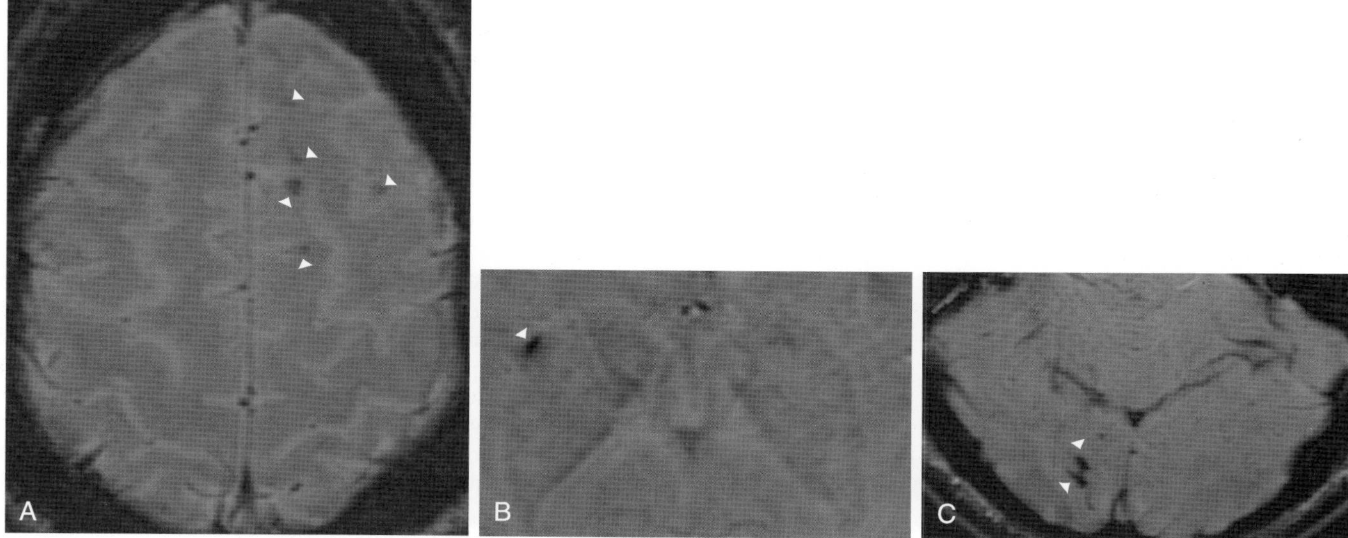


**Fig. 40.72 Diffuse Axonal Injury.** Magnetic resonance image from a 42-year-old assault victim. Susceptibility-weighted images reveal multiple hypointense areas *(arrowheads)* in the left frontal lobe **(A)**, right external capsule **(B)**, and right occipital lobe **(C)**. These are areas of microbleeds associated with axonal injury.

history and thorough neurological examination. In equivocal cases or in the academic/research setting, functional imaging has shown value in the evaluation of various movement disorders. Nevertheless, structural imaging is frequently obtained in patients presenting with movement disorders, and it is therefore necessary to discuss the potential structural imaging findings in the most common parkinsonian syndromes and other common movement disorder syndromes.

This discussion is available online at http://www.expertconsult.com. Refer to Chapter 96 on movement disorders.

## Degenerative Disorders Primarily Causing Dementia

***Age-related involutional changes.*** The aging brain displays multiple potential changes that usually are of no clinical significance but should be distinguished from pathological processes (Fig. 40.78). Many of these findings appear on CT, but, in general, MRI is more sensitive as to their extent and nature. Cerebral volume loss is commonly seen in the elderly brain (prevalence is 50% in the eighth decade), even in the absence of neurological signs or symptoms. Atrophy involves the hemispheres, mostly the frontal lobes, as revealed by prominence of the sulci, but enlargement of the cisterns, sylvian fissures, and third and lateral ventricles is also frequent.

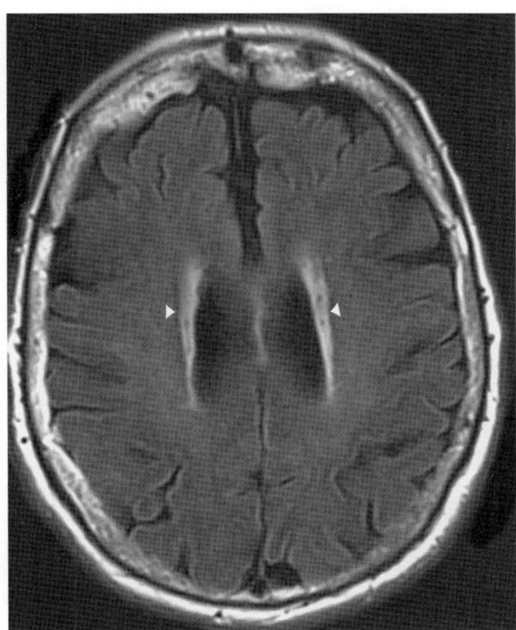

**Fig. 40.78 Normal Aging.** Magnetic resonance image of a cognitively intact 85-year-old person. There is linear T2 hyperintense signal bordering the bodies of the lateral ventricles. It has a smooth outer margin *(arrowheads)*, most likely representing ependymal cell loss and gliosis. Faint ground-glass T2 hyperintensity is seen in the white matter, likely due to microvascular changes. Note the mild frontal lobe atrophy. There is some thickening and fatty marrow transformation of the calvarium.

T2 hyperintense signal changes in the hemispheres are another common finding. A typical pattern is "capping" of the frontal horns, with or without additional signal changes along the borders of the lateral ventricles, seen as a T2 hyperintense lining that has a smooth outer margin. These findings are believed to be related to ependymal cell loss and gliosis. Scattered T2 hyperintense areas of signal change that are of variable size and shape are also commonly found within the cerebral hemispheric white matter in both PV and subcortical locations. These patches of abnormal signal may be due to dilation of periarteriolar spaces or to ischemic demyelination and gliosis and can result from hypertension, narrowing of small vessels, hypoxia, hypoperfusion, or small emboli. In many individuals these are asymptomatic, and their clinical prognostic significance as well as their relation to the more extensive symptomatic microangiopathy, leukoaraiosis, and Binswanger disease has been debated.

Normal aging at times may also be accompanied by iron deposition in the brain. This appears as symmetrical hypointense signal on susceptibility sensitive sequences, the most commonly affected structures being the globus pallidus, substantia nigra, red nuclei, and dentate nuclei. Iron deposition in the putamen may later occur.

Enlargement of the perivascular spaces may be noted at any age, but it is seen more commonly in the elderly. These enlarged spaces follow CSF signal characteristics and are often seen in the basal ganglia region at the level of the anterior commissure, but also in the hemispheres within the centrum semiovale. They should not be mistaken for chronic lacunar ischemic lesions.

For further discussion of the imaging characteristics of perivascular spaces, see the section "Nonneoplastic Congenital Cystic Lesions," available at http://www.expertconsult.com.

***Alzheimer disease.*** CT and MR imaging may provide helpful findings in AD, in addition to excluding other pathologies that can also lead to cognitive decline, such as stroke or tumors (Masdeu and Pascual). Atrophy begins in the entorhinal cortex, eventually involving the rest of the anterior and medial part of the temporal lobes and progressing through the limbic structures to the neocortex. Insular cortex is affected early, while paracentral cortex is resistant to the disease. The temporal horns and sylvian fissures are frequently enlarged. It is important to remember that volume loss occurs in the aging brain; at times, patients with marked atrophy are asymptomatic, whereas patients with mild or moderate AD may have little volume loss, at least by visual inspection. Computerized volumetric analysis of the hippocampal formation and other brain regions is a more precise way to measure atrophy. Various volumetric methods have been developed to study cerebral volume loss in AD and other dementias (Nestor et al., 2008). Measurement of cortical thickness has been suggested as a biomarker of atrophy. Calculation of cortical thickness average in multiple regions of interest has been used to predict development of dementia in cognitively intact individuals (Dickerson et al., 2011). Both open-source and commercial software packages are available to quantify regional brain atrophy, such as FreeSurfer (http://surfer.nmr.mgh.harvard.edu), the Functional Imaging of the Brain Software Library (http://www.fmrib.ox.ac.uk/fsl), and NeuroQuant (CorTechs Labs, LaJolla, CA). eFig. 40.79 demonstrates a case of AD, where the NeuroQuant volumetric analysis reveals the typical findings of significantly reduced hippocampal volume and resultant enlargement of the inferior portion of the lateral ventricle. PET findings, more helpful than MRI to characterize AD, are discussed in Chapter 42.

***Frontotemporal lobar degeneration, including Pick disease.*** Frontotemporal lobar degeneration (FTLD) is a category of dementing illness with different clinical subtypes: behavioral-type FTLD and primary progressive aphasia (PPA). Within the PPA type, three subtypes are distinguished: nonfluent/agrammatic, semantic, and logopenic. Formerly, *Pick disease* was a term used for the clinical syndromes now encompassed by FTLD, but it is currently used to refer to only one of the several types of pathology that cause these conditions. FTLD subtypes, just like AD, cannot be diagnosed with structural neuroimaging, but CT and MRI show changes that can assist in differentiating them from each other and other dementias, as well as excluding other etiologies (Masdeu and Pascual, 2016). A characteristic finding in these dementias is atrophy of the frontal and temporal lobes, which may be asymmetrical or symmetrical. Semantic dementia causes most often prominent asymmetrical atrophy of the left temporal pole (eFig. 40.80). Primary progressive prosopagnosia affects the right temporal lobe (eFig. 40.81). When frontotemporal dementia is advanced, gyral atrophy may be so prominent that it has been termed *knife-edge atrophy* (eFig. 40.82).

## Neurocutaneous Syndromes

Structural neuroimaging features of the neurocutaneous syndromes (NF, hamartoma, neurofibroma, tuberous sclerosis [Bourneville disease], cortical tubers, subependymal nodules, white matter lesions, von Hippel-Lindau disease, Sturge-Weber syndrome) are discussed in the online version of this chapter, available at http://www.expertconsult.com. Refer to Chapter 99 for further review of this topic.

## Congenital Anomalies of the Brain

This topic is available in the online version of the chapter at http://www.expertconsult.com.

## Nonneoplastic Congenital Cystic Lesions

Nonneoplastic congenital cystic lesions are discussed online at http://www.expertconsult.com.

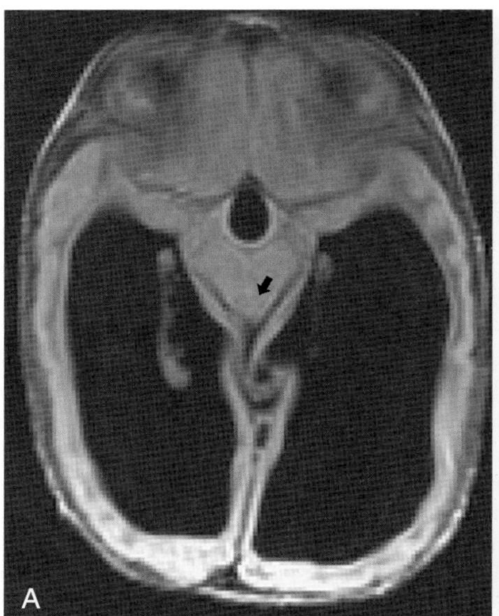


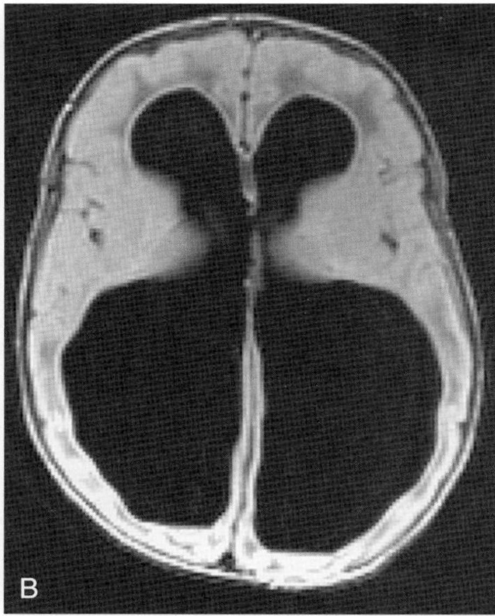


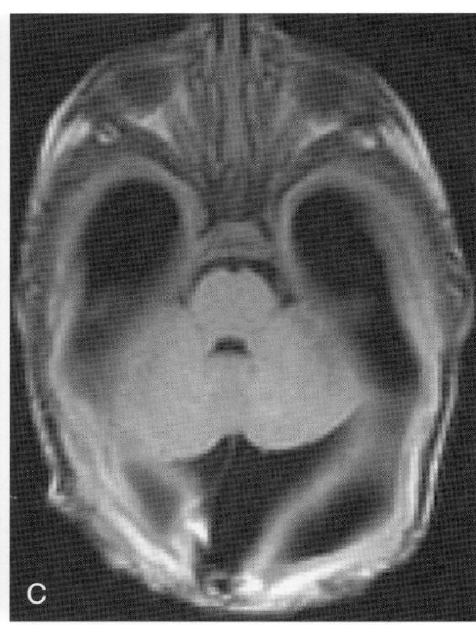


**Fig. 40.99 Obstructive Hydrocephalus. A–C,** In this case of congenital obstructive hydrocephalus, the cerebral aqueduct appears stenotic *(small arrow)*. There is extreme dilatation of the third and lateral ventricles, with the cerebral tissue being extremely thinned. The fourth ventricle is normal in size.

### Vascular Malformations

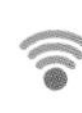

The various vascular malformations (AVMs, cavernous malformations, developmental venous anomaly [DVA], and capillary telangiectasia) are discussed in the online version of this chapter, available at http://www.expertconsult.com. See Chapters 66 and 67 for further review.

### Cerebrospinal Fluid Circulation Disorders

Abnormalities in CSF and intraspinal cord flow cause changes in the brain or spinal cord that are readily identifiable by CT or MRI. Hydrocephalus is an abnormal intracranial accumulation of CSF that interferes with normal brain function (see Chapter 88). It should be distinguished from dilation of the ventricles and subarachnoid space due to decreased brain volume, which can be normal or pathological and has been called *hydrocephalus ex vacuo*. We will avoid using this term, because true hydrocephalus often requires treatment by shunting. Hydrocephalus may follow increased CSF production or impaired resorption. Resorption occurs not only via the pacchionian granulations in the venous sinuses but also through the brain lymphatic system. Traditionally, two main types of hydrocephalus are distinguished: obstructive and nonobstructive. Nonobstructive hydrocephalus is due to increased CSF production, as with choroid plexus papillomas in children. Depending on whether CSF flow from the ventricular system to the subarachnoid space is intact or impeded, we can distinguish between communicating and noncommunicating types of obstructive hydrocephalus. Some processes increase CSF ICP but not the volume of intracranial CSF, causing the syndrome of idiopathic intracranial hypertension (known as *pseudotumor cerebri*). Interruption of CSF circulation can also happen at the craniocervical junction, where pathologies that interfere with the return of CSF from the spinal subarachnoid space to the intracranial compartment, as happens in the Chiari malformations, can arise. Finally, CSF intracranial volume may be abnormally reduced, causing the syndrome of intracranial hypotension.

***Obstructive, noncommunicating hydrocephalus.*** Depending on the site of obstruction, various segments of the ventricular system will enlarge. Obstruction at the foramen of Monro causes unilateral or bilateral enlargement of the lateral ventricles. Aqueductal stenosis, which may be congenital, leads to enlargement of the third and lateral ventricles, but the fourth ventricle is normal in size (Fig. 40.99). Obstruction of the foramina of Luschka and Magendie results in enlargement of the third, fourth, and lateral ventricles. Other possible imaging findings include thinning and upward bowing of the corpus callosum. In third ventricle enlargement, the optic and infundibular recesses are widened. When the evolution of the hydrocephalus is rapid, transependymal CSF flow induces a T2 hyperintense signal (best seen on FLAIR sequences) along the walls of the involved ventricular segments, and in the case of the lateral ventricles, most pronounced at the frontal horns.

***Normal-pressure hydrocephalus.*** In this type of hydrocephalus, there is enlargement of the ventricles, most pronounced for the third and lateral ventricles (Fig. 40.100). The subarachnoid spaces at the top of the convexity are typically compressed, but the larger sulci, such as the interhemispheric sulcus and the sylvian fissure, may be dilated as well as the ventricles (Kitagaki et al., 1998). In this case, the cross-sections of the dilated sulci often have the appearance of a "U" rather than the appearance of a "V" characteristic of atrophy. These morphological findings are more helpful than flow studies. Increased CSF flow in the cerebral aqueduct may cause a hypointense "jet-flow" sign on all sequences. Quantitative CSF flow studies (cine phase-contrast MR imaging) are frequently used for evaluation of patients with suspected normal-pressure hydrocephalus. However, the distinction between using MRI to diagnose normal-pressure hydrocephalus versus determining the probability of clinical improvement from shunt placement should be kept in mind, as studies seem to show that MRI may be better at the former than the latter. Although CSF flow studies had been thought to help to predict shunt responsiveness (Bradley et al., 1996), later studies have challenged this view (Dixon et al., 2002; Kahlon et al., 2007). Traditionally it has been hypothesized that in this condition there is a problem with CSF absorption at the level of the arachnoid granulations, since normal-pressure hydrocephalus has been observed as a late complication after meningitis or subarachnoid hemorrhage that caused meningeal involvement/scarring. But this syndrome, often associated with vascular disease in older people, may also be the result of decreased superficial venous compliance and a

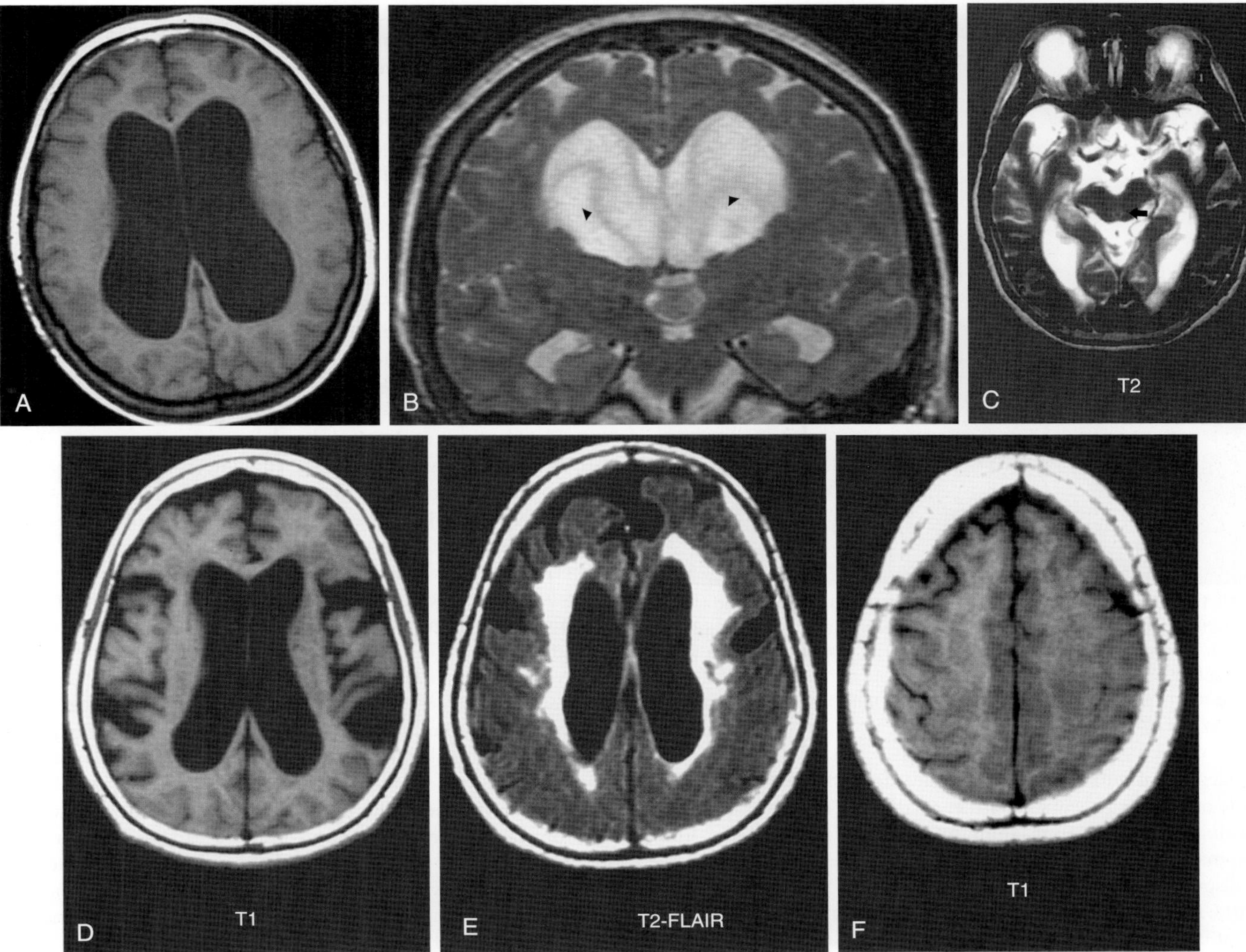


**Fig. 40.100 Two Cases of Normal-Pressure Hydrocephalus.** In the first case (**A**) axial noncontrast T1-weighted images demonstrate significant enlargement of the ventricles, which is clearly out of proportion to the size of the superficial cerebrospinal fluid (CSF) spaces. The parietal sulci appear somewhat effaced. **B**, Coronal T2-weighted image also exhibits prominent ventricular enlargement. Note intraventricular artifact due to CSF pulsation *(arrowheads)*, indicating hyperdynamic flow. The second case demonstrates communicating hydrocephalus. Images **C–F** are axial sections of the MRI from a 71-year-old woman with progressive gait and cognitive impairment, as well as urinary incontinence. Note the low signal in the sylvian aqueduct, owing to a flow void from high-velocity CSF flow through this structure (**C**, *arrow*). Although basal cisterns (**C**) and interhemispheric and sylvian fissures (**D, E**) are dilated, sulci in the high convexity (**F**) are compressed. Trans-ependymal reabsorption of CSF, suggested by the homogeneous high signal in the periventricular white matter (**E**), need not occur in all cases of symptomatic hydrocephalus. In addition to the compressed sulci in the convexity, the U-shape of some of the dilated sulci (**E**, *white arrows*) is helpful to make the diagnosis.

reduction in the blood flow returning via the sagittal sinus (Bateman, 2008). The term *normal pressure* is a misnomer because long-term monitoring of ventricular pressure has shown recurrent episodes of transient pressure elevation.

***Chiari malformation.*** Depending on associated structural abnormalities, different types of Chiari malformation are distinguished. In the most common, type 1 Chiari, there is caudal displacement of the tip of the cerebellar tonsils 5 mm or more below the level of the foramen magnum. Most often this malformation is accompanied by a congenitally small posterior fossa. However, acquired forms of tonsillar descent also exist, either due to space-occupying intracranial pathology or to a low-pressure environment in the spinal canal, such as after lumboperitoneal shunt placement. In typical Chiari 1, the ectopic cerebellar tonsils are frequently peg shaped, but otherwise the cerebellum is of normal morphology. There is usually crowding of the structures at the level of the foramen magnum. The 5-mm diagnostic cutoff value has been selected in adults, as this condition tends to be symptomatic and clinically significant at this or higher measured values. If the tonsils are caudal to the level of the foramen magnum by less than 5 mm, the term *low-lying cerebellar tonsils* is used; this is frequently an asymptomatic incidental finding. When evaluating younger patients or children, it is to be remembered that the considered "normal" position of the cerebellar tonsils is different in the various age groups. In the first decade, 6 mm below the foramen magnum is considered the upper limit of normal, and with increasing age, there is an "ascent" of the tonsils, with a 5-mm cutoff value in the second and

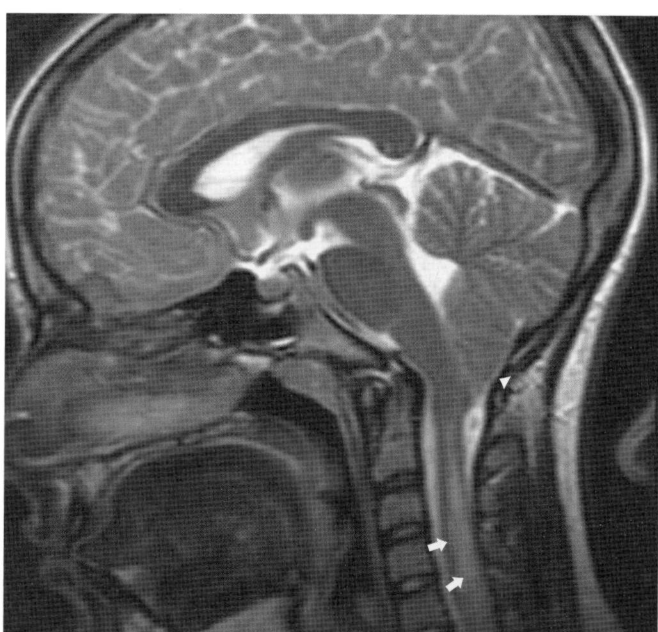

**Fig. 40.101 Chiari Type 1 Malformation.** Sagittal T2-weighted image demonstrates caudal displacement of the cerebellar tonsil through the foramen magnum into the cervical spinal canal *(arrowhead)*. The tonsil is characteristically peg-shaped. There is a prominent longitudinal hyperintense cavity in the visualized cervical spinal cord segment, consistent with a syrinx *(arrows)*.

third decades, 4 mm up to the eighth decade, and 3 mm in the ninth decade of life (for review see Nash et al., 2002). Tonsillar ectopia and crowding at the foramen magnum interfere with return of CSF from the spinal to the intracranial subarachnoid space. This may lead, by still-disputed mechanisms, to syrinx formation in the spinal cord (Fig. 40.101). If there is imaging evidence of a Chiari malformation on brain MRI, it is essential to image the cervical and thoracic cord to rule out a syrinx.

In Chiari type 2 malformation, there is a developmental abnormality of the hindbrain and caudal displacement not only of the cerebellar tonsils but also the cerebellum, medulla, and fourth ventricle. The cervical spinal nerve roots are stretched/compressed, and there is often a spinal cord syrinx present. Other abnormalities include lumbar or thoracic myelomeningocele; hydrocephalus is often present as well. Chiari type 3 malformation is an even more severe developmental abnormality, with cervical myelomeningocele or encephalocele.

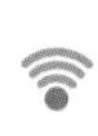

For a description of idiopathic intracranial hypertension (pseudotumor cerebri) and of the imaging sequelae of intracranial hypotension, see the online version of this chapter at http://www.expertconsult.com.

### Orbital Lesions

The structural neuroimaging of orbital lesions is discussed online at http://www.expertconsult.com.

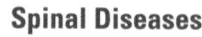

## Spinal Diseases

### Spinal Tumors

Tumors affecting the spinal region can be classified according to their predominant location, intrinsic to the vertebral column itself or within the spinal canal. Spinal canal tumors may be intramedullary or extramedullary. Intramedullary tumors involve the spinal cord parenchyma, whereas extramedullary tumors are outside the spinal cord but within the spinal canal. Depending on their relation to the dura, extramedullary tumors may be classified as intradural or extradural. As tumors grow, they can spread to other compartments. For example, metastases in the vertebral bodies often extend to the epidural space and cause spinal cord compression. Tumors in pre- and paravertebral locations may also extend to the extradural space, either through the vertebral bodies, as happens with metastatic lung cancer, or through the neural foramina, as in lymphoma.

***Vertebral metastases, extradural tumors.*** In the majority of cases, tumors involving the vertebrae are metastatic in origin. Half of all vertebral metastatic tumors are from lung, breast (Fig. 40.106), and prostate cancer. Kidney and gastrointestinal tumors, melanoma, and those arising from the female reproductive organs are other common sources. Of all structural neuroimaging techniques, MRI is the imaging modality of choice to evaluate vertebral metastases, with sensitivity equal to and specificity better than bone scan (Mechtler and Cohen, 2000). MR imaging protocols for the evaluation of vertebral metastases typically include T1-weighted images with and without gadolinium, T2-weighted images, and STIR sequences. Typically, osteolytic metastases appear as hypointense foci on noncontrast T1-weighted images, hyperintense signal on T2 and STIR sequences, and enhance on postcontrast images. The enhancement may render the previously T1 hypointense metastatic foci isointense, interfering with their detection. Therefore, precontrast T1-weighted images should always be obtained as well. Osteoblastic metastases, such as seen in prostate cancer, are hypointense on T2-weighted images. Besides the vertebral bodies, metastases preferentially involve the pedicles. With marked involvement, the vertebral body may collapse.

Extradural tumors most commonly result from spread of metastatic tumors to the epidural space, directly from the vertebral body or from the prevertebral/paravertebral space. These mass lesions in the epidural space initially indent the thecal sac, and, as they grow, they displace and eventually compress the spinal cord or cauda equina. If spinal cord compression is long-standing and severe enough, T2 hyperintense signal change may appear in the involved cord segment as a result of edema and/or ischemia secondary to compromised local circulation. An example of tumor spread from a paravertebral focus is lymphoma, which may extend into the spinal canal through the neural foramen. When intraspinal extension is suspected in a patient with lymphoma, MRI is the study of choice (Fig. 40.107). In cases of epithelial tumors, by the time of presentation, plain radiographs reveal the intraspinal extension with more than 80% sensitivity, but in patients with lymphoma, plain radiographs are still normal in almost 70% of cases (Mechtler and Cohen, 2000).

In the smaller group of extradural primary spinal tumors, multiple myeloma is the most common in adults. Involvement of the vertebral bone marrow may occur in multiple small foci, but diffuse involvement of an entire vertebral body is also possible. Myelomatous lesions are hypointense on T1-, hyperintense on T2-weighted images, and highly hyperintense on STIR sequences. There is marked enhancement after gadolinium administration.

***Extramedullary intradural spinal tumors.*** This group of tumors includes leptomeningeal metastases, meningiomas, nerve sheath tumors, embryonal tumors (teratoma), congenital cysts (epidermoid, dermoid), and lipoma.

***Leptomeningeal metastases.*** Leptomeningeal metastases result from tumor cell infiltration of the leptomeningeal layers (pia and arachnoid). Non-Hodgkin lymphoma, leukemia, breast and lung cancer, melanoma, and gastrointestinal cancers are the most common sources of metastases. Leptomeningeal seeding also occurs from primary CNS tumors such as malignant gliomas, ependymoma,

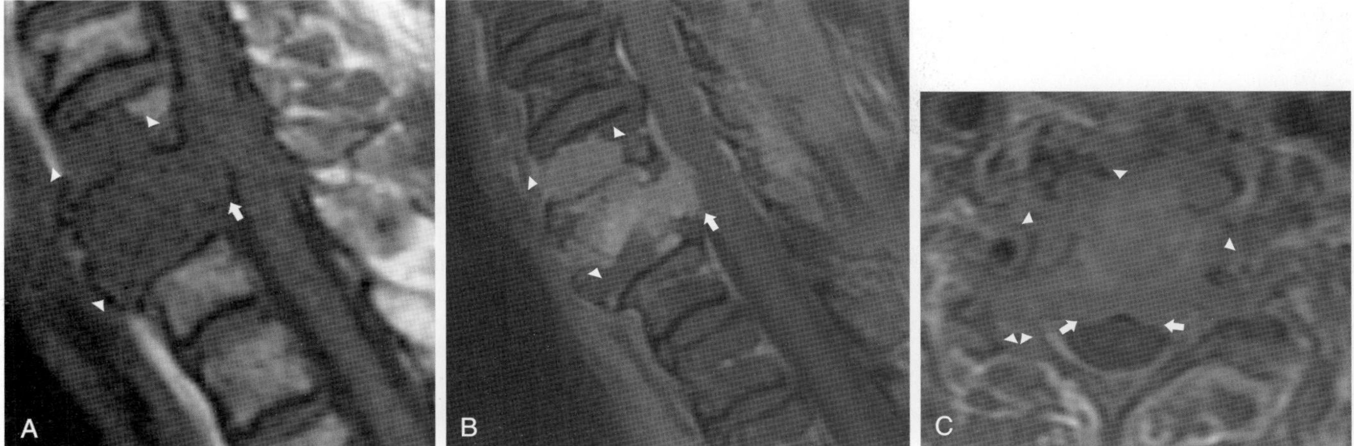


**Fig. 40.106 Spinal Metastasis.** MRI from a 52-year-old woman with breast cancer. **A,** Sagittal T1-weighted image reveals hypointense signal in two adjacent vertebral bodies *(arrowheads)*. Metastatic mass extends beyond the vertebral bodies into the epidural space *(arrow)*. **B,** Sagittal T1-weighted, fat-suppressed post-contrast image better delineates the extent of the tumor. **C,** Axial postcontrast image demonstrates tumor spread toward the pre- and paravertebral space *(arrowheads)*, into the epidural space *(small arrows)* and into the pedicle *(double arrowheads)*.

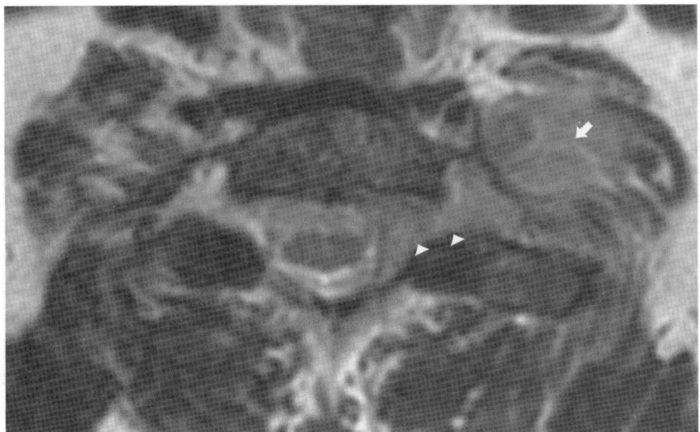

**Fig. 40.107 Lymphoma.** A left paravertebral tumor *(arrow)* extends through the left neural foramen into the cervical spinal canal *(arrowheads)*.

and neuroblastomas. The optimal imaging modality to detect leptomeningeal seeding is gadolinium-enhanced MRI, which reveals linear or multifocal nodular enhancing lesions along the surface of the spinal cord or nerve roots. The diagnostic yield can be improved by using higher doses of gadolinium.

***Spinal meningiomas.*** Most (90%) spinal meningiomas are intradural, but extradural extension also occurs. The tumors displace/compress the spinal cord or nerve roots. MRI signal characteristics can be variable: they often exhibit isointense signal to the spinal cord on both T1- and T2-weighted images, but T2 hypointensity may also be seen. Similar to intracranial meningiomas, these tumors enhance in an intense homogeneous fashion (Fig. 40.108). In patients with NF type 2, the entire spine should be imaged because multiple meningiomas may be present.

Nerve sheath tumors and embryonal tumors that belong to this group of spinal tumors are described in the online version of this chapter, available at http://www.expertconsult.com.

***Intramedullary tumors.*** The most common primary spinal cord tumors are astrocytomas and ependymomas, representing 80%–90% of all primary malignancies. For best structural assessment of intramedullary tumors (primary and metastatic), MR imaging with and without gadolinium should be obtained.

***Ependymoma.*** Ependymomas are more common in males and in about 50% of cases involve the lower spinal cord in the region of the conus medullaris and cauda equina. The myxopapillary type arises from the ependymal remnants of the filum terminale. Ependymomas are usually well demarcated and may exhibit a T1 and T2 hypointense pseudocapsule. This is important from a surgical standpoint, because these tumors may usually be removed with minimal injury to the surrounding cord parenchyma. The involved cord is expanded. On T1-weighted images, ependymomas are usually isointense to the spinal cord or, rarely, hypointense. On T2-weighted images, they are usually hyperintense relative to the spinal cord. The tumor may have a hemorrhagic component as well, in which case the signal characteristic is usually heterogeneous, depending on the stage of the hemorrhage. Ependymomas are often associated with a rostral or caudal cyst, which is hypointense on T1- and hyperintense on T2-weighted images. With gadolinium, intense homogeneous enhancement is seen within the solid portion of the tumor.

***Astrocytoma.*** Astrocytomas occur in both the pediatric and adult populations. Their peak incidence is in the third to fifth decades of life. They have a preference for the thoracic cord segments. Up to three quarters are low grade. They exhibit T1 hypointensity and appear hyperintense on T2-weighted images. Although the tumor margin is usually poorly defined, subtotal resection is often possible. A cyst or syringomyelic cavity is associated with spinal cord astrocytoma in up to 50% of cases. Contrary to intracranial low-grade gliomas, spinal astrocytomas typically enhance, often in a heterogeneous fashion (Fig. 40.110).

***Intramedullary metastases.*** Lung and breast cancer are the most common sources of intramedullary metastases, but lymphoma, colorectal cancer, and renal cell cancer may also metastasize to the cord. Metastases have some preference for the conus medullaris but may be multiple in 10% of cases and involve other cord segments as well. Their signal intensity varies; mucus-containing breast or colon cancer metastases can be hyperintense on noncontrast T1-weighted images. On postcontrast images, intense enhancement is seen, which may be homogeneous or ringlike. Associated edema is frequently seen as surrounding T1 hypointensity and T2 hyperintensity. The cord may be expanded to variable degrees.

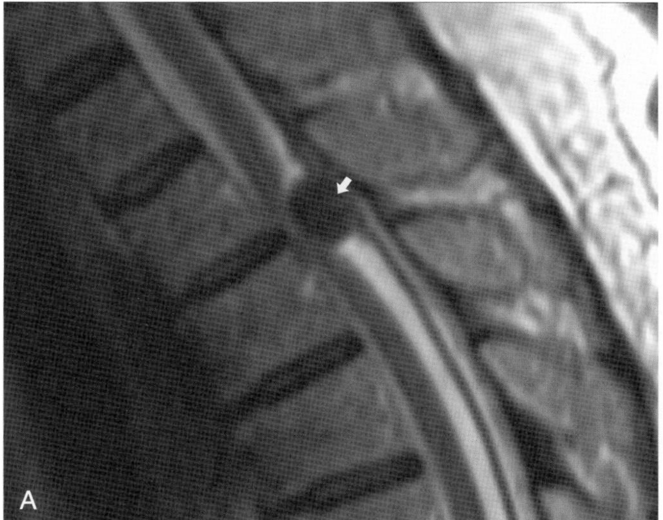


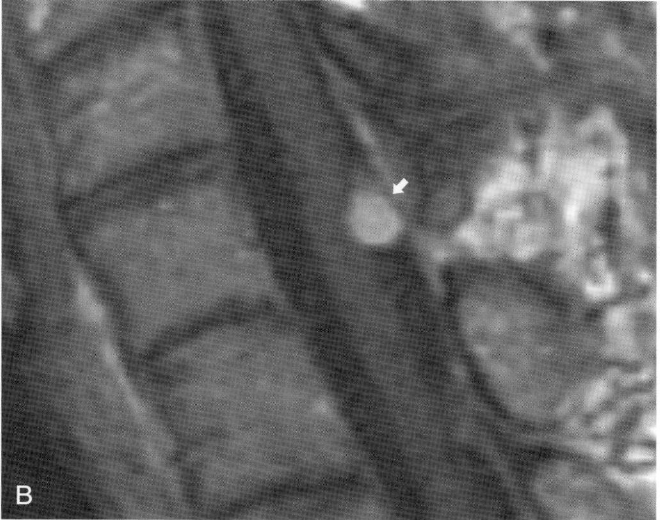


**Fig. 40.108 Two Cases of Meningioma. A,** Sagittal T2-weighted image demonstrates a hypointense extramedullary dural-based mass lesion that causes marked spinal cord compression *(arrow)*. **B,** Sagittal T1-weighted postcontrast image reveals an extramedullary dural-based mass lesion in a similar location. The mass enhances homogeneously *(arrow)*.

## Vascular Disease

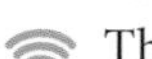

This section is available online at http://www.expertconsult.com. Refer to Chapter 69.

## Infection

Infections of the spine may involve the disk spaces as well as the vertebral bodies. Neurological emergency occurs when the infection proceeds to the epidural space, leading to abscess formation that can result in spinal cord compression.

***Diskitis and osteomyelitis.*** The most common pathogen responsible for diskitis and osteomyelitis is *Staphylococcus aureus*. The most common route of transmission is hematogenous, and in these cases the lumbar spine is involved most frequently, usually at the L3/4 or L4/5 levels. Contiguous spread of infection may also occur, and postoperative causes (such as after instrumentation) have been documented as well. In adults the diskitis/osteomyelitis complex generally begins with infection of the subchondral bone marrow inferior to the cartilage endplate. Infection of the subchondral region of a vertebral body results in subsequent perforation of the vertebral endplate, leading to infection of the intervertebral disk, or diskitis. The infected disk decreases in height and in conjunction with spread of infection through the disk, the adjacent vertebral body is infected. In children, a direct hematogenous route to the disk can cause diskitis to occur before the development of osteomyelitis. Diskitis and osteomyelitis are typically hypointense relative to normal disks and vertebrae on T1-weighted images and hyperintense on T2-weighted images, indicating edema. On STIR, markedly hyperintense signal correlates with the signal changes on T1 and T2. There is destruction of the endplates and, therefore, the endplate/disk margin is poorly seen. With gadolinium, there is enhancement of the infected marrow and irregular peripheral enhancement at the periphery of the involved disk (Fig. 40.112). Pathological fractures of the infected vertebrae may also be seen.

***Epidural abscess, paravertebral phlegmon.*** The pathologies of epidural abscess and paravertebral phlegmon are most commonly seen as complications of diskitis and osteomyelitis. Since epidural abscess and resultant spinal cord compression represent a neurological emergency, besides the affected vertebral bodies and disks, it is important to always evaluate the epidural space for abscess and the paraspinal tissues for phlegmon (purulent inflammation and diffuse infiltration of soft or connective tissue) if diskitis and/or osteomyelitis are seen. Epidural abscess may be missed on conventional T1- and T2-weighted images because its signal characteristics may blend in with its surroundings. The central portion of the abscess may exhibit hyperintensity similar to CSF on T2-weighted images while exhibiting iso- to hypointense signal relative to the spinal cord on T1-weighted images. With gadolinium administration, however, intense enhancement is noted (Fig. 40.113). Just as may occur with compression due to epidural tumors, the compressed spinal cord segment may exhibit T2 hyperintense signal alteration. Phlegmon in the paravertebral tissues also enhances peripherally with gadolinium. This paravertebral infectious process is also well seen on STIR sequences as hyperintensity against the hypointense signal of the fat-suppressed bone marrow background.

## Noninfectious Inflammatory Disorders

***Multiple sclerosis.*** MS (see Chapter 80) commonly affects the spinal cord. Simultaneous cerebral demyelinating lesions are usually seen in the same patient (Matsushita et al., 2010). On MRI studies of the spinal cord in MS patients, the cervical segments are most commonly involved (Fig. 40.114). The lesions are hyperintense on T2-weighted images and are seen even more conspicuously on sagittal STIR sequences. The lower signal-to-noise ratio of STIR makes this sequence less specific than T2-weighted images for cord lesions, but it is more sensitive. STIR is generally useful only in the sagittal plane, and findings on this sequence should always be correlated with T2 images. Lesional signal changes with either technique are patchy and segmental, often discretely overlapping with the dorsal, anterior, or lateral columns of the spinal cord. The lateral and dorsal columns are affected most frequently. The signal changes are usually in the peripheral regions of the cord, but individual lesions may intersect with the central cord gray matter as well. In MS, the lesions typically do not span more than two vertebral lengths rostrocaudally and tend to involve less than half of the cross-section of the cord. Following administration of gadolinium, active cord lesions may exhibit homogeneous or open-ring enhancement. Large active MS lesions may cause swelling, with local expansion of the cord. In patients with a severe clinical picture or a long-standing history of MS, varying degrees of spinal cord atrophy may be seen. In less severe cases, volumetric analysis may reveal atrophy not detectable by visual inspection.

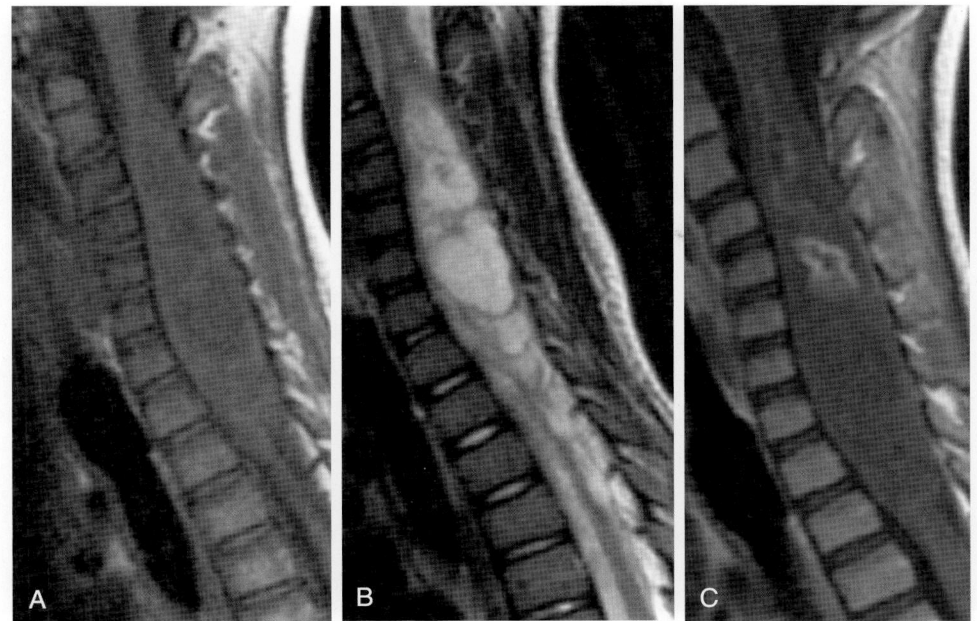


**Fig. 40.110 Astrocytoma. A,** Sagittal T1-weighted image reveals prominent expansion of the cervical and upper thoracic cord due to a T1 hypointense intramedullary tumor. **B,** Sagittal T2-weighted image demonstrates the hyperintense mass. **C,** Sagittal T1-weighted postcontrast image reveals a patchy heterogeneous pattern of enhancement.

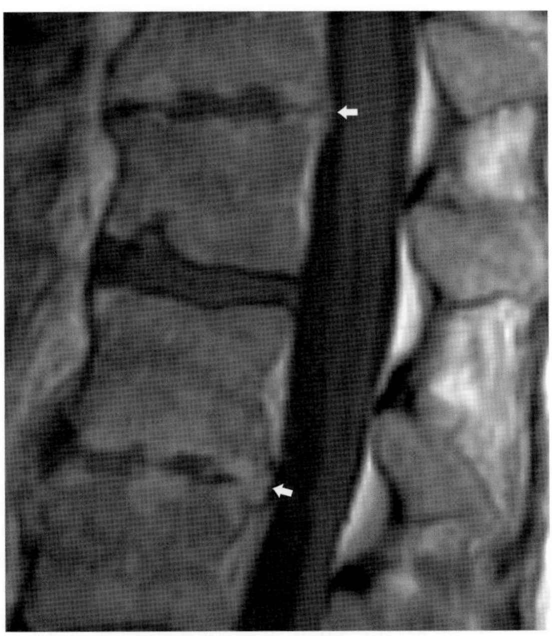

**Fig. 40.112 Diskitis and Osteomyelitis.** Two levels are involved *(arrows)*. Sagittal T1-weighted postcontrast image demonstrates decreased disk height and destruction of the adjacent endplates. With gadolinium, there is irregular enhancement of the infected marrow.

***Neuromyelitis optica.*** Acute spinal cord involvement presents with bright spotty T2 lesions with corresponding T1 prolongation, spanning at least three vertebral segments, known as longitudinally extensive transverse myelitis (LETM; Fig. 40.115). The central gray matter along the central canal of the spinal cord is the preferred area of involvement, as it corresponds to the most prominent expression of the AQP4 antigen (Dutra et al., 2018; Wingerchuk et al., 2015). Following contrast administration, patchy or lens-shaped enhancement of the aforementioned lesions in sagittal view can be distinctive for NMO (see Fig. 40.115, *C*). Although the LETM pattern is characteristic of NMOSD, 7%–14% of myelitis attacks in AQP4-IgG-seropositive patients do not meet the LETM definition. Therefore, NMOSD must also be considered in the differential diagnosis in patients presenting with short myelitis lesions (Wingerchuk et al., 2015). In the chronic phase, sharply demarcated extensive atrophy with or without T2 signal changes are visible.

***Acute disseminated encephalomyelitis.*** The widespread demyelinating lesions in this condition commonly involve the spinal cord as well. Diffuse or multifocal T2 hyperintense signal changes with variable degrees of cord swelling may be seen (Fig. 40.116). There is a variable amount of enhancement after gadolinium administration.

***Transverse myelitis.*** Transverse myelitis is an inflammatory disorder of the spinal cord that involves the gray as well as the white matter. The inflammation involves one or more (typically 3–4) cord segments and usually more than two-thirds of the cross-sectional area of the cord (Fig. 40.117). Transverse myelitis etiologies include viral infection, postviral or post-vaccine autoimmune reactions, vasculitis, mycoplasma infection, syphilis, antiparasitic and antifungal drugs, and even intravenous heroin use (Sahni et al., 2008). Brain MRI abnormalities suggestive of MS and a history of clinically apparent optic neuritis exclude the diagnosis of idiopathic transverse myelitis. The imaging modality of choice is MRI. Acutely, there is T2 hyperintense signal change and cord swelling. In more severe cases, hemorrhage and necrosis may also occur. Following gadolinium administration, diffuse or multifocal patchy enhancement is seen. In the subacute and chronic stages, the swelling and enhancement subside, and the T2 hyperintense signal decreases in extent. In the chronic stage, there may be a variable amount of faint residual T2 hyperintensity. In more severe cases, focal cord atrophy or myelomalacia may be seen.

Spinal sarcoidosis and vacuolar myelopathy are described online at http://www.expertconsult.com. 

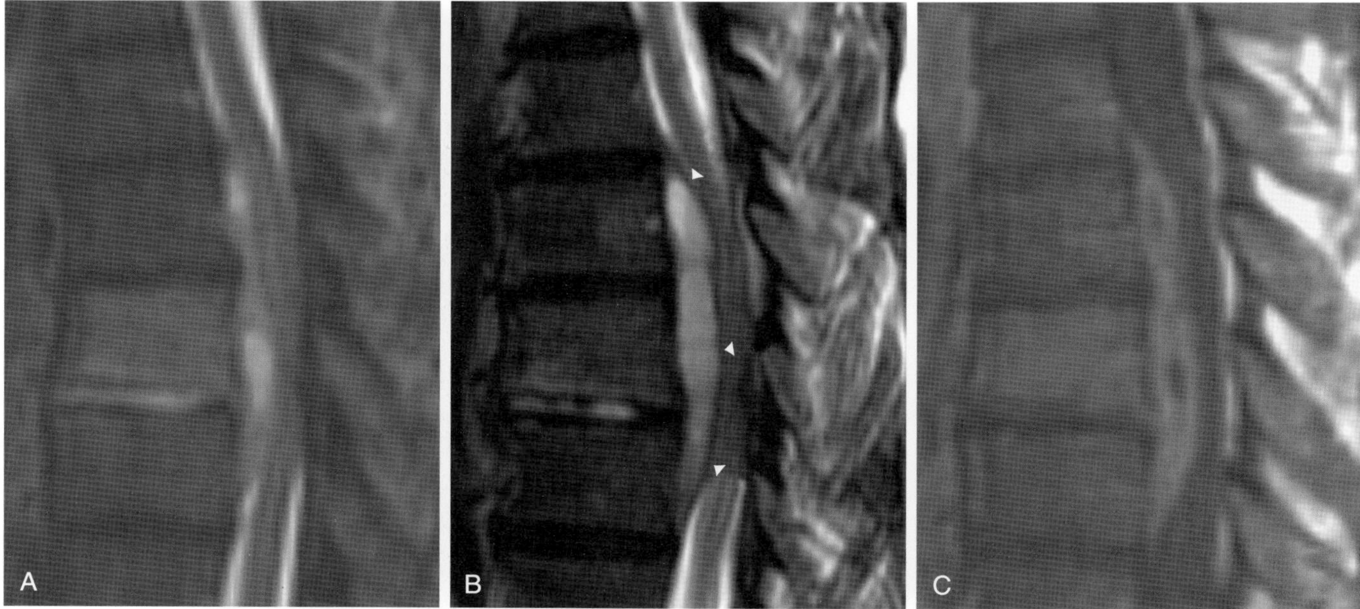


**Fig. 40.113 Diskitis, Osteomyelitis, and Epidural Abscess. A,** Sagittal fat-suppressed image reveals hyperintense signal in the involved disk and hyperintense edema in the vertebral body marrow. Note associated hyperintense epidural collection that displaces the spinal cord. **B,** Sagittal T2-weighted image reveals the diskitis and involvement of the inferior endplate of the vertebral body above. The epidural abscess is hyperintense, and the hypointense contour of the dura is well seen *(arrowheads).* **C,** Sagittal T1-weighted postcontrast image demonstrates intense enhancement of the abscess.

## Trauma

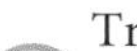

Traumatic lesions to the spine are discussed online, available at http://www.expertconsult.com.

## Metabolic and Hereditary Myelopathies

Here we group metabolic disorders that potentially cause myelopathy, as well as hereditary and degenerative diseases that result in myelopathy by progressive loss of spinal neurons and/or degeneration of spinal cord pathways. Some of the pathologies result in characteristic signal alterations of the spinal cord, such as that seen in subacute combined degeneration due to vitamin $B_{12}$ deficiency. Others (most degenerative diseases) do not alter the signal characteristics but cause cord atrophy, with or without atrophy of other CNS structures.

The most common entities belonging to this group of myelopathies (subacute combined degeneration, adrenomyeloneuropathy, SCA, Friedreich ataxia, amyotrophic lateral sclerosis, and hereditary spastic paraplegia) are discussed online at http://www.expertconsult.com.

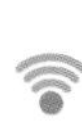

## Degenerative Spine Disease

Degenerative changes are very commonly seen on neuroimaging studies of the spine. These changes may involve the intervertebral disks, the vertebral bodies, and the posterior elements (facet joints, ligamentum flavum) in various combinations.

***Degenerative disk disease.*** In young people, the intervertebral disks have a fluid-rich center (nucleus pulposus) that appears hyperintense on T2-weighted images (Fig. 40.127). With aging, the nucleus pulposus loses water, becoming progressively more hypointense, and the disk flattens. This phenomenon is no longer considered to be abnormal but an age-related involutional change. However, the often concurrent weakening of the annulus fibrosus raises the chance of annular tear and resultant disk abnormalities.

The nomenclature of disk abnormalities (Fardon and Milette, 2001) is complex (Fig. 40.128). A *disk bulge* is symmetrical presence of disk tissue "circumferentially" (50%–100%) beyond the edges of the ring apophyses. On sagittal views, disk bulges have a "flat-tire" appearance. Disk bulges are not categorized as herniations and in the majority of cases do not have any clinical significance.

The term *disk protrusion* refers to extension of a disk past the borders of the vertebral body. A disk protrusion (1) is not classifiable as a bulge, and (2) any one distance between the edges of the disk material beyond the disk space is *less than* the distance between the edges of the base when measured in the same plane. We distinguish between focal and broad-based disk protrusions depending on whether the base of protrusion is less or more than 25% of the entire disk circumference. Disk protrusions may or may not be clinically significant. Whether they affect the neural structures depends on multiple factors. In a congenitally narrow spinal canal, even a small disk protrusion may result in spinal cord or cauda equina compression. In a normal spinal canal, a central disk protrusion may not do anything other than indent the thecal sac. A protrusion of the same size, however, may cause nerve root compression when situated in the lateral recess (Fig. 40.129) or neural foramen (paracentral or lateral disk protrusion).

*Disk extrusion* refers to a herniation in which any one distance between the edges of the disk material beyond the disk space is *greater than* the distance between the edges of the base measured in the same plane. It occurs when the inner content of the disk, the nucleus pulposus, herniates through a tear of the outer annulus fibrosus. If the extruded disk material loses its continuity with the disk of origin, it is referred to as a *sequestrated* or *free fragment.*

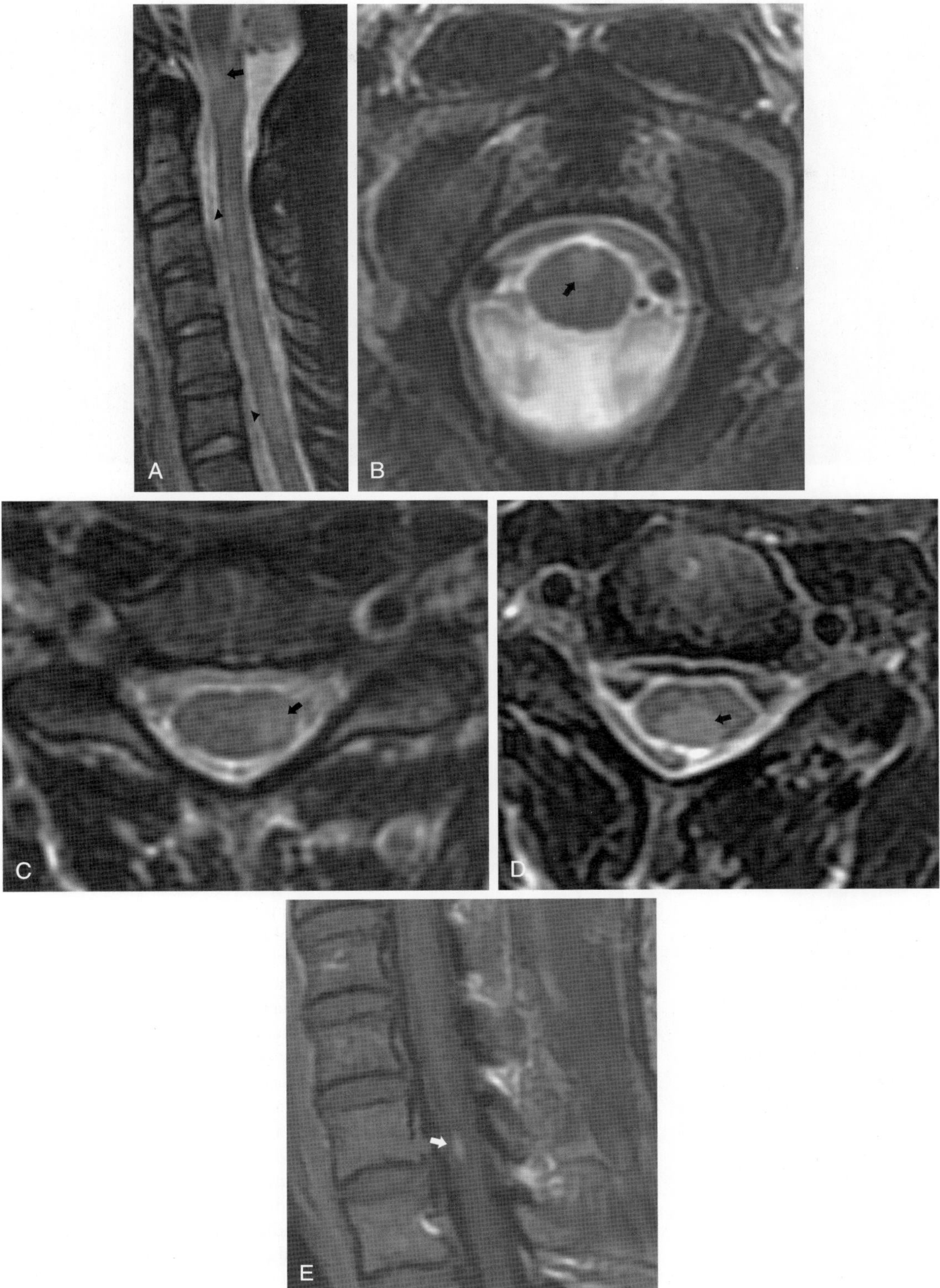


**Fig. 40.114 Multiple Sclerosis. A,** Sagittal fat-suppressed image reveals multiple hyperintense demyelinating lesions in the spinal cord parenchyma *(arrowheads)*, including at the cervicomedullary junction *(arrow)*. On axial T2-weighted images, hyperintense demyelinating lesions are seen in the **(B)** anterior, **(C)** lateral, and **(D)** posterior columns of the cord *(arrows)*. **E,** Sagittal T1-weighted postcontrast image reveals an enhancing lesion in the cord parenchyma *(arrow)*.

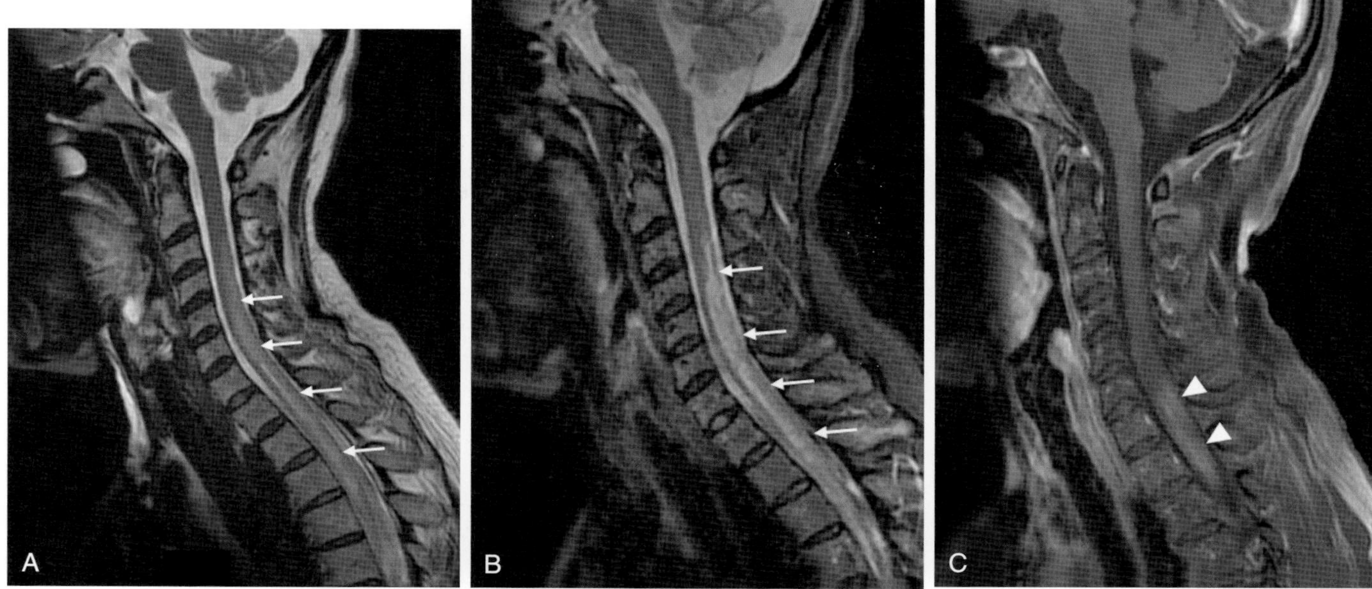


**Fig.40.115 Neuromyelitis Optica.** In sagittal T2 **(A)** and STIR sequence **(B)**, longitudinally extensive transverse myelitis (LETM) is present, extending from C2 to T5 *(arrows)*. Following contrast administration **(C)**, lens-shaped enhancement *(arrowheads)* is noted, extending from C6 to T2.

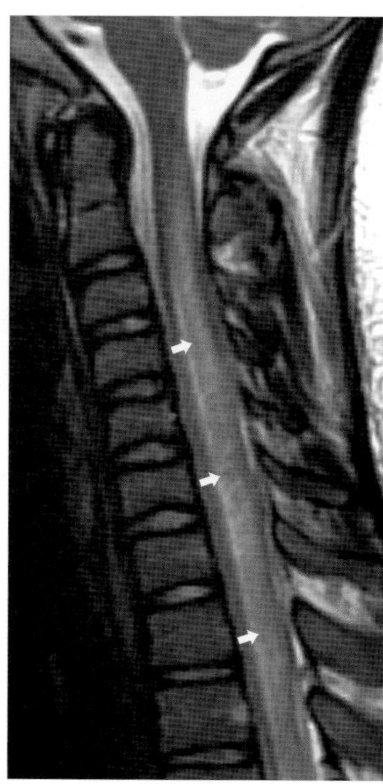

**Fig. 40.116 Acute Disseminated Encephalomyelitis (ADEM).** Sagittal T2-weighted image shows a diffuse hyperintense lesion spanning the length of the cervical cord *(arrows)*. Note the enlarged caliber of the cord, which is due to swelling.

Sometimes it is difficult to determine whether continuity exists or not. The term *migration* is used when there is displacement of disk material away from the site of extrusion, regardless of whether it is sequestrated or not, so it may be applied to displaced disk material irrespective of its continuity with the disk of origin (Fig. 40.130). On T2-weighted images, an annular tear may be appreciated as a dotlike or linear hyperintensity against the hypointense background of the annulus fibrosus. This is sometimes also referred to as a *high intensity zone* (HIZ).

Disk herniation frequently reaches considerable size and clinical significance owing to compression of the exiting/descending nerve roots of the spinal cord (Fig. 40.131). Disk protrusions and extrusions/herniations may compromise the spaces to various degrees. As a general guide, spinal canal or neural foraminal stenosis of less than one-third of their original diameter is mild, between one- and two-thirds is moderate, and stenosis involving more than two-thirds of the original caliber is considered severe.

Disk abnormalities are most common in the lumbar spine, particularly at the L4/5 and L5/S1 levels, and second most common at the cervical levels C5/6 and C6/7. These regions represent the more mobile parts of the spinal column.

***Degenerative changes of the vertebral bodies.*** The bone marrow of the vertebral bodies undergoes characteristic changes with age that are well demonstrated by MRI. In younger people, it is largely red marrow composed of hemopoietic tissue. In this age group, the only area of fatty conversion, appearing as a linear T1 hyperintensity, is at the center of the vertebral body around the basivertebral vein. In people older than 40 years, additional foci of fatty marrow changes appear T1 hyperintense in other regions of the vertebral body. The size and extent of these fatty deposits increases with advancing age.

In degenerative disk disease, characteristic degenerative changes often occur in the adjacent vertebral body endplates as well, seen as linear areas of signal change in these regions (Fig. 40.132). The process of degenerative endplate changes has been thought to occur in stages which have their characteristic MRI signal change patterns. These patterns were traditionally referred to as *Modic type 1, 2,* and *3 endplate changes* (for review, see Rahme and Moussa, 2008). This nomenclature has been largely abandoned. The most common change, formerly Modic type 2, is a linear hyperintensity in the endplate region of variable width on T1- as well as T2-weighted images, with corresponding hypointense signal loss on STIR sequences.

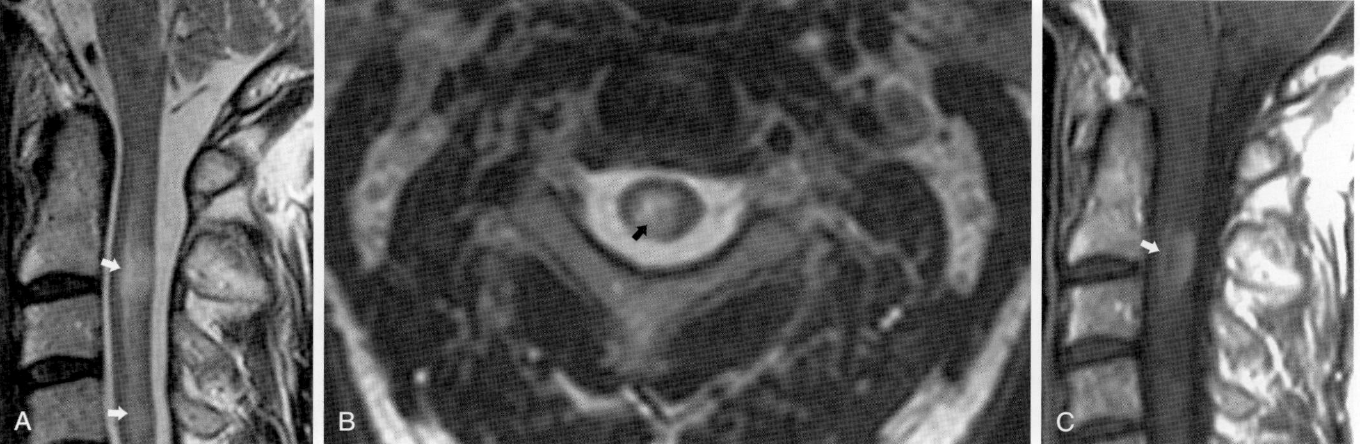


**Fig. 40.117 Transverse Myelitis.** A, Sagittal T2-weighted image demonstrates a longitudinal hyperintense spinal cord lesion spanning three vertebral segments *(arrows)*. B, On an axial T2-weighted image, the lesion involves more than two-thirds of the cord's cross-sectional area *(arrow)*. C, Sagittal T1-weighted postcontrast image shows an enhancing area within the lesion *(arrow)*.

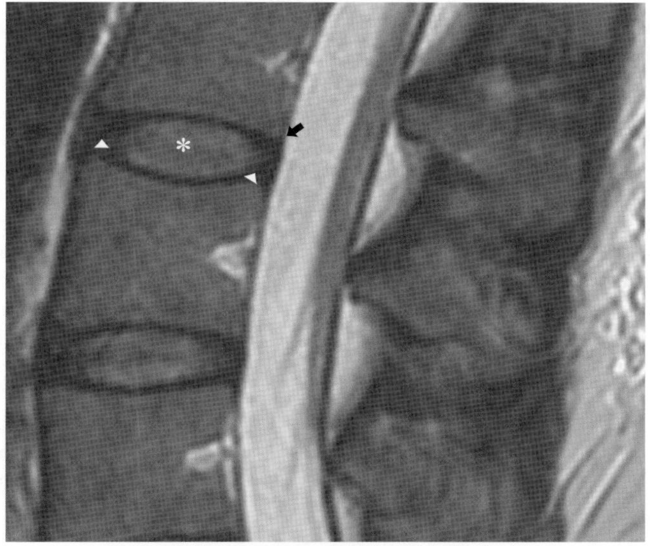

**Fig. 40.127 Normal Intervertebral Disks.** Sagittal T2-weighted image demonstrates normal disk height. Note the T2 hyperintense nucleus pulposus *(asterisk)* and the hypointense annulus fibrosus *(arrowheads)*. The disk does not extend beyond the borders of the vertebral body *(arrow)*.

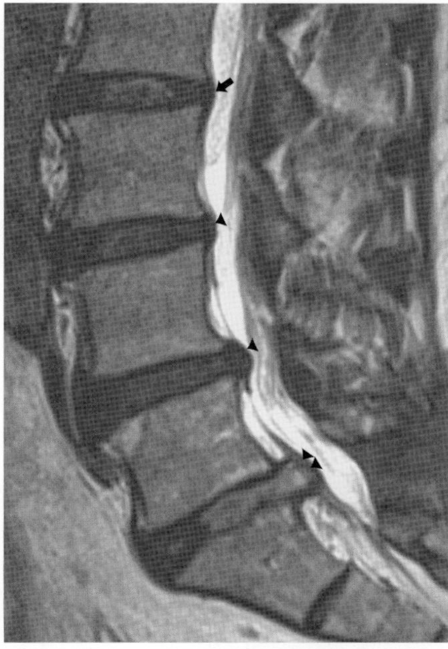

**Fig. 40.128 Disk Bulge, Protrusion, and Herniation.** Sagittal T2-weighted image demonstrates examples for all stages of disk pathology. Going from rostral to caudal, a disk bulge *(arrow)*, a small and more prominent protrusion *(arrowheads)*, and a herniation *(double arrowhead)* are seen.

These changes have been attributed to degenerative fat deposition in these regions.

Besides signal changes, vertebral bodies may also undergo morphological changes. In cases of disk protrusion or extrusion, the bone of the vertebral body may grow along the disk and form osteophytes or spurs. These may contribute to the narrowing of spaces and compromise of the neural elements. Large osteophytes may fuse across vertebral bodies, forming spondylotic bars.

***Degenerative changes of the posterior elements.*** Facet joint arthropathy and ligamentum flavum hypertrophy are common findings in degenerative disease of the spine. In facet arthropathy, the synovial surface of the joint becomes poorly defined, and hyperintense synovial fluid may accumulate. The joint becomes hypertrophied. Sometimes the synovial fluid accumulation results in outpouching of the synovium, which emerges from the joint, forming a synovial cyst. When prominent enough, this cyst may compromise the diameter of the spinal canal and (rarely) compress the neural elements (Fig. 40.133). Hypertrophy of the T2 hypointense ligamentum flavum is also frequent and may contribute to compromise of the spaces and neural elements.

***Spondylolysis, spondylolisthesis.*** Spondylolysis and spondylolisthesis are pathological changes that often occur together and are most common in the lumbar spine. *Spondylolysis* refers to a defect in the pars interarticularis of the vertebral arch, resulting in separation of the articular processes from the vertebral body. A traumatic etiology is common, but it may happen in the setting of advanced degenerative disease as well. A common cause is stress microfractures resulting from episodes of axial loading force on the erect spine, such as when landing after a jump, diving, weightlifting, or due to rotational forces. This abnormality can be visualized with CT or MRI. On sagittal views, the pars defect is well seen; on axial images, the spinal canal may appear slightly elongated at the level of the spondylolysis.

*Spondylolisthesis* is shifting of one vertebral body relative to its neighbor, either anteriorly (anterolisthesis) or posteriorly (retrolisthesis). It is often associated with spondylolysis (Fig. 40.134). Four grades of spondylolisthesis are distinguished, depending on the degree of shifting. *Grade I spondylolisthesis* refers to shifting over less than one-fourth of a vertebral body's anteroposterior diameter; grade II is shifting over one-fourth to one-half the diameter; grade III is up to three-fourths; and the most severe, grade IV, is shifting over the full vertebral body diameter.

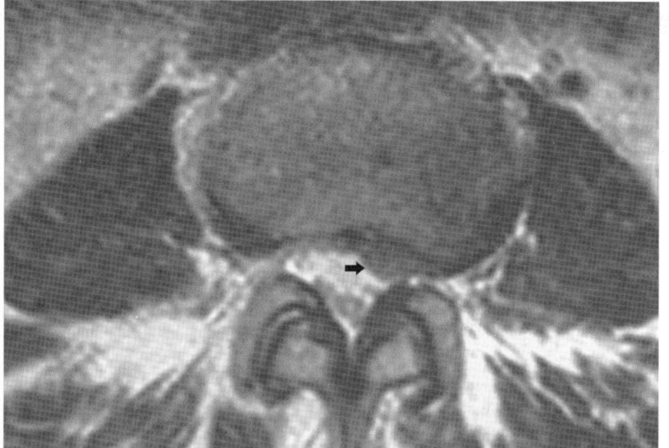

**Fig. 40.129 Disk Protrusion.** Axial T2-weighted image shows a left paracentral disk protrusion *(arrow)* that indents the thecal sac and narrows the left lateral recess.

Isolated spondylolysis results in elongation of the spinal canal, whereas spondylolisthesis causes segmental spinal canal narrowing, the extent of which depends on the degree of listhesis. In severe cases, there is compression of the spinal cord or cauda equina, and the changes also frequently cause narrowing of the neural foramina and compromise of the exiting nerve roots at the involved level.

## INDICATIONS FOR COMPUTED TOMOGRAPHY OR MAGNETIC RESONANCE IMAGING

Structural neuroimaging studies are probably the most commonly ordered diagnostic tests in both inpatient and outpatient neurological practice. Imaging greatly helps with the diagnosis of various neurological diseases and does so in a relatively quick and noninvasive way. This section (available online at http://www.expertconsult.com) summarizes the most common indications for obtaining a neuroimaging study in clinical neurological practice. Selection of the imaging study should be guided by the patient's history and objective findings on neurological examination, as opposed to shooting in the dark and obtaining "all-inclusive" imaging studies of the entire neuraxis. The availability and cost of the various techniques should also be factored into the decision of what tests to obtain in a given clinical situation.

### Neuroimaging in Various Clinical Situations

This section, including a summary (eTable 40.3) on selection of imaging modalities in various clinical situations, based on the current American College of Radiology (ACR) Appropriateness Criteria, is available online at http://www.expert-consult.com.

*The complete reference list is available online at https://expertconsult.inkling.com/.*

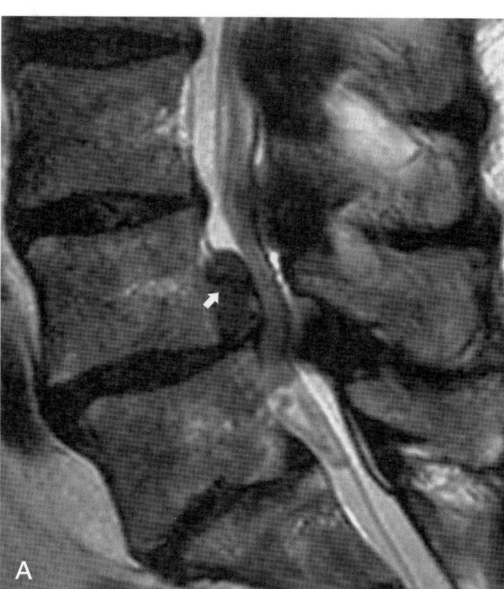

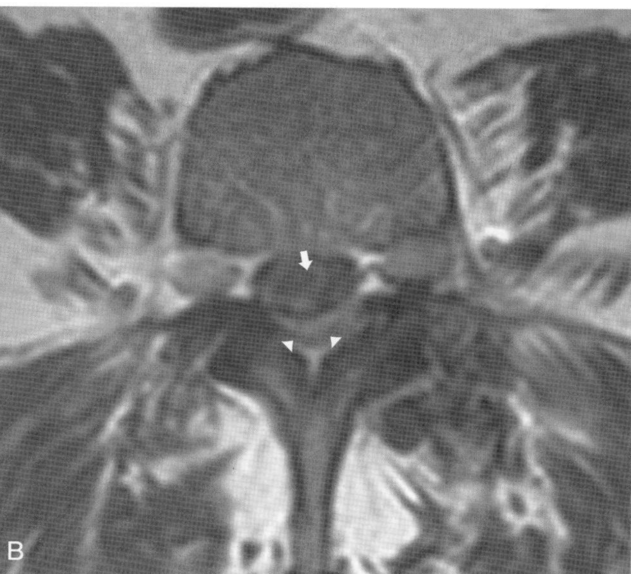

**Fig. 40.130 Disk Migration. A,** Sagittal T2-weighted image shows disk material that did not stay at the level of the disk of origin but migrated cranially *(arrow)*. **B,** Axial T2-weighted image demonstrates the migrated disk material *(arrow)* and the compressed thecal sac *(arrowheads)*.

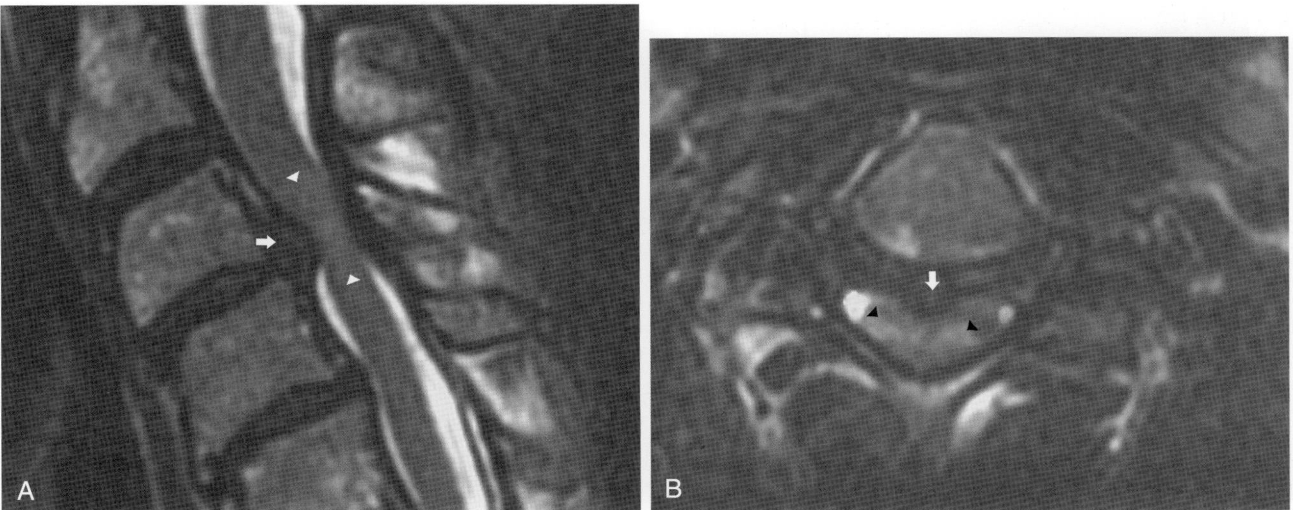


**Fig. 40.131 Disk Herniation, Spinal Cord Compression. A,** Sagittal T2-weighted image demonstrates a disk herniation at the C3–C4 level that compresses the cervical spinal cord *(arrow)*. Note the hyperintense signal abnormality in the compressed cord parenchyma *(arrowheads)*. **B,** Axial T2-weighted image shows the herniation, which has a central component *(arrow)*. The hyperintense signal change in the cord is also well seen *(arrowheads)*.

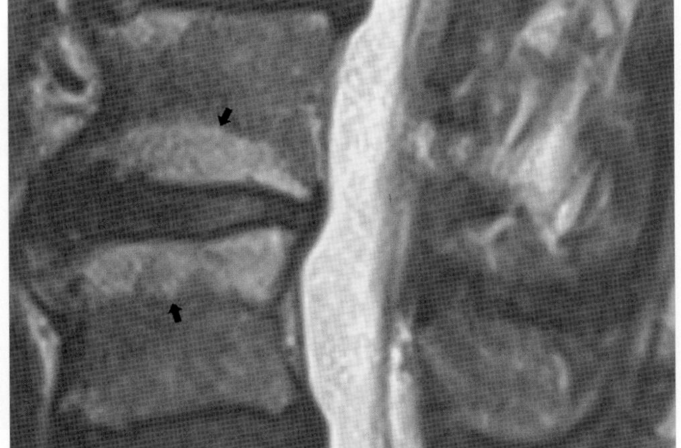

**Fig. 40.132 Degenerative Endplate Change.** Sagittal T2-weighted image reveals hyperintense bands of signal change parallel with the disk space in the endplate region of the adjacent vertebral bodies *(arrows)*.

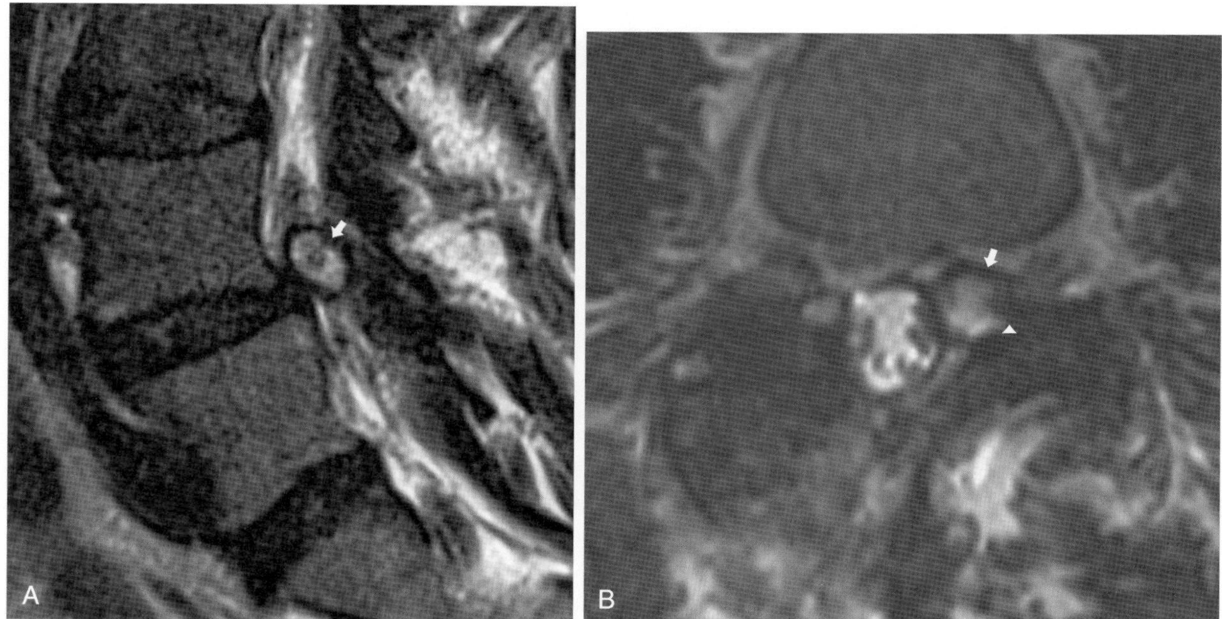


**Fig. 40.133 Synovial Cyst. A,** Sagittal T2-weighted image demonstrates a hyperintense cyst with hypointense rim in the spinal canal *(arrow)*. **B,** Axial T2-weighted image reveals that this cyst *(arrow)* arises from the left facet joint *(arrowhead)*, consistent with a synovial cyst. It narrows the left lateral recess and neural foramen.

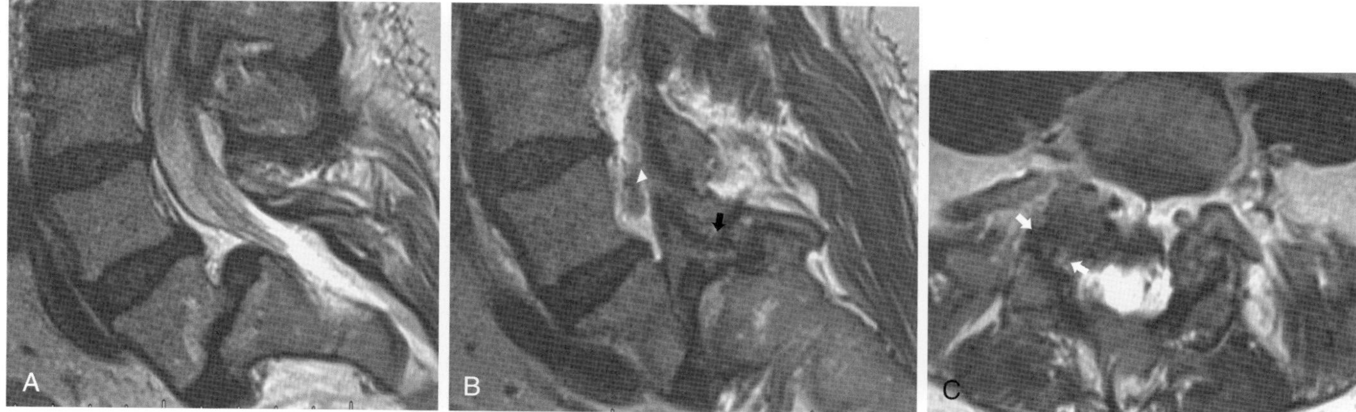


**Fig. 40.134 Spondylolysis, Grade 2 Anterolisthesis. A,** Sagittal T2-weighted image demonstrates grade 2 anterolisthesis of the L5 vertebral body on S1. **B,** Sagittal T2-weighted image reveals separation of the L4/L5 facet joint *(arrowhead)* and forward displacement of the L5 articular process *(arrow)*. **C,** Axial T2-weighted image also reveals the spondylolysis *(arrows)*.

# 41

# Vascular Imaging: Computed Tomographic Angiography, Magnetic Resonance Angiography, and Ultrasound

*Peter Adamczyk, David S. Liebeskind*

## OUTLINE



## COMPUTED TOMOGRAPHIC ANGIOGRAPHY

Computed tomographic angiography (CTA) is a relatively rapid, thin-section, volumetric, helical CT technique performed with a time-optimized bolus of contrast medium to enhance visualization of the cerebral circulation. This approach may be tailored to illustrate various segments of the circulation, from arterial segments to the venous system. The ongoing development of multidetector CT scanners has advanced CTA, with increasing numbers of detectors used to further improve image acquisition and visualization.

### Methods

Helical CT scanner technology, providing uninterrupted volume data acquisition, can rapidly image the entire cerebral circulation from the neck to the vertex of the head within minutes. Typical CT parameters use a slice (collimated) thickness of 1–3 mm with a pitch of 1–2, which represents the ratio of the table speed per rotation and the total collimation. Data are acquired as a bolus of iodinated contrast medium traverses the vessels of interest. For CTA of the carotid and vertebral arteries in the neck, the helical volume extends from the aortic arch to the skull base. Typical acquisition parameters are 7.5 images per rotation of the x-ray tube, 2.5-mm slice thickness, and a reconstruction interval (distance between the centers of two consecutively reconstructed images) of 1.25 mm. For CTA of the circle of Willis and proximal cerebral arteries, the data acquisition extends from the skull base to the vertex of the head. Typical acquisition parameters for this higher spatial resolution scan are 3.75 images per rotation, 1.25-mm slice thickness, and an interval of 0.5 mm. A volume of contrast ranging from 100 to 150 mL is injected into a peripheral vein at a rate of 2–3 mL/sec and followed by a saline flush of 20–50 mL. Adequate enhancement of the arteries in the neck or head is obtained approximately 15–20 seconds after injection of the contrast, although this may vary somewhat in each case. Image acquisition uses automated detection of bolus arrival and subsequent triggering of data acquisition. The resulting axial source images are typically postprocessed for two-dimensional (2D) and three-dimensional (3D) visualization using one or more of several available techniques, including multiplanar reformatting, thin-slab maximum-intensity projection (MIP), and 3D volume rendering. More recent CT with 320 detector rows enables dynamic scanning, providing both high spatial and temporal resolution of the entire cerebrovasculature (four-dimensional [4D] CTA). The cervical vessels are imaged by acquisition of an additional helical CT scan analogous to 64-detector row CT. An increasing spectrum of clinical applications utilizing this advanced technique remains under investigation (Diekmann et al., 2010).

### Limitations

#### Contrast-Induced Nephropathy

Careful consideration must be made for performing contrast-enhanced CT studies in patients with renal impairment. Exposure to all contrast agents may result in acute renal failure, called *contrast-induced nephropathy* (CIN), which is typically reversible but may potentially result in adverse outcomes. The incidence of renal injury appears to be associated with increased osmolality of contrast agents, which have been steadily declining with the newer generations of nonionic agents. Due to the perceived risk of CIN, many centers require that pre-imaging serum creatinine levels be taken and extra caution used with patients who have a creatinine level above 1.5 gm/dL or an estimated glomerular filtration rate below 60 mL/min/1.73 $m^2$. Treatment for this condition relies on prevention of this disorder, and agents such as *N*-acetylcysteine and intravenous (IV) saline and/or sodium bicarbonate may reduce the incidence of CIN. Avoidance of volume depletion and discontinuation of potential nephrotoxic agents, such as nonsteroidal anti-inflammatory drugs or metformin, is often recommended for patients prior to the procedure. Patients who are on hemodialysis should undergo dialysis as soon as possible afterwards to reduce contrast exposure (Kim et al., 2010). For patients who undergo CTA on an emergent basis and cannot take these precautionary steps, there is emerging evidence that the risk of CIN remains low. A 2017 systematic review evaluating ischemic stroke patients undergoing both CTA with CT perfusion (CTP) studies found that the overall rate of acute kidney injury (AKI) was 3% and the overall rate of hemodialysis was 0.07%. There was no difference in AKI among these patients with and without chronic kidney disease (odds ratio [OR] = 0.63; 95% confidence interval [CI] = 0.34–1.12). When adjusting for baseline creatinine, there was no difference in AKI between patients undergoing CTA/CTP and those who underwent noncontrast scans (OR = 0.34; 95% CI = 0.10–1.21). These findings suggest that the current contrast exposure involved with CTA may not be associated with a statistically significant increase in the risk of AKI in stroke patients, including those with known chronic renal impairment (Brinjikji et al., 2017).

### Metal Artifacts

Metallic implants, such as clips, coils, and stents, are generally safe for CT imaging, but it should be noted that they may lead to severe streaking artifacts, limiting image evaluation. These artifacts occur because the density of the metal is beyond the normal range of the processing software, resulting in incomplete attenuation profiles. Several processing methods for reducing the artifact signal are available, and operator-dependent techniques such as gantry angulation adjustments and use of thin sections to reduce partial volume artifacts may help decrease this signal distortion. Generally, knowledge of the composition of metallic implants may help in determining the potential severity of artifacts on CT. Cobalt aneurysm clips produce a lot more artifacts than titanium clips. For patients with stents, careful consideration must be made in evaluating stenosis, as these implants may lead to artificial lumen narrowing on CTA. The degree of artificial lumen narrowing decreases with increasing stent diameter. Lettau et al. evaluated patients with various types of stents and found that CTA may be superior to magnetic resonance angiography (MRA) at 1.5 tesla (1.5 T) for stainless steel and cobalt alloy carotid stents, whereas MRA at 3 T may be superior for nitinol carotid stents (Lettau et al., 2009). Data remain limited for patients undergoing intracranial stent placement, but, compared with digital subtraction angiography (DSA), inter-reader agreement for the presence of in-stent stenosis is noted to be inferior.

## Applications

### Extracranial Circulation

***Carotid artery stenosis.*** In evaluating occlusive disease of the extracranial carotid artery, CTA complements DSA and serves as an alternative to MRA (Fig. 41.1). In the grading of carotid stenosis using the North American Symptomatic Carotid Endarterectomy Trial (NASCET) criteria, Randoux and colleagues (2001) found that the rate of agreement between 3D CTA and DSA was 95%. In addition, CTA was significantly correlated with DSA in depicting the length of the stenotic segment. In reference to DSA, multiple studies have demonstrated a sensitivity of 77%–100% and a specificity of 95%–100% for CTA in detecting severe (70%–99%) stenosis (Binaghi et al., 2001). Data for moderate (50%–69%) stenoses remain less reliable (Wardlaw et al., 2006). For detection of a complete occlusion, the sensitivity and specificity have been found to be 97% and 99%, respectively (Koelemay et al., 2004). Saba et al. (2007) evaluated the use of multidetector CTA and carotid ultrasound in comparison to surgical observation for evaluating ulceration, which is a severe complication of carotid plaques. CTA was found to be superior, with 93.75% sensitivity and 98.59% specificity compared with carotid ultrasound, which demonstrated 37.5% sensitivity and 91.5% specificity. Furthermore, another study found that plaque ulceration on CTA had a high sensitivity (80.0%–91.4%) and specificity (92.3%–93.0%) for the prediction of intraplaque hemorrhage, an important marker of atherosclerotic disease progression, as defined on magnetic resonance imaging (MRI; U-King-Im et al., 2010).

Fibromuscular dysplasia (FMD), which often involves a unique pattern of stenoses in the cervical vessels, may be detected by CTA, although no large studies have evaluated the sensitivity and specificity for detection. This disorder, which characteristically demonstrates a string-of-beads pattern of vascular irregularity on angiography, has been reliably demonstrated on carotid artery evaluations from case reports. This may potentially reduce the need for more invasive angiographic imaging in the future, although further studies in this area are required (de Monye et al., 2007).

Currently, either CTA or MRA is used to evaluate suspected carotid occlusive disease, with the choice of method determined by clinical conditions (e.g., pacemaker), accessibility of CT and MR scanners, and additional imaging capabilities (CT or MR perfusion brain imaging). In contrast to occlusions due to atherosclerosis or dissection, the absence of opacification on CTA may be seen during pseudo-occlusion. This phenomenon may occur due to sluggish or stagnant flow in the patent artery produced by a distal intracranial occlusion. Retrospective studies on patients who underwent mechanical thrombectomy have demonstrated a sensitivity ranging from 82% to 96% and a specificity ranging from 70% to 86% for the detection of pseudo-occlusions on CTA compared with DSA. The presence of an intracranial internal carotid artery (ICA) bifurcation (carotid-T) occlusion was more frequently associated with

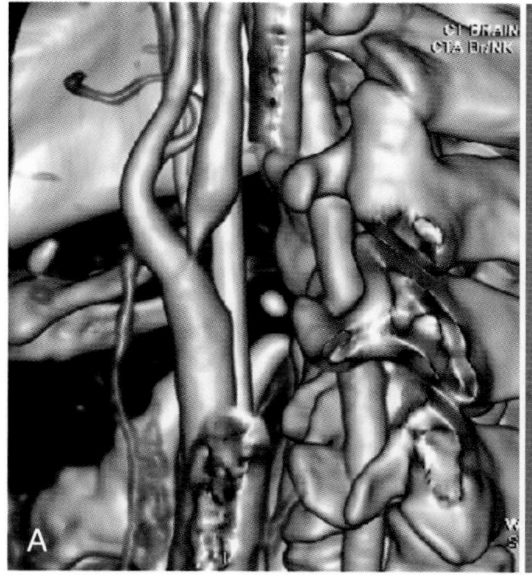


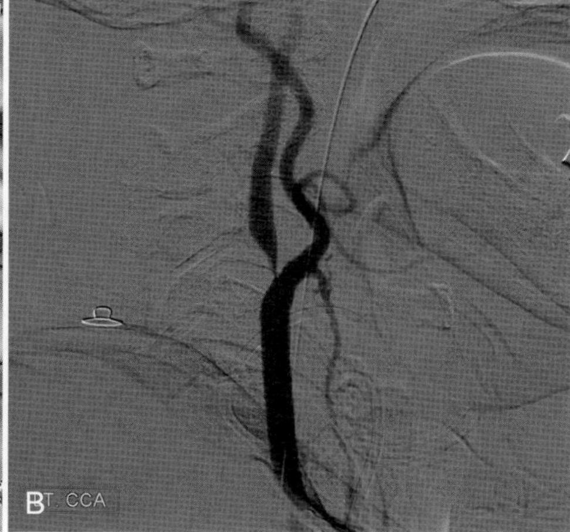


**Fig. 41.1 Computed Tomographic Angiography *(CTA)* Compared With Digital Subtraction Angiography (DSA) in a Patient With Proximal Internal Carotid Artery (ICA) Stenosis. A,** Three-dimensional reconstructed CTA image of left ICA reveals severe stenosis distal to the ICA bifurcation. **B,** DSA confirms severe stenosis seen on CTA due to an atherosclerotic plaque.

pseudo-occlusions rather than true occlusions. (Kappelhoff et al., 2018; Rocha et al., 2018) Clinicians should be acquainted with this potential finding as it may impact planning for acute endovascular stroke therapy.

***Carotid and vertebral dissection.*** Dissections of the cervicocephalic arteries, including the carotid and vertebral arteries, remain an important cause of ischemic strokes in young adults. CTA findings include demonstration of a narrowed eccentric arterial lumen in the presence of a thickened vessel wall, with occasional detection of a dissecting aneurysm. In subacute and chronic dissection, CTA has been shown to detect a reduction in the thickness of the arterial wall, recanalization of the arterial lumen, and reduction in the size or resolution of the dissecting aneurysm. Compared with DSA, CTA of the anterior and posterior circulations (pc) has been found to have a sensitivity of 51%–100% and a specificity of 67%–100% (Provenzale et al., 2009; Pugliese et al., 2007). CTA is likely superior to MRI in evaluating aneurysms of the distal cervical ICA, a common site of dissection, because MRI findings are often complicated by the presence of flow-related artifacts. CTA depiction of dissections at the level of the skull base may be complicated in some cases because of beam hardening and other artifacts that obscure dissection findings, including similarities in the densities of the temporal and sphenoid bones with the dissected vessel.

## Intracranial Circulation

***Acute ischemic stroke.*** CTA is a reliable alternative to MRA for evaluating arterial occlusive disease near the circle of Willis in patients with symptoms of acute stroke (Fig. 41.2). The rapid imaging time has resulted in a significant escalation in the use of this modality during acute strokes (Vagal et al., 2014). A large database of acute stroke patients across multiple community and academic hospitals in Los Angeles and Orange counties found that the proportion of ischemic stroke patients undergoing CTA steadily increased from 4% in 2005 to 26% in 2012 (Powers et al., 2018; Sanossian et al., 2017). CTA shows clinically relevant occlusions of major cerebral arteries and enhancement caused by collateral flow distal to the site of occlusion. Several published studies have noted sensitivities ranging from 92% to 100% and specificities of 82%–100% for the detection of intracranial vessel occlusion. (Latchaw et al., 2009; Nguyen-Huynh et al., 2008). Bash et al. (2005) have suggested that CTA has a higher sensitivity when directly compared with 3D time-of-flight MRA (TOF-MRA), with sensitivities of 100% and 87%, respectively.

CTA source images (CTA-SI) may be used to provide an estimate of perfusion by taking advantage of the contrast enhancement in the brain vasculature that occurs during a CTA, possibly making it unnecessary to perform a separate CTP study with a second contrast bolus. In normal perfused tissue, contrast dye fills the brain microvasculature and appears as increased signal intensity on the CTA-SI. In ischemic brain regions with poor collateral flow, contrast does not readily fill the brain microvasculature. Thus, these regions demonstrate low attenuation. The hypoattenuation seen on CTA-SI correlates with abnormality on diffusion-weighted MRI (DWI), and they have been found to be more sensitive than noncontrast CT scans in the detection of early brain infarction (Camargo et al., 2007). The sensitivity of CTA-SI and DWI when directly compared has been found to be similar in detecting ischemic regions, but DWI is better at demonstrating smaller infarcts and those in the brainstem and posterior fossa. Such findings may be useful for patients with symptoms of acute infarction who cannot undergo MRI (Latchaw et al., 2009).

In addition to anatomical pathology and perfusion status, CTA imaging may potentially be used for prognostication in patients undergoing acute stroke intervention. The 10-point Clot Burden Score (CBS) was devised as a semiquantitative analysis of CTA to help determine prognosis in acute stroke (Fig. 41.3). The CBS subtracts 1 or 2 points each for absent contrast opacification on CTA in the infraclinoid ICA (1), supraclinoid ICA (2), proximal M1 segment (2), distal M1 segment (2), M2 branches (1 each), and A1 segment (1). The CBS applies only to the symptomatic hemisphere. A CBS below 10 was associated with reduced odds of independent functional outcome (OR 0.09 for a CBS of 5 or less; OR 0.22 for CBS 6–7; OR 0.48 for CBS 8–9; all vs. CBS 10). The quantification of intracranial thrombus extent with the CBS predicts functional outcome, final infarct size, and parenchymal hematoma risk acutely (Puetz et al., 2008). An increased CBS is correlated with good clinical outcomes with a sensitivity of 58% and a specificity of 77% (Dehkharghani et al., 2015). This scoring system requires external validation and may be useful for patient stratification in future stroke trials.

The Alberta Stroke Program Early CT Score (ASPECTS) is a 10-point analysis of the topographic CT scan score used in patients with middle cerebral artery (MCA) stroke (Fig. 41.4 and Box 41.1). Segmental assessment of MCA territory is made, and 1 point is removed from the initial score of 10 if there is evidence of infarction in the following regions: putamen, internal capsule, insular cortex, anterior MCA cortex, MCA cortex lateral to insular ribbon, posterior MCA cortex, anterior MCA territory immediately superior to M1, lateral MCA territory immediately superior to M2, and posterior MCA territory immediately superior to M3. An ASPECTS score of 7 or less predicts a worse functional outcome at 3 months and symptomatic hemorrhage. The ASPECTS scoring system can be similarly applied to CTA-SI and, compared with noncontrast CT, has been found to be more reliable in predicting the final infarct size, particularly in early time windows (Bal

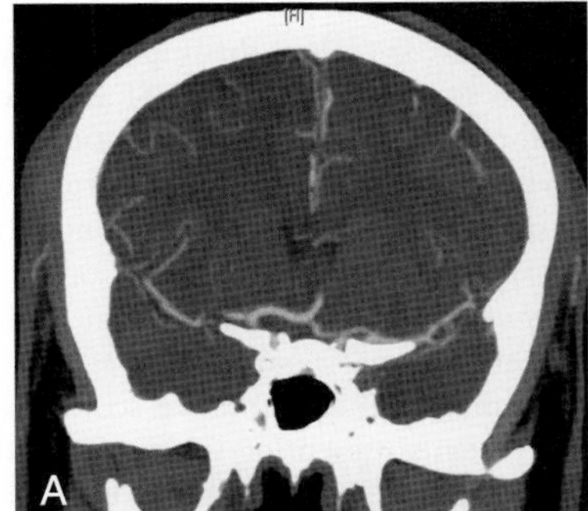


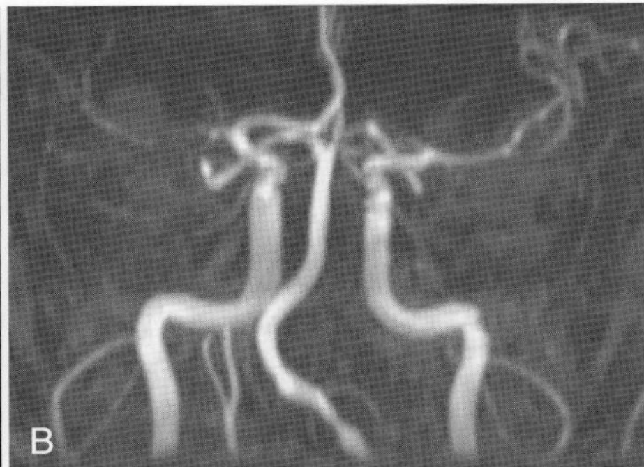


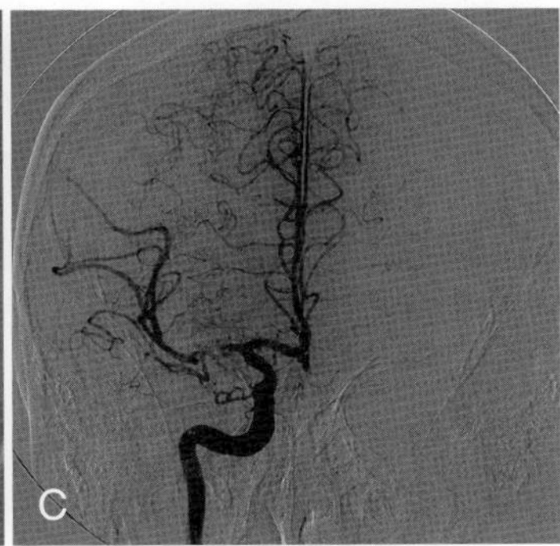


**Fig. 41.2 Right Middle Cerebral Artery (MCA) Stenosis in a Patient Who Subsequently Received Intracranial Stent Placement. A,** Coronal image from computed tomographic angiography (CTA) shows focal distal M1 segment stenosis prior to stenting. **B,** 1.5 T 3D time-of-flight magnetic resonance angiography (MRA) demonstrates a focal flow gap of the right M1. MRA overestimates degree of stenosis when compared with CTA. **C,** Digital subtraction angiography image after stent placement reveals right MCA restenosis.

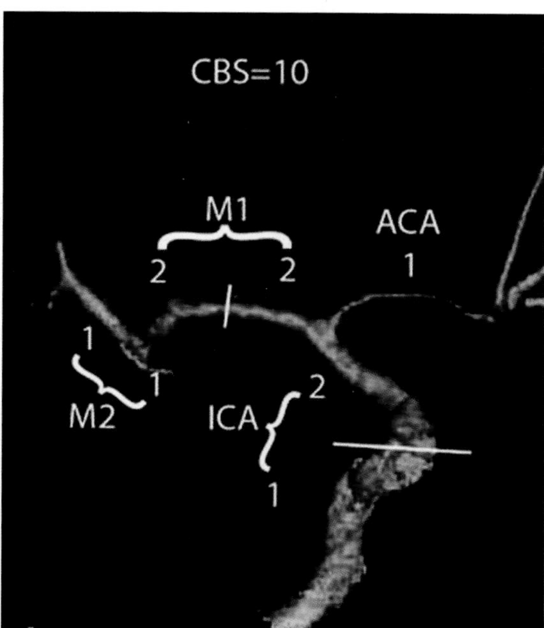


**Fig. 41.3 The Clot Burden Score (CBS) on Computed Tomographic Angiography (CTA).** This is a 10-point imaging-based score where two points are subtracted for thrombus found on CTA in the supraclinoid internal carotid artery *(ICA)* and each of the proximal and distal segments of the middle cerebral artery trunk. One point is subtracted for thrombus in the infraclinoid ICA and A1 segment and for each M2 branch. *ACA*, Anterior Cerebral Artery.

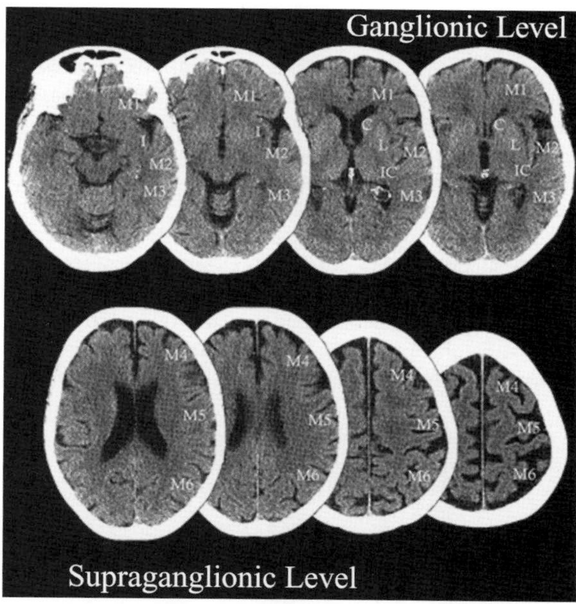


**Fig. 41.4** Axial noncontrast head computed tomography (CT) demonstrating middle cerebral artery territory regions defined by the Alberta Stroke Program Early CT Score (ASPECTS). *C*, Caudate, *I*, insular ribbon, *IC*, internal capsule, *L*, lentiform nucleus.

et al., 2012). Kawiorski et al. (2016) evaluated acute stroke patients receiving IV thrombolysis and/or thrombectomy and found that CTA-SI-ASPECTS was a reliable predictor of a poor clinical outcome despite successful revascularization with a sensitivity of 35% and a specificity 97% (positive predictive value [PPV] 86%; negative predictive value [NPV] 7%). Subsequent studies on patients undergoing endovascular

**BOX 41.1 Alberta Stroke Program Early Computed Tomography Score (ASPECTS)***

**ASPECTS Territories**

Caudate
Putamen
Internal capsule
Insular cortex
M1—Anterior MCA cortex
M2—MCA cortex lateral to insular ribbon
M3—Posterior MCA cortex
M4—Anterior MCA territory immediately superior to M1
M5—Lateral MCA territory immediately superior to M2
M6—Posterior MCA territory immediately superior to M3

*This is a 10-point quantitative scoring system for patients with acute MCA-territory strokes. Segmental assessment of MCA territory is made, and 1 point is removed from the initial score of 10 if there is evidence of infarction in that region.
*MCA,* Middle cerebral artery.

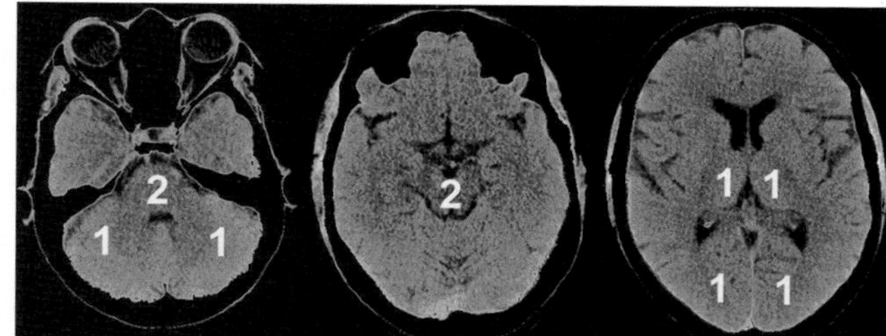


**Fig. 41.5** Cerebral map defining the posterior circulation Acute Stroke Prognosis Early Computed Tomography Score (pc-ASPECTS) territories. From 10 points, 1 or 2 points each *(as indicated)* are subtracted for early ischemic changes or hypoattenuation on computed tomographic angiography source images in left or right thalamus, cerebellum, or posterior cerebral artery territory, respectively (1 point); and any part of midbrain or pons (2 points).

treatment have demonstrated that CTA SI-ASPECTS correlates with follow-up MR DWI better than noncontrast CT ASPECTS and was better able to predict favorable functional outcomes (Park et al., 2018; Sallustio et al., 2017). This scoring method may serve to reliably predict futile recanalization and remains a valuable tool for treatment decisions regarding the indication of revascularization therapies.

Puetz et al. (2010) sought to determine whether CTA-SI ASPECTS could be combined with the CBS system for improved prognostication. A 10-point ASPECTS score based on CTA-SI and the 10-point CBS were combined to form a 20-point score for patients presenting acutely with stroke who received thrombolysis treatment. For patients with a combined score of 10 or less, only 4% were functionally independent, and mortality was 50%. In contrast, 57% of patients with scores of 10 or greater were functionally independent, and mortality was 10%. Additionally, parenchymal hematoma rates were 30% versus 8%, respectively. A similar semiquantitative scoring system for CTA-SI was devised for patients presenting with acute basilar artery occlusion and termed the *pc-ASPECTS* (Fig. 41.5). This 10-point scoring system subtracts 1 or 2 points each for areas of hypoattenuation in the left or right thalamus, cerebellum, or posterior cerebral artery (PCA) territory, respectively (1 point), or any part of the midbrain or pons (2 points). Median follow-up pc-ASPECTS was lower in patients with a CTA-SI pc-ASPECTS less than 8 than in patients with a CTA-SI pc-ASPECTS of 8 or higher, respectively. Hemorrhagic transformation rates were 27.3% versus 9.5%, respectively, for patients who received thrombolysis. The results indicate that such analysis can predict a larger final infarct extent in patients with basilar artery occlusion. Larger prospective trials are required for validation, but the systematic acute evaluation of CTA along with CTA-SI may potentially be used to help guide future stroke treatments (Puetz et al., 2009).

Whole-brain dynamic time-resolved CTA or 4D CTA is a novel technique capable of generating time-resolved cerebral angiograms from skull base to vertex. This modality offers additional hemodynamic information on leptomeningeal collateral status as well as the extent of any retrograde flow. Unlike a conventional cerebral angiogram, this technique also visualizes simultaneous pial arterial filling in all vascular territories (Menon et al., 2012). Due to the increased sensitivity for collateral flow, 4D CTA has been shown to more closely outline intracranial thrombi than conventional single-phase CTA, which may potentially assist neurointerventional treatment planning, and prognostication (Frölich et al., 2013).

Significant advancements have recently been made in the treatment of acute ischemic stroke. An increasing proportion of acutely presenting stroke patients are receiving successful recanalization with mechanical thrombectomy devices. However, treatment is often time dependent, requiring an ideal imaging selection tool that is able to accurately detect salvageable brain rapidly with widespread availability. Cerebrovascular collateral status at baseline has been found to be an important determinant of future clinical outcomes among patients with acute ischemic stroke undergoing mechanical thrombectomy. CTA is increasingly recognized as a valid tool for assessing collateral flow and predicting clinical outcomes in these patients. A higher rate of patients with good collaterals on CTA have improved functional outcomes compared with those with poor collaterals (Sallustio et al., 2017). One study found that the evaluation of collateral flow was noted to be consistent by both CTA and conventional angiography and remains the strongest predictor of clinical outcome (Nambiar et al., 2014).

Multiple methods have been ascribed for the assessment of collateralization on CTA in acute ischemic stroke patients, but there is no clear consensus yet on the optimal scoring system. The most common methods utilize the presence and extent of leptomeningeal vascular enhancement in the symptomatic hemisphere relative to the asymptomatic side. One such scoring system adapted from conventional angiography is the modified American Society of Interventional and Therapeutic Neuroradiology/Society of Interventional Radiology (ASITN/SIR) system that assigns a score of 0 for nonexistent or barely visible pial collaterals on the ischemic site during any point in time, 1 for partial collateralization of the ischemic site until the late venous phase, 2 for partial collateralization of the ischemic site before the venous phase, 3 for complete collateralization of the ischemic site by the late venous phase, and 4 for complete collateralization of the ischemic site before the venous phase. A higher modified ASITN/SIR score is associated with better collateral flow on the symptomatic side. In comparing multiple CTA-based collateral scores with CTP scans among patients with emergent large vessel occlusions, one study found that modified ASITN/SIR collateral scores demonstrated good correlation with early infarct core (rho = −0.696, $P < .001$) and mismatch ratio (rho = 0.609, $P < .001$; Seker 2016).

Multiphase CT angiography (mCTA) is an imaging technique that can be helpful in identifying patients that will benefit from mechanical thrombectomy by quickly evaluating the degree and extent of pial arterial filling in the whole brain in a time-resolved manner. Imaging of the brain vasculature from the skull base to the vertex is attained in three phases after contrast material injection. The first phase is composed of angiography from the aortic arch to the vertex on a multidetector CT scanner. Imaging acquisition during this phase is timed to occur during the peak arterial phase in the healthy brain tissue and is triggered by bolus monitoring. Imaging acquisition during the second and third phases occurs from the skull base to the vertex in the equilibrium/peak venous and late venous phases in the healthy brain. The two additional phases of mCTA use no additional contrast material. One collateral scoring system adapted for mCTA is the ASPECTS on collaterals system, which includes a six-point scale that also assigns a higher value for better collateral flow in the ischemic region. A score of 0 is assigned if no vessels are visible in any phase. A score of 1 indicates that only a few vessels are visible in the ischemic territory on any phase. A score of 2 is given if there is a two-phase delay associated with reduced prominence and extent of peripheral vascular filling or if there is a single-phase delay associated with ischemic regions with no vascular enhancement. A score of 3 is assigned for a delay on two phases or a single-phase delay associated with significantly reduced number of vessels in the ischemic territory. A score of 4 indicates that contrast delay is present on one phase, but the prominence and extent of peripheral vascular enhancement remains unchanged. A score of 5 is given if there is no delay in enhancement of pial vessels on all phases. The six-point scale can be further trichotomized into a descriptive categorization of collaterals as being poor (0–1), intermediate (2–3) or good (4–5).

Interrater reliability using this technique has been noted to be excellent among readers (Menon et al., 2015). Furthermore, the interpretation of mCTA can easily be adopted as one study demonstrated a high interrater agreement between stroke neurology trainees and an experienced neuroradiologist (Yu et al., 2016). When compared with single-phase CTA, mCTA has been shown to be superior in both interrater reliability as well as the ability to predict clinical outcomes in patients undergoing acute reperfusion therapy. Poor collaterals noted on mCTA have been shown to be an independent predictor of development of malignant MCA infarction (Flores et al., 2015). The interpretation of collaterals on mCTA has been compared with standard CTP imaging, as described elsewhere. Investigators have demonstrated that mean $T_{max}$, cerebral blood flow, and cerebral blood volume values on CTP correspond with different score categories on mCTA (D'Esterre et al., 2017). The use of mCTA may provide a viable alternative for CTP in the evaluation of acute ischemic stroke patients in centers where such modality is not available or where time constraints may deter performing additional imaging. In addition to collateral assessment, mCTA has also been found to be useful in better identifying distal vessel occlusions due to delayed distal opacification, termed the "delayed vessel sign." When compared with single-phase CTA, the use of later phases may significantly improve the sensitivity and time to interpretation in identifying such occlusions (Byrme et al., 2017).

***Intracranial stenosis.*** CTA offers a more readily available and less costly alternative to DSA in the evaluation of intracranial atherosclerotic disease (ICAD). The sensitivities for detection of intracranial stenoses range from 78% to 100%, with specificities of 82%–100% (Latchaw et al., 2009). The Stroke Outcomes and Neuroimaging of Intracranial Atherosclerosis (SONIA) study more recently evaluated CTA findings of intracranial atherosclerosis against DSA in a prospective blinded multicenter setting. Based on DSA stenosis defined as 50%–99%, the PPV of CTA was only 46.7% and the NPV was 73.0%. For DSA stenosis defined as 70%–99%, the PPV of CTA was 13.3% and the NPV was 83.8% (Liebeskind et al., 2014). CTA is considered to be superior to transcranial Doppler (TCD) ultrasound in detecting intracranial stenoses with a high false-negative rate noted for Doppler ultrasound (Suwanwela et al., 2002). Studies also suggest that CTA has a higher sensitivity when directly compared with 3D TOF-MRA. Bash et al. (2005) found that CTA had a sensitivity of 98%, while MRA had a sensitivity of 70% for detection of intracranial stenosis. Additionally, CTA may be superior to both MRA and DSA in detecting pc stenoses when slow or balanced flow states were present, possibly owing to a longer scan time, which allows for more contrast to pass through a critical stenosis. Although previous studies noted decreased accuracy with the presence of atheromatous calcifications, the sensitivity and specificity of CTA for stenosis quantification remains consistent when appropriate window and level adjustments are made to account for frequently associated blooming artifacts.

***Cerebral venous thrombosis.*** The diagnosis of cerebral venous thrombosis (CVT) was previously often made with conventional angiography and more recently by MRI techniques. Magnetic resonance venography (MRV) is commonly considered the most sensitive noninvasive test in diagnosing CVT. However, given the prolonged imaging time and often limited availability, CTA has been studied as a potential alternate means of detecting CVT. Spiral CT with acquisition during peak venous enhancement has been implemented with single-section systems but remains limited in spatial and temporal resolution. One study directly comparing CTV with MRV demonstrated a sensitivity and a specificity of 75%–100%, depending on the sinus or venous structure involved (Khandelwal et al., 2006). Multidetector-row CTA (MDCTA) offers higher spatial and temporal resolution, which allows for high-quality multiplanar and 3D reformatting. Two small studies found 100% specificity and sensitivity with MDCTA when compared with MRV. The venous sinuses could be identified in 99.2% and the cerebral veins in 87.6% of cases. MDCTA may be equivalent to MRV in visualizing cerebral sinuses, but further studies are needed to evaluate the diagnostic potential of MDCTA in specific types of CVT, such as cortical venous thrombosis, thrombosis of the cavernous sinus, and thrombosis of the deep cerebral veins. The advantages of MDCTA include the short examination duration and the possible simultaneous visualization of the cerebral arterial and venous systems with a single bolus of contrast. MDCTA visualizes thrombus via contrast-filling defects and remains less prone to flow artifacts. A potential problem with this technique lies in the fact that in the chronic state of a CVT, older organized thrombus may show enhancement after contrast administration and may not produce a filling defect, leading to a false-negative result. The addition of a noncontrast CT with the MDCTA is sometimes used to remove another potential to obtain false-negative results from the presence of a spontaneously hyperattenuated clot that could be mistaken for an enhanced sinus. This phenomenon is known as the *cord sign* and may be seen in 25%–56% of acute CVT cases (Gaikwad et al., 2008; Linn et al., 2007).

***Intracerebral hemorrhage.*** Patients presenting acutely with intracerebral hemorrhage (ICH) within the first few hours of symptom onset are known to be at increased risk for hematoma expansion. However, only a fraction of such patients arrive at a hospital within this time frame, so alternative means of identifying potential hemorrhage expansion have been sought because it is an important predictor of 30-day mortality. One such prognostic marker has been identified on CTA: the *spot sign*, defined as tiny, enhancing foci seen within hematomas, with or without clear contrast extravasation. The predicting hematoma growth and outcome in ICH using contrast bolus CT (PREDICT) investigation was a multicenter prospective study that validated the CTA spot sign as an independent predictor of hematoma expansion. The CTA spot sign demonstrated an excellent interrater agreement with a sensitivity of 51% and specificity of 85%, with a PPV of 61% and a NPV of 78% (Demchuk et al., 2012; Huynh et al., 2013). A more recent meta-analysis of 29 studies observed similar findings with a pooled sensitivity of 62% and a specificity of 88%. The spot sign was significantly associated with increased risk of hematoma expansion, a higher risk of in-hospital death, poor discharge outcomes, and increased 3-month mortality (Xu, 2018).

Later image acquisition may improve detection for the spot sign, and this marker is seen more frequently in the venous phase compared with the arterial phase of CTA evaluation. Ciura et al. (2014) noted that when a 90-second delayed CTA acquisition was added, the sensitivity increased from 55% to 64%. However, the presence of significant hematoma expansion and higher total hematoma enlargement were observed more frequently among spot sign–positive patients with earlier phases of image acquisition (Rodriguez, 2014). The timing of CTA evaluation relative to the onset of the patient's symptoms also has a significant impact in the detection of this radiographic marker. One systematic review demonstrated that the frequency of the spot sign significantly decreased from 39% within 2 hours of onset to 13% beyond 8 hours. Additionally, there was a significant decrease in hematoma expansion in spot-positive patients as onset-to-CTA time increased with PPVs decreasing from 53% to 33% (Dowlashahi et al., 2016).

***Cerebral aneurysms.*** DSA has been the standard imaging method for diagnosis and preoperative evaluation for patients with ruptured and unruptured cerebral aneurysms. However, DSA is invasive and subject to complications resulting from catheter manipulation. Thus, in patients at greater risk for cerebral aneurysms, the use of noninvasive techniques such as CTA to screen for aneurysms is particularly attractive.

The main disadvantages of CTA are radiation exposure, the use of iodinated contrast material, difficulty in detecting very small aneurysms, and imaging artifacts from endovascular coils in treated aneurysms. CTA has diagnostic limitations for determining the presence of a residual lumen and the size/location of the remnant neck of a treated aneurysm because of the streak artifacts caused by clips, coils, flow diverters, and other embolization-related devices.

In general, the accuracy of CTA is felt to be at least equal if not superior to that of MRA (Figs. 41.6 and 41.7) in most circumstances, and in some cases, its overall accuracy approaches that of DSA (Latchaw et al., 2009). CTA can provide quantitative information, such as dome-to-neck ratios and aneurysm characterization, such as the presence of mural thrombi or calcium, branching pattern at the neck, and the incorporation of arterial segments in the aneurysm. The incorporation of 3D volume-rendered images in particular provided a surgically useful display of the aneurysm sac in relation to skull base structures (see Fig. 41.7). Additionally, 3D CTA may help identify cerebral veins, which generally display more anatomical variation than arteries. The presence of an unexpected vein or the lack of collateral drainage from a region drained by a vein that may need to be sacrificed during surgery can alter the approach to resection of an aneurysm. This anatomical information may permit more informed selection for a therapeutic procedure (surgery versus endovascular coiling) and in planning the treatment approach.

For the detection of cerebral aneurysms, a meta-analysis of eight studies demonstrated that CTA had a pooled sensitivity of 99% and a specificity of 94% on a per-patient basis. On a per-aneurysm basis, the pooled sensitivity was 96% and the specificity was 91% (Feng, 2016). Interrater agreement has been noted to be high when evaluating aneurysm features, such as location, side, maximum diameter, and dome of the intracranial aneurysm. The level of agreement has been observed to be lower during assessment of neck diameter, presence of multiple aneurysms, and aneurysm morphology. The degree of interrater agreement increases with rater seniority emphasizing the importance of interpretation experience (Maldaner et al., 2017). Phillipp et al. (2017) conducted a large single-center retrospective evaluation demonstrating a lower sensitivity of 57.6% for smaller aneurysms less than 5 mm and 45% for aneurysms originating from the ICA. The limited sensitivity of conventional CTA for the detection of very small aneurysms and aneurysms adjacent to the skull can be significantly improved by using subtracted CTA, which offers bone-free visualization. Chen et al. (2017) evaluated subtracted 320 detector-row volumetric CTA for the detection of small aneurysms less than 3 mm and found sensitivity, specificity, and accuracy were 96.9%, 99.2%, and 98.6%, respectively, on a per-aneurysm basis. In contrast to typical aneurysms located near the base

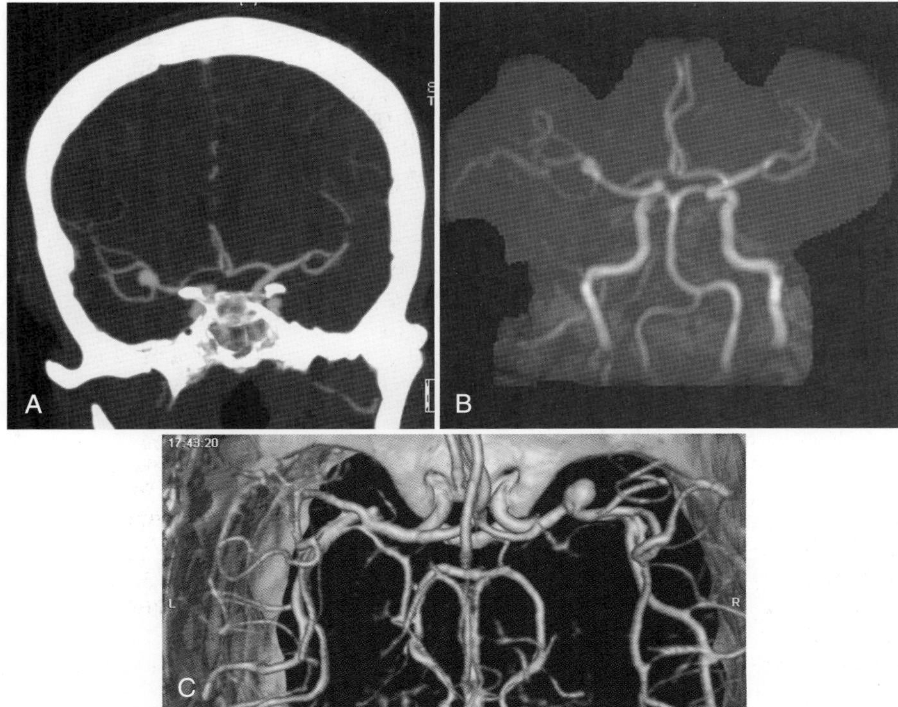


**Fig. 41.6 Right Middle Cerebral Artery Aneurysm Seen on Both Computed Tomographic Angiography (CTA) and Magnetic Resonance Angiography (MRA). A,** Coronal section on CTA reveals aneurysm in right middle cerebral artery bifurcation. **B,** MRA also displays aneurysm with less definition. **C,** Three-dimensional reconstruction of CTA better defines saccular appearance of this aneurysm.

of the brain, distal aneurysms such as mycotic and oncotic aneurysms may be more difficult to detect on CTA. One study found a lower sensitivity of 45.5% and a specificity of 90.0%, indicating DSA should be considered when strong clinical suspicion exists for such aneurysms (Walkoff et al., 2016). For patients presenting with a nontraumatic subarachnoid hemorrhage and a negative CTA, causative vascular pathology has been identified with subsequent DSA in 9%–13% of cases (Heit et al., 2016). However, in specific cases of perimesencephalic subarachnoid hemorrhage, which are rarely associated with a ruptured aneurysm, CTA has been noted to have a NPV as high as 100%, suggesting that follow-up DSA may not be warranted in these patients (Mortimer et al., 2016).

Postoperative aneurysms typically require follow-up imaging to exclude the presence of residual aneurysm, new aneurysmal growth, or recanalization. For the detection of treated aneurysms, one meta-analysis found that CTA had a sensitivity and specificity of 92.6% and 99.3%, respectively, using multidetector CTA. Although DSA remains the gold standard, CTA may present a promising, cost-effective, noninvasive alternative for long-term evaluation (Thaker et al., 2011). However, Pradilla et al. (2012) noted that, in a tertiary center, CTA had limited accuracy, particularly with small aneurysms, with a 20.5% false-positive rate most often in the anterior communicating artery or basilar artery bifurcation regions. Additionally, they noted a 21.6% false-negative rate most commonly in the cavernous segment ICA and MCA regions. There is an increasing utilization of flow diversion and intrasaccular embolization devices for the treatment of intracranial aneurysms, which pose new challenges for follow-up evaluation with CTA due to increased metallic artifacts and limited visualization of aneurysmal contrast opacification. Several small studies have noted technical feasibility and reliability in using this modality for subsequent assessment, but further prospective investigation is warranted (Raoult et al., 2018; Saake et al., 2012).

A common sequela of aneurysmal subarachnoid hemorrhage is the development of cerebral vasospasm. TCDs are more commonly employed for surveillance, while DSA remains the gold standard for confirming this condition. However, CTA may offer high diagnostic accuracy as one meta-analysis demonstrated a pooled sensitivity of 79.6% and a specificity of 93.1% (Greenberg et al., 2010). This modality may offer a sufficient alternate means of evaluation, especially for patients who may not have sufficient bone windows for ultrasound evaluation.

***Cerebral vascular malformations.*** A cerebral arteriovenous malformation (AVM) requires DSA for accurate spatial and temporal assessment of blood flow to the feeding arteries, nidus, and draining veins. CTA has been found to have sensitivities of 87% and 96% for ruptured and unruptured AVMs, respectively. For large AVMs (>3 cm), the overall sensitivity was found to be 100%. Importantly, the sensitivity for identifying associated aneurysms was 88%, making this a useful adjunct imaging modality (Gross et al., 2012). The use of 4D CTA allows for improved accuracy in the diagnosis and classification of shunting patterns using the Spetzler-Martin grading system for AVMs. Moreover, cross-sectional imaging and perfusion data obtained from this modality may assist in treatment planning (Willems et al., 2011).

Limited data exist for CTA in the identification of a dural arteriovenous fistula (DAVF), but recent investigations have demonstrated that 4D CTA may correctly reveal the angioarchitecture and differentiate the various patterns of venous drainage. (Beijer et al., 2013). Tian et al. (2015) reported that 4D CTA may be used for the follow-up assessment of patients who underwent transarterial DAVF embolization. Despite differences in temporal and spatial resolutions, the intermodality agreement between 4D CTA and DSA has been found to be excellent in determining shunt location, identification of drainage veins, and fistula occlusion after treatment. This modality may

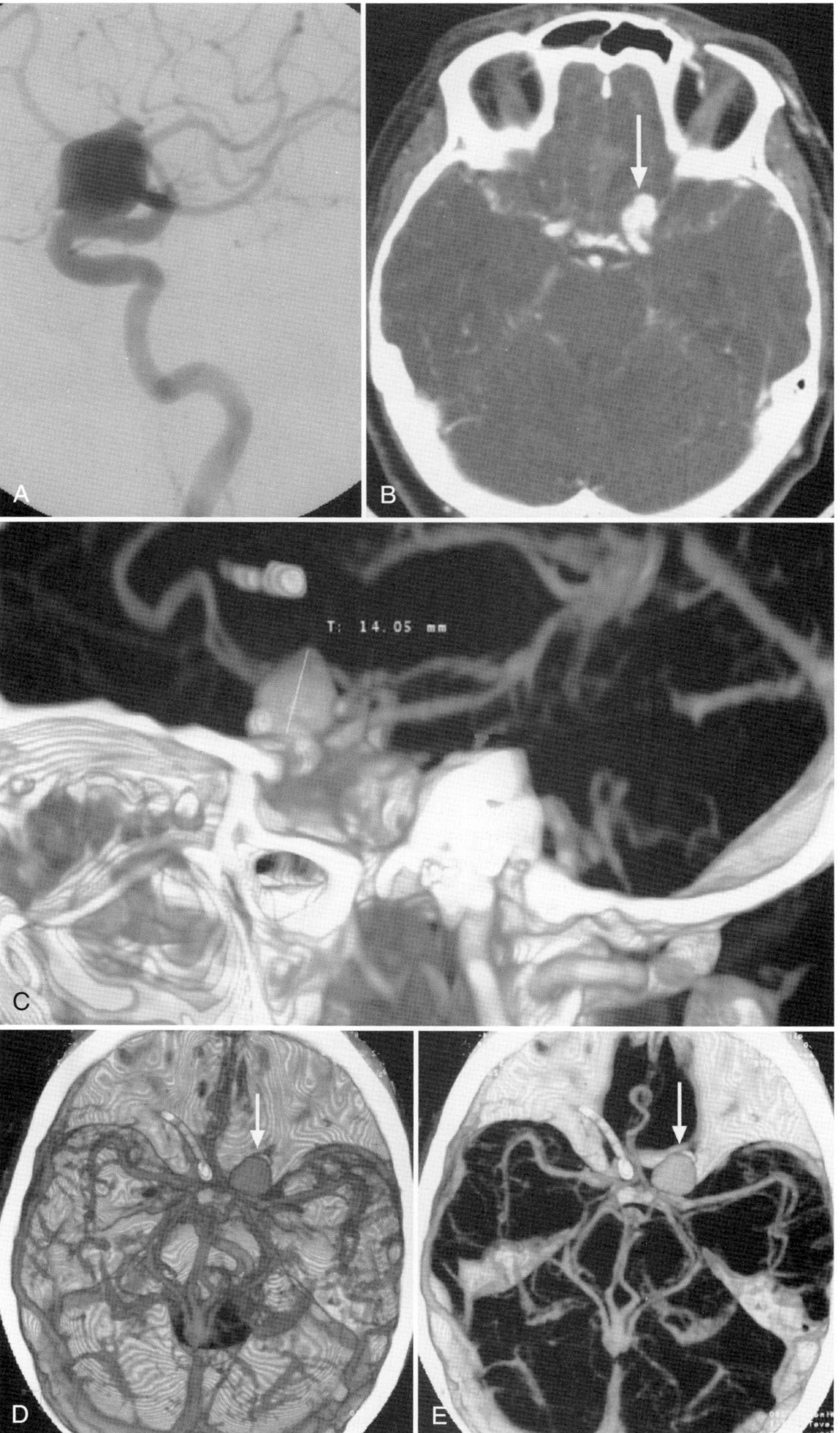


**Fig. 41.7 Left Internal Carotid Artery (ICA) Aneurysm.** Comparison of computed tomographic angiography (CTA) postprocessed images with catheter angiography. **A,** Catheter angiography lateral view, following left ICA injection, shows aneurysm *(arrow)* originating from supraclinoid portion of ICA. **B,** CTA axial source image reveals lobulated aneurysm *(arrow)*. **C–E,** CTA three-dimensional (3D) volume-rendered images with transparency feature for user-selected tissue regions (called *4D angiography*). **C,** Lateral view from left side of patient demonstrates relationship of the aneurysm, measuring 14 mm from neck to dome, to the anterior clinoid process. **D,** View of aneurysm *(arrow)*, skull base, and circle of Willis from above. **E,** Same view as **D** of aneurysm *(arrow)* but edited to remove most of skull base densities and improve visibility of vessels.

offer a potentially feasible alternative for follow-up evaluation. A retrospective review of eight studies evaluating 4D CTA for the detection of both AVMs and DAVFs noted a pooled sensitivity of 77% with a specificity of 100%. The use of 4D CTA offers a practical, minimally invasive alternative for evaluating these cerebrovascular pathologies and may reduce the need for DSA, which carries a risk of important complications (Biswas et al., 2015).

***Brain death.*** The absence of cerebral circulation is an important confirmatory test for brain death, and CTA is emerging as an important alternative means of testing. No clear consensus exists regarding the optimal criteria for determining brain death on CTA. Frampas et al. (2009) described a 4-point score with points subtracted based on the lack of opacification of the cortical segments of the MCAs and internal cerebral veins. This method was used to prospectively evaluate 105 patients who were clinically brain dead and was found to have a sensitivity of 85.7% and a specificity of 100%. A meta-analysis evaluating 12 studies determined that if the CTA criterion for brain death was complete lack of opacification of intracranial vessels, then the pooled sensitivity was 62% for the venous phase and 84% for the arterial phase imaging. The sensitivity of CTA was higher when the criterion for brain death included the absence of opacification of internal cerebral veins, either alone (99%) or in combination with lack of flow to the distal MCA branches (85%; Kramer et al., 2014). This appears to be a possible alternative means of detecting cerebral circulatory arrest, and given that it is a fast and noninvasive technique, it may become a useful confirmatory test (Escudero et al., 2009; Frampas et al., 2009).

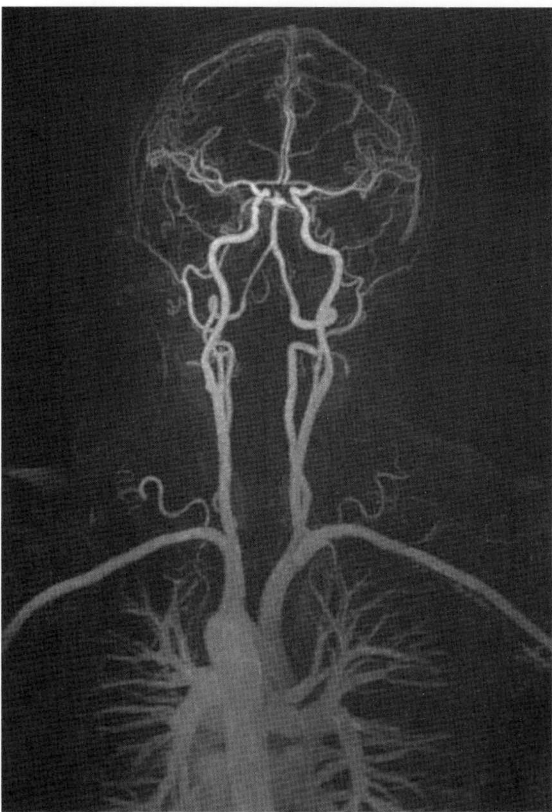

**Fig. 41.8** Three-dimensional contrast-enhanced magnetic resonance angiography of the cerebrovascular system.

## MAGNETIC RESONANCE ANGIOGRAPHY

### Methods

Numerous techniques are used in the acquisition of MRA images. In general, TOF-MRA and phase-contrast (PC) MRA do not use a contrast bolus and generate contrast between flowing blood in a vessel and surrounding stationary tissues. In 2D TOF-MRA, sequential tissue sections (typically 1.5 mm thick and approximately perpendicular to the vessels) are repeatedly excited, and images are reconstructed from the acquired signal data. This results in high intravascular signal and good sensitivity to slow flow. In 3D TOF-MRA, slabs that are a few centimeters thick are excited and partitioned into thin sections less than 1 mm thick to become reconstructed into a 3D data set. A 3D TOF-MRA has better spatial resolution and is more useful for imaging tortuous and small vessels, but because flowing blood spends more time in the slab than that in a 2D TOF-MRA section, a vessel passing through the slab may lose its vascular contrast upon exiting the slab.

In TOF-MRA, stationary material with high signal intensity, such as subacute thrombus, can mimic blood flow. PC-MRA is useful in this situation because the high signal from stationary tissue is eliminated when the two data sets are subtracted to produce the final flow-sensitive images. This technique provides additional information that allows for delineation of flow volumes and direction of flow in various structures from proximal arteries to the dural venous sinuses. In the 2D PC-MRA technique, flow-encoding gradients are applied along two or three axes. A projection image displaying the vessel against a featureless background is produced. Compared with the 2D techniques, 3D PC-MRA provides higher spatial resolution and information on flow directionality along each of three flow-encoding axes. The summed information from all three flow directions is displayed as a speed image, in which the signal intensity is proportional to the magnitude of the flow velocity. The data set in TOF-MRA or PC-MRA may be used to visualize the course of vessels in 3D by mapping the hyperintense signal from the vessel-containing pixels onto a desired viewing plane using a MIP algorithm, thus producing a projection image. MIP images are generated in several viewing planes and then evaluated together to view the vessel architecture. A presaturation band is applied and represents a zone in which both flowing and stationary nuclei are saturated by a radiofrequency pulse that is added to the gradient recalled echo (GRE) pulse sequence. The downstream signal of a vessel that passes through the presaturation zone is suppressed because of the saturation of the flowing nuclei. Presaturation bands may be fixed or may travel, keeping the same distance from each slab as it is acquired. In general, the placement of presaturation bands can be chosen so as to identify flow directionality and help distinguish arterial from venous flow.

Contrast-enhanced MRA (CE-MRA) uses scan parameters that are typical of 3D TOF-MRA but uses gadolinium to overcome the problem of saturation of the slow-flowing blood in structures that lie within the 3D slab (Fig. 41.8). The scan time per 3D volume is 5–10 minutes, and data are acquired in the first 10–15 minutes after the bolus infusion of a gadolinium contrast agent (0.1–0.2 mmol/kg). Presaturation bands usually are ineffective at suppressing the downstream signal from vessels when gadolinium is present. In 3D CE-MRA, the total scan time per 3D volume (usually about 30–50 partitions) is reduced to 5–50 seconds (Fain et al., 2001; Turski et al., 2001). Data are acquired as the bolus of the gadolinium contrast agent (0.2–0.3 mmol/kg and 2–3 mL/sec infusion rate) passes through the vessels of interest, taking advantage of the marked increase in intravascular signal (first-pass method). Vessel signal is determined primarily by the concentration of the injected contrast, analogous to conventional angiography. Because 3D CE-MRA entails more rapid data acquisition, and hence higher temporal resolution, than TOF-MRA, spatial resolution may be reduced. The most common approaches to synchronizing the 3D data acquisition with the arrival of the gadolinium bolus in the arteries are measurement of the bolus arrival time for each patient using a small (2 mL) test dose of contrast followed by a separate synchronized manual 3D acquisition by the scanner operator (Fain et al., 2001). Another method rapidly and repeatedly acquires 3D volumes (<10 sec per volume) in the neck, beginning at the time of contrast bolus injection to ensure that at least one 3D volume showing only arteries will be acquired (Turski et al., 2001). Subtraction of preinjection source images from arterial phase images, termed *digital subtraction MRA*, is sometimes used to increase vessel-to-background contrast.

The advent and increasing availability of MRI scanners with 3.0 T or even higher field strengths (up to 7 T) in selected centers may also be used to improve MRA by capitalizing on higher signal-to-noise ratios and parallel imaging (Nael et al., 2006). Parallel imaging at 3 T or greater can be used to improve spatial resolution, shorten scan time, reduce artifacts, and increase anatomical coverage in first-pass CE-MRA. Recent investigation with 7 T TOF-MRA demonstrated that such ultrahigh field strength allows vivid depiction of the large vessels of the circle of Willis with significantly more first- and second-order branches and can even distinguish diseased diminutive vessels in hypertensive patients (Hendrikse et al., 2008a; Kang et al., 2009). The time-resolved or dynamic CE-MRA, also known as 4D MRA, is a more recent contrast-enhanced vascular imaging method under investigation that uses novel processing techniques to achieve subsecond temporal resolution while maintaining high spatial resolution. Dynamic MRA scans may be obtained up to 60 times faster and with higher spatial resolution at 3 T. The resulting images may attain the diagnostic performance of conventional DSA, allowing for better characterization of various vascular lesions (Hope et al., 2010; Parmar et al., 2009; Willinek et al., 2008).

## Limitations

### Nephrogenic Systemic Fibrosis

Clinicians should be aware that a rare but serious complication of contrast-enhanced MRI studies includes the development of nephrogenic systemic fibrosis (NSF). This condition is characterized by widespread thickening and hardening of the skin, with the potential for rapid systemic progression and immobility over several weeks. Although the precise mechanism remains unclear, NSF was first noted in 1997 and occurs exclusively in patients with renal failure. The majority of reported cases involved exposure to a gadolinium chelate within 2–3 months prior to disease onset in dialysis-dependent patients. A large percentage of cases have been specifically associated with gadodiamide (Omniscan), with a possible dose-dependent effect, although it should be noted that cases have been reported with all gadolinium agents. Careful consideration must be made for gadolinium administration in patients with renal impairment (glomerular filtration rate <30 mL/min/1.73 $m^2$), especially those on dialysis. The risks and benefits should be carefully discussed prior to any contrast-enhanced procedures, and the dose of gadolinium should be minimized. Additionally, for patients on hemodialysis, prophylactic dialysis is generally recommended as soon as possible, ideally within 3 hours after contrast administration (Kuo et al., 2007).

### Metal Implant Contraindications

Limitations due to the presence of metallic materials (clips, stents, coils, flow diverters) remain a common concern in patients undergoing vascular imaging. Aneurysm clips made from martensitic stainless steels remain a contraindication for MRI procedures because excessive magnetic forces may displace these implants and cause serious injury. However, most clips are now made of metals that are nonferromagnetic, and all patients with any metallic implants require screening to determine whether they are safe to undergo an MRI study. For the majority of coils and stents that have been tested, it is unlikely that these implants would be moved or displaced as a result of exposure to MRI systems operating at 1.5 T or even 3 T. Additionally, it is often unnecessary to wait an extended period of time after a procedure to perform an MRI study in a patient with an implant made of nonferromagnetic material unless there are concerns associated with MRI-related heating. Dental materials, including wires and prostheses, do not appear to pose a risk, although they may result in artifacts on MRI. Artifacts from metal may have varied appearances on MRI, depending on the type or configuration of the piece of metal. Artifact sizes may increase at 3 T compared with 1.5 T, depending on the implant type and composition, but these distortions may be substantially reduced by optimizing imaging parameters. Patients who are deemed unsafe for MRI upon screening may be considered for CT evaluation (Olsrud et al., 2005).

## Applications

### Extracranial Carotid and Vertebral Circulation

***Time-of-flight magnetic resonance angiography.*** ICA stenosis grading methods used in the landmark NASCET (North American Symptomatic Carotid Endarterectomy Trial) and ECST (European Carotid Surgery Trial) trials remain the most widely applied methods and were determined by DSA (European Carotid Surgery Trialists' Collaborative Group, 1998; Ferguson et al., 1999). However, DSA has the drawback of being an invasive and costly modality. MRA has become increasingly used as a noninvasive imaging alternative for carotid stenosis as it avoids the radiation and iodinated contrast exposure associated with both DSA and CTA. Furthermore, images are often higher in quality and less operator dependent when compared with ultrasound imaging. Despite these advantages, TOF-MRA remains relatively insensitive to slow flow and may be associated with increased scan times and signal voids, resulting in decreased quality images and overestimation of stenoses. Compared with 2D TOF-MRA, the 3D TOF-MRA method is less likely to overestimate the degree of stenosis, particularly if original (Fig. 41.9) or reformatted source images are evaluated rather than the MIP images (Norris and Rothwell, 2001).

In a 2008 meta-analysis of 37 studies, TOF-MRA was noted to have a sensitivity of 91.2% with a specificity of 88.3% for the detection of high-grade (70%–99%) ICA stenosis. For the detection of ICA occlusions, the sensitivity of TOF-MRA was 94.5% and the specificity was 99.3%. For moderately severe (50%–69%) stenoses, TOF-MRA had a sensitivity of only 37.9% and a specificity of 92.1% (Debrey et al., 2008). These results were similar to a 2014 study that determined that 3D TOF-MRA had a sensitivity of 91.7% and a specificity of 98.5% for high-grade stenoses. For ICA occlusions, 3D TOF-MRA was found to be highly sensitive (100%), with a specificity of 98.7% (Weber et al., 2015). These results suggest that TOF-MRA may serve as a useful imaging alternative to DSA for the detection of high-grade carotid stenoses.

Atherosclerotic narrowing of the vertebral artery commonly involves the origin or distal intracranial portion. For TOF-MRA evaluation of posterior-circulation cerebrovascular disease, the vertebral origins usually are not evaluated for the same reasons the common carotid origins are not evaluated. However, sequential 2D TOF-MRA of the neck is useful in determining whether proximal occlusion is present and in demonstrating flow direction in the vertebral arteries in patients with suspected subclavian steal. A 2D TOF study obtained with no presaturation band shows flow enhancement in both vertebral arteries, whereas a study obtained with a superiorly located walking presaturation band shows flow only in the vertebral artery with normal anterograde flow. While published data remain limited for evaluation of vertebral artery stenosis, a small study investigating 1.5 T TOF-MRA noted a sensitivity of 94% and a specificity of 96% for greater than 29%

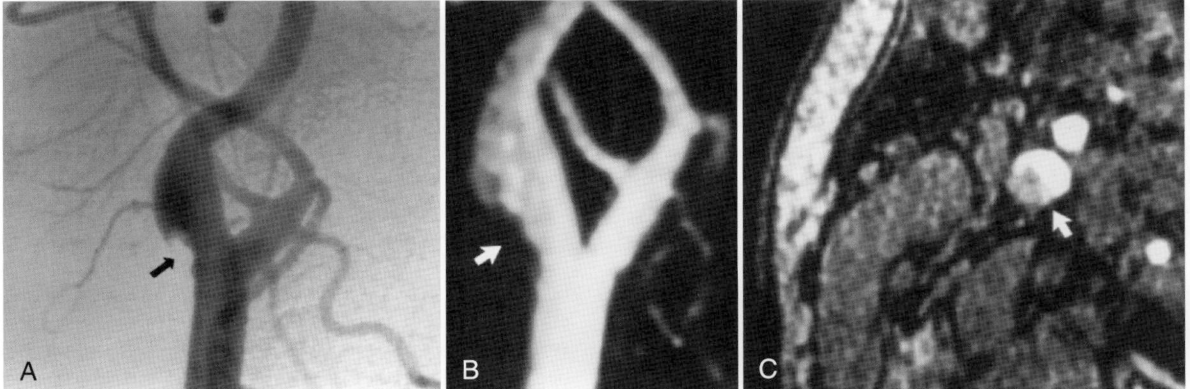

**Fig. 41.9 Carotid Stenosis.** Comparison of magnetic resonance angiogram and source image to catheter angiogram. **A,** Catheter angiogram of the right carotid system shows narrowing *(arrow)* at the origin of the internal carotid artery. Findings suggest intraluminal thrombus. **B,** Three-dimensional (3D) time-of-flight (TOF) angiogram demonstrates similar narrowing *(arrow)*. **C,** Axial 3D TOF source image at the site of stenosis shows clearly that the lumen is narrowed *(arrow)* by approximately 50%. In this case, there is agreement between the narrowing shown on source image and that detected by the maximum-intensity projection image **(B)**.

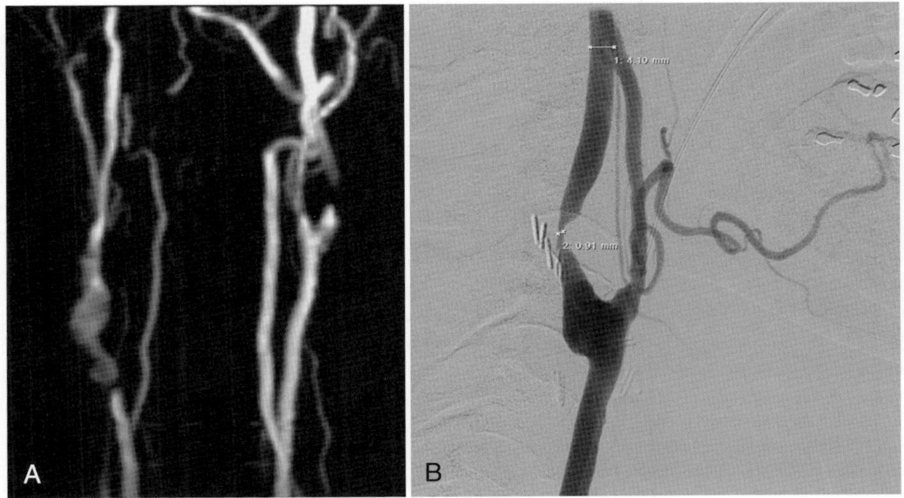

**Fig. 41.10 Carotid Stenosis.** Comparison of contrast-enhanced magnetic resonance angiography (CE-MRA) with conventional catheter angiography. **A,** CE-MRA reveals flow gap in proximal left internal carotid artery suggestive of high-grade stenosis. **B,** Digital subtraction angiography of the left carotid system confirms greater than 70% stenosis.

stenosis when compared with DSA. For greater than 49% stenosis, the sensitivity and specificity were similar, at 95% and 96%, respectively. In this investigation, 22% of patients had an overestimated degree of stenosis (Sadikin et al., 2007). Although TOF-MRA may be fairly accurate, evaluation for stenosis may be more reliable with CE-MRA.

The evaluation of cervical artery dissection is more commonly performed with MRI in combination with CE-MRA as will be described later. However, TOF-MRA may be a viable alternative for patients who are contraindicated from contrast imaging. Using combined MRI and CE-MRA as a gold standard, TOF-MRA has demonstrated a sensitivity of 93%–97% and a specificity of 96%–98% for the detection of cervical artery dissection (Coppenrath et al., 2013).

***Three-dimensional contrast-enhanced magnetic resonance angiography.*** Compared with 2D and 3D TOF-MRA, 3D CE-MRA delineates carotid arterial stenosis better (Fig. 41.10). Surface morphology (e.g., ulcerated plaque), nearly occluded vessels (e.g., "string sign"), and arterial occlusions are more easily identified (Etesami et al., 2012; Weber et al., 2015). Additional advantages of 3D CE-MRA include greater anatomical coverage (Fig. 41.11) and more accurate identification of intraplaque hemorrhage, a marker for disease progression. When compared with pathology, Qiao et al. (2011) noted that 3 T CE-MRA demonstrated a sensitivity of 90% and a specificity of 98% for intraplaque hemorrhage evaluation. For high-grade stenosis, which can cause intravascular flow gaps on TOF-MRA MIP images, the addition of CE-MRA to the imaging protocol provides sensitivity and specificity values equivalent to CTA in determining the severity of stenosis (relative to DSA as the reference standard).

A 2008 systematic review of 21 CE-MRA studies found that for the detection of high-grade (≥70%–99%) ICA stenoses, CE-MRA had a sensitivity of 94.6% with a specificity of 91.9%. For the detection of complete ICA occlusions, CE-MRA demonstrated a sensitivity of 99.4% and a specificity of 99.6%. However, for moderately severe ICA stenoses (50%–69%), CE-MRA had a fair sensitivity of 65.9%, with a specificity of 93.5% (Debrey et al., 2008). A more recent 2018 investigation of 3D CE-MRA observed that the sensitivities to mild (1%–49%), moderate (50%–69%), and severe (≥70%) stenoses were 85.5%, 100%, and 100%, respectively. The corresponding specificities were 95.3%, 98.6%, and 99.5%, respectively (Cui et al., 2018).

The ability to detect an FMD pattern of stenoses by MRA in the carotid vessels remains uncertain. This disorder may not be as well delineated on TOF-MRA due to limited resolution, although no large comparative studies with CE-MRA have been performed. In one series evaluating FMD in the renal arteries, Willoteaux et al. (2006) found the sensitivity and specificity of CE-MRA to be 97% and 93%, respectively. These findings suggest that using CE-MRA to identify FMD in the cervical vessels may be possible, although further studies are required.

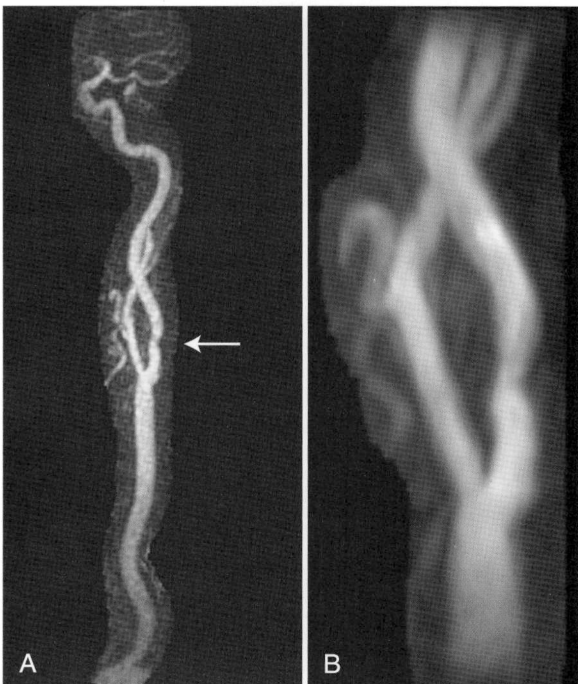

Fig. 41.11 Similar appearance of mild stenosis *(arrow)* of left internal carotid artery on oblique maximum-intensity projection images. A, Three-dimensional (3D) contrast-enhanced magnetic resonance angiography (CE-MRA). B, 3D time-of-flight (TOF)-MRA. Note the greater coverage of the carotids afforded by CE-MRA compared with TOF-MRA. *(From Bowen, B.C., 2007. MR angiography versus CT angiography in the evaluation of neurovascular disease. Radiology 245, 357–361.)*

For evaluation of posterior-circulation cerebrovascular disease, a 3D TOF-MRA study typically covers the vertebrobasilar system from the C2 level to the tip of the basilar artery (Fig. 41.12). The 3D CE-MRA techniques can display both the origins and distal intracranial portions of the vertebral arteries in a single acquisition and are particularly useful in evaluating vertebral artery segments with partial or complete signal loss caused by slow flow and in-plane saturation effects. The accuracy of 3D CE-MRA measurements of stenosis at the vertebral artery is less than that of carotid bifurcation measurements because of the smaller size of the vertebral origins. Choi et al. (2010) observed that the sensitivity and specificity of CE-MRA was 100% and 80.4%, respectively, with a false-positive rate of 52.5%.

In patients with carotid or vertebral artery dissection, CE-MRA is often complemented by MRI with fat-saturation sequences that aid in the detection and characterization of dissecting hematoma, associated dissecting aneurysm, and the length and caliber of the residual patent lumen, especially at the skull base (Fig. 41.13). Subacute hyperintense thrombus is better seen if fat suppression is implemented on thin T1-weighted images to eliminate the high signal intensity from perivascular adipose tissue. Serial MRA examinations are required to evaluate for recanalization of the vessel following the dissection (Fig. 41.14) and also to evaluate for dissecting aneurysms that may occasionally develop as the hematoma resolves.

The MRA assessment of vascular stenosis after placement of a metallic stent is limited by turbulence and susceptibility effects. Stent geometry, the relative orientation of the magnetic field, and alloy composition contribute to signal intensity alterations within the stent lumen (Fig. 41.15). As with CTA, artificial lumen narrowing is commonly noted within the stent, especially with decreasing stent diameters (see Fig. 41.15), but this effect may be decreased in 3 T CE-MRA compared with 1.5 T CE-MRA. Lettau et al. (2009) also noted that there is less of this effect in most nitinol stents than in stents made of stainless steel or cobalt alloy.

## Intracranial Circulation

TOF-MRA may be used to detect stenosis or occlusion of the proximal intracranial arteries. Initially, accuracy was limited by technical

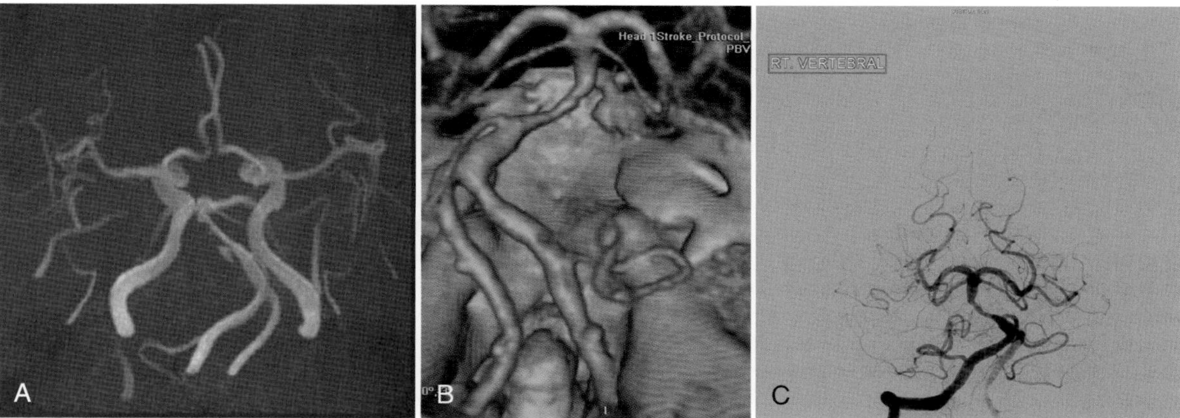


Fig. 41.12 Basilar artery stenosis seen on both magnetic resonance angiography (MRA) and computed tomographic angiography (CTA). A, A 3 T time-of-flight-MRA reveals moderate luminal narrowing in mid to distal portion of basilar artery. B, Three-dimensional reconstruction of CTA images reveals a 1-cm area of irregular narrowing in the basilar artery, with 65% stenosis. C, Digital cerebral angiography most accurately depicts the stenotic region with high temporal and spatial resolution.

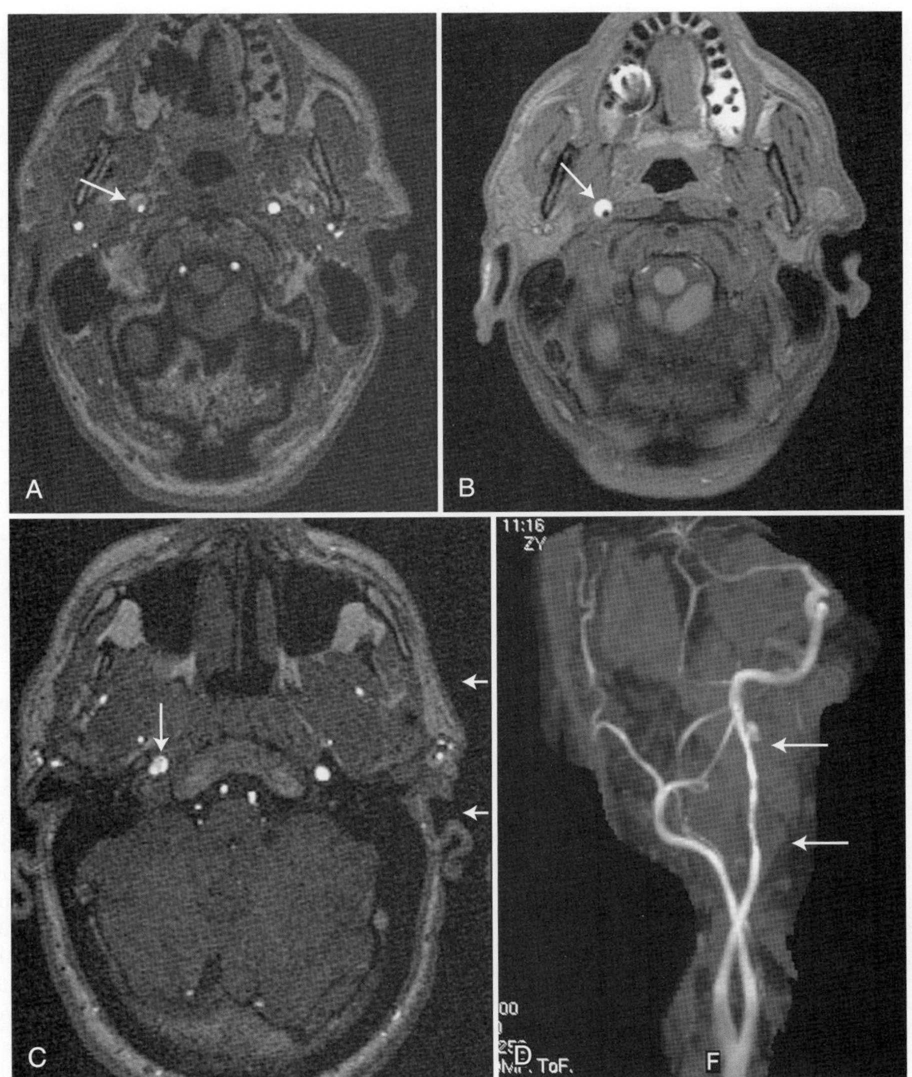

**Fig. 41.13** Right internal carotid artery dissection (see all arrows) with intramural hematoma causing severe narrowing of the residual patent lumen as well as pseudoaneurysm at the skull base. **A,** Three-dimensional (3D) time-of-flight (TOF) axial source image. **B,** Fat-suppression T1-weighted axial image at C1–C1 shows the narrowed cervical carotid lumen with flow and the thickened wall with unsuppressed hyperintensity consistent with subacute hematoma *(arrows)*. **C,** 3D TOF axial source image at the level of the carotid canal entrance shows outpouching of pseudoaneurysm *(arrow)*. **D,** Oblique maximum-intensity projection image displays the length of the narrowed lumen *(between arrows)*, ending at the carotid canal and the pseudoaneurysm *(large arrow)*. (*From Bowen, B.C., 2007. MR angiography versus CT angiography in the evaluation of neurovascular disease. Radiology 245, 357–361.*)

shortcomings such as long echo time (TE), lower spatial resolution, and single thick-slab acquisition. These resulted in a decrease in vascular signal due to intravoxel phase dispersion, susceptibility effects, and saturation effects. Signal loss was typically evident in the petrous, cavernous, and supraclinoid segments of the ICA and in the proximal M1 segment of the MCA. Second- and third-order branches of the cerebral arteries were poorly shown. Later studies reported that normal vessels and completely occluded vessels could be graded correctly when compared with DSA results, but stenotic segments were only correctly graded (as either < or >50% narrowing) about 60% of the time. Subsequently, technical improvements in the 3D TOF method (variable flip angle, magnetization transfer suppression, multiple thin-slab acquisitions, and higher spatial resolution [512 matrix or greater]) improved the accuracy of stenosis grading, resulting in sensitivities and specificities ranging from 80% to 100% and 89% to 95%, respectively (Baradaran, 2017).

The current approach to evaluating the intracranial arteries uses a multislab 3D TOF acquisition that covers the head from the foramen magnum extending superiorly to the areas of interest. Each slab has a transaxial orientation and may or may not have a superiorly located presaturation band. The axial source images and the reprojected MIP images (Fig. 41.16) are reviewed in conjunction with other MR images. In the setting of acute infarction with the potential for thrombolytic treatment, protocols often include a rapidly acquired 2D PC-MRA study of the circle of Willis instead of the more time-consuming 3D TOF study. Other clinical settings in which MRA complements routine MRI include sickle cell disease, moyamoya syndrome, hemifacial spasm, and trigeminal neuralgia. Flow dynamics (magnitude and direction) in the circle of Willis are more easily determined with the PC method, especially when vessel diameters are 1 mm or more. A promising technique under investigation utilizes the distal:proximal signal intensity ratio (SIR) on TOF-MRA to obtain a measurement of fractional flow across a stenotic vessel region. This measurement technique, used in coronary artery disease, reflects blood flow velocity through a stenotic segment and represents a novel marker of hemodynamic impairment. Diminished signal intensities distal to the stenotic site have been associated with delayed ipsilateral perfusion and an elevated risk of future territorial strokes (Lan et al. 2016; Liebeskind et al. 2015).

The simplest type of 3D CE-MRA technique uses scan parameters typical of 3D TOF-MRA acquisitions with scan times of 5–10 minutes per 3D volume. Under these steady-state conditions, visibility of the small intracranial arteries is greater after IV gadolinium administration; however, the intracranial veins also show a much greater increase in visibility. Consequently, the MIP images become cluttered with veins, resulting in greater difficulty in identifying and delineating specific arteries. With dynamic 3D CE-MRA, as used for extracranial carotid imaging, temporal resolution is improved, and visibility of the arteries is greater than that of veins. Some investigators have suggested the use of region-of-interest MIP postprocessing to further exclude veins from intracranial artery displays. Despite the limits placed on spatial resolution by the dynamic 3D CE-MRA technique, Parker and colleagues (1998) have shown that, in theory, imaging with a TR of 7–10 ms (e.g., scan time approximately 1 minute per 3D volume) and a T1 relaxation time of 25–50 ms for flowing blood containing gadolinium (first-pass arterial concentration of approximately 5–10 mM) can produce images of the intracranial arteries (≈0.5 mm diameter) with vascular contrast comparable to that produced by the steady-state 3D CE-MRA technique. When compared with TOF-MRA, another study found that 3D CE-MRA had greater specificity (97% vs. 89%) in detecting >50% stenosis (Nael et al., 2014). Dynamic 3D CE-MRA may play a prominent future role in evaluating intracranial arterial steno-occlusive disease, but the accuracy, reproducibility, and reliability of CE-MRA measurements compared with those of DSA and TOF-MRA warrant further delineation.

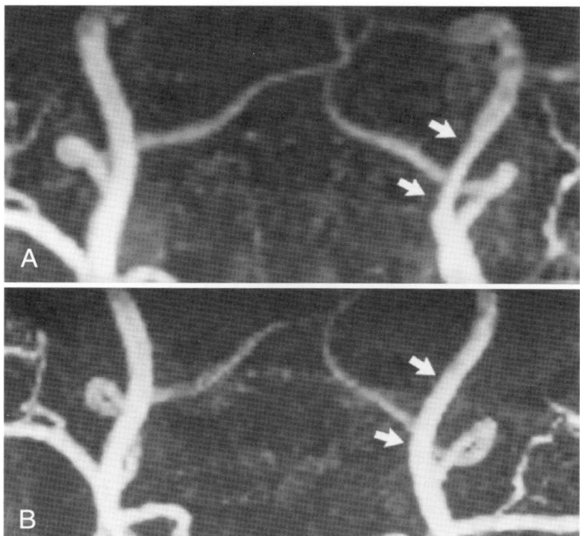


**Fig. 41.14** Resolution of Carotid Dissection Followed with Magnetic Resonance Angiography (MRA). **A,** MRA produced by the three-dimensional time-of-flight technique shows a segmental stenosis *(arrows)* involving the distal cervical portion of the left internal carotid artery. **B,** Repeat study obtained after anticoagulant therapy demonstrates return to normal caliber of the internal carotid artery segment *(arrows)*.

***Subclavian steal syndrome.*** *Subclavian steal syndrome* describes the reversal of normal direction of flow in the vertebral artery ipsilateral to a severe stenosis or occlusion occurring between the aortic arch and vertebral artery origin. DSA remains the standard in visualizing disease in the great vessels, along with abnormal retrograde filling of the affected vertebral artery. Given the invasive nature of DSA, Doppler sonography is often used, but this study may be limited by lack of visualization of the relevant pathology in the subclavian artery. Therefore, MRA offers a reliable comprehensive means to test patients with suspected subclavian steal syndrome. PC-MRA methods encode direction of flow and can accurately depict subclavian stenosis along with reversal of flow in the vertebral artery. Although TOF-MRA does not possess true flow-encoded information, flow direction can be deduced with suppression of flow from a single direction by a saturation pulse that allows for selective arterial or venous MRI, with reversal of flow presenting as a flow void. This finding may also be seen with severe stenosis or occlusion but may be distinguished by anatomical imaging of vessel patency, such as with 3D CE-MRA.

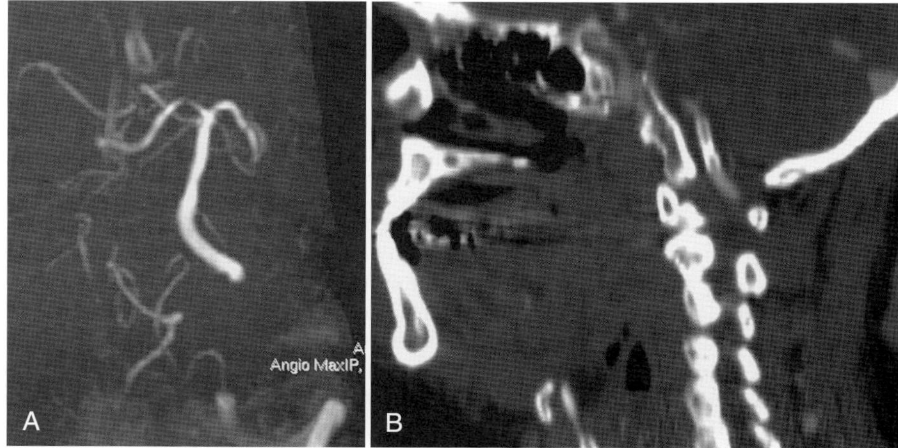


**Fig. 41.15 Stent Device in the Distal Left Vertebral Artery. A,** Coronal time-of-flight magnetic resonance image demonstrates loss of enhancement in the distal portion of the stent placement, suggesting a severe stenosis. **B,** Axial images of the neck after contrast administration is unable to accurately determine the degree of residual luminal narrowing. Widening the window settings results in overestimation of stenosis, and a later digital subtraction angiography demonstrated only mild stenosis.

However, 3D CE-MRA has a potential disadvantage in the lone evaluation of subclavian steal syndrome because it does not possess inherent flow-encoded information. However, the low-resolution 2D TOF localizer acquisition that is often performed beforehand has been shown to provide the same information as a formal TOF-MRA sequence (Sheehy et al., 2005).

***Acute ischemic stroke.*** MRA is considered less accurate than CTA and DSA for the evaluation of occlusive intracranial disease. However, when combined with the detailed parenchymal anatomy on brain MRI, significant information may be obtained to better prognosticate and guide further treatment (Marks et al., 2008; Torres-Mozqueda et al., 2008). TOF-MRA, rather than CE-MRA, is more commonly utilized for patients with acute stroke and has a sensitivity and specificity of 81% and 98%, respectively, for the detection of occlusion (Bash et al., 2005). However, the use of CE-MRA may be preferred as it has been noted to be superior in localizing vessel occlusion within a shorter acquisition time while providing a larger coverage, including extracranial vessels, and a more accurate assessment of collateral status (Boujan et al., 2018). The use of dynamic MRA for acute ischemic stroke remains under investigation but has shown promise as an accurate surrogate of collateral circulation seen on conventional angiography. This modality offers a fast and reliable means to assess cerebral hemodynamics and collateral circulation in patients with acute ischemic stroke that may be of benefit for those patients undergoing screening for potential thrombectomy treatment (Hernández-Pérez et al., 2016). Overall, MRA is implemented less often for stroke patients who present in early time windows amenable for acute intervention due to its prolonged imaging time relative to CTA. However, advances are being made to optimize rapid combined MRI and MRA stroke protocols, making this an increasingly used modality for potential thrombolytic or thrombectomy candidates.

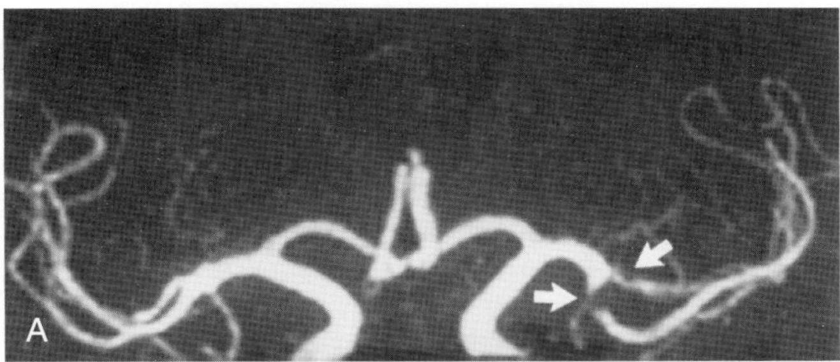


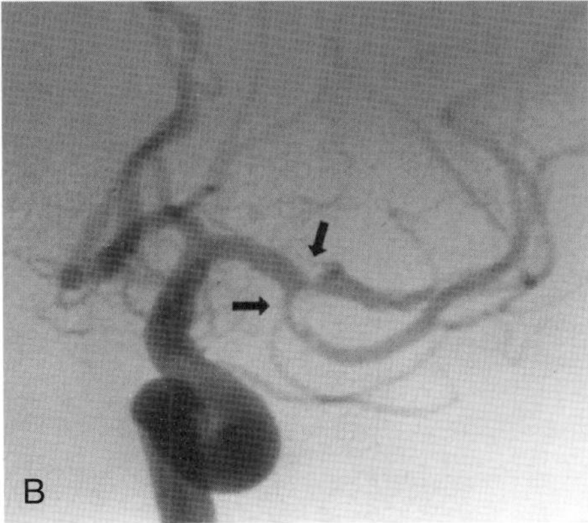


**Fig. 41.16 Proximal Middle Cerebral Artery (MCA) Stenosis (Same Patient as in Fig. 41.4). A,** Coronal projection magnetic resonance angiogram was produced from the axial source images shown in Fig. 41.4. Coronal view shows better than the axial view (Fig. 41.4, *C*) that there is stenosis *(arrows)* involving both M2 branches of the MCA. **B,** Catheter angiography confirms the presence of both stenoses *(arrows)*.

***Cerebral aneurysms.*** MRA has become increasingly used for noninvasive screening and surveillance of aneurysmal disease (Fig. 41.17). The most thoroughly investigated MRA technique for cerebral aneurysms is 3D TOF-MRA, but its main disadvantages are long scanning times, limitations in detecting very small aneurysms, difficulty establishing the relationship of the aneurysm to adjacent (and surgically important) osseous anatomy, and occasional uncertainty in distinguishing between patent lumen, high-grade stenosis, and occlusion. In general, noninvasive imaging evaluation includes a review of T1- and T2-weighted (fast) spin-echo images and T2*-weighted gradient echo images, in addition to the source images and MIP images from the MRA acquisition.

A 2017 meta-analysis of 18 studies comprising 3463 patients found that TOF-MRA demonstrated a pooled sensitivity and specificity of 89% and 94%, respectively. Additionally, the sensitivity for aneurysms greater than 3 mm is higher (89%) compared with the sensitivity for detecting smaller aneurysms ≤3 mm (78%). Unruptured aneurysms are more likely to be detected than aneurysms on studies with subarachnoid hemorrhage present (Haifeng et al., 2017). False-positive and false-negative aneurysms are more commonly depicted at the skull base and MCA. False-positive aneurysms are often attributable to infundibula and arterial loops (Cho et al., 2011). The addition of 3D reconstructions has been shown to increase diagnostic performance, and studies performed on 3 T demonstrated a trend toward

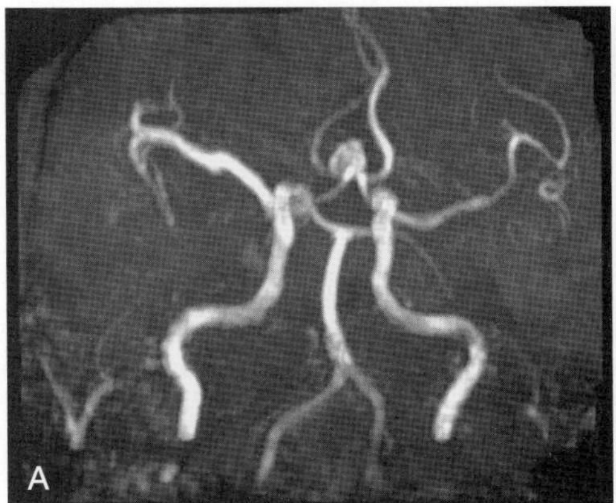


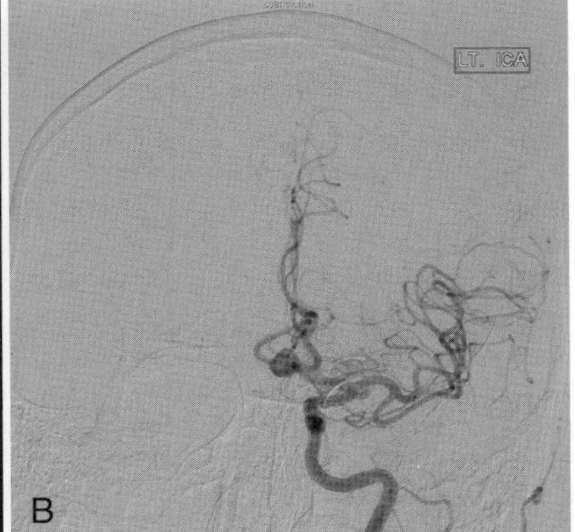


**Fig. 41.17 Anterior Communicating Artery Aneurysm. A,** A three-dimensional time-of-flight magnetic resonance angiogram on 1.5 T reveals a lobulated, saccular aneurysm arising from the junction of the A1 and A2 segments. **B,** Digital subtraction angiogram prior to coil embolization also demonstrates this anterosuperiorly directed aneurysm.

better accuracy (Sailer et al., 2014). For patients presenting with subarachnoid hemorrhage, 3 T TOF-MRA with 3D volume rendering was found to have a sensitivity of 97.6% and a specificity of 93.1% compared with DSA. For the prediction of the correct treatment planning strategy based on aneurysm anatomy, MRA demonstrated a sensitivity of 94% and a specificity of 100%, suggesting that it may serve both as a useful screening and treatment planning tool (Chen et al., 2012).

Compared with TOF MRA, CE-MRA is generally considered more accurate in assessing the sac shape, aneurysm neck detection, and visualization of branches originating at the sac or neck (Cirillo et al., 2013). When compared with DSA, one study found that the sensitivity was higher in CE-MRA (96%) compared with TOF-MRA (92%) with an identical specificity of 98% (Levent, 2014). Although MRA demonstrates similar sensitivity and specificity to CTA for detection of intracerebral aneurysms ≥5 mm in diameter, they have lower sensitivity for aneurysms less than 5 mm (Villablanca et al., 2002). Despite the lower sensitivity of MRA for smaller aneurysms, the results of the International Study of Unruptured Intracranial Aneurysms (ISUIA; Wiebers et al., 2003) suggest that this may not significantly impact management of these aneurysms during initial screening because small incidental aneurysms, especially in the anterior circulation, have a lower rupture risk and are more likely to be monitored.

In addition to screening, MRA imaging has emerged as a common noninvasive means for surveillance after endovascular treatment for detecting aneurysm recurrences, although the data remain mixed regarding its accuracy (Fig. 41.18). One meta-analysis evaluated 16 studies that compared 1.5 T TOF-MRA and 1.5 T CE-MRA with DSA in the follow-up of coiled intracranial aneurysms. Pooled sensitivity and specificity of TOF-MRA for the detection of residual flow within the aneurysmal neck or body were 83.3% and 90.6%, respectively. Pooled sensitivity and specificity of CE-MRA for the detection of residual flow were 86.8% and 91.9%, respectively, but they were not found to be significantly different (Kwee and Kwee, 2007). A prospective analysis was performed to compare TOF-MRA and CE-MRA at 1.5 T and 3 T with a reference standard of DSA in the evaluation of previously coiled intracranial aneurysms. For the detection of any aneurysm remnant, the sensitivity was 90%, 85%, 88%, and 90% for 1.5 T TOF, 1.5 T CE, 3 T TOF, and 3 T CE-MRA, respectively. These sensitivities dropped to 50%, 67%, 50%, and 67%, respectively, for the detection of only larger (class 3 and 4) aneurysm remnants because several of these remnants were underclassified as smaller remnants by MRA. CE-MRA at 1.5 T and 3 T had a better sensitivity for larger remnants than TOF-MRA, which may be related to greater flow-related artifacts within larger aneurysm remnants on TOF-MRA compared with the luminal

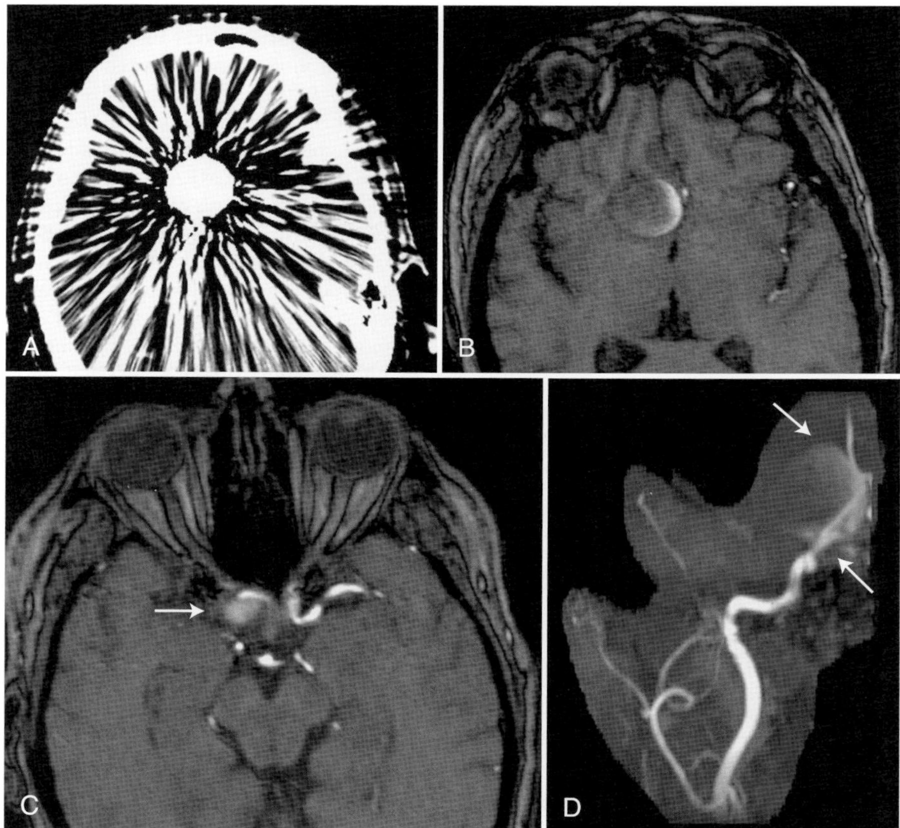


**Fig. 41.18 Right Ophthalmic Artery Aneurysm Following Coil Embolization. A,** Computed tomographic angiography source image nondiagnostic for residual lumen due to streak artifacts. **B,** Three-dimensional time-of-flight magnetic resonance angiogram (3D TOF-MRA) axial source image at level of aneurysm dome reveals central and eccentric hypodensity due to packed coils and peripheral hyperintensity due to flow-related enhancement in residual lumen. **C,** 3D TOF-MRA axial source image at level of aneurysm neck also shows evidence of flow through patent neck remnant *(arrow).* **D,** Coronal maximum-intensity projection image demonstrates continuity of flow into neck and dome remnants of coiled aneurysm *(arrows).* (*From Bowen, B.C., 2007. MR angiography versus CT angiography in the evaluation of neurovascular disease. Radiology 245, 357–361.*)

contrast-filling characteristics of aneurysms on CE-MRA. Specificities of these four MRA techniques for detecting any aneurysm remnant were 52%, 65%, 52%, and 64%, respectively. Specificities improved to 85%, 84%, 85%, and 87%, respectively, for the detection of larger (class 3 and 4) aneurysm remnants, reflecting the difficulty in detecting smaller remnants with MRA. Regarding the detection of any aneurysm growth since previous comparison angiograms, sensitivities for these MRA techniques were 28%, 28%, 33%, and 39%, respectively, and specificities were 93%, 95%, 98%, and 95% (Kaufmann et al., 2010). Artifacts from coil embolization are generally smaller on 3 T MRA versus 1.5 T MRA because a shorter echo-time at 3 T negates artifact enlargement. These artifacts may potentially lead to artificially smaller aneurysm remnants on 1.5 T MRA that should be considered when imaging treated patients (Schaafsma et al., 2014). Although CE-MRA is more likely than TOF-MRA to classify larger aneurysm remnants appropriately, TOF-MRA better identifies the location of coil masses and may be more advantageous if suboptimal CE-MRA contrast bolus is given. Therefore, the advantage of CE-MRA over TOF-MRA remains uncertain, and consideration for both examinations may be made in the follow-up of patients with coiled intracranial aneurysms. Lavoie et al. (2012) found that the sensitivity on MRA for treated aneurysms remains limited for aneurysms <6 mm, and the authors recommended that recurrent aneurysms should still be confirmed with DSA before planning retreatment. Furthermore, another study found that despite the high reported sensitivity and specificity of MRA, real-world experience led to a change in treatment strategy for 30.1% of patients with an aneurysm on MRA for various reasons, including size and location discrepancies or detection of a benign vascular variant (Tomycz et al., 2011). 4D MRA has been investigated for assessment of the blood inflow zone and the inflow velocity profile of aneurysms treated with coil embolization. These characteristics may help determine the risk of coil compaction and recanalization after treatment (Futami, 2014).

The emerging use of flow diverters for the primary treatment of aneurysms has created diagnostic challenges when evaluating residual aneurysm filling on MRA due to significant imaging artifacts that are produced. The sensitivity in detecting aneurysm occlusion with flow diverters on 3D TOF-MRA has been reported to be 50%–57%. Diagnostic evaluation is improved on CE-MRA, which has demonstrated a sensitivity of 83%–96%, with a specificity ranging from 85% to 100% (Attali et al., 2016; Binyamin et al., 2017; Boddu et al., 2014). Intrasaccular flow disruption devices pose an even greater diagnostic challenge due to significant signal loss related to the radiofrequency shielding effect around the device. Few studies exist, but the sensitivity has been reported to be as low as 25% for both TOF-MRA and CE-MRA, prompting recommendations to use DSA as a standard for follow-up imaging (Nawka et al., 2018; Timsit et al., 2016). Although MRA cannot yet completely replace DSA, it has certainly proven to be a valuable adjunctive imaging option for aneurysm evaluation.

***Venous disorders.*** Imaging of the cerebral venous system differs from approaches tailored to the arterial system because of the lower velocity of venous flow and the morphology of the venous sinuses. For suspected dural sinus occlusion resulting from thrombosis or tumor invasion, the primary technique has traditionally utilized 2D TOF-MRA in conjunction with spin-echo imaging. To establish the diagnosis of venous thrombosis, lack of visualization of a vein or sinus on the source images and angiogram must be accompanied by identification of the clot on the spin-echo images at the location of the suspected occlusion (Fig. 41.19). With the 2D TOF technique, optimal flow enhancement in a section is achieved when it is perpendicular to the flow direction. This condition is best approximated using coronal

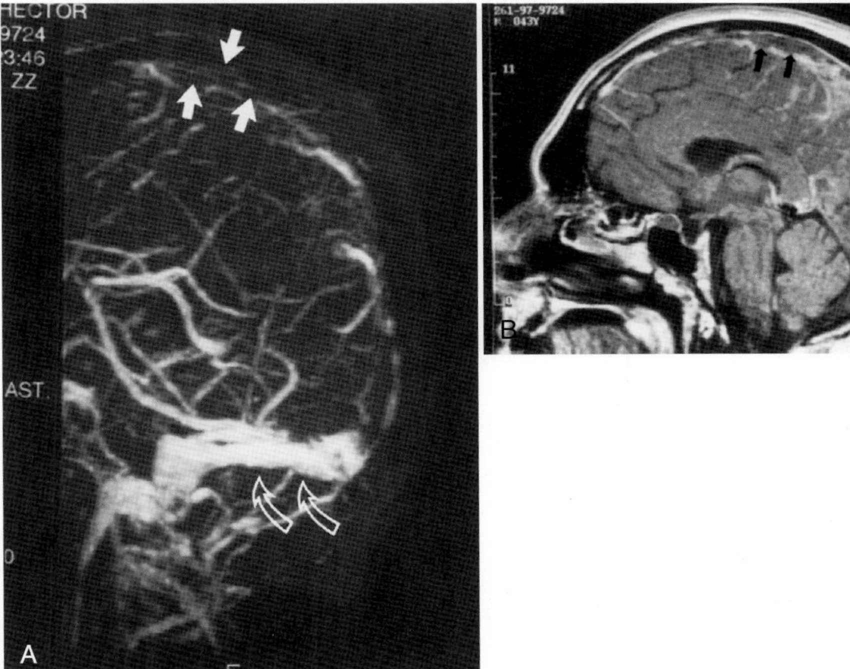

**Fig. 41.19 Acute Superior Sagittal Sinus Thrombosis. A,** Magnetic resonance angiogram (lateral view) produced from 80 sequential two-dimensional time-of-flight coronal sections covering posterior half of the head. Flow-related signal is observed in transverse *(open arrows)* and sigmoid sinuses but not in superior sagittal sinus *(closed arrows)* or straight sinus. Short segments of vessels projecting over posterior course of superior sagittal sinus represent patent superficial cerebral veins lateral to the sinus. **B,** Postgadolinium midsagittal T1-weighted image shows hypointense signal in superior sagittal sinus and enhancing margins. Combined with the results in **A,** findings are consistent with the presence of intraluminal thrombus.

sections to image the sagittal, straight, and transverse sinuses (along with the internal cerebral veins, basal veins of Rosenthal, and to a lesser degree, the vein of Galen). The acquisition of coronal sections can be augmented by the acquisition of oblique sagittal sections to allow better flow enhancement in the posterior portions of the transverse sinuses and the cortical veins draining into the superior sagittal sinus. With the 2D TOF-MR venography technique, arterial signal is reduced or eliminated by an axial presaturation band placed across the upper neck below the skull base. A common diagnostic pitfall of the technique is the presence of flow gaps in the transverse sinus. Ayanzen and colleagues (2000) observed these gaps in 31% of patients with normal MRI findings. Flow gaps were not observed in the superior sagittal, straight, or dominant transverse sinuses, so gaps occurring in these locations should raise suspicion of venous obstruction. The authors found that the nondominant transverse sinuses (90% of gaps) or codominant transverse sinuses (10%) that demonstrated the flow gaps were hypoplastic yet patent by DSA.

Alternative techniques for demonstrating cerebral veins and dural venous sinuses lack the robustness of the 2D TOF technique. The 3D TOF technique suffers from saturation effects and hence frequent signal loss in the veins and dural sinuses. The 2D PC technique is limited by gradient heterogeneity, eddy currents, aliasing artifacts, and lower spatial resolution. Although the PC technique can be useful in differentiating very slow flow in the dural sinuses from thrombosis, it was found to be inferior to the 2D TOF technique and a contrast-enhanced 3D FLASH (fast low-angle shot) MRA technique in displaying the normal septal veins, internal cerebral veins, and the basal veins (Kirchhof et al., 2002). Both the 3D FLASH technique and a 3D magnetization-prepared, rapid-acquisition gradient echo MRI technique (Liang et al., 2001) are contrast-enhanced methods and reportedly are superior to the 2D TOF technique in depicting normal venous structures, especially in overcoming the flow gap artifact. However, these contrast-enhanced techniques have two potential limitations: (1) both techniques involve rapid acquisition (1–2 minutes per 3D volume), so the intensity of the intravascular signal depends on the timing of the contrast infusion relative to data acquisition, and (2) chronic thrombus may enhance with gadolinium and mimic a patent lumen. Consequently, these two contrast-enhanced techniques should be viewed as adjuncts to the 2D TOF technique.

***Vascular malformations.*** Traditional MRA methods (2D and 3D TOF-MRA and PC-MRA) have played a secondary role to DSA in evaluating intracranial AVMs because of a lack of consistent and complete demonstration of all components of an AVM: feeding arteries, nidus, and draining veins. For this reason, and because of the general impression that TOF-MRA adds little to the spin-echo MRI findings useful for preliminary staging of an AVM (nidus size and location and central versus peripheral pattern of venous drainage in the Spetzler-Martin Grading Scale) before definitive DSA, many investigators have considered TOF-MRA of AVMs superfluous (Table 41.1). PC techniques

**TABLE 41.1 Spetzler-Martin Grading System***

| LESION SIZE | | LOCATION | | VENOUS DRAINAGE | |
|---|---|---|---|---|---|
| Small (<3 cm) | 1 | Noneloquent site | 0 | Superficial only | 0 |
| Medium (3–6 cm) | 2 | Eloquent site† | 1 | Any deep | 1 |
| Large (>6 cm) | 3 | | | | |

*Assigns cumulative points based on arteriovenous malformation characteristics, with higher scores indicating increased surgical risk.
†Eloquent areas include sensorimotor, language, visual, thalamus, hypothalamus, internal capsule, brainstem, cerebellar peduncles, and deep cerebellar nuclei.

have been used by some investigators to estimate blood flow velocities and volume flow rates in the largest arteries supplying the AVM. A high-resolution 3D gradient echo technique based on the paramagnetic property of deoxyhemoglobin has been used to detect cerebral veins with submillimeter resolution, resulting in greater sensitivity in identifying the presence of small AVMs. But compared with TOF-MRA, the technique provides poorer detection of feeding arteries and is markedly limited in its delineation of nidus size and shape when there are susceptibility artifacts from nearby bone, air, or blood products (hemosiderin). High-resolution, real-time, auto-triggered, elliptic, centric-ordered 3D CE-MRA (Farb et al., 2001) and lower-resolution time-resolved 2D CE-MRA have also been applied to the evaluation of AVMs and the results compared with those of TOF-MRA and intra-arterial DSA. In an initial investigation, Farb and colleagues found that their 3D CE-MRA technique was superior to 3D TOF-MRA, particularly in depicting nidus and draining veins. The 3D CE-MRA technique consistently showed AVM components and their spatial relationships on MIP images and was equivalent to DSA in depicting AVM components in 70%–90% of cases (total patients = 10), based on blinded independent assessments by two experienced neuroradiologists.

Several small studies prospectively examined 4D CE-MRA at 3 T for evaluating AVM and found that 4D CE-MRA yielded 100% accuracy in identifying the Spetzler-Martin classification (nidus size, venous drainage, eloquence) of cerebral AVMs when compared with DSA. One study demonstrated a 93% rate of detection of feeding arteries using 4D MRA alone. Moreover, the combined use of selective ASL provided additional functional or anatomical information in 4 of 16 cases (25%), enabling the detection of a cross-filling feeding artery that was not identified by 4D MRA without selective arterial spin labeling (ASL) technique, and improved sensitivity to 96% (Kukuk et al., 2010). For patients who underwent AVM treatment with radiosurgery, embolization, and/or surgical resection, 4D MRA has been found to be a useful technique for the evaluation of residual pathology, with a noted sensitivity of 73.7% and a specificity of 100% (Noguiera et al., 2013; Soize et al., 2014). Although 4D MRA appears to represent a promising noninvasive alternative to DSA, it currently suffers from low spatial resolution and vessel superposition, making differentiation of arterial feeders of the nidus difficult (Hadizadeh et al., 2008; Machet et al., 2012).

Dural AVFs most commonly involve the cavernous, transverse, and sigmoid sinuses along the skull base. Arterial feeders not seen on spin-echo MR are sometimes detected on 3D TOF-MRA, but much less often than on catheter angiography. Transverse and sigmoid sinus occlusion and dilated cortical veins are detected better by MRA than spin-echo imaging, yet neither technique achieves the accuracy of catheter angiography. Traditional 3D TOF-MRA is useful in detecting cavernous sinus fistulas because flow enhancement in the cavernous sinus and contiguous veins can provide evidence of the fistula (Fig. 41.20). This finding must be regarded with caution because venous flow signal may occasionally be observed in the cavernous sinus and inferior petrosal sinus of patients without clinical evidence of carotid-cavernous fistula. Farb et al. (2009) compared the use of 3 T time-resolved MRA for the diagnosis and classification of a cranial dural AVF with DSA. Patients underwent a commercially available contrast-enhanced time-resolved imaging of contrast kinetics (TRICKS) MRA (trMRA) technique that combines $k$-space segmentation into central, mid, and peripheral zones with superimposed elliptic centric-view ordering. High temporal resolution is obtained by sampling the central zones of the $k$-space at a more frequent rate than peripheral zones. The high spatial and temporal resolution allows for identification of dural AVFs by identifying both early opacification of a dural sinus and reflux into the connecting cortical veins if present. In 93% (39/42) of dural

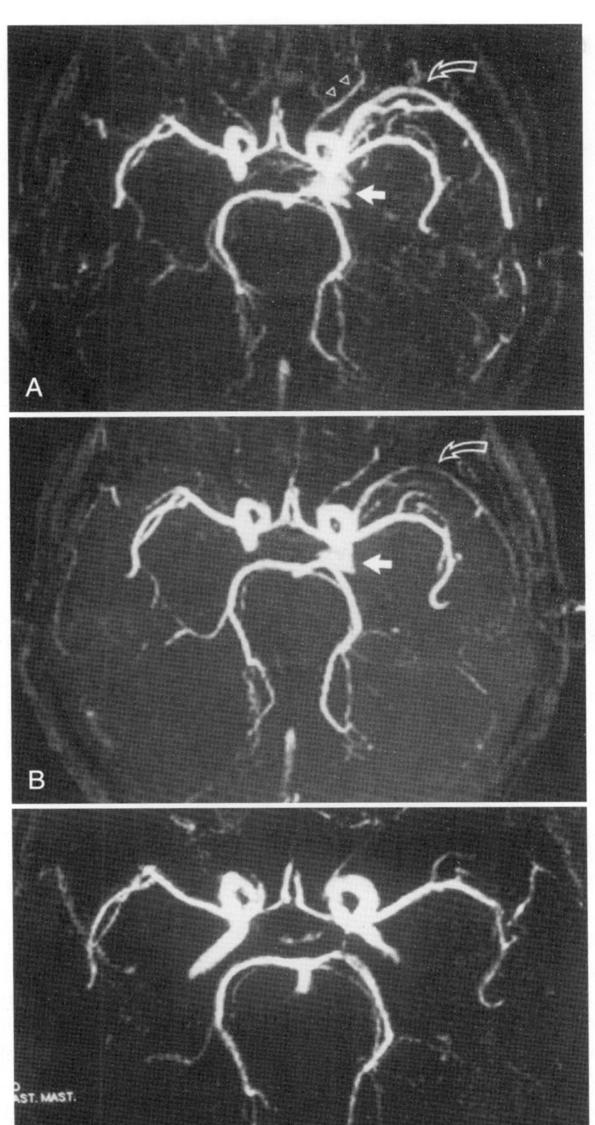

**Fig. 41.20 Spontaneous Resolution of a Left Carotid-Cavernous Dural Arteriovenous Fistula (AVF).** Magnetic resonance angiograms (axial maximum-intensity projection images) of sellar region and circle of Willis were acquired with three-dimensional time-of-flight technique (no gadolinium enhancement). The studies, performed at the time of clinical presentation (**A**), 3 months later (**B**), and 3 years later (**C**) show progressive resolution of venous drainage from the AVF. Flow-related signal in left cavernous sinus *(closed arrow)*, sphenoparietal sinus *(open arrow)*, and cerebral veins results from shunting of high-flow-rate arterial blood through fistula. Note progressive decrease in signal in the sphenoparietal sinus. Flow-related signal in the left orbit is caused by the ophthalmic artery *(arrowheads)*, not the superior ophthalmic vein, which was found by catheter angiography to be thrombosed at the time of presentation.

AVF cases, investigators had unanimously correct interpretations of the trMRA to correctly identify or exclude all fistulas and accurately classify them when found. The small series suggests that trMRA may be a reliable technique in the screening and surveillance of DAVFs in certain clinical situations, but further validation studies are required (Farb et al., 2009).

The diagnostic imaging features of venous malformations (angiomas, developmental venous anomalies) are well shown on postgadolinium T1-weighted spin-echo images. These features include the radially oriented collection of small vessels (medullary veins) that produce a caput medusa or spoke-wheel configuration. This is contiguous with a large trunk vein that drains into either subependymal or superficial cerebral veins or a dural sinus. The 2D TOF technique and the PC method with low anticipated maximum blood flow velocity often display these slow-flow malformations without the use of gadolinium and allow determination of flow direction. However, the 3D TOF technique, which provides greater spatial resolution, requires gadolinium to avoid saturation effects. Cavernous malformations and capillary telangiectasias do not show flow enhancement on MRA studies, and the former are usually identified on spin-echo and gradient echo images by the heterogeneous signal intensity caused by blood products from prior hemorrhage.

## Spine Disorders

Spinal MRA is used as an adjunct to MRI to improve the visibility of the millimeter-sized intradural vessels and to help differentiate abnormal ones from normal ones. The combined MR examination provides better characterization of spinal vessels and thus more effective noninvasive screening for vascular lesions (e.g., dural AVFs) than MRI alone (Saraf-Lavi et al., 2002). The improved screening facilitates decisions regarding invasive catheter angiography for definitive diagnosis and endovascular treatment. The combined MR examination also allows the largest normal vessels to be localized noninvasively before surgical or endovascular procedures that carry a risk of cord injury. Studies have also shown that patients undergoing catheter angiography following MRA require half the fluoroscopy time and half the volume of iodinated contrast if the level and side of the fistula have been identified on a screening MRA (Luetmer et al., 2005). MRA and CTA are reported to have similar sensitivities in screening for the level of the artery of Adamkiewicz (Yoshioka et al., 2003).

Enhancement of the intradural vessels with gadolinium contrast agents has been found necessary for optimal detection on MRA. The 3D CE-MRA technique with steady-state conditions (i.e., TOF pulse sequence parameters) detects the largest intradural veins in healthy volunteers: the posterior and anterior median veins and the great medullary veins draining from the surface of the cord to the epidural space. This technique, and to a lesser extent the 3D PC technique, also detects the abnormally enlarged and tortuous veins draining dural AVFs (Fig. 41.21) and intramedullary AVMs. In detecting the presence of dural AVFs, the steady-state 3D CE-MRA technique combined with spin-echo MRI had a sensitivity ranging from 80% to 100%, a specificity of 82%, and an accuracy of 81%–94% in a randomized blinded review by three neuroradiologists of 11 control subjects and 20 patients with proven dural AVFs (Saraf-Lavi et al., 2002). More importantly, in determining the vertebral level of the fistula, the correct level was predicted in 73% of cases by combined MRA and MRI, representing a significant improvement over MRI alone. Improved noninvasive localization of the fistula level potentially expedites the subsequent invasive catheter angiography study.

Preliminary studies of spinal vascular malformations using time-resolved or fast 3D CE-MRA indicate that such first-pass studies may provide better depiction of the dural AVF in the neural foramen because of diminished extradural venous enhancement and improved visibility of the feeding arteries of AVMs (Binkert et al., 1999). A retrospective review of 31 first-pass CE-MRA studies noted a pooled sensitivity and specificity of 100% and 82%, respectively. In comparison, a review of 15 time-resolved CE-MRA studies noted a pooled sensitivity and specificity of 100% and 80%, respectively.

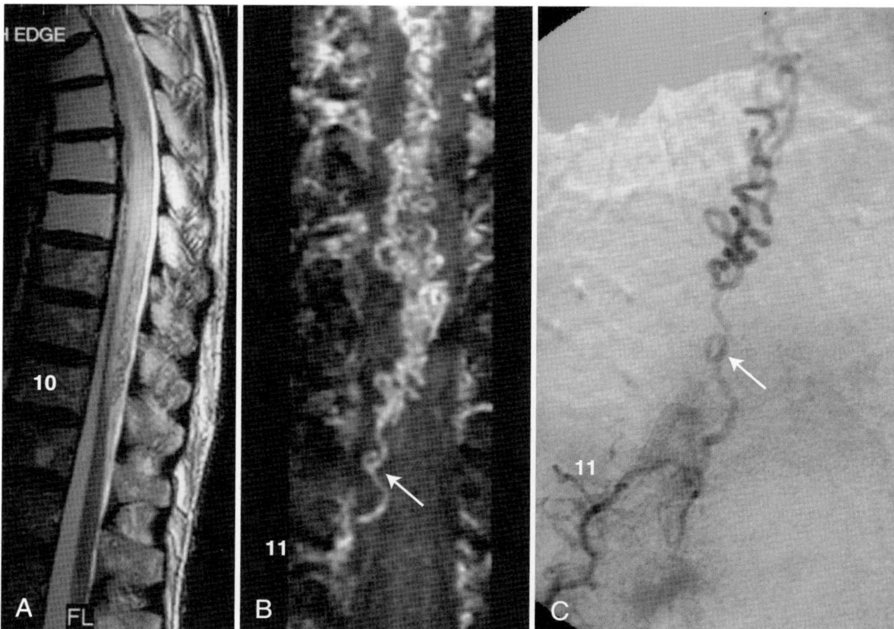


**Fig. 41.21 Spinal Dural Arteriovenous Fistula (AVF). A,** Sagittal T2-weighted fast-spin-echo image of thoracic spine shows hyperintensity of spinal cord and vertebra above T8, as well as serpentine "intradural flow voids" in a patient with a history of radiation therapy for lung carcinoma and progressive myelopathy. **B,** Coronal maximum-intensity projection image from three-dimensional steady-state contrast-enhanced magnetic resonance angiography of the same thoracic region reveals an enlarged, tortuous vessel *(arrow)* extending from approximately the right T11 foramen to abnormal vessels on the cord surface. Findings are typical for a dural AVF and are confirmed by subsequent catheter angiography. **C,** Anteroposterior view shows the enlarged vessel *(arrow)* to be the medullar vein draining from the fistula in the T11 foramen to the coronal venous plexus on the cord surface. (*From Bowen, B.C., 2007. MR angiography versus CT angiography in the evaluation of neurovascular disease. Radiology 245, 357–361.*)

Both modalities demonstrated excellent interobserver agreement, although there were more instances of ambiguity in fistula localization on first-pass CE-MRA. The similar findings suggest that both techniques may be comparable for the diagnosis and localization of spinal DAVFs (Mathur et al., 2017). Time-resolved 3 T CE-MRA has also been investigated for presurgical localization of the artery of Adamkiewicz prior to reimplantation of the feeding intercostal artery, lumbar artery, or both during aortic aneurysm repair. Bley et al. (2010) identified the artery of Adamkiewicz and the location of the feeding intercostal and/or lumbar artery with high confidence in 88% of cases (68 patients). The artery of Adamkiewicz and the anterior spinal artery were identified and differentiated from the great anterior radiculomedullary vein, even in patients with substantially altered hemodynamics from aortic disease.

## Intracranial Vessel Wall Imaging

MRA remains limited to the evaluation of the vessel lumen, often leading to findings that are nonspecific for disease etiology. High-resolution intracranial vessel wall (IVW) MRI techniques have been developed to subtract the signal of flowing blood in the vessel lumen. This process permits direct visualization of the vessel wall, enabling better delineation of various pathologies. IVW-MRI may serve as a complementary tool to luminal imaging techniques to improve diagnostic specificity of conditions such as vasculitis, reversible cerebral vasoconstriction syndrome (RCVS), and ICAD.

The small caliber and tortuous course of the intracranial arteries pose a challenge in accurately depicting the normal vessel wall and differentiating pathological states. Although some protocols have used 1.5 T scanners, the use of 3 T is preferred due to the higher signal-to-noise ratio, providing superior delineation of various vessel wall pathologies. IVW-MRI requires suppression of the MR imaging signals from luminal blood and cerebrospinal fluid (CSF). Various blood-suppression techniques have been described, and they often exploit flowing blood to achieve separation from the stationary vessel wall. Alternate techniques depend on the particular longitudinal relaxation time (T1) of blood, but these techniques typically rely on flow as well to some degree. Multiple tissue-weighting sequences have been investigated for IVW-MRI. Most examinations utilize a pre- and postcontrast T1-weighted vessel wall sequence. It is possible to use a proton-density-weighted sequence instead, as it provides a higher signal-to-noise ratio. However, contrast enhancement may be less conspicuous, and CSF signal intensity often approaches vessel wall intensity. High-resolution T2-weighted imaging has also shown some promise for VWI. Investigators have often utilized multicontrast protocols, as the variable pattern and degree of contrast enhancement on different sequences may enable better overall characterization of vessel wall pathology. Peripheral pulse gating is a potentially useful adjunctive technique, particularly when imaging dilated intracranial arteries or large aneurysms. Artifacts related to slow flow may be reduced with improved blood suppression by gating to the point of maximum flow in the vessel.

Accurate interpretation of IVW-MR relies on visualization of the vessel wall in both short- and long-axis planes. This may be achieved using multiplanar 2D or 3D acquisitions. 2D sequences may be obtained in multiple orthogonal planes while focusing on a specific vessel of interest. However, due to the inherent tortuosity of intracranial vessels, these images may be susceptible to partial volume averaging effects that may limit visualization of the arterial wall. Vessel obliquity, slice thickness, and in-plane resolution are all factors that will affect wall measurements and the sharpness of the vessel wall borders. Various 3D acquisition techniques are commercially available, and the variable refocusing pulse flip angle (VRFA) fast-spin-echo sequences represents one of the most widely used and reported techniques. Blood suppression with 3D sequences differs from 2D techniques and exploits intravoxel dephasing. Luminal blood contains spins traveling at varying velocities from laminar flow. Intravoxel phase dispersion with signal loss occurs as these spins travel through magnetic field gradients at varying rates between the time of excitation and readout. A diffusion-sensitizing gradient preparation may be added to exploit the intravoxel dephasing effect for 3D sequences. 3D techniques offer advantages over 2D acquisitions by providing increased brain coverage and enabling isotropic resolution that can be reformatted into multiple planes. This approach reduces total scan time and provides more flexibility as any imaged vessel may be visualized in any reformatted plane. Optimal protocols may include both 2D and 3D sequences.

IVW imaging protocols may be performed rapidly. At 3 T with a 2D sequence and a voxel size of 2.0 × 0.4 × 0.4 mm the scan duration may be approximately 5–7 minutes for a 2- to 4-cm-thick section of tissue. At 3 T with a 3D sequence and a voxel size of 0.5 mm isotropic, it is possible to cover the intracranial vessels up to third-order branches in 7–10 minutes (Mandel, 2017). The use of IVW-MRI remains largely investigational for most disease pathologies. Further prospective evaluation of IVW-MRI is needed to better depict imaging findings at various stages of disease and more accurately characterize underlying pathophysiology.

Various applications of this imaging technique remain under active investigation. In contrast to evaluating the degree of plaque-related stenosis for ICAD, IVW-MRI directly evaluates plaque composition, including the degree and pattern of wall thickening at the site of disease that may result in more accurate stroke risk stratification. The typical appearance of ICAD on IVW-MRI is an eccentric, outward remodeling lesion with heterogeneous T2 signal and juxtaluminal T2 hyperintensity with heterogeneous mild-moderate enhancement. An increased volume of the lipid-rich necrotic core, which appears isointense on T1-weighted imaging and hypointense on fat-saturated T2-weighted imaging, has been associated with higher rates of plaque rupture. The presence of intraplaque hemorrhage, which appears as intraplaque T1 hyperintensity greater than 150% of the signal intensity of internal reference muscle tissue, has been demonstrated to be an important risk factor for plaque vulnerability, with increased rates of thromboembolic stroke. In patients with multifocal disease, culprit lesions enhance more prominently than nonculprit lesions (Kesav et al., 2019; Lee et al., 2018b).

In contrast to ICAD, vasculopathy from moyamoya disease often demonstrates minimal to no circumferential enhancement without outward remodeling. Vessel wall inflammation and edema seen with central nervous system (CNS) vasculitis has been described on IVW-MRI as showing thickening and multifocal, homogeneous, smooth, intense, concentric enhancement of the vessel wall unlike the nonconcentric and heterogenous enhancement seen in atherosclerotic disease. For patients with RCVS, which reflects a noninflammatory vasospasm, IVW-MRI studies show minimal smooth thickening of the vessel wall that is concentric with minimal to no enhancement. IVW-MRI has also been used for the evaluation of intracranial dissection and typically includes visualization of a curvilinear hyperintensity on T2-weighted images, reflecting an intimal flap that separates the true lumen from the false lumen. The vessel wall abnormality may have a layered appearance on contrast-enhanced T1-weighted images with enhancement along the luminal and peripheral margins of the artery wall. Intramural hematoma often appears as hyperintensity on T1-weighted images for acute dissections, although signal characteristics of intramural blood evolve over time.

There is more published experience with IVW-MRI in the setting of ischemic disease compared with hemorrhagic conditions. However, there is growing interest in the use of IVW-MRI for the evaluation of intracranial aneurysms and its various components, including the vasa vasorum, the aneurysm wall, and mural hematoma. IVW-MRI has been reported to more accurately measure wall thickness and depict the presence of thick peripheral wall enhancement. These features may aid in identifying a culprit lesion associated with subarachnoid hemorrhage among patients with multiple aneurysms (Larsen et al., 2018; Mossa-Basha et al., 2016). Ongoing investigations continue to further evaluate aneurysm characteristics on IVW-MRI that are predictive of aneurysm growth and rupture.

## ULTRASOUND

### Methods

Although the physics and underlying methodology of ultrasound techniques comprise a complex topic, ultrasound studies are often reported in the relatively simplistic terms of flow-velocity measurements and associated diagnoses of steno-occlusive lesions in the cerebral circulation. Comprehending the physical basis of such findings may provide the clinician with an even greater appreciation for subtle findings and insight on the strengths and limitations of these ultrasound techniques (Kremkau, 2006).

Most diagnostic ultrasound devices operate at frequencies of 2–10 MHz and evaluate acoustic properties of blood and tissue to obtain both hemodynamic and anatomical information for vessels. Transducers for Doppler ultrasonography, using a single element, may continuously transmit and receive (continuous-wave Doppler) acoustic information to accurately identify flow velocities or intermittently emit and receive a series of short pulses of sound (pulsed-wave Doppler) to sample a specific depth or a time window for recording. Many hemodynamic parameters are obtained, such as flow direction, peak systolic velocity, and end-diastolic flow velocity, along with several indirect or derived parameters, such as width or spread of the spectral band of velocities, flow acceleration time (systolic acceleration slope), pulsatility, and resistivity index. An embolic particle passing through the Doppler sample volume has acoustic impedance that can be distinguished from surrounding blood, resulting in transient high-intensity signals called *microembolic signals* (MES). Individual vessels also have characteristic spectral appearances primarily caused by distal peripheral resistance and specific spectral patterns, particularly very high- or low-resistance signals, and provide indirect clues about hemodynamics and potential pathological conditions both proximally and distally.

In brightness-mode (B-mode) imaging, the transducer is swept in a single plane to produce a 2D structural and anatomical display of a slice of tissue based on its acoustic properties (Tegeler et al., 2005). These are static images, but the image can be updated 15–30 times per second, so it appears to be moving in real time. Duplex ultrasonography makes use of both pulsed-wave Doppler ultrasound and B-mode imaging to obtain both hemodynamic and anatomical information (Fig. 41.22). Color-flow imaging (CFI) uses Doppler flow-velocity information obtained from multiple sample volumes within the image, which is then color-coded based on the speed and direction of flow and overlaid onto the appropriate anatomical site in the grayscale B-mode image (Fig. 41.23; Tegeler et al., 2005). Modern transducers for extracranial high-resolution B-mode carotid imaging

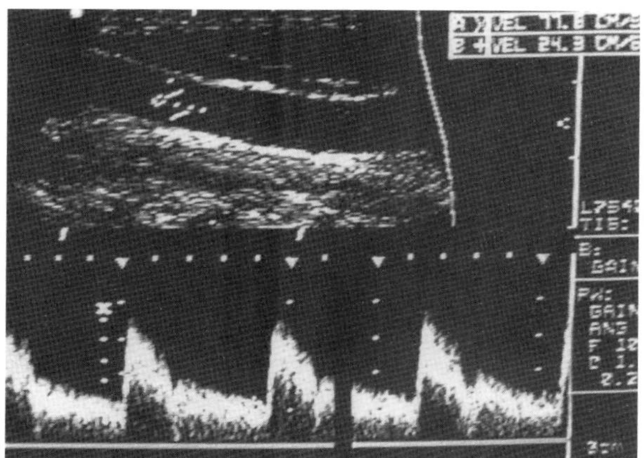

**Fig. 41.22 Duplex Ultrasonography.** Combined Doppler velocity spectral display and brightness-mode image-guided placement of the sample volume.

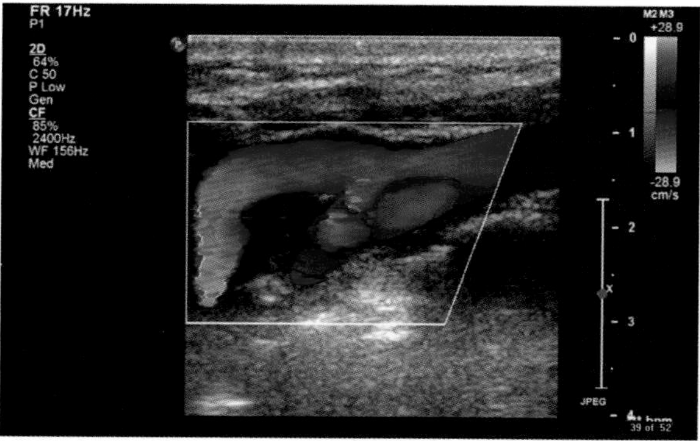


**Fig. 41.23 Color-Flow Imaging.** Duplex color-flow imaging superimposes the color-coded velocity information onto the brightness-mode image of the carotid bifurcation, internal carotid artery, and external carotid artery.

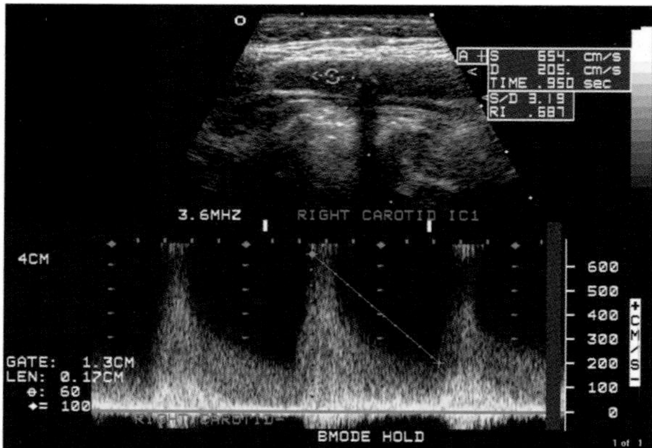


**Fig. 41.24 Doppler Ultrasound with Tight Stenosis.** Spectral display of duplex Doppler flow velocities suggesting 75%–90% internal carotid artery stenosis, with high systolic (654 cm/sec) and diastolic velocities (205 cm/sec) and spectral broadening.

operate at frequencies of 7.5–10.0 MHz, whereas those used for transcranial CFI operate at 2–3 MHz. Power Doppler imaging (PDI) is a variation of CFI that uses the integrated intensity or amplitude of power in the Doppler spectrum to provide information regarding the amount of blood flow detected at each point, rather than the mean velocity.

## Techniques

### Carotid Ultrasonography

Duplex examination of the carotid arteries must include Doppler flow-velocity sampling of the proximal, mid, and distal common carotid arteries (CCAs), proximal and distal Internal Carotid Arteries (ICAs), and the External Carotid Arteries (ECAs) bilaterally. The proximal great vessels (innominate and subclavian arteries) are also studied if they can be visualized. If disease is detected, additional Doppler sampling of the vessel proximal to, at the point of, and distal to the stenosis should be included. Sampling should be across the entire vessel diameter to avoid missing a high-velocity jet along the vessel wall. Sampling should be done using a standard angle of insonation or at least within a standard range of angles. Most sonographers try to sample at a 60-degree angle, but any angle between 45 and 60 degrees is acceptable. Enough of the study should be videotaped to allow review of both the spectral display and the audible signals from all target vessels or regions of abnormality. Transducer frequencies for Doppler interrogation usually are between 4.0 and 7.5 MHz.

As a result of predictable hemodynamic changes as stenosis develops, duplex Doppler ultrasound can be used to estimate the severity of stenosis. Very mild degrees of stenosis have little hemodynamic effect and cause little change in flow velocity or in the Doppler spectral waveform. Progressive stenosis first causes increased peak-systolic velocity across the narrowed segment. Additional narrowing causes a further increase in the peak-systolic velocity and a disturbed flow pattern, or *turbulence*, emerges (Fig. 41.24). Severe stenosis prevents adequate blood-flow volume across the lesion, even though the peak-systolic and end-diastolic velocity values are both increased. In very tight carotid stenosis approaching occlusion, peak-systolic and end-diastolic velocity values may increase even further or may begin to decrease as critical narrowing is reached.

These changes in velocity and pattern of flow are used to estimate the severity of stenosis. Most criteria used for interpretation are based primarily on the peak-systolic velocity, end-diastolic velocity, and ratios of velocities in the ICA and CCA. The ratio of velocities is helpful because the velocity in the stenotic segment remains high when compared with the velocity proximal or distal to the stenosis even when cardiac dysfunction exists. Any set of criteria should serve as a guideline for interpretation of velocity data and should not be considered as hard, inflexible rules. Interpreters also must consider the overall clinical picture in every patient and exercise judgment and flexibility in reaching conclusions. Current ultrasound laboratories should strive for an accuracy of approximately 90% for identification of tight carotid stenosis, as documented by a program of ongoing quality assurance.

High-resolution carotid B-mode real-time imaging should be done with transducers having frequencies greater than 5 MHz and preferably exceeding 7 MHz. Imaging should include visualization of the CCA, CCA bifurcation, ICA, ECA (including anterior, lateral, posterior, and transverse views), or a circumferential scan at each level to include all these views. Real-time recording of these images allows for the study of pulsation patterns and movement of intimal flaps or complex plaques. Measurements of the plaque thickness and residual lumen are performed frequently. Plaque severity can be classified by thickness, with minimal (1.1–2.0 mm), moderate (2.1–4.0 mm), and severe (>4.0 mm) categories. The posterolateral approach is usually optimal for measurements of plaque formation and residual lumen because plaques most often occur on the posterior wall of the carotid bifurcation and ICA, and B-mode imaging is most accurate when the sound beam is at 90 degrees to the interface being imaged.

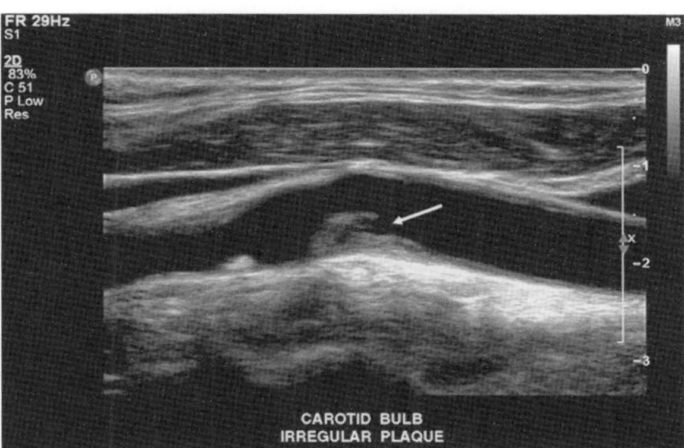


**Fig. 41.25 Atherosclerotic Plaque.** Longitudinal B-mode image of an atherosclerotic plaque in the region of the carotid bifurcation and proximal internal carotid artery, with possible crater formation *(arrow)*.

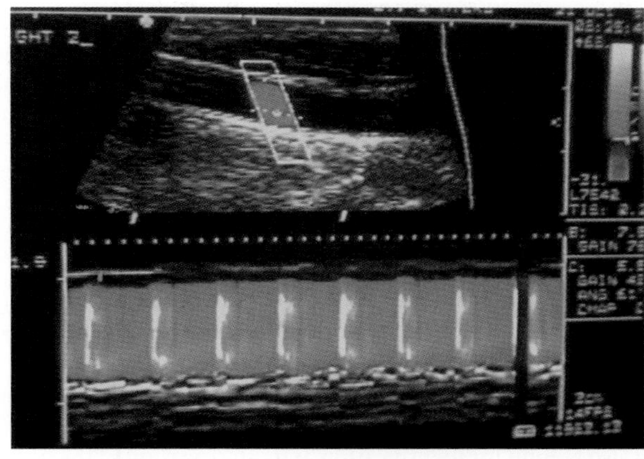

**Fig. 41.26 Volume Flow Rate.** Measurement of volume flow rate using color velocity imaging quantification with a color M-mode display of the flow velocities across the common carotid artery and tracking of the vessel diameter. Flow volume is in milliliters per minute.

High-resolution B-mode imaging also has a unique ability to evaluate the specific features of atherosclerotic plaques (Fig. 41.25; Tegeler et al., 2005). Identifiable characteristics include the distribution of plaque (concentric, eccentric, length), surface features (smooth, irregular, crater), echodensity presence of any calcification producing acoustic shadowing, and texture (homogeneous, heterogeneous, or intraplaque hemorrhage). The presence of hypoechoic plaques and the presence of plaques that are quite heterogeneous with prominent hypoechoic regions (complex plaque) identify an increased risk of stroke. High-resolution B-mode imaging is more accurate than Doppler ultrasound testing for defining atherosclerosis of the vessel wall early in the course of the disease. Measurement of the intima-media thickness, which increases in the early stages of plaque formation, has been correlated with the risk of cardiovascular disease and has been used as a surrogate endpoint for clinical therapeutics (Polak, 2005; van den Oord et al., 2013). The sensitivity of B-mode imaging for detection of surface ulceration is approximately 77% in plaques causing less than 50% linear stenosis and 41% for plaques causing more than 50% linear stenosis, with no significant differences between B-mode carotid imaging and arteriography. Although associated with a somewhat worse outcome, surface irregularity or crater formation appears to be a less important morphological risk factor than echodensity and heterogeneity.

Advantages of CFI include rapid determination of the presence and direction of blood flow, with more accurate placement of the Doppler sample volume and determination of the angle of insonation. Absence of color filling in what appears to be the vessel lumen provides clues about the presence of a hypoechoic plaque, and the contour of the color column can provide information about surface features. If a crater or ulcer is open to the lumen, color further details the surface architecture. Newer instruments with sensitive CFI designed to detect very low-flow velocities are able to accurately differentiate critical stenosis from total occlusion (87%–100% sensitivity, 84% specificity vs. angiography), negating the need for conventional angiography (Sitzer et al., 1996). The addition of CFI improves the understanding of many unusual anatomical configurations, such as kinks or coils. Although difficult to quantify accurately, CFI probably adds approximately 5% to the overall diagnostic accuracy of carotid duplex ultrasound.

The addition of PDI offers more potential to improve the accuracy in some difficult situations. In the setting of high-grade stenosis, PDI improves the identification of stenosis and the measurement of residual lumen and may improve the visualization of plaque surface features, even in the presence of calcification.

Conventional criteria for reporting carotid stenosis use flow velocity to estimate the linear percent stenosis. However, increased flow velocity may be seen in other conditions, such as a hyperperfusion state seen in anemia that might be misconstrued as stenosis. To avoid such mistakes, various methods have been devised to evaluate volume flow rate in the extracranial cerebral vessels. Processing techniques, such as color velocity imaging quantification (CVI-Q), may be implemented, and normal volume flow rate values (330 mL/min for women and 375 mL/min for men) have been defined. Use of the CCA volume flow rate in patients with carotid stenosis reveals characteristic decreases in the rate with progressive stenosis. In some laboratories, measurement of CCA volume flow rate is a standard part of the carotid evaluation for patients whose flow velocity suggests 75% or greater carotid stenosis (Fig. 41.26); this technique may better delineate hemodynamic changes (Tan et al., 2002). There appears to be an acceptable correlation between results of CVI-Q and Doppler-based methods (Likittanasombut et al., 2006), and diminished extracranial cerebral volume flow rate may identify an increased risk for recurrent stroke (Han et al., 2006).

Contrast-enhanced ultrasound (CE-US) is a more recent technique for the evaluation of high-risk atherosclerotic carotid lesions. The high temporal and spatial resolution capabilities allow better distinction of macrovascular morphology and the visualization of intraplaque neovascularization. The contrast agents administered for CE-US are approved by the US Food and Drug Administration (FDA) for use in cardiac imaging but currently remain off-label for use in the carotid artery. Using CTA as a reference, ten Kate et al. (2013) noted that CE-US had higher sensitivity (88% vs. 29%) than color Doppler ultrasound. Three-dimensional carotid ultrasound is another emerging technique that utilizes postprocessing imaging software to semiautomatically reconstruct 3D plaque volume and surface identified in B-mode and with the aid of color (Makris et al., 2011). Further applications of these techniques remain under investigation.

The optimal noninvasive imaging method for determining the severity of carotid artery stenosis remains uncertain. MRA and CTA are being used with rapidly increasing frequency to determine the degree of stenosis. Although duplex carotid ultrasound should not be used as the sole method for definitive diagnosis of carotid disease, this inexpensive imaging technique remains a valid screening tool. A systematic review of published studies comparing carotid ultrasound with DSA showed that for distinguishing severe stenosis (70%–99%), duplex carotid ultrasound had a pooled sensitivity of 86% and a pooled specificity of 87%. For recognizing occlusion, duplex carotid ultrasound had a sensitivity of 96% and a specificity of 100% (Nederkoorn et al., 2003). Another study found high concordance rates among CTA, contrast-enhanced MRA, and ultrasound for patients with asymptomatic carotid stenosis (Nonent et al., 2004). However, a study comparing ultrasound and MRA to DSA determined that ultrasound alone would have misassigned 28% of patients to receive carotid endarterectomy (CEA), whereas ultrasound combined with CE-MRA reduced this misassignment rate to 17% (Johnson et al., 2000).

### Vertebral Ultrasonography

Because pc cerebrovascular disease is quite common, study of the vertebral arteries is considered part of the routine extracranial duplex ultrasound examination. The same techniques described for use in the carotid arteries can be used to study the vertebral arteries and the proximal subclavian or innominate arteries. As such, there should be duplex Doppler and B-mode imaging of these arterial segments. CFI is also helpful for identification and interrogation of the vertebral arteries. The vertebral artery can virtually always be evaluated in the pretransverse and intertransverse cervical segment of C5–C6, whereas the origin can only be studied on the right in 81% of cases and on the left in 65% of cases. Because there is mostly a low-resistance distal vascular bed, the vertebral artery usually shows a low-resistance Doppler spectral pattern similar to that seen with the ICA. Unlike the carotid arteries, there are no widely accepted criteria for stenosis in the extracranial vertebral artery. As with the carotid system, spectral analysis provides insight into proximal and distal disease. Another confounding factor is contralateral occlusive disease, associated with increased carotid volume flow, which may result in an overestimation of the severity of stenosis. One study noted that ultrasound evaluation of the vertebral arteries had a sensitivity and specificity of 40.7% and 100%, respectively, for the detection of symptomatic atherosclerotic disease in stroke patients. The low sensitivity likely precludes this modality from becoming a sufficient screening tool, but this study may serve as a reasonable alternative for monitoring pc disease in patients who may have difficulty undergoing CT or MR imaging (Tábuas-Pereira et al., 2017). Given the variable factors associated with carotid duplex sonography, it has been recommended that each laboratory validate its own Doppler criteria for clinically relevant stenosis and undergo certification by an independent organization, such as the Intersocietal Commission for Accreditation of Vascular Laboratories Essentials and Standards for Accreditation in Noninvasive Vascular Testing. Studies have shown that the accuracy of duplex ultrasound examination is much better from accredited versus nonaccredited laboratories (Latchaw et al., 2009).

### Transcranial Doppler Ultrasonography

Most commercially available TCD ultrasonography instruments use a low-frequency 2-MHz probe to allow insonation through the cranium. These pulsed-wave Doppler instruments have an effective insonation depth range of 3.0–12.0 cm or more that can be evaluated by increments of 2–5 mm. At an insonation depth of 50 mm, the sample volume is usually 8–10 mm axially and 5 mm laterally. TCD probes also differ from the 4- to 10-MHz transducers used to monitor the progress of intraoperative neurosurgical procedures (Unsgaard et al., 2002). Advantages of TCD include the maneuverability of the relatively small probes, the Doppler sensitivity, and—compared with transcranial color-coded duplex (TCCD) and MRA—the relatively low price of instruments.

Routine TCD testing relies on three natural acoustic windows to study the basal segments of the main cerebral arteries. Insonation through the temporal bone window allows detection of flow through the MCA M1 segment and the anterior cerebral artery A1 segment. Normal blood flow direction is toward the probe in the MCA and away from it in the anterior cerebral artery. The supraclinoid ICA is also detected but may occasionally be difficult to distinguish from the MCA. Depending on the position of the window, the probe usually has to be tilted frontally to detect these vessels. A posterior (or occipital) tilt of the probe enables insonation of the PCAs. The occipital window takes advantage of the foramen magnum's opening into the skull. Flow in the distal vertebral artery and proximal to mid-portions of the basilar artery can be detected; its direction is away from the probe in these arterial segments. A considerable degree of natural variation occurs in the position and caliber of these arteries, making insonation occasionally difficult. The ophthalmic artery and carotid siphon can be studied through the orbital window. Flow in the ophthalmic artery is toward the probe and has a high resistance pattern. Flow in the ICA siphon can be either toward or away from the probe, depending on the insonated segment. The power output of the instrument must be decreased when insonating through the orbital window because prolonged exposure to high-intensity ultrasound has been associated with cataract formation.

Flow velocities change with age and differ among men and women. Normal values are available. Repeated measurements of flow velocities are highly reproducible. Thus, based on the general knowledge of the location of intracranial arteries and flow direction, a comprehensive map of the basal arteries can be generated. This map is clinically useful because common pathological conditions affecting the intracranial arteries (e.g., atherosclerosis, sickle cell disease, vasospasm associated with aneurysmal subarachnoid hemorrhage) often affect arterial segments that can be insonated. Convexity branches of the cerebral arteries are beyond the reach of TCD.

### Transcranial Color-Coded Duplex Ultrasonography

Examinations performed with 2.25-MHz phased array and 2.5-MHz 90-degree sector transducers enable color-coded imaging of intracranial arterial blood flow in red and blue, respectively, indicating flow toward and away from the probe. The main advantages of TCCD ultrasonography is the ability to visualize and positively identify the insonated vessel, thus increasing the ultrasonographer's confidence, and the ability to correct for the angle of insonation. In addition, TCCD provides a limited B-mode image of intracranial structures.

## Applications

### Acute Ischemic Stroke

TCD studies obtained within hours from the onset of symptoms of stroke in the carotid territory may reveal stenosis or occlusion of the distal intracranial ICA or proximal MCA in 70% of patients. When compared with DSA, TCD is more than 85% sensitive and specific in detecting supraclinoid ICA or MCA M1 segment lesions. The use of contrast-enhanced color-coded duplex sonography can be especially useful in this context. The use of TCD in the early hours of stroke may also provide important prognostic information. Patency of the MCA by TCD testing within 6 hours of the onset of stroke symptoms is an independent predictor of a better outcome (Allendoerfer et al., 2006).

Transcranial power motion-mode Doppler (PMD-TCD) is a technique that along with spectral information simultaneously displays real-time flow signal intensity and direction over 6 cm of intracranial space. One study compared PMD-TCD with CTA and found a sensitivity of 81.8% and a specificity of 94% for detecting an acute arterial occlusion. The sensitivity for detecting MCA occlusions was 95.6%, and the specificity was 96.2%. For the anterior circulation, PMD-TCD demonstrated a sensitivity of 100% and a specificity of

94.5%. For the pc, sensitivity was 57.1% and specificity was 100% (Brunser et al., 2009).

TCD can also help in monitoring the effect of thrombolytic agents. Testing before and after the administration of tissue plasminogen activator (tPA) can assess the agent's efficacy in obtaining arterial patency and ascertain continued patency during the days after treatment. Ultrasound energy has also been observed to accelerate enzymatic fibrinolysis, possibly by allowing increased transport of drug molecules into the clot and promoting the motion of fluid throughout the thrombus. This observation has led to studies that allow for real-time monitoring of vessel recanalization while potentially providing additional therapeutic benefit from the ultrasound energy (Alexandrov et al., 2004). One meta-analysis found that complete recanalization rates were higher in patients receiving a combination of TCD with IV tPA than in patients treated with IV tPA alone (37.2% vs. 17.2%; Tsivgoulis et al., 2010). Administration of microbubbles and/or lipid microspheres remains under investigation and may help transmit energy momentum from an ultrasound wave to residual flow to promote further recanalization, thereby enhancing the effect of ultrasound on thrombolysis (Alexandrov et al., 2008; Molina et al., 2009). Early studies initially noted increased rates of symptomatic intracranial hemorrhage, highlighting the need to determine the minimum and safe amounts of ultrasound energy necessary to enhance thrombolysis (Eggers et al., 2008; Rubiera and Alexandrov, 2010). Several studies have demonstrated equivalent ICH rates, but additional operator-independent devices, different microbubble-related techniques, and other means of improving sonothrombolysis are being evaluated (Barreto et al., 2013; Bor-Seng-Shu et al., 2012). Investigations remain ongoing for more conclusive evidence of efficacy, while rapid advancements in the designs of therapeutic TCD devices may herald a new therapeutic option for acute ischemic stroke patients treated with IV thrombolysis.

### Recent Transient Ischemic Attack or Stroke

Compared with other available methods, ultrasound testing offers a safe, accurate, noninvasive, and less expensive method for evaluating extracranial cerebrovascular disease. It is considered the initial test of choice for identifying significant carotid stenosis in patients with recent transient ischemic attack (TIA) or stroke. For the carotid territory, this should include duplex ultrasonography, with or without CFI. Reports should address the severity of stenosis based on Doppler flow-velocity measurements. There also must be information provided about the presence of any plaque, as well as the morphology, based on high-resolution B-mode imaging. Additional helpful ultrasound tools include PDI and volume flow-rate measurement. Results of carotid ultrasound testing must then be integrated with other available testing modalities if additional information is needed. At present, this often means a combination of ultrasound and MRA or CTA, with DSA reserved for those in whom the results of the preceding tests are technically inadequate, equivocal, or contradictory. The combination of ultrasound and MRA is more cost-effective than the use of routine DSA in this setting. However, the best algorithm for evaluation may vary, depending on the services and expertise available at each medical center.

MCA or basilar artery occlusion is associated with an absence or severe reduction of Doppler signal at the appropriate depth of insonation at a time when signals from the other ipsilateral basal cerebral arteries are detectable. Follow-up studies often show spontaneous recanalization of previously occluded segments. The latter can be detected within hours from the onset of symptoms, with the majority of symptomatic occlusions being recanalized within 2 days and followed by a period of hyperperfusion.

Collateral flow patterns associated with severe cervical carotid stenosis or occlusion can also be detected by TCD. They include retrograde flow of the ophthalmic artery and anterior or posterior communicating artery flow toward the hemisphere distal to the stenosed or occluded ICA. Among patients with symptomatic carotid occlusions, one study found that compared with DSA, TCD detection of collateral flow via the major intracerebral collateral branches had a sensitivity of 82% and a specificity of 79% in the anterior portion of the circle of Willis. In the posterior communicating artery, TCD demonstrated a sensitivity of 76% and a specificity of 47% (Hendrikse et al., 2008b). Lesions causing stenosis of the V4 segment of the vertebral artery and the proximal basilar artery can be imaged by TCD. Focal increases of the peak-systolic and mean velocities to 120 cm/sec and 80 cm/sec or more, respectively, at depths of insonation corresponding to these arterial segments are considered significant. Velocities often exceed 200 cm/sec, with lesions causing more than 50% stenosis. Compared with DSA, the sensitivity of TCD is approximately 75% in detecting vertebrobasilar stenotic lesions, and its specificity exceeds 85%. Frequent variation in the size and course of the vertebrobasilar trunk and its contribution of collateral flow to the anterior cerebral circulation are the main reasons for these relatively low figures. Contrast media and TCCD imaging can be particularly helpful in this setting (Stolz et al., 2002).

MESs detected by TCD correspond to gaseous microbubbles or emboli composed of platelets, fibrinogen, or cholesterol moving in intracranial arteries. Such MES can be detected spontaneously or with provocative stimuli, such as the Valsalva maneuver. In patients with extracranial carotid disease, these signals are associated with a history of recent TIAs or cerebral infarction in the distribution of the insonated artery, and they correlate with the presence of ipsilateral severe stenosis and plaque ulceration. They are detected mainly during the week following symptoms of cerebral ischemia and resolve afterward. MES can also be detected in subjects with cardiac prosthetic valves but often correspond to gaseous microbubbles in that setting. They are less common in adequately anticoagulated patients with atrial fibrillation. The clinical impact of microembolus detection studies remains limited at this time. The presence of these signals in an arterial territory is useful in identifying proximal "active" lesions. This is especially relevant when a symptomatic patient has more than one potential lesion, such as cervical carotid stenosis and atrial fibrillation, or a suboptimal history. In this situation, laboratory data can help identify the specific cause of cerebral infarction. In addition, because the presence of MES is predictive of future cerebral ischemic events in the insonated artery's territory, detecting these signals may affect therapeutic decisions. In the future, microembolus detection studies may be useful in monitoring the effect of antithrombotic agents (Markus et al., 2010).

Microemboli monitoring is also of interest in the context of potential carotid revascularization procedures. MESs have been reported in 43% of patients with symptomatic carotid stenosis and 10% of patients with asymptomatic carotid stenosis. MESs were reported in 25% of the patients with symptomatic versus 0% of patients with asymptomatic intracranial stenosis. The presence of MES has been found to be associated with a higher risk of ischemic events in patients with spontaneous carotid artery dissections (Brunser et al., 2017). Among patients with aortic embolism, patients with plaques 4 mm or larger demonstrated MES more frequently than patients with smaller plaques. MES has been shown to be useful for risk stratification in patients with carotid stenosis, but data from published studies remain insufficient to reliably predict future events in patients with intracranial stenosis, cervical artery dissection, and aortic embolism (Best et al., 2016; Ritter et al., 2008).

## Extracranial Stenotic Lesions

Ultrasound remains a safe and noninvasive method for monitoring patients with carotid or vertebral artery disorders. Periodic evaluation can be helpful for assessing the progression or regression of existing plaques or the development of new lesions, whether symptomatic or asymptomatic. The timing of follow-up carotid testing must be individualized, depending on the severity and type of lesions and/or the onset of new or recurrent symptoms. The identification of asymptomatic carotid stenosis has become an important clinical mandate since the Asymptomatic Carotid Atherosclerosis Study (ACAS) showed the benefit of CEA in asymptomatic patients with 60%–99% stenosis, when compared with treatment with 325 mg of aspirin daily (Executive Committee for the Asymptomatic Carotid Atherosclerosis Study, 1995). Yet, it is not cost-effective to screen the entire population, even with ultrasound. Asymptomatic individuals with cervical bruits should be studied, even though bruits are often due to another cause. Patients with multiple risk factors probably warrant study, but the clinical utility of this has not yet been confirmed. Practice guidelines are being developed for carotid screening in high-risk individuals to identify stenosis that may need clinical treatment or intervention (Qureshi et al., 2007). If vessel disease is identified, stenosis of less than 50% might be initially restudied in 12–24 months, whereas lesions with 50%–75% stenosis and uncomplicated plaques might be restudied in 6–12 months. For 50%–75% stenosis with complicated plaque features or for more than 75% stenosis, an initial restudy at 3–6 months is appropriate. Lack of progression for several years should result in lengthened intervals before restudy. When evidence of asymptomatic progression is present, a shorter interval is recommended. The development of new symptoms should prompt urgent re-evaluation. After CEA, repeat ultrasound is often done at approximately one month after surgery and then yearly to identify potential restenosis.

Large population studies, such as the Atherosclerosis Risk in Communities and the Cardiovascular Health Study, have documented the association between risk factors and intima-media thickening in the wall of the carotid artery on B-mode imaging. This may represent an early stage in the development of atherosclerosis; the presence of significant thickening correlates with the risk of heart attack and abnormalities on MRI of the brain. Further investigations remain ongoing regarding the clinical utility of identifying increased intima-media thickness values, but it has been suggested that B-mode imaging for evaluation of intima-media thickness should be used clinically to identify patients at high risk for coronary or cerebrovascular events or to assess responses to risk factor modification (Polak, 2005). The hope is that such early identification of atherosclerotic changes will allow interventions to prevent later development of clinical events.

## Intracranial Stenotic Lesions

Intracranial atherosclerotic plaques are dynamic lesions that may increase in degrees of stenosis or regress over relatively short periods of time. TCD enables noninvasive monitoring of these lesions. It is often obtained at baseline in conjunction with DSA, CTA, or MRA and is subsequently repeated during the follow-up period (Fig. 41.27). Several studies have found that TCD exhibits good accuracy compared with DSA for the detection of greater than 50% of intracranial stenosis. Zhao et al. (2011) noted that TCD had a

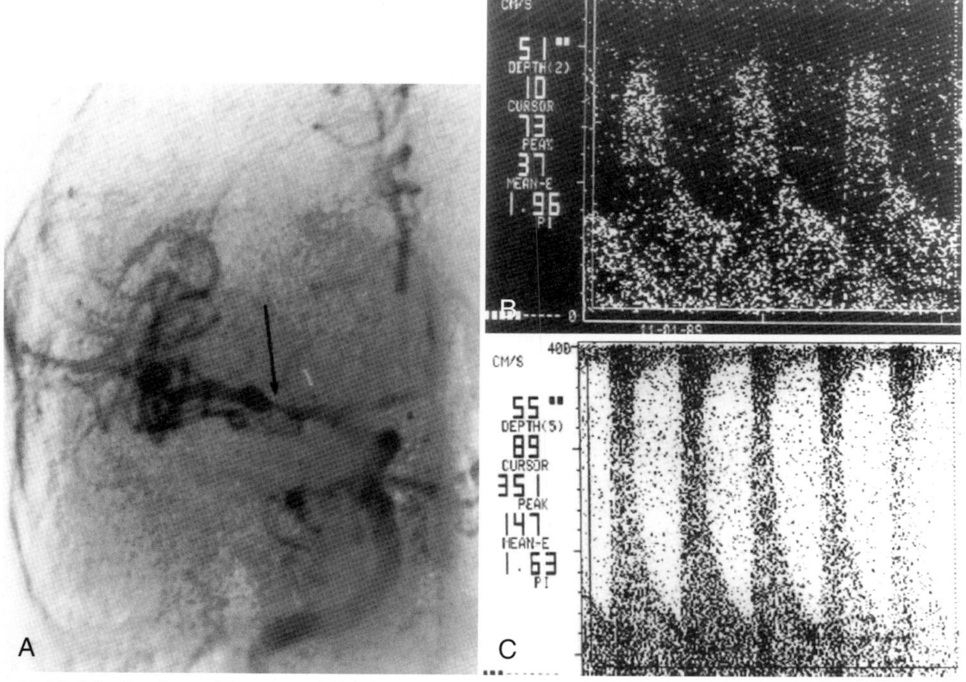


**Fig. 41.27** Monitoring of Intracranial Atherosclerotic Lesions. **A,** Cerebral angiogram shows an area of stenosis *(arrow)* in the M1 segment of the right middle cerebral artery. **B,** The first transcranial Doppler study obtained within 48 hours of angiography shows a corresponding peak-systolic velocity of 188 cm/sec. **C,** Repeat transcranial Doppler study 34 months later shows a further increase of the peak-systolic velocity to approximately 350 cm/sec. (*Reprinted with permission from Schwarze, J.J., Babikian, V., DeWitt, L.D., et al., 1994. Longitudinal monitoring of intracranial arterial stenoses with transcranial Doppler ultrasonography. J Neuroimaging 4, 182–187.*)

sensitivity and specificity of 78% and 93%, respectively, in the MCA, using mean flow velocity greater than 100 cm/sec. Using the criteria of mean flow velocities greater than 80 cm/sec in the basilar and vertebral arteries, TCD demonstrated a sensitivity and specificity of 69% and 98%, respectively. Using peak systolic velocity =120 cm/sec, You et al. (2009) found that TCD had a sensitivity and specificity of 96.7% and 93.9%, respectively, in the carotid siphon. Furthermore, Saqqur et al. (2010) noted that in patients with positional neurological changes, TCD had a 94% sensitivity and a 100% specificity in predicting neurological symptoms with testing using a criteria of mean flow velocity decrease of greater than 25%. While TCD monitoring enables detection of new atherosclerotic plaques, clinical experience is limited, and further prospective investigations are needed to make recommendations regarding the frequency and timing of follow-up studies.

## Aneurysmal Subarachnoid Hemorrhage

Vasoconstriction of intracerebral arteries is the leading cause of delayed cerebral infarction and mortality after aneurysmal subarachnoid hemorrhage. Vasospasm is clinically detected 3 or 4 days after the hemorrhage and usually resolves after day 12. Although the exact cause of vasospasm remains unknown, its presence correlates with the volume and duration of exposure of an intracranial artery to the blood clot. Laboratory and animal models indicate that blood breakdown products can lead to vasoconstriction. The detection of vasospasm is important because it may potentially be treated with medications, hemodynamic management, and endovascular interventions. These treatments are not without risk, so the ability to detect and monitor vasospasm noninvasively has considerable clinical importance. Although vasospasm can be angiographically detected in 30%–70% of patients with aneurysmal subarachnoid hemorrhage, only 20%–40% develop clinical signs of cerebral ischemia. Thus, the presence of vasospasm is not a sufficient condition for the development of a clinical focal ischemic deficit. Several factors, including the severity of spasm, presence of collateral flow, condition of the patient's intravascular volume, and cerebral perfusion pressure, are considered mitigating factors. TCD has been widely adopted for the daily monitoring of patients with aneurysmal subarachnoid hemorrhage due to its portability to the bedside and its noninvasive nature. A survey of vascular neurosurgeons and neuroradiologists across 32 countries noted that daily screening for vasospasm was a common practice among US (70%) and non-US (53%) practitioners (Hollingworth et al., 2015). TCD studies show an increase in the flow velocities of basal cerebral arteries, usually starting on day 4 after subarachnoid hemorrhage and peaking by days 7–14 (Fig. 41.28). Although a diffuse increase in velocities is often detected in patients with severe hemorrhage, arterial segments in close proximity to the subarachnoid blood clot usually have the highest velocities.

Severe vasospasm in an arterial segment can be associated with reduced regional cerebral blood flow in the artery's distal territory. There is a linear inverse relationship between the severity of vasospasm and the amplitude of flow-velocity increase in an arterial segment. This is valid until the vasoconstriction is so severe that the flow volume is reduced, flow velocities drop, and the TCD signal becomes difficult to detect. The linear relationship can also be affected by several factors, including the presence of hyperperfusion. Angiographic studies confirm the presence of at least some degree of MCA vasospasm when the mean flow velocities are higher than 100 cm/sec, but values below 120 cm/sec are not usually considered clinically significant. Mean velocities in the range of 120–200 cm/sec correspond to 25%–50% angiographically determined diameter reduction; values exceeding 200 cm/sec correspond to more than 50% luminal narrowing (Sloan et al., 1999). The 200 cm/sec threshold and rapid flow-velocity increases exceeding

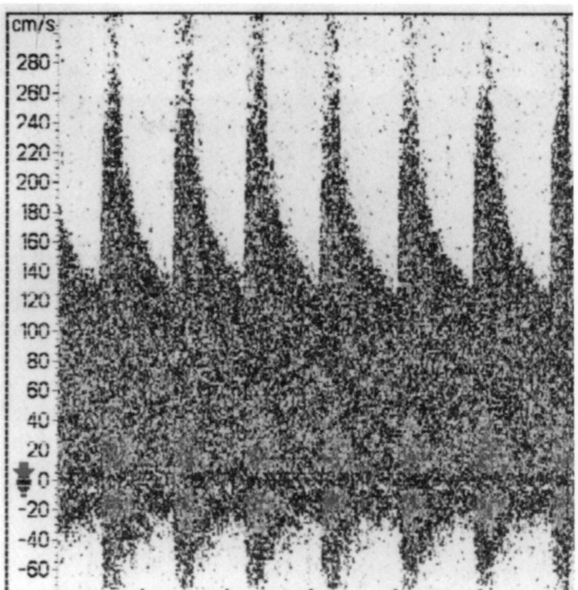


**Fig. 41.28 Subarachnoid Hemorrhage.** Temporal bone window; depth of insonation of 56 mm. Increased flow velocities indicating moderate to severe vasospasm in the middle cerebral artery M1 segment.

50 cm/sec on consecutive days are associated with subsequent infarction. TCD is also used to monitor the effects of endovascular treatment of vasospasm. Flow velocities decrease after successful angioplasty or papaverine infusion. Persistent increases after treatment indicate either extension of vasospasm to new arterial segments or hyperemia in the treated arterial segment and may constitute a valid reason for repeat cerebral angiography.

The accuracy of TCD in detecting vasospasm depends to some degree on the location of the involved arterial segment. A recent meta-analysis of 15 studies noted a pooled sensitivity of 66.7%, with a specificity of 89.5% for the detection of vasospasm in the MCA (Mastantuono et al., 2018). Basilar artery vasospasm is detected with an approximate sensitivity of 75% and specificity of 80% (Sloan et al., 1999). However, for vasospasm of the ACA and PCA, sensitivity of TCD is notably inferior (Sloan et al., 2004). Several factors, including the effects of hyperemia, increased intracranial pressure (ICP) and blood pressure changes, the presence of vasospasm in convexity branches not accessible by TCD, and difficulties in assessing vasospasm by angiography contribute to these findings. Because of these limitations in accuracy, the combined use of TCD and single-photon emission computed tomography (SPECT) or xenon-enhanced CT has been advocated, with the expectation that it will provide a more comprehensive and accurate assessment of the clinical condition. Overall, however, TCD is considered to have acceptable accuracy for the evaluation of vasospasm in aneurysmal subarachnoid hemorrhage. It is a useful tool with limitations that must be taken into consideration in the clinical setting.

## Cardiopulmonary Shunt Detection

Paradoxical embolism via a right-to-left cardiopulmonary shunt remains an important cause of stroke in younger patients. A patent foramen ovale (PFO) is a common source of right-to-left circulatory shunting that occurs in approximately 25% of the general population. Patients with suspected cerebrovascular ischemia secondary to paradoxical embolism may undergo a TCD "bubble" study. Microparticle contrast agents or simple agitated saline with microbubbles may be peripherally injected while continuous TCD monitoring of the MCA is performed for MES detection. The Valsalva maneuver by the patient is often elicited a few seconds after contrast injection to ensure arrival of the microbubbles into the right atrium. This technique increases the right atrial pressure and facilitates the travel of microbubbles into the left atrium if a shunt is present. TCD monitoring is typically performed up to 40 seconds while the patient remains in supine and/or sitting positions. Larger shunts with higher MES counts are associated with an increased risk of ischemic strokes (Lee et al., 2018a). In comparison with transesophageal echocardiograms, TCD has been shown to have a pooled sensitivity and specificity of 96.1% and 92.4%, respectively, based on a meta-analysis of 35 studies (Katsanos et al., 2016). A more recent study noted a sensitivity and specificity of 100%, confirming that TCD represents an optimal screening test for the detection of cardiopulmonary shunts in younger patients with cryptogenic strokes (Palazzo et al., 2019). When acoustic bone windows are absent, TCD monitoring in the cervical internal carotid arteries or vertebral arteries has been demonstrated to be a valid substitute (Perren et al., 2016).

## Cerebrovascular Reactivity

Cerebrovascular reactivity testing evaluates the presence of abnormal cerebral hemodynamic changes to potentially identify patients at an increased risk of recurrent stroke. Both IV acetazolamide administration and carbon dioxide inhalation are used to assess cerebrovascular reactivity. In patients with exhausted cerebrovascular reactivity reserves, flow velocities fail to adequately increase after the IV administration of acetazolamide or have a decreased response to hypercapnia and hypocapnia. Multiple studies have demonstrated that an impaired TCD cerebrovascular reactivity in patients with severe ICA stenosis or occlusion is independently associated with an increased risk of ipsilateral ischemic events (Reinhard et al., 2014). Further investigation is necessary to determine whether such testing can reliably identify patients who might benefit from a revascularization procedure.

## Sickle Cell Disease

An occlusive vasculopathy characterized by a fibrous proliferation of the intima often involves the basal cerebral arteries of patients with sickle cell disease. Cerebral infarction is a common complication of this vasculopathy and has a frequency of approximately 5%–15%. As in all patients with anemia, flow velocities are diffusely increased in individuals with sickle cell anemia. Additional focal velocity increases in the basal cerebral arteries can be detected in some subjects. A time-averaged mean of the maximum velocity of 200 cm/sec or greater in the distal ICA and proximal MCA identifies neurologically asymptomatic children at an increased risk for first-time stroke (Adams et al., 1998). In addition to standard insonation techniques with the TCD probe, extending the submandibular approach to include infrasiphon portions of the ICA increases the sensitivity to better identify sickle cell patients with potential sources of cerebral infarction (Gorman et al., 2009). Periodic red blood cell transfusion is associated with a 90% reduction in the rate of stroke. Expert guidelines from the National Heart, Lung, and Blood Institute strongly recommend that children with sickle cell disease between ages 2 and 16 receive annual TCD examinations (Yawn et al., 2014). Discontinuation of transfusion therapy can result in a reversal of abnormal blood-flow velocities and stroke (STOP 2 Trial, 2005). A 2012 review determined that treating children with transfusions based on TCD results was both clinically effective and cost-effective (Cherry et al., 2012). Despite national recommendations and its proven efficacy, TCD screening rates continue to remain low and underutilized (Reeves et al., 2016).

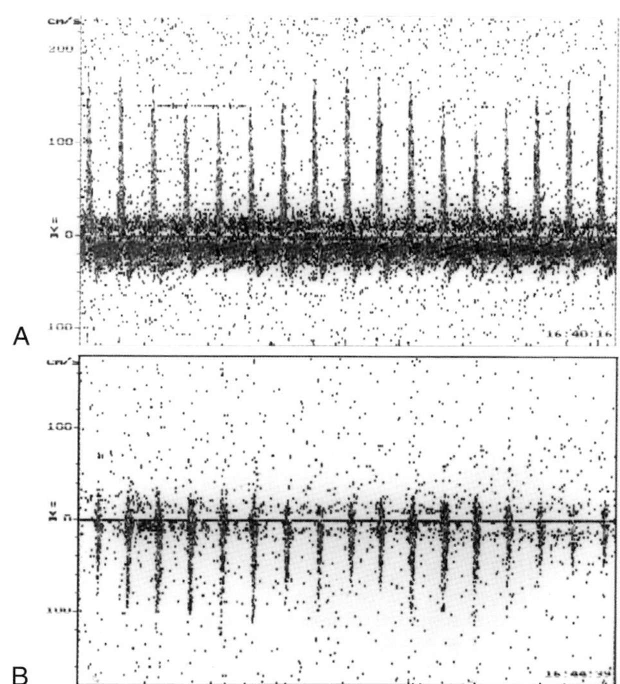

**Fig. 41.29 Raised Intracranial Pressure.** Reverberating flow pattern (**A**) and small systolic spikes (**B**) seen in a patient with markedly increased intracranial pressure.

## Brain Death

A characteristic pattern of changes can be detected by TCD in patients with increased ICP. Early findings consist of a mild decrease in the diastolic flow velocity and an increase in the difference between peak-systolic and end-diastolic velocities. When ICP increases further and reaches the diastolic blood pressure level, flow stops during diastole, and the corresponding flow velocity drops to zero; flow continues during systole, and spiky systolic peaks are observed. A further increase in ICP is associated with a reverberating flow pattern, with forward flow in systole and retrograde flow in diastole (see Fig. 41.28). The net volume of flow decreases and can reach zero. At cerebral perfusion pressure values close to zero, either small systolic spikes are observed (Fig. 41.29) or no signal at all is detected. This corresponds to a complete arrest of flow as demonstrated by cerebral angiography. The pattern of TCD changes is not specific to a particular neurological disease and can occur in a variety of conditions associated with increased ICP.

These changes are also observed in patients clinically diagnosed as brain dead. Multiple case series have generally reported good correlations between TCD confirmation of cerebral circulatory arrest and clinical confirmation of brain death. Furthermore, this study remains useful as an ancillary test for brain death confirmation because it is safe, noninvasive, and easily performed at the bedside. A 2016 meta-analysis of 22 studies noted a sensitivity of 76% and a specificity of 74.3% for TCD assessment when compared with clinical brain death criteria (Chang et al., 2016). Although TCD is helpful in detecting cerebral circulatory arrest, it cannot be recommended as the sole diagnostic test for the diagnosis of brain death. The latter must be established based on the clinical presentation and neurological

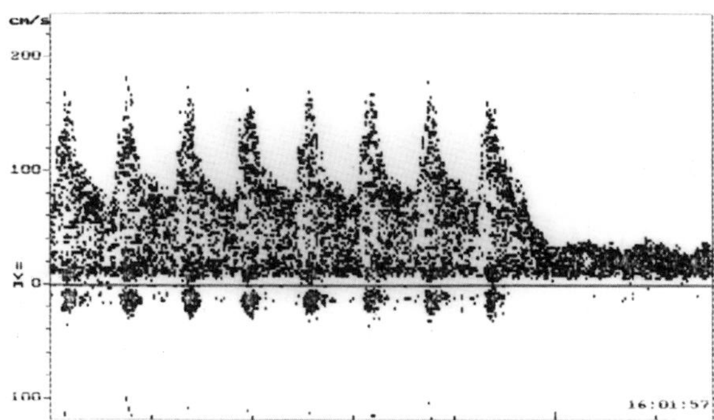


**Fig. 41.30 Carotid Endarterectomy.** At clamp insertion, the peak-systolic flow velocity decreases from approximately 175 cm/sec to 35 cm/sec.

examination findings. TCD and other laboratory tests can help confirm the clinical impression.

## Periprocedural Monitoring

CEA and carotid artery stenting (CAS) remain important interventions for certain cases of asymptomatic and symptomatic carotid stenosis. Monitoring is often performed to identify and correct periprocedural events that can lead to cerebrovascular complications. Monitoring tests currently in use for CEA include electroencephalography. These tests are useful in detecting cerebral hypoperfusion or its consequence, cerebral ischemia, and investigations remain ongoing to determine their effectiveness in reducing the perioperative stroke rate. TCD monitoring during CEA shows a consistent pattern of flow-velocity changes in the ipsilateral MCA. The most significant changes occur at the time of carotid clamping, with persistent and severe flow-velocity decreases to less than 15% of pre-clamp values in up to 10% of patients (Fig. 41.30). Patients with velocities decreasing to this level usually are considered candidates for shunting. Although definitive TCD criteria for shunting have not yet been established, a post-clamp peak-systolic or mean flow-velocity decrease to less than 30% of the pre-clamp value is often considered an acceptable criterion. A 2017 meta-analysis noted that MCA velocity changes on intraoperative TCD had a pooled specificity and sensitivity of 84.1% and 49.7%, respectively, for the prediction of perioperative strokes (Udesh et al., 2017).

TCD monitoring also has the unique capability of detecting microembolism as it occurs. This provides a considerable edge to TCD when compared with other monitoring techniques because the majority of

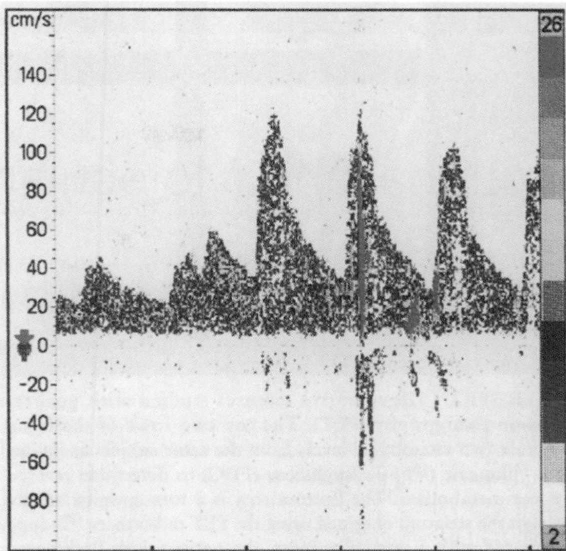


**Fig. 41.31 Carotid Endarterectomy.** At clamp release, flow velocities are restored, and microembolic signals are seen.

perioperative infarcts are thought to be secondary to cerebral embolism. Microemboli are detected at specific stages of surgery; dissection, clamp insertion and release, and the immediate postoperative period are the high-risk periods (Fig. 41.31). The presence of solid and gaseous microemboli in patients undergoing CEA and/or carotid stenting has been associated with procedure-related acute ipsilateral ischemic strokes on MRI and postoperative cognitive decline (Skjelland et al., 2009). One study evaluating patients who underwent CEA under TCD monitoring found that low MCA mean blood-flow velocity (≤28 cm/sec) during carotid dissection was significantly associated with new postoperative neurological deficits in patients with 10 or greater MES during carotid dissection. This combined evaluation resulted in improved specificity and PPV when compared with either criterion used alone (Ogasawara et al., 2008). TCD remains a relative newcomer to the field of periprocedural monitoring and provides useful information for potentially averting cerebrovascular complications.

*The complete reference list is available online at https://expertconsult.inkling.com/.*

42

# Functional and Molecular Neuroimaging

Karl Herholz, Stefan Teipel, Sabine Hellwig, Sönke Langner, Michel Rijntjes, Stefan Klöppel, Cornelius Weiller, Philipp T. Meyer

## OUTLINE



Structural imaging modalities such as computed tomography (CT) and magnetic resonance imaging (MRI) are essential techniques for evaluating various central nervous system (CNS) disorders, providing superb structural resolution and tissue contrast. On the other hand, functional and molecular imaging modalities—such as functional MRI (fMRI), positron emission tomography (PET), and single-photon emission computed tomography (SPECT)—visualize brain functions that are not necessarily related to brain structure, most notably cerebral blood flow (CBF), metabolism, receptor binding, and pathological deposits. The techniques are particularly valuable for mapping brain functions or depicting disease-related molecular changes that occur independently of or before structural changes. The principles of fMRI, PET, and SPECT and their applications in clinical neurosciences are discussed in this chapter. Regarding applications of PET and SPECT, the focus is on dementia, parkinsonism, brain tumors, epilepsy, and autoimmune encephalitis. These applications are particularly well established and important in clinical practice. Localization of brain function as a main focus of fMRI research is utilized in presurgical mapping, whereas fMRI research is increasingly also addressing functional brain networks and their changes in neurological diseases.

## FUNCTIONAL NEUROIMAGING MODALITIES

### Functional Magnetic Resonance Imaging

Today, fMRI is a standard technique in neuroscience brain imaging. It relates to the blood oxygen level–dependent (BOLD) effect, which is due to a transient and local excess of oxygenated blood resulting from changes in regional CBF and neuronal activity. Oxygenated hemoglobin is used here as an intrinsic contrast agent and serves as a surrogate marker of neuronal oxygen consumption and activity.

One approach to studying the integrity of functional neuronal networks uses experimental stimuli (e.g., words that have to be read) either in a block design (series of words for 20–30 seconds alternating by rest blocks of similar length over several minutes) or event-related tests (≈30–40 stimuli of each type presented in a counterbalanced order, each followed by some baseline period). Experiments are often conducted with multiple subjects, which requires stereotactic normalization into a standard space. Time series are analyzed using univariate analyses within the general linear model (GLM), enabling inferences on local effect sizes. Resulting visualizations illustrate regions with task-specific statistically significant differences in brain activation. More recently multivariate analyses, such as partial least squares, enable inferences on network connectivity on the whole-brain level. Complementary approaches use graph theory analysis to elucidate the network features during task condition or resting state (see later) and their alteration through brain disease or assessment of effective connectivity using causal inference modes, such as dynamic causal modeling, Granger causality, or Bayesian learning networks.

Parallel to task-related MRI, resting-state fMRI (Rs-fMRI) has been developed for applications in dementia research (Fox et al., 2005; Thomas et al., 2014). Analysis of spontaneous fluctuations of the BOLD signal during resting-state conditions has revealed consistent networks of intrinsic connectivity that partly map with functional networks activated during task performance, such as motor networks, language networks, attention networks, or deactivated during task performance, such as the default mode network (DMN) involving medial temporal lobe, superior parietal, and prefrontal lobe areas. Analysis of resting-state intrinsic connectivity networks typically involves analysis of correlations with seed regions or network analysis using multivariate techniques such as independent component analysis. Rs-fMRI analyses have been used in the analysis of prodromal or manifest stages of dementia due to the more limited requirements for patients' compliance in comparison with task-based fMRI. However, the high interscanner and longitudinal variability of resting-state networks (in comparison with task-elicited functional networks) limits their utility for individual diagnostic or prognostic applications.

## Arterial Spin Labeling

Arterial spin labeling (ASL) is an MRI technique that provides estimates of cerebral perfusion at the tissue level noninvasively and without the administration of contrast media. The main physiological parameter that can be measured by ASL is the CBF. ASL imaging techniques provide quantitative parametric imaging maps of CBF for visual and region-of-interest (ROI)–based analysis (Grade et al., 2015; Haller et al., 2016).

ASL was first introduced in the early 1990s (Detre et al., 1992; Williams et al., 1992). However, its main drawback is its inherent low signal-to-noise ratio (SNR; Golay et al., 2004). Although ASL is possible with 1,5 tesla (T) MR systems, low SNR increases the necessary scan time and therefore makes the technique sensitive to motion artifacts. Recent advances in coil technology and increasing field strength of the MR systems have led to a rapidly growing interest in ASL in clinical and preclinical imaging (Haller et al., 2016).

In contrast to other MR-based techniques for the evaluation of tissue perfusion (e.g., dynamic contrast-enhanced MRI [DCE-MRI]), ASL uses the water molecules of the blood as an endogenous contrast agent to estimate tissue perfusion. ASL is based on the strategy of magnetically labeling the protons in blood molecules before they flow into the tissue of interest. According to the spin labeling technique used, ASL can be divided into three different types: pulsed ASL (PASL), pseudo-continuous ASL (pCASL), and continuous ASL (CASL). Currently the most used types of ASL are pCASL and PASL.

Important technical parameters for ASL acquisition are positioning of the labeling plane below the brain, labeling duration, and the post-labeling delay (PLD) or inflow-time of the postlabeling period. This delay describes the time between the end of the labeling period and the start of the imaging period. It describes the time allowed for the labeled blood to enter the tissue of interest within the imaging volume. The PLD depends on the blood velocity, which is correlated with the subject's age. Because older patients have a decreased velocity, the recommended PLD is 1500 ms for pediatric patients and 1800 and 2000 ms for healthy adults below and above 70 years of age, respectively. For adult patients, a PLD of 2000 ms is recommended.

There is also a need for background suppression and prevention of patient motion during image acquisition to reduce noise and artifacts masking the signal difference, thus subsequently hindering image analysis. Image readout of ASL was traditionally based on fast echo planar imaging (EPI) techniques. Recently more advanced three-dimensional (3D) acquisition techniques have been proposed (e.g., 3D gradient and spin echo [GRASE] or 3D rapid acquisition relaxation enhanced [RARE] techniques). Compared with two-dimensional (2D) techniques, 3D readout has superior SNR and allows the acquisition of the entire volume of interest within one shot, thus reducing the slice-dependent variations of the perfusion signal observed in 2D techniques (Vidorreta et al., 2013).

## Positron Emission Tomography

The concept of modern PET was developed during the 1970s (Phelps et al., 1975). The underlying principle of PET and also of SPECT is to image and quantify a physiological function or molecular target of interest in vivo by noninvasively assessing the spatial and temporal distribution of the radiation emitted by an intravenously injected or inhaled target-specific probe (radiotracer). Importantly, PET and SPECT tracers are administered in a nonpharmacological dose (micrograms or less), so they neither perturb the underlying system nor cause pharmacological effects. Because of their ability to enable the visualization of molecular targets and functions on a macroscopic level with unsurpassed sensitivity down to a picomolar concentration, PET and SPECT are also called molecular imaging techniques. (See Cherry, 2003, for a textbook on PET and SPECT physics.) (See Table 42.1 for a glossary of PET and SPECT tracers.)

In the case of PET, a positron-emitting radiopharmaceutical is injected or inhaled by the subject. The emitted positron travels a short distance in tissue (effective range <1 mm for common PET radionuclides) before it encounters an electron; the positron and electron combine, yielding a pair of two 511-keV annihilation photons emitted in opposite directions and detected quasi-simultaneously by a PET detector ring surrounding the patient. 3D PET image datasets of the distribution of the PET tracer and its target are then generated by standard image reconstruction algorithms. To actually gain quantitative PET images (i.e., radioactivity/tracer concentration per unit tissue), the acquired data are corrected for scatter and random coincidences and photon attenuation by tissue absorption (e.g., using low-dose CT in the case of a PET/CT scanner). The spatial resolution of modern PET systems is about 3–5 mm. Thus PET is susceptible to partial volume effects if the size of the object or lesion is less than twice the scanner's resolution (as a rule of thumb). Today's PET systems are either constructed as hybrid PET/CT or, more recently, PET/MRI systems. Although the clinical utility of the latter still needs to be defined, integrated PET/MRI allows for the comprehensive, synchronous imaging of multiple morphological, functional, and molecular parameters in a single scanning session.

Commonly used radionuclides in neurological PET research studies are carbon-11 ($^{11}$C, half-life = 20.4 minutes), oxygen-15 ($^{15}$O, physical half-life = 2.03 minutes), and fluorine-18 ($^{18}$F, half-life = 109.7 minutes), which are all produced in cyclotrons. Although the relatively long half-life of $^{18}$F allows for the shipping of $^{18}$F-labeled tracers from a cyclotron site to a distant clinical PET site, this is not possible for shorter-lived isotopes. Thus only $^{18}$F-labeled radiopharmaceuticals are widely available and have been used clinically.

The most frequently used PET radiopharmaceutical is the glucose analog [$^{18}$F]2-deoxy-2-fluoro-d-glucose ([$^{18}$F]FDG). It was originally developed to assess cerebral glucose metabolism and is now also widely used as a tumor imaging agent in oncology. With the rate of glucose metabolism being closely related to maintenance of ion gradients and transmitter turnover (in particular, glutamate), [$^{18}$F]FDG represents an ideal tracer for the assessment of neuronal function and its changes (Sokoloff, 1977). After uptake in cerebral tissue by specific glucose transporters, [$^{18}$F]FDG is phosphorylated by hexokinase. Since [$^{18}$F]FDG-6-P is not a substrate for transport out of the cell and cannot be metabolized further, it is irreversibly trapped in cells. Therefore the distribution of [$^{18}$F]FDG in tissue imaged by PET (started 30–60 minutes after injection to allow for sufficient uptake; 5–20 minute scan duration) closely reflects the regional distribution of cerebral glucose metabolism. It is highest in neocortical areas, basal ganglia, and thalamus; intermediate in hippocampus, amygdala, brainstem and cerebellum; and lowest in white matter. There is an age-related decline of cerebral glucose metabolism, most prominently in frontal cortex (Zuendorf et al., 2003). For clinical use, normal plasma glucose levels and standard resting-state conditions (low noise level and low ambient light) should be maintained during tracer accumulation to avoid changes in the metabolic pattern by regional brain activation (Varrone et al., 2009).

Neuronal function is closely related to synaptic function, which involves the release of synaptic vesicles. Recently tracers have been

**TABLE 42.1 Glossary: Clinically Relevant Positron Emission Tomography and Single-Photon Emission Computed Tomography Tracers**

| Abbreviation | Tracer | Target Process/Structure |
|---|---|---|
| [$^{99m}$Tc]ECD | [$^{99m}$Tc]ethylcysteinate dimer | Cerebral blood flow |
| [$^{18}$F]FDG | [$^{18}$F]2-fluoro-2-deoxy -d-glucose | Cerebral glucose metabolism |
| [$^{18}$F]FDOPA | [$^{18}$F]6-fluoro-L-DOPA | Dopamine synthesis, amino acid transport |
| [$^{18}$F]FET | [$^{18}$F]O-(2-fluoroethyl)-L-tyrosine | Amino acid transport |
| [$^{18}$F]FLT | [$^{18}$F] 3′-deoxy-3′-fluorothymidine | Proliferation |
| [$^{123}$I]FP-CIT | [$^{123}$I]N-ω-fluoropropyl-2β-carbomethoxy-3β-(4-iodophenyl)nortropane | Dopamine transporter |
| [$^{99m}$Tc]HMPAO | [$^{99m}$Tc]hexamethylpropyleneamine oxime | Cerebral blood flow |
| | [$^{18}$F]florbetaben, BAY-949172, NeuraCeq | Amyloid beta |
| | [$^{18}$F]florbetapir, AV-45, Amyvid | Amyloid beta |
| | [$^{18}$F]flortaucipir, AV-1451 | Fibrillary tau |
| | [$^{18}$F]flutemetamol, GE-067, Vizamyl | Amyloid beta |
| [$^{11}$C]MET | L-[methyl-$^{11}$C]methionine | Amino acid uptake |
| [$^{11}$C]PIB | [$^{11}$C]Pittsburgh compound B | Amyloid beta |

developed to image the synaptic vesicle protein SV2A (Chen et al., 2018). This could provide a molecular marker for synaptic function that is complementary to functional imaging with [$^{18}$F]FDG and fMRI.

A large number of other PET tracers have been used in clinical research over the past decades, and a few have established clinical diagnostic utility. They are mentioned in the respective disease chapters. Generally the clinical interpretation of PET images is done by qualitative visual inspection, often supported by voxel-wise statistical analyses in comparison to normal subjects. However, PET also provides quantitative regional data, which are mainly used for research. The highest levels of quantitative accuracy employ mathematical modeling of tracer kinetics in tissue in relation to an arterial or reference tissue input function. However, such research techniques require dedicated expertise, software, and often also equipment for measuring plasma activity and tracer metabolites (Carson, 2005) and are not usually required for the clinical use of PET.

## Single-Photon Emission Computed Tomography

The first SPECT measurements were performed in the 1960s (Kuhl and Edwards, 1964). SPECT employs gamma-emitting radionuclides that decay by emitting a single gamma ray. Typical radionuclides employed for neurological SPECT are technetium-99m ($^{99m}$Tc; half-life = 6.02 hours) and iodine-123 ($^{123}$I; half-life = 13.2 hours). Gamma cameras are used for SPECT acquisition, whereby usually two detector heads rotate around the patient's head to acquire 2D planar images (projections) of the head from multiple angles (e.g., in three-degree steps). Whereas radiation collimation is achieved by coincidence detection in PET, hardware collimators with lead septa are placed in front of the detector heads in the case of SPECT scanners. Finally, 3D image data reconstruction is done by conventional reconstruction algorithms. With combined SPECT/CT systems, a low-dose CT transmission scan can replace less accurate calculated attenuation correction.

The different acquisition principles imply that SPECT possesses a considerably lower sensitivity than PET. Thus rapid temporal sampling (image frames of seconds to minutes) as a prerequisite for pharmacokinetic analyses is the strength of PET, whereas a single SPECT acquisition usually takes 20–30 minutes. Furthermore, the spatial resolution of modern SPECT is only about 7–10 mm, deteriorating with increasing distance between object and collimator (i.e., higher resolution for cortical than subcortical structures; distance between patient and collimator should be minimized for optimal resolution). Thus SPECT is more susceptible to partial volume effects than PET, which can be a particular drawback when it comes to imaging small structures or lesions (e.g., brain tumors). Nevertheless, brain-dedicated SPECT instruments have been proposed that allow for optimized spatial and temporal sampling and pharmacokinetic data quantification (Meyer et al., 2008). The important advantages of SPECT over PET are the lower costs and broader availability of SPECT systems and radionuclides. Although $^{123}$I-labeled tracers (e.g., [$^{123}$I]FP-CIT ([$^{123}$I]ioflupane, DaTSCAN) for dopamine transporter [DAT] imaging) can easily be shipped over long distances, technetium-99m can be eluted onsite from molybdenum-99 ($^{99}$Mo)/$^{99m}$Tc generators and used for labeling commercially available radiopharmaceutical kits.

The two most widely used CBF tracers are hexamethylpropyleneamine oxime ([$^{99m}$Tc]HMPAO) and ethylcysteinate dimer ([$^{99m}$Tc]ECD). Owing to their lipophilic nature and thus high first-pass brain extraction, both radiotracers are rapidly taken up by the brain. They are quasi-irreversibly retained after conversion into hydrophilic compounds (enzymatic deesterification of [$^{99m}$Tc]ECD; instability, and possibly interaction with glutathione in the case of [$^{99m}$Tc]HMPAO). Differences in uptake mechanisms may explain slight differences in biological behavior (e.g., in stroke), with [$^{99m}$Tc]HMPAO being more closely correlated to perfusion, whereas [$^{99m}$Tc]ECD uptake is also influenced by metabolic activity. Despite the fact that cerebral radiotracer uptake is virtually complete within just 1–2 minutes of injection, SPECT acquisition is usually started after 30–60 minutes to allow for sufficient background clearance.

Given the fact that the CBF is closely coupled to cerebral glucose metabolism and thus to neuronal function (with a few rare exceptions), [$^{99m}$Tc]HMPAO and [$^{99m}$Tc]ECD are used to assess neuronal activity indirectly. However, since cerebral autoregulation is also affected by many other factors (e.g., carbon dioxide level) and possibly diseases, cerebral glucose metabolism represents a more direct and less variable marker of neuronal activity. Given the technical limitations mentioned earlier, [$^{18}$F]FDG PET is generally preferred to CBF SPECT; therefore the following sections of this chapter primarily refer to PET studies. One important exception, however, is the use of ictal CBF SPECT in the assessment of patients with epilepsy.

# CLINICAL APPLICATIONS

## Overview of Dementia

Dementia is one of the main challenges to human health. Its importance is increasing worldwide due to the overall increase in life expectancy. Although the diagnosis of dementia is made by clinical assessment, the diagnosis of specific diseases causing dementia increasingly relies on imaging. The most prevalent cause of dementia is Alzheimer disease, which is characterized by deposits of the pathological proteins beta-amyloid and tau. Current research criteria for AD define the presence of the disease based on the detection of specific biomarkers (i.e., amyloid accumulation and tau) as detected in CSF or by PET (Jack et al., 2018). Notably, under this definition, Alzheimer *disease* (AD) does not imply presence of dementia at the time of diagnosis but indicates a disease process that will eventually lead to Alzheimer dementia. A positive test for amyloid and tau in the absence of cognitive impairment is an indicator of preclinical AD, or of prodromal AD, known as mild cognitive impairment (MCI). These conceptual developments can rely on molecular imaging techniques based on PET disease-defining biomarkers of AD. Thus detection of amyloid deposits in vivo by PET enables earlier diagnosis and improved distinction from other diseases causing dementia, such as frontotemporal dementia (FTD), dementia with Lewy bodies (DLB), and vascular dementia (VD). The different patterns of cortical functional deficits associated with these diseases are detected by functional imaging techniques, with [$^{18}$F]FDG PET being the most firmly established technique and various methods to assess CBF (SPECT, PET, ASL MRI) as potential alternatives. Typically these deficits also affect communication between brain areas, which increasingly is being studied by techniques for the analysis for brain networks, in particular by resting-state fMRI. PET and SPECT imaging of specific transmitter systems, which are impaired in AD (cholinergic) and DLB (dopaminergic and cholinergic), can provide further information for diagnosis, prediction, and the monitoring of therapy.

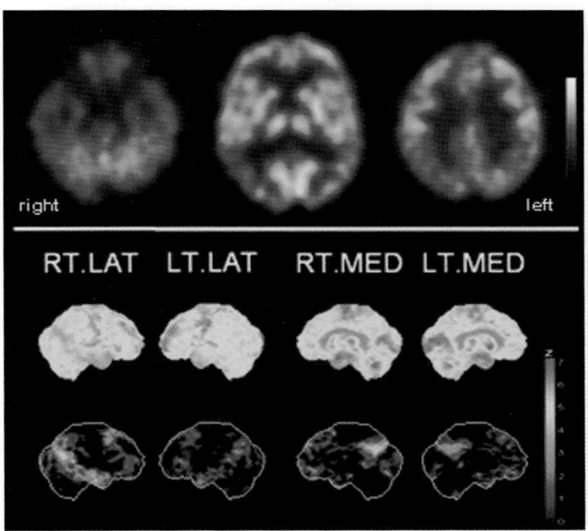


**Fig. 42.1** [$^{18}$F]FDG positron emission tomography (PET) in early Alzheimer disease. Early disease stage is characterized by mild to moderate hypometabolism of temporal and parietal cortices and posterior cingulate gyrus and precuneus. Distinct asymmetry is often noticed, as in this case. As disease progresses, frontal cortices also become involved. *Upper panel,* Transaxial PET images of [$^{18}$F]FDG uptake (color coded, see color scale on right with higher values at the top; orientation in radiological convention as indicated). *Lower panel,* Results of voxel-based statistical analysis using Neurostat/3D-SSP. Three-dimensional stereotactic surface projections of [$^{18}$F]FDG uptake *(upper row)* and statistical deviation of the individual's examination (as z-score) from age-matched healthy controls *(lower row)*. Data are color coded in rainbow scale (see lower right for z scale). Given are right and left lateral *(RT.LAT and LT.LAT)* and mesial views *(RT.MED and LT.MED)*. *(From Neurostat/3D-SSP analysis based on Minoshima, S., Frey, K.A., Koeppe, R.A., Foster, N.L., Kuhl, D.E., 1995. A diagnostic approach in Alzheimer's disease using three-dimensional stereotactic surface projections of fluorine-18-FDG PET. J Nucl Med. 36 [7], 1238–1248.)*

## Alzheimer Disease

### [$^{18}$F]2-deoxy-2-fluoro-d-glucose Positron Emission Tomography

The early and accurate diagnosis of dementia is of crucial importance for appropriate treatment (including possible enrollment into clinical trails and avoidance of possible side effects of treatments), for prognosis, and for adequate counseling of patients and caregivers. The diagnostic power of [$^{18}$F]FDG PET in this situation is well established (Bohnen et al., 2012) and reflected in clinical guidelines (Filippi et al., 2012; Frey et al., 2016). [$^{18}$F]FDG PET has also been included as a biomarker of neuronal damage in current diagnostic research criteria (McKhann et al., 2011). In clinical practice, [$^{18}$F]FDG PET studies are interpreted by qualitative visual readings. To achieve optimal diagnostic accuracy, these readings should be supported by voxel-based statistical analyses in comparison with aged-matched normal controls (Herholz et al., 2002; Minoshima et al., 1995). PET studies should always be interpreted with parallel inspection of a recent CT or MRI scan to detect structural defects (e.g., ischemia, atrophy, subdural hematoma), which can cause regional hypometabolism.

The typical finding in AD dementia is bilateral hypometabolism of the temporal and parietal association cortices, with the temporoparietal junction being the center of impairment. As the disease progresses, frontal association cortices also become involved (Figs. 42.1 and 42.2). The magnitude and extent of the hypometabolism increase with progressing disease, although there is relative sparing of the primary motor and visual cortices, basal ganglia, and cerebellum (often used as reference regions). The degree of hypometabolism is closely correlated with the severity of dementia (Salmon et al., 2005).

Cortical hypometabolism is bilateral but often asymmetrical, corresponding to predominant clinical symptoms (language impairment if the dominant hemisphere is most affected or visuospatial impairment if the nondominant hemisphere is most affected). Voxel-based statistical analyses consistently show that the posterior cingulate gyrus and precuneus are also affected; this is an important diagnostic clue even in the early stages of AD (Minoshima et al., 1997). The hippocampus is most affected by AD pathology, in particular by pathological tau deposits and atrophy, but hypometabolism appears less pronounced than in temporoparietal cortex (Herholz et al., 2018; Villain et al., 2008). This may be due to limitations of PET spatial resolution, although relative functional hyperactivity has also been discussed (Apostolova et al., 2018). A clear reduction of hippocampal metabolism in patients was observed as compared with selected control patients who remained stable over at least 4 subsequent years (Mosconi et al., 2005).

The logopenic variant, primary progressive aphasia (lvPPA), which is characterized by most prominent deficits in word retrieval and sentence repetition, is commonly also caused by AD (Rabinovici, et al., 2008). LvPPA patients typically show a strongly leftward asymmetric hypometabolism of the temporoparietal cortex (Gorno-Tempini et al., 2011; Lehmann et al., 2013; Madhavan et al., 2013; Fig. 42.3). Patients with posterior cortical atrophy (PCA), another nonamnestic presentation of AD with predominant visuospatial and visuoperceptual deficits, typically exhibit pronounced

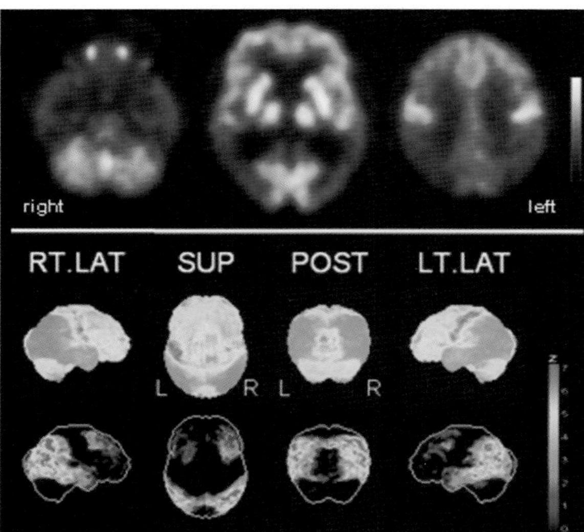


Fig. 42.2 [$^{18}$F]FDG positron emission tomography (PET) in advanced Alzheimer disease. Advanced disease stage is characterized by severe hypometabolism of temporal and parietal cortices and posterior cingulate gyrus and precuneus. Frontal cortex is also involved, while sensorimotor and occipital cortices, basal ganglia, thalamus, and cerebellum are spared. Mesiotemporal hypometabolism is also apparent. *Upper panel,* Transaxial PET images of [$^{18}$F]FDG uptake. *Lower panel,* Results of voxel-based statistical analysis using Neurostat/3D-SSP. Given are right and left lateral (*RT.LAT and LT.LAT*), superior (*SUP*), and posterior (*POST*) views (see Fig. 42.1 for additional details). *(From Neurostat/3D-SSP analysis based on Minoshima, S., Frey, K.A., Koeppe, R.A., Foster, N.L., Kuhl, D.E., 1995. A diagnostic approach in Alzheimer's disease using three-dimensional stereotactic surface projections of fluorine-18-FDG PET. J Nucl Med. 36 [7], 1238–1248.)*

hypometabolism of occipital association cortex (Lehmann et al., 2013; Spehl et al., 2015; Fig. 42.4).

A meta-analysis of [$^{18}$F]FDG-PET cross-sectional case-control studies ($n$ = 562 in total) revealed a very high sensitivity (96%) and specificity (90%) of [$^{18}$F]FDG PET for the diagnosis of AD in patients with dementia (Bohnen et al., 2012). In [$^{18}$F]FDG PET studies with autopsy confirmation in patients with memory complaints, the pattern of temporoparietal hypometabolism as assessed by visual readings alone showed a high sensitivity of 84%–94% for detecting pathologically confirmed AD, with a specificity of 73%–74% (Foster et al., 2007; Silverman et al., 2001). Visual inspection of [$^{18}$F]FDG PET was found to be of similar accuracy as a clinical follow-up examination performed 4 years after PET. Moreover, when [$^{18}$F]FDG PET disagreed with the initial clinical diagnosis, the PET diagnosis was considerably more likely to be congruent with the pathological diagnosis than the clinical diagnosis (Jagust et al., 2007).

Patterns of hypoperfusion observed with CBF SPECT in AD are similar to metabolic deficits on [$^{18}$F]FDG PET; but according to meta-analyses (Dougall et al., 2004) and direct comparisons (Herholz et al., 2002), their accuracy is inferior. There are increasing numbers of techniques to provide CBF mapping as replacement of FDG PET, including ASL MR and imaging early uptake of amyloid and tau tracers (see the following section). Studies in selected patient series suggest similar accuracy as [$^{18}$F]FDG PET, but larger studies are still needed to confirm the robustness of these findings.

## Amyloid Imaging

Several PET radiopharmaceuticals that bind to fibrillary beta-amyloid plaques have been developed and brought to clinical application in the past 20 years. Initially, carbon-11–labeled Pittsburgh compound B ([$^{11}$C]PIB) was used, demonstrating cortical binding in patients with AD (Klunk et al., 2004) and in many patients with MCI (Nordberg et al., 2013). Subsequently, $^{18}$F-labeled radiopharmaceuticals (see Table 42.1) were developed that enabled broader clinical application. Common to all amyloid tracers is a relatively high level of nonspecific binding to white matter, which is even more pronounced with the $^{18}$F-labeled compounds than with [$^{11}$C]PIB. Thus a negative scan is characterized by an image showing activity in white matter surrounded by low activity in gray matter, whereas a positive scan shows high uptake in cortical areas also (Fig. 42.5).

The first $^{18}$F-labeled amyloid marker was [$^{18}$F]FDDNP (Small, Kepe et al., 2006), which, however, did not match the specificity of [$^{11}$C]PIB. Since then several $^{18}$F-labeled amyloid markers with better specificity have been developed and licensed for commercial distribution as radiopharmaceuticals. These include [$^{18}$F]flutemetamol (Vandenberghe et al., 2010), which is chemically related to [$^{11}$C]PIB; the stilbene-derivatives [$^{18}$F]florbetapir (Wong et al., 2010); and [$^{18}$F]florbetaben (Sabri et al., 2010). Kinetic properties differ, resulting in recommended imaging times after the intravenous administration of around 60 minutes for [$^{18}$F]florbetapir and 90–120 minutes for [$^{18}$F]flutemetamol and [$^{18}$F]florbetaben. All licensed tracers have undergone formal trials to demonstrate validity, comparing in vivo imaging in terminally ill patients with postmortem assessments of beta amyloid in the patients' brains. Athough the general principle of comparing cortical uptake with white matter for visual analysis is the same for all tracers, recommendations differ slightly about color scales for display and for cases when cortical uptake is visible in only part of the brain. Formal training is required for readers.

Although visual analysis provides a binary distinction between positive and negative scans, *regional analysis* can provide measures of the magnitude of the amyloid load. Values are typically calculated as ratios relative to a *reference region*, which should represent a brain area devoid of fibrillary amyloid. Such regions include the pons, cerebral white matter, and cerebellar cortex. For practical reasons, the whole cerebellum is also frequently used (Pontecorvo et al., 2017). Some limitations must be kept in mind. Although cerebellar cortex is largely free of fibrillary amyloid until the very late stages of AD, it may contain diffuse and vascular amyloid, and therefore show some moderately variable tracer binding. The pons is a relatively small region in the brainstem that may represent relatively low total counts, causing some statistical variation. White matter is subject to high nonspecific binding, which may change in disorders affecting white matter and spillover effects from cortex in case of high cortical amyloid load; but it appears to be very stable in AD even under disease progression and has, therefore, been advocated for longitudinal studies (Brendel et al., 2015; Landau et al., 2015).

Most frequently standardized uptake value ratios (SUVRs) are being used for regional quantification. However, values in normal subjects and patients and also thresholds separating these groups differ among tracers and among reference regions used for calculation. Therefore the concept of centiloids has been introduced (Klunk et al., 2015) to provide standardization of uptake measures.

Although late uptake mostly represents tracer binding, it is not completely independent of nonspecific tracer delivery by CBF, which dominates the initial regional uptake immediately after tracer injection and influences slow washout from nonspecific binding. Images of initial tracer uptake or so-called $R_1$ maps yielded by relatively simple kinetic analyses have been shown to be very similar to [$^{18}$F]FDG scans in patients with dementia, indicating that they also have diagnostic potential (Meyer et al., 2011; Rostomian et al., 2011).

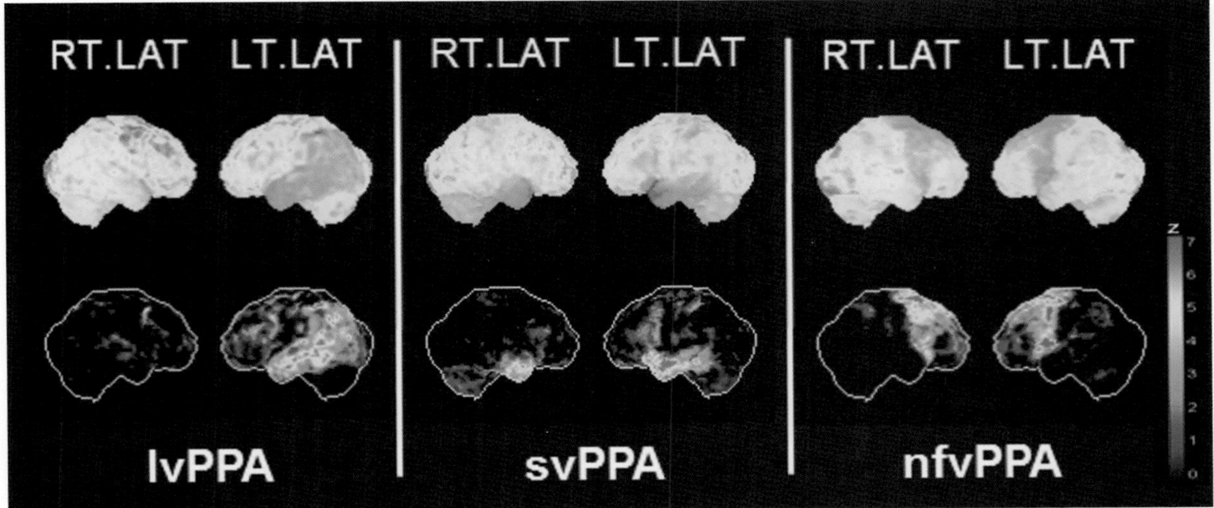


**Fig. 42.3** [18F]FDG positron emission tomography (PET) in the different variants of primary progressive aphasia (PPA). [18F]FDG PET scans in logopenic variant PPA *(lvPPA)* are characterized by a leftward asymmetric temporoparietal hypometabolism, whereas the semantic variant PPA *(svPPA)* involves the most rostral part of the temporal lobes. Patients with the nonfluent variant PPA *(nfvPPA)* typically show leftward asymmetric frontal hypometabolism with inferior frontal or posterior frontoinsular emphasis. Results of voxel-based statistical analysis using Neurostat/3D-SSP. Given are right and left lateral (*RT.LAT and LT.LAT*) views (see Fig. 42.1 for additional details).

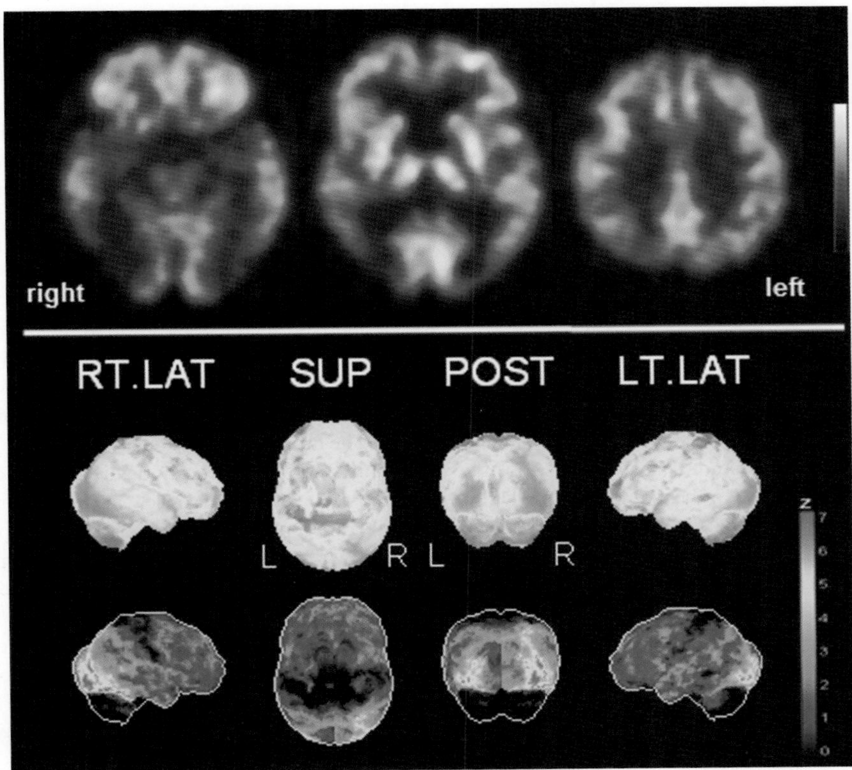


**Fig. 42.4** [18F]FDG positron emission tomography (PET) in posterior cortical atrophy (PCA). Patients with PCA usually show a rightward asymmetric temporoparietal hypometabolism with strong involvement of the lateral occipital cortex. Results of voxel-based statistical analysis using Neurostat/3D-SSP. Given are right and left lateral (*RT.LAT and LT.LAT*), superior (*SUP*), and posterior (*POST*) views (see Fig. 42.1 for additional details).

Kinetic modeling, including early and late phases of tracer uptake, provides the most accurate measures of tracer binding (van Berckel et al., 2013). However, this does require longer scanning times and has not been widely used in multicenter studies.

Studies indicate that up to 30% of patients clinically diagnosed with Alzheimer dementia may not have positive amyloid scans (Jack et al., 2016). Pathological diagnoses have been obtained in few of them, suggesting that they do not actually have AD but other forms

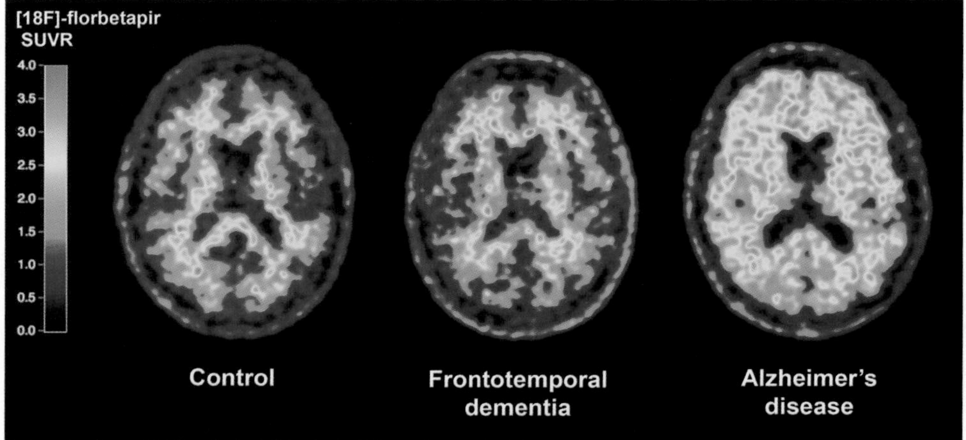


**Fig. 42.5** [$^{18}$F]florbetapir positron emission tomography (PET) demonstrating nonspecific white-matter uptake in a normal control subject *(left)* and patient with frontotemporal dementia (FTD) *(middle)* as well as cortical binding to amyloid in a patient with Alzheimer disease (AD) *(right)*. *SUVR*, Standardized uptake value ratio.

of neurodegenerative dementia. The clinical syndrome of MCI is even more heterogeneous. The frequency of amyloid positivity, indicating that symptoms are an early sign of AD, varies considerably depending on clinical subtype and ApoE4 genotype. Several studies indicate that more than 50% of MCI patients with a positive amyloid scan and signs of neuronal dysfunction on FDG or severe hippocampal atrophy will progress to dementia within the following 2–3 years (Vos et al., 2015). In contrast, the vast majority (about 90%) of MCI patients with normal amyloid and normal FDG scans will not progress to dementia in that time period. Patients with inconsistent findings (one normal and one abnormal FDG or amyloid scan) have an intermediate prognosis. Furthermore, in a real-life memory clinic population (i.e., various, possibly mixed etiologies of MCI), amyloid PET seems to be a better predictor of conversion to Alzheimer dementia than [$^{18}$F]FDG PET (Frings et al., 2018). Tau PET scans (see later) will likely add further prognostic information and may be particularly useful for monitoring the progression of AD (Jack et al., 2018; Johnson et al., 2016).

Several caveats must be kept in mind with the diagnostic use of amyloid PET scans. The frequency of positive scans in normal controls and in patients with other diseases increases substantially with age (Ossenkoppele et al., 2015), reaching 40% in 80-year-old subjects without cognitive deficits. Longitudinal studies suggest that a positive scan in a cognitively normal subject may indicate preclinical AD, but cognitive decline will likely be protracted over many years or even decades and thus not be clinically relevant to subjects of older ages. On the other hand, a positive scan in a patient with dementia does not always mean that the patient has AD. Amyloid deposition may be present as an incidental finding in elderly patients with other neurodegenerative or cerebrovascular disease. Especially in DLB, additional fibrillary amyloid deposition is a frequent finding (Siderowf et al., 2014; see "Dementia with Lewy Bodies," later). Cerebral amyloid angiopathy without AD is rare but also associated with positive amyloid PET scans (Farid et al., 2017).

There is no close correlation between amyloid deposition and cognition, either in normal subjects or in patients with dementia, albeit the laterality of amyloid load may coincide with predominant clinical symptoms (e.g., left- and rightward asymmetry in lvPPA and PCA, respectively; Frings et al., 2015). Thus one cannot use the intensity of amyloid deposition in patients with positive scans as a marker of clinical impairment. When controls are compared with AD patients, a bimodal distribution of uptake with clearly separate peaks is found (Nordberg et al., 2013). However, in patients with MCI and in elderly normal subjects, borderline findings are not uncommon and can cause diagnostic uncertainty.

Deposition of beta amyloid in the brain is inversely related to its concentration in CSF. Thus, as diagnostic markers, analysis of CSF amyloid and amyloid PET provide similar information (Palmqvist et al., 2015). Initial brain deposition of amyloid as oligomers cannot be detected by current PET tracers but may be toxic to neurons. Thus experimental research is ongoing to develop tracers for the detection of oligomeric amyloid (Meier et al., 2018).

The main genetic factor influencing the deposition of amyloid in the brain is apolipoprotein E4. Carriers of that gene typically show more intense accumulation, which starts at a younger age (long before symptoms appear; Jansen et al., 2015) and is associated with an increased risk of AD. Further genetic factors have been identified in genome-wide association studies (GWAS), but they have less effect (Ramanan et al., 2015).

There is much less variation in the regional distribution of amyloid in the brain than the variation observed with [$^{18}$F]FDG and other tracers. Uptake is highest in prefrontal cortices and the posterior cingulate cortex, followed by temporal, parietal, and occipital association cortices. The hippocampus is relatively spared. Typical and atypical clinical manifestations, which can be distinguished on [$^{18}$F]FDG PET and are often related to age at onset, show the same pattern on amyloid PET. Only rare genetically dominant forms of familial AD appear to be associated with earlier and greater amyloid deposition in the basal ganglia than sporadic cases (Villemagne et al., 2009).

Amyloid PET has been recognized as an imaging biomarker for clinical trials in AD. It is used to confirm the presence of amyloid and thus the diagnosis at entry. It is of particular relevance for interventions such as active and passive immunization, to remove amyloid deposits. In these studies, amyloid is also usually used as an outcome marker to demonstrate the biological drug effect (Salloway, et al., 2018). Some immunization agents have resulted in reduced binding of tracer after treatment; it is hoped that with larger studies at early stages of AD, this may translate into better cognitive outcomes. Obviously the development of a clinically effective treatment reducing brain amyloid would boost the diagnostic importance of amyloid imaging. Even at present, without such treatments, amyloid PET can contribute substantially to earlier and more accurate diagnosis with a substantial impact on patient management (Hellwig et al., 2019).

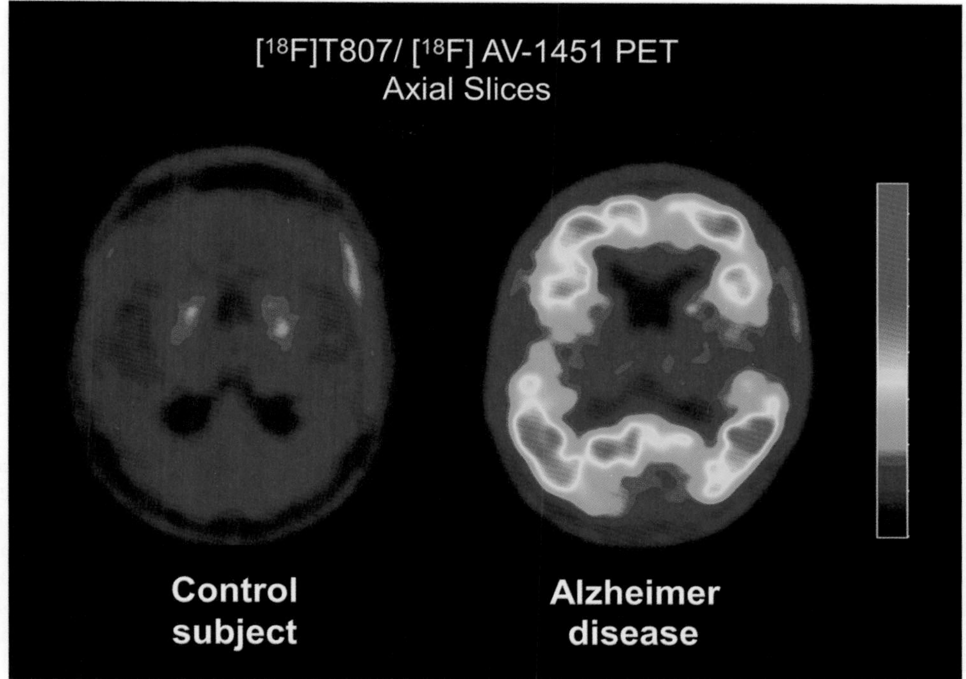


**Fig. 42.6** [18F]flortaucipir positron emission tomography (*PET*) demonstrating low uptake in normal control subject *(left)* and binding to pathological tau deposits in frontal and temporoparietal association cortices in a patient with Alzheimer disease. *(Courtesy Prof. Alexander Drzezga, University of Cologne, Germany.)*

## Other Imaging Methods in Positron Emission Tomography

AD is also characterized by pathological deposits of tau protein. Although their density is much lower than that of amyloid and they are primarily localized intracellularily, they can be visualized in vivo by PET (Leuzy et al., 2019). Among the first generation of $^{18}$F-labeled tau radiopharmaceuticals, [$^{18}$F]flortaucipir has been used most widely; it has been shown that it is related to symptoms and severity and that it can be used for staging and the monitoring of disease progression (Villemagne et al., 2015).

In normal elderly controls, increased tracer uptake is found in the hippocampal area even in the absence of amyloid. In patients with positive amyloid scans, tau spreads from the mesial temporal areas to other parts of the temporal lobe and then further on to other cortical areas in accordance with pathological Braak stages (Cho et al., 2018; Fig. 42.6). However, it has also been noted that first-generation tracers may show off-target binding (e.g., with [$^{18}$F]THK5351 to monoamine oxidase B [MAO-B]). It is expected that second-generation tracers will show less off-target binding (Okamura et al., 2018). The performance of tau tracers in other neurodegenerative diseases (e.g., tau-positive FTD, PSP, and CBD) still awaits detailed investigation, which will also clarify whether tau tracers can support differential diagnosis.

The most prominent neurotransmitter deficit in AD is the loss of cholinergic fibers, most of which originate from the nucleus basalis of Meynert in the basal forebrain with widespread cortical projections (Geula and Mesulam, 1989). Research studies have linked cholinergic degeneration with neuropsychological deficits and cognitive reserve (Garibotto et al., 2013). There has been a long-standing effort to develop flourine-18–labeled ligands for nicotinergic receptors, which also decline as cholinergic fibers are lost. Although past ligands have been plagued by very slow kinetics, more recent developments look promising for clinical application (Sabri et al., 2018).

There is substantial research interest in immunological mechanisms associated with AD and other neurodegenerative diseases (Kreisl et al., 2018). PET tracers have been developed to image activated microglia, which are the intrinsic immune cells of the brain. These are mostly ligands to the mitochondrial translocator protein 18D (TSPO), which is expressed in activated microglia (Rupprecht et al., 2010). Although moderately increased binding has been observed in manifest and prodromal AD, tracers have also shown substantial limitations related to nonspecific or low binding depending on a TSPO polymorphism, as yet preventing their routine clinical use. Related research is targeting activated astrocytes, which may play a role at an early stage of AD (Carter et al., 2019).

Traumatic brain injury is a risk factor for AD. Possible pathophysiological mechanisms are being explored using tau and the imaging of microglia (Folkersma et al., 2011; Mohamed et al., 2019). With regard to the imaging of nigrostriatal integrity for the differential diagnosis of AD, see "Dementia with Lewy Bodies," further on.

## Resting-State Functional Magnetic Resonance Imaging

Resting-state fMRI is used mostly as a research tool in AD. A large majority of studies have targeted the DMN, consistent with the notion that the components of the DMN are those typically found to be affected in resting state [$^{18}$F]FDG PET studies in MCI and early AD dementia. Using seed-based analysis or multivariate (e.g., independent component) analysis, reduced connectivity of DMN components was found in AD dementia patients compared with healthy controls and with a similar regional distribution, albeit less pronounced in amnestic MCI cases compared with healthy controls (Badhwar et al., 2017).

The diagnostic use of resting-state fMRI-based assessment of functional connectivity demonstrates declining connectivity when AD and MCI are compared with controls and reached more than 80% accuracy in single-center studies typically involving less than 50 patients per group and lacking cross-validation of accuracy levels (Koch et al., 2012). When machine learning was employed with cross-validation, the diagnostic accuracy of resting-state connectivity for MCI patients versus controls reached up to 80% accuracy; however, when applied to multicenter data, the levels of cross-validated accuracy fell below 80% (Teipel et al., 2017). In summary, the diagnostic use of resting-state fMRI for the separation of MCI or AD dementia patients from healthy controls is not sufficiently validated.

## Mild Cognitive Impairment

The syndrome of MCI (Petersen et al., 1999, 2018) represents a risk state for dementia. Patients may progress to manifest dementia in subsequent years but may also remain cognitively stable; a small proportion may even become normal. Patients with positive amyloid scans are now regarded as having prodromal AD, or "MCI due to AD" (Dubois and Albert, 2004), and they have a higher probability of progressing to dementia than patients with a negative scan, who do not have prodromal AD. [$^{18}$F]FDG PET is now regarded as an indicator of neuronal dysfunction (Albert et al., 2011), and an abnormal [$^{18}$F]FDG PET also indicates an increased probability for progression to dementia, as demonstrated in multiple studies (Drzezga et al., 2005; Mosconiet al., 2008). MCI patient in whom both amyloid and [$^{18}$F]FDG PET are abnormal will progress to dementia within 2 years with a probability of 40%–50% (Vos et al., 2015).

In cohort studies, although most cognitively normal healthy controls at risk for AD (ApoE ε4 carrier and/or positive maternal family history) showed normal FDG PET individually, they exhibited a significantly reduced glucose metabolism in those cortical areas typically affected by AD dementia preceding the possible onset of AD dementia by decades (Reiman et al., 2004). Follow-up studies in subjects at risk for AD also demonstrated that the subsequent decline in cerebral glucose metabolism in AD-typical regions was significantly greater compared with subjects who were not at risk (Mosconi et al., 2009).

Studies with fMRI have suggested differences in the functional connectivity pattern between MCI patients who remained stable and those who converted to AD dementia during clinical follow-up in areas of the DMN and beyond (Binnewijzend et al., 2012). Some studies showed parallel effects of treatment of cognitive tasks and task-related increases in functional network activity with short-term interventions, such as a single dose or 4 weeks of a cholinesterase inhibitor, but this was not consistently found after longer-term treatment (McGeown et al., 2010).

Interstingly, fMRI studies suggest a nonlinear course of hyper- and hypoactivation across the healthy aging MCI–mild AD dementia continuum. Thus hippocampal hyperactivity during memory performance was associated with a higher risk of subsequent cognitive decline (Bakker et al., 2012). Other studies have interpreted hyperactivation during still intact task performance as a compensatory mechanism. However, in more advanced stages of MCI this may be a marker of network pathology, possibly as an effect of or even driving cortical amyloid accumulation (Yamamoto et al., 2015). These findings underscore the potential of fMRI studies in AD to uncover pathogenetic mechanisms of disease beyond the use of a diagnostic or prognostic biomarker.

## Dementia with Lewy Bodies

DLB is associated with pathological cortical deposits of α-synuclein. The typical [$^{18}$F]FDG PET pattern observed in DLB resembles the pattern observed in AD with additional hypometabolism of the primary visual cortex and the occipital association cortex (Albin et al., 1996; Fig. 42.7). The latter has been linked with the occurrence of typical visual hallucinations in DLB patients (particularly in those with relatively preserved posterior temporal and parietal metabolism; Imamura et al., 1999). Occipital hypometabolism was found to be a valuable diagnostic feature to distinguish clinically diagnosed patients with AD from those with DLB (sensitivity 83%–92%, specificity 91%–93%; Higuchi et al., 2000; Ishi et al.,1998: Lim et al., 2009). This was substantiated in a study with autopsy confirmation (sensitivity 90%, specificity 80%; Minoshima et al., 2001). Recent studies have demonstrated that regional metabolism of the hippocampus (Ishii et al., 2007; Mosconi et al., 2008) and mid- to posterior cingulate gyrus (so-called cingulate island sign; Lim et al., 2009) is relatively preserved in DLB compared with AD, offering a high specificity for DLB. However, differences between AD and DLB may be hard to appreciate in the routine clinical examination of individual patients.

In this situation, PET or SPECT examinations of nigrostriatal integrity (most notably [$^{123}$I]FP-CIT SPECT) can be very helpful in differentiating between AD and DLB (McKeith et al., 2007). A recent meta-analysis indicated a pooled sensitivity and specificity of [$^{123}$I] FP-CIT SPECT for DLB of 87% and 94%, respectively (Papathanasiou et al., 2012). Furthermore, in a direct comparison of [$^{18}$F]FDG PET and DAT SPECT, the latter was found to be superior for the differential diagnosis of DLB versus AD (Lim et al., 2009). In line with this, striatal DAT loss is defined as an indicative biomarker in the current diagnostic criteria for DLB, whereas occipital hypometabolism is a supportive biomarker (McKeith et al., 2017). Of note, nigrostriatal projections may also be damaged in FTD (Rinne et al., 2002) and atypical parkinsonian syndromes with dementia (e.g., PSP and CBD; see below). Concerning a possible prodromal stage of DLB, it has been shown that primary visual cortex hypometabolism is associated with clinical core features of DLB in nondemented memory clinic patients (Fujishiro et al., 2012). Those who converted to DLB during follow-up showed a more pronounced lateral occipital and parietal hypometabolism (Fujishiro et al., 2013).

DLB is clinically distinguished from Parkinson disease (PD) with dementia (PDD) by the so-called 1-year rule. In line with the notion that both diseases most likely represent manifestations of the same disease spectrum (the Lewy body disease spectrum; Lippa et al., 2007), [$^{18}$F]FDG PET studies in PDD (Peppard et al., 1992; Vander Borght et al., 1997) found very similar results to those in DLB. In fact, in a direct comparison of both groups there were only minor differences, if any (Yong et al., 2007). PDD is associated with marked reductions in cholinergic activity (Bohnen et al., 2003; Hilker et al., 2005) greater than those seen in AD. The pathology of PDD is mixed but often includes cortical Lewy body deposition (with or without evidence of AD pathology); therefore there has been considerable interest in whether agents that bind to aberrantly folded protein can be used to image DLB or PDD. However, according to a recent meta-analysis, about two-thirds of DLB patients but only one-third of PDD patients have a positive amyloid-beta PET scan (Donaghy et al., 2015), suggesting a differential contribution of amyloidbeta to the manifestation of cognitive impairment and its timing in PD and DLB (reviewed in Meyer et al., 2014). In fact, it appears likely that patients with PDD who demonstrate [$^{11}$C]PiB uptake have concurrent amyloid plaques, as suggested by a relationship to ApoE4 allele and CSF Aβ42 levels (Maetzler et al., 2009) as well as recent postmortem (Burack et al., 2010) and in vitro (Fodero-Tavoletti et al., 2007) studies. However, the pattern of amyloid deposition varies between PD and AD, suggesting that amyloid may play a different role in these illnesses (Campbell et al., 2013).

Recent [$^{18}$F]FDG PET studies also support the notion that PD with MCI (PD-MCI) represents a prodromal stage of PDD (Litvan et al., 2012): Similar to the pattern observed in PDD, PD-MCI patients typically exhibit a decreased temporoparietal, occipital, precuneus, and frontal metabolism as compared with healthy controls

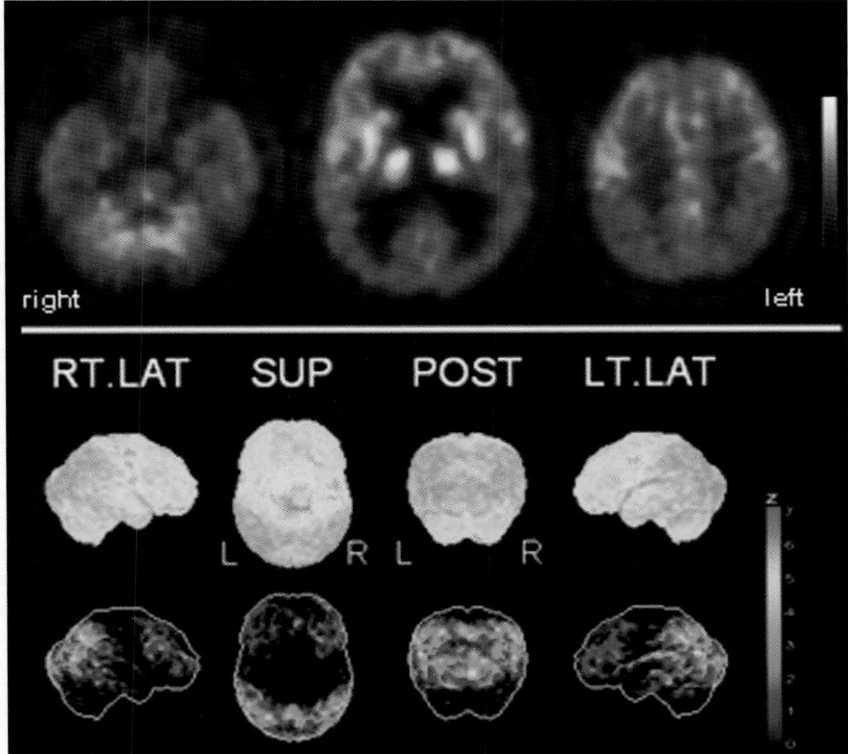


Fig. 42.7 [$^{18}$F]FDG positron emission tomography (PET) in dementia with Lewy bodies (DLB). This disorder affects similar areas as those affected by Alzheimer disease (AD). Occipital cortex is also involved, which may distinguish DLB from AD; in turn, the mesiotemporal lobe is relatively spared in DLB. A very similar if not identical pattern is observed in Parkinson disease with dementia (PDD). *Upper panel*, Transaxial PET images of [$^{18}$F]FDG uptake. *Lower panel*, Results of voxel-based statistical analysis using Neurostat/3D-SSP. Given are right and left lateral (*RT.LAT and LT.LAT*), superior (*SUP*), and posterior (*POST*) views (see Fig. 42.1 for additional details).

and, to a lesser extent, to PD patients without MCI (Garcia-Garcia et al., 2012; Hosokai et al., 2009; Pappata et al., 2011). These changes are more pronounced in multidomain compared with single-domain MCI (Huang et al., 2008; Lyoo et al., 2010) and correlate with overall cognitive performance across patients with PD, PD-MCI, and PDD (Garcia-Garcia et al., 2012; Meyer et al., 2014). Conversion from PD to PDD was predicted by hypometabolism in posterior cingulate, occipital cortex, Brodmann area [BA](BA18/19), and caudate nucleus, whereas hypometabolism of the primary visual cortex (BA17) was also observed in cognitively stable PD patients. A high predictive value of posterior cortical hypometabolism for conversion within 4 years was also observed by Pilotto et al. (2018). Converters showed a widespread metabolic decline in several cortical and subcortical areas on follow-up imaging (Bohnen et al., 2011).

As in other neurodegenerative disorders, there has been great interest in the possibility of an inflammatory component to the pathogenesis and progression of diseases of the Lewy body disease spectrum. TSPO ligands show activated microglia in the substantia nigra of PD patients (Ouchi et al., 2005), which in DLB extend into associative cortices (Edison et al., 2013).

Resting-state fMRI studies in PD with cognitive decline or dementia and DLB have found consistently reduced functional connectivity in nonmotor networks, most prominently including the DMN and frontoparietal networks (Wolters et al., 2018). DLB patients showed increased task-related deactivation in DMN components in comparison with controls. This was different from AD patients, who showed decreased task-related DMN deactivation compared with controls. These findings suggest a similar regional distribution but different mechanisms of cognitive networks compared with AD patients. Preliminary evidence from cross-sectional data in cognitively unimpaired PD patients suggests that such functional changes may precede cognitive decline in PD (Tessitore et al., 2012). Resting-state fMRI, however, is not sufficiently validated as a biomarker to provide individual prediction of PD-associated cognitive decline.

## Frontotemporal Lobar Degeneration

Frontotemporal lobar degeneration (FTLD) refers to a heterogeneous group of syndromes characterized by predominant deficits in behavior, language, and executive functions; these deficits are caused by a progressive degeneration of frontal and/or temporal lobes. FTLD comprises the major clinical syndromes of behavioral variant frontotemporal dementia (bvFTD) with prominent behavioral/cognitive symptoms like disinhibition, apathy, or executive deficits (Rascovsky et al., 2011) and primary progressive aphasia (PPA), which also has several subtypes (see later; Gorno-Tempini et al., 2011). The underlying pathology is diverse, including deposits of tau, transactive response DNA binding protein 43 kDa (TDP43), or fused in sarcoma (FUS) protein, but it is not associated with amyloid pathology. Although associations between clinical syndromes have been described, these syndromes as well as pathologies may overlap considerably (Mann and Snowden, 2017).

BvFTD is usually associated with a bilateral, often asymmetrical frontal hypometabolism, which is most pronounced in the mesial (polar) frontal cortex (Fig. 42.8; Garraux et al., 1999; Salmon et al., 2003).

The striatum, thalamus, and temporal and parietal cortices are also affected, though to a lesser extent (Garraux, et al., 1999; Ishii et al., 1998 ). Despite the fact that bvFTD and AD affect overlapping cortical areas, the predominance of frontal and temporoparietal deficits, respectively, is usually very apparent and allows for a clear distinction between FTD and AD. In line with this, a voxel-based statistical analysis provided a diagnostic accuracy of 90% (sensitivity 98%, specificity 86%) for separating FTD (bvFTD and svPPA) and AD in an autopsy-confirmed study, which was clearly superior to clinical diagnosis alone (Foster et al., 2007). Consequently, frontal or anterior temporal hypoperfusion or hypometabolism was incorporated as a criterion for probable bvFTD into the revised diagnostic criteria (Rascovsky et al., 2011). A pathological [$^{18}$F]FDG PET can be helpful in the clinical diagnosis of bvFTD (Kipps et al., 2009), but its sensitivity may be limited in cases without corresponding atrophy on MRI (Kerklaan et al., 2012). Amyloid scans are typically negative (Herholz et al., 2014; Rabinovici et al., 2011).

Patients with semantic dementia or semantic variant PPA (svPPA) typically show a predominant hypometabolism of the rostral temporal lobes, which is usually asymmetric leftward (see Fig. 42.3; Diehl, Grimmer et al., 2004; Rabinovici et al., 2008). This pattern distinguishes patients with svPPA from those with lvPPA, who present a more posterior temporoparietal hypometabolism (as a nonamnestic AD manifestation; see earlier). Patients with nonfluent variant PPA (nfvPPA) exhibit a left frontal hypometabolism, especially in inferior frontal or posterior frontoinsular regions (see Fig. 42.3; Josephs et al., 2010; Nestor et al., 2003; Rabinovici et al., 2008 ).

Resting-state fMRI is still a research tool in FTLD. In bvFTD, resting-state fMRI revealed altered connectivity in cortical networks, predominantly the salience network (Filippi et al., 2013; Sturm et al., 2018), including dorsal anterior cingulate and anterior insular cortices that subserve detection of salient stimuli depending on their homeostatic, emotional, or cognitive relevance. Similarly, resting-state fMRI studies in PPA variants showed network alterations in connectivity that corresponded with the clinical phenotype of language impairment. For example, people with primary progressive apraxia of speech had reduced connectivity of the right supplementary motor area and left posterior temporal gyrus relative to the rest of the speech and language networks (Botha et al., 2018), underscoring the key role of the supplementary motor area in this syndrome.

With respect to diagnostic usefulness, preliminary analyses suggest that in combination with structural imaging markers, the measurement of resting-state fMRI connectivity may improve the diagnostic classification of patients with AD dementia and bvFTD (Bouts et al., 2018; Hafkemeijer et al., 2015). However, group differences were found in functional connectivity between anterior midcingulate cortex and frontoinsular regions in FTD mutation carriers compared with noncarriers (Dopper et al., 2014). The identification of presymptomatic carriers of the FTD mutation using resting-state fMRI reached only chance-level accuracy (Feis et al., 2018). Studies found reductions of functional connectivity in distinct intrinsic networks, but discrimination from the longitudinal course of patients with AD dementia was poor (Hafkemeijer et al., 2017).

## Vascular Dementia

VD is a frequent consequence of stroke, especially when it presents as multi-infarct dementia. Without preceding stroke, VD seems to be rather rare in North America and Europe and more prevalent in Japan. In agreement with CT and MRI, PET may show defects of [$^{18}$F]FDG uptake corresponding to ischemic infarcts, not sparing regions that are usually well preserved in AD. Thus defects in basal ganglia, thalamus, and cerebellum can provide important diagnostic clues. Cerebral glucose metabolism was reported to be globally reduced in VD (Mielke et al., 1992), but without absolute quantification this finding cannot be reliably assessed. Subcortical white-matter changes, as frequently seen on MRI in elderly patients without a history of stroke, are associated with the slowing of motor and attentional functions and increase the risk for dementia; however, they are rarely the sole cause of dementia (Ylikoski et al., 1993).

Changes in DMN connectivity have been studied in people with subcortical vascular cognitive impairment using resting-state fMRI, with decreased connectivity reported in anterior cingulate and parahippocampal gyrus (Chen et al., 2016); but these results are based on small samples and there are only few studies so far. Also, current trial protocols for treatment studies in vascular cognitive impairment use fMRI endpoints as surrogate markers for intervention effects on neuronal network integrity (Leijenaar et al., 2018), with one study showing effects of attention process training on cerebellar resting state activity in people with vascular cognitive impairment (Pantoni et al., 2017). The localization of the effect was not predefined, rendering this outcome inconclusive. In summary, fMRI analyses in vascular cognitive decline are just beginning. One reason for this is the poor definition of vascular cognitive decline. A likely confounder will be a high rate of AD comorbidity in older people with suspected vascular cognitive decline, which would require prior exclusion of AD-type pathology using amyloid PET or CSF analysis.

## Parkinsonism

An early and correct differential diagnosis of parkinsonism is of paramount therapeutic and prognostic importance, given the possible treatment options and good prognosis in patients without nigrostriatal degeneration (e.g., drug-induced parkinsonism, essential tremor, vascular parkinsonism) and the limited responsiveness to L-dopa and more rapid progression to disability and death in patients with atypical parkinsonism syndromes (APS) compared with PD (Kempster al., 2007; O'Sullivan et al., 2008). However, postmortem studies suggest that the clinical diagnosis of PD, as the most frequent cause of parkinsonism, is incorrect in about 25% of patients (Tolosa et al., 2006). Frequent misdiagnoses include secondary parkinsonism and the APS entities multiple system atrophy (MSA), progressive supranuclear palsy (PSP), and corticobasal degeneration (CBD). In turn, cumulative clinicopathological data suggest that about 30% of MSA and PSP and up to 74% of CBD patients are not correctly diagnosed even at a late stage (Ling et al., 2010). Against this background, SPECT and PET are used with two aims: first to identify patients with progressive nigrostriatal degeneration, which is the common pathological feature in PD, MSA, PSP, and CBD; and second to differentiate between these patient groups.

### Imaging of Nigrostriatal Integrity

Accurate diagnosis of neurodegenerative parkinsonism can be achieved by imaging nigrostriatal function (Benamer et al., 2000; Benitez-Rivero et al., 2013; Marshall et al., 2009): In PD, [$^{18}$F]FDOPA uptake (as a marker of dopamine synthesis and storage), DAT binding (most notably [$^{123}$I]FP-CIT SPECT), and vesicular monoamine transporter type 2 (VMAT2) binding (e.g., with [$^{11}$C]DTBZ) are all reduced in a similar pattern, with a rostrocaudal gradient in which the posterior striatum is maximally affected and the caudate nucleus is relatively spared (Fig. 42.9). The degree of abnormality is typically asymmetrical, in keeping with clinical findings, but even patients with clinically unilateral disease have evidence of bilateral striatal dopamine denervation on PET or SPECT (Marek et al., 1996). With disease progression, uptake of all tracers declines according to an exponential function. The rostrocaudal gradient of involvement is maintained throughout the course of the illness

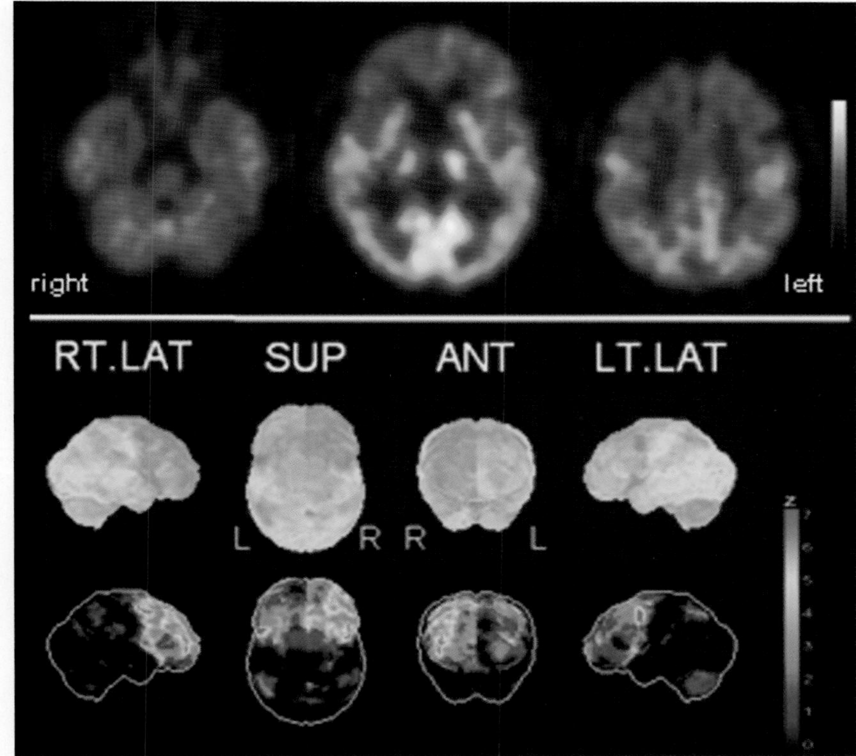


Fig. 42.8 [$^{18}$F]FDG positron emission tomography (PET) in behavioral variant frontotemporal dementia (bvFTD). Bifrontal hypometabolism is usually found in FTD, often in a somewhat asymmetrical distribution, as in this case. At early stages, frontomesial and frontopolar involvement are most pronounced, while parietal cortices can be affected later in disease course. *Upper panel*, Transaxial PET images of [$^{18}$F]FDG uptake. *Lower panel*, Results of voxel-based statistical analysis using Neurostat/3D-SSP. Given are right and left lateral (*RT.LAT and LT.LAT*), superior (*SUP*), and posterior views (see Fig. 42.1 for additional details).

but the asymmetry between sides lessens over time (Nandhagopal et al., 2009). Because the symptoms of PD do not become manifest until loss of approximately 50% of nigral neurons or 80% of striatal dopamine, imaging may be used to detect preclinical abnormalities in individuals at high risk for developing parkinsonism. These include persons exposed to the selective nigral toxin N-methyl-4-phenyl-1,2,3,6-tetrahydropridine (MPTP; Calne et al., 1985), twins of persons with PD (Piccini et al., 1999), family members from pedigrees with dominantly inherited PD (Adams et al., 2005; Nandhagopal et al., 2008), and individuals with rapid-eye-motion (REM) sleep behavior disorder (Albin et al., 2000). Interestingly, heterozygous mutation carriers from kindreds with recessively inherited PD also demonstrate imaging evidence of dopamine denervation (Hilker et al., 2001; Khan et al., 2002, 2005).

Among numerous different radiotracers proposed for imaging nigrostriatal integrity, the SPECT ligand [$^{123}$I]FP-CIT has gained the most widespread acceptance as an approved SPECT tracer in Europe and the United States. Trials have demonstrated that [$^{123}$I]FP-CIT SPECT offers excellent diagnostic specificity for identifying neurodegenerative parkinsonism (>95%), with diagnostic sensitivity depending on the inclusion of either patients with clinically well-established diagnoses (97%, ET vs. neurodegenerative parkinsonism; Benamer, Patterson et al., 2000) or patients with clinically "uncertain" parkinsonian syndromes (CUPS) or tremor (78%; Marshall, Reininger et al., 2009). The lower apparent sensitivity in the latter study was due to the inclusion of patients with *scans without evidence of dopaminergic deficit* (SWEED) who were clinically diagnosed with neurodegenerative parkinsonism. Lower rates of SWEED (10%–15%) have also been observed in clinical therapy trials including clinically certain cases; but accumulating evidence (e.g., stable clinical and imaging follow-up, no response to dopaminergic treatment) suggests that SWEED patients do not suffer from neurodegenerative parkinsonism (Mareket al., 2014). Larger studies also underline the diagnostic value of [$^{123}$I]FP-CIT SPECT in secondary parkinsonism-like schizophrenia and possible drug-induced parkinsonism (normal DAT binding; Tinazzi et al., 2014) or vascular parkinsonism (normal, homogenously reduced, or focal DAT defects; Benitez-Rivero et al., 2013). The actual clinical impact of DAT imaging on the management of patients with CUPS was highlighted by multicenter studies (Catafau et al., 2004; Kupsch et al., 2012). For instance, in one of these studies (Catafau et al., 2004), 36% and 54% of patients with clinically suspected decreased and normal nigrostriatal intergrity showed a normal and pathological [$^{123}$I] FP-CIT SPECT, respectively, which led to changes in the clinical management in 72% of cases.

### Differential Diagnosis of Neurodegenerative Parkinsonism

However, DAT imaging does not allow for a reliable differential diagnosis between PD, MSA, PSP, and CBD (Meyer and Hellwig, 2014). Instead, [$^{18}$F]FDG PET has gained acceptance as the method of choice. It surpasses the diagnostic accuracies of other commonly used techniques such as the imaging of cardiac sympathetic innervation (e.g., using [$^{123}$I]metaiodobenzylguanidine ([$^{123}$I]MIBG) scintigraphy) or

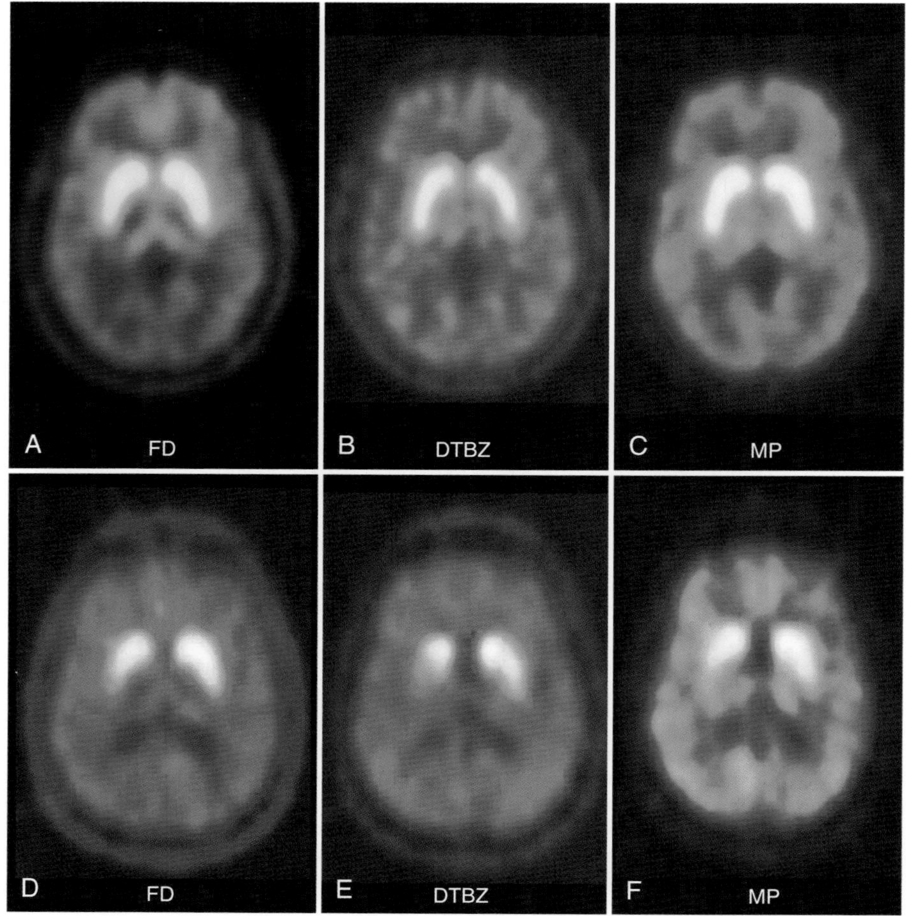


**Fig. 42.9** *Upper panel,* Physiological striatal [$^{18}$F]FDOPA (*FD*) uptake, VMAT2 ([$^{11}$C]*DTBZ*), and DAT ([$^{11}$C]-methylphenydate, *MP*) binding in a healthy control. *Lower panel,* Asymmetrical reduction of uptake in a patient with PD, with activity reduction of all three tracers in the posterior putamen and relative sparing of the caudate nucleus. *(Courtesy Vijay Chandran and A. Jon Stoessl, University of British Columbia, Canada.)*

of striatal dopamine D2/D3 receptors (e.g., using [$^{123}$I]iodobenzamide ([$^{123}$I]IBZM); Meyer and Hellwig, 2014). Assessment of regional CBF changes with SPECT may also be used for this purpose (e.g., Eckert et al., 2007). However, since [$^{18}$F]FDG PET is technically superior and also widely available, the focus here is on [$^{18}$F]FDG PET.

[$^{18}$F]FDG PET shows disease-specific alterations of cerebral glucose metabolism (e.g., Eckert et al., 2005; Juh et al., 2004; Hellwig et al., 2012; Teune et al., 2010). In scans of PD patients, major abnormalities may not appear initially. On closer inspection and especially on voxel-based statistical analyses, PD is characterized by a posterior temporoparietal, occipital, and sometimes frontal hypometabolism (especially in PD with MCI and PDD) and relative hypermetabolism of putamen, globus pallidus, sensorimotor cortex, pons, and cerebellum (Fig. 42.10). Interestingly, temporo-parieto-occipital hypometabolism may also been seen in nondemented PD patients (Hellwig et al., 2012; Hu et al., 2000), indicating an increased risk of subsequent development of PDD (see "Dementia and Mild Cognitive Impairment," earlier). Conversely, MSA patients show a marked hypometabolism of striatum (posterior putamen; especially in MSA-P), pons, and cerebellum (especially in MSA-C; Fig. 42.11). In PSP, regional hypometabolism is consistently noted in medial, dorsolateral, and ventrolateral frontal areas (pronounced in anterior cingulate gyrus as well as supplementary motor and premotor areas), caudate nucleus, (medial) thalamus and upper brainstem (Fig. 42.12). Recently proposed MDS-PSP criteria set a framework to diagnose several PSP-predominant types (Hoglinger et al., 2017), which can be expected to also differ on [$^{18}$F]FDG PET. For example, respective functional domains have been linked to predominant regional hypometabolism of bilateral anterior cingulate gyrus (vertical gaze palsy; Amtage et al.,2014), thalamus (repeated unprovoked falls; Zwergal et al., 2011), midbrain (gait freezing; Park et al., 2009) and left medial and dorsolateral frontal lobe (nonfluent aphasia; Roh et al., 2010). Finally, CBD is characterized by a usually highly asymmetric hypometabolism of frontoparietal areas (particularly parietal), motor cortex, middle cingulate gyrus, striatum and thalamus contralateral to the most affected body side (Fig. 42.13). The aforementioned results gained from categorical comparisons fit the results gained from spatial covariance analyses. These were employed to detect abnormal disease-related metabolic patterns in PD, MSA, PSP, and CBD, which were demonstrated to be highly reproducible and to correlate with disease severity and duration; thus they allow for prospective discrimination between cohorts (Eckert et al., 2008; Ma et al., 2007; Niethammer et al., 2014; Poston et al., 2012). The expression of two distinctive spatial covariance patterns characterizes PD: one related to motor manifestations (PDRP) and one to cognitive manifestations (PDCP). The PDRP is already significantly increased in the ipsilateral ("presymptomatic") hemispheres of patients with hemiparkinsonism (Tang et al., 2010a). Finally, using [$^{18}$F]FDG PET and CBF SPECT, it was demonstrated that PDRP is also increased in REM sleep behavior

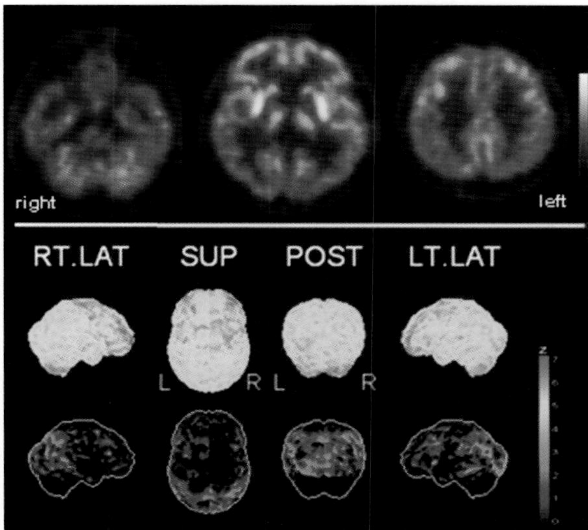


**Fig. 42.10** [$^{18}$F]FDG positron emission tomography (PET) in Parkinson disease (PD) is typically characterized by (relative) striatal hypermetabolism. Temporoparietal, occipital, and sometimes frontal hypometabolism can be observed in a significant fraction of PD patients without apparent cognitive impairment. Cortical hypometabolism can be fairly pronounced, possibly representing a risk factor for the subsequent development of Parkinson disease with dementia (PDD). *Upper panel,* Transaxial PET images of [$^{18}$F]FDG uptake. *Lower panel,* Results of voxel-based statistical analysis using Neurostat/3D-SSP. Given are right and left lateral (*RT.LAT and LT.LAT*), superior (*SUP*), and posterior (*POST*) views (see Fig. 42.1 for additional details). *(From Neurostat/3D-SSP analysis based on Minoshima, S., Frey, K.A., Koeppe, R.A., Foster, N.L., Kuhl, D.E., 1995. A diagnostic approach in Alzheimer's disease using three-dimensional stereotactic surface projections of fluorine-18-FDG PET. J Nucl Med. 36 [7], 1238–1248.)*

disorder, being a significant predictor of phenoconversion to PD or DLB (Holtbernd et al., 2014). Thus covariance patterns of cerebral glucose metabolism represent very interesting biomarkers for early diagnosis and therapy monitoring in parkinsonism (Hirano et al., 2009).

PSP and CBD may be considered to represent different manifestations of a disease spectrum with several common clinical, pathological, genetic, and biochemical features (Kouri et al., 2011). This issue becomes even more complex if one considers that FTD is often caused by PSP and CBD pathology (see earlier; Kertesz et al., 2005). Consequently the clinical diagnosis of CBD is notoriously inaccurate (Ling, et al., 2010; Wadia and Lang, 2007 ) and imaging results in patients with clinically diagnosed PSP and CBD may be very similar. For instance, findings can be fairly asymmetric not only in CBD but also in PSP, whereby an asymmetric PSP presentation is related to an asymmetric metabolism in motor cortex, cingulate gyrus, and thalamus (Amtage et al., 2014). However, the aforementioned group analysis (Amtage et al., 2014) and the few available studies with postmortem verification (Zalewski et al., 2014) imply that asymmetric frontoparietal hypometabolism is suggestive of CBD. Taken together, these observations indicate that additional studies with postmortem verification are needed to define reliable PET criteria, particularly in tauopathies.

Several larger, in part, prospective studies have investigated the applicability of [$^{18}$F]FDG PET for the differential diagnosis of parkinsonism. They unanimously found a very high accuracy (>90%) of [$^{18}$F]FDG PET for the distinction between PD and APS, which was largely independent of analytic methods, patient groups (with or without CBD and/or PDD/DLB), and symptom duration (Eckert et al., 2005; Garraux et al., 2013; Hellwig et al., 2012; Juh et al., 2004; Tang et al., 2010b; Tripathi et al., 2013). Consistently, a preliminary meta-analysis of currently available studies with inclusion of multiple disease groups yielded a diagnostic sensitivity and specificity for visual PET readings—supported by voxel-based statistical analyses—for the diagnosis of APS of 91.4% and 90.6%, respectively. Diagnostic specificity of [$^{18}$F]FDG PET for diagnosing MSA, PSP, and CBD was consistently shown to be high (>90%, as requested for a confirmatory test), whereas sensitivity was more variable (>75%; Meyer et al., 2017). However, given the clinical and imaging ambiguity, it may be advisable to use a combined PSP/CBD tauopathy category for PET readings, which reaches a sensitivity and specificity of 87% and 100%, respectively (Hellwig et al., 2012).

## Additional Observations in Parkinson Disease Using Other Positron Emission Tomography Imaging Methods

Postural instability and gait disturbances in PD are less responsive to dopaminergic therapy. PET studies show an association of these features with cholinergic dysfunction. PD patients with falls have lower thalamic cholinergic activity than nonfallers despite comparable nigrostriatal dopaminergic activity (Bohnen et al., 2009). Reduction in gait speed correlates with a reduction in cortical cholinergic activity (Bohnen et al., 2013). Amyloid deposits have also been associated with postural instability and gait dysfunction (Muller et al., 2013).

PET has been used to investigate depression in PD, with surprising results. Using the selective serotonin transporter (SERT) ligand [$^{11}$C]DASB, Guttman and colleagues demonstrated widespread reductions in SERT in PD patients compared with healthy controls, compatible with loss of serotonergic fibers (Guttman et al., 2007). In PD patients with depression, however, SERT binding was increased, particularly in dorsolateral and prefrontal cortex (Boileau et al., 2008); SERT binding correlated with clinical ratings of depression. Although not anticipated, this finding is reminiscent of major depression, where SERT binding is increased in those subjects with negativistic dysfunctional attitudes (Meyer et al., 2004). Additional studies are warranted.

## Brain Tumors

Gliomas are the most frequent intraparenchymal tumors of the brain. Their histological classification and grading have recently been revised, now also including prognostically relevant molecular markers (International Agency for Research on Cancer et al., 2016). Most imaging studies have been conducted prior to this revision, but the main results still remain valid.

As in other malignancies, increased glucose metabolism is associated with proliferative activity and aggressiveness in brain tumors. In fact, the imaging of brain tumors was the first oncological application of [$^{18}$F]FDG PET (Di Chiro et al., 1982). However, opposed to other body regions, the use of [$^{18}$F]FDG PET in brain tumor imaging is compromised by lack of contrast due to the high physiological uptake of [$^{18}$F]FDG in normal gray matter. Thus accurate tumor delineation is not feasible with [$^{18}$F]FDG PET alone and PET/MRI coregistration is mandatory for [$^{18}$F]FDG PET interpretation. Due to this limitation of [$^{18}$F]FDG PET, other radiotracers with little physiological brain uptake—in particular, amino acid tracers [$^{18}$F]FET, [$^{18}$F]FDOPA and [$^{11}$C]MET—are increasingly used (Herholz et al., 2012). However, virtually all other imaging methods depend on changes of transport at the blood–brain barrier (BBB), and [$^{18}$F]FDG is the only tracer mainly reflecting tumor metabolism. Since cerebral uptake of amino acid tracers is mediated by the carrier (i.e., largely independent of a BBB leak), these tracers allow for a high tumor-to-brain contrast and accurate

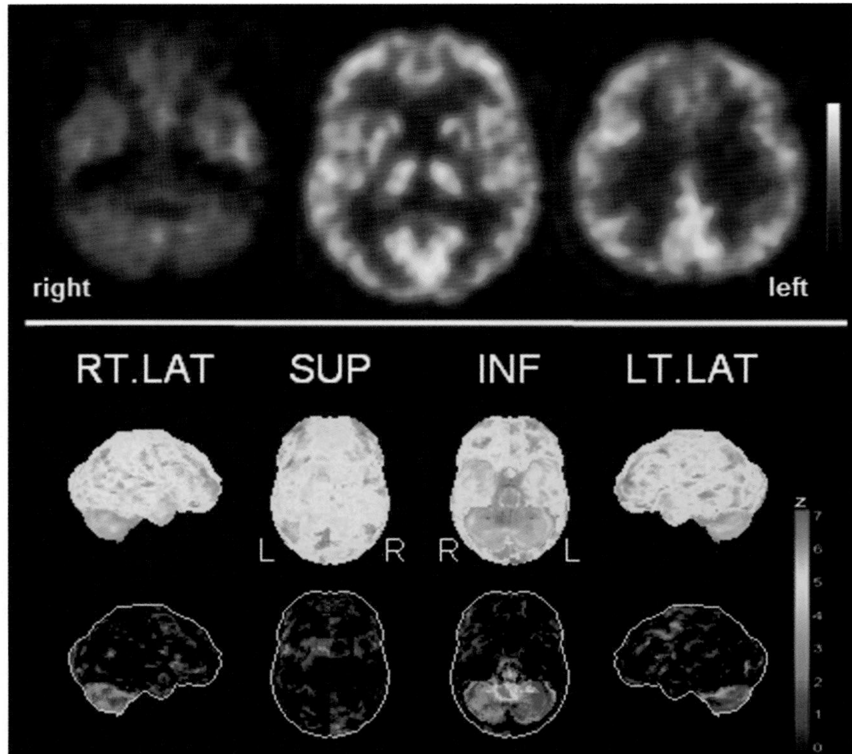


Fig. 42.11 [18F]FDG positron emission tomography (PET) in multiple system atrophy (MSA). In contrast to Alzheimer disease (AD), striatal hypometabolism is commonly found in MSA (see left striatum), particularly in those patients with striatonigral degeneration (SND, or MSA-P). In patients with olivopontocerebellar degeneration (OPCA or MSA-C), pontine and cerebellar hypometabolism is particularly evident. *Upper panel:* Transaxial PET images of [18F]FDG uptake. *Lower panel:* Results of voxel-based statistical analysis using Neurostat/3D-SSP. Given are right and left lateral (*RT.LAT and LT.LAT*), superior (*SUP*), and inferior (*INF*) views (see Fig. 42.1 for additional details).

tumor delineation even in the majority of low-grade gliomas (LGGs) without contrast enhancement on CT or MRI.

High-grade gliomas (HGGs; WHO grades III–IV) show a significantly higher [18F]FDG uptake than LGGs; (WHO grades I–II) and normal white matter (Figs. 42.14 and 42.15; Delbeke et al., 1995; Meyer et al., 2001; Padma et al., 2003). Oligodendrogliomas show higher uptake of astrocytomas of the same grade (Derlon et al., 2000). Common causes of false-positive [18F]FDG PET scans include brain abscesses, inflammatory changes, pituitary adenomas, and childhood brain tumors (e.g., juvenile pilocytic astrocytomas, choroid plexus papillomas, and gangliogliomas). Nevertheless, [18F]FDG PET may also be a helpful method for tumor grading in childhood CNS tumors (Borgwardt et al., 2005). [18F]FDG uptake is also a predictor of overall survival in patients with gliomas (Alavi et al., 1988; De Witte et al., 2000; Kim et al., 1991; Padma et al., 2003; Patronas et al., 1985). Primary CNS lymphoma (PCNSL) usually show very high [18F]FDG uptake, even exceeding normal gray matter, making [18F]FDG PET a powerful method for the detection of cerebral lymphoma (Fig. 42.16). Moreover, [18F]FDG uptake was found to be an independent predictor of progression-free survival in PCNSL (Kasenda et al., 2013).

Some limitations of FDG in gliomas can be overcome by PET studies using large neutral amino acid tracers like [18F]FET and [11C]MET, which are transported by the symmetric A-type carrier and avidly taken up by most LGG (~80%) and virtually all HGG (>90%) tumors, while physiological brain uptake is low (see Figs. 42.14 and 42.15). [18F]FDOPA can also be used as an amino acid for glioma imaging, but high physiological uptake in the basal ganglia due to conversion and storage as [18F]fluoro-dopamine must be considered when scans are being interpreted (Bell et al., 2015). Amino acids such as [18F]fluciclovine, transported by the asymmetric ASC transporter, provide even better contrast because of their very low uptake in normal brain (Tsuyuguchi et al., 2017); however, total uptake in tumors is also lower than with FET and MET.

Amino acid PET is very highly sensitive in detecting and delineating gliomas (Galldiks and Langen, 2015). A recent meta-analysis described the high accuracy of [18F]FET PET in differentiating between neoplastic and nonneoplastic brain lesions (sensitivity 82%, specificity 76%; Dunet et al., 2012). In rare instances false-positive findings can be caused by acute inflammatory processes, focal status epilepticus, gliosis, surrounding hematomas, and reperfused ischemia (Hutterer et al., 2013). It has been shown that amino acid PET significantly improves biopsy planning and tumor delineation for surgical resection compared with MRI or [18F]FDG PET, with amino acid PET typically showing larger tumor volumes (Pauleit et al., 2009; Pirotte et al., 2004, 2006; see Fig. 42.15). Furthermore, complete resection of tissue with increased PET tracer uptake ([11C]MET or [18F]FDG) was associated with better survival in HGG, whereas resection of areas with contrast enhancement on MRI was not (Pirotte et al., 2009).

Concerning grading, most studies showed a higher amino acid uptake of HGG compared with LGG. However, considerable overlap between groups prohibits a reliable distinction. This situation is further complicated by the observation that oligodendrogliomas show higher amino acid uptake than corresponding astrocytomas (Glaudemans et al., 2013; Herholz et al., 2012). Consequently the prognostic value of

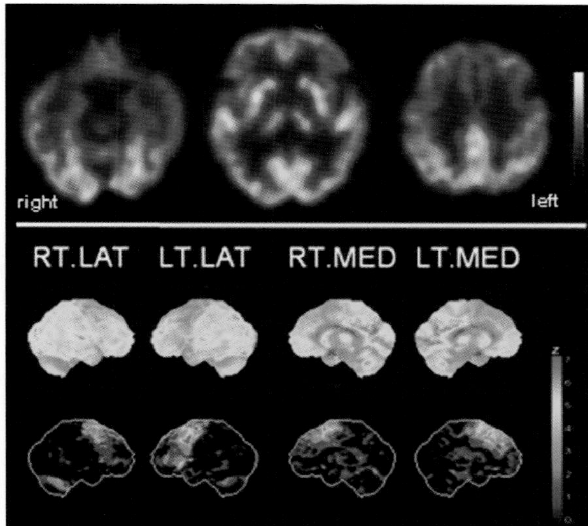


**Fig. 42.12** [$^{18}$F]FDG positron emission tomography (PET) in progressive supranuclear palsy (PSP). Typical finding in PSP include bilateral hypometabolism of mesial and dorsolateral frontal areas (especially supplementary motor and premotor areas). Thalamic and midbrain hypometabolism is usually also present. In line with overlapping pathologies in frontotemporal dementia (FTD) and PSP, patients with clinical FTD can show a PSP-like pattern and vice versa (see Fig. 42.3). *Upper panel,* Transaxial PET images of [$^{18}$F]FDG uptake. *Lower panel,* Results of voxel-based statistical analysis using Neurostat/3D-SSP. Given are right and left lateral (*RT.LAT and LT.LAT*) and mesial (*RT.MED and LT.MED*) views (see Fig. 42.1 for additional details). *(From Neurostat/3D-SSP analysis based on Minoshima, S., Frey, K.A., Koeppe, R.A., Foster, N.L., Kuhl, D.E., 1995. A diagnostic approach in Alzheimer's disease using three-dimensional stereotactic surface projections of fluorine-18-FDG PET. J Nucl Med. 36 [7], 1238–1248.)*

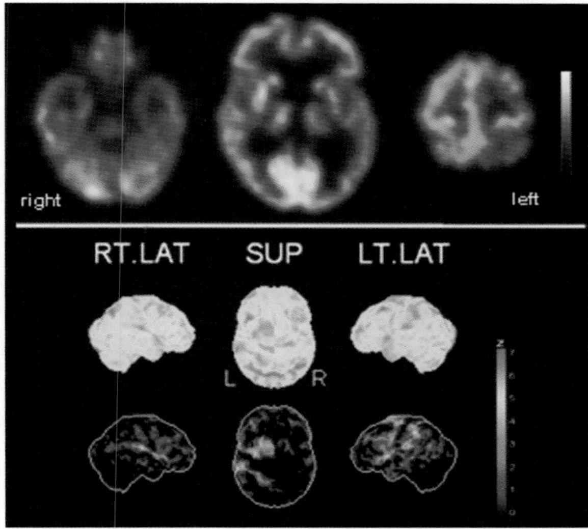


**Fig. 42.13** [$^{18}$F]FDG positron emission tomography (PET) in corticobasal degeneration (CBD). In line with the clinical presentation, CBD is characterized by a highly asymmetrical hypometabolism of frontoparietal areas (including the sensorimotor cortex; often most pronounced parietal), striatum, and thalamus. *Upper panel,* Transaxial PET images of [$^{18}$F]FDG uptake. *Lower panel.* Results of voxel-based statistical analysis using Neurostat/3D-SSP. Given are right and left lateral (*RT.LAT and LT.LAT*) and superior (*SUP*) views (see Fig. 42.1 for additional details). *(From Neurostat/3D-SSP analysis based on Minoshima, S., Frey, K.A., Koeppe, R.A., Foster, N.L., Kuhl, D.E., 1995. A diagnostic approach in Alzheimer's disease using three-dimensional stereotactic surface projections of fluorine-18-FDG PET. J Nucl Med. 36 [7], 1238–1248.)*

amino acid uptake is inferior to [$^{18}$F]FDG PET in mixed populations (Pauleit et al., 2009). However, the initial uptake and kinetic course of [$^{18}$F]FET uptake was found to be highly predictive of tumor grade (Calcagni et al., 2011; Popperl et al., 2006): HGGs usually show an early peak with a subsequent decrease of [$^{18}$F]FET uptake, whereas LGGs commonly show a delayed and steadily increasing [$^{18}$F]FET uptake. These kinetic patterns were also found to predict malignant transformation and prognosis in patients with LGG (Galldiks et al., 2013; Jansen et al., 2014). Within groups of LGG, lower amino acid uptake is also associated with a better prognosis (Floeth et al., 2007; Smits et al., 2008). There is often considerable heterogeneity within gliomas with regard to local tumor proliferation and malignancy. PET can localize the most malignant tumor parts, which should be selected for histological assessment by biopsy in order to provide accurate tumor grading (Goldman and Pirotte, 2011).

Planning radiation therapy is another important application. Clinical trials will investigate whether amino acid PET for the definition of gross tumor volume and for radiation treatment can improve outcome (Oehlke et al., 2016). This is particularly relevant after surgery, when the specificity of MRI is compromised by postoperative changes (Grosu et al., 2005; Hirata et al., 2018). Hypoxic tumor tissue is resistant to radiation therapy. Research studies have demonstrated that PET with tracers based on agents that bind to hypoxic tissue, such as [$^{18}$F]FMISO, can identify hypoxic tissue in gliomas and thus potentially guide radiotherapy (Bekaert et al., 2017).

Differentiation between benign treatment-associated changes (radiation necrosis and pseudoprogression in particular) and residual

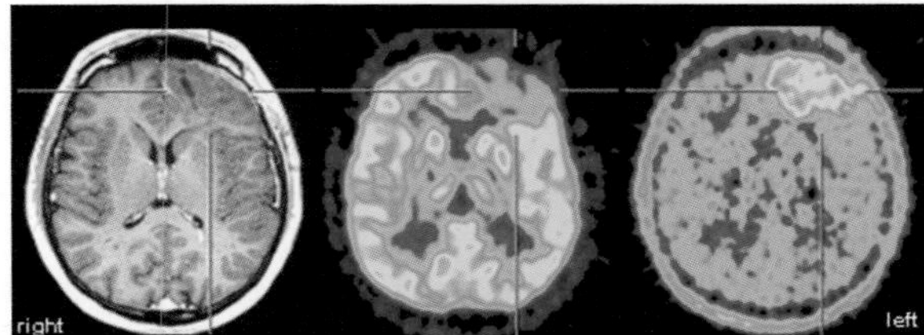


**Fig. 42.14** [$^{18}$F]FDG and [$^{18}$F]FET positron emission tomography (PET) in a left frontal low-grade oligodendroglioma (World Health Organization grade II). [$^{18}$F]FDG uptake *(middle)* of low-grade gliomas is usually comparable to white-matter uptake, prohibiting a clear delineation of tumor borders. In contrast, the majority of low-grade gliomas (particularly oligodendrogliomas) show intense and well-defined uptake of radioactive amino acids such as [$^{18}$F]FET *(right)* even without contrast enhancement on MRI *(left)*. *(Courtesy Karl-Josef Langen, MD, Institute of Neuroscience and Medicine, Research Center Juelich, Germany.)*

or recurrent tumor is of paramount importance. Since the specificity of CT and MRI is compromised by contrast enhancement due to nonneoplastic posttherapeutic changes, PET imaging is frequently used. However, the merit of [$^{18}$F]FDG PET is controversial, since earlier studies provided highly variable results with sensitivity and specificity ranging from 40% to 100% (Herholz et al., 2012; Langleben et al., 2000). False-negative results are relatively frequent and may occur due to very recent radiation therapy, pretreatment low [$^{18}$F]FDG uptake (e.g., in LGG or metastases with low [$^{18}$F]FDG avidity), masking by physiological uptake, and small tumor volumes. Conversely, intense inflammatory reaction after radiation therapy (especially stereotactic) and

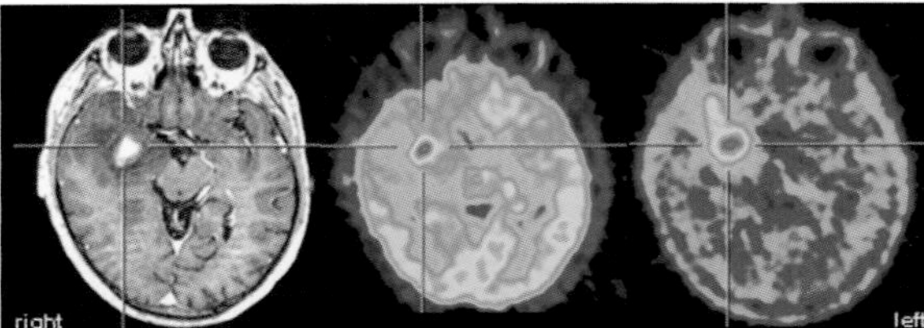


**Fig. 42.15** [$^{18}$F]FDG and [$^{18}$F]FET positron emission tomography (PET) in a right mesial temporal high-grade astrocytoma (World Health Organization grade III). In contrast to low-grade gliomas, high-grade tumors usually have [$^{18}$F]FDG uptake *(middle)* that is distinctly higher than white matter and sometimes even above gray matter, as in this case. Nevertheless, the [$^{18}$F]FET scan *(right)* clearly depicts a rostral tumor extension that is missed by [$^{18}$F]FDG PET, owing to high physiological [$^{18}$F]FDG uptake by adjacent gray matter. Tumor delineation is also clearer on [$^{18}$F]FET PET than on magnetic resonance imaging *(left)*. *(Courtesy Karl-Josef Langen, MD, Institute of Neuroscience and Medicine, Research Center Juelich, Germany.)*

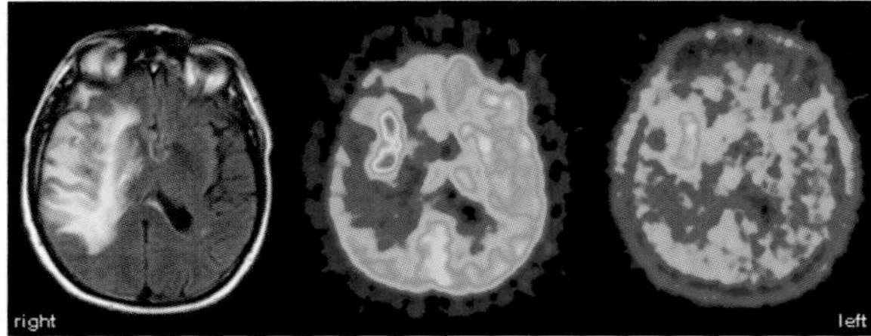


**Fig. 42.16** [$^{18}$F]FDG and [$^{18}$F]FET positron emission tomography (PET) in a primary central nervous system lymphoma (PCNSL). PCNSL usually show a very intense [$^{18}$F]FDG uptake *(middle)*, whereas the metabolism of surrounding brain tissue is suppressed by extensive tumor edema (see magnetic resonance image, *left*). [$^{18}$F]FET uptake *(right)* of cerebral lymphoma can also be high. *(Courtesy Karl-Josef Langen, MD, Institute of Neuroscience and Medicine, Research Center Juelich, Germany.)*

seizure activity may result in false-positive findings. If tumor uptake exceeds the expected background uptake in adjacent brain tissue, it is crucial to carefully evaluate the accuracy of PET/MRI coregistration (Fig. 42.17). Under these conditions, the sensitivity and specificity of [$^{18}$F]FDG PET in differentiating between tumor recurrence (gliomas and metastases) and radiation necrosis is about 75% to 80% and 85% to 90%, respectively (Chao et al., 2001; Gomez-Rio et al., 2008; Wang et al., 2006; ). As in the case of primary tumors, the shortcomings of [$^{18}$F]FDG PET may be overcome by amino acid PET (see Fig. 42.17). The reported sensitivity and specificity of amino acid PET range from 75% to 100% and 60% to 100%, respectively (Glaudemans et al., 2013; Galldiks et al., 2012; Nihashi et al., 2013). Finally, PET has also been used successfully to assess response following drug treatment (Roelcke, Wyss et al., 2015), but appropriate PET criteria and the clinical role of PET still requires further definition.

The assessment of proliferation is of particular interest in the case of brain tumors. Thymidine-based tracers [$^{11}$C]thymidine and [$^{18}$F]fluorothymidine ([$^{18}$F]FLT) are incorporated into DNA in proliferating tumors and have been used to assess proliferation. However, uptake of these tracers in lesions with an intact BBB is very low, and high uptake is observed only in tumors with BBB damage. Thus dynamic scanning is required to measure tracer incorporation into DNA. This has been used successfully to distinguish between recurrent tumors and radiation necrosis (Spence et al., 2009), but the results were not superior to those from [$^{18}$F]FDG PET (Enslow et al., 2012).

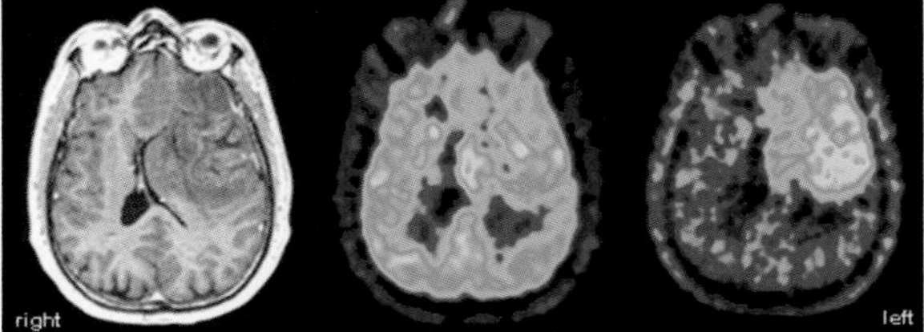


**Fig. 42.17** [$^{18}$F]FDG and [$^{18}$F]FET positron emission tomography (PET) in a recurrent high-grade astrocytoma (World Health Organization grade III). [$^{18}$F]FDG uptake *(middle)* is clearly increased above expected background in several areas of suspected tumor recurrence on magnetic resonance image *(left)*, confirming viable tumor tissue. Compared with [$^{18}$F]FDG PET, [$^{18}$F]FET PET *(right)*, more clearly and extensively depicts the area of active tumor. *(Courtesy Karl-Josef Langen, MD, Institute of Neuroscience and Medicine, Research Center Juelich, Germany.)*

[$^{11}$C]Methionine has also been used for the imaging pituitary tumors and monitoring their treatment, with dopamine receptor ligands as a possible alternative (Bergstrom et al., 1991). More recently there has been considerable interest in imaging of somatostatin receptors (SSTRs) in brain tumors, including meningiomas and gliomas, using $^{68}$Ga-DOTA-conjugated peptides such as [$^{68}$Ga]DOTA-TATE or [$^{68}$Ga]DOTA-TOC (Rachinger et al., 2015). Interestingly, in meningioma, the expression of SSTRs seems to increase with increasing tumor grade (Barresi et al., 2008; Wang et al., 2013). Thus SSTR PET may serve as a selection criterion for radionuclide treatment with beta-emitting SSTR ligands (e.g., [$^{177}$Lu]DOTA-TATE or [$^{90}$Y]DOTA-TOC), but the overall benefit of this theranostic approach still requires further validation (Seystahl et al., 2016). Experimental studies include endothelial receptor imaging and theranostic approaches using longer-lived isotopes such as $^{66}$Cu and $^{89}$Zr (Jansen et al., 2017).

Magnetic resonance spectroscopy (MRS) has been suggested in addition to MRI to help in the characterization of brain tumors by detecting metabolic alterations that may be indicative of the tumor class (Callot et al., 2008). MRS emerged as a clinical research tool in the 1990s; it has not yet entered broad clinical practice, although it is frequently used at some instituations. Of the principal metabolites that can be analyzed, *N*-acetylaspartate (NAA) is present in almost all neurons. Its decrease corresponds to neuronal death or injury or the replacement of healthy neurons by other cells (e.g., tumor). Choline-containing compounds increase whenever there is cellular proliferation. Creatine is a marker of overall cellular density. Myoinositol is a sugar that is present only in glia. Lactate concentrations reflect hypoxic conditions as well as hypermetabolic glucose consumption. The most frequently studied chemical ratios to distinguish tumors from other brain lesions with MRS are choline/creatine, choline/NAA and lactate/creatine. Specifically, a choline/NAA ratio greater than 1 is indicative of neoplasm. The differentiation between astrocytomas of WHO grades II and III is especially difficult. MRS in conjunction with structural MRI has been used to differentiate cystic tumor from brain abscess (Chang et al., 1998), LGG versus gliomatosis cerebri, and edema versus infiltration (Nelson et al., 2002). Positive responses to radiotherapy or chemotherapy may be associated with a decrease in choline (Lichy et al., 2005; Murphy et al., 2004).

## Epilepsy

In drug-refractory focal epilepsy, surgical resection of the epileptogenic focus offers an excellent chance of a seizure-free outcome or at least reduced seizure frequency, making epilepsy surgery the treatment of choice in these patients. Accurate localization of the seizure focus as a prerequisite for successful surgery is commonly accomplished by a comprehensive presurgical evaluation including neurological history and examination, neuropsychological testing, interictal and ictal electroencephalography (EEG), depth recordings, high-resolution MRI, and video-EEG monitoring. To circumvent the necessity for invasive EEG recordings or to target their location for invasive EEG recordings, [$^{18}$F]FDG PET and CBF SPECT are often used to gain information about the location of the focus of seizure onset. In contrast to the aforementioned PET and SPECT indications, in which PET is superior to SPECT, both modalities are equally essential and often complementary in the presurgical assessment of patients with drug-refractory focal epilepsy (Goffin et al., 2008). In general, PET and SPECT are of particular diagnostic value if the surface EEG and MRI yield inconclusive or normal results (Casse et al., 2002; Knowlton et al., 2008; Willmann et al., 2007). Several neurotransmitter receptor ligands (most notably [$^{11}$C]/[$^{18}$F]flumazenil) have been proposed for imaging in epilepsy. However, their availability is still very restricted and their superiority compared with [$^{18}$F]FDG PET and ictal SPECT has not been validated (Goffin et al., 2008).

Because of their rapid, virtually irreversible tissue uptake, CBF SPECT tracers such as [$^{99m}$Tc]ECD and [$^{99m}$Tc]HMPAO (stabilized form) can be used in combination with video-EEG monitoring to image the actual zone of seizure onset. To do so, the patient is monitored by video EEG and the tracer is administrated as fast as possible after seizure onset or EEG discharges to capture the associated CBF increase. For rapid tracer administration and radiation safety reasons, the radiotracers should be stored in a shielded syringe pump and injected via remote control from the surveillance room. Actual SPECT acquisition can then be done at a later time (preferably within 4 hours after injection), when the patient has recovered and is cooperative.

Although ictal SPECT alone may show a well-defined region of hyperperfusion corresponding to the seizure onset zone, it is recommended to acquire an additional interictal SPECT scan (also under EEG monitoring) to exclude seizure activity. By comparing both scans, even areas with low ictal CBF increases or CBF increases from an interictally hypoperfused state to an apparent "normal" perfused ictal state can be reliably defined. In addition to visual inspection, computation of parametric images of CBF changes (e.g., ictal—interictal difference images), which are overlaid onto a corresponding MRI, are optimal for focus localization. Such analyses (most notably subtraction ictal SPECT coregistered to MRI [SISCOM]) significantly improve the accuracy and interrater agreement on localization of the seizure focus with ictal SPECT, particularly in frontoparietal neocortical epilepsy (Lee et al., 2006; O'Brien, et al., 1998; Spanaki et al., 1999 Fig. 42.18). The area with the most intense and extensive ictal CBF increase is commonly assumed to represent the seizure onset zone. However, depending on the time gap between seizure onset and cerebral tracer fixation, ictal SPECT depicts not only the onset zone but also the propagation zone. Therefore accurate knowledge regarding the timing of tracer injection is crucial for the interpretation of ictal SPECT. In patients with temporal lobe epilepsy (TLE), CBF increases may propagate to various cortical areas during seizure progression—including the contralateral temporal lobe, insula, basal ganglia, and frontal lobe—reflecting seizure semiology (Shin et al., 2002). In patients with focal dysplastic lesions, distinct ictal perfusion patterns have been observed with seizure propagation, during which the area of most intense CBF increase may migrate away from the seizure onset zone (Dupont et al., 2006). This underlines the need for rapid tracer injection after seizure onset to localize the actual onset zone. A delay not exceeding 20–45 seconds enables optimal localization results (Lee et al., 2006; O'Brien et al., 1998). At later time points, a so-called postictal switch occurs, leading to hypoperfusion of the onset zone. Within 100 seconds from seizure onset, about two-thirds of ictal SPECT studies can be expected to show hyperperfusion; after that (>100 seconds postictally), hypoperfusion will be observed (Avery et al., 1999).

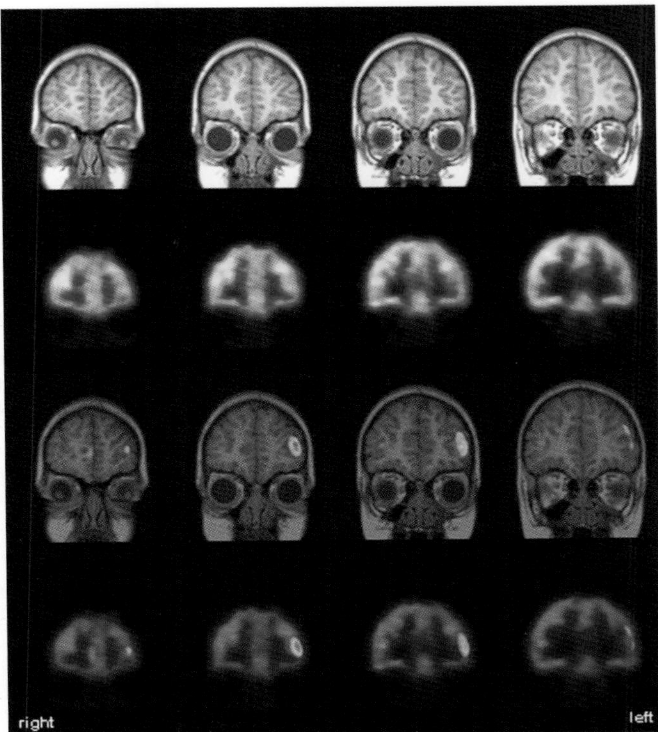


**Fig. 42.18** [$^{18}$F]FDG positron emission tomography (PET) and ictal [$^{99m}$Tc]ECD SPECT in left frontal lobe epilepsy. This patient's magnetic resonance imaging (MRI) scan *(top row)* was normal, whereas [$^{18}$F] FDG PET showed extensive left frontal hypometabolism *(second row)*. Additional ictal and interictal [$^{99m}$Tc]ECD SPECT scans were performed for accurate localization of seizure onset. Result of a SPECT subtraction analysis (ictal-interictal; blood flow increases above a threshold of 15%, maximum 40%) was overlaid onto MRI and the [$^{18}$F]FDG PET scan (*third and fourth rows*, respectively), clearly depicting the zone of seizure onset within the functional deficit zone given by [$^{18}$F]FDG PET.

The diagnostic sensitivity of ictal SPECT to correctly localize the seizure focus (usually with reference to surgical outcome) is about 85% to 95% in TLE and 70% to 90% in extratemporal lobe epilepsy (ETLE; Devous et al., 1998; Newton et al., 1995; Weil et al., 2001; Zaknun et al., 2008). Focus localization can also be successful by postictal tracer injection, capturing postictal hypoperfusion. However, localization accuracy will be lower (about 70%–75% in TLE and 50% in ETLE; Devous et al., 1998; Newton et al., 1995). In contrast, interictal SPECT to detect interictal hypoperfusion is insufficient for focus localization (sensitivity about 50% in TLE; of no diagnostic value in ETLE; Newton et al., 1995; Spanaki et al., 1999; Zaknun et al., 2008).

In contrast to ictal SPECT, [$^{18}$F]FDG PET studies are performed in the interictal state to image the functional deficit zone, which shows abnormal metabolism between seizures and is generally assumed also to contain the seizure onset zone. The etiology of this hypometabolism is not fully understood and probably relates to functional (e.g., surround inhibition of areas of seizure onset and propagation as a defense mechanism) and structural changes (e.g., neuronal or synaptic loss due to repeated seizures). Hypometabolism appears to increase with the duration, frequency, and severity of seizures and usually extends considerably beyond the actual seizure onset zone, occasionally involving contralateral mirror regions (Kumar and Chugani, 2013). A direct comparison of ictal perfusion abnormalities detected by SISCOM and interictal [$^{18}$F]FDG PET hypometabolism in TLE patients demonstrated high concordance, suggesting that seizures are generated and spread in metabolically abnormal regions (Bouilleret et al., 2002). To ensure an interictal state, the patient should ideally be seizure free for at least 24 hours before PET and be monitored by EEG after [$^{18}$F]FDG injection to rule out possible subclinical epileptic activity. Side-to-side asymmetry may be calculated by ROI analysis to support visual interpretation, whereby an asymmetry ≥10% is commonly used as a threshold for regional pathology. Furthermore, voxel-wise statistical analyses are strongly recommended: Visual analysis by an experienced observer is at least as accurate in TLE patients (Fig. 42.19), but accuracy and interobserver agreement of focus localization is considerably improved by additional voxel-wise statistical analyses in ETLE (Drzezga et al., 1999; Fig. 42.20). Finally, PET/MRI coregistration is very helpful for detecting PET abnormalities in regions with apparently normal anatomy (e.g., caused by subtle focal cortical dysplasia, FCD) and to disclose the extent of PET findings in relation to structural abnormalities (e.g., in epileptogenic tumors or tuberous sclerosis; Lee and Salamon, 2009). However, if structural abnormalities and the accompanying hypometabolism are extensive (e.g., infarction, contusion, surgery), ictal SPECT may be preferred to image the area of seizure onset. [$^{18}$F]FDG PET may nevertheless be helpful to evaluate the functional integrity of the remaining brain regions.

In meta-analyses, the sensitivity of [$^{18}$F]FDG PET for focus lateralization (rather than localization given the extent of hypometabolism) in TLE was reported to be around 86%, whereas false lateralization to the contralateral side of the epileptogenic focus rarely occurs (<5%; Casse et al., 2002; Willmann et al., 2007). Consequently presurgical unilateral temporal hypometabolism predicts a good surgical outcome (Engel class I–II) in 82% to 86% of total TLE cases and even 80% and 72% in TLE patients with normal MRI and nonlocalized ictal scalp EEG, respectively (Casse et al., 2002; Willmann et al., 2007). In contrast, asymmetrical thalamic metabolism (particularly in reverse direction to temporal lobe asymmetry) and extratemporal cortical hypometabolism (in particular of the contralateral hemisphere) are associated with poor postoperative seizure control (Choi et al., 2003; Newberg et al., 2000; ). In ETLE, the sensitivity of [$^{18}$F]FDG PET is lower, providing a seizure focus localization in about 67% of ETLE patients (Casse et al., 2002; Drzezga et al., 1999; ). Again, correct localization by [$^{18}$F]FDG PET was demonstrated to be a significant predictor of a good surgical outcome in patients with neocortical epilepsy (Yun et al., 2006).

Few large-scale studies have directly compared ictal SPECT with interictal [$^{18}$F]FDG PET. Comparing rates of correct lateralization provided by [$^{18}$F]FDG PET and [$^{99m}$Tc]HMPAO SPECT in patients with good surgical outcomes revealed that the overall performance of [$^{18}$F]FDG PET was slightly better (86% vs. 78%), mainly because of higher accuracy in TLE cases (90% vs. 83%; 64% vs. 62% in ETLE; Won et al., 1999). In FCD patients, [$^{18}$F]FDG PET showed a corresponding focal hypometabolism in 71%, whereas SPECT revealed an ictal hyperperfusion in 60% of cases. However, unlike the extent of lesion resection and pathological features, neither PET nor SPECT predicted good surgical outcome in FCD (Kim et al., 2009). In patients with ETLE (the majority of cases) and inconclusive scalp EEG and MRI, the sensitivity/specificity (with respect to surgical outcome) of PET and SPECT were 59%/79% and 50%/72%, respectively (Knowlton et al., 2008). Finally, in pediatric patients, [$^{18}$F]FDG PET was found to be particularly valuable in TLE (correct lateralization/localization: 96%/73%), whereas ictal CBF SPECT with SISCOM was more accurate in ETLE (92%/85%; Kim et al., 2009).

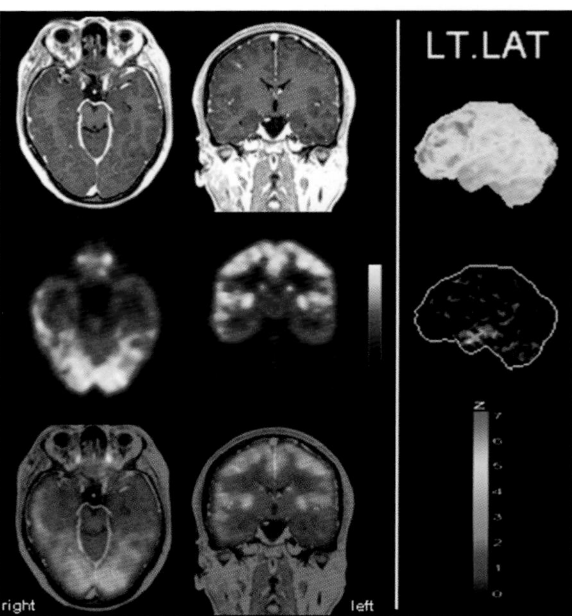


**Fig. 42.19** [$^{18}$F]FDG positron emission tomography (PET) in left temporal lobe epilepsy. Diagnostic benefit of [$^{18}$F]FDG PET is greatest in patients with normal magnetic resonance imaging (MRI) *(left panel, top row)* in which [$^{18}$F]FDG PET still detects well-lateralized, temporal lobe, hypometabolism (*second row*, left temporal lobe hypometabolism). As in this patient with left mesial temporal lobe epilepsy, the area of hypometabolism often extends to the lateral cortex (functional deficit zone; *third row*, PET/MRI fusion). *Right panel*, Results of voxel-based statistical analysis of [$^{18}$F]FDG PET scan using Neurostat/3D-SSP. Given are left lateral (*LT.LAT*) views (*top image*, [$^{18}$F]FDG uptake; *bottom image*, statistical deviation of uptake from healthy controls, color coded as z-score; see Fig. 42.1 for additional details). *(From Neurostat/3D-SSP analysis based on Minoshima, S., Frey, K.A., Koeppe, R.A., Foster, N.L., Kuhl, D.E., 1995. A diagnostic approach in Alzheimer's disease using three-dimensional stereotactic surface projections of fluorine-18-FDG PET. J Nucl Med. 36 [7], 1238–1248.)*

## Presurgical Brain Mapping

Since its first description in 1992 (Ogawa, 2012), fMRI based on BOLD contrast has gained an important role in presurgical brain mapping. Task-based BOLD fMRI enables the evaluation of the spatial relationship between an intracranial lesion and different cortical functional areas (e.g., primary motor cortex or lateralization of essential language areas; Stippich, 2015).

Contrary to research fMRI studies, presurgical clinical fMRI is usually based on a simple block design and the control condition is usually rest or visual fixation. A major limitation of clinical fMRI is that despite recent initiatives (e.g., by the American Society of Functional Neuroradiology [ASFNR]; Neuroradiology, 2019), official recommendations or guidelines for the performance, evaluation, and interpretation of presurgical fMRI examinations are lacking (Szaflarski et al., 2017) and only a few studies are evaluating larger patients samples under standardized fMRI conditions (Krings et al., 2001; Tyndall et al., 2017).

Large randomized controlled trials demonstrating a beneficial effect of presurgical fMRI on patient outcome are lacking (Buchbinder, 2016) because they are very difficult to accomplish. However, there are multiple small-sample-size studies of patients with brain tumors in the literature demonstrating that preoperative fMRI alters surgical management significantly (Pillai, 2010).

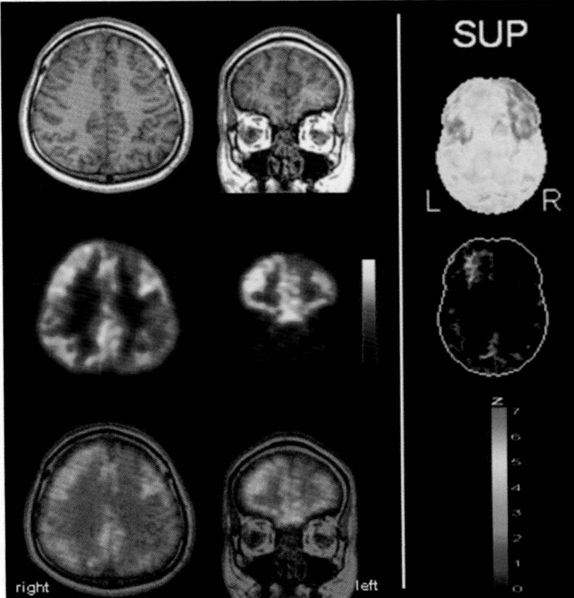


**Fig. 42.20** [$^{18}$F]FDG positron emission tomography (PET) in left frontal lobe epilepsy. Despite a normal magnetic resonance imaging (MRI) scan *(left panel, top row)*, [$^{18}$F]FDG PET *(second row)* depicts a circumscribed area of left frontal hypometabolism (i.e., functional deficit zone; *third row*, PET/MRI fusion). Additional voxel-based statistical analysis of [$^{18}$F]FDG PET scan is strongly recommended in extratemporal lobe epilepsy to improve sensitivity and reliability *(right panel*, results of a Neurostat/3D-SSP analysis. Given are views from superior of *(SUP)* [$^{18}$F]FDG uptake *(top)* and of statistical deviation of uptake from healthy controls, color coded as z-score *(bottom)*; see Fig. 42.1 for additional details.

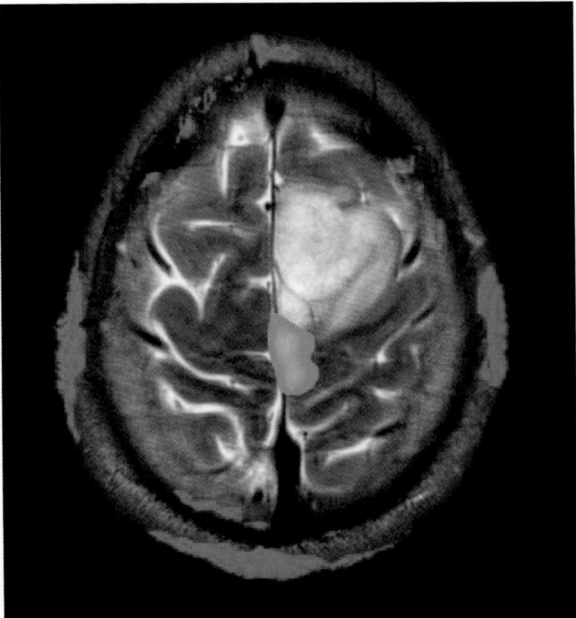

**Fig. 42.21** Localization of the motor cortex activation of the right foot *(green)* in a patient with a left frontal intra-axial tumor (anaplastic astrocytoma, World Health Organization grade II). Generated by block design (Black et al., 2017) using the vendor's software with threshold 10 for activated clusters and z-value 6. Functional magnetic resonance imaging (fMRI) data *(green)* and gradient field mapping *(purple)* acquired prior to fMRI fused with the axial T2-weighted dataset.

## Sensorimotor Mapping

Mapping of the motor and somatosensory cortices with fMRI is an established technique to identify the cortical representation of the foot (Fig. 42.21), hand, and tongue. Typical paradigms are repetitive flexion of the foot, thumb-to-finger opposition, and movement of the tongue with the mouth closed (Krings et al., 2001). Success rate for motor paradigms in larger cohort studies are between 85% and 95% (Krings et al., 2001; Tyndall et al., 2017) and up to 100% in studies with smaller patient samples (Petrella et al., 2006). Inadequate compliance (e.g., head motion artifacts) beside tumor-associated neurological deficits is the main reason for paradigm failures (Tyndall et al., 2017). This emphasizes the necessity of adequate patient preparation before performing fMRI examinations.

Multiple studies have demonstrated that fMRI results correlate well with direct electrocortical stimulation (ECS; Buchbinder, 2016; Wray et al., 2012). Direct comparison of accuracy of both techniques, however, is difficult. This can be related to multiple factors: for example, methodological effects. Activation may vary with statistical and electrical thresholds in fMRI and ECS, respectively. It also has to be kept in mind that there is a displacement of the fMRI activation focus from the parenchymal activation due to the BOLD signal in the veins draining the activated area. Other important factors that affect the BOLD signal, especially in tumor patients, may be an alteration in neurovascular coupling due to tumor-related compression or alteration of the perfusion situation of the activated area and medication effects (Silva et al., 2018). In patients with frontal lobe epilepsy, fMRI activation of motor areas is reduced after seizures on the side of the focus (Woodward et al., 2014).

Compared with language mapping, motor paradigms demonstrate a higher rate of significant activation of the particular cortical area. This effect is independent of 1,5 T or 3 T magnetic field strength of the MR system used (Buchbinder, 2016). To increase diagnostic accuracy, fMRI results can be combined with diffusion tensor imaging (DTI) tractography for mapping the corticospinal tract in relation to the fMRI activation. Preoperative fMRI may predict a postsurgical neurological deficit or deterioration based on the spatial relationship of fMRI activation and the brain lesion. Krishnan, et al., 2004 demonstrated that a resection closer than 5 mm to the fMRI locus increases the risk of neurological deficit. Other small-sample-size studies have shown that a distance greater than 10 mm between the fMRI locus and the lesion significantly reduces the risk of a postoperative neurological deficit (Haberg et al., 2004). However, a precise safe lesion-to-activation margin is not defined in the literature and may also be dependent on the histology of the lesion (Hadjiabadi et al., 2018).

Especially in patients who are unable to cooperate with task-based paradigms, resting-state fMRI (rs-fMRI) for sensorimotor mapping is promising (Dierker et al., 2017; Hadjiabadi et al., 2018) but does not yet a provide a valid method to guide clinical decisions.

## Language Mapping

Although the intracarotid amobarbital procedure (IAP), also known as the Wada test, is an invasive technique and language or memory testing is not standardized in IAP, it is still considered the preoperative gold standard (Szaflarski et al., 2017), especially in patients with epilepsy.

A fMRI-based language mapping can be used to detect lateralization and location of language areas and is an increasingly accepted alternative method (Fig. 42.22). As in sensorimotor mapping, standardized paradigms and recommendations for presurgical language mapping have not yet been defined (Buchbinder, 2016). However, a

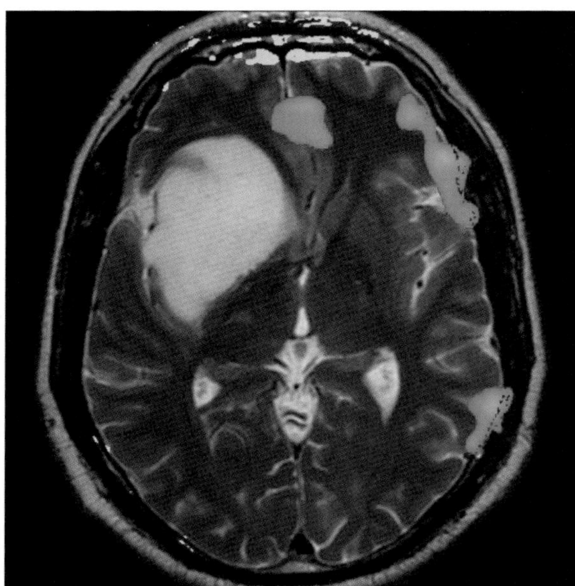

**Fig. 42.22** Clinical functional magnetic resonance imaging (fMRI) for the evaluation of language lateralization in a right-handed patient with a right insular tumor (diffuse astrocytoma, World Health Organization grade II): activation of Broca and Wernicke areas lateralized to the left hemisphere.

recent initiative of the ASFNR has proposed a collection of language paradigms (Black et al., 2017) and an algorithm of how to perform fMRI. Because language processing is more complex than the execution of simple motor tasks, the use of two or more paradigms is recommended (Black et al., 2017; Rutten et al., 2002). The ASFNR algorithm recommends the use of three different paradigms, with each paradigm leading to the activation of different language areas. Language mapping should start with sentence completion (SC), the overall most robust paradigm (Zaca et al., 2013). This should be followed by silent word generation (SWG), which is better than SC in testing for language lateralization. Compared with vocalization, covert word generation reduces head motion and thus motion artifacts. The choice of the third paradigm depends on the patient's neurological condition and ability to cooperate (Black et al., 2017). The authors also provide a dedicated algorithm for the examination of pediatric patients.

Of all semantic paradigms, SWG has been most extensively compared with the Wada test (Black et al., 2017; Buchbinder, 2016; Stippich, 2015; Woermann et al., 2003; ) and direct ECS. In a relatively large series of 100 patients with epilepsy, Woermann and coworkers demonstrated 91% concordance between the Wada test and SWG for language lateralization (Woermann et al., 2003). For SWG and object naming (ON), another very robust speech paradigm, there is evidence in the literature for good correlation between the locus of activation in fMRI and ECS with up to 100% sensitivity (Black et al., 2017; Buchbinder 2016). In its recent guidelines, the American Association of Neurology considers fMRI an option for the detection of language lateralization in patients with mesial temporal lobe epilepsy (MTLE), TLE in general, and ETLE. However, this recommendation has only evidence level C, and the authors emphasize that in each individual case the advantages and disadvantages of fMRI must be thoroughly discussed (Szaflarski et al., 2017). In patients undergoing anterior temporal lobe resection, fMRI has a positive predictive value of 60% to 81% for predicting postoperative language deficits (sensitivity 100%; specificity 33%–45%). Although the evaluation of memory encoding by fMRI is not as yet well validated, language fMRI demonstrating activation asymmetry to the left hemisphere may predict verbal memory outcome after left medial temporal lobe surgery (Szaflarski, Gloss et al., 2017).

## Paraneoplastic and Autoimmune Disorders

The role of molecular imaging in inflammatory diseases of the brain is increasingly recognized. Aside from still rather experimental approaches (e.g., including TSPO ligands to image microglial activation), the use of [$^{18}$F]FDG PET has gained widespread clinical use for the diagnosis and follow-up of paraneoplastic and autoimmune disorders of the CNS. As described in more detail in Chapters 81 and 82 (for recent reviews see also Graus et al., 2016; Stich and Rauer, 2014), these disorders can be divided into paraneoplastic disorders of the CNS associated with well-characterized antineuronal or onconeuronal antibodies directed against intracellular antigens on the one side and, on the other side, autoimmune encephalitis with antibodies against cell surface or synaptic antigens (possibly associated with malignant tumors). Paraneoplastic diseases with onconeuronal antibodies often lead to irreversible damage, the progression of which is most effectively attenuated by treating the underlying immunogenic tumor. In contrast, autoimmune encephalitis associated with antibodies against surface antigens may be reversible and effectively treated with antibody depletion and immunosuppression. In both situations, cerebral [$^{18}$F] FDG PET may be very helpful to confirm the clinical suspicion and exclude other possible diagnoses (e.g., neurodegenerative dementia in cases of rapid cognitive decline), especially if the results of antibody testing (which may take weeks) are not yet available or are negative. In addition, whole-body PET/CT is employed for tumor screening.

In our experience, the clinical manifestation most often referred for [$^{18}$F]FDG PET is limbic encephalitis (LE). LE is clinically characterized by the subacute onset of neuropsychiatric symptoms such as memory deficits, personality changes, confusion, and complex partial seizures: LE may occur in both paraneoplastic or autoimmune encephalitis. Patients with paraneoplastic LE often show Anti-Hu and Anti-Ma2 antibodies (typically observed in small cell lung cancer [SCLC] and testicular tumors, respectively), whereas the frequency of associated malignancies is much more variable in autoimmune encephalitis depending on possibly observed antibodies (e.g., AMPA receptor, SCLC, breast cancer or thymoma in 70%; $GABA_B$ receptor, SCLC or neuroendocrine tumors in 50%; LGI1, thymoma in <20% of patients; Graus et al., 2016; Stich and Rauer, 2014), PET imaging findings are typically characterized by a considerable, often asymmetric mesiotemporal (Fig. 42.23) and possibly also striatal brainstem and cerebellar hypermetabolism. The latter may correspond to an inflammatory involvement (coinciding with clinical symptoms) or a relative preservation of cerebral metabolism in these structures, which cannot be accurately distinguished in clinical settings without absolute quantification of regional cerebral glucose metabolism. In contrast, association cortices often show variable hypometabolism, which is often pronounced in the posterior cingulate cortex and precuneus (possibly due to deafferentation caused by mesiotemporal pathology, resembling findings in AD) and frontal areas (Baumgartner et al., 2013). In parallel to clinical recovery, the aforementioned changes may resolve. However, mesiotemporal hypermetabolism may also turn into hypometabolism, signifying irreversible postinflammatory damage.

Another disorder frequently referred for PET imaging is anti–*N*-methyl-D-aspartate (NMDA)-receptor encephalitis, which is most common in young women and often associated with ovarian teratoma (in up to 50% of females <45 years of age). Typical presentations involve acute psychiatric symptoms, leading to a multistage process including memory deficits, diminished level of consciousness, movement

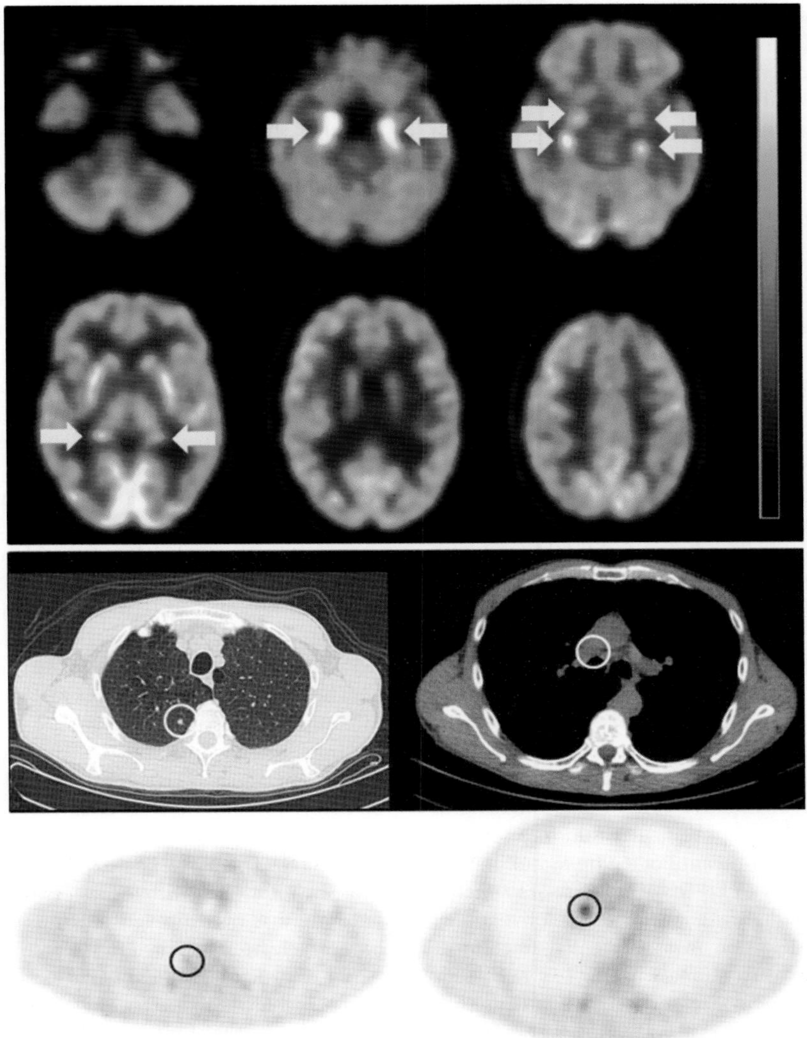

**Fig. 42.23** Paraneoplastic limbic encephalitis in small-cell lung cancer. Case of a 68-year-old male presenting with classical paraneoplastic limbic encephalitis associated with anti-Hu antibodies. *Upper panel,* Cerebral [$^{18}$F]FDG positron emission tomography (PET) revealed strongly increased hypermetabolism of bilateral mesial temporal lobes *(arrows)* accompanied by a mild hypometabolism of the left-sided association cortices. *Lower panel,* Whole-body [$^{18}$F]FDG PET/computed tomography (CT) revealed a 5-mm spiculated solitary pulmonary nodule in the right upper lobe of the lung with mild hypermetabolism and a strongly hypermetabolic mediastinal lymph node (*circles; upper row,* low-dose CT, lower row: [$^{18}$F]FDG PET). Patient was curatively treated by upper lobe resection and lymhadenectomy, verifying small-cell lung cancer (pT1a N2) on histopathology.

disorders, seizures, and autonomic dysfunction (Graus et al., 2016; Stich and Rauer, 2014). [$^{18}$F]FDG PET findings in anti–NMDA receptor encephalitis include relative frontotemporal hypermetabolism (Leypoldt et al., 2012) and parietal and occipital hypometabolism (Leypoldt et al., 2012; Solnes et al., 2017). In the authors' experience, findings in anti–NMDA receptor encephalitis may be fairly heterogeneous, including focal areas of relative cortical hypo- and hypermetabolism. Furthermore, the extent of cortical abnormalities usually corresponds with clinical severity and may resolve completely with successful treatment even in severe cases of long standing (Endres et al., 2015; Leypoldt et al., 2012). Of note, the aforementioned cortical PET findings are not specific for anti–NMD receptor encephalitis and may also occur in cases of encephalitis associated with other antibodies against surface or synaptic antigens (e.g., the voltage-gated potassium channel (VGKC) complex; Solnes et al., 2017). In line with the aforementioned results, a preliminary study detected a significant association between [$^{18}$F]FDG PET findings and autoantibody type. Although patients with antibody against intracellular targets showed mesiotemporal hypermetabolism, this was rarely true in patients with antibodies against surface antigens (NMDA receptor and/or voltage-gated potassium channel (VGKC) complex). Finally, patients with the clinical diagnosis of LE but negative autoantibody testing exhibited abnormal findings on [$^{18}$F]FDG PET, mostly including mesiotemporal hypermetabolism (Baumgartner et al., 2013).

Only a few studies have conducted a systematic comparison between [$^{18}$F]FDG PET and MRI for diagnosing LE (Baumgartner et al., 2013) and autoimmune encephalitis (Solnes et al., 2017). These studies strongly suggest that [$^{18}$F]FDG PET is superior to MRI in depicting CNS involvement (abnormal findings in 78%–100% vs. 42%–63% of cases, respectively), which may be particularly true for anti–NMDA receptor encephalitis. In contrast, recent consensus guidelines for the diagnosis of autoimmune encephalitis (Graus et al., 2016) define a role for cerebral [18F]FDG PET only as an alternative to MRI in diagnosing "definite autoimmune LE," whereas only MRI is considered as a diagnostic criterion for "possible autoimmune encephalitis" and "autoantibody negative but probable autoimmune encephalitis", and neither MRI nor PET is considered for diagnosing "anti–NMDA receptor encephalitis." Given this inconsistency and subsequent controversy (Morbelli et al., 2016), it is probably advisable to use cerebral [18F]FDG PET in questionable cases and as an adjunct to whole-body PET/CT (see later).

Paraneoplastic cerebellar degeneration (PCD) is typically associated with antibodies directed against intracellular antigens (e.g., Anti-Yo and Anti-Ri in breast or ovarian cancer or SCLC). If such patients are imaged during the early phase of the disorder, [18F]FDG PET may show bilateral cerebellar hypermetabolism. However, in most cases PCD is associated with reduced metabolism, which may be difficult to distinguish from other types of cerebellar degeneration (e.g., MSA and SCA).

At least as important as the role of [18F]FDG PET for the confirmation of suspected CNS involvement is its use for diagnosing occult malignancies (see Fig. 42.23). Guidelines of the European Federation of Neurological Societies (EFNS; Titulaer et al., 2011) state that the nature of the antibody and, to a lesser extent, the clinical syndrome determine the risk and type of an underlying malignancy. According to these guidelines, screening is preferentially done by conventional structural imaging: CT for SCLC and thymoma; mammography/MRI for breast cancer; ultrasound/CT/MRI for ovarian carcinoma/teratoma and testicular tumors. [18F]FDG PET or PET/CT is recommended as a second-line modality in case of negative conventional imaging in the aforementioned malignancies except testicular tumors and ovarian teratoma, "other tumors," and if no antibodies are found. In fact, it has been shown that whole-body [18F]FDG PET possesses a higher sensitivity for detection of occult malignancies than conventional imaging and provides tumor detection in a substantial fraction of patients with preceding negative conventional imaging (e.g., PET sensitivity and specificity of 75% and 87%, respectively, in patients with negative whole-body CT; Hadjivassiliou et al., 2009; for review see also Basu and Alavi, 2008). As acknowledged by the EFNS authors, data on hybrid PET/CT were still limited at the time the guidelines were prepared (Titulaer et al., 2011). However, combined whole-body PET/CT has gained widespread use even in smaller institutions and provides fast and highly accurate combined molecular and conventional imaging in a single session. A recent meta-analysis showed that the sensitivity and specificity of [18F]FDG PET and PET/CT for the detection of underlying malignancies is about 89%, and 83% in neurological paraneoplastic syndromes, with PET/CT providing a significantly higher specificity than stand-alone PET (Sheikhbahaei et al., 2017). Thus combined whole-body [18F]FDG PET/CT may be chosen as the method of choice for tumor screening, particularly in classical paraneoplastic syndromes and suspected autoimmune encephalitis with a high risk for [18F]FDG-avid cancers (see also (Hadjivassiliou et al., 2009). As a practical approach to [18F]FDG PET scanning, it must be emphasized that a dedicated brain scan can easily be added to a whole-body scan (usually from the base of the skull to proximal thighs) and vice versa. Therefore, to avoid treatment delay and additional radiation exposure by repeated scans and [18F]FDG injections, a dedicated brain PET scan should be liberally added in patients with suspected encephalitis schedule for whole-body [18F]FDG PET/CT, whereas a whole-body scan (usually with lose-dose CT) may be added in those patients scheduled for a first brain PET scan, even if the assumed likelihood of an occult malignancy is limited. Finally, given that paraneoplastic manifestations may precede clinical and imaging tumor manifestation by years, it has been recommended to repeat tumor screening by imaging for up to 4 years if results remain negative (Titulaer et al., 2011).

## Ischemic Stroke

Ischemic stroke is caused by severe disruption of local CBF. The severity, duration, and extent of this disruption has been imaged by various techniques, most notably and accurately by [15O]water PET (Baron et al., 1987). Although they are the most important factors to determine ultimate infarct size, they can rarely be assessed in clinical practice because of time and logistic constraints.

Thrombolysis is an efficient therapeutic method for the reperfusion of tissue but it must be applied within a critical time window depending on the severity of the initial impairment, usually within 3 or no more than 6 hours after symptom onset. It can salvage tissue that is not yet infarcted but is being affected by critical hypoperfusion, often called the "penumbra." Thus the use of imaging to determine whether such tissue exists in order to initiate thrombolysis is likely to be effective has been a major topic of research over many years (Leigh et al., 2018; Sobesky et al., 2005). Current recommendations put a priority on essential structural imaging to avoid loss of time and reserve more complex functional procedures, such as diffusion- and perfusion-weighted MRI, to patients with occluded large anterior circulation vessels for mechanical thrombectomy between 6 and 24 hours from last known symptom-free state (Powers et al., 2018).

The ischemic insult induces a vast range of secondary metabolic and molecular changes in affected tissue. Some of these changes—including impairment of the cerebral metabolic rate of oxygen ($CMRO_2$), glucose metabolism (Heiss et al., 1992), disruption of the BBB, loss of GABA receptors (Heiss et al., 2001), and inflammatory response with microglial activation—are accessible by in vivo imaging (Gerhard et al., 2005). There may be therapeutic potential to improve stroke outcome by interfering with secondary damage due to such mechanisms, but none has been proven yet; thus the related imaging techniques have largely been confined to research.

CT or structural MRI is used to localize the resulting structural lesion. It may include gray matter as well as fiber tracts. The latter are often most important for functional deficits. Their severity and extent can be assessed by DTI. The structural lesions may also cause a dysfunction in remote noninfarcted but connected areas. The concept of "diaschisis" as a temporary disturbance of function through disconnection was introduced by von Monakow (1906). Functional imaging of CBF or glucose metabolism has been used to identify functionally impaired areas (Herholz and Heiss, 2000), and in recent years the analysis of functional network changes by fMRI and electrophysiological methods has added deep insight into functional mechanisms that may worsen or ameliorate neurological symptoms after stroke (Grefkes and Fink, 2014).

Lesions of the motor cortex or the corticospinal tract are associated with spastic paresis. Motor activation studies show an increase of activated brain areas involving midline premotor areas and contralesional motor areas. These may contribute to residual function via nonpyramidal tracts, such as the cortico-rubro-spinal system (Grefkes and Ward, 2014) but patients who recover typically also show recovery of the more restricted normal activation pattern. Thus there is some evidence that the reduction of inhibitory transcallosal projections from the lesioned to the nonlesioned hemisphere may contribute to increased activation in the nonlesioned hemisphere and, vice versa, increased activation there may functionally inhibit some areas in the lesioned hemisphere that were not directly damaged by the ischemic insult (Heiss and Thiel, 2006). These observations may open new therapeutic avenues by targeted inhibition of contralateral areas using electrical and transcranial magnetic stimulation (Grefkes and Fink, 2016).

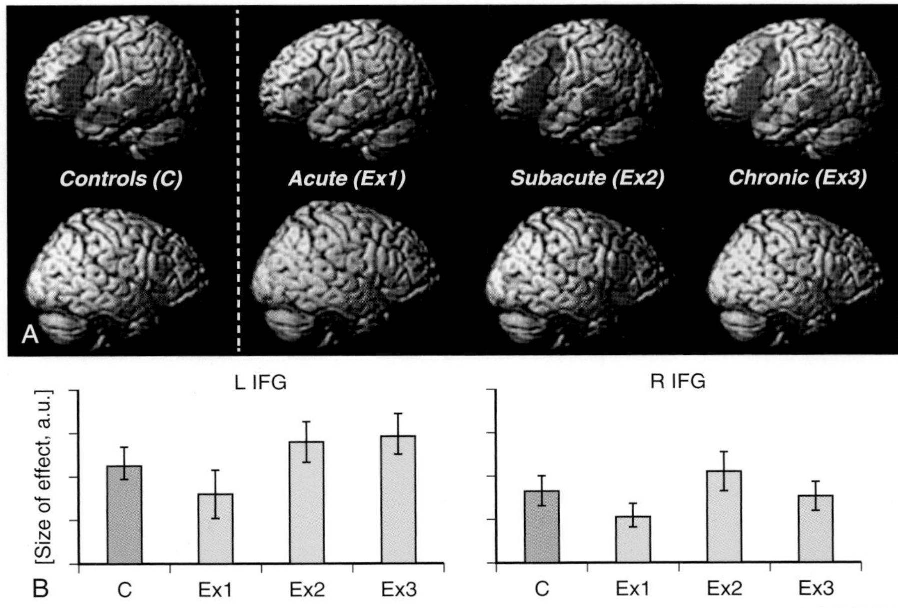


**Fig. 42.24 A,** Dynamics of language-specific (speech [SP] contrasted with reversed speech [REV]) fMRI activation in healthy control subjects (first column, a single functional magnetic resonance imaging [fMRI] exam) and in 14 patients with acute aphasia (columns 2–4, representing the three exams). Activation is shown for the left hemisphere in *the top* row and for the right hemisphere in the *bottom row.* Note that there is little or no left hemispheric activation in the acute stage. This is followed by a bilateral increase in activation in the subacute stage, peaking in the right hemisphere homolog of the Broca area. In the chronic phase, consolidation and gradual normalization emerged, with a "reshift" to the left hemisphere. **B,** Parameter estimates extracted in the left and right inferior frontal gyri (*R IFG and L IFG*), indicating a continuous increase of activation in the L IFG over time but a biphasic course in the R IFG. *(Modified from Saur, D., Lange, R., Baumgaertner, A., Schraknepper, V., Willmes, K., Rijntjes, M., 2006. Dynamics of language reorganization after stroke. Brain 129 [Pt 6], 1371–1384.)*

Language deficits result from lesions to the Broca and Wernicke areas as well as associated fiber bundles, most prominently the arcuate fasciculus. In the acute phase, a nearly complete abolition of language function is reflected by little if any activation in brain regions that are activated by language tasks in normal controls (Lange et al., 2006; Rijntjes, 2006; Saur et al., 2006; Rijntjes and Weiller, 2013; Fig. 42.24). Recovery of perfusion and metabolism in those areas and restitution of the associated networks are strong indicators of recovery, whereas the activation of contralateral areas may precede recovery but by itself cannot support language function (Thiel Kessler et al., 1998). Inhibition of contralesional inferior frontal gyrus by transcranial magnetic stimulation (TMS) may enhance naming abilities in chronic stroke (Thiel Hartmann et al., 2013), opening future perspectives for advanced functional therapy by brain–machine interfacing (Ramos-Murguialday et al., 2013).

Diffuse white-matter lesions contribute to cognitive impairment after stroke and limit the potential for recovery. Impairment of the default mode network (DMN) and loss of the normal anticorrelation with task-associated networks is associated with impairment of cognition, whereas restitution is related to behavioral recovery. In the acute stroke phase, 2–3 days poststroke, patients with neglect show a downregulation of the whole attention system. This includes noninfarcted structures of the visuospatial attentional system, such as the right lateral occipital cortex, while left hemispheric areas may provide a better compensation, as is the case in extinction (Umarova et al., 2011).

The functional stages of language recovery may be used to influence the therapeutic regimen. During the hyperacute stage, no activation and no function is observed; most likely, specific treatment might be useless at this stage. Still, the therapist should see the patients, detect changes (e.g., worsening in behavioral tests) and support the patient by indicating that he or she is there to start treatment when appropriate. Subsequent recovery of activation could possibly be modulated by pharmacological or functional intervention. Pariente et al. (2001) found a correlation between intake of a selective serotonin reuptake inhibitor (SSRI) and increased activity of BOLD in the motor cortex of chronic stroke patients. The fluoxetine in motor recovery of patients with acute ischaemic stroke (FLAME) study built on this and showed improved recovery through an SSRI when administered within the first 10 days after stroke (Chollet et al., 2011).

## Coma and Consciousness

Coma is associated with large decrease (30%–60%) in global glucose metabolism, which can be measured with [$^{18}$F]FDG PET using techniques for the calculation of metabolic rates (see Positron Emission Tomography, earlier). Midline brain structures are most critical for basic consciousness functions, whereas lateral associative cortices support more specific cognitive functions (Laureys and Schiff, 2012). Severe impairment of association cortices in the dominant hemisphere can preclude meaningful interaction, although conscious awareness may still be maintained if midline structures are intact (Bruno et al., 2012). The most severe metabolic reductions were observed in persistent vegetative states, probably reflecting Wallerian and transsynaptic degeneration (Rudolf et al., 1999). Thus functional imaging techniques, also including resting-state and activation fMRI, have widely been used to explore whether comatose or vegetative patients actually are in a minimally conscious state with potential for recovery (Naccache, 2018; Owen et al., 2006). These investigations have provided deep insights into the biological foundations of consciousness and offer perspectives for the improved prediction of recovery (Stender et al., 2014).

Functional imaging has also provided insight into the central processing of pain (Wiech, 2016). This includes top-down mechanisms for the modulation of pain, which have been studied using fMRI with pharmacological intervention (e.g., Eippert et al., 2009). The network originates in the dorsolateral prefronal cortex, which is potentially accessible for therapeutic modulation by TMS (Krummenacher et al., 2010). The system is mediated by endogeneous opioids, and changes in the opioid system have been observed in chronic pain using PET with opioid ligands (Jones et al., 2004). A comprehensive analysis of pain perception and placebo analgesia will probably require the analysis of the interaction between descending and ascending networks (Buchel et al., 2014).

*The complete reference list is available online at www.expertconsult.com.* 

43

# Ocular Functional and Structural Investigations

*Robert Mallery, Devin Mackay, Sashank Prasad*

## OUTLINE



Functional and structural investigations that assess the integrity of the visual system are of utmost importance for diagnosing and monitoring ophthalmic or neurological disorders that affect vision. These investigations complement the ophthalmic and fundus examinations, allowing precise quantitative baseline and serial assessments. Structural investigations include fundus imaging, fluorescein angiography (FA), optical coherence tomography (OCT) imaging, and orbital ultrasound. Functional investigations include assessment of the visual field with perimetry and electrodiagnostic studies, such as electroretinography (ERG) or visual evoked potentials (VEPs), to assess function of the retina and optic nerve, respectively.

## INVESTIGATIONS OF RETINAL AND OPTIC NERVE STRUCTURE

Ocular imaging modalities complement the fundus examination and allow enhanced assessment and documentation of anatomical changes within the visual pathways. Photography, FA, and orbital ultrasound have long served as the principal modalities for retinal and optic nerve imaging. More recently, OCT has emerged as a major breakthrough in ocular imaging, permitting a more detailed characterization of retinal and optic nerve pathologies.

### Fundus Imaging

Fundus imaging, which includes modalities used to capture two-dimensional (2D) images, serves as an indispensable method to recognize and record abnormalities evident on fundus examination, leading to an improved ability to diagnose, treat, and monitor retinal and neurological disease.

#### Color Fundus Photography

Standard fundus cameras, which are typically found in ophthalmology clinics, require pupillary dilation to capture images of the macula (central retina), optic disc, and retinal periphery. Dilation is needed to overcome the technical limitations of these cameras, which require the incident light beam projected on the fundus to follow a different optical path through the cornea and lens than the reflected imaging beam in order to avoid reflections from the cornea and lens. Newer nonmydriatic cameras have become available that capture high-quality images of the central retina or optic nerve in patients with pupils as small as 3–4 mm (Fig. 43.1, *A–C*). Two-dimensional retinal images may also be obtained with scanning laser ophthalmoscopy (SLO), which generates an image based on the amount of light reflected by a single wavelength of infrared laser. Newer cameras utilizing multiple scanning lasers and pseudo-coloration (e.g., Optos plc, Dunfermline, Scotland, UK) are capable of capturing ultra-widefield retinal views of up to 200 degrees; they have particular utility for assessing disorders that affect the retinal periphery (see Fig. 43.1, *D*).

Fundus photography is primarily used to document and allow scrutiny of the ocular fundus, relying on the discernment of disease pathology by an experienced specialist who interprets the images, similar to the interpretation of a fundus examination performed during ophthalmoscopy. Although not yet routinely used, automated image analysis methods to detect abnormalities in retinal images have also been developed (Abràmoff et al., 2010).

In the context of waning proficiency with direct ophthalmoscopy, due to limited training, interest has recently been spurred in the development of nonmydriatic fundus cameras in settings such as emergency departments and neurology offices (Bruce et al., 2011; Mackay et al., 2015). Nonmydriatic fundus photography offers significant advantages over direct ophthalmoscopy: it offers a much wider field of view (45 vs. 5 degrees), circumvents the technical barriers of direct ophthalmoscopy, and yields images that can be used to monitor a patient's visual or neurological disorder—images that can be shared with consulting specialists or the patients themselves to educate them regarding their condition. Disadvantages include limited availability, lack of portability of tabletop devices, and cost.

Recent technological advances have facilitated the development of handheld nonmydriatic fundus cameras that yield a relatively wide field of view and may be used in critically ill patients, but cost and availability limit their use. Fundus photography devices that attach to the built-in cameras of smartphones have also generated considerable interest, offering many of the advantages of fundus photography and great portability. However, they can be difficult to use, especially without pupillary dilation, and image quality tends to be considerably inferior to that from tabletop cameras.

There has been growing interest in the use of fundus photography to research neurological disorders. Changes in retinal vascular caliber associated with cerebrovascular disease and cognitive impairment can

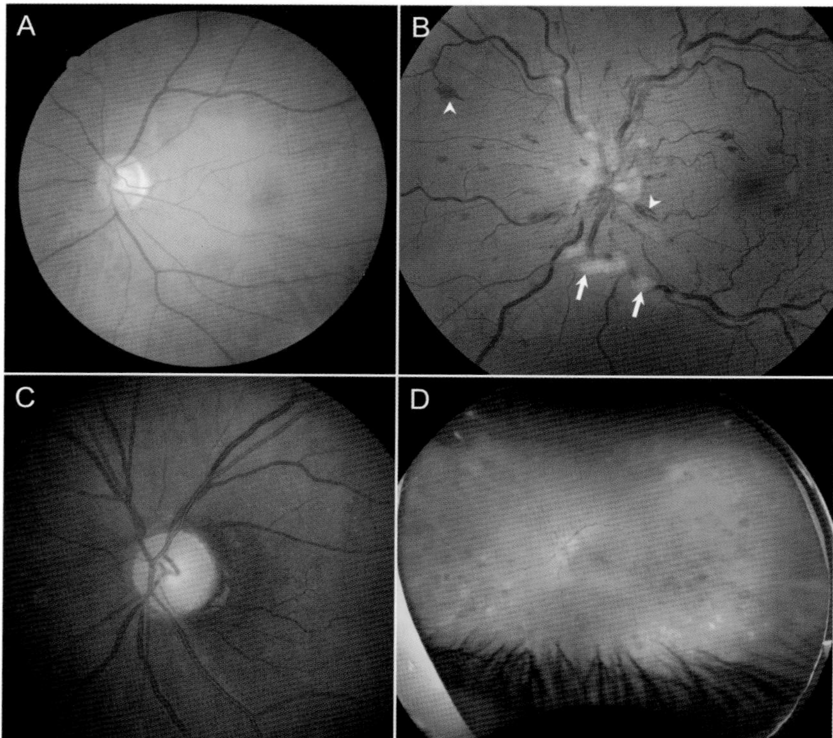


**Fig. 43.1 Fundus Photography. A,** Normal fundus image of the macula obtained by a nonmydriatic fundus camera without pupillary dilation. **B,** Central retinal vein occlusion with peripapillary and midperipheral retinal hemorrhages in the nerve fiber layer *(arrowheads)*, cotton-wool spots in the peripapillary retina *(arrows)*, and optic disc edema. **C,** Optic disc pallor in a patient with autosomal dominant optic atrophy from a mutation in the *OPA1* gene. **D,** Pseudo-color wide-field image (Optos plc, Dunfermline, Scotland, UK) showing peripheral retinal whitening, hemorrhages, and optic disc edema in a patient with acute retinal necrosis related to varicella zoster.

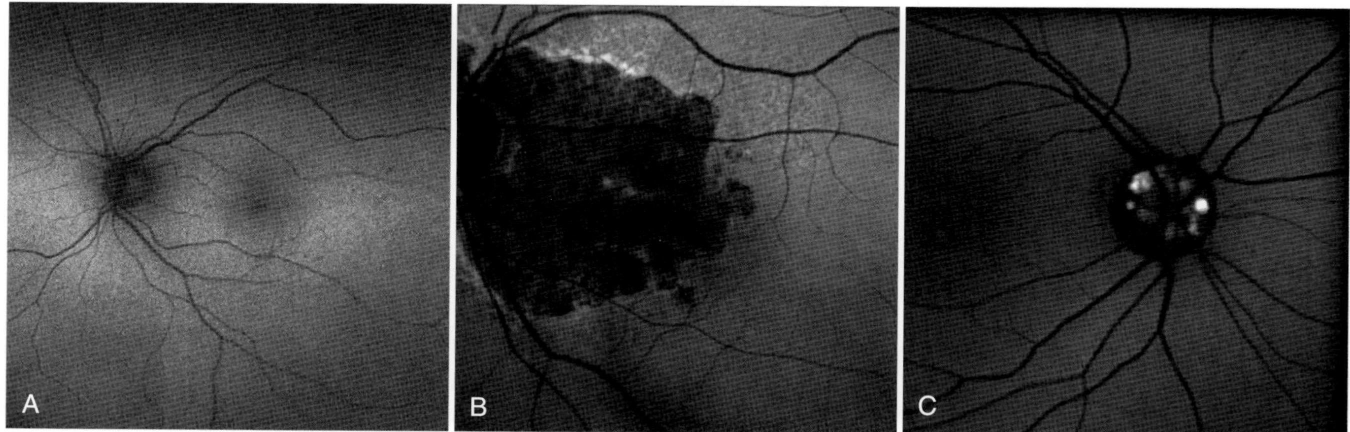


**Fig. 43.2 Fundus Autofluorescence Imaging. A,** Normal pattern of fundus autofluorescence. **B,** Geographic atrophy involving the central and nasal macula of a patient with age-related macular degeneration appears as a well-demarcated zone of hypofluorescence. **C,** Optic disc drusen appear as hyperfluorescent foci on the optic nerve. *(A and B courtesy Rachel Huckfeldt, MD, PhD.)*

be analyzed with fundus photography. These findings raise the possibility that routine fundus photography may eventually play a role in the early identification of medical and neurological conditions (Rodenbeck and Mackay, 2019).

## Fundus Autofluorescence Imaging

Autofluorescence imaging records the light emitted by native fluorophores in the retina after excitation by light of a blue or green wavelength. The principal naturally occurring fluorophore is lipofuscin, contained within cytoplasmic granules of retinal pigment epithelial cells. Images may be captured by a properly equipped fundus camera, an SLO-OCT machine, or a wide-field SLO. A normal fundus autofluorescence (FAF) image shows a low-intensity background autofluorescence with reduced intensity in the foveal region related to the absorption of blue light by macular luteal pigment (Fig. 43.2, *A*). The optic nerves and blood vessels, which contain no fluorophores, appear very dark. Changes in the normal pattern of FAF most often occur in retinal diseases that disrupt retinal pigment epithelium (RPE) cells (see Fig. 43.2, *B*). Autofluorescence

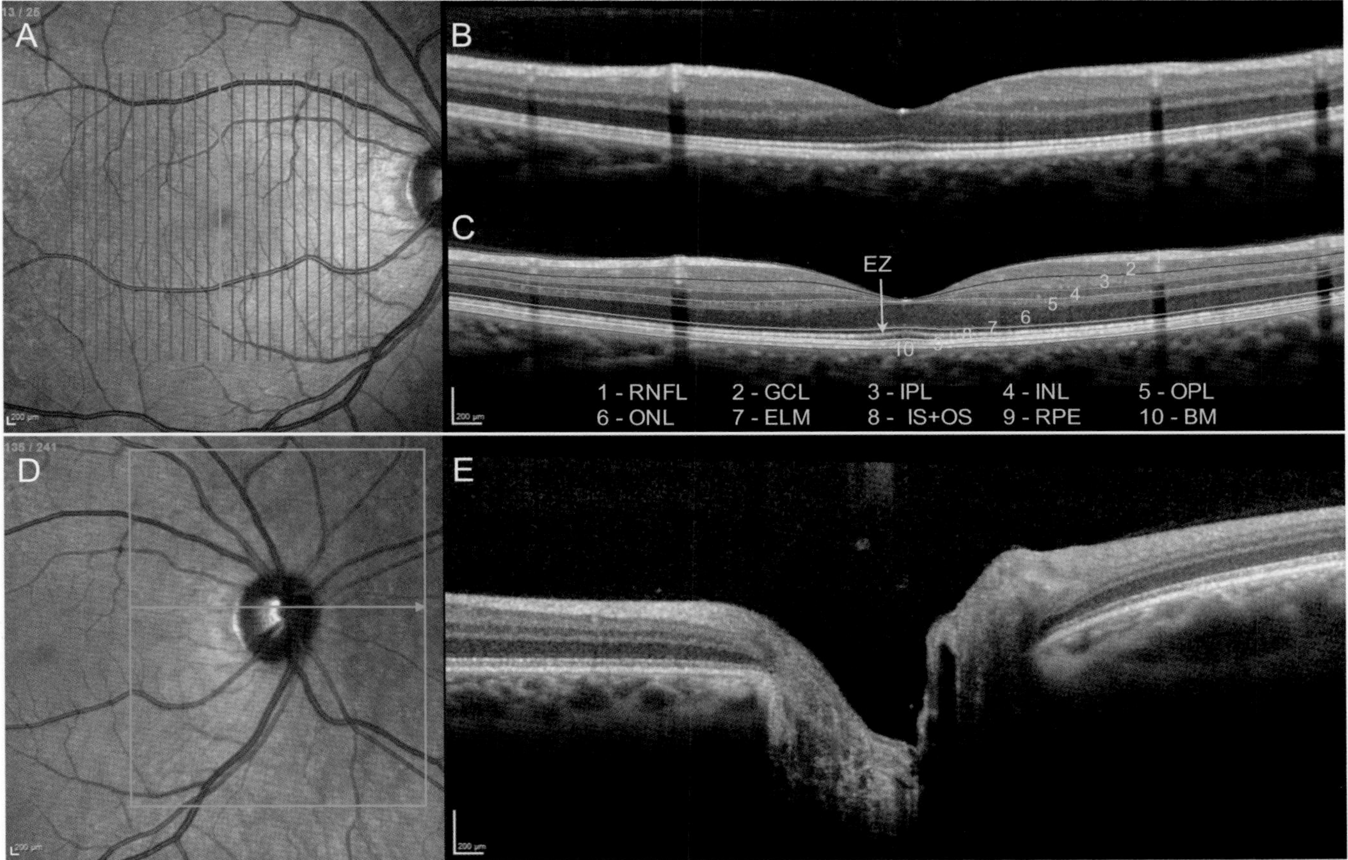


**Fig. 43.3** **Normal Optical Coherence Tomography B-scans of the Macula and Optic Nerve Head. A,** Adjacent B-scans are performed to complete a volume scan of the macula. **B,** Central B-scan through the anatomical fovea. **C,** Retinal layers determined by automated segmentation. The ellipsoid zone (EZ) line *(arrow)* corresponds to the ellipsoid zone of photoreceptor inner segments. **D** and **E,** B-scan showing the cross section of a normal optic nerve. *BM*, Bruch membrane; *ELM*, external limiting membrane; *EZ*, ellipsoid zone; *GCL*, ganglion cell layer; *INL*, inner nuclear layer; *IPL*, inner plexiform layer; *IS+OS*, photoreceptor inner and outer segments; *ONL*, outer nuclear layer; *OPL*, outer plexiform layer; *RNFL*, retinal nerve fiber layer; *RPE*, retinal pigment epithelium

imaging is also useful for identifying optic disc drusen at or slightly below the surface of the optic nerve head (see Fig. 43.2, *B* and *C*).

## Optical Coherence Tomography Imaging

OCT is an imaging modality, often described as the light equivalent of ultrasound, which utilizes the backscatter of near-infrared light and the concept of low-coherence interferometry to generate a cross-sectional image of biological tissue (Fujimoto and Swanson, 2016). The first clinical OCT device designed for retinal imaging became available in 1996, and OCT imaging of retinal disease had been widely adopted by the early 2000s. Collection of adjacent cross-sectional images with very high spatial resolution makes OCT essentially a three-dimensional (3D) imaging modality (Fig. 43.3, *A*). The retinal layers are evident as alternating bands of hyper- or hyporeflective signal depending upon the cellular characteristics of that layer (see Fig. 43.3, *B*), and the thickness of individual retinal layers can be assessed through automated image segmentation algorithms (see Fig. 43.3, *C*). Older-generation time-domain OCT devices had a limited axial spatial resolution of approximately 10 μm, but newer-generation spectral-domain OCT devices have a resolution below 5 μm because of higher image acquisition speeds (up to 80,000 A-scans per second) that reduce motion artifact and allow better characterization of deeper retinal layers. OCT cross-sectional images of the retina (see Fig 43.3, *A–C*) or optic nerve (see Fig. 43.3, *D* and *E*) demonstrate retinal and optic nerve pathology in exquisite detail. In addition, growing evidence suggests that optic nerve and retinal changes measured longitudinally with serial OCT studies are important biomarkers for several neurological disorders.

### Optical Coherence Tomography for Assessing Retinal Disorders

OCT imaging is an indispensable component of the diagnosis and monitoring of retinal disorders in which pathology is evident by morphological changes in the retina. It is also extremely valuable to distinguish cases of subtle macular pathology from other causes of visual loss, such as retrobulbar optic neuropathy.

***Retinal artery occlusion.*** The retinal arterioles originating from the central retinal artery give rise to capillary networks supplying the inner retinal layers, including the retinal nerve fiber layer, ganglion cell layer (GCL), inner plexiform layer (IPL), and most of the inner nuclear layer (Salzmann, 1912; Tan et al., 2012). The outer retinal layers, which include the photoreceptors, receive oxygen through diffusion from the retinal choriocapillaris, which is supplied by posterior ciliary arteries originating from the ophthalmic artery. Thus an acute central or branch retinal artery occlusion results in cytotoxic edema in the inner retinal layers that is evident as hyperreflective signal change and thickening (Fig. 43.4, *A* and *B*). In areas with

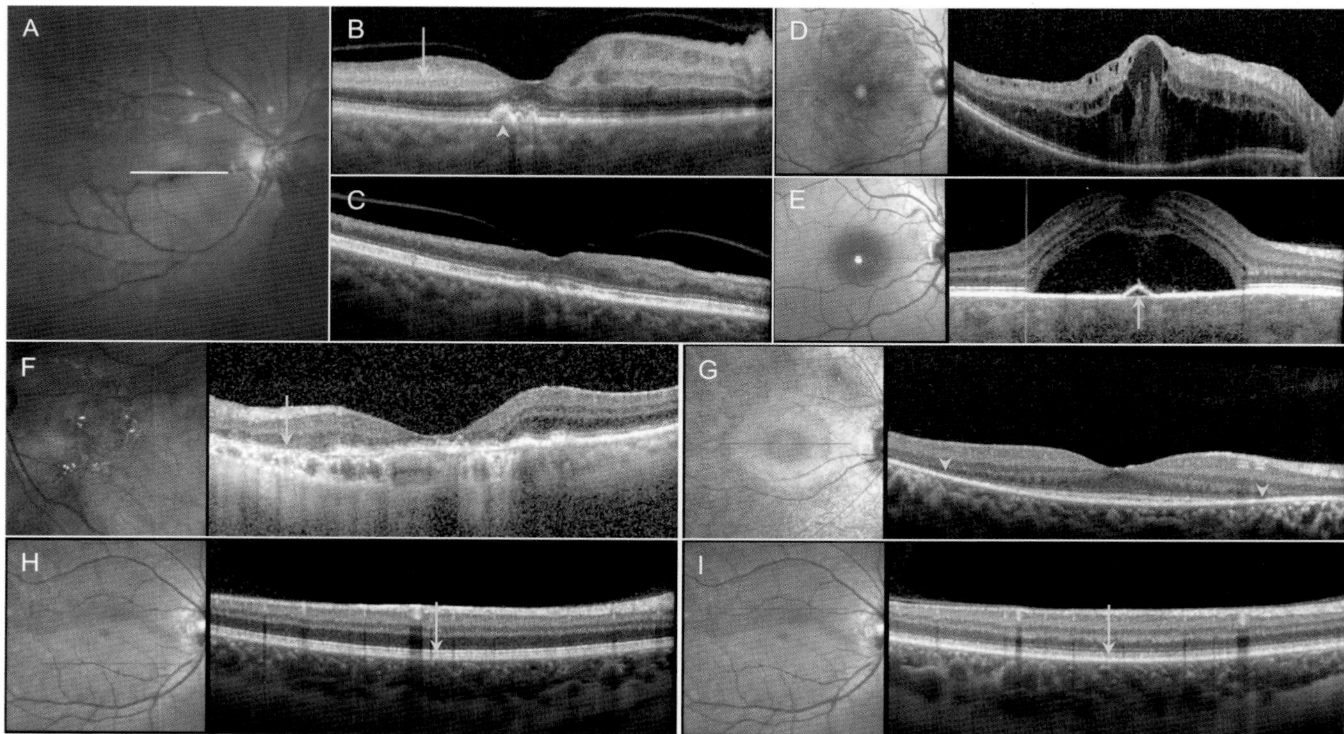


**Fig. 43.4 Examples of Optical Coherence Tomography Imaging of Retinal Disorders.** **A,** Fundus photograph showing retinal ischemia from a central retinal artery occlusion. **B,** Optical coherence tomography (OCT) within 1 day of visual loss showing increased hyperreflective signal *(arrow)* and thickening within the inner retinal layers, sparing the outer retina. This patient also has subfoveal drusen *(arrowhead)* from age-related macular degeneration. **C,** OCT 3 months later showing thinning of all inner retinal layers. **D,** Diabetic macular edema with retinal thickening and cystoid spaces related to intraretinal fluid. **E,** Central serous chorioretinopathy in a patient with blurred vision in the right eye. Detachment of pigment epithelium is seen as a small hyporeflective space between the retinal pigment epithelium (RPE) and basement membrane *(arrow)* along with a larger subfoveal neurosensory retinal detachment. **F,** In this patient with age-related macular degeneration, geographic atrophy extends from the fovea toward the optic nerve nasally (left side of OCT image) with thinning of the outer nuclear layer *(arrow)* and loss of the underlying external limiting membrane (ELM), photoreceptor layers, and RPE. **G,** OCT from a 10-year-old boy with X-linked retinitis pigmentosa shows attenuation of photoreceptor layers in the peripheral macula *(arrowheads)* with preserved architecture centrally *(arrow)*. **H** and **I,** OCT of a patient with acute zonal occult outer retinopathy causing an inferior visual field defect and a normal fundus examination. **H,** OCT B-scan of the unaffected inferior macula shows normal appearance of the RPE and photoreceptor layers. **I,** B-scan of the affected superior macula shows indistinct photoreceptor layers and RPE. *(D–F, Courtesy Rachel Huckfeldt, MD, PhD.)*

permanent injury, atrophy ensues over weeks, with loss of thickness of the retinal layers extending beyond the GCL into the inner nuclear layer, which includes the bipolar cell soma (see Fig. 43.4, *C*). The outer retinal layers that receive oxygen through diffusion from the retinal choroid are preserved in an isolated occlusion of a central or branch retinal artery. In contrast to the optic atrophy that ensues following occlusion of a central retinal artery, optic atrophy from primary optic neuropathies is characterized by selective thinning of the retinal nerve's fiber layer and GCL without involvement of the deeper inner retinal layers.

***Cystoid macular edema.*** Cystoid macular edema may result from retinal pathology (e.g., neovascularization from age-related macular degeneration [AMD], diabetic retinopathy, retinal vein occlusion, epiretinal membrane, retinitis pigmentosa [RP]) or from edema originating at the optic disc (e.g., papilledema, anterior ischemic optic neuropathy, neuroretinitis). Macular edema is also a rare complication of fingolimod use for the treatment of multiple sclerosis (MS), occurring in about 2 per 1000 patients (Kappos et al., 2010). Macular edema, which may be somewhat difficult to appreciate on fundal examination, is easily detected on OCT, where it appears as hyporeflective intraretinal cystoid spaces with retinal thickening (see Fig. 43.4, *D*). Lipid exudates are evident as hyperreflective foci.

***Central serous chorioretinopathy.*** Central serous chorioretinopathy (CSCR) is a cause of acute or subacute painless loss or distortion of central vision originating from subfoveal neurosensory retinal detachment or pigment epithelial detachment. Men are affected more frequently than women, most often between 30 and 50 years of age (Daruich et al., 2015; Haimovici et al., 2004). The cause is not fully understood, but increasing evidence suggests that hyperpermeability of the choriocapillaris endothelium results in secondary dysfunction of the retina pigment epithelium and accumulation of fluid beneath the neurosensory retina or retina pigment epithelium. CSCR is more likely to develop in patients treated with exogenous corticosteroids, those with type-A behavioral traits, or in patients experiencing an acute stress (Bouzas et al., 2002; Yannuzzi, 1987). It may also worsen following administration of corticosteroids if another type of inflammatory choroiditis is suspected or if it is mistaken for optic neuritis. OCT demonstrates a sensorineural retinal detachment and

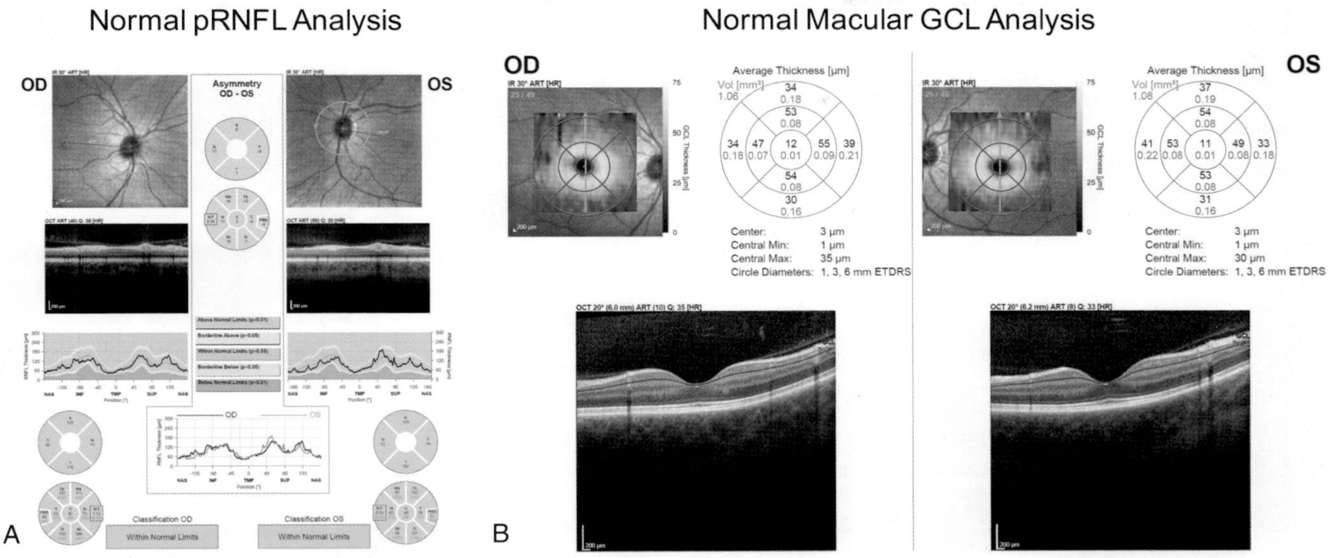

Fig. 43.5 **Normal Optic Nerve Optical Coherence Tomography Segmentation Analysis. A,** An optical coherence tomography (OCT) B-scan with a diameter of 12 degrees (3.4–3.5 mm depending upon axial eye length) is obtained from each eye, and the thickness of the retinal nerve fiber layer (highly reflective most superficial retinal layer) at each radial location is compared with the age-adjusted normal range. The thickness of the peripapillary retinal nerve fiber layer *(pRNFL)* is given as a global average by quadrant (superior, temporal, inferior, nasal), and by sector (superior-temporal, superior-nasal, nasal, inferior-nasal, inferior-temporal, temporal, and the papillomacular bundle). **B,** Segmentation of the macular volume OCT allows assessment of the macular ganglion cell layer *(GCL),* displayed as a thickness color map. The normal GCL has the topography of an annulus owing to the displacement of retinal ganglion cells away from the fovea, which has the greatest concentration of cone photoreceptors. The global integrity of the GCL may be given by either average thickness (μm) or total macular GCL volume (mm$^3$). OD - right eye; OS - left eye.

in the majority of cases also demonstrates a component of pigment epithelial detachment (see Fig. 43.4, *E*).

***Geographic atrophy.*** Geographic atrophy (GA) consists of outer retinal atrophy within the macula and is a feature of late-stage AMD as well as inherited maculopathies such as ABCA-4–related retinopathy (Stargardt disease). In AMD, GA results in central visual loss, with OCT showing attenuation of the outer nuclear layer (ONL), external limiting membrane (ELM), ellipsoid zone (EZ), retinal pigment epithelium (RPE), and choriocapillaris accompanied by subretinal drusenoid deposits (see Fig. 43.4, *F*; Arya et al., 2018).

***Retinitis pigmentosa.*** RP refers to a group of inherited retinopathies that cause progressive visual loss as a result of degeneration of rod and cone photoreceptors. Patients typically develop peripheral visual loss and nyctalopia during early stages, followed by gradual development of central visual loss. Fundus changes may include peripheral "bone spicule" pigment accumulation, atrophy of the RPE, and retinal arteriolar attenuation. OCT imaging assists in the diagnosis, as fundus features may be nonspecific or bland early in the disease course. Characteristic OCT findings include attenuation of the RPE, EZ, ELM, ONL, and OPL, often progressing from the outer to the central macula over time (see Fig. 43.4, *G*; Battaglia Parodi et al., 2016).

***Acute zonal occult outer retinopathy.*** Acute zonal occult outer retinopathy (AZOOR) is a retinal disease presenting with rapid onset of a visual scotoma due to loss of retinal function with minimal changes on fundus examination. Visual loss is typically accompanied by photopsias due to photoreceptor dysfunction. Variants of AZOOR include the acute idiopathic blind spot enlargement syndrome (AIBSES). This disease may relate to the retinal white dot syndromes, a group of inflammatory disorders of the choroid, RPE, and outer retina. OCT is particularly useful, as the fundus examination shows minimal if any changes initially, and the first changes are detected with alterations of the EZ on OCT (see Fig. 43.4, *H* and *I*). ERG localizes the dysfunction to the RPE-photoreceptor layers. Over time, patients develop visible atrophic changes in the RPE, and OCT demonstrates thinning of the photoreceptor layers, RPE, and choroid. In the AIBSES these structural changes occur in the peripapillary region.

### Optical Coherence Tomography for Assessing Optic Neuropathies

OCT has utility for the diagnosis and monitoring of optic neuropathies and optic disc edema through both cross-sectional imaging of the optic nerve structure and evaluation of the inner retinal layer thicknesses using automated segmentation algorithms. Topographically oriented quantitative data on the thickness of the peripapillary retinal nerve fiber layer (pRNFL), as well as that of the macular GCL or combined macular GCL and inner plexiform layer (GCIPL), can provide information regarding the presence of optic neuropathy or optic disc edema and make it possible to monitor changes in optic nerve structure quantitatively. A normal analysis of the pRNFL and macular GCL is shown in Fig. 43.5.

The relationship between pRNFL and macular GCL/GCIPL thinning in optic neuropathy provides insight into the timing of the optic neuropathy. In acute retrobulbar optic neuropathies without optic disc edema, pRNFL thickness is typically normal at presentation. Initial changes become evident as thinning of the macular GCL/GCIPL within a few weeks, whereas pRNFL thinning occurs in a delayed fashion once axon retraction has occurred.

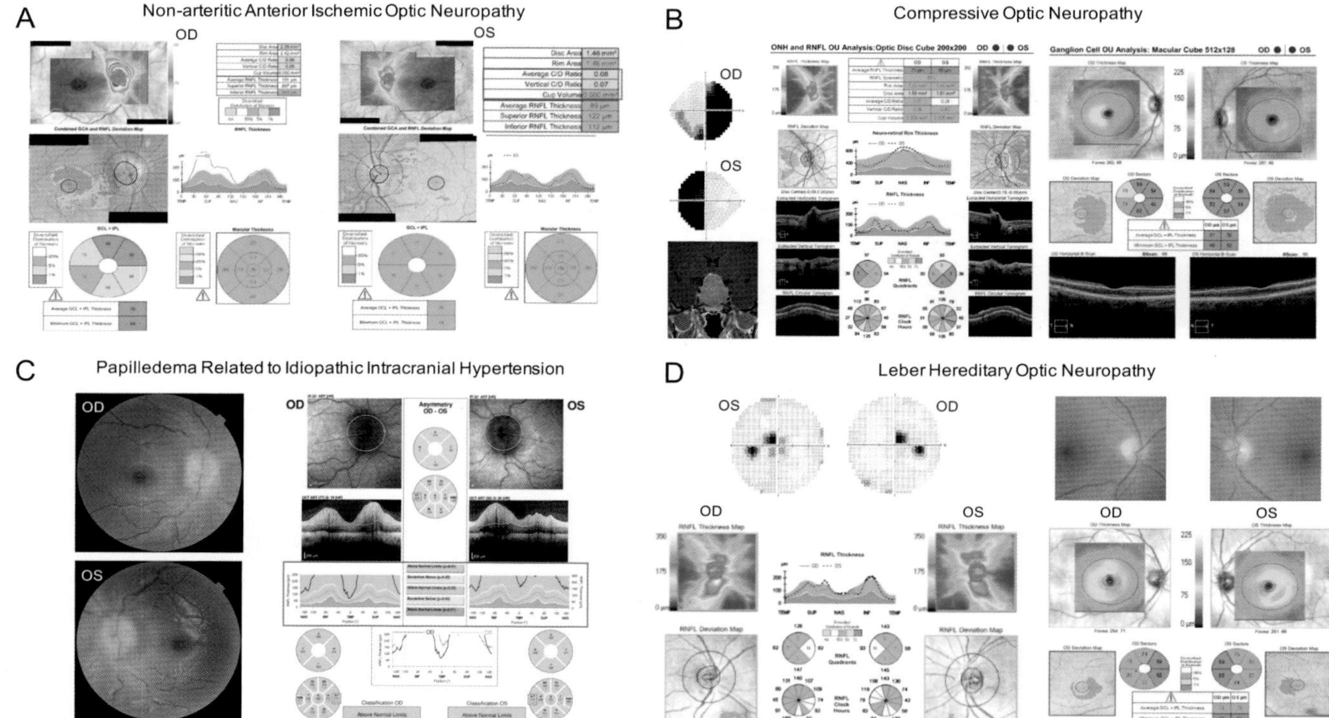


**Fig. 43.6 Examples of Optical Coherence Tomography Findings in Optic Neuropathies. A,** Combined peripapillary retinal nerve fiber layer (pRNFL), combined macular ganglion cell layer, and inner plexiform layer (GCIPL) analysis for a patient with nonarteritic anterior ischemic optic neuropathy (NAION) affecting the right eye (OD), with superior optic disc edema causing inferior and central visual field loss. There is thickening of the superior pRNFL and thinning of the superior and nasal macular GCIPL. Optical coherence tomography (OCT) of the unaffected left eye (OS) demonstrates a small cup size *(red box)*, which is a risk factor for NAION. **B,** Optic nerve OCT for a patient with compression of the optic chiasm by a nonfunctioning pituitary macroadenoma, causing a dense bitemporal hemianopia. pRNFL analysis *(left)* shows thinning greatest temporally OD and temporally and inferiorly OS. Macular GCIPL analysis shows thinning that is greatest nasally OD and more diffuse OS indicating compression on the optic chiasm and left optic nerve. **C,** Optic nerve OCT in a patient with papilledema from idiopathic intracranial hypertension (IIH). Fundus photographs show chronic grade 3 papilledema. pRNFL thickness analysis shows marked thickening of the pRNFL in both eyes (average 365 μm OD and 357 μm OS; normal 99 μm). **D,** Thirty-eight-year-old woman with Leber hereditary optic neuropathy (LHON) due to the 14484/ND6 mutation (OD 2 months prior, OS 1 months prior). This patient's visual fields show localized central scotomas. pRNFL analysis shows thickening nasally but otherwise normal-range values. GCIPL thickness map shows thinning nasal to the fovea in each eye within the region served by the papillomacular bundles. In the right eye, thinning is progressing inferiorly and temporally in a sequence characteristic of LHON.

***Glaucoma.*** Glaucoma, the most common optic neuropathy, results in gradual loss of the visual field (typically peripheral before central); the fundal examination is characterized by the development of optic disc cupping with preservation of the neuroretinal rim. OCT enables the measurement of pRNFL thickness and demonstrates thinning in the superior, inferior, and nasal quadrants. The pattern of pRNFL thinning varies by glaucoma subtype: in primary open angle glaucoma (POAG), pRNFL thinning tends to be greater inferiorly and inferotemporally compared with pseudoexfoliation glaucoma, where there is greater thinning superiorly and superonasally (Baniasadi et al., 2016). OCT has also led to greater appreciation that glaucoma results in early macular ganglion cell damage, which may be overlooked (Hood et al., 2013).

***Nonarteritic anterior ischemic optic neuropathy.*** OCT may be a useful accompaniment to the fundal examination in nonarteritic anterior ischemic optic neuropathy (NAION) by more precisely measuring the degree of optic disc edema in each clock-hour sector of the optic nerve head (Fig. 43.6, *A*—right eye). As NAION typically involves sectoral visual loss, there is a high degree of topographic correlation between the region of visual field loss, the region of the macula with GCL/GCIPL thinning, and the sector of the optic disc with the greatest degree of pRNFL thickening acutely and pRNFL atrophy chronically. OCT may also assist in following the resolution of optic disc edema and precisely measuring the optic disc and cup size in the fellow eye (a small cup size is a risk factor for NAION; see Fig. 43.6, *A*—left eye). The authors have observed GCL/GCIPL thinning as early as 10 days from onset of visual loss in NAION.

***Compressive optic neuropathy.*** Compressive optic neuropathy may result in either optic atrophy or optic disc edema, depending on the location of the compressive lesion. Optic disc edema may occur initially with intraorbital lesions or lesions within the optic canal, but compressive intracranial lesions typically cause only optic atrophy. In cases such as compression by pituitary adenoma, normal pRNFL with intact macular GCL/GCIPL thickness indicates a better prognosis for recovery of vision following decompression of the optic nerve or chiasm (Danesh-Meyer et al., 2008, 2015; Moon et al., 2011;

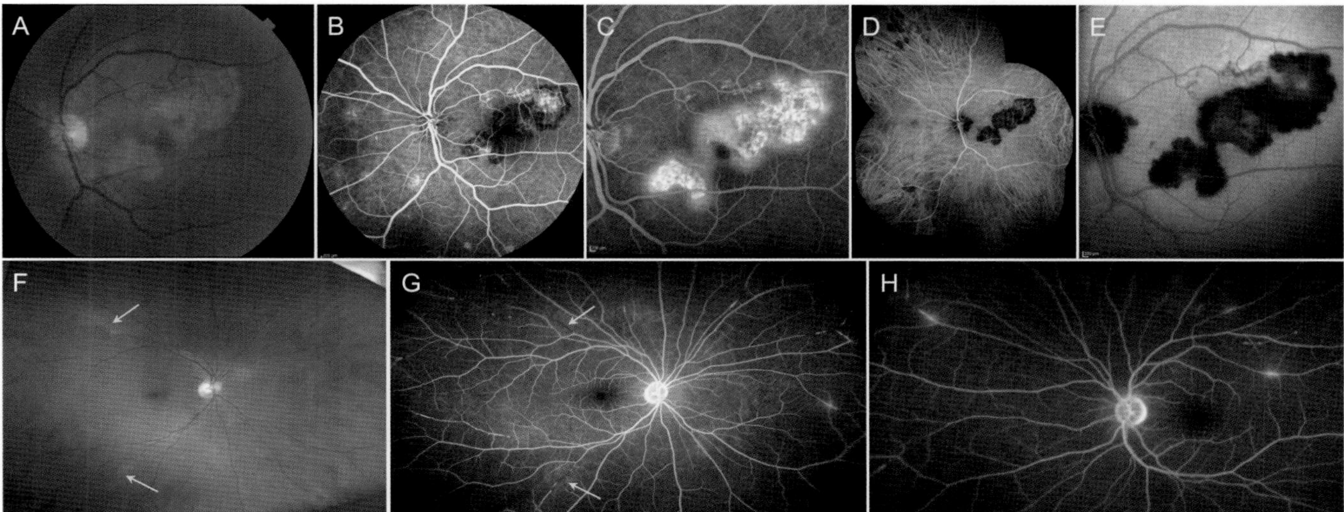


**Fig. 43.7 Examples of Fluorescein Angiography and Indocyanine Green Angiography. A–E,** Twenty-six-year-old man presenting with headache, blurred vision in the left eye, and multifocal strokes related to cerebral vasculitis. **A,** Color photography shows a placoid yellow-white retinal lesion involving the macula. **B,** Fluorescein angiography (FA) at 46 seconds (early) shows early blockage of the choroid by the lesion. **C,** FA at 13 minutes (late) shows staining of the lesion related to leakage of fluorescein. **D,** Early-phase indocyanine green angiography (ICGA) montage shows hypofluorescence of the lesion due to blockage. **E,** Late-phase ICGA (15 minutes) shows persistent hypofluorescence (blockage) due to the different molecular size of ICG and lack of extravasation from disrupted vessels. **F–H,** Forty-year-old man with confusion and headaches related to Susac syndrome. **F,** Wide-field Optos pseudo-color image shows two peripheral branch retinal artery occlusions associated with areas of retinal ischemia *(arrows)*. **G,** Numerous midsegment branch retinal arteriolar occlusions are evident on Optos FA (01:12) *(arrows)*. **H,** Late-phase FA images from the left eye show areas of vessel wall hyperfluorescence, which are characteristic of Susac syndrome.

Ohkubo et al., 2012). pRNFL and macular GCIPL thinning related to compression of the optic chiasm by a pituitary macroadenoma is shown in Fig. 43.6, *B*.

***Papilledema.*** OCT can be utilized to monitor the severity of papilledema by measuring the average and sectoral thicknesses of the peripapillary RNFL (see Fig. 43.6, *C*); it has been shown to correlate well with Frisen grade (OCT Sub-Study Committee for NORDIC Idiopathic Intracranial Hypertension Study Group et al., 2014; Rebolleda and Muñoz-Negrete, 2009; Scott et al., 2010). It may also be useful for excluding subtle papilledema in cases where the optic nerve appears congenitally crowded or there is uncertainty based on the fundus examination. OCT may also identify whether a reduction in the thickness of the pRNFL is related to an improvement of papilledema from effective treatment of intracranial hypertension (in which case the macular GCL/GCIPL thickness will be preserved) or to loss of retinal ganglion cells (RGCs) and consequent axonal atrophy of RGCs (in which case pRNFL improvement occurs with thinning in the macular GCL/GCIPL). Volumetric measurement of the optic nerve head and assessment of other features of the optic nerve, such as anterior deflection of Bruch's membrane, may also have utility for monitoring or diagnosing papilledema (Malhotra et al., 2018; Sibony et al., 2014; Wang et al., 2012). With OCT, chorioretinal folds and retinal wrinkles caused by optic disc edema can also be better assessed. In the Idiopathic Intracranial Hypertension Treatment Trial (IIHTT), full-thickness chorioretinal folds had the strongest correlation with opening pressure on elevated lumbar puncture, whereas other forms of peripapillary retinal wrinkles were the result of disc edema rather than distortion of the posterior globe from a pressurized optic nerve sheath (Sibony et al., 2015).

***Leber hereditary optic neuropathy.*** Leber hereditary optic neuropathy (LHON) is the prototypical mitochondrial optic neuropathy and results in sequential loss of the central visual field related to one of several mitochondrial DNA point mutations. Patients present with central or cecocentral scotomas, and fundus examination is characterized initially by hyperemic optic discs with fullness or pseudoedema of the peripapillary RNFL and peripapillary telangiectasias. These changes may be subtle or not apparent initially on fundus examination. OCT imaging demonstrates several features of this condition that may be helpful for early diagnosis (see Fig. 43.6, *D*). OCT reveals mild peripapillary RNFL thickening, which evolves to temporal pRNFL thinning chronically. Macular GCL/GCIPL segmentation demonstrates central thinning nasal to the fovea, which progresses inferiorly, temporally, and then superiorly before more widespread GCL/GCIPL thinning becomes evident (Balducci et al., 2016). The initial GCL/GCIPL thinning may be evident prior to the development of symptoms, offering the potential to identify a window when therapy could be effective.

***Optic disc drusen.*** OCT is increasingly used for the assessment of buried optic disc drusen in order to distinguish pseudopapilledema from true papilledema. Enhanced depth imaging (EDI)-OCT protocols that increase the depth of penetration by moving the imaging device closer to the eye and recording an inverted retinal image are superior to standard spectral domain OCT imaging for this purpose. EDI-OCT identifies optic disc drusen as signal-poor cores surrounded by short hyperreflective bands (Fig. 43.7) and may be more sensitive than orbital ultrasound (Merchant et al., 2013). A consensus protocol for the assessment of optic disc drusen using OCT has outlined a standardized approach in order to avoid misinterpretation of OCT findings (Malmqvist et al., 2018).

### Utility of Optical Coherence Tomography in Neurological Disorders

The retina and optic nerve are the only parts of the central nervous system that can be visualized directly. OCT has been demonstrated to

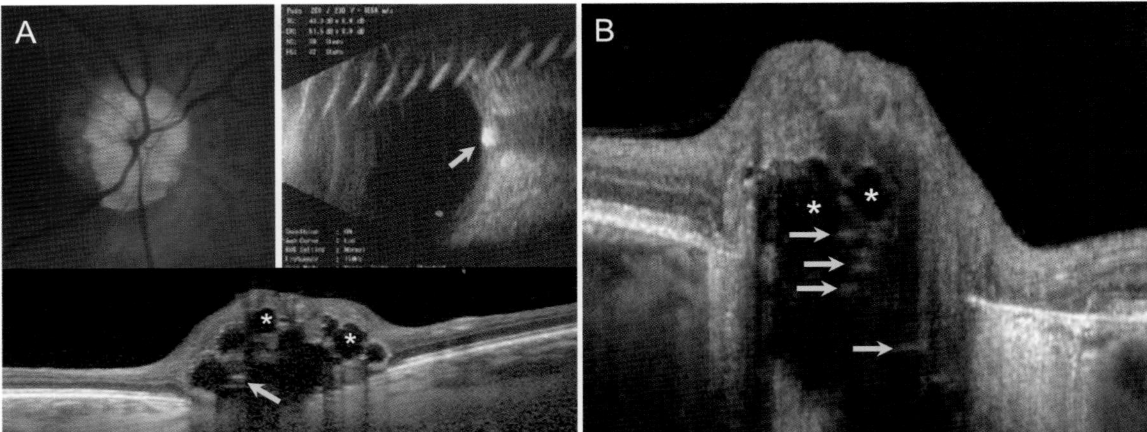


**Fig. 43.8 Enhanced Depth Imaging–Optical Coherence Tomography of Optic Disc Drusen. A,** When visible, optic disc drusen appear as refractile bodies on the optic nerve head *(upper left)*. Orbital ultrasound *(upper right)* demonstrates hyperechoic signal at the optic nerve head *(arrow)*. Enhanced depth imaging–optical coherence tomography *(bottom)* allows greater depth of penetration, and optic nerve head drusen appear as signal-poor regions within the optic nerve head *(asterisks)* surrounded by hyperreflective bands *(arrows)*. **B,** Hyperreflective bands *(arrows)* surrounding hyporeflective drusen cores in another patient with buried optic disc drusen. *(A Images courtesy Lasse Malmqvist, MD, PhD and Steffen Hamman, PhD, FEBO.)*

detect retinal changes that occur in neurological disorders; therefore it may serve as useful clinical and research tool for finding biomarkers of disease progression.

***Multiple sclerosis.*** MS is commonly associated with optic neuritis, which can present subacutely or acutely with optic disc edema if the anterior optic nerve is inflamed. Chronically, both anterior and retrobulbar optic neuritis results in pRNFL and macular GCL/GCIPL thinning from neuroaxonal loss secondary to demyelination. It has been shown that macular GCL/GCIPL and peripapillary RNFL thickness may also be reduced in patients with MS and no prior history of optic neuritis, with proposed mechanisms including subclinical inflammation or primary RGC and axonal degeneration. Change in pRNFL and macular GCL thickness mirror other markers of visual and global MS disability (Fisher et al., 2006; Galetta et al., 2012; Gordon-Lipkin et al., 2007; Petzold et al., 2017; Ratchford et al., 2013; Walter et al., 2012).

***Alzheimer disease.*** Postmortem studies of retinas in Alzheimer disease (AD) have shown loss of parafoveal RGCs and peripheral RGCs, with an increase in midperipheral retinal astrocytes in patients with AD (Blanks et al, 1996a, 1996b). Although the results of OCT studies have varied, superior and inferior pRNFL thinning and macular GCL seem to correlate with the degree of cognitive impairment in patients with mild cognitive impairment (MCI) or AD (Ascaso et al., 2014; Cunha et al., 2017; Kwon et al., 2017; Mutlu et al., 2018; Sánchez et al., 2018; Wang et al., 2015). Although the range of normal macular GCL thickness or peripapillary RNFL thickness may be too great to distinguish normal patients from those with MCI or AD, an accelerated thinning of pRNFL or macular GCL in patients with clinically diagnosed MCI or AD may serve as a useful biomarker for monitoring the efficacy of therapies targeted at preventing neuronal loss.

***Parkinson disease.*** Although there are many explanations for the development of visual symptoms in patients with Parkinson disease, one underappreciated explanation is impaired foveal visual processing as evidenced by changes in VEP measurements, pattern ERG, reduction in contrast sensitivity, and alterations in color perception. Changes in pattern ERG and contrast sensitivity are somewhat specific for RGC dysfunction, which may be driven by changes in dopaminergic amacrine cells that alter the receptive field organization of RGCs (Bodis-Wallner, 2009; Bodis-Wallner and Tzelepi, 1998; Djamgoz et al., 1997). Reported retinal changes measured by OCT in PD patients include thinning within the pRNFL, macular GCL, and combined outer nuclear and photoreceptor layers (Inzelberg et al., 2004; Kaur et al., 2015; Roth et al., 2014; Sari et al., 2015).

## Retinal Angiography

FA and indocyanine green angiography (ICGA) are techniques used to image the retinal and choroidal circulations following intravenous injection of a fluorescent dye. FA utilizes fluorescein sodium dye injected through an antecubital vein. White light from a flash is then passed through a blue excitation filter. Blue light with a wavelength of 465–490 nm is absorbed by unbound fluorescein molecules that fluoresce and emit light of a longer wavelength (520–530 nm). The emitted light is captured using a barrier filter and recorded as digital images. Images from the FA are time stamped in relation to the time of injection. Filling of the choroidal circulation via the short posterior ciliary arteries normally begins within 12–15 seconds in adult patients and may occur sooner in children. Central retinal artery filling usually begins 1–3 seconds later. The retinal arteries, arterioles, and capillaries fill during the early arteriovenous (AV) phase, followed by laminar (late AV phase) filling of the retinal veins. Peak total fluorescence occurs at about 30 seconds followed by recirculation phases. A perifoveal capillary-free zone is normally seen due to blockage of choroidal fluorescence by xanthophyll pigment and tightly packed RPE cells. Fluorescein is normally absent from the retinal vessels by 10 minutes, although some structures, including the peripapillary sclera and Bruch's membrane, continue to fluoresce. ICGA is based on principles similar to those governing FA, but ICG is almost completely bound, with little diffusion through the fenestrations of the choriocapillaris. It also fluoresces in the near-infrared range (795–805 nm), which allows it to better penetrate through

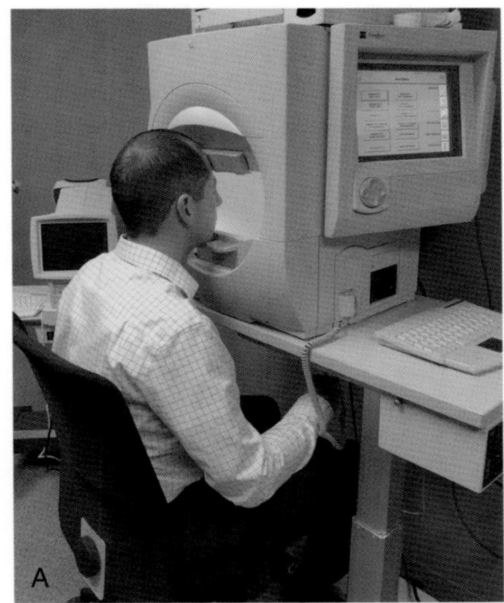


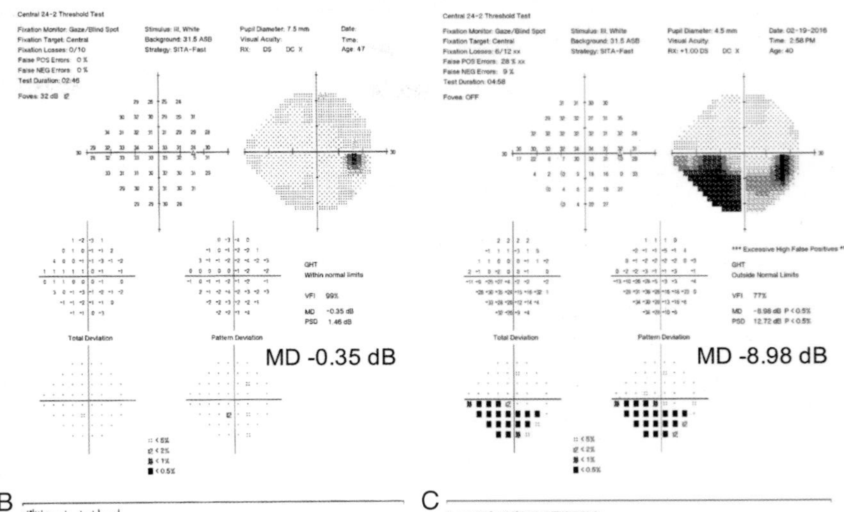


**Fig. 43.9 Standard Automated Perimetry. A,** A test subject seated at a Humphrey Field Analyzer II (Zeiss). **B,** Sample normal visual field analysis report for the 24-2 Swedish interactive thresholding algorithm (SITA) fast testing procedure showing detection threshold plot *(upper left)*, gray-scale plot *(upper right)*, total deviation plot *(lower left)*, and pattern deviation plot *(lower right)*. Overall performance is measured by the mean deviation score. **C,** 24-2 SITA standard report for a patient with an inferior arcuate defect in the right eye related to nonarteritic anterior ischemic optic neuropathy.

substances that might block fluorescein transmission, including pigment, fluid, lipid, and blood.

Abnormalities on FA or ICGA are characterized in terms of hypofluorescence (due to vascular filling defect or blocking), hyperfluorescence (due to fluorescein leakage, staining, pooling, or window defects), or autofluorescence seen prior to fluorescein/ICG injection (see Fig. 43.7).

### Orbital Ultrasound

Orbital ultrasound may be utilized to better assess the ocular structure, particularly when a slit lamp or fundus examination cannot fully assess the relevant anatomy. Frequency transducers generate high-frequency sound waves (in the range of 12–20 MHz for posterior pole imaging and 30–50 MHz for anterior segment ultrasound biomicroscopy) that are reflected back by tissue. The echoes returning to the transducer are translated into either a time-amplitude scan (A-scan), consisting of a series of spikes corresponding to tissue interface zones, or a brightness-amplitude scan (B-scan), consisting of cross-sectional 2D images. Orbital ultrasound is commonly used to calculate axial eye length for cataract surgery, measure the size of choroidal tumors, assess for foreign bodies or globe integrity in the setting of trauma, identify retinal detachment, and assess the posterior pole in the setting of dense cataract or vitreous hemorrhage. In neuro-ophthalmic practice, orbital ultrasound may be useful to distinguish between papilledema and pseudopapilledema by identifying buried optic disc drusen, which appear as hyperreflective foci due to their calcium content (Fig. 43.8, *A*).

## INVESTIGATIONS OF VISUAL FUNCTION

Perimetric assessment of the visual field and electrodiagnostic studies of retinal and optic nerve function are the principal modalities used in conjunction with the ophthalmic or neuro-ophthalmic examination to assess visual function.

### Perimetric Assessment of the Visual Field

#### Standard Automated Perimetry

Standard automated perimetry (SAP) is the most utilized form of automated visual field testing and measures threshold values for detecting nonmoving (static) light stimuli. The Humphrey Field Analyzer (HFA; Carl Zeiss, Jena, Germany) and Octopus perimeters (Haag-Streit, Köniz, Switzerland) are the most commonly used such devices (Donahue, 1999). In SAP, the patient places his or her head in a chin rest in the center of the testing bowl and is instructed to maintain fixation on a central target (Fig. 43.9, *A*). Near refractive error is corrected with lenses and the contralateral eye is occluded. The perimeter projects brief light stimuli at defined locations within the visual field and the patient responds with a handheld button when a light stimulus is seen. Thresholds at each test location in the visual field are derived from either a staircase method (full threshold test) or proprietary algorithms, such as the Swedish interactive testing algorithm (SITA; HFA), to reduce test time. Threshold values are compared with those of age-matched controls to generate a total deviation map. The pattern deviation map is then calculated to better identify regions of focal visual field loss (see Fig. 43.9, *B*). The most commonly used automated static visual field algorithms assess the central 24–30 degrees of vision, which is sufficient to identify most neurological causes of visual loss (Szatmáry et al., 2002).

Automated static perimetry is adept at quantifying central visual loss, has been well validated over decades of use, is widely available in eye care providers' offices, and does not take long to perform. However, patients with inattention or cognitive impairment and slow response time may be produce unreliable results. Moreover, this technique cannot effectively evaluate the far peripheral vision, and it is limited in characterizing vision in patients with severe central visual loss.

#### Goldmann Kinetic Perimetry

Kinetic perimetry utilizes moving targets of varying size and intensity to assess the full extent of a patient's visual field. Hans Goldmann

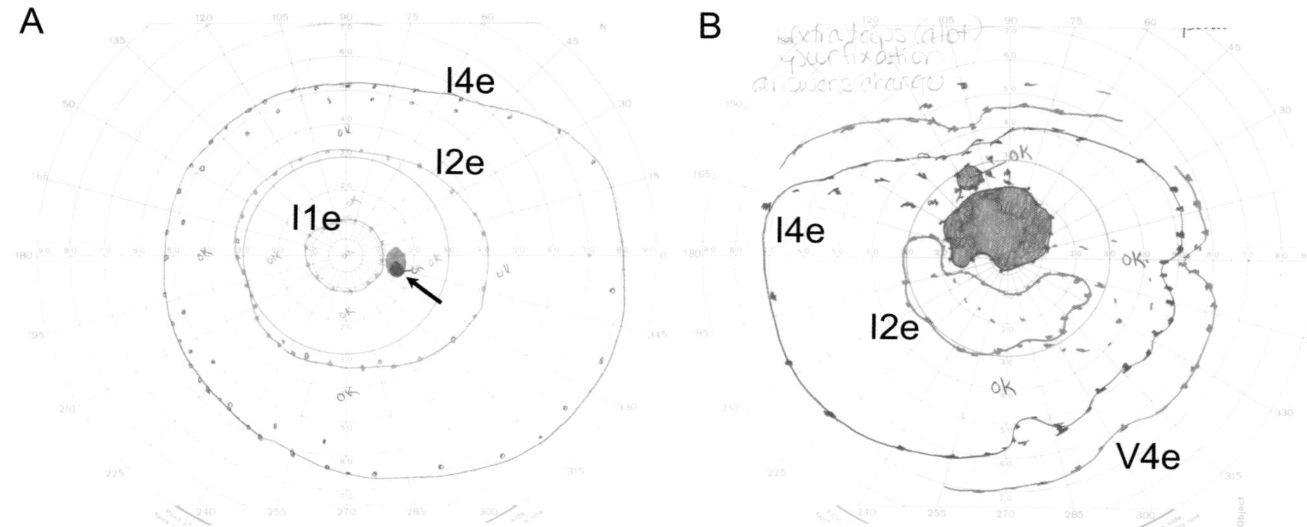


**Fig. 43.10 Goldmann Kinetic Perimetry. A,** Goldmann visual field (GVF) of a patient's right eye shows no visual loss and a normal span for the I4e, I2e, and I1e isopters. The physiological blind spot to the I2e and I4e isopters is mapped as a shaded region *(arrow)*. The V4e stimulus was seen throughout the location of the physiological blind spot. **B,** GVF of the left eye of a patient with Leber hereditary optic neuropathy and visual acuity of 20/150. He has a large cecocentral scotoma to the V4e and I4e isopters and a remaining island of I2e isopter inferiorly and temporally.

invented the Goldmann kinetic perimeter in 1945, and it remains the standard form of kinetic perimetry. However, today it is performed less commonly than automated perimetry owing to the need for a skilled perimetrist or physician to administer the test and map the patient's visual field. Although it is a time-intensive test, Goldmann perimetry provides exquisite characterization of the topography of the visual field, and the interaction of the perimetrist with the patient makes Goldmann perimetry advantageous in patients with poor central vision or inattention.

The test is performed in a semispherical white bowl with standard background illumination of 1000 asp. A topographical map of the patient's visual field is created by presenting circular light stimuli that vary in size and intensity. An isopter is created for each stimulus and encloses the region of the visual field in which that stimulus is detected. Although stimuli of larger size and light intensity are identified in the periphery, stimuli that are small and dim are detected only centrally. Scotomata, including the physiological blind spot, are represented as shaded regions within the isopter. Six stimulus sizes are available, ranging from size 0 (0.0625 $mm^2$) to size V (64 $mm^2$). Light intensity is adjusted by an amount represented by an Arabic number (1–4) and letter (a–e). A decrease in the Arabic number by 1 represents an attenuation of the light by 5 dB, and a decrease in the letter by 1 represents an attenuation of 1 dB. A combination of the I1e, I2e, I4e, III4e, and V4e isopters is most frequently used. A normal and an abnormal GVF are shown in Fig. 43.10. The Octopus 900 perimeter (Haag-Streit, Switzerland) is the modern equivalent of the Goldmann perimeter and is able to perform both manual and semiautomated kinetic perimetry in addition to versions of SAP.

## Microperimetry

Newer fundus-based perimeters, termed microperimeters, serve exclusively to test the central visual field and may be particularly well suited for assessing visual loss related to retinal disorders or optic neuropathies causing central scotomata (Altpeter et al., 2013; Midena et al., 2007; Sato et al., 2013; Wu et al., 2015). These microperimeters utilize a scanning-laser ophthalmoscope to track the retina and target visual field stimuli directly onto specific locations of the macula, eliminating the effects of eye movements and poor visual fixation that typically affect the sensitivity of standard perimetry (Fig. 43.11). Fundus-based perimeters often display a distribution of the patient's fixation and calculate a preferred retinal locus and fixation instability, measures that can be useful for understanding visual function with respect to structural abnormalities of the retina (Wu et al., 2015). Newer fundus-based perimeters are capable of assessing up to 30 degrees of the visual field (the same as for standard automated perimeters; Montesano et al., 2019).

## Tangent Screen

The tangent screen method of visual field testing can be performed in an office setting using a white stimulus against a black background. The stimulus is moved from a nonseeing area of the peripheral vision toward the center at multiple radial locations in order to map the region of intact visual field based on the patient's responses. This method may be useful when automated or kinetic perimetry cannot be performed reliably or when there is suspicion for a nonorganic constriction of the visual fields. In physiological visual field constriction, the span of the visual field on the tangent screen measured at 2 m is double the span measured at 1 m and with half the stimulus size. In nonorganic visual field constriction, the span of the visual field constriction does not expand appropriately; this configuration is referred to as nonphysiological "tubular" constriction. A modified tangent screen test using a laser pointer stimulus can be performed quickly and is more sensitive than confrontation visual field testing to identify visual field defects detected by SAP (Lee et al., 2003).

# Electrodiagnostic Studies

Electrodiagnostic tests, including the electroretinogram (ERG) and the VEP, provide objective data on the function of the retina and optic nerve, respectively, and play an important role in the diagnosis and monitoring of conditions affecting these elements of the visual system.

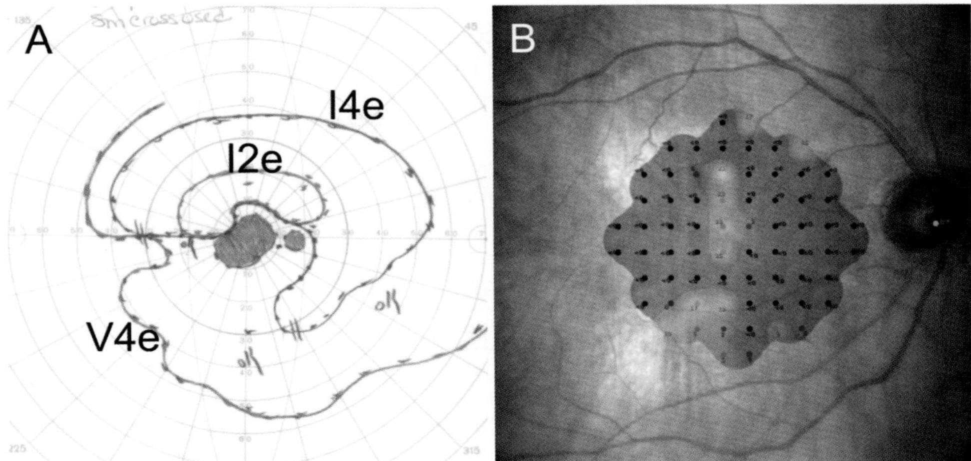


**Fig. 43.11 Central Island of Vision Revealed by Microperimetry.** **A,** Goldmann visual field (GVF) of a 52-year-old man with nonarteritic anterior ischemic optic neuropathy of the right eye and visual acuity of 20/50. GVF shows a central and inferior defect with an altitudinal quality nasally, but there is a large scotoma to the V4e (largest and brightest) test stimulus. **B,** Microperimetry (MAIA perimeter, Centervue) shows a preserved island of vision within the scotoma, explaining this patient's disproportionately good visual acuity. Test points of a 10-2 test grid are localized to the retina using scanning laser ophthalmoscopic eye tracking to compensate for retinal movement and avoid fixation losses.

## Electroretinography

The full-field ERG assesses retinal function by measuring the electrical potential generated by the photoreceptors and other retinal neurons following stimulation by light. This response, which is recorded by an electrode resting on the corneal surface, is a summed response across the retina. Within-normal results thus do not exclude focal pathology. Parameters including the state of retinal adaptation (dark adapted/scotopic versus light-adapted/photopic), stimulus wavelength and intensity, and stimulus dynamics (isolated flash versus flicker) determine the relative contributions of rods versus cones. After 30 minutes of dark adaptation, scotopic responses are recorded, beginning with a dim flash to elicit a rod-only response from "on" bipolar cells (Fig. 43.12, *A*—left) followed by brighter flashes to elicit a mixed rod-cone response. Components of the resulting responses include the a-wave, which is a negative deflection resulting from hyperpolarization of photoreceptors, and a larger b-wave arising from the subsequent depolarization of bipolar cells and Müller cells. Oscillatory potentials, which are wavelets on the ascending limb of the b-wave, represent the inhibitory effect of inner retinal amacrine cells. After 10 minutes of light adaptation to suppress rod responses, photopic cone-drive responses to a single bright flash and a 30-Hz flicker are recorded (see Fig. 43.12, *A*—right).

The pattern of responses and any abnormalities provide insight into retinal function and underlying pathophysiology. For example, rod-driven responses are more impaired than cone responses in rod-cone dystrophies, whereas cone responses are selectively impaired in dystrophies affecting only cone function (see Fig. 43.12, *B* and *C*). An extinguished ERG without recordable responses can be seen in advanced RP or in cancer-associated retinopathy. An electronegative ERG occurs when the b-wave amplitude is smaller than the a-wave and is associated with impaired photoreceptor to bipolar cell signaling. This finding can be associated with central retinal artery occlusion and inherited retinal degenerations including congenital stationary night blindness. It may also be a clue that occult vision loss is related to melanoma-associated retinopathy (MAR; see Fig. 43.12, *D*). Prolongation of the implicit time, which is the time to peak response, can have clinical significance. Finally, isolated abnormalities of oscillatory potentials can be seen in conditions that affect inner retinal amacrine cells such as early diabetic retinopathy or mild central retinal vein occlusion.

### Multifocal Electroretinogram

Multifocal ERG (mfERG) is used to evaluate macular function by simultaneously recording a distribution of retinal responses across the macular region while the patient fixates on an array of flickering hexagons. mfERG may be useful in disorders such as RP where only macular function is preserved, and it may be the key to diagnosis of early cone-rod dystrophies (occult macular dystrophy) or autoimmune retinopathies in which the fundal appearance may be normal. This test can also be useful in distinguishing retinal (especially macular) from optic nerve pathology.

### Visual Evoked Potentials

VEPs are generated in the visual cortex as a response to a visual stimulus. A flash or pattern-reversal stimulus is presented on an electronic screen or via light-emitting diode (LED) goggles, and the response is recorded using occipital scalp electrodes. The variability in the responses of normal individuals limits the clinical utility of the flash VEP, but flash VEP may still provide visual information in infants, small children, or patients with poor fixation otherwise unable to cooperate with more sensitive testing methods. Pattern VEP, using most often a black and white checkerboard stimulus that reverses in a regular phase frequency, is the preferred study in most adults and elicits a more robust and reproducible response. The pattern reversal stimulus maintains constant luminance and preferentially stimulates RGCs that respond to orientation and edge detection.

At least 100 sequential visual stimuli are presented to generate an average waveform and reduce noise. The P100 waveform is the basis for interpretation of the VEP response. It is a positive (downward) deflection on the electrographic tracing that occurs at approximately 100 ms from the time of stimulus presentation in normal subjects. The latency of the P100 waveform peak is measured in each eye individually and compared with the fellow eye and with normative control data from the laboratory in which the test was performed. Amplitude is recorded but is less informative. Variables known to prolong the P100

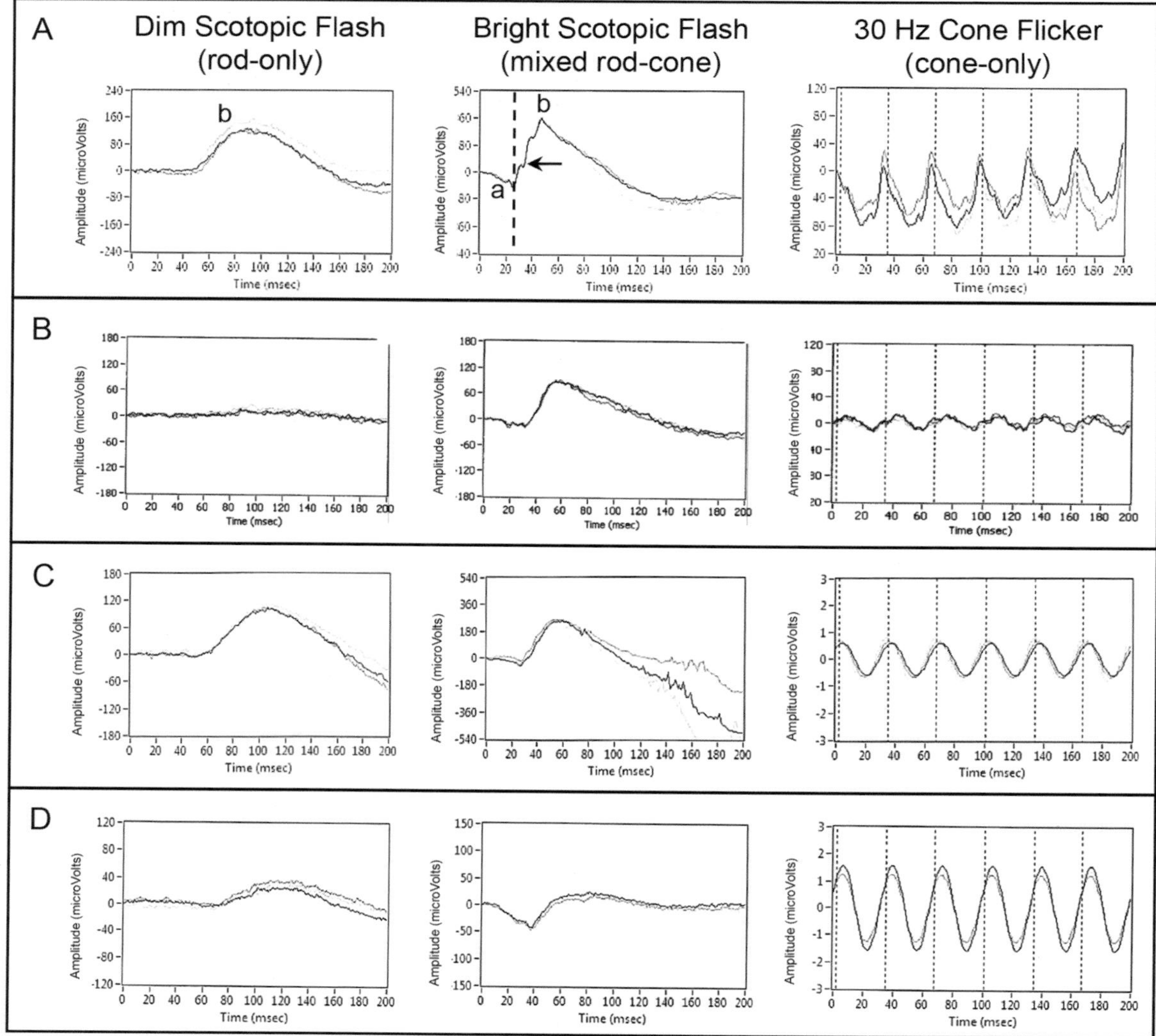


**Fig. 43.12 Examples of Normal and Abnormal Full-field Electroretinogram Responses. A,** Normal electroretinogram (ERG) responses. An a-wave is not measured after the dim scotopic flash. Oscillatory potentials *(arrow)* are seen in the ascending b-wave following the bright scotopic flash. **B,** In retinitis pigmentosa, impaired rod function results in abnormal rod-only responses. A secondary involvement of cones also leads to depressed photopic responses. As disease advances, all responses may become extinguished. **C,** In achromatopsia, a retinal dystrophy in which cone function is impaired, the cone flicker response is essentially absent. The rod-driven dim flash response remains normal, and intact rod function results in a minimally depressed mixed rod-cone signal. **D,** Electronegative ERG in melanoma-associated retinopathy. Following the bright scotopic flash, the a-wave is larger than the b-wave. There is a marked reduction in the dim scotopic response. *(ERG tracings courtesy Rachel Huckfeldt, MD, PhD.)*

latency in normal patients include advancing age, male gender, smaller pattern-reversal stimulus check size, and smaller pupillary diameter (resulting in less retinal luminance). Visual acuity, level of alertness, size of the stimulus field, and variability in scalp electrode placement also influence P100 waveform characteristics (American Clinical Neurophysiology Society, 2006).

VEPs may be useful in the detection of optic nerve disease that is subtle enough to evade detection through examination of the pupils, visual fields, visual acuity, and optic disc appearance. Prolongation of the P100 waveform latency more than 2.5–3 standard deviations above the control mean is considered abnormal and is an indication of optic nerve damage (American Clinical Neurophysiology Society, 2006). Although VEPs are sensitive to optic nerve dysfunction, they are not specific to the exact cause. Glaucoma, compressive, ischemic, toxic, nutritional, and hereditary causes of optic neuropathy may all be associated with P100 waveform abnormalities. Acute optic neuritis often causes severe abnormalities of the P100 waveform, and although the VEP most often subsequently improves, it generally remains delayed even with seemingly full clinical visual recovery. For this reason, in the appropriate clinical context, the finding of a delayed P100 latency in a patient with a clinically isolated syndrome other than optic neuritis can help prove dissemination of lesions in time and space to suggest a diagnosis of MS (Asselman et al., 1975; Leocani et al., 2018). The relatively high sensitivity of VEPs also supports their use in ruling out an optic neuropathy; normal pattern-reversal VEPs in the setting of profound monocular visual loss, normal neuroimaging, and a normal funduscopic examination strongly indicates nonorganic visual loss.

## CONCLUSION

Ocular structural and functional investigations are a tremendous aid in the diagnosis and management of patients with visual loss due to ophthalmic and neurological disorders. Clinicians benefit greatly from understanding the fundamental methods, uses, and limitations of these diagnostic tests. Often a combination of various investigations serves to optimally identify and characterize retinal and neuro-ophthalmic disorders affecting vision.

*The complete reference list is available online at https://expertconsult.inkling.com/.* 

# 44

# Neuropsychology

Jane S. Paulsen, Carissa Gehl

## OUTLINE



*Neuropsychology* is the scientific study of neural correlates for cognition and behavior, with a specific clinical interest in patients presenting with a range of medical, neurological, and psychiatric illnesses. Neuropsychologists are specialized clinicians who receive extended fellowship training (with available board certification) in functional neuroanatomy, neurobiology, psychopharmacology, neurological illness or injury, neuroimaging, psychometric and statistical principles of neurocognitive measures, and clinical psychology. Neuropsychological evaluation refines neuroimaging and neurological examinations by operating from a biopsychosocial framework to determine the extent to which cognition and behavior are affected by brain dysfunction. Neuropsychologists aim to characterize and objectively quantify abilities ranging from simple sensory and motor functions to complex "higher cognitive abilities" that include cognitive processing speed, attention, language, visuoperception, constructional praxis, memory, executive functioning (behavioral, cognitive, and motivational aspects), and emotional/personality functioning.

In this chapter, we begin by explaining the goals and utility of neuropsychology and describing the neuropsychological evaluation. Guidelines are then suggested for brief cognitive screenings that may be useful for neurologists in clinical settings. Finally, the typical patterns of cognitive impairments associated with major neurological disorders are discussed.

## GOALS OF NEUROPSYCHOLOGY

When neural damage is present or cognitive changes are observed, a neuropsychological evaluation is appropriate. The prominent neuropsychologist Arthur Benton (1975) best described neuropsychology as "a refinement of clinical neurological observation [that] serves the function of enhancing clinical observation [and] is closely allied to clinical neurological evaluation and in fact can be considered to be a special form of it" (p. 68). Neuropsychological assessment aims to extend the neurological examination by: (1) providing important information for differential diagnosis and prognosis; (2) identifying the cognitive, emotional, and behavioral deficits of disease or injury and characterizing their severity; (3) intervention and functional needs such as guiding treatment by using test results to select effective rehabilitation strategies, determining functional capacity and decision-making abilities for level-of-care decisions, driving and work capacity, assessing medication cognitive side effects, and establishing candidacy for surgical procedures; and (4) monitoring cognitive changes and treatment effectiveness across time. Neuropsychological assessment is also frequently used in forensic settings and for neuroscience research, but discussion on these topics is beyond the clinical focus of this chapter (Schoenberg et al., 2011).

Before the advent of neuroimaging in the 1970s and 1980s, one of the main goals of neuropsychology was lesion localization. Today,

TABLE 44.1 **Neuropsychological Characteristics of Cortical Versus Subcortical Dementia Using Alzheimer Disease and Huntington Disease as Examples**

| | Alzheimer Disease (Cortical Dementia) | Huntington Disease (Subcortical Dementia) |
|---|---|---|
| **Learning and Memory** | | |
| Episodic memory | Impaired encoding/consolidation<br>Poor delayed recall and recognition memory | Impaired information retrieval<br>Recognition memory is better than delayed recall |
| Retrograde amnesia | Severe, temporally graded, retrograde amnesia | Mild, nongraded, retrograde amnesia |
| Priming | Impaired | Preserved |
| Implicit procedural/motor learning | Preserved | Impaired |
| Implicit cognitive skill learning | Preserved | Impaired |
| Attention/concentration | Relatively preserved | Poor auditory and visual attention |
| Processing speed | Relatively intact | Very slow |
| **Executive Functioning** | | |
| Set shifting | Better able to shift focus | Difficulty with perseveration |
| Working memory | Mild deficits in ability to manipulate information, but preserved phonological loop and visuospatial sketchpad | Early notable deficits in phonological loop, visuospatial sketchpad, and ability to manipulate information |
| **Language and Semantic Knowledge** | | |
| Speech | Preserved | Dysarthric and slow |
| Fluency | More impaired semantic fluency than phonemic fluency | Severe and equal impairment in phonemic and semantic fluency |
| Naming | Impaired; more semantic errors (e.g., calling a lion "an animal") | Relatively preserved; more perceptual errors (e.g., calling a bucket "a cup") |
| Structure of semantic knowledge | Tend to focus on concrete perceptual information | Able to focus on abstract conceptual knowledge |

*Adapted from Salmon, D.P., Filoteo, J.V., 2007. Neuropsychology of cortical versus subcortical dementia syndromes. Semin Neurol 27, 7–21.*

neuropsychology has shifted toward differential diagnosis when lesions may not be evident or in conditions with no clear biomarkers. For example, neuropsychologists assist in the early identification of various dementias, since they are primarily diagnosed based on patterns of clear cognitive declines and behavioral disturbances: Table 44.1 gives a comparison of cortical versus subcortical dementias as an example. Neuropsychological testing is also useful for diagnosing "non-neurological" conditions that can affect cognitive functioning or masquerade as neurocognitive disease, such as dementia of depression or somatoform disorders. Exaggerated and manufactured symptoms can also be clearly identified through the use of stand-alone and embedded measures of symptom and performance validity.

Another goal of neuropsychology is to accurately describe cognitive deficits and their severity. Even when the cause of cognitive dysfunction is clear (e.g., traumatic brain injury) or lesions are evident on imaging, the cognitive and behavioral manifestations of neural damage can be heterogeneous. The interaction among symptom onset, etiology, and patient characteristics results in a wide range of individual variability in cognitive deficits. For instance, the neuropsychological profiles of stroke and tumor patients can be very dissimilar even after matching for lesion location (tumor patients show notably less severe language deficits in the left hemisphere, presumably due to the acute versus chronic etiologies; Anderson et al., 1990). Repeated neuropsychological evaluations are also useful for monitoring the decline of neurodegenerative diseases over time, given the potential for varying degrees of disease progression across patients.

In addition to offering information regarding the diagnosis and clinical manifestation of neuroanatomical dysfunction, neuropsychological assessment is unique in its ability to guide treatment and assist with decisions regarding functional needs. Neuropsychologists are capable of utilizing objective test data to thoroughly assess patients' abilities to make legal, financial, and healthcare decisions; their need for supervision; their ability to live independently and to return to work (Demakis, 2012). Neurocognitive assessments may also be used to guide treatment plans by identifying cognitive deficits for specific rehabilitation strategies. For example, patients with behavioral disinhibition and poor emotional regulation due to lesions in the orbitofrontal cortex can be targeted for behavioral modification strategies and training in self-monitoring (Sohlberg and Turkstra, 2011). Neuropsychological assessments are also useful for evaluating patients' candidacy for certain surgical procedures. Neurosurgeons considering a temporal lobectomy for refractory epilepsy often call on neuropsychologists to conduct Wada testing to localize language, memory, or motor functioning in order to minimize postoperative cognitive losses. Neuropsychological assessment is also used prior to the placement of a deep brain stimulator to help predict post-surgical outcomes.

Lastly, neurocognitive testing is useful for monitoring treatment effectiveness and patients' recovery from acquired brain injuries. For instance, neuropsychologists use their expertise to determine whether a coma patient has progressed into a vegetative or minimally conscious state (Giacino and Whyte, 2005). Accurate monitoring is vital, given the differences in clinical outcomes for each level of consciousness and the danger of making erroneous decisions regarding the withdrawal of treatment. Treatment effectiveness can also be monitored using repeat assessments to determine whether medical, pharmacological, and rehabilitation interventions are having their desired cognitive effects. Monitoring treatment effectiveness leads to more efficient utilization of resources by updating treatment plans as necessary.

## NEUROPSYCHOLOGICAL EVALUATION

Depending on the referral question and clinical setting, neuropsychological assessments can range from quick bedside assessments to

**BOX 44.1 Heaton Adaptation of Halstead–Reitan Neuropsychological Test Battery**

Tactual performance test
Finger oscillation test
Category test
Seashore rhythm test
Speech sounds perception test
Aphasia screening test
Sensory-perceptual examination
Grip strength test
Tactile form recognition test
Wechsler adult intelligence scale—revised
Wechsler memory scale—revised

*Adapted from Heaton, R.K., Grant, I., Matthews, C.G., 1991. Comprehensive Norms for Expanded Halstead-Reitan Battery: Demographic Corrections, Research Findings, and Clinical Applications. Psychological Assessment Resources, Odessa, FL.*

extended evaluations that include formal standardized testing and a comprehensive clinical interview. A complete neuropsychological interview covers the onset and course of the patient's cognitive and mood problems, current functional capacity, developmental background, medical, psychiatric, and family history, academic performance, vocational achievements, and social background. Information obtained from collateral sources such as caregivers or spouses about the patient's medical and psychosocial history can also be critical because many patients lack insight into their deficits. Besides gathering patient-reported information, the goals of the neuropsychological interview are to develop hypotheses about the patient's cognitive status and to establish rapport that will elicit their best performance on testing. Behavioral observations made during the interview and testing are also an important source of information that can influence test selection and interpretation. After a clinical interview is completed, the following cognitive domains are assessed: sensory, motor, intellectual functioning, processing speed, attention, language, visuoperception, constructional praxis, memory, executive functioning (behavioral, cognitive, and motivational aspects), functional capacity, and emotional/personality functioning.

## Test Administration

Early approaches to neuropsychological evaluation tended to use a fixed battery approach requiring that the same tests are administered to every patient in a standardized manner. One example of a fixed battery is the Halstead–Reitan battery (Box 44.1), for which comprehensive norms have been published by Heaton and colleagues (Heaton et al., 1991). While this approach had the benefit of providing comprehensive assessment of cognitive functioning, the length of the battery (up to 8 hours), which was not tolerated by all patients, was not always necessary to address the referral question, and is often incompatible with the limited reimbursement schedules in managed care. For these reasons, the flexible battery (or hypothesis-driven battery) is more commonly used today.

The flexible battery approach allows neuropsychologists to develop a test battery based on the referral question, patient's history, and clinical interview. In the flexible battery approach, a brief set of basic tests is initially administered, and additional tests of more specific abilities are used to conduct in-depth follow-up assessments based on each patient's needs. For an example of this, see the Iowa-Benton method as illustrated in Fig. 44.1 (Tranel, 2008). Considerations when selecting tests include age, primary language, level of education, ethnicity/cultural factors, reading level, expected level of global cognitive impairment (to avoid ceiling or floor effects in testing), and physical disabilities (Smith et al., 2008). Although this approach is more tailored to the individual needs of the patient (and is therefore briefer), it can be less comprehensive than the fixed-battery approach. Most neuropsychologists' approaches fall somewhere between the use of a set battery and a completely individualized examination.

## Test Interpretation

The interpretation of cognitive test results is central to the role of the neuropsychologist and differentiates neuropsychology from all other disciplines. Accurate interpretation of neuropsychological test results depends on a comprehensive understanding of the neuroanatomical correlates of cognition, neurological disease processes, *and* psychometric testing principles. One cannot simply administer a test, look at the score, and declare that the score indicates intact/impaired cognitive functioning. Test interpretation requires an understanding of test validity and reliability, sensitivity and specificity, likelihood ratios, and score distributions to avoid over- or underdiagnosing cognitive deficits. Substantial intraindividual differences exist in cognitive abilities, and a small number of poor test performances within a larger battery of tests is common among the general population. Cognitive test performances are also impacted by extra-neurological factors such as the number of tests administered, where cut scores are placed, the probability of certain test scores occurring, and the demographic characteristics of the patient (Iverson and Brooks, 2011). Proper test interpretation requires that all of these variables are considered and that conclusions are based on recognizable patterns of test results rather than the interpretation of test scores in isolation.

Neuropsychological test interpretation is also dependent on an understanding of the scientific and theoretical concepts that underlie cognitive tests. No cognitive test measures a single isolated aspect of cognitive functioning. Most neuropsychological tests engage multiple cognitive abilities simultaneously. To illustrate, verbal memory tests (e.g., word list memory tasks) assess memory functioning, but they are also dependent on the patient's attention, processing speed, and executive functioning. Therefore, an impaired score on a verbal memory task does not necessarily indicate a primary memory impairment. It is the neuropsychologist's task to determine which cognitive deficits are actually causing impaired test performances by analyzing the patient's overall pattern of results across the test battery and by comparing the neuropsychological profile to known patterns of disease. If a score on a verbal memory test does reflect a primary memory deficit, then the neuropsychologist determines whether the impairment is due to a deficit in encoding, storage, or retrieval, since the type of memory impairment may be indicative of different disease processes or lesion locations. Neuropsychologists use a similar method of analysis when assessing performances in other cognitive domains.

Test interpretation also requires the integration of neuropsychological test scores with findings from the clinical interview, the patient's history, the neurological examination, neurophysiology and neuroimaging data, and relevant literature. Raw test scores must be compared to an appropriate reference standard. Several reference standards are used in interpreting neuropsychological test scores, including the use of normative data, cut scores, and comparisons with an individual's own prior testing results.

Inferences about individual patients' neuropsychological test scores are often derived by comparing test scores to normative data that are typically collected by test developers as a standardization sample. Normative data are useful for accounting for variables that are likely to influence test performance (e.g., demographic factors) so that accurate and appropriate conclusions are drawn. Confounding variables are accounted for by stratifying test scores according to

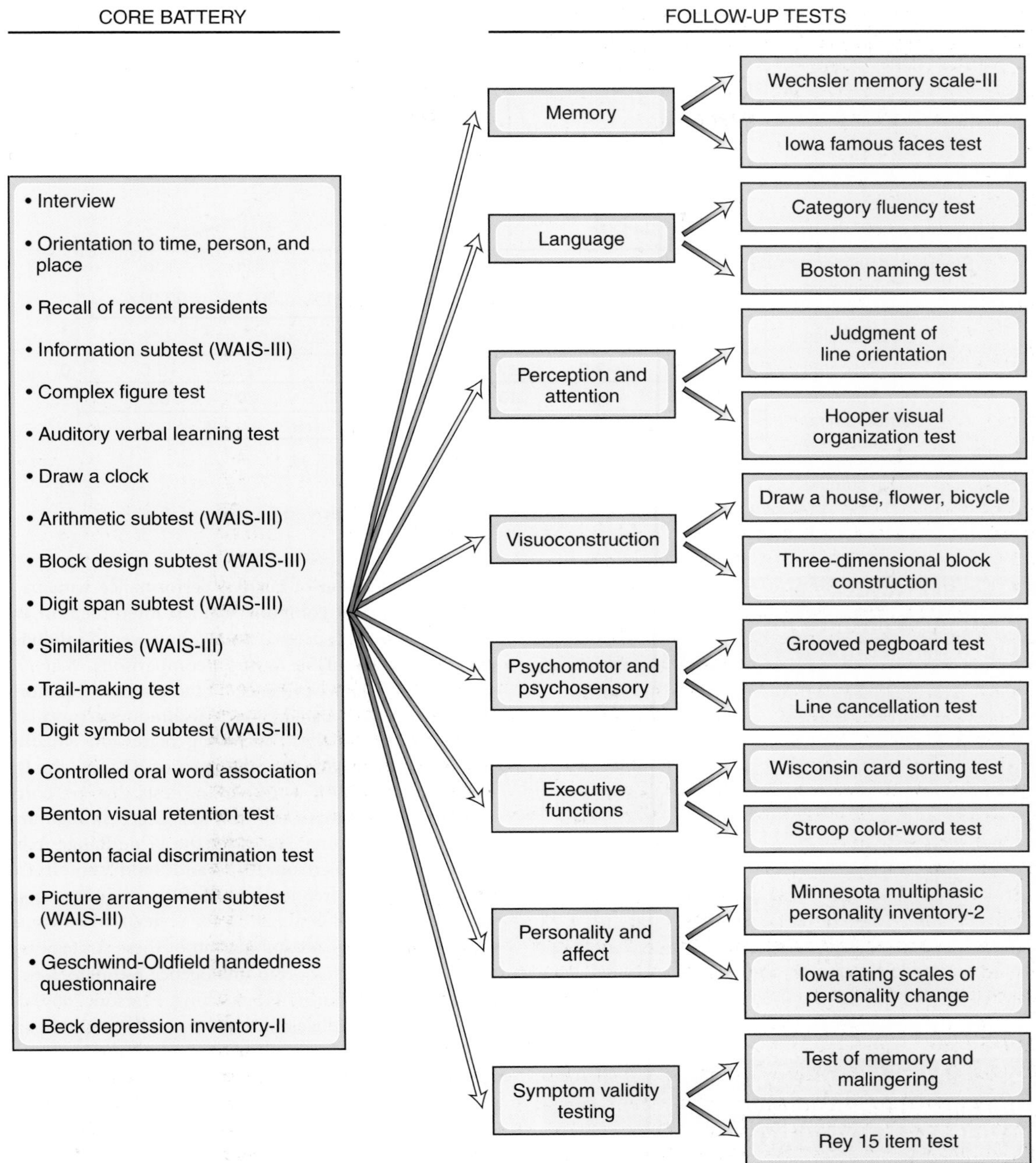


**Fig. 44.1** Example of a Flexible Battery Approach. (*Adapted from Tranel, D., 2008. Theories of clinical neuropsychology and brain-behavior relationships. In: Morgan, J.E., Ricker, J.H. (Eds.), Textbook of Clinical Neuropsychology. Taylor & Francis, New York, pp. 25–37.*)

sex, age, and level of education. An individual's raw score is compared with the distribution of scores from his or her peer group to determine where it falls within the range of expected performances. Fig. 44.2 and Table 44.2 show a normal distribution and interpretive guidelines for use in neuropsychological interpretation. The usefulness of normative data depends strongly on the size and representativeness of the standardization sample. Clinical interpretation can also be greatly affected by the goodness-of-fit between the individual patient and the standardization sample. Furthermore, it is important to use the most recent norms available, because cohort effects may lead to differences between current patients and those from whom data were collected years ago. When appropriate norms are not available, there is a danger of over- or underdiagnosis of cognitive impairment.

Another approach to test interpretation is the use of cut scores. Tests that rely on cut scores often measure performances with low base rates or deficits very few healthy people demonstrate. Some tests are straightforward in their capability to measure abilities that are largely intact in normal subjects but impaired in disordered patients. For example, most people are able to bisect a line without difficulty, but patients with left-sided visuospatial neglect typically identify the midpoint of the line to be to the right of center. Cut scores are useful with brief tests of cognitive screening, such as the Mini-Mental State Examination (MMSE). It is critical to remain current with normative

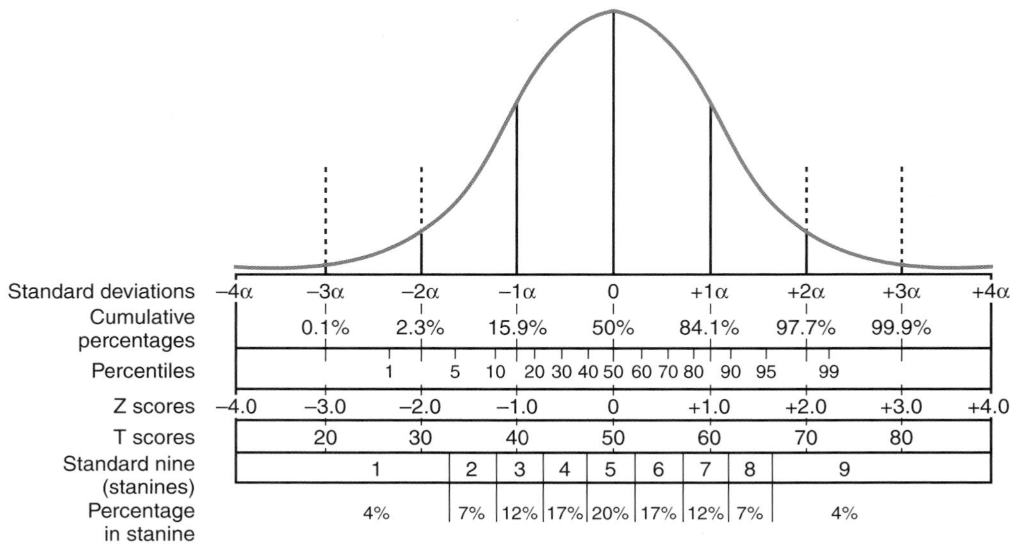


**Fig. 44.2** The Normal Curve and Its Relationship to Derived Scores.

**TABLE 44.2 Descriptive Terms Associated With Performance Within Various Ranges of the Normal Distribution**

| Qualitative Terms | Standard Deviation Score (i.e. Z-Score) | T-Score | Percentile Rank |
|---|---|---|---|
| Severely impaired | <−2.20 | <29 | <2 |
| Moderately impaired | −2.20 to −1.60 | 29–34 | 2–5 |
| Mildly impaired | −1.59 to −1.33 | 35–37 | 6–9 |
| Below average | −1.32 to −0.68 | 38–42 | 10–24 |
| Average | −0.67 to +0.67 | 43–57 | 25–75 |
| Above average | +0.68 to +1.59 | 58–66 | 76–94 |
| Superior | +1.60 to +2.20 | 67–72 | 95–98 |
| Very superior | >+2.20 | >72 | >98 |

Note: The patient's educational history and premorbid level of functioning should be taken into consideration in applying any qualitative label.

**TABLE 44.3 Mini-Mental State Examination Cutoff Scores for Detection of Alzheimer Disease Varying by Ethnicity**

| Cohort Age | Prevalence of MCI | Confidence Interval |
|---|---|---|
| 60–64 | 6.7% | 3.4–12.7 |
| 65–69 | 8.4% | 5.2–13.4 |
| 70–74 | 10.1% | 7.5–13.5 |
| 80–84 | 25.2% | 16.5–36.5 |

*MCI*, Mild cognitive impairment.

standards, however, as even these very brief screening tests vary greatly with persons varying in education and ethnicity. See Table 44.3 for MMSE cutoff scores for detection of Alzheimer disease varying by ethnicity (Spering et al., 2012). One recent study of over 10,450 Medicare recipients suggested that claims data and cognitive performances were poorly matched, with less than half being identified by both measures, suggesting that healthcare providers underestimated dementia diagnoses in Black and Hispanic populations, compared with Whites (Chen, 2019).

The comparison of current performance with past test scores is another important component of test interpretation, especially if cognitive decline is suspected. Rarely, however, do individuals have previous test data available for these comparisons. When no previous test scores are available, evidence of the patient's premorbid intellectual functioning is estimated. Several techniques are available for estimating premorbid intellect, including regression equations that utilize demographic variables as predictors of IQ (e.g., the Barona formula; Barona et al., 1984), word reading tests that are correlated with IQ (e.g., the North American Adult Reading Test; Blair and Spreen, 1989 or the Word Reading Test from the Wide Range Achievement Test; Wilkinson and Robertson, 2017), and "hold" subtests from intelligence measures that are frequently used as proxies for premorbid functioning (e.g., see Lezak et al., 2012, for review). Most contemporary neuropsychologists use a combination of these strategies, either formally (e.g., Oklahoma Premorbid Intelligence Estimate-3, Schoenberg et al., 2002; Test of Premorbid Functioning, Pearson, 2009) or informally.

Ultimately, feedback about the results of the neuropsychological evaluation, along with diagnostic impressions and treatment recommendations, is communicated to the referring physician and the patient. Some form of written report is typical in neuropsychological evaluations, and these tend to vary in length and level of detail (e.g., <1–15 pages). A common structure for a neuropsychological report includes sections summarizing the patient interview, collateral interview, medications, medical history, social background, behavioral observations, neuropsychological battery, neuropsychological test results and interpretation, final diagnostic impressions, and treatment recommendations.

## BRIEF MENTAL STATUS EXAMINATION

Before referring a patient for a neuropsychological evaluation, the neurologist typically has either clinical or historical evidence of cognitive concerns. This might come from patient self-report or collateral report, an informal mental status examination, or a brief objective screening measure of mental status. Although many mental status examinations are conducted in a nonstandard manner, neurologists are encouraged to use formal cognitive screening measures to develop a standardized method of mental status examination so comparisons across time and patients can be reliably made. One purpose

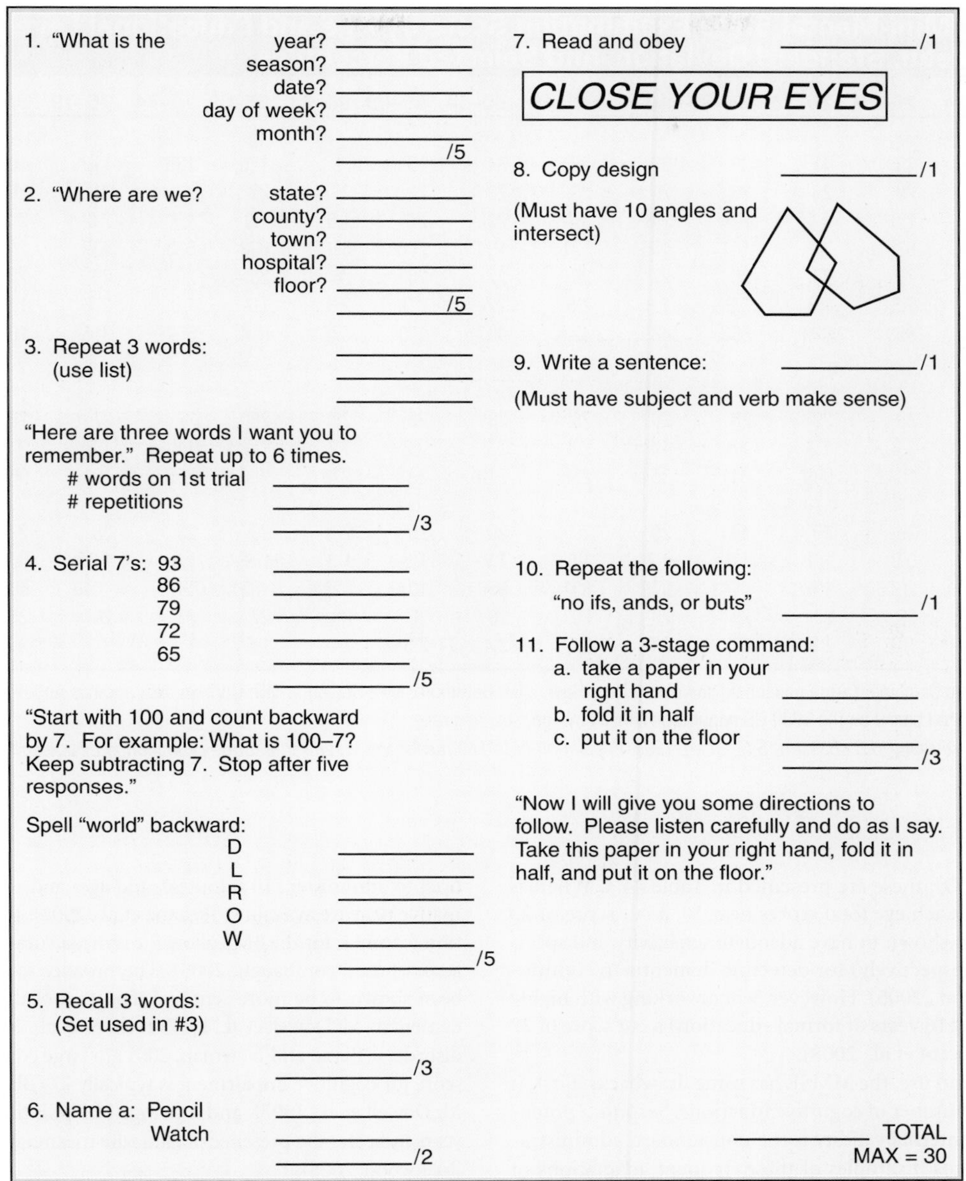

1. "What is the year? ______
season? ______
date? ______
day of week? ______
month? ______
______ /5

2. "Where are we? state? ______
county? ______
town? ______
hospital? ______
floor? ______
______ /5

3. Repeat 3 words: ______
(use list) ______
______

"Here are three words I want you to remember." Repeat up to 6 times.
# words on 1st trial ______
# repetitions ______
______ /3

4. Serial 7's: 93 ______
86 ______
79 ______
72 ______
65 ______
______ /5

"Start with 100 and count backward by 7. For example: What is 100–7? Keep subtracting 7. Stop after five responses."

Spell "world" backward:
D ______
L ______
R ______
O ______
W ______
______ /5

5. Recall 3 words: ______
(Set used in #3) ______
______
______ /3

6. Name a: Pencil ______
Watch ______
______ /2

7. Read and obey ______ /1

CLOSE YOUR EYES

8. Copy design ______ /1

(Must have 10 angles and intersect)

9. Write a sentence: ______ /1

(Must have subject and verb make sense)

10. Repeat the following:
"no ifs, ands, or buts" ______ /1

11. Follow a 3-stage command:
a. take a paper in your right hand ______
b. fold it in half ______
c. put it on the floor ______
______ /3

"Now I will give you some directions to follow. Please listen carefully and do as I say. Take this paper in your right hand, fold it in half, and put it on the floor."

______ TOTAL
MAX = 30

**Fig. 44.3** Mini–Mental State Examination. (*Reprinted with permission from Folstein, M.F., Folstein, S.E., McHugh, P.R., 1975. Mini-Mental State: a practical method for grading the cognitive state of patients for the clinician. J. Psychiatr. Res. 12, 189–198.*)

of cognitive screening measures is to determine the need for a more extended evaluation of neuropsychological functioning. Given the limited scope of cognitive screening measures and the psychometric considerations noted earlier, it is not recommended that cognitive screening measures be used as a final summation of a patient's cognitive status. Scores from cognitive screeners must be considered in conjunction with clinical observation and judgment to determine whether a referral for neuropsychological evaluation is necessary, since many patients may pass a cognitive screen but still have suspected deficits that warrant more sensitive neuropsychological testing. The Patient Protection and Affordable Care Act of 2010 suggests conducting an annual wellness visit for all Medicare patients, including a cognitive assessment. The Alzheimer's Association describes many suggested screening questionnaires on their website and provides validated assessment tools recommended to primary care physicians (https://www.alz.org).A few suggested objective screening measures of cognitive functioning that may be useful for neurologists to administer are briefly described in the following.

## Mini–Mental State Examination

One of the most widely used mental status examinations is the MMSE (Folstein et al., 1975), a 30-point standardized screening tool for assessing orientation, attention, short-term recall, naming, repetition, simple verbal and written commands, writing, and construction (Fig. 44.3). The MMSE has been used in a variety of settings (e.g., community, institutions, general hospitals, specialty clinics), with many different neurological and psychiatric conditions (e.g., dementia, stroke, depression), across age ranges, and with different cultural and ethnic subgroups. Demographic variables such as age and education have been shown to systematically influence MMSE scores, so normative data or cut scores should account for these variables. One example of appropriate norms comes from the Epidemiologic Catchment Area

**TABLE 44.4 Mini-Mental State Examination Score by Age and Educational Level, Number of Participants, Mean, Standard Deviation, and Selected Percentiles**

| Age (Years) | 18–24 | 25–29 | 30–34 | 35–39 | 40–44 | 45–49 | 50–54 | 55–59 | 60–64 | 65–69 | 70–74 | 75–79 | 80–84 | ≥85 | Total |
|---|---|---|---|---|---|---|---|---|---|---|---|---|---|---|---|
| **Educational Level** | | | | | | | | | | | | | | | |
| 0–4 years | 17 | 23 | 41 | 33 | 36 | 28 | 34 | 49 | 88 | 126 | 139 | 112 | 105 | 61 | 892 |
| Mean | 22 | 25 | 25 | 23 | 23 | 23 | 23 | 22 | 23 | 22 | 22 | 21 | 20 | 19 | 22 |
| *SD* | 2.9 | 2.0 | 2.4 | 2.5 | 2.6 | 3.7 | 2.6 | 2.7 | 1.9 | 1.9 | 1.7 | 2.0 | 2.2 | 2.9 | 2.3 |
| 5–8 years | 94 | 83 | 74 | 101 | 100 | 121 | 154 | 208 | 310 | 633 | 533 | 437 | 241 | 134 | 3223 |
| Mean | 27 | 27 | 26 | 26 | 27 | 26 | 27 | 26 | 26 | 26 | 26 | 25 | 25 | 23 | 26 |
| *SD* | 2.7 | 2.5 | 1.8 | 2.8 | 1.8 | 2.5 | 2.4 | 2.9 | 2.3 | 1.7 | 1.8 | 2.1 | 1.9 | 3.3 | 22 |
| 9–12 years or high school diploma | 1326 | 958 | 822 | 668 | 489 | 423 | 462 | 525 | 626 | 814 | 550 | 315 | 163 | 99 | 8240 |
| Mean | 29 | 29 | 29 | 28 | 28 | 28 | 28 | 28 | 28 | 28 | 27 | 27 | 25 | 26 | 28 |
| *SD* | 2.2 | 1.3 | 1.3 | 1.8 | 1.9 | 2.4 | 2.2 | 2.2 | 1.7 | 1.4 | 1.6 | 1.5 | 2.3 | 2.0 | 1.9 |
| College experience | 783 | 1012 | 989 | 641 | 354+ | 259 | 220 | 231 | 270 | 358 | 255 | 181 | 96 | 52 | 5701 |
| Mean | 29 | 29 | 29 | 29 | 29 | 29 | 29 | 29 | 29 | 29 | 28 | 28 | 27 | 27 | 29 |
| *SD* | 1.3 | 0.9 | 1.0 | 1.0 | 1.7 | 1.6 | 1.9 | 1.5 | 1.3 | 1.0 | 1.6 | 1.6 | 0.9 | 1.3 | 1.3 |
| **Total** | 2220 | 2076 | 1926 | 1443 | 979 | 831 | 870 | 1013 | 1294 | 1931 | 1477 | 1045 | 605 | 346 | 18,056 |
| Mean | 29 | 29 | 29 | 29 | 28 | 28 | 28 | 28 | 28 | 27 | 27 | 26 | 25 | 24 | 28 |
| *SD* | 2.0 | 1.3 | 1.3 | 1.8 | 2.0 | 2.5 | 2.4 | 2.5 | 2.0 | 1.6 | 1.8 | 2.1 | 2.2 | 2.9 | 2.0 |

Data from the Epidemiologic Catchment Area household surveys in New Haven, CT; Baltimore, MD; St. Louis, MO; Durham, NC; and Los Angeles, CA, between 1980 and 1984. The data are weighted based on the 1980 US population census by age, sex, and race.

*Adapted from Crum, R.M., Anthony, J.C., Bassett, S.S., et al., 1993. Population-based norms for the Mini-Mental State Examination by age and educational level. JAMA 269, 2386–2391.*

study (Crum et al., 1993); these are presented in Table 44.4. Whereas many intact individuals achieve total scores near 30, a cut score of 23 on the MMSE has been shown to have adequate sensitivity and specificity (86% and 91%, respectively) for detecting dementia in community samples (Cullen et al., 2005). However, when working with highly educated patients (i.e., ≥16 years of formal education) a cut score of 27 is recommended (O'Bryant et al., 2008).

Despite its widespread use, the MMSE has some drawbacks. First, it only assesses a limited number of cognitive functions. Second, a potential threat to the test's internal validity is the nonstandard administration of some of the items. Examples of these frequent adaptations of the MMSE include the use of nonorthogonal (i.e., semantically related) word stimuli for registration and recall, nonstandard scoring of serial 7's, and nonstandard inclusion of spelling *world* backward. Another drawback of the MMSE is that it has "ceiling effects" that can miss cognitive impairments in high-functioning individuals. The MMSE also has difficulty differentiating individuals with mild cognitive impairment (MCI) from controls and those with dementia (Mitchell, 2009). Finally, because this test relies on a single total score, partial administration of the measure (e.g., due to sensory impairments of the patient) provides no information about cognitive status. This same limitation is true for the Montreal Cognitive Assessment (MoCA). The MMSE is now copyrighted and is available for purchase.

## Modified Mini-Mental State Examination

Some of the criticisms of the MMSE led to the development of the Modified Mini-Mental State Examination (3MS) (Teng and Chui, 1987), a 14-item extension of the MMSE that assesses orientation (self, time, place), attention (simple and complex), memory (recall and recognition), language (naming, verbal fluency, repetition, following commands, writing), construction, and executive functioning (similarities). It remains relatively brief to administer (10 minutes), and age- and education-corrected normative data are available (Tschanz et al., 2002). Regression-based prediction formulas for the 3MS allow for more accurate assessments of change across time (Tombaugh, 2005). The broader scoring range (0–100) has been shown to be more sensitive than that of the MMSE in identifying dementia (McDowell et al., 1997; Tschanz et al., 2002) and other cognitive disorders (Bland and Newman, 2001) in large community samples. A cut score for cognitive impairment is typically 77 (Bland and Newman, 2001; McDowell et al., 1997), and a change of 5 points over the course of 5–10 years indicates the presence of clinically meaningful decline (Andrew and Rockwood, 2008).

## Montreal Cognitive Assessment

The MoCA was originally developed as a screening tool to correct the shortcomings of the widely used MMSE, which demonstrated an insensitivity to mild cognitive impairment (Nasreddine et al., 2005). The MoCA also improved upon the MMSE by probing more cognitive domains, including executive functioning, immediate and delayed memory, visuospatial abilities, attention, working memory, language, and orientation to time and place (Fig. 44.4 for example). Including more cognitive domains reduces the likelihood that impairments or disorders will be overlooked (e.g., executive dysfunction, a hallmark symptom of vascular dementia). The total score ranges from 0 to 30 points, and a cut score of 26 has demonstrated very good specificity (by correctly identifying 87% of healthy participants) and excellent sensitivity when differentiating MCI (90%) and Alzheimer disease (AD) (100%) from healthy comparisons. More important, the positive predictive value of the MoCA is 89% for both MCI and AD. Since its inception as a screening measure for MCI, other studies have found the MoCA to outperform the MMSE in screening for general cognitive impairment in Parkinson disease (PD) (Hoops et al., 2009; Nazem

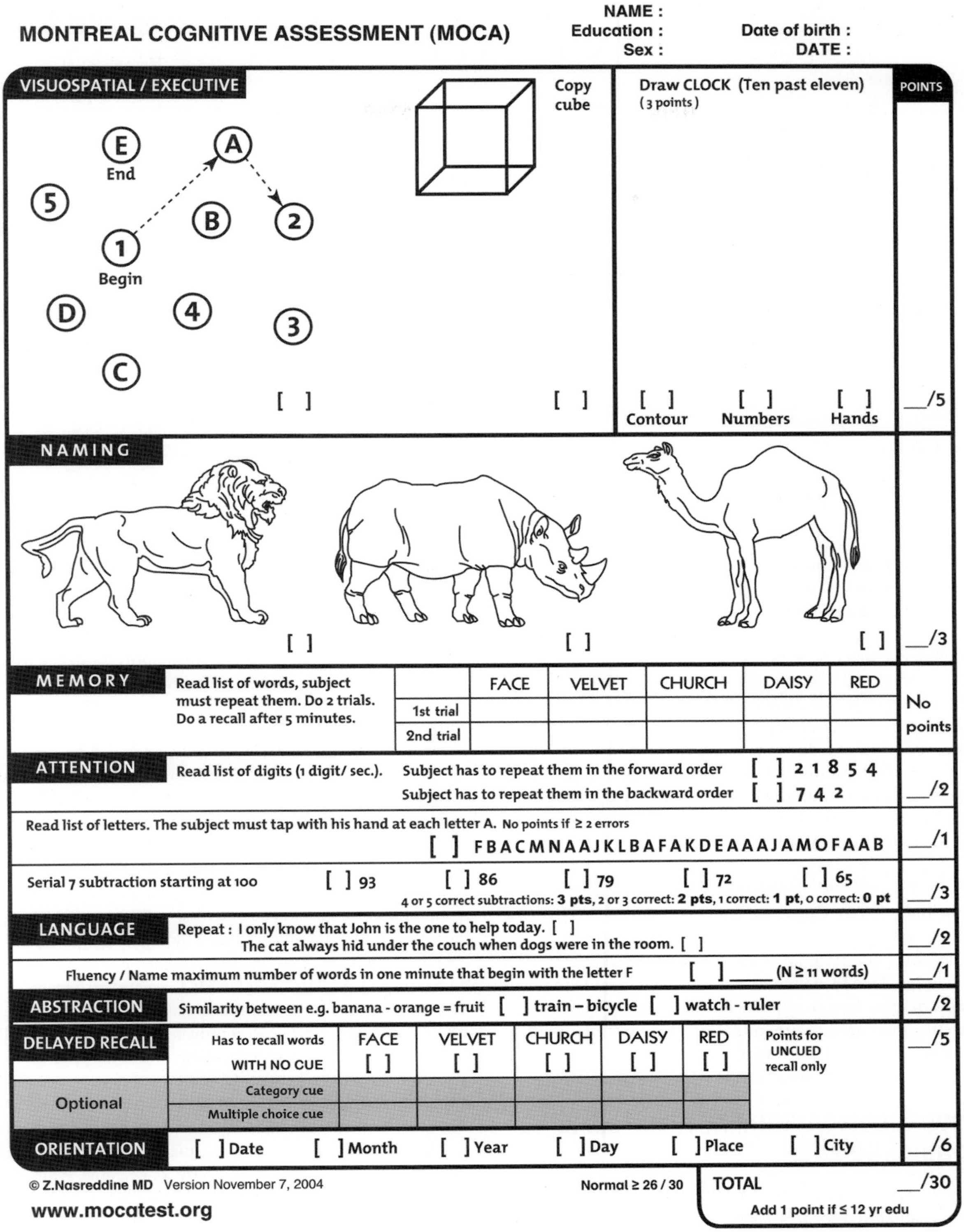

**MONTREAL COGNITIVE ASSESSMENT (MOCA)**

NAME :
Education :
Sex :
Date of birth :
DATE :

| | | POINTS |
|---|---|---|
| VISUOSPATIAL / EXECUTIVE | (E) End, (A), (B), (1) Begin, (2), (3), (4), (5), (C), (D) [ ]; Copy cube [ ]; Draw CLOCK (Ten past eleven) (3 points) [ ] Contour [ ] Numbers [ ] Hands | ___/5 |
| NAMING | [ ] [ ] [ ] | ___/3 |

| MEMORY | Read list of words, subject must repeat them. Do 2 trials. Do a recall after 5 minutes. | FACE | VELVET | CHURCH | DAISY | RED | No points |
|---|---|---|---|---|---|---|---|
| | 1st trial | | | | | | |
| | 2nd trial | | | | | | |

| | | POINTS |
|---|---|---|
| ATTENTION | Read list of digits (1 digit/ sec.). Subject has to repeat them in the forward order [ ] 2 1 8 5 4<br>Subject has to repeat them in the backward order [ ] 7 4 2 | ___/2 |
| | Read list of letters. The subject must tap with his hand at each letter A. No points if ≥ 2 errors<br>[ ] FBACMNAAJKLBAFAKDEAAAJAMOFAAB | ___/1 |
| | Serial 7 subtraction starting at 100 [ ] 93 [ ] 86 [ ] 79 [ ] 72 [ ] 65<br>4 or 5 correct subtractions: **3 pts**, 2 or 3 correct: **2 pts**, 1 correct: **1 pt**, 0 correct: **0 pt** | ___/3 |
| LANGUAGE | Repeat : I only know that John is the one to help today. [ ]<br>The cat always hid under the couch when dogs were in the room. [ ] | ___/2 |
| | Fluency / Name maximum number of words in one minute that begin with the letter F [ ] ___ (N ≥ 11 words) | ___/1 |
| ABSTRACTION | Similarity between e.g. banana - orange = fruit [ ] train – bicycle [ ] watch - ruler | ___/2 |

| DELAYED RECALL | Has to recall words WITH NO CUE | FACE [ ] | VELVET [ ] | CHURCH [ ] | DAISY [ ] | RED [ ] | Points for UNCUED recall only | ___/5 |
|---|---|---|---|---|---|---|---|---|
| Optional | Category cue | | | | | | | |
| | Multiple choice cue | | | | | | | |

| ORIENTATION | [ ] Date | [ ] Month | [ ] Year | [ ] Day | [ ] Place | [ ] City | ___/6 |
|---|---|---|---|---|---|---|---|

© Z.Nasreddine MD Version November 7, 2004
www.mocatest.org

Normal ≥ 26 / 30 **TOTAL** ___/30
Add 1 point if ≤ 12 yr edu

**Fig. 44.4** Montreal Cognitive Assessment. *(Reprinted with permission from Nasreddine, Z.S., Phillips, N.A., Bedirian, V., et al., 2005. The Montreal Cognitive Assessment, MoCA: a brief screening tool for mild cognitive impairment. J. Am. Geriatr. Soc. 53, 695–699.)*

et al., 2009), vascular dementia after acute stroke (Dong et al., 2010), and Huntington disease (HD) (Videnovic et al., 2010) as a measure sensitive to early stages of different types of dementia.

Although the MoCA has demonstrated its utility as a cognitive screener, there are a few caveats worth noting. First, some studies have demonstrated that its reliability is notably low in nonclinical populations (Bernstein et al., 2011), which indicates that it should primarily be used only to detect suspected cognitive impairment in clinical patients. Additionally, the original cut score of 26 used to identify impairment was developed without fully accounting for other variables that affect test

TABLE 44.5 **Montreal Cognitive Assessment Score by Age and Education**

| | YEARS OF EDUCATION | | | | | | TOTAL BY AGE | |
|---|---|---|---|---|---|---|---|---|
| | <12 | | 12 | | >12 | | | |
| Age Group (Years) | No. | Mean (SD) Median | No. | Mean (SD) Median | No. | Mean (SD) Median | No. | Mean (SD) Median |
| <35 | 20 | 22.80 (3.38) 23 | 65 | 24.46 (3.49) 25 | 122 | 25.93 (2.48) 26 | 207 | 25.16 (3.08) 26 |
| 30–40 | 37 | 22.84 (3.18) 23 | 106 | 23.99 (2.93) 24 | 264 | 25.81 (2.64) 26 | 408 | 25.07 (2.95) 25 |
| 35–45 | 55 | 22.11 (3.33) 23 | 177 | 23.02 (3.67) 24 | 355 | 25.38 (3.05) 26 | 588 | 24.37 (3.51) 25 |
| 40–50 | 77 | 21.36 (3.73) 22 | 227 | 22.26 (3.94) 23 | 418 | 25.09 (3.16) 26 | 723 | 23.80 (3.80) 24 |
| 45–55 | 77 | 20.75 (3.80) 21 | 216 | 21.87 (3.95) 22 | 461 | 24.70 (3.24) 25 | 755 | 23.48 (3.84) 24 |
| 50–60 | 62 | 19.94 (4.34) 20 | 172 | 22.25 (3.46) 22 | 424 | 24.34 (3.38) 25 | 659 | 23.37 (3.78) 24 |
| 55–65 | 60 | 19.60 (4.14) 20 | 143 | 21.58 (3.93) 22 | 369 | 24.43 (3.31) 25 | 573 | 23.20 (3.96) 23 |
| 60–70 | 57 | 19.30 (3.79) 19 | 113 | 20.89 (4.50) 21 | 246 | 24.32 (3.04) 25 | 418 | 22.69 (4.12) 23 |
| 65–75 | 38 | 18.37 (3.87) 19 | 67 | 20.57 (4.79) 21 | 122 | 24.00 (3.35) 24 | 228 | 22.05 (4.48) 23 |
| 70–80 | 14 | 16.07 (3.17) 17 | 23 | 20.35 (4.91) 20 | 42 | 23.06 (3.47) 24 | 79 | 21.32 (4.78) 22 |
| Total by education | 230 | 20.55 (4.04) 21 | 608 | 22.34 (3.97) 23 | 1306 | 24.81 (3.20) 25 | 2148 | 23.65 (3.84) 24 |

*SD*, Standard deviation.

*Adapted from Rossetti, H.C., Lacritz, L.H., Cullum, C.M., Weiner, M.F., 2011. Normative data for the Montreal Cognitive Assessment (MoCA) in a population-based sample. Neurology 77, 1272–5.*

performance (e.g., age, education, sex, and race) and the score has also been shown to identify a high number of false positives in certain populations. Rossetti and colleagues (2011) attempted to correct these problems by conducting a normative study of the MoCA in an ethnically diverse sample of healthy participants, as presented in Table 44.5. They found that 66% of their sample fell below the cut score of 26, indicating "impairment," and that many of the MoCA items had high failure rates.

The MoCA is free to clinicians (http://www.mocatest.org) and has been translated into 31 different languages and dialects. As of September 2020, completion of a 1-hour online training and certification regarding administration, scoring, and interpretation of the MoCA is required prior to clinicians using it in their clinical practice. See their website for more details.

### Telephone Interview for Cognitive Status—Modified

The Telephone Interview for Cognitive Status—Modified (mTICS) is a relatively brief screening instrument designed to quickly and accurately assess cognition over the telephone, although it can also be used in face-to-face settings. This 13-item measure is heavily weighted toward immediate and delayed free recall, which might make it particularly useful in detecting mild AD impairments (Duff et al., 2009; Lines et al., 2003) such as amnestic MCI (Fig. 44.5). Age-, education-, sex-, and race-corrected normative data are available (Hogervorst et al., 2004).

## NEUROPSYCHOLOGICAL CHARACTERISTICS OF NEUROLOGICAL DISEASE

In this section we briefly address the neurocognitive sequelae of some of the major neurological disorders. Although many of these disorders have psychiatric characteristics as well, these will only be briefly discussed. Please see Chapter 9 for a more comprehensive discussion on the psychiatric aspects of neurological disorders.

### Mild Cognitive Impairment

A major focus in dementia has been detecting cognitive impairment associated with neurodegenerative diseases at the earliest time to maximize the potential impact of treatments to slow disease progression. The diagnostic term MCI was defined by Petersen and colleagues (1999) as the presence of subjective memory complaints, a measured deficit in a cognitive domain of approximately 1.5 standard deviations below normative means, otherwise intact cognition, no functional impairments, and the absence of dementia. MCI diagnosis typically requires the utilization of neuropsychological tests to quantify the deficit using normative data. The Diagnostic and Statistical Manual of Mental Disorders, fifth edition (DSM-V) (APA, 2013) diagnosis of mild neurocognitive disorder is essentially MCI (Petersen et al., 2009). The American Academy of Neurology recently updated the practice guidelines for MCI (Petersen, 2018). The term *amnestic MCI* describes a syndrome where memory impairment is the first, and most prominent, cognitive expression of deficit and is most likely to progress to AD. Nonamnestic MCI is used to describe patterns of cognitive dysfunction when other cognitive domains are prominent (such as language, visuospatial, executive, motor learning) and may be more likely to progress into other dementias. MCI is common and its prevalence increases with age and lower educational level (see Table 44.6 for prevalence by cohort age). Despite over 14 clinical trials conducted, no pharmacotherapy has shown benefit. A review of pharmacological treatment in MCI revealed no benefit, although exercise training and cognitive training may improve cognitive performances (Petersen, 2018). Practice Recommendations are shown in Table 44.6.

Patients of memory disorder clinics with MCI progress to dementia at a rate of 10% to 15% per year (Farias et al., 2009), and community-dwelling adults at an annual rate of 6% to 10% per year (Petersen et al., 2009), but more than 25% revert back to normal cognitive baseline at follow-up. Predictors of conversion to dementia are diverse. Findings are mixed regarding the relation between severity of cognitive symptoms and likelihood of conversion to dementia (Guo et al., 2013). Additional factors that have been shown to be predictive of conversion to MCI include impaired olfaction (Conti et al., 2013), use of preclinical staging of AD (Vos et al., 2013), genetic factors such as the presence of the *APOE* gene, reduced hippocampal and entorhinal cortex volume, hypometabolism in tempoparietal regions, and other biomarkers of AD. In contrast, factors such as bilingualism (Bialystok et al., 2014), advanced education, and healthy lifestyle behaviors (Lojo-Seoane et al., 2014) have been found to be protective factors regarding reduced progression to dementia.

At autopsy, less than one-quarter of MCI cases showed "pure" AD; MCI diagnosis was usually associated with comorbid neuropathologies.

**Modified Telephone Interview for Cognitive Status (mTICS)**

1. What is your name?________________________________ /2
2. What is your telephone number?________________________________ /2
3. What is today's date (month, date, year, season, day)? (5 points maximum, 1 point per correct response)
   Month: ______________________ /1
   Date: ______________________ /1
   Year: ______________________ /1
   Season: ______________________ /1
   Day: ______________________ /1 /5
4. I'm going to read you a list of 10 words. Please listen carefully and try to remember them. When I am done, tell me as many as you can in any order. Ready? (10 points maximum, 1 point per correctly recalled word)

| | |
|---|---|
| Cabin | |
| Pipe | |
| Elephant | |
| Chest | |
| Silk | |
| Theatre | |
| Watch | |
| Whip | |
| Pillow | |
| Giant | |
| TOTAL | |

/10

5. Please count backwards from 20 to 1. /2
   20 19 18 17 16 15 14 13 12 11 10 9 8 7 6 5 4 3 2 1
6. Please take 7 away from 100. Now continue to take away 7 from what you have left over until I ask you to stop. (5 points maximum, 1 point per correct response)
   93: ________ /1
   86: ________ /1
   79: ________ /1
   72: ________ /1
   65: ________ /1 /5
7. What do people usually use to cut paper?____________________ /2
8. What is the prickly green plant found in the desert?____________________ /2
9. Who is president of the United States now?____________________ /2
10. Who is the vice president of the United States now?____________________ /2
11. What word is opposite of east?____________________ /2
12. Please say this: "Methodist Episcopal" /2
    Correct response (circle one): YES NO
13. Please tap your finger 5 times on the part of the phone you speak into.
    (2 points if they tap 5 times, 1 point if they tap more or less than 5 times) /2
14. Please repeat the list of 10 words I read earlier.

| | |
|---|---|
| Cabin | |
| Pipe | |
| Elephant | |
| Chest | |
| Silk | |
| Theatre | |
| Watch | |
| Whip | |
| Pillow | |
| Giant | |
| TOTAL | |

/10

TOTAL: /50

**Fig. 44.5** Modified Telephone Interview for Cognitive Status. (*Data from Welsh, K.A., Breitner, J.C.S., Magruder-Habib, K.M., 1993. Detection of dementia in the elderly using telephone screening of cognitive status. Neuropsychiatry Neuropsychol. Behav. Neurol. 6, 103–110.*)

Among a group that maintained a diagnosis of MCI to death, mixed AD neuropathological changes were more frequent that pure AD neuropathological changes (55% vs. 22%). A majority (74%) of research participants who died with MCI were without primary AD neuropathologies, Lewy body disease, or hippocampal sclerosis, and exhibited significant cerebrovascular pathologies (Abner, 2017).

## Alzheimer Disease

Alzheimer disease–related dementia is the most common type of dementia, with prevalence rates of 11% in those of 65 years and older (Hebert et al., 2013; Illán-Gala, 2018; Jack, 2019) and 68% in memory disorder clinics (Paulino Ramirez Diaz et al., 2005). Clinical diagnosis of probable AD requires core clinical criteria (McKhann, 2011). Definitive diagnosis requires postmortem neuropathological examination of brain tissue for the hallmark signs of plaques and neurofibrillary tangles in the hippocampal and entorhinal regions (Braak and Braak, 1991); however, premortem diagnostic criteria are widely employed. DSM-V (APA, 2013) changed the terminology for diagnosis of dementia in AD to "major neurocognitive disorder due to Alzheimer disease," with specified criteria being evidence of significant cognitive decline from a previously higher level of functioning and the cognitive impairments interfering with everyday functioning. The diagnosis is considered probable AD if there is objective evidence of decline in memory and one other cognitive domain, insidious onset and gradual progression of symptoms, and no evidence of other etiology. Evidence of a genetic mutation associated with AD would also result in probable AD diagnosis. However, autosomal dominant cases such as *APP*, *PSEN1*, or *PSEN2* are rare and account for less than 1% of AD patients (Storandt et al., 2014).

The brief bedside examinations mentioned earlier in this chapter have some degree of utility in detecting cognitive changes, but their comparatively limited scope, low sensitivity, and susceptibility to ceiling effects make them better suited for screening purposes. Complaints about "memory problems" are what often lead to a clinical evaluation of possible AD. Cognitive decline begins 7.5 years prior to diagnosis on average (Wilson et al., 2012). Though the presence of biomarkers for dementia has taken a leading role in AD research, the presence of biomarker abnormality without evidence of cognitive decline has a lower risk for dementia than if cognitive deficits are present (Jack et al., 2013). Similarly, neuropsychological assessment for measuring AD-related declines has been demonstrated to have better sensitivity than magnetic resonance imaging (MRI) for tracking disease progression (Schmand et al., 2014). Consistent with patient report and behavioral observations of rapid forgetting of new information, performances across a comprehensive battery of neuropsychological assessment measures are likely to identify stark memory deficits for information mediated both verbally (e.g., lists, stories, paired associates) and visually (e.g., concrete or abstract figures), including an atypical lack of a primacy effect for information presented early in lists (Salmon and Bondi, 2009). Recognition memory is also likely to be significantly impaired, and intrusion errors are common (e.g., adding extra words to delayed-recall trials on word-list memory tasks). Other cognitive deficits are seen in a number of other domains, including language functions (e.g., paraphasias, naming), semantic knowledge, visuospatial abilities, and executive functions such as motor planning (Weintraub et al., 2012). Impaired awareness of their own cognitive deficits, known as anosognosia or impaired metacognition, is also common (Rosen et al., 2014). Even though impaired memory is a cardinal feature of AD, it is important to keep in mind that other neurodegenerative dementia syndromes can also result in memory decline and that a nonmemory cognitive deficit may be the primary cognitive

**TABLE 44.6 Practice Guidelines for Mild Cognitive Impairment: Assessment**

- Objective cognitive assessment should be conducted for anyone who reports subjective cognitive decline; do not assume it is normal aging
- Medicare Annual Wellness visits require an assessment to detect cognitive impairment
- Objective screening for MCI should use validated assessment tools with acceptable diagnostic accuracy and positive screens should be referred for neuropsychological assessment
- Evidence for functional impairment limiting independence must be obtained to ascertain MCI from dementia
- Clinicians who lack the necessary experience should refer patients to a specialist in cognition
- Modifiable risk factors should be assessed, such as medication side effects, sleep apnea, depression, and other medical conditions
- Counsel patients and families that there are no acceptable biomarkers at this time
- Serial assessments over time are required to monitor for changes in cognitive status

*MCI,* Mild cognitive impairment.

presentation of AD, possibly reflecting posterior cortical atrophy. Given the pattern of deficits in AD, it is not surprising that measures of semantic fluency, delayed free recall, and global cognitive status demonstrate the highest levels of sensitivity and specificity for detecting patients with early AD (Salmon et al., 2002). Although memory deficits are usually glaring compared with other deficits in AD, general and progressive cognitive decline is common and shows an eightfold increase in rate of decline approximately 3 years prior to death (Wilson et al., 2010; Yu et al., 2013). As dementia progresses to moderate stages, learning and memory performances are likely to produce floor effects on many standardized neuropsychological measures, and more profound deficits are apparent in other cognitive domains. Deficits in praxis also begin to develop. These pervasive declines in late AD often make formal neuropsychological testing unnecessary or impossible.

According to the 2018 National Institutes of Aging—Alzheimer's Association (NIA-AA) research framework (Jack, 2016, 2018). AD is no longer defined by the clinical consequences of the disease, but by its underlying pathology, measured by biomarkers. Evidence of amyloid-beta (AB) and phosphorylated tau protein (p-tau) deposition assessed with positron emission tomography (PET) and/or cerebrospinal fluid (CSF) analysis is recommended to diagnose AD in a living person. The classification is described by amyloid/tau/neurodegeneration (AT[N]). Regardless of the presence of clinical symptoms, both AB and p-tau are required for classification as AD, whereas AB deposition alone is an early sign, labeled "AD pathologic change". The 2018 research framework also identifies a staging for clinical severity, ranging from cognitively unimpaired (CU), to MCI and dementia. Validity of these criteria as well as standardization of protocols for the AT(N) classification is ongoing. Three biologically defined diagnostic entities were recommended: AD continuum (abnormal amyloid regardless of tau status), AD pathological pathologic change (abnormal amyloid but normal tau), and AD (abnormal amyloid and tau). Carandini and colleagues (2019) retrospectively analyzed 628 participants referred for dementia for classification according to new criteria and reported that 94% of persons with a clinical diagnosis of AD showed biomarkers in the AD continuum. Additionally, however, the AD biomarkers also detected in 26% of frontotemporal dementia, 49% of Lewy body dementia, 25% of atypical parkinsonism, and 45% of vascular dementia as residing within the AD continuum. Jack and his colleagues (2019) estimated the prevalence of the three biologically defined diagnostic categories using over 5000 participants from the Mayo Clinic Study of Aging and found that the prevalence of AD defined by biological abnormality was up to three times greater than that defined using traditional clinical diagnoses of probable AD. Efforts to provide blood-based tests for widespread usage in primary care and to standardize the application of this framework are ongoing (Palmqvist, 2019). The Food and Drug Administration (FDA) of the United States has approved five medications to treat the cognitive symptoms of AD.

## Vascular Dementia

Cerebrovascular disease frequently leads to cognitive impairment, and vascular factors have garnered significant attention as a modifiable risk factor for dementia. So-called silent brain infarcts, or asymptomatic vascular pathology, are found in up to 35% of individuals with vascular disease (Slark et al., 2012) and are known to double the risk of vascular dementia (VaD) or major neurocognitive disorder due to vascular disease, as described in the DSM-V. Extracerebellar lacunar, large vessel, or strategically placed infarcts and hemorrhage lead to varying degrees of cognitive impairment, and small-vessel disease is the most frequently observed vascular pathology that leads to cognitive decline. Recently, the term *vascular cognitive impairment* (VCI) has been introduced to encompass all cognitive changes attributable to cerebrovascular pathology (i.e., from MCI due to vascular events to VaD; Rincon and Wright, 2013; Sachdev et al., 2014). Cognitive changes can occur abruptly and in a stepwise pattern with coinciding cerebrovascular accidents (CVAs), or they may fluctuate or remain static. Neuroimaging is likely to detect lesions that are a result of a CVA, and enhances diagnostic certainty, but imaging is not required to accurately identify dementia with a vascular etiology. Neurological evidence of cerebrovascular pathology (e.g., history of strokes, sensorimotor changes consistent with stroke) in combination with cognitive changes is considered indicative of VaD and the estimated prevalence is 8%–12% (Jellinger, 2013).

The clinical presentation of VaD varies depending on the number of infarcts, severity of neural damage following stroke, and location of the CVA. Although many VaD patients may acknowledge "memory problems," which may lead to suspicions of AD, further questioning reveals that these complaints are quite different from those typically seen in AD. If VaD results from a discrete stroke, then the primary cognitive impairment will likely be functionally related to the area of infarct, resulting in focal deficits and a heterogeneous presentation for VaD. Many patients do not experience a notable stroke preceding the onset of VaD, and may not present to memory disorder clinics because their primary symptoms are often dysexecutive in nature (e.g., the patient "just can't figure things out anymore"), with accompanying apathy and/or depression being common (Weintraub et al., 2012). Particularly in the frontal regions, increasing lacunae are associated with a higher probability of depression, apathy, atypical behaviors, and other neuropsychiatric symptoms (Kim et al., 2013). Impaired executive functioning is also strongly related to the presence of metabolic syndrome, a significant risk factor for VaD (Falkowski et al., 2014).

Classic dementia symptoms might be reported (e.g., difficulty remembering names, appointments, medications) but changes in

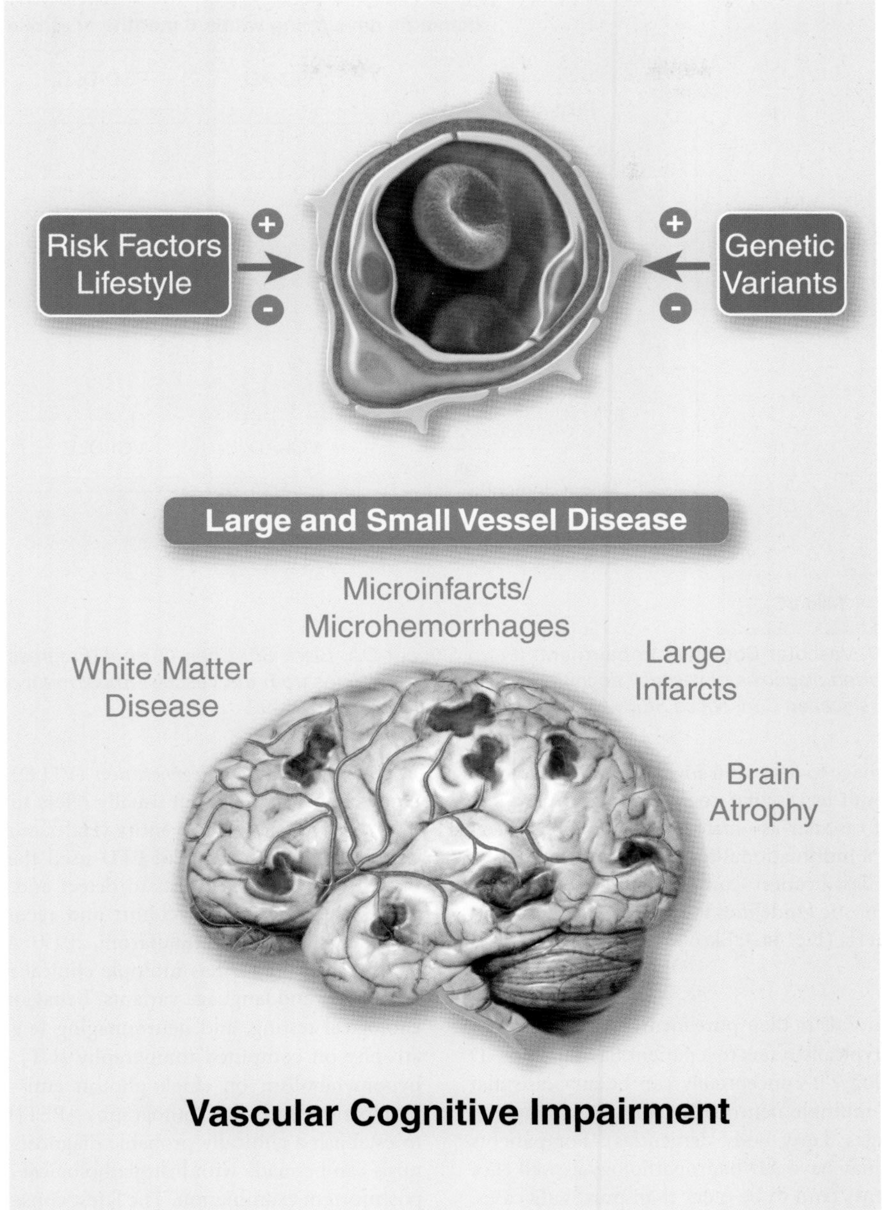


**Fig. 44.6** Vascular Dementia. (*From Iadecola et al., J Am Coll Cardiol 2019; 73(25):3326–44.*)

instrumental activities of daily living that require complex organizational and problem-solving skills (such as managing finances or following directions) are likely more prominent in a patient with early VaD than in one with early AD. Depression and apathy are hallmark symptoms and there is evidence that vascular factors are etiologically linked to late-life depression (Taylor et al., 2013). Upon first inspection, VaD may initially be cognitively indistinguishable from other dementias in many ways. However, a detailed neuropsychological examination and behavioral observations are likely to reveal a unique pattern of deficits in VaD, referred to as the subcortical profile. VaD patients tend to have better long-term verbal memory than their AD counterparts, worse executive functioning, and slowed processing speed, particularly on motor tasks. Impaired complex attention is also prominent (Benedet et al., 2012) and VaD tends to have a rapid initial onset. Free recall might occasionally appear similar in VaD and in AD, but patients with VaD significantly outperform their AD counterparts on tests of recognition memory (Tierney et al., 2001). Better recognition memory suggests encoding processes are relatively intact in VaD patients compared with AD patients, but information retrieval is deficient. This retrieval deficit appears to be quite common in subcortical dementias, with which VaD appears to have several components in common. Patients with VaD also perform more poorly on phonemic fluency tasks relative to semantic fluency tasks, which suggests greater executive dysfunction due to disruption of the frontal subcortical circuitry, rather than degeneration in the temporal lobes.

A presidential advisory from the American Heart Association and American Stroke Association was published to identify metrics to define optimal brain health in adults. Ideal health behaviors include nonsmoking, physical activity at goal levels, healthy diet consistent with current guidelines, and body mass index below 25 kg/m$^2$ Ideal health factors include untreated blood pressure below 120/80 mm Hg, untreated total cholesterol less than 299 mg/dL, and fasting blood glucose less than 100 mg/dL (Gorelick, 2017). As depicted in Fig. 44.6, risk factors and lifestyle as well as genetic variants can

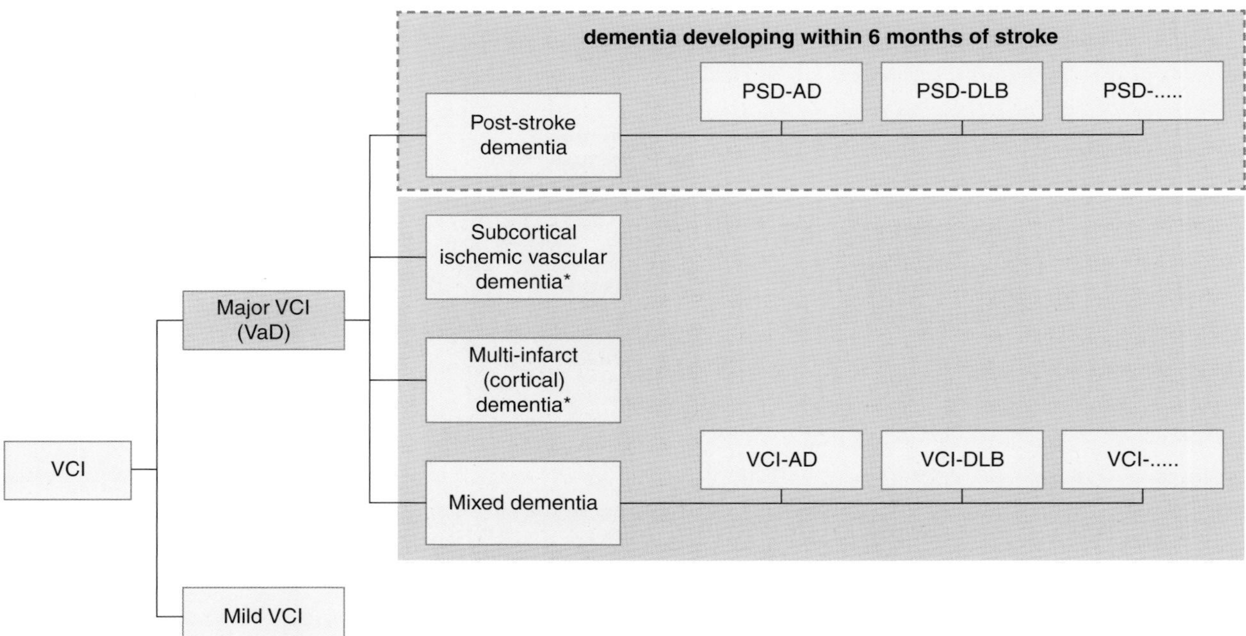


**Fig. 44.7 Vascular Cognitive Impairment.** (*From Skrobot OA, Black SE, Chen C, et al. Progress toward standardized diagnosis of vascular cognitive impairment: guidelines from the Vascular Impairment of Cognition Classification Consensus Study. Alzheimers Dement 2018;14: 280–92*)

either promote or delay damage to large and small cerebral blood vessels, which subsequently result in vascular cognitive impairment and dementia. Classifications of vascular-associated cognitive impairment were recently addressed by a multinational focus group, the Vascular Impairment of Cognition Classification Consensus Study (VICCCS), convened to proposed diagnostic guidelines for VCI and to standardize research and clinical criteria (Fig. 44.7; Skrobot et al., 2018).

## Mixed Dementia

More common than AD and VaD in their pure forms is mixed dementia. While mixed dementia typically refers to a patient having both AD and cerebrovascular pathology, it conceptually can be any case that involves the coexistence of multiple neuropathologies (e.g., amyloid, small-vessel ischemic changes, Lewy body dementias). For patients diagnosed with VaD, 30% may have AD neuropathology as well (Lee et al., 2011) and these patients tend to be older than pure VaD cases. Across dementia autopsy studies, 21%–80% of cases had mixed AD and vascular pathology (Jellinger, 2013; Wilson et al., 2012). In older patients (>90 years), having both AD and vascular pathology at autopsy was more likely if they had been diagnosed with mixed dementia rather than AD alone (James et al., 2012). The vast majority of mixed dementia cases are AD and vascular pathology but 5% of cases are AD and Lewy body disease. Persons with multiple pathologies are three times more likely to develop dementia than others with only one identifiable diagnosis (Schneider et al., 2007). There is evidence that mixed dementia cases are more globally impaired than similarly staged AD patients (Dong et al., 2013). While this may result from interactive effects, there is evidence that vascular and amyloid burden combine independently to impact cognitive impairment (Park et al., 2013).

## Frontotemporal Dementia

Frontotemporal dementia (FTD) is another common type of dementia and is in fact the second most common in those younger than age 65 (Arvanitakis, 2010). It is less common in older adults and is frequently misdiagnosed as AD (Beber and Chaves, 2013). The term *frontotemporal lobar degeneration* (FTLD) is also frequently used in connection with FTD but usually refers to the pathological aspects of FTD and not the clinical entity (Hales and Hu, 2013). A consortium developed for the study of FTD used the NIH-EXAMINER battery of neuropsychological tests to detect and track cognitive changes in a presymptomatic FTD cohort and recommend its usage for endpoints in clinical trials (Staffaroni, 2019). According to DSM-V (APA, 2013) criteria, FTD has multiple clinical manifestations that include behavioral and language variants. Behavioral observations, neuropsychological testing, and neuroimaging (e.g., frontal or temporal lobe atrophy on computed tomography [CT] or MRI, hypoperfusion or hypometabolism on single-photon emission tomography [SPECT] or positron emission tomography [PET]) are used in combination to establish a clinically probable diagnosis of FTD. A definitive diagnosis can be made with histopathological evidence through biopsy or postmortem examination. The latest consensus clinical diagnostic criteria (Rascovsky et al., 2011) define possible FTD as the presence of progressive behavioral and/or cognitive deterioration and three of the following: behavioral disinhibition, apathy or inertia, loss of empathy, perseverative or compulsive behaviors, hyperorality or dietary change, and neuropsychological testing demonstrating executive impairments with intact memory and visuospatial abilities. Probable FTD requires that the patient meet criteria for possible FTD and also has evidence of functional decline and neuroimaging consistent with frontal and anterior temporal atrophy or dysfunction.

Although cognitive deficits are clearly evident on formal testing, the earliest and most common complaints for the behavioral variant of FTD are related to changes in personality and behavior. Increases in impulsivity, poor judgment, stereotypic behaviors, lack of hygiene, and loss of appropriate social behaviors are all prominent. Euphoria and disinhibition are particularly predictive of FTD compared with other dementias (Perri et al., 2014) while apathy is a nonspecific symptom that can occur in all dementias. A formerly mild-mannered and conscientious patient who develops the behavioral variant of FTD may present as overly frank, crass, and uncaring. The patient is usually indifferent to their behavior, but spouses and adult children are usually embarrassed by his or her conduct. Many of these behavioral issues may have underlying cognitive components. Impaired metacognition, or a deficit in monitoring and appreciating behavior, is typical and much more severe than is seen in AD (Rosen et al., 2014). Social impairments likely reflect an inability to cognitively recognize emotions or perspectives in others. Deficits on cognitive testing typically involve impaired executive functions such as mental flexibility, planning deficits, slowed word/design generation, and multiple response errors. Phonemic fluency also tends to be more impaired than semantic fluency. As the disease progresses, even simple go/no go tasks are difficult. Despite the array of cognitive deficits in FTD, memory and visuospatial functioning tend to be well preserved, and some suggest that a lack of deficits in these domains might be one of the best ways to differentiate FTD from other diseases such as AD (Weintraub et al., 2012).

The language variants of FTD are different clinical entities than the behavioral variant (Harciarek and Cosentino, 2013). Confrontation naming, word finding, speech production, comprehension, and/or syntax all gradually worsen over the course of disease. Memory functioning and visuospatial skills are relatively spared. The proposed DSM-V diagnostic criteria suggest that the language variant of FTD be divided into four subtypes: primary progressive aphasia (PPA), semantic variant, nonfluent/agrammatic variant, and logopenic/phonologic variant (APA, 2013). All of these variants except possibly the semantic variant involve some aspect of anomia or impaired object naming that is worse than AD (Reilly et al., 2011) but have otherwise unique neuropsychological profiles. PPA is characterized primarily by the insidious and gradual decomposition of expressive language functions such as word finding, object naming, grammar, and speech production that also affects comprehension later in the disease process (Weintraub et al., 2012). The semantic variant of FTD involves impaired single-word comprehension, object and/or person knowledge, and dyslexia in the presence of spared single-word repetition, motor speech production, and syntax. These patients may appear to have intact expressive and comprehension language functions but are unable to define vocabulary words or concepts. Nonfluent/agrammatic FTD results in impaired motor speech production, grammatical errors, and comprehension of complex sentences, with intact single-word comprehension and object knowledge. Lastly, the logopenic/phonologic variant presents with deficits in spontaneous word retrieval and repetition of sentences and phrases, while single-word comprehension, object knowledge, and motor speech and grammar production are spared. Neuropsychological testing is ideally suited for specifically characterizing deficits and parsing out the complexity of FTD variants and their specific cognitive profiles. Efforts to differentiate semantic from nonfluent FTD suggest that dual streams of speech processing models may underlie the distinct language presentation with the lexical-conceptual stream subserving the semantic FTD (i.e., ventral tracts that connect the temporal, orbitofrontal, and occipital lobes) and the motor stream impacting the nonfluent FTD (Fridriksson, 2016) and involving striatal connections.

Clinical care for both the cognitive and the behavioral components of FTD are essential for patients and families. Publications are available for healthcare providers and families that offer strategies to help minimize the distressing symptoms associated with FTD (Barton et al., 2016; de Wit et al., 2019; Merrilees et al., 2018; Possin et al., 2017).

## Parkinson Disease and Parkinson-Plus Syndromes

PD is diagnosed upon observation of the cardinal motor signs: reduced movement or speed of movement, rigidity, tremor, and disorders of gait, balance, and posture. PD is also associated with a host of non-motor symptoms, including anxiety, depression, apathy, hallucinations, sleep disruption, sensory changes, autonomic and gastrointestinal dysfunction, fatigue, and cognitive impairments that may progress to dementia (Hoogland et al., 2019). Cognitive decline is common and occurs quickly in PD; over 25% convert from normal cognition to MCI within 3 years of diagnosis and over 20% convert from MCI to dementia without 3 years of follow-up (Saredakis et al., 2019). The prevalence of dementia in PD has been reported from 40% to over 75%. Parkinson disease with dementia (PDD) and dementia with Lewy bodies (DLB) have been collectively classified as *Lewy body dementias*, given their shared α-synuclein pathology (Lim et al., 2013). Incidence peaks at 70–79 years and decreases after that (Savica et al., 2013), making both PDD and DLB two of the young dementias (along with FTD) that do not increase in prevalence with advanced age. The neuropsychological findings in the two disorders are largely similar, so they are often distinguished by differences in the onset of signs and symptoms (Sezgin et al., 2019a, 2019b; Weintraub et al., 2012). The cognitive symptoms of PDD often develop at least 2 years after the onset of motor signs (e.g., bradykinesia, gait instability, tremor, rigidity), while the cognitive symptoms in DLB tend to precede motor features or occur within 1 year of the manifestation of motor signs (Gealogo, 2013; Sezgin et al., 2019a, 2019b). Motor signs develop more quickly in DLB when compared with the insidious onset of PDD signs and symptoms. Although the time course of cognitive symptoms and motor signs in DLB and PDD may serve as a helpful heuristic, caution should be used when differentiating these dementias from one another based on onset alone, since subtle cognitive declines can be detected early in the course of PDD (Tröster, 2008).

The neuropsychological profiles of PDD and DLB are similar. There is considerable heterogeneity in the presentation and progression of cognitive deficits, with some patients displaying only minor cognitive slowing. Rapidly fluctuating attention and level of alertness is a signature symptom (Lee et al., 2012) along with abnormal rapid eye movement (REM) sleep behaviors and anosmia. Overall, the neuropsychological profile of PDD includes bradyphrenia and significant executive and visuospatial impairments (Ballard et al., 2013). Executive dysfunction—including impairments in decision making and planning—may be among the earliest signs of cognitive decline in PDD. Language problems such as decreased verbal fluency, poor comprehension, and difficulty producing complex sentences can occur frequently. Regardless of domain, patients with Parkinson disease generally perform better on neuropsychological testing than Alzheimer patients. It has been noted that the visuospatial deficits common in Parkinson disease may account for some impairments observed on neuropsychological testing (Toner et al., 2012). Psychiatric manifestations, including mood disturbances, anxiety, apathy, and psychosis, are also common in PDD (Ballard et al., 2013). Similar psychiatric problems are also observed in patients with DLB, with the most striking symptom in these patients being well-formed visual hallucinations (Weintraub et al., 2012). These hallucinations are typically not frightening to the patient. They can be any visual object but often take human or animal form. Severity of visuospatial deficits predicts likelihood of visual hallucinations (Perri et al., 2014). Importantly, both PDD and DLB patients have strong adverse reactions to antipsychotic medications that make their use contraindicated in this group.

In addition to characterizing the cognitive sequelae of PD and the effects of pharmacological treatment, neuropsychologists are often called upon to evaluate candidates for deep brain stimulation (DBS) of the subthalamic nucleus. DBS in this region is known to result in potential global cognitive decline (Witt et al., 2013) in preoperatively intact patients and may be contraindicated in PDD or DLB patients who are already cognitively impaired. Furthermore, older PD patients

**TABLE 44.7 Practice Guidelines for Mild Cognitive Impairment: Management**

- Wean from medications that contribute to cognitive impairment (when feasible) and treat modifiable risk factors potentially impacting cognition
- Counsel patients and families that no FDA medications are approved and no pharmacological or dietary agents have been shown to be effective
- A diagnosis of MCI does not mandate an offer of cholinesterase inhibitors. If a clinician chooses to prescribe these, the patient must be informed that this is not backed by empirical evidence
- All patients and families can be informed of participation in current clinical trials (e.g., Trial Match, ClinicalTrials.gov)
- Clinicians should recommend regular exercise (2–3/wk) as part of an overall approach to management
- Clinicians should always counsel patients and families to discuss long-term planning topics such as advance directives, driving safety, finances, and estate planning
- Always assess for behavioral and neuropsychiatric symptoms in MCI and treat with pharmacological and nonpharmacological approaches
- Cognitive interventions can be recommended for persons with MCI

*FDA,* Food and drug administration; *MCI,* mild cognitive impairment.

with MCI prior to DBS may be at greater risk for postoperative declines (Halpern et al., 2009). Systematic review of neuropsychological instruments used in subthalamic nucleus deep brain stimulation in PD patients is shown in Table 44.7 (Barbosa et al., 2019) and may be helpful for clinicians to utilize in their practice (Barbosa et al., 2019). Finally, it is important to note that neuromodulation techniques are growing in popularity for treatment of mood and cognition in PD. Repetitive transcranial magnetic stimulation has been suggested as a method to improve cognitive functions (or delay cognitive decline in PD), although replication is warranted prior to widespread usage (Randver et al., 2018; Trung et al., 2019).

## Huntington Disease

The diagnosis of HD is dependent upon the manifestation of an unequivocal extrapyramidal movement disorder, although cognitive (Paulsen et al., 2014) and behavioral deficits can be the most debilitating aspect of the disease, place the greatest burden on HD families (Nehl and Paulsen, 2004), and can be present in the absence of motor dysfunction (Paulsen and Long, 2014) (Figs. 44.8 and 44.9). HD is characterized by insidious and progressive cognitive, emotional-behavioral, and motor symptoms. The symptom presentation for any given individual can include one or all of the HD domains. Cognitive symptoms can include forgetfulness, inattention, executive dysfunction, slowed psychomotor speed, negative emotion recognition, and deficits in time discrimination and production. Emotional-behavioral symptoms may include apathy, depression, aggression, disinhibition, anxiety, and obsessive and perseverative behaviors. In response to findings illustrating the prominence of cognitive outcomes in HD, Brooks and Dunnett (2013) reviewed animal models of basal ganglia cognitive impairments suggesting that translation of cognitive outcomes may provide readouts that better track disease for interventional studies. Additionally, readers are referred to a recent review that provides an excellent characterization of the human cognitive profile of HD (Snowden, 2017). Unawareness of symptoms in HD has been widely recognized and it can be important for clinicians to monitor symptoms and to provide education concerning them when possible (Andrews et al., 2018).

In a large study of over 1000 research participants with the gene expansion for HD, longitudinal cognitive declines were evident in every test examined (19 tests), with the earliest declines in the Symbol Digit Modality Test, the Smell Identification Test, the Stroop Word Identification Test, and the Trail Making Test evident in a subgroup decades before motor diagnosis (Paulsen et al., 2013, 2014). All cognitive measures examined showed significant changes in the subgroup with the greatest proximity to motor diagnosis, whereas 9 of 10 cognitive measures showed significant change in the intermediate group (7–15 years from motor diagnosis). The cognitive profile of HD is

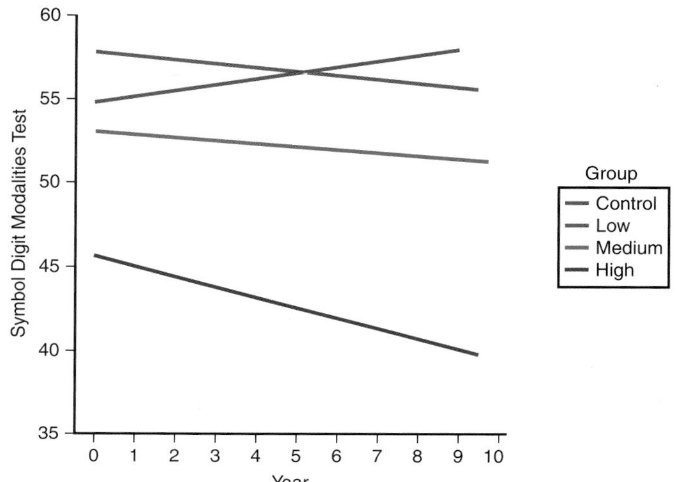


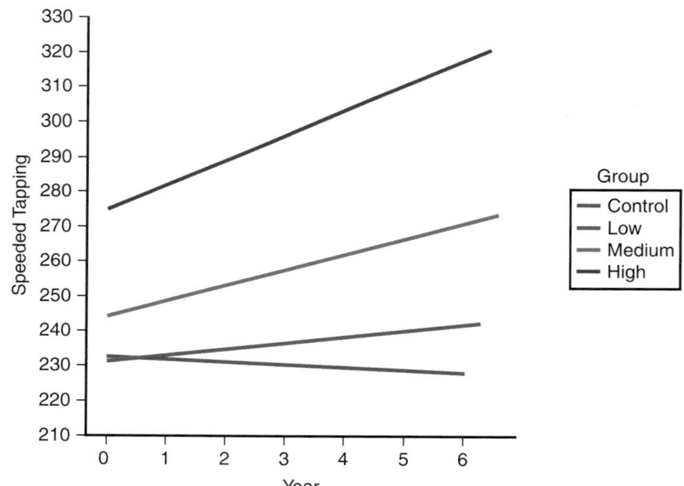


**Fig. 44.8** The upper graph shows the fitted curves (based on a linear mixed effects regression fitted model) of the Symbol Digit Modalities Test by year for progression groups (Control, Low probability of near-future diagnosis, Medium probability, High probability). The lower graph shows the fitted curves for speeded tapping. *(From Paulsen, J.S., Smith, M.M., Long, J.D., 2013. PREDICT-HD investigators and coordinators of the Huntington Study Group. J. Neurol. Neurosurg. Psychiatry 84, 1233–1239, with permission from BMJ Publishing Group Ltd.)*

characterized by bradyphrenia, and impairments in executive function, attention, working memory, emotion recognition, smell identification, and the perception and production of time (Paulsen et al., 2013, 2014; Rowe et al., 2010). One author proposed that poor attention in HD may be due to an inability to automatize task performance, which results in the diversion of cognitive resources to tasks that are normally automatic in healthy people (Thompson et al., 2010). This premise is consistent with the well-known deficit patients with HD have with procedural learning and memory (Holl et al., 2012) as well as automated behavior such as the Stroop reading task. Memory problems are also frequently reported by patients with HD and their families. Objective deficits in learning and memory have been widely reported, with these patients displaying a typical subcortical profile of reduced learning with difficulty in retrieval and improvement with recognition cues. Additionally, emotion recognition declines regardless of modality (i.e., facial expression, verbal intonation), especially for fear, anger, and disgust (Brune et al., 2011; Eddy et al., 2011; 2012; Johnson et al., 2007; Snowden et al., 2008). The cognitive processing retardation is a sensitive (but nonspecific) indicator of dysfunction in most diseases of the basal ganglia and some recent authors have attempted to disintegrate cognitive processing speed, motor slowing, and executive abilities (Maroof et al., 2011; O'Rourke et al., 2011). Similarly, efforts have been made to separate the syntax deficits from working memory in HD (Sambin et al., 2012) to determine whether difficulties in language processing may be secondary to word retrieval, working memory, or a direct syntactical role of the striatum.

Given the known pathology of the striatum and its frontosubcortical connections in HD, attention has only recently been shifted to the importance of the tail of the caudate and its connections with hippocampal-dependent cognition. Careful assessments of spatial memory require further exploration as indicators of HD disease progression (Johnston et al., 2019; Harris et al., 2019).

## Multiple Sclerosis

Cognitive impairment is a common and debilitating symptom of multiple sclerosis (MS). Based on objective neuropsychological testing, it is now recognized that up to 70% of individuals with MS have cognitive impairment (Benedict & Zivadinov, 2011). Although cognitive impairment is significantly greater in the progressive forms, MCI may be observed at the earliest stages of disease even before the MS diagnosis (Amato et al., 2006; Jonsson et al., 2006). Slowed processing speed and executive dysfunction are the most prominent neuropsychological deficits in MS (Parmenter et al., 2007). A large collaborative research group recently reported cognitive impairments of over 1000 MS patients across the subtypes of MS (Ruano et al., 2017). Overall prevalence of cognitive impairment was 46.3%; 34.5% in patients with a clinically isolated syndrome (CIS), 44.5% in relapsing remitting MS, 79.4% in secondary progressive MS, and 91.3% in primary progressive MS. The authors concluded that cognitive impairment is present in all MS subtypes and differences seem to be more associated with patient age and physical disability. Across studies, cognitive impairment is a good predictor of both clinical and cognitive deterioration over time (Damasceno et al., 2019).

Individual differences in the microscopic and macroscopic pathology of the disease lead to variability depending on the location of sclerotic plaques (e.g., subcortical white matter versus spinal cord), though consistent correlations between brain lesion magnitude and severity of cognitive dysfunction have been reported (Benedict et al., 2002). Although deficits vary, the typical cognitive profile of MS has been described as a subcortical one, similar to PD or HD, given the deficits outlined above. Depression and other disturbances of emotional functioning occur in nearly half of these patients (Siegert and Abernethy, 2005). Psychiatric disturbances have also been linked with additional cognitive disability (Feinstein, 2004). Depression in MS has also been found to be related to cognitive deficits, particularly speeded attention and executive functioning (Arnett et al., 2002). Recent efforts have been made to encourage common cognitive assessment tools being used across sites, clinics, countries, and MS cohorts. Early tools lacked robust executive assessments and the Minimal Assessment of Cognitive Functioning in MS (MACFMS) was developed, validated, and normed (Benedict et al., 2006). Given the time (90 minutes) and training commitment of the tool, a shorter assessment was needed. The Brief International Cognitive Assessment in MS (BICAMS; Langdon et al., 2012) was designed for administration in 15 minutes. Ongoing efforts involve the development of computerized assessments and single tests (Benedict et al., 2017) for clinical trials in MS (Langdon et al., 2012). Treatment strategies have expanded significantly, and include pharmacological strategies as well as dietary and exercise training and cognitive rehabilitation (Sailer et al., 2019).

## Epilepsy

Epilepsy, or seizure disorder, is well known to result in significant psychiatric and cognitive comorbidities. Traditionally, these comorbid issues were viewed as epiphenomena of epilepsy but the emerging view is that there is a bidirectional relationship (Helmstaedter et al., 2017). Evidence suggests that neuropsychological deficits in epilepsy are likely related to a variety of factors such as the cumulative effect on the brain of seizure disorder, interictal activity, and negative side effects of antiepileptic drugs (AEDs). Diagnosis of epilepsy is based on electroencephalographic studies. Most successful treatments are pharmacological though about 30% of patients fail to respond to standard treatment. The cognitive effects of epilepsy are unique for each patient, because there is no single cognitive profile associated with any epilepsy subtype; this is largely due to the fact that epilepsy is not a single disease process but rather any number of etiologies affecting different cortical substrates that result in seizures (Korczyn et al., 2013). In general, there are known associations of increased cognitive decline with earlier onset age of seizures and significant discrepancies in intellectual functions (van Iterson et al., 2014) that vary according to the location of the seizure foci, frequency of seizures, duration of seizure disorder, and antiepileptic drug effects (Jokeit and Schacher, 2004; Lee and Clason, 2008). Given the heterogeneity of cognitive deficits in epilepsy, neuropsychological testing is particularly indicated to provide an accurate characterization of patients' unique cognitive deficits. Common data elements for epilepsy have been identified and clinicians should make an effort to utilize the recommended tasks: American National Adult Reading Test, Wechsler Adult Intelligence Scale, Wechsler Abbreviated Scale of Intelligence, Trail Making Test, Wisconsin Card Sorting Test, Grooved Pegboard, Boston Naming Test, Controlled Oral Word Association Test, Animal Naming, Rey Auditory Verbal Learning Test (Loring et al., 2011; Hermann et al., 2017).

Memory deficits are one of the most common clinical manifestations of cognitive impairment in epilepsy, likely due to the high incidence of seizures originating in the medial temporal lobes. There is general support for left temporal lobe epilepsy (TLE) resulting in verbal memory impairment (Brown et al., 2014), but there are mixed findings regarding right TLE specifically resulting in visual memory impairments. There is evidence that left TLE results in greater disruption of cortical connective networks than right TLE and this may support greater memory deficits in left TLE than right TLE (Zulfi et al., 2014). In addition to memory, executive functioning and visuoconstructional abilities can be mildly impaired in both left and right TLE compared

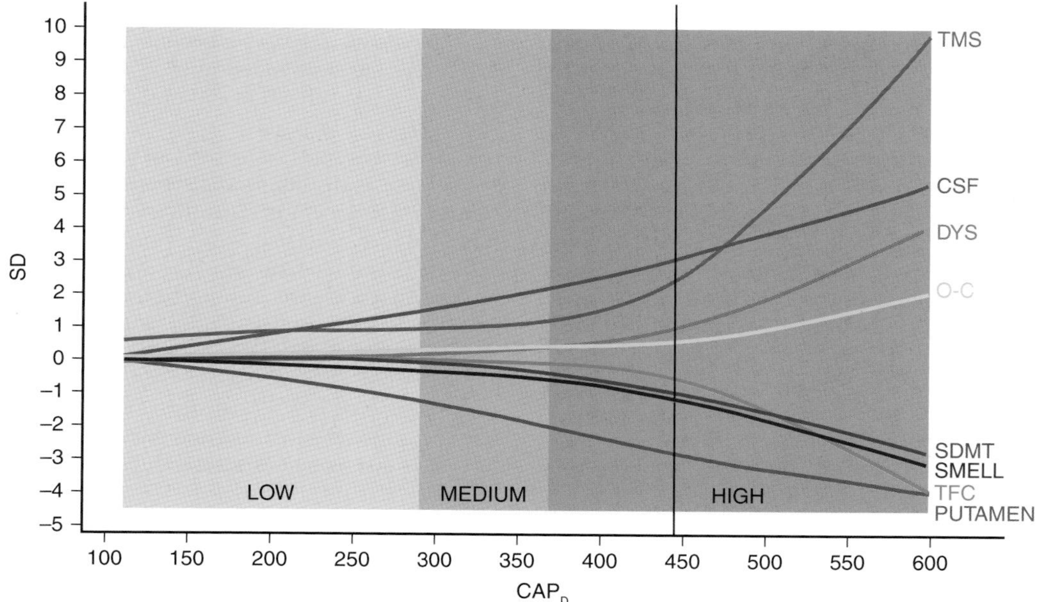


**Fig. 44.9** Data-derived model of premanifest Huntington disease. Scaled fitted spline curves of key variables plotted over CAP$_D$ (CAG-corrected age). *Blue colors* indicate variables that decrease and *red colors* indicate variables that increase. Vertical axis is in standard deviation *(SD)* units. *TMS,* Total motor score; *CSF,* cerebrospinal fluid; *DYS,* dysrhythmia; *O-C,* obsessive–compulsive; *SDMT,* Symbol Digit Modalities Test; *SMELL,* University of Pennsylvania Smell Identification Test (UPSIT); *TFC,* total functional capacity. (*From Paulsen, J.S., Long, J.D., Johnson, H.J., et al., the PREDICT-HD Investigators and Coordinators of the Huntington Study Group, 2014. Clinical and biomarker changes in premanifest Huntington disease show trial feasibility: a decade of the PREDICT-HD study. Front. Aging Neurosci. 6, 78.*)

with healthy individuals, with earlier age of onset being associated with worse deficits. It should be noted that many forms of epilepsy—such as benign rolandic, absence, and juvenile myoclonic epilepsies, to name just a few—are thought to have little to no progressive effect on cognitive functions (Avanzini et al., 2013).

Neuropsychological evaluation is an integral part of neurosurgical treatments for pharmaco-resistant epilepsy (Helmstaedter, 2004). Preoperative evaluations and Wada testing provide useful information about the localization and lateralization of seizure-induced cognitive impairment. Assessment of patients' cognitive reserve can be useful for predicting postoperative outcomes (e.g., better memory performance at baseline usually means greater memory loss after resection). Postoperative testing is also useful for treatment planning and quality control following resection, and ultimately refines the effectiveness of surgical procedures. It should be noted that the evidence is mixed whether resective surgery significantly improves cognitive functioning (Hallböök et al., 2013; Smith et al., 2014). Neuropsychological test batteries for surgery candidates are usually very extensive. Given the frequency of temporal lobectomy surgery relative to other procedures, most batteries are heavily focused on assessing memory and language functioning, given the deleterious effects these areas can have on quality of life impairments, but executive functioning, attention, cognitive efficiency, and visuospatial abilities are also examined. Wada testing is still considered the gold standard for determining how the nonepileptic hemisphere will function in isolation, but functional MRI (fMRI) is gaining acceptance as an alternative for language mapping (Barnett et al., 2014). Other indications for improved prognosis include early seizure onset (due to the increased potential for cortical reorganization) and left-handedness. Ultimately, neuropsychological assessment in Wada testing can help reduce the potential for post-surgical disconnection syndromes, aphasia, and functional loss due to unexpectedly poor contralateral compensation.

In addition to the cognitive aspects of epilepsy, psychiatric and behavioral disorders are prevalent (McCagh et al., 2009). Depression is the most common mood disorder, with 42% of epilepsy patients reporting symptoms (Helmstaedter and Witt, 2012). Rates of depression do not differ between TLE and FLE, though TLE patients with comorbid depression or interictal psychosis have more complicated courses and neuropathological differences than TLE patients without psychiatric comorbidities (Kandratavicius et al., 2012). Increased anxiety in patients does not appear to be directly associated with the neuropathology of epilepsy, but rather the unpredictability of seizures, social consequences of epilepsy, and societal stigmatization (Mensah et al., 2007). There is also the phenomenon known as forced normalization, where the successful pharmacological management of seizures results in onset of psychotic symptoms. It is hypothesized in these cases that the uncontrolled seizures provided a type of electroconvulsive therapy to suppress a pre-existing psychotic condition.

A landmark paper reviewing the intersection of cognition, brain structure, and epilepsy can be found in JINS (Hermann, 2017), where leaders in the field review historical research and progress in clinical care for epilepsy over the past 50 years.

## Traumatic Brain Injury

Traumatic brain injury (TBI) is one of the most common forms of neurological damage in the United States, resulting in more than 53,000 deaths a year, particularly in young males (Coronado et al., 2011). Prevalence studies estimate that over 5.3 million people in the United States and over 7.7 million in Europe have persistent impairments secondary to TBI. In cases of moderate to severe injury, impairments in several cognitive domains can occur, depending on what caused the injury, the severity of the injury, site of the lesion, premorbid cognitive and personality factors, and treatment received after the injury. Advances in knowledge regarding the various cognitive

**TABLE 44.8 Common Neurocognitive Sequelae of Moderate to Severe Traumatic Brain Injury**

| Cognitive Domain | Clinical Manifestation of Impairment |
|---|---|
| Attention | Difficulty with sustained attention<br>Poor concentration<br>Psychomotor impersistence |
| Memory | Problems with acquiring and retaining new verbal or nonverbal information<br>Problems in retrieving verbal and nonverbal memories |
| Speed of information processing | Slowed sensorimotor skills and information processing |
| Executive functioning | Problems in convergent and divergent reasoning<br>Poor judgment<br>Difficulty planning<br>Problems in self-monitoring and self-correcting behavior |
| Awareness of symptoms | Difficulty recognizing deficits<br>Unrealistic expectations concerning the recovery of functions<br>Problems related to poor treatment compliance |
| Language and communication | Problems in word comprehension<br>Impaired reading, spelling, and writing ability<br>Tendency to become fragmented in free speech |
| Integrative functions | Problems in adequate or time-efficient execution of various perceptual-motor-spatial-sequential tasks |

sequelae of TBI have allowed for better diagnostic clarity. Staging the severity of TBI is based on signs and symptoms that occur at the time of the injury. Methods for such staging include the Glasgow Coma Scale Total Score, with scores greater than or equal to 13 being mild, scores 9–12 called moderate, and scores less than or equal to 8 being severe. Alternatively, mild TBI, otherwise referred to as "concussion," reflects loss of consciousness less than 30 minutes and retrograde or anterograde amnesia less than 30 minutes surrounding the injury. Injuries associated with greater than 30 minutes of loss of consciousness or retrograde or anterograde amnesia of greater than 30 minutes are diagnosed with moderate or severe TBI. Beyond these established methods for staging the severity of TBI, neuropsychological testing can be used to increase understanding about functional capacity and rehabilitation needs by measuring the classic cognitive deficits that result from head injury.

The range of deficits following parenchymal damage can vary significantly, so neuropsychological assessment is frequently warranted. Damage to the frontal cortex is common due to the morphology of the skull and frequency of anterior impacts during falls and motor vehicle accidents. For example, a circumscribed TBI involving the ventromedial prefrontal cortex can produce changes in social cognition and emotion recognition that result in behavioral issues (Spikman et al., 2013) associated with misinterpretation of social cues or lowered frustration tolerance. There is also evidence of a general pattern of executive impairment following TBI resulting from disruption of white matter structural networks in the brain (Caeyenberghs et al., 2014). This combination of social, behavioral, and executive dysfunction is often called the *frontal lobe syndrome* and is common in TBI. A less severe TBI might only lead to subtle deficits in attention or processing speed (Rackley et al., 2012), though fatigue is also a common comorbidity (Zgaljardic et al., 2014). Despite individual clinical variability, several common neurobehavioral sequelae of moderate to severe TBI can be identified (Table 44.8). Cognitive recovery is protracted for moderate to severe TBIs, with most improvements occurring in the first year but measurable recovery of cognitive functioning still occurring several years after the injury. However, even after a prolonged length of time, individuals do not necessarily return to preinjury levels.

Cognitive sequelae of concussion, or mild TBI, have become a major focus of research and public education campaigns with particular emphasis on sports-related concussion and blast-related TBIs sustained by soldiers in Iraq and Afghanistan. Mild TBI can be further subdivided into: uncomplicated, with a recognized change in mental status without observed structural abnormalities; and complicated, where there is an acute change in mental status and visible structural abnormalities are observed on neuroimaging. While complicated mild TBI has traditionally been believed to result in worse outcomes, research has demonstrated there is no substantial difference between complicated and uncomplicated TBI on measures of cognitive functioning and self-reported symptoms at 1 month post-injury (Iverson et al., 2012a; Lange et al., 2012).

The latest consensus statement on treatment of concussion (McCrory et al., 2013) states that 90% of adults with mild TBI resolve within 10 days, that neuropsychological assessment is recommended to assist with management, and that while acute rest is recommended, there is limited research support for the efficacy of this intervention. Comparing moderate and severe classifications of TBI with mild TBI suggests that milder TBI typically results in no lingering deficits (Jamora et al., 2012; Vanderploeg et al., 2014; Winardi et al., 2014); the vast majority of mild TBI cases will make a full recovery. Some individuals report a constellation of symptoms following mild TBI that include headaches, fatigue, irritability, depression, and poor concentration. This is commonly referred to as the post-concussive syndrome (PCS) and is associated with pre-existing mood and anxiety symptoms, as well as mood changes surrounding the injury, and negative beliefs regarding cognitive effects of TBI (Kit et al., 2014; Lange et al., 2014). Some controversy has occurred about the interpretation of research following mild TBI, however, and it is recommended that care is taken when reading articles claiming a "systematic review" or a "scoping review" (Iverson et al., 2019). It is suggested that all individuals with TBI have a careful examination of PCS severity and cognitive consequences and that follow-up assessment is planned by 1 year to document the persistence or absence of cognitive impairment as well as the existence of post-concussive syndrome (i.e., headache, fatigue, inattention, mood, and anxiety changes). Within the individual patient, this controversy can be improved via careful measurement of cognitive as well as psychiatric sequelae (Stein et al., 2016). Treatment for patients with persisting PCS frequently involves education and setting factual expectations about the normal course of recovery from their injury and prognosis, with earlier education leading to generally better outcomes.

Additionally, though clinical lore stipulates that there is increasing neurological damage with a history of multiple concussions, there is mixed evidence supporting this proposition (Iverson et al., 2012b), though a history of more severe TBI may negatively affect health outcomes (Dams-O'Connor et al., 2013). It is likely that outcomes following all severity levels and frequencies of TBI will continue to increase in precision as TBI is better evaluated and described. The mandate for better evaluation of concussion and TBI will continue as we learn about repetitive head impact exposure (RHIE) from sports-related injuries and consequences of war, including biological and blast injuries.

## Challenges and Recommendations for Future Research

The fields of investigation into neuropsychological measurement, interpretation, and treatments that might impact adults with brain injury, degeneration, and dysfunction has advanced widely over the past few decades. With the advances in technology including wearable devices, computerized assessments facilitating preconscious as well as conscious assessments of brain functions, neuroimaging of structure, function, static and dynamic connectivity including multimodal and multiplexed imaging platforms, as well as therapeutic advances in genome editing and pharmaceutical developments, the field is likely to undergo an unprecedented explosion of clinical applications over the next few decades.

*The complete reference list is available online at https://expertconsult.inkling.com/.* 

45

# Neurourology

*Jalesh N. Panicker, Ranan DasGupta, Amit Batla*

## OUTLINE



Urogenital dysfunction can result from a variety of neurological disorders, and the impact of lower urinary tract (LUT) dysfunction on a patient's health, dignity, and quality of life is increasingly becoming recognized. The investigation and management of disorders of urogenital function have traditionally been regarded as the preserve of urologists. More recently, neurologists and specialists in rehabilitation have become involved in assessment as well as with the range of effective nonsurgical treatments. Mechanical obstruction of urinary outflow, bladder stones, and other intravesical pathology are still considered to be within the surgical domain. However, problems of neuronal control of the bladder may present to physicians or urologists, and there has been a concomitant increased awareness among treating clinicians about the investigative approach and treatment options in cases of urogenital dysfunction. This has, in turn, led the clinical specialists to increasingly inquire about their patients' symptoms of disordered urogenital function and take an active interest in *uroneurology*—bladder dysfunction viewed from a neurological perspective. This chapter describes what a neurologist needs to know for the management of patients with neurogenic urogenital and bowel problems. Urodynamic, neurophysiological, and radiological investigations and available treatment options are described.

## THE LOWER URINARY TRACT AND ITS NEUROLOGICAL CONTROL

The LUT, consisting of the bladder and urethra, performs two roles in health: storage of urine and emptying at appropriate times. Control of the detrusor and urethral sphincters in these two mutually exclusive states depends on both local spinal reflexes and central cerebral control. The pontine micturition center, which receives input from higher centers (including the hypothalamus and cortical areas such as the medial prefrontal cortex) via the periaqueductal gray of the midbrain, is responsible for switching between these two states. Intact neural circuitry between the pontine micturition center and the LUT ensures coordinated activity between the detrusor and the sphincters.

The frequency of micturition in a person with a bladder capacity of 400–600 mL is once every 3–4 hours, and voiding takes 2–3 minutes. This means that for more than 98% of life, the bladder is in a *storage phase.* Switching to a *voiding phase* is initiated by a conscious decision, which is determined by the perceived state of bladder fullness and an assessment of the social appropriateness of doing so. Connections between the pons, the sacral spinal cord, and the peripheral innervation to the LUT must be intact for these functions to be effective. During the storage phase, sympathetic and pudendally mediated contraction of the internal and external urethral sphincters, respectively, maintains continence. Inhibition of the parasympathetic outflow prevents detrusor contractions (Fowler et al., 2008). When it is deemed appropriate to void, the pontine micturition center is no longer tonically inhibited and reciprocal activation-inhibition of the sphincter-detrusor is reversed. Relaxation of the pelvic floor and external and internal urethral sphincters accompanied by parasympathetically mediated detrusor contraction results in effective bladder emptying. Intact neural circuitry between the pontine micturition center and the bladder ensures coordinated activity between the detrusor and sphincter muscles. Fig. 45.1 reviews the innervation of the bladder.

Functional brain imaging studies—initially positron emission tomography (PET) and today functional magnetic resonance imaging (fMRI) using different paradigms comprising LUT or pelvic floor tasks—have helped to identify different cortical, subcortical, and brainstem regions involved in the higher control of urinary storage and voiding in humans. The initial PET experiments of Blok and colleagues identified the brain centers activated during attempted micturition (Blok et al., 1997, 1998). In patients able to void during the scanning, activity was shown in a region of the medioposterior pons called the *Mregion*. In those subjects unable to void, a distinct region in the ventrolateral pontine tegmentum was activated, the *Lregion*. Although it had been demonstrated in cats that separate pontine nuclei exist for the storage and voiding phases of bladder activity, subsequent experiments have failed to consistently demonstrate activity in this distinct L region. In the cortex, the PET scans showed significant activity in the right inferior frontal gyrus and the right anterior cingulate gyrus during voiding that was not present during the withholding phase. Nour and associates then corroborated these findings with their own PET study of 12 healthy male volunteers. Their study showed activity in a number of brain areas, including the cerebellum (Nour et al., 2000). Other areas that show "activation" in fMRI during bladder filling include the anterior cingulate gyrus and right insula. Functional MRI has shown that the medial prefrontal cortex, which is responsible for complex cognitive and socially appropriate behavior, plays an important role in voiding. A recent article reviews the contribution of functional imaging studies to the current understanding of the central neural control of LUT functions (Griffiths, 2015).

## THE LOWER BOWEL AND ITS NEUROLOGICAL CONTROL

Similar to the bladder, the lower bowel also exists mostly in the storage mode. Continence is maintained by a combination of the acute anorectal angle, puborectalis contraction, and internal anal sphincter tone; these are determined by sympathetic activity. In health, defecation can be delayed if necessary by contraction of the external anal sphincter and pelvic floor musculature, which requires sensory feedback from the anorectum. The process of defecation involves a series of neurologically controlled actions that begin in response to the conscious sensation of a full rectum. When this is perceived and if judged to be appropriate, defecation is initiated by maneuvers to raise the intraabdominal pressure and by straining down, causing descent of the pelvic floor. The internal anal sphincter pressure falls as a result of the rectoanal inhibitory reflex, and the pubococcygeus and striated external sphincter relax. Functional imaging has been applied to evaluate central processing of different types of gastrointestinal stimulation. Hobday and associates used fMRI to identify the brain centers involved in the processing of anal (somatic) and rectal (visceral) sensation in healthy adults (Hobday et al., 2001). Rectal stimulation resulted in activation of the somatosensory cortex, insula, anterior cingulate, and prefrontal cortex; anal canal stimulation produced similar regions of activity, although anterior cingulate activity was absent and primary somatosensory activation was slightly more superior in location. The activation of the cingulate cortex with rectal stimulation may signify the function of the limbic system in the processing of visceral stimuli.

The processing of rectal sensation is relevant in bladder function because, unlike other gut organs, it has an important sensory role, and the rectum is a visceral organ that contains both unmyelinated C fibers

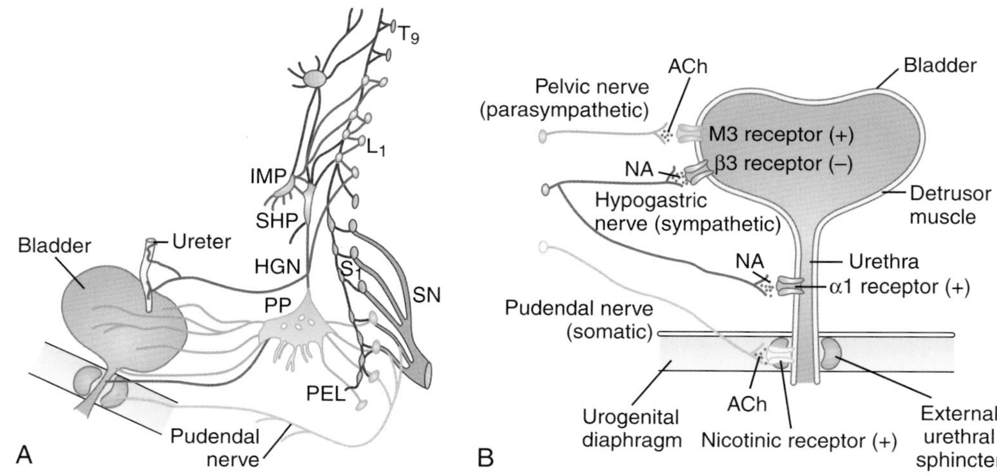


**Fig. 45.1 Innervation of the Lower Urinary Tract. A,** Sympathetic fibers (shown in *blue*) originate in the T11–L2 spinal cord segments and running through the inferior mesenteric ganglia (inferior mesenteric plexus *[IMP]*) and hypogastric nerve *(HGN)* or through the paravertebral chain to enter pelvic nerves at the base of the bladder and urethra. Parasympathetic preganglionic fibers (shown in *green*) arise from the S2–S4 spinal cord segments and travel in sacral roots and pelvic nerves *(PEL)* to ganglia in the pelvic plexus *(PP)* and bladder wall. This is where the postganglionic nerves that supply parasympathetic innervation to the bladder arise. Somatic motor nerves (shown in *brown*) that supply the striated muscles of the external urethral sphincter arise from S2–S4 motor neurons and pass through pudendal nerves. **B,** Efferent pathways and neurotransmitter mechanisms that regulate lower urinary tract. Parasympathetic postganglionic axons in pelvic nerve release acetylcholine *(ACh)*, which produces bladder contraction by stimulating M3 muscarinic receptors in bladder smooth muscle. Sympathetic postganglionic neurons release noradrenaline *(NA)*, which activates $\beta_3$-adrenergic receptors to relax bladder smooth muscle and activates $\beta_1$-adrenergic receptors to contract urethral smooth muscle. Somatic axons in pudendal nerve also release ACh, which produces contraction of external sphincter striated muscle by activating nicotinic cholinergic receptors. $L_1$, First lumbar root; $S_1$, first sacral root; *SHP*, superior hypogastric plexus; *SN*, sciatic nerve; $T_9$, ninth thoracic root. *(From Fowler, C.J., Griffiths, D., de Groat, W.C., 2008. The neural control of micturition. Nat Rev Neurosci 9, 453–466.)*

and thinly myelinated Aδ afferents. In contrast, the anal canal has a somatic innervation from the pudendal nerve. The study by Hobday and associates (2001) has highlighted the differences in its cortical representation from that of the rectum. The various brain imaging studies of visceral stimulation, including the foregoing report, have been reviewed (Derbyshire, 2003).

Lower gastrointestinal stimuli predominantly activate the prefrontal and orbitofrontal cortices, as well as the insula, with variability in cingulate activation.

## SEXUAL FUNCTION AND ITS NEUROLOGICAL CONTROL

Physiological sexual responses in men and women has been divided classically into four phases: excitement, plateau, orgasm, and resolution. Excitation occurs in response to both physical and psychological stimulation and results in clitoral or penile tumescence. Homologous to achieving an erection in men is vaginal lubrication in females. The plateau phase is accompanied by the various physical changes of high sexual arousal in anticipation of orgasm. Orgasm, an intensely sensory event, usually is associated with rhythmic contraction of the pelvic floor and culminates with ejaculation in men. During resolution, the increased genital blood flow resolves. A modification of this model of sexual response was the three-phase model proposed by Kaplan, consisting of desire, arousal, and orgasm.

There has been a shift in contemporary literature with regard to viewing sexual response in physiological terms as a motivation/incentive–based cycle involving a complex network of cognitive, motivational, emotional, and autonomic components (Basson, 2015).

In summary, the components of the neural control are as follows:

a. The cognitive component with recognition of potentially sexual stimuli, with focused attention on motor imagery. This leads to activation of the right lateral orbitofrontal cortex, of the right and the left inferior temporal cortices, of the superior parietal lobules, and of areas belonging to the neural network mediating motor imagery (inferior parietal lobules, left ventral premotor area, right and left supplementary motor areas, cerebellum).
b. The motivational component processes the direct behavior to a sexual goal, including the perceived urge to express overt sexual behavior with correlates in the anterior cingulate cortex, claustrum, posterior parietal cortex, hypothalamus, substantia nigra, and ventral striatum.
c. The emotional component is the brain activity underlying pleasure from the mental excitement and the perception of bodily changes, especially those of the genital response with correlates in the left primary and secondary somatosensory cortices, the amygdala, and the right posterior insula.
d. The autonomic and neuroendocrine component includes various responses (e.g., genital, cardiovascular, respiratory, changes in hormonal plasma levels), leading subjects to a state of physiological readiness for sexual behavior. The neural corelates are in the anterior cingulate cortex, anterior insulae, putamen, and hypothalamus.

Studies using functional brain imaging have highlighted some key areas associated with sexual functioning—for example, the role of the hypothalamus in reproductive function, regulation of human sexuality, and regulation of erection through the medial preoptic area, or the roles of the insula and claustrum in autonomic regulation and visceral sensory processing. The other areas involved in sexual arousal are lateral occipitotemporal, inferotemporal, parietal, orbitofrontal, medial prefrontal, insular, anterior cingulate, and frontal premotor cortices as well as, for subcortical regions, the amygdala, claustrum, hypothalamus, caudate nucleus, thalami, cerebellum, and substantia nigra. Most studies included visual sexual stimuli, which were seen to activate the amygdala and thalami more in men than in women. There are no differences in the areas that show increased activity in response to sexual arousal in heterosexual or homosexual humans. Ejaculation is associated with decreased activation throughout the prefrontal cortex.

### Male Sexual Response

Erection results from increased blood flow into the corpora cavernosa caused by relaxation of the smooth muscle in the cavernosal arteries and a reduction in venous return. The major peripheral innervation determining this is parasympathetic, which arises from the S2–S4 segments and travels to the genital region in the pelvic nerves. Sympathetic input also is important: the sympathetic innervation of the genital region originates in the thoracolumbar chain (T11–L2) and travels through the hypogastric nerves to the confluence of nerves that lies on either side of the rectum and the LUT—the pelvic plexus.

The pelvic plexus also receives input from the pelvic nerves. It is from the pelvic plexus that the cavernous nerves, which innervate the corpora cavernosa, arise. Although erection is induced by parasympathetic activity, nitric oxide has been identified as important in causing relaxation of the corporeal blood vessels and the increase in penile blood flow that causes erection. Psychogenic erection requires cortical activation of spinal pathways. The preservation of this type of responsiveness in men with low spinal cord lesions suggests that sympathetic pathways can mediate it. Reflex erections occur as a result of cutaneous genital stimulation. Preservation of reflex erections in men with lesions above T11 indicates that the response is the result of spinal reflexes, with afferent signals conveyed in the pudendal nerve, the S2–S4 roots, and efferent signals through the same sacral roots. In health, reflex and psychogenic responses merge and are thought to reinforce one another. In men, orgasm and ejaculation are not the same process: ejaculation is the release of semen, and orgasm consists of the sensory changes accompanied by pelvic floor contractions. Ejaculation involves the emission of semen from the vas and seminal vesicles into the posterior urethra and closure of the bladder neck. The latter processes are under sympathetic control, whereas the contraction of the pelvic floor muscles is under somatic nerve control, innervation being from the perineal branch of the pudendal nerve. After ejaculation, a period of resolution is necessary before sexual activity can be reinitiated.

### Female Sexual Response

The neurological control of sexual function in women is less well understood than that in men, but similarities exist: the main parasympathetic innervation is from the pelvic nerves, the sympathetic innervation from the hypogastric nerves, and bilateral somatic innervation from the pudendal nerves. The finding of acetylcholinesterase-positive nerves around blood vessels in the vagina points to parasympathetic control of vaginal vasodilation and secretomotor function. It seems likely that increased vaginal blood flow, erection of the cavernous tissue of the clitoris and around the outer part of the vagina, and lubrication are brought about through neural mechanisms similar to those that control erection in men. The lubrication that occurs as part of sexual arousal results from transudation through the vaginal walls and fluid from the Bartholin glands.

During orgasm, a series of synchronous contractions of the sphincter and vaginal muscles may occur. As many as 20 consecutive contractions have been registered, lasting for 10–50 seconds. The accompanying sensory experience is generally described as an intensely pleasurable pelvic event (Huynh et al., 2013).

## NEUROGENIC LOWER URINARY TRACT DYSFUNCTION

Lesions of the nervous system can result in characteristic changes in LUT functions depending upon the level of the lesions in the neurological axis; the phrase "neurogenic bladder" is an oversimplification of LUT dysfunction occurring following neurological disease. Depending upon the site of lesion in the neuraxis, different patterns of dysfunction may occur (Fig. 45.2; Panicker et al., 2015).

Suprapontine and infrapontine–suprasacral lesions result in involuntary spontaneous or induced contractions of the detrusor muscle (known as detrusor overactivity), which can be identified during the filling phase of urodynamics. Bladder emptying can be affected following infrapontine lesions. Following spinal cord injury (SCI), simultaneous contraction of the urethral sphincters and detrusor may occur during attempted voiding, known as *detrusor–sphincter dyssynergia,* which results in incomplete bladder emptying and abnormally high bladder pressures. Following lesions of the conus medullaris or cauda equina, voiding dysfunction can occur due to poorly sustained detrusor contractions and possibly nonrelaxing urethral sphincters (see Fig. 45.2).

### Cortical Lesions and Dementia

#### Lower Urinary Tract Dysfunction

It has been known since the 1960s that anterior regions of the frontal lobes are critical for bladder control. Following frontal lobe injuries—such as intracranial tumors, damage after rupture of an aneurysm, penetrating brain wounds, and prefrontal lobotomy (leukotomy)—the typical clinical picture of frontal lobe incontinence is of a patient with severe urgency and frequency of micturition and urge incontinence but without dementia; the patient is socially aware and embarrassed by the incontinence. Micturition is normally coordinated, indicating that the disturbance is in the higher control of these processes. Urinary retention has also been uncommonly described in patients with brain lesions. A small number of case histories have described patients with right frontal lobe disorders who had urinary retention and in whom voiding was restored once the frontal lobe disorder had been treated (Fowler, 1999).

Urinary incontinence develops in some patients after stroke. Urinary incontinence at 7 days following stroke predicts poor survival, disability, and institutionalization independent of level of consciousness. It has been suggested that incontinence in such cases is the result of severe general loss of function or that persons who become incontinent may be less motivated to recover both continence and general function. Urodynamic studies in incontinent patients have been carried out, and the general conclusion drawn from studying patients with disparate cortical lesions is that voiding is most often normally coordinated. The most common cystometric finding is that of detrusor overactivity. It has not been possible to demonstrate a correlation between any particular lesion site and urodynamic findings, though urinary incontinence is most often associated with strokes occurring

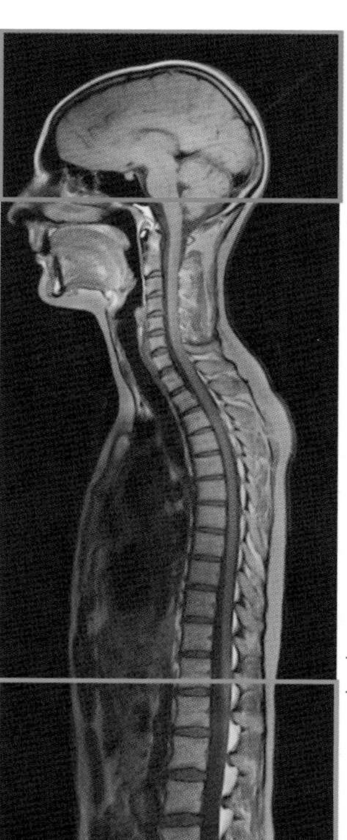



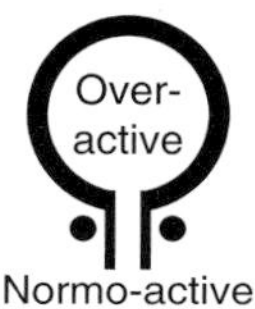

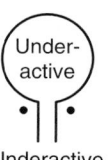

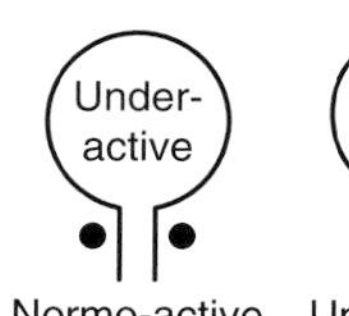

**Fig. 45.2 Patterns of Lower Urinary Tract Dysfunction Following Neurological Disease.** The pattern of lower urinary tract dysfunction following neurological disease is influenced by the site of the lesion. The *blue box* denotes the region above the pons and the *green box* denotes the sacral cord and infrasacral area. Figures on the right show the expected dysfunctional states of the detrusor–sphincter system. *PVR,* Postvoid residual. *(Requires permission from Panicker, J.N., Fowler, C.J., Kessler, T.M., 2015. Lower urinary tract dysfunction in the neurological patient: clinical assessment and management. Lancet Neurol 14[7], 720–732.)*

anteriorly. Patients with hemorrhagic stroke are more likely to have detrusor underactivity in urodynamics compared with patients with ischemic stroke, who more often have detrusor overactivity (Han et al., 2010). Small vessel disease of the white matter (leukoaraiaosis) is associated with urgency incontinence. It is increasingly becoming clear that this is an important cause of incontinence in the functionally independent elderly (Tadic et al., 2010).

The cause of urinary incontinence in dementia is probably multifactorial. Not all incontinent older adults are cognitively impaired, and not all cognitively impaired older adults are incontinent. In a study of patients with progressive cognitive decline, incontinence was observed to occur in more advanced stages of Alzheimer disease, whereas it may occur earlier on in the course of patients who have dementia with Lewy bodies (Ransmayr et al., 2008).

A much less common cause of dementia is normal pressure hydrocephalus, where incontinence is a cardinal feature. Improvement in urodynamic function has been demonstrated within hours of lumbar puncture in patients with this disorder.

### Bowel Dysfunction

Additional text is available at http://expertconsult.inkling.com.

### Sexual Dysfunction

Before functional imaging experiments, all that was known about human cerebral control and sexuality came from observations of patients with brain lesions, particularly those affecting temporal or frontal regions. These areas can be affected by disorders that cause epilepsy or others due to trauma, tumors, cerebrovascular disease, or encephalitis. It has long been observed that sexual dysfunction is more common in men and women with epilepsy. Although various sexual perversions and occasionally hypersexuality have been described in patients with temporal lobe epilepsy, the picture most commonly seen is that of sexual apathy. From studies comparing sexual dysfunction in generalized epilepsy with that in focal temporal lobe epilepsy, the evidence is sufficient to suggest that the deficit is a result of the specific temporal lobe involvement rather than a consequence of epilepsy, psychosocial factors, or antiepileptic medication. The problem is usually that of a low or absent libido, of which patients may not complain.

The role of hormonal dysfunction has yet to be fully determined. On the basis of measurements of sex hormones and pituitary function, it has been suggested that the hyposexuality of temporal lobe epilepsy results from a subclinical hypogonadotropic hypogonadism and that the dysfunction of medial temporal lobe structures may dysmodulate hypothalamopituitary secretion (Murialdo et al., 1995). Erectile dysfunction (ED) with preservation of libido can also occur in men with temporal lobe damage with or without epilepsy and may be characterized by the loss of nocturnal penile tumescence. Surgery for epilepsy rarely restores erectile function, although a survey of operated patients showed a higher level of satisfaction with sexual function among those who were free of seizures. Sexual dysfunction is not uncommon after head injury, particularly in patients who demonstrate cognitive damage. Hypersexual behavior may occur after frontal lobe damage. Lesions of the frontal lobes, the basal-medial part in particular, may lead to loss of social control, which may also affect sexual behavior.

## Basal Ganglial Lesions and Parkinsonism

### Parkinson Disease

Bladder symptoms in Parkinson disease (PD) correlate with neurological disability (Araki and Kuno, 2000) and stage of disease; both findings appear to support a link between dopaminergic degeneration and symptoms of urinary dysfunction. In line with current thinking about the staging of PD in terms of underlying neuropathology (Braak et al., 2004), it appears that bladder dysfunction does not occur until some years after the onset of motor symptoms and that the dysfunction is correlated with the extent of dopamine depletion (Sakakibara et al., 2001c). This means that the underlying pathological process is likely to have extended into the neocortex and explains why the clinical context in which bladder dysfunction is seen in PD is common in patients with cerebral symptoms as well as with the adverse effects of long-standing treatment with dopaminergic agents.

Thirty-eight to 71% of PD patients report lower urinary tract symptoms (LUTS) (Andersen, 1985; Berger et al., 1987). Storage symptoms are the most common problem, which is seen in more than 60% of PD patients; these symptoms have a considerable impact on quality of life (Araki et al., 2000a; Campos-Sousa et al., 2003; Sakakibara et al., 2001b). Nocturia (56.7%) is the most common symptom, followed by urinary urgency; together, these are the commonest nonmotor symptoms in PD. The most common abnormality in urodynamic studies is detrusor overactivity (Araki et al., 2000b). It has been demonstrated that the overactive bladder symptom score (OABSS) in PD relates to poor performance of frontal lobe executive function, rapid-eye-movement (REM) sleep behavior disorder, and a higher Hoehn and Yahr score (Xu et al., 2019). This may reflect the fact that OAB symptoms are integral to the neurodegenerative process in PD. It is thought that neuronal loss in the substantia nigra may disinhibit the normal effect of basal ganglia on the micturition reflex, resulting in detrusor overactivity. Dopaminergic stimulation through D1 dopamine receptors provides the main inhibitory influence on the micturition reflex (Yoshimura et al., 2003) in health. However, this is poorly reflected with dopaminergic stimulation in patients with PD.

Overactive bladder (OAB) is currently believed to be the main urological symptom in PD. Many patients with PD have nocturnal polyuria (NP), which may be a significant cause of nocturia and may be associated with excessive production of urine at night, perhaps related to the loss of circadian rhythm in PD (Batla et al., 2016; Batla and Panicker, 2012; Suchowersky et al., 1995). NP would not be expected to improve with antimuscarinics directed to improve the symptoms of OAB. In addition to neurogenic bladder dysfunction, prostatic enlargement may occur concomitantly in some men with PD and contribute to bladder dysfunction. Pelvic floor weakness, stress incontinence, and bradykinesia of the pelvic floor muscles, causing "pseudo-dyssynergia," may be other key factors to consider. A study evaluating the management of benign prostatic obstruction in men with PD highlights the importance of proper patient selection involving neurological and urological input before proceeding with transurethral resection of the prostate (Roth et al., 2009).

Other factors that may contribute to LUTS in PD include associated vascular disease, cervical spondylosis and myelopathy, diabetes mellitus, congestive cardiac failure or pedal edema, and the use of diuretic drugs. These may be commonly associated and difficult to dissect out from inherent bladder dysfunction in PD. Sleep disturbances and disturbed circadian rhythm may be closely associated with nocturia (Cochen De Cock et al., 2010; Gomez-Esteban et al., 2006; Menza et al., 2010). Sleep apnea has been proven to be contributory to nocturia (Saunders and Schuckit, 2006). The management must hence be individualized and should also aim to address the associated features.

### Multiple System Atrophy

MSA must be suspected if bladder symptoms dominate the clinical picture at onset of a parkinsonian condition. As many as 41% of MSA patients present with LUTS and 97% have LUTS during the disease course (Sakakibara et al., 2001d, 2010, 2011; Sammour et al., 2009). These include daytime frequency (45% of women, 43% of men), nighttime frequency (65% of men, 69% of women), urinary urgency

(64% of men), and urgency incontinence (66% of women, 75% of men) (Saunders, 2006).

Although it is well known that patients with MSA of the cerebellar dominant type (MSA-C) show severe autonomic dysfunction, there is poor correlation between the severity of motor dysfunction and urinary dysfunction in MSA-C (Yamamoto et al., 2019). The bladder dysfunction in MSA-P appears much earlier and is more disabling as compared with that in PD. Although OAB symptoms of urgency and frequency occur in both conditions, patients with MSA are more likely to have a high (>100 mL) postvoid residual (PVR; Hahn and Ebersbach, 2005), detrusor–sphincter dyssynergia, an open bladder neck at the start of bladder filling on videocystometrogram (Sakakibara et al., 2001a), and a neurogenic electromyogram (EMG) of the anal sphincter (Kirby et al., 1986; Palace et al., 1997; Roth et al., 2009; Tison et al., 2000).

### Pure Autonomic Failure

Although not affecting basal ganglia predominantly, pure autonomic failure (PAF) is a synucleinopathy similar to MSA. Neurodegeneration is mainly in the postganglionic autonomic neurons with Lewy bodies confined primarily to the neurons of the autonomic ganglia. Nocturia and voiding dysfunction are common and bladder emptying is often affected. Bladder dysfunction in PAF appears to be as common as but less severe than that in in MSA, which could possibly reflect slower progression of the disease (Sakakibara et al., 2000). Orthostatic hypotension, ED, and constipation are also common.

### Bowel Dysfunction

Additional text is available at http://expertconsult.inkling.com.

### Sexual Dysfunction

Experimental evidence from animals and humans shows that dopaminergic mechanisms are involved in determining libido and inducing penile erection. The cause of ED in PD is unclear, but it is a significant problem; in one study it was shown to affect 60% of a group of men with PD as compared with 37.5% of age-matched healthy controls. ED usually affects men later in the course of PD, with onset years after the diagnosis of neurological disease has been established. A survey of relatively young patients with PD (mean age 49.6 years) and their partners revealed a high level of sexual dysfunction, with the most severely affected couples being those in which the patient was male.

ED may be the first symptom in men with MSA, predating the onset of any other neurological symptoms by several years. The disorder appears chronologically to be distinct from the development of postural hypotension. The reason for the apparently early selective involvement of neural mechanisms for erection is not known. Preserved erectile function in a man with parkinsonism strongly contradicts the diagnosis of MSA. The available literature on female sexual problems in movement disorders is limited (Jacobs et al., 2000; Oertel et al., 2003).

Hypersexuality—due to compulsive sexual behavior in some patients with PD treated with dopamine agonists and L-dopa as part of an impulse control disorder (Giovannoni et al., 2000)—is a well-recognized phenomenon. The DOMINION study, which systematically assessed 3090 individuals with PD for impulse control disorders, found that such disorders were present in 13.6% of the patients; specifically, pathological gambling in 5.0%, compulsive sexual behavior in 3.5%, compulsive buying in 5.7%, and binge-eating disorder in 4.3% (Weintraub et al., 2010).

## Brainstem Lesions

Voiding difficulty is a rare but recognized symptom of a posterior fossa tumor and has been reported in series of patients with brainstem disorders (Fowler, 1999). In an analysis of urinary symptoms in 39 patients who had had brainstem strokes, lesions that resulted in micturition disturbance were usually situated dorsally (Sakakibara et al., 1996)—a finding consistent with the known location of the brainstem centers involved with control of the bladder. The proximity in the dorsal pons between the pontine micturition center and the medial longitudinal fasciculus means that a disorder of eye movements, such as an internuclear ophthalmoplegia, is highly likely in patients with a pontine disorder causing difficulty in voiding.

## Spinal Cord Lesions

### Bladder Dysfunction

Spinal cord disorders are the most common cause of neurogenic bladder dysfunction. Transspinal pathways connect the pontine micturition centers to the sacral cord. Intact connections are necessary to affect the reciprocal activity of the detrusor and sphincter, which are needed to switch between storage and voiding. After disconnection from the pons, this synergistic activity is lost, resulting in detrusor–sphincter dyssynergia.

Initially after acute SCI, there is usually a phase of neuronal shock of variable duration characterized clinically by complete urinary retention, with urodynamics demonstrating an acontractile detrusor. Gradually, over the course of weeks, new reflexes emerge to reinitiate bladder emptying and cause detrusor contractions in response to low filling volumes. The neurophysiology of this recovery has been studied in cats, and it has been proposed that after SCI, C fibers emerge as the major afferents, forming a spinal segmental reflex that results in automatic voiding. It is assumed that the same pathophysiology occurs in humans. In support of this assumption is the observed response to intravesical capsaicin (a C-fiber neurotoxin) in patients with acute traumatic SCI or chronically progressive spinal cord disease from multiple sclerosis (MS). The abnormally overactive, small-capacity bladder that characterizes spinal cord disease causes patients to experience urgency and frequency. However, patients with complete transection of the cord may not complain of urinary urgency. If detrusor overactivity is severe, incontinence is highly likely. Poor neural drive on the detrusor muscle during attempts to void, together with an element of detrusor–sphincter dyssynergia, contributes to incomplete bladder emptying. This difficulty may exacerbate the symptoms of the OAB. Although the neurological process of voiding may have been as severely disrupted as the process of storage, the symptoms of difficulty with emptying can be minor compared with those of urge incontinence. Only on direct questioning may the patient admit to having difficulty initiating micturition, an interrupted stream, or possibly a sensation of incomplete emptying.

Because bladder innervation arises more caudally than innervation of the lower limbs, any form of spinal cord disease that causes bladder dysfunction is likely to produce clinical signs in the lower limbs as well unless the lesion is limited to the conus. This rule is sufficiently reliable to be of great value in determining whether a patient has a neurogenic bladder caused by spinal cord disease.

### Spinal Cord Injury

After SCI, bladder dysfunction can be of such severity as to cause ureteric reflux, hydronephrosis, and eventual upper urinary tract damage. Before the introduction of modern treatments, renal failure was a common cause of death after SCI. The bladder problems of persons with SCI, therefore, must be managed aggressively to lessen the possibility of upper tract disease and provide the patient with adequate bladder control for a fully rehabilitated life. People with SCI are often young and otherwise fit; it may be best for them to undergo surgery on the LUT with a view to fulfilling these two aims rather than to be treated medically.

## Multiple Sclerosis

The pathophysiological consequences for the bladder of progressive MS affecting the spinal cord are similar to those of SCI, but the medical context of increasing disability is such that management must be quite different. Estimates of the proportion of patients with MS who have LUTS vary according to the severity of the neurological disability in the group under study, but a figure of about 75% is frequently cited (Marrie et al., 2007). Several studies have shown that urinary incontinence is considered to be among the worst aspects of the disease, with 70% of a self-selected group of patients with MS responding to a questionnaire classifying the impact bladder symptoms had on their life as "high" or "moderate" (Hemmett et al., 2004). A strong association has been recognized between bladder symptoms and the presence of clinical spinal cord involvement, including paraparesis and upper motor neuron signs on examination of the lower limb in patients with MS. A similar observation has been made in patients with a similar condition, acute disseminated encephalomyelitis (ADEM; Panicker et al., 2009).

Considering the multitude of symptoms in MS, not surprisingly, LUTS may be overlooked in the clinical management of MS. The North American Research Committee on MS questionnaire survey found that of more than 5000 patients with MS in North America with troublesome urinary symptoms, only 43% had been referred to urological services and 51% had been treated with antimuscarinic medications (Mahajan et al., 2010). Recently, a screening tool for patients with bladder problems related to MS has been developed and validated; it is called the Actionable Bladder Symptom Screening Tool (Burks et al., 2013). It must be remembered as well that there may be several factors contributing to LUTS in MS (Table 45.1).

Often incomplete bladder emptying and an OAB coexist, with residual urine exacerbating symptoms. Whereas the symptoms of an OAB are a reliable indicator of underlying LUT dysfunction detrusor overactivity (DO), patient reports of incomplete bladder emptying are often not. In a cohort of patients studied by Betts et al. (1993), patients who thought they did not empty their bladders were found to most often be correct; however, only half of those who thought they did were wrong. It is for this reason that measurement of the PVR volume is such a critical investigation in the management of LUTS in patients with MS (Fowler et al., 2009).

A particular problem in MS is that neurological symptoms may worsen acutely when the patient has an infection and pyrexia, including urinary tract infection (UTI). As MS progresses, it is not uncommon for recurrent infections to result in deficits that accumulate and lead to progressive neurological deterioration (Buljevac et al., 2002).

## Bowel Dysfunction

Additional text is available at http://expertconsult.inkling.com.

## Sexual Dysfunction

***Male sexual dysfunction.*** The level and completeness of a spinal cord lesion determine erectile and ejaculatory capability after SCI. With a complete cervical lesion, psychogenic erections are lost, but the capacity for spontaneous or reflex erections may be intact. With low spinal cord lesions, particularly if the cauda equina is involved, little or no erectile capacity may be retained. Theoretically, a lesion below spinal level L2 leaves psychogenic erections intact, but in practice it is uncommon for men with such a lesion to have erections adequate for intercourse. Psychogenic erections are more likely to be preserved in incomplete lesions. Preservation of ejaculatory function after a spinal cord lesion is unusual. Although earlier studies indicated a much lower figure, it is now known that 60%–65% of men with MS have ED, often coexisting with urinary symptoms, with urodynamically demonstrable overactivity in a majority of those affected. Typically, in the early stages of MS, the chief complaint is of difficulty maintaining an erection. With advancing neurological disability, erectile function may cease, and difficulty with ejaculation may develop or become manifest. A study of pudendal evoked potentials in men with MS found that those with severely delayed latencies (i.e., with more severe spinal cord disease) were more likely to be unable to ejaculate. Although it has been said that a diagnosis of MS should be considered in a young man presenting with impotence, this possibility seems unlikely in the absence of clinical spinal cord disease. In one series, only a single patient had erectile difficulties at the time of the first symptoms of MS, and neurological disease did not develop subsequently in any of the men who presented with ED.

***Female sexual dysfunction.*** Studies of women with SCI at different levels, both complete and incomplete, have advanced current understanding of the neural pathways involved in female sexual response. It has been hypothesized that the sensory experience of orgasm may have an autonomic basis, because orgasmic capacity is preserved in a proportion of affected women, particularly those with higher cord lesions (Sipski et al., 2001); fMRI studies in SCI patients suggest preservation of vagal pathways. Sexual dysfunction in women with MS is common (affecting 50%–60%) although probably underdiagnosed, with the incidence increasing with worsening disability. Neurogenic problems during intercourse include decreased lubrication and reduced orgasmic capacity. A double-blind randomized placebo-controlled crossover study of sildenafil citrate in treating females with sexual dysfunction due to MS did not show any overall benefit with this drug, which has been shown to be far more effective in men with MS (Dasgupta et al., 2004). In women with advanced disease, additional problems may include lower limb spasticity, loss of pelvic sensation, genital dysesthesia, and fear of incontinence (Hulter and Lundberg, 1995).

**TABLE 45.1 Diagnostic Findings in Patients with Suspected Neurogenic Bladder Dysfunction**

| | Suprapontine Lesion | Infrapontine–Suprasacral Lesion | Infrasacral Lesion |
|---|---|---|---|
| Examples | Stroke, PD | SCI, MS | Conus medullaris tumor, cauda equina syndrome, peripheral neuropathy |
| History/bladder diary | Urgency, frequency, urgency incontinence | Urgency, frequency, urgency incontinence, hesitancy, interrupted stream | Hesitancy, interrupted stream |
| PVR urine | PVR urine <100 mL | ±Elevated PVR | PVR urine >100 mL |
| Uroflowmetry | Normal flow | Interrupted flow | Poor/absent flow |
| Urodynamics | Detrusor overactivity | Detrusor overactivity<br>Detrusor–sphincter dyssynergia | Detrusor underactivity, sphincter insufficiency |

*MS*, Multiple sclerosis; *PD*, Parkinson disease; *PVR*, postvoid residual; *SCI*, spinal cord injury.
*From Panicker, J.N., Fowler, C.J., 2010. The bare essentials: uro-neurology. Pract Neurol 10, 178–185.*

## Impaired Sympathetic Thoracolumbar Outflow

The fibers that travel from the thoracolumbar sympathetic chain emerge from the T10–L2 spinal levels and course through the retroperitoneal space to the bifurcation of the aorta, from which they enter the pelvic plexus. Loss of sympathetic innervation of the genitalia causes disorders of ejaculation, with either failure of emission or retrograde ejaculation; the ability to experience the sensation of orgasm may be retained. The sympathetic thoracolumbar fibers are susceptible to injury following radical retroperitoneal lymph node dissection or spine surgery such as transperitoneal anterior lumbar discectomy and interbody fusion; complaints of loss of ejaculation are common after these surgeries.

## Conus and Cauda Equina Lesions

The cauda equina consists of the sacral somatic efferent and afferent fibers together with the parasympathetic outflow. Damage to the cauda equina leaves the detrusor decentralized rather than denervated, as the postganglionic parasympathetic innervation remains unaffected. This distinction may explain why LUT dysfunction following cauda equina injury is unpredictable and why even detrusor overactivity has been described (Podnar, 2014).

Inability to evacuate the bowel may be a severe problem; manual evacuation may be necessary for the long term. Additional denervation of the anal sphincter can result in incontinence of flatus and feces. Damage to the cauda equina results in sensory loss, and both men and women complain of perineal sensory loss and loss of erotic genital sensation. No effective treatment is available for these problems. In men, ED is also a complaint (Podnar et al., 2006).

## Disturbances of Peripheral Innervation

### Diabetic Neuropathy

Bladder involvement was once considered an uncommon complication of diabetes, but the increase in use of techniques for studying bladder functions has shown that such involvement is common although often asymptomatic. Bladder dysfunction does not occur in isolation, and other symptoms and signs of generalized neuropathy are necessarily present in affected patients. The onset of the bladder dysfunction is insidious, with progressive loss of bladder sensation and impairment of bladder emptying over years, eventually culminating in chronic low-pressure urinary retention (Hill et al., 2008). Urodynamic studies demonstrate impaired detrusor contractility, reduced urine flow, increased PVR volume, and reduced bladder sensation. It seems likely that vesical afferent and efferent fibers are involved, causing reduced awareness of bladder filling and decreased bladder contractility.

Diabetes is the most common cause for ED. Surveys of andrology clinics have found that 20%–31% of men attending such clinics are diabetic. The prevalence of ED increases with age and the duration of diabetes. The problem is also known to be associated with severe retinopathy, a history of peripheral neuropathy, amputation, cardiovascular disease, raised levels of glycosylated hemoglobin, and the use of antihypertensive medications such as beta-blockers. A large population study of men with early-onset diabetes reported that 20% had ED. Whether its pathogenesis in diabetic patients results mainly from neuropathy or involves a significant microvascular contribution or whether the two processes are codependent is not yet resolved. Age-matched studies of women with and without diabetes suggest that diabetic women may also be affected by specific disorders of sexual function, including decreased vaginal lubrication and capacity for orgasm.

### Amyloid Neuropathy

Autonomic manifestations are common; in Familial Amyloid polyneuropathy (FAP) these include ED, orthostatic hypotension, bladder dysfunction, distal anhidrosis, and abnormal pupils. LUTS generally appear early on and are present in 50% of patients within the first 3 years of the disease. Patients most often complain of difficulty in bladder emptying and incontinence (Andrade, 2009). Often, however, bladder dysfunction may be asymptomatic and uncovered only during investigations. Urodynamic studies have demonstrated reduced bladder sensation, underactive detrusor, poor urinary flow, and opening of the bladder neck. Bladder wall thickening may be seen on ultrasound scanning. As many as 10% of patients with FAP type I (link to additional text below) may proceed to end-stage renal disease (Lobato, 2003) and may complain of polyuria. Urinary incontinence has been shown to be associated with higher mortality after liver transplantation (Adams et al., 2000).

Reduced libido and ED are common and phosphodiesterase inhibitors may have the adverse effect of accentuating orthostatic hypotension and should therefore be used with caution.

Additional text is available at http://expertconsult.inkling.com. 

### Immune-Mediated Neuropathies

Approximately a quarter of all patients with Guillain-Barré syndrome have bladder symptoms. These usually occur in the patients with more severe neuropathy and appear after limb weakness is established. Both detrusor areflexia and bladder overactivity have been described.

### Autoimmune Autonomic Ganglionopathy

Patients with autoimmune autonomic ganglionopathy present with a rapid onset of severe autonomic failure, with orthostatic hypotension, gastrointestinal dysmotility, anhidrosis, bladder dysfunction, ED, and sicca symptoms; they may also have ganglionic acetylcholine receptor (AChR) antibodies. Bladder dysfunction generally manifests with voiding difficulty and incomplete emptying. The severity and distribution of autonomic dysfunction appear to depend on the level of antibody titers (Gibbons and Freeman, 2009).

## Myotonic Dystrophy

Although myotonic activity has not been found in the sphincter or pelvic floor of patients with myotonic dystrophy, bladder symptoms may be prominent and difficult to treat, presumably because bladder smooth muscle is involved. With advancing disease, megacolon and fecal incontinence may also become intractable problems.

## Urinary Retention

Urinary retention may occur in different neurological conditions (Table 45.2) and arises either due to an impairment of contractility of the detrusor or a failure of relaxation of the sphincter (Panicker, 2017) such as opiates (Panicker et al., 2012) those with anticholinergic properties (e.g. antipsychotics, antidepressants, respiratory agents with anticholinergic effects and antimuscarinic agents for the bladder) and alpha-adrenoceptor agonists may be associated with different degrees of voiding dysfunction, ranging from incomplete bladder emptying to complete urinary retention (Verhamme et al., 2008)

Urinary retention or symptoms of obstructed voiding in young women in the absence of overt neurological disease have long puzzled urologists and neurologists alike; in the absence of any convincing organic cause, the condition was once thought to be due to hysteria. The typical clinical picture is that of a young woman in the age range of 20–30 years who presents with retention and a bladder capacity greater than 1 L. Although patients retaining such quantities of urine may be uncomfortable, they do not have the sensation of extreme urgency that might be expected. Many affected women have previously experienced an interruption of the urinary stream but are unaware that this is abnormal; therefore a voiding history can be misleading unless it

**TABLE 45.2 Differential Diagnosis for Urinary Retention in a Patient in Whom a Structural Urological Lesion Has Been Excluded** (Panicker, 2017)

| Urogenital Symptoms in Neurological Patients |
|---|
| 1. Lesions of the conus medullaris or cauda equina: |
| Compressive lesions |
| Spinal fracture |
| Intervertebral disc prolapse |
| Space-occupying lesions: tumor, granuloma, abscess |
| Noncompressive lesions |
| Vascular: infarction, arteriovenous malformation with vascular steal |
| Inflammation: myelitis, meningitis retention syndrome |
| Infection: herpes simplex, varicella zoster, cytomegalovirus, Elsberg syndrome (viral aseptic meningitis) |
| 2. Other neurological conditions: |
| Spina bifida |
| Multiple system atrophy |
| Autonomic failure (e.g., pure autonomic failure, autonomic neuropathies) |
| 3. Miscellaneous: |
| Medications (e.g., opiates, anticholinergics, retigabine) |
| Fowler syndrome (females) |
| Radical pelvic surgery |

is taken carefully. Other clinical neurological features or findings on laboratory investigation that would support a diagnosis of MS are lacking, and MRI of the brain, spinal cord, and cauda equina is normal. The lack of sacral anesthesia makes a cauda equina lesion improbable. An association between this syndrome and polycystic ovaries was mentioned in the original description of the syndrome (Panicker et al., 2018). In some young women with urinary retention, concentric needle electrode examination of the striated muscle of the urethral sphincter reveals complex repetitive discharges and myotonia-like activity or decelerating bursts. Sometimes known as Fowler syndrome, this condition had long been managed only by treating the symptoms. However, it is now known that these patients respond particularly favorably to sacral neuromodulation (SNM) and sphincter injections of botulinum toxin (Datta et al., 2008; Panicker et al., 2015).

## DIAGNOSTIC EVALUATION

### History

History taking forms the cornerstone of evaluation and should address both storage and voiding dysfunction. Patients with storage dysfunction complain of frequent micturition, nocturia, urgency, and urgency incontinence, collectively known as OAB symptoms (Abrams et al., 2002). Patients experiencing voiding dysfunction report hesitancy for micturition, a slow and interrupted urinary stream, the need to strain to pass urine, and double voiding. Patients may be in complete urinary retention. The history of voiding dysfunction is often unreliable and patients may be unaware of incomplete bladder emptying. Therefore the history should be supplemented by a measurement of the PVR, usually by bladder scan (see the section titled "Bladder Scan" further on).

#### Bladder Diary

The bladder diary supplements the history taking and records the frequency of micturition, volumes voided, episodes of incontinence, and fluid intake over the course of a few days (Fig. 45.3).

### Physical Examination

Findings on clinical examination are useful to assess whether a patient's urogenital complaints are neurological in origin. As the spinal segments in the spinal cord that innervate the bladder and genitalia are distal to those that innervate the lower limbs, bladder disturbances have generally been shown to correlate with lower limb deficits. The possible exceptions are lesions of the conus medullaris and cauda equina, where findings may be confined to saddle anesthesia and absence of sacral cord–mediated reflexes such as the anal reflex or bulbocavernosus reflex. The additional findings of akinetic rigidity, cerebellar ataxia, and postural hypotension should raise suspicion for MSA, a condition characterized by early and severe urinary incontinence and ED.

Findings of peripheral neuropathy would suggest that a lesion of the peripheral innervation may be responsible for symptoms such as ED. As the neuropathy progresses, the innervation of the detrusor becomes affected, resulting in voiding dysfunction. Clear evidence for peripheral neuropathy is likely to appear before the innervation of the bladder becomes involved.

The neurological examination is complete only after an inspection of the lumbosacral spine. Congenital malformations of the spine can sometimes present with pelvic organ symptoms in adulthood; dimpling, a tuft of hair, a nevus, or a sinus in the sacral region may prove to be of relevance.

| | Time / Volume (mL) | | | | | | Total Fluid intake | Episodes of leakage |
|---|---|---|---|---|---|---|---|---|
| Day 1 | Time | 6 AM | 10 AM | 12:30 PM | 3:30 PM | 5 PM | 1700 | 4 |
| 26/4/2009 | Volume | 160 | 120 | 130 | 190 | 140 | | |
| Time out of bed (am) - 6 AM | Time | 7 PM | 8:45 PM | 2:30 AM | 4 AM | | | |
| | Volume | 150 | 170 | 200 | 180 | | | |
| Time to bed (pm) - 9 PM | Time | | | | | | | |
| | Volume | | | | | | | |

**Fig. 45.3** Bladder diary, recorded over 24 hours, demonstrating increased day- and nighttime urinary frequency, low voided volumes, and incontinence. These findings are seen in patients with detrusor overactivity. *(From Panicker, J.N., Kalsi, V., de Seze M., 2010. Approach and evaluation of neurogenic bladder dysfunction. In: Fowler, C.J., Panicker, J.N., Emmanuel, A. (Eds.), Pelvic Organ Dysfunction in Neurological Disease: Clinical Management and Rehabilitation. Cambridge University Press, New York.)*

### Investigations

Table 45.3 presents an overview of the assessments that a neurological patient undergoes after reporting LUT dysfunction (Panicker et al., 2015)

#### Screening for Urinary Tract Infections

Patients presenting with LUTS should be screened for UTIs. Combined rapid tests of urine using reagent strips ("dipstick" test) have a negative

**TABLE 45.3 Assessment of the Neurological Patient Reporting Lower Urinary Tract Symptoms**

| | Essential | Desirable | Required in Specific Situations |
|---|---|---|---|
| Bedside | History taking<br>Bladder diary | LUT-specific symptoms and quality-of-life questionnaires | |
| Noninvasive tests | Urinalysis<br>Bladder scan or in-out catheterization to measure PVR<br>Ultrasonography | Uroflowmetry<br>Blood biochemistry | Urine culture<br>Urine cytology |
| Invasive tests | - | - | (Video) urodynamics, cystoscopy, pelvic neurophysiology, renal scintigraphy |

*LUT*, Lower urinary tract; *PVR*, postvoid residual.
*From Panicker J.N., Fowler, C.J., Kessler, T.M., 2015. Lower urinary tract dysfunction in the neurological patient: clinical assessment and management. Lancet Neurol 14(7), 720–732.*

productive value for excluding UTI of nearly 98%. However, the positive predictive value for confirming infection is only 50% (Fowlis et al., 1994); hence, if abnormal, a urine sample should be sent to the lab for culture.

## Bladder Scan

As the extent of incomplete bladder emptying cannot be predicted from history or clinical examination, it is pertinent to estimate the PVR urine. This is most commonly carried out using a portable bladder scanner (Figs. 45.4, *A* and *B*), or by "in-out" catheterization, especially in patients who perform intermittent self-catheterization (ISC). It is recognized that a single measurement of a PVR volume is often not representative. Ideally, therefore, a series of measurements should be made over the course of 1 or 2 weeks.

## Ultrasound Scan

In patients known to be at risk of upper tract disease, surveillance ultrasonography should be performed periodically to evaluate for evidence of damage such as upper urinary tract dilatation or renal scarring. Ultrasound may also detect complications of neurogenic bladder dysfunction such as bladder stones.

## Urodynamic Studies

Urodynamic studies examine the function of the LUT. Included under the heading of urodynamics are noninvasive measurement of urine flow rate and residual volume and tests involving catheterization, including filling cystometry and pressure flow studies, videocystometry, and urethral pressure profilometry.

***Uroflowmetry.*** Uroflowmetry is a valuable noninvasive investigation, particularly when combined with an ultrasound measurement of the PVR volume. A commonly used design for a flow meter consists of a commode or urinal into which the patient passes urine as naturally as possible. In the base of the collecting system is a spinning disk; flow of urine onto this disk tends to slow its speed of rotation, which a servomotor holds constant. The urinary flow is calculated based on the rotation speed, and time taken to reach maximum flow; (Fig. 45.5). It is important that the patient perform the test with a comfortably full bladder, containing, if possible, a volume of at least 150 mL; privacy is essential, and a spurious result may be obtained if the subject is not fully relaxed.

***Cystometry.*** Cystometry evaluates the pressure–volume relationship during nonphysiological filling of the bladder and during voiding. The detrusor pressure is derived by subtraction of the abdominal pressure (measured using a catheter in the rectum) from the intravesical pressure (measured using a catheter in the bladder). The rate of filling is recorded by the machine, which pumps sterile water or saline through the catheter in the bladder. For speed and convenience, most laboratories use filling rates of from 50 to 100 mL/ min. This nonphysiological rapid filling does mean that the full bladder capacity can be reached usually within 7 or 8 minutes. First sensation of bladder filling may be reported

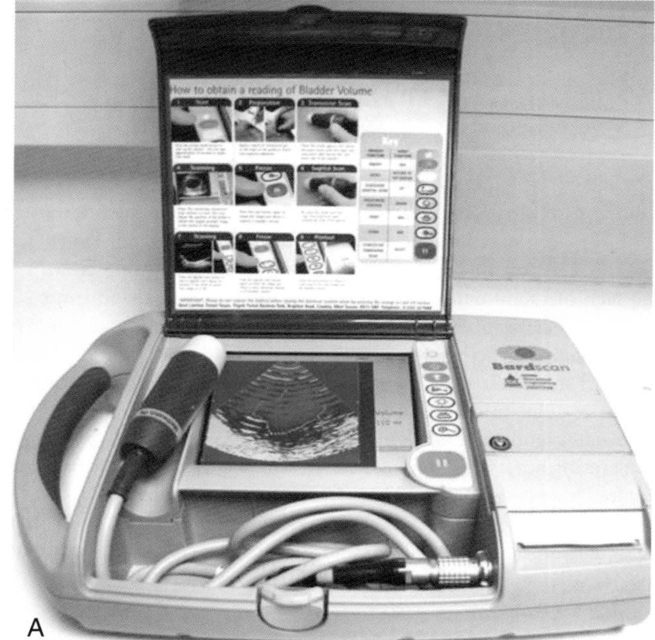


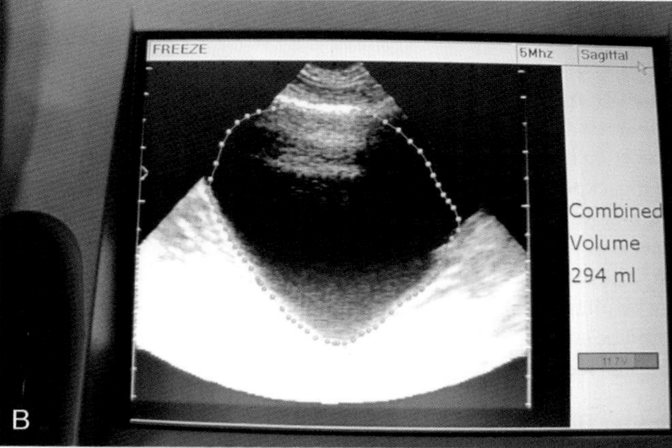


**Fig. 45.4** A small portable ultrasound machine (**A**) that can be used to measure postvoid residual urine (**B**).

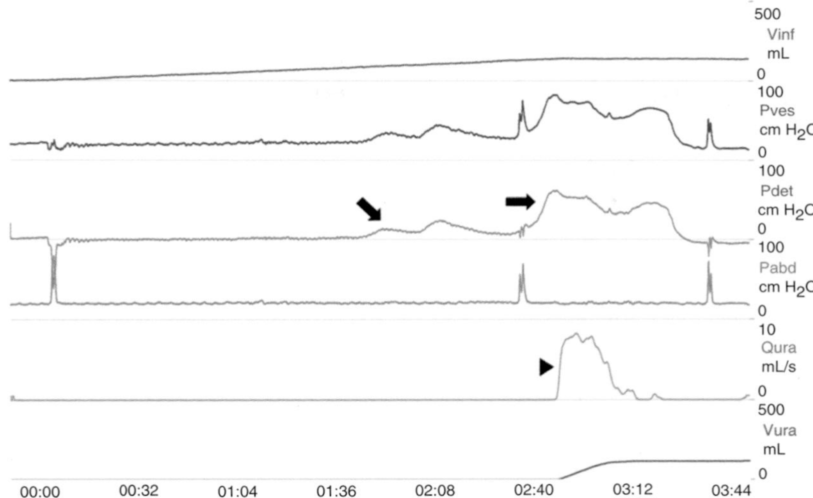


**Fig. 45.5 Filling Cystometry Demonstrating Detrusor Overactivity.** The *red trace (Pabd)* is the intraabdominal pressure recorded by the rectal catheter; the *dark blue trace (Pves)* is the intravesical pressure recorded by the bladder catheter. The *pink trace (Pdet)* is the subtracted detrusor pressure *(Pves–Pabd). Green traces* represent volume infused *(Vinf)* during the test and the volume voided *(Vura)*; the *orange trace* represents urinary flow *(Qura)*. The *black arrow* demonstrates detrusor overactivity, and the *black arrowhead* indicates associated incontinence. *(From Panicker, J.N., Fowler, C.J., 2010. The bare essentials: uro-neurology. Pract Neurol 10, 178–185.)*

at around 100 mL and full capacity is reached between 400 and 600 mL. In healthy subjects, the bladder expands to contain this amount of fluid without an increase of pressure more than 15 cm $H_2O$. A bladder that behaves in this way is said to be "stable." The main abnormality sought during filling cystometry in patients with a neurological disease is the presence of detrusor overactivity (see Fig. 45.5). This is a urodynamic observation characterized by involuntary detrusor contractions, which may be spontaneous or provoked. It should be emphasized that on urodynamics, detrusor overactivity of neurogenic origin is indistinguishable from other causes for detrusor overactivity. When bladder filling has been completed, the patient voids into the flow meter with the bladder and rectal lines still in place. Valuable information can be obtained by measuring detrusor pressure and urine flow simultaneously.

When cystometry is carried out using a contrast filling medium and the procedure visualized radiographically, the technique is known as *videocystometry*. This gives additional information about morphological changes that are consequent to neurogenic bladder dysfunction in the presence of vesicoureteric reflux. Urologists and urogynecologists have found videocystometry useful for detecting sphincter or bladder neck incompetence in genuine stress incontinence and the opportunity to inspect the outflow tract during voiding is of great value in patients with suspected obstruction.

The urethral pressure profile is measured using a catheter-mounted transducer that is run slowly through the urethra by a motorized armature. The test can be performed in men or women and is called *static* if no additional maneuvers such as coughing or straining are performed. It has been found to be helpful in the assessment of women with obstructed voiding or urinary retention, some of whom have abnormally high urethral pressures.

A general criticism of cystometric studies is that, valuable as they may be in demonstrating the underlying pathophysiology of a patient's urinary tract, the findings contribute little to elucidating the underlying cause of the disorder. "Urodynamic diagnosis" is therefore a meaningless term. The study provides information about the safety and efficiency of bladder filling and emptying. It is valuable for assessing risk factors for upper urinary tract damage and planning management. In addition, it is helpful in identifying concomitant urological conditions such as bladder outflow obstruction or stress incontinence.

The necessity to perform a complete urodynamic study in all patients with a suspected neurogenic bladder is a subject of debate. Patients with SCI, spina bifida, and possibly advanced MS should undergo urodynamic studies because of the higher risk for upper tract involvement and renal impairment, although ultrasound is a less invasive method for monitoring. Guidelines underlying the key role of urodynamics for baseline evaluation, management, and follow-up of a neurogenic bladder in these patient groups have been published. However, in other conditions such as early MS, stroke, and PD, some authors have recommended to restrict the initial evaluation to noninvasive tests on the basis that the risk for upper urinary tract damage is less (Fowler et al., 2009). In the absence of evidence-based medicine data comparing these two models of management, the decision to perform complete baseline urodynamics would depend upon local resources and recommendations.

### Pelvic Neurophysiology Testing

There are clinical situations where neurophysiology tests evaluating the pelvic somatic motor and sensory innervation may be useful in the evaluation of patients reporting unexplained pelvic organ or perineal complaints.

## Assessing Motor Innervation

### Electromyography

Pelvic floor EMG was first introduced as part of urodynamic studies for assessing the extent of relaxation of the urethral sphincter during voiding, with the aim of recognizing detrusor–sphincter dyssynergia. However, it is now rarely recorded in view of the technical difficulties in obtain a good-quality EMG signal specifically from the urethral sphincter in the environment in which urodynamic studies are performed and the availability of videocystometry that allows the outlet to be visualized.

Concentric needle EMG studies of the pelvic floor performed separately from urodynamics have however been useful for assessing innervation in certain scenarios. Electromyography has been used to demonstrate changes of reinnervation in the urethral or anal sphincter in a few neurogenic disorders. The motor units of the pelvic floor and sphincters fire tonically so they may be captured conveniently using a trigger and delay line and subjected to individual motor unit analysis.

***Sphincter electromyography in the evaluation of suspected cauda equina lesions.*** Lesions of the cauda equina are an important cause of pelvic floor dysfunction. Most often, EMG of the external anal sphincter demonstrating changes of chronic reinnervation, with a reduced interference pattern and enlarged polyphasic motor units (>1 mV amplitude), can be found in patients with long-standing cauda equina syndrome (Podnar et al., 2006). Although EMG may demonstrate pathological spontaneous activity 3 weeks or more after injury, these changes of moderate to severe partial denervation or complete denervation often become lost in the tonically firing motor units of the sphincter.

***Sphincter electromyography in the diagnosis of multiple system atrophy.*** Neuropathological studies have shown that the anterior horn cells in the Onuf nucleus are selectively lost in MSA, which results in changes in the sphincter muscles that can be identified by EMG. The anal sphincter is most often studied and, as compared to the changes of chronic reinnervation in patients with cauda equina syndrome described earlier, the changes of reinnervation in MSA tend to result in prolonged duration motor units, presumably because the progressive nature of that disease precludes motor unit "compaction." These changes can be detected easily, but it is important to include measurement of the late components of the potentials (Fig. 45.6).

Although the value of sphincter EMG in the differential diagnosis of parkinsonism has been widely debated, a body of opinion exists that maintains that a highly abnormal result in a patient with mild parkinsonism is of value in establishing a diagnosis of probable MSA (Vodusek, 2001). This correlation is important not only for the neurologist but also for the urologist, because inappropriate surgery for a suspected prostate enlargement as the cause of bladder troubles can then be avoided.

***Sphincter electromyography in the investigation of urinary retention in young women.*** Isolated urinary retention in young women has long been a mystery, as the neurological examination is normal and investigations such as MRI exclude a neurological cause of voiding dysfunction. A characteristic abnormality, however, can be found on urethral sphincter EMG, consisting of complex repetitive discharges, akin to the "sound of helicopters" and decelerating bursts, a signal somewhat like myotonia and akin to the "sound of underwater recording of whales." It has been proposed that this abnormal spontaneous activity results in impairment of relaxation of the urethral sphincter, which may cause urinary retention in some women and obstructed voiding in others. This condition, now known as Fowler syndrome, is also characterized by elevated urethral pressures.

### Assessing Sensory Innervation

***Pudendal somatosensory evoked potentials.*** Pudendal somatosensory evoked potentials (SEPs) are typically recorded from the scalp using surface electrodes following electrical stimulation of the dorsal nerve of the penis or clitoris (Fig. 45.7). The test assesses the integrity of the afferent sensory pathway in the pudendal nerve, S2,3,4 nerve roots, sacral spinal cord, and posterior column of the spinal cord. Results are compared with latencies of the tibial evoked potentials. The SEPs may be abnormal when a spinal cord lesion is the cause of sacral sensory loss or neurogenic detrusor overactivity. The finding of an abnormal pudendal SEP and normal tibial SEP would suggest an isolated lesion of the conus medullaris, cauda equina, or pudendal nerve.

### Assessing the Sacral Reflex Arc

The "bulbocavernosus" reflex (penile-cavernosus reflex) assesses the afferent and efferent pathways consisting of the pudendal nerve, sacral roots, and sacral spinal cord (S2, S3, and S4 segments). The dorsal nerve of the penis (or clitoris) is electrically stimulated and recordings are made from the bulbocavernosus muscle or external anal sphincter, usually with a concentric needle (Fig. 45.8). Testing may therefore be of value in the assessment of the sacral roots in patients with bladder dysfunction suspected to be secondary to cauda equina damage or damage to the lower motor neuron pathway.

## COMPLICATIONS ARISING FROM NEUROGENIC LOWER URINARY TRACT DYSFUNCTION AND THE RISK FOR DEVELOPING UPPER TRACT DAMAGE

Detrusor overactivity and reduced bladder wall compliance may result in raised intravesical pressure, which can in turn lead to structural changes in the bladder wall such as trabeculations and diverticula. Patients with a neurogenic bladder are also prone to a variety of genital UTIs such as cystitis, pyelonephritis, and epididymo-orchitis, and also to bladder stones.

Detrusor overactivity and Detrusor sphincter dyssynergia (DSD) can result in high pressures within the LUT, which in turn may affect the upper urinary tract (kidney and ureter), resulting in vesicoureteric reflux, hydronephrosis, and in some instances renal impairment and even end-stage renal disease. For reasons that are not understood

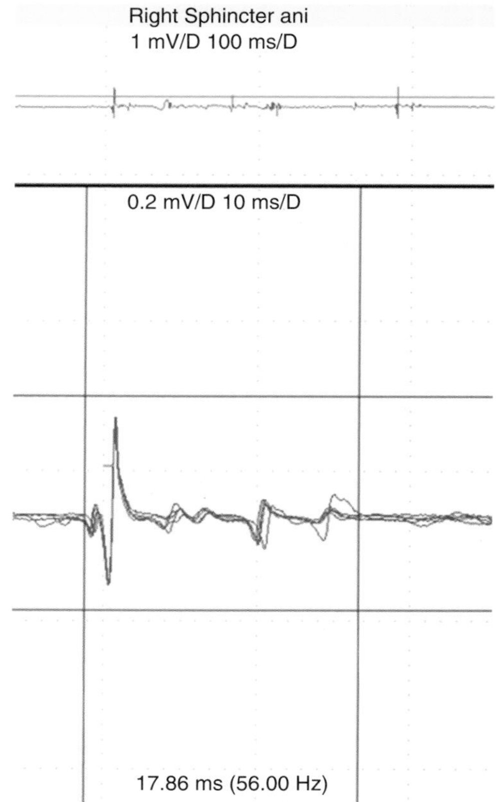


**Fig. 45.6** Concentric needle electromyography (EMG) of the external anal sphincter from a 64-year-old male presenting with parkinsonism and urinary retention. Duration of the motor unit is 17.9 ms (normal <10 ms); prolonged motor units suggest chronic reinnervation. The mean duration of motor unit potentials during the study was 22.9 ms. This EMG is compatible with a diagnosis of multiple system atrophy.

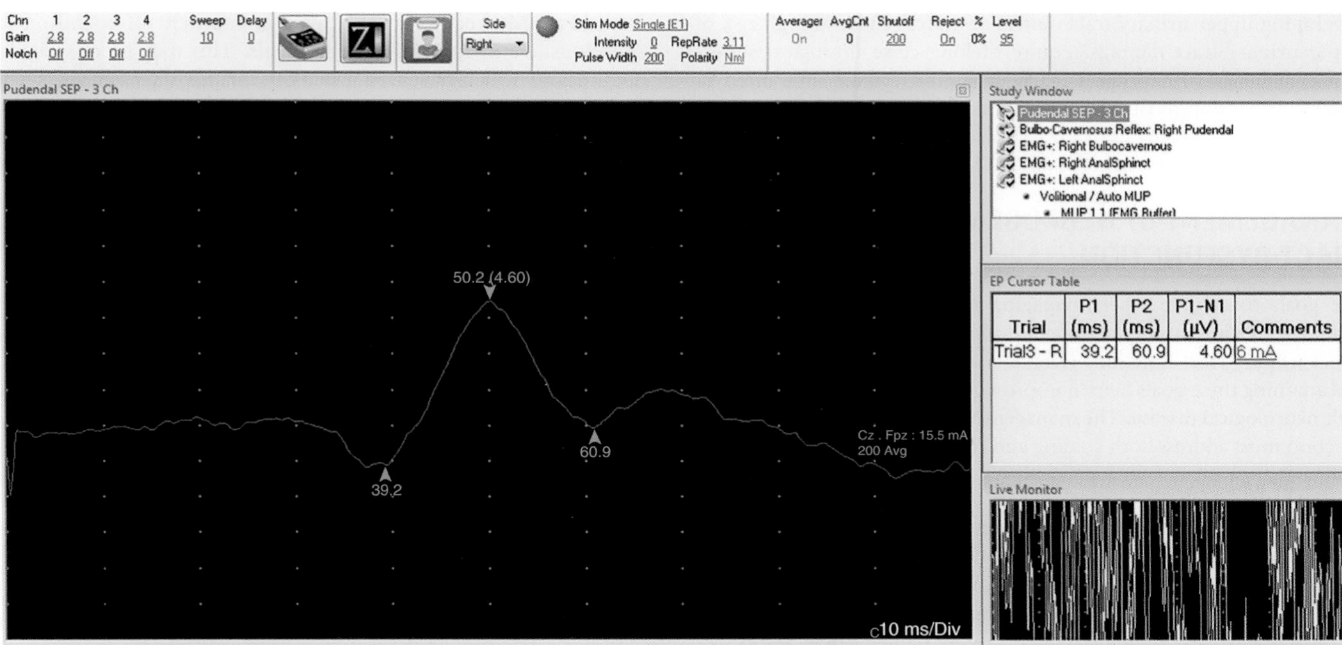


**Fig. 45.7** Pudendal cortical somatosensory evoked potential in a 38-year-old male (height 180 cm). A stimulation of 15 mA of the dorsal penile nerve at the shaft at the base of the penis was delivered at a rate of 3.1 Hz. The cortical response (P40) was recorded using Cz′-Fz montage.

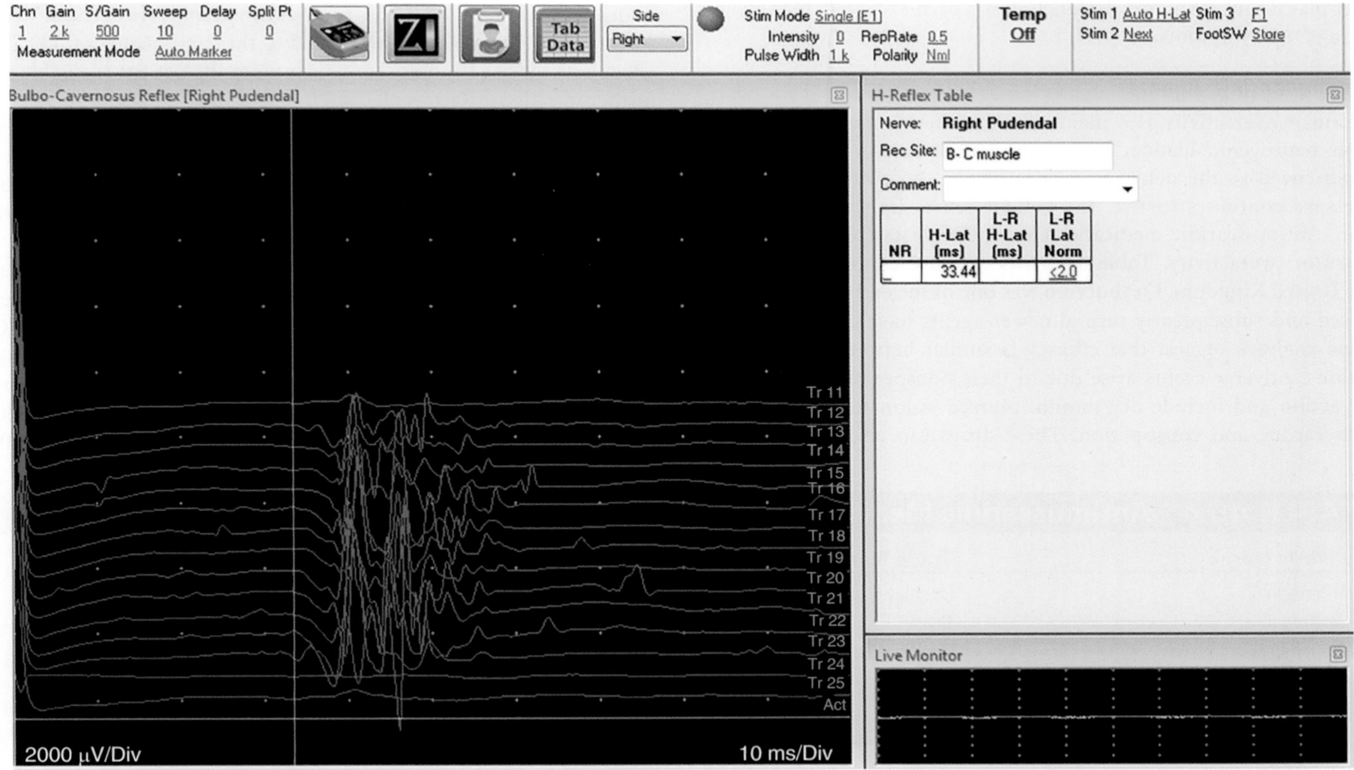


**Fig. 45.8** Bulbocavernosus reflex (BCR). Stimulation at the base of the penis (1-ms pulse delivered at 2 Hz). The response was recorded from the bulbocavernosus muscle using a concentric needle. The first response appeared at 10 mA; BCR latency (onset latency) was 33.4 ms.

fully, patients with SCI or spina bifida are more likely to develop these problems compared to patients with slowly progressive non-traumatic neurological disorders such as MS and PD (Castel-Lacanal et al., 2015; Lawrenson et al., 2001).

The risk for upper urinary tract damage is highest in patients who have raised intravesical pressure due to detrusor overactivity, low bladder compliance, and a competent bladder neck. The management of neurogenic LUT dysfunction should include a risk assessment of developing upper urinary tract damage: whereas those at high risk of upper urinary tract damage require lifelong close urological supervision, patients with progressive neurological disease and often at lowrisk, the group most often being followed up by neurologists, are much more troubled by poor LUT control than dangerously high urinary tract pressures (Panicker et al., 2015)

## MANAGEMENT OF NEUROGENIC LOWER URINARY TRACT DYSFUNCTION

The goals to achieve when managing neurogenic LUT dysfunction include achieving urinary continence, preventing UTIs and preserving upper urinary tract functions (Drake et al., 2016; Groen et al., 2016), and attaining these goals help in improving the quality of life of patients with neurological disease. The management of neurogenic bladder dysfunction must address both voiding and storage dysfunction.

### General Measures

Nonpharmacological measures are generally effective in the early stages when symptoms are mild. A fluid intake of around 1–2 L/day is suggested, although this should be individualized, and it is often helpful to assess fluid balance by means of a bladder diary (Hashim and Abrams, 2008). Caffeine reduction may reduce urgency and frequency, especially in patients drinking coffee or tea in excess. Bladder retraining, whereby patients void by the clock and voluntarily "hold on" for increasingly longer periods, aims to restore the normal pattern of micturition. Pelvic floor exercises and neuromuscular stimulation may play a role, if voiding dysfunction has been excluded, for ameliorating OAB symptoms.

### Antimuscarinic Agents

Detrusor overactivity is a major cause of incontinence in patients with neurogenic bladder disorders. The sensation of urgency is experienced as the detrusor muscle begins to contract, and if the pressure continues to rise, the patient senses impending micturition. Antimuscarinic medications are the mainstay of treatment for detrusor overactivity. Table 45.4 lists the medications available in the United Kingdom. Oxybutynin was one of the earlier drugs introduced and subsequently several newer agents have been marketed. Meta-analyses suggest that efficacy is similar between these medications. Adverse events arise due to their nonspecific anticholinergic action and include dry mouth, blurred vision for near objects, tachycardia, and constipation. These drugs can also block central muscarinic M1 receptors and cause impairment of cognition and consciousness in susceptible individuals. This may be mitigated by medications which have low selectivity for the M1 receptor, such as darifenacin, or restricted permeability across the blood–brain barrier, such as trospium. The PVR urine may increase following treatment and it should be monitored by repeat bladder scans, especially if initial beneficial effects are short-lasting. In many patients, there may also be underlying voiding dysfunction and often it is the judicious use of antimuscarinic medication with a clean ISC, which is the most effective management for neurogenic bladder dysfunction (Fig. 45.9; Fowler et al., 2009).

***Beta-3 receptor agonists.*** The beta-3 receptor agonist mirabegron has recently been licensed for managing OAB symptoms. Although devoid of the adverse effects reported with antimuscarinic agents, side effects do occur, affecting the cardiovascular system; these include palpitations, raised blood pressure, and, rarely, atrial fibrillation. Studies suggest that mirabegron is efficacious in neurological patients (Krhut et al., 2018).

### Botulinum Toxin

Botulinum toxin was introduced on the basis that it blocks synaptic release of acetylcholine from the parasympathetic nerve endings and produces a paralysis of detrusor muscle (and indeed a demonstrable increase in bladder capacity has been reported in the various studies). However, accumulating evidence indicates that the mechanism of action is more complex and may actually involve the afferent innervation as well. Botulinum toxin type A injected into the detrusor muscle under cystoscopic guidance has been shown to improve detrusor overactivity, symptoms of an OAB related to this, and quality of life. The effect lasts for 8–11 months, at which point the patient is eligible for further injections (Kalsi et al., 2007).

There is high-quality evidence for the efficacy of detrusor injections of botulinum toxin A in the treatment of neurogenic DO (Fowler, 2011). Studies also suggest that patients receiving botulinum toxin injections have fewer UTIs and reduced catheter bypassing (urethral leakage when using an indwelling catheter). Few adverse events have been reported, but the need for ISC in these groups of patients is an important consideration. In the registration study described earlier, 30% of the 200-U group and 42% of the 300-U group required ISC, compared with 12% of the placebo group (Fowler, 2011). Pivotal phase III studies of onabotulinumtoxin A have shown clear benefit in managing neurogenic detrusor overactivity. There was no clinically relevant benefit in efficacy or duration of effect between dosages of 300

**TABLE 45.4 Antimuscarinic Medications Available in the United Kingdom**

| Generic Name | Trade Name | Dose (mg) | Frequency |
|---|---|---|---|
| Darifenacin | Emselex | 7.5–15 | Once daily |
| Fesosterodine | Toviaz | 4–8 | Once daily |
| Oxybutynin IR | Ditropan, Cystrin | 2.5–20 | bid–qid |
| Oxybutynin ER | Lyrinel XL | 5–20 | Once daily |
| Oxybutynin transdermal | Kentera | 3.9/24 h | One patch twice weekly |
| Propantheline | Pro-Banthine | 15–120 | tid (1 h before food) |
| Propiverine | Detrunorm | 15–45 | qd–qid |
| Solifenacin | Vesicare | 5–10 | qd |
| Tolterodine IR | Detrusitol | 2–4 | bid |
| Tolterodine ER | Detrusitol XL | 4 | qd |
| Trospium | Regurin | 20–40 | bid (before food) |
| Trospium ER | Regurin XL | 60 | Once daily |

*bid,* Twice daily; *ER,* extended release; *IR,* immediate release; *qd,* once daily; *qid,* four times daily; *tid,* three times daily.
*From Fowler, C.J., Panicker, J.N., Drake, M., et al., 2009. A UK consensus on the management of the bladder in multiple sclerosis. J Neurol Neurosurg Psychiatry 80, 470–477.*

U and 200 U, whereas the likelihood of developing urinary retention requiring self-catheterization was dose dependent (Cruz et al., 2011; Ginsberg et al., 2012). Based on these studies, onabotulinumtoxin A is now licensed for use in neurogenic detrusor overactivity in several countries.

Intradetrusor injections of botulinum toxin have revolutionized the management of the neurogenic bladder, being a less invasive yet highly effective option for managing detrusor overactivity. It must be remembered, however, that patients must be counseled about the risk of performing a clean ISC, due to the resultant voiding dysfunction and raised PVR volume. Therefore patients being considered for this should be shown how to perform a clean ISC and demonstrate the ability and willingness to do so should this become necessary after the injections.

## Peripheral Nerve Stimulation

Electrical stimulation of peripheral nerves such as the sacral nerve roots, tibial nerve, pudendal nerve, and dorsal penile or clitoral nerves has been shown to be effective in managing the OAB. The mechanism by which this results in suppression of detrusor overactivity is uncertain; however, it seems this is by the modulation of sacral afferent nerves and spinal cord mediated reflexes through inhibitory interneurons.

## Percutaneous Tibial Nerve Stimulation

PTNS is an effective option for managing mild/moderate OAB symptoms and a typical treatment course would consist of stimulating the nerve intermittently for 30 minutes over 12 sessions, typically weekly, through a fine-gauge stainless steel needle using a fixed frequency, variable current strength electrical signal. The treatment has been found to be effective in neurological patients reporting OAB symptoms and does not worsen voiding difficulties or increase the PVR, unlike other treatments such as antimuscarinic agents or botulinum toxin (Gobbi et al., 2011). Effects are relatively short lived and the need to return for maintenance top-up treatments is influenced by the degree of improvement of LUTS (Salatzki et al., 2019). Transcutaneous tibial nerve stimulation (TTNS) involves stimulating the nerve using a cutaneous electrode which may be performed at home and has been shown to be safe and effective in patients with MS and stroke experiencing urgency incontinence. In a study of 73 patients, 12 sessions per week of PTNS were found to be a safe and effective treatment for OAB. Responders to treatment returning for maintenance PTNS more often reported significant improvements in nocturia and perceived benefits over time, compared to those not returning for maintenance treatment (Salatzki et al., 2019). The advantages of tibial nerve stimulation are the minimal or noninvasiveness of the treatment, and almost nonexistent adverse events.

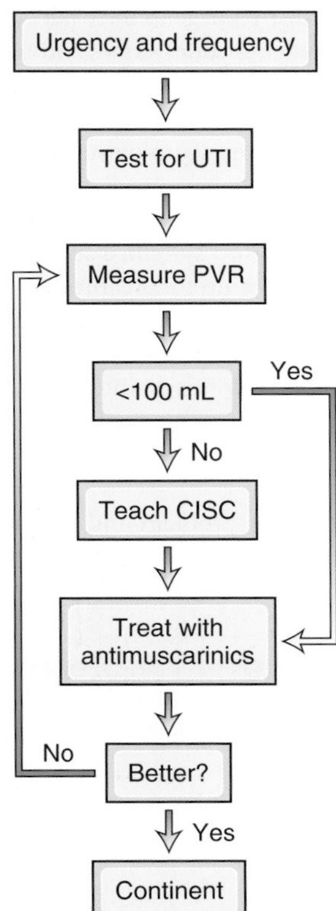


**Fig. 45.9** Algorithm for the management of neurogenic lower urinary tract dysfunction. *CISC*, Clean intermittent self-catheterization; *PVR*, postvoid residual; *UTI*, urinary tract infection. *(From Fowler, C.J., Panicker, J.N., Drake, M., et al., 2009. A UK consensus on the management of the bladder in multiple sclerosis. J Neurol Neurosurg Psychiatry 80, 470–477.)*

## Sacral Neuromodulation

An extradural sacral nerve stimulator can be highly effective in lessening detrusor overactivity refractory to antimuscarinic medications. Implanting the stimulator is a two-stage procedure, the first being a test phase with a stimulating lead inserted through the S3 foramen and connected to an external stimulator. During this test phase, it is noted whether the patient's symptoms reduced significantly as judged by bladder diaries and measurement of residual volumes, and if so the patient is eligible for a permanent stimulator. This is implanted in a subcutaneous pocket and connected to the stimulating lead. The stimulator is continuously active, although its efficacy can be maintained at a subsensory level so that patients are not aware of its chronic action. The permanent stimulators are expensive, and patient selection is crucial in order to minimize the need for revision procedures.

SNM has been tried in small numbers of patients with MS with limited success, but being a progressive neurological condition, it may lose its efficacy as the disease progresses. Moreover, currently available implants are not MRI compatible and therefore it is likely that the procedure would be an option only in patients whose MS has a benign indolent course and reporting bladder symptoms that are not responsive to less invasive treatments. A systematic review of SNM for neurogenic LUT dysfunction concluded that the number of patients investigated so far is low, and there is a lack of randomized controlled trials, which would be needed before further guidance can be issued (Kessler et al., 2010). Interestingly, it has been shown that in patients with SCI, early SNM prevented the development of neurogenic detrusor overactivity and high detrusor pressures compared with the control patients who did not receive early intervention (Sievert et al., 2010).

In patients with Fowler syndrome the mainstay of treatment had been indefinite intermittent or indwelling catheterization; however, SNM has been shown to restore voiding in these women (Datta et al., 2008).

## Surgery

Surgery can be subdivided according to whether the underlying problem relates primarily to the bladder and/or to the bladder outlet in male patients.

For bladder outflow obstruction, there are a plethora of new treatments alongside the traditional transurethral resection of the prostate, such as laser enucleation of the prostate, prostatic implants (e.g., UroLift), and vaporization; also less-invasive modalities such as prostate artery embolization have been reported now, with early reports comparing these with transurethral prostatectomy (Ray et al., 2018).

The role of these therapies in the neurological patient remains to be fully evaluated.

In terms of surgical intervention for incontinence, these are summarized in Table 45.5. A surgical procedure to rectify a disorder causing incontinence in an otherwise fit and healthy person often is highly successful. Even after SCI, a surgical option might be the best solution for long-term bladder management. This, however, does not apply to patients with progressive neurological disease causing incontinence. For example, at a time when the bladder is becoming unmanageable by intermittent catheterization and an antimuscarinic medication, the patient with MS may only just be managing to remain independent. A multidisciplinary approach will help ascertain whether urinary diversion (e.g., ileal conduit) is actually better for an individual patient rather than augmentation cystoplasty. With the advent of botulinum toxin for the bladder, some of these debilitating symptoms can now be better controlled with less-invasive procedures, and the reduction in the number of augmentation cystoplasty procedures is corroboration of this. While the relative simplicity of intravesical botulinum toxin has led to its widespread adoption, the individual patient's dexterity and other mobility needs (for instance, whether wheelchair or bed bound) will also shape a decision to focus on the bladder (Biers et al., 2012). At the time of writing there is also ongoing discussion about the risks associated with surgical mesh products (initially being discussed for prolapse surgery), and this may have implications for the use of these products in neurological patients also.

### Management of Voiding Dysfunction

There lacks a consensus regarding the figure of residual volume at which ISC should be initiated. However, in general, as patients with a neurogenic bladder have reduced bladder capacity, a volume of more than 100 mL, or more than one-third of bladder capacity, is taken as the amount of residual urine that contributes to bladder dysfunction (Fowler et al., 2009). The widespread use of ISC has greatly improved management of neurogenic bladder dysfunction. Incomplete emptying can exacerbate detrusor overactivity, and an OAB constantly stimulated by a residual volume responds by contracting and producing symptoms of urgency and frequency, thus making antimuscarinic medications less effective. Sterile intermittent catheterization was first introduced in the 1960s, but subsequently a clean rather than sterile technique was found to be adequate. Intermittent catheterization is best performed by the patients themselves, who should be taught by someone experienced with this method such as a nurse continence advisor. Neurological lesions affecting manual dexterity, weakness, tremor, rigidity, spasticity, impaired visual acuity, and cognitive impairment may make it impossible for the patient to self-catheterize; in which case, it may be performed by the partner or care assistant. The incidence of symptomatic UTIs is low when performed regularly.

Reflex voiding using trigger techniques and the Credé maneuver (nonforceful smooth even pressure applied from the umbilicus toward the pubis) are usually not recommended as they may result in high detrusor pressure and incomplete bladder emptying during voiding (Fowler et al., 2009). Suprapubic vibration using a mechanical "buzzer" has been demonstrated to be effective in patients with MS with incomplete bladder emptying and detrusor overactivity; however, its effect is limited (Prasad et al., 2003). Alpha-blockers relax the internal urethral sphincter in men and there is evidence that they improve bladder emptying and reduce PVR volumes (O'Riordan et al., 1995). However, this is not consistently seen in clinical practice unless there is concomitant bladder outlet obstruction. Botulinum toxin injections into the external urethral sphincter may improve bladder emptying in patients with SCI who have significant voiding dysfunction (Naumann et al., 2008).

#### Permanent Indwelling Catheters

There comes a point when the patient is no longer able to perform self-catheterization or when incontinence is refractory to management, at which time an indwelling catheter may become necessary. The immediate solution is a urethral indwelling catheter, held in place by an inflatable balloon in the bladder proximal to the catheter opening. The long-term ill effects of these devices are well known. One of the major problems may be catheter bypassing, which occurs when strong detrusor contractions produce a rapid urine flow that cannot drain sufficiently quickly. A common response to this would be to use a wider-caliber catheter, with the effect that the bladder closure mechanism becomes progressively stretched and destroyed. The detrusor contraction may be of sufficient intensity to extrude the 10- or 20-mL balloon from the bladder, causing further damage to the bladder neck and resulting in a totally incompetent outlet. Bladder stones and recurrent infections are also more likely in patients with an indwelling catheter.

A preferred alternative to a urethral catheter is a suprapubic catheter. This can be inserted by a urologist; however, extreme care is required as these patients often have small, contracted bladders and this contributes to the risk of bowel perforation during catheter placement. Although by no means a perfect system, a suprapubic catheter is a better long-term alternative to a urethral catheter as it preserves urethral integrity, and helps to promote perineal hygiene and sexual functions.

The option of intermittent bladder drainage using a catheter valve, as opposed to continuous drainage into a leg bag, depends upon whether the bladder has a reasonable capacity to store urine.

#### External Devices

If incontinence is the major problem and the bladder empties completely, some men are able to wear an external device such as a penile sheath.

**TABLE 45.5 Urological Procedures That May Be Performed to Treat Various Causes of Incontinence**

| | |
|---|---|
| Stress incontinence: pelvic floor weakness | Bladder neck suspension<br>TVT<br>TOT |
| Stress incontinence: sphincter incompetence | Artificial sphincter |
| Urgency incontinence (detrusor overactivity) | Botulinum toxin<br>Sacral neuromodulation<br>Augmentation cystoplasty<br>Possibly myomectomy |
| Intractable incontinence | Urinary diversion with stoma |

*TOT*, Transobturator tape; *TVT*, tension-free vaginal tape.

### Management of Nocturia

***Desmopressin.*** Desmopressin, a synthetic analog of arginine vasopressin, temporarily reduces urine production and volume-determined detrusor overactivity by promoting water reabsorption at the distal and collecting tubules of the kidney. It is useful for the treatment of urinary frequency or nocturia in patients with MS, providing symptom relief for up to 6 hours (Bosma et al., 2005). It is also helpful in managing NP, characterized by increased production of urine in the night. This may be seen in patients with PD and also various neurological conditions associated with dysautonomia and orthostatic hypotension. However, it should be prescribed with caution in patients over the age of 65 or with dependent leg edema, and should not be used more than once in 24 hours for fear of fluid overload and hyponatremia.

### Referral to a Specialist Urology Service

Adoption of a care pathway that includes evaluating LUTS, risk assessment for upper tract impairment, and regular review after instituting treatment provides the practicing neurologist a framework to manage LUT dysfunction in their patients with progressive non-traumatic neurological disorders. There are situations, however, where specialist urology services should be involved early in the care of these patients (Box 45.1; Panicker et al., 2015)

### Stepwise Approach to Neurogenic Bladder Dysfunction

The treatment options offered to a patient should reflect the severity of bladder dysfunction, which generally parallels the extent of neurological disease (Fig. 45.10). However, beyond a certain point, incontinence may become refractory to all treatment options and it is at this stage that a long-term indwelling catheter should be offered.

### Urinary Tract Infections in Neurological Patients

Recurrent UTIs, defined as more than two UTIs in 6 months, or more than three in a year, commonly occur in neurological patients and are an important cause for hospital admissions. It is important to distinguish recurrent infections from persisting infections as undertreatment of the latter may result in chronic infections. A high PVR can predispose to UTIs and the incidence of symptomatic UTIs often falls when intermittent catheterization is performed regularly.

It is important to establish whether the UTIs relate to incomplete bladder emptying (e.g. bladder outflow obstruction, reduced detrusor contractility, etc.) or a structural abnormality (foreign body in bladder, bladder stone, tumor, etc.), and for this reason the input of a urologist would be valuable.

**BOX 45.1 Red Flags That Should Prompt Referral to Specialist Urology Services**

- Presence of hematuria
- Recurrent urinary tract infections
- Pain suspected to originate from the urinary tract
- Increased risk for upper urinary tract damage or findings of upper tract damage or renal impairment in imaging or blood tests
- Suspicion of concomitant local pathologies (e.g., bladder outlet obstruction due to prostate enlargement in men or stress incontinence in women)
- Lower urinary tract symptoms refractory to conservative treatment suggest the consideration of more invasive treatments such as intradetrusor injections of botulinum toxin A or surgery, or when suprapubic catheterization as appropriate

*From Panicker, J.N., Fowler, C.J., Kessler, T.M., 2015. Lower urinary tract dysfunction in the neurological patient: clinical assessment and management. Lancet Neurol 14[7], 720–732.*

In individuals with proven recurrent UTIs and when no urological structural abnormality has been identified, it would be reasonable to initiate non-antibiotic options such as cranberry extract tablets or D-mannose. Prophylactic low-dose antibiotics for a finite duration may be required; rotating between antibiotics is one approach for minimizing antibiotic resistance developing (Phe et al., 2016). The presence of asymptomatic bacteriuria alone in a neurological patient performing ISC should not be an indication for antibiotics (Fowler et al., 2009). The value of cranberry juice in preventing UTIs in neurogenic patients is debatable.

## MANAGEMENT OF NEUROGENIC SEXUAL DYSFUNCTION

The first step is providing an opportunity for patients and their partners to openly discuss their sexual dysfunction. There are several barriers to discussing sexual dysfunction in clinic (Tudor et al., 2018). This can often be broached during the consultation while discussing concomitant bladder or bowel troubles. An explanation of the neurological basis for sexual dysfunction often relieves anxiety about the problem and removes assumptions that the problem is essentially psychological in origin.

There are several contributing factors to sexual dysfunction in the context of neurological disease (Box 45.2; Foley and Werner, 2000). Primary sexual dysfunction results from the neurological lesion affecting the neural pathways responsible for the control of sexual functions. For example, lesions in the spinal cord may cause loss of tactile sensations from the genitalia. Dysfunction can arise secondary to different physical disabilities such as spasticity or pain consequent to the neurological disease. Lastly, the psychological and emotional changes that ensue after a neurological disease can also contribute to

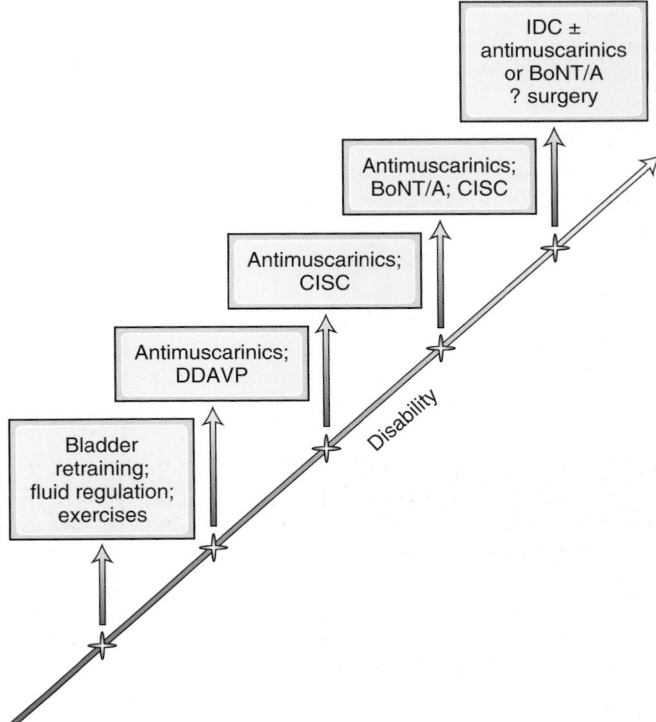


**Fig. 45.10** Stepwise approach to neurogenic bladder dysfunction and its relation to the progression of disabilities (see text for details). *BoNT/A*, Botulinum toxin A; *CISC*, clean intermittent self-catheterization; *DDAVP*, desmopressin; *IDC*, indwelling catheter.

sexual difficulties. A holistic approach to managing sexual dysfunction involves addressing all these contributory factors.

## Management of Erectile Dysfunction

Sexual dysfunction in men most commonly manifests with ED. The evidence generally points to spinal cord involvement as the major cause of ED in neurological conditions such as MS. Cord involvement may initially result in a partial deficit, so that ED is variable, with preserved nocturnal penile erections and erections on morning waking. It is only in the past 20–25 years that neurological teaching has recognized the error of the view that "if a man can get an erection at any time, ED is likely to be psychogenic." With increasing neurological disability, there may be a total failure of erectile function and also difficulty with ejaculation. Few men with complete SCI can ejaculate and difficulty with ejaculation may become apparent when ED is successfully treated. The treatment of ED was transformed by the introduction of phosphodiesterase type 5 inhibitors. These act to increase nitric oxide release in the corpora cavernosa and thereby induce penile erections. The first such agent was sildenafil (Viagra) and clinical studies have demonstrated that the optimal dose should be taken up to 1 hour before anticipated sexual activity. These are not aphrodisiacs, and intimacy and stimulation, which promote nitric oxide release, are required for these medications to be effective. The medications have few side effects, and these relate to its vasodilator action and commonly include headache, flushing, dyspepsia, and nasal congestion. Given their known pharmacology, these medications increase the hypotensive effects of organic nitrates, leading to excessive vessel dilatation and therefore hypotension; they are absolutely contraindicated in patients receiving nitrates to treat angina. Of relevance to neurological patients, they should be used with caution in patients with orthostatic hypotension.

After the introduction of sildenafil, two other medications with similar mechanism of action were introduced (Table 45.6). All three medications are generally well tolerated, but there are some differences to be considered. Sildenafil and vardenafil are effective after 30–60 minutes, respectively, from administration and last for up to 4 hours. By contrast tadalafil is effective from 30 minutes after administration but its peak efficacy is expected after approximately 2 hours. Efficacy is maintained for up to 36 hours and may, therefore, mean less planning and pressure to have sexual intercourse to a schedule. A fatty meal may affect the absorption of sildenafil and vardenafil, with potential bearing on efficacy.

The use of oral agents is now established as first-line treatment, and alternative approaches are available if found to be ineffective. Prostaglandin $E_1$ (alprostadil) can be injected directly into the penis and acts by relaxing the smooth muscle of the cavernosal vessels. Adverse effects include penile pain, groin pain, hypotension, prolonged erection (priapism), and in some instances, penile fibrosis when used long term. Intraurethral therapy of alprostadil (medicated urethral system for erection, or MUSE) was introduced to obviate the need for self-injection. Efficacy rates of 75%–69% have been reported, but adverse effects include burning and irritation of the urethra, making the therapy unpopular.

Vacuum constriction devices are overall the most economical therapy for ED. A plastic tube is placed around the penis and air is pumped out of the chamber, creating a vacuum, thereby drawing blood into the penis and resulting in penile engorgement. Tumescence is maintained by placing one or more tension bands around the base of the turgid penis. These bands may be left in situ for as long as 30 minutes and the device may be reused. Though highly efficacious, satisfaction rates are generally only 55%. They are cumbersome and give an unnatural erection. They also require manual dexterity, and the patient may have to shave the pubic hair to facilitate the creation of a seal for the vacuum. Side effects include petechiae, pain, numbness or coldness, delayed ejaculation, and sense of trapped ejaculate. Generally, this type of therapy is preferred for older patients who are in stable relationships.

Implantation of a penile prosthesis can be offered as a third-line option. However, their use in patients with neurological disease is limited because, with increasing sensory loss, there is a risk of erosion of the prosthesis. Also, they may interfere with performing catheterization should the neurological patient be in urinary retention.

**BOX 45.2 Potential Factors Predisposing to Sexual Dysfunction in Neurological Disease**

**Primary**

Lesions in the central nervous system impairing sexual function

**Secondary**

Fatigue
Difficulties in attention and concentration
Bladder/bowel incontinence
Physical immobility: muscle weakness
Leg spasms
Dysesthesia/allodynia
Other factors: incoordination, tremor, pain

**Tertiary**

Depression, anxiety
Anger, guilt, and fear
Altered self-image, low self-esteem
Relationship with the partner, change in family role

**Others**

Medications used in the treatment of multiple sclerosis: antidepressants, baclofen, gabapentin
Use of a urethral indwelling catheter

## Management of Ejaculatory Dysfunction

Impaired ejaculation is a problem reported by many men with spinal cord lesions. There is, as yet, no medical intervention that restores ejaculatory function, although a small proportion of patients report some

**TABLE 45.6 Phosphodiesterase Type 5 Inhibitors available in United kingdom for the Treatment of Erectile Dysfunction**

| | GENERIC NAME | | |
|---|---|---|---|
| | Sildenafil | Vardenafil | Tadalafil |
| Available doses | 25, 50, 100 mg | 5, 10, 20 mg | 10, 20 mg |
| Starting dose | 50 mg/day | 10 mg/day | 10 mg/day |
| Time to onset of action | 30–60 min | 30 min | 30 min |
| Duration of effect | 4 h | 4 h | 36 h |
| Interaction with fatty meals | Yes | Yes | No |

improvement of "erotic sensitivity" with yohimbine. This is an alkaloid derived from the bark of the African tree *Pausinystalia yohimbe* and the South American herb quebracho, *Aspidosperma quebracho-blanco.* Available as an oral preparation, it is principally a monoamine oxidase inhibitor that stimulates release of norepinephrine. Yohimbine can be used 1–2 hours before intercourse. Its main side effects include rise in blood pressure and increased frequency of micturition. It may also have an anxiogenic effect. Midodrine, an α-1 agonist, has recently been shown to improve ejaculation in men with SCI (Soler et al., 2007).

Infertility caused by ejaculatory failure can be managed by means quite different from those that would be suggested for ejaculatory difficulties. Patients should be referred to a center that specializes in this problem; such centers usually exist in association with a spinal cord unit.

### Sexual Dysfunction in Women

Until recently, sexual dysfunction in women has been generally neglected by mainstream clinical practice. Sexual dysfunction has significance for both the affected woman and her partner and often is an underlying strain in a relationship. The success of sildenafil in treating ED in men led to a placebo-controlled randomized study of its effect in women (Dasgupta et al., 2004). The only benefit seemed to be a slight, but significant, improvement in vaginal lubrication explained by the vasodilatory action of sildenafil. However, this was not associated with an improvement in orgasmic function or on quality of life. Anesthetic gels or pain modulation may be useful for women with dyspareunia. Despite available help, sexual dysfunction remains underrecognized and undertreated. Although 43% women with MS reported sexual dysfunction in a study, they were quite dissatisfied with the management offered to them (Mahajan et al., 2014).

## MANAGEMENT OF FECAL INCONTINENCE

Additional text is available at http://expertconsult.inkling.com. 

*The complete reference list is available online at https://expertconsult.inkling.com.* 

46

# Sexual Dysfunction in Neurological Disorders

*Frédérique Courtois, Dany Cordeau*

OUTLINE



Neurological disorders have many effects on sexual function that are often dismissed by rehabilitation professionals. They have been classified into primary, secondary, and tertiary impacts. Primary impacts refer to the direct effects of the neurological lesion on sexual function. Secondary impacts refer to their effects on other body functions involved in sexuality as well as the side effects of medications. Tertiary impacts refer to psychosocial aspects that reduce access to social contacts, thus interfering with sexual relationships.

This chapter explores these various aspects, starting with a review of the neural innervation of the male and female genitals, followed by a review of the primary, secondary, and tertiary impacts of neurological conditions on sexual function as well as a discussion of their treatment.

## THE NEUROPHYSIOLOGY OF HUMAN SEXUAL RESPONSES

### The Neurophysiology of Male Sexual Responses

#### Erection

Erection is a reflex receiving excitatory and inhibitory influences from the brain (Andersson, 2011; Courtois et al., 2013a; Giuliano, 2011; Tajkarimi and Burnett, 2011).

Reflexogenic erection arises from genital stimulation mediated by the spinal segments S2-S4 (Fig. 46.1). Sensory fibers run through the dorsal penile nerve, synapse with the preganglionic pelvic nerves, run through the pelvic plexus, and synapse with the postganglionic cavernous nerves (Courtois et al., 2013a; Tajkarimi and Burnett, 2011; Yang and Bradley, 1999a, 1999b). Nitric oxide (NO) release from the cavernous nerves and from the penile epithelium triggers a cascade of events, transforming GTP into cGMP, and resulting in relaxation of the smooth penile muscles and vasodilation of the penile arteries, leading to tumescence (Clement and Giuliano, 2015; Giuliano, 2011; Lue, 2000). Sporadic stimulation of the perineal nerves during tumescence triggers contractions of the bulbospongiosus and ischiocavernosus muscles (Fig. 46.2), increasing the internal penile pressure during erection and maximizing penile rigidity (Courtois et al., 2013a; Tajkarimi and Burnett, 2011).

Erection can also arise from psychogenic stimuli originating from the brain and feeding into the sacral pathway (facilitating or inhibiting reflex) or running through the thoracolumbar (TL) pathway exiting the T11-L2 segments and running down the paravertebral sympathetic chain that feeds into the pelvic plexus (Courtois et al., 2013a; Giuliano, 2011; Tajkarimi and Burnett, 2011).

#### Ejaculation

Ejaculation consists of emission and expulsion. Emission involves contractions of the internal reproductive organs, which release their content into the prostatic urethra and create the semen (see Fig. 46.1; Courtois et al., 2013a; Giuliano and Clément, 2005a, 2005b). Expulsion involves rhythmic contractions of the perineal muscles.

Emission is controlled by TL innervation, receiving inputs from the sacral pathway, which activates the sympathetic splanchnic nerves synapsing in the celiac and mesenteric ganglia with the hypogastric nerves innervating the internal reproductive organs (see Fig. 46.1). As semen is collected in the prostatic urethra (see Fig. 46.1), stimulation of urethral stretch receptors initiates expulsion controlled by the sacral spinal segments and mediated by the perineal nerves (Courtois et al., 2013a; Giuliano and Clément, 2005a, 2005b; McMahon et al., 2004).

These phases of ejaculation are orchestrated by a spinal generator of ejaculation (SGE), located in the L3-L4 spinal segments (Chehense et al., 2017; Truitt and Coolen, 2002 ), which coordinates the events from the sensory inputs of erection, to the intraspinal connections between the sacral and TL pathways, to emission and expulsion (Borgdoff et al., 2008; Truitt and Coolen, 2002; Tuitt et al., 2003).

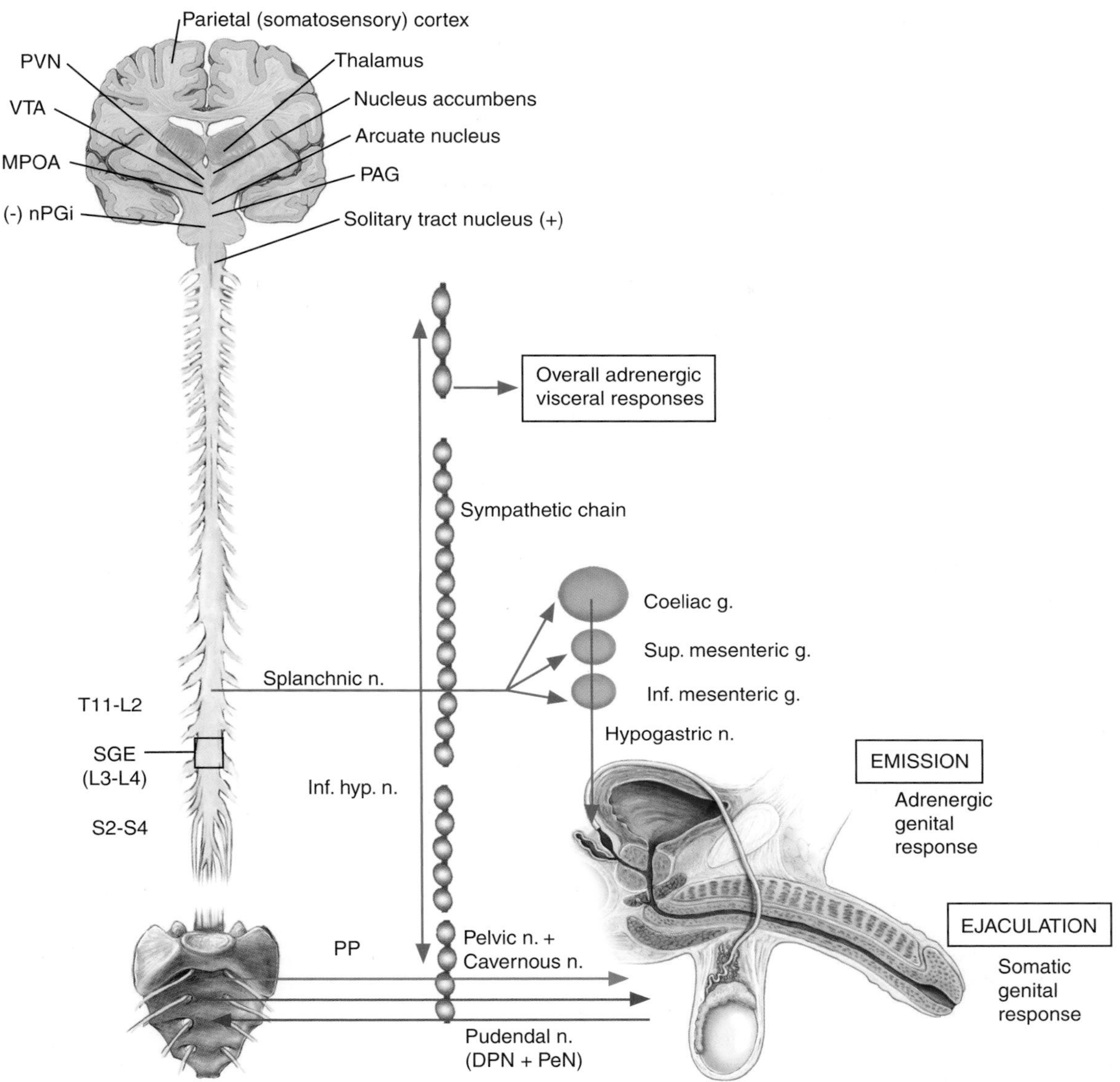


**Fig. 46.1 Innervation of the Male Genital and Reproductive System.** Sensory inputs from genital stimulation are conveyed through the dorsal penile nerve (afferent pudendal nerve) to the sacral segments S2-S4 of the spinal cord, where they synapse with the preganglionic pelvic nerve, running through the pelvic plexus and synapsing with the postganglionic cavernous nerve within the penile wall. Psychogenic inputs can also travel from the brain (1) to the sacral segments to enrich erection or (2) through the thoracolumbar segments T11-L2 running through the splanchnic nerves and descending the inferior sympathetic chain (inferior hypogastric nerve) to feed into the pelvic plexus and trigger psychogenic erection. At the threshold of ejaculation, intraspinal connections between the sacral and thoracolumbar segments trigger emission through activation of the splanchnic nerves, synapsing in the coeliac and mesenteric ganglia with the postganglionic hypogastric nerve. Emission, consisting of contraction of the internal reproductive organs (ampulla of the vas deferens, seminal vesicles, prostate gland), leads to the release of semen in the prostatic urethra, which stretches its receptors and initiates the expulsion reflex of ejaculation. The expulsion reflex is controlled by the sacral segments of the spinal cord, mediating the contraction of the bulbospongiosus and ischiocavernous muscles through the perineal nerve. The sequence of events between erection, emission, and ejaculation is coordinated by the spinal generator of ejaculation *(SGE)* located in the lumbar segments L3-L4 of the spinal cord. Orgasm, which usually accompanies ejaculation, is initiated by activation of the entire sympathetic chain at the time of emission (in addition to activation of the hypogastric nerve responsible for emission), triggering the overall adrenergic visceral responses (e.g., hypertension, tachycardia, hyperventilation, red skin spots) in addition to the adrenergic and somatic genital responses. *DPN,* Dorsal penile nerve; *MPOA,* medial preoptic area of the hypothalamus; *g.,* ganglia; *hyp.,* hypogastric; *Inf.,* inferior; *n.,* nerve; *nPGi,* nucleus paragigantocellularis; *PAG,* periaqueductal gray; *PeN,* perineal nerve; *PP,* pelvic plexus; *PVN,* paraventricular nucleus; *sup.,* superior; *VTA,* ventrotegmental area.

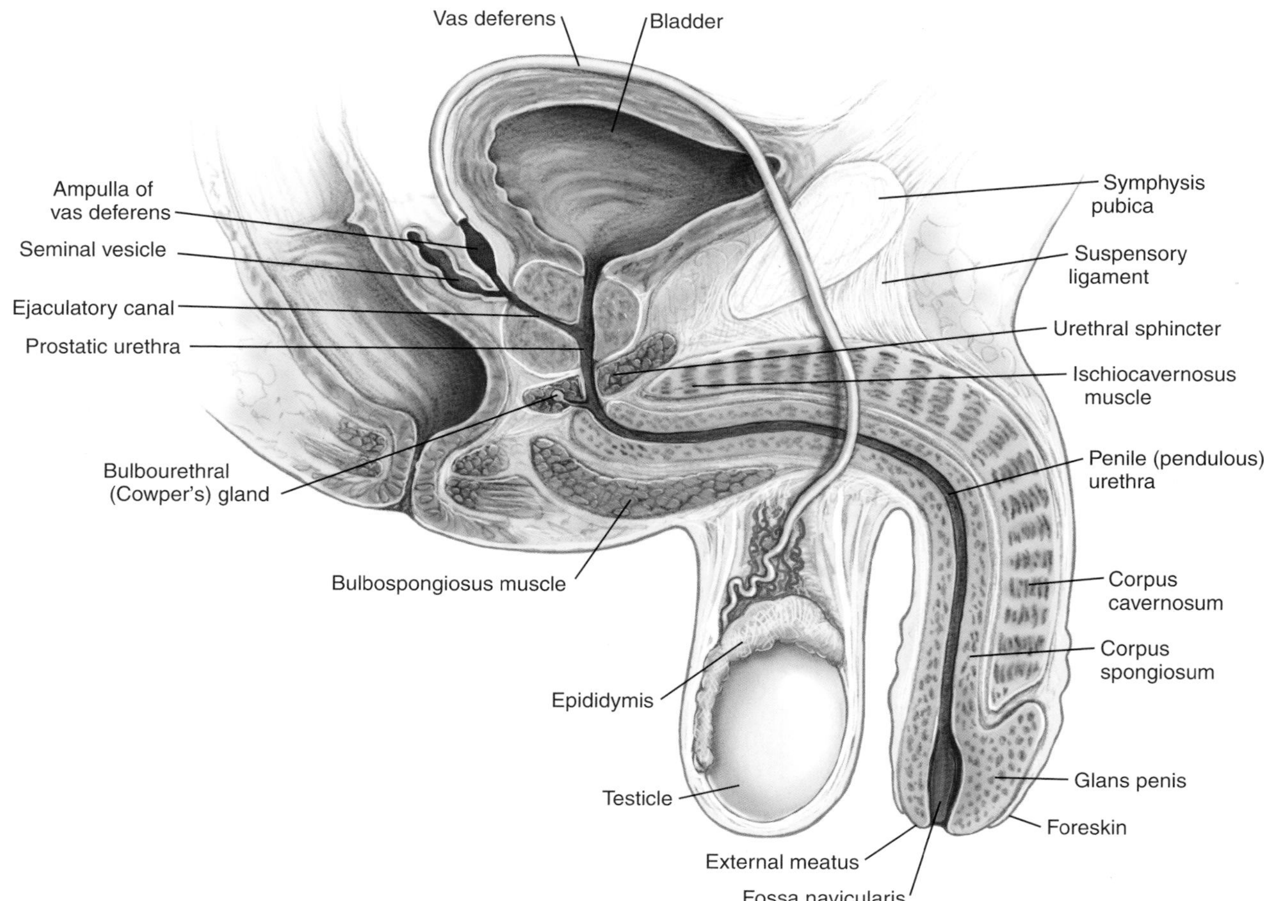


**Fig. 46.2** Anatomy of the Male Genital and Reproductive System.

### Orgasm

Orgasm is characterized by cardiovascular responses (tachycardia, hypertension, hyperventilation), muscular contractions, and sympathetic discharge (sweating, shivering, red skin spots; Masters and Johnson, 1966). Orgasm is suggested to be a nonpathological equivalent of autonomic dysreflexia (AD) normally submitted to supraspinal inhibition (Courtois et al., 2008b, 2011b, 2013a; Courtois and Charvier, 2015). The neural control involves the sympathetic fibers (see Fig. 46.1) synapsing with the hypogastric nerves responsible for emission and suggested to also activate the overall sympathetic chain that stimulates the collective response of orgasm (hypertension, tachycardia, hyperventilation, and so on; Courtois et al., 2011b, 2013a).

## The Neurophysiology of Female Sexual Responses

### Anatomy of the Female Genitalia

Recent ultrasonography and magnetic resonance imaging (MRI) reveal that the clitoris is composed not only of a glans (Fig. 46.3) but is also prolonged by a short body attached to the suspensory ligament and extending into the vestibular bulbs (bulbospongiosus cavities; Buisson and Foldès, 2008; Caruso et al., 2011; Foldès and Buisson, 2009; O'Connell et al., 2008) that shape the labia majora and the crura (ishiocavernous cavities) running laterally. The urethral opening is surrounded by erectile tissue, which, combined with the clitoris and the vaginal opening, forms the clitoro-urethro-vaginal complex involved in female orgasm (Buisson and Foldès, 2008; Buisson and Jannini, 2013; Foldès and Buisson, 2009; Jannini et al., 2010). The vestibular bulbs and crura surrounding the anterolateral vaginal wall support the existence of the G spot (Grafenberg, 1950), better known as the previously mentioned clitoro-urethro-vaginal complex (Fig. 46.4; Battaglia et al., 2010; Buisson and Jannini, 2013; Caruso et al., 2011; Gravina et al., 2008).

Although these findings have been criticized by some authors (Puppo and Puppo, 2015), others have suggested that the ultrasonographic and imaging findings of the female clitoral anatomy support the orgasms described by females, including clitoral, vaginal, urethral, and cervico-uterine orgasm. Multiple pathways from the genitals to the brain (Rees et al., 2007) also support these possible expressions of female orgasm.

### Arousal and Plateau Phase

The female sexual response has been classically described as consisting of four phases: arousal, plateau, orgasm, and resolution (Masters and Johnson, 1966) in addition to desire. Although this description is still useful for the assessment of females with neurological disorders, these several phases involve more complex interactions with motivational, emotional, experiential, and developmental factors (Basson, 2015).

The arousal phase consists of clitoral erection, congestion of the labia majora and minora, and vaginal lubrication. These responses are controlled by reflexes (see Fig. 46.4) conveyed through the dorsal clitoral nerve synapsing in the sacral segments S2-S4 with the parasympathetic preganglionic pelvic nerve, running through the utero-vaginal plexus, and synapsing with the postganglionic cavernous nerves (Courtois et al., 2013b, 2013c; Giuliano et al., 2002; Rees et al., 2007).

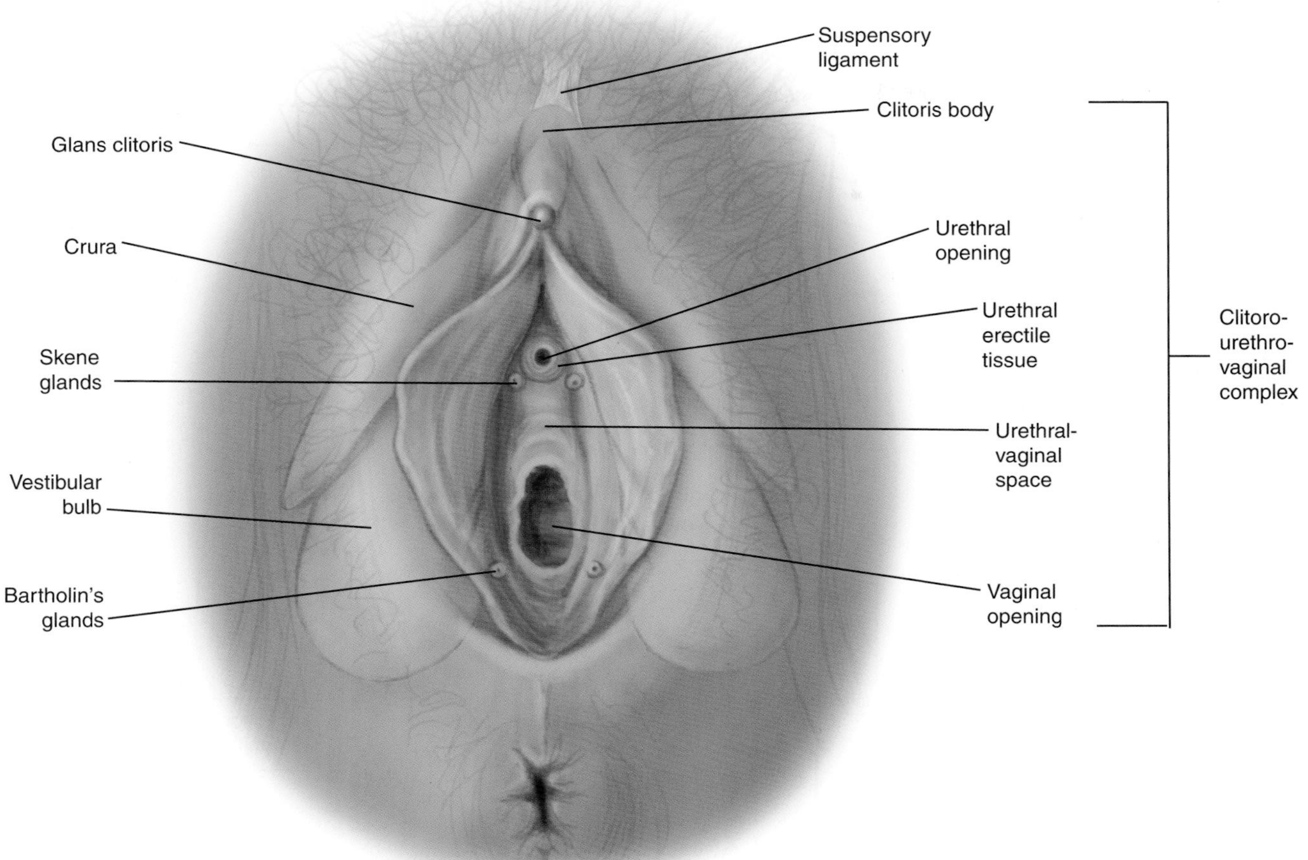


Fig. 46.3 Anatomy of the Clitoris.

Vaginal lubrication results from vasodilation and vasocongestion of the vaginal epithelium, triggering a pressure gradient that stimulates the transudation of plasma from the vaginal wall into its lumen (Cuzin, 2012; Giuliano et al., 2002).

Sexual arousal also stimulates contractions of the uterine ligaments, resulting in anterior elevation of the uterus and functionally elongating the vagina (allowing stronger but painless thrusts). Bartholin gland (see Fig. 46.4) secretions provide a mucous lining that prevents irritation during intercourse (Courtois et al., 2013b, 2013c; Masters and Johnson, 1966).

The plateau phase follows, with maximal congestion of the clitoral structure and contraction of the suspensory ligament embedding the clitoral glans under its prepuce (allowing stronger nonaversive stimulation). Maximal congestion of the vestibular bulbs stimulates the G spot (see Fig. 46.3), facilitating vaginal orgasm (Courtois et al., 2013b, 2013c; Masters and Johnson, 1966).

Sexual arousal can also be activated by psychogenic stimuli feeding into the sacral pathway or synapsing with the TL pathway, traveling through the paravertebral sympathetic chain, and feeding into the utero-vaginal plexus.

## Orgasm and Resolution

Orgasm is characterized by rhythmic contractions of perineal muscles perceived as clitoral, vulvar, vaginal, and anal pulsations and by various signs of autonomic discharge, including hypertension, tachycardia, hyperventilation, flushing, shivering, red skin spots, and the like (Courtois et al., 2011b; Graziottin and Gambini, 2015; Masters and Johnson, 1966). Given the resemblance between these responses in males and females (see Figs. 46.1 and 46.4), the neural pathways governing climax in females is suggested to be identical to emission and ejaculation—that is, involving the concurrent activation of the hypogastric nerves and sympathetic chain (Courtois et al., 2013b, 2013c).

Following orgasm, the resolution phase clears out vasocongestion and brings cardiovascular and autonomic responses back to normal (Masters and Johnson, 1966).

## Brain Regulation of Sexual Responses

Brain structures control sexual reflexes through excitatory or inhibitory influences (Hubscher et al., 2004, 2010; Johnson et al., 2011) and modulate sexual desire and arousal (Georgiadis and Kringelbach, 2012; Karama et al., 2002; Kim et al., 2006; Moulier et al., 2006; Parada et al, 2016, 2018; Poeppl et al., 2014; Ponseti et al., 2006; Redouté et al., 2005; Sescousse et al., 2010; Stoléru et al., 2012) as well as participating in the perceptual, cognitive-emotional, and rewarding effects of orgasm (Cacioppo et al., 2012; Georgiadis et al., 2006, 2009; Georgiadis and Kringelbach, 2012; Stoléru et al., 2012).

The medial preoptic area (MPOA; Marson, 2004; Marson and McKenna, 1994), the paraventricular nucleus (PVN), and the arcuate nucleus of the hypothalamus exert excitatory influences on sexual reflexes, whereas the nucleus paragigantocellularis (nPGI) exerts tonic

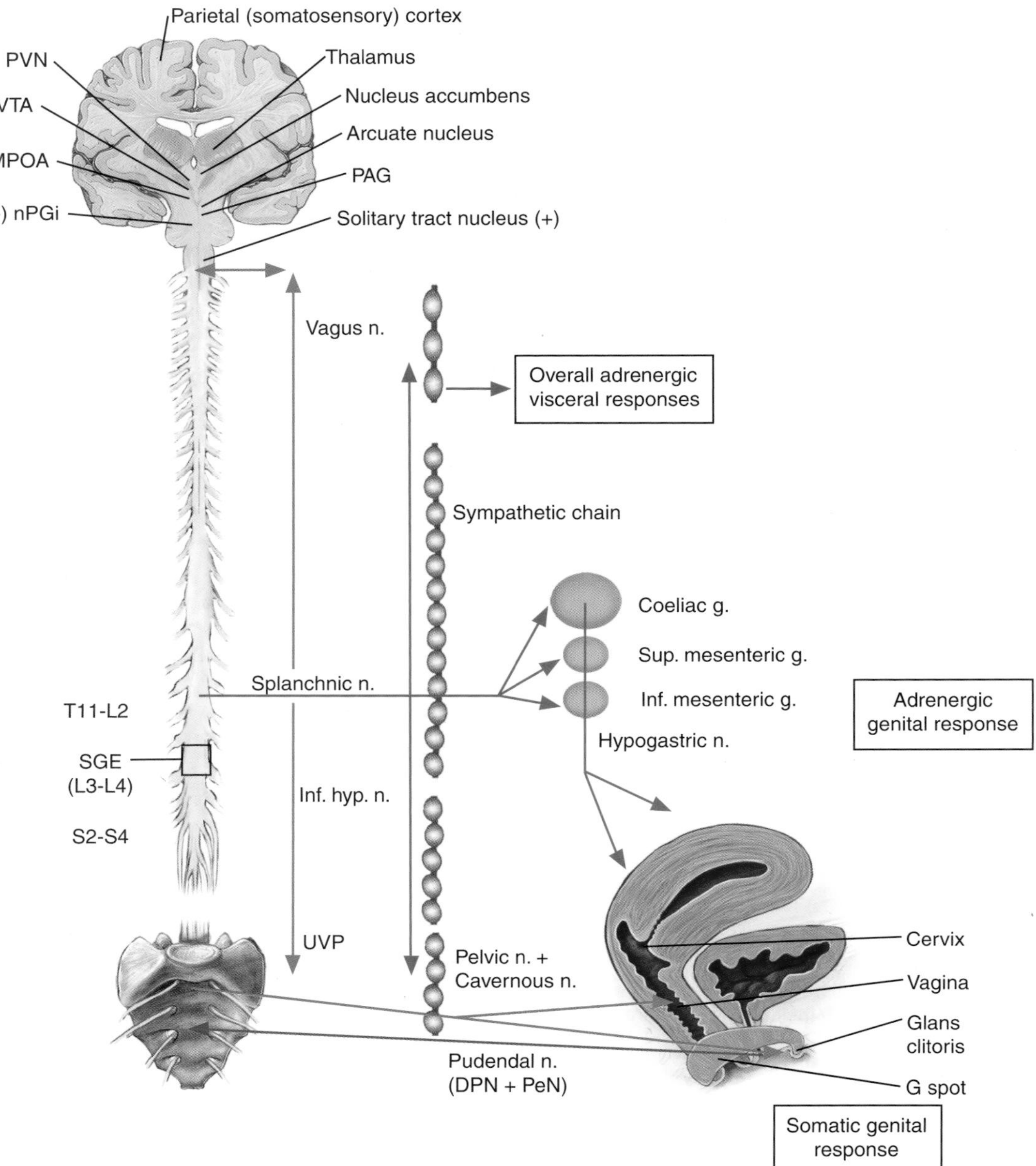


**Fig. 46.4 Innervation of the Female Genital and Reproductive System.** Genital stimulation of the glans clitoris, G spot, and vagina are conveyed through the dorsal clitoral nerve (afferent pudendal nerve) to sacral segments S2-S4 of the spinal cord, where they synapse with the preganglionic pelvic nerve, running through the uterovaginal plexus and synapsing with the postganglionic cavernous nerve to initiate clitoral erection and vaginal lubrication. Deeper stimulation of the vagina and cervix is conveyed through thoracolumbar segments T11-L2 running through the splanchnic nerves and descending the inferior sympathetic chain (inferior hypogastric nerve) feeding into the uterovaginal plexus to trigger clitoral erection and vaginal lubrication. Psychogenic inputs can further travel from the brain (1) to the sacral segments, (2) the thoracolumbar segments T11-L2 descending the inferior sympathetic chain (inferior hypogastric nerve), feeding into the uterovaginal plexus, or (3) the vagus nerve innervating the genitals. At the threshold of orgasm, intraspinal connections are believed to be established, as in males, between the sacral and thoracolumbar (TL) segments to activate (1) the hypogastric nerve innervating the uterus and responsible for uterine contractions and (2) the entire sympathetic chain responsible for the overall adrenergic visceral responses (e.g., hypertension, tachycardia, hyperventilation, red skin spots) in addition to the adrenergic and somatic genital responses of climax. The spinal generator of ejaculation *(SGE)*, which is also identified in females, may presumably participate in the coordination of events. *DPN,* Dorsal penile nerve; *g.,* ganglia; *hyp.,* hypogastric; *Inf.,* inferior; *MPOA,* medial preoptic area of the hypothalamus; *n.,* nerve; *nPGi,* nucleus paragigantocellularis; *PAG,* periaqueductal gray; *PeN,* perineal nerve; *PVN,* paraventricular nucleus; *sup.,* superior; *UVP,* uterovaginal plexus; *VTA,* ventrotegmental area.

inhibition (see Figs. 46.1 and 46.4). Excitatory inputs from the MPOA can be conveyed through connection with the PVN and the periaqueductal gray (PGA), both inhibiting the inhibitory nPGI (Meston et al., 2004).

Sexual interest or desire (Ruesink and Georgiadis, 2017) and sexual arousal during manual stimulation of the genitals (Georgiadis et al., 2010; Hostege et al., 2003; Ruesink and Georgiadis, 2017) or visual erotic stimulation (Bocher et al., 2001; Ferretti et al., 2005; Karama et al., 2002; Kim et al., 2006; Moulier et al., 2006; Poeppl et al., 2014; Ponseti et al., 2006; Ruesink and Georgiadis, 2017; Stoléru et al., 2012; Walter et al., 2008) are associated with activity in the orbitofrontal cortex and insula, the frontal (motor) cortex, the parietal (sensory) cortex, the occipital (visual) cortex, and to some extent the temporal cortex. The basal ganglia, limbic system, and, in particular, the amygdala are also activated during manual stimulation of the genitals (Georgiadis and Holstege, 2005; Georgiadis et al., 2009; Georgiadis and Kringelbach, 2012; Ruesink and Georgiadis, 2017; Stoléru et al., 2012) or in response to visual erotic stimulation (Ferretti et al., 2005; Georgiadis and Kringelbach, 2012; Hamann et al., 2004; Karama et al., 2002; Poeppl et al., 2014; Ponseti et al., 2006; Redouté et al., 2000; Ruesink and Georgiadis, 2017; Stoléru et al., 2012). In females, independent but overlapping cortical representations of the clitoris, vagina, cervix, and breast are found on the homunculus of the parietal lobe (Komisaruk et al., 2011). Generalized arousal, and that characterizing climax, is associated with activity in the thalamus, whereas visceral perception is associated with activity in the ventroposterior thalamus (Ferretti et al., 2005; Georgiadis et al., 2010; Hostege et al., 2003; Karama et al., 2002; Kim et al., 2006; Moulier et al., 2006; Poeppl et al., 2014; Ponseti et al., 2006; Redouté et al., 2000; Stoléru et al., 2012; Walter et al., 2008). Cardiovascular activity and respiratory events (Georgiadis et al., 2009) are recorded in the brainstem and muscular spasms in the cerebellum. Cerebellar projections participate in the cardiovascular (Georgiadis et al., 2009) and motor aspects of orgasm (Georgiadis et al., 2007; Hostege et al., 2003). Ventrolateral pontine area activity is partly responsible for climactic pelvic floor contractions (Huynh et al., 2013).

The emotional and phenomenological experiences of orgasm are associated with deactivation of the prefrontal, temporal, and entorhinal cortex and explain the hedonic and satiety experience of climax (Bianchi-Demicheli and Ortigue, 2007; Georgiadis et al., 2009; Hostege et al., 2009; Ruesink and Georgiadis, 2017). Similar deactivation of the amygdala but activity in limbic structures (PVN, MPOA, nucleus accumbens, hippocampus; Bianchi-Demicheli and Ortigue, 2007; Georgiadis et al., 2009) explains the euphoric and emotional state of orgasm (Bianchi-Demicheli and Ortigue, 2007; Hostege et al., 2003). Further connections between limbic structures, the ventrotegmental area (VTA), and the mesodiencephalic zone containing dopamine neurons are held to be responsible for the rewarding effect of climax (Hostege et al., 2003).

Most brain areas, except for the brainstem and cerebellum, are deactivated at the very moment of orgasm (Georgiadis et al., 2006, 2009), suggesting a transient removal of supraspinal inhibition (Courtois et al., 2011b, 2013a).

## THE IMPACT OF NEUROLOGICAL CONDITIONS ON SEXUAL FUNCTION

### Spinal Cord Lesions

Of all neurological conditions, spinal cord lesions (SCLs) are the most studied with respect to sexual function (Alexander et al., 2017a; Bors and Comarr, 1960; Brackett et al., 2010; Courtois et al., 2013d; Courtois and Charvier, 2015; Comarr, 1970; deForge et al., 2005, 2006; Everaert, et al., 2010; Sipski et al., 2005, 2006; Sipski-Alexander et al., 2017; Soler et al., 2007a, 2007b, 2008; Whipple et al., 2002). The severity of the sexual deficits varies according to the level and completeness of the lesion, higher lesions being associated with better sexual reflexes (Fig. 46.5) and lower lesions with major losses (Fig. 46.6) (Alexander et al., 2017a; Courtois et al., 2013d; Everaert et al., 2010; Sipski-Alexander et al., 2017). Detailed assessment of remaining function despite the injury is recommended as a first step to treatment and may use the international standards of autonomic function as a guide (Alexander et al., 2017b; Krassioukov et al., 2012; Prévinaire et al., 2017).

#### Primary Impacts of Spinal Cord Lesions on Male Sexual Function

***Erection.*** Men with higher lesions generally maintain reflexogenic erections, but they have poor psychogenic erections unless the lesion is incomplete (see Fig. 46.5). Tetraplegic and paraplegic men whose lesions are above the sacral segments are capable of reflexogenic erection, the quality of which is superior for tetraplegic than paraplegic men (Courtois et al., 2013d, 2015; Everaert et al., 2010; Prévinaire et al., 2017). Men with lower lesions (see Fig. 46.6) have sacral damage and lose reflexogenic erection unless the lesion is incomplete. In most cases they maintain psychogenic erections, but these are often of poor quality. The remaining potential with reflexogenic (genital) or psychogenic stimulation may or may not be of sufficient quality (e.g., duration, stability, rigidity) to complete intercourse (Brackett et al., 2010a, 2010b; Hess and Hough, 2012; Lombardi et al., 2015 ). In such cases, various treatment options are available (see section "Treatment Options for the Primary Impact of Neurologic Conditions on Sexual Function" later).

***Ejaculation.*** Ejaculation requires preserved intraspinal connections between the sacral and TL pathways (see Fig. 46.5). Males with lesions above T10 maintain the potential for ejaculation (Bors and Comarr, 1960; Comarr, 1970) but sometimes require vibrostimulation (Biering-Sorensen et al., 2012; Chéhensse et al., 2013; Courtois and Charvier, 2015; deForge et al., 2005), sometimes in association with additional midodrine (Courtois et al., 2015; Soler et al., 2007b).

Males with lesions within the TL segments (i.e., T11-L2) or between the sacral and TL segments (i.e., L3-S1) lose the intraspinal connections necessary for emission. Lower thoracic lesions (T11-T12) have a better prognosis than upper lumbar lesions (L1-L2). Lower sacral lesions (e.g., conus terminalis) can present psychogenic emissions (see Fig. 46.6); however, they are generally dribbling and premature (Courtois and Charvier, 2014).

Males with higher lesions (above T10) can experience anterograde and expulsive ejaculation but also retrograde ejaculation. Lower lesions damage the perineal muscles, leading to dribbling ejaculation (Courtois et al., 2013d).

***Orgasm.*** From 50% to 65% of males with SCLs report orgasm (Alexander and Marson, 2018; Sipski et al., 2006), mostly during ejaculation, although often retrograde ejaculation (Soler et al., 2018). Orgasm can be perceived in the absence of ejaculation (Sipski et al., 2006). In several cases, reports of orgasm in males (and females) with spinal cord injury (SCI) were recorded during functional magnetic resonance imaging (fMRI), documenting the activity in the sacral and TL spinal segments (Alexander et al., 2017a). Orgasm intensity is sometimes attenuated (Cardoso et al., 2009; Dahlberg et al., 2007) but can also be heightened (or aversive) during AD (Courtois et al., 2008a, 2008b, 2011). In normal physiology, orgasm is accompanied by hypertension, tachycardia, hyperventilation, and autonomic discharge (piloerection, red spots on skin), which also characterizes AD. When hypertension exceeds 180 mm Hg or ejaculation is accompanied by headache, AD treatment is considered (Courtois et al., 2012).

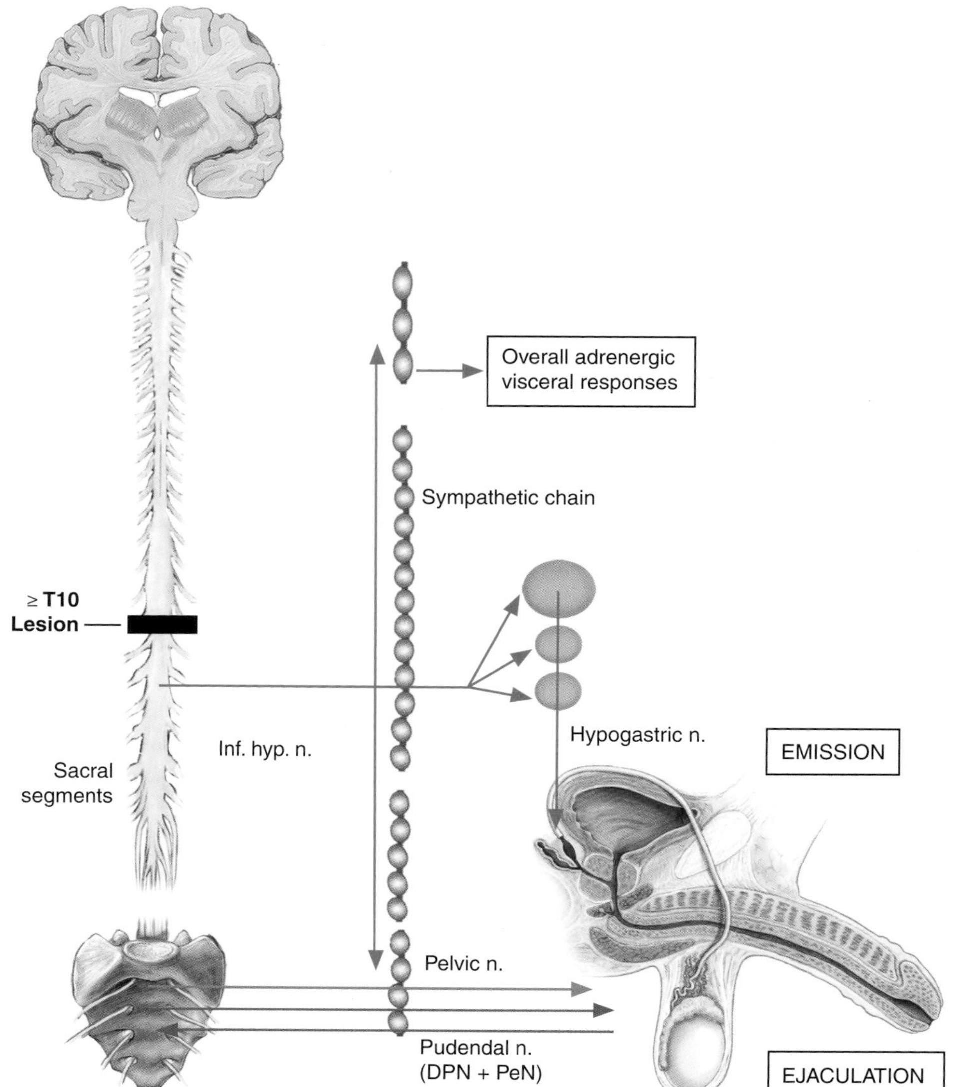


**Fig. 46.5 Sexual Function Following Higher Spinal Lesions (≥10) in Males.** Tetraplegic and paraplegic men with lesions located anywhere above the sacral segments are capable of reflexogenic erection but not psychogenic erection unless the lesion is incomplete. Males with lesions located anywhere above T10 maintain the potential for ejaculation as the intraspinal connections between the sacral and thoracolumbar pathway are preserved and can mediate emission and expulsion through multisegmental reflexes. Orgasm is also possible as the entire sympathetic chain can be activated during emission. *DPN,* Dorsal penile nerve; *n.,* nerve; *PeN,* perineal nerve.

Although orgasm is reported with psychogenic stimulation in lower lesions, ejaculation is more often lacking pleasurable sensations in such cases (Courtois and Charvier, 2014).

## Primary Impacts of Spinal Cord Lesions on Female Sexual Function

***Arousal.*** Females with lesions above T10 maintain response to stimulation of the clitoris, vulva, vagina, G spot, and cervix, allowing clitoral erection, labial congestion, and vaginal lubrication (Courtois et al., 2013c; Komisaruk et al., 2004; Sipski et al., 1995a, 1995b, 1997, 2005; Whipple et al., 1996, 2002). Females with higher lesions (Fig. 46.7) maintain vaginal lubrication with genital stimulation; females with lower lesions (Fig. 46.8) show better vaginal lubrication with psychogenic lubrication (Sipski et al., 1995b, 1997).

***Orgasm.*** Orgasm can be achieved with clitoral, vaginal, or cervical stimulation (see Fig. 46.4) even with complete lesions but usually associated with higher levels of injury (Alexander and Rosen, 2008; Komisaruk et al., 2004; Sipksi et al., 1995a, 2017; Whipple et al., 2002). Reports of orgasm are supported by fMRI (Alexander et al., 2017b) and positron emission tomography (PET) showing activity in the hypothalamus (PVN) and in the brainstem's nucleus solitarius (Komisaruk et al., 2004; Whipple et al., 2002). These findings suggest possible retrograde transmission of sympathetic activity during orgasm to these hypothalamic and brainstem nuclei as well as sympathetic plasticity in females with SCLs (Alexander and Marson, 2018; McLachlan, 2007). Orgasm, in contrast, is seldom achieved with psychogenic stimulation unless the lesion is incomplete, ruling out phantom as opposed to actual orgasm (Whipple et al., 1996). In general, females with lower motor neuron (LMN) lesions have greater

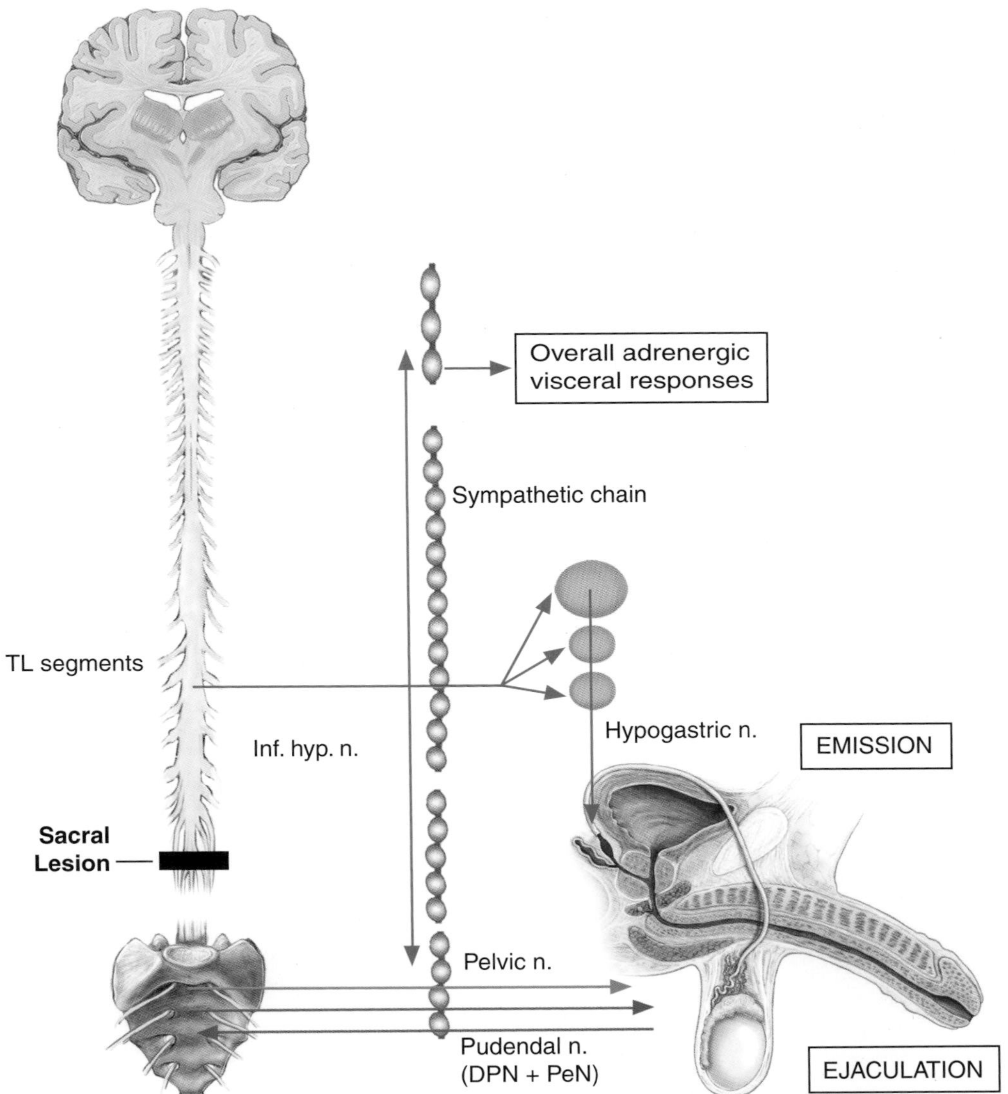


**Fig. 46.6 Sexual Function Following Lower (Sacral) Lesions in Males.** Males with lower spinal lesions have damaged sacral segments and lose reflexogenic erection unless the lesion is incomplete. They can, however, maintain psychogenic erection mediated through the thoracolumbar *(TL)* pathway. Expulsive ejaculation is lost due to the damaged sacral segments but dribbling (often premature) emission is possible. *DPN,* Dorsal penile nerve; *n.,* nerve; *PeN,* perineal nerve.

difficulties achieving orgasm than females with upper motor neuron (UMN) lesions (Sipski-Alexander et al., 2017).

### Secondary Impacts of Spinal Cord Lesions on Sexual Function

Secondary effects of SCLs on sexual function encompass bladder and bowel incontinence (Anderson et al., 2007), especially problematic for females (Cramp et al., 2015) and during oral sex, as urinary incontinence is present in 49% of females with SCLs (Elmelund et al., 2019). Other secondary effects involve uncontrolled spasticity, which limits the possible positions during intercourse (Hess and Hough, 2012; Kreuter et al., 2011); AD; limited mobility; neurogenic pain; and the side effects of medication including antispastic drugs, painkillers, antidepressants, and sleeping pills (Calabro and Bramanti, 2014; Hess and Hough, 2012; Kreuter et al., 2011). Counseling with these aspects of injury and regular revisions of medications are recommended.

Recovery from the state of spinal shock can extend over a period of 18 months (Ditunno et al., 2004), thus reducing sexual reflexes. Pressure ulcers can develop and interfere with sexual positions, so that skin inspection after sexual activity should be encouraged (Hess and Hough, 2012).

Aside from SCL, conditions such as diabetes, hyperlipidemia, and metabolic syndrome are possible contributors to sexual dysfunction; they should not be underestimated or overlooked (Lombardi et al., 2010).

### Tertiary Impacts of Spinal Cord Lesions on Sexual Function

Tertiary effects of SCI concern psychosocial impacts such as depression, anxiety, relationship issues, concerns with sex role, self-confidence, self-esteem, body image, anger, frustration, and social isolation, thus jeopardizing sexual adjustment (Hess and Hough, 2012; Kreuter et al., 2011; Lombardi et al., 2010). These should all be addressed during sex

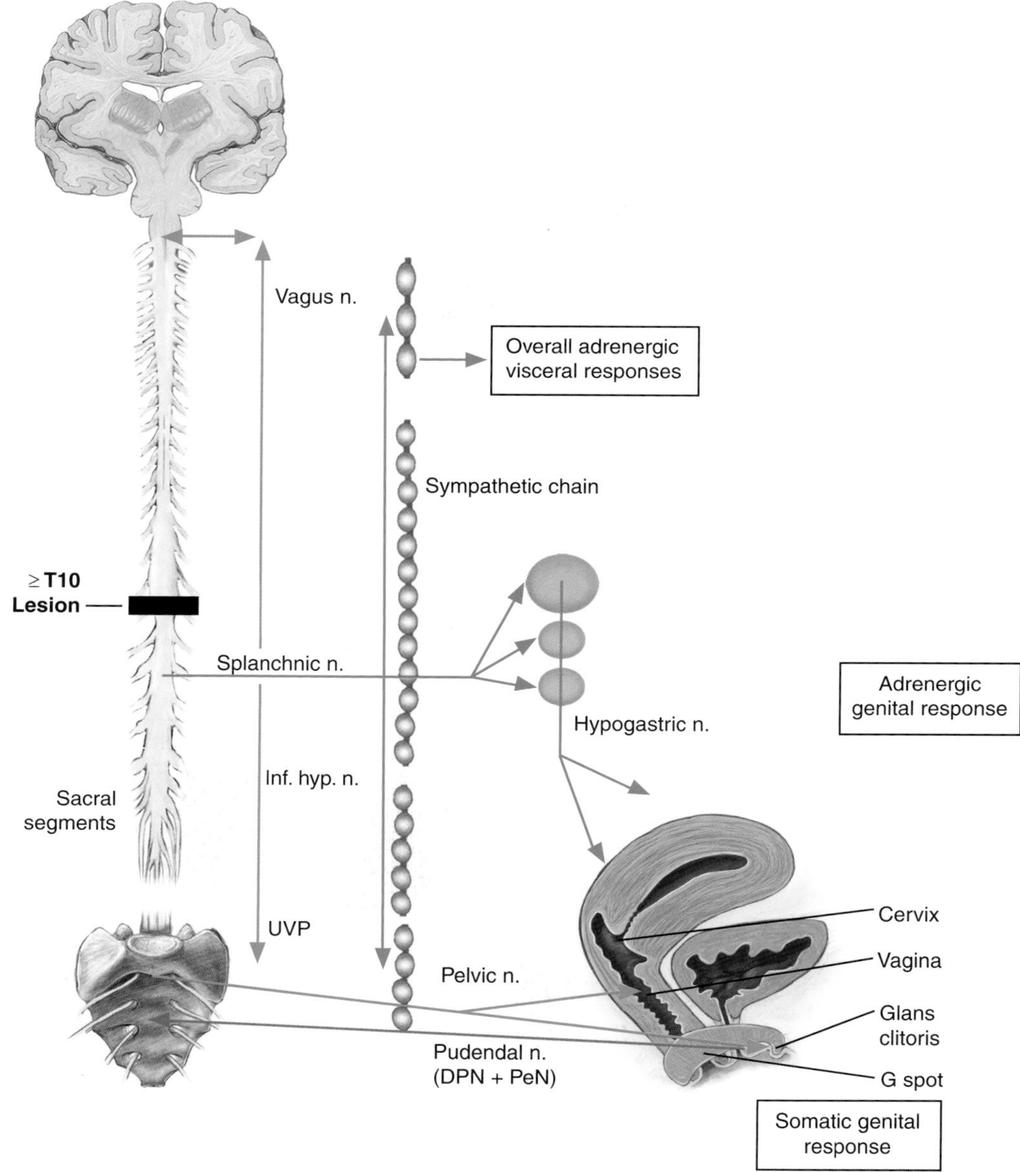


**Fig. 46.7 Sexual Function Following Higher Spinal Lesions (≥10) in Females.** Females with lesions located anywhere above the sacral segments are capable of erection of the clitoris and vaginal lubrication but not psychogenic responses unless the lesion is incomplete. They may also show reflex responses to deeper vaginal and cervical stimulation. Orgasm is possible as the entire sympathetic chain can be activated during genital stimulation and because genital responses can be mediated through the vagus nerve. *DPN,* Dorsal penile nerve; *n.,* nerve; *PeN,* perineal nerve; *UVP,* uterovaginal plexus.

therapy or psychotherapy and not only during active rehabilitation but also following hospital discharge, when new stressors arise.

## Multiple Sclerosis

### Primary Impacts of Multiple Sclerosis on Sexual Function

The primary effects of multiple sclerosis (MS) include impaired genital sensation, decreased sexual desire, and other sexual dysfunctions. Erectile, ejaculatory, and orgasmic dysfunctions are reported in 50% to 75% of males with MS (Crayton and Rossman, 2006). Females are 1.87 times more at risk of reporting sexual dysfunctions than healthy controls (Zhao et al., 2018). Overall, females with MS complain of a lack of desire, inadequate vaginal lubrication, dyspareunia, and delayed orgasm (Çelik et al., 2013; Lew-Starowicz and Rola, 2013; Orasanu et al., 2013; Sacco et al., 2001; Tepavcevic et al., 2008; Zivadinov et al., 2003). Results from the number of lesions and lesion locations are not necessarily associated with sexual dysfunction (Solmaz et al., 2018), although lesions to the brain, brainstem, spinal cord, pyramidal tract, and autonomic pathways have been reported as having impacts on sexual function. Lesions to the limbic system and cognitive centers are also described as affecting the emotional and gratifying experience of sexuality (Barak et al., 1996; Rees et al., 2007). Lesions disrupting the hypothalamic–pituitary–gonadal circuit are described as altering the hormonal control of sexual reflexes (DasGupta and Fowler, 2003), but hormonal levels (thyroid, estrogens, testosterone) are not always associated with sexual dysfunction (Solmaz et al., 2018).

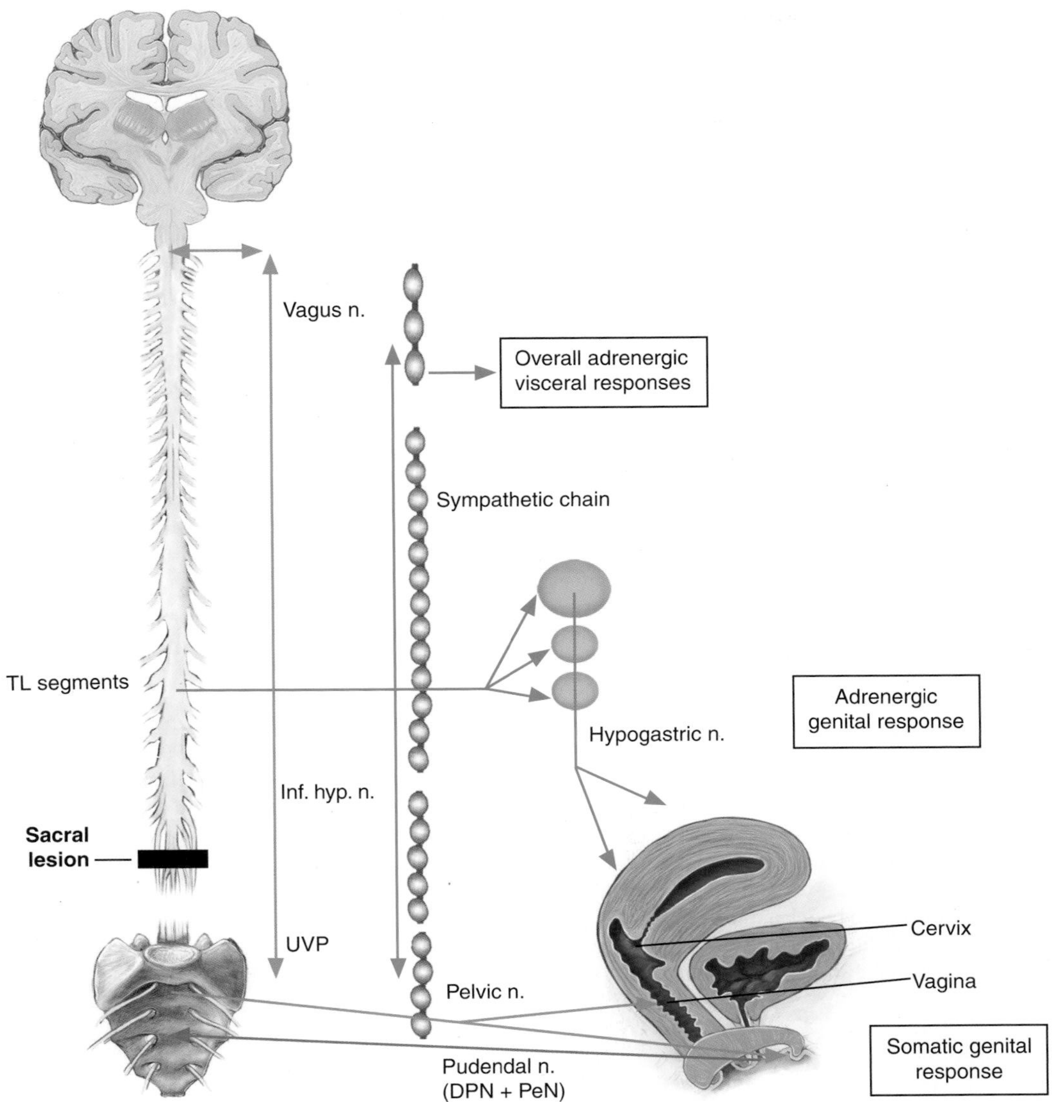


**Fig. 46.8 Sexual Function Following Lower (Sacral) Lesions in Females.** Women with lesions that damage the sacral segments may not respond to clitoral or G spot stimulation mediated through the sacral segments but may respond to deeper vaginal and cervical stimulation mediated through the thoracolumbar *(TL)* segments. They may also respond to psychogenic stimulation mediated through the TL segments. *DPN,* Dorsal penile nerve; *n.,* nerve; *PeN,* perineal nerve; *UVP,* uterovaginal plexus.

Age and duration of MS correlate with sexual disorders (Bartnik et al., 2017; Lew-Starowicz and Rola, 2013; Tepavcevic et al., 2008; Zorzon et al., 2003), and subtypes of MS also affect sexual dysfunction (Young et al., 2016). Any given status can deteriorate with time (Çelik et al., 2013; Kisic-Tepavcevic et al., 2015).

## Secondary Impacts of Multiple Sclerosis on Sexual Function

Secondary effects of MS include chronic fatigue, muscle tightness or weakness, spasticity, bladder and bowel dysfunction, incoordination or reduced mobility, pain, and side effects of medications (Bronner et al., 2010; Çelik et al., 2013; Demirkiran et al., 2006; Lew-Starowicz and Rola, 2013; Lombardi et al., 2011; Tepavcevic et al., 2008; Wang et al., 2018; Zivadinov et al., 2003). Up to 91% of these patients (mostly females) are bothered by incontinence and sexual difficulties (Wang et al., 2018). Pain, fatigue, incontinence, and level of disability are all associated with sexual dysfunction in MS patients (Bartnik et al., 2017; Kisic-Tepavcevic et al., 2015; Wang et al., 2018; Young et al., 2016).

Females with MS report burning sensations and memory impairments (Çelik et al., 2013; Orasanu et al., 2013). In men, erectile dysfunction is linked with urinary symptoms and ejaculatory dysfunction with advanced disability (DasGupta and Fowler, 2003).

Side effects of medications including those for disease progression or symptom management can have negative effects on sexuality (Crayton and Rossman, 2006).

## Tertiary Impacts of Multiple Sclerosis on Sexual Function

Tertiary effects of MS involve concerns with body image, feeling of anger due to being less sexually attractive, or because of dependency on others. Diminished self-confidence, concerns about sexually gratifying one's partner, fear of rejection, difficulty in communicating with the partner, guilt, anxiety, depression (Çelik et al., 2013; Foley et al., 2013; Orasanu et al., 2013), declining quality of the relationship (Blackmore et al., 2011; Lew-Starowicz and Rola, 2013; McCabe, 2004), and inadequate cognitive performance (Tepavcevic et al., 2008) are also described. Depression and anxiety significantly contribute to sexual dysfunctions in MS patients (Bartnik et al., 2017; Hösl et al., 2018; Solmaz et al., 2018).

## Stroke

### Primary Impacts of Stroke on Sexual Function

Stroke is associated with a high rate of hypoactive sexual desire among patients (Choi-Kwon and Kim, 2002) and their spouses (Korpelainen et al., 1999).

A diminished frequency of intercourse is described and partly attributed to the decrease in sexual desire (Jung et al., 2008); it tends to worsen with time (Choi-Kwon and Kim, 2002).

Erectile and ejaculatory dysfunction (Jung et al., 2008; Tamam et al., 2008), as well as decreased vaginal lubrication and a diminished capacity to reach orgasm, are reported (Tamam et al., 2008).

More patients with right hemispheric lesions complain of decreased sexual desire and diminished frequency of intercourse than patients with left hemispheric lesions. Erectile dysfunctions are associated with lesions to the right occipitoparietal cortex and thalamus, and the left insula and temporoparietal cortex, which are involved in the integration of visual and somatosensory information and arousal states (Winder et al., 2017). Hypersexuality is described (Cheasty et al., 2002) following temporal and thalamic lesions (Spinella, 2004); changes in sexual orientation have been reported in cases involving infarction of the left middle cerebral artery (Jawad et al., 2009).

Some authors refute the association between the lesion site per se and sexual dysfunctions (Bugnicourt et al., 2014; Choi-Kwon et al., 2002; Tamam et al., 2008) except for ejaculation disorders, which are more frequently found with lesions to the right cerebellum; decreased sexual desire is reported in association with left lesions to the basal ganglia (Jung et al., 2008). Conversely, some authors have suggested that an insult to either hemisphere can be related to sexual difficulties but for different reasons. Examples include aphasia in the case of left hemispheric lesions and visuospatial disorders with right hemispheric lesions (Boller et al., 2015).

### Secondary Impacts of Stroke on Sexual Function

Secondary effects of stroke encompass limitations of movement and position (Korpelainen et al., 1999) and heminegligence playing a role in poor sexual experience. Decreased interest in sexual activity is associated with decreased sensitivity, pain, and fatigue related to stroke but is also related to aging and changes in life stages (Nilsson et al., 2017)

Age and comorbidities, including hypertension and/or diabetes, have negative effects on sexual function; moreover, antihypertensive medications can disrupt sexual reflexes (Bugnicourt et al., 2014; Choi-Kwon and Kim, 2002; Winder et al., 2017).

### Tertiary Impacts of Stroke on Sexual Function

Tertiary effects of stroke include depression and anxiety, contributing to hypoactive sexual desire and sexual dysfunction (Bugnicourt et al., 2014; Korpelainen et al., 1999). Performance anxiety, poor self-image, and body transformations, as well as fear of experiencing a new stroke add to the dysfunctions (Lever and Pryor, 2017). On the positive side, stroke may increase feelings of intimacy (Nilsson et al., 2017)

Emotional incontinence can heighten the symptoms of depression and contribute to lower desire (Choi-Kwon and Kim, 2002). Fear of rejection, of erectile failure, and an incapacity to discuss sexual issues can heighten symptoms of anxiety (Duits et al., 2009; Korpelainen et al., 1999; Tamam et al., 2008). Level of disability, altered daily functioning, and dependence on others (Tamam et al., 2008) further contribute to diminished self-esteem as well as sexual dysfunction.

## Traumatic Brain Injury

### Primary Impacts of Traumatic Brain Injury on Sexual Function

Sexual dysfunctions following TBI include hypoactive sexual desire, erectile dysfunction, orgasmic disorder, diminished frequency of sexual activity, and decreased sexual satisfaction (Bivona et al., 2016; Mazaux et al., 2002; Moreno et al., 2013; Ponsford, 2003; Strizzi et al., 2015; War et al., 2014). Inappropriate sexual touch, sexual exhibitionism, and sexual aggression (abuse) also appear following TBI and correlate with younger age and more severe injury (Turner et al., 2015). Older age, more severe injury, and gender (in females) are associated with greater dysfunction (Goldin et al., 2014).

Frontal and diencephalic lesions as well as septal and limbic lesions are associated with hypersexuality and inappropriate sexual behaviors and also with more fantasies, more experiences, and higher levels of arousal (Moreno et al., 2013). Hyposexual desire is also reported in frontal lesions, right hemispheric lesions being associated with better sexual function. Medial frontal lesions tend to involve more hyposexuality and hypoactive desire than bilateral temporal lesions, and limbic lesions may lead to hypersexuality (Bélanger, 2009).

Pituitary deficits following TBI (40%–54%) suggest possible dysfunction due to hormonal deficits (Bondanelli et al., 2004; Kelly et al., 2000).

### Secondary Impacts of Traumatic Brain Injury on Sexual Function

Hemiplegia, sensory and visual deficits, tremor, spasms, incontinence, joints limitations, gait problems, diminished mobility, fatigue, pain, cognitive and communication deficits, memory impairments, attention deficits, lack of initiative and interest have all been described as contributing to sexual dysfunction (Borgaro et al., 2003; Downing et al., 2013; Goldin et al., 2014; Turner et al., 2015). Diminished motor speed and decreased (sustained) attention correlate with lower sexual drive as well as erectile and ejaculatory dysfunction in males with TBI (War et al., 2014). Females report a lower frequency of sexual activity but also mention that sex is less important to them than to males (Goldin et al., 2014). Patients may or may not be aware of their deficits, which can further contribute to poor sexual adjustment (Bélanger, 2009). Females report poorer body image, diminished self-esteem, and feeling of no longer being attractive (Downing et al., 2013; Turner et al., 2015).

Side effects of medications can contribute to sexual dysfunction (Borgaro et al., 2003; Howes et al., 2005; Parcell et al., 2006; Ponsford, 2003).

Although lesion location suggests links between sexual dysfunction and TBI, such problems often appear later, suggesting secondary (or tertiary) deficits. Inappropriate sexual behaviors may be among the manifestations of impulsivity and lack of self-control often resulting from TBI (Bélanger, 2009).

### Tertiary Impacts of Traumatic Brain Injury on Sexual Function

Depression and anxiety reduce social contacts and psychological readiness for sexual activity (Bivona et al., 2016; Borgaro et al., 2003; Howes et al., 2005; Moreno and McKerral, 2017; Parcell et al., 2006; Ponsford, 2003; Turner et al., 2015). Loss of self-control, generating impulsive behaviors, makes social contacts even more problematic, whereas less social participation is associated with more inappropriate behaviors (Turner et al., 2015). Conversely, better social participation correlates with better sexual functioning. Emotional regression, frequent mood changes, and mental rigidity impair sexual relationships (Bélanger, 2009). Less communicative facial expressions or, conversely, difficulty in interpreting nonverbal communications can render a couple's interactions difficult. Memory loss and attention deficits reduce the individual's capacity for sensuous experiences (Bélanger, 2009).

## Parkinson Disease

### Primary Impacts of Parkinson Disease on Sexual Function

Parkinson disease (PD) is associated with decreased (although sometimes increased) libido, arousal disorder, erectile dysfunction, vaginismus, orgasmic dysfunction, abnormal sexual fantasies, decreased frequency of intercourse, and sexual dissatisfaction, particularly for males (Bhattacharyya and Rosa-Grilo, 2017; Buhmann et al., 2017; Meco et al., 2008). Some authors suggest that PD patients do not have more dysfunctions than non-PD patients matched on other variables, suggesting that comorbidities might explain the complaints (Ferrucci et al., 2016). Sexual dysfunction nevertheless varies with progression of the disease, evolves with age, and is associated with a late onset and advanced stages of the disease (Bronner et al., 2015; Meco et al., 2008; Özcan et al., 2015, 2016; Varanda et al., 2016).

Dopamine deficiency (Bartels and Leenders, 2009) in the brainstem, limbic system (Meco et al., 2008), nucleus accumbens (Meco et al., 2008), and cerebral cortex is suggested to affect the emotional experience and rewarding effect of sexuality. Further release of dopamine from the MPOA and PVN (normally inhibiting the nPGI) and oxytocin release from the pituitary gland are suggested to alter the expression of genital reflexes (Meco et al., 2008). Conversely, lesions to the amygdala and mesencephalic tegmentum projecting to the lumbosacral spinal neurons may alter sexual desire, arousal, and genital reflexes (Meco et al., 2008; Rees et al., 2007), whereas testosterone deficits may diminish erectile function (Bronner, 2011). fMRI findings suggest that hypersexual behaviors in PD patients (Weintraub and Claassen, 2017), usually associated with dopaminergic therapy, appear to be linked with activity in the limbic system, ventral striatum, and the cingulate and orbitofrontal cortices as well as in the temporal, occipital, somatosensory, and prefrontal cortices, all of which suggest mediation through the emotional, cognitive, autonomic, visual, and motivational aspects of sexuality (Politis et al., 2013).

PD patients generally respond well to treatment with dopaminergic drugs (dopamine agonists, levodopa; Bartels and Leenders, 2009; Schapira, 2008), which can also positively affect nonmotor components of the disease, such as restless leg syndrome, sleep disorder, sweating, and pain (Schaeffer and Berg, 2017). However, such therapy can also have a negative effect on the stability of relationships (Buhmann et al., 2017) as well as undesirable effects on hypersexual behaviors (Bartels and Leenders, 2009; Bhattacharyya and Rosa-Grilo, 2017; Bronner et al., 2015; Schapira, 2008; Weintraub and Nirenberg, 2013) as a general form of compulsive behaviors (e.g., compulsive gambling, shopping, binging eating; Morgante et al., 2016; Weintraub and Claassen, 2017). Treatment-mediated hypersexuality seems to be more easily triggered by visual cues, which stimulate increased desire and hedonic responses (Politis et al., 2013), and more readily affect younger patients, those with PD appearing at younger age, with an earlier diagnosis of bipolar disorder, compulsive personality traits, or a history of substance abuse or gambling (Weintraub and Nirenberg 2013)

### Secondary Impacts of Parkinson Disease on Sexual Function

PD is associated with pain, cramps, numbness, tingling sensations, and fatigue (Bartels and Leenders, 2009), interfering with sexual adjustment (Bronner, 2011). Functional deficits to cortical areas can damage the perceptual olfactory and visuospatial cues of sexual arousal (Bartels and Leenders, 2009). Motor symptoms interfere with the physical demands of intercourse, and tremor can disturb orgasm (Bronner, 2011). Fine motor function is required for sexual caresses and facial muscle coordination for kissing, both of which can be altered (Bronner, 2011), and incontinence can discourage sexual approaches.

Side effects of medications decrease libido or delay orgasm (Hand et al., 2010), and dopamine therapy can produce unexpected hypersexuality (Klos et al., 2005, Meco et al., 2008) as well as compulsive behaviors (Bronner, 2011; Meco et al., 2008). Inappropriate sexual behaviors can have legal effects when extreme, but their effect is modulated by the dosage of medication that is used (Klos et al., 2005; Meco et al., 2008). Dopamine agonists can cause involuntary erections (Meco, 2008), the frequency of which decreases with lower dosages (Meco et al., 2008). Conversely, gastrointestinal dysfunction in PD patients can diminish the absorption of some drugs (e.g., phosphodiesterase type 5 [PDE5] inhibitors) (Bronner, 2011).

### Tertiary Impacts of Parkinson Disease on Sexual Function

Psychological impacts include depression and anxiety, but also concerns with body image, especially in hemiplegic patients who lack facial expression and symmetry. These effects can contribute to sexual difficulties (Bronner, 2011; Meco et al., 2008; Özcan et al., 2015). Patients report fear of not meeting their partner's sexual expectations; they tend to avoid sexual activities and withdraw from their relationships (Buhmann et al., 2017).

# TREATMENT OPTIONS FOR THE PRIMARY IMPACT OF NEUROLOGICAL CONDITIONS ON SEXUAL FUNCTION

There is a general consensus in the literature regarding the lack of information, poor professional support, and the rarity of interventions that are offered for the sexual concerns of patients with various neurological conditions. Although efforts have been made to help patients with SCL, lack of resources remains a deep concern for patients with stroke (Calabrò and Bramanti, 2014; Dusenbury et al., 2017; Kautz and Van Horn, 2017; Lever and Pryor, 2017; Nilsson et al., 2017; Richards et al., 2016; Rosenbaum et al., 2014; Stein et al., 2013), TBI (Downing and Ponsford, 2018), and PD (Bronner and Korczyn, 2017).

Treatment options depend on the assessment of the presence (or absence) of remaining sexual, TL, and perineal reflexes (Alexander et al., 2017b; Cordeau et al., 2014; Pukall et al., 2007). Hormonal levels should also be assessed and Doppler evaluation provided as appropriate. Finally, the various comorbidities known to be associated with sexual dysfunctions (e.g., diabetes, metabolic syndrome) should be noted.

## Treatments for Erectile Dysfunction

### Natural Potential

Because neurological lesions (SCL, MS, spinal bifida) can maintain either sexual reflexes or psychogenic responses, patients should be encouraged to try various sources of genital or psychogenic stimulation.

### Rehabilitation by Stimulation of the Bulbocavernous Reflex

Diminished perineal muscle activity (SCL, MS) can be responsible for poor erectile function or vulvar congestion. Training with the bulbocavernous reflex or Kegel exercises may maximize tumescence, rigidity, and vulvar congestion (Courtois et al., 2013d).

### Phosphodiesterase Inhibitors and Other Oral Treatments

PDE5 inhibitors have been shown to be effective treatments for erectile dysfunction in various neurological conditions (Bernard et al., 2016; Greenberg et al., 2019; Jia et al., 2016; Lombardi et al., 2015),). Pharmacological restoration of erectile function does not necessarily guarantee an improvement in quality of life and is not necessarily associated with treatment adherence (Bernard et al., 2016; Biering-Sørensen et al., 2012).

PDE5 inhibitors include sildenafil (Viagra; 25, 50, and 100 mg) acting within 30 minutes to 1 hour and lasting 2–4 hours. Taladafil (Cialis; 10 and 20 mg) lasts from 1 to 2 days but is also available in daily doses (2.5 and 5 mg). Vardenafil (Levitra, Staxyn) (5, 10, and 20 mg) acts within 15–60 minutes and lasts from 4 to 6 hours. Avanafil (Stendra; Vivus) a newcomer, has fewer side effects. These side effects, which are not frequent, include headaches, dyspepsia, flushing, myalgia, low back pain, and rhinitis (Montorsi et al., 2010; Smith et al., 2013). Contraindications involve some blood diseases and the concomitant use of nitrates.

PDE5 inhibitors may be less effective in patients with lower SCLs or with comorbidities (e.g., diabetes). Degenerative disease may require increases in dosages or treatment combinations (Bronner, 2011; DasGupta and Fowler, 2003; Meco et al., 2008).

### Intracavernous Injections

Intracavernous injections (ICI; Greenberg et al., 2019; Porst et al., 2013) include papaverine, alprostadil, and Bi-Mix and Tri-Mix. Doses are gradually increased (in 0.1-mL steps) until they are adequate. Priapism, defined as an erection lasting more than 3 hours, requires treatment, starting with ice packs or ejaculation, followed by aspiration of blood with or without concomitant injection of alpha-adrenergic drug (ephedrine, phenylephrine).

Minor side effects include bruising, and penile fibrosis (subsiding with cessation of treatment). ICIs are effective for SCLs (Courtois et al., 2013d) and other neurogenic conditions (Crayton and Rossman, 2006; DasGupta and Fowler, 2003 ) but require manual dexterity.

### Intraurethral Medication

Prostaglandin capsules (MUSE) in the urethra showed significant results (Guay et al., 2000) but are disappointing clinically (Mulhall et al., 2001). Recently developed alprostadil cream (Vitaros), applied on the glans penis or within urethral meatus, show positive effects on erectile function (Cai et al., 2019).

### Penile Rings and Vacuum Devices

Penile rings of various sizes placed around the base of the penis limit the penile venous outflow and benefits erection as well as maximizing penile rigidity. There is no contraindication, although the concomitant use of anticoagulants may warrant caution. Side effects include delayed or absent ejaculation, bruising, pain, and tingling sensations. The penis may become cold and bluish. Patients must be warned not to wear the rings for more than 20 or 30 minutes.

Penile rings accompany vacuum devices (e.g., Erect Aid) in applying negative pressure for erection. Although useful, they are not necessarily well accepted (Biering-Sørensen et al., 2012).

### Penile Prostheses

Severe erectile dysfunction or failure of other treatments may require penile prosthesis (Courtois et al., 2013d; Trost et al., 2013; Zermann et al., 2006). Semirigid two- and three-piece prostheses are available. The semirigid types are not suited for neurological patients and the two- and three-piece types require fine manual dexterity.

### Other Developing Treatments

Novel treatments are currently investigated for erectile dysfunction but are not yet tested on neurological populations. Among these treatments, injections of platelet-rich plasma, injections of stem cells, external prosthetic devices, and shock-wave therapy have been explored (Scott et al., 2019; Sokolakis et al., 2019). Only the last of these is backed by some scientific evidence but with heterogeneous protocols and generally limited to mild and to vasculogenic ED (Rizk et al., 2018; Sokolakis et al., 2019).

## Treatment of Ejaculation Disorders

### Penile Vibrostimulation

Penile vibrostimulation (PVS; Ferticare) is the first treatment for anejaculation in SCL (Biering-Sorensen et al., 2012; Courtois et al., 2013d). It can be combined with oral midodrine (5–30 mg; Courtois et al., 2008a, 2008b; Soler et al., 2007, 2008), an alpha-stimulating drug administered 45 minutes before vibrostimulation.

When midodrine and PVS fail, rectal probe electroejaculation (EEJ) can be offered (Seager and Halstead, 1993) for fertility only. Other fertility methods (Fode et al., 2012) include microepididymal sperm aspiration (MESA) and testicular sperm extraction (TESE) followed by intrauterine injections (IUI), in vitro fertilization (IVF), or intracytoplasmic sperm injections (ICSI).

### Selective Serotonin Receptor Inhibitors for Premature Ejaculation

Premature ejaculation can develop in some neurological conditions (SCL, PD) and is treated with selective serotonin reuptake inhibitors (SSRIs), particularly paroxetine (Paxil; 10–40 mg), sertraline (Zoloft; 50–200 mg), fluoxetine (Prozac; 20–40 mg; Jian et al., 2018; Jin et al., 2018; Waldinger, 2007, 2018). Dapoxetine, a short-acting SSRI (Abu El-Hamd and Abdelhamed, 2018; Buvat et al., 2009; Porst and Burri, 2019; Pryor et al., 2006; Russo et al., 2016; Simsek et al., 2014), is available in Europe but not in North America.

## Treatments for Sexual Dysfunction in Females

### Natural Potential and Lubricants

Females with neurological conditions can maintain reflexogenic or psychogenic response and should be encouraged to explore their differential effects. Specific attempts on the clitoris, vagina, and cervix should be encouraged, along with explorations of the breast. Females also benefit from questionnaire completion on body sensations (Courtois et al., 2011a, 2013c), increasing their perception of sexual tension.

### Rehabilitation by Kegel Exercises

The effects of Kegel exercises on sexual function in females with neurological conditions have been suggested but not formally tested (Courtois et al., 2013c).

### Vacuum Device, Vibrostimulation, and Sex Toys

Clitoral vacuum devices have been shown to significantly improve sexual desire, arousal, lubrication, sexual sensations, orgasm, and sexual satisfaction in females with SCL and MS (Alexander et al., 2018; Courtois et al., 2013c). Vibrostimulation significantly improves their potential for orgasm. Results with the vacuum device are maintained for 4 weeks after treatment, whereas vibrostimulation is effective only during active treatment. Vacuum devices initially designed for clitoral stimulation can also be used to explore nipple sensations. Sexual aids and commercial vibrators (sex toys) can be incorporated and explored as treatment strategies (Courtois et al., 2011a; Crayton and Rossman, 2006).

### Phosphodiesterase Inhibitors

PDE5 inhibitors show inconsistent results with females, although vaginal and clitoral congestion has been shown in animals (Gragasin et al., 2004; Kim et al., 2003) and with cadaveric tissues (D'Amati et al., 2002;

Uckert et al., 2005). Clinically, PDE5 inhibitors improve lubrication, but not necessarily sexual satisfaction (Alexander et al., 2011; DasGupta and Fowler, 2003; Mayer et al., 2005; Munarriz et al., 2003). They can thus be offered on an individual basis to assess its potential efficacy (Alexander et al., 2018).

### Hormonal and Other Drug Therapy

Hormonal treatment is not specifically recommended, although testosterone or testosterone patches have been used off label to treat sexual arousal disorders in females (Alexander et al., 2017) and flibanserin treatment has shown positive results on sexual desire and satisfaction but negative side effects including dizziness and drowsiness (Terrier and Terrier, 2016).

Symptoms of vaginal dryness (SCL, MS, PD) and dyspareunia can be treated with water-based, silicone-based, glycerin-based, oil-based, or hybrid lubricants, which—except for the water-based—are not always suitable for condoms or sex toys (Hess and Hough, 2012). Topical, oral, ring, or suppository estrogen therapy can also be used and improve hypoactive sexual desire (Crayton and Rossman, 2006; DasGupta and Fowler, 2003). Intravaginal (Labrie et al., 2009) or transdermal testosterone therapy (Wiermann et al., 2006) produces inconsistent results (Davis et al., 2008), as do flibanserin (a serotonin agonist; Katz et al., 2013) and bremelanotide (a melatonin agonist; Diamond et al., 2006).

## TREATMENT OPTIONS FOR SECONDARY IMPACT EFFECTS OF NEUROLOGICAL CONDITIONS ON SEXUAL FUNCTION

Treatment of secondary effects focuses on body functions that interfere with sexuality. Adaptive devices (e.g., intimate rider), pillows, cushions can be used to support the body and reduce the physical demands of intercourse. Sexual activities in the wheelchair, with the arms removed, can facilitate movements. Specific positions (e.g., side ways) can relieve pressure and prevent fatigue (Hess and Hough, 2012).

Stretching muscles with massages can reduce spasticity (Zencius et al., 1990) during foreplay (Hess and Hough, 2012), and while sexual stimulation can trigger spasms, ejaculation and orgasm relieve spasticity (Biering-Sorensen et al., 2005; Courtois et al., 2004; Sonksen et al., 2001).

Finding adequate positions to relieve pressure on the abdomen, avoiding G spot or anal stimulation, may reduce urinary incontinence (Bronner et al., 2010; Çelik et al., 2013; Cramp et al., 2015; Orasanu et al., 2013).

Planning sexual activities (e.g., morning rather than evening, following rather than preceding pain medication) may alleviate pain and fatigue (Çelik et al., 2013; Orasanu et al., 2013).

Side effects of medications may be reduced by diminishing the doses of antispastic, anticonvulsive, and antidepressive drugs, painkillers, muscular relaxants, and sleeping pills (Hess and Hough, 2012). Discontinuing dopamine treatment or using alternatives may eliminate hypersexuality and compulsive behaviors in PD patients (Bronner, 2011; Weintraub and Nirenberg, 2013).

Comorbidities (cardiovascular disease, diabetes, hormonal deficiency; Biering-Sorensen et al., 2012; Lombardi et al., 2010), bladder infections, and severe constipation should all be explored. Recovery from surgery, new episodes of degenerative disease, spinal shock, and intensive rehabilitation should also be considered as potential contributors to sexual dysfunction.

Strategies should encourage sexual gratification with other forms of stimulation including engaging in more frequent kissing, hugging, caressing the body, achieving longer and stronger foreplay, increased tenderness, observing the partner's satisfaction, becoming more open to sexual fantasies, talking about feelings (Bronner and Korczyn, 2017; Buhmann et al., 2017; Hess and Hough, 2012), using sex toys, substitution devices (Borisoff et al., 2010), and assistive devices (straps, handles, dildos; Hess and Hough, 2012; Kreuter et al., 2011).

## TREATMENT OPTIONS FOR TERTIARY EFFECTS OF NEUROLOGICAL CONDITIONS ON SEXUAL FUNCTION

Tertiary effects should assess the access and motivation for sexual activities. Readiness for sexuality should be assessed by rehabilitation professionals or when patients manifest explicit concerns (Ferreiro-Velasco et al., 2005; Hess and Hough, 2012; Kreuter et al., 2008). Information and education on the impact of the neurological condition on sexual functioning should be provided (Bélanger, 2009).

Treatments with mindfulness training, pelvic and yoga exercises are largely used for females with generally positive results for sexual dysfunctions (Mosalanejad et al., 2018; Stephenson and Kerth, 2017; Vilarinho, 2017), and positive impacts on quality of life, fatigue, and pain (Nejati et al., 2016; Vilarinho, 2017).

Current and past psychiatric conditions such as depression, anxiety, and alcohol or drug abuse (Lombardi et al., 2010) should be evaluated. Social isolation should be avoided by attending social clubs, peer groups, web chats, and web dating. Social skill training may be provided for behavior and communication problems (TBI, PD).

Cognitive behavioral therapy can help to modulate stress and anxiety, anger, rejection, and catastrophization. Modeling and role play can reinforce acceptable behaviors and inhibit unacceptable ones (Bélanger, 2009). Relationship issues may be reinforced by overt signs of affection, intimacy, and empathy (Bélanger, 2009; Moreno et al., 2013). Strategies must be repeated in order to develop new functional repertoires (Bélanger, 2009).

Education programs can be provided individually, in group meetings or through documentation (Bélanger, 2009; Courtois et al., 2013c, 2013d; Moreno et al., 2013). Printed guides and internet materials are available for equipment (e.g., intimate rider, vacuum devices) and positioning (e.g., internet videos by Mitchell Tepper for SCL).

## CONCLUSION

Individuals with neurological conditions have sexual concerns that deserve proper information, assessment, and treatment of the primary, secondary, and/or tertiary consequences.

## CONFLICT OF INTEREST

The authors declare no conflict of interest.

### Acknowledgment

The authors wish to thank Anabelle Grenier-Genest PhD(c) and Geneviève Leblanc MA(c) for their help in preparing this chapter and Thomas Lefebvre for the figures.

*The complete reference list is available online at https://expertconsult.inkling.com/.* 

47

# Neuroepidemiology

*Mitchell T. Wallin, Kathryn C. Fitzgerald*

## OUTLINE



Neurological disorders as a group are the leading cause of disability worldwide, and their contribution to the overall burden from all health conditions is increasing (GBD 2016 Neurology Collaborators, 2019). Aging of the population, population growth, and the ongoing epidemiological transition are occurring in many countries and regions, and surveillance of the burden of neurological disorders is required to optimize healthcare planning and resource allocation. Epidemiology is the scientific discipline that provides the tools to assess and quantitate the burden of disease.

A useful definition of *epidemiology* is "the science of the natural history of diseases." This concept is based on the Greek roots of the word: *logos*, from *legein*, "to study"; *epi* "[what is] on"; *demos*, "the people." In epidemiology, the unit of study is a person affected with a disorder of interest. Therefore a definitive diagnosis is the essential prerequisite. This is why the neurologist must be part of any inquiry into the epidemiology of neurological diseases.

After diagnosis, the most important question is the frequency of a disorder. Much of this type of information has been based on case series—that is, the series of cases encountered by individual practitioners, clinics, or hospitals. With such data, however, whether taken as numerator alone (case series) or compared with all admissions (relative frequency), it is difficult to ensure that what has been included is representative of the total population. Accordingly, case material must be referenced to its proper denominator, its true source: the population at risk.

## POPULATION-BASED RATES

Ratios of cases to population, together with the period to which they refer, constitute the population-based rates. Those commonly measured are the incidence rate, the mortality rate, and the so-called prevalence rate. They ordinarily are expressed in unit-population values. For example, a total of 10 cases among a community of 20,000 represents a rate of 50 per 100,000 population, or 0.5 per 1000.

The *incidence* or *attack rate* is the number of new cases over a defined study period divided by the population at risk. This is usually given as an annual incidence rate in cases per 100,000 population per year. The date of onset of clinical symptoms typically dictates the time of accession, although occasionally the date of first diagnosis is used. The *(point) prevalence rate* is more properly called a *ratio*, but it refers to the number of those affected, both old and new cases, at one point in time within the community per unit of population. The *lifetime prevalence rate* refers to the proportion of persons manifesting a disorder of interest during the period of their lives up to the survey date. It is typically reported per 1000 of the population at risk. If no change in case-fatality ratios occurs over time and no change in annual incidence rates (and no migration) occurs, then the average annual incidence rate times the average duration of illness in years equals the point prevalence rate. When numerator and denominator for a rate each refer to an entire community, their quotient is a crude rate for all ages. When both terms of the ratio are delimited by age or sex, these are age- or sex-specific rates, respectively. Such rates for consecutive age groups, from birth to the oldest group of each sex, provide the best description of a disease within a community. In comparing morbidity or mortality rates between two communities for an age-related disorder (such as stroke or epilepsy), differences in crude rates may be observed solely because of differences in the age distributions of the denominator populations. This can be avoided by comparing only the individual age-specific rates between the two, but it rapidly becomes unwieldy. Methods exist for adjusting the crude rates for all ages to permit such comparisons. One such method involves taking community age-specific rates and multiplying them by the proportion of a "standard" population within the same age group. The sum of all such products provides an age-adjusted (to a standard) rate, or a rate for all ages adjusted to a standard population. One common standard in the United States is its population for a given census year. The *mortality* or *death rate* is the number of deaths in a population in a period with a particular disease as the underlying cause, such as an annual death rate per 100,000 population. Deaths by cause, based on standard death certificates, are provided by official government agencies. At times, deaths listed as other than underlying cause on the certificate are added to give a count of total deaths for the disease. The standardized mortality ratio (SMR) is the observed number of deaths in the study group of interest divided by the expected number of deaths based on the standard population rates applied to the study group. The great advantage of death rates is their current availability over time and geographical area for many disorders, whereas morbidity rates require specific community surveys. Geographical distributions from death data are especially informative because most population studies available are, of necessity, spot surveys that may tell little about areas that were not investigated. Most often, too, the numbers are larger by orders of magnitude than those that prevalence studies can provide. The principal disadvantage, and it is a major one, is the question of diagnostic accuracy. In clinical practice, the diagnostic code used for morbidity and mortality rates is a three- or four-digit number representing a specific diagnosis in the *International Statistical Classification of Diseases, Injuries and Causes of Death* (ICD), which is revised periodically. The ICD is the world's standard tool to code disease. The changes in the 10th revision (ICD-10) were major. ICD-10 was published in 1992 and adopted for use in the United States in 1999 but not fully implemented in most health systems until 2015. It introduced the innovation of an alphanumerical coding scheme of one letter followed by three numbers (e.g., I63.1, cerebral infarction due to thrombosis of precerebral arteries). One drawback of the ICD system of classification is that different diseases are often subserved under the same primary code. To provide a more refined classification for individual diseases, several disciplines have published specialty-related expansions of the primary ICD structure. ICD-10-NA is the expansion of the codes relating to neurological diseases, so that virtually every known neurological disease or condition has a unique alphanumerical identifier (St. Germaine-Smith et al., 2012). An initial version of ICD-11 was published in 2018; it will undergo translation into national languages (WHO, 2019). The expectation is that ICD-11 will be available for use in 2022. Lack of space here precludes attention to community survey methods, risk factors and analytic epidemiology, treatment comparisons, and statistical methods—all intrinsic aspects of epidemiology. This chapter highlights the descriptive epidemiological analysis for a few major neurological diseases selected as representative of those most likely to be encountered in clinical neurology.

## CEREBROVASCULAR DISEASE

Stroke (see Chapter 68) is the leading cause of disability among major neurological conditions worldwide (GBD 2016 Neurology Collaborators, 2019) and a major cause of disability in the United States (GBD 2016 Stroke Collaborators, 2019). There are approximately 800,000 strokes annually in the United States. Recent epidemiological studies have subdivided stroke into subarachnoid hemorrhage (SAH) or hematoma, intracerebral hemorrhage, and cerebral infarction. Subdural hemorrhage is not included in this category. Cerebral infarction is the most common type of stroke in developed countries, making up more than 70% of cases. Intracerebral hemorrhages account for approximately 10%–15% of strokes, and SAHs make up less than 5%; the remainder are of undetermined etiology.

### Mortality Rates

Since the late 1960s, US stroke death rates have declined by 75% overall. The largest declines in stroke mortality were seen in white men and the smallest in black men. Similar decreasing rates in stroke mortality are reported for other countries, including Japan, Australia, New Zealand, Canada, and all of Western Europe.

Quality improvement (QI) programs in hospitals have been shown to improve mortality outcomes. The Florida–Puerto Rico Collaboration to Reduce Stroke Disparities (CreSD) (Gardener, 2019) registry tracks Medicare beneficiaries in hospitals and is part of a national QI initiative by the American Heart Association; its outcomes were compared with those of non-QI hospitals. For the period 2010–2013 in patients treated for a stroke at CreSD hospitals, there were no differences in risk-adjusted in-hospital mortality by race or ethnicity. Blacks had a lower 30-day mortality rate versus Whites (odds ratio, 0.86) but a higher rate of 30-day readmission (hazard ratio, 1.09) and 1-year mortality (odds ratio, 1.13).

In 2016, stroke was the second largest cause of death globally (5.5 million deaths) after ischemic heart disease (GBD 2016 Stroke Collaborators, 2019). The age-standardized stroke mortality rates decreased by 36.2% from 1990 to 2016. These death rates also declined for all but one region from 1990 to 2016, with the greatest decrease in the high-income Asia Pacific region (−66.3%) and no significant change in southern Sub-Saharan Africa (−3.8%).

The geographic differences in stroke mortality within the United States are notable, with the highest rates since the 1940s in the southeastern region. The so-called stroke belt states of Georgia, North Carolina, and South Carolina have consistently demonstrated mortality rates above the US average. The Centers for Disease Control and Prevention (CDC) examined this issue by assessing stroke mortality at the county level between 2014 and 2016 (Fig. 47.1). The concentration of stroke mortality rates in the highest two quintiles within the southeastern region validates the persistence of this trend. The Reasons for Geographic and Racial Difference in Stroke (REGARDS) Study was launched in 2001 to clarify the demographic differences in stroke. Recent data from this project have shown that elevated depressive symptoms in conjunction with high levels of perceived stress were more strongly associated with several parameters of metabolic health than only one of these psychological constructs in a large, diverse cohort of adults (Gowey, 2019).

### Morbidity Rates

Like mortality rates, stroke incidence has declined rapidly over the past 50 years in high-income countries. Within the past 20 years, however, the decline in incidence rates in industrialized countries has attenuated (Thrift, 2017). In 2010, an estimated 11.6 million incident ischemic strokes and 5.3 million incident hemorrhagic strokes occurred worldwide, with the majority (63% of ischemic strokes and 80% of hemorrhagic strokes) occurring in low- and middle-income countries (Krishnamurthi, 2013). Stroke incidence increases logarithmically with increasing age but with a lesser increase beyond age 74. In recent years, the annual stroke incidence rate in Europe and North America has been between 100 and 350 per 100,000 population, and mostly near 150.

The most recent worldwide trends in stroke incidence were reported from the Global Burden of Disease Group (GBD 2016 Stroke Collaborators, 2019). The highest age-standardized incidence rates for stroke were observed in East Asia (China 354 per 100,000 person-years) and Eastern Europe (Estonia 335 per 100,000 person-years). The lowest incidence rates were in central Latin America (El Salvador: 97 per 100,000 person-years). Regarding stroke

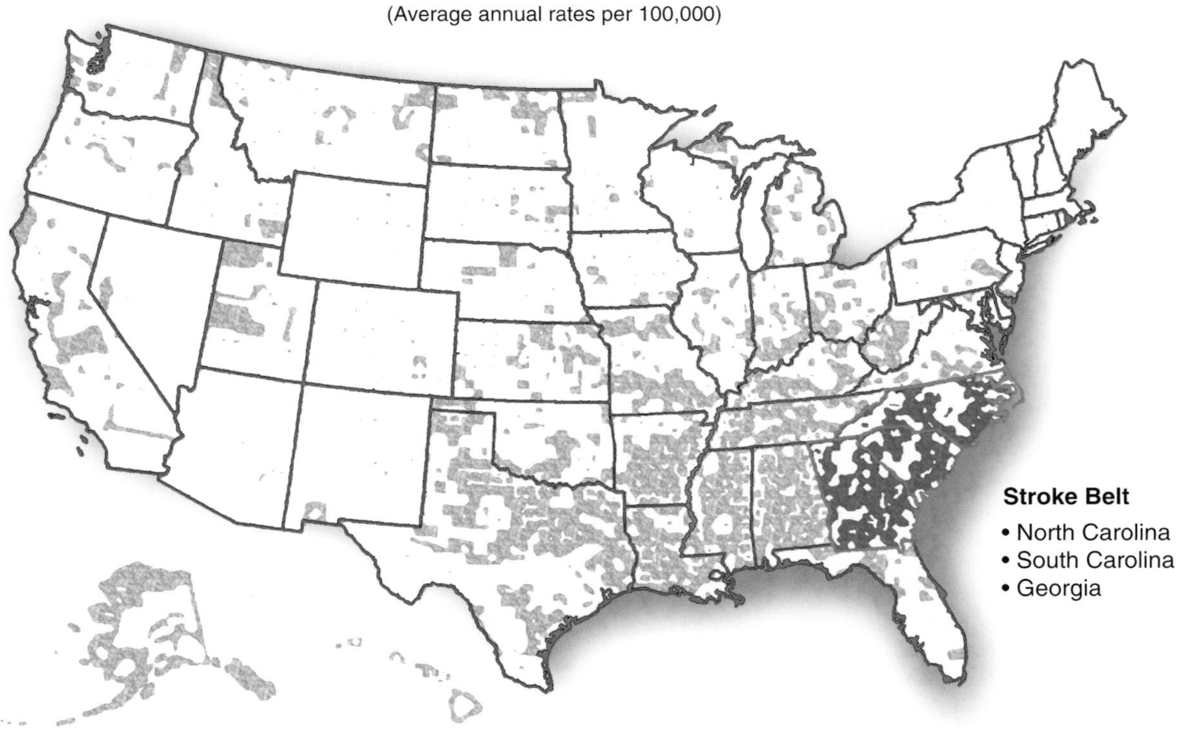


**Fig. 47.1** Age-specific stroke death rates per 100,000 population for stroke among persons above 35 years of age in the United States at the county level, 2000–2006. (*Data from the National Vital Statistics System and the US Census Bureau.*)

subtypes, ischemic stroke incidence rates declined more precipitously in southern Latin America (−38.0%), and the largest increase occurred in East Asia (17.5%). For hemorrhagic stroke, incidence rates decreased in all regions of the world. The largest declines were seen in the high-income Asia Pacific (−32.5%) area, and the smallest in southern Sub-Saharan Africa (−5.1%). In contrast to the 8% global decline in the age-standardized incidence of stroke between 1990 and 2016, rates increased by 0.3%, albeit nonsignificantly, in the group of middle-income countries.

The Greater Cincinnati and Northern Kentucky Stroke Study was the first large metropolitan-based study of stroke trends among a racially diverse population (Madsen, 2017). The incidence for stroke between 1993 and 2010 in the study population was assessed to identify temporal trends. Incidence rates for all strokes decreased in men over the time interval but were stable for women. Incidence rates for intracerebral hemorrhage and SAH were stable in both men and women. Overall decreases in stroke incidence over time are driven by a decrease in ischemic stroke in men. In the United States, the age-adjusted prevalence of stroke was 2.7% in 2006 and remained relatively stable at 2.5% between 2013 and 2016 (Benjamin, 2019). Breakdown by race revealed the highest rates among Native American/Alaska Native people (5.9%), followed by Black people (3.9%); the lowest rates were found in Asian/Native Hawaiian/Other Pacific Island people (1.5%). Between 2006 and 2010, the age group above 65 years of age had stroke prevalence rates 10-fold greater than those in the 18- to 44-year-old group.

## Transient Ischemic Attacks

Although clearly a subset of cerebrovascular disease, transient ischemic attacks (TIAs) have generally been excluded from most morbidity and mortality surveys of stroke. As with incidence and prevalence rates for stroke, a marked increase in TIA rates occurs with age. To better elucidate time trends in TIA, an analysis of incident TIAs from 1998 to 2000 and 2009 to 2011 in northern Portugal was assessed (Felgueiras et al., 2020). Crude annual TIA incidence rates had a nonsignificant increase from 67 to 74 per 100,000 between periods; however, men below age 65 showed a significantly increased risk for TIA (incident relative risk: 1.79). A higher TIA risk in men has been demonstrated in other studies as well. Recent population-based incidence studies for TIA have reported slightly lower rates from 0.26 per 1000 person-years in China to 40 per 100,000 in New Zealand (Barber, 2016).

The new tissue-based definition of TIA takes into account recent neuroimaging findings and also provides a much shorter duration for the diagnosis (Albers et al., 2002). Studies that have used this new definition have shown a heterogeneous response in the frequency of diffusion-weighted magnetic resonance imaging (DW-MRI) signal in patients presenting with TIA symptoms (Brazzelli et al., 2014). This calls into question the utility of using MRI in population-based studies until the variability in responses can be understood. If the new definition were to be used in epidemiological studies, the estimated annual incidence of TIA would be lowered by 33% and the incidence of ischemic stroke increased by 7% (Ovbiagele et al., 2003). However, a major underascertainment of TIA is probable in all surveys unless one directly questions the entirety of the subject population. This may also give spuriously high frequencies for completed stroke after TIA because only a retrospective history of TIA occurrence is given in many studies of stroke.

## PRIMARY NEOPLASMS

Three large centralized US databases that provide descriptive epidemiological data on primary brain tumors have been created (see Chapter 71). These databases are the Central Brain Tumor Registry of the United States (CBTRUS); the Surveillance, Epidemiology, and End Results (SEER) database; and the National Cancer Database (NCDB). According to the CBTRUS database, an estimated 86,970 new cases of primary malignant and nonmalignant brain and other central nervous system (CNS) tumors are expected to be diagnosed in the United States in 2019 (Ostrom, 2018). The lifetime risk of developing a CNS tumor is estimated to be 0.62% in the United States (SEER, 2017). Little is known of the causes of most primary brain tumors, but their epidemiological features may provide clues for more definitive studies.

Within the CNS, approximately 85% of primary tumors have been intracranial and 15% intraspinal. For the brain, the major groupings are the gliomas (40%–50%, of which approximately half are glioblastomas) and the meningiomas (15%–20%). Pituitary adenomas plus schwannomas, especially acoustic, add another 15%–20%. The most common spinal cord tumors are neurofibroma and meningioma, followed by ependymoma and angioma.

### Mortality Rates and Survival

Between 2011 and 2015, the average annual mortality rate in the United States was 4.37 per 100,000, with 77,375 deaths attributed to primary brain malignancies and other CNS tumors. The 5-year relative survival rate in the United States following diagnosis of a primary brain malignancy or other CNS tumor (including lymphomas and leukemias, tumors of the pituitary and pineal glands, and olfactory tumors of the nasal cavity) is 33.8% for males and 36.4% for females (Ostrum, 2018).

Reported 5-year survival ratios for the period 1995–2008 have been 69% for clinically diagnosed meningioma. The relative 5-year survival rate for children younger than 15 years of age with brain and other CNS tumors is now 70.9%, compared with 35% some 30 years ago (CBTRUS, 2012; Parker et al., 1997). The 5-year survival for oligodendrogliomas between 2000 and 2013 was 77.1 years for males and 81.1 years for females. The more aggressive anaplastic oligodendroglioma had corresponding 5-year survival estimates of 55.5 years for males and 54.7 years for females (Achey, 2017).

Glioblastoma is the most common primary brain tumor in adults, with a uniformly poor prognosis. Median survival for glioblastoma remains approximately 1 year after diagnosis. Overall 5-year survival from SEER registries for glioblastoma between 1995 and 2008 was 4.7 years. Several studies from cancer registries have indicated that the 5-year survival rate, typically reported at 4%–10% over the past 30 years, may be too optimistic (Tran and Rosenthal, 2010). Series from Canada, Sweden, and the United States that reviewed clinical and histological data from registries found that in half of all reported cases of glioblastoma, the tumor had been misclassified and on close inspection was found to be a less aggressive tumor (McLendon and Halperin, 2003). Corrected 5-year survival rates are more likely to be in the range of 2%–3%. Recent treatment trials for glioblastoma using temozolomide and radiation have shown some promise in improving survival (Perry, 2017).

The Global Burden of Disease 2016 collaborators evaluated brain and CNS cancer mortality in regions around the globe (GBD 2016 Brain and Other CNS Cancer Collaborators, 2019). Age-standardized death rates for brain and other CNS cancers were the highest in central Europe, tropical Latin America, and Australasia. Country-level age-standardized death rates were highest for Palestine (8.3 per 100,000 person-years) and Albania (7.2 per 100,000 person-years). The countries with the most brain and CNS cancer deaths overall were China, India, and the United States.

### Morbidity Rates

In the United States between 2011 and 2015, brain and other CNS tumors (malignant and nonmalignant) were the most common cancers in persons aged 0–14 years, with an average annual age-adjusted incidence rate of 5.65 per 100,000 population. Moving up to the group aged 15–39 years, brain and other CNS tumors constituted the second leading cancer group, with an average annual age-adjusted incidence of 11.20 per 100,000 population. Finally, brain and other CNS tumors were the eighth most common cancers among persons above 40 years of age, with an average annual age-adjusted incidence of 44.5 per 100,000 population. The most recent overall incidence estimate for all primary brain tumors in the United States is 19.9 per 100,000 population for 2004–2008 (CBTRUS, 2012). For children 0–19 years of age, the rate was 4.9 per 100,000 person-years and for adults above 20 years of age it was 25.9 per 100,000 population. Fig. 47.2, *A* displays the overall primary brain tumor incidence rates by age group and histological behavior. The distribution of CNS tumors by site is presented in Fig. 47.2, *B*. The meninges, at 34%, are the most frequent site for tumors. As a group, the major lobes of the brain (frontal, temporal, parietal, and occipital) account for 22% of brain tumors. The pituitary is the location for nearly 15% of tumors and the pineal for 0.5%. The spinal cord and cauda equina account for 3% of tumors in the CNS.

The GBD collaborators have shown that the number of incident cases of brain cancer and CNS tumors has increased across all geographical regions between 1990 and 2016 with the exception of Eastern Europe, where incident cases are stable (GBD 2016 Brain and Other CNS Cancer Collaborators, 2019). Age-standardized incidence rates were highest in Western Europe, East Asia, and Central Europe. They were lowest in Oceania and Sub-Saharan Africa. Specific countries with the highest age-standardized incidence rates included the Nordic countries (Finland's 13.2 per 100,000 person-years to Iceland's 20.8 per 100,000 person-years) and Luxembourg (16.2 per 100,000 person-years). In this study, the mortality-to-incidence ratio decreased in countries with higher levels of economic development, which is likely related to the specialized imaging and therapy required to diagnose and treat brain tumors. Overall there is great heterogeneity in incidence rates worldwide; this requires further study.

Although some CNS tumors have a clear genetic character, less than 5% can be attributed to inheritance. Many risk factors have been implicated in human brain tumors, the vast majority of which are unsubstantiated by scientific evidence. High-dose irradiation leads to an increased incidence of primary brain tumors, but the association of higher brain tumor risk with low doses of radiation is more controversial.

## CONVULSIVE DISORDERS

*Epilepsy* is defined as recurrent seizures (i.e., two or more distinct seizure episodes) that are unprovoked by any immediate cause or diagnosis of an epilepsy syndrome (see Chapter 101). In 2017, the International League Against Epilepsy (ILAE) updated the classification system for seizures; they are divided into those of (1) focal, (2) generalized, and (3) unknown onset, with subcategories of motor and nonmotor and with retained or impaired awareness for focal seizures (Fisher, 2017). Within the localization-related and generalized groups,

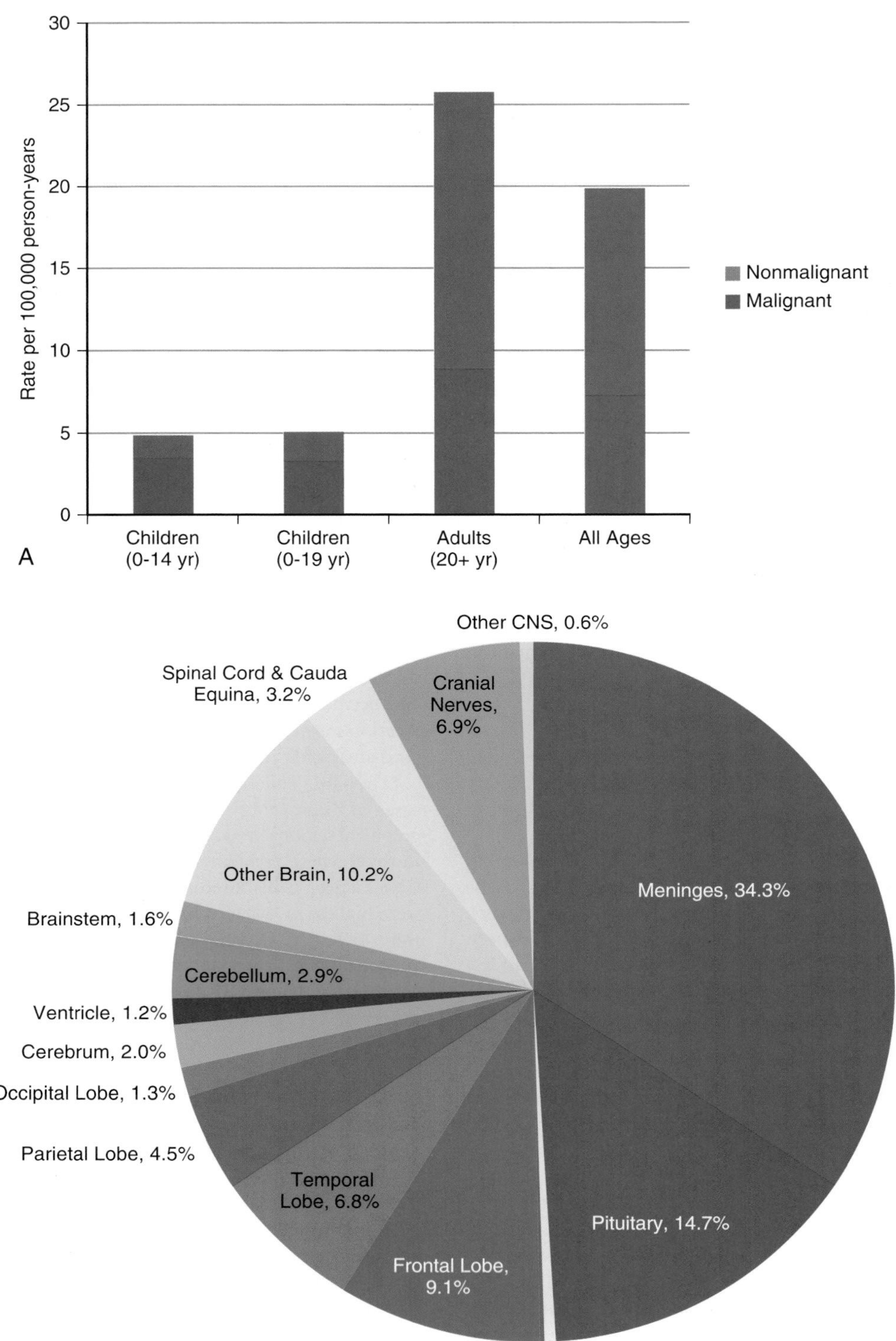


**Fig. 47.2** Central nervous system malignancy incidence rates by age (years) at diagnosis: Surveillance, Epidemiology, and End Results (SEER); Central Brain Tumor Registry of the United States (CBTRUS). **A,** Incidence rates are standardized by age to the United States 2000 standard population. **B,** Histological classification of central nervous system brain tumors (CBTRUS, 2012). *CNS,* Central nervous system. *(Data from Central Brain Tumor Registry of the United States, Hinsdale, IL. Available at: http://www.cbtrus.org. Accessed March 2019.)*

further subdivisions into symptomatic (known cause), idiopathic (presumed genetic origin), and cryptogenic (no clear cause) are recognized. The major clinical types of seizures within the localization groups include tonic-clonic, clonic, myoclonic, epileptic spasms, and nonmotor (absence) seizures. *Status epilepticus* is defined as any seizure lasting for 30 minutes or longer, or recurrent seizures for more than 30 minutes during which the patient does not regain consciousness.

Epidemiological studies of epilepsy have often suffered from lack of agreement on definitions and classifications. Consensus guidelines have been published to assist in the standardization of such studies, but a new, simplified, etiology-oriented classification system will likely be needed in light of new genetic and imaging developments.

## Mortality Rates

The GBD Epilepsy Collaborators assessed the worldwide burden of epilepsy between 1990 and 2016 (GBD 2016 Epilepsy Collaborators, 2019). In 2016, age-standardized mortality rates of idiopathic epilepsy were 1.7 per 100,000 population for women and 2.09 per 100,000 population for men. Between 1990 and 2016, age-standardized mortality rates of idiopathic epilepsy decreased significantly in 74 countries, mostly from Western and Central Europe, Australasia, high-income North America, high-income Asia Pacific, Latin America, the Caribbean, North Africa, and the Middle East. On the other hand, mortality rates climbed over the same period in 22 countries predominantly from western Sub-Saharan Africa, Europe, and Southeast Asia.

Reported mortality rates with epilepsy are on average two to three times greater than those in the general population. Population-based studies with long-term follow-up give SMRs between 2 and 4, which appear to be the more accurate estimates. Recent reports from low- and middle-income countries reveal SMRs for epilepsy in the range of 4–6, with a high burden of death in young adults with active epilepsy (Ngugi et al., 2014). As opposed to high-income countries, there is a significant proportion of deaths in low- and middle-income countries from epilepsy-related causes that could be prevented by access to basic medical care of seizures. As to evaluating cause of death, the proportionate mortality (PMR) is frequently used. The PMR for conditions related to epilepsy ranges between 1% and 13% for population-based studies (Hitiris et al, 2007). Etiologies include status epilepticus and seizure-related causes (PMR 0%–10%), sudden unexplained death in epilepsy (SUDEP; PMR 0%–4%), suicide (PMR 0%–7%), and accidents (0%–12%). Causes of death unrelated to epilepsy include ischemic heart disease (PMR 12%–37%), cerebrovascular disease (PMR 12%–17%), cancer (PMR 18%–40%), pneumonia (PMR 0%–7%), suicide (PMR 0%–12%), and accidents (0%–4%).

With epilepsy, overall death rates in most studies are greater for men than those for women. Mortality is increased in the early years after diagnosis, largely due to the underlying cause of symptomatic epilepsy. Mortality is also increased for all patients with refractory epilepsy.

Epilepsy-related mortality has peaks in early childhood and early adulthood, after which rates tend to stabilize before rising once again in old age. Patients with idiopathic and cryptogenic epilepsy have the lowest long-term mortality rates, with SMRs of approximately 2, whereas those with symptomatic epilepsy with underlying neurological disease have the highest mortality rates, with reported SMRs of 11–25. Deaths attributed to epilepsy itself account for less than 50% of deaths of any cause in persons with the disorder; specific etiological disorders or factors include status epilepticus, accidents due to seizures, treatment-related factors, suicide, aspiration pneumonia, and SUDEP. A large population-based epilepsy cohort in Sweden found an 11-fold increased risk of premature mortality compared with general population and sibling controls (Fazel et al., 2013). Of these deaths, 16% were due to external causes such as motor vehicle accidents and suicide. Psychiatric comorbidity was strongly associated with external causes of death.

SUDEP is generally considered to be the most common cause of epilepsy-related death, with a relative frequency of 1 per 1000 epilepsy cases (Opeskin and Berkovic, 2003). Risk factors that have been consistent across studies include male sex, generalized tonic-clonic seizures, early age of onset of seizures, refractoriness to treatment, and being in bed at the time of death. Proposed mechanisms for SUDEP include central apnea, acute neurogenic pulmonary edema, and cardiac arrhythmia precipitated by seizure discharges acting via the autonomic nervous system. Other causes of death in epilepsy can be classified as those in which epilepsy is secondary to an underlying disease (e.g., cerebrovascular disease) or is an unrelated disorder (e.g., ischemic heart disease). Mortality data were similar in configuration to those for age-specific prevalence data, but rates were 1000-fold lower. This finding suggests that 0.1% of the patients with epilepsy die each year of causes directly related to their epilepsy.

Status epilepticus affects 105,000–152,000 persons annually in the United States (DeLorenzo et al., 1996). Status epilepticus represents a neurological emergency, and despite improvements in treatment, the mortality rate is still high. Population-based studies have reported 30-day case-fatality ratios between 8% and 22%. Short-term fatality after status epilepticus is associated with the presence of an underlying acute etiological disorder. Fatality ratios are lowest in children (short-term mortality rate 3%–9%) and highest in the elderly (short-term mortality rate 22%–38%). Case-fatality ratios for those surviving the initial 30 days after status epilepticus are 40% within the following 10 years.

## Morbidity Rates

Fig. 47.3 also shows morbidity measures for epilepsy in Rochester, Minnesota, by age group. The age-specific incidence of epilepsy was high during the first year of life, declined during childhood and adolescence, and then increased again after age 55. The cumulative incidence of epilepsy was 1.2% through age 24 and steadily increased to 4.4% through age 85 years. Age-specific prevalence increased with advancing age; nearly 1.5% of the population older than 75 years had active epilepsy.

In 2016 there were 45.9 million patients globally with all-active epilepsy, both idiopathic and secondary (GBD 2016 Epilepsy Collaborators, 2019). The proportion of this total with active epilepsy was 24 million. The global age-standardized prevalence of all-active epilepsy was 621.5 per 100,000 population. It varied from a low of 311.0 per 100,000 population in Japan to a peak of 1287.7 per 100,000 population in Cape Verde. The global age-standardized prevalence of idiopathic epilepsy was 326.7 per 100,000, with the highest prevalence estimates in eastern, western, and southern Sub-Saharan Africa, Central Asia, Central America, Andean Latin America, and Southeast Asia.

Surveys from developing countries are fewer and less rigorous and report much higher incidence rates, ranging between 43 and 190 cases per 100,000. Within industrialized countries, temporal trends in epilepsy over the past 30 years have shown a decrease in incidence in children and an increase in incidence for the elderly. Improved prenatal care and immunization may explain the changes for the former and perhaps longer life expectancy with more concomitant CNS disease for the latter. The overall prognosis for controlling seizures is good, with more than 70% of patients achieving long-term remission. Age-specific incidence rates for epilepsy from several surveys showed a sharp decrease from maximal rates in infancy to adolescence and thereafter a slow decline for new cases throughout life. In other studies, rates were essentially constant after infancy or showed an irregular rise with age.

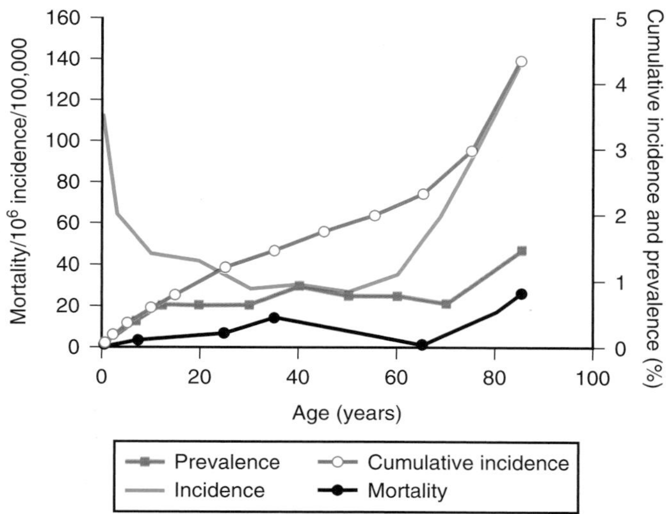


**Fig. 47.3** Measures of epilepsy (Rochester, Minnesota, 1935–1984): age-specific incidence per 100,000 person-years; cumulative incidence (percent); age-specific prevalence (percent); and age-specific mortality per 100,000 person-years. *(From Hauser, W.A., Annegers, J.F., Rocca, W.A., 1996. Descriptive epidemiology of epilepsy: contribution of population-based studies from Rochester, Minnesota. Mayo Clin Proc. 71, 576–586.)*

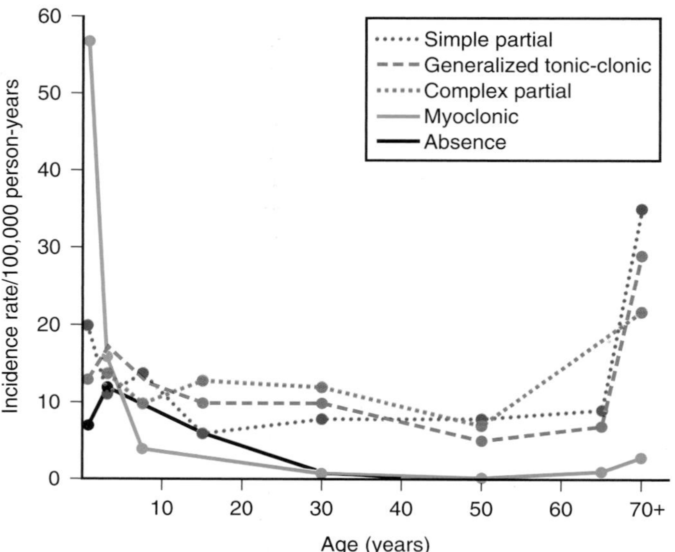


**Fig. 47.4 Epilepsy.** Average annual age-specific incidence rates per 100,000 population by clinical type of seizure—absence, myoclonic, generalized, simple, complex partial. *(From Kurtzke, J.F., Kurland, L.T., 2004. The epidemiology of nervous system disease. In: Joynt, R.J., Griggs, R.J. (Eds.) Baker and Joynt's Clinical Neurology on CD-ROM. Lippincott Williams & Wilkins, London.)*

In Rochester, Minnesota, however, the configuration was U-shaped, with a marked increase in incidence rates at the age of 75 years and older (Fig. 47.4). This configuration reflects generalized tonic-clonic disorders together with absence and myoclonic seizures for the left arm of the U and complex partial and generalized tonic-clonic epilepsies for the right arm. Myoclonic seizures were the major type diagnosed during the first year of life; they were also the most common in the age group but rarely occurred after 4 years of age. Absence (petit mal) seizures peaked in the age group from 1 to 4 years and did not begin in patients older than 20 years. Both complex partial and generalized tonic-clonic seizures had fairly consistent incidence rates of 5–15 per 100,000 in persons 5–69 years of age, after low maxima at ages 1–4 years; for age 70 and older, the rates of each were sharply higher. Rates of generalized tonic-clonic seizures had a similar configuration for both primary and secondary seizures. Simple partial seizures increased only slightly with age.

### Febrile Seizures

In the United States and Europe, the risk of a child's developing febrile seizures has been about 2%, ranging between 1% and 4%. Surveys from Japan and the Mariana Islands showed rates of 7% and 11%, respectively. As with epilepsy in general, a male preponderance of 1.2 to 1 for febrile convulsions was observed. In most studies, recurrent febrile seizures occur in approximately one-third of the cases, and overall the risk of subsequent epilepsy is approximately 2%–4% for simple and 11% for complex febrile seizures.

## MULTIPLE SCLEROSIS

### Mortality Rates and Survival

Over the past 50 years, mortality for multiple sclerosis (MS; see Chapter 80) has declined steadily in North America and Western Europe while it remained stable or increased in Eastern Europe. For example, a recent population-based study conducted in Ontario from 1996 to 2013 found the prevalence of MS to increase by 69% (from 157 per 100,000 population in 1996 to 265 per 100,000 in 2013). However, incidence remained largely stable during this time period and MS mortality decreased by 33% (from 267 per 100,000 population in 1996 to 180 per 100,000 in 2013; Rotstein et al., 2018). There is some variability in mortality data within population-based cohort studies, but overall average time to death from MS onset ranges between 24 and 45 years (Scalfari et al., 2013). SMRs range from 1.3 to 2.9 for MS compared with the general population.

As to cause of death, approximately 50% of patients with MS die of complications related to their disease. Koch-Henriksen and colleagues (1998) in Denmark as well as Smestad and colleagues (2009) in Norway attributed more than half of all deaths in a large population cohort to MS or its complications. An overall SMR of 2.5 for all causes was calculated for the Norwegian cohort (Smestad et al., 2009). Infections were the most common cause of death; survival was age dependent and not related to disease course. In a large registry of over 32,000 US-based MS patients, male sex, longer disease duration, and greater disability were associated with an increased risk of mortality (Cutter et al., 2015).

As more patients with MS survive to older ages, however, a greater proportion of them can be expected to die of causes unrelated to MS and thus will not be coded as dying from MS (underlying cause). This last point is supported by an analysis of contributory causes of death for patients with MS in Denmark and the United States. The estimated 25-year survival of the population with MS in Rochester, Minnesota, was 76.2%, compared with 87.7% for the general US White population of similar age and gender. Survival for men was less than that for women. This survival figure was slightly greater than that from earlier estimates for Rochester. The Danish National MS Registry data provided a median survival of 30 years from onset of the disease. Median survival times for US World War II veterans from MS disease onset were 43 years for White females, 30 years for Black males, and 34 years for White males (Wallin et al., 2000). The male rates did not differ significantly, and when relative survival ratios were calculated, none of the three groups were significantly different, indicating that the excess for the White females was attributable more to gender than to disease.

In addition, there has been growing interest in comorbidity as a contributor to mortality. A Danish study found a higher risk of death in people with MS following a diagnosis of psychiatric, cerebrovascular, cardiovascular, and lung disease as well as diabetes, cancer, and Parkinson disease comorbidity; the study also reported a highly significant diagnostic delay of comorbidity in people with MS and postulated that the delayed diagnoses contributed to an excess risk of death associated with comorbidity (Thormann et al., 2017).

## Morbidity Rates

The prevalence surveys for Europe and the Mediterranean basin from the later 20th century appear to separate into clusters within two zones: one to the north, with rates of 30 per 100,000 and higher, considered to represent high frequency, and the other to the south, with rates less than 30 per 100,000 but greater than 4 per 100,000 population, classified as medium frequency.

The northernmost parts of Scandinavia and the Mediterranean basin were medium-prevalence regions in 1980. More recent surveys of Italy and its islands, however, have documented prevalence rates of 60 per 100,000 and higher; therefore this country is now clearly within the high-frequency band (Kurtzke, 2005). This increase in prevalence appears to be recent, because some of the earlier Italian surveys with lower rates were well done. This change is not limited to Italy—indeed, all of Europe from northernmost Norway to the Mediterranean regions now falls in the high-frequency zone, as documented by Pugliatti et al. (2006).

Although, clearly, intra- and international diffusion of this disease has occurred in recent years, the general worldwide distribution of MS may still be described within three zones of frequency or risk. As of 2004, the high-risk zone, with prevalence rates of 30 per 100,000 population and above, included essentially all of Europe, the United States, Canada, Israel, and New Zealand, plus southeastern Australia and easternmost Russia. These regions are bounded by areas of medium frequency, with prevalence rates between 5 and 29 per 100,000, consisting now of Russia from the Ural Mountains into Siberia as well as the Ukraine. Also, in the medium zone still fall most of Australia and perhaps Hawaii, all of Latin America, the North African littoral, and White people in South Africa; even northern Japan seems now to be of medium prevalence. Low-frequency areas, with prevalence rates below 5 per 100,000, still comprise all other known areas of Asia, Africa, Alaska, and Greenland (Kurtzke, 2005).

In recent years, the classical definitions of low-, medium-, and high-prevalence countries may be shifting. For example, countries located in the Far East and South Asia were traditionally considered to be in a low-prevalence region for MS; however, emerging evidence suggests that prevalence may be increasing in these regions. A recent review of 68 studies conducted in East Asia, Southeast Asia, and South Asia found that MS prevalence in these regions ranged from 0.77 per 100,000 population in Hong Kong to 85.8 per 100,000 in Iran (Eskandarieh et al., 2016; Schiess et al., 2016). MS prevalence in Iran, the United Arab Emirates, and Japan may be increasing (Etemadifar et al., 2014a, 2014b). Continuing advances in MS epidemiology and the development of MS registries across countries, including those traditionally considered to be low-prevalence regions, will facilitate more accurate classifications of low-, medium-, and high-prevalence areas in the coming years.

A recent comprehensive review of 101 MS studies of the Americas, Europe, Asia, Africa, and Australia/New Zealand estimated the median worldwide prevalence of MS to be 112.0 (range 5.2–335) cases per 100,000 person-years (Melcon et al., 2014). In the United States, the 2010 estimated 10-year MS prevalence was 309.2 per 100 000 population and represented 727,344 individuals living with MS; the estimated prevalence for 2017 was 339.7 per 100,000 (totaling 913,925 persons with MS). Consistent with global estimates, MS prevalence in the United States was higher in women (450.1 per 100,000) relative to men (159.7 per 100,000), representing a sex ratio of 2.8 (Fig. 47.5).

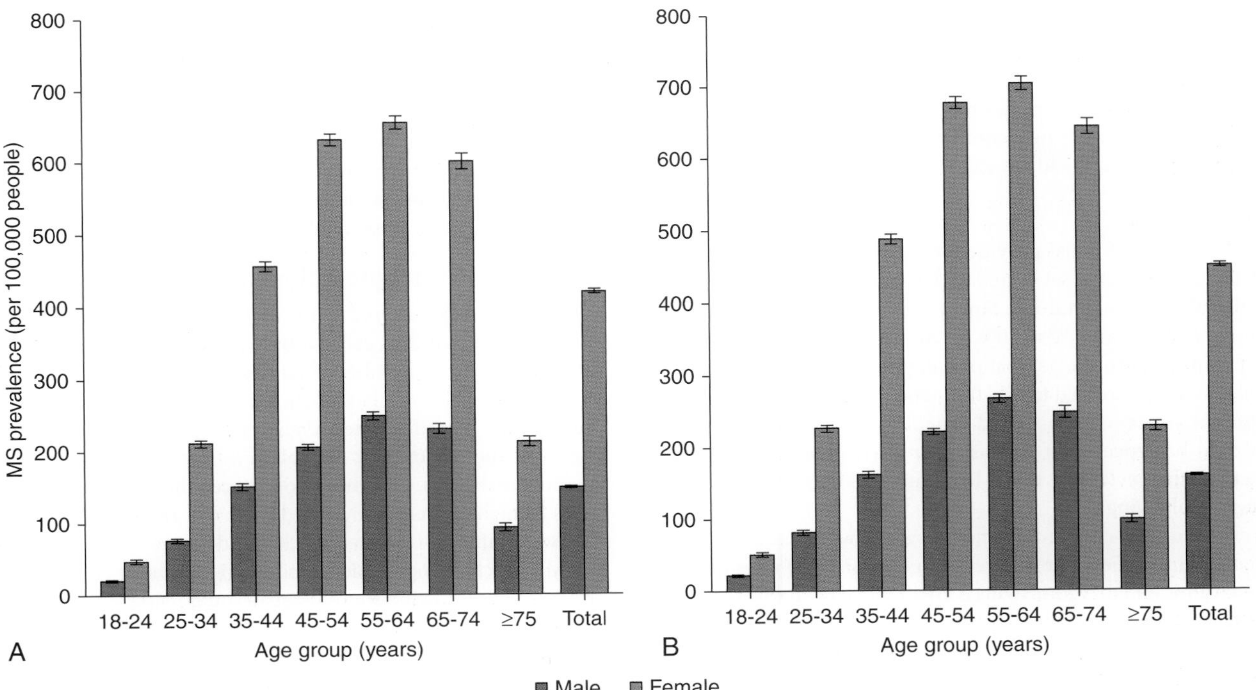


**Fig. 47.5** Age group–specific 2010 multiple sclerosis prevalence estimates for men are in blue (current figure) and women are in green (current figure) in the United States (higher bound) rates in Europe (adjusted to the 2010 US Census). (A) Lower estimate based on adjusments; (B) Upper esimate based on adjustments. *(From Wallin M.T., Culpepper W.J., Campbell J.C., et al., 2019. The prevalence of MS in the United States: A population-based estimate using health claims data. Neurology. 92, e1029–e1040.)*

Prevalence was highest among 55- to 64-year-olds, and a decreasing north-south prevalence gradient in the United States was observed (Wallin et al., 2019). With respect to incidence, the annual incidence rate for MS in high-risk areas at present is approximately 3–6 per 100,000 population, whereas in low-risk areas it is approximately 1 per 1,000,000. Medium-risk areas have an incidence near 1 per 100,000. In Denmark during the years 1939–1945, age-specific incidence rates rose rapidly, from essentially zero in childhood to a peak at about age 27 of more than 9 per 100,000 for females and almost 7 per 100,000 for males. Beyond age 40, little difference between the sexes was seen; in both, rates declined equally to 0 by age 65. The most recent evidence indicates that women of all races in the United States now have incidence rates three times higher than those of men, and Black/African-American people have the highest incidence rates compared with all other groups (12.1 per 100,000 among Black/African-Americans vs. 9.3 per 100,000 among Whites and 6.9 per 100,000 among other races). The incidence rates for Hispanic people (8.2 per 100,000), Asian people (3.3 per 100,000), and Native American people (3.1 per 100,000) are in the moderate to high range (Wallin et al., 2012). Theses incidence rates are comparable to estimated incidence rates of MS reported from Canadian provinces such as Ontario, Manitoba, and British Columbia (Rotstein et al., 2018; Marrie et al, 2010; Kingwell et al., 2015)

The US World War II veteran series showed a markedly elevated risk for residents who lived in the northern region of the country. This was seen for both sexes among White people and for Black men, with a north-to-south difference of almost 3 to 1. Veterans of the Vietnam War and later conflicts still showed a gradient, but it was much less (Wallin et al., 2004). All southern states then were calculated to lie within the high-frequency zone, with prevalence rates that were estimated at well over 30 per 100,000 population. In the Canadian province of Ontario, MS prevalence and incidence were not consistently associated with latitude; most of the population resides within the 42nd and 46th parallels, which is a limited range and may have dampened the ability of studies to find an effect of latitude.

For all races and both sexes, the north-to-south difference was only 2 to 1. This is not a "regression to the mean" with a decreased prevalence in the north but rather reflects an even greater increase in the south. This diffusion is in accord with the intra- and international changes for Europe, as already noted.

## Genetic Studies

Family studies in MS have provided a means of assessing environmental factors against a set genetic background. Such studies have shown that the risk for multiple family members with MS is 3%–4% for primary relatives and 20%–30% for monozygotic twins. This finding is in contrast with the general population prevalence of approximately 0.1%. The increased family frequency may be related to shared environment as opposed to shared genetic factors because close relatives would be expected to share similar environmental influences. However, further evidence that MS is under some genetic control includes the following:

1. An excess of MS-concordant monozygous twins has been found in most twin studies. The difference in concordance rates between monozygotic and dizygotic twins is attributable primarily to genetic factors. Moreover, a recent study found no evidence for genetic, epigenetic, or transcriptome differences in identical twins discordant for MS (Baranzini et al., 2010). The maximum concordance rate for MS in monozygotic twins in high-risk areas is approximately 30%. Modern estimates of the heritability of MS using genome-wide approaches estimates that the heritability of MS as explained by common variation to be approximately 38%.
2. Variation in the human leukocyte antigen (HLA) genes of the major histocompatibility complex (MHC) presents the strongest genetic risk factor for MS and includes both class II risk alleles (HLA-DRB1*15:01, HLA-DRB1*13:03, HLA-DRB1*03:01, HLA-DRB1*08:01 and HLA-DQB1*03:02) and class I protective alleles (HLA-A*02:01, HLA-B*44:02, HLA-B*38:01 and HLA-B*55:01) (Moutsianas et al., 2015). Specifically, variation in the DQB*06:02–HLA-DRB1*15:01 haplotype confers the largest genetic risk for MS. Large-scale studies have also suggested interactions involving pairs of class II alleles (HLA-DQA1*01:01, HLA-DRB1*15:01 and HLA-DQB1*03:01-HLA-DQB1*03:02) in MS risk. A greater burden of HLA risk alleles is highly associated with earlier age of onset ($P$ = 6.6E-10); as expected, this result was largely driven by the DQB*06:02–HLA-DRB1*15:01 haplotype, which reduced MS age of onset by 0.72 years. The interplay between MHC alleles via epistasis within racial groups could be a factor but has not been extensively studied.
3. Recently genome-wide association studies (GWAS) including over 40,000 MS patients have implicated 200 non-MHC genetic variants that contribute to the risk for MS (International Multiple Sclerosis Genetics Consortium, 2017). In addition to the 200 validated susceptibility alleles, 192 suggestive effects were also identified; the combined estimate of MS heritability when both validated and suggestive alleles are considered extends to 48%. The study confirmed known associations between variants in interleukin-2 *(IL-2RA)* and interleukin 7 *(IL-7RA)* receptor genes as risk factors for MS. Newer gene loci have relatively low risk ratios (<1.5) for determining MS susceptibility. As in the case of other complex genetic diseases, many more genes will be discovered but will probably not add significantly to the models of disease risk for individual patients; however, such studies can also implicate novel genes or biological processes potentially contributing to MS risk. For example, risk variants are associated with gene-expression enrichment in T cells as well as B cells, whose critical role in MS has emerged more recently. Notably, limited studies have evaluated the genetic contribution to MS risk among those not of European descent. One study of 800 Black/African-Americans (considered to be a relatively small study from a genetic association study perspective) found a large degree of overlap between identified risk alleles in both White and Black/African-Americans but several candidate variants for subsequent validation (Isobe et al., 2015). The genetic contribution to MS risk in other populations has not been well described.

## Migration in Multiple Sclerosis

If the risk for MS is altered by moves to or from different risk areas, MS must have an acquired, exogenous, environmental cause or major precipitating factor. A number of studies of both morbidity and mortality in migrants show clearly that such moves do change the risk. Several studies have identified a tendency for immigrants to retain much but not all of the risk of their birthplace if they have come from high- or medium-risk areas. Evidence also surfaced that migrants from low-risk areas to high-risk areas increased their risk for MS. A large case-control series among US veterans clearly demonstrated a change in risk for MS by changing residence between birth and entry into military service. Those moving south decreased their risk; those moving north increased it. These findings also indicated that the time when such moves are critical is well after birth but also well before clinical onset, suggesting for the north-to-south moves an acquisition of the disease midway between birth and age at service entry, or at about age 10–15.

Kurtzke and associates (1998) identified North African immigrants among 7500 patients with MS in a nationwide survey in France in 1986. A total of 260 had emigrated from North Africa, mostly between

1960 and 1965. Two-thirds were from Algeria, where virtually its entire European population had emigrated in 1962 at the end of the Algerian war for independence. The migrants were younger in 1986 and at onset of MS than the French-born persons with MS. The 225 with onset more than 1 year after migration presumably acquired their MS in France. They provided an age-adjusted (to the US 1960 population) MS prevalence rate 1.5 times that for all of France. If the latter is 50 per 100,000 population, their estimated adjusted rate is 77. At each year of age at immigration, there was a mean interval of 13 years and a minimum of 3 years to clinical onset from either age 11 or age at immigration if that was older than 11. The other 27 migrants with presumed acquisition in North Africa had an estimated adjusted prevalence of 17 per 100,000, the same as expected in their native lands. Disease frequencies that are higher among immigrants than among natives are typical of the former's exposure to a new infection. The study also suggested that 3 years of exposure from age 11 were needed for immigrants from medium-risk areas to acquire MS, and that susceptibility extended to about age 45 or so. These findings are also consistent with more recent migration studies conducted in Scandinavia (Berg-Hansen et al., 2015). For example, the prevalence of MS among first-generation Iranian immigrants was not significantly different from that of the total Norwegian population (standardized prevalence ratio [SPR]: 0.70; 95% confidence interval [CI]: 0.46–1.03). Second-generation Pakistani immigrants were at a markedly higher prevalence of MS (SPR: 1.62; 95% CI: 0.88–2.76) when compared with first-generation Pakistani immigrants (SPR 0.13, 95% CI: 0.05–0.28). Similar findings were noted among South Asian immigrant populations in Sweden (Ahlgren et al, 2010, 2012).

Other studies of migrants from high- to low-risk areas also suggest a critical age for risk retention. This is exemplified by a series of northern European immigrants to South Africa. Their MS prevalence rate for immigration under age 15 was 13 per 100,000, the same as for the native-born English-speaking White South Africans. For all older age groups at immigration, the prevalence rate was 30–80 per 100,000, the same as in their high-risk lands of birth. For those with onset after immigration, the intervals between immigration and clinical onset were some 20–30 years for those younger than 15 years of age and approximately 10–12 years for those 15 years or older. These findings support the existence of a long "incubation" or "latency" period between the acquisition of MS and clinical onset. They also indicate that young children are much less susceptible to MS, despite their living in high-risk areas such as northern Europe.

## Epidemics of Multiple Sclerosis

The Faroe Islands, in the North Atlantic Ocean between Iceland and Norway, are a semi-independent unit of the Kingdom of Denmark. As of June 1999, we had found 70 native-born Faroese with onset of MS in the 20th century. Of these, 15 had lived for 3 or more years off the islands before onset and were excluded from the native resident series as having likely acquired their disease while living overseas in high-risk MS lands, a decision fostered by the finding that their periods of overseas residence correlated with age at onset. The remaining 55 comprised the native resident series: 14, most of whom had lived less than 2 years overseas, with such periods uncorrelated with time of onset; and 41 who had not lived off the islands before onset. Of these 55, no patient had clinical onset before July 1943, when symptoms began in one man. With a minimum exposure period of 2 years needed to acquire MS, 1941 was the most recent year for the disease to have been introduced into the Faroes. Between 1943 and 1949, a total of 17 patients had symptom onset in this populace of 26,000. There were four others who were also at least age 11 by 1941 whose onsets occurred between 1950 and 1961. These 21 patients constituted a type 1 point source epidemic of MS. Annual incidence rates rose steeply from 0 to more than 10 per 100,000 in 1945 and 1946 and then fell almost as steeply with the short tail as noted. Age at first exposure ranged from 11 to 45 and at onset from 15 to 48.

We divided the other 33 patients (the 34th heralded a possible epidemic V) according to when they reached age 11, which then provided three more (type 2) epidemics of 10, 10, and 13 patients each—epidemics II, III, and IV (data as of 1991 are shown in Fig. 47.6) (Kurtzke and Heltberg, 2001).

We concluded that the disease was introduced into the Faroe Islands by the British troops who had occupied the islands for 5 years starting in April 1940, most of whom had been billeted within the villages scattered across most of the islands where the patients had lived during the war. What was probably introduced was an infection that was transmitted to the Faroese population at risk from a large proportion of the British troops (because of its scattering), who were asymptomatic carriers (because they were healthy troops). We called this infection the *primary MS affection* (PMSA), which we defined as a single, specific, widespread, systemic but unknown infectious disease (that may be totally asymptomatic). PMSA produces clinical neurological MS (CNMS) in only a small proportion of the affected population after an incubation period averaging 5–6 years in virgin populations and perhaps 15–20 years in high-risk endemic areas. Using this hypothesis, transmissibility is limited to part or all of this systemic phase, which ends by the usual age at onset of MS symptoms. The PMSA-affected persons of the first population cohort of Faroese transmitted the disease to the next Faroese population cohort, those who reached age 11 in the period when the first cohort was transmissible. Included in the second Faroese cohort were the epidemic II cases of CNMS, and this cohort similarly transmitted PMSA to the third population cohort with its own (epidemic III) cases, and from them to the fourth cohort with its epidemic IV. Thus, PMSA seems to be a geographically delimited, specific (but unknown), age-limited, transmissible, persistent infection that is acquired principally during the hormonally active years of age and one that only rarely leads to clinical MS. To seek evidence for an infectious origin of the type I epidemic of MS in the Faroe Islands, we examined data from the Danish National Health Service from 1900 to 1977 (Wallin et al., 2010). eFig. 47.7 shows the monthly count of three of these diseases and the troop units. The rise in the incidence of acute infectious gastroenteritis and paradysentery clearly seems to correlate with the introduction and later surge in British troop levels during World War II.

Speaking to these findings, Kurtzke concluded that "Primary multiple sclerosis affection itself may have been manifest there (Faroes) as a newly introduced cause of acute infectious gastroenteritis and is possibly the underlying cause of multiple sclerosis in general" (Kurtzke, 2013). More detailed data supporting that view have been published (Kurtzke, 2014).

# MOVEMENT DISORDERS

Movement disorders as a group (see Chapters 24 and 95) span multiple unique conditions within neurology. The most common adult-onset movement disorder is essential tremor. A recent review estimated the pooled prevalence of essential tremor to be 2.2% for all ages (Louis et al., 2014); the study estimated that approximately 7.23–7.63 individuals in theUnited States are living with essential tremor. There was a marked increase in essential tremor with increasing age, with the highest pooled rate of essential tremor occurring among individuals older than 65 years.

Parkinson disease (PD) has received the most attention in epidemiological studies among movement disorders and is the focus of this section. Idiopathic PD must be distinguished from other neurodegenerative diseases and parkinsonism related to other causes. An accurate diagnosis of PD can be made clinically and is based on symptomatic bradykinesia, muscular rigidity, rest tremor, and postural instability.

The cause of PD remains unclear. Age is the most important risk factor for developing the disease. Genetic studies have linked dopa-responsive parkinsonism to a variety of mutations in seven genes; GWAS have also identified 41 susceptibility loci implicating genes involved in lysosomal and innate immune function as mechanistic players in PD (Chang et al., 2017; Li et al., 2019). Environmental risk factors that appear to be protective in developing PD include intake of caffeine and smoking as well as moderate physical exercise (Fang et al., 2018). Weaker associations have been shown between PD and head injury, exposure to pesticides, and potentially vagotomy. Metabolic abnormalities include diabetes and insulin resistance;, and an overall higher burden of comorbidities may be associated with an increased risk of PD (Pupillo et al., 2016; Xu et al., 2011).

## Morbidity Rates

The prevalence of PD ranges between 100 and 200 per 100,000 population in most studies from Western nations. Prevalence increases with increasing age, with rates for those older than aged 80 between 3% and 6%. In terms of age at onset, the onset of PD is uncommon before 60 years of age (Van Den Eeden et al., 2003). For example, a population-based study from the United Kingdom reported that 5.4% of PD cases had their onset at less than 50 years of age and 33% at less than age 65 (Wickremaratchi et al., 2009). The sex ratio for PD prevalence has been mixed, with some studies showing a higher proportion of males with the disease and some showing no significant sex difference. However, a recent population-based study conducted in Olmsted County, Minnesota, found that the age-standardized prevalence of PD among males was 2.5 times higher than in females and that the observed sex difference increased with age (Savica et al., 2018).

Recent prospective incidence studies have reported PD age-adjusted annual rates per 100,000 population as between 10 and 18 cases (Van Den Eeden et al., 2003; de Lau et al., 2006). Incidence rates are slightly higher for men than for women in many studies of Western countries, with a male-to-female rate of about 1.5.

The rates by sex for PD among Asian countries have been similar. As in the case of prevalence rates, incidence rates for PD rise exponentially with increasing age. Incidence rates have been relatively stable in studies that have tracked trends over several decades. In Olmsted County, Minnesota, the incidence of PD remained relatively stable between 1935 and 2005 (Rocca et al., 2001; Savica et al., 2013). For the most recent period, 1991–2005, incidence rates in men ranged between 27.0 per 100,000 person-years and for women 15.4 per 100,000 person-years (eFigs. 47.8 –47.10). Consistent with previous findings, there were no significant birth cohort effects in this population (Savica et al., 2013).

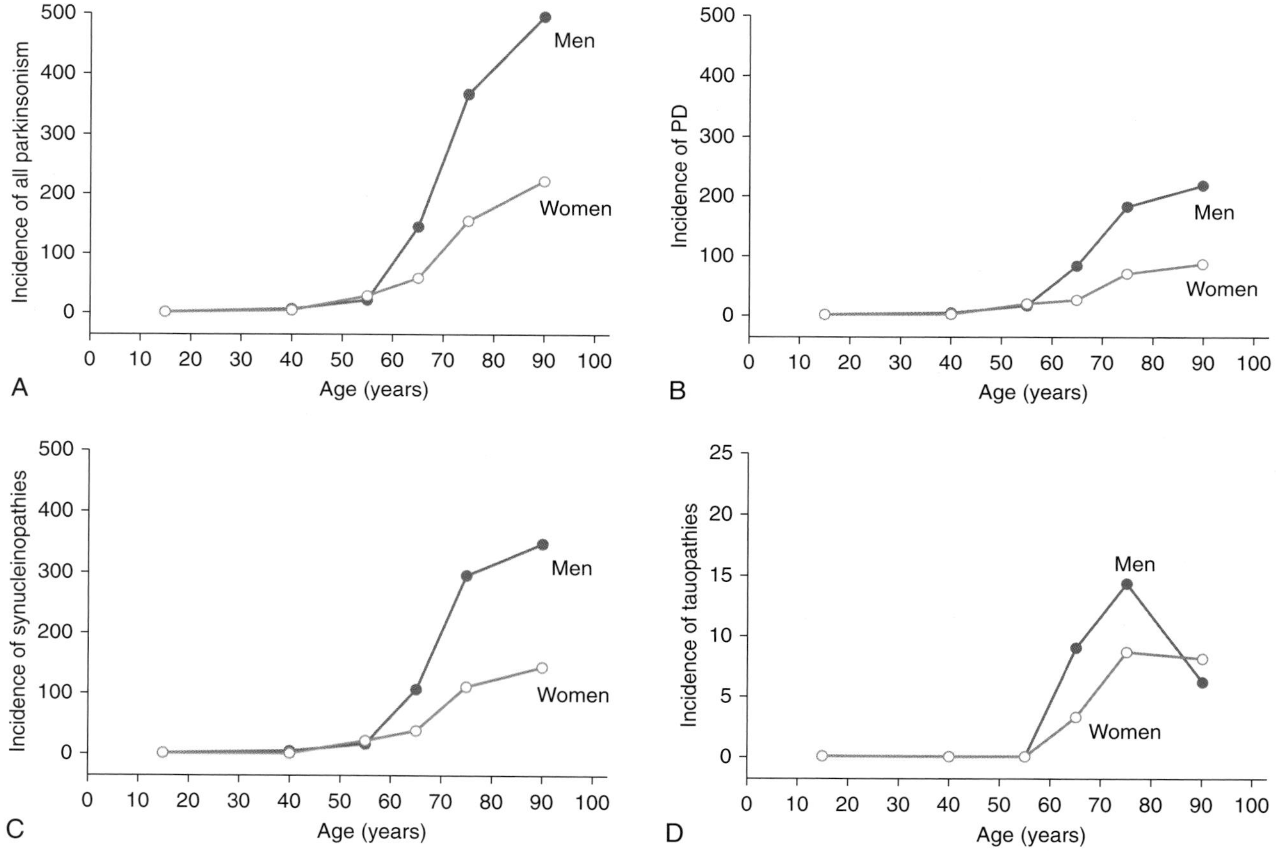

**Fig. 47.6** Age- and sex-specific incidence rates for synucleinopathies and tauopathies manifesting with parkinsonism. Incidence is calculated per 100 000 person-years. **A**, All parkinsonism. **B**, Parkinson disease *(PD)*. **C**, Synucleinopathies. **D**, Tauopathies. The scale for incidence was reduced for tauopathies (the y-axis values range from 0 to 25 per 100 000 person-years). *(From Savica R., Grossardt B.R., Bower J.H., et al., 2013. Incidence and pathology of synucleinopathies and tauopathies related to parkinsonism. JAMA Neurol. 70 [7], 859–66.)*

These results suggest that no major environmental risk agents were introduced into the population during the period of study.

### Mortality Rates

PD has generally been shown to increase mortality in a number of studies, with risk ratios for death between 0.8 and 3.5. Studies evaluating incident PD with long follow-up have produced the best data on mortality. In one population-based study in Sweden, the SMR for patients with PD was 1.58 and was also higher among women relative to men (2.09 vs. 1.33; Backstrom et al., 2018). In this population, estimated survival in idiopathic PD was 9.6 years, assuming an age of onset of 71.6 years. Recent studies with follow-up extending beyond 10 years have shown the relative risk for death due to PD to range between 1.4 and 2.5. Patients who developed PD in the Physicians Health Study had a 2.3 relative risk of dying after adjustment for age at onset and smoking (Driver et al., 2008). This study matched controls on comorbidities and found that PD patients were at increased risk for dying from stroke, psychiatric disease, and cardiac disease but were less likely to die from cancer. The risk of PD death was apparent across all categories of PD duration. The SMR in this study at 5 years after disease onset was 0.9; by 20–30 years after onset, it was 1.3. A similar study of male health professionals found that the risk of death due to PD increased with time from diagnosis and ranged from 1.1 during the first 5 years from diagnosis to 3.5 after 10 years. Another Spanish cohort study with a 20-year follow-up found that older age at onset and symptoms of akinesia and rigidity at onset were independent predictors of mortality (Duarte et al., 2013); another recent Swedish study found that in PD patients within 2 years of diagnosis, cognitive impairment early in the disease and cerebrospinal fluid (CSF) leukocytosis were predictors of reduced survival (Backstrom et al., 2018). Additionally, treatment with dopamine agonists had a protective effect on survival. Overall, PD independently increases the risk for death. It will be important to confirm modifiable risk factors for mortality in the preventive care of patients with PD.

## SELECTED INFECTIONS AND NEUROLOGICAL DISEASE

### Human Immunodeficiency Virus Infection

Infection with the human immunodeficiency virus (HIV; see Chapter 76) has become a global epidemic since the virus was first identified in 1981 as the cause of the acquired immunodeficiency syndrome (AIDS). The virus is a member of the retrovirus family and selectively infects T-helper cells ($T_H4$, $CD4^+$), causing a defect in cell-mediated immunity. It is spread through contact with blood and bodily fluids. After acute infection, most people enter an asymptomatic period of 8–10 years before the viral infection manifests clinically through immune dysregulation (Harrison and McArthur, 1995). Despite recent advances in treatment and prevention, the scope of the HIV epidemic remains daunting. In 2017, some 36.9 million people worldwide were living with HIV, and there were 1.8 million new HIV infections globally (UNAIDS, 2018). The infection killed 940,000 people in 2017 and has been the cause of death for greater than 25 million since the first AIDS cases were identified (UNAIDS, 2018). During the first 6 months of 1996, the first reported decline in AIDS mortality rates occurred in the United States (CDC, 1997). This decline occurred in all racial and ethnic groups and in all regions of the United States. Mortality rates have continued to decline in many HIV-infected cohorts after the introduction of highly active antiretroviral therapy (HAART) in 1996. Notably, a 51% reduction in AIDS-related deaths has occurred since the peak in 2004. For example, the 940,000 AIDS-related deaths occurring in 2017 are in contrast to the 1.4 million deaths in 2010 and 1.9 million deaths in 2004 (UNAIDS, 2018). Rates of new HIV infection continue to decline in many countries, and it is now clear that the HIV pandemic has passed its peak. A large portion of people living with HIV are located in low- and middle-income countries. In eastern and southern Africa, there were 19.6 million people living with HIV (53%); there were 6.1 million (16%) living in western and central Africa, 5.2 million (14%) in Asia and the Pacific, and 2.2 million (6%) living in Western and Central Europe and North America (UNAIDS, 2018). In the United States, the prevalence of HIV as well as the risk for new infections is highest among racial and ethnic minorities. Specifically, Blacks/African-Americans are more likely to be living with HIV and have a higher risk of new HIV infection relative to other races/ethnicities (CDC 2017, 2018). For example, in 2017, some 13% of the US population is estimated to be Black/African-American; however, 16,694 of the 38,739 (43%) new HIV diagnoses in the United States and dependent areas were among this subgroup. Collectively, despite the availability of effective HIV prevention tools and methods as well as large-scale efforts to increase HIV treatment in the past 5 years, new infections among adults remain a significant global burden. Continued surveillance, data sharing, and the targeting of control efforts will be required to reduce the burden of HIV/AIDS.

HIV disease can produce a variety of effects on both the CNS and the peripheral nervous system (PNS; Price, 1996). A useful way of classifying these complications is to use the temporal profile of HIV infection on the immune system. Box 47.1 illustrates a simplified classification scheme. Early neurological complications include acute aseptic meningitis, acute and chronic demyelinating polyneuropathy, and multiple mononeuropathy. These early complications are autoimmune in nature and occur at $CD4^+$ cell counts above 200/mm$^3$. Late complications typically appear when a severe depression in cellular immunity occurs, with $CD4^+$ cell counts below 200/mm$^3$. Most of these disorders are opportunistic infections (e.g., cryptococcal meningitis) or represent reactivation of a prior infection (e.g., toxoplasmosis and progressive multifocal leukoencephalopathy [PML]). In the late 1980s and early 1990s, we had also personally encountered notable frequencies of tuberculosis and neurosyphilis among AIDS patients; these excesses have since disappeared. In Sub-Saharan Africa, tuberculosis and malaria remain at excessively high frequencies among the HIV-infected. HIV dementia, distal sensory polyneuropathy, and vacuolar myopathy are directly related to the late stages of HIV infection itself. Other complications affecting the nervous system involve the metabolic and toxic effects of treatment, including zidovudine myopathy and nucleoside neuropathy. Six AIDS-indicator neurological illnesses are defined by the CDC: HIV dementia, CNS cryptococcal infection, cytomegalovirus (CMV) infection, primary CNS lymphoma, CNS toxoplasmosis,

**BOX 47.1 Neurological Complications of Human Immunodeficiency Virus Infection**

**Early Complications ($CD4^+$ Cell Count >200/mm$^3$)**

Acute aseptic meningitis
Demyelinating polyneuropathy (acute and chronic)
Mononeuritis

**Late Complications ($CD4^+$ Cell Count <200/mm$^3$)**

Cryptococcal meningitis
CMV encephalitis or polyradiculopathy
Cerebral toxoplasmosis
PML
Primary CNS lymphoma
HIV dementia
Sensory neuropathy
Vacuolar myelopathy

*CMV*, Cytomegalovirus; *CNS*, central nervous system; *HIV*, human immunodeficiency virus; *PML*, progressive multifocal leukoencephalopathy

and PML. The CDC records data on these illnesses primarily if they represent the initial AIDS diagnosis. Occurrence of these illnesses during the course of HIV infection must therefore be studied in other series. One such population is that of the HIV Outpatient Study, which is a prospective cohort study of 7155 patients in 10 US HIV clinics. Hospitalization rates for HIV-infected patients declined for the years 1994–2005, due predominantly to reductions in AIDS opportunistic infections including neurological illnesses (Buchacz et al., 2008).

In addition to the risk of serious AIDS-defining illnesses in the CNS, CNS-relevant comorbidity including both neurological and psychiatric comorbidities represents another noteworthy complication of HIV infection. For example, major depressive disorder (MDD) is extremely common in people with HIV (up to 40% of patients) and contributes substantially to excess HIV-associated morbidity and mortality (Cook et al., 2007; Nanni, et al., 2015; Orlando et al., 2002). In people with HIV, MDD is linked with mortality, poor antiretroviral adherence, missed clinical follow-up visits, and HIV progression (Belenky et al., 2014; Croxford et al., 2017; Lesko et al., 2017; Mills et al., 2018; O'Donnell et al., 2016; Pence et al., 2018; Todd et al., 2017). Although variable, estimates of the incidence of attempted and completed suicide are at least double in people with HIV relative to those without HIV (Thames et al., 2011). Although the most serious outcome associated with depression in people with HIV is the twofold increase in mortality, a potential increase in the risk of neurocognitive impairment (NCI) associated with depression may be an additional critical concern. Severe NCI is a driver of reductions in daily functioning in people with HIV and lower quality of life in this population (Doyle et al, 2012; Marquine et al., 2018; Thames et al., 2011). NCI serves as a reliable predictor of everyday functioning, including financial and medication management, driving, multitasking, and vocational functioning (Heaton et al., 2004; Scott et al., 2011; Waldrop-Valverde et al., 2010). Studies suggest that cognitive difficulties among people with HIV may remain despite persistent viral suppression. Furthermore, though not well-established, some studies have suggested that the rate of NCI accrual in people with HIV may be accelerated relative to people without HIV. For example, one longitudinal study of women living with HIV demonstrated modest decrements in neurocognitive performance relative to women without HIV (Rubin et al., 2019). When decrements were present, they were largest in the domain of verbal learning and memory.

## West Nile Virus Infection

The West Nile virus (WNV) is a mosquito-borne flavivirus that was initially isolated in 1937 from a symptomatic patient in Uganda (Tyler, 2014). The virus was rarely studied until 1999, when it first appeared in New York City as the cause of a naturally acquired meningitis and encephalitis. Over the next several years, a dramatic westward spread of WNV across the United States was recognized. Most human infections occur through the bite of an infected mosquito of the *Culex* genus during the summer months. Wild birds—particularly crows, sparrows, and jays—serve as the natural reservoir. Symptoms begin after an average incubation period of approximately 1 week. WNV is now the leading cause of arboviral encephalitis in the United States. The WNV strain predominant in the United States at present (NA/WN02) differs from the initial emergent isolate in 1999 (NY99).

A spectrum of clinical presentations may be seen with WNV infection, but approximately 80% of cases remain asymptomatic. Among symptomatic cases, West Nile fever is the most common illness. This has traditionally been characterized by fever, rash, and lymphadenopathy. Headache, fatigue, and gastrointestinal (GI) symptoms are also variably present. In a proportion of symptomatic cases, neurological illness develops, which may manifest as aseptic meningitis, encephalitis, or acute flaccid paralysis. Using arboviral surveillance data managed by the CDC, 2150 cases of WNV infection were reported from 45 states and the District of Columbia in 2016; the median age of infection was 57 years (interquartile range [IQR] = 44–68 years) and 1326 cases were male (Burakoff et al., 2018). Of the 2150 WNV infections, 1130 (61%) of cases were classified as being neuroinvasive, with 468 (36%) cases of aseptic meningitis, 689 (53%) cases reported as encephalitis, and 78 (6%) as acute flaccid paralysis. Overall, the incidence of neuroinvasive WNV infection–associated disease was 0.41 per 100,000 population, which is similar to the incidence observed from 2002 to 2015 in the United States. The case-fatality rate was also similar to that reported in the previous decade. Limited studies have evaluated long-term outcomes of WNV-associated neuroinvasive disease; one follow-up survey of New York City residents with WNV meningitis or encephalitis did find that only 37% had achieved a full recovery at 1 year (Klee et al., 2004). Deficits were found in physical, cognitive, and functional performance.

Evidence for WNV human disease continues to be detected in all geographic regions of the United States, with the highest rates in the West Central States; South Dakota (4.04 per 100,000 population), North Dakota (3.17), Nebraska (1.84), Wyoming (1.37), and Colorado (1.06) had the highest incidence rates in the United States in 2016. The two major risk factors for neuroinvasive disease are increasing age and immunosuppression; WNV infection is also slightly more common in men than in women (61% vs. 39% in 2016). Therapy for WNV infection is primarily supportive because no treatment has been found to be effective in altering morbidity or mortality rates. Preventive efforts constitute the major focus of controlling this illness. These involve environmental control of mosquito breeding areas, using insect repellents and wearing protective clothing, and screening the blood supply. Horses remain the major animal vector for WNV, and an effective vaccine for horses has been in use for several years. Vaccine trials for human WNV are under way, and a safe and effective vaccine for humans is expected to be developed soon. In view of the high recurrence rates from 1999 to 2004, the transmission of WNV will continue to be an issue for many years to come.

## Neurocysticercosis

Neurocysticercosis (NCC) is caused by an infection of the human CNS by the larval stage of the pork tapeworm *Taenia solium* (Garcia and Del Brutto, 2005). Currently the most common parasitic disease of the human CNS, NCC has become a major public health problem for most of the developing world as well as for industrialized countries with high immigration rates of people from endemic countries in Latin America, Asia, and Africa. It is the most common cause of symptomatic epilepsy worldwide. Current estimates of the number of individuals with epilepsy due to NCC are 0.45–1.35 million in Latin America, 1 million in India, and 0.31–4.6 million in Africa (Coyle et al., 2012).

NCC has become an increasingly important emerging infection in the United States. The number of cases of imported NCC is higher in the United States than in all other developed countries combined; one study estimates that between 1320 and 5050 new cases of NCC occur every year in the United States (Serpa et al., 2012). There was an estimated 33,060 cysticercosis-related hospitalizations in theUnited States from 1998 to 2011, representing a hospitalization rate of 8.03 per 1 million population (O'Keefe et al., 2015). These numbers have been driven largely by the influx of immigrants from endemic regions into the United States and the ease of international travel; at the same time, widespread access to neuroimaging has permitted easier diagnosis. Among large case series (i.e., $N > 20$), a total of 1494 patients with NCC were reported in the United States between 1980 and 2004 (Wallin and Kurtzke, 2004). In 2012, estimates of reported cases of NCC had reached 4632. Although accurate incidence data regarding NCC in the United States are not readily available, previous reports have estimated the incidence to range from 0.20 to 0.60 cases per 100,000 population; incidence among individuals of Hispanic ethnicity are generally higher, at 1.5–5.8 cases per 100,000 (Serpa et al., 2012). eTable 47.1 lists the 13 largest case 

series that were published on NCC within the United States from 1980 to 2012. Collectively, these reports are largely concentrated in the southwestern United States, but they include NCC cases from every region of the country. In the case series, a slight male bias was observed, and the average age ranged between 24 and 44 years. Prior to 2004, common onset symptoms for NCC patients within the United States included seizures (66%), hydrocephalus (16%), and headaches (15%). A majority of these patients presented (presented) with parenchymal disease (91%); whereas ventricular cysts, subarachnoid cysts, and spinal cysts were the presenting manifestations in the remaining patients. In contrast, the case series from New Mexico (Figueroa et al., 2011) found that 30% were extraparenchymal; the series from Houston found that 54% had parenchymal disease, while 20% had intraventricular disease, 12% had subarachnoid disease, and 12% had calcifications only (Serpa et al., 2011).

Treatment with antiparasitic drugs has been shown to be beneficial in the early stages of parenchymal NCC. Seizures are typically controlled with standard anticonvulsants. However, therapy directed at the parasite varies according to the stage, location, and number of parasites within the CNS. An increasing number of NCC cases have been reported in the US literature over the past 50 years. NCC is reportable in Arizona, California, New Mexico, Oregon, Texas, and Alaska. A national reporting network would be helpful in the control and eventual eradication of this disease. Because neurologists in the United States are often involved in the diagnosis and management of NCC, they must become familiar with this disorder.

## OVERVIEW OF THE FREQUENCY OF NEUROLOGICAL DISORDERS

What follows are the best estimates of the numerical impact of neurological diseases. The data refer primarily to White people in Western countries. Some modifications of the cited references have been made, but the authors have not found reasons to change most of these figures. For the 66 disorders listed in Tables. 47.2 and 47.3, the average annual incidence rates add up to greater than 2500 per 100,000 population, or

**TABLE 47.2 Most Common Neurological Disorders: Incidence**

| Disorder | Rate |
|---|---|
| Herpes zoster | 400 |
| Migraine | 250 |
| Brain trauma | 200 |
| Other severe headache | 200* |
| Acute cerebrovascular disease | 150 |
| Head injury without brain trauma | 150* |
| Transient postconcussive syndrome | 150 |
| Lumbosacral herniated nucleus pulposus | 150 |
| Lumbosacral pain syndrome | 150* |
| Neurological symptoms (with no defined disease) | 75 |
| Epilepsy | 50 |
| Febrile seizures | 50 |
| Dementia | 50 |
| Meniere disease | 50 |
| Transient ischemic attacks | 40 |
| Mononeuropathies | 40 |
| Polyneuropathy | 50 |
| Bell palsy | 25 |
| Single seizures | 20 |
| Parkinsonism | 20 |
| Cervical pain syndrome | 20* |
| Persistent postconcussive syndrome | 20 |
| Alcoholism | 20* |
| Meningitides | 15 |
| Encephalitides | 15 |
| Sleep disorders† | 15 |
| Subarachnoid hemorrhage | 15 |
| Cervical herniated nucleus pulposus | 15 |
| Peripheral nerve trauma | 15 |
| Blindness | 15 |
| Metastatic brain tumor | 10 |
| Benign brain tumor | 10 |
| Deafness | 10 |

Approximate average annual incidence rates per 100,000 population, all ages.
*Cited rates are 10% of actual rates, as proportions of patients likely to need care by a physician competent in neurology.
†Narcolepsies and hypersomnias (with sleep apnea).
*Modified from Kurtzke, J.F., 1982. The current neurologic burden of illness and injury in the United States. Neurology 32, 1207–1214.*

**TABLE 47.3 Less Common Neurological Disorders: Incidence**

| Disorder | Rate* |
|---|---|
| Cerebral palsy | 9.0 |
| Congenital malformations of central nervous system | 7.0 |
| Malignant primary brain tumor | 7.0 |
| Mental retardation, severe | 6.0 |
| Mental retardation, other | 6.0† |
| Metastatic cord tumor | 5.0 |
| Tic douloureux | 4.0 |
| Multiple sclerosis | 3.0‡ |
| Optic neuritis | 3.0† |
| Dorsolateral sclerosis | 3.0 |
| Functional psychosis | 3.0† |
| Spinal cord injury | 3.0 |
| Motor neuron disease | 2.0 |
| Down syndrome | 2.0 |
| Guillain-Barré syndrome | 2.0 |
| Intracranial abscess | 1.0 |
| Benign cord tumor | 1.0 |
| Cranial nerve trauma | 1.0 |
| Acute transverse myelopathy | 0.8 |
| All muscular dystrophies | 0.7 |
| Chronic progressive myelopathy | 0.5 |
| Polymyositis | 0.5 |
| Syringomyelia | 0.4 |
| Hereditary ataxias | 0.4 |
| Huntington disease | 0.4 |
| Myasthenia gravis | 0.4 |
| Acute disseminated encephalomyelitis | 0.2 |
| Charcot-Marie-Tooth disease | 0.2 |
| Spinal muscular atrophy | 0.2 |
| Familial spastic paraplegia | 0.1 |
| Wilson disease | 0.1 |
| Malignant primary cord tumor | 0.1 |
| Vascular disease of cord | 0.1 |

*Approximate average annual incidence rates per 100,000 population, all ages.
†Cited rates are 10% of actual rates, as proportions of patients likely to need care by a physician competent in neurology.
‡Rate for high-risk areas.
*Modified from Kurtzke, J.F., 1982. The current neurologic burden of illness and injury in the United States. Neurology 32, 1207–1214; and from Kurtzke, J.F., Kurland, L.T., 1983. The epidemiology of neurologic disease, in: Baker A.B., Baker, L.H. (Eds.), Clinical Neurology, vol. 4. Harper & Row, Philadelphia.*

**TABLE 47.4 Most Common Neurological Disorders: Prevalence**

| Disorder | Rate |
|---|---|
| Migraine | 2000* |
| Other severe headache | 1500† |
| Brain trauma | 800 |
| Epilepsy | 650 |
| Acute cerebrovascular disease | 600 |
| Lumbosacral pain syndrome | 500† |
| Alcoholism | 500† |
| Sleep disorders‡ | 300 |
| Meniere disease | 300 |
| Lumbosacral herniated nucleus pulposus | 300 |
| Cerebral palsy | 250 |
| Dementia | 250 |
| Parkinsonism | 200 |
| Transient ischemic attacks | 150 |
| Febrile seizures | 100 |
| Persistent postconcussive syndrome | 80 |
| Herpes zoster | 80 |
| Congenital malformations of central nervous system | 70 |
| Single seizures | 60 |
| Multiple sclerosis | 60§ |
| Benign brain tumor | 60 |
| Cervical pain syndrome | 60† |
| Down syndrome | 50 |
| Subarachnoid hemorrhage | 50 |
| Cervical herniated nucleus pulposus | 50 |
| Transient postconcussive syndrome | 50 |
| Spinal cord injury | 50 |

Approximate point prevalence rates per 100,000 population, all ages.
*Cited rate is 20% of actual prevalence rate, as a proportion of patients likely to need care by a physician competent in neurology.
†Cited rates are 10% of actual rates, as proportions of patients likely to need care by a physician competent in neurology.
‡Narcolepsies and hypersomnias (with sleep apnea).
§Rate for high-risk areas.
*Modified from Kurtzke, J.F., 1982. The current neurologic burden of illness and injury in the United States. Neurology 32, 1207–1214.*

**TABLE 47.5 Less Common Neurological Disorders: Prevalence**

| Disorder | Rate |
|---|---|
| Tic douloureux | 40 |
| Neurological symptoms without defined disease | 40 |
| Mononeuropathies | 40 |
| Polyneuropathies | 40 |
| Dorsolateral sclerosis | 30 |
| Peripheral nerve trauma | 30 |
| Other head injury | 30* |
| Acute transverse myelopathy | 15 |
| Metastatic brain tumor | 15 |
| Chronic progressive myelopathy | 10 |
| Benign cord tumor | 10 |
| Optic neuritis | 10 |
| Encephalitides | 10 |
| Vascular disease of spinal cord | 9 |
| Hereditary ataxias | 8 |
| Syringomyelia | 7 |
| Motor neuron disease | 6 |
| Polymyositis | 6 |
| Progressive muscular dystrophy | 6 |
| Malignant primary brain tumor | 5 |
| Metastatic cord tumor | 5 |
| Meningitides | 5 |
| Bell palsy | 5 |
| Huntington disease | 5 |
| Charcot-Marie-Tooth disease | 5 |
| Myasthenia gravis | 4 |
| Familial spastic paraplegia | 3 |
| Intracranial abscess | 2 |
| Cranial nerve trauma | 2 |
| Myotonic dystrophy | 2 |
| Spinal muscular atrophy | 2 |
| Guillain-Barré syndrome | 1 |
| Wilson disease | 1 |
| Acute disseminated encephalomyelitis | 0.6 |
| Dystonia musculorum deformans | 0.3 |
| Primary malignant cord tumor | 0.1 |

Approximate point prevalence rates per 100,000 population, all ages.
*Cited rate is 10% of actual rate, as a proportion of patients likely to need care by a physician competent in neurology.
*Modified from Kurtzke, J.F., 1982. The current neurologic burden of illness and injury in the United States. Neurology 32, 1207–1214; and from Kurtzke, J.F., Kurland, L.T., 1983. The epidemiology of neurologic disease. In: Baker A.B., Baker, L.H. (Eds.), Clinical Neurology, vol. 4. Harper & Row, Philadelphia.*

2.5%. Included in these tables are eight disorders for which only one-tenth of the incident cases were thought to require neurological attention: the two vertebrogenic pain syndromes, nonmigrainous headache, head injury without brain trauma, alcoholism, psychosis, mental retardation, and deafness. Total blindness numbers were taken as an estimate for the proportion of all visually impaired patients the neurologist might encounter. Even if all headaches, trauma, vertebrogenic pain, vision loss, deafness, and psychosis are excluded from consideration, it is estimated that more than 1100 new cases of neurological disease will appear each year in every 100,000 members of the population, or more than 1 case for every 100 people (Tables 47.4 and 47.5).

Neurological practice, of course, varies widely among countries and even within the United States. The concept of the neurologist as a physician who is directly responsible for both acute and chronic care of patients with neurological diseases has evolved only over the past three decades in the United States. But such responsibilities, as well as provisions for continuity of care, are explicit statements in the current special requirements for residency training programs in neurology and child neurology. Regardless of the type of practice a given country deems appropriate for neurologists, patients with neurological disease will continue to require care. The data in Tables 47.2 through 47.5 could therefore well serve as at least a basis for the rational allocation of available resources for teaching, research, and care of patients with neurological disorders in any country.

*The complete reference list is available online at https://expertconsult.inkling.com/.*

# 48

# Clinical Neurogenetics

*Brent L. Fogel, Daniel H. Geschwind*

## OUTLINE



## GENETICS IN CLINICAL NEUROLOGY

Since the discovery of the structure of deoxyribonucleic acid (DNA) and the elucidation of the genetic mechanisms of heredity, clinical neurology has benefited from advances in genetics and neuroscience. This clinically relevant basic research has permitted dissection of the cellular machinery supporting the function of the brain and its connections while establishing causal relationships between such dysfunction, human genetic variation, and various neurological diseases. In the modern practice of neurology, the use of genetics has become widespread, and neurologists are confronted daily with data from an ever-increasing catalog of genetic studies relating to conditions such as developmental disorders, dementia, ataxia, neuropathy, and epilepsy, to name but a few. The use of genetic information in the clinical evaluation of neurological disease has expanded dramatically over the past decade. More efficient techniques for discovering disease genes have led to a greater availability of genetic testing in the clinic. Approximately one-third of pediatric neurology hospital admissions are related to a genetic diagnosis, and with the widespread use of next-generation sequencing technology, essentially every gene is now available for testing by the practicing neurologist (Rexach et al., 2019). In conjunction with the precision health movement, this increase in availability of information across the genome is leading to new avenues of diagnostic testing, extending beyond the consideration of only rare neurological disease toward more common disorders. Neurogenetics now touches every aspect of neurology, and while the clinical focus still remains primarily on disease-causing mutations, we can begin to anticipate what the future may hold for a broader appreciation of the role of genetics in all neurological disorders.

As neuroscience and genetic research have progressed, we have been led to a deeper understanding of the sources and nature of human genetic variation and its relationship to clinical phenotypes. In the past there has been a tendency to consider genetic traits as either present or absent, and correspondingly, patients were either healthy or diseased; this is the traditional view of Mendelian, or single-gene, conditions. Although certain relatively rare neurological diseases—Friedreich ataxia or Huntington disease (HD), for example—can be traced to a single causal gene, the common forms of other diseases such as Alzheimer dementia (AD), stroke, epilepsy, or autism usually arise from an interplay of multiple genes, each of which increases disease susceptibility and likely interacts with environmental factors. Subsequently, the realm of the "sporadic" and the "idiopathic" has been challenged by the identification of genetic susceptibility factors, which has sparked a flurry of investigation into a variety of genes and genetic markers that confer a risk of illness yet are not wholly causative. Disease status may lie on the end of a continuum of individual variation and thus can be considered a quantitative rather than purely qualitative trait (Plomin et al., 2009). So, rather than using what might be considered an arbitrary cutoff point, such as a specific number of senile plaques or neuritic tangles that define affected or unaffected patients, one might instead think in terms of a continuum of pathology that relates to different levels of burden or susceptibility.

As we continue to discover more genes involved either directly or indirectly in neurological disease pathogenesis, the amount of information available to the clinician grows, as do the challenges in interpreting this in a meaningful way for an individual patient. Much of this information, particularly with respect to genetic risk, is not a matter of a positive or negative result, but instead is a feature to be incorporated into the clinical framework supporting an overall diagnosis. While modern neurologists need not also be geneticists, it is essential that they possess a firm understanding of the basics of human genetics in order to be fully prepared to confront the litany of diagnostic information available today. This is becoming more true as the use of clinical exome and genome sequencing becomes increasingly widespread. In this chapter we will discuss these essential basics and present examples of how genetic information has informed our understanding of disease definition and etiology, show how it is utilized in the practice of neurology today, and how it will be used even more extensively in the future. Given the massive acceleration in technology, from microarrays to the methods enabling complete and efficient human genome sequencing, this future is close at hand and the era of genomic medicine is well underway.

## GENE EXPRESSION, DIVERSITY, AND REGULATION

The basic principles of molecular genetics are outlined in Fig. 48.1 and Table 48.1, and more detailed descriptions can be found elsewhere (Alberts et al., 2015; Griffiths et al., 2002; Lodish et al., 2016; Strachan and Read, 2019). To briefly summarize, DNA, found in the nucleus of all cells, comprises the raw material from which heritable information is transferred among individuals, with the simplest heritable unit being the gene. DNA is composed of a series of individual nucleotides, all of which contain an identical pentose (2′-deoxyribose)-phosphate backbone but differ at an attached base that can be adenine (A), guanine (G), thymine (T), or cytosine (C). A and G are purine bases and pair with the pyrimidine bases T and C, respectively, to form a double-stranded helical structure which allows for semiconservative bidirectional replication, the means by which DNA is copied in a precise and efficient manner. In total, there are approximately 3.2 billion base pairs in human DNA. By convention, a DNA sequence is described by listing the bases as they are expressed from the 5′ to 3′ direction along the pentose backbone (e.g., 5′-ATGCAT-3′), as this is the order in which it is typically used by the cellular machinery, also called the *sense strand* (compare with RNA, later). The opposite paired, or *antisense*, strand is arranged antiparallel (3′–5′) and can also be referred to when discussing sequence; however, by convention this is generally not done unless that strand is also transcribed into RNA.

The expression of a gene is tightly and coordinately regulated (see Fig. 48.1), an important consideration for understanding the molecular mechanisms of disease. The typical gene contains one or more *promoters*: DNA sequences that allow for the binding of a cellular protein complex that includes RNA polymerase and other factors that faithfully copy the DNA in the 5′–3′ direction in a process known as *transcription*. The resulting single-stranded molecule contains a ribose sugar unit in its backbone and thus the resulting molecule is termed *ribonucleic acid*, or RNA. RNA also differs from the template DNA by the incorporation of uracil (U) in place of thymine (T), as it also pairs efficiently with adenine, and thymine serves a secondary role in DNA repair that is not necessary in RNA. The sequence of the RNA matches the sense DNA strand and is therefore complementary to (and hence derived from) the antisense strand.

Transcribed coding RNA must be processed to become protein-encoding *messenger RNA* (mRNA), a term used to differentiate these RNAs from all other types of RNA in the cell. To become mature, RNA is stabilized by modification at the ends with a 7-methylguanosine 5′ cap and a long poly-A 3′ tail. A further critical stage in the maturation of the RNA molecule involves a rearrangement process termed *RNA splicing* (Fig. 48.2). This is necessary because the expressed coding sequences in DNA, called *exons*, of virtually every gene are discontinuous and interspersed with long stretches of generally nonconserved intervening sequences referred to as *introns*. This, along with other mechanisms, likely plays an evolutionary role in the development of new genes by allowing for the shuffling of functional sequences (Babushok et al., 2007). Nascent RNA molecules are recognized by the *spliceosome*, a protein complex that removes the introns and rejoins the exons. Not every exon is utilized at all times in every RNA derived from a single gene. Exons may be skipped or included in a regulated manner through alternative splicing, which occurs in nearly 95% of all genes to create different isoforms of that mRNA. This is especially prominent in the nervous system, where alternative splicing is not only prevalent but also highly conserved (Raj and Blencowe, 2015), reflecting critical aspects of normal neuronal function and links to human disease. The dynamic nature of this observation is critical to a complete understanding of cellular gene expression. DNA is essentially a storage molecule, and with few exceptions in the absence of mutagens, its sequence remains static and, aside from epigenetic events, is therefore limited to a genetic regulatory role as a transcriptional rheostat. Current estimates place the number of individual human protein-coding genes at roughly 21,000 (Salzberg, 2018), so it is difficult to reconcile biological and clinical diversity with simple variations in expression. Alternative splicing provides a means of dramatically elevating this diversity by enabling a single gene to encode multiple proteins with a wide array of functions. Supporting this, early analysis of RNA complexity in human tissues suggested that there were at least seven alternative splicing events per multi-exon gene, generating over 100,000 alternative splicing events (Pan et al., 2008), with more recent estimates raising that number to over 300,000 across the genome (Salzberg, 2018). Because alternative splicing and other forms of RNA processing can be subject to complex layers of temporal and spatial regulation, particularly in the human brain (Licatalosi and Darnell, 2010; Raj and Blencowe, 2015; Ward and Cooper, 2010), it is a robust source for both biological diversity and disease-causing mutations (see Polymorphisms and Point Mutations).

### DNA to RNA to Protein

The central dogma of genetics has been that DNA is transcribed into RNA that is then translated into protein—the "business" end of the process. So, following its transcription from DNA in the nucleus, mRNA is transported out of the nucleus to the cytoplasm, and possibly to a specific subcellular location depending on the mRNA, where it can be deciphered by the cell. This takes place via interaction with a complex known as the *ribosome*, which binds the mRNA and converts its genetic information into protein via the process of *translation*. The ribosome initiates translation at a pre-encoded start site and converts the mRNA sequence into protein until a designated termination site is reached. Sequence information is read in three-nucleotide groups called *codons*, each of which specifies an individual amino acid. With the four distinct bases, there are mathematically 64 possible codons,

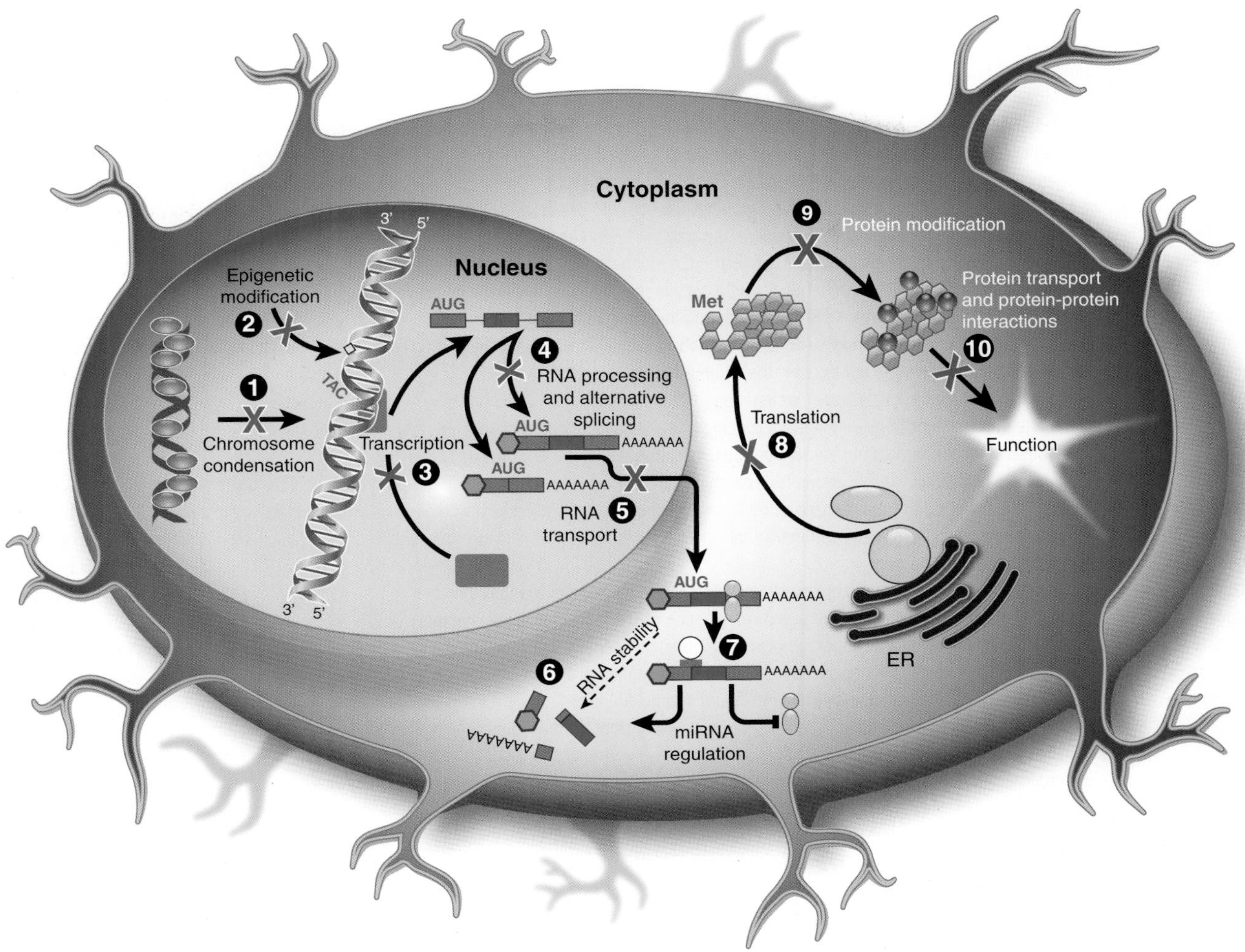


**Fig. 48.1 Neuronal Gene Expression and Regulation.** A generic human neuron is depicted. **(1)** Deoxyribonucleic acid (DNA) bound to histones forms transcriptionally inactive chromatin, which can be relieved through the action of various proteins and enzymes. **(2)** Epigenetic modifications *(yellow)* are heritable changes to the DNA or its associated histones that alter gene expression without changing the DNA sequence and can result from various environmental stimuli or perturbations. **(3)** Active DNA is bound by *RNA* polymerase in a process regulated by protein factors, and the genetic information contained within the DNA is converted to RNA via the process of transcription. An example of a three-nucleotide codon *(red)* is shown on the antisense DNA strand being converted to its complement on the sense strand of the RNA. **(4)** Nascent RNA undergoes processing to become messenger RNA (mRNA) with the addition of a 5′ cap structure *(green)* and a poly-A tail, as well as undergoing RNA splicing which removes noncoding sequences and can generate transcript diversity through the use of alternative exons (see text). **(5)** Mature mRNA is exported from the nucleus to the cytoplasm and/or to a specific subcellular location. **(6)** Over time, mRNA is subject to degradation within the cell, and its inherent stability can be dynamic, changing in relation to the state of the cell. **(7)** Short noncoding RNAs, called *micro-RNAs* (miRNAs) *(purple)*, can target cellular protein complexes *(white)* to specific mRNAs and regulate their activity by promoting degradation or blocking translation (see text). **(8)** The mRNA is bound by ribosomes (either free or associated with the endoplasmic reticulum *[ER]*) and undergoes translation into protein. The three-nucleotide codon *(red)* directs the incorporation of a single amino acid into the newly synthesized protein (in this example methionine, met). **(9)** The protein undergoes post-translational chemical modifications *(purple)* to generate a functional protein for use by the cell. **(10)** Mature protein interacts with other proteins and/or is transported to its site of activity within the cell. All direct steps in this pathway are potential sites for disease-modifying therapies *(red X's)*, depending on the gene in question.

but these have an element of redundancy and code for only 20 different amino acids and 3 termination signals (UAG, UGA, and UAA), also called *stop codons*. The *start codon* is ATG and codes for methionine. These amino acids are joined by the ribosome to synthesize a protein. This protein, which may undergo further modification, will ultimately carry out a programmed biological function in the cell. Regulation of this process is highly coordinated and important in learning, for example, where activity-dependent translation at the synapse underlies some aspects of synaptic plasticity, which may go awry in certain disorders such as fragile X syndrome and autism (Morrow et al., 2008). In other cases, such as repeat-associated non-ATG (RAN) translation, specific mutations causing disruption of this fundamental process can be an important mechanism underlying neurological disease (Zu et al., 2018; see Repeat Expansion Disorders).

| TABLE 48.1 | Glossary of Genetic Terminology |
|---|---|
| Allele | Alternate forms of a locus (gene) |
| Anticipation | Earlier onset and/or worsening severity of disease in successive generations |
| Antisense | Nucleic acid sequence complementary to mRNA |
| Chromosome | Organizational unit of the genome consisting of a linear arrangement of genes |
| *Cis*-acting | A regulatory nucleotide sequence present on the molecule being regulated |
| Codon | A three-nucleotide sequence representing a single amino acid |
| Complex disease | Disease exhibiting non-Mendelian inheritance involving the interaction of multiple genes and the environment |
| De novo | A mutation newly arising in an individual and not present in either parent |
| Diploid | A genome having paired genetic information; half-normal number is haploid |
| DNA | Deoxyribonucleic acid; used for storage, replication, and inheritance of genetic information |
| Dominant | Allele that determines phenotype when a single copy is present in an individual |
| Endophenotype | Subset of phenotypic characteristics used to group patients manifesting a given trait |
| Epigenetic | Relating to heritable changes in gene expression resulting from DNA, histone, or other modifications that do not involve changes in DNA sequence |
| Exome | Portion of the genome representing only the coding regions of genes |
| Exon | Segment of DNA that is expressed in at least one mature mRNA |
| Expressivity | The range of phenotypes observed with a specific disease-associated genotype |
| Frameshift | DNA mutation that adds or removes nucleotides, affecting which are grouped as codons |
| Gene | Contiguous DNA sequence that codes for a given mRNA and its splice variants |
| Gene therapy | A technique designed to treat disease through the modification or replacement of a gene or its product(s). |
| Genome | A complete set of DNA from a given individual |
| Genotype | The DNA sequence of a gene |
| Haplotype | A group of alleles on the same chromosome close enough to be inherited together |
| Hemizygous | Genes having only a single allele in an individual, such as the X chromosome in males |
| Heteroplasmy | A mixture of multiple mitochondrial genomes in a given individual |
| Heterozygous | Genes having two distinct alleles in an individual at a given locus |
| Homozygous | Genes having two identical alleles in an individual at a given locus |
| Intron | Segment of DNA between exons that is transcribed into RNA but removed by splicing |
| Kilobase | 1000 bases or base-pairs |
| Linkage disequilibrium | The co-occurrence of two alleles more frequently than expected by random chance, suggesting they are in close proximity to one another |
| Locus | Location of a DNA sequence (or a gene) on a chromosome or within the genome |
| Lyonization | The process of random inactivation of one of the pair of X chromosomes in females |
| Marker | Sequence of DNA used to identify a gene or a locus |
| Megabase | 1,000,000 bases or base-pairs |
| Meiosis | Process of cellular division that produces gametes containing a haploid amount of DNA |
| Mendelian | Obeying standard single-gene patterns of inheritance (e.g., recessive or dominant) |
| Microarray | A glass or plastic support (e.g., slide or chip) to which large numbers of DNA molecules can be attached for use in high-throughput genetic analysis |
| Missense | DNA mutation that changes a given codon to represent a different amino acid |
| Mitosis | Process of cellular division during which DNA is replicated |
| Nonsense | DNA mutation that changes a given codon into a translation termination signal |
| Penetrance | The likelihood of a disease-associated genotype to express a specific disease phenotype |
| Phenotype | The clinical manifestations of a given genotype |
| Polygenic risk score | A number derived based on variation observed across multiple genetic loci weighted to enhance prediction of complex disease |
| Polymorphism | Sequence variation among individuals, typically not considered to be pathogenic |
| Precision health | A medical model promoting health care through the utilization of genomic, clinical, environmental, lifestyle, and other personal data to develop treatment and/or risk prevention strategies unique to the individual patient |
| Probe | DNA sequence used for identifying a specific gene or allele |
| Promoter | DNA sequences that regulate transcription of a given gene |
| Protein | Functional cellular macromolecules encoded by a gene |
| Recessive | Allele that determines phenotype only when two copies are present in an individual |
| Relative risk | The ratio of the chance of disease in individuals with a specific genetic susceptibility factor over the chance of disease in those without it |
| Resequencing | A method of identifying clinically relevant genetic variation in a candidate gene of interest by comparing the sequence in individuals with disease to a reference sequence |
| RNA | Ribonucleic acid; expressed form of a gene, called *messenger* or *mRNA* if protein coding |
| Sense | Nucleic acid sequence corresponding to mRNA |
| Silent | DNA mutation that changes a given codon but does not alter the corresponding amino acid |
| SNP | Single nucleotide polymorphism |
| Splicing | RNA processing mechanism where introns are removed and exons joined to create mRNA; in alternative splicing, exons are utilized in a regulated manner within a cell or tissue |
| *Trans*-acting | A regulatory protein that acts on a molecule other than that which expressed it |
| Transcription | Cellular process where DNA sequence is used as template for RNA synthesis |
| Transcriptome | The complete set of RNA transcripts produced by a cell, tissue, or individual |
| Translation | Cellular process where mRNA sequence is converted to protein |

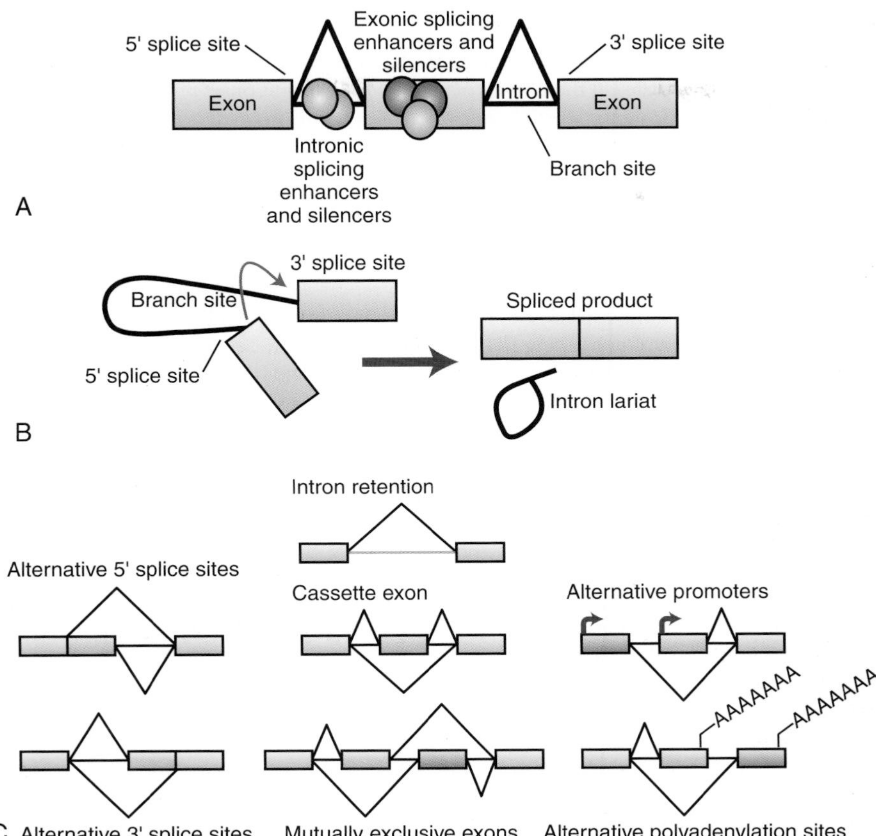


**Fig. 48.2** RNA Splicing. **A,** A generic precursor RNA is shown, consisting of three exons *(blue)* with intervening introns *(dark lines)*. Representative sequences recognized by the protein complexes that mediate splicing are shown (5′ and 3′ splice sites and the branch site). Binding of these complexes may be influenced either positively or negatively by regulatory sequences and their associated proteins *(circles)* located in either the introns or exons. Splicing pattern is shown by angled lines spanning introns. **B,** Splicing occurs via the complex-mediated association of the 5′ splice site and the branch site, with subsequent attack of the 3′ splice site by the upstream exon *(arrow)*, which joins it to the downstream exon and releases the intron. **C,** Possible alternative splicing patterns for various messenger RNAs are shown. Constitutive exons are in *blue*. Alternatively utilized exons are shown in *orange or purple*. A retained intron is shown by an *orange line*.

Over the past decade, the discovery of several classes of functional non-protein-coding RNAs has added additional complexity to our understanding of how the genetic code is manifest at the level of cellular function. Of these, microRNAs (miRNAs) are increasingly being recognized as vital players in gene regulation and neurological disease (Weinberg and Wood, 2009). Nascent miRNA molecules are processed to form short (approximately 22-nucleotide) RNA duplexes that target endogenous cellular machinery to specific coding RNAs and induce post-transcriptional gene silencing through a diverse repertoire including RNA cleavage, translational blocking, transport to inactive cell sites, or promotion of RNA decay (Filipowicz et al., 2008; Weinberg and Wood, 2009). Depending on the cell and the context, miRNA activity can result in specific gene inactivation, functional repression, or more subtle regulatory effects, and may involve multiple RNAs in a given biological pathway (Flynt and Lai, 2008). Estimates suggest that miRNAs may regulate 30% of protein-coding genes, implicating these molecules as important targets for future research into the biology of neurological disease (Filipowicz et al., 2008; Weinberg and Wood, 2009).

For a specific disease-related gene, the DNA sequence present within an individual is referred to as their *genotype*, and the expression of that code often results in a feature (or features) that can be observed or measured, known as the *phenotype*. Genes are further organized into higher-order structures termed *chromosomes*, which together compose the entire set of DNA, or *genome*, of the individual. The human genome is diploid, meaning we possess 23 pairs of chromosomes, 22 autosomes, and 1 sex chromosome. Consequently, normal individuals possess two copies (or alleles) of every autosomal gene, one from the mother and one from the father. Because there are two distinct sex chromosomes, X and Y, genes on these chromosomes are expressed in a slightly different manner, discussed in more detail later for the sex-linked disorders.

It is important to emphasize that most genes are not simply "on" or "off." In reality, cells maintain strict regulatory control over their genes. Some genes, such as those required for cell structure or maintenance, must be expressed constitutively, but genes with specific precise functions may only be needed in certain cells at certain times under certain conditions. Potential levels of regulation are depicted in Fig. 48.1 and include virtually every stage of gene expression. Initially, genes can be regulated at the level of transcription, ranging from the regulated binding of histone proteins, which leads to chromosome condensation, inactivating genes, to the coordinated activity of protein factors that activate or repress gene transcription in response to cell state, environmental conditions, or other factors. Once expressed, the RNA is subject to processing regulation, particularly through alternative splicing, as already discussed. Transport of the mRNA and its translation provide additional steps for cellular regulation. Last, the final protein can be subject to control via post-translational modifications or interactions with other proteins. To operate, all these levels of regulation require *trans-acting* factors, such as proteins, which stimulate or repress a particular step, as well as *cis-acting* elements, sequences recognized and bound by the regulatory factors.

*Epigenetics*, or the study of heritable changes in gene expression that do not involve changes in the DNA sequence itself, is emerging as an important aspect of both gene regulation and neurological disease (Qureshi and Mehler, 2013). These changes can involve several mechanisms including methylation of the DNA, modification of histone proteins, chromatin remodeling, expression of noncoding RNAs, and RNA editing, all of which may occur in response to a variety of intracellular or environmental signals (Qureshi and Mehler, 2013). Disruption of epigenetic mechanisms can cause Mendelian neurological disease (see Imprinting), as can impairment of the function of factors that mediate these epigenetic mechanisms (Qureshi and Mehler, 2013). Epigenetics may also play a role in sporadic disease, as a recent study reported the H1 haplotype of the *MAPT* gene to be differentially methylated in a dose-dependent manner in patients with progressive supranuclear palsy (Li et al., 2014), suggesting an epigenetic mechanism for the disease risk associated with the presence of that haplotype. Further studies investigating the role of these pathways genome-wide in clinical populations will likely uncover more associations with disease and disease risk (Qureshi and Mehler, 2013).

These detailed levels of regulation provide a dynamic and expansive capability to precisely control cellular function, essential for growth, development, and survival in an unpredictable environment. This also provides many potential points at which disease can arise from disrupted regulation, however. Consequently, a defective gene could cause disease directly through its own action or indirectly by disrupting regulation of other cellular pathways. For example, the forkhead box P2 (FOXP2) transcription factor regulates the expression of genes thought to be important for the development of spoken language (Konopka et al., 2009). Mutations in this gene cause an autosomal-dominant disorder characterized by impairment of speech articulation and language processing (Lai et al., 2001). However, other mutations in this gene are responsible for approximately 1%–2% of sporadic developmental verbal dyspraxia (MacDermot et al., 2005), likely via downstream effects. Mutation of the methyl-CpG-binding protein 2 (MECP2), which regulates chromatin structure, causes the neurodevelopmental disorder Rett syndrome, but other mutations in this gene can cause intellectual disability (ID) or autism (Gonzales and LaSalle, 2010). Similarly, the RBFOX1 protein (also called ataxin 2 binding protein 1, or A2BP1), a neuron-specific RNA splicing factor (Underwood et al., 2005) predicted to regulate a large network of genes important to neurodevelopment (Fogel et al., 2012; Yeo et al., 2009; Zhang et al., 2008), causes autistic spectrum disorder when disrupted (Martin et al., 2007) but has also been implicated as a susceptibility gene associated with both primary biliary cirrhosis (Joshita et al., 2010) and hand osteoarthritis (Zhai et al., 2009), presumably due to downstream effects or specific effects in non-neural tissues. This concept of genes acting on other genes will be explored further later (see Common Neurological Disorders and Complex Disease Genetics).

In addition to the complexity of regulatory mutations that affect gene expression by altering RNA or protein levels or by disrupting RNA splicing, there are certain mutations that do not cause protein dysfunction but instead have effects restricted to the RNA itself. For example, RNA inclusions are found in several forms of triplet repeat disorders (see Repeat Expansion Disorders) including myotonic dystrophy type 1 and the fragile X-associated tremor/ataxia syndrome (FXTAS; Garcia-Arocena and Hagerman, 2010; Paulson, 2018). The latter is particularly interesting from a genetic standpoint, because a disorder of late-onset progressive ataxia, tremor, and cognitive impairment occurs in carriers of *FMR1* alleles of intermediate sizes, which are not full fragile-X-causing mutations (Garcia-Arocena and Hagerman, 2010). FXTAS is a dominant gain-of-function disease that occurs via an entirely different mechanism than the recessive loss-of-function disease that is fragile X syndrome (Garcia-Arocena and Hagerman, 2010; Penagarikano et al., 2007). FXTAS pathogenicity appears related to repeat-associated non-AUG-initiated translation of a cryptic polyglycine protein (Todd et al., 2013), an example of a rapidly emerging mechanism in several RNA-mediated neurodegenerative disorders, including DM1 myotonic dystrophy, C9orf72-mediated amyotrophic lateral sclerosis (ALS) and frontotemporal dementia (FTD), and several others (Cleary and Ranum, 2013; Mohan et al., 2014; Zu et al., 2018). Primary disorders of RNA still represent relatively uncharted territory and it is likely that more RNA-specific diseases will be identified. This is particularly exciting for many reasons, not the least of which is that certain classes of these disorders may be amenable to therapy (Nakamori and Thornton, 2010; Wheeler et al., 2009).

## TYPES OF GENETIC VARIATION AND MUTATIONS

### Rare versus Common Variation

As dictated by the principles of natural selection, most genetic variation is not deleterious, and the induced phenotypic variability can be beneficial as a source on which evolution may act. From a clinical standpoint, it is helpful to dichotomize genetic variation into common and rare variation, while accepting that genetic variation is likely a continuum, and the choice of cutoff could be considered arbitrary. Rare genetic variants are of low frequency in the population (<1% frequency), either because they are deleterious and selected against or because they are new and most often benign. Common genetic variation (>1%–5% population frequency), on the other hand, is adaptive, neutral, or not deleterious enough to be subject to strong negative selection; such variants are referred to as *polymorphisms*. The preeminent genetic model has been that common disease susceptibility is related to common genetic variation, and more rare forms of disease are caused by rare genetic variants, so-called mutations, which act in a Mendelian fashion. In contrast, common variants or polymorphisms may increase susceptibility for disease, but each variant alone is not sufficient to cause disease. Instead, hundreds or thousands of variants necessarily act in combination to lead to disease risk, which is termed "*polygenic risk*" (Wray et al., 2019; see Common Neurological Disorders and Complex Disease Genetics).

### Polymorphisms and Point Mutations

The most prevalent form of genetic polymorphism is the *single nucleotide polymorphism* (SNP), which occurs on average every 300–1000 base pairs in the human genome. Most of these SNPs are relatively benign on their own and do not directly cause disease, so for the purposes of this initial discussion, we will concern ourselves primarily with mutations: rare genetic variants sufficient to cause disease. Pathogenic mutations can occur in numerous ways and vary from single nucleotide changes to gross rearrangements of chromosomes (Fig. 48.3). Owing to the large volume of DNA in the human genome, heritable mutations can arise spontaneously in the germline over time through errors in DNA replication or from DNA damage by metabolic or environmental sources, despite the constant surveillance of extensive cellular preventive proofreading and repair mechanisms. Thus, mutations

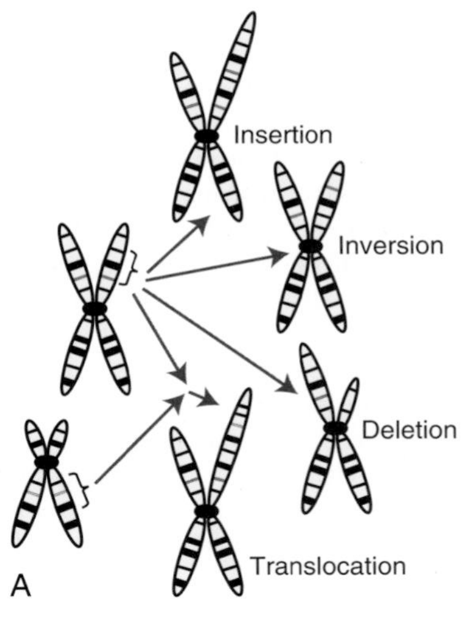


**Normal**

| | | | | | | | | | | | |
|---|---|---|---|---|---|---|---|---|---|---|---|
| Protein | Ser | Val | Ile | Asp | Arg | Ser | Pro | Cys | Leu | Gln | Ala |
| RNA | AGC | GUA | AUC | GAU | CGC | UCU | CCG | UGC | UUG | CAG | GCU |
| DNA | TCG | CAT | TAG | CTA | GCG | AGA | GGC | ACG | AAC | GTC | CGA |

**Point mutation - missense**

| | | | | | | | | | | | |
|---|---|---|---|---|---|---|---|---|---|---|---|
| Protein | Ser | Val | Ile | Asp | **Gly** | Ser | Pro | Cys | Leu | Gln | Ala |
| RNA | AGC | GUA | AUC | GAU | **G**GC | UCU | CCG | UGC | UUG | CAG | GCU |
| DNA | TCG | CAT | TAG | CTA | **C**CG | AGA | GGC | ACG | AAC | GTC | CGA |

**Point mutation - nonsense**

| | | | | | | | | | | | |
|---|---|---|---|---|---|---|---|---|---|---|---|
| Protein | Ser | Val | Ile | Asp | Arg | Ser | Pro | **STOP** | | | |
| RNA | AGC | GUA | AUc | GAU | CGC | UCU | CCG | UG**A** | UUG | CAG | GCU |
| DNA | TCG | CAT | TAG | CTA | GCG | AGA | GGC | AC**T** | AAC | GTC | CGA |

**Point mutation - silent**

| | | | | | | | | | | | |
|---|---|---|---|---|---|---|---|---|---|---|---|
| Protein | Ser | Val | Ile | Asp | Arg | Ser | Pro | Cys | Leu | Gln | Ala |
| RNA | AGC | GUA | AUC | GAU | CGC | UC**G** | CCG | UGC | UUG | CAG | GCU |
| DNA | TCG | CAT | TAG | CTA | GCG | AG**C** | GGC | ACG | AAC | GTC | CGA |

**Frameshift - insertion**

| | | | | | | | | | | | | |
|---|---|---|---|---|---|---|---|---|---|---|---|---|
| Protein | Ser | Val | Ile | Asp | Arg | Ser | **Ser** | **Val** | **Leu** | **Ala** | **Gly** | |
| RNA | AGC | GUA | AUC | GAU | CGC | UC**C** | **UCC** | **GUG** | **CUU** | **GCA** | **CCC** | **U** |
| DNA | TCG | CAT | TAG | CTA | GCG | AG**G** | AGG | CAC | GAA | CGT | CCG | A |

**Frameshift - deletion**

| | | | | | | | | | | | |
|---|---|---|---|---|---|---|---|---|---|---|---|
| Protein | Ser | Val | Ile | Asp | Arg | Ser | **Arg** | **Ala** | **Cys** | **Arg** | — |
| RNA | AGC | GUA | AUC | GAU | CGC | UC-**C** | **CGU** | **GCU** | **UGC** | **AGG** | **CU** |
| DNA | TCG | CAT | TAG | CTA | GCG | AG-G | GCA | CGA | ACG | TCC | GA |

B

$CAG_{(N)}$

$CAG_{(N+X)}$

C

**Fig. 48.3 Genetic Mutations. A,** Categories of chromosomal aberrations. Paired homologous chromosomes are shown, with various anomalies indicated. An insertional translocation is depicted; other common types include reciprocal translocations and centric fusions (Robertsonian translocations). **B,** Types of point mutations. A generic deoxyribonucleic acid sequence is shown *(boxed)* along with its corresponding messenger RNA (mRNA) sequence. Codons are indicated, as are their translation into protein (designed by the standard three-letter code). Mutations are in *purple*, as are the corresponding alterations in the mRNA and protein if present. Note that silent point mutations do not alter the protein sequence. **C,** Repeat expansion disorders. An example mRNA is shown with a CAG-codon (polyglutamine) repeat region indicated. In the expanded form, an additional number of repeats are present which may perturb the function of the protein produced and/or lead to cell damage via the expanded polyglutamine region (see text for details).

can be inherited from the parent or occur de novo in the germline. An example of a common de novo variant is trisomy 21, which causes Down syndrome (discussed further in Chromosomal Analysis and Abnormalities). The smallest pathogenic alterations, termed *point mutations*, involve a change in a single nucleotide within a DNA sequence. A point mutation can result in one of three possible effects with respect to protein: (1) a change to a different amino acid, called a *missense mutation*; (2) a change to a termination codon, called a *nonsense mutation*; or (3) creation of a new sequence that is *silent* with regard to protein sequence but alters some aspect of gene regulation, such as RNA splicing or transcriptional expression levels. Nonsense mutations can cause premature truncation of a protein, a potentially disastrous effect, often leading to production of a nonfunctional protein. Missense mutations, in contrast, can affect a protein in different ways depending on the chemical properties of the new amino acid and whether the change is located in a region of functional importance.

It is often not possible to determine the outcome of specific missense changes, or even nonsense ones, without experimental evidence. The term "mutation" thus should be reserved only for those changes known to cause disease, with the typical description of such alterations being "variants." For example, genome sequencing demonstrates that more than 100 nonsense variants may exist per genome, and the vast majority are expected to be relatively benign (Lupski et al., 2010; see Genome/Exome Sequencing in Clinical Practice, Disease Gene Discovery, and Gene Therapy). In many cases, the pathogenicity of rare missense variants is not immediately discernible, and without strong statistical or functional evidence, labeling such genetic variation a mutation is premature and may be misleading. As our knowledge of normal human genetic variation grows, it is likely that most of these, including even some variants thought previously to cause rare Mendelian diseases, will be reclassified as benign genetic variation. This is not surprising, as even a complete knockout of one allele caused by a premature stop codon *(haploinsufficiency)* may have no discernible effect on gene function for a majority of genes in the human genome (Lupski et al., 2010; Ng et al., 2009; Shen et al., 2013; Yngvadottir et al., 2009). In some cases, Mendelian diseases may even require combinations of variants in more than one gene (Margolin et al., 2013) before a phenotype is observed, further illustrating the challenge of predicting pathogenicity.

Occasionally, silent coding or noncoding variants may cause disease if they damage sequences important for gene expression (e.g., transcriptional and/or RNA processing regulatory elements). It has been estimated that up to half of all disease-causing mutations impact RNA splicing, which can have dire consequences given the importance of splicing to regulated gene expression. Such is the case for FTD with parkinsonism, linked to chromosome 17 (FTDP-17), where in some populations, the most common mutations disrupt splicing, causing a pathogenic imbalance in tau isoforms (D'Souza and Schellenberg, 2005). As for noncoding mutations, given the large volume of such sequences in the human genome—perhaps up to 96%—and our still imprecise ability to predict sequences required for regulation or to interpret identified sequence changes without direct experimentation (Thusberg et al., 2011), the majority of these mutations likely go unrecognized. Advances in next-generation sequencing and bioinformatic technologies are beginning to examine larger populations of patients globally for both coding and noncoding variants and are expected to expand our understanding of the role of these types of mutation in human disease.

### Structural Chromosomal Abnormalities and Copy Number Variation

Small deletions and insertions can occur through slippage and strand mispairing at regions of short, tandem DNA repeats during replication. If the deletion or insertion is not a multiple of three, a *frameshift* will result, which leads to the translation of an altered protein sequence from the site of the mutation. On a larger scale, errors of chromosomal replication or recombination can result in inversions, translocations, deletions, duplications, or insertions (Stankiewicz and Lupski, 2010). When the region of deletion or duplication is greater than 1 kb, this is referred to as a *copy number variation* (CNV). CNV is far more common than previously suspected, and it is estimated that at least 4% of the human genome varies in copy number (Conrad et al., 2010; Redon et al., 2006), much of which is commonly observed in the population and benign (Conrad et al., 2010). However, some rare CNVs such as the recurrent chromosome 17p12 duplication underlying most cases of Charcot-Marie-Tooth (CMT) type 1A (Shchelochkov et al., 2010) or the alpha-synuclein triplication that can cause Parkinson disease (PD; Singleton et al., 2003) are pathogenic and act in a Mendelian fashion. Even though such changes may be extensive, they may not be pathogenic if they do not disrupt expression of any key genes. This is particularly true for balanced translocations where genetic material is rearranged between chromosomes, yet no significant portion is actually lost. Although an individual with such a condition may be normal, if the germline is affected their offspring may receive unbalanced chromosomal material and consequently develop a clinical phenotype (Kovaleva and Shaffer, 2003), which may be quite severe. CNVs will be discussed in greater detail when we consider common and complex disease genetics (see Copy Number Variation and Chromosomal Microarray Analysis).

### Repeat Expansion Disorders

Most mutations thus far discussed pass from parent to offspring unaltered, and in large affected families, the identical mutation can potentially be traced back generations. In contrast, there is a specific class of mutation, the repeat expansion (Paulson, 2018; Table 48.2), which is unstable and can present with earlier onset and increasing severity in successive generations, a process known as *anticipation*. There are several examples of diseases caused by expanded repeats in coding sequence (e.g., the common dominant spinocerebellar ataxias [SCAs], HD), as well as examples in noncoding sequence (e.g., fragile X syndrome, myotonic dystrophy) and within an intron (e.g., Friedreich ataxia). Interestingly, virtually all these disorders show neurological symptoms that can include such features as ataxia, ID, dementia, myotonia, or epilepsy, depending on the disease. The most common repeated sequence seen in these diseases is the CAG triplet, which codes for glutamine. Its expansion is seen in a variety of the SCAs including SCA types 1, 2, 3, 6, 7, 17, and dentatorubropallidoluysian atrophy (DRPLA). In addition to protein-specific effects, these disorders likely share a common pathogenesis due to the presence of the enlarged polyglutamine repeat regions. Furthermore, recent studies have shown that bidirectional transcription may occur from these repeat regions in many of the disorders, through a process termed RAN translation, producing polypeptide proteins which may disrupt metabolism, induce toxic cellular effects, and lead to disease (Zu et al., 2018). In some disorders, the phenotype can be quite different depending on the number of repeats, such as in the *FMR1* gene, where more than 200 CCG repeats cause fragile X syndrome, but repeats in the premutation range of 60–200, from which fully expanded alleles arise, can result in FXTAS or premature ovarian failure (Oostra and Willemsen, 2009). Although, in general, the underlying mutation is similar, each specific repeat expansion has distinct effects on its corresponding gene, and thus in addition to varying phenotypes, they may also show very different inheritance patterns, as illustrated later (see Disorders of Mendelian Inheritance).

## CHROMOSOMAL ANALYSIS AND ABNORMALITIES

The DNA coding for an individual gene is generally too small to be visualized microscopically, but it is possible to observe the chromosomes as they condense during mitosis as part of cell division (Griffiths et al., 2002; Strachan and Read, 2019). Traditionally, various staining techniques (e.g., Giemsa) are applied, producing a detailed pattern of banding along the chromosomes that is then photographed and aligned for comparative analysis. This arrangement and analysis of the chromosomes is known as a *karyotype* (Fig. 48.4). Through these methods, it is possible to visually identify large chromosomal deletions, duplications, or rearrangements. If high-resolution banding techniques are employed, structural alterations as small as 3 Mb (3 million base pairs) can be detected. More sophisticated techniques can also be employed, such as fluorescent in situ hybridization (FISH). In this method, a short DNA sequence, or probe, that corresponds to a chromosomal region of interest is hybridized with the patient's DNA and detected visually via excitation of a fluorescent label. FISH can improve on visual resolution by 10- to 100-fold and is in common use for detection of a large number of well-defined genetic syndromes (Speicher and Carter, 2005) such as 15q duplication syndrome, DiGeorge syndrome (22q11 deletion), and Smith-Magenis syndrome (17p11 deletion).

More recent technological developments involving microarray technology (Geschwind, 2003) permit screening of the entire genome at high resolution (from kilobase to single nucleotide level) and are rapidly replacing techniques based on microscopic analysis. This technology is responsible for the emerging appreciation for the structural chromosomal variation in humans mentioned earlier, most of which is submicroscopic. We will first focus on chromosomal alterations that can be detected microscopically, and discuss small or rare structural variants subsequently (see Copy Number Variation and Chromosomal Microarray Analysis).

The most common chromosomal abnormalities encountered clinically involve sporadic aneuploidy, either a deletion leaving one chromosome, or a monosomy, or a duplication leaving three chromosomes, or a trisomy (Strachan and Read, 2019). This occurs most frequently via nondisjunction, whereby chromosomes fail to separate during meiosis in the production of the gametes. The majority of aneuploidies are lethal, although there are a few that are viable and will be briefly discussed. Monosomy X (45,XO), also called Turner syndrome, is seen in approximately 1 of every 5000 births and results in sterile females of small stature with a variety of

**TABLE 48.2 Selected Repeat Expansion Disorders**

| Disease | Locus | Gene Symbol | Protein Name | Protein Function | Normal Repeat* | Repeat Location† | Expanded Repeat‡ |
|---|---|---|---|---|---|---|---|
| ALS | 9p21.2 | *C9orf72* | C9orf72 protein | Unknown | ≤23 GGGGCC | Promoter | ≥700 |
| FTD | | | | | | 5′ UTR | |
| DM1 | 19q13.2-q13.3 | *DMPK* | Dystrophia myotonica protein kinase | Ser/Thr protein kinase | ≤34 CTG | 3′ UTR | ≥50 |
| DM2 | 3q13.3-q24 | *ZNF9* | Zinc finger protein 9 | Translational regulation | ≤26 CCTG | Intronic | ≥75 |
| DRPLA | 12p13.31 | *ATN1* | Atrophin-1 | Transcription | ≤35 CAG | Coding | ≥48 |
| FRAXA | Xq27.3 | *FMR1* | Fragile-X mental retardation protein | Translational regulation | ≤40 CGG | 5′ UTR | >200 |
| FXTAS§ | | | | | | | 60–200§ |
| FRDA | 9q13 | *FXN* | Frataxin | Mitochondrial metabolism | ≤33 GAA | Intronic | ≥66 |
| HD | 4p16.3 | *HTT* | Huntington | Unknown | ≤26 CAG | Coding | ≥36 |
| SBMA | Xq11-q12 | *AR* | Androgen receptor | Transcription | ≤34 CAG | Coding | ≥38 |
| SCA1 | 6p23 | *ATXN1* | Ataxin-1 | Transcription | ≤38 CAG | Coding | ≥39 |
| SCA2 | 12q24 | *ATXN2* | Ataxin-2 | RNA processing | ≤31 CAG | Coding | ≥32 |
| SCA3 | 14q24.3-q31 | *ATXN3* | Ataxin-3 | Protein quality control | ≤44 CAG | Coding | ≥52 |
| SCA6 | 19p13 | *CACNA1A* | $Ca_V2.1$ | Calcium channel | ≤18 CAG | Coding | ≥20 |
| SCA7 | 3p21.1-p12 | *ATXN7* | Ataxin-7 | Transcription | ≤19 CAG | Coding | ≥36 |
| SCA8¶ | 13q21 | *ATXN8* | Ataxin-8 | Unknown | ≤50 CAG | Coding | ≥80 |
| | | *ATXN8OS* | None | Unknown | ≤50 CTG | Noncoding | ≥80 |
| SCA10 | 22q13 | *ATXN10* | Ataxin-10 | Unknown | ≤29 ATTCT | Intronic | ≥800 |
| SCA12 | 5q31-q33 | *PPP2R2B* | Protein phosphatase 2 regulatory subunit B, beta | Mitochondrial morphogenesis | ≤32 CAG | 5′ UTR | ≥51 |
| SCA17 | 6q27 | *TBP* | TATA box-binding protein | Transcription | ≤42 CAG | Coding | ≥49 |

*In some instances, normal/abnormal repeat length is an estimate due to adjacent polymorphic sequences.
†Location of repeat region within the expressed mRNA.
‡Does not include alleles with known incomplete penetrance.
§Premutation alleles for FRAXA result in the FXTAS phenotype.
¶SCA8 involves bidirectional expression from two overlapping reading frames.
*ALS*, Amyotrophic lateral sclerosis; *DM*, myotonic dystrophy; *DRPLA*, dentatorubralpallidoluysian atrophy; *FRAXA*, fragile X syndrome; *FRDA*, Friedreich ataxia; *FTD*, Frontotemporal dementia; *FXTAS*, fragile X-associated tremor/ataxia syndrome; *HD*, Huntington disease; *SBMA*, spinal and bulbar muscular atrophy; *SCA*, spinocerebellar ataxia; *UTR*, untranslated region.

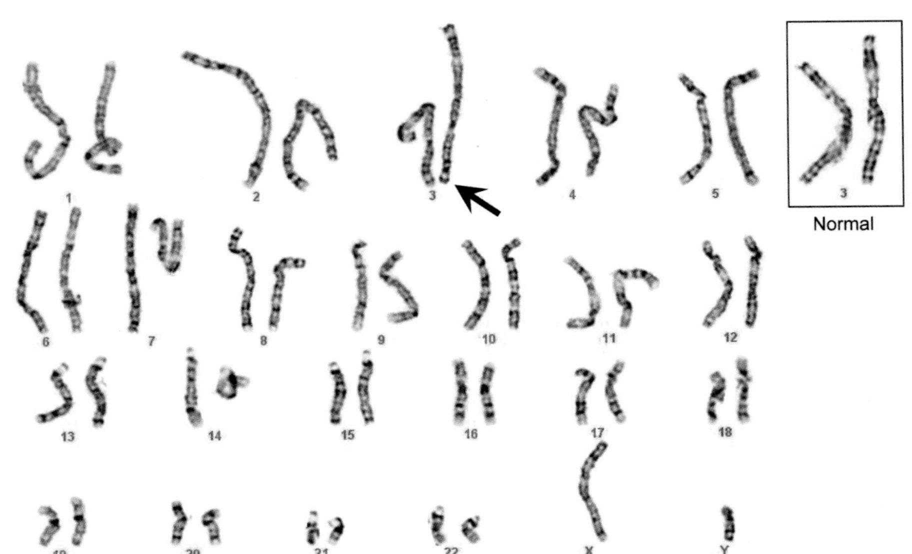


**Fig. 48.4 Abnormal Male Karyogram.** Patient is a male child with a clinical diagnosis of autism. Metaphase chromosomes were isolated from peripheral blood leukocytes and high-resolution GPG (G-Bands by Pancreatin using Giemsa) banding was performed to visualize structural features. A deletion of the telomeric region of the long arm of chromosome 3 was detected *(arrow)*, consistent with a diagnosis of 3q29 microdeletion syndrome. A normal chromosome 3 pair is shown for comparison *(insert)*. Analysis of the parents showed this to be a de novo deletion. *(Photo courtesy of F. Quintero-Rivera, UCLA Clinical Cytogenetics Laboratory.)*

mild physical deformities including webbing of the neck, multiple nevi, and hand and elbow variations, with a very specific cognitive profile in patients with the full deletion (Strachan and Read, 2019). Individuals with additional copies of the X chromosome are also seen. While both females (47,XXX) and males (47,XXY) may have varying degrees of learning disabilities, especially involving language and attention (Geschwind et al., 2000), the males are referred to as having Klinefelter syndrome (KS) due to a phenotype also involving gynecomastia and infertility. XYY males have cognitive profiles similar to XXY males but several studies have suggested more severe social and behavioral problems in some individuals, especially increased aggression, which is rare in KS. Trisomy 21 (47, +21), or Down syndrome, includes profound intellectual impairment, flat faces with prominent epicanthal folds, and a predisposition to cardiac disease. At 1 in approximately 700 births, this is the most common genetic cause of ID and is associated with advanced maternal age at the time of conception. The other aneuploidies which can survive to term (trisomy 13 [47, +13], Edwards syndrome; trisomy 18 [47, +18], Patau syndrome) have much more severe phenotypes with drastically decreased viability, and death generally occurs within weeks to months after birth.

## DISORDERS OF MENDELIAN INHERITANCE

In this section we will consider genetic disorders caused by mutation of a single gene. Associating a clinical disease phenotype to the mutation of a specific gene has long been the goal of clinically based, or translational, neuroscience. It is expected that a more complete knowledge of the effects of genetic variants on gene function, coupled with environmental influences and lifestyle, will eventually lead to an understanding of the basis of disease etiology as well as more accurate diagnosis and better treatments, both for common and rare disease, a concept known as precision health (Rexach et al., 2019). The ability to determine the genetic nature of most single-gene disease is ultimately based upon the laws of inheritance devised by Mendel in the late 1800s (Griffiths et al., 2002). To summarize these findings in a clinical context, the assumption is made that a phenotypic trait (or in this example, a disease) is caused by the alteration of a single gene. It is important to emphasize that this assumption does not always hold true, particularly for the more complex genetic diseases, as we will discuss later, but it is still true for many diseases seen by neurologists, and more than 5000 Mendelian conditions have been identified to date (OMIM, 2019). Now, if we accept the premise that a given disease is caused by a single gene, we know that for any individual, the gene exists as a pair of alleles with one copy from each parent. However, the alleles may not be equal, and one member of the pair may control the phenotype despite the presence of the other copy. In this case, we say that allele is *dominant* over the other, the latter of which is labeled as *recessive*. Depending on the gene and the mutation, as discussed later, a disease allele may be either dominant or recessive. Next, during the development of the gametes, these alleles segregate randomly in a process independent from all other genes. Therefore, the chance of a child receiving a particular allele is entirely random. If these laws all hold true, the observed inheritance of the clinical disease in families will follow a specific pattern that can be used to identify the nature of the causative gene. Although diseases showing Mendelian inheritance are either rare conditions or rare forms of common conditions (e.g., early-onset AD or PD), identification of such genes is a seminal biological advance that can have enormous impact on our understanding of these neurological conditions.

### Autosomal Dominant Disorders

Diseases involving autosomal genes that require mutation of only one allele are defined as dominant. In most cases, the affected individual has two distinct alleles of a gene (in this case, one normal and one pathogenic) and is described as being *heterozygous*. Often these pathogenic mutations impart new functionality, referred to as a *toxic gain of function*, meaning that the phenotype is produced as a result of the expression of the mutated protein. Other disease mechanisms in dominantly inherited conditions include: (1) *haploinsufficiency*, where inactivation of a single allele is sufficient to produce disease despite the presence of another normal copy, and (2) *dominant negative* effects, where a mutated protein disrupts function of the normal protein transcribed from the other nonmutant allele.

*Autosomal dominant inheritance* is characterized by direct transmission of the disorder from parent to child (Fig. 48.5). Affected individuals are seen in all generations, and a vertical line can be drawn on the pedigree to illustrate the passage of the disorder. Since only one deleterious copy of the disease gene is necessary, risk of transmission from an affected parent is 50%. Since the disorder is autosomal, there is no sex preference, and both males and females can present with the disease. One caveat involves the concept of *penetrance*, or the percent likelihood that a trait will manifest in a person with a specific genotype. A dominant gene is considered to have complete penetrance if all individuals with a given mutation develop disease. In practice, however, many autosomal dominant genes show varying degrees of penetrance or expressivity, most likely due to the influence of other genes and environmental factors.

There are over 500 examples of diseases with neurological phenotypes that show autosomal dominant inheritance (OMIM, 2019).

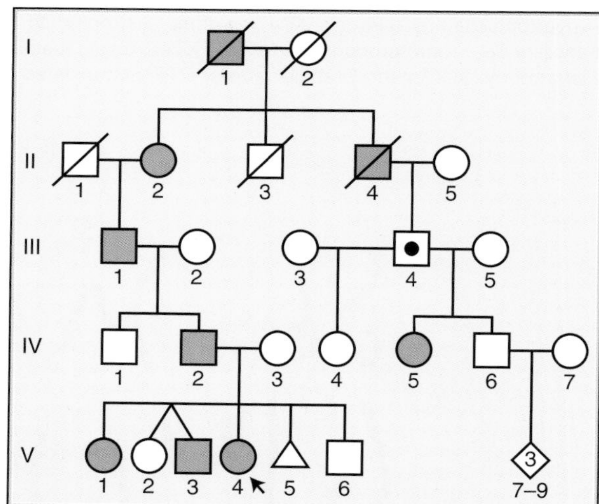


**Fig. 48.5 Autosomal Dominant Inheritance.** A pedigree diagram is shown, using standard nomenclature. Generations are numbered consecutively on the left, and individuals are numbered within each generation. Males are depicted as squares and females as circles. Affected persons are indicated by filled icons. Death is indicated by a diagonal line. A union producing offspring is indicated by horizontal lines. A diamond represents individuals (n) of unknown sex. A triangle represents a spontaneous abortion. Individuals V-2 and V-3 illustrate the diagramming of dizygotic twins. The proband of the pedigree is indicated by an arrow. An autosomal dominant pedigree demonstrates vertical transmission of disease without a sex preference. On average, 50% of offspring are affected. Individual III-4 represents a case of incomplete penetrance *(dark circle)* where the individual carries the mutation but does not manifest disease. Anticipation (see text) would be illustrated by increasing severity/onset in patients III-1, IV-2, and V-4.

These conditions include hyperkalemic periodic paralysis (voltage-gated sodium channel $Na_V1.4$ on chromosome 17, often caused by missense mutations), HD (Huntington on chromosome 4, caused by CAG repeat expansion), SCA type 3 (ataxin-3 on chromosome 14, caused by CAG repeat expansion), CMT type 1B (myelin protein zero on chromosome 1, often caused by missense mutations), early-onset familial AD (presenilin-1, often caused by missense mutations), FTD with parkinsonism (microtubule-associated protein tau on chromosome 17, often caused by missense or splicing mutations), tuberous sclerosis type 1 (hamartin on chromosome 9, often caused by nonsense mutations and frameshifts), neurofibromatosis type 1 (neurofibromin on chromosome 17, caused by point mutations, frameshifts, and splicing mutations), and familial ALS (superoxide dismutase-1 on chromosome 21, caused by missense mutations), to name a few. Even rare Mendelian forms of more common syndromes such as epilepsy or sleep disorders (e.g., familial advanced sleep-phase syndrome) have been identified. More detailed lists can be found using the recommended online resources (Table 48.3).

**TABLE 48.3 Selected Online Clinical Neurogenetics Resources**

| Category | Resource |
|---|---|
| Disease-specific and gene-specific resources | GeneCards: The Human Gene Database<br>The Crown Human Genome Center at The Weizmann Institute of Science, Rehovot, Israel<br>http://www.genecards.org<br>GeneReviews<br>University of Washington, Seattle, WA, USA<br>US National Center for Biotechnology Information<br>http://www.ncbi.nlm.nih.gov/books/NBK1116/<br>Neuromuscular Disease Center<br>Washington University, St. Louis, MO, USA<br>http://neuromuscular.wustl.edu/<br>Online Mendelian Inheritance in Man<br>Johns Hopkins University, Baltimore, MD, USA<br>http://omim.org/ |
| Clinical genetic testing and clinical trials resources | ClinicalTrials.gov<br>US National Institutes of Health<br>http://clinicaltrials.gov/<br>The Genetic Testing Registry<br>US National Center for Biotechnology Information<br>http://www.ncbi.nlm.nih.gov/gtr/ |
| Genomic variation and other genome resources | ClinVar Database<br>US National Center for Biotechnology Information<br>https://www.ncbi.nlm.nih.gov/clinvar/<br>DECIPHER<br>The Deciphering Developmental Disorders (DDD) Study<br>The Wellcome Sanger Institute, Cambridge, UK<br>https://decipher.sanger.ac.uk/<br>ExAC (Exome Aggregation Consortium)<br>The Broad Institute, Cambridge, MA, USA<br>http://exac.broadinstitute.org/<br>Genotype-Tissue Expression Project (GTEx)<br>US National Institutes of Health<br>https://gtexportal.org/home/<br>GnomAD (Genome Aggregation Database)<br>The Broad Institute, Cambridge, MA, USA<br>https://gnomad.broadinstitute.org/<br>GWAS Catalog<br>US National Human Genome Research Institute<br>The European Bioinformatics Institute<br>US National Center for Biotechnology Information<br>https://www.ebi.ac.uk/gwas/home<br>The Human Gene Mutation Database<br>The Institute of Medical Genetics at Cardiff University, Cardiff, UK<br>http://www.hgmd.cf.ac.uk/ac/index.php<br>IGSR: The International Genome Sample Resource<br>Providing ongoing support for the 1000 Genomes Project data<br>http://www.internationalgenome.org/home<br>University of California, Santa Cruz (UCSC) Genome Bioinformatics<br>University of California, Santa Cruz, Santa Cruz, CA, USA<br>http://genome.ucsc.edu/ |

*GWAS*, Genome-wide association study.

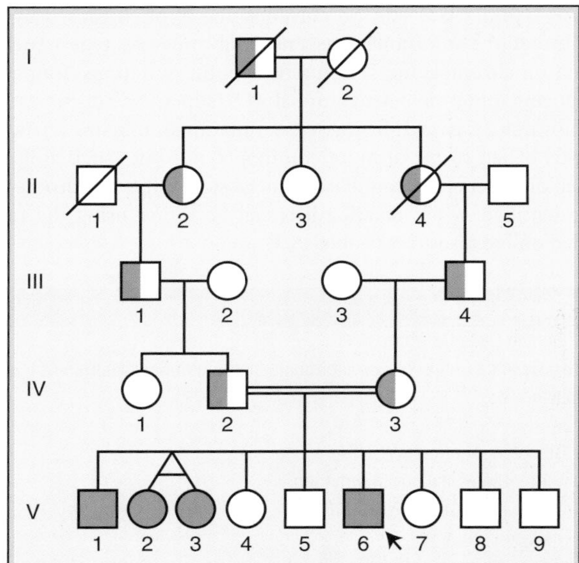


**Fig.48.6** Autosomal Recessive Inheritance. A pedigree diagram is shown, using standard nomenclature as described in Fig. 48.5. Carriers of disease are indicated by half-filled icons. The proband of the pedigree is indicated by an arrow. Individuals V-2 and V-3 illustrate the diagramming of monozygotic twins. Consanguineous mating is indicated by a doubled line. An autosomal recessive pedigree demonstrates indirect transmission of disease without a sex preference, often in a single generation (occasionally described as horizontal). On average, 25% of offspring of two carriers are affected.

## Autosomal Recessive Disorders

Disease involving autosomal genes that require mutation of both alleles is defined as *recessive*. An unaffected individual who harbors one disease-causing allele is referred to as a *carrier* of that allele. For some disorders, a mild phenotype can be seen in these individuals, who are then described as symptomatic carriers. An individual with two identical alleles (in this case both pathogenic) is described as being *homozygous*. Alternatively, if they possess two different pathogenic alleles, this is described as being *compound heterozygous*. In general, autosomal recessive mutations modify the function of the protein in a negative way, meaning that the phenotype is produced because of the absence of the mutated protein. This is referred to as a *loss of function*.

*Autosomal recessive inheritance* is characterized by lack of intergenerational transmission, in contrast to dominantly inherited disorders (Fig. 48.6). Affected individuals are seen in single generations, often separated by one or more unaffected generations. Because two deleterious copies of the disease gene are necessary, transmission requires both parents to be either affected or carriers. In the most common scenario when both parents are carriers, the risk of an affected child is 25% (50% from each parent). As with all autosomal disorders, there is no sex preference, and both males and females can present with the disease. In families showing this mode of inheritance, it is important to ask about consanguinity. In rare cases of families with considerable inbreeding, recessive alleles may be so common as to cause disease in successive generations, creating a *pseudodominant* pattern of inheritance.

As mentioned for the autosomal dominant disorders, diseases that share this mode of inheritance may have very distinct types of underlying mutations. Over 700 disorders with autosomal recessive inheritance show neurological symptoms (OMIM, 2019). Examples include Friedreich ataxia (frataxin on chromosome 9, caused by intronic GAA repeat expansion), spinal muscular atrophy type 1 (survival of motor neuron 1 on chromosome 5, caused by deletion of exon 7), Wilson disease (ATPase, $Cu^{2+}$ transporting, beta-polypeptide on chromosome 13, often caused by missense mutations), Tay-Sachs disease (hexosaminidase A on chromosome 15, commonly caused by frameshift, splicing, or nonsense mutations), glycogen storage type II or Pompe disease (acid alpha-glucosidase gene on chromosome 17, often caused by point mutations, splicing mutations, and exon deletions), phenylketonuria (phenylalanine hydroxylase on chromosome 12, often caused by missense mutations), and ataxia-telangiectasia (ataxia-telangiectasia mutated on chromosome 11, often caused by point mutations and splicing mutations). More detailed lists can be found using the recommended online resources (see Table 48.3).

It is important to note that the severity of recessive mutations can have a dramatic impact on phenotype expressivity, often to the point where the two conditions can no longer be recognized as the same disease. For example, severe mutations in the glycogen branching enzyme *(GBE1)* cause glycogen storage disease type IV, a devastating metabolic disorder often leading to death in infancy, while less severe mutations result in a late-onset progressive neuromuscular condition known as adult polyglucosan body disorder (Klein, 2013). Furthermore, there are examples of genes that can exhibit both dominant and recessive phenotypes, depending on the type and location of the mutation in question. For example, heterozygous inframe deletions and missense mutations in the *SPTBN2* gene cause an adult-onset pure cerebellar ataxia termed SCA type 5 (SCA5), while homozygous truncating mutations cause a more severe infantile-onset disorder of ataxia and cognition (Cho and Fogel, 2013; Elsayed et al., 2014; Lise et al., 2012). This adds another layer of complexity to the study of phenotypic expressivity caused by mutations within specific genes, and many more examples are being detected as clinical exome and genome sequencing are used more broadly in varying clinical populations.

## Sex-Linked (X-Linked) Disorders

The sex chromosomes in humans are referred to as the X and Y chromosomes, the latter of which programs the individual to be male. There are as yet no known Y-linked diseases, so we will focus on the X chromosome. As males only possess a single X chromosome, they are *hemizygous* for all its genes, and consequently any pathogenic mutation is expressed by default. Because of this, dominance of X-linked genes applies with respect to whether female carriers express disease. This is complicated by the observation that although females possess two X chromosomes, no single cell expresses genes from both; instead, one chromosome is randomly and permanently inactivated during development via a process known as *lyonization*. Therefore, all women inherently possess cells of two different genotypes, or are *mosaic*, for the X chromosome. This can be clinically relevant insofar as disproportionate activation of an abnormal X chromosome could potentially lead to clinical phenotypes in female carriers of recessive X-linked disorders. Usually, though, skewing occurs, so that the pathogenic allele is less expressed than the other normal allele, although the mechanism for this is unclear.

Recessive X-linked transmission is characterized by the presence of disease in males only (Fig. 48.7). Affected males cannot pass the disease on to their sons, but all their daughters must inherit the abnormal X chromosome and are, therefore, *obligate carriers*. A carrier female has a 50% chance of passing the disease allele to a child, but all males receiving it will be affected. Dominant X-linked transmission (see Fig. 48.7) is similar, except carrier females are affected and transmit the disease to 50% of their children irrespective of their sex. Affected males usually show a more severe phenotype, or may even exhibit lethality, and transmit the disease to all of their daughters and none of their sons.

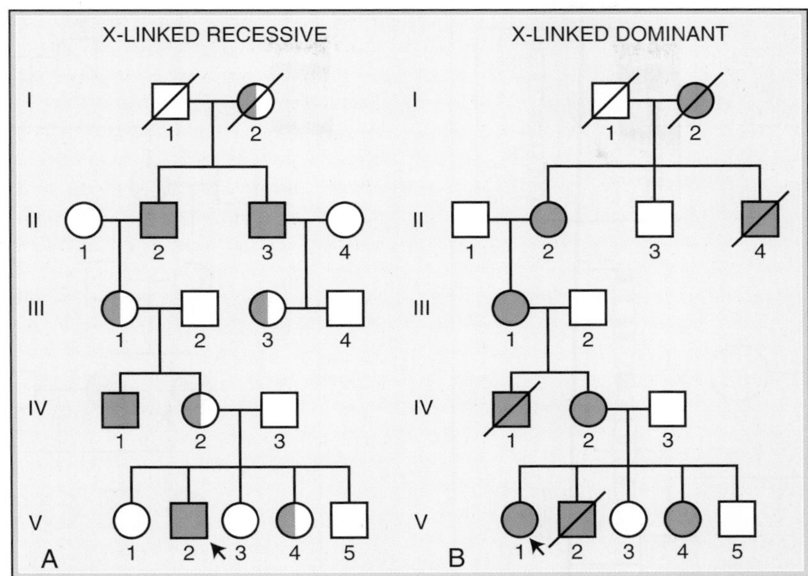


**Fig. 48.7** **X-linked Inheritance. A,** X-linked recessive disease. A pedigree diagram is shown using standard nomenclature as described in Fig. 48.5. Carriers of disease are indicated by half-filled icons. The proband of the pedigree is indicated by an arrow. Disease manifests only in hemizygous males. Fathers cannot pass the disease to their sons, but all daughters of an affected male are obligate carriers of disease. Carrier females have a 50% chance to pass on the disease gene and can have affected sons. In some cases, a female carrier can be mildly symptomatic, usually due to nonrandom lyonization. **B,** X-linked dominant disease. A pedigree diagram is shown using standard nomenclature as described in Fig. 48.5. The proband of the pedigree is indicated by an arrow. Disease manifests in heterozygous females (although severity may be affected by lyonization). The mutant gene is either lethal in males (as shown here) or has a much more severe phenotype. Affected females pass on the disease 50% of the time.

Over 100 X-linked disorders with neurological phenotypes are known (OMIM, 2019). The majority of these X-linked disorders are recessive, and, as seen for the autosomal diseases, mutation type varies widely among the different disorders. Some examples include X-linked adrenoleukodystrophy (ATP-binding cassette subfamily D member 1, commonly caused by missense and frameshift mutations), Duchenne muscular dystrophy (dystrophin, commonly caused by deletions), Emery–Dreifuss muscular dystrophy-1 (emerin, often caused by nonsense mutations), Menkes disease (ATPase, $Cu^{2+}$-transporting, alpha-polypeptide, commonly caused by frameshifts, nonsense mutations, and splicing mutations), Fabry disease (alpha-galactosidase A, commonly caused by point mutations, gene rearrangements, and splicing mutations), and Pelizaeus-Merzbacher disease (proteolipid protein-1, often caused by duplications and missense mutations). X-linked dominant disorders include Rett syndrome (methyl-CpG-binding protein-2, often due to missense and nonsense mutations), fragile X-associated disorders (fragile X mental retardation protein, due to repeat expansion), incontinentia pigmenti (inhibitor of kappa light polypeptide gene enhancer in B cells, kinase gamma [IKBKG], often due to deletions), and Aicardi syndrome (gene unknown). More detailed lists can be found using the recommended online resources (see Table 48.3).

## MENDELIAN DISEASE GENE IDENTIFICATION BY LINKAGE ANALYSIS AND CHROMOSOME MAPPING

As mentioned previously, patterns of inheritance can be utilized to locate genes responsible for disease. Historically, genes showing Mendelian patterns of inheritance were physically mapped and identified through linkage analysis (Altshuler et al., 2008; Pulst, 2003; Fig. 48.8). In this technique, one attempts to find a known region of DNA, termed a *marker*, which is co-inherited (segregates) with the disease being studied and subsequently uses the location of that marker to find the disease gene. Although, in principle, two points on the same chromosome theoretically segregate independently from one another, the recombination process that mediates this (termed *crossing-over* because maternal and paternal chromosomes swap segments during gamete formation) is statistically more likely to separate points that are far apart from one another than those that are close. Segments of DNA that segregate together are described as being linked. If the degree of linkage exceeds that expected by chance, the regions are said to be in *disequilibrium* and are therefore in close proximity. By using naturally occurring DNA polymorphisms as locational markers, the physical mapping of an unknown disease gene is possible, although the mapped region will likely contain other genes as well. Depending on the size of the family, the generational distance of affected individuals sampled, and the density of the markers being used, the region containing the disease gene is narrowed down to a size more amenable to further detailed analysis. Subsequent analysis, usually DNA sequencing of likely candidate genes, is then performed to locate a mutation that segregates with the affected members of the original family. Many genes important to neurological disease have been identified in this way, including the genes for HD, Duchenne muscular dystrophy, Wilson disease, neurofibromatosis type 1, Von Hippel–Lindau syndrome, torsion dystonia 1, Friedreich ataxia, myotonic dystrophy type 1, hyperkalemic periodic paralysis, familial advanced sleep-phase syndrome, and many others. Although still useful clinically for large families, utilization of this technique is not possible for many diseases because of small family sizes and/or lack of power due to insufficient generational separation between affected individuals in the pedigree. Recent advances in next-generation sequencing technology have allowed for the utilization of entire exomic or genomic sequences for mapping, using the known mutation frequency in population control databases

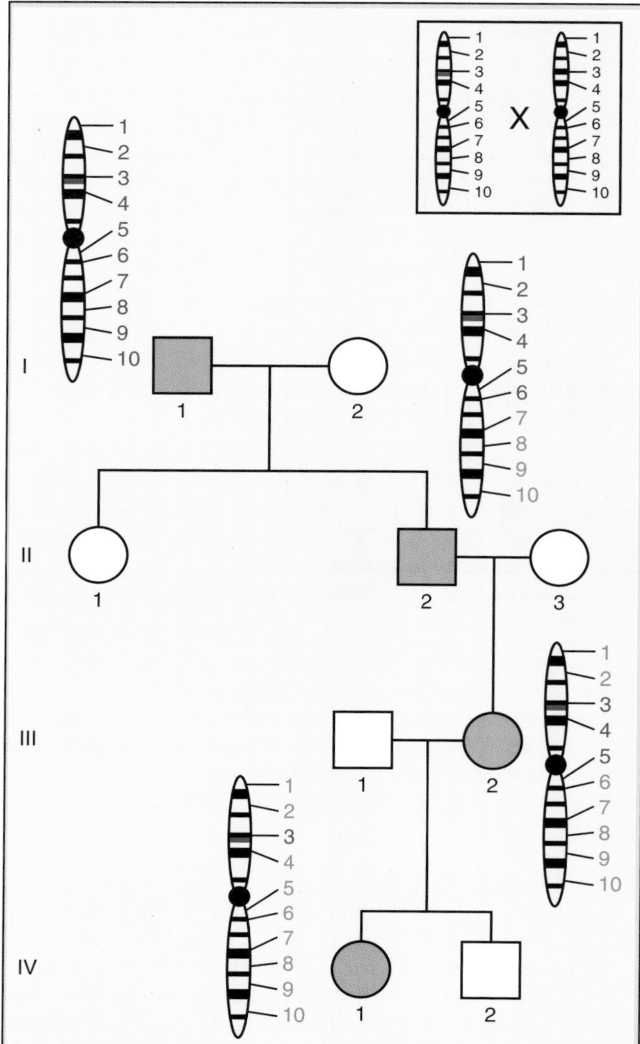


Fig. 48.8 **Linkage Analysis.** A pedigree is depicted as in Fig. 48.5, showing autosomal dominant inheritance of disease *(filled icons)*. Transmission of the chromosome containing the mutant gene *(purple line)* is illustrated for all affected individuals. Numbers represent the location of specific chromosomal markers (e.g., single nucleotide polymorphisms or other sequences). *Purple numbers* represent markers originally from the mutant chromosome in individual I-1. With each mating, there is potential crossing over between regions of homologous chromosomes *(inset)*, likely resulting in the separation of markers spaced far apart along the chromosome. In this example, examination of all affected individuals shows the disease segregates with marker 3, and the two are therefore in linkage disequilibrium, suggesting they are near one another. Once identified, the marker location can be used to select candidate genes for sequencing to identify the causative gene and mutation in the family.

for comparison, allowing for disease gene identification in families of smaller size (see Genome/Exome Sequencing in Clinical Practice, Disease Gene Discovery, and Gene Therapy).

## NON-MENDELIAN PATTERNS OF INHERITANCE

In rare instances, pedigree analysis of affected families has revealed patterns of inheritance that do not conform to the classic Mendelian patterns

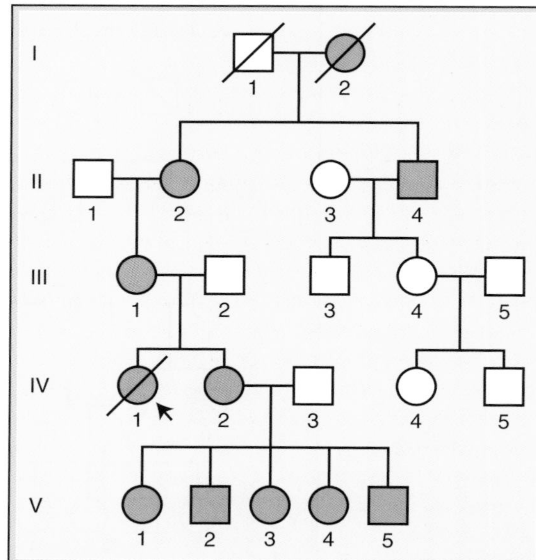


Fig. 48.9 **Mitochondrial (Maternal) Inheritance.** A pedigree diagram is shown using standard nomenclature as described in Fig. 48.5. As the mutant gene is carried in the mitochondrial genome, disease is passed on to all the offspring of affected females (see text). Males can be affected but cannot pass on disease. Severity and onset of the disease may be affected by heteroplasmy, the proportion of abnormal mitochondria per cell, as illustrated by a severe phenotype seen in patient IV-1 *(arrow)*.

thus far described and, therefore, must result from other mechanisms. In this section, we will discuss the more common and clinically relevant ways in which single-gene disorders can be transmitted in a non-Mendelian fashion: mitochondrial inheritance, imprinting, and uniparental disomy. It is important to recognize that this is not all-inclusive. Other examples exist, such as developmental events that can potentially lead to disease or syndromic conditions through formation of a *mosaic*, an individual with cells of different genotypes derived from a common cell, or a *chimera*, an individual who contains cells of different distinct genotypes (e.g., from separate fertilizations). Such rare events will not be discussed further. Additionally, the non-Mendelian heritability of diseases that are *polygenic*, or involve multiple genes, and other forms of complex disorders will be discussed in later sections.

### Mitochondrial Disorders

Mitochondria are double-membraned organelles responsible for energy production within the cell via the process of oxidative phosphorylation, which relies on the transfer of electrons through a chain of protein complexes within the inner mitochondrial membrane. Disruption of mitochondrial function can lead to a variety of diseases with multisystem involvement, including prominent neurological symptoms (DiMauro and Hirano, 2009; Zeviani and Carelli, 2007). Mitochondria possess their own genome with 37 genes. Because mitochondria are cytoplasmic and the majority of cytoplasm within the zygote is derived from the egg and not the sperm, disorders involving mitochondrial DNA are inherited through the maternal line (Fig. 48.9). A single cell contains many mitochondria which all replicate independently of the nuclear DNA, so it is possible that a mutation in the mitochondrial genome may be present in some of the mitochondria but not others, a condition termed *heteroplasmy*. This proportion can affect whether a disease is expressed and, if so, what tissues are affected if a minimum threshold of abnormal mitochondria is reached. Heteroplasmy may also change over time as cells divide and the mitochondria are redistributed. Some examples of such disorders include MELAS (mitochondrial encephalomyopathy, lactic acidosis, and stroke-like episodes, caused by point mutations within the gene encoding mitochondrial $tRNA^{LEU}$), MERRF (myoclonic epilepsy with ragged red fibers, caused by point mutations within the gene-encoding mitochondrial $tRNA^{LYS}$), and LHON (Leber hereditary optic neuropathy, most often caused by point mutations in either of two mitochondrial genes encoding complex I subunits, ND4 or ND6).

Because the mitochondria themselves contain only a few genes, the majority of mitochondrial proteins, including the machinery responsible for the replication and repair of the mitochondrial genome, are all encoded by nuclear genes. Since these genes are located within the nuclear genome, despite the fact that their mutation gives rise to dysfunctional mitochondria, the disease will show a Mendelian pattern of inheritance. Some examples include infantile-onset SCA (twinkle on chromosome 10, autosomal recessive, caused by missense mutations), progressive external ophthalmoplegia A2 (adenine nucleotide translocator 1 on chromosome 4, autosomal dominant, caused by missense mutations), and CMT type 2A2 (mitofusin-2 on chromosome 1, autosomal dominant, often caused by missense mutations). Interestingly, various mutations, commonly missense, of the nuclear gene DNA polymerase gamma (POLG) on chromosome 15, which encodes the polymerase responsible for both replication and repair of the mitochondrial genome, cause a wide variety of diverse phenotypes with different modes of inheritance (Hudson and Chinnery, 2006). These include the autosomal recessive Alpers syndrome of encephalopathy, seizures, and liver failure, an autosomal dominant form of chronic progressive external ophthalmoplegia, and autosomal recessive phenotypes of cerebellar ataxia and peripheral neuropathy, among others.

## Imprinting

For most genes, expression is controlled by distinct cellular processes that operate irrespective of the gene's parental origin. However, for some genes, expression in the offspring differs, depending on whether the allele was maternally or paternally inherited, and such genes are described as being imprinted (Spencer, 2009). *Imprinting* arises from epigenetic modifications such as DNA or histone methylation, which are parent-specific alterations that do not change the actual DNA sequence (Fig. 48.10). One example of this is sex-specific DNA methylation that occurs for some genes during the formation of gametes. In the offspring, the methylated gene is bound by histone proteins forming transcriptionally inactive heterochromatin. This allows all gene expression to be driven by the allele derived from the other parent. This can be dynamic, depending on the gene, and the magnitude of differential expression between the alleles can vary based on stage of development, tissue type, and possibly other factors. Deletion of an imprinted region or defective imprinting in gametogenesis can lead to disease, as illustrated by observations involving chromosome 15q (Lalande and Calciano, 2007; Zoghbi and Beaudet, 2016). In this example, differential methylation affects the expression of multiple genes, and loss of maternal patterning can lead to Angelman syndrome, characterized by intellectual impairment, epilepsy, ataxia, and inappropriate laughter, while loss of the paternal pattern causes Prader-Willi syndrome, associated with intellectual impairment, obesity, and behavioral problems. The most common mechanism involves de novo deletion of the imprinted region from one parent, although in some cases, defective imprinting can also occur during gametogenesis. In the majority of cases, defective imprinting occurs spontaneously and is therefore unlikely to recur in families; however, imprinting defects can rarely be due to small deletions involving sequences important for regulating parent-specific methylation.

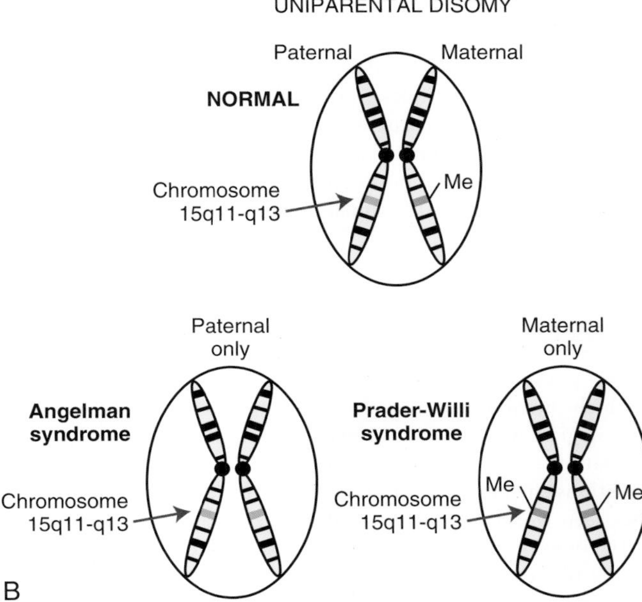


**Fig. 48.10 Epigenetics in Human Disease. A,** Imprinting. Gene expression on human chromosome 15q11-q13 is subject to epigenetic regulation via imprinting. The region contains the loci for two neurological diseases, Prader–Willi syndrome and Angelman syndrome (see text). When inherited from the father, gene expression occurs from the Prader-Willi locus *(blue arrow)*, and this also inactivates genes at the Angelman locus via a presumed antisense-RNA mechanism *(dashed arrow)*. In contrast, when inherited from the mother, a specific site on the chromosome called the *imprinting center (circle)* becomes methylated (Me). This methylation causes transcriptional inactivation of the genes within the Prader-Willi locus *(X)*, which correspondingly allows transcription from genes at the Angelman locus *(purple arrow)*. If imprinting does not properly occur, either Angelman or Prader–Willi syndrome will arise depending on whether the maternal or paternal expression pattern is absent. **B,** Uniparental disomy. During gamete/zygote formation, errors in chromosomal segregation or chromosomal rearrangement can result in retention of all or part of a chromosome inherited from the same parent. Although there is no loss of genetic information, the epigenetic imprinting pattern is lost, and therefore correct gene expression patterns are not retained. For chromosome 15q11-q13, for example, this can give rise to Angelman or Prader–Willi syndrome, depending on whether the duplicated chromosome is that of the father or the mother, respectively.

## Uniparental Disomy

*Uniparental disomy* arises when pairs of chromosomes are inherited from the same parent, either in their entirety or in large segments due to segregation errors or chromosomal rearrangement (Kotzot, 2008; see Fig. 48.10). The uniparentally inherited chromosomes can be identical (isodisomic) or different (heterodisomic). In families where the parents lack underlying chromosomal abnormalities, these events usually occur spontaneously and are unlikely to recur. Disease can result from effects related to loss of chromosomal imprinting, pairing of an autosomal recessive mutation, pairing of an X-linked recessive mutation in a female child, or from the generation of a mosaic trisomy. The disorders most commonly associated with this mechanism are the Prader-Willi and Angelman syndromes, discussed previously for imprinting disorders, which can arise from maternal and paternal uniparental disomy, respectively, due to a loss of the imprinting pattern from the missing parental allele. Down syndrome can also rarely result from a mosaic trisomy. There are several examples in the literature of single cases where an autosomal recessive disease arose in a child from uniparental disomy pairing an abnormal allele from a carrier parent, including disorders such as abetalipoproteinemia, Bloom syndrome, autosomal recessive deafness-1A, spinal muscular atrophy, cystic fibrosis, and others (Zlotogora, 2004).

## COMMON NEUROLOGICAL DISORDERS AND COMPLEX DISEASE GENETICS

To this point, we have focused on Mendelian neurological disease, in which mutations of a single gene are sufficient to cause disease. Neurological diseases with Mendelian inheritance are rare in most populations, and account for less than 5% of those with common conditions such as AD. Yet, many of the common neurological diseases seen worldwide have significant genetic contributions (Table 48.4). For example, twin studies have shown high heritability (≥60%) for AD (Gatz et al., 2006) and autism (Abrahams and Geschwind, 2008; Freitag, 2007), increased relative risk is seen in first-degree relatives of probands with ALS (approximately 10-fold; Fang et al., 2009) and epilepsy (about 2.5-fold; Helbig et al., 2008), and a variety of studies support a degree of heritability in PD (Belin and Westerlund, 2008) and cerebrovascular disease (Matarin et al., 2010). But even when family history is present, the mode of inheritance is not clear, and no major disease-causing Mendelian mutations are usually identified in the majority of cases. So, in contrast to the single-gene Mendelian disorders previously discussed, these common complex genetic conditions appear to be genetically heterogeneous and multifactorial, likely involving interplay between multiple genes, each with small effect size, and environmental factors, none of which are sufficient to be causal, but each of which increases susceptibility to the disorder. This is the basis of the "common disease–common variant" (CDCV) model, which has driven most research into common genetic diseases (Schork et al., 2009). The alternative model is that rather than common SNPs, multiple inherited rare variants of small to intermediate effect size, or de novo mutations with large effect size, underlie genetic risk for common disorders. The difficulty with assessing this latter proposition is that until the very recent advent of efficient genome or exome sequencing, genome-wide identification of such rare variants was not feasible. In contrast, efficient genome-wide assessment of common variation has been possible for several years and has been applied to numerous neurological disorders (for examples see eTable 48.5, available online).  Still, while the exact forms of genetic variation underlying most complex disease are not known, major advances are being made to elucidate their basic genetic architecture (the types of mutations, and the relative contributions of common and rare variation) and there are several large-scale initiatives underway worldwide to investigate genomic contributions at a broader level in many common neurological disorders. Here we discuss examples of strategies currently being used, starting with genome-wide screening for common variation.

### Common Variants and Genome-Wide Association Studies

As already discussed, genetic linkage provides a means of localizing a disease gene to a specific region of a chromosome by using a DNA marker that tracks with affected individuals within families. Linkage analysis, while not without value in genetically complex disease, is less powered than genetic association studies for identification of common variation in complex genetic disease. Genetic association studies assess whether one or more of a defined set of genetic variants are increased or decreased in a disease versus a control population. If a genetic variant is observed in individuals with disease significantly more often or less than expected by chance, that variant is said to be associated with the disease. When one or a few genes are studied, this is a candidate-gene association study. When common variants from across the entire genome are studied in this manner, the result is a genome-wide association study, or GWAS (Mullen et al., 2009; Simon-Sanchez and Singleton, 2008; Fig. 48.11). Original genetic association studies were conducted with a small number of candidate genes, but advances in technology have permitted GWAS in thousands of subjects in a wide variety of human diseases,

**TABLE 48.4 Estimated Heritability of Selected Neurological Diseases**

| Disease | Heritability* | Method | Reference |
|---|---|---|---|
| Alzheimer dementia | 60%–80% | Twin studies | (Gatz et al., 2006) |
| Amyotrophic lateral sclerosis | 21% | Genome-wide complex trait analysis | (Keller et al., 2014) |
| Autism | 70%–90% | Twin studies | (Abrahams and Geschwind, 2008) |
| Epilepsy | 80%† | Twin study | (Kjeldsen et al., 2003) |
| Frontotemporal dementia | 42%‡ | Family history data | (Rohrer et al., 2009) |
| Ischemic stroke | 34%–42%§ | Genome-wide complex trait analysis | (Bluher et al., 2015) |
| Multiple sclerosis | 25%–76% | Twin studies | (Hawkes and Macgregor, 2009) |
| Parkinson disease | 34%–40% | Twin study | (Wirdefeldt et al., 2011) |
| Restless legs syndrome | 40%–90% | Twin studies | (Caylak, 2009) |

*Unless otherwise indicated, percent heritability refers to the proportion of variation attributable to genetic causes

†Varies per syndrome.

‡Estimation based on likelihood of having an affected family member.

§Varies by age of onset.

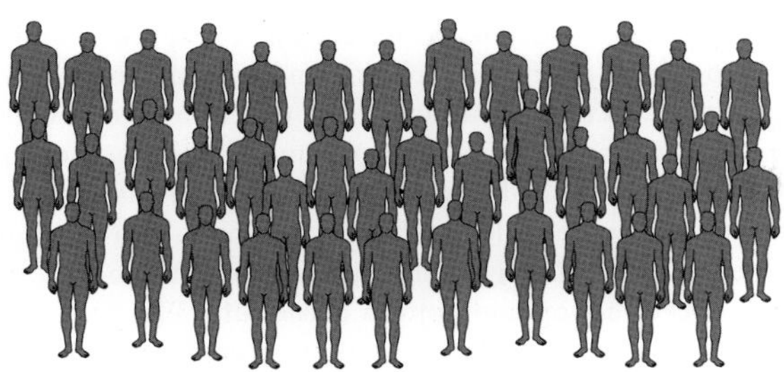
#1 Select population (cases and controls) for study
#2 Genotyping
Single Nucleotide Polymorphism (SNP)
...ACGTCAGTGGCATA...Major allele
...ACGTCAGTCGCATA...Minor allele
#3 Analysis – Is either SNP associated with disease phenotype?

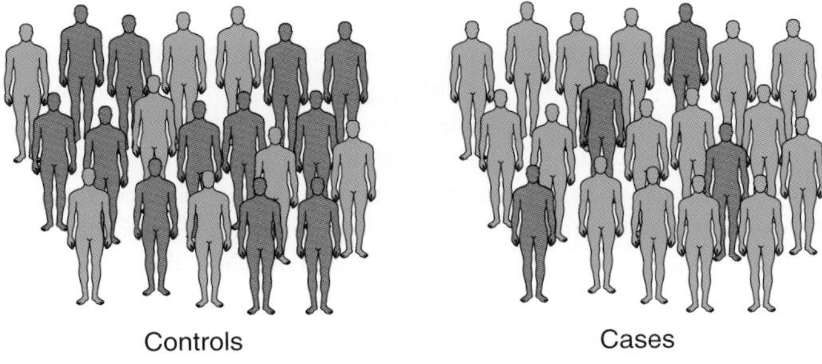
Controls
Cases
Patients with major allele are more likely to have disease
odds ratio > 1.0

**Fig. 48.11 Genome-Wide Association Study.** A genome-wide association study (GWAS) for disease is performed by genotyping a selected population of cases and controls using microarray or other technology for single nucleotide polymorphisms *(SNPs)* across the genome. In this example, a sample SNP is depicted, with major and minor alleles illustrated as *green or red,* respectively. Detailed computational analysis is performed to determine whether any individual SNPs are associated with the disease state greater than by chance. In this example, the major allele *(green)* is associated with the disease and more likely to be present in cases than controls, reflected in an odds ratio above 1.0. Note that while the SNP in question may be involved in the disease, it may also be a marker near an involved gene.

including dozens of neurological conditions (for examples see eTable 48.5, available online) and the GWAS catalogue website, which keeps an up-to-date open resource (see Table 48.3).

Although the SNPs themselves may directly influence the disease under study, most often this is not the case, and SNPs are best thought of as markers for the location of a gene(s) or region relevant to the disease. In fact, most common alleles of the second major type of common genetic variation, CNVs, are mostly captured by SNPs (Conrad et al., 2010) and can be identified by the common SNP genotyping platforms, allowing GWASs to evaluate the contribution of common inherited CNVs as well as SNPs. Further discussion of the use of this technology (including Box 48.2) is available at http://expertconsult.inkling.com.

For the most common neurodegenerative dementia, AD, GWASs have benefited from large numbers of available cases and expanded the loci known to be associated with disease beyond the apolipoprotein E locus to include other neuronal molecules such as BIN1 and PICALM, which are involved in clathrin-mediated endocytosis and intracellular trafficking, and the apolipoprotein CLU (Harold et al., 2009; Lambert et al., 2009; Naj et al., 2011; Seshadri et al., 2010). The most recent GWAS meta-analysis in AD involved almost 95,000 individuals diagnosed with late-onset AD, and confirmed 20 previous loci, while identifying 5 new loci (Kunkle et al., 2019). In PD, recent GWASs in large cohorts of European and Japanese patients identified alpha-synuclein (SNCA) and LRRK2 as susceptibility loci (Edwards et al., 2010; Lill et al., 2012; Satake et al., 2009; Sharma et al., 2012; Simon-Sanchez et al., 2009), which is notable because both genes also give rise to autosomal dominant forms of parkinsonism. The tau protein (*MAPT*), another gene responsible for autosomal dominant forms of parkinsonism, was also found to be associated with disease in European populations (Edwards et al., 2010; Lill et al., 2012; Sharma et al., 2012; Simon-Sanchez et al., 2009). Together these results suggest a commonality between Mendelian and sporadic forms of this disorder.

The cost of SNP genotyping is dropping to the point where GWASs for most common neurological diseases will number in the hundreds of thousands if not millions over the next several years. This low-cost genotyping has fueled the growth of direct-to-consumer genetic testing companies, which commonly utilize findings from such studies to generate risk profiles for their consumers. Consequently, it is important that physicians have a clear understanding of the meaning of these risk profiles and GWAS results so as to be able to differentiate common variants associated with disease from disease-causing mutations. A potential error to be avoided in the clinical interpretation of GWAS data is directly equating the findings to the future development of the disease. It must be reiterated that the finding of an association with a common variant does not equal the finding of a disease gene. By definition, these common variants must have low penetrance; otherwise, they would not be so common in normal individuals, and they would likely act in a more Mendelian way. Furthermore, such variants might be associated with disease modifiers—for example, genes acting either upstream or downstream in pathways where disruption or dysregulation can lead to the disease, or perhaps genes involved in the production or regulation of factors involved in such pathways. Instead of directly causing disease, such modifier genes confer a risk of disease, the magnitude of which is sometimes not directly quantifiable because it involves interaction with other genes and the environment. Therefore, for most conditions, reported GWAS information cannot be directly translated into a clinical setting, because the presence of the variant does not necessarily lead to the disease in most cases, particularly for the more rare disorders. As an example, one of the strongest and best-known identified associations, the apolipoprotein E ε4 allele detected in sporadic AD, with an odds ratio of 4 (Coon et al., 2007), has such an inconsistent predictive value that it is not recommended for routine use in disease prediction nor as a typical part of most clinical dementia evaluations (Knopman et al., 2001). Despite this, commercial organizations do market direct-to-consumer tests for this and other genetic variations associated with disease. As the public has become more aware of the impact of genetics on health and disease, there has been a growing desire for pre-emptive screening, particularly for individuals with family members afflicted with common disease (Sweeny et al., 2014). In response to this need, genetic variation screening tests are often marketed as a means of assessing the potential for future development of disease. Given the caveats discussed, there is no definitive means at present to accurately define an individual's risk of disease based on the presence of one or more associated common variants, and attempting to do so may place patients at unnecessary risk (Bellcross et al., 2012; Brownstein et al., 2014). It is important for the physician to be aware of this insofar as patients may contact them regarding such testing, and it should be emphasized that any positive results would have unclear predictive value.

There are examples of clinically important allelic variants identified by other methods, particularly with regard to pharmacogenomics, so such expectations for GWAS in neurological disease are not unfounded. One such illustration is the variation seen in the cytochrome P450 isoenzyme CYP2C9, which is responsible for the metabolism of a number of clinically relevant pharmaceutical agents, in particular the anticoagulant warfarin (Sanderson et al., 2005).

The major allele CYP2C9*1 is seen in more than 95% of Asian and African populations, but multiple variants commonly exist in European and Caucasian populations, including CYP2C9*2 and CYP2C9*3, both of which reduce warfarin metabolism (Sanderson et al., 2005). In one study, 20% of patients carried either CYP2C9*2 or CYP2C9*3 and required a mean reduction of their warfarin dosage by 27% to maintain an optimal therapeutic range, reflected by an increased relative risk of bleeding of about 2.3 (Sanderson et al., 2005). Although the relative risk in this example is still greater than typically seen in most GWASs (ranging from 1.1 to 1.3), it demonstrates how common variant risk information can potentially affect the care of an individual patient. As we discover more regarding the nature of complex genetic disease, new ways of utilizing this information clinically will likely be determined. In the meantime, the value of GWAS data, especially from a pharmacogenomic research perspective, is significant; it can help identify new genes, pathways, and biological networks related to disease that may have therapeutic benefit (Box 48.1). A recent example identified loci responsible for accelerating or delaying the onset of HD by years (GeM-HD Consortium, 2015), suggesting the possibility of developing disease-modifying therapies targeting the related pathways, once identified.

## BOX 48.1 Pharmacogenetics and Personalized Medicine

In addition to contributing to disease susceptibility, genetic variation can have other medically applicable roles. One of the most highly anticipated benefits for genetic research is the capability of tailoring medical or pharmacological therapies to target a patient's disease based on their individual genotype, a key concept of precision health. The initial application of this concept is in the optimization of drug effects and minimization of toxic side effects based on genotype, termed pharmacogenetics (Chan et al., 2011; Holmes et al., 2009). Although this field has not yet advanced to the point of routine clinic use, there are several examples of the potential utility and the benefit to patients we may hope to see in the near future (Chan et al., 2011).

- In stroke, genetic variation has been found to impact patient response to antiplatelet agents and anticoagulants (Meschia, 2009; see main text) and influence statin-associated myopathy (Link et al., 2008; Meschia, 2009). In a recent GWAS analysis, an association was demonstrated between a SNP in the *SLCO1B1* gene, which encodes a membrane protein that mediates liver uptake of various drugs including statins, and myopathy (odds ratio [OR] 4.3 when heterozygous and 17.4 when homozygous; Link et al., 2008), clearly reflecting a need to modify statin treatment in such patients.
- In epilepsy, GWAS analysis has identified the HLA-A*3101 allele as associated with carbamazepine-induced hypersensitivity reactions in patients of Northern European (OR = 12.4, 95% confidence interval 1.27–121.03; McCormack et al., 2011) and Japanese (OR = 10.8, 95% confidence interval 5.9–19.6; Ozeki et al., 2011) descent, suggesting a need to consider individual genotype when selecting antiepileptic medications.
- In Parkinson disease, patients with the *COMT*$^{HH}$ genotype, reflecting a homozygous SNP that modulates catechol-O-methyltransferase activity, show a more clinically effective response to entacapone during a L-dopa challenge (Corvol et al., 2011), suggesting genotyping may play a useful role in the management of an individual patient's drug therapies.

A number of practical issues will have to be solved before such testing can achieve widespread use in the clinic, particularly determinations of the clinical benefit relative to cost-effectiveness in specific diseases and populations (Chan et al., 2011; Holmes et al., 2009; Meschia, 2009; Swen et al., 2007); however, recent rapid advancements in technology, such as next-generation DNA sequencing, may prove beneficial in this arena (Chan et al., 2011). In fact, some diagnostic laboratories are already offering this information to patients as part of routine diagnostic testing that utilizes genomic sequencing.

Lastly, as GWASs expand and we are able to capture a sufficiently large proportion of genetic risk, prediction based on scores composed of the additive effects of common genetic variation becomes possible. *Polygenic risk scores* (PRS) are based on summing the weighted effects of thousands of individual SNPs associated with disease risk at some nominal, non–genome-wide significance threshold. In many common medical conditions, ranging from hyperlipidemia to obesity, the difference between the top and bottom deciles of a PRS are as large as those observed with Mendelian mutations (Khera et al., 2018, 2019). In AD, for example, although these scores are not yet useful for population-level diagnostics, the difference between the lowest and highest deciles corresponds to approximately a 10-year difference in age of onset (Chasioti et al., 2019). As PRS scores are refined, they can be used to explore potential mechanistic overlap between disorders (Brainstorm Consortium et al., 2018), and to serve as essential components in disease risk assessment algorithms, especially for enhancing the efficiency and effectiveness of surveillance and screening, as well as stratification for treatment.

## Rare Variants and Candidate Gene Resequencing

So far, common variation is only able to explain a small percentage of genetic risk for common neurological disease. The other major model that attempts to explain what is currently referred to as the missing heritability (Manolio et al., 2009) in complex genetic disease implicates rare variants with medium to high penetrance instead of more common ones with low penetrance (Schork et al., 2009; Fig. 48.12). *Rare variants* are defined as DNA alterations that are found in less than 1% of most populations or, in some cases,

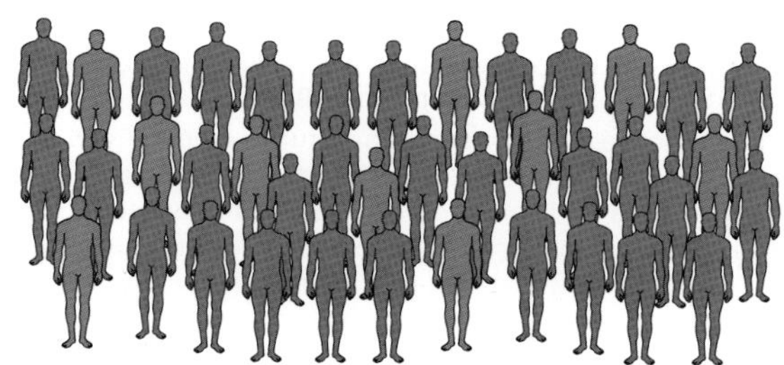

Common disease, common variant
(variant identifiable by GWAS)

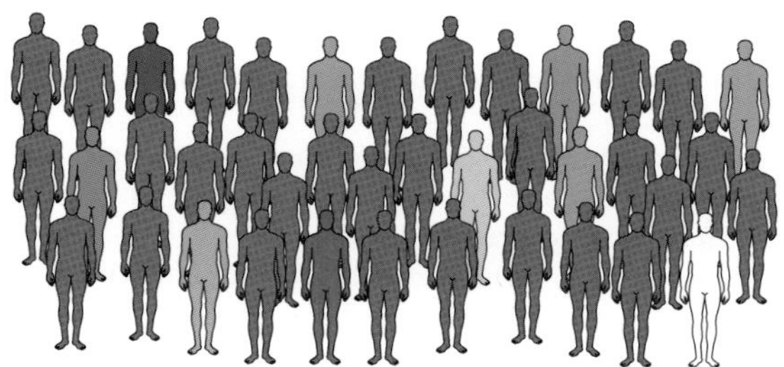

Common disease, rare variant
(variant too rare to be identifiable by GWAS)

**Fig. 48.12 Models of Causal Variants in Complex Disease.** In the common disease–common variant model, risk of disease is imparted by the presence of one or more gene variants present in 5% or more of the population *(red)*. Such variants are amenable to detection by genome-wide association studies *(GWAS)*. Conversely, in the common disease–rare variant model, disease is caused by rare genetic variants present in less than 1% of the population or only in specific families *(various colors)*. Such variants would not be amenable to detection by GWAS, since they would not be represented in large enough numbers to generate statistical significance. Note that both models are not mutually exclusive, and both may contribute to common disease.

are "private" and only seen in specific affected families. In this model, one or more rare variants, alone or in combination with common variants, produce the disease in question. A GWAS is not well suited to detect these variants, because they are rare and most likely to be relatively recent mutations that do not segregate on common haplotypes measured in these studies. Even when they do, they do not occur at high enough frequency in the general population to provide statistical power for their detection using current sample sizes. Detection generally requires resequencing of potentially involved candidate genes in a defined population of patients and controls. One major difficulty of such investigations is that the baseline level of rare variation among normal humans was not clearly established until recently. Studies such as the 1000 and 100,000 Genomes Projects (https://www.genomicsengland.co.uk/), the UK10K project (Consortium UK et al., 2015), the Exome Aggregation Consortium (ExAC; Kobayashi et. al., 2017), and the Genome Aggregation Database (gnomAD; Lek et al., 2016; see Table 48.3) catalog normal human variation in hundreds of thousands of individuals, allowing researchers to better define this class of rare variants and develop more effective strategies for their detection. There is expected to be a significant rare-variant burden across all common neurological diseases, and WGS (see below) will be necessary to detect such variants. In ALS, it is estimated that a significant proportion of the risk is imparted by low-frequency variants in the 1% frequency range (Chasioti et al., 2019). WGS has also identified many new risk genes in AD (Cruchaga et al., 2014; Jin et al., 2014). Similar architecture is likely in other dementias, where rare but non-Mendelian low- to moderate-effect-size risk variants, such as the A152T mutation in *MAPT*, contribute to disease risk (Coppola et al., 2012; Labbe et al., 2015; Lee et al., 2013).

An early example of the sequencing-based rare variant approach involves the developmental disorder autism, where sequencing of the gene contactin-associated protein-like 2 (*CNTNAP2*) in 635 patients with autism spectrum disorder (ASD) and 942 controls found 13 rare variants unique to patients, including one which was seen in 4 patients from 3 unrelated families (Bakkaloglu et al., 2008). Recessively inherited mutations in *CNTNAP2* in an Amish family with a syndromic form of autism with epilepsy provided the most convincing evidence for the causal role of mutations in this gene (Strauss et al., 2006). Interestingly, this same gene illustrates that the common disease–rare variant and CDCV hypotheses are not mutually exclusive, since common variants in this gene modulate language function in ASD and other conditions (Alarcon et al., 2008; Vernes et al., 2008). Integrating genetic and clinical data from human studies with other investigative approaches to understanding gene function (i.e., animal disease models) can better define mechanisms of disease pathogenesis and may suggest novel treatment strategies (Penagarikano et al., 2011; Penagarikano and Geschwind, 2012). Next-generation DNA sequencing (see Genome/Exome Sequencing in Clinical Practice, Disease Gene Discovery, and Gene Therapy) will allow the analysis of many whole exomes and whole genomes to better understand to what extent common and/or rare variants contribute to many common neurological diseases, ranging from autism (Ramaswami and Geschwind, 2018) to dementia (Carmona and Guerreiro, 2018; Patel et al., 2019; Pottier et al., 2019).

## Copy Number Variation and Chromosomal Microarray Analysis

The majority of variation and disease-causing mutations discussed to this point have centered around single base-pair changes in DNA sequence. However, as previously described in Structural Chromosomal Abnormalities and Copy Number Variation, the CNV (Beckmann et al., 2007; Stankiewicz and Lupski, 2010; Wain et al., 2009; Zhang et al., 2009; see Fig. 48.14) actually represents more total real estate in our genome. Advances in methods such as the advent of the microarray indicate that such changes occur quite commonly (at $10^{-4}$–$10^{-6}$ per locus per generation) compared with single-nucleotide changes ($10^{-8}$ per base pair per generation on average) (Lupski, 2007). Overall, CNVs are estimated to represent at least 4% (Conrad et al., 2010) and potentially up to 13% of the total human genome (Redon et al., 2006; Stankiewicz and Lupski, 2010). The high frequency of these events may reflect an evolutionary advantage of CNVs as a mechanism for producing genetic diversity (Zhang et al., 2009) but such frequency also implies that clinically relevant CNVs are quite likely to occur de novo, more frequently than point mutations (Table 48.6). CNVs can potentially cause disease in numerous ways, including disruption of a gene's coding region (which could cause a dominant effect or release a recessive effect on the homologous allele) or by altering regulated gene expression via positive or negative dosage effects. If the CNV itself results in the disease phenotype, it could be transmitted as a Mendelian disorder, as is the case for CMT type 1A. Such CNVs may be examples of rare variants in the common disease model. Alternatively, their contribution may be more subtle and insidious, with low penetrance and variable expressivity contributing to the risk of a complex genetic disease, such as in autism (Bucan et al., 2009).

CNVs can be detected via essentially the same microarray technology used to detect SNPs, with only a few minor adjustments. In this case, DNA probes corresponding to specific chromosomal regions are placed on an array and hybridized with differentially fluorescent-labeled genomic DNA from the individual being studied and from a reference genomic DNA sample, a technique termed *array comparative genomic hybridization* (CGH) but more commonly called *chromosomal microarray analysis* (CMA) (Fig. 48.13, *A*). The average ratio of fluorescence is normalized across the array and then evaluated for each probe. If both samples hybridize to a given probe equally, the corresponding DNA region is present equally in both samples. However, if the DNA sample being studied hybridizes more or less intensely than the reference sample, it must contain either more or less of the chromosomal region in question, thus indicating a CNV at that location. The minimum size of a CNV that can be detected by this method is limited to the genomic distance between the minimum number of probes needed to observe a statistically significant signal change, but is usually on the order of kilobases for the highest resolution arrays. The same microarrays used to genotype SNPs in GWASs may also be used to detect CNVs, incorporating both intensity and inheritance data. Array CGH essentially produces a molecular karyotype capable of detecting genomic structural changes with much finer detail than routine microscopic methods. In most major diagnostic labs, this method has replaced microscopic karyotyping and FISH, the latter of which is now used for confirmation. Next-generation sequencing methods, in particular WGS, will likely eventually supersede these methods for clinical diagnostics, as it has a much higher resolution and can more accurately determine CNV boundaries (see Genome/Exome Sequencing in Clinical Practice, Disease Gene Discovery, and Gene Therapy).

Some examples of clinically relevant CNVs are seen in Mendelian disorders, including adult-onset autosomal-dominant leukodystrophy (autosomal dominant, caused by duplication of the lamin B1 gene on chromosome 5), CMT type 1A (autosomal dominant, most frequently caused by duplication of the peripheral myelin protein 22 on chromosome 17), hereditary liability to pressure palsies (autosomal dominant, most commonly due to deletion of the peripheral myelin protein 22 on chromosome 17), spastic paraplegia type 4 (autosomal dominant,

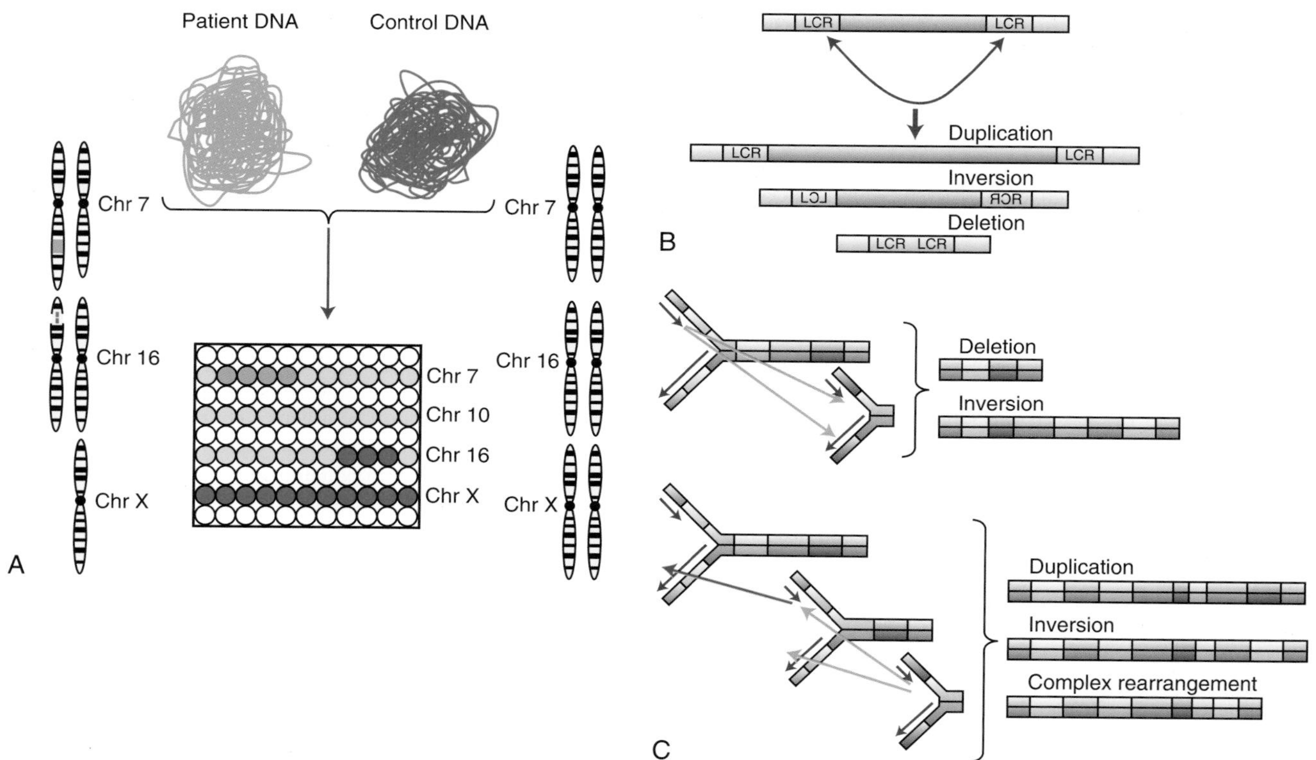


**Fig. 48.13 Copy Number Variation. A,** Copy number variation can be detected via comparative genomic hybridization or chromosomal microarray analysis, shown here. In this example, patient genomic deoxyribonucleic acid *(DNA)* and an equal amount of control DNA is hybridized to a microarray platform containing representative probes spanning the genome at a specified resolution, usually at the kilobase level. In the illustration, patient DNA is fluorescently labeled *green,* and control DNA is labeled *red.* Following hybridization, regions present in equal amounts are *yellow,* whereas regions duplicated in the patient are *green,* and deletions are *red.* In this example, the patient possesses two copy number variations (CNVs), a duplication on chromosome 7 (illustrated by the increased *green signal* at that locus on the array) and a deletion on chromosome 16 (with corresponding increased *red signal* at the locus). The patient also has Turner syndrome (monosomy X) reflected by the increased *red signal* across the entire chromosome. Chromosome 10 is shown as an example of a chromosome that does not differ between the samples *(yellow).* **B,** Introduction of CNVs by the nonallelic homologous recombination (NAHR) mechanism. NAHR occurs when genomic instability is introduced by the presence of low copy repeat *(LCR)* regions greater than 1 kilobase in size with more than 90% homology. Pairing of nearby regions during DNA replication can lead to deletions, duplications, or inversions as illustrated. **C,** Introduction of CNVs by the fork stalling and template switching (FoSTeS) mechanism. FoSTeS occurs when replication on the lagging strand stalls during DNA replication and resumes at an adjacent replication fork. The structural variation introduced depends on whether the reinitiation occurs upstream or downstream of the original fork and whether it occurs on the lagging or leading strand. Examples of how deletions, duplications, or inversions might result are shown *(orange arrows).* Furthermore, if more than one FoSTeS event occurs *(purple arrow),* a complex structural rearrangement could result.

occasionally caused by deletion of the spastin gene on chromosome 2), juvenile PD 2 (autosomal recessive, occasionally caused by deletions or duplications in parkin on chromosome 6), and Williams syndrome (autosomal dominant, caused by deletion of several contiguous genes on chromosome 7).

CNVs are also particularly important for neurodevelopmental disorders, with de novo CNVs present in more than 5% of patients with ID (Koolen et al., 2009) or ASD (Bucan et al., 2009; Marshall et al., 2008; Pinto et al., 2010; Sebat et al., 2007). Based on these findings, chromosomal microarray is now clinically indicated in children with a wide range of neurodevelopmental disabilities including ID and ASD (Miller, D.T., et al., 2010). Such studies have revealed several potential new autism candidate genes as well as novel biological pathways for future study of disease pathogenesis (Bucan et al., 2009; Pinto et al., 2010). Remarkably, de novo CNVs are also associated with schizophrenia (Stefansson et al., 2008; Walsh et al., 2008), especially childhood-onset forms, and some of the same CNVs observed in ASD are also observed in schizophrenia (Cantor and Geschwind, 2008), suggesting some shared liability between what were previously considered clinically distinct conditions.

## GENOME/EXOME SEQUENCING IN CLINICAL PRACTICE, DISEASE GENE DISCOVERY, AND GENE THERAPY

The identification of disease genes and their mutations hinges on the capability to sequence DNA to assess for detrimental alterations. Initially, the standard method of DNA sequencing technology most commonly in use was called *Sanger sequencing.* Although effective and accurate, the high throughput of this method was severely limited by reaction time and length of read, which is less than 1 kilobase, limiting use for single-gene testing or small-gene panels. More recently, another technology has taken hold for high-throughput diagnostic testing (Lee et al., 2019). Termed *next-generation sequencing* (Lee et al., 2019; Mardis, 2013; McGinn and Gut, 2013; Metzker, 2010; Rexach et al., 2019), this method can rapidly generate large amounts of high-quality DNA sequence information in a relatively inexpensive and efficient manner (Table 48.7). The sequence of the human genome was derived using Sanger sequencing over a 13-year period, and subsequent Sanger sequencing of human genomes took roughly a year, but next-generation sequencing can now accomplish the same feat in hours. Therefore, it has become possible to

**TABLE 48.6 Selected Neurological Diseases Caused by Copy Number Variation**

| Disease | Locus | Variation | Gene* | Inheritance† |
|---|---|---|---|---|
| Alzheimer dementia | 21q21 | Duplication | *APP* | Complex |
| Amyotrophic lateral sclerosis | 5q12.2-q13.3 | Deletion | *SMN1* | Complex |
| Angelman syndrome | 15q11-q12 | Maternal deletion | *UBE3A* | Sporadic |
| Aniridia | 11p13 | Deletion | *AN* | Sporadic |
| Ataxia with oculomotor apraxia type 2 | 9q34.13 | Deletion | *SETX* | Mendelian |
| Autism spectrum disorder | 2p16.3 | Deletion | *NRXN1* | Complex |
| | 15q11-q13 | Deletion or duplication | *Many* | Complex, sporadic |
| | 16p11.2 | Deletion or duplication | *Many* | Complex, sporadic |
| | 22q13.3 | Deletion | *SHANK3* | Complex |
| | Xp22.33 | Deletion | *NLGN4* | Complex |
| Autosomal dominant leuko-dystrophy | 5q23.2 | Duplication | *LMNB1* | Mendelian |
| Charcot-Marie-Tooth type 1A | 17p12 | Duplication | *PMP22* | Mendelian |
| Charcot-Marie-Tooth type 4B2 | 11p15.4 | Deletion | *SBF2* | Mendelian |
| CHARGE syndrome | 8q12.1 | Deletion | *CHD7* | Sporadic |
| Cri du chat syndrome | 5p15.2-p15.3 | Deletion | *Many* | Sporadic |
| DiGeorge and velocardiofa-cial syndrome | 22q11.2 | Deletion | *Many* | Sporadic |
| Duchenne/Becker muscular dystrophy | Xp21.2 | Deletion or duplication | *DMD* | Mendelian |
| Epilepsy | 15q13.3 | Deletion | *CHRNA7* | Complex |
| Hereditary neuropathy with liability to pressure palsies | 17p12 | Deletion | *PMP22* | Mendelian |
| Miller-Dieker syndrome | 17p13.3 | Deletion | *LIS1* | Sporadic |
| Neurofibromatosis type 1 | 17q11.2 | Deletion or duplication | *NF1* | Sporadic |
| Parkinson disease | 4q21 | Duplication or triplication | *SNCA* | Mendelian |
| Pelizaeus-Merzbacher disease | Xq22.2 | Deletion or duplication | *PLP1* | Mendelian |
| Potocki-Lupski syndrome | 17p11.2 | Duplication | *RAI1* | Sporadic |
| Prader-Willi syndrome | 15q11-q12 | Paternal deletion | *Many* | Sporadic |
| Rett syndrome and variants | Xq28 | Deletion or duplication | *MECP2* | Sporadic |
| Rubinstein-Taybi syndrome | 16p13.3 | Deletion or duplication | *CREBBP* | Sporadic |
| Schizophrenia | 2q31.2 | Deletion | *RAPGEF4* | Complex |
| | 2q34 | Deletion | *ERBB4* | Complex |
| | 5p13.3 | Deletion | *SLC1A3* | Complex |
| | 12q24 | Deletion | *CIT* | Complex |
| Silver-Russell syndrome | 11p15 | Duplication | *Many* | Complex |
| Smith-Magenis syndrome | 17p11.2 | Deletion | *RAI1* | Sporadic |
| Sotos syndrome | 5q35 | Deletion | *NSD1* | Sporadic |
| Spinal muscular atrophy | 5q13 | Deletion | *SMN1* | Mendelian |
| Tuberous sclerosis | 16p13.3 | Deletion or duplication | *TSC2* | Sporadic |
| WAGR syndrome | 11p13 | Deletion | *Many* | Sporadic |
| Williams-Beuren syndrome | 7q11.23 | Deletion | *ELN* | Sporadic |
| Other microdeletion/dupli-cation syndromes with developmental delay and/or mental retardation | 1q41-q42 | Deletion | *Many* | Sporadic |
| | 2q37 | Deletion | *Many* | Sporadic |
| | 3q29 | Deletion or duplication | *Many* | Sporadic |
| | 7q11.23 | Duplication | *Many* | Sporadic |
| | 17q21.3 | Deletion or duplication | *Many* | Sporadic |
| | 22q11.2 | Duplication | *Many* | Complex |

*If a single causative or strong candidate gene is known. If multiple genes are suspected to be involved, this is indicated.

†Inheritance is described as sporadic if the variation typically arises de novo in patients, complex if it most commonly increases disease susceptibility (rare familial mutations may also occur), and Mendelian if it is typically inherited.

*Table adapted from Fanciulli et al. (2010), Lee and Scherer (2010), Stankiewicz and Lupski (2010), Wain et al. (2009) with additional data from online public databases of genomic variation (listed in Table 48.3) as needed.*

**TABLE 48.7 Comparison of DNA-Sequencing Technologies for Genome Sequencing**

| | Sanger | Next-Generation |
|---|---|---|
| Technology | Dye-terminator | Massively parallel* |
| Approximate read length (bases) | 500–800 | 50–100† |
| Current clinical use | Gene mutation analysis | Exome, genome, and gene mutation analysis |
| Number of individual genomes sequenced and published | 1‡ | Many |
| Estimated clinical cost per gene sequenced | US$Hundreds to thousands | US$0.05 or less |
| Estimated cost per genome§ | US$Millions | ~US$800 |
| Estimated time per genome§ | Years | Hours |

*A number of commercial platforms exist which utilize variations in this technology.
†Most common, varies per specific platform used.
‡Not including the Human Genome Project reference genome.
§Not including bioinformatic analysis.

rapidly interrogate an individual patient's DNA on a genome-wide level for disease-causing mutations. Several different technologies exist under the next-generation sequencing umbrella and cannot be fully described here (for details, see Mardis, 2013; Metzker, 2010; McGinn and Gut, 2013). The same technology can also be applied to mRNA to study gene expression and/or alternative splicing on a genome-wide basis. This technology has dramatically reduced the cost of sequencing an entire genome to less than a fraction of 1% of the cost of Sanger technology (Mardis, 2013; Metzker, 2010; McGinn and Gut, 2013), and as costs are becoming comparable to other forms of current clinical testing, we are beginning to see diagnostic laboratories offer clinical genome sequencing. Although this technology brings new questions regarding data storage, analysis, and quality control, the translation to use in a clinical setting has already begun, adding new powerful technology to the clinician's repertoire, capable of assessing genetic variation on a genome-wide scale (Coppola and Geschwind, 2012). The first example of the clinical utility of this approach was demonstrated by Lupski and colleagues, who sequenced the genome of the proband in a family with a previously undiagnosed form of CMT disease type 1 (Lupski et al., 2010). By comparing the proband's genome sequence with the human genome reference sequence, over 3.4 million SNPs and 234 CNVs were detected and subsequently pared down using a more detailed analysis until compound heterozygous mutations were identified in the *SH3TC2* gene on chromosome 5, a gene previously shown to cause a different form of CMT, CMT type 4C (Lupski et al., 2010). The new mutations identified within this single family revealed an unexpected level of complexity and highlighted an observation that has become more common as more clinical exome sequencing has been performed,—namely, that genomic sequencing methods may be clinically necessary to identify many disease-causing mutations, even in known disease genes, as they lead to unexpected phenotypic variation distinct from the classically reported presentations of the disease.

Although extremely powerful, the complexities of data interpretation and analysis present a formidable challenge to the routine use of genome sequencing in the clinic. As an initial step in the transition of this technology to the clinical arena, a significant reduction in cost, data volume, and degree of analysis can be achieved by selecting only genomic regions containing protein-coding information for sequencing, a process called *whole exome sequencing* (WES; Choi et al., 2009; Hedges et al., 2009; Ng et al., 2009; Rexach et al., 2019). These coding sequences are initially enriched from a pool of total genomic DNA and then subjected to next-generation sequencing. Although this method is unable to detect relevant noncoding events, and is limited in its ability to observe structural events such as CNV, it still proves useful as a means of evaluating Mendelian disorders caused by coding mutations, which are considered to represent up to 85% of disease-causing mutations (Cooper et al., 1995), although this is likely an overestimate. The utility of the technique was illustrated by early reports using this technology to detect novel mutations causing distal arthrogryposis type 2A (Freeman-Sheldon syndrome; Ng et al., 2009), to confirm an unanticipated diagnosis of congenital chloride diarrhea (Choi et al., 2009), and to elucidate the gene underlying postaxial acrofacial dysostosis (Miller syndrome; Ng et al., 2010). In the past few years, the use of exome sequencing has dramatically increased for the identification of disease genes both in individual families and in populations of patients with disease. Some recent examples of the effectiveness of this method include the discovery of *MATR3* (Johnson et al., 2014), *PFN1* (Wu et al., 2012), and *VCP* (Johnson et al., 2010) in familial ALS, *ADA2* in early-onset stroke (Zhou et al., 2014), *GNAO1* in epileptic encephalopathy (Nakamura et al., 2013), *KCND3* in SCA22 (Lee et al., 2012), *TGM6* in SCA35 (Wang et al., 2010), *KCNT1* in nocturnal frontal lobe epilepsy (Heron et al., 2012), *ATP1A3* in alternating hemiplegia of childhood (Heinzen et al., 2012), and numerous studies identifying novel or published mutations in known disease genes associated with classic or variant presentations. Next-generation sequencing is now the most common tool used for large-scale sequencing and gene discovery, with over 20,000 publications in the last 5 years. Clinically, its comprehensive and unbiased nature coupled with its relative low cost has established next-generation sequencing, namely exome sequencing, as the most effective diagnostic test for evaluating clinically heterogeneous diseases (see Clinical Approach to the Patient with Suspected Neurogenetic Disease) such as xeroderma pigmentosum (Ortega-Recalde et al., 2013), CMT disease (Choi et al., 2012), or SCA (Fogel et al., 2014a; Sailer et al., 2012; Sawyer et al., 2014).

Next-generation methods also make possible the concomitant examination of the mitochondrial genome as well as the exome or genome (Dinwiddie et al., 2013; Picardi and Pesole, 2012). This can be clinically useful, as mitochondrial dysfunction can arise from mutations in both the mitochondrial and nuclear genomes. Furthermore, in addition to identification of Mendelian mutations, this technology also allows for a more detailed exploration of complex genetic variation. In studies of common disease, it may prove a more effective means of assessing the contributions of rare variants than other methods such as a GWAS (Cirulli and Goldstein, 2010). Additionally, it may also identify novel types of variation such as double- and triple-nucleotide polymorphisms, which generate amino acid changes more than 90% and 99% of the time, respectively, and occur at 1% the density of SNPs (Rosenfeld et al., 2010). Future studies will have to further assess the contribution of such novel DNA changes to human disease, but the current findings confirm that next-generation sequencing technology will be able to uncover new types of functional genomic variation.

Genome sequencing may also provide new information regarding environmental contributions to disease. For example, genome sequencing was reported from a pair of monozygotic twins who were discordant for multiple sclerosis (MS; Baranzini et al., 2010). No significant genomic, transcriptional, or epigenetic changes were found to explain disease disconcordance between these twins (Baranzini et al., 2010), suggesting there may be other critical genetic or epigenetic factors not examined by this study, or that key differences may lie in other cell types, or that as-yet-undetermined environmental factors are contributing to disease—conclusions that would not be possible to establish without next-generation sequencing technology.

Lastly, new therapies directed at specific gene targets are beginning to enter the clinic. Drugs called anti-sense oligonucleotides, which alter the expression of specific disease-associated RNAs, are now available for spinal muscular atrophy (Finkel et al., 2017) and Duchenne muscular dystrophy (Lim et al., 2017), offering treatment options to patients who previously had none, with dramatic results in some cases (Finkel et al., 2017). Drugs that reintroduce working copies of dysfunctional genes, termed gene replacement therapies, are also being introduced for disorders such as *RPE65*-mediated retinal dystrophy (Ledford, 2017; Russell et al., 2017), spinal muscular atrophy (Mendell et al., 2017), and X-linked adrenoleukodystrophy (Eichler et al., 2017) with more in preclinical development or approaching clinical trial. This emphasizes the need for early and precise genetic diagnoses and supports the use of genomic diagnostic techniques such as next-generation sequencing to achieve this (Rexach et al., 2019).

## FUTURE ROLE OF SYSTEMS BIOLOGY IN NEUROGENETIC DISEASE

The complex relationship between genetic risk variants, even when they are inherited in a Mendelian fashion, and clinical features, or the relationship of these mutations to disease pathophysiology, present significant challenges to the use of genetics for diagnosis and therapeutics. There are many diseases, including virtually all neurodegenerative disorders, where knowledge of the specific causative gene has not immediately yielded new curative therapies but has instead raised many new questions regarding the underlying molecular etiology of the disease. Although there is hope for development of gene-specific therapies in the near future for a small percentage of these conditions (Rexach et al., 2019), for the remainder, research into the underlying mechanisms is essential to uncover new therapeutic targets. Toward that goal, the technologies discussed have made greater amounts of information available for scientific analysis than ever before. For example, microarrays can be used to study not only genome-wide genetic variation via SNPs, as described earlier, but also variations in gene expression (Fig. 48.14). For this method, the array platform contains probes that are complementary to genome-wide mRNA sequences, and the study is performed by hybridizing the array with fluorescently labeled mRNA collected from either patients or controls. The intensity of the fluorescent signal can be used to determine and compare the relative levels of expression for each gene across the samples. Similar techniques can also be used to evaluate RNA splicing with probes that correspond to all the exons in a given gene and then assessing samples for their alternative usage in cases and controls. Next-generation sequencing can also be used to study RNA expression and splicing on a genome-wide scale in individual tissues or even in single cells (Gandal et al., 2018; Wang et al., 2018). With the availability of data encompassing both genetic variation and gene expression in clinically evaluated patients and controls, it becomes possible to incorporate and synthesize the totality of this information together in ways that assess phenotype, genetic variation, and gene expression simultaneously in a more comprehensive way. This field of study, known as *systems biology*, strives to use these sets of information to develop detailed genetic pathways to identify related genes and genetic programs relevant to disease (Geschwind and Konopka, 2009; see Fig. 48.14). Such integrative analysis, a critical aspect to the concept of precision health (Ashley, 2015; Rexach et al., 2019), has begun to accelerate our understanding of disease pathogenesis and generate new insights into more effective treatment strategies, which will only improve as we learn more and the techniques improve.

One example of this type of systems biology approach involves using gene expression data, such as from microarray studies, to group individual genes according to their degree of coexpression, forming functionally related gene expression modules. These modules are then graphed according to the interconnectivity of their members, which produces a network of correlations centered around one or more key genes, termed *hubs*, which functionally drive the association either directly or indirectly. Further assessment of these hub genes and their connections can identify potentially important genes and biological pathways affected in disease. Such techniques have been applied to the study of AD (Miller et al., 2008, 2010). Epilepsy (Winden et al., 2011), HIV-associated dementia (Levine et al., 2013), ALS (Saris et al., 2009), chronic fatigue syndrome (Presson et al., 2008), hereditary cerebellar ataxia (Fogel et al., 2014b), and schizophrenia (Torkamani et al., 2010), and have already led to new therapeutic targets (Swarup et al., 2019). In one of these examples, the observance of shared molecular disease underpinnings between humans and mice with drastically differing phenotypes (Fogel et al., 2014b) led to the observation of a new phenotype in patients (Becherel et al., 2019). These various systems biology studies illustrate the versatility of such an approach and the potential impact these studies can have on research into complex disease pathogenesis.

## ENVIRONMENTAL CONTRIBUTIONS TO NEUROGENETIC DISEASE

Although this chapter has principally dealt with the molecular aspect of neurogenetic disease, the contributions of the environment cannot be overlooked, particularly for complex genetic disease. Aside from perhaps the few Mendelian disorders with complete penetrance, all genetic disorders are likely influenced either directly by environmental factors or indirectly by the influence of the environment on other aspects of the patient's genetic background. Despite this, we still know very little regarding the precise role of the environment in the development of neurogenetic disease, and this is therefore an important area requiring further study (Reis and Roman, 2007). Monozygotic twin studies and animal studies have both indicated that environmental influences can affect the development/severity of Mendelian genetic disease, as well as more complex disorders, but precisely how this occurs in a genetically susceptible individual remains a mystery. Many suggestions have been postulated for various disorders, including exposures to diverse physical, chemical, or biological insults, but an overall comprehensive picture has yet to develop. For example, MS is a complex neurological disease that likely results from a combination of genetic susceptibility and environmental contributions, all of which may act independently of one another (Banwell et al., 2011; Handel et al., 2010), and is one of the most well-studied neurological disorders for environmental influence. Several environmental factors have been postulated to play a role in the development of MS. These include vitamin D levels, which may explain epidemiological findings that MS risk is associated with geographical location in childhood and month of birth; exposure to Epstein–Barr virus, which is associated with increased MS risk if it occurs after the age of 15 years; and smoking, which appears to increase MS risk and can worsen established disease course (Banwell et al., 2011; Handel et al., 2010). Similarly, in Parkinson disease, studies examining prior environmental exposures have found links to air pollution and pesticides (Lee et al., 2016; Narayan et al., 2017). If such environmental influences could be linked to specific molecular and/or cellular events that may trigger disease in genetically susceptible individuals, it would have a dramatic impact on our understanding of disease pathogenesis, our treatment of established patients, and our recommended preventive strategies to reduce disease. The influx of new genetic information identifying risk factors for complex disease is expected to stimulate research into the impact of the environment on these variants (Traynor, 2009), ideally translating into improvements in our understanding of the environmental effects on neurogenetic disease.

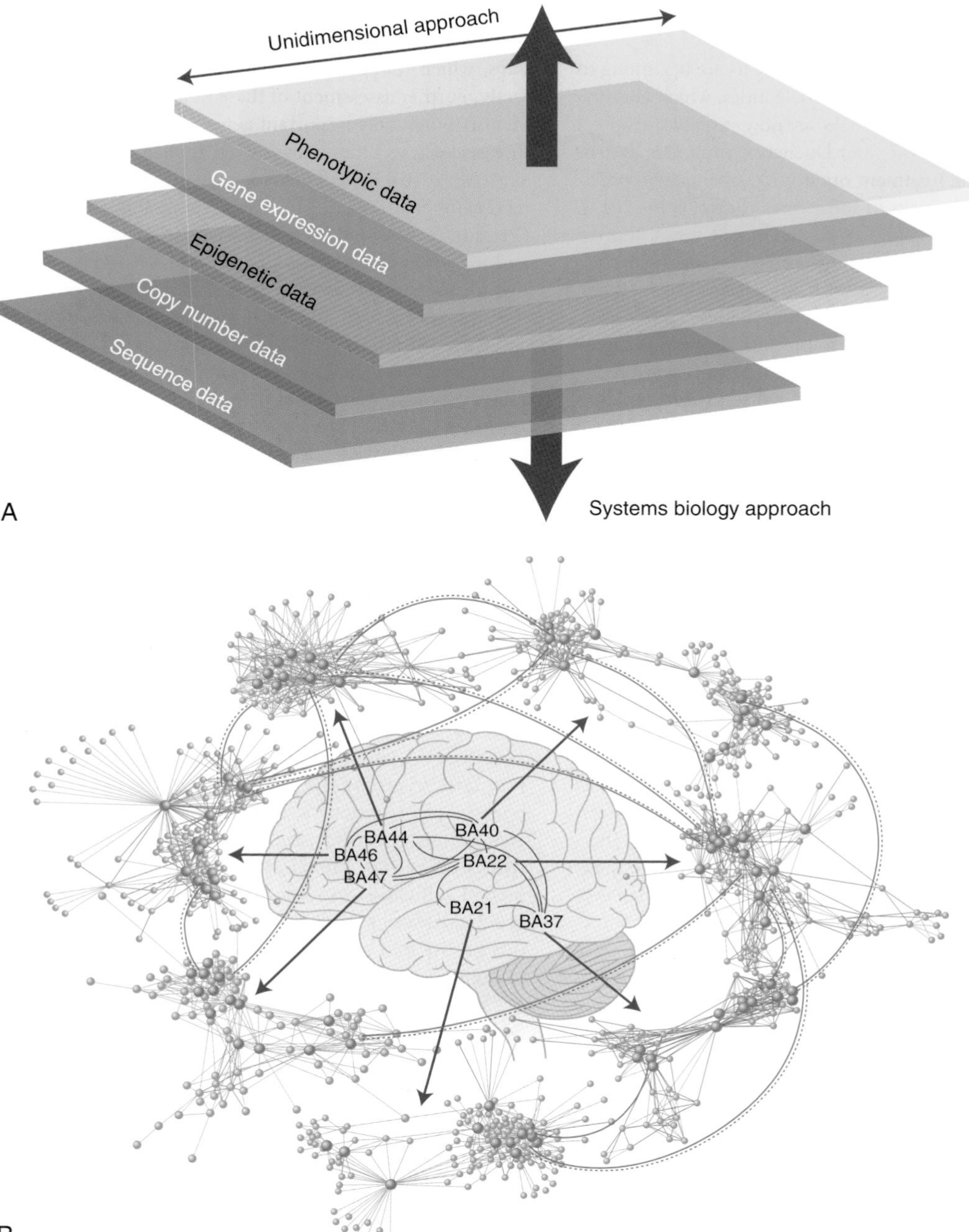


**Fig. 48.14 A Systems Biology Approach to Human Disease Allows Integration of Multiple Layers of Data. A,** Typical experimental approaches to neurological diseases are one-dimensional and, most commonly, efforts focus on a single layer of information such as genetic data (e.g., sequence variants), genomic data (e.g., gene expression changes), or clinical data (e.g., phenotypes). The systems biology approach considers all these aspects simultaneously, using comprehensive databases to explore the relationships between the individual data sets by identifying higher-level structure. This multidimensional use of the data sets (e.g., via network analysis) links the different types of information. **B,** An example using a systems-based approach to study regional gene expression in the brain, using network-based analysis and imaging data to provide insights into brain connectivity. This is a stylized visualization of the combination of diffusion tensor imaging of language areas, with gene expression and weighted gene coexpression network analysis to reveal integration of gene coexpression across brain areas (*BA*, Brodmann area), as well as novel brain region wiring. The *green lines* and *dashed red lines* indicate information flow in both directions and can be extrapolated to suggest excitatory and inhibitory interconnections. Each gene is depicted as a node *(green or purple)*, with hub genes (those with the most connections to other genes) represented by *purple nodes. Blue lines* indicate positive correlations, and *red lines* indicate negative correlations. *Lines between BAs* indicate real and potential interactions through white matter tracts. This integration of network analysis, gene expression data, and imaging demonstrates relationships among key genetic factors in distinct regions and their role in regional brain connectivity in both normal individuals and those with disease. *(With permission from Geschwind, D.H., Konopka, G., 2009. Neuroscience in the era of functional genomics and systems biology. Nature 461, 908–915.)*

## GENETICS AND THE PARADOX OF DISEASE DEFINITION

Research into the genetics of neurological disease has established an alternative standard to the clinical or pathological definition of a disease, the genetic diagnosis. However, these standards are not equivalent, and to fully understand the difference, we must consider the meaning of a genetic diagnosis. Currently, pathology is thought of as a gold standard for diagnosis, but it is not available antemortem in many cases. A clinical diagnosis is limited by the homogeneity of the disease in question and the sensitivity and specificity of its clinical features. Although genetic testing can often provide a definitive answer to diagnosis, one of the potential paradoxes that has emerged from our identification of disease genes, and subsequent clinical and pathological correlations, is that the relationship between genetic susceptibility and clinical diagnosis is far from simple. This is true for virtually all Mendelian diseases and becomes even more complicated when complex diseases are considered.

In Mendelian disorders, X-linked adrenoleukodystrophy is a prime example of this paradox. In a single family, all with the same mutation, neurological phenotypes may range from an inflammatory cerebral demyelination to a noninflammatory distal axonopathy to a behavioral phenotype similar to attention-deficit/hyperactivity disorder (ADHD) or ASD (Moser et al., 2005), despite all family members carrying the identical genetic diagnosis. With regard to complex disease, FTD spectrum disorders provide another salient example, as families with the same mutations can have vastly different clinical features ranging from purely psychiatric to motor neuron disease, parkinsonism, cortical basal degeneration, progressive supranuclear palsy, or dementia, either singly or in combination (van Swieten and Heutink, 2008). A similar scenario can be observed in epilepsy, where broad seizure phenotypes are seen in some familial forms of epilepsy (Helbig et al., 2008). Conversely, identification of Mendelian mutations can lead to a broadening of disease definition, as has been the case in Friedreich ataxia, where adults with a distinct late-onset phenotype are now frequently identified (Bhidayasiri et al., 2005), or in adult polyglucosan body disease, a progressive myeloneuropathy discovered to be the adult form of glycogen storage disease type IV, which can lead to fatal liver complications in children (Lossos et al., 2009). What is further remarkable is that genetic findings in certain Mendelian forms of PD question the notion of pathology as the gold standard. Here, certain families with mutations in the *LRRK2* gene lack Lewy body pathology, yet have clear dopamine-responsive PD (Zimprich et al., 2004). This raises the question of what the gold standard *is*, as the absence of Lewy bodies would not be consistent with a pathological PD diagnosis. Seen from this perspective, it is clear that pathology, genetic findings, or clinical phenotypes cannot be interpreted in isolation, and it is the combination of these characteristics that defines a disease. As we gather more genetic information about neurological disorders in the coming years, our definitions of these diseases will certainly expand and change. Identifying disease-causing mutations and/or establishing a genetic risk profile will provide further knowledge regarding disease etiology, with implications for counseling, further diagnostic workup, and eventually for treatment—described in greater detail next.

## CLINICAL APPROACH TO THE PATIENT WITH SUSPECTED NEUROGENETIC DISEASE

In this chapter we have outlined the current state of clinical neurogenetics and the techniques available to neurologists and neuroscientists to better understand and study genetic disease for the benefit of patients. A consistent theme has been that, in the near future, most neurological diseases will be described on a genomic level, and large amounts of detailed genetic information will become available to the clinician, particularly with the availability of exome and genome sequencing. This raises the important question of how the clinical neurologist is to synthesize all this newly available genetic information regarding Mendelian disorders and common disease and apply that to patients in the clinic on a daily basis. We hope this overview will provide some basic tools to utilize and interpret such information in a meaningful way. In this section, we will deal with the four major clinical areas impacted most by this new genetic knowledge: (1) evaluation and diagnosis, (2) genetic counseling, (3) prognosis, and (4) treatment.

### Evaluation and Diagnosis

Evaluation and diagnosis benefit from the arsenal of genetic testing available for single-gene disorders and for genomic variation. Many commercial laboratories offer testing for Mendelian disease genes, and in some settings, genetic testing has become as routine as other common blood tests. However, because genetic testing carries additional implications for a patient and their family, particularly with regard to heritability of disease, it is important that it be used appropriately and that patients be fully educated prior to such testing. Important points to consider for genetic testing are summarized in Table 48.8. Although how the testing is incorporated into a clinical evaluation strategy will vary by disease, a general principle is that most genetic disease is diagnosed clinically via a thorough history (including family history) and physical examination. A complete evaluation for nongenetic causes should be performed as appropriate prior to any genetic testing, so that possible treatments can be initiated in a timely manner. Genetic testing should only be used to confirm a clinical suspicion, not for screening purposes, because currently this is low yield and not cost-effective in the majority of cases (Fogel et al., 2013, 2016). Specialist referral to a tertiary center is appropriate for all cases where a diagnostically useful clinical phenotype cannot be established. Genetic counseling (see later) should be provided, by either a physician or a licensed genetic counselor, prior to testing to ensure that patients understand the nature of the test and the possible results. When testing is ordered, it should be based on phenotype and supported by mode of inheritance if this can be determined. Testing of an asymptomatic minor is never indicated for a genetic disease where there is no treatment or cure. Knowledge of the disease status without chance for treatment may have many negative consequences.

The types of single-gene testing available vary by laboratory and gene (Table 48.9). The most comprehensive (and expensive) testing type commonly available is full individual gene sequencing, where all coding regions, as well as approximately 50 bases in each intron/exon junction, are sequenced for the presence of mutation. This will detect all coding point mutations and splice-site mutations as well as small insertions and deletions, but will miss more fine-grained structural variation, including that affecting noncoding regions. Importantly, novel coding mutations that are clinically interpretable can be detected using this approach. Targeted sequence analysis (also called *select exon testing*) consists of specific sequencing reactions designed to only detect one or a few previously identified mutations. This will not detect any sequence variations outside of the limited region of the gene being searched. Although Sanger sequencing methods are still used significantly for single-gene testing, next-generation sequencing is being utilized more and more often due to practical reasons primarily related to improved cost and time. For repeat disorders, there are specific tests to identify the relevant expansions using either polymerase chain reaction (PCR) or Southern blotting, a hybridization-based DNA sizing technique. Larger deletions or duplications (e.g., CNVs) can be detected by quantitative PCR methods or, more commonly, by CMA. Overall, interpretation of CNV results can be challenging, particularly if the CNV is not observed in databases

**TABLE 48.8 The Neurogenetic Evaluation and the Clinical Utilization of Genetic Testing**

| | |
|---|---|
| Establish the phenotype | All patients in whom a genetic diagnosis is suspected require a thorough physical examination and clinical history including a detailed family history. Differential diagnosis is established based on phenotype. Genetic etiologies should be considered in all cases where there is a positive family history of disease. |
| Rule out nongenetic etiologies | With the exception of suspected genetic diseases with known disease-modifying treatments, patients should be fully evaluated for nongenetic causes of disease prior to the initiation of genetic testing, as these are generally more amenable to curative or disease-modifying treatment. |
| Order genetic testing based on phenotype | Genetic testing should not be used as a screening tool. Physicians suspecting a hereditary disorder but unable to arrive at a diagnostically useful clinical phenotype should refer these patients for further evaluation at a tertiary center specializing in such cases. |
| Use disease biomarkers when available | Cost management should be maintained through the use of biomarker testing whenever possible, with genetic testing as the confirmatory step in diagnosis to obtain the genotype for symptomatic (or disease-modifying, if available) therapies, clinical trials, research studies, and genotype–phenotype clinical correlations. |
| Avoid using genetic panels as screening tools | Routine screening patients with disease- or inheritance-based multigene panels should be discouraged in clinical practice, as this is not a cost-effective use of patient resources. There is, however, a role for focused panels (particularly those based on less expensive next-generation sequencing technology) in specific disorders with heterogeneous phenotypes. |
| Provide genetic counseling | Genetic counseling (by a physician, geneticist, or genetic counselor) should be provided to all patients for whom genetic testing is recommended. Follow-up counseling should be provided to all patients with a positive gene test and offered to family members who may be at risk or disease carriers. Any and all ethical concerns should be fully addressed. |
| Utilize best available technology in challenging cases | Exome and/or genome sequencing may be an appropriate clinical consideration for patients with suspected genetic disease and negative focused genetic and nongenetic evaluations, particularly for disorders with heterogeneous phenotypes. Sequencing of parents and/or other affected family members may improve diagnostic yield. |

of normal human variation. Here, the parents will often need to be evaluated to determine whether the CNV in question is inherited or de novo. Such findings may require interpretation by a specialist and/or further testing to determine the likelihood of pathogenicity. As always, it is important to be aware of the type of testing being ordered; for example, in copy number testing, a negative result for deletions or duplications does not exclude point mutations elsewhere in the gene.

With the availability of next-generation sequencing, many companies now offer broad genetic panels, covering dozens, hundreds, or even thousands of genes based on general phenotypes or modes of inheritance for a particular symptom, which have appeal because they are simple to order and often advertised as a molecular means of differentiating between overlapping phenotypes. For some disorders this may be an effective strategy if the specific phenotype in question is only due to a defined set of genes (Fogel, 2018; Nemeth et al., 2013; Rexach et al., 2019). In contrast, for many clinically heterogeneous phenotypes, this has the potential to do a disservice to the patient, as variants observed in the tested genes may be overemphasized where obvious mutations in genes untested could remain overlooked (Fogel, 2018; Rexach et al., 2019). Over time, the clinical use of WES and WGS will likely significantly reduce the usage of most multigene panels, given these tests are vastly more comprehensive and cost-effective (Coppola and Geschwind, 2012; Fogel, 2018; Fogel et al., 2014a, 2016; Rexach et al., 2019) and, in fact, many gene panels in current use are already performed by filtering exome data, for practical reasons such as lower cost (Fogel, 2018; Rexach et al., 2019). Genome sequencing is the more comprehensive method and capable of detecting more types of mutation, as well as structural variation, but its widespread use will hinge on the development of accurate and efficient bioinformatic techniques for translating the expected massive genomic variation per patient (millions of SNPs and hundreds of CNVs across the whole genome) into clinically meaningful results (Fogel, 2018; Rexach et al., 2019). In general, interpretation of these genetic results may be straightforward, for example, if no rare variants are present in relevant genes or if known pathogenic changes are found. In contrast, interpretation may be complicated, if rare or novel sequence "variants of uncertain significance" are identified. Inconclusive results may require interpretation by a specialist, and/or further testing to determine the likelihood of pathogenicity. Sequencing of the parents along with the patient, when possible, can be extremely informative. The public availability of large data sets of human variation has also helped tremendously in recognizing rare polymorphisms (Lek et al., 2016) coupled with the establishment of guidelines to aid the process of determining variant pathogenicity and to create uniformity in reporting among clinical laboratories (Richards et. al., 2015). However, in many cases, clinicians may still be left with uncertainty, although there is evidence that through continued bioinformatic analysis, over time the nature of these variants may be resolved (Ewans et al., 2018).

Common diseases must be approached in a different manner, because detailed phenotype alone cannot always predict whether a condition is due to mutation of a single gene. Still, the goal remains to develop strategies incorporating known genetic information into a systematic protocol designed to maximize diagnostic capability while minimizing cost and unnecessary testing (Lintas and Persico, 2009). Tests such as CMA are clinically available to search genome-wide for disease-causing CNVs and are recommended for sporadic causes in disorders such as ID or autism, where CNVs have been found responsible for a reasonable percentage of disease (Geschwind and Spence, 2008; Miller et al., 2010). Use of such testing in sporadic adult-onset disease is less clear, so the physician is advised to refer to current published guidelines for the disease in question before ordering. We should note that clinical exome sequencing is appropriate in the principal evaluation of sporadic neurodevelopmental cases, including ID and congenital anomalies (Lee et al., 2014; Yang et al., 2013, 2014). Overall, the clinical examination should always be used to precisely define the patient's phenotype, which will in turn suggest the most high-yield conditions for genetic testing. This systematic approach is of immense benefit in resource management; the education of current and future physicians should include discussions on the implementation and utilization of such strategies in clinical practice (Fogel et al., 2013) for both rare and common disease.

TABLE 48.9 **Types of Genetic Testing**

| Type of Test | Sequence Variant(s) Identified | Sequence Variant(s) Missed or Not Accurately Determined |
|---|---|---|
| Gene sequencing (coding region only) | Point mutations*<br>Frameshifts<br>Splicing mutations†<br>Polymorphisms | Noncoding variants‡<br>Copy number variations§<br>Repeat expansions |
| Select exon sequencing (targeted mutation analysis) | Known predefined variants<br>*Target region only*¶<br>Point mutations*<br>Frameshifts<br>Splicing mutations†<br>Polymorphisms | *Variants outside target region*¶<br>Point mutations*<br>Frameshifts<br>Splicing mutations†<br>Polymorphisms<br>Noncoding variants‡<br>Copy number variations§<br>Repeat expansions |
| Repeat expansion testing# (targeted mutation analysis) | Repeat expansion in the specific gene tested | Point mutations*<br>Frameshifts<br>Splicing mutations†<br>Polymorphisms<br>Noncoding variants‡<br>Copy number variations§ |
| Gene copy number variation (deletion/duplication testing) | Copy number variation§ of gene tested | Point mutations*<br>Frameshifts<br>Splicing mutations†<br>Polymorphisms<br>Noncoding variants‡<br>Repeat expansions |
| Chromosomal microarray analysis** (comparative genomic hybridization) | Genome-wide copy number variations†† | Point mutations*<br>Frameshifts<br>Splicing mutations†<br>Polymorphisms<br>Noncoding variants‡<br>Repeat expansions |
| Clinical exome sequencing** | Point mutations*<br>Frameshifts<br>Splicing mutations†<br>Polymorphisms | Noncoding variants‡<br>Copy number variations§<br>Repeat expansions‡‡ |
| Clinical genome sequencing** | Point mutations*<br>Frameshifts<br>Splicing mutations†<br>Polymorphisms<br>Noncoding variants‡<br>Copy number variations§ | Repeat expansions‡‡ |

*Includes missense, nonsense, and silent mutations.
†Includes only those involving splice sites and exonic splicing regulatory sequences.
‡Includes promoter mutations and noncoding splicing regulatory elements.
§Arbitrarily defined here as any deletion/duplication/insertion larger than detectable by Sanger sequencing.
¶Size and number of region(s) targeted varies per individual test.
#Targeted mutation analysis using either polymerase chain reaction (PCR) and/or Southern blot is preferred, as sequencing may be inaccurate due to the large size of many repeat regions.
**Genome-wide testing method.
††Minimum size of CNVs detected and density of genomic coverage may vary by platform.
‡‡Potentially detectable by genomic sequencing methods with appropriate read lengths.

## Genetic Counseling

Establishing a precise genetic diagnosis will definitively establish the means of inheritance of a disorder and is extremely useful in genetic counseling and family planning, particularly for disorders that show incomplete penetrance. However, unlike other tests typically ordered by physicians, a positive diagnosis carries implications not only for individual patients but also for the entire family. Genetic counseling, therefore, should be provided in all cases where genetic testing is recommended, by an experienced neurologist, a geneticist, or a licensed genetic counselor. Follow-up counseling should also be provided to all patients with a positive test result and, in many cases, offered to other family members who may be at risk for disease or as carriers. Physicians must be aware of the various ethical implications involved in such testing (Ensenauer et al., 2005). One area of particular importance in this regard involves considerations of genetic testing in asymptomatic individuals, especially minors. This stems in part from concerns that have been raised regarding risks of depression and suicide in asymptomatic individuals diagnosed with fatal genetic disease, although this is not well established, and further study will be important for determining best practices. For minors, standard practice dictates that unless there is disease-modifying therapy available, they should not be tested if asymptomatic until they reach an age to consent to such testing and are properly counseled as to the implications. Counseling regarding prenatal testing and assisted reproduction are other topics of relevance to patients of reproductive age. Current reproductive medicine techniques such as in vitro fertilization and preimplantation genetic testing, by assuring that offspring will not harbor the mutation in question, can aid couples concerned about the risk for passing on inherited conditions. Other ethical considerations may also apply, depending on the disease and specific family/patient circumstances.

## Prognosis and Treatment

A confirmed genetic diagnosis can contribute clinically useful data concerning patient prognosis, as it allows information from published case studies to be utilized in the care of an individual patient. This can aid in the identification of specific clinical features to focus on for surveillance in the development of a particular genetic disorder, such as cognitive decline in a patient with isolated chorea found to have HD, or cardiac testing in an autistic patient with chromosome 15q duplication. A genetic diagnosis may also alert the clinician to potential life-threatening comorbidities such as adrenal insufficiency in X-linked adrenoleukodystrophy or cardiomyopathy in Friedreich ataxia. Review of case studies in a particular disorder may help answer questions regarding life expectancy or future disability, such as years of disease prior to loss of ambulation in the various SCAs. Lastly, there are important positive psychological aspects to establishing a definitive diagnosis, particularly for patients who have undergone many fruitless clinical evaluations.

Although the majority of genetic diseases are not curable, therapies do exist for many of them with more in development, including potentially disease-modifying gene therapies. Defining the genetic etiology of a patient's disease allows for utilization of the published literature on these as well as other symptomatic treatments and pharmacotherapy that may benefit a specific condition. Phenylketonuria is an excellent example of this, since dietary restriction of phenylalanine initiated soon after birth will prevent cognitive impairment and enable virtually normal development (Burgard et al., 1999). More important, new clinical trials are being developed frequently and can be offered to patients with an established diagnosis. Many disease-based patient registries exist to facilitate this.

The ultimate goal of translational neuroscience is to utilize advances in our understanding of disease at the molecular level to aid in the treatment of patients in the clinic. Recent new treatments, which take advantage of the molecular aspects of these disorders, show promise in the clinic and the laboratory. Such treatments include enzyme replacement therapy for metabolic disorders such as the severe fatal glycogen storage disorder Pompe disease, where use of recombinant acid α-glucosidase in 18 infants prior to 6 months of age enabled all to live to the age of 18 months, a 99% reduction in death, as well as reducing their risk of death or invasive ventilation by 92% compared with historical controls (Kishnani et al., 2007). Work in animal models has suggested potential new pharmacological treatments, such as a recent research study which demonstrated that the use of histone-deacetylase inhibitors can unsilence expanded frataxin alleles in a Friedreich ataxia mouse model, restoring wild-type gene expression levels and reversing cellular transcription changes associated with frataxin deficiency (Rai et al., 2008), leading to the use of such compounds in clinical trials (Gottesfeld et al., 2013). As described previously, targeted molecules have been designed to correct specific disease-causing biological defects, as shown by recent work with antisense oligonucleotides (ASOs) designed to alter gene expression. In spinal muscular atrophy, disease occurs due the loss of functional protein from the *SMN1* gene. However, a second gene exists, *SMN2*, capable of producing the same protein but typically at a level 10% that of *SMN1*, due to alternative splicing. By using an ASO designed to alter this splicing to increase the amount of functional protein from *SMN2*, 51% of treated infants gained motor milestones compared with to 0% of controls (Finkel et al., 2017). Such techniques may markedly exceed the therapeutic benefit of other available options, such as in Duchenne muscular dystrophy (Lim et al., 2017), where patients can otherwise expect only moderate short-term benefit (up to 2 years) from the gold standard treatment, glucocorticosteroids (Manzur et al., 2008; Wood et al., 2010). Novel treatments aimed at genetic modification of disease are also in development, such as RNA interference techniques to specifically degrade and thus silence the disease allele in a rat model of SCA type 3, resulting in a reduction in neuropathological changes in the brain (Alves et al., 2008). Further molecular analysis suggests such strategies are viable for further preclinical studies (Rodriguez-Lebron et al., 2013). More recently, targeted viral-mediated gene therapy strategies designed to restore dopamine expression (Palfi et al., 2014) or modulate the production of GABA (LeWitt et al., 2011) in PD, or introduce nerve growth factor into the brains of patients with AD (Rafii et al., 2014), have shown some success in early clinical trials and support the further testing of such strategies for these and other disorders. Stem cell therapies, although in their infancy, have also shown early promise in the restoration of gene function in X-linked adrenoleukodystrophy (Cartier et al., 2009) and in the generation of functional oligodendrocytes in patients with Pelizaeus-Merzbacher disease (Gupta et al., 2012), whose cells are incapable of myelinating axons. Lastly, as discussed earlier, gene replacement therapies offer the potential to restore the missing function brought on by genetic mutation (Eichler et al., 2017; Ledford, 2017; Mendell et al., 2017; Russell et al., 2017). The incorporation of new technologies such as next-generation sequencing and the use of systems biology approaches to disease are expected to lead to additional new innovations. With these advances, the future of clinical neurogenetics is full of promise and stands poised to answer the challenge stated most eloquently by Bernard Baruch (1870–1965): "There are no such things as incurables; there are only things for which [medicine] has not found a cure."

*The complete reference list is available online at https://expertconsult.inkling.com.* 

49

# Neuroimmunology

*Tanuja Chitnis, Samia J. Khoury*

## OUTLINE



The past decade has seen a rich interaction between the fields of neurology and immunology. This has provided further insight into the mechanisms of immunologically mediated neurological diseases and given rise to new therapies for many neuroimmunological diseases, including multiple sclerosis (MS). To understand and effectively employ these emerging neuroimmunologically based therapies, a solid grasp of immunology is required. Here we provide an overview of the major components of the immune system and highlight important advances in the field of neuroimmunology, with a focus on relevant disease processes and treatment strategies.

## IMMUNE SYSTEM

The function of the immune system is to protect the organism against infectious agents and prevent reinfection by maintaining immunological memory. Additionally, the immune system performs tumor surveillance, promotes healing, and prevents damage mediated by dying cells.

The immune system normally does not react to self-antigens, a state known as *tolerance*, except in the setting of autoimmune disease. An overactive immune system may mediate ongoing immune-mediated damage, so a delicate balance must be maintained between the protective effects of the immune system and potential deleterious effects.

The normal functions of the immune system and the disorders resulting from its dysfunction are listed in Box 49.1.

### Adaptive and Innate Immunity

The immune system has two functional divisions: the innate immune system and the adaptive immune system. The innate immune system acts nonspecifically as the body's first line of defense against pathogens. However, this type of response, if perpetuated, would result in unwanted nonspecific damage to the host. Therefore a secondary, antigen-specific response develops and leads the attack. This is mediated by T cells and B cells, which are equipped with antigen-specific receptors. The effector cells release mediators and trigger other components of the immune system to eliminate the target. Subpopulations of T and B cells develop and maintain immunological memory, which facilitates a more rapid response in the case of recurrent infection.

The innate immune system consists of the following components:

1. Skin—The exterior surface of the body, primarily the skin, is the body's primary defense against foreign pathogens. Many inflammatory cells and antigen-presenting cells (APCs) line the epidermis and serve as the first line of defense.
2. Phagocytes are cells capable of phagocytosing foreign pathogens. They include polymorphonuclear cells, monocytes, and macrophages. These cells are present in the blood as well as in organs. Phagocytes recognize cell components or pathogen-associated molecular patterns (PAMPs) of a variety of microorganisms through families of pattern recognition receptors (PRRs) expressed on their cell surface. PRRs allow phagocytes to attach nonspecifically and phagocytose pathogens, which are then killed via intracellular

**BOX 49.1 Normal Functions and Disorders of the Immune System**

**Normal Functions**

Immunity against microorganisms and pathogens
Wound healing
Tumor surveillance

**Disorders Resulting From Immune System Dysfunction**

Autoimmunity
Immune-mediated disorders
Bystander damage
Graft rejection

lysosomes. Families of PRRs include the Toll-like receptors (TLRs) and the nucleotide-binding oligomerization domain (NOD) receptors.

3. Natural killer (NK) cells—NK cells recognize cell surface molecules on virally infected or tumor cells. They subsequently bind to the infected cells and kill them via cell-mediated cytotoxicity.
4. Acute-phase proteins—C-reactive protein is a model acute-phase protein whose concentration increases in response to infection. C-reactive protein binds to cell surface molecules on a variety of bacteria and fungi and acts as an opsonin, essentially increasing recognition of pathogens by phagocytic cells.
5. Complement system—The complement system is a cascade of serum proteins whose overall function is to enhance and mediate inflammation. The complement system has the intrinsic ability to lyse the cell membranes of many cells including bacteria. It functions in concert with components of both the innate and adaptive immune systems and can also act as an opsonin, facilitating phagocytosis. The complement cascade can be directly activated by certain microorganisms through the alternative pathway, or it can be activated by particular antibody subtypes through the classical pathway.

The adaptive immune response consists of the following components:

1. Antibodies—Otherwise known as *immunoglobulins* (Igs), antibodies are able to specifically recognize a variety of free antigens. Igs are produced by B cells and are present on their cell surface. In addition, Igs are secreted in large amounts in the serum. Antibodies recognize specific microbial and other antigens through their antigen-binding sites and bind phagocytes via their Fc receptors, thereby facilitating antigen removal. Some subclasses of Ig are capable of activating complement via their Fc portion, thereby lysing their targets.
2. B cells—The primary function of B cells is to produce antibody. Antigen binding to B cells stimulates proliferation and maturation of that particular B cell, with subsequent enhancement of antigen-specific antibody production, resulting in the development of antibody-secreting plasma cells. Most B cells express class II major histocompatibility complex (MHC) antigens and have the ability to function as APCs.
3. T cells, or thymus-derived cells, have the ability to recognize specific antigens via their T-cell receptors (TCRs). T cells may be classified into two main groups: T-helper ($T_H$) cells expressing CD4 antigen on their cell surface, and T-cytotoxic ($T_C$) cells expressing CD8 on their surface. CD4 T cells recognize antigen presented in association with MHC class II on the surface of APCs. CD4 T cells help to promote B-cell maturation and antibody production and produce factors called *cytokines* to enhance the innate or nonspecific immune response. CD8 T cells recognize antigen in association with MHC class I antigen on the surface of most cells and play an important role in eliminating virus-infected cells. Cytotoxic T cells are capable of damaging target cells via the release of degrading enzymes and cytokines. Responses in which the T cell plays a major role are termed *cell-mediated immunity* (CMI). T-cell–macrophage interactions often lead to delayed reactions, termed *delayed-type hypersensitivity* (DTH).
4. APCs are required to present antigen to T cells. They are found primarily in the skin, lymph nodes, spleen, and thymus. Unlike B cells that can recognize free antigen, T cells are only capable of recognizing antigen in the context of self-MHC molecules. APCs process antigen intracellularly and present antigen peptide in the groove of their MHC class II molecules. The primary APCs are macrophages, monocytes, dendritic cells, and Langerhans cells.

## Principal Components of the Immune System

Cells of the immune system arise from the pluripotent stem cells in the bone marrow and diverge into the lymphoid or myeloid lineages. The myeloid lineage primarily contains cells with phagocytic functions such as neutrophils, basophils, eosinophils, and macrophages. The lymphoid lineage consists of T cells, B cells, and NK cells.

### Monocytes and Macrophages

Bone marrow–derived myeloid progenitor cells give rise to monocytes (mononuclear phagocytes of the reticuloendothelial system) that serve important immune functions. They constitute about 4% of the peripheral blood leukocytes and are morphologically identified by an abundant cytoplasm and a kidney-shaped nucleus. Their cytoplasm contains many enzymes, which are important for killing microorganisms and processing antigens. Monocytes differentiate into tissue-specific macrophages including Kupffer cells of the liver and brain microglia.

### Natural Killer Cells

NK cells make up about 2.5% of peripheral blood lymphocytes and are synonymous with large granular lymphocytes because of their large intracytoplasmic azurophilic granules and high cytoplasm-to-nucleus ratio. NK cells are activated primarily in response to interferons and are involved in the elimination of virally infected host cells; they also play a role in tumor immunity. Unlike cytotoxic $CD8^+$ T cells, NK cells lack immunological memory and have the ability to kill a wide variety of tumor and virus-infected cells without MHC restriction (see the discussion of the function of MHC genes) or activation. NK cells lack the cell surface markers present on B cells and T cells. $NK1.1^+$ T cells are a subset of cells sharing characteristics of both NK cells and T cells. These cells express the $\alpha/\beta$ TCR and the NK1.1 receptor and secrete large amounts of interferon gamma (IFN-$\gamma$) or interleukin 4 (IL-4) in response to TCR stimulation.

### T Lymphocytes

T cells originate from the thymus. Differentiation of T cells occurs in the thymus, and every T cell that leaves the thymus is conferred with a unique specificity for recognizing antigens. T cells that recognize self-antigens are generally either deleted or rendered tolerant within the thymus, a process called *central tolerance*.

T cells may be divided into two groups on the basis of expression of either the $CD4^+$ or $CD8^+$ marker. Functionally, $CD4^+$ T cells are involved in DTH responses and also provide help for B-cell differentiation (and hence are termed *helper T cells*). In contrast, $CD8^+$ T cells are involved in class I restricted lysis of antigen-specific targets (and hence are termed *cytotoxic T cells*). T cells with suppressor or regulatory activity can express either CD4 or CD8.

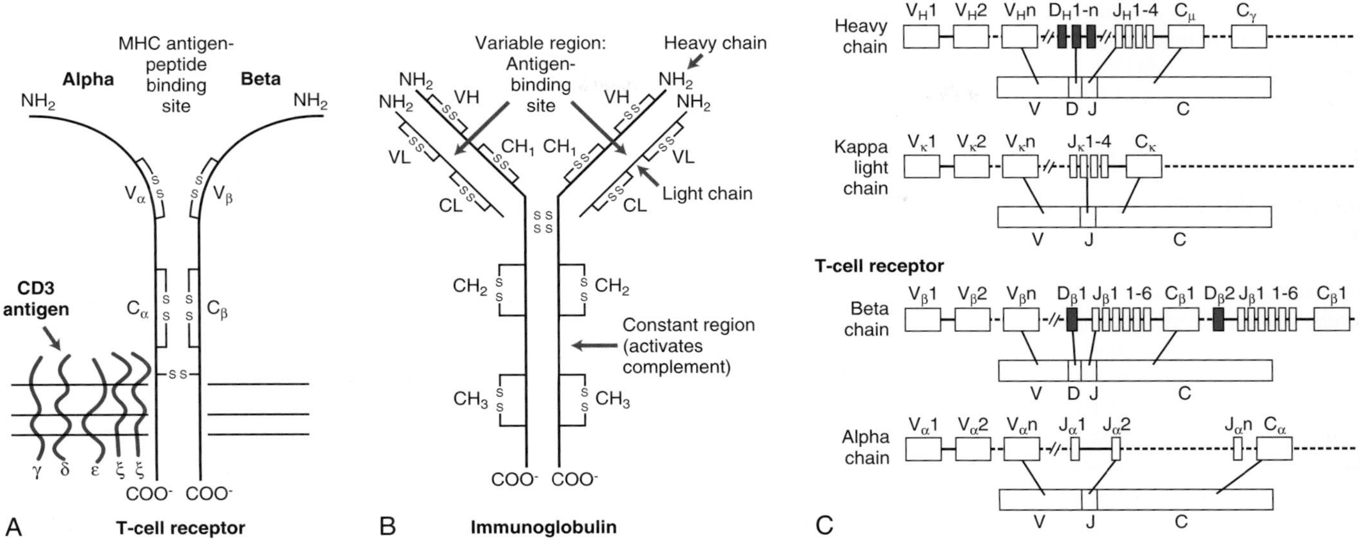


**Fig. 49.1 Molecular and Genetic Organization of the T-Cell Receptor (TCR) and Immunoglobulin (Ig) Molecule.** A and B, Structural organization of the TCR and Ig molecule. The TCR is a heterodimer consisting of two chains, $\alpha$ and $\beta$; the Ig molecule consists of two heavy and light chains. Both molecules are stabilized by interchain and intrachain disulfide bonds. Variable-region domains are located at the amino terminal, and constant-region domains are located on the carboxy terminal. The antigen-binding site on the Ig molecule is located between the variable-region domains of the heavy and light chains. The variable region of the TCR recognizes foreign peptides in the context of self-*MHC* (major histocompatibility complex) molecules. The TCR is also associated with the CD3 antigen (consisting of g, d, e, and z-z chains) to form the TCR complex. C, Organization of the gene families of Ig and TCR. The common feature of the four gene pools is that they contain a number of variable *(V)* gene segments that are separated from the constant *(C)* region genes by the joining *(J)* genes. In the case of the TCR $\beta$ chain and the Ig heavy-chain gene, additional diversity *(D)* genes are present. During ontogeny, one of the *V* gene segments is juxtaposed to the J segment through a process of chromosomal rearrangement to form the *V(D)J* gene. This, along with the constant region genes, is transcribed to form messenger RNA and then protein.

## T-Cell Receptors

The TCR consists of two glycosylated polypeptide chains, alpha ($\alpha$) and beta ($\beta$), of 45,000 and 40,000 Da molecular weight, respectively. This heterodimer of an $\alpha$ and $\beta$ chain is linked by disulfide bonds. Amino acid sequences show that each chain consists of variable (V), joining (J), and constant (C) regions closely resembling Igs (Fig. 49.1). There are about $10^2$ TCR-variable genes grouped by homology into a small number of families, compared with $10^3$ or greater for Igs (see later discussion). The principles governing generation of diversity in the TCR are very similar to those for Ig genes. T cells can only recognize short peptides that are associated with MHC molecules. In contrast, the Ig receptor can recognize peptides, whole proteins, nucleic acids, lipids, and small chemicals.

T cells also express a variety of nonpolymorphic antigens on their surfaces. The most abundantly expressed is CD45, comprising 10% of lymphocyte membrane proteins. CD45 exists as a number of isoforms that differ in the molecular weight of their extracellular domains as a result of RNA splicing. These isoforms can be distinguished serologically. The low molecular weight (CD45RO) isoforms define activated, or memory, T-cell populations.

## B Lymphocytes

B cells are the precursors of antibody-secreting cells. The cells develop in the bone marrow and during their ontogeny acquire Ig receptors that commit them to recognizing specific antigens for the rest of their lives. B cells normally express IgM on their cell surfaces but switch to other isotypes as a consequence of T-cell help, while maintaining antigen specificity (see later discussion). Following antigenic challenge, T lymphocytes assist (help) B cells directly (cognate interaction) or indirectly by secreting helper factors (noncognate interaction) to differentiate and form mature antibody-secreting plasma cells.

## Immunoglobulins

Immunoglobulins are glycoproteins that are the secretory product of plasma cells. Their biochemical structure and genomic organization are shown in Fig. 49.1. All Ig molecules share a number of common features. Each molecule consists of two identical polypeptide light chains (kappa [$\kappa$] or lambda [$\lambda$]) linked to two identical heavy chains. The light and heavy chains are stabilized by intrachain and interchain disulfide bonds. According to the biochemical nature of the heavy chain, Igs are divided into five main classes: IgM, IgD, IgG, IgA, and IgE. These may be further divided into subclasses depending on differences in the heavy chain.

Each heavy and light chain consists of variable and constant regions. The amino terminus is characterized by sequence variability in both the light and the heavy chain, and each variable heavy- and light-chain unit acts as the antigen-binding site (the Fab portion). The carboxy terminal of the heavy chain (also known as the *Fc portion*) is involved in binding to host tissue and fixing complement. This part of the molecule is important for antibody-dependent, cell-mediated cytotoxicity by cells of the reticuloendothelial system and for complement-mediated cell lysis.

Classes of Igs differ in their ability to fix complement. In humans, IgM, IgG1, and IgG3 antibodies are capable of activating the complement cascade. Different Ig classes also differ in their transport properties and ability to bind to phagocytes. Fc binding to Fc receptors (FcRs) present on macrophages, dendritic cells, neutrophils, NK cells, and B cells initiates signaling within the cell only when the receptors are cross-linked by immune complexes containing more than one IgG molecule. Different FcRs mediate different cellular responses, some being predominantly stimulatory, while others are inhibitory.

## Genetics of the Immune System

### Antigen Receptor Gene Rearrangements

During B- and T-cell development, multiple gene rearrangements occur to form their respective antigen receptors, the Ig and the TCR. Diversity of the antigen receptors is due to diversity in their principal components, the V gene segment and the J gene segments. One of the many V gene segments is juxtaposed by chromosomal rearrangements with one of the J segments (and when present, with the diversity [D] segment) to form the complete variable region gene. Recombinational inaccuracies at the joining sites of the V, D, and J regions further increase the diversity of the antigen receptors.

C gene segments are present in all receptors. The V, D, J, and C gene segments along with the intervening noncoding gene segments between the J and C regions are initially transcribed into mature RNA. Through a process of RNA splicing, the noncoding gene segments are excised, and the V(D)JC messenger RNA (mRNA) is translated into protein. After binding antigen, B cells undergo somatic mutations that further increase the diversity and the affinity of antigen binding (affinity maturation). This phenomenon does not occur in T cells. During isotype switching in B cells, further rearrangements lead to recombination of the same variable region gene with new constant region genes (see Fig. 49.1).

### Major Histocompatibility and Human Leukocyte Antigens

MHC gene products or the human leukocyte antigens (HLAs) serve to distinguish self from nonself. In addition, they serve the important function of presenting antigen to the appropriate cells. The MHC class I gene product contains an MHC-encoded α chain, and a smaller non-MHC-encoded $\beta_2$-microglobulin chain. The MHC class II gene product consists of two polypeptide chains, α and β, which are noncovalently linked. Both class I and class II proteins are stabilized by intrachain disulfide bonds. Class I antigens are expressed on all nucleated cells, whereas class II antigens are constitutively expressed only on dendritic cells, macrophages, and B cells, and are expressed on a variety of activated cells including T cells, endothelial cells, and astrocytes.

In humans, class I molecules are HLA-A, B, and C, whereas the class II molecules are HLA-DP, DQ, and DR. Several alleles are recognized for each locus; thus the HLA-A locus has at least 20 alleles, and HLA-B has at least 40. The number of alleles for the D region appears to be as extensive as that for HLA-A, HLA-B, and HLA-C. In view of the extensive polymorphisms present, the chances of two unrelated individuals sharing identical HLA antigens are extremely low. The reason for the extensive diversity and evolutionary pressure that lead to this are not fully understood.

Class I antigens regulate the specificity of cytotoxic CD8$^+$ T cells, which are responsible for killing cells bearing viral antigens or foreign transplantation antigens (Fig. 49.2). The target cells share class I MHC genes with the cytotoxic cell. Thus the cytotoxic cell that is specific for a particular virus is capable of recognizing the antigenic determinants of the virus only in association with a particular MHC class I gene product. The function of class II MHC gene products appears to be to regulate the specificity of T-helper cells, which in turn regulate DTH and antibody response to foreign antigens. Similarly, an immunized T-cell population will recognize a foreign antigen only if it is presented on the surface of an APC that shares the same class II MHC antigen specificity as the immunized T-cell population. Thus the functional specificity of the T-cell population is restricted by the MHC molecules they recognize. CD8$^+$ T cells (cytotoxic) and CD4$^+$ T cells (helper) are referred to as *MHC class I* and *MHC class II restricted T cells*, respectively (Fig. 49.3).

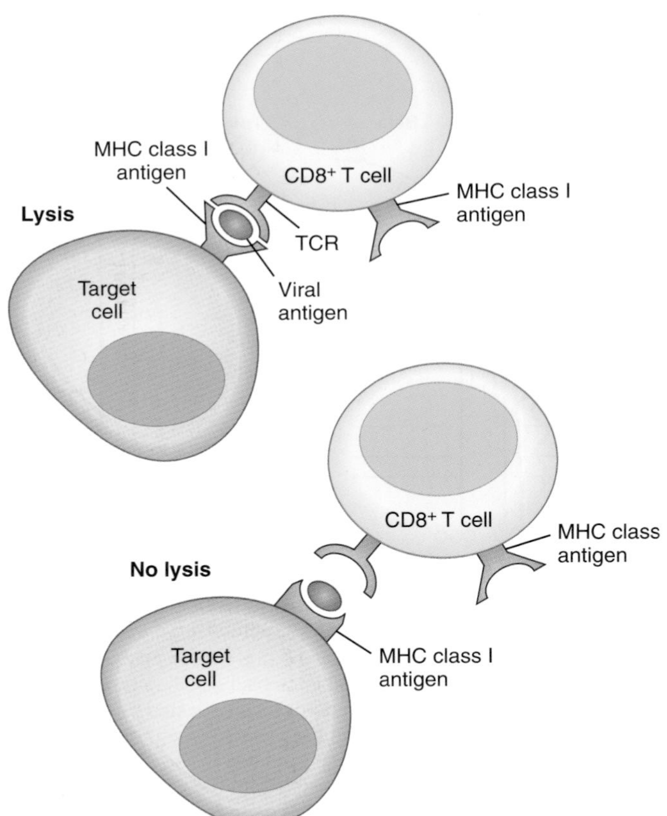


**Fig. 49.2 The Phenomenon of Major Histocompatibility Complex *(MHC)* Restriction.** For antigen-specific cytolysis of virus-infected targets to occur, T cells should be sensitized to the virus and share the same class I human leukocyte antigen (HLA) with the target cell. In the lower part of the figure, the MHC class I antigen expressed on the CD8$^+$ T cell is different from the MHC class 1 antigen expressed on the target cell; therefore lysis does not occur. *TCR,* T-cell receptor.

The analysis of the three-dimensional structure of the class I and class II molecules has confirmed the notion that these molecules are carriers of immunogenic peptides that are processed by APCs and presented on the cell surface (Fig. 49.4). Both MHC class I and class II molecules share similarities in crystal structure that allow them to accept and retain immunogenic peptides in grooves, or pockets, and present them to T cells.

# ORGANIZATION OF THE IMMUNE RESPONSE

## Initiation of the Immune Response

### Antigen Presentation

One of the crucial initial steps in the immune response is the presentation of encountered antigens to the immune system. Antigens are carried from their site of arrival in the periphery by way of lymphatics or blood vessels to the lymph nodes and spleen. There, antigens are then taken up by cells of the monocyte-macrophage lineage and by B cells, processed intracellularly, and presented not as whole molecules but as highly immunogenic peptides.

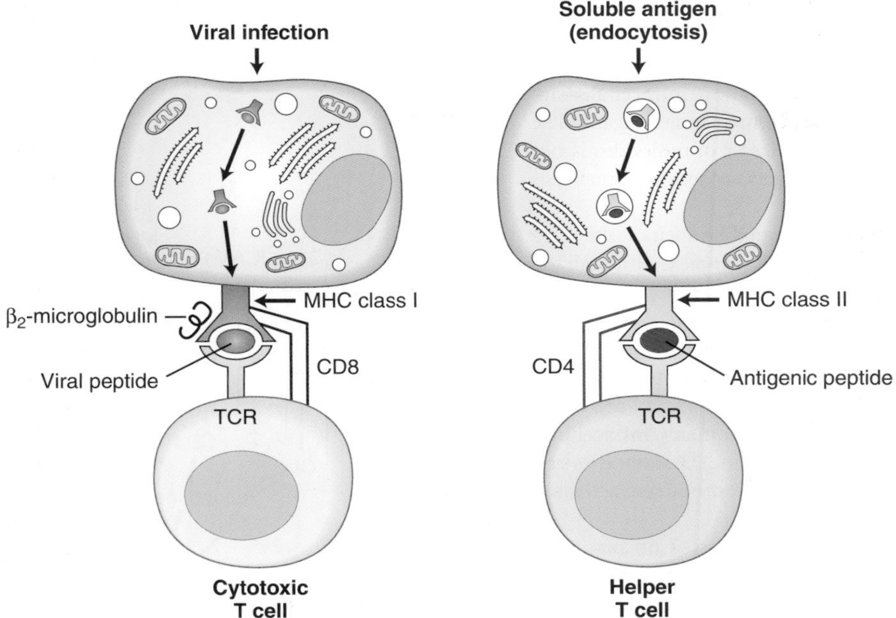


**Fig. 49.3 Antigenic Recognition of Cytotoxic and Helper T Cells.** The cytotoxic T cell recognizes viral peptides associated with human leukocyte antigen-A (HLA-A), HLA-B, or HLA-C molecules. The coreceptor for the helper T cell is the CD4 molecule. *MHC,* Major histocompatibility complex; *TCR,* T-cell receptor.

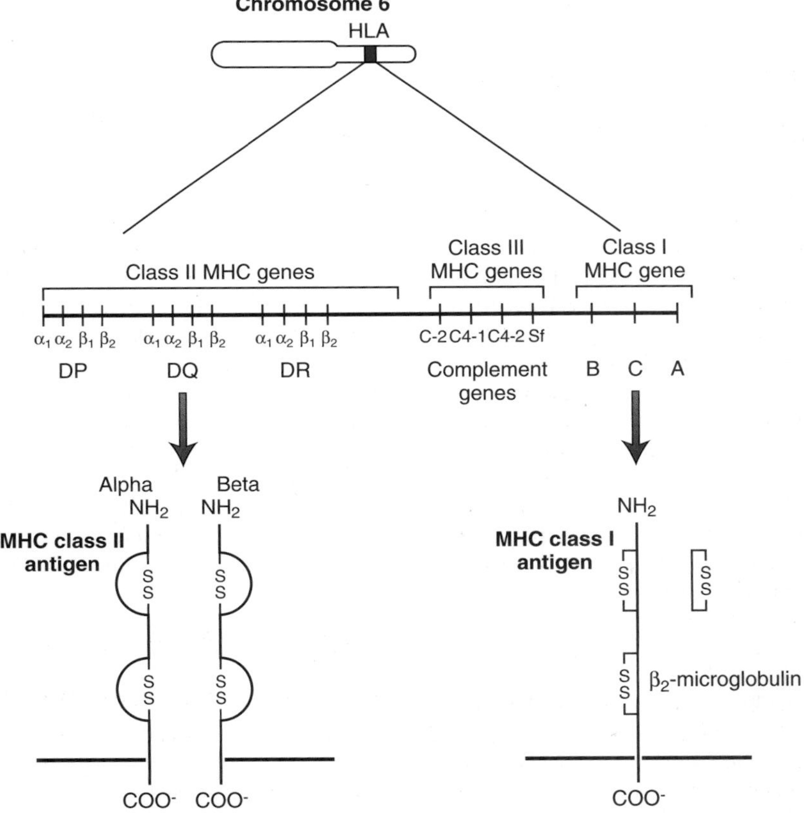


**Fig. 49.4 Schematic Diagram of the Human Leukocyte Antigen *(Hla)* Complex in Humans, Located on Chromosome 6.** The HLA class I gene (HLA-A, -B, and -C) codes for a single heavy-chain molecule. The $\beta_2$-microglobulin is coded by genes on a different chromosome. The HLA class II genes (*DR, DP,* and *DQ*) form the $\alpha\beta$ heterodimer. The HLA class III genes include those encoding for members of the complement family of proteins. *MHC,* Major histocompatibility complex.

## Accessory Molecules for T-Cell Activation

The interaction of MHC-peptide complex with T cells, although necessary, is insufficient for T-cell activation. Other classes of molecules are involved in T-cell antigen recognition, activation, intracellular signaling, adhesion, and trafficking of T cells to their target organs. The distinction between the functions of these classes of molecules is not absolute, and many may be involved in interactions between other cells of the immune system.

***CD3.*** Molecules whose primary role is signaling include the CD3 molecule. The CD3 molecule is part of the TCR complex. Although the TCR interacts with the MHC-peptide complex on APCs, the signals for the subsequent enactment of T-cell activation and proliferation are delivered by the CD3 antigen. The cytoplasmic tail of the CD3 proteins contains one copy of a sequence motif important for signaling functions, called the *immunoreceptor tyrosine-based activation motif* (ITAM). Phosphorylation of the ITAM initiates intracellular signaling events. In experimental situations, anti-CD3 antibodies can nonspecifically activate these intracellular signals, producing activated T cells in the absence of antigen.

***CD4 and CD8.*** CD4 or CD8 antigens are expressed on mature T cells and serve an accessory role in signaling and antigen recognition. CD4 binds to a nonpolymorphic site on the MHC class II β chain, and CD8 binds to the α3 domain of the MHC class I molecule. Signals for cell division that are delivered to the nucleus are mediated by second messengers. When the receptor binds its ligand, it causes the activation of protein kinases. These kinases add phosphate groups to other proteins that ultimately signal the cell to divide. CD4, CD8, and CD3 on T cells and CD19 on B cells are examples of receptors that are linked to kinases. CD4 is the cell surface receptor for human immunodeficiency virus (HIV-1), and the fact that certain non-T cells such as microglia and macrophages can express low levels of CD4 may explain the propensity of the virus for the central nervous system (CNS).

***Costimulatory molecules.*** Costimulatory molecules serve as a "second signal" to facilitate T-cell activation. Costimulatory pathways that are critical for T-cell activation include the B7-CD28 and CD40-CD154 pathways. Members of the integrin families including vascular cell adhesion molecule 1 (VCAM-1), intercellular adhesion molecule (ICAM-1), and leukocyte function antigen 3 (LFA-3) can provide costimulatory signals, but they also play critical roles in T-cell adhesion, facilitate interaction with the APCs, mediate adhesion to nonhematopoietic cells such as endothelial cells, and guide cell traffic (Fig. 49.5).

The B7-CD28 interaction is one of the most extensively studied costimulatory systems. The B7 molecules are expressed on APCs, and their expression is induced in activated cells. There are two forms of B7, B7-1 (CD80) and B7-2 (CD86), that share some homology but have different expression kinetics. The B7 molecules interact with their ligand, CD28, which is constitutively expressed on most T cells. Binding of the CD28 molecule mediates intracytoplasmic signals that increase expression of the growth factor, IL-2, and enhance expression of the anti-apoptotic molecule, Bcl-$x_L$. An alternate ligand for B7 is CTLA-4, which is homologous to CD28 in structure, but in contrast to CD28, CTLA-4 functions to inhibit T-cell activation. Costimulatory molecules may deliver either a stimulatory (positive) or inhibitory (negative) signal for T-cell activation (Brunet et al., 1987). Examples of molecules delivering a positive costimulatory signal for T-cell activation include the B7-CD28 and CD40-CD154 pathways. Examples of molecular pathways delivering a negative signal for T-cell activation include B7-CTLA-4 and PD1-PD ligand (Khoury and Sayegh, 2004). The delicate balance between positive and negative regulatory signals can determine the outcome of a specific immune response.

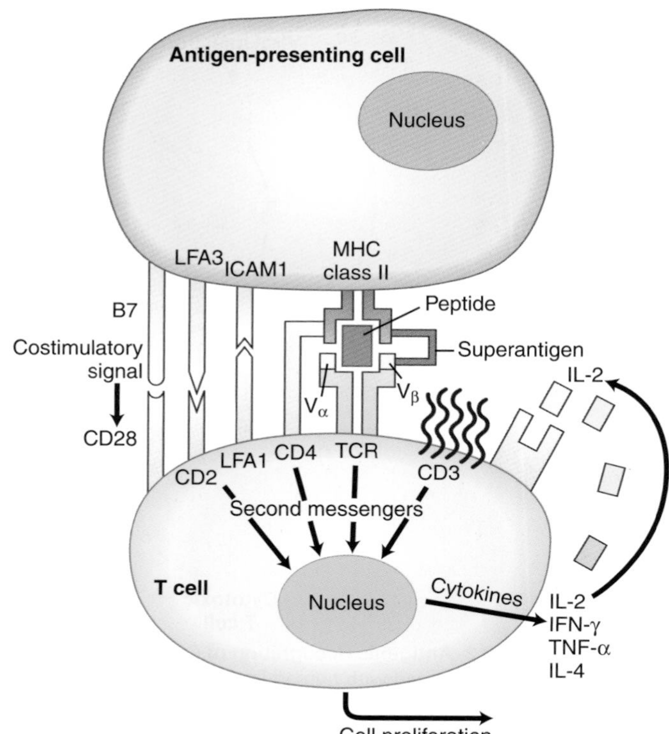


**Fig. 49.5** Antigen-Driven Activation of Helper T Cells. Proliferation of T cells requires the delivery of a number of concordant signals. Along with stimulation through the T-cell receptor–*CD3* complex, the presence of appropriate costimulatory signals via *CD28* antigen, adhesion molecules, leukocyte function antigen 1 *(LFA1)* and *CD2*, and the coreceptor molecule CD4 are essential for T-cell activation and proliferation. The membrane events of antigen recognition lead to activation of second messengers. The second messengers signal the nucleus and cell to divide and secrete cytokines. Interleukin 2 *(IL-2)* acts as an autocrine growth stimulator, thereby amplifying the response. *ICAM*, Intercellular adhesion molecule; *IFN-γ*, interferon γ; *MHC*, major histocompatibility complex; *TCR*, T-cell receptor; *TNF-α*, tumor necrosis factor alpha.

***Cell migration.*** Molecules primarily involved in cell migration into tissues include chemokines, integrins, selectins, and matrix metalloproteinases (MMPs). Chemokines constitute a large family of chemoattractant peptides that regulate the vast spectrum of leukocyte migration events through interactions with chemokine receptors. The integrin family includes VCAM-1, ICAM-1, LFA-3, CD45, and CD2 and mediates adhesion to endothelial cells and guiding cell traffic. L-selectins facilitate the rolling of leukocytes along the surface of endothelial cells and function as a homing receptor to target peripheral lymphoid organs. The MMPs are a family of proteinases secreted by inflammatory cells; MMPs digest specific components of the extracellular matrix, thereby facilitating lymphocyte entry through basement membranes including the blood-brain barrier (BBB).

## Accessory Molecules for B-Cell Activation

Like T cells, B cells require accessory molecules that supplement signals mediated through cell-surface Igs. Signaling molecules whose functions are likely to be analogous to CD3 are linked to Ig. Unlike T cells that may only respond to peptide antigens, B cells can respond to proteins, peptides, polysaccharides, nucleic acids, lipids, and small chemicals. B cells responding to peptide antigens are dependent on T-cell help for proliferation and differentiation, and these antigens are termed *thymus-dependent* (T-dependent). Nonprotein antigens do not

**TABLE 49.1 An Abridged List of Cytokines Involved in Interactions Between the Immune and Nervous Systems**

| Cytokine | Cell Source | Cells Principally Affected | Major Functions |
|---|---|---|---|
| IL-1 | Most cells; macrophages, microglia | Most cells; T cells, microglia, astrocytes, macrophages | Costimulates T- and B-cell activation<br>Induces IL-6, promotes IL-2 and IL-2R transcription<br>Endogenous pyrogen, induces sleep |
| IL-2 | T cells | T cells, NK cells, B cells | Growth stimulation |
| IL-3 | T cells | Bone marrow precursors for all cell lineages | Growth stimulation |
| IL-4 | T cells | B cells, T cells, macrophages | MHC II up-regulation<br>Isotype switching (IgG1, IgE) |
| IL-6 | Macrophages, endothelial cells, fibroblasts, T cells | Hepatocytes, B cells, T cells | Inflammation, costimulates T-cell activation<br>MHC I up-regulation, increases vascular permeability<br>Acute phase response (Shwartzman reaction) |
| IL-10 | Macrophages, T cells | Macrophages, T cells | Inhibition of IFN-γ, TNF-α, IL-6 production<br>Down-regulation of MHC expression (macrophages) |
| IL-12 | Macrophages, dendritic cells | T cells, NK cells | Costimulates B-cell growth, CD4+ $T_H1$ cell differentiation, IFN-γ synthesis, cytolytic function |
| IL-17 | T cells | Neutrophils, T cells, epithelial cells, fibroblasts | Host defense against gram-negative bacteria, induction of neutrophilic responses<br>Induction of proinflammatory cytokines |
| IFN-γ | T cells, NK cells | Astrocytes, macrophages, endothelial cells, NK cells | MHC I and II expression<br>Induces TNF-α production, isotype switching ($IgG_2$)<br>Synergizes with TNF-α for many functions |
| TNF-α | Macrophages, microglia (T cells) | Most cells, including oligodendrocytes | Cytotoxic (e.g., for oligodendrocytes), lethal at high doses<br>Up-regulates MHC, promotes leukocyte extravasation<br>Induces IL-1, IL-6, cachexia; endogenous pyrogen |
| Lymphotoxin (TNF-β) | T cells | Most cells (shares receptor with TNF-α) | Cytotoxic (at short range or through contact)<br>Promotes extravasation |
| TGF-β | Most cells; macrophages, T cells, neurons | Most cells | Pleiotropic, antiproliferative, anticytokine<br>Promotes vascularization, healing |

*IFN-γ*, Interferon gamma; *Ig*, immunoglobulin; *IL*, interleukin; *MHC*, major histocompatibility complex; *NK*, natural killer; *TGF-β*, transforming growth factor beta; *TNF-α*, tumor growth factor alpha; *TNF-β*, tumor growth factor beta.

require T-cell help to induce antibody production and are therefore T-independent.

The interaction between B cells and T-helper (CD4+) cells requires expression of MHC class II by B cells and is antigen dependent. In addition, a number of other molecules mediate adhesion between T and B cells and induce signaling for B-cell activation. These include B7 expressed on B cells interacting with CD28 on T cells and CD40 on B cells interacting with CD154. Interaction of T-helper and B cells occurs in the peripheral lymphoid organs, initially in the primary follicles and later in the germinal centers of the follicle. Activation of B cells induces activation of transcription factors (c-Fos, JunB, NFκB, and c-Myc), which in turn promote proliferation and Ig secretion. Cytokines elicited from the T-helper cell induce isotype switching in B cells, producing stronger and long-lived memory responses, in contrast to weak IgM responses to T-independent antigens.

Further generation of high-affinity antibody-producing B cells and memory B cells occurs in the germinal center of lymphoid follicles through a process called *affinity maturation*. As the amount of available antigen lessens, B cells that do not express high-affinity receptors for antigen are eliminated by apoptosis. Some B cells lose the ability to produce Ig but survive for long periods and become memory B cells.

## Regulation of the Immune Response

### Cytokines

Cytokines play a major role in regulating the immune response. Cytokines are broadly divided into the following categories, which are not mutually exclusive: (1) growth factors: IL-1, IL-2, IL-3, and IL-4 and colony-stimulating factors; (2) activation factors, such as interferons (α, β, and γ, which are also antiviral); (3) regulatory or cytotoxic factors, including IL-10, IL-12, transforming growth factor beta (TGF-β), lymphotoxins, and tumor necrosis factor alpha (TNF-α); and (4) chemokines that are chemotactic inflammatory factors, such as IL-8, MIP-1α, and MIP-1β.

Cytokines are necessary for T-cell activation and for the amplification and modulation of the immune response. A limited representation of the cytokines that participate in the immune response is shown in Table 49.1. Secretion of IL-1 by macrophages results in stimulation of T cells. This leads to synthesis of IL-2 and IL-2 receptors and finally to the clonal expansion of T cells. Only activated T cells express the IL-2 receptor (CD25); therefore the cytokine-induced expansion favors antigen-activated cells only. T-cell activation causes secretion of interferon gamma (IFN-γ), which induces expression of MHC class I and class II molecules on many cell types including APCs. This in turn increases the T-cell response to the antigen. Secretion of IL-2 also results in activation of NK cells that mediate lysis of tumor cell targets. In addition, IL-3 is released, resulting in stimulation of hematopoietic stem cells. The signal for differentiation of B cells to form antibody-secreting cells involves clonal expansion and differentiation of virgin memory B cells. IL-4 and B-cell differentiation factors secreted by T cells induce differentiation and expansion of committed B cells to become plasma cells.

IFN-α and IFN-β are both type I interferons. IFN-α is produced by macrophages, whereas IFN-β is produced by fibroblasts. Both inhibit viral replication by causing cells to synthesize enzymes that interfere with viral replication. Also they can inhibit the proliferation of lymphocytes by unknown mechanisms.

Although the emphasis has been on factors that cause expansion and differentiation of lymphocytes, there are cytokines that can down-regulate immune responses. Thus IFN-α and IFN-β, in addition to possessing antiviral properties, can modulate antibody response by virtue of their antiproliferative properties. Similarly, TGF-β (a cytokine produced by T cells and macrophages) also can decrease cell proliferation. IL-10, a growth factor for B cells, inhibits the production of IFN-γ and thus may have antiinflammatory effects.

CD4$^+$ T-helper cells differentiate into $T_H1$ or $T_H2$ phenotypes, as well as a more recently described $T_H17$ subset, which secrete characteristic cytokines and stimulate specific functions. $T_H1$ cells secrete IFN-γ, IL-2, and TNF-α. These cytokines exert proinflammatory functions and, in $T_H1$-mediated diseases such as MS, promote tissue injury. IL-2, TNF-α, and IFN-γ mediate activation of macrophages and induce DTH. $T_H1$ cell differentiation is driven by IL-12, a cytokine produced by monocytes and macrophages. In contrast, the $T_H2$ cytokines IL-4, IL-5, IL-6, IL-10, and IL-13 promote antibody production by B cells, enhance eosinophil functions, and generally suppress CMI. $T_H3$ cells secrete TGF-β, which inhibits proliferation of T cells and inhibits activation of macrophages. Cytokines of the $T_H1$ type may inhibit production of $T_H2$ cytokines and vice versa. More recently, a subset of T cells that predominantly produce IL-17 have been described (Yao et al., 1995). These cells are believed to represent a distinct subset from IFN-γ-producing $T_H1$ cells, evidenced by the dependence of $T_H$ IL-17 cells on IL-6 and TGF-β for differentiation (Bettelli et al., 2006; Mangan et al., 2006; Veldhoen et al., 2006) and IL-23 for expansion (Aggarwal et al., 2003; Langrish et al., 2005), as opposed to $T_H1$ cells, which are dependent on IL-12 and IL-2, respectively, for differentiation and expansion. Both $T_H1$ and $T_H2$ cytokines have been shown to suppress the development of $T_H17$ cells (Harrington et al., 2005; Park et al., 2005). $T_H17$ cells facilitate the recruitment of neutrophils and participate in the response to gram-negative organisms. These cells may also play a role in the initiation of autoimmune disease. $T_H17$ cells produce a range of cytokines and may produce IL-10, IL-21, and IL-9 (classic $T_H17$), or IL-23, IFN-γ, and GM-CSF (alternative $T_H17$) that are more pathogenic (Peters et al., 2011). Interestingly, recent data showed that modest increase in sodium chloride concentration induces SGK1 expression in T cells with increased IL-23R expression and $T_H17$ cell generation in vitro (Wu et al., 2013), suggesting that increased dietary salt intake might represent an environmental risk factor for the development of autoimmune diseases through the induction of pathogenic $T_H17$ cells (Kleinewietfeld et al., 2013).

Another effector T-cell subset, $T_H9$ cells, has recently been described (Dardalhon et al., 2008; Veldhoen et al., 2008). Driven by the combined effects of TGF-β and IL-4, $T_H9$ cells produce large amounts of IL-9 and IL-10. It has been shown that IL-9 combined with TGF-β can contribute to $T_H17$ cell differentiation, and $T_H17$ cells themselves can produce IL-9 (Elyaman et al., 2009).

Traditionally, $T_H$ cell subsets have been distinguished by their patterns of cytokine production, but identification of distinguishing surface molecule markers has been a major advance in the field. Tim (T cell, immunoglobulin and mucin-domain containing molecules) represents an important family of molecules that encode cell-surface receptors involved in the regulation of $T_H1$ and $T_H2$ cell–mediated immunity. Tim-3 is specifically expressed on $T_H1$ cells and negatively regulates $T_H1$ responses through interaction with the Tim-3 ligand, galactin-9, also expressed on CD4$^+$ T cells (Monney et al., 2002; Sabatos et al., 2003; Zhu et al., 2005). Tim-2 is expressed on $T_H2$ cells (Chakravarti et al., 2005), and appears to negatively regulate $T_H2$ cell proliferation, although this has not been fully established. Tim-1 is expressed on $T_H2$ cells > $T_H1$ cells, and interacts with Tim-4 on APCs to induce T-cell proliferation (Meyers et al., 2005).

### Chemokines

Chemokines are a recently discovered and extensively studied group of molecules that aid in leukocyte mobility and directed movement. Chemokines may be grouped into two subfamilies based on the configuration and binding of the two terminal cysteine residues. If the two residues participating in disulfide bonding are adjacent, they are termed the *C-C family* (e.g., MCP, MIP-1α, RANTES). Those separated by one amino acid, are C-X-C family members (e.g., IL-8), where X indicates a nonconserved amino acid. Two chemokine receptors, CCR-5 and CXCR-4, can act as coreceptors for strains of HIV. Chemokines are produced by a variety of immune and nonimmune cells. Monocytes, T cells, basophils, and eosinophils express chemokine receptors, and these receptor-ligand interactions are critical to the recruitment of leukocytes into specific tissues.

## Termination of an Immune Response

The primary goal of the immune response is to protect the organism from infectious agents and generate memory T- and B-cell responses that provide accelerated and high-avidity secondary responses on reencountering antigens. It is desirable to terminate these responses once an antigen has been cleared. In parallel, the immune system must constantly function to prevent autoimmune activation and to maintain self-tolerance. A number of systems operate to prevent uncontrolled responses. Here we discuss termination of individual components of the immune response. Following is a discussion of the mechanisms that maintain self-tolerance, many of which are also involved in immune-response termination.

### B-Cell Inhibition

In most instances, an antigen is cleared either by cells of the reticuloendothelial system or through the formation of antigen–antibody complexes. These complexes can themselves result in the inhibition of B-cell differentiation and proliferation through binding of the Fc receptor to the CD32 (FcγRIIB) receptor on the surface of the B cell.

### Immunoglobulin

The variable regions of the Ig and the TCR molecule represent novel proteins that can act as antigens. Antigenic variable regions are called *idiotopes*, and responses against such antigens are called *anti-idiotypic*. Niels Jerne's network hypothesis postulates that anti-idiotypic responses serve to regulate the immune response; however, the extent to which this operates is unclear.

### T Cells

Termination of the T-cell immune response is mediated by several mechanisms including anergy, deletion, and suppressor cell activity. Anergy or functional unresponsiveness occurs when there is insufficient T-cell activation. Repeated stimulation of T cells may lead to activation-induced cell death through apoptosis. Cytokine-mediated regulation can also serve to terminate the immune response, notably by secretion of $T_H2$ and $T_H3$ cytokines. Regulatory cells (discussed in the following section) generally inhibit the immune response through secretion of cytokines, through cytotoxic mechanisms, or by modulation of the function of APCs.

A combination of the above-described mechanisms cooperate to maintain self-tolerance, particularly peripheral tolerance, and are discussed later.

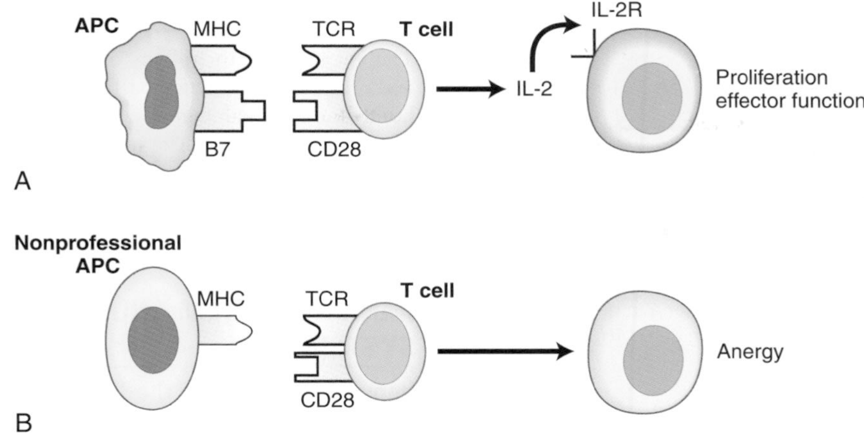


**Fig. 49.6 A Two-Signal Model of T-Cell Activation.** Activation of the T-cell receptor *(TCR)* by an antigen major histocompatibility complex *(MHC)* provides signal 1, which is sufficient to induce the T cell to enter the cell cycle and begin blast transformation, which is characterized by an increase in cell size. Signal 2, the costimulatory signal, can be provided to the T cell through interaction of CD28 with molecules of the B7 family found on the surface of bone marrow–derived antigen-presenting cells *(APCs)*. **A,** In this instance, TCR signals are complemented, enabling the T cell to proliferate, produce cytokines, and develop mature effector functions. **B,** In the absence of a second signal, T-cell activation is abortive, and the cell becomes anergic. Signal 2 might not be delivered if the APC does not express a costimulatory ligand on its surface, perhaps because a nonprofessional APC, such as an epithelial cell, is presenting antigen. *IL,* Interleukin.

## SELF-TOLERANCE

An organism's ability to maintain a state of unresponsiveness to its own antigens is termed *self-tolerance.* Self-tolerance is maintained through three principal mechanisms: deletion, anergy, and suppression. Self-tolerance may be broadly categorized as either central or peripheral tolerance. Similar mechanisms may also be used to induce tolerance to a foreign antigen or terminate an immune response.

### Central Tolerance

Bone marrow stem cells migrate to the thymus, thereby becoming thymocytes, or T cells. In this location, T-cell VDJ germline genetic elements recombine to create $\alpha$ and $\beta$ chains, which in turn form the TCR. Thymocytes then undergo a process of education that involves positive and negative selection. Positive selection of thymocytes occurs in the thymus cortex when the cells are in the double negative stage, $CD4^-$ $CD8^-$. The cortex contains dendritic and epithelial cells that present MHC antigens to the developing thymocytes. T cells with receptor having no affinity to MHC will fail to receive signals needed for maturation and will die in situ. Those with low affinity toward MHC survive and become single-positive thymocytes depending on their affinity toward MHC I ($CD8^+$) or MHC II ($CD4^+$). In the thymus medulla, thymocytes that display a high affinity toward self-antigen are deleted by apoptosis, a process called *negative selection.* Most T-cell education occurs in the thymus; however, extrathymic sites may exist.

### Peripheral Tolerance

Self-reactive lymphocytes may escape central tolerance; therefore peripheral mechanisms exist to maintain self-tolerance. This is termed *peripheral tolerance.* Peripheral tolerance is maintained through clonal anergy or clonal deletion. It is not clear to what extent each of these mechanisms functions in maintaining human self-tolerance; however, extensive research has been done to elucidate the mechanisms through which anergy and deletion work. In addition, self-tolerance may be maintained despite the presence of antigen-responsive lymphocytes. It is postulated that this is due to the presence of suppressor T cells or other factors that may interfere with a successful lymphocyte response.

### Anergy Due to Failure of T-Cell Activation

In normal circumstances, an APC presents antigen as a peptide + MHC complex (signal one). In the absence of signal one, the T cell dies because of neglect. If signal one is presented in the absence of costimulatory signals (signal two), the T cell becomes anergic. An example of this situation occurs when an antigen is presented by nonprofessional APCs that lack the appropriate costimulatory molecules (Fig. 49.6). However, when a T cell is activated, it up-regulates the expression of an alternate costimulatory molecule, CTLA-4. CTLA-4 engagement by CD80 and CD86 on the surface of APCs sends a negative signal to the T cell, inhibiting cell growth and proliferation. Animals deficient for CTLA-4 expression on their T lymphocytes have an uncontrolled lymphoproliferative phenotype with autoreactivity (Waterhouse et al., 1995).

### Apoptosis

Apoptosis is the process in which a cell undergoes programmed cell death. As opposed to necrosis, when interruption of the supply of nutrients triggers cell death, apoptosis may be triggered by various signals including withdrawal of growth factors, cytokines, exposure to corticosteroids, and repeated exposure to antigens. Mediators of apoptosis include the Bcl family of genes, which are mostly antiapoptotic, and the Fas family of genes, which are proapoptotic. Activated T cells also express Fas ligand (CD95L or FasL) and Fas (CD95); ligation of Fas and FasL induces apoptosis of the T cells.

Repeated stimulation with an antigen may also induce apoptosis via the Fas/FasL pathway, a process termed *activation-induced cell death* (AICD). Therefore an autoreactive T lymphocyte may encounter large doses of self-antigen in the periphery and consequently may be deleted by AICD. Mice lacking Fas or FasL develop a lupus-like syndrome (Zhou, et al., 1996), and mutations in the Fas gene were associated with an autoimmune disease with lymphoproliferation in humans (Drappa, et al., 1996).

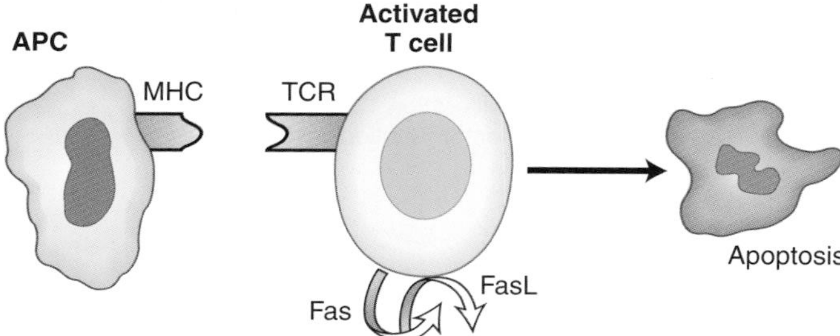


**Fig. 49.7** Activation of the T cell leads to coexpression of the death receptor *Fas* (CD95) and its ligand *(FasL)*, resulting in death of the cell and neighboring cells. *APC,* Antigen-presenting cell; *MHC,* major histocompatibility complex; *TCR,* T-cell receptor.

IL-2 is the prototypical growth factor, inducing clonal expansion of antigen-stimulated lymphocytes; paradoxically, disruption of the IL-2 gene leads to accumulation of activated lymphocytes and autoimmune syndromes (Sadlack, et al., 1993). This is because IL-2 induces the transcription and surface expression of Fas ligand (FasL). Interactions of Fas with FasL lead to cell death (Fig. 49.7). Therefore IL-2 plays a dual role in T-cell regulation, reflecting a possible role for cytokine concentration and timing of exposure. Other cytokines that mediate apoptosis and cell death are TNF-α and IFN-γ. Complete absence of either of these cytokines results in deficient T-cell apoptosis, inability to terminate the immune response, and uncontrolled autoimmune disease.

### Regulatory T Cells

Regulatory T cells ($T_{reg}$) function to down-regulate CD4 and CD8 T-cell responses. Regulatory T cells can be of the $CD4^+$ or $CD8^+$ subtypes. Regulatory T cells can be generated under similar conditions used to generate anergic cells, and it has been postulated that they are the same entity (Lombardi et al., 1994). Several populations of regulatory or suppressor T cells have been described in humans. $CD4^+$ regulatory T cells were initially identified by expression of CD4 and high levels of CD25 (Baecher-Allan et al., 2001; Dieckmann et al., 2001; Levings et al., 2001; Stephens et al., 2001; Yagi et al., 2004). Most Tregs also express GITR, CD103, CTLA-4, lymphocyte activation gene 3 (LAG-3), and low levels of CD45RB, although no single marker is specific for Tregs. The expression of the transcription factor Foxp3 correlates with regulatory function of $CD4^+$ T cells in mice (Littman and Rudensky, 2010) and deletion of Foxp3 results in loss of suppressive phenotype. In humans, immune dysfunction/polyendocrinopathy/enteropathy/X-linked (IPEX) syndrome is an autoimmune syndrome consisting of lymphoproliferation lympho-proliferation, thyroiditis, insulin-dependent diabetes mellitus, enteropathy, and other immune disorders. Most cases of IPEX syndrome are caused by mutations in *FOXP3*.

Other types of regulatory T cells include $CD8^+CD28^-$ T cells (Koide and Engleman 1990), IL-10-producing $T_H2$ cells (Bacchetta, Bigler et al. 1994), and TGF-β-producing $T_H3$ cells (Kitano et al., 2000; Levings et al., 2001; Roncaro and Levings, 2000). In humans, there is little evidence for antigen-specific suppressor cell responses. Regulatory T cells suppress T-cell proliferation through a variety of mechanisms, including the production of immunosuppressive cytokines ($T_H2$ or TGF-β) or through T–T cell interactions, including the expression of inhibitory molecules such as CTLA-4. Regulatory cells play an important role in the control of the immune response in autoimmune disorders, and the function of regulatory T cells may be enhanced by immunomodulatory therapies.

## THE GUT MICROBIOME

The gut is home to trillions of commensal bacteria, viruses, fungi, and protozoa. Commensal bacteria have co-evolved with humans and homeostasis is maintained with beneficial effects for both (Forbes, Bernstein et al. 2018). The microbiome has a large influence on the immune system, and changes in the microbiome have been reported in many diseases although the exact mechanisms by which these changes affect human health are still unknown. This in an area of active investigation.

## IMMUNE SYSTEM AND CENTRAL NERVOUS SYSTEM

### Immune Privilege in the Central Nervous System

Immunological reactions in the CNS differ from those in the rest of the body because of its unique architecture, cellular composition, and molecular expression. The CNS has been termed an *immunologically privileged site* because of the relative improved survival of allografts within this region. Indeed, the same factors that play a role in immunological tolerance in the CNS play a role in immune-mediated diseases involving the CNS, infections of the CNS, tumor survival, and therapies.

Important factors relevant to immunological responses in the CNS are: (1) absence of classic lymphatic drainage, limiting the immunological circulation; (2) the BBB, which limits the passage of immune cells and factors; (3) the low level of expression of MHC factors, particularly MHC II in the resident cells of the CNS; (4) low levels of potent APCs, such as dendritic or Langerhans cells; and (5) the presence of immunosuppressive factors such as TGF-β (Wilbanks and Streilein, 1992) and CD200 (Webb and Barclay, 1984).

The CNS was long-thought to lack a lymphatic system; however, the recent discovery of lymphatic vessels within the CNS dural sinuses (Aspelund et al., 2015; Louveau et al., 2015). has opened new areas of investigation into the trafficking of cerebral immune cells. Monocyte-derived CNS resident cells, termed *microglia,* play an important role in immune surveillance in these areas. The BBB is composed of tight junctions between endothelial cells and a layer of astrocytic foot processes that prevent entry of inflammatory cells and other factors into the CNS. Entry of inflammatory cells across the BBB is facilitated by up-regulation of adhesion molecules ICAM-1 and VCAM-1 on endothelial cells. T cells must be activated before crossing the BBB. Entry is facilitated by expression of receptors for adhesion molecules, including α4-integrin.

The CNS houses cells that are capable of antigen presentation under certain conditions in vitro, but to what extent this occurs in vivo remains under debate. In the CNS, endogenous expression of MHC class I and class II on APCs, such as microglia, is low, and in oligodendrocytes and astrocytes it is almost undetectable. Neurons express MHC class I only when damaged and in the presence of IFN-γ (Neumann et al., 1995). Expression of MHC antigens on both microglia and astrocytes is enhanced by the presence of cytokines, TNF-α, and IFN-γ. Under certain conditions, microglial cells may play a role as APCs in the nervous system (Perry, 1994). More recently, populations of perivascular dendritic cells capable of antigen presentation have been identified in rodents (Greter et al., 2005), with analogous populations demonstrated in humans; however, their role in human disease is unclear.

Immune privilege in the CNS is also influenced by the constitutive expression of a number of immunoregulatory factors, some of which are common to immune privilege in the anterior chamber of the eye. Anterior chamber immune privilege is due in part to expression of

TGF-β in the aqueous of the eye. In the CNS, TGF-β is produced by astrocytes and microglia and may play a role in down-regulating immune responses locally. Neurons are also capable of producing TGF-β, which in animal models has been shown to facilitate the differentiation of regulatory T cells (Liu, et al., 2006). Increased expression of Fas ligand in the CNS compared with the peripheral nervous system (PNS) may increase apoptosis of T cells, thereby down-regulating the immune response (Moalem et al., 1999). Some CNS tumors express large amounts of TGF-β, which may play a role in protecting them from immune surveillance. CNS tumors may also express Fas or Fas ligand, facilitating protection from immune surveillance. Some populations of neurons express a cell surface marker named *CD200*. CD200 is a nonsignaling molecule but serves to inhibit activation of cells including microglia and macrophages that express the CD200 receptor (CD200R) (Hoek et al., 2000; Wright et al., 2000). CD200 has been shown to down-regulate inflammatory responses in models of MS (Liu et al., 2010) and uveitis (Broderick et al., 2002, Banerjee and Dick, 2004). Fractalkine (CXCL1) is a chemokine that is constitutively expressed on some populations of neurons. Interaction with its receptor, CX3CR1, present on microglia and NK cells, serves to down-regulate microglial-mediated neurotoxicity both in vitro and in animal models of Parkinson disease and amyotrophic lateral sclerosis (ALS) (Cardona et al., 2006). In the animal model of MS, absence of fractalkine or its receptor resulted in a reduction of NK cells in the CNS and exacerbation of disease, supporting the view that NK cells play an inhibitory role in CNS inflammation (Huang et al., 2006).

### Neuroglial Cells and the Immune Response

Neuroglial cells including microglia and astrocytes participate in immune responses within the CNS, and there is increasing evidence that these cells play a central role in initiating and propagating immune-mediated diseases of the CNS.

Microglia are derived from bone marrow cells during ontogeny (Hickey and Kimura, 1988) and reside within the CNS as three principal types of cells: perivascular microglia, parenchymal microglia, and Kolmer cells, which reside in the choroid plexus. Microglia have mitotic potential and can differentiate from bone marrow–derived cells to perivascular microglia and parenchymal microglia. Compared with macrophages, microglia are relatively radioresistant. Microglia may exist either in a resting (ramified) form or activated or phagocytic forms within the CNS. Activated microglia express higher levels of MHC class II and produce higher levels of proinflammatory cytokines including TNF-α, IL-6, and IL-1, as well as nitric oxide and glutamate. Microglia express chemokine receptors and various PRRs, including TLRs. PRRs recognize PAMPs expressed by a variety of microbes, and interaction results in microglial activation. The primary functions of microglia are immune surveillance for foreign antigens and phagocytic scavengers of cellular debris. Microglia, particularly perivascular microglia, may also participate in antigen presentation within the CNS under certain conditions. Microglia play a role in regulating the programmed elimination of neural cells during brain development and, in some cases, enhance neuronal survival by producing neurotrophic and antiinflammatory cytokines. Microglia may also play a role in neuroregeneration and repair. However, there is overwhelming evidence that microglia play a deleterious role in several neurodegenerative diseases: MS, ALS, Parkinson disease, and HIV-associated dementia. Their role in Alzheimer disease (AD) is less clear. Overactivation of microglia, possibly by microbes or other environmental factors through PRRs, may result in chronic proinflammatory milieu in the CNS, leading to progressive neurodegeneration. Strategies to down-regulate such responses are under investigation (Block et al., 2007).

Astrocytes play multiple roles in the CNS, including their role in the glia limitans at the BBB and physical support of neuronal and axonal structures, as well as provision of growth factors. Astrocytes secrete cytokines including TGF-β and are also influenced by IL-1 and interferons to divide and express proteins such as costimulatory molecules and TLRs on their surfaces. There is increasing evidence against the role of astrocytes in antigen presentation within the CNS. Astrocytes play a critical role in converting glutamate to glutamine, a less toxic substance, so impairment of astrocyte function may result in increased glutamate-mediated neurotoxicity. Astrocytes also produce chemo-kines, including stromal-derived factor-1 (SDF-1), which plays a significant role in HIV-associated dementia.

Cells of the CNS not only respond to inflammatory stimuli but also are also capable of producing cytokines and other inflammatory factors, often directly under the influence of lymphocytes. These observations led to the conclusion that the brain is not an immunologically sequestered organ but that it interacts, produces immunologically active factors, and is closely involved with the systemic immune response.

## PUTATIVE MECHANISMS OF HUMAN AUTOIMMUNE DISEASE

Why does autoimmune disease occur? It largely results as a culmination of interactions between genetic predisposition, environmental factors, and failure of self-tolerance maintenance mechanisms. Some diseases such as MS are termed *immune-mediated* because no definitive autoantigen has been demonstrated. Other diseases are clear cases of molecular mimicry such as Gd1b-mediated axonal neuropathy, in which the self-antigen attacked by the immune system is similar to that of an environmental antigen (in this case the Penner O:19 serotype of *Campylobacter jejuni*). Thus autoimmune diseases may be mediated by heterogeneous mechanisms, and in some cases more than one mechanism may be operating.

Autoimmune diseases may be classified as T- or B-cell mediated. Some, such as myasthenia gravis (MG), are mediated through a combination of both. In many B cell–mediated diseases, an autoantigen has been identified, to which the B cell produces autoantibodies. Examples are MG, in which sera from patients contain antibodies to the α subunit of the acetylcholine receptor, and Lambert-Eaton syndrome, in which symptoms are caused by antibodies targeting calcium channels. In contrast to T-cell–mediated diseases, identification of autoantigens in antibody-mediated diseases may be easier, because B cells react to whole proteins, whereas the determinants recognized by T cells tend to be APC-processed small peptides of 10–20 amino acids. Thus for T-cell–mediated diseases such as MS, inflammatory demyelinating polyneuropathy, and polymyositis, there is little evidence demonstrating a causal relationship between an autoantigen and autoimmune disease. In addition, T-cell reactivity to autoantigens does not necessarily guarantee disease, because autoreactivity to some self-antigens is seen in healthy individuals. Thus the only conclusive evidence that can indicate causality between an antigen and T-cell–mediated autoimmune disease would be the reversal of the disease process by removal of the putative autoreactive T-cell repertoire. Although this has been feasible in some animal models, establishing the efficacy of such a strategy is difficult in most human T-cell–mediated diseases.

### Genetic Factors

Genetic makeup plays a role in susceptibility to autoimmune diseases. In particular, an association between certain MHC haplotypes and disease has been noted. MS is linked to the HLA-DR2 allele, and the relative risk of having this allele in the Northern European population is 3.8. MG has been linked to HLA-DR3. However, the presence of the allele does not guarantee disease. In general, the relative risk of developing disease among individuals who carry the antigen may be calculated by the following formula:

$$\frac{[\text{number of patients carrying the HLA antigen}] \times [\text{number of controls lacking the antigen}]}{[\text{number of patients lacking the HLA antigen}] \times [\text{number of controls carrying the antigen}]}$$

Association of a particular HLA haplotype with autoimmune disease may be due to the ability of a particular MHC molecule to bind and present autoantigen to the T cell, as in MS where the MHC class II allele, DRB1*1501, has been shown to be effective in presenting myelin basic protein (MBP peptide) to T-cell clones isolated from MS patients (Wucherpfennig et al., 1995). Conversely, if an MHC molecule does not bind a particular self-antigen in the thymus, the developing T cell will not recognize that antigen as self and will escape negative selection. Therefore certain MHC haplotypes have an association with disease, whereas others protect against disease. Disease linkage tends to be with class II genes of the MHC rather than class I, suggesting a key role for T-cell autoimmunity.

Association of a particular HLA-haplotype with disease may be due to its linkage to another locus or disease susceptibility gene. *Linkage disequilibrium* refers to the increased chance of inheriting two alleles together because they are genetically linked, as opposed to inheriting them together as separate random events.

Sex is one of the most important genetic determinants associated with autoimmune disease. Many autoimmune diseases are more frequent in females; systemic lupus erythematosus (SLE) is 10 times more common in women, and MS twice as common. Evidence from animal models has shown that females are more resistant to infections and reject foreign skin grafts sooner than their male counterparts. This is especially true during periods of high estrogen availability. Estrogen levels decrease after ovulation or during pregnancy, and this is associated with a progesterone surge. The lowering of estrogen ensures immunological tolerance toward the sperm and subsequently toward the fetus. Therefore estrogen's effects on the immune system may predispose women toward autoimmune diseases. This is reflected in experimental disease models of autoimmunity. Only female (NZB × NZW)F1 mice develop the SLE-like disease, and this is abrogated by androgen treatment. Similarly, in experimental autoimmune encephalomyelitis (EAE), an experimental model for MS, female SJL mice are more susceptible to disease induction and are protected with testosterone (Dalal et al., 1997). Preliminary studies testing the effectiveness of a testosterone gel in males with MS have shown encouraging results but require additional validation. Initial studies investigating estriol effects in women with MS have shown a potent effect on reduction of new lesion formation, evident on gadolinium-enhanced magnetic resonance imaging (MRI) (Sicotte et al., 2002). Independent of sex hormones, the XY sex chromosome complement induces increased severity of EAE, with an increased expression of TLR-7 on CNS neurons (Du et al., 2014).

### Environmental Factors

Environmental factors may play a role in the pathogenesis of autoimmune diseases. Molecular mimicry is one of the mechanisms implicated. In this situation, an environmental antigen resembling a self-antigen elicits an immune response to both itself and the self-antigen. The environmental antigen involved in molecular mimicry may be a superantigen. Superantigens have the property of stimulating all T cells that express a given TCR variable gene family, regardless of their exact specificity, because of direct TCR-superantigen interaction. They are usually of bacterial or viral origin and bind as intact molecules to MHC.

In many cases of molecular mimicry, the environmental antigen is a pathogen, and autoimmune disease follows the pathogen-caused disease. The classic example of this is streptococcal-induced endocarditis. Neurological diseases caused by this mechanism include streptococcal-induced chorea, Gd1b axonal neuropathy, Semple rabies vaccine–induced encephalomyelitis, and the anti-Hu paraneoplastic syndrome. Several studies have demonstrated that both adult (Ascherio and Munger 2007) and pediatric (Alotaibi et al., 2004; Pohl et al., 2006; Banwell et al., 2007; Lunemann et al., 2008) MS patients more frequently demonstrate evidence of a remote infection with Epstein-Barr virus (EBV) than controls, implicating a role for this virus in disease pathogenesis. Interestingly, epitopes of EBV resemble MBP, supporting a role for molecular mimicry in disease pathogenesis (Lang et al., 2002). However, despite these associations, it is clear that the majority of persons are infected with EBV without autoimmune sequelae. Recent studies have integrated risk factors in the pathogenesis of MS and found that the relative risk of MS among DR15-positive women with elevated (>1 : 320) anti-EBNA-1 titers was ninefold higher than that of DR15-negative women with low (<1 : 80) anti-EBNA-1 titers (De Jager et al., 2008).

It is possible that once an inflammatory reaction proceeds, the tissue injury may expose other self-antigens that were previously unrecognized by the immune system. For unknown reasons, peripheral tolerance mechanisms may fail, and an autoimmune reaction ensues. The spreading of the autoimmune reaction from one antigen to another is termed *determinant spreading* or *epitope spreading*. Epitope spreading may play a role in perpetuating immune-mediated reactions and therefore in causing chronic diseases. Therapies that inhibit molecular mimicry or epitope spreading may be useful in preventing autoimmune diseases.

## NEUROIMMUNOLOGICAL DISEASES

Immune-mediated disorders occur at all levels of the nervous system. Disorders of the CNS and PNS, including the peripheral nerve, neuromuscular junction, and muscle, have been described. Some of these disorders are clearly autoimmune, in that a clear autoantigen has been identified, whereas others are immune-mediated. In this section, we identify neurological immune-mediated diseases and highlight immunological features pertinent to pathogenesis and treatment. A full description of each disease may be found in other sections of this book.

### Multiple Sclerosis

MS is a heterogeneous disease and is characterized by neurological deficits disseminated in time and space. It is a major cause of disability in the adult population in North America. Women are predominantly affected, in a ratio of 2 : 1. The disease is characterized by a varying array of neurological deficits. There are four main disease types, classified on the basis of the clinical disease course: relapsing-remitting (RR), secondary progressive (SP), primary progressive (PP), and progressive relapsing (PR). RR disease affects 65% of patients and is characterized by onset of neurological deficits that remit over a period of weeks to months. After 15 years, most RR patients go on to have an SP form of disease in which neurological deficits become fixed and accumulate. PP patients accumulate permanent neurological deficits from the onset of disease, whereas patients with PR disease have a combination of progressive and stepwise deficits. Disease onset generally occurs in the early 20s for RR disease and in the mid-30s for PP disease, although childhood-onset MS is becoming increasingly recognized.

MS is a complex polygenic disease. Monozygotic twins carry a concordance rate of 27%, whereas dizygotic twins of the same sex display a 2.3% concordance rate. The incidence for first-degree relatives of MS patients is 2% to 5%, whereas the incidence for the general population is under 0.1%. Genetic linkage studies have been performed, and several regions of interest have been found, but the most robust association remains with the HLA region. There is an increased incidence of MS in patients with the HLA-DR2 (DR1501) haplotype (Haines et al., 1998; Sawcer and Goodfellow, 1998; Stewart et al., 1981).

More recently, a large genome-wide study identified single nucleotide polymorphism of IL-2R and IL-7R alleles as risk alleles for MS (Hafler et al., 2007). A report in 2013, now identifies 110 established MS risk variants at 103 discrete loci outside of the MHC (International MS Genetics et al., 2013). MS remains most prevalent among people of Northern European descent. There is a lower prevalence in other populations, such as Arabic and Mediterranean people, but among those with disease, there is a higher incidence of other disease-associated haplotypes such as DR4 and DR6.

Although genetic factors play an important role in pathogenesis, migration and other studies have demonstrated that environment also plays a critical role. Epidemiological studies have shown that residence in certain geographical areas and migration to these areas before the age of 15 increases the incidence of MS. In addition, there is a diminishing north-to-south gradient in MS prevalence in the Northern Hemisphere, with an opposite trend in the Southern Hemisphere. This led to the hypothesis and demonstration of an inverse association between sunlight exposure and MS (van der Mei et al., 2003).

An extension of this hypothesis has led to exploration of the role of vitamin D in MS, since vitamin D is metabolized in the skin by ultra-violet (UV) irradiation. A prospective study in army recruits found that 25-hydroxyvitamin D levels in the highest quintile (above 99.1 nmol/L) were associated with a lower risk of MS (odds ratio [OR], 0.38) (Munger et al., 2006). Treatment of animal models of MS with vitamin D ameliorates disease, and several studies have shown that the active form of vitamin D, calcitriol, can down-regulate proinflammatory dendritic cells (DC) and reduce $T_H1$ lymphocyte responses while promoting anti-inflammatory $T_H2$ lymphocyte responses (Adorini et al., 2004; Griffin et al., 2001; Penna and Adorini, 2000; Penna et al., 2007).

Studies exploring the therapeutic effects of vitamin D in MS have been reported but were mostly small studies with methodological limitations and a meta-analysis showed no significant association between high-dose vitamin D treatment and risk of MS relapses (James et al., 2013). EBV exposure appears to be a strong environmental risk factor for MS as described above. Other environmental risk factors include smoking (Ascherio et al., 2012) and childhood obesity (Chitnis et al., 2016; Hedstrom et al., 2014). Increasing evidence suggest that several of these risk factors may have a sex-specific effect, as described in Table 49.2.

Pathologically, MS is characterized by inflammatory infiltrates in the CNS white matter, with resultant demyelination and axonal transections (Trapp, et al., 1998) producing sclerotic plaques. Inflammation is generally perivenular, and lesions typically occur in the periventricular subcortical white matter, corpus callosum, optic nerve, brainstem, cerebellum, and spinal cord. Cortical lesions have also been described. The pathology of MS lesions has been classified into four distinct subtypes with the following predominant features: (1) cellular infiltration, (2) antibody deposition, (3) oligodendrocyte apoptosis, and (4) oligodendrocyte death without apoptosis (Lucchinetti et al., 2000). Observations to date show a single subtype of lesion in each patient, raising the possibility of distinct MS disease pathogenetic

**TABLE 49.2 Selected Genetic, Environmental, and Lifestyle Factors With Potentially Sexually Dimorphic Effects on Multiple Sclerosis Disease Susceptibility and Progression**

| | |
|---|---|
| Smoking | Risk of MS increased in female smokers only, but statistical significance in men could be affected by low *N* |
| | Potential mechanisms may include an interaction between sex and smoking to yield increased levels of mature peripheral functioning T cells (OKT3+) in female smokers. |
| | F:M ratio in MS parallels that in smoking; but the high F:M ratio in smoking may be driven both by decreasing rates in males or increased rates in females (Kotzamani, Panou et al. 2012) |
| Vitamin D | A functional synergy between 1,25(OH) D(3) and 17-β estradiol has been observed, mediated through estrogen receptor α, mainly in women and secondarily in men (Correale et al., 2010; Disanto et al., 2011; Nashold et al., 2009), such that Vitamin D seems to play an immunomodulatory role in MS mainly in women |
| Uric acid | Urate, an antioxidant, is significantly lower in females than males in all types of MS |
| Sunlight | Worse consequences of sunlight deprivation in women than in men |
| Westernizing gender norms | Rapid increases for girls of time spent indoors as a result of rapid urbanization, rises in female education, and participation in the workforce. |
| | Reproductive choices (see above) |
| Diet and metabolism | Overweight/obesity at ages 18–20 may double the risk of MS, but not overweight/obesity in childhood (ages 5 or 10), or adulthood. |
| | Only among female adults, obesity at MS onset may be associated with a twofold increased OR of a relapsing course at onset. |
| | Since adipocytes produce estrone, this may represent an important source of inflammatory signaling in both men and women |
| EBV exposure | Anti-Epstein-Barr VCA immunoglobulin G levels may be positively correlated with female sex and HLA DR2 |
| Genetics/Epigenetics | Genome-wide association studies have historically controlled for sex, ignoring a potential effect of SNPs in one sex |
| | Maternal parent of origin effect in transmission of disease risk, as well as of the HLA-DRB1*1501 risk allele, even when mother not affected (reviewed in Bove and Chitnis, 2013). |
| | The HLA-DRB5*0101–HLA-DRB1*1501–HLA-DQA1*0102–HLA-DQB1*0602 extended haplotype is more common in female than in male patients, has a higher F:M ratio in MS subjects than in controls, and in families with two generations of MS, females in the latest generation have an increased frequency of HLA-DRB1*15; these findings suggest a sex-specific interaction between genes and environment, leading to epigenetic regulation |

*See Bove and Chitnis, Clinical Immunology Review 2013.*

types. Activated microglia have been demonstrated in non-lesion, or otherwise normal-appearing white matter (NAWM), and may play a role in axonal damage and disease progression.

It is clear that the immune system plays a central role in mediating CNS damage in MS. Oligoclonal bands are commonly observed in the CNS of MS patients; however, the target of these antibodies has yet to be elucidated. Cell-mediated immunity, primarily involving T-helper cells, is believed to play an important role in initiating the disease, and immunological studies have substantiated the presence of activated T cells in MS. Most of the therapies for MS also target T cells. No clear autoantigen has been described in MS, and it therefore remains an immune-mediated disease rather than an autoimmune disease. Reactivity to various myelin antigens, including MBP, proteolipid protein (PLP), and myelin oligodendrocyte protein (MOG) has been investigated. MBP-reactive T cells are present in normal individuals; however, MS patients have a higher frequency of activated MBP-reactive T cells in the peripheral blood and the cerebrospinal fluid (CSF) (Zhang et al., 1994). More recently, a separate entity characterized by MOG antibodies and MOG-reactive T cells has been described, which is likely separate from MS. MOG antibody-associated diseases are more frequent in children and are characterized by optic neuritis, acute disseminated encephalomyelitis, and transverse myelitis (Reindl and Rostasy, 2015).

The immunopathogenesis of MS is thought to involve activation of myelin-specific T cells via molecular mimicry or by a superantigen presumably in the periphery. These cells are believed to predominantly be of the $T_H1$ phenotype, as evidenced by increased production of IL-12 (the major inducer of $T_H1$ cytokines) by APCs in the peripheral blood of MS patients with active disease, and the observation that a clinical trial of IFN-γ worsened MS. These cells then cross the BBB and get reactivated in the CNS when they are presented with their cognate antigen. Perivascular dendritic-like cells have been shown to play a role in T-cell reactivation in animal models of MS (Greter et al., 2005), but their role in the human disease is unclear. Adhesion molecules and their ligands are expressed on T cells and endothelial cells to facilitate passage through the BBB. VCAM-1 and its ligand, VLA-4, are up-regulated in T cells during chronic disease, thus perpetuating inflammation, and VLA-4 antibody therapy (natalizumab) has recently been shown to be effective in reducing MS relapses and lesion formation.

Invasion of activated T cells into the brain and reactivation within the CNS initiates a cascade of cytokines. IL-2, IFN-γ, and TNF-α activate macrophages, which in turn elicit nitric oxide and TNF-α. In experimental models, myelin damage is mediated by nitric oxide lipid peroxidation, direct TNF-α damage, and complement-induced pore formation. As mentioned previously, $T_H2$ cytokines can induce B-cell activation and antibody production that further damage myelin. Each of these steps in the pathogenesis may be targeted for therapeutic intervention (see Fig. 49.1).

There is mounting evidence indicating that T cells play a key role in the relapsing-remitting phase of MS. However, it is increasingly evident that that disease progression in MS occurs through distinct mechanisms (Weiner 2009). Epitope spreading may occur within the CNS, and in animal models can be facilitated by microglia, macrophages, and dendritic cells (McMahon et al., 2005). Activated microglia are found in progressive forms of the disease and have been associated with axonal damage and demyelination (Kutzelnigg et al., 2005). B-cell follicles have been demonstrated at autopsy in patients with chronic MS (Serafini et al., 2004) and may play a role in facilitating an autonomous inflammatory response within the CNS. Cortical demyelination is also associated with progressive forms of MS (Kutzelnigg et al., 2005).

A number of immune-mediated autoimmune disorders of the nervous system are available for study in laboratory animals. Besides allowing for the analysis of the immunoregulatory network, they have been critical in designing immunotherapies. Two major animal models exist that mimic the clinical manifestations of MS. These are EAE and Theiler murine encephalomyelitis virus-induced disease (TMEV-IDD). Although animal models are not identical to the human disease, each model may represent certain pathogenic aspects of MS.

EAE is a T-cell–mediated autoimmune demyelinating disease of the CNS. The disease can be induced in a number of experimental laboratory animals, including primates, by subcutaneous injection of whole-brain homogenate or of a purified preparation of MBP, PLP, or MOG emulsified in adjuvant. By altering the immunization protocols and animal strains, a relapsing-remitting or a chronic form of the disease may be induced. Various EAE models have demonstrated that mice with a $T_H1$ cytokine profile are more susceptible to EAE than wild-type mice, whereas animals with a $T_H2$ (IL-4, IL-10) cytokine profile are generally resistant to disease development (Chitnis et al., 2001). Transfer of $T_H17$-producing cells induces a more severe form of EAE than transfer of $T_H1$ cells (Jager, et al., 2009).

TMEV-IDD is induced by injecting TMEV picornavirus into the cerebral hemisphere. The virus infects neurons and glial cells. In some strains of mice, the host is unable to clear the virus, resulting in encephalitis and death; in other cases, the virus is cleared completely, and the host is resistant to demyelination. In TMEV-IDD-susceptible strains of mice, the virus is partially cleared, saving the host from death but inciting an immune response that results in demyelination. Thus the damage induced by the virus is due to a failure of the host to mount a fully protective response, which predisposes the pathogen to persistence, resulting in immunopathology. TMEV-IDD is a T-cell–mediated disease; although the exact immunological mechanisms inducing demyelination remain unclear, damage may be a result of epitope spreading (Miller, et al., 1997). Studies in both EAE and TMEV have contributed vastly to our understanding of MS, and these models offer a system for testing new therapeutics.

There are currently 15 approved medications for MS (Table 49.3). Details of available therapies in MS are discussed in Chapter 80. Here, we discuss the immunological mechanisms of currently used medications, as well as experimental therapeutic strategies.

β-Interferon (IFN-β) is available in three different forms: subcutaneous IFN-β-1b (Betaseron and Extavia), subcutaneous IFN-β-1a (Rebif), or intramuscular IFN-β-1a (Avonex). Interferons have many properties, including suppressing proliferation of viruses and T cells. The mechanisms of IFN-β action in MS has been attributed to several different mechanisms. Interferon-associated increased production of IL-10 by macrophages down-regulates the number of $T_H1$ cells. IFN-β has also been shown to decrease production of IL-12 by dendritic cells, potential CNS APCs, further inhibiting $T_H1$ cell formation. In addition, IFN-β modulates adhesion molecule expression, primarily by facilitating the conversion of cell-associated VCAM-1 into soluble VCAM-1. These drugs also down-regulate costimulatory molecule expression, thus decreasing T-cell activation and migration to the CNS (Yong 2002).

Glatiramer acetate (GA), also known as *copolymer-1* or *Copaxone*, is another class of drug used in the treatment of MS. In contrast to IFN-β, GA is a synthetic molecule that was originally designed to resemble MBP. It is composed of random repetitive sequences of the amino acids glutamic acid, lysine, alanine, and tyrosine (G-L-A-T). Its mechanism of action is unclear; however, it is thought to bind with high affinity to the MHC groove, leading to the generation of GA-specific T cells. Several studies have suggested that GA-specific T cells display a $T_H2$ bias (Duda et al., 2000), and animal models have demonstrated that these cells can migrate to the CNS and ameliorate

**TABLE 49.3 Approved Medications for Multiple Sclerosis**

| Generic (Brand) Name and Mode of Administration | Indications(s) | Side Effects | Chemical Structure |
|---|---|---|---|
| Glatiramer acetate, Copaxone<br>Daily SQ injection | To reduce relapse frequency in patients with relapsing-remitting multiple sclerosis (MS) and patients who have experienced a first clinical episode and have MRI features consistent with MS | Injection site reactions, lipoatrophy with prolonged use | Synthetic polymer |
| IM IFN-β-1a, Avonex<br>Weekly IM injection | To slow accumulation of physical disability and decrease frequency of clinical exacerbations in patients with relapsing forms of MS and patients who have experienced a first clinical episode and have MRI features consistent with MS | Flu-like symptoms, injection site reactions, neutropenia, anemia, liver function test abnormalities | Interferon beta-1 alpha |
| SC IFN-β-1a, Rebif<br>Three times weekly SQ injections | To slow accumulation of physical disability and decrease frequency of clinical exacerbations in relapsing forms of MS | Flu-like symptoms, injection site reactions, neutropenia, anemia, liver function test abnormalities | Interferon beta-1-alpha |
| IFN-β-1b, Betaseron<br>Every other day SQ injections | To reduce the frequency of clinical exacerbations in patients with relapsing forms of MS and patients who have experienced a first clinical episode and have MRI features consistent with MS | Flu-like symptoms, injection site reactions, neutropenia, anemia, liver function test abnormalities | Interferon beta-1-beta |
| Fingolimod, Gilenya<br>Daily oral tablet | To reduce frequency of clinical exacerbations and delay accumulation of physical disability in patients with relapsing forms of MS | Risk of herpes virus infections, bradycardia, macular edema, and changes on pulmonary function test. | Sphingosine-1-phosphate receptor blocker |
| Natalizumab, Tysabri<br>Monthly IV infusions | As monotherapy for relapsing forms of MS; to delay accumulation of physical disability and reduce frequency of clinical exacerbations | PML brain infection (risk 1:1000) | α4-integrin adhesion molecule blocker |
| Mitoxantrone, Novantrone<br>IV chemotherapy | To reduce neurological disability and/or the frequency of clinical relapses in secondary (chronic) progressive, progressive relapsing or worsening relapsing-remitting MS | Cardiomyopathy, increased risk of secondary lymphoid malignancies | Cytotoxic chemotherapy; synthetic antineoplastic anthracenedione |
| Teriflunomide, Aubagio<br>Daily oral tablet | To reduce frequency of relapses in relapsing-remitting MS | Hepatotoxicity, bone marrow suppression, peripheral neuropathy | Pyrimidine synthesis inhibitor |
| Dimethyl fumarate, Tecfidera<br>Twice daily capsule | To reduce frequency of relapses in relapsing-remitting MS | Flushing, gastro-intestinal side effects, lymphopenia | Dimethyl fumarate |
| Ocrelizumab, Ocrevus<br>Every 6-monthly infusion | To reduce frequency of relapses in relapsing-remitting MS; slows progression in primary progressive MS | Infusion reactions; risk of infection | B-cell antibody |
| Cladribine<br>2 weeks of oral pills/year | To reduce frequency of relapses in relapsing-remitting MS | Potential cancer risk; risk of infection | Purine synthesis modulator |

*IV*, Intravenous; *MRI*, magnetic resonance imaging; *MS*, multiple sclerosis.

EAE disease through a local down-regulation of the immune responses (Aharoni et al., 1997). It has also been demonstrated that GA-specific T cells protect from optic nerve crush injuries, possibly mediated by the production of brain-derived neurotrophic factor (BDNF) (Kipnis et al., 2000).

Natalizumab, an α4β1-integrin antibody (Tysabri), is approved for the treatment of relapsing forms of MS and effectively blocks T- and B-cell migration across the BBB by interfering with binding of α4β1 to VCAM-1 on the surface of endothelial cells. However, blockade of CNS immune surveillance has produced profound adverse effects, as evidenced by the development of progressive multifocal leukoencephalopathy (PML).

Fingolimod (Gilenya) was the first oral therapy approved for MS (Cohen et al., 2010, Kappos et al., 2010), and is the first US Food and Drug Administration (FDA)–approved therapy for pediatric MS (Chitnis et al., 2018). It is a structural analogue of sphingosine and interacts with sphingosine-1-phosphate receptors causing retention of CCR7+ naïve and central memory T cells in lymph nodes.

Dimethyl fumarate (Tecfidera) was recently approved for the treatment of relapsing forms of MS. It is metabolized to monomethyl fumarate and both activate the nuclear factor (erythroid-derived 2)-like 2 (Nrf2) pathway in vitro. The mechanism of action is unknown but presumed to effect inhibition of NF-κB-dependent genes, thus reducing inflammation.

Teriflunomide is another oral agent recently approved for MS. It is a pyrimidine synthesis inhibitor and blocks proliferation of blasting T cells.

Altered peptide ligands (APL) resembling MBP have been used in phase 1 trials for MS with little success. Two concurrent trials were initiated using the same compound, CGP77116. One showed an increased number of lesions on MRI in some patients after the initiation of treatment (Bielekova et al., 2000). In the other trial, 9% of patients developed allergic-type reactions associated with a $T_H2$ deviation (Kappos et al., 2000). Both trials were stopped because of safety concerns.

Alemtuzumab (Campath-1H) targets the CD52 receptor present on lymphocytes and monocytes. Phase 2 studies have shown potent effects in MS, with depletion of peripheral lymphocytes. However, a quarter of treated patients develop autoimmune thyroid disease, and, rarely, immune thrombocytopenic purpura, suggesting that Campath enhances immune dysregulation in a subset of patients (Coles et al., 2008; Jones et al., 2009). Daclizumab blocks the IL-2R α chain (CD25) present in the high-affinity IL-2 receptor on T cells, thus inhibiting T-cell replication and making more IL-2 available to the low-affinity CD25 receptor present on NK cells, which induces a regulatory NK cell population (Bielekova et al., 2006).

Rituximab, an antibody that primarily targets activated B cells, has recently been shown to reduce disease activity in relapsing-remitting (Hauser et al., 2008) and a subset of primary progressive MS patients (Hawker et al., 2009). Interestingly, open-label studies have suggested that rituximab treatment is effective in patients with neuromyelitis optica, which is increasingly thought of as an antibody-mediated disease. Ocrelizumab is a secondary generation B-cell antibody, which is now approved for relapsing-remitting as well as primary progressive MS (Hauser et al., 2017a, 2017b)). Another therapy currently under investigation is CTLA-4Ig, which blocks B7-CD28 costimulatory signals on T cells and may induce T-cell anergy in vivo.

Cladribine is a synthetic analog of the purine adenosine; however, unlike adenosine, it resists degradation and interferes with the cell's ability to process DNA (Giovannoni et al., 2010). It was approved by the FDA for relapsing forms of MS in 2018.

Many therapeutic strategies that have been used in the past nonspecifically target components of the immune response. Nonspecific strategies include cyclophosphamide and mitoxantrone, which depress bone marrow production of cells, including T cells. Cyclophosphamide may also function by inducing a cytokine switch, with a decrease in IL-12 and an increase in IL-4, IL-5, and TGF-β (Comabella et al., 1998).

## Acute Disseminated Encephalomyelitis

Acute disseminated encephalomyelitis (ADEM) is a monophasic demyelinating disease associated with vaccination or a systemic viral infection; it can affect both adults and children. ADEM was originally described in association with rabies and smallpox vaccines, both of which were prepared with neural tissues, suggesting a parallel with EAE, the animal model of MS. These vaccines have since been modified, using non-neural human diploid cell lines. ADEM has not been associated with any vaccines that are currently administered in the United States. The parainfectious variant of ADEM has been associated with measles infection, rubella, mumps, and several other viruses. Viral or bacterial epitopes resembling myelin antigens have the capacity to activate myelin-reactive T-cell clones through molecular mimicry (Wucherpfennig et al., 1995) and can thereby elicit a CNS-specific autoimmune response. Thus, it has been suggested that microbial infections elicit a cross-reactive antimyelin response through molecular mimicry, resulting in ADEM. Myelin peptides have been shown to resemble several viral sequences, and in some cases, cross-reactive T-cell responses have been demonstrated. MBP is the prototypical inducer of EAE, but other myelin proteins like MOG and PLP have also been extensively studied. Examples of cross-reactive T cells with MBP antigens include HHV-6 (Tejada-Simon et al., 2003), coronavirus (Talbot et al., 1996), influenza virus hemagglutinin (Markovic-Plese et al., 2005), and EBV (Lang et al., 2002). PLP shares common sequences with *Haemophilus influenzae* (Olson et al., 2001). Semliki Forest virus (SFV) peptides mimic MOG (Mokhtarian et al., 1999).

The lesions in ADEM resemble those of MS; however, they are characterized by inflammatory infiltrates as well as demyelination, which are limited to the perivascular space, unlike in MS where the demyelination is far more diffuse. The most likely mechanism by which this disease occurs is molecular mimicry. Experimental evidence has shown that T cells isolated from patients with ADEM are 10 times more likely to react with MBP than controls, likening this disease to EAE in animal models (Pohl-Koppe et al., 1998). We have recently found that 30% of patients with ADEM demonstrate serum antibodies to MOG, which were absent in MS patients (O'Connor et al., 2007), and are part of the MOG-antibody associated disease syndrome. Because of the monophasic nature of ADEM, it appears that the immunological response occurs acutely, but in contrast to MS, further amplification of inflammation within the CNS is suppressed.

MRI demonstrates multifocal white matter lesions involving the cerebrum, brainstem, cerebellum, and spinal cord, which may or may not enhance with gadolinium. Lesions generally resolve over time. CSF is characterized by normal pressure, moderately elevated cell count (5–100/μL), moderately elevated protein (40–100 mg/dL), and normal glucose. The presence of red blood cells may indicate a diagnosis of hemorrhagic leukoencephalitis. Oligoclonal bands may very rarely be present, and these cases should be followed for the development of MS.

Acute episodes of ADEM should be treated with intravenous corticosteroids. The usual dose is 1 g/day of methylprednisolone for 5 days in adults. Refractory cases have been treated with plasmapheresis or cyclophosphamide. Cases that are suspicious for MS should be followed with MRI.

## Neuromyelitis Optica

Neuromyelitis optica spectrum disorder (NMOSD), or Devic disease, is a rare subtype of demyelinating disease characterized by clinical episodes of optic neuritis and transverse myelitis and demonstration of contiguous lesions in the spinal cord (Wingerchuk et al., 2006). It was originally considered to be a form of MS; however, increasing evidence demonstrates a distinct pathogenesis and response to treatment. The presence of serum antibodies targeting the aquaporin-4 water channel present on the surface of the glia limitans at the BBB has been shown to be a sensitive and specific marker of NMOSD (Lennon et al., 2004). Injection of aquaporin-4 antibodies into animal models of disease have demonstrated enhanced complement deposition around blood vessels, loss of aquaporin-4, and astrocyte and myelin damage (Kutzelnigg et al., 2005). This study, as well as others, indicates increasing recognition of the role of glial pathology in MS. Intravenous steroids are typically used for acute relapses, and are administered at a dose of 20–30 mg/kg (up to 1 g/day) for a 3- to 5-day period. Plasmapheresis may be used as first- or second-line treatment for acute attacks, and five exchanges are administered every other day or as tolerated. NMO titers may be reduced following plasmapheresis, suggesting that the antibody is linked to relapses. Intravenous immunoglobulin (IVIG; up to 2g/kg divided into 2–5 doses) has been used as third-line therapy by some investigators. Prophylactic therapies used for NMO include rituximab (anti-CD20 antibody), azathioprine, mycophenolate mofetil, and mitoxantrone. Eculizumab is a long-acting humanized monoclonal antibody which targets the C5 complement, thereby inhibiting the cleavage of C5 into C5a and C5b, and terminal complement system, including the formation of MAC. It was approved for treatment of NMOSD in 2019. Some MS therapies including beta-interferon, fingolimod, and natalizumab may worsen disease in NMO patients, reinforcing that immune mechanisms may be distinct in these two diseases.

## Myelin Oligodendrocyte Protein Antibody-Associated Diseases

Anti-MOG antibodies have been reported in the serum of 18% to 35% of children with an acute demyelinating syndrome, and approximately 5% of adults (McLaughlin et al., 2009, Waters et al., 2015). The disease occurs throughout the age spectrum but is more common in children, with a sex ratio of approximately 3:1.

Children with MOG antibodies in the serum present with a variety of clinical syndromes that include, but are not limited to, ADEM, multiphasic ADEM, optic neuritis, ADEM followed by optic neuritis, recurrent optic neuritis, encephalitis or meningitis (often associated with seizures), transverse myelitis, and NMO spectrum disorder (Reindl and Rostasy, 2015). The phenotype seems to follow an age-related spectrum, with ADEM and optic neuritis being the most common presentations in children, while NMO and transverse myelitis are the most common in adults (Fernandez-Carbonell et al., 2016, Jurynczyk et al., 2017). Rarely, cases of typical MS have been associated with MOG antibodies. For relapsing cases of MOG antibody–associated demyelinating syndrome, IVIG, mycophenolate mofetil, azathioprine, and rituximab are the most commonly used immunomodulatory treatments, with approximately 50% efficacy (Hacohen et al., 2018).

## Immune-Mediated Neuropathies

The immune-mediated neuropathies are a large and heterogeneous group of diseases. We shall focus on acute inflammatory demyelinating polyneuropathy (AIDP) and chronic inflammatory demyelinating polyneuropathy (CIDP), which may be defined by the time to peak disability; in the former, 4 weeks, and in the latter, 2 months. Although AIDP and CIDP share many characteristics, the question of whether one is a continuum of the other is still under debate. AIDP or Guillain-Barré syndrome (GBS) usually presents with symmetrical ascending weakness and may be associated with autonomic dysfunction and respiratory depression. Sensory systems may be involved and may present with paresthesias or numbness. Demyelination and axonal damage may be involved to varying degrees. If the patient's symptoms continue to progress beyond 4 weeks, the illness is termed *CIDP*.

AIDP is the most common acute paralytic disease in the Western world, with a mean annual incidence of 1.8 per 100,000 persons. There is an increasing incidence with age. Mortality was generally due to respiratory failure and has now been significantly reduced with the introduction of positive-pressure ventilation. Epidemics have been found, most notably in northern China, where a high incidence has been associated with *C. jejuni* infections (McKhann, et al., 1993).

AIDP or GBS is characterized pathologically by an endoneurial lymphocytic, monocytic, and macrophage infiltrate. Several autoantibodies to myelin glycolipids have been identified; including GM1, GD1a, and GD1b. Antibody-mediated demyelination due to complement fixation has been identified in pathology specimens. In some cases, axonal damage is present and is believed to be a result of bystander damage. Activation of calcium-dependent processes within the nerve, including calpain activation, has been shown in animal models to augment axonal degeneration (O'Hanlon et al., 2003). GBS is primarily an antibody-mediated disease, as evidenced by the fact that many patients improve after treatment with plasmapheresis, and that serum from GBS patients causes demyelination after transfer into experimental animals and peripheral nerve cultures. The Miller-Fisher variant of GBS is characterized by ophthalmoplegia, ataxia, and areflexia and is associated with the presence of GQ1b antibodies in the serum.

The occurrence of AIDP has been linked to many infectious diseases, including *C. jejuni*, herpesvirus, *Mycoplasma pneumoniae*, and many other bacterial and viral infections, as well as vaccinations. The incidence of infection has been reported to be 90% in the 30 days before occurrence of GBS. *C. jejuni* is one of the most commonly identifiable agents, and molecular mimicry and host susceptibility play a role in disease pathogenesis. Autoantibodies not present in controls have been identified in the sera of GBS patients associated with *C. jejuni*, including autoantibodies to the gangliosides GM1, GD1a, GD1b, and GQ1b (Sheikh, et al., 1998).

In contrast to AIDP, in CIDP no specific autoantibodies have yet been discovered. The histopathological picture is similar to AIDP; however, most studies identify fewer inflammatory infiltrates. Nerve biopsy reveals mixed demyelination and axonal changes. Onion bulbs may be present, indicating attempts at remyelination. There is little laboratory evidence that this disease is antibody mediated, but, paradoxically, patients do improve with plasmapheresis. There is indirect evidence that CIDP is T-cell mediated; however, this area is still under investigation.

Treatment of AIDP involves supportive care and cardiac and respiratory monitoring. Plasmapheresis or IVIG has been used for acute treatment of AIDP and has been shown to be equally effective in shortening recovery time. Plasmapheresis is a short-term immunotherapy that nonspecifically removes antibodies from the circulation. IVIG is an immunomodulating agent commonly used in the treatment of allergic and autoimmune diseases. It works in part through the presence of Fc fragments that interact with the inhibitory Fc receptor Fc$\gamma$RIIB, which is also induced on macrophages following IVIG administration (Samuelsson et al., 2001). Additionally, IVIG may displace low-affinity autoantibodies from the nerve. High-dose steroids have not been found to be effective in AIDP.

In contrast with AIDP, CIDP responds well to high-dose oral corticosteroids. Both plasmapheresis and IVIG are also used with success. Immunosuppressants such as cyclosporin A, cyclophosphamide, azathioprine, and rituximab have had positive outcomes in refractory cases but require further testing in controlled studies. Future therapies for AIDP or CIDP may target complement activation or inhibition of axonal calpain activation.

## Autoimmune Myasthenia Gravis

Myasthenia gravis is a disorder of the neuromuscular junction. It is an autoimmune disorder, and 80% to 90% of cases have detectable autoantibodies to the $\alpha$ subunit of the acetylcholine receptor (AChR). MG is characterized by fluctuating weakness and fatigability, primarily in muscles innervated by the cranial nerves, but may occur in skeletal and respiratory muscles. MG has a biphasic age distribution. Most cases occur in women between the ages of 20 and 40 years, the remainder in older patients, with an equal sex distribution. Thymomas occur in 10% to 15% of cases; most are in the older age group. Some 75% of patients will have a thymic abnormality, 85% being thymic hyperplasia. MG is often associated with other autoimmune diseases, thyroid disorders, rheumatoid arthritis (RA), pernicious anemia, and SLE. A similar syndrome, Lambert-Eaton, is associated with antibodies against the presynaptic voltage-gated calcium channel, generally in the setting of small cell cancer of the lung.

Autoimmune MG is caused by the presence of $\alpha_1$ nicotinic acetylcholine receptor (nAChR) antibodies and is a B cell–mediated disease. Eighty to ninety percent of patients have detectable autoantibodies. These are polyclonal and may be of any IgG subtype. Transfer of serum from myasthenic patients to experimental animals results in neuromuscular blockade. The mechanism by which antibody mediates neurological symptoms is controversial. Possible mechanisms include neuromuscular blockade or damage to the AChR from complement-mediated damage after attachment of the IgG antibody. However, there is poor correlation between serum antibody titers and disease course and severity.

Although the B cell is the effector cell producing antibodies, experimental evidence has shown that autoreactive T cells are necessary for the disease to occur (Yi and Lefvert, 1994). Removal of the thymus results in improvement of disease in 80%–90% of myasthenic patients. The role of thymic abnormalities remains unclear, and patients with thymomas have antibodies to additional skeletal muscle proteins such as the ryanodine receptor and titin, as well as the neuromuscular junctional protein, MuSK. Patients may also display symptoms of neuromyotonia. Antibodies directed towards $\alpha_3$-nAChR are associated with autoimmune autonomic neuropathy.

A large body of research is targeted at understanding the reasons for the failure of T-cell and subsequent failure of B-cell tolerance in MG. Both normal and myasthenic thymus glands contain myoid cells and epithelial cells that express the AChR. T cells expressing the $V\beta5.1^+$ TCRs are overrepresented, both in the core of germinal centers and in perifollicular areas of hyperplastic thymuses, suggesting a role in the autoimmune response (Truffault et al., 1997). Failure of central or thymic tolerance may play an important role in disease pathogenesis.

Genetic factors play a role in the pathogenesis of autoimmune MG, but monozygotic twins demonstrate less than 50% concordance rate. There is a moderate association of MG with the HLA antigens B8 and DRw3 in young women. The stronger association with HLA-DQw2 remains controversial. There is an unusually high incidence of other autoimmune diseases such as SLE, RA, and thyroid diseases in first-degree relatives of myasthenic patients, suggesting the presence of shared autoimmune genes.

Therapies in MG are targeted toward alleviating symptoms with acetylcholinesterase inhibitors and using strategies to reduce the damage being done by the immune system. Thymectomy is recommended for patients 15–65 years old, with 80%–90% remission rate (Durelli et al., 1991). The thymus plays an important role in T-cell education in the developing human; therefore prepubertal thymectomy is discouraged. A variety of anticholinesterase inhibitors provide temporary symptomatic relief in most patients. Pyridostigmine bromide (Mestinon) and neostigmine bromide (Prostigmin) are the most commonly used agents and must be taken daily.

MG is an antibody-mediated disease and therefore responds to therapies that nonspecifically target antibodies. Both plasmapheresis and treatment with IVIG are used for acute MG exacerbations or in preparation for surgery (Gajdos et al., 1997). Because the autoantigen is known in MG, investigational therapies may target specific molecules, such as the B-cell surface Ig or the TCR, and deliver immunotoxins.

Corticosteroids are used at various stages of treatment and have multiple effects on the immune system, including reducing AChR antibody levels. Immunosuppressives such as cyclosporine, azathioprine, and mycophenolate are used to augment treatment when symptoms are not adequately controlled by the previously mentioned methods, but the decision to use such agents must balance the need and the side effects. Rituximab has also been used in severe generalized MG. Eculizumab, which is a long-acting humanized monoclonal antibody targeting C5 complement, was approved by the FDA for the treatment of MG in 2017.

## Inflammatory Muscle Diseases

Polymyositis (PM), dermatomyositis (DM), and inclusion body myositis (IBM) are all inflammatory and presumably immune-mediated diseases of the muscle and the surrounding connective tissue. Each has its own unique clinical and immunohistological features. Both PM and DM are more common in females, whereas IBM is more common in males. DM in adults is associated with an increased risk of cancer, and therefore a full cancer screening should be part of patient management.

PM is thought to result from a multitude of causes, including systemic autoimmune connective-tissue disorders and viral and bacterial infections. PM is characterized histopathologically by an endomysial inflammatory infiltrate containing predominantly $CD8^+$ T cells. There is relative sparing of blood vessels. In one subtype of PM, T cells with $\gamma\delta$ receptors have been identified surrounding non-necrotic muscle fibers (Hohlfeld et al., 1991).

In contrast, DM is characterized by perifascicular atrophy. There is hypoperfusion and subsequent degeneration of the muscle fibers in the periphery of the fascicle, secondary to microvascular damage. Damage to capillaries, resulting in muscle fiber ischemia, is mediated by complement. Immunofluorescence studies have revealed immune-complex deposition within the endothelium, indicating that this is an antibody-mediated disease; therefore the disease differs from PM (Kissel et al., 1986).

As with PM, IBM is mediated by $CD8^+$ T cells. However, in contrast to PM, the muscle biopsy in IBM may also demonstrate the presence of characteristic autophagic "rimmed" vacuoles. Amyloid deposits may be demonstrated in the muscle, similar to those seen in AD, suggesting similarities in pathogenesis of these two diseases (Askanas et al., 1992).

Various autoantibodies directed against nuclear and cytoplasmic cell components are found in up to 30% of inflammatory myopathies. Most are nonspecific for connective-tissue disease. Viruses including coxsackie B are implicated in the pathogenesis of disease, and both PM and DM patients may have anti-Jo-1 antibodies to the viral enzyme, histidyl-tRNA synthetase (Mathews and Bernstein, 1983). More recently, the presence of B cells, and in particular antibody-secreting plasma cells with V-D-J rearrangements, has been demonstrated in muscle biopsies from both IBM and PM and to a lesser extent in DM (Greenberg et al., 2005).

The mainstay of treatment of PM and DM is corticosteroids. Dosages may vary from 60 to 100 mg/day of prednisone, and duration is determined by clinical outcome. Alternative treatment options for the inflammatory myositis diseases include IVIG, methotrexate, azathioprine, cyclophosphamide, cyclosporine, and in extreme cases, total lymphoid or whole-body irradiation (Mastaglia et al., 1998). A recent study of rituximab in polymyositis in over 200 adults and children with PM/DM, suggested a benefit (Oddis et al., 2013). Mortality rates vary between 15% and 35% and are generally due to cardiac or respiratory failure. Because there is a higher incidence of malignancy with PM and DM, screening for breast, lung, hematological, ovary, stomach, and colon carcinoma should be performed on patients with these diagnoses. IBM may be more resistant to corticosteroid therapy and is often diagnosed after an assumed PM fails to respond to treatment.

## Alzheimer Disease and Amyotrophic Lateral Sclerosis

It may seem strange to include AD and ALS in a chapter on neuroimmunology. These diseases have traditionally been considered neurodegenerative, but recent studies and therapies have suggested a role for the immune system in disease pathogenesis and protection.

Amyloid-β plaques and neurofibrillary tangles consisting of hyperphosphorylated tau protein are the hallmarks of AD. Clearance of amyloid plaques consisting of amyloid-β fibrils is considered a primary goal of therapy. Amyloid plaques are often surrounded by activated microglia and reactive astrocytes, and are associated with complement activation, leading to the hypothesis that the immune response participates in the clearance of amyloid deposits. Further studies in animal models of AD demonstrated that immunization with amyloid-β peptide resulted in the induction of amyloid-β-specific antibodies, which enhanced the clearance of amyloid plaques (Janus et al., 2000; Morgan et al., 2000). Passive transfer of amyloid-β-specific antibodies yielded similar results. Amyloid plaque clearance is believed to occur through either microglial- and complement-mediated clearance or through direct antibody-amyloid interactions. These studies led to a clinical trial investigating an amyloid-β vaccine administered in conjunction with an adjuvant, which enhanced $T_H1$ responses. Although cognitive testing results were favorable, 6% of patients developed meningoencephalitis, which is generally believed to be a result of T-cell responses to amyloid-β (Gilman et al., 2005; Orgogozo et al., 2003). Thus, induction of an antibody and microglial-mediated clearance of amyloid in the absence of a prominent $T_H1$ response is the current goal of therapy. An intriguing study has recently demonstrated that nasal administration of glatiramer acetate (Copaxone), which induces a predominantly $T_H2$ cellular response, to a murine model of AD resulted in the clearance of amyloid-β plaques in association with activated microglia, but in the absence of antibody formation (Frenkel et al., 2005). Recently, phase III trials of monoclonal antibodies against Aβ, bapineuzumab, aducanumab, and solanezumab, failed to significantly improve clinical outcomes in patients with mild to moderate AD (Doody et al., 2014; Salloway et al., 2014; Sevigny et al., 2016). Future immunotherapeutic strategies for AD include modified vaccines and strategies to induce activation of microglial cells in the absence of deleterious side effects.

In ALS, a new avenue of investigation has emerged: exploring the role of microglia in disease pathogenesis and, in particular, on disease progression. Pathological analysis and neuroimaging using positron electron tomography (PET) studies have demonstrated activated microglia in areas of severe motor neuron loss. Studies in the animal model of ALS have demonstrated that the presence of the SOD1 mutation in microglia enhanced disease progression (Boillee et al., 2006). However, the use of minocycline, which acts in part by inhibiting microglial activation, did not show benefit in human ALS. Cyclooxygenase-2 (COX-2) inhibitors have reduced disease severity in animal models of ALS but have been ineffective in humans. More recent therapeutic trials to date include studies of masitinib, NP001 (modulator of NFκB function on monocytes), and celecoxib. Of these, only masitinib—a tyrosine kinase inhibitor targeting microglia and mast cells—has demonstrated positive results. Interim analysis showed that masitinib met both its primary and secondary endpoint, a change in the ALS function rating scale revised score, while the latter included respiratory function and combined assessment of function and survival (Petrov et al., 2017). Edavarone is a free radical scavenger with antioxidant effects that was approved for ALS in the United States in 2017 based on a small randomized controlled clinical trial with people with early-stage ALS in Japan.

## IMMUNE RESPONSE TO INFECTIOUS DISEASES

The immune response within the CNS must carefully balance the need to eliminate the pathogen and the risk of inducing bystander damage to the delicate and vital nervous tissues. This is believed to be the reason the CNS immune response deviates from that in the rest of the body, and it remains an immune-privileged site. The result is that many pathogens are not completely eliminated and may persist to cause further symptoms. Examples of this are CNS syphilis, Lyme neuroborreliosis, herpes zoster, HIV, and *Mycobacterium tuberculosis.* Lyme *Borrelia burgdorferi* incites IFN-γ production, with correspondingly low levels of IL-4 in the CSF, thus predisposing the CNS tissue to bystander damage.

The portal of entry and site of replication of the pathogen plays a critical role in elimination of the infection. In the case of viral meningitis, the portal of entry is the mucosal membrane, usually the nasopharynx. This incites a strong local immune response to the proliferating organism, and by the time the virus disseminates to the leptomeninges, a sufficient immune response has been mounted in the periphery to eliminate the pathogen. However, in the case of viral encephalitis, the CNS invasion is so sudden that the peripheral immune system has insufficient time to react, and the weak CNS immune response is often inadequate, resulting in a poor outcome.

HIV-associated dementia (HAD) is a clinical disorder characterized by cognitive, behavioral, and motor dysfunction in AIDS patients. HIV infection of the brain is characterized by multinucleated giant cells, astrogliosis, microglial nodules, and neuronal loss in the cortex and basal ganglia. The HIV protein, gp120, can bind directly to CXCR4 on neurons, resulting in neuronal signaling and apoptosis. Neurodegeneration is also thought to occur through production of neurotoxic factors by HIV-infected microglia and astrocytes. HIV infection results in production of proinflammatory cytokines (IL-6, IL-1, and TNF-α), nitric oxide, and MMPs by microglia, as well as increased glutamate by dysfunctional astrocytes. Astrocyte production of SDF-1 (CXCR4 ligand)—which is subsequently cleaved by MMP-2 to produce a truncated protein, c-SDF—is neurotoxic in vitro. In summary, glial-mediated neurotoxicity plays a significant role in the pathogenesis of HAD and is an active area of investigation.

## TUMOR IMMUNOLOGY

The immunological response to tumors has elicited much interest in the past 10 years. This field provides opportunities for understanding the cause and immunological features of tumors and venues for treatment.

The body uses a mechanism called *tumor immunosurveillance* to prevent the formation of tumors or inhibit further growth. The main effector cells are CTLs, NK cells, and TNF-α-producing macrophages. Tumor-reactive antibodies have also been identified in patients but are thought to play a lesser role. It has been recognized that tumors express tumor-specific antigens that may be recognized by the previously mentioned cells. However, tumor cells may escape the body's natural surveillance mechanisms, resulting in cancer. Tumor cells escape surveillance mechanisms by masking or modulating antigens on their surface, down-regulating class I and II molecules (thereby inhibiting antigen presentation), and expressing immunosuppressant factors.

Tumors in the CNS have similar abilities to evade the immune system, and it has been shown that some gliomas produce high levels of TGF-β, an immunosuppressant. Down-regulation of class II MHC may also occur, but this remains controversial. It has recently been established that gliomas may express high levels of FasL, allowing for local apoptosis of Fas-bearing cells including lymphocytes. Increased expression of the inhibitory costimulatory molecule B7H1 on gliomas has been shown to play a role in down-regulating T-cell (Wintterle et al., 2003). Glioma patients have been shown to express increased frequencies of $CD4^+CD25^+Foxp3^+$ regulatory T cells. Treatment with daclizumab (anti-CD25 antibody) in a murine model of glioma reduced regulatory T-cell function and enhanced host tumor immunity, so daclizumab therapy in CNS tumors merits additional investigation.

Additional therapies are being designed to exploit the body's natural tumor immune surveillance mechanisms. One avenue of research is vaccination with killed tumor cells or tumor antigens. Another technique employs genetic engineering to transfect tumors with plasmids bearing genes for costimulatory molecules to enhance the tumor APC ability. Injection of cytokines such as IL-2 and TNF-α, which enhance lymphocyte and NK function, has been attempted with variable results. Dendritic cells pulsed with tumor antigens to induce NK cell–mediated tumor killing is a promising new therapy for CNS gliomas and is under investigation.

Overall, strategies to enhance host tumor immunosurveillance and reduce inhibitory responses mediated by CNS tumors are promising new avenues of treatment.

### Paraneoplastic Syndromes

*Neurological paraneoplastic disorders* are defined as neurological syndromes arising in association with a distant cancer. These are mediated by antibodies produced by the immune system in reaction to a tumor antigen, which cross-react with neural tissue. It is likely that aberrant, primitive, or hamartomatous antigens are expressed by the tumor cells. Enhanced cellular infiltrates are found in tumors associated with paraneoplastic syndrome compared to those not associated with a paraneoplastic syndrome. Therefore one can postulate that the immune system is more active in these situations. Cancers associated with paraneoplastic syndromes are generally associated with a better outcome. Several autoantibodies associated with paraneoplastic syndromes have been identified. The anti-Hu antibody arises in association with small-cell cancer of the lung and cross-reacts with neurons; it is linked to a syndrome of encephalomyelitis and/or sensory neuropathy. Similarly, anti-Yo antibody produces cerebellar degeneration due to cross-reactivity with Purkinje cell cytoplasm and is associated with breast and ovarian cancer. Opsoclonus-myoclonus syndrome is associated with anti-Ri antibody and is found in cases of cancer of the ovary and breast. Cases of paraneoplastic and immune-mediated brainstem and limbic encephalitis have recently been reported to be caused by antibodies targeting LGI1, a neuronal-secreted protein that interacts with presynaptic ADAM23 and postsynaptic ADAM22 (Lai et al., 2010). NMDA receptor encephalitis typically presents with seizures and psychiatric symptoms, but a recent case report describes a patient presenting with optic neuritis and transverse myelitis mimicking neuromyelitis optica (Kruer et al., 2010). Antibodies directed against voltage-gated potassium channels (VGKC) are also associated with acquired neuromyotonia, or Isaac syndrome, and Morvan syndrome, characterized by neuromyotonia and insomnia. Lambert-Eaton myasthenic syndrome is caused by antibodies directed against the P/Q type of voltage-gated calcium channels and is generally found in the setting of small-cell cancer of the lung. The same antibodies have also been associated with cases of lung cancer–associated cerebellar ataxia. Stiff person syndrome is associated with antibodies to glutamic acid decarboxylase (GAD), and both autoimmune and paraneoplastic forms, principally associated with breast cancer, have been described.

## ANTIBODY-ASSOCIATED NEUROLOGICAL SYNDROMES

In the past 10 years, more sophisticated techniques have led to greater insights into the study of antibodies in CNS diseases. Antiphospholipid (APL) syndrome, or Hughes syndrome, results in CNS symptoms that include chorea, strokes, bleeding, migraine headaches, and epilepsy (Asherson 2006). These result in part from the underlying systemic problems of coagulopathy and thrombocytopenia, but more direct effects of autoantibodies directed against neuronal antigens have been implicated both in APL syndrome and in CNS lupus. One study found that antibodies directed against the NR2A and NR2B subunits of the NMDA receptor were found in a subset of patients with CNS lupus and could facilitate apoptotic death of neurons (DeGiorgio et al., 2001).

Recently, antibodies against the N-methyl-D-aspartate subtype of ionotropic glutamate receptors (N-methyl-D-aspartate receptor [NMDAR] antibodies) have been reported, predominantly in young women who developed a subacute-onset encephalopathy, commonly associated with a prominent movement disorder and frequently an underlying ovarian teratoma (Dalmau et al., 2007), although two recent reports suggest a much higher incidence of non-paraneoplastic cases in children (Dale et al., 2009; Florance et al., 2009). Additional reports have confirmed these findings, and the mainstay of treatment in patients with NMDAR antibody-associated syndromes includes removal of underlying tumors, and immunotherapy with either steroids, IVIG, or plasmapheresis acutely. In patients with refractory disease, chronic immunosuppression with rituximab or mycophenolate mofetil is used. Other neuronal antibodies including those to the AMPA receptor, the GABAB receptor, LGII, and Caspr2 have been recently associated with neuropsychiatric syndromes, increasing the potential role for immunotherapy in these antibody-associated disorders.

Sydenham chorea is associated with *Streptococcus pyogenes* (β-hemolytic streptococcal) infections, and there is considerable evidence for a causative role of antibodies that cross-react with streptococcal antigens and neurons in the basal ganglia. This association has led to the postulation that molecular mimicry mechanisms related to streptococcal infections may result in other movement disorders, including Tourette syndrome and the clinical entity of pediatric autoimmune neuropsychiatric disorders associated with streptococcal infection (PANDAS), which encompasses tics and obsessive-compulsive disorder in children. Evidence for an immune-mediated mechanism is inconclusive (Harris and Singer, 2006).

Antibodies directed against glutamate receptor 3 (GluR3) are associated with Rasmussen encephalitis, a form of severe intractable epilepsy localized to one hemisphere and partially responsive to immunotherapy. The presence of antibodies directed against voltage-gated potassium channels in a small group of patients with intractable epilepsy has been demonstrated (Majoie et al., 2006), and, more recently, other antibodies, including GAD65 and CRMP-5 as well as VGKC, have been described in patients with chronic epilepsy, with some response to immunotherapy (Quek et al., 2012). Besides SLE chorea, there are many autoimmune movement disorders, such as antiphospholipid syndrome, anti-NMDAR encephalitis, Hashimoto's thyroiditis, opsoclonus-myoclonus syndrome, stiff person syndrome, progressive encephalomyelitis with rigidity, ataxia, and other hypokinetic and hyperkinetic movement disorders associated with a variety of antibodies.

## IMMUNOLOGY OF CENTRAL NERVOUS SYSTEM TRANSPLANT

Recently, there has been much research in the field of CNS transplantation, with the use of fetal dopaminergic striatal cells, various types of genetically engineered cells, and the potential of stem cell transplantation. A major factor in the survival of these grafts is their lack of immunogenicity in the relatively immune-privileged site of the CNS. Therefore transplant grafts in the CNS tend to have longer survival times than peripheral grafts; however, this is not absolute, and rejection can undoubtedly occur.

Factors that influence CNS graft survival are type of graft (xenogeneic, allogeneic, genetically modified tissue, or stem cell populations); location of the graft, with the periventricular areas being the most susceptible to rejection; presence of APCs within the graft, which can be eliminated in purified grafts; and host immunosuppression.

Immunosuppressive strategies currently under investigation include the immunophilins, daclizumab, and cyclosporine. Successful immunosuppression must be balanced against the risk of graft toxicity.

Neural stem cells (NSCs) are increasingly being investigated in neurodegenerative diseases (Gincberg et al., 2012). In addition to their effects on repair, studies in the animal model of MS found that these cells suppress disease (Einstein et al., 2003, 2007; Pluchino et al., 2003, 2006; Yang et al., 2009) through immunomodulatory mechanisms. Some studies suggested that NSCs can directly inhibit T-cell proliferation in response to concanavalin A (ConA) or to MOG peptide (Einstein et al., 2003; Pluchino et al., 2005) by inducing T-cell apoptosis (Pluchino et al., 2005; Yang et al., 2009) or through nitric oxide– and PGE2-mediated T-cell suppression (Wang et al., 2009). Neural stem cells can express costimulatory molecules, CD80 and CD86, particularly after exposure to the proinflammatory cytokines, IFN-γ and TNF-α (Imitola et al., 2004). Thus, NSCs are not conventional immune cells, but under certain conditions, they can interact with immune cells.

Mesenchymal stem cells (MSCs) are also being investigated for treatment of neurological diseases, including MS and ALS. Their therapeutic benefit is thought to be by induction of immune tolerance and the release of molecules fostering tissue repair. There are phase II trials of MSCs in MS ongoing.

## SUMMARY

The field of immunology has progressed significantly in the past 30 years. This knowledge is currently being applied to immune-mediated diseases in neurology. In this rich environment, we can expect many advances in the field of neuroimmunology, including new therapies and better strategies for the treatment of neurological diseases.

*The complete reference list is available online at https://expertconsult.inkling.com/.* 

50

# Neuroendocrinology

*Paul E. Cooper, Stan H.M. Van Uum*

## OUTLINE



Neuroendocrinology, in its broadest sense, is the study of the coordinated interaction of the nervous, endocrine, and immune systems to maintain the constancy of the internal milieu (homeostasis). This chapter concentrates on the functions of the hypothalamus and its interaction with the pituitary gland.

## NEUROPEPTIDES, NEUROTRANSMITTERS, AND NEUROHORMONES

One of the features of the neuroendocrine system is that it uses neuropeptides as both neurotransmitters and neurohormones. The term *neurotransmitter* is applied traditionally to a substance that is released by one neuron and acts on an adjacent neuron in a stimulatory or inhibitory fashion. The effect is usually rapid, brief, and confined to a small area of the neuronal surface. In contrast, a *hormone* is a substance that is released into the bloodstream and usually travels to a distant site to act over seconds, minutes, or hours to produce its effect over a large area of the cell or over many cells. *Neuropeptides* can act in either fashion. For example, the neuropeptide vasopressin, produced by the neurons of the supraoptic and paraventricular nuclei, is released into the bloodstream and has a hormonal action on the collecting ducts in the kidney. Vasopressin is also released within the central nervous system (CNS), where it acts as a neurotransmitter. Similarly, the neuropeptide substance P acts as a neurotransmitter in primary sensory neurons that convey pain signals and as a neurohormone in the hypothalamus.

The influence of neurohormones and neuropeptides on the brain can be divided into two broad categories: organizational and activational. *Organizational effects* occur during neuronal differentiation, growth, and development and bring about permanent structural changes in the organization of the brain and therefore brain function. An example of this is the structural and organizational changes brought about in the brain by prenatal exposure to testosterone. *Activational effects* are those that change preestablished patterns of neuronal activity, such as an increased rate of neuronal firing caused by exposure of a neuron to substance P or vasopressin.

Numerous neuropeptides are found in the brain, where they have a wide variety of effects on neuronal function (Table 50.1). Current understanding of all the actions of neuropeptides in the nervous system is far from complete.

## NEUROPEPTIDES AND THE IMMUNE SYSTEM

It has been known for many years that stress, through activation of the hypothalamic-pituitary-adrenal (HPA) axis, modulates the function of the immune system (Tsigos and Chrousos, 2002; Wrona, 2006). Infections in the periphery convey information to the CNS through humoral (cytokines and bacterial toxins) and neuronal routes to bring about behaviors that enhance survival (McCusker and Kelley, 2013). Certain peptides and their receptors, once thought to be unique to either the immune or the neuroendocrine system, are actually found in both.

Cytokines—interleukins (IL)-1, -2, -4, and -6 and tumor necrosis factor (TNF)—are synthesized by glial cells in the CNS in response to cell injury. IL-1 and the other cytokines, through their ability to stimulate the synthesis of nerve growth factor, may be important promoters of neuronal damage repair. Circulating cytokines have been thought to

**TABLE 50.1 Neuropeptides Found in the Brain and Their Effects on Brain Function**

| Neuropeptide | Central Nervous System Function and Selected Function Outside the Central Nervous System |
|---|---|
| **Hypothalamic Peptides Modulating Pituitary Function** | |
| Corticotropin (ACTH)-releasing hormone (CRH) | Regulation of ACTH secretion |
| | Integration of behavioral and biochemical responses to stress |
| | Modulatory effects on learning and memory |
| Growth hormone-releasing hormone (GHRH) | Regulation of growth hormone secretion |
| Growth hormone release-inhibiting hormone (somatostatin) | Regulation of growth hormone secretion |
| Ghrelin | Regulation of growth hormone secretion |
| | Regulation of feeding |
| Thyrotropin-releasing hormone (TRH) | Regulation of thyroid-stimulating hormone secretion |
| | May be involved in depression |
| | Enhances neuromuscular function (in the periphery) |
| | Stimulates prolactin release |
| Gonadotropin-releasing hormone (luteinizing hormone-releasing hormone; GnRH) | Regulates gonadotropin secretion |
| | Influences sexual receptivity |
| Prolactin-releasing peptide | Stimulates prolactin secretion |
| Neurotensin | Endogenous neuroleptic |
| | Regulates mesolimbic, mesocortical, and nigrostriatal dopamine neurons |
| | Thermoregulation |
| | Analgesia |
| Neuropeptide Y | Stimulates hunger, food intake, and drinking |
| | Sexual behavior |
| | Locomotion |
| | Memory |
| Agouti-related protein | Stimulate hunger and food intake |
| Orexins (hypocretins) | Stimulate CRH and antidiuretic hormone (ADH) |
| | Inhibit GHRH |
| | Stimulate GnRH |
| | May stimulate preovulatory prolactin release |
| | Inhibit TRH release |
| | Inhibit hunger and food intake |
| **Pituitary Peptides** | |
| Prolactin | Maternal behavior |
| | Mood |
| | Anxiety |
| Growth hormone | |
| Thyroid-stimulating hormone | |
| Follicle-stimulating hormone | |
| Luteinizing hormone | Elevated levels may promote neurodegeneration |
| Pro-opiomelanocortin | |
| ACTH | |
| ACTH-like intermediate lobe peptides | |
| β-Endorphin | Analgesic mechanisms |
| | Feeding |
| | Thermoregulation |
| | Learning and memory |
| β-Lipotropic hormone | Skin tanning |
| Melanocyte-stimulating hormone (α- and γ-) | Weight loss |
| | Skin tanning |
| | Increased sexual desire |
| | Anti-inflammatory effect |
| | Important mediator of leptin control on energy homeostasis |
| Oxytocin | Anxiety and mood |
| | Active/passive stress coping |
| | Maternal behavior, aggression |
| | Pair bonding |
| Vasopressin | Active/passive stress coping |

*Continued*

**TABLE 50.1 Neuropeptides Found in the Brain and Their Effects on Brain Function—cont'd**

| Neuropeptide | Central Nervous System Function and Selected Function Outside the Central Nervous System |
|---|---|
| | Anxiety<br>Spatial memory<br>Social discrimination, social interaction<br>Pair bonding<br>Activation of the hypothalamic-pituitary-adrenal (HPA) axis |
| Neurophysins | |
| **Brain–Gastrointestinal Tract Peptides** | |
| Vasoactive intestinal polypeptide | Cerebral blood flow<br>Potent anti-inflammatory factor |
| Somatostatin | |
| Insulin | Feeding behavior<br>Modulatory effect on learning and memory<br>Hunger |
| Glucagon | Inhibition of feeding |
| Pancreatic polypeptide | |
| Gastrin | |
| Cholecystokinin | Feeding behavior<br>Satiety<br>Modulates dopamine neuron activity<br>Facilitates memory processing (especially under stress) |
| Tachykinins (e.g., substance P) | Substance P colocalizes with serotonin and is involved in nociception |
| Secretin | Modulates motor and other functions in brain, facilitating GABA |
| Thyrotropin-releasing hormone | |
| Bombesin | Thermoregulation<br>Inhibition of feeding<br>Modulatory effect on learning and memory |
| Orexins (hypocretin) | Gastric and gastrointestinal motility and secretion<br>Pancreatic hormone release<br>Regulation of energy homeostasis<br>Feeding behavior<br>Locomotion and muscle tone<br>Wakefulness/sleep |
| Galanin | Modulates release of gonadotropin-releasing hormone, prolactin, insulin, glucagons, growth hormone, and somatostatin<br>Affects feeding, sexual behavior, and anxiety<br>Potent anticonvulsant effects |
| Leptin | Satiety factor |
| **Growth Factors** | |
| Insulin-like growth factors (IGF) 1 and 2 | |
| Nerve growth factors | Axonal plasticity |
| **Opioid Family** | |
| Endorphins | Analgesia |
| Enkephalins (met-, leu-) | Analgesic mechanisms<br>Feeding<br>Temperature control<br>Learning and memory<br>Cardiovascular control |
| Dynorphins | |
| Kytorphin | |
| **Neuropeptides Modulating Immune Function** | |
| ACTH | |
| Endorphins | |
| Interferons | |

*Continued*

**TABLE 50.1 Neuropeptides Found in the Brain and Their Effects on Brain Function—cont'd**

| Neuropeptide | Central Nervous System Function and Selected Function Outside the Central Nervous System |
|---|---|
| Neuroleukins | |
| Thymosin | |
| Thymopeptin | |
| **Other Neuropeptides** | |
| Atrial natriuretic factors | Possibly a role in cerebral salt wasting |
| Bradykinins | Cerebral blood flow |
| Calcitonin gene-related peptide (CGRP) | Migraine and other vascular headaches<br>Movement of water into the gastrointestinal lumen<br>Vasodilatation of microvascular beds |
| **Other Neuropeptides** | |
| Angiotensin | Hypertension<br>Thirst |
| Synapsins | |
| Calcitonin | |
| Sleep peptides | Regulation of sleep cycles |
| Orexins (hypocretin) | Sleep-wake regulation<br>Narcolepsy<br>Energy homeostasis |
| Carnosine | |
| Pituitary adenylate cyclase–activating polypeptide (PACAP) | Migraine and other vascular headaches |
| **Precursor Peptides** | |
| Pro-opiomelanocortin | |
| Proenkephalins (A and B) | |
| Calcitonin gene product | |
| Vasoactive intestinal polypeptide gene product | |
| Proglucagon | |
| Proinsulin | |

This is only a partial list of all of the neuropeptides that have been found in the brain, and not all of the putative functions are listed.
*ACTH,* Adrenocorticotropic hormone; *GABA,* γ-aminobutyric acid.

play a role in the hypothalamus to activate the HPA axis in response to inflammation elsewhere in the body (see the section titled "Fever," later in this chapter) and inhibit the pituitary-thyroid and pituitary-gonadal axes in response to systemic disease.

Several other hormones and neuropeptides have modulatory effects on immune function. Similarly, immunocompetent cells contain hormones and neuropeptides that may affect neuroendocrine and brain cells (Table 50.2). There is accumulating evidence that stress and the psyche-brain-immune network plays a role in psychiatric disease (Bottaccioli et al., 2018). The overall ability of the psyche to influence immunological function and therefore disease outcome is less clear.

## NONENDOCRINE HYPOTHALAMUS

### Temperature Regulation

The hypothalamus plays a key role in ensuring that body temperature is maintained within narrow limits by balancing the heat gained from metabolic activity and the environment with the heat lost to the environment (Nakamura, 2011; Romanovsky, 2007). A theoretical schema of the mechanisms of hypothalamic temperature regulation is depicted in Fig. 50.1. Although numerous neurotransmitters and peptides can alter body temperature, their physiological roles remain unclear.

Hypothalamic injury can cause disordered temperature regulation. One potentially serious consequence is the hyperthermia that may occur when the preoptic anterior hypothalamic area is damaged or irritated by ischemia, subarachnoid hemorrhage, trauma, or surgery. In some patients, the marked impairment of heat loss mechanisms and the resulting hyperthermia may be fatal. In those individuals who survive, temperature control usually returns to normal over a period of days to weeks. Chronic hyperthermia of hypothalamic origin is extremely uncommon; it may occur with continued impairment of the ability to dissipate heat adequately or with difficulty sensing temperature elevations. Chronic hypothalamic hyperthermia does not respond to salicylates and other antipyretics because it is not mediated by prostaglandin. Hypothermia, both acute and chronic, can be due to hypothalamic injury, the most common causes being head trauma, infarction, and demyelination. Other entities to be considered in the differential diagnosis are severe hypothyroidism, Wernicke disease, and drug effect. Some patients with no apparent hypothalamic structural abnormalities may have episodes of recurrent hypothermia. The cause of this syndrome is unclear, although the response of some patients to anticonvulsant agents and of others to clonidine or cyproheptadine suggests a possible neurotransmitter abnormality. Agenesis of the corpus callosum in association with episodic hyperhidrosis and hypothermia (Shapiro syndrome) is caused in some individuals by an abnormally low hypothalamic "set point." These symptoms

TABLE 50.2 Immunoregulatory Effects of Several Hormones and Peptides

| Hormone or Peptide | Immunocompetent Cell in Which Hormone Is Found | Comments |
|---|---|---|
| **Inhibitory** | | |
| Glucocorticoids | | Inhibit lymphokine synthesis, inflammation |
| Corticotropin (ACTH) | B lymphocytes | Stimulated by corticotropin-releasing hormone; inhibited by cortisol |
| | | Macrophage activation, synthesis of IgG and γ-interferon |
| Chorionic gonadotropin | T cells | Stimulated by thyrotropin-releasing hormone; inhibited by somatostatin |
| | | Activity of T cells and natural killer cells |
| α-Endorphin | | IgG synthesis, T-cell proliferation |
| Somatostatin | Mononuclear leukocytes, mast cells | T-cell proliferation, inflammatory cascade |
| Vasoactive intestinal peptide | Mononuclear leukocytes, mast cells | T-cell proliferation and migration in Peyer patches |
| | | Potent anti-inflammatory effect |
| α-Melanocyte-stimulating hormone | | Fever, prostaglandin synthesis, secretion of interleukin 2 |
| | | Impairs function of antigen-producing cells and T cells |
| | | Anti-inflammatory effects |
| **Stimulatory** | | |
| Estrogens | | Lymphocyte proliferation and secretion |
| Growth hormone | T lymphocytes | Stimulated by growth hormone |
| | | Thymic growth, lymphocyte reactivity |
| Prolactin | Mononuclear cells | Thymic growth, lymphocyte proliferation |
| **Stimulatory** | | |
| Thyrotropin (TSH) | T cells | Stimulated by thyrotropin-releasing hormone; inhibited by somatostatin |
| | | IgG synthesis |
| β-Endorphin | | Activity of T, B, and natural killer cells |
| Substance P | | Proliferation of T cells and macrophages, inflammatory cascade |
| Corticotropin (ACTH)-releasing hormone | | Lymphocyte and monocyte proliferation and activation |
| **Not Known to Be Stimulatory or Inhibitory** | | |
| Enkephalins | B lymphocytes | |
| Vasopressin | Thymus | |
| Oxytocin | Thymus | |
| Neurophysin | Thymus | |

*ACTH*, Adrenocorticotropic hormone; *IgG*, immunoglobulin G; *TSH*, thyroid-stimulating hormone
*Modified from Reichlin, S., 1993. Neuroendocrine-immune interactions. N Engl J Med 329, 1246–1253.*

may respond to clonidine (a centrally acting $\alpha_2$-adrenergic agonist). A similar condition associated with hyperthermia (so-called reverse Shapiro syndrome) has been found to respond with normalization of temperature to low-dose L-dopa, higher doses causing hypothermia. Large lesions in the posterior hypothalamus may impair both heat production (by altering the set point) and heat loss (by damaging the outflow from the preoptic anterior hypothalamic area). This results in poikilothermia, a condition in which body temperature varies with the environmental temperature.

## Fever

Classical teaching has been that inflammatory cells in the periphery (primarily monocytes) release cytokines in response to infection and inflammation. These cytokines were thought to act on the hypothalamus to induce the production of prostaglandin $E_2$ ($PGE_2$) and cause elevation of the body temperature set point. The body then used its normal physiological mechanisms of vasoconstriction, vasodilation, sweating, and shivering to maintain this new higher set point (i.e., fever). This view of the mechanism by which bacterial infections cause fever is probably incorrect. Bacterial endotoxic lipopolysaccharide (LPS) does appear to work in the periphery to cause macrophages to release a variety of factors; however, the initial signal to the brain probably travels by vagal afferents to the preoptic anterior hypothalamus via norepinephrine, which activates the cyclooxygenase isoenzyme COX-2 to generate and release $PGE_2$. The slower or second febrile increase in $PGE_2$ is due to COX-2 activation by IL-1β produced locally in the brain, not to circulating factors (Blatteis et al., 2000). Acetylsalicylic acid and acetaminophen reduce fever by inhibiting cyclooxygenase, thereby reducing the levels of $PGE_2$ within the hypothalamus.

In otherwise healthy persons, extreme elevations of body temperature (as high as 41.1°C [106°F]) can sometimes be tolerated without serious effects. However, hyperthermia associated with prolonged exertion, heatstroke, malignant hyperthermia, neuroleptic malignant

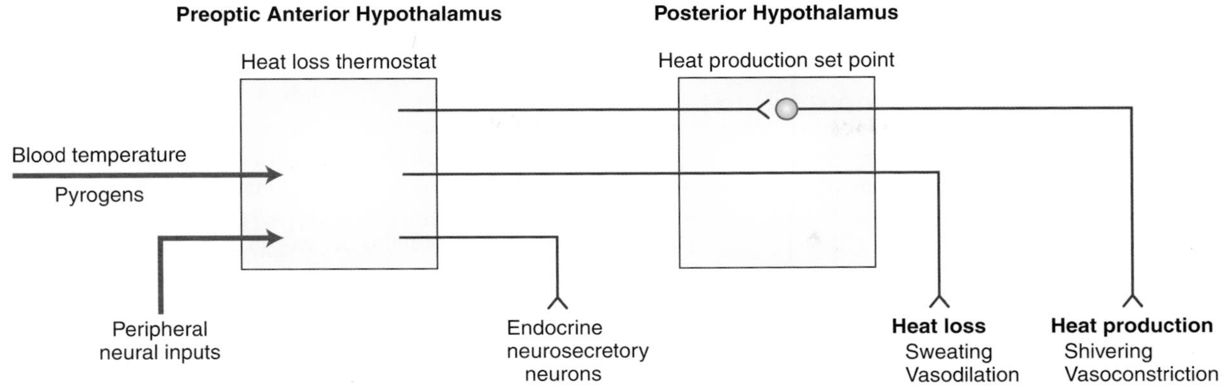


**Fig. 50.1 Schematic Representation of Hypothalamic Temperature Regulation Mechanisms.** The preoptic anterior hypothalamus functions as a thermostat and contains mechanisms for the regulation of heat loss. The posterior hypothalamus integrates heat production mechanisms. Lesions of the preoptic anterior hypothalamus result in hyperthermia; lesions of the posterior hypothalamus cause hypothermia or poikilothermia. *(Reprinted with permission from Cooper, P.E., Martin, J.B., 1983. Neuroendocrine disease. In: Rosenberg, R.N. (Ed.), The Clinical Neurosciences, Churchill Livingstone, New York.)*

syndrome (NMS), hyperthyroidism, pheochromocytoma crisis, and some drugs may have serious and even fatal consequences. Exertional hyperthermia occurs with prolonged physical activity, particularly in hot, humid weather. It usually decreases athletic performance initially and can cause muscle cramps or heat exhaustion. When severe, it may result in heatstroke, a syndrome characterized by hyperthermia, hypotension, tachycardia, hyperventilation, hypoglycemia, and a decreased level of consciousness. Seizures are common in heatstroke and can further exacerbate the elevated body temperature. Even in the face of early and vigorous treatment, deaths continue to occur.

### Drug-Induced Hyperthermia

Drug-induced hyperthermic syndromes include anticholinergic poisoning, sympathomimetic poisoning, malignant hyperthermia, NMS, and serotonin syndrome. In *malignant hyperthermia*, a syndrome associated most often with the use of various general anesthetic agents and muscle relaxants, an inherited defect leads to excessive release of calcium from sarcoplasmic reticulum, stimulating severe muscle contraction (see Chapters 98 and 109). The *neuroleptic malignant syndrome* is characterized by diffuse muscular rigidity, akinesia, and fever accompanied by a decreased consciousness level and evidence of autonomic dysfunction—namely, labile blood pressure, tachyarrhythmias, excessive sweating, and incontinence. NMS can be associated with the administration of major tranquilizers (primarily those that work by blocking dopamine receptors); with rapid withdrawal from dopaminergic agents including entacapone; and less commonly with the administration of tricyclic antidepressants. It appears to result from an alteration of temperature control mechanisms in the hypothalamus. As part of treatment, the withdrawal of all neuroleptics is mandatory. In addition to general supportive measures and cooling, the use of bromocriptine—a dopamine agonist (2.5–10 mg four times daily, increasing by 7.5 mg daily in divided doses to a maximum of 60 mg daily) can be helpful. Hypotension, psychosis, and nausea are possible side effects. An alternative is dantrolene (50–200 mg/day orally, or 2 to 3 mg/kg intravenously (IV) per day to a maximum of 10 mg/kg/day).

The *serotonin syndrome* is characterized by mental status changes, neuromuscular symptoms, autonomic dysfunction, and gastrointestinal (GI) dysfunction. In addition to tremor and rigidity (seen also in NMS), other features may include shivering, myoclonus, and hyperreflexia. Nausea, vomiting, and diarrhea are common in serotonin syndrome but uncommon in NMS. Treatment entails withdrawal from the offending drug and general supportive care.

## Appetite

Given free access to food and water, most animals maintain their body weight within narrow limits. With a change in energy intake/expenditure (a change in the size or number of individual meals that is not balanced by an equal and opposite change in energy use), the animal experiences a change in weight. One possible model of nutrient balance is depicted in Fig. 50.2. The four components of energy balance are (1) the afferent system, (2) the CNS processing unit, (3) the efferent system, and (4) the absorption of food from the gut and its metabolism in the liver. Defects at any point in these systems may lead to weight loss or weight gain (Wynne et al., 2005).

In response to a meal or to starving, hormonal and neural signals are generated in the periphery. Some are of short duration and others of long duration. Some relate to satiety, others relate to feeding behavior, and still others relate to "thinness and fatness." Leptin is secreted by fat cells in the periphery and is sensed in the brain. Leptin seems to be most important if the levels fall below normal. In that circumstance it stimulates hunger. High levels of leptin tend not to suppress hunger. Neurons in the hypothalamus release the pro-opiomelanocortin (POMC) segment alpha-melanocyte–stimulating hormone (α-MSH), which suppresses appetite. Neurons that release agouti-related peptide (AgRP) also corelease neuropeptide Y (NPY) and γ-aminobutyric acid (GABA), both of which stimulate appetite (Lowell, 2019). Ghrelin, a stimulator of growth hormone (GH) release, is released from the stomach in the fasting state. Ghrelin activates NPY and agouti-related protein in the hypothalamus, leading to increased feeding and the deposition of energy into body fat. Peripheral insulin seems to mediate a satiety signal in the ventromedial hypothalamus. Destruction of the ventromedial hypothalamus, in both animals and humans, leads to obesity. Lesions in the paraventricular nucleus have a similar effect (Harrold et al., 2012). Overeating (hyperphagia) is only one of the mechanisms that produce hypothalamic obesity; more efficient handling of calories by the eater is probably another important factor. Hypothalamic lesions can also cause weight loss. Lesions in the dorsomedial nucleus lead to a reduction in body weight and fat stores, as do lesions in the lateral hypothalamus. Oral motor and meal-size responses may be dependent on centers in the caudal brainstem modulated by the hypothalamus.

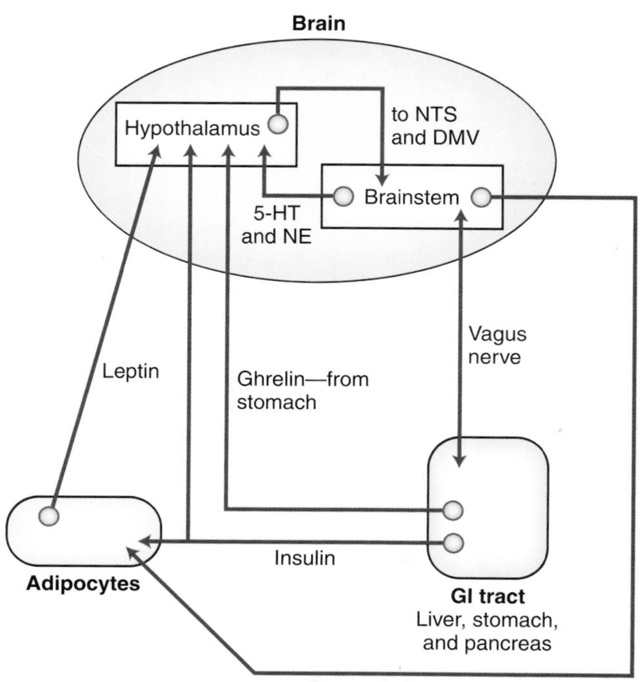


**Fig. 50.2 Sympathetic Nervous System.** In the regulation of energy balance, the brain is the central processing unit. It receives afferent neuronal signals from the vagus nerve via the brainstem as well as hormonal signals—ghrelin (from the stomach), insulin (from the pancreas), and leptin (from adipocytes). The brainstem also has input to the hypothalamus via norepinephrine (*NE*; from the locus ceruleus) and serotonin, or 5-hydroxytryptamine (*5-HT*; from the raphe nuclei). These afferent signals are interpreted both in the brainstem (in the nucleus tractus solitarius *[NTS]*) and in the hypothalamus (in the ventromedial nucleus). The ventromedial nucleus of the hypothalamus communicates with the lateral hypothalamic area and the paraventricular nucleus by means of pro-opiomelanocortin-cocaine/amphetamine-regulated transcript, an anorexigenic peptide (the release of which is stimulated by insulin and leptin), and by NPY/agouti-related protein, an orexigenic peptide (the release of which is stimulated by ghrelin and inhibited by leptin and insulin)—or through the parasympathetic nervous system. Output from the lateral hypothalamic area (LHA) and paraventricular nucleus (PVN) is either via the sympathetic nervous system, which leads to energy expenditure through physical activity, activation of $\beta_2$-adrenergic receptors, and uncoupling proteins in the adipocyte to cause energy release through lipolysis, or through the parasympathetic nervous system. Output via the vagus nerve leads to increased insulin secretion, which causes adipogenesis and energy storage. For a more complete explanation of this control of energy balance, the interested reader is directed to the article by Lustig (2001). *DMV*, Dorsal motor nucleus of the vagus; *GI*, gastrointestinal.

Meal size and food intake are influenced by many different stimuli. Sensory cues such as the sight, aroma, and taste of food are major factors in dietary obesity. A decrease in blood glucose or in the oxidation of fatty acids in the liver stimulates the act of eating. Stomach distention gives rise to neural and hormonal signals that reduce food intake. GI peptides—such as cholecystokinin (CCK), bombesin, and glucagon—inhibit feeding by their actions on the autonomic nervous system, particularly the vagal nucleus (Sam et al., 2012). Increased fatty acid oxidation leads to higher levels of 3-hydroxybutyrate, which then acts on the hypothalamus to reduce food intake. Interference with any of these sensing systems in the CNS can lead to obesity. NPY infused into the ventromedial nucleus of the hypothalamus induces obesity, perhaps by inhibiting sympathetic drive and stimulating insulin release. Although this may explain obesity with hypothalamic lesions, obesity related to eating highly palatable food is probably not related to central changes in NPY.

In animals, the *ob*, *db*, and *fa* genes play a role in the ability of adipose tissue to regulate feeding through a circulating factor. When the product of the *ob* gene, leptin, is administered peripherally to a genetically obese (ob/ob) mouse deficient in leptin, the animal reduces its intake of food, with a resulting decrease in body weight. The role of leptin in appetite regulation is complex. Leptin does not reverse the obesity seen in db/db mice and in obese humans. In these groups, serum leptin concentrations are higher than in subjects of normal weight, suggesting an insensitivity to the effects of endogenously secreted leptin.

When α-MSH binds to its receptor in the hypothalamus, it causes satiety. Up to 5% of obese children have been found to have an abnormality of the α-MSH receptor $MC_4R$ as a cause of their obesity (Lustig, 2001).

The orexins (hypocretins) are neuropeptides that play a role in energy balance and arousal (Ferguson and Samson, 2003). Narcolepsy is caused by failure of orexin-mediated signaling. Orexins are found in the hypothalamus, where they regulate sleep/wake cycles (Baumann and Bassetti, 2005), and in the GI tract, where they excite secretomotor neurons and modulate gastric and intestinal motility and secretion (Kirchgessner, 2002; Parker and Bloom, 2012).

Anorexia nervosa and bulimia nervosa are clinical eating disorders of unknown etiology seen primarily in young women and girls. Anorexia nervosa is characterized by reduced caloric intake and increased physical activity associated with weight loss, a distorted body image, and a fear of gaining weight. Bulimia nervosa is characterized by episodic gorging followed by self-induced vomiting or laxative and diuretic abuse or dieting and exercise to reduce weight. Initially these syndromes were considered to be neuroendocrine in origin; then, for many years, they were assumed to be purely psychiatric. Although malnutrition produces changes in neuroendocrine function, disturbances in corticotropin-releasing hormone (CRH), opioids, NPY, vasopressin, oxytocin, CCK, ghrelin, and leptin as well as the monoamines—serotonin, dopamine, and norepinephrine—have been found in patients with eating disorders (Barbarich et al., 2003; Ogiso et al., 2011). These neurotransmitters play a role not only in appetite but also in mood and impulse control. The abnormalities have been found to persist, in some instances, long after recovery. Autoantibodies have been implicated in the eating abnormalities seen in this condition (Smitka et al., 2013). Furthermore, patients with anorexia nervosa seem to have an increased total daily energy expenditure because of their increased physical activity. All of this suggests a complex interaction between the psyche and the endocrine system as a cause of these syndromes.

## Emotion, Libido, and Sexual Differentiation

Experimental and clinical data support the hypothesis that interaction of the frontal and temporal lobes and the limbic system is necessary for normal emotional function. Lesion and stimulation experiments in cats have shown that rage reactions can be provoked from the hypothalamus. In humans, electrical stimulation of the septal region produces feelings of pleasure or sexual gratification, whereas lesions of the caudal hypothalamus or manipulation of this area during surgery may cause attacks of rage. The amygdala (with its rich input from polysensory areas and limbic-associated areas and its output to the hypothalamus) and other subcortical areas are important structures through which the external environment can influence and cause emotional responses. In depression, activation of the HPA axis has been recognized, but the story is more complex than this simple observation.

Data have shown that depressed patients with suicidal ideation have less activation of the HPA axis, whereas those who commit suicide have a more active axis. Unfortunately, many of these data are derived from peripheral tests that primarily examine pituitary function rather than assessing true hypothalamic function.

Libido, like other feelings, requires the participation of both hypothalamic and extrahypothalamic sites. In most instances of hypothalamic disease, loss of libido is caused by the impaired release of gonadotropin-releasing hormone (GnRH) and a subsequent decrease in testicular testosterone in men. In women, libido is related more to adrenal androgens and in menstruating women to ovarian androgens. Adrenal androgen levels may be low in women with corticotropin (i.e., adrenocorticotropic hormone [ACTH]) deficiency and secondary adrenal insufficiency. Hypersexuality associated with hypothalamic disease is rare and may occur with or without a subjective increase in libido. The melanocortins (ACTH and α-, β-, and γ-MSH) may play a role in the motivational aspects of sexual behavior as well as having a sildenafil-like effect on penile and vaginal blood flow, albeit through a central rather than a peripheral mechanism. Melanocortinergic agents may be useful in the treatment of sexual dysfunction in both males and females (Shadiack et al., 2007).

Current understanding of the human hypothalamus in relation to normal development, sexual differentiation, and behavior is expanding gradually. Sexual differentiation of the genitals occurs during the first 2 months of pregnancy, whereas sexual differentiation of the brain does not occur until the second half of pregnancy. Gender identity appears to result from the developing brain being exposed to testosterone, resulting in a male direction if exposed or a female direction if not. In addition to brain differences related to gender, there are brain differences related to sexual orientation (Swaab, 2007)

It has been known for some time that oxytocin, the classical posterior pituitary hormone that has effects on uterine contraction and milk letdown, works in the brain to promote social affiliation in humans. This brain effect is important for parent-infant bonding and romantic attachments (Feldman, 2012). It also offers hope for the treatment of some of the behavioral aspects of frontotemporal dementia (Tampi et al., 2017).

### Biological Rhythms

Most endocrine rhythms are circadian—that is, a complete cycle takes approximately 24 hours. Although longer and shorter cycles do occur, the circadian rhythms have been studied most extensively. In many animals, light plays an important role in regulating circadian rhythms. Nerve fibers project from the optic chiasm to the suprachiasmatic and arcuate nuclei of the hypothalamus. The hypothalamus is responsible for the hormonal rhythms, such as cortisol and GH secretion, and for the behavioral rhythms, such as sleep/wake cycles and estrous activity. Although patients with hypothalamic disease often have disturbances in their biological rhythms, these are usually of less clinical importance than other problems caused by such lesions, and this is seldom if ever a presenting complaint.

## ENDOCRINE HYPOTHALAMUS: THE HYPOTHALAMIC-PITUITARY UNIT

### Functional Anatomy

In humans, discernible hypothalamic-pituitary tissue begins to develop during week 5 of embryonic life. The Rathke pouch, a diverticulum of the buccal cavity, forms and expands dorsally to contact and invest the diverticulum that develops from the floor of the third ventricle. By week 11, the buccal tissue has lost its connection with the foregut and has flattened to form the primitive anterior pituitary, whereas the neural tissue from the floor of the third ventricle is forming the posterior pituitary. Residual Rathke pouch tissue is postulated to give rise to the craniopharyngiomas that can occur in this region. Rarely, ectopic functional pituitary tissue in the oropharynx can cause signs and symptoms of hyperpituitarism.

**TABLE 50.3 Hypothalamic Peptides Controlling Anterior Pituitary Hormone Release**

| Pituitary Hormone | Hypothalamic Factor |
|---|---|
| Growth hormone (somatotropin) | Growth hormone–releasing hormone (GHRH)<br>Growth hormone releasing–inhibiting hormone (somatostatin) |
| Prolactin | Prolactin-releasing factors (PRFs)<br>Prolactin releasing–inhibiting factor: dopamine and possibly the precursor of gonadotropin-releasing hormone (GnRH) |
| Thyrotropin | Thyrotropin-releasing hormone (TRH)<br>Thyrotropin releasing–inhibiting factor: somatostatin can do this but has not been confirmed to do so physiologically |
| Pro-opiomelanocortin is cleaved to form corticotropin (ACTH) | Corticotropin-releasing hormone (CRH) |
| Luteinizing hormone (LH) and follicle-stimulating hormone (FSH) | Gonadotrophin-releasing hormone (GnRH) |

*ACTH*, Adrenocorticotropic hormone.

The hypothalamus, despite its small size, is the region of brain with the highest concentrations of neurotransmitters and neuropeptides. Beginning with the pioneering work of Ernst and Berta Scharrer and Geoffrey Harris in the 1940s, the hypothalamus has been assigned a central role in regulating anterior pituitary function. In addition to the identified hypophysiotropic hormones (Table 50.3), other peptides with putative regulatory functions are found in high concentration in the hypothalamus: neurotensin, substance P, CCK, NPY, vasoactive intestinal polypeptide, and the opioid peptides. The hypothalamus also is rich in acetylcholine, norepinephrine, dopamine, serotonin, histamine, and GABA. In many neurons, these neurotransmitters colocalize with peptides, although this colocalization and presumptive co-release have uncertain physiological significance. In patients with nonfunctioning pituitary or parapituitary tumors, symptoms produced by compression of neural structures adjacent to the pituitary gland are a common presentation. Understanding these symptoms requires knowledge of the anatomy of the region (Fig. 50.3).

Tumor erosion of the floor of the sella turcica may lead to cerebrospinal fluid (CSF) rhinorrhea. Conversely, sinusitis or sphenoid sinus mucocele can invade the sella, resulting in anterior pituitary dysfunction. Expansion of pituitary tumors into the cavernous sinus can produce palsies of the third, fourth, fifth, and sixth cranial nerves. The development of such deficits is especially common with the sudden expansion of pituitary tumors that occurs in pituitary apoplexy. Carotid aneurysms or ectatic carotid arteries in the cavernous sinus may expand medially and mimic pituitary adenomas by enlarging the sella and causing anterior pituitary hypofunction. Appropriate evaluation with computed tomography (CT) or magnetic resonance imaging (MRI) can identify these conditions.

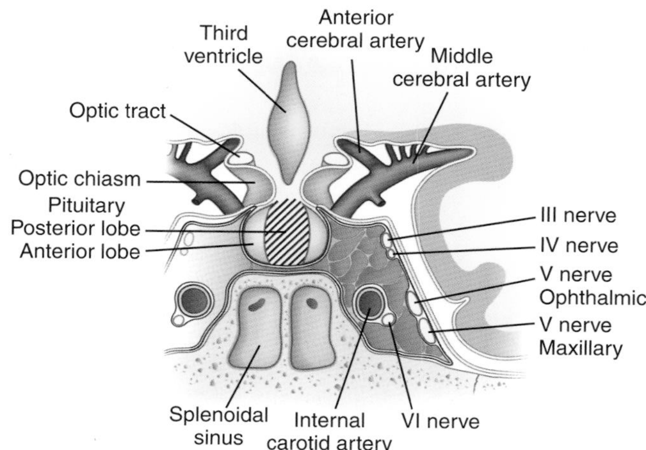


**Fig. 50.3 Diagrammatic Representation of the Anatomical Relations of the Pituitary Fossa and Cavernous Sinus.** The lateral wall of the sella turcica is formed by the cavernous sinus. The sinus contains the carotid artery, two branches of the fifth cranial nerve (the ophthalmic and maxillary nerves), third nerve (oculomotor), fourth nerve (trochlear), and sixth nerve (abducens). The optic chiasm and optic tract are located superior and lateral, respectively, to the pituitary. *(Drawing by B. Newberg. Modified from Makwell, A.K., 1973. Gray's Anatomy, 35th ed. Saunders, Philadelphia.)*

The dura overlying the sella is sensitive to pain, and stretching of this structure by expanding pituitary tumors gives rise to headache referred to the vertex and retro-orbital area. In some cases, especially if intracranial pressure is elevated, the dura may herniate into the sella, where continued pulsation of the CSF over time leads to remodeling and expansion of the sella. This produces the radiological finding of the empty sella syndrome, another cause of which is lymphocytic hypophysitis. The pituitary gland becomes a thin ribbon of tissue along the walls of the normal-sized or expanded sella, and the sella contains mostly CSF. Only rarely can evidence of impairment of pituitary function be found in such patients. In cases of marked hydrocephalus, accompanying pituitary-hypothalamic dysfunction can be seen, presenting most commonly in females as amenorrhea.

Expansion of pituitary tumors out of the sella tends to lead to compression of the anterior and inferior crossing fibers of the optic chiasm (see Chapter 16). These fibers subserve vision in the superior temporal quadrants. Therefore pituitary adenomas typically cause bitemporal superior quadrantanopias. Lesions such as craniopharyngiomas that impinge on the posterior and superior fibers of the optic chiasm tend to manifest with bitemporal inferior quadrantanopias. Nevertheless, owing to the variability of the positioning of the optic chiasm and the tendency for tumors to be asymmetrical in their growth, parasellar lesions result in a wide variety of field defects. Because pressure on the optic chiasm preferentially affects the fibers subserving color vision, these visual field defects may be missed on bedside confrontation testing with the fingers. A better bedside test is to look for subtle color desaturation in the affected visual field.

## Blood Supply

The superior and inferior hypophysial arteries are the pituitary's major source of blood (Fig. 50.4). The posterior pituitary gland is supplied principally by the inferior hypophysial arteries and drained by the inferior hypophysial veins. The superior hypophysial artery forms a primary capillary plexus in the median eminence of the hypothalamus. From here, blood flows into the long hypophysial portal veins, which carry it to the anterior pituitary. Although some blood from the anterior pituitary drains into the cavernous sinus, some drains into the posterior pituitary and some returns to the median eminence by way of the long portal veins, which are capable of bidirectional blood flow. This vascular anatomy provides a potential mechanism for the important feedback loops necessary for the regulation of hypothalamic-pituitary function.

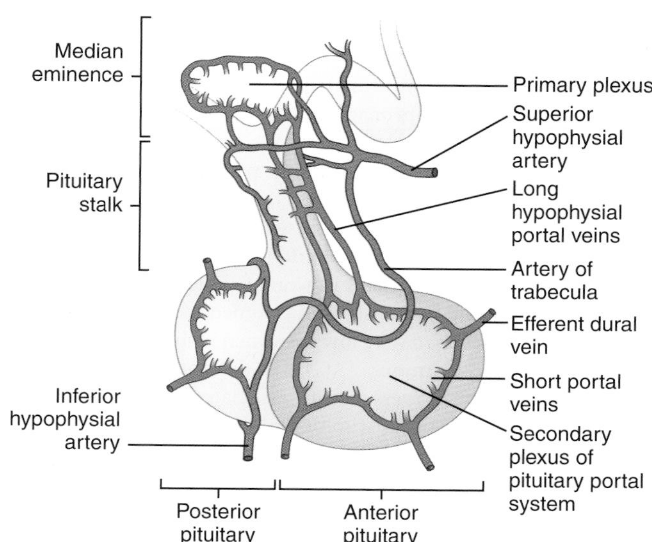


**Fig. 50.4 Blood Supply of the Median Eminence and Pituitary Gland.** *(Reprinted with permission from Cooper, P.E., Martin, J.B., 1983. Neuroendocrine disease. In: Rosenberg, R.N. (Ed.), The Clinical Neurosciences, Churchill Livingstone, New York.)*

# ANTERIOR PITUITARY

## Hypothalamic Control of Anterior Pituitary Secretion

The hypothalamus produces hypophysiotropic substances that control the secretion of anterior pituitary hormones. Five neuropeptides and one neurotransmitter (dopamine) are known to be important physiological regulators of pituitary function (see Table 50.3). In addition, several neurotransmitters affect pituitary hormone release, although their physiological role remains uncertain. Since their discovery in 1998, the orexins (hypocretins) have been found to regulate virtually all the hypothalamic-pituitary axes as well as to participate in the coordination of anterior pituitary function with sleep, arousal, and general metabolism. This is well reviewed in an article by López et al. (2010).

## Abnormalities of Anterior Pituitary Function

### Hypofunction

The causes of pituitary insufficiency are summarized in Box 50.1. In general the symptoms of hypopituitarism (Table 50.4) are those of the secondary failure of end-organ function. Because the associated changes usually develop slowly and some autonomous end-organ function remains, the symptoms are often less severe than those that occur with primary end-organ disease. The term *Simmonds disease* is applied to panhypopituitarism of the anterior pituitary gland. When this syndrome develops in the postpartum period after an episode of pituitary infarction, it is called *Sheehan syndrome*.

Intrauterine growth is independent of GH. Therefore, although GH-deficient children are of normal size at birth, they subsequently fail to grow. Insulin-like growth factors (IGFs) 1 and 2 are important mediators in human somatic growth. IGF-1 production in the liver is dependent on GH, whereas IGF-2 is relatively insensitive to GH. True GH deficiency is rare. It may manifest in an isolated fashion or as part

**TABLE 50.4 Clinical Syndromes of Anterior Pituitary Dysfunction**

| Hormone | Excess Secretion | Deficient Secretion |
|---|---|---|
| Growth hormone | *In children:* Gigantism | *In children:* Growth failure and tendency to hypoglycemia |
| | *In adults:* Acromegaly | Increased body fat, decreased exercise capacity, and decreased bone density |
| Prolactin | *In children:* Delayed puberty | |
| | *In adults:* *Women:* Amenorrhea, galactorrhea, and infertility *Men:* Impotence, infertility, and (rarely) galactorrhea | *In adults:* *Women:* Inability to breastfeed and possible infertility |
| Luteinizing hormone and follicle-stimulating hormone | *In children:* Precocious puberty *In adults:* Infertility, hypogonadism, polycystic ovary syndrome | *In children:* Delayed puberty *In adults:* Amenorrhea, infertility, erectile dysfunction |
| Thyrotropin (TSH) | Hyperthyroidism Hyperprolactinemia (due to excessive TRH stimulation) | Hypothyroidism |
| Pro-opiomelanocortin | Cushing disease, Nelson syndrome | Hypoadrenalism; glucocorticoids affected more severely than mineralocorticoids |

*TSH,* Thyroid-stimulating hormone.

of general pituitary failure. Apparent GH deficiency may result from an isolated deficiency of growth hormone–releasing hormone (GHRH) or from a lack of GH receptors in the liver, leading to failure of IGF-1 production (resulting in Laron dwarfism). GH opposes insulin action; in children especially, its deficiency may be associated with episodes of fasting hypoglycemia.

Pituitary insufficiency of GH in children may manifest as delayed or absent puberty. Onset of puberty depends to some extent on the achievement of a critical body mass. Thus anything that delays growth—such as GH deficiency, adrenal insufficiency, or hypothyroidism—delays puberty. If breasts or sexual hair growth have not started to develop in girls by age 14 or if testicular enlargement and sexual hair growth have not occurred in boys by age 15, puberty should be considered delayed. Luteinizing hormone (LH) or follicle-stimulating hormone (FSH) deficiency may occur as part of generalized pituitary failure, from isolated GnRH deficiency, or as a result of high prolactin levels inhibiting their release from the pituitary.

One cause of hypopituitarism is *pituitary apoplexy*, a term that should be reserved for infarction of or hemorrhage into the normal pituitary gland or into a pituitary adenoma. To be classified as true apoplexy, the hemorrhage should be of sufficient severity to produce signs of compression of parasellar structures or evidence of meningeal irritation. A sudden expansion of the pituitary gland may lead to chiasmal compression or cranial nerve palsies. Rupture of the necrotic gland into the CSF may be clinically indistinguishable from subarachnoid hemorrhage due to rupture of a berry aneurysm or an arteriovenous malformation. Hypotension, aggravated by coexisting ACTH

**BOX 50.1 Causes of Pituitary Insufficiency**

Pituitary aplasia
- Complete
- Monohormonal

Trauma
- Head injury
- Surgery
- Radiotherapy
- Compression by cysts or tumors

Pituitary apoplexy
Pituitary infarction
Hypophysitis
- Infection
- Granulomatous disease
- Autoimmune disease

Hypothalamic failure
Drugs
- Opioids

Cancer chemotherapy

deficiency, may further complicate the picture. The diagnosis can usually be made readily by CT scanning (although apoplexy may be missed on CT slices 1-cm thick) or MRI. Treatment includes admission to hospital; close clinical observation with general supportive measures; corticosteroid replacement; and, in case of worsening neurological symptoms, surgical decompression by an experienced pituitary surgeon (Rajasekaran et al., 2011).

### Hyperfunction

***Precocious puberty.*** Development of secondary sexual characteristics before age 8 in girls and age 9 in boys is considered abnormal. In approximately one-fifth of affected girls and one-half of affected boys, the cause of precocious puberty is a neurological lesion. Various types of tumors have been associated with the development of precocious puberty—including hamartoma, teratoma, ependymoma, optic nerve glioma, glioma, and neurofibroma—either alone or as part of von Recklinghausen syndrome. Tumors are most commonly located in the posterior hypothalamus, pineal gland, or median eminence, or they put pressure on the floor of the third ventricle. The cause of precocious puberty in these circumstances has not been clearly delineated. However, some of these tumors may be an ectopic source of GnRH or of human chorionic gonadotropin, a placental peptide with LH- and FSH-like activity.

In the investigation of precocious puberty, LH and FSH levels as well as human chorionic gonadotropin should be measured along with testosterone (in males) and estradiol (in females). An MRI study of the head is mandatory. If LH and FSH levels are in the adult range and the head imaging result is negative, it is most likely that the precocious puberty is idiopathic. Very high human chorionic gonadotropin levels suggest ectopic production. If LH and FSH levels are low, adrenal, ovarian, testicular, or exogenous causes must be sought.

Chronic administration of long-acting analogs of GnRH results in an initial stimulation of LH and FSH secretion, followed by complete inhibition. This effect on LH and FSH release can be used to stop and prevent progression of hypothalamic precocious puberty.

***Hyperprolactinemia.*** Probably the most common abnormality of pituitary function encountered by the neuroendocrinologist is hyperprolactinemia; its causes are summarized in Box 50.2. Prolactin levels in excess of 200 ng/mL (normal <25 ng/mL) if not caused by pregnancy are usually due to excessive production of the hormone by

## BOX 50.2 Causes of Hyperprolactinemia

Drugs
- Dopamine receptor blockers
- Phenothiazines such as chlorpromazine
- Butyrophenones such as haloperidol
- Metoclopramide
- Reserpine
- α-Methyldopa
- Monoamine oxidase inhibitors
- Tricyclic antidepressants (unusual, probably idiosyncratic)
- Benzodiazepines (unusual, probably idiosyncratic)
- Verapamil
- Cocaine
- Fluoxetine
- Amoxapine

Hormones
- Estrogens
- Thyrotropin-releasing hormone (as can occur in primary hypothyroidism)
- Pituitary tumor
- Prolactin-secreting adenoma
- Interference of flow of dopamine down the pituitary stalk by a large pituitary or parapituitary tumor

Chest wall stimulation

Chronic skin disease (e.g., severe acne) chronic skin disease and tumours of the chest wall should be indented slightly—they are subforms of chest wall stimulation

Tumors of chest wall

Chronic renal failure

Cirrhosis

Ectopic production

Hypothalamic disease

Pseudocyesis

Idiopathic

a pituitary adenoma. In premenopausal women, the development of amenorrhea secondary to direct inhibition of LH and FSH by prolactin leads to early investigation and diagnosis of prolactin-secreting tumors at the microadenoma (<10 mm in diameter) stage. In men, the insidious onset of reduced libido usually means that these tumors are found late, often only after they have produced signs and symptoms of optic nerve compression. Galactorrhea, a rare accompaniment of elevated prolactin in men, is seen frequently in women with hyperprolactinemia.

Serum prolactin levels increase after generalized tonic-clonic seizures and complex partial seizures due to temporary lack of hypothalamic dopaminergic inhibition of prolactin release, but they show no change after virtually all cases of psychogenic, absence, or simple or complex partial seizures of frontal lobe origin. After a seizure, prolactin levels peak at 15–20 minutes and then decrease to baseline levels within 60 minutes. The increase should be at least two times baseline. Caution should be exercised in interpreting early-morning prolactin levels because a 50%–100% increase in prolactin is normal just before waking. Furthermore, prolactin elevations are far from specific for epilepsy, and some tendency for the elevation to attenuate in patients with frequent seizures has been observed.

Because prolactin secretion is under strong inhibitory control by the hypothalamus (owing to the secretion of dopamine), anything that interferes with the free flow of blood down the pituitary portal veins can reduce the exposure of the pituitary to the dopamine released by the hypothalamus. This results in raised peripheral blood prolactin levels. In patients with this condition, prolactin levels commonly range from 50 to 150 ng/mL (usually <100 ng/mL; normal is <25 ng/mL); such elevations can be seen, for example, in patients with granulomatous disease involving the pituitary stalk. However, probably the most common situation in which this occurs is in patients in whom the pituitary stalk is "kinked" by a nonsecretory pituitary adenoma. In such circumstances, this may lead to the erroneous assumption that the pituitary adenoma is secreting prolactin, and long-term therapy with bromocriptine might be undertaken. We have seen such patients whose tumors continued to grow despite normalization of prolactin levels. The mistake with these patients is to assume that a prolactin-secreting macroadenoma would result in a moderately elevated prolactin level. Patients with macroadenomas that secrete prolactin usually have prolactin levels above 200 ng/mL, and not infrequently in excess of 1000 ng/mL.

## BOX 50.3 Common Clinical Signs and Symptoms of Acromegaly

Headache—nonspecific, tension-type, felt at the vertex and behind the eyes

Impaired glucose tolerance or diabetes mellitus

Enlargement of hands and feet

Enlargement of the jaw, with increased spacing between the teeth and malocclusion

Hypertension

Menstrual irregularities

Soft-tissue growth
- Thick skin
- Dough-like feel to palm (e.g., during handshake)
- Carpal tunnel syndrome

Arthralgia and osteoarthritis

Proximal muscle weakness

Hyperhidrosis

Patients taking neuroleptic medications may also have elevated prolactin levels; occasionally the elevation is enough to cause galactorrhea or amenorrhea. In such patients it may be uncertain whether symptoms are secondary to drug-induced hyperprolactinemia or to a microadenoma. In the ideal situation, serum prolactin levels are measured before starting the patient on these medications. Our practice is to perform an MRI study of the pituitary to look for a tumor. Occasionally we will perform dynamic pituitary testing with thyrotropin-releasing hormone and metoclopramide. In most patients, drug-induced hyperprolactinemia responds normally to stimulation with these agents. The treatment of drug-induced hyperprolactinemia is difficult if the causative drug cannot be stopped. Some patients may benefit from the use of atypical antipsychotics with reduced or no action at dopamine receptors (at normal therapeutic doses).

***Gigantism and acromegaly.*** The presence of excessive amounts of circulating GH before closure of the epiphyses leads to gigantism. If the epiphyses have closed, the only tissue still capable of responding to GH will grow, leading to the clinical syndrome of acromegaly; its clinical features are summarized in Box 50.3. Of particular note for the neurologist and neurosurgeon is the frequent complaint of headache and symptoms related to carpal tunnel syndrome. It is not uncommon to find patients with acromegaly in whom surgery for carpal tunnel release was performed bilaterally 3–5 years before diagnosis of their disease.

Most cases of gigantism and acromegaly are due to excess GH production by a pituitary adenoma. Rare cases of ectopic GH production have been described. Excessive GHRH production by pancreatic tumors can cause acromegaly. Excess production of GHRH by the hypothalamus could theoretically cause an identical clinical syndrome.

**BOX 50.4 Common Clinical Features of Cushing Disease**

- Truncal obesity—arms and legs tend to be thin; excess fat deposition in preauricular and supraclavicular fat pads
- Hypertension
- Impaired glucose tolerance and diabetes mellitus
- Menstrual irregularities or amenorrhea
- Excessive hair growth
- Acne
- Proximal myopathy
- Abdominal striae (purplish)
- Osteoporosis
- Thin skin with excessive bruising

***Cushing disease and Nelson syndrome.*** The term *Cushing syndrome* refers to the clinical picture resulting from exposure to excessive corticosteroids, either endogenous or exogenous. If the clinical manifestations are caused by excessive production of ACTH from the pituitary, the condition is referred to as *Cushing disease*. Common clinical features of Cushing disease are listed in Box 50.4. The syndrome of hyperpigmentation and local compression of parapituitary structures that occurs in approximately 10% of patients with Cushing disease who have been treated with bilateral adrenalectomy is called *Nelson syndrome*. Given the generally good results from surgery on the pituitary gland in Cushing disease, bilateral adrenalectomy is seldom required today and Nelson syndrome is quite uncommon.

The diagnosis of Cushing syndrome, although simple in theory, is often quite difficult in practice (Findling and Raff, 2005). It is also often difficult for tests to distinguish between true Cushing syndrome and so-called pseudo-Cushing syndrome due to alcoholism, depression, and eating disorders.

As a screening test, the most sensitive and specific screening tool is an 11 p.m. salivary cortisol determination. Unfortunately, this test may not be readily available in many clinical centers, and 24-hour urine collections for urinary free cortisol are still used. The sensitivity and specificity of the 24-hour collection can be increased by doing two collections on consecutive days. A third screening test is the 1-mg overnight dexamethasone suppression test. For years now, the 2-day low-dose dexamethasone suppression test has been pivotal in the diagnosis of Cushing disease. For this test, 0.5 mg of dexamethasone is given every 6 hours for eight doses; during the second 24 hours of administration, the normal response is suppression of cortisol production as reflected by reduced urinary levels of 17-ketogenic steroids or urinary free cortisol and of serum ACTH and cortisol. Patients with Cushing disease usually show a similar suppression only when the dose of dexamethasone is increased to 2 mg every 6 hours for eight doses. The formal dexamethasone suppression test is cumbersome, requiring 6 consecutive days of collection of urine for urinary-free cortisol levels. Various modifications of this test may be useful and less cumbersome. More detailed discussion can be found in the literature, both for the screening (Findling and Raff, 2005) and diagnosis (Lindsay and Nieman, 2005) of Cushing syndrome.

In Cushing disease, ACTH levels are usually in the normal range or moderately elevated. Failure of cortisol to suppress on high-dose dexamethasone and unmeasurable ACTH levels is seen with primary adrenal problems such as adenoma or carcinoma. Ectopic ACTH production is not usually suppressible; the ACTH levels tend to be much higher than those seen in typical pituitary Cushing disease, although many exceptions to these rules have been found. In well-documented cases of ectopic ACTH production and primary adrenal problems, results of the dexamethasone suppression test have been compatible with a diagnosis of pituitary ACTH production. Intermittent excess ACTH production also can give rise to false-negative results in patients who actually have Cushing disease—so-called cyclic Cushing disease.

Even when all test results point to a pituitary source for the excessive ACTH production, care must be taken in diagnosing the patient as having Cushing disease. An abnormality of the sella may or may not be present on MRI. Intermediate-lobe cysts or clefts may mimic the appearance of adenoma on MRI. In such cases simultaneous sampling from the petrosal sinuses bilaterally and from the inferior vena cava can help localize the excessive ACTH production.

The pituitary glands of some patients with biochemical Cushing disease do not show adenoma formation but demonstrate evidence of hyperplasia of the cells that secrete ACTH. Although this picture can be due to ectopic production of CRH, the hypothalamic peptide that stimulates release of ACTH, or to excessive release of CRH from the hypothalamus, such etiologies affect less than 0.3% of patients with Cushing disease who have pituitary surgery.

***Excessive secretion of thyroid-stimulating hormone.*** Elevated levels of thyroid-stimulating hormone (TSH) are seen most commonly with primary hypothyroidism. The resulting pituitary hypertrophy infrequently can be of sufficient magnitude to cause visual field defects. Hyperthyroidism due to excessive TSH secretion is a rare (accounting for less than 1% of all pituitary tumors) but well-recognized entity, and these tumors are usually large and readily visible on CT and MRI.

Pituitary resistance to thyroid hormone may also produce a clinical picture of hyperthyroidism with high-normal or mildly elevated TSH levels. Unlike TSH-secreting tumors, which are relatively autonomous, the TSH levels in patients with pituitary resistance usually respond well to stimulation with thyrotropin-releasing hormone or to suppression with dexamethasone or dopamine.

***Gonadotropin-secreting tumors.*** Many pituitary tumors formerly classified as nonfunctioning are actually gonadotropin- or gonadotropin subunit–producing tumors. The usual presentation is a macroadenoma in an elderly man; however, they occur in persons of all ages and both genders, with a male preponderance.

Many of these tumors secrete only FSH; only rarely do they secrete LH alone. Some may secrete both LH and FSH and others secrete biologically inactive gonadotropin subunits: the $\alpha$ subunit, LH-$\alpha\beta$ subunit, or FSH-$\beta$ subunit. Most clinical radioimmunoassays used to measure LH and FSH require the $\alpha$ and $\beta$ subunits to be associated before they register in the assay. As a result, subunit secretion is not detected in such assays. FSH levels are usually elevated in patients with FSH-secreting tumors, and testosterone or estradiol levels are almost always low. In patients with LH-secreting tumors, LH levels are usually elevated, and estradiol or testosterone levels may be high. Despite high sex steroid levels, these patients often have no clinical gonad-related symptoms. Patients with tumors that secrete both LH and FSH usually have normal or high sex steroid levels, but again, they are often clinically asymptomatic. Because subunits are biologically inactive, they do not interfere directly with hormonal function. However, by means of pressure effects on the pituitary, subunit-secreting tumors can cause hypopituitarism.

Long-standing primary hypogonadism that is not replaced adequately may cause pituitary enlargement secondary to gonadotroph hyperplasia. Rarely, this may lead to gonadotroph tumor development. Most of the time, the pituitary enlargement is asymptomatic and regresses in response to sex steroid replacement.

An overall review of pituitary dysfunction can be found in the article by Levy (2004).

**TABLE 50.5 2017 Classification of Pituitary Adenomas from the World Health Organization**

| Tumor |
|---|
| Somatotroph adenoma |
| Lactotroph adenoma |
| Thyrotroph adenoma |
| Corticotroph adenoma |
| Gonadotroph adenoma |
| Null cell adenoma |
| Plurihormonal adenoma |

### Pituitary Tumors and Pituitary Hyperplasia

Pituitary tumors account for approximately 15% of all intracranial tumors. Although most are benign, they can be locally invasive. Only rarely is true malignancy evidenced by metastases. The World Health Organization (WHO) revised the classification of pituitary tumors in 2017 (Lopes, 2017); seven adenoma types are identified (Table 50.5). Hyperplasia of various cellular elements of the pituitary is relatively rare and usually seen only in cases of ectopic hypothalamic-releasing hormone production (Ironside, 2003).

Most pituitary tumors that have been removed surgically and examined have been found to be monoclonal in origin. This finding suggests that a majority of pituitary tumors arise from a single cell in which a mutation either activated a proto-oncogene or inactivated a tumor suppressor gene. Around 2% of pituitary adenomas occur in a familial setting in the absence of any other tumor and are referred to as familial isolated pituitary adenomas (FIPAs). Some 15%–30% of such families harbor inactivating germline mutations in the aryl hydrocarbon receptor–interacting protein (AIP) gene, which is associated with early onset and aggressive macroadenomas, most of which secrete somatotropin (GH; Williams et al., 2014). Almost half of pituitary tumors show aneuploidy (usually more or [rarely] fewer than the normal number of chromosomes). The significance of this to tumor formation is uncertain. The cell cycle inhibitory proteins p14ARF and $p16^{INK4a}$ are coded for by the *CDKN2A* (cyclin-dependent kinase inhibitor) gene. This gene has been found to have reduced expression in a majority of human pituitary tumors. *PTTG* (pituitary tumor-transforming gene) expression is increased in certain human pituitary tumors, but whether these changes in gene expression play a role in tumor induction or are the result of tumor formation is unclear.

The G proteins are a family of proteins comprising α, β, and γ subunits that bind to guanine nucleotides. A variety of mutations involving single-amino-acid substitutions in the portion of the Gs gene that encodes the Gs α subunit have been identified in nearly 40% of GH-secreting tumors. These mutations inhibit the breakdown of the α subunit, thereby mimicking the effect of specific growth factors and leading to increased adenylate cyclase activity and elevated intracellular levels of cyclic adenosine monophosphate. Nevertheless, no single mutation or alteration of function seems to explain tumor formation in more than the occasional case. Somatostatin inhibits the production of both GH and cyclic adenosine monophosphate, which may be the mechanism by which it shrinks GH-secreting pituitary tumors.

Although some pituitary tumors are due to genetic abnormalities, it is possible that a majority are not "tumors" in the usual sense but rather represent an excessive response to normal trophic factors that has failed to normalize once the growth stimulus has returned to normal.

The new WHO classification of pituitary tumors has identified that although pituitary adenomas have a low probability for recurrence, adenomas with elevated proliferative activity and special subtypes—sparsely granulated somatotroph adenoma, lactotroph adenoma in men, silent corticotroph adenoma, Crooke cell adenoma, and plurihormone PIT-1 positive adenoma—have a high probability for recurrence (Lopes, 2017).

### Other Tumors

Gliomas, meningiomas, chordomas, teratomas, and dermoid and epidermoid tumors all can occur in the region of the sella turcica, and local compressive effects may produce a clinical picture resembling that of a primary pituitary tumor. The pituitary gland is the site of metastatic deposits in 4% of cancer patients. Usually these metastases are asymptomatic; when symptoms do occur, however, they are most often related to the disturbance of posterior pituitary function.

Craniopharyngiomas are only one-third as common as pituitary tumors. They are thought to arise from residual rests of Rathke pouch tissue. Most commonly found in a suprasellar location, they also occur anywhere along the pituitary-hypothalamic axis, including within the sella. Craniopharyngiomas can appear at any age; however, approximately one-third of cases arise before the age of 15 years. Because these tumors produce no hormones, patients usually present with signs of local compression, especially of the visual system, or with hypothalamic dysfunction such as growth failure or diabetes insipidus (DI). Almost half of affected children show evidence of growth failure. Three-fourths of patients, both adults and children, have visual symptoms, and these are more common in patients requiring complex treatment (Yeun et al., 2014).

### Hypophysitis

Hypophysitis from infection or granulomatous disease such as sarcoidosis can result in hypopituitarism. Lymphocytic hypophysitis, a sterile inflammation of the pituitary of probable autoimmune origin, is seen almost exclusively in women, particularly during pregnancy. It usually causes hypopituitarism, although it can cause hyperprolactinemia and may be a cause of the empty sella syndrome.

## POSTERIOR PITUITARY

### Physiology

#### Vasopressin

Vasopressin, or antidiuretic hormone (ADH), an essential hormone in fluid and electrolyte homeostasis, is synthesized in the magnocellular neurons of the supraoptic and paraventricular nuclei as a large precursor molecule, which is cleaved enzymatically to yield vasopressin and neurophysin. The function of this latter peptide is unknown.

Four vasopressin-containing pathways have been recognized in the brain: (1) hypothalamic-neurohypophysial, (2) paraventricular nucleus to the zona incerta of the median eminence, (3) paraventricular nucleus to the limbic system (amygdala), and (4) paraventricular nucleus to the brainstem and spinal cord. The best-characterized of these is the hypothalamic-neurohypophysial (hypophysial-portal) pathway. Virtually all of the neurons from the supraoptic nuclei contribute to this pathway, whereas only a portion of paraventricular nuclei terminate in the posterior pituitary. Some of the vasopressin-containing fibers from the paraventricular nuclei appear to be more involved in ACTH regulation than in fluid balance. Vasopressin-containing fibers also project widely outside the hypothalamus, where (as some evidence suggests) they may participate in memory.

## Oxytocin

Oxytocin, like vasopressin, is synthesized in magnocellular neurons of the supraoptic and paraventricular nuclei as a large precursor molecule that is cleaved into oxytocin and a specific neurophysin. Many of the physiological stimuli of vasopressin also result in oxytocin release; although this occurs in supraphysiological doses, oxytocin does have ADH-like properties. Its physiological role in these circumstances remains obscure. The only specific stimulus that causes the release of oxytocin but not vasopressin is suckling. Oxytocin's role in normal lactation and parturition in the human remains to be clearly defined. Oxytocin receptors are found in the limbic system, particularly in the amygdala; for this reason oxytocin has been implicated in emotion. Lim and Young (2006) have shown that it plays a role in a variety of complex social behaviors in mammals as well as helping to regulate the response to stress.

### Thirst and Drinking

Certain cells of the anterior hypothalamus are sensitive to changes in the osmolality of the blood and to the levels of angiotensin II bathing them. The organum vasculosum of the lamina terminalis (OVLT) and the subfornical organ (SFO) are outside of the blood-brain barrier and therefore are capable of rapidly detecting changes in osmolality and levels of angiotensin II. They relay information to the median preoptic nucleus (MnPO), and it is these neurons that signal the cells of the supraoptic and paraventricular nuclei to alter their secretion of vasopressin (Lowell, 2019). The hypothalamic cells that sense osmolality are most sensitive to osmotic substances that do not diffuse freely into cells, such as sodium, sucrose, and mannitol. Substances such as urea produce less osmotic stimulation because they diffuse freely. Glucose, in addition to diffusing freely, actually inhibits ADH release. These cells respond with marked increases in ADH secretion not only to increased osmolality, and hence dehydration, but also to hypotension.

Water homeostasis cannot be maintained by antidiuresis alone but also requires thirst and the drinking behavior induced by it. A drinking center is thought to be located near the feeding center in the lateral hypothalamus. Angiotensin may play an important role in stimulating drinking in humans and animals.

### Sodium Homeostasis and Atrial Natriuretic Peptide

Sodium homeostasis is extremely important for the organism's normal functioning. Most of the regulation of body sodium takes place in the kidney. Sodium reabsorption is under control of the renin-angiotensin-aldosterone system. In normal physiological circumstances, aldosterone, the principal mineralocorticoid produced by the adrenal gland, is affected in only a minor way by ACTH.

The SFO contains neurons that are sensitive to angiotensin II and stimulate sodium appetite through projections to the ventrolateral area of the bed nucleus of the stria terminalis. Neurons in the nucleus tractus solitarius (NTS)' secrete aldosterone and work with angiotensin II on SFO neurons to stimulate sodium appetite.

The human heart has been shown to synthesize and secrete atrial natriuretic peptide, which has diuretic, natriuretic (serving to increase urinary sodium excretion), and vasorelaxant properties. In addition to atrial natriuretic peptide, the brain contains brain natriuretic peptide and C-type natriuretic peptide. Judging from the pattern of their distribution in the brain, these substances may have important roles in the central control of the cardiovascular system. The natriuretic peptides seem to act as natural antagonists to the central actions of angiotensin II.

## Diabetes Insipidus

DI is a clinical syndrome characterized by severe thirst, polydipsia, and polyuria. Central DI must be distinguished from nephrogenic DI (an inability of the kidney to respond to ADH) and from compulsive water drinking (Baylis, 1995). Distinguishing between these entities is normally done using a water deprivation test. A urine osmolality of greater than 750 mmol/L after water deprivation excludes the diagnosis of DI. Central DI is characterized by an increase in osmolality to greater than 750 mmol/L after administration of desamino-D-arginine-vasopressin (DDAVP). In nephrogenic DI, little change in osmolality occurs after DDAVP administration. The polyuria induced by chronic compulsive water drinking may produce a renal tubular concentrating defect because of medullary washout—that is, the loss of sodium and other solutes from around the loops of Henle. This can make it difficult to differentiate partial DI of central or renal cause from polydipsia. Treatment by gradual fluid restriction, with or without DDAVP, can be used to reverse the medullary washout, thereby increasing the sensitivity of the test. Fenske et al. (2018) recommend the direct measurement of hypertonic saline-stimulated plasma copeptin in patients with hypotonic polyuria as being more accurate than the water deprivation test.

The water deprivation test must be strictly supervised by a health professional familiar with the technique. Severe and potentially fatal dehydration can occur rapidly in patients with complete DI, especially children. Similarly, patients with compulsive water drinking who are given DDAVP and allowed access to water can drink themselves into hyponatremic coma.

### Etiology

Approximately one-third of patients with central DI have no demonstrable disease of the hypothalamic–posterior pituitary unit. The remaining patients have damage to the supraoptic-hypophysial-portal pathway from trauma, surgery, tumors, inflammatory lesions (which may be granulomatous or infectious), or vascular lesions. In patients with polyuria, the urine should be examined to ensure that a solute diuresis, as with hyperglycemia, has not occurred, or that a type of nephrogenic DI has not been induced by hypokalemia, hypercalcemia, or lithium carbonate therapy. In the acute care setting on a neurosurgical ward, administration of mannitol may be one of the more common causes of polyuria. The investigation of DI has been well summarized by Diederich and colleagues (2001).

### Management

Patients with DI excrete mainly water; therefore water replacement alone is the mainstay of their management. Patients who are alert and have intact thirst mechanisms should be given free access to water. Only if urine output exceeds 7 L/day is treatment necessary. In most circumstances, DDAVP given as a nasal solution or as an oral or sublingual tablet is the treatment of choice. To avoid water intoxication, underreplacement is preferable in these patients, who should be allowed to modulate their water balance by drinking.

Management problems may occur when an unconscious patient's fluid needs are being calculated; that is, the clinician should be aware that the urine in DI is electrolyte poor. Thus, the electrolyte requirements of such a patient are little different from those of other patients. The bulk of the urinary replacement should be given as 5% dextrose in water. The administration of 5% dextrose in 0.2 NaCl or solutions with even higher salt concentrations presents a high solute load to the kidney and tends to exacerbate the polyuria.

## Syndrome of Inappropriate Antidiuretic Hormone Secretion

### Etiology and Pathophysiology

The syndrome of inappropriate ADH secretion (SIADH) is characterized by low serum sodium, high urine sodium, and the relative or absolute hyperosmolarity of urine to serum. Before making the diagnosis, the physician must exclude all of the following: (1) dehydration, (2) edema-forming states such as congestive heart failure, (3) primary renal disease, (4) adrenal or thyroid insufficiency, and (5) the use of medications that cause salt loss in urine (e.g., diuretics).

The initial clue to the diagnosis of SIADH is the low serum sodium (Reynolds et al., 2006). Measured serum osmolality must also be low to exclude the artifactual hyponatremia that occurs with hyperlipidemia and hyperproteinemia, in which the sodium concentration in the plasma water is actually normal. The urine osmolality in SIADH is not always above the serum osmolality, but the urine is less than maximally dilute, which excludes the dilutional hyponatremia of water intoxication. Causes of SIADH are listed in Box 50.5.

### Clinical Features

The clinical features of SIADH are nonspecific and are related to the hypo-osmolality of the body fluids. The more rapidly this condition develops, the more symptomatic the patient. Serum sodium less than 115 mmol/L is almost always associated with confusion or obtundation, and seizures can occur. With milder hyponatremia, the symptoms may be nonspecific, including fatigue, general malaise, loss of appetite, and some clouding of consciousness (Bhardwaj, 2006).

### Treatment

For asymptomatic or mildly symptomatic SIADH-induced hyponatremia, the mainstay of treatment is restriction of fluid. Intake should be reduced to insensible losses (approximately 800 mL/day). Obtundation by itself does not necessitate more aggressive treatment of hyponatremia. In patients with severe hyponatremia complicated by seizures, however, a more rapid *partial* correction can be undertaken. Diuresis is induced with furosemide (1 mg/kg IV), and urinary losses are replaced with 3% sodium chloride through a central line at a rate of 0.1 mL/kg/min, to which appropriate amounts of potassium are added (to counter urinary losses). Considerable controversy exists over the rate at which serum sodium can be raised safely. An expert consensus panel suggests that the serum sodium level be raised by no more than 10 to 12 mmol/L during the first 24 hours of treatment and by less than 18 mmol/L over 48 hours (Verbalis et al., 2007). Patients must be monitored carefully to avoid acute elevation to hypernatremic or even normonatremic levels; it is also important to avoid a change of more than 25 mmol/L in 48 hours, which seems to be dangerous and can cause the syndrome of osmotic demyelination, one form of which is central pontine myelinolysis (Tisdall et al., 2006). The interested reader is referred to the excellent clinical practice guideline on the diagnosis and treatment of hyponatremia by Spasovski et al. (2014).

Prolonged fluid restriction is often poorly tolerated by these patients, who may quickly become noncompliant. In cases where the underlying cause of the SIADH cannot be eliminated or corrected, the drug demeclocycline, a tetracycline, in a dose of 300–600 mg twice a day, can be used to induce a temporary nephrogenic DI, thus alleviating the necessity for fluid restriction. Antagonists of the vasopressin receptor in the kidney (e.g., lixivaptan and tolvaptan) may be more effective than demeclocycline at managing SIADH. Conivaptan, a vasopressin receptor antagonist, is approved by the US Food and Drug Administration (FDA) for the treatment of hyponatremia caused by SIADH. To date, it seems to have low side effects and good efficacy.

**BOX 50.5 Causes of Syndrome of Inappropriate Antidiuretic Hormone Secretion**

**Disorders of the Nervous System**
Tumor, usually parapituitary and large
Trauma, often to the pituitary stalk
Surgery in the region of the pituitary/hypothalamus
Metabolic encephalopathy
Infections (meningitis, encephalitis)
Vascular (e.g., stroke)
Subdural hematoma
Hydrocephalus
Guillain-Barré syndrome
Acute intermittent porphyria

**Drugs**
Carbamazepine
Chlorpromazine
Chlorpropamide
Cisplatinum
Clofibrate
Cyclophosphamide
Oxytocin
Selective serotonin reuptake inhibitors
Thiazide diuretics
Tricyclic antidepressants
Vasopressin (e.g., in overtreatment of diabetes insipidus)
Vinblastine
Vincristine

**Disorders of the Chest**
Pneumonia
Tuberculosis
Cystic fibrosis
Pneumothorax
Empyema
Asthma

**Endocrine Causes**
Hypoadrenalism
Hypothyroidism—unusual cause of syndrome of inappropriate antidiuretic hormone secretion

**Ectopic Production of Antidiuretic Hormone**
Carcinoma—lung, gastrointestinal tract, and genitourinary tract (especially kidney)
Mesothelioma
Lymphoma and leukemia
Thymoma
Sarcoma
Idiopathic

## Cerebral Salt Wasting

Some patients with hyponatremia do not have SIADH secretion with resultant retention of renal free water. Instead, they have an inappropriate natriuresis. Hyponatremia, accompanied by renal sodium loss and volume depletion, occurs in patients with primary cerebral tumors, carcinomatous meningitis, subarachnoid hemorrhage, head trauma, and after intracranial surgery and pituitary surgery. Unlike patients with SIADH, these patients respond to vigorous sodium and water replacement, and their condition actually is worsened by fluid restriction. This inappropriate natriuresis that accompanies intracranial disease (so-called cerebral salt wasting) may be caused either by a natriuretic hormone such as atrial natriuretic peptide or by an alteration of the sympathetic neural input to the kidney.

It is critical to distinguish between these patients and those with SIADH because the treatment for SIADH worsens the hyponatremia

**TABLE 50.6 Common Tests of Pituitary Function**

| Test | Comments |
|---|---|
| Insulin hypoglycemia (regular insulin, 0.1 U/kg IV fasting) | Adequate hypoglycemia is associated with a rise in growth hormone, ACTH, and to a lesser extent, prolactin. It is probably the most physiological stressor of the hypothalamic-pituitary-adrenal axis. The test should not be used in patients with epilepsy or unstable angina |
| Gonadotropin-releasing hormone (2 μg/kg IV to a maximum of 100 μg) | Stimulates LH and FSH release directly at the pituitary. May be used to test LH and FSH reserve. Cannot reliably distinguish between pituitary and long-standing hypothalamic problem |
| Thyrotropin-releasing hormone (7 μg/kg IV to a maximum of 400 μg) | Stimulates release of thyroid-stimulating hormone and prolactin from pituitary. Failure of prolactin to respond to thyrotropin-stimulating hormone is very suggestive of autonomous secretion by an adenoma, but exceptions do occur |
| Metyrapone test (750 mg q 4 h for six doses; collect 24-h urine the day before, day of, and day after the test) | Metyrapone blocks the production of cortisol in the adrenal gland, resulting in increased ACTH secretion. This is an alternative to insulin hypoglycemia as a test of the hypothalamic-pituitary-adrenal axis |
| L-Dopa (500 mg PO) | L-Dopa can be used to stimulate growth hormone release (probably by increasing growth hormone–releasing hormone). It is a less potent stimulus than insulin-induced hypoglycemia but can be used as an alternative |
| Corticotropin-releasing hormone (CRH; 1 μg/kg to a maximum of or 100 μg IV) | Stimulates release of cortisol and ACTH. ACTH is sampled at −5, 0, 15, and 30 minutes and cortisol at −5, 0, 30, and 45 minutes. |

*ACTH*, Adrenocorticotropic hormone (corticotropin); *FSH*, follicle-stimulating hormone; *IV*, intravenously; *LH*, luteinizing hormone; *PO*, orally.

of cerebral salt wasting. Differentiation is best done by a careful assessment of volume status using clinical and laboratory examinations to detect signs of volume depletion. If the diagnosis is uncertain, fluid restriction should be instituted. Then, if the natriuresis persists in the face of volume restriction, the syndrome of cerebral salt wasting should be suspected and appropriate therapy initiated. Because either syndrome can develop in patients undergoing pituitary surgery, it is very helpful to know the patient's presurgical weight. This makes it much easier to determine his or her postsurgical volume status.

## APPROACH TO THE PATIENT WITH HYPOTHALAMIC-PITUITARY DYSFUNCTION

### History and Physical Examination

Patients with suspected hypothalamic or pituitary disorders should be questioned specifically about dysfunction of the nonendocrine aspects of the hypothalamus: appetite, body temperature, sleep/wake cycles, emotion, libido, and autonomic nervous system function. Such symptoms may point to a hypothalamic rather than a pituitary location. A careful functional inquiry should also cover clinical aspects of the hyperfunction and hypofunction of each of the anterior and posterior pituitary hormones.

Because of the proximity of the optic nerves to the hypothalamic-pituitary unit, a careful examination of the visual fields is essential (see Chapter 16).

### Assessment by Imaging Studies

MRI has generally replaced CT as the investigation of choice in the diagnosis of pituitary and parapituitary lesions. The use of MRI with gadolinium contrast is associated with a detection rate for pituitary tumor of 82%–94%. Angiography is reserved primarily for demonstrating the blood supply of suspected meningiomas, and very often this information can be gathered from CT angiography.

### Endocrinological Investigation

Not every patient with hypothalamic-pituitary disease requires a full battery of pituitary tests. In general, the endocrinological investigation is aimed at determining the extent of pituitary functional damage, if any, and—in patients whose blood levels of hormones are elevated or in whom excessive hormonal secretion is suspected on the basis of clinical features—determining whether the hormones in question respond normally to physiological suppressors and stimulators.

No single endocrine test can provide all the answers about pituitary function. Conclusions are based on a synthesis of evidence gained from clinical examination, endocrine tests, and MRI. Endocrine testing is used to determine residual pituitary function after surgery or radiotherapy. Table 50.6 summarizes some of the more common pituitary tests and their use.

## Treatment of Pituitary Tumors

### Medical Management

***Prolactinoma.*** Hyperprolactinemia of whatever cause can often be suppressed by a dopamine agonist, but such suppression is not diagnostic of a prolactinoma. Bromocriptine (2.5–7.5 mg/day in divided doses) or cabergoline (0.5 mg once or twice a week) usually normalizes serum prolactin. In up to 25% of patients on bromocriptine and 10%–15% on cabergoline, however, prolactin levels will fail to normalize, and a 50% or greater reduction in tumor size will not be achieved. Maximum shrinkage of tumors usually occurs within 6 months—often within 6–8 weeks. Experience indicates that bromocriptine is safe to use to restore fertility. Once pregnancy occurs, the bromocriptine can be stopped with little risk of expansion of the prolactinoma during the remainder of the pregnancy and immediate postpartum period. Bromocriptine appears to cause growth of fibrous tissue in prolactinomas. This fibrous tissue may make such tumors more difficult to remove surgically, resulting in lower rates of surgical success. Use of bromocriptine and cabergoline at high doses in patients with Parkinson disease has been associated with valvular fibrosis of the heart. This is not usually an issue with low-dose treatment of pituitary tumors but should be kept in mind if higher doses are used or if symptoms of this condition develop. Baseline echocardiography with regular follow-up can be used to achieve early detection of any cardiac valve abnormalities. A recent meta-analysis has confirmed that low-dose cabergoline in hyperprolactinemia is associated with an increased prevalence of tricuspid regurgitation (Stiles et al., 2019), although the clinical significance of this is uncertain.

In patients with aggressive prolactin-secreting tumors that fail to respond to conventional treatment, a recent case report suggests that the addition of everolimus to the treatment may be helpful (Zhang et al., 2019)

***Cushing disease.*** Results with long-term medical therapy of Cushing disease have been disappointing. Cyproheptadine temporarily lowers ACTH levels in some patients, but it is rarely effective for long and commonly associated with somnolence and increased appetite. Drugs such as metyrapone and ketoconazole, which block corticosteroid synthesis, can be used to lower cortisol levels and improve the patient's clinical status before surgery. Ketoconazole can be used to control cortisol levels over the long term, but patients must be monitored closely for side effects (Castinetti et al., 2014). Mifepristone (RU-486) in high doses has been shown to provide control in patients with Cushing disease and diabetes mellitus that had been refractory to other medications. Pasireotide, a somatostatin receptor antagonist, has recently been shown to reduce cortisol secretion in the majority of Cushing disease patients.

***Acromegaly.*** Until the development of a long-acting somatostatin analog (octreotide), the outcome of medical therapy for acromegaly, like that for Cushing disease, was disappointing. Bromocriptine in doses of 20–60 mg/day could reduce GH levels and cause tumor shrinkage, but it seldom normalized GH levels. Octreotide can normalize GH levels when it is given by subcutaneous injection every 8 hours or when used in a long-acting form given once monthly. The analog can be combined with bromocriptine if necessary to achieve maximal suppression and tumor shrinkage. For those patients who fail to respond to long-acting octreotide, pegvisomant (a GH receptor blocker) can be added to the regimen to normalize IGF-1 levels. Most patients treated with pegvisomant will require continuing therapy with octreotide. Patients who fail to respond to octreotide may respond to pasireotide. The Endocrine Society has a helpful guideline for treatment of acromegaly (Katznelson et al., 2014). Also, emerging data suggest that pathology and imaging characteristics may be able to identify those patients most appropriate for medical management (Ezzat et al., 2019).

***Thyroid-stimulating hormone–secreting and gonadotropin-secreting tumors.*** Most patients with TSH-secreting and gonadotropin-secreting tumors are treated surgically, sometimes followed by radiotherapy. TSH-secreting tumors respond to octreotide with a decrease in hormone production; however, little if any tumor shrinkage is achieved. Early reports suggest that octreotide can reduce levels of α-subunit secretion in gonadotropin-secreting tumors, as can bromocriptine. Surgery remains the treatment of choice for TSH-secreting adenomas, but if it is unsuccessful or contraindicated, treatment with a somatostatin analog, sometimes combined with methimazole, and/or radiation therapy should be considered (Malchiodi et al., 2014).

### Surgery

In a medically fit patient with an accessible lesion, surgery is the treatment of choice for all nonsecretory pituitary and parapituitary lesions causing symptoms or signs or showing signs of growth on serial imaging. For secretory tumors, surgery offers the possibility of rapid and complete cure. It is the preferred treatment when serious compression of parapituitary structures occurs. Surgical cure rates have been reported to be greater than 80% in cases of microadenoma, although these rates may well be lower when strict endocrine criteria for cure are applied and with follow-up periods of 15 years. In the hands of an experienced neurosurgeon, pituitary surgery is associated with low rates of morbidity and mortality. In tumors that secrete prolactin or GH, medical management is now achieving results that are sometimes better than those being achieved by surgery. Depending on the availability of surgery and the skill of the surgeon, for prolactinomas and GH-secreting tumors, surgery may no longer be the first choice but instead be used only in those patients who fail medical therapy.

### Radiotherapy

Conventional radiotherapy is used primarily as an adjunct to surgery and medical therapy, most commonly in the treatment of acromegaly, although octreotide and pegvisomant are reducing its need. It also is used in surgical failures in cases of Cushing disease. It is rarely used in treating microprolactinoma in North America, although it can be used with larger tumors. Recurrence of nonsecreting adenomas after partial removal is usually effectively prevented by radiotherapy. The major problems with conventional radiotherapy are the long delay in onset of its effect (often 18 months or longer), its tendency to provide only incomplete efficacy in secretory tumors, and the high frequency of eventual development of panhypopituitarism.

Proton beam therapy, external beam radiation therapy using a linear accelerator (LINAC), and the Gamma Knife permit a dose of radiation to be given at the pituitary gland that is 20–25 times greater than with conventional radiotherapy techniques. At the same time, radiation doses to other brain areas are limited. Unfortunately these techniques are available in only a few centers. Furthermore, the tumor must be farther than 5 mm from the chiasm. The reported results compare favorably with those of transsphenoidal surgery, but the tumors that are best suited for this type of treatment are also those that are the best suited for transsphenoidal surgery.

### Treatment of Hypopituitarism

Vasopressin, ACTH, and TSH are the pituitary hormones critical to health and well-being. The management of vasopressin deficiency has already been discussed. ACTH deficiency is managed by glucocorticoid replacement; mineralocorticoid supplementation is seldom necessary in patients with ACTH deficiency. Most patients require 5 mg of prednisone (or 20 mg of hydrocortisone) each morning, and some require an additional 2.5 mg of prednisone (or 10 mg of hydrocortisone) in the evening. With the development of mild intercurrent illness, the dose of steroid should be doubled. Corticosteroid replacement in the glucocorticoid-deficient patient with serious illness or undergoing surgery consists of hydrocortisone sodium succinate, 10 mg/h IV around the clock or 50 to 100 mg IV every 8 hours. As the patient recovers, the dose is slowly tapered to maintenance levels.

TSH deficiency is managed by levothyroxine (L-thyroxine) replacement. TSH levels, either suppressed or elevated, cannot be used to determine the adequacy of replacement in patients with pituitary-hypothalamic disease. Resolution of the clinical signs and symptoms of hypothyroidism is the important goal. In patients who receive adequate replacement, so that tri-iodothyronine ($T_3$) levels in the upper half of the therapeutic range are achieved, thyroxine ($T_4$) levels are often at or above the upper limit of normal.

Gonadotropin deficiency is usually managed by administration of testosterone or estrogen. This therapy, however, does not restore fertility. In patients for whom fertility is sought, a consultation with a reproductive endocrinologist and administration of various substitution therapies for LH and FSH may allow induction of fertility.

GH deficiency in children is treated by the administration of synthetic GH. GH-deficient adults do not routinely receive GH replacement. The evidence suggests that muscle strength, wound healing, and lean body mass all are improved by treatment with synthetic GH. A guide to the appropriate selection of patients who might benefit from GH replacement therapy can be found in the Endocrine Society's clinical practice guideline (Molitch, 2006). No therapy is available for prolactin deficiency.

## NEUROENDOCRINE TUMORS

Many endocrine cells distributed throughout the body are capable of taking up and decarboxylating amine precursors and synthesizing biogenic amines and polypeptide hormones. These cells are referred to as *a*mine *p*recursor *u*ptake and *d*ecarboxylation (APUD) cells. APUD cells are found in the pituitary gland, adrenal gland, peripheral autonomic ganglia, lung, GI tract, pancreas, gonads, and thymus. Tumors arising from APUD cells as a class generally produce symptoms through the secretion of biogenic amines (norepinephrine, epinephrine, dopamine, serotonin) or hormones. APUD cell tumors—insulinomas, gastrinomas, vasoactive intestinal polypeptide-secreting tumors (VIPomas), medullary carcinomas of the thyroid, pheochromocytomas, and carcinoid tumors—can manifest as clinical emergencies. Of these, only pheochromocytomas and carcinoid tumors are discussed here.

## Pheochromocytomas

Pheochromocytomas are rare tumors that arise most commonly (85%–90% of the time) from the catecholamine-producing cells of the adrenal medulla; they can also arise from extra-adrenal chromaffin tissue in the cervical and thoracic regions and from the abdomen, where they are referred to as paragangliomas. A majority of these tumors develop spontaneously; however, they can be part of other syndromes such as multiple endocrine neoplasia types II and IIb, von Hippel-Lindau disease, neurofibromatosis, ataxia-telangiectasia, tuberous sclerosis, and Sturge–Weber syndrome.

Pheochromocytomas secrete predominantly norepinephrine, epinephrine, and some dopamine. These compounds are responsible for the most common signs and symptoms of pheochromocytoma: throbbing headache, sweating, palpitations, pallor, nausea, vomiting, and tremor. Pheochromocytomas also are capable of secreting other neuropeptides that can be responsible for different clinical symptoms. Pheochromocytoma should be suspected in patients with progressive or malignant hypertension; hypertension of early onset without family history; hypertension resistant to conventional therapy; paradoxical worsening of hypertension in response to treatment with beta blockers; a history of pressor response provoked by anesthesia, labor or delivery, or angiography; or a family history of pheochromocytoma. We screen for pheochromocytoma by collecting two consecutive 24-hour urine specimens for fractionated metanephrines (metanephrine and normetanephrine) and catecholamines (epinephrine, norepinephrine, and dopamine). For catecholamines, these collections should be done around the time when the patient is symptomatic; however, this is not required for metanephrines as their secretion is stable. The completeness of the 24-hour collection should be confirmed by an analysis of urinary creatinine. Sensitivity and specificity of testing can be enhanced by adding an assay of plasma metanephrines and/or catecholamines. The interested reader is referred to the clinical guideline by Lenders (2014).

Tumor localization can usually be achieved by CT of the adrenals. If a wider search is necessary, MRI may be more helpful. Radiolabeled metaiodobenzylguanidine ($^{123}$I-MIBG), an iodinated guanethidine derivative, is taken up by chromaffin tissue, and its use with single-photon emission computed tomography (SPECT) can be helpful in localizing nonadrenal tumors and metastases. Some centers have been using indium 111–labeled pentetreotide, an analog of somatostatin, to localize somatostatin receptors on these tumors; 6-[$^{18}$F]-fluorodopamine positron emission tomography (PET) and [$^{11}$C]hydroxyephedrine PET are complementary techniques for tumor localization (Eriksson et al., 2005).

Patients with pheochromocytoma should be managed in centers with previous experience in treating this type of tumor. Suitable preoperative preparation is necessary to prevent hypertensive or hypotensive crisis during surgery. For benign tumors, complete surgical removal is the treatment of choice. For malignant tumors, palliative management using a variety of treatments is indicated.

## Carcinoid Tumors

Carcinoid tumors arise from enterochromaffin cells in the GI tract, pancreas, or lungs and only rarely from the thymus or gonads. When carcinoid tumors release biogenic amines directly into the systemic circulation, bypassing the liver, the *carcinoid syndrome* results. This syndrome is characterized by episodes of flushing, often with accompanying diarrhea or asthma. Later in the syndrome, fibrosis of the endomyocardium may develop. Carcinoid tumors may be a source of ectopic ACTH, CRH, or GHRH secretion.

The diagnosis is made by finding elevated urinary 5-hydroxyindoleacetic acid levels. As in pheochromocytoma, carcinoids also secrete peptides (e.g., kallikrein, substance P, neurotensin) and other amines (e.g., histamine, dopamine), and some of these substances may be responsible for the flushing that occurs in the syndrome. To localize these tumors, [$^{11}$C]5-hydroxytryptophan and [$^{11}$C] L-dihydroxyphenylalanine can be useful in PET scans.

Surgery is the treatment of choice, but by the time the tumors become symptomatic, they often are incurable because liver metastases are required for the appearance of symptoms. Serotonin antagonists may be used to relieve some of the symptoms, and octreotide may successfully manage carcinoid crisis. Radiolabeled octreotide is being used in some centers for palliative management of these tumors.

*The complete reference list is available online at https://expertconsult.inkling.com/.*

# INDEX

Note: Page numbers followed by "*f*" indicate figures, "*t*" indicate tables, and "*b*" indicate boxes.

## C

## D

## F

## M

## O

## S

## V

## W

## X

BRADLEY *and* DAROFF'S

# NEUROLOGY

## IN CLINICAL PRACTICE

*We dedicate this book to our families in acknowledgement of their understanding and support.*

EIGHTH EDITION

# BRADLEY *and* DAROFF'S NEUROLOGY IN CLINICAL PRACTICE

**Volume II**

**Joseph Jankovic, MD**
Professor of Neurology
Distinguished Chair in Movement Disorders
Director of Parkinson's Disease Center and Movement Disorders Clinic
Department of Neurology
Baylor College of Medicine
Houston, TX, United States

**John C. Mazziotta, MD, PhD**
Vice Chancellor of UCLA Health Sciences
Dean, David Geffen School of Medicine
CEO UCLA Health
University of California, Los Angeles
Los Angeles, CA, United States

**Scott L. Pomeroy, MD, PhD**
Bronson Crothers Professor of Neurology
Director, Intellectual and Developmental Disabilities Research Center
Harvard Medical School
Chair, Department of Neurology
Neurologist-in-Chief
Boston Children's Hospital
Boston, MA, United States

**Nancy J. Newman, MD**
LeoDelle Jolley Professor of Ophthalmology
Professor of Ophthalmology and Neurology
Instructor in Neurological Surgery, Emory University School of Medicine
Director, Section of Neuro-Ophthalmology
Emory Eye Center
Emory University
Atlanta, GA, United States

For additional online content visit ExpertConsult.com

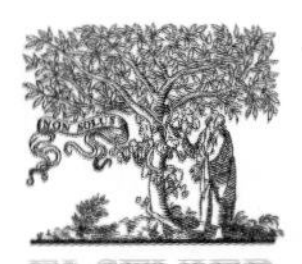

ELSEVIER Edinburgh London New York Oxford Philadelphia St Louis Sydney 2022

First edition 1991
Second edition 1996
Third edition 2000
Fourth edition 2004
Fifth edition 2008
Sixth edition 2012
Seventh edition 2016



**Notices**

Practitioners and researchers must always rely on their own experience and knowledge in evaluating and using any information, methods, compounds or experiments described herein. Because of rapid advances in the medical sciences, in particular, independent verification of diagnoses and drug dosages should be made. To the fullest extent of the law, no responsibility is assumed by Elsevier, authors, editors or contributors for any injury and/or damage to persons or property as a matter of products liability, negligence or otherwise, or from any use or operation of any methods, products, instructions, or ideas contained in the material herein.

**ISBN: 978-0-323-64261-3**

*Content Strategist:* Melanie Tucker
*Content Development Specialist:* Joanne Scott
*Project Manager:* Andrew Riley
*Design:* Margaret Reid
*Illustration Manager:* Paula Catalano
*Illustrator:* Joe Chovan
*Marketing Manager:* Claire McKenzie

Printed in India

Last digit is the print number: 9 8 7 6 5 4 3

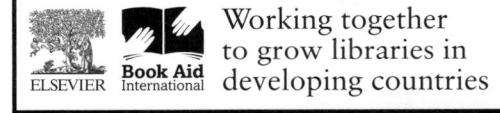

# CONTENTS

# PREFACE

From the very beginning, *Neurology in Clinical Practice* has served as a textbook of neurology that comprehensively covers the clinical neurosciences and provides, not only a description of neurological diseases and their pathophysiology, but also a practical approach to their diagnosis and management. Following the publication of the last edition our colleague, Dr. Robert Daroff, decided to step down. In recognition of his distinguished contributions from the inception, the book has been renamed as *"Bradley and Daroff's Neurology in Clinical Practice"*. We are delighted that Dr. Nancy Newman has joined the current team of editors. With her many scientific contributions to the field of neuro-ophthalmology and her long-standing commitment to excellence in neurologic education she is eminently qualified to continue Dr. Daroff's legacy.

In the preface to the 1991 first edition of this book, we forecast that major technological and research advances would soon reveal the underlying cause and potential treatment of an ever-increasing number of neurological diseases. This prediction has been realized. The three decades since that initial prediction have been marked with the excitement of new discoveries resulting from the blossoming of neurosciences. Advances in genetics, molecular biology, pharmacology, imaging, and surgery have revolutionized our approach to neurological disorders. Pathogenesis-targeted therapies, coupled with improved symptomatic management, have improved outcomes and changed the course of patients with many neurological diseases. Therapies are now available that slow the course of diseases such as multiple sclerosis and other neuroimmune disorders, neurologic and systemic neoplasms, and spinal muscular atrophy which until the past several years were relentlessly progressive. Advances in neuroimaging now enable the precise identification of functional regions and fine neuroanatomy of the human brain in health and disease. The important and challenging problems of neuroprotection are being addressed in both neurodegenerative disorders and acute injuries to the nervous system, such as stroke, hypoxic brain injury, and trauma. In line with this effort, basic science progress in areas of neuroplasticity and neural repair is yielding important results that should translate into disease-modifying therapies in the near future. New advances in immunology and the study of gut flora have important implications in the understanding of gut-brain interaction of many neurological disorders including Parkinson's disease.

When the first edition of this textbook was published, there was essentially no effective means of treating acute ischemic stroke. Today we have numerous opportunities to help such patients, and campaigns continue to educate the general public about the urgency of seeking treatment when stroke symptoms occur. These and other advances have changed neurology to a field in which interventions are increasingly improving the outcomes for patients with disorders that were previously considered to be untreatable.

The advent of teleneurology and wearables are increasingly used to assess neurologic symptoms and signs and to enhance access to medical providers. Teleneurology is now used by nearly all subspecialties, with a particular emphasis on patients who need intraoperative monitoring, critical care neurology, and stroke interventions.

To the benefit of patients, clinical neuroscience has partnered with engineering. Neuromodulation has become an important part of clinical therapy for patients with Parkinson's disease and other movement disorders, and has applications in pain management and seizure control. Along these same lines, brain-controlled devices are already helping to provide assistance to individuals whose mobility or communication skills are compromised. Recent advances in optogenetics have led to development of techniques that allow exploration and manipulation of neural circuitry, which likely have therapeutic applications in a variety of neurologic disorders.

Age-related neurodegenerative diseases, such as Alzheimer disease and Parkinson disease, are increasingly prevalent and represent a growing health and socioeconomic burden. A search for biomarkers that reliably identify a preclinical state and track progression of disease is an important goal for many neurodegenerative disorders. The costs in terms of suffering and hardship for patients and their families are too immense to quantify. As such, there is an urgent need for basic and clinical neuroscience to make progress in finding ways to delay the onset and slow progression of neurodegenerative disorders and, ultimately, prevent them.

There are startling new advances changing the neurosciences. The engineering of nanotechnologies into strategies to treat patients with neurological disorders is just beginning. Advances in genetics, including whole exome and whole genome sequencing, allow for not only discoveries of new genes, but also new disease mechanisms. Novel imaging techniques provide insights into connectivity deficits in sensory and motor networks that are associated with several neurological disorders. Innovative neurosurgical techniques and robotics are increasingly being utilized in enhancing function and optimizing quality of life of patients with neurological disorders.

We still have a long way to go to reach the ultimate goal of being able to understand and treat all neurological diseases. Neurology remains an intellectually exciting discipline, both because of the complexity of the nervous system and because of the insight that the pathophysiology of neurological disease provides into the workings of the brain and mind. Accordingly, we offer the eighth edition of *Neurology in Clinical Practice* as the updated comprehensive and most authoritative presentation of both the art and the science of neurology.

For this edition, the text has been rewritten and updated, and over 60 new authors have been added to the cadre of contributors. New chapters have been added covering ocular functional and structural investigations, cerebral palsy and palliative and end of life care, and chapters have been reorganized and consolidated. The eighth edition includes an interactive online version housed on *www.expertconsult.com*, which can be also downloaded for offline use on phones or tablets. The electronic version of the text contains even more video and audio material, as well as additional illustrations and references.

This new and expanded volume would not have been possible without the contributions of many colleagues throughout the world. We are deeply grateful to them for their selfless devotion to neurological education. We are also grateful to our Elsevier partners, Lucia Gunzel, Senior Content Development Manager, Joanne Scott, Deputy Content Development Manager and Melanie Tucker, Senior Acquisitions Editor, Neuroscience and Neurology who were key in drawing this project together. Additionally, we thank Andrew Riley, Senior Project Manager, without whose energy and efficiency we would not have achieved the high quality of production and rapidity of publication of this work. We also gratefully acknowledge the contributions of our readers, whose feedback regarding the print and online components of *Bradley and Daroff's Neurology in Clinical Practice* has been invaluable in refining and enhancing our educational goals. Finally, we wish to express our deep appreciation to our families for their support throughout this project and over the many decades of our shared lives.

**Joseph Jankovic, MD**
**John C. Mazziotta, MD, PhD**
**Scott L. Pomeroy, MD, PhD**
**Nancy J. Newman, MD**

# LIST OF CONTRIBUTORS

The editor(s) acknowledge and offer grateful thanks for the input of all previous editions' contributors, without whom this new edition would not have been possible.


**Bassel W. Abou-Khalil, MD**
Professor of Neurology
Director of Epilepsy Division, Neurology
Vanderbilt University Medical Center
Nashville, TN, USA

**Peter Adamczyk, MD**
Neurosciences Department Chair
Eden Medical Center
Castro Valley, CA, USA

**Bela Ajtai, MD, PhD**
Attending Neurologist
DENT Neurologic Institute
Amherst, NY, USA

**Jeffrey C. Allen, MD**
Director, Pediatric Neuro-oncology and Neurofibromatosis Programs
Department of Pediatrics, Division of Pediatric Hematology-Oncology
NYU Langone Medical Center
New York, NY, USA

**Brandon Ally, PhD**
Assistant Professor
Department of Neurology
Vanderbilt University
Nashville, TN, USA

**Andrea A. Almeida, MD**
BA Sports Neurology Fellow
Clinical Lecturer, Neurology
University of Michigan
Ann Arbor, MI, USA

**Anthony A. Amato, MD**
Vice-Chairman Neurology
Brigham and Women's Hospital;
Professor of Neurology
Harvard Medical School
Boston, MA, USA

**Michael J. Aminoff, MD, DSc, FRCP**
Distinguished Professor
Department of Neurology
School of Medicine
University of California
San Francisco, CA, USA

**Nicolaas C. Anderson, DO, MS**
Assistant Professor
Department of Neurology
Baylor College of Medicine
Houston, TX, USA

**Tetsuo Ashizawa, MD**
Professor
Department of Neurology
Houston Methodist Research Institute
Houston, TX, USA

**Hatim Attar, MD**
Assistant Professor of Neurology
Department of Neurology
Medical College of Wisconsin and Zablocki VA Medical Center, Milwaukee, WI
Milwaukee, WI, USA

**Alon Y. Avidan, MD, MPH**
Director, UCLA Sleep Disorders Center
Director, UCLA Neurology Clinic
University of California at Los Angeles
David Geffen School of Medicine at UCLA
Los Angeles, CA, USA

**Joachim M. Baehring, MD, DSc**
Associate Professor
Departments of Neurology, Neurosurgery and Medicine
Chief
Section of Neuro-Oncology
Yale Cancer Center
Yale School of Medicine
New Haven, CT, USA

**Asim K. Bag, MD**
Associate Member
Department of Diagnostic Imaging,
St. Jude Children's Research Hospital
Memphis, TN, USA

**Laura J. Balcer, MD, MSCE**
Professor of Neurology and Population Health
Vice Chair, Department of Neurology
NYU Langone Medical Center
New York, NY, USA

**Leomar Y. Ballester, MD, PhD**
Assistant Professor
Co-Director, Molecular Diagnostics Laboratory
Department of Pathology and Laboratory Medicine
Department of Neurosurgery
University of Texas Health Science Center at Houston, TX, USA

**Robert W. Baloh, MD**
Professor, Department of Neurology
Division of Head and Neck Surgery
University of California School of Medicine
Los Angeles, CA, USA

**Elizabeth Barkoudah, MD**
Program Director, Neurodevelopmental Disabilities Residency
Program Director, Children with Disabilities HMS Student Clerkship
Co-Director Cerebral Palsy and Spasticity Center
Department of Neurology
Boston, MA, USA

**Roger A. Barker, BA, MBBS, MRCP PhD**
Professor of Clinical Neuroscience
Honorary Consultant Neurologist
Department of Clinical Neurosciences
University of Cambridge
Addenbrooke's Hospital
Cambridge, UK

**Ryan Barmore, MD**
Adjunct Clinical Postdoctoral Associate
Neurology
University of Florida
Gainesville, FL, USA

**J.D. Bartleson, MD, FAAN**
Emeritus Professor of Neurology
Mayo Clinic
College of Medicine and Science
Rochester, MN, USA

**Amit Batla, MBBS MD DM (Neurology) FRCP**
Honorary Consultant Neurologist
National Hospital for Neurology and Neurosurgery and Royal Free London Hospital
UCL Queen Square Institute of Neurology, London, UK

**John David Beckham, MD**
Associate Professor
Departments of Medicine, Neurology, and Immunology and Microbiology
University of Colorado Anschutz Medical Campus
Aurora, CO, USA

**Leigh Beglinger, PhD**
Neuropsychologist
Elks Rehab System
Boise, ID, USA

**David H. Benninger, PD Dr**
Senior Consultant and Lecturer in Neurology
Department of Clinical Neurosciences
University Hospital of Lausanne (CHUV)
Lausanne, Switzerland

**Joseph R. Berger, MD, FACP, FAAN, FANA**
Professor of Neurology and Associate Chief of the Multiple Sclerosis Division
Perelman School of Medicine
University of Pennsylvania
Philadelphia, PA, USA

**José Biller, MD, FACP, FAAN, FAHA, FANA**
Professor and Chairman
Department of Neurology
Loyola University Chicago Stritch School of Medicine
Maywood, IL, USA

**David F. Black, MD**
Assistant Professor of Neurology and Radiology
Mayo Clinic
Rochester, MN, USA

**Nicholas Boulis, MD**
Associate Professor
Department of Neurosurgery, Emory University
Atlanta, GA, USA

**Michael P. Bowley, MD, PhD**
Staff Neurologist
Massachusetts General Hospital
Instructor
Harvard Medical School
Boston, MA, USA

**Sherri A. Braksick, MD**
Assistant Professor
Department of Neurology
Senior Associate Consultant
Neurosciences ICU
Mayo Clinic
Rochester, MN, USA

**Helen M. Bramlett, PhD**
Professor, Neurological Surgery
University of Miami Miller School of Medicine
Research Health Scientist, Research Service
Bruce W. Carter Department of Veterans Affairs Medical Center
Miami, FL, USA

**Steven M. Bromley, MD**
Director
Bromley Neurology
Audubon, NJ, USA

**Joseph Bruni, MD, FRCPC**
Consultant Neurologist
St. Michael's Hospital;
Associate Professor of Medicine
University of Toronto
Toronto, ON, Canada

**John C.M. Brust, AB, MD**
Professor of Neurology
Columbia University College of Physicians and Surgeons
New York, NY, USA

**W. Bryan Burnette, MD, MS**
Associate Professor
Pediatrics and Neurology
Vanderbilt University School of Medicine,
Nashville, TN, USA

**Carol Camfield, MD**
Professor Emeritus
Pediatrics
Dalhousie University
Halifax, NS, Canada

**Peter Camfield, MD**
Professor Emeritus
Pediatrics
Dalhousie University
Halifax, NS, Canada

**Alan Carson, MB, ChB, MD, FRCPsych, FRCP, MPhil**
Consultant Neuropsychiatrist
Senior Lecturer in Psychological Medicine
Department of Clinical Neurosciences
University of Edinburgh
Edinburgh, United Kingdom

**Dimitri Cassimatis, MD**
Associate Professor of Medicine
Emory University School of Medicine
Atlanta, GA, USA

**Robert Cavaliere, MD**
Assistant Professor
The Ohio State University
Columbus, OH, USA

**David A. Chad, MD**
Staff Neurologist
Reliant Medical Group
Saint Vincent Hospital
Worcester, MA, USA

**Vijay Chandran, MBBS, DM**
Clinical Fellow
Pacific Parkinson's Research Centre
University of British Columbia
Vancouver, BC, Canada

**Gisela Chelimsky, MD**
Professor of Paediatrics
The Medical College of Wisconsin
Milwaukee, WI, USA

**Thomas Chelimsky, MD**
Professor of Neurology
The Medical College of Wisconsin
Milwaukee, WI, USA

**Tanuja Chitnis, MD**
Professor of Neurology
Harvard Medical School
Boston, MA, USA

**Sudhansu Chokroverty, MD, FRCP**
Professor and Co-Chair
Program Director of Clinical Neurophysiology and Sleep Medicine
NJ Neuroscience Institute at JFK
Clinical Professor, Robert Wood Johnson Medical School
New Brunswick, NJ, USA

**Ugonma N. Chukwueke, MD**
Center for Neuro-Oncology
Dana-Farber Cancer Institute
Boston, MA, USA

**Paul E. Cooper, MD, FRCPC, FAAN**
Professor of Neurology,
Schulich School of Medicine and Dentistry and
University Hospital, London Health Sciences Centre,
London, ON, Canada

**Dany Cordeau, RN, PhD(c)**
Registered Nurse
Department of Sexology
Université du Québec à Montréal
Montreal, QC, Canada

**Frédérique Courtois, PhD**
Chair, Full Professor
Department of Sexology
Université du Quéébec à Montréal
Montreal, QC, Canada

**Claire J. Creutzfeldt, MD**
Harborview Comprehensive Stroke Center
University of Washington
Seattle, WA, USA

**Josep Dalmau, MD, PhD**
ICREA Research Professor
Hospital Clinic, IDIBAPS/University of Barcelona
Barcelona, Spain, Adjunct Professor
Neurology
University of Pennsylvania
Philadelphia, PA, USA

**Robert B. Daroff, MD**
Professor and Chair Emeritus
Department of Neurology
Case Western Reserve School of Medicine
University Hospitals Case Medical Center
Cleveland, OH, USA

**Ranan DasGupta, MBBChir, MA, MD, FRCS(Urol)**
Consultant Urological Surgeon
Department of Urology
Imperial College Healthcare NHS Trust
London, UK

**Mariel B. Deutsch, MD**
Behavioral Neurology and Neuropsychiatry Fellow
V.A. Greater Los Angeles Healthcare System
David Geffen School of Medicine at UCLA
Los Angeles, CA, USA

**Michael W. Devereaux, MD**
Professor of Neurology
University Hospitals Case Medical Center
Case Western Reserve University
Cleveland, OH, USA

**Melissa DiBacco, MD**
Postdoctoral Clinical Research Fellow
Department of Neurology – Epilepsy Division
Boston Children's Hospital
Boston, MA, USA

**W. Dalton Dietrich, PhD**
Scientific Director
The Miami Project to Cure Paralysis
Professor of Neurological Surgery, Neurology, Cell Biology and Biomedical Engineering
University of Miami
Leonard M. Miller School of Medicine Center
Miami, FL, USA

**Pradeep Dinakar, MD, MS, MBA, FAAP**
Director, Interventional Pain Program
Boston Children's Hospital
Pain Management Center
Mass General Brigham
Assistant Professor of Anesthesiology
Harvard Medical School Boston, MA, USA

**Bruce H. Dobkin, MD**
Professor of Neurology
University of California Los Angeles
Los Angeles, CA, USA

**Richard L. Doty, BS, MA, PhD**
Director, Smell and Taste Center
Hospital of the University of Pennsylvania
Professor, Otorhinolaryngology: Head and Neck Surgery
University of Pennsylvania, Perelman School of Medicine
Philadelphia, PA, USA

**Gary R. Duckwiler, MD**
Professor and Director Interventional Neuroradiology
Director, INR Fellowship Program
Co-Director UCLA HHT Center of Excellence
David Geffen School of Medicine at UCLA
Los Angeles, CA, USA

**Ronald G. Emerson, MD**
Attending Neurologist and Director Intraoperative Monitoring Program
Hospital for Special Surgery
New York, NY, USA

**Michelle T. Fabian, MD**
Assistant Professor
Icahn School of Medicine at Mount Sinai
New York, NY, USA

**Alireza Faridar, MD**
Assistant professor
Neurology
Houston Methodist
Houston, TX, USA

**Conor Fearon, BE, MB, BCh, BAO**
Clinical Fellow
Department of Neurology
University of Toronto
Toronto, ON, Canada

**Marcia V. Felker, MD**
Clinical Assistant Professor of Pediatric Neurology
Indiana University School of Medicine
Riley Hospital for Children
Indianapolis, IN, USA

**Richard D. Fessler, MD, PhD**
Neurosurgery Resident
Rush University Medical Center
Chicago, IL, USA

**Richard G. Fessler, MD, PhD**
Professor, Neurosurgery
Rush University Medical Center,
Chicago, IL, USA

**Kathryn C. Fitzgerald, ScD**
Assistant Professor of Neurology and Epidemiology, Johns Hopkins University, Baltimore, MD, USA

**Laura Flores-Sarnat, MD**
Adjunct Research Professor of Clinical Neurosciences and Paediatrics
University of Calgary and Alberta Children's Hospital Research Institute
Calgary, AB, Canada

**Brent L. Fogel, MD, PhD**
Associate Professor of Neurology and Human Genetics
David Geffen School of Medicine
University of California, Los Angeles
Los Angeles, CA, USA

**Brent P. Forester, MD, MSc**
Associate Professor of Psychiatry
Chief, Division of Geriatric Psychiatry
McLean Hospital, Harvard Medical School, Belmont, MA, USA

**Jennifer E. Fugate, DO**
Assistant Professor of Neurology
Divisions of Critical Care and Cerebrovascular Neurology
Mayo Clinic
Rochester, MN, USA

**Martin J. Gallagher, MD, PhD**
Associate Professor of Neurology
Vanderbilt University School of Medicine
Nashville, TN, USA

**Sharon L. Gardner, MD**
Associate Professor, Pediatrics
Stephen D Hassenfeld Childrens Center For Cancer and Blood Disorders
New York University Langone Medical Center
New York, NY, USA

**Jarred Garfinkle, MDCM, MSc, FRCPC**
Neonatologist, Department of Pediatrics
McGill University/Montreal Children's Hospital Montreal, QC, Canada

**Ivan Garza, MD**
Assistant Professor of Neurology
Department of Neurology
Mayo Clinic
Rochester, MN, USA

**Claudio Melo de Gusmao, MD**
Clinical Director, Movement Disorders Program
Neurology
Boston Children's Hospital
Boston, MA, USA

**Carissa Gehl, PhD**
Clinical Associate Professor
Department of Psychiatry
University of Iowa
Iowa City, IA, USA

**Christopher D. Geiger, DO**
Assistant Professor
Department of Neurology
Case Western Reserve School of Medicine
University Hospitals Cleveland Medical Center
Cleveland, OH, USA

**David S. Geldmacher, MD**
Professor
Department of Neurology
University of Alabama at Birmingham
Birmingham, AL, USA

**Carter Gerard, MD**
Neurosurgery Resident
Rush University Medical Center
Chicago, IL, USA

**Daniel H. Geschwind, MD, PhD**
David Geffen School of Medicine
University of California, Los Angeles
Los Angeles, CA, USA

**Michael D. Geschwind, MD, PhD, FAAN, FANA**
Professor, Michael J. Homer Family Chair in Neurology
Department of Neurology, Memory and Aging Center
University of California, San Francisco
San Francisco, CA, USA

**Katherine A. Gifford, PhD**
Assistant Professor of Neurology
Vanderbilt University Medical Center
Nashville, TN, USA

**K. Michael Gibson, PhD**
Professor of Pharmacotherapy
College of Pharmacy and Pharmaceutical Sciences
Washington State University
Spokane, WA, USA

**Meredith R. Golomb, MD, MSc**
Associate Professor
Division of Child Neurology
Department of Neurology
Indiana University School of Medicine
Indianapolis, IN, USA

**Rachel Goode, MD**
Assistant Professor of Pediatrics
Department of Pediatrics
Vanderbilt University Medical Center
Nashville, TN, USA

**Jonathan Graff-Radford, MD**
Assistant Professor of Neurology
Mayo Clinic College of Medicine
Rochester, MN, USA

**Olivia Groover, MD**
Assistant Professor of Neurology
Emory University
Atlanta, GA, USA

**Jeffrey T. Guptill, MD, MA, MHS**
Professor of Neurology
Director, Duke University School of Medicine, Faculty
Duke Clinical Research Unit
Durham, NC, USA

**Cecil D. Hahn, MD, MPH**
Associate Professor
Paediatrics (Neurology)
University of Toronto
Director
Critical Care EEG Monitoring Program
The Hospital for Sick Children
Toronto, ON, Canada

**Christine Hall, PhD**
Adjunct Professor
Department of Psychology
Emory University
Atlanta, GA, USA

**Mark Hallett, MD**
Chief, Human Motor Control Section
National Institute of Neurological Disorders and Stroke
National Institutes of Health
Bethesda, MD, USA

**Aline I. Hamati, MD**
Clinical Assistant Professor of Pediatric Neurology
Indiana University School of Medicine
Riley Hospital for Children
Indianapolis, IN, USA

**David Hart, MD**
Director, Neurosurgery Spine
The Neurological Institute
University Hospitals Case Medical Center
Associate Professor of Neurological Surgery
Department of Neurological Surgery
Case Western Reserve University
Cleveland, OH, USA

**Sabine Hellwig, MD**
Neurologist
Assistant in Psychiatry
Department of Psychiatry and Psychotherapy
University Hospital Freiburg
Freiburg, Germany

**Karl Herholz, MD**
Professor in Clinical Neuroscience
Division of Neuroscience and Experimental Psychology
University of Manchester
Manchester, UK

**Alan Hill, MD, PhD**
Professor, Pediatrics
University of British Columbia
Child Neurologist
British Columbia's Children's Hospital
Vancouver, BC, Canada

**Benjamin D. Hill, PhD**
Assistant Professor
Psychology Department/CCP
University of South Alabama
Mobile, AL, USA

**Fred H. Hochberg, MD**
Visiting Scientist, Neurosurgery
University of California at San Diego
San Diego, CA, USA

**Kristin Huntoon, PhD, DO**
University of Texas
MD Anderson Cancer Center
Houston, TX, USA

**Jason T. Huse, MD, PhD**
Associate Professor
Departments of Pathology and Translational Molecular Pathology
University of Texas MD Anderson Cancer Center
Houston, TX, USA

**Monica P. Islam, MD, FAES, FACNS**
Associate Professor of Clinical Pediatrics
Section of Child Neurology
Nationwide Children's Hospital
The Ohio State University College of Medicine
Columbus, OH, USA

**Michael Iv, MD**
Clinical Associate Professor, Radiology
Stanford University
Stanford, CA, USA

**Reza Jehan, MD**
Professor
Department of Radiological Sciences
David Geffen School of Medicine at UCLA
Los Angeles, CA, USA

**Joseph Jankovic, MD**
Professor of Neurology
Distinguished Chair in Movement Disorders
Director of Parkinson's Disease Center and Movement Disorders Clinic
Department of Neurology
Baylor College of Medicine
Houston, TX, USA

**S. Andrew Josephson, MD**
Carmen Castro Franceschi and Gladyne K. Mitchell
Neurohospitalist Distinguished Professor and Chair
Department of Neurology
University of California, San Francisco
San Francisco, CA, USA

**Tudor G. Jovin, MD**
Neurology
Cooper University Hospital
Camden, NJ, USA

**Min K. Kang, MD**
Assistant Clinical Professor
Department of Neurology
University of California, San Francisco
San Francisco, CA, USA

**Matthias A. Karajannis, MD, MS**
Chief, Pediatric Neuro-Oncology Service
Attending Physician
Department of Pediatrics
Memorial Sloan Kettering Cancer Center
New York, NY, USA

**Carlos S. Kase, MD**
Professor of Neurology
Emory University School of Medicine
Atlanta, GA, USA

**Bashar Katirji, MD**
Director, Neuromuscular Center and EMG Laboratory
University Hospitals Cleveland Medical Center
Professor
Department Neurology
Case Western Reserve University School of Medicine
Cleveland, OH, USA

**Kevin A. Kerber, MD**
Professor
University of Michigan Health System
Ann Arbor, MI, USA

**Geoffrey A. Kerchner, MD, PhD**
Global Development Leader
Product Development Neuroscience
F. Hoffman-La Roche, Ltd.
Basel, Switzerland

**Ryan Khanna, MD**
Neurosurgery Resident
Rush University Medical Center
Chicago, IL, USA

**Samia J. Khoury, MD**
Director of Abou-Haider Neuroscience Institute
Professor of Neurology
American University of Beirut Medical Center
Beirut, lebanon;
Visiting Professor of Neurology
Harvard Medical School
Boston, MA, USA

**Howard S. Kirshner, BA, MD**
Professor and Vice Chairman
Department of Neurology
Vanderbilt University Medical Center
Nashville, TN, USA

**Stefan Klöppel, MD**
Head of Memory Clinic
Department of Psychiatry and Psychotherapy
University Medical Center Freiburg
Freiburg, Germany

**Anita A. Koshy, MD**
Assistant Professor
Department of Neurology
Department of Immunobiology
University of Arizona, College of Medicine
Tucson, AZ, USA

**Stephen C. Krieger, MD**
Associate Professor of Neurology
Corinne Goldsmith Dickinson Center for MS
Icahn School of Medicine at Mount Sinai
New York, NY, USA

**Abhay Kumar, MD**
Assistant Professor
Neurology
Saint Louis University
Saint Louis, MO, USA

**John F. Kurtzke, MD, FACP, FAAN**
Professor Emeritus, Neurology
Georgetown University;
Consultant, Neurology
Veterans Affairs Medical Center
Washington, DC, USA

**Jeffrey S. Kutcher, MD, FAAN**
Director, Kutcher Clinic for Sports Neurology
Brighton, Michigan
Park City, UT, USA

**Sheng-Han Kuo, MD**
Assistant Professor
Department of Neurology
College of Physicians and Surgeons
Columbia University
New York, NY, USA

**Anthony E. Lang, MD, FRCPC**
Professor
Department of Medicine, Neurology
University of Toronto
Director of Movement Disorders Center and the Edmond J. Safra Program in Parkinson's Disease
Toronto Western Hospital
Toronto, ON, Canada

**Patrick J.M. Lavin, MB, BCh, BAO, MRCPI**
Professor, Neurology and Ophthalmology
Department of Neurology
Vanderbilt University Medical School
Nashville, TN, USA

**Alice Lawrence, PT, MD**
Assistant Professor of Pediatrics
Department of Pediatrics
Vanderbilt University Medical Center
Nashville, TN, USA

**Marc A. Lazzaro, MD**
Assistant Professor of Neurology and Neurosurgery
Director, Neurointerventional Fellowship Training Program
Medical Director, Telestroke Program
Medical College of Wisconsin and Froedtert Hospital
Milwaukee, WI, USA

**Sönke Langner**
Department of Diagnostic Radiology and Neuroradiology, University Medicine, Greifswald, Germany

**David S. Liebeskind, MD, FAAN, FAHA**
Professor of Neurology
Neurology Director, Stroke Imaging
Co-Director, UCLA Cerebral Blood Flow Laboratory
Director, UCLA Vascular Neurology Residency Program;
Associate Neurology Director, UCLA Stroke Center
UCLA Department of Neurology
Los Angeles, CA, USA

**Chih-Chun Lin, MD, PhD**
Movement Disorders fellow
Department of Neurology
College of Physicians and Surgeons
Columbia University
New York, NY, USA

**Eric Lindzen, MD, PhD**
Jacobs Neurological Institute School of Medicine and Biomedical Sciences
State University of New York at Buffalo
Buffalo, NY, USA

**Alan H. Lockwood, MD, FAAN, FANA**
Emeritus Professor
Neurology and Nuclear Medicine
University at Buffalo
Buffalo, NY, USA

**Glenn Lopate, MD**
Professor of Neurology
Department of Neurology
Washington University School of Medicine
Saint Louis, MO, USA

**Fred D. Lublin, MD**
Saunders Family Professor of Neurology;
Director, The Corinne Goldsmith Dickinson Center for MS
Icahn School of Medicine at Mount Sinai
New York, NY, USA

**Michael J. Lyerly, MD**
Associate Professor
Director, Birmingham VA Medical Center Stroke Center
Department of Neurology
University of Alabama at Birmingham
Birmingham, AL, USA

**Robert L. Macdonald, MD, PhD**
Professor of Neurology
Vanderbilt University Medical Center
Nashville, TN, USA

**Devin D. Mackay, MD**
Associate Professor of Neurology, Ophthalmology and Neurosurgery
Director of Neuro-Ophthalmology
Indiana University School of Medicine
Indianapolis, IN, USA

**Robert Mallery, MD**
Assistant Professor
Neurology
Brigham and Women's Hospital
Boston, MA, USA

**Joseph C. Masdeu, MD, PhD**
Graham Family Distinguished Chair in Neurological Sciences
Director, Nantz National Alzheimer Center and Neuroimaging
Houston Methodist Neurological Institute
Houston Methodist Hospital
Houston, TX, USA

**John C. Mazziotta, MD, PhD**
Vice Chancellor of UCLA Health Sciences
Dean, David Geffen School of Medicine
CEO UCLA Health
University of California, Los Angeles
Los Angeles, CA, USA

**Mario F. Mendez, MD, PhD**
Director, Behavioral Neurology Program, and Professor Neurology and Psychiatry
David Geffen School of Medicine at UCLA
Director, Neurobehavior
V.A. Greater Los Angeles Healthcare System
Los Angeles, CA, USA

**Philipp T. Meyer, MD, PhD**
Medical Director and Professor
Department of Nuclear Medicine
Medical Center - University of Freiburg
Faculty of Medicine, University of Freiburg
Freiburg, Germany

**Dominique S. Michaud, ScD**
Professor, Department of Public Health and Community Medicine
Tufts University School of Medicine
Boston, MA, USA

**Amanda Miller, LMSW**
Social Worker
University of Iowa Huntington's Disease Society of America Center of Excellence
University of Iowa Carver College of Medicine
Iowa City, IA, USA

**Karl E. Misulis, MD, PhD**
Professor of Clinical Neurology and Clinical Biomedical Informatics
Director of Neurology Hospitalist Service
Vanderbilt University School of Medicine
Nashville, TN, USA

**Hiroshi Mitsumoto, MD, DSc**
Director
Eleanor and Lou Gehrig MDA/ALS Research Center
The Neurological Institute
New York, NY, USA

**Brian Murray, MB, BCh, BAO, MSc**
Consultant Neurologist
Hermitage Medical Clinic
Old Lucan Road
Dublin, Ireland

**E. Lee Murray, MD, FACP**
Clinical Assistant Professor of Neurology
University of Tennessee Health Science Center
Memphis, TN, USA
Attending Neurologist
West Tennessee Neuroscience
Jackson, TN, USA

**Evan D. Murray, MD**
Assistant in Neurology/ Instructor in Neurology
Department of Neurology
McLean Hospital/ Massachusetts General Hospital/ Harvard Medical School
Belmont, MA, USA;
Director, Traumatic Brain Injury Service
Manchester VA Medical Center
Manchester, NH, USA

**Fadi Nahab, MD**
Associate Professor of Neurology and Pediatrics
Emory University
Atlanta, GA, USA

**Ruth Nass, MD**
Professor of Child Neurology, Child and Adolescent Psychiatry, and Pediatrics
New York University Langone Medical Center
New York, NY, USA

**Lakshmi Nayak, MD**
Assistant Professor of Neurology, Harvard Medical School
Center for Neuro-Oncology, Dana-Farber/ Brigham and Women's Cancer Center
Boston, MA, USA

**Nancy J. Newman, MD**
LeoDelle Jolley Professor of Ophthalmology
Professor of Ophthalmology and Neurology
Instructor in Neurological Surgery, Emory University School of Medicine
Director, Section of Neuro-Ophthalmology
Emory Eye Center
Emory University
Atlanta, GA, USA

**Thanh N. Nguyen, MD**
Neurology, Radiology
Boston Medical Center
Boston University School of Medicine
Boston, MA, USA

**Raul G. Nogueira, MD**
Neurology
Marcus Stroke and Neuroscience Center
Grady Memorial Hospital
Emory University School of Medicine
Atlanta, GA, USA

**John G. Nutt, MD**
Professor of Neurology
Oregon Health & Science University
Portland, OR, USA

**Marc R. Nuwer, MD, PhD**
Department Head, Clinical Neurophysiology
Ronald Reagan UCLA Medical Center;
Professor, Neurology
David Geffen School of Medicine at UCLA
Los Angeles, CA, USA

**D. David O'Banion, MD FAAP**
Assistant Professor of Pediatrics, Developmental and Behavioral Pediatrics, Neurology
Emory University School of Medicine
Children's Healthcare of Atlanta Pediatrics Institute
Atlanta, GA, USA

**Michael S. Okun, MD**
Adelaide Lackner Professor of Neurology and Neurosurgery
UF Center for Movement Disorders and Neurorestoration
Gainesville, FL, USA

**Justin J.F. O'Rourke, PhD**
Clinical Neuropsychologist
South Texas Veterans Healthcare System
San Antonio, TX, USA

**Claudia R. Padilla, MD**
Behavioral Neurology and Neuropsychiatry Fellow
David Geffen School of Medicine
University of California at Los Angeles
Neurobehavior Unit
VA Greater Los Angeles Healthcare System
Los Angeles, CA, USA

**Jalesh N. Panicker, MD, DM, MRCP(UK)**
Consultant and Honorary Senior Lecturer
Department of Uroneurology
The National Hospital for Neurology and Neurosurgery and UCL Institute of Neurology
London, UK

**Leila Parand, MD**
Behavioral Neurology Fellow
David Geffen School of Medicine
University of California at Los Angeles
V.A. Greater Los Angeles Healthcare System
Los Angeles, CA, USA

**Jane S. Paulsen, PhD**
Professor
Department of Neurology
University of Wisconsin-Madison
Madison, WI, USA

**Phillip L. Pearl, MD**
Director of Epilepsy and Clinical Neurophysiology
William G. Lennox Chair, Department of Neurology
Boston Children's Hospital
Professor of Neurology, Harvard Medical School
Boston, MA, USA

**Zhongxing Peng-Chen, MD**
Neurologist
Movement Disorder Specialist
Neurología
Universidad del Desarrollo, Hospital Padre Hurtado
Facultad de Medicina Clínica Alemana
Santiago, Chile

**David L. Perez, MD, MMSc**
Assistant Professor of Neurology
Departments of Neurology and Psychiatry
Massachusetts General Hospital
Harvard Medical School
Boston, MA, USA

**Ronald C. Petersen, PhD, MD**
Professor of Neurology
Cora Kanow Professor of Alzheimer Disease Research
Department of Neurology
Mayo Clinic College of Medicine
Rochester, MN, USA

**Ronald F. Pfeiffer, MD**
Professor
Department of Neurology
Oregon Health & Science University
Portland, OR, USA

**Robert D.S. Pitceathly, MBChB, PhD**
MRC Clinician Scientist and Honorary Consultant Neurologist
Department of Neuromuscular Diseases
University College London Queen Square Institute of Neurology and
The National Hospital for Neurology and Neurosurgery
London, UK

**Scott L. Pomeroy, MD, PhD**
Bronson Crothers Professor of Neurology
Director, Intellectual and Developmental Disabilities
Research Center
Harvard Medical School
Chair, Department of Neurology
Neurologist-in-Chief
Boston Children's Hospital
Boston, MA, USA

**Sashank Prasad, MD**
Associate Professor of Neurology
Harvard Medical School
Chief, Division of Neuro-Ophthalmology
Brigham and Women's Hospital
Director, Harvard-Brigham and Women's-Massachusetts
General Hospital Neurology Residence Program
Boston, MA, USA

**Bruce H. Price, MD**
Chief, Department of Neurology
McLean Hospital
Associate Neurologist
Massachusetts General Hospital
Associate Professor of Neurology
Harvard Medical School
Boston, MA, USA

**Raymond S. Price, MD**
Associate Professor of Clinical Neurology and Neurology Residency Program Director
Perelman School of Medicine
University of Pennsylvania
Philadelphia, PA, USA

**Louis J. Ptáček, MD**
Distinguished Professor
Department of Neurology
University of California, San Francisco
San Francisco, CA, USA

**Alejandro A. Rabinstein, MD**
Professor
Department of Neurology
Consultant
Neurosciences ICU
Mayo Clinica
Rochester, MN, USA

**Vijay Ramaswamy, MD, PhD, FRCPC**
Assistant Professor and Staff Neuro-Oncologist
Division of Haematology/Oncology
Departments of Medical Biophysics and Paediatrics
Hospital for Sick Children and University of Toronto
Toronto, ON, Canada

**Tyler Reimschisel, MD, MHPE**
Founding Associate Provost for Interprofessional Education
Research and Collaborative Practice
Case Western Reserve University and Cleveland Clinic
Cleveland, OH, USA

**Bernd F. Remler, MD**
Professor of Neurology and Ophthalmology
Departments of Neurology and Ophthalmology
Medical College of Wisconsin
Chief, Section of Neurology, Zablocki VA Medical Center, Milwaukee, WI
Milwaukee, WI, USA

**Michel Rijntjes, MD**
Department of Neurology and Neuroscience
University Medical Center Freiburg
Freiburg, Germany

**E. Steve Roach, MD**
Professor of Neurology
University of Texas Dell Medical School
Austin, TX, USA

**Carrie E. Robertson, MD**
Assistant Professor
Department of Neurology
Mayo Clinic
Rochester, MN, USA

**Maisha T. Robinson, MD, MS**
Departments of Neurology and Family Medicine
Mayo Clinic
Jacksonville, FL, USA

**Michael Ronthal, MbBCh, FRCP, FRCPE, FCP(SA)**
Professor of Neurology Emeritus
Department of Neurology
Beth Israel Deaconess Medical Center
Harvard Medical School
Boston, MA, USA

**Karen L. Roos, MD**
John and Nancy Nelson Professor of Neurology
Department of Neurology
Indiana University School of Medicine
Indianapolis, IN, USA

**Ashley M. Roque, MD**
Assistant Professor
Department of Neuro-Oncology
Mount Sinai Hospital
New York, NY, USA

**Gary A. Rosenberg, MD**
Professor of Neurology
Director, UNM Center for Memory and Aging
University of New Mexico Health Sciences Center
Albuquerque, NM, USA

**Myrna R. Rosenfeld, MD, PhD**
Senior Investigator
Neuroimmunology Program
Hospital Clinical/IDIBAPS
Barcelona, Spain
Adjunct Professor, Neurology
University of Pennsylvania
Philadelphia, PA, USA

**Janet C. Rucker, MD**
Bernard A. and Charlotte Marden Professor
Departments of Neurology and Ophthalmology
New York University School of Medicine
New York, NY, USA

**Sean D. Ruland, DO**
Professor
Department of Neurology
Loyola University Chicago Stritch School of Medicine
Maywood, IL, USA

**Delaram Safarpour, MD, MSCE**
Assistant Professor of Neurology
Department of Neurology
Oregon Health and Science University
Portland, OR, USA

**Donald B. Sanders, MD**
Professor of Neurology
Duke University Medical School
Durham, NC, USA

**Harvey B. Sarnat, MS, MD, FRCPC**
Professor
Departments of Paediatrics, Pathology (Neuropathology)
and Clinical Neurosciences
University of Calgary, Cumming School of Medicine
Calgary, AB, Canada

**Jeffrey L. Saver, MD, FAHA, FAAN, FANA**
Professor of Neurology
Senior Associate Vice Chair for Clinical Research
Department of Neurology
Director, UCLA Comprehensive Stroke and Vascular Neurology Program
David Geffen School of Medicine at UCLA
Los Angeles, CA, USA

**Komal T. Sawlani, MD**
Assistant Professor
Department of Neurology
Case Western Reserve University School of Medicine
Cleveland, OH, USA

**Anthony H.V. Schapira, MD, DSc, FRCP, FMedSci**
Chairman and Professor of Clinical Neurosciences
Department of Clinical and Movement Neurosciences
University College London Queen Square Institute of Neurology
London, UK

**David Schiff, MD**
Harrison Distinguished Teaching Professor
Departments of Neurology, Neurological Surgery, and Medicine
University of Virginia School of Medicine
Charlottesville, VA, USA

**Michael J. Schneck, MD, FACP, FAAN, FAHA, FANA**
Professor Department of Neurology Loyola University Chicago
Stritch School of Medicine
Maywood, IL, USA

**Kirsten M. Scott, MRCP, PhD**
Neurology Registrar
Department of Neurology
Addenbrooke's hospital
Cambridge, UK

**Meagan D. Seay, DO**
Assistant Professor
Department of Ophthalmology and Visual Sciences
Assistant Professor
Department of Neurology
University of Utah
Moran Eye Center
UT, USA

**D. Malcolm Shaner, MD, FAAN**
Clinical Professor of Neurology
Department of Neurology
David Geffen School of Medicine, UCLA
Kaiser Permanente West Los Angeles Medical Center
Los Angeles, CA, USA

**Kaveh Sharzehi, MD, MS**
Assistant Professor of Medicine
Department of Medicine
Division of Gastroenterology and Hepatology
Oregon Health & Science University
Portland, OR, USA

**Ashkan Shoamanesh, MD, FRCPC**
Assistant Professor of Medicine (Neurology)
Director, Hemorrhagic Stroke Research Program
Marta and Owen Boris Chair in Stroke Research and Care
McMaster University / Population Health Research Institute
Hamilton, ON, Canada

**Reet Sidhu, MD**
Director, Developmental Neurology Program
Assistant Professor of Pediatrics, Neurology
Emory University School of Medicine
Children's Healthcare of Atlanta Pediatrics Institute
Atlanta, GA, USA

**Jonathan H. Smith, MD, FAHS**
Associate Professor of Neurology
Department of Neurology
Mayo Clinic
Scottsdale, AZ, USA

**Laura A. Snyder, MD, FAANS**
Attending Neurosurgeon
Barrow Neurological Institute
Phoenix, AZ, USA

**Yuen T. So, MD, PhD**
Professor of Neurology
School of Medicine
Stanford University
Palo Alto, CA, USA

**Marylou V. Solbrig, MD**
Formerly Professor
Departments of Medicine (Neurology) and Medical Microbiology
University of Manitoba
Winnipeg, MB, Canada

**Siddharth Srivastava, MD**
Instructor of Neurology
Department of Neurology
Boston Children's Hospital
Harvard Medical School
Boston, MA, USA

**Martina Stippler, MD, AANS, FACS**
Director of Neurotrauma
Department of Neurosurgery Harvard Medical School
Beth Israel Deaconess Medical Center
Boston, MA, USA

**Jon Stone, MB ChB FRCP PhD**
Honorary Professor (University of Edinburgh)
Department Clinical Neurosciences
Western General Hospital
Edinburgh, UK

**Jerry W. Swanson, MD, MHPE**
Professor of Neurology
Department of Neurology
Mayo Clinic College of Medicine and Science
Rochester, MN, USA

**Viktor Szeder, MD, PhD, MSc**
Associate Clinical Professor
Department of Radiological Sciences
David Geffen School of Medicine at UCLA
Los Angeles, CA, USA

**Lee A. Tan, MD**
Assistant Professor
Department of Neurosurgery
UCSF Medical Center
San Francisco, CA, USA

**Satoshi Tateshima, MD, DMSc**
Professor
Division of Interventional Neuroradiology
Department of Radiological Sciences
Ronald Reagan UCLA Medical Center
David Geffen School of Medicine at UCLA
Los Angeles, CA, USA

**Boon Lead Tee, MD, MSc**
Assistant Professor
Department of Neurology
Memory and Aging Center
University of California, San Francisco
San Francisco, CA, USA

**Stefan J. Teipel, MD**
Head of Section for Gerontopsychosomatic and Dementia Diseases
Deputy DZNE Site Speaker Rostock
Greifswald and Head of the Section for Clinical Research
Clinic for Psychosomatic and Psychotherapeutical Medicine
Section of Gerontopsychosomatic
Universitiy Medicine Rostock
German Center for Neurodegenerative Diseases, Site Rostock/Greifswald
Rostock, Germany

**Reena P. Thomas, MD PhD**
Clinical Assistant Professor
Division of Neuro-Oncology
Department of Neurology
Stanford University
Stanford, CA, USA

**Philip D. Thompson, MBBS PhD FRACP**
Emeritus Professor of Neurology
Department of Medicine
University of Adelaide
Adelaide, SA, Australia

**Matthew J. Thurtell, MBBS, MSc, FRACP**
Associate Professor, Ophthalmology and Neurology
Director, Neuro-Ophthalmology Service
Department of Ophthalmology and Visual Sciences
Department of Neurology
University of Iowa
Iowa City, IA, USA

**Robert L. Tomsak, MD, PhD**
Professor of Ophthalmology and Neurology
Wayne State University School of Medicine
Specialist in Neuro-ophthalmology
Kresge Eye Institute
Detroit, MI, USA

**Bryan Tsao, MD, MBA, FAAN, FANA**
Professor and Chair
Department of Neurology
Loma Linda University Health
School of Medicine
Loma Linda, CA, USA

**Chris Turner, FRCP PhD**
Consultant Neurologist
Queen Square Centre for Neuromuscular Diseases
The National Hospital for Neurology and Neurosurgery
Queen Square
London, UK

**Kenneth L. Tyler, MD**
Louise Baum Endowed Chair
Chairman of the Department of Neurology
University of Colorado School of Medicine
Aurora, CO, USA

**Stan H.M. Van Uum, MD, PhD, FRCPC**
Professor of Medicine,
Schulich School of Medicine and Dentistry,
St. Joseph's Health Care
London, ON, Canada

**Ashok Verma, MD, DM, MBA, FAAN, FANA**
Professor of Neurology
Staff Neurologist, Miami VA Medical Center
Director, Neuromuscular Medicine Fellowship Training Program
Medical Director, Bruce W. Carter VAMC ALS Program
Department of Neurology
University of of Miami Miller School of Medicine
Miami, FL, USA

**Michael Wall, MD**
Professor of Ophthalmology and Neurology
University of Iowa, College of Medicine
Iowa City, IA, USA

**Mitchell T. Wallin, MD, MPH**
Associate Professor of Neurology, Department of Neurology,
George Washington University & University of Maryland
Washington, DC, USA

**Leo H. Wang, MD, PhD**
Associate Professor of Neurology
Department of Neurology
University of Washington School of Medicine
Seattle, WA, USA

**Karin Weissenborn, MD, FRCP**
Associate Professor
Clinic for Neurology
Hannover Medical School
Hannover, Germany

**Cornelius Weiller, MD**
Director and Chair
Department of Neurology and Clinical Neuroscience Medical Faculty
University Hospital Freiberg
Freiberg, Germany

**Patrick Y. Wen, MD**
Center for Neuro-Oncology
Dana-Farber Cancer Institute
Boston, MA, USA

**Mark A. Whealy, MD**
Assistant Professor of Neurology
Department of Neurology
Mayo Clinic Rochester
Rochester, MN, USA

**Eelco F.M. Wijdicks, MD PhD**
Professor of Neurology
Consultant Neurosciences intensive Care Unit
Division of Neurocritical Care and Hospital Neurology
Mayo Clinic
Rochester, MN, USA

**Stephen M. Wilson, PhD**
Associate Professor
Department of Hearing and Speech Sciences
Vanderbilt University Medical Center
Nashville, TN, USA

**Daniel Winkel, MD**
Assistant Professor of Neurology
Department of Neurology
Emory University School of Medicine
Atlanta, GA, USA

**Oleg Y. Yerstein, MD**
Director
Center for Memory and Cognitive Disorders
Lahey Hospital and Medical Center
Los Angeles, CA, USA

**Osama O. Zaidat, MD, MS**
Neuroscience Institute
Bon Secours Mercy Health System
St Vincent Hospital
Toledo, OH, USA

# VIDEO TABLE OF CONTENTS

51

# Management of Neurological Disease

*Joseph Jankovic, John C. Mazziotta, Nancy J. Newman, Scott L. Pomeroy*

## OUTLINE



How an experienced neurologist uses the history of the patient's illness, the neurological examination, and investigations to diagnose neurological disease is discussed in Chapters 1–33. This chapter presents some general principles guiding the management of neurological disease. Chapters 52–56 cover individual areas of neurological management such as pain management, neuropharmacology, intensive care, neurosurgery, neurological rehabilitation, and managing the transition from childhood to adulthood. Chapter 114 covers palliative and end-of-life care. Details about the management of specific neurological diseases are presented in Chapters 57–113. Many aspects of management are common to all neurological disorders; these management considerations are the subject of this chapter.

## PRINCIPLES OF NEUROLOGICAL MANAGEMENT

Once a neurological diagnosis has been established, it is necessary to develop a management plan. In addition to disease-specific treatments, steps must be taken to provide support for the patient, family, and caregivers. Communicating bad news should be done with compassion, with a goal to offer as much hope as realistically possible (discussed further in Chapter 114). If a genetic diagnosis is made, genetic counseling should be offered to support the patient and also to address the potential for disease occurrence in other family members. A detailed discussion of genetic diagnosis and management is provided in Chapter 48.

At present, many neurological diseases are "incurable." This does not mean, however, that such diseases are not treatable and that nothing can be done to help the patient. Help that can be provided short of curing the disease ranges from treating the symptoms, to providing support for the patient and family, to end-of-life care (Box 51.1).

Unfortunately, a physician who is fixated on the need to cure disease may simply strive to make the diagnosis of an as-yet incurable disease and then give no thought to patient management. Such a physician will tell the patient that he or she has an incurable disease, so coming back for further appointments is pointless. The aphorism "To cure sometimes, to relieve often, to comfort always" originated in the 1800s with Dr. Edward Trudeau, founder of a tuberculosis sanatorium. Any other attitude is not only an abrogation of the physician's responsibility to care for the patient but also leaves the patient without the many modalities of assistance that can be provided even to those with incurable diseases. The neurologist who accepts the responsibility for treating the patient will review with the patient and family all the issues listed in Box 51.1. In fact, it is usually necessary to spend *more* time with the patient with an incurable disease than with one for whom effective treatment is available. In addition to providing all the practical help available, the compassionate neurologist should share the grief and provide consolation for the patient and family; both are essential aspects of patient management.

## EVIDENCE-BASED MEDICINE IN NEUROLOGY

No treatment should be given to a patient without a good rationale. Although there is growing emphasis on evidence-based medicine, it should be acknowledged that this approach has some limitations.

Subjects selected for double-blind placebo-controlled studies must meet criteria strictly defined by inclusion/exclusion, and they may not represent the population for whom the treatment will eventually be prescribed. Such patients, for example, may not necessarily have exactly the same demographic or clinical characteristics as those of the well-defined study population, and they may be taking other medications that could affect the response. For these and other reasons, the findings from controlled trials may often not be generalizable. Furthermore, most double-blind placebo-controlled drug trials are relatively short-term studies, and it is not until a long-term open-label trial has taken

**BOX 51.1 Types of Help That a Physician Can Provide to Patients with Any Disease**

Curative treatment
Modification of disease progression/arrest of the disease
Symptomatic treatment:
- Relief of symptoms
- Circumventing the effects of the disease

Treatment of secondary effects of the disease:
- Psychological
- Social
- Family

Definition of the prognosis
Genetic counseling
End-of-life care

place that efficacy and adverse effects are better understood. Moreover, the cumulative experience of a seasoned physician—whose clinical judgment relies not only on the published evidence-based literature but also on personal and often empirical experience—can be of great importance in the management of a specific patient. It would be wrong if this resource were to be disregarded in areas where the relevant literature is not definitive or available. Absence of evidence (usually because the appropriate studies have not yet been done or published) does not mean that support for a specific intervention or application is lacking.

## GOALS OF TREATMENT

In defining the goals of treatment, it is important to separate neurological impairment from disability. *Neurological impairment* (the presence of abnormal neurological signs) allows a diagnosis to be made. Impairment may cause *disability*. For instance, a stroke may cause a hemiplegia, which is the impairment. The hemiplegia may cause difficulty in walking, which is the disability. The patient may be concerned about the abnormal neurological signs but to a greater degree wants correction of the disability. It may not be possible to correct the underlying stroke lesion or reverse the hemiparesis or other neurological deficits, but symptomatic treatment such as providing physical therapy, a walker, and a wheelchair can mitigate these disabilities. The functional state of a stroke patient who has benefitted from neurological rehabilitation may be gratifying as compared with the state of untreated patients.

Amyotrophic lateral sclerosis (ALS) is perhaps the disease that epitomizes the role of symptomatic care. Patients with ALS often report being told by their doctor that they have ALS and are likely to die within 3 years; therefore, because nothing can be done for them, they should go home, put their affairs in order, and prepare to die. A doctor who dispenses such advice is not only uncaring but also leaves the patient without hope and without the symptomatic treatment that could help the patient to circumvent the disabilities attending the disease. The psychological support of a caring neurologist who is familiar with the disease can be of great help to the patient and family (Chiò et al., 2004). An increasing number of lay organizations and support groups are available to provide information and services. Patients will often have found these by searching the internet, but the physician should keep available the addresses and contact information of key organizations to give those who need them.

Symptomatic treatment depends on the nature of the disease. It can consist of arresting an attack of a disease such as multiple sclerosis (MS); circumventing the effects of the disease, as with antispasticity medications; or end-of-life care for a patient approaching death. This last is sometimes called *palliative care*, but in fact every treatment short of cure, even in the early stages of a disease, is palliative. There is no "cookbook" approach to the management of any neurological disorder; therapy must be individualized, and the selection of the therapeutic strategy must be guided by the specific impairment and tailored to the needs of the individual patient.

### Arresting an Attack

Many neurological diseases cause episodic attacks. These include strokes, migraine, MS, epilepsy, paroxysmal dyskinesias, and periodic paralyses; in some of these diseases, treatment may prevent or halt the attacks. Although it does not cure the underlying disease, aborting the attacks is of great help to the patient. Triptan-class drugs may arrest a migraine, and valproate, a beta-blocker, or a calcium channel blocker will reduce the frequency of the attacks (see Chapter 102). Status epilepticus can usually be arrested by intravenous antiepileptic drugs, and the frequency of epileptic attacks can be reduced by the use of chronic oral anticonvulsant drugs (see Chapter 100). Intravenous and intra-arterial thrombolytics may terminate and potentially reverse an otherwise disastrous "brain attack" (cerebral ischemia; see Chapter 64).

### Slowing Disease Progression

Examples of treatments that slow the progress of neurological disease are numerous. A malignant cerebral glioma is almost universally fatal, but high-dose corticosteroids, neurosurgical debulking, radiotherapy, and chemotherapy may slow tumor growth and prolong survival (see Chapters 73–75). The beta-interferons, glatiramer, natalizumab, or mitoxantrone or other immunomodulatory drugs may reduce relapses and slow the progression of MS (see Chapter 79). Liver transplantation in familial amyloid polyneuropathy may slow or arrest disease progression (see Chapter 106). Riluzole may slow the progression of ALS (see Chapter 97). Despite many efforts to slow the progression of Parkinson disease (PD), no neuroprotective therapy has proved to be effective, although certain monoamine oxidase-B inhibitors and dopamine agonists delay the onset of levodopa-related motor complications.

### Relieving Symptoms

Symptomatic treatment is available for many neurological diseases. Relief of pain, although not curative, is the most important duty of the physician and can be accomplished in many ways (see Chapter 52). Baclofen and tizanidine can reduce spasticity, particularly in spinal cord disease, without affecting the disorder itself. Injections of botulinum toxin provide marked relief in patients with dystonia, spasticity, and other disorders manifested by abnormal muscle contractions. High-dose corticosteroid therapy reduces the edema surrounding a brain tumor, temporarily relieving headache and neurological deficits without necessarily affecting tumor growth. In PD, dopaminergic drugs partly or completely relieve symptoms for a time without affecting the progressive degeneration of substantia nigra neurons (see Chapter 95). The physician–patient relationship and the placebo response are both important tools used by the experienced neurologist to help relieve a patient's symptoms (Murray and Stoessl, 2013).

### Circumventing Functional Disability

In neurological diseases such as Alzheimer disease, PD, and ALS, the clinical course is usually progressive. Other disorders, such as stroke and spinal cord injury, have an acute onset, and the damage occurs before the neurologist first sees the patient. Although some recovery is expected, substantial functional deficits often persist. In both situations, many ways to circumvent the functional disability and the resultant handicap are available.

Neurological rehabilitation is the discipline that concentrates on restoration of function (see Chapter 55). Physical and occupational therapy help the patient to strengthen weak muscles, retrain the nervous system to compensate for lost function, increase mobility, and reduce spasticity. Some authorities believe that cognitive or behavioral therapy may similarly reeducate undamaged cortical areas to compensate for the effects of brain injury and stroke. Orthopedic procedures can be beneficial for rehabilitation; transfer of the tibialis posterior tendon to the dorsum of the foot can correct a footdrop in appropriate cases. Surgical release of the Achilles tendon and iliotibial contractures in boys with Duchenne muscular dystrophy can delay loss of the ability to walk by 2 years or more.

Aids and appliances such as ankle-foot orthoses to prevent footdrop as well as canes, walkers, and wheelchairs can increase mobility and limit handicap. Changes to the home and work environment—a ramp or stair lift, widening of doors to allow wheelchair access, rails for the bath and toilet, replacement of the bath with a shower and shower chair—can be of great help. Only the ingenuity of clinicians and biomechanical engineers, the availability of technology, and the associated cost limit the scope of such appliances. Cochlear implants are commonly in clinical use for persons who were born deaf. Computer-controlled motorized body and lower-limb braces may allow paraplegic patients to walk (Hochberg et al., 2006).

The range of options available to help a patient with a severe and chronic neurological disease can be illustrated by reference to ALS. In the early stages, the patient may simply need enlarged handles on tools, pens, and utensils to compensate for a weak hand grip or a cane to help with walking. Later, the patient may need a wheelchair and home adaptation. Speech therapy, a communication board, or a computer with specialized software can help when speech is severely impaired. Weight loss and choking from dysphagia may necessitate a percutaneous gastrostomy. An incentive spirometer and an artificial cough machine can protect respiratory function (see the section titled "Respiratory Failure," later). If the patient decides not to use a ventilator, end-of-life counseling and hospice will be are needed.

Management of disabilities in patients with progressive neurological diseases may tax the neurologist's knowledge and ingenuity, but the beneficial effect of symptomatic therapy for patients and families makes the effort worthwhile and demonstrates that no neurological disease is untreatable. Collaboration with colleagues in other fields (e.g., pulmonary medicine, physical therapy, biomedical engineering, hospice care) is essential for optimal care.

## PRINCIPLES OF SYMPTOM MANAGEMENT

### Treatment of Common Neurological Symptoms

Several symptoms—such as pain, weakness, dysphagia, and respiratory failure—are common to many different neurological diseases. This section outlines the general principles that govern the management of these symptoms. Chapters 52, 53, and 55 provide more complete discussions. Specific treatment for individual diseases is found in the relevant chapters in Volume II of this book.

#### Pain

The first step in pain management is to diagnose the source of the pain and assess the prognosis of the disease (see Chapter 52). Consider, for example, a patient with incapacitating pain in one leg from carcinoma infiltrating the lumbosacral plexus on one side. This patient's life expectancy may be measured in weeks or months, and progressive plexus damage will produce leg paralysis. Destructive procedures and narcotics are justified in this situation. Surgical interruption of pain pathways is considered the final choice to relieve pain from carcinomatous infiltration of the lumbosacral plexus. Such procedures include surgical or chemical posterior rhizotomy, contralateral anterolateral spinothalamic tractotomy in the midthoracic region, and stereotactic contralateral thalamotomy. Tachyphylaxis for narcotics can occur, and the oral dose of narcotics required to control pain may rise rapidly in patients who live for several months. This does not appear to occur with morphine administered by an intrathecal or epidural spinal catheter using a subcutaneous infusion pump.

Narcotics should not be used for patients with nonmalignant chronic pain syndromes such as painful polyneuropathies or low back pain because of the development of tachyphylaxis and the risk of producing drug dependency without pain control (Manchikanti et al., 2012). Biofeedback, hypnosis, and acupuncture may help some patients to control their pain. Antidepressant drugs are of benefit in many chronic pain syndromes by blocking the neurochemical transmitter mechanisms of central nervous system pain pathways as well as treating depression. Many patients are resistant to taking anti-depressant drugs for pain because they insist that the pain is real and not due to depression; the effectiveness of antidepressant drugs for pain control is a point that must be clarified in such instances. Sometimes a single drug may be effective, but frequently a combination of a selective serotonin reuptake inhibitor (SSRI) and a tricyclic antidepressant (TCA) is better.

#### Sensory Loss, Paresthesias, and Burning Pain

Occasionally sensory loss produces an intolerable positive sensation termed *anesthesia dolorosa* that may respond to a combination of a TCA with either carbamazepine, gabapentin, pregabalin, or an SSRI. Paresthesias generally result from damage to the large-diameter myelinated axons in the peripheral nerves or posterior columns of the spinal cord. Patients who complain of burning sensations from small-fiber peripheral neuropathies are often helped by a TCA, an SSRI, pregabalin, or a combination of these.

#### Weakness

The management of weakness, considered more fully in Chapter 55, is a major component of neurological rehabilitation. Choice of treatment depends on the extent, severity, and prognosis of the patient's weakness. For example, weakness of flexion of the ankle due to Charcot-Marie-Tooth disease may be treated with a triple arthrodesis of the foot. Such a procedure, however, would not be appropriate to overcome the footdrop caused by a more rapidly progressive condition such as ALS. For such patients, an ankle-foot orthosis is best. Most neuromuscular conditions benefit from exercise, although fatigue may limit the amount of exercise that can be tolerated. Myasthenia gravis, however, is worsened by exercise. Weakness due to upper motor neuron disease can be addressed by physical and occupational therapy to promote the use of alternative neuronal pathways. Medications such as baclofen, tizanidine, and botulinum toxin injections reduce spasticity and may improve function in upper motor neuron disorders.

#### Ataxia

Ataxia can result from cerebellar dysfunction or sensory deafferentation. A weighted cuff (wrist weight) placed on an ataxic limb may lessen kinetic tremor; the added inertia reduces the amplitude of the

**BOX 51.2 Types of Neurological Disease Associated with Respiratory Failure**

Acute neurological disease
Brainstem damage
High cervical cord injury
Subacute or chronic neurological disease
Bulbar palsy with airway compromise
Motor neuron degenerations (e.g., amyotrophic lateral sclerosis)
Neuropathies (e.g., Guillain-Barré syndrome)
Neuromuscular junction diseases (e.g., myasthenia gravis)
Muscle diseases (e.g., muscular dystrophy)

involuntary movement during feeding and other activities of daily living that require coordinated movement. Gait ataxia is best managed with the use of mobility aids such as a cane, walker, wheelchair, and other measures designed to prevent fall-related injuries. Displacing the center of gravity forward improves the gait of elderly patients, whose loss of postural reflexes causes retropulsion and falls. Increasing the height of the heels on shoes and lowering the walker so that the patient must stoop forward displaces the center of gravity forward.

## Slowness of Movement or Abnormal Involuntary Movements

Along with rest tremor and rigidity, slowness of movement (bradykinesia) is one of the clinical hallmarks of PD and other parkinsonian disorders. Bradykinesia usually responds to dopaminergic therapy. Conversely, excessive involuntary movements, such as chorea and stereotypies, typically decrease with drugs that deplete dopamine or block dopamine receptors. Postural tremors (e.g., essential tremor) often remit with beta-blockers, primidone, and topiramate.

Botulinum toxin injections are considered the treatment of choice for most focal dystonias and may also be effective for movement disorders including tremors, tics, and conditions associated with abnormal muscle contractions. Stereotactic surgery, particularly high-frequency deep brain stimulation, is now an established therapeutic strategy in patients with severe movement disorders that continue to be troublesome or disabling despite optimal medical therapy.

## Aphasia and Dysarthria

The treatment of language disorders is, in principle, very similar to that of limb weakness. Speech therapy can improve aphasia by retraining contralateral speech and nonspeech areas of the brain to compensate for the effects of damaged speech centers. If the lesion is limited, some aspects of language function may be preserved and thus provide an immediate mechanism for communication. For instance, an aphasic patient may be able to communicate through writing. With speech therapy, dysarthric patients can learn to slow their delivery and emphasize words, thereby improving the clarity of speech.

## Respiratory Failure

Respiratory failure may develop in several neurological diseases (Box 51.2; see also Chapter 53). Patients with chronic neuromuscular diseases often complain of respiratory distress when they are close to respiratory failure. Patients with a weak diaphragm experience dyspnea when lying supine because the abdominal contents prolapse into the chest, thereby lowering the patient's vital capacity and tidal volume. A neurologist or pulmonary specialist who is relatively inexperienced in neurological problems affecting respiration may underestimate the warning signs of potentially fatal respiratory failure. This is particularly true in myasthenia gravis and Guillain-Barré syndrome. Blood gas measurements do not change until late in the development of respiratory failure in chronic neuromuscular diseases. By the time evidence of hypoxia and hypercapnia appears in the blood, the patient may be bordering on acute respiratory collapse. Reduced vital capacity, patient distress, and a good knowledge of the disease are better ways of judging impending respiratory failure (Hutchinson and Whyte, 2008). A patient with Duchenne muscular dystrophy and a vital capacity of 600 mL may survive for several years without dyspnea. A patient with myasthenia gravis who has a vital capacity of 1200 mL but is anxious, sweating, and complaining of dyspnea is at serious risk for the development of fatal respiratory paralysis. With borderline respiratory function, sleep or sedation may produce carbon dioxide retention and narcosis, leading to further respiratory suppression and death.

***Ethical considerations in the treatment of respiratory failure.*** Respiratory failure was once invariably fatal but is now commonly treated by noninvasive positive-pressure ventilation in the early stages and by intubation and positive-pressure ventilation in the terminal stages (Radunovic et al., 2013). The treatment of chronic progressive respiratory failure in neuromuscular diseases such as ALS and muscular dystrophy is highly challenging. Moreover, cultural differences in different countries must be recognized. For example, in Japan, it is established practice to provide the ALS patient with a tracheostomy and positive-pressure ventilation when signs of early respiratory failure appear. In Western countries, many patients consider life on a ventilator unacceptable, and the neurologist must discuss quality-of-life issues with the patient and family before proceeding to intubation.

Ideally, decisions about life-support measures should be made long before the patient is in acute respiratory distress because it is more difficult to make these decisions when death is imminent. Patients and families require considerable counseling by the neurologist and may benefit from speaking with others who have experienced the situation, such as a patient on a ventilator or a person who has lost a relative to ALS. Many patients cannot make a definitive decision about life-support measures and so defer the decision until the emergency occurs.

In these matters, the decision of a competent patient or the healthcare surrogate (in cases of an incompetent patient or one with whom communication is impossible) holds primacy. For instance, a 40-year-old patient with ALS may request respiratory support to see a child graduate or marry, even though there is no likelihood of recovery. On the other hand, a request to continue ventilator support for a 90-year-old patient with cancer and severe dementia cannot be considered to be in the best interest of the patient, and the physician should convey the hopelessness of the situation and the patient's unnecessary suffering to the next of kin. Patients who decide against ventilator support should provide a living will or terminal care document to their physician and next of kin and legally grant to a designated person (the healthcare surrogate) the power of attorney to make medical management decisions for them if they become incompetent. Even if patients have prepared living wills, they will be taken by emergency services to a hospital emergency department and be intubated unless proper arrangements are in place for end-of-life care at home, usually through hospice services.

For patients who decide to request ventilator support, health insurance and economic matters must be considered. Although the availability of insurance to cover the cost of ventilator care is paramount in the United States, in Japan the health insurance system pays for the cost of 24-hour home ventilatory care for all ALS patients.

The patient with a tracheostomy may still be able to talk using a valved tracheostomy tube or a partially inflated cuff, but many such patients lose bulbar functions and must use communication devices such as computers or letter boards. Many of the conditions listed in

Box 51.2 also cause limb paralysis, which further impairs the ability to communicate. Quality of life usually becomes an issue when ventilator dependency becomes permanent. In many patients, the prognosis becomes clear within a relatively short time, as with stroke and coma. Because the patient is unconscious, the healthcare surrogate or, if such a person is not designated, the next of kin must decide, with the advice of the doctor, whether to continue respiratory support. If the healthcare surrogate or family of an unconscious patient requests that respiratory support be discontinued, it is standard medical practice in most parts of the world to end it. The legal and ethical issues are more complex with an awake and competent patient who requests that the ventilator be switched off. Although the legal systems in many parts of the world accept that such requests fall under the right of the patient to refuse medical treatment, involvement of a hospital ethics committee is strongly recommended.

## LEGAL ISSUES

There are serious practical and legal aspects patients and families must face when they or their relative is diagnosed with certain types of neurological disorders. Perhaps the most common is the question of whether the patient can drive. Most states have laws that govern particular circumstances. For example, some states require physicians to report to regulatory agencies (e.g., Department of Public Health, Motor Vehicle Department) any patient who has a seizure or alteration in consciousness, motor control, or vision if these symptoms are likely to recur. Failure to do so puts the patient and physician at risk for criminal and civil prosecution. As public debate on such matters evolves, there may soon be similar laws related to cognitive function and judgment. Certain types of employment may also have specific restrictions (e.g., for airline pilots, commercial drivers, construction workers). Neurologists must be completely familiar with these rules and policies in the state where they practice.

It is often very difficult for the physician to inform patients that they will be reported because of their diagnosis and/or symptoms. Frequently the patient will object and ask that this not be done, as it would result in significant practical and economic hardship. Losing the privilege of driving is also associated with a loss of personal freedom and independence. Nevertheless, it is the neurologist's responsibility and duty to explain the reasons for such decisions, the consequences of not doing so, and the associated risks. It is prudent to give examples. Tell the patient what could happen if he or she had a seizure while driving: that the patient or others could be injured or killed; and that if the patient were killed, his or her family would be liable for the financial consequences. When there is a realistic chance of alleviating the patient's disability, indicate that with proper treatment, the restrictions may be dropped and the privilege reinstated.

## IMPLICATIONS FOR CLINICAL PRACTICE

The numerous and multifaceted aspects of modern management of neurological disease presented in this chapter serve to underscore an expanded role for the neurologist in clinical practice. Improved diagnostic methods identify affected persons more often and earlier, and patients with serious or even fatal disease are living longer, so that the physician–patient relationship may be prolonged. It is essential for today's clinical neurologists to recognize that their scope of practice involves much more than diagnosis. Although a correct diagnosis is essential, the clinician's proper focus is on the treatment and management of the patient and the disease.

*The complete reference list is available online at https://expertconsult.inkling.com/.* 

52

# Pain Management

*Pradeep Dinakar*

## OUTLINE



## DEFINITION AND CHALLENGE

Pain is the most common neurological complaint. Chronic pain constitutes a major public health burden. Over 116 million patients suffer with chronic pain. The economic burden of chronic pain is quite significant, at an annual cost of 560–635 billion dollars in direct treatment costs and lost productivity (Institute of Medicine, 2011). Given the enormous nature of this challenge, chronic pain management warrants a multidisciplinary approach with collaboration among multiple specialties including neurology, anesthesiology, physiatry, physical therapy, psychiatry, psychology, and primary care physicians. Treatment of acute and chronic pain conditions including headaches, facial pain conditions including trigeminal neuralgia (TN), peripheral neuropathy, and chronic pain caused by damage or malfunction in the central and peripheral nervous systems is still a major task and challenge facing most neurologists in their daily work.

Pain is classified as acute and chronic pain on the basis of duration of symptoms. Acute pain is defined by the International Association for the Study of Pain as an unpleasant sensory and emotional experience associated with, or resembling that associated with actual or potential tissue damage (Raja, 2020). *Acute pain* is caused by injury, surgery, illness, trauma, or painful medical procedures. It generally lasts for a short period of time and usually disappears when the underlying cause has been treated or has healed. Acute pain usually has a protective role biologically. However, if untreated, acute pain may lead to chronic pain problems. *Chronic pain* is a persistent pain state not associated with the inciting event and exists beyond the normal course of healing. Chronic pain lacks a biological protective role. Acute pain is usually a symptom of the underlying disease condition and chronic pain is a disease condition in itself, presenting with symptoms of refractory pain, functional and psychological impairment, and disability.

Neurologists are traditionally well trained in anatomical localization and differential diagnosis of a variety of pain-related neurological disorders. The successful treatment of chronic pain conditions, however, requires more than an accurate diagnosis; the treating physician must be familiar with the newer multimodal and multidisciplinary aspects of pain management, including pharmacological therapy, physical therapy and rehabilitation, psychological care, interventional pain management, complementary and alternative medicine techniques, and surgical treatment. Along with an excellent understanding of the anatomical localization of pain conditions and with incorporation of multimodal management in clinical practice, the neurologist is in a unique position to offer the best possible comprehensive care in chronic pain management.

In this chapter, we first outline the anatomical basis of chronic pain conditions and some recent developments in molecular pain research. The second portion of the chapter illustrates the multidisciplinary approach to pain management, incorporating recent developments in pharmacological treatment and interventional pain management techniques for treating common chronic pain conditions. The last section of the chapter discusses some common pain conditions seen in daily neurology practice.

## ANATOMY AND PHYSIOLOGY OF THE PAIN PATHWAYS

Nociceptor receptors are found in skin, connective tissue, blood vessels, periosteum, and most of the visceral organs. These nociceptors are formed by peripheral endings of sensory neurons with various morphological features. Noxious stimuli are transduced into depolarizing current by specialized receptors congregated in the nociceptor terminals. Cutaneous nociceptors include: (1) high-threshold mechanical nociceptors (HTMs) associated with small-diameter myelinated axons (Aδ fibers), (2) myelinated mechanothermal nociceptors (MTs) (Aδ fibers), and (3) polymodal nociceptors associated with unmyelinated axons (C fibers). Polymodal nociceptors respond to mechanical, chemical, and thermal stimuli. The afferent fibers that convey nociceptive information are thinly myelinated Aδ fibers with conduction velocities of about 15 m/s and unmyelinated C fibers with conduction velocities of 0.5–2 m/s. Stimulation of afferent Aδ nociceptive fibers causes a sharp, well-localized pain sensation. Activation of nociceptive C fibers is associated with dull burning or aching and poorly localized pain. Because pain impulses are conducted by small, slowly conducting nerve fibers, conventional nerve conduction velocity (NCV) studies that measure the speed of conduction of large myelinated fibers are not sensitive to abnormal function of small-diameter fibers. It is very common that patients with small-fiber neuropathy have normal NCV tests.

Most primary afferent fibers that innervate tissues below the level of the head have cell bodies located in the dorsal root ganglion (DRG) of the spinal nerves. Visceral nociceptive afferent fibers (Aδ, C fibers) travel with sympathetic and parasympathetic nerves whose cell bodies are also found in the DRG.

Axons of DRG neurons send the primary nociceptive afferents through the dorsal roots to the most superficial layers of the dorsal horns (Rexed laminae I and II) and to some of the deep laminae (Rexed V). The Aδ fibers conveying input from HTMs and MTs terminate primarily in laminae I and V; C fibers mainly terminate in lamina II. Neurotransmitters related to pain conduction include excitatory amino acids and neuropeptides, particularly substance P (Geracioti et al., 2006). The second-order neurons in the dorsal horn include cells that respond only to noxious stimuli (nociceptive specific neurons) and others (wide dynamic range [WDR] neurons) that respond to both nociceptive and non-nociceptive sensory stimuli.

Axons of most of the second-order sensory neurons associated with pain sensation cross in the anterior white commissure of the spinal cord and ascend as the spinothalamic tract in the opposite anterolateral quadrant. This tract is somatotopically organized, with sacral elements situated posterolaterally and cervical elements more anteromedially. In humans, most of the spinothalamic tract projects to the ventral posterolateral (VPL) nucleus of the thalamus as the neospinothalamic pathway, which is related to fast and well-localized pain sensation. Axons from the third-order sensory neurons in the VPL directly project to the primary sensory cortex. Some of the fibers in the spinothalamic tract synapse with neurons of the periaqueductal gray (PAG, spinoreticular pathway) and other brainstem nuclei. Fibers from these brainstem neurons join with fibers from the spinothalamic tract to project to the central or laminar nuclei of the thalamus and constitute the paleospinothalamic tract, which is related to slow and poorly localized pain and emotional response to pain stimulation.

Multiple areas of the cerebral cortex are involved in the processing of pain sensation and the subsequent behavioral and emotional responses. Recent functional magnetic resonance imaging (fMRI) and positron emission tomography (PET) scan studies indicate that the primary and secondary somatosensory cortex, thalamus, PAG matter, supplemental motor, inferior prefrontal, and insular cortex are activated in response to painful stimulation. It is now believed that the primary sensory cortex (SI) seems to play a role in basic pain processing, while secondary sensory cortex (SII) and insula are involved in higher functions of pain perception. Emotional aspects of pain perception are mediated by the anterior cingulate cortex and the posterior insula and parietal operculum.

### Central Modulation of Nociception

Nociceptive transmissions are modulated at the spinal level by both local neuronal circuits and descending pathways originating in the brainstem through the dorsal horns and the spinothalamic projections. Intrasegmental and intersegmental projections arising from cells located in the Rexed laminae I and II modulate both presynaptic and postsynaptic elements of primary nociceptive afferent terminals in the spinal cord. Activation of non-nociceptive afferent fibers may suppress nociceptive transmission in the dorsal horn. This is the major component of circuitry models referred to as the *gate control theory of pain transmission*. The development and widespread use of the spinal cord stimulator is based on this theory.

Descending inhibitory systems appear to have three functionally interrelated neurotransmitter mechanisms: the opioid, the noradrenergic, and the serotonergic systems. Opioid precursors and their respective peptides (β-endorphin, methionine [met]-enkephalin, leucine [leu-] enkephalin, and dynorphin) are present in the amygdala, hypothalamus, PAG, raphe magnus, and the dorsal horn. Noradrenergic neurons project from the locus ceruleus and other noradrenergic cell groups in the medulla and pons. These projections are found in the dorsolateral funiculus. Stimulation of these areas produces analgesia, as does the administration (direct or intrathecal) of $\alpha_2$-receptor agonists such as clonidine (Khodayar et al., 2006). Many serotonergic neurons are found in the raphe magnus. These neurons send projections to the spinal cord via the dorsolateral funiculus. Administration of serotonin to the spinal cord produces analgesia, and pharmacological blockade or lesion of the raphe magnus can reduce the effects of morphine. The antinociceptive effects of antidepressants such as tricyclics and newer serotonin-norepinephrine reuptake inhibitors such as duloxetine and milnacipran are believed to reduce pain by increasing serotonin and norepinephrine concentrations in descending inhibitory pain pathways.

### Opioid Receptors

Opioids are the core pharmacological treatment for acute pain. They act via receptors on cell membranes. Opioid receptors are coupled to G proteins and are thus able to effect protein phosphorylation via the second messenger system and change ion channel conductance. Presynaptically, activation of opioid receptors inhibits the release of neurotransmitters involved in pain, including substance P and glutamate. Postsynaptically, activation of opioid receptors inhibits neurons by opening potassium channels that hyperpolarize and inhibit the neuron.

Currently, there are five proposed classes of opioid receptors: μ, δ, κ, σ, and ε. μ receptors are the main functional target of morphine and morphine-like drugs; they are present in large quantities in the PAG matter in the brain and the substantia gelatinosa in the spinal cord. μ receptors are also found in the peripheral nerves and skin. Activation of μ receptors results in analgesia, euphoria, respiratory depression, nausea, vomiting, and decreased gastrointestinal (GI) activity, as well as the physiological syndromes of tolerance and dependence. Two distinct subgroups of the μ receptors have been identified: $\mu_1$, found supraspinally, and $\mu_2$, found mainly in the spinal cord. The $\mu_1$ receptor is associated with the pain-relieving effects of opioids, whereas $\mu_2$ receptors mediate constipation and respiratory depression.

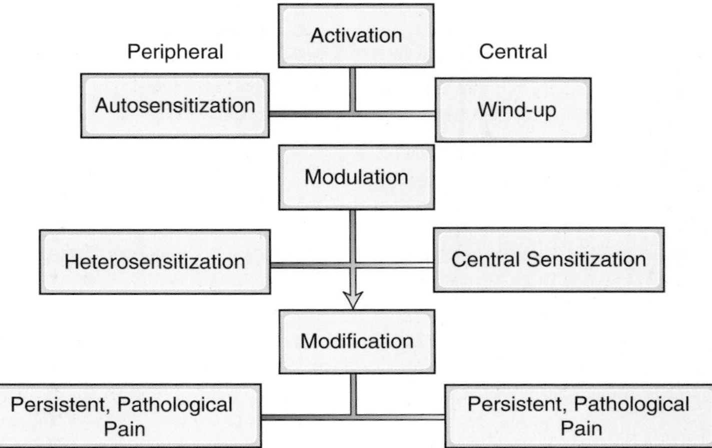


**Fig. 52.1** Neuronal Plasticity Changes of the Somatosensory System With Exposure to Repeated Noxious Stimuli. *(With permission from Woolf, J.W., Salter, M., 2000. Neuronal plasticity: increasing the gain in pain. Science 288 [5472], 1765–1769.)*

The δ receptor has central and peripheral distribution similar to the μ receptors. Studies have shown that δ-opioid agonists can provide relief of inflammatory pain and malignant bone pain. Meanwhile, peripherally restricted κ-opioid agonists have been developed to target κ-opioid receptors located on visceral and somatic afferent nerves for relief of inflammatory, visceral, and neuropathic chronic pain. The potential analgesic effects, combined with a possible lower abuse rate and fewer side effects than μ-receptor agonists, make δ- and peripherally restricted κ-opioid receptor agonists promising agents for treating pain (Vanderah, 2010).

### Neuronal Plasticity and Chronic Pain

Activity-dependent plasticity is secondary to repeated stimuli of the nociceptive pathway. This occurs both in the peripheral and central nervous system (CNS) and determines the gain of the pain system through activation, modulation, and modification (Woolf et al., 2000). This presents clinically as pain hypersensitivity.

*Activation* is the initial process, following repeated painful stimuli, which affects both the peripheral nervous system as *autosensitization* and the CNS as a *wind-up* phenomenon (Fig. 52.1). Autosensitization is the secondary reduced threshold of the nociceptors and is a rapid and readily reversible phenomenon. This is secondary to protein conformational changes from the repeated painful stimuli.

On the other hand, wind-up is a dorsal horn neuron phenomenon that results early after exposure to chronic repetitive noxious stimuli. Postsynaptic depolarization in the spinal cord in response to afferent stimulation can induce removal of magnesium blockade in *N*-methyl-D-aspartate (NMDA) receptors such that glutamate now induces a depolarization upon receptor binding. It is responsible for the temporal summation of inputs (see Fig. 52.1). This process is short-lived and potentially reversible (Katz and Rothenberg, 2005).

Ongoing repeated exposure to painful stimuli causes the second set of changes, namely *modulation*. These are primary sensory and/or dorsal horn changes secondary to phosphorylation of receptor and/or ion channels or regulatory proteins. This phenomenon increases the membrane excitability of the peripheral nociceptors and is called *heterosensitization*. Activation of the intracellular pathways of serine/threonine and tyrosine is seen here.

Modulation happening in the CNS is called *central sensitization*. This is either related to phosphorylation of the NMDA receptor or happens independently of the NMDA receptor. This is a key process for longer-lasting changes in the excitability of the dorsal horn neurons (see Fig. 52.1).

The final process in the pain pathway, *modification*, causes persistent pathological pain. This process results in gene alteration for both constitutively expressed and new genes. A fibers express C-fiber markers, resulting in tactile stimulus contributing to pain hypersensitivity. Prolonged exposure to pain results in sensory neuron loss, C fiber more than A fiber. This results in central reorganization of the A fibers and their functional synaptic contact at the C-fiber areas, resulting in refractory chronic pain.

Clinically, the real meaning of *peripheral* and *central sensitization* is the enhanced and prolonged pain perception consequent on minor stimulations, or sometimes without peripheral stimulation. Once peripheral and central sensitizations are involved, the pain is usually more difficult to treat. It is now believed that peripheral and central sensitization may be involved in a wide variety of chronic pain conditions, such as reflex sympathetic dystrophy, tension headache, carpal tunnel syndrome, pain after spinal cord injury (SCI) (Carlton et al., 2009), and even in pain conditions previously thought to be mainly nociceptive in nature, such as fibromyalgia, epicondylalgia, and osteoarthritis (Gwilym et al., 2009).

The clinical challenge in chronic pain involves not only pain localization and diagnosis but also factoring in the role of peripheral and central sensitization, and presenting a comprehensive multidisciplinary approach to chronic pain.

## MULTIDISCIPLINARY APPROACH TO PAIN MANAGEMENT

Management of acute pain is usually achieved with oral, intravenous (IV), regional, epidural, and intrathecal administration of both opioid and nonopioid analgesics. Acute pain presents as a symptom of the underlying disease condition and improves with healing of the primary problem. Chronic pain, on the other hand, is a disease in itself without a biologically protective role. It has bio-psycho-socio-economic influences on its development (Dinakar and Ross, 2013a). The evaluation of chronic pain must identify all associated comorbidities and a treatment plan for chronic pain must include treating the comorbidities as well. A multimodal approach results in the best possible outcome

**TABLE 52.1 Multimodal Treatment Options for Chronic Pain Management**

| Multimodal Treatment Modalities | Types |
|---|---|
| Medications | Antiinflammatory medications (NSAIDs, Tylenol), muscle relaxants, opioids, neuropathic medications (anticonvulsants, TCA, SNRI), SSRI, NMDA antagonist, alpha 2 agonist, topical medications |
| Rehabilitation | Physical therapy, occupational therapy, TENS, bracing |
| Psychology | Cognitive behavioral therapy, biofeedback, relaxation therapy, support groups |
| Interventional pain management | Epidural injections, facet joint injections, peripheral nerve block, major joint/bursa injections |
| Implantable therapies | Spinal cord stimulator therapy and intrathecal pumps |
| Complementary and alternative treatments | Acupuncture, chiropractic manipulation, massage, craniosacral therapy |
| Nutrition counseling | Weight loss, bone density |
| Vocational counseling | Return to work |

*NMDA*, *N*-methyl-D-aspartate; *NSAIDs*, nonsteroidal anti-inflammatory drugs; *SNRI*, selective serotonin/norepinephrine reuptake inhibitor; *SSRI*, selective serotonin reuptake inhibitor; *TCA*, tricyclic antidepressant; *TENS*, transelectrical nerve stimulation.

(Table 52.1). Simultaneous use of multiple modalities of pain management (Fig. 52.2) is needed for the best possible treatment outcome as opposed to using them sequentially. Barriers to chronic pain management include pharmacological factors (analgesic overuse, underuse, abuse, polypharmacy), failure to identify psychological or rehabilitative problems, and lack of social support. Identifying these is of utmost importance in a successful pain management plan.

## PHARMACOLOGICAL MANAGEMENT OF CHRONIC PAIN

In recent years, several different adjunct analgesics have been used to treat chronic pain syndromes, including nonsteroidal antiinflammatory drugs (NSAIDs), antidepressants, anticonvulsants, local anesthetics, topical agents, baclofen, and NMDA receptor antagonists. Tricyclic antidepressants and anticonvulsants are the first-line drugs in the treatment of neuropathic pain. If a patient does not respond to treatment with different agents within one drug class, agents from a second drug class may be added. When all first-line options have been exhausted, narcotic analgesics may be considered, but with the risks of tolerance, dependence, addiction, and opioid hyperalgesia, this is being increasingly discouraged for chronic pain that is not related to malignancies. The World Health Organization's (WHO) analgesic ladder for cancer pain (World Health Organization. Cancer pain relief. World Health Organization; Geneva, 1990) is a good guide for pharmacological management of chronic noncancer pain (Fig. 52.3).

### Nonsteroidal Antiinflammatory Drugs

NSAIDs, including aspirin, are the most widely used analgesics. Traditionally, NSAIDs are considered weak analgesics and used extensively for headaches, arthritis, and a wide range of minor aches and postsurgical pain conditions.

NSAIDs are powerful inhibitors of prostaglandin synthesis through their effect on cyclooxygenase (COX). Prostaglandins are not thought to be important pain mediators, but they do cause hyperalgesia by sensitizing peripheral nociceptors to the effects of various mediators of pain and inflammation such as somatostatin, bradykinin, and histamine. Thus, NSAIDs are used primarily to treat pain that results from inflammation and hyperalgesia. Table 52.2 lists commonly used NSAIDs.

Acetaminophen is not strictly an antiinflammatory medication. Its peripheral and antiinflammatory effects are weak, but it shares many properties of NSAIDs. It readily crosses the blood–brain barrier, and its action resides primarily in the CNS, where prostaglandin inhibition produces analgesia and antipyresis.

Common side effects of NSAIDs include GI toxicity, stomach ulcers, and gastric bleeding. Renal dysfunction can occur with prolonged and excessive use of NSAIDs. Particularly at risk from excessive use of NSAIDs are elderly patients with renal dysfunction, congestive heart failure, ascites, or hypovolemia. Other adverse effects of NSAIDs include hepatic dysfunction or necrosis, asthma, vasomotor rhinitis, angioneurotic edema, urticaria, laryngeal edema, or even cardiovascular collapse. Because of the wide availability of acetaminophen and its potential toxicity (especially liver toxicity), in 2009 the US Food and Drug Administration (FDA) proposed a decrease in the maximum daily dose of acetaminophen from 4000 to 3250 mg, reducing the maximum individual dose from 1000 to 650 mg. They relegated 500-mg tablets to prescription status and mandated new labeling on acetaminophen packaging (Krenzelok, 2009). Acetaminophen is a potential cyclooxygenase 2 (COX-2)–selective inhibitor. It may also increase cardiovascular risks.

Cardiovascular risks of NSAIDs, especially COX-2 inhibitors, have become a major focus of attention in recent years. Suggestions that the use of COX-2 inhibitors may decrease prostacyclin ($PGI_2$) levels, with relatively unopposed platelet thromboxane $A_2$ generation that may lead to increased thrombotic risk, have cautioned against the use of such agents. Rofecoxib (Vioxx) was withdrawn from the market in September 2004 owing to increased cardiovascular risks. A recent study found that the hazard ratio (95% confidence interval) for death was 1.70, 1.75, 1.31, 2.08, 1.22, and 1.28 for rofecoxib, celecoxib, ibuprofen, diclofenac, naproxen, and other NSAIDs, respectively (Gislason et al., 2009). Even though limited long-term data on cardiovascular risk associated with nonselective NSAIDs have been available, and some contradictory warnings and recommendations have been published recently by the American Heart Association, FDA, and independent experts (Gluszko and Bielinska, 2009), the general suggestion is that both NSAIDs and selective COX-2 inhibitors should be avoided or used with extreme caution if a patient has a high cardiovascular risk and a history of heart failure.

### Antidepressants

Tricyclic antidepressants are probably the most commonly used adjunct analgesics in the management of chronic pain (Dworkin et al., 2010) (Table 52.3). Even though this class does not have analgesic indications, the tertiary amines (amitriptyline, imipramine, doxepin, and clomipramine) and the secondary amines (nortriptyline and desipramine) are extensively used in chronic pain with associated low mood. Amitriptyline is the prototype antidepressant used in this context. Clinical efficacy of tricyclics for neuropathic pain has been demonstrated by numerous well-controlled double-blind

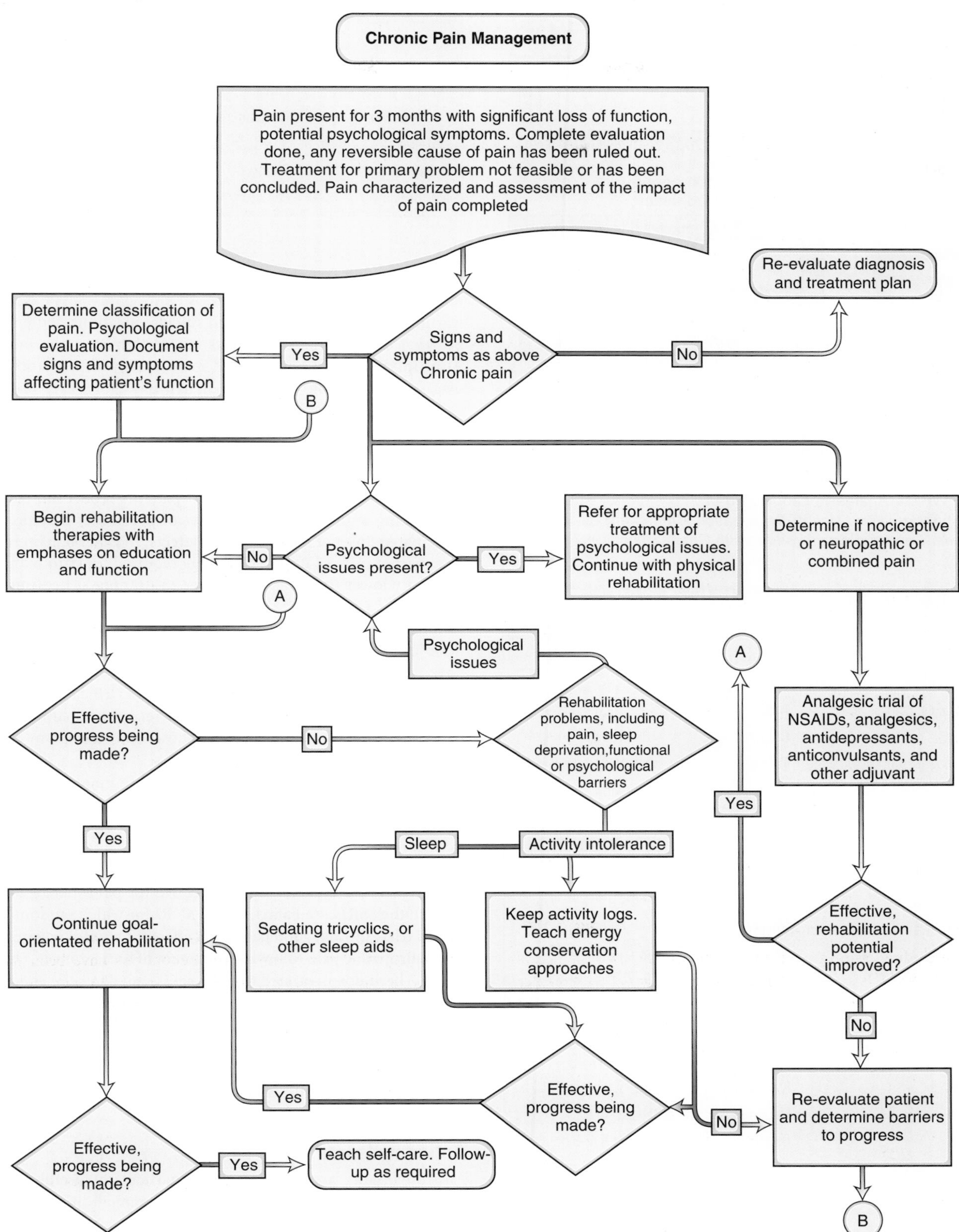


**Fig. 52.2** Overview of the Multidisciplinary Approach to Chronic Pain. *NSAIDs,* nonsteroidal antiinflammatory drugs. *(With permission from Ross, E.L., 2003. Pain Management: Hot Topics, first ed. Hanley & Belfus.)*

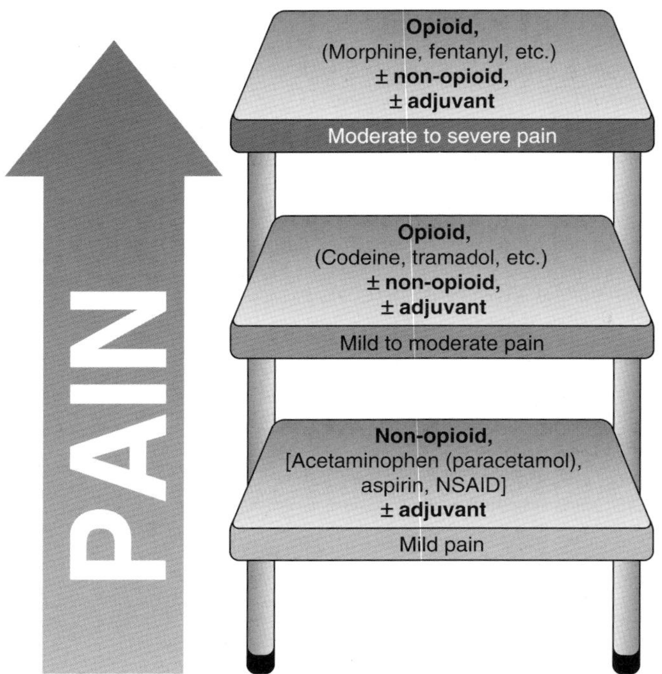


**Fig. 52.3** WHO's Analgesic Ladder. *NSAID,* nonsteroidal antiinflammatory drug. *(From World Health Organization. Traitement de la douleur cancéreuse. Geneva, Switz: World Health Organization; 1987.)*

**TABLE 52.2 Commonly Used Oral Nonsteroidal Antiinflammatory Drugs**

| Generic Name | Trade Name | Adult Dosage |
|---|---|---|
| Acetaminophen | Tylenol | 325–650 mg q 4–6 h |
| Acetylsalicylic acid | Aspirin | 325–1000 mg q 4–6 h |
| Celecoxib | Celebrex | 100–200 mg q 12-24 h |
| Choline magnesium trisalicylate | Trilisate | 750–1000 mg q 8–12 h |
| Diclofenac sodium | Voltaren | 25–75 mg q 8–12 h |
| Diflunisal | Dolobid | 250–500 mg q 8–12 h |
| Etodolic acid | Lodine | 200–400 mg q 6–8 h |
| Fenoprofen calcium | Nalfon | 200 mg q 4–6 h |
| Flurbiprofen | Ansaid | 50 mg q 4–6 h |
| Ibuprofen | Motrin | 200–800 mg q 6–8 h |
| Indomethacin | Indocin | 20–50 mg q 8–12 h |
| Ketoprofen | Orudis | 25–75 mg q 6–8 h |
| Ketorolac | Toradol | 10 mg q 6–8 h |
| Meclofenamate sodium | Meclomen | 50–100 mg q 4–6 h |
| Meloxicam | Mobic | 7.5–15 mg QD |
| Naproxen | Naposyn | 220–500 mg q 8–12 h |
| Piroxicam | Feldene | 10–20 mg QD |
| Salsalate | Disalcid | 500 mg q 4–6 h |
| Sulindac | Clinoril | 150–200 mg q 12 h |
| Tolmetin | Tolectin | 20–400 mg q 8 h |

clinical studies for both neuropathic and somatic pain. Clinicians must be familiar with the possible side effects of amitriptyline, especially in elderly patients. These adverse effects include sedation, dry mouth, constipation, urinary retention, glaucoma, orthostatic hypotension, and cardiac arrhythmias. All antidepressants have the FDA warnings of worsening mood and suicidal ideations. Patients should be warned about the side effects before they start the medication. Amitriptyline should be avoided in patients with a history of heart disease (conduction disorders, arrhythmias, or heart failure) and closed-angle glaucoma. To routinely get a baseline ECG looking for long QT syndrome prior to starting a tricyclic antidepressant (TCA) might be beneficial in preventing cardiac arrhythmias. Amitriptyline should be started at a relatively low dose (10 mg) at bedtime and slowly titrated up as tolerated. Most patients report improved sleep after taking amitriptyline. The onset of pain relief may precede the anticipated onset of antidepressant effects. In general, pain relief may be expected in 7–14 days. The dosage required for pain management is usually lower than for depression; 25–100 mg at bedtime is often effective. If the patient cannot tolerate this dose or is not a good candidate for amitriptyline, other tricyclics such as nortriptyline or desipramine may be considered. These secondary amines generally have fewer anticholinergic effects and are therefore better tolerated than tertiary amines. However, their clinical efficacy is not as well established as that for amitriptyline. A recent trial comparing amitriptyline, topiramate and placebo showed no change in efficacy in pediatric migraines (Power et al. 2017).

**TABLE 52.3 Tricyclic Antidepressants Commonly Used for Pain Management**

| Generic Name | Trade Name | Adult Dosage Range (mg/day) |
|---|---|---|
| Amitriptyline | Elavil | 10–150 |
| Desipramine | Norpramin | 10–150 |
| Doxepin | Sinequan | 10–200 |
| Imipramine | Silenor | 50-150 |
| Nortriptyline | Pamelor | 10–150 |

The main advantage of the selective serotonin reuptake inhibitors (SSRIs) is the favorable side-effect profile. However, SSRIs are clearly less effective than tricyclic antidepressants. The NNT (number needed to treat to reach 50% pain relief) is 6.7 versus 2.4 (Coluzzi and Mattia, 2005). It seems that selective serotonin/noradrenaline reuptake inhibitors (SNRI) are relatively more effective for pain management than most of the SSRIs. Venlafaxine is an SNRI for which randomized controlled trials showed good pain relief effect for painful polyneuropathy and neuropathic pain following treatment of breast cancer. Duloxetine has also been demonstrated to have significant analgesic effects in diabetic polyneuropathy and fibromyalgia. Milnacipran is another SNRI; randomized double-blind placebo-controlled studies found that milnacipran is effective in controlling pain and improving global status, fatigue, and physical and mental function in patients with fibromyalgia (Arnold et al., 2010). Nausea, hyperhidrosis, and headache are the most common adverse events.

## Anticonvulsants

Anticonvulsants are believed to be particularly useful in treating lancinating, electrical, or tic-like pain. These medications may be also beneficial in patients with neuropathic pain who do not respond to antidepressants. The older generation of anticonvulsants includes carbamazepine, valproic acid, clonazepam, and phenytoin. The newer generation of anticonvulsants includes topiramate, oxcarbazepine, lamotrigine, pregabalin, tiagabine, zonisamide, and levetiracetam. All anticonvulsants used in pain have FDA warnings for mood changes, worsening depression, and suicidal ideation, predominantly in adolescents and young adults.

Carbamazepine was perhaps the most popular agent used for TN. However, carbamazepine may cause serious side effects such as sedation, nausea, vomiting, bone marrow suppression, hyponatremia, hepatic dysfunction, and serious drug–drug interaction. Carbamazepine should be started at 100 mg at night and titrated up slowly, especially for the elderly.

Valproic acid has been proven to be effective in reducing the frequency of migraine attacks (Vikelis and Rapoport, 2010). Some studies found that valproates may provide significant pain relief in patients with postherpetic neuralgia and diabetic neuropathy. However, negative results have also been reported. Common side effects include tremor, ankle swelling, sedation, and GI discomfort. Weight gain and hair loss may be a major cosmetic concern, especially for younger patients. Valproate should not be used for children younger than 2 years of age because of hepatotoxicity. Generally, valproate is not the first-line choice for neuropathic pain.

Gabapentin modulates the function of the $\alpha_2$-$\delta$ subunit of voltage-dependent calcium channels in the dorsal horn of the spinal cord to decrease the release of excitatory neurotransmitters such as glutamate and substance P. The analgesic efficacy of gabapentin has been demonstrated in several types of nonmalignant neuropathic pain. Its high safety profile, few drug–drug interactions, and proven analgesic effect in several types of neuropathic pain have made gabapentin the recommended first-line co-analgesic for treating a variety of neuropathic pains, especially in the medically ill and in elderly patients. The most common adverse effects are drowsiness, dizziness, and unsteadiness. Gabapentin should be started at a dose of 100–300 mg at bedtime. If titrated carefully, gabapentin is usually well tolerated up to 3600 mg daily. However, gabapentin has a nonlinear pharmacokinetic profile: the rate of bioavailability decreases as the dose increases.

Pregabalin is a $\gamma$-aminobutyric acid (GABA) analog with a structure and mechanism of action similar to gabapentin. It has antiepileptic, analgesic, and anxiolytic activity. Pregabalin has been approved by the FDA for the management of neuropathic pain associated with diabetic neuropathy, postherpetic neuralgia, and fibromyalgia (Straube et al., 2010). Food does not significantly affect the extent of absorption. Pregabalin is not protein bound and exhibits a plasma half-life of about 6 hours. Hepatic metabolism is negligible, and most of the oral dose (95%) appears unchanged in the urine. At a dose of 300 mg/day, about 45% of diabetic neuropathy patients had 50% pain relief. This means that pregabalin has an NNT of 2.2 for diabetic neuropathy. Pregabalin seems to be more effective than gabapentin and other anticonvulsants for neuropathic pain. Common side effects of pregabalin include dizziness, sedation, dry mouth, and peripheral edema.

Oxcarbazepine is a keto derivative of carbamazepine, with better tolerability. It can block sodium-dependent action potentials. The medication does not induce hepatic enzymes and has fewer drug-drug interactions than carbamazepine. Multiple open studies have suggested that oxcarbazepine may be effective for the treatment of neuropathic pain. However, a double-blind controlled study did not find significant difference between oxcarbazepine and placebo for the treatment of pain due to diabetic neuropathy (Grosskopf et al., 2006).

Lamotrigine is an antiepileptic drug that stabilizes neural membranes by blocking the activation of voltage-sensitive sodium channels and inhibiting the presynaptic release of glutamate. Multiple open studies have supported the use of lamotrigine in neuropathic pain. However, controlled studies found no efficacy of lamotrigine for the treatment of neuropathic pain (Breuer et al., 2007; Rao et al., 2008). Lamotrigine is ineffective for prevention of migraine.

Topiramate has proven its efficacy and safety in the prophylactic treatment of episodic migraine in a number of randomized controlled clinical trials (Naegel and Obermann, 2010). Even though open studies and case reports continue to support the use of topiramate in the treatment of various kinds of neuropathic pain, controlled studies failed to reveal any benefit of topiramate for the treatment of neuropathic pain. The mechanisms of action include blockade of sodium channels, enhancement of GABA inhibition, and attenuation of kainate-induced responses at glutamate receptors. The starting dose is usually small (e.g., 25 mg twice a day for an adult). It may be incrementally increased weekly by 50 mg/day up to 200 mg/day. Topiramate may induce memory loss, word-finding difficulties, disorientation, and sedation. The other common adverse effects are renal calculi, tremors, dizziness, ataxia, headaches, fatigue, and GI upset. Topiramate may also induce significant weight loss. This medication may be more helpful in obese pain patients.

Tiagabine, zonisamide, and levetiracetam are among the group of new anticonvulsants. Some uncontrolled and case studies have reported positive effects of these medications for neuropathic pain. However, controlled double-blind studies have not been reported.

### Systemic Local Anesthetic Therapies

Systemic administration of local anesthetics has been used to treat neuropathic pain syndrome. Clinical trials have provided some evidence that lidocaine and mexiletine are superior to placebo for neuropathic pain (Carroll et al., 2008). Intravenous lidocaine is used for the treatment of refractory neuropathic pain. If a patient has a positive response to IV lidocaine therapy, a trial of oral mexiletine may be considered. However, mexiletine has a relatively high rate of adverse effects such as nausea, vomiting, tremor, dizziness, unsteadiness, and paresthesias. Given the limited number of supportive studies, lidocaine, mexiletine, and other oral local anesthetics should only be used as second-line agents for neuropathic pain that has failed to respond to anticonvulsants or antidepressants.

### Topical Analgesics

Double-blind placebo-controlled studies have confirmed the efficacy of the 5% lidocaine patch for the treatment of postherpetic neuralgia (Lin et al., 2008) and for those patients with trigger points in myofascial pain syndrome (Affaitati et al., 2009). However, the lidocaine patch may not be effective in treating pain due to traumatic rib fractures (Ingalls et al., 2010). Minimal systemic absorption occurs. The patch is usually applied 12 hours per day, with minimal systemic side effects. Topical lidocaine ointment in various concentrations (up to a compounded formulation of 10%) may offer a cost-effective alternative.

Capsaicin is the spicy ingredient in chili pepper. It can deplete substance P from the terminals of afferent C fibers, potentially leading to decreased pain perception. Capsaicin creams are effective in reducing postsurgical pain in cancer patients. When applied topically, it may initially release substance P and cause severe burning pain. Pain related to the use of capsaicin gradually decreases over a few days if the cream is applied regularly. A lower-concentration cream (0.025%) or the application of a topical local anesthetic may help some patients decrease the initial burning pain and tolerate the medication better. A recent study found that topical capsaicin might effectively decrease pain in patients with chronic migraine (Papoiu and Yosipovitch, 2010). It is important to warn patients not to get any trace of the cream on mucous membranes, since this causes severe pain.

### Muscle Relaxants

Baclofen is a $GABA_B$ receptor agonist with powerful antinociceptive effects in experimental animal models and established efficacy for

**TABLE 52.4 Commonly Used Opioids**

| | | EQUI-ANALGESIC DOSAGE* | | AVERAGE ADULT DOSAGE | |
|---|---|---|---|---|---|
| **Generic Name** | **Trade Name** | **Oral** | **Parenteral** | **Oral or Transdermal** | **Parenteral** |
| Codeine | | 30 mg q 3–4 h | 10 mg q 3–4 h | 30 mg q 3–4 h | 10 mg q 3–4 h |
| Fentanyl patch | Duragesic | N/A | N/A | 25 μg/h patch q 72 h | N/A |
| Hydrocodone | Lortab, Lorcet | 10 mg q 3–4 h | N/A | 10 mg q 3–4 h | N/A |
| Hydrocodone ER | Zohydro | N/A | N/A | 10–40 mg q 12 h | N/A |
| Hydromorphone | Dilaudid | 7.5 mg q 3–4 h | 1.5 mg q 3–4 h | 6 mg q 3–4 h | 1.5 mg q 3–4 h |
| Meperidine | Demerol | 300 mg q 2–3 h | 100 mg q 3 h | 200 mg q 3 h | 100 mg q 3 h |
| Methadone | Dolophine | 20 mg q 6–8 h | 10 mg q 6–8 h | 10 mg q 6–12 h | 5 mg q 8–12 h |
| Morphine | | 30 mg q 3–4 h | 10 mg q 3–4 h | 30 mg q 3–4 h | 10 mg q 3–4 h |
| Morphine SR | MS Contin | N/A | N/A | 15 mg q 12 h | N/A |
| Oxycodone | Percocet | N/A | N/A | 5 mg q 3–4 h | N/A |
| Oxycodone | OxyContin | N/A | N/A | 10 mg q 8–12 h | N/A |

*ER*, Extended release; *N/A*, not applicable; *SR*, sustained release.
*The equi-analgesic dosage is the dose of different narcotics needed to achieve the same analgesic effects. Example, 7.5 mg of oral hydromorphone q 3 h has analgesic effects equal to 1.5 mg intravenous hydromorphone q 3–4 h or 30 mg oral morphine q 3–4 h.

chronic pain. It may be most useful in blocking the lancinating or episodic types of pain and reducing allodynia. It is commonly used for TN, together with carbamazepine. Baclofen may be started in doses of 5 mg, 2–3 times a day, and may be escalated to doses of 80–100 mg given in divided doses. Common side effects include CNS symptoms such as dizziness and drowsiness, as well as GI symptoms. Baclofen is a highly hydrophilic agent and has poor penetration of the blood–brain barrier. Intrathecal baclofen could be a promising adjuvant therapy to enhance the effect of other intrathecal medications such as morphine or clonidine or spinal cord stimulation (SCS) for chronic pain. Benzodiazepines including diazepam and lorezepam are very helpful GABA agonists that help with muscle relaxation and anxiolysis. Flexeril and tizanidine are newer muscle relaxants that are commonly used. Orphenadrine (Norflex), which is an antihistamine, is an uncommonly used muscle relaxant.

### *N*-Methyl-D-Aspartate Receptor Blockers

NMDA receptors are involved in the development of central sensitization associated with chronic refractory pain syndromes. NMDA antagonists may modulate CNS function, offering a novel approach to treating chronic neuropathic pain. Intravenous anesthetic doses of ketamine may induce serious side effects such as vivid hallucinations and psychosis. However, double-blind placebo-controlled studies have confirmed that low-dose IV ketamine may provide significant pain relief for complex regional pain syndrome (CRPS) type 1 without significant psychomimetic side effects (Sigtermans et al., 2009). Methadone has the properties of both μ-opioid receptor agonist and NMDA antagonist. Evidence indicates that methadone has similar analgesic efficacy to that of morphine, but adverse effects due to prolonged half-life—particularly respiratory depression, cardiac arrhythmia, and sudden death—make it critical for providers to be familiar with methadone's pharmacological properties before considering methadone as an analgesic therapy for chronic pain. Amantadine is a noncompetitive NMDA antagonist. Dextromethorphan, the D-isomer of the codeine analog levorphanol, is a weak, noncompetitive NMDA receptor antagonist. Memantine is an NMDA antagonist used for the treatment of Alzheimer disease. All three of these medications possess some analgesic properties. Current data are too scant or too weak, however, to recommend clinical use of any of these drugs for chronic pain management.

### Opioid Analgesics

Opioids are the major class of analgesics used in the management of moderate to severe pain. These medications produce analgesia by binding to specific receptors both within and outside the CNS. However, their use in pain not related to malignancy is still controversial. Opioid analgesics should be used with caution for chronic nonmalignant pain.

Opioids are classified according to the activity on the opioid receptors as full agonists, partial agonists, or mixed agonists–antagonists. Commonly used full agonists include hydrocodone, codeine, morphine, oxycodone, hydromorphone, methadone, and fentanyl. Buprenorphine is a partial agonist. It has lower intrinsic efficacy than other full opioid agonists and displays a ceiling effect to analgesia. Mixed agonist–antagonists include pentazocine, butorphanol tartrate, dezocine, and nalbuphine hydrochloride. These medications block opioid analgesia at one type of receptor (μ) while simultaneously activating other opioid receptors (κ). Mixed agonist–antagonists should not be used together with full agonists, because they may cause withdrawal syndrome and increased pain. Table 52.4 lists commonly used narcotics and their equi-analgesic dosage.

*Equi-analgesic dosage* means the dose of different narcotics needed to reach the same analgesic effects. The middle two columns of Table 52.4, for example, indicate that 7.5 mg of oral hydromorphone every 3 hours may have analgesic effects equal to 1.5 mg of IV hydromorphone every 3–4 hours or 30 mg of oral morphine every 3–4 hours.

Narcotics are also classified as mild to strong according to their potency. Codeine is the prototype of the mild opioid analgesics. The duration of action (2–4 hours) is similar to that of aspirin and acetaminophen. It is commonly used together with NSAIDs when NSAIDs alone have proven ineffective. Hydrocodone, oxycodone, propoxyphene, and meperidine are other mild opioid analgesics. Meperidine is likely to cause dysphoria, or less commonly to cause myoclonus, encephalopathy, and seizures. These toxic effects result from metabolites such as normeperidine that accumulate with repeated doses. Meperidine should be avoided in patients who require chronic treatment. Morphine and hydromorphone are the prototypes of high-potency opioid analgesics. Morphine has a relatively rapid onset, especially when administered parenterally, and a short duration of action, about 2–4 hours. Sustained-release oral preparations (e.g., MS Contin and Kadian, with duration of action of 12 and 24 hours, respectively) are useful for patients requiring chronic opioid therapy.

Route of administration is important to consider when choosing opioids. Oral administration of opioids is the preferred route, because it is the most convenient and cost-effective. Oral opioids are available in tablet, capsule, and liquid forms and in immediate and controlled-release formulations. Patients should be informed not to break the controlled-release tablets, since this can cause immediate release and cause a potential overdose. If patients cannot take medication orally, other less-invasive routes such as transdermal or rectal routes should be tried. Intramuscular administration of narcotics should be avoided because this route is often painful and inconvenient, and absorption is unreliable. Intravenous administration may be more expensive and is not practical for most chronic pain patients.

The advantage of transdermal administration is that it bypasses GI absorption. Both fentanyl and buprenorphine are commercially available for transdermal administration. Fentanyl patches come in five sizes, delivering medication at 12, 25, 50, 75, and 100 μg/h. Each patch contains a 72-hour supply of fentanyl, passively absorbed through the skin during this period. Plasma levels rise slowly over 12–18 hours after the patch placement. This dosage form has an elimination half-life of 21 hours. Unlike IV fentanyl, transdermal administration of fentanyl is not suitable for rapid dose titration. It is often used for patients with chronic pain and already on opioids. As with other long-acting analgesics, all patients should be provided with oral or parenteral short-acting opioids for breakthrough pain.

Intrathecal analgesia may be considered when pain cannot be controlled by oral, transdermal, subcutaneous, or IV routes because side effects such as confusion and nausea further limit dose titration. Documentation of the failure of maximal doses of opioids and adjunct analgesics administered through other routes should precede consideration of intrathecal analgesia. For patients with chronic pain who have failed or cannot tolerate other treatment modalities, before implantation of a permanent pump, a trial of single intrathecal injections, epidural injection, or continuous epidural administration is usually needed. If there is significant pain relief without major side effects during the trial, the patient may be a candidate for permanent implantation of an intrathecal delivery system. Morphine is the intrathecal drug most commonly used for pain relief. The main indication of the long-term intrathecal opioids is intractable pain in the lower part of the body. With proper selection and screening, good to excellent pain relief is expected in up to 90% of patients.

Physicians need to be familiar with side effects of opioids before prescribing these medications. Common side effects of opioids include constipation, sedation, nausea, vomiting, and respiratory depression due to overdoses. Occasionally, opioids may cause myoclonus, seizures, hallucinations, confusion, sexual dysfunction, sleep disturbances, and pruritus. Constipation is a common problem associated with opioid administration. Tolerance to the constipating effects of opioids hardly ever occurs during chronic therapy. Some patients are too embarrassed to tell the physician about constipation problems, so physicians should always ask patients about this. Mild constipation can usually be managed by an increase in fiber consumption and the use of mild laxatives such as milk of magnesia. Severe constipation may be treated with a stimulating cathartic drug (e.g., bisacodyl, standardized senna concentrate, MiraLAX, and similar drugs). Tapentadol is a novel centrally acting analgesic with two modes of action, μ-opioid agonist and norepinephrine reuptake inhibition. It was approved by the FDA for treatment of acute pain in 2008. Multiple double-blind controlled studies found tapentadol's analgesic effects similar to those of morphine and oxycodone. However, tapentadol has fewer GI side effects such as nausea and vomiting (Daniels et al., 2009; Smit et al., 2010). Owing to its dual mechanism of action and better GI tolerability, there is potential for off-label use in chronic pain.

Transitory sedation is common if opioid doses are increased substantially, but tolerance also usually develops rapidly. Reducing the opioid dose, switching to another opioid, or use of CNS stimulants such as caffeine, dextroamphetamine, or methylphenidate may help increase alertness. Nausea and vomiting may be managed with antiemetics chosen according to the modes of action (e.g., metoclopramide, chlorpromazine, haloperidol, scopolamine, hydroxyzine). Patients receiving long-term opioid therapy usually develop tolerance to the respiratory-depressant effects of these agents. However, respiratory depression is often due to an overdose, or when pain is abruptly relieved and the sedative effect of the opioid is no longer opposed by the stimulating effect of pain. To reverse respiratory depression, opioid antagonists (e.g., naloxone) should be given incrementally in doses that improve respiratory function but do not reverse analgesia, to avoid reoccurrence of severe pain.

Accumulation of normeperidine, a metabolite of meperidine, may cause seizures, especially in patients with chronic renal insufficiency. Therefore, meperidine is only indicated for acute use; chronic use should be avoided. Tramadol is a synthetic narcotic, most commonly used for mild pain. Tramadol may decrease the seizure threshold and induce seizures, so it should be avoided in patients with a history of seizures. It should not be used with tricyclic antidepressants. The recommended dosage of tramadol is 50 mg every 6 hours as needed for pain.

Tolerance and physical dependence should be expected with long-term opioid treatment and not confused with psychological dependence or drug abuse, which is characterized by compulsive use of narcotics. Patients may crave narcotics and continue to consume them despite physiological or social damage consequent to their use. *Tolerance* of opioids may be defined as the need to increase dosage requirements over a period of time to maintain optimum pain relief. For most pain patients, the first indication of tolerance is a decrease in the duration of analgesia for a specific dose. Patients with stable disease do not usually require increasing doses. Increasing the dosage requirement is most consistently correlated with a progressive disease that produces more intense pain. *Physical dependence* on opioids is revealed when opioids are abruptly discontinued or when naloxone is administered; it typically manifests as anxiety, irritability, chills and hot flashes, joint pain, lacrimation, rhinorrhea, diaphoresis, nausea, vomiting, abdominal cramps, and diarrhea. The mildest form of the *opioid abstinence syndrome* may be manifested as viral flu-like syndromes. For short-acting opioids (i.e., codeine, hydrocodone, morphine, hydromorphone), the onset of withdrawal symptoms may occur within 6–12 hours and peak at 12–72 hours after discontinuation. For opioids with long half-lives (i.e., methadone and transdermal fentanyl), the onset of the withdrawal syndrome may be delayed for 24 hours or more after drug discontinuation. If a rapid decrease or a discontinuation of opioids is possible because the pain has been effectively eliminated, the opioid abstinence syndrome may be avoided by withdrawal of the opioid on a schedule that provides half the prior daily dose for each of the first 2 days and then reduces the daily dose by 25% every 2 days thereafter until the total dose (in morphine equivalent) is 30 mg/day. The drug may be discontinued after 2 days on the 30-mg/day dose, according to 1992 guidelines from the American Pain Society. Transdermal clonidine (0.1–0.2 mg/day) may reduce anxiety, tachycardia, and other autonomic symptoms associated with opioid withdrawal.

Diminishing opioid analgesic efficacy and increased pain during the course of opioid therapy is quite common. It is traditionally considered

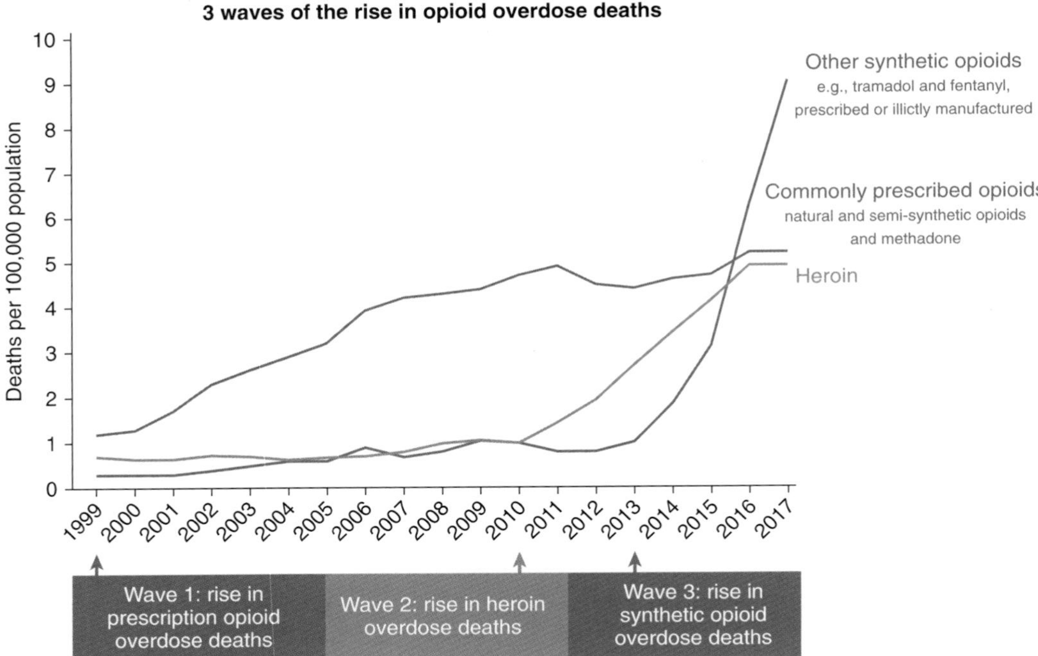


**Fig. 52.4 Waves of Opioid Overdose Deaths Since the 1990s.** (From CDC/NCHS (2020). National Vital Statistics System, Mortality. CDC WONDER, Atlanta, GA: US Department of Health and Human Services, CDC: https://wonder.cdc.gov/.

a result of opioid tolerance but could also be the result of opioid-induced hyperalgesia (OIH), which occurs when prolonged administration of opioids results in a paradoxical increase in atypical pain that appears to be unrelated to the original nociceptive stimulus. The mechanism of OIH is still unclear. However, opioid receptor desensitization, upregulation of spinal dynorphin, and enhanced activity of excitatory transmitters such as NMDA are believed to be involved the pathogenesis of OIH (Silverman, 2009). Clinically, it is difficult to distinguish opioid tolerance and OIH. However, the issue of opioid-induced pain sensitivity should also be considered when an adjustment of opioid doses is being contemplated because opioid treatment is failing to provide the expected analgesic effects and/or there is an unexplainable pain exacerbation following a period of effective opioid treatment. Quantitative sensory testing of pain may offer the most appropriate way of diagnosing hyperalgesia. With OIH, an increased opioid dose is not always the answer. Office-based detoxification, reduction of opioid dose, opioid rotation, and the use of specific NMDA receptor antagonists are all viable treatment options for OIH.

## Opioid Crisis—The Three Waves of Opioid Overdosing

Chronic pain has been a devastating condition affecting more than 116 million people in the United States. Most treatment options have not been very effective and their effects plateau over time. This has resulted in the overuse of pain medications, including NSAIDs and opioids for management of refractory chronic pain. The use of opioids has been particularly troubling given that the prescription medications bear similarities to street drugs such as heroin, which are easily available. The statistics from the Center for Disease Control (CDC) shows that from 1999 to 2017, more than 700,000 people have died from a drug overdose, of which 400,000 are from opioid overdosing (Scholl et al., 2018). In 2017, 68% of those deaths (70,200) have involved an opioid and there has been a sixfold increase in opioid-related deaths since 1999. On average, 130 Americans die from an opioid overdose on a daily basis (CDC National Center for Health Statistics, 2017). The states with the highest rates of overdose death in 2017 include West Virginia (57.8 per 100,000), Ohio (46.3 per 100,000), Pennsylvania (44.3 per 100,000), the District of Columbia (44.0 per 100,000), and Kentucky (37.2 per 100,000) (Scholl et al., 2018). This epidemic has resulted in increasing waves of opioid overdose deaths over the last 30 years (Fig. 52.4). The first wave began in the 1990s (Kolodny et al., 2015) with prescription opioids, including natural/semi-synthetic opioids such as methadone. The second wave began in 2010 with heroin and the third wave in 2013 with synthetic opioids, particularly with illicitly manufactured fentanyl (IMF). Unfortunately the IMF is combined with heroin, counterfeit pills, and cocaine (Rudd et al., 2016; Scholl et al., 2018).

## Opioid Overdose Prevention

The CDC has mounted a phenomenal effort in gathering data on opioid overdose; tracking trends; supporting healthcare systems, providers, and law enforcement; and raising awareness among consumers. The past CDC programs that have focused on opioid overdose and injury prevention include the following: Data-Driven Prevention Initiative (**CDC-RFA-CE16-1606**), Prescription Drug Overdose Prevention for States (**CDC-RFA-CE15-1501**), Enhanced State Surveillance of Opioid-Involved Morbidity and Mortality (**CDC-RFA-CE16-1608**), Cooperative Agreement for Emergency Response: Public Health Crisis Response—Opioid Epidemic (**CDC-RFA-TP18-1802**), and Core State Violence and Injury Prevention Program (**CDC-RFA-CE16-1602**).

## Overdose Data to Action

The CDC empowers states, local communities, and tribes with resources and collaborates with them to bring awareness to address this rapidly progressing crisis. The CDC runs drug monitoring programs, regulates controlled substances, licenses healthcare providers, responds to drug overdose outbreaks, and runs public insurance programs such as Medicaid and Workers Compensation. The Overdose Data to Action (OD2A), which was built on prior CDC programs, is a 3-year collaboration with state, county, and city health departments, starting in September 2019, where high-quality big data on opioid overdoses are obtained and used to prevent further waves of this epidemic from happening. Information from emergency departments regarding overdoses, and overdose death–related information, including death certificates, toxicology, and medical examiner reports, are collected. The health departments can then tailor their surveillance efforts to specifically address the local needs for increased comprehensiveness. Based on this, the data are put into action for prevention by improving the prescription drug monitoring programs (PDMPs), improving state-local integration and legislation, and improving provider and health system support.

### Enhanced State Opioid Overdose Surveillance

This program funds the states to increase timely reporting of nonfatal opioid overdoses through surveillance of the emergency departments and emergency medical services data. The information surrounding fatal opioid overdoses is reported through the state unintentional drug overdose reporting system (SUDORS).

### Prescription Drug Monitoring Programs

This state-level real-time intervention helps improve opioid prescription practices and protects patients at risk. Healthcare providers can see patients prescription histories and providers are mandated to look at this prior to prescribing controlled medications. Since its inception this program has caused a positive change in opioid prescription practices, reduced patient use of multiple providers, and resulted in a decrease in substance abuse treatment admissions.

### Center for Disease Control Guidelines for Opioid Prescription

In 2016 the CDC published revised opioid prescribing guidelines (Dowell et al 2016) for chronic pain outside of active cancer, and palliative and end-of-life care using the GRADE framework (Grading of Recommendations Assessment, Development, and Evaluation). Twelve recommendations were made. The goal of these guidelines was to improve prescription practices among providers leading to better patient care. The three main focus areas as described by the CDC include the following (www.cdc.gov/drugoverdose/prescribing/guideline.html):

1. Determining when to initiate or continue opioids for chronic pain:
   - Selection of nonpharmacological therapy, nonopioid pharmacological therapy, opioid therapy
   - Establishing treatment goals
   - Discussion of risks and benefits of therapy with patients
2. Opioid selection, dosage, duration, follow-up, and discontinuation:
   - Selection of immediate-release or extended-release and long-acting opioids
   - Dosage considerations
   - Duration of treatment
   - Considerations for follow-up and discontinuation of opioid therapy
3. Assessing risk and addressing harms of opioid use:
   - Evaluation of risk factors for opioid-related harms and ways to mitigate patient risk
   - Review of PDMP data
   - Use of urine drug testing
   - Considerations for co-prescribing benzodiazepines
   - Arrangement of treatment for opioid use disorder

## INTERVENTIONAL PAIN MANAGEMENT

Interventional pain management techniques have grown rapidly since the 1990s and have become a major tool in treating acute and chronic pain. The American Society of Interventional Pain Physicians has developed evidence-based guidelines for improving compliance and the quality of care. Numerous reports have been published to investigate the long-term efficacy of interventional pain management techniques and have provided critical evidence indicating that these techniques may be useful (Manchikanti et al., 2009).

Traditionally, neurosurgeons have utilized surgical techniques to destroy part(s) of the peripheral and central nervous systems to interrupt conduction of painful information into the CNS. These techniques include resection of peripheral nerves, dorsal root ganglia, the dorsal root entry zone, the spinal thalamic tract, entire spinal cord, nuclei of the thalamus, and the sensory cortex, as well as the pituitary gland. Although these techniques may provide temporary pain relief, the pain may quickly become even worse than presurgical levels because of subsequent deafferent pain that is more difficult to treat than most somatic pain. As a result, surgical resection techniques are not commonly used anymore. Instead, modern interventional pain management techniques emphasize the importance of accurate delivery of medications such as corticosteroids or local anesthetics to suppress inflammation and block conduction of painful information, respectively. Selective destruction of nerve tissue with heat generated by radiofrequency energy or freezing the nerve tissue with liquid nitrogen (cryotherapy) has largely replaced surgical resections. Nerve stimulation techniques have also evolved concomitant to neuroscientific developments in our understanding of the mechanisms of pain. Table 52.5 lists commonly used interventional pain management techniques and their indications (Dinakar and Ross, 2013b).

**TABLE 52.5 Commonly Used Interventional Pain Management Techniques and Indications**

| Name of Procedure | Indication |
|---|---|
| Celiac plexus block | Pancreatic cancer, chronic pancreatitis |
| Diskography | Diagnosis of anatomical localization of discogenic pain |
| Epidural corticosteroid injection | Lumbar, cervical, or thoracic radiculopathy |
| Facet joint block/medial branch block | Lumbar, cervical, or thoracic facet joint syndrome |
| Facet joint rhizotomy/radiofrequency lesioning | Lumbar or cervical facet joint syndrome |
| Gasserian ganglion block<br>Maxillary nerve block | Trigeminal neuralgia |
| Greater occipital nerve block<br>Lesser occipital nerve block<br>Superficial cervical plexus block | Occipital neuralgia |
| Intravenous regional block | CRPS |
| Lumbar sympathetic block | CRPS of the legs |
| Percutaneous disk decompression | Lumbar or cervical disk herniation |
| Sacroiliac joint injection | Sacroiliac joint pain |
| Sphenopalatine ganglion block | Headache and facial pain |
| Spinal cord stimulator | CRPS, PVD, low back pain, angina |
| Stellate ganglion block | CRPS of arm, neck, and head; headache |
| Suprascapular nerve block | Shoulder pain |
| Vertebroplasty | Vertebral fracture |
| Motor cortex stimulation | Neuropathic pain |
| Deep brain stimulation | Neuropathic pain |

*CRPS,* Complex regional pain syndrome; *PVD,* peripheral vascular disease.

### Greater Occipital Nerve Block

Greater occipital nerve block is indicated for occipital neuralgia, commonly seen in patients after whiplash injury, falls on the back of the head, and other closed-head injuries. Patients are often misdiagnosed as having tension headache or migraine. These patients may have continuous headaches in the occipital, parietal, and sometimes the frontal region. The headaches may increase several times a week and may be accompanied by nausea and vomiting. This condition is easily confused with migraine attacks, but physical examination may reveal positive tenderness over the greater occipital nerve. Palpation of the greater occipital nerve often makes the headache worse.

Greater occipital nerve block is the easiest interventional procedure for neurologists to perform in the office. For the procedure, one can palpate the posterior occipital protuberance, move 1.5–2 cm laterally, feel for the occipital artery pulsation and groove, then inject 2–3 mL of 0.5% bupivacaine with 20 mg of triamcinolone or 20 mg of Depo-Medro down to the bone, and fan out (Fig. 52.5). Along with the greater occipital nerve block, a lesser occipital or superficial cervical plexus block is done in a similar fashion over the posterior border of the middle third of the sternocleidomastoid. Care must be taken to remain subcutaneous and to avoid intravascular structures (Fig. 52.6).

For patients with occipital neuralgia after whiplash injuries, a greater occipital nerve block may provide immediate headache relief in 90% of patients and last for an average of 28 days. More rigorous clinical trials are needed to confirm the clinical efficacy of occipital nerve block for occipital neuralgia and cervicogenic headache (Ashkenazi et al., 2010). More research and education are warranted to increase clinician awareness of the existence of occipital neuralgia and cervicogenic headache, inasmuch as most neurologists seem more interested in examining the 12 pairs of cranial nerves than the greater occipital nerves, and are better trained in these.

### Botox Injections of the Head and Neck

Botox is an acetylcholine release inhibitor and blocks the neuromuscular junction, relieving spasticity. It has multiple overall body indications, including migraine headaches, upper and lower extremity spasticity, and cervical dystonia. Botox is injected intramuscularly and done every 3 months. The maximum dose in adults is 360 units. In children under 18 years the safety and efficacy has not been established. The injection can be done with electromyography (EMG) guidance in extremity spasticity. In a 2019 Cochrane systematic review

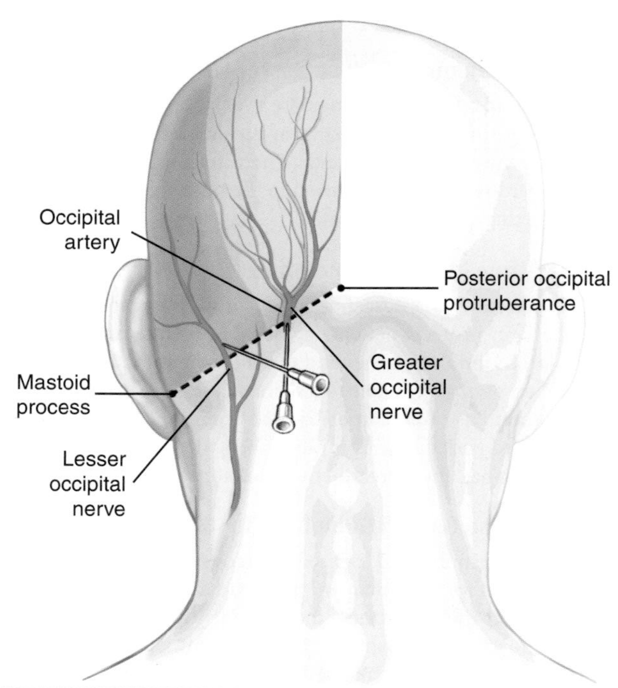


**Fig. 52.5** Occipital Nerve Block. *(With permission from Keel, J.C., Bodas, A.V., 2011. Interventional pain management I: epidural, ganglion and nerve block. In: Vacanti, C., Segal, S. [Eds.], Essential Clinical Anesthesia. Cambridge University Press, Cambridge, pp. 907–918.)*

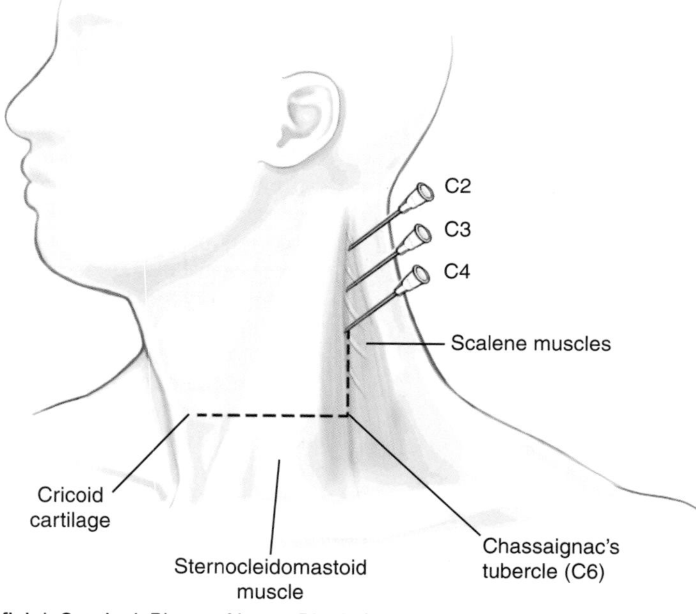


**Fig. 52.6** Superficial Cervical Plexus Nerve Block (Lesser Occipital Nerve Block). *(With permission from Keel, J.C., Bodas, A.V., 2011. Interventional pain management I: epidural, ganglion and nerve block. In: Vacanti, C., Segal, S. [Eds.], Essential Clinical Anesthesia. Cambridge University Press, Cambridge, pp. 907–918.)*

and meta-analysis of botulinum toxin for the prevention of migraine, botulinum toxin reduces migraine frequency by 2 days/month and has a favorable safety profile (Herd et al., 2019). Refer to the section on chronic migraine headaches for further details of the use of Botox.

## Sphenopalatine Ganglion Block for Headache and Facial Pain

The sphenopalatine ganglion is a small triangular structure located in the pterygopalatine fossa, posterior to the middle turbinate and inferior to the maxillary nerve. It is covered by a thin layer (about 1–5 mm) of connective tissue and mucous membrane. Anesthetization of the sphenopalatine ganglion can be accomplished via the transnasal approach. The patient is placed supine on the treatment table with the nose pointed at the ceiling. A cotton applicator soaked with 2%–4% lidocaine is inserted into the nose on the side of headache. To avoid mechanical discomfort, the cotton applicator should not be inserted deeply into the upper posterior wall of the nasopharynx. A slow drip of 2–4 mL of lidocaine over a 2- to 4-minute period into the nose through the cotton applicator often achieves the goal of a sphenopalatine ganglion block, with the local anesthetic flowing down to the back of the nasopharynx by gravity. Sphenopalatine ganglion blocks have been reported to be effective in the relief of a wide variety of pain conditions of the head, including acute migraine attacks, cluster headache, atypical facial pain, head and facial reflex sympathetic dystrophy (RSD), and postdural puncture headache (Cohen et al., 2009). Intranasal sphenopalatine ganglion block is safe and easy to perform in the clinic and may be helpful for neurologists without special training in interventional pain management techniques to treat an acute headache attack. Other methods for sphenopalatine ganglion block, such as a lateral approach with fluoroscopic guidance, or endoscopic sphenopalatine ganglion block, have also been used. However, special training and equipment are needed.

## Gasserian Ganglion Lesions for Trigeminal Neuralgia

The first choice for treatment of TN is carbamazepine. It can be used with other medication such as baclofen. Gasserian ganglion blocks and rhizhotomies are indicated when patients fail other medication treatments. These procedures include radiofrequency thermocoagulation, balloon compression, and glycerolysis. Radiofrequency thermocoagulation is the most commonly used procedure. This procedure is often performed by neurosurgeons, interventional pain specialists, or interventional radiologists with special training. The treatment requires inserting a radiofrequency needle through the face and foramen ovale into the base of the skull under the guidance of fluoroscopy, CT, or CT fluoroscopy (Fig. 52.7). After the needle reaches the Gasserian ganglion, radiofrequency energy is applied to induce thermocoagulation; 87%–91% of patients experience immediate pain relief. In a 5-year follow-up, 50% of patients still had good pain relief. Common side effects include corneal anesthesia, masticator weakness, and anesthesia dolorosa. Recently, stereotactic radiosurgery (SRS) for TN has been used more widely because of its noninvasive nature. Significant pain relief was achieved in 73% at 1 year, 65% at 2 years, and 41% at 5 years follow-up (Kondziolka et al., 2010). However, this procedure may be more costly than other procedures already mentioned.

## Stellate Ganglion Block

The stellate ganglion is a sympathetic ganglion innervating the ipsilateral upper extremity, the neck, and the head. The structure is usually located in front of the junction between the C6 vertebral body and the transverse process. Stellate ganglion block is primarily indicated for CRPS of the head, neck, and upper extremities. Uncontrolled clinical reports indicate this procedure provides effective pain relief or may even reverse the course of early-stage CRPS type I. Other indications include vascular insufficiency of the arm and acute herpes zoster infection.

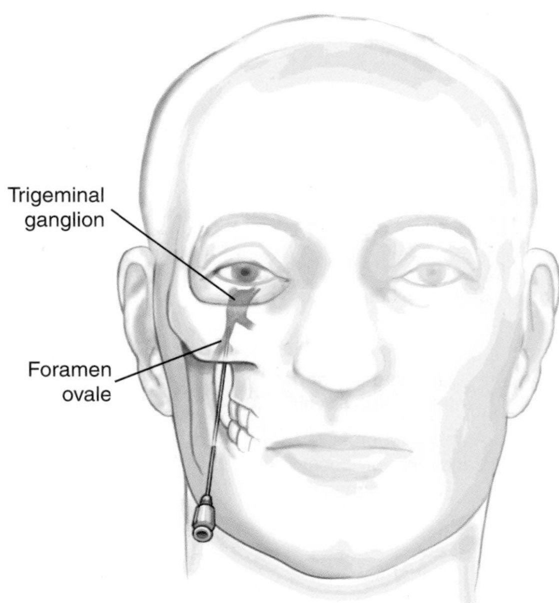


**Fig. 52.7** Trigeminal Nerve Block. *(With permission from Keel, J.C., Bodas, A.V., 2011. Interventional pain management I: epidural, ganglion and nerve block. In: Vacanti, C., Segal, S. [Eds.], Essential Clinical Anesthesia. Cambridge University Press, Cambridge, pp. 907–918.)*

Technically, this block is achieved by inserting a needle through the neck to the front of the junction between the C6 vertebral body and the transverse process (Fig. 52.8). Traditional hand palpation technique without guidance of fluoroscopy bears significant risks of injecting local anesthetics into critical structures in the neck such as the carotid and vertebral arteries or intrathecal space. Incorrectly located injections of local anesthetics may lead to loss of consciousness, seizures, paralysis, cardiac arrest, and death. Current use of fluoroscopic guidance for stellate ganglion block dramatically decreases the possibility of serious side effects and increases the rate of success.

## Epidural Corticosteroid Injection

Pain specialists have used epidural corticosteroid injection (ESI) for decades to treat back and neck pain. The procedure is further divided into cervical, thoracic, and lumbar ESI (LESI), with the purpose of treating pain originating from different spinal regions. The procedure is performed either blindly or with the help of fluoroscopy guidance. A Tuohy needle is inserted in a similar fashion to a spinal tap but the needle stops short in the epidural space. Loss of resistance to saline or air is used to confirm needle position in the epidural space (Fig. 52.9).

By 1995, there were at least 12 double-blind placebo-controlled studies investigating the clinical efficacy of LESI for low back pain (LBP). Of these studies, only six yielded positive results, while the other studies did not support the use of LESI for LBP. Actually, several of these studies exhibited the critical flaw of treating "low back pain" as a single entity. It is now realized that LBP is a clinical syndrome that may be caused by a variety of pathologies in the lumbar spine and adjacent organs. It is not reasonable to treat LBP with ESI, regardless of the cause. More recent well-designed placebo-controlled studies have provided clinical evidence that LESI decreases lumbar radicular pain caused by lumbar disk herniation (Roberts et al., 2009). The pain-relieving effect of LESI may last up to 3 months. Corticosteroids appear

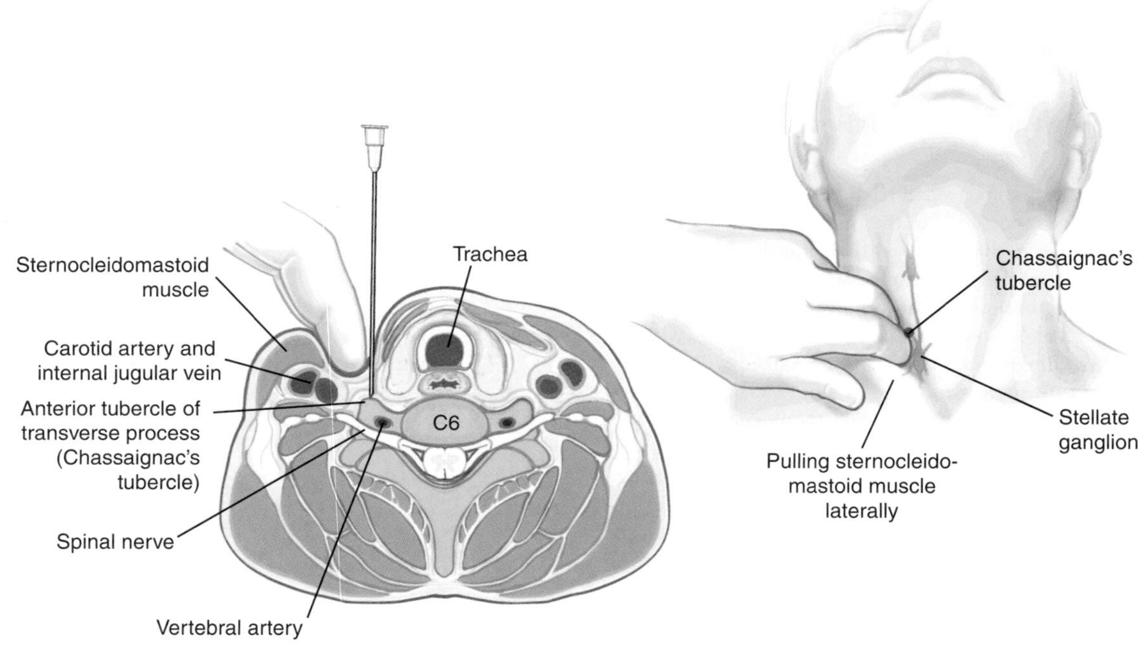


**Fig. 52.8 Stellate Ganglion Block.** *(With permission from Keel, J.C., Bodas, A.V., 2011. Interventional pain management I: epidural, ganglion and nerve block. In: Vacanti, C., Segal, S. [Eds.], Essential Clinical Anesthesia. Cambridge University Press, Cambridge, pp. 907–918.)*

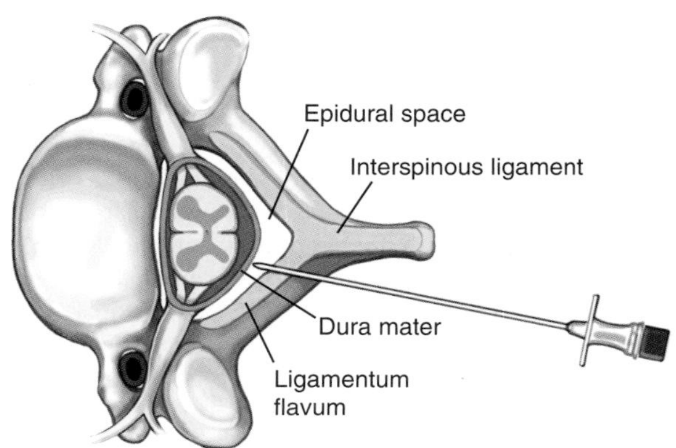


**Fig. 52.9 Epidural Steroid Injection.** *(With permission from Keel, J.C., Bodas, A.V., 2011. Interventional pain management I: epidural, ganglion and nerve block. In: Vacanti, C., Segal, S. [Eds.], Essential Clinical Anesthesia. Cambridge University Press, Cambridge, pp. 907–918.)*

to speed the rate of recovery and return of function, allowing patients to reduce medication levels and increase activity while waiting for the natural improvement expected in most spinal disorders. Recent studies also support the use of LESI for pain relief in patients with spinal stenosis (Lee et al., 2010).

Past the age of 60, more than 90% of the normal population has a variety of degenerative spine changes, including disk herniation, spinal stenosis, and foraminal stenosis. The majority of persons with these changes, however, do not have pain. It is now believed that the pain in patients with disk herniation and associated radiculopathy is not purely due to mechanical compression but is more likely due to chemical inflammation. A recent study provided convincing evidence for the role of inflammatory mediators in the pathogenesis of lumbar radicular pain and LBP in patients with lumbar degenerative diseases. In the study, the immunoreactivity of an array of cytokines was measured in lavage samples and compared with clinical response to the therapeutic injection. Ten subjects underwent repeated epidural lavage sampling 3 months after the steroid injection. It was found that interferon gamma (IFN-$\gamma$) was the most consistently detected cytokine. IFN-$\gamma$ immunoreactivity was also highly correlated with reduction of pain 3 months after the epidural steroid injection. In subjects reporting significant pain relief (>50%) from the injection, mean IFN-$\gamma$ immunoreactivity was significantly greater than that in patients experiencing no significant relief. The IFN-$\gamma$ immunoreactivity in repeated lavage samples decreased to trace residual concentrations in patients who reported pain relief from the steroid injection. These results suggest that IFN-$\gamma$ may be part of a biochemical cascade triggering pain in lumbar radicular pain (Scuderi et al., 2009). Other chemical substances such as phospholipase $A_2$, which is responsible for the liberation of arachidonic acid from cell membranes and starting the cascade of formation of inflammatory mediators such as prostaglandin E (PGE), are also believed to play a major role in pathogenesis of LBP. ESI has been proven to suppress the functional activity of inflammatory mediators such IFN-$\gamma$ and phospholipase $A_2$ (Scuderi et al., 2009) to decrease inflammation in the epidural space and surrounding nerve roots. With the support of evidence from both basic science and clinical studies, it is current common practice to offer patients with lumbar radicular pain due to disk herniation a trial of LESI before considering a surgical treatment for lumbar disk herniation. The procedure often prevents back surgeries. As long as pain is relieved and the patient is free of neurological deficits, a herniated disk should be left alone without further treatment.

In summary, a trial of epidural steroid injections in adults can be offered for adults with persistent radiculopathy from a herniated disc for short-term pain relief or for those who are poor surgical candidates or who would like to defer surgery. There is poor evidence for suggesting use in acute lumbar radiculopathy, spinal stenosis, nonspecific back pain, and back pain from unrelated conditions.

## Lumbar Facet Joint Block

The lumbar facet joint block procedure is indicated for lumbar facet joint pain syndrome. Lumbar facet joint syndrome may be found in up to 35% of patients with LBP. Clinically, this syndrome may mimic lumbar radiculopathy (sciatica). Patients may complain of LBP, often on one side, with pain radiating down the back or front of the thigh. Clinical examination may reveal tenderness on either or both sides of the lumbar spine over the lumbar facet joints. Lumbar spine extension and lateral rotation to the painful side may increase LBP because this maneuver increases pressure on the lumbar facet joints. The straight leg raising test is often negative. Traditionally, pain specialists have performed intrajoint corticosteroid injections, but over the past decade, this procedure has largely been replaced by a diagnostic medial branch (nerve innervating the lumbar facet joints) block with a small amount of local anesthetic. If the patient has significant pain relief (more than 50%) after two consecutive diagnostic medial branch blocks, facet joint rhizotomy with radiofrequency destruction of the medial branch will be performed to denervate the lumbar facet joints. A recent systematic literature review found moderate evidence to support the clinical efficacy and use of radiofrequency rhizotomy for lumbar facet joint syndrome (Datta et al., 2009).

## Percutaneous Disk Decompression

Over 300,000 spine surgeries are performed each year in the United States. A majority of these surgeries are conducted for lumbar and cervical disk herniation. Traditional neurosurgical and orthopedic techniques for lumbar disk herniation include laminectomy, diskectomy, and fusion. A significant number of patients end up with so-called failed back surgery syndrome. Recurrent disk herniation, epidural abscess, scar tissue formation around nerve roots, facet joint syndrome, and muscle spasm may contribute to the clinical features of this syndrome. According to the recent literature, up to 100,000 new cases of failed back surgeries are produced every year in the United States alone as the result of spine surgeries. To avoid possible complications of open surgery, minimally invasive techniques for disk decompression have been developed. These techniques include chymopapain, the Nucleotome system, laser diskectomy, nucleoplasty, and Disc Dekompressor.

Chymopapain is a proteolytic enzyme from the papaya fruit that may induce enzymatic decompression of the nucleus pulposus of a herniated disk. Initial clinical reports were highly positive, but serious side effects such as anaphylactic shock, transverse myelitis, and even death caused chymopapain to be largely replaced by other techniques.

Percutaneous Nucleotome was developed by a Japanese orthopedic surgeon, Dr. Hijikata, in 1975. This procedure inserts a 7-mm-diameter tube into the annulus and removes the disk material with specially designed forceps. The procedure has a reported success rate of 72%. However, because of the large diameter of the cannula, this technique is no longer commonly used. In 1986, Ascher and Choy introduced YAG laser diskectomy, a procedure still being used by spine surgeons, neurosurgeons, and some interventional pain specialists. This technique utilizes an 18-gauge probe and generates laser energy to evaporate part of the nucleus pulposus. It decreases the intradiscal pressure, with a reported success rate for back pain relief of 78%–80%. Heat generated by the laser energy may cause patients to experience severe pain during the procedure and increased muscle spasm afterward.

Over the past decade, two new percutaneous disk decompression techniques have been reported. Introduced in 2000, DISC Nucleoplasty utilizes a unique plasma technology called *Coblation* to remove tissue from the center of the disk. During the procedure the DISC Nucleoplasty SpineWand is inserted into the center of the disk, where a series of channels are created to remove tissue from the nucleus. Disc Dekompressor was introduced in 2003. This procedure uses a 1.5-mm percutaneous lumbar diskectomy probe to aspirate the disk material. It is minimally invasive with less risk for nerve root damage. This technique is indicated for patients with contained disk herniation and lumbar radiculopathy. Observational studies suggest both Nucleoplasty and Disc Dekompressor may be potentially effective, minimally invasive treatments for patients with symptomatic contained disks. However, prospective randomized controlled trials are needed to confirm their clinical efficacy and to determine ideal patient selection for these procedures (Gerges et al., 2010).

## Spinal Cord Stimulation

SCS (dorsal column stimulation) uses an array of electrodes placed in the epidural space immediately behind the spinal cord to stimulate the dorsal column of the spinal cord. The exact mechanism of SCS is unclear. However, it is believed that the gate-control theory of pain conduction plays a major role. When the dorsal column of the spinal cord is stimulated, it may attenuate the conduction of the pain signal on the spinothalamic tract through collateral inhibition. Inhibitory neurotransmitters such as GABA may also be involved.

As noted earlier in the chapter, patients should have a trial of SCS prior to permanent implantation. During the trial, a percutaneous lead is inserted through the skin into the epidural space. Once the tip of the lead reaches the appropriate level, it is connected to an external pulse generator. When the stimulator is turned on, the patient may feel tingling and numbness. If the painful area is covered by the stimulation, the pain is decreased by more than 50%, and the patient is satisfied with the stimulation, a permanent implantation may be considered. The procedure of permanent implantation of the SCS is performed by pain specialists or neurosurgeons in an operating room. It requires percutaneous insertion of an electrode into the epidural space under the guidance of fluoroscopy. The tip of the electrode is threaded up to the appropriate level in the epidural space immediately behind the dorsal column for the treatment of the related pain condition (Fig. 52.10). The other end of the electrode is connected through a subcutaneous tunnel to an internal pulse generator buried under the skin in the low back or abdominal wall. The strength of the stimulation can be changed through a remote control. Common complications of SCS implantation include infection, migration of the electrodes, and failure of pain relief even after a "satisfied" trial. Serious complications such as spinal cord compression or epidural abscesses are rare.

SCS is indicated for failed back surgery syndrome, CRPS, and unremitting pain due to peripheral vascular disease. Multiple studies have found that SCS may also improve pain due to refractory angina and improve circulation in the coronary arteries. Some authors have reported treatment success with SCS for severe peripheral neuropathy, postherpetic neuralgia, chronic knee pain following total knee replacement, central pain in multiple sclerosis (MS), and painful spasms of atypical stiff limb syndrome (Ughratdar et al., 2010). The value of SCS for amputation stump pain, phantom-limb pain, and SCI is yet to be established. Patients seeking SCS treatments usually have failed all other conservative treatments such as medication, physical therapy, and nerve blocks with anesthetics and/or corticosteroids. SCS is not indicated for severe depression and contraindicated for patients with a cardiac pacemaker or defibrillators.

## Intrathecal Drug Delivery Systems

For patients with chronic severe pain, especially malignant pain, who are unable to tolerate the side effects of oral or IV medications, intrathecal delivery of medication offers a useful alternative. The technique of intrathecal delivery of medication has evolved since 1979. There are two kinds of pumps available in the United States: Codman and Medtronic intrathecal pumps. The pump is usually implanted

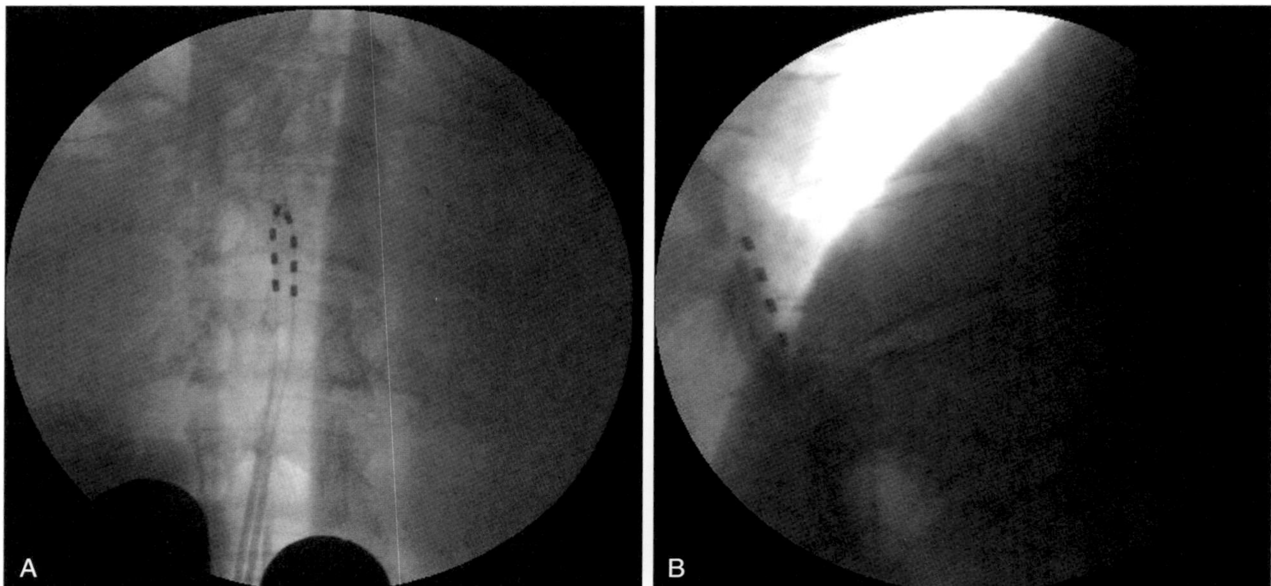


**Fig. 52.10** (A) Radiograph of thoracolumbar spinal cord stimulation leads. (B) Radiograph of lumbosacral leads. *(With permission from Gonzalez, C.D., Dinakar, P., Ross, E.L., 2011. Interventional pain management II: implantable and other invasive therapies. In: Vacanti, C., Segal, S. [Eds.], Essential Clinical Anesthesia. Cambridge University Press, Cambridge, pp. 919–924.)*

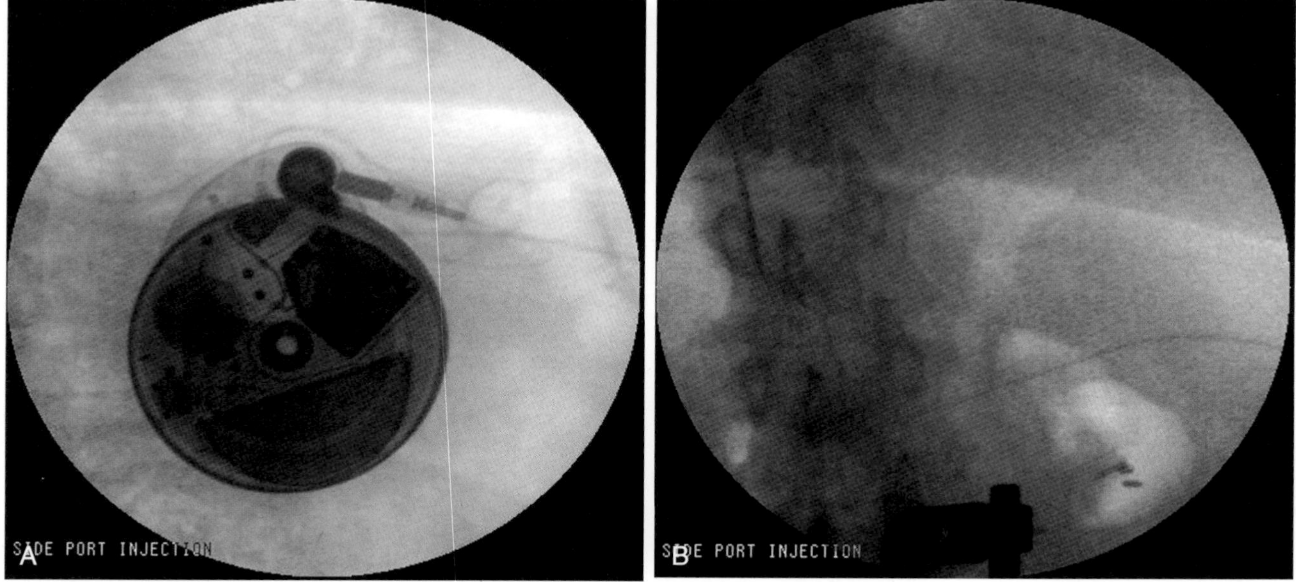


**Fig. 52.11 (A) Programmable Intrathecal Pump and (B) Intrathecal Catheter Radiographs.** *(With permission from Gonzalez, C.D., Dinakar, P., Ross, E.L., 2011. Interventional pain management II: implantable and other invasive therapies. In: Vacanti, C., Segal, S. [Eds.], Essential Clinical Anesthesia. Cambridge University Press, Cambridge, pp. 919–924.)*

subcutaneously in the abdominal wall. The pump contains about 18–50 mL of medication. It is connected to one end of a small-diameter tube that runs to the intrathecal space. The pump continuously delivers small amounts of medication directly into the lumbar cerebrospinal fluid (Fig. 52.11). The Codman pump has fixed delivery rates of 0.5 or 1 mL/day. The concentration of medication must be changed in order to change the daily dose of medication. Medtronic pumps are programmable with an external magnetic control to adjust the dosage and time of medication delivery.

Commonly used medications for pain management include morphine, hydromorphone, bupivacaine, clonidine, and ziconotide, a novel peptide that functions as a calcium channel blocker. Ziconotide was approved by the FDA in 2004 for treating intractable severe chronic pain, but its serious side effects have called the clinical use of this medication into question (Ziconotide, 2008). Baclofen is a $GABA_B$ agonist. It has been used through an intrathecal delivery system for the treatment of severe spasticity and may also decrease the pain related to spasticity. Even though intrathecal opioid treatment was initially approved by the FDA for the treatment of patients with malignant pain, over the past decade intrathecal opioids have been used extensively for nonmalignant pain such as failed back surgery syndrome. A retrospective cohort study with 3-year follow-up found a favorable outcome for intrathecal opioids. Some patients are able to eliminate oral opioids, although some increase in intrathecal opioid dosing may be required (Atli et al., 2010).

### Motor Cortex Stimulation

Motor cortex stimulation (MCS) has been used for the treatment of central and neuropathic pain syndromes since 1991. It has been used to treat medically unresponsive central and neuropathic pain including that due to thalamic, putaminal, and lateral medullary infarction, traumatic trigeminal neuropathy (not idiopathic TN), facial postherpetic neuralgia, brachial plexopathy, neuropathic pain after an SCI, phantom-limb pain, and CRPS. MCS has shown particular promise in the treatment of intractable neuropathic facial pain and central pain syndromes such as thalamic pain syndrome (Levy et al., 2010).

The MCS leads are surgically placed on the dura, with the target selected on the primary motor cortex based on somatotopic anatomical landmarks. The optimal stimulation level is that which provides the best pain relief yet does not cause a seizure, pain from dural stimulation, or EMG activity. Cortical stimulation is not indicated for patients with a history of seizures. Personality disorders such as severe depression or psychotic disorders must be screened out prior to using this procedure.

The precise mechanism for MCS in relieving pain remains unknown, but studies have demonstrated that it leads to an increase in cerebral blood flow in the ipsilateral thalamus, cingulate gyrus, orbitofrontal cortex, and midbrain. The extent of pain relief correlates best, however, with anterior cingulate gyrus blood flow. Rostroventromedial medulla (RVM) and the descending serotonergic pathway acting on the spinal 5-HT (1A) receptor may also contribute to spinal antinociception induced by M1 stimulation.

## PSYCHOLOGICAL THERAPY IN CHRONIC PAIN MANAGEMENT

Associated comorbid psychological problems are not uncommon in chronic pain patients. Addressing them in a multidisciplinary approach with psychopharmacology and psychological pain coping skills is of utmost importance for a successful treatment outcome. A pain clinic must have a full-time psychologist for serial assessments of their patients for mood-related issues, opioid abuse, and assessment of whether patients are candidates for implantable devices. The various types of psychological approaches are listed in Table 52.6.

**TABLE 52.6 Psychotherapy for Chronic Pain Management**

| Therapy | Description |
|---|---|
| Hypnosis and visualization | The patient is taught to visualize relaxing mental images such as a secluded beach, or peaceful meadow. This helps to decrease anxiety, and facilitates deep relaxation |
| Guided imagery | Directed visualization focusing on specific psychological issues utilizing pain-decreasing images |
| Biofeedback | Relaxation technique that measures a physiological phenomenon such as muscle tension and provides an audible or visual feedback indicating a state of relaxation |
| Cognitive-behavioral therapy | This teaches various techniques such as distraction training, cognitive restructuring, role-playing, or mental imagery |
| Group therapies | When well planned and with appropriate patient dynamics, group therapy is very helpful. The interaction is planned to share important breakthroughs in insight, as well as to discuss progress with treatment and different strategies for overcoming everyday obstacles to improvement |
| Family therapy | Patients and their families often feel angry at each other. The family can be a significant stressor but is an important source of support that is needed for progress. This approach attempts to bring insight on how to provide support without enabling continued disability |

*With permission from Ross, E.L., 2003. Pain Management: Hot Topics, first ed. Hanley & Belfus.*

## REHABILITATION IN CHRONIC PAIN MANAGEMENT

Rehabilitation helps achieve meaningful functional recovery and improved quality of life. It helps patients work through their chronic pain and overcome deconditioning. Most common approaches are physical therapy, occupational therapy, bracing, and the use of the transelectrical nerve stimulation (TENS) unit (Table 52.7).

## COMMON PAIN SYNDROMES

### Trigeminal Neuralgia

*Trigeminal neuralgia* (TN), or *tic douloureux*, is characterized by paroxysmal lancinating attacks of severe facial pain. TN has an incidence of approximately 4/100,000, with a large majority of cases occurring spontaneously. Both genders experience TN, but there is a slight female predominance, and the diagnosis is most common over the age of 50. Classic TN is characterized by abrupt onset and termination of unilateral brief electric shock-like pain. Pain is often limited to the distribution of one or two (commonly the second and third) divisions of the trigeminal nerve. Trivial stimuli including washing, shaving, smoking, talking, and/or brushing the teeth (*trigger factors*) can evoke the pain. Some areas in the nasolabial fold and/or chin may be particularly susceptible to stimulation (*trigger areas*). In individual patients, pain attacks are stereotyped, recurring with the same intensity and distribution. Most TN patients are symptom free between attacks, and clinical examination is usually normal. Attacks of TN occur in clusters, and remissions can last for months.

The cause of TN pain attacks is unknown. Compression of the trigeminal nerve by benign tumors and vascular anomalies may play a role in the development of clinical symptoms. Studies of surgical biopsy specimens from TN patients who had presumed vascular compression demonstrate evidence of inflammation, demyelination, and close apposition of axons (leading to the possibility of ephaptic transmission between fibers). The *ignition hypothesis* of Devor proposes that a trigeminal nerve injury induces physiological changes that lead to a population of hyperexcitable and functionally linked trigeminal primary sensory neurons. The discharge of any individual neuron in this group can quickly spread to activate the entire population, resulting in a sudden synchronous discharge and a sudden jolt of pain characteristic of a TN attack.

The diagnosis of TN is based primarily on a history of characteristic paroxysmal pain attacks. The White and Sweet criteria are still commonly used worldwide (Box 52.2). In the majority of TN patients, the

**TABLE 52.7 Rehabilitation in Chronic Pain**

| Rehabilitative Therapy | Description of Treatment and Goals |
|---|---|
| Modalities such as heat, ice, ultrasound | These are temporary, short-lasting therapies and therefore should only be used as adjuvant to an active rehabilitation |
| Stretching | Mild and controlled stretching prepares the patient for further activity. Care should be taken to avoid injuring tight muscles that have not been active for a long period of time |
| Cardiovascular exercise | Chronic pain patients are often much deconditioned. A general aerobic program can increase endurance and activity tolerance. Aerobic exercise has antidepressant effects |
| Work conditioning | This is a specific program used to prepare for return to work. A job description is obtained, and the goals of therapy should lead to the physical demands of that type of work |
| Strength training | This is usually focused on the portion of a chronic pain patient that is significantly weakened by the original insult. This approach is also used to train alternate muscle to supplement the site of original injury. Care should be taken to keep the goals realistic and avoid further injury |
| Orthotics and prosthetics | Adaptive aids are often very useful for return to function. The benefits of truly understanding a patient's impairments and creatively designing adaptive aids can be extremely helpful in enhancing function |

*With permission from Ross, E.L., 2003. Pain Management: Hot Topics, first ed. Hanley & Belfus.*

**BOX 52.2 White and Sweet Criteria for Trigeminal Neuralgia**

1. The pain is paroxysmal.
2. The pain may be provoked by light touch to the face (trigger zones).
3. The pain is confined to the trigeminal distribution.
4. The pain is unilateral.
5. The clinical sensory examination is normal.

*From Powers, S.W., Coffey, C.S., Chamberlin, L.A., et al.; CHAMP Investigators, 2017. Trial of amitriptyline, topiramate, and placebo for pediatric migraine. N Engl J Med. 376 (2), 115–124.*
*Dowell, D., Haegerich, T.M., Chou, R., 2016. CDC guideline for prescribing opioids for chronic pain—United States, 2016. JAMA. 315 (15), 1624–1645.*

clinical examination, imaging studies, and laboratory tests are unremarkable (*classic TN*). In a smaller group, TN is secondary to other disease processes affecting the trigeminal system (*symptomatic TN*). Because a significant percentage of patients have symptomatic TN resulting from other disease processes, diagnostic MRI studies should be part of the initial evaluation of any patient with TN symptoms. Special attention should be paid to MS plaques, tumor, and subtle vascular anomalies that may be the source of root compression. Recent studies found that high-resolution three-dimensional (3D) MRI reconstruction and magnetic resonance cisternography may provide alternative tools for better identifying the presence of neurovascular compression and even measuring the volume of neurovascular compression at the cerebellopontine angle and predict the prognosis after initial treatment (Tanaka et al., 2009).

Carbamazepine is the first choice for treatment of TN; both controlled and uncontrolled studies confirm its clinical efficacy. Carbamazepine monotherapy provides initial symptom control in as many as 80% of TN patients. Of those initially responding to the drug, approximately 75% will continue to have long-term control of pain attacks. Controlled studies demonstrate that baclofen and lamotrigine are superior to placebo for treatments of TN. In the experience of many clinicians, baclofen is just as effective as carbamazepine and often better tolerated. A recent study found that oxcarbazepine may be effective for those who were unresponsive to the treatment of carbamazepine (Gomez-Arguelles et al., 2008). Pregabalin may also be potentially effective. If a patient is not satisfied with single medication therapy, adding another oral medication may offer additional benefits. IV lidocaine or phenytoin could be effective for some severe refractory cases of TN. However, these treatments carry additional risks and require close cardiovascular monitoring. Opioid analgesics have not been proven effective for TN and should be avoided.

Posterior fossa exploration and microvascular decompression (MVD) is assumed to directly treat the cause of TN. However, this is a complex and invasive therapy with a possibility of death. With the availability of other less-invasive procedures, MVD is infrequently used and is only reserved for younger and healthier patients. Several studies have demonstrated that trigeminal radiofrequency rhizotomy successfully controls symptoms in over 85% of TN cases. The technique is minimally invasive. To heat the Gasserian ganglion, a radiofrequency needle is inserted through the foramen ovale under the guidance of fluoroscopy. The procedure can be finished in less than 30 minutes in experienced hands. A few patients experience sensory loss and dysesthesia (analgesia dolorosa) in the distribution of the damaged trigeminal fibers with this procedure. SRS employs computerized stereotaxic methods to concentrate ionizing radiation on the trigeminal root entry zone. Several studies have demonstrated the high clinical efficacy and relative safety of this new technique. It is currently recommended as a first-line noninvasive surgical technique in many pain centers, especially for frail or elderly patients (Zahra et al., 2009).

## Low Back Pain

LBP is the most common condition seen in pain clinics. Approximately 60%–80% of the US population will experience back pain some time during life. Neurologists are often consulted for the diagnosis and treatment of LBP. It is critical for clinicians to appropriately examine the patients and make a diagnosis before treatment is rendered. Common causes of LBP include muscle strain, lumbar disk herniation, lumbar radiculopathy, lumbar facet joint syndrome, sacroiliac (SI) joint syndrome, and lumbar spinal stenosis.

Patients with acute muscle strain in the low back often have histories of acute injury. Physical examination may reveal tenderness or muscle spasms. NSAIDs, muscle relaxants, massage therapy, physical therapy, and acupuncture often provide effective pain relief. However, many times muscle pain in the low back is secondary to injuries in deeper tissues, such as lumbar disk herniation or lumbar radiculopathy.

Acute lumbar disk herniation after injury may cause severe LBP. Patients often complain of severe shooting or stabbing pains in the low back, with frequent radiation pain down the dorsomedial part of the foot when the L5 nerve root is involved, or the lateral part of the foot or the small toe when the S1 nerve root is involved. The straight leg raising test is often positive. Detailed neurological examinations may find decreased sensation to pinprick in the area innervated by L5 and/or S1 nerve root(s). Patient may also have mild weakness on the tibialis anterior (L5), or peroneus longus and brevis muscles (S1). These patients usually have severe tenderness and spasm over the lumbar paraspinal muscles. Lumbosacral MRIs may reveal disk herniation at L4–L5 and/or L5–S1 level(s). EMG/NCV tests may not detect a lumbar radiculopathy. NSAIDs, muscle relaxants, and physical therapy may help some patients with acute disk herniation and lumbar radiculopathy. If patients fail these treatments, LESIs may offer fast and effective pain relief if the nerve roots are not severely mechanically compressed. Surgery is suggested for those with moderate to severe focal neurological deficit, including numbness and/or weakness of relevant muscles or bowel or bladder dysfunction. Surgery may also be indicated for severe pain that lasts for more than 3 months and does not respond to aggressive pain management if disk herniation is demonstrated by MRI or computed tomography (CT) studies.

*Lumbar facet joint syndrome* is found in up to 35% of patients with LBP. It is frequently associated with arthritis or injuries in lumbar facet joints. Patients may complain of pain in the low back, either bilateral or unilaterally. Pain may occasionally radiate down the back or front of the thigh but only up to the knee joint at the most. Physical examination may find positive tenderness over the lumbar paraspinal muscles and facet joints. Back extension and lateral rotation to the side of the pain often increases the back pain. Results of a straight leg raising test are negative. Neurological examination should be normal unless there is a coexistent lumbar radiculopathy or other neurological condition. Diagnosis of facet joint syndrome is clinical. MRI and CT reports of facet joint arthropathy do not correlate with clinical findings. Single-photon emission CT (SPECT) images can be more specific for facet joint arthropathy. Often these changes are age related. NSAIDs should be tried for patients with lumbar facet joint syndrome before they are considered for diagnostic medial branch blocks or intra-joint corticosteroid injections.

*Sacroiliac (SI) joint syndrome* is another major source of LBP. The patient may have pain in one side of the low back, with occasional pain radiating down to the hip or thigh. Pain is often increased when these patients try to walk upstairs. Physical examination may find tenderness over the SI joint, and the Patrick test or single-leg standing often exacerbate SI joint pain. NSAIDs are the first-line medication for SI joint inflammation. SI joint corticosteroid injection can provide temporary pain relief. Radiofrequency lesions to denervate the SI joint have been reported effective; however, more studies are needed to confirm clinical efficacy of this treatment.

*Lumbar spinal stenosis* is a common age-related change. The majority of seniors older than 60 years of age have varying degrees of spinal stenosis due to disk herniation, osteophytes, or degenerative spondylolisthesis. Preexisting congenital lumbar canal stenosis predisposes to the development of this syndrome. Fortunately, fewer than 30% of those with spinal stenosis have clinical pain. Patients often have pain in the low back, with pain radiation down the back of both legs. Standing or walking may worsen pain. Patients often walk with a hunched back and sit down after walking a short distance to relieve pain (neurogenic claudication). The pain usually takes minutes to disappear, compared to seconds with vascular claudication. On physical examination, patients often have less tenderness over the lumbar spine than those with acute lumbar disk herniation. A straight leg raising test may be normal. The condition must be distinguished from vascular claudication. Patients may try NSAIDs first. LESIs may provide short-term pain relief for this group of patient for weeks or none based on recent trials. In a recent 2014 randomized study for the treatment of lumbar spinal stenosis, epidural injection of glucocorticoids plus lidocaine offered minimal or no short-term benefit as compared with epidural injection of lidocaine alone (Fridely et al. 2014) If a patient has severe pain and refuses surgery, chronic narcotic treatment often provides adequate pain control but runs a risk of the development of tolerance and addiction.

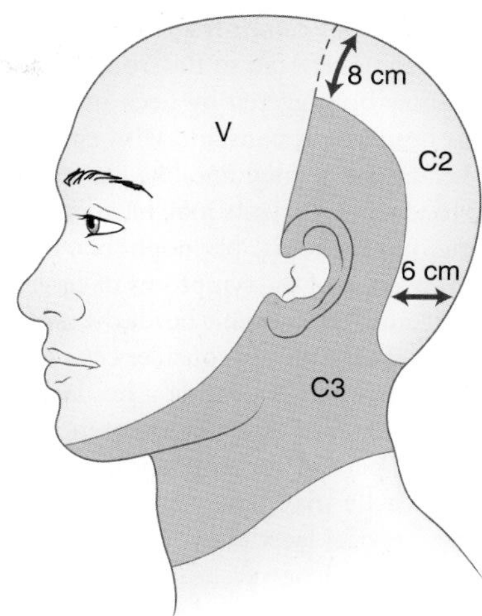


**Fig. 52.12 Pain Referral From C2 and C3 Nerve Roots.** The C2 pain dermatome consists of an occipital parietal area 6–8 cm wide, extending paramedially from the subocciput to the vertex. The C3 pain dermatome is a craniofacial area, including the scalp around the ear, the pinna, the lateral cheek over the angle of the jaw, the submental region, and the lateral and anterior aspects of the upper neck. *(With permission from Poletti, C.E., 1996. Third cervical nerve root and ganglion compression: clinical syndrome, surgical anatomy, and pathological findings. Neurosurgery 39, 941–948.)*

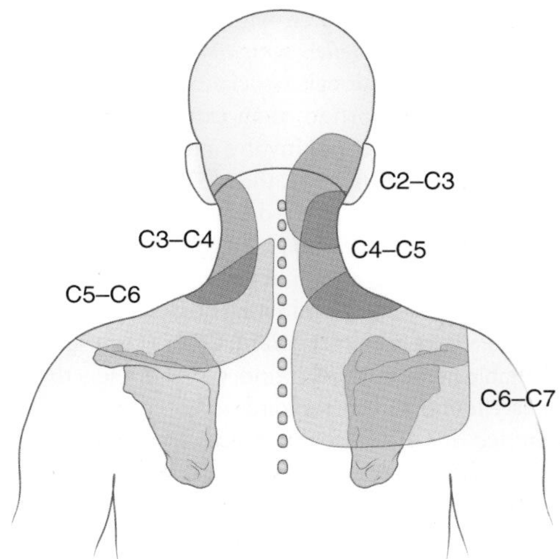


**Fig. 52.13 Pain Referral Pattern From the Cervical Facet Joints.** Injection of contrast medium into the cervical facet joints in normal volunteers induced pain in the head, neck, and shoulder area. Of note, injection of C2–C3 facet joints can cause pain in the occipital area. *(With permission from Dwyer, A., Aprill, C., Bogduk, N., 1990. Cervical zygapophyseal joint pain patterns. I: a study in normal volunteers. Spine 15, 453–457.)*

## Cervicogenic Headache

*Cervicogenic headache* refers to head pain originating from pathology in the neck. It is believed that pain from the C2–C3 nerve dermatome can radiate to the head and face (Fig. 52.12). An earlier study found that pain from the C2–C3 and C3–C4 cervical facet joints can also radiate to the occipital area (Fig. 52.13). The term *cervicogenic headache* was first introduced by Sjaastad and colleagues in 1983. However, the concept of cervicogenic headache is controversial and not well accepted by the majority of neurologists. The International Headache Society (2004) published its first diagnostic criteria in 1998 and revised it in 2004. Patients with cervicogenic headache often have histories of head and neck trauma. Pain may be unilateral or bilateral. Pain is frequently localized to the occipital area, but it may also be referred to the frontal, temporal, or orbital regions. Headaches may be triggered by neck movement or sustained neck postures. This headache is constant, with episodic exacerbations. Typical migraine headaches or migraine-like exacerbations can also be triggered by these headaches. Patients may have other symptoms, such as nausea, vomiting, photophobia, phonophobia, and blurred vision. Owing to significant overlap of the symptoms of cervicogenic headache and migraine without aura, cervicogenic headache is often misdiagnosed as migraine. Clinicians should always consider cervicogenic headache in the differential diagnoses when evaluating a headache patient. History of head/neck injury and detailed examination of the occipital and upper cervical area should be part of the evaluation for headache. Patients with cervicogenic headache may have tenderness over the greater or lesser occipital nerve, cervical facet joints, and muscles in the upper or middle cervical region. Cervicogenic headache does not respond well to migraine medications. Treatment should be focused on removal of the pain source from the occipital-cervical junction. Initial therapy is directed to physical therapy modalities and NSAIDs. Interventional treatment such as greater occipital nerve block, cervical facet joint block, superficial cervical plexus block, and botulinum toxin injections may provide effective pain relief (Zhou et al., 2010).

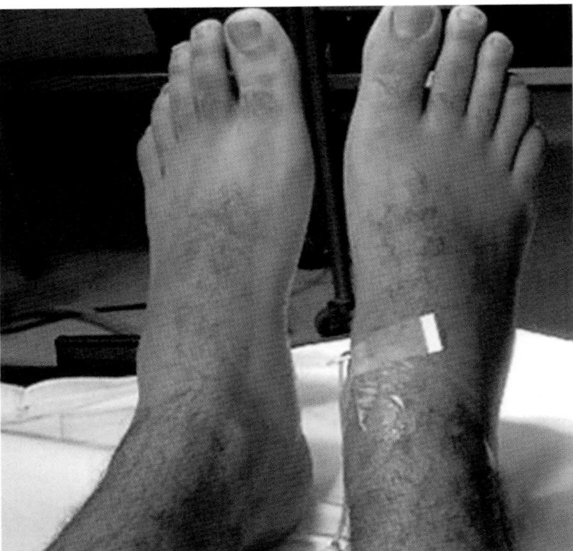

**Fig. 52.14 Complex Regional Pain Syndrome I.** The right foot and ankle are mildly swollen and reddish in comparison with the left foot and ankle. The intravenous access was used for a Bier block.

## Complex Regional Pain Syndrome

Terminology describing the CRPSs has evolved over the last century. The term *causalgia* was first coined by Weir Mitchell in the 1870s for severe progressive distal limb pain with major nerve injury. In 1946, Evans introduced the term *reflex sympathetic dystrophy* (RSD); it was later defined by the International Association for Study of Pain (IASP) as "continuous pain in a portion of an extremity after trauma, which may include fracture but does not involve a major nerve, associated with sympathetic hyperactivity." In 1994, the IASP introduced the term *complex regional pain syndrome* (CRPS), describing a painful condition that includes regional pain, sensory changes (e.g., allodynia), abnormalities of temperature, abnormal sudomotor activity, edema, and abnormal skin color changes that occur after an initiating noxious event such as trauma. Two types of CRPS have been recognized: *CRPS I* corresponds to RSD, in which no definable nerve lesion is found. *CRPS II* refers to the cases with a definable nerve lesion and corresponds to the earlier term of *causalgia*.

The mean age of CRPS patients ranges from 36 to 46 years, with women predominating (60%–81%). It is caused typically by an injury such as a fracture (16%–46%), strain or sprain (10%–29%), postsurgery (3%–24%), and contusion or crush injury (8%–18%). Clinical features of CRPS often include pain, edema, autonomic dysfunction such as change in temperature or color in the involved limbs, motor dysfunction, and psychological abnormalities such as depression (Fig. 52.14). Schwartzman and Maleki reported the pattern of spreading of CRPS in three stages. In the early stage, CRPS often involves only one limb with pain, minor edema, and increased skin temperature. CRPS may spread from one limb to the others. In the later stage, CRPS could involve the full body and the four extremities with severe pain, edema, cold and cyanotic limbs, joint contracture, and atrophy of muscles and bones.

Excruciating pain is the cardinal feature of CRPS. Pain is often described as burning, aching, pricking, or shooting. Severity of pain is not proportional to the initial injury, and pain is not limited to the area of the injury or a specific nerve distribution. Patients may feel severe pain to minor pain stimulation such as a safety-pin prick (hyperalgesia). A light touch to skin (innocuous stimulation) may cause severe long-lasting pain (mechanical allodynia). A cooling stimulus such as a drop of alcohol may be perceived as painful (thermal allodynia). Decreased temperature and pinprick sensations in the affected limb are common.

Edema of the affected limb is present in the majority of patients. It could be very mild in the early stage of CRPS, mimicking mild cellulitis. However, in the late stage, edema may be so severe that a Doppler test is needed to rule out the possibility of deep vein thrombosis (DVT).

Autonomic dysfunction may manifest as changes of skin color and temperature, as well as sweating abnormalities. The affected area may be reddish at one time and then become blue, purple, or pale over a course of minutes to hours. Livedo reticularis is common in CRPS. *Livedo* is a descriptive term used to describe the red, nonblanchable (i.e., does not turn white when pressed) network pattern (reticulated) in the skin. About 60% of patients may report excessive sweating in the affected limbs. Temperature asymmetry between the affected and unaffected sides may exceed 1°C.

Motor dysfunctions in CRPS include mild weakness, decreased range of motion, tremor, dystonia, and myoclonus. Dystrophic manifestations are seen in the form of increased or decreased nail and hair growth in the affected extremity, hyperkeratosis or thin glossy skin, and osteoporosis of the underlying bones.

Diagnosis of CRPS is clinical. According to IASP, if a patient has the above-mentioned features, a diagnosis of CRPS may be made if other clinical conditions such as infection or DVT are ruled out. EMG/NCV tests are not sensitive to CRPS and frequently cause severe pain to patients. A triple-phase bone scan may reveal abnormal absorption in the affected limbs (increased or decreased), though it is not a primary diagnostic procedure for CRPS.

The pathophysiology of CRPS is not completely understood. Multiple mechanisms are considered in the generation and maintenance of CRPS. Increased systemic calcitonin gene-related peptide (CGRP) levels may contribute to neurogenic inflammation, edema, vasodilatation, and increased sweating. Elevated neuropeptide concentrations may lead to pain and hyperalgesia. Immunological mechanisms (e.g., altered expressions of human leukocyte antigen [HLA], substance P, cytokines, and interleukins) are believed to contribute to the pathogenesis of clinical symptoms such as edema. Upregulation of adrenergic receptors and functional coupling between sympathetic efferent and sensory afferent fibers may provide the basis of the sympathetic nervous system abnormalities in the pathogenesis of CRPS. The central mechanisms in CRPS may include central sensitization in the spinal cord, brainstem, or thalamus, cortical reorganization in the primary somatosensory cortex, and disinhibition of the motor cortex.

The goals of treatment for CRPS are pain relief, functional recovery, and psychological improvement. However, treatment of CRPS remains a challenge. There is little if any evidence for the efficacy of any treatment modality. In the early stages of CRPS treatment, occupational and physical therapies are often used.

Patients diagnosed with CRPS for over 2 months should also undergo a psychological evaluation—which includes psychometric testing—to identify and treat psychological disorders such as anxiety, depression, or personality disorders. Counseling, behavioral modification, biofeedback, relaxation therapy, group therapy, and self-hypnosis should be considered. The goal of psychotherapy is to improve patient motivation and coping skills.

Tricyclic antidepressants, antiepileptics, and narcotics such as methadone are commonly used empirically for CRPS, even though clinical controlled studies have not proven their efficacy. A recent review article summarized the evidence derived from randomized controlled trials pertaining to the treatment of CRPS. The review reported clinical improvement with dimethyl sulfoxide, steroids, epidural clonidine, and intrathecal baclofen. Only bisphosphonates appear to offer clear benefits for patients with CRPS (Tran et al., 2010). NMDA receptor modulation is a major interest of current research. It has been reported that subanesthetic infusions of ketamine might offer a promising therapeutic option in the treatment of appropriately selected patients with intractable CRPS (Schwartzman et al., 2009). A recent preliminary study reported that IV immunoglobulin treatment could potentially decrease pain in CRPS patients (Goebel et al., 2010). Other infusion treatments currently used include IV lidocaine infusion. However, more studies are needed to further establish the safety and efficacy of these novel approaches.

Minimally invasive techniques have been used extensively for the treatment of CRPS. Techniques include sympathetic block, intravenous regional block (IVRB), somatic nerve block, epidural drug administration, intrathecal drug delivery, and neurostimulation. Stellate ganglion blocks in early-stage CRPS may significantly decrease pain and hasten clinical recovery. It may also prevent the recurrence of CRPS after reoperation of the affected extremity. In a double-blind study, IVRB with bretylium provided significantly longer analgesia than lidocaine. Good pain relief is reported with the use of epidural delivery of clonidine and ketamine and also with intrathecal baclofen and morphine. An early study with 2-year follow-up reported that SCS results in a long-term pain reduction and improvement in health-related quality of life. However, a more recent randomized study with 5-year follow-up found no extra benefit in terms of pain relief for those with a combination of SCS and physical therapy, compared to those with physical therapy alone (Kemler et al., 2008). The author shares the same experience and opinion with the cited report. It seems that most RSD patients feel better immediately after the SCS implantation. However, the SCS itself may have difficulty stopping the spread of RSD, and once RSD spreads out of the area initially covered by the SCS, the pain is no longer "under control."

## Poststroke Pain Syndrome

Lesions at any level of the neuroaxis (generally affecting spinothalamocortical afferent sensory pathways) including the medulla, pons, midbrain, thalamus, subcortical white matter, and the cortex may produce central poststroke pain syndrome (PSP). However, the thalamus and brainstem are common sites for PSP; 8%–16% of thalamic strokes may lead to chronic pain. The frequency of pain after a geniculothalamic artery stroke is even higher (13%–59%).

The pathogenesis of PSP is not yet known. However, it has been suggested that hyperexcitation in the damaged sensory pathways, damage to the central inhibitory pathways, or a combination of the two may be responsible for the onset of PSP. Pain is the cardinal symptom and is described as spontaneous, severe, paroxysmal, and burning. Patients with thalamic pain syndrome also have hyperalgesia and allodynia in the affected limbs. Right-sided lesions predominate among reported cases of the thalamic pain syndrome.

Patients reporting pain due to brainstem infarction usually have involvement of pontine or medullary structures. Patients with midbrain infarction seldom complain of pain. Transitory eye and nose pain may be an initial symptom of pontine infarction. About 25% of patients with dorsolateral medullary infarction develop ipsilateral facial pain, especially when the lesion involves the spinal trigeminal tract. Facial allodynia is also common. Some patients may experience pain in the contralateral limbs and trunk.

Treatment of central PSP remains a challenge. Tricyclic antidepressants are still a choice of treatment. Gabapentin and lamotrigine have been used to treat central PSP syndrome in open-labeled studies. Selective posterior rhizotomy has been reported to decrease painful spasticity in the lower limbs of hemiplegic patients after a stroke. It has been reported that chronic MCS therapy provides pain relief for some poststroke patients (Brown and Pilitsis, 2006). SRS of the pituitary and deep brain stimulation (DBS) have been used to treat PSP syndrome with some success (Pickering et al., 2009).

Some 40%–60% of patients develop shoulder pain after a stroke. The mechanism of shoulder pain is not clear, but a strong association exists between pain and an abnormal shoulder joint examination, ipsilateral sensory abnormalities, and arm weakness. These patients usually have significant tenderness over the shoulder joint. It is postulated that the pain is due to inflammation in the joint secondary to immobilization and joint contracture (*frozen shoulder syndrome*). The majority of shoulder pain may be resolved or improved for 6 months following a stroke with intensive physical/occupational therapy. Antiinflammatory medications may be used. Suprascapular nerve or brachial plexus block can provide temporary pain relief to prepare for physical therapy. Proper positioning of the shoulder, range-of-motion activities, and avoidance of immobilization may further help prevent or alleviate shoulder pain.

## Spinal Cord Injury and Pain

There are about 240,000 patients with SCIs in the United States; 86% of individuals with SCI report pain at 6 months post-discharge, with 27% of these individuals reporting pain that impacts most of their daily activities. Patients can have pain both at and below the level of spinal injury. Pain intensity is not associated with the magnitude or location of the lesion, occurrence of myofascial pain syndrome, or onset of pain. However, pain is usually more severe in patients with gunshot injuries.

Pain after SCI originates from different sources, including neuropathic, musculoskeletal, and visceral pain. Neuropathic pain after SCI is further divided into central and segmental pain. Central neuropathic pain often begins within weeks or months after injury. It is generally described as a burning, sharp, or shooting pain. Patients feel pain at or below the level of injury in areas where there is partial or complete loss of sensation to touch. Central pain is believed to be due to differentiation caused by SCI. Astrocytic activation in the spinal cord, upregulation of chemokines, hyperexcitability of wide–dynamic range neurons in the spinal dorsal horn rostral to the lesion, and loss of GABAergic interneurons in laminae I–III of the spinal cord dorsal horn (Meisner et al., 2010) have been suggested to cause the neuropathic pain that follows SCI. Segmental pain often occurs around the border of the injury and usually develops within the first few months after an injury. Allodynia and hyperalgesia are common. Nerve root entrapment could lead to severe segmental pain. Patients may describe stabbing or sharp pain or a band of burning pain at the level of injury. Syringomyelia with a cyst ascending from the level of the SCI may occasionally cause central pain.

Musculoskeletal pain in this group of patients may be due to muscle spasms below the level of SCI and arthritis in disused joints. Pain is generally described as dull or aching. It is usually worsened by movement and eased with rest. Visceral pain may begin a short time following SCI and could be related to constipation and urinary retention due to sphincter dysfunction. It may occur in the abdomen above or below the level of injury. This pain is often described as cramping, burning, and constant.

Pain management after SCI is difficult. Pharmacological and rehabilitative procedures are effective in only about 38% of patients. However, the initial work-up should target identifying the pain source. Different kinds of pain may respond differently to treatments. For neuropathic pain, medications such as gabapentin, amitriptyline, and nortriptyline may ease the pain in some patients. Intravenous lidocaine may provide temporary pain relief. Intrathecal baclofen therapy may reduce chronic musculoskeletal pain associated with spasticity and improve the patient's quality of life. Intrathecal morphine and clonidine offer limited help to relieve the pain. DBS has been reported to be effective in some cases, but there is insufficient evidence to validate its routine use. Limited evidence exists for use of MCS (Previnaire et al., 2009). SCS lacks long-term efficacy for the relief of spasticity and pain in SCI and is believed not to be cost-effective. Dorsal root entry zone lesions and dorsal rhizotomy have also been used with limited success. Appropriate management of bowel or bladder dysfunction may help ease visceral pain. If an ascending syrinx is present, surgical drainage may be effective in relieving the pain.

## Pain in Multiple Sclerosis

Pain is a common symptom in multiple sclerosis (MS). The prevalence of pain in this disease is higher than initially expected; some studies estimate it to be up to 86% (Bermejo et al., 2010), depending on the sample and specific questions used to assess the incidence and severity of pain. Osterberg et al. (2005) studied pain syndromes in 429 patients with definite MS, and 58% reported pain during the course of their disease; 100 (28%) had central pain, including 18 patients (5%) with TN. The majority of patients (87%) with central pain had symptoms located in the legs, while 31% were in the arms. Pain was mostly bilateral (76%) and constant. Aching, burning, and pricking were common qualities. Other reported pain syndromes in MS include the Lhermitte sign, dysesthetic pain, back pain, headache, and painful tonic spasms. Chronic pain in MS was found to have no significant relationship to gender, age of onset, disease duration, or disease course. Chronic pain can have a significant negative impact on functions in persons with MS, such as the ability to engage in household work and psychological functioning. Chronic pain is significantly related to anxiety and depression in females. In the long-term care facility, residents with MS are more physically disabled and experience more frequent pain and a higher prevalence of pressure ulcers and depression than residents without MS.

Though pain affects a high percentage of patients with MS, its pathophysiology is unknown, and few studies have been conducted to investigate the treatment of pain in MS. The following principles are currently recommended for treatment of MS-related pain:

1. For pain directly related to MS, such as TN, carbamazepine is the first choice. Lamotrigine, gabapentin, oxcarbazepine, and other anticonvulsants may also be used. Painful "burning" dysesthesia may be treated with tricyclic antidepressants or carbamazepine. Further options include gabapentin or lamotrigine.
2. Pain related to spasticity may improve with adequate physiotherapy. Drug treatment includes antispastic agents like oral baclofen or tizanidine. In severe cases, intrathecal baclofen and botulinum toxin injections merit consideration.
3. Pain due to subcutaneous injections of β-interferons or glatiramer acetate may be reduced by optimizing the injection technique and by local cooling. Systemic side effects of interferons (e.g., myalgias) could be reduced by paracetamol or ibuprofen.

Cannabis is legally used in some states in the United States to treat pain. European studies indicate that cannabis-based medicines are effective in reducing pain and sleep disturbance in patients with MS-related central neuropathic pain and are mostly well tolerated (Rog et al., 2005; Thaera et al., 2009). Oral ketamine, an NMDA receptor antagonist, has also been reported to be effective in the treatment of pain and allodynia associated with MS.

## Phantom-Limb Pain and Stump Pain

*Phantom-limb pain* describes the pain in a body part that is no longer present, which occurs in 50%–80% of all amputees. Pain can have several different qualities, such as stabbing, throbbing, burning, or cramping. It seems to be more intense in the distal portions of the phantom limb. This pain may be related to a certain position or movement of the phantom and may be elicited or exacerbated by a range of physical factors (e.g., changes in weather or pressure on the residual limb) and psychological factors (e.g., emotional stress). It is more likely to occur if the individual had chronic pain before the amputation. Pain in the phantom is often similar to the pain felt in the limb before amputation. Phantom pain is most common after the amputation of an arm or leg, but it may also occur after the surgical removal of other body parts such as breast, rectum, penis, testicle, eye, tongue, or teeth. About 30% of persons with amputation report the feeling of *telescoping*, the retraction of the phantom toward the residual limb, and in many cases the disappearance of the phantom into the limb. This may be accompanied by a shrinking of the limb. Recent evidence suggests that telescoping is associated with more phantom-limb pain.

Phantom-limb pain is commonly confused with pain in the area adjacent to the amputated body part. This pain is referred to as *residual-limb* or *stump pain*. Patients may report severe "knife-stabbing" or sharp pain at the end of the amputated limb. Formation of a neuroma or pressure lesions of the stump may exacerbate stump pain. Physical examination may reveal the existence of a neuroma; it is usually very sensitive to touch or pressure. However, stump pain may coexist with phantom-limb pain.

Changes along the neuroaxis may contribute to the experience of phantom-limb pain. Spinal mechanisms are characterized by increased excitability of the dorsal horn neurons, reduction of inhibitory processes, and structural changes at the central nerve endings of the primary sensory neurons, interneurons, and the projection neurons. Supraspinal changes related to phantom-limb pain involve the brainstem, thalamus, and cortex. Reorganization of the somatosensory cortex of the human cerebral cortex in amputees has been supported by findings from several imaging studies. People with arm or hand amputations show a shift of the mouth into the hand representation in the primary somatosensory cortex (Woodhouse, 2005). Studies in human amputees have shown that reorganizational changes also occur at the thalamic level and are closely related to the perception of phantom limbs and phantom-limb pain. Neuroma in the stump may be more responsible for stump pain than phantom-limb pain. However, abnormal input originating from a neuroma in the residual limb may increase the amount of central reorganization, enhancing the chance of phantom-limb pain. Psychological factors play a role in the modulation of phantom-limb pain; the pain may be exacerbated by stress. Patients who lack coping strategies, fear the worst, or receive less social support tend to report more phantom-limb pain.

Treatment for phantom-limb pain is difficult. Although tricyclic antidepressants and sodium channel blockers are treatments of choice for neuropathic pain, no controlled studies exist of these agents for phantom-limb pain. Opioids, calcitonin, and ketamine have proven to be effective in reducing phantom-limb pain in controlled studies. Transcutaneous electrical nerve stimulator (TENS) may have a minor effect. A maximum benefit of about 30% has been reported from treatments such as local anesthesia, far-infrared rays, sympathectomy, dorsal root entry-zone lesions, cordotomy, rhizotomy, neurostimulation methods, or pharmacological interventions such as anticonvulsants, barbiturates, antidepressants, neuroleptics, and muscle relaxants. Use of a myoelectric prosthesis may alleviate cortical reorganization and phantom-limb pain, and DBS has also been reported to treat phantom-limb pain. Mirror therapy has been studied, but, to date, there is only circumstantial evidence for the effectiveness of mirror therapy in treating phantom pain; more studies are needed to support its clinical use.

## SUMMARY

Treatment of chronic pain conditions remains a challenge. However, recent advances in basic scientific research and clinical studies have provided clinicians with more insight regarding the mechanism and clinical features of chronic pain conditions. Advances in clinical technologies have provided new hope in the treatment of some refractory pain conditions previously regarded as impossible. With a combination of multidisciplinary pain treatment modalities, a majority of pain conditions may be alleviated or managed. The future of pain management requires more physicians, including neurologists, to contribute diagnostic and therapeutic skills to fulfill the needs of patients.

### Center for Disease Control and Prevention Opioid Guidelines

Centers for Disease Control and Prevention recommendations for prescribing opioids for chronic pain outside of active cancer, palliative, and end-of-life care.

Determining When to Initiate or Continue Opioids for Chronic Pain

1. Nonpharmacologic therapy and nonopioid pharmacologic therapy are preferred for chronic pain. Clinicians should consider opioid therapy only if expected benefits for both pain and function are anticipated to outweigh risks to the patient. If opioids are used, they should be combined with nonpharmacologic therapy and nonopioid pharmacologic therapy, as appropriate.
2. Before starting opioid therapy for chronic pain, clinicians should establish treatment goals with all patients, including realistic goals for pain and function, and should consider how therapy will be discontinued if benefits do not outweigh risks. Clinicians should continue opioid therapy only if there is clinically meaningful improvement in pain and function that outweighs risks to patient safety.
3. Before starting and periodically during opioid therapy, clinicians should discuss with patients known risks and realistic benefits of opioid therapy and patient and clinician responsibilities for managing therapy.

Opioid Selection, Dosage, Duration, Follow-up, and Discontinuation

4. When starting opioid therapy for chronic pain, clinicians should prescribe immediate-release opioids instead of extended-release/long-acting (ER/LA) opioids.
5. When opioids are started, clinicians should prescribe the lowest effective dosage. Clinicians should use caution when prescribing opioids at any dosage, should carefully reassess evidence of individual benefits and risks when increasing dosage to 50 morphine milligram equivalents (MME) or more per day, and should avoid increasing dosage to 90 MME or more per day or carefully justify a decision to titrate dosage to 90 MME or more per day.
6. Long-term opioid use often begins with treatment of acute pain. When opioids are used for acute pain, clinicians should prescribe the lowest effective dose of immediate-release opioids and should prescribe no greater quantity than needed for the expected duration of pain severe enough to require opioids. Three days or less will often be sufficient; more than 7 days will rarely be needed.
7. Clinicians should evaluate benefits and harms with patients within 1–4 weeks of starting opioid therapy for chronic pain or of dose escalation. Clinicians should evaluate benefits and harms of continued therapy with patients every 3 months or more frequently. If benefits do not outweigh harms of continued opioid therapy, clinicians should optimize therapies and work with patients to taper opioids to lower dosages or to taper and discontinue opioids.

Assessing Risk and Addressing Harms of Opioid Use

8. Before starting and periodically during continuation of opioid therapy, clinicians should evaluate risk factors for opioid-related harms. Clinicians should incorporate into the management plan strategies to mitigate risk, including considering offering naloxone when factors that increase risk for opioid overdose, such as history of overdose, history of substance use disorder, higher opioid dosages (≥50 MME/day), or concurrent benzodiazepine use are present.
9. Clinicians should review the patient's history of controlled substance prescriptions using state prescription drug monitoring program (PDMP) data to determine whether the patient is receiving opioid dosages or dangerous combinations that put him or her at high risk for overdose. Clinicians should review PDMP data when starting opioid therapy for chronic pain and periodically during opioid therapy for chronic pain, ranging from every prescription to every 3 months.
10. When prescribing opioids for chronic pain, clinicians should use urine drug testing before starting opioid therapy and consider urine drug testing at least annually to assess for prescribed medications as well as other controlled prescription drugs and illicit drugs.
11. Clinicians should avoid prescribing opioid pain medication and benzodiazepines concurrently whenever possible.
12. Clinicians should offer or arrange evidence-based treatment (usually medication-assisted treatment with buprenorphine or methadone in combination with behavioral therapies) for patients with opioid use disorder.

All recommendations are category A (apply to all patients outside of active cancer treatment, palliative care, and end-of-life care) except recommendation 10 (designated category B, with individual decision making required); detailed ratings of the evidence supporting the recommendations are provided in the full guideline publication.

*From Friedly, J.L., Comstock, B.A., Turner, J.A., Heagerty, P.J., Deyo, R.A., Sullivan, S.D., et al., 2014. A randomized trial of epidural glucocorticoid injections for spinal stenosis. N Engl J Med. 371 (1), 11–21; Herd, C.P., Tomlinson, C.L., Rick, C., Scotton, W.J., Edwards, J., Ives, N.J., et al., 2019. Cochrane systematic review and meta-analysis of botulinum toxin for the prevention of migraine. BMJ Open. 9 (7), e027953.*

***The complete reference list is available online at https://expertconsult.inkling.com/.*** 

53

# Neurointensive Care

*Alejandro A. Rabinstein, Sherri A. Braksick*

## OUTLINE



Neurocritical care is a discipline devoted to the application of critical care principles to seriously ill patients with acute neurological or neurosurgical conditions and has become one of the most rapidly growing subspecialties of neurology in recent years. Neurological-neurosurgical (or neuroscience) intensive care units (NICUs) are staffed by clinicians with solid knowledge of the principles of intensive care unit (ICU) management (mechanical ventilation, hemodynamic monitoring, nutrition, infection control and antibiotic prescription, general postoperative care, etc.) and specific interest in the treatment of acute neurological and neurosurgical diseases. In-depth knowledge of acute neurology is the sine qua non to mastery of the job.

Patients admitted to a NICU have central or peripheral nervous system dysfunction as a consequence of a primary neurological condition or as a complication of systemic illness. The most common diagnoses encountered in the NICU are acute ischemic strokes, intracerebral hemorrhage (ICH), subarachnoid hemorrhage (SAH), traumatic brain injury (TBI), brain tumors, elevated intracranial pressure (ICP; from any of the previous or other conditions), spinal cord injury, central nervous system (CNS) infections (meningitis, encephalitis, brain abscesses), status epilepticus, neuromuscular respiratory failure, and postoperative care (either after open neurosurgery or an endovascular procedure). Management of each of these conditions demands specific training that focuses on neurological recovery. Principles of general ICU care are applicable but must be adjusted accordingly.

## CLINICAL ASSESSMENT OF CRITICALLY ILL NEUROLOGICAL PATIENTS

The practice of neurology in the ICU demands specific clinical skills for timely and effective patient assessment. Since it is often impossible to gather direct history from the patient and the neurological examination must necessarily be more focused, attention to detail becomes crucial. Time for examination is very limited in neurological emergencies, and patients are often unconscious, sedated, acutely distressed, or confused and agitated. Physical findings may change rapidly, but a proficient physical examination remains central to determining diagnosis and prognosis in these critically ill patients.

The neurological examination for a NICU patient should always begin by defining the level and content of consciousness. *Level of consciousness* describes the patient's degree of arousal or wakefulness. Scales are useful for facilitating communication and monitoring changes over serial examinations; the Glasgow Coma Scale (GCS) is the most widely used (Teasdale et al., 1974). However, it loses accuracy in patients who are intubated or develop cerebral ptosis (inability or only partial ability to open the eyes [by contracting the frontalis muscle] because a brain lesion impairs control of eye-opening mechanisms) and fails to provide information on brainstem function and respiratory status. The FOUR Score addresses these shortcomings, has been validated in various patient populations, and merits consideration as an alternative (Wijdicks et al., 2005; Fig. 53.1). For patients with localized structural brain diseases, the National Institutes of Health (NIH) Stroke Scale may be used to grade and track focal neurological deficits.

In patients with altered consciousness, the results of one of these scales should be complemented with documentation of additional neurological features. A detailed description of movements of the eyes, gaze deviation, brainstem reflexes (pupillary light reactions, corneal, oculocephalic, oculovestibular, gag, cough), spontaneous movements and motor responses to pain, lateralizing signs, and breathing pattern must be recorded. In patients with delirium, the clinician must note the predominant behavioral abnormalities, degree of motor activity, and ability to interact with the environment. It is always important to dedicate special attention to any abnormal or adventitious movements, since seizures in critically ill patients may

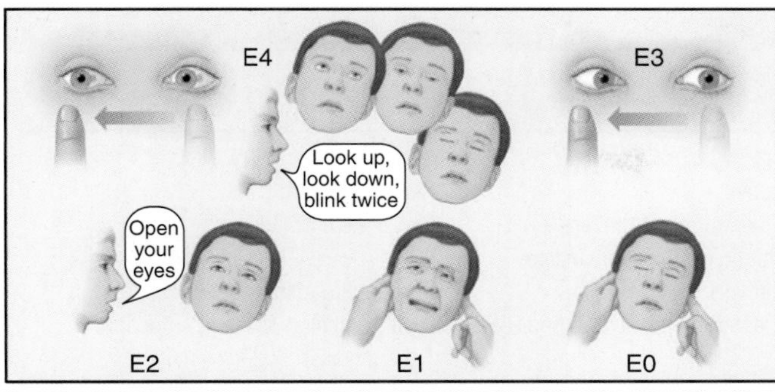


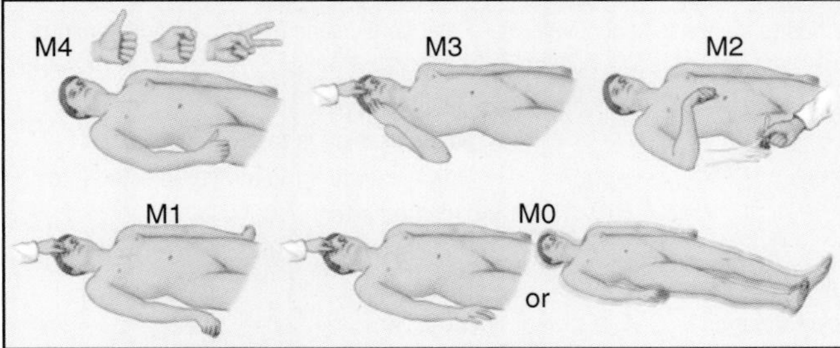


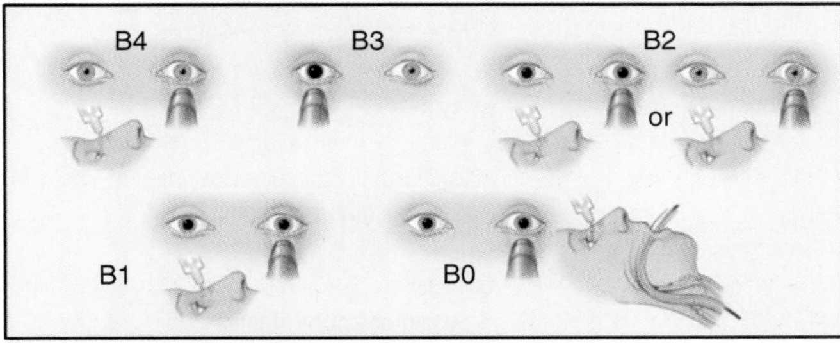


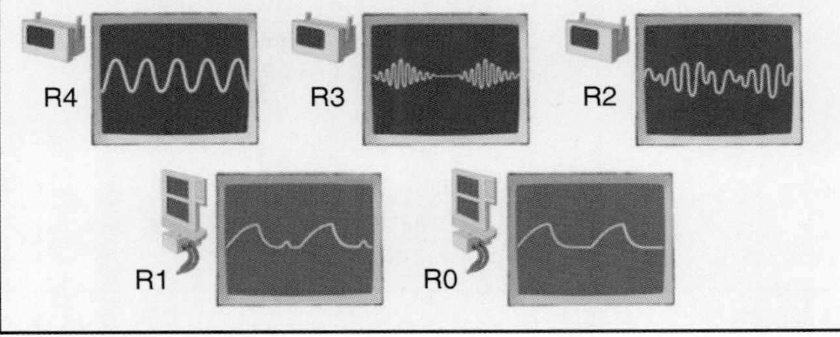


**Fig. 53.1** The FOUR Score: Scale for Assessing Coma in the Neurological-Neurosurgical Intensive Care Unit. *E: eye examination. E4,* eyelids open or opened and eyes tracking and eyelids blinking to command; *E3,* eyelids open but eyes not tracking; *E2,* eyelids closed but open to loud voice; *E1,* eyelids closed but open to pain; *E0,* eyelids remain closed with pain. *M: motor response. M4,* thumbs up, fist, or peace sign to command; *M3,* localizing to pain; *M2,* flexion response to pain; *M1,* extensor response to pain; *M0,* no response to pain or generalized myoclonic status. *B: brainstem reflexes. B4,* pupillary and corneal reflexes present; *B3,* one pupil dilated and fixed; *B2,* pupillary or corneal reflexes absent; *B1,* pupillary and corneal reflexes absent; *B0,* absent pupillary, corneal, and cough reflexes. *R: respiration. R4,* not intubated, with regular breathing pattern; *R3,* not intubated, with Cheyne-Stokes breathing pattern; *R2,* not intubated, with irregular breathing pattern; *R1,* intubated, breathing above the ventilator rate; *R0,* intubated, breathing at ventilator rate or apnea.

present with very subtle motor manifestations (e.g., nystagmoid eye movements). Fundoscopy may also offer valuable information and should be attempted; however, to avoid confounding future pupillary evaluations, mydriatic agents should not be administered. The reader is referred to Chapters 4 and 5 for further information relative to clinical evaluation of comatose and delirious patients.

Another essential aspect of the examination in critically ill patients is evaluating neuromuscular respiratory weakness. Timely recognition of signs of impending neuromuscular respiratory failure may avoid potentially devastating complications. Among them, use of accessory muscles and paradoxical breathing pattern are most indicative of problems. *Paradoxical breathing* is defined as the loss of synchronicity in chest and abdominal movements during respiration (i.e., abnormal sinking of the abdomen during inspiration) and represents an unequivocal sign of diaphragmatic failure (Rabinstein and Wijdicks, 2003b).

It is important to integrate the information provided by the neurological examination with data from the general systemic examination, vital signs monitoring, and other physiological variables, including laboratory results. Alterations in heart rate, respiration, and blood pressure (BP), for example, often result from brain herniation.

## MONITORING IN THE NEUROLOGICAL INTENSIVE CARE UNIT

### Systemic Monitoring

Systemic monitoring in the NICU typically includes cardiac telemetry, frequent scheduled noninvasive BP measurements (by automatic cuff inflation) or continuous invasive arterial BP recording, pulse oximetry, and core body temperature. Continuous arterial BP monitoring is accomplished by inserting an indwelling cannula into a medium-caliber artery (e.g., radial arterial line). The invasiveness of the procedure is justified by the precise real-time information it provides. Continuous arterial BP monitoring is especially recommended in patients treated with induced hypertension (e.g., symptomatic vasospasm SAH), cases requiring very strict BP control to avoid hemorrhagic complications (e.g., ruptured arteriovenous malformations), patients with hypotension (e.g., shock), compromised cerebral perfusion pressure (CPP; e.g., TBI with raised ICP), or autonomic instability (e.g., Guillain-Barré syndrome [GBS]). Arterial lines provide the additional advantage of eliminating the need for repeated arterial punctures to measure arterial blood gases. However, although generally safe, placement of an arterial line may be complicated by local infection, leading to bacteremia, or thrombosis with a risk of digital ischemia. Careful attention to proper technique and adherence to strict sterile conditions during placement and manipulation of the catheter are mandatory (Tegtmeyer et al., 2006).

The most accurate method of measuring core body temperature is a pulmonary artery catheter thermistor, but since most patients in the NICU do not require pulmonary artery catheter insertion, bladder or rectal probes are most frequently used. Bladder and rectal probes correlate well with pulmonary artery catheter thermistor readings, but there is a lag in the detection of temperature changes by the probes. The site of temperature recording becomes particularly important in patients treated with cooling measures. Thus monitoring esophageal temperatures is recommended when certain intravascular cooling devices are being used.

Central venous catheters allow monitoring of central venous pressure while also providing access for fluid and drug administration. They are, however, a frequent source of infection. Rigorous sterile techniques at the time of catheter insertion, cutaneous antisepsis with chlorhexidine (rather than povidone-iodine), topical application of anti-infective ointment or a chlorhexidine-impregnated dressing to the insertion site, and catheters with an anti-infective surface may reduce the risk of catheter-related bloodstream infection (Safdar et al., 2002). The role of pulmonary artery catheters in ICUs is shrinking as studies consistently demonstrate that their use is associated with higher rates of complications without improving patient outcome (Richard et al.,

TABLE 53.1 **Brain Monitoring Methods**

| Method | Spatial Resolution | Temporal Resolution | Purpose | Advantages | Disadvantages |
|---|---|---|---|---|---|
| ICP | Global | Continuous | Measure intracranial pressure | Reliable<br>Quantitative<br>Allows monitoring of CPP and calculation of secondary indices | Invasive<br>Risk of infection<br>Risk of hemorrhage |
| Jugular oximetry ($SjvO_2$) | Global | Continuous | Measure adequacy of hemispheric oxygenation | Quantitative<br>Allows monitoring of $AVDO_2$ and $O_2ER$ | Susceptible to artifacts<br>Local complications (e.g., infection, thrombosis) |
| EEG | Global | Continuous | Monitoring electrical brain activity<br>Detection of seizures | Technique well standardized<br>Only method to diagnose nonconvulsive seizures | Qualitative<br>Relatively insensitive to secondary insults |
| SSEP | Global | Continuous | Monitoring integrity of sensory pathways | Technique well standardized<br>Simple | Qualitative<br>Fairly insensitive to secondary insults |
| Bedside Xe-133 CBF | Regional | Discontinuous | Measure hemispheric CBF | Quantitative | Only accurate if radiotracer injected into carotid artery<br>Radioactivity |
| Laser Doppler flowmetry | Local | Continuous | Measure cortical CBF | Accurate<br>Dynamic information | Qualitative<br>Invasive<br>Susceptible to artifacts<br>Monitors only 1–2 $mm^3$ of tissue |
| Thermal diffusion flowmetry | Local | Continuous | Measure cortical CBF | Simple<br>Dynamic information | Qualitative<br>Invasive<br>Monitors small volume of tissue |
| TCD | Regional | Continuous | Measure CBF velocities | Simple<br>Noninvasive<br>Allows measuring PI, VMR | Qualitative, indirect assessment of CBF, technically challenging. |
| Brain tissue $Po_2$ | Local | Continuous | Measure cerebral oxygenation | Quantitative<br>Sensitive<br>Probes also measure brain temperature | Invasive<br>Susceptible to artifacts<br>Monitors small volume of tissue |
| NIRS | Local | Continuous | Measure cerebral oxygenation | Noninvasive | Measures only relative changes<br>Susceptible to artifacts |
| Microdialysis | Local | Discontinuous | Measure cerebral metabolism | Sensitive<br>Quantitative | Invasive<br>Complicated technique<br>Labor intensive<br>Unclear which is the best parameter to monitor |

*$AVDO_2$,* Arteriovenous oxygen difference; *CBF,* cerebral blood flow; *CPP,* cerebral perfusion pressure; *EEG,* electroencephalogram; *ICP,* intracranial pressure; *NIRS,* near-infrared spectroscopy; *$O_2ER$,* oxygen extraction rate; *PI,* pulsatility index; *$Po_2$,* partial pressure of oxygen; *TCD,* transcranial Doppler; *$SjvO_2$,* jugular venous oxygen saturation; *SSEP,* somatosensory evoked potentials; *VMR,* vasomotor reactivity.

2003; Sandham et al., 2003; Wheeler et al., 2006). Newer devices for hemodynamic monitoring have become available. For instance, the Pulse index Continuous Cardiac Monitoring (PiCCO) system integrates static and dynamic hemodynamic data using a combination of transcardiopulmonary thermodilution and pulse contour analysis (Litton and Morgan, 2012); others, such as the Non-invasive Volume Management to Guide Clinical Decision Making (NICOM) device, use proprietary formulas to determine cardiac parameters (e.g., stroke volume, stroke volume variation, etc.) that correlate with thermodilution-obtained clinical information (Squara et al., 2007). Although these devices are pathophysiologically sound, their value in improving patient care remains to be firmly established in critical care patients in general and neurocritical care patients in particular.

## Brain Monitoring

The neurological examination may lack sensitivity in critically ill patients who have depressed levels of consciousness due to brain disease or from the effect of sedative medications. Brain monitoring methods developed and refined over the past several decades may provide additional valuable information in these cases. These techniques offer real-time data, unlike imaging modalities that represent only "snapshots" of the patient's condition at certain points in time. Therefore brain monitoring techniques are better suited to assess dynamic changes in the neurological status of critically ill patients.

Multiple brain monitoring methods are now available. They are most useful when they are applied in combination, a practice known as *multimodality monitoring* (Diedler and Czosnyka, 2010). It is important to be aware, however, that the endpoints of most studies validating the use of brain monitoring methods have been surrogate physiological measures rather than actual assessments of patients' functional outcome. In fact, there is no class I evidence proving that the use of multimodality brain monitoring results in improved clinical outcomes. Currently the clinical application of brain monitoring techniques is restricted to large centers, especially those treating numerous TBI patients.

Methods for cerebral monitoring are divided into three main categories according to their spatial resolution: global, regional, and local brain monitoring (Table 53.1). Global brain monitoring techniques

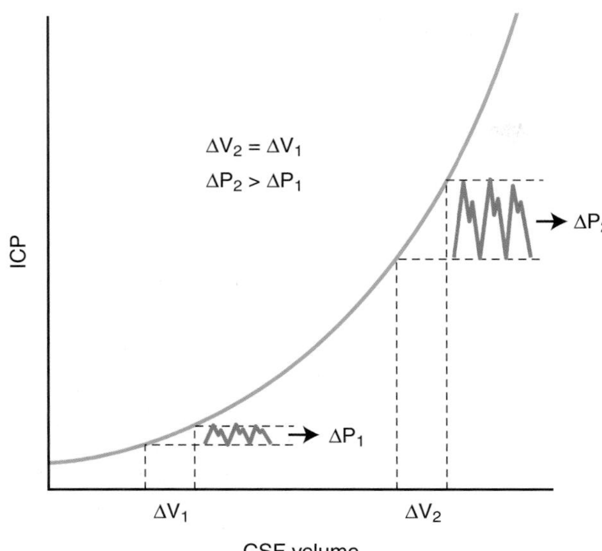


**Fig. 53.2 Relationship Between Pressure and Volume Changes in the Intracranial Compartment.** *CSF,* Cerebrospinal fluid; *ICP,* intracranial pressure; *P,* pressure; *V,* volume.

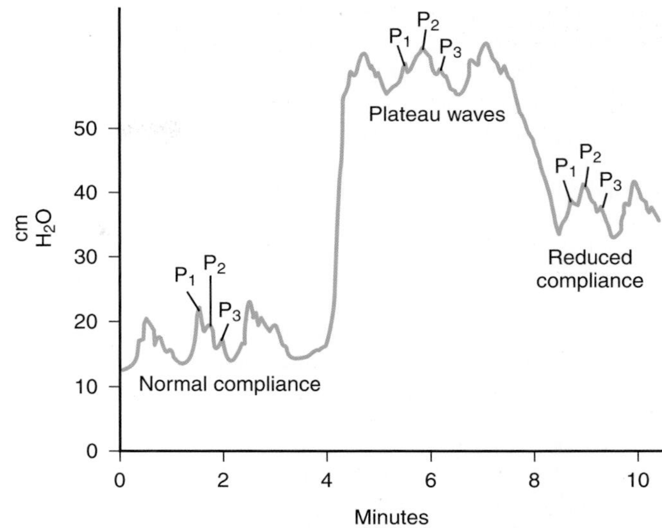


**Fig. 53.3 Intracranial Pressure Tracings in the Setting of Normal and Reduced Compliance.** Plateau waves (Lundberg A waves) is seen in the center of the figure.

measure ICP, CPP, electrical potentials, and venous oxygen saturation. Regional and local brain monitoring methods include cerebral blood flow (CBF), CBF velocities (BFVs), brain tissue metabolism, temperature, and oxygenation.

## GLOBAL BRAIN MONITORING TECHNIQUES

### Intracranial Pressure Monitoring

The intracranial space is occupied by three constituent compartments: the brain (accounting for 80%–90% of the intracranial volume), the blood, and the cerebrospinal fluid (CSF). Under normal conditions, local CNS pressure gradients are equilibrated if the craniospinal CSF circulation is patent. Because the skull is rigid, any expansion of one of these compartments must be compensated by a reduction in size of the others (a physiological principle known as the *Monro-Kellie doctrine*) if ICP is to remain constant. If these compensations are insufficient, ICP rises. Small increases in intracranial volume can initially be accommodated with little or no effect on the ICP, but as more volume is added, intracranial compliance falls until it reaches a critical point beyond which a minimal increase in volume causes an exponential rise in ICP. This pressure-volume relationship is depicted in Fig. 53.2. In other words, as long as CSF circulation is not obstructed and there remains a pressure gradient from the subarachnoid space to the dural venous sinuses, the initial physiological response to an increase in brain volume is a reduction in the CSF and venous blood volumes by shifting these fluids out of the intracranial space. Once these compensatory mechanisms are exhausted, the system becomes noncompliant and further increases in intracranial volume compromise arterial blood flow and eventually lead to the herniation of brain tissue.

Normal ICP in a supine individual is less than 15 mm Hg when measured at the level of the foramen of Monro (typically referenced to the tragus). Levels exceeding 20–25 mm Hg define a generally accepted threshold of raised ICP, which deserves treatment. Knowing the actual ICP is a prerequisite to determining CPP, which is defined by the relationship between mean ICP and mean arterial pressure (MAP) as follows: CPP = MAP − ICP.

It has also been argued that the main purpose of ICP monitoring is maintenance of adequate CPP because the latter may be more related to secondary ischemic injury (Rosner et al., 1995). The relative importance of ICP and CPP as main targets of therapy remains a matter of debate.

ICP is pulsatile and the pressure waveforms provide useful information beyond numbers measured. ICP waveforms are made of three distinct components: heart pulse waves, respiratory waves, and slow vasogenic waves (Lundberg B waves), each with a characteristic frequency. The normal ICP waveform consists of three peaks (Fig. 53.3). $P_1$, the first and generally the tallest peak, is also known as the "percussion wave." $P_2$ (the tidal wave) and $P_3$ (the dicrotic wave) are normally smaller peaks, and the notch between them corresponds to the dicrotic notch of the arterial waveform.

ICP can be monitored using intraparenchymal, intraventricular, epidural, or subdural devices. Intraventricular monitoring remains the gold standard because of its precision. It consists of a ventricular catheter connected to an external transducer that allows continuous ICP readings, as long as the catheter is clamped. Advantages of this technique are the feasibility of repetition measurements and that the measurement corresponds to the transmitted systolic BP. As ICP increases, $P_2$ and $P_3$ rise and eventually surpass $P_1$. Ultimately, with continued elevation of ICP, the waveform loses distinct peaks and assumes a triangular morphology. Intracranial pathology leading to sustained elevations of ICP may produce *plateau waves*, also known as *Lundberg* (see Fig. 53.3). These waves reflect a sudden dramatic rise in ICP to levels of 40–100 mm Hg, often lasting 5–20 minutes. Plateau waves indicate critically low intracranial compliance leading to marked changes in ICP, even with very small variations in intracranial volume. Although their pathophysiology is not fully elucidated, plateau waves are thought to be generated by brief episodes of decreased CPP (often caused by systemic hypotension), leading to exaggerated cerebral vasodilation, increased blood volume, and increased ICP (Rosner and Becker, 1984). This further decreases CPP and contributes to a detrimental cycle unless broken by a sudden surge of hypertension (Cushing response) or another therapeutic intervention, such as hyperventilation, to cause cerebral arteriolar vasoconstriction.

ICP can be monitored using intraparenchymal, intraventricular, epidural, or subdural devices. Intraventricular monitoring remains the gold standard because of its precision. It consists of a ventricular catheter connected to an external transducer that allows continuous ICP readings as long as the catheter is clamped. Advantages of this technique are the feasibility of repetitive calibration to achieve accurate and reliable ICP measurements and allowing external drainage of CSF for the treatment of raised ICP. Hence, ventricular monitoring is indicated in patients with hydrocephalus and is often preferred in those with refractory intracranial hypertension. Major drawbacks are the difficulty of inserting a catheter in patients with brain edema and small ventricles, a higher risk of infection (the rate of ventriculitis is 3%–8% and it increases with duration of the ventriculostomy; Flibotte et al., 2004; Holloway et al., 1996; Martinez-Manas et al., 2000), risk of bleeding at the time of catheter placement (especially in patients with underlying coagulopathy or recent use of antithrombotics), and system malfunction (dampening of the waveform may be caused by apposition of the catheter tip against the ventricular wall or obstruction of the catheter by a blood clot or air bubble). Furthermore, ICP monitoring by ventricular catheters allows continuous monitoring of ICP only if the catheter is clamped. Spikes of raised ICP may go undetected by ventricular catheters that are open to drain. Risks may be minimized by careful placement of the catheter and maintenance of the system under strict sterile conditions, use of antibiotic prophylaxis (e.g., cefazolin 2 g every 8 hours from the time of catheter insertion until 24–48 hours after its removal, or use of antibiotic-impregnated catheters; Flibotte et al., 2004), and withdrawal of the catheter as soon as possible (Holloway et al., 1996). Exchange of the catheter every 5 days, although a common practice, does not appear to decrease the risk of infection (Holloway et al., 1996; Lozier et al., 2002); in fact, repeated catheter insertions have been found to be associated with a higher risk of ventriculitis (Arabi et al., 2005).

Intraparenchymal fiberoptic monitors are also quite accurate. As compared with intraventricular catheters, the measurements provided by intraparenchymal monitors differ on average by ±2 to 5 mm Hg. Advantages of this monitoring system include simple and safe insertion technique, easy maintenance, continuous ICP measurements, relative lack of substantial drift (even after several days), and low risk of infection. Disadvantages include high cost; technical complications (e.g., breakage of the optical fiber); and, most importantly, inability to drain CSF. Epidural and subdural monitors are less reliable and therefore rarely used. ICP can be estimated using noninvasive techniques such as transcranial Doppler (TCD) to measure changes in arterial or venous blood flow velocity or analyze the pulse waveform, displacement of the tympanic membrane, or diameter of the optic nerve sheath by transorbital ultrasound or magnetic resonance imaging (MRI). Ultrasound technology is an attractive tool as there are essentially no adverse effects with this method, but its use can be substantially limited by technique and provider experience. These methods are not currently precise enough to be used clinically for ICP management decisions but may be useful in the future, particularly for screening and selecting patients for invasive monitoring.

Measuring ICP can provide additional useful information because it allows the calculation of secondary indices about cerebral physiology. For example, the cerebrovascular pressure reactivity index (PRx), a moving correlation coefficient between mean ICP and slow fluctuations in MAP (Czosnyka et al., 1997), reflects the ability of smooth muscle within cerebral arteriolar walls to react to changes in transmural pressure. An increase in pressure normally causes cerebral arterial and arteriolar vasoconstriction, which leads to decreased cerebral blood volume and thus decreased ICP. PRx estimates CBF autoregulation status (although it is not synonymous), and its value ranges from −1 to +1. Positive values indicate impaired autoregulation and have been correlated with clinical outcomes in TBI (Sorrentino et al., 2012). Another example of an ICP-derived index is RAP, the correlation between the amplitude of ICP to the mean pressure. RAP close to 0 indicates little or no change in the mean ICP in response to increases in volume, which indicates good pressure-volume compensatory reserve. When RAP is close to +1, the amplitude varies directly with ICP, suggesting low compensatory reserve and a shift to the right on the intracranial compliance curve (Czosnyka and Pickard, 2004).

The previous Brain Trauma Foundation recommendations for ICP monitoring in patients with severe TBI, a GCS sum score below 9, and an abnormal computed tomography (CT) scan or a normal CT scan with two or more of the following criteria—age older than 40, unilateral or bilateral motor posturing, and systolic BP less than 90 mm Hg—have been less emphasized in the most current management guideline (Brain Trauma Foundation, 2016) due to the lack of high-quality evidence to support them. A recent study in South America evaluated the benefit of ICP monitoring—where patients were treated based on their clinical examination and neuroimaging as compared with those with an ICP monitor to target a normal ICP measurement—and found no difference in clinical outcome (Chestnut et al., 2012). The ideal patient who requires ICP monitoring following TBI has yet to be determined, and the decision to place an invasive ICP monitor is at the discretion of the treating neurosurgeon. In patients without TBI, some experts advocate monitoring ICP in comatose patients with a large intracranial mass lesion (hematoma, abscess, large infarctions, etc.) causing a radiologically documented tissue shift. Patients with SAH, ICH, or cerebellar ischemic or hemorrhagic strokes producing acute hydrocephalus typically have their ICP monitored once a ventriculostomy has been placed, although the catheter is often placed primarily for drainage purposes.

### Jugular Bulb Oximetry

Jugular bulb oximetry measures the oxygen saturation of venous blood returning from the brain (normal 50%–65%) by means of a fiberoptic catheter (Feldman and Robertson, 1997). The main goal of jugular venous oxygen saturation ($SjvO_2$) monitoring is to provide a continuous measure of the changing balance between cerebral oxygen delivery and cerebral oxygen consumption. Simultaneous determination of $SjvO_2$ using the jugular bulb catheter and arterial oxygen saturation ($SaO_2$) allows for the calculation of the intracranial arteriovenous oxygen difference ($AVDO_2$; normal 24%–42%). Cerebral oxygen consumption can be calculated as the product of $AVDO_2$ and CBF. The cerebral oxygen extraction rate ($O_2ER$) is derived from the ratio of cerebral oxygen consumption to cerebral oxygen delivery.

Jugular venous desaturations denote relative reductions of global cerebral oxygenation. $SjvO_2$ below 50% for 15 minutes or more is deemed indicative of ischemia. $SjvO_2$ monitoring has been mostly tested in patients with severe TBI. In these patients, jugular venous desaturations have previously been shown to correlate with the occurrence of secondary brain insults and poor outcome (Gopinath et al., 1994; Robertson et al., 1995). High $SjvO_2$ should not simply be equated with hyperemia; it may also be associated with poor outcome in comatose patients, possibly indicating lack of oxygen utilization after extensive neuronal death (Cormio et al., 1999). Favorable experience with jugular bulb oximetry has been reported in patients with SAH and ICH

(Heran et al., 2004), but interpreting $SjvO_2$ may be difficult in patients with severe unilateral hemispheric lesions. This technique is also used to monitor cerebral oxygenation during neurosurgical procedures.

Therapeutic interventions in response to information provided by jugular bulb oximetry have been proposed, including adjustment of the degree of hyperventilation, timing and intensity of osmotherapy, adjustment of MAP, and treatment of anemia (Macmillan and Andrews, 2000). There is no proof, however, that these interventions improve functional outcome; therefore jugular bulb oximetry is an uncommonly utilized monitoring method. As shown by the negative results observed in studies testing therapies guided by pulmonary artery catheters, the clinical value of aggressive interventions aimed at optimizing physiological parameters must be proven before we incorporate these into clinical practice.

Advantages of the jugular bulb catheter as a monitoring modality include the practicality of continuous bedside monitoring, the ability to confirm the oximeter reading by drawing blood through the catheter, and the numerous physiological parameters that can be derived from the $SjvO_2$ to ascertain cerebral oxygen balance. Disadvantages of the catheter include its susceptibility to positioning artifacts and the complications associated with catheter insertion, including carotid puncture, infection, accidental misplacement, and jugular thrombosis (Coplin et al., 1997, 1998; Latronico et al., 2000).

### Electroencephalography

Continuous bedside electroencephalography (EEG) monitoring is based on four of its major neurobiological features (Jordan, 1995): (1) its close relationship to cerebral metabolic rate, (2) its sensitivity in detecting hypoxic-ischemic neuronal dysfunction at an early stage, (3) its obvious primacy as a monitor of seizure activity, and (4) its value in cerebral localization. Continuous EEG recording has been advocated as a valuable tool for monitoring critically ill neurosurgical and neurological patients.

Despite the fact that the technical aspects of EEG application in the NICU do not differ greatly from the standard routine EEG, some factors are relatively unique to the ICU setting. The main differences are the many sources of electrical artifact (ventilators, intravenous pumps, dialysis machines, suctioning equipment) and the patient's inability to cooperate secondary to various degrees of encephalopathy. In addition, continuous bedside EEG monitoring requires EEG interpreters available to view the recording, frequently throughout the day, and specially trained nurses or technicians capable of recognizing meaningful changes in the tracing.

Status epilepticus is the most common indication for EEG monitoring because the clinical ascertainment of ongoing seizure activity is often obscured by the effect of sedatives and analgesic agents. The EEG is essential for monitoring the effects of treatment, especially when barbiturates or general anesthetics are administered to achieve a burst-suppression pattern. Detection of nonconvulsive seizures and nonconvulsive status epilepticus (NCSE) can be accomplished only by EEG monitoring. Timely diagnosis of NCSE is important because delayed recognition may be associated with increased mortality (Young et al., 1996).

Nonconvulsive seizures have been reported in up to one-third of unselected NICU patients, frequently involving the presence of NCSE (Jordan, 1995). Continuous EEG monitoring has documented nonconvulsive seizures after severe TBI, ischemic stroke, poor-grade SAH, ICH, encephalitis, and after termination of generalized convulsive status epilepticus (DeLorenzo et al., 1998; Dennis et al., 2002; Vespa et al., 1999,Viarasilpa et al., 2018). These events might exacerbate excitotoxic injury in vulnerable brains and have been associated with high mortality (Young et al., 1996). But although their prognostic value is fairly well established, the impact of aggressive treatment of nonconvulsive seizures on clinical outcome remains to be determined (Hirsch, 2004), as seizures may represent severe brain injury associated with a poor outcome independent of the presence of electrographic abnormalities.

Continuous EEG monitoring has also been used as an aid for the early detection of ischemia in patients with SAH who are at high risk for vasospasm (Claassen et al., 2006; Vespa et al., 1997), but there is not enough information to recommend continuous EEG for this indication. Intracortical EEG (based on the use of deep electrodes) may be substantially superior to scalp EEG for detecting changes related to secondary neurological insults in patients with various forms of acute brain injury (Waziri et al., 2009). Furthermore, recurrent cortical spreading depolarizations may exacerbate local brain hypoxia and cause a shift toward anaerobic metabolism in patients with TBI or SAH (Bosche et al., 2010; Sakowitz et al., 2013), but the value of monitoring for these changes with intracortical EEG remains to be conclusively determined.

Continuous EEG can also be useful for the recognition of nonconvulsive seizures and NCSE in patients with persistent coma of unknown cause (Claassen et al., 2013; Oddo et al., 2009). EEG may also help in the evaluation of toxic and metabolic encephalopathy. In these cases, EEG serves to substantiate the diagnosis by showing diffusely slow low-amplitude activity and often triphasic waves, but does not distinguish between various causes of the condition. EEG can also be used as a confirmatory test of brain death (Wijdicks, 2001). After cardiac arrest, near-complete suppression, burst-suppression, nonreactive alpha or theta rhythms (alpha or theta coma), status epilepticus, and generalized periodic complexes are considered malignant patterns (Rossetti et al., 2007; Synek, 1990). Although valuable for the prognostication of anoxic-ischemic encephalopathy, EEG data should not be interpreted in isolation in these patients (Wijdicks et al., 2006).

A position statement authored by the Critical Care Continuous EEG Task Force recommends continuous video EEG monitoring for many indications, including the detection of nonconvulsive seizures in patients with persistent encephalopathy and for the early detection of ischemia. The identified EEG abnormalities along the ictal-interictal continuum often seen on prolonged EEG monitoring have been shown to correlate with worse clinical outcome; however, as previously mentioned, the utility of treating these identified EEG abnormalities (secondary injury or a manifestation of the severity of the primary brain injury) is of unclear benefit (Herman et al., 2015). As technology advances, quantitative EEG will likely become more routinely used in interpretation of critical care EEG.

## REGIONAL/FOCAL BRAIN MONITORING TECHNIQUES

### Regional Cerebral Blood Flow Monitoring

A major focus in neurointensive care is to ensure that patients maintain adequate CBF. Unfortunately, CBF is not easily measured. Normal CBF in adult individuals ranges from 45 to 60 mL/100 g/min, and it is higher in the gray matter than in the white matter. Values below 10 mL/100 g/min are considered indicative of ischemia. Determinants of CBF include the status of brain metabolism, $Paco_2$, systemic BP, hematocrit, and cardiac output. Most of these determinants can be therapeutically manipulated by interventions such as the use of sedatives, changes in the ventilator setting, volume expansion, administration of vasoactive agents, blood transfusions, and inotropic medications. When information offered by CBF monitoring techniques is being interpreted, it is essential to understand the concept that CBF may be inappropriately low (i.e., metabolic demands exceed supply of blood flow, resulting in ischemia), appropriately low (i.e., metabolic demands are reduced and result in a coupled reduction in blood flow and oxygen consumption), inappropriately high (i.e., cerebral hyperemia), or appropriately high (i.e., situations of increased metabolic demand, such as seizures or fever). There are regional and local techniques for CBF monitoring. Regional modalities include (1) bedside xenon-133 intravenous injection technique, (2) stable xenon CT scan, (3) single-photon emission computed tomography (SPECT), (4) positron emission tomography (PET), (5) perfusion-weighted imaging by magnetic resonance imaging (PWI-MRI), and (6) CT perfusion scans.

The main disadvantage of most of these techniques is that they require transportation of the patient from the ICU to the location of the scanner. Consequently, they provide information about the status of CBF only at certain points in time, and CBF is a highly dynamic variable that may fluctuate extensively over time. The bedside xenon-133 technique is the only regional CBF monitoring modality that permits repeated testing in the NICU. However, it requires injection of small doses of the radioactive isotope. The xenon-CT technique involves transporting the patient to the CT scanner and administering nonradioactive xenon gas by inhalation. The inhaled gas can create a euphoric sensation, thus making this technique less desirable in agitated patients. SPECT, PET, MRI perfusion, and CT perfusion are valid options for assessing brain perfusion at a certain point in time. PET also allows measurement of the oxygen extraction fraction, which, when elevated, is a reliable indicator of hemodynamic failure and early ischemia. MRI scanning provides greater anatomical information and has the advantage of displaying areas of ischemia on diffusion-weighted imaging. CT perfusion is becoming increasingly available and offers quantifiable perfusion data. However, cumulative exposure to radiation limits the number of CT perfusion scans that can be safely performed for monitoring purposes.

Local CBF monitoring techniques include laser Doppler flowmetry and thermal diffusion flowmetry. Laser Doppler flowmetry is based on assessing the Doppler shift of low-power laser light captured by the moving red blood cells (red cell flux). It produces the continuous real-time flow output, which is linearly related to CBF, thus providing reliable information on local perfusion with excellent dynamic resolution. The main disadvantages of this technique, however, are its invasiveness (requires insertion of the probe via a burr hole), its susceptibility to movement artifact, its small sample volume (1–2 $mm^3$), and the qualitative nature of the information provided (this technique does not enable the quantification of CBF, and only relative changes can be assessed). Thermal diffusion flowmetry is used to estimate cortical blood flow by measuring changes in the temperature gradient between two thermistors within a probe applied to the cortex. Advantages include its simplicity and continuous measurement without using ionizing radiation. However, this technique can monitor only a 4- to 5-mm region of tissue, does not provide absolute measures of CBF, and has not been sufficiently standardized to be recommended for clinical practice.

TCD ultrasonography and various brain oxygenation monitoring techniques represent indirect measures of CBF monitoring.

## Transcranial Doppler Ultrasonography

TCD ultrasonography is a noninvasive technique used to evaluate mean CBF velocity in the large intracranial arteries at the level of the circle of Willis. TCD is easy to learn and use, noninvasive, and safe. It measures CBF velocity rather than CBF, and the linear relationship between CBF and BFV depends on the angle of insonation and a constant vessel diameter. Still, TCD provides a wealth of useful clinical information including the presence or absence of blood flow, its velocity (systolic, diastolic, and mean), and direction. It also allows calculation of the pulsatility index (PI = peak systolic velocity minus end-diastolic velocity divided by mean BFV), which represents the downstream resistance to blood flow. Increases in BFV are observed in patients with cerebral vasospasm, hyperventilation (which produces vasoconstriction), and anemia. Cerebral vasospasm may be distinguished from hyperdynamic status by measuring the hemispheric index or Lindegaard ratio (ratio of middle cerebral artery to extracranial internal carotid artery mean BFV; Lindegaard et al., 1989). A ratio greater than 3 is considered indicative of vasospasm; a low ratio is more suggestive of hyperemia. TCD also enables assessment of vasomotor reactivity (Ng et al., 2000). Impairment of vasomotor reactivity is well established as pointing to a poor prognosis in patients with TBI and may portend the occurrence of symptomatic vasospasm in patients with SAH (Czosnyka et al., 1997; Frontera et al., 2006b). TCD may also be used as a confirmatory test for the diagnosis of brain death (severely diminished mean cerebral BFV associated with absent diastolic flow, reversed flow, and severely elevated PI).

The diagnosis of cerebral vasospasm in patients with SAH remains the main indication of TCD monitoring in the NICU. Vasospasm in the territory of the middle cerebral artery is suspected when the mean BFV is greater than 120 cm/sec with a hemispheric index greater than 3 or an increment greater than 50 cm/sec within a 24-hour period (Suarez et al., 2002). A specialized headset enables continuous monitoring of BFV and may be a useful adjunct in monitoring patients at high risk for vasospasm. TCD monitoring in patients with cerebral vasospasm has generally good correlation with angiographic vasospasm and is comparable to conventional angiography in the prognostication of delayed ischemia in these patients, although neither technique is uniformly diagnostic (Rabinstein et al., 2004). The use of TCD as a noninvasive and safe test that can be performed at the bedside makes it an attractive tool for monitoring a critically ill neurological patient, but clinicians should be mindful that this modality is very dependent on technique, and only staff who are adequately trained and who routinely perform this study should complete the examination.

## Evoked Potentials

Evoked potentials have a more restricted role in the NICU (Moulton et al., 1998). The median nerve somatosensory evoked potential (SSEP) has been mostly used. Bilateral absence of the N20 response 1–3 days after cardiopulmonary resuscitation accurately predicts a poor chance of recovery of awareness (Zandbergen et al., 2006). Unfortunately, the presence of these responses after anoxic brain injury lacks meaningful prognostic value. The widespread use of therapeutic hypothermia after cardiac arrest may potentially confound the results of an SSEP study; therefore this test is best completed once patients have been returned to normothermia.

Continuous monitoring of brainstem evoked potentials and SSEPs is now technically feasible. However, the very few studies conducted using these modalities failed to demonstrate any value in the early recognition of secondary insults.

## Techniques for the Monitoring of Local Cerebral Oxygenation

Brain tissue oxygen probes and near-infrared spectroscopy (NIRS) allow assessment of local oxygenation. Brain tissue oxygen may be measured by invasive probes such as the Licox catheter. Apart from tissue partial pressure of oxygen ($Po_2$), this catheter enables the measurement of brain temperature. Brain tissue $Po_2$ measures the diffusion of dissolved plasma oxygen across the blood-brain barrier (rather than CBF, arterial delivery of oxygen, or brain metabolism) in a relatively small area of brain tissue ($\approx$15 $mm^3$) (Rosenthal et al., 2009). Factors that determine brain tissue $Po_2$ include $Pao_2$, arterial $Paco_2$, systemic BP, and CBF. Normal brain tissue $Po_2$ values range

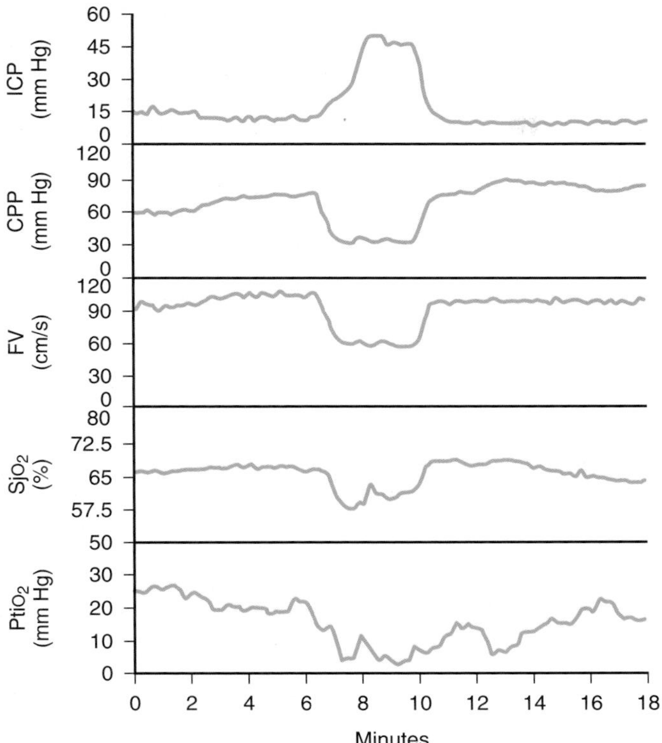


**Fig. 53.4 Example of Multimodality Monitoring in a Patient with Traumatic Brain Injury.** Notice the evidence of local and regional hypoxia, with elevation of intracranial pressure leading to reduction in cerebral perfusion. *CPP,* Cerebral perfusion pressure; *FV,* flow velocities on transcranial Doppler; *ICP,* intracranial pressure; *PtiO$_2$,* oxygen pressure in brain tissue; *SjO$_2$,* oxygen saturation in jugular blood.

from 20 to 30 mm Hg. The major disadvantages of brain oxygen probes include their invasiveness, limited spatial resolution, and susceptibility to artifacts (due to inappropriate calibration and head movement, among other factors). Its use has been recommended by experts in various major centers for patients with severe head injuries and poor-grade SAH (Maloney-Wilensky et al., 2009). It is best used when applied in the setting of multimodality monitoring, along with jugular oximetry and perhaps microdialysis (Andrews et al., 2008; Fig. 53.4).

NIRS is based on the property of a near-infrared light (700–1000 nm) to pass through tissues while being both scattered and absorbed. The absorption of a near-infrared light is proportional to the local concentration of certain chromophores, most notably hemoglobin. Thus, the absorption of near-infrared light changes according to the oxygenation state of hemoglobin. The probes illuminate up to a volume of 10 mL of brain tissue. All measurements are expressed as absolute concentration changes from a baseline zero at the start of the measurement. Normal values of oxygenated hemoglobin are reported to be 60% to 80%, and ischemic threshold is estimated to be below 47% saturation (Casati et al., 2006). However, the accuracy and reliability of this technique have been questioned and studies offer conflicting results. NIRS is susceptible to extraneous light, motion artifact, and signal drift. The measurement may also become unreliable when it is obtained through intracranial hematomas or through blood in the CSF. NIRS should be used to detect trends within an individual patient and should not be used in isolation to make management decisions; rather, it should be combined with other brain-monitoring methods.

### Microdialysis

The basic concept of microdialysis involves inserting a fine catheter into the brain parenchyma, then perfusing the catheter with a physiological solution such as Ringer lactate, thereby facilitating the exchange of molecules between the perfusate and the extracellular fluid across a dialysis membrane within the catheter tip. The dialysate is sampled under sterile conditions at hourly or other regular intervals and put through a microdialysis analyzer at the bedside. Insertion artifacts make measurements unreliable for the first hour after placement (Bellander et al., 2004).

Microdialysis enables the monitoring of brain pH, lactate and pyruvate, glucose, glycerol, glutamate, urea, and potentially other soluble molecules of interest (Bellander et al., 2004; Vespa et al., 1998). A lactate/pyruvate ratio greater than 25 seems to be the most sensitive parameter to detect brain ischemia, while increased glutamate and decreased glucose concentrations may be additional markers (Andrews et al., 2008; Bellander et al., 2004). Rises in glycerol are believed to reflect phospholipid breakdown as a result of cell membrane damage. Cerebral microdialysis has been employed in the NICU to identify secondary insults after severe brain trauma and to monitor for cerebral vasospasm and delayed cerebral ischemia in poor-grade SAH (Schmidt et al., 2011).

Several aspects of microdialytic analysis remain controversial, such as where to place the catheter (Andrews et al., 2008), whether the lactate/pyruvate ratio alone or in combination with other parameters is a better indicator of early cerebral ischemia, and why there has been no correlation between microdialysis measures and clinical outcome in some studies. Other problems are the invasiveness and labor intensiveness of the technique. This technique can offer very valuable information to advance our understanding of the pathophysiology of acute brain injury. Its usefulness to guide clinical practice still needs to be fully demonstrated.

## PRINCIPLES OF MANAGING CRITICALLY ILL NEUROLOGICAL PATIENTS

### Analgesia and Sedation

Analgesia and sedation are essential practices in neurointensive care. It is always challenging to avoid confounding the neurological examination while keeping the patient comfortable. Distinguishing agitation from the psychomotor manifestations of pain may be a difficult task in acutely ill neurological patients. Anxiety and pain lead to stress responses characterized by a hyperdynamic circulation, increased metabolic rate, and hyperkinesis. When pain is the cause of restlessness, the abnormal behavior may be more refractory to sedative medications. In those cases, appropriate and timely use of analgesics may result in correction of the abnormal behavior.

Whenever a patient is agitated in the NICU, an organic cause for the agitation should be sought. Confusion and restlessness are often seen in patients with acute strokes (especially those involving the right parietal lobe or the territory of the left posterior cerebral artery), early after SAH, in TBI with bifrontal damage, and in certain postictal states. On the other hand, patients with neuromuscular respiratory failure may become extremely anxious as they fail to achieve adequate ventilation and gas exchange. Drug withdrawal and side effects from medications are other common causes of agitation in the NICU. Infectious, metabolic, and endocrine derangements should also be investigated in agitated critically ill patients.

The ideal sedative agent in the NICU would be one that can achieve sedation rapidly and allow for fast and reliable reversal of its effect to allow for an accurate neurological examination. Propofol is one of the most commonly used drugs because it fulfills these criteria to a great extent. Propofol crosses the blood-brain barrier within minutes of administration and is a markedly effective hypnotic agent. Another advantageous pharmacokinetic property of propofol is that its clearance is not significantly altered by liver or renal failure, which is often a problem with benzodiazepines and opiates. Propofol lacks amnestic and analgesic properties, so adequate analgesia should be ensured in patients receiving this drug.

Awakening is typically seen within minutes of discontinuation of the infusion, but time to awakening may be significantly prolonged when the drug has been used in large doses for several days, because propofol is redistributed to the fat tissue from which it is only slowly released. Hypotension is the most common side effect of propofol infusion, especially when administered as a bolus. Falls in BP are more frequent and pronounced in patients who are hypovolemic. Other adverse effects include caloric overload (1 mL of propofol contains 1 kilocalorie), hypertriglyceridemia (and rarely pancreatitis), and withdrawal myoclonus (often confused with seizures). Propofol can also be used to treat elevated ICP and status epilepticus (Parviainen et al., 2006). However, administration of high doses of propofol for prolonged periods of time (i.e., >4–5 mg/kg/h for more than 48 hours) can cause the *propofol infusion syndrome* (Kam and Cardone, 2007). This is a serious complication characterized by metabolic acidosis, rhabdomyolysis, refractory bradycardia, myocardial depression, and, when most severe, cardiac arrest (Iyer et al., 2009). Even strict surveillance for these manifestations may fail to prevent this life-threatening complication. Consequently propofol should be used with great caution for the treatment of recalcitrant intracranial hypertension and status epilepticus, indications in which high doses of the medication are often necessary for up to several days to achieve the therapeutic goal.

Midazolam and lorazepam are the two most commonly used benzodiazepines in the NICU. The advantages of midazolam are its rapid effect and short duration of action (half-life 1.9 hours); it has only one active metabolite. Clearance is fast, but accumulation may occur after 3 days of continuous infusion. Patients who receive midazolam for several days can be expected to exhibit delayed awakening. Clearance of midazolam is diminished by hepatic and renal failure. Lorazepam has a much longer half-life (14 hours), which leads to a much slower emergence from sedation. However, lorazepam can produce severe metabolic acidosis from propylene glycol toxicity (Arroliga et al., 2004) and is therefore often avoided as a continuous infusion, although it remains a valuable medication in the management of acute seizures. The main side effect of benzodiazepines is respiratory depression in patients who are not mechanically ventilated. They can also induce hypotension in patients with reduced intravascular volume. Generally the risk of withdrawal symptoms is small with intravenous formulations. However, abrupt cessation of clonazepam after long-term use may result in withdrawal seizures. Benzodiazepines are effective in the treatment of status epilepticus, but pharmacoresistance emerges over time and requires a progressive increase in the rate of infusion of the drug. Benzodiazepines do not have a significant effect on ICP.

Unlike propofol, benzodiazepines have an effective antidote in flumazenil, which is a benzodiazepine receptor antagonist with little or no agonist activity and a half-life of 0.5–1.3 hours. Its administration is free of negative cardiovascular effects but may be complicated by the occurrence of seizures. The risk of seizures after administration of flumazenil is relatively small except in patients with a history of epilepsy or with a significantly reduced seizure threshold. Therefore caution should be exercised when this medication is administered to patients with acute brain disease.

Dexmedetomidine is a selective alpha-2 adrenergic receptor agonist. It produces effective sedation while preserving the patient's alertness. Patients sedated with this medication are often easily aroused, so adequate neurological assessment may be performed without the need to temporarily discontinue the sedative infusion. The most common adverse effect of dexmedetomidine is systemic hypotension, and bradycardia is also common. The drug has a short elimination half-life of approximately 2 hours, although that may be prolonged in patients with liver failure. Caution is recommended when this medication is used in patients with severe preexistent bradycardia or abnormal cardiac conduction, in patients with a severely depressed cardiac ejection fraction, and in those who are hypovolemic or hypotensive at the time of infusion.

Haloperidol is the drug of choice for patients with signs of psychosis. Intravenous doses of haloperidol may achieve successful control of agitated psychotic behavior within 20 minutes. The drug is fairly safe, but its use can be complicated by the appearance of extrapyramidal signs and (rarely) by neuroleptic malignant syndrome. Haloperidol should be used with caution in patients with prolongation of the QT interval. New-generation antipsychotics (atypical antipsychotics such as risperidone, olanzapine, and quetiapine) are also useful in the management of agitation and delirium. However, they can be administered only by the enteric route, although some are available as an oral-dissolving tablet, and their therapeutic effect is slower; hence their effect is limited in patients with extreme agitation.

Opioids represent the mainstay of analgesic treatment in acutely ill neurological patients. Options include morphine, fentanyl, sufentanil, alfentanil, remifentanil, oxycodone, and codeine. They all produce analgesia, a reduced level of consciousness, and respiratory depression. Hypotension may occur in hypovolemic patients or when high doses of these medications are being used. Fentanyl is preferred to morphine because it provokes fewer cardiovascular side effects and does not produce histamine release. Codeine is a much less potent agent, and its role is limited in the NICU. The action of opioids may be reversed by using naloxone, a competitive antagonist. Hypertension and cardiac arrhythmias are potential side effects of naloxone use. For milder forms of pain, nonsteroidal anti-inflammatory agents (e.g., ketorolac), tramadol, and acetaminophen may be helpful options. Table 53.2 summarizes key pharmacokinetic and pharmacodynamic information for the most commonly used sedative and analgesic agents in the NICU.

Often, nonopioid medications are desired in patients with brain injury for two principal reasons. First, the development of somnolence after opioid administration may affect a patient's neurological examination and lead to unnecessary tests. Second, in patients with intracranial mass lesions and decreased intracranial compliance, the development of hypoventilation and secondary intracranial vasodilation may lead to increased ICP and thus increase the possibility of herniation if the respiratory status is not closely monitored and/or controlled.

## Airway and Ventilatory Assistance

Acutely ill neurological patients often develop respiratory failure because of their inability to oxygenate or to sustain their ventilatory needs. The most common causes for oxygenation failure in NICU patients are cardiogenic and neurogenic pulmonary edema. However, sudden hypoxia should always raise the suspicion for pulmonary embolism (PE). Aspiration pneumonia occurs frequently because patients with a depressed level of consciousness and impaired cough reflex may be unable to protect the airway. Atelectasis may be a cause of hypoxia in patients with neuromuscular weakness. Ventilatory insufficiency resulting in hypercapnia from upper airway collapse is encountered in patients with neuromuscular respiratory failure or coma.

At the time of endotracheal intubation, the two main complications in neurological patients are a rise in ICP and exacerbation of hypoxia.

TABLE 53.2 **The Most Commonly Used Sedatives and Analgesics in the Neurological-Neurosurgical Intensive Care Unit**

| Drug | Therapeutic Class | Main Advantages | Main Disadvantages |
|---|---|---|---|
| Propofol | Sedative | Rapid sedation<br>Rapid clearance<br>Anticonvulsive<br>Reduces ICP | Expensive<br>Respiratory depression<br>Accumulates over time<br>Hypotension<br>May lower CBF<br>Hypertriglyceridemia<br>Hypercaloric<br>Lack of amnestic/analgesic properties<br>Infusion syndrome |
| Midazolam | Sedative | Rapid sedation<br>Rapid clearance<br>Anticonvulsive<br>Amnestic and anxiolytic properties | Expensive<br>Respiratory depression<br>Clearance reduced in renal or liver failure<br>Contraindicated in untreated glaucoma |
| Lorazepam | Sedative | Cheaper<br>Otherwise similar to midazolam | Longer duration of action<br>Risk of metabolic acidosis (propylene glycol)<br>Otherwise similar to midazolam |
| Dexmedetomidine | Sedative | Relative preservation of arousal<br>Minimal respiratory depression<br>Analgesic and anxiolytic properties | Expensive<br>Hypertension/hypotension<br>Possible bradycardia |
| Haloperidol | Neuroleptic | Rapidly effective treatment for agitation<br>No respiratory depression | Risk of extrapyramidal signs and NMS<br>QTc prolongation |
| Opioids | Analgesics | Rapidly effective analgesia | Respiratory depression<br>Sedation<br>Constipation<br>Urinary retention<br>Emesis<br>Hypotension<br>Histamine release (morphine)<br>Cerebral vasodilation (due to pH and $CO_2$ changes) |
| NSAIDs | Analgesics | Lack of sedation<br>Antiinflammatory | May increase risk of bleeding<br>Possible renal toxicity |
| Tramadol | Analgesic | Less respiratory depression than opioids | Less potent than opioids<br>May lower seizure threshold |

*CBF,* Cerebral blood flow; *ICP,* intracranial pressure; *NMS,* neuroleptic malignant syndrome; *NSAIDs,* nonsteroidal anti-inflammatory drugs.

Rapid-sequence intubation is the safest approach for patients with increased ICP (Wijdicks and Borel, 1998). It proceeds in three phases: (1) preoxygenation to prevent worsening hypoxia during intubation—this can be achieved by providing effective bag-valve-mask (AMBU) ventilation; (2) pretreatment with drugs to mitigate the hemodynamic changes that may increase ICP upon intubation (e.g., lidocaine, thiopental); and (3) sequential administration of a potent sedative (e.g., propofol) and, when necessary, a rapid-acting nondepolarizing neuromuscular blocking agent (e.g., rocuronium, vecuronium). Succinylcholine should be avoided because it may increase ICP due to widespread muscle fasciculations, increased central venous pressure, and hypercarbia; it can also produce dangerous hyperkalemia in patients with underlying muscle disease. In cases of TBI, it is essential to maintain in-line stabilization of the cervical spine. When cervical spine injury is suspected, fiberoptic-assisted intubation is often preferred and should be completed by a physician with experience in this technique.

The essential goal of mechanical ventilation is to assist the patient to achieve adequate gas exchange. There are two basic forms of mechanical ventilation: volume control and pressure control. *Volume-control ventilation* delivers a consistent preset volume of air with each ventilator breath. *Pressure-control ventilation* delivers a preset amount of pressure to the patient, with varying degrees of volume depending on the amount of resistance in the system.

The modes of volume-control ventilation most frequently used in neurological and neurosurgical patients are assist/control (A/C) and synchronized intermittent mandatory ventilation (SIMV). In A/C ventilation, the ventilator will always deliver the preset air volume. In control mode, breaths are initiated by the machine and not influenced by the patient. The rate of these controlled breaths is determined in the ventilatory settings. In assist mode, the ventilator will deliver extra breaths of the same predetermined tidal volume every time the patient generates sufficient negative pressure during an attempted inspiration. In SIMV, the ventilator delivers breaths with full preset volume up to a prescribed rate. If the patient's inspiratory effort exceeds such a preset rate, all additional breaths initiated by the patient (spontaneous breaths) will have a volume determined by the extent of the negative inspiratory pressure produced by the patient. The volume of this spontaneous breath may be adjusted by setting a support function on the ventilator called *pressure support.* Thus, pressure support is used in conjunction with SIMV to augment the patient's negative inspiratory force and increase the efficiency of the independent breaths produced by the patient. SIMV is well tolerated by patients and avoids deconditioning of respiratory muscles. Its main disadvantages include the possibility of developing high peak airway pressures, a high rate of gas delivery in the early phase of inspiration (which may not be tolerated by agitated patients), and insufficient treatment of hypoxia in severely hypoxemic patients.

A newer mode of ventilation that is similar to SIMV is mandatory minute ventilation (MMV), which allows the patient to take spontaneous breaths with a preset amount of pressure support. When a preset minute ventilation (MV) is met solely by patient effort, the ventilator will not deliver any assisted breaths. However, if the patient's effort is not enough to achieve the set MV, the ventilator will then deliver the necessary breaths, each with a preset tidal volume, to ensure that the MV is met. With this mode of ventilation, the ventilator adjusts the number of breaths given per minute based on the patient's performance and theoretically should protect the patient from hypoventilation.

Pressure-control ventilation differs from volume control mode in that inspiratory and expiratory airway pressures are consistently regulated at the expense of variation in the delivered volume. Pressure-control ventilation is used most frequently in patients who are sedated and paralyzed and is overall an uncommon ventilatory mode in the NICU. It requires setting the fraction of inspired oxygen ($FIO_2$), the ventilatory rate, and the pressure difference between inspiration and expiration.

In pressure-support ventilation (PSV), all breaths are triggered by the patient. The ventilator delivers a particular level of pressure support each time a breath is initiated; this pressure is delivered at the onset of inspiration. When the flow rate reaches 20% of its initial value, gas flow is terminated. This mode is often fairly comfortable for the conscious patient as it closely approximates the flow characteristics of a normal breath. Since patients on a pressure-support ventilator may become hypopneic, they should be closely monitored with the help of apnea alarms. For patient safety, mechanical ventilators have a back-up "apnea ventilation" setting to automatically trigger controlled breaths if patients on PSV become apneic.

Regardless of the ventilatory mode used, oxygenation depends upon the $FIO_2$ and the level of positive end-expiratory pressure (PEEP) provided. Increasing the $FIO_2$ increases the oxygen available for absorption by the pulmonary capillaries. Very high levels of $FIO_2$ (>0.6) may result in pulmonary oxygen toxicity, and the use of PEEP allows for tapering of the $FIO_2$ in many cases. The basic goal of PEEP is to prevent microatelectasis by keeping alveoli from collapsing at the end of expiration. This improves the efficiency of gaseous exchange by maximizing recruitment of lung units. The main danger of PEEP use is increasing intrathoracic pressure to levels that compromise venous return, which may result in hypotension unless intravascular filling pressures are augmented by volume expansion. High levels of PEEP may rarely produce tension pneumothorax. Finally, it is important to monitor the ICP when positive airway pressure is applied. Patients with decreased intracranial compliance may develop increases in ICP as intrathoracic pressure rises and imposes resistance to venous return. However, for the most part, relatively high levels of PEEP are well tolerated by euvolemic patients with intracranial hypertension.

Weaning from mechanical ventilation is usually achieved in critically ill neurological patients by decreasing the rate of mandatory breaths on SIMV or, more commonly, by using PSV. In fact, both methods can be combined in practice. A patient on SIMV can have the set rate decreased as clinical improvement occurs. If the patient has adequate spontaneous tidal volumes and no apneas, he or she may be switched to PSV, which consists of pressure support at the onset of inspiration and PEEP to prevent alveolar collapse and improve oxygenation. Subsequently, the amount of pressure support may be weaned until extubation is deemed safe.

In patients with acute brain disorders, level of consciousness may be a limiting factor when considering extubation. Despite successful weaning, the stuporous patient may be considered unsafe for extubation because of concerns about airway safety. Keeping patients intubated once they have fulfilled the ventilatory criteria for extubation is a common but questionable practice. In patients with TBI, this practice may be associated with a higher risk of ventilator-associated complications (Coplin et al., 2000). Thus the safety of extubation in patients with adequate respiratory function but a persistently depressed level of consciousness is a problem that demands further research (Manno et al., 2008). Additionally, it is not uncommon for patients with acute brain injury who subsequently require intubation for various reasons to be unable to follow commands, which is often considered necessary prior to extubation outside of a NICU. This should not preclude a trial of extubation if other weaning parameters have been met in a neurologically injured patient.

Patients with neuromuscular respiratory failure are commonly encountered in a NICU, and ventilator weaning in these patients requires special consideration. For patients who are intubated due to myasthenic crisis, some intensivists will perform a T-piece trial prior to extubation to make sure that the patients are able to tolerate a period without pressure support prior to extubation. If this method is used, the length of the trial should not be excessive (as this may cause unnecessary fatigue), and a period of recovery on pressure support prior to extubation should be considered. On a study of patients recovering from myasthenic crisis, the presence of atelectasis and intubation for more than 10 days predicted extubation failure (Seneviratne et al., 2008).

Patients with GBS also pose a challenge with regard to ventilatory weaning. A protracted recovery course is expected in patients with GBS and respiratory failure; many will require tracheostomy placement as a result. In these patients, the timing of ventilatory weaning may be difficult to determine. Therefore careful monitoring during weaning trials is necessary, as a change from fully controlled or partially controlled (SIMV) ventilation may not initially be successful.

Patients who fail extubation and those who are considered unsafe for an extubation trial will require a tracheostomy. The timing of a tracheostomy varies according to the patient's primary condition. The risk of local airway complications, such as acquired tracheal stenosis, increase with longer duration of endotracheal intubation. In addition, tracheostomy is more comfortable for patients than endotracheal intubation and provides better access for effective pulmonary toileting. The most common indications for tracheostomy in the NICU are persistent stupor or coma, severe impairment of cough reflex, and prolonged neuromuscular respiratory failure. Percutaneous tracheostomy has become the standard procedure in most ICUs. It is important to bear in mind that tracheostomies are reversible. Also, specially modified tracheostomy tubes that allow patients to vocalize and communicate are now available.

## Pulmonary Complications

The main respiratory complications in critically ill neurological patients are pneumonia (either induced by aspiration or ventilator associated), PE, atelectasis, and pulmonary edema (either cardiogenic or neurogenic). Aspiration is common in patients with a depressed level of consciousness, seizures, or bulbar weakness. Patients who have been intubated for over 48 hours may develop ventilator-associated pneumonia, manifested by increased amount of thick secretions, fever, leukocytosis, new radiographic abnormalities, and increased $PaO_2$:$FIO_2$ ratio. Aspiration pneumonia should prompt coverage for anaerobes and gram-negative organisms. Coverage for ventilator-associated pneumonia will depend on the organisms and antibiotic susceptibility most prevalent in each ICU.

Sudden development of unexplained hypoxia should be considered possible PE until proven otherwise. Patients with critical neurological illness are especially predisposed to the development of venous thromboembolism because of prolonged immobility. Tachypnea is often prominent in patients with PE. However, quadriparetic patients with high cervical lesions cannot develop this response; oxygen desaturation associated with tachycardia may be the only manifestation in these patients. The differential diagnosis in cases of acute tachypnea and oxygen desaturation includes plugging of the airway by secretions. However, these patients typically also develop hypercapnia due to hypoventilation. If hypoxia is not resolved by airway suctioning and the situation remains unexplained after an emergent chest radiograph (to exclude new infiltrates, pneumothorax, or lobar collapse), the patient

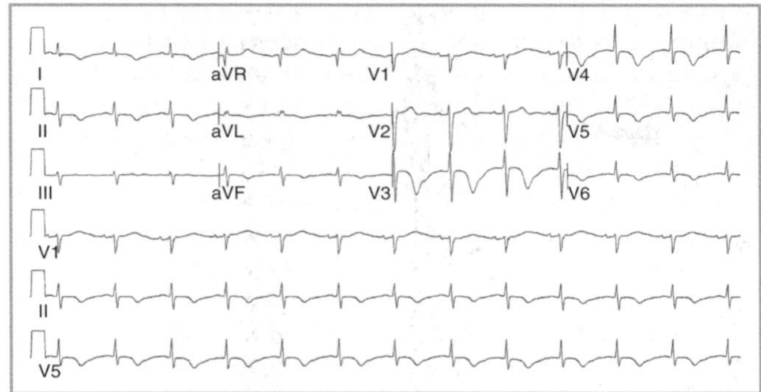


**Fig. 53.5 Electrocardiographic Changes in a Patient with an Acute Aneurysmal Subarachnoid Hemorrhage.** Notice diffuse repolarization abnormalities in the precordial leads.

should undergo specific studies to rule out PE. At present, CT angiography is the diagnostic modality of choice. The possibility of deep venous thrombosis (DVT) should also be investigated by venous Doppler of the lower extremities. The treatment of venous thromboembolism may be particularly challenging in acutely ill neurological patients. Patients with large ischemic strokes or intracranial hemorrhages are at increased risk for complications from intravenous heparin. When systemic anticoagulation is deemed strictly contraindicated, insertion of an inferior vena cava filter may be a reasonable alternative. Patients with massive PE may require endovascular maneuvers to mechanically remove the clot or provide intra-arterial infusion of a thrombolytic agent.

Atelectasis is very common in patients receiving mechanical ventilation. Large areas of atelectasis or lobar collapse may produce profound hypoxia. Mucous plugging of the airway is common among critically ill patients. Increased levels of PEEP are often used to treat collapsed lung regions. Physical measures including suctioning, postural drainage, and external percussion may be effective, but bronchoscopic suction and lavage are necessary in severe cases.

Interpretation of pulmonary edema is more complex in critically ill neurological patients than in the general population of ICU patients. Although most cases of pulmonary edema will be due to cardiac failure, neurogenic pulmonary edema may occur after acute SAH, TBI, and other neurological catastrophes associated with massive surges of central sympathetic output. Neurogenic pulmonary edema is successfully treated using high levels of PEEP. Cardiogenic pulmonary edema should be treated by ameliorating cardiac workload (through diuresis and vasodilation) and providing adequate levels of supplemental oxygen.

## Cardiovascular Care and Blood Pressure Management

Cardiac disorders are common in critically ill neurological patients, and they may precede or accompany the neurological illness. They are often related to the massive catecholamine release associated with the acute brain insult (Banki et al., 2005). The most common forms of cardiac complications in the NICU are acute coronary syndrome, cardiac arrhythmias, and congestive heart failure.

### Acute Coronary Syndrome

Electrocardiographic (ECG) and clinical abnormalities suggestive of myocardial ischemia are fairly common in patients with acute brain injury (e.g., large ischemic stroke, SAH, large intraparenchymal hematoma, TBI with contusions, status epilepticus). Typical ECG abnormalities in patients with acute brain damage include nonspecific ST segment changes, symmetrically inverted T waves (Fig. 53.5), and sometimes ST segment elevation across all the precordial leads. Most often, these neurogenic ECG changes are not restricted to a coronary territory, unlike those related to coronary ischemia. Elevation of serum troponin levels should be considered indicative of myocardial injury, whereas elevation of serum creatinine kinase is much less specific in patients with acute brain damage (Woodruff et al., 2003). Yet troponin elevation is seen in patients with SAH as an expression of ventricular dysfunction secondary to the neurogenic (adrenergic-induced) injury (Deibert et al., 2003).

It is always difficult to define optimal hemodynamic goals in patients with coexistent myocardial ischemia and acute neurological conditions that require maintenance of adequate CPP, such as acute ischemic stroke and SAH at risk for vasospasm. In these patients, lowering the BP to the levels commonly used as goals in most patients with acute myocardial ischemia may further compromise cerebral perfusion and precipitate infarction in areas of ischemic penumbra. Anticoagulation or intravenous glycoprotein IIb/IIIa inhibitors may be contraindicated early in patients who have had an extensive ischemic stroke, in those with large intraparenchymal hematomas, or shortly after a neurosurgical procedure. Percutaneous coronary angioplasty and stenting may be considered, but limitations on the use of heparin intraprocedurally and aspirin and clopidogrel after the intervention may increase the risk of procedural complications or acute in-stent thrombosis. Induced diuresis is indicated to reduce afterload in patients with depressed left ventricular ejection fraction, but it should be closely monitored; hypovolemia may induce cerebral ischemia in patients with vasospasm or areas of ischemic penumbra.

### Cardiac Arrhythmias

Cardiac arrhythmias in acutely ill neurological patients may be due to preexisting cardiac disease. They may also be responsible for the acute neurological disorder, as occurs in patients with atrial fibrillation presenting with embolic stroke. Conversely, arrhythmias and conduction abnormalities may be due to acute brain disease. Decreased heart rate viability, increased risk for arrhythmias, and even increased risk for sudden death have been documented in patients with insular strokes (Abboud et al., 2006). Cardiac arrhythmias may also develop as a complication of seizures, and dysregulation of autonomic function may provoke life-threatening arrhythmias in patients with GBS.

Profound bradycardia in the ICU may be seen in the context of autonomic dysreflexia, after carotid stenting (from stretching of the carotid body), and with increasing ICP (Cushing reflex). Cases of symptomatic bradycardia with hemodynamic compromise should be treated emergently with intravenous atropine. Immediately after controlling the emergency, treatment should focus on the underlying cause of the bradycardia. *Autonomic dysreflexia* is a severe complication of high cervical spinal cord lesions, typically consisting of profound bradycardia and extreme hypertension, often precipitated by distention of the viscera, manipulations (e.g., bladder catheterizations), or a change in body position (e.g., turning). Autonomic dysreflexia caused by high spinal cord injuries does not have an effective treatment, so episodes of autonomic imbalances must be prevented by carefully avoiding the situations that precipitate them. The bradycardia observed after carotid stenting is transient, and in most cases hemodynamic stability can be preserved with adequate fluid therapy. Bradycardia due to increased ICP demands immediate treatment of the primary problem. The patient should be emergently assessed for the possibility of hydrocephalus. If the rise in ICP is secondary to cerebral edema, then osmotherapy, corticosteroids, or hyperventilation should be instituted as needed.

Tachycardias in the NICU are most commonly supraventricular. They include paroxysmal supraventricular tachycardia, atrial fibrillation, and atrial flutter. Treatment does not vary from that applied to other critically ill patients. When sustained ventricular tachycardia occurs, patients should be investigated for the possibility of myocardial ischemia, underlying cardiac disease, or prolonged QT interval.

### Congestive Heart Failure

Administration of large amounts of intravenous fluids may precipitate volume overload and pulmonary edema in patients with underlying cardiac insufficiency. This is common among patients with SAH who receive hemodynamic augmentation therapy for symptomatic vasospasm. It is also a frequent complication in patients with acute ischemic stroke aggressively treated with fluids to maximize collateral flow in an attempt to preserve an area of ischemic penumbra. Cautious induced diuresis is indicated in these patients when the degree of pulmonary edema is severe enough to produce hypoxemia.

*Apical ballooning syndrome* is a characteristic form of cardiomyopathy seen after acute neurological insults (Lee et al., 2006). Sudden sympathetic hyperstimulation of the myocardium causes a specific pattern of myocardial stunning (Prasad et al., 2008), and its diagnosis depends on echocardiographic demonstration of apical hypokinesis or akinesis with sparing of basal segments. Consequently the heart takes on the form of an octopus-catcher pot (*takotsubo* in Japanese, hence the name *takotsubo cardiomyopathy* that is sometimes given to this condition). Patients with apical ballooning syndrome have reductions in left ventricular ejection fraction and may develop acute congestive heart failure with pulmonary edema. The presentation may also mimic myocardial ischemia. Cardiac function typically returns to baseline after 2 or 3 weeks (Lee et al., 2006; Prasad et al., 2008), and conservative management with supportive care is often all that is needed. Yet in the most severe cases, a temporary cardiac assist device such as an intra-aortic balloon pump may be necessary.

### Blood Pressure Management

BP management represents one of the most crucial aspects of neurocritical care. The three main goals of BP management in critically ill neurological and neurosurgical patients are to ensure adequate cerebral perfusion, prevent intracranial bleeding, and avoid exacerbation of cerebral edema. These goals must often be balanced in individual cases in which the risk of hypoperfusion and worsening ischemia coexists with the danger of new or enlarging hemorrhage and progression of brain swelling. Although guidelines and practice parameters have been published to guide BP treatment in various acute neurological conditions (Table 53.3), there are still areas of debate in regard to what should be considered optimal BP targets in patients with some of the most common disorders treated in the NICU.

**Acute ischemic stroke.** Sudden and profound reductions of BP are associated with neurological decline in patients with acute ischemic stroke (Oliveira-Filho et al., 2003). This is likely related to insufficient perfusion in areas already affected by ischemic penumbra. In fact, elevation of BP appears to be a protective physiological response that occurs after occlusion of a cerebral vessel, as suggested by the spontaneous resolution of hypertension in patients who achieve successful recanalization (Mattle et al., 2005). Furthermore, low BP (diastolic BP <70, systolic BP <155, or MAP <100 mm Hg) on initial evaluation in the emergency department and greater BP fluctuations within the first 3 hours have been shown to correlate with increased 90-day mortality in patients with acute cerebral ischemic infarction (Stead et al., 2005, 2006).

Current practice guidelines advocate a very conservative approach to treating hypertension after acute ischemic stroke. With regard to patients who are ineligible for thrombolysis, antihypertensive therapy is recommended only for those with a systolic BP higher than 220 mm Hg or diastolic BP higher than 120 mm Hg (Jauch et al., 2013). Intermittent doses of intravenous labetalol or hydralazine or continuous infusion of nicardipine are the preferred treatment options; when diastolic BP exceeds 140 mm Hg, sodium nitroprusside should be infused instead. The initial objective of treatment should be to reduce the BP by 10%–15%. However, it is important to acknowledge that this permissive approach to hypertension is not based on direct evidence from randomized trials. Some data actually indicate that modest BP reduction within 36 hours after an ischemic stroke could actually be beneficial (Potter et al., 2009). An optimal arterial BP target probably exists on an individual basis and likely depends on stroke mechanism and other characteristics such as severity and chronicity of preexisting hypertension, autoregulation status, and comorbidities such as cardiac disease. In patients eligible for thrombolytic therapy, BP management should be more aggressive to limit the risk of hemorrhagic complications associated with use of the fibrinolytic agent. The BP should be below 185/110 mm Hg before thrombolysis is begun. After administration of the fibrinolytic drug, BP must be strictly maintained below 180/105 mm Hg. Failure to control the BP according to this parameter has been repeatedly shown to be associated with increased risk of symptomatic intracranial hemorrhagic and poor functional outcome. Additionally, in patients who undergo endovascular therapy and have complete reperfusion or clot retrieval (Thrombolysis In Cerebral Infarction - TICI 3), the role of permissive hypertension is not well defined, and BP elevations may encourage hyperperfusion to ischemic tissue, further emphasizing the importance of an individualized approach to poststroke BP management. The current guideline from the American Heart Association recommends maintenance of BP less than 180/105 mm Hg in the first 24 hours following endovascular therapy (Powers et al., 2018)

**TABLE 53.3 Guidelines for Blood Pressure Management in the Most Common Conditions Treated in the Neurological-Neurosurgical Intensive Care Unit**

| Diagnosis | Recommendation |
|---|---|
| Acute ischemic stroke | Establish and maintain BP <185/110 mm Hg prior to receiving intravenous thrombolysis<br>Keep <180/105 mm Hg if thrombolysis<br>Treat only BP >220/120 mm Hg if no thrombolysis<br>Keep <180/105 mm Hg following endovascular clot retrieval |
| Intracerebral hemorrhage | Keep SBP <180 and MAP <130 mm Hg<br>(ideal SBP <160 mm Hg) |
| Subarachnoid hemorrhage | Keep SBP <160 mm Hg before aneurysm treated<br>Do not lower BP after aneurysm treated |
| Traumatic brain injury | Keep adequate MAP to maintain CPP 60–70 mm Hg<br>Suggested SBP goals: >100 mm Hg (ages 50–69 yr) or >110 mm Hg (ages 15–49 yr) |

*BP,* Blood pressure; *CPP,* cerebral perfusion pressure; *MAP,* mean arterial pressure; *SBP,* systolic blood pressure.

There is limited but promising evidence suggesting that pharmacological elevation of BP may be beneficial for certain patients with acute ischemic stroke (Mistri et al., 2006). Further research is needed to determine the safety of this intervention and to indicate which patients could be optimal candidates for this type of aggressive hemodynamic treatment.

**Intracerebral hemorrhage.** The treatment of hypertension in patients with spontaneous (hypertensive) intraparenchymal hematomas is more controversial. There is abundant (Fogelholm et al., 1997; Leira et al., 2004; Terayama et al., 1997) although not uniform (Brott et al., 1997; Jauch et al., 2006; Qureshi et al., 1999) evidence that extreme hypertension is associated with greater risk of hematoma expansion, a major determinant of poor outcome and increased mortality in ICH (Davis et al., 2006). Meanwhile, solid demonstration that areas of hypoperfusion are frequently present around parenchymal hematomas (Kidwell et al., 2001; Mayer et al., 1998; Rosand et al., 2002) has supported the argument that aggressive BP reduction could precipitate ischemia in these regions. However, this theoretical risk is not substantiated by studies showing decreased oxygen extraction fraction in the hypoperfused perihematoma tissue (as opposed to the increased oxygen extraction that would be expected in areas of ischemic penumbra; Kate et al., 2014; Zazulia et al., 2001) and preserved CBF in those regions after acute BP reduction (Powers et al., 2001). However, current guidelines advise keeping the systolic blood pressure (SBP) below 140 mm Hg if there is suspicion of intracranial hypertension; furthermore, ICP monitoring should be considered to target therapy to maintain CPP between 50 and 70 mm Hg (Hemphill et al., 2015). A large randomized clinical trial, INTERACT2, compared intensive BP lowering (target SBP ≤140 mm Hg) with conventional antihypertensive treatment (target SBP ≤180 mm Hg) for hypertensive patients with spontaneous ICH and found no difference in poor outcome (death or major disability) between the groups (52% in the intensive arm vs. 55.6% in conventional arm, $P = .056$) (Anderson et al., 2013). There was no evidence of harm from aggressive BP lowering in this trial, but the results should be interpreted with caution considering that only 33% of patients in the intensive arm had reached the goal BP within 1 hour. An ordinal analysis of the functional outcome scores indicated a favorable shift with intensive BP lowering. Therefore there may be a modest improvement in functional outcome when an SBP equal to or less than 140 mm Hg is being targeted in patients with acute spontaneous ICH. An additional study, ATACH II, demonstrated that more intensive BP lowering (goal SBP 110–139 mm Hg) did not improve outcome and suggested that the more rigorous BP goal, as opposed to a more lenient BP target, resulted in more renal adverse events (Qureshi et al., 2016). In sum, neurointensivists generally agree that BP should be controlled following ICH, but the goal BP range is not uniform and is dependent on many different patient characteristics and on balancing the risk of hematoma expansion with systemic hypoperfusion from excessive BP restriction.

***Subarachnoid hemorrhage.*** In patients with acute aneurysmal SAH, in order to prevent rebleeding, it is often recommended to keep a systolic BP below 160 mm Hg until the ruptured aneurysm is secured. It should be noted that this widespread practice of aggressive BP lowering is not based on solid scientific data. After the aneurysm is secured, BP should not be lowered, since these patients are at risk for delayed ischemia from vasospasm, and they will often "autoaugment" their BP when vasospasm occurs. Hemodynamic augmentation therapy, often including the use of vasopressors, is indicated in patients with symptomatic vasospasm (Connolly et al., 2012).

***Traumatic brain injury.*** Maintenance of an adequate CPP is one of the principal therapeutic goals in the intensive care of severe TBI patients, since secondary ischemic insults are known to have a major detrimental impact on prognosis (Sarrafzadeh et al., 2001). It is advisable to keep the CPP within the range of 60–70 mm Hg, although it is unclear whether raising the MAP or lowering the ICP should be the main therapeutic strategy to achieve this goal (Brain Trauma Foundation, 2016). Patients with intact autoregulation tolerate higher CPPs better, and it is possible that by monitoring autoregulation status (with PRx, for example), an "optimal CPP" for individual patients may be determined (Aries et al., 2012); however, this is still an area of active research. Additionally, maintenance of SBP above 100 mm Hg (ages 50–69 years) or above 110 mm Hg (ages 15–49 years) for patients with severe TBI has been suggested as reasonable (Brain Trauma Foundation, 2016). Aggressive fluid resuscitation is the mainstay of hemodynamic treatment in TBI. Vasopressors should be reserved for patients with persistent hypotension after aggressive fluid replacement.

## Fluid and Electrolytes

Acute renal failure in acutely ill neurological or neurosurgical patients is most commonly iatrogenic. Mannitol can rapidly cause prerenal azotemia when adequate hydration is not provided to compensate for the fluid lost from osmotic diuresis. This complication can be reliably avoided by adjusting the fluid intake to prevent negative fluid balance while monitoring serum osmolality. If serum osmolality exceeds 320 mOsm/kg, mannitol infusion is typically withheld to protect renal function. If continuation of osmotherapy is indispensable, mannitol may be continued with relatively low risk of kidney failure as long as concomitant aggressive hydration is provided. Hypertonic saline may be a valuable alternative in these cases; it is a safer choice than mannitol in patients with chronic renal insufficiency but does require the use of a central line. Radiocontrast-induced nephropathy can often be prevented by preemptive hydration, *N*-acetylcysteine, and bicarbonate infusion (Merten et al., 2004; Tepel et al., 2000). Acute interstitial nephritis from drug toxicity (e.g., antibiotics) and (less commonly) pyelonephritis (in patients with chronic indwelling catheters) are also causes of acute renal failure in the NICU.

When renal failure is established, it is essential that the neurointensivist cooperates with the consulting nephrologist to maximize the safety of renal replacement therapy (dialysis). Sudden fluid shifts and changes in BP that would be inconsequential in other patients may have dramatic detrimental effects in patients with cerebral edema or cerebral hypoperfusion. In patients with renal failure, it is also important to closely monitor the free levels of anticonvulsive drugs. These patients have a heightened risk of developing toxic complications from decreased drug elimination and rapid clearance of the anticonvulsant during dialysis may increase the risk of seizures.

Hyponatremia is the most common electrolyte imbalance encountered in critically ill neurological patients. The two most common mechanisms of hyponatremia in these patients are cerebral salt-wasting syndrome (CSWS) and the syndrome of inappropriate secretion of antidiuretic hormone (SIADH; Rabinstein and Wijdicks, 2003a). Both mechanisms produce hypotonic hyponatremia with high concentration of urinary sodium (secondary to increased sodium excretion in CSWS and increased water reabsorption in SIADH). In fact, determination of extracellular fluid volume remains the only reliable distinguishing feature between these two conditions: SIADH is a state of volume *expansion*, while CSWS is a state of volume *depletion* (Table 53.4).

**TABLE 53.4 Clinical and Laboratory Features of Cerebral Salt-Wasting Syndrome and Syndrome of Inappropriate Secretion of Antidiuretic Hormone**

| Variable | CSWS | SIADH |
|---|---|---|
| Extracellular fluid volume | ↓ | ↑ |
| Body weight | ↓ | ↑ |
| Fluid balance | Negative | Positive |
| Urine volume | ↔ or ↑ | ↔ or ↓ |
| Tachycardia | + | – |
| Hematocrit | ↑ | ↔ |
| Albumin | ↑ | ↔ |
| Serum bicarbonate | ↑ | ↔ or ↓ |
| Blood urea nitrogen | ↑ | ↔ or ↓ |
| Serum uric acid | ↔ or ↓ | ↓ |
| Urinary sodium | ↑ | ↑ |
| Sodium balance | Negative | Neutral or positive |
| CVP/PCWP | ↓ | ↔ or slightly ↑ |

↔, Absent or minor variable change; ↓, decreased; ↑, increased; *CSWS*, cerebral salt-wasting syndrome; *CVP*, central venous pressure; *PCWP*, pulmonary capillary wedge pressure; *SIADH*, syndrome of inappropriate secretion of antidiuretic hormone.

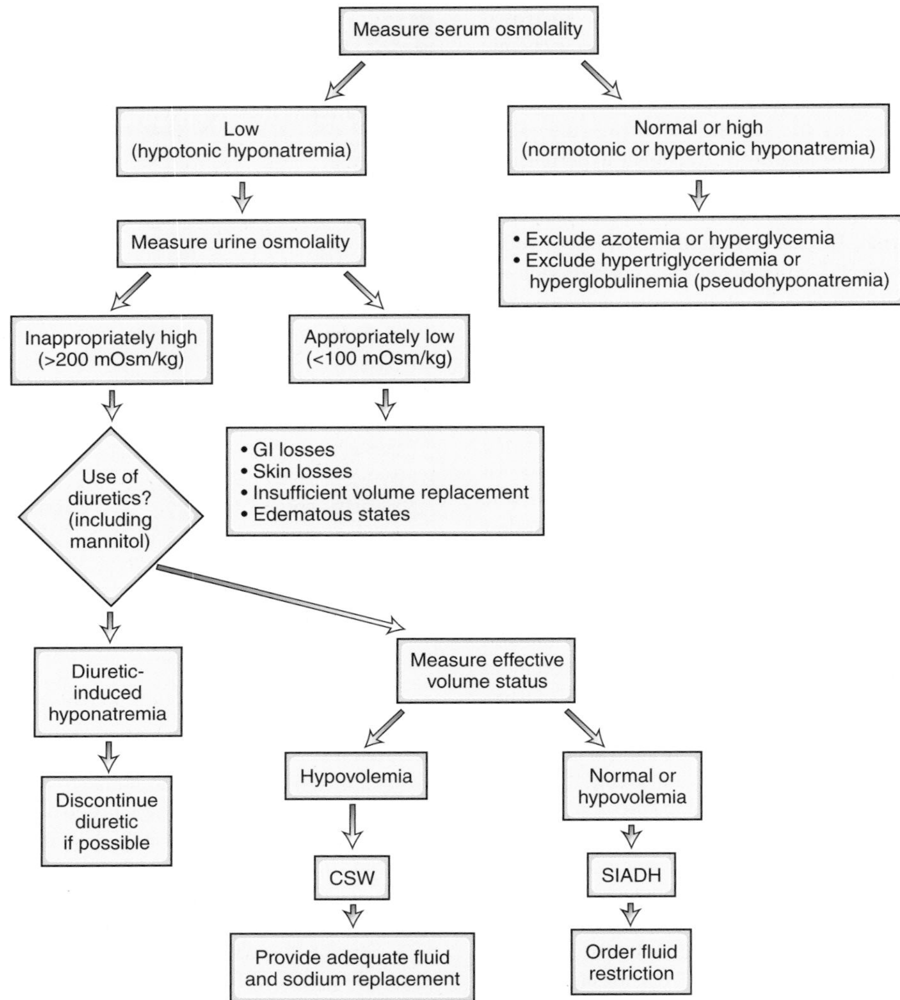


**Fig. 53.6** Algorithm for the Diagnosis and Management of Hyponatremia in Critically Ill Neurological Patients. *CSW*, Cerebral salt-wasting; *SIADH*, syndrome of inappropriate secretion of antidiuretic hormone.

The practical importance of this concept needs to be highlighted because fluid restriction—adequate therapy for SIADH—may be enormously deleterious in patients with CSWS, particularly in those with concurrent SAH-related vasospasm. Symptomatic acute hyponatremia requires tightly controlled infusion of hypertonic saline. Excessively rapid correction of profound chronic hyponatremia may precipitate severe osmotic myelinolysis. The rate of correction should not exceed 10 mmol/L over any 24-hour period to avoid this potentially devastating complication (Laureno and Karp, 1997). Fig. 53.6 presents an algorithm for the diagnosis and management of hyponatremia in critically ill neurological patients.

Hypernatremia in the NICU is most often produced by therapeutic interventions (e.g., mannitol without sufficient fluid replacement, infusion of hypertonic saline) or diabetes insipidus (DI). Focal brain lesions (most frequently tumors or trauma) or surgery involving the sellar/suprasellar region are the typical causes of DI. Profound DI is also seen at the time of brain death. Diagnosis of DI hinges on the finding of polyuria (characteristically >250–300 mL/h for ≥2 consecutive hours) with very dilute urine (specific gravity <1.010, urine osmolality <250 mOsm/kg). Treatment demands aggressive fluid replacement. Central DI responds rapidly to administration of vasopressin or desmopressin acetate (DDAVP). Vasopressin is a short-acting (within 2–4 hours) drug, and the recommended dose is 2–5 U subcutaneously or intramuscularly every 4 hours. Desmopressin acetate has a longer duration of action and should be administered cautiously in postsurgical patients because, in those cases, DI tends to resolve spontaneously within days or even hours of its presentation. The recommended dose is 0.5–4 µg given intravenously or subcutaneously every 12 hours. Serum and urine osmolalities and serum electrolytes should be checked every 2–4 hours in every patient with DI until stability is established.

## Nutrition and Metabolic Derangements

Adequate nutrition is essential for the recovery of critically ill patients, including those with primary acute neurological conditions. Depressed levels of consciousness and abnormal swallowing function are very prevalent in NICU patients who, consequently, often require tube feedings. Meanwhile, gastroparesis is also common and may increase the risk of aspiration in patients receiving enteral nutrition. This potential risk demands close monitoring of gastric residuals and positioning of the feeding tube in the distal part of the stomach or first portion of the duodenum. Agents that promote gastric motility (e.g., metoclopramide) may be added in the most severe cases (Booth et al., 2002).

Daily caloric requirement is calculated using the Harris Benedict equation to estimate basal energy expenditure (BEE):

$$\text{For men}: \text{BEE} = 665 + (13.75 \times W) + (5 \times H) - (6.78 \times A)$$

$$\text{For women}: \text{BEE} = 665 + (9.56 \times W) + (1.85 \times H) - (4.68 \times A)$$

For both equations, $W$ is body weight in kilograms, $H$ is height in centimeters, and $A$ is age in years. This is often operationally translated into approximately 25–30 kcal/kg/day. Nutritional requirement may be adjusted to the particular disease and nutritional status indicators. For instance, sepsis may require increasing nutritional support by 30%, whereas high-calorie feeding should be avoided in GBS and myasthenia gravis. Adequacy of nutritional support is better assessed using prealbumin (half-life of 2–3 days) rather than albumin (half-life of 20 days). It is highly advisable to work closely with a nutritionist specialized in critical care patients in order to make adequate adjustments.

Enteral feeding is preferred whenever possible to help maintain the integrity of the intestinal mucosal lining. It is recommended to start feeding patients early (ideally within 48 hours of admission); early feeding has been associated with a trend toward better survival and less disability in patients with TBI (Yanagawa et al., 2002). The optimal timing of percutaneous gastrostomy in neurological patients has not been sufficiently studied. There is some evidence that gastrostomy should be performed in patients with dysphagia from stroke persisting after 14 days (Norton et al., 1996).

Hyperglycemia is the most frequent metabolic derangement in critically ill neurological patients. There is solid evidence that hyperglycemia activates neurotoxic oxidative and inflammatory responses after acute ischemia. In patients with acute ischemic stroke, hyperglycemia has been associated with increased risk of hemorrhagic transformation and hyperacute worsening and lower rates of recanalization after thrombolysis (Alvarez-Sabin et al., 2004; Leigh et al., 2004; Ribo et al., 2005). It has also been found to correlate with infarct expansion and worse functional outcome (Baird et al., 2003; Bruno et al., 2002). Similarly, functional recovery is poorer in hyperglycemic patients with ICH and SAH (Frontera et al., 2006a; Passero et al., 2003). Intensive insulin therapy to maintain strict normoglycemia is no longer recommended for critically ill patients, after this practice led to increased mortality in a large randomized trial (Finfer et al., 2009). However, strict blood sugar control could decrease the rate of critical illness polyneuropathy (Van den Berghe et al., 2005). In the NICU, intensive insulin therapy carries the risk of inducing neuroglycopenia (with the ensuing risk of energy failure), which may occur in patients with acute brain insults even with serum glucose concentrations within the usual normal range (Godoy et al., 2010; Oddo et al., 2008). Therefore the treatment of hyperglycemia must proceed with particular caution in patients with acute brain disease, and serum glucose concentrations below 100 mg/dL should be avoided.

## Fever and Infections

Fever in a patient with acute brain disease demands prompt diagnostic investigation to determine its cause and symptomatic treatment to avoid the deleterious impact of hyperthermia on the injured brain. Experimental models have consistently shown that even mild hyperthermia worsens cerebral damage after ischemia or trauma (Baena et al., 1997; Dietrich et al., 1996; Kim et al., 1996). Fever has been associated with poor functional outcome in patients with ischemic infarction (Reith et al., 1996; Wang et al., 2000; Greer et al., 2008), ICH (Schwarz et al., 2000), SAH (Oliveira-Filho et al., 2001), and TBI (Jiang et al., 2002). Increased metabolic expenditure, exacerbation of excitotoxicity, and elevated ICP may be responsible for the detrimental effects of hyperthermia (Rossi et al., 2001; Thompson et al., 2003).

Fever is very prevalent among NICU patients. Disturbances in central thermoregulation occur frequently in patients with acute brain insults (Rabinstein and Sandhu, 2007), but infections are also a common cause of fever in the NICU and should always be excluded (Commichau et al., 2003). Pneumonia, urinary tract infection, and bloodstream infection are the most frequent infectious complications. Ventriculitis must always be ruled out in patients with ventriculostomy. Thus the appearance of fever in an NICU patient should be evaluated with cultures of blood, urine, respiratory secretions (ideally collected by bronchoalveolar lavage), and CSF (always in patients with ventriculostomy and when deemed clinically indicated in others). Chest radiography and microscopic analysis of the urine are also pertinent. CT scan of the sinuses may be added to the diagnostic evaluation in febrile patients who have been intubated for several days. CT of the abdomen and pelvis is sometimes necessary to detect abscesses, pancreatitis, or cholecystitis. The skin should be thoroughly searched for signs of cellulitis or phlebitis. Osteomyelitis and discitis must be included in the differential diagnosis of fever after spinal surgery.

When an infection is suspected, empirical antibiotic therapy is reasonable. It should cover for the most likely responsible organisms, depending on the patient's risk factors and the local microbiological resistance patterns of the ICU. Empirical antibiotics may be discontinued after 2–3 days if no infection is documented. It is always prudent to consider changing indwelling catheters (central venous, arterial, bladder, ventricular) in persistently febrile patients.

Drug reactions, DVT, ethanol withdrawal, pancreatitis, and gout are relatively common causes of noninfectious fever in the NICU. Drug fever is most frequently caused by phenytoin in neurological patients. Signs of anticonvulsant hypersensitivity or drug reaction with eosinophilia and systemic symptoms (DRESS) syndrome (rash, lymphadenopathy, hepatomegaly, eosinophilia, elevation of liver transaminases) must be readily recognized, since failure to discontinue the culprit medication promptly may lead to the devastating consequence of Stevens-Johnson syndrome (Schlienger and Shear, 1998).

Detailed physical examination, venous Doppler, and measurement of liver and pancreatic enzymes should be performed in NICU patients with fever of unclear cause. In chronically immobile patients (especially those with spinal cord injury), heterotopic ossification may rarely be a cause of persistent fever; it may be suspected by marked elevation of the C-reactive protein and sedimentation rate and confirmed by bone scintigraphy.

Central fever is a very common occurrence in the NICU and occurs as a consequence of the primary brain injury. Learning to recognize it can be very useful for avoiding overutilization of tests and antibiotics. Central fever is more likely to occur within the first 2–3 days of admission to the NICU and tends to be persistent. Patients with central fever often have prolonged hyperthermia with failure to return to normal body temperature, as opposed to the spikes of fever followed by normothermia typically observed with infections. The combination of negative cultures, absence of infiltrate on chest x-ray, primary diagnosis of SAH, intraventricular hemorrhage, or tumor, and onset of fever within the first 72 hours of admission predicted that the fever was central with a 90% probability in a large cohort of NICU patients (Hocker et al., 2013). In patients with SAH, central fever is associated with an increased risk of vasospasm (Oliveira-Filho et al., 2001; Rabinstein et al., 2007). Especially among patients with TBI, high fevers may be accompanied by other manifestations of *paroxysmal sympathetic hyperactivity* (tachycardia, hypertension, diaphoresis, dystonia; Rabinstein, 2007).

Multiple measures can be used to normalize body temperature in febrile patients. Antipyretic medications (acetaminophen, ibuprofen) are sufficient in milder cases. However, mechanical cooling methods must be added in patients with more severe or refractory hyperthermia. Ice packs, air- or water-circulating cooling blankets, and effective cooling vests are alternative methods of conductive cooling (Seder and Van der Kloot, 2009). Endovascular cooling devices may offer greater control of temperature modulation but require placement of a central venous catheter (Seder and Van der Kloot, 2009). Patients should be monitored for the appearance of shivering, which can be treated with skin counterwarming devices such as warming gloves; it can also be treated with medications such as buspirone, meperidine (in patients without high risk for seizures), magnesium infusion, or dexmedetomidine in patients who are awake. In severe cases, however, neuromuscular paralysis may be necessary.

## Hematological Complications

The risk of DVT is increased in immobilized patients. The incidence of clinical DVT after acute ischemic stroke ranges between 1% and 5%, and clinical PE occurs in 0.5%–3.5% of these patients (Kamphuisen et al., 2005). However, the incidence of subclinical DVT is much higher when assessed by ultrasound, venography, or nuclear scans (Kamphuisen et al., 2005). The risk of DVT is also increased after craniotomy (Hamilton et al., 1994), ICH (Lacut et al., 2005), and in patients with severe neuromuscular weakness. The main diagnostic test for DVT is noninvasive bedside vascular ultrasound (venous Doppler). Physical examination is relatively insensitive to detect DVT in acutely ill hospitalized patients. When PE is suspected, spiral CT angiography of the chest should be performed.

Early mobilization should be promoted in all patients. Options for the prevention of thromboembolic complications in immobilized patients include intermittent pneumatic compression and antithrombotics. Intermittent pneumatic compression should be used in all immobilized patients. Evidence supports the use of prophylactically dosed subcutaneous anticoagulants for most patients with acute ischemic stroke (Jauch et al., 2013; Kamphuisen et al., 2005) and after craniotomy (Iorio and Agnelli, 2000). There is more debate regarding the management of thromboprophylaxis in patients with ICH or large ischemic cerebral infarction, although the current recommendation is to initiate subcutaneous prophylactic low-molecular-weight heparin or unfractionated heparin after stability of the hemorrhage has been demonstrated (1–4 days after hemorrhage; Hemphill et al., 2015). Enoxaparin (40 mg/day) was found to be superior to unfractionated heparin (5000 U bid) in one randomized controlled trial of patients with acute ischemic stroke (Sherman et al., 2007). In cases of documented DVT with a high risk of hemorrhagic complications from anticoagulation, placement of a Greenfield filter in the inferior vena cava is a valuable alternative.

The optimal hematocrit level in critically ill neurological patients has not been adequately studied and probably varies according to the underlying primary disease process. Mild hemodilution may improve the rheological properties of the cerebral circulation, but excessive anemia may compromise oxygen delivery. Transfusions are indicated only for general critically ill patients when the hemoglobin concentration is lower than 7 g/dL. The appropriateness of this conservative practice in patients with acute brain damage (who may be particularly sensitive to local or regional hypoxia) remains to be established. Yet transfusions have been associated with worse outcomes in patients with SAH (Festic et al., 2013).

Thrombocytopenia in the NICU is most commonly associated with exposure to heparin or other drugs (e.g., valproic acid, antibiotics). Heparin-induced thrombocytopenia may be diagnosed by the presence of circulating serum antibodies to platelet factor 4 and confirmed with a serotonin release assay (a functional measure of platelet activity). Discontinuation of heparin results in prompt normalization of the platelet count. In patients with heparin-induced thrombocytopenia who still have an indication for continuing therapeutic anticoagulation, a direct thrombin inhibitor (recombinant hirudin or argatroban) should be used instead of heparin.

*The complete reference list is available online at https://expertconsult.inkling.com/.* 

54

# Principles of Neuroendovascular Therapy

*Thanh N. Nguyen, Tudor G. Jovin, Raul G. Nogueira, Osama O. Zaidat*

## OUTLINE



Neuroendovascular therapies consist of minimally invasive, catheter-based interventions for disorders affecting blood vessels (arteries and veins) of the brain and spine that are performed from within the vessel. For the past decade, the field of neuroendovascular therapies has been characterized by continuous and substantial growth through transformative technological advancements and multidisciplinary collaboration. Previously inaccessible lesions have become treatable with minimally invasive techniques; abnormalities that were once deemed too complex for standard endovascular therapies are now treated with new-generation devices. In parallel with technological advances, increased operator experience has improved safety and efficacy. Although basic neuroangiography techniques such as cerebral angiography were developed by the Portuguese neurologist Egaz Moniz, the majority of developments within the field of therapeutic neuroendovascular procedures have occurred over the past three decades. Digital subtraction angiography and flat-panel fluoroscopy systems have led to improved imaging capabilities and allow characterization of vascular anatomy with exquisite detail. Imaging of the parenchymal tissue has also become feasible in the neuroangiography suite through the use of cone-beam computed tomography (CT) technology. The introduction of the detachable platinum coil for aneurysm represents a paradigm shift in aneurysm treatment by introducing a minimally invasive treatment option to open surgical treatments that were hitherto not amenable to endovascular approaches. Following this landmark moment, endovascular therapy for aneurysms has continued to evolve at breathtaking pace as stent, balloon, flow-diverter, and more recently, intrasaccular devices have emerged with safer, faster, and more effective results. However, the most disruptive effect on the field was brought by the advent of technologies allowing endovascular treatment for acute ischemic stroke due to proximal large vessel occlusion with high rates of effective reperfusion that have been shown to translate into unprecedented clinical benefit when tested in multiple randomized clinical trials enrolling patients up to 24 hours after last seen well. Revascularization strategies for moderate to severe carotid stenosis consisting of carotid angioplasty and stenting (CAS) typically with the aid of embolic protection devices and the development of intracranial angioplasty and stenting have expanded treatment options for cerebrovascular conditions caused by atherosclerotic disease. Embolization techniques and new liquid embolic agents have expanded the role of neurointervention through embolization methods for arteriovenous malformations (AVMs), tumors, and chronic subdural hematomas (SDHs). Potential future approaches such as intraarterial (IA) of chemotherapy, IA stem cells, implantable stents for neuromonitoring (Oxley, 2016), and endovascular cerebrospinal fluid (CSF) shunts (Heilman, 2019) may further expand the landscape of neuroendovascular therapies.

## ISCHEMIC STROKE

### Large Vessel Occlusion

Stroke is the fourth leading cause of death and the most common reason for disability worldwide (Kochanek et al., 2011, Feigin et al., 2016). The majority of ischemic strokes result from vessel occlusion secondary to thromboembolic or atheromatous processes. Timely reperfusion of ischemic brain tissue is the most effective therapeutic strategy. Time-based intravenous (IV) thrombolysis was initially restricted to a narrow 3-hour time window based on the NINDS trials (National Institute of Neurological Disorders and Stroke rt-PA Stroke Study Group, 1995) and subsequently extended in clinical practice (although not approved by the US Food and Drug Administration [FDA]) based on the Third European Cooperative Acute Stroke Study demonstrating a smaller but definite benefit of IV thrombolysis in the 3–4.5 hours after symptom onset (Hacke et al., 2008). Recent studies have shown when physiological data derived from advanced imaging studies (magnetic resonance imaging [MRI] or CT perfusion imaging) capable of identifying the presence of mismatch between the infarcted territory relative to the entire "at-risk" territory supplied by the occluded vessel, a small benefit of IV tissue plasminogen activator (tPA) could be demonstrated up to 9 hours from last seen well (Ma et al., 2019). Another approach (Thomalla et al., 2018) using specific MRI diffusion-weighted imaging (DWI)–fluid-attenuated inversion recovery (FLAIR) mismatch signatures as a surrogate for time also demonstrated benefit of IV thrombolysis. Nonetheless, the main restrictions on IV recombinant tissue plasminogen activator (rtPA) remain the relatively narrow time window, limited effect on proximal arterial occlusions, need for advanced imaging in later time windows, and its nontargeted systemic mode of delivery. Coupled with a relative lack of public awareness, these factors have limited the use of IV thrombolysis to less than 5% of eligible candidates (Barber et al., 2001). To improve reperfusion, many techniques have evolved, including adjunctive focused ultrasound therapy in IV rtPA and endovascular catheter-based therapies.

## Endovascular Revascularization Therapy

In 2015, five randomized clinical trials demonstrated benefit of endovascular thrombectomy compared with medical management for patients with acute ischemic stroke due to large vessel occlusion presenting in the 6–12-hour time window (Berkhemer et al., 2015, Campbell et al., 2015, Goyal et al., 2015, Jovin et al., 2015, Saver et al., 2015). Although some of these trials used time windows of up to 12 hours, the vast majority of patients enrolled were randomized within 6 hours of time last seen well. These findings were further supported by two other completed randomized trials conducted in the early time window: THRACE (Trial and Cost Effectiveness Evaluation of Intra-Arterial Thrombectomy in Acute Ischemic Stroke) (Bracard, 2016) and RESILIENT (EndoVascular Treatment with Stent-retriever and/or Thromboaspiration vs. Best Medical Therapy in Acute Ischemic Stroke) (Martins, 2019). The landmark DAWN (DWI or CT perfusion (CTP) assessment with Clinical Mismatch in the Triage of Wake-Up and Late Presenting Strokes undergoing Neurointervention) and DEFUSE 3 (Endovascular Therapy Following Imaging Evaluation for Ischemic Stroke 3) trials demonstrated the benefit of thrombectomy in patients presenting beyond 6 hours and up to the 24 hours from last seen well, which represents a change in paradigm for acute stroke care worldwide (Nogueira, 2018, Albers et al., 2018). Patients who, based on time constraints, were previously not considered candidate for thrombectomy, are now being evaluated for the presence of vessel occlusion and presence of salvageable brain up to 24 hours from last seen well as standard of care. Although inclusion criteria varied across the several randomized endovascular acute stroke trials, adequate patient selection to avoid both overtreatment and undertreatment is critical. From a pathophysiological perspective, what explains the clinical benefit seen with reperfusion therapies in acute stroke due to large vessel occlusions is the concept of mismatch between tissue that is already infarcted (ischemic core) and the entire tissue at risk of undergoing infarction. Subtracting the former from the latter yields tissue that is functionally impaired and imminently threatened to undergo infarction due to ongoing hypoperfusion but is structurally intact and thus potentially salvageable (penumbra). It is believed that the larger the mismatch, the stronger the clinical benefit with reperfusion. Consequently, selection algorithms are determined not only by clinical but also by imaging criteria and time of symptom onset determines risk/benefit stratification. Parenchymal imaging with CT or MRI is used to quantify infarct size and assess for presence of hemorrhage. CT angiography (CTA), MR angiography (MRA), or catheter angiography are used to confirm large vessel occlusion, whereas CT and MRI perfusion imaging can assess potentially salvageable tissue in the ischemic penumbra. Because the extent of neurological deficit measured by the National Institutes of Health Stroke Scale (NIHSS) is a rough estimate of the extent of tissue at risk, it can be used in conjunction with imaging-based assessment of ischemic core to assess for the presence of mismatch (Box 54.1). The constellation of clinical deficit that is out of proportion to the size of the infarct observed on imaging is indicative of mismatch and is predictive of benefit with reperfusion therapies (clinical-infarct mismatch) (Dávalos et al., 2004).

## Intraarterial Thrombolysis

Compared with IV approaches, IA administration of thrombolytics via a microcatheter positioned in the cerebral vasculature affords rapid local delivery of greater therapeutic treatment concentrations to the vascular occlusion site. The technique entails performing a catheter-based cerebral angiogram to confirm the point of occlusion. Under fluoroscopic guidance, a microcatheter is advanced through a larger guide catheter to the clot. Once positioned, a thrombolytic agent is injected as intermittent control angiograms are performed. Recanalization of the occluded vessel is then evaluated using an established scoring method such as the Treatment in Cerebral Ischemia (TICI) method (Zaidat et al., 2013).

Clinical studies have been performed using streptokinase, urokinase, rtPA, recombinant prourokinase, and reteplase. These agents differ in fibrin selectivity, stability, half-life, and mechanism of action (Nguyen, 2011a; Schellinger et al., 2001). The Prolyse in Acute Cerebral Thromboembolism II (PROACT II) trial demonstrated the effectiveness of IA prourokinase when given within 6 hours of acute stroke caused by middle cerebral artery occlusion (Furlan et al., 1999). Patients were randomized to IA recombinant prourokinase and IV heparin or heparin alone. The primary clinical outcome of minimal or no disability at 90 days (modified Rankin Scale [mRS] score ≤2) was achieved in 40% of the treatment group and 25% of the controls. The Middle Cerebral Artery Embolism Local Fibrinolytic Intervention Trial (MELT) Japan randomized 114 acute stroke patients with M1/M2 occlusion into control treatment versus IA urokinase within 6 hours of symptoms onset (Ogawa et al., 2007). The primary clinical outcome of mRS of 2 or less at 90 days was achieved in 49.1% of the treatment group and 38.6% of the controls.

The Interventional Management of Stroke (IMS) study investigators compared acute stroke patients treated with a bridging IV rtPA dose (0.6 mg/kg) followed by IA rtPA, with historical controls given only the traditional IV dosing regimen from the NINDS trial. The IMS I study was an open-label, single-arm, feasibility study using a microcatheter to infuse up to 22 mg of IA rtPA over 2 hours (IMS Study Investigators, 2004). The prospective randomized IMS III trial using early-generation IA treatment methods including IA t-PA, and ultrasound-enhanced local thrombolysis with the use of the EKOS MicroLysUS (EKOS Corp., Bothell, WA) microinfusion catheter, which incorporates sonographic technology to increase permeability and penetration of the intraluminal clot (IMS II Trial Investigators, 2007), and first-generation thrombectomy devices was stopped for futility and showed no significant difference in functional independence between combined IV/IA therapy as compared with IV tPA; however, similar safety outcomes were demonstrated (Broderick et al., 2013). Future research on the role of IA thrombolysis in the era of new-generation mechanical thrombectomy devices is needed (Zaidi, et al., 2019).

## Mechanical Thrombectomy

Narrow time windows, limited efficacy, and the risk of hemorrhage associated with thrombolytic agents prompted the design and application of mechanical thrombectomy devices. Endovascular clot retrieval provides potential for rapid flow restoration, with a decreased incidence of clot fragmentation and distal embolism (Nogueira et al., 2009b). Catheter-based, retrieval/aspiration systems began to be used in acute stroke patients who were either ineligible for or had failed IV rtPA administration; initially they were used in conjunction with thrombolytic infusion.

***Mechanical Embolus Removal in Cerebral Ischemia device.*** The first device to have received FDA approval for clot retrieval was the Mechanical Embolus Removal in Cerebral Ischemia (MERCI) device (Concentric Medical Inc., Mountain View, CA). The retriever is a flexible tapered nitinol wire with radiopaque helical loops at the distal tip (Fig. 54.1). Results from the single-arm MERCI and Multi MERCI trial demonstrated the efficacy of the MERCI system in restoring the patency of occluded intracranial vessels within 8 hours of acute ischemic stroke (Smith et al., 2005, 2008). Although no control group was available for comparison, safety and efficacy data compared with historical controls were encouraging. Some 48% of occluded vessels were recanalized, a rate significantly higher than that of the control arm in the PROACT II trial (18%) (Furlan et al., 1999; Nogueira et al., 2009b). After adjuvant therapy (IA rtPA, angioplasty, snare), the rate of recanalization was 60.3%. The overall rates of good outcome (mRS score ≤2) and mortality were 27.7% and 43.5%, respectively, with a procedural complication rate of 7.1%. Furthermore, successful revascularization was found to be an independent predictor of decreased mortality and favorable neurological outcome at 90 days. Similar results were noted in the Multi MERCI trial, which included patients treated with IV tPA prior to thrombectomy and used a modified version of the original MERCI device. These trials are of historical importance because the MERCI device has been discontinued.

**BOX 54.1 National Institutes of Health Stroke Scale**

1A. Level of consciousness (0–3)
1B. Month/age (0–2)
1C. Commands eyes open/closed (0–2)
2. Best gaze (0–2)
3. Visual (0–3)
4. Facial palsy (0–3)
5. Best motor arm (0–4)
6. Best motor leg (0–4)
7. Limb ataxia (0–2)
8. Sensory (0–2)
9. Best language (0–3)
10. Dysarthria (0–2)
11. Neglect (0–2)

Normal/near normal examination (0–1)
Minor stroke (1–4)
Moderate stroke (5–15)
Moderate/severe stroke (15–20)
Severe stroke (>20)

***Distal Catheter Aspiration Systems.*** The Penumbra System (Penumbra Inc., Alameda, CA) was the first aspiration device through which a thromboembolic clot could be retrieved following acute ischemic stroke (Fig. 54.2). The device removes thrombus via aspiration and extraction with or without mechanical disruption. Multiple aspiration catheters of varying luminal diameters are available for use in the cervical and intracranial vasculature, depending on vessel caliber. The aspiration device is advanced coaxially to the level of the thrombus through a guide catheter. When positioned immediately proximal to the target lesion, an aspiration pump is connected to the reperfusion catheter or manual aspiration is applied. The separator is then advanced through the catheter into the distal clot and repeatedly retracted and advanced, to clear the catheter tip during aspiration (Fig. 54.3). A multicenter, prospective, single-arm, phase I trial of the Penumbra reperfusion catheter was designed to assess safety and efficacy (Bose et al., 2008). Recanalization (Thrombolysis in Myocardial Infarction [TIMI] score of 2 or 3) was achieved in all vessels in which the device was deployed. A secondary endpoint of mRS score of 2 or less or improvement of NIHSS score by 4 or better was achieved in 45% of patients. The Penumbra device received FDA approval in 2008, and since then newer-generation large-bore reperfusion catheters have been introduced to allow improved aspiration of the clot. The separator clot disruption device has since been abandoned.

The Contact Aspiration vs Stent Retriever for Successful Revascularization (ASTER) and the COMPASS (A Direct Aspiration First Pass Technique) trial were two multicenter randomized trials comparing aspiration thrombectomy versus stent retriever thrombectomy as first-line approaches for large vessel occlusion (Lapergue et al., 2017, Turk et al., 2019). Patients with large vessel occlusion presenting within 6 hours of symptom onset were randomly assigned to a first-line strategy consisting of either direct aspiration or stent retriever. Both studies showed that direct or contact aspiration first pass was not inferior to stent retriever as first-line therapy (Lapergue et al., 2017, Turk et al., 2019).

***Stent retriever.*** Retrievable stent devices designed to retrieve the occlusive thrombus emerged as favorable methods for acute stroke thrombectomy (Fig. 54.4) after two such devices in a head to head head-to-head comparison against the MERCI device showed superior rates of recanalization and better clinical outcomes (Saver et al., 2012, Nogueiraa). Both the Solitaire FR (Medtronic, Irvine, CA) and Trevo Retriever (Stryker Neurovascular) devices subsequently received FDA approval. Subsequently,

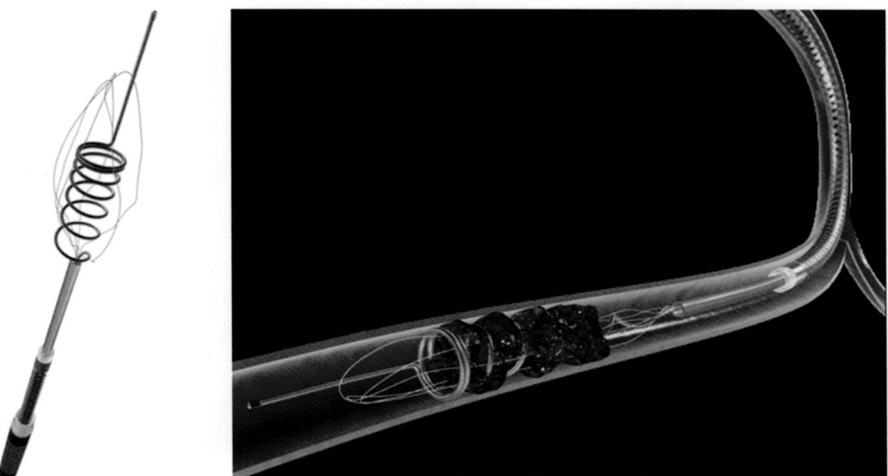

**Fig. 54.1** Mechanical Embolus Removal in Cerebral Ischemia (MERCI) clot retrieval device *(left)* and diagram demonstrating mechanism of action *(right)*. Spiral loops and suture material are designed to engage the clot and mechanically remove it from the vessel. *(Picture courtesy Concentric Medical Inc.)*

a third stent retriever, EmboTraP (Cerenovus, Miami, Fl), was approved by the FDA following the 228 patient clinical trial (ARISE II: Analysis of Revascularization in Ischemic Stroke with EmboTrap) demonstrating TICI ≥2b rate of 80% and mRS 0–2 of 67% at 90 days (Zaidat, 2018a).

In the wake of the negative IMS 3 and MR RESCUE (Mechanical Retrieval and Recanalization of Stroke Clots Using Embolectomy) trials, the higher rates of recanalization observed with newer-generation devices, particularly with stent retrievers, prompted an international effort to reappraise the benefit of thrombectomy in a new era of endovascular stroke therapy. Nine completed randomized trials revealed overwhelming efficacy for acute ischemic stroke thrombectomy for large vessel occlusion in early and extended time windows.

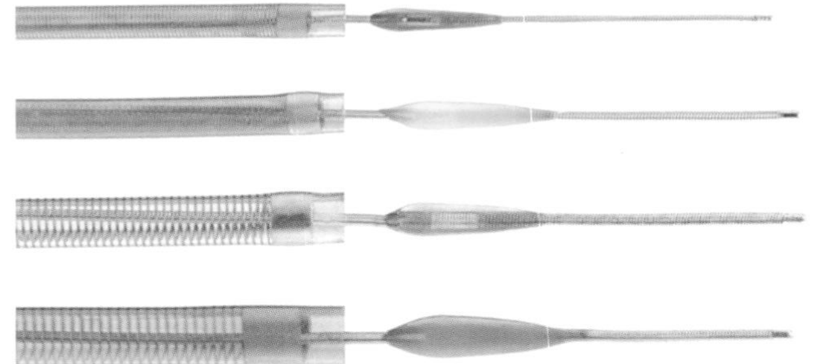

**Fig. 54.2 Penumbra Reperfusion Catheters and Separator Wires of Different Sizes.** Wire is used to fragment clot as the catheter provides suction/aspiration. *(Picture courtesy Penumbra Inc.)*

## MR CLEAN, ESCAPE, EXTEND-IA, SWIFT PRIME, REVASCAT, Thrace Trials

The Multicenter Randomized CLinical trial of Endovascular treatment for Acute ischemic stroke in the Netherlands (MR CLEAN) study was a randomized clinical trial in acute ischemic stroke patients with large vessel occlusion (Berkhemer et al., 2015). Patients were randomized to best medical management with or without IA therapy using the new class of mechanical thrombectomy devices (retrievable stent) within 6 hours of symptom onset. Patients were eligible with NIHSS score of as low as 2 and a large vessel occlusion on the head CT angiogram; however, the median NIHSS of patients enrolled in this trial was 17. The trial demonstrated positive outcome in favor of IA therapy over best medical management alone.

After the release of the MR CLEAN trial results at the World Stroke Congress in 2014, all subsequent mechanical thrombectomy randomized trials in the early time windows with the exception of RESILIENT were stopped due to potential lack of equipoise for continued enrollment.

An individual-level meta-analysis comprising 1287 patients enrolled in MR CLEAN, SWIFT PRIME (Solitaire with the Intention for Thrombectomy as PRIMary Endovascular Treatment), ESCAPE (Endovascular Treatment for Small Core and Proximal Occlusion

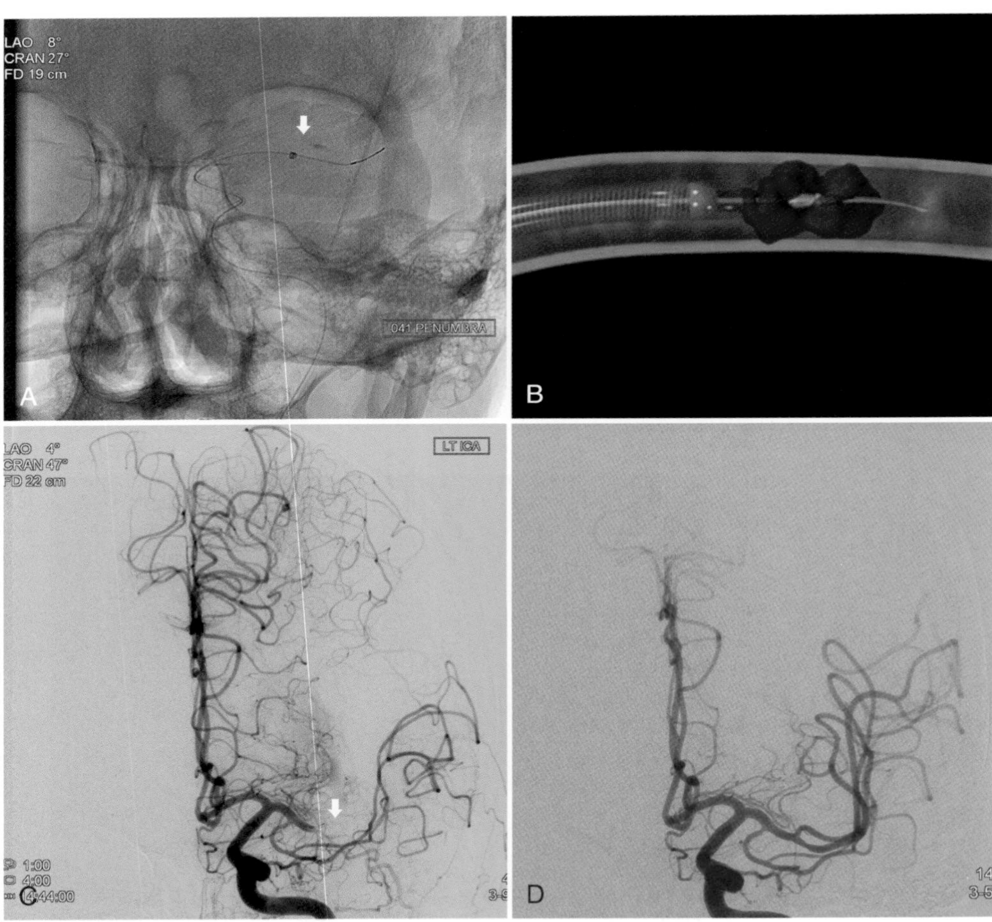


**Fig. 54.3** An anteroposterior view shows a Penumbra aspiration catheter positioned within the left middle cerebral artery as indicated by the catheter tip *(arrow)* with Separator wire **(A)**. An artistic illustration depicts the process of clot removal with aspiration **(B)**. Angiogram images of a left middle cerebral artery occlusion before **(C)** and after thromboaspiration **(D)** show complete vessel recanalization. *(Courtesy Penumbra Inc.)*

Ischemic Stroke), EXTEND IA (Extending the Time for Thrombolysis in Emergency Neurological Deficits- Intra-Arterial), and REVASCAT (Extending the Time for Thrombolysis in Emergency Neurological Deficits- Intra-Arterial) confirmed the overwhelming benefit of endovascular therapy for stroke, translating into a number needed to treat (NNT) of 3 to reduce poststroke disability. Patients allocated to thrombectomy achieved a modified Rankin Score of 0–2 (signifying independence in activities of daily living) in a significantly higher proportion than patients allocated to medical therapy (which in the vast majority of cases included IV tPA) (291/633–42% vs. 171/645–26.5%, respectively, $P < .00001$). The rates of symptomatic intracerebral hemorrhage did not differ significantly between the two groups (4.4% vs. 4.3%, respectively) and neither did the rates of mortality (15.3% vs. 18.9%).

## Mechanical Thrombectomy in the Delayed Window, 6–24 Hours

### DAWN Trial

Prior to the publication of DAWN, no evidence existed with regards to clinical benefit in patients presenting later than 6 hours from time last known well, with evidence of proximal large vessel occlusion and substantial mismatch. Available data suggest that these patients may comprise approximately 30% of all patients with acute stroke due to proximal large vessel occlusion (Jadhav et al., 2018) and thus represent a significant proportion of patients potentially eligible for thrombectomy. The DAWN trial was a randomized trial of patients with occlusion of the internal carotid artery (ICA) or proximal middle cerebral artery who could be randomized 6–24 hours from the time last seen well and with mismatch between the severity of the clinical deficit (NIHSS) and infarct volume assessed by means of automated software based on CT perfusion or MRI (clinical infarct mismatch). Patients were randomized to thrombectomy with the Trevo device in addition to standard of care versus standard of care alone largely consisting of antiplatelet therapy and general supportive care for stroke in the ICU setting. The primary endpoints were the mean score for disability on the utility-weighted mRS and the rate of functional independence. The trial was stopped prematurely due to an interim analysis that allowed stopping based on efficacy yielded results that met prespecified endpoints. Favorable clinical outcome as defined by mRS ≤2 was achieved more often in patients who underwent thrombectomy compared with medical management (49% vs. 13%, 95% confidence interval [CI] 24%–44%). There were no safety concerns. There were no differences in the rates of symptomatic intracranial hemorrhage (6% vs. 3%, $P = .5$) or 90-day mortality (19% vs. 18%, $P = 1$) between the thrombectomy and control groups, respectively (Nogueira et al., 2018).

### DEFUSE 3 Trial

The release of the DAWN trial results prompted an interim analysis by the DEFUSE 3 investigators. DEFUSE 3 was a randomized trial comparing patients with proximal large vessel occlusion and mismatch as determined by CT perfusion or MRI, treated with best medical management or mechanical thrombectomy. Key inclusion criteria included NIHSS 6 or greater, middle cerebral artery or ICA occlusion, and symptom randomization between 6 and 16 hours from time last seen well. Patients were selected based on an imaging profile demonstrating an

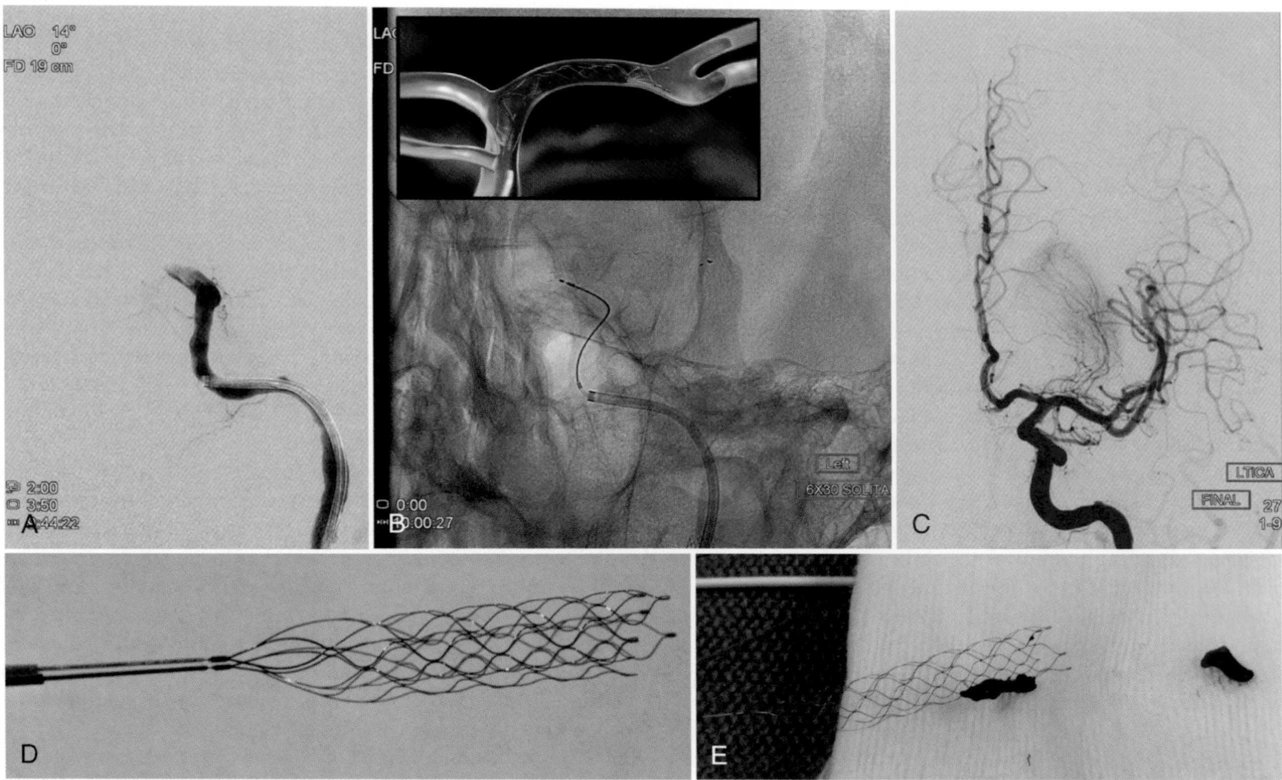


**Fig. 54.4** A left internal carotid artery angiogram shows complete occlusion of the terminal segment which extends into the left middle cerebral artery **(A)**. Fluoroscopy imaging shows a guide sheath positioned in the left internal carotid artery, a coaxially introduced microcatheter extending into the internal carotid artery terminal segment, and a retrievable stent design thrombectomy device (Solitaire FR) deployed within the left middle cerebral artery **(B)**. An artistic depiction of the device is shown in the inset. After mechanical clot removal, complete revascularization of the left internal carotid artery and middle cerebral artery is observed on an angiogram **(C)**. The Solitaire FR is an example of a retrievable stent design thrombectomy device **(D)**. Thrombus can be observed adherent to the device after thrombectomy **(E)**. *(© Medtronic. Used with permission.)*

infarct volume of less than 70 mL assessed by DWI MRI or CT perfusion and ratio of volume of ischemic tissue at risk (assessed by MR or CT perfusion as <30% contralateral cerebral blood flow [CBF]) to infarcted tissue ratio of 1.8. Similar to DAWN, DEFUSE 3 demonstrated better outcomes for patients treated with thrombectomy compared with standard medical management (mRS 0–2; 45% vs. 17%, $P < .001$). An individual-level pooled analysis of patients from DAWN, DEFUSE 3, and other three trials that randomized patients beyond 6 hours from symptoms onset revealed no increased incidence in symptomatic intracranial hemorrhage (sICH) between treatment and control and a treatment effect that is equivalent to that seen in patients randomized in the early time window (adjusted odds ratio [OR] for the distribution of mRS treatment vs. control of 2.77 (95% CI 1.95–3.94), $P < .0001$) vs. 2.49 (95% CI 1.76–3.53), $P < .0001$, respectively (Jovin et al., 2019).

### Multicenter Registries of Mechanical Thrombectomy

Two retrospective multicenter registries, TRACK (The TREVO Stent-Retriever Acute Stroke [TRACK] Registry) and North American Solitaire Acute Stroke Registry (NASA), demonstrated good clinical outcome with the stent retriever in real world clinical practice with favorable reperfusion rates of 80% and 88%, respectively; good clinical outcome defined as modified Rankin score 2 or less was seen in 48% and 42%, respectively (Zaidat et al., 2014 Zaidat, 2018a,b). The NASA study also coined the notion of first pass effect, defined as achieving complete recanalization with a single thrombectomy device pass (Zaidat, 2018b). In the NASA study, later confirmed by other thrombectomy studies (Ducroux et al., 2019), first-pass effect was found to be significantly associated with better clinical outcome.

The clinical effectiveness of thrombectomy has been more recently confirmed by two large prospective registries. The Systematic Evaluation of Patients Treated with Stroke Devices for Acute Ischemic Stroke (STRATIS) registry enrolled 984 patients (mean NIHSS 17.3; IV tPA use 64%) with large vessel occlusion strokes who were treated with the Solitaire or Mindframe Capture devices (Medtronic, Irvine, CA) within 8 hours from stroke onset at 55 US sites. The rates of successful reperfusion (TICI ≥ 2b), SICH, 90-day good outcome (mRS 0–2), and mortality were 87.9%, 1.4%, 56.5%, and 14.4%, respectively (Muell-er-Kronsat et al., 2017). The Trevo Registry recruited 2008 acute ischemic stroke patients (mean NIHSS 15.5; IV tPA use 52.3%) across 76 centers in 12 countries. Unlike STRATIS, the Trevo registry had no limits in terms of baseline stroke severity, premorbid mRS, occlusion site, or duration of symptoms. The rates of successful reperfusion (TICI ≥ 2b), SICH, 90-day good outcome (mRS 0–2), and mortality were 92.8%, 1.7%, 55.3%, and 13.9%, respectively (Binning et al., 2018).

Subanalysis of the NASA registry evaluated the role of the balloon guide catheter in reperfusion for patients treated with the Solitaire stent retriever. The balloon guide catheter is a catheter placed at the cervical carotid or vertebral artery. Once the clot is ready for retrieval, the balloon mounted on the outside of the catheter is inflated to arrest antegrade flow as the clot is retrieved with concomitant aspiration at the guide catheter. In multiple nonrandomized registries, the use of the balloon guide catheter was associated with improved reperfusion and clinical outcome compared with patients who were treated with conventional guide catheter (Nguyen, 2014, Zaidat, 2019, Nguyen, 2019, Baek et al., 2019).

### Intracranial Angioplasty and Stenting in Acute Stroke

Mature fibrinous clots can be difficult to treat pharmacologically, and thrombi adherent to the vascular intima or associated with underlying atheromatous disease can present a challenge for mechanical thrombectomy. Percutaneous transluminal angioplasty (PTA) and stenting procedures have been successful in acute coronary revascularization. Recanalization with angioplasty and stenting has been used in the absence of clot dissolution or extraction (Levy et al., 2009; Zaidat et al., 2008a). Several studies reported improvement in clinical outcome following angioplasty and local thrombolytic administration in the setting of acute stroke (Nogueira et al., 2008; Jovin et al., 2015; Ringer et al., 2001). A single-arm prospective trial of primary intracranial stenting for acute stroke demonstrated promising results. The authors reported 100% TIMI 2–3 recanalization in a cohort of 20 patients treated with intracranial stenting. Self-expanding stents (Wingspan [Boston Scientific, Natick, MA]; Enterprise [Cordis Neurovascular, Miami Lakes, FL]) designed exclusively for cerebral indications facilitated access and navigation through tortuous craniocervical anatomy. Although adjuvant IA antiplatelet therapy was used in 50% of patients, the authors reported only a 5% rate of symptomatic intracranial hemorrhage. At 1 month, 60% of patients had mRS scores of 3 or less, and 45% had mRS scores of 1 or less. These results suggest a potential role for this therapy in select acute stroke patients. Treatment for acute large vessel occlusion (LVO) stroke with balloon-mounted stents as second-line approach after failed thrombectomy in patients with presumed intracranial atherosclerotic disease (ICAD) has been shown to have reperfusion rates and clinical outcomes comparable to thrombectomy, although the rates of sICH and mortality were higher in this cohort of high-risk patients (Gross et al., 2019). Nonetheless, the need for immediate antiplatelet agent administration to prevent stent thrombosis, with their ensuing hemorrhagic risk especially in those patients who receive IV tPA, are potential limitations of this technology. Larger randomized studies are needed, to assess the safety and efficacy of this treatment modality.

**BOX 54.2 Patients at High Risk for Carotid Endarterectomy**

Defined as having significant comorbidities and/or anatomical risk and would be poor candidates for carotid endarterectomy (CEA) in the opinion of a surgeon.

Significant comorbid conditions include but are not limited to:

1. Congestive heart failure class III/IV
2. Left ventricular ejection fraction <30%
3. Unstable angina
4. Contralateral carotid occlusion
5. Recent myocardial infarction
6. Previous CEA with recurrent stenosis
7. Prior radiation treatment to the neck; and
8. Other conditions that were used to determine patients at high risk for CEA in the prior carotid angioplasty followed by stenting (CAS) trials

### Carotid Artery Disease

Extracranial carotid artery disease and its management have remained a long-standing focus in efforts targeting stroke prevention. Indications and outcomes for carotid endarterectomy (CEA) have been extensively studied in the setting of large-vessel extracranial steno-occlusive disease. Multicenter randomized clinical trials demonstrated that, compared with medical therapy alone, CEA in addition to aspirin reduces the incidence of stroke and death in both symptomatic and asymptomatic patients with severe carotid stenosis, with dramatic differences in treatment effect according to asymptomatic versus symptomatic status and in the latter group, according to timing of surgery.

The two landmark randomized controlled trials that enrolled symptomatic carotid stenosis patients were the North American Symptomatic Carotid Endarterectomy Trial (NASCET) and the European Carotid Surgery Trial (ECST) (Barnett et al., 1998; European Carotid Surgery Trialists' Collaborative Group, 1996). The NASCET investigators showed that CEA reduced the risk of ipsilateral stroke (9%) at 2 years, compared with best medical therapy (26%) in patients harboring carotid stenoses of 70%–99%. A more modest yet still significant reduction in the 5-year rate of ipsilateral stroke was evident in patients with 50%–70% stenosis

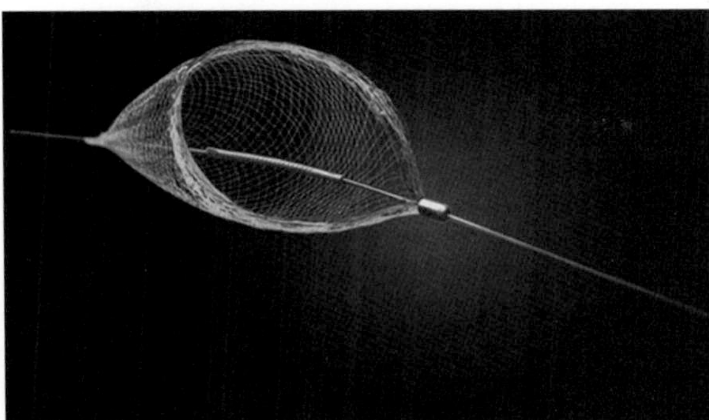

**Fig. 54.5 Over-the-Wire Distal Embolic Protection Device.** Filter is positioned in distal cervical internal carotid artery (beyond stenotic segment) to prevent embolic debris from reaching intracranial circulation.

(Box 54.2). The overall perioperative stroke and death rate for patients treated with CEA was 5.8%. Using a different measurement criterion for quantifying luminal stenosis on angiography, the ECST arrived at a similar result. Data demonstrated that surgically treated patients with stenosis greater than 80% had a lower estimated risk of death or major stroke when compared with those managed medically. A subsequent meta-analysis that included all NASCET and ECST patients revealed that the strongest benefit from revascularization is within the first 2 weeks of the index event (Rothwell et al., 2003). There is still considerable debate regarding the optimal timing of intervention within those 2 weeks. Although mounting evidence indicates that the risk of intervention is highest in the first 48 hours post index event, this does not necessarily imply that revascularization should be preferentially performed outside of this time frame when the risk of recurrent events without revascularization is also highest. There is a paucity of natural history data on the risk of recurrent stroke ultra-early after index event in patients with ipsilateral high-grade carotid stenosis. However, prospective studies have estimated that the ultra-early risk of neurological deterioration may be as high as 5%–21% within the first 48–72 hours.

The Asymptomatic Carotid Atherosclerosis Study (ACAS) and the Asymptomatic Carotid Surgery Trial (ACST) addressed indications for CEA in asymptomatic patients (Executive Committee for the ACAS, 1995; Halliday et al., 2004). Both studies demonstrated that compared with those treated with best medical therapy, the 5-year incidence of ipsilateral stroke or death was reduced in the CEA group. The 5-year stroke and death rate was 11% for patients in the medical therapy cohort, while the stroke risk was 5.1% for patients treated with CEA.

Based on these results, the American Heart Association guidelines recommend CEA for symptomatic patients with 50%–99% stenosis if the perioperative risk of stroke or death is less than 6%, and for asymptomatic patients with stenosis of 60%–99% if the perioperative risk of stroke or death is less than 3% (Biller et al., 1998; Kernan et al., 2014; Sacco et al., 2006 ).

Based on observed lower rates of ipsilateral stroke in asymptomatic patients in the era of modern medical therapy compared with those noted during ACAS and ACST, the concept of revascularization treatment (with stenting or endarterectomy) for asymptomatic carotid disease, regardless of severity is being reevaluated in the ongoing Carotid Revascularization Endarterectomy versus Stenting Trial (CREST) II trial (Heck et al., 2017).

## Carotid Artery Angioplasty and Stenting

CAS evolved because of a need for alternative, less-invasive treatment modalities for patients deemed poor operative candidates on the basis of anatomical or clinical parameters. In addition, the less-invasive nature of the stenting procedure makes it an appealing alternative to surgery for many patients.

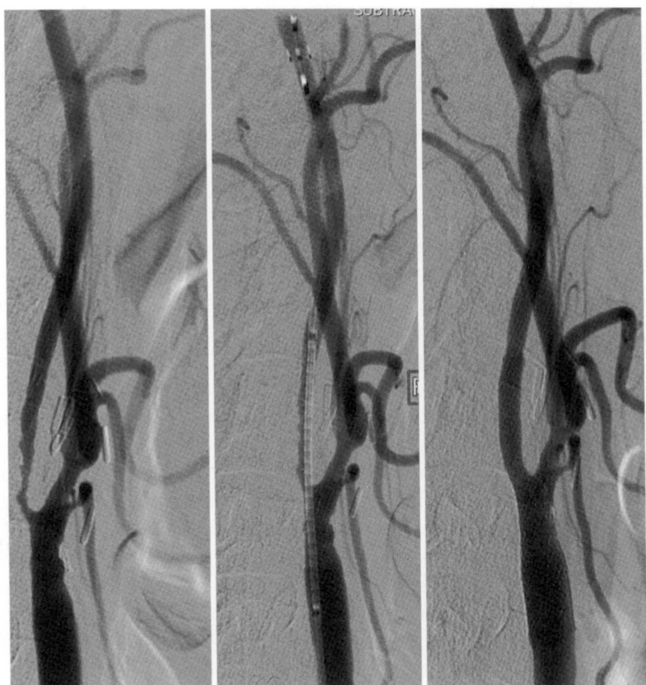

**Fig. 54.6** Lateral angiogram demonstrating critical proximal internal carotid artery stenosis *(left)*. Embolic protection device is opened in distal cervical internal carotid artery (top of picture, *middle*). Following balloon dilatation, stent is positioned across stenotic segment *(middle)*. Lateral angiogram showing stent deployed in distal common and proximal internal carotid artery, with minimal residual stenosis *(right)*.

***Angioplasty and stenting procedure.*** In anticipation of carotid artery angioplasty and stenting, dual antiplatelet therapy is initiated prior to the intervention to decrease the risk of thromboembolic complications. Most procedures are performed awake or under monitored anesthesia care, allowing for continuous neurological assessment. Placement of an embolic protection system is generally attempted, to mitigate the effects of distal embolization. Distal protection is most commonly achieved with over-the-wire distal filters sized to the diameter of the native cervical ICA that are navigated past the stenotic lesion (Fig. 54.5). Such devices allow continuous cerebral perfusion through pores in the filter baskets. Following angioplasty and stenting, the device is collapsed and withdrawn and embolic material retrieved. Alternatively, proximal flow control systems such as balloon occlusion devices may be used to prevent anterograde flow within the ICA. Any displaced material can be aspirated prior to balloon deflation. However, temporary carotid occlusion may not be well tolerated in all patients, limiting the applicability of this strategy.

Once embolic protection is achieved, balloon pre-dilatation of tight stenoses can help ensure safe advancement of a self-expanding stent past the target lesion. Balloon inflation is done slowly to lessen the incidence of thromboembolism. Communication with an anesthesiologist is critical to address bradycardia which can occur with balloon inflation at the level of the carotid bulb, and later, to lower blood pressure after carotid revascularization to prevent reperfusion hemorrhage. Stent diameter is calibrated to the common carotid artery diameter and length is measured to traverse the entire lesion with a margin of several millimeters both proximally and distally. Tapered stents are available to accommodate the larger diameter of the common carotid artery and the smaller lumen of the ICA. Depending on residual stenosis and distal perfusion, post-stent balloon dilatation may be undertaken (Fig. 54.6).

***Clinical trials.*** Since the advent of CAS procedures, multiple clinical trials have demonstrated that carotid stenting procedures are feasible in most patients with carotid stenosis. Over the recent 20 years the procedure has undergone a significant maturation process and most studies have attested to the decreasing incidence of adverse events with this procedure over time (Lichtman, et al., 2017). Studies have demonstrated benefit of CAS over CEA in high-risk surgical patients and equivalent benefits in lower-risk candidates.

The largest randomized trial conducted in North America, the prospective CREST enrolled a total of 1326 symptomatic patients with greater than 50% stenosis and 1176 asymptomatic patients with greater than 60% stenosis deemed good candidates for either CEA or CAS (Hobson et al., 2004). Primary endpoints included death, stroke, and myocardial infarction (MI) at 30 days or ipsilateral stroke at 1 year. Based on the rates of the primary endpoint achieved in each arm, (7.2% with stenting vs. 6.8% with endarterectomy) carotid artery stenting was found to be equivalent to CEA. Furthermore, both the incidence of death, MI, or stroke at 30 days and the incidence of periprocedural major (disabling) stroke were nonsignificant between the two arms (5.2% vs. 4.5%) and (0.9% vs. 0.7%), respectively. Although the overall incidence of stroke was significantly higher in the CAS arm (4.1% vs. 2.3%, $P = .01$), the incidence of MI was significantly lower in the CAS arm, compared with the CEA arm (1.1% vs. 2.3%, $P = .03$). Cranial nerve palsies were also significantly more common in the CEA arm. Long-term follow-up suggested that the incidence of ipsilateral stroke after the periprocedural period (≈4 years of follow-up) was similar between the two arms (2.0% vs. 2.4%). Subgroup analyses indicated effect modification by age such that patients 69 years of age or younger had lower rates of the primary endpoint with CAS, whereas those aged 70 or older had higher rates with CEA (Brott et al., 2010). During the periprocedural period, rates of the primary endpoint did not differ significantly between the stenting group and the endarterectomy group among symptomatic patients (6.7% vs. 5.4%; hazard ratio [HR] for stenting, 1.26; 95% CI, 0.81–1.96) or among asymptomatic patients (3.5% vs. 3.6%; HR, 1.02; 95% CI, 0.55–1.86). These results have justified expansion of indications for CAS procedures to include non–high-risk patients.

The International Carotid Stenting Study (ICSS), also known as *CAVATAS II*, is a European trial in symptomatic carotid stenosis patients. It was designed to revisit the questions raised in the original investigation while using stents in all percutaneous procedures (CAVATAS, 2001; Ederle et al., 2010). Initial results were published at the same time the CREST data were revealed. ICSS enrolled 1713 patients and demonstrated that the incidence of stroke, death, or procedural MI was significantly elevated in the stenting group (8.5%) compared with the endarterectomy group (5.2%). There was an increased number of cranial nerve palsies in the CEA group.

The conflicting initial results generated by the CREST study, which was performed in the United States, and the European ICSS trial raised further questions regarding the indications for these two procedures. However, it must be noted that the studies were designed differently. Although CREST evaluated both symptomatic and asymptomatic patients, ICSS examined only those with symptoms. Furthermore, as perhaps the most significant difference between the two trials, ICSS allowed participation of less experienced operators compared with CREST with no "lead-in time" allowed into the trial.

Equivalence between CAS and CEA based on the CREST cohort was reported at 10 years results (Brott et al., 2016). and noninferiority of CAS compared with CEA has been demonstrated in the randomized asymptomatic ACST trial, further supporting the use of CAS as a viable alternative to CEA along the wide spectrum of carotid stenosis patients, who based on anatomical and clinical grounds are deemed suitable for stenting.

The Carotid Revascularization and Medical Management for Asymptomatic Carotid Stenosis Trial (CREST-2) is an ongoing trial which will assess whether CEA or CAS, in addition to intensive medical therapy, is superior to intensive medical therapy alone in the primary prevention of stroke in patients with high-grade asymptomatic carotid stenosis (Howard et al., 2017). There are two components to CREST-2. One trial compares CEA to intensive medical therapy versus intensive medical therapy alone. The other trial compares carotid stenting in addition to intensive medical therapy versus intensive medical therapy alone. CAS and CEA are not compared against each other in CREST. Of note, the effects of carotid revascularization on cognition will also be evaluated (Norling et al., 2019).

## Intracranial Atherosclerotic Disease

ICAD is a common etiology of cerebrovascular disease, responsible for at least 9% of all ischemic strokes (Sacco et al., 1995). The Warfarin-Aspirin Symptomatic Intracranial Disease (WASID) trial and subset analyses demonstrated that patients who had suffered an ischemic cerebrovascular event and harbored more than 70% stenosis of a referable intracranial artery were at a high risk for recurrent stroke (Chimowitz et al., 2005). A reported 23% of enrolled patients experienced a subsequent ipsilateral stroke over the course of the next year despite state-of-the-art medical therapy at the time the trial was conducted (Chimowitz et al., 2005). This high event rate occurred regardless of whether or not patients had failed antithrombotic therapy at the time of their qualifying event (Turan et al., 2009).

The development and widespread success of angioplasty and stenting for peripheral and coronary atheromatous disease have promoted adaptation of these techniques to treat lesions in the cerebral vasculature. Modern imaging modalities and technological advancements in catheter and device design have enabled endovascular treatment of ICAD.

### Intracranial Angioplasty

Balloon angioplasty was the first percutaneous transluminal technique evaluated for ICAD. In a large retrospective study reported on 120 patients with intracranial stenosis treated by primary angioplasty (Marks et al., 2006), the periprocedural stroke and death rate was 5.8% and a total yearly event rate of 3.2%. This and other investigations have reported posttreatment residual vessel stenosis in the range of 40% (Marks et al., 2006; Terada et al., 1996, Nguyen et al., 2011c). High incidences of angiographic vessel dissection have been documented, although they have rarely been noted to manifest as clinical events (Marks et al., 2006; Mori et al., 1998; Wojak et al., 2006). Durability of primary angioplasty has also been questioned, with reported retreatment rates near 20% (Siddiq et al., 2008). Mori et al. (1998) investigated lesion-specific features that predicted successful angioplasty and low restenosis rates. They determined that short segment, concentric narrowing, and subtotal angiographic occlusion correlated with the lowest incidence of restenosis following PTA. By contrast, features that portended poor outcome or higher rates of restenosis were eccentricity, extreme angularity, length greater than 10 mm, or excessive tortuosity of the proximal vessel segment. In addition, the success rate was significantly lower for lesions treated more than 3 months from the time of stroke.

Experience in the coronary literature indicated that the shortcomings of primary angioplasty (plaque dislodgement, acute elastic recoil, vessel dissection, recurrent stenosis) could be overcome by subsequent stent deployment (George et al., 1998). These concepts were translated directly to the intracranial vasculature.

### Intracranial Angioplasty and Stenting

Several early case reports described angioplasty and stenting of cerebral vessels using coronary artery techniques (Chow et al., 2005; Gomez et al., 2000; Yu et al., 2005). Device rigidity and vascular tortuosity rendered navigation difficult, resulting in periprocedural morbidity and mortality rates greater than those of angioplasty alone (Chow et al., 2005; Gomez et al., 2000; Jiang et al., 2004; Kim et al., 2004; Levy et al., 2001; Yu et al., 2005). The multicenter nonrandomized Stenting in Symptomatic Atherosclerotic Lesions of Vertebral and Intracranial Arteries (SSYLVIA) trial reported the safety and efficacy of a balloon-mounted stent (Neurolink, Guidant Corporation, Indianapolis, IN) designed specifically for craniocervical application; 43 patients with symptomatic intracranial disease and 18 with extracranial vertebral artery stenoses were evaluated. Successful stent placement was achieved in 95% of patients. The investigators reported a 6.6% periprocedural stroke rate and an additional 7.3% incidence of stroke at 1-year follow-up. However, angiographic restenosis was documented in 35% of patients and was symptomatic in more than one-third of these individuals (SSYLVIA Study Investigators, 2004). Based on these data, the FDA granted the stent a humanitarian device exemption (HDE) for the treatment of high-risk patients with significant intracranial and extracranial atherosclerotic disease who had failed medical therapy. Another study, using the Apollo intracranial balloon-mounted stent, documented a 91.7% rate of technical success (MicroPort Medical, Shanghai, China) in patients harboring stenosis greater than 50% (Jiang et al., 2004). The primary endpoint, ischemic stroke in the target lesion arterial territory or any stroke/death within 30 days, occurred at a rate of 4.3 per 100 patient-years. A restenosis rate of 28% was reported.

The Wingspan stent is the first self-expanding system designed for ICAD application (Fig. 54.7). A hybrid of nickel and titanium (nitinol) metal construct allows navigation of small and tortuous intracranial vessels. The FDA granted an HDE approval for the Wingspan Stent System with Gateway PTA balloon catheter (Boston Scientific) for symptomatic ICAD referable to an intracranial vessel with greater than 50% stenosis and refractory to medical therapy. Endorsement was predicated on a safety study conducted in Europe and Asia (Bose et al., 2007). In that initial investigation, technical success was achieved in 98% of patients, and the 6-month death or ipsilateral stroke rate was 7%, with an all-cause stroke rate of 9.7%. In the National Institute of Health (NIH) Multicenter Wingspan Intracranial Stent Registry Study, 129 patients with symptomatic 70%–99% intracranial stenosis were enrolled. The technical success rate was 97%. The frequency of any stroke, intracerebral hemorrhage, and death within 30 days or ipsilateral stroke beyond 30 days was 14% at 6 months (Zaidat et al., 2008b). The reported frequency of angiographic restenosis was 25%.

In-stent restenosis has decreased following cardiac angioplasty and stenting procedures with the advent of drug-eluting stents (Regar et al., 2002). Although this new generation of stents has been shown to be useful in reducing neointimal hyperplasia, no platforms have been designed and approved for use in the small and tortuous intracranial vessels. However, it has been reported that placement of drug-eluting stents in the intracranial circulation is feasible, with a lower incidence of restenosis and similar safety profile compared with bare metal stents (Gupta et al., 2016).

***Angioplasty/stenting procedure.*** After a microcatheter is advanced past the lesion, an exchange-length microwire is used to advance, in series, the balloon angioplasty and stent catheters to the level of stenosis. The lesion is initially dilated with a PTA balloon typically sized to 80% of the native vessel luminal diameter, using the slow inflation technique advocated by Connors and Wojak (1999). After initial vessel dilation, the balloon catheter is exchanged for the self-expanding stent system, which is deployed across the stenotic lesion. Poststenting balloon dilation is discouraged by the manufacturer. Balloon-mounted design intracranial stents are also delivered over a wire but with the stent mounted over the balloon in a single device (Fig. 54.8). Following angioplasty and stenting, with self-expanding stents, residual stenosis (30%) tends to be less than that observed following PTA alone (40%) but more severe than that noted after balloon-mounted stent deployment (Fiorella and Woo, 2007; Henkes et al., 2005). Follow-up angiograms have demonstrated restenosis rates exceeding 30%, presumably due to elastic recoil, neointimal hyperplasia, and vascular remodeling (Garas et al., 2001). Coating stents with antiproliferative agents such as sirolimus has been effective in reducing restenosis rates in the cardiology literature (Ong et al., 2006). Some studies have demonstrated encouraging results for the treatment of ICAD patients with drug-eluting stents (Gupta et al., 2006; Qureshi et al., 2006).

#### *Intracranial atherosclerotic disease clinical trials*

SAMMPRIS trial. The Stenting and Aggressive Medical Management for Preventing Recurrent Stroke in Intracranial Stenosis (SAMMPRIS) study was a large randomized investigation comparing intracranial angioplasty and stenting with intensive medical management to optimal medical management alone (Chimowitz et al., 2011; Derdeyn et al., 2014). Patients with 70%–99% intracranial stenosis who suffered a stroke or transient ischemic attack (TIA) within 30 days of enrollment were randomized to either aggressive medical therapy alone or aggressive medical therapy plus angioplasty and stenting (PTAS) with the Wingspan Stent system (Stryker Neurovascular). The primary endpoint was stroke or death within 30 days. Enrollment was halted after 451 patients were enrolled and interim analysis showed the 30-day rate of stroke or death was 14.7% in the PTAS group and 5.8% in the group receiving medical management alone ($P$ = .002). These results showed higher than expected risk of early stroke following PTAS and lower than expected stroke with aggressive medical therapy

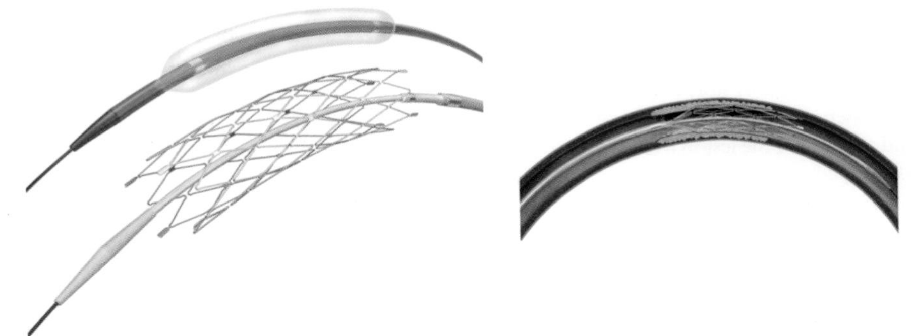

**Fig. 54.7** Gateway balloon and Wingspan stent *(left)*. Stent deployment across an intracranial stenotic lesion with resultant opening of vessel lumen *(right)*. *(Pictures courtesy Boston Scientific.)*

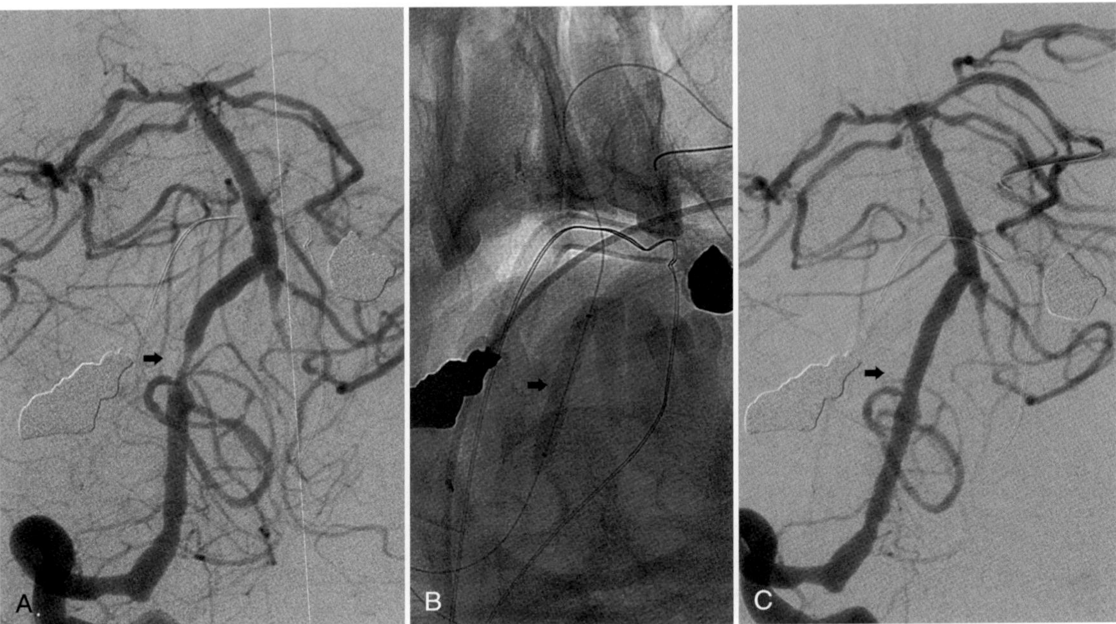


**Fig. 54.8** In a patient with recurrent posterior circulation strokes, anteroposterior angiogram shows diffuse intracranial atherosclerotic disease and severe narrowing of a right vertebral artery intracranial segment *(arrow)* resulting in 70% stenosis and occlusion of the contralateral vertebral artery **(A)**. A balloon mounted intracranial stent was implanted **(B)**. Angiogram following angioplasty and stenting shows no residual stenosis **(C)**.

alone. This study was important in illustrating the benefit of aggressive medical therapy, the limitations of the Wingspan stent system with need for improved device design, and insight to patient selection for future studies. Following the SAMMPRIS trial results, the FDA narrowed the indications for the use of the Wingspan Stent system to patients who meet criteria that include having two or more ipsilateral cerebral ischemic events despite aggressive medical management, who have made a good recovery from prior strokes, and who have evidence of 70%–99% stenosis in the intracranial artery related to the strokes.

**VISSIT trial.** The VISSIT (Vitesse Intracranial Stent Study for Ischemic Stroke Therapy) trial was a randomized clinical trial evaluating the role of balloon mounted stenting compared with medical management in patients with symptomatic intracranial stenosis greater than 70%. This study was halted after release of the SAMMPRIS study and also demonstrated lower rates of stroke and death with medical management compared with intracranial balloon mounted stenting (Zaidat et al., 2015).

**Wingspan Stent System Post Market Surveillance trial.** The Wingspan Stent System Post Market Surveillance (WEAVE) trial was an FDA-mandated trial to assess safety of the Wingspan Stent System in the treatment of symptomatic intracranial atherosclerosis (Alexander et al., 2019). FDA on-label criteria include age 22–80 years, symptomatic ICAD 70%–99%, baseline mRS score of 3 or less, two or more strokes in the vascular territory of the stenotic lesion with at least one stroke while on medical therapy, and stenting of the lesion 8 days or more after the last stroke. The trial was stopped early after interim analysis of 152 patients demonstrated lower periprocedural stroke, bleed, and death rate (2.6%, 4/152 patients) than expected of the 4% procedural primary event threshold for the interim analysis of the study. The authors concluded that with proper patient selection following on-label usage guidelines, the Wingspan stent could demonstrate low periprocedural complication for patients with symptomatic ICAD. Because of its single-arm design, despite the low rates of stroke noted when the procedure is performed more than 8 days post index event, the WEAVE trial does not provide information regarding the benefit of this procedure compared with medical therapy only based on timing of intervention. Although the periprocedural stroke rate in WEAVE was low, the risk of recurrent stroke is highest in the first week after the index event. Further clarification of optimal timing of intracranial stenting relative to the index event should be provided by randomized trials.

## Extracranial Vertebral Artery Disease

Extracranial vertebral artery atherosclerotic disease, including vertebral artery origin stenosis, has been implicated as a common cause of posterior circulation stroke (20% of all posterior circulation strokes) (Caplan et al., 1992). Just as with other large extra or intracranial arteries, the mechanism of stroke from vertebral artery origin atherosclerotic disease may be thromboembolism, hemodynamic failure, or the coexistence of both. The variability of vertebral artery supply to the posterior circulation, including artery dominance, hypoplasia, and termination as the posterior inferior cerebellar artery, requires a thorough evaluation of vascular anatomy when considering stroke mechanism and recurrence risk. Most of the procedural data addressing extracranial vertebral artery stenting derive from single-arm studies. Consistent with results from other reports, the Society of Vascular and Interventional Neurology (SVIN) research consortium study, one of the largest reports to date of stenting for vertebral ostial disease, reported a 1-month incidence of stroke of 1/148 patients (0.8%) and 15% incidence of restenosis at 6 months post procedure (Edgell et al., 2013). The clinical benefit of this approach is difficult to assess given that prospective data on the natural history of this disease are scarce.

A preplanned pooled individual patient data analysis of 354 patients across three randomized controlled trials comparing stenting with medical treatment in patients with symptomatic vertebral stenosis was recently published. The analysis comprised 179 patients from Vertebral Artery Ischaemia Stenting Trial (VIST) (148 with

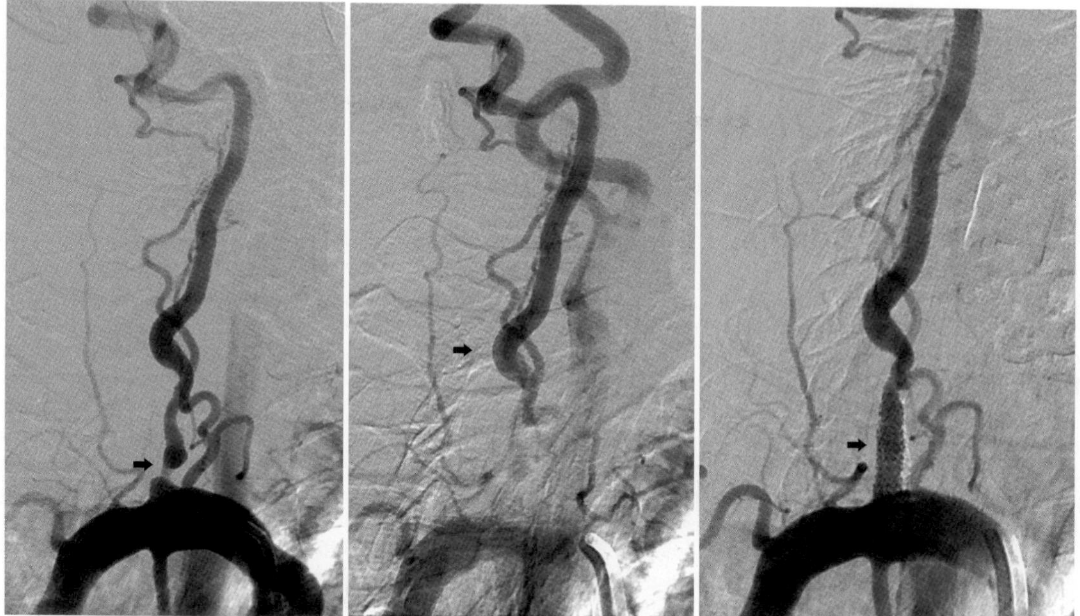

**Fig. 54.9** Anteroposterior projection angiogram of a right subclavian artery shows severe atherosclerotic stenosis of the right vertebral artery origin *(arrow, left)*. Attenuated contrast washout within the right vertebral artery *(arrow, center)* illustrates severe hemodynamic compromise from the stenosis. Normal lumen caliber and antegrade flow is restored after endovascular therapy with angioplasty and stenting *(arrow, right)*.

extracranial stenosis and 31 with intracranial stenosis), 115 patients from Vertebral Artery Stenting Trial (VAST) (96 with extracranial stenosis and 19 with intracranial stenosis), and 60 patients with intracranial stenosis from SAMMPRIS (no patients had extracranial stenosis). In the three trials, 168 patients (46 with intracranial stenosis and 122 with extracranial stenosis) were randomly assigned to medical treatment and 186 to stenting (64 with intracranial stenosis and 122 with extracranial stenosis). In the stenting group, the periprocedural stroke or death rate was higher for intracranial stenosis than for extracranial stenosis (16% vs. 1%, $P < .0001$). During 1036 person-years of follow-up, the HR for any stroke in the stenting group compared with the medical treatment group was 0.81% (CI 0.45–1.44; $P = .47$). For extracranial stenosis alone, the HR was 0.63 (95% CI 0.27–1.46), and for intracranial stenosis alone it was 1.06 (0.46–2.42; $P = .395$). [Markus et al., 2019.] Pending confirmatory studies, stenting might be a reasonable alternative for symptomatic extracranial vertebral stenosis but should be reserved for only medically refractory cases of intracranial vertebral artery disease (Fig. 54.9).

## HEMORRHAGIC STROKE

### Cerebral Aneurysms

Aneurysms represent a common cerebrovascular pathology, with a reported adult prevalence of 0.2%–9% worldwide (Inagawa and Hirano, 1990). Autopsy studies suggest 2% rate of intracranial aneurysms in a large autopsy series, of which multiple aneurysms are seen in 22% of cases (McCormick and Nofzinger, 1965). Vessel degeneration and hemodynamic factors contribute to changes in sheer stress and flow patterns that ultimately may result in aneurysmal enlargement or rupture.

Most unruptured aneurysms remain undetected, but an increasing number of incidental aneurysms are being discovered during cerebral imaging studies (Wakhloo et al., 2008; Wiebers et al., 2003). Although patients harboring intracranial aneurysms may present with symptoms resulting from mass effect or thromboembolism, the most common and perilous clinical manifestation is that of subarachnoid hemorrhage (SAH). It is estimated that 10 of every 100,000 intracranial aneurysms rupture annually. Aneurysmal rupture carries an approximately 50% mortality rate, with 10%–20% of survivors failing to regain long-term functional independence (Ellegala and Day, 2005; Hop et al., 1997; Schievink, 1997).

### Ruptured Aneurysms

Following rupture of an intracranial aneurysm, recurrent hemorrhage occurs at a high frequency. Jane et al. (1985) documented that the incidence of rebleeding among patients with SAH and untreated aneurysms was 50% in the first 6 months and 3% per year thereafter. Patients presenting with higher clinical grade and larger aneurysms are at higher risk of rehemorrhage. Because of the high risk of subsequent rupture, virtually every ruptured aneurysm requires urgent treatment.

### ISAT

The randomized prospective multicenter International Subarachnoid Aneurysm Trial (ISAT) compared the efficacy of endovascular treatment with that of surgery in patients with ruptured intracranial aneurysms suitable for either treatment modality (Molyneux et al., 2002, 2009). A total of 2143 patients were randomized. Recruitment was terminated after a planned interim analysis demonstrated reduced disability in the endovascular treatment group. In an intention-to-treat analysis, the proportion of patients who were dead or disabled at 1 year was significantly lower in the endovascular therapy group compared with the surgical cohort. In addition, the risk of perioperative seizures was lower following coiling. The investigators noted that the low rates of late rebleeding and potential periprocedural complications associated with retreatment in the endovascular group were unlikely to alter the treatment benefit at 1 year. They concluded that endovascular coil embolization of ruptured intracranial aneurysms when a patient has a good clinical grade (World Federation of Neurosurgical Societies grades I–III) and the aneurysm anatomy is suitable for endovascular treatment is more likely than not to lead to independent survival at 1 year than those receiving neurosurgical treatment. Results may be generalized to good-grade patients harboring anterior circulation aneurysms. Statistical comparisons were difficult in poor-grade patients and those with posterior circulation aneurysms, because the vast majority of these individuals were not randomized due to treating physicians' overwhelming preference for endovascular therapy.

### Barrow Ruptured Aneurysm Trial

The Barrow Ruptured Aneurysm Trial (BRAT) was a single-center study undertaken to compare the safety and efficacy of microsurgical clipping and endovascular coil embolization for the treatment of acutely ruptured cerebral aneurysms (McDougall et al., 2012; Spetzler et al., 2013). Patients were assigned to therapy in an alternating fashion, resulting in 238 patients assigned to surgical clipping and 233 patients assigned to endovascular coil embolization. Despite patients in the clipping group having a higher degree of aneurysm obliteration and lower rate of recurrence and retreatment; at the 1-year and 3-year follow-ups, coil embolization resulted in fewer poor outcomes than surgical clipping. There was no recurrence of SAH in either group.

To address issues regarding incomplete occlusion and recanalization following endovascular therapy, long-term rerupture rates after treatment for aneurysmal SAH were investigated in the ISAT. At 10 years, more patients allocated to endovascular coiling were alive and independent compared with patients in the neurosurgical clipping group (OR 1.34, 95% CI 1.07–1.67). Rebleeding was more likely after endovascular coiling than after neurosurgical clipping, but the risk was small and probability of disability-free survival significantly greater in the endovascular group compared with the neurosurgical group (Molyneux et al., 2015).

### Trial Unruptured Aneurysms

The decision matrix for treatment of incidentally discovered unruptured aneurysms is based on natural history data and the risk/benefit stratification for the applicable treatment modalities.

***Natural history.*** Rupture rates for intracranial aneurysms vary with size and location, as reported by the International Study of Unruptured Intracranial Aneurysms (ISUIA) and Unruptured Cerebral Aneurysms (UCAS) and the natural course of unruptured cerebral aneurysms in a Japanese cohort (International Study of Unruptured Intracranial Aneurysms Investigators, 1998; Morita et al., 2012; Wiebers et al., 2003). The prospective observational arm of the ISUIA study investigated 2686 unruptured, untreated cerebral aneurysms. Individuals with no history of SAH who harbor incidental aneurysms located in the anterior circulation (ICA, anterior communicating or anterior cerebral artery, middle cerebral artery) had 5-year cumulative rupture rates of 0%, 2.6%, 14.5%, and 40% for aneurysms of less than 7 mm, 7–12 mm, 13–24 mm, and 25 mm or greater, respectively. Rupture rates for aneurysms of the same sizes located at the posterior communicating artery or in the posterior circulation were 2.5%, 14.5%, 18.4%, and 50%, respectively. Patients with a prior history of SAH resulting from rupture of an aneurysm distinct from that being studied had a 5-year cumulative rupture rate of 1.5% for aneurysms less than 7 mm in the anterior circulation, compared with 3.4% for aneurysms of the same size located at the posterior communicating artery or in the posterior circulation. Aneurysms greater than 7 mm in this cohort had similar rupture rates to the group with no prior history of SAH (Wiebers et al., 2003). In the UCAS Japanese study, 6697 aneurysms were studied with a follow-up period of 11,660 aneurysm-years showing an overall annual rate of rupture of approximately 1% per year with increased rate with size to 1.13, 3.35, 9.09, and 76.26 for aneurysm size of 5–6, 7–9, 10–24, and 25 mm or greater, respectively (Morita et al., 2012).

***Management considerations.*** Based on available prospective natural history data, incidental single less than 5-mm aneurysms with no other associated risk factors (young, A-comm [anterior communicating], P-comm [posterior communicating] or basilar, irregular shape, daughter sac, documented growth, family history, multiple aneurysms, SAH history, hypertension, smoking) may be managed expectantly with serial imaging. However, patient-specific desires or the presence of risk factors may encourage consideration of surgical or endovascular treatment even in this cohort (Broderick et al., 2009, Eskey et al., 2018). Quantitative hemodynamic analysis using computer-generated flow models to predict aneurysmal growth and rupture can be considered in decision making (Chien et al., 2009). Although these methods hold promise, further development and application to large patient cohorts are required to develop reliable algorithms that predict rupture risk in the clinical setting. According to the ISUIA data, aneurysms located in the posterior circulation and those in patients who have experienced prior SAH carry a significant 5-year cumulative rupture risk and warrant treatment consideration (Wiebers et al., 2003).

***Unruptured intracranial aneurysm trials.*** The question of whether a patient with an unruptured, asymptomatic intracranial should be treated has not been answered in randomized clinical trial. The Trial of Endovascular Aneurysm Management was an international, prospective, randomized clinical trial comparing patients with unruptured intracranial aneurysm to endovascular coiling versus medical management with primary outcome to evaluate safety and efficacy of treatment. The trial was halted in 2009 due to low recruitment (Raymond et al., 2011).

The CURES (Canadian UnRuptured Endovascular versus Surgery) trial is a randomized trial comparing the results of surgical clipping and endovascular treatment of unruptured aneurysms (Darsaut et al., 2011). Primary endpoints in this trial look at a composite of aneurysm obliteration, major saccular aneurysm remnant or recurrence, or intracranial hemorrhage at 1 year after treatment.

Individualized algorithms must be tailored to specific clinical and anatomical factors when selecting an appropriate treatment paradigm (Raja et al., 2008). Several retrospective studies document low morbidity and mortality rates for surgical clipping with experienced neurosurgeons (Bederson et al., 2000; Deruty et al., 1996; Komotar et al., 2008a; Moroi et al., 2005; Raaymakers et al., 1998). In 2003, Ogilvy and Carter retrospectively reviewed a series of 604 unruptured aneurysms in an attempt to identify risk factors associated with outcome following surgical treatment. The authors found patient age, aneurysm size, and location within the posterior circulation to be independent predictors of poor outcome with open surgical clipping (Ogilvy and Carter, 2003).

Data on the endovascular treatment of unruptured intracranial aneurysms suggest low morbidity and mortality rates across all aneurysm locations. Large studies indicate morbidity of 3%–10% (Johnston et al., 2001; Pierot et al., 2008; Wiebers et al., 2003,). Johnston et al. (2001) compared the safety of endovascular coiling and microsurgical clipping in 2069 patients treated in California between 1990 and 1998. In-hospital mortality and discharge to an alternate facility (rather than home) were significantly less frequent in the endovascular cohort. Mortality was 0.5% in the endovascular group and 3.5% in the open surgical cohort. These results are striking given that the investigation was conducted during the relatively early development of endovascular coiling technology. More recent data from the ISUIA study suggest that endovascular morbidity and mortality is lower at 1 year than that reported for open surgical treatment in both patients with (7.1% vs. 10.1%) and without (9.8% vs. 12.6%) prior SAH (Wiebers et al., 2003). Furthermore, outcome following endovascular procedures appeared

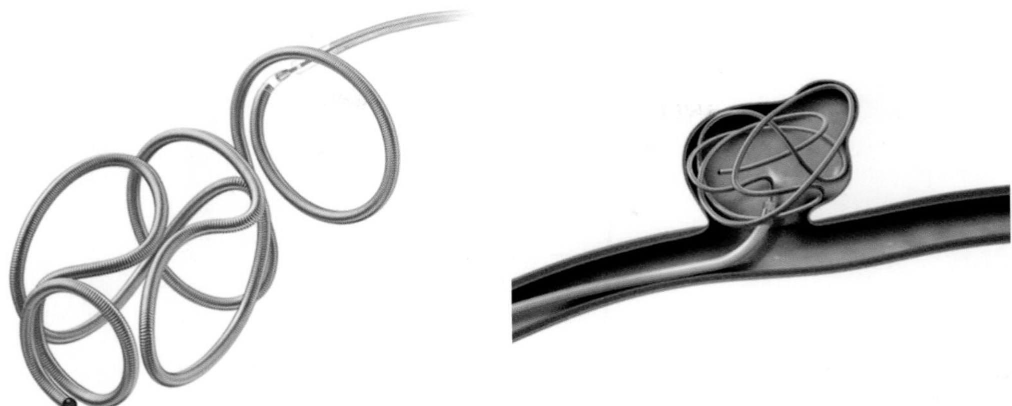

**Fig. 54.10** Three-dimensional coil *(left)* and diagrammatic depiction of coil deployment through a microcatheter positioned in an aneurysm *(right)*. *(Pictures courtesy Stryker Neurovascula.)*

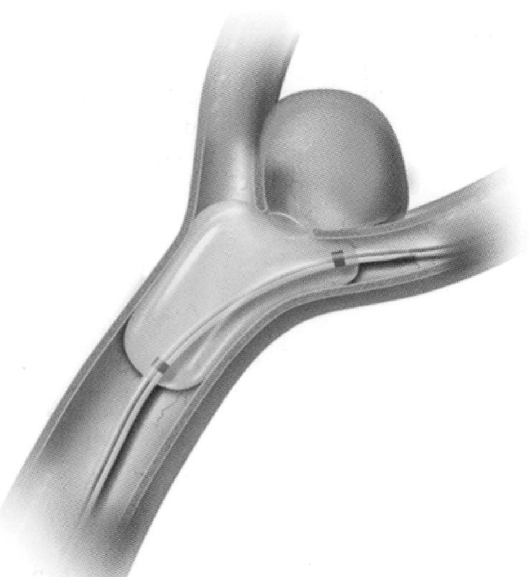

**Fig. 54.11** Diagram demonstrating balloon remodeling technique with HyperForm balloon (Medtronic, Irvine, CA) prior to coil placement. Balloon is positioned across the neck of aneurysm to temporarily prevent coil herniation into parent vessel.

to be less dependent upon patient age. However, direct comparisons were not generated because the endovascular cohort was relatively small given that physician preference led to coil embolization treatment of a greater percentage of older medically ill patients and those with aneurysms located in the posterior circulation.

In an unruptured aneurysm study comparing 1388 patients who underwent clipping, and 3551 who underwent coiling from the Premier Perspective database, patients treated with microsurgical clipping had significantly higher likelihood of discharge to long-term care, ischemic complications, hemorrhagic complications, postoperative neurological complications, and ventriculostomy when compared with patients treated with coiling (McDonald et al., 2013).

## Endovascular Treatment Modalities

***Coil embolization.*** Since 1990, when Dr. Guglielmi first introduced electrolytically detachable platinum microcoils, rapid technological advancements have resulted in more efficacious endovascular treatment of complex aneurysms (Guglielmi et al., 1992). Improved detachment mechanisms, stretch-resistant coils, three-dimensional complex shapes (Piotin et al., 2003; Wakhloo et al., 2007), varying degrees of softness, and coil lattice incorporating a bioabsorbable polymer (Hetts et al., 2014; Linfante et al., 2005; Murayama et al., 2003) or hydrogel (Benkok et al., 2018; White et al., 2008), smaller coil sizes (Nguyen et al., 2015) have been designed to minimize procedural complications, expand the endovascular treatment indications for patients with brain aneurysms, and help to prevent delayed recanalization.

Although CTA or MRA are often used for aneurysm diagnosis and treatment planning, digital subtraction angiography is the "gold standard" for diagnosis, angioarchitecture of the aneurysm, and treatment planning. Angiography is used if CTA or MRA does not elucidate the SAH etiology. In the event that no aneurysm or vascular malformation is discovered after a complete intracranial angiogram, it is important to assess the ascending cervical and posterior deep cervical branches of the subclavian artery and the bilateral external carotid arteries for the presence of a dural arteriovenous fistula (DAVF). Spinal angiography may also be indicated if there are prominent cervical or back symptoms with large burden of spinal SAH to detect for the presence of spinal aneurysms (Renieri, et al., 2018). Delayed repeat angiography is often warranted in cases with a comprehensive negative initial study and a suspicious pattern of SAH.

In the event an aneurysm is identified following diagnostic cerebral angiography, aneurysm morphology and regional vascular anatomy are assessed to determine the safety and feasibility of coil embolization. Coiling involves placement of the initial framing coil into the aneurysm dome under real-time digital subtraction fluoroscopy. Additional filling coils of various shapes, softness, and successively diminishing sizes are deployed until complete angiographic occlusion is obtained (Fig. 54.10).

***Balloon remodeling.*** Initially described by Moret et al. (1997), the balloon remodeling technique provides an ability to effectively treat broad-neck aneurysms by protecting the parent vessel from coil prolapse. Positioned within the parent artery, a small balloon occlusion microcatheter is intermittently inflated and deflated across the aneurysm neck (Figs. 54.11 and 54.12). This provides temporary structural support against which coils are then deployed through a second microcatheter located within the aneurysm sac. Anterograde flow is completely reestablished within the parent artery after successive balloon deflations. Balloon remodeling can lead to higher coil packing density and more effective parent vessel reconstruction. In a review of their initial experience, the Moret group documented complete angiographic occlusion in 20 of 21 broad-necked cerebral aneurysms treated via balloon-assisted coil embolization. They reported sustained occlusion without recanalization at 4 months or greater angiographic follow-up. The authors noted complication rates that were no greater

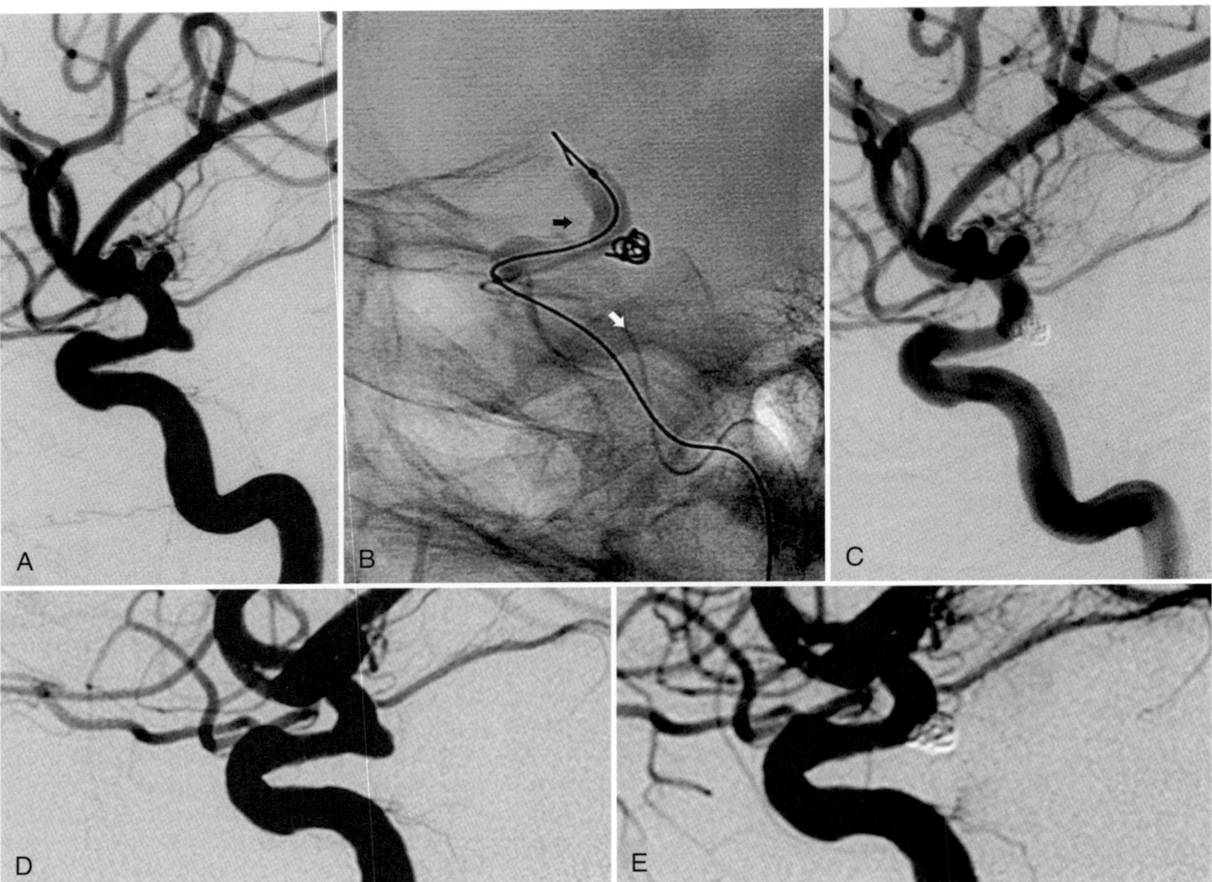


**Fig. 54.12** Lateral oblique projection angiogram shows a right internal carotid artery supraclinoid segment aneurysm in a patient with subarachnoid hemorrhage **(A)**. A balloon *(arrow)* inflated within the right internal carotid artery across the aneurysm neck supports coil embolization **(B)**. Complete occlusion of the aneurysm was achieved **(C)**. Pretreatment and posttreatment lateral projection angiograms show the treatment result **(D, E)**.

than those experienced with primary coil embolization (Moret et al., 1997). These results have been corroborated by several other clinical series (Layton, 2007; Lefkowitz et al., 1999; Malek et al., 2000).

Balloon-assistance has greatly facilitated the endovascular treatment of wide-neck ruptured cerebral aneurysms in the acute phase, allowing for mechanical coil support and vessel remodeling without the need for antiplatelet therapy that is typically necessary with stent assisted coiling. Balloon-assisted coiling also provides what oftentimes can be a life-saving opportunity for immediate hemostasis in the event of procedure rupture, allowing time for the neurointerventionist to stop the bleeding by packing the aneurysm with coils or other materials while the balloon inflated in the parent artery prevents entry of blood into the aneurysm. In a large series of ruptured aneurysms treated by coiling, use of a hemostatic balloon across the aneurysm neck was associated with better clinical outcomes in the setting of inadvertent intraprocedural aneurysm rupture compared with no balloon use (Nguyen et al., 2008). This adjunctive technique extends the indication for endovascular aneurysm treatment to cases with less favorable anatomy.

***Stent-assisted coil embolization.*** In some challenging broad-neck cerebral aneurysms, balloon remodeling may not be sufficient to prevent coil protrusion into the parent vessel. In such cases an endoluminal/endovascular approach uses a permanently deployed intracranial stent as supportive scaffolding. Nitinol self-expanding stents with either open- or closed-cell configuration have been designed exclusively for this use (Higashida et al., 2005) (Fig. 54.13). A stent is deployed across the aneurysm neck and then the coiling microcatheter is placed into the sac through the stent interstices. An alternative method is to first position the coiling microcatheter within the aneurysm dome and then "jail" the distal tip in position through subsequent stent deployment. With either strategy, stent placement precedes positioning and detachment of the coils within the aneurysm (Figs. 54.14 and 54.15). Clinical studies have documented favorable results, with initial occlusion rates greater than 80% (Jankowitz et al., 2019; Lylyk et al., 2005) and complete or near-complete angiographic occlusion at 12 months. Studies have reported the use of complex stent-assisted techniques such as telescoping/overlapping multiple stents for the treatment of fusiform aneurysms (Crowley et al., 2009) and Y-stent configurations for bifurcation aneurysms (Chow et al., 2004). Stent-assisted coil embolization is generally reserved for the treatment of unruptured aneurysms. Most physicians are reluctant to deploy stents in the setting of SAH, due to the requirement of dual antiplatelet therapy associated with its use.

## Alternative Treatments

Incomplete occlusion and subsequent recanalization rates following coil embolization have raised concerns regarding the durability of endovascular treatment for cerebral aneurysms with unfavorable geometry (Debrun et al., 1998; Fernandez Zubillaga et al., 1994; Guglielmi et al., 1992; Raymond et al., 2003). Risk factors for aneurysm recurrence after coiling include wide neck aneurysms (≥4 mm), large aneurysms (≥10 mm), aneurysm presentation in ruptured state, and incomplete aneurysm occlusion at the time of treatment (Raymond et al., 2003,

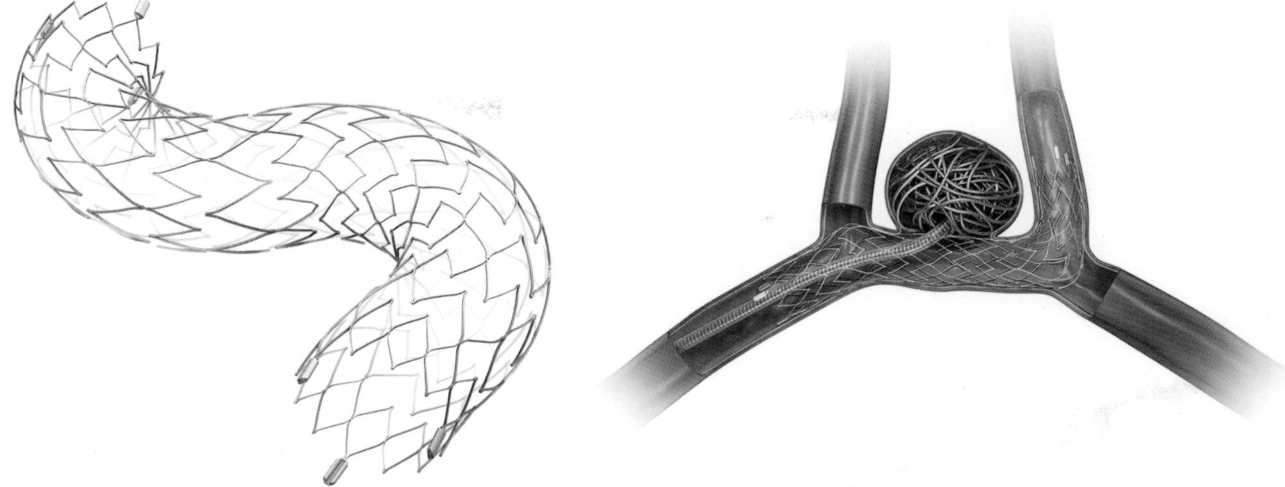

**Fig. 54.13** Picture of the Atlas Neuroform stent with open-cell hybrid design *(left)* and diagrammatic depiction of stent-assisted anterior communicating artery aneurysm coil embolization through a microcatheter positioned in an aneurysm *(right)*. Note that stent provides permanent scaffolding for stabilization of coil mass. *(Neuroform Atlas™ Stent Conformability, Images courtesy Stryker; 2018 Copyright © Stryker.)*

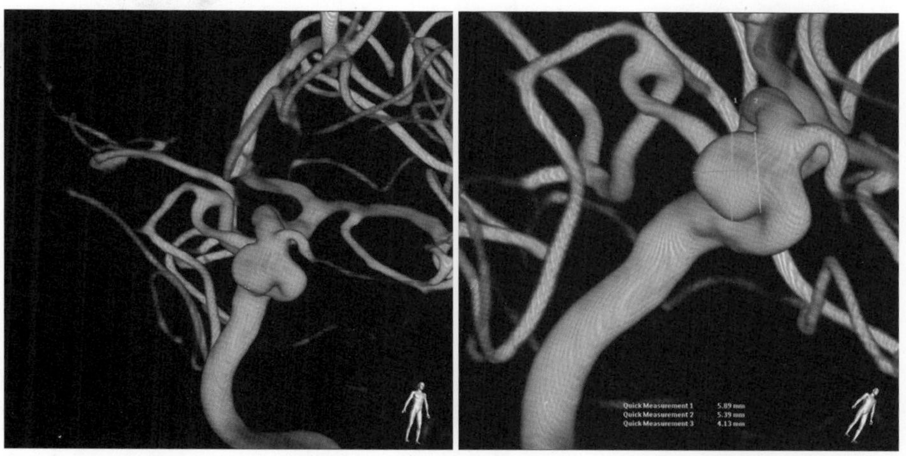

**Fig. 54.14** Three-dimensional reconstruction of a left superior hypophyseal region aneurysm *(left)*. Measurements *(right)* demonstrate cranial-caudal (1), transverse (3) dimensions of aneurysm and size of the neck (2).

Nguyen, 2007). Experimental models have demonstrated that coils occupy less than 40% of aneurysmal volume. Therefore residual flow may remain even in tightly packed lesions (Piotin et al., 2000, 2003). This has prompted the development of novel techniques such as liquid embolic agents and flow-diverting devices.

***Flow diversion.*** The advent of endovascular *flow-diversion devices* represents a paradigm shift in the treatment strategy for large, broad-neck aneurysms. Circumferential, endoluminal, parent-vessel reconstruction may allow for complete aneurysmal occlusion in the absence of direct endovascular embolization. The Pipeline Embolization Device (PED; Medtronic, Irvine, CA) is engineered to reconstruct a segmentally diseased vessel (Fig. 54.16). Lylyk et al. (2009) detailed a large initial experience with the PED; 53 patients with 63 wide-necked aneurysms were treated. The study reported a mean follow-up time of 5.9 months. Complete occlusion was achieved in 95% of aneurysms, and no major complications were encountered. The Pipeline for Uncoilable or Failed Aneurysms: Results from a Multicenter Clinical Trial (PUFS) was a multicenter, prospective, single-arm study of the PED (Becske et al., 2013). In this study, 108 patients with unruptured large wide-neck aneurysms of the ICA were enrolled. Angiographic evidence of complete aneurysm occlusion was observed in 73.6% of treated aneurysms, and six (5.6%) patients experienced a major ipsilateral stroke or neurological death. Given the high complexity of these aneurysms, the authors concluded that the occlusion rate and safety profile of this treatment offered an acceptable alternative treatment. The PED became the first FDA-approved flow-diverter device for the treatment of brain aneurysms.

***Intrasaccular flow disruptors.*** The Woven EndoBridge (WEB) device is an intrasaccular device developed for the endovascular treatment of wide-neck bifurcation aneurysms (see Fig. 54.18). These aneurysms are often located at the middle cerebral artery, basilar artery, or anterior communicating artery and can be difficult to treat, most often requiring adjunctive balloon- or stent-assisted coiling to achieve satisfactory aneurysm occlusion. Sometimes, these patients are referred for surgical clipping if the anatomy is thought to not be amenable for coiling. The Woven EndoBridge Intrasaccular Therapy (WEB-IT) Study was a prospective study evaluating the safety and efficacy of the WEB device for the treatment of wide-neck bifurcation aneurysms (Arthur et al., 2019). There were 148 patients who received the WEB device, of which one patient developed delayed parenchymal hemorrhage 3 weeks after treatment. There were no primary safety events between 30 days and 1 year. At 1-year follow-up, 54% of

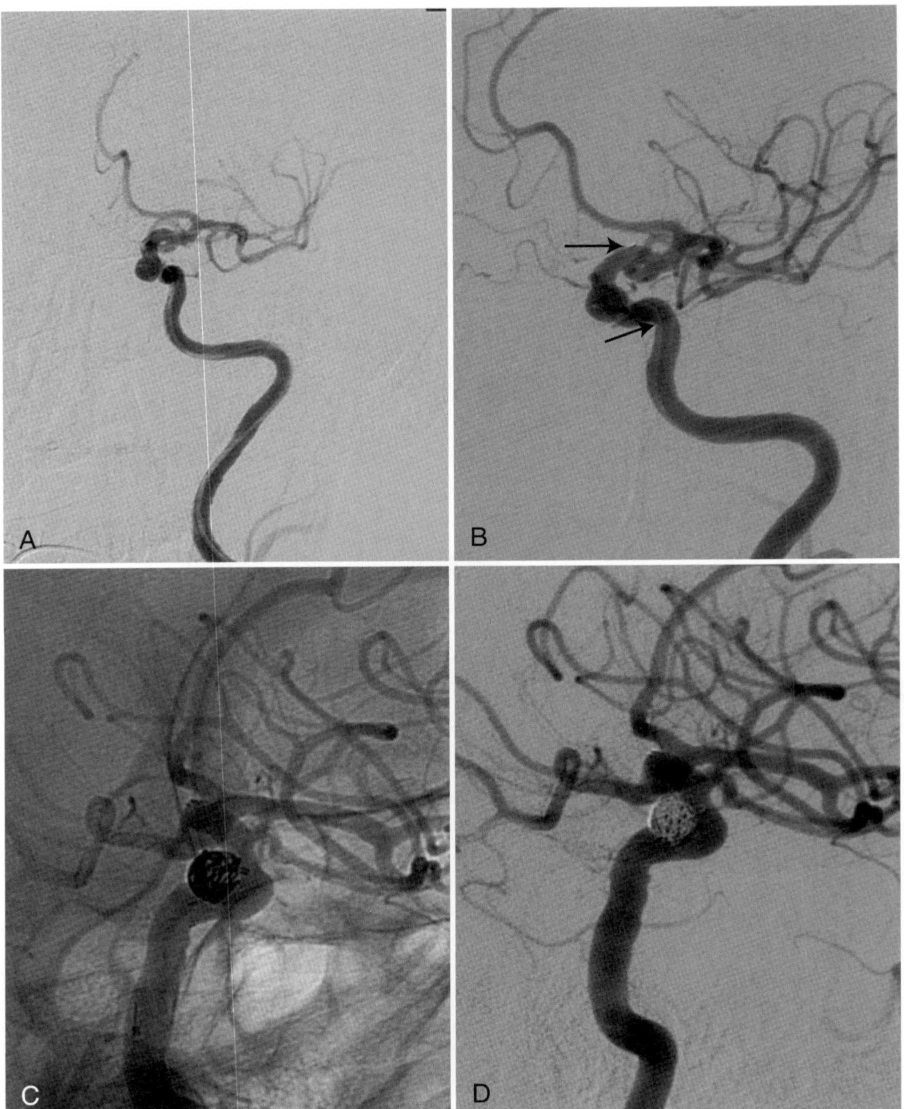


**Fig. 54.15** Same aneurysm seen in Fig. 54.12. Large size of aneurysm neck compared with dome led to stent-assisted coiling technique being used. **(A)** Working projection oblique angiogram demonstrating stent tines positioned across neck of aneurysm. **(B)** *Arrows* point to proximal and distal stent tines. **(C)** Unsubtracted view demonstrating stent position and coil mass. **(D)** Postintervention angiogram in working projection showing no residual aneurysmal neck and no filling within coil mass.

patients had complete aneurysm occlusion; adequate occlusion was achieved in 85% of patients. The authors concluded that WEB can be a good option for patients with wide-neck bifurcation aneurysms that is as effective as currently available therapies.

## Management of Cerebral Vasospasm

Cerebral vasospasm, a delayed reversible narrowing of the intracranial vasculature, is the leading cause of stroke, morbidity, and mortality following treatment of aneurysmal subarachnoid hemorrhage (aSAH). Occurring most frequently between 3 and 14 days after aSAH, vasospasm causes a decrease in blood flow and a resultant lowering of cerebral perfusion pressure (Janardhan et al., 2006; Macdonald et al., 2007). Medical treatments include oral nimodipine and hypertensive therapy to enhance cerebral oxygenation in the setting of vasoconstriction. Despite maximal medical measures, 15% of patients who initially survive aSAH experience stroke or death secondary to vasospasm (Mayberg, 1998). For vasospasm refractory to medical management or in patients with treatment contraindications, endovascular therapy has emerged as an alternative or supplementary therapeutic modality (Newell et al., 1992). Both balloon angioplasty and IA vasodilator infusion have established roles in the management of medically intractable vasospasm. More recently, reports have emerged describing the successful use of retrievable stents for vasospasm. Although each of the endovascular methods has its advantages and disadvantages, the optimal method and timing of endovascular treatment remain controversial.

### Balloon Angioplasty

A technique first applied by Zubkov et al. (1984), PTA commonly results in permanent mechanical reversal of cerebral vasospasm. Proposed mechanisms for smooth-muscle dysfunction include endothelial denudation, collagen fiber stretching, and rupture of internal elastic lamina (Chan et al., 1995; Honma et al., 1995; Macdonald et al., 1995; Yamamoto et al., 1992).

If severe vasospasm is encountered on angiography, percutaneous balloon angioplasty may be performed. A balloon catheter is advanced over a microguidewire to the vessel narrowing. The balloon is slowly

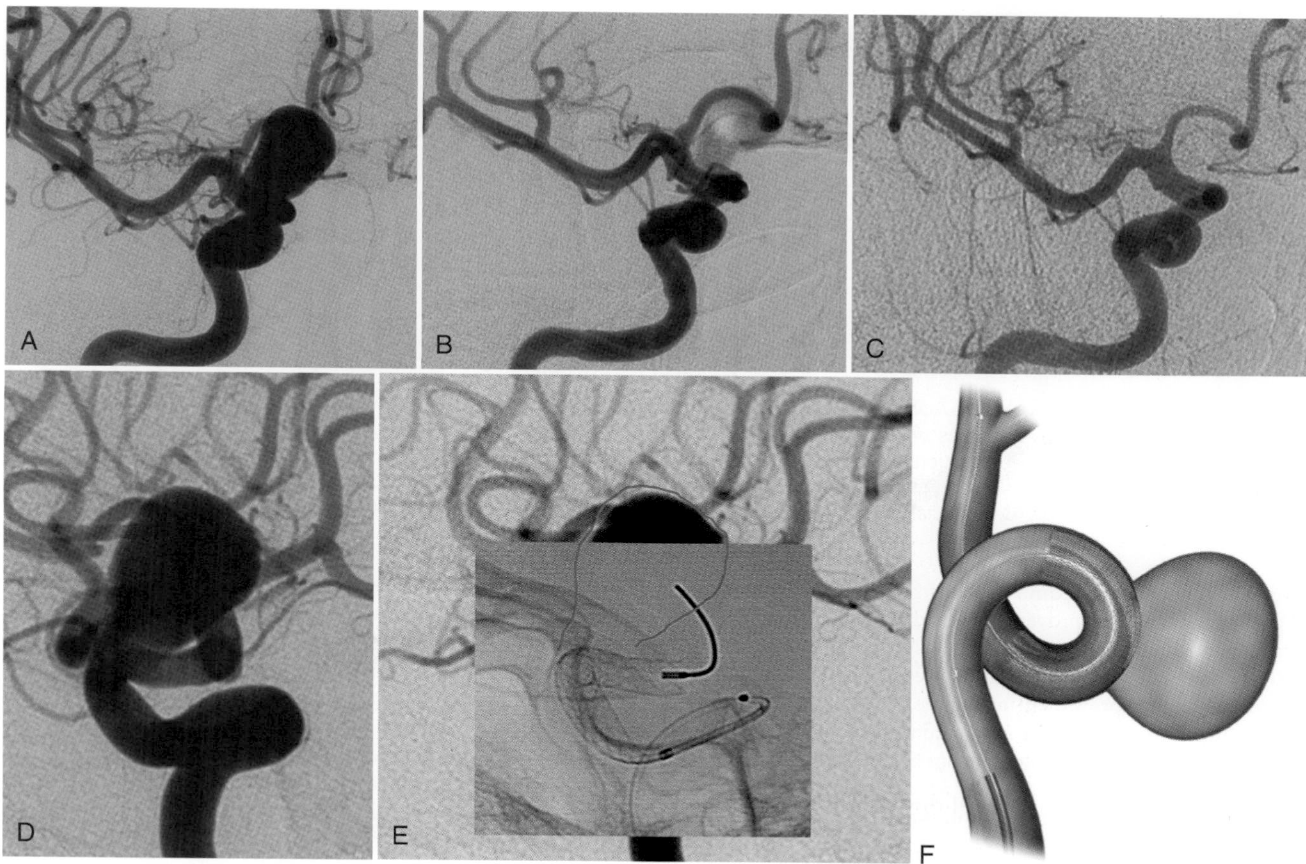

**Fig. 54.16** A large right internal carotid artery aneurysm treated with a Pipeline Embolization Device at initial angiogram **(A)**, immediately after implant **(B)**, and at 6-month follow-up **(C)**, shows progressive and complete obliteration of the aneurysm. A lateral view angiogram shows the aneurysm **(D)** with fluoroscopy imaging of the device being deployed across the aneurysm neck **(E)**. An artistic depiction of the device shows the low porosity of the dense mesh device across the aneurysm neck **(F)**. *(© Covidien. Used with permission.)*

inflated over the length of the accessible spastic segment to increase vessel caliber. Balloon angioplasty is generally restricted to larger proximal vessels of the circle of Willis and, less commonly, the smaller immediately more distal branches. Balloon angioplasty can also be effectively used to open proximal vessels and facilitate catheterization of small distal vessels previously inaccessible to microcatheters. This permits potential for subsequent injection of IA vasodilators in the respective distal vascular territories (Fig. 54.17).

An analysis of six retrospective series reporting treatment of cerebral vasospasm by balloon angioplasty demonstrated a mean clinical improvement of 65% (Komotar et al., 2008b). Eskridge et al. (1998) conducted a study examining 50 patients and 170 arterial segments; 61% of patients demonstrated sustained clinical improvement within 72 hours of balloon angioplasty treatment. In a 2005 literature review, Hoh and Ogilvy (2005) found an overall clinical improvement in 62% of patients treated for vasospasm with balloon angioplasty. Rosenwasser et al. (1999) sought to ascertain the time period during which balloon angioplasty was maximally effective. The authors determined that 70% of patients treated within 2 hours of symptom onset demonstrated clinical improvement. By contrast, only 40% of those treated beyond the 2-hour window sustained recovery. Rates of angiographic vasospasm resolution were similar between the two cohorts, indicating that earlier treatment of patients with medically resistant cerebral vasospasm results in superior clinical outcome despite similar radiographic results. Preemptive balloon angioplasty has been advocated for vasospasm prophylaxis in high-risk patients (Muizelaar et al., 1999). A multicenter phase II study published in 2008 that evaluated prophylactic balloon angioplasty in patients with Fisher grade III SAH demonstrated no significant difference in Glasgow Outcome Score when compared with patients treated with standard-of-care therapy. Although a statistically significant decrease in the need for therapeutic angioplasty was reported, four procedure-related vessel perforations and three resultant deaths were documented in the prophylaxis cohort (Zwienenberg-Lee et al., 2008).

### Intraarterial Vasodilators

IA vasodilator therapy is often used to treat mild to moderate clinical vasospasm or disease affecting the more distal intracranial vasculature. A vasodilatory agent can be injected through a microcatheter advanced to a more selective distal target vessel. Some data regarding efficacy of IA pharmacological therapy for the treatment of cerebral vasospasm with papaverine have been accumulated. An opium alkaloid and nonspecific smooth muscle–cell relaxant, papaverine causes vasodilation through cyclic adenosine and guanosine monophosphate phosphodiesterase inhibition and has a half-life of nearly 2 hours. Investigations have documented incidences of immediate angiographic vasospasm relief ranging between 57% and 90% (Firlik et al., 1997; Kassell et al., 1992; Milburn et al., 1998). However, due to the temporary effect of this medication, often mandating repeat treatment sessions, papaverine has been abandoned.

Concerns regarding the toxicity profile and short effect of papaverine have prompted the off-label use of IA calcium channel antagonists in the treatment of cerebral vasospasm (Smith et al., 2004). Feng et al. (2002) reported a 45% increase in vessel diameter and 33% clinical

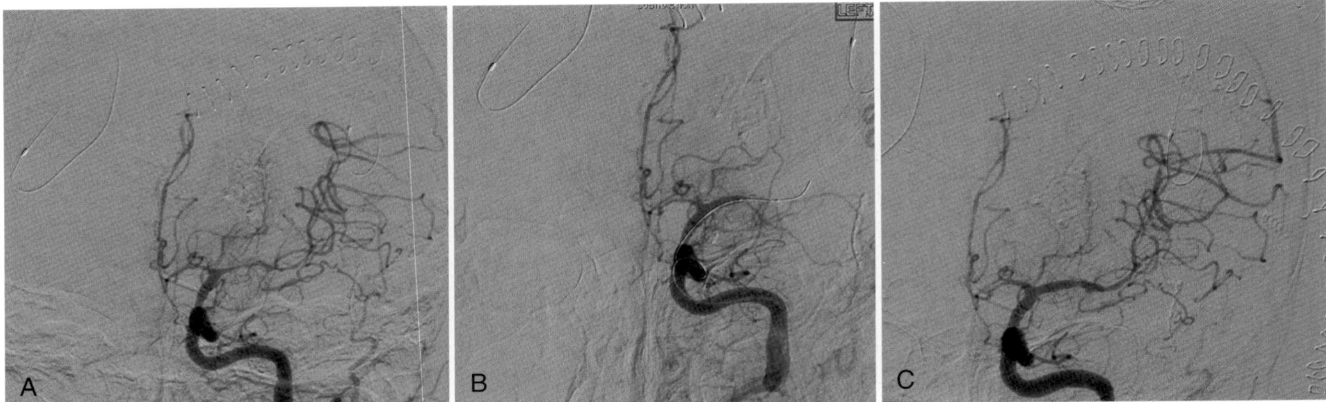


**Fig. 54.17** **A**, Anteroposterior (AP) angiogram demonstrating severe narrowing of M1 segment of left middle cerebral artery and moderate stenosis of A1 segment of left anterior cerebral artery. **B**, Hyperglide balloon positioned across narrowed middle cerebral artery segment. Note two radiopaque markers that confirm position of balloon. **C**, Postdilatation AP angiogram demonstrating an increase in caliber of proximal left middle cerebral artery.

improvement following verapamil administration. Similarly, neurological and radiographic improvement was demonstrated in patients receiving IA nicardipine (Badjatia et al., 2004, Nogueira, 2009a). Biondi et al. (2004) demonstrated a 43% rate of vessel dilation and a 76% incidence of clinical improvement in the first 24 hours following IA administration of nimodipine. The most significant shortcoming associated with the use of IA vasodilator therapy is the transitory efficacy. Repeat endovascular instillation is often necessary (Hoh and Ogilvy, 2005). Bridging IA to maintenance IV infusion of milrinone can help to reduce risk of vasospasm relapse of these patients and lessen the intensive requirement of triple H therapy (Lannes et al., 2012).

## CEREBRAL ARTERIOVENOUS MALFORMATIONS

A brain AVM is an aggregate of arterial and venous communications with no intervening capillary network. Studies suggest that the incidence of brain AVMs is 1.21 per 100,000 person-years (Stapf et al., 2002). Despite their congenital nature, cerebral AVMs may become symptomatic at any time, with a mean presentation age of 31 (Hofmeister et al., 2000). Over 50% of AVMs manifest with rupture (Brown et al., 1996; Hofmeister et al., 2000), yielding an annual hemorrhage rate between 2% and 4% (Gross and Du, 2013; Kondziolka et al., 1995; Ondra et al., 1990). Although the resultant blood pattern is most often intracerebral, subarachnoid, or intraventricular hemorrhage may occur. AVM rupture accounts for approximately 2% of all intracranial hemorrhages (Stapf et al., 2001, 2002). The risk of rebleeding in patients who initially present with rupture may approach 6%–17% during the first year before stabilizing to a baseline level after 3 years (Forster et al., 1972; Graf et al., 1983; Mast et al., 1997). Several demographic and anatomical factors, including age, deep brain location, and deep venous drainage, have been associated with hemorrhage at presentation in patients harboring brain AVMs (Stapf et al., 2006a; Turjman et al., 1995). As many as 35% of patients present with seizures or ischemic symptoms secondary to regional vascular steal phenomenon (Sekhon et al., 1997).

Uncertainty about the natural history of unruptured AVMs and about optimal management options led to initiation of A Randomized Trial of Unruptured Brain Arteriovenous Malformations (ARUBA). This multicenter trial compared a treatment strategy consisting of endovascular, microneurosurgical, radiosurgical, or a combination of these therapies with that of conservative management (Stapf et al., 2006b). Enrollment was stopped early when an interim analysis of a mean follow-up of 33.3 months showed that the event rate in the treatment group was significantly higher at 30.7% versus 10.1% in the medical management group (Mohr et al., 2014). The interim analysis included data from 223 participants enrolled at 39 sites worldwide. The enrolled patients will continue to be followed for a minimum of 5 years to determine if there is a difference in stroke and death in the two arms over time. The study was not powered to detect differences between the various treatment modalities.

AVM angioarchitecture has been characterized as plexiform or fistulous, depending on the rate and degree of vascular shunting. Hemodynamic changes often produce arterial aneurysms and venous stenoses or varices. Changes in flow dynamics and sheer stress often lead to proximal aneurysms in the circle of Willis. These lesions should be treated independently either by endovascular or surgical techniques. Feeding artery and intranidal aneurysms are directly dependent on the nidal flow pattern of the AVM and represent high-risk features effectively addressed by embolization.

The modern management of cerebral AVMs relies upon the combination of four distinct therapeutic modalities: endovascular embolization, microneurosurgery, and/or stereotactic radiosurgery. Spetzler-Martin Scale is often used to predict the outcome dependent on the AVM nidus size, location, and type of drainage (deep versus superficial). Endovascular management of brain AVMs focuses on eliminating high-risk angiographic features such as aneurysms and high-flow fistulae, in addition to minimizing the lesion size or associated technical challenges prior to definitive radiosurgical or operative procedures. When an AVM harbors a relatively small number of feeding arteries and draining veins, endovascular cure may be achievable.

In response to the ARUBA trial, the Trial of Brain AVM study is a pragmatic, prospective, multicenter randomized controlled trial and ongoing registry which offers a care trial context for brain AVM treatment including conservative management, radiosurgery, endovascular embolization, and surgical resection. The study includes two nested randomized trials and a multimodality prospective registry (Magro et al., 2018).

### Embolization Procedure

A detailed superselective diagnostic cerebral angiogram is necessary to determine the angioarchitecture and flow patterns associated with an AVM prior to endovascular treatment. Penetration of the nidus with embolic material, rather than simple occlusion of the feeding vessels, decreases the incidence of recanalization via flow through collateral channels (Vinuela et al., 1986). Procedural staging reduces

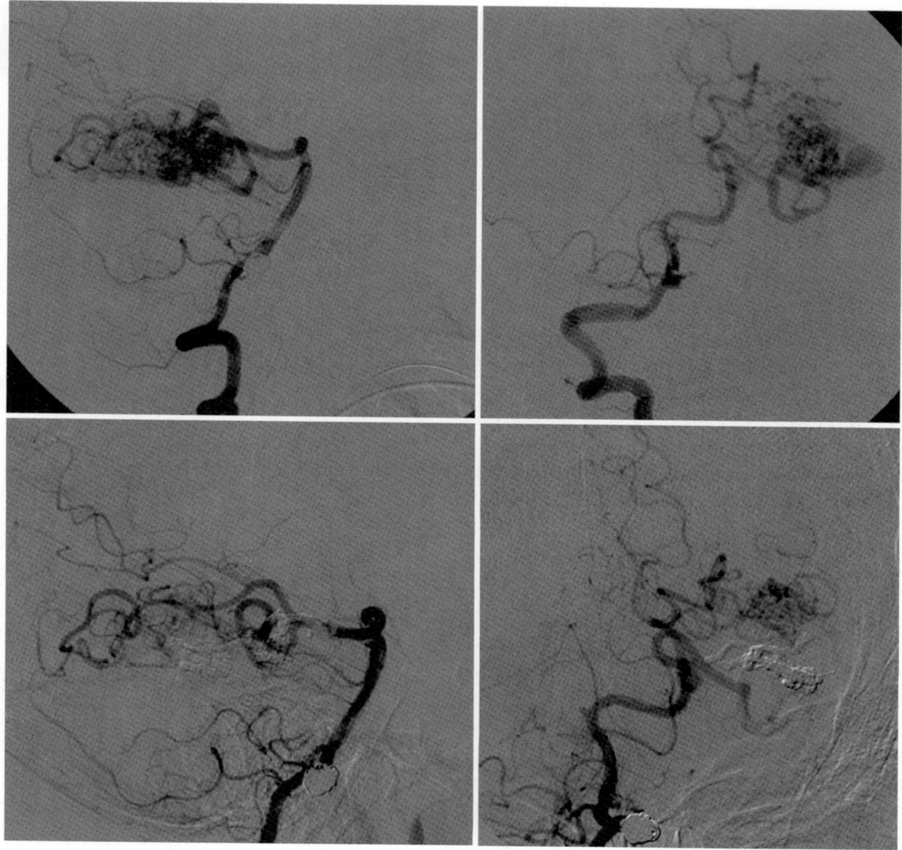

**Fig. 54.18** Anteroposterior *(left)* and lateral *(right)* angiograms before *(upper)* and after *(lower)* embolization of a 3-cm arteriovenous malformation (AVM) at the inferior and middle left temporal gyri. AVM was supplied by two inferior temporal branches of the posterior cerebral artery. Following *n*-butyl cyanoacrylate embolization to superior branch and Onyx-34 to inferior branch, there was approximately 25% reduction in total nidal volume, with no opacification of a lateral perinidal aneurysm. This patient received radiotherapy after embolization and in long-term follow-up had complete obliteration of the AVM.

the likelihood of edema or hemorrhagic complications secondary to normal perfusion breakthrough (Andrews and Wilson, 1987; Spetzler et al., 1987). Superselective Wada testing with sodium amytal allows for functional assessment in an awake patient. Infusion may reveal vascular supply to eloquent cortical tissue via *en passage* vessels not apparent on angiographic assessment (Purdy et al., 1991).

Under constant, real-time, roadmap guidance, an over-the-wire or flow-guided microcatheter is advanced to a distal intracranial position. Biplane superselective angiography is obtained and carefully analyzed for *en passage* vascular segments or cerebral capillary blush (Fig. 54.18). Several agents have been used for AVM embolization, discussed next.

## Polyvinyl Alcohol

Polyvinyl alcohol (PVA) particles (Boston Scientific) were the first material approved by the FDA for intravascular use. Dependent on flow, they are sized to the caliber of the target vessel. Consequently, the microcatheter lumen must be able to accommodate the particle diameter and prevent occlusion secondary to aggregation. Particle embolization occurs in a slower fashion than liquid embolic occlusion. Often, low-flow shunts are disconnected first, leading to increased pressure in the remaining feeding arteries and nidal vessels and rendering the AVM susceptible to rupture. Transient and permanent morbidity rates of 14.3% and 8.6%, respectively, have been reported following particle treatment (Schumacher and Horton, 1991). Nidal recanalization is the most significant failing associated with particle embolization. In a large series, Sorimachi et al. (1999) reported a 43% rate of enlargement following particle embolization and an 80% nidal recanalization rate in completely occluded lesions.

## *n*-Butyl Cyanoacrylate

*n*-Butyl cyanoacrylate (nBCA) (TRUFILL; Cordis Neurovascular) is an adhesive liquid monomeric agent that polymerizes and solidifies upon contact with an ionic solution such as blood (Debrun et al., 1997). Administration results in chronic inflammation, fibrosis, and vessel occlusion (Kish et al., 1983; Klara et al., 1985; Wikholm et al., 2001). The safety of nBCA in AVM embolization was assessed in a prospective randomized noninferiority trial demonstrating that nBCA was equivalent to PVA in achieving target embolization volume goal and reduction in feeding vessel number. The rates of permanent occlusion were more favorable in the nBCA group, with very low incidences of recanalization (*n*-BCA Trial Investigators, 2002). These results led to FDA approval for this indication. More recent investigations confirm that nBCA embolization results in complete, durable vessel occlusion. Yu et al. (2004) reported no recanalization at 17- to 32-month follow-up in a series of AVMs treated with nBCA. Wikholm et al. (2001) demonstrated a lack of recanalization at 5-year follow-up. Achieving nidal penetration requires modification of polymerization and viscosity parameters according to the hemodynamic characteristics of the lesion. Such factors are adjusted by varying the relative concentrations of Ethiodol and nBCA in the treatment mixture. Some groups advocate changing the pH of the solution with an organic acid such as glacial acetic acid to lengthen polymerization time (Lieber et al., 2005). Outcomes following nBCA embolization by experienced operators are favorable. In a series of 103 patients, Liu et al. (2000) reported transient and permanent complications of 4.9% and 1.9%, respectively, as well as two deaths. Gobin et al. (1996) documented morbidity and mortality rates of 12.8% and 1.8%, respectively.

### Ethylene Vinyl Alcohol Copolymer

Ethylene vinyl alcohol copolymer was first proposed for the treatment of AVMs by (Taki et al. (1990). Subsequently, many groups have reported on its use as a liquid embolic agent (Jahan et al., 2001; Murayama et al., 1998). Slow solidification permits prolonged controlled injections, with allowance for continuous assessment and deeper nidal penetration with each catheterization (Katsaridis et al., 2008; Murayama et al., 1998). Onyx was first tested in a phase I investigation conducted by Jahan et al. (2001). The group demonstrated a 63% volume reduction in 23 AVM patients with 129 targeted feeding artery pedicles. They reported a 12% transient and 4% permanent associated morbidity. Van Rooij and colleagues (2007) treated 44 patients with Onyx, embolizing 138 pedicles in 52 sessions. They documented an average volume reduction of 75%, with complete occlusion of seven lesions. A morbidity rate of 8.5% and a mortality rate of 3.2% were reported. Other large single-center case series have assessed potential for complete AVM occlusion with Onyx embolization. Katsaridis et al. (2008) reported a 54% rate of complete occlusion, with an associated morbidity and mortality of 3.7% and 1.4%, respectively, per embolization session. Using a combination of Onyx and nBCA therapy (Onyx as the first-line agent), Mounayer et al. (2007) reported a 49% complete occlusion rate, with similar incidences of complications (8.5% morbidity, 3.2% mortality).

Although it has revolutionized the way many groups treat brain AVMs, Onyx Liquid Embolic System (LES) carries inherent limitations and disadvantages. It can be used only with dimethylsulfoxide (DMSO)-compatible catheters. This prohibits the use of most flow-guided microsystems that facilitate access to small distal intracranial vessels. In addition, dimethyl sulfoxide (DMSO) can be angiotoxic if injected too rapidly into the cerebral vasculature (Jahan et al., 2001). Furthermore, limited opacification may prevent adequate visualization of reflux into small vessels supplying viable cortical tissue (van Rooij et al., 2007). Onyx AVM embolization requires increased fluoroscopy and procedure times compared with nBCA (Velat et al., 2008).

### Stereotactic Radiotherapy

Stereotactic radiosurgery is intended to induce progressive occlusion of an AVM by using high-dose targeted radiation. A radiation source, such as a Gamma Knife, delivers precise focused treatment using a navigation system. The AVM exposed to radiation undergoes endothelial damage and thickening of the intimal layer, which leads to thrombosis of the nidal vessels. This progressive obliteration of the AVM takes approximately 2–3 years, with a median of approximately 20 months (Wowra et al., 2009). Successful obliteration with radiosurgery depends on several factors including nidus volume and vessel density, radiation dose, and lesion location (Starke et al., 2008). This therapy offers a noninvasive intervention; however, complete obliteration may require up to 5 years and associated parenchymal radiation injury can complicate outcomes. Radiotherapy is one of several approaches to AVM treatment which can be an adjunctive or singular treatment for selected patients.

## CEREBRAL ARTERIOVENOUS FISTULAS

### Cranial Dural Arteriovenous Fistulas

Cranial DAVFs are direct shunts between arteries and venous sinuses or cortical veins with no transitional capillary network. The mean age of presentation is 50–60 years, without gender predilection or evidence for familial inheritance (Zipfel et al., 2009). Although most are presumed to be idiopathic, DAVFs may be associated with trauma, craniotomy, or venous thrombosis (Berenstein et al., 2001; Nguyen et al., 2011b). These lesions account for 6% of supratentorial and 35% of posterior fossa vascular malformations (Newton and Cronqvist, 1969). DAVFs present with symptoms according to anatomical localization and their pattern of venous drainage. Lesions draining into the cavernous sinus often result in proptosis, chemosis, ophthalmoplegia, or increased ocular pressure (Ito et al., 1983; Kim et al., 2002; van Dijk et al., 2004). By contrast, those with venous egress into the transverse or sigmoid sinus frequently present with pulsatile tinnitus (Brown et al., 1994). Posterior fossa DAVFs may cause lower cranial nerve deficits or brainstem findings (Borden et al., 1995; Kim et al., 2002). Lesions draining into the superior sagittal sinus can manifest with nonspecific cortical symptoms such as hydrocephalus, seizures, focal neurological deficit, or mental status change (Hirono et al., 1993; Hurst et al., 1998; Kim et al., 2002).

**BOX 54.3 Borden and Cognard Classification Systems**

**Borden Classification System**

Type I: dural arteriovenous fistula drainage into a dural venous sinus or meningeal vein with normal anterograde flow. Usually benign clinical behavior

Type II: anterograde drainage into dural venous sinus and onward, but retrograde flow is into cortical veins. May present with hemorrhage

Type III: direct retrograde flow of blood from fistula into cortical veins, causing venous hypertension with a risk of hemorrhage

**Cognard Classification System**

Type I: normal anterograde flow into a dural venous sinus

Type IIa: drainage into a sinus, with retrograde flow within the sinus

Type IIb: drainage into a sinus, with retrograde flow into cortical vein(s)

Type II a + b: drainage into a sinus, with retrograde flow within the sinus and cortical vein(s)

Type III: direct drainage into a cortical vein, without venous ectasia

Type IV: direct drainage into a cortical vein, with ectasia >5 mm and three times larger than the diameter of the draining vein

Type V: direct drainage into spinal perimedullary veins

*From Borden, J.A., Wu, J.K., Shucart, W.A., 1995. A proposed classification for spinal and cranial dural arteriovenous fistulous malformations and implications for treatment. J Neurosurg 82, 166–179; and Cognard, C., Gobin, Y.P., Pierot, L., et al., 1995. Cerebral dural arteriovenous fistulas: clinical and angiographic correlation with a revised classification of venous drainage. Radiology 194, 671–680.*

The natural history of DAVFs is influenced by cortical venous drainage (CVD), which, if present, increases the risk of intracranial hemorrhage and nonhemorrhagic neurological deficits (Borden et al., 1995; Cognard et al., 1995; Zipfel et al., 2009). The impact of CVD has been reflected in the angiographic classification systems of Borden and Cognard (Box 54.3), both of which categorize fistulas with cortical venous reflux as high-grade dangerous lesions (Borden et al., 1995; Cognard et al., 1995). Other associated angiographic features, such as venous ectasias and varices, have been correlated with poor outcome. More recent studies report that individuals who present with symptoms of cortical venous hypertension have a substantially higher risk of new neurological events than those who present incidentally or with symptoms consistent with increased dural sinus drainage (Soderman et al., 2008; Strom et al., 2009).

MRI can reveal the presence of a DAVF through flow voids or edema secondary to venous hypertension. Furthermore, dilated vessels may be evident on either CTA or MRA. However, catheter angiogram

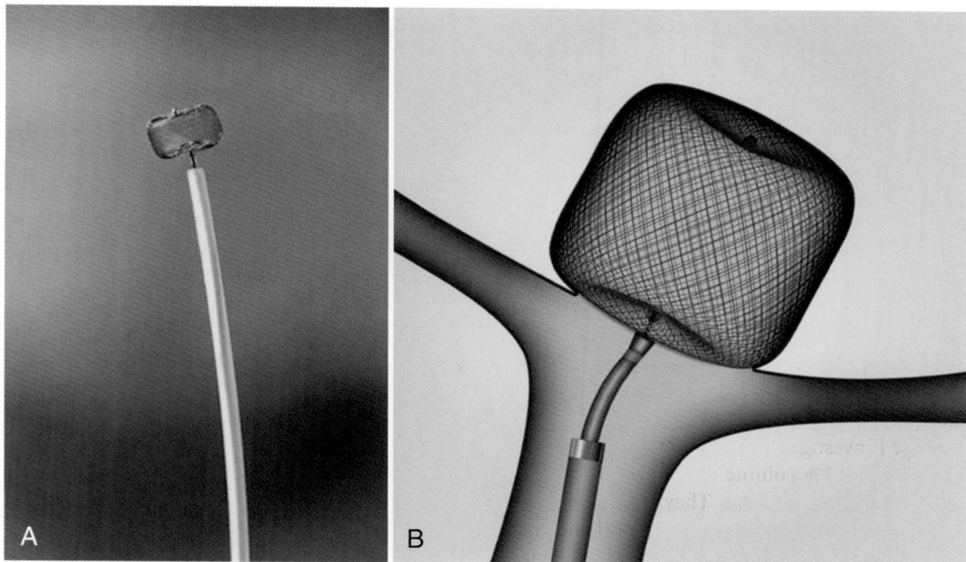


**Fig. 54.19** Woven EndoBridge Device, an intrasaccular aneurysm device (A), deployed via a microcatheter (B). *(Pictures courtesy Microventio.)*

remains the most accurate method of diagnosis and is critical in the assessment of lesional angioarchitecture and venous outflow pattern. Data suggest that lesions with dangerous CVD be addressed urgently (Duffau et al., 1999; van Dijk et al., 2002). Although angiographically benign fistulas may be managed conservatively, those with persistent clinical manifestations often warrant treatment for symptomatic relief.

Treatment options include endovascular occlusion, surgical disconnection, and stereotactic radiosurgery. Embolization, which is the preferred treatment option at most institutions, may be achieved through a transarterial or transvenous access route. Liquid embolic agents such as Onyx or nBCA are typically used alone or in conjunction with thrombogenic coils to attain fistula occlusion. Complete embolization via infiltration of the venous pouch and outflow tract is the ultimate objective. However, partial treatment with selective CVD disconnection is indicated in cases where normal venous drainage through an affected sinus precludes total fistula obliteration. Surgical treatment is typically reserved for lesions not amenable to endovascular therapy or select anterior cranial fossa DAVFs supplied by ethmoidal branches of the ophthalmic artery. Stereotactic radiosurgery is an effective treatment modality used either alone or in conjunction with endovascular therapy (Guo et al., 1998; Pollock et al., 1999). However, obliteration occurs over the course of several years, with an inherent interim risk of hemorrhage and neurological events according to the natural history of the specific lesion (Fig 54.19).

### Carotid-Cavernous Fistulas

Carotid-cavernous fistulas (CCFs), abnormal arteriovenous communications in the cavernous sinus, represent a subset of cranial arteriovenous fistulas (Fig. 54.20). These lesions may be classified on the basis of etiology (traumatic or spontaneous) or angioarchitecture (direct or indirect). The Barrow classification system (Barrow et al., 1985) segregates lesions according to their arterial supply (Box 54.4).

The classic presentation of direct CCFs is the sudden onset of exophthalmos, conjunctival injection, and a cephalic bruit. Associated cranial nerve palsies and visual decline are common. Indirect CCFs typically have a more gradual onset and mild presentation but may manifest in a similar clinical fashion. Proposed etiologies include pregnancy, sinusitis, trauma, and cavernous sinus thrombosis (Kwan et al., 1989).

Axial CT and MRI may reveal proptosis, flow voids, an enlarged cavernous sinus, or a prominent superior ophthalmic vein. Digital subtraction angiography is essential in classifying the CCF and elucidating the precise fistulous site and pattern of venous drainage. Injection of the vertebral artery while manually compressing the ipsilateral common carotid artery (in the presence of a posterior communicating artery) aids in localization, as the reduced flow facilitates visualization of the fistula.

Direct CCFs can be approached through transarterial or transvenous access. The standard endovascular treatment of direct CCFs had been transarterial disconnection with a detachable balloon. However, technical problems forced removal of this device from the US market. Current strategies use detachable coils, liquid embolic agents, and covered stents via either a transarterial or transvenous approach (Fig. 54.21). The transvenous route usually involves a posterior approach through the inferior petrosal sinus (IPS). However, if the IPS is occluded or absent, the superior ophthalmic vein (via the angular branch of the facial vein), inferior ophthalmic vein, superior petrosal sinus, pterygoid plexus, or sphenoparietal sinus may be used for access. A temporary balloon can be inflated in the ICA, across the communication, to assist with visualization and protect the integrity of the vessel lumen. Endovascular occlusion with parent-vessel preservation may not be achievable or necessary for direct CCFs caused by extensive injury to the ICA or those associated with significant steal. In such circumstances, occlusion of the parent artery may be the best (or only) viable management option. In rare reports, spontaneous closure of the direct CCF can be seen if the shunt is small (Naragum et al., 2018).

Indirect fistulas may thrombose without vascular intervention (Higashida et al., 1986). However, persistent indirect CCFs are embolized through arterial or venous access routes (listed earlier) in the manner previously described for cranial DAVFs.

## SPINAL VASCULAR MALFORMATIONS

Spinal vascular malformations are a rare and underdiagnosed entity that, if not treated properly, can result in progressive spinal cord symptoms with considerable associated morbidity (Krings and Geibprasert, 2009). A majority of the lesions occur in males and are located in the thoracic or lumbar region of the spinal cord. DAVFs frequently cause

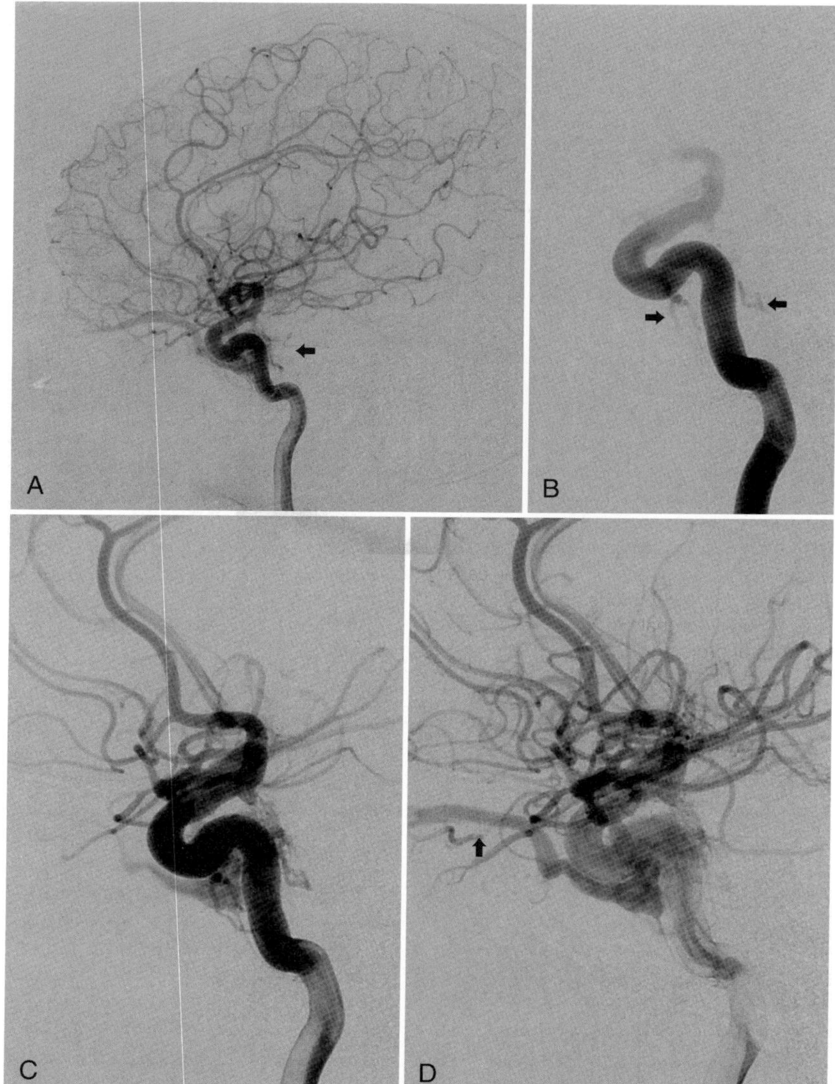


**Fig. 54.20** A lateral projection right internal carotid artery angiogram shows a carotid-cavernous fistula *(arrow)* (**A**). A magnified lateral projection angiogram shows the fistula with indirect supply from inferolateral and meningohypophyseal trunk arteries *(arrows)* in the early arterial phase (**B**), with rapid filling of the cavernous sinus in mid-arterial phase (**C**), and venous outflow through the superior ophthalmic vein *(arrow)* (**D**).

### BOX 54.4 Grading Scale for Carotid-Cavernous Fistulas

Type A (direct): direct communication between the internal carotid artery (ICA) and the cavernous sinus. Usually arises as a result of traumatic laceration or aneurysmal rupture and presents with high flow rate.

Type B (indirect): supplied only by the dural branches of the ICA. Most often arises spontaneously and presents with a lower flow rate.

Type C (indirect): supplied only by dural branches of the external carotid artery (ECA). Most often arises spontaneously and presents with a lower flow rate.

Type D (indirect): supplied by dural branches of the ICA and ECA. Most often arises spontaneously and presents with a lower flow rate.

gradual ascending paraparesis or bowel and bladder dysfunction, whereas intramedullary spinal cord malformations typically present with hemorrhage. Although MR studies may reveal flow voids or conus medullaris edema, spinal digital subtraction angiography is necessary for diagnosis, characterization of lesional angioarchitecture, and treatment planning (Fig. 54.22).

The arterial supply to the spinal cord is derived from a single anterior spinal artery (ASA) and paired posterior spinal arteries (PSAs). The ASA originates from both vertebral arteries, typically just proximal to the vertebrobasilar junction. It courses through the anterior sulcus of the spinal cord and receives tributaries from radiculomedullary branches of the segmental arteries. The most robust anastomotic supply is provided in the cervical lower thoracic and lumbar regions, with a paucity of radicular connections at the upper thoracic levels. One such anastomotic branch, the artery of lumbar enlargement or artery of Adamkiewicz, provides the main arterial supply to the spinal cord from the lower thoracic region to the conus medullaris. It most often originates from a radicular vessel on the left, between the T8 and L4 levels (McCutcheon et al., 1996). The PSAs originate more proximally from the bilateral vertebral arteries. The paired vessels course along the posterolateral aspect of the spinal cord and anastomose with multiple radiculopial branches of the segmental arteries, which enter the dura

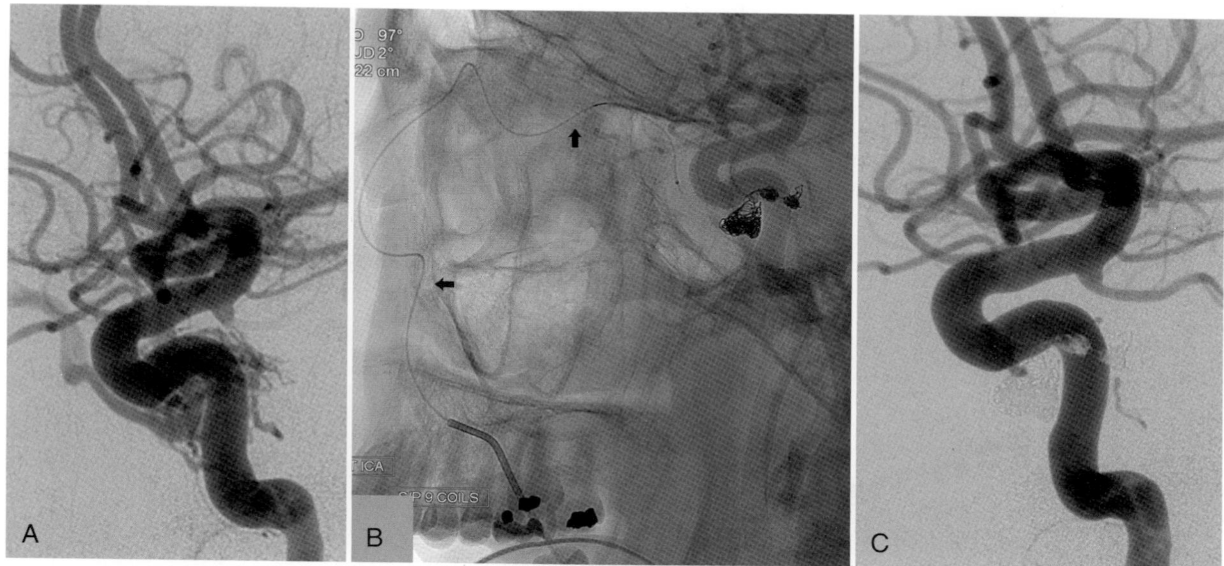


**Fig. 54.21** A lateral projection right internal carotid artery angiogram shows the pretreatment carotid-cavernous fistula **(A)**. A transvenous approach was used by microcatheterization of the cavernous sinus via the facial and superior ophthalmic veins *(arrows)*, to achieve complete coil embolization of the fistula **(B)**. Posttreatment lateral projection angiogram shows obliteration of the fistula **(C)**.

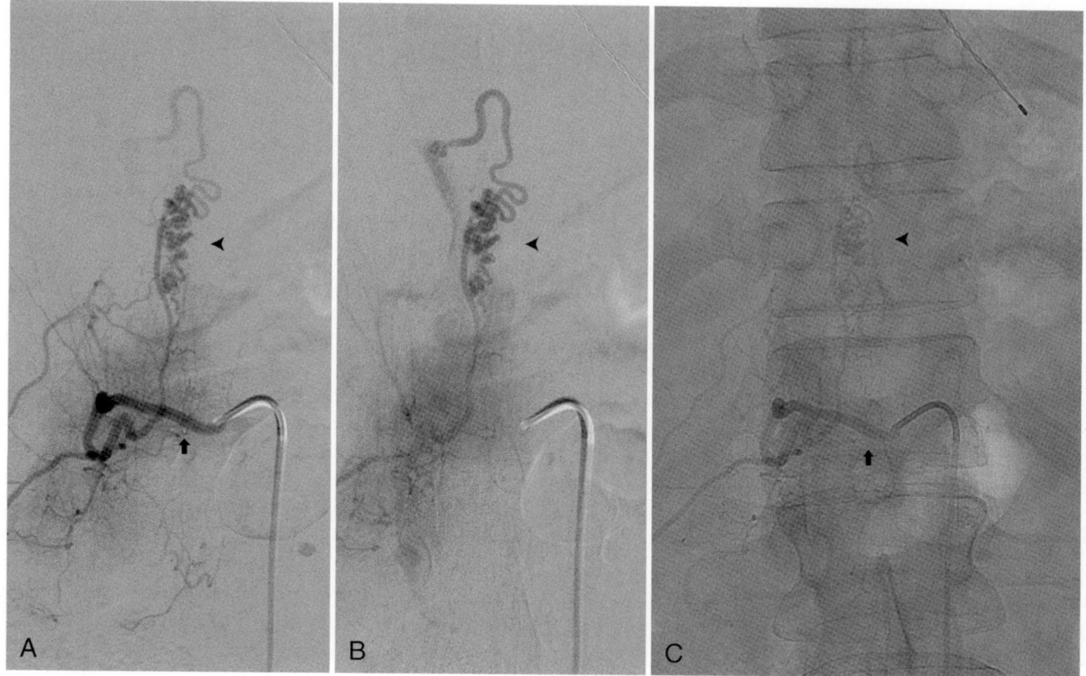


**Fig. 54.22** Frontal projection angiogram of the right T12 segmental artery *(arrow)* in early arterial phase shows arteriovenous shunting from a spinal dural arteriovenous fistula *(arrowhead)* **(A)**. Late arterial phase shows further characterization of venous outflow **(B)**. The unsubtracted angiogram image shows the relationship of the vascular anatomy to the spinal column **(C)**.

through the nerve root sheaths. Classification schemes for spinal vascular malformations are based upon this arterial anatomy (Kim and Spetzler, 2006; Spetzler et al., 2002).

## Spinal Dural Arteriovenous Fistula (Type I)

These lesions represent the most common type of spinal vascular malformation and may be supplied by one (type 1a) or multiple (type 1b) dorsal radiculomedullary vessels, which form a fistulous connection with the coronal venous plexus upon entering the dura at the root sleeve (Anson and Spetzler, 1992; Kim and Spetzler, 2006; Sivakumar et al., 2009). They occur most frequently in men older than 50 years of age and classically present with progressive myelopathy secondary to chronic venous hypertension. Endovascular treatment consists of embolization of the fistulous origin, including the proximal portion of

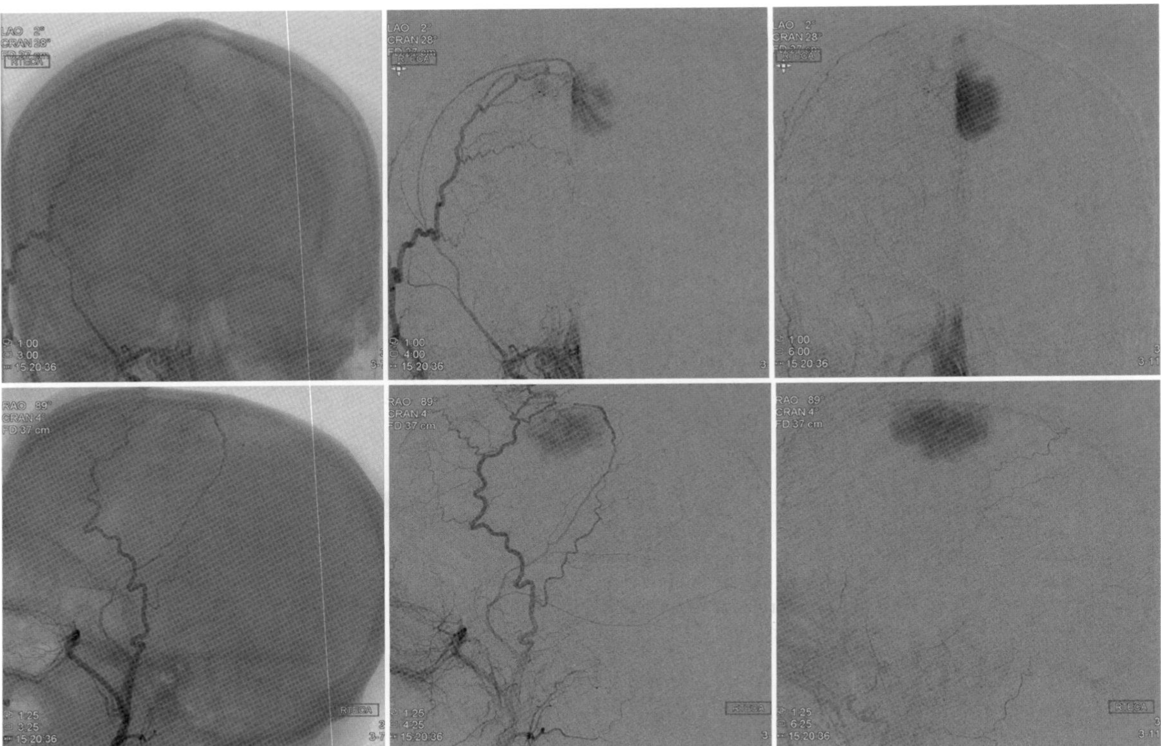

**Fig. 54.23** Anteroposterior *(top row)* and lateral *(bottom row)* right external carotid artery angiograms show a left parasagittal meningioma with right middle meningeal artery supply. Characteristic features include a dural-based location and a hypervascular appearance with a homogenously intense and prolonged vascular stain.

the draining vein (van Dijk et al., 2002). Open surgical disconnection may be used to achieve a similar result.

### Glomus Arteriovenous Malformation (Type II)

Similar to intracranial AVMs, these lesions are supplied by perforating branches of the anterior or PSAs and drain into the venous plexus surrounding the spinal cord (Kim et al., 2006; Spetzler et al., 2002; Wakhloo et al., 2008). A high-pressure, high-flow nidus may be diffuse or compact and is often associated with a feeding artery or intranidal aneurysms. These lesions most frequently occur in younger men and women and frequently present with hemorrhage. Embolization is usually used as an adjunct to surgical resection.

### Juvenile/Metameric Arteriovenous Malformation (Type III)

Found predominantly in children and young adults, these lesions are fed by multiple arterial pedicles and affect bone and soft tissue in addition to spinal cord parenchyma (Kim and Spetzler, 2006; Spetzler et al., 2002) (Wakhloo et al., 2008). Involvement of an entire metamere including skin, soft tissue, bone, and spinal cord parenchyma is referred to as *Cobb syndrome*. Multimodality therapy is frequently indicated because of the complex nature of these malformations.

### Perimedullary Arteriovenous Malformation (Type IV)

Vascular supply to these intradural extramedullary fistulas is derived from either the anterior (most commonly) or PSAs. They occur most frequently between the ages of 30 and 60 and often present with progressive neurological deficits (Anson and Spetzler, 1992; Heros et al., 1986). The treatment paradigm is dependent on the angioarchitecture of the lesion, including the number of feeding pedicles and rate of fistulous flow. Surgical disconnection has been successfully used for low-flow fistulas supplied by a single feeding artery, while a combination of endovascular and surgical techniques has commonly been used for the management of more complex lesions.

## TUMOR EMBOLIZATION

Preoperative embolization of extracranial head and neck or intracranial tumors is a useful adjunct to microsurgical resection. Tumors most commonly treated by this means are meningiomas (Figs. 54.23 and 54.24), glomus tumors, juvenile nasopharyngeal angiofibromas, hemangioblastomas, sarcomas, head and neck squamous cell carcinomas, and choroid plexus tumors (Eskridge et al., 1996; Scholtz et al., 2001). These lesions are often vascular, so preoperative embolization can ease complete resection by diminishing surgical time and intraoperative blood loss (Gruber et al., 2000; Manelfe et al., 1986). Many cranial-base tumors are characterized by vascular pedicles that are medially located with respect to the operative approach (Rosen et al., 2002). In such cases the surgical corridor is often narrow and deep, which amplifies the difficulty of resection. In addition to improving operative safety and visualization, preoperative embolization is believed to reduce transmitted forces to adjacent neural tissues during surgical resection by causing ischemic necrosis and a resultant softening of the tumor mass (Yoon et al., 2008). In selected patients who are not suitable candidates for surgery, embolization can be used for palliation, with a goal of size and tumor growth reduction. Because the primary blood supply is most frequently derived from the external carotid artery, a thorough understanding of the head, neck, and intracranial vascular anatomy is critical.

### Clinical Evidence

Several large case series document angiographic, histological, and surgical benefit following meningioma embolization (Dean et al., 1994;

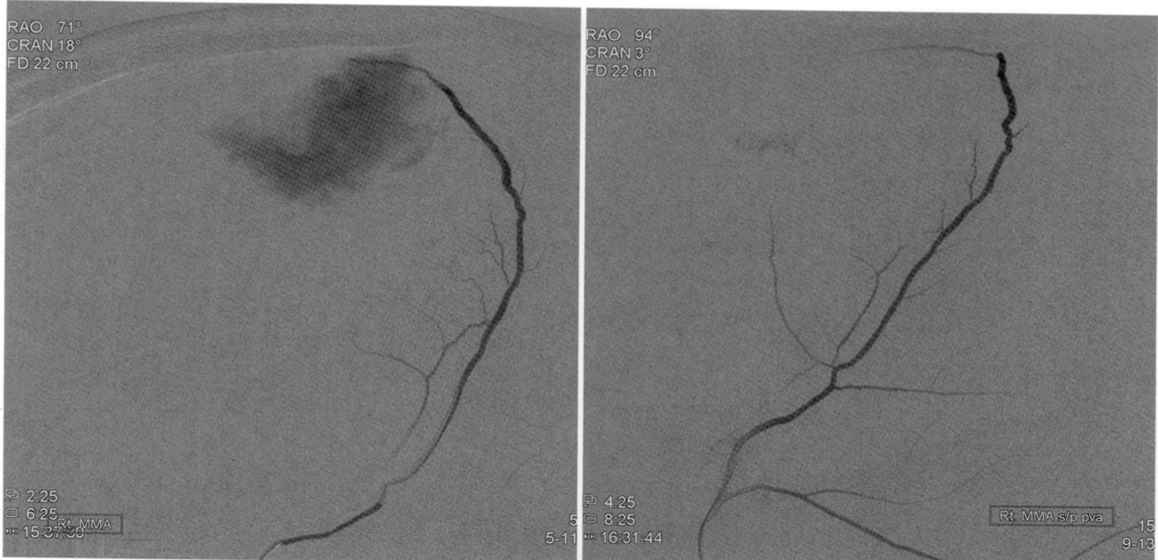


**Fig. 54.24** Superselective right middle meningeal artery lateral oblique angiogram shows the left parasagittal meningioma before *(left)* and after *(right)* embolization with polyvinyl alcohol particles. Nonvisualization of the tumor blush after treatment is consistent with complete devascularization of the middle meningeal artery supply to the tumor.

Gruber et al., 2000; Manelfe et al., 1986; Masoud et al. 2017; Wakhloo et al., 1993; Yoon et al., 2008). Endovascular treatment of juvenile nasopharyngeal angiofibromas has been shown to reduce both perioperative blood loss and the duration of surgical resection (Davis, 1987; Economou et al., 1988; Roberson et al., 1979). Other reports question the benefit, citing no differences in operative time, blood loss, or clinical outcome (Bendszus et al., 2000). Some groups reserve preoperative embolization for difficult skull-base lesions, referencing complication rates deemed unacceptable for straightforward surgical resections (Rosen et al., 2002). The optimal timing of resection following tumor embolization has been debated. Some operators contend that timing of surgery does not affect outcome, but others have advocated delayed resection to allow for interval tumor necrosis. A comparative retrospective analysis of 50 patients who underwent preoperative embolization for meningioma resection indicated that delaying resection more than 24 hours after embolization can decrease intraoperative blood loss (Chun et al., 2002). Other groups have suggested that the optimal interval between embolization and resection is between 7 and 9 days, because this permits maximal tumor softening (Kai et al., 2002). However, a significantly long interval between particulate embolization and surgical resection may allow for recanalization of blood vessels supplying the tumor.

Significant neurological deficits have been reported following preoperative tumor embolization. Causes include distal vessel occlusion, reflux of embolic agents, cranial nerve injury, and tumor swelling or hemorrhage following devascularization (Bendszus et al., 2005; Carli et al., 2010; Marangos and Schumacher, 1999). Therefore potential benefits of embolization must be weighed against the risk of adverse outcome. Patients harboring large hypervascular tumors supplied primarily by external carotid artery branches that are located in anatomical regions difficult to access surgically likely derive the greatest benefit from preoperative embolization.

### Subdural Hemorrhage Embolization

Chronic SDH is a collection of blood under the dural layer covering the brain but external to the brain and arachnoid membrane. In the setting of chronic SDH, the blood components are hypodense or isodense to the brain and are thought to have developed over 3 weeks from presentation (Fiorella and Arthur, 2019). The initiation, development, and progression of SDH is related to a cycle of chronic inflammation and angiogenesis. There is an initial hemorrhage, followed by fibrinolysis, the breakdown products of which trigger inflammation. This, in turn, incites angiogenesis of the dural layer with growth of capillaries which leak blood, which can lead to progressive enlargement of the hematoma. As the hematoma enlarges, patients can present with a variety of neurological manifestations including chronic headaches, altered mental status, seizure, gait impairment, focal neurological deficit, or cognitive decline with dementia.

Treatment of patients with chronic SDH can range from conservative management for the asymptomatic patient, to surgical resection for patients with 10-mm or greater diameter of the hematoma associated with midline shift. Recurrent subdural hemorrhage after surgical evacuation is not uncommon, estimated in 10%–20% of patients. Antithrombotic agents are often withheld or reversed in the setting of subdural hemorrhage and surgery, which is associated with prothrombotic risks to the patient. Recently, embolization of the middle meningeal artery has emerged as an alternative or adjunct treatment for chronic SDH with excellent results in several case series. A meta-analysis review comparing embolization and conventional surgery demonstrated lower hematoma recurrence in the embolization group compared with conventional treatment group (2% vs. 27.7%) (Srivatsan et al., 2019). Although these results are promising, a randomized controlled trial comparing medical management versus embolization as single treatment or adjunct to surgery will be important in establishing the effectiveness and safety of this promising new treatment.

## IDIOPATHIC INTRACRANIAL HYPERTENSION

Idiopathic intracranial hypertension (IIH), or pseudotumor cerebri, is a commonly diagnosed disorder with a limited understanding of the underlying pathophysiology. Patients can present with debilitating headaches, vision loss, findings of papilledema, and elevated CSF pressure. Surgical therapies for those patients who experience progressive visual decline despite maximum medical therapy include optic nerve sheath fenestration and ventricular shunt placement. Many patients

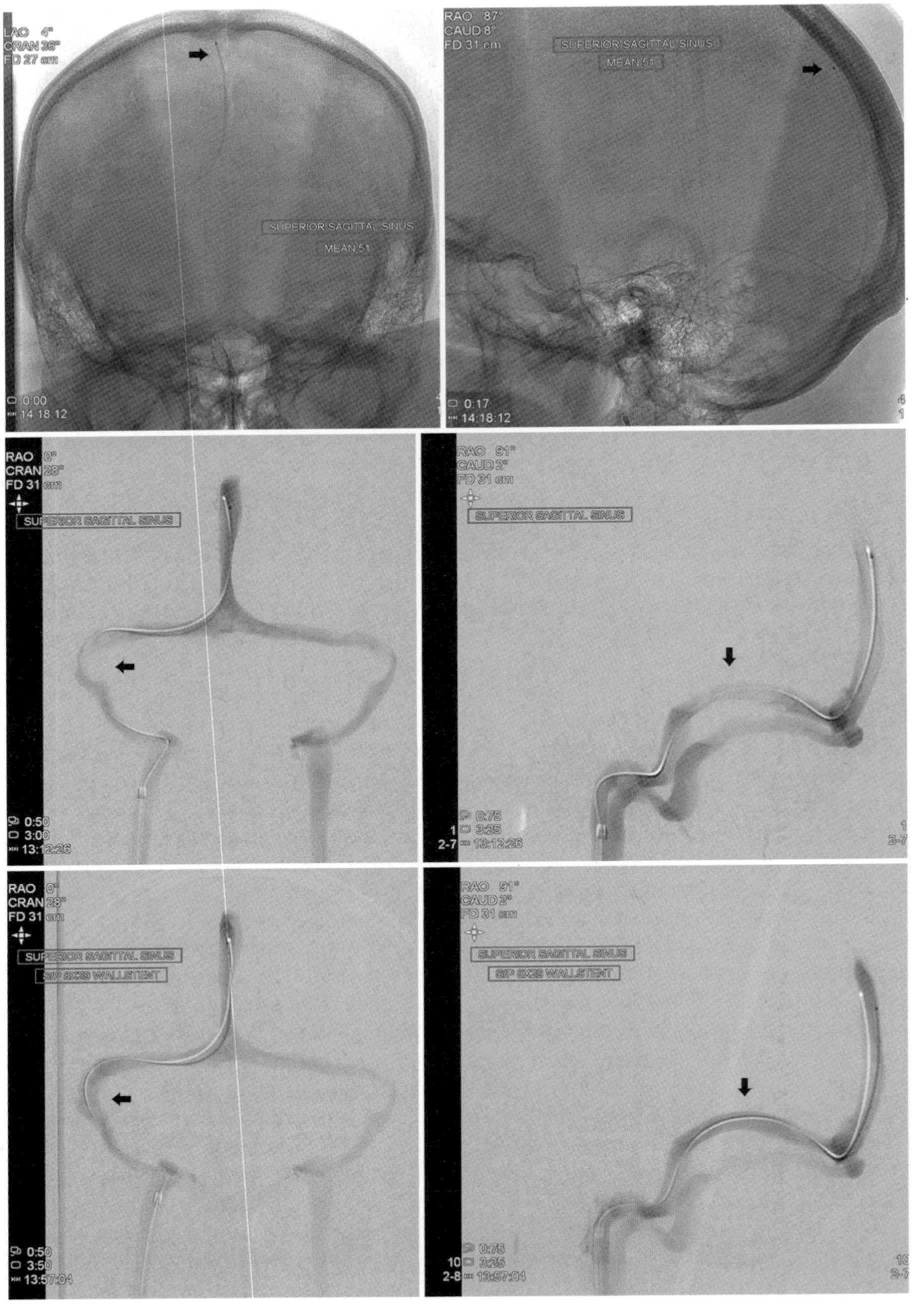

**Fig. 54.25** Anteroposterior and lateral projection images show microcatheterization *(arrows)* of the superior sagittal sinus for venous pressure manometry *(top row)*. Anteroposterior and lateral projection venograms show bilateral transverse sinus narrowing before treatment *(arrow, middle row)* and improved lumen caliber and antegrade flow following right transverse sinus stenting *(arrow, bottom row)*. Mean venous pressures improved from 51–17 mm Hg within the superior sagittal sinus following treatment.

have a finding of dural sinus narrowing, which has generated considerable interest in the potential role of endovascular reconstructive therapy with stent implantation. In some cases of IIH, transvenous manometry testing shows a dramatic pressure gradient across the focal dural sinus narrowing, suggesting a venous outflow obstruction as a component of the pathophysiology. Although the hydrodynamic disequilibrium in IIH is not well understood, this may represent a self-perpetuating cycle of progressive dural sinus incompetence that leads to venous outflow obstruction and the resulting intracranial pressure (Lazzaro et al., 2012). Few reports describe safety and efficacy of endovascular therapy for IIH, and scientific validation is needed. In selected patients with progressive visual threat despite maximum medical therapy, and findings of a substantial pressure gradient across a focal dural sinus narrowing, endovascular stent implantation (Fig. 54.25) can be considered to reduce the risk of vision loss.

*The complete reference list is available online at https://expertconsult.inkling.com/.*

55

# Neurological Rehabilitation

*Bruce H. Dobkin*

OUTLINE



## GOALS AND STRUCTURE OF REHABILITATION

Rehabilitation training focuses on reducing physical and cognitive impairments and their related disabilities and limitations on activity in an effort to increase functional independence and health-related quality of life. Training of movements and skills involves an active learning process as well as self-management techniques that draw on motivation, guidance, goal setting, progressive practice, feedback, and social support. National guidelines for neurological rehabilitation with an emphasis on stroke care have been created in many countries. A guideline developed by members of the American Stroke Association offers a comprehensive review of service organization and interventions (Winstein et al., 2016a).

### Aims

Neurological rehabilitation involves multidisciplinary services—preferably a collaborative team effort that includes patients, caregivers, and families—designed to improve functional and cognitive skills such as walking and language, reduce dependence in personal care and other home and community activities, lessen the burden of care on family and society, and prevent and manage medical and psychosocial complications. Rehabilitation practices address the links between disease pathology, physical and cognitive deficits/impairments, related disabilities, home and community activity, participation in daily life, handicap, and health-related quality of life.

Neurorehabilitation assessment identifies the most productive focus for interventions and the most appropriate setting in which better outcomes can be achieved within expected time frames. Clinical evaluation initiates a treatment program that is continually revised in light of successive assessments. Both short- and long-term goals take into account the amount of likely neurological recovery and the amount of residual disability. Progressive goal setting is a technique to encourage the patient as each short-term objective is achieved while also serving to monitor efficacy and identify emerging confounders of gains. Short-term goals must be relevant, motivating, explicit, attainable, measurable, and agreeable to the patient.

To achieve these aims, the rehabilitation process differs from the usual medical model of care by including personnel from multiple disciplines, problem-solving strategies that include methods to engage mechanisms of neuroplasticity, disease-related standardized outcome measures, and the organization of home and community services to meet the patient's needs.

## Rehabilitation Team Strategies

A team approach to inpatient and outpatient care best manages the diverse problems faced by disabled patients and their families. An interdisciplinary approach is oriented toward problem solving to improve functional outcomes rather than being bound by individual disciplines. For example, training procedures for motor and cognitive learning or behavioral modification are reinforced by all members of an interdisciplinary group using agreed-on strategies. The inpatient care milieu—comprising a team of physical, occupational, and speech therapists as well as nurses, social workers, neuropsychologists, and physicians—emphasizes the mitigation of disability and is one of rehabilitation's most powerful tools. Studies of inpatient stroke rehabilitation, for example, support the team approach as an efficient way to organize services for patients with functional disabilities. With traumatic brain injury (TBI) or spinal cord injury (SCI), the special needs of affected patients suggest that interdisciplinary inpatient and outpatient care will lead to fewer medical and psychosocial complications.

### Physicians

An understanding of the underlying disorder—including the mechanisms of disability, potential outcomes, and natural history of the disease being managed—is critical in planning any rehabilitation program. This expertise may be provided by the growing number of neurologists with expertise in neurorehabilitation who can bring principles from their increasing storehouse of knowledge to bear on recovery and by rehabilitation physicians or physiatrists, who also have broad experience in musculoskeletal, orthopedic, and cardiopulmonary rehabilitation issues. Orthopedists, urologists, psychiatrists, plastic surgeons, neurosurgeons, and podiatrists are often consulted during rehabilitation and for the long-term management of disabled patients.

The clinician superimposes the contributions of neurological, musculoskeletal, cardiopulmonary, and other impairments on a map of the patient's functional abilities and disabilities. For example, does tender musculoligamentous tissue cause pain, limit movement, or exacerbate spasticity? Does a medication or metabolic abnormality lessen concentration, the ability to learn, or endurance for exercise? Physicians tend to be the facilitators of the multidisciplinary team, especially during inpatient care. Here, the physician may conduct a weekly team conference that reviews the patient's progress in reaching the functional goals that will permit a discharge to the home. To do this well, the physician must help build the team's infrastructure and understand the practices of its disciplines. Rehabilitation physicians should serve as clinician-scientists as well. The physician can encourage therapists to weigh, formulate, and test strategies. Drawing on current literature and collaborating with basic and clinical researchers, the neurological rehabilitation specialist can optimally assess and develop interventions and creative solutions.

Physicians should explain to both patient and primary care doctor the indications for medications, measures for secondary prevention of complications, management of risk factors for recurrence or exacerbation of the disease, and the type and duration of rehabilitative interventions. Increasingly, doctors must address the risks and possible benefits of not only medications and usual rehabilitative approaches to care but also potential research interventions such as cellular transplantation. During outpatient care, physicians must provide informed counseling about exercise and home practice for motor and cognitive retraining. The clinician reviews the details of what the patient is practicing to improve walking, the functional use of an affected upper extremity, language and memory skills, and socialization. Education should be offered about how task-specific practice may alter the brain's adaptive representations of these activities and improve the patient's abilities even years after the neurological illness began. For patients with chronic diseases that progress, such as multiple sclerosis (MS), practice is perhaps even more important because it may spur gradual neural reorganization to maintain function. Clinicians can encourage patients to increase their strength, speed, and precision of multijoint movements, and to build cardiovascular fitness. The physician should also monitor outcomes with serial tests of targeted activities to best determine the optimal dose of a treatment. For example, if the gait pattern is suboptimal, the clinician can test walking speed for 50 feet or the distance walked in 2 minutes to reassess progress in mobility at each visit. By documenting the effects of treatment, the physician can best outline the continuing goals of rehabilitation to patients and insurers.

The internet offers access to many sites from which to develop educational materials as well as lectures and articles about recovery and experimental interventions that physicians and the therapy team can offer to patients.

### Rehabilitation Nursing

Traditionally, the nursing role has been one of providing care and support during a phase of illness and doing for others the things they would normally do for themselves. During inpatient rehabilitation, nurses encourage greater independence in self-care, manage a bowel and bladder program that may include intermittent bladder self-catheterization, and teach skin care and pressure sore management. Their extended contact with patients allows nurses to address the carryover of skills from physical and occupational therapy sessions, teach problem solving, and recognize impending medical complications. A nurse practitioner can be a valuable asset to the physician and team on a busy inpatient service where patients have complex medical illnesses.

### Physical Therapists

Physical therapists (PTs), or physiotherapists relate voluntary motor control and patterns of multijoint movements, sensory appreciation, range of motion of joints, strength, balance, and endurance to the training needs for bed and wheelchair mobility, standing up, walking, and functional mobility during activities. PTs bring expertise to the team in wheelchair design, assistive devices, and orthoses. They manage compensatory strategies for carrying out activities of daily living (ADLs) such as the use of a walker and offer interventions to lessen specific impairments. PTs play a primary role in managing musculoskeletal and radicular pain, contractures, spasticity, and deconditioning.

Two broad categories of physical therapy—therapeutic exercise and the so-called neurophysiological and neurodevelopmental techniques—were the bulwark of the approaches used by therapists in the past (Box 55.1). Newer concepts related to practice-induced neuroplasticity, motor control, and skills learning have taken greater hold, beginning in the past decade.

***Exercise and compensatory functional training.*** Most therapy programs emphasize education about impairments and disabilities, compensatory techniques for ADLs and mobility, and repetitive exercises to build from less complex to more functional multijoint movements. Traditional exercise programs employ repetitive passive and active joint-by-joint exercises and resistance exercises

**BOX 55.1 Practices in Physical Therapy**

Therapeutic exercise and reeducation
Resistance exercises
Fitness training
Neurofacilitation techniques:
- Proprioceptive neuromuscular facilitation
- Bobath technique
- Others

Motor control approaches:
- Motor skill learning

Shaping more complex, accurate movements:
- Task-oriented practice
- Forced use
- Massed practice, including constraint of one limb or robotic-assisted devices

Compensatory training:
- Biofeedback
- Musculoskeletal manipulation techniques
- Orthotics (e.g., ankle-foot orthosis), assistive devices (e.g., quad cane)

in anatomical planes to optimize strength and range of motion. The approach aims to prevent the complications of immobilization such as contractures, muscle atrophy, and spasticity. In the therapeutic exercise approach to stroke, SCI, and other upper motor neuron (UMN) diseases, residual motor skills in affected and unaffected extremities are used to compensate for impairments. The acquisition of self-care and mobility skills may take precedence over the quality of movement as long as the patient's safety can be ensured. Upper and lower extremity orthoses and assistive devices tend to be used early to promote functional compensation. PTs also use breathing and general conditioning exercises and teach energy conservation techniques, particularly to reduce the energy cost of a pathological gait.

***Conditioning and strengthening.*** Light resistance exercises for any UMN or lower motor neuron (LMN) disease—from stroke and SCI to amyotrophic lateral sclerosis (ALS), the postpolio syndrome, and the muscular dystrophies—are generally safe and effective in improving strength and sometimes function. Strength can be increased without inducing spasticity in patients with UMN and other neuromuscular diseases without injuring muscle tissue. Concern about falls, disability, and muscle atrophy in older adults has led to many studies showing that a strengthening program can benefit any sedentary person. Initial resistance training can lead to an increase in strength without any improvement in muscle bulk, probably by augmenting the amount of supraspinal input recruited to the task. Thus strengthening can be considered a form of motor learning. Isometric resistance exercises are probably the safest approach for weak patients and can be performed without equipment. For example, flexing the elbow of one arm about 60 degrees and pressing down on that forearm with the palm of the other arm to reach an equilibrium of tension in each arm will enhance strength in the shoulder girdle, elbow flexors and extensors, and forearm groups. To build muscle mass requires the subject to perform one or two sets of 8–15 repetitions three times a week against 50% or more of the maximum resistance manageable in a single lift. Pool therapy can be used to augment fitness and strengthening exercises. Patients may work against the resistance of the water, for example, by repeatedly flexing, extending, abducting, and adducting each leg at the hip while standing on the other or by using swim strokes. Practicing walking in a pool allows the patient to make use of the water's buoyancy, but the refraction of light within the water may make visual cues for foot placement less reliable.

Fitness training is valuable in UMN, extrapyramidal, and LMN diseases. Repetitive exercise, at least in animal models of stroke and SCI, also has induced potential reparative biological effects such as neurogenesis and increased expression of neurotrophic factors (Voss et al., 2010). This finding may be used to motivate patients. Executive functions may also improve with aerobic training. Treadmill walking and stationary recumbent biking can be aerobic workouts across diseases in persons with fair motor control of hip flexors and knee extensors.

***Schools of neurophysiology.*** Many schools of physical therapy have developed approaches that focus on enhancing the movement of paretic limbs affected by UMN lesions. These approaches may be especially valuable when motor therapies are initiated in patients with profound weakness. Techniques include using sensory stimuli and reflexes to facilitate or inhibit muscle tone and single- and whole-limb muscle movements in and out of mass actions called synergies. Most approaches try to sequence therapy in a progression reminiscent of the neurodevelopmental evolution in infants from reflexive to more complex movements. The emphasis is on normal postural alignment before any movement. Some techniques permit mass movement patterns early in treatment; others inhibit spastic overflow synergistic movements. For example, mobility activities may proceed in a developmental pattern from rolling onto the side with arm and leg flexion on the same side, followed by extension of the neck and legs while prone, then lying prone while supported by the elbows, and then doing static and weight-shifting movements while crawling on all fours. These mat activities are followed by efforts for sitting, standing, and finally walking. This progression is used most often in children with cerebral palsy, but some therapists also apply it to stroke and TBI rehabilitation.

The *Bobath hands-on approach* is a particularly popular neurodevelopmental technique. It aims to facilitate normal movement and desired automatic reactions and to restore postural control while inhibiting abnormal tone and reflex activity using specific motor patterns. Bobath therapists avoid provoking mass flexor synergies from the shoulder, elbow, and wrist or extensor synergies at the knee and ankle. The coordination of patterns of muscle group activity is viewed as more important than the actions of individual muscles. Use of Bobath techniques has led to equivalent outcomes or, in several small trials, modestly inferior outcomes to other approaches (van Vliet et al., 2005).

***Motor learning approaches.*** Movement science and the bases for learning motor skills have become key concepts for understanding normal movement and analyzing motor dysfunction. The motor control approach may incorporate techniques to eliminate unnecessary muscle activity and provide feedback about performance and practice during specific, often real-world tasks. In rehabilitation settings, little attention has been paid to whether training procedures—not what is taught but how it is taught—can optimize gains in cognitive skills, motor functions, self-care, and community activities. The essence of therapy for any disability, as with the acquisition of any novel motor or cognitive skill, is practice. Although a practice session can have a powerful effect, such effects are only temporary. Practice that improves performance during a training session may not lead to long-term learning. The goal of practice should be a permanent effect. Research studies of interventions, however, rarely include deliberate reinforcement strategies or dose–response curves to establish how much practice is needed to achieve a retraining goal. For example, practice of functional activities using the hemiparetic arm for reaching and grasping items, including the contextual interference of intermixing other tasks such as pointing and touching during learning, may lead to better retention over time than blocks of repetitive practice of the same task.

***Task-oriented practice.*** Motor learning emphasizes visual, verbal, and other sensory feedback to perform movements necessary to complete motor tasks; this contrasts with neurophysiological techniques, which rely on cutaneous, proprioceptive, and other sensory stimuli to elicit facilitation and inhibition of movement patterns. The latter approach is used mostly when a patient has very poor motor control. A key aim of the PT is to put the patient in the best position to be able to practice progressively. Constraint-induced therapy (CIT) for the upper extremity was one of the first well-defined procedures to encourage repetitive task-oriented movement and has been shown to be better than usual care (minimal practice) and as good as other types of progressive, task-specific practice. Body weight–supported treadmill training (BWSTT) for walking seemed task specific but failed to produce better results than the same intensity of over ground training. Training in a virtual reality (VR) environment can be another task-oriented approach to improve motor control for particular tasks or skills. A review of repetitive task training across 36 pairs of intervention versus control therapies for hemiparetic stroke found good evidence that patients improve for at least 6 months after an adequate amount of repetitive practice in their use of the upper extremity and in ambulation (French et al., 2016). The intensity of practice is moot. A trial that compared patients with upper extremity impairment more than 6 months poststroke found no difference in improvement on Action Research Arm Test (ARAT) scores in groups that practiced daily for 4 weeks at a dose of 3200 versus 9600 or as many task-specific repetitions as able (Lang, et al., 2016).

***Assistive equipment.*** Canes and walkers improve stability through a lever arm that can share the body's weight between the leg and device, keep the pelvis level during stance on the weak leg, and generate a joint moment to assist the hip abductors and reduce loading on the knee. Devices must be fitted properly. For example, handgrips should be at a height that allows approximately 20–30 degrees of elbow flexion. The cane should swing forward with the involved limb and bear the most weight during stance on that leg.

Wheelchairs are of two main types, companion operated and patient operated. The latter can be manual or power assisted. Lightweight and very lightweight patient- or companion-operated wheelchairs must be fitted with at least a dozen characteristics in mind (Box 55.2). Severe spasticity, poor head or trunk control, the amount of upper extremity function, and the types of work and sports engaged in may necessitate additional modifications. Very lightweight wheelchairs tend to be most manageable and durable for the patient with paraplegia. Models with power-assisted wheels or a power assist wheel attached to the mid lower frame have become more affordable and are practical for use by patients with weakness or pain in the upper extremities. Motorized wheelchairs can be maneuvered by joystick switches and chin or sip-and-puff mouth controls. The high cost of custom-designed wheelchairs means that therapists, vendors, patients, and families must work together to obtain what is most appropriate and cost-effective. Wheelchairs also require maintenance. A wobbly front wheel or poorly aligned main rear wheel adds to the energy cost of mobility and may cause shoulder and wrist injuries. Most rehabilitation centers that manage patients with myelopathies offer a wheelchair clinic and have close links to suppliers of durable medical equipment.

## Occupational Therapists

Occupational therapists (OTs) facilitate the practical management of disability so that their clients can participate more fully in daily care and community activities. The philosophical foundation of OT is that purposeful activity helps prevent and remediate dysfunction and elicits maximal adaptation. Goal-oriented tasks are meant to be culturally meaningful and important to the needs of clients and their families.

### BOX 55.2 Wheelchair Characteristics

- Frame:
  - Material
  - Weight
  - Foldable structure
- Seat:
  - Weight, width, depth, angle
  - Sling or cushioned, inserts
  - Cushion (foam, air, fluid, gel, gelfoam)
- Back:
  - Weight, fixed or reclining, headrest
  - Flexible, custom-molded; foam or gel inserts
- Armrests:
  - Weight (fixed or adjustable)
  - Fixed, removable, swing-away
  - Arm troughs, clear plastic lap board, power controls
- Leg and footrest:
  - Weight, adjustment from edge of seat, knee flexion angle
  - Fixed, removable, swing-away; straps
- Rear wheels:
  - Materials (alloys, plastic)
  - Tires (width, tread; pneumatic or solid)
  - Camber for speed and turning radius
- Handrims:
  - Power-assisted
- Front casters
- Brakes (locking, backsliding)
- Anti-tip bars
- Power supply, hand or mouth power control system
- Fully powered or power assist

Activities include daily life and work skills, exercise, recreation, and crafts. Occupational therapy is also concerned with improving the patient's interaction with the environment and maximizing his or her role in society in terms of relationships, occupation, and personal standing. The OT implements a program to enable patients to learn or relearn specific activities, develop new or compensatory skills, adapt their behavior to what is feasible, make adjustments to increase the accessibility of their environment, and perform leisure activities.

Adaptive aids can improve independence, ranging from simple devices (e.g., a thickened grip to better grasp cutlery or a pen) to complex ones (e.g., use of an environmental control unit). Some adaptive aids for daily living are listed in Box 55.3. Patients with progressive cognitive or motor impairments often benefit from at least a yearly OT reassessment for additional adaptive aids. Hemicuff and Bobath slings are used to reduce shoulder subluxation and prevent pain in patients with upper limb paralytic disorders (Fig. 55.1). A balanced forearm orthosis can support the upper arm and allow a modest biceps and triceps contraction to swing the arm over a table, which may be especially effective for the patient with a level C5 SCI. For patients with stroke and brain injury, OTs work closely with the neuropsychologist to address visuospatial inattention, memory loss, apraxia, difficulties in problem solving, and the skills needed for return to school or employment. Some OTs manage dysphagia and interpret modified barium swallow (MBS) studies.

Task-oriented and motor learning strategies have gained attention in formal occupational therapy research. Using this approach, the OT presents activities in a way that elicits the retention and transfer of particular skills for use in a functional setting. Practice in object-related tasks, rather than simple repetition of reaching and grasping of items

**BOX 55.3 Adaptive Aids for Daily Living**

**Feeding**
Utensil: thickened handle, cuff holder
Dish: food guard, suction holder
Cup: no-spill covers, holders

**Bathing**
Shower seat, transfer bench
Washing: mitt, long-handled scrub brush
Safety: grab bars

**Dressing**
Hook-and-loop closures for shoes, pants
Button hook, zipper pull
Low clothes rods in closet
Long-handled comb or brush

**Toileting**
Safety rails, raised seat, commode

**Mobility**
Prefabricated ramp
Powered stair lift
Wheelchair, standing wheelchair
Transfer devices and ceiling-mounted track lifts
Automobile and van: access for wheelchair, hand controls

**Communication**
Cellular smartphone with internet access

**Computer Workstation**
Environmental controls by electronic switches
Communication: voice-to-print, print-to-voice synthesis
Interface adaptations: keyboard, microswitch, voice activation

**Miscellaneous**
One-handed jar opener
Doorknob extension for better grip
Book holder, page turner (electronic or mouth stick)
Holder for one-handed cutting
Long-reach jaw grabbers ("lazy tongs")

that have no significance for the client, may provide more concrete sensory information and offer rewards that motivate performance. In many instances, OT strategies evolve from problems requiring a pragmatic solution that arise in daily living. For example, adaptive equipment and an OT educational intervention in stroke patients to remediate their lack of confidence and increase the amount of information patients have available to them has reduced the barriers to outdoor mobility and participation in the community. Controlled trials of OT strategies to improve ADLs after stroke have many methodological problems, so the efficacy of any specific approach is moot (Legg et al., 2017).

### Speech and Cognitive Therapists

Speech and language therapists are trained in many aspects of communication and cognition, including phonetics and linguistics, attention and memory, audiology, and developmental psychology; they provide expertise in the investigation and management of dysphagia. These therapists treat primarily patients with dysarthria, dysphonia, aphasia, and cognitive dysfunction that interferes with daily activities.

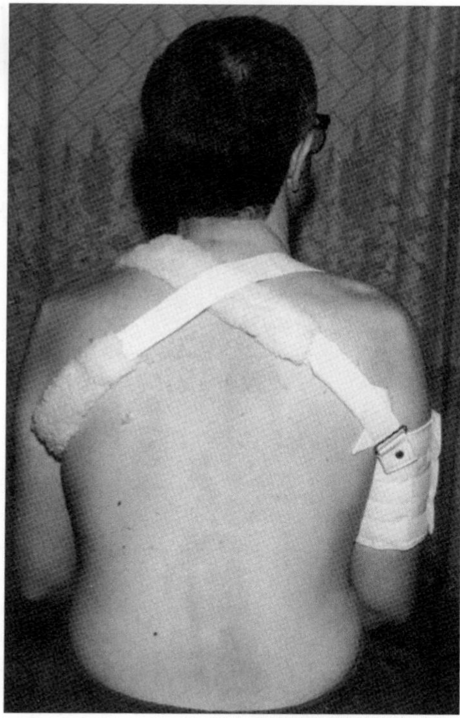

**Fig. 55.1** A cuff support to prevent pain and lessen the subluxation of the glenohumeral shoulder joint in a patient with left hemiplegia after stroke.

Interventions to improve the patient's speech intelligibility, volume, and fluency include exercises for the affected oromotor structures. For example, patients may be trained to slow their articulation, use shorter sentences, maximize breath support, extend jaw motion, adjust placement of the tongue, and exaggerate articulatory movements. Communication aids include voice amplification and computer assistive and voice recognition devices. These therapists also provide guidance for persons with swallowing difficulties; assessment may include the MBS study during videofluoroscopy.

Treatment for aphasia generally is based on clinical evaluation of the patient's cognitive and linguistic assets and deficits. The therapy plan is fine tuned according to standardized language and neuropsychological test results, knowledge of the cortical and subcortical structures damaged, and the ongoing response to specific therapies. Speech therapists attempt to circumvent, deblock, or help the patient compensate for defective language behaviors. Stimulation-facilitation approaches, listed in Box 55.4, are commonly employed. Views on the value of speech therapy for aphasia vary. Most randomized controlled trials (RCTs) demonstrate a significant benefit for aspects of expression and comprehension in moderately impaired subjects. The amount of practice is a key variable for enhancing outcomes for any particular approach. With this in mind, many home computer-based programs are available to retrain planning, sequencing, memory, expression of single words and short phrases, comprehension of short phrases, and naming. Their efficacy is modest at best.

### Recreational Therapists

Recreational therapists involve patients on an inpatient unit in group games, crafts, cooking, playing with pets, and other activities to help them socialize, practice skills, and enjoy the physical and emotional value of recreation despite their disabilities. In addition, the recreational therapist joins with the PT and the OT to teach patients how to reintegrate into

**BOX 55.4 Stimulation-Facilitation Approaches for Aphasia Therapy**

- Gestural expression and pointing
- Word-to-picture matching
- Yes/no response reliability
- Oral-motor imitation
- Phoneme, then word repetition
- Verbal cueing for words and sentence completion
- Contextual cueing
- Phonemic and semantic word-retrieval strategies
- Priming for responses
- Auditory processing at phrase level and then sentence level
- Word-, phrase-, then sentence-level reading
- Melodic stimulation
- Graphic tasks: tracing, copying, word completions
- Calculations
- Pragmatic linguistic and nonlinguistic conversational skills
- Psychosocial supports

the home and community. Outpatient recreational activities carried out in a wheelchair or with one hand also foster socialization and fitness. More than 200 local, national, and international organizations have developed rules and equipment for at least 75 sports and recreational activities—such as wheelchair tennis and basketball, upper extremity bicycling, and downhill skiing—that take into account a range of functional abilities.

### Psychologists

Neuropsychologists with skills in clinical psychology help define and manage cognitive impairments and mood and behavioral disorders. Detailed psychometric testing is fundamental to establishing a rehabilitation program for a patient with cognitive impairment. However, these tests of aspects of memory, learning, perception, language, and executive function do not represent the range of cognitive skills needed for real-world activities. The neuropsychologist often takes the lead in the management of mild to severe brain injury resulting from trauma or stroke and plays an important role in counseling patients, caregivers, and staff. When he or she is working with amnestic patients after TBI, the neuropsychologist may design operant conditioning paradigms or a token economy to reinforce appropriate social interactions, awareness of deficits, and learning. The neuropsychologist also develops relaxation techniques for anxiety states and behavioral approaches for the management of chronic pain.

### Social Workers

Social workers deal with the psychosocial aspects of disability and provide counseling and often brief psychotherapy. Their concerns extend to the ability of the patient and family to cope with disability in and out of the hospital. They play a key role in apprising the rehabilitation team about family issues, supports needed for best management of the disabled patient, and appropriate care services in the community. The close interactions of social workers and patients or caregivers during inpatient rehabilitation often provide valuable insight into the dynamics of family involvement and the adequacy of resources. Social workers serve as liaisons to private and government agencies and to case managers from insurance companies. Smooth discharge planning from an inpatient service requires their assistance.

### Orthotists and Bracing

Expertise in the manufacture, selection, and application of orthotic devices is another key component of a rehabilitation service. The PT or OT works with an orthotist to select external devices that modulate directional forces from the body and joints in a controlled manner. Although many orthotic devices are mass produced, the expertise of a trained orthotist is invaluable in choosing and constructing orthoses and supervising their fitting and adjustment. Orthoses include ankle and ankle-knee braces, finger-wrist and shoulder splints, spinal braces, collars, and corsets. The material most often used in manufacture of these devices is a malleable type of plastic, but light metals may be used when large biomechanical forces have to be managed. The effects of pressure, shear forces, and heat retention with sweating must also be considered during fitting to protect the skin.

With shortened inpatient rehabilitation stays, especially after stroke, ankle-foot orthoses (AFOs) that fit inside a shoe tend to be used early to more quickly assist foot clearance and knee control during ambulation in patients with a central or peripheral lesion. Observation of gait is usually enough to determine the need for a trial with an AFO in a patient with hemiparesis or foot drop. Indications include inadequate dorsiflexion for initial heel contact or for toe clearance during early and midswing, excessive hip hiking during swing, mediolateral subtalar instability during stance, tibial instability during stance, and uncontrolled foot placement caused by sensory loss. An orthosis also may be needed after operative heel cord lengthening. If the knee of the hemiplegic person buckles during stance, angling the AFO in slight plantar flexion will extend the knee earlier. Dorsiflexing the AFO by 5 degrees can decrease knee hyperextension and help prevent the snapping back that causes instability and pain in midstance. Ankle inversion may necessitate greater rigidity and longer anterior foot trim. The AFO worn in a shoe ought to improve weight bearing on the affected leg, increase single-limb stance time, and perhaps lessen postural sway. This may improve safety, especially on uneven surfaces and in terms of walking velocity. Fig. 55.2 shows a thermoplastic AFO that fits in a shoe to limit plantar flexion and rotation and help control the knee. Orthoses may be static, such as a rest splint worn at night, or dynamic, with joints that may be lockable or free moving. Fig. 55.3 shows a thermoplastic AFO with a hinged joint that enables flexibility on rising to stand and at heel strike to start the stance phase of the gait cycle. Toe clawing can be managed with a metatarsal pad that spreads the toes. Some patients who have foot drop from a neuropathy, such as Charcot-Marie-Tooth disease or diabetes, may find that a fashionable boot with a flat heel that fits snugly above the ankle can improve gait by lessening its steppage quality yet allowing toe clearance. An orthotist can assess the potential for shoe modifications and inserts to improve balance and pressure points. Multiple small trials in patients with hemiplegic stroke show that walking activity increases and impairments in walking and balance decrease with the use of an AFO.

A metal double-upright brace offers greater rigidity for mediolateral foot instability and allows more versatility in adjustments for the amount of plantar flexion and dorsiflexion, but it can be expensive, heavy, and cosmetically unappealing to the hemiplegic patient. Metal bracing systems are used more often by selected subjects with paraplegia from spinal injuries and in those with polio. The lightweight knee-ankle-foot orthosis (KAFO) with locking metal knee joints shown in Video 55.1 allows the hemiplegic person to prevent snapping back of the knee in the stance phase as well as to clear the foot and enable heel strike at the end of the swing phase. Such devices can also assist patients with severe polyneuropathy, muscular dystrophy, meningomyelocele, or SCI. Reciprocal gait orthoses (RGOs) with wire cables that link flexion of one hip to extension of the opposite hip are available for paraplegics. The Walkabout (Polymedic, Inc.) acts as an RGO. Short-distance ambulation for exercise can also be aided in the patient with SCI by variations on a KAFO and walker, but at high energy cost.

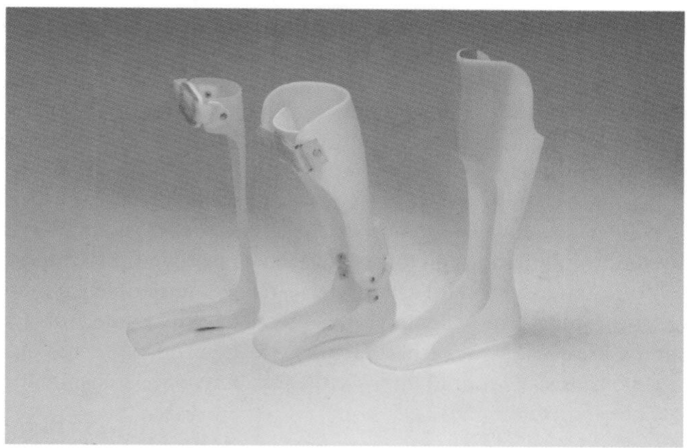

**Fig. 55.2** These fabricated ankle-foot orthoses are designed for ankle and knee control in a hemiparetic patient. The narrowest one on the left can assist foot drop due to a peripheral neuropathy. A wider lateral flange with hook-and-loop straps across the front of the ankle, like the orthotic at the far right, provides greater ankle and knee control. The thermoplastic hinged ankle orthotic in the middle includes a heel stop to allow about 5 degrees of dorsiflexion for standing up and in the early stance phase of gait.

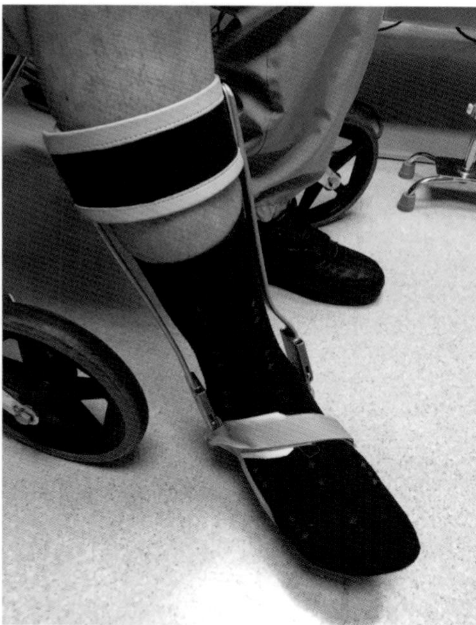

**Fig. 55.3** This patient has a marked right hemiplegia and hemisensory impairment. The lightweight double-upright brace fixes his ankle optimally and enables him to lock his knee. The supplemental video shows a safe if abnormal gait pattern—initial swing from the hip with slight hiking is followed by a flat foot landing without a heel strike or subsequent toe-off phase. The leg and foot are rotated outward. In midstance, the knee locks but does not hyperextend sharply.

Static orthoses allow no motion of the primary joint. Solid wrist-hand orthoses are usually set between neutral and 30 degrees of extension. However, based on small trials after stroke, upper limb orthoses have not been shown to improve arm or hand function, increase range of motion, or lessen the incidence of pain. Dynamic orthoses use elastic, wire, or powered levers that compensate for

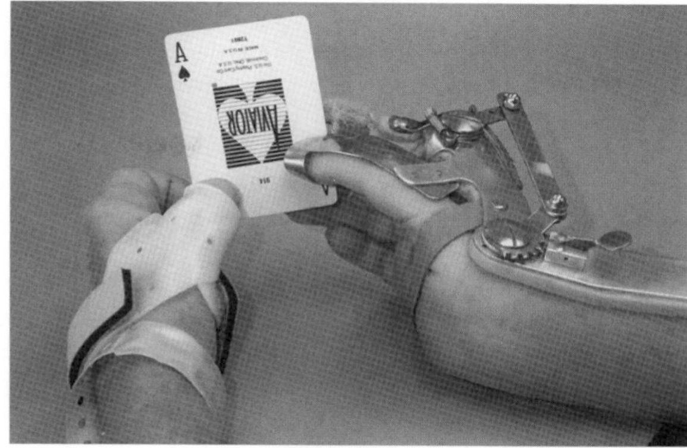



**Fig. 55.4** This card-playing patient with a C6 spinal cord injury uses a molded thumb-opposition splint to pinch better with the right hand and a lightweight metal tenodesis orthotic that pinches the thumb to the next two fingers when he dorsiflexes his wrist.

weakness or an imbalance in strength and allow some controlled movement. Fig. 55.4 shows the paretic left hand of a patient with a level C6 SCI holding a playing card with the aid of a thumb opposition splint. The weaker right hand needs wrist extension to mechanically oppose the thumb to the second and third digits. Such custom-made devices can be produced with lightweight metals and plastics.

## Stages of Rehabilitation Services

### Service Provision

The way in which services are organized depends to some extent on the disease being managed. The most fundamental differentiation is between acute-onset diseases with different pathophysiological characteristics such as brain and spinal cord trauma and stroke; chronic conditions such as cerebral palsy and polio, in which disability may increase with aging and overuse of muscles and joints; and progressive disorders such as MS, muscular dystrophies, ALS, and Parkinson disease (PD). Service provision should also be driven by the philosophy underlying rehabilitation: to return the patient home and optimize home and community activities as soon as possible. The speed with which this is done depends as much on the services available in the community and the capacity of the family and caregivers to look after the patient as it does on the severity of the disability. Some tension arises between inpatient services in which all of the necessary ingredients are gathered under one roof, which appeals to patients and families, and community services, which are less centralized but support patients in their own environment. Most important is the smooth interface between these two settings when patients are discharged from an inpatient service.

***Inpatient rehabilitation unit.*** The most efficient rehabilitation setting is an inpatient unit designed and staffed specifically for this purpose. In the United States, approximately 1200 inpatient sites are covered under Medicare. The benefits of dedicated units for stroke management have been convincingly demonstrated. Patients managed in stroke units are significantly less likely to die than those cared for on ordinary wards. Death, institutionalization, and dependency all are significantly less common in stroke unit patients, in part because of a reduction in secondary complications of stroke and a milieu dedicated to managing disability. Early functionally oriented therapies by an organized team tend to enable patients to become independent enough to return home sooner than sporadic therapy that does not articulate specific attainable goals for mobility, self-care, and family training. These benefits persist for up to 5 years after discharge and improve patients' quality of life. With inpatient stroke rehabilitation in the United States usually starting within 8 days of onset and with the average length of stay less than 20 days, planning is imperative. Several studies of TBI also suggest the benefit of coordinated care starting during the inpatient stay.

The role of inpatient rehabilitation units in managing progressive conditions such as MS and PD is much less well defined, although some evidence suggests a benefit in progressive MS. Inpatient care may also return patients home at a higher level of functioning after implantation of a deep brain stimulator for PD or after an exacerbation of walking disability caused by a hip fracture in a patient with a chronic hemiparesis.

***Community-based services.*** Although community-based rehabilitation appears to have a number of advantages from the perspective of the disabled patient, few studies have addressed its efficacy. This lack may relate at least in part to the methodological difficulties in defining the training team's level of expertise; the patient's level of disability; the amount of caregiver support; and the frequency, duration, and type of therapy. One large randomized stroke trial compared rehabilitation at home after an average 12-day inpatient stay with another week of inpatient care followed by hospital-based outpatient treatment. Patients who lived alone were either independent in transfers when they left the hospital or needed to be assisted by a caregiver. Similar outcomes 12 months after a stroke were achieved at lower cost because of less use of hospital beds by the early discharge group. An intention-to-treat randomized trial with 250 subjects showed that rehabilitation in an inpatient unit after a brief stay in an acute stroke unit or general medical ward produced better outcomes in moderate to severely disabled patients (Barthel Index [BI] score <50) compared with rehabilitation treatment in the community. No differences in quality of life were found, and levels of activity outside the home were not measured. Smaller trials confirm similar positive outcomes at 3–6 months following home care as compared with various forms of outpatient care, with the home group having fewer in-hospital days and greater gains in instrumental ADLs. Community-based trials to increase activity have also shown modest functional gains—greater frequency of feedback and reinforcement may be a critical element (Dean et al., 2012).

A day treatment program may be available for persons with residua from a TBI. In one trial, 100 patients who were unable to work for 1–2 years after TBI received a range of interventions during group therapy for a mean of 190 days. The investigators found a significant reduction in physical disability, increased self-awareness and emotional self-regulation, and more effective participation in interpersonal activities. At 1 year after completion, 72% lived independently and 57% were employed.

A brief stint of outpatient therapy for a well-defined goal, such as to improve transfers in a patient who declines from MS or to make walking safe again after an illness that causes deconditioning in a patient with chronic hemiparesis, is an invaluable means for patients to maintain their highest level of independence and avoid placement in a nursing home. A few therapy sessions a week for a few weeks plus a home program may accomplish this when provided for a task-specific goal that may lessen burdens on caregivers.

Specialized rehabilitation centers may offer better care for patients with high cervical SCIs and severe TBI or difficult neurobehavioral impairments. Such patients may require specialized orthopedic and plastic surgery procedures, cognitive and behavioral management, wheelchairs with special seating needs, custom orthotics and prosthetics, rehabilitation engineering, functional electrical stimulation devices for walking and upper extremity movement, neuroprostheses, communication aids and environmental controllers for quadriparetic patients, driving assessments, and work and school accommodations months after onset.

Telerehabilitation services may prove especially useful in supporting patients who live far from available services or are too disabled to leave home. Limitations on formal postacute rehabilitation services by Medicare and insurers also call for new strategies to remotely monitor and give feedback to patients as they practice in the home and community. Wearable sensors that recognize the type, quantity, and quality of skills practice should improve the feasibility of telerehabilitation (Dobkin and Dorsch, 2017).

## Measurement Tools

Outcome measurement is essential to demonstrate the effectiveness of inpatient or outpatient rehabilitation services, of an intervention for an individual, and for clinical trials that aim to develop better evidence-based practices. Neurorehabilitation employs measurement tools to characterize the impairments, disabilities, activities, and psychosocial needs of patients as well as to monitor interventions, assess outcomes, and document services. To provide a comprehensive assessment of the impact of disease, outcomes may be considered at four levels: pathophysiology and related impairments, disability and level of functional activity, handicap and ability to participate, and health-related quality of life. Each outcome level addresses distinct aspects of the disease process. The relationships among them are complex. The first two levels entail physician-oriented outcomes, whereas those at the third and fourth levels are more accurately called *patient-based outcomes*, although only the fourth incorporates the patient's perspective. Rehabilitation is especially interested in measurements of the impact of disease, as contained within the World Health Organization (WHO) International Classification of Impairments, Disabilities, and Handicaps. The focus is on the consequences of the disease or health condition rather than the disease alone (i.e., a classification of disablements and functioning). A classification available on the WHO website (http://www.who.int/icidh/) emphasizes whether people actually perform the tasks, especially those that require a lot of time and energy. The dimensions of the WHO classification also include personal and environmental factors that affect functioning. The emphasis on activities, participation, and contextual factors interacting with impairments and disabilities may influence the design of new measurement tools.

Two generic measures of the assistance needed to perform basic ADLs are the 10-item BI, which can be totaled to a maximum score of 20 or 100, and the 18-item functional independence measure (FIM), which includes a modestly responsive cognitive component for a total of 126 points. The FIM (Box 55.5) is used more often in the United States, especially for studies with large numbers of subjects, than in Europe or Asia. A comprehensive system of inpatient unit documentation in the United States often includes the Uniform Data System for Medical Rehabilitation (UDS). The UDS program allows inpatient units to compare their patient population across diseases to other sites for FIM change scores, length of stay, and descriptive data. In many respects, the BI and FIM reflect the level of care needed by patients. These and most scales have floor or ceiling effects and variable sensitivity to change, especially if used during outpatient care.

The primary outcome for most walking trials is short-distance walking speed (10–15 m) and distance walked in a fixed time, such as 2 or 6 minutes, using a stopwatch. This test is very useful to monitor changes in gait during outpatient care as well. The results provide

**BOX 55.5 Components of the Functional Independence Measure**

**Self-Care**
Eating
Grooming
Bathing
Dressing upper body
Dressing lower body
Toileting

**Sphincter Control**
Bladder management
Bowel management

**Mobility and Transfers**
Bed-to-chair and wheelchair-to-chair transfer
Toilet transfer
Tub and shower transfer

**Locomotion**
Walking or wheelchair use
Climbing stairs

**Communication**
Comprehension
Expression

**Social Cognition**
Social interaction
Problem solving
Memory

**Burden-of-Care Rating**
7 = Complete independence (timely, safely)
6 = Modified independence (device)
5 = Supervision
4 = Minimal assistance (subject contributes 75% or more)
3 = Moderate assistance (subject contributes at least 50%)
2 = Maximal assistance (subject contributes at least 25%)
1 = Total assistance (subject contributes 0% up to 25%)

little insight into what patients actually do every day. Gait analysis for cadence, speed, and stance and swing times can be monitored in a laboratory by pressure sensors embedded in a mat and by reflective markers whose successive position during the gait cycle are captured by cameras. The Kinect (Microsoft) system is also being used for analyses.

Over 140 different outcome measures were reported in 243 post-stroke arm rehabilitation trials that were included in a Cochrane review. The Fugel-Meyer Assessment (FMA) for upper extremity, which grades a series of selective arm and hand movements (cannot, partial, and full) was included in 33% as an impairment scale. The ARAT grades task-related actions for functional ability and was used in 23%. These were followed by the modified Ashworth Scale for hypertonicity, the Motor Activity Log for frequency of use of the arm, the FIM, goniometers to test range of motion, the Wolf Motor Function Test for timed tasks using the arm and hand, and dynamometry for strength across a joint. Robotic devices are poised to offer angular velocities and many other measurements during specified movements. Recent deep learning techniques show that ordinary frontal and sagittal cameras can record movements using automated joint markers with remarkable accuracy outside of a laboratory.

There is a critical need for real-world activity monitoring and outcome measurement tools. Recent mobile health devices with wearable accelerometers, gyroscopes, and global positioning satellite data that employ clever algorithms offer the possibility to measure the type, quantity, and quality of daily walking, cycling, exercise, community participation, and upper limb purposeful actions (Dobkin and Dorsch, 2017). Wearables are showing that self-reports about activity and actual activity may differ significantly (Waddell and Lang, 2018).

Measurement tools to assess health-related quality of life tend to be disease specific, beyond the Medical Outcomes Scale-36. For example, the Stroke Impact Scale is an ordinal tool for self-reported domains of activity, mood, and participation. The National Institutes of Health Toolbox website (http://www.healthmeasures.net/explore-measurement-systems/nih-toolbox) includes most such scales.

### Self-Management Goals

Self-efficacy is an important goal for a disabled person as it is for anyone. The rehabilitation process ought to build the individual's confidence in his or her ability to develop and meet planned goals, as self-efficacy increases as self-management proceeds successfully. This holds for practice of skills, compensatory adaptations, and all health-related behaviors, such as use of medications, finances, management of mood and psychosocial stressors, and dealing with barriers in daily life. Behavioral training for this goal should include education about the effects of practice and exercise that are relevant to the person, goal setting, identification of possible barriers, problem solving, feedback about performance, tailored instruction, decision making, and ongoing personal or social support by therapists, family, and friends (Dobkin, 2017).

## BIOLOGICAL BASES FOR REHABILITATIVE INTERVENTIONS

The potential to enhance neurological recovery by manipulating the biological adaptability of the brain, spinal cord, and peripheral nerves has become remarkably relevant to clinical practice. Basic neuroscience studies suggest that physical and cognitive training, extrinsic stimulation by diverse means such as transcranial direct cortical stimulation and intermittent hypoxia (Hayes et al., 2014), and pharmacological interventions (Wang et al., 2011), along with natural biological reactions to injury, could enhance the restoration of motor and cognitive functions. Box 55.6 lists some of the potential mechanisms that contribute to changes in impairments and disabilities. These are not discrete mechanisms. They overlap, and many depend on each other over time and location in the central nervous system (CNS) after injury and with training. In addition, biological therapeutic approaches such as use of cellular implants may enhance these mechanisms (Tornero et al., 2013). Although care must be taken in extrapolating from animal studies of recovery to their implications for human interventions, at least a few of these potential mechanisms suggest how latent pathways and repetitive skills practice may improve outcomes.

The combination of mutable neuronal assemblies that represent movements and sensation and multiple representational maps in parallel, distributed CNS systems offers a sound basis for developing rehabilitation interventions. Specific circuits and distributed network functions can be activated selectively by intrinsic and extrinsic stimuli. In patients, this reorganization can be assessed structurally by anatomical and diffusion tensor imaging using magnetic resonance imaging

**BOX 55.6 Mechanisms That May Support Recovery of Function**

**Network Plasticity**

Recovery of neuronal excitability:
- Resolve cell and axon ionic disequilibrium and conduction block
- Resolve edema, resorb blood products
- Reversal of diaschisis

Increased activity in neurons adjacent to injured ones and in partially spared pathways

Representational adaptations in neuronal assemblies:
- Expansion of representational maps
- Recruitment of cells not ordinarily involved in an activity

Recruitment of parallel and subcomponent pathways:
- Altered activity in distributed cortical and subcortical networks
- Activation of pattern generators (e.g., for stepping)
- Recruitment of networks not ordinarily involved in an activity

Modulation of excitability by neurotransmitters

Use of alternative behavioral strategies

**Neuronal Plasticity**

Altered efficacy of synaptic activity:
- Activity-dependent unmasking of previously ineffective synapses
- Learning tied to activity-dependent changes (e.g., long-term potentiation, long-term depression) in synaptic strength in peri-injury and remote regions
- Increased neuronal responsiveness from denervation hypersensitivity
- Delayed decline in number of neurons (e.g., from apoptosis)
- Change in number or variety of receptors
- Change in neurotransmitter release and uptake

Regeneration and sprouting from injured and uninjured axons and dendrites:
- Angiogenesis
- Expression of developmental regeneration-associated genes for cell viability, growth, and remodeling proteins
- Modulation by neurotrophic factors, neurotransmitters, and signaling molecules
- Dendritic spine remodeling
- Inhibition of growth cone extension (e.g., myelin-associated glycoprotein, Nogo receptor activation, chondroitin)
- Actions of chemoattractants and inhibitors in the milieu for growth cone function and targeting

Remyelination from oligodendrocyte precursors

Neurogenesis and gliogenesis with cell migration

**Cellular Transplantation**

Local implantation of stem cells or neuronal, glial, oligodendrocyte precursors

Cellular injection into spinal fluid

Intravenous bone marrow stem cell injection

Cellular bridge (may include a gel or neuromodulating matrix in region of myelo/encephalomalacia)

(MRI), physiologically by functional MRI (fMRI) activation, and connectivity studies (Grefkes and Fink, 2014) as well as by transcranial magnetic stimulation (TMS) and positron emission tomography using glucose and neurotransmitter markers.

The molecular processes induced by injury and by activity in neurons, axons, and dendrites are under intense investigation. Morphological changes such as axonal regeneration over short distances, dendritic arborization, and synaptogenesis have been observed after brain and cord injuries. When inputs from one pathway to the dendritic tree of a neuron are lost, intact axons can sprout and form synapses on denervated receptors. Although this occurs regularly in animal injury models—within, for example, corticorubral, corticoreticular, and propriospinal fibers—a remarkable number of typically crossed corticospinal tract fibers appear to recross at spinal segments under the central canal to innervate interneurons ipsilateral to their origin. The net effect of these changes in the weight of inputs could have a positive or detrimental effect on neural function. Can such changes be manipulated? Signaling molecules include neurotrophic factors and those that act at the axon growth cone, many of which are also involved in learning and memory, so they are also being pursued in studies of neurodevelopmental and neurodegenerative disorders.

Genetic studies may become of value in identifying patients who have polymorphisms in a single nucleotide that affects memory, learning, cortical morphology, and other critical functions. If patients are predisposed to lower levels of brain catecholamines as a result of enzyme activity (catechol-*O*-methyltransferase Val vs. Met polymorphism) or have higher or lower neurotrophic factor activity (e.g., brain-derived neurotrophic factor [BDNF] Val vs. Met polymorphism), these differences may be amplified after brain injury, potentially affecting outcomes. Medications could be used in a more focused fashion with genetic screening to identify persons most likely to benefit.

## NEUROMEDICAL COMPLICATIONS THAT INTERFERE WITH REHABILITATION

Neurological and systemic complications often interfere with progress during inpatient and outpatient rehabilitation. With shorter acute hospital and inpatient rehabilitation stays, physicians, nurses, and therapists must anticipate, recognize, and treat medical conditions that may impede progress in the rehabilitation process. Some of these problems will arise from new medications, neurological impairments, immobility, transient infections and metabolic abnormalities, and underlying systemic illness. In addition, patients and caregivers must be trained to prevent errors of omission and commission that arise in using medication, performing daily care, and managing risk factors such as hypertension that lead to late morbidity.

As noted, most but not all studies suggest that specialized stroke, SCI, and TBI hospital programs appear to lead to better early outcomes than with treatment on general medical units. Differences in morbidity, mortality, and length of hospital stay have been associated with more organized services. For example, protocols that use prophylactic subcutaneous heparin, hold oral intake until completion of a screening test for safety of swallowing, avoid indwelling bladder catheters, and assess postvoid residuals by ultrasound examination to avoid unnecessary intermittent catheterizations or overfilling, can reduce medical complications.

### Frequency of Complications

#### Complications in Patients with Stroke

Medical complications often interfere with a patient's ability to participate in therapy (Table 55.1). Medical and neurological complications occur at rates of approximately 4 and 0.6 per patient, respectively, during an average course of inpatient rehabilitation. Side effects during the adjustment of new medications are especially prevalent, including orthostatic hypotension from antihypertensives or dialysis, drowsiness from anticonvulsants and analgesics, and a statin-induced myopathy with normal serum creatine kinase. Across inpatient rehabilitation centers, 5%–15% of patients must be transferred back to an acute hospital setting.

**TABLE 55.1 General Frequency of Inpatient Stroke Rehabilitation Neuromedical Complications**

| Complication | Percent of Patients |
|---|---|
| Urinary tract infection | 40 |
| Musculoskeletal pain | 30 |
| Depression | 30 |
| Urine retention | 25 |
| Falls | 25 |
| Fungal rash | 20 |
| Hypertension | 20 |
| Hypotension | 15 |
| Incipient pressure sores | 15 |
| Hypoglycemia or hyperglycemia | 15 |
| Azotemia | 15 |
| Toxic-metabolic encephalopathy | 10 |
| Pneumonia | 10 |
| Arrhythmia | 10 |
| Congestive heart failure | 5 |
| Angina | 5 |
| Thrombophlebitis | 5 |
| Allergic reaction | 5 |
| Gastrointestinal bleeding | 5 |
| Pulmonary embolus | <5 |
| Myocardial infarction | <5 |
| Decubitus ulcer | <5 |
| Recurrent stroke | <5 |
| Seizure | <5 |

### Complications in Patients with Spinal Cord Injury

Medical complications of a somewhat different nature are common in the acute and chronic phases after SCI (see Chapter 63). In the generally younger patients, chronic comorbid systemic medical problems are less common than in patients with stroke. Prior substance abuse and emotional and behavioral disorders, however, are much more likely to complicate therapy. In the first 6 weeks after SCI, reparative operative procedures affect what can be done in rehabilitation. Approximately half of patients undergo spinal fusion and internal fixation. Acute spinal care also entails the use of external stabilization techniques such as a halo vest and Philadelphia collar for cervical injuries and a custom-molded or fitted, thoracolumbar fixation device. These braces limit head and trunk mobility, which makes self-care tasks that involve balance, management of the lower extremities, and intermittent bladder self-catherization more difficult. Lower extremity fractures, especially of the femur, occur in about 5% of patients with acute SCI, which can further limit mobility and increase the risk of deep venous thrombosis and skin breakdown. Table 55.2 lists the complications found during a prospective clinical trial of methylprednisolone for acute SCI in 487 patients.

Early morbidity is greater with cervical and upper thoracic injuries and with complete lesions than with lower-level or incomplete lesions. Ventilatory dysfunction, aspiration, dysautonomia with upright hypotension or paroxysmal hypertension, a neurogenic bowel with impactions, a neurogenic bladder with retention and infections, a catabolic state, and gastric atony are especially likely to complicate early inpatient rehabilitation. Hypercalciuria or hypercalcemia related to immobilization may also necessitate therapy. Central and musculoskeletal pain and grief reactions warrant immediate attention.

**TABLE 55.2 Medical Complications Within 6 Weeks of Acute Spinal Cord Injury**

| Complication | Percent of Patients |
|---|---|
| Urinary tract infection | 46 |
| Pneumonia | 28 |
| Decubitus ulcer | 18 |
| Paralytic ileus | 9 |
| Arrhythmia | 6 |
| Sepsis | 6 |
| Thrombophlebitis | 5 |
| Wound infection | 4 |
| Gastrointestinal hemorrhage | 3 |
| Pulmonary embolus | 3 |
| Congestive heart failure | 1 |

### Complications in Patients with Traumatic Brain Injury

Systemic and neurological complications are common after serious TBI (see Chapter 62). The older patient carries more systemic comorbidity, whereas the younger patient may have alcohol or drug abuse as a comorbid condition. Unrecognized fractures and heterotopic ossification (HO) as a cause of pain, in addition to other bodily injuries, may complicate rehabilitation along with any of the complications that may accompany stroke and SCI. Physicians must also monitor for pituitary–hypothalamic dysfunction with endocrinopathies and disorders of homeostasis including cerebral salt wasting and inappropriate secretion of antidiuretic hormone as well as cerebral hygromas and obstructive hydrocephalus. Ventricular enlargement develops in 30%–70% of patients with severe TBI. Most have hydrocephalus ex vacuo. In the patient with enlarging ventricles who reaches an early plateau or declines in mobility and cognition, a diagnosis of symptomatic normal- or high-pressure hydrocephalus must be considered.

## Management of Neuromedical Complications

### Dysphagia

Neurogenic dysphagia is the potential cause of a pulmonary infection in any patient with stroke, TBI, motor neuron disease, MS, advanced PD, cervicomedullary disorders such as a syrinx, Guillain-Barré syndrome, myasthenia gravis, and most neuromuscular diseases. Indeed, swallowing disorders affect 10% of acutely hospitalized older adults and 30% of nursing home residents. Even transient dysphagia can lead to malnutrition, dehydration, aspiration pneumonia, and airway obstruction with asphyxiation. It increases the patient's risk of death and institutionalization. Chapter 15 discusses management.

The natural history of recovery from dysphagia after stroke and TBI is favorable. For example, a British study diagnosed dysphagia in 30% of 357 conscious patients within 48 hours of a unilateral hemispheric stroke; the patients were rated as having impaired deglutition if they exhibited delayed and prolonged swallowing or if they coughed on 10 mL of water. At 1 month only 2% and at 6 months only 0.4% of survivors were still impaired. Symptoms and signs that suggest a risk of aspiration include lethargy, coughing or a hoarse and gurgly voice after feeding, slow eating or drinking (<10 mL of water per second drunk from a cup), dysphonia, and poor oropharyngeal movement. The limitations of bedside indicators have led to the use of the MBS with videofluoroscopy as the method of choice to rule out silent aspiration. The relationship between small-volume aspiration as seen on MBS and clinical complications is uncertain, however, and requires clinical judgment. The MBS also visualizes the effects of dietary texture and compensatory techniques. In attentive stroke rehabilitation inpatients, coughing or a wet-hoarse quality of the voice noted within 1 minute of continuously swallowing 90 mL of water from a cup had a sensitivity of 80% and specificity of 54% for aspiration detected by an MBS study. The bedside test had a sensitivity of 88% and specificity of 44% for large-volume aspiration, which may be clinically more significant. Fiberoptic endoscopy also can identify mechanisms of dysphagia and can be performed at the bedside.

The FOOD Trial Collaboration (Dennis et al., 2005) reported that early placement of a nasogastric tube to feed aphagic patients after stroke improved nutrition and reduced deaths and poor outcomes compared with no enteral feeding, but early use of percutaneous gastrostomy caused a 1% absolute increase in complications. Gastrostomy may not lessen the risk of reflux aspiration any more than a nasopharyngeal feeding tube for patients with persisting aphagia.

### Skin Ulcers

Education in skin management during rehabilitation provides an important opportunity for preventing later morbidity and mortality. Ischemia of the skin and underlying tissues occurs particularly in weight-bearing areas adjacent to bony prominences. The American Model Systems data for patients hospitalized within 24 hours of traumatic SCI showed that pressure sores subsequently developed in 4%, and 13% of these were graded as severe. The lesions occurred over the sacrum, heel, scapula, foot, and greater trochanter of the hip. Lower-grade skin lesions developed over the genitals. Sores related to sitting most often are located over the ischial tuberosities, where tissue pressure can exceed 300 mm Hg on an unpadded seat. A foam pad 2 inches thick decreases the local pressure to 150 mm Hg. Even with the use of cushions designed to distribute pressure evenly over weight-bearing skin surfaces, pressures in the sitting position are far above the pressures of 11–33 mm Hg in the capillaries and venules. Raising the head of the bed by only a few inches increases shearing forces especially over the sacrum.

A standard classification for degrees of integument breakdown, prophylactic measures, and wound care is available from the Agency for Health Care Policy and Research in Washington, DC. Rubor, induration, and blistering are signs that precede a break in the skin. Pressure relief by turning and repositioning is the best approach, performed every half hour after a complete SCI and every 2–3 hours in patients with intact sensation after stroke or other disabling injuries. Patients must develop a skin care program based on their general health, nutrition, continence, toughness of their skin, most commonly used positions, type of wheelchair seat, presence of old skin scars, and other factors.

### Contractures

Across studies, approximately 15% of patients with SCI admitted for rehabilitation and 80% admitted after moderate to severe TBI lost more than 15% of the normal range of motion of at least one joint. Hemiparetic patients with stroke fall between these extremes. Adhesive capsulitis of the shoulder develops within several months in the hemiplegic person with little motor control. Contractures are found especially in the lower extremities in neuromuscular diseases, affecting at least 70% of outpatients with Duchenne muscular dystrophy. Contractures limit functional use of a limb and impair hygiene, mobility, and self-care. Serious contractures can cause pressure sores, pain, and, especially in youngsters, emotional distress when odd postures distort the body. After an acute UMN lesion, proper positioning of the arm in abduction and hand in extension and of the leg in hip abduction with knee flexed and ankle in neutral position can protect the affected extremities. Passive ranging of joints through their full usual degrees of movement for a few minutes once or twice a day will lessen the opportunity for adhesions and contractures to develop. Any source of pain will increase muscle tone and predispose to contractures. Serial casting and surgeries are occasionally necessary for contractures that interfere with skin care or functional use of a limb.

### Heterotopic Ossification

HO—or ectopic bone formation—below the neurological level of injury may cause functional impairment in up to 20% of patients with SCI, usually in the first 4 months after injury. Patients with a complete lesion, pressure sores, spasticity, and age older than 30 years may be at greatest risk. After TBI, HO especially tends to affect the proximal joints of comatose patients. During rehabilitation of less-responsive and cognitively impaired or aphasic patients, pain caused by undetected musculoskeletal injury and HO can add greatly to their agitation and limit their participation. HO develops when multipotential connective tissue cells transform into chondroblasts and osteoblasts, presumably under the influence of locally induced growth factors. The hips, knees, and shoulders are affected most often. Swelling, erythema, and decreasing range of motion are among the first clinical signs. A three-phase technetium 99m–labeled methylene diphosphonate bone scan reveals focal uptake before radiographic visualization of bone. Early treatment with disodium etidronate suppresses mineralization of the osteoid. Range-of-motion exercises, aspirin, nonsteroidal anti-inflammatory drugs (NSAIDs), and a wedge resection of mature heterotopic bone can decrease pain and immobility.

### Dysautonomia

Bed rest, dehydration, cardiac and antihypertensive medications, antidepressants, and autonomic reflex dysfunction from diabetes mellitus contribute to postural hypotension in the patient with stroke and TBI. Supine and standing blood pressures should be checked as mobilization proceeds during rehabilitation. Autonomic reflexes may fail in patients with SCI levels above T6. Symptomatic postural hypotension is common in the first weeks after injury and may persist in quadriplegic patients.

Initial therapies for OH include gradual reconditioning of postural reflexes on a tilt table, sleeping in a reverse Trendelenburg position to prevent overnight diuresis, wearing full compression leg hose, and application of an abdominal binder. In the inpatient setting, fluid loading with saline or albumin may aid the effort to compensate for venous pooling, decreased cardiac output, and impaired vasoconstriction and venoconstriction from interruption of sympathetic outflow. Fludrocortisone increases the intravascular volume and peripheral vascular resistance. The dosage can be pushed gradually to 0.5 mg/day. Salt tablets should be added to the diet. Hypokalemia and edema with pressure sores can complicate use of mineralocorticoids. While the patient is upright, ephedrine 25–100 mg up to every 3 hours; ergotamine 2 mg up to several times daily; or midodrine up to 10 mg three times a day can be tried. Droxydopa can also be titrated upward in combination with a mineralocorticoid.

Episodic autonomic hyperreflexia related to uninhibited sympathetic outflow may affect 50%–90% of SCI patients with high-level SCI, usually beginning several months after injury. It is caused by visceral and joint pain, HO, pressure sores, bowel and bladder distention, fecal impaction, urinary infection and cystitis, ingrown toenails, pregnancy and labor, venous thrombosis, and late development of a syrinx. Wearing tight clothing, assuming a particular supine position, or oropharyngeal suctioning can also cause bradyarrhythmias. Often it has no evident precipitating cause. Hypertension, headache, diaphoresis, anxiety, reflexive bradycardia, nasal congestion, flushing above and pallor below the SCI level, extensor spasms, and piloerection can result. The instigating agent must be removed. Acute therapies include upright positioning, search for an unemptied bladder or rectum using lidocaine on a catheter or finger when probing, and treatment of blood pressure that exceeds 180/100 mm Hg. A beta-blocker such as labetalol; a short-acting calcium channel blocker; vasodilators such as hydralazine; and occasionally phenoxybenzamine, prazosin, clonidine, or nitroglycerin usually lower the pressure safely. Some quadriplegic patients have very labile responses to antihypertensive drugs and suddenly become hypotensive with these treatments. For frequent bouts of hypertension, maintenance therapy includes low dosages of any of these oral agents but with dosage adjustments based on the finding of supine hypertension coupled with sitting hypotension. For paroxysmal bradycardia, propantheline or a pacemaker may be needed. Scopolamine and propantheline can prevent bouts of sweating.

### Bowel and Bladder Dysfunction

Urinary incontinence occurs in up to 60% of patients in the first week after a stroke, but function tends to improve without a specific medical treatment. This likelihood must be considered in the context of an incidence of urinary dribbling and involuntary emptying of approximately 30% in the population of healthy, noninstitutionalized adults older than 65 years of age. Across studies, about 18% of those who were incontinent at 6 weeks after a stroke were still so at 1 year. By the end of inpatient rehabilitation, the incidence was about 10% in patients with a motor-only stroke and about 30% of those with large hemispheric strokes. A Cochrane Database Systematic Review of the prevention and treatment of urinary incontinence after stroke found insufficient evidence for most physical, behavioral, and pharmacological interventions, but specialist management tended to reduce the number of urinary tract infections.

After SCI, the bladder detrusor reflex may not return for 6 weeks to 12 months. In the absence of spontaneous bladder emptying, intermittent catheterization is done on a schedule that prevents the accumulation of more than 400 mL. Patients should measure their output from time to time and develop a voiding schedule that takes into account variations in fluid intake and the use of alcohol and caffeine. Catheters can be washed, stored in a plastic bag, and reused. If sensorimotor impairments persist, nearly all patients with an SCI lesion that spares the S2 to S4 micturition center will develop dyssynergia between the detrusor and the external sphincter. These uncoordinated contractions lead to incontinence and intermittent outlet obstruction. Urodynamic studies and an intravenous pyelogram are indicated as a baseline and to assist in therapy, especially in patients with SCI (Chapters 47 and 63). Obstruction can cause recurrent infections, urosepsis, vesicourethral reflux, urolithiasis, and hydronephrosis.

Patients should learn the signs of bladder fullness, such as sweating, changes in temperature, increased spasticity, and an increase in heart rate. Some palpate the area of the bladder to determine fullness. Once awareness of fullness develops, the person can aid in initiating or completing micturition by tapping over the bladder, rubbing the skin over the pubis or on the inner thighs, pressing on the abdominal wall (Credé maneuver), and bearing down or coughing. These maneuvers are particularly helpful in those with an LMN bladder with an open sphincter. Most patients with SCI also learn the signs of an early bladder infection, such as a change in clarity or odor as well as more spasms, and work out a system with their physician to obtain a culture and antibiotics as needed.

Pharmacological treatment can be understood in relation to problems in bladder filling, storage, and emptying with any neurological disease (Table 55.3). Urodynamic studies often aid in the choice of drug trial. The goals are continence and regular emptying that is achieved without high intravesicular pressure and with less than 100 mL of residual volume after voiding. After stroke many males who have an enlarged prostate benefit from an alpha-blocker. If the goal of micturition is not achieved, several alternatives to the use of an indwelling catheter on a long-term basis are available. To prevent inadequate emptying at low pressure at the price of external sphincterotomy and resultant incontinence, long-term intermittent catheterization can be used in combination with anticholinergic medications or bladder infusion of botulinum toxin to partially paralyze detrusor function. This procedure has become increasingly accepted as an effective alternative in the management of low intravesicular pressure. An external collecting device can be used to ensure dryness. The patient must be trained to adjust fluid intake and the timing of catheterization to meet the flexible needs of community living. The absence of an effective external collecting device for female patients makes it necessary to continue long-term intermittent catheterization in women with paralysis of detrusor function. A waterproof undergarment may be worn between catheterizations to avoid embarrassment. The difficulties of this regimen cause many women to choose constant indwelling catheter drainage despite its drawbacks. Augmentation enterocystoplasty, reservoirs, conduits, and electrical stimulation techniques are less often needed. The VOCARE Bladder System for patients with UMN SCI allows patients to stimulate sacral nerves that have been implanted with electrodes to empty the bladder and bowel. Other neuromuscular and spinal cord stimulation devices that are also usually externally controlled continue to be refined. Implantable flexible sensors and stretchable electronics that can detect changes in organ dimension in a way that does not affect organ function—along with developments in the field of optogenetics, wireless data, and energy transfer—may enable new technologies for bladder and sphincter control.

**TABLE 55.3 Pharmacological Manipulation of Bladder Dysfunction**

| Medication | Indication(s) | Mechanism of Action |
|---|---|---|
| Bethanechol, 25 mg bid–50 mg qid | Difficulty emptying | Increases detrusor contraction |
| Prazosin, 1 mg bid–2 mg tid or tamsulosin, 0.4 mg/day | Outlet obstruction<br>Prostatic hypertrophy | Alpha-blockade of external sphincter; decreases tone |
| Hyoscyamine, 0.125 mg hs–0.25 mg tid; oxybutynin 2.5 mg hs–5 mg qid | Urge incontinence | Relaxes detrusor, increases internal sphincter tone, decreases detrusor contractions |
| Tolterodine, 2 mg/day or imipramine, 25–100 mg hs | Frequency<br>Enuresis | |

*bid*, Twice daily; *hs*, at bedtime; *qid*, four times daily; *tid*, three times daily.

The optimal management of spina bifida in children includes self-catheterization. Through cartoons and drawings, children can be taught how to prevent germs from growing in the bladder. Intermittent self-catheterization of the bladder usually can begin by age 5 years or by the time the child starts school.

Bowel evacuation can be brought under control in a majority of persons with SCI or other causes of myelopathy or cauda equina injury. The goals include continence, the prevention of impaction and discomfort caused by inadequate elimination, prevention of rectal bleeding, and a reasonable amount of time for bowel care. Some people with SCI can identify a signal of rectal distention, such as sweating or an increase in spasticity. It is particularly useful to establish a fixed time, usually after a meal, for evacuation. Once a pattern has been established with stimulatory suppositories, patients often get by with dilatation of the anal sphincter, either digitally or by a glycerin suppository. Those who cannot develop enough intraabdominal pressure to defecate may need manual evacuation several times a week.

### Fatigue

Although most commonly associated with MS, various forms of fatigue occur in all patients with central and peripheral neurological diseases. Fatigue may encompass malaise, lack of energy, and depression. Underlying mechanisms may include disease-related autonomic, endocrine, and inflammatory dysregulation, as may occur in MS. Cognitive processing effort that is increased by the presence of cerebral lesions may induce a form of fatigue in carrying out mental and physical activities. One of the least recognized forms of fatigue that will interfere with ADLs occurs with repetitive use of muscles. This fatigability especially affects overused girdle muscles during walking but can be so insidious in the course of a motor activity that patients do not realize why they employ a slow gait with short stride. Clinically, this fatigability can often be detected by testing strength immediately before and after 10 leg lifts by a supine or prone subject or after a 30-m walk. It arises from problems as diverse as the more familiar fatigability found in myasthenia gravis and in lumbar stenosis with intermittent compression of cauda equina roots. Contributors include impaired drive of motor units from the motor cortex due to less cortical excitability or greater inhibition, loss of corticospinal projections, conduction blocks along the descending projections, spinal mechanisms of reciprocal inhibition, disruption of firing rates of fast and slow motor units, and muscle atrophy.

Strengthening and conditioning exercises as well as use of techniques for energy conservation may lessen motor fatigability. Medications such as antidepressants, modafinil, and methylphenidate or noradrenergic modulation may reduce symptomatic fatigue.

***Acquired myopathy.*** Proximal weakness of the shoulder and hip girdle muscles arises from a sedentary lifestyle and disuse of the arm and leg muscles for antigravity and other actions. Such paresis can be superimposed on muscles affected by UMN or LMN disease and not uncommonly occur in neurodegenerative diseases such as PD. Once the difficulty is recognized, a program of even light resistance exercise can reverse much of the negative impact of weakness on gait, balance, and arm functions.

Medications such as the statins may cause an insidious myopathy without elevated muscle enzymes that induces weakness and greater fatigability. Walking and balance are most affected, but this may not be appreciated in the person who already has a neurological cause of paresis. A variety of genetic predispositions have been identified but no one cause has been found.

By 4–8 months after stopping any one of the statins, strength will gradually recover.

### Central Neurogenic Pain

A major source of disability can be pain from a thalamoparietal stroke or SCI. One of the most common complaints a year or more after SCI is burning pain at and below the level of the lesion. Approximately half of these patients gauge their symptoms as moderate or severe. Some patients need only assurance that the pain does not represent a serious complication or a warning signal of another stroke. Others will need the help of the physician in setting goals and identifying interventions to moderate the severity, frequency, and duration of the pain, also taking into consideration the usual time of day for pain onset. Tricyclic antidepressants and selective serotonin reuptake inhibitors, pregabalin, carbamazepine, clonidine, gabapentin, lamotrigine, benzodiazepines, and baclofen are among the drugs that diminish dysesthetic or lancinating pain in some patients. Occasionally, methadone in doses from 5 to 20 mg tid may reduce the pain. Intrathecal clonidine, baclofen, and morphine can be efficacious when other approaches fail (see Chapter 52).

### Sleep Disorders

During rehabilitation, insomnia, sleep apnea, and excessive daytime sleepiness can interfere with attention and learning. Stimulants, alcohol, medications, pain, anxiety, depression, and chronically poor sleep habits contribute. Central and obstructive sleep apneas have been associated with a higher risk of stroke. Pharyngeal muscle weakness and impaired neural control during sleep of the nasopharyngeal and pharyngolaryngeal muscles caused by a stroke or TBI contribute to the risk of obstructive apnea. Up to one-third of stroke inpatients may have a sleep disorder. Polysomnography is indicated when the inpatient rehabilitation team observes a hypersomnolent, confused, and snoring or apneic patient. One study found an average of 52 sleep-disordered breathing events per hour in selected subjects within 1 year of stroke. The number of oxygen desaturation events and the oximetry measures during sleep-disordered breathing correlated with poorer functional recovery scores at 1 and 12 months after stroke. Management with a continuous-pressure breathing mask and related devices is similar to usual management (see Chapter 101).

### Spasticity and Upper Motor Neuron Syndrome

Spasticity is found in less than 20% of hemiplegic patients after stroke. Patients with bilateral weakness from TBI, especially if hypoxic injury occurred, are likely to have signs of spasticity as well. After SCI, spasticity is more prominent with incomplete than with complete motor and sensory impairments, especially with cervical and upper thoracic lesions.

The most important UMN problems that cause disability are the decrement in motor control associated with dyssynergic patterns of muscle activation and the coactivation of agonist and antagonist groups during movements; these problems are associated with paresis, slow movements, loss of dexterity, and fatigability with repetitive contractions. Spasticity per se does not produce weakness or these other aspects of impaired motor control. Exaggerated cutaneous and autonomic reflexes and involuntary flexor and extensor spasms are the most disabling episodic problems associated with spasticity. During rehabilitation, the most visually striking signs associated with the UMN syndrome tend to be treated and sometimes overtreated. These include hyperreflexia; flexor synergy of the elbow, wrist, and fingers; plantar flexion of the ankle; and the dystonic postures, rigidity, and eventually contractures that may accompany profound paresis.

***Mechanisms.*** Clinical signs of hypertonicity can also be the consequence of interactions between central and peripheral factors. The mechanical velocity-dependent resistance to passive movement at a joint arises from the elastic and viscous properties of muscle, tendon, and connective tissue as well as from reflexively mediated stiffness. Some investigators have proposed that secondary changes in muscle—such as an increase in connective tissue and loss of muscle fibers or change in their properties—explain at least some of this increased stiffness. Hyperexcitability of motoneurons probably plays a larger role in this resistance but especially leads to hyperreflexia and clonus. A number of ill-defined mechanisms may alter membrane properties and thus reorganize spinal circuits both morphologically and physiologically, leading to hypertonicity. A variety of neurotransmitters act within these systems, although their net effects are uncertain. In addition, 5-hydroxytryptamine (5-$HT_{2C}$) receptors have been shown to increase 400% in the spinal cord of those with chronic severe SCI, leading to cutaneous stimulated spasms. Thus drug interventions produce hard-to-predict changes in muscle tone and the incidence and severity of spasms.

***Assessments.*** For routine assessments and for clinical trials of antispasticity interventions, a number of measures of hypertonicity have been used. The Ashworth Scale (Table 55.4) has had good interrater reliability in studies of stroke, SCI, and MS. The relationship between this descriptor score and disability is not so evident, however, and its utility as a measure of outcome is moot (Fleuren et al., 2010). Hypertonicity, clonus, and spasms vary in relation to positioning of the limbs, posture, and activities. A clenched, plegic hand may lead to disability if pain or maceration of the palm develops, but a treatment that lowers the Ashworth Scale score is unlikely to improve motor control. Other measurement techniques require instrumentation.

***General treatment.*** Therapists can usually manage pathologically increased tone, spasms, and poor range of motion in patients with hemiplegia by aiming to maintain normal length of the muscle and soft tissue across a joint, eliminating shoulder and other sources of pain, and helping patients to avoid abnormal flexor and extensor patterns at rest and during movement. Splinting to extend the wrist and the long finger flexor muscles is a common practice in the first month after stroke. In randomized trials, however, this intervention has not clearly reduced the likelihood of a wrist contracture without the use of other modalities. Spasms and dystonic postures should be treated more aggressively when they interfere with nursing care and perineal hygiene or evolve into contractures and pressure sores. Treatment is often needed for patients with myelopathies, who may endure painful spasms or involuntary flexor or extensor trunk and leg movements during transfers and after minor cutaneous stimulation. Measures to lessen hypertonicity can be useful when hypertonicity appears to restrain voluntary upper or lower limb movements through the cocontraction of agonist and antagonist groups. In most cases, however, upper extremity flexor postures during voluntary movement may best be explained by abnormal muscle contraction evoked by action. For example, the typical synergistic response to attempted shoulder abduction causes flexion torques at the elbow, probably because the usual coactivation that stiffens the elbow to stabilize it fails as a result of an imbalance in strength of the opposite extensor action. Passive abduction of the shoulder often enables more successful voluntary reach by elbow and wrist extension.

Hypertonicity and spasms have potential value. For example, spasms can decrease muscle atrophy and bone demineralization and increase venous return. An extensor thrust can provide the rigidity needed for weight-bearing stance. Learning to induce an extensor spasm can assist bed transfers in patients with myelopathy. Determining how and when hypertonicity interferes with a patient's activities is the most useful way to determine whether an intervention is needed. Bouts of clonus and flexor and extensor spasms during ambulation, driving, wheelchair push-up pressure releases, transfers, self-care activities, bed mobility, sleep, and sexual activities can be counted over the course of a day or week. Any intervention should aim to greatly lessen recurrences.

Noxious sensory inputs can exacerbate hypertonicity and trigger flexor and extensor spasms and dystonic postures. A painful shoulder can cause the hemiplegic arm to flex at the elbow and wrist. Even an ordinarily innocuous stimulus like tight clothing or sunburn can abruptly increase tone, much as it can cause autonomic dysreflexia in the patient with a cervicothoracic SCI. Treatable pain stimuli include bowel and bladder distention, urinary tract infection, epididymitis, joint pain especially on range of motion, unrecognized fractures, pressure sores, ingrown toenails, and deep venous thrombosis (DVT). Repetitive resistance exercises, although generally useful during rehabilitation, can increase flexor or extensor tone, especially if the exercise brings out associated movements. Selective serotonin reuptake inhibitors used for managing anxiety and depression can exacerbate spasms, presumably via upregulation of 5-$HT_{2C}$ receptors. The only way to make this diagnosis is to taper off the possibly offending drug and see if improvement follows by 2–3 weeks after cessation.

**TABLE 55.4 Clinical Measures of Spasticity**

| Score | Measure |
|---|---|
| **Ashworth Scale** | |
| 1 | No increase in tone |
| 2 | Slight increase, producing a catch when joint is moved in flexion or extension |
| 3 | More marked increase in tone but easily flexed |
| 4 | Considerable increase, passive movement difficult |
| 5 | Affected part rigid in flexion or extension |
| **Spasm Scoring Scale** | |
| 0 | No spasms |
| 1 | Mild spasms induced by stimulation |
| 2 | Spasms less than 1/h |
| 3 | Spasms more than 1/h |
| 4 | Spasms more than 10/h |

An overall approach to the management of pathological hypertonicity and spasms includes reversing any noxious stimulus, using physical interventions before adding drug trials, and reserving more invasive techniques such as nerve blocks and orthopedic or neurosurgical procedures for a few recalcitrant situations.

***Physical modalities.*** Slow stretching movements and daily passive range-of-motion exercises will reduce motion-sensitive symptoms of spasticity and the risk of contractures. Static stretching with splints probably will not prevent contractures when motor control is absent. Serial casting can reduce stretch reflex activity and contractures as the joint angle gradually increases. Muscle cooling, tendon vibration, pressure exerted over a tight muscle belly, postural adjustments, loading a limb by weight bearing on an extended arm or, for paraplegics, standing in a support frame, electrical stimulation, and electromyographic biofeedback (BFB) can complement a stretching program.

***Pharmacotherapy.*** Controlled trials of antispasticity agents have varied widely in the target symptoms managed and the outcome assessments used. Functional gains related to locomotion and voluntary use of the upper extremity usually are marginal in any UMN disease. A medication that prevents disabling spasms, however, may improve quality of life. Table 55.5 lists useful first- and second-line drugs.

After an SCI, about 25% of patients are discharged with an antispasticity agent, and half are still using medication by 1 year. Patients with American Spinal Injury Society (ASIA) grades A and D (see Chapter 63) are less likely to have been treated than those with grades B and C. Baclofen, tizanidine, and clonidine are especially useful in reducing clonus and extensor spasms caused by a myelopathy. The latter two drugs are $\alpha_2$ agonists that inhibit the excitatory influences of peripheral sensory inputs on motoneurons. Thus they are especially useful in persons whose spasms are associated with noxious sensory inputs. Medications with short-lasting effects, such as tizanidine, may be especially useful in limiting spasms during sleep or brief activities like transferring from wheelchair to bed. Baclofen, dantrolene, and the benzodiazepines can cause muscular weakness and difficulty with weight bearing during gait in hemi- and paraparetic persons. Children with cerebral palsy and patients with hemiplegic stroke often need their extensor tone to ambulate on a paretic leg. Dantrolene tends to be most useful in managing hypertonicity of the upper extremity after

**TABLE 55.5 Dosages of Medications for Symptomatic Spasticity**

| Drug | Dosage |
|---|---|
| **First-Line Agents** | |
| Diazepam | 2 mg bid–15 mg qid |
| Dantrolene | 25 mg bid–100 mg qid |
| Baclofen | 5 mg bid–40 mg qid |
| Clonidine | 0.05 mg/day–0.2 mg tid |
| Tizanidine | 2 mg bid–8 mg qid |
| Gabapentin | 400 mg tid–900 mg qid |
| **Occasionally Useful Additions** | |
| Intrathecal baclofen | 50–150 μg trial dosages; intrathecal infusion with pump |
| L-Dopa or carbidopa | 25 or 100 mg bid, respectively |
| Phenytoin | Serum concentration 10–20 μg/dL |
| Phenobarbital | Serum concentration 10–30 μg/dL |
| Cyproheptadine | 4 mg bid–8 mg qid |
| Chlorpromazine | 10 mg/day–50 mg tid |
| Dronabinol | 2.5 mg/day–2.5 mg tid |

*bid,* Twice daily; *qid,* four times daily; *tid,* three times daily.

stroke and TBI. Less than 0.5% of users develop hepatotoxicity after several months of intake. L-Dopa may be of additive value to lessen spasms in selected adults after stroke or SCI. All these drugs can also cause sedation, confusion, or hypotension; may add to bowel and bladder dysfunction; and can produce other central and systemic side effects. Great care must be taken in using them in the patient who has neurogenic dysphagia or a pseudobulbar palsy and is at risk for aspiration. Cyproheptadine blocks constitutively active 5-$HT_{2C}$ receptors to help reduce spasms and can be remarkably effective after a profound SCI, yet is little used clinically (Murray et al., 2010). Whenever a drug appears to be useful, it is worth tapering the dosage down from time to time so that the patient can help to reassess its usefulness.

For refractory spasms and pain, intrathecal baclofen or clonidine, given by an implanted programmable pump infusion, generally has replaced surgical myelotomy, intrathecal morphine, and electrical spinal stimulation. These strategies are usually reserved for persons with myelopathy but are sometimes also used to treat selected patients after stroke or TBI (Creamer et al., 2018). Intrathecal baclofen or clonidine has also replaced selective dorsal rhizotomy, except in some children with spastic diplegia from cerebral palsy. The functional effects on mobility and self-care are more difficult to discern, but some patients achieve modestly better walking speeds with intrathecal agents.

Recent experience with spinal cord electrical stimulation protocols suggests that spasms and marked hypertonicity may be diminished when combined with standing and stepping practice.

***Chemical injections.*** Chemical agents such as phenol have been injected into the lumbar theca, nerve, motor point, or muscle to lessen inappropriate muscle cocontraction, spasms, and dystonic postures. Because motor point blocks can partially spare voluntary movement and may reduce reciprocal inhibition when given to an antagonist muscle, they could improve some aspects of motor control. Intramuscular infiltrative injections of 50% ethanol or botulinum toxin reduce focal resistance to passive movement for approximately 3 months.

Botulinum injections have seemed most efficacious for the wrist and finger flexors and plantar flexors of the ankle. Interpretation of the results of clinical trials using botulinum toxin requires attention to how well the outcome measure reflects clinical effectiveness for an important problem. Is a change in ease of passive range of motion, as in the Ashworth Scale, as meaningful as an increase in functional use of the limb? A few trials in children with cerebral palsy and spastic diplegia reveal modest 10% increases in walking speed after injections. The great majority of studies for stroke, SCI, and MS report a 1- or 2-point decrease in the Ashworth Scale score for 3 months. The clinical meaning of such change is that with the wrist and finger flexors loosened, the hand was easier to keep open passively, or the arm became easier to manage when, for example, the patient tried to put it through a shirt sleeve. No functional gains are usually found (Shaw et al., 2011). After stroke, early prophylactic treatment of the upper extremity with a botulinum toxin did not prevent onset of spasticity any more often than did placebo. Treatment with any of the commercial botulinum toxins (equivalent dosing differs by brand) should include passive or active range of motion and treatments for pain to try to maintain better range of motion.

***Surgical interventions.*** A variety of surgical procedures—including tendon lengthening, tenotomy, and tendon transfer—can correct deformities induced by spasticity and improve function. A gait analysis with electromyography (EMG) can help determine which of these procedures may aid mobility. Physical therapy must follow any surgery. Tenotomy of the hip adductors and iliopsoas and tendon lengthening of the hamstrings, Achilles, and toe or finger and wrist flexors are among the more common interventions. Lower extremity surgeries are performed most often in children with cerebral palsy, although the data are difficult to interpret in terms of meaningful clinical gains. Achilles tenotomies for Duchenne muscular dystrophy and a variety of foot surgeries, including triple arthrodesis, for Charcot-Marie-Tooth disease may be beneficial.

Posterior rhizotomy has been carried out, especially in children with spastic diplegia. Selective division of posterior nerve rootlets of the second lumbar to the second sacral level is based on intraoperative EMG responses of lower extremity muscles to posterior nerve rootlet stimulation. Youngsters with the most dramatic functional improvements are bright, ambulatory patients with spastic diplegia who have minimal fixed contractures and good strength. Some clinicians argue that such patients would do well with any intensive therapy. Indeed, controlled trials suggest that the intervention is no better than routine physical therapy in terms of functional walking.

## THERAPIES FOR IMPAIRMENTS AND DISABILITIES

For problems of mobility and use of the upper extremities, therapeutic exercise and neurodevelopmental approaches are merging with strategies related to engaging neural systems for activity-dependent plasticity, motor control, and motor and cognitive learning. Success in motor retraining during rehabilitation requires attention to the movement components of a task; residual sensory and motor control; how performance and learning is reinforced; the patient's mood, motivation, attention, and memory for carryover of what is taught; minimizing environmental distractions and physical barriers; family and community support; and creative problem solving. All can influence how motor and cognitive programs are built, shaped, and refined as the patient acquires a new skill. Overall, trials suggest that repetitive practice of related motor sequences aimed at a defined functional goal will lead to better gains, especially for walking and increased use of a paretic arm and hand. Improvements may make use of spared neural networks but often mixed with compensatory behaviors. A wide variety of well-specified approaches to therapy have gained and sometimes lost momentum as the results of well-designed clinical trials have been published. The Canadian Partnership for Stroke Recovery maintains an ongoing evidence-based review of clinical trials of rehabilitation interventions that includes over 2400 randomized trials (www.

ebrsr.com). About two dozen types of neurological rehabilitation interventions have also been examined by the Cochrane Database for Systematic Reviews.

## Early Mobilization and Intensive Therapy

Recent studies primarily in stroke have tried to initiate specific rehabilitation strategies as early as feasible, preferably within the first week after onset of new impairment, to incorporate and drive spontaneous gene expression and molecular and immune cascades that have been associated with neural repair in animal injury models (Carmichael and Dobkin, 2016). Two large randomized trials failed to observe differences in outcomes, however. In the Active Mobility Very Early After Stroke (AMOBES) trial, 2 weeks of intensive PT for 45 minutes a day starting within 72 hours of onset of stroke, did not lessen impairment (Yelnik et al., 2017). In Very early mobilisation within 24 h of stroke onset (AVERT), mobilizing the experimental group within 24 hours after onset did not prove better than routine care, although the mean time to mobilization was only 4 hours less (Bernhardt et al., 2015). The early group spent a mean of 21 more minutes per day out of bed.

## Mobility and Gait

Visual observation of the gait cycle for temporal asymmetries of the legs and for the kinematics at the hip, knee, and ankle during the stance and swing phases reveals deviations that the clinician can identify and target to help train patients. The timing of loading the stance leg and unloading the swing leg after it approaches 10 degrees of hip extension for toe-off (Fig. 55.5), for example, provides proprioceptive information that is important for driving reciprocal stepping movements. Table 55.6 lists components of the gait cycle that are often used in kinematic and kinetic gait analyses. The therapist identifies and tries to modify serious deviations that interfere with the safety and energy requirements of ambulation as the patient walks on a flat surface. Temporal features of the gait cycle—such as the symmetry of each leg's stride length, time in stance and swing phases, and overall cadence and walking speed—are other key targets for management. These parameters have been enhanced by stationary bicycling, treadmill walking, and rhythmic auditory stimulation, which may help entrain the timing of more automatic stepping.

The threshold velocity for home ambulation is approximately 40 cm/sec (45 cm/sec = 1 mile per hour [mph]), if patients have hip flexion and knee extension at least against gravity. Therapy ought to aim for faster walking speeds and for more energy-efficient distances to permit unlimited community activities. Community ambulation requires a walking velocity of approximately 80 cm/sec, or more than 1.5 mph. Therefore, task-oriented training over ground or on a treadmill ought to try to exceed 1.5 mph as patients progress. In contradistinction to this outcome goal, typical disability measures such as the FIM and the BI assess only the level of independence to walk 15–45 meters at any velocity. During inpatient stroke rehabilitation, daily feedback simply about walking speed over 10 meters led to significantly higher walking speeds upon discharge compared with no feedback (Dobkin et al., 2010).

The notion of task-oriented training led to many small trials of treadmill training, circuit training around obstacles, bicycling, and related walking activities for patients with hemiplegic stroke and lower extremity weakness or abnormal gait patterns from SCI, TBI, MS, and other entities. The specificity of the training aims to improve walking safety and velocity, leg strength, and fitness to reduce the energy cost of walking. The addition of partial body weight support to treadmill training (BWSTT) has been tested in patients with stroke, SCI, Parkinson disease (PD), MS, and cerebral palsy. Subjects wear a chest harness that is attached to an overhead lift. The amount of weight borne by the lower extremities is adjusted to optimize the stance and swing phases of gait.

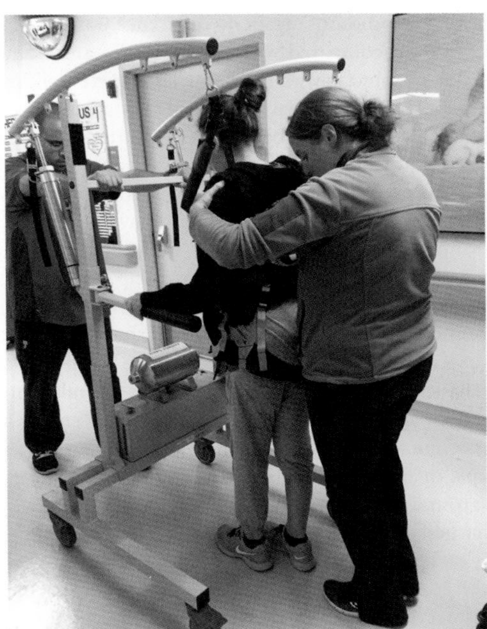

Fig. 55.5 This rolling walker with a pneumatic lift attached to a harness partially unloads the body's weight, here by 80 lb, on the legs to prevent knee buckling and enable stepping. This woman with a cervical spinal cord injury would not be able to practice hip flexion for stepping without such support.

**TABLE 55.6 Easily Observed Components of the Gait Cycle**

| Gait Phase | Component |
|---|---|
| **Stance** | |
| Pelvis | Lateral and horizontal shift to the stance leg |
| Hip | Extension to approximately 10 degrees |
| Knee | Slight flexion upon loading |
| | Extension at midstance |
| | Flexion at foot push-off |
| Ankle | Dorsiflexion to 10 degrees at heel contact |
| | Dorsiflexion as the lower leg moves over the foot |
| | Plantar flexion to 20 degrees with a propulsive rocker motion of the foot for push-off |
| **Swing** | |
| Pelvis | Drop at toe-off, then forward rotation |
| Hip | Flexion to 20 degrees to "shorten" the leg |
| Knee | Flexion to 65 degrees to "shorten" the leg, then extension just before heel contact |
| Ankle | Dorsiflexion to 10 degrees for heel strike |

One or more therapists may manually assist the lower extremities and pelvis during step training to optimize the step pattern. BWSTT allows repetitive practice guided by the verbal and physical cues of the therapist to improve components of the step cycle. The Locomotor Experience Applied Post Stroke (LEAPS) trial randomized 400 subjects who still walked less than 0.8 m/sec at 2 months after stroke (Duncan et al., 2011). It compared usual care to BWSTT with over-ground practice and to progressive strengthening and balance exercises in the home for 36 sessions. Improvements were significant for both supervised home-based exercise and for BWSTT compared with usual care when started at 2 months. When the usual care group received the same amount of

BWSTT starting at 6 months, again no difference was found in walking speed at 12 months compared with early BWSTT and home exercise. The proportion of subjects with moderate and severe walking disability did not differ in gains. The trial confirmed that progressive, challenging, mobility-related exercise is better than less structured therapies, but BWSTT was equivalent to other more common strategies. The gains with home-based exercise that did not emphasize walking raise the issue of the context of training—home treatment may encourage practice in a more meaningful environment. Other well-designed trials of more chronically and not severely hemiparetic participants suggest a modest benefit (Mehrholz et al., 2017a). Applied to cerebral palsy (CP), MS, PD, and after numerous examples of ASIA Impairment Scale graded A-D SCI (Dobkin et al., 2006a), BWSTT has shown no better results for independent walking, walking speed, or distance than similar intensity of a more conventional intervention. The technique may enable more stepping per session in a safe environment and seem task-specific, in keeping with concepts of motor relearning, but it still is not different enough from over-ground training to reveal a benefit. A commercially available overhead harness attached to a track that allows walking over ground also enables safe practice of stepping. Both techniques are best reserved for those who are highly disabled in taking steps to help get them started.

Peroneal nerve stimulation to dorsiflex and clear the foot during swing is the oldest approach to aid over-ground gait, with a variety of newer and possibly more efficient devices commercially available (Fig. 55.6). The stimulators produce walking speeds similar to what an AFO provides (Everaert et al., 2013). In patients with paraplegia, peroneal stimulation also aids reflexive hip and knee flexion during swing.

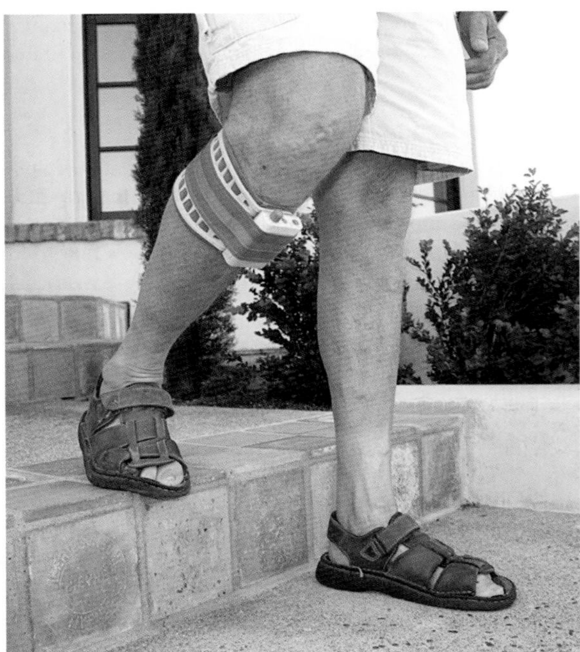

**Fig. 55.6** Stimulation of the peroneal nerve under the cuff on the right leg is in response to a signal from an accelerometer, leading to dorsiflexion from toe-off to heel strike to help clear the hemiparetic leg (WalkAide from Innovative Neurotronics, Inc.).

## Task-Oriented Therapies for Upper Extremity Recovery

### Functional Strengthening During Tasks

Conventional therapies often include functional strengthening with resistance exercise during practiced tasks and hands-on cues to improve the quality of movements as patients perform everyday tasks. A stroke trial that randomized 288 subjects to one or the other plus a standard conventional program for 6 weeks soon after the acute stroke found no differences in the significant amount of improvement of both on the ARAT and WMFT (Hunter, et al., 2018).

The Interdisciplinary Comprehensive Arm Rehab Evaluation (ICARE) trial primarily compared three interventions for motor stroke and moderate weakness at a mean of 45 days after onset: structured, task-oriented upper extremity training (Accelerated Skill Acquisition Program [ASAP]; $n = 119$); dose-equivalent occupational therapy ($n = 120$); and monitoring-only occupational therapy ($n = 122$) (Winstein et al., 2016b). ASAP was a best-practice synthesis of motor training approaches and schedules for purposeful, skilled movement execution—task specific, intense, engaging, and, unlike prior trials, a collaborative, self-directed, and patient-centered intervention. It included 30 one-hour treatment sessions (three times a week for 10 weeks). A constraint or mitt worn on the less affected hand was available but not mandated. Results were better but equivalent in all groups.

## Constraint-Induced Upper Extremity Therapy

CIT is a task-oriented strategy that calls for forced use of the affected upper extremity to overcome what is theorized to be "learned nonuse" of the paretic limb. The strategy limits the use of the unaffected hand by placing it in a sling or glove to force actions by the affected arm, along with gradual shaping of a variety of functional movements through considerable practice.

The first rendition of this approach for the upper extremity provided a course of 6 hours of practice with the affected arm on a series of functional tasks combined with restraint of the unaffected one throughout the day for 2 weeks. The key requirement for participation has been the ability to dorsiflex the wrist and extend several fingers of the paretic arm at least 10 degrees. The key treatment focus is as much practice as tolerated of progressively more complex and difficult tasks (shaping) that involve reaching in various planes to grasp or pinch items of different weights and sizes. The most important aspect of this approach is massed practice.

Several randomized inpatient trials for hemiparetic stroke have found modest or no benefit from CIT compared with an equal intensity of conventional therapy (Dromerick et al., 2009). A well-powered multicenter randomized trial called Extremity Constraint-Induced Therapy Evaluation (EXCITE) entered patients who had sustained a first stroke within 3–9 months of enrollment (Wolf et al., 2006). They received 2 weeks of training for 6 hours daily, a home practice program, and wore a mitt on the unaffected hand during formal therapy and at home. Statistically significant and clinically relevant improvements in paretic arm functional skills were found, measured by the Wolf Functional Motor Test (timed tasks dropped from a mean of 78–35 seconds to perform, with normal being <10 seconds) and by perceived daily use. The control group received no training or restraint. The improvements persisted up to 1 year and were not influenced by age, gender, or initial level of paretic arm function.

Modified CIT strategies eliminated or reduced the use of the restraining mitt and decreased the intensity of formal practice with a therapist from 6 hours to 1–3 hours a day over 2–4 weeks of training for stroke, CP, and MS. Based on over 50 clinical trials, the technique modestly lessens arm motor impairment and may increase use of the affected hand, but it does not reduce disability (Corbetta et al., 2015). Benefits accrue only to those who already have some selective motor control of the hand.

## Bimanual Upper Extremity Therapy

Bimanual training is based on the hypothesis that in-phase voluntary movements of the intact arm may facilitate interlimb coordination to improve the paretic arm. The substrate for this bilateral motor control includes the primary, premotor, and supplementary motor cortices and may involve both excitation and disinhibition. Several techniques and devices have been developed to aid proximal and distal upper limb training. For example, the Bi-Manu-Track (Reha-Stim, Berlin, Germany) aims to promote bilateral elbow pronation-supination and wrist flexion-extension as well as unilateral movements and can accommodate neuromuscular electrical stimulation to facilitate these movements. Hundreds of repetitive movements can be made in four directions in highly impaired subjects with stroke. Small trials suggest a modest gain in proximal and distal strength and some aspects of motor control in chronic hemiparetic patients with mild to moderate impairment after 20–30 hours of bilateral arm training with or without special devices. The bimanual approach is not clearly better than primarily unilateral practice with the affected arm (Wu et al., 2011).

### Virtual Reality Training

VR training can proceed in an immersive or nonimmersive environment. Multiple commercial software training programs have been developed, some enabled by the Kinect and headsets such as the Oculus. The goal is to better motivate pleasure during interactive video gaming so as to increase compliance and repetition of movements. Whether in the home or a laboratory, measurements of movement patterns can be integrated with the training and reinforcement paradigms that are provided as reaching and hand tasks are carried out. For example, walking on a treadmill surrounded by a complex indoor or outdoor environment aims to restore visual flow and lessen the influence of distracters while motivating patients to walk along nature trails or test their balance. VR systems have also been combined with electromechanical exoskeletons for the arms or legs and functional neuromuscular stimulation. Many small clinical trials for stroke and an adequately powered comparison of VR versus conventional therapy for the upper extremity (Brunner et al., 2017) suggest good compliance but so far no gains in functional use of the hand or in ADLs beyond more conventional therapy (Laver et al., 2017) Similar equivalent results have been found for VR to improve walking and balance after stroke, MS, PD, and TBI (Porras et al., 2018). Small clinical trials have also revealed encouraging but limited results for cognitive rehabilitation assessment and for the treatment of attention and spatial memory deficits and apraxia. The technology is rapidly improving—less expensive, smaller, more flexible. This may enable better VR interventions with more emphasis on cognitive-motor interactions during retraining.

### Mirror Therapy and Imagery

Observing another person make a movement activates mirror neurons; imagining a movement evokes activity in cell recordings and by fMRI in some of the same neurons in the primary and nonprimary motor regions and parietal lobe as with performing the movement. This form of practice is routinely used by athletes and dancers before a performance to reactivate in working memory the representation of a motor memory. A Cochrane analysis indicated evidence for the effectiveness of mirror therapy for improving upper extremity motor function, motor impairment, ADLs, and pain, at least as an adjunct to conventional rehabilitation for people after stroke. Action-observation therapy shows modest benefit for task practice with the affected upper extremity after stroke. As for many meta-analyses of rehabilitation interventions, major limitations were small sample sizes and lack of reporting of methodological details, resulting in uncertain evidence quality (Thieme et al., 2018). The level of residual motor function necessary, the capacity for imagery in patients with brain lesions, the necessary intensity of practice, and efficacy are works in progress.

### Instrumented Biofeedback

Biofeedback includes a variety of instrumented techniques that try to make the subject aware of physiological information that can be used to better perform an activity. Across controlled trials of ambulation in selected patients after stroke, electromyographic BFB using a visual or auditory cue may increase ankle dorsiflexion. BFB also can be combined with EMG-triggered neuromuscular stimulation. A minimal voluntary movement such as slight wrist extension of a paretic hand fires low-amplitude motor units. If this reaches the gain that is preset, radial nerve stimulation is triggered for increased motor unit activity of the extensors. The strategy has led to very modest gains in handgrip. Biofeedback may also improve performance during training, but not necessarily when visual or auditory guidance is withdrawn. For example, the Balance Master (Neurocom, Inc.) provides continuous visual feedback on the position of the center of gravity when patients stand on its force plate. The system detects postural sway and asymmetries of weight distribution on each leg and patients get feedback when they shift in ways that improve symmetry. However, meta-analyses of trials find that improved postural control on the force plate does not carry over to a significant increase in symmetry of stance or improved gait performance over ground.

### Acupuncture

In China and Korea, a variety of acupuncture methods are widely used after stroke. Controlled trials and meta-analyses of these trials using sham acupuncture compared with traditional treatment have not shown clear benefit on impairment, ADLs, functional use of a hand, or quality of life (Yang et al., 2016). Reports of techniques that lessen focal musculoskeletal pain and hypertonicity are frequent.

### Visual Field Deficits

The most common compensatory methods include saccadic visual search training into the affected field of vision, attentional cues to that field, and prisms. Computer-based training has been used to stimulate the border areas of a field cut to gain a few degrees of possibly restored vision or to enable blindsight training. These techniques, plus transcranial direct cortical stimulation, may compliment other forms of cueing, especially when spatial inattention is also present.

### Electromechanical Robotic-Assistive Devices and Exoskeletons

Electromechanical and robotic-assistive exoskeletons that provide passive and active movement of the paretic arm and leg aim to increase the intensity and reproducibility of reaching and grasping or overground stepping. Their commercial appearance has preceded evidence from controlled trials of efficacy for increasing voluntary movement or lessening disability. Portable exoskeleton devices aim to work in concert with the subject's limited voluntary movements or automatically carry out a movement such as a step. So many technology groups have been developing models that a yearly Cybathlon lets makers compete in Switzerland across standard tasks that are important to disabled persons. Commercial devices employ impedance-, counterbalance-, EMG-, and adaptive-based controllers that adjust forces and kinematics to assist movements based on the patient's performance. One goal is to decrease mechanical loading on the paretic leg and improve kinematics and energy cost of walking at faster speeds than otherwise feasible. For persons with paraplegia, at least five commercial devices enable standing up and slow walking over ground with good stability. Myoelectric controlled AFOs and KAFOs may use artificial muscle fibers. These engineered devices are a work in progress—limited by cosmetics, power source, weight, and flexibility—but they are also advancing rapidly.

#### Upper Extremities

Over 100 active, passive, and haptic mechanical robotic devices have been developed for the paretic arm (Pawel et al., 2014). A passive device, the

Therapy Wilmington Robotic Exoskeleton (T-WREX), was designed to support the paretic arm against gravity, measure arm motion, and trace hand grasp as the user interacts with computer games. After 24 sessions, patients assigned to the device or to an equal intensity of tabletop exercises had equally modest gains. A commercial device with an adjustable suspension, the ArmeoSpring, has not been studied in a controlled trial. Such devices may yet show better outcomes based on their built-in entertainment value for repetitive practice and feedback about results. The first in its class to reach commercial development was the MIT-MANUS, which manipulated a patient's paretic elbow and shoulder much as a therapist might provide hand-over-hand therapy for reaching in a single plane. Power and control at the shoulder have improved with this robotic training, consistent with the greater intensity of practice using those muscle groups, but the device did not offer better outcomes than active therapy for reaching (Volpe et al., 2008). A multicenter Veterans' Administration trial of a more complex three-part device (InMotion, Bionik Labs, Inc.) for the arm in multiple planes, as well as wrist and hand incorporated the principles of the MIT-MANUS technology and visual feedback during tasks. The robotic assist was equal in effectiveness to the same amount of intensive conventional therapy in moderately impaired patients; meta-analysis of trials of robotic-assisted and electromechanical upper extremity devices reveal equal or modest improvements in impairment and arm function over conventional therapy at the same intensity (Mehrholz et al., 2018). One potential advantage of these devices is that the antigravity support for shoulder abduction, as provided by, for example, the ArmeoSpring reduces synergy-dependent coupling between the shoulder and elbow and wrist of the paretic arm during practice. The use of virtual environments, types and intensities of practice paradigms, and levels of assisted movement are all works in progress. A lightweight, cosmetically acceptable exoskeleton that can enable motion control of the shoulder, elbow, wrist, and hand for reaching, grasping, and feeding seems more feasible than in the past, given the gains in materials, actuators, and achievements of prosthetic limbs.

## Mobility

Commercially available robotic-assistive stepping devices for use on a treadmill have been available for 20 years. One is the Lokomat (Hokoma AG, Volketswil, Switzerland). The Lokomat attaches each thigh and lower leg to a motorized exoskeleton while fixing the hips in its frame. Reference trajectories based on the gait of healthy subjects are adjusted by on-line optimization that adapts the parameters of the trajectory of the hip and knee to minimize the measured forces of interaction. The Lokomat has not been superior in over-ground training for stroke, SCI, and MS (Lo and Triche, 2008) and especially not for patients who are already able to ambulate, even if slowly (Mehrholz et al., 2017b). The clinical efficacy of a stereotypical assisted-step pattern with relatively unvarying sensory inputs may not enable motor learning, even with available forms of feedback, but could supplement over-ground practice. For neural repair trials after SCI, such practice may be the only feasible form of practice to aid axonal targeting and spinal cord modifications for voluntary movement.

Commercially available bilateral trunk-to-foot exoskeletons enable a paraplegic person to stand and take steps at a slow casual cadence (e.g., Ekso Bionics (Richmond, CA, USA), ReWalk Robotics (Yokneam Ilit, Israel), HAL (Hybrid Assistive Limb, Cyberdyne, Tsuluba, Japan)). Devices include a battery backpack and use foot pressure and joint angle sensors to enable alternating stance and swing. They have been touted as a means to train hemiplegic patients as well, but efficacy is unclear and they may face some of the same conceptual problems that treadmill robotics incur in terms of being able to foster motor learning.

Partial limb electromechanical devices are growing in number to assist a particular aspect of movement in moderately impaired persons. For example, the Honda Stride Management Assist exoskeleton is a hip-only powered device that straps from the low back to the thigh. It improved walking speed and endurance compared with conventional gait therapy in chronic hemiplegic persons after stroke (Jayaraman et al., 2019). Several single-motor knee and elbow joint assists weigh as little as 1.5 kg. A heavier Bionic Knee (AlterG) straps from the upper thigh to the lower leg and foot. Such devices may come to enable more practice repetitions or help compensate for a key impairment—for example, in knee control regardless of pathology.

## Functional Neuromuscular Stimulation

Functional neuromuscular stimulation (FMS) systems activate one or more muscle groups synchronously or sequentially to enable single- and multijoint movements. Surface and intramuscular electrical stimulation systems have become more widely available in the past 5 years, but despite extensive study and commercial development, they have not come into sustained use. The discontinued FreeHand provided hand grasp and release in C5 and C6 tetraplegic patients. Electrode wires were implanted in the appropriate muscle of one forearm, and a controller device at the opposite shoulder allowed patients to complete upper limb grasp, pinch, and release after training. The first commercial wireless surface electrode-driven device for grasping was the Bioness System, which has found some use in quadriplegic patients with at least C5 intact and in hemiplegic patients with poor hand function (Fig. 55.7). The external control unit operates from a button managed by the patient for the level of output that allows grasp, holding, or release. Small studies suggest that the combination of task-oriented training and assisted grasping in patients who cannot otherwise incorporate the hand may provide better outcomes than either strategy alone, but it also can act as a prosthesis for grasp when the proximal arm is capable of reaching.

Functional Neuromuscular Stimulation (FNS) systems can also aid standing and ambulation. Peroneal nerve stimulation to aid foot dorsiflexion to clear the foot during the swing phase can increase step length and walking speed in hemiparetic persons. A growing number of commercial devices are available that use an accelerometer to switch on the below-the-knee stimulus. Used alone or combined with other assistive and bracing devices such as an RGO, these systems can allow walking as an exercise and in some instances permit stepping for indoor

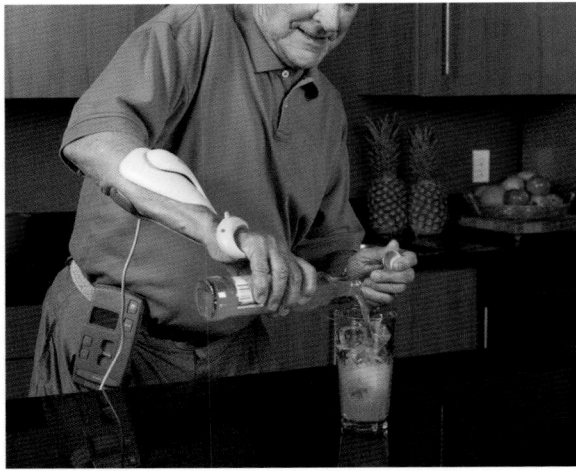

**Fig. 55.7** The hemiparetic right arm is assisted by an orthosis with functional neuromuscular stimulation that helps dorsiflex the wrist and produce a palmar grasp or finger pinch (Bioness, Inc.). Its practical usefulness depends on the ability to lift and extend the proximal arm.

distances. However, a lengthy strengthening and fitness program must precede the use of these devices by paraplegic patients. The first commercial device to assist stepping, the Parastep System (Sigmedics, Inc. New York, USA), used six surface electrodes to stimulate the gait cycle as subjects held a rolling walker. Stimulation of the quadriceps muscles and push-off with the arms permitted standing up. Constant stimulation maintained standing. A button on the walker was pressed to stop the quadriceps firing and to stimulate the peroneal nerve to initiate a triple flexion response for swing. The patient released the button after the hip flexed, which fired the quadriceps stimulator for stance.

Patients with a complete UMN SCI may exercise with a bicycle ergometer. Bilateral surface electrodes are placed over the quadriceps, hamstrings, and gluteal muscles to sequentially activate leg forces on the pedals. As muscle strength increases, contractions are made against greater ergometer resistance to increase muscle bulk and aerobic fitness. Clinical trials suggest that FNS exercise in sets of 10–15 repetitions against an increasing load resistance of 1–15 kg over 12 weeks will increase muscle bulk, improve strength, and reduce fatigability for the FNS activity. Although psychological and other physiological benefits (possibly focal increases in bone density, greater fitness) have been attributed to FNS in paraplegic subjects, long-term home programs require much motivation.

## Noninvasive Brain Stimulation

Subthreshold cortical electrical stimulation at an optimal frequency and amplitude aims to increase cortical excitability and synaptic efficacy during training. Possible mechanisms include reinforcement by Hebbian plasticity, modulation of neurotransmitters, remote effects on excitation-inhibition, and molecular mechanisms of neural repair. Repetitive transcranial magnetic stimulation (rTMS) and transcranial direct cortical stimulation (over the primary motor cortex, combined with upper extremity rehabilitation) as well as ulnar and median peripheral nerve stimulation have led to modest increases in motor control and arm or hand function in small controlled trials after stroke (Elsner et al., 2016). Forms of vagal nerve stimulation are also evolving, combined with physical or other specific therapies. Greater motor gains are made in patients with incomplete subcortical corticospinal tract lesions. rTMS also has been used to inhibit a cortical region to improve activation of the homologous contralateral hemisphere. An RCT of motor cortex stimulation via an epidural electrode placed over primary motor cortex combined with arm therapy found no overall better functional gains than by the same therapy alone after stroke (Levy et al., 2016). Somewhat better function was likely in more mildly paretic subjects. More studies are needed to determine how to best use these interventions to augment conventional treatments for motor skills. Noninvasive brain stimulation is also being tested with some success to reduce dysphagia, in aphasia to lessen dysnomia (Fridriksson et al., 2018), and for hemineglect.

### Invasive Neural Stimulators

Spinal cord stimulators have been placed over the dorsal spinal cord in the epidural space to reduce some types of central pain and severe hypertonicity with spasms after SCI. Recent case studies suggest that in persons with paraplegia but some sparing of descending pathways (e.g., SCI graded AIS B), the combination of an optimized pattern of lumbosacral stimulation of the dorsal horns plus lengthy training of stepping can lead to independent slow over-ground walking with assistive devices (Wagner et al., 2018). The primary movement elicited is voluntary hip flexion for swing alternating with knee extension for stance. Possibly, the rhythmic stimulation lowers the threshold for motor neuron firing and enables latent supraspinal inputs to become effective. The notion of increasing the excitability of motor pools in the cervical region is also being tested in persons with very poor motor function after stroke and SCI.

Nerve cuffs placed around a portion of a peripheral nerve can provide a permanent electrochemical interface to selectively initiate or record electrical signals or modulate the nerve's responses. Their initial experimental use has been for ankle dorsiflexor stimulation during walking, but they have become applicable for sacral nerve stimulation for bowel and bladder emptying.

## Neural Prostheses and Brain–Computer Interfaces

Up to 2 million Americans and many others worldwide may be without any voluntary control due to ALS, a locked-in syndrome after stroke or trauma, MS, cerebral palsy, or muscular dystrophy. To aid these highly disabled persons to manage their surroundings and communicate, a variety of brain–computer interfaces (BCIs) have been developed and tested. The devices use surface and intracortical neural signals from defined regions of the brain to drive, for example, an FNS system or a computer mouse. Signals are acquired from field potentials over the surface of the scalp, dura, or subdural regions or from the spike potentials of small clusters of neurons picked up by microelectrode arrays from motor cortex or cognitive planning regions. Selected signals such as the amplitude of an evoked potential, a specific rhythm from sensorimotor cortex, or the firing rate of cortical spikes are digitized and processed by algorithms to extract specific features. A translation algorithm converts the particular electrophysiological features chosen to simple commands to a device such as a word processor or keyboard, a website, an upper extremity–like robotic device, or an exoskeletal neuroprosthesis for reaching and gripping as well as environmental controls. The error rate, often in the range of 10%–20%, can be frustrating to a patient who tries to make binary changes in the amplitude of a cortical signal to choose a letter or word. Rapid improvements in signal processing and interfaces offer greater utility for paralyzed patients. BCIs also show some promise as tools to increase training-related neural adaptations, monitored by functional connectivity imaging, for motor control when combined with rehabilitation (Ramos-Murguialday et al., 2013).

## Pharmacological Adjuncts

A stroke or other brain injury that diminishes the availability of a neurotransmitter projection system from the brainstem may degrade synaptic adaptation and learning during rehabilitation. Neurotransmitters and neuromodulators given in pharmacological dosages could be supplied to augment neural activity within a network during a specific motor or cognitive task. It takes much study to find a drug with a dose–response ratio that produces positive effects with no adverse effects. Human clinical trials of drug interventions have had underpowered sample sizes. Investigators often screen 10–20 subjects for every one who meets entry criteria. Early after onset of hemiplegic stroke, varying support persists for fluoxetine and citalopram as adjuncts for early motor gains (FOCUS Trial Collaboration, 2019), but larger trials are ongoing. Dextroamphetamine (Goldstein et al., 2018) and ropinirole have failed to show efficacy inadequately powered trials. For inpatients and outpatients, *N*-of-1 experiments with simple outcome measures for short-term trials that alternate placebo versus active medication can be safe and occasionally beneficial.

### Regenerative and Cellular Agents

Many animal studies have pursued manipulation of many of the biological regenerative processes in Table 55.6.Trophic factors and antibodies to dendritic growth inhibitors, including anti-nogo-A antibodies (Kucher et al., 2018) soon after SCI and myelin-associated glycoprotein monoclonal antibodies after stroke (Cramer et al., 2017) have been found to be safe but not yet effective for neural repair. Recently completed dose–response safety trials of cellular therapies for stroke, SCI, and TBI offer a basis for continuing to pursue this strategy with circumspection. Modified bone marrow–derived mesenchymal stem cells (SB623) were implanted via stereotactic intracranial injection into patients (6–60 months poststroke) along the circumference of the infarct. Some of the subjects had sustained motor improvements that began shortly after the injections. The same cell line was used in large randomized trials in patients with stroke and with TBI. There was no primary or secondary benefit for chronic stroke impairment. FMA scores were modestly but significantly higher in TBI patients who received cells. Prior to this, small controlled trials failed to reveal any effect of partially differentiated neural and glial precursors in patients with stroke and SCI.

About 30 trials involving mainly autologous cell therapy have been published in SCI, mostly using stem cells and less often Schwann cells and olfactory ensheathing cells, but without much success,. Animal models suggest that a bridging strategy may be most suitable after a complete SCI. For example, spinal neural stem cells have been injected into the area of myelomalacia in macaques with a gel or other matrix that contains three to five key regeneration-associated gene activators (Rosenzweig et al., 2018). Injured descending corticospinal inputs were shown to synapse with these and, remarkably, the implanted cells grew axons over long distances to make synaptic contacts below the lesion in the ventral gray matter. Hand motor outcomes also improved.

At conferences and on websites but not in peer-reviewed published reports, clinicians at hospitals in China and at least 100 sites around the world have built stem-cell spas to treat a broad range of neurological and other diseases. They claim to use fetal, olfactory ensheathing glia, bone marrow stromal, and fat-derived autologous stem cells for cerebrospinal fluid or intravenous injection or implantation in uncontrolled and poorly documented experimental therapies in patients. The sites offer hope at $10,000–$50,000 for their services. These unpublished interventions tend to be based on a misinterpretation of preclinical experiments in rodents. The US Food and Drug Administration has recently been challenging or closing these commercial entities and China is increasing its scrutiny, but most of the exploitation takes place outside of the United States. Clinicians should encourage patients to read the educational materials about participating in neural repair experiments, such as the guidelines available at http://www.icord.org.

### Mobile Health and Wireless Sensing Devices

Smartphones, web-based telerehabilitation, and wearable accelerometers and gyroscopes with pattern-recognition algorithms that can calculate the type, quantity, and quality of movements in the community are becoming available under the rubric of mHealth endeavors (Dobkin, 2017). These technologies will enable feedback about performance via continuous monitoring of gait or use of an upper extremity, may improve compliance with exercise and skills learning by enabling self-management behavioral paradigms, and will offer ratio and continuous scaled outcome measures for clinical trials and daily care. Simpler devices that serve as step monitors—worn on the wrist, trunk or on one leg—already provide some insight into daily activities, but ankle sensors are more reliable for a slow and irregular gait. Therapists will be able to deploy the more sophisticated wearable sensors to remotely progress the intensity and type of therapy by knowing what the patient is practicing outside of formal sessions. Ground truth about skills practice, activity, and participation at home and in the community should become feasible

## THERAPIES FOR COGNITIVE AND BEHAVIORAL DISABILITIES

### Overview of Cognitive Therapy

Cognitive and behavioral disorders are common with stroke, TBI, MS, PD, and other degenerative diseases. Box 55.7 lists some of the cognitive impairments dealt with by the rehabilitation team. These impairments can seriously impede gains in mobility, ADLs, and community reintegration. Prospective studies of patients with an acute stroke reveal that 15%–35% have greater memory impairments 3 months to 1 year after onset than age-matched controls. Cognitive and behavioral dysfunction, especially from diffuse axonal injury, is especially common after TBI. Greater severity and longer duration of impairments are associated with a lower Glasgow Coma Scale (GCS) score on acute admission and longer duration of posttraumatic amnesia (PTA). Up to half of patients with an SCI have cognitive impairments from an associated TBI that may not be obvious early in postinjury care.

**BOX 55.7 Cognitive Impairments Managed During Rehabilitation**

**Language**
Aphasia
Affective expression

**Attention**
Alertness
Speed of mental processing
Awareness of disability and impairment
Focused attention on a single stimulus
Sustained attention to a task
Selective attention during distraction
Divided or alternating attention between tasks (for multitasking)

**Memory**
Retrograde, antegrade
Immediate, delayed, cued, and recognition recall

**Learning**
Visual, verbal, and procedural or skill

**Perception**
Visual
Auditory
Visuospatial

**Executive**
Planning
Initiation
Organization skills
Maintaining goal or intention
Conceptual reasoning
Hypothesis testing and ability to shift responses
Self-appraisal
Self-monitoring

**Intelligence**
Verbal
Performance
Problem solving
Abstract reasoning

The amount and rate of recovery of neuropsychological function vary with the sophistication of the measures used; type and severity of impairment; type, severity, and distribution of lesions; time since onset; and age at onset and follow-up. More subtle factors such as the interactions of diseases, associated sensorimotor and cognitive impairments, and premorbid intellect and education can affect the efficacy of a particular therapeutic approach. Comparisons between interventions are often confounded by the intensity and duration of treatment, lack of specification of the treatment methods, personal interactions between the therapist and patient, and the family's ability to reinforce desired behaviors.

After the cognitive and behavioral problems have been identified, general management approaches include training in particular functional adaptive or compensatory skills, behavioral modification, and remediation of specific cognitive processes. In the adaptive approach, therapy tries to circumvent the effects of cognitive impairments on targeted daily activities. Repetition, cues (both internal and environmental), and cognitive assistive devices are used for training. Learning to do a particular task usually does not generalize to other tasks that are not closely related. Behavioral modification techniques most often are used in acute and transitional living settings for patients with TBI. Rewards are given for accomplishing a task or reducing antisocial actions. In the cognitive remediation approach, the subcomponents or hierarchical organization of a given cognitive skill are addressed. The strategy assumes that at least some of the parallel and hierarchical neural networks for cognitive processes are understood. More often, techniques emphasize interventions meant to boost intact domains to help compensate for more impaired ones.

A modest number of studies suggest a benefit with use of a particular approach or combination of approaches for a specified set of cognitive impairments compared with no treatment or a placebo or psychosocial intervention as well as with conventional training in ADLs (Cicerone et al., 2011). The data for efficacy are strongest for some of the rehabilitation strategies to manage attention, memory, and social communication as well as visuospatial, aphasia, and apraxia training. Techniques usually merge as the rehabilitation team experiments with interventions that address the most deleterious problems. Outpatients with a TBI are the most likely group to need multimodality programs that stress training in task-specific skills by remediative techniques, awareness of impairments and limitations, and an emphasis on the skills needed for independent living and work.

## Aphasia

The incidence of language disorders has varied across studies of patients with stroke and TBI. Chapter 13 provides details about specific disorders. In a British health district of 250,000 people, new cases of stroke-induced aphasia for 1 year numbered 202. By 1 month after stroke, 165 survivors were potential candidates for speech therapy. A prospective community-based Danish study of acute stroke found that 38% of 881 patients were aphasic on admission, with 20% of the admissions rated as severe on the Scandinavian Stroke Scale. Nearly half of the patients with severe aphasia died soon after stroke onset, and half of those with mild aphasia recovered by 1 week. Only 18% of community survivors were still aphasic at the time of their rehabilitation hospital discharge. Up to 28% received early speech therapy as needed. Patients were retested over the subsequent 6 months; 95% with mild aphasia reached their best level of recovery at 2 weeks, those with moderate aphasia peaked at 6 weeks, and patients with severe aphasia reached best language function within 10 weeks. Only 8% of those with severe aphasia fully recovered by 6 months on the scoring system used. The best predictor of recovery was less severe aphasia close to the time of the stroke.

### Treatments

Some 20%–50% of aphasic patients have partial features of the traditional aphasia subtypes (see Chapters 13 and 14). For rehabilitation therapy, the broadly defined features used to classify patients often do not address in enough detail the underlying disturbances of language, so they may not be optimal for directing treatment. A neurolinguistic assessment of aphasia aims to specify the types of representations or units of language (e.g., simple words, word formation, sentences, discourse) that are abnormally processed during speech, auditory comprehension, reading, and writing. For each unit, the therapist ascertains how the disturbance affects linguistic forms such as phonemes, syntactic structures, and semantic meanings.

Speech therapists most often attempt to find ways for the patient to circumvent, unblock, or help compensate for defective language function by using a great variety of stimulation-facilitation techniques (see Table 55.4). These include visual and verbal cueing techniques such as picture matching and sentence completion tasks, along with frequent repetition and positive reinforcement as the patient approaches the desired responses. Phoneme-based treatment, for example, would aim to lessen anomia by increasing phonological production and reduce nonword repetition. Strategies for therapeutic training have also been drawn from hypotheses about activity-dependent adaptations and learning. Since action words and the actions themselves have overlapping neural networks, language tasks perhaps ought to be practiced within relevant physical activities. Massed practice, avoidance of learned nonuse of words due to prior failures, and linking words to actions and daily relevance has been advocated to maximize Hebbian-type plasticity. Constraint-induced language therapy, in which intensive training of either nouns or verbs with an emphasis on phonemic cues, led to increased use of the taught words but not of untrained words (Berthier et al., 2009).

Initial treatments often use tasks that relate to self-care, the immediate environment, and emotionally positive experiences. To prevent withdrawal and isolation, it is especially important to quickly find a way to obtain reliable verbal or gestural "yes-no" responses. Behavioral techniques, particularly for patients with TBI, can be used to improve skills in maintaining eye contact, initiating and staying on a topic, turn taking during conversation, adapting to listener needs, and using speech to warn, assert, request, acknowledge, or comment. Beyond the stimulation-facilitation approach to therapy, a variety of theoretical models for therapy have been proposed, such as the modality, linguistic, processing, functional communication, and minor hemisphere mediation models.

Specific therapy techniques have been designed for defined aphasia syndromes and neurolinguistic impairments as well. For example, the efficacy of melodic intonation therapy (MIT) has been especially good in nonfluent aphasia (van der Meulen et al., 2014). In MIT, therapists and patients melodically intone multisyllabic words and commonly use short phrases while the therapist taps the patient's left hand to mark each syllable. Gradually, the continuous voicing and tapping are withdrawn. MIT works best in persons with Broca aphasia who exhibit sparse or stereotypical nonsense speech and good auditory comprehension. If a single sound, word, or phrase overwhelms any other attempted output, the Voluntary Control of Involuntary Utterance Program can help the patient gain control over perseverative intrusions. Some mute or nonfluent aphasics can acquire a limited but useful repertoire of gestures using, for example, American Sign Language. Comprehension in persons with the global and Wernicke forms of aphasia has been managed with the Sentence Level Auditory Comprehension Program. It trains patients to discriminate consonant-vowel-consonant words that are the same or differ by only one phoneme (e.g., "bill, pill, fill"). They then try to associate the word sounds with the written word and later try to identify the target word embedded in a sentence. For persons with global aphasia, nonverbal communication using pantomime has decreased limb apraxia and improved auditory comprehension through a technique called *visual action therapy*. Use of an electronic device that provides delayed auditory feedback by about 200 msec after the aphasic person voices each phoneme can be tried as a means to improve awareness of paraphasic errors and intelligibility. Recent case studies also suggest that focal cortical stimulation using TMS may be able to activate or deactivate a node in the language network to enhance the effectiveness of simultaneous training. Smartphone and tablet apps for practice are widely available; up to 80% of aphasic persons have used one or more that offer gamification to increase adherence and feedback about performance.

### Outcome Measures for Aphasia

Local conventions dictate assessment and measurement tools, and these vary by native language. A US and Canadian group of experts recommended the following instruments. For language: the Western Aphasia Battery Revised (WAB-R) (74% consensus); for emotional well-being: General Health Questionnaire (GHQ)-12 (83% consensus); for quality of life: Stroke and Aphasia Quality of Life Scale (SAQOL-39).

### Pharmacological Adjuncts

A few studies suggest that intensive therapy combined with a drug that enhances vigilance or learning may benefit patients who have adequate language comprehension. Piracetam, a derivative of γ-aminobutyric acid (GABA) but with no GABA activity, may facilitate cholinergic and aminergic neurotransmission. A randomized placebo-controlled trial included 50 moderately aphasic patients who had a stroke a mean of 10 months before starting the 6-week intervention of 10 hours of speech therapy weekly. The drug-treated group had a significantly better total score on the Aachen Aphasia Test, although the clinical impact is not clear. In a randomized trial of 24 patients, use of piracetam also was associated with some language subtest gains and higher cerebral blood flow in left hemisphere language regions during a word repetition task. Other cholinergic agents have improved naming in patients with moderately severe Wernicke aphasia or dysnomia, especially by reducing perseveration. Amphetamines, memantine (Berthier et al., 2009), and dopaminergic agents have improved aspects of language in some small studies but not all. Short-term trials of such agents can be carried out in combination with language therapy and standardized tests in individual patients to look for responsiveness.

### Outcomes of Trials

A meta-analysis of 57 trials of speech therapy in persons with stroke-induced aphasia found significant benefits for patients who received treatment at all stages of recovery, with the greatest improvement found for therapy in higher doses (Brady et al., 2016). Treatments of more than 2 hours per week gave greater gains than lesser amounts of therapy. In another meta-analysis, treatments given for approximately 100 hours over 11 weeks were more efficacious than when given for 45 hours over 22 weeks. Persons with severe aphasia showed larger gains when their management included treatment by a speech-language pathologist. In the Rotterdam Aphasia Therapy Study-3, a total of 4 weeks of intensive cognitive-linguistic treatment initiated within 2 weeks of stroke was not more effective than no language treatment for the recovery of poststroke aphasia. On the other hand, a 3-week course of intensive (15 hours a week) speech and language therapy using individualized one-on-one linguistic and communicative-pragmatic approaches and computer self-training resulted in significantly greater verbal communication during everyday activities in 78 chronically impaired persons with stroke compared with 78 randomly assigned controls (Breitenstein et al., 2017). Treatments for aphasia typically average 45–60 minutes and are provided up to three times a week in community practices. The family must continue at home to practice word finding, longer phrasing, and social communication, optimally for at least 5 hours a week.

## Apraxia

Many forms of apraxia have been defined (see Chapter 11). Up to 25% of patients will have an ideational or ideomotor apraxia after stroke that affects the sequential performance of tasks and knowledge of how to use a limb or deploy objects. This disability interferes with ADLs; but with both left and right cerebral lesions, some recovery is likely over several months. Oromotor apraxia often accompanies nonfluent aphasia. Most approaches are compensatory rather than building on an understanding of the cognitive bases for the impairment. Practice of limb gesturing and structured behavioral training, training in specific strategies for necessary ADLs that use relatively errorless learning, and sensory cues lead to moderately positive effects on praxis and may generalize to untrained but related ADLs. Theoretically driven therapies such as strategies that activate the action-observation system of mirror neurons can be explored as well.

## Attentional Disorders

Sustained, focused, alternating, and divided attention are often disorders affected by the frontal lobe and diffuse injuries induced after stroke by TBI and MS; they disconnect thalamic-basal ganglia-frontal pathways from mass effect or vasospasm and with any toxic-metabolic complication such as a urinary tract infection. Real-time feedback about performance (during visual, verbal, sequential, and environmental tasks), reinforcement paradigms as varied as praise and earned tokens, and compensatory strategies to manage increasingly complex tasks are often part of the rehabilitation of attention. Cognitive processes associated with increasingly difficult attentional demands have been a focus of treatments. These include processing speed, flexibility, interference and distraction thresholds, and use of working memory. However, computer programs for attention that emphasize gains in processing speed and reaction times usually have not generalized to improved focused or divided attention. The entire rehabilitation team must develop and reinforce attentional strategies across ADLs in the hope that the approaches will generalize. Aspects of attention often improve rather spontaneously during inpatient rehabilitation. Severe impairment may continue in patients with TBI or hydrocephalus. Clinical trials of specific approaches for persistent difficulties during outpatient care do not point to the greater efficacy of any particular strategy.

## Memory Disturbances

Memory disturbances can have a profoundly negative influence on compensation and new learning in the patient undergoing neurorehabilitation. The therapy team depends on teaching that can be encoded and retrieved. Patients with TBI, a remarkably large percentage of those with stroke, and those with degenerative neurological diseases such as MS and PD are most frequently affected by problems in working, recent, prospective, and remote memory. Clinical trials of therapies are complicated by variation in the severity of the amnestic syndrome, time since onset, and difficulties in "teasing out" spared and affected components of implicit and explicit memory processes as well as in specifying the exact nature of the treatment strategy.

### Frequency of Memory Disturbance Across Diseases

The frequency of and risk factors for memory loss and dementia caused by one or more strokes have become increasingly appreciated

(Kalaria, 2012). The prevalence of memory disturbance in population- and community-based studies is nine times greater in the first year after a stroke than in an age-controlled group, and it doubles in each subsequent year. Other studies find a risk of memory dysfunction of approximately 20% at 3 months after a stroke. The frequency of dementia rises with increasing age and varies with the definition used. Even a mild aphasia may affect verbal memory and can interfere with verbal learning during rehabilitation.

Memory impairments after TBI have been related to the time between injury and assessment, to the nature of the memory task, and to the severity of the injury. Tasks that require divided attention are especially useful to tease out executive dysfunction caused by a TBI. Natural history studies have reported varying outcomes. For example, in a group of 102 patients with TBI (ages 10–60 years) who were hospitalized for any period of unconsciousness, for PTA lasting for more than 1 hour, or for evidence of cerebral trauma, the TBI group performed significantly worse on the Wechsler Memory Scale and the Selective Reminding Test 1 month later than did a control group. Those who could not follow a command for the longest times beyond 24 hours after injury scored below the control subjects on more subtests of the Wechsler Memory Scale. Tests that required storage of new information for later use were superior to tests of orientation and short-term memory in their ability to reveal memory deficits. At 1 year, patients performed better than they had at 1 month after onset. Many patients who were hospitalized for serious TBI are found later on to underestimate their memory and emotional impairments even as they acknowledge physical and other cognitive problems. Without insight or concern, they deny having the impairment and withdraw or become angry with attempts at rehabilitation. The rehabilitation team must provide the counseling and insight therapy needed to overcome this.

### Treatments

Clinical evidence from RCTs neither supports nor denies the effectiveness of cognitive rehabilitation techniques for memory and other impairment stroke, TBI, or MS; however, many strategies for the diverse types of patients, impairments, and disabilities have been tried with limited benefit for quality of life in some patients (das Nair et al., 2016; Kumar et al., 2017). Most rehabilitative efforts aim to help patients encode new information and to recognize and retrieve declarative memories of facts and events. Previous exposure to verbal and especially to nonverbal information, with cues and prompts, can allow many amnestic patients after TBI to recall that information, a phenomenon called *priming*. Priming does not require semantic processing for encoding. It is specific to the properties of the input and relies on perceptual representations stored by modality-specific memory subsystems such as those that process word forms and visual objects. Tests of recognition memory are especially sensitive methods for detecting residual memory in patients with severe amnesia. This implicit memory neocortical mechanism can even support the rapid acquisition of novel verbal and nonverbal material. It is relatively independent of the hippocampal and diencephalic structures that relate to amnesia. Priming seems especially useful during rehabilitation to enhance procedural memory for skill acquisition. The best training paradigm for implicit learning in markedly amnestic patients after TBI appears to be errorless learning rather than trial-and-error learning. The latter tends to produce better consolidation of what has been learned in healthy and mildly affected subjects.

Cognitive remediation of amnestic disorders aims to train patients to use the theoretical subcomponent processes that underlie declarative and nondeclarative memory. Therapists can then take a restorative or compensatory approach to affect particular memory skills for functionally important activities. For example, therapists may address attentional impairments that could interfere with memory training by strategies for improving focused, sustained, selective, alternating, and then divided attention. Impairments in encoding and recall of information are then addressed. This approach uses associative and external cues that are meant to prompt an action after increasingly longer intervals have passed, as well as external aids, rehearsal, and visual imagery.

After a moderate to severe TBI, repetitive paper-and-pencil or electronic drills on names, appointments, orientation, and daily routines may have little impact on daily functional recall and memory outside of the training session. Learning to make associations and "chaining" tasks in a sequence has had better results for daily activities. External aids such as calendars, lists, appointment diaries, and pagers have been shown in clinical trials to be better than no aids. The devices listed in Box 55.8 may improve daily activities if patients can be reminded to use them. Apps for smartphones can enable intermittent reminders by phone or email or social media, provide checklists, and take a person through the steps of a task.

Computers have been used extensively in cognitive remediation and skill training. Although software programs abound for working on reaction times, aspects of attention, language, problem solving, and other cognitive tasks, almost no data demonstrate the efficacy of such programs. Some patients have learned tasks such as data entry, database management, and word processing by taking advantage of preserved cognitive abilities, including the ability to respond to partial cues and acquire procedural information, even in the presence of a marked amnestic syndrome. However, this knowledge often does not generalize to even modest changes in the tasks. Through procedural memory, verbal and visual mnemonic strategies have been used to teach subjects a computer graphics program. Cooking and vocational tasks were taught with an interactive guidance system that cued each subtask to build up to the desired task.

There is still insufficient good-quality evidence to support the role of any particular set of cognitive rehabilitation interventions—as compared with no intervention or conventional rehabilitation—to improve return to work, independence in ADLs, community integration, or quality of life in adults with TBI. A growing number of animal and human studies suggest that aerobic exercise itself can improve aspects of cognition, including memory, reaction times, and attention. Such training ought to be part of the attempt to improve executive functioning and build self-esteem and self-management skills.

### Pharmacological Adjuncts

Studies of single subjects and small groups suggest that the drugs listed in Box 55.9 may benefit some patients with amnestic and attentional impairments. TBI may lead to damage in a particular neurotransmitter system; presynaptic cholinergic neurotransmission was abnormal in a human postmortem study of TBI.

### Outcomes

Although memory-related processes are found to improve over the first 3 months after a stroke, reports on the natural history of ongoing cognitive sequelae suggest that both inpatient and outpatient rehabilitation efforts must include ongoing attention to the need for compensatory aids and other strategies for these patients. After mild TBI, memory usually recovers by 3 months. However, this varies with the test used to measure severity, the time from injury to testing, and the comparison group. The patients who exhibit the greatest impairment at 1 year after a serious TBI initially are unable to follow a command for more than a day and have PTA for more than 14 days as well as a GCS score of 8 or less. At 1 year after a severe closed head injury, patients followed in the Traumatic Coma Data Bank had greater impairments in verbal and visual memory and in other neurobehaviors, such as

## BOX 55.8 Aids and Strategies for Memory Impairment

**External**

***Reminders by Others***

Tape recorder or portable voice organizer
Notes written by hand or entered into smartphone calendar

***Time Reminders***

Alarm clock, phone call, smartphone app
Personal organizer or diary
Calendar or wall planner
Orientation board

***Place Reminders***

Labels
Codes (colors, symbols)

***Person Reminders***

Name tags
Clothes that offer a cue

***Organizers***

Lists
Personal organizer or diary
Numbered series of reminders
Items grouped for use
Calendar and event alarm on smartphone or tablet

**Internal**

Mental retracing of events
Visual imagery
Alphabet searching
Associations to what is already recalled
Rehearsal
First-letter mnemonics
Chunking or grouping of items

## BOX 55.9 Possibly Useful Medications for Attentional and Memory Dysfunction

**Cholinergic Agonists**

Physostigmine
Donepezil, rivastigmine
Metrifonate
Cytidine diphosphocholine
Choline and lecithin precursors

**Catecholamine Agonists**

Dextroamphetamine
Methylphenidate
L-Dopa
Amantadine
Bromocriptine and other dopamine receptor agonists
Desipramine

**Modafinil**

**Serotonergic Agonists**

***N*-Methyl-D-Aspartate Receptor Agonists**

Ampakines
Memantine

**Nootropics**

Pramiracetam
Piracetam

**Neuropeptides**

Vasopressin and analogs

naming to confrontation and block construction, compared with normal controls. Selective rather than global cognitive impairments were likely at 1 year. Memory was disproportionately impaired compared with overall intellectual functioning in 15% of the moderately injured and 30% of the severely injured patients. After moderate to severe TBI, children plateau in recovery by 1 year after onset, with little change in the next 2 years, and do not catch up to their peers in terms of memory, problem-solving ability, and academic performance. Late changes do evolve in some. In a long-term outcome study of mostly young adults, Wilson and colleagues reassessed 26 patients who had a TBI resulting in 1 hour to 24 weeks of coma, followed by rehabilitation. After 5–10 years, 58% were unchanged, 31% performed better, and 11% did worse on the Rivermead Behavioral Memory Test and Wechsler Memory Scale. Many had to rely on memory aids.

## Hemineglect

Hemineglect can arise from injury to any node in the cortical-limbic-reticular network, which directs attention and integrates the localization and identification of a stimulus and its importance to the person.

### Frequency

Community-based studies of stroke survivors detect visual neglect in 10%–30% of patients. The neglect is modestly associated with poorer ADL scores and slower recovery, although severe neglect is rare beyond 6 months. Right-sided inattention, when looked for, has been detected in 15%–40% of nonaphasic patients with acute left cerebral infarcts, although it is clinically the most prominent after right brain injury. Patients with anosognosia, visual neglect, tactile extinction, motor impersistence, or auditory neglect have the lowest BI scores at 1 year even after the data are adjusted for initial ADL scores and for post-stroke rehabilitation. During rehabilitation, patients with left hemiplegia and neglect tend to improve on the motor portion of the FIM more than those with neglect and anosognosia.

Recovery across reports has been most rapid in the first 2 weeks, regardless of the side of stroke. By 3 months, most patients have little visual neglect. Severe visual neglect and anosognosia in the first week tend to predict some level of persistent impairment at 6 months. Many patients have more subtle and lingering impairments that depend on the test used to detect them. For example, early after a right hemisphere stroke, a group of patients showed a strong and consistent rightward attentional bias in addition to an inability to reorient their attention leftward. Twelve months later, the attentional bias continued, but now the patients could fully reorient to left hemispace when performing line bisection and cancellation tasks.

### Treatments

The initial choice of an intervention may depend on the proposed mechanism of unilateral neglect or hemispatial inattention. For example, the patient can be treated for an underaroused right hemisphere that has difficulty processing sensory inputs. After a right brain injury, a powerful bias of the left hemisphere for attention to contralateral space could lead to an imbalance, necessitating intervention to lessen the bias. A selective inability to disengage from inputs from ipsilateral

**BOX 55.10 Interventions for Hemineglect**

- Multisensory visual and sensory cues, then fading cues
- Verbal elaboration of visual analysis
- Environmental adaptations (bed position, red ribbon at left book margin)
- Computer training
- Video feedback
- Monocular and binocular patches
- Prisms
- Left limb movement in left hemispace
- Head and trunk midline rotation
- Vestibular cold caloric stimulation
- Contralesional cervical nerve stimulation
- Repetitive transcranial magnetic stimulation of unaffected hemisphere
- Reduction of hemianopic defects by a few degrees
- Pharmacotherapy trials; rotigotine

space may need to be addressed. Other strategies may have to be developed if the mental representation of contralesional space has been degraded or if a unilateral impairment in the activation of motor programs delays or prevents the intention to move to the contralesional side. rTMS and transcranial direct cortical stimulation have been used with some success to inhibit or disinhibit one side of the brain after stroke and lessen hemineglect (Fasotti and van Kessel, 2013).

If the initial theory-based intervention is not successful, then others should be tried. Box 55.10 lists some of the traditional and clever ways clinicians have tried for the management of hemineglect. For example, prisms have been used to transform sensorimotor coordinates and passive prostheses can be worn during tabletop activities. A 10-degree prism that shifts objects to the right in a patient with left hemi-inattention causes the patient to reach to the left when the glasses are removed. After adaptation to wearing the prism for 5 minutes, the patient's internal visual and proprioceptive map apparently realigns in the direction opposite to the optical deviation.

Spatial and visual cues, visuomotor feedback, and combined training of visual scanning and reading, copying, and describing pictures and figures are more commonly employed strategies. A variety of attempts have been made with some success to help patients recalibrate or realign the workspace or frame of reference that is at the center of a task. Noradrenergic and dopaminergic stimulants including guanfacine, methylphenidate, modafinil, bromocriptine, and rotigotine may modulate vigilance for tasks and are worth trying in recalcitrant cases (Gorgoraptis et al., 2012).

## Behavioral Disorders

A great variety of behavioral changes can follow any hypoxic-ischemic injury or TBI. Alterations in personality have been reported in up to 75% of patients 1–15 years after a TBI and tend not to improve spontaneously beyond 2 years after onset. Box 55.11 lists some of the more common changes. Agitated motor and verbal behaviors after TBI, although not easy to define or treat, are found in more than 10% and restlessness in 35% of patients during acute inpatient rehabilitation. As cognition improves, agitation declines, but directed and nondirected aggressive, impulsive behavior may evolve. Persistent aggression and emotional dyscontrol suggest premorbid mood and behavioral disorders.

Interventions include a medical assessment for exacerbating problems such as pain and drug-induced confusion, behavioral modification with positive and consistently applied reinforcements, a structured milieu for the most impaired, instruction in formal problem-solving techniques, individual and group psychotherapy, and medication (possibly useful drugs are listed in Box 55.12). Interventions to improve self-awareness of deficits in self-regulation and self-monitoring have

**BOX 55.11 Potential Changes in Behavior and Personality After Traumatic Brain Injury and Cerebral Hypoxia**

Disinhibition
Impulsivity
Aggressiveness
Irritability
Lability
Euphoria
Paranoia
Lack of self-criticism and insight
Irresponsibility and childishness
Egocentricity
Selfishness
Sexual inappropriateness
Self-abuse
Poor personal care habits
Apathy, indifference
Indecision
Lack of initiation
Blunted emotional responses
Poor self-worth
Passive dependency

**BOX 55.12 Drug Interventions for Aggressive Behavior, Restlessness, and Episodic Dyscontrol**

Anticonvulsants (carbamazepine, valproate, gabapentin)
Beta-blockers (e.g., propranolol)
Lithium
Antidepressants (e.g., amitriptyline, fluoxetine)
Stimulants (e.g., methylphenidate, pemoline)
Neuroleptics (e.g., risperidone)
Benzodiazepines (e.g., clonazepam)
Clonidine
Calcium channel blockers

not been successful in small trials of patients with TBI. When a focused program of rehabilitation is provided, improvements have been reported even years after the onset of TBI. Some patients who exhibit hypoarousal improve with stimulants such as methylphenidate and amphetamine, modafinil, or dopamine agonists. Aggressive behavior is sometimes decreased by dopaminergic or noradrenergic receptor blockade. Beta-blockers can decrease irritability. A randomized trial of propranolol with dosage escalation to 420 mg/day showed a reduction in the intensity of agitation but not the frequency of episodes compared with placebo. Hypomanic behavior may respond to lithium or anticonvulsant medications that are used in the management of bipolar disorders. Anticonvulsants such as carbamazepine sometimes prevent outbursts related to episodic dyscontrol.

## Affective Disorders

### Incidence

Depression is very common after stroke and mild TBI. The community-based Framingham Study diagnosed depression in 47% of 6-month stroke survivors, with no difference found in the incidence between those with left- and right-sided lesions, compared with 25%

of age- and sex-matched controls. In a population-based cohort of Swedish stroke patients whose mean age was 73 years, the prevalence of major depression was 25% at hospital discharge, 30% at 3 months after stroke, 16% at 1 year, 19% at 2 years, and 29% at 3 years. In this and many other studies, a left anterior infarct, dysphasia, and living alone contributed to the prediction of depression upon discharge. At 3 months, greater dependence in ADLs and relative social isolation were associated with depression. Few social contacts at 1 and 2 years contributed.

Anxiety is another stroke-related affective disorder. Although less often studied, a generalized anxiety disorder was present in 28% of recent stroke victims and was associated with greater social isolation and greater dependence in ADLs. Apathy was found in approximately one-fourth of patients within 10 days of a stroke, associated with greater cognitive impairment, poorer ability to perform ADLs, and some cases of major but not minor depression. Depressed people with an SCI report spending more time in bed and fewer days out of the house. They receive more help with personal care than better-adjusted patients with SCI at 2–7 years after injury. Suicide rates may be two to four times those in the general population within 5 years of SCI. Anxiety and depression can also arise from a posttraumatic stress disorder associated with the event that led to the SCI. After TBI, 25%–60% are diagnosed with depression. Late-onset depression has been associated with premorbid psychiatric history and lower psychosocial function. Poor social adjustment can cause long-term depression and anxiety.

### Treatment

Clinicians should manage mood disorders aggressively, especially when progress in rehabilitation falls short of expectations. Psychosocial support, individual and group therapy, and support groups appear to help across diseases. In general, patients with depression respond to all classes of antidepressant medications and can be managed with the same judicious care in finding the optimal dose that is necessary for managing the elderly. For example, by 6 weeks after initiation of fluoxetine or citalopram therapy, two-thirds of depressed subjects after a stroke recover compared with 15% of those given a placebo. The same medications can help alleviate pseudobulbar emotional incontinence with its involuntary weeping, grimacing, and laughing. Close clinical monitoring for adverse reactions to the antidepressants is important during inpatient and outpatient rehabilitation. Such reactions include sedation, insomnia, constipation, inability to void, reduced salivation, orthostatic hypotension, cardiac arrhythmias, anxiety, extrapyramidal symptoms, and a serotonin syndrome.

## FUNCTIONAL OUTCOMES WITH REHABILITATION

The most important outcomes for the rehabilitation team include the degree of independence in ADLs and community living. Thus functional measures that reflect the level of care needed and the quality of life achieved by people with neurological disabilities are used in outcome studies more often than measures of change in sensorimotor and cognitive impairments. The scores on the FIM at admission for inpatient rehabilitation and at discharge offer an interesting snapshot of clinical status of a large number of patients with stroke, TBI, and SCI from American institutions that participate in the Uniform Data System for Medical Rehabilitation (Table 55.7). Over the past 25 years, data reveal that the time from onset of neurological illness to transfer for rehabilitation has dropped about 50%. The length of stay in rehabilitation has followed a similar decline, driven by fiscal concerns. In the United States, Medicare also limits the number of outpatient sessions for all therapies to about 15 per year. These declines may put a greater burden of care on families and lead to the need for more efficient rehabilitation strategies.

**TABLE 55.7 Summary of Inpatient Rehabilitation for First Admissions for Stroke, Traumatic Brain Injury, and Nontraumatic and Traumatic Spinal Cord Injury**

| | Stroke | TBI | NTSCI | TSCI |
|---|---|---|---|---|
| Onset to rehab admission (days) | 9.2 | 14.0 | 11.8 | 21.1 |
| Admission FIM | 59.7 | 60.5 | 68.5 | 73.3 |
| Discharge FIM | 87.9 | 90.5 | 95.2 | 101.3 |
| LOS (days) | 14.3 | 13.5 | 13.1 | 12.4 |
| Discharge (%): | | | | |
| Community | 77.9 | 78.6 | 81.6 | 91.0 |
| Long-term care | 8 | 6.8 | 5.2 | 2.8 |

*FIM*, Functional independence measure; *LOS*, length of [inpatient rehabilitation] stay; *NTSCI*, nontraumatic spinal cord injury; *TBI*, traumatic brain injury; *TSCI*, traumatic spinal cord injury

Accessed from the National Uniform Data System for all of 2013; 427,595 admissions for all causes.

### Stroke

A meta-analysis of 36 trials carried out before 1992 showed that the average patient who received a program of focused stroke rehabilitation or a particular procedure performed better than approximately 65% of the patients in the comparison group. Larger treatment effect sizes were associated with earlier timing of the intervention and younger age. This trend has continued over the past 15 years. Interventions for a well-defined disability (e.g., functional use of an affected hand, walking, swallowing, speech intelligibility, community activities) as well as impairments in areas such as muscle strength and fitness show a moderate benefit from rehabilitation services of optimized intensity and specificity.

Rehabilitation studies of patients with stroke generally show that 50% of 6-month survivors have no motor impairment, 70%–80% can walk 150 feet alone, and 50%–70% are independent in ADLs based on the BI. These gains in subjects with the best outcomes do not imply that they can walk or function efficiently in the community. Most studies suggest that 50%–75% of survivors do not return to their prestroke level of activities in the community.

Prospective and retrospective studies of recovery of motor impairment suggest that many patients recover about 70% of arm and leg movement within about 3 months based on their initial Fugl-Meyer score (Krakauer, et al., 2015). Such improvements are presumably from recovery of primarily corticospinal networks that enable selective movements, primarily against gravity; further motor gains, then, may primarily arise from compensatory movements. The findings are still controversial but do fit with clinical observations. Proportional recovery of aphasia within certain domains has also been reported.

#### Ambulation

A community-based population study in Copenhagen prospectively followed 800 survivors of acute stroke. On admission, 51% were unable to walk, 12% walked with assistance, and 37% were independent. In the same facility, all who needed rehabilitation received services for an average total stay of 35 ± 41 days. At discharge, 22% could not walk, 14% walked with human assistance, and 64% of survivors walked independently by BI criteria. Recovery of ambulation correlated directly with leg strength. About 80% of those who initially were nonwalkers reached their best walking function within 6 weeks, and 95% achieved this within 11 weeks. If patients walked with assistance at stroke onset, 80% reached their best function within 3 weeks and 95% within 5 weeks. With rehabilitation, 34% of the survivors who had been dependent and 60% of those who initially needed assistance achieved independent walking for at least 150 feet.

Life table analysis of patients from different impairment groups reveals a somewhat different pattern of gains. During their rehabilitation, 90% of patients with a pure motor (M) deficit become independent in walking 150 feet by week 14 after stroke onset, but only 35% of those with motor and proprioceptive or sensory (SM) loss by week 24 and 3% of those with motor, sensory, and hemianopic deficits (SMH) by week 30. The probability of walking more than 150 ft with assistance increases to 100% with M impairment by week 14. It increases to 90% in those with SM loss by week 26 and in those with SMH deficits by 28 weeks. At 1 month and 6 months after stroke for all survivors, 50% and 85%, respectively, of M subjects recover walking, 48% and 72% of SM subjects recover, and 16% and 38% of SMH subjects walk without human assistance.

Although many patients become independent in gait, stroke patients who need rehabilitation most often have self-selected walking speeds that peak in 3–6 months at one-third to one-half of normal for age. Speed is a good reflection of the overall gait pattern and, as noted earlier, reflects general capabilities for walking in the home and community.

## Self-Care Skills

In the Copenhagen Stroke Study, ADLs measured by the BI were assessed weekly in the hospital and at 6 months. Some 20% of survivors had a severe disability and 8% a moderate disability after a mean hospital stay of 37 days. Functional recovery peaked by 13 weeks after stroke onset in 95%. The highest BI score was reached within 13 weeks by those with moderate impairments and within 20 weeks in those with severe impairments by the Scandinavian Stroke Scale. A BI score greater than 60 is associated with a home discharge. Using the impairment grouping schema, the cumulative probability of reaching a BI score greater than 60 and greater than 90 at 6 months after stroke is 95% and 70%, respectively, 85% for M subjects, 62% for SM subjects, and 52% and 35% for SMH patients. Similarly, approximately 65% of inpatients during rehabilitation achieve a BI score greater than 95 by 15 weeks if they have only M deficits and by 26 weeks with SM loss. Only 10% score that high with SMH deficits after 18–30 weeks. However, 100% achieve a score greater than 60 by 14 weeks with M loss only, 75% by 23 weeks with SM deficits, and 60% by 29 weeks with SMH loss.

For patients admitted for stroke rehabilitation, the admission BI or FIM score predicts later burden of care. The FIM score on admission positively correlates with discharge FIM and negatively correlates with length of stay, except in patients under age 50. The largest FIM change over time occurs in patients with admission FIM scores of 40–80. Patients with admission scores greater than 80 and age younger than 55 years routinely return home. A score of less than 40 and age older than 65 leads to a nursing home discharge for 60%.

Much of self-care depends on making use of the unaffected hand and trying to incorporate the affected one. If no recovery of wrist and finger extension has evolved by 4 weeks after hemiplegic stroke, functional dexterity of the hand rarely develops (Houwink et al., 2013). Poor voluntary control correlates with less residual corticospinal tract by diffusion tensor imaging. When selective flexion and extension are present, gains in use of the hand may evolve for as long as patients practice specific tasks such as reaching into their workspace to grasp and perform key and pincer pinches. Patients must work on accuracy, precision, speed, and endurance. For example, putting a key into a lock at home, if difficult to perform, should be done 20–30 times a day in sets of 10 until this becomes a more functional movement.

## Spinal Cord Injury

An improvement from ASIA A (sensorimotor complete) and B (sensory present) grades of injury to ASIA C (less than useful motor return) injury occurred in only about 10% of patients during inpatient rehabilitation after a cervical or thoracic SCI. These patients tend to regain some sensorimotor function one level below the initial level of impairment. Gains may be a bit better for these ASIA-level patients with conus and cauda equina injuries.

A clinical trial of GM1 ganglioside found the following changes in 760 patients assessed between 72 hours and 26 weeks after they suffered a traumatic SCI of the cervical or thoracic cord (Geisler et al., 2001). Approximately 80% of patients with a central cord injury became able to walk at least 25 feet. Only 4% of ASIA A patients at onset recovered any ability to walk, whereas 40% of ASIA B subjects regained this function. At least 70% of ASIA C subjects recovered unlimited walking. ASIA A patients almost never recovered normal bowel and bladder function. Approximately 15% of subjects with incomplete injuries recovered these functions. The drug, of note, did not alter outcomes compared with a placebo.

Self-care skills depend especially on the level and completeness of an SCI. For ASIA A patients, the absence of recovery of movement two levels below a cervical traumatic SCI injury at 8 weeks predicts little likelihood of gains. Any movement one level below anticipates ongoing gains in strength in the muscles at that level. For ASIA B patients, no motor gains by 16 weeks after SCI markedly diminishes the likelihood that useful motor function will develop. ASIA C patients, however, are highly likely to continue to make gains in motor function. For patients with complete lesions at C4 or above, ventilatory support and assistive devices are needed along with physical help. With C5 intact, self-feeding is achieved with devices such as a balanced forearm orthosis and wrist splints with attachments for utensils. Patients can use a power-assisted wheelchair with a hand control. With C6 intact, wrist extension allows the thumb and fingers to oppose, but a tenodesis orthosis may be needed. Upper extremity dressing, self-catheterization, manual wheelchair propulsion, and sliding board transfers are feasible. With C7 intact, these activities are performed more efficiently and use of a suppository for the bowel program is feasible. With C8 intact, long finger flexion permits most ADLs to be accomplished from a wheelchair.

The strength of the lower extremities determines the amount of work that must be performed by the upper extremities for support, which in turn determines the energy cost and feasibility of ambulation. A study using the ASIA motor score found that patients with incomplete tetraplegia who had an ASIA lower extremity motor score of 10 or more (the maximum normal score is 50 for five muscle groups of each leg on a five-point scale of strength) at 1 month after injury became community ambulators with crutches and orthoses by 1 year. They subsequently achieved nearly effortless community ambulation if the lower extremity motor score improved to at least 30. This finding was confirmed in the SCI Locomotor Trial (Dobkin et al., 2006a). By comparison, scores of 20 or less were associated with limited ambulation at slower average velocities, higher heart rates, greater energy expenditure, and greater peak axial loads on assistive devices. Walking speeds gradually increased with a lower extremity motor score of 20–30, and highest speeds were obtained above 40. Paraparetic community ambulators usually need to have pelvic control with at least movement against gravity in the hip flexors and one knee extensor, so that they at most require one KAFO to step with a reciprocal pattern.

Patients need encouragement and resources to be able to return to work or school. Those with education beyond high school are far more likely to return to work and stay employed. Aging with SCI poses problems for many. One-fourth of patients who sustained their injuries 20 or more years earlier evolve a greater need for physical assistance over time, especially for help with transfers.

### Traumatic Brain Injury

In general, after moderate to severe TBI, self-care and mobility improve from admission for inpatient rehabilitation to discharge, and gains are maintained or continue to increase for approximately 6 months. The Citicoline Brain Injury Treatment Trial found that 35% of subjects in the drug and placebo groups had favorable improvements on the Glasgow Outcome Scale-Extended by 180 days postinjury (Zafonte et al., 2012). About 50% in most studies return to work at 6 months. Socialization and leisure activities generally do not return to premorbid levels.

In a series of 243 consecutive admissions to a rehabilitation unit, a significant inverse relationship was found between the GCS score and the duration of coma, along with a strong positive relationship between the duration of coma and PTA. Of 119 patients with diffuse axonal injury, no one in a coma for more than 2 weeks or with PTA for more than 12 weeks had a good recovery by the GCS outcome score at 1 year after injury. Two-thirds of the small subgroup with coma for more than 2 weeks improved to moderate disability when the coma lasted 2–4 weeks; only one-third achieved this level if in coma for more than 4 weeks. Among patients with PTA for less than 2 weeks, 80% had a good recovery. Half of those with PTA lasting 2–8 weeks were moderately disabled at 1 year after admission. At another inpatient facility, patients who had a GCS score of 3–7 within 24 hours of onset of TBI had lower admission and discharge FIM scores for motor and cognitive function during their rehabilitation. In many communities, approximately 10% of patients return to former jobs, and less than 30% are employed 2 years after severe TBI. In a Cochrane analysis, moderate to strong evidence supports the benefit of multidisciplinary inpatient and outpatient rehabilitation after moderate to severe TBI (Turner-Stokes, 2015).

### Parkinson Disease

Patients with PD can reduce their symptoms and improve their function with focused physical and occupational rehabilitation therapies to maintain range of motion, flexibility, proximal strength, mobility, freezing, safety, and fitness. Speech therapy can improve prosody, breath support for speaking, and intelligibility. Most trials involve outpatients, but a 4-week inpatient crossover study found that quality of life improved for at least 3 months post intervention, with possible gains in motor skills (Ferrazzoli et al., 2018) Outpatients have also been trained to increase the speed of a skilled movement such as buttoning, although with more practice than normal controls need. In another trial, twice-a-week practice for 3 months in whole-body movements such as sitting, kneeling, standing up, and throwing, along with problem solving for these activities, improved the speed of movements needed for mobility in moderately disabled PD patients. A randomized crossover study compared regular activity with 1 hour of repetitive stretching, endurance, balance, gait, and fine motor exercises in moderately disabled patients. Exercises were performed three times a week for 4 weeks, with a progressive increase in the number of repetitions. The total United Parkinson Disease Rating Scale score and the ADL and motor subscores, particularly the bradykinesia and rigidity components, significantly improved with exercise. Without an ongoing formal exercise program, these gains were lost 6 months later. Walking to auditory cues and treadmill training have lessened hypokinesia and bouts of freezing and cueing will increase stride length. Gait-specific training, compared with general exercise and no exercise, improves cadence, step length, and speed but does not lessen freezing (Ni et al., 2018).

### Multiple Sclerosis

Evaluating the impact of rehabilitation in MS presents difficulties because it is a chronic condition continuing over many decades that is variable, unpredictable, and subject to spontaneous improvement in many patients. In a disease with a clinical course up to 40 years in duration, about 50% of affected persons will use aids for walking and about 25% will require a wheelchair by 15 years after onset. Thus plenty of opportunities arise for rehabilitative interventions for specific disabilities, education, and monitoring to prevent unnecessary complications. Although physical activity and exercise training may have beneficial effects on mobility and hand function (Haselkorn et al., 2015), heterogeneity both in the magnitude and pattern of change is expected given the heterogeneity of disease course. The effect of an extended outpatient rehabilitation program on symptom frequency, fatigue, and functional status has been modest. Although not yet studied by a scientific design, a day program may include general physical fitness exercises, practice in ADLs, group recreation, gardening, and local travel to help maintain or build self-care and community skills along with psychosocial supports for clients and caregivers.

### Other Diseases

Critical illness–related polyneuropathy and myopathy associated with sepsis, organ transplantation, and prolonged disease have become a common cause of diffuse weakness, deconditioning, and disability necessitating inpatient rehabilitation. Exercise management is similar to that for patients with Guillain-Barré syndrome. As soon as feasible, these patients need to enter a milieu that encourages them to assist themselves, stay out of bed, and do light resistance exercises throughout the day. Patients are encouraged to work their arms and legs against the resistance of a stretchable rubber exercise band for 10–15 repetitions in various planes every hour, even when resting in bed, or to do isometric exercises with a family member. Nearly all patients with critical illness–induced weakness improve their strength from movement only against gravity at admission to offering resistance in proximal muscles within 3 weeks of the inpatient stay.

#### Aging with Neurological Disabilities

Aging is associated with a variety of musculoskeletal and central and peripheral nervous system changes that can worsen the impairments and disabilities of people who have had neurological diseases and injuries earlier in life. These degradations in signal processing along with relative inactivity can diminish the neural representations for skills that had been regained through rehabilitation and compensatory training and problem solving. Patients should be encouraged to maintain their fitness and strength with exercise and to practice motor and cognitive skills they wish to maintain.

## FUTURE DIRECTIONS

Well-designed clinical trials for theory-based interventions are leading to more evidence-based practices. These trials provide a solid armamentarium of therapies for specific needs and many of these training-related interventions for cognitive, sensory, and motor skills are likely to be applicable across diseases. Traditional therapies, however, are limited to making use of spared neural connections. At present, rehabilitation is less successful for more highly disabled persons, including those with minimal sensorimotor control of the hand, without movement against gravity of one or both legs for walking, with hemineglect plus hemisensorimotor loss, with no social communication skills, or with other profound impairments that markedly limit quality of life. Neurological rehabilitation must come to include biological, cellular, and molecular signaling interventions for circuit repair and activation, direct brain or spinal cord focal stimulation to excite or inhibit specific circuits, drugs that activate learning during training, and more refined exoskeletons and brain–machine interfaces that support flexible arm and leg movements across ADLs. Functional and structural imaging and genetic analysis may serve as biomarkers to help apply interventions where they can be most successful. These novel cellular, molecular, physiological, and engineered strategies will aim to augment rehabilitation training from onset of pathology and throughout life.

*The complete reference list is available online at https://expertconsult.inkling.com/.* 

# Transition to Adult Care for Youth with Chronic Neurological Disorders

*Peter Camfield, Carol Camfield*

## OUTLINE



Youth with chronic neurological disorders eventually need to move to adult health care. Transition is a process beginning in early adolescence to help these youth to be successful in managing their disorder in adulthood. Transfer is the process of passing responsibility for health care from a pediatric to adult healthcare provider. This chapter reviews the goals of transition and why the process may be difficult. Listed are special issues that may be encountered in transition/transfer for youth with chronic neurological disorders. The evidence for the value of transition programs is reviewed along with current guidelines for transition/transfer programs. Current models for transition/transfer programs are described with the caveat that the evidence base for these programs is somewhat limited.

Most children with chronic neurological disorders become adults with chronic neurological disorders. As treatments in pediatrics have improved, many who previously died in childhood now live well into adulthood. For example, prior to steroids and ventilatory support, boys with Duchenne muscular dystrophy died by the end of the teenage years but now, on average, they survive into the their 40s. As adolescence comes to an end, youth with neurological disorders move from pediatric to adult care. While this seems like a simple process, it is often complex and anxiety provoking for the patient, family, and healthcare system.

The move from pediatric to adult care ideally involves two concepts—transition and transfer, terms that are often used interchangeably but have different connotations. "'Transition' is the purposeful, planned process that addresses the medical, psychosocial, and educational/vocational needs of adolescents and young adults with long-term conditions as they move from child-centered to adult-oriented healthcare systems (Blum, 1993). Transition should begin in early adolescence and continue after transfer. 'Transfer' is the formal event when the health care of a young person moves from children's to adults' services" (Blum, 1993). Transfer is usually at an age determined arbitrarily by the healthcare system and rarely is based on the developmental stage and abilities of the patient or needs of the family.

The goals of transition are at minimum threefold (Nandakumar et al., 2018). First, educate youth at a level that they can understand about their disorder and its clinical course and treatment. Youth need to learn to become skilled in managing all aspects of their disorder with good adherence to medication and treatment protocols. They need to learn how to explain their personal healthcare concerns to adult healthcare providers, their peers, and other community members. Second, patients need to learn about and accept lifestyle changes that are imposed by their illness. For example, youth with uncontrolled epilepsy are not permitted to drive automobiles and their alcohol consumption should be modest. Third, transition/transfer programs need to initiate and, if possible, cement an ongoing relationship between the young person with a chronic neurological disorder and their adult care team.

## WHY IS TRANSITION SOMETIMES DIFFICULT?

There are several reasons why the goals of transition may be complicated to achieve. Pediatric care is very family-centered: children are accompanied to healthcare visits by their parents and a great deal of the visit may be devoted to parental issues. Adult care is typically focused on the individual. The patient sees the adult physician by him/herself and communication with the family is expected to happen separately by the patient. Children with chronic neurological disease are often physically and emotionally dependent on their parents, rarely attend pediatric visits by themselves, and may not be encouraged to explain their medical or social problems to healthcare workers—it is easier and quicker to ask the parents to do the communication, since they always have. The neurological disorder may have been explained to the parents long before the child could understand, and the explanation not repeated as the child approaches adulthood. The relationship between pediatric specialists and families of children with chronic neurological disorders has often spanned more than a decade and is close and trusting. Parents and pediatricians are reluctant to change. We suspect that the greater the complexity of the pediatric disorder, the greater is parental anxiety about transfer to adult care. In addition, many youth with neurological disorders have multiple healthcare problems that have been cared for in a multidisciplinary clinic—a model of care that is uncommon in adult medicine.

Intellectual disability (ID) accompanies many pediatric neurological disorders and adds additional complexity to transition/transfer. Adult physicians may be uncomfortable with ID, their offices and waiting rooms too small or unsatisfactory in other ways for a large adolescent with ID accompanied by several caregivers. The youth with ID may be loud and intimidating to others in the waiting room and too heavy to lift onto an examining table. A Delphi study of 134 general internists in the United States identified 8 adult physician concerns:

lack of training in congenital and childhood-onset conditions, lack of family involvement, difficulty meeting patients' psychosocial needs, need for a super specialist for complex disorders such as congenital heart disease, lack of adolescent training, facing disability/end-of-life issues shortly after transfer, financial pressures limiting visit time, and families' high expectations (Peter et al., 2009).

The transfer to adult care means a change for the entire family and the model of multidisciplinary care is uncommon—health care is likely to become fragmented with multiple appointments in different settings with adult specialists who may have little experience or knowledge with the young person's specific disorder. Pediatricians may have communicated to the family their doubt about the ability of the adult care system to offer comprehensive care, while adult physicians may view pediatric care as smothering and overindulgent.

Transition preparation and transfer occur during important stages of social and emotional development of adolescents when mature peer relationships, personal identity, and sense of life goals are cemented. Youth with chronic neurological disease are often unable to become completely independent. Their sense of self-identity and self-worth are likely to be disrupted along with poor development of close peer relationships. Normal stages of sexual development are difficult to achieve when the youth is dependent on others for much of their care. Milestones of independence may be hard to achieve, especially driving, which may be curtailed because of epilepsy, physical disability, or cognitive problems.

## WHAT HAPPENS WITHOUT A TRANSITION PROGRAM?

It is tempting to dismiss the above concerns and simply expect that the patient and family will eventually adapt to adult care. While there are limited systematic studies of the value of transition programs, there are a few that strongly indicate that poor transition leads to poor adult health outcomes. The most poignant examples come from experiences of youth who have had kidney transplants and then been transferred to adult care. A UK study found that between 2000 and 2006, of nine youth simply transferred to adult care, six rejected their graft shortly after transfer and had to go back on dialysis (Harden et al., 2012). Presumably these "disasters" were the result of poor adherence to anti-rejection medications. Following the introduction of a transition program, there were no lost grafts in the next 12 patients. A similar result was noted in British Columbia where it was possible to show that the cost of an extensive transition program was considerably less than the cost of a few patients going back onto dialysis (Prestidge, 2012).

For youth with juvenile diabetes, poor control of serum glucose leads directly to many adult health problems including loss of vision and cardiovascular disease. A meta-analysis in 2017 identified 18 controlled trials about transition involving 3382 youth with type 1 diabetes (Schultz and Smaldone, 2017). Even though Hemoglobin A1c (HgA1c) levels (a marker of overall glucose levels) remained unchanged, there were consistent findings that transition programs lead to fewer episodes of ketoacidosis and hypoglycemia.

It is possible to speculate about the effect of poor transition/transfer programs for youth with neurological disorders. Examples might be epilepsy, attention deficit disorder (ADD), and cerebral palsy. For those with epilepsy, poor medication compliance would lead to more frequent seizures, episodes of status epilepticus, emergency room visits and hospitalizations, and sudden unexpected death (SUDEP; Nabbout et al., 2019). Those without contact with adult epilepsy services would be unlikely to use newer treatments and might not be considered for epilepsy surgery. For patients with ADD, poor compliance might lead to more automobile accidents, higher rates of unemployment,

**TABLE 56.1 NICE Guidelines for Generic Transition Programs**

| |
|---|
| Age-banded clinic |
| Meet adult team before transfer |
| Promotion of health self-efficacy |
| Written transition plan |
| Appropriate parental involvement |
| Key transition worker for each person |
| Coordinated healthcare team |
| Holistic life skills training |
| Transition manager for clinical team |

*National Institute for Health and Care Excellence (NICE), 2016. Transition from Children's to Adults' Services for Young People Using Health or Social Care Services, Guideline 43. London: National Institute for Health and Care Excellence (NICE),. https://www.nice.org.uk/guidance/ng43/evidence/full-guideline-pdf-2360240173 (accessed February 17, 2019.)*

and more sexual misadventure (Barkley et al., 2006). For those with cerebral palsy, poor attendance at rehabilitation sessions could lead to decreased ambulation.

There are no randomized controlled trials that establish the value of transition programs for chronic neurological disorders. In order to justify the "extra" expenses involved in transition programs, there is a strong need for systematic studies that examine health outcomes and costs (Nabbout et al., 2019).

## GUIDELINES FOR TRANSITION PROGRAMS

A variety of guidelines have suggested the essential elements of transition/transfer programs. None of these guidelines are strongly evidence based; however, this is a field where randomized clinical trials are few and extremely difficult to carry out (Wright et al., 2018). We outline three of these guidelines—they each have different emphases and some communality.

The National Institute for Health and Care Excellence (NICE) guidelines suggested nine key elements for transition (Table 56.1; NICE, 2016). A very helpful study from the UK prospectively evaluated these elements by studying 374 intellectually normal youth with chronic illness (150 with type 1 diabetes, 106 with cerebral palsy, and 118 with autism spectrum disorder with an associated mental health problem) (Colver et al., 2018). Following transfer to adult care, the investigators assessed the participants once/year for the following 3 years using a mixture of personal interviews and standardized questionnaires. Only three of the nine NICE items were associated with satisfactory transition, assessed with "measures of satisfaction with services, mental wellbeing, participation and autonomy in appointments." The three key items were appropriate parental involvement, promotion of health self-efficacy, and meeting the adult team before transfer. Appropriate parental involvement was evaluated simply by asking parents and youth separately if they thought that their level of involvement was appropriate. The concept of "involvement" considered if the parent attended a typical clinic visit and if the youth or parent did most of the talking. Promotion of health self-efficacy was assessed in several ways but most directly by the youth answering the question "Have you received enough help to increase your confidence in managing your condition?" Meeting the adult team before transfer could be in a joint clinic with both pediatric and adult healthcare professionals, an appointment with the adult physician in the pediatric center, or an appointment in the adult clinic. For each of these the youth would be accompanied by a key worker from the pediatric

**TABLE 56.2 Child Neurology Foundation Eight Best Practices for Transition**

1. Discuss with the youth and family before the youth's 13-year-old birthday, the expectation of future transition to the adult care system.
2. Assess by age 12 years of age, self-management skills and re-evaluate these on a yearly basis.
3. Yearly transition planning sessions should address the youth's medical condition including current medications and potential side effects; signs and symptoms of concern; genetic counseling and reproductive implications of the condition; issues of puberty and sexuality; driving, alcohol, substance use and other risks; and emotional or psychological concerns and wellness.
4. If appropriate, beginning by 14 years of age, discuss with caregivers the youth's expected legal competency (possible need for legal guardianship and powers of attorney). If the youth's expected legal competency is unclear, assessment of that capacity should be made yearly.
5. A comprehensive transition plan should be developed by age 14 in collaboration with the youth, caregivers, healthcare providers, school personnel, vocational professionals, community services providers, and legal services regarding all aspects of health, financial, and legal care. This is usually the responsibility of the primary care provider.
6. The child neurology team is responsible for the neurological component of the comprehensive transition plan and should update it annually.
7. Adult providers should be identified in collaboration with the youth and caregivers prior to the anticipated time of transfer. A medical transfer packet needs to be prepared for the adult provider and provided to the youth; it includes the transition plan and medical summary with pertinent history, diagnostic evaluations, previous drug trials, current medications, and protocol for emergency care.
8. The child neurology team should communicate directly with the new adult provider to ensure smooth completion of the transition process, which is finalized after the first appointment. It is recommended that the child neurologist be available both to the youth and the adult provider for continuity and support.

*Brown, L.W., Camfield, P., Capers, M., et al., 2016. The neurologist's role in supporting transition to adult health care: a consensus statement. Neurology 87, 835–840.*

clinic. The findings of this study suggest key features for any transition program.

The Child Neurology Foundation developed a position statement about principles for transition for youth with neurological problems (Table 56.2; Brown et al., 2016). This position statement was endorsed by the Child Neurology Society, the American Academy of Neurology, and the American Academy of Pediatrics. The eight principles were based on a literature review and the opinions of a wide variety of "stake holders." One of the complex issues considered is the responsibility/role of the pediatric neurologist for transition for patients with complex, multidisciplinary problems. It is suggested that the primary care physician is most responsible to assemble the group of adult specialists who are required.

An Ontario, Canada, task force involved a very wide variety of interested parties and developed an approach for transition for youth with epilepsy (Table 56.3; Andrade et al., 2017). This guideline points out the importance of re-evaluation of the youth's disease prior to transfer.

Two large Delphi studies have attempted to define key elements for transition programs for youth with chronic illness, regardless of the disease (Fair et al., 2016; Suris and Akre, 2015). Table 56.4 compares many of the recommendations of the NICE, Child Neurology, Ontario, and the Delphi studies.

**TABLE 56.3 Ontario Seven Steps for Transition for Youth with Epilepsy**

Step 1 (Ages 12–15 years): Introduce the concept of transition
Step 2 (Ages 12–17 years): Explore financial, community, and legal support
Step 3 (Ages 16–17 years): Determine transition readiness of patients and parents
Step 4A (Ages 12–19 years): Identify and address risk factors for unsuccessful transition in adolescents with epilepsy and normal intellect
Step 4B (Ages 12–17 years): Identify and address risk factors for unsuccessful transition in adolescents with epilepsy and intellectual disability
Step 5 (Ages 16–19 years): Re-evaluate the epilepsy diagnosis
Step 6 (Ages 16–17 years): Identify obstacles for continuing treatment of drug-resistant epilepsies
Step 7 (Ages 17–18 years): Prepare the Pediatric Discharge Package

*Andrade, D.M., Bassett, A.S., Bercovici, E., et al., 2017. Epilepsy: transition from pediatric to adult care. Recommendations of the Ontario epilepsy implementation task force. Epilepsia 58, 1502–1517.*

## Special Issues for Transition for Neurological Problems

There are many special challenges for the transition of youth with neurological problems. Many of these are outlined below with one or two examples offered in each category.

1. Concomitant intellectual disability (ID)
   ID is associated with many pediatric neurological disorders and completely changes the nature of transition. While people who work with patients with ID hope to make them become independent, there are limits and adult supervision will nearly always be necessary. It is unreasonable to expect that those with ID will entirely assume responsibility for and control of their healthcare needs. With ID, it is parents and caregivers who need to "adapt" to the adult healthcare model. The majority of youth with ID are still living with their parents in mid-adulthood (Gray et al., 2014). These parents know the evolution of their child's disorder and are able to communicate any significant change. Eventually many with ID end up in institutional care, and there is a real hazard that no one will know the early diagnoses and clinical course. The net effect for the adult neurologist is that the patient with ID may be accompanied by a caretaker who does not know the patient well and is unable to compare the current situation with the past. This is most unfortunate as new treatments emerge. Bigby in Australia coined the term "well known by no one" (Bigby, 2008). She followed patients with ID from a large institution who were placed in small options community centers. Their parents aged or died, their siblings moved away or lost interest, and there was a high turnover in staff at the small centers. Within a few years no one knew much about these patients—they were "well known by no one." Finding a way to avoid this sad evolution is important for the process of transition/transfer for patients with ID.
2. Unusual, rare neurological disorders
   Many youth who transition to adult care have rare neurological disorders with complex evolutions and treatments. As an example, children with alternating hemiplegia may have partial control of their movement disorder with medications such as flunarizine, a calcium channel blocker not likely familiar to the adult neurologist. Patients may then develop epilepsy in adulthood with attacks that may be difficult to distinguish from their movement disorder. To offer appropriate care, the adult neurologist will need detailed knowledge of the adult manifestations of alternating hemiplegia. The patient with a

**TABLE 56.4 Key Components for Transition Programs**

| | CNF* | NICE Guidelines† | Delphi 2015‡ | Delphi 2016§ | Ontario Guideline¶¶ | UK Follow-Up Study¶ |
|---|---|---|---|---|---|---|
| Age-banded clinic | | X | | | | |
| Meeting adult team before transfer | | X | | | | X |
| Promotion of health self-efficacy | X | X | X | X | | X |
| Written pediatric transition program, including transfer summary | X | X | X | | X | |
| Appropriate parental involvement | | X | X | | | X |
| Key transition worker | | X | X | | | |
| Coordinated heathcare team | X | X | | | | |
| Holistic life skills training | | X | | X | | |
| Transition manager | | X | X | | | |
| Start transition program at early age | X | | X | | | |
| Seeing patient alone | | | X | | | |
| Identifying adult provider | X | | X | | | |
| Ensuring that first appointment takes place | | | X | | | |
| Informing primary healthcare providers | X | | X | | | |
| Assessing risk behaviors | X | | X | | X | |
| Understanding characteristics of conditions and complications | X | | | X | X | |
| Adhering to medications and/or other treatment | X | | | X | | |
| Attending most medical appointments | | | | X | | |
| Having a medical (health) home | X | | | X | | |
| Avoiding unnecessary hospitalizations | | | | X | | |
| Understanding health insurance options and community supports | X | | | X | X | |
| Having a social network of friends | | | | X | | |
| Rethink diagnosis and reinvestigate, if appropriate, prior to transfer | | | | | X | |
| Identify obstacles for patients with drug resistant epilepsy | | | | | X | |

*CNF*, Child Neurology Foundation; *NICE*, National Institute for Health and Care Excellence.

**Brown, L.W., Camfield, P., Capers, M., et al., 2016. The neurologist's role in supporting transition to adult health care: a consensus statement. Neurology 87, 835–840.*

*†National Institute for Health and Care Excellence (NICE), 2016. Transition from Children's to Adults' Services for Young People Using Health or Social Care Services, Guideline 43. London: National Institute for Health and Care Excellence (NICE). https://www.nice.org.uk/guidance/ng43/evidence/full-guideline-pdf-2360240173 (accessed February 17, 2019.)*

*‡Suris, J.C., Akre, C., 2015. Key elements for, and indicators of, a successful transition: an international Delphi study. J Adolesc Health 56, 612–618.*

*§Fair, C., Cuttance, J., Sharma, N., et al., & International and Interdisciplinary Health Care Transition Research Consortium. International and interdisciplinary identification of health care transition outcomes. JAMA Pediatr 170, 205–211.*

*¶¶Andrade, D.M., Bassett, A.S., Bercovici, E., et al., 2017. Epilepsy: transition from pediatric to adult care. Recommendations of the Ontario epilepsy implementation task force. Epilepsia 58, 1502–1517.*

*¶Colver, A., McConachie, H., Le Couteur, A., et al., 2018. Transition Collaborative Group. A longitudinal, observational study of the features of transitional healthcare associated with better outcomes for young people with long-term conditions. BMC Med 16, 111.*

*Adapted from Camfield, P.R., Andrade, D., Camfield, C.S., et al., 2019. How can transition to adult care be best orchestrated for adolescents with epilepsy? Epilepsy Behav 93, 138–147.*

rare neurological disorder and their family who have been through a thorough transition program should understand and be able to communicate the expected evolution of the disorder. They should be well connected to disease support groups so that they can learn about and request new treatments. For example, the gene defect for alternating hemiplegia has been known for several years and it is reasonable to expect that new therapies will emerge.

3. Disorders that evolve in adult life in an unexpected way

Children with some benign familial infantile seizure disorders have remission from their seizures very early in life and yet years later in adulthood develop significant movement disorders that should lead to a neurological assessment. Familiarity with the early diagnosis and an awareness of its evolution should lead to better care. Lennox-Gastaut syndrome in childhood is defined by tonic seizures during sleep, other seizure types, and an interictal Electroencephalogram (EEG) showing slow spike and wave plus bursts of generalized, low-voltage fast activity. In adulthood, the EEG features vanish and the tonic seizures in sleep are difficult to recognize. But treatment with specific medications may still be valuable. Most of these patients have ID, but their parents and other caretakers can carry with them the original correct diagnosis of Lennox-Gastaut syndrome and its expected evolution.

4. Fragile problems that may deteriorate suddenly—metabolic disease
Increasingly, children with metabolic disorders live on into adulthood. Many of these patients have metabolic crises that are lethal if not treated appropriately. For example, boys with ornithine transcarbamylase deficiency have intermittent severe hyperammonemia crises, often precipitated by minor infections. Prompt intensive intervention may be lifesaving. Knowing the impending symptoms and what treatment works best for this young person is critical for adult care. The patient and family need to very vigilant and their ability to communicate the issues in an adult emergency room are important issues to deal with in a transition program.
5. Drugs and treatments that are unfamiliar to adult neurology
Dravet syndrome is an example of a pediatric disorder that is increasingly treated successfully with medications that are unlikely to be familiar to adult neurologists. Stiripentol has a synergistic effect with valproic acid and clobazam. Both cannabidiol and fluphenazine have recently been shown to be effective. Youth with Dravet syndrome will arrive at the doors of adult care with these medications—a good transition program will be needed to be sure that optimal care continues.
Dietary therapy for childhood neurological disorders is not uncommon. Epilepsy and glucose transmitter disorders are treated with the ketogenic diet. Phenylketonuria is managed with a complex low phenylalanine diet and many metabolic disorders have special dietary restrictions. There are very few adult diet treatment centers and few adult dietitians familiar with these special diets.
6. Disorders that were previously lethal in childhood but now have treatment
The adult evolution of these "new" disorders is completely unknown. An example is early-onset spinal muscular atrophy that was previously nearly always lethal by age 2 years. With intrathecal nusinersen treatment, some of these children are close to normal at age 2–4 years and presumably will continue to respond. Their adult care needs are completely unknown.
7. Disorders that require lifelong care but are relatively easily managed
ADD is typically diagnosed in childhood and usually responds to stimulant medication. Perhaps half of these patients continue with ADD in adult life with problems especially related to impulsiveness, including traffic accidents, unplanned pregnancies, and substance abuse. Transition programs need to emphasize the need for lifelong treatment and adult care needs to be more comprehensive than just a series of prescriptions.
8. Disorders that start in childhood but often have their most serious manifestations in adulthood
Neurofibromatosis is often diagnosed in childhood with few manifestations—perhaps mild cognitive problems only. Yet, in adulthood early strokes and a variety of cancers may develop. Tuberous sclerosis is another example which may present in childhood with difficult to control epilepsy, but in adulthood severe hypertension and renal failure may dominate the clinical problems.
9. Disorders that may remit leaving serious comorbidities
A variety of pediatric neurological disorders will have remission of their cardinal symptoms but persistence of comorbidities. Childhood absence epilepsy is a good example. Absence seizures remit in the majority in relatively early childhood, yet the adult social outcome is often very unsatisfactory, possibly in part related to poor treatment of associated ADD. Another example is the brain tumor that may be successfully treated in childhood but leaving the patient with long-term cognitive problems and a social outcome that is less successful than sibling controls. Finding appropriate adult care for these patients may be challenging because the primary neurological diagnosis has vanished.
10. Disorders that benefit from multidisciplinary care
Children with cerebral palsy are often treated in pediatric multidisciplinary clinics that include, amongst others, neurologists, rehabilitation physicians, orthopedic experts, physiotherapists, speech and language pathologists, occupational therapists, therapeutic dietitians, and social workers. In adult care such coordinated clinics are unusual, yet there is evidence that gait problems increase in adulthood.

## HOW IS TRANSITION BEST ORCHESTRATED?

The process of transition should ideally begin several years before the time of transfer—most authors suggest that it should start by age 11–13 years. Many centers use a generic program that applies potentially to all children with chronic illness. Two examples are ReadySteadyGo from the UK and Good2Go from Canada (ReadySteadyGo, 2019; Good2Go, 2019). These programs have a "core" curriculum that encourages children and adolescents with chronic disease to learn about their disease, incrementally take responsibility for their own health care, and develop a sense of how to advance their own self-advocacy. The Good2Go program includes a "MyHealthPassport," a wallet-sized summary of their illness (diagnosis and treatment) prepared by the youth and assisted by the healthcare team (MyHealthPassport, 2019). The ReadySteadyGo program includes five steps that begin at about age 11 years and are completed at the time of the first adult clinic visit. Each step begins with a short questionnaire which helps to identify subjects that need to be addressed. Both of these programs use a "ready for transition" questionnaire to help the youth and professionals to know if this young person is prepared for adult care. There are a number of other transition readiness questionnaires available such as the TRAC questionnaire (Wood, 2014), which has 20 questions in five categories—managing medications, appointment keeping, tracking health issues, talking with providers, and managing daily activities. Some centers have added disease-specific modules to these generic transition programs.

### Transfer

Eventually the young person needs to move on to adult care, often at an age that is determined administratively, rather than by readiness. There are three important steps just prior to transfer. First, the diagnosis needs to be as definite and precise as possible. Many patients have an etiological diagnosis defined by an initial evaluation which has not been updated for many years before transfer. New developments in genetics and imaging may lead to a different or refined diagnosis with implications for treatment in adulthood. Some of these investigations are best carried out in the pediatric center. For example, sedation for an magnetic resonance imaging (MRI) scan for patients with ID is routine in a pediatric center but difficult to arrange in an adult hospital. We suspect that genetic evaluations are currently often more familiar to pediatric neurologists than their adult counterparts. In addition to treatment issues, a precise diagnosis may end the diagnostic "odyssey" for families.

Secondly, the pediatric service needs to generate a detailed summary of the diagnostic workup, clinical course, and past treatment. Medical and social factors should be included. Details of such a summary for epilepsy have been published (Camfield et al., 2012). Preparation of this summary is time consuming and may not be adequately remunerated, but it is essential for ongoing care. The summary should be given to the adult service and a copy presented to and reviewed with the patient and family.

Next, an appropriate adult service needs to be identified that is willing to accept the patient for long-term care. The actual "hand off" may take place in several ways as outlined below, although we suspect that a simple referral note with the detailed summary is the most common form of transfer, an approach that is probably suboptimal. Some form of formal transition/transfer clinic is likely to most effective.

Thirdly, is a key issue—the identification of a "medical home." Many youth with chronic neurological problems are cared for by several pediatric specialty services. Pediatric neurologists may provide more than strictly neurological care and multidisciplinary clinics provide well-coordinated care. The model of care in adult neurology is more likely to have a more neurological focus and coordination of care between services is less common than in pediatrics. A primary care provider who is willing to coordinate the adult care is essential. It is not always easy to find such a person who is willing to be the "quarterback" and also be trusted by the patient and family. Because pediatric neurology services often provide extensive non-neurological care, the young person's primary care physician has played a minor role in care through the childhood years, and therefore may not be knowledgeable about the specific illness. Bringing the primary care physician into the center of care should be accomplished before transfer to adult specialty services. Pediatric neurologists need to be sure that transfer to adult care includes transfer to each of the appropriate adult services for comprehensive care.

Transition clinics exist for many specific neurological disorders—epilepsy provides several examples, although none has been extensively evaluated (Camfield et al., 2019). A first group of models involves a joint pediatric–adult epilepsy clinic attended simultaneously by a pediatric neurologist, adult epileptologist, and an adult epilepsy nurse specialist (Appleton et al., 1997; Camfield et al., 2019). Patients and caregivers are seen several times in this clinic to be sure that they have developed sufficient knowledge, communication, and disease management skills to cope successfully with the adult epilepsy service. A major advantage of this type of clinic is reassurance to all that information about the child's epilepsy is fully communicated to the adult service. A practical problem may be reimbursement when a patient is seen at the same time by both the pediatric and adult neurologists. Nonetheless, we are of the opinion that such clinics provide the best care.

A second, compelling model is entirely run by epilepsy nurse specialists (Jurasek et al., 2010). The adult and pediatric nurse specialists meet jointly with parents and the patient and over a series of visits ensure good knowledge about a wide variety of topics related to living with epilepsy. Then the patient moves on to the adult epilepsy service with the adult epilepsy nurse providing continuity. This program yields a great deal of patient and parent satisfaction.

A third model provides a series of services to youth with epilepsy that they access independently without their parents—"La Suite" (Camfield et al., 2019). Services include social work, sport coach, educators, make up specialists, hairdressers, as well as special medical clinics such as dermatology, primary care physicians (community care), gynecology, endocrinology, occupational and physiotherapy, and nutrition.

### Reality Check

All transition/transfer programs described to date have been developed and implemented within major academic centers. While the principles of transition should be universal, they may be much easier to implement in larger centers. It is unclear how practical these concepts are in the setting of the private practice of a solitary pediatric or adult neurologist.

While the need for transition/transfer programs is compelling, very little data have been generated to date to demonstrate their effectiveness in achieving the overall goal of care for young people with a chronic neurological disorder that leads to an independent adulthood with a successful and fulfilling life.

## CONCLUSION

If a neurological problem is likely to persist into adulthood, some form of transition program and a well-orchestrated transfer program is indicated. Transition programs may be generic or disease specific. Transfer includes a detailed summary of the pediatric course of the disorder and a clear identification of the appropriate adult healthcare providers. A joint pediatric/adult transition clinic may be the most effective model. More comprehensive evaluation of transition programs is needed to make them more captivating for funding agencies.

*The complete reference list is available online at https://expertconsult.inkling.com/.* 

57

# Palliative and End-of-Life Care in Neurological Disease

*Maisha T. Robinson, Claire J. Creutzfeldt*

## OUTLINE



## INTRODUCTION

Neuropalliative care represents both a growing subspecialty among neurologists as well as a set of palliative care skills that are relevant to all clinicians caring for patients with serious, chronic, advanced, or terminal neurological diseases (Brizzi and Creutzfeldt, 2018; Creutzfeldt et al., 2016; Dallara and Tolchin, 2014; Robinson and Barrett, 2014). Patients with neurological disease have high symptom burden, experience functional and cognitive disability, and typically a decline over time, as well as significant caregiver needs. Palliative medicine is a specialty that focuses on maximizing quality of life through timely and careful assessment and alleviation of symptoms and other sources of suffering, conversations around goals of care, and caregiver support. Incorporating a palliative approach to care in the management of patients with a variety of neurological conditions promotes patient- and family-centered care that aligns with their goals.

## COMMUNICATING DIFFICULT NEWS

Clear and effective communication is a cornerstone of high-quality care and a prerequisite for developing a trusting patient–physician relationship. Skilled and compassionate communication can ease the burden of a symptom or diagnosis and make a challenging situation more manageable (Barnett, 2002). Neurologists come into their profession with a wide variety of communication skills. As we consider the biomedical and physiological as well as the psychosocial effects of an illness on the patient and their families, it is important that we consider a set of basic tools for all clinicians (Table 57.1).

As neurologists accompany patients and their families on a journey, that in some cases may last only hours to days after a catastrophic illness, and in other cases years and even decades, the expectations are rarely for a cure. Instead, a variety of challenges may occur such as increasing symptom burden and disability, changing social roles, loss of personhood, and struggles with finding meaning and hope in the face of prognostic uncertainty. Patients and their families will need to consider their values in the setting of the neurological disease and plan for what may happen in the future. Serious illness conversations are necessary at various time points along this journey to ensure correct information exchange, trust building, and, most importantly, that patients receive medical care that matches their values. Multiple professional societies, including the American Academy of Neurology (AAN) and the Accreditation Council for Graduate Medical Education (ACGME), emphasize communication with patients and families as key components and milestones of neurology training, yet few neurologists receive formal training during residency (Creutzfeldt et al., 2009; Lemmon and Strowd, 2016). One sign of inadequate communication is the lack of advance care planning for patients with neurological diseases; for example, recent studies suggest that only one in five patients with advanced dementia and less than half of well, able stroke survivors have advance directives (Johnson et al., 2019; Sleeman et al., 2013). Even though we know that timely, honest, and iterative serious illness conversations improve patient and family quality of life (Detering et al., 2010; Temel et al., 2010), it is rarely, if ever, easy to have them. Barriers to these conversations include deficits in skills and knowledge, time constraints, and discomfort as well as a feeling that giving bad news diminishes hope or could end a trusting patient–physician relationship (Lakin et al., 2016). Research and practice, however, suggest that these skills can be learned, and clinicians' comfort levels can substantially increase (Arnold et al., 2015; Back et al., 2007); that these conversations do not need to be long, can be divided up, and may allow for additional billing codes (CMS, 2016); and that early, skilled conversations about prognosis reduce anxiety, improve quality of life, and can strengthen relationships with providers (Curtis et al., 2001; Lautrette et al., 2007). Knowing better (a) when and (b) how to have these conversations will enhance the patient and family experience of care as well as the work life of healthcare clinicians.

### a. Serious Illness Conversation Triggers

During the course of a serious illness, expected and unexpected events occur that may serve as a signpost for providers, but also for patients

**TABLE 57.1 Basic Communication Skills**

| | |
|---|---|
| Authentic and active listening | Communicate with empathy and compassion |
| Narrative competence to elicit the patient's story | Communicate prognosis for quantity and quality of life |
| Effectively elicit individual treatment goals and engage in shared decision making | Effectively share information with the patient and family using terms they understand |

**TABLE 57.2 Serious Illness Conversation Triggers**

**General**

*Proactive* with every diagnosis; "Surprise Question": would you be surprised if the patient died within the next year?

*Reactive* to concerns raised by patient or family about their quality of life, appropriateness of care, or caregiver strain

*Reactive* to a previously agreed on time-limited trial (Quill and Holloway, 2011)

**A New Event or Intervention (*proactive* when event is anticipated, *reactive* when it is occurring)**

Any hospitalization—*proactive* (this is a "captive audience") or *reactive* (this hospitalization may present a complication of the underlying illness or a "next stage" on the disease trajectory)

Need for a change in treatment: for example, switching a chemotherapy agent or considering artificial nutrition

Actual or anticipated change in living situation (increased assistance at home, move to assisted living or Skilled Nursing Facility)

**A New Loss**

Loss of ability to work, loss of ability to drive (or concerns with driving), loss of mobility (as indicated by falls or a need for assistive device), loss of independence (as indicated by needing assistance with dressing, meals, toileting, or bathing)

**A New Symptom**

New behavioral symptom, such as anger, social withdrawal, hallucinations, wandering

Sleeping more than 16 h/day

and their families if appropriately prepared, to consider a new or repeated conversation about the "status quo" in terms of their disease, their treatment, and their goals for next steps. Such a trigger may also serve as a prompt to consider a referral to a palliative care specialist, depending on the specific needs of the patient and family, the skillset of the primary team, and the local resources available. Examples of such triggers are listed in Table 57.2. In addition to these triggers, setting up routine times to revisit such conversations should be considered. Ample examples exist in clinical practice where opportunities for serious illness conversations were missed and discussions around life and death had to be held in a crisis situation, when the patient was unable to participate and a trusted clinician was not available.

## b. Serious Illness Conversation Skills

Serious illness communication invariably occurs at many levels, including a cognitive and an affective (emotional) level. Delivering serious news therefore requires a delicate balance of compassionate information delivery and attention to emotions. The theory is that when emotions are not brought to the surface by acknowledging or supporting them, the patient's ability to absorb any more information is restricted. Sometimes, emotions hide behind a cognitive statement. For example,

**TABLE 57.3 Responding to Emotions**

| | |
|---|---|
| Name | I can see that this is very...; People often feel ... in this situation |
| Understand | I can only imagine how ... this must be |
| Respect | I am so impressed by your commitment to your mother |
| Support | We will work through this together |
| Explore | Tell me more; tell me what's going through your mind |

*Back, A., Arnold, R.M., Tulsky, J.A., 2009. Mastering Communication with Seriously Ill Patients Balancing Honesty with Empathy and Hope. Cambridge University Press, Cambridge, England; New York, p. 1 online resource (x, 158 pages).*

**TABLE 57.4 Key Considerations During Clinic Visits With Patients With Serious Neurological Diseases**

**Information regarding the disease**
- What does this mean for the patient? For the family?

**Symptom management**
- What are the common symptoms that may arise? What are options for treatments?

**Mood and coping**
- Monitor for adjustment and mood disorders
- Encourage a support system

**Progression of disease and prognostication**
- What is the typical trajectory of this disease?

**Advance care planning**
- Living will, healthcare surrogate, residential plan, estate/financial planning

telling a patient he or she has amyotrophic lateral sclerosis (ALS) may elicit an immediate question "How long do I have?" or "How can you be so sure?" While the cognitive answer to this question may need to be addressed in some way during this conversation, the emotions in this question need to be considered first: "I know this was not what we had been hoping for" (see Table 57.3 for other examples). The following 5-step roadmap can be used when conducting a serious illness conversation and has been adapted from a variety of valuable resources (Back et al., 2007) and at www.vitaltalk.org.

1. Prepare: Before going in to a meeting, the clinician should take a moment to "get ready" by asking what this news will mean to the patient or family and who needs to hear it: Is the patient alone? Are the people the patient would want in the room—family members, faith representatives, friends? What needs to be considered during this conversation (Table 57.4)? Preparing also means having a place that is quiet and where everyone can sit down.
2. Assess: Before giving information, it is important to "know the audience" and to ensure that all participants in the room, even if it is just the clinician and the patient, are on the same page. Ask the patient/family what they have heard already. This not only allows them to tell their story the way they understand it but also helps the actively listening clinician understand their coping strategies and their emotional state and then calibrate the information given in the next step.
3. Inform: Tell the news in one simple sentence. Short and concise is usually better than long-winded and should be followed by a pause that allows step 4.
4. Expect and Respond: Sensitive diagnostic acumen is needed to read and recognize an emotion. Examples of how to respond to patients'

or families' emotional cues are listed in Table 57.3. Steps 3 and 4 will often be repeated as more detail is desired. Sometimes, it can be helpful to ask the patient's permission to provide more detail. Not everyone needs or desires the same amount of information.

5. Ask: The final "Ask" allows the clinician to ensure that the patient/family understood. One way to gage a patient's understanding might be to ask how he or she will be explaining all of this to family members after leaving this meeting.

## INCORPORATING PALLIATIVE CARE INTO SPECIFIC DISEASE CATEGORIES

### Demyelinating Disease/Autoimmune

Multiple sclerosis (MS) is the most common demyelinating disease and can lead to chronic disability through an often protracted course of disease. Functional challenges due to limited mobility, bowel and bladder dysfunction, pain, and spasticity impact quality of life (Borreani et al., 2014). One of the most significant symptoms that affects a majority of patients with MS is fatigue (Brenner and Piehl, 2016; Miller and Soundy, 2017). The management involves pharmacological and nonpharmacological approaches with aerobic, resistance, and endurance training. Yoga and intentional energy conservation and fatigue management interventions also have demonstrated efficacy in improving fatigue; amantadine and modafinil may be beneficial (Miller and Soundy, 2017). In addition to the physical symptoms, psychological suffering due to social isolation, depression, and anxiety is common (Borreani, et al., 2014; Figved et al., 2005), as are sleep disturbances (Bamer et al., 2008; Marrie et al., 2015). These symptoms can negatively contribute to overall well-being and can increase the risk of suicide (Brenner and Piehl, 2016). Therefore supportive care for these primarily younger individuals with MS is needed in parallel with disease-modifying therapies.

The ideal timing of palliative care intervention in MS is unclear but opportunities exist for both generalized palliative care and specialized palliative care. Specific times along the course of disease that may be appropriate for palliative care integration include when progressive and disabling disease requires consideration of a change in residential location, when pain and other symptoms emerge, and when discussions about advance care planning are needed (Strupp et al., 2014). Patients with advanced MS desire prognostic information from their physicians (Buecken et al., 2012). Destigmatization of palliative care and increased education about palliative care services may increase palliative care consultations in this patient population (Strupp, et al., 2014).

Neuromyelitis optica (NMO), an autoimmune disease of the central nervous system, is often more disabling than MS due to the severity of transverse myelitis and motor involvement, and patients tend to have a high symptom burden related to neuropathic pain, intractable nausea and vomiting, weakness, bowel and bladder dysfunction, and fatigue (Qian et al., 2012). Pain may be more severe in patients with NMO due to the severity of attacks and progressive disability as compared to patients with MS (Kanamori et al., 2011). Mood disorders are also common in this population (Chavarro et al., 2016).

### Malignant Brain Tumors

Patients with high-grade gliomas have an overall poor prognosis and a limited life expectancy, necessitating a palliative approach to care from the time of diagnosis (Walbert, 2014). A suggested framework for care begins with the recognition of the patient's psychological needs and the challenges of coping with a new and devastating diagnosis (Philip et al., 2018). Understanding that the disease course may involve notable improvements in the imaging and functional status but also setbacks and expected decline requires clinicians to routinely reassess the psychological state of their patients (Philip et al., 2018). Physical symptoms such as gait instability, motor impairments, seizures, and headaches are common as are cognitive changes secondary to the consequences of radiation and chemotherapy or disease progression (Gofton et al., 2012). In the later stages of the disease, patients may become drowsier and lose the ability to communicate or develop motor deficits such as hemiparesis or focal weakness (Walbert, 2014).

Caregiver needs increase as their loved one's functional and cognitive status decline and the patient becomes more dependent on the caregiver (Giammalva et al., 2018). Mitigating caregiver burnout involves increased communication between the clinician and the caregiver and addressing their concerns about the future (Pace et al., 2017).

Despite the known incurable nature of high-grade gliomas, studies have revealed low rates of advance care planning as defined by code status documentation and advance directive completion (Kuchinad et al., 2017). Hospice referrals in this population tend to be late, with over half of the patients in one cohort being enrolled within 30 days of death (Diamond et al., 2016) and a median hospice length of stay of 21 days in another cohort (Kuchinad, et al., 2017).

### Acute Neurology—Cerebrovascular Disorders/Stroke, Neuroscience Intensive Care Unit

The role of palliative care in acute neurology can begin at the time of presentation and continue throughout the course of disease. In patients who have a stroke with severe functional impairments, cognitive deficits, or multiple medical comorbidities, a palliative approach should involve establishing goals of care based on prognostic data and patient preferences, aligning treatment options with those goals, and addressing the potential outcomes (Holloway et al., 2014). Given the uncertainty that often clouds the initial days post-stroke, the use of best case, worst case, and most-likely case scenarios can provide patients and family members with much-needed and much-desired prognostic information (Creutzfeldt, et al., 2016). Time-limited trials may offer another strategy in the case of prognostic uncertainty (Holloway, Arnold, 2014). This option allows family members and the medical team to assess the patient's response to aggressive interventions prior to another decision point in the future.

Among those with severe and disabling deficits, some may choose a plan of care that focuses on comfort and quality of life and withhold or withdraw life-prolonging interventions such as cardiopulmonary resuscitation, enteral feeding, mechanical ventilation, surgery for decompression or cerebrospinal fluid shunting, vasopressor treatment, and measures to reduce elevated intracranial pressure (Holloway, Arnold, 2014). In these situations, compassionate end-of-life care involving symptom management, anticipatory guidance, caregiver support, and psychosocial support should be delivered by the primary providers, a palliative care team, or hospice services.

As the majority of patients who are admitted to neurological intensive care units were previously healthy, conversations about goals and preferences for life-sustaining care may not have been had prior to the precipitating event (Frontera et al., 2015). Identifying surrogate decision makers early is crucial for patients with acute neurological disease as patients may not be able to engage in critical discussions regarding potential therapeutic options and life-prolonging measures. Providing support for family members and caregivers is necessary during the time when they are often tasked with making decisions about life-sustaining care without significant input from the patient (Creutzfeldt et al., 2015; Tran et al., 2016).

Stroke should not be thought of as an event, but as a disease, with continued impact after the acute setting due to high mortality with long-term disability, high symptom burden, complex care transitions, and caregiver strain. For stroke survivors, physical disability may be the most obvious contributor to quality of life but other post-stroke symptoms may arise and further impact a person's psychological and physical state. Symptoms including mood disorders, neuropathic pain, sexual dysfunction, sleep-disordered breathing, fatigue, and seizures should be assessed and addressed by providers in the post-stroke period (Creutzfeldt et al., 2012). Advance care planning should be part of regular conversation at post-stroke clinic visits (Johnson, Ulrich, 2019).

### Movement Disorders

Patients with Parkinson disease (PD) and parkinsonian disorders such as multiple system atrophy (MSA) and progressive supranuclear palsy (PSP) have a wide range of palliative needs including motor and nonmotor symptom management, care planning, maintenance of communication, and caregiver burden. Focus groups and interviews with PD patients highlighted their unmet needs and categorized them into several themes, including physical challenges and subsequent limitations in social engagement, loss of one's prior identity and relationship roles, anticipatory grief about the loss of independence, and the expected progression of physical and possibly cognitive dysfunction, coping with the disease, and a desire for more PD education and prognostic information from the care team (Boersma et al., 2016).

Pain, anxiety, depression, speech difficulties, fatigue, constipation, stiffness, and cognitive concerns are common, bothersome symptoms in patients with PD, and the severity of these symptoms is similar in PD patients compared to patients with metastatic cancer (Boersma, et al., 2016; Miyasaki, 2013; Miyasaki et al., 2012) . The Edmonton Symptom Assessment Scale—PD is available for routine assessment of symptoms in this patient population (Miyasaki, Long, 2012). The atypical parkinsonian disorders are also appropriate for palliative care due to the more rapid decline and decreased responsiveness to dopaminergic therapy as compared to PD (Wiblin et al., 2017).

Caregivers of patients with PD can benefit from palliative care. They experience social isolation, financial concerns, and communication challenges due to dysarthria and cognitive decline that can negatively impact their quality of life (Boersma et al., 2017; Miyasaki and Kluger, 2015). They desire more information about the disease trajectory and medications at the time of a loved one's diagnosis and throughout the disease in order to feel better prepared for their responsibilities (Boersma, et al., 2017).

### Dementia

The palliative needs of patients with dementia and their caregivers center around goals of care, effective symptom management, residential environment, and advance care planning. Early in the disease course, while cognition remains relatively intact, and a person has the capacity to make medical decisions, detailed conversations are encouraged about the trajectory of the disease and likely decision points that will occur along the disease course. Understanding the patient's values and eliciting preferences for life-prolonging measures and end-of-life care is paramount. The nature of shared decision making with the patient, family, and care team is expected to shift over time yet the goal is to prioritize the patient's preferences, if possible (van der Steen et al., 2014). As the disease progresses, tools to assess pain and other symptoms in a nonverbal manner should be used.

In advanced dementia, treatment intensity preferences regarding hospitalizations, invasive procedures, artificial nutrition and hydration, and antibiotics need to be discussed with the goal of improving quality of life and managing symptoms while minimizing suffering (van der Steen, et al., 2014). Specific discussions about the possibility of decreased oral intake during the endstage of the disease and a plan for feeding need to occur before the patient loses the ability to participate in these decisions. Enteral feeding with percutaneous endoscopic gastrostomy (PEG) tubes is not recommended in patients in the advanced stage of dementia as PEG tubes have not been shown to reduce aspiration, improve wound healing, functional status, or increase survival (Sampson et al., 2009). Rather, hand feeding and comfort feeding are encouraged.

At the end of life, hospice services improve symptom management and reduce the likelihood of increased healthcare utilization in people with dementia. Family members of people with dementia report satisfaction with the quality of care and the dying experience with hospice enrollment (Teno et al., 2011).

### Neuromuscular Diseases

Neuromuscular diseases, with ALS being the most common and well-studied condition from a palliative care standpoint, lead to disability that impacts independence and quality of life. Palliative considerations at the time of diagnosis in patients with ALS include coping with the disease and mood, planning for the expected functional decline, advance care planning, and caregiver support.

Throughout the disease course, symptom management is a primary focus of care as patients with ALS experience pain, depression, anxiety, sialorrhea, spasticity, dysarthria, weakness, and cognitive dysfunction, which can affect up to 50% of people (Giordana et al., 2011). As the disease progresses, concerns about respiratory status become more salient.

Early discussions about preferences for life-prolonging interventions such as tracheostomy and mechanical ventilation are necessary to facilitate appropriate planning and respiratory support depending on the decision. While many patients utilize noninvasive positive pressure ventilatory support, which has demonstrated a survival benefit and improvement in quality of life, tracheostomy is uncommon in patients with ALS (Miller et al., 2009). Fewer than 5% of patients elect to undergo this intervention but rates vary across the world and tend to be influenced by providers (Albert et al., 1999; Bradley et al., 2001). If patients decide to proceed with a tracheostomy, comprehensive conversations regarding the respiratory and caregiving support are needed. Caregivers of patients on mechanical ventilation report worse quality of life than the patients themselves (Miller, et al., 2009). PEG tube placement is more common than tracheostomy. Enteral feedings in patients with dysphagia can stabilize weight and may have a survival benefit (Miller, et al., 2009). A primary consideration for the timing of PEG tube placement is respiratory status. A functional vital capacity greater than 50% is recommended for the procedure (Miller, et al., 2009).

## GOALS OF CARE

Goals-of-careconversations are based on the premise that we all have different values around the way we want to live and what is important to us if we get very sick. Eliciting person-centered values should be considered as routine as a physical exam and, similarly, needs to be revisited at regular intervals and after certain events (see Table 57.2). These conversations may start by considering one's position or location on a rough roadmap (Fig. 57.1) and envisioning next steps: "As you look to the future, what's most important?" Some people recommend asking the patient about their bucket list (Periyakoil et al., 2018) or what currently brings them joy. Open-ended questions help the patient think about his or her values. Depending on the situation, these questions can be more specifically geared towards a situation ("If your illness became very serious" or "If you got sick suddenly"), a treatment (artificial nutrition and hydration or intensive care unit admission), or

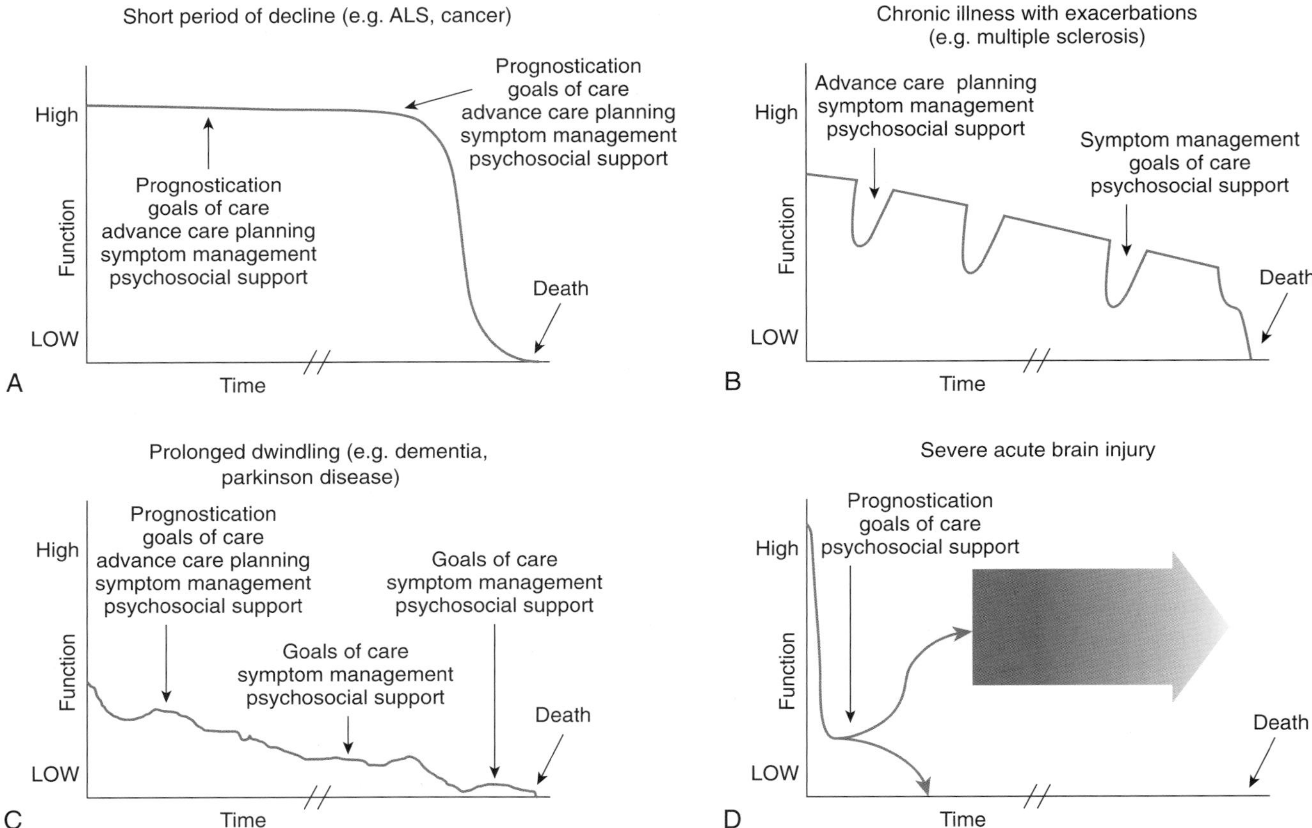


**Fig. 57.1 Palliative Care Considerations Along the Disease Trajectories.** *ALS*, Amyotrophic lateral sclerosis. *(Adapted from Creutzfeldt, C.J., Kluger, B.M., Holloway, R.G., 2019. Neuropalliative Care: A Guide to Improving the Lives of Patients and Families Affected by Neurologic Disease. Springer, Cham, Switzerland.)*

an outcome ("What level of disability might you consider acceptable?" or "Where might you draw the line?"). Sometimes, the patient may ask for something that is not possible or unlikely to lead to the desired outcome. We can still align with the patient, for example by using an 'I wish' statement ("I wish I could turn this around" or "I, too, am hoping for a miracle"), which implicitly acknowledges that this won't happen. Aligning with a patient's hopes allows us to refocus on a realistic goal ("I also think we need to prepare for the situation where that would not work").

## ADVANCE CARE PLANNING

Advance care planning involves a series of conversations and the documentation of the discussions regarding one's preferences for care at the end of life (Sudore et al., 2017). It is meant to be performed in advance of when it is needed and not at the end of life. Discussions should include the role of a healthcare surrogate, the designation of one, and preferences for life-prolonging measures at the end of life.

An ideal surrogate is a person who is familiar enough with the medical issues and who is willing to honor the outlined wishes for treatment intensity at the end of life. Advance directives are typically used when a person has either an end-stage or terminal condition or is in a persistent vegetative state with no reasonable chance of recovery. Unique to patients with neurological diseases, who may have PEG tubes or tracheostomies in the setting of a neurodegenerative condition, specific attention should be given to discussions about the continuation or discontinuation of artificial nutrition and hydration and mechanical ventilation at the end of life. Ideally, these discussions happen before patients undergo these life-prolonging procedures. As part of the broader advance care planning discussion, outpatient code status should be discussed as should the options of Physician Orders for Life-Sustaining Treatment (POLST) and Medical Orders for Life-Sustaining Treatment (MOLST).

These conversations involve patients and their clinicians and caregivers. When the paperwork has been completed, instructions should be given about when to review the documentation in the future to ensure that the documents continue to reflect one's preference. It is suggested that advance directives are reviewed every 10 years or if a new serious diagnosis has been made, if a loved one dies, if one's medical condition declines, or if a person gets divorced and the prior spouse is the designated healthcare surrogate. If the designated healthcare surrogate has a serious medical or neurodegenerative condition, this should also prompt a review of the advance directive. Copies of the document should be distributed to the healthcare surrogates and to the clinician or hospital where care is primarily provided.

## CAREGIVER AND FAMILY SUPPORT

Neurological illness affects not only the patient but also their family, friends, and community. Because most of our patients spend most of their lives at home, and a large proportion of them need assistance, this role is typically assumed by the spouse, parent, child, or other family member or friend. Family caregivers provide the majority of long-term care for chronically disabled older adults, and this care is associated with reduced morbidity and mortality as well as improved quality of life compared to patients who are alone (Dickens et al., 2004;

Hillman, 2013). While caregiving is overall considered a positive, rewarding, and meaningful experience, these "informal" (or unpaid) caregivers also face substantial physical, psychosocial, emotional, and financial challenges that can lead to significant strain, isolation, and even burnout. It is important to carefully assess caregiver needs at the patient's clinic visit ("Who do YOU have to support you?"; "How are you taking care of yourself and your own needs?"), to provide emotional and informational support to family members, and to consider different resources for caregivers that are often available through the local support organizations (Alzheimer disease foundation, or stroke support groups: more at www.stroke.org.

## TRANSITION TO HOSPICE CARE

Hospice guidelines for neurological disease offer general considerations about when to refer a patient to hospice. In the United States, Medicare guidelines suggest that a person is appropriate for hospice if the life expectancy is 6 months or less, if the disease progresses in its normal fashion. Given the challenges of prognostication in neurological disease, the accuracy of a 6-month prognosis is difficult. Disease-specific hospice enrollment guidelines for dementia, stroke, coma, and ALS exist and they focus on the nuances of the particular disease course. However, general circumstances for a person with an advanced neurological disease that should prompt hospice consideration include: a rapid or progressive permanent functional decline that results in a need for significant assistance with activities of daily living, a loss of approximately 10% of body weight in the prior 6 months, frequent hospitalizations, recurrent infections, and multiple comorbidities. These signs may suggest that a person is progressing toward the end of life.

## SUMMARY

Patients with neurological diseases have high palliative care needs that necessitate an integrated approach to care. Palliative care involves communicating difficult news, establishing goals of care and reviewing them throughout the disease course, managing symptoms to maximize function and reduce suffering, engaging in advance care planning discussions, and offering hospice care at the end of life. Incorporating palliative care techniques into the management plans for neurological patients can improve the quality of life for them and for their caregivers. Neurologists and other clinicians who care for patients with neurological conditions should be competent in primary palliative care skills to facilitate patient-centered and goal-oriented care.

*The complete reference list is available online at https://expertconsult.inkling.com/.* 

58

# Neurological Complications of Systemic Disease: Adults*

*S. Andrew Josephson, Michael J. Aminoff*

## OUTLINE



*Chapter 58 discusses neurological complications of systemic disease in adults; additional details can be found elsewhere (Aminoff and Josephson, 2021). Chapter 59 discusses the same subject in children. Some disorders are discussed in both chapters but with a different emphasis.

## CARDIAC DISORDERS AND THE NERVOUS SYSTEM

Neurological complications are an important cause of morbidity in patients with cardiac disease. Cardiogenic emboli may result from cardiac disease or its treatment, and cardiac dysfunction can cause global cerebral hypoperfusion, which—depending on its severity and duration—leads to syncope, stroke, anoxic-ischemic encephalopathy, or death.

### Cardiogenic Embolism

Cardiogenic emboli are most prevalent in patients with atrial fibrillation with or without mitral stenosis, intramural thrombi, prosthetic cardiac valves, infective endocarditis, atrial flutter, and sick sinus syndrome. Other causes include recent myocardial infarction (MI), left atrial thrombus or turbulence, atrial myxoma, mitral annulus calcification and prolapse, hypokinetic left ventricular segments, and dilated cardiomyopathy. (Chapter 59 discusses emboli from congenital heart disease, a consideration in young people with valvular heart disease.)

Echocardiography is an important investigative procedure in patients with suspected cardiogenic emboli. Transesophageal echocardiography is preferable to the transthoracic approach in the evaluation of suspected atrial diseases such as myxoma or thrombus, in examination of the aortic arch, and in the diagnosis of a patent foramen ovale. Transesophageal echocardiography is an important method for visualizing the ventricular apex, characterizing mitral or aortic valvular disease, and delineating left ventricular thrombus.

Transesophageal echocardiography is an appropriate method for investigating people younger than 60 years of age with suspected cardiogenic emboli who may need anticoagulation or surgery and in those with no clear source demonstrated on transthoracic echocardiography when suspicion for an embolic source is high. Some have suggested that transesophageal echocardiography is appropriate in all patients with cryptogenic stroke (Katsanos et al., 2016).

Embolus formation is more likely when atrial fibrillation is associated with valvular heart disease. The incidence of stroke among patients with atrial fibrillation, with or without rheumatic heart disease, is increased 17-fold or 5-fold, respectively. Atrial fibrillation in the absence of cardiovascular disease or other predisposing illness carries a considerably lower risk of neurological complications. The neurological prognosis for paroxysmal rather than chronic atrial fibrillation has not been definitively established.

Anticoagulation has established benefit in reducing the risk of stroke in persons with atrial fibrillation. Consensus supports the use of long-term therapy for atrial fibrillation in most cases. Although warfarin was traditionally the oral anticoagulant of choice, both oral direct thrombin inhibitors (e.g., dabigatran) and oral factor Xa inhibitors (e.g., rivaroxaban, apixaban) have emerged as effective and commonly used alternatives for anticoagulation in nonvalvular atrial fibrillation (Ruff et al., 2014). Risk stratification systems are helpful in deciding whether anticoagulation is warranted (Stroke Risk in Atrial Fibrillation Working Group, 2008). Aspirin (325 mg/day) is the recommended agent when anticoagulation is contraindicated. Recent studies suggest that addition of clopidogrel (75 mg/day) may also be worthwhile when anticoagulation cannot occur, although with a higher risk of bleeding over aspirin alone (Connolly et al., 2009).

Standard practice is to start warfarin at least 3 weeks before elective cardioversion in patients with atrial fibrillation of more than 2 days' duration. Anticoagulation therapy is then continued at least until a normal rhythm has been maintained for 4 weeks. Myocardial infarcts—especially apical, anterolateral, or large infarcts—carry a risk of embolic stroke. In most cases, the stroke occurs within a week, but the risk persists for approximately 2 months. Therefore it is recommended to use heparin for those patients who are not on thrombolytic therapy after MI and to continue anticoagulation for 3 months if they have an increased risk of embolism. The groups with increased risk are those with congestive heart failure, previous emboli, a mural thrombus, left ventricular dysfunction, substantial wall motion abnormalities, or atrial fibrillation.

Emboli are an important cause of death in people with rheumatic valvular disease. The risk of embolism increases in the presence of atrial fibrillation or intra-atrial thrombus or in patients with a history of emboli; long-term warfarin is the recommended treatment. Addition of low-dose aspirin (50–100 mg/day) is recommended for recurrent systemic emboli or left atrial thrombus despite adequate warfarin therapy.

Mitral valve prolapse is a common anomaly, especially in young women, and is a recognized source of cerebral emboli. The risk of embolism is relatively small, and long-term warfarin therapy is the recommended treatment for persons who have had previous embolic phenomena or are in atrial fibrillation. Aspirin therapy (50–325 mg/day) is the recommended treatment for patients with mitral valve prolapse and transient cerebral ischemic attacks of uncertain nature.

Patent foramen ovale is common in asymptomatic subjects and does not seem to be a risk factor for cryptogenic ischemic stroke or transient ischemic attacks (TIAs), especially when they are small or occur as an isolated cardiac abnormality. Those that are large or associated with an atrial septal aneurysm are at higher risk of causing stroke, but treatment with aspirin, warfarin, or percutaneous closure is equally effective for stroke prophylaxis. Secondary prevention after incident stroke of unknown etiology should involve percutaneous closure of patent foramen ovale only if the patient is less than 60 years of age, the infarct appears embolic, and the patent foramen ovale is moderate to large in size provided that a thorough workup has excluded other potential causes of stroke (Ahmed et al., 2018).

Among patients with a history of cardiogenic emboli, recurrent stroke is more likely in those with cardiac valve disease and congestive heart failure. Nevertheless, the main cause of death in such patients is from the heart disease itself rather than neurological complications. The conversion of a cerebral infarct into a hemorrhage is a concern when patients with stroke from cardiogenic emboli are anticoagulated. The concern is especially justified in patients with large infarcts or when imaging studies suggest preexisting hemorrhagic transformation or a large number of asymptomatic microhemorrhages. With small infarcts, it is good practice to initiate anticoagulation therapy when initial computed tomography (CT) shows no evidence of major hemorrhagic transformation; with large infarcts, anticoagulation should be delayed for 3 to 7 days.

### Syncope

Transitory global cerebral ischemia secondary to cardiac arrhythmia often causes syncope. Nonspecific premonitory symptoms—such as visual disturbances, paresthesias, and lightheadedness—may precede the syncope. Syncope usually is associated with loss of muscle tone, but prolonged ischemia causes tonic posturing and irregular jerking movements that are easily mistaken for seizures. The syncopal patient is pale, and postictal confusion is absent or short lived, usually lasting less than 30 seconds. Obstructed outflow from aortic stenosis or left atrial tumor or thrombus is one cardiac cause of syncope. Other causes are arrhythmias, especially from ventricular tachycardia or fibrillation; chronic sinoatrial disorder or sick sinus syndrome; and paroxysmal tachycardia. Placement of implantable loop recorders or external event recorders allows the recording of electrocardiographic data during spontaneous syncopal events. This strategy increases the diagnostic rate and permits appropriate treatment to be instituted.

Arrhythmia is detectable in 25% to 46% of patients with syncope, and another 24% to 42% will be in sinus rhythm during a clinical event, which is therefore not attributable to a disturbance of cardiac rhythm (McKeon et al., 2006). Additional causes of syncope are central and peripheral dysautonomias, postural hypotension, and endocrine and metabolic disorders. (Discussions of vasovagal syncope and the syndrome of prolonged QT interval may be found in Chapter 2.)

## Cardiac Arrest

Brain function is critically dependent on the cerebral circulation. The brain receives approximately 15% of total cardiac output. Ventricular fibrillation, pulseless ventricular tachycardia, or asystole leads to circulatory failure, which can cause irreversible anoxic-ischemic brain damage if it lasts for more than a critical time. The prognosis generally depends on age, the duration of the arrest before institution of cardiopulmonary resuscitation, the initiation of therapeutic hypothermia when appropriate, and the interval before the initiation of defibrillating procedures. The prognosis is better when the cause of circulatory arrest is ventricular fibrillation rather than asystole.

The pathophysiology of neurological damage secondary to transitory interruption of cerebral blood flow is unclear. Suspected mechanisms are the accumulation of intracellular calcium, increased extracellular concentrations of glutamate and aspartate, and increased concentrations of free radicals.

In the mature brain, gray matter is generally more sensitive to ischemia than white matter, and the cerebral cortex and deep nuclei are more sensitive than the brainstem. (The white matter of the premature brain has increased sensitivity to injury; see Chapter 110.) Cerebral or spinal regions lying between the territories supplied by the major arteries (watershed areas) are especially vulnerable to ischemic injury.

The severity of neurological complications of circulatory arrest correlates with the duration of the arrest. Brief arrests (<5 minutes in duration) cause temporary loss of consciousness and may lead to impaired cognitive function. A demyelinating encephalopathy may occur up to 10 days later, even in those who initially seem to recover fully. Characteristic of the encephalopathy are increasing cerebral dysfunction with cognitive disturbances and pyramidal or extrapyramidal abnormalities that may lead to a fatal outcome. Thus some patients regain consciousness after several hours, with the subsequent development of progressive neurological deficits affecting cognitive and cortical function, including intellectual decline, seizures, visual agnosia, cortical blindness, amnestic syndromes, and personality changes. Less common residua are the locked-in syndrome, parkinsonism and other extrapyramidal syndromes, abnormal ocular movements, bilateral brachial paresis, and action myoclonus. Spinal cord dysfunction is uncommon and usually involves the watershed region around T5; flaccid paraplegia with sensory loss, areflexia, and sphincter dysfunction are the immediate findings.

Prolonged cardiac arrest causes widespread and irreversible brain damage characterized by prolonged coma, which leads to a persistent vegetative state. Prolonged coma and loss of brainstem reflexes indicate a poor prognosis for survival or useful recovery. Therapeutic hypothermia initiated rapidly after the arrest may improve the neurological outcome (Hessel, 2014). Absence of the pupillary response to light and absence of motor recovery better than extensor posturing at 72 hours are perhaps the most useful clinical guides to prognosis (see Chapter 5 for further discussion). These features of the clinical examination, along with measurement of neuron-specific enolase and recording of median-derived somatosensory evoked potentials (to determine whether the N20 component is absent bilaterally), can be helpful in prognostication, although these same tests and time frames may not apply in patients treated with hypothermia (Rossetti et al., 2010).

## Complications of Cardiac Catheterization and Surgery

Cardiac catheterization in adults causes large cerebral emboli in less than 1% of cases; for unexplained reasons, these emboli more often involve the posterior than the anterior circulation. The frequency of large cerebral emboli after percutaneous transluminal coronary angioplasty is less than 1% and may involve either the carotid or vertebral circulation. The risk of stroke, however, is greater in patients with acute MI treated by angioplasty.

Hypoxia and emboli are the usual causes of "post-pump" encephalopathy, seizures, and cerebral infarction after cardiac surgery. The type of surgery, symptomatic cerebrovascular disease, diabetes mellitus, and advanced age are important risk factors for neurological complications (Boeken et al., 2005). Ascertaining the degree of functionally significant cerebrovascular disease is an essential part of the preoperative evaluation. The causes of postoperative psychosis or encephalopathy are metabolic disturbances, medication, infection, and multiorgan failure. Intracranial infection should be suspected when behavioral disturbances develop several weeks postoperatively in patients receiving immunosuppressive agents. The usual causes of postoperative seizures are focal or generalized cerebral ischemia, electrolyte or metabolic disturbances, and multiorgan failure. Intracranial hemorrhage is a rare complication of cardiopulmonary bypass. Cognitive changes after cardiac bypass surgery are detectable in more than half of such patients at discharge, and many of these changes persist indefinitely (Saczynski et al., 2012). However, the previously described late cognitive decline that occurs years following cardiac bypass surgery is similar to that found in age-matched patients with coronary artery disease managed without surgery (Selnes et al., 2008). Compression or traction injuries to the brachial plexus, especially the lower trunk, and the phrenic and recurrent laryngeal nerves may occur during cardiac surgery. Cerebral air embolism may require high-flow or even hyperbaric oxygen therapy combined with aggressive resuscitation.

Other common early complications of cardiac transplantation are organ rejection followed by cardiac failure and the side effects of immunosuppressive drugs. Infection (meningitis, meningoencephalitis, or cerebral abscess) secondary to immunosuppressive therapy is the most important late complication. The infecting organisms include *Aspergillus*, *Toxoplasma*, *Cryptococcus*, *Candida*, *Nocardia*, and viruses including the JC virus. An increased risk of lymphoma and reticulum cell sarcoma has been observed in patients on long-term immunosuppressive agents. Primary central nervous system (CNS) lymphoma may be difficult to distinguish clinically or radiologically from infection, and biopsy may be necessary (see Chapters 71 and 73).

Stroke occurs in approximately 5% of patients undergoing coronary artery bypass surgery. The risk is increasing because of the higher number of procedures in older patients with more severe vascular disease; it is also increasing in complicated combined procedures such as bypass surgery plus valve replacement (Tarakji et al., 2011). Other risk factors include proximal aortic atherosclerosis, hypertension, diabetes, and female gender. The mechanism is either embolic or, less commonly, a watershed infarction from hypoperfusion. A history of previous stroke also increases the risk, but a carotid bruit or radiological evidence of atherosclerotic disease of the carotid artery does not. Carotid endarterectomy preceding cardiac surgery is not justified.

Those few patients who fail to recover consciousness after surgery despite the absence of any metabolic cause have probably suffered diffuse cerebral ischemia or hypoxia. Hemispheric or multifocal infarction (Fig. 58.1) is responsible in some cases. In evaluating patients with postoperative neurological deficits, diffusion-weighted magnetic resonance imaging (MRI) is more sensitive than CT to ischemic change and may reveal multiple small embolic infarcts (Chalela et al., 2007).

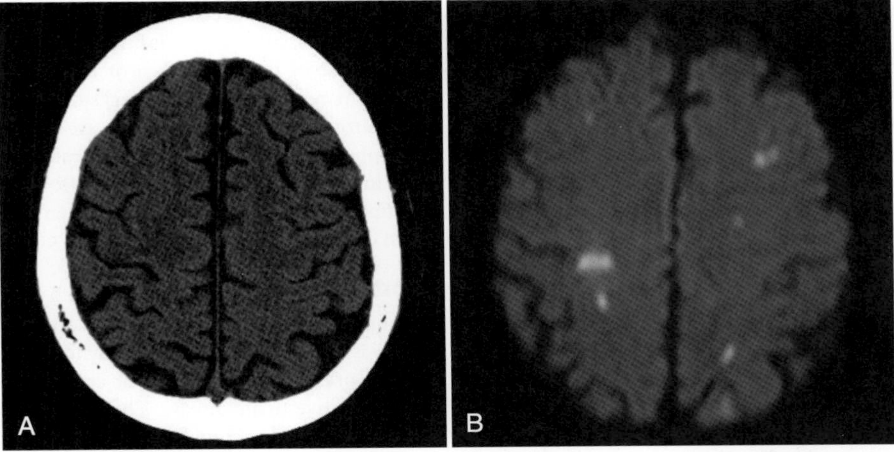


**Fig. 58.1 A,** Noncontrast computed tomography (CT) scan of brain performed 3 days after coronary artery bypass to evaluate confusion and left-sided weakness in a 76-year-old man. **B,** Multiple bilateral ischemic lesions can be seen on diffusion-weighted magnetic resonance imaging that are not conspicuous on CT scan.

## Neurological Complications of Medication

Infectious and neoplastic complications of immunosuppressive agents have already been discussed in previous sections. Other adverse effects associated with corticosteroid treatment are behavioral disturbances, psychoses, postural tremor, cataracts, osteoporotic fractures, and proximal weakness with type II muscle fiber atrophy. Benign intracranial hypertension may occur during treatment with or on withdrawal of corticosteroids. Neurological complications of cyclosporine and other calcineurin inhibitors include tremor, seizures, focal deficits, paresthesias, encephalopathy, and ataxia; the cerebral imaging appearance may be that of the posterior reversible encephalopathy syndrome (PRES). Sirolimus is an alternative immunosuppressant in solid-organ transplantation and appears to have less neurotoxicity than the calcineurin inhibitors.

Among antiarrhythmic agents, amiodarone causes tremor, sensorimotor peripheral neuropathy, myopathy, ataxia, optic neuropathy, and pseudotumor cerebri. Procainamide may unmask latent myasthenia gravis or precipitate a lupus-like syndrome with secondary vascular occlusive complications that are probably associated with lupus anticoagulant and antiphospholipid antibodies. Quinidine has neurological side effects similar to those of procainamide; it also causes headache, tinnitus, and syncope.

Lidocaine and related agents may cause seizures, tremor, paresthesias, and confusional states. Calcium channel–blocking agents occasionally cause encephalopathy, as may cefepime and rarely other members of the cephalosporin class of antibiotics. Beta-blockers are associated with mental status changes, paresthesias, and disturbances of neuromuscular transmission, whereas digoxin and thiazide diuretics are associated with an encephalopathy and disturbances of color vision.

## Infective Endocarditis

The incidence of infective endocarditis has increased due to the abuse of intravenous substances and the increasing use of prosthetic cardiac valves. The overall incidence of neurological complications of infective endocarditis is approximately 25% to 35%, but it varies with the type of infecting organism. Such complications are the initial sign or major complaint in 25% to 50% of patients and are associated with a substantially higher mortality rate. Neurological manifestations are especially common in patients with mitral valve abnormalities and consist of embolic or hemorrhagic stroke and infections such as meningitis or brain abscess.

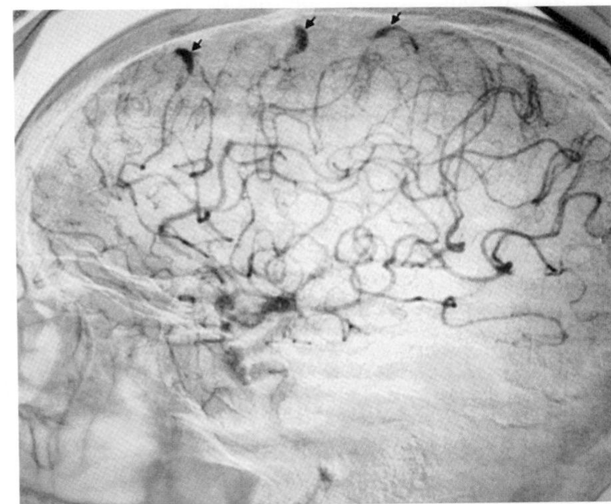

**Fig. 58.2 Carotid Angiogram, Lateral View With Subtraction.** The patient was a 48-year-old man with multiple peripheral mycotic aneurysms *(arrows)*, which were verified at autopsy.

Cerebral mycotic aneurysms (Fig. 58.2) are recognized complications of infective endocarditis and may result in intracranial hemorrhage. They are generally more distally located than noninfective berry aneurysms. The pathogenesis of mycotic aneurysms is unclear. The most likely cause is impaction of infected material in the vasa vasorum of the artery, with resulting destruction of the arterial wall. Intraluminal occlusion of the vessel by infected material, with subsequent aneurysmal formation, is a less likely mechanism but has been documented in some cases. Mycotic aneurysms may be clinically silent and sometimes resolve with antibiotic therapy. They are less common but occur earlier in acute than subacute bacterial endocarditis. Their natural history is unknown.

Intracranial hemorrhage is also caused by septic arteritis, which destroys the vessel wall without causing aneurysm; it also leads to the hemorrhagic transformation of cerebral septic infarctions. Angiography distinguishes intracranial hemorrhage from mycotic aneurysm and septic arteritis.

Intracranial bleeding from a ruptured mycotic aneurysm can be the initial feature of an underlying cardiac disorder or may occur during the management of a recognized infective endocarditis. Every patient with infective endocarditis who has a subarachnoid hemorrhage requires catheter-based angiography.

Embolization of infected material causes cerebral microabscesses and meningitis. Multiple septic emboli may cause meningoencephalitis or a diffuse encephalopathy characterized by a confusional state, headache, meningismus, and an inflammatory cerebrospinal fluid (CSF) profile. The basis of these symptoms is probably multifactorial, including infection, vascular occlusion, metabolic abnormalities, and sometimes mycotic aneurysms.

Antibiotic therapy to resolve the cardiac infection is the mainstay of treatment and is important in preventing neurological complications (Heiro et al., 2000). Neurological abnormalities usually resolve. Patients with progressive or persistent neurological deficits or abnormalities on CSF examination require imaging studies. Findings suggestive of mycotic aneurysm necessitate vascular imaging. Once mycotic aneurysms have ruptured, curative surgical or endovascular treatment is necessary to prevent repeated rupture. Management of unruptured mycotic aneurysms is less clear; many advocate conservative management with antibiotics and serial imaging. Owing to the risk of hemorrhagic transformation of embolic infarcts or rupture of an unrecognized mycotic aneurysm, anticoagulants are usually withheld from patients with infective endocarditis and cerebral embolism until after appropriate antibiotic therapy.

## DISEASES OF THE AORTA

The aorta supplies blood to the CNS and peripheral nervous system (PNS). Several neurological syndromes result from aortic disease, depending on the site and severity of obstruction.

Spinal cord ischemia may result from congenital aortic abnormalities such as coarctation, acquired disorders such as aortic aneurysm or occlusive atherosclerotic disease, and following aortic surgery or aortography. The level of myelopathy depends on the site of aortic disease. In general, aortic pathology that causes spinal cord ischemia is above the origin of the renal arteries; obstruction at a more distal point is less likely to affect the segmental vessels that feed the spinal cord. Risk factors for spinal cord ischemia during aortic surgery include the presence of dissection, extensive thoracoabdominal disease, and a long cross-clamp time. The thoracic cord is more susceptible to ischemia than the cervical and lumbosacral regions. When spinal cord ischemia complicates aortic surgery, drainage of CSF via a lumbar catheter may be effective in limiting neurological dysfunction, but the evidence is incomplete (Khan and Stansby, 2012).

Spinal cord ischemia from aortic disease usually causes a complete transverse myelopathy or an anterior spinal artery syndrome. Clinical features include weakness, loss of sphincter control, and impaired pain and temperature appreciation below the level of myelopathy. Spasticity, hyperreflexia, and bilateral extensor plantar responses eventually replace the initial flaccidity and areflexia. The existence of a true posterior spinal artery syndrome is doubtful because the posterior spinal arteries have multiple feeding vessels along their length. Occasional reports of a clinical disorder resembling progressive spinal muscular atrophy have been attributed to cord ischemia from aortic disease, especially affecting the anterior horn cells.

Neurogenic claudication may be caused by ischemia of the nerve roots or cauda equina (as from a protruded lumbar disk in spinal stenosis), by intermittent cord ischemia from spinal vascular malformations, or by aortic disease. Pain, weakness, or a sensory disturbance develops in one or both legs during walking or in relation to certain postures. Rest or change of posture relieves the symptoms. Extension of the spine often exacerbates the symptoms, so patients may prefer a posture that includes forward flexion at the hips. The distinction between neurogenic claudication and the intermittent claudication of peripheral vascular disease is important because their treatments differ.

Disease of the aortic arch or its main branches may also lead to transient cerebral ischemic attacks or strokes. Estimates of the risk of embolization from the aortic arch are low. Transesophageal echocardiography is an important means of evaluating the aortic arch, although less invasive means such as CT or MR angiography are gaining favor. Antiplatelet drugs remain the treatment of choice for cerebral embolism due to aortic arch disease.

### Aortic Aneurysms

An unusually high incidence of dissecting aneurysm of the ascending aorta is associated with Marfan syndrome, in which a dilated aortic root is present. Dissecting aortic aneurysms also occur in the absence of connective tissue disease. The neurological features usually consist of acute cerebral or spinal cord deficits from ischemia, the former often due to extension of the dissection into the carotid arteries. Acute chest pain often is an associated symptom.

Thoracic aortic aneurysms suggest a syphilitic etiology. Left recurrent laryngeal nerve palsy may result from compression or traction of the nerve, especially when the aneurysm involves the aortic arch. Horner syndrome is a rare finding caused by pressure on the sympathetic trunk and superior cervical ganglion. Cerebral emboli are a complication of thoracic aortic aneurysms.

Atherosclerosis is the usual cause of abdominal aortic aneurysms. Compression of the femoral or obturator nerve is usually due to a hematoma and rarely to the aneurysm itself. Injury to the lumbosacral plexus and nerves may occur at surgery, as may spinal cord ischemia. Occlusive disease of the terminal aorta sometimes leads to an ischemic monomelic neuropathy characterized by pain and loss of all sensation in the distal portion of the leg. Disturbances of micturition and sexual function may also result from aortic aneurysms.

### Aortitis

The causes of aortitis include syphilis, Takayasu disease, irradiation, transient emboligenic aortoarteritis, rheumatic fever, ankylosing spondylitis, reactive arthritis, and several connective tissue diseases. The latter group includes giant cell arteritis (see Chapter 102), rheumatoid arthritis, systemic lupus erythematosus (SLE), and scleroderma. Neurological complications occur when arteries that perfuse neural tissues are involved or in relation to a secondary aortic pathological process or lesion such as an aneurysm.

Takayasu disease (pulseless disease) is primarily a disease of young Asian women. Nonspecific symptoms are fever, weight loss, myalgias, and arthralgia. Obstruction of the major vessels of the aortic arch causes loss of pulses in the neck and arms, hypertension, and aortic regurgitation. Less common signs and symptoms are headache, seizures, transient cerebral ischemic attacks, and stroke (Bond et al., 2017). The diagnosis is established by the clinical features, and corticosteroids are the treatment of choice. Despite the severe vascular involvement, the clinical neurological course is often good in patients who receive appropriate treatment, which sometimes includes revascularization procedures.

Transient emboligenic aortoarteritis is a rare inflammatory process of uncertain etiology affecting the aorta and other central elastic arteries but sparing the more peripheral vessels. It causes stroke or TIAs in young people.

### Coarctation of the Aorta

Congenital coarctation of the aorta is a narrowing of the thoracic aorta just after the origin of the left subclavian artery. Acquired coarctation may follow irradiation during infancy; the narrowing is in the irradiated region. A narrowed segment that is atypically located for congenital coarctation and unrelated to previous irradiation suggests Takayasu disease.

Headache occurs in more than 25% of patients with coarctation. Subarachnoid hemorrhage may occur with rupture of an associated cerebral aneurysm. Episodic loss of consciousness (of uncertain basis) occurs as well. Spinal cord dysfunction occurs when the lower part of the cord becomes ischemic owing to insufficient flow in vessels arising from the aorta beyond the narrowed segment. Neurogenic intermittent claudication may result from the "stealing" of blood from the cord by retrograde flow through the anterior spinal artery, a part of the collateral circulation that bypasses the narrowed segment. Marked enlargement of collateral vessels within the spinal canal may compress the cervicothoracic cord, causing myelopathy. Enlargement of the anterior spinal artery or one of its feeders may lead to aneurysmal distention and rupture, resulting in spinal subarachnoid hemorrhage. Treatment involves surgical correction of the underlying coarctation.

### Subclavian Steal Syndrome

Occlusion of either the innominate or the left subclavian artery before the origin of the vertebral artery reverses the direction of blood flow in the vertebral artery on the affected side. This reversal of flow is often asymptomatic but may cause ischemia in the posterior cerebral circulation. Neurological features are weakness, vertigo, visual complaints, and syncope. The underlying cause is a small or occluded contralateral vertebral artery on a congenital or acquired basis. Typically, the pulse diminishes or disappears in the affected arm, and systolic pressure decreases by at least 20 mm Hg compared with the opposite arm. Reconstructive surgery or endovascular repair is sometimes helpful but is unnecessary in most patients.

### Complications of Aortic Surgery

Spinal cord infarction remains the most serious neurological complication of aortic surgery. CSF drainage and distal aortic perfusion may be important adjuncts to corrective surgery for thoracic and thoracoabdominal aortic aneurysms, significantly reducing the incidence of paraplegia and paraparesis (Bilal et al., 2012), although the evidence is incomplete (Khan and Stansby, 2012). Other complications are neuropathy, radiculopathy, postsympathectomy neuralgia after surgical division of the sympathetic chain, and disturbances of penile erection or ejaculation with surgical division of the superior hypogastric plexus.

## CONNECTIVE TISSUE DISEASES AND VASCULITIDES

Neurological complications may be direct consequences of connective tissue diseases or may be secondary to other organ involvement or to treatment. (The adverse effects of corticosteroids and immunosuppressive agents are discussed earlier in this chapter and in other sections.) Autoimmune inflammatory responses, especially necrotizing vasculitis, characterize connective tissue disorders. The mechanism of vasculitis is uncertain but may involve the deposition of immune complexes in vessel walls or cell-mediated immunity and the release of lymphokines; autoantibodies may also be important in some instances. The common direct CNS manifestations of connective tissue diseases are cognitive or behavioral changes and focal neurological deficits. Peripheral neuropathies also occur and may take the form of a vasculitic neuropathy, distal axonal polyneuropathy, compression neuropathy, sensory neuronopathy, trigeminal sensory neuropathy, acute or chronic demyelinating polyneuropathy, or plexopathy.

The cause of vasculitic neuropathy is nerve infarction from occlusion of the vasa nervorum. A mononeuropathy multiplex develops that becomes more confluent with increasing nerve involvement until it resembles a distal symmetrical polyneuropathy. Nerves in watershed regions that lie between different vascular territories, such as the midthigh or mid- to upper arm, are more likely to be involved. Both large and small fibers are affected. Treatment with corticosteroids, often in conjunction with other immunosuppressive therapy, is usually effective, but intravenous immunoglobulin or rituximab may be helpful in resistant cases (Gwathmey et al., 2014).

### Polyarteritis Nodosa, Churg-Strauss Syndrome, and Overlap Syndrome

Peripheral neuropathy occurs in up to 60% of patients with polyarteritis nodosa, Churg-Strauss syndrome, or overlap syndrome. A painful mononeuropathy multiplex, at least in polyarteritis nodosa, usually develops during the first year. As more nerves are affected, the deficits become more confluent and may resemble a length-dependent polyneuropathy. A few patients exhibit only patchy hypesthetic areas; in others, a secondary polyneuropathy (e.g., from renal failure) may develop. A plexopathy, radiculopathy, or cauda equina syndrome can also occur. Electrophysiological studies and nerve histology are often abnormal even in the absence of clinical evidence of peripheral nerve involvement.

CNS involvement usually occurs later than peripheral involvement in the course of the disease. Common features are headache, which sometimes indicates aseptic meningitis, and behavioral disturbances such as cognitive decline, acute confusion, and affective or psychotic disorders. The electroencephalogram (EEG) sometimes shows diffuse slowing, but neuroimaging studies are generally normal. Focal CNS deficits are uncommon but are typically sudden in onset and may be caused by cerebral infarction or hemorrhage. Angiography may not show the underlying vasculitis, and tissue biopsy may be needed to establish the diagnosis (Fig. 58.3). Ischemic or compressive myelopathies from extradural hematomas are rare complications.

The 6-month survival rate for patients with untreated polyarteritis nodosa is only 35%. Prompt diagnosis and treatment are critical. Weight loss, fever, cutaneous abnormalities, and arthralgias are common, and hypertension and renal, cardiac, pulmonary, or gastrointestinal (GI) involvement may occur. Laboratory studies show multiorgan involvement and immunological abnormalities. Common abnormalities are an increased erythrocyte sedimentation rate (ESR), anemia, and peripheral leukocytosis. Hepatitis B surface antigen, hypocomplementemia, and uremia each occur in at least 20% of cases.

Patients with Churg-Strauss syndrome often have asthma and a marked peripheral eosinophilia; perinuclear anti-neutrophil cytoplasmic antibodies (p-ANCA) elevations are present in over half of such cases. Nerve or muscle biopsy often shows the necrotizing vasculitis, and angiography reveals segmental narrowing or aneurysmal distention, especially in the renal, mesenteric, or hepatic vessels.

Treatment for these conditions is with corticosteroids combined with cyclophosphamide or rituximab and has reversed the poor prognosis of this disease. With adequate combined therapy, approximately 60% of patients do well. Some are able to discontinue treatment by 2 years, although a subset will require lifelong therapy.

### Giant Cell Arteritis

Headache is the most common initial complaint of patients with giant cell arteritis; some also complain of masticatory claudication. The temporal and other scalp arteries are often erythematous, tender, and nodular but may be normal. A more serious presenting manifestation is acute transitory or permanent blindness affecting one or both eyes; arteritic ischemic optic neuropathy is the cause. Other CNS complications are rare, but neuropsychiatric disturbances, stroke, diplopia, or

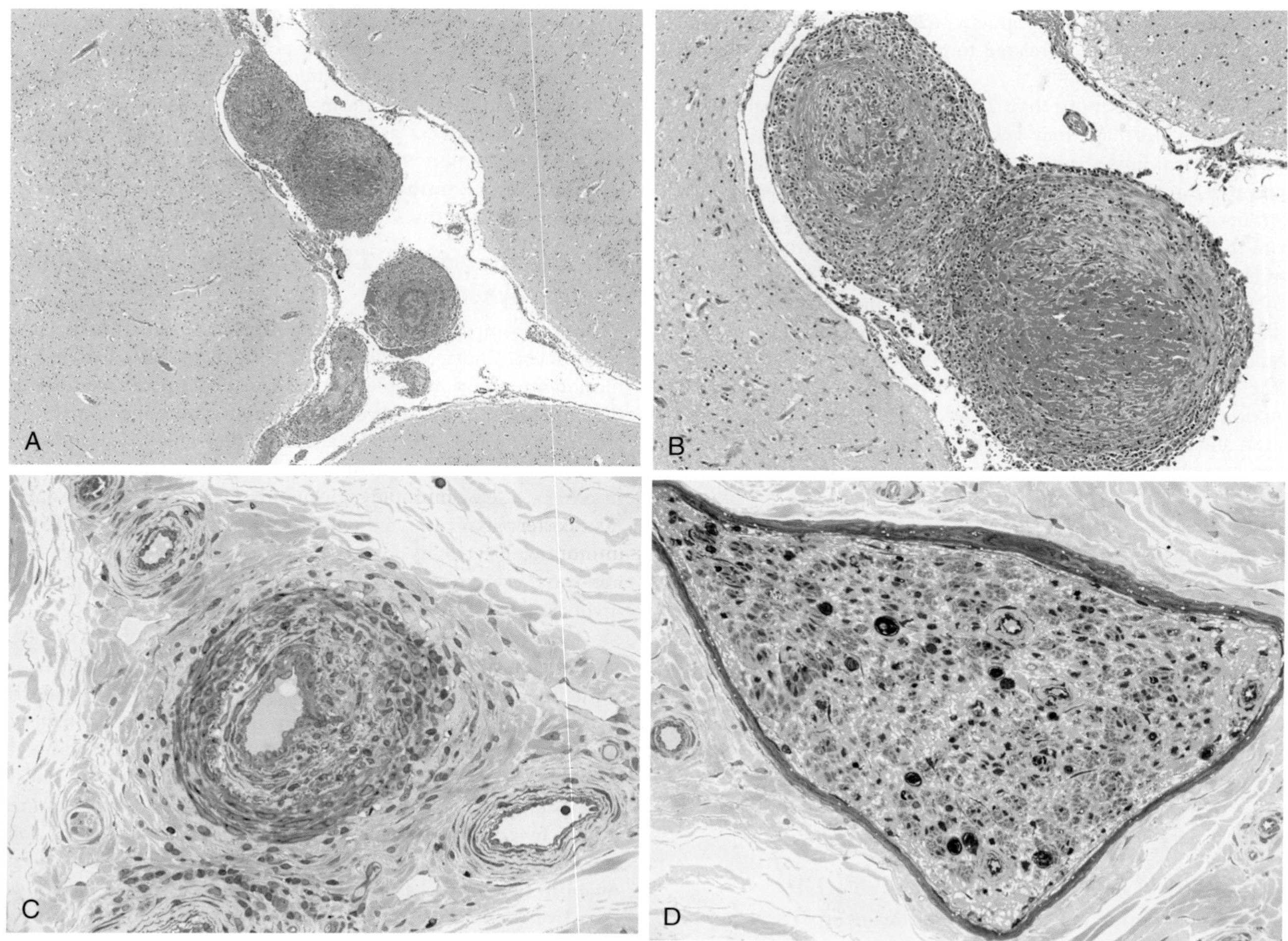


**Fig. 58.3 Histopathological Features of Polyarteritis Nodosa. A,** Medium magnification of hematoxylin and eosin image of polyarteritis nodosa involving the medium-sized vessels in the leptomeninges. **B,** Higher magnification shows characteristic necrotizing vasculitis with predominant lymphocytic infiltrates in the vascular walls. Polyarteritis nodosa is commonly accompanied by peripheral nerve involvement, highlighted here (**C**) in toluidine blue–stained sections with lymphocytic infiltrates in the vascular wall and (**D**) severe axonal loss in a nearby nerve fascicle. *(Courtesy Eric J. Huang MD, PhD.)*

seizures may occasionally be the presenting feature. Peripheral neuropathies occur in up to 15% of patients, and half of these are generalized.

The ESR is typically elevated, often markedly, and polymyalgia rheumatica and anemia are often associated findings. When giant cell arteritis is suspected, high-dose corticosteroid treatment should be started immediately while waiting to perform a temporal artery biopsy; any delay increases the risk of vision loss. Treatment is monitored by the clinical response and the ESR, but the corticosteroid dose should be increased if clinical signs of disease activity appear regardless of test results. With time, the corticosteroid dose can be tapered, but treatment should continue for 18 to 24 months. Tocilizumab has recently been studied as a corticosteroid-sparing alternative treatment agent (Mariano and Frishman, 2018).

## Granulomatosis With Polyangiitis

Neurological involvement occurs in up to 50% of patients who have granulomatosis with polyangiitis. Direct involvement of the brain may occur by vasculitis or by the extension of granulomas from the upper respiratory tract. Among patients with neurological complications, peripheral neuropathy is most common. The neuropathy is usually a mononeuropathy multiplex, but symmetrical polyneuropathies sometimes occur. Cranial neuropathy may also occur (usually involving cranial nerves [CN] II, VI, and VII), and multiple cranial neuropathies sometimes develop. Other neurological features include an external ophthalmoplegia (due to orbital pseudotumor), cerebrovascular events (e.g., stroke and venous sinus obstruction), seizures (e.g., from metabolic causes, sepsis, or vasculitis), basal meningitis, and cerebritis. Treatment includes corticosteroids, often in conjunction with other immunosuppressive agents such as cyclophosphamide or methotrexate.

## Isolated Angiitis of the Nervous System

A description of isolated angiitis (granulomatous angiitis) of the CNS is provided in Chapter 69, and that of the PNS is discussed in Chapter 106.

## Rheumatoid Arthritis

Rheumatoid arthritis is the most common connective tissue disease. A discussion of juvenile rheumatoid arthritis can be found in Chapter 59. Systemic vasculitis occurs in up to 25% of adult patients, but CNS involvement is rare. Pathological involvement of the cervical spine (Fig. 58.4) or atlantoaxial dislocation may cause a myelopathy, headaches, or hydrocephalus or lead to brainstem and cranial nerve signs from compression or vertebral artery involvement. Special care with

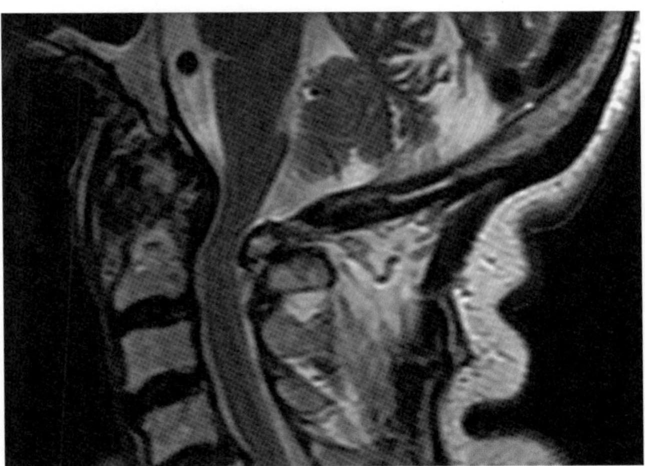

**Fig. 58.4** Magnetic resonance imaging of the craniocervical region in a 65-year-old woman with rheumatoid arthritis and progressive myelopathy. T2-weighted midsagittal image of the cervical spine demonstrates pannus formation at the C1 spinal level, causing severe narrowing of the foramen magnum.

maneuvers requiring hyperextension of the neck, such as endotracheal intubation, is essential in patients with rheumatoid arthritis. Surgical fixation of subluxation is usually unnecessary unless displacement is marked or an associated myelopathy is severe or progressive. The risk of a fatal outcome with a relatively minor whiplash injury is a consideration.

Peripheral nerve involvement is common in rheumatoid arthritis. A distal sensory or sensorimotor polyneuropathy is the usual presentation; clinical or electrophysiological evidence of sensory dysfunction may be found in up to 75% of patients. Mononeuropathy multiplex and entrapment or compression neuropathies are also common. Compression injuries to the median nerve in the carpal tunnel, medial plantar nerve in the tarsal tunnel, ulnar nerve in the cubital tunnel or canal of Guyon, or the fibular (peroneal) nerve at the fibular head may also occur.

Several antirheumatic agents have adverse effects on the neuromuscular system. Gold treatment causes peripheral neuropathy in up to 1% of cases. Its onset is rapid, and the evolution of weakness and the CSF profile may suggest Guillain-Barré syndrome. Chloroquine can cause neuropathy, myopathy, or both, and D-penicillamine causes disturbances of taste, an inflammatory myopathy, and a reversible form of myasthenia gravis. Commonly used tumor necrosis factor-alpha (TNFα) inhibitors can lead to opportunistic CNS infections and a demyelinating disorder resembling multiple sclerosis.

## Systemic Lupus Erythematosus

Neurological involvement occurs during the course of SLE in as many as 75% of patients, often during the first year. Neurological complications may lead to a fatal outcome. The mechanism of CNS involvement is unknown. Neither the presence of antineuronal and other autoantibodies nor the deposition of antibody in the choroid plexus correlates with CNS involvement.

The most common neurological manifestations are episodic affective or psychotic disorders that may be difficult to distinguish from corticosteroid-induced mental changes. Cognitive dysfunction is often temporary. The clinical and imaging features may mimic those of multiple sclerosis (Magro Checa et al., 2013). Treatment is empirical, depending on presentation and the probable underlying pathophysiology. Disturbances of consciousness sometimes occur, especially in patients with systemic infections. Focal neurological deficits may result from stroke. The pathogenesis of stroke in SLE includes cardiac valvular disease, thrombosis associated with antiphospholipid antibodies, and, less commonly, cerebral vasculitis. Anticoagulant therapy may prevent stroke recurrence in patients with the antiphospholipid antibody syndrome. Dyskinesias, especially chorea, occur in some patients with SLE, but underlying structural pathology of the basal ganglia is rare; chorea is associated with the presence of antiphospholipid antibodies. The probable causes of generalized or partial seizures are microinfarcts, metabolic disturbances, and systemic infections. (The pediatric aspects of SLE are discussed in Chapter 59.)

PNS involvement occurs less often and is usually characterized by a distal sensory or sensorimotor polyneuropathy (Florica et al., 2011) that is sometimes subclinical but can be detected by sensory threshold testing; it is related to reduced intraepidermal nerve fiber density (Tseng et al., 2006). Other forms of neuropathy include an acute or chronic demyelinating polyneuropathy that resembles Guillain-Barré syndrome or chronic inflammatory demyelinating polyneuropathy (CIDP), single or multiple mononeuropathies, and optic neuropathy. Corticosteroids, immunosuppressive agents, high-dose intravenous immunoglobulin, and plasmapheresis are beneficial in treating neuropathies caused by necrotizing vasculitis but have less certain value in other circumstances.

## Sjögren Syndrome

Sjögren syndrome may be a primary disorder or secondary to other connective tissue diseases. The main features are xerostomia and xerophthalmia. Women are more often affected than men. Definitive diagnosis requires a positive result on the Rose Bengal dye test for keratoconjunctivitis, evidence of diminished salivary gland flow, abnormalities on biopsy of a minor salivary gland, and an abnormal test result for ss-A and ss-B antibodies. CNS complications are not common but include psychiatric disturbances, late-onset migrainous episodes, aseptic meningitis, meningoencephalitis, focal signs, and an acute or chronic myelopathy. Cranial MRI may show small hyperintense subcortical lesions.

Polyneuropathy is the most common peripheral manifestation, but mononeuropathy multiplex may also occur (Streifler and Molad, 2014). Sensory neuronopathy is unusual but is more characteristic of Sjögren syndrome than other connective tissue diseases (Berkowitz and Samuels, 2014).

## Progressive Systemic Sclerosis

Progressive systemic sclerosis (i.e., scleroderma) occasionally affects the nervous system. The usual syndromes are a distal sensorimotor polyneuropathy, entrapment mononeuropathy, trigeminal neuropathy, myopathy, or myositis (Streifler and Molad, 2014). A rare scleroderma-like illness, nephrogenic systemic fibrosis, is an exceedingly rare complication of gadolinium administration in patients with underlying renal dysfunction, especially those who are undergoing dialysis.

## Behçet Disease

The combination of uveitis and oral and genital ulcers defines Behçet disease, a disorder of unknown cause. Aseptic meningitis or meningoencephalitis occurs in 20% of cases. Other findings may include focal or multifocal neurological signs caused by ischemic disease of the brain or spinal cord related to small vessel inflammatory disease; the brainstem is frequently involved. Cerebral venous sinus thrombosis is another possible complication (Shi et al., 2018). The CSF commonly shows a mild pleocytosis, and the protein concentration may be increased. Peripheral nerve involvement is rare and takes the form of polyneuropathy or mononeuropathy multiplex. Treatment is with corticosteroids. Anticoagulation is used to treat cerebral venous sinus thrombosis (see Chapter 64).

### Relapsing Polychondritis

Relapsing polychondritis is an infrequently diagnosed inflammatory condition of cartilage, such as that of the ears, nose, trachea, ribs, and joints. Episodes of ear or nose inflammation typically last 1 to 4 weeks and then either resolve completely or leave deformities secondary to the destruction of cartilage. The disorder affects both genders equally, with peak age at incidence between 30 and 60 years. Eye inflammation, especially episcleritis or conjunctivitis, may be associated with the attacks. Systemic vasculitis or features of other connective tissue disorders may develop. The diagnosis requires a typical clinical picture of chondritis confirmed by biopsy. The ESR is usually elevated. Although autoimmunity against type II collagen may play a role in pathogenesis, only half of affected patients have serological evidence of anti–type II collagen antibodies.

Auditory or vestibular dysfunction occurs in nearly half of patients. The pathological mechanism usually is otic rather than inflammation of CN VIII. Other cranial neuropathies, such as optic or facial neuropathy, may be associated. The cause of headache, when it occurs, more often involves extracranial chondritis than intracranial inflammation. Aseptic meningitis, which may be recurrent, and vasculitic meningoencephalitis are sometimes associated neurological conditions.

Corticosteroid therapy is the traditional treatment. The efficacy of other anti-inflammatory or immunosuppressive drugs is difficult to assess because of the remitting and relapsing pattern of the disease.

## RESPIRATORY DISEASES

Ventilation requires the integrity of the CNS and PNS to support its coordinated motor activity. Diseases of the forebrain, brainstem, and spinal cord can cause abnormal ventilatory patterns or ventilatory arrest, and diseases of the motor unit cause hypoventilation and ventilatory failure. This section is concerned with the neurological consequences of respiratory abnormalities rather than neurological causes of ventilatory disturbances.

### Hypoxia

The neurological manifestations of hypoxia depend on its rate of onset, duration, and severity. Acid-base imbalance may complicate hypoxia, leading to other hematological and biochemical changes that affect cerebral function. The precise mechanisms responsible for the neurological abnormalities are complex and not completely understood.

Headache, disorientation, confusion, and depressed cognitive function characterize the encephalopathies caused by chronic pulmonary insufficiency. Postural tremor, myoclonus, asterixis, and brisk tendon reflexes are common examination findings, and papilledema is sometimes present. These encephalopathies are due not only to cerebral hypoxia but also to hypercapnia, which leads to cerebral vasodilatation, increased CSF pressure, and altered pH of the CSF.

Sleep apnea syndromes cause chronic nocturnal hypoxia and become symptomatic as excessive daytime sleepiness and sometimes as cognitive dysfunction. Many affected patients are obese and plethoric and snore heavily. Sleep apnea is an independent and potentially modifiable risk factor for ischemic stroke. A summary of treatment appears in Chapter 101.

Headache, lassitude, anorexia, nausea, difficulty in concentration, and disturbances of sleep characterize high-altitude sickness. Symptoms begin within hours or days of ascending higher than 10,000 ft. At even higher altitudes, consciousness may be disturbed; coma develops in severe cases and may eventuate in death. Cerebral edema of uncertain cause is the major underlying feature that causes papilledema, retinal hemorrhages, cranial neuropathies, focal or multifocal motor and sensory deficits, and behavioral disturbances. Corticosteroids or carbonic anhydrase inhibitors such as acetazolamide avert or relieve the syndrome, along with return to lower altitudes.

### Hypercapnia

Ventilatory impairment causes hypercapnia along with hypoxemia; the neurological manifestations of each are difficult to distinguish.

### Hypocapnia

The hypocapnia that results from hyperventilation causes cerebral vasoconstriction, a shift of the oxyhemoglobin dissociation curve that reduces the peripheral availability of oxygen, and an alteration in the ionic balance of calcium. The clinical features are lightheadedness, perioral paresthesias, visual disturbances, headache, unsteadiness, tremor, nausea, palpitations, muscle cramps, carpopedal spasms, and loss of consciousness.

Hyperventilation occurs in hepatic and diabetic coma, with some brainstem lesions, with cardiopulmonary diseases, as a result of acidosis from certain drugs, and on an iatrogenic basis in patients being ventilated mechanically. Episodic hyperventilation often occurs without an identifiable systemic disease.

## SYSTEMIC INFLAMMATORY RESPONSE SYNDROME

Neurological complications may occur when infection and trauma have induced a systemic inflammatory response affecting the microcirculation to multiple organs. For example, in patients with sepsis and multiorgan (including respiratory) failure, an axonal neuropathy sometimes develops that comes to attention during attempts to withdraw ventilatory support. The neuropathy, called *critical illness polyneuropathy*, resolves only slowly as the critical illness subsides.

Corticosteroids and neuromuscular blocking drugs may induce a myopathy, especially in patients with obstructive airway diseases. Its highest prevalence is among asthmatic patients who require ventilatory support in addition to corticosteroids and also have received neuromuscular blocking agents. It sometimes occurs in patients who have received either corticosteroids or neuromuscular blockers but not both. Muscle biopsy may show muscle fibers with specific loss of myosin (thick filaments). This *critical illness myopathy* is often characterized by a low level of serum creatine kinase, in contrast to most other myopathies.

Encephalopathy complicates sepsis and most often occurs in patients with acute respiratory distress syndrome. The pathogenesis is multifactorial and relates to impairment of the cerebral microcirculation, cerebral edema, disruption of the blood–brain barrier, direct cerebral infection, toxins produced by infecting organisms, metabolic abnormalities, oxidative stress, mitochondrial dysfunction, prolonged inflammatory processes, and the effects of medication (Schmutzhard and Pfausler, 2017). The encephalopathy tends to fluctuate in severity, is often worse at night, and may be associated with marked EEG abnormalities. Treatment is the correction of factors responsible for the underlying sepsis; no specific treatment exists for the encephalopathy.

## SARCOIDOSIS

Sarcoidosis, a disorder of unknown cause, involves many organ systems and has many different clinical presentations. It is more common in people of African descent than in Whites and occurs more often in women than in men. Discovery of the pulmonary disease is often incidental on routine chest x-ray examination. The prevalence of neurological involvement in any series varies with case selection and diagnostic criteria but may be as high as 10%. The nervous system may be involved directly by the disease or involvement may be secondary to

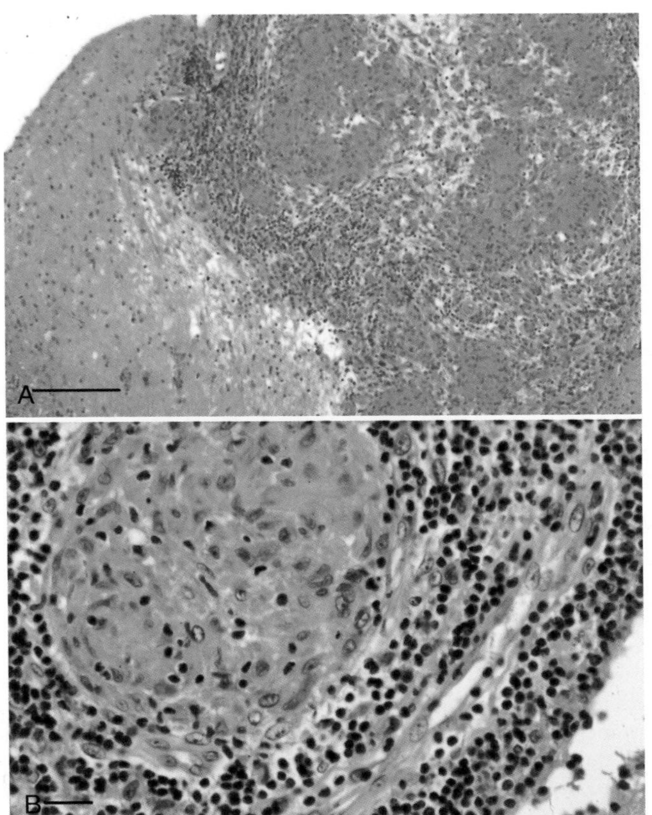

**Fig. 58.5 Brain Biopsy Section Stained with Hematoxylin and Eosin.** **A,** Low-magnification photomicrograph showing dense granulomatous inflammation involving leptomeninges, with underlying gliotic cerebral cortex in a patient with neurosarcoidosis (scale bar, 50 μm). **B,** High-magnification photomicrograph showing Virchow-Robin space involvement by a collection of epithelioid histiocytes (granulomatous inflammation) and lymphocytes in a patient with neurosarcoidosis (scale bar, 20 μm). *(From Aminoff, M.J., Josephson, S.A. [Eds], 2014. Aminoff's Neurology and General Medicine, fifth ed. Elsevier, San Diego.)*

opportunistic infections associated with abnormalities of the immune system. The following discussion considers only direct involvement (Fig. 58.5).

Cranial neuropathies from chronic basal meningitis constitute the most common neurological manifestation of sarcoidosis. Most often affected is the facial nerve, sometimes bilaterally. Increased intracranial pressure from a space-occupying lesion, meningeal involvement, or obstructive hydrocephalus may cause papilledema. Visual changes may be due to direct involvement of the optic nerves or their meningeal covering or to uveitis. Unilateral or bilateral recurrent laryngeal, trigeminal, or auditory nerve involvement may also occur, and multiple cranial neuropathies are possible as well.

Disturbances of the hypothalamic region are associated with diabetes insipidus, abnormalities in thermoregulation, amenorrhea, impotence, and hypoglycemia as well as disturbances of sleep, obesity, personality changes, and evidence of hypopituitarism. Other neurological features depend on the distribution of intracranial or intraspinal meningeal or parenchymal involvement. Diffuse meningoencephalitis causes cognitive abnormalities or affective disorders. An enlarging granuloma may mimic a cerebral tumor and lead to seizures and focal neurological deficits.

Peripheral nerve involvement may take the form of a symmetrical polyneuropathy or an asymmetrical mononeuropathy multiplex. This may result from polyradicular involvement via extension of meningeal sarcoidosis or from direct involvement of the nerves by sarcoid granulomas. Muscle granulomas may cause clinical features of a myopathy and commonly occur in clinically unaffected muscles.

Neurosarcoidosis often remits spontaneously, but progressive neurological disease occurs in approximately 30% of cases. The diagnosis of neurosarcoidosis is difficult in the absence of systemic disease, especially cutaneous or pulmonary involvement. Whole-body CT or positron emission tomography (PET) scans may identify subclinical systemic tissue involvement. Histological confirmation often requires biopsy of seemingly unaffected tissue (e.g., muscle or conjunctiva) if other lesions are not accessible. Neither the tuberculin skin test, urinary calcium levels, nor the blood concentration of angiotensin-converting enzyme definitively establishes the diagnosis, and each has limited sensitivity and specificity.

The recommended treatment is with corticosteroids, but its long-term value is not established. The initial dose of prednisone is 1 mg/kg/day, which is adjusted according to clinical response. Irradiation of a focal lesion is beneficial in some cases. Refractory cases of neurosarcoidosis may respond to a variety of immunosuppressive agents including cyclophosphamide, methotrexate, and infliximab (Joubert et al., 2017). Useful surgical measures are the excision of focal enlarging granulomas and the placement of a shunt to relieve hydrocephalus.

## HEMATOLOGICAL DISORDERS WITH ANEMIA

Anemia often causes nonspecific behavioral symptoms such as lassitude, lightheadedness, inattentiveness, irritability, headache, and unsteadiness. Iron-deficiency anemia is associated with pica, restless legs syndrome, idiopathic intracranial hypertension, and an increased risk of stroke or TIAs due to thrombocytosis. Severe anemia may rarely cause focal neurological deficits in patients with preexisting cerebral atherosclerotic disease. Pancytopenia may cause hemorrhagic CNS complications.

### Megaloblastic Anemia

Vitamin $B_{12}$ deficiency causes myelopathy, encephalopathy, optic neuropathy, peripheral neuropathy, or some combination of these disorders. The neurological complications do not necessarily correlate with the presence or severity of associated megaloblastic anemia. Folic acid can mask the anemia without preventing the neurological complications. Nitrous oxide anesthesia or recreational abuse may unmask a subclinical cobalamin deficiency (Patel et al., 2018). Folic acid fortification of the grain supply in the United States began in 1994 to prevent spina bifida; consequently, anemia is no longer a reliable marker of vitamin $B_{12}$ deficiency. Increased serum levels of homocysteine and methylmalonic acid may indicate intracellular vitamin $B_{12}$ deficiency even in the setting of normal serum vitamin $B_{12}$ levels.

Vitamin $B_{12}$ is absorbed exclusively by the terminal ileum using intrinsic factor, and deficiency occurs in patients with ileal resection or urinary intestinal diversion. Some patients have an autoimmune condition that leads to a loss of intrinsic factor, which is identified by the presence of anti–parietal cell antibodies or intrinsic factor antibodies. Treatment with intramuscular injections of vitamin $B_{12}$ corrects the deficiency, often with arrested progression or reversal of the neurological changes. The extent of residua correlates with the severity and duration of symptoms before treatment.

### Sickle Cell Disease

Sickle cell disease, the result of a genetic point mutation in the beta-globin gene, causes a vasculopathy of both large and small vessels (Connes et al., 2013). Sickled cells adhere to the vascular endothelium, and a cascade of activated inflammatory cells and clotting factors leads to a nidus for thrombus formation. Hypoxia, infection, inflammation, dehydration, and acidosis increase sickling.

The most common neurological complication of sickle cell disease is stroke, which occurred more often in children than in adults before the routine use of transfusion therapy. Other complications are convulsions, intracranial (usually subarachnoid) hemorrhage, behavioral disturbances, and alteration in consciousness. The cause of intracranial hemorrhage cannot always be determined despite detailed investigation, but rupture of an aneurysm, which may be treated by surgical or endovascular means, is sometimes responsible. Blindness sometimes results from proliferative retinopathy; retinal detachment or infarction also occurs. Spinal cord infarction is rare.

### Thalassemias

Extramedullary hematopoiesis occurs in the liver, spleen, and lymph nodes of patients with severe forms of beta-thalassemia. It may also occur in the spinal epidural space, causing a compressive myelopathy. Treatment includes local irradiation, surgical decompression, corticosteroids, and repeated blood transfusions. Bone marrow hypertrophy also causes facial deformity, nerve root compression, and auditory impairment. Surgical decompression or radiation therapy is sometimes beneficial.

### Acanthocytic Syndromes

Acanthocytes, or spiny red cells, are associated with abetalipoproteinemia (see Chapter 84), neuroacanthocytosis (see Chapter 95), and McLeod syndrome (see Chapter 95).

## PROLIFERATIVE HEMATOLOGICAL DISORDERS

### Leukemias

Leukemic infiltration of the nervous system, hemorrhage, infection, electrolyte disturbances, hyperviscosity, and adverse effects of treatment cause the neurological complications of leukemia. Localized leukemic deposits are more likely to affect the brain than the spinal cord; peripheral nerve involvement is rare.

The clinical features of meningeal leukemia are headache, nausea and vomiting, somnolence, irritability, convulsions, and coma. Obstructive or communicating hydrocephalus with increased intracranial pressure, papilledema, or meningismus may be associated. Cranial neuropathies and spinal radiculopathies are common; their multifocal distribution suggests the possibility of meningeal leukemia. Examination of the CSF shows abnormal leukemic cells, especially if cytospin techniques are used, but a normal examination result does not exclude the diagnosis of meningeal leukemia. Treatment consists of intrathecal and systemic chemotherapy.

Intracerebral hemorrhage is more common than subarachnoid or subdural hemorrhage. It tends to occur when the platelet count is less than 20,000/mL. The hemorrhage is often multifocal and ranges in severity from microscopic to fatal. Spinal subdural or subarachnoid hemorrhage is less common than intracranial bleeding but is a potentially serious complication of lumbar puncture, sometimes requiring surgical decompression.

A hyperviscosity syndrome occurs when the high white blood cell count markedly increases resistance to blood flow, impairing the transit of blood through the microcirculation. It is characterized by headache, somnolence, impaired consciousness, stroke or TIAs, and visual disturbances. Venous sinus thrombosis, nonbacterial thrombotic endocarditis, and disseminated intravascular coagulation (DIC) (discussed later) may also occur. The most common cause of this syndrome is an increase in the concentration of circulating gamma globulins, discussed in the following section. When this is caused by a high serum leukocytosis, urgent leukapheresis is the treatment of choice.

Infection is a common complication of chemotherapy or corticosteroid therapy. The use of broad-spectrum antibiotics often encourages infection by unusual organisms. Progressive multifocal leukoencephalopathy is an uncommon complication of leukemia and its treatment (see Chapter 77).

### Plasma Cell Dyscrasias

The basis for the classification of plasma cell dyscrasias is the protein synthesized. Complicating these disorders are paraneoplastic syndromes (see Chapter 81) and an increased susceptibility to CNS infections.

#### Myelomatosis

Multiple myeloma, the most common plasma cell dyscrasia, is associated with a monoclonal immunoglobulin G (IgG) or immunoglobulin A (IgA) paraprotein in the serum, urine, or both. The clinical features are pain, fracture, and destruction of bone. Tumor infiltration of the vertebrae may cause compression of the spinal cord or nerve roots. Back pain is conspicuous, and radicular pain is common; cord or root dysfunction may also be present. Treatment by local irradiation and high-dose corticosteroids prevents or minimizes residual neurological deficits, but urgent decompressive surgery is usually required if there is cord compression. Cranial involvement is less common than spinal involvement. Cranial neuropathies—especially of CN II, V, VI, VII, and VIII—may occur. A reversible optic neuropathy of uncertain etiology, but probably not due to nerve infiltration, has been described.

Increased intracranial pressure does not necessarily indicate intracranial infiltration; intracranial hypertension sometimes occurs without evidence of intracranial myeloma or hyperviscosity syndromes.

Peripheral neuropathy is a recognized complication of myeloma. This may be a symmetrical axonal sensory or sensorimotor polyneuropathy or a predominantly motor neuropathy resembling CIDP. These can occur with either osteolytic or osteosclerotic myeloma. Treatment with cytotoxic agents and plasmapheresis sometimes slows or reverses the neuropathy, as may the irradiation of bone lesions. Tumor infiltration of nerves can lead to an asymmetrical neuropathy that has the features of mononeuropathy multiplex. Amyloidosis is sometimes associated with myeloma and causes a neuropathy characterized by dysautonomia, marked loss of pain and temperature appreciation, and weakness. In addition, thalidomide and related compounds used to treat myeloma may also lead to a length-dependent sensory neuropathy, often with autonomic involvement.

The POEMS syndrome consists of *p*olyneuropathy, *o*rganomegaly, *e*ndocrinopathy, *M* protein, and *s*kin changes in patients with plasma cell dyscrasia. A markedly elevated serum vascular endothelial growth factor (VEGF) level is often present. The POEMS syndrome is most often associated with osteosclerotic myeloma but also occurs with osteolytic myeloma accompanied by only minor sclerotic changes; it also occurs in patients without myeloma. Osteosclerotic myeloma is usually considered a variant of solitary or early multiple myeloma but may be a distinct entity. The neuropathy is a distal sensorimotor polyneuropathy with both axonal degeneration and segmental demyelination. Other clinical features are papilledema, lymphadenopathy, hepatosplenomegaly, impotence, gynecomastia, amenorrhea, glucose intolerance, peripheral edema, ascites, pleural effusions, and skin changes including cutaneous pigmentation, thickening, and hypertrichosis. Corticosteroids, cyclophosphamide, and the irradiation of solitary osteosclerotic lesions may be beneficial. Hematopoietic stem cell transplantation following high-dose chemotherapy may be used in cases of severe disease.

The causes of other neurological manifestations are infections related to immunodeficiency, hypercalcemia, uremia, and hyperviscosity. The characteristic features of the hyperviscosity syndrome are headache, visual disturbances, and encephalopathy. Funduscopic examination reveals hemorrhages, exudates, and venous engorgement.

### Waldenström Macroglobulinemia

Waldenström macroglobulinemia is a plasma cell dyscrasia associated with IgM gammopathy. Neurological complications are common. A progressive sensorimotor polyneuropathy occurs. The cause is the binding of monoclonal immunoglobulin M (IgM) to peripheral nerves or lymphocytic infiltration of the nerves. Other neurological complications relate to hyperviscosity or a bleeding tendency resulting from platelet abnormalities. Presentation is with a diffuse encephalopathy or focal neurological deficits. Fatigue, lassitude, lethargy, confusion, altered consciousness, and seizures are common. Visual, auditory, and vestibular disturbances also occur.

Neurological examination shows pyramidal, cerebellar, or brainstem abnormalities. Funduscopic examination may reveal papilledema, venous engorgement, hemorrhages, and exudates. Plasmapheresis relieves symptoms caused by hyperviscosity and helps attenuate the peripheral neuropathy in some cases; B-cell-depleting therapies such as rituximab may also be useful.

### Monoclonal Gammopathy of Undetermined Significance

Many patients with a monoclonal gammopathy have no evidence of serious underlying pathology, but a malignant plasma cell dyscrasia may eventually develop in some cases. CIDP is the characteristic polyneuropathy associated with monoclonal gammopathy of undetermined significance. IgM autoantibodies that react with myelin-associated glycoproteins or with other target antigens may be present in the blood. Treatment with cycles of cyclophosphamide and prednisone, plasmapheresis, high-dose intravenous immunoglobulin, or rituximab may provide benefit.

### Amyloidosis

Amyloidosis may occur as a familial disorder with dominant inheritance. Portuguese, Japanese, Swedish, and other varieties occur. The main neurological complication is a small-fiber sensory neuropathy with marked impairment of pain and temperature appreciation and lesser involvement of other sensory modalities (see Chapter 106). An associated dysautonomia is conspicuous. Weakness develops later.

Both primary and secondary nonfamilial amyloidosis occurs. Primary amyloidosis occurs in the absence of other disorders (except multiple myeloma), whereas secondary amyloidosis occurs in association with such disorders as chronic infection. Peripheral neuropathy is a common feature of primary but not secondary amyloidosis. Characteristic of the neuropathy is a progressive sensory or sensorimotor polyneuropathy with autonomic involvement or carpal tunnel syndrome. Cranial neuropathy is uncommon; CN III, V, and VII are most often affected. Cardiovascular and renal dysfunction is common, and other organ systems may be involved. The clinical features and presence (in most cases) of a monoclonal protein in the serum suggest the diagnosis. A variety of treatments are available, many with limited success (Rajkumar and Gertz, 2007). Patients with neurological manifestations of transthyretin amyloidosis may benefit from inotersen treatment or liver transplantation (Benson et al., 2018). Death usually results from systemic complications.

Accumulation of beta-2 microglobulin–associated amyloid in patients undergoing long-term hemodialysis may cause carpal tunnel syndrome, a cervical myelopathy, or a cauda equina syndrome. Surgical decompression may be helpful in such circumstances.

### Cryoglobulinemia

Cryoglobulins are proteins that precipitate in the cold and dissolve when heated. They are classified as monoclonal IgM, IgG, IgA, or light chains (type 1), mixed but with one monoclonal immunoglobulin (type 2), and polyclonal without any monoclonal protein (type 3).

Primary cryoglobulinemia occurs in the absence of other disease. Secondary cryoglobulinemia occurs in association with disorders such as myelomatosis or macroglobulinemia with monoclonal protein production or in disorders with polyclonal protein production, such as vasculitis or other chronic inflammatory diseases. Cryoglobulinemia is associated with TIAs, strokes, and a peripheral neuropathy that is probably ischemic in origin. The extent to which the neurological complications are due to the cryoglobulinemia, as opposed to the accompanying vasculitis, is unclear. Treatment with corticosteroids, plasmapheresis, or both may be beneficial.

### Lymphoma

Neurological complications of lymphoma can be due to direct spread of tumor, compression of the nervous system by extrinsic tumor, and paraneoplastic syndromes (see Chapter 80). They may also result from irradiation or chemotherapy, thrombocytopenic hemorrhage, or opportunistic infections. Primary CNS lymphoma is a known complication of immunosuppression and occurs most often in patients with acquired immunodeficiency syndrome (see Chapter 77) and less frequently in transplant recipients; it is also increasingly found in immunocompetent patients.

### Polycythemia

The thrombotic and hemorrhagic complications of polycythemia often affect the nervous system. Occlusion of small or large arteries or venous channels may cause cerebral infarctions, which are sometimes recurrent. Possible causes of the thrombotic tendency are increased blood viscosity, thrombocytosis, and possibly chronic DIC. Intracranial hemorrhage is caused by abnormalities of clot retraction, thromboplastin generation, and platelet function. Spinal cord infarction is rare. Patients with polycythemia often complain of headache, poor concentration, unsteadiness, tinnitus, blurred vision, dysesthesias, and other nonspecific symptoms. The basis of such symptoms is unclear, but disturbances in the retinal circulation may account for the visual complaints. Intracranial hypertension and chorea may occur with polycythemia. Chorea reverses when the underlying hematological disorder is treated. Low-dose aspirin (75–100 mg/day) is recommended for the prophylaxis of thrombotic complications in those patients who do not have a history of major bleeding.

## HEMORRHAGIC DISEASES

### Hemophilia

Intracranial hemorrhage is a major cause of death in patients with hemophilia. Hemorrhages may be epidural, subdural, subarachnoid, or intracerebral and may occur spontaneously or follow trivial head injury. Neurological symptoms may not develop for several days after injury. The severity of bleeding generally correlates with the severity of coagulopathy. Spinal subdural or epidural hemorrhage may occur but is uncommon; the clinical features are back or neck pain and a progressive painful paraparesis or quadriparesis. Surgical decompression is necessary to preserve neurological function. Replacement of the deficient factor VIII is required to perform any invasive procedures.

Peripheral neuropathies secondary to compression of individual nerves by intramuscular or retroperitoneal hematomas are a common complication. Urgent operative decompression may be needed to preserve function.

Seizures may result from brain injury caused by previous intracranial hemorrhage. Their control with anticonvulsant agents helps to prevent further bleeding.

### Other Hemorrhagic Disorders

Other coagulopathies are associated with a lower frequency of neurological complications than hemophilia, but complications are similar to those already described.

#### Disseminated Intravascular Coagulation

DIC is characterized by thrombotic occlusion of small vessels and concomitant hemorrhagic complications, because clotting factors (including fibrinogen and factors V and VIII) and platelets are consumed in the thrombotic process. DIC occurs in association with primary brain disease, diseases of other organs, septicemia, immune-mediated disorders, diabetic ketoacidosis, neoplastic disease, and obstetrical complications. Several organs may be affected, the brain most commonly. The underlying cause, rate of onset, and severity of DIC influence the clinical features, as do the organs affected and the predominance of thrombosis or hemorrhage.

Neurological features fluctuate in severity. Encephalopathy is common and varies in severity from a mild confusional state to coma. Comatose patients may recover completely, indicating the need for aggressive management. The prothrombin time is usually prolonged, the serum level of fibrin degradation products is increased, and thrombocytopenia may be present. The serum fibrinogen concentration is sometimes normal but is usually depressed. Neuroimaging may show multifocal cerebral hematomas and infarctions. The underlying cause of the DIC determines the treatment to be given. Heparin may limit thrombotic complications but can worsen hemorrhagic complications; its value is uncertain. The same is true of antiplatelet agents, antithrombin concentrates, and transfusions.

#### Thrombocytopenia

Thrombocytopenia, caused by the reduced production or increased breakdown of platelets, may lead to hemorrhage. Intracerebral hemorrhage is usually from capillaries and characterized first by clinically silent petechial hemorrhages and later by symptomatic hematomas. Spinal or peripheral nerve involvement by hemorrhage is uncommon. Platelet transfusions arrest further bleeding. Corticosteroids may be beneficial when platelet function is abnormal; splenectomy or intravenous immunoglobulin is sometimes required.

#### Thrombotic Thrombocytopenic Purpura

Thrombotic thrombocytopenic purpura is a rare disorder that often has a fatal outcome. It has been related most commonly to a severe deficiency in ADAMTS13, the specific von Willebrand factor–cleaving protease, resulting from autoimmunity. Less commonly, it is related to mutation (Upshaw-Schulman syndrome) of the *ADAMTS13* gene (Joly et al., 2017). The clinical features are thrombocytopenic purpura, hemolytic anemia, fever, neurological abnormalities, and renal disease. The neurological features may include headache, mental changes, altered state of consciousness, seizures, and focal deficits. MRI may reveal infarctions or white matter abnormalities. Treatment options are plasmapheresis (supplying deficient ADAMTS13) and administration of corticosteroids, rituximab, and other immune modulators. Bortezomib is a promising adjunct to plasmapheresis for refractory or relapsed disease in patients unresponsive to rituximab. Salvage splenectomy may be necessary.

#### Iatrogenic Hemorrhagic Disorders

In patients receiving heparin or warfarin, intracranial or spinal hemorrhage may develop. The bleeding may be parenchymal, subarachnoid, subdural, or extradural. It can occur spontaneously or after injury and cause the acute or subacute onset of a neurological deficit. Treatment includes reversal of the coagulopathy, definition of the pathology by neuroimaging studies, and urgent decompressive surgery if necessary. Intramuscular hemorrhage may cause a plexopathy or peripheral neuropathy that also may require urgent decompression.

## ANTIPHOSPHOLIPID ANTIBODY SYNDROMES

Antiphospholipid antibodies (the lupus anticoagulant and anticardiolipin antibodies) are detectable in several disorders, but especially in SLE, Sneddon syndrome (Fig. 58.6), and other connective tissue disorders (Wijetilleka et al., 2012). These antibodies occur in patients taking certain medications (e.g., phenothiazines, phenytoin, propranolol, amoxicillin), with some infections and obstetrical complications, and as an incidental finding in healthy people. The presence of antiphospholipid antibodies—together with other antibodies and antibody complexes of different immunoglobulin subtypes (Uthman et al., 2019)—increases the risk of thrombotic disease. The cause of cerebral ischemia is either arterial or venous occlusion. Visual abnormalities include amaurosis fugax and ischemic optic neuropathy or retinopathy. The occurrence of migraine-like headaches may be fortuitous. An acute ischemic encephalopathy characterized by confusion, obtundation, quadriparesis, and bilateral pyramidal signs may occur. Dementia, chorea, transient global amnesia, transverse myelopathy, Guillain-Barré syndrome, and seizures are other possible manifestations. The condition may simulate multiple sclerosis clinically and on MRI (Uthman et al., 2019).

The pathogenesis of the thrombotic tendency is not established. The presence of antiphospholipid antibodies does not require immunosuppression. Secondary prevention in patients with antiphospholipid antibody syndrome who have experienced a stroke typically involves anticoagulation.

## LIVER DISEASE

In patients with acute hepatic failure, the development of severe cerebral edema is common (Fig. 58.7). Several other neurological manifestations occur with chronic hepatic disorders.

### Portal-Systemic Encephalopathy

Chronic liver disease causes a portal-systemic encephalopathy characterized by an abnormal mental status. Points to emphasize are that (1) the encephalopathy may have an insidious onset, delaying its clinical recognition and treatment; (2) a flapping tremor (asterixis) may be the only other neurological sign; and (3) liver function test results, other than the fasting arterial ammonia concentration, do not always correlate with the severity of the clinical disturbance. Focal neurological signs may be present but have no prognostic significance (Cadranel et al., 2001). EEG abnormalities also correlate with the severity of encephalopathy. MRI may show abnormal signal intensity in the basal ganglia on T1-weighted images (Fig. 58.8). The mechanism of the encephalopathy is unknown. Treatment is discussed in Chapter 83.

### Chronic Non-Wilsonian Hepatocerebral Degeneration

In some patients with chronic liver disease, a permanent neurological deficit develops, even in the absence of previous portal-systemic encephalopathy. The neurological features are similar to those of Wilson disease (see Chapter 95): intention tremor, ataxia, dysarthria,

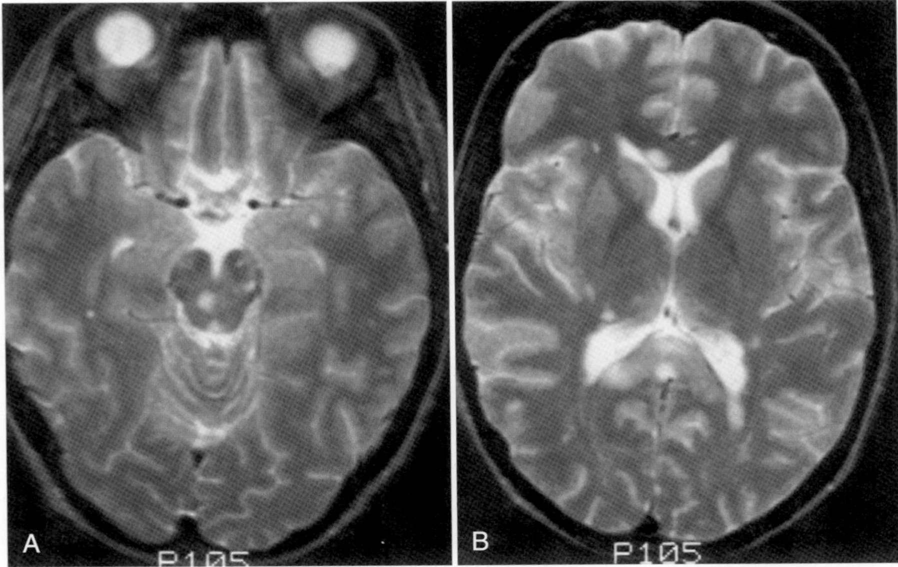


**Fig. 58.6** This Patient was A 27-Year-Old Woman with Sneddon Syndrome (Livedo Reticularis and Cerebro-Vascular Disease). T2-weighted magnetic resonance imaging scans show multiple foci of high signal intensity in the mesencephalon (**A**) as well as in the corpus callosum and periventricular white matter (**B**).

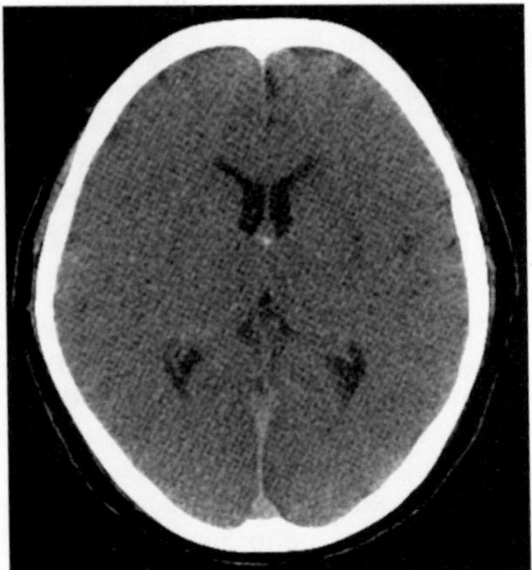

**Fig. 58.7** This Patient was An 81-Year-Old Woman with Anoxic Injury Following Choking on Food Despite Multiple Failed Attempts at A Heimlich Maneuver. Computed tomographic scan without contrast shows severe diffuse cerebral edema.

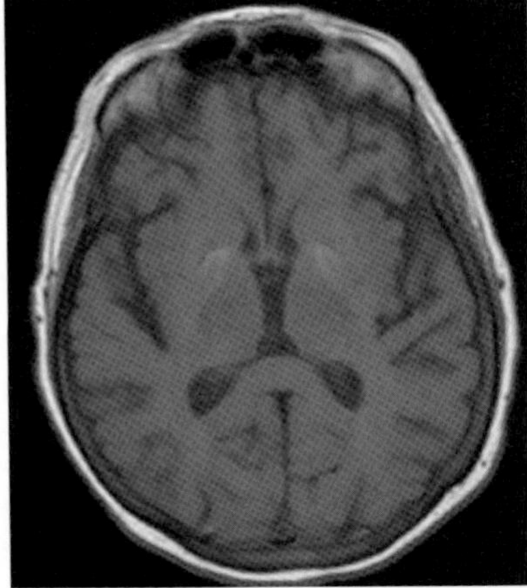

**Fig. 58.8 This 67-Year-Old Woman Had Chronic Liver Disease Related to Hepatitis C.** T1-weighted magnetic resonance imaging scan obtained without contrast shows bright signal in the region of the globus pallidus bilaterally.

and choreoathetosis are common. As with portal-systemic encephalopathy, the severity of the neurological disorder correlates best with the fasting arterial ammonia level but not the more commonly measured random venous serum ammonia levels. Neuroimaging findings may be abnormal. Specific treatment is not available.

### Liver Transplantation

The neurological consequences of liver transplantation are similar to those of transplantation of other organs. The earliest postoperative disturbances are caused by organ rejection (with worsening hepatic encephalopathy), cerebral anoxia, cerebrovascular disease, or the side effects of immunosuppressant drugs, especially cyclosporine and tacrolimus. Seizures are common and may result from metabolic disturbances, cerebrovascular disease, CNS infections, or adverse effects of treatment. Coagulopathies may also develop and can cause fatal cerebral hemorrhage. The causes of late complications are usually infections (e.g., PML, human herpesvirus 6 limbic encephalitis) or malignancies affecting the nervous system.

## PANCREATIC ENCEPHALOPATHY

The association of acute pancreatitis with a transitory encephalopathy is not established. The signs and symptoms are nonspecific and similar to those of other metabolic encephalopathies.

## GASTROINTESTINAL DISEASES

Nutritional deficiency is the usual cause of neurological complications of GI disorders (see Chapter 84). Several different dietary components are simultaneously deficient, and a single responsible nutrient is rarely defined.

### Gastric Surgery

Neurological complications occur in 10% to 15% of patients after gastric resection. Because of the loss of gastric intrinsic factor, impaired vitamin $B_{12}$ absorption may be responsible in part for neuropathy or myelopathy

(Majumder et al., 2013). However, postgastrectomy neuropathy does not usually respond to vitamin $B_{12}$ replacement alone. The myopathy that sometimes occurs is probably caused by vitamin D deficiency.

Gastric plication (bariatric surgery) has been associated with encephalopathy, myelopathy, polyneuropathy, Wernicke syndrome, and a nutritional amblyopia, but the precise nutritional deficiencies responsible remain to be established. Complications are especially likely in the context of recurrent vomiting. Appropriate vitamin supplementation and monitoring after surgery are essential to prevent these deficits.

### Small-Bowel Disease

Neuropathy and myelopathy are associated with the malabsorption syndromes caused by small-bowel disease, biliary atresia, or blind loop syndrome, or with previous extensive GI resection. The findings may include pigmentary retinal degeneration, external ophthalmoplegia, dysarthria, peripheral neuropathy, and pyramidal and cerebral signs in the limbs. Ataxia may be an especially conspicuous feature; therefore the neurological disorder resembles a spinocerebellar degeneration with an associated polyneuropathy. Vitamin E deficiency causes the disorder in many cases and responds to intravenous supplementation.

### Celiac Disease

Chronic gluten enteropathy may cause a progressive and sometimes fatal CNS disorder that includes some combination of encephalopathy, myelopathy, and cerebellar disturbance. Peripheral neuropathy may be an associated, relatively underrecognized finding (Thawani et al., 2015). An axonal neuropathy also occurs alone and without a measurable vitamin deficiency; restriction of dietary gluten leads to the gradual resolution of neuropathic symptoms.

### Whipple Disease

Whipple disease is a multisystem disorder caused by infection with the bacillus *Tropheryma* whippelei. The clinical features are steatorrhea, abdominal pain, weight loss, arthritis, lymphadenopathy, and a variety of systemic complaints. Neurological involvement is rare but may occur in the absence of GI symptoms. The most common neurological feature is dementia (Rossi et al., 2005). Less common are cerebellar ataxia, seizures, myoclonus, clouding of consciousness, visual disturbances, papilledema, supranuclear ophthalmoplegia, myelopathy, and hypothalamic dysfunction. A characteristic movement disorder, oculomasticatory myorhythmia, is peculiar to Whipple disease; pendular vergence oscillations of the eyes with concurrent contractions of the masticatory muscles occur and persist during sleep. Oculofacial-skeletal myorhythmia is also pathognomonic. When present, it resembles oculomasticatory myorhythmia but also involves nonfacial muscles. Postmortem examination shows abnormalities of the gray matter of the hypothalamus, cingulate gyrus, basal ganglia, insular cortex, and cerebellum.

Small-intestine biopsy establishes the diagnosis. Patients with neurological involvement also show cells that stain positively with periodic acid–Schiff stain in the CSF and brain parenchyma (Fig. 58.9). Polymerase chain reaction analysis of intestinal tissue or CSF is sometimes helpful but has a low sensitivity. Treatment is prolonged, with antibiotics such as trimethoprim-sulfamethoxazole, penicillin, tetracycline, or erythromycin. Patients who have a compatible clinical syndrome should receive treatment even when the biopsy result is negative.

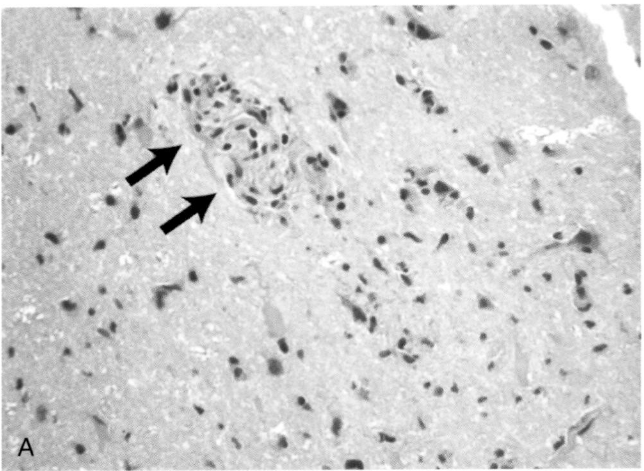


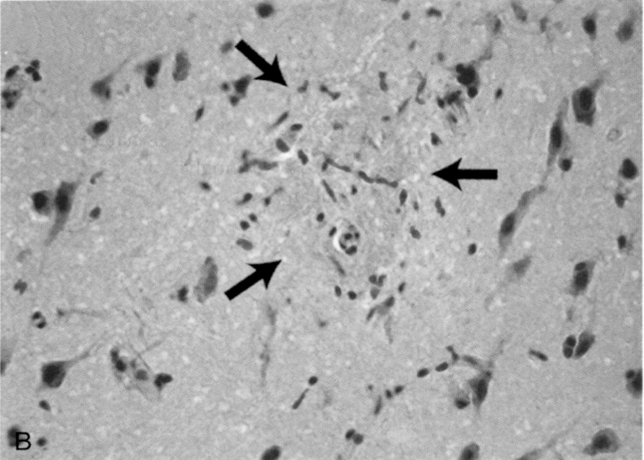


**Fig. 58.9 Brian Biopsy of the Left Putamen in a Patient with Whipple Disease. A,** Stained with hematoxylin and eosin (100×), the lesions *(arrows)* are seen as mild areas of increased cellularity around blood vessels and in neuropil; they consist predominantly of small macrophages or reactive microglial cells. **B,** With hematoxylin and eosin (200×), a single lesion *(arrows)* in the gray matter neuropil is seen. It resembles a neuritic plaque but is composed of microglial cells and macrophages disrupting the neuropil. *(With permission from Mohamed, W., Neil E., Kupsky, W.J., et al., 2011, Isolated intracranial Whipple's disease—report of a rare case and review of the literature. J Neurol Sci 308, 1–8.)*

## RENAL FAILURE

### Overview of Related Neurological Complications

Renal failure is associated with several neurological manifestations. Uremic encephalopathy is discussed in Chapter 83. Its clinical features resemble those of other metabolic encephalopathies, and its severity does not correlate well with any single laboratory abnormality. The mechanism of encephalopathy is not established but has been attributed to the accumulation of toxic organic acids in the CNS or to direct toxic effects on the CNS of parathyroid hormone. It may be associated with asterixis and myoclonus; muscle twitches and seizures may also occur (Brouns and De Deyn, 2004). Chorea may result from dysfunction of the basal ganglia. Stroke incidence increases in chronic renal failure. Ischemic stroke may relate to atherosclerosis, thromboembolic disease, or hypotension during dialysis. Atherosclerosis is generally more diffuse than in the age-matched general population, probably because of a combination of traditional risk factors and factors related to the renal failure, such as the accumulation of endogenous guanidino compounds. Hyperhomocysteinemia also is common; this condition, of uncertain etiology, may predispose affected persons to ischemic stroke; it responds to enhanced dialysis over superflux membranes (Brouns and De Deyn, 2004). The incidence of intracranial hemorrhage is increased; hypertension, uremic platelet dysfunction, polycystic kidney disease, and the use of anticoagulation or antiplatelet agents are probable risk factors.

A length-dependent, symmetrical, sensorimotor polyneuropathy is a common complication of uremia. It usually worsens over several months but may progress more rapidly until the patient is profoundly disabled. Dysesthesias, muscle cramps, and restless legs are common early features. The neuropathy may stabilize or improve with long-term dialysis. Renal transplantation produces progressive improvement over the following year or longer, and complete recovery is possible. The accumulation of metabolites with a molecular weight of 500 to 2000 Da is the probable cause of the neuropathy, but the precise pathogenesis is not established.

Autonomic dysfunction leads to postural hypotension, sudomotor abnormalities, impotence, and GI disturbances. Dysautonomia may be important in the development of hypotension during hemodialysis, but other factors such as volume depletion and rapid fluid shifts are undoubtedly involved as well.

Uremic optic neuropathy causes a rapidly progressive vision loss that responds to hemodialysis and corticosteroid treatment. Isolated peripheral mononeuropathies occur in uremic patients from compression or entrapment or from intramuscular hemorrhage. Hyperkalemia is sometimes responsible for a flaccid quadriparesis that responds to electrolyte correction. Treatment with aminoglycoside antibiotics in uremic patients can lead to cochlear, vestibular, or neuromuscular junction disturbances, and a myopathy sometimes results from electrolyte disturbances, corticosteroid treatment, or the end-stage kidney disease itself (Lacerda et al., 2010).

### Neurological Complications of Dialysis

Hemodialysis requires an arteriovenous shunt in the forearm that sometimes causes a carpal tunnel syndrome attributed either to ischemia and venous congestion or to beta-2 microglobulin amyloidosis.

The probable cause of dialysis disequilibrium syndrome is a shifting of water into the brain. Headache, irritability, agitation, somnolence, seizures, muscle cramps, and nausea occur during or after hemodialysis or peritoneal dialysis. Less common features are exophthalmos, increased intraocular pressure, increased intracranial pressure, and papilledema.

In patients undergoing dialysis for longer than 1 year, a progressive encephalopathy called *dialysis dementia syndrome* may develop. Hesitancy of speech, leading to speech arrest, is a characteristic early feature. Intellectual function declines with time, and delusions, hallucinations, seizures, myoclonic jerking, asterixis, gait disturbances, and other neurological abnormalities ultimately develop. Death usually occurs within 6 to 12 months of onset of signs and symptoms. Increased cerebral concentrations of aluminum at postmortem examination previously suggested aluminum intoxication as the cause of dialysis dementia. Dialysis dementia has become much less common since the removal of aluminum from dialysates (Seifter and Samuels, 2011). Deferoxamine, a chelating agent that binds aluminum, treats dialysis dementia, but the optimal duration of treatment is unclear. Deferoxamine may actually exacerbate or precipitate encephalopathy in patients with very high serum aluminum concentrations, and it also causes visual and auditory disturbances.

Another cause of encephalopathy in patients undergoing dialysis is Wernicke encephalopathy. Dialysis removes thiamine, a water-soluble vitamin; thiamine supplementation, initially via an intravenous route, is therefore essential.

### Neurological Complications of Renal Transplantation

The placement of the transplanted kidney close to the inguinal ligament increases the risk of retraction injury or hematoma formation around the femoral nerve. The result can be a postoperative femoral neuropathy, which often resolves completely. Retraction or hematoma also causes dysfunction of the ipsilateral lateral femoral cutaneous nerve. Stroke occurs in 5% to 8% of renal transplant recipients; underlying causes may relate to hypertension, diabetes, and accelerated atherosclerosis. The neurological complications associated with long-term immunosuppressive treatment are the same as those for transplantation of other organs.

Headache, confusion, or convulsions in patients with evidence of acute graft rejection are a feature of rejection encephalopathy. In most cases, onset of this condition is within 3 months of transplantation; complete recovery occurs rapidly after treatment of the acute rejection episode. A possible cause is cytokine production related to the rejection process.

## ELECTROLYTE DISTURBANCES

### Sodium

Serum sodium concentration determines serum osmolarity. Rapid changes in serum sodium concentration cause CNS dysfunction by altering the osmotic equilibrium between the brain and body fluids. The typical clinical features are disturbances of cognition and arousal that can progress to coma. Myoclonus, asterixis, and tremulousness are common. Seizures, when they occur, often are refractory to anticonvulsant medications until the underlying sodium disturbance has been corrected. Focal signs and symptoms (e.g., hemiparesis) may manifest during hyponatremia without any demonstrable structural basis, but they may also indicate a prior or subclinical focal abnormality that is aggravated by the metabolic disturbance.

Focal abnormalities associated with hypernatremia may reflect subdural hemorrhage. The cause of hemorrhage is brain shrinkage from osmotic forces, with secondary tearing of blood vessels. Hypernatremia, a common consequence of dehydration, may develop in patients receiving inadequate parenteral fluid replacement. It also occurs with diabetes insipidus, pathological involvement of the hypothalamic thirst center by tumor, and excessive salt intake.

Hyponatremia, defined as a serum sodium concentration less than 132 mEq/L, is associated with hypo-osmolarity except in patients with hyperlipidemia or hyperglycemia. It occurs in several pathological states: excessive salt loss from the kidney or GI tract, impaired water excretion, the syndrome of inappropriate secretion of antidiuretic hormone (SIADH), adrenocortical insufficiency, and iatrogenic water intoxication. Many medications can lead to hyponatremia, including diuretics (e.g., hydrochlorothiazide), antidepressants (e.g., amitryptiline), antipsychotics (e.g., haloperidol), antiepileptics (e.g., oxcarbazepine), and antineoplastic agents (e.g., cyclophosphamide). Often thought to be secondary to SIADH in patients with acute brain syndromes (e.g., subarachnoid hemorrhage), hyponatremia in this instance is more likely to be the result of salt wasting by the kidneys ("cerebral salt wasting") than of SIADH; patients have a reduced plasma volume rather than a normal or increased plasma volume as expected with SIADH. In such cases, fluid restriction further exacerbates the hypovolemia, which may cause cerebral ischemia; sodium supplementation is necessary to avoid the complications of severe hyponatremia.

Rapid correction of hyponatremia may cause central pontine myelinolysis, a disorder initially associated with alcoholism or malnutrition but now more often iatrogenic in origin. Neurological deterioration due to central pontine myelinolysis may obscure or follow the resolution of hyponatremic encephalopathy. Spastic or flaccid quadriparesis, pseudobulbar palsy, and decreased states of consciousness characterize severe cases. In some patients, the clinical features are minimal compared with the abnormalities seen on MRI. Central pontine myelinolysis is usually prevented when hyponatremia is corrected slowly, at a rate of less than 8 to 12 mEq/L/day, especially in patients in whom hyponatremia is of long standing.

### Potassium

The difference in the concentrations of intracellular and extracellular potassium creates the resting membrane potential of nerve and muscle cells. Disturbances of serum potassium adversely affect cardiac and neuromuscular function. The hereditary periodic paralyses are discussed in Chapters 98 and 109.

Hyperkalemia usually causes cardiac arrhythmia before neurological function is disturbed. The arrhythmia is sometimes associated with rapidly progressive flaccid paralysis and depressed tendon reflexes. Weakness, which may last for several hours, may be preceded by burning paresthesias and is sometimes accompanied by mental changes. The underlying cause, the severity of the hyperkalemia, and the electrocardiographic findings determine the treatment.

Hypokalemia usually causes neuromuscular disturbances rather than encephalopathy. Mild hypokalemia causes myalgia, fatigability, and proximal weakness while sparing the bulbar muscles. Severe hypokalemia causes rhabdomyolysis and myoglobinuria, and hypokalemic alkalosis causes tetany. All signs and symptoms remit when normokalemia is reestablished.

### Calcium

Hypercalcemia is associated with metastatic bone disease, myeloma, paraneoplastic syndromes, primary or secondary hyperparathyroidism, vitamin D intoxication, and the milk-alkali syndrome. The main CNS complication is an encephalopathy, characterized by altered state of consciousness, apathy or agitation, depression or mania, headache, and, in rare instances, seizures, which may be a result of vascular occlusive complications. PNS manifestations include muscle weakness and fatigability, especially in patients with hyperparathyroidism, in whom a myopathy may develop.

Hypocalcemia may follow thyroid or parathyroid surgery and is a recognized feature of hypoparathyroidism, malabsorption syndromes, vitamin D deficiency, and acute pancreatitis. Tetany is the main manifestation of hypocalcemia. Perioral and distal limb paresthesias are initial features and are followed by muscle cramps, a feeling of muscle spasms, and then actual spasm of the hands and feet (carpopedal spasms).

CNS complications of hypocalcemia are focal or generalized seizures and an encephalopathy characterized by hallucinations, delusions, psychosis, altered states of consciousness, and cognitive impairment. The seizures respond poorly to anticonvulsant drugs but stop after correction of the hypocalcemia. Other CNS complications are parkinsonism or chorea that responds to correction of the calcium abnormality, intracranial hypertension (in patients with hypoparathyroidism), and myelopathy.

### Magnesium

Intracellular magnesium is involved in the activation of several enzymatic reactions, and extracellular magnesium is important in synaptic transmission.

The cause of hypomagnesemia is reduced intake or impaired absorption of magnesium or excessive loss from diuretics, kidney disorders such as renal tubular acidosis, alcoholism, and diabetic acidosis. Serum concentrations do not accurately reflect the severity of magnesium depletion because magnesium is predominantly an intracellular ion.

The neurological complications of hypomagnesemia are similar to those of hypocalcemia, and the two often coexist. The possibility of concurrent hypomagnesemia should be considered in the management of hypocalcemia, especially when parenteral calcium supplementation fails to provide the expected response. The cause of complaints of weakness in patients with hypomagnesemia may be magnesium deficiency alone or with other electrolyte abnormalities. The treatment of hypomagnesemia is with magnesium sulfate given orally unless an absorptive defect or urgency to correction (e.g., status epilepticus) necessitates intramuscular or intravenous administration.

The cause of hypermagnesemia is either excessive intake or impaired excretion of magnesium. The usual cause is renal failure or magnesium administration to treat preeclampsia. Clinical features are drowsiness and diminished responsiveness, confusion, and depressed or absent tendon reflexes. Other features are hypotension, respiratory depression, and weakness from impaired neuromuscular transmission. Severe hypermagnesemia results in coma and may be fatal.

## PITUITARY DISEASE

### Pituitary Adenomas

The initial features of prolactin-secreting pituitary adenomas are amenorrhea and galactorrhea in women and impotence in men. Often, however, symptoms of increased intracranial pressure originating in the sella region develop before prolactinoma becomes a consideration. The treatment choices are transsphenoidal surgery and administration of dopaminergic agonists such as cabergoline or bromocriptine. Radiation therapy can be used as an adjunct after incomplete resection or when surgery or medications are either unhelpful or not feasible. Tension pneumocranium is a rare complication of transsphenoidal surgery. Impaired mental status, seizures, and headaches—sometimes associated with systemic hypertension and bradycardia—occur in the early postoperative period and necessitate surgical drainage of the pneumocranium. Serum sodium measurements exclude the possibility of iatrogenic central diabetes insipidus postoperatively (see later).

Growth hormone–secreting pituitary tumors cause acromegaly; gigantism occurs in children and enlargement of the jaw, extremities, and skull in adults. Approximately 50% of patients have a myopathy, which improves over many months when the underlying hormonal disorder is treated. Carpal tunnel syndrome in patients with acromegaly results from hypertrophy of the transverse carpal ligament. Symptoms usually resolve 2 to 3 months after surgical excision of the pituitary tumor, but electrophysiological abnormalities may persist longer. In patients with acromegaly, a mild (usually subclinical) polyneuropathy may also develop.

### Cushing Disease and Syndrome

The cause of Cushing disease is excessive secretion of adrenocorticotropic hormone from the pituitary gland. The clinical features are truncal obesity, hypertension, acne, hirsutism, osteoporosis, diabetes mellitus, and menstrual irregularities. Mental changes are common and include anxiety, agitation, insomnia, depression, euphoria, mania, and psychosis. Proximal muscle weakness and wasting are common, especially in the legs. Muscle biopsy shows type II fiber atrophy, a characteristic feature of patients who receive long-term corticosteroid therapy (see Chapter 109); electromyographic findings are generally normal and the serum creatine kinase levels may be normal. The constellation of clinical features that constitutes Cushing syndrome is also a feature of the paraneoplastic syndrome of ectopic secretion of adrenocorticotropic hormone (ACTH) and occurs in association with adrenal adenomas and after long-term corticosteroid treatment.

An enlarging pituitary adenoma may cause a visual field defect (Fig. 58.10). Treatment of Cushing disease by bilateral adrenalectomy sometimes leads to rapid expansion of the underlying pituitary adenoma (Nelson syndrome), with compression of other cranial nerves,

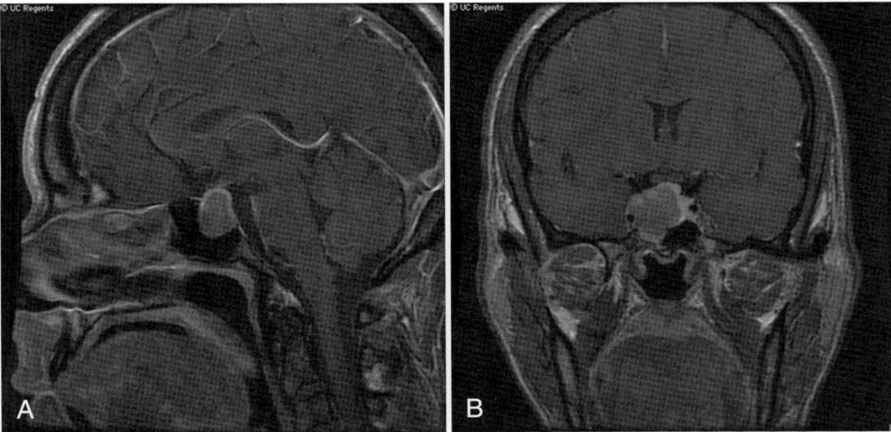


**Fig. 58.10** T1-Weighted magnetic Resonance Imaging with Gadolinium Enhancement. **A,** Sagittal view. **B,** Coronal view. A heterogeneously enhancing mass arises out of the sella turcica and extends up to involve the region of the optic chiasm. Surgery confirmed a growth hormone–secreting pituitary adenoma.

especially CN III. Intracranial hypertension is a recognized complication of Cushing syndrome and occurs particularly after resection of the pituitary adenoma.

### Hypopituitarism

Hypopituitarism results from diseases of the pituitary gland or hypothalamus. The neurological features depend on the severity of secretory impairment and on the hormones affected. Common features are apathy and intellectual decline, which are often difficult to attribute to a single hormonal deficiency because of the concurrent dysfunction of several glands.

## DIABETES INSIPIDUS

Central diabetes insipidus, the inability to conserve water, results from disorders of the hypothalamus or pituitary gland or from interruption of the neurohypophyseal tract. Transitory central diabetes insipidus is often a complication of head injury, intracranial surgery, or injury to the territory of the anterior cerebral artery and may occur without explanation in previously well patients. Synthesis of vasopressin occurs in the hypothalamus, from where it is transported to the posterior pituitary gland. The main neurological feature is an encephalopathy of variable severity, ranging from irritability to somnolence and ultimately to coma; many of these symptoms are likely a result of hypernatremia. Hypotension and hyperthermia also occur. Treatment is with vasopressin or a long-acting vasopressin analog. The cause of nephrogenic diabetes insipidus is impaired renal responsiveness to vasopressin, often secondary to medication effect; treatment involves removal of the offending agent.

## THYROID DISEASE

### Hyperthyroidism

The features of hyperthyroidism are anxiety, restlessness, irritability, emotional lability, impaired concentration, headaches, mental slowing, and insomnia. Elderly patients may become depressed and lethargic, a condition designated *apathetic hyperthyroidism*. An enhanced physiological tremor and generalized hyperreflexia are common. Hyperthyroidism itself may cause seizures or can trigger a preexisting seizure disorder. Chorea and paroxysmal choreoathetosis also occur. Treatment of hyperthyroidism typically leads to improvement in these neurological complications, but anticonvulsants may be needed for seizures and antidopaminergic agents (e.g., tetrabenazine or deutetrabenazine) for chorea.

Confusion and agitation leading to coma characterize thyrotoxic crisis or storm. Additional features include fever, cardiac arrhythmias, diarrhea and vomiting, and other systemic disturbances. Treatment often requires management in the intensive care unit and, in addition to antithyroid agents, consists of hydration and cooling, beta-blocking drugs, corticosteroids, and in some cases plasmapheresis. Thyroid surgery is sometimes necessary.

Dysthyroid orbitopathy (ophthalmic Graves disease) characterized by exophthalmos and ophthalmoplegia is common. Orbital edema—particularly involving the extraocular muscles and infiltration by inflammatory cells—leads to orbital fullness, conjunctival edema and hyperemia, proptosis, and some limitation of ocular movement. The cause of eyelid retraction may be sympathetic overactivity affecting the superior tarsal muscle in the upper lids and fibrosis of the levator palpebrae muscle. The occasional occurrence of optic neuropathy relates to infiltration of the optic nerve, crowding of the orbital apex, and enlargement of the extraocular muscles. Dysthyroid orbitopathy may occur in patients without a history of thyroid disease or clinical signs of hyperthyroidism. Treatment options include corticosteroids, other immunosuppressive drugs, radiation therapy, orbital decompression, and restoration of a euthyroid state.

Compression of the recurrent laryngeal nerve or cervical sympathetic fibers by an enlarged thyroid gland, commonly neoplastic, may lead to vocal cord paralysis or Horner syndrome, respectively.

Several neuromuscular disorders are associated with hyperthyroidism. Most common is a proximal myopathy accompanied by fasciculations. Its mechanism is unknown, but the severity of myopathy does not correlate with the severity of thyroid abnormality. Serum creatine kinase levels are generally normal. Improvement occurs with treatment of the underlying thyroid disorder. Hyperthyroidism and myasthenia gravis often coexist, since both are immune-mediated disorders (see Chapter 108). Treatment of one disorder, however, does not have any predictable effect on the other.

Thyrotoxic periodic paralysis is similar to familial hypokalemic periodic paralysis (see Chapters 98 and 109). It is most common in persons of Asian descent, and the hyperthyroidism may be clinically silent. Episodes of weakness occur after activity or after meals with high carbohydrate content. Potassium administration treats the acute attacks, and nonselective beta-blockers can help to alleviate the acute attack;

both may prevent the recurrence of paralytic attacks (Falhammar et al., 2013). Correction of the thyroid disorder cures the periodic paralysis.

### Hypothyroidism

Mental changes are common in hypothyroidism. Apathy, somnolence, and impaired concentration are typical and are often attributed to depression. Confusion, delirium, and psychosis (myxedema madness) may also occur and remit with treatment of the underlying thyroid disorder; therefore the level of serum thyroid-stimulating hormone (TSH) should be measured in patients presenting for the evaluation of cognitive decline. In severe hypothyroidism, decreased states of consciousness are associated with hypotension, hypothermia, respiratory failure, hypoglycemia, and other metabolic derangements; untreated, the disorder progresses to coma and sometimes death.

Other features of hypothyroidism are an increased incidence of seizures, truncal ataxia due to cerebellar degeneration, hearing loss, and cranial neuropathies. Structural changes in the vocal cords cause voice hoarseness rather than neurological disease. The neurological complications of hypothyroidism usually resolve with thyroid replacement, especially if the deficiency is not of long-standing.

The PNS is often involved in hypothyroidism. Most common is a proximal myopathy accompanied by myalgia and muscle stiffness. The affected muscles may be enlarged and exhibit myoedema (transient local mounding of a muscle in response to percussion).

Carpal tunnel syndrome occurs in as many as 30% of these patients and usually responds to correction of the thyroid disorder. Screening most patients with carpal tunnel syndrome for occult hypothyroidism is reasonable. Less common is a sensory or sensorimotor neuropathy, for which evidence implicates both segmental demyelination and axonal degeneration. Slow relaxation of tendon reflexes may also be noted. An association with myasthenia gravis is recognized but is less common than the association with hyperthyroidism.

### Hashimoto Thyroiditis

Hashimoto thyroiditis is a chronic autoimmune-mediated thyroiditis; it is probably related to both genetic and environmental factors. An association exists with myasthenia gravis and less clearly with giant cell arteritis and vasculitic peripheral neuropathy. In addition, a relapsing encephalopathy may occur in association with Hashimoto thyroiditis along with high titers of antithyroglobulin and antithyroperoxidase antibodies, commonly termed *Hashimoto encephalitis.* Confusion, altered level of consciousness, and seizures are common presenting features. Tremulousness occurred in 80%, transient aphasia in 80%, and myoclonus in 65% of the patients in the series reported by Castillo et al. (2006). Gait ataxia (affecting 65% of the patients) and sleep abnormalities (reported by 55%) are also common. The EEG is diffusely abnormal, and the CSF protein concentration is increased, sometimes without an associated pleocytosis but often accompanied by markers of inflammation including an elevated Ig index or unique CSF oligoclonal bands. Brain MRI results may be abnormal but are often unremarkable. The diagnosis should be a consideration even in the presence of a normal serum TSH concentration and ESR. Treatment is with corticosteroids. The long-term prognosis is good, but relapses are expected and steroid-sparing immunosuppressive drugs are often necessary.

## PARATHYROID DISEASE

### Hyperparathyroidism

Neurological manifestations of hyperparathyroidism are common. They are essentially those of hypercalcemia (described earlier in the chapter). A mild proximal myopathy also may occur and improves with surgical treatment of the parathyroid disorder. A clinical syndrome that mimics amyotrophic lateral sclerosis may also occur.

### Hypoparathyroidism

Hypoparathyroidism commonly follows thyroidectomy or has an idiopathic basis. The etiological disorder in pseudohypoparathyroidism is peripheral resistance to the effects of parathyroid hormone rather than deficiency of hormone secretion. The neurological manifestations of these disorders relate primarily to the effects of hypocalcemia on the nervous system. Intracranial calcification is common in patients with hypoparathyroidism, occurring especially in the basal ganglia and deep cerebellar nuclei. These calcifications are usually asymptomatic, but they can occasionally lead to seizures, falls, and progressive mental changes. Intracranial hypertension may also be associated with hypoparathyroidism; correction of the underlying metabolic disorder reverses the condition.

## ADRENAL GLANDS

### Pheochromocytoma

Pheochromocytoma is associated with neurofibromatosis and von Hippel-Lindau disease (see Chapter 99). The initial features of pheochromocytoma are those of paroxysmal excessive catecholamine secretion: headache, hyperhidrosis, palpitations, cardiac arrhythmias, tremulousness, and anxiety. Most patients have hypertension, which can be severe, occasionally leading to intracranial hemorrhage. Seizures occur in approximately 5%. Malignant pheochromocytomas are rare, and metastatic tumors may respond to radiation therapy.

### Addison Disease

Adrenal failure results from diseases of the pituitary or adrenal gland or from adrenal suppression from long-term use of exogenous corticosteroids. The major features are generalized weakness, fatigability, lassitude, depression, headache, weight loss, anorexia, and hyperpigmentation of the skin. Increased intracranial pressure may be present. Adrenal failure is a feature of X-linked adrenoleukodystrophy.

## DIABETES MELLITUS

### Peripheral Nervous System

In developed countries, diabetes is the most common cause of polyneuropathy (see Chapter 106). The mechanism of neuropathy is not established but may be either metabolic or vascular. Between 10% and 20% of newly diagnosed diabetic patients exhibit evidence of neuropathy. Prediabetes, as diagnosed by a glucose tolerance test demonstrating insulin resistance, can be associated with a painful sensory polyneuropathy. The diagnosis of diabetes should be excluded in all patients presenting with an otherwise idiopathic sensory-predominant neuropathy.

Diabetic polyneuropathy features both axonal degeneration and demyelination. It may be asymptomatic; depressed tendon reflexes and impaired vibratory sense in the legs will suggest the diagnosis. Symptoms are more common in the feet than in the hands. The initial symptom is pain, paresthesia, or numbness. Profound weight loss sometimes precedes the development of an acute painful neuropathy. Progressive neuropathy is characterized by distal sensory loss and weakness in the limbs as well as by areflexia. Severe impairment of pain and temperature appreciation occasionally develops and results in distal ulceration and arthropathy (acrodystrophic neuropathy).

Autonomic neuropathy is an important feature of diabetes mellitus. Clinical features range from lack of symptoms to a syndrome that includes postural hypotension, abnormal cardiovascular and thermoregulatory control, and erectile dysfunction. Other possible clinical features are pupillary abnormalities, gastroparesis, diarrhea from intestinal dysmotility, and a blunted response to hypoglycemia.

Diabetic polyradiculoneuropathy is characterized by pain and asymmetrical limb weakness usually involving the thighs and often accompanied by weight loss. A diabetic plexopathy or polyradiculopathy accounts for most cases of diabetic amyotrophy. A painless lower-limb motor-predominant neuropathy is likely another variant of this syndrome (Garces-Sanchez et al., 2011). Symptoms are rapidly progressive but stabilize after a few weeks; gradual but often incomplete recovery occurs over the following months or years.

The typical syndrome of diabetic thoracoabdominal polyradiculopathy consists of nonradicular truncal pain, which initially may suggest intraabdominal or intrathoracic pathology necessitating surgical exploration. Sensory loss and weakness are mild.

Diabetic mononeuropathy multiplex has a vascular basis. Simple mononeuropathies also are common in diabetic patients. Entrapment neuropathies, especially carpal tunnel syndrome, occur with an increased incidence. Cranial neuropathies—usually isolated involvement of CN III, IV, and VI—cause a painful extraocular palsy. Sparing of the pupillary reflex differentiates a diabetes-induced palsy of cranial nerve III from compressive lesions. Disturbances of cranial nerve VII cause unilateral facial weakness.

A specific treatment for diabetic neuropathy is not available, but complete control of the diabetes is imperative. In recipients of pancreatic islet transplants, diabetic neuropathy may stabilize or even regress (Lee et al., 2005). Painful neuropathies may respond to standard pharmacological measures to treat neuropathic pain (see Chapter 52). Care of the feet is important, especially in patients with sensory neuropathy, to prevent ulceration.

## Central Nervous System

Stroke is more common in persons with diabetes than in the general population, partially because of an increased incidence of hypertension and atherosclerosis in the former. Diabetes increases stroke severity and mortality and predisposes affected persons to deep subcortical infarctions. Hyperglycemia at the time of acute stroke leads to worse outcome and increased hemorrhage following thrombolytic therapy, but lowering blood glucose in the setting of acute stroke does not clearly improve these outcomes.

Diabetic ketoacidosis, an important cause of morbidity and mortality, may be the presenting feature of previously unrecognized diabetes. Severe hyperglycemia and a metabolic acidosis cause an osmotic diuresis that dehydrates the patient. Clinical presentation includes an altered state of consciousness that progresses to coma. Focal or lateralizing signs are usually absent unless the patient has underlying brain disease. The pathogenesis of diabetic coma is poorly understood and probably multifactorial. Serum hyperosmolality and acidosis are probably important contributing factors. Postmortem examination in some patients with severe diabetic ketoacidosis shows evidence of DIC, which contributes to the altered level of consciousness. Potential contributory factors are other metabolic derangements, infection, vascular occlusive phenomena, and cerebral edema.

An acute medical complication such as an infection or MI often precipitates nonketotic hyperosmolar coma in diabetic patients. Affected patients are typically elderly persons who have mild disease. Hyperglycemia and hyperosmolality occur without significant ketosis. Progressive obtundation is the principal feature, but seizures and focal deficits may develop. Some patients develop chorea and other hyperkinetic movement disorders typically associated with hyperintensity of the putamen and caudate on T1-weighted MRI. Treatment of diabetic ketoacidosis and nonketotic hyperosmolar coma includes fluid, potassium, and phosphate replacement as necessary and correction of hyperglycemia by the administration of insulin. Cerebral edema may complicate therapy; often, it is an incidental CT finding.

## Hypoglycemia

Hypoglycemia can cause an acute metabolic encephalopathy with initial features of tremulousness, anxiety, confusion, stupor, or coma, depending on the level of hypoglycemia. Later features are brainstem dysfunction and transitory focal neurological deficits that resemble those associated with stroke but either resolve or alternate from side to side. Seizures are sometimes the only manifestation of hypoglycemia. Administration of glucose reverses the symptoms. Severe hypoglycemic cerebral injury causes MRI abnormalities localized to the basal ganglia, cerebral cortex, substantia nigra, and hippocampus, suggesting a particular vulnerability of these areas. Neuromuscular syndromes resembling a peripheral sensorimotor polyneuropathy or lower motor neuron degeneration occur in patients with insulinomas or those who receive excessive insulin for therapeutic purposes.

*The complete reference list is available online at https://expertconsult.inkling.com/.* 

59

# Neurological Complications of Systemic Disease: Children

*Aline I. Hamati, Marcia V. Felker*

## OUTLINE



This chapter addresses a complex and diverse topic: the neurological complications of systemic disease in children. Although some clinical features are similar in children and adults, others vary according to the child's age and stage of development.

## CARDIAC DISORDERS AND THE NERVOUS SYSTEM

### Congenital Heart Disease

Children with congenital heart disease (CHD) are at risk for neurological complications, including cerebrovascular accidents (CVAs), cerebral abscess, seizures, developmental delay, and cognitive impairment. The neurological complications, seen in as many as 25% of children with CHD, are the most common extracardiac complications of CHD. The many advances in the treatment of CHD and early correction in the first year have reduced the occurrence of developmental disabilities caused by long-term exposure to hypoxia and the neurological complications of uncorrected CHD. The focus has now shifted to neurological injury caused by cardiac surgery and cardiac transplantation.

#### Cerebral Dysgenesis and Malformations

Cerebral dysgenesis is a consideration to explain neurological symptoms in children with CHD. Autopsy studies reveal a 10%–29% prevalence of cerebral malformations. Patients with hypoplastic left heart syndrome are at a higher risk for associated brain dysgenesis. In one series of 41 patients with hypoplastic left heart syndrome, 29% had associated brain malformations of variable severity, 27% had microcephaly, 21% had immature cortical mantle, and the remainder had other malformations, including one with holoprosencephaly. Other reports include agenesis of the corpus callosum, Dandy-Walker syndrome, and aqueductal stenosis. Lutterman and colleagues (1998) described the association of moyamoya disease and structural CHD, including ventricular septal defect (VSD), aortic and mitral valve stenosis, and tetralogy of Fallot (TOF).

#### Chromosomal and Genetic Disorders

The combination of CHD and neurological disorders, mainly developmental delay, is sometimes a manifestation of genetic conditions combining both cardiac and central nervous system (CNS) involvement.

Such conditions include trisomy 21, trisomy 13, trisomy 18, cri du chat syndrome (5p deletion), CHARGE association, Williams syndrome, DiGeorge syndrome/velocardiofacial syndrome, and RASopathies. Our understanding of the role of genetics in CHD has improved at a rapid pace during the past few years, with the use of chromosomal microarray and next generation sequencing (NGS), leading to the rapid discovery of numerous pathogenic copy number variants (CNVs) and gene mutations. Chromosomal microarray analysis, also known as *array-based comparative genomic hybridization* (CGH), has recently become an extremely valuable diagnostic tool, allowing the detection of subtle genomic imbalances that were undetected by conventional chromosome analysis. Lu et al. (2008) studied 101 patients with CHD with or without other malformations, such as cleft palate, club foot, and polydactyly, and array-based CGH detected significant abnormalities in 21.8% of patients. Richards et al. (2008) and other studies reported similar findings and encouraged screening patients with CHD and developmental delay with chromosomal microarray analysis. Bachman et al. (2013) showed the clinical utility of CGH as a first-tier test in the evaluation of neonates with CHD. More recently Page et al. (2019) used whole exome sequencing (WES) in 829 non-syndromic TOF patients and found genetic variants in almost 7% of patients, most frequently seen in the NOTCH1 locus.

## Neurological Complications Unrelated to Intervention and Cardiac Surgery

### Cerebrovascular Accidents in Uncorrected Congenital Heart Disease

The incidence of stroke (CVA) in children with CHD unrelated to surgery or endocarditis is 1.5%–2%. The most commonly associated cardiac anomalies are TOF and dextroposition of the great arteries. Children with cyanotic CHD or right-to-left shunt have a higher incidence of stroke because of relative anemia, which leads to increased blood viscosity. Stroke may be arterial or venous in origin and either embolic or thrombotic. Cardiogenic stroke can result from emboli arising from the right heart or systemic venous circulation through a right-to-left shunt (paradoxical emboli) or from an intracardiac arterial embolic source. It also can result from cerebral venous thrombosis secondary to the combination of polycythemia, venous stasis, and central venous hypertension. Hemiplegia is the most frequent clinical finding; other presenting features include sudden alteration in consciousness, seizures, and dysphasia or aphasia. Brainstem infarcts are rare; common clinical features are ataxia, dysphagia, cranial nerve palsies, and weakness.

Patients with acyanotic CHD and left-to-right shunt, such as atrial septal defect (ASD), VSD, and patent ductus arteriosus (PDA), are not usually at risk for cardiogenic emboli because of the protection provided by the pulmonary vascular bed. Stroke can occur in rare cases if the direction of the shunt flow reverses.

Congenital stenosis of the great vessels (e.g., aortic stenosis, pulmonary artery stenosis, coarctation of the aorta) contributes to the occurrence of CVA and neurological complications. The usual causes are bacterial endocarditis, arrhythmias, chronic hypoxia, and cerebral aneurysms, with their known association with coarctation of the aorta.

Infants who have CHD are at risk for intraventricular-periventricular hemorrhage because of vascular immaturity and systemic hemodynamic instability. Cranial ultrasound examination shows hemorrhage in 24% of term infants with CHD and an increased incidence of cerebral atrophy and linear echodensities in the basal ganglia and thalamus.

### Brain Abscess

The incidence of brain abscess is higher in cyanotic CHD. Earlier report rates were 2%–6%. In recent years, the incidence of brain abscess has decreased markedly because of earlier corrective surgery and more aggressive treatment of dehydration and infections. The occurrence of brain abscess is now largely confined to the developing world, where CHD goes uncorrected. TOF is the most common underlying cardiac lesion, followed by transposition of the great arteries. Brain abscesses are rare before the age of 2 years. In 75% of the cases, the lesion is supratentorial; in 20%, multifocal. The most common early presentation, often subtle, consists of headache in 50% of patients, vomiting in 72% of patients, personality change, and irritability. In some cases, the clinical onset can be abrupt, with seizures as the first clinical manifestation. Focal neurological signs and visual disturbances occur. Early on, as many as 75% of patients are afebrile. Eventually, papilledema and coma can occur. Computed tomography (CT) and magnetic resonance imaging (MRI) establish the diagnosis by revealing areas of hypodensity with contrast ring enhancement surrounded by edema. The usual causative organisms are mixed aerobic and anaerobic streptococci, staphylococci, *Haemophilus*, and occasionally gram-negative bacteria. Early detection at the stage of cerebritis allows a conservative approach with high-dose broad-spectrum antibiotic therapy for 3–6 weeks. Surgery sometimes is required, by either direct resection or CT-guided aspiration, depending upon the location of the abscess.

### Infective Endocarditis

The implementation of subacute endocarditis prophylaxis before dental and surgical procedures in patients with CHD has greatly reduced the incidence of bacterial endocarditis, but it has not improved mortality, which remains at 11.1% (Dolgner et al., 2018). Approximately one-third of cases of infective endocarditis are associated with neurological complications. These include cerebral embolization, usually in the middle cerebral artery (MCA) territory, meningitis, brain abscess, and seizures (Fig. 59.1). Cerebral mycotic aneurysms complicate 1.2%–5% of cases of infective endocarditis and carry a high mortality rate of 60%. The risk of hemorrhagic transformation of septic infarctions is high and associated with a mortality rate of 80%–90%.

### Cognitive Impairment

Children with CHD, predominantly the cyanotic type, are at an increased risk for intellectual impairment and behavioral problems. Studies have shown that 25% of children with cyanotic CHD required special education, and 23.7% of adolescents with CHD had behavioral problems (Easson et al., 2018). Mean IQ scores in cyanotic CHD usually are in the mid-90s. Also noted is an early delay in gross motor skills in infancy, but there has been improvement over time. Hence, developmental quotients, influenced by gross motor scores, are inaccurate in this population. The most significant factors contributing to developmental delays are chronic hypoxia, white matter gliosis, and small cortical scars, even in the absence of demonstrable emboli.

## Neurological Complications of Intervention and Cardiac Surgery

The risk of neurological complications with cardiac catheterization in infants and children is low. The incidence of seizures is 1%. Rare complications are focal paresthesias and injuries of the lumbar plexus or femoral nerve caused by localized hematoma.

The mortality rate associated with cardiac surgery has dramatically fallen in the past 20 years and is now less than 10%. As the mortality rate continues to decline, the emphasis is now on finding measures to improve morbidity. The incidence of neurological complications after cardiac surgery in children ranges between 2% and 25%. Neurological monitoring should be implemented during and after cardiac surgery to detect these types of complications earlier. Neuromonitoring strategies, such as the use of intraoperative monitoring with near-infrared

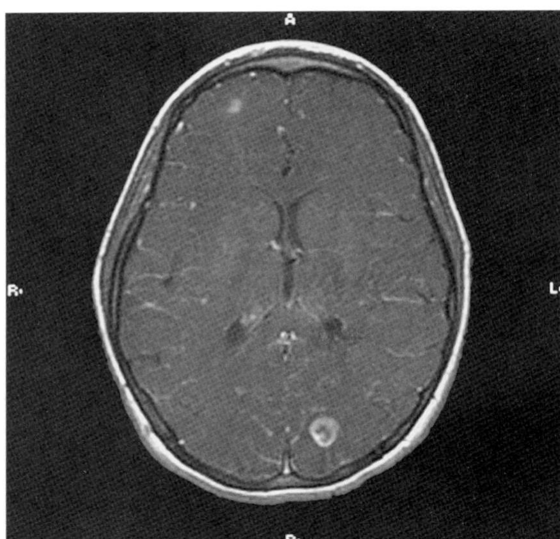


**Fig. 59.1** Magnetic resonance image of brain of a 12-year-old girl with congenital heart disease, subacute endocarditis, and brain abscess. The patient presented with fever, headaches, and diplopia.

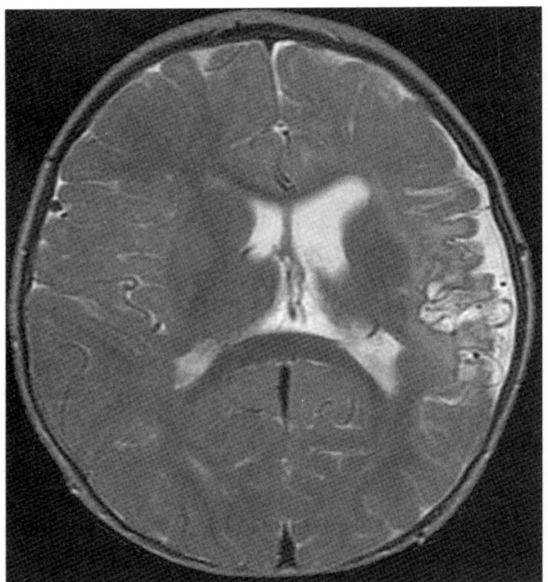

**Fig. 59.2** Magnetic resonance image of a 13-month-old child with tetralogy of Fallot and stroke in the middle cerebral artery distribution.

spectroscopy or NIRS to estimate cerebral oxygenation (Khan and Frazer, 2012) and the use of continuous electroencephalogram (EEG) and transcranial Doppler (TCD) ultrasound, may hold promise for early detection of neurological complications, but future studies are needed.

Fallon and associates (1995) reviewed data for 523 cardiac surgery patients and found neurological events or deficits in 31 patients in the immediate postoperative period. Seizures occurred in 16, pyramidal signs (hemiparesis-quadriparesis) in 11, extrapyramidal signs in eight, and neuro-ophthalmic deficits (gaze palsies, visual field defects) in six. Six patients were unconscious, and four demonstrated miscellaneous neurological changes, such as development of Horner syndrome secondary to brachial plexus injury, vocal cord palsy, isolated bulbar palsy, and transient ischemic episodes. A period of low perfusion pressure, either intraoperatively or postoperatively, was present in more patients who had an adverse neurological event than in those who were normal. The likely pathogenesis of CNS injury is microembolization and ischemia during bypass or the development of intracranial hemorrhage (Du Plessis, 1999). Corrective surgery for coarctation of the aorta is especially associated with CVAs.

Seizures are the most common complication after cardiac surgery, seen in up to 15% of children postoperatively. The prognosis varies with the underlying cause. Other complications include delayed recovery of mental status (thought to be caused by hypoxic-ischemic reperfusion injury), and movement disorders such as choreoathetosis, oculogyric crisis, and Parkinsonism.

A postoperative encephalopathy, characterized by choreoathetosis and developmental delay, is a well-defined complication after cardiac surgery in children, but not after cardiac surgery in adults. The incidence has dropped from 18% to 0.6% in recent reports (du Plessis et al., 2002). A mild transitory form can follow cardiac surgery in infants. The severe form occurs in children who undergo such surgery after infancy. In the severe postpump choreoathetosis, the early mortality rate approaches 40%. Most of the patients have residual involuntary movements and severe long-term neurological disturbances years later. The mild form is associated with cognitive and behavioral disturbances despite complete resolution of choreoathetosis. The mechanisms underlying the pathogenesis remain unclear, with the usual proposed explanations being deep hypothermia and intraoperative hypoxic injury (Wessel et al., 1995). Brain imaging in these cases usually reveals nonspecific changes such as cerebral atrophy. Neuropathological data are limited; however, the external globus pallidus is the most consistent locus of injury, with evidence of gliosis, neuronal loss, nerve fiber degeneration, and capillary proliferation (Kupsky et al., 1995).

Open heart surgery is associated with several risk factors for stroke (Fig. 59.2). The risks include altered intravascular endothelial surfaces, thrombus formation facilitated by the use of prosthetic devices, gaseous emboli originating from the cardiopulmonary bypass, global hypoperfusion, inflammatory cascades and microvascular inflammatory changes, and occurrence of a prothrombotic state during surgery, owing to consumptive coagulopathy and decreased protein C and antithrombin levels. Silvey et al. (2018) found increasing rates of thrombosis in CHD patients.

Spinal cord injury occurs especially after aortic coarctation repair. Peripheral neuromuscular complications include plexopathies (mostly brachial), pressure palsies (peroneal and ulnar nerves), myopathy, "critical care neuropathy," and polyneuropathy developing after withdrawal of neuromuscular blocking agents. Dittrich et al. (2003) reviewed data for 90 patients younger than 1 year of age who underwent cardiac surgery. These patients had no brain anomalies or syndromes associated with delayed mental development, but 32% had evidence of psychomotor impairment.

## Cardiac Transplantation

In the past decades, the number of cardiac transplantation procedures performed worldwide has increased. Although the survival rate has steadily improved, the potential for significant complications remains. Such complications include graft rejection, graft arteriosclerosis, infections, malignancies, pneumonia, pericarditis, gastrointestinal hemorrhages, and drug toxicity, leading to an overall perioperative mortality rate of approximately 9%.

Perez-Miralles and associates (2005) reported neurological complications after cardiac transplantation in 13.7% of patients. Other studies, however, have reported an incidence of 50%–70%, mostly in the perioperative period.

In the series of Cemillan and colleagues (2004), 48% of transplant recipients suffered neurological complications, such as encephalopathy

(16.6%), seizures (13.6%), neuromuscular disorders (10.6%), headaches (10.6%), CVA (10.1%), psychiatric problems (2.2%), and CNS infections (2.2%). Signs and symptoms of cyclosporine toxicity include tremor, seizures, and encephalopathy.

### Acquired Heart Disease

Several acquired heart diseases are associated with neurological complications. The most common entities are cardiomyopathies, arrhythmias, and hypertension. Ventricular dilatation and hypokinesia cause stasis of intraventricular blood, resulting in thrombus formation and embolic stroke. Furthermore, poor ejection fraction can lead to arrhythmias and syncope. In rheumatic heart disease, the source of emboli to the brain is either vegetations or septic emboli due to infective endocarditis. Sydenham chorea occurs in 10%–25% of patients with rheumatic heart disease.

Cardiac arrhythmias cause neurological symptoms secondary to impaired cerebral perfusion. These include dizziness, syncope, transient ischemic episodes, confusion, dementia, and abnormal behavior. Convulsive syncope occurs in severe cases associated with some degree of cerebral anoxia. Embolic strokes from arrhythmias are more likely to occur during or after surgical manipulation at the time of heart surgery or in the postoperative period.

The most important neurological complication of hypertension in children is hypertensive encephalopathy. This entity is discussed later in the "Hypertension" section.

## CONNECTIVE TISSUE DISEASES AND VASCULITIDES

### Polyarteritis Nodosa

Polyarteritis nodosa (PAN) is rare in childhood and occurs most frequently in the fifth and sixth decades of life. Early reports of infantile PAN probably were severe cases of Kawasaki disease. PAN is a necrotizing vasculitis of small- and medium-sized arteries. The etiology is unknown, but an association with hepatitis B and C is recognized in adults. In children, severe PAN-like vasculitis may follow cytomegalovirus (CMV) and parvovirus B19 infections. An association with a preceding group A or B streptococcal infection is questionable. Furthermore, some cases of PAN have followed drug exposure.

Signs and symptoms of systemic illness, such as weight loss, fatigue, and anorexia, can be prominent. Other manifestations include fever, arthralgias, rash, edema, petechiae, myalgia, painful subcutaneous nodules in the calf and foot, and livedo reticularis. Gastrointestinal-vessel involvement causes abdominal pain, ulcers, and bleeding. Renal, cardiac, and pulmonary involvement can occur, with the potential for renal or heart failure. Hypertension is common. Guirola et al. (2014) describe a patient presenting with hypertension, seizures, and posterior reversible encephalopathy syndrome (PRES) who was eventually diagnosed with PAN.

Neurological manifestations can develop in 50%–70% of children and occur in 10% of children at presentation. Mononeuritis multiplex, a characteristic feature of the disease in adults, is much less frequent in children. A comparison of 15 pediatric and 22 adult patients with PAN found neurological involvement in 40% of pediatric patients and 59% of adults (Erden et al., 2017). Focal neurological deficits secondary to ischemia, infarction, and hemorrhage are common. The signs and symptoms include unilateral blindness, visual field defect, seizures, headache, encephalopathy, cognitive decline, cranial neuropathies (III, IV, VI, and VII nerves), and aseptic meningitis. In the brain, changes are mainly seen in the small meningeal arteries (Nadeau, 2002). Catastrophic intracranial hemorrhage with altered sensorium at presentation has been described in a child with PAN (Srinivasaraghavan et al., 2013). Eleftheriou et al. (2013) reviewed 69 children with PAN. The most frequent clinical features at presentation were fever (87%), myalgia (83%), and skin lesions (88%). Neurological involvement at presentation was present in 10% of children and included motor mononeuritis multiplex in 4%, sensory neuropathy in 4%, meningitis/encephalitis in 4%, cranial nerve palsy in 6%, and stroke in 10%.

Confirmation of the diagnosis is either by the histopathological demonstration of the characteristic vascular lesions of necrotizing angiitis or by radiological documentation of aneurysms. MRI, magnetic resonance angiography (MRA), and angiography reveal segmental arterial narrowing and ischemic injuries. Aneurysms are common in visceral arteries and are rare intracranially. In the presence of a peripheral neuropathy, muscle or nerve biopsy (of the sural nerve) also may be diagnostic. Common laboratory features include leukocytosis, anemia, elevation in erythrocyte sedimentation rate, and increased C-reactive protein level and serum immunoglobulin (Ig) levels. Antineutrophil cytoplasmic antibodies (ANCAs) and circulating immune complexes may be present. Detection of rheumatoid factor and antinuclear antibody (ANA) is rare.

Corticosteroid therapy improves life expectancy and decreases the incidence of hypertension and renal complications. In severe cases, lack of response to steroids is an indication for use of oral or intravenous-pulse cyclophosphamide. Plasmapheresis has not improved survival. Methotrexate, azathioprine, mycophenolate mofetil, intravenous immunoglobulin (IVIG), and more recently tumor necrosis factor (TNF) inhibitors (infliximab) and anti-CD20 monoclonal antibodies (rituximab) have been used successfully in children (Gedalia and Cuchacovich, 2009).

Identification of certain *CECR1* mutations that lead to ADA2 deficiency, often associated with stroke in early-onset PAN-like patients, has resulted in improved treatment of some causes of PAN with anti-TNF treatments (Caorsi et al., 2017).

### Kawasaki Disease

Kawasaki disease is one of the most common vasculitides affecting small- and medium-sized arteries in childhood, typically diagnosed between 6 months and 5 years of age. There is an increased incidence in Asians and Pacific Islanders (McCrindle et al., 2017). Some early reports of infantile PAN, in which the patient died of a ruptured or thrombosed coronary artery aneurysm, were probably severe cases of Kawasaki disease. Some 85% of affected patients are younger than 5 years of age. The etiology is unknown, but an infectious cause is thought possible. Current etiological hypotheses include a novel RNA virus that enters the upper respiratory tract and causes an inflammatory cascade. Tropospheric wind patterns transporting a substance that leads to disease when inhaled by genetically predisposed children is also a hypothesis. Single-nucleotide polymorphisms in six genes have been associated with the disease (McCrindle et al., 2017).

The criteria for the diagnosis of complete Kawasaki disease include the presence of unexplained fever for at least 5 days, with at least four of the following physical features: (1) nonpurulent conjunctivitis, (2) cervical lymphadenopathy, (3) rash, (4) mucosal changes (redness and fissuring of the lips, "strawberry tongue"), and (5) changes in the extremities (erythema and edema of palms and soles, with desquamation). Up to one-third of patients develop myocarditis, coronary artery aneurysms, and, less often, pericarditis or valvular disease. Aneurysms smaller than 8 mm usually resolve, whereas those larger than 8 mm rarely resolve and are usually associated with stenosis. Incomplete Kawasaki disease, presenting with unexplained fever and neurological features, without initial typical physical features, was reported in children as young as 2 months of age (Ma et al., 2018).

Neurological complications in Kawasaki disease are reported in 1%–30% of patients (Rodriguez-Gonzalez et al., 2018). The most common neurological manifestations consist of extreme irritability, probably caused by aseptic meningitis, sensorineural hearing loss, facial nerve palsy, headaches, and encephalopathy. Cerebral infarction, seizures, polyneuropathy, myositis, other cranial neuropathies, retinal vasculitis, subdural effusions (Chou et al., 2016) are rare complications. Arterial ischemic stroke has been described in 10 pediatric patients with KD (Sabatier et al., 2013). Muneuchi and associates (2006) described a single patient with a silent right cerebellar infarct and suggested the need to consider the possibility of brain lesions in all children with Kawasaki disease with or without neurological symptoms. Diffuse microhemorrhages with multifocal white matter injury on MRI were described in a pediatric patient with severe KD (Gitiaux et al., 2012). Few reported patients with KD had mild encephalopathy and reversible restricted diffusion of the splenium of the corpus callosum or MERS and hyponatremia (Takanashi et al., 2012). A child with incomplete Kawasaki disease had a left MCA stroke that responded well to IVIG and aspirin (Nikkhah, 2018).

Treatment consists of a single dose of IVIG at 2 g/kg and is usually accompanied by high-dose aspirin (80–100 mg/kg of body weight per day in the United States and 30-50 mg/kg of body weight in Western Europe and Japan) typically until the patient is afebrile for 3–7 days, and then the dose is decreased to 3–5 mg/kg/day and continued until the inflammatory markers and thrombocytosis have resolved and the echocardiogram is normal. Failure of IVIG treatment occurs in 10%–20% of patients, and alternative agents are used (McCrindle et al., 2017).

## Henoch-Schönlein Purpura

Henoch-Schönlein purpura (HSP) is a leukocytoclastic multisystem IgA-mediated vasculitis, one of the most common in childhood (Barut et al., 2016). The characteristic features are arthralgia, abdominal pain, and nonthrombocytopenic purpura mostly involving the buttocks and lower extremities. Fever, fatigue, and edema are common. Nephritis occurs in 40% of patients.

Neurological complications are estimated to occur in 1 out of 14 patients with HSP, but they are mostly mild (Bérubé et al., 2014). Headache is the most common neurological symptom, sometimes caused by hypertension. However, CNS vasculitis can occur with the potential for development of ischemia and hemorrhage. Seizures, facial palsy, paralysis, chorea, Guillain–Barré syndrome, visual abnormalities, ataxia, and central and peripheral neuropathy are also reported. HSP complicated by posterior reversible leukoencephalopathy syndrome or PRES has been described (Fidan et al., 2016; Fuchigami et al., 2010). In some cases, manifestations of CNS vasculitis can precede or follow the rash. Imaging studies can show ischemic lesions most of the time involving two or more vessels, intracerebral hemorrhage, brain edema, and sagittal sinus thrombosis (Garzoni et al., 2009). Permanent sequelae from CNS manifestations are rare in children, though adults may suffer more serious sequelae (Bérubé et al., 2014). The long-term outcome of HSP depends on the degree of renal involvement.

## Takayasu Arteritis

*Takayasu arteritis* is a chronic granulomatous large-vessel vasculitis affecting the aorta and its major branches. In 75% of cases, the onset of symptoms is between the ages of 11 and 30 years. However, onset in persons as young as 5 months of age has been described. Greater than 80% of the patients are female and more likely to be of Japanese origin. Takayasu arteritis is the most common large-vessel vasculitis in children, with overall mortality reports of 3% during the first year and around 50% of morbidity within 5 years from diagnosis (Fan et al., 2019).

The examination reveals loss of radial pulses, and sometimes a carotid bruit is present. Other clinical manifestations are hypertension, fever, back pain, dyspnea, chest pain, claudication, weight loss, transitory visual loss, myalgias, arthralgias, abdominal pain, and congestive heart failure. Brunner et al. (2010) reviewed 241 pediatric cases of Takayasu arteritis. The most frequent problem at presentation was hypertension (83%), followed by headaches (31%). Aeschlimann et al. (2017) saw headache, dizziness, stroke/TIA, and syncope as the top neurological symptoms in their cohort of 27 children. Fan et al. (2019) described carotid artery involvement in 43% of the patients, and stroke occurred in 6% of 101 reported patients. Diagnosis is based on characteristic angiographic findings in the aorta and its major branches. MRI/MRA are useful both in diagnosis and in monitoring disease activity by detecting early smooth-muscle thickening and signs of vascular inflammation of the vessel walls.

Cerebral hypoperfusion secondary to stenosis of the carotid and vertebral arteries and complications of hypertension cause the neurological complications. The signs and symptoms include visual loss, vertigo, syncope, seizures, hemiplegia, and headaches. Recurrent chorea has recently been reported (Lopes et al., 2015). Treatment consists of corticosteroids and immunosuppressive agents, such as methotrexate and cyclophosphamide. A small series revealed the usefulness of anti-TNF agents. Recent reviews suggested improved mortality and morbidity with biological agents (Aeschlimann et al., 2017). Management of hypertension is critical, and antiplatelet agents are useful in preventing thrombosis. Surgical intervention, angioplasty, and stent placement are sometimes required.

## Churg-Strauss Syndrome

Churg-Strauss syndrome, or eosinophilic granulomatosis with polyangiitis (EGPA), affects middle-aged males and is rare in children. However, cases have been reported in children as young as 2 years of age. Churg-Strauss is an antineutrophil cytoplasmic antibody (ANCA)-associated vasculitis of small and medium vessels. The clinical picture consists of asthma symptoms, eosinophilia, fever, allergic rhinitis, pulmonary infiltrates, sinus problems, purpura, skin nodules, and cardiac and renal involvement. Histopathological examination reveals vasculitis of small arteries and veins associated with necrotizing extravascular granulomas and eosinophilic infiltrates. The disease is associated with prominent eosinophilia and high IgE levels. ANCA are seen in only 25% of pediatric cases.

Neurological manifestations consist mainly of neuropathy, with evidence of mononeuritis multiplex, polyneuropathy, and cranial neuropathy. The optic nerve is the most frequently affected cranial nerve in this disorder. CNS features are less common, but focal neurological deficits occur secondary to infection and hemorrhage, and pseudotumor cerebri is reported. Neurological symptoms have been reported to continue despite treatment. Reports of pediatric cases without clear respiratory features except rash and polyneuropathy highlight the importance of imaging in suspected cases (Yener et al., 2018). Treatment options include high-dose corticosteroids, cyclophosphamide, methotrexate, IVIG, mycophenolate mofetil, rituximab, interferon-α, and plasmapheresis. Other biological therapies, such as omalizumab, are being used in resistant pediatric cases with good success (Iglesias et al., 2014).

## Juvenile Idiopathic Arthritis

Juvenile idiopathic arthritis (JIA), previously called juvenile rheumatoid arthritis or JRA, is a heterogeneous group of seven inflammatory arthropathies in children. The age at onset must be younger than 16 years. For definitive diagnosis, objective evidence of arthritis is required in one or more joints for 6 weeks or longer and the exclusion of other causes for the arthritis. Systemic JIA is characterized by daily fever for at least 2 weeks, rash, arthritis, lymphadenopathy, or pericarditis, but overall the presentation of JIA is much more heterogeneous than adult rheumatoid arthritis (Mahmud and Binstadt, 2019).

The neurological complications of the systemic form include acute encephalopathy, which can be lethal as a result of the macrophage activation syndrome (Ueno et al., 2002). The cause of this syndrome is disruption of the macrophage–lymphocyte interaction, causing uncontrolled proliferation of highly activated macrophages and T lymphocytes, with consequent sepsis-like symptoms often resulting in multiple organ failure. High-grade fever, hepatosplenomegaly, pancytopenia, consumption coagulopathy, and low erythrocyte sedimentation rate are other features. Macrophage activation syndrome is seen in 5%–8% of cases (Barut et al, 2017). Treatment is with high-dose steroids and cyclosporine (Stabile et al., 2006).

Reye syndrome has been described in affected patients secondary to the use of acetylsalicylic acid. Other neurological manifestations include myelopathy secondary to cervical arthritis. Myelopathy from atlantoaxial dislocation is rare in children. Motor and sensory neuropathies, such as entrapment neuropathies, are uncommon in children. One-third of patients have high serum creatine kinase concentration; however, evidence of proximal weakness or histological evidence of myositis is uncommon.

The management of JIA is usually with nonsteroidal anti-inflammatory agents. There is a growing pool of disease modifying antirheumatic drugs. The advances in treatment with biological agents such as etanercept, infliximab, and others have led to significant improvement in the treatment of JIA (Barut et al., 2017).

## Systemic Lupus Erythematosus

Systemic lupus erythematosus (SLE) is an episodic multisystem autoimmune disease characterized by the presence of ANA, especially antibodies to double-stranded DNA.

SLE accounts for 4.5% of patients seen in pediatric rheumatology clinics. The onset of SLE is uncommon before adolescence. In childhood, the ratio of affected girls to boys is 4.5:1.

The clinical features of SLE are constitutional (fever, weight loss), cutaneous (malar butterfly rash), musculoskeletal (myopathy, arthralgias), cardiac (pericarditis, myocarditis, endocarditis), vascular (Raynaud phenomenon, livedo reticularis), and renal manifestations (glomerulonephritis, nephrotic syndrome, hypertension). Gastrointestinal, pulmonary, and ocular signs and symptoms also may be features. Neurological symptoms have been used as diagnostic criteria for SLE, including seizures, psychosis, mononeuritis multiplex, myelitis, peripheral or cranial neuropathy, and acute confusional state (Petri et al., 2012). Neurological involvement occurs in 30%–60% of children with SLE during the course of their illness, though recent papers from Turkey and Singapore indicate less neurological involvement in some populations (Sahin et al., 2018; Tan et al., 2015). Patients with CNS involvement usually have a more severe clinical course. Possible neurological complications of SLE include vertigo, sensorineural hearing loss, aseptic meningitis, stroke, transverse myelopathy, and peripheral neuropathy with predominantly sensory deficits. Other less commonly reported complications include ataxia, generally associated with a good recovery (Joubert et al., 2018), chorea (Torreggiani et al., 2013), and myositis (Ghosh and Gupta, 2005). Parkinsonism has been reported in 10 patients, and changes in basal ganglia on brain imaging are inconsistent (Khubchandani et al., 2007). Corticosteroid-related myopathy can complicate the course of the disease. Ophthalmoplegia, diplopia, sudden blindness, or ptosis can occur, and findings of papilledema, optic neuritis, retinal hemorrhage, and vasculitis ("cotton wool spots") have been described. Neuromyelitis optica spectrum disorders

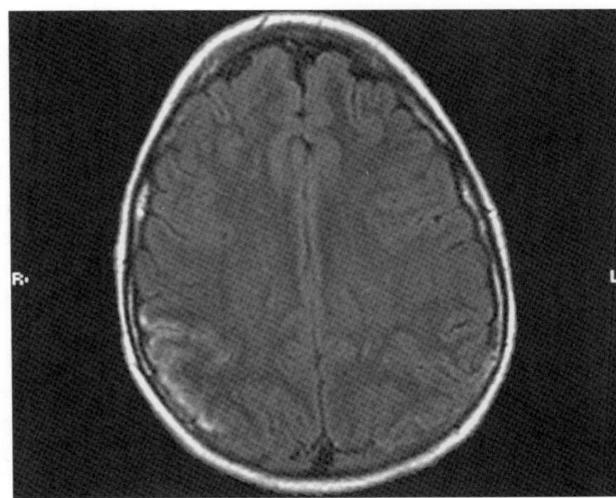


**Fig. 59.3** Magnetic resonance image of brain of a 16-year-old girl with lupus, antiphospholipid antibodies, Addison disease, and hypertension. Laminar necrosis of the right parietal region is evident.

are being increasingly recognized (Yang et al., 2018). Muscal et al. (2010) and others (Emeksiz et al., 2016) have described pediatric lupus patients presenting with seizures, altered mental status, and MRI findings suggestive of PRES. Pseudotumor cerebri has been reported as the first manifestation of SLE (Raeeskarami et al., 2016).

Overall prevalence of symptoms include: recurrent headaches in 71%, migraine 36%, cognitive disorders 55%, isolated seizures 47%, epilepsy 15%, acute confusional state 35%, dysesthesia or paresthesia 14%, transient ischemic attacks (TIAs) 12%, and CVA 8% (Gosh and Gupta, 2005).

Neuropsychiatric abnormalities range in reports from 24.5% to more thn 50% of patients (Balci et al., 2019; Lynall, 2018). The most common clinical manifestations of neuropsychiatric lupus are depression, memory problems, fatigue, emotional lability, trouble with concentration, and psychosis. Psychiatric assessment is important in the evaluation of children with SLE. Many of the neuropsychiatric symptoms associated with lupus are felt to be multifactorial and are not associated with brain imaging abnormalities (Lynall, 2018).

Vasculitis in SLE is rare and affects small arterioles and venules. Perivasculitis is more common. CVAs occur mainly in patients with hypertension or severe renal and cardiac disease (Fig. 59.3) and have been associated with positive results on serological tests for syphilis and the presence of lupus anticoagulant (LA). Gattorno and colleagues (1995) found that 79% of pediatric patients with SLE had anticardiolipin antibodies (aCLs), and 42% had LA. These patients were at high risk for the development of deep vein thrombosis and other antiphospholipid antibody (APA)-related pathology. A statistically significant correlation also has been found between APA and neurological manifestations, such as vascular events, seizures, and psychosis. Other antibody systems, such as antiribosomal P antibodies, antineuronal antibodies, or lymphocytotoxic antibodies, also may be associated with an increased risk for neurological involvement.

Laboratory abnormalities include high erythrocyte sedimentation rate, anemia, leukopenia, thrombocytopenia, low CH50, and low C3 and C4. ANAs are present in almost all patients. Antibodies to double-stranded DNA are pathognomonic for SLE and are present in almost all patients with active disease. Antibodies to extractable nuclear antigen (Sm, Ro/SS-A, La/SS-B, RNP) and antihistone antibodies are strongly associated with SLE. Anti-Sm is highly specific for the disease. The MRI abnormalities in neuropsychiatric lupus include small periventricular and subcortical white matter lesions, cortical atrophy, ventricular dilatation, and infarction. Data from newer imaging techniques, such as diffusion tensor imaging (DTI), magnetization transfer imaging (MTI), and quantitative volumetric studies, are very promising in detecting CNS damage and could be used as biomarkers in clinical trials (Hughes et al., 2007).

The usual treatment of the CNS manifestations of SLE is high-dose oral or intravenous corticosteroids after an infectious process has been ruled out. Cyclophosphamide is used in the management of severe neuropsychiatric lupus unresponsive to other modalities. Some centers use azathioprine as an alternative therapy. Unfortunately, no published neuropsychiatric lupus treatment trials in children exist, and there continue to be calls for larger trials (Groot et al., 2017). It remains unclear whether children require earlier or more aggressive treatment programs to prevent long-term neurological sequelae. In patients who have APA and platelet counts greater than 70,000/mm$^3$, low-dose aspirin therapy is recommended. Anticoagulation with heparin followed by warfarin is required for patients with CVA and antiphospholipid antibodies.

## Granulomatosis with Polyangiitis (Wegener)

Granulomatosis with polyangiitis (GPA), formerly known as Wegener granulomatosis, is characterized by the triad of (1) granulomatous vasculitis of small vessels in the upper and lower respiratory tract, (2) focal segmental glomerulonephritis, and (3) disseminated necrotizing vasculitis. It occurs mostly in middle-aged adults. In the young, onset is in the second decade. In some series, 3.3% of patients had disease onset before age 20.

Clinical manifestations include sinus problems, pulmonary disease (cough and hemoptysis), and glomerulonephritis. Nonspecific complaints of fever, malaise, and weight loss are frequent at onset.

Nervous system involvement occurs less frequently in children than in adults, with a recent meta-analysis revealing up to 24.6% of pediatric GPA patients had neurological symptoms at presentation (Iudici et al., 2016). Neurological manifestations may include seizures, sensorineural hearing loss, myopathy, stroke, hemorrhage, dural venous thrombosis, pachymeningitis, cerebritis, and myelopathy. Neuropathy, including mononeuritis multiplex and polyneuropathy are common symptoms in adults but seen in only 2% of a recent Italian cohort of children (Calatroni et al., 2017).

The cause of neurological symptoms is either direct invasion of paranasal tissues by the granulomatous process or metastasis to CNS sites not contiguous with the upper airway or necrotizing vasculitis. Orbital pseudotumors cause exophthalmos and ophthalmoplegia. Involvement of the optic nerve, seventh and eighth cranial nerves, chiasm, and pituitary gland can occur. Pituitary involvement causes diabetes insipidus.

The most helpful diagnostic laboratory test in GPA is the demonstration of cytoplasmic-staining antineutrophil cytoplasmic antibody (c-ANCA) to proteinase-3 (PR3) antigen. A definitive diagnosis requires tissue diagnosis by biopsy of lung, skin, or kidney.

Induction therapy with corticosteroids in combination with cyclophosphamide leads to remission in more than 90% of patients with GPA. Maintenance therapy includes methotrexate, azathioprine, leflunomide, trimethoprim-sulfamethoxazole, etanercept, and rituximab.

## Behçet Disease

Definitive diagnosis of Behçet disease requires recurrent oral ulcerations (aphthous or herpetiform) plus two of the following: recurrent genital ulcerations, ocular lesions (uveitis or retinal vasculitis), skin lesions (erythema nodosum, pseudofolliculitis, papulopustular lesions, acneiform nodules), and a positive pathergy test (skin reaction to a needle prick).

Several review studies have documented Behçet disease in childhood and adolescence. It may occur in neonates born to mothers with the disease. The disease is more common in Turkey and other countries in the Middle East. In a large Turkish Behçet population of 728 patients, 3.6% of the patients were pediatric, with a preponderance of male patients in those with neuro-Behçet's. The pediatric Behçet patients were more likely to have venous sinus thrombosis (88.5%) than parenchymal brain disease (11%), in contrast to adult patients (Uluduz et al., 2011).

The reported incidence of CNS involvement (neuro-Behçet) in children ranges from 5% to 15%. According to Saip and colleagues (2005), headache is the most common neurological symptom. Other neurological complications include encephalomyelitis, seizures, brainstem and basal ganglia involvement, aseptic meningitis, pseudotumor cerebri, and dural sinus thrombosis. Psychiatric manifestations include depression, psychosis, and dementia. A few children have suffered acute focal and generalized myositis. Vasculitis of both the arterial and venous systems, associated with thrombosis and arterial aneurysms, can occur. Children are more likely to present with isolated neuro-ophthalmological symptoms, making the diagnosis difficult (Mora et al., 2013).

Treatment includes corticosteroids, sulfasalazine, colchicine, and immunomodulating agents, such as methotrexate, cyclosporine, azathioprine, interferon-α, infliximab, and other bilological agents. Thalidomide is useful in treating isolated mucocutaneous Behçet disease. Azathioprine is one of the first choices for treatment of severe uveitis.

## Sjögren Syndrome

Sjögren syndrome is a chronic inflammatory autoimmune disease that can be either isolated or seen in conjunction with other connective tissue diseases, such as SLE, JIA, or dermatomyositis. The disease mainly affects females and can occur in children. The typical sicca symptoms of dry eyes (xerophthalmia) and dry mouth (xerostomia) are secondary to infiltration of the salivary and lacrimal glands with lymphocytes and plasma cells. Tubular interstitial nephropathy also occurs. Child-specific diagnostic criteria for Sjögren syndrome have been recommended, as children are less likely to have sicca symptoms and more likely to have symptoms such as parotitis and neurological and nephrological symptoms (Yokogawa et al., 2016).

The neurological problems in Sjögren syndrome include aseptic meningitis, infarction, optic neuritis, myelopathy, seizures, encephalopathy, behavioral changes, and motor and sensory neuropathy. Neuromyelitis optica has been reported in a case of primary pediatric Sjögren syndrome (Kornitzer et al., 2016). Several reports have highlighted Sjögren syndrome presenting with an acute febrile encephalopathy (Matsui et al., 2016).

The main laboratory features are nonspecific anemia, leukopenia, and hypergammaglobulinemia. Several autoantibodies are positive, including ANA, anti-SSA, anti-SSB, and rheumatoid factor. Lymphocytic infiltration of the salivary glands of the lower lip is characteristic of Sjögren syndrome and confirms the diagnosis. Treatment is symptomatic. Corticosteroids are useful in severe cases. Marino et al. (2017) reported successful treatment of Sjögren syndrome and neuromyelitis optica with tocilizumab.

## Primary Angiitis of the Central Nervous System

Primary angiitis of the CNS (PACNS) was initially called *granulomatous angiitis*. PACNS is felt to be one of the most common forms of CNS vasculitis; however, prevalence and incidence studies are limited. PACNS is divided into subtypes based on the size of the vessels involved and the presence of progression. A large-vessel, angiography-positive subtype without progression consists of a monophasic form of the disease with good response to steroids; it is more common in boys. The progressive large-vessel, angiography-positive form of PANCS also occurs more often in boys and is associated with focal deficits on presentation. Small-vessel, angiography-negative forms of PANCS are seen more often in girls and present most often with seizures (Twilt et al., 2016). Further clinical manifestations of PACNS include headaches, TIAs, encephalopathy, visual loss, hemiparesis, and neurocognitive changes.

Angiography is diagnostic, showing small- and medium-sized vessel beading or alternating segmental narrowing and ectasia. Cerebrospinal fluid (CSF) analysis shows increased proteins and mild pleocytosis. Inflammatory blood markers are positive. Raised intracranial pressure also occurs. MRI can reveal bilateral or unilateral multifocal T2 hyperintensities in both white and gray matter.

Early diagnosis and treatment with corticosteroids and immune modulating treatments have reduced the high morbidity previously reported and the frequency of recurrences, though more studies are needed (Twilt et al., 2016).

## RESPIRATORY DISORDERS

### Periodic Breathing and Apnea

The *periodic breathing* pattern, more common in premature infants, consists of characteristic cyclic episodes during sleep, when brief apneic pauses of 5–10 seconds interrupt regular breathing, followed by a burst of rapid respiration. Infants who become hypoxic require supplemental oxygen. Neurological complications do not occur unless hypoxic periods are prolonged and severe. The definition of *apnea* is cessation of breathing for more than 20 seconds. The incidence of associated bradycardia increases with the duration of the apnea and correlates with the severity of hypoxia. Apnea can be idiopathic (idiopathic apnea of prematurity) or can be caused by intraventricular hemorrhage, seizures, obstruction, atelectasis, pneumonia, sepsis, meningitis, phrenic nerve paralysis, gastroesophageal reflux, hypovolemia, and heart failure. Apnea of prematurity treatment with caffeine has been a standard treatment, and new data suggest that early caffeine therapy is associated with better neurodevelopmental outcomes in patients born earlier than 29 weeks of gestation (Lodha et al., 2019).

Undiagnosed obstructive sleep apnea (OSA) can lead to failure to thrive, pulmonary hypertension, and systemic hypertension. It also can cause long-term deleterious effects on neuronal and intellectual functioning, with behavioral changes, restlessness, aggressive behavior, memory problems, and poor test performance. Increasing evidence supports the association of OSA and symptoms of attention-deficit/hyperactivity disorder (ADHD). Some of the neurobehavioral deficits are not totally reversed with treatment of the apnea (Li et al., 2016).

### Bronchopulmonary Dysplasia

Bronchopulmonary dysplasia (BPD) is a chronic lung disease of infancy that follows mechanical ventilation and oxygen therapy for acute respiratory distress or hyaline membrane disease in premature newborns. Multiple studies have shown that the neurological outcome of infants with BPD is closely associated with the presence of complications of prematurity, such as intraventricular hemorrhage, periventricular leukomalacia, seizures, and prolonged ventilatory support, leading to the gross and fine motor delays and cerebral palsy seen in this population. The presence of severe BPD alone, however, poses an additional risk for neuromotor sequelae that include mild spasticity, microcephaly, and behavioral problems (Majnemer et al., 2000). When compared with a matched cohort of preterm peers, children with prematurity and BPD exhibited a higher frequency of subtle neurological signs, such as involuntary movements, poor coordination, clumsiness, poor postural control, synkinesias, and dyspraxia, and an increased need for special education. A comprehensive review of 450 extremely preterm children with BPD found these effects persisted 10 years later, with these children more likely to have dysfunction in the cognitive, language, executive function, and social skills realms (Sriram et al., 2018).

In an earlier report, a syndrome characterized by rapid, random, jerky movements similar to chorea and restless movements similar to akathisia involving the limbs, neck, trunk, tongue, and mouth developed in a series of 10 premature infants with severe BPD. The movements, which began in the third month, were exacerbated by respiratory failure and were attenuated during sleep. The natural history was either partial or complete resolution or a static course. One patient had histopathological evidence of neuronal loss and astrocytosis in the basal ganglia and thalamus.

### Cystic Fibrosis

The neurological complications in cystic fibrosis (CF) result from chronic hypoxia and hypercapnia, leading to lethargy, somnolence, and sometimes coma. Brain abscess occurs in a small number of adolescents and adults with CF, usually in association with advanced pulmonary disease and paranasal sinus disease.

Increased intracranial pressure, characterized by a bulging fontanelle and irritability, may occur in malnourished infants with CF after initiation of nutritional therapy. The cause is unclear but may involve intrathoracic obstruction of venous return. Vitamin A deficiency must be excluded in this setting.

Patients with CF and pancreatic insufficiency frequently suffer from vitamin E deficiency, with the potential for development of spinocerebellar degeneration with ataxia, dysarthria, areflexia, and proprioceptive loss. Neuropathological studies reveal posterior column degeneration. Peripheral neuropathy, ophthalmoplegia, diminished visual acuity, tremor, and weakness may be neurological manifestations of CF. The use of indwelling intravenous catheters can result in venous thrombosis and cerebral thromboembolism. Other contributing factors for thrombotic complications include associated diabetes, chronic inflammation, acquired thrombophilia due to hepatic insufficiency, and cholestasis. In addition, patients with CF have an increased risk for right-to-left shunting because of chronic cough and secondary pulmonary hypertension.

Chiari type I malformation seems to be more common in patients with CF than in the general population. Needleman and colleagues (2000) described five children and adolescents with CF and Chiari type I malformations with swallowing dysfunction, syncope, numbness, headaches, and recurrent emesis.

### Sarcoidosis

Sarcoidosis is an idiopathic, chronic, multisystem, granulomatous disease, uncommon in children. It predominantly affects females and African American children. In 3%–15% of published cases, the patients were younger than 15 years of age.

The clinical presentation varies between younger (before 4 years of age) and older children (8–15 years) and is different from that in the adult population (Yanardag et al., 2006). Children younger than 4 years of age present mainly with a maculopapular rash, uveitis, and arthritis. In the 8- to 15-year-old age group, signs and symptoms include fever, cough, lymphadenopathy, malaise, ocular lesions, and abnormalities on the chest radiograph. In 1985, Edward Blau described families with autosomal dominant granulomatous disease similar to early-onset sarcoidosis. Recent data have suggested that Blau syndrome and early-onset sarcoidosis may represent the same disease. They both share the same genetic mutations in the NOD2 (nucleotide binding oligomerization domain 2), also known as *CARD 15* (capsule recruitment domain family member 15). CNS abnormalities, known as *neurosarcoidosis*, occur in 30% of children, compared with 5%–10% of affected adults. CNS complications include encephalopathy, seizures, cranial neuropathy (with nerve VII most frequently affected), optic neuritis, mass lesions, obstructive hydrocephalus, basilar granulomatous meningitis, aseptic meningitis, peripheral neuropathy, headaches, myelopathy, and pituitary–hypothalamic lesions. Reports of symptomatology in children are somewhat wide-ranging. Baumann et al. (2003) found children are more likely to develop seizures and space-occupying lesions and less likely to develop cranial nerve palsies. Rao et al. (2016) found seizures in 24.5% of their pediatric sarcoid cohort, cranial neuropathies in 21%, and papilledema or optic neuritis in 15.6%.

Sarcoid granulomas are more commonly located in the cerebral hemispheres than in the posterior fossa. They probably result from extension of the inflammatory process through the Virchow-Robin spaces. The MRI appearance of neurosarcoid mass lesions is nonspecific. The lesions have a higher density than that of the brain and enhance with contrast. White-matter sarcoid lesions seen on T2-weighted images can resemble the tumefactive demyelinating lesions seen in multiple sclerosis.

Histologically, the diagnostic feature of sarcoidosis is the presence of noncaseating granuloma. Serum levels of angiotensin-converting enzyme (ACE) are elevated in 80% of children with sarcoidosis. Most patients have hypercalcemia and hypercalciuria.

Corticosteroids are the standard treatment for sarcoidosis, but other immunosuppressants are gaining popularity.

## HYPERTENSION

The causes of hypertension in children include renal disease, aortic coarctation, collagen vascular disease, hemolytic-uremic syndrome (HUS), Cushing syndrome, steroid use, and immunosuppressive therapy. It also occurs in association with neurofibromatosis type I, von Hippel-Lindau syndrome, and Guillain-Barré syndrome.

Neurological complications develop in more than 40% of patients with malignant hypertension: stroke, encephalopathy, fever, opisthotonos, muscle twitching, myoclonus, and cranial neuropathies.

Hypertensive encephalopathy occurs with a rapid and severe rise in blood pressure. It is mostly seen with HUS, acute glomerulonephritis, and medication use. Initial clinical features are headache, projectile emesis, fatigue, and meningismus, followed by rapid onset of encephalopathy and generalized seizures. Whereas retinal arteriolar spasm is a more characteristic sign, papilledema is seen in only one-third of cases.

Prompt management and safe reduction of blood pressure are very important in the management of hypertensive encephalopathy. Antiepileptic medications are used to treat persistent seizures, but chronic therapy usually is not required.

PRES is a syndrome characterized by headaches, seizures, and reversible subcortical vasogenic edema. It can also be associated with visual loss, hallucinations, lethargy, and transitory motor deficits. The first description of this syndrome was in patients receiving cyclosporine. PRES can be seen with multiple etiologies, most often hypertension, but also with chronic renal failure and chemotherapy in the absence of hypertension. Recent reviews revealed that acute lymphoblastic leukemia (ALL) induction chemotherapy regimens were the most predisposing factors for PRES (Kim et al., 2012). Brain imaging reveals increased T2 and fluid-attenuated inversion recovery signals, predominantly involving the posterior parietal-occipital regions, affecting both white and gray matter (Fig. 59.4). Similar findings can be seen in other parts of the brain. A case report of isolated posterior fossa involvement during induction chemotherapy for ALL was described (Shimizu et al., 2013), and, more recently, spinal cord involvement in two children with PRES was reported (Lucchesi et al., 2017). It is postulated that dysfunction in cerebral autoregulation causes perivascular edema that compresses surrounding microvessels, leading to proliferative endarteritis. This process increases the patient's vulnerability to infarction and petechial hemorrhage. Vasospasm, endothelial dysfunction, and an inflammatory state could be the explanation in the absence of hypertension. Cases of PRES have been reported in pediatric lupus, influenza A infections, and in association with severe infections, sepsis, and shock (Bartynski et al., 2009).

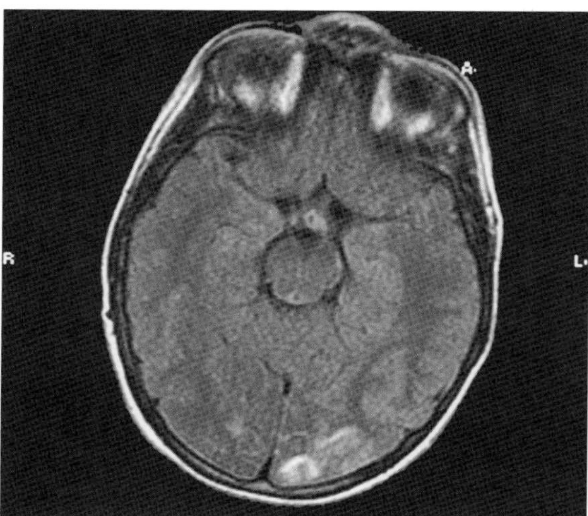


**Fig. 59.4** Magnetic resonance image of brain of a 6-year-old boy with end-stage renal disease and hypertensive encephalopathy (i.e., posterior reversible leukoencephalopathy syndrome). Bilateral occipital high signal intensity is more pronounced on the left side.

Some reports of PRES in children with cancer have described irreversible MRI changes. In 3 out of 11 patients in one series, epilepsy developed despite clinical and radiographic evidence of recovery, requiring chronic antiepileptic drug therapy (Morris et al., 2005).

## HEMATOLOGICAL DISORDERS

### Hemolytic Disease of the Newborn and Kernicterus

Hemolytic disease of the newborn, or erythroblastosis fetalis, is caused by Rh incompatibility, A and B incompatibility, or other blood group incompatibility (C, E, Kell, and Duffy). The use of RhoGAM or human anti-D globulin within 72 hours of delivery or abortion has reduced the risk of initial sensitization of Rh-negative mothers.

In affected infants, jaundice develops within the first few hours of life. Serum bilirubin concentrations exceed safe limits within 48 hours. Unconjugated bilirubin can reach the CNS and injure neurons, mainly basal ganglia (globus pallidus and subthalamic nucleus), cerebellar vermis, dentate nuclei, hippocampi, and cranial nerve nuclei, especially the oculomotor and eighth cranial nerves, leading to the occurrence of kernicterus, or nuclear jaundice.

The clinical features include lethargy, poor feeding, rigidity, opisthotonos, high-pitched cry, fever, and convulsions. Approximately half of patients with kernicterus die. The survivors typically have choreoathetoid cerebral palsy, high-frequency deafness, and mental retardation. Fortunately, the classic clinical picture of kernicterus is rare with improved nursery care and early treatment of jaundice. However, recent studies have focused on the assessment of minor bilirubin neurotoxicity manifested later in childhood in more subtle ways, such as learning deficits and mild motor, cognitive, and behavioral disorders. Phototherapy and exchange transfusion are the major modes of therapy.

Bilirubin-induced neurological dysfunction (BIND) and acute bilirubin encephalopathy (ABE) are terms that have been used in the literature to describe the neurological sequelae of hyperbilirubinemia. More recently, Le Pichon et al. (2017) proposed the use of kernicterus spectrum disorders (KSDs) as a systematic nomenclature to help unify and promote more research.

## Hemorrhagic Disease of the Newborn

The cause of hemorrhagic disease of the newborn is a transitory deficiency of vitamin K-dependent factors. This may be due to poor placental transfer of vitamin K, marginal vitamin K content in breast milk, or maternal use of medications that interfere with vitamin K stores or function (e.g., phenytoin). Bleeding starts in the first postnatal week. The neurological complications are caused by subarachnoid or intraparenchymal hemorrhage. Administration of vitamin K intramuscularly at birth prevents hemorrhagic disease of the newborn.

## Neonatal Polycythemia

The definition of neonatal polycythemia is a central hematocrit of 65% or higher. Hypoglycemia, hypocalcemia, and thrombocytopenia are often associated. Concurrent hypoglycemia increases the risk of a poor outcome.

The hyperviscosity may cause arterial or venous thrombosis. It can also lead to increased cerebrovascular resistance and diminished cerebral blood flow. Ischemic lesions are often complicated with hemorrhage. Neurological complications include stroke, developmental delay, tremor, spastic diplegia, hemiparesis, monoparesis, mental retardation, and learning deficits. Lethargy, poor feeding, tremor, and jitteriness are common clinical findings. Treatment consists of partial exchange transfusion, adequate hydration, and correction of associated metabolic disorders.

## Sickle Cell Disease

Sickle cell disease (SCD) is the most common hematological disorder associated with CVAs. The incidence of stroke in SCD ranges from 7% to 33% (Fig. 59.5). The prevalence of silent infarcts was 21.8% among 266 patients in the Cooperative Study of SCD (Kinney et al., 1999). Silent infarcts occur in the distribution of small vessels. The most common underlying lesion is an intracranial arterial stenosis or obstruction, often seen in the proximal middle cerebral and anterior cerebral arteries, leading to a vasculopathy and moyamoya syndrome. Sickled erythrocytes cause chronic injury to the vessel endothelium, resulting in a narrow lumen. Subarachnoid hemorrhage and intraparenchymal hemorrhage can also occur and are commonly attributed to the association of aneurysms with cerebral vasculopathy. Spontaneous acute epidural, subgaleal hematomas, and extradural hematomas are rare complications of sickle cell crises (Dahdaleh et al., 2009; Hettige et al., 2015).

The most common neurological signs are hemiparesis, speech abnormalities, focal seizures, gait dysfunction, headaches, and neurocognitive deficits. Seizures occur in 12%–14% of patients with SCD. Triggering factors include CNS infections, chest syndrome, trauma, hypertension, nephrotic syndrome, and nocturnal hypoxemia. In the Cooperative Study of SCD, seizures were an independent risk factor for silent infarction. A small cohort of patients with SCD complicated with reversible posterior leukoencephalopathy syndrome has been described during painful crisis and acute chest syndrome and after blood transfusion (Khademian et al., 2009; Kolovou et al., 2013).

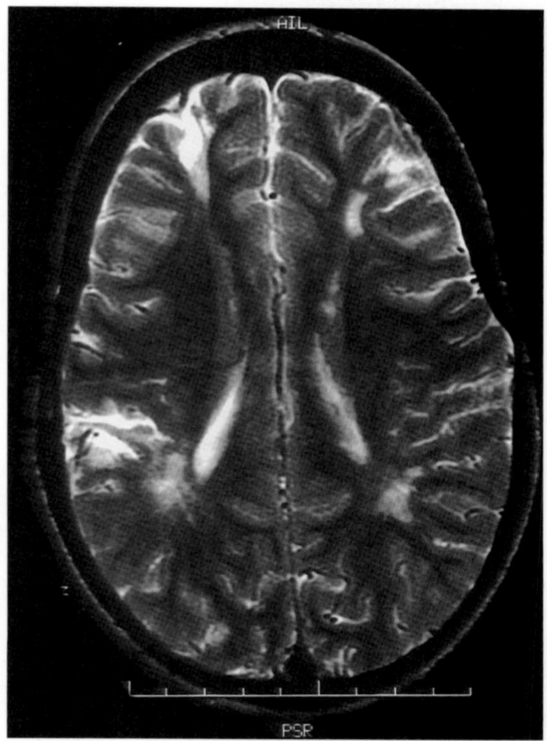


**Fig. 59.5** Magnetic resonance image of brain of an 8-year-old girl with sickle cell disease shows multiple cortical and subcortical infarcts.

Prengler and co-workers (2005) evaluated 76 patients with SCD with TCD studies and perfusion MRI. All patients with seizures had decreased cerebral perfusion ipsilateral to an electroencephalographic abnormality, suggesting that a complex mechanism of large- and small-vessel disease and hypoperfusion plays a role in the pathogenesis of seizures.

The Stroke Prevention Trial in Sickle Cell Anemia (STOP) reported in 1998 that long-term transfusion therapy to decrease the levels of hemoglobin S to less than 20%–30% reduced the risk of stroke in high-risk patients (Adams et al., 1998). The follow-up trial (STOP 2) showed that the risk reverts to former status if transfusion is discontinued (Adams et al., 2005). Silent cerebral infarction is the most frequent neurological complication in patients with SCD. It is reported in as many as 28% of children with SCD who have suffered a clinically evident stroke and is associated with lower cognitive scores and poor academic achievement (Kwiatkowski et al., 2009). The silent cerebral infarct multicenter clinical trial (SIT) showed that blood- transfusion therapy reduced the incidence of infarct recurrence in SCD children who had silent cerebral infarcts, and more research is needed to identify children with silent cerebral infarcts, so transfusion therapy can be offered (DeBaun et al., 2014). Hydroxyurea has shown efficacy in preventing stroke in earlier studies. The pediatric hydroxyurea phase III clinical trial (BABY HUG) showed that hydroxyurea can be given to children 9–18 months of age without significant toxicity (Wang et al., 2011); however, the Stroke with Transfusions Changing to Hydroxyurea (SWiTCH) trial was closed prematurely concluding that transfusion and chelation therapy remain a better way of preventing stroke in SCD (Ware et al., 2012). Therefore, the role of hydroxyyrea for primary and secondary prevention of silent cerebral infarcts has not been fully established.

The potential benefit of TCD ultrasound screening for cerebral vasculopathy and stroke risk in children with SCD was first recognized in the early 1990s. The current standard of care for stroke prevention in children with SCD is TCD screening every 6 months between 2 years and 16 years of age followed by regular blood-transfusion therapy when TCD measurement is above a threshold indicating a high stroke risk (Adams et al., 1998; Jordan et al., 2012).

Children with SCD are susceptible to infections with *Streptococcus pneumoniae*, *Haemophilus influenzae*, and *Mycoplasma pneumoniae*, which can involve the CNS. Sinus venous thrombosis, posterior reversible leukoencephalopathy, and acute demyelination are other complications. Moyamoya disease is a relatively uncommon neurovascular complication of SCD and is a risk factor for stroke and transient ischemic episodes despite prophylactic blood transfusion. Encephaloduroarteriosynangiosis (EDAS) procedures constitute an effective treatment option for moyamoya disease and have had promising results (Fryer et al., 2003).

Partial exchange transfusion is standard therapy in the setting of occlusive crisis and ischemic injury. Indications for anticoagulation are dissection and sinus venous thrombosis, especially with coexistent prothrombotic abnormalities and recurrent stroke. Emerging prophylactic regimens include citrulline, arginine, aspirin, and overnight oxygen supplementation (Kirkham et al., 2006). Bone marrow transplantation offers a potentially curative therapy for patients with SCD and protection from progressive CNS and pulmonary disease (Walters et al., 2010).

### Hemophilia

Studies show that 42% of patients with hemophilia B and 34% of patients with hemophilia A suffer neurological complications. These include intracranial hemorrhage, peripheral nerve lesions due to intramuscular hemorrhage after minor injuries, and spontaneous hematoma formation in the groin or other closed anatomical spaces. Femoral nerve involvement is the most commonly reported complication. Other affected nerves are the lumbosacral plexus, median nerve, radial nerve, and lateral cutaneous nerve. Hemophilic pseudotumor in the spinal canal and cranium has been described and spinal epidural and subdural hematomas presenting as back pain and torticollis (Cuvelier et al., 2006).

Klinge and associates (1999) reported the incidence of intracranial hemorrhage in 42.5% of patients with hemophilia A or B. Bleeding occurred within 1 week of birth in 41% of cases. Trauma, the most important factor, occurred in 57% of cases either during birth (30%) or later (27%). Sixty-three percent had seizures, and one of the 33 patients died. Psychomotor retardation occurred in 59% of cases and cerebral palsy in 45% of cases. Nelson and colleagues (2000) evaluated the incidence and sequelae of 2- to 5-mm focal white-matter hyperintensities on T2-weighted images in hemophiliac patients and reported no correlation with neurological factors; the investigators concluded that the findings were incidental.

### Thrombotic Thrombocytopenic Purpura

Thrombotic thrombocytopenic purpura (TTP) shares many features with HUS. This disorder occurs mainly in adults. It is rare in children but could be congenital or acquired. The diagnosis requires at least two major criteria (thrombocytopenia, Coombs-negative microangiopathic hemolytic anemia, neurological dysfunction) and two minor criteria (fever, renal dysfunction, circulating thrombi). Congenital TTP was recently found to be secondary to a severe deficiency in ADAMTS13 (a disintegrin and metalloproteinase with thrombospondin type 1 repeats, member 13), inherited in congenital TTP or secondary to anti-ADAMTS13 antibodies in acquired TTP. Diagnosis now includes rapid techniques for ADAMTS13 assays. The microangiopathy of TTP can affect any organ but predominantly targets the CNS, kidneys, pancreas, heart, and adrenal glands. Purpura is the initial manifestation in more than 90% of cases. Thrombosis of small arterioles, venules, and capillaries leads to cerebral microinfarctions. Petechial hemorrhages occur in the gray matter.

Neurological symptoms consist of lethargy, headache, confusion, and visual and speech disturbances. Corticosteroids are useful in mild cases. Plasma exchange, performed in severe cases, has improved survival. Recently, rituximab has been used in refractory or relapsing cases (Cuker, 2016). Recombinant ADAMTS13 or BAX930 was found to be safe, nonimmunogenic, and well tolerated in 15 patients with congenital TTP and may become a revolutionary treatment for congenital and immune-mediated TTP (Scully et al., 2017).

### Hemolytic-Uremic Syndrome

HUS frequently follows an episode of gastroenteritis caused by an enteropathogenic strain of *Escherichia coli* (O157:H7). However, it also follows *Shigella*, *Salmonella*, *Campylobacter*, and viral infections. The organisms release a toxin called *verotoxin*, causing endothelial injury. The syndrome is more common in children younger than 4 years of age and is the most frequent cause of acute renal failure in young children.

Involvement of the CNS is found in around 30% of children with HUS and usually predicts a severe outcome and may include encephalopathy, coma, seizures, stroke, behavioral changes, and blindness (Eriksson et al., 2001).

## GASTROINTESTINAL DISORDERS

### Hepatic Encephalopathy

Hepatic encephalopathy can complicate liver failure, whether acute, subacute, or chronic. The most common causes of liver failure in children are fulminant viral or autoimmune hepatitis, drug ingestion (acetaminophen, salicylates, valproic acid), Reye syndrome, mitochondrial diseases, galactosemia, tyrosinemia, and Wilson disease.

Understanding of the pathogenesis, which probably is multifactorial, is incomplete. The role of ammonia as a main causative agent has been widely studied. In 10% of patients with hepatic encephalopathy, however, serum ammonia levels are normal. Implicated agents include γ-aminobutyric acid (GABA), mercaptans, β-phenylethanolamine, tyramine, and octopamine. Ammonia has a direct effect on the neuronal membranes. Both ammonia and GABA cause postsynaptic inhibition.

Clinically evident encephalopathy in children with chronic liver disease appears to be less common than in adults. However, it is possible that encephalopathy is underdiagnosed in children because of its more subtle manifestations. Fifty percent of children with chronic liver disease can develop minimal hepatic encephalopathy or MHE as is evident on neuropsychological tests and showed higher mean diffusivity on DTI, which could become a useful tool in diagnosing MHE (Srivastava et al., 2017). Irritability and lethargy are the most common signs. The neurological examination may demonstrate pyramidal signs changing to hypotonia, focal findings, early parkinsonian syndrome, ataxia, tremor, and dysarthria. Asterixis is a characteristic flapping tremor seen in hepatic encephalopathy, but it can also be seen in other metabolic encephalopathies. Seizures can occur in 10%–30% of patients.

Hepatic encephalopathy progresses over four stages. The signs and symptoms in stages 3 and 4 are similar in both adults and children. Stages 1 and 2 carry certain modifications in the pediatric population.

Stage 1: Mild confusion, irritability, excessive crying, sleep disturbances, mental slowing, and short attention span

Stage 2: Excessive sleepiness, moderate confusion, personality changes, inappropriate behavior, intermittent periods of disorientation, and inability to perform mental tasks

Stage 3: Profound confusion, stupor, delirium, hyper-reflexia, and an extensor plantar response sign

Stage 4: Coma with or without decerebrate or decorticate posturing (4a: response to pain present, 4b: no response to pain).

Intracranial hypertension and cerebral edema are invariably present in stage 4, potentially leading to poor cerebral perfusion, anoxic injury, and brainstem herniation. The last is the most common cause of death seen on postmortem examination.

Coagulopathy and thrombocytopenia, although uncommon, can cause intracranial hemorrhage.

The EEG reveals very early slowing of the alpha rhythm, progressing to delta frequencies with evolution of the encephalopathy. Triphasic waves may be seen at a late stage and usually portend a poor prognosis. More recently Press et al. (2017) found that spectral EEG analysis was useful in improving assessment of hepatic encephalopathy grade in children with acute liver failure. Brain imaging reveals edema and atrophy. T1 hyperintensity of globus pallidus is suggestive of CNS involvement in hepatic encephalopathy and may become a screening tool in the management of children with chronic liver disease (Hanquinet et al., 2017). Spectroscopy shows elevation in glutamine. The CSF contains elevated concentrations of glutamine and α-ketoglutarate.

Management includes ammonia-lowering measures with protein restriction, lactulose, polyethylene glycol (PEG), l-ornithine-l-aspartate (LOLA), and bowel decontamination with neomycin or rifaximin. Flumazenil, a benzodiazepine receptor antagonist, reduces the severity of hepatic encephalopathy. Probiotics, acarbose, and L-carnitine may also be helpful (Foster et al., 2010). Management of cerebral edema involves restriction of fluids, use of hyperosmolar agents, and hyperventilation. Interest has been increasing in the design of liver support devices such as cleansing devices or bioartificial liver support systems. The use of disease-specific therapies, such as *N*-acetylcysteine for acetaminophen toxicity, and the correction of metabolic disturbances and coagulopathy are very important measures in the management of hepatic encephalopathy.

### Liver Transplantation

Advances in medical and surgical techniques in liver transplantation have improved long-term post-transplantation survival, with reported 5-year survival rates of 80%–90%. Congenital biliary atresia is the most common reason for liver transplantation in children. Other causes are biliary micronodular cirrhosis, viral hepatitis, Alagille syndrome, and several rare genetic disorders.

Neurological problems occur in 48% of pediatric orthotopic liver transplant recipients, including seizures, mental status changes, and even coma. Three-fourths of comatose patients had significant intracerebral hemorrhage on brain imaging. Neurological complications constitute a significant source of mortality and morbidity in these patients. Ghaus and associates (2001) reviewed data for 41 adults and pediatric patients who underwent liver transplantation. Encephalopathy occurred in 62%, with either immediate or delayed onset. Seizures (multifocal myoclonus, focal, or status epilepticus) occurred in 11% and were associated with the presence of encephalopathy. Three patients had neuropathy. Other complications were headache, tremor, fatigue, restlessness, enuresis, dizziness, critical illness myopathy, and detached retina. Erol et al. (2007) found seizures to be the most common neurological complications of liver transplantation. Ghosh P.S. et al. (2012) recently reviewed 65 children with liver transplantation; 30.7% had neurological complications. Delayed neurological complications (16.9%) were more frequent than early complications (13.8%), with seizures being the most common. Brain imaging can reveal atrophy, mild cerebral edema, bilateral basal ganglia T1 hyperintensities, hypoxic injury, subarachnoid hemorrhage, intracerebral hemorrhage, focal cerebritis, meningitis, and PRES. Drug toxicity may occur with the use of cyclosporine, tacrolimus, or corticosteroids, in addition to the development of infections (from *Candida albicans*, *Pseudomonas aeruginosa*, *Staphylococcus aureus*, vancomycin-resistant enterococci, *Mycobacterium tuberculosis*, and other opportunistic pathogens, such as *Aspergillus fumigatus* and *Listeria monocytogenes*). Limbic encephalitis, associated with human herpesvirus 6, has been described after liver transplantation and can present with confusion, amnesia, and seizures (Vinnard et al., 2009).

## ENDOCRINE DISORDERS

### Thyroid Disorders

#### Hypothyroidism

The clinical features of thyroid deficiency depend on the age at onset. Congenital hypothyroidism is the most common treatable cause of mental retardation. In the last decade, the incidence has nearly doubled to 1 in 2000 live births, due to the lowering of newborn screen thresholds (Wassner et al., 2017). The historic most common cause of congenital hypothyroidism worldwide, iodine deficiency, is occurring less often due to widespread salt iodization programs. Other congenital hypothyroidism causes include thyroid dysgenesis, thyroid-stimulating hormone (TSH) receptor blocking antibody, defective synthesis of thyroxine, TSH deficiency, TSH unresponsiveness, thyroid hormone unresponsiveness, and use of radioiodine during pregnancy.

Clinical evidence of hypothyroidism is difficult to appreciate in the newborn period. Many of the classic features, such as large tongue, umbilical hernia, hoarse cry, facial puffiness, cold mottled hands and feet, hypotonia, constipation, feeding problems, somnolence, and apnea, only develop with time. Prolongation of physiological jaundice may be one of the earliest signs. The anterior and posterior fontanelles are large. A delay in diagnosis results in delayed subsequent linear growth, anemia, sensorineural hearing loss, cardiomegaly, and pericardial effusion. Retardation of physical and mental development becomes apparent by 3–6 months of age. Myxedema may involve the skin of the eyelids, backs of the hands, and genitalia. All affected children have hypotonia except for those with Kocher-Debré-Semelaigne syndrome, in which generalized muscular hypertrophy, predominating in the calf muscles, gives the patient an athletic appearance. Newborn screening programs detect these disorders in the United States and much of Western Europe, providing early detection and treatment. Despite the eradication of severe mental retardation, the intelligence quotient (IQ) of treated infants is 6–19 points lower than that of controls. The need for special education increases fourfold in affected children. Sensorineural hearing loss, attention problems, and various neuropsychiatric problems can persist and may not be reversible with postnatal therapy (Morin et al., 2002).

Acquired hypothyroidism can develop at any age, and can result from tumors, irradiation, infections, drugs, autoimmune processes, trauma, iodine deficiency and iodine excess. It is often associated with multiple hypothalamic–pituitary hormone deficiencies and could be a component of genetic syndromes such as Pendred syndrome and septo-optic dysplasia. Neurological complications include dementia, psychosis, seizures, ataxia, coma, myopathy, and length-dependent peripheral neuropathy (Katzberg et al., 2016). Deep tendon reflexes may show a delayed relaxation time.

Hashimoto thyroiditis is the most frequent form of thyroiditis in children. It affects 1.2% of school-aged children and is the most common cause of hypothyroidism and thyroid enlargement in patients older than 6 years.

Hashimoto encephalopathy is a steroid-responsive encephalopathy that manifests with acute to subacute evidence of cognitive impairment (80%), variable psychiatric symptoms (90%–100%) including psychosis and suicidal ideation, alteration in consciousness, hallucinations (visual mostly), involuntary movements, seizures, myoclonus, tremor, opsoclonus, chorea, ataxia, dystonia, speech disturbances, stroke-like episodes, and myelopathy. Hashimoto encephalopathy can also develop gradually in a relapsing-remitting pattern with slow progressive cognitive decline and psychiatric signs. The literature contains many pediatric cases with this condition (Alink et al., 2008). Most affected patients are adolescent females. Most of the published cases presented with seizures, generalized tonic-clonic in 80% of the cases. Neuropsychiatric features, such as agitation, restlessness, apathy, social isolation, and minor personality and behavioral changes, could be seen at presentation. The diagnosis requires the clinical triad of neuropsychiatric symptoms, detection of antimicrosomal or antithyroglobulin antibodies, and the exclusion of other causes. The most frequently detected antibodies are antithyroid peroxidase (almost 100%), antithyroglobulin (70%), and to a lesser extent, TSH receptor-blocking antibodies. Recently, α-enolase, a novel autoantigen, was described and appears to be highly relevant for Hashimoto encephalopathy (Ochi et al., 2002). Recent Japanese studies showed that autoantibodies against the amino ($NH_2$) terminal of α-enolase (NAE) were found to be 50% sensitive and 91% specific, suggesting that anti-NAE antibodies may be useful diagnostic biomarkers for Hashimoto encephalopathy (Kishitani et al., 2013). The initial antithyroid antibody titers can be normal or mildly elevated in children; therefore, follow-up titers are required in patients clinically suspected to have Hashimoto encephalopathy (Lee et al., 2018).

The proposed mechanism of pathogenesis is an autoimmune cerebral vasculitis, perhaps related to immune complex deposition, leading to cerebral hypoperfusion (Marshall and Doyle, 2006). Some patients have antithyroid antibodies in the CSF, and 60% show mild to moderate elevation of CSF protein levels. MRI findings are normal in most pediatric patients; however, some children show nonspecific prolongation of T2-weighted signals in the subcortical white matter. Spectroscopy studies in a few pediatric patients revealed evidence of hypoperfusion, mainly in the frontotemporal regions (Watemberg et al., 2006). The EEG often reveals diffuse slowing of the background. The symptoms in Hashimoto encephalopathy can occur even if the patient is euthyroid. Hypothyroidism is observed in 52% of the reported pediatric patients (Alink and de Vries, 2008). The condition does not respond to thyroxine replacement. Most children show a dramatic response to a short course of high-dose corticosteroids, with a slow taper over weeks to months. Full recovery was described in 55% of reported cases. Incomplete recovery is associated with neuropsychological difficulties, seizures, and behavioral problems. Cases with multiple recurrences or cases failing to respond to a short course of corticosteroids are placed on long-term treatment with prednisone, azathioprine, cyclophosphamide, hydroxychloroquine (Plaquenil), methotrexate, mycophenolate mofetil (CellCept), periodic IVIG, or plasma exchange, usually with good success.

### Hyperthyroidism

Neonatal hyperthyroidism is usually transient and results from the transplacental passage of maternal TSH receptor-stimulating antibodies. It occurs in 2%–3% of mothers with Graves disease. When it becomes permanent, the usual cause is a germline mutation in the TSH receptor. When the condition goes untreated, craniosynostosis and developmental delay occur.

Hyperthyroidism in childhood is rare, but largely due to Graves disease. Neurological symptoms include emotional lability, irritability, short attention span, anxiety, restlessness, tremor, excessive sweating, lid lag, impairment of convergence, muscular weakness, brisk reflexes, and chorea (Srinivasan et al., 2015). Exophthalmos, tachycardia, and hypertension may also be present. Thyrotoxic periodic paralysis and the association with myasthenia gravis are less common in children. An infant with giant omphalocele who was treated with iodine dressings in preparation for surgery developed thyrotoxicosis, rather than the typical reports of hypothyroidism with excessive iodine exposure (Malhotra et al., 2016)

## Parathyroid Disorders

Hypoparathyroidism is the result of parathyroid hormone (PTH) deficiency secondary to either aplasia or hypoplasia of the parathyroid gland as seen with some genetic syndromes (DiGeorge syndrome), *PTH* gene mutations, PTH receptor defects (pseudohypoparathyroidism), autoimmune parathyroiditis, infiltrative lesions, and removal or damage to the parathyroid glands surgically. The end result is hypocalcemia. The neurological signs and symptoms of hypocalcemia include muscular pain, cramps, tetany, apnea, seizures, numbness, stiffness, and increased intracranial pressure with headaches and vomiting. Calcifications, mostly in the basal ganglia (most commonly in the globus pallidus), but also in the cortex and cerebellum, can be seen and are usually asymptomatic; however, rare cases of intracranial calcifications presenting as a movement disorder and seizures have been described (Ghosh, K., et al., 2012). Recombinant human PTH is being explored as a treatment option (Desanctis et al., 2018).

Hyperparathyroidism results in hypercalcemia and can manifest with muscular weakness, anorexia, nausea, vomiting, encephalopathy, polydipsia, polyuria, and weight loss. Headaches, seizures, and psychiatric symptoms may also be features. Sporadic primary hyperparathyroidism is rare in children, but does occur more commonly than hereditary primary hyperparathyroidism, which is generally due to multiple endocrine neoplasia type I (Nicholson et al., 2016).

## Adrenal Gland Dysfunction

### Addison Disease

Addison disease is the most common cause of adrenal insufficiency. The initial description was a complication of tuberculosis. Currently, the most frequent cause is an autoimmune destruction of the gland. It can also follow prolonged use of steroids, adrenal hemorrhage, infection, and tumor. Addison disease can be seen in adrenoleukodystrophy. A recent case series found that only 3 out of 48 patients with confirmed X-linked adrenoleukodystrophy presented with symptoms of Addison disease; however, this number increased to 6 out of 48 patients in the follow-up (Tran et al., 2017). Signs and symptoms of Addison disease include anorexia, muscular weakness, fatigue, weight loss, hypotension, and headaches. Pigmentation of the skin in the face and hands increases secondary to excessive secretion of corticotropin (or adrenocorticotropic hormone [ACTH]).

### Cushing Syndrome

Cushing syndrome results from high cortisol caused by excessive function of the adrenal cortex. The syndrome may be ACTH dependent, as with pituitary tumors or ectopic production of ACTH, or ACTH independent, as with primary pigmented nodular adrenocortical disease, bilateral adrenal hyperplasia, McCune-Albright syndrome, or other genetic causes (Stratakis, 2016). The clinical manifestations are cushingoid appearance, moon facies, buffalo hump, purple striae in the skin overlying hips and abdomen, and hypertension. The neurological problems consist of weakness, headache, proximal myopathy, emotional lability, and decline in school performance.

### Excess Mineralocorticoid Secretion

Primary aldosteronism and pheochromocytoma result in increased secretion of aldosterone. Primary aldosteronism is rare in pediatrics and is typically associated with familial cases. Multiple genetic disorders associated with familial aldosteronism are being recognized (Scholl et al., 2018). Hypertension, headaches, fatigue, dizziness, visual disturbances, muscle weakness, tetany, and intermittent paralysis can occur.

### Pituitary Disorders

Panhypopituitarism can occur with septo-optic dysplasia (de Morsier syndrome), holoprosencephaly, and Laurence-Moon-Biedl syndrome. The neurological symptoms depend on the deficient hormones and specific features of the genetic conditions. Diabetes insipidus manifests with irritability, polyuria, and polydipsia. If left untreated, the disorder progresses to coma and death.

Pituitary adenomas can cause headaches, visual disturbances, hydrocephalus, cranial nerve palsies, and seizures. Growth hormone-secreting adenomas cause gigantism in children and adolescent acromegaly. Clinical features include headaches, visual disturbances, myopathy, and carpal tunnel syndrome.

### Diabetes Mellitus

Diabetes mellitus type 1 (DM1) is the most common endocrine disorder of childhood. The chronic complications of diabetes mellitus have been increasingly studied. The incidence of diabetic neuropathy with onset of DM1 in childhood reaches 28%–40% after 20 years of symptoms and 70% after 30 years. Clinical diabetic neuropathic pain (DNP) is uncommon in children and adolescents but is detectable by neurophysiological studies.

Nery Ferreira and colleagues (2005) evaluated 48 children with DM1 for periods ranging from 5 to 10 years. Neurological complaints, such as lower extremity pain and numbness, were reported by 6.3% of patients. Almost 65% exhibited abnormalities on examination consistent with neuropathy: absence of deep tendon reflexes and vibration sensation. Sixty percent showed changes in motor and sensory nerve conduction. El Bahri-Ben Mrad and colleagues (2000) reported a 10% incidence of clinical neuropathy, compared with 29% with neurophysiological evidence, predominantly in the legs. Jaiswal and colleagues (2017) studied 2000 youth with diabetes and found peripheral neuropathy in 7% of the type 1 cases and 22% of the type 2 cases, highlighting the need for early monitoring and interventions.

A longitudinal epidemiological study of the evolution of diabetic microvascular disease and autonomic function revealed a substantial prevalence of microvascular and neurological abnormalities (Karavanaki and Baum, 1999). Reduced pupillary adaptation in darkness was noted in 7.9% of patients and impaired vibration sensation in the lower extremities in 6.2%. Low sensory nerve conduction and autonomic dysfunction were findings in 25% of newly diagnosed diabetic children in whom the disease was not yet under good control (Solders et al., 1997). Turgut and associates (2004) suggested that monitoring of the dorsal sural sensory nerve action potential (SNAP) is a sensitive method for detection of peripheral neuropathy in early stages of diabetes in children.

Nordwall and co-workers (2006) found evidence of subclinical neuropathy in 59% of children and adolescents with a duration of diabetes longer than 3 years despite intensive insulin treatment and good control. Nerve conduction studies (NCV) are the gold-standard method for detection of subclinical diabetic neuropathy, but they are invasive. Vibration sensation thresholds (VSTs) and thermal discrimination thresholds (TDTs) are alternative easier screening tools (Louraki et al., 2012).

Cranial neuropathies (III, IV, and VI) are rare in children. Polyradiculopathy, a well-documented complication of diabetes in adulthood, rarely occurs in diabetic children and adolescents. Carpal tunnel syndrome is uncommon. The incidence of stroke is higher in diabetic children than in the general population.

Diabetic ketoacidosis is the most serious complication of diabetes and the most common cause of death. Cerebral edema develops in 1% of the cases and occurs rarely in diabetics older than 20 years. The attributed etiology of cerebral edema is retention of intracellular osmolytes in the brain during hydration, causing a shift of water into the intracellular space. Signs of cerebral edema include agitation, confusion, lethargy, headache, emesis, and incontinence (Muir et al., 2004). Stroke can occur in patients with diabetic ketoacidosis as a result of a prothrombotic tendency in these patients. Brain herniation, venous thrombosis, and cerebral hemorrhage can also occur (Lee et al., 2011).

Prevention of cerebral edema is by gradual rehydration over 48 hours and avoidance of hypotonic fluids. Treatment consists of mannitol, fluid restriction, and hyperventilation.

Rare cases of extrapontine and central pontine myelinosis have been described after treatment of diabetic ketoacidoses and were attributed to rapid correction of hyperosmolality (Sivaswamy and Karia, 2007). Hypoglycemia, a known complication of diabetic treatment, usually occurs at night or during early morning hours. Shehadeh and co-workers (1998) reported that 32% of pediatric diabetic patients experienced at least one severe hypoglycemic episode. Variable neurological signs and symptoms, including confusion, tremor, seizures, behavioral changes, blurred vision, transitory hemiparesis, and coma, occurred in all of the cases. One patient had permanent hemiparesis.

## RENAL DISORDERS

### Renal Failure

Acute or chronic renal failure leads to multiple metabolic and vascular derangements that can affect the CNS and peripheral nervous system.

Uremic encephalopathy manifests early on with fatigue, drowsiness, restlessness, and reduced attention span. These symptoms can fluctuate. Mild headaches can present, but mainly during dialysis. Severe headaches usually occur with concomitant hypertension. With the progression of azotemia, anorexia and generalized weakness develop. Dysarthria, cramps, fasciculations, twitching, and asterixis may appear. Psychiatric symptoms include confusion, hallucinations, and frank psychosis. Myoclonic jerks, seizures, stupor, and coma occur in severe untreated cases.

Other features may include transient focal neurological signs, such as transient loss of vision (uremic amaurosis). Cranial nerve palsies, hearing loss, gait disturbances, ataxia, tremor, monoplegia, and hemiplegia may also develop and sometimes are associated with ischemic injuries caused by hypertensive encephalopathy, ischemic stroke, or intracerebral hemorrhage.

Overt clinical distal motor and sensory symmetric mixed polyneuropathy, affecting mainly the legs, is unusual in early childhood. Reduced peroneal motor nerve conduction velocities, however, are common in children on dialysis, even without clinical evidence of neuropathy. Autonomic dysfunction leading to postural hypotension occurs. Neuropathy is manifested early on with restless legs syndrome, characterized by a pricking sensation and pruritus. Other features may include marked hypersensitivity to touch and a burning sensation in the feet known as *burning feet syndrome*. The neuropathy can evolve into weakness; loss of deep tendon reflexes, mainly at the knees and ankles; and distal sensory loss. Histopathological changes consist of degeneration and segmental demyelination.

Psychometric studies have shown intellectual impairment in most patients with renal failure on dialysis, with deficits in academic skills, executive function, attention, and visual and verbal memory (Chen et al, 2018). Future studies are needed to assess cognitive remediation approaches in this vulnerable population (Javalkar et al., 2017). Hypertensive encephalopathy can occur in end-stage renal disease. Myoclonic jerks, focal or generalized seizures, and status epilepticus occur frequently in renal failure. Uremic seizures usually are myoclonic or generalized. The presence of focal seizures, therefore, suggests a structural brain lesion or coexisting pathology. The myoclonic jerks are nonrhythmical. They may be symmetrical or asymmetrical, stimulus-sensitive, and occasionally generalized. Rapid metabolic changes in blood pH and electrolytes and a rapid fall in urea levels are common antecedents. Myoclonus is best left untreated unless it is disabling. Clonazepam, levetiracetam, and valproic acid are the drugs of choice. The doses of anticonvulsant drugs will need adjustment, and frequent blood level monitoring is important in the management of seizures in patients with renal failure.

## Complications of Dialysis

### Headaches

Headaches occur in up to 70% of patients on dialysis (Antoniazzi et al., 2003b). Approximately half of such patients have evidence of a migrainous disorder. The International Headache Society has defined criteria for the headaches related to hemodialysis. The headache must begin during hemodialysis and terminate within 24 hours (Antoniazzi et al., 2003a).

Severe headaches can be associated with hypertension and cerebral hemorrhage. Subdural hemorrhage occurs in 1%–3%.

### Dialysis Disequilibrium Syndrome

Single or recurrent seizures, encephalopathy, and psychosis are the main features of the dialysis disequilibrium syndrome. Symptoms vary from restlessness and headache to coma and death. It is difficult to reverse and has a very high mortality rate. This disorder is more common in children than in adults and more frequently follows hemodialysis than peritoneal dialysis. It is more likely to occur with initiation of dialysis in severely uremic patients and rapid dialysis protocol. Onset may be as early as 3 hours and as late as 48 hours after dialysis. The cause is osmotic gradient leading to flow of water into the brain, with the end result of cerebral edema.

### Progressive Dialysis Dementia

Progressive dialysis dementia, first recognized in adult patients on chronic dialysis in the 1960s, was attributed to the aluminum content of the dialysate. Affected patients had high levels of aluminum in the brain, muscle, and bone. It has become less common since the removal of aluminum from diasylates and is now a rare complication of dialysis, with an estimated prevalence of 0.4%–1.1% in patients less than 45 years of age (Kurella et al., 2006)

Presenting features are dysarthria, speech apraxia, and personality changes. Eventually, dementia occurs, with severe myoclonus and seizures. The early symptoms can be intermittent, worsening during dialysis. Similar presentations were described in children whose renal failure started in infancy and who had received aluminum hydroxide orally but were not dialyzed.

## Renal Transplantation

Recent advances in surgical techniques and immunosuppression have greatly enhanced the outcome in renal transplantation and graft survival. Mir et al. (2005) analyzed data for 72 pediatric renal transplant recipients and reported hypertension in 31.9%, acute rejection in 27.8%, chronic rejection in 13.9%, and CMV infections in 20.8% of patients.

Rejection encephalopathy manifests with headaches, confusion, fever, irritability, and seizures. Symptoms develop within 3 months of transplantation in more than half of affected patients. Infections contribute significantly to transplantation-associated mortality and morbidity, developing in more than 80% of transplant recipients; of these, 5%–10% are in the nervous system (meningitis, brain abscess). Three-fourths of intracerebral infections after renal transplantation are caused by *Listeria*. The causative organisms are *L. monocytogenes*, *Cryptococcus*, and *Toxoplasma gondii*. Aspergillosis is a more common cause of brain abscess. Infections with CMV and EBV rarely produce encephalitis.

CNS post-transplantation lymphoproliferative disorder is rare but its incidence is increasing. It often occurs late and is associated with Epstein-Barr virus infection (Rego Silva et al., 2018). It can manifest with focal neurological abnormalities, seizures, or increased intracranial pressure. Neurotoxicity secondary to the use of immunosuppressive agents, such as cyclosporine, tacrolimus, and long-term corticosteroids, is frequent. Clinical features include seizures, hypertensive encephalopathy, myalgia, tremor, and fatigue.

Qvist and colleagues (2002) studied neurodevelopmental outcomes in 33 school-aged children who underwent transplantation before the age of 5 years; their mean IQ was 87. Neuropsychiatric testing was impaired in 6%–24%. The children with learning problems had a greater number of hypertensive crises and seizures and a higher incidence of prematurity. Six of seven children attending a special school had evidence of brain infarcts on MRI. No significant difference existed in mean serum aluminum levels between these patients and the children who had received transplants and demonstrated normal school performance. Earlier age of dialysis onset and a longer time on dialysis (>9 months) were associated with lower IQ scores (Molnar-Varga et al., 2016).

*The complete reference list is available online at https://expertconsult.inkling.com/.* 

60

# Basic Neuroscience of Neurotrauma

W. Dalton Dietrich, Helen M. Bramlett

OUTLINE



Traumatic brain injury (TBI) is a leading cause of death and disability among children and young adults. In addition, head injury in older adults, as a result of falls, is a growing clinical concern. To investigate the pathophysiology of brain injury and develop novel therapeutic strategies to treat this condition, experimental models of TBI have been established. Although no experimental model completely mimics the human condition, individual models produce many features of human brain injury (Ma et al., 2019). Based on these models, therapeutic strategies directed at specific pathomechanisms have been initiated. This chapter reviews the basic science of neurotrauma and summarizes the various experimental strategies used to investigate and treat TBI.

## EXPERIMENTAL MODELS OF TRAUMATIC BRAIN INJURY

Severe closed-head injury produces a range of cerebral lesions, which may be divided into four general categories: (1) diffuse axonal injury, (2) vascular lesions including subdural hematoma, (3) contusion, and (4) neuronal degeneration in selectively vulnerable regions. In a recent review of animal models of head injury, Estrada-Rojo et al. (2018) provide an in-depth discussion of the utility of each model as well as the limitations. Fluid percussion (FP) and controlled cortical impact models are both brain deformation injury models, whereas weight-drop models are considered unconstrained in head movement and may more closely mimic human TBI. Other models have specifically targeted brain trauma that occurs in combat situations, including high-velocity penetrating and blast injuries. An emphasis has recently been placed on developing these types of TBI in large-animal models, which may closely mimic the human condition (Dai et al., 2018). In an attempt to investigate the effects of mechanical deformation on specific cell types, in vitro models of stretch-induced injury have also been developed.

### Percussion Concussion

The FP injury model produces a brief 22-ms deformation of the exposed cortex. A craniotomy is performed, and a plastic modified Luer-Lok injury tube is attached to the exposed dura and sealed. A Plexiglas cylinder filled with sterile saline is attached to the injury tube via a metal fitting. A pendulum is released on the other end and at impact produces a pressure wave that results in a bolus injection of saline onto the exposed dura. By varying the distance of the pendulum swing, several degrees of injury severity—mild (1.1–1.5 atm), moderate (2.0–2.3 atm), and severe (2.4–2.6 atm)—can be studied in a reproducible fashion. This is an important model characteristic because of the heterogeneous nature of human TBI and the possibility that treatment strategies may vary with injury severity. The central, lateral, and parasagittal FP models are characterized by brief behavioral responsiveness (e.g., coma), metabolic alterations, changes in local cerebral blood flow (LCBF), blood–brain barrier (BBB) permeability, and behavioral deficits. The central FP model tends to involve variable and small contusions in the vicinity of the fluid pulse as well as scattered axonal damage mostly limited to the brainstem. In contrast, lateral and parasagittal FP is characterized by a lateral cortical contusion that is remote from the impact site. Evidence of axonal damage is seen throughout the white matter tracts in the ipsilateral cerebral hemisphere, and tissue tears are seen at gray matter/white matter interfaces. Hippocampal damage is pronounced in the lateral and parasagittal FP injury models, with little brainstem damage. The FP injury model thus produces a range of disorders including contusion, widespread axonal injury, and selective neuronal necrosis.

Another commonly used rodent TBI model is controlled cortical impact injury. In this model, a bone flap is removed and the impact device is vertically driven into the cerebral cortex to produce tissue displacement. This model produces a well-demarcated cortical contusion with variable degrees of hippocampal involvement depending on velocity and deformation depth. An advantage of the controlled cortical impact model is that it can be used in mice and allows the testing of genetically altered mice to help determine the cause-and-effect relationships between gene expression and cell injury.

### Acceleration Concussion

Inertial acceleration models can produce pure acute subdural hematomas and diffuse axonal injury. These models accelerate the head of the animal in one plane followed by a rapid deceleration, resulting in movement of the brain within the cranial cavity. The inertial acceleration models are designed to mimic motor vehicle accidents. Tissue-tear hemorrhages occur in the central white matter, and gliding contusions occur in the parasagittal gray matter/white matter junctions. These models are characterized by a variable period of coma and axonal damage in the upper brainstem and cerebellum. For the impact acceleration model, the animal is placed on a foam bed with a metal disk attached to the exposed skull. A weight is then dropped from a specified height to produce brain injury. This model also produces prolonged coma and widespread axonal damage. However, these models are characterized by variable and somewhat uncontrolled skull fractures.

Human head injury is never as pure as an experimental model, and the total human injury condition may not be addressed adequately with a single animal model. Therefore the use of complicated models in assessing pathomechanisms after TBI can provide valuable data. Many of these studies have added secondary insults such as hypotension (shock), hypoxia, or hyperthermia after the primary injury to more adequately mimic human head trauma. However, this added component to the model can result in complex data interpretation. Thus, once a particular feature of human brain injury has been produced in an experimental model, the pathogenesis of the injury can be critically investigated.

### Military Models

The incidence of brain injury is currently estimated to be as high as 40%–70% of combat casualties. Advancements in protective body armor have limited the number of high-velocity impact injuries to the brain, but the use of improvised explosive devices has caused blast injury to become more prevalent. Military-relevant models have only recently been developed, and much work is needed to fully explore pathomechanisms induced by these models (Kovacs et al., 2014; Bolouri and Zetterberg, 2015). Two models of significance are the penetrating ballistic brain injury (PBBI) model and a blast injury model using a metal tube with a small amount of plastic explosive at one end. The PBBI model mimics a bullet wound by expanding and contracting a balloon that has been inserted into the brain. Injury severity and placement of the probe can be varied so that different types of bullet injuries can be studied. PBBI produces robust histopathological damage and increases in intracranial pressure (ICP) and hemorrhage. In addition, sensorimotor deficits are observed in this model, along with seizure activity. Blast injury models that can mimic whole-body blast or local blast injury have been developed (Hernandez et al., 2018). This type of trauma produces cognitive deficits as well as ultrastructural and oxidative damage to the hippocampus. Axonal damage is also present, as indicated by increases in phosphorylated neurofilament proteins. These military-relevant injury models have the potential to provide valuable information for managing and treating combat casualties.

### In Vitro Models

A shortcoming of animal models is that they preclude a critical assessment of individual cell responses to trauma. In animal experiments, for example, the cellular response to injury may be a consequence of both primary and secondary events initiated by a complex cascade of cellular interactions. To critically investigate the consequences of injury on a specific cell type in the absence of confounding cellular and systemic factors, several in vitro cell culture models have been developed. Models range from scratching the culture with a pipette tip to inducing cellular deformation by stretching cultured cells. Most recently, these models have incorporated multiple cell types including neurons, astrocytes/glia, and endothelial cells in order to study cellular interactions after injury (Kumaria, 2017).

Using these approaches, investigators have found that trauma induces a wide range of primary cellular alterations. Astrocytic responses include hyperplasia, hypertrophy, and increased glial fibrillary acidic protein content. Increases in intracellular calcium occur, which are blocked by specific receptor antagonists. Traumatized astrocytes also produce interleukins (ILs) and neurotrophic factors. Neonatal cortical neurons that are stretched undergo delayed depolarization that depends on the activation of specific receptor populations. Combined mechanical trauma and metabolic impairment in vivo also induces *N*-methyl-D-aspartate (NMDA) receptor–dependent neuronal cell death and caspase-3–dependent apoptosis. In vitro experimental approaches provide novel data concerning intracellular signaling cascades, mechanisms underlying cellular responses to trauma, and the role of specific cell types in the pathophysiology of brain trauma (Campos-Pires et al., 2018, Morrison et al., 2011).

## NEURONAL DAMAGE AFTER TRAUMATIC BRAIN INJURY

### Temporal Patterns of Neuronal Death

The neuropathological sequelae of experimental and human TBI have been well described (Blennow et al., 2012). In experimental TBI, temporal patterns of neuronal damage have also been characterized. As early as 6 hours after cortical contusion injury, the contused tissue appears edematous and pyknotic neurons are apparent at the injury site. By 8 days, a cortical cavity surrounded by a border containing necrotic tissue, a glial scar, or both has developed. The temporal profile of neuronal damage after parasagittal FP brain injury has also been assessed with light and electron microscopy. As early as 1 hour after impact, dark shrunken neurons indicative of irreversible damage are seen in cortical layers overlying the gliding contusion, which displays BBB breakdown to protein tracers. Ultrastructural studies demonstrate that early BBB dysfunction results from mechanical damage of small venules in vulnerable regions, including the external capsule. In some brain regions, focal sites of acute neuronal damage are associated with extravasated protein, whereas neuronal damage in other regions appears to occur without overt BBB breakdown. Astrocytic swelling is observed early after injury, with increased glial fibrillary acidic protein immunoreactivity apparent at later times in some areas, demonstrating histopathological damage (Fig. 60.1). In terms of neuroprotection, the acuteness of this damage limits the potential for therapeutic interventions directed against the early neuronal and glial response to TBI.

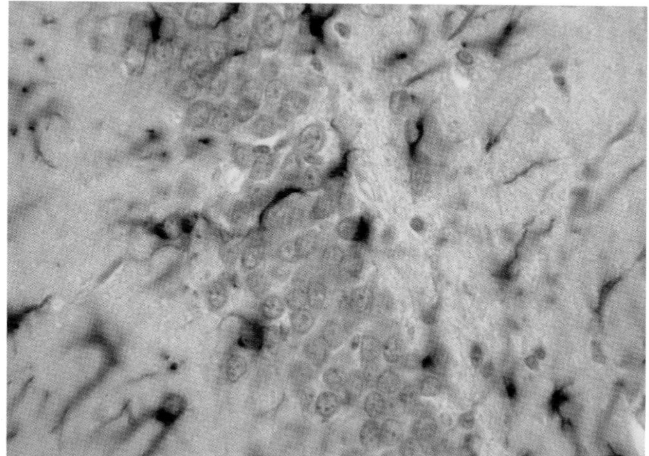

**Fig. 60.1** Three days after fluid percussion injury, glial fibrillary acidic protein-positive astrocytes and processes are prominent in the hippocampus (×1200).

More subacute patterns of neuronal injury have been documented in various TBI models. At 3 days after moderate parasagittal FP brain injury, scattered necrotic neurons are present throughout the frontoparietal cerebral cortex remote from the impact site (Fig. 60.2). In addition, selective neuronal damage is seen in the CA3 and CA4 hippocampal subsectors, the dentate hilus, and lateral thalamus ipsilateral to the trauma. These patterns of selective neuronal damage are associated with a well-demarcated contusion overlying the lateral external capsule. Ultrastructural changes consistent with apoptosis have been described after TBI; therefore delayed patterns of neuronal cell death may involve necrotic and programmed cell death processes. Additional nonapoptotic cell death mechanisms have also been identified, including necroptosis and pyroptosis, both being demonstrated in models of TBI. Some studies have shown that, should apoptosis fail to execute, these alternative nonapoptotic forms of cell death may be activated (Tait et al., 2014). In addition to these cell death mechanisms in some TBI studies, autophagy has been associated with various forms of cell death in other conditions (Zhang and Wang, 2018). Numerous interconnections between autophagy and the other cell death mechanisms have been described in models of TBI. Pyroptosis, a caspase 1–dependent form of cell death, is an inflammatory type of cell death associated with cell swelling and rapid membrane breakdown. In this cell death

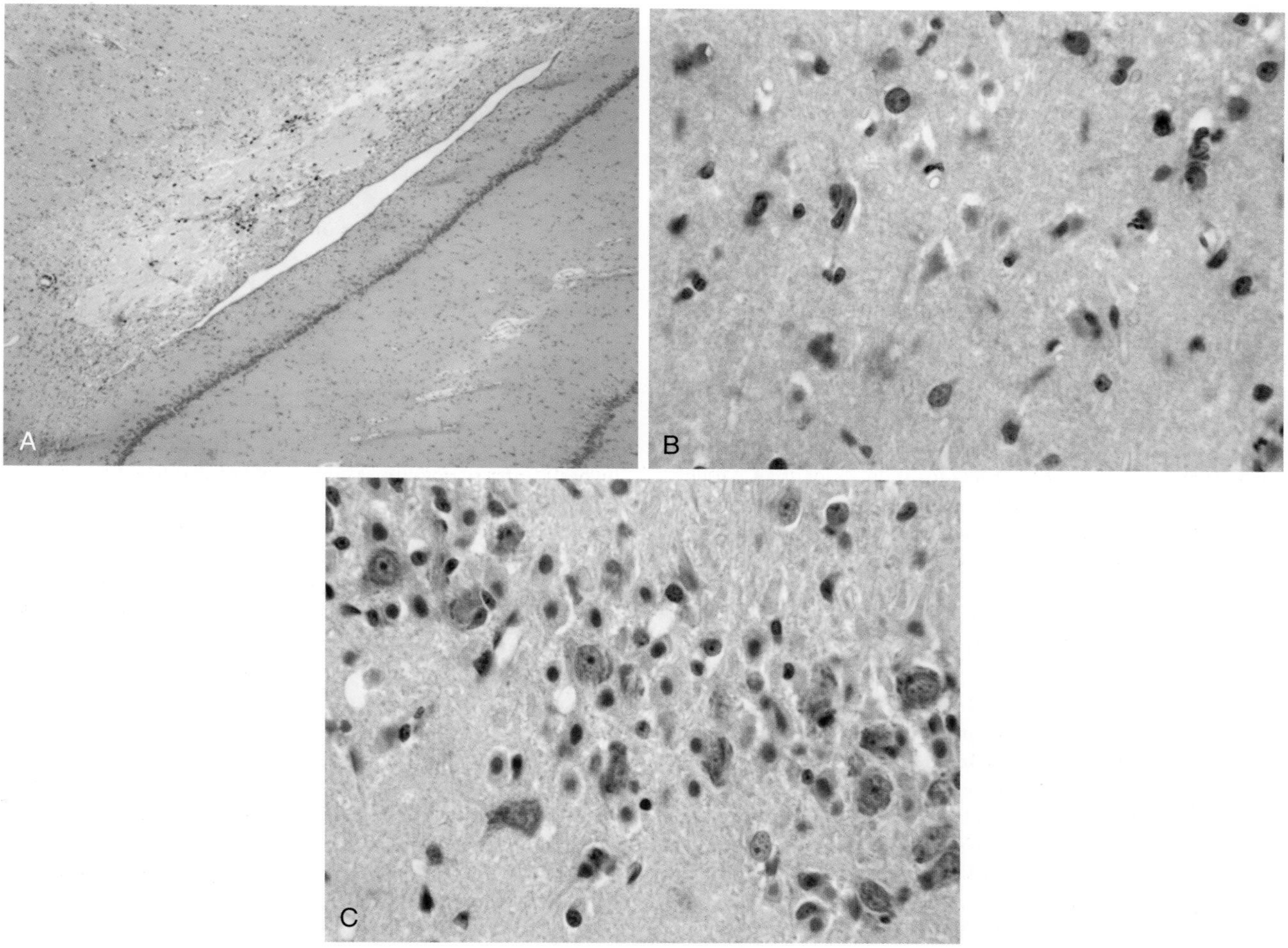

**Fig. 60.2 Photomicrographs of Rat Brain 3 Days After Fluid Percussion Injury. A,** Focal contusion at gray/white interface (×120). **B,** Damaged cortical neurons overlying the contusion (×1200). **C,** Damaged and eosinophilic neurons in CA3 hippocampus (×1200).

mechanism, caspase-1 is activated by a multiprotein complex termed the inflammasome that also responds to molecular and biochemical toxins and viral RNA. Recent evidence in models of TBI has shown that inflammasome-induced pyroptotic cell death occurs in models of TBI and can lead to neuronal inflammatory cell death (de Rivero Vaccari et al., 2018). Finally, all other cell death mechanisms—commonly termed *caspase-independent cell death* (Tait and Green, 2008), resulting from mitochondrial membrane permeabilization—have also been described in models of TBI and have additional distinct morphological and biochemical characteristics. It is important to understanding the underlying cellular molecular mechanisms of cell death after TBI because they present potentially new targets for therapeutic intervention that may reduce the degree of both cell death and axonal damage, thus improving functional outcomes. Continued investigations into underlying factors that lead to these distinct cell death mechanisms and new therapeutic interventions that target cell vulnerability in models of TBI could lead to new improvements and acute neuroprotection as well as reducing TBI-induced progressive neural degenerative disorders.

## Selective Neuronal Vulnerability

Damage to the hippocampus is commonly reported in autopsy studies of head-injured patients. Clinical and experimental studies describe cognitive abnormalities thought to be associated with hippocampal dysfunction. In an acceleration model of brain injury in nonhuman primates, CA1 hippocampal histopathological damage was reported in the majority of animals. CA1 damage was not produced by secondary global ischemia, elevated ICP, or seizure activity alone. In this regard, CA1 hippocampal damage is not routinely reported in other TBI models, including cortical contusion and moderate FP injury. However, midline FP injury followed by a delayed sublethal global ischemic insult leads to CA1 neuronal damage. The studies indicate the importance of injury severity on outcome and the vulnerability of the posttraumatic brain to secondary insults. Finally, the dentate gyrus, bilateral dentate hilus, and CA3 hippocampus have also been reported to be selectively damaged in FP models.

Thalamic damage after brain injury is described in clinical and experimental studies. In human brain injury, the loss of inhibitory thalamic reticular neurons is proposed to underlie some forms of attention deficits. In radiographic studies of patients with TBI using magnetic resonance imaging, relationships between injury severity, lesion volume, ventricle-to-brain ratio, and thalamic volume have been reported. Patients with moderate to severe injuries have smaller thalamic volumes and greater ventricle-to-brain ratios than patients with mild to moderate injuries. Decreased thalamic volumes suggest that subcortical brain structures may be susceptible to transneuronal degeneration after cortical damage. Focal damage to thalamic nuclei seen after long-term (Bramlett and Dietrich, 2015) FP injury may result from progressive circuit degeneration after axonal damage, neuronal cell death, or lack of neurotrophic delivery.

## Progressive Damage

Only recently has the progressive nature of the histopathological consequences of TBI been appreciated (Bramlett and Dietrich, 2015). At 2 months after moderate parasagittal FP injury, significant atrophy of the cerebral cortex, hippocampus, and thalamus is apparent in histological sections (Fig. 60.3, *A*). Progressive tissue loss in the cortex and hippocampus at various times up to 1 year after lateral FP injury has been reported. Similar findings have been found in a model of controlled cortical impact injury. At 3 weeks and 1 year after injury, analysis demonstrated a significant hemispheric volume loss and expansion of the ipsilateral lateral ventricle. Thus atrophy of gray matter structures is associated with significant enlargement of the lateral ventricle.

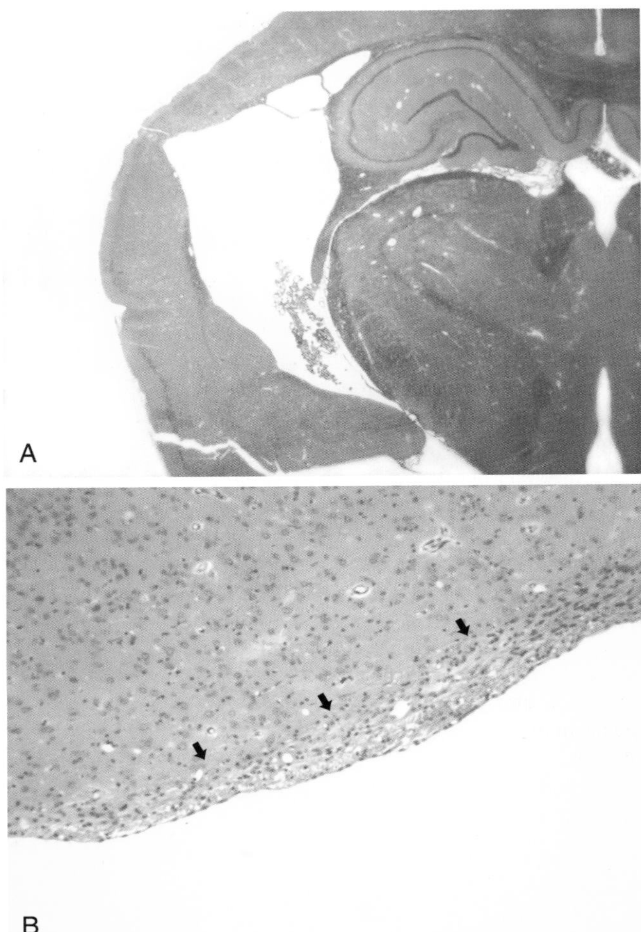


**Fig. 60.3 Photomicrographs of Rat Brain 1 Year After Fluid Percussion Injury (×30).** **A,** Brain shows gross atrophy with marked expansion of lateral cortex. **B,** Severe loss of white matter in external capsule *(arrows)* (×300).

Ventricular expansion not associated with hydrocephalus or increased ICP is felt to be a sensitive indicator of structural damage and an indirect measure of white matter atrophy. Indeed, ventricular size has been correlated with memory disturbances; patients with the highest ventricular volumes demonstrated significantly lower memory scores. Recent findings provide direct evidence of progressive white matter damage after FP brain injury (Bramlett and Dietrich, 2015). At 1 year after TBI, severe atrophy of specific tracts including the external capsule and cerebral peduncle was documented (see Fig. 60.3, *B*). This white matter vulnerability may result from direct trauma-induced axonal damage as well as recently described oligodendrocyte vulnerability after TBI. In experiments where long-term survival has been evaluated in both animal models and human tissue, patterns of chronic microglial activation have been identified; this underlines the progressive nature of the inflammatory response after TBI (Smith et al., 2013; Younger et al., 2019). The importance of a progressive injury cascade after TBI in terms of other neurological conditions merits consideration. For example, if mild head trauma leads to a progressive reduction in neuronal reserve, would the person who sustained such trauma be more susceptible than others to neurodegenerative processes associated with aging? Recent findings indicate that TBI may also be a risk factor for the development of age-associated neurodegenerative disorders including Alzheimer disease, Parkinson disease, amyotrophic lateral sclerosis, and multiple sclerosis (Wilson et al., 2017). The observation that pathological processes which potentially affect long-term outcome may be active days or even months after injury provides new targets to improve outcome after central nervous system (CNS) injury. This new way of assessing and treating acute injuries is also important as we think about how TBI may enhance the vulnerability of the aging brain and underlying mechanisms responsible for syndromes including chronic traumatic encephalopathy (CTE) (Esopenko and Levine, 2015). Transgenic models of neurodegenerative diseases are now being produced and investigated to clarify novel injury cascades that may underlie the increased vulnerability of the postinjured brain to patterns of progressive injury (Kokiko-Cochran et al., 2016).

## Secondary and Repetitive Damage

A challenging problem faced by medical personnel responsible for the health care of amateur and professional athletes and the military is recognizing and managing mild head injury. Returning an injured athlete to competition when the brain needs time to recover is an obvious concern. Also, a basic understanding of posttraumatic consequences that affect the vulnerability of the brain to secondary or repeated head injury remains unknown. This is a clinically important issue because TBI is often associated with respiratory suppression, resulting in secondary hypoxic insults. Experimental studies have documented the detrimental consequences of secondary insults after mild to moderate TBI (Simon et al., 2016). The effects of secondary hypoxia on histopathological and behavioral outcome were investigated. Secondary hypoxia induced immediately after moderate FP injury resulted in significantly greater cortical and hippocampal CA1 damage and sensorimotor and cognitive deficits than were found in normoxic animals. Mild hypotension (shock) after TBI was reported also to worsen traumatic outcome. Taken together, these findings point to the enhanced vulnerability of the posttraumatic brain to mild secondary insults.

Clinical studies indicate that patients with mild head injury may be at risk if they have a subsequent head injury (secondary impact syndrome). Animal models have been developed to investigate the behavioral and pathological changes associated with repetitive head injury. The consequences of single and repetitive injuries induced 24 hours apart were assessed. Repetitive head injury led to greater functional impairment and structural damage than was found in the single-injury group. At the cellular level, repeated mild injury in an in vitro hippocampal cell culture model has shown elevations of neuron-specific enolase and S-100β compared with a single insult. Repetitive injury in transgenic mice that expressed mutant human Aβ precursor protein produced elevated Aβ levels and increased Aβ deposition, thus linking TBI to the mechanisms of Alzheimer disease. Besides an increase in Aβ levels, TBI leads to the accumulation of key proteins that are known to form pathological aggregates in neurodegenerative diseases including CTE. The development of tauopathies following TBI as seen in postmortem tissue provide evidence for this disease (Goldstein et al., 2012; Fig. 60.4). The known risk of developing neurodegenerative disease later in life is greater after repetitive brain trauma and makes this type of investigation extremely important (Smith et al., 2013).

## Axonal and Dendritic Injury

Traumatic axonal injury exists as a spectrum involving widespread areas of the brain in experimental models of TBI (Johnson et al., 2013). This pattern of white matter pathology can evolve from focal axonal alterations to complete transection of the axon. Reactive axonal changes using monoclonal antibodies targeted at neurofilament subunits or β-amyloid precursor protein have been characterized after FP brain injury and controlled cortical impact injury (Fig. 60.5). Within 1–2 hours of injury, reactive axonal change is most conspicuous in brainstem regions, including the pontomedullary junction. This

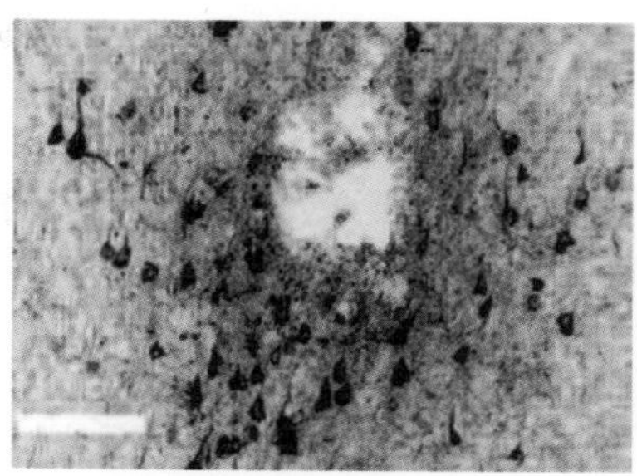

**Fig. 60.4** Phosphorylated tau neuropathology with perivascular neurofibrillary degeneration in the frontal cortex of a 21-year-old male amateur football player with a history of repetitive subconcussive injury. Scale bar, 100 μm. *(Adapted from Goldstein, L.E., Fisher, A.M., Tagge, C.A., Zhang, X.L., et al., 2012. Chronic traumatic encephalopathy in blast-exposed military veterans and a blast neurotrauma mouse model. Sci Transl Med 4, 134ra60.)*

pattern of axonal damage seen in experimental models is in contrast to the human condition, in which callosal and subcortical white matter axonal damage predominates. In contrast, moderate parasagittal brain injury leads to widespread axonal damage in forebrain regions that represent reversible, irreversible, and delayed axonal perturbations. In more recent studies, evidence for circuit dysfunction in gray matter structures such as the cerebral cortex has also been emphasized (McGinn and Povlishock, 2015). These findings may explain some of the transient and delayed functional consequences of TBI.

In addition to axonal damage, studies indicate that TBI also leads to significant changes in neuronal dendrites. A common feature of damage of injured neurons is loss of microtubule-associated protein 2 (MAP2) antigenicity. MAP2 is an important microtubule cross-linking protein that is found predominantly in somatodendritic environments, so changes in MAP2 may reflect damage to dendrites. Using this strategy, evidence of dendritic damage not necessarily associated with neuronal death has been obtained that may participate in some of the functional consequences of TBI.

Evidence for neurodegeneration following severe controlled cortical impact injury in the mouse has been shown using silver staining. This marker identifies degenerating neurons and processes. Both hippocampal and cortical neurodegeneration is observed as late as 72 hours and continues to 7 days in select brain regions. This degeneration is associated with calpain-mediated proteolysis of cytoskeletal proteins and decreases in growth-associated protein 43 (GAP-43) expression, which may inhibit the brain's response to elicit an attempt at plasticity to restore function.

## Importance of Gender

Recent clinical and experimental data have emphasized the importance of gender in the consequences of TBI and the contributions of sex hormones, including progesterone and estrogen (Brotfain et al., 2016; Spani et al., 2018). In a study of 334 patients with TBI, female patients had a better predicted outcome at the time of discharge from an inpatient rehabilitation program. However, a meta-analysis of eight previous studies in which outcome was reported separately for men and women reported a worse outcome in women than in men. The impact of gender on TBI is an understudied area of clinical neurotrauma and should be emphasized in future trials.

In experimental models of TBI, gender also appears to influence traumatic outcome. The hemodynamic consequences of brain injury and contusion volume were significantly less in female than in male rats. In this study, ovariectomy 10 days before TBI removed the volume differences between male and female rats. Thus, intact females appear

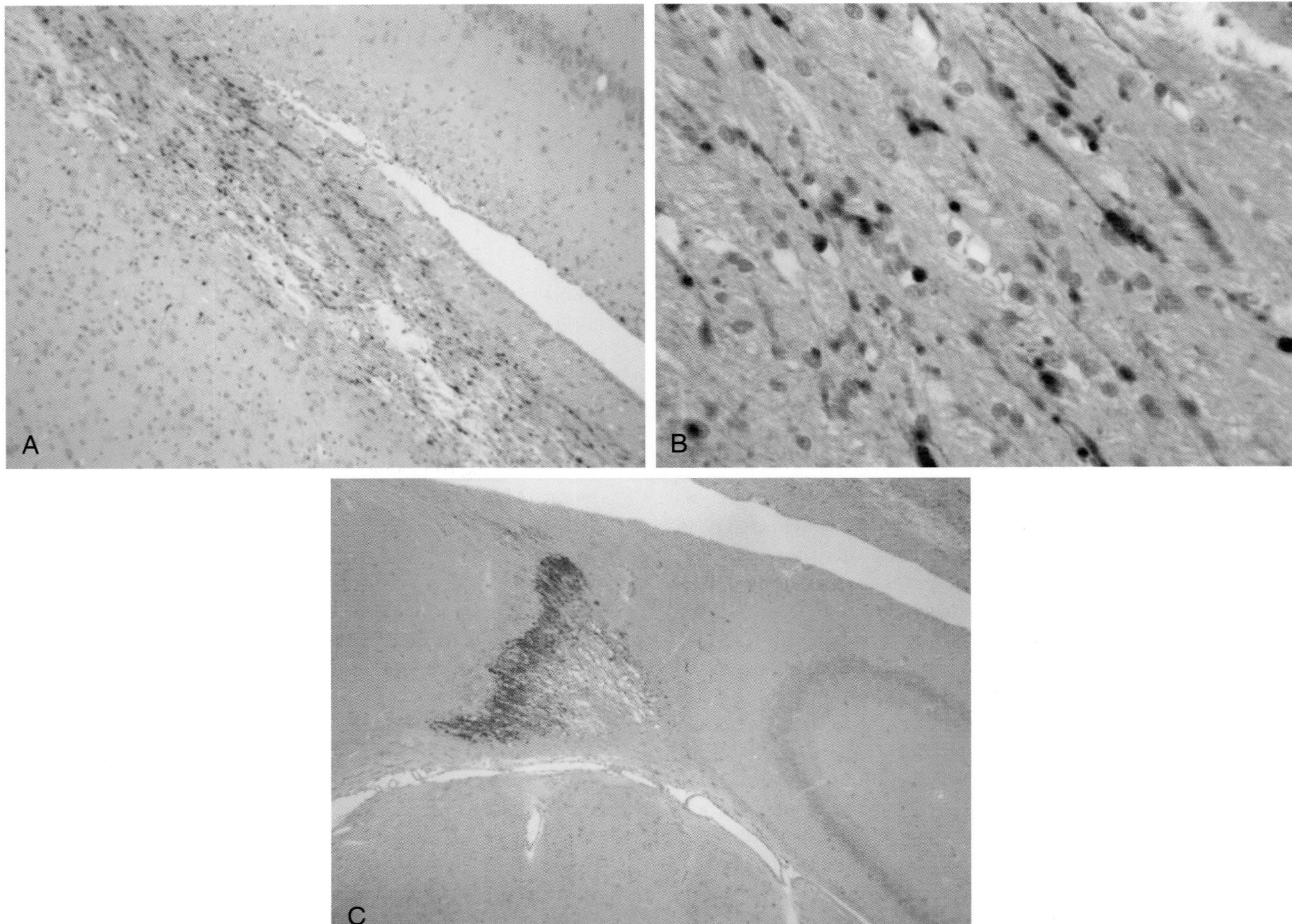


**Fig. 60.5** β-Amyloid Precursor Protein Immunoreactivity After Traumatic Brain Injury. **A,** Large numbers of immunoreactive profiles in external capsule (×120). **B,** High magnification of axonal swellings (×1200). **C,** Dense reactive profiles within the fimbriae of hippocampus, consistent with primary axotomy (axonal shearing) (×120).

to have an endogenous neuroprotective mechanism that reduces the detrimental consequences of TBI. In terms of testing neuroprotective strategies in models of TBI, gender differences must be assessed.

In this regard, two randomized double-blind placebo-controlled phase III clinical trials—Progesterone for the Treatment of Traumatic Brain Injury (ProTECT) and the Study of the Neuroprotective Activity of Progesterone in Severe Traumatic Brain Injuries (SyNAPSe)—were conducted. However, both trials were negative, possibly due to three critical trial design factors. Because of the overwhelming preclinical data on the neuroprotective effects of hormones (Howard et al., 2017), further clinical studies are needed.

## BASIC MECHANISMS OF INJURY

### Primary Injury Mechanisms

Two major types of forces are responsible for brain injury: one localized at the impact site and a second characterized by rotational forces. Depending on the force and location of the primary impact, head trauma can produce acute damage to blood vessels and axonal projections. Contact phenomena generate superficial or contusional hemorrhages through coup and countercoup mechanisms. Direct injury is commonly superficial, and the coup–countercoup hemorrhages may be adjacent or central.

Axonal shearing is a common lesion of the cerebral white matter that occurs particularly in acceleration-deceleration injury. Only recently has morphological evidence of axonal shearing (primary axotomy) become available in FP models. Ultrastructural evidence demonstrates the tearing or shearing of axons in nonhuman primates exposed to lateral acceleration. Perturbations of the axolemma leading to the accumulation of cytoskeletal components and organelles or activation of intracellular mediators of injury, such as calpain activation, may represent secondary injury processes that can be treated.

Shearing strains may also damage blood vessels and cause petechial hemorrhages, deep intracerebral hematomas, and brain swelling. Mechanical damage to small venules, resulting in focal BBB breakdown and platelet accumulation, is reported immediately after FP injury. Vascular damage leads to the formation of hemorrhagic contusions. Early vascular damage may increase neuronal vulnerability by causing posttraumatic perfusion deficits and extravasation of potentially neurotoxic blood-borne substances.

### Secondary Injury Mechanisms

In head-injured patients, the extent of neurological recovery depends on the contribution of posttraumatic secondary insults. In the clinical setting, secondary insults include hypotension, hypoxia, hyperglycemia, anemia, sepsis, and hyperthermia. Experimental evidence indicates increased susceptibility of the posttraumatic brain to secondary insults. For example, after midline FP brain injury, CA1 hippocampal vulnerability is enhanced with superimposed secondary ischemia. An important area of research regarding the treatment of brain injury involves the characterization of secondary injury processes, which may be targeted for intensive care management or pharmacotherapy.

A high frequency of hypoxic or ischemic brain damage occurs in patients who die as a result of nonmissile head injury. Hypoxic damage in the form of hemorrhagic infarction and diffuse neuronal necrosis is most common in arterial boundary zones between the major cerebral arteries. Hypoxic damage is also common in patients who have experienced an episode of intracranial hypertension. A significant correlation between hypoxic brain damage and arterial spasm in patients with nonmissile TBI has been reported. Posttraumatic hypoxia aggravates the consequences for the BBB of FP brain injury.

Posttraumatic hemodynamic impairments represent another injury mechanism. Clinical and experimental investigations report moderate reductions in LCBF after TBI. After moderate parasagittal FP brain injury, widespread reductions in LCBF range from 40% to 80% of control. In contrast, severe FP injury leads to LCBF reductions that reach ischemic levels. Focal reductions in LCBF are associated with subarachnoid and intracerebral hemorrhage and local platelet accumulation. Reductions in LCBF result from the mechanical occlusion of cerebral vessels, the release of vasoactive substances, or possibly as a secondary consequence of reductions in neuronal activity or metabolism. Injury severity is therefore a critical factor in determining the hemodynamic and histopathological consequences of experimental TBI.

Cortical spreading depolarization (CSD) is caused by ionic changes within tissue resulting in waves of depressed electrical activity. CSDs are not necessarily harmful to tissue unless there is damage present. It was previously thought that CSDs could only be induced experimentally; however, spontaneous self-propagating waves within damaged tissue, known as *peri-infarct depolarizations* and similar to CSDs, have been reported (Lauritzen and Strong, 2017). The incidence of CSD has been well described in the literature on experimental focal ischemia, and CSD is associated with increasing amounts of neuronal damage within the cerebral cortex. However, the presence of CSDs in the human brain-injured population had remained controversial until recently because of the inability to measure the phenomenon adequately. Although it does not occur in all acutely injured individuals, the incidence is higher in younger patients. Such findings have resulted in a new initiative to document the occurrence of CSDs after TBI and study their relationship to outcome.

Hypotension and shock are present in a significant number of patients with TBI. In severely injured patients, outcome is correlated with reduced mean arterial blood pressure. Hemorrhagic hypotension after FP injury results in a more severe histopathological outcome than that due to TBI alone. The increased sensitivity of the posttraumatic brain to moderate levels of hypotension may result from deficits in autoregulation, which have been reported in patient and experimental studies. Hypotensive periods that may occur during surgical procedures and anesthesia may produce secondary insults and be hazardous to the head-injured patient.

Many patients experience fever after head injury, and clinical data indicate that brain temperature may be higher than core or bladder temperature (Bao et al., 2014). Experimentally, posttraumatic brain hyperthermia induced artificially 24 hours after trauma increases mortality rate and aggravates histopathological outcome, including contusion size and axonal pathology. Recent data have shown that hyperthermia after mild TBI can augment inflammatory events as well as cerebral vascular perturbations (Truettner et al., 2018). In the clinical setting, posttraumatic hyperthermia may represent a secondary injury mechanism that might negate the beneficial effects of a therapeutic agent.

A significant debilitating consequence of TBI is the development of seizures (Zimmerman et al., 2016). Some 40%–50% of patients with moderate to severe TBI develop epilepsy, and brain injuries account for 20% of symptomatic epilepsy cases. Trauma-induced mechanisms of reduced seizure threshold include damage to specific neuronal populations and circuits, increased BBB damage, and aberrant mossy-fiber sprouting of dentate granule cells. Importantly, posttraumatic epilepsy has been shown to worsen outcome and aggravate cognitive problems in some clinical studies. Unfortunately, chronic seizures after brain injury are poorly controlled by available antiepileptic drugs (Szaflarski et al., 2014).

Significant advances are also being made in the identification and testing of biomarkers that can potentially help clarify the pathogenesis of TBI. Strategies such as serum blood biomarkers as well as neuroimaging are helping to bridge the gap between experimental studies and the clinic (Manivannan et al., 2018).

## THERAPEUTIC INTERVENTIONS DIRECTED AGAINST PATHOPHYSIOLOGICAL PROCESSES

The treatment of TBI has been investigated using a variety of animal models; new therapies have been initiated, some of which have been tested in patients. Several reviews summarize the agents that have been investigated in TBI (Hawryluk and Bullock, 2016). The problem of TBI involves injury pathways that are common to other brain injuries, including cerebral ischemia. However, the pathogenesis of TBI is unique in other ways and necessitates therapeutic approaches specifically targeted at brain trauma (Fig. 60.6). The present discussion is limited to several of the major therapeutic strategies currently being assessed experimentally and clinically (Stein et al., 2015).

### Glutamate Antagonists

Excitatory amino acid neurotransmitters have been implicated in the pathophysiology of TBI. Microdialysis techniques have documented elevated levels of extracellular excitatory amino acids, whereas *N*-methyl-D-aspartic acid (NMDA) receptor antagonists, including

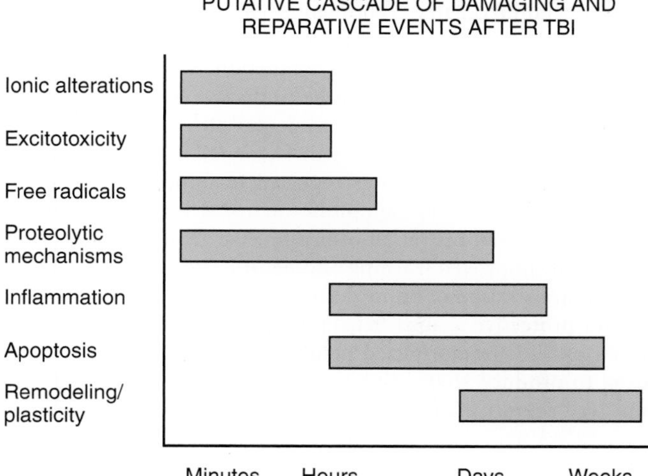


**Fig. 60.6** Paradigm for several time-dependent pathomechanisms and reparative events that may be targeted for therapeutic interventions. *TBI*, Traumatic brain injury. *(Adapted from Dirnagl, U., Iadecola, C., Moskowitz, M.A., 1999. Pathobiology of ischemic stroke: an integrated review. Trends Neurosci 22, 391–397.)*

MK-801 (dizocilpine), provide behavioral and histopathological protection against brain trauma. The role of glutamate antagonists in treating CNS system injury has been reviewed, and clinical stroke trials have been held. However, trials of the competitive NMDA antagonist MK-80I were withdrawn because of harmful side effects. Nevertheless, topiramate, an inhibitor of glutamate release, is being evaluated for its effects in reducing seizures.

### Free-Radical Scavengers

The genesis of oxygen free radicals has also been implicated in the pathophysiology of TBI. Experimental FP injury increases the production of these radicals, and inhibitors of free-radical scavengers have been reported to be protective in brain injury models. Sensitive indicators of hydroxy radical production and microdialysis have detected elevations in extracellular hydroxy radical production after FP injury. The free-radical scavenger superoxide dismutase (SOD) reduces BBB opening and the genesis of brain edema after TBI. Transgenic mice that overexpress human copper-zinc SOD1 are protected against brain trauma. Clinical trials using polyethylene glycol SOD and free-radical scavengers have been initiated in brain trauma, but with little success.

The reason for these negative results is not known, although questions regarding brain penetration and a limited therapeutic window have been discussed. In one experimental study, treatment with a potent inhibitor of lipid peroxidation and an antioxidant provided significant neuroprotection in an FP model when treatment was delayed 30 minutes but not 3 hours after TBI. Based on neurochemical and treatment studies, the therapeutic window for treatments that target free-radical reactions and lipid peroxidation after moderate TBI seems to be limited. Whether these treatments may protect against secondary insults remains to be investigated.

### Neurotrophic Factors

A unique problem of brain trauma is diffuse axonal injury. Axonal injury leading to circuit disruption may not only produce immediate functional consequences but also affect trophic signaling between neuronal populations. Addition of trophic factors after TBI may help maintain neuronal survival and promote both circuit reorganization and functional recovery. Neurotrophins have been shown to be neuroprotective by in vitro and in vivo models of neuronal injury. After experimental TBI, delayed treatment with basic fibroblast growth factor significantly reduced histopathological damage and improved cognitive function. Several neurotrophic factors have also been shown to be protective when administered exogenously to animals after experimental TBI. For example, posttraumatic infusion of nerve growth factor (NGF) into the injured cortex or lateral ventricle was reported to improve learning and memory and to decrease apoptotic neuronal loss in the septa of rats. Systemic administration of insulin-like growth factor 1 (IGF-1) after TBI improved learning and neuromotor function. In contrast, administration of brain-derived neurotrophic factor (BDNF) was not protective against behavioral or histopathological defects caused by TBI. Immortalized neural stem cells retrovirally transduced to produce NGF when transplanted into the injured brain improved cognitive and neuromotor function and rescued hippocampal CA3 neurons. Therefore an important direction of future research will be to use engineered cell lines to produce neurotrophins that could synthesize and locally release factors that enhance plasticity and circuit reorganization. If experimental studies continue to show a benefit of neuroprotection on neuronal injury and behavioral outcome in TBI models, this may be an important direction for future clinical trials in brain trauma.

### Protection by Nitric Oxide–Related Species

In the nervous system, nitric oxide (NO) may serve as a neurotransmitter, a signal between cells, and an autocrine signal within a given cell. After brain injury, an increase of neuronal calcium triggers constitutive NO synthase (cNOS) activity, leading to release of NO that may enhance excitotoxicity. Studies of mutant mice deficient in neuronal (nNOS) or endothelial NOS (eNOS) activity have demonstrated that whereas nNOS exacerbates ischemic injury, eNOS protects against it.

Therapeutic strategies directed at the NO pathway have been reported in models of brain injury. Data indicate that FP injury leads to the acute activation of cNOS, and that the selective inhibition of nNOS by 3-bromo-nitroindazole protects histopathologically and behaviorally. In addition, inhibition of inducible NOS (iNOS) with aminoguanidine (a selective iNOS inhibitor) also improved histopathological outcome. However, work using iNOS knockout mice has shown a beneficial effect of iNOS in brain injury. Thus, whereas early iNOS activity after brain trauma may contribute to secondary injury mechanisms, later or chronic activation may participate in reparative processes. As novel strategies are developed to target NO-mediated cell injury, these points regarding what processes should be targeted and when they should be inhibited are critical. Additional studies using mutant mice deficient in nNOS, eNOS, or iNOS activity will be important to advance this area of investigation.

## INFLAMMATION

Inflammation is a host defense mechanism initiated by injury or infection through which blood-derived leukocytes (neutrophils, monocytes and macrophages, T cells) and soluble factors (cytokines, chemokines, complement) try to restore tissue homeostasis (Thelin et al., 2017). Although evidence supports the beneficial role of inflammatory processes in acute injury, including the production of neurotrophic factors, inflammation is also thought to contribute to the resulting neuropathology and secondary necrosis that occur after trauma. Brain trauma is associated with the production and release of proinflammatory cytokines, including tumor necrosis factor (TNF)-α, interleukin (IL)-1β, and IL-6. The inhibition of cytokines such as IL-1β and TNF-α has been reported to decrease lesion size and improve behavioral outcome after TBI. Cytokine receptor antagonist (ra) drugs may also show promise in treating TBI. A report on mice treated with an IL-1ra showed a decrease in histopathological damage and lesion volume, with an improvement in behavioral recovery. Treatment with the potent anti-inflammatory cytokine IL-10 was reported to improve outcome as well. However, absolute TNF-α inhibition in the form of knockout mice has yielded conflicting results regarding pathological and neurological outcomes. Again, these studies emphasize the diverse actions of cytokines and both the good and bad consequences of overexpression and inhibition. More recent studies have identified a novel upstream regulator of cytokine activity that is active after CNS injury. This molecular complex, known as the inflammasome, is upregulated after TBI, SCI, and stroke (de Rivero Vaccari et al., 2016). Current research has demonstrated that by blocking the inflammasome after injury, improvement in behavior as well as reductions in histopathological damage are observed. This novel therapeutic approach of targeting the innate immune response after injury may prove beneficial in the clinical setting.

### Antiapoptotic Agents

Apoptosis is a mode of cell death in both physiological and pathological processes. Evidence of apoptotic cell death has also been observed after TBI. After FP injury, apoptotic cells have been identified in the ipsilateral cortex, hippocampus, and thalamus as soon as 4 hours after injury, and immunocytochemical markers for caspase-3, -8, and -9 activation have been reported (Fig. 60.7). The effects of FP injury on the expression of the bcl-2 protein, which regulates developmental programmed cell death, have also been investigated. Evidence of apoptosis of oligodendroglia in long tracts undergoing wallerian degeneration has been reported after spinal cord injury. Therefore demyelination of tracts after brain or spinal cord trauma may result from apoptotic death of oligodendrocytes. Importantly, indicators of apoptotic cell death have also been observed in human tissues.

Although the molecular events leading to apoptosis are not fully understood, the family of cysteine proteases (caspases) plays an active role in its pathogenesis. In reference to neuroprotection, in vitro studies have demonstrated that protease inhibitors specific to caspase-3 inhibit apoptosis. Whereas some experimental data indicate that inhibition of caspase-3 improves outcome after TBI, other studies suggest that this approach has limitations. Current emphasis is on more upstream apoptotic processes, in contrast to targeting caspase activation to attenuate damage. Calpain inhibition may target not only apoptotic cell death by regulating caspase activation but also cytoskeletal protein degradation (Wang et al., 2018). More research is needed to clarify the various pathways involved in apoptotic cell death and determine which pathways may be most sensitive to therapeutic interventions. Using agents specific to apoptosis, other recently defined cell death mechanisms, or in combination with agents that target necrosis is a potential research direction.

## Therapeutic Hypothermia

Numerous studies have demonstrated that although mild to moderate hypothermia is neuroprotective in models of TBI, mild hyperthermia worsens outcome (Dietrich and Bramlett, 2016). After brain trauma, hypothermia has been shown to improve histopathological and behavioral outcomes and to influence a wide range of injury processes. Microdialysis studies report that posttraumatic hypothermia reduces the acute surge in levels of extracellular glutamate and hydroxy free radicals after injury. Posttraumatic hypothermia protects against BBB dysfunction. Hypothermia attenuates progressive cortical atrophy and subsequent ventricular enlargement. The ability of any therapeutic intervention to provide long-term protection is an important requirement for the advancement of any therapeutic strategy to the clinical setting.

As previously discussed, a significant number of patients with TBI sustain a secondary insult that may include hypotension, hypoxia, or hyperthermia. This fact has led to the use of complicated models to test novel neuroprotective agents before clinical trials. This point is important because experimental therapeutic strategies are commonly tested in simple models of brain injury as

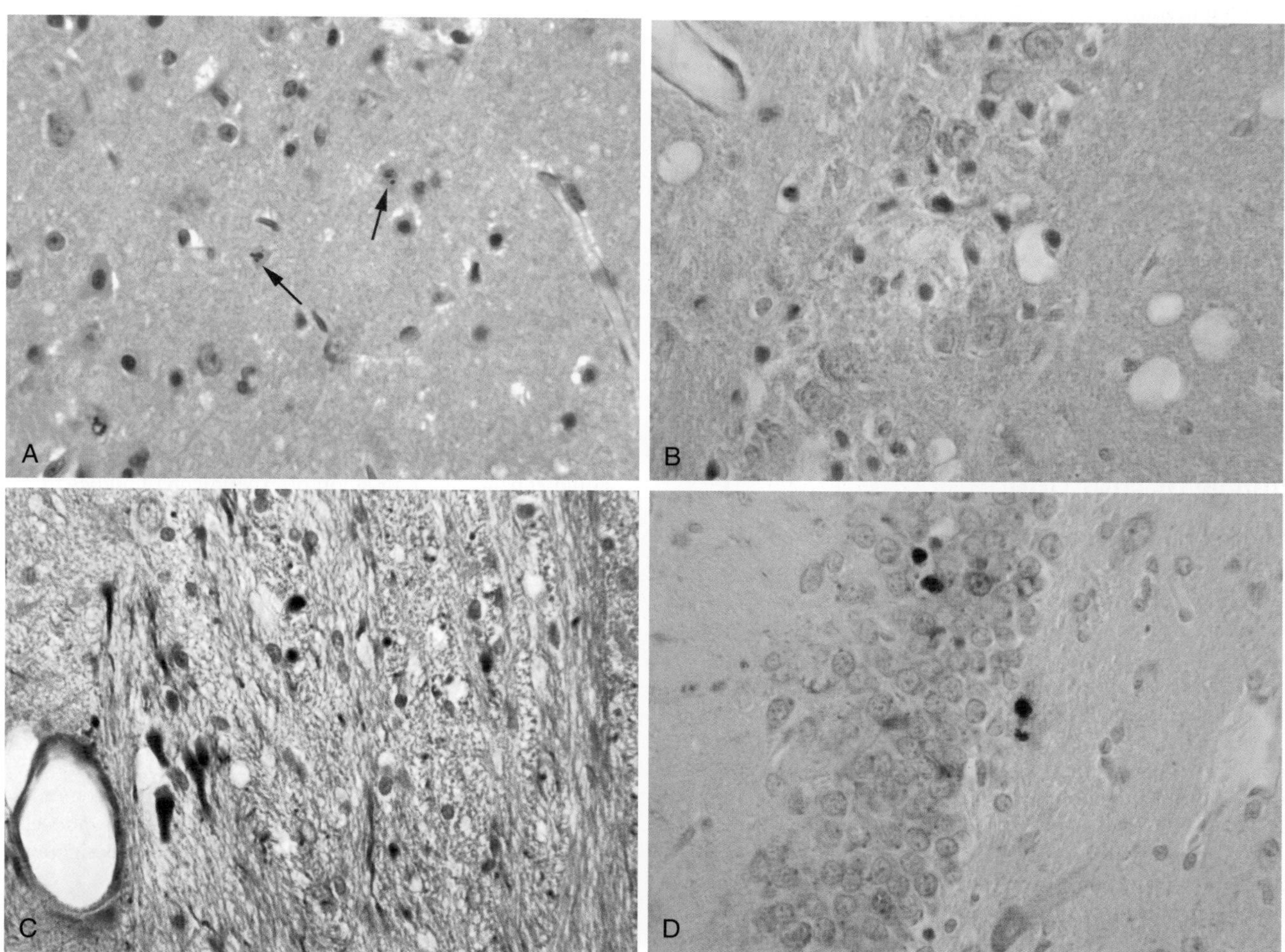


**Fig. 60.7** Histopathological and immunohistochemical evidence of apoptotic cell change 1 day after traumatic brain injury. **A,** Hematoxylin and eosin–stained section showing apoptotic bodies (×1200). **B,** Caspase-8 immunoreactivity (×1200). **C,** Caspase-9 immunoreactivity in the thalamus (×1200). (arrows) **D,** Immunohistochemistry of active caspase-3 in dentate gyrus (×1200).

proof of concept (Simon et al., 2016). In this regard, posttraumatic hypothermia followed by a controlled rewarming period has been evaluated in TBI models complicated by secondary hypoxia. Taken together, these studies showed that hypothermia was protective in complicated models, but the degree of protection depended on injury severity, duration of hypothermic period, and the rewarming procedure.

The use of moderate levels of hypothermia (>32°C) also improves outcome in patient studies. Systemic hypothermia (32°C–33°C) begun within 6 hours of injury (Glasgow Coma Scale score 4–7) resulted in no cardiac or coagulopathy-related complications, a lower seizure frequency, and more patients in the good recovery to moderate disability category. In other head trauma studies, therapeutic hypothermia attenuated intracranial hypertension but did not affect the frequency of delayed intracerebral hemorrhage. Results from three multicenter TBI trials failed to demonstrate a protective effect of hypothermia on traumatic outcome, but a subgroup analysis in one showed that patients who came into the emergency room hypothermic and had hematomas evacuated while still hypothermic demonstrated a reduced rate of poor outcome (Andrews et al., 2018; Clifton et al., 2012). In the more recent Prophylactic Hypothermia Trial to Lessen Traumatic Brain Injury (POLAR) randomized clinical trial, early prophylactic hypothermia compared with normothermia after severe TBI was reported to have failed to improve neurological outcome at 6 months (Cooper et al., 2018). Obviously more experimental and clinical studies are needed to determine what factors are most important in providing protection when hypothermic strategies fail. Temperature is known to affect many pathophysiological processes after TBI, and this characteristic may be advantageous because of the multifactorial nature of trauma pathomechanisms. The cooling and rewarming periods are also important variables in determining the extent of neuroprotection. In TBI studies, prolonged periods of hypothermia (i.e., >24 hours) may therefore be necessary to protect the brain from primary and secondary injury processes. In a multicenter TBI trial from China, long-term cooling (5 days) was significantly better than short-term cooling (2 days) in terms of improved outcome in patients. Because brain temperature can be elevated compared with bladder temperature in head-injured patients, normothermia or mild hypothermia should be maintained during critical postinjury periods.

## RECOVERY OF FUNCTION

### Environmental Enrichment

The effect of environmental enrichment (EE)—which exposes animals to a complex, highly stimulatory, and social environment—has been studied in a number of TBI models (Hannan, 2014). Using a midline FP injury model that produced no noticeable histopathology, EE was reported to improve cognitive function. In addition, EE has been shown to decrease overall contusion volume and improve performance in the Morris water maze task. The effects of EE have been suggested to be reflected in changes in dendritic arborization. Recent experimental studies have reported that animals raised with EE have larger contusion injuries and greater sensorimotor deficits after mild TBI compared with standard laboratory cage-reared animals. However, the sensorimotor deficit improved at a much more rapid pace in the EE animals compared with age-matched controls. Future studies combining EE with neuroprotective and reparative strategies will probably be needed to maximize improvement in outcome.

### Reparative and Transplantation Strategies

After a variety of acute CNS system injuries, there is a massive proliferation of stem or progenitor cells (Yu et al., 2016). The identification and origin of the fate of these cells is an area of intensive investigation. In a model of FP injury, the total number of proliferating cells as identified with 5-bromo-deoxyuridine, a marker of mitotic activity, was shown to significantly increase in areas of the subventricular zone and hippocampus. In that study, proliferating cells did not express cell markers and therefore appeared not to have begun to differentiate. Targeting this endogenous proliferative response to injury may be one way of enhancing recovery following TBI.

In contrast to attempts to enhance endogenous reparative events, providing new cells from exogenous sources is an alternative approach and may be necessary when neuronal loss and axonal injury are severe. Neural transplantation has been explored in TBI models (Lemmens and Steinberg, 2013). Fetal cortical tissue transplanted into the injury cavity improved motor function and transiently attenuated cognitive dysfunction alone and in combination with NGF infusion. Although the reestablishment of normal adult neural circuitry has not been demonstrated with fetal tissue grafts, one mechanism for improved function may be neuroprotection by release of trophic factors from the grafts. Recent studies have also attempted to provide cellular replacement and host-graft integration using self-renewing cell lines (Dekmak et al., 2018). Using transplanted immortalized neural progenitor cells transduced with the mouse *NGF* gene to secrete NGF, improved neuromotor and cognitive function, and reduced hippocampal CA3 cell death have been reported. Continued study in this exciting field may establish transplantation procedures relevant to clinical strategies to promote recovery after TBI.

## SUMMARY AND FUTURE DIRECTIONS

Continued experimental studies directed at investigating the pathogenesis of TBI will enhance our understanding of the neuroscience of brain trauma. Clarifying what injury processes dominate the injury cascade will improve strategies directed at brain protection. Development of novel genetic mouse models of disease should also allow researchers to elucidate cause-and-effect relationships between specific pathomechanisms and cell death. The continued emphasis on determining how various factors, including age and gender, affect traumatic outcome should enhance the translation of experimental findings to patients. The relationship between early head injury and increased incidence of neurodegenerative disease is an important area for investigation as well. Determining what genetic and environmental factors may interact to enhance the susceptibility of the posttraumatic brain to age-related disease processes is of utmost importance. Also, scientists from different laboratories need to assist in replicating exciting data that will promote the design of successful clinical trials. Finally, the testing of combination therapies targeting multiple pathomechanisms must be encouraged. Strategies to protect vulnerable neurons, inhibit secondary injury mechanisms, and promote reparative processes must be considered in experimental studies. Continued communication between scientists involved in brain injury research and clinicians responsible for treating this patient population and designing clinical trials will advance efforts toward these goals.

*The complete reference list is available online at https://expertconsult.inkling.com/.*

61

# Concussion in Sports and Performance

Jeffrey S. Kutcher

## OUTLINE



## EPIDEMIOLOGY

Sports-related concussion (SRC) is a type of mild traumatic brain injury (mTBI) that continues to garner increasing concern worldwide (Covassin et al., 2012; De Beaumont et al., 2007; King et al., 2014). In the United States alone, estimates of sports and recreation-related concussion range from 1.6 to 3.8 million annually (Giza et al., 2013). Concussion occurs in 9% of all US high school sports injuries (Armstrong, 2014; Gessel et al., 2007; Kutcher et al., 2010) and, because many of the clinical findings are subjective, it is among the most difficult injuries in sports medicine to diagnose, assess, and manage. Despite the frequency and possible consequences of repeated head trauma, concussions are often underreported.

## DEFINITION OF CONCUSSION

Agreement on the definition of concussion has come into focus over time (Conidi, 2012; King et al., 2014). Historically, concussion has been described as a "low velocity" injury leading to a transient disturbance of function rather than structure (McCrory et al., 2005, 2009, 2012, 2017). In 2001, the first International Conference on Concussion in Sport expanded the definition to include the common clinical presentations of SRC (Aubry et al., 2002). In the most recent iteration of the international consensus effort, the definition was further specified to be "a traumatic brain injury induced by biomechanical forces" that "may be caused either by a direct blow to the head, face, neck or elsewhere on the body with an impulsive force transmitted to the head" (McCrory, 2017). Additionally, the following common clinical features were described as potentially useful for defining the nature of SRC:

1. "SRC typically results in the rapid onset of short-lived impairment of neurological function that resolves spontaneously. However, in some cases, signs and symptoms evolve over a number of minutes to hours" (Aubry et al., 2002; McCrory et al., 2005, 2009, 2012).
2. "SRC may result in neuropathological changes, but the acute clinical signs and symptoms largely reflect a functional disturbance rather than a structural injury and, as such, no abnormality is seen on standard structural neuroimaging studies" (McCrory et al., 2017).
3. "SRC results in a range of clinical signs and symptoms that may or may not involve loss of consciousness. Resolution of the clinical and cognitive features typically follows a sequential course. However, it is important to note that in some cases symptoms may be prolonged" (Aubry et al., 2002; McCrory et al., 2009, 2012).

This definition is well accepted and widely cited in the medical literature. However, the intense focus on concussion in the public eye, particularly in the realm of popular sport, has created an environment in which the term *concussion* is often used incorrectly to describe either the actual injury mechanism itself, persistent symptoms that outlive the underlying concussion pathophysiology, tissue-level structural changes to the brain, or long-term neurodegenerative processes. Each of these instances is distinct from concussion, and care should be taken to apply the term correctly.

### Definition of *Sport* and *Athlete*

Considering SRC as a clinical entity distinct from non-SRC is supported not by the underlying pathophysiology, which is identical in the two scenarios, but by the populations themselves and the unique injury and disease risk profiles that are incurred as a result of the physical activities involved. As such, SRC applies to a wide and diverse set of circumstances. The term *sport* should be applied broadly to include any athletic or performance-based endeavor. As well, the term *athlete* should be used to include any individual with a physical performance–based vocation, hobby, or pursuit. In this way, SRC applies to the population of individuals participating in traditional sports (either as professionals, amateurs, or recreational athletes), performance arts, or military/police professions.

## PATHOPHYSIOLOGY

A more complete understanding of the pathophysiology of concussion and how it leads to the clinical effects also continues to be elucidated. The primary elements of the pathophysiological process of concussion include the neurometabolic cascade (abrupt neuronal depolarization, subsequent release of excitatory neurotransmitters, ionic shifts, and changes in glucose metabolism), altered cerebral blood flow (CBF), and impaired axonal function.

### Neurometabolic Cascade

The metabolic cascade of concussion has been well studied and characterized in both animal models and humans. After exposure to a clinically relevant biomechanical force, neuronal cell membranes undergo disruptive stretching, which leads to transient ionic dysequilibrium (Choe et al., 2012; Farkas et al., 2006; Giza and DiFiori, 2011; Giza and Hovda, 2001; Shrey et al., 2011). There is also an initial depolarization of neuronal membranes, which results in glutamate release and a dramatic rise in extracellular potassium leaking through the cell membrane (Choe et al., 2012; Giza and DiFiori, 2011; Giza and Hovda, 2001; Shrey et al., 2011). The release of glutamate, in turn, activates *N*-methyl-D-aspartate (NMDA) and 2-amino-3-(5-methyl-3-oxo-1,2-oxazol-4-yl) propanoic acid (AMPA) receptors, which results in the accumulation of intracellular calcium and sodium (Choe et al., 2012; Giza and DiFiori, 2011; Giza and Hovda, 2001; Osteen et al., 2004; Shrey et al., 2011). This ionic flux drives an upregulation of the ATP-dependent sodium-potassium pumps as the cell attempts to restore normal resting membrane potential (Choe et al., 2012; Giza and DiFiori, 2011; Giza and Hovda, 2001; Shrey et al., 2011). The process also augments cerebral glucose demand, leading to a cellular energy crisis. Additionally, increased intracellular calcium subsequently causes mitochondrial dysfunction and protease activation, which can initiate apoptosis (Choe et al., 2012; Giza and DiFiori, 2011; Giza and Hovda, 2001; Shrey et al., 2011; Sullivan et al., 2005). Neurons are then forced to use the glycolytic pathway instead of aerobic metabolism, leading to lactate accumulation (Giza and Hovda, 2001; Shrey et al., 2011). Lactate accumulation leads to acidosis, which worsens ionic dysequilibrium, membrane permeability, and cerebral edema (Shrey et al., 2011). In human studies, a significant correlation between increased glutamate levels and derangements in lactate, potassium, and brain tissue pH and $CO_2$ levels has been found (Giza and Hovda, 2001; Shrey et al., 2011; Yuen et al., 2009). Ultimately, cellular glucose stores become exhausted.

### Cerebral Blood Flow

Given the derangement of the neurometabolic cascade, a calcium ion–induced vasoconstriction occurs, which in turn reduces CBF. CBF is tightly coupled to cerebral glucose metabolism and neuronal activity. A 50% reduction from normal CBF has been seen in studies using experimental fluid percussion injury in mice (Giza and Hovda, 2001). Although this posttraumatic decrease in CBF does not reach the 85% reduction seen in ischemia, it potentiates the energy crisis (Giza and Hovda, 2001). Decreased CBF and glucose delivery result in a state of "metabolic depression" as the brain's energy demand is not met by the vascular energy supply. Metabolic depression has been demonstrated to last several days in animal models and weeks in humans (Giza and Hovda, 2001; Willer and Leddy, 2006). This complex cascade and energy-deficient state is thought to render neural tissue more susceptible to further injury.

### Axonal Dysfunction

Axonal injury has been well described with severe TBI as well as reversibly in mTBI/concussion (Barkhoudarian et al., 2011; Giza and Hovda, 2001; Makdissi et al., 2014). Biomechanical forces applied to neural tissue can lead to damaged and dysfunctional axons (Armstrong, 2014; Choe et al., 2012; Giza and Hovda, 2001). Axonal transport is disrupted and axonal swelling can then occur. Calcium influx also destabilizes microtubules 6–24 hours after initial injury (Giza and Hovda, 2001). Partial breakage of microtubules occurs, leading to undulations in axonal morphology, which then evolves to periodic swelling (Barkhoudarian et al., 2011; Buki and Povlishock, 2006; Choe et al., 2012; Tang-Schomer et al., 2012). Molecular studies in mice have shown predominant damage at the axonal level with minimal impact on the neuronal cell bodies and myelin sheaths (Barkhoudarian et al., 2011; Spain et al., 2010).

### Synaptic Plasticity and Neural Activation

There have been suggestions that alterations of neuronal plasticity occur after concussive injury. Remodeling of synaptic structures occurs throughout a lifetime and maximally during development. During this critical period, cortical inhibitory γ-amino butyric acid (GABA)ergic interneurons play an influential role in plasticity (Chattopadhyaya, 2011; Choe et al., 2012). Some studies have suggested that there is a period of impaired neural activation after concussive injuries (Choe et al., 2012). The measure of the brain's ability to manipulate its structure and function based on environmental stimulation is known as *experience-dependent plasticity* (Giza et al., 2011; McFarlane and Glenn, 2015). Studies have shown an increase in cortical thickness, proliferation of dendritic branching, larger neurons, and improved cognition in rats that were reared in an enriched environment (Giza et al., 2005; Ip et al., 2002; McFarlane and Glenn, 2015). These rats, which also endured moderate fluid percussive injury, failed to develop the aforementioned indicators of increased plasticity (Giza et al., 2005; Ip et al., 2002; McFarlane and Glenn, 2015). Therefore there may be a period of time following a concussive injury where the brain is less responsive to external stimuli (Giza et al., 2005, 2011; McFarlane and Glenn, 2015).

## INITIAL EVALUATION AND DIAGNOSIS

The clinical syndrome produced by a concussion may take several hours to develop (McCrory et al., 2017). Given that, it is important to recognize that the role of the medical provider at a sporting event or practice is to triage for safety and screen for emergent neurological injury rather than to diagnose concussion per se. The likelihood of concussion is best clarified over the days following the injury. During this time, if concussion is suspected, the patient should not be allowed to participate in any activity involving the risk of impact.

If, after an biomechanical insult, a patient is unconscious or unresponsive, safety concerns should immediately be addressed. A focused physical examination is important to exclude other critical diagnoses, including cervical spine injury. Transfer to the emergency room (ER) should occur with any open injury, convulsive activity, altered mental status, persistent Glasgow Coma Scale (GCS) score less than 15, or focal neurological deficit. After an emergent situation has been ruled out, the evaluation for concussion begins, with screening for specific signs and symptoms (Table 61.1).

Previously, concussion was both diagnosed and then further graded based on the presence and duration of loss of consciousness as well as the presence of specific symptoms (i.e., disorientation/confusion). However, loss of consciousness occurs in less than 10% of concussions and does not predict the duration or severity of injury. More recently, previously used scales and grading systems have been abandoned in favor of more individualized approaches.

Symptoms from concussion may present directly after the traumatic force is applied or several hours later. In the acute setting, it is difficult to rely solely on the clinical evaluation, since the complexity

**TABLE 61.1 Common Symptoms of Sports-Related Concussion**

| Somatic | Cognitive | Neurobehavioral |
|---|---|---|
| Headache | Disorientation/confusion | Lethargy/fatigue |
| Dizziness | Feeling "in a fog" or "hazy" | Drowsiness |
| Photophobia | Lack of attention/focus | Hypersomnia/ insomnia |
| Phonophobia | Distractibility | Sadness/depression |
| Blurred vision/diplopia | Memory deficits | Anger |
| Nausea | | Nervousness/ irritability |
| | | "Not feeling right" |
| **Physical** | **Cognitive** | **Neurobehavioral** |
| Loss of consciousness | Disorientation/confusion | Personality changes |
| Loss of awareness | Memory impairment | Irritability/violent outburst |
| Blank stare/dazed look | Slowed reaction time or processing speed | Depression |
| Seizure | Attention deficit | Emotional lability |
| Vomiting | Impaired comprehension | |
| Dysarthria/slurred speech | Problems with concentration | |
| Ataxia/discoordination | | |

of the brain creates significant variability in the type and severity of concussion presentations (Kutcher et al., 2013). Therefore meaningful diagnostic and management tools—including objective measures of eye movement, clinical reaction times, and balance as well as neurocognitive tests—may be helpful. Standardized assessment tools may provide a structure for the evaluation of concussion (Harmon et al., 2013). Graded symptom checklists may also be helpful. These tools can help to document the clinical presentation, can aid in diagnosis, and serve to document recovery.

Several assessment tools exist, including the Standardized Assessment of Concussion (SAC), the Standardized Concussion Assessment Tool (SCAT5; McCrory et al., 2017), and the Military Acute Concussion Evaluation (MACE; Coldren et al., 2010; Eckner et al., 2010; Kutcher et al., 2010). Most tools include aspects that track concussion symptoms, cognitive performance, and balance. It is important to note that some of these tools have not been standardized for use in children or adolescents. Cognitive evaluation usually includes the assessment of orientation, immediate memory, and delayed recall as well as concentration, learning, and attention. The physical examination usually includes assessments of speech fluency, cranial nerve examination, pronator drift, and gait.

Training in the proper use of concussion tests is important. Assessment tools should never be the sole decision makers for diagnosis and are most appropriately used as supplemental information to a comprehensive concussion evaluation based on salient features from the history and clinical examination. An individualized approach should be taken in each case (Harmon et al., 2013).

## In-Office/Outpatient Evaluation

The hallmark of concussion diagnosis lies in a thorough history and physical examination. If the clinician is seeing a patient for the first time, video footage of the event may be helpful, providing important information regarding the mechanism of the injury and the presence of acute signs (Makdissi et al., 2014). The history should include a detailed account of the injury, symptoms, and course, including the following:

- Mechanism of injury
- Loss of consciousness/posttraumatic amnesia/retrograde amnesia
- Signs and symptoms directly after the injury and during the following days
- Current symptoms, including headache, nausea, dizziness, cognitive or mood changes, sleep dysfunction
- Physical and cognitive exertion levels between injury and presentation

Further details about the number of prior concussions, specific symptoms associated with each one, time to resolution, prior neuroimaging, and any treatments should then be elucidated. Information about all prior head, face, or neck injuries is also relevant, since patients do not always recognize that a concussion has occurred.

The physical examination is critical and should be thorough. Common neurological examination findings in concussion include the following:

1. Nystagmus
2. Saccadic eye movements with smooth pursuit
3. Changes in gait
4. Truncal ataxia/increased postural sway and/or gait ataxia
5. Balance abnormalities
6. Mental status changes—amnesia/memory deficits, confusion/disorientation, emotional lability

Nystagmus, incoordination, and deficits in balance are most commonly seen. Balance and vestibular deficits can persist for up to 10 days after concussion (Peterson et al., 2003; Willer and Leddy, 2006). It is important to note that it can be difficult to attribute examination findings to concussion versus a more malignant injury, such as an intracranial hemorrhage. It is extremely important to keep in mind the timing of these findings. Any worsening of the clinical presentation—whether in the first few hours or even days later, especially despite proper rest and management—should warrant further evaluation with neuroimaging.

It is extremely important to apply comprehensive neurological principles throughout the evaluation and management process in order to develop a full differential diagnosis. Common concurrent and/or alternative diagnoses include but are not limited to migraine headache, mood disorders, peripheral vestibular dysfunction, and cervical strain. Care should be taken that patients are not assumed to be concussed based on a symptom checklist alone.

## Neuropsychological Testing

Cognitive deficits associated with concussion are typically subtle and may exist in multiple domains. In some cases, cognitive deficits may outlast subjective symptoms (Makdissi et al., 2014). In some studies, neuropsychological testing was found to be more sensitive than the clinical examination (Harmon et al., 2013). However, many factors can influence test results, including environment, motivation, fatigue, and practice effects. It is important to note that different modes of testing, such as computer-based tests versus traditional neuropsychological tests, may produce different results since they measure different neurocognitive constructs.

Ideally, postinjury results should be compared with preinjury results when available. Formal neuropsychological testing is recommended in any case where there is prolonged recovery or uncertainty about recovery (Harmon et al., 2013; Makdissi et al., 2014). It must be noted that neuropsychological testing is only one component of assessment and should never be used as the sole basis for management decisions.

## Neuroimaging

Neuroimaging should be used to evaluate for additional injury, such as fracture or intracranial hemorrhage. As mentioned earlier, open injury, convulsive activity, altered mental status, and a persistent GCS score less than 15 should trigger an emergent response with neuroimaging. Any clear deterioration in consciousness should raise suspicion of a structural head injury. Similarly, structural head injury should be considered in any case where there is continued unexplained clinical deterioration, worsening of symptoms, or emergence of new focal neurological deficits.

Conventional imaging such as computed tomography of the head and magnetic resonance imaging (MRI) of the brain are usually normal after an uncomplicated concussive injury (Makdissi et al., 2014). Advanced neuroimaging modalities may reveal microstructural or functional neurobiological changes and have been utilized to better quantify the functional disturbances of the concussed brain (Choe et al., 2012). Both magnetic resonance spectroscopy (MRS) and positron emission tomography (PET) demonstrate cerebral metabolism and have been used to quantify physiological changes that occur in concussion. Diffusion tensor imaging (DTI) is an advanced MRI technique that measures fractional anisotropy and thus evaluates axonal integrity. Axonal damage on DTI has been seen after concussive injury in adult, adolescent, and pediatric patients (Barkhoudarian et al., 2011; Lipton et al., 2008; McCrory et al., 2013a; Niogi et al., 2010; Wilde et al., 2008). Some of these studies also demonstrated subtle deficits in cognitive ability that correlated to these changes seen on DTI (Barkhoudarian et al., 2011; McCrory et al., 2013a; Niogi et al., 2010; Wilde et al., 2008). Functional MRI (fMRI) provides real-time feedback on cerebral metabolism during motor or cognitive tasks. The main limitation of this technique is that it reveals only regions of the brain that are active in the specific cognitive task being studied. These advanced modalities have been used mainly for research purposes; no clear clinical application for them has yet been found. Investigations involving their sensitivity and specificity in concussion diagnosis and ability to estimate the severity of injury continue.

## ACUTE AND SUBACUTE MANAGEMENT

The care of athletes with concussion begins prior to any practice or competition by establishing a clinical action plan. If a concussion is suspected, the athlete should be removed from play immediately. If the athlete is unresponsive, a careful assessment of airway, breathing, and circulation (the ABCs) should follow, as well as an evaluation for cervical spine injury. Emergency transfer should also occur if any of the following signs or symptoms is noted:

- Worsening mental status (lethargy, inability to arouse, progressive confusion)
- Worsening symptoms (intractable vomiting, increased severity of headache)
- Cranial nerve paralysis (particularly extraocular muscles and/or fixed, dilated pupil)
- Focal neurological deficit (motor weakness, sensory deficit)
- Seizure

Once a concussion has been diagnosed, the athlete should not participate for the remainder of that day. He or she should also be monitored for the duration of the game or practice and for at least 3–4 hours afterward (Armstrong, 2014; Kutcher et al., 2010). The athlete may have to be monitored longer if signs and symptoms change or worsen. Return to sports participation must be ruled out until the athlete has been evaluated and cleared by a licensed healthcare provider, preferably a physician trained in the assessment and management of concussion. Specific instructions should be given regarding follow-up and the potential for neurological deterioration, including specific written instructions regarding signs and symptoms to look for.

Clinical attention should then focus on symptom management. The concussed athlete should be instructed to avoid any physical or cognitive exertion that significantly heightens symptoms. Relative physical and cognitive rest in the early stages is important to limit overall morbidity, as both physical and cognitive activity (computer use, schoolwork, and video games) can worsen symptoms (Makdissi et al., 2014; McCrory et al., 2012). Although an initial brief period of rest may be important in the management of acute concussion, there is limited evidence that further rest is beneficial in cases where clinical features are prolonged beyond the typical 7–10 days (Blume et al., 2011; McCrory et al., 2013b). Evidence now suggests that an active rehabilitation program is beneficial in the management of concussion (Makdissi et al., 2013, McCrory et al., 2017).

In the acute setting (0–6 hours), medications that can alter mental status—such as narcotics, benzodiazepine medications, and other central nervous system (CNS) depressants—should be avoided. During this time, treatment options for headaches are limited. Acetaminophen is most often recommended because it does not increase bleeding risk. Approximately 6–10 hours after injury, the administration of anti-inflammatory medication may be given. At this stage, overall nutrition, hydration, and sleep should also be emphasized.

Headache is the most common symptom reported in concussion, often requiring active treatment. Most headaches are described as steady, aching, or of the tension type, commonly with associated features such as photophobia/phonophobia or nausea/vomiting. Most respond to anti-inflammatory medications during the acute phase and then usually resolve. Typical strategies for headache management should be used, emphasizing regular sleep, frequent meals, good hydration, and avoidance of triggers. Primary characteristics of posttraumatic headache can be used to guide treatment. Similar medications typically used for primary headache disorders can be used to manage disabling or prolonged posttraumatic headaches. Many different medications have been used to help manage posttraumatic headache. There is, however, insufficient evidence to support the use of specific pharmacological interventions in the treatment of postconcussion headache (Blume et al., 2011). The choice of medication and therapy will depend on the patient's symptoms, history, and comorbidities.

Given the typical mechanism of SRC and the possibility of concurrent cervical injury, the clinician should evaluate the neck and paraspinal musculature for cervicogenic or other factors contributing to headache. Modalities such as ice, massage, physical therapy, and manual medicine are commonly used. If the patient demonstrates cervical or occipital tenderness, trigger point injections or superficial nerve blocks can be administered by experienced providers in the appropriate circumstances.

Vertigo and/or dizziness are also common complaints in concussion. Typical medications used for these complaints should be used cautiously since they may cloud the neurocognitive examination and impair the neurological assessment. Vestibular physical therapy is another viable treatment option and studies have demonstrated good results (Fife and Giza, 2013).

Nausea may occur independently, or as an associated feature of a headache, vertigo, or dizziness. Antiemetics may be used, but only for severe attacks, since they may also undermine neurocognitive assessment.

Both hypo- and hypersomnia sleep disturbances are commonly found. A lack of restorative sleep may contribute to worsening of other concussion symptoms, such as headache, depression, and cognitive impairments. Sleep hygiene techniques should be implemented as first-line treatment, including regimenting sleep schedule, avoiding daytime naps, and removing distracting factors (television, phones, and computer) from the bedroom. Caffeine use should be restricted and aerobic activity encouraged earlier in the day. A sleep diary may be helpful to determine prebedtime activities, sleep environment, and the use of caffeine or alcohol. Sleep aids such as sedative-hypnotics should be avoided, especially in the acute phase. Melatonin can be used to help improve sleep latency and efficiency if sleep hygiene techniques do not provide adequate improvement. However, data to support its use are lacking.

Transient mood disturbances are commonly seen including depression, irritability, or lability. Pharmacological treatment is usually avoided in the early stages. Cognitive restructuring comprising education, reattribution of symptoms, and reassurance has been shown to diminish the likelihood of developing chronic symptoms (Armstrong, 2014; Blume et al., 2011). If mood disturbance persists beyond 6–12 weeks, either as part of a postconcussion syndrome (PCS) or as a manifestation of an exacerbated mood disorder, additional treatment should be considered.

### Return to School, Work, or Cognitive Activity

There are no standardized guidelines regarding how athletes should return to academic or cognitive activities. Patients may require cognitive rest and possibly academic accommodations while recovering from a concussion. Return to full cognitive activity should occur in a stepwise fashion and each plan should be individualized, taking into account the specific classwork and activities that may make symptoms worse or delay recovery.

### Return to Physical Activity

The complex nature of the return-to-play decision should be understood and respected, as the role of the clinician is to recommend when it is reasonable for their patient to return to an activity that likely imparts continued injury risk. Understanding the sport or activty in question and the risk it carries is essential to providing comprehensive care.

When the clinical features of the injury have begun to resolve, the patient may be considered for beginning a specifically defined return-to-activity process. The patient does not have to be completely free of concussion-related symptoms. Rather, the clinical decision should be made that being exposed to simple activity is unlikely to produce an intolerable increase in symptoms. At this stage, medication use should be minimal or absent.The physical examination should be normal.

Return to participation can then be progressively implemented and should involve a gradual, stepwise increase in physical demands, followed by noncontact sport-specific activities (Table 61.2). The purpose of this approach is to determine whether the injury is still present though not producing symptoms at rest. With each stage, enough time should elapse, typically 24 hours, for the patient to experience any symptoms of the concussion that have been produced by that particular challenge (Kutcher et al., 2010). This progression should be started only with the guidance of a licensed healthcare provider trained in the evaluation and management of concussions. Ideally, the exertional test itself should be supervised and used to guide further activity recommendations. The process should begin with basic cardiovascular activity, such as 20–30 minutes on a stationary bicycle, with enough of an exertion level (e.g., sustained heart rate [HR] of 140–160 BPM) to induce an increase in metabolic demand (Kutcher et al., 2010). If the challenge is tolerated, the athlete can continue to proceed through the protocol as presented in Table 61.2. As the athlete progresses, close monitoring for signs or symptoms is required when making the decision to progress. During the final stage, it is important to simulate game conditions as much as possible prior to full return to play. If any symptoms occur during a specific stage, the progression should be paused and the athlete should be allowed to recover. Once symptoms resolve, the patient may repeat the same level or return to the previous level at the clinician's discretion. A more conservative approach should be taken in cases where there is uncertainty about the patient's ability to provide a history or if the exertion is unable to be supervised. An athlete with a history of prior prolonged concussion recovery may require a more conservative approach, with an elongated amount of time spent at each exertional level. Additional considerations or further evaluation with formal neuropsychological testing can be used prior to full clearance to aid with these special circumstances. Finally, medical clearance should be given before full return to participation occurs.

Unfortunately there is very limited evidence on the clinical effect of return-to-play guidelines. The best available evidence on prognosis after sport concussion suggests that most athletes recover within 7–10 days (King et al., 2014; McCrory et al., 2005, 2012). Some findings have indicated that younger athletes have slightly longer recovery periods. Consequently, individuals supervising athletes of high school age or younger should manage these patients more conservatively.

## RISK INVOLVED WITH PREMATURE RETURN TO PARTICIPATION

The brain may be vulnerable to further injury during concussion as the complex metabolic cascade of concussion is thought to render neurons more susceptible to physiological perturbations. Some studies have suggested there is an increased risk of sustaining a second injury within

**TABLE 61.2 Protocol for Return to Participation**

| Stage of Rehabilitation | Functional Exercise | Objective of Each Stage |
|---|---|---|
| No activity | Complete physical rest | Recovery |
| Light cardiovascular activity | Stationary bike, walking, swimming, light skating | Increased HR and CBF |
| Sport-specific activity | Interval training, conditioning drills, running or skating drills, ball work, sprints, etc. | Fluctuation in HR, adding cognitive function to activity, adding movement |
| Noncontact practice | Complex training drills, noncontact team practices | Increased cognitive load, assess coordination and processing speed |
| Full-contact practice | Participation in normal training activities—only with medical clearance | Assess functional skills, assess for recurrence of symptoms by applying smaller magnitude of forces, ensuring self-confidence and readiness to play |
| RTP | Full participation in game play | |

*CBF*, Cerebral blood flow; *HR*, heart rate; *RTP*, return to play.

*Adapted from McCrory, P., Meeuwisse W., Johnston, K., et al., 2009. Consensus Statement on Concussion in Sports, 3rd International Conference on Concussion in Sport held in Zurich, November 2008. Clin J Sport Med 19(3), 185–200.*

the first 7–10 days (Choe et al., 2012; Guskiewicz et al., 2003; Makdissi et al., 2014), although these cases may also represent recrudescence of the original injury. Early vulnerability after concussion has also been described as a potential risk for catastrophic outcomes. Although controversial, second-impact syndrome (SIS) has been described (Shrey et al., 2011). SIS is felt to be a rare form of additional injury that occurs prior to the complete resolution of a previous concussion. Both animal and human studies support the concept of postconcussive vulnerability, showing that a second traumatic force before the brain has fully recovered may result in cerebrovascular dysregulation, causing massive cerebral edema and subsequent brain herniation. However, diffuse cerebral swelling has also been reported in pediatric patients after a single mTBI (Kutcher et al., 2010). Interestingly, studies have linked a mutation in the *CACNA1A* calcium channel subunit gene that is associated with familial hemiplegic migraine and cases of fatal malignant brain edema or SIS (Choe et al., 2012; Kors et al., 2001; Kutcher et al., 2010). Additionally, almost all of the suspected cases of SIS have occurred in athletes younger than age 20, with the majority being 17 years old or younger (Kutcher et al., 2010). This may imply a unique susceptibility to SIS in younger populations.

## LONG-TERM EFFECTS

### Postconcussion Syndrome

Based on systematic reviews, prospective cohort studies, and animal models, the majority of concussions resolve within 7–10 days (Guskiewicz et al., 2003, 2007; Makdissi et al., 2013). However, some patients may go on to have a more prolonged symptoms course. In these cases, individuals are thought to have a PCS. It is important to understand that PCS is not a prolonged concussion but rather a separate clinical entity. The risks of developing PCS are not well defined. Symptoms are typically subjective and often vague, making diagnosis difficult. The clinical features vary, but commonly include headache, dizziness, nausea, memory disturbance, confusion, fatigue, depression, sleep problems, difficulty concentrating, and mental "fogginess" (Armstrong, 2014; Kutcher et al., 2010; Makdissi et al., 2013). The Diagnostic and Statistical Manual of Mental Disorders – 4th Edition (DSM-IV) criteria for PCS require that symptoms last at least 3 months. PCS symptoms are nonspecific, however, and have been reported in healthy athletic populations as well in patients with other illnesses, psychiatric conditions, and other injuries (Makdissi et al., 2013). Multiple factors including genetic makeup, medical history, and psychosocial stressors play significant roles. Some studies have demonstrated no correlation between concussion severity and the likelihood of developing persistent PCS (McCrory et al., 2013b). A prior history of headaches, learning disabilities, and psychiatric disorders, however, has been shown to play a role in persistent symptoms.

The assessment of PCS requires a detailed history and physical examination. Vestibular, sleep, mood, and cognitive function as well as cervical spine function should be assessed. Consideration should be given to neuroimaging to investigate for a structural injury. Although there are limited data to support its recommendation, formal neuropsychological testing can be performed to quantify cognitive deficits and identify other factors impacting cognition.

Numerous medications are available to treat PCS (Makdissi et al., 2013). Fann et al. (2000) demonstrated an improvement of symptoms with the use of sertraline in a small cohort of volunteers that were diagnosed with major depression and PCS (Makdissi et al., 2013). One study demonstrated that amitriptyline reduced headache symptoms in post-mTBI patients without depression (Willer and Leddy, 2006). Small studies of patients with headaches and presumed PCS demonstrated moderate to good results with antimigraine medications (amitriptyline, propranolol, intravenous dihydroergotamine (DHE), and metoclopramide, valproic acid) (Makdissi et al., 2013; Willer and Leddy, 2006). However, these studies have not been confirmed in larger randomized trials. Medications should be limited to cases that do not resolve with an initial conservative approach. Choice of pharmacological treatment should be individualized.

Other treatment modalities may be used in combination with pharmacological agents. However, there are limited data using these techniques in PCS. Manual or physical therapy can help in treating cervicogenic headache or myofascial pain. Anxiety, depression, panic attacks, or other emotional/psychological problems may benefit from meditation, cognitive behavior therapy, psychotherapy, or biofeedback. Those with persistent cognitive deficits or changes in memory may benefit from cognitive therapy. Persistent vestibular symptoms may be addressed with vestibular therapy (Blume et al., 2011; Fife and Giza, 2013; Makdissi et al., 2013). Finally, there is evidence suggesting that a progressive, well-measured, and monitored exercise rehabilitation program can be useful in cases of PCS (Blume et al., 2011; Leddy et al., 2011; Makdissi et al., 2013).

### Chronic Traumatic Encephalopathy

The long-term brain health effects of traumatic forces, especially repetitive impacts, continue to be elucidated. There is evidence in the professional athlete population suggesting neurocognitive impairments with multiple concussions or longer exposure to contact sports (Choe et al., 2012; Guskiewics et al., 2007). There is additional concern that repetitive brain trauma may be a risk factor for developing chronic traumatic encephalopathy (CTE). Historically, CTE, previously termed "dementia pugilistica," was first described in retired boxers who demonstrated similar motor, behavioral, and cognitive impairments (Critchley, 1957; Kors et al., 2001; Martland, 1928).

Two distinct clinical patterns of CTE have been described (Johnson, 1969; McCrory, 2007, 2011; McCrory et al., 2013b). In approximately 70% of cases, dysarthria, pyramidal problems, and cognitive deficits predominate, including difficulties in memory, insight, orientation, and information processing speed. The second pattern consists of pyramidal problems, dysarthria, but relatively spared cognitive abilities (Johnson, 1969; McCrory, 2011; McCrory et al., 2013b). Other common symptoms that may occur include agitation, depression, aggression, poor judgment, social withdrawal, and paranoia.

There have been recent cases of professional contact sport athletes thought to have CTE whose autopsy revealed pathological findings of variable degrees of tau deposition manifesting as neurofibrillary tangles, suggesting a degenerative process (Choe et al., 2012; Gavett et al., 2011; McKee et al., 2009; Shrey et al., 2011). The exact mechanism that leads to their accumulation is not known (Shrey et al., 2011) and it should be emphasized that no causal relationship between abnormal tau deposition and any one clinical effect has been determined. Additionally, in slightly less than half of CTE cases, neuritic β-amyloid plaques have been found (Johnson et al., 2010; Jordan et al., 1997; McCrory et al., 2013b; McKee et al., 2009; Shrey et al., 2011). The pathogenesis of β-amyloid deposits is not entirely clear and the exact role played by β-amyloid is also unclear, where in some cases it has been found to be pathogenic, and in others, neuroprotective (Johnson et al., 2010; Shrey et al., 2011). A number of common pathological features of CTE have also been shown, including fenestrated septum pellucidum, cerebral atrophy, enlarged ventricles, and reduced pigmentation of the substantia nigra and locus ceruleus (McKee et al., 2009).

It is important to note that there are no published epidemiological, prospective, or cross-sectional studies of CTE. Most of the published studies have been pathological case series or case reports, making it impossible to determine the causality or risk factors with any certainty

(McCrory et al., 2013b). Additionally, the extent to which age-related changes, genetic risk, use of alcohol or drugs, or coexisting psychiatric or dementing illnesses contribute is yet to be established. Beyond the ranks of professional contact sport athletes, it is unknown whether there is any long-term risk involved with youth contact or collision sports. At this point, further prospective and longitudinal studies are needed in order to truly determine the causal relationships.

## WHEN TO RETIRE AN ATHLETE

There are no evidence-based guidelines for disqualifying or retiring an athlete from a sport due to concerns regarding traumatic brain injury (Harmon et al., 2013). When retirementis are being considered, it is imperative that each case be carefully reviewed and an individualized approach be taken. With that, there are scenarios that should raise concern. Any athlete who shows objective evidence for chronic or persistent cognitive deficits should retire from contact sport in order to minimize the severity of chronic neurobehavioral impairments (Giza et al., 2013). Athletes with subjective persistent neurobehavioral impairment should also be counseled about the potential for developing permanent impairments. Finally, retirement should be considered when an athlete begins to sustain concussive injuries or experience concussive-type symptoms with forces of a lesser degree of magnitude or when subsequent concussions are followed by a prolonged recovery.

## PREVENTION

Helmets do well to prevent structural impact injuries but have not been shown to reduce the incidence or severity of concussions (Harmon et al., 2013). Evidence suggests the use of a properly fitted helmet does not eliminate but may mildly reduce risk of concussion in rugby and hockey (Armstrong, 2014; Hollis et al., 2009; Kemp et al., 2008). There are insufficient data to support the use of protective headgear in soccer, and there is no compelling evidence that mouth guards protect athletes from concussion (Armstrong, 2014; Giza et al., 2013; Hollis et al., 2009; Kemp et al., 2008).

With modification and enforcement of sport rules, the primary prevention of some injuries may be possible (Harmon et al., 2013). The duration of injuries and the development of PCS are also important prevention outcomes. Prevention can occur only when athletes, parents, coaches, officials, and healthcare providers are educated. Studies have shown that athletes, parents, and coaches lack the knowledge needed to make informed decisions regarding concussions. Concussion education should include at least the following:

- Signs and symptoms of concussion
- Proper fit and use of equipment
- Player respect, sport-specific technique, sport rules
- Symptom reporting and assessment
- Training in assessment tools
- Testing and treatment options
- Guidelines for return to participation
- Risks in repetitive injuries or returning too soon

Still, research on injury prevention and evidence-based management should remain a high priority.

*The complete reference list is available online at https://expertconsult.inkling.com/.*

# 62

# Craniocerebral Trauma

*Martina Stippler, Anil Mahavadi*

## OUTLINE



## EPIDEMIOLOGY

Traumatic brain injury (TBI) is a silent epidemic in developed nations and one of the leading causes of death and disability, accounting for almost one-third of all trauma-related deaths. In the United States, a TBI occurs every 7 seconds and results in a death every 5 minutes. More than 50,000 Americans die of TBI annually, and approximately 5.3 million live with TBI-related disabilities such as cognitive deficits and impairments in memory, judgment, and perception. TBI is most prevalent in the young, and the elderly have the worst outcomes. Although only 10% of TBI occurs in the old, they account for 50% of TBI-related deaths.

Although 50% of all TBI cases are due to road traffic, falls are the most common cause in the elderly. Assaults, sports, and recreational injuries are more frequent in children and young adults. The socioeconomic burden of TBI is tremendous because of the loss of productivity among young members of society.

Diagnosis, treatment, and outcome vary significantly by the mechanism, severity, and morphology of the underlying injury. Whereas mild TBI is rarely brought to medical attention, severe TBI requires diagnosis and treatment as soon as possible to prevent or limit secondary injury and maximize the chances for a good outcome. Despite major advances in the trauma response system and neurocritical care for severe TBI, outcomes are still poor. Only one-third of patients can resume normal occupational and social activities with or without minor deficits. About 40% remain disabled, unable to return to their preinjury level of employment and social function; they may also be dependent on others for daily living activities. Even today, one-third of TBI patients die as a result of their injuries.

## CLASSIFICATION

TBI is classified by mechanism, severity, and morphology 50B-1(Table 62.1).

### Mechanism

**Blunt injury is** the most common mechanism; it includes both low- and high-velocity impacts. These injuries may be from a direct blow (e.g., a club) or a rapid deceleration force (e.g., falling or striking the windshield in a car crash). Motor-vehicle collisions and falls cause most of the severe TBIs.

Gunshot wounds are the most prevalent **penetrating injuries** (Fig. 62.1), accounting for 35% of deaths from TBI under the age of 45 years in the United States. Self-inflicted injuries—for example, with nail guns—can also lead to penetrating injuries (Testerman and Dacks, 2007; Fig. 62.2). Gunshot wounds are the most lethal type of brain injury, 90% resulting in death. They cause soft tissue damage, often comminuted depressed skull fractures, and direct injury to the brain tissue from the missile. Beyond the laceration along the bullet path, further damage is done by shock waves, especially with high-velocity weapons. Depending on the type of penetrating injury, contamination may be a concern. However, bullet fragments are considered sterile due to their exposure to heat from the firearm and are not routinely removed.

Vascular injury can occur with any type of TBI but is more common with penetrating trauma (25%–36% incidence) than with blunt injuries (<1%). Traumatic aneurysms, or pseudoaneurysms, can develop when all layers of the vessel wall rupture and surrounding cerebral tissue forms the aneurysmal wall. Such pseudoaneurysms can present as delayed subarachnoid hemorrhage (SAH) and can lead to death or severe disability. Therefore patients with penetrating injuries routinely undergo a cerebral angiogram to screen for traumatic pseudoaneurysm. A follow-up angiogram within the first months after a penetrating injury is recommended (du Trevou and van Dellen, 1992).

**Blast** is a rare mechanism of injury in civilian life but is common in combat. With ongoing militarily conflicts, blast injury has become more frequent among US military personnel. American military members returned from deployment to Iraq or Afghanistan have self-reported a 12% to 20% incidence of mild TBI; explosions are recognized as a common injury mechanism (Wolf et al., 2009). Blast injuries occur as a direct result of supersonic waves of intense air (primary blast injury), from objects put in motion by the blast that hit people (secondary blast injury), and by a person being forcefully put in motion by the blast (tertiary blast injury) (DePalma et al., 2005; Kocsis and Tessler, 2009). The brain is obviously vulnerable to secondary and tertiary blast injury, but whether primary blast forces directly injure the brain is controversial (Taber et al., 2006). The severity of blast exposure

**TABLE 62.1 Overview of Classification of Traumatic Brain Injury**

| | | | |
|---|---|---|---|
| Mechanism | Blunt | | High velocity (MVC) |
| | | | Low velocity (fall, assault) |
| | Penetrating | | GSW |
| | | | Other (stab wounds, etc.) |
| | Blast | | Explosive devices |
| Severity | Mild | | GCS 14–15 |
| | Moderate | | GCS 9–13 |
| | Severe | | GCS 3–8 |
| Morphology | Skull fracture | Vault | Linear versus stellate |
| | | | Depressed/nondepressed |
| | | | Open/closed |
| | | Basilar | With/without CSF |
| | | | With/without CN palsy |
| | Intracranial lesions | Focal | Epidural |
| | | | Subdural |
| | | | Intracerebral |
| | | Diffuse | Mild concussion |
| | | | Classic concussion |
| | | | Diffuse axonal injury |

*CN,* Cranial nerve; *CSF,* cerebrospinal fluid; *GCS,* Glasgow Coma Scale; *GSW,* gunshot wound; *MVC,* motor vehicle collision.

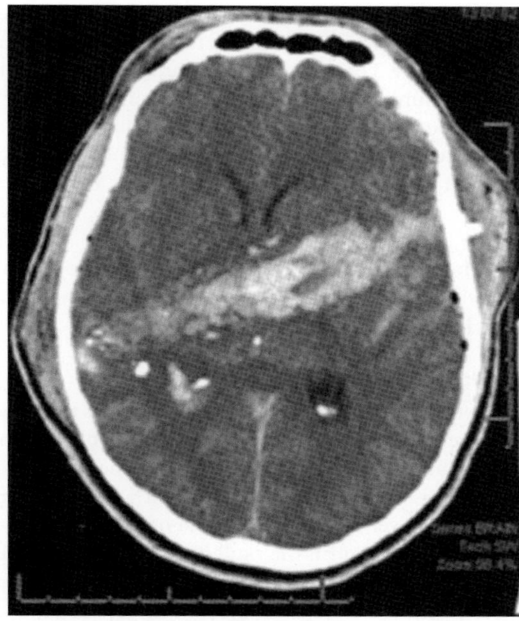

**Fig. 62.1 Picture of a Gunshot Wound to the Head—a Penetrating injury.** The bullet leaves a path of destructions marked by blood, bone, and bullet fragments. Brain tissue around the bullet path is also damaged by the propagating pressure wave. However, this is not visible on computed tomography (axial computed tomography).

needed to cause persistent symptoms is not clear (Hicks et al., 2010). Until research produces a definitive answer, one should consider the possibility that primary blast energy might cause an isolated mild TBI.

The severity of injury resulting from exposure to blast can range from mild to fatal. Displacement, stretching, and shearing forces of the primary blast wave can affect the brain directly and lead to such sequelae as concussion, hemorrhage, severe edema, or diffuse axonal injury (DAI). Systemic acute air embolism from pulmonary disruption

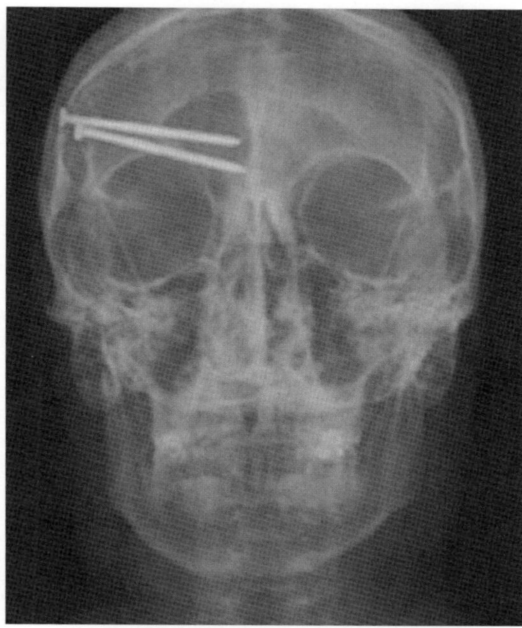

**Fig. 62.2** Another form of penetrating injury is shown on this anteroposterior x-ray of the skull, with two nails from a nail gun stuck in the skull and penetrating the right frontal lobe. This patient was neurologically intact on presentation. The difficulty in such a case is that bleeding can occur deep in the brain when the nails are removed. This patient was also at high risk for developing pseudoaneurysm later on.

is believed to occlude the blood vessels of the brain or spinal cord and lead to stroke (Guy et al., 2000; Wolf et al., 2009). Reports from war zones suggest that brain swelling occurs within hours after a blast injury and that the risk of mortality can be decreased by early decompressive craniectomy (DC). Others have found that cerebral vasospasm occurs more often after a blast injury than with blunt TBI and leads to a worse outcome than severe blunt TBI. Blast exposure on the mild end of the spectrum has led to somatic, behavioral, psychological, and cognitive symptoms similar to postconcussion syndrome. There is well-recognized overlap between posttraumatic stress disorder and blast injury, and misdiagnosis can occur in both directions.

## Severity

There are different ways to stratify TBI by severity, and all are arbitrary. The most commonly used is the Glasgow Coma Scale (GCS), which was first published in 1974 by Graham Teasdale and Bryan K. Jennett, two neurosurgeons at the University of Glasgow (Teasdale and Jennett, 1974). The GCS assesses level of consciousness. It consists of three subscores: eye opening (maximal score 4), verbal response (maximal score 5), and motor response (maximal score 6). Despite some shortcomings, it has excellent interrater agreement (weighted kappa >0.75) for verbal and total scores and intermediate agreement (weighted kappa 0.4–0.75) for motor and eye scores (Holdgate et al., 2006). Today it has been widely adopted by emergency medicine services and physicians to communicate the severity of injury in a consistent way. However, it is not designed to detect focal neurological deficits and is not a replacement for a thorough neurological examination.

A GCS score of 15 to 13 is considered to indicate mild TBI, and a score greater than or equal to 8 is a universally accepted definition of coma and severe head injury. Scores between 13 and 8 are classified as moderate. It is true that moderate and severe TBIs are rare. Mild TBI is eight times more common than moderate and severe TBIs. Moderate

**TABLE 62 2 Factors to Consider Regarding the Need for Computed Tomography in Head-Injured Patients**

| |
|---|
| Indications for urgent CT include the following: |
| • Evidence of skull fracture—basal, depressed, or open |
| • Abnormal results of neurological examination |
| • Seizure |
| • Vomiting more than once |
| • High-risk mechanism (e.g., ejection from vehicle; injury to pedestrian or cyclist vs. car occupant) |
| • Decreasing GCS score or persistently decreased GCS score below 15 |
| Indications for lower threshold for CT scan include the following: |
| • Age >60 yr |
| • Persistent anterograde amnesia |
| • Retrograde amnesia >30 min |
| • Coagulopathy |
| • Fall >5 stairs or >3 ft |
| • Intoxication (examination unreliable) |
| • LOC >30 min |
| • Mechanism and location of injury |
| • Social factors (e.g., abusive situation at home, language barriers precluding an accurate history) |

*CT*, Computed tomography; *GCS*, Glasgow Coma Scale; *LOC*, loss of consciousness.

and severe TBIs are seen equally often. One can imagine that the GCS score shows a significant ceiling effect in patients with mild TBI; therefore more sensitive measures exist for this purpose. The two most often used are the Cantu system (Cantu, 1996) and the American Academy of Neurology system (1997) (Table 62.2)

**Mild TBI** is extremely common. In North America, between 1.5 and 2 million patients visit an emergency department each year for head trauma, with 70% to 90% of cases having mild TBIs. Because this number does not include the many people who choose not to seek medical attention, the true prevalence of mild TBI is difficult to ascertain.

Despite its high incidence, no objective test to diagnose mild TBI currently exists. Diagnosis is hampered by the lack of obvious injuries on computed tomography (CT) or conventional magnetic resonance imaging (MRI) and is usually based solely on clinical symptoms. Preliminary studies are investigating brain injury biomarkers to diagnose mild TBI (Dash et al., 2010; Hergenroeder et al., 2008; Kochanek et al., 2008). Although initial progress has been promising, these markers are not yet used in the clinical setting (Unden and Romner, 2009; Springborg et al., 2009). Others have shown that an integrated approach with magnetoencephalography and diffusion tensor imaging (DTI) is more sensitive than conventional CT and MRI in detecting subtle neuronal injury in mild TBI and postconcussion syndrome (Huang et al., 2009).

A **concussion** is defined as injury to the brain caused by a hard blow or violent shaking, producing a sudden and temporary impairment of brain function, such as a brief loss of consciousness or disturbance of vision and equilibrium. A concussion is equivalent to a mild TBI with negative CT findings. The annual incidence of such concussions in the United States is 128 per 100,000 population (Ropper and Gorson, 2007). The characteristic loss of consciousness is believed to result from rotational forces exerted on the upper midbrain and thalamus, impairing the function of reticular neurons. Headache, nausea, dizziness, irritability, and impaired ability to concentrate can persist for days after the event. Persistence of these symptoms for weeks is called *postconcussion syndrome* and can last from 1 month to a year.

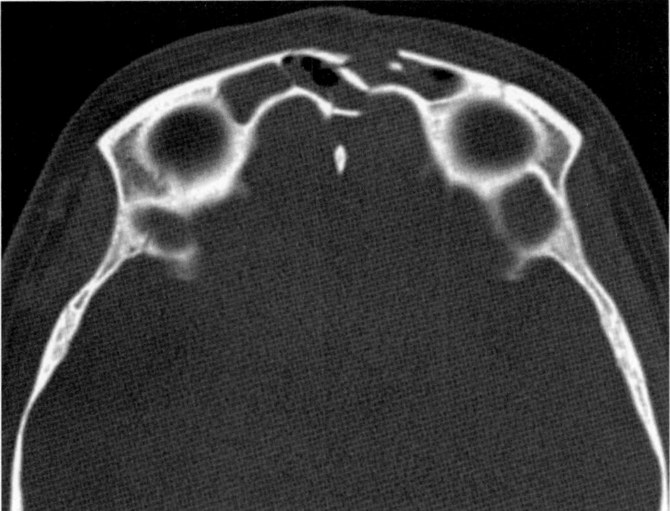

**Fig. 62.3** A Depressed Skull Fracture Penetrating the Frontal Sinus (Axial Computed Tomography).

Patients with severe TBI (GCS score ≤8) often have injuries in at least one other organ system (Saul and Ducker, 1982). There is also a 5% incidence of associated spinal fractures. About one-quarter of patients with a severe TBI undergo neurosurgical intervention. Early diagnosis of TBI improves outcome by reducing secondary injury, which can develop subsequent to the impact and includes edema, hypoxia, hypertension, ischemia, and elevated intracranial pressure (ICP) (Chestnut et al., 1993a, 1993b).

## Morphology

TBI can also be classified by the underlying morphology. Thus, TBI can be subdivided between injuries to the skull itself and intracranial injuries, which can be focal or diffuse (see Table 62.1).

### Skull Fractures

There are two types of skull fractures. **Linear** fractures traverse the full thickness of the skull from the outer to the inner table; they are usually fairly straight and involve no bone displacement. The common method of injury is blunt force trauma, in which the energy from the blow is transferred over a wide surface area of the skull. They can be located in the calvarium or in the skull base. Skull base fractures are associated with cranial nerve (CN) palsy. Depending on their location, CN VII (temporal bone) and CN VI (clivus) are at risk. These fractures are also prone to cause cerebrospinal fluid (CSF) leaks (Fig. 62.3). **In depressed skull fractures, the** method of injury is similar to that in linear skull fractures but in this case the inner and outer tables are more shattered and pieces are displaced into the brain (Fig. 62.4); they may or may not lacerate the dura. **The presence of skull fractures has** consistently been associated with a higher incidence of intracranial lesions, neurological deficits, and poorer outcome (Bullock et al., 2006a). Hence cranial fractures are important indicators of intracranial injuries, and CT scanning should be performed in all patients with a known or suspected cranial fracture to rule out serious intracranial pathology. A large study of patients with TBIs found that 71% of 850 patients with cranial fractures had an intracranial lesion (e.g., contusion or hematoma), compared with only 46% of 533 patients without cranial fractures.

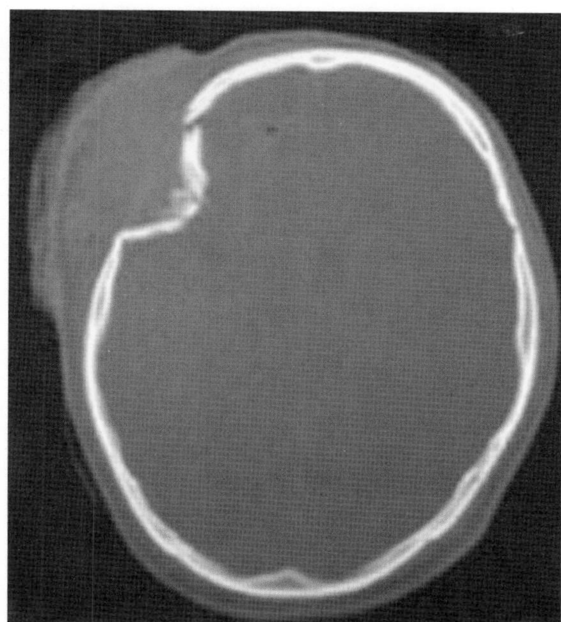

**Fig. 62.4** A Depressed Skull Fracture (Axial Computed Tomography).

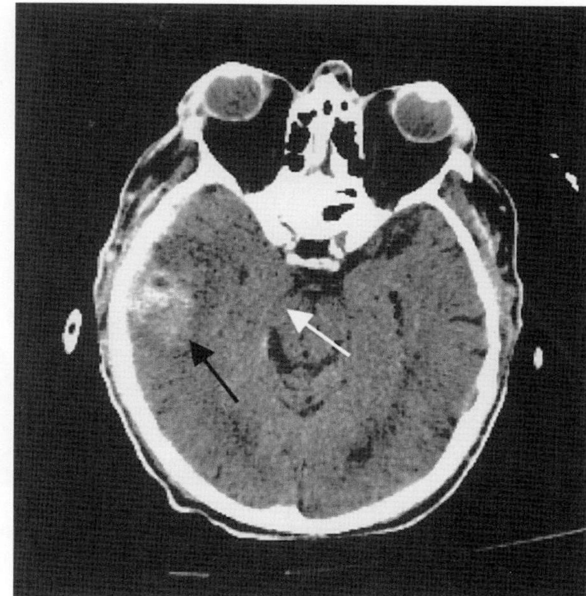

**Fig. 62.5** Temporal lobe contusions *(black arrow)* must be followed closely because even a slight enlargement can cause uncal herniation *(white arrow)*, often without an increase in intracranial pressure (axial computed tomography).

## Intracranial Injuries

**Contusions** occur when the brain moves within the skull enough to collide with the skull, causing bruising of the brain parenchyma (hemorrhage and edema). The most common locations are the frontal and temporal poles because these areas most often strike the bony surfaces of the skull base. Often, a second injury (countercoup) is seen diagonally across the site of the direct impact (coup injury) when the accelerated brain strikes the skull on the opposite site. In contrast to concussion, contusions are visible on a CT scan of the head. The edema surrounding the contusion has lower signal intensity than brain on CT (Fig. 62.5). Hemorrhages have higher CT signal intensity and are commonly multiple bright areas of variable size. Progression of contusions is common, with delayed hemorrhage occurring over the first 24 hours in 25% of cases. However neurosurgical intervention is rare.

**An epidural hematoma (EDH)** is bleeding between the dura and the skull. The peak incidence of this is in the second decade, and the mean age of TBI victims with EDH is between 20 and 30 years. Traffic-related accidents, falls, and assaults account for 53% of EDH in adults; falls account for half of the EDHs in children. Most (70%–90%) EDHs are associated with a skull fracture and bleeding from a lacerated artery or indirect bleeding from bone. In a systematic review, arterial bleeding was identified as the source of the EDH in 36% of adults. Rupture of the middle meningeal vein, the diploic veins, or the venous sinuses can also cause EDH. The most common location of EDH is temporal. Because the temporal bone is thinner than the rest of the skull, it breaks more easily, often resulting in a laceration of the middle meningeal artery (Bullock et al., 2006b; Fig. 62.6).

**Subdural hematoma** (SDH) develops between the brain parenchyma and the dura (Fig. 62.7). It occurs when the brain moves within the skull enough to tear a surface vein, also called a bridging vein, which runs from the brain surface to the dural venous sinus. The most common locations are the frontal and parietal convexities. On a CT scan, an acute SDH typically appears as a bright (hyperdense) extra-axial crescent-shaped, homogeneous collection of fluid that conforms to the cerebral surface. Unlike an EDH, its spread is not limited by suture lines; it can spread over the whole convexity, but it almost never crosses the midline. An SDH can be acute or chronic. Herein, "acute SDH" is defined as an SDH diagnosed within 14 days of TBI. Chronic SDH may be of mixed density or isodense to gray matter. In these cases, it can be identified by its mass effects, including sulcal effacement, inward buckling of the gray-white interface, and the presence of midline shift.

In studies conducted after the introduction of CT, the incidence of SDH was estimated to be 11% of all patients with TBI. The most common injuries involving traumatic SDH are motor vehicle collisions in the younger population and falls in those above 75 years of age. Between 37% and 80% of patients with acute SDH present with an initial GCS score of 8 or less, and dilated pupils are seen preoperatively in 50% of these patients. Mortality among patients who arrive at the hospital in a coma and undergo surgical evacuation is between 57% and 68%.

**Traumatic subarachnoid hemorrhage (tSAH),** seen with mild and severe TBI alike, refers to microhemorrhages into the subarachnoid space from crushed or ruptured smaller vessels. CT scans show hyperdense linear areas in superficial brain sulci (Fig. 62.8). In contrast to aneurysmal SAH, the blood is superficial in the cortex and not present in the basal cisterns. In some instances, for example, if blood is found in the sylvian fissure, a vascular study (CT angiography, four-vessel digital subtraction angiography) is needed to rule out an aneurysmal rupture. Most of the time, traumatic SAH indicates a more severe underlying brain injury and is seen in conjunction with DAI, SDH, or EDH. It has been shown that the presence of traumatic SAH is an independent factor for poor outcome. This finding could reflect a more extensive underlying injury that CT or conventional MRI cannot detect, or it could be attributable to a less recognized phenomenon: posttraumatic vasospasm. The incidence of posttraumatic vasospasm in patients with a mean GCS score of 7 (range 3–15) is similar to that following aneurysmal SAH (see Chapter 51C). Posttraumatic vasospasm is often overlooked. But one study found that hemodynamically significant vasospasm may exist in 44% of patients with SAH. The highest risk of developing hemodynamically significant vasospasm is found on day 3. Younger patients and patients with GCS scores less than or equal to 8 were more likely to develop posttraumatic vasospasm.

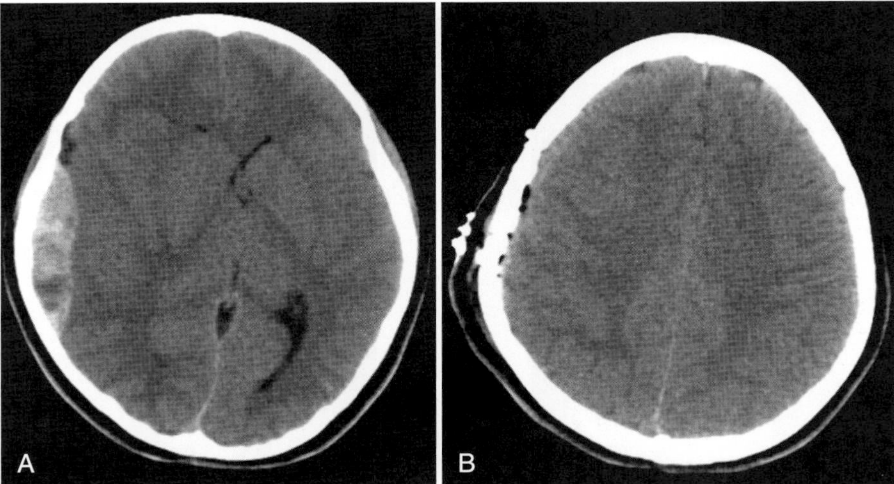


**Fig. 62.6 A,** A right frontoparietal epidural hematoma—typical lenticular hyperdense lesion in the epidural space with mass effect and midline shift. Note the absence of sulci, consistent with brain damage in children. **B,** Postoperative result. Air is visible under the bone flap.

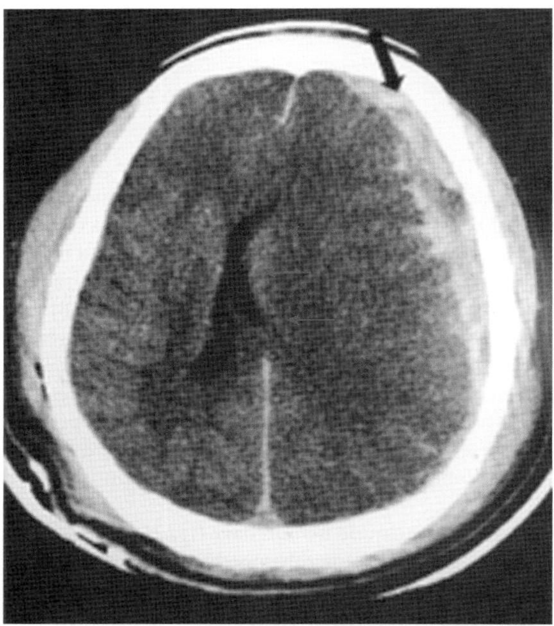

**Fig. 62.7 Left-sided Acute Subdural Hematoma (SDH).** Notice the concave shape along the convexity in contrast to the convex shape seen in epidural hematoma. This patient was comatose on arrival in the emergency room and taken emergently to the operating theater for a left-sided craniotomy and evacuation of the SDH. Also seen is significant subfalcine herniation *(red arrows)* (axial computed tomography).

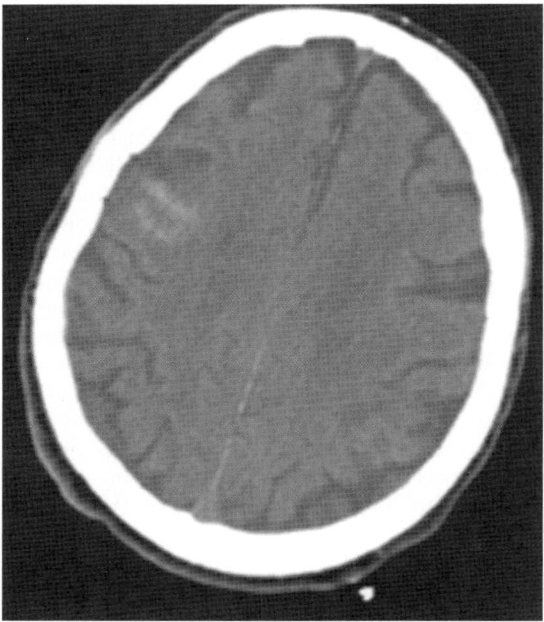

**Fig. 62.8** Axial computed tomography scan of a 35-year-old trauma patient with a traumatic subarachnoid hemorrhage in the right frontal gyrus.

**Diffuse axonal injury** is a very common severe head injury associated with significant morbidity. It is characterized clinically by rapid progression to coma in the absence of specific focal lesions. Adam classified DAI as mild, moderate, or severe. The duration of coma after a TBI correlates with the severity of DAI. Patients who survive the most severe form rapidly lapse into coma and remain unconscious, vegetative, or severely disabled.

DAI is a result of shearing, stretching, and/or angular forces pulling on axons and small vessels. Impaired axonal transport leads to focal axonal swelling and may result in axonal disconnection. The most common locations are the corticomedullary (gray matter/white matter) junction (particularly in the frontal and temporal areas), internal capsule, deep gray matter, upper brainstem, and corpus callosum.

MRI is more sensitive than CT in detecting DAI. Gradient echo MRI is most sensitive to areas of hemorrhage, and fluid-attenuated inversion recovery images are best for visualizing nonhemorrhagic lesions. DTI is a new imaging technology that is more sensitive to DAI than is conventional MRI. With DTI, the connectivity and integrity of neuronal tracts can be investigated. DTI is important when a tissue–such as the neural axons in white matter of the brain–have an internal structure. Water molecules will then diffuse more rapidly in the direction aligned with the internal structure and more slowly as they move perpendicular to the preferred direction. With this information, injury to the white matter (diffusion anisotropy) can be detected and neural tracts followed through the brain (Fig. 62.9). DTI measurements

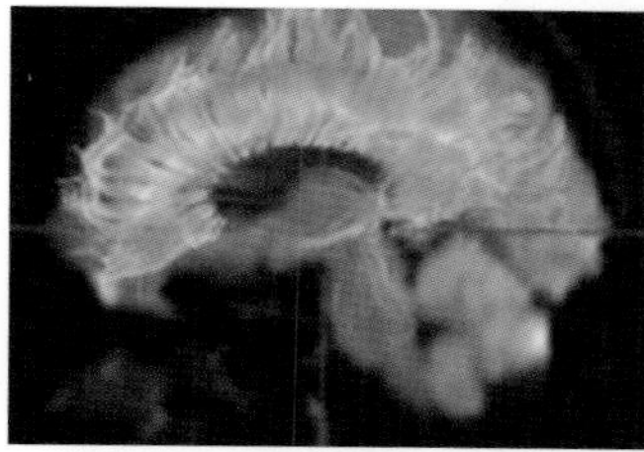

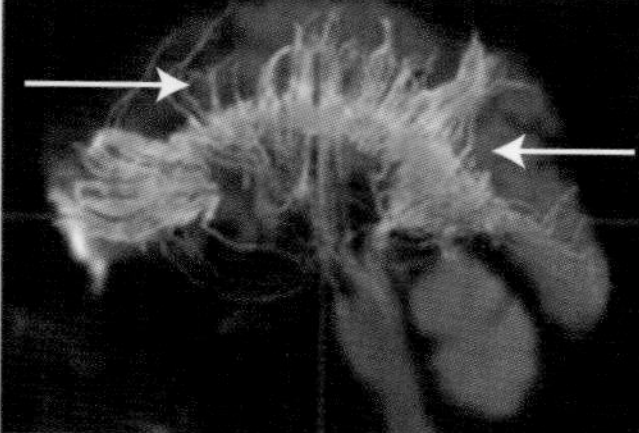

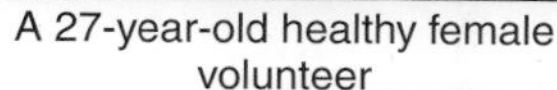

A 27-year-old healthy female volunteer

A 26-year-old male with DAI

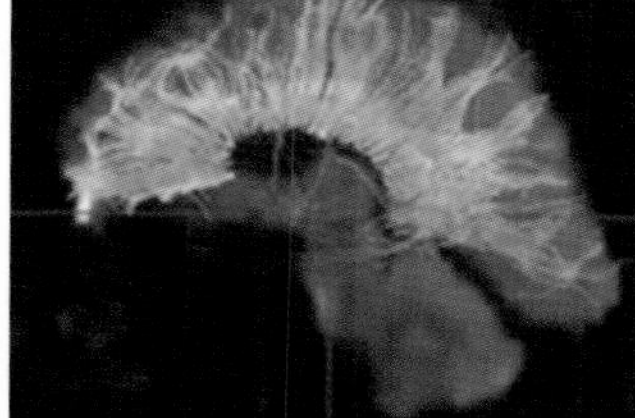

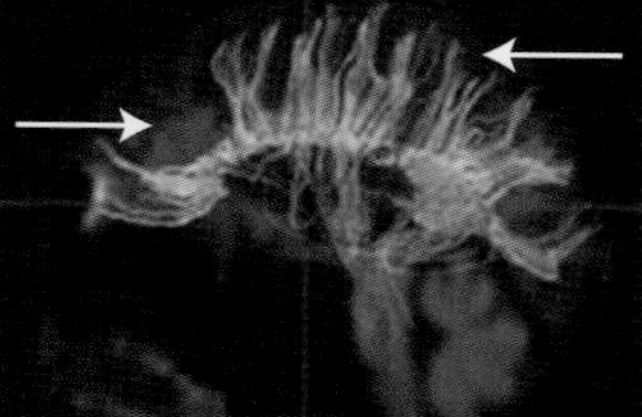

A 36-year-old healthy male volunteer

A 34-year-old male with DAI

**Fig. 62.9 Two Examples of Diffuse Axonal Injury (DAI).** Diffusion tensor imaging fiber tractography from the seed area around the corpus callosum on the left side midsagittal image. Fewer fibers extent to the frontal, parietal, and occipital regions in the DAI patients as compared with normal volunteers. *(Sugiyama, K., Kondo, T., Higano, S., Endo, M., Watanabe, H., Shindo, K. et al., 2007. Diffusion tensor imaging fiber tractography for evaluating. Brain Inj. 21, 413–19.)*

correlate with injury severity (acute GCS score) and outcome (Rankin score at discharge) (Li and Feng, 2009; Sugiyama et al., 2007).

## PATHOPHYSIOLOGY

Following primary brain injury, a cascade of cellular and biochemical events occurs in the initial minutes and extends into the subsequent weeks, leading to secondary neuronal degeneration (secondary brain injury) and, ultimately, neuronal impairment or cell death. Since the invention of the GCS, it has been possible to quantitate the degree of TBI in survivors so that they could be classified in terms of those that would go on to a full recovery and those who would remain disabled for life. The main drivers of such outcomes were thought to be secondary injuries (Kassi 2018). Much of the research concerning TBI is directed at affecting the mechanisms of secondary brain injury. These mechanisms include free-radical species, excitatory amino-acid toxicity, hypoxia, impaired cerebrovascular autoregulation, hyperthermia, blood-brain barrier breakdown, and hypercalcemia. Hypoxia and hypoperfusion are recognized as leading contributors to secondary brain injury. A single hypotensive episode in which systolic blood pressure falls below 90 mm Hg has been associated with worse outcomes after severe TBI (Chesnut, Marshall et al. 1993). All of these factors contribute to brain swelling, which leads to increased ICP, which further exacerbates secondary injury.

**Cerebrovascular dysregulation,** often seen after TBI, is thought to contribute to secondary brain ischemia. One study found that cerebral blood flow (CBF) that was decreased (<20 mL/100 g per minute) in the initial 24 hours after injury was associated with poor outcome.[3 4] Increased CSF levels of endothelin-1 are also implicated in cerebrovascular dysregulation. Elevated CBF is often seen, especially in children and younger trauma patients. An increase in cerebral perfusion pressure (CPP) can be detrimental for such patients. Multimodal monitoring with a CBF probe, cerebral oximetry, or transcranial Doppler can help to identify these patients so that elevated ICP can be treated appropriately.

**Diffuse cerebral swelling** after TBI may be a significant contributor to elevated ICP, which can result in further ischemia and brain damage. This swelling is thought to result from blood-brain barrier disruption (vasogenic edema), osmolar changes, and edema at the cellular level (cytotoxic or cellular edema). Hypoxia, hypoperfusion, inflammation, and oxidative stress can also contribute to cerebral swelling. Osmolar shifts occur primarily in areas of necrosis, where the osmolar load increases with the degradation of neurons. As reperfusion and recovery occur, water is drawn into the area secondary to the high osmolar load, and the surrounding neurons become edematous. Cellular swelling independent of osmolar load occurs primarily in astrocyte foot processes and is thought to be brought on by excitotoxicity and the uptake of glutamate.

After a TBI, excitotoxicity occurs upon the release of excessive amounts of excitatory amino acids such as glutamate, resulting in neuronal injury. Excitotoxic damage occurs in two phases: (1) sodium-dependent neuronal swelling followed by (2) delayed calcium-dependent neuronal degeneration. These effects are mediated through the activation of *N*-methyl-D-aspartate (NMDA) and glutamate receptors, leading to a rise in the intracellular calcium-mediated activation of proteases and lipases, which facilitates neuronal degeneration and necrotic cell death. In contrast to necrotic cell death, apoptosis or programmed cell death is marked not by swelling and dissolution of cell membranes but rather by DNA fragmentation and the formation of apoptotic cell bodies associated with neuronal shrinkage. Apoptosis is a cellular event triggered by intrinsic mechanisms (initiated in the mitochondria) or extrinsic mechanisms (the tumor necrosis factor superfamily of cell-surface death receptors), which activate a cascade of enzymes called caspases and lead to cell termination. Apoptosis is thought to contribute to secondary neuronal injury after a TBI event. Animal studies have shown that developing neurons are more susceptible than mature neurons to excitotoxic injury, probably because more calcium is transmitted via the NMDA-mediated calcium channel in the immature brain.[7] However, although the administration of NMDA antagonists following TBI in immature rats led to decreased excitotoxic-mediated neuronal death, apoptotic cell death increased. The role of excitotoxicity and apoptosis following trauma to the developing brain warrants further investigation.

Preclinical studies have also recently begun giving insights into inflammation (dependent processes such as spreading depolarization and tissue loss) as another disease process responsible for amplifying the initial TBI injury. After the initial insult, an inflammatory milieu is created secondary to leftover debris from damaged cells. As part of the subsequent inflammatory response, microglial cells are drawn to this damaged region and, while attempting to phagocytose debris, are activated into a "proinflammatory phenotype" (Lampron et al., 2015). Subsequent to such activation, for reasons yet to be determined, the response escalates into death of the microglia by a destructive process, pyroptosis, which can exacerbate cell loss (Lee et al., 2018). Indeed, the interaction between proinflammatory microglia and the microenvironment of the injured brain may explain why the region immediately adjacent to injury, known as the penumbra, is lost in the weeks following the initial insult (Lee et al., 2018). Additionally, such microglial death results in the persistence of injury-induced debris, which may lead to the development of TBI-induced autoantibodies (Zhang et al., 2014) and contribute to a state of chronic inflammation that lasts for years after the primary injury (Cole et al., 2018; Ramlackhansingh et al., 2011; Tomaiuolo et al., 2012). Evidence for an inflammatory disease component to TBI is also found in the CSF, where interleukin-6 (IL-6), IL-8, and soluble adhesion molecules (sP-selectin and intercellular adhesion molecule [sICAM-1]) were increased following TBI (Scott Gentleman 2017/8 Minocycline trial). As our understanding of the underlying disease processes grows, techniques to manage them will also have to evolve.

## TREATMENT

### Evaluation

Early intervention is essential if TBI care is to succeed. As in any emergency situation, the ABCs (airway, breathing, and circulation) also apply to TBI. Another priority of prehospital care is to optimize perfusion and oxygenation so as to prevent hypoxia and hypertension. Once in the emergency room, further measures can be taken, if necessary, to achieve adequate cardiopulmonary function. Next, a neurological examination is performed to triage patients accordingly. The GCS score is widely used to convey the severity of TBI. However, a low GCS score upon arrival in the emergency room may be the result of sedation in the field. Only after the patient has been weaned from sedation can the severity of injury be accurately assessed. Trauma patients with altered mental status, pupillary asymmetry, and flexion or extension posturing are at high risk for a SDH or an EDH compressing the brain and brainstem and must be evaluated with a CT scan of the head. CT is central to acute TBI diagnosis. The two externally validated rules for when to require a CT scan after mild TBI are the Canadian CT Head Rule (CCTHR) (Stiell et al., 2001) and the New Orleans Criteria (NOC) (Haydel et al., 2000). These rules have 100% sensitivity for neurosurgical lesions and 83% to 98% sensitivity for nonoperative lesions. The CCTHR has greater specificity and hence has led to fewer CT scans than the NOC (Levine, 2010). Neither addresses the presence of coagulopathy and anticoagulation, which others deem to be important risk factors for intracranial hemorrhage (Cohen et al., 2006; Ivascu et al., 2008). These criteria were updated in 2007 by the World Health Organization Task Force on mild TBI and the Neurotraumatology Committee of the World Federation of Neurosurgical Societies (Fabbri et al., 2004) and in 2008 by the Centers for Disease Control and Prevention and the American College of Emergency Physicians. All in all, research findings agree on several indications for urgent CT scanning of the head after a minor TBI (see Table 62.2).

Depending on CT findings, TBI patients will undergo emergency surgery or nonoperative management. Neurocritical care and any therapeutic intervention, operative or nonoperative, have one goal: the prevention of secondary injury, which, unlike the irreversible primary injury, can be limited.

### Management of Diffuse Injuries

Patients with complicated **mild TBI** (positive CT findings) **and moderate TBI** are admitted to the ICU and followed with serial neurological examinations. Intracranial complications are uncommon after a mild TBI;, in 6% to 12% of patients, however, CT shows abnormalities (Ibanez et al., 2001; Smits et al., 2005) in the form of a contusion, SAH, SDH, or EDH. As of now, another CT scan is obtained within 12 to 24 hours as standard of care in many hospitals. However, studies of 1 million emergency department visits for mild TBI have found that neurosurgical intervention was required in only 0.13% to 0.3% of these patients (Fabbri et al., 2004; Haydel et al., 2000; Jeret et al., 1993; Miller et al., 1996; Nagy et al., 1999). Over the past several years, evidence has suggested that the routine use of follow-up CT scans in patients with complicated mild TBI may not be necessary (Fabbri et al., 2008; Huynh et al., 2006; Nagy et al., 1999; Sifri et al., 2006; Velmahos et al., 2006). Most of these cases are nonoperative, and the patient can be discharged to home after a short observation period (Thiruppathy and Muthukumar, 2004). The only exception is an EDH, which can present

**TABLE 62.3 Grading of Concussion**

| Grade | Cantu System | American Academy of Neurology System |
|---|---|---|
| 1 (Mild) | A. PTA <30 min<br>B. No LOC | A. Transient confusion<br>B. No LOC<br>C. Symptoms resolved in <15 min |
| 2 (Moderate) | A. LOC <5 min, or<br>B. PTA >30 min | As above, but symptoms last >15 min (still *no* LOC) (PTA is common) |
| 3 (Severe) | A. LOC ≥5 min, or<br>B. PTA ≥ 24 h | *Any* LOC, whether brief (seconds) or prolonged |

*LOC*, Loss of consciousness; *PTA*, posttraumatic amnesia.

with a lucid interval after a brief loss of consciousness and then progress to coma and death (Levine, 2010).

**Concussions** are graded according to the severity of symptoms: presence or absence of loss of consciousness and time (more or less than 15 minutes) for resolution of symptoms (Table 62.3). Data to guide the treatment of concussion are lacking. Clinical experts suggest a benefit from the use of mild analgesics for headache, avoidance of narcotics, the use of meclizine or promethazine, and vestibular exercise for dizziness. Brief seizures may occur immediately after the initial impact and can easily be mistaken as a sign of a severe head injury.

Because 10% of all head **injuries are sports** related, return to play after concussion is an important issue. The American Academy of Neurology (1997), the Canadian Academy of Sports Medicine (2000), and several international symposia (McCrory et al., 2009) have developed guidelines for return to play after TBI, based mostly on expert opinion. Because no consensus has been reached regarding the most appropriate set of guidelines, the return-to-play decision remains in the realm of clinical judgment on an individualized basis. All guidelines agree that because of the potentially increased vulnerability of the brain to a second injury, a symptomatic player should never return to play. This sensitivity may outlast the symptoms, which tend to resolve within 1 week. Evidence indicates that after a concussion, metabolic equilibrium, and oxygen consumption of neurons are abnormal for several months. This suggests an initial and rapid phase of functional recovery, driven by compensatory mechanisms, followed by a prolonged neuronal recovery period during which subtle deficits in brain functioning are present but not apparent to standard clinical assessment tools (Ellemberg et al., 2009). The Balance Error Scoring System (BESS), Sensory Organization Test (SOT), and King-Devick test can be used to detect these deficits, but all have been found to be limited in their ability to differentiate more subtle deficits (Bell et al., 2011; Kontas et al., 2017; Mucha et al., 2014). The widely used Post-Concussion Symptom Scale (PCSS) is a self-reported scale used to determine concussion-related symptoms. Respondents quantify the severity of different postconcussive symptoms such as memory impairment, difficulty concentrating, etc., on a scale of 0 to 6 at successive time points postconcussion. Higher PCSS scores have been found to correspond to changes in activation patterns on functional MRI (fMRI) and poorer performance on cognitive tests (Chen et al., 2007). However, the subjective nature of the test, wide variability in test results, and the fact that a large number of healthy respondents also report high symptom scores means that this test should not be used in isolation (Dessy et al., 2017; Iverson and Lange, 2003). More recently, the vestibular and oculomotor screening (VOMS) assessment has been increasingly used due to its increased sensitivity, as it focuses on a more comprehensive examination of the vestibular system, which is commonly affected in concussion and mild TBI (Akin et al., 2017; Heitger et al., 2009; Kontas et al., 2017;

**TABLE 62.4 Guidelines for the Management of Sport-Related Concussion***

| Symptoms | First Concussion | Second Concussion |
|---|---|---|
| *Grade 1:* No loss of consciousness, transient confusion, resolution of symptoms and mental abnormalities in <15 min† | Remove from play<br>Examine at 5-min intervals<br>May return to play if symptoms disappear and results of mental function examination return to normal within 15 min | Allow return to play after 1 wk if there are no symptoms at rest or with exertion |
| *Grade 2:* As above but with mental symptoms for ≥15 min | Remove from play and disallow play for rest of day<br>Examine for signs of intracranial lesion at sidelines and obtain further examination by a trained person on same day<br>Allow return to play after 1 wk if neurological examination is non-concerning | Allow return to play after 2-wk period of no symptoms at rest or with exertion<br>Remove from play for season if imaging shows abnormality |
| *Grade 3:* Any loss of consciousness | Perform thorough neurological examination in hospital and obtain imaging studies when indicated<br>Assess neurological status daily until postconcussive symptoms resolve or stabilize<br>Remove from play for 1 wk if loss of consciousness lasts seconds or for 2 wk if it lasts minutes; must be asymptomatic at rest and with exertion to return to play | Withhold from play until symptoms have been absent for at least 1 mo |

*These guidelines reflect consensus opinion, are not evidence-based, and are under revision. Adapted from the American Academy of Neurology guidelines.

†Testing includes orientation, repetition of digit strings, recall of word list at 0 and 5 min, recall of recent game events, recall of current events, pupillary symmetry, finger-to-nose and tandem-gait tests, Romberg test, and provocative testing for symptoms with a 4-yd (3.5-m) sprint, five push-ups, and five knee bends.

Mucha et al., 2014). Deficits in the vestibulospinal and vestibulo-ocular systems have been associated with prolonged recovery and can dictate how long before a patient can return to baseline performance (Corwin et al., 2015; Kontos et al., 2017; Lau et al., 2011). Depending on the grade of the concussion, the athlete may resume play within 1 week or 1 month (Mayers, 2008; Table 62.4). An objective measure of postural stability increases the sensitivity to ongoing neurological impairment in the return-to-play decision-making process and minimizes the consequences of mitigating factors such as practice effects and motivation. During recovery after a concussion, it is important to emphasize to the athlete that physical and cognitive rest are required as long as the athlete is symptomatic. As knowledge grows regarding the role of the vestibular and oculomotor systems in concussion, rehabilitation techniques are moving toward early return to activity and attempting to avoid prolonged rest (Alsalaheen, et al., 2010; Ciuffreda et al., 2008; Kontos et al., 2017; Schneider et al., 2014; Thiagarajan et al., 2014).

Management of nonoperative **severe TBI** is directed by the evidence-based *Guidelines for the Management of Severe Traumatic Brain Injury*. The most recent (third) edition was published in 2007 by the Brain Trauma Foundation (Povlishock and Bullock, 2007; Table 62.5). With severe TBI, **ICP-guided therapy** is the fundamental principle underlying all treatment. Patients with a GCS score less than or equal to 8 qualify for ICP monitoring. The gold standard remains the external ventricular drain (EVD), which allows both ICP measurement and CSF drainage to reduce ICP. Other, more expensive options are fiberoptic or microscopic strain-gauge devices, which are placed in the brain parenchyma. These devices cannot be recalibrated during monitoring and have a negligible drift. Subarachnoid, subdural, and epidural monitors measure ICP via a fluid-coupled or pneumatic mechanism and are less accurate than an EVD.

An escalating protocol should be followed to control ICP (Table 62.6), using sedation **hyperosmolar therapy** in the form of mannitol and hypertonic saline and hyperventilation. Currently, patients with increased ICP initially receive a continuous 3% saline infusion and 250-mL boluses if needed. Mannitol is reserved for emergency situations such as an acutely dilated pupil and imminent brain herniation. Serum sodium can be elevated safely to 155 mEq/L and a serum osmolality of 320 mOsm/kg. Beyond those levels, renal failure can develop. If hypertonic saline administration is stopped suddenly, rebound intracranial hypertension is a risk but can be avoided by tapering the hypertonic saline solution over 48 hours.

The *TBI Guidelines* recommend striving for a CPP above 60 mm Hg, a change from the goal of 70 mm Hg in the second edition published in 2000. Although maintaining CPP this high is helpful in patients with posttraumatic vasospasm, it can be harmful in patients with cerebral hyperemia. Multimodality monitoring can be helpful to identify this subpopulation with hyperemia. Vasoactive pharmacological agents must be used with caution. They may have effects on cerebral vasomotor tone, causing vasoconstriction in the brain, and should be used only if the patient's neurological status worsens and CPP cannot be maintained with intravenous fluids alone.

**Hyperventilation** has the potential to reduce ICP via reflex vasoconstriction in the presence of hypocapnia. The vasoconstriction leads to decreases in CBF, overall cerebral fluid volume, and therefore ICP. The potential dangers associated with inducing hypocapnia are related to the resultant vasoconstriction. Excessive hypocapnia may lead to ischemia secondary to insufficient CBF. Therefore it is not recommended in the first 24 hours after TBI or prophylactically. Individual autoregulation of CBF with respect to hypocapnia varies widely and is difficult to predict. The measurement of brain tissue oxygenation can help to guide hyperventilation.

**Paralysis** is less frequently used to lower ICP because of a higher incidence of ventilator-associated pneumonia and longer hospital stays.

ICP that remains elevated despite maximal medical treatment is an indication for **decompressive craniectomy (DC)**. Depending on the underlying pathology, one side of the skull or the frontal bone bilaterally (Kjellberg procedure) is removed to give the swollen brain more room. Clinical trials analyzing the effectiveness of unilateral or bilateral DC, as either an early or late tier treatment, have demonstrated that although surgical decompression can be a useful option

**TABLE 62.5 Guidelines for the Management of Severe Traumatic Brain Injury**

| Topic | Level 1 | Level 2 | Level 3 |
|---|---|---|---|
| Blood pressure and oxygenation | Insufficient data | Avoid systolic blood pressure <90 mm Hg | Avoid hypoxia ($Pao_2$ <60 mm Hg or $O_2$ saturation <90%) |
| Hyperosmolar therapy | Insufficient data | Mannitol is effective for control of raised ICP at doses of 0.25 g/kg to 1 g/kg body weight | Restrict mannitol use prior to ICP monitoring in patients with signs of transtentorial herniation |
| Prophylactic hypothermia | Insufficient data | Insufficient data | Pooled data indicate that prophylactic hypothermia is not significantly associated with decreased mortality as compared with normothermic controls |
| Infection prophylaxis | Insufficient data | Periprocedural antibiotics for intubation should be administered to reduce the incidence of pneumonia<br>Early tracheostomy should be performed to reduce days on mechanical ventilation with pneumonia | To reduce infection, routine ventricular catheter exchange or prophylactic antibiotic use for ventricular catheter placement is not recommended |
| Deep venous thrombosis prophylaxis | Insufficient data | Insufficient data | Intermittent pneumatic compression stockings are recommended<br>Low-molecular-weight heparin or low-dose unfractionated heparin should be used in combination with mechanical prophylaxis |
| Indications for ICP monitoring | Insufficient data | ICP should be monitored in all salvageable patients with a GCS score of 3–8 after resuscitation and an abnormal CT scan | ICP monitoring is indicated in patients with severe TBI with a normal CT scan if >40 yr of age with blood pressure <90 mm Hg |
| ICP pressure-monitoring technology | N/A | N/A | N/A |
| ICP thresholds | Insufficient data | Treatment should be initiated with ICP >20 mm Hg | A combination of ICP values and clinical and brain CT findings should be used to determine the need for treatment |
| Cerebral perfusion thresholds | Insufficient data | Aggressive attempts to maintain CPP above 70 mm Hg with fluids and pressors should be avoided because of the risk of adult respiratory distress syndrome | CPP of <50 mm Hg should be avoided<br>The CPP value to target lies within the range of 50–70 mm Hg. Patients with intact pressure autoregulation tolerate higher CPP values. Ancillary monitoring of cerebral parameters that include blood flow, oxygenation, or metabolism facilitates CPP management |
| Brain oxygen monitoring and thresholds | Insufficient data | Insufficient data | Jugular venous saturation (<50%) or brain tissue oxygen tension (<15 mm Hg) are treatment thresholds |
| Anesthetics, analgesics, sedatives | Insufficient data | Prophylactic administration of barbiturates to induce burst suppression electroencephalogram is not recommended. High-dose barbiturate administration is recommended to control elevated ICP refractory to maximum standard medical and surgical treatment. Hemodynamic stability is essential before and during barbiturate therapy. Propofol is recommended for the control of ICP but not for improvement in mortality or 6-mo outcome | N/A |

**TABLE 62.5 Guidelines For The Management Of Severe Traumatic Brain Injury—cont'd**

| Topic | Level 1 | Level 2 | Level 3 |
|---|---|---|---|
| Nutrition | Insufficient data | Patients should be fed to attain full caloric replacement by day 7 postinjury | N/A |
| Antiseizure prophylaxis | Insufficient data | Anticonvulsants are indicated to decrease the incidence of early PTS (within 7 days of injury) | N/A |
| Hyperventilation | Insufficient data | Prophylactic hyperventilation ($Paco_2$ of 25 mm Hg or less) is not recommended | Hyperventilation is recommended as a temporizing measure for the reduction of ICP. Hyperventilation should be avoided during the first 24 hours after injury, when cerebral blood flow is often critically reduced. If hyperventilation is used, jugular venous oxygen saturation ($SjO_2$) or brain-tissue oxygen tension ($PbtO_2$) measurements are recommended to monitor oxygen delivery |
| Steroids | The use of high-dose methylprednisolone is associated with increased mortality and is contraindicated | N/A | N/A |

*CT,* Computed tomography; *CPP,* cerebral perfusion pressure; *ICP,* intracranial pressure; *GCS,* Glasgow Coma Scale; *PTS,* posttraumatic seizures; *TBI,* traumatic brain injury.

for intractable ICP, it is not without risk. The DC in diffuse traumatic brain injury (DECRA) trial evaluated early bifrontotemporoparietal decompressive craniotomy. It demonstrated that although this approach was beneficial for reducing ICP, it was associated with a lower 6-month score on the Extended Glasgow Outcome Scale (EGOS) and a greater number of complications in subjects such as those with bilateral blown pupils (Cooper et al., 2011). However, this trial was later criticized for including patients with only a short duration of elevated ICP, inadequately controlling for multicenter enrollment and not standardizing rehabilitation care (Honeybul et al., 2013; Kassi et al., 2019). The Rescue ICP randomized trial showed that DC as a late-stage treatment was effective at reducing mortality and increasing independent living at home as compared with medical management in TBI patients with intractable ICP. However, this improvement came at the cost of higher rates of being in a vegetative state and dependency on others for care in the surgical cohort (Hutchinson et al., 2016). Furthermore, there was a statistically significant difference in favorable outcome rates between trial and control subjects at 12 months but not at 6 months, suggesting that the benefits of DC may be delayed. One systematic review found that 1 out of 10 patients with DC may experience complications, including subdural effusion, hydrocephalus, and infection (Kurland et al., 2015). Other studies suggest that this rate may be even higher (Ban et al., 2010; Gopalakrishnan et al., 2018). Complications such as posttraumatic hydrocephalus are higher in patients after DC, possibly as a result of disturbances of CSF dynamics and normal physiological function after DC. Bilateral DC is sometimes performed but can also be associated with an unfavorable outcome in 46% of cases (Bao et al., 2010). Some patients suffer delayed neurological deterioration, described as the "syndrome of the trephined," in which brain function is thought to be impaired by the atmospheric pressure. Given the potential for poor outcomes, the risks and benefits of DC must be weighed carefully in deciding on the appropriate course of action.

**Hypothermia** is an alternative therapy that should be reserved for patients with persistent intracranial hypertension refractory to other medical or surgical interventions. A recent meta-analysis of all prospective TBI clinical trials found that therapeutic moderate hypothermia (32°–34°C, 89.6°–93.2°F) resulted in less mortality (relative risk [RR] 0.51; 95% confidence interval [CI] 0.33, 0.79) and an increased likelihood of a good outcome (RR 1.91; 95% CI 1.28, 2.85) compared with normothermia during acute care but that the risk of pneumonia increased (RR 2.37; 95% confidence interval [CI] 1.37, 4.10) (Peterson et al., 2008). Problems associated with hypothermia include increased bleeding risk, arrhythmias, and increased susceptibility to infection and sepsis.

The *Guidelines for the Management of Severe Traumatic Brain Injury (TBI)* recommend the use of **high-dose barbiturate** to control elevated ICP only after maximum standard medical and surgical treatment have failed. High-dose barbiturate therapy has shown to be effective in lowering ICP, but it has never been shown to improve outcome. High-dose pentobarbital, for example, has the potential benefit of suppressing cerebral metabolism and thus decreasing oxygen demand. Barbiturates have the added benefit of neuroprotection through mechanisms such as the inhibition of free-radical lipid peroxidation and neuronal membrane disruption. However, clearance of barbiturates from the body varies among patients, and titration of therapy based on serum levels is difficult. Instead, continuous electroencephalographic monitoring can be used to titrate barbiturate infusions to achieve burst suppression. Barbiturate therapy also has major disadvantages. It is associated with serious cardiac side effects, potentially leading to both myocardial depression and hypotension and thus offsetting any ICP-lowering effect it may have. The ability to perform a valid neurological examination is also lost when barbiturates are used to control ICP. Additionally, barbiturate therapy may result in immune suppression leading to sepsis.

**TABLE 62.6 Elevated ICP Management**

1. Verify ICP
   - Check if EVD is still patent
   - Check to see if EVD waveform is present and adequate
   - Check to see if EVD ICP correlates with intraparenchymal monitor if present
2. Check for 30-degree head elevation
3. Loosen cervical collar if in place
4. Open EVD for ICP >20 mm Hg for 10 min and then close and transduce ICP
   - Repeat once
   - If ICP >20 mm Hg, keep open at 15 mm Hg above midbrain and proceed with ICP module
5. Treat temperature >37.5°C with 650 mg of acetaminophen once
6. Sedation
   - Titrate propofol to a Ramsay score of 4
     Do not exceed 5 mg/kg/h for more than 24 h
   - Check potassium, triglycerides, creatine kinase, and urinalysis for myoglobinuria q 8 h for 24 h
   - If maximal dose of propofol is reached and ICP >20 mm Hg
     - Start fentanyl drip at 0.8 μg/kg/h
     - Apply bispectral index (BIS) monitor
     - Titrate fentayl drip to a bispectral index of 30 or to a maximum of 5 μg/kg/h
     - Start chlorhexidine gluconate (Peridex) with a loading infusion of 1 μg/kg over 10 min

   Continue maintenance infusion of 0.2 to 0.7 μg/kg/h
6. Hyperosmolar therapy
   - 3% hypertonic saline bolus of 250 mL
     - Before administering 3% hypertonic saline bolus, check if Na <130 mEq/L
   - In emergency, administer mannitol 1–0.5 mg/kg bolus once
     - Check sodium and serum osmolality q 4 h × 2 after every bolus
   - Start 3% hypertonic saline drip at 0.5 mL/h if ≥ three 3% hypertonic saline boluses within 6 h
     - Check sodium and serum osmolality q 2 h while on drip
     - If sodium >160 mEq/L or serum osmolality >320 sOsm/L, call physician
     - If serum sodium has increased to >10 mEq/L within the last 24 h, call physician
     - If CBF > 35 mL/min/100 g white matter or >80 mL/min/100 g gray matter refer to CBF module high flow
7. If core body temperature ≥37.5°C, start normothermia protocol
8. Hyperventilation
   - Do not hyperventilate in the first 24 hours (goal of $Paco_2$ of 35–40 mm Hg)
   - If $PbtO_2$ is <20 mmHg, go to hypoxia module
   - If CBF <18 mL/min/100 g white matter or <67 mL/min/100 g gray matter, go to CBF module
   - If $PbtO_2$ and CBF are optimized, hyperventilate to 33–35 mm Hg
9. Radiology
   - Refractory ICP > 20 mm Hg despite intervention, obtain portable head CT without contrast immediately if no head CT since ICP is elevated despite maximal therapy
10. Consider surgery
11. Induce pentobarbital coma
    - Only for diffuse noneoperative injuries
    - Only with attending approval
    - Order continuous EEG monitoring if not already in place
    - Have norepinephrine drip ready at the bedside for MAP < 80 mm Hg/CPP < 60 mm Hg
    - Pentobarbital bolus/loading: 10 mg/kg once over 60 min, then 5 mg/kg qh × 4 or until burst suppression
    - Pentobarbital maintenance dose: 1 mg/kg/h titrated to burst suppression

*CBF*, Cerebral blood flow; *CPP*, cerebral perfusion pressure; *EEG*, electroencephalography; *EVD*, external ventricular drain; *ICP*, intracranial pressure; *MAP*, mean arterial pressure; *$PbtO_2$*, Brain tissue oxygen.

**Hemodynamic management** can be challenging after a severe TBI. Hypo-osmolar solutions should be avoided because they lead to an increase in ICP, and hyperosmolar treatments of elevated ICP such as mannitol can actually lower CPP. Normal saline is commonly used to achieve euvolemia. A hypertonic saline bolus with a 3% sodium solution is optimal for patients who are volume depleted, need to be resuscitated, or have elevated ICP. The advantage of hypertonic saline is that it remains intravascular longer than normal saline and has an osmolar mechanism of action similar to that of mannitol but without the diuretic effects. Other theoretical benefits of hypertonic saline include improvements in vasoregulation, cardiac output, immune modulation, and plasma volume expansion.

**Multimodality monitoring** is more frequently used now, at least in centers specializing in TBI. Besides ICP, other factors monitored in patients with severe TBI include partial brain-tissue oxygen tension ($PbtO_2$), CBF, microdialysis variables, bispectral index, and cerebral oximetry. ICP measurements alone are only surrogate measures of CBF, brain oxygenation, and cerebral metabolism. A combination of ICP, CBF, and $PbtO_2$ can lead to a better understanding of brain pathophysiology after TBI.

The ability to limit secondary brain injury after a severe TBI relies on ensuring the delivery of an adequate supply of oxygen and metabolic substrate to the brain and to detect TBI as early as possible. Once the ICP rises, it may be too late to intervene. By measuring **$PbtO_2$**, or brain tissue oxygen, directly, compromise in oxygen delivery should be detected earlier than by relying on ICP alone. Several studies have investigated the relationship between outcome and focal $PbtO_2$, which can be measured with the Licox monitor. It was found that the likelihood of death increased with the duration of time that $PbtO_2$ was less than 15 mm Hg, prompting one to ask whether oxygen-directed therapy will improve outcome; this has not been shown so far. The benefits of hyperoxemia after TBI are also unclear. Although mild hyperoxemia is beneficial in TBI patients, a study of 3420 patients found worse outcomes with extreme hyperoxemia ($O_2$ of 487 mm Hg). The detrimental effects of hyperoxemia have been demonstrated in patients with ischemic brain injury not due to TBI, but whether the same pathophysiological process of postreperfusion hyperoxemia is harmful in TBI remains to be determined (Davis et al., 2009).

Transcranial cerebral oximetry is a noninvasive technique for monitoring changes in **cerebral oxygenation.** The method relies on the measurement of absorption of light at multiple wavelengths with near-infrared spectrum, which allows the transmission of photons through skin, bone, brain, and CSF. The values obtained with near-infrared spectroscopy represent primarily the oxygenation status of the chromophores of the venous compartment (75%) or the cerebral vascular bed (arterial 20%, capillary 5%). Changes in transcranial cerebral oximetry result from changes in the balance between the cerebral oxygen supply and oxygen consumption. The Near Infrared Spectroscopy (NIRS) light emitter and a receiver are usually placed at the lateral forehead. Scalp edema and forehead abrasion can interfere with cerebral oximetry.

Knowing about $PbtO_2$ and CBF can help the treating physician to prevent secondary injury more effectively. Regional CBF can be measured with thermal diffusion probes along with $PbtO_2$ measurements. The latest edition of the *Guidelines for the management of severe traumatic brain injury* has commented on their usefulness of these catheters the first time. High ICP can be secondary to malignant brain edema due to decreased cerebral perfusion or hyperemia; treatment of high ICP would be very different. Treatment of high ICP due to malignant brain edema would entail hyperosmolar therapy to decrease the edema and increase CBF to maintain brain perfusion. Treatment of high ICP due to hyperemia would entail lowering CCP with aggressive hyperventilation.

The metabolic state of the brain can also be assessed with cerebral microdialysis, which monitors **energy metabolites** over extended periods, but only in a small focal volume of the brain. The threshold for abnormal metabolism is evidenced by the lactate/pyruvate ratio of 40. Microdialysis showed that in patients with severe TBI, tight systemic glucose control is associated with reduced cerebral extracellular glucose availability and increased prevalence of brain energy crisis (microdialysis glucose <0.7 mmol/L with a lactate/pyruvate ratio >40), which in turn correlates with increased mortality. Moreover, intensive insulin therapy may impair cerebral glucose metabolism after severe brain injury (Oddo et al., 2008). The combined use of microdialysis variables and $PbtO_2$—in addition to ICP, mean arterial pressure (MAP), and CPP—was found to have the best predictive accuracy for outcome after severe TBI (Low, 2009).

One conundrum that remains unsolved, even with multimodality monitoring, is the value of continuous information versus global information about the condition of the brain. Although $PbtO_2$ and CBF probes provide continuous information about these variables, they reflect only a very small portion of the brain. Positron emission tomography and xenon-enhanced CT can provide global information about the metabolic status of the brain and blood flow, but only at a given time.

Most patients with a severe TBI have **associated comorbidities** that can also lead to secondary brain injury. Hypoxia from adult respiratory distress syndrome or ventilator-associated pneumonia and hyperthermia from infection or sepsis are the most common. Comatose patients are at high risk for deep vein thrombosis and pulmonary embolism. Sequential compression stockings can be used for the first 48 hours after TBI. After the first 48 hours, subcutaneous heparin or low-molecular-weight heparin can be used safely.

Hyperthermia following a severe TBI is common, potentiates secondary injury, and worsens neurological outcome. Induced normothermia (36.5°C–37.5°C) via an intravascular cooling catheter is effective prophylaxis to reduce fever burden (Puccio et al., 2009).

No class 1 evidence yet exists to guide the decision for blood transfusion (whether and when) after a severe TBI. Although intuitively it makes sense that increasing a patient's hematocrit will lead to increased oxygen delivery to the brain, this benefit has not been clearly shown. Over recent years, evidence has emerged that blood transfusion may actually have a negative effect after TBI, even after controlling for anemia as a possible confounder (Carlson et al., 2006); stored blood has decreased deformability and may, in fact, exacerbate ischemia.

## Management of Focal Injuries

Patients with focal TBI and axial or extra-axial bleeding with mass effect are treated surgically. Sometime patients with mass lesion without signs of mass effect and controlled ICP may be managed nonoperatively with intracranial monitoring and serial imaging. However, the development of mass effect can result in secondary brain injury, posing the risk of further neurological deterioration, herniation, and death. This condition necessitates emergent neurosurgical intervention. Traumatic SAH rarely causes any mass effect or warrants neurosurgical intervention. Patients with severe TBI and only traumatic SAH on CT scan are managed nonoperatively with intracranial monitoring and serial imaging.

Various surgical techniques have been advocated to evacuate intracranial hemorrhages. The most commonly used is craniotomy with or without subtemporal DC. Sometimes a large decompressive hemicraniectomy is performed at the same time if the brain appears swollen intraoperatively. Preoperative CT can help to predict malignant brain swelling. More midline shift than one would expect from the extra-axial hematoma, effacement of basal cisterns and sulci, and loss of gray-white matter differentiation are warning signs.

Between 22% and 50% of patients with EDH are comatose on admission or immediately before surgery. Additionally, 47% of patients with an EDH have a lucid interval (i.e., they awaken after initial unconsciousness and then deteriorate neurologically), which may obscure the development of an EDH. A patient with an EDH can go from normal neurological status to coma within minutes. Most often, the patient becomes agitated and restless and may have an episode of emesis because of the increased ICP. This is generally followed by focal neurological signs such as hemiparesis, seizures, pupillary dilation, decrease in consciousness, and, in the worst-case scenario, decortication. Because of the strong association between skull fractures and EDH, screening x-rays of the skull can help to identify the risk for an EDH. The guidelines for the surgical management of acute epidural hematomas, published in 2006, list the following criteria for surgical evacuation of an EDH (Bullock et al., 2006c):

- An EDH greater than 30 $cm^3$ should be evacuated regardless of the GCS score.
- An EDH less than 30 $cm^3$ in volume and less than 15-mm thick, with less than 5-mm midline shift in patients with a GCS score less than or equal to 8 without focal deficit can be managed nonoperatively with serial CT scanning and close neurological observation in a facility with neurosurgical coverage.

Regarding timing, emergent surgical evacuation is strongly recommended for comatose (GCS score ≤8) patients with an acute EDH. Emergent craniotomy for evacuation also is indicated if an EDH thicker than 1 cm develops or leads to neurological symptoms. The mortality for patients in all age groups and GCS scores who require surgery for evacuation of EDH is approximately 10% compared with 5% in the pediatric population.

The 2006 *Guidelines for the Surgical Management of SDH* give the following criteria for cases of SDH (Bullock et al., 2006):

- An acute SDH thicker than 10 mm or causing a midline shift greater than 5 mm on CT scans should be surgically evacuated regardless of the patient's GCS score.
- A comatose patient (GCS score ≤8) with an SDH less than 10-mm thick and midline shift less than 5 mm should undergo surgical evacuation of the lesion if the GCS score decreased by 2 or more points between the time of injury and hospital admission, the pupils are asymmetric or fixed and dilated, or ICP exceeds 20 mm Hg.
- ICP monitoring should be performed in all comatose (GCS score ≤8) patients with an acute SDH.

The GCS score, pupillary examination, comorbidities, CT findings, age, and, in delayed decisions, ICP, influence the decision to evacuate an acute SDH. Neurological deterioration over time is common and can also influence the decision to operate. Although the time from neurological deterioration to surgery influences outcome, optimal timing of surgery is difficult to pinpoint because most patients who undergo early surgery for SDH also have a more severe injury and worse outcome than patients undergoing delayed evacuation. The magnitude of preoperative midline shift also seems to correlate with unfavorable outcome (Nelson et al., 2010). Age is an independent predictor of outcome in patients with SDH: Age older than 65 years is statistically correlated with poorer outcome. A study showed that at 3 months after SDH evacuation, patients between 18 and 30 years of age had 25% mortality, whereas those aged 50 years and older had 75% mortality.

Isolated linear **fractures** are usually of little clinical significance unless they are near or traverse a suture or they involve a venous sinus groove or vascular channel. In those cases, complications may include suture diastasis, venous sinus thrombosis, and EDH. Although rare, a growing linear skull fracture can develop in young children, especially if the parietal bone is fractured. CSF pulsation and pressure then prevent the bone from healing and cause enlargement of the fracture. A tear in the dura under the fracture is usually the underlying cause. Surgical obliteration of the CSF leak is needed so that the skull fracture can heal.

Patients with simple ("closed") **depressed cranial fractures** may be treated nonoperatively if there is no clinical or radiographic evidence of dural penetration (pneumocephalus), significant intracranial hematoma, depression greater than 1 cm, frontal sinus involvement, cosmetic deformity, or gross wound contamination. Compound (open) depressed skull fractures are associated with infections and the development of late epilepsy. They undergo surgical debridement and elevation to decrease the possibility of infection. Also, any neurological deficit that can be associated with the skull fracture, whether open or closed, is an indication for surgery. The *Guidelines for Surgical Management of Depressed Cranial Fractures* recommend the routine administration of antibiotics.

As stated earlier, it is important to consider a patient's medication history when TBI is being evaluated. Use of anticoagulants, specifically new oral anticoagulants (NOACs), which directly inhibit thrombin and factor Xa, can increase the risk of intracranial hemorrhagic complications. These medications are a superior alternative to warfarin but are more difficult to reverse when acute TBI treatment is necessary (Zeeshan et al., 2018). Only within the last 3 years has the US Food and Drug Administration approved two new reversal agents, idarucizumab and andexanet alfa, which have been found to be effective at reversing the effects of anticoagulation safely and rapidly (Connolly et al., 2016; Pollack et al., 2017). However, the clinical benefit, especially in non–life threatening hemorrhage, has yet to be determined, as the reversal is present for only about 2 hours after the infusion and no patients needing neurosurgical intervention were evaluated.

Another potential cause of bleeding events during TBI management is coagulopathy (Maegele, 2013; Zhang et al., 2012). Changes in coagulation test values such as prothrombin time (PT) and partial thromboplastin time (PTT) are typically used to determine the presence of such pathologies. However, these tests have not been found to be perfectly sensitive or specific in determining which TBI patients can progress to having intracranial hemorrhage (Kurland et al., 2012). Thromboelastography (TEG) is an alternative technique that can assess for coagulopathies in TBI patients much more accurately than traditional coagulation tests as it measures whole-blood viscoelastic properties (Rao et al,. 2017; Martin et al., 2018).

## LATE COMPLICATIONS

Late complications from head injury include seizures, hormonal disturbances, posttraumatic hydrocephalus, postconcussion syndrome, and psychosocial problems. **Posttraumatic seizures** (PTSs) can be categorized as early (<7 days after TBI) or late (>7 days after TBI). Early PTSs are seen in 30% of all patients with a severe TBI and in about 1% of those with mild or moderate TBI. The estimated incidence of late-onset PTS is 13% within 2 years after severe TBI. PTSs are more common in children and after penetrating head injuries (50%). Anticonvulsants are used to prevent early seizures but should not be given for more than 7 days because this practice does not decrease the frequency of late PTSs.

**Posttraumatic hormonal disturbances** can contribute to fatigue and impede recovery after a TBI. Hypopituitarism occurs in approximately 25% of patients with a severe TBI. It may be underrecognized due to its subtle clinical manifestations. Most common are deficiencies in growth hormone, gonadotropin, and corticotropin levels. A routine neuroendocrine evaluation should be included in all follow-up examinations of patients with a severe TBI.

**Posttraumatic communicating hydrocephalus** has an incidence of 14% in severe head injuries.

**Postconcussion syndrome** has an incidence of 4%–59%. The entire spectrum of TBI severity is associated with a risk for psychiatric conditions and long-standing neurological deficits. Functional MRI has shown that working memory recruitment is different even 1 year after mild TBI compared with healthy controls (McAllister et al. 2006; Fig. 62.10). Therefore thorough neurocognitive assessment after these patients are released from an acute care hospital is imperative to offer them the best chance for recovery. Approaches used to treat neurocognitve deficits have included cognitive and behavioral therapy along with pharmacological treatment.

Psychosocial problems such as decreased social contact, anxiety, depression, and loneliness create a major challenge for the majority of TBI victims and can lead to aggression and substance abuse and hinder community reentry. Psychosocial problems are a persistent long-term problem and can interfere with rehabilitation. Individuals who experience a severe TBI are vulnerable to a loss of friendships and social support, which leads to social isolation, fewer leisure activities, and new dependence on others. This situation is aggravated by a lack of opportunity to establish new social contacts and friends. Clinicians such as psychiatric social workers, psychologists, or psychiatrists may have to be called upon more often to provide the psychological services that may be necessary for many of these patients.

## OUTCOME

Outcome after severe TBI remains poor; approximately one-third die, and 25% survive with severe disabilities. A number of factors play an important role in predicting outcome. One study retrospectively analyzed 846 cases of severe TBI to clarify the prognostic effects of multiple factors (Jiang et al., 2002). One year after injury, GCS score, age, pupillary response and size, hypoxia, hyperthermia, and ICP were associated with outcome, indicating that prevention of hypoxia and hyperthermia and control of high ICP may be useful ways of improving the outcome of patients with severe head injury. A GCS score of 3 on presentation has been recognized as a poor prognostic factor. Mortality approaches 100% in the presence of bilateral fixed dilated pupils.

Age in itself is an independent predictor of outcome. With or without surgery, outcome in the elderly is worse than in the young. Different age thresholds have been named in the literature. Depending on the statistical analysis performed, one study found worse outcomes above 39 and 65 years of age. Multiple regression analysis showed that every 10 years above this threshold increase in age led to a 10% increase in mortality. Even with timely and satisfactory surgery, unexplained clinical deterioration occurs in patients 70 years of age or older.

For people 65 years of age and older, falls are the leading cause of TBI-related death, accounting for 40% of all TBI deaths in that age group. Additionally, falls can cause other injuries such as hip fractures, which can impede independent living and increase the risk of premature death. An epidemiological study over 10 years showed that fall-related TBI increased by 126% and the related case fatality rate decreased from 32% to 18%, meaning that more elderly people are living with TBI disabilities. However, rehabilitation efforts in the elderly have been poor because of the often negative attitude (ageism) toward the recovery potential in this group. Despite their relative disadvantages, the elderly might see improved outcomes with rehabilitation programs intended for their age group.

Some CT findings can predict outcome. The length, width, depth, and location of SDH and EDH; number, volume, and location of

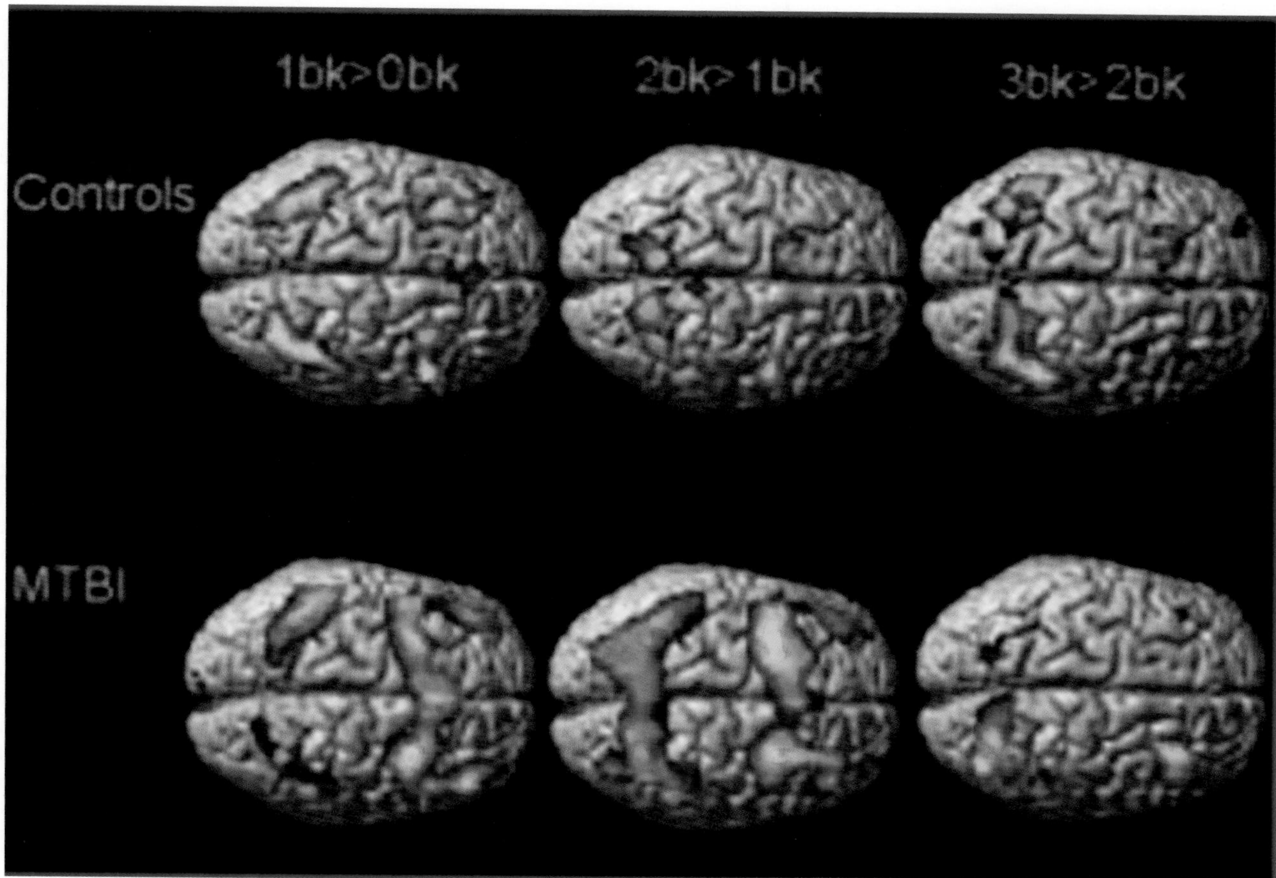


**Fig. 62.10** Surface-rendered projection of areas of activation as a function of working memory (WM) processing load for mild traumatic brain injury (TBI) and control groups. Note increased activation in bilateral frontal and parietal regions, consistent with activation of WM circuitry in both groups. The mild TBI group showed significantly more activation associated with the moderate processing load condition (2 back–1 back), and very little further left hemispheric increase in activation at the higher processing load condition (3 back–2 back). Controls show more of a bilateral stepwise increase in activation in response to increases in processing load (2 back–1 back; 3 back–2 back). *(From McAllister, T.W., Flashman, L.A., McDonald, B.C., Saykin, A.J., 2006. Mechanisms of working memory dysfunction after mild and moderate TBI: Evidence from functional MRI and neurogenetics. J. Neurotrauma. 23, 1450–67.)*

contusions; compression of ventricles and the basal cistern; and presence or absence of traumatic SAH are all relevant. The most important CT-defined predictor of outcome is the magnitude of the midline shift (Nelson et al., 2010).

Finally, the facility where patients with TBI are treated affects outcome. Patient with severe TBI treated in American College of Surgeons (ACS)–designated level 1 trauma centers have better survival rates and outcomes than those treated in ACS-designated level 2 centers (DuBose et al., 2008).

It is very important to provide goal-concordant care for patients with severe TBI, especially as it is difficult to predict outcome and many interventions currently can prolong life but have not been shown to improve functional outcome. Patients may consider some forms of functional or cognitive disability as worse than death, and simply understanding the terminal nature of their disease or having an end-of-life (EOL) discussion with their physician can steer patients away from preferring life-extending therapies (Lilley et al., 2018; Mack et al., 2010; Rubin, 2015). Elderly patients in particular ofen prefer no treatment over treatment that would leave them with cognitive disabilities.

However, physicians are often reluctant to initiate EOL conversations, and the TBI patient is often unable to vocalize his or her preferences for treatment; therefore the burden of deciding between palliative care versus life-extending care is often falls on the surrogate decision maker (Pino et al., 2016). Lack of formal training in goal-of-care and EOL discussion often cited as one of the barriers. Medical schools and governing bodies have recognized that and have begun paying more attention to goal-concordant care. Shared decision making (SDM)—where disease prognosis and treatment risks and benefits are communicated to patients and their family members using cartoons, symbols, and other cues called decision aids (Muehlschlegel et al., 2015)—is an example of a potential workaround to this problem.

As treatments improve and patients live longer with TBI deficits, transparent communication between surrogate decision makers, providers, and—to the extent possible—patients, will become a necessary part of the TBI management protocol. The following five-step process has been suggested: (1) collection of evidence, (2) information sharing, (3) critical appraisal, (4) recommendation and decision, and (5) assessment and follow-up. Using this framework, the physician can better understand the patient's values and preferences while building rapport with the family, determining any bias-inducing information, and recommend decisions through an every-10-year SDM model with appropriate follow-up at the end. Another communication tool specially developed for emergency situations and surgeons is the "Best Case/Worst Case" tool, which has been shown to facilitate the discussion around EOL values and care (Kruser et al., 2017).

## FUTURE OF TRAUMATIC BRAIN INJURY

The improvement of neurological outcome after TBI over the last three decades can be attributed only to faster recognition and earlier treatment of secondary injury. To this date there is no medication that can improve TBI outcome and most therapeutic clinical trials in TBI have failed.

An important but poorly understood feature of TBI is spatiotemporal **progression or "blossoming" of a hemorrhagic contusion**. Between 25% and 50% of 'traumatic hemorrhagic contusions'? show evidence of progression during the acute postinjury period on serially obtained CT scans. The fact that such contusions and hematomas are possibly preventable makes this an attractive therapeutic target once the molecular mechanisms responsible for blossoming of hemorrhagic contusions are clarified (Simard et al., 2009).

Given the overlap of symptoms and mechanisms of mild TBI and posttraumatic stress disorder, an **objective diagnosis for mild TBI** is needed. Functional and metabolic imaging or brain-injury proteins may offer a solution. Such a tool could help to diagnose patients correctly and also propel mild TBI research.

The establishment of markers in brain injury, such as protein **biomarkers in TBI** care, could help in the diagnosis, triage, management, and prognosis for the very heterogeneous population of TBI victims. Doing so also may help to identify patients with TBI of similar severity so that they can be allocated appropriately to TBI trials. S-100Beta, a calcium binding protein expressed primarily by astrocytes, has the potential to serve as a good screening biomarker because of its high sensitivity for abnormal findings on CT scans of the head. Initially S-100B was used to see which patients with mild TBI should have a head CT; this was the first attempt to introduce biomarkers in clinical TBI care (Unden and Romner, 2009). An analysis showed that if blood test results require less time than imaging and if head CT scan rates for patients with isolated mild TBI are relatively high, S-100B will lower costs (Ruan et al., 2009).

A safe and effective neuroprotective treatment for acute-stage TBI has yet to be found. The search for a "magic bullet" drug targeting a single receptor for the treatment of TBI has failed thus far for a variety of reasons. The pathophysiology of ischemic brain injury and TBI involves several mechanisms leading to neuronal injury, including excitotoxicity, free-radical damage, inflammation, necrosis, and apoptosis.

In 2007 a randomized clinical trial of **progesterone** for acute TBI showed that intravenous administration of progesterone had no serious side effects and showed signs of benefit, especially in patients with moderate TBI (Wright et al., 2007). In 2009, a prospective randomized double-blind placebo-controlled clinical trial found a good safety profile for **cyclosporin A** infusion when given at the chosen dose of 5 mg/kg and infused over 24 hours during the early phase after severe TBI (Mazzeo et al., 2009). Because of its ability to preserve mitochondrial integrity in experimental brain injury models, cyclosporin A was recently proposed for use in humans after TBI to provide improved behavioral outcomes as well as significant histological protection. However, a phase 2 clinical trial assessing cyclosporin A in TBI (NCT02496975) was recently withdrawn due to the biphasic dose-response that was exhibited.

A new body of research around stem cell transplantation as a viable neuroprotective and neurorestorative therapy is slowly gaining ground. Mesenchymal stem cells have already been found to possess anti-inflammatory properties and have been applied successfully to animal TBI models (Hasan et al., 2017). Human fetal neural stem cells (hNSCs) have been shown to modulate the proinflammatory nature of microglia and the engraftment of transplanted hNSCs into surrounding parenchyma in a penetrating injury rat brain model has also been demonstrated (Cao et al., 2016; Spurlock et al., 2017). Tests in animal models with spinal cord injuries (SCIs) have demonstrated functional improvement after grafting transplanted hNSCs (Rosenzweig et al., 2018). hNSCs are already being used in clinical trials for amyotrophic lateral sclerosis (ALS), where they have been shown to improve survival and function in patients compared with historical controls (Goutman et al., 2018). It is only a matter of time before similar trials for TBI are initiated. Although the mechanism of action is yet to be completely elucidated, preliminary research indicates that the modulation of succinate may play a role (McGinley et al., 2018; Peruzzotti-Jametti et al., 2018).

Finally, **supplemental magnesium** has been considered because it affects many of the processes involved in secondary injury positively and consistently improves outcome in animal models of TBI. In 2007, a randomized controlled trial investigated the use of magnesium sulfate for neuroprotection after TBI. This study, however, found that infusions of magnesium given to patients for 5 days beginning within 8 hours after a moderate or severe TBI were not neuroprotective and might even have a negative effect in the treatment of significant head injury (Temkin et al., 2007).

*The complete reference list is available online at https://expertconsult.inkling.com/.* 

# 63

# Spinal Cord Trauma

Ryan Khanna, Richard D. Fessler, Laura Snyder, Richard G. Fessler

## OUTLINE



Spinal cord injury (SCI) is a major problem in today's clinical practice. It is a condition presently handled by a multidisciplinary team of neurologists, neurosurgeons, neurointensivists, physiatrists, anesthesiologists, and trauma surgeons. Even though newer diagnostic techniques and our growing understanding of the pathophysiology and management of SCIs enable us to treat these patients more effectively, traumatic insult to the spinal cord often leads to a permanent disabling condition. This can be an overwhelming burden on patients and their families. With a higher incidence of injuries occurring in the younger population, over time SCIs can be a great economic burden on society and the healthcare system as well.

## EPIDEMIOLOGY

The annual incidence of SCI worldwide is between 11.5 and 57.8 cases per million persons (Ackery et al., 2004). In the United States, the annual incidence is approximately 40 cases per million, with approximately 12,000 new cases diagnosed a year. There is a bimodal age distribution, with the highest frequency occurring between 15 and 29 years of age and the second occurring at 65 years of age and older (van den Berg et al., 2010b). The leading cause of death in patients with SCI relates to respiratory complications (van den Berg et al., 2010). In North American trauma centers, approximately 1 in 40 patients admitted suffers from an acute SCI (Burney et al., 1993). The present estimation of SCI victims is reported to be 259,000 (Spinal Cord Injury Information Network, 2009). The two most common causes of SCIs are motor vehicle collisions and falls (van den Berg et al., 2010). Other causes of SCI include work-related injuries, sports and recreational injuries, and violence. Typically, SCIs occur more commonly in males than females by a factor of 3 or 4 (Sekhon and Fehlings, 2001). The cost associated with care of SCI patients can range from $1.25 to $25 million, but lifetime direct and indirect costs average $1.6 million for paraplegia and $3 million for tetraplegia per individual (Krueger et al., 2013; Radhakrishna et al., 2014 ).

## PATHOPHYSIOLOGY

When the spinal cord suffers trauma, the initial insult causes immediate damage, but, over time, an acute inflammatory process coupled with astrogliosis contributes to secondary insults to the spinal cord while serving some neuroprotective and neurorestorative functions. Thus SCI is a biphasic process, and understanding the mechanisms of this process is essential for developing effective therapeutic treatment options for SCIs.

Primary injury mechanisms include shearing, laceration, acute stretching, and sudden acceleration-deceleration events that lead to disruption of axons, blood vessels, or cell membranes. There are few instances where the spinal cord is transected completely. Most injuries often leave a "subpial rim" of demyelinated or dysmyelinated axons that act as a substrate for which regeneration can potentially occur. There can also be acute swelling of the cord contributing to cord ischemia. However, at times there may be no visible injuries seen either radiographically or histopathologically. Elevated levels of cytokines, including tumor necrosis factor alpha (TNF-α) and interleukin 1-beta (IL-1β), appear within minutes of the injury. Furthermore, cytotoxic levels of glutamate can be present, owing to dumping of glutamate stores and dysfunction of astrocyte glutamate transporters. This immediate phase of injury can last up to 2 hours after the insult.

Secondary injuries are divided into acute, intermediate, and chronic stages. The acute phase is divided into an early acute phase and a subacute phase. The biochemical processes occurring in the early acute phase of injury are targeted for neuroprotective therapies. Ionic homeostasis is desynchronized during this period and contributes to apoptosis and necrotic cell death. In particular, $Ca^{2+}$ deregulation leads to a variety of damaging processes such as mitochondrial dysfunction. This in turn leads to low adenosine triphosphate (ATP) levels. Without enough ATP to sustain energy-dependent transporters such as the $Na^+$/$K^+$-ATPase membrane transporter, ionic homeostasis is further disrupted. This disruption of ionic homeostasis leads to failure of the $Na^+$/$K^+$/glutamate pump, which conceivably leads to elevated levels of glutamate. Glutamate in turn acts on a variety of glutamate receptors such as *N*-methyl-D-aspartate (NMDA), alpha-amino-3-hydroxy-5-methyl-4-isoxazolepropionic acid (AMPA), and kainite receptors, leading to an influx of $Na^+$ and $Ca^{2+}$. Free radical reactions create membrane damage via lipid peroxidation, further promoting cell lysis, dysfunction of organelles, and calcium deregulation. Free radical production peaks at 12 hours post injury and continues to have an active presence for another week before returning to preinjury levels at 4–5 weeks. The primary mediator of free radical injury is the peroxynitrite radical (Xiong et al., 2007). In rats the peroxynitrite radical has been shown to cause apoptosis (Bao and Liu, 2003). Antioxidants and inhibitors of peroxynitrite radicals have shown promise as neuroprotective elements. One such compound, methylprednisolone (MPSS), had been previously used because of its suspected role in the inhibition of lipid peroxidation; however, its routine use is currently no longer recommended (Nesathurai, 1998). Following injury to the spinal cord, the blood–brain barrier has a higher permeability due to injured endothelial cells and astrocytic processes and inflammatory mediators that increase vascular permeability. Animal studies show the peak vascular permeability occurring at 24 hours and tapering off over a 2-week period (Noble and Wrathall, 1989). In humans, the time course is suspected to be the same. Two mediators upregulated to increase vascular permeability are TNF-α and IL-1β. Other compounds found to have negative effects on the permeability of the blood–brain barrier include reactive oxygen species (ROS; e.g., nitric oxide), histamine, matrix metalloproteinases, and elastase.

Despite the inflammatory response exerting deleterious effects, it is crucial in maintaining an environment for regenerative growth and removing cellular debris. Spinal cords taken from autopsy specimens of patients suffering from SCIs were used to study the changes occurring at the cellular level by Fleming et al. in 2006. This study showed the presence of neutrophils at the injured sites within 4 hours post injury. After peaking between 1 and 3 days post injury, they remained present for as long as 10 days. Microglial cells were also shown to be an important component of the early inflammatory process. They became activated and increased in number during the first 3 days post injury. Like the neutrophils, their presence correlated with areas of increased tissue damage. During the following 5- to 10-day period post injury, the predominant cell population transitioned to the activated microglia and macrophages. It is believed that the secretion of oxidative and proteolytic enzymes by neutrophils, activated microglia, and macrophages during the first 3 days post injury imparts a high degree of secondary injury to the spinal cord (Kroner et al., 2019; Wu et al., 2019). Noncellular mediators that contribute to this process include TNF-α, interferons, and interleukins, as discussed. Inhibition of TNF-α has been found to promote recovery following SCI (Bethea et al., 1999). However, TNF-α has been found to be neuroprotective in vitro (Cheng et al., 1994) and in studies with TNF-α–deficient mice (Kim et al., 2001). Thus the exact role of TNF-α in SCI must be better defined before future therapeutic modalities can capitalize on the manipulation of this mediator.

Cell death following SCI occurs by one of two mechanisms: apoptosis or necrosis. Potentially, a newly discovered mechanism of cell death known as necroptosis can cause a programmed necrotic event to occur (Galluzzi and Kroemer, 2008). Numerous studies investigating the therapeutic effect of inhibiting the initiation of apoptotic mechanisms, such as initiation of the caspase cascade, have shown promise in animal models.

The subacute period lasts from 2 days to 2 weeks. It is during this time that the phagocytic response is responsible for removing cellular debris. The removal of growth-inhibiting compounds found in myelin debris can potentially have some beneficial effects on the efforts of axonal recovery (Donnelly and Popovich, 2007). Astrocytes also reach peak numbers in the subacute period. They form a scar that prevents axonal regeneration in rodent studies. The presence of the astroglial scar is less obvious in humans (Hagg and Oudega, 2006). Despite suspected negative effects on healing, they have important roles in ionic homeostasis and reestablishing the blood–brain barrier, thus limiting the immigration of immune cells and edema.

The intermediate phase is observed between 2 weeks and 6 months post injury and is characterized by maturation of the astrocytic scar and continual axonal regeneration. Following this period, SCIs enter a chronic phase. During the chronic phase, there is maturation and stabilization of the astrocytic scar, formation of syrinx and cavities, and wallerian degeneration. This is the period where most therapies target remyelination and the plasticity of the nervous system.

## CLINICAL PRESENTATION

The majority of SCIs occur in the cervical spine (55%; Sekhon and Fehlings, 2001). Other injuries are evenly divided among the thoracic, thoracolumbar, and lumbar regions. The most frequent injuries suffered are incomplete tetraplegia followed by complete paraplegia, complete tetraplegia, and incomplete paraplegia.

In general, SCIs can be categorized into complete injuries and incomplete injuries. In complete injuries, there is an absence of motor, sensory, and bowel and bladder function below the level of injury. There is some preservation of neurological function with incomplete injuries. At present, SCIs are graded using the American Spinal Injury Association/International Medical Society of Paraplegia (ASIA/IMSOP) Impairment Scale (Box 63.1) in conjunction with motor grading provided by the Medical Research Council Muscle Grading System (Table 63.1). This grading system provides a standard method by which clinicians and researchers can classify SCIs. In defining the level of the injury, the most caudal segment at which there is normal motor and sensory function is taken into account. This may differ from the level in the vertebral column where the injury occurred. A recent update to this scale in 2019 allows for notation of a deficit likely due to a preexisting neurological deficit with a "*" and allows for notation of a zone of partial preservation (ZPP) for injuries that lack either voluntary anal contraction or deep anal pressure sensation.

**BOX 63.1 ASIA/IMSOP Impairment Scale**

**Grade A**
Complete
No motor or sensory function is preserved in the sacral segments S4 and S5.

**Grade B**
Incomplete
Sensory but not motor function is preserved below the neurological level and extends through sacral segments S4 and S5.

**Grade C**
Incomplete
Motor function is preserved below the neurological level, and a majority of key muscles below the neurological level have a muscle grade of less than 3.

**Grade D**
Incomplete
Motor function is preserved below the neurological level, and a majority of key muscles below the neurological level have a muscle grade of 3 or greater.

**Grade E**
Normal motor and sensory functions are normal.

*Modified and reprinted with permission from the American Spinal Injury Society (ASIA) and International Medical Society of Paraplegia (IMSOP).*

**TABLE 63.1 Medical Research Council Muscle Grading System**

| Grade | Physical Examination Finding |
|---|---|
| 5 | Full ROM against full resistance |
| 4+ | Full ROM against nearly full resistance |
| 4 | Full ROM against moderate resistance |
| 4– | Full ROM against some resistance |
| 3 | Full ROM against gravity |
| 2 | Full ROM with gravity eliminated |
| 1 | Partial or trace muscle contraction |
| 0 | No muscular contraction |

*ROM*, Range of motion.
*Modified from Aids to the Examination of the Peripheral Nervous System, 1986. Baillière Tindall on behalf of the Guarantors of Brain, London.*

## SPINAL CORD INJURY SYNDROMES

### Central Cord Syndrome

Central cord syndrome is present in 9% of all traumatic cord injuries and is the most common of the spinal cord syndromes. This is a condition first reported by Thornburn in 1887 and then popularized by Schneider et al. in 1954. Hyperextension in the cervical spine, with some preexisting cervical spondylosis, is usually responsible for this type of injury. Imaging the cervical spine in patients with central cord syndrome will reveal stenosis from spondylosis, fracture subluxation, or sequestered disk, with no spinal stenosis. Schneider proposed that these injuries resulted from acute compression from preexisting bone spurs anteriorly and hypertrophied ligamentum flavum posteriorly and contributed to hematomyelia and central cord necrosis (Fig. 63.1). Schneider witnessed weakness in the upper extremities greater than the lower extremities, as well as a variable degree of sensory disturbances and loss of bladder control. It was proposed that involvement of the anterior horn cells led to weakness in the arms greater than the legs, secondary to the topography of the corticospinal tracts. Because of their good recovery, Schneider was in favor of taking a more conservative approach toward treating these patients. Correlations of magnetic resonance imaging (MRI; Quencer et al., 1992) and histopathology (Jimenez et al., 2000; Martin et al., 1992) fail to suggest hematomyelia from Schneider's hypothesis. There is in fact minimal disruption of the central gray matter. Axonal disruption and swelling are more widespread in the white matter.

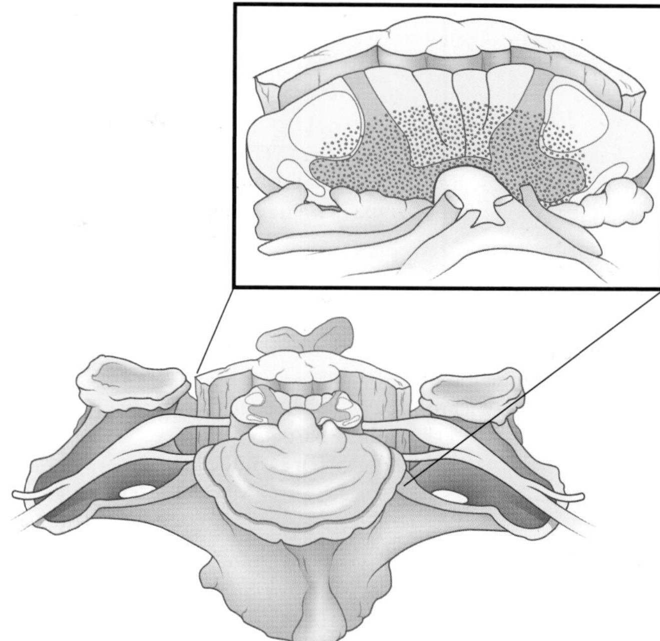

**Fig. 63.1 Central Cord Syndrome.** Described classically as injury to corticospinal tracts supplying arm and hand function, which is topographically located medial to the fibers supplying the lower extremity. *(Reprinted with permission from Tator, C.H., 1994. Classification of spinal cord injury based on neurological presentation. In: Narayan, R.J., Wilberger, J.E., Jr., Povlishock, J.T. (Eds.), Neurotrauma. McGraw-Hill, New York, pp. 1059–1073.)*

### Anterior Cord Syndrome

Anterior cord syndrome occurs with injuries to the ventral two-thirds of the cord, while sparing the posterior column (Fig. 63.2). It is present in 2.7% of all traumatic SCIs (McKinley et al., 2007). Motor function is lost distal to the site of the injury. Spinothalamic function may be disrupted, leading to loss of pain and temperature sensation in certain areas. Because the posterior columns remain intact, the sensations of vibration, position, and crude touch will not be affected. Occasionally patients feel hyperesthesia and hypoalgesia below the level of the lesion. Although this syndrome is classically described for anterior spinal artery compromise, in the setting of trauma it is due to flexion injuries or retropulsed disk or bone. Anterior cord syndrome carries a worse prognosis than other cord syndromes.

### Posterior Column Syndrome

Posterior column syndrome is a rare condition with an incidence of less than 1%. This syndrome has been linked to neck hyperextension injuries. Injuries occur to the posterior aspect of the cord (Fig. 63.3). Because the posterior columns are injured, there is usually a loss of vibration and position sense, with retained spinothalamic

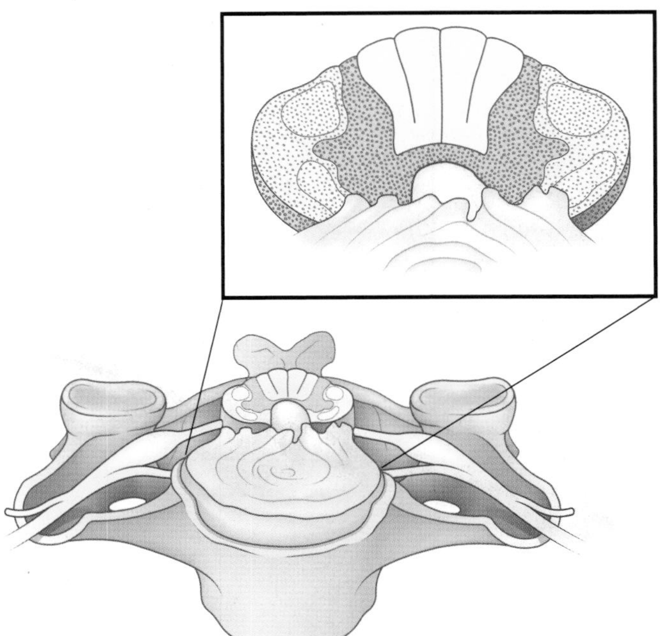

**Fig. 63.2 Anterior Cord Syndrome.** Anterior cord damage results in injury to corticospinal and spinothalamic tracts. There is preservation of dorsal columns. *(Reprinted with permission from Tator, C.H., 1994. Classification of spinal cord injury based on neurological presentation. In: Narayan, R.J., Wilberger, J.E., Jr., Povlishock, J.T. (Eds.), Neurotrauma. McGraw-Hill, New York, pp. 1059–1073.)*

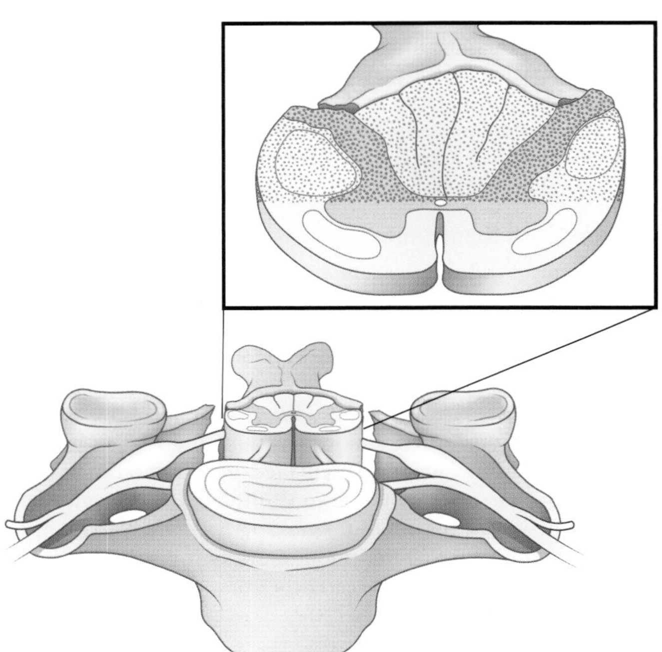

**Fig. 63.3 Posterior Cord Syndrome.** Posterior cord damage results in dorsal columns injury and preservation of spinothalamic tracts. *(Reprinted with permission from Tator, C.H., 1994. Classification of spinal cord injury based on neurological presentation. In: Narayan, R.J., Wilberger, J.E., Jr., Povlishock, J.T. (Eds.), Neurotrauma. McGraw-Hill, New York, pp. 1059–1073.)*

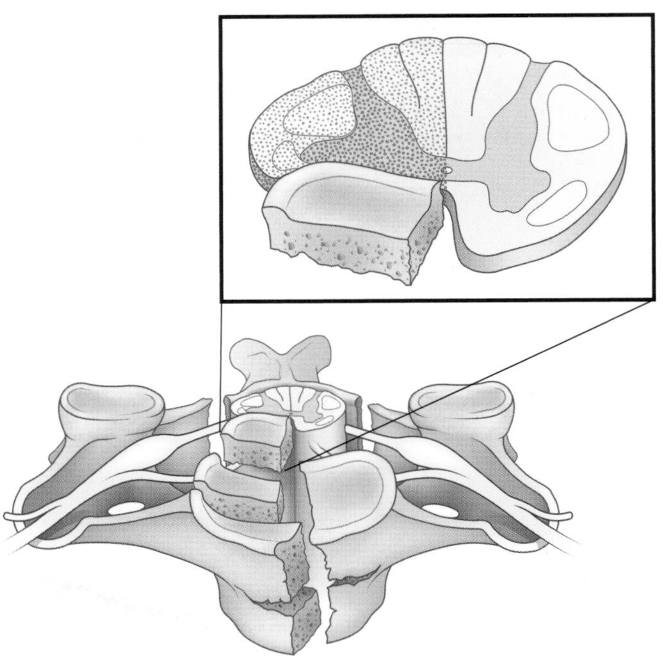

**Fig. 63.4 Brown-Séquard Syndrome.** Corticospinal tracts, dorsal columns, and spinothalamic tracts are injured from hemisection of the cord. Spinothalamic tracts cross in the ventral white commissure to the opposite side of the cord and course rostrally. Dorsal column and corticospinal tracts are impaired on the ipsilateral side. *(Reprinted with permission from Tator, C.H., 1994. Classification of spinal cord injury based on neurological presentation. In: Narayan, R.J., Wilberger, J.E., Jr., Povlishock, J.T. (Eds.), Neurotrauma. McGraw-Hill, New York, pp. 1059–1073.)*

function of pain and temperature sensation. Occasionally, motor function can be affected as well. Although this syndrome has been previously mentioned in the literature, it was omitted from the International Standards for Neurological and Functional Classification of SCI and is not currently recognized as a separate syndrome. This syndrome can also be seen in the context of pernicious anemia.

## Brown-Séquard Syndrome

Brown-Séquard syndrome accounts for 1%–4% of all traumatic SCIs. Injuries affect the lateral half of the cord (Fig. 63.4). It occurs most frequently in the cervical spine and is usually due to penetrating injuries and (less commonly) blunt trauma including disk herniations. In cases of blunt trauma, Brown-Séquard syndrome usually occurs in the context of hyperextension injuries, although it has been observed in flexion injuries, locked facets, and compression-related injuries. Below the level of the lesion, it classically manifests with ipsilateral pyramidal deficit, loss of ipsilateral tactile discrimination, position sense, and vibratory sensation, and loss of pain and temperature sensation on the contralateral aspect of the body one to two dermatomes below the level of the injury.

However, this classic presentation of Brown-Séquard syndrome rarely occurs. More frequently, patients presenting with Brown-Séquard syndrome present with a variation of the classic syndrome, termed Brown-Séquard plus (Taylor and Gleave, 1957). With Brown-Séquard plus, there is asymmetrical hemiplegia as well as hypoalgesia more prominent on the less paretic side. Patients presenting with a clinical picture consistent with a classic Brown-Séquard syndrome injury have a worse prognosis than patients presenting with a variation

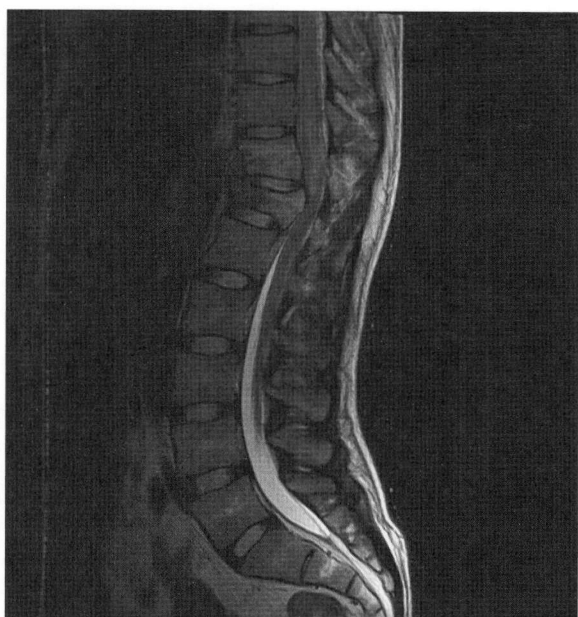

**Fig. 63.5 Conus Medullaris Syndrome.** T2 sagittal magnetic resonance imaging study showing a T12 burst fracture resulting in conus medullaris syndrome.

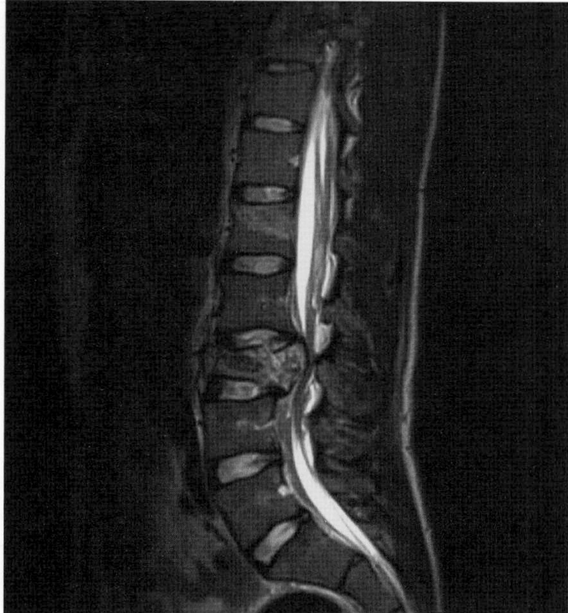

**Fig. 63.6 Cauda Equina Syndrome.** T2 sagittal magnetic resonance imaging study showing an L3 burst fracture resulting in cauda equina syndrome.

of the syndrome, but the overall prognosis is good. Brown-Séquard has the best functional motor recovery when compared with other clinical spinal cord syndromes. Most subjects obtain bowel and bladder continence. Patients having predominantly more weakness in the upper extremities compared with the lower extremities have a favorable outcome in regard to ambulating. The symptoms of Brown-Séquard syndrome may appear instantaneously or in a delayed fashion. Furthermore, they may occur in conjunction with other spinal cord syndromes.

## Cervicomedullary Syndrome

Cervicomedullary syndrome injuries appear in the upper cervical cord and extend to the medulla. Because of its location, the clinical manifestations of this syndrome include respiratory compromise, hypotension, tetraparesis (often mimicking a central cord syndrome with arms affected more than legs), hyperesthesia, and the onion-skin or Déjerine pattern of sensory loss over the face. Lower medullary and high cervical cord injuries will tend to affect the perioral distribution, whereas a more caudal cervical segment will tend to affect the peripheries of the face. This occurs as sensory fibers enter the trigeminal tract and descend to various levels depending on their somatotropic origin, then synapse in the adjacent nucleus. Fibers from the anterior face synapse more rostrally in the trigeminal tract while fibers from the hindface synapse more caudally, adjacent to the sensory input of C2–3. Mechanisms of injury for this syndrome include a variety of injuries to the atlantoaxial complex as well as injuries resulting from compression via burst fractures or herniated disks.

## Conus Medullaris Syndrome

There is high probability that injuries to the thoracolumbar region can involve the conus medullaris. The conus medullaris represents the transition of the spinal cord from the central nervous system to the peripheral nervous system. The location of this region is highly variable—between the T12 and L1 disk space to the middle third of L2 in the majority of the population (Fig. 63.5).

The lumbar parasympathetic fibers, sacral sympathetic fibers, and sacral somatic nerves originate in the conus medullaris. The classic presentation entails lower-extremity weakness, absent lower-limb reflexes, and saddle anesthesia. There is usually mixed upper motor neuron (UMN) and lower motor neuron (LMN) involvement. Loss of the bulbocavernosus and anal reflexes is permanent, differentiating conus medullaris syndrome from SCIs that have a return of these reflexes within 48 hours of the injury. Patients typically have an areflexic bowel and bladder (low-pressure, high-capacity bladder). The most common injuries to the vertebral column resulting in this condition are burst fractures or fracture-dislocation. There is no strong clinical evidence favoring surgical intervention over nonsurgical intervention for conus medullaris injuries. Furthermore, if surgical intervention is performed, there is no compelling evidence to suggest that earlier decompression affects functional outcome.

## Cauda Equina Syndrome

The cauda equina is defined as the region of the neuroaxis occupied by the filum terminale. The only neurological structures in this region include the lumbar and sacral roots. Injuries in this location are typically a pure LMN injury (Fig. 63.6). Findings often include absent bulbocavernosus reflex, absent deep tendon reflexes, flaccid urinary bladder, and reduced lower-extremity muscle tone. It is differentiated from conus medullaris syndrome by the presence of asymmetrical weakness and the absence of UMN involvement (Table 63.2). Like conus medullaris syndrome, burst fracture and fracture-dislocation are the most common vertebral column injuries associated with this condition. Cauda equina injuries have better recoveries owing to the resiliency of the roots to injuries and the greater regeneration capacity of the roots compared with the spinal cord. However, the sacral roots are very delicate, and injuries to them may be permanent. In general, cauda equina syndrome in the setting of herniated disk pathology is treated early (within 24 hours) if possible, to prevent residual symptoms (Kennedy et al., 1999). However, functional outcome in a traumatic setting is similar to conus medullaris syndrome. There is no strong evidence correlating functional outcome to surgical decompression, nor is there any evidence that suggests cauda equina injuries fare better with early versus late decompression.

**TABLE 63.2 Similarities and Differences Between Conus Medullaris Syndrome and Cauda Equina Syndrome**

| Conus Medullaris Syndrome | Cauda Equina Syndrome |
|---|---|
| Upper and lower motor neuron involvement | Lower motor neuron involvement |
| Symmetrical motor impairment | Asymmetrical motor impairment |
| Vertebral column injuries between T12 and L2 | Vertebral column injuries distal to L2 |
| Absent deep tendon reflexes | Absent deep tendon reflexes |
| Permanent areflexic bladder | Permanent areflexic bladder |
| Absent bulbocavernosus reflex | Absent bulbocavernosus reflex |

## TRANSIENT SPINAL CORD SYNDROMES

Transient spinal cord syndromes have been documented in the literature, with multiple reported incidents occurring in contact sports. The term "burning hand syndrome" was initially coined to describe a severe burning sensation in the upper extremities occurring in athletes who suffer injuries in contact sports. It is likely related to lesions of the spinothalamic tract in central cord injuries. Because the most medial fibers of the spinothalamic tract provide pain and temperature sensation to the hands and fingers, injuries to these fibers would explain the dysesthesias of the hand, so this syndrome is most suggestive of a mild central cord syndrome. Although it has been noted to occur with central cord syndrome, it can occur in isolation. Unilateral burning pain down the arm to the hand can signify root injury and has been termed a "burner" or "stinger"; they typically last seconds to hours but rarely longer than 24 hours. Stingers occur more frequently with baseline cervical stenosis, which leads to a narrow intervertebral foramen. Traction or direct trauma to the brachial plexus can mimic cervical root injury. A positive Spurling test can suggest compression of the nerve root as the cause of symptoms.

An estimated 7.3 out of 10,000 football participants suffer a cervical cord neuropraxia (Torg et al., 1997). Cervical cord neuropraxia is typically described as any motor or sensory complaints in any extremity lasting 15–30 minutes, but some cases can last up to 24–48 hours (Bailes, 2005). This injury is typically due to hyperextension, hyperflexion, or axial loading of the cervical spine. Cervical cord neuropraxia has been attributed to local anoxia and elevation of intracellular calcium (Torg et al., 1995). Bailes described "pathophysiologically similar to cerebral contusions, spinal cord concussion has become accepted to define those instances in which sufficient forces result in temporary inhibition of spinal cord impulse transmission without causing structural damage to the vertebral column or spinal cord, and is known to occur in athletes." Bailes also concluded that "a single episode of temporary spinal cord dysfunction in an athlete with spinal stenosis will substantially increase the risk of future catastrophic SCI." In his series, patients who returned to contact sport activities with no effacement of cerebrospinal fluid (CSF) around the cord or any radiographic abnormalities suggestive of cord damage encountered no further episodes of recurrent transient SCI with a mean follow-up period of 40 months.

## SPINAL SHOCK

Spinal shock was initially described as arterial hypotension following SCIs. The definition has evolved to include permanent extinction of tendon reflexes. Additional modifications to the definition have since revised it to include all findings related to the physiological and

**TABLE 63.3 Similarities and Differences Between Neurogenic and Hypovolemic Shock**

| Neurogenic Shock | Hypovolemic Shock |
|---|---|
| Hypotension | Hypotension |
| Bradycardia | Tachycardia |
| Areflexia | Normal reflexes |
| Responsive to pressors | Responsive to volume replacement |

anatomical transection of the spinal cord that results in depressed spinal reflexes for a limited period of time.

The severity of the injury correlates with the severity of spinal shock. An injury alters reflexes that occur closest to the insult first, with those more distal from the transection presenting later. Thus high-level cervical injuries may have retention of sacral reflexes, such as a preserved bulbocavernosus and anal wink. The observation that a proximal-to-distal spread of reflex depression occurs on the order of minutes suggests a physiological explanation for these changes. It has been hypothesized that the loss of supraspinal input leading to hyperpolarization of neurons is responsible for this physiological change. There have been additional observations that an upward spread of reflex depression, the Schiff-Sherrington phenomenon, is not uncommon. It is important to delineate blood pressure drops from circulatory shocks from those of spinal shock (Table 63.3). As there is loss of sympathetic tone, there is pooling of blood in the venous system and a loss of sympathetic tone in the cardiovascular system. On the one hand, circulatory shock requires volume replacement, and on the other hand, spinal shock requires vasopressors. As spinal shock resolves, muscle spindle reflexes return in a caudal-to-cranial direction, except at the level of injury. Over time, a spastic syndrome results.

There is no uniform consensus on what constitutes the cessation of spinal shock. Most references define the end of spinal shock with a return of certain reflexes. However, not all reflexes are uniformly depressed in each patient; reflexic changes are individualized. The resolution of spinal shock occurs over a period of days to months, so there is a slow transition from spinal shock to spasticity that occurs on a continuum. It has been proposed that this transition comprises four phases (Ditunno et al., 2004). The first phase occurs from 0 to 24 hours following the injury and is characterized by areflexia or hyporeflexia. During this period, the first pathological reflex to appear is the delayed plantar reflex, followed by a series of cutaneous reflexes such as the bulbocavernosus, abdominal wall, and cremasteric reflex. Impaired sympathetic control can lead to bradyarrhythmias, atrioventricular conduction block, and hypotension. Motor neuron hyperpolarization explains the changes that occur. Phase 2 occurs between day 1 and day 3 post injury. Cutaneous reflexes are more prominent during this period, but deep tendon reflexes remain mute. It is not unusual for elderly individuals and children to experience recovery of deep tendon reflexes during this time. The Babinski sign may become apparent in the elderly as well. Denervation supersensitivity and receptor upregulation account for these changes in the second phase. The next phase occurs between 4 days and 1 month post injury. Deep tendon reflexes usually recuperate by day 30. There is great disagreement about when these reflexes appear. The recovery of the Babinski response closely parallels the return of the ankle jerk reflex. There is also diminution of the delayed plantar reflex. Autonomic changes such as bradyarrhythmias and hypotension begin to subside. This time period is reflected by axon-supported synapse growth. The fourth phase is dominated by hyperactive reflexes and occurs from 1 to 12 months after injury. Vasovagal hypotension and bradycardia generally resolve in 3–6 weeks, but orthostatic hypotension may take 10–12 weeks before it disappears. Episodes of malignant hypertension or autonomic dysreflexia (AD) begin to appear during this time period. Soma-supported synapse growth accounts for these findings.

## MECHANISMS AND TYPES OF INJURIES

### Cervical Spine Fractures

#### Atlanto-Occipital Dissociation

Atlanto-occipital dissociations occur from high-energy impact and frequently lead to death. When the diagnosis is missed, subjects can have poor outcomes. These injuries result in laceration of the pontomedullary or spinomedullary junctions and are more common in children because of the horizontal orientation of their atlanto-occipital joint. Atlanto-occipital dissociations are classified into three types based on the dislocation of the condyles in relation to the atlas: type I, anterior; type II, vertical; and type III, posterior (Traynelis et al., 1986). Patients who survive this injury can present with cranial neuropathy or weakness. The diagnosis in survivors can be made by measuring the dislocation on lateral cervical x-rays. Additional findings on x-rays include prevertebral soft-tissue swelling. However, studies with computed tomography (CT) and MRI are recommended in patients with suspected atlanto-occipital dissociation. When craniocervical subarachnoid blood is present, atlanto-occipital dissociation should be suspected. The diagnosis of this injury requires prompt reduction and stabilization in a halo vest, followed by fixation by occipital-cervical fusion. Traction can cause further deterioration and should be avoided. Thus any collar placed on these patients in the field should be removed. Sandbags can be used on either side of the patient's head and neck to stabilize them until a halo can be placed.

#### Occipital Condyle Fractures

Occipital condyle fractures were first described by Bell in 1817 and have been more frequently diagnosed in head injuries since the introduction of CT. They tend to occur with high-energy compression shear forces. The frequency of occipital condyle fractures has been reported as high as 16.4% of patients who undergo high-energy blunt craniocervical trauma (Bloom et al., 1997). Patients can present with a complaint of subtle neck discomfort, but when associated with traumatic brain injury or atlanto-occipital dissociation, more severe presentation may occur. Thus the variety of presentations seen include low Glasgow Coma Scale values, retropharyngeal soft-tissue swelling, occipitocervical tenderness, reduced craniocervical motion, and lower cranial neuropathy.

The classification described by Anderson and Montesano (1988) is still widely used nowadays. According to their classification, there are three types of occipital condyle fractures: (1) a unilateral impacted fracture resulting in comminuted elements, (2) a linear basilar skull fracture that extends into the condyle, and (3) avulsion fractures of the condyle. Type III injuries warrant a high degree of caution because they may have associated atlanto-occipital dissociation and can bear instability with alar and tectorial membrane disruption. For this reason, they are treated more aggressively with halo immobilization followed by occipital-cervical stabilization. External immobilization should be considered for type I and II injuries.

#### Atlantoaxial Injuries

Injuries to the atlas can involve the anterior arch, posterior arch, the lateral masses, and the transverse process. The most notable of the atlas fractures is the Jefferson fracture, which is a burst fracture involving the anterior and posterior ring of C1. The transverse ligament provides stability of the odontoid in relation to the atlas, and injuries to the transverse ligament can occur with atlas fractures. Transverse ligament disruption can be detected by x-ray or MRI. When isolated injuries to the atlas are discovered, treatment with external immobilization by hard collar for 8–12 weeks is sufficient. Atlantoaxial injuries with disruption of the transverse ligament on MRI require a halo brace or surgical stabilization.

Fractures of the axis occur in the odontoid process, pars interarticularis, vertebral body, lateral masses, or spinous process. Vertebral body and spinous process fractures are conservatively treated with external immobilization, unless they continue into the odontoid process. The most common injuries to C2 involve the odontoid process. Injuries to the spinal cord result from instability from translational displacement of C1 on C2. Treatment strategies involve preserving axial rotation of the neck, which can be up to 60 degrees at this level. The most widely used classification of odontoid fractures is the Anderson and D'Alonzo classification. Type I fractures involve the upper portion of the odontoid. Type II fractures involve the base of the odontoid. A subgroup of these fractures is known as type IIA, which is a comminuted fracture at the base of the odontoid with associated free fragments. Type III fractures descend into the vertebral body. Type I and type III odontoid fractures are treated with external rigid immobilization with cervical collar for 8–12 weeks. There is less blood supply at the base of the odontoid, which factors into lower fusion rates and avascular necrosis for type II than either type I or type III fractures. Furthermore, odontoid fractures occurring in patients older than 50 years of age have a 21-fold risk of nonunion (Lennarson et al., 2000). Thus strong consideration should be given to treating patients with type II odontoid fractures with halo bracing for 8–12 weeks. If no fusion is seen, surgical stabilization is necessary. For patients with type II fractures who are older than 50 years of age and have displacement greater than 5 mm, or with a comminuted component at the base of the odontoid (type IIA), surgical stabilization should be considered as the first treatment option. Halo bracing can be associated with a number of complications in patients older than 70, including respiratory distress, dysphagia, and pin-site complications (Horn et al., 2006). Usually, early surgical treatment with an odontoid screw can preserve C1/C2 rotation. Surgical stabilization following failed nonunion of odontoid fractures with nonoperative treatment requires a C1/C2 fusion limiting rotation.

Pars interarticularis fractures of C2 are commonly called hangman's fractures, named after injuries associated with judicial hangings. However, the compression and hyperextension mechanism seen in the classic hangman's fracture contrasts from the distraction and hyperextension mechanism seen in judicial hangings. Two classification schemes exist: the Francis grading system and the modified Effendi system. The Francis grading system classifies hangman's fractures into five categories depending on the degree of displacement and angulation of C2 on C3. Grade I fractures have less than 3.5 mm of displacement and less than 11 degrees of angulation; grade V have complete disruption. The alternative to the Francis system is the modified Effendi system, which accounts for the underlying mechanism. Type I fractures involve axial loading and hyperextension and usually involve little or no displacement. The primary mechanism underlying type II fractures is axial loading and rebound flexion. These injuries have disruption of the C2–C3 disk complex and posterior longitudinal ligament, with significant translation and angulation. Light traction can be applied to reduce the amount of displacement. A subgroup of type II injuries involving flexion and distraction has been categorized as type IIA. These fractures occur in a more oblique angle, producing little subluxation but significant angulation. There is complete avulsion of the C2–C3 disk, and traction should be avoided because it can produce displacement. Type III fractures entail primary flexion with rebound hyperextension. These injuries are associated with facet dislocation and anterolisthesis. In general, hangman's fractures are associated with a low frequency of injury to the spinal cord and nerve root. Instability can occur at C2–C3. When these injuries are associated with C1 fractures, there is a higher incidence of neurological deficits and instability from a greater underlying mechanism causing combined injuries. Because most cases fuse on their own, a rigid cervical collar or halo orthosis is usually sufficient to treat a hangman's fracture. A small subset involving severe angulation or disruption of the C2–C3 disk complex requires consideration of surgical stabilization as a primary treatment option. Anterior cervical discectomy and fusion of C2–C3 or C1–C3 posterior fixation and fusion are both reasonable options depending on the morphology and mechanism of the fracture. Cases of failed conservative management should also undergo surgical intervention.

Trauma is one of the many causes of atlantoaxial rotatory subluxation. These injuries are seen more commonly in children because the combination of ligamentous laxity and unique facet joint structure predispose them to the initial insult producing overrotation and subluxation. Neck spasm, inflammation, and bony fragments may prevent the neck from returning to its neutral position. Typical presentations include neck discomfort and limited rotation of the neck. The head is maintained with rotation to one side, termed a cock-robin position. Asymmetry of the shoulders may be noted. Cases left untreated can present with continual pain and deformity. Changes in the voice and difficulties opening the mouth may be observed. When suspected, a timely diagnosis and rapid initiation of treatment can deliver a successful outcome. In early presentations of atlantoaxial rotatory subluxation, a trial of conservative measures with cervical immobilization, muscle relaxants, and antiinflammatory medications can be attempted. For cases presenting 2 weeks after injury, traction in conjunction with benzodiazepines, followed by external immobilization for 3 months is necessary. If after successful reduction there is recurrence, another attempt at closed reduction can be attempted. If these measures fail, open reduction and atlantoaxial fusion is necessary.

### Subaxial Cervical Spine Injuries

Blunt trauma to the neck can frequently lead to subaxial spine injuries that vary in severity and treatment depending on the type of injury. Subaxial spine injuries are divided into categories based on suspected mechanisms of injury. The Allen and Ferguson classification system categorizes subaxial injuries six groups: (1) flexion-compression, (2) vertical compression, (3) flexion-distraction, (4) extension-compression, (5) extension-distraction, and (6) lateral flexion.

Flexion-compression injuries are most often due to ventral axial loading. The prototypical cause of this injury is the classic diving injury. As a result of the forces directed on the body, there are compressive fractures seen in the anterior vertebral body. Posterior element fractures can occur in up to 50% of cases. There can be mild distraction of the facets and disruption of the posterior ligaments. With intact facets, these injuries are stable and can be treated with external immobilization. Vertical compression fractures lead to burst fractures. Surgery is warranted for retropulsion of bony elements into the canal leading to neurological deficits. Mechanical stability must be assessed for each of these cases. Teardrop fractures represent the extreme variant of these injuries and result from severe hyperflexion and axial forces. They appear as a fractured vertebral body with associated retrolisthesis and posterior ligamentous disruption and dislocation. These are highly unstable fractures and require surgical stabilization. Lateral flexion injuries may lead to unilateral vertebral body or posterior arch injuries. They are usually stable and can be treated with external immobilization. Flexion-distraction injuries typically involve minimal osseous injury, with a predominance of ligamentous injury. They vary in severity from hyperflexion strain to bilateral jumped facets. Thus MRI can typically be used to evaluate the extent of these injuries that is not obvious on lateral C-spine x-rays. A significant number of subjects who are diagnosed with jumped facets have neurological deficits; 21% of patients diagnosed with unilateral jumped facets are neurologically intact (Shapiro, 1993), compared with only 10% of patients diagnosed with bilateral jumped facets (Wolf et al., 1991). Treatment of locked facets begins with attempts at closed reduction with traction. Failed attempts warrant an open reduction. Once reduced, stabilization is required, with surgical fixation being the preferred method. Compressive-extension injuries can cause vertebral arch and laminar fractures and may lead to instability and a need for surgical stabilization. Extension-distraction injuries are common in falls and can produce central cord syndrome in the setting of trauma in an elderly patient with baseline cervical spondylosis. No fractures or ligamentous injuries may be present, but buckling of the ligamentum flavum is sufficient to damage the cord. Surgical decompression is beneficial to these patients and will be covered further in the "Surgical Management" portion of this chapter.

### Thoracolumbar Injuries

In general, the thoracic and lumbar spine is divided into three segments: an anterior column, middle column, and posterior column. The anterior column extends from the anterior longitudinal ligament to the middle of the vertebral body. The middle column is defined as the portion between the middle of the vertebral body to the posterior longitudinal ligament. The posterior column is the remaining extent of the vertebrae. A CT scan can provide precise information regarding the extent of injury. There are four major categories of thoracolumbar spine fractures (Fig. 63.7). Compression fractures involve compression of the anterior body, leading to wedging. Compression of the anterior and middle column is seen in burst fractures. With burst fractures, radiographic indications for surgery are typically loss of vertebral height of 50%, 30 degrees of kyphosis, or 50% canal compromise from retropulsion of elements. There may be neurological deficits associated with retropulsion. Seat belt injuries involve the middle and posterior column. Patients are generally neurologically intact. However, these injuries are typically deemed unstable fractures and should be treated with surgical stabilization. In fracture-dislocation injuries, involvement of all three columns is seen. The radiographic appearance of these injuries suggests a flexion-rotation, sheer, or flexion-distraction mechanism. These fractures are highly unstable and require surgical intervention.

## Penetrating Spinal Cord Injuries

The majority of penetrating SCIs are due to gunshot wounds to the spine and second only to automobile accidents in causing spinal cord–related disability. Stab wounds to the spine are less commonly seen and present with Brown-Séquard features. When making an evaluation of gunshot injuries to the spine, the trajectory of the bullet must be considered in addition to the physical location of the bullet. It is important to assess whether bowel penetration and contamination are present. The destructive nature of a bullet is related to direct injury from the bullet itself, the shock waves it creates, and temporary cavitation. These factors are dependent on the size and velocity of the missile. On examination, injuries can present one level higher than the observed location of the bullet. CT scan can assess for instability and be more helpful than MRI, which can also be safely done. MRI will not typically influence acute treatment decisions unless an evolving hematoma is present. There has been debate over whether patients benefit from laminectomy and bullet removal with incomplete injuries. The National Institute of Disability and Rehabilitation Research suggests that there is no benefit from these measures.

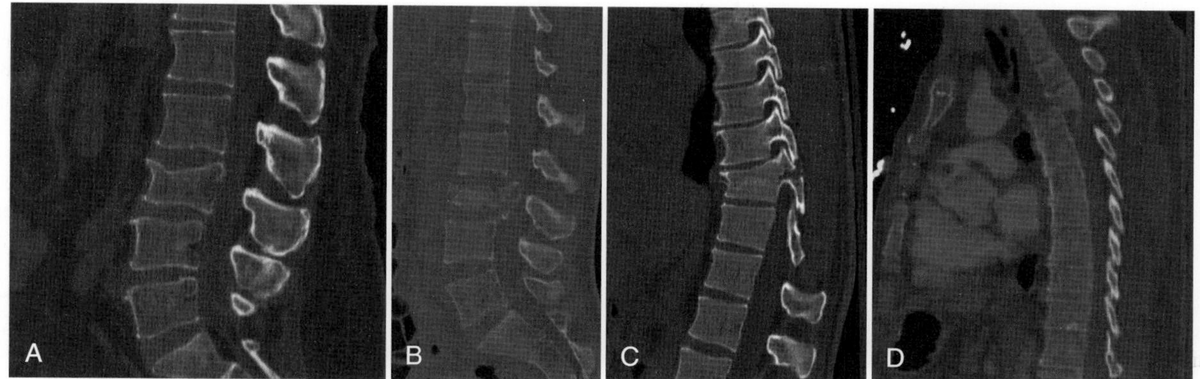


**Fig. 63.7** Computed Tomography of Various Thoracolumbar Fractures. **A,** Compression fracture. **B,** Burst fracture. **C,** Seat belt injuries. **D,** Fracture-dislocation.

## MANAGEMENT OF ACUTE SPINAL CORD INJURIES

### Management in the Field

Initial evaluation of patients should begin with standard Advance Life Support Trauma protocol to address airway, breathing, and circulation. Trauma patients with significant multiple injuries, neurological deficits, loss of consciousness or altered mental status, or posterior midline tenderness should be treated as having SCI until further evaluation can be safely done at the hospital. They should be placed in a rigid cervical collar with sand bags on either side of the head. These patients should be carefully transported on a backboard and log rolled when turning to avoid any additional injuries. The head is typically taped down on the backboard. To avoid potential injury, intubation should be done with the chin lift method, not the jaw thrust technique.

### Initial Hospital Assessment

Once the patient arrives at the hospital, a more detailed history and physical can be obtained. Paramedics are usually helpful in providing a detailed summary of events compiled from multiple sources at the scene of the injury. The history should focus on the timing and the potential mechanisms of injury. Information regarding the forces to the spine can be inferred from a clear description of the details of the event. The trauma team should repeat assessment of airway, breathing, and circulation while the patient is connected to monitors. Nasogastric tube and Foley catheters can be placed at this time. Blood work should include a basic metabolic panel, complete blood cell count, coagulopathy panel, type and screen, and toxicology panel. A detailed physical examination to determine the completeness and level of injury is essential. This will include an evaluation of muscle stretch reflexes as well as the abdominal cutaneous, cremasteric, and sacral reflexes. Rectal tone should be assessed in all patients. Radiographic imaging should be done to assess location of injuries. Based on the clinical manifestations and imaging findings, a decision should be made regarding immediate closed reduction, emergent decompression and stabilization, or conservative management.

### Radiographic Evaluation

#### Current Guidelines

In awake and obtunded patients, initial radiographic evaluation of the spine should be performed with a high-quality CT scan of the cervical spine, and, if this is unavailable, three-view cervical spine plain radiographs should be performed (Ryken et al., 2013). The decision to obtain cervical spine imaging is based on the NEXUS (National Emergency X-Radiography Utilization Study) criteria (Hoffman et al., 2000), a set of five screening assessments created to help guide physicians in making a decision to exclude low-risk/low-yield patients from undergoing cervical radiography. Awake, asymptomatic patients who meet all the criteria in Box 63.2 can bypass imaging. This study reported a 99% sensitivity and a 12.9% specificity in diagnosing SCIs when using these criteria. The Canadian C-Spine Rule was noted to be superior to the NEXUS criteria in terms of sensitivity and specificity for alert, stable patients in whom cervical spine injury is a concern (Stiell et al., 2003). Screening criteria include high-risk factors, low-risk factors, and ability to actively rotate the neck. Using the Canadian C-Spine Rule, patients older than age 65 who are subject to a "dangerous mechanism" or experience paresthesias (high-risk criteria) should receive plain radiography. Those not meeting any of the high-risk criteria are assessed further. If this subgroup of patients has delayed pain in the neck, has posterior neck tenderness, cannot tolerate sitting or ambulatory position at any time after injury, or are involved in an accident that is more than a simple rear-end motor vehicle collision (low-risk criteria), then imaging should be obtained. If they lack any of the listed findings, they are further assessed for their ability to rotate the head. High-quality CT scan, or three-view plain radiography of the cervical spine should be obtained for patients incapable of rotating their head 45 degrees in either direction.

**BOX 63.2 NEXUS Criteria**

No posterior midline cervical spine tenderness
No evidence of intoxication
A normal level of alertness
No focal neurological deficit
No painful distracting injuries

*NEXUS,* National Emergency X-Radiography Utilization Study.

#### Plain Radiography

Typical plain radiography of the cervical spine should include anteroposterior (AP), open odontoid, and lateral views with flexion-extension. An adequate lateral C-spine x-ray should visualize the area between the occiput and the top of T1. A so-called swimmer's view may be helpful to view the caudal portion of the cervical spine. Four lines should be drawn on a lateral C-spine x-ray to evaluate for subluxation or fractures: (1) anterior vertebral body line, (2) posterior vertebral body line, (3) spinal laminar line, and (4) posterior spinous line (Fig. 63.8). Findings showing more than 3.5 mm of subluxation or kyphotic angulation greater than 11 degrees to adjacent vertebral body segments can imply instability. Subluxation on the order of 25% or 50%, respectively, suggests unilateral or bilateral jumped facets. Mild

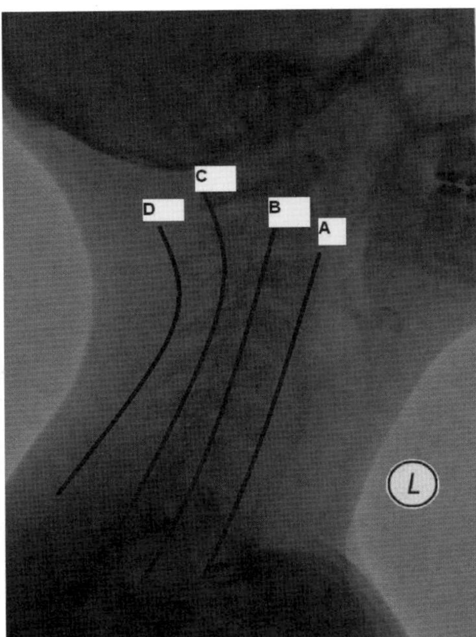


**Fig. 63.8 Evaluation of Alignment of the Cervical Spine.** (*A*) Anterior vertebral body line. (*B*) Posterior vertebral body line. (*C*) Spinal laminar line. (*D*) Posterior spinous process.

flexion-distraction injuries can be suggested by enlargement of the interspinous distance. The atlantodental interval (ADI) is a measure taken from the anterior margin of the dens to the closest portion of the anterior arch of C1. A value greater than 3 mm can suggest transverse ligament disruption. The Powers ratio is defined as a ratio of the distance from the basion to the posterior arch of the atlas divided by the distance from the opisthion to the anterior arch of the atlas. Atlanto-occipital dissociation can be suggested with a Powers ratio greater than 1. Prevertebral soft-tissue swelling should also be noted on the lateral C-spine x-rays. The upper limit of normal at the level of C3 is 4 mm. The amount of lateral mass overhang of C1 on C2 seen on the odontoid views can be measured to assess the integrity of the transverse ligament. A sum of lateral mass overhang greater than 7 mm is suggestive of transverse ligament disruption.

Complete x-rays of the whole spine should be performed if any abnormalities of the spine are detected on imaging, because noncontiguous spine injuries are seen in 10.5% of cases (Vaccaro et al., 1992). Plain radiographs of the thoracic and lumbar spine should include AP and lateral films to assess for alignment, kyphosis, disk height, and fractures. Thoracic fractures can be missed on x-rays and may require a CT or MRI if injury is suspected in this region. Scoliosis films can detect present deformity and sagittal imbalance but more importantly can be used as a baseline study for assessing progressive posttraumatic kyphosis.

### Computed Tomography

Thin-cut axial CT scans of the spine with sagittal reconstructions are more sensitive for diagnosing fractures of the spine. In particular, fractures in the occipitocervical region or at the cervicothoracic junction are better visualized with CT scan. Computed tomography angiography (CTA) can be used to assess for vertebral artery injuries with fractures involving the foramen transversarium from C1 to C6. Dynamic CT studies can be used to assess for atlantoaxial rotatory subluxation.

### Magnetic Resonance Imaging

MRI is a sensitive test to evaluate for ligamentous injury, disk disruption, cord compression, or hematomas of the spine. Obtunded trauma patients who cannot undergo flexion-extension films for cervical spine clearance can have an MRI of the cervical spine if obtained within 24 hours of injury to evaluate for ligamentous injury, particularly with short tau inversion recovery (STIR) sequences. The transverse ligament can also be evaluated for injury with MRI. Fat-suppression sequences can be helpful in diagnosing vertebral dissection. When there is a diagnosis of jumped facets of the cervical spine, MRI can be helpful in detecting disk herniations that may alter management strategies.

## SCIWORA

Spinal cord injuries without radiographic abnormalities (SCIWORAs) were first diagnosed in 1982 before the MRI era (Pang and Wilberger, 1982). Since the advent of MRI, there has been a broad spectrum of injuries present in SCIWORA patients that range from normal MRI imaging to complete cord disruption or abnormal disk pathology. SCIWORAs are more commonly encountered in the pediatric population. The incidence of SCIWORAs in cases of traumatic myelopathy of children between 1 and 17 years of age has been estimated at 34.8% (Pang, 2004). Reasons to suggest a higher incidence in the pediatric population center around the laxity of ligaments, expandability of the intervertebral disk, and the biological and anatomical differences noted in the spine between children and adults. Other considerations include the proportionally larger size of children's heads and the lack of development of paravertebral muscles. Since the advent of the MRI, the definition of SCIWORA has been revised to exclude compressive lesions found on MRI, but not intraneuronal lesions. Some practitioners feel that any spinal cord lesions should be excluded in the definition.

## TREATMENT OF SPINAL CORD INJURIES IN THE ACUTE SETTING

Contemporary hospitals are equipped with intensive care units (ICUs) with dedicated subspecialized care to treat SCIs. Aggressive medical management in the ICU setting has led to reduced morbidity and mortality and improved patient care. Despite the emergence of these centers, there are still significant numbers of patients who are not monitored for cardiovascular and respiratory function in a critical care setting. Systemic alterations in blood pressure can lead to altered perfusion and further damage to the spinal cord from secondary injuries. Global hypoxemia secondary to decreased inspiratory and vital capacity leads to further risk of spinal cord ischemia.

### Cardiovascular Management in the Intensive Care Unit Setting

Cardiovascular disease is a significant contributor to death in acute and chronic SCI patients. Hypotension, cardiac arrhythmias, and AD in the acute stage result from loss of supraspinal sympathetic influence. To gain an appreciation of this topic, a thorough understanding of neuroanatomy and pathophysiology is needed.

Sympathetic preganglionic neurons supplying the heart arise from T1 to T6 and synapse on postganglionic neurons in the middle cervical and stellate ganglia. There can be an impairment of sympathetic control with high thoracic or cervical cord injuries. In general, complete cervical injuries are associated with the highest risk of needing vasopressor support (Ploumis et al., 2010). With unopposed parasympathetic activity from the vagus nerve, bradycardia, hypotension, and other arrhythmias result. Lesions higher than T6 will also affect the supraspinal influence to the splanchnic bed, as well as the vascular supply to the lower extremity. As a result of the denervated sympathetic vascular bed, there is potential for upregulation or hypersensitivity of denervated peripheral α-adrenoreceptors. Furthermore, there is evidence to suggest that there is decreased presynaptic norepinephrine uptake. Following the obvious disruption of descending cardiovascular pathways that takes place with acute injuries, there are a series of known changes in the autonomic system that contribute to abnormal cardiovascular control. They include (1) morphological changes in the preganglionic sympathetic neurons, (2) the formation of inappropriate connections, (3) altered responsiveness and transmission of signal to vascular smooth muscle, and (4) abnormal spinal efferents.

Significant cardiovascular abnormalities have been correlated with the severity of the injury. Two abnormalities commonly reported are bradycardia and hypotension. Hypotension responds well to volume, although some patients require pressors to maintained elevated mean pressures. Bradycardia can be life threatening and require atropine. The 2-week period following an injury is the time when patients are most susceptible to cardiovascular instability, either from cardiac arrhythmias or episodes of hypotension requiring intervention.

Studies have demonstrated that aggressive medical management of hypotension may be beneficial in improving neurological recovery. One particular study focused on keeping mean arterial pressure (MAP) elevated greater than 85 mm Hg and early open or closed reduction for bilateral jumped facets (Wolf et al., 1991). This study showed a favorable outcome with these measures. Another study has shown beneficial neurological outcome for patients receiving invasive hemodynamic monitoring and given volume and pressor support to maintain adequate cardiac output and MAP greater than 90 mm Hg (Levi et al., 1993). A study performed under a prospective setting tested the hypothesis that MAP parameters greater than 85 mm Hg during the first several days of injury were associated with better outcomes (Vale et al., 1997). This study's authors noted that 9 of 10 ASIA A cervical injury patients required pressors versus 9 of 29 patients with complete thoracic injuries. In addition, 3 of 10 ASIA A cervical injury patients regained ambulatory capacity at the 1-year follow-up point, while 2 of 10 patients regained bowel and bladder control. The incomplete cervical injury group had 23 of 25 and 22 of 25 patients recover ambulatory capacity and bladder function, respectively. They further grouped patients into an early, middle, or late period when surgical intervention was performed and found no statistical correlation between timing of surgery and neurological outcome. Their study stressed the importance of aggressive volume resuscitation and blood pressure control in influencing outcome.

A low resting blood pressure and orthostatic hypotension is common following cervical and high thoracic injuries. Although it is generally accepted that reduced sympathetic output to the cardiovascular system leads to a low baseline blood pressure in SCI patients, orthostatic hypotension is an incompletely understood phenomenon. It is possible that there is excessive pooling of blood in the viscera and organs secondary to a lack of a reflex vasoconstrictor activity from an ineffective baroreceptor response. Furthermore, with the absence of muscular activity in the lower extremity, there is less recirculation of blood in the venous pool. Additional explanations include reduced plasma volumes from hyponatremia and a cardiac deconditioned patient.

Current recommendations based on the 2013 American Association of Neurological Surgeons and the Congress of Neurological Surgeons (AANS/CNS) guidelines focus on providing acute critical care for patients who have suffered SCI. This entails transferring these patients to ICU centers, preferably with dedicated SCI units for cardiac and hemodynamic monitoring where cardiac arrhythmias and neurogenic shock can be detected in a timely fashion and treated appropriately. The primary treatment for hypotension is fluid resuscitation to restore preload. Once intravascular volume is restored, pressors should be initiated to keep MAP greater than 85 mm Hg for 1 week. Pressors should be used with invasive monitoring such as an arterial line and central venous catheters to allow for accurate readings. Dopamine has α-adrenergic, β-adrenergic, and dopaminergic agonist activity. It can counteract hypotension and bradycardia by increasing heart rate and contractility, thus increasing cardiac output. However, the α-mediated vasoconstriction effects are variable. Phenylephrine is a pure α-agonist useful in restoring systemic vascular resistance and increasing MAP. It is less potent than norepinephrine. With a lack of β-adrenergic activity, it can potentially cause reflex bradycardia due to increased end-systolic volume. Patients being treated with phenylephrine may have a difficult time with fluid resuscitation because of the increased partition coefficient of intravascular volume. Norepinephrine is a more logical choice than phenylephrine because of its combined α- and β-adrenergic agonist properties. Preload is restored through decreased venous capacitance. Norepinephrine has some inotropic activity to counteract hypotension and bradycardia. Epinephrine is used in refractory cases because of its potent effects in causing renal, splanchnic, and peripheral ischemia. Vasopressin is usually used in conjunction with norepinephrine and dopamine in septic patients; its role in SCI is yet to be defined. Milrinone and dobutamine can be used to promote cardiac output, but their vasodilatory effects make them less than ideal agents for treating hypotension. No individual pressor is considered the "gold standard" for treating hypotension in the setting of SCI, and each case should be considered individually (Ploumis et al., 2010).

## Respiratory Management in the Intensive Care Unit Setting

Respiratory derangements in SCI patients depend on the extent and level of injury. The innervation of the diaphragm from the phrenic nerve is supplied by C3, C4, and C5. Injuries at or above the C2 level require immediate ventilatory support. Patients with injuries between C3 and C5 may need initial ventilatory support, but as inflammation subsides in the cord, they may regain ventilatory strength and have effective recruitment of accessory muscles. Age and preexisting comorbidities can greatly affect outcomes. Patients can still require ventilatory support with injuries below C5. Optimal function of the diaphragm is also dependent on intact intercostal and abdominal function (Schilero et al., 2018). There is a restrictive respiratory pattern encountered in SCI patients that can result from immobilization or additional physical injuries in the trauma patient such as contusion, pneumothorax, hemothorax, and flail chest; all these can lead to additional compromise. One study has shown a decrease in functional vital capacity (FVC) and expiratory flow rate immediately after injury (Ledsome and Sharp, 1981). Patients with FVC less than 25% had a greater chance of requiring ventilatory support. The authors attributed hypoxemia ($Pao_2 < 80$ mm Hg) to a ventilation/perfusion mismatch. They found supplemental oxygen to be beneficial in treating hypoxemia. Other challenges of the restrictive respiratory patterns associated with SCI are decreased compliance, increased effort in breathing, and difficulties in clearing secretions and producing an effective cough. Thus additional complications such as retained secretions, atelectasis, and pneumonia occur.

In acute SCI patients, atelectasis is the most common respiratory-related complication. It can progress to significant pneumonia and respiratory failure. Certain measures can prevent and treat atelectasis, including intermittent positive-pressure breathing (IPPB), inflation by inflating bags. Bronchospasm can result from autonomic changes in acute injury. Ipratropium has been shown to increase FVC in approximately half of patients with tetraplegia. Larger tidal volumes (>20 mL/kg) have been shown to decrease atelectasis. Chest physiotherapeutic techniques including manually assisted cough, mechanical insufflation-exsufflation, therapeutic bronchoscopy, and bronchial lavage can also be beneficial following acute injury to promote lung expansion and promote secretion clearance. Aggressive measures taken by the respiratory therapist have been shown to decrease the incidence of pneumonia and bronchoscopy use in the acute period. Warm air, bronchodilators, and mucolytics can help to improve respiratory status. The intrapulmonary percussive ventilator is a device that delivers high-frequency pulsations to loosen secretions and provide aerosolized medications to the lungs. Manually assisted coughing with a provider or via a device can clear bronchopulmonary secretions. Additional measures include a rotational bed and postural drainage. Although suctioning is widely used and a mainstay of treatment, it can complicate matters by causing hypoxia, hypotension, infection, tracheal mucus drainage, vagus nerve stimulation, and increased mucus production. Its effectiveness can be limited by patient fears and anxieties.

Pneumonia is a common complication related to the use of mechanical ventilation, with a risk of 1%–3% per day of mechanical ventilation (Ball et al., 2001). The culprits of ventilator-associated pneumonia occurring within the first 4 days are usually *Haemophilus influenzae* and *Staphylococcus pneumoniae*. Only when *Pseudomonas aeruginosa* is suspected should double coverage with antipseudomonal β-lactam agents and aminoglycosides be considered. Prevention of aspiration and monitoring for its effects are essential for optimal care. Patients with diabetes can have preexisting gastric atony. A nasogastric tube is needed to treat an ileus. Patients on tube feeds require monitoring of their gastric residual content after feeding.

*Respiratory failure* is defined as a $Pco_2$ greater than 50 mm Hg or $Po_2$ less than 50 mm Hg on room air, or the requirement of ventilatory support in the setting of a high cervical injury. It is prevalent in 40% of subjects with C1–C4 injuries, 25% of subjects with C5–C8 injuries, and 9.9% of subjects with thoracic injuries (Jackson and Groomers, 1994). Patients with injuries in the high cervical cord may suffer neurological deterioration in subsequent days as the injury ascends superiorly in the cord. There is no standard protocol in providing ventilatory support to this group of patients, but simple principles can be used. Patients with high cervical injuries (C1–C3) will typically need full ventilatory support with controlled mechanical ventilation permanently. SCI patients who are alert and maintain the capacity to initiate respiratory effort may require intubation, especially when FVC decreases to less than 10–15 $cm^3/kg$. Patients with low FVC may have difficulties producing an effective cough and compromised bronchial hygiene. They do not require controlled ventilatory settings that promote ventilator dyssynchrony. Instead, they can benefit from pressure support modes to reduce ventilation/perfusion mismatches. In addition, patients who are likely to be full-time ventilator dependent may use techniques such as glossopharyngeal or "frog" breathing to have brief periods of ventilator independence.

Invasive respiratory support can incapacitate an individual's defense mechanisms. The clearing mechanism of the cilia and the cough reflex become impaired. In addition, speech can be affected. Because of this, it may be beneficial to use noninvasive support. Patients with intact respiratory musculature but with decreased compliance from associated injuries may benefit from noninvasive support such as bilevel positive airway pressure (BiPAP) or continuous positive airway pressure (CPAP).

There is considerable debate over where to place tidal volume for SCI patients. Higher tidal volumes can be used to prevent atelectasis. Typically, tidal volume averages no higher than 6–8 mL/kg are used to avoid barotrauma, but one study suggested that tidal volumes as high as 20 mL/kg are needed to avoid atelectasis and prevent prolonged weaning times (Peterson et al., 1997). Regardless, tidal volumes can be progressively increased in a manner to resolve atelectasis on chest x-ray. Peak pressure should never exceed 40 mm Hg.

Patients requiring long-term ventilatory support may require a tracheostomy to avoid subglottic stenosis and sinusitis. Tracheostomy is easier to tolerate, facilitates improved pulmonary hygiene, produces less dead space and less airway resistance, and creates more favorable conditions for weaning off a ventilator. Furthermore, tracheostomy allows for earlier initiation of rehabilitation. The decision to place a tracheostomy should not extend past 2 weeks. In the event anterior cervical surgery is performed, a time period of 2 weeks between surgery and tracheostomy placement is suggested. When there are higher comorbidities such as baseline respiratory disease, acquired pneumonia, ASIA and B injury, smoking history, age older than 60, or C4 level or higher, early tracheostomy placement should be considered.

## Medical Management

Secondary injuries that occur in the spinal cord lead to deleterious and unwanted permanent damage. Steroids have been studied extensively as pharmacotherapy to hinder unwanted sequelae and have raised much debate. Early animal models suggested benefit in impeding secondary injury, and this has translated into clinical studies in humans to assess steroid efficacy and safety. To date, results from these studies have not led to US Food and Drug Administration (FDA) approval of steroids in the treatment of SCIs. For many years, administration of methylprednisolone was commonplace following SCI; however, the guidelines from 2013 developed by the AANS and CNS have a level 1 recommendation against "the administration of [methylprednisolone] for treatment of acute SCI" because there is no class I or II evidence supporting its benefit. The class III evidence supporting its benefit is inconsistent and subject to selection bias, while there is class I, II, and III evidence of its deleterious effects in SCI (Hurlbert et al., 2013).

There have been at least six prospective randomized trials studying steroid effects, with great controversy in interpretation of the methods and results from these studies. The National Acute Spinal Cord Injury Study (NASCIS) I trial compared two sets of patients receiving methylprednisolone (Bracken et al., 1985). One group received 100 mg of methylprednisolone followed by 25 mg every 6 hours for 10 days. The other arm used doses with 10 times that magnitude. Patients were followed up to 1 year after treatment, and results failed to show any significant difference between the two arms despite lacking a placebo. Following this study, NASCIS II was performed to include three groups: a placebo group, an opiate antagonist group using naloxone, and a methylprednisolone group that received a 30 mg/kg bolus over an hour, followed by 5.4 mg/kg/h for the next 23 hours (Bracken et al., 1990). Patients receiving methylprednisolone before 8 hours after injury were separated from patients receiving treatment after 8 hours following their injury. The authors suggested that patients with acute SCIs treated within 8 hours of the accident benefited; post-hoc analysis suggested that patients with acute SCIs treated within 8 hours of the accident had significant improvement in sensory and motor function from methylprednisolone (Witiw, 2015). Although the entire patient sample consisted of 487 patients, this study showed encouraging results from a subgroup of patients receiving treatment within 8 hours of injury. This was not the case for patients receiving treatment 8 hours after injury. Since that time, there have been many critical analyses of the methods, statistical analysis, and scientific interpretation of the study. One of the most critical arguments stems from the lack of functional measures to assess outcome. Independent chart analysis shows that the placebo group treated within 8 hours of injury had similar recovery patterns to the corresponding methylprednisolone group for the first 6 weeks. Afterwards, the recovery plateaued. Most clinicians feel that incomplete injuries that show functional improvement at 6 months continue an ongoing trend of recovery. Chart analysis also showed that the placebo group treated within 8 hours of injury did worse than the group treated with placebo 8 hours after injury. In addition, the placebo group treated after 8 hours from the onset of injury had similar results to the methylprednisolone group treated within 8 hours of the injury. The study lacked any information regarding the timing or type of surgical interventions that were performed for these patients. Statistical tools have been criticized as being excessive, confusing, and difficult to replicate by professional statisticians. Furthermore, data from this study have never been made available for independent review. Only one study has attempted to model the NASCIS II study (Otani et al., 1994). Their results mirrored the NASCIS II data. Although results were published as class I–level evidence, their methodology was not well reported, and they deviated from classical standards of a prospective randomized double-blinded study. NASCIS III attempted to evaluate the effects of methylprednisolone administered in a 24-hour versus 48-hour setting (Bracken et al., 1997). An added treatment arm received 48 hours of tirilazad, a medication with antioxidant properties. All patients received a bolus of 30 mg/kg followed by 5.4 mg/kg/h for the 24- and 48-hour methylprednisolone groups, or 2.5 mg of tirilazad every 6 hours. The authors noted neurological improvement at the 6-week and 6-month postinjury period for the 48-hour methylprednisolone group if medication was given between 3 and 8 hours post injury. Randomization bias was noted in NASCIS III, and there were no criteria established for a minimal motor deficit needed for participation in the study. Patients who had no motor deficits were included in the study, complicating matters. In addition, patients with the 48-hour MPSS protocol had higher rates of infection. However, a recent meta-analysis in 2017 conducted by AOSpine showed that a "high-dose 24-hour regimen of MPSS confers a small positive benefit on long-term motor recovery," so controversy still remains (Fehlings, 2017).

Potential side effects related to methylprednisolone use in SCI patients include pulmonary embolism (PE), sepsis, pneumonia, gastrointestinal hemorrhage, and wound infection. Steroids have been demonstrated to increase the risk of major complications (Dimar et al., 2010).

GM-1 ganglioside, nimodipine, naloxone, and tirilazad mesylate have all been studied, but GM-1 ganglioside is the only other medication tested through clinical trials. In vitro studies have been promising, showing neuritic sprouting and reduced apoptosis. Clinical trials were performed to test its effects in the clinical setting. A small single-center prospective, randomized, placebo-controlled study showed significant motor improvement at 1 year. A follow-up study with a large multimember prospective, randomized, placebo-controlled study failed to confirm these results. Thus this agent has not been recommended for use in clinical practice by the AANS and CNS (Hurlbert et al., 2013)

Three additional agents considered to have neuroprotective effects were studied prospectively with randomized double-blinded clinical trials. Thyroid-releasing hormone (TRH) has been tested in humans for its antagonistic effect on secondary injury mediators. Only one clinical trial tested this hypothesis in humans (Pitts et al., 1995). This study showed a statistically significant improvement for patients with incomplete SCI who received TRH, but the study was limited in statistical power by virtue of its small study size. Gacyclidine is an NMDA receptor antagonist known to compete against glutamate. Studies have not shown a significant benefit for incomplete cervical injuries at 1 year post injury (Tadie et al., 1999). Nimodipine has been studied for its ability to impede calcium-dependent injury in the secondary stages. Despite animal studies showing benefit, human controlled trials failed to show any benefit (Petitjean et al., 1998). Naloxone and tirilazad mesylate were both studied with no difference in motor scores between groups.

Currently, riluzole in acute SCI is being studied. Riluzole is a sodium channel–blocking anticonvulsant drug that is approved for use in amyotrophic lateral sclerosis (ALS) by the FDA and modulates excitatory neurotransmission with neuroprotective effective. Because it has been shown to improve survival in the setting of ALS, it was studied in preclinical SCI studies with results suggestive of functional motor recovery. Because of this, a randomized, double-blinded multicenter trial of riluzole (Riluzole in Acute Spinal Cord Injury Study [RISCIS]) is currently ongoing, studying its neuroprotective effects in SCI (Fehlings, 2016).

### Nutritional Support

The nutritional requirements of acute SCI patients are vastly different from those of trauma patients without SCI. Immediately following an injury, especially in cases of high cervical injury, there is a period of reduced metabolic activity. However, there is a catabolic cascade that occurs. The resting energy expenditure (REE) of head injury patients may be 140%–200% of the predicted normal basal energy expenditure (BEE), whereas the REE of SCI patients is approximately 56%–90% of the predicted normal BEE. Indirect calorimetry has been advocated as a more accurate measure to assess caloric needs of this population. Muscle mass is lost during this period from denervation, promoting a negative nitrogen balance. Achieving nitrogen balance is an unrealistic goal and should not be the objective.

Compromised gastrointestinal and immune integrity alter normal physiology and factor into the timing of initiating a diet. It is generally acceptable to provide early nutritional support to meet caloric requirements, counteract losses of muscle mass, and maintain gastrointestinal and immune integrity. There has also been evidence to refute fears that early feeding leads to increased septic complications (Dvorak et al., 2004), but the clinician should always be cognizant of a paralytic ileus, which can promote aspiration in light of cervical immobilization and swelling.

## STABILIZATION AND SUPPORT

### Nonsurgical Management

Spinal orthoses have been used to apply external forces to the spine to correct or prevent deformity and provide indirect stabilization of the spine while allowing the bone to fuse. Spinal immobilization techniques have been practiced throughout history and have been shown to be effective in achieving bony fusion. Although bracing and bed rest often provide the desired result in the long term, this is not always a practical method of achieving fusion. Medical complications associated with bed rest include PE, hospital-acquired infections, pressure ulcers and skin breakdown, and detrimental psychological effects. Furthermore, bed rest may be financially taxing and require prolonged hospital stays. Bed rest also limits early rehabilitation. For these reasons, in every case, the decision to brace is based on multiple factors and may not be dependent on the types of fractures present. Furthermore, the orthoses chosen must restrict movement, provide spinal realignment, and maintain trunk support. In general, orthoses are worn for a 3-month period to allow proper promotion of bony fusion.

Spinal orthoses of the cervical spine range from soft collars and Minerva braces to external splinting techniques such as the halo vest. The cervical soft collar provides negligible resistance to motion and is primarily used as a reminder to patients to limit motion or for comfort by providing support to the cervical musculature. Hard cervical collars (Aspen, Miami J, Philadelphia) take into account the base of the skull, jaw, and shoulder to provide resistance for the cervical spine. Cervicothoracic orthoses (Yale, Somi, 4-poster, Guilford) provide a three-point bending movement as a means to restrict motion in the mid-to-low cervical region. They provide added resistance to flexion, extension, and rotation compared with conventional hard collars but inadequate prevention of lateral flexion. They can also be uncomfortable to wear. When cervical collars are worn, they may produce a parallelogram-like bracing effect seen as a ventral and dorsal translation of the head. Halo bracing is still considered the most effective method of restricting motion (flexion-extension, lateral bending, and rotation) in the cervical spine. They reduce the parallelogram-like bracing effects at the expense of a snaking effect. The snaking effect is demonstrated with segmental movement in each single cervical level but with minimal overall movement between the occiput and lower cervical spine. The Minerva jacket is fitted by an orthotics expert and provides contact support through a thermoplastic shell, which is fitted around with a circumferential headband extending down to the thorax. These devices are known for minimizing the snaking effect but have the disadvantage of being in direct contact with the skin and causing skin breakdown, discomfort, warmth, and limited mobility of jaw movements. The halo device lacks direct contact with skin and soft tissue, leading to less skin breakdown. It also allows the jaw to be free so that easier speaking and eating may occur. Halo devices are associated with pin-site infection and require tightening of pins.

Thoracolumbosacral orthoses are useful for compression fractures and nonoperative burst fractures; they mainly target fractures between T10 and L2. In principle, they apply a three-point fixation. The Jewitt device uses one posterior pad on the midthoracic region and two anterior pads on the sternum and pubic symphysis. This device is useful in limiting flexion and extension motion but ineffective in limiting rotation and lateral bending. Because sternal fixation is the most cephalad region of support for this brace, the amount of segmental motion above T6 can be increased. Thus the Jewitt brace is contraindicated for fractures superior to T6. Custom-molded clamshell thermoplastic devices provide the added benefit of limiting lateral bending and rotation and distributing pressure over a wider surface area. They can be used for fractures extending from T3 to L3. Lumbosacral orthoses have been used to treat fractures distal to this region and are less effective. Their use is controversial because their effectiveness is limited by the inadequate effective fixation of the pelvis to manage low fractures. Lengthening the brace downward toward the inguinal region or distal to the iliac crest can prevent an individual from sitting. As a result, some lumbosacral orthoses include a hip spica cast to provide partial compensation of movement.

Closed reduction has been used to provide spinal realignment in the setting of facet fracture, jumped facets, subluxation, or spinal deformity as a primary means of realignment before open reduction is attempted. Successful reduction of jumped facets can be safely done. It has been shown that patients who undergo successful closed reduction can have better outcomes than those patients requiring surgery (Papadopoulos et al., 2002). Patients must be awake and cooperative and provide a reliable neurological examination. Traction is performed with the patient in supine position. The head is placed in Gardner Wells tongs or a halo ring attached to a set of weights by a rope suspended off the side of the bed via a pulley mechanism. A distracting force is applied with progressive weights. The initial weight for traction is usually 3 lbs multiplied to the level of injury in the cervical spine. Weight is added in 5- to 10-lb increments, spinal alignment is checked with fluoroscopy, and a neurological examination is performed at 10- to 15-minute intervals. In general, there is no defined upper limit of traction that should be applied. Subjective neck pain and objective neurological deficit should discourage any further traction. Furthermore, if the weight applied shifts the patient in bed, traction should be halted. Once spinal realignment is achieved, the patient may either be locked into the halo vest or taken to the operating room in traction, where surgical stabilization can be achieved.

## Surgical Management

Indications for surgery include decompression, stabilization, and correction of deformity. In a general sense, White and Panjabi define *spinal stability* as the "ability of the spine under physiological loads to limit patterns of displacement so as not to damage or irritate the spinal cord or nerve roots and, in addition, to prevent incapacitating deformity or pain due to structural changes" (White and Panjabi, 1990). The initial radiographic workup may suggest spinal instability, but more often, clinical judgment based on history and physical examination in conjunction with follow-up imaging can help to establish a more definitive diagnosis of spinal instability. For acute fractures and dislocations, the timing of events in relation to the presentation and the completeness of the injury should be noted. Prospective randomized trials done with animals show neurological improvement with early surgical decompression for SCI (Rabinowitz et al., 2008). In a systemic review of the literature, early decompression was found to have better neurological outcomes than late decompression if done within 24 hours of the injury (La Rosa et al., 2004), and recent guidelines suggest "early surgery be offered as an option for adult acute SCI patients regardless of level" (Fehlings, 2017). Surgery in the early period has been shown to be safe when there are stable hemodynamic parameters with monitoring and expert surgical and anesthesia staff are present (Fehlings and Perrin, 2006). Favorable results in motor recovery and cost-effectiveness have been recorded for decompression of disk herniation and fractures causing central cord syndrome (Guest et al., 2002).

Cervical pathology contributing to traumatic central cord syndrome are divided into one of three categories: (1) cervical spondylosis in the setting of segmental spinal stenosis or anterior pathology from disk/osteophyte complex; (2) fracture subluxations; and (3) disk sequestration with no evidence of spinal stenosis. Previously the timing of such decompression was controversial, but there is increasing evidence stating that early decompression (within 24 hours) is associated with improved outcomes. Surgical Timing in Acute Spinal Cord Injury Study (STASCIS), the largest multicenter, international, cohort study for acute SCI, was published. The study recruited 313 patients, out of which 182 patients underwent early (<24 hours) decompression with a mean of 14.2 ± 5.4 hours until the surgery while 121 patients in the delayed group underwent decompressive surgery with a mean time of 48.3 ± 29.3 hours until the surgery. The study concluded that improvement was 2.8 times more likely in the early group (Fehlings et al., 2012). Another study out of Pakistan demonstrated that they too had improved outcomes with early decompression (Umerani et al., 2014). A meta-analysis of 18 studies demonstrated "early" spinal surgery was significantly associated with a higher total motor score improvement, neurological improvement rate, and shorter length of hospital stay; however, due to the heterogeneity of the studies, the evidence cannot be described as "robust" (van Middendorp et al., 2013).

The Spine Study Trauma Group attempted to provide a standard protocol to guide physicians in treating thoracolumbar fractures. As a result, the Thoracolumbar Injury Severity Score (TLISS) and Thoracolumbar Injury Classification and Severity Score (TLICS) were introduced (Tables 63.4 and 63.5). The TLISS is an algorithm that assigns a score based on mechanism of injury, posterior ligamentous injury, and neurological deficits (Vaccaro et al., 2005). There was concern that substantial variability existed among observers as they attempted to postulate the mechanisms of injury and assign an additive score for this category. TLICS was then created to focus on fracture morphology (Lee et al., 2005).

**TABLE 63.4 Thoracolumbar Injury Severity Score**

| Parameter | Points |
|---|---|
| **Mechanism of Injury** | |
| Compression: | |
| Simple compression | 1 |
| Lateral angulation >15 degrees | 1 |
| Burst | 1 |
| Translational/rotational | 3 |
| Distraction | 4 |
| **Neurological Involvement** | |
| Intact | 0 |
| Nerve root | 2 |
| Cord, conus medullaris: | |
| Incomplete | 3 |
| Complete | 2 |
| Cauda equina | 3 |
| Posterior ligamentous complex: | |
| Intact | 0 |
| Injury suspected/indeterminate | 2 |
| Injured | 3 |
| ***MANAGEMENT*** | ***Points*** |
| Nonoperative | 0–3 |
| Nonoperative or operative | 4 |
| Operative | ≥5 |

**TABLE 63.5 Thoracolumbar Injury Classification and Severity Score**

| Parameter | Points |
|---|---|
| **Morphology** | |
| Compression fracture | 1 |
| Burst fracture | 2 |
| Translational/rotational | 3 |
| Distraction | 4 |
| **Neurological Involvement** | |
| Intact | 0 |
| Nerve root | 2 |
| Cord, conus medullaris: | |
| Incomplete | 3 |
| Complete | 2 |
| Cauda equina | 3 |
| Posterior ligamentous complex: | |
| Intact | 0 |
| Injury suspected/indeterminate | 2 |
| Injured | 3 |
| ***MORPHOLOGY*** | ***Points*** |
| Nonoperative | 0–3 |
| Nonoperative or operative | 4 |
| Operative | ≥5 |

Patients with compression fractures of the thoracolumbar spine not requiring open surgical intervention may qualify for vertebral augmentation procedures. *Vertebroplasty* is a percutaneous procedure that uses a specially formulated acrylic bone cement injected into a fractured vertebra to provide stabilization. *Kyphoplasty* is a procedure that uses an inflatable percutaneous balloon to restore height and reduce complications from cement leakage. There is a theoretical restoration of vertebral body height and reduction of kyphotic deformity with this procedure. In general, patients qualifying for vertebroplasty must have acute or subacute fractures and no posterior vertebral body breech. Two prospective randomized trials failed to show any improvement of pain with vertebroplasty (Buchbinder et al., 2009; Kallmes et al., 2009), although recent evidence suggests those with severe pain who are treated less than 6 weeks from fracture onset are good candidates for vertebroplasty (Chandra et al., 2018). Although kyphoplasty has been shown to reduce local kyphotic deformity, there does not seem to be a positive effect seen on a global scale (Korovessis et al., 2008; Pradhan et al., 2006).

## LONG-TERM MANAGEMENT OF SPINAL CORD INJURIES

### Spinal Cord Injury and Bladder Function

The bladder maintains storage and release of urine through influences from the central nervous system. In the past, renal failure has been a leading cause of death in the SCI patient. With improved management of urological dysfunction in SCI patients, mortality has been greatly reduced. Specific objectives for a bladder management program entail efficient storage and emptying while maintaining low pressures and preventing overdistention of the bladder. These measures can prevent complications from high intravesicular pressure. It is to the patient's benefit to maintain a bladder regimen that allows them to integrate into society. Urinary tract infections (UTIs) should be prevented.

In SCIs, neurogenic bladders are classified according to the location of the lesion. A LMN lesion is localized below the conus medullaris. In this situation, the bladder detrusor is areflexic or hyporeflexic but maintains a normal or underactive external sphincter. With this type of injury, there is still coordination between the bladder detrusor and the sphincter. Additional characteristics depend on the extent of involvement of the peripheral fibers and whether there is predominance of afferent or efferent fibers. With peripheral fiber loss, an absent sacral reflex (bulbocavernosus and cremasteric reflexes) may be observed. A purely motor neurogenic bladder will have preserved sensation. With afferent loss, there is impaired emptying consequent to diminished or absent sensation, and this can lead to chronic overdistention. Findings on urodynamic studies would reveal a low bladder pressure, absent electromyographic (EMG) activity, and altered functional bladder outlet mechanisms (eFig. 63.9, *A*).  As a result, a high postvoid residual would be expected. In UMN lesions, the sacral arc is preserved, but pontine modulation is disrupted. There is discoordination between the detrusor and sphincter, which is known as *detrusor–external sphincter dyssynergia* (DESD; Table 63.6). With a preserved sacral reflex, there is urinary incontinence from reflexic contraction of the bladder when filling occurs and meets a certain threshold. Detrusor overactivity can be seen in suprasacral spinal lesions. When coupled with DESD, high intravesicular pressures result. As a result, urodynamic studies will confirm a baseline spontaneous activity of the bladder as well as simultaneous firing of the detrusor and external sphincter (see eFig. 63.9, *B*).  High intravesicular pressure and postvoid residuals occur from this abnormal activity. A highly compliant bladder, seen in lower motor injuries, can lead to overdistention injuries and require clean

TABLE 63.6 Differences Between Atonic Bladder and Detrusor External Sphincter Dyssynergia

| Atonic Bladder | Detrusor External Sphincter Dyssynergia |
|---|---|
| Areflexic or hyporeflexic bladder | Detrusor overactivity |
| Localized below the conus medullaris | Occur from lesions above the conus medullaris |
| Coordination between bladder detrusor and sphincter | Incoordination between bladder detrusor and sphincter |
| Low bladder pressures | High bladder pressures |

intermittent catheterization (CIC) to counteract the unwanted phenomenon. However, with a poorly compliant bladder, high pressures can lead to injuries in the upper urinary tract. A detrusor leak-point pressure (DLPP) determined from urodynamic studies will indicate the pressure at which leakage occurs in the bladder. This value is typically 40 cm $H_2O$. Vesicoureteral reflux from high DLPP can also complicate matters by causing UTI, pyelonephritis, or ischemic injuries. Chronically, this can lead to renal scarring.

In the hospital setting, spinal shock will predominate and will manifest as an areflexic, acontractile bladder usually lasting 6–12 weeks, but it can last up to 1 year. During this time, Foley catheterization or CIC is used to maintain integrity of the urinary system. CIC should be performed every 4 hours to keep volumes in the bladder less than 500 mL. For long-term management, intermittent catheterization is the preferred method to drain the bladder, owing to the high complication rates from long-term use of indwelling catheters, which include infection, cancer, renal stones, alterations in bladder compliance, strictures, and diverticula. Indwelling catheters may be a temporary option for patients who lack motivation or have limited hand function and are unable to receive adequate care by the caregiver. LMN injuries may be treated by physical measures such as the Valsalva or the Credé maneuvers. The Valsalva maneuver increases intraabdominal pressure, whereas the Credé maneuver applies manual direct pressure to the suprapubic area. Reflex voiding involves suprapubic tapping as a method to stimulate the sacral reflux arc in supraspinal lesions to facilitate voiding. However, this is used in conjunction with transurethral sphincterotomy to allow bladder drainage at low pressures in order to avoid upper tract injuries.

Currently, the medications used to inhibit bladder overactivity include anticholinergics (oxybutynin, tolterodine), tricyclic antidepressants (TCAs; e.g., imipramine), and antispasmodic medications (baclofen, tizanidine). Intravesicular therapy with botulinum toxin A has been used and avoids the undesirable side effects associated with systemic pharmacological agents. The effects of botulinum A can last for 16–36 weeks to prevent bladder overactivity, lower bladder pressures, and alter maximum bladder capacity. This agent can also be used in the external sphincter.

A variety of surgical options exist when primary bladder management methods fail. Electrical stimulation of the sacral roots (S2–S4) promotes bladder contraction. Selective posterior sacral root rhizotomy can suppress hyperreflexic detrusor activity. Augmentation enterocystoplasty is a bladder augmentation procedure known to increase total bladder capacity by using the bowel to augment the bladder. Complications known to arise from this procedure include changes in bowel habits and metabolic derangements. An alternative method to accomplish augmentation entails detrusor myomectomy caused by the formation of a diverticula by weakening the muscle from an excision in the submucosa. Considerations for this procedure are made for patients with intractable detrusor hyperactivity, a lack of motivation for self-catheterization, a desire to convert from reflux voiding to self-catheterization, or high risk for developing upper urinary tract complications. Cutaneous conduits and urinary diversion have been used for detrusor overactivity. They provide external drainage of urine through the abdominal wall to an external collecting device. This is accomplished by connecting the ureters to an intestinal segment which is externalized. The ileal conduit does not serve as a storage reservoir, and there is no metabolic derangement because there is only transient exposure of urine to the absorptive surface. Continent urinary diversions contain a reservoir that is attached to the urethra instead of the bladder or can be accessed through an abdominal stoma which is catheterized. Metabolic derangements can occur with prolonged contact of urine with the surface of the bowel. These procedures are useful for females and patients with structural abnormalities of the urethra or bladder, bladder cancer, and incontinence that prevents proper care of perineal decubiti. In general, females have more technical difficulties with intermittent catheterization and have no external incontinence devices like the male condom catheter. They also experience urethral erosion from catheterization. Transurethral sphincterotomy is the preferred surgical method in patients with DESD refractory to anticholinergic medications. It is typically used for a male with quadriplegia or a high thoracic injury that affects hand function. Females are unable to have an external drainage device and thus do not qualify for this procedure.

## Spinal Cord Injury and Bowel Function

Bowel dysfunction in SCI can lead not only to the inconvenience and embarrassment of fecal incontinence but also to significant physical distress. Common symptoms noted in these patients include infection, ileus, gastric ulcers, gastroesophageal reflux disease (GERD), volvulus, stercoral perforation, dyspnea, worsening spasticity, AD, constipation, diarrhea, nausea, pain, distention, hemorrhoids, loss of appetite, impaction, fecal incontinence, and delayed and unanticipated evacuation. Despite defecation occurring in SCI patients, more energy and time are required, and this can be both physically and emotionally taxing; assistance is often needed in half of this population. Manual stimulation and manual disimpaction are required in a great majority of patients. Not surprisingly, higher-level injury, complete injury, and nonambulatory states correlate with toilet dependency.

Following SCI, there is a disruption of the extrinsic influences of the nervous system on the bowel. Initial studies evaluating bowel dysfunction in SCI patients showed decreased compliance and deficient postprandial motor and myoelectrical response in the colon (Glick et al., 1984). The term *neurogenic bladder* evolved to account for either an LMN bowel syndrome producing areflexia or a UMN syndrome producing hyperreflexia (Stiens et al., 1997). The LMN syndrome results from injury of the conus medullaris, cauda equina, or pelvic nerves, with decreased influence from the parasympathetic system. Thus this injury pattern reduces peristalsis leading to slow stool movement and constipation. Furthermore, a denervated external anal sphincter (EAS) leads to fecal incontinence. A lesion proximal to the conus medullaris results in UMN bowel syndrome or hyperreflexic bowel, and this in turn leads to increased tone in the colonic wall, anus, and EAS. Reflex coordination and stool propulsion remain preserved from intact connections between the spinal cord and colon. Thus, with a tight EAS present, constipation predominates. This theory of UMN and LMN syndromes was tested as researchers characterized the motility of the bowel in more detail. Resting motility of the colon was present in lower levels of contractility than in normal subjects that was independent of the level or completeness of injury (Fajardo et al., 2003). Furthermore, a postprandial motor response was confined to the descending colon in SCI patients with lower levels of contractility than in normal subjects. Despite the efforts of research, there continues to be a great void in our understanding of the pathophysiological basis of bowel dysfunction in SCI patients (Holmes et al., 2019).

A bowel management program in SCI patients involves diet modifications, monitoring adequate fluid intake, management of medications, and physical means to stimulate or promote defecation. Therapy should target satisfying the specific objectives of each individual. A few important principles are kept in mind when developing an individualized bowel management program. The goal of therapy is a well-formed fecal mass with appropriate volume and consistency. A regular elimination pattern is also preferred. The bowels should initiate propulsive motility when needed. If the bowel is able to achieve adequate filling, evacuation of stool should be spontaneous. Complete evacuation of stool contents should be the goal.

The methods to treat constipation in this population are difficult because the pathophysiological mechanisms are not well defined. Physical measures include manual disimpaction and anorectal stimulation. In terms of diet, a well-balanced meal should consist of a wide variety of ingredients and good proportions of carbohydrates, proteins, and fats. The use of laxatives should be limited. Fiber and probiotic supplements should be used to enhance stool consistency. Scheduled emptying and deposition of suppositories will also lead to a regular frequency of evacuation. If these methods do not work, then medications are supplemented to the existing regimen. This includes macrogol, high doses of psyllium, prokinetics, digestive enzymes, and many other agents combined to provide a customized treatment for each individual. Transanal irrigation can be used if medications are not effective. Randomized trials comparing this intervention to other traditional conservative bowel management programs showed transanal irrigation to be beneficial in reducing constipation, reducing fecal incontinence, and improving quality of life (Christensen et al., 2006). When conservative measures fail, an enterostomy should be considered. Presently, two other surgical interventions are gaining attention and have been noted to improve bowel function in the SCI population: the sacral anterior root stimulator and the Malone anterograde continence enema (MACE).

## DELAYED POSTTRAUMATIC SPINAL CORD SYNDROMES

### Posttraumatic Syringomyelia

Syringomyelia is found in 21%–28% of SCI patients (Brodbelt and Stoodley, 2003). Cystic changes are found in approximately 30%–50% of all SCI patients. There have been many proposed mechanisms but no unified theory behind the formation of the initial cystic structure. The formation has largely been attributed to hematomyelia, inflammatory responses leading to edema in the cord, ischemia, or arachnoiditis. Enlargement, on the other hand, is generally thought to be due to changes in the compliance of the subarachnoid space or from spinal stenosis, arachnoid adhesions, or persistent cord compression impairing CSF circulation. Correlations exist between the presence of uncorrected kyphosis and stenosis and severity of symptoms. The cystic cavity, acting as a one-way valve, creates imbalance of CSF flow into the cavity. The proposed "slosh mechanism" attributes the growing collections to be secondary to the influences of respirations and blood pressure on CSF pressure.

Although present in a significant portion of SCI patients, only 3%–4% of these patients suffer from symptoms related to syringomyelia. Symptoms of the syrinx can occur from 3 to 34 months following injury. Injury to the spinothalamic tracts leads to pain and a dull, aching, or burning sensation at or above the level of injury. There may also be a dissociated sensory loss (loss of pain and temperature sensation without loss of light touch or proprioception). Measures that increase intraabdominal pressure, such as sneezing, coughing, or straining, can increase the pain. Positional changes such as sitting can also increase pain. The intensity of pain is highly variable. Because a syrinx is typically unilateral, asymmetrical dysreflexia and ascending weakness may appear. Hyperhidrosis, AD, Horner syndrome, dysphagia, cardiopulmonary dysfunction, and bulbar signs and symptoms can present. Following an injury, spasticity can be more severe in those patients with syrinx. Although the condition is progressive in most patients, some may have stable or resolving symptoms and radiographic appearance of the syrinx.

Although this problem is easy to diagnose with modern imaging, it is difficult to treat. Currently, 80% of patients who undergo a form of surgical intervention to treat their syrinx will have persistent or deteriorating findings on follow-up imaging. Modern day therapies focus on one of four surgical options: shunting procedures, lysis of adhesions, correction of deformity or decompression, and cord transsection. Correction of deformity or decompression is usually the preferable option, with good results in reducing the size of the syrinx. The timing of surgery is controversial. Surgery is typically performed on those patients who are deteriorating neurologically or have increasing pain. Some clinicians believe that a symptomatic posttraumatic syrinx should be treated once it is diagnosed, because symptoms are often irreversible. Arachnolysis and duraplasty are another option that is preferable over shunting and serves to untether and decompress the spinal cord. Arachnoid adhesions prevent flow of CSF from occurring in the subarachnoid space. Surgery is focused on leaving the arachnoid intact while removing arachnoid scarring. The majority of cases will have a small rim of arachnoid scarring left. Caution should be exercised to prevent blood products from entering the cord. Artificial dural substrate is preferred to prevent scarring as well. Aspiration of a syrinx cavity in a posttraumatic patient is not recommended.

Shunt, although a viable option, produces mixed results. Shunting should be reserved for situations in which patients fail arachnolysis and duraplasty or where tethering is not found. Syringoperitoneal or syringopleural shunts are commonly placed, although syringosubarachnoid shunts are becoming more common. Subarachnoid-to-peritoneal shunts have been used but with no evidence to support benefits. The shunt is typically placed on the caudal portion of the syrinx in a cranial trajectory, with the entry into the dorsal root entry zone or the posterior median sulcus to minimize spinal cord damage. Ultrasonography may be useful intraoperatively to locate the syrinx. For syringosubarachnoid shunts, the distal end must not be placed in a region occupied by arachnoiditis. Shunt failure rates are high; approximately half report failure. Myelotomies, cord transections, and percutaneous aspirations provide no long-term solution.

Medical therapies are aimed at treating the symptoms. Antispasmodic agents can be used when spasticity creates significant pain or functional disability or interferes with quality of life. TCAs (amitriptyline) and anticonvulsants (gabapentin) help with the neuropathic pain. Anticholinergics can reduce excessive secretions and sweating.

### Neuropathic Pain

Neuropathic pain from SCI can be disabling. It can affect quality of life by limiting sleep and activities of daily living and causing functional disability. Furthermore, the prognosis for a resolution of the pain syndrome is poor. It is estimated that 65%–85% of those suffering from SCI will suffer from neuropathic pain and that a third of these patients will suffer from severe pain (Siddall et al., 2003). The discrepancy in estimates appears to be related to the nonuniform nomenclature used in the literature. Only recently has the International Association for the Study of Pain (IASP) established a Spinal Injury Pain Task Force. In general, four types of pain are considered. Pain is divided into visceral and musculoskeletal, as well as two major neuropathic categories. Musculoskeletal pain is often related to mechanical instability of the spine or muscle spasm. The first type of neuropathic pain deals with a dermatomal pattern at the level of the injury, and the second type is more diffuse and occurs below the level of the injury. One study shows prevalence of neuropathic pain post SCI at 53% (Burke et al., 2017). There appears to be no correlation between completeness or level of injury and the development of postoperative pain.

The mechanism behind the development of pain is unclear. Traditional efforts to understand the cause of neuropathic pain have focused on the region in close proximity to the level of injury. However, contemporary views suggest that more "downstream" or "upstream" changes occur in the nerve roots or the brain. When incomplete injuries occur, transmission of nociceptive impulses can theoretically still occur through various residual pathways. Even in complete injuries, residual sensory pathways exist that may not be evaluated with standard physical examination and may serve as these residual pathways. Studies have shown that injections of local anesthetic at the rostral end of the injuries can bring pain relief (Davis et al., 1954; Pollock et al., 1951). More recent investigations have shown an increased sensitivity of nerve cells close to the level of injury. These nerve cells have a higher amount of background activity, greater amount of responsiveness to stimuli, and a longer duration of firing. Additional changes are suggested to occur at the molecular level and include changes to the level and function of neurotransmitters and their receptors. Glial activation occurs following injury, leading to increased secretion of prostaglandins and various cytokines. Structural changes are known to occur, with restructuring of connections in the dorsal horn. More recent work has focused on thalamocortical dysrhythmia and the plasticity and reorganizational changes that occur in the brain.

The methods of treating neuropathic pain are broad, but principles center around treating the underlying causes of pain. If this is not possible, treatment should focus on palliative measures. Symptomatic treatment is necessary for at-level and below-level neuropathic pain. Surgical options should always focus first on decompressing nervous tissue, untethering the spinal cord, or dealing with a syrinx formation. If these measures do not provide a satisfactory remedy to the pain, then disconnecting the site of abnormal activity is the next appropriate step. Lesions in the dorsal root entry zone can be used to destroy an area of hyperactive nerve cells in the dorsal horn cells in close proximity to the level of the injury. Most studies suggest that 50%–85% of patients have a good amount of relief of pain from this procedure (Siddall, 2009). Electrophysiological techniques such as intramedullary recording of C-fiber evoked electrical hyperactivity may aide in targeting the lesion. Finally, some patients may benefit from cordotomy or cordomyelotomy.

Pharmacological agents are at best a modest means of controlling pain. Only a third of patients have 50% pain reduction. Local and parenteral administration of lidocaine has been shown to be beneficial in treating neuropathic pain, but local administration is generally not long-lasting. NMDA antagonists such as ketamine work by reducing excitability, but ketamine, like lidocaine, confers no long-term relief and is not administered orally. Opioids, antiepileptics, and antidepressants increase inhibitory signals and limit excitability of neurons transmitting pain signals. Two randomized controlled studies show improvement of neuropathic pain following administration of parenteral morphine (Attal et al., 2002) and alfentanil (Elde et al., 1995). The evidence for using oral and transdermal varieties of narcotics is limited. Current recommendations for pharmacological treatment are directed at symptomatic relief and include first-line agents such as systemic lidocaine, gabapentin, and pregabalin. Although a randomized study failed to show benefit from the use of gabapentin in treating neuropathic pain (Rintala et al., 2007), pregabalin has been shown to be of benefit (Vraken et al., 2008). Other new agents that may be considered include lamotrigine and topiramate; topiramate in particular has had encouraging results (Harden et al., 2002). Second-line agents include TCAs, alone or in combination with antiepileptics. TCAs have been shown to have benefit in a subgroup of patients with depression. Both valproate and carbamazepine have been used to treat this condition as well. Third-line treatment options include ketamine, opioids, intrathecal baclofen and morphine, selective serotonin reuptake inhibitors (SSRIs), clonidine, or other antiepileptics. SSRIs are not proven to work. In patients with localized symptoms, topical lidocaine therapy may provide relief. Intrathecal medications have shown some promise. Intrathecal morphine and clonidine have provided short-term pain relief by acting on the opioid receptors of the dorsal horn of the spinal cord. Although intrathecal baclofen works well to treat spasticity, its role in neuropathic pain is still to be determined. A variety of neurostimulation modalities have been used but without good data proving efficacy. These include transcutaneous electrical nerve stimulation (TENS) and acupuncture, which have been shown to help with below-level neuropathic pain (Norrbrink, 2009). Spinal cord stimulators have been shown to be beneficial for at-level neuropathic pain and incomplete injuries (Ciono et al., 1995). Deep brain stimulators do not show good long-term results (Finnerup et al., 2001), and transcranial and epidural stimulation have mixed results (Nguyen et al., 1999).

## Spasticity

Spasticity has been shown to affect more than 80% of SCI patients (Levi et al., 1995). It typically takes several months after the injury for symptoms to become obvious. The initial signs of spasticity include some early reflexes such as tendon reflex, flexor withdrawal reflex, and a Babinski sign. Over time, the threshold to bring about a reflex response decreases, so that even ephemeral stimuli can produce long-lasting flexor contraction. Extensor reflexes present later, and cocontraction of combined flexor/extensor response becomes prominent. Spasms triggered by bladder distention or heat/cold sensations can cause severe pain and create enough intensity to expel an individual from their wheelchair. The symptoms of spasticity are debilitating and lead to a reduced quality of life by limiting activities of daily living, affecting sleep, causing pain, predisposing to unnecessary decubitus ulcers, infections, and contractures, creating a burden on caregivers, and limiting rehabilitation efforts.

For a short time following injury, there is flaccid paralysis and loss of deep tendon reflexes. Over time, changes occur which lead to spasticity. Hyperactivity of gamma motor neurons creates hypersensitivity of the stretch reflex. Following an injury, there is an initial period of downregulation of neuronal membrane receptors. This is followed by upregulation of receptors, which leads to hypersensitivity. Axonal sprouting occurs over time, explaining the temporal changes that occur with spasticity. This mechanism contributes to prolongation of the time-to-peak for excitatory postsynaptic potentials (EPSPs) and the disruption of balance between excitatory and inhibitory input. Alterations occur in the excitatory and inhibitory pathways. A phenomenon known as *postactivation depression* occurs normally as neurotransmitters become depleted. There is a reduction of postactivation depression as well as presynaptic inhibition following SCI. Normally Ia-reciprocal inhibition prevents simultaneous firing of antagonistic muscles. In SCI, this inhibition is reduced, leading to coactivation of antagonistic muscles. Other well-documented mechanisms that play a large role in spasticity include enhancement in the excitability of motor neurons and interneurons. Motor neuronal excitability arises from activation of persistent inward currents and alternations in the monoaminergic drive from the brainstem to the spinal cord. Altered muscular properties also lead to increased tone. Muscle fibers change, along with accumulation of connective tissue and fibrosis, which decreases the elastic properties of muscle. There is also atrophy and loss of muscle fibers and sarcomeres. Alterations in the contractile properties thus become evident.

The management of spasticity centers around reducing unwanted symptoms that limit quality of life. Treatment modalities are multidisciplinary and include physical therapy and rehabilitation, pharmacological interventions (oral and intrathecal), and surgical options. Physical techniques should target passive muscle stretching, with a goal of reducing muscle tone and maintaining flexibility and a wide range of motion. Orthoses can resist contractures and prevent muscle shortening. Treating muscle spasms pharmacologically is often difficult. Medications used to treat spasticity work by suppressing neuronal activity. Although they can benefit the aforementioned exaggerated responses, they can also amplify the negative symptoms—loss of finger dexterity, weakness, and selective use of specific muscle groups. Pharmacological treatments generally fall into three categories: $\gamma$-aminobutyric acid (GABA)-ergic agents that act on interneurons; $\alpha_2$-adrenergic agent; and peripheral-acting drugs that act at the neuromuscular level. Diazepam and baclofen work on the $GABA_A$ and $GABA_B$ receptors, respectively. Diazepam opens chloride channels and hyperpolarizes the presynaptic Ia afferent neurons. In turn, this affects the monosynaptic and polysynaptic reflexes. Diazepam is comparatively more useful in treating the hyperactive reflexes and painful spasms that follow SCI than those associated with stroke or multiple sclerosis. Clonazepam has a lower risk of dependence and causes less sedation. It can be used for nocturnal spasms. Baclofen, on the other hand, acts on both the presynaptic and postsynaptic terminals, affecting both monosynaptic and polysynaptic reflexes as well. On the presynaptic channel, it reduces the influx of calcium. On the postsynaptic channel, it allows the outflow of potassium. Baclofen is effective in reducing flexor spasms and is considered a first-line agent. Functional measures have not been shown to improve with either of the two GABAergic medications. Clonidine works by enhancing $\alpha_2$-adrenergic–mediated presynaptic inhibition of sensory afferents. Ultimately this leads to suppression of the polysynaptic reflexes of the spine. Clonidine has been shown to improve walking in the incomplete SCI population. Tizanidine is an $\alpha_2$-adrenergic agonist that inhibits release of excitatory amino acids from the presynaptic terminals and works on controlling muscle spasms. It has additional effects on glycine, another molecule with inhibitory properties. Dantrolene is a peripheral-acting drug that works by inhibiting calcium from the sarcoplasmic reticulum. It is less useful in SCI because it leads to weakness, although it does reduce muscle tone, tendon reflexes, and clonus while increasing range of motion. Less common medications include cyproheptadine and cannabis. Intrathecal medications are useful when individuals fail to respond to oral agents or are unable to tolerate the side effects of oral agents. Injections are used for the purpose of chemodenervation of local nerves and reserved for individuals with focal spasticity. The injections accomplish nerve block, motor point block, or chemical neurolysis. Agents used include phenol, ethanol, and botulinum toxin. Phenol and ethanol work in the short term by blocking sodium channels. The long-term effects are aimed at denaturing proteins and promoting fibrosis of the neural tissue, interrupting nerve conduction and hence the reflex arc. Patients who receive this therapy have preservation of motor strength, but there is some permanent denervation with each injection. Botulinum toxin has been hailed as the first choice for treating focal spasticity but can produce weakness in the treated muscle. Despite most SCI patients having generalized spasticity, botulinum toxin has the potential to be effective in facilitating rehabilitation and improving function when combined with other treatments. The effects of botulinum toxin appear in 24–72 hours after administration and have a duration of approximately 3 months.

It is necessary to make mention that not all surgical treatment options for spasticity apply to SCIs. Selective rhizotomy, although helpful for cerebral palsy, is not useful in SCI. With the exception of intrathecal baclofen pumps, most of the surgical treatment options are aimed at the muscle and tendon. Tenotomy is used in cases of severe spasticity. Tendon-lengthening procedures and tendon transfer can reduce tension on the intrafusal fibers. Electrical stimulation can reduce the amount of spasticity and can be applied to the muscles, peripheral nerves, and epidural space or in the spinal cord. Electrical fields have also been used to modulate the rate of firing of motor neurons.

## AUTONOMIC DYSREFLEXIA

Acute episodes of AD are characterized by acute elevations in blood pressure coupled with bradycardia, although tachycardia has been known to occur. They usually occur with injury at T6 and above. Systolic blood pressure elevations of 20–30 mm Hg signify a dysreflexic episode. Cervical or high thoracic injuries can place a baseline systolic blood pressure 15–20 mm Hg lower; thus dysreflexic episodes can typically mimic healthy or slightly elevated blood pressure readings. Sympathetic discharge is the source behind these episodes. The symptoms of a rise in blood pressure have varied consequences, from being asymptomatic (mild discomfort, headache, blurred vision) to being life threatening (seizures, intracranial or subarachnoid hemorrhage, death, retinal detachment). Vasoconstriction occurs from sympathetic activation, so dry, pale skin is often observed below the lesion. Above the lesion, intact baroreceptor reflexes initiate a parasympathetic response responsible for bradycardia, as well as sweating, piloerection, and flushing above the level of injury. Once an episode has occurred, the risk for another episode occurring in the next 24–72 hours is increased. A higher percentage of cases exists in high injuries and complete SCIs. In SCI, supraspinal input in the form of inhibitory and excitatory vasomotor pathways to the sympathetic preganglionic neurons are disrupted, and thus unstable blood pressures are found to occur. Stimulation of the urinary bladder or colon has been known to trigger these events. Symptoms are usually brief, either from termination of the episode by treatment or the self-limiting nature of the episode. Alterations have been suspected to occur in the spinal and peripheral autonomic circuits.

The clinical guidelines used for treating a patient with acute episodes of AD focus on an algorithm, with monitoring of blood pressure and heart rate after each step. The first step in caring for a patient suffering from an acute episode of AD should be to place the patient in a sitting position. Second, the patient needs to be inspected for areas of constriction (including clothing). Third, an indwelling catheter should be placed to relieve bladder distention. If a Foley catheter is in place, potential regions of kinks or obstruction should be investigated. Systolic blood pressure is measured after this step, and if the value is greater than 150 mm Hg, a fast-acting short-duration antihypertensive agent is considered. Usually, nifedipine, nitrates, and captopril have been shown to be beneficial in the acute setting. To date, only nifedipine has been studied in controlled trials for AD. Once blood pressure is within an acceptable range (<150 mm Hg), fecal disimpaction can begin. If neither indwelling catheterization nor bowel disimpaction alleviate symptoms, other potential causes should be sought after, but an admission to the hospital is likely needed first to stabilize the patient's blood pressure. After control of symptoms, the patient should be observed for 2 hours to make sure another episode does not recur.

Because bladder distention and irritation are the most common stimulators of AD, good preventive medicine requires routine urological follow-up and enrollment in bladder management programs. A bladder management program that focuses on intermittent catheterization or indwelling catheter ensures proper emptying measures. Urological examinations with cystoscopy or urodynamic studies may be done annually. Ultimately, measures to reduce bladder afferent stimulation may be necessary. The effects of botulinum toxin on bladder detrusor to increase bladder capacity and reduce bladder sphincter dyssynergia, facilitating emptying, has been studied and noted to have positive effects for up to 9 months (Schurch et al., 2000). This can be a safe and effective option for patients who use clean intermittent self-catheterization and do not respond to anticholinergic medications. Anticholinergics and sacral denervation are unproven therapies, with no strong evidence to support efficacy.

## DEEP VENOUS THROMBOSIS AND THROMBOEMBOLISM IN SPINAL CORD INJURY

Deep venous thrombosis (DVT) and PE continue to be major contributors to significant morbidity and mortality in this population. SCI patients are prone to develop DVT because of stasis, hypercoagulable state, and intimal injury. The current incidence is noted to be less than the period before the early 1990s when subcutaneous heparin was not widely used. Prospective analysis of DVT in SCI before the use of prophylactic anticoagulation for a 21-day postinjury period was measured to be 62% (Geerts et al., 1994). Despite widespread use of DVT prophylaxis, screening for DVT in this population still detects a significant number of positive findings. In one prospective study screening prophylactic anticoagulation, the incidence of DVT during a 21-day period was 45.3% (Germing et al., 2009). PE is reported in 8%–14% of all SCI patients (Chiou-Tan et al., 2003; Geerts et al., 2004).

The clinical manifestations of DVT and PE are not always present or obvious, so screening by diagnostic testing is the preferred method to detect these lesions. Screening for DVT in SCI patients can significantly reduce morbidity and mortality. Currently there are no formal guidelines to dictate when to obtain screening for DVTs, although the optimal period of testing is thought to be during the first 13 weeks post SCI (Furlan and Fehlings, 2007). Ultrasound venography is currently used to identify DVT, and chest CTA is used to identify PE. The sensitivity of these tests is related to the size of the lesion.

Current guidelines published in 2017 found a trend toward lower risk of DVT using enoxaparin and no significant differences in rate of DVT, PE, bleeding, and mortality between patients treated with different types of low-molecular-weight heparin or between low-molecular-weight heparin and unfractionated heparin. Combined anticoagulant and mechanical prophylaxis initiated within 72 hours of SCI resulted in lower risk of DVT that treatment commenced after 72 hours of injury (Arnold et al., 2017). Pneumatic compression stockings and gradient elastic stockings have been shown to reduce the incidence of DVTs in SCI patients (Winemiller et al., 1999). Rotating beds, commonly used to prevent decubitus ulcers and provide even distribution of respiration, have also proven effective in preventing DVT (Becker et al., 1987). Inferior vena cava filters have shown a benefit in reducing the risk of PE, but there has also been some suggestion that they may increase the risk of DVT (Gorman et al., 2009).

DVT and PE ultimately require anticoagulation for treatment. The traditional methods of anticoagulation for DVT include intravenous heparin with a transition to warfarin for a period of 3–6 months. In some centers where the cost of hospitalization may be prohibitive, enoxaparin may be used in the outpatient setting to bridge the patient to warfarin.

## FUTURE DIRECTIONS

Current therapies target SCIs from a multitude of perspectives. Prospective trials to assess early versus late decompression in SCI are ongoing. Researchers have been investigating the use of an oscillating field stimulator in neural regeneration. This investigational device is built on the observation that neurons migrate toward the negative pole in an electrical field. Oscillation in the polarity of the electrical field promotes growth in both directions. The device has been assessed for safety in phase I trials and awaits further trials to test its efficacy (Shapiro et al., 2005). CSF drainage as a method of reducing ischemic paraplegia in patients undergoing thoracoabdominal aortic aneurysm surgery has been shown to improve outcomes (Coselli et al., 2002).

Hypothermia as a neuroprotective therapy has been studied extensively in animals and recently in human trials. On a biochemical, histological, and molecular level, hypothermia has been shown to reduce apoptosis, damage from oxidative stress, vasogenic edema, neutrophil and macrophage invasion, and extracellular glutamate concentration. Preclinical studies have demonstrated these neuroprotective effects with improvements in locomotive and urinary outcomes of animals with SCI treated with hypothermia (Grulova et al., 2013). However, the risks associated with hypothermia include unwanted cardiac arrhythmias, sepsis and infection, and coagulopathy. Retrospective analysis has been done showing no additional risks in patients undergoing 48 hours of hypothermia to a target temperature of 33°C (Levi et al., 2009).

Pharmacological advances are also on the horizon. Two medications currently approved for other medical conditions that are being tested in SCI subjects are minocycline and riluzole. Minocycline has been used for years in the treatment of a variety of dermatological conditions, but it has been noted to have neuroprotective effects in dealing with apoptosis and inhibition of microglial activation. Riluzole has been found to block voltage-sensitive sodium channels and prevent calcium-mediated release of glutamate. Only recently has it been shown to enhance growth of sensory neurons.

New pharmacological arenas are currently being explored to expand upon the available treatment options for SCIs. One area of interest in SCI research deals with the regenerative capacity of neurons. It is well recognized that neurons possess the capacity to regenerate, but the presence of inhibitory molecules prevents regeneration from occurring. Of interest is a molecule contained within myelin, known as *Nogo*, which blocks axonal growth. Anti-Nogo antibodies have been used in animal studies to show functional recovery and axonal sprouting. Additional targets of therapy include the Rho Guanosine Triphosphatase (Rho GTPase). Rho GTPase has been found to be the central mediator of axonal growth inhibitors. BA-210 is a bacterial toxin known to inhibit Rho GTPase. It is added with a fibrin sealant to form a compound called *Cethrin*. Cethrin has been designed to be delivered to the dura at the time of spinal surgery. Initial clinical trials have shown promise for motor improvement in SCI, without significant side effects (Onose et al., 2009).

The latest addition to SCI therapies is cell transportation therapy. Transplantation of activated autologous macrophages has been considered a potential therapeutic modality, based on the knowledge that macrophages are present in abundance following nerve injury in the peripheral nervous system. Macrophages are thought to be essential in clearing cellular debris and secreting growth factors and cytokines that may promote axonal growth. A nonrandomized study has shown it to be safe, with an encouraging efficacy profile (Knoller et al., 2005).

Schwann cells have also been targeted for their potential to encourage axonal growth and provide a myelin highway to reestablish axonal conduction. Researchers have also attempted to capitalize on the regenerating properties of olfactory ensheathing cells. Recently, transplantation of adult neural precursor cells in rats was seen to promote remyelination and functional recovery (Karimi-Abdolrezaee et al., 2006).

Currently, multiple centers are also performing trials of mesenchymal stem cell (MSC) transplantation. However, encouraging preclinical studies in animal models were followed by weak and conflicting results in clinical trials (Cofano et al., 2019). The use of MSC remains safe, with no studies showing harm, but ongoing trials are needed to help researchers improve clinical knowledge and provide benefit to the patients. Although many of these innovative treatments require substantial further trials before becoming mainstream, researchers and clinicians feel hopeful that in the future they will be able to provide new life to SCI victims.

*The complete reference list is available online at https://expertconsult.inkling.com/.*

64

# Trauma of the Nervous System: Peripheral Nerve Trauma

*Bryan Tsao, Kevin Cronin, Brian Murray*

## OUTLINE



Historical interest in peripheral nervous system (PNS) trauma dates back many centuries. Leonardo Da Vinci made detailed anatomical drawings of the brachial plexus, believing this complex of nerves existed to ensure continued function of the upper extremity should one of its elements be severed (e.g., by a sword thrust) (Murray and Wilbourn, 2002). By 1885, Duchenne, Erb, and Klumpke all had recorded their landmark descriptions of various brachial plexus injuries. The US Civil War and both World Wars provided the substrate for the systematic study of peripheral nerve injuries by 19th-century American neurologist Weir Mitchell and 20th-century neurosurgeon Barnes Woodhall, respectively; their work led to the advent of nerve injury classification systems by Sir Herbert Seddon, Sir Sydney Sunderland, and George E. Omer.

Today, up to 5% of all admissions to level I trauma centers have a peripheral nerve, nerve root, or plexus injury (Noble et al., 1998). While regeneration is much more effective and efficient in the PNS than the central nervous system (CNS), the outcome is rather variable and much depends on the severity and site of the injury. In general, injuries to the upper extremity are more common than those to the lower extremity, accounting for two-thirds of all peripheral nerve injuries. Of the four major PNS plexuses—cervical, brachial, lumbar, and sacral—the brachial plexus is by far the most commonly affected.

This chapter begins with a review of relevant neuroanatomy. Then the common mechanisms that cause peripheral nerve injury in adults are examined, and an approach to the diagnosis and management of such injuries is presented. Next, current surgical techniques used in nerve repair are described, followed by a look at new therapeutic technologies.

## ANATOMY OF THE SPINAL NERVES OF THE PERIPHERAL NERVOUS SYSTEM

The PNS is composed of those neural elements that extend between the CNS (in this case the spinal cord) and their target organs (Fig. 64.1). The peripheral motor system axons (somatic efferents) originate from the anterior horn cells and exit the spinal cord to form the ventral (anterior) rootlets. Muscle spindle fusimotor efferents and afferents travel with these fibers. Axons of the peripheral sensory system (somatic afferent) extend from specialized sensory organs within skin, muscle, tendon–muscle junctions, and viscera to their cell bodies, the dorsal root ganglia (DRG), which lie within the bony intervertebral foramen. These sensory fibers make up the dorsal (posterior, somatic afferent) rootlets that enter the posterior horn of the spinal cord. The mixed spinal nerves are formed when anterior and posterior rootlets combine within the neural foramen just distal to the DRG at the point where the dura ends. The short spinal nerve then divides into two branches: (1) a large anterior branch (ventral ramus) that extends forward to supply the trunk muscles and gives rise to the roots of the plexus, and (2) a small posterior branch (dorsal ramus) that extends backward to supply motor fibers to paravertebral muscles and ferry sensory fibers from posterior longitudinal ligaments, intervertebral discs, dura mater, facet joints, and the skin of the neck and back. Autonomic sympathetic axons communicate and travel with the mixed spinal nerves via the rami communicantes.

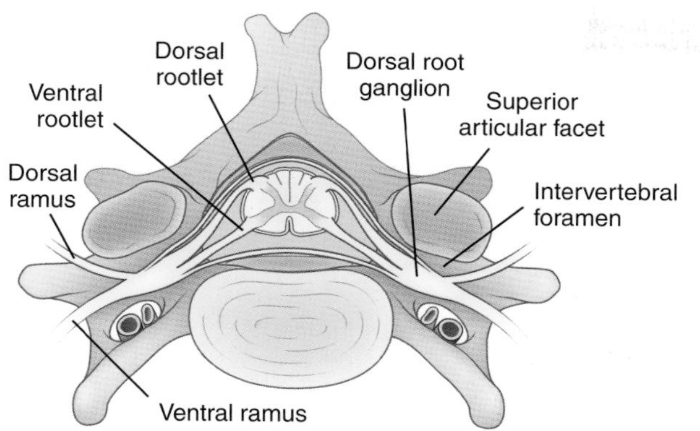


**Fig. 64.1 Anatomy of a Spinal Nerve.** Dorsal and ventral rootlets combine within the intervertebral foramen to form mixed spinal nerves, which further divide on exiting the foramen into the dorsal and ventral rami. *(Image courtesy of Cleveland Clinic, 2006. Illustrator, David Schumick, BS, CMI.)*

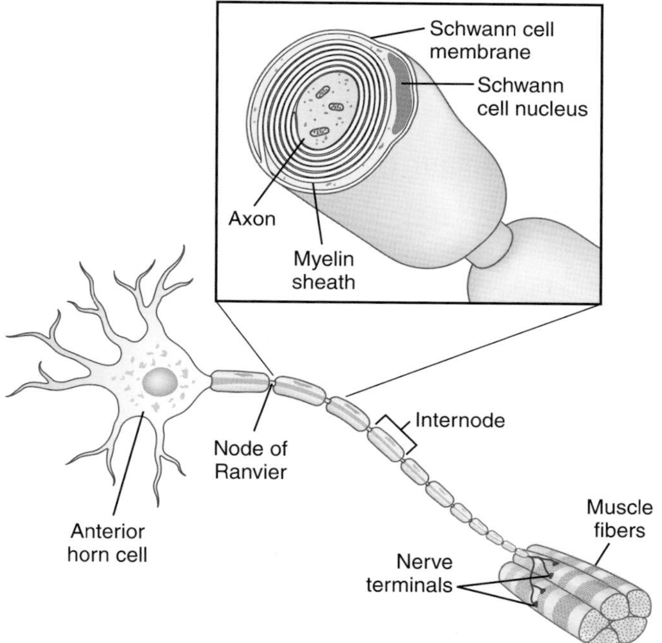


**Fig. 64.2 Anatomy of a Peripheral Nerve.** The motor nerve cell body lies within the anterior horn of the spinal cord. A single axon extends from the anterior horn cell to its target muscle, making contact at the neuromuscular junction. Local support cells called *Schwann cells* generate a myelin sheath that is laid down at regular intervals around the axon; each interval is called an *internode*, and the intervening gap is called the *node of Ranvier*.

## Axon

The core element of the nerve is the *axon*, a thin tube of axoplasm that extends from the nerve cell body to the target organ. Unmyelinated axons are partially ensheathed by invaginations of the Schwann cell membrane, whereas myelinated axons are enveloped in concentric lamellae of myelin composed of compacted spiraled Schwann cell membrane to form a sheath (Fig. 64.2). The *myelin sheath* is laid down in segments called *internodes*, each derived from one Schwann cell. The small gap of uncovered axoplasm between sheaths is called the *node of Ranvier*, the site where the largest part of ion flow takes place to transmit the action potential. In *saltatory conduction*, action potentials leap from node to node, rather than traveling in a continuous conduction process along the entire length of the axolemma. In this way, a myelinated large-caliber axon in human adults may conduct electrical impulses at more than 70 m/sec, whereas a small unmyelinated axon may conduct as slowly as 0.5 m/sec (Kimura, 2005).

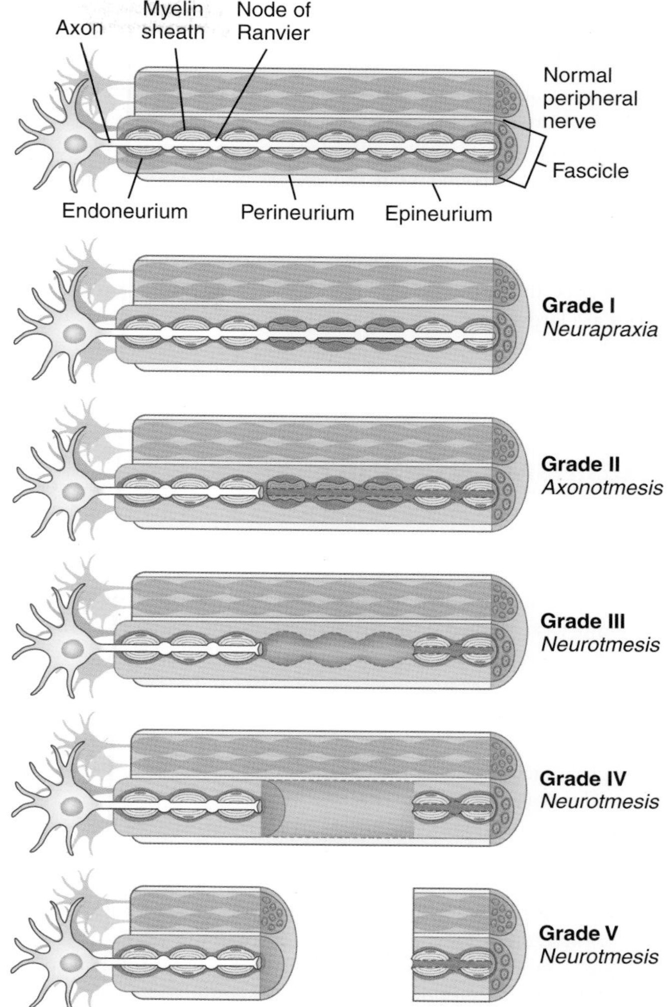


**Fig. 64.3** Classification of Peripheral Nerve Trauma (see text). *(Image courtesy of Cleveland Clinic, 2006. Illustrator, David Schumick, BS, CMI.)*

## Peripheral Nerve Trunks

The connective tissue within a peripheral nerve trunk is composed of the endoneurium, perineurium, and epineurium (Fig. 64.3). These tissues provide structure, tensile strength, and elasticity.

The *endoneurium* is a thin layer of collagenous connective tissue that surrounds individual nerve fibers and is continuous with the fine layer of connective tissue of the nerve roots. In the nerve trunk, bundles of myelinated and unmyelinated nerve fibers are arranged into *fascicles* (or funiculi). These fascicles, which vary greatly in size and number, are arranged in an intertwining pattern (sometimes called the *Sunderland plexus*) in the more proximal portion of the nerve trunk but are arrayed in a more parallel pattern in the distal parts of the nerve. Each fascicle is surrounded by *perineurium*, which consists of perineurial cells that interlock to form tight cell junctions, creating the blood–nerve barrier that maintains an immunologically privileged endoneurial environment. A typical spinal nerve trunk consists of a variable number of fascicles separated by inter- and extrafascicular *epineurium* that constitutes an extension of the dura mater. Finally, the nerve trunk melds into surrounding structures via a loose layer of protective areolar tissue, or the *mesoneurium*, which allows the nerve passive movement in the transverse and longitudinal planes.

Peripheral nerves have an abundant and anastomotic blood supply. The arterial arrangement is composed of extraneural arteries (arteriae nervorum) that enter the nerve proper at various sites and angles along the length of the nerve. Longitudinally arranged arterioles travel along the interfascicular epineurium before they branch off to pierce the perineurium. The endoneurial or intraneural capillaries are larger in diameter than typical capillaries in other organs and resemble end arterioles in size, although they are surrounded only by pericytes. Venous drainage is conducted along postcapillary venules.

## CLASSIFICATION OF NERVE TRAUMA

Based on observations made in Great Britain during the Second World War, Seddon devised a three-tiered classification system for nerve trauma (Table 64.1; see Fig. 64.3). In this system, the mildest form of injury is due to a transient focal block in conduction along the nerve fiber; injury is confined to the myelin sheath and spares the axon. He called this *neurapraxia* (Greek for "nonaction of nerve"). This type of injury has an excellent prognosis for complete and spontaneous recovery within a 6-week period. Indeed, many patients return to normal within hours. A clinical example of neurapraxia is wrist drop secondary to prolonged external pressure that compresses the radial nerve at the spiral groove of the humerus.

Seddon's second grade of injury, *axonotmesis* (Greek for "cutting of the axon"), involves injury not only to the myelin sheath but also to the axon itself, so that, as noted by Seddon in 1942, "the sheath and the more intimate supporting structures of the nerve have not been completely divided, which means that the nerve as a mass of tissue is still in continuity." Axonotmesis is common in crush injuries and displaced bone fractures, and complete recovery is less certain than with neurapraxia. It triggers the process of wallerian degeneration and regeneration, the success of which depends in part on the preservation of connective tissues such as endoneurium and perineurium.

Seddon's most severe type of injury, called *neurotmesis* (a "cutting of the nerve"), entails damage to myelin, axons, and various layers of connective tissue. Seddon originally used this term to describe complete nerve transection in which "the injury produces a lesion which is in every sense complete," but later amended the definition to "describe the state of a nerve that has either been completely severed or is so seriously disorganized by scar tissue that spontaneous regeneration is out of the question." This is common after laceration or ischemic injuries and portends the worst prognosis for clinical recovery, often necessitating surgical intervention.

A second classification system for nerve trauma was devised by Sunderland to include additional information regarding the degree of injury to connective tissue. This system is divided into five grades: grades I and II are identical to Seddon's neurapraxia and axonotmesis, respectively (see Table 64.1 and Fig. 64.3). However, Sunderland subdivided Seddon's neurotmesis into three further levels of injury: grade III entails injury to the myelin sheath, axon, and endoneurium, with sparing of the perineurium and epineurium; grade IV describes an injury to all nerve trunk elements except the epineurium; and grade V entails complete transection of all neural and connective tissue elements of the nerve trunk. Only Sunderland's classification system is used in the rest of this chapter.

**TABLE 64.1 Nerve Trauma Classifications**

| | CLASSIFICATION | | |
|---|---|---|---|
| **Injured Tissue(s)** | **Seddon** | **Sunderland** | **Modification (MacKinnon)** |
| Myelin | Neurapraxia | Grade I | — |
| Myelin, axon | Axonotmesis | Grade II | — |
| Myelin, axon, endoneurium | Neurotmesis | Grade III | — |
| Myelin, axon, endoneurium, perineurium | Neurotmesis | Grade IV | — |
| Myelin, axon, endoneurium, perineurium, epineurium | Neurotmesis | Grade V | — |
| Combination | | | Grade VI |

Modifications to these two systems have been devised, largely with the surgeon in mind. A further grade (grade VI) has been proposed to highlight the fact that some injuries may feature a combination of Sunderland grades (e.g., some areas may be grade III and others grade IV) affecting different fascicles within a segment of nerve.

## PERIPHERAL NERVE DEGENERATION AND REGENERATION

Large myelinated peripheral axons may respond to injury or disease in three ways: segmental demyelination, wallerian degeneration, and axonal degeneration. Segmental demyelination and wallerian degeneration are relevant to traumatic nerve injury and are discussed in more detail in this chapter, whereas axonal degeneration is more characteristically seen in metabolic and toxic nerve disorders such as diabetes mellitus and renal failure (see Chapter 107).

### Segmental Demyelination

Segmental demyelination occurs when a focal segment of nerve is subjected to a relatively mild compressive or traction force. The nerve segments that lie distal and proximal to the site of injury are not affected and function normally. Conduction across the injured segment is impaired, however, when distortion of the myelin sheath causes degeneration of one or several internodes, thereby reducing the ability of the sheath to act as an electrical insulator. If the myelin is only slightly damaged, the only local consequence may be a widening of the node of Ranvier that causes a slowing of conduction velocity across the nerve segment. Focal demyelination of axons within a nerve fascicle may affect some but not all fibers, resulting in asynchronous conduction across the affected nerve segment. In this case, impulses eventually reach their destination after a delay measured in milliseconds, but the slowing may affect certain nerve functions that rely on highly synchronous firing (e.g., deep tendon reflexes, vibration sense), resulting in paresthesia.

More severe compression may involve most or all myelinated nerve fibers at the injury site and several internodes. In this situation, blockade of conduction across that segment results in weakness or sensory disturbance. Study of nerve segments that have been subjected to tourniquet compression reveals that the nodes of Ranvier located at the edge of the tourniquet are subjected to greater pressure and are deformed to a greater degree than the segment lying directly beneath the tourniquet. This pressure gradient causes the underlying axon and myelin to telescope into neighboring segments, which greatly distorts

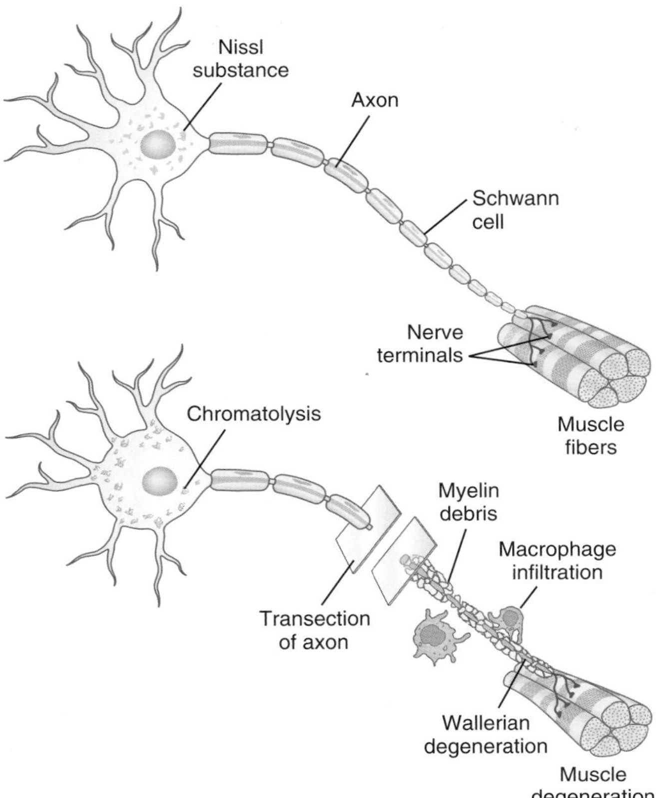


**Fig. 64.4 Wallerian Degeneration.** After axotomy, the axon and the myelin sheath distal to transection begin to degenerate. Within a few days, macrophages are recruited into the injury site; they digest debris. Changes also occur proximal to the site of the injury. A degree of wallerian degeneration takes place up to the first encountered node of Ranvier, and the cell body undergoes chromatolysis, which represents a switch in function of the cell body from axon maintenance to axon regeneration. If regeneration does not take place, the target tissue is not reinnervated, and degeneration of the target organ eventually occurs.

the paranodal segment of myelin, resulting in conduction slowing or demyelinating conduction block.

## Wallerian Degeneration

Injury to a peripheral nerve triggers a complex process that involves the axon, its cell body, its cellular connections, and the surrounding connective tissues. Wallerian degeneration follows grade II to grade V injuries and can be divided into changes that involve the segments of nerve distal and proximal to the zone of injury (Fig. 64.4).

### Distal Segment Changes

After nerve injury, the earliest changes occur in the axon distal to the site of injury, where there is disruption of retrograde and anterograde flow of signals within the axon (Menorca et al., 2013; Scheib and Hoke, 2013). Rapid inflow of extracellular ions such as calcium and sodium occurs through the disruption in the axonal plasma membrane, which activates a cascade of events that shares features with programmed cell death or apoptosis. Axonal injury also leads to recruitment of leukocytes and initiates the cytokine-mediated signaling cascade and changes in the neighboring non-neuronal cells. This in turn triggers the synthesis of neurotrophins, chemokines, extracellular matrix molecules, proteolytic enzymes, and interleukins (Radtke and Vogt, 2009). The entire axonal process of wallerian degeneration takes approximately 1 week. By day 3, the Schwann cells retract from the node of Ranvier, and activated Schwann cells and macrophages begin to digest myelin. The process of neuronal degeneration quickly undergoes a transition to neuronal regeneration from the proximal stump. The transition of Schwann cells from myelin-manufacturing cells to repair cells is significantly affected by upregulation of c-Jun protein (Scheib and Hoke, 2013). Schwann cell proliferation facilitates sprouting of new nerve branches from the injured axon terminus and initiates the sequence of events that lead to rebuilding of neural contacts to distal muscles.

### Proximal Segment

Depending on the severity of injury, a limited degree of axon breakdown extends proximally from the site of injury up to the level of the first node of Ranvier. Although very proximal injury may lead to apoptosis of the cell body itself (e.g., after a proximal arm amputation), the more common consequence of axonal injury is for the cell body to go through the process of chromatolysis. This involves the breakup and dispersion of the rough endoplasmic reticulum, the eccentric displacement of the cell nucleus, and increased nuclear expression of transcription factors that switch the pattern of gene expression from axon maintenance to protein synthesis (Scheib and Hoke, 2013).

## Nerve Regeneration

The method of nerve regeneration depends on the type of injury sustained: remyelination after grade I lesions and collateral axon sprouting and proximal-to-distal nerve regeneration after grade II to grade V lesions.

With focal demyelinating lesions, recovery of function occurs as the Schwann cell divides and initiates remyelination. Conduction, and thereby strength, is re-established within a few weeks or months, but the new myelin sheath usually is thinner and has several internodes for each original internode.

When only some of the axons supplying a muscle are damaged, the intact motor axons produce sprouts that reinnervate the denervated muscle fiber; this is referred to as *collateral sprouting*. These nerve sprouts originate from the nodes of Ranvier (nodal sprouts) or the nerve terminals (terminal sprouts) as early as 4 days from the time of injury. By adopting denervated muscle fibers, collateral innervation increases the size of the remaining motor units and results in increased contractile force. Clinical recovery due to collateral sprouting takes 3–6 months from the time of injury. During this same period, compensatory hypertrophy of muscle fibers that have retained their axons occurs, although the muscle as a whole atrophies. Enhanced synchronization of motor unit firing contributes to improved strength.

In contrast with partial or mild nerve injury, in which the surviving motor axon begins the process of collateral sprouting almost immediately, in severe or complete injury, neuronal regeneration starts from the proximal stump only after wallerian degeneration is completed. Schwann cells play a key role in neuronal regeneration. They dedifferentiate and upregulate the expression of adhesion molecules and neurotrophins (i.e., cadherins, immunoglobulin superfamily factors, laminin), which promote the migration of nerve sprouts that form at the regenerating axon tip. These sprouts then form cords aligned around the original basal lamina tubes of the myelinated axons (bands of Büngner) that provide a pathway along which new axons are destined to grow (Geraldo and Gordon-Weeks, 2009). The contribution of axon regeneration to clinical recovery overlaps with collateral sprouting at approximately 3 months, but axon regeneration is the main recovery mechanism from 6 to 24 months after the injury, depending in part on the distance the nerve must grow to reach its target muscle.

The tip of the axon sprout, called the *growth cone*, travels by way of *filopodia* and *lamellipodia* (Fig. 64.5). *Neurotropism*, the term used to describe guidance of a regenerating axon, is accomplished by

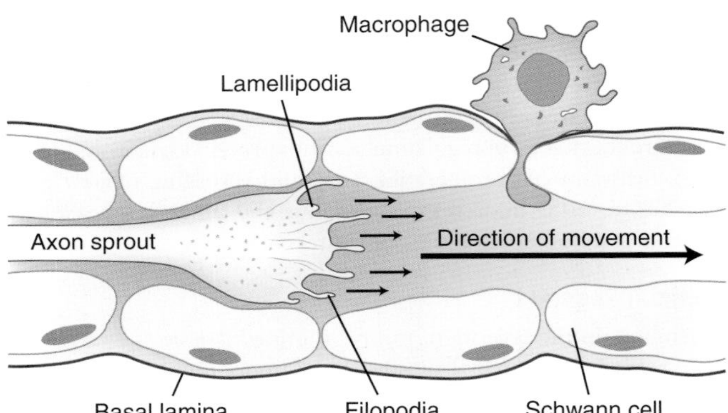


**Fig. 64.5 Schematic Diagram of Axonal Regeneration.** An axon sprout grows out from the proximal stump and proceeds toward the degenerated distal axon stump via the bands of Büngner (formed by proliferating Schwann cells and bounded by intact basal lamina). Macrophages migrate through basal lamina into the injury site to phagocytose myelin ovoids and axonal debris, clearing the way for the axon sprout to progress distally. The motile tip of the axon sprout is called the *growth cone*, which bears receptor-rich lamellipodia (sheet-like) and filopodia (finger-like). These structures are guided through the bands of Büngner to their target by multiple signals in the microenvironment.

guidance molecules (i.e., semaphorins, ephrins, netrins, slits) that act to attract or repulse the growth cone to prevent misdirected growth of axon sprouts. To pass through endoneurial tubules plugged with cellular debris, the growth cone secretes plasminogen activators that dissolve cell–cell and cell–matrix adhesions. Axonal sprouts grow from the proximal to the distal stump at a rate of approximately 1–2 mm/day (or approximately 1 inch/month). This rate of regrowth varies depending on the location of the lesion; with proximal lesions, growth may be as fast as 2–3 mm/day, while that with distal lesions is about 1 mm/day.

Peripheral axons and non-neuronal cells contain growth-inducing and trophic molecules that provide the fertile milieu required for nerve regeneration. These include the neurotrophins (nerve growth factor, brain-derived neurotrophic factor, neurotrophins 3 and 4), glial cell line–derived neurotrophic factors (neurturin, artemin, persephin), insulin-like neurotrophic factor, interleukin-6, leukemia inhibitory factor, ciliary neurotrophic factor, fibroblast growth factors, and several transcription factor activators (Scheib and Hoke, 2013; Tucker and Mearow, 2008).

The condition of the endoneurial tube at the injury site determines the efficiency of nerve regeneration. If the tube is intact, regrowth of the proximal axon has a greater chance of success. With severe or complete disruption of the endoneurial tube, the proximal axon may stray into the surrounding connective tissue, which increases the chance of disorganized nerve sprouts or neuroma formation. Misplaced axons within a neuroma are subject to ectopic hyperexcitability that results from the accumulation of sodium channels and this in turn generates neuropathic pain. Once the advancing axon has crossed the injury gap and entered the distal endoneurial tube, the nerve has a reasonably good chance of successfully reaching its target end organ. If it takes the axon longer than 4 months to reach the gap, however, the distal endoneurial diameter shrinks to perhaps 3 μm or less, further impeding complete recovery. Nevertheless, some degree of reinnervation can occur for up to 2 years after injury.

Successful axon regeneration also relies on the presence of a viable end organ. Denervated muscle fibers quickly undergo atrophy, and collagen deposition occurs within the endomysium and perimysium, but the overall muscle architecture, along with end-plate integrity, is maintained for at least 1 year after nerve injury. Irreversible muscle fibrosis and degeneration, however, often has occurred by 2 years. Sensory cross-reinnervation is common, and pacinian and meissnerian corpuscles (mediating rapidly adapting light touch) and Merkel cells (mediating slow-adapting touch and pressure) are able to survive in a denervated state for a period of years. Thus, even late reinnervation on the order of 2–3 years may restore useful protective sensory function to a limb.

## MECHANISMS OF TRAUMATIC NERVE INJURY

### Compression

Compressive nerve injuries most commonly affect large-caliber myelinated nerve fibers in nerves that cross over bony surfaces or between rigid structures. Such injuries can be broadly divided into acute compression injuries (e.g., Saturday night palsy; compression of the radial nerve against the spiral groove) and chronic compression injuries (e.g., median neuropathy located at or distal to the wrist and seen in carpal tunnel syndrome). Acute compression neuropathies are more pertinent to the assessment of the traumatic nerve injury. Experimental histological models have shown that the compressed segment of nerve intussuscepts into a neighboring segment of axon. Most typically they occur in patients who have been sedated or unconscious in a single position for an extended period but they occur with relatively little injury in patients with hereditary neuropathy with liability to pressure palsies (HNPP). Because the primary underlying pathophysiology is that of demyelinating conduction block, an excellent recovery generally can be expected in the following days to weeks. A similar problem can be recognized in the postoperative setting. In classic postoperative brachial plexopathy, the patient awakens from general anesthesia with complete upper limb paralysis due to compression and stretch of brachial plexus elements between the clavicle and first rib while the arm is extended and hyperabducted intraoperatively. Electrophysiological examination may reveal a combination of upper trunk demyelinating conduction block and a lesser component of axon loss. The deficit characteristically reduces to a pure upper trunk distribution within the first few days, and within 2–3 months has fully resolved.

Mechanical compression may lead to secondary ischemic injury, as in the case of acute compartment syndromes that compromise nerve microcirculation while sparing distal-extremity pulses. When the intracompartmental pressure exceeds intra-arterial pressure, nerve (and muscle) ischemia results in axon-loss lesions of variable severity. An example is the medial brachial fascial compartment syndrome after axillary arteriography or axillary regional block. Severe or irreversible single or multiple axon-loss mononeuropathies can occur within 4 hours if untreated by immediate exploration of the puncture site and decompression (Tsao and Wilbourn, 2003).

### Stretch and Traction

Peripheral nerves are vulnerable to serious injury from excessive stretch or traction. As the stretching force increases, the elastic properties of the nerve are overcome, and myelin sheaths, axons, and connective tissue may rupture. In addition, it has been shown in an in vivo rat sciatic model that an 8% elongation of a nerve increases intraneural pressure to the point that blood flow is reduced by half.

An important example of a closed traction or stretch injury is neonatal Erb-Duchenne palsy due to excessive traction forces applied to the infant's C5–C6 roots and fibers of the upper trunk of the brachial plexus during a difficult delivery. Significant axonal injury characteristically occurs, which may leave the child with permanent paralysis of upper arm flexors and forearm supinators, causing the arm to be held in the "waiter's tip" position.

Sufficient stretch produced by distraction of the neck from the shoulder results in avulsion injury of the intraspinal rootlets from the spinal cord. Avulsion injuries most often are due to motor vehicle and motorcycle accidents. The typical scenario is that of a motorcycle rider being thrown off the motorcycle; the head and shoulder strike the pavement, laterally flexing the neck away from the shoulder, stretching the brachial plexus, and pulling the rootlets out of the spinal cord. Another example is a heavy object falling from a height onto a person's shoulder. Avulsion particularly affects the intra- and extraforaminal portions of the cervical root fibers and the proximal brachial plexus fibers. Lesions of the lumbosacral plexus and roots are uncommon. The prognosis with avulsion of motor and preganglionic sensory fibers is poor. Avulsion is associated with particularly severe and lasting neuropathic pain.

### Laceration

In laceration, the nerve is partly or completely severed by a sharp object. Common laceration injuries are knife wounds and injuries from broken glass, metal shards, chainsaw blades, wood splinters, and animal bites. In general, the sharper the injurious object, the neater the injury and the shorter the distance between proximal and distal nerve stumps. Shorter distance means a greater likelihood of a satisfactory functional recovery. An iatrogenic example is the inadvertent transection of branches of the spinal accessory nerve during surgical removal or biopsy of a mass in the posterior triangle of the neck.

### Crush

A crush injury may arise from a sudden significant force applied to the nerve from a blunt object such as a surgical clamp, lead pipe, baseball bat, or motor vehicle component. Mild degrees of crush may cause a predominantly demyelinating conduction-block injury, but axon loss usually is prominent in most cases. Experimental work on animal nerves using smooth-tipped forceps has shown that axon and myelin debris is displaced longitudinally by the crush force. The myelin is thinned out directly under the crush force and is thicker at the edges, thus creating the histological appearance of "tadpoles swimming away" from the crush site; the Schwann cell and its membranes remain intact. After removal of the crush force, axon and myelin tissues flow back into the crush site. Nerve regeneration may be quite satisfactory if the distance between the proximal and distal healthy margins is not too great and continuity of the axon structure is maintained. Neuroma formation, however, is common at injury sites with longer wounds.

### Gunshot

It is important to distinguish between low-velocity and high-velocity gunshot injuries. Low-velocity weapons more often are used in the civilian setting, and their missiles typically cause laceration, compression, and stretch injuries to localized segments of nerve and tissue. High-velocity weapons are used in both military and civilian settings. Missiles fired from such weapons are surrounded by a high-pressure gas zone, and the associated explosive force causes extensive damage to both local and distant nerves, together with other tissues such as muscle, bone, organs, and blood vessels. As a consequence, all grades of nerve injury may occur concurrently within and around the wound site. Although neurotmesis lesions may be clearly apparent on first inspection of the wound, the very real likelihood of additional areas of neurapraxia and axonotmesis must be considered. Therefore, it is vital in these patients to perform serial clinical evaluations and electrophysiological studies after the injury, prior to making the decision to attempt graft repair.

### Radiation

A delayed adverse effect of radiotherapy includes nerve injury; pathogenesis is proposed to be due to an initial intermittent microvascular endothelial inflammatory response and then a fibrotic phase.

The field of original radiation therapy is related to the site of the neuropathy. Cranial irradiation—for example, for Hodgkin lymphoma—can lead to delayed onset of focal or grouped cranial neuropathies, such as facial palsy, hypoglossal palsy, recurrent laryngeal nerve palsy, or combinations thereof.

One of the most frequently encountered radiation-induced nerve injuries is that to the infraclavicular brachial plexus (initially involving the lateral cord) after radiotherapy of the axillary chain of lymph nodes for breast cancer. Supraclavicular brachial plexus involvement is seen less often but may follow mantle radiation (or delivery of a downward cone beam) for lymphoma of the cervical, peritracheal, or supraclavicular regions (Gu et al., 2014). A delay in onset between 6 months and 35 years after therapy is typical, and the neuropathy most commonly starts with paresthesia in the index or middle finger, followed by weakness in muscles mainly derived from the lateral cord. Progression over time is the rule, often over a few months to 5 years; a flail deformity eventually may develop in the involved limb. This form of plexopathy is initially characterized by the development of persistent proximal demyelinating conduction block, which actually portends a poor prognosis and makes this plexopathy considerably different from the neurapraxias associated with acute compression injuries. Myokymic discharges are useful electrodiagnostic indicators of radiotherapy-induced nerve injury. Sometimes it may be difficult to determine whether a progressive neuropathy is due to prior radiotherapy or to relapsing disease (e.g., lymphoma) but modern imaging techniques such as positron emission tomography (PET) imaging have been invaluable in that regard. It is now recognized that there can be cases of a transient rather than chronic progressive radiation-associated neuropathy, as has been demonstrated with cases of a lumbosacral plexopathy after treatment of testicular disease and acute transient brachial plexopathy after breast disease therapy (Delanian et al., 2012).

### Cold Injury

Peripheral nerves are especially prone to damage from excessively cold temperatures ("frostbite" and "trench foot"). In frostbite, tissue freezing occurs through formation of ice crystals in both superficial and deep tissues. The severity of the injury depends on the duration of exposure, the environmental temperature, the wind chill factor, patient factors (physical fitness) and ranges from mild partial skin freezing to complete tissue mummification (Golden et al., 2013; Imray et al., 2009). Trench foot can occur in an extremity that is both damp and exposed to prolonged cold environs (1°C–10°C) leading to vasoconstriction. Actual frostbite occurs at freezing temperatures (typically less than −2°C). Duration of freezing is directly related to severity of injury, but other factors play a part, including body habitus, history of smoking, nutrition, and poor fitness. Indeed, there can be a significant lack of self-reporting or recognition of an evolving frostbite injury, as may occur through psychological factors (Sullivan-Kwantes and Goodman, 2017) or if the sufferer has encephalopathy (as may occur in mountain sickness). With transient or mild exposure, the underlying nerve pathophysiology is primarily that of demyelinating conduction block, but continued exposure to low ambient temperatures causes increasingly severe degrees of axon injury. The endoneurium becomes particularly edematous, thus raising intraneural pressure to the point at which blood flow is compromised, thereby further compounding the injury. If the cold-induced injury is not complete, function is restored in the order it was lost—for example, recovery of first sensory and then motor modalities.

### Electrical

A severe neurological injury may follow contact with a high-voltage electric current in the home or workplace, or from a lightning strike. Damage is produced mainly by heating, which may cause the tissues to explode. With high-voltage (>1000 V) injuries, frank necrosis of all tissues including nerve may develop, with subsequent loss of the limb or part thereof. Low-voltage (<1000 V) events are associated with a better prognosis, and the injury may or may not include cutaneous burns. Most peripheral nerve injuries occur in association with third- and/or fourth-degree electrical burns and include axonal mononeuropathies, polyneuropathies, and plexopathies, which may be either early or delayed in onset (by months) and are frequently bilateral. High-voltage electrical injuries can lead to secondary traumatic injury in up to 15% of cases if the person is bodily thrown by the energy force against a hard object. Injury to vascular structures, muscle, bone, and other soft tissues can also be present and compartment syndromes are possible (Sanford and Gamelli, 2014). The median and ulnar nerves most frequently are affected. Symptoms and signs may be similar to those of focal compression neuropathies, occurring at sites of minimal limb cross-sectional area where nerves cross bony protuberances. Joule's law predicts that heat production will be maximal at such sites, and it has been proposed that perineurial fibrosis may occur at these sites, giving rise to neuropathies that may be relieved by surgical decompression (Kwon et al., 2013).

### Injection

One of the most severe forms of peripheral nerve injury is that due to injection of drug (prescribed or illicit). Unfortunately, these injuries are relatively common and are a direct effect of needle insertion into the nerve or (more often) are due to the drug itself or its associated buffer and solvent. The presence of drug in and around a nerve may stimulate an intense inflammatory reaction that may lead to extensive epineurial scarring and distortion of the architecture of the nerve trunk. In general, an intact blood–nerve barrier (i.e., an intact perineurial–endoneurial border) will prevent diffusion of drug or toxin into the nerve fibers themselves. Direct intrafascicular injection of drug into nerve, however, may cause severe endoneurial fibrosis with neural ischemia and axon loss (Farber et al., 2013). The radial and sciatic nerves are the most frequently affected, but injection injuries also have been described in the median, femoral, and ulnar nerves. The first symptom often is immediate onset of pain, paresthesia, and paralysis, but in some affected persons, the onset apparently is delayed. Patients who fail to show signs of recovery within 3–5 months or who have persistent pain may benefit from surgical intervention.

## EVALUATION OF NERVE TRAUMA

### Clinical and Electrodiagnostic Examination

The clinical assessment of traumatic nerve injury should ascertain an account of the injury itself (including the exact circumstance) with details regarding the localization, severity, and particularly the precise time it occurred (Box 64.1 and Table 64.2). The electrodiagnostic examination confirms the site of injury and its underlying pathophysiology and severity and may uncover additional information such as subclinical abnormalities or evidence of early recovery. All these elements determine if and when surgical repair is required and provide a timeline for any interventions. For example, if a period of 4 years has elapsed from the time of injury, it is very unlikely that any significant motor recovery will take place despite surgical intervention. The reduction in ability to regenerate following neurorrhaphy or grafting results from several mechanisms. First, the proximal stumps (motor neuron axons) lose the ability to grow. Second, the distal stump loses

**BOX 64.1 Important Elements of the History in Patients with Peripheral Nerve Injury**

- Patient's age and "handedness"
- Exact time (as near as possible) injury occurred, stated as the date and time, not as a phrase such as "3 days ago Monday")
- Time interval between injury and initial evaluation
- Description of injury (to differentiate among laceration, compression, traction, etc.); presence of associated injury (e.g., head trauma, vascular repair, compartment syndromes)
- Description of motor weakness (maximum at onset? progressive? improving? if so, over what time period?)
- Absence or presence of pain or sensory changes
- Any recovery of sensorimotor function
- Presence of systemic disease (e.g., diabetes, preexisting peripheral neuropathy, entrapment neuropathy)
- Score on a quantitative pain scale (i.e., Visual Analog Scale)

**TABLE 64.2 Neurological Examination in Patients with Peripheral Nerve Injury**

| Feature/ Component | Focus/ Description |
|---|---|
| Wound | Open or closed, other tissues or vascular structures involved, presence of infection |
| Estimated distance from injury site and target organ | |
| Cranial nerves | Routine, plus assessment for Horner syndrome (partial ptosis, miosis, and variable degree of anhidrosis for preganglionic lesions) or cranial nerve deficits often associated with brachial plexus injury (including spinal accessory nerve) |
| Skin | Should be closely examined for trophic and atrophic changes, including vasomotor instability |
| Motor | Should contain a reliable and consistent measure of motor function (e.g., British Medical Research Council, Louisiana State University Medical Center grading scale) |
| Sensory | Should provide quantitative data of both large- and small-fiber function (e.g., touch-pressure via von Frey filaments, Weber two-point discrimination, protective sensibility or appreciation for pain, cold, warmth, or pressure) |
| Deep tendon reflexes and presence of Tinel sign over nerve distal to injury | |

the ability to support and guide axonal growth. Finally, atrophy in muscle and tendon contractures often limits the impact of the few axons that can reinnervate functioning neuromuscular junctions. Regarding mechanism, intraoperative transection of a nerve by a scalpel is likely to portend a better prognosis than is possible with a laceration by a chain saw. Early (at <3 months) return of motor and sensory function is a good prognostic sign and supports grade I lesions. Elderly patients and those with metabolic disorders such as diabetes and renal failure are less likely to enjoy good functional outcome after nerve injury.

Determining the distance from the injured nerve segment to its muscle helps establish prognosis. For example, if the target muscle is

3 inches from the injury site on the nerve, a good outcome over the next 3 months is reasonably likely. The reverse is true with nerve injuries that occur at a great distance from the target muscle; an axon-loss lower-trunk brachial plexus injury may be 30 inches or more from target intrinsic hand muscles, so any spontaneous recovery would have to occur by means of collateral sprouting. The presence of the *Tinel sign*, a tingling induced by mechanical distortion of the distal terminus of a regenerating axon (elicited by tapping the nerve with a finger or tendon hammer), supports ongoing axon regeneration; conversely, absence of the Tinel sign distal to a nerve lesion after 4–6 weeks have elapsed is strong evidence against axon regeneration.

The electrodiagnostic examination consists of nerve conduction studies (NCSs) and needle electromyography (EMG). The two main components of the NCSs are assessment of sensory nerve action potentials (SNAPs) and compound muscle action potentials (CMAPs). When the study is performed to assess for complex lesions of the brachial plexus or lower-extremity nerve lesions, it is essential that the electrodiagnostician examine particularly relevant NCSs and an expanded EMG in addition to those done in routine studies (Ferrante and Wilbourn, 2002).

Timing of the electrodiagnostic examination is important and has both practical and prognostic implications. If it is performed too early (<5 days) after the injury, sufficient time may not have elapsed for electrodiagnostic signs of motor axon loss to develop, and the physician cannot judge whether a nerve lesion is caused primarily by demyelinating conduction block or by axon loss. In the case of a severe axon-loss injury, CMAPs and SNAPs will be entirely normal for the first 2 days despite the presence of an obvious clinical deficit and the patient's inability to voluntarily recruit motor unit potentials (MUPs) during EMG examination (an electrodiagnostic observation known as *axon discontinuity conduction block*). By day 3, however, wallerian degeneration should cause some loss of the distal CMAP amplitude, and by day 7, the CMAP may have reached its nadir, being further diminished or even absent. By day 5, the SNAP amplitude also is decreasing; it reaches its nadir at day 10 or 11 (the reason for the earlier loss of CMAP amplitude relates to the failure of neuromuscular junction transmission). Finally, after at least 3 weeks, clear evidence of active denervation in the form of fibrillation potentials should be observed during EMG. An important EMG feature is the early appearance of MUPs of low amplitude, increased duration, and increased polyphasia, the so-called reinnervational or "nascent" MUPs that fire at slow to moderate rates. These represent electrodiagnostic evidence of early axon collateral sprouting and may be found as early as 10 days from the time of injury, but usually are more evident after 1–3 months.

If the lesion is due to focal demyelinating conduction block (grade I injury), and nerve stimulation is applied both distal and proximal to the lesion site, the examiner should detect a lower proximal than distal CMAP amplitude. The difference in proximal and distal CMAP amplitude and the reduction in distal MUP voluntary recruitment on EMG are proportional to the amount of motor fibers blocked. Even with primarily demyelinating lesions, a limited amount of axon loss (i.e., fibrillation potentials) may occur if some axons at the site of the conduction block have incurred injury (Wilbourn, 2002).

## Imaging Studies

In trauma cases, plain films of skull base, spine, and long bones may disclose fractures at sites that may compromise local nerve structures. Myelography, sometimes with computed tomography (CT), but now most commonly with gadolinium-enhanced magnetic resonance imaging (MRI) of the spine is used to diagnose nerve root avulsions; contrast material may be seen passing through the torn meningeal sheaths of avulsed nerve roots (pseudomeningoceles). Radiology confirmation of nerve root avulsion may be confounded by localized hematoma formation within or around the neural foramina, which may prevent extravasation of contrast material, thereby obscuring the typical appearance of pseudomeningoceles.

MR neurography is the term used to refer to MR imaging of the PNS. It uses a combination of high-resolution T1-weighted sequences for anatomical studies and fluid-sensitive, T2-weighted sequences that allow better distinction of nerve versus surrounding tissue to facilitate the assessment of pathological changes. Diffusion-weighted, T2-weighted, and short tau inversion recovery (STIR) images are based on the longitudinally oriented water diffusion properties of nerves as opposed to surrounding tissues. Images are ideally obtained in axial and longitudinally oriented planes (Chhabra et al., 2018; Cortes et al., 2013; Stoll et al., 2013). Nerve injury does not have a large impact on the T1-weighted signal intensity of a nerve, but the caliber and shape may be affected. Signal hyperintensity, however, can be seen on T2-weighted and STIR images of traumatized nerve segments; abnormal high signal intensity is seen both at and distal to the injury site (Fig. 64.6). This MRI modality can detect neuroma formation at nerve repair sites, and it may even be possible to identify which fascicles within a nerve trunk are injured and which are spared. These signal changes may be transient in cases of mild nerve injury or may be prolonged (up to many years) in severe preganglionic brachial plexus avulsion injuries. Despite breakdown in the blood–nerve barrier, standard gadolinium diethylenetriamine pentaacetic acid (Gs-DTPA) enhancement is not always seen in cases of nerve trauma, which may be explained by the fact that the contrast may be rapidly washed out of the endoneurial space. A new form of gadolinium (Gf) appears to be superior in detection of blood–nerve barrier breakdown and may continue to show enhancement until regeneration occurs (Stoll et al., 2013). Signal hyperintensity may be seen in denervated muscle on T2-weighted and STIR images occurring within 48 hours and peaking 2–4 weeks later. This signal change will persist if nerve discontinuity prevents reinnervation, but if a muscle is denervated for more than a year, there are often T1-weighted MRI features of fatty replacement and atrophy.

While MR neurography can be performed on both 1.5 T and 3.0 T scanners, the more powerful MRI scanners (3.0 T) offer enhanced resolution due to increased signal-to-noise ratio. Another technique, diffusion tensor imaging (DTI) and tractography of peripheral nerves (also performed on 3.0 T MRI), is based on the principle that water molecules have anisotropic diffusion properties (or a preferred orientation) in white-matter fiber tracts, compared with isotropic diffusion (equal in all directions) in surrounding tissues. The data generated by DTI is quantitative and is referred to as fractional anisotropy (FA) and apparent diffusion coefficient (ADC). FA values decrease with axonal degeneration and increase with axonal regeneration. The post-processing algorithms that produce images are not identical to standard anatomical MR images but they can show changes such as thinning or distortion (Hiltunen et al., 2005; Sheikh, 2010; Simon and Kliot, 2014).

A number of imaging and interpretation pitfalls may arise in MR neurography, such as pulsation artifact from a nearby vessel and "magic angle" artifact, causing some T2 hyperintensity, as often occurs in the sciatic nerve at the greater sciatic notch and the lateral femoral cutaneous nerve of thigh at the anterior superior iliac spine (Chhabra et al., 2018). Furthermore, a meta-analysis of published research on the specificity and sensitivity of MR neurography showed heterogeneous results, indicating a need for further well-designed studies to establish standard criteria to apply to MR neurography, in terms of both performance and interpretation (Kwee et al., 2014).

Ultrasonography of peripheral nerve and muscle is a relatively inexpensive and accessible diagnostic method for providing further information in the assessment of nerve injury (Heinen et al., 2019;

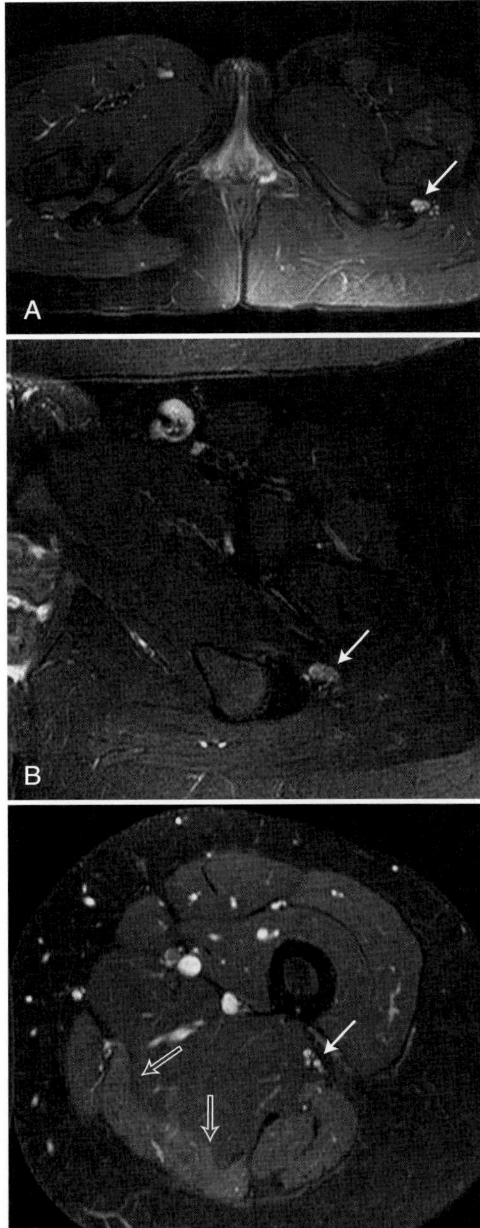


**Fig. 64.6** Magnetic resonance neurography images from a 23-year-old woman 1 month after she was diagnosed with a compressive left sciatic neuropathy due to prolonged compression (alcohol-induced coma). **A**, Large field-of-view axial T-weighted image with fat suppression demonstrates marked T2 signal hyperintensity in left sciatic nerve *(solid arrow)*. Large field of view allows comparison with normal right side, which can be useful in cases of subtle T2 signal hyperintensity to differentiate from normal nerve signal. **B**, Small field-of-view axial T2-weighted image with fat suppression demonstrates same changes in left sciatic nerve as in **A** *(solid arrow)* but with improved spatial resolution, allowing for detection of small mass lesions and subtle signal changes. **C**, Small field-of-view axial T1-weighted image obtained after injection of intravenous contrast demonstrates minimal nerve enhancement *(solid arrow)* and enhancement of hamstring musculature *(open arrows)*. Note that although most regions of T2 signal hyperintensity also enhance, signal changes may be subtler than on T2-weighted images. Contrast-enhanced images are most useful for detecting small mass lesions and characterizing solid versus cystic lesions. (*MR images courtesy of Joshua Polster, MD, Diagnostic Radiology, Cleveland Clinic.*)

Stoll et al., 2013; Umans et al., 2010; Visser, 2010; Zaidman et al., 2013). Normal nerves are hypoechoic and are surrounded by echogenic connective tissues; injured nerve, however, reveals altered echogenicity due to edema, and one may be able to detect axonal swelling, neuroma formation, or discontinuity. Although the resolution of ultrasound imaging is below that of MRI, this test can be performed in the office setting, has the advantage of real-time imaging, can assess long segments of nerve, and is of particular use in patients who cannot tolerate MRI. Ultrasonography enables more dynamic observation of in vivo nerve segments (e.g., retroepicondylar subluxation of the ulnar nerve) and focal structural changes that accompany nerve injury.

## SURGICAL REPAIR OF NERVE TRAUMA

The surgical repair of peripheral nerve injuries is a demanding discipline. Thorough knowledge of the anatomy involved and the pathophysiology of nerve healing are prerequisites for surgeons engaging in this area. Many factors in nerve injury are already disposed against a good outcome, and therefore it is paramount that the surgical interventions undertaken to repair nerves are performed to the highest degree of excellence possible.

Historically the repair of injured nerves was postulated by Galen in the first century AD, but it was Paulus of Aegina who first described repairing a nerve in a battle wound in the 7th century. The routine practice of nerve repair did not really become commonplace until the latter part of the 20th century, however. Pioneers such as Narakas, Millesi, Brunelli, McKinnon, and Oberlin drove this now burgeoning field with a combination of original laboratory research and careful clinical follow-up of nerve repair procedures, which has provided us with the knowledge base which now informs our clinical decision making.

The factors that influence outcome in nerve injury and repair are well described and must be fully understood to prognosticate honestly and accurately with patients. They are largely beyond the control of both the surgeon and the patient, and include the following: older age; proximal injuries; crush, stretch, avulsion, radiation, electrical, injection, and cold injuries; and smoking. Concomitant vascular and/or orthopedic factors also play a role. Are there good prognostic factors? Probably not really, as all nerve injuries carry the long-term prospect of incomplete recovery. However, it can be readily seen that of serious nerve injuries, a clean sharp cut to the distal part of a noncritical peripheral nerve during infancy is one with the best prognosis.

### Indications for and Timing of Surgical Repair

A treatment algorithm for nerve injuries has been proposed by Spinner and Kline (2000) and is presented in Fig. 64.7. Surgical intervention is not indicated in patients with grade I/neurapraxia injuries because spontaneous full recovery is expected. However, for axon loss lesions (grades II–VI), the algorithm divides peripheral nerve injury into two major categories: open and closed. The open category is further divided into early repair (within 72 hours) and delayed primary repair, which involves limited initial exploration to tack the proximal and distal nerve stumps to an adjacent structure such as fascia, to allow easier identification at the time of definitive repair, carried out within 3–4 weeks (usually using nerve grafts). The closed category is subdivided into delayed repair and nonsurgical management. The basic techniques used in surgical repair are illustrated in Fig. 64.8.

#### Open Injuries

***Primary repair.*** The vast majority of peripheral nerve injuries are related to limb lacerations and penetrating trauma. The patient presents with a laceration and neuropathy as well as possible damage to

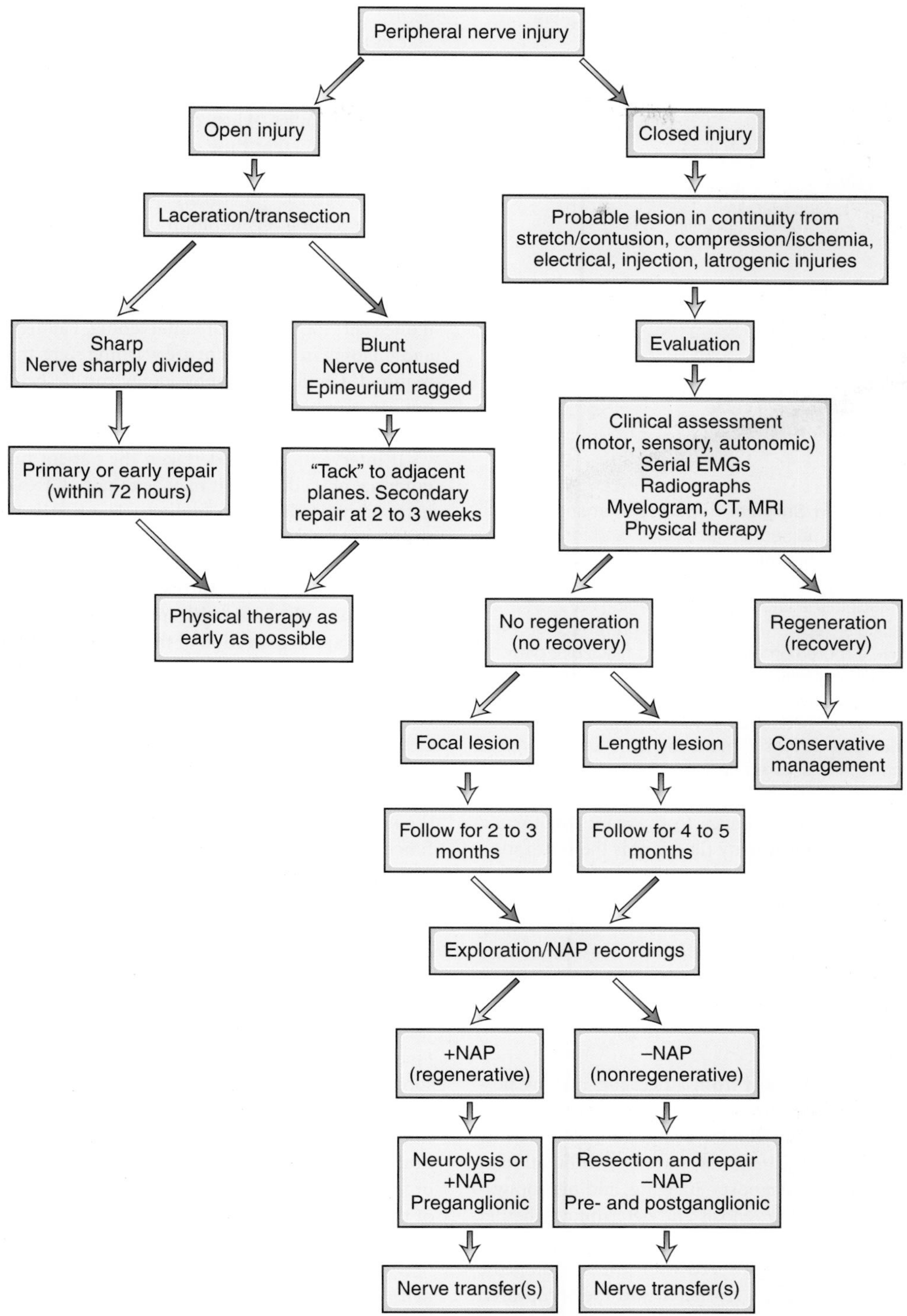


**Fig. 64.7** Diagnostic Treatment Algorithm for Peripheral Nerve Trauma (see Surgical Repair of Nerve Trauma section) *(Adapted from Dubuisson, A., Kline, D. G., 1992. Indications for peripheral nerve and brachial plexus surgery. Neurol Clin 10, 935–951.)*

tendons, vessels, and joints. Most lacerations are sustained due to sharp objects penetrating the skin: broken glass, knife blades, or even surgical iatrogenic injury. These are grade V/neurotmesis injuries. Thankfully, this usually means that the nerves are cleanly cut and can be repaired accurately with relative ease. This exploration and repair should be performed as quickly as possible by an experienced peripheral nerve surgeon, ideally within 72 hours. Expert anatomical knowledge and meticulous careful dissection are key to identifying the nerve ends. Sharp injuries rarely require debridement and accurate opposition of the nerve ends can usually be achieved using appropriate magnification and microsurgical instruments and sutures. Where debridement of the injured nerve ends is necessary this should be minimized to prevent excessive tension at the repair site.

***Delayed primary repair.*** More complex open injuries where there are elements of severe crush, nerve stretch, tissue loss, and concomitant orthopedic or vascular injury are thankfully rarer. For example,

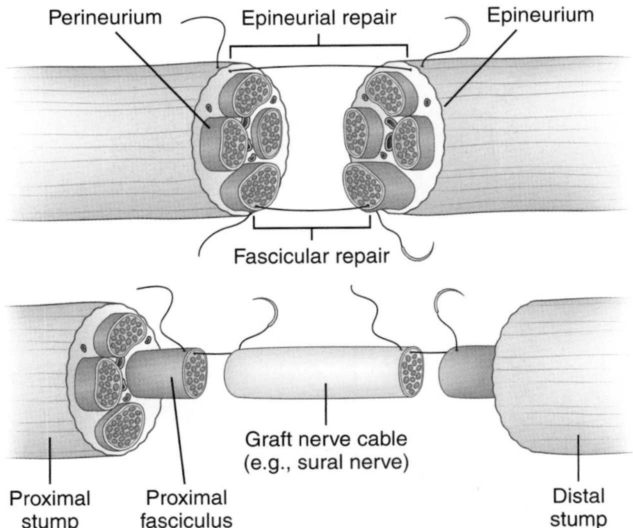


**Fig. 64.8 Basic Techniques in Surgical Repair.** Schematic diagram illustrating basic concepts of epineural, fascicular, and graft repair. Direct end-to-end neurorrhaphy of small distal nerves is usually carried out using an epineurial repair approach *(upper panel)*, which entails placing sutures through epifascicular epineurium and bringing nerve stumps into approximation. Fascicular repair *(upper panel)* is preferred for more proximal nerves that have a more complex interlaced fascicular pattern. Stumps are approximated using sutures that have been placed through the perineurium. Graft repairs *(lower panel)* are performed when direct end-to-end neurorrhaphy would cause excessive tension on the repair site. Graft material is harvested from a "nonessential" sensory nerve (e.g., sural nerve), which is then sutured between fascicles.

a chainsaw injury will cause severe damage to the skin, soft tissues, vascular supply, and skeleton. The priority therefore is the restoration of vascular supply, skeletal stabilization, and debridement of devitalized and contaminated tissue. The nerve injury should be defined at the time of primary exploration and the nerve ends tacked to surrounding structures with a view to delayed primary repair some weeks later, once the wounds are healed. In such circumstances primary nerve repair will not be possible and nerve grafts will be required.

### Closed Injuries

Closed injuries are less straightforward from a decision-making perspective. Open injuries are almost always grade V/neurotmesis injuries, but closed injuries can be any Sunderland grade and it can be difficult to ascertain which type a patient may have. A combination of clinical history, clinical recovery, diagnostic imaging, and neurophysiology informs the clinician of the prognosis and determines whether the patients should be managed operatively or nonoperatively. For example, a motorcyclist injured at high speed with severe orthopedic injuries, a flail anesthetic upper limb, a Horner syndrome, a ruptured subclavian artery, and MRI evidence of meningoceles has undoubtedly suffered a severe avulsion injury of the brachial plexus. Early exploration and nerve transfer are indicated. Conversely, a patient who has sustained a low-velocity shoulder dislocation with axillary nerve palsy with some evidence of early recovery and positive neurophysiology warrants careful observation until recovery is complete.

It is necessary to operate urgently on a closed nerve injury in certain well-described situations. For example, a supracondylar fracture in a child with median nerve symptoms requires urgent manipulation or open reduction. Similarly, complex elbow fractures with ulnar nerve palsy or unreduced shoulder dislocations with axillary nerve palsy require urgent attention. Compartment syndrome causes severe neurological symptoms and urgent fasciotomy is indicated for both the sake of the muscle compartment and the nerves that run through it.

Outside of these emergency situations, each case has to be managed individually, taking into account all the factors outlined above. It is vital to remember, when managing a peripheral motor nerve injury nonoperatively, that time is of the essence. We know that motor end plates in denervated muscle start to disappear from about 10 months, never to return, potentially permanently paralyzing that muscle. Allowing for the regeneration distances involved, it is therefore very important to make a decision on surgical intervention before it is too late. This is generally between 3 and 6 months. If in doubt it is better to look and see than wait and see, as the motor end plates will be gone if one waits too long before intervening. Failure to see clinical recovery and ongoing improvement are warning signs that intervention may be required. Clinical neurophysiology can be helpful in such situations but can also be overly optimistic; the decision on intervention should be weighted toward the clinical progress of the patient.

If intervention is undertaken the patient must be apprised of the potential procedures that may be required. Exploration of the affected nerve may produce two findings. The first is a ruptured nerve. This will require either nerve grafts or possibly nerve transfer repair. The second situation is a lesion of the nerve in continuity. In this situation the nerve is intact as a continuous structure but obviously is not functioning normally. This may represent any of the grade II, III, IV or VI injuries. Careful dissection of the nerve away from scar tissue (external neurolysis) may help identify normal or abnormal ultrastructure under magnification. A longitudinal incision through the scarred outer layer (epineurotomy) may help release scarred but functional internal fascicles from within the nerve. Visible fascicular structure over the course of the nerve suggests a less severe injury; thickened scar tissue in the substance of the nerve suggests the opposite. Proximal stimulation of the nerve producing distal muscle contraction indicates physiological function across the nerve and is a positive sign. The SNAPs can also be mapped across the injured segment, giving further information. If the appearance and neurophysiology of the nerve are encouraging, then the nerve can be left alone after external neurolysis in the hope that spontaneous recovery will ensue. If the appearance and neurophysiology are not positive, then the nerve should be micro-dissected under high magnification (internal neurolysis) to reveal any continuity in the fascicles, and the neurophysiology repeated. If this shows improvement (something I have never seen) then the nerve can be left to recover spontaneously. In my experience the internal architecture of the nerve in such situations is so severely disrupted that nerve transmission cannot occur. Such nerves need to be cut back proximally and distally to healthy pouting soft fascicles and the defect grafted with donor nerve or a nerve transfer needs to be done. In severe injuries large segments of the nerve may be damaged and the defects may therefore be large, lessening the chance of a successful nerve graft.

***Primary neurorrhaphy.*** In the vast majority of cases primary neurorrhaphy is a simple and straightforward procedure. Most nerve injuries are caused by penetrating trauma, which usually cleanly severs the nerve. The severed ends are usually lying close to each other and easy to locate. Careful dissection will reveal the injured nerve ends and the repair can begin. There is usually no nerve tissue missing and a tension-free anastomosis can be easily performed under the microscope. It is very important to avoid excessive resection of the nerve ends. Even with minimal debridement the gap obviously widens and there is some tension imparted to the repair. Inspection of the nerve ends allows the surgeon to judge how to orientate the nerve ends accurately to restore, in as far as possible, the original anatomy. There are several clues to be found that will help. First, the shape of the laceration may be useful. Oblique lacerations are easily orientated owing to the obvious way the ends "fit" back together. Transverse lacerations are more difficult to orient but the fascicular patterns and the blood vessel anatomy in the epineurium provide excellent clues as to how the nerve should line up.

The repair itself usually requires the careful insertion of micro-sutures to maintain the alignment of the opposed nerve ends. It is vital that the sutures are inserted into the adventitial tissues and not into neural tissue. This can be quite challenging in smaller nerves, as the adventitia can be very flimsy and getting a bite is difficult. As a general rule the sutures used should be of small gauge (8/0, 9/0, 10/0). The number used should be just enough to hold the nerve ends orientated toward each other with a small gap between the nerve ends and no pouting fascicles. This can be achieved by as few as two sutures in a small nerve such as a digital nerve or as many sutures as may be required to repair a large sciatic nerve laceration. I have personal preference for tying the sutures loosely, allowing some play in the repair, which makes inserting subsequent sutures easier and ultimately allows a more accurate repair, as the nerve is not pulled excessively tightly toward one part of the repair. The repair can be augmented by the use of fibrin glue but the evidence for the efficacy of this is scant.

When the nerve ends are ragged, such as in a power saw injury, it is obviously necessary to debride the damaged ends of the injured nerves. This can make the nerve repair difficult, as it is hard to avoid applying excessive tension across the repair. There are several techniques that can be employed to reduce the tension and allow a tension-free repair. First, mobilization of the nerve ends proximally and distally will reduce tension. This is usually sufficient unless the gap is too big. In certain situations the anatomical path of the nerve can be altered to reduce tension. The most obvious example of this is the ulnar nerve at the elbow, where it can be transposed anteriorly out of the cubital tunnel, with a consequent gain in length, allowing tension-free repair. A more radical example (thankfully rare) is to shorten the underlying bone. The best illustration of this is when re-implanting an amputated arm at humeral level. Radically shortening the humerus will provide the opportunity to repair the vessels and the nerves directly without tension or grafts.

***Nerve grafting.*** When the nerve defects are too big and the techniques above are not applicable, then nerve grafts provide the best solution. There is good evidence to support the use of entubulation devices/constructs for smaller nerve gaps of up to 2 cm, but nerve grafts still remain the gold standard even for these short defects. For larger defects, autologous nerve grafts provide the only proven practical method of restoring nerve continuity. Nerve grafting essentially involves taking a donor nerve from another part of the patient's anatomy and using it to bridge the gap in the injured nerve. The common donor nerves used are the sural nerve, the lateral antebrachial nerve and the anterior branch of the medial antebrachial nerve. In some circumstances other nerves such as the superficial radial nerve can be used if the proximal radial nerve has been injured. These donors are small-caliber nerves and often several "cables" of nerve graft are used to bridge gaps in larger-diameter nerves. The nerve grafts are nonvascularized and function as protein-based guides to allow nerve regeneration across the defect in the injured nerves. Nerve grafts may be vascularized in rare situations, such as the use of the whole length of the ulnar nerve based on the ulnar collateral branch of the brachial artery (only available when the C8/T1 nerve roots are avulsed) but this is seldom used in clinical practice. The donor sites are chosen to minimize secondary difficulties for the patients. The areas of permanent sensory loss are minimal. However, the patients must be apprised of this sensory loss and also of the risk of painful neuromata and even chronic pain in the distribution of the donor nerve.

The technique of nerve grafting is straightforward. Essential to the process is the cutting back of the injured nerve ends until healthy pouting fascicles are seen. The defect in the nerve is then measured with all the joints in maximum extension so that the repair can never be placed under strain during rehabilitation (Fig. 64.9). The donor cables are cut to length and inserted between the injured nerve ends using a combination of micro-sutures and fibrin glue (Figs. 64.10 and 64.11). Obviously smaller gaps are preferred but large defects in excess of 10 cm can still be successfully bridged with functional recovery, especially in children. Motor recovery is less likely with larger gaps due to the loss of motor end plates over time, as the slow pace of nerve regeneration takes its toll. Sensory recovery and improvement can still occur years after the grafting procedure. Because of the donor site morbidity and the limited availability of nerve graft donor sites there has been much research into the development of alternatives. Nerve allograft with temporary immune suppression, autologous vein and muscle, and a variety of synthetic alternatives have been proposed; however, as yet none have proved to be superior to autologous nerve graft.

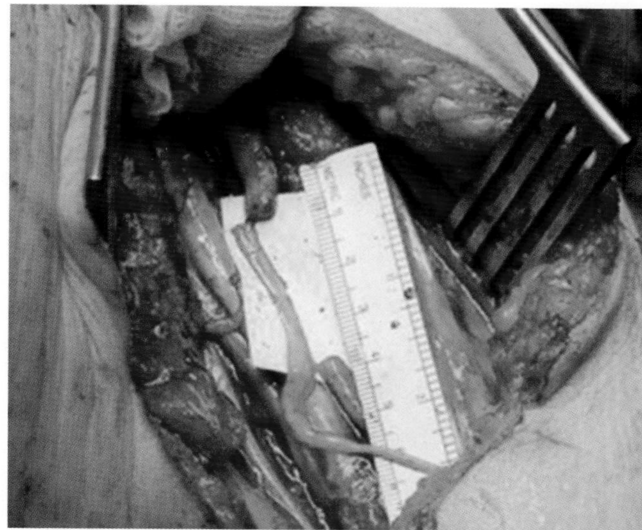

**Fig. 64.9 A 3-cm. Nerve Gap after Neuroma Resection of Element of Brachial Plexus.** Sural nerve graft laid across gap in preparation for graft repair. (*Image courtesy of Kevin Cronin, Mater Misericordiae University Hospital.*)

Overall, a satisfactory functional outcome is achieved in about 50% of nerve graft cases. This is an approximate figure, however, and many factors are involved. For example, at one major nerve trauma center, good functional recovery of motor function was observed in 68% to 75% of median and 80% of radial nerve injuries that were repaired by nerve grafting (Kim et al., 2001a, 2001b). Retrospective review of functional outcomes after repair of sciatic nerve injuries at the same center reported good outcomes after repair of tibial, but not peroneal (<36%), division injuries.

***Nerve transfer.*** Nerve transfer may be defined as the use of a functioning nerve or part of a functioning nerve to restore function in an injured nerve. This technique was initially proposed in the early 20th century, mainly in relation to facial nerve injury, but it never came into common use. The publication of the techniques of partial spinal accessory to suprascapular nerve transfer and partial ulnar nerve to biceps nerve transfer in the latter part of the 20th century, however, established nerve transfer as the new powerhouse in the treatment of nerve injury and especially brachial plexus injury.

Nerve transfer has distinct advantages in terms of short re-innervation distances and rapid recovery of motor function, obviating the potential loss of motor end plates that may occur while waiting for

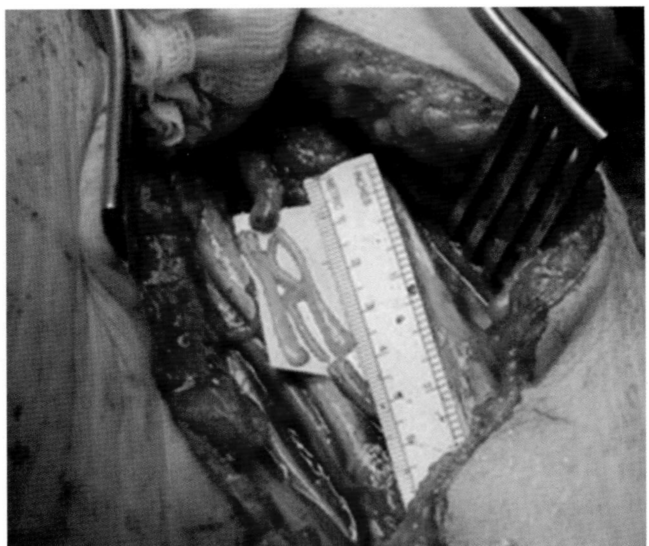

**Fig. 64.10** Sural nerve graft divided into three cables and laid across gap in preparation for graft repair. (*Image courtesy of Kevin Cronin, Mater Misericordiae University Hospital.*)

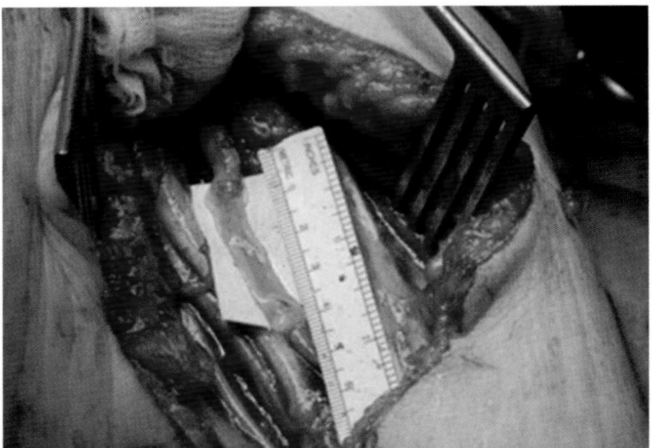

**Fig. 64.11** Completed nerve graft repair having used a combination of sutures and fibrin glue. (*Image courtesy of Kevin Cronin, Mater Misericordiae University Hospital.*)

a nerve graft to regenerate. It has definite disadvantages in that the patient will lose some function in the donor nerve and the patient will have to relearn how to operate the re-innervated muscle using a different nerve. In my experience the advantages by far outweigh the disadvantages and the outcomes in terms of functional muscle strength are much superior to nerve grafting in brachial plexus injuries. Partial spinal accessory to suprascapular nerve can restore excellent strength in shoulder abduction and external rotation, Oberlin/Double Oberlin transfer usually restores powerful elbow flexion (via transfer of a nerve fascicle of the ulnar nerve to the musculocutaneous nerve), and partial radial nerve to axillary nerve transfer can restore function to the deltoid. Intercostal nerve and medial pectoral nerves can be used for a variety of targets in brachial plexus injury. Beyond that, nerve transfers are now used more extensively in facial reanimation, spinal injury, to correct foot drop, and to power free microvascular muscle transfers. They have not replaced nerve grafting but have added hugely to the options peripheral nerve surgeons have when faced with difficult nerve injuries.

Optimization of functional outcome does not rest purely upon surgical technique but also upon an effective rehabilitation tailored to the particular injury and type of surgery performed. Initial therapy, which follows postoperative immobilization (varying from a few days to weeks), is aimed at reduction of pain and edema together with graded range-of-motion mobilization to promote nerve gliding and reduce adhesions. Electrical muscle stimulation is sometimes employed to promote motor recovery but there is limited evidence for efficacy (Novak and von der Heyde, 2013).

## MANAGEMENT OF NEUROPATHIC PAIN ASSOCIATED WITH NERVE TRAUMA

Neuropathic pain is defined as pain caused by a lesion or disease of the somatosensory system. In the case of peripheral nerve trauma, therefore, this pain is likely (but not obligatorily) to be experienced in the territory of injured elements of the PNS. The individual peripheral sensory nerve fibers involved in transmission of pain and sensory disturbances are Aβ, Aδ, and C fibers. The central pathway is relayed via the ascending spinothalamic tract to the thalamus and ultimately to the somatosensory cortex (Colloca et al., 2017). Based upon his observations in the American Civil War, Silas Weir Mitchell coined the term *causalgia* to describe a particular type of progressive pain resulting from injury to a nerve within the distribution of that nerve and unassociated with damage to non-neural tissue. This typical superficial burning pain may be accompanied by a deeper crushing or tearing sensation. Allodynia (pain evoked by nonpainful stimuli) and hyperalgesia (pain that is more intense than expected from a painful stimulus) are characteristic. The entity known as complex regional pain syndrome-2 (CRPS-2) is a combination of such pain with additional apparent features of sensory, autonomic, trophic, and motor abnormalities that may occur in the setting of nerve injury (as opposed to type-1 where there is no apparent injury) (Marinus et al., 2011). The incidence of causalgia ranges from 1% to 12%, with a predilection for the median nerve. The pain usually occurs within the first few weeks of injury, although this may be delayed up to 1 month. Most cases of causalgia resolve after 6–12 months but may rarely continue indefinitely. With nerve root avulsion injuries, patients may suffer a severe pain syndrome that is notoriously difficult to treat. A vivid description of this deafferentation pain was provided by a physician who suffered a brachial plexus avulsion injury himself when he was struck by a window cleaner falling from the fourth floor of a building as he was passing: "The pain is continuous; it does not stop either day or night. It is either burning or compressing (like a vise) or dragging (a sense of weight) in character, or a combination of all these at the same time" (Murray and Wilbourn, 2002). Undoubtedly, patients frequently suffer significant pain as a consequence of nerve injury. Nonetheless, there remains considerable debate as to the validity of CRPS as a distinct pathophysiological entity. Legitimate concerns remain about potential misdiagnosis, risk of opiate overuse, litigation, and inappropriate use of procedures (Bass and Yates, 2018; Clark et al., 2018).

### Pharmacological Options

A pharmacological strategy is to establish effective longer-acting anti epileptic or antidepressant monotherapy, while breakthrough pain is judiciously treated with shorter-acting medications. First-line treatments include pregabalin, gabapentin, duloxetine, and various tricyclic antidepressants and all are backed by strong evidence of efficacy in drug studies. Combinations of these agents at moderate doses may be superior to monotherapy with a high dose agent that is causing unacceptable side effects. Weaker evidence is present for the use of capsaicin cream, lidocaine patches, and tramadol, and thus these types of agents are considered second-line therapies. The weakest evidence is for strong opioids, antiepileptics (other than $\alpha_2\delta$ type) and botulinum toxin A, all of which are third-line options. There is a lack of published evidence of efficacy of cannabinoids, selective serotonin reuptake inhibitors (SSRIs), *N*-methyl-D-aspartate (NMDA) antagonists, mexiletine, and topical clonidine (Colloca et al., 2017).

### Interventional Strategies

Refractory neuropathic pain (e.g., after avulsion of preganglionic posterior nerve roots) can be treated through a variety of interventions. These approaches can involve nerve blocks, ablation of pain pathways (e.g., neurectomy, nerve lesioning) or neuromodulation (e.g., implantation of electrodes in the PNS and CNS). Neurectomy can be used to treat painful end-neuromas via an incision proximal to the site of the neuroma. It is most effective when applied to root avulsion. For this procedure, the dorsal root entry zone (DREZ) is exposed above and below the level of avulsion. Various means have been devised to destroy the dorsal horn, but the most common technique uses high-radiofrequency ablation. The electrode is inserted at 1- to 2-mm intervals between the rootlets for individual lesioning (Awad et al., 2013).

## MOVEMENT DISORDERS AFTER NERVE TRAUMA

Albeit relatively rare, a variety of peripherally derived movement disorders can arise after nerve trauma, including dystonia, tremor, tics, and myoclonus (Jankovic, 2009). Coexistent psychological distress can lead the clinician to assume a functional origin, but this would appear to account for only a significant minority of cases. A systematic review of this limited literature has shown that dystonia (fixed more often than mobile) is the most common movement disorder (a little over 70%) and that the timing of onset of the involuntary movement after trauma generally was less than 1 year. Pain (allodynia, hyperalgesia), sensory disturbance (hypoalgesia, hypoesthesia), and CRPS-2 were frequently present. Therapeutic interventions, including botulinum toxin, pharmacotherapy, deep brain stimulation, and nerve decompression, often met with little success (van Rooijen et al., 2011).

## FUTURE DIRECTIONS IN TREATMENT OF NERVE TRAUMA

Although the PNS has the inherent capacity for regeneration, functional recovery after injury—with or without surgery—remains suboptimal. A clear need exists for improved understanding and therapeutics that can be used to enhance the outgrowth of axons and provide guidance cues in the distal nerve. Improvements in graft products are necessary to provide not only a scaffold for axonal growth but also to promote this growth. Tissue engineered nerve grafts (TENGs) are being evaluated in human short-gap nerve repair, often achieving results that approach those of standard nerve grafting. Acellular nerve grafts (ANGs) are a form of allograft from which the cellular immunogenic elements have been removed. Biological conduits include arteries, veins, empty epineural sheath, and muscle, whereas artificial conduits include resorbable and nonresorbable synthetic polymers and/or extracellular matrix components. Stem cell–derived Schwann cells hold promise in improving nerve regeneration and management of neuropathic pain (Patel et al., 2018). Neurophysiological, neuropsychological, and functional neuroimaging studies have identified reorganization of central motor and sensory pathways in the aftermath of peripheral nerve injury and repair. Chronic denervation leads to extensive reorganization of representational maps within the sensory and motor cortex, including a limited degree of reorganization within subcortical structures (Hua et al., 2013; Ma et al., 2018). Further study into the dynamic relationship between central reorganization and peripheral nerve regeneration may lead to more refined rehabilitative therapy.

*The complete reference list is available online at https://expertconsult.inkling.com/.* 

65

# Ischemic Cerebrovascular Disease

*José Biller, Michael J. Schneck, Sean Ruland*

## OUTLINE



## EPIDEMIOLOGY AND RISK FACTORS

There are approximately 795,000 new or recurrent strokes annually in the United States (610,000 being first events and 185,000 being recurrent events) (Benjamin et al., 2019) Despite declining stroke incidence, 7 million Americans above the age of 20 are estimated to have experienced a stroke. (Benjamin et al., 2019). Approximately 88% of these strokes are ischemic and 8%–12% of ischemic strokes result in death within 30 days. Despite gradual declines in overall stroke death rates in many industrialized countries, stroke remains a leading cause of death and disability worldwide. Stroke mortality is particularly high in Eastern Europe and Asia (World Health Organization, 2004). By 2020, 19 of 25 million annual stroke deaths will be in developing countries (Lemogoum et al., 2005). Of survivors, approximately 30% require assistance with activities of daily living, 20% require assistance with ambulation, and 16% require institutional care.

Steep decreases in stroke incidence and mortality have occurred in industrialized nations. The reduction in stroke mortality in the United States has been attributed to a declining stroke incidence, and lower case-fatality rates, suggesting a trend in declining stroke severity (Benjamin et al., 2019). However, the declining stroke incidence has been reversing with the aging of the population, greater awareness of stroke symptoms, and better diagnostic tools. Furthermore, despite a decrease in developed countries, stroke mortality and incidence are increasing in developing nations. Socioeconomic factors, dietary and lifestyle behaviors, different risk factor patterns, and environmental conditions may explain the different stroke incidences observed in different parts of the world.

Risk factors classified as modifiable and nonmodifiable increase the risk for ischemic stroke (Table 65.1). Nonmodifiable stroke risk factors include older age, male gender, ethnicity, family history, and prior history of stroke. Modifiable risk factors may be subdivided

**TABLE 65.1 Risk Factors for Ischemic Stroke**

| Nonmodifiable | Modifiable |
|---|---|
| Age | Arterial hypertension |
| Gender | Transient ischemic attacks |
| Race/ethnicity | Prior stroke |
| Family history | Asymptomatic carotid bruit/stenosis |
| Genetics | Cardiac disease |
| | Aortic arch atheromatosis |
| | Diabetes mellitus |
| | Dyslipidemia |
| | Cigarette smoking |
| | Alcohol consumption |
| | Increased fibrinogen |
| | Elevated homocysteine |
| | Lack of physical activity |
| | Low serum folate |
| | Elevated anticardiolipin antibodies |
| | Oral contraceptive use |
| | Obesity |

into behavioral and nonbehavioral factors. Behavioral factors include lack of physical activity, tobacco use, alcohol abuse and illicit drug use. Nonbehavioral factors include low socioeconomic status, arterial hypertension, dyslipidemia, heart disease, and carotid artery disease. Sickle cell disease is also a modifiable nonlifestyle risk factor because exchange therapy can reduce the associated stroke risk. Potentially modifiable risk factors include diabetes mellitus (DM), hyperhomocysteinemia, and left ventricular hypertrophy. Less well-documented risk factors include blood markers (e.g., C-reactive protein), ankle-brachial blood pressure ratios, silent cerebral infarcts, white-matter hyperintensities on magnetic resonance imaging (MRI), and degree of carotid artery intima-media thickness. There are also data implicating hemostatic and microcirculatory disorders in stroke as well as circadian and environmental factors.

## Risk Factors for Stroke

The incidence of stroke increases steeply with advancing age. Increasing age is the most powerful stroke risk factor. Stroke incidence doubles each decade past 55 years of age. Half of all strokes occur in people older than 75 years. Women have higher stroke case-fatality rates as compared with men. Men age 45–75 have higher stroke rates than women; thereafter, stroke rates are higher in women; overall, females have a higher lifetime stroke risk than males (Benjamin et al., 2019). With an estimated 20% of the population being older than 65, greater than 10 million octogenarians, and an increasing life expectancy in the United States, it is predicted that the annual number of strokes will reach 1 million by the middle of the 21st century. Compared to Whites, African-Americans have approximately a twofold-increased risk of first-ever stroke. The rate of cerebral infarction is higher in African-Americans and Hispanic Americans than in Whites; this could be partially explained by the higher prevalence of DM and arterial hypertension in these groups. African-Americans may have higher rates of intracranial atherosclerotic occlusive disease compared with Whites, but this may actually reflect ascertainment bias. Native Americans have a particularly high stroke incidence (6.79 per 100 person-years), predominantly ischemic strokes (Benjamin et al., 2019). Furthermore, the stroke incidence and case-fatality rates are also markedly different among the major ethnic groups in Auckland, New Zealand. Maori and Pacific Islands people have a higher mortality rate within 28 days of stroke when compared with Europeans, especially men. Chinese, Koreans, and Japanese also may have increased rates of intracranial hemorrhage and intracranial atherosclerotic cerebrovascular disease compared to Whites. In comparison with the United States and Western Europe, where hemorrhagic stroke represents 20% or less of all stroke subtypes, 40% of the stroke subtypes are hemorrhagic (intracerebral or subarachnoid hemorrhage) in Japan. Conversely, in India, where ischemic stroke accounts for 80% of all strokes, 10%–15% of strokes occur in people younger than 40 years and are mostly related to intracranial atherosclerosis.

## Heredity and Risk of Stroke

An increased risk is seen with a history of stroke among first-degree relatives. Genetic factors have been linked with ischemic stroke, but specific genetic variants remain largely unknown (Boehme et al., 2017; Chinnery et al., 2010). There are a number of genetic causes of stroke. Some inherited diseases, such as the hereditary dyslipoproteinemias, predispose to accelerated atherosclerosis. There are also a number of common genetic variant point mutations associated with increased stroke risk (Boehme et al., 2017). Several inherited diseases are associated with nonatherosclerotic vasculopathies, including Ehlers-Danlos (especially type IV) syndrome, Marfan syndrome, hereditary hemorrhagic telangiectasia (HHT) (Rendu-Osler-Weber disease), and Sturge-Weber syndrome. Familial atrial myxomas, hereditary cardiomyopathies, and hereditary cardiac conduction disorders are examples of inherited cardiac disorders that predispose to stroke. Deficiencies of protein C and S or antithrombin (AT) are examples of inherited hematological abnormalities that can cause stroke. Finally, rare inherited metabolic disorders that can cause stroke include mitochondrial encephalomyopathy lactic acidosis, and stroke-like episodes (MELAS), Fabry disease, and homocystinuria. The presence of the apolipoprotein epsilon-2 allele in elderly individuals and deletion of the gene for the angiotensin-converting enzyme may increase stroke risk, but the association with stroke subtype is unclear. The Siblings With Ischemic Stroke Study (SWISS) demonstrated a relationship between age and stroke in probands and sibs, and the lack of a tight association among ischemic stroke subtypes (Adams et al., 1993) within families (Meschia et al., 2005, 2006; Wiklund et al., 2007).

## Common Modifiable Risk Factors

At least 25% of the adult population has *arterial hypertension*, defined as systolic blood pressure (SBP) greater than or equal to 140 mm Hg or diastolic blood pressure (DBP) greater than or equal to 90 mm Hg. According to the 7th Report of the Joint National Committee on Prevention, Detection, Evaluation and Treatment of Hypertension (JNC7), *prehypertension* is defined as SBP between 120 and 139 mm Hg or DBP between 80 and 89 mm Hg (Chobanian et al., 2003). The report from the Eighth Joint National Committee (JNC8) recommended treatment of a blood pressure goal of SBP less than 150 mm Hg and DBP less than 90 mm Hg in patients greater than or equal to 60 years old without DM and chronic kidney disease and SBP less than 140 mm Hg and DBP 90 mm Hg in all other adults greater than or equal to 18 years (James et al., 2014). The 2017 American Heart Association (AHA)/American College of Cardiology (ACC) hypertension guidelines expanded the definition of arterial hypertension to greater than {130/80} mm Hg, resulting in approximately 63% of the middle aged (45–75 year-old) US population and 55% of the Chinese population meeting those definitions (German et al., 2019; Whelton et al., 2017) (Table 65.2). The European 2018 hypertension guidelines made similar recommendations though the goal blood pressure for persons greater than 65 years old remained less than {140/90} mm Hg and less than {160/90} mm Hg for those age 80 or older (Whelton et al.,

**TABLE 65.2 ACC/AHA 2017 Guideline for the Management of High Blood Pressure in Secondary Stroke Prevention in Adult Patients**

| Population | BP Goal | Agents and Timing of Therapy |
|---|---|---|
| Adult with stroke or TIA | SBP <130<br>DBP <80 (long term) | • Thiazide-type diuretic (preferably a long-acting agent), ACE-I or ARB, or in combination<br>• Restart anti-HTN medication a few days after the index event for patients previously on medication<br>• For patients not previously on drugs with established BP ≥140 mm Hg or DBP ≥ 90 mm Hg start therapy a few days after event<br>• For patients not previously treated with SBP <140 mmHg or DBP <90 mm Hg the benefit of anti-HTN drugs is less clear |

*ACE-I*, Angiotensin-converting enzyme inhibitor; *ARB*, angiotensin II type 1 receptor blocker; *BB*, beta-blocker; *BP*, blood pressure; *CCB*, calcium-channel blocker; *DBP*, diastolic blood pressure; *HTN*, hypertensive; *SBP*, systolic blood pressure; *TIA*, transient ischemic attack.

*From Whelton, P.K., Carey, R.M., Aronow, W.S. et al., 2017. ACC/AHA/AAPA.AC.ACPM/AphA, ASH, ASPC, NMA/PCNA. Guideline for the prevention, detection, evaluation and management of high blood pressure in adults. Circulation 139, e426–e433.*

2018). Unfortunately, arterial hypertension remains poorly treated worldwide. Arterial hypertension predisposes to ischemic stroke by aggravating atherosclerosis and accelerating heart disease, increasing the relative risk for stroke three-to fourfold. The risk is greater for patients with isolated systolic hypertension and elevated pulse pressure. Arterial hypertension is also the most important modifiable risk factor for stroke. Lowering blood pressure in stroke survivors helps prevent recurrent stroke and is more important than the specific agent used, although there is some suggestion that beta-blockers are less effective than other agents based on meta-analyses (Lindholm et al., 2005). Blood pressure treatment that results in a modest reduction in SBP of 10–12 mm Hg and 5–6 mm Hg diastolic is associated with a 38% reduction in stroke incidence (MacMahon and Rodgers, 1996). The Systolic Hypertension in the Elderly Program showed a 36% reduction in nonfatal plus fatal stroke over 5 years in the age 60-and-older group when isolated systolic hypertension was treated. Treating systolic hypertension also slows the progression of carotid artery stenosis. The PROGRESS trial evaluated the effects of perindopril and indapamide on the risk for stroke in patients with previous stroke or transient ischemic attack (TIA). Regardless of blood pressure at entry, patients clearly benefited from treatment (PROGRESS Collaborative Group, 2001).

About 171 million people worldwide have type 2 DM. It is estimated that these numbers will grow to 366 million people worldwide by 2030. DM increases the ischemic stroke risk two- to fourfold. In addition, DM increases morbidity and mortality after stroke. Macrovascular disease is the leading cause of death among patients with DM. Stroke secondary to DM may be caused by cerebrovascular atherosclerosis, cardiac embolism, or rheological abnormalities. The excess stroke risk is independent of age or blood pressure status. DM associated with arterial hypertension adds significantly to stroke risk. There is a fourfold increase in the relative risk of cardiovascular events among patients with DM and hypertension. Diabetic persons with retinopathy and autonomic neuropathy appear to be a group at particularly high ischemic stroke risk. High insulin levels increase the risk for atherosclerosis and may represent a pathogenetic factor in cerebral small-vessel disease. Presently, no evidence exists that tighter diabetic control over time decreases the stroke risk.

High total cholesterol and high low-density lipoprotein (LDL) concentration are correlated with atherosclerosis. Dyslipidemia is a recognized risk factor for ischemic stroke. Meta-analyses have suggested that ischemic stroke risk increases with increasing serum cholesterol, and the reduction in stroke risk associated with 3-hydroxy, 3-metthyl-glutaryl coenzyme A reductase inhibitor (statin) therapies is related to reduction in LDL (Amarenco et al., 2004; Tirschwell et al., 2004). Reduction of LDL with statins is an established therapy to reduce cardiovascular risk. Statins benefit stroke survivors as well. Lipid-lowering agents may slow atherosclerotic plaque progression and may even cause plaque regression.

The Myocardial Ischemia Reduction with Aggressive Cholesterol Lowering (MIRACL) showed a 50% relative risk reduction (RRR) ($P$ = .045) in stroke among high-risk coronary disease patients (Schwartz et al., 2001). The Anglo-Scandinavian Cardiac Outcomes Trial-Lipid Lowering Arm (ASCOT-LLA) study demonstrated a favorable trend for fatal and nonfatal stroke, with a 27% RRR in patients at low risk for coronary events (Hazard Ration (HR) 0.73; 95% confidence interval [CI], 0.56–0.96; $P$ = .0236) (Sever et al., 2003).

The Heart Protection Study (HPS) of patients at high risk with DM, coronary artery disease, or other atherosclerotic vascular disease showed an overall reduction in stroke risk (Heart Protection Study Collaborative Group, 2004). Subsequently, the Stroke Prevention by Aggressive Reduction in Cholesterol Levels (SPARCL) study (SPARCL Investigators, 2006) was a study of 4731 patients who had suffered either a stroke or TIA, had no known coronary heart disease, had LDL cholesterol (LDL-C) levels of 100–190 mg/dL, and who were randomized to placebo or 80 mg of atorvastatin. A 56mg/dL reduction in LDL treatment was noted in patients on atorvastatin. During a median follow-up of 4.9 years, 11.2% of atorvastatin-treated patients and 13.1% of placebo patients had a fatal or nonfatal stroke for an adjusted HR of 0.84 (95% CI, 0.71–0.99). A small increase in hemorrhagic stroke was reported in the atorvastatin group. Moreover, recent studies evaluating withdrawal of statins after acute ischemic stroke showed a higher incidence of death or dependency at 90 days (Blanco et al., 2007). Current guidelines of the AHA and proposed modifications of the NCEP-III guidelines suggest that all patients at risk for stroke or who have had an atherosclerotic cerebral infarction should be treated to a goal LDL-C level of below 70 mg/dL (Grundy et al., 2004; Sacco et al., 2006). The 2013 ACC/AHA guideline on the management of blood cholesterol recommended that all ischemic stroke and TIA patients should be treated with a statin regardless of the initial LDL-C, and this was confirmed by the 2018 ACC guideline (Grundy et al., 2018; Stone et al., 2013). The 2018 guideline recommends a high-intensity statin to achieve a goal LDL-C less than 70 mg/dL (1.8 mmol/L) for patients with clinical atherosclerotic cardiovascular disease (ASCVD), including stroke or TIA. DM patients without clinical ASCVD, age 40–75 with LDL-C ≥70 mg/Dl, should be treated with moderate-intensity statins and, for DM patients with multiple risk factors or age 50–75 years, a high-intensity statin may be reasonable as these DM patients should be treated as if they had clinical ASCVD. Ezetimibe may be added when the LDL-C remains above that goal, especially for patients at very high risk of ASCVD. The PCSK9 (proprotein convertase subtilisin/kexin type 9) inhibitors evolocumab and alirocumab are monoclonal antibodies that block the activity of PCSK9, which results in reduction of the degradation of LDL receptors, thereby increasing liver clearance of LDL-C. In the FOURIER trial (Further Cardiovascular Outcomes Research with PCSK9 Inhibition in Subjects with Elevated Risk), evolocumab was associated with lower incidence of myocardial infarction (MI), stroke, and cardiovascular revascularization, but did not clearly demonstrate a mortality benefit (Sabatine et al., 2017). The 2018 ACC guideline notes that, for patients who do not achieve that goal on maximally tolerated statin (or who are statin intolerant) following addition of ezetimibe therapy, therapy with a PCSK9 inhibitor is reasonable though the safety of these new drugs beyond 3 years and the cost-effectiveness is less certain (Grundy et al., 2018).

Atrial fibrillation (AF), the most common sustained cardiac arrhythmia in the general population, affects about 1% of adults, is the most common cause for cardioembolic stroke, and is a risk factor for future cardiovascular disease. An estimated 1–2 million Americans have chronic nonvalvular atrial fibrillation (NVAF), a condition that is associated with an overall increased stroke risk approximately five- to sixfold, and a mortality rate approximately twice that of age- and sex-matched individuals without AF. Its prevalence increases with age and is 0.5% for patients aged 50–59 years and 8.8% for those aged 80–89 years. Approximately 70% of individuals with AF are between 65 and 85 years of age. NVAF is associated with a substantial risk for stroke. Heart failure, arterial hypertension, DM, prior stroke or TIA, and age older than 75 years increase the risk for embolism in patients with NVAF. High-risk patients have a 5%–7% yearly risk for thromboembolism. The CHADS2 Score represents a validated quantification of risk, with congestive heart failure, hypertension, age older than 75 years, and a history of DM being assigned 1 point; stroke or TIA is assigned 2 points (Gage et al., 2001). Ischemic stroke rates increase from 1.9 to 18.2 events per 100 patient-years with CHADS 2 scores of 0 and 6, respectively. Left atrial enlargement also increases the risk for stroke in men. Likewise, left ventricular hypertrophy as demonstrated by electrocardiography (ECG) in men with preexisting ischemic heart disease is a major stroke risk factor. The $CHA_2DS_2$-VASc score for AF stroke risk assessment is an updated scoring system that is significantly better at stratifying patients into risk groups as compared with the CHADS2 score (Camm, 2010; Olesen et al., 2011). Additionally, the HAS-BLED score defines those AF patients with significantly greater hemorrhagic risk if placed on anticoagulants (Pisters et al., 2010; Table 65.3).

Cigarette smoking is the leading cause of preventable death in the United States. Cigarette smoking is a major risk factor for coronary artery disease, stroke, and peripheral arterial disease, an independent risk factor for ischemic stroke in men and women of all ages, and a leading risk factor of carotid atherosclerosis in men. The risk for stroke in smokers is two to three times greater than in nonsmokers. The mechanisms of enhanced atherogenesis promoted by cigarette smoking are incompletely understood but include reduced capacity of the blood to deliver oxygen, cardiac arrhythmias, increased blood coagulability, and triggering of arterial thrombosis and arterial spasm. Tobacco also increases carotid artery plaque thickness. More than 5 years of smoking cessation may be required before a reduction in stroke risk approaches that of never-smokers. Switching to pipe or cigar smoking is of no benefit. Counseling, nicotine replacement products, varenicline (a nicotinic receptor partial agonist), and bupropion are efficacious smoking cessation treatments.

There is a J-shaped association between alcohol consumption and ischemic stroke; light to moderate use (up to two drinks a day for men

**TABLE 65.3 (a) $CHA_2DS_2$-VASc AND (b) HAS-BLED Scores**

**(a) Adjusted Stroke Rate According to the $CHA_2DS_2$VASC Score**

| $CHA_2DS_2$-VASc Score | Patients ($n$ = 7329) | Adjusted Stroke Rate (%/year) |
|---|---|---|
| 0 | 1 | 0% |
| 1 | 422 | 1.3% |
| 2 | 1230 | 2.2% |
| 3 | 1730 | 3.2% |
| 4 | 1718 | 4.0% |
| 5 | 1159 | 6.7% |
| 6 | 679 | 9.8% |
| 7 | 294 | 9.6% |
| 8 | 82 | 6.7% |
| 9 | 14 | 15.2% |

**(b) HAS-BLED Risk Assessment Score**

| Letter | Clinical Characteristic | Points Awarded |
|---|---|---|
| H | Hypertension | 1 |
| A | Abnormal renal and liver function (*) | 1 or 2 |
| S | Stroke | 1 |
| B | Bleeding | 1 |
| L | Labile INRs | 1 |
| E | Elderly (age >65 years) | 1 |
| D | Drugs or alcohol (*) | 1 or 2 |
| Maximum 9 points | | |

Score of >3 indicates high risk.
*INRs*, International normalized ratios.
* *1 point each.*
*(a) From Camm, A.J., Kirchof, P., Lip, G.Y.H., et al., 2010. Guidelines for the management of atrial fibrillation: The task force for the management of atrial fibrillation of the European Society of Cardiology (ESC). Eur. Heart J. 31(19), 2360–2429.*
*(b) From Pisters, R., Lane, D.A., Nieuwlaat, R., et al., 2010. A novel user-friendly score (HAS-BLED) to assess 1-year risk of major bleeding in patients with atrial fibrillation. Chest 138(5), 1093–1100.*

and one for women) evenly distributed throughout the week elevates High-density lipoproteins (HDL) concentration and is associated with reduced risk, whereas heavy alcohol consumption is associated with an increased risk for total stroke. Heavy drinking may precipitate cardiogenic embolism. Alcohol consumption also increases the risk for hemorrhagic stroke. Furthermore, active drinkers have a higher frequency of obstructive sleep apnea (OSA) with more severe hypoxemia. Elimination or reduction of alcohol consumption is recommended for heavy drinkers. Restriction of alcohol consumption to fewer than two drinks daily for men and less than one drink daily for nonpregnant women is recommended for light to moderate drinkers.

The prevalence of obesity (body mass index [BMI] of 30 kg/m$^2$ or higher) in the United States has increased. More than 61% of adult Americans are overweight, and 27% are obese. Obesity, particularly abdominal, is an important risk factor for cardiovascular disease. There is some evidence that physical activity can reduce the risk for stroke. Regular exercise lowers arterial blood pressure, decreases insulin resistance, increases HDL cholesterol, and is associated with lower cardiovascular morbidity and mortality.

Numerous studies have established an association between OSA and stroke; moreover, the severity of OSA is much higher in stroke patients than in controls. Habitual snoring increases the risk for stroke and adversely affects the outcome of patients admitted to the hospital with stroke. Whether or not treatment of OSA reduces the risk of recurrent stroke is unclear (Tomfohr et al., 2012). The Sleep for Stroke Management and Recovery Trial (Sleep-SMART) is a randomized trial designed to investigate whether continuous positive airway pressure (CPAP) for OSA can prevent recurrent stroke and cardiovascular events (Brown, 2019). Mounting evidence also suggests that inflammation, lipoprotein(a) concentration, impaired fibrinolysis, and increased thrombotic potential are important nontraditional cardiovascular risk factors.

Atherosclerotic lesions of the carotid artery bifurcation are a common cause of stroke. Asymptomatic carotid artery disease carries a greater risk for vascular death from coronary artery disease than from stroke. Asymptomatic carotid artery stenosis of less than 75% carries a stroke risk of 1.3% annually; with stenosis of greater than 75%, the combined TIA and stroke rate is 10.5% per year, with most events occurring ipsilateral to the stenosed carotid artery. Plaque composition may be an important factor in the pathophysiology of carotid artery disease. Plaque structure rather than degree of carotid artery stenosis may be a more critical factor in determining stroke risk. Ultrasonographic carotid artery plaque morphology may identify a subgroup of patients at high risk for stroke. Ulcerated, echolucent, and heterogeneous plaques with a soft core represent unstable plaques at high risk for producing thromboembolism. Over 74% of patients with major stroke and ipsilateral carotid stenosis have been shown to have thrombotically active plaque surface characteristics (Spagnoli et al., 2004).

Patients who suffer TIAs are at threefold greater risk than normal controls for stroke or vascular death. Symptomatic carotid artery stenosis of greater than 70% carries an annual stroke risk of approximately 15%. Approximately 10%–15% of those experiencing a stroke have TIAs before their stroke. Patients with hemispheric TIAs are at greater risk for ipsilateral stroke than patients with retinal TIAs. Recurrent stroke is greatest early after the first stroke. Those who suffer a recurrent stroke have a higher mortality than patients with first stroke. If the recurrence is contralateral to the first stroke, prognosis for functional recovery is poor. The risk for stroke recurrence is also increased by the presence of underlying dementia.

The aorta is the most frequent site of atherosclerosis. Protruding atheroma may be the cause of otherwise unexplained TIAs or strokes. Aortic-arch atheromatosis detected by transesophageal echocardiography (TEE) is an independent risk factor for cerebral ischemia; the association is particularly strong with mobile and thick atherosclerotic plaques more than 4 mm in thickness (French Study of Aortic Plaques in Stroke Group, 1996). The prevalence of ulcerated plaques was 16.9% among patients with cerebrovascular diseases, compared to 5.1% among patients with other neurological diseases. Remarkably, ulcerated plaques were found in 61% of patients with cryptogenic cerebral infarcts, compared to 22% of cerebral infarcts with a known cause.

## Other Risk Factors for Stroke

Hemostatic factors may be important in assessing the risk for cerebrovascular events. Elevated hematocrit, hemoglobin concentration, and increased blood viscosity may be indicators of ischemic stroke risk. Elevation of plasma fibrinogen is an independent risk factor for the development of cerebral infarction. Epidemiological studies have shown a correlation between elevated plasma fibrinogen levels and both ischemic stroke incidence and mortality. An elevated plasma fibrinogen level may reflect progression of atherogenesis. Plasminogen activator inhibitor-1 excess and factor VII are independent risk factors for coronary heart disease. Compared with White Americans, Black Americans have higher mean levels of fibrinogen, factor VIII, von Willebrand factor, and AT, and lower mean levels of protein C. Fibrinogen levels are closely correlated with other stroke risk factors such as cigarette smoking, arterial hypertension, diabetes, obesity, hematocrit levels, and spontaneous echocardiographic contrast. Antiphospholipid (aPL) antibodies are a marker for an increased thrombosis risk, including TIAs and stroke, particularly in those younger than 50 years. In older patients, the presence of aPL (either lupus anticoagulant [LA] or anticardiolipin [aCL]) antibodies among patients with ischemic stroke predicts neither subsequent vascular occlusive events over 2 years nor a differential response to aspirin or warfarin therapy. As such, routine screening for aPL in older patients with ischemic stroke is not warranted (Levine et al., 2004). Activated protein C (APC) resistance due to the factor V Leiden mutation is associated with deep venous thrombosis (DVT) in otherwise healthy individuals with additional prothrombotic risk factors. An overall association of the factor V Leiden mutation and arterial thrombosis has not been found. As opposed to homozygous mutations, heterozygous factor V Leiden and prothrombin gene mutations have no clear association with increased stroke risk (Fields and Levine, 2005). Elevated von Willebrand factor is a risk factor for MI and ischemic stroke. Elevated levels of fasting total homocysteine (normal 5–15 mM), a sulfhydryl-containing amino acid, have been associated with an increased risk for stroke and thrombotic events in case-controlled studies. Metabolism of homocysteine requires vitamin $B_6$ (pyridoxine), vitamin $B_{12}$ (cobalamin), folate, and betaine. Plasma homocysteine concentrations may be reduced by the administration of folic acid alone or in combination with vitamins $B_6$ and $B_{12}$. Conversely, serum folate concentrations of 9.2 nM or less have been associated with elevated plasma levels of homocysteine, and a decreased folate concentration alone may be a risk factor for ischemic stroke, particularly among Blacks. However, folic acid supplementation does not have a major impact on stroke reduction (Lee et al., 2010).

Stroke is uncommon among women of childbearing age. The relative risk for ischemic stroke is increased among users of high-dose estrogen oral contraceptives, particularly with coexistent arterial hypertension, cigarette smoking, and increasing age. Based on an odds ratio (OR) of 1.93, the incidence is increased to 8.5/100,000, which translates into a number needed to harm of 24,000 women to cause one ischemic stroke (Gillum et al., 2000). Thus, for a healthy young woman without any other stroke risk factors, the risk associated with oral contraceptives is small. New agents containing lower doses of estrogen and progestin have reduced the frequency of oral contraceptive–related cerebral infarction. Two postmenopausal hormone replacement studies with equine estrogen (Premarin) showed no benefit in reducing the incidence of stroke in a cohort of women with coronary heart disease (Hulley et al., 1998). The Women's Estrogen for Stroke Treatment study of estradiol replacement in postmenopausal women after stroke also failed to show a reduction in recurrent stroke (Viscoli et al., 2001). In addition, the Women's Health Initiative (WHI), a prospective randomized trial of estrogen therapy in healthy postmenopausal women, was halted prematurely because the risks outweighed the benefits. Absolute excess risks per 10,000 person-years attributable to estrogen plus progestin were sevenfold for coronary heart disease events, eightfold for strokes, eightfold for pulmonary thromboembolism, and eightfold for invasive cancers, whereas absolute risk reductions per 10,000 person-years were sixfold for colorectal cancers and fivefold for hip fractures (Rossouw et al., 2002). The risk for thrombosis associated with pregnancy is high in the postpartum period. The risk for cerebral infarction is increased in the 6 weeks after delivery but not during pregnancy.

A diurnal and seasonal variation of ischemic events occurs. Circadian changes in physical activity, catecholamine levels, blood pressure, blood viscosity, platelet aggregability, blood coagulability, and fibrinolytic activity may explain the circadian variations of myocardial and cerebral infarction. An early-morning peak occurs for all subtypes of stroke. Rhythmometric analyses support the notion that stroke is a chrono-risk disease, in which cold temperatures also represent a risk factor. A history of recent infection, particularly of bacterial origin and within 1 week of the event, is also a stroke risk factor. A number of reports suggest that *Chlamydia pneumoniae*, a causative organism of respiratory infections, may have a role in carotid and coronary atherosclerosis. Some studies have also identified an association with chronic infections with *Helicobacter pylori* and cytomegalovirus.

## PATHOPHYSIOLOGY OF CEREBRAL ISCHEMIA

Except for the lack of an external elastica lamina in the intracranial arteries, the morphological structure of the cerebral vessels is similar to those in other vascular beds. The arterial wall consists of three layers: the outer layer, or adventitia; the middle layer, or media; and the inner layer, or intima. The intima is a smooth monolayer of endothelial cells providing a nonthrombotic surface for blood flow. One of the major functions of the endothelium is active inhibition of coagulation and thrombosis.

The brain microcirculation comprises the smallest components of the vascular system, including arterioles, capillaries, and venules. The arterioles are composed primarily of smooth-muscle cells around the endothelial-lined lumen and are the major sites of blood flow resistance. The capillary wall consists of a thin monolayer of endothelial cells. Nutrients and metabolites diffuse across the capillary bed. The venules are composed of endothelium and a fragile smooth-muscle wall and function as collecting tubules. The cerebral microcirculation distributes blood to its target organ by regulating blood flow and distributing oxygen and glucose to the brain, while removing by-products of metabolism.

A cascade of complex biochemical events occurs seconds to minutes after cerebral ischemia. Cerebral ischemia is caused by reduced oxygen delivery to the microcirculation. Ischemia causes impairment of brain energy metabolism, loss of aerobic glycolysis, intracellular accumulation of sodium and calcium ions, release of excitotoxic neurotransmitters, lactate elevation with local acidosis, free radical production, cell swelling, overactivation of lipases and proteases, and cell death. Many neurons undergo apoptosis after brain ischemia. Ischemic brain injury is exacerbated by leukocyte infiltration and development of brain edema. These biochemical changes have been the targets for many strategies aimed at neuroprotection.

Complete interruption of cerebral blood flow (CBF) causes suppression of the electrical activity within 12–15 seconds, inhibition of synaptic excitability of cortical neurons after 2–4 minutes, and inhibition of electrical excitability after 4–6 minutes. Normal CBF at rest in the normal adult brain is approximately 50–55 mL/100 g/min, and the cerebral metabolic rate of oxygen is 165 mmol/100 g/min. There are ischemic thresholds in experimental focal brain ischemia. When blood flow decreases to 18 mL/100 g/min, the brain reaches a threshold for electrical failure. Although these neurons are not functioning normally, they do have recovery potential. The second level, known as the *threshold of membrane failure*, occurs when blood flow decreases to 8 mL/100 g/min. Cell death rapidly results. These thresholds mark the upper and lower limits of the ischemic penumbra. The ischemic penumbra, or area of "misery perfusion," is the area of the ischemic brain between these two flow thresholds in which there are some neurons that are functionally silent but structurally intact and potentially salvageable.

## PATHOLOGY OF ISCHEMIC STROKE

The pathological characteristics of ischemic stroke depend on the stroke mechanism, the size of the obstructed artery, and the collateral blood flow availability. There may be advanced changes of atherosclerosis visible within arteries. The brain surface in the area of infarction appears pale. With ischemia caused by hypotension or hemodynamic changes, the arterial border (or watershed) zones are most vulnerable. A wedge-shaped area of infarction in the center of an arterial territory may result if there is occlusion of a main artery in the presence of collateral blood flow. In the absence of collateral blood flow, the entire territory supplied by an artery may be infarcted. With occlusion of a major artery such as the internal carotid, there may be a multilobar infarction. There may be evidence of flattening of the gyri and obliteration of the sulci caused by cerebral edema. A lacunar infarction with a size of 1.5 cm or less in subcortical areas or in the brainstem may be barely visible in the macroscopic analysis of the cut brain. Small emboli to the brain tend to lodge at the junction between the cerebral cortex and the white matter. Reperfusion of the infarct may occur, leading to hemorrhagic transformation.

The microscopic changes after cerebral infarction are well documented. These observed changes depend on the age of the infarction. They do not occur immediately and may be delayed up to 6 hours after onset. There is neuronal swelling initially, which is followed by shrinkage, hyperchromasia, and pyknosis. Chromatolysis appears, and the nuclei become eccentric. Swelling and fragmentation of the astrocytes and endothelial swelling occur. Neutrophil infiltrates appear as early as 4 hours after the ischemia and become abundant by 36 hours. Within 48 hours, the microglia proliferate and ingest myelin breakdown products and form foamy macrophages. Later there is neovascularization. The necrotic elements are gradually reabsorbed, and a cavity consisting of glial and fibrovascular elements forms. In a large infarction, there are three distinct zones: an inner area of coagulative necrosis; a middle zone of vacuolated neuropil, leukocytic infiltrates, swollen axons, and thickened capillaries; and an outer marginal zone of hyperplastic astrocytes and variable changes in nuclear staining.

## CLINICAL SYNDROMES OF CEREBRAL ISCHEMIA

A number of syndromes result from central nervous system (CNS) ischemia (Brazis et al., 2011).

### Transient Ischemic Attacks

An estimated 400,000 individuals experience a TIA each year in the United States. The true frequency of TIA may be far greater due to under-reporting. The 2014 AHA statistical update suggested that there may be as many as 5 million possible TIAs annually in the United States.

A TIA is a prognostic indicator of stroke, with one-third of untreated TIA patients having a stroke within 5 years. About 1 in 10 patients with TIA experience a stroke in the next 3 months. The interval from the last TIA is an important predictor of stroke risk; of all patients who subsequently experience stroke, 21% do so within 1 month and 51% do so within 1 year. In one series, patients with TIA had a 3-month stroke risk of 10.5%, similar to the recurrence rate following a stroke. Furthermore, 50% occurred within 48 hours of TIA onset (Johnston et al., 2000). Cardiac events are the principal cause of death in patients who have had a TIA. The 5%–6% annual mortality rate after TIA is mainly caused by MI.

A TIA is a temporary and "non-marching" neurological deficit of sudden onset; attributed to focal ischemia of the brain, retina, or cochlea; and lasting less than 24 hours. Most TIAs last only a few minutes. Episodes that last longer than 1 hour are usually due to small infarctions. With the advent of diffusion-weighted magnetic resonance imaging (DW-MRI), the time-based definition of TIA is inadequate because infarctions are frequently evident on DW-MRI in patients whose clinical manifestations resolved completely within a few hours. Thus, a "tissue-based" modification of the TIA definition has been proposed that includes any transient episode, regardless of duration, associated with a clinically appropriate imaging lesion defined as a stroke (Albers et al., 2002). Patients with TIA and DW-MRI lesions are at greater early risk for experiencing a subsequent stroke than patients without a lesion (Coutts et al., 2005). The ABCD2 score is a risk stratification score in patients with TIAs based on age, blood pressure (≥140/90 mm Hg), clinical features, TIA duration, and diabetes (Table 65.4). ABCD2 scores of 4 or greater indicate a moderate to high stroke risk and justify prompt hospital admission (Johnston et al., 2007).

The onset of TIA symptoms is sudden, reaching maximum intensity almost immediately. To qualify as a TIA, an episode should also be followed by complete clinical recovery. TIAs involving the carotid circulation should be distinguished from those involving the vertebrobasilar circulation. Headaches often occur in patients with TIAs. As such, migraine with aura may sometimes be indistinguishable from TIA.

Agreement between physicians to define the likelihood of a TIA is poor (Castle et al., 2010). The following symptoms are considered typical of TIAs in the carotid circulation: ipsilateral amaurosis fugax, contralateral sensory or motor dysfunction limited to one side of the body, aphasia, contralateral homonymous hemianopia, or any combination thereof. The following symptoms represent typical TIAs in the vertebrobasilar system: bilateral or shifting motor or sensory dysfunction, complete or partial vision loss in the homonymous fields, or any combination of these symptoms. Perioral numbness also occurs. Isolated diplopia, vertigo, dysarthria, and dysphagia can also occur but are not clinically diagnostic of a TIA unless they occur in combination with one another or with any of the other symptoms just listed (Box 65.1). Older patients with isolated vertebrobasilar symptoms and a significant history of cardiovascular risk factors should, however, be evaluated for possible TIA or stroke, because they are at substantially higher risk for cerebrovascular events (Norrving et al., 1995).

Occlusive disease in the subclavian arteries or the innominate artery can give rise to extracranial steal syndromes. The most well-defined syndrome is subclavian steal syndrome (SSS). In SSS, reversal of flow in the vertebral artery is caused by a high-grade subclavian artery stenosis or occlusion proximal to the origin of the vertebral artery from the aortic arch or innominate artery, with resultant symptoms of brainstem ischemia, usually precipitated by actively exercising the ipsilateral arm. The left side is involved most frequently. With innominate artery occlusion, the origin of the right carotid is also subject to reduced perfusion pressure. Subclavian artery or innominate artery stenosis can be suspected by a reduced or delayed radial pulse and diminished blood pressure in the affected arm relative to the contralateral arm. A subclavian steal may be symptomatic or asymptomatic. Many patients have angiographic evidence of reversed vertebral blood flow without ischemic symptoms. Transcranial Doppler (TCD) ultrasonography may detect transient retrograde basilar blood flow during an ischemic forearm challenge. Retrograde vertebral artery flow is a benign entity. Brainstem infarction is an uncommon complication of the SSS.

Transient global amnesia (TGA) is characterized by a reversible antegrade and retrograde memory loss, except for a total amnesia of events that occur during the attacks and inability to learn newly acquired information. During the attacks, patients remain alert without motor or sensory impairments and often ask the same questions repeatedly. Patients are able to retain personal identity and carry on complex activities. TGA most commonly affects patients 50 years and older. Men are affected more commonly than women. The attacks begin abruptly without warning. A typical attack lasts several hours (mean, 3–6 hours) but seldom longer than 12 hours. Onset of TGA may follow physical exertion, sudden exposure to cold or heat, or sexual intercourse. Although many conditions have been associated with transient amnesia, in most instances, TGA is of primary or unknown cause. TGA has been associated with epilepsy, migraine, intracranial tumors, overdose of diazepam, cardiac arrhythmias secondary to digitalis intoxication, and as a complication of cerebral and coronary angiography. Many reports have suggested a vascular causal factor. Bilateral hippocampal and parahippocampal complex ischemia in the distribution of the posterior cerebral arteries (PCAs) or cortical spreading depression of migrainous origin in these areas are potential mechanisms. Acute confusional migraines in children and TGA have a number of similar features. Others have suggested an epileptic causal factor for a minority of patients. Venous hypertension with transient hypoxemia in the context of incompetent internal jugular vein valves has also been suggested as a possible mechanism for TGA (Nedelmann et al., 2005). Transient amnesias have been divided into pure TGA,

**TABLE 65.4 ABCD2 Score**

| | |
|---|---|
| **A**ge 60 or older | 1 point |
| **B**lood pressure ≥{140/90} | 1 point |
| **C**linical: | |
| Unilateral weakness | 2 points |
| Speech impairment | 1 point |
| **D**uration: | |
| 60 min or more | 2 points |
| <60 min | 1 point |
| **D**iabetes mellitus | 1 point |

*From Johnston, S.C., Rothwell, P.M., Nguyen-Huyn, M.N., et al., 2007. Validation and refinement of scores to predict very early stroke risk after transient ischemic attack. Lancet 369, 283–292.*

**BOX 65.1 Recognition of Carotid and Vertebrobasilar Transient Ischemic Attacks**

**Symptoms Suggestive of Carotid Transient Ischemic Attacks**

Transient ipsilateral monocular visual loss (amaurosis fugax)
Contralateral body weakness or clumsiness
Contralateral body sensory loss or paresthesias
Aphasia with dominant hemisphere involvement
Various degrees of contralateral homonymous visual field defects
Dysarthria (not in isolation)

**Symptoms Suggestive of Vertebrobasilar Transient Ischemic Attacks**

Usually bilateral weakness or clumsiness, but may be unilateral or shifting
Bilateral, shifting, or crossed (ipsilateral face and contralateral body) sensory loss or paresthesias
Bilateral or contralateral homonymous visual field defects or binocular vision loss
Two or more of the following symptoms: vertigo, diplopia, dysphagia, dysarthria, and ataxia

**Symptoms Not Acceptable as Evidence of Transient Ischemic Attack**

Syncope, dizziness, confusion, urinary or fecal incontinence, and generalized weakness
Isolated occurrence of vertigo, diplopia, dysphagia, ataxia, tinnitus, amnesia, drop attacks, or dysarthria

probable epileptic amnesia, and probable transient ischemic amnesia. In contrast to patients with TIAs, the prognosis of persons with pure TGA is benign, with no apparent increased risk for vascular endpoints. Recurrences are uncommon. Extensive evaluations are not usually required, except to distinguish TGA from TIA or seizures. Treatment with platelet antiaggregants is not indicated in most patients unless there is a suspicion for transient ischemic amnesia. The use of prophylactic calcium channel blockers may be justified in patients with a potential migrainous causal factor.

Drop attacks are characterized by the sudden loss of muscle tone and strength. The attacks cause unexpected falling. Consciousness is preserved. Most attacks occur while standing or walking and often follow head or neck motion. Drop attacks have been considered a symptom of vertebrobasilar ischemia, but many of these patients have other coexistent disorders that could otherwise explain their symptoms. In rare instances, drop attacks may be caused by ischemia of the corticospinal tracts or reticular formation. However, isolated drop attacks are seldom a manifestation of vertebrobasilar occlusive disease. In most instances these attacks are secondary to akinetic seizures, high cervical spine or foramen magnum lesions, postural hypotension, Tumarkin otolithic crises (in Meniere disease), or near syncope of cardiac origin.

The causes of TIA are similar to those of stroke (see below). Preceding TIAs occur frequently in patients with brain infarction. In published series, TIAs occurred before 25%–50% of atherothrombotic infarcts, in 11%–30% of cardioembolic infarcts, and in 11%–14% of lacunar infarcts.

Crescendo episodes of cerebral ischemia that increase in frequency, severity, or duration must be treated as neurological emergencies. The *capsular warning syndrome* is characterized by restricted, stereotyped, repeated episodes of capsular ischemia causing contralateral symptoms involving the face, arm, and leg. Occasionally, "stuttering TIAs" may be confused with epileptic events. When capsular infarction develops, it is usually a lacunar-type stroke and involves a single penetrating vessel. Occasionally, striatocapsular or anterior choroidal artery territory infarction occurs. These may be lacunar in origin but sometimes are associated with carotid artery disease. Typically these patients are refractory to conventional forms of therapy.

The treatment of patients with TIAs depends on a careful history and detailed physical examination. The neurovascular examination may disclose a well-localized bruit in the mid- or upper cervical area. Bruits arise when normal laminar blood flow is disturbed. However, the presence of a cervical bruit does not necessarily indicate underlying carotid artery atherosclerosis. Correlation with vascular imaging shows only a 60% concordance with cervical auscultation in predicting the presence of stenosis. Radiated cardiac murmurs, hyperdynamic states, nonatherosclerotic carotid arterial lesions, and venous hums can produce cervical murmurs. The absence of a bruit has little diagnostic value; the bruit may disappear when the stenosis is advanced. Conversely, a cervical bruit may be heard contralateral to an internal carotid artery occlusion or reflect ipsilateral external carotid artery disease.

Different types of microemboli (e.g., cholesterol crystals, platelet fibrin, calcium, and other forms of debris) can be seen in the retinal arterioles during or between attacks of transient monocular visual loss. Engorgement of conjunctival and episcleral vessels, corneal edema and rubeosis irides, and anterior-chamber cell flare are indicative of an underlying ischemic oculopathy. Asymmetrical hypertensive retinal changes noted on funduscopy are suggestive of a high-grade carotid artery stenosis or occlusion on the side of the less severely involved retina. Venous stasis retinopathy may occur with high-grade carotid artery stenosis or occlusion and is characterized by diminished or absent venous pulsations, dilated and tortuous retinal veins, peripheral microaneurysms, and blossom-shaped hemorrhages in the mid-peripheral retina. Retinal microvascular abnormalities correlate with an increased incidence of lacunar strokes (Yatsuya et al., 2010). Corneal arcus senilis may be less obvious or absent on the side of low perfusion.

Many conditions can resemble a TIA. Subdural, intracerebral, or subarachnoid hemorrhage, space-occupying lesions, seizures, hypoglycemia, migraine, syncope, and labyrinthine disorders are among the diverse conditions in the differential diagnosis. Symptoms of a transient neurological dysfunction that resolve incompletely should lead the physician to question the diagnosis of TIA. Similarly, a migration or "march of symptoms" from one part of the body to another is rare during a TIA and more indicative of a focal seizure or migraine. Fortification phenomena or scintillating bright visual symptoms are suggestive of migraine. In rare instances, involuntary limb-shaking movements can occur, but in general, involuntary movements reflect convulsive activity rather than a TIA.

## Carotid Artery System Syndromes

### Carotid Artery Syndromes

*Amaurosis fugax* is a sudden onset of transient monocular visual loss. A curtain or shade pattern of vision loss, moving superiorly to inferiorly, is described in only 15%–20% of patients. Less commonly, a concentric vision loss, presumed to be caused by diminished blood flow to the retina, is described. Most attacks are spontaneous and unrelated to positional changes. The duration is usually 1–5 minutes and rarely lasts more than 30 minutes. It is typically painless. After an episode of amaurosis fugax, the vision is usually fully restored, although some patients may have permanent vision loss caused by a retinal infarction (see Chapter 16).

### Middle Cerebral Artery Syndromes

Amaurosis fugax is the sole feature that distinguishes the carotid artery syndrome from a middle cerebral artery (MCA) syndrome. An MCA infarction is one of the most common manifestations of cerebrovascular disease. The clinical picture varies and depends on whether the site of the occlusion is in the stem, superior division, inferior division, or lenticulostriate branches of the MCA, and the extent of collateral blood flow.

When the stem is occluded, there is usually a large hemispheric infarction with contralateral hemiplegia, hemianesthesia, homonymous hemianopia, and conjugate ipsilateral eye deviation. Global aphasia occurs if the dominant hemisphere is involved, and hemineglect with nondominant lesions. The difference between an upper-division MCA infarction and an MCA stem lesion is that the hemiparesis usually affects the face and arm more than the leg with upper division infarction. A Broca-type aphasia is common in upper-division infarcts of the dominant hemisphere because of the preferential involvement of the anterior MCA branches. Impaired prosody may be seen with anterior nondominant MCA infarcts. With lower-division MCA syndromes, a Wernicke-type aphasia is seen with dominant hemisphere infarction and behavioral disturbances are seen with nondominant infarction. A homonymous hemianopia may be present. A lenticulostriate branch occlusion may cause a subcortical infarction with involvement of the internal capsule, producing pure motor hemiparesis. These syndromes are variable and depend on the presence of collaterals or whether brain edema is present.

Alexia with agraphia may occur with left-sided angular gyrus involvement. Gerstmann syndrome, which consists of finger agnosia, acalculia, right-left disorientation, and agraphia, may be seen with dominant-hemisphere parietal lesions. The aphasias with dominant-hemispheric infarctions may be of the Broca, Wernicke,

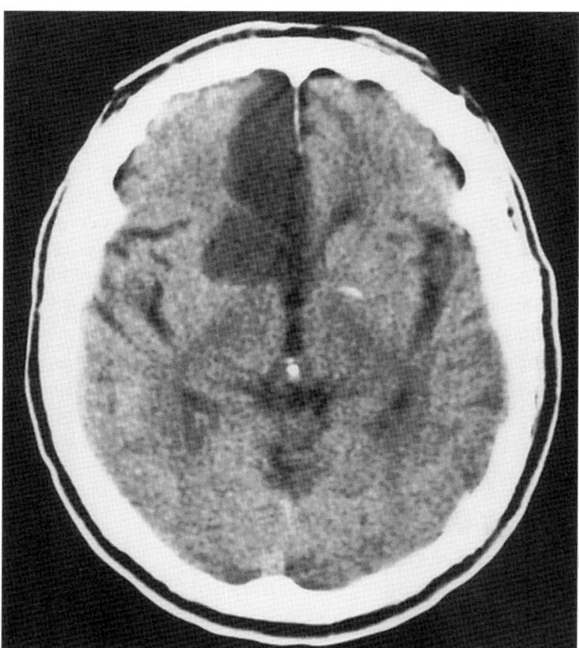

**Fig. 65.1** Nonenhanced axial computed tomographic scan of a 63-year-old man with left-sided weakness and abulia demonstrates a right anterior cerebral artery (ACA) territory infarction. More superior images showed the entire ACA distribution was infarcted.

conduction, transcortical, or global type, depending on the site and extent of involvement. Anosognosia, the denial of hemiparesis, is most commonly associated with right hemispheric strokes. Nondominant infarction may cause hemi-inattention, tactile extinction, visual extinction, anosognosia, anosodiaphoria, apraxia, impaired prosody, and (rarely) acute confusion and agitated delirium. A contralateral homonymous hemianopia or contralateral inferior quadrantanopia can occur with infarctions in either hemisphere.

## Syndromes of the Anterior Cerebral Artery and Related Blood Vessels

Anterior cerebral artery (ACA) territory infarctions are uncommon in isolation (Fig. 65.1). They occur in patients with vasospasm after subarachnoid hemorrhage caused by ACA or anterior communicating artery aneurysm. Excluding these causes, the percentage of acute cerebral infarcts that are in the ACA territory is less than 3%. The characteristics of ACA infarction vary according to the site of involvement and the extent of collateral blood flow. Contralateral weakness involving primarily the lower extremity and, to a lesser extent, the arm is characteristic of infarction in the territory of the hemispheric branches of the ACA. Other characteristics include abulia, akinetic mutism (with bilateral mesiofrontal damage), impaired memory or emotional disturbances, transcortical motor aphasia (with dominant hemispheric lesions), deviation of the head and eyes toward the lesion, paratonia (gegenhalten), discriminative and proprioceptive sensory loss (primarily in the lower extremity), and sphincter incontinence. An anterior disconnection syndrome with left arm apraxia due to involvement of the anterior corpus callosum can be seen. Pericallosal branch involvement can cause apraxia, agraphia, and tactile anomia of the left hand. Infarction of the basal branches can cause memory disorders, anxiety, and agitation. Infarction in the medial lenticulostriate artery territory (artery of Heubner) causes more pronounced weakness of the face and arm without sensory loss due to this artery's supply of portions of the anterior limb of the internal capsule. Bilateral simultaneous infarctions in the ACA territory are unusual and may mimic space-occupying midline lesions.

The anterior choroidal artery syndrome is often characterized by hemiparesis caused by involvement of the posterior limb of the internal capsule, hemisensory loss caused by involvement of the posterolateral nucleus of the thalamus or thalamocortical fibers, and hemianopia secondary to involvement of the lateral geniculate body or the geniculocalcarine tract. The visual field defect with anterior choroidal artery syndrome infarcts is characterized by a homonymous defect in the superior and inferior visual fields that spares the horizontal meridian. Rarely, left spatial hemineglect with right hemispheric infarctions, and a mild language disorder with left hemispheric infarctions, may occur. With bilateral infarctions in the anterior choroidal artery territory, there can be pseudobulbar mutism and a variety of other features including facial diplegia, hemisensory loss, lethargy, neglect, and affect changes.

## Lacunar Syndromes

Ischemic strokes resulting from small-vessel or penetrating artery disease (lacunes) have unique clinical, radiological, and pathological features. Lacunar infarcts occur in the deep regions of the brain or brainstem that range in diameter from 0.5 to 15 mm. They result from occlusion of the penetrating arteries, chiefly from the anterior choroidal, middle cerebral, posterior cerebral, and basilar arteries. They can also be the result of occlusion of penetrating artery origin by atherosclerosis of the parent artery or by microembolism. Lacunes may be single or multiple, symptomatic or asymptomatic. At least 20 lacunar syndromes have been described and are predictive of lacunar infarcts. The five best recognized syndromes are (1) pure motor hemiparesis, (2) pure sensory stroke, (3) sensorimotor stroke, (4) homolateral ataxia and crural paresis (ataxic hemiparesis), and (5) dysarthria–clumsy hand syndrome. Multiple lacunes may be associated with acquired cognitive decline. Headaches are an uncommon feature.

Pure motor hemiparesis is often caused by an internal capsule, basis pontis, or corona radiata lacune and is characterized by a contralateral hemiparesis or hemiplegia involving the face, arm, and leg, accompanied by mild dysarthria. There should be no aphasia, apraxia, or agnosia, and there are no sensory, visual, or other higher cortical disturbances. Pure sensory stroke is the least predictive syndrome of lacunar infarction but may be due to a lacune involving the ventroposterolateral nucleus of the thalamus. However, cortical infarcts of the postcentral gyrus may present with a similar syndrome. Pure sensory stroke is characterized by paresthesia, numbness, and a unilateral hemisensory deficit. Sensory-motor stroke is often caused by a lacuna involving the posterior limb of the internal capsule and thalamus; large striatocapsular infarcts also can cause a similar syndrome. It is characterized by a contralateral motor deficit with a superimposed hemisensory deficit. Homolateral ataxia and crural paresis are often caused by a lacuna either in the posterior limb of the internal capsule or the basis pontis is characterized by weakness, predominantly in the contralateral lower extremity, and ipsilateral incoordination of the arm and leg. Dysarthria–clumsy hand syndrome is often caused by a lacuna involving the deep areas of the basis pontis and is characterized by supranuclear facial weakness, dysarthria, dysphagia, loss of fine motor control of the hand, and Babinski sign.

## Vertebrobasilar System Syndromes

The areas of the cerebellum supplied by the posterior inferior cerebellar artery (PICA) are variable (see Chapter 21.). There are several different patterns of PICA territory infarctions. If the medial branch territory is affected, involving the vermis and vestibulocerebellum, the clinical findings include prominent vertigo, ataxia, and nystagmus. If

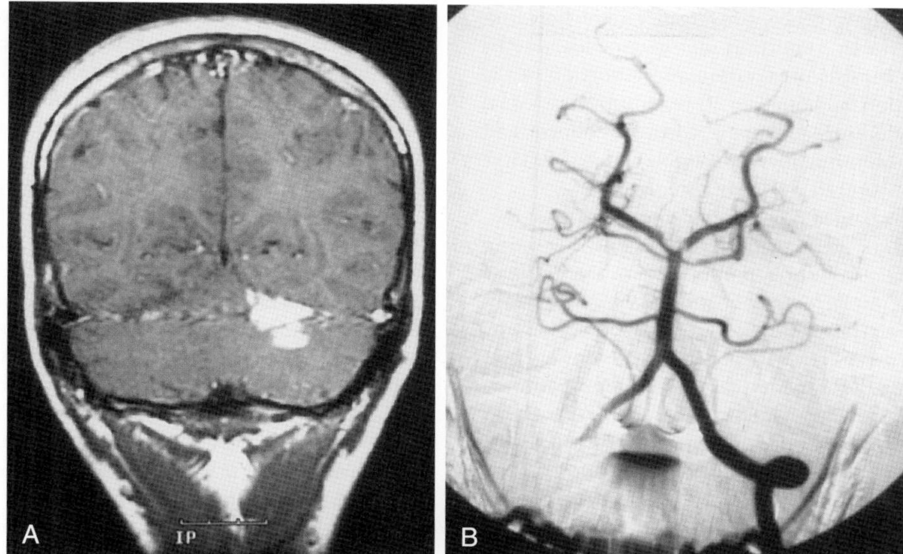

**Fig. 65.2** A 15-year-old boy had vomiting, tinnitus, and unsteadiness. **A,** T1 coronal postgadolinium magnetic resonance imaging shows enhancing lesions in the superior aspect of the left cerebellar hemisphere consistent with superior cerebellar artery infarct. **B,** Anteroposterior view. Left vertebral artery injection shows a filling defect of the basilar apex also involving the proximal left superior cerebellar artery, consistent with thromboembolus.

the lateral cerebellar hemisphere is involved, patients can have vertigo, gait ataxia, limb dysmetria, nausea, vomiting, conjugate or dysconjugate gaze palsies, miosis, and dysarthria. If the infarction is large, altered consciousness or confusion may occur as a result of cerebellar edema causing obstructive hydrocephalus or brainstem compression. Herniation downward through the foramen magnum or upward through the tentorial notch may occur, leading to compression of vascular and parenchymal structures. Although a PICA occlusion can be the cause of Wallenberg (lateral medullary) syndrome, this syndrome is more often due to an intracranial vertebral artery occlusion.

The anterior inferior cerebellar artery (AICA) syndrome causes a ventral cerebellar infarction. The signs and symptoms include vertigo, nausea, vomiting, and nystagmus caused by involvement of the vestibular nuclei. There may be ipsilateral facial hypalgesia and thermoanesthesia and corneal hypesthesia because of involvement of the trigeminal spinal nucleus and tract. Ipsilateral deafness and facial paralysis occur with involvement of the lateral pontomedullary tegmentum. An ipsilateral Horner syndrome due to compromise of the descending oculosympathetic fibers is present. Contralateral trunk and extremity hypalgesia occurs, and involvement of the lateral spinothalamic tract causes thermoanesthesia. Finally, ipsilateral ataxia and asynergia follow involvement of the cerebellar peduncle and cerebellum.

Infarction in the territory of the superior cerebellar artery (SCA) produces a dorsal cerebellar syndrome (Fig. 65.2). Vertigo may be present, although it is less common with SCA infarcts than with the other cerebellar syndromes. Nystagmus is caused by involvement of the medial longitudinal fasciculus and the cerebellar pathways. An ipsilateral Horner syndrome due to involvement of the descending sympathetic tract may be present. Ipsilateral ataxia and asynergia and gait ataxia follow involvement of the superior cerebellar peduncle, brachium pontis, superior cerebellar hemisphere, and dentate nucleus. There is an intention tremor caused by involvement of the dentate nucleus and superior cerebellar peduncle. Choreiform dyskinesias may be present ipsilaterally. Contralaterally, there is hearing loss due to lateral lemniscus disruption and trunk and extremity hypalgesia and thermoanesthesia caused by spinothalamic tract involvement.

Weber syndrome is caused by infarction in the distribution of the penetrating branches of the PCA affecting the cerebral peduncle, especially medially, with damage to the fascicle of cranial nerve (CN) III and the corticospinal fibers. The resultant clinical findings are contralateral hemiplegia of the face, arm, and leg secondary to corticospinal and corticobulbar tract involvement, and ipsilateral oculomotor paresis including a dilated pupil. A slight variation of this syndrome is Foville syndrome, in which the supranuclear fibers for horizontal gaze are interrupted in the medial peduncle, causing conjugate gaze palsy to the opposite side. Benedikt syndrome is caused by a lesion affecting the ventral mesencephalic tegmentum, with involvement of the red nucleus, brachium conjunctivum, and fascicle of CN III. This syndrome is due to infarction in the distribution of the penetrating branches of the PCA to the midbrain. The clinical manifestations are ipsilateral oculomotor paresis, usually with pupillary dilation and contralateral involuntary movements including intention tremor, hemiathetosis, or hemichorea. Claude syndrome is caused by lesions that are more dorsal in the midbrain tegmentum than with Benedikt syndrome. There is dorsal red nucleus injury, which results in more prominent cerebellar signs without the involuntary movements. Oculomotor paresis occurs. Nothnagel syndrome is characterized by an ipsilateral oculomotor palsy with contralateral cerebellar ataxia. Infarction in the distribution of the penetrating branches of the PCA to the midbrain is the cause. Parinaud syndrome can result from infarctions in the midbrain territory of PCA penetrating branches. This syndrome is characterized by supranuclear paralysis of upward gaze, convergence-retraction nystagmus, pupillary light-near dissociation, and bilateral lid retraction (see Chapter 21). Parinaud syndrome occurs more characteristically as a result of mass effect from pineal region mass lesions.

Top of the basilar syndrome (see Chapter 21) is caused by infarction of the midbrain, thalamus, and portions of the temporal and occipital lobes. It is often due to embolic occlusion of the rostral basilar artery. Associated behavioral abnormalities include somnolence, peduncular hallucinosis, memory disturbances, or agitated delirium. Ocular findings include unilateral or bilateral paralysis of upward or downward gaze, impaired convergence, convergence-retraction nystagmus, abnormalities of ocular abduction due to pseudoabducens palsy, Collier sign (which consists of elevation and retraction of the upper eyelids), skew deviation, and oscillatory eye movements. Visual defects may be present, including hemianopia, cortical blindness, and Balint syndrome. Pupillary abnormalities are variable and may be large or small, reactive or fixed. Motor deficits may also occur.

Although there are many named pontine syndromes, the most useful categorization is based on neuroanatomical divisions. Locked-in syndrome is the result of bilateral ventral pontine lesions that produce quadriplegia, aphonia, and impairment of horizontal eye movements. Wakefulness and normal sleep/wake cycles are maintained because the reticular formation is spared. The patient can move his or her eyes vertically and blink, because the supranuclear ocular motor pathways lie more dorsally. In some patients with symptomatic basilar artery occlusive disease, there may be a herald hemiparesis that suggests a hemispheric lesion. However, within a few hours, there is progression to bilateral hemiplegia and CN findings associated with the locked-in syndrome.

Occlusion of the AICA can lead to the lateral inferior pontine syndrome. Associated findings include ipsilateral facial paralysis, impaired facial sensation, conjugate gaze paralysis, deafness, tinnitus, and ataxia. Contralateral to the lesion, there is hemibody impairment to pain and temperature that in some instances includes the face. There may be horizontal and vertical nystagmus as well as oscillopsia. The medial inferior pontine syndrome is caused by occlusion of a paramedian branch of the basilar artery. With this syndrome, there is ipsilateral paralysis of conjugate gaze, abducens palsy, nystagmus, and ataxia. Contralateral to the lesion, there is hemibody impairment of tactile and proprioceptive sensation and hemiparesis. An occlusion of the AICA may lead to the total unilateral inferior pontine syndrome, a combination of those symptoms and signs seen with the lateral and medial pontine syndromes.

The lateral pontomedullary syndrome can occur with occlusion of the vertebral artery. The manifestations are a combination of the medial and lateral inferior pontine syndromes.

Occlusion of the paramedian branch of the midbasilar artery can lead to ipsilateral impaired sensory and motor function of the trigeminal nerve with limb ataxia, characteristics of the lateral midpontine syndrome. Ischemia of the medial midpontine region is caused by occlusion of the paramedian branch of the midbasilar artery and can lead to ipsilateral limb ataxia. Contralateral eye deviation and hemiparesis occur. Although there are predominant motor symptoms, variable impaired touch and proprioception may also occur. The lateral superior pontine syndrome may occur with occlusion of the SCA and produces ipsilateral Horner syndrome, horizontal nystagmus, conjugate gaze paresis, occasional deafness, and severe ataxia of the limbs and gait. Contralateral to the lesion, there is hemibody impairment to pain and temperature, skew deviation, and impaired tactile, vibratory, and proprioceptive sensation in the leg greater than in the arm.

The lateral medullary syndrome (Wallenberg syndrome) is most often due to occlusion of the intracranial segment of the vertebral artery (eFig. 65.3). Less commonly, it is caused by occlusion of the PICA. This syndrome produces an ipsilateral Horner syndrome; loss of pain and temperature sensation in the face; weakness of the palate, pharynx, and vocal cords; and cerebellar ataxia. Contralateral to the lesion, there is hemibody loss of pain and temperature sensation. The medial medullary (Dejerine) syndrome is less common and may be caused by occlusion of the distal vertebral artery, a branch of the vertebral artery, or the lower basilar artery. Vertebral artery dissection, dolichoectasia of the vertebrobasilar system, and embolism are less common causes of the medial medullary syndrome. The findings with this syndrome include an ipsilateral lower motor neuron paralysis of the tongue and contralateral hemiparesis. The face is often spared. In addition, there is contralateral hemibody loss of tactile, vibratory, and position sense. Occlusion of the intracranial vertebral artery can lead to a total unilateral medullary syndrome (Babinski-Nageotte) or a combination of the medial and lateral medullary syndromes.

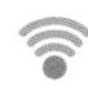

## Posterior Cerebral Artery Syndromes

The manifestations with PCA territory infarctions depend on the site of the occlusion and the availability of collateral blood flow. Occlusion of the precommunal P1 segment causes midbrain, thalamic, and hemispheric infarction. Occlusion of the PCA in the proximal ambient cisternal segment before branching in the thalamogeniculate pedicle causes lateral thalamic and hemispheral symptoms. Occlusions also may affect a single PCA branch, primarily the calcarine artery, or cause a large hemispheric infarction of the PCA territory. Unilateral infarctions in the distribution of the hemispheral PCA branches may produce a contralateral homonymous hemianopia caused by infarction of the striate cortex, the optic radiations, or the lateral geniculate body. There is partial or complete macular sparing if the infarction spares the occipital pole. The visual field defect may be limited to a homonymous quadrantanopia. A superior homonymous quadrantanopia is due to infarction of the striate cortex inferior to the calcarine fissure or the inferior optic radiations in the temporo-occipital lobes. An inferior homonymous quadrantanopia is the result of an infarction of the striate cortex superior to the calcarine fissure or the superior optic radiations in the parieto-occipital lobes.

More complex visual changes may occur, including formed or unformed visual hallucinations, visual and color agnosias, or prosopagnosia. Finally, some alteration of sensation with PCA hemispheral infarctions occurs, including paresthesias or altered position, pain, and temperature sensations. Infarction in the distribution of the callosal branches of the PCA involving the left occipital region and the splenium of the corpus callosum produces alexia without agraphia (Fig. 65.4). Patients can write, speak, and spell normally but are unable to read. The ability to name letters and numbers may be intact, but there can be inability to name colors, objects, and photographs. Right-hemispheric PCA territory infarctions may cause contralateral visual-field neglect. Amnesia may be present when infarctions involve the left medial temporal lobe or when there are bilateral mesiotemporal infarctions. In addition, an agitated delirium may occur with unilateral or bilateral penetrating mesiotemporal infarctions. Large infarctions of the left posterior temporal artery territory may produce an anomic or transcortical sensory aphasia.

Infarctions in the distribution of the penetrating branches of the PCA can cause aphasia (if the left pulvinar is involved), akinetic mutism, global amnesia, and Dejerine-Roussy syndrome. In the latter syndrome, the patient has contralateral sensory loss to all modalities, severe dysesthesias on the involved side (thalamic pain), vasomotor disturbances, transient contralateral hemiparesis, and choreoathetoid or ballistic movements. A number of syndromes that can result from infarctions in the distribution of the penetrating branches of the PCA to the midbrain were previously discussed with the midbrain syndromes.

Bilateral infarctions in the distribution of the hemispheric PCA branches may cause bilateral homonymous hemianopias. Bilateral occipital or occipitoparietal infarctions can cause cortical blindness, often with denial or unawareness of blindness (Anton syndrome). Balint syndrome, seen with bilateral occipital or parieto-occipital infarctions, consists of optic ataxia, optic apraxia (paralysis of voluntary fixation), with inability to look to the peripheral field and disturbance of visual attention, and simultanagnosia.

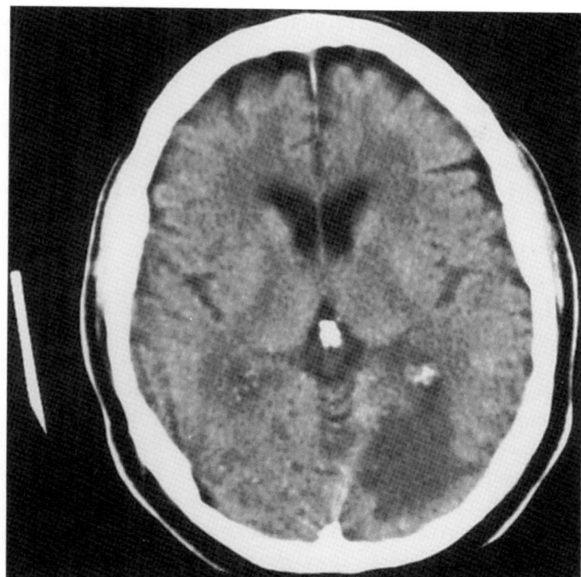

**Fig. 65.4** A 77-year-old man had alexia without agraphia, right homonymous hemianopia, and antegrade amnesia. Nonenhanced axial cranial computed tomography demonstrates an area of decreased parenchymal attenuation in the left occipitoparietal region.

### Syndromes of Thalamic Infarction

The main thalamic blood supply comes from the posterior communicating arteries and the perimesencephalic segment of the PCA. Thalamic infarctions typically involve one of four major vascular regions: posterolateral, anterior, paramedian, and dorsal. Posterolateral thalamic infarctions result from occlusion of the thalamogeniculate branches arising from the P2 segment of the PCA. Three common clinical syndromes may occur: pure sensory stroke, sensorimotor stroke, and the Dejerine-Roussy syndrome. Anterior thalamic infarction results from occlusion of the polar or tuberothalamic artery. Bilateral thalamic infarction may occur with an anatomical variant whereby the rostral mesencephalon and paramedian thalami receive flow from a single thalamic perforating artery known as the artery of Percheron 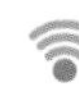 (eFig 65.5), which is typically present contralateral to an absent P1 segment of a PCA. An absent or atretic P1 segment may occur as a normal variant when the PCA has a persistent fetal pattern arising directly from the intracranial internal carotid artery. The main clinical manifestations of thalamic infarction consist of neuropsychological disturbances, emotional-facial paresis, occasional hemiparesis, and visual-field deficits. Left-sided infarcts are associated with dysphasia, whereas neglect is seen primarily in patients with right-sided lesions. Paramedian thalamic infarctions result from occlusion of the paramedian, thalamic, and subthalamic arteries. The main clinical manifestations include the classic triad of decreased level of consciousness, memory loss, and vertical-gaze abnormalities. Dorsal thalamic infarctions result from occlusion of the posterior choroidal arteries. These infarctions are characterized by the presence of homonymous quadrantanopia or horizontal sectoranopias. Involvement of the pulvinar may account for thalamic aphasia.

### Watershed Ischemic Syndromes

Watershed infarcts occur in the border zone between adjacent arterial perfusion beds. During or after cardiac surgery or after an episode of sustained and severe arterial hypotension that can happen after cardiac arrest, prolonged hypoxemia, or bilateral severe carotid artery disease, ischemia may occur in the border zones between the major circulations. Watershed infarctions may be unilateral when there is hemodynamic failure in patients with underlying unilateral severe arterial stenosis or occlusion. Border zone infarcts also may be caused by microembolism or hyperviscosity states.

Ischemia in the border zone or junctional territory of the ACA, MCA, and PCA may result in bilateral parieto-occipital infarcts. There can be visual manifestations, including bilateral lower altitudinal–field defects, optic ataxia, cortical blindness, and difficulty in judging size, distance, and movement. Ischemia between the territories of the ACA and MCA bilaterally may result in bi-brachial cortical sensorimotor impairment ("person in a barrel") and impaired saccadic eye movements caused by compromise of the frontal eye fields. Ischemia in the border zone between the MCA and PCA may cause bilateral parietal-occipital infarctions. Initially there is cortical blindness that may improve, but defects such as dyslexia, dyscalculia, dysgraphia, and memory defects for verbal and nonverbal material may persist.

Watershed infarcts are also recognized between the territorial supply of the PICA, AICA, and SCA. Watershed infarctions may also involve the internal border zone in the centrum semiovale adjacent to and slightly above the body of the lateral ventricles.

## DIAGNOSIS AND TREATMENT OF THREATENED ISCHEMIC STROKE

Ischemic strokes may result from (1) large-artery atherosclerotic disease resulting in stenosis or occlusion, (2) intrinsic small-vessel or penetrating artery disease (lacunes), (3) cardiogenic or artery-to-artery embolism, (4) nonatherosclerotic vasculopathies, (5) hypercoagulable disorders, and (6) undetermined causes. The most recognized mechanistic classification is the TOAST (Trial of Org 10172 in Acute Stroke Treatment) classification (Madden et al., 1995). However, a rigid classification of ischemic stroke subtypes is often difficult because of the frequent occurrence of mixed syndromes.

## LARGE-ARTERY ATHEROTHROMBOTIC INFARCTIONS

Large-artery atherothrombotic infarctions almost always occur in patients who already have significant risk factors for cerebrovascular atherosclerosis (see Table 65.1). Atherothrombosis is multifactorial, comorbidities frequently overlap, and risk factors are often additive. After a stroke, there is a 25% chance of a fatal thrombotic event in 3 years. Many of these deaths are due to MI. The mechanism of large-artery atherothrombotic infarction is often artery-to-artery embolization or thrombosis in the setting of preexisting atherostenosis commonly with plaque rupture or ulceration. (Fig. 65.6). In situ thrombosis occurs in the proximal carotid artery, distal vertebral artery, and lower or middle basilar artery. Atherosclerotic involvement of the intracranial vertebrobasilar system frequently occurs in tandem and is the common pathological mechanism associated with the syndrome of vertebrobasilar territory infarction; this may also arise in association with hypercoagulable states. Hypoperfusion secondary to hemodynamic alterations also may trigger these events. The pathogenesis of stroke due to intracranial arterial stenosis is similar to stroke due to extracranial arterial disease (Qureshi and Caplan, 2014).

In patients with vascular risk factors, the cholesterol-rich fatty streak may progress to a fibrous plaque that can evolve into a complicated plaque with intraplaque hemorrhage, extensive necrosis, calcification, and subsequent thrombosis (Fig. 65.7). The infiltration of the fibrous cap by inflammatory cells may contribute to the rupture of the atherosclerotic carotid artery plaque. Atherosclerosis is often segmental and asymmetrical, and earlier lesions tend to occur in areas

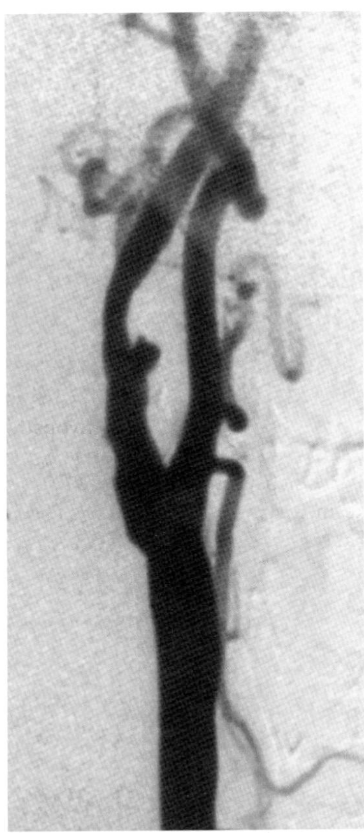

**Fig. 65.6** Right common carotid angiogram shows 17% right internal carotid artery stenosis (North American Symptomatic Carotid Endarterectomy Trial criteria) just superior to a large carotid ulceration. *(Courtesy Vincent Mathews, MD.)*

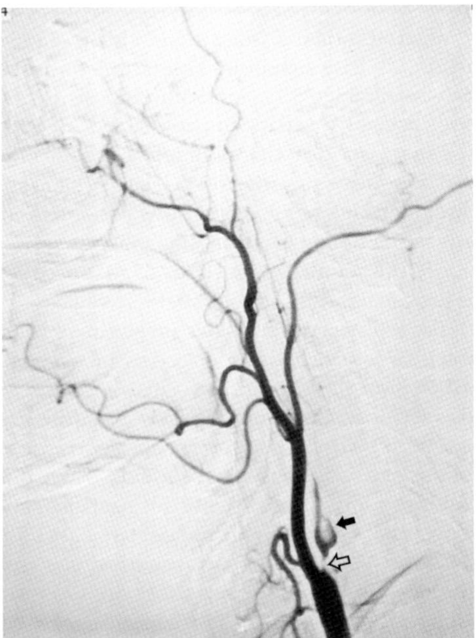

**Fig. 65.7** Left carotid angiogram (lateral view) shows severe stenosis *(open arrow)* of origin of the left internal carotid artery, with an intraluminal thrombus *(closed arrow)*. The artery was occluded in other images. *(Courtesy Vincent Mathews, MD.)*

of low shear stress, such as the outer aspect of the carotid artery bulb. Atherosclerosis primarily affects larger extracranial and intracranial vessels, particularly the bifurcation of the common carotid artery and proximal internal carotid artery, the carotid siphon, MCA stem, origin (V1) and intracranial segment (V4) of the vertebral arteries, and basilar artery. The distribution of cerebral atherosclerosis may vary by race and ethnicity. Intracranial involvement may be more prevalent among Blacks and Asians than in Whites, but this may also reflect ascertainment biases.

## SMALL-VESSEL OR PENETRATING ARTERY DISEASE

Lacunes usually occur in patients with long-standing arterial hypertension, current cigarette smoking, and DM. The most frequent sites of involvement are the putamen, basis pontis, thalamus, posterior limb of the internal capsule, and caudate nucleus. Multiple Lacunar infarctions or Lacunar infarcts are strongly associated with arterial hypertension and DM. Available evidence suggests that structural changes of the cerebral vasculature caused by arterial hypertension are characterized by fibrinoid angiopathy, lipohyalinosis, and microaneurysm formation. Accelerated hypertensive arteriolar damage of the small penetrating arteries is common among patients with lacunar infarction. However, microatheroma of the ostium of a penetrating artery, arterial or cardiac embolism, or hemorheological changes can be operative in some cases. Microatheromas are associated with the majority of lacunes greater than 50 μm. The mere association of a lacunar syndrome in a patient with arterial hypertension and DM is insufficient for a diagnosis of lacunar infarct, and other causes of ischemic stroke must be excluded. In particular, the presence of sensorimotor stroke, limb weakness, and sudden onset in a patient with AF, and large striatocapsular infarctions, should be distinguished from lacunar infarcts, because they frequently have potential cardioembolic sources or coexistent severe carotid or MCA stenosis, and they often present with signs and symptoms of cortical dysfunction (Arboix et al., 2010). Control of hypertension, intensive statin therapy, and platelet antiaggregants are essential in the management of patients with lacunar infarcts.

## CARDIOGENIC EMBOLISM

Cardioembolic strokes are associated with substantial morbidity and mortality and account for approximately 15%–20% of all ischemic strokes. These emboli may be composed of platelet, fibrin, platelet-fibrin, calcium, microorganisms, or neoplastic fragments. The most common etiology of cerebral embolism in older individuals is AF, accounting for half to two-thirds of cardiogenic emboli. Other cardiac conditions with high embolic potential include acute MI, infective endocarditis, rheumatic mitral stenosis, mechanical prosthetic heart valves, dilated cardiomyopathy, and cardiac tumors. Low or uncertain embolic risk disorders include mitral valve prolapse, mitral annulus calcification, aortic valve calcification, calcific aortic stenosis, remote MI, left ventricular aneurysm, hypertrophic cardiomyopathy, patent foramen ovale (PFO), atrial septal aneurysm (ASA), atrial flutter, valvular strands, and a Chiari network.

Congenital heart disease is the most common cardiac disorder causing ischemic stroke in children. With the increased survival of many children with congenital heart disease, strokes are being seen with increased frequency. Children with congenital heart disease and a low hemoglobin concentration are at special risk for arterial strokes; those with a high hematocrit are more likely to experience cerebral venous thrombosis. Emboli from cardiac sources may be silent or cause severe neurological deficit or death. Although most types of heart disease may

**BOX 65.2 Sources of Cardioembolism**

Acute myocardial infarction
Left ventricular aneurysm
Dilated cardiomyopathy
Cardiac arrhythmias
Atrial fibrillation
Sick sinus syndrome
Valvular heart disease
Rheumatic mitral valve disease
Calcific aortic stenosis
Mitral annulus calcification
Mitral valve prolapse
Infective endocarditis
Nonbacterial thrombotic endocarditis
Prosthetic heart valves
Filamentous strands of the mitral valve
Giant Lambl excrescences
Aneurysms of the sinus of Valsalva
Intracardiac tumors (atrial myxoma, rhabdomyoma, papillary fibroelastoma)
Intracardiac defects with paradoxical embolism
Patent foramen ovale
Atrial septal aneurysm
Atrial septal defect
Cyanotic congenital heart disease
Fontan procedure or its modifications (cavopulmonary anastomosis)
Mitochondrial encephalomyopathy (mitochondrial encephalopathy, lactic acidosis, and stroke-like episodes; myoclonic epilepsy and ragged-red fibers; Kearns-Sayre syndrome)
Coronary artery bypass grafting
Ventricular-inhibited pacing
Heart transplantation
Artificial hearts
Cardioversion for atrial fibrillation
Balloon angioplasty
Ventricular support devices
Extracorporeal membrane oxygenator

produce cerebral embolism, certain cardiac disorders are more likely to be associated with emboli (Box 65.2).

Cardioembolic cerebral infarctions are often large, multiple, bilateral, and wedge shaped. Sudden unheralded focal neurological deficits that are worse at onset are often presenting manifestations of a cardioembolic infarction. Any vascular territory may be affected. Reliable clinical determination of a cardioembolic source of stroke may be hampered by a variety of problems. Identification of a potential embolic cardiac source is not by itself sufficient to diagnose a brain infarct as cardioembolic because (1) many cardiac problems coexist with potential stroke etiologies, (2) cardiac arrhythmias may occur after arrhythmogenic lesions such as parieto-insular and brainstem infarcts, (3) brain imaging differentiation between cardioembolic and other causes of cerebral infarction is not always reliable, and (4) cardiac changes detected by echocardiography are prevalent in control populations.

An embolic stroke occurs in approximately 1% of hospitalized patients with acute MI. Left ventricular thrombi are commonly associated with recent anterior wall transmural MI. Echocardiographic studies have demonstrated that approximately one-third to one-half of acute *anterior* MIs but less than 4% of acute *inferior* MIs develop left ventricular thrombi. Almost all episodes of embolism occur within 3 months following acute MI, with 85% developing in the first 4 weeks. A decreased ejection fraction is an independent predictor of stroke following MI. Although the prevalence of left ventricular thrombi in individuals with left ventricular aneurysms is high, the frequency of systemic embolism is low. Dilated cardiomyopathy may result from arterial hypertension or a variety of inflammatory, infectious, immune, metabolic, toxic, and neuromuscular disorders. The global impairment of ventricular performance predisposes to stasis and thrombus formation. Patients commonly have signs of impaired left ventricular systolic function, and less than half have diastolic heart failure. Occasionally, patients have concomitant AF. Embolism occurs in approximately 18% of patients with dilated cardiomyopathy not receiving anticoagulants. Patients with idiopathic hypertrophic subaortic stenosis may also present with stroke. Thromboembolism occurs in patients with congestive heart failure. Mitochondrial disorders, (see Chapter 93) are seldom associated with dilated cardiomyopathies, but cerebral infarction is a complication of mitochondrial encephalomyopathies (MELAS, myoclonic epilepsy and ragged-red fibers, and Kearns-Sayre syndrome). Stroke in Kearns-Sayre syndrome is likely secondary to embolism. Apical aneurysms also complicate Chagas cardiomyopathy, with resultant cerebral embolism.

Most cases of mitral stenosis are due to rheumatic heart disease. Emboli occur in 9%–14% of patients with mitral stenosis, with 60%–75% causing stroke or TIA. Embolism may be the first manifestation of mitral stenosis, particularly if it is associated with AF. Aortic valve calcification, with or without stenosis, is not a major stroke risk factor, but cases have been described. Cerebral embolism is a rare but described occurrence in patients with bicuspid aortic valves. Individuals with mitral annular calcification (MAC) have a twofold risk for stroke compared with those without MAC, but stroke rates are low. Mitral valve prolapse affects 3%–4% of adults and, when uncomplicated, does not increase stroke risk. Cerebral ischemic events appear to occur more commonly among men older than 50 years who have auscultatory findings of a systolic murmur and thick mitral valve leaflets on echocardiography. Thromboembolic phenomena complicating infective endocarditis may be systemic (left-sided endocarditis) or pulmonary (right-sided endocarditis). Vegetations are detected by transthoracic echocardiography (TTE) in most patients and are associated with an increased risk for embolism. TEE is the gold standard, with detection rates of better than 90%. Systemic emboli may occur in nearly half of patients with nonbacterial thrombotic endocarditis, a condition characterized by the presence of multiple small, sterile thrombotic vegetations most frequently involving the mitral and aortic valves. The risk for thromboembolism is higher with mechanical prosthetic heart valves than with bioprosthetic heart valves. Thromboemboli are more common with prosthetic heart valves in the mitral position than in the aortic position. The rate of embolism in patients with mechanical heart valves receiving anticoagulant therapy is 4% per year in the mitral position and 2% per year in the aortic position. Filamentous strands attached to the mitral valve may represent a risk for cerebral embolism, particularly in young patients, but the risk for recurrent cerebral ischemia is incompletely understood. The association between cerebral embolism and giant Lambl excrescences or aneurysms of the sinus of Valsalva is low.

The incidence of thromboembolism in patients with AF is 4%–7.5% per year. Patients with NVAF, the leading source of cardioembolic infarctions in older adults, have a five- to sixfold increase in stroke incidence, with a cumulative risk of 35% over a lifetime. Patients with rheumatic AF have a 17-fold increase in stroke incidence. However, individuals younger than age 65 with lone AF have a low embolic potential, particularly when heart failure, hypertension, DM, and previous history of stroke or TIA are absent. Stroke patients with AF are also at high risk for death during the acute phase of stroke and

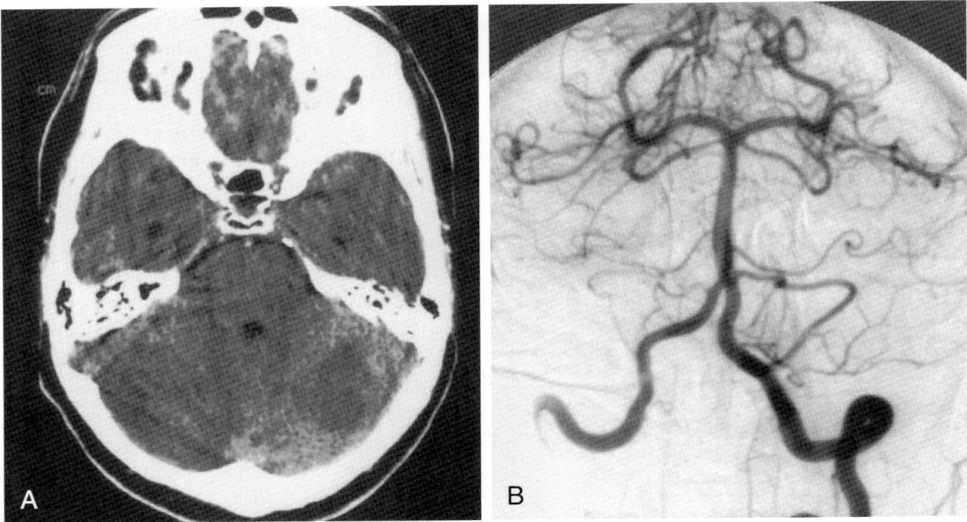


**Fig. 65.8** A, Nonenhanced axial computed tomographic scan shows bilateral cerebellar and pontine infarcts. B, Anteroposterior view of vertebrobasilar angiogram shows a large filling defect on the basilar artery, consistent with partial thrombosis. *(Courtesy Vincent Mathews, MD.)*

during the subsequent year. The prevalence of AF increases with age, from 0.2 cases per 1000 patients aged 30–39 years to 39 cases per 1000 patients aged 80–89 years. The proportion of strokes caused by AF also steadily increases from 6.7% of all strokes in patients aged 50–59 years to 36.2% in those aged 80–89 years. The risk for embolism is increased among patients with AF and hyperthyroidism, who also have an increased sensitivity to warfarin.

Embolism also may occur in the setting of the sick sinus syndrome. Patients at greatest risk for embolization have brady-tachyarrhythmias; left atrial spontaneous echocardiographic contrast and decreased atrial ejection force increase stroke risk. Patients with sick sinus syndrome may experience embolism even after pacemaker insertion. Ventricular-inhibited (VVI) pacing is associated with a higher risk for embolic complications than atrial or dual-chamber pacing. The risk for thromboembolism is also higher among patients in chronic atrial flutter.

Atrial myxomas are rare cardiac tumors complicated by postural syncope and systemic and embolic manifestations. Atrial myxomas and can result in stroke due to embolism of myxomatous material or thrombus. Embolic complications are a presenting symptom in one-third of patients with atrial myxoma. Recurrent emboli before surgery are common. Peripheral and multiple cerebral arterial aneurysms also have been diagnosed years after the initial embolic manifestations from atrial myxoma. Treatment consists of prompt surgical resection of the cardiac mass. Cardiac rhabdomyomas are associated with tuberous sclerosis; embolism is unusual. Mitral valve papillary fibroelastoma, an uncommon valvular tumor, is complicated rarely by stroke.

A paradoxical embolism via a right-to-left shunt through a PFO or atrial septal defect during transient increases in right atrial pressure and can be responsible for cerebral ischemic events. A PFO is present in 35% of subjects without stroke between the ages of 1 and 29 years, in 25% of people between the ages of 30 and 79 years, and in 20% between the ages of 80 and 99 years. A PFO is more common in patients with stroke than in matched controls. Patients with no identifiable cause for ischemic stroke and PFO tend to have larger PFOs with more extensive right-to-left shunting than patients with stroke of determined cause. Platelet antiaggregants, oral anticoagulants, transcatheter closure of the PFO, or surgical closure of the PFO have been recommended. Cerebrovascular complications of percutaneous PFO closure can include air embolism or thromboembolism, AF, infective endocarditis, or delayed cardioembolic stroke due to thrombus formation around the device. While early catheter-based closure trials failed to show a benefit for PFO closure, four more recent randomized studies established the benefit of PFO closure in patients 60 years old or less with cryptogenic stroke (Diener et al., 2018; Kuijpers et al., 2018). The ROPE score uses age, absence of hypertension and diabetes, and prior stroke or TIA as risk factors. A cutoff of 7 points identifies those with a high likelihood of a PFO being associated with cryptogenic stroke (Kent et al., 2013). Only one PFO-closure trial, however, used the ROPE score for patient selection (Mas et al., 2017). Various studies have found no difference in the time to primary endpoints between aspirin and warfarin, but limited data are available regarding the direct oral anticoagulants (DOACs). Only one study has reported that the coexistence of PFO and ASA increases the risk for embolic stroke (Messe et al., 2004). PFO and ASA also have been associated with mitral valve prolapse. Strokes are sometimes severe, but recurrences are uncommon in the context of PFO-related stroke. Pulmonary arteriovenous malformations can also be a source of paradoxical embolism causing cerebral ischemia and occur in 15%–20% of patients with HHT.

Spontaneous echocardiographic contrast is associated with elevated fibrinogen levels and plasma viscosity and is a potential stroke risk factor. Spontaneous echocardiographic contrast is highly associated with previous stroke or peripheral embolism in patients with AF or mitral stenosis and increased left atrial size. The risk for cerebrovascular events is increased in adults with cyanotic congenital heart disease in the presence of arterial hypertension, AF, history of phlebotomy, and particularly with microcytosis.

Cerebral ischemia is a rare complication following cardiac catheterization. Stroke occurs after coronary artery bypass grafting (CABG) with a frequency between 1% and 5% (Fig. 65.8 and 65.9). Two-thirds of strokes occur by the second postoperative day and predominantly involve the cerebral hemispheres; brainstem/cerebellar infarcts and lacunar strokes are less common. The cause is multifactorial; hypoperfusion, ventricular thrombus, and emboli are probable causal factors, although embolic causes are the most likely mechanisms. Clamp manipulation during surgery also may favor the release of aortic atheromatous debris. Epiaortic ultrasound studies demonstrate an increased stroke rate associated

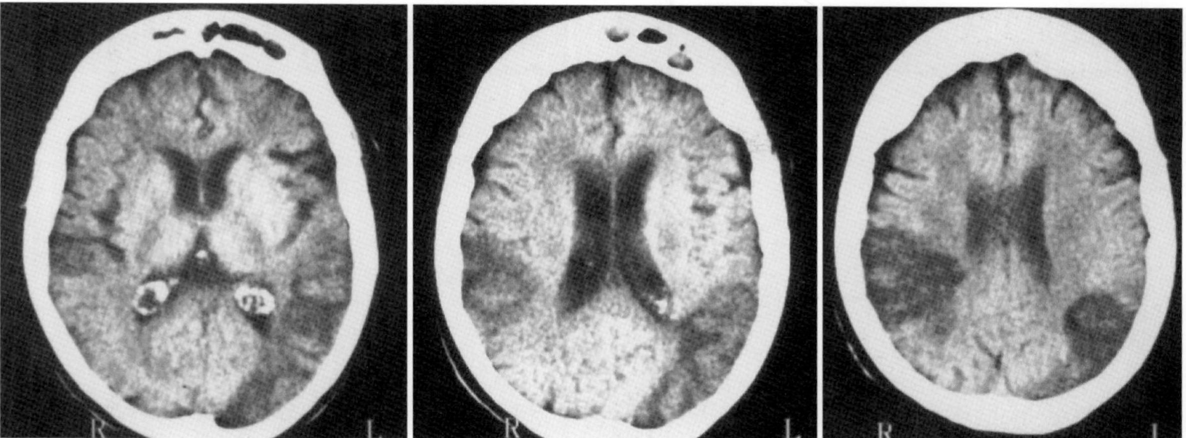


**Fig. 65.9** An 80-year-old woman remained unresponsive, with left-sided hemiplegia and right-sided hemiparesis after coronary artery bypass grafting and aortic valve replacement. Nonenhanced axial computed tomography demonstrates large left temporo-parieto-occipital and right frontoparietal infarctions.

with increasing severity of aortic atherosclerosis. Strokes following CABG relate to carotid artery stenosis. Carotid artery occlusion, but not carotid artery stenosis, increases the stroke risk for stroke following CABG. Thromboembolic phenomena can complicate cardiac surgery using cardiopulmonary bypass with deep hypothermia and cardiac arrest. Stroke is a potential complication of cardioversion for AF. Cerebral embolism may also complicate valvuloplasty; the risk is greater for aortic rather than mitral valvuloplasty. Strokes may follow heart transplantation, the use of ventricular support systems and artificial hearts, and the use of the extracorporeal membrane oxygenator. Stroke following inadvertent placement of left-sided heart pacemaker leads is an unusual complication. Ischemic myelopathy is a rare complication of the intraaortic balloon pump. Aortic dissection or hematoma may lead to an occlusion of a major radicular branch or local occlusion of the artery of Adamkiewicz.

## NONATHEROSCLEROTIC VASCULOPATHIES

Although the majority of arterial disorders leading to stroke are caused by atherosclerosis, several nonatherosclerotic vasculopathies can be responsible for a minority of ischemic strokes. These include cervicocephalic arterial dissections, traumatic cerebrovascular disease, radiation vasculopathy, moyamoya, fibromuscular dysplasia (FMD), and cerebral vasculitis (Boxes 65.3 and 65.4). Together, these conditions represent 5% of all ischemic strokes. They are relatively more common in children and young adults.

### Dissections

Cervicocephalic arterial dissections are one of the most frequent nonatherosclerotic vasculopathies causing ischemic stroke in young adults. A dissection is produced by subintimal penetration of blood with subsequent longitudinal extension of the intramural hematoma between vascular layers. Most dissections involve the extracranial segment of the internal carotid artery or extracranial vertebral arteries. Intracranial carotid and vertebrobasilar dissections are less common; intracranial dissections are usually subintimal and may follow trivial trauma, closed head trauma, basilar skull fracture, or penetrating injuries. The recurrence rate of extracranial cervicocephalic arterial dissections is approximately 1% per year. The risk for recurrent dissections is higher in younger patients, those with a history of FMD, and in patients with family history of arterial dissections.

Cervicocephalic arterial dissections have been reported after blunt or penetrating trauma and also are associated with FMD, Marfan syndrome, Turner syndrome (Muscat et al., 2001), Williams syndrome (Vanacker and Thijs, 2009), Ehlers-Danlos syndrome type IV, pseudoxanthoma elasticum, coarctation of the aorta, Menkes disease, $\alpha_1$-antitrypsin deficiency, cystic medial degeneration, reticular fiber deficiency, accumulation of mucopolysaccharides, hereditary hemochromatosis (Gallerini et al., 2006), osteogenesis imperfect type I, adult polycystic kidney disease, elevated arterial elastase content, lentiginosis, atherosclerosis, extreme vessel tortuosity, moyamoya syndrome, hyperhomocyteinemia (Arauz et al. 2007), the 677TT genotype of the 5,10-methylenetetrahydrofolate reductase gene (MTHFR 677TT), pharyngeal infections, sympathomimetic drug abuse, luetic arteritis, and styloid process length (Raser et al. 2011). Most cervicocephalic arterial dissections occur either spontaneously or in relation to minor trauma (Debette and Leys, 2009).

Dissection of the cervicocephalic vessels may cause transient retinal, hemispheric, or posterior fossa ischemia; Horner syndrome; hemicranial or neck pain; CN palsies; cerebral infarction; or subarachnoid hemorrhage (when the dissection involves an intracranial vessel due to the absence of an external elastic lamina beyond penetration through the dura). Ischemic symptoms result from arterial occlusion or secondary embolization. In addition to a postganglionic Horner syndrome, neuro-ophthalmological manifestations of internal carotid artery dissections may also include central retinal artery occlusion, ophthalmic artery occlusion, ischemic optic neuropathy, homonymous hemianopia, and ocular motor nerve palsies (CN III, IV, and VI). In addition to a first-order neuron Horner syndrome, other neuro-ophthalmological manifestations of vertebrobasilar dissections include diplopia, nystagmus, oscillopsia, ocular misalignment, skew deviation, ocular motor nerve palsies (CN III, IV, and VI), lateral gaze palsy, internuclear ophthalmoplegia, and homonymous visual-field defects.

Cervicocephalic arterial dissections should be considered in the differential diagnosis of ischemic stroke in any young adult, particularly when traditional risk factors are absent. Diagnosis is based on vascular imaging. High-resolution MRI with T1 fat suppression sequences and magnetic resonance angiography (MRA), computed tomographic angiography (CTA), and extracranial and TCD ultrasound have largely replaced contrast angiography for the diagnosis of cervicocephalic arterial dissections (eFig. 65.10).

Features on arteriography include the "pearl-and-string" sign; double-lumen sign; short, smooth, tapered occlusion; or pseudoaneurysm

**BOX 65.3 Selected Nonatherosclerotic Vasculopathies**

Cervicocephalic arterial dissections
Traumatic cerebrovascular disease
Radiation-induced vasculopathy
Moyamoya disease
Fibromuscular dysplasia
Vasculitis
Migrainous infarction

formation (eFig. 65.11) MRI demonstrates the intramural hematoma within the false lumen of the dissected artery (Fig. 65.12). MRA, CTA, or ultrasound studies can help in the monitoring of the course of dissection.

Although the optimal antithrombotic regimen after cervicocephalic dissections is uncertain, reasonable therapeutic interventions have included immediate anticoagulation with heparin, followed by a 3- to 6-month course of warfarin or platelet antiaggregants. Angioplasty and stenting or surgical correction is reserved for selected individuals with pseudoaneurysms or those who have multiple recurrent events following adequate medical therapy. Although anticoagulants are often empirically used, their value in patients with extracranial cervicocephalic arterial dissections has not been established. Anticoagulation should be withheld in patients with intracranial dissections (particularly involving the vertebrobasilar circulation) because of the risk for subarachnoid hemorrhage. No benefit of anticoagulants was seen in the Cervical Artery Dissection in Stroke Study (CADISS), a randomized multicenter open-treatment trial comparing anticoagulant and antiplatelet therapies for acute (within 7 days) symptomatic extracranial carotid or vertebral artery dissection (Markus et al. 2019). However, this trial was stopped prematurely due to slow recruitment.

## Trauma

Trauma is a leading cause of cerebrovascular mortality in the United States (see Chapter 62). Blunt or penetrating traumatic cerebrovascular disease may result in cervicocephalic arterial dissection, arterial thrombosis, arterial rupture, pseudoaneurysm formation, or development of an arteriovenous fistula. Internal carotid artery thrombosis also may follow maxillary and mandibular angle fractures. Carotid artery trauma may cause hematoma formation of the lateral neck, retinal or hemispheric ischemia, and post-ganglionic Horner syndrome. Patients with carotid arterial injuries with a Glasgow Coma Scale score of 8 or less do poorly regardless of treatment (see Chapter 5). A thorough evaluation of the airway, oropharynx, and esophagus is needed. Vascular imaging is indicated in most instances; thereafter, surgical repair or angioplasty may be needed (Nuñez et al., 2004).

## Radiation Vasculopathy

Injury to the endothelial cells by high-intensity radiation may cause accelerated atherosclerotic changes, particularly in the presence of hyperlipidemia. These changes may occur months to years after completion of radiation therapy. Radiation vasculopathy correlates with radiation dose and age at time of radiation therapy. Lesions develop in locations that are unusual for atherosclerosis and may involve the extracranial or intracranial vessels. Patients who receive therapeutic radiation therapy for lymphoma, Hodgkin disease, or thyroid carcinoma are at risk for involvement of the extracranial circulation. Radiation vasculopathy can also affect small and large intracranial

**BOX 65.4 Classification of Cerebral Vasculitides**

Infectious vasculitis:
- Bacterial, fungal, parasitic
- Spirochetal (syphilis, Lyme disease)
- Viral, rickettsial, mycobacterial
- Cysticercosis, free-living amebae

Necrotizing vasculitides:
- Classic polyarteritis nodosa
- Granulomatosis with polyangiitis
- Allergic angiitis and granulomatosis (Churg-Strauss)
- Necrotizing systemic vasculitis-overlap syndrome
- Lymphomatoid granulomatosis

Vasculitis associated with collagen vascular disease:
- Systemic lupus erythematosus
- Rheumatoid arthritis
- Scleroderma
- Sjögren syndrome

Vasculitis associated with other systemic diseases:
- Behçet disease
- Ulcerative colitis
- Sarcoidosis
- Relapsing polychondritis
- Kohlmeier-Degos disease (malignant atrophic papulosis)

Giant cell arteritides:
- Takayasu arteritis
- Temporal (cranial) arteritis

Hypersensitivity vasculitides:
- Henoch-Schönlein purpura
- Drug-induced vasculitides
- Chemical vasculitides
- Essential mixed cryoglobulinemia

Miscellaneous:
- Vasculitis associated with neoplasia
- Vasculitis associated with radiation
- Cogan syndrome
- Dermatomyositis polymyositis
- X-linked lymphoproliferative syndrome
- Thromboangiitis obliterans
- Kawasaki syndrome
- Primary angiitis of the central nervous system
- Amyloid-beta related angiitis

*From Biller, J., Sparks, L.H., 1993. Diagnosis and management of cerebral vasculitis. In: Adams Jr., H.P. (Ed.), Handbook of Cerebrovascular Diseases. Marcel Dekker, New York, p. 150.*

arteries following irradiation of intracranial neoplasms. Intracranial arterial stenosis also may follow stereotactic radiosurgery.

## Moyamoya Disease

Moyamoya disease is a chronic progressive nonatherosclerotic, noninflammatory, nonamyloid occlusive intracranial vasculopathy of unknown cause. There is fibrocellular intimal thickening, smooth muscle cell proliferation, and increased elastin accumulation, resulting in stenosis of the supraclinoid intracranial internal carotid arteries. There is also thinning of the media and a tortuous and often multilayered internal elastic lamina. Thrombotic lesions may be seen in major cerebral arteries. There are also numerous perforating and anastomotic branches around the circle of Willis. Intracranial aneurysms may be seen at the circle of Willis or in the peripheral vessels. Moyamoya disease is

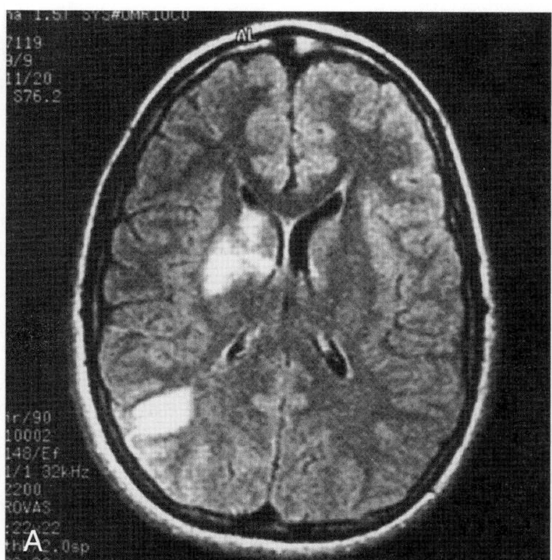


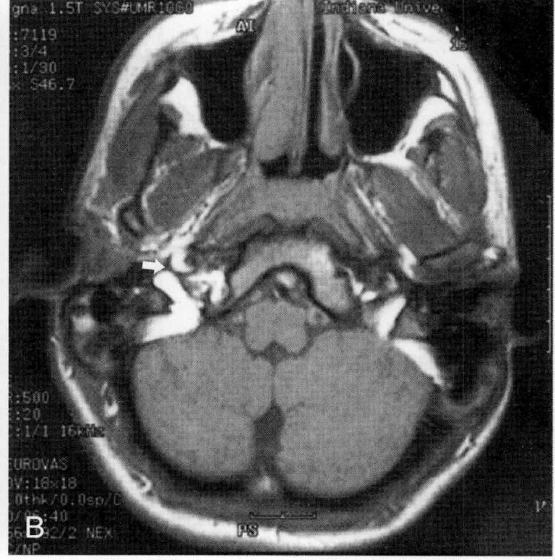


**Fig. 65.12** A 16-year-old boy collapsed to the ground after experiencing right eye pain and left-sided weakness. **A,** Axial T2-weighted magnetic resonance imaging of the brain shows ischemic areas in the right basal ganglia and right posterior parietal region, associated with a crescent sign *(arrow in B)* of high signal consistent with intraluminal blood products on the right internal carotid artery suggestive of a dissection.

sometimes distinguished from moyamoya syndrome associated with a number of different putative causes. Cases have been associated with neonatal anoxia, trauma, basilar meningitis, tuberculous meningitis, leptospirosis, cranial radiation therapy for optic pathway gliomas, neurofibromatosis type 1, tuberous sclerosis complex, encephalotrigeminal angiomatosis (Sturge-Weber syndrome), phakomatosis pigmentovascularis type IIIb, brain tumors, FMD, polyarteritis nodosa, Marfan syndrome, Turner syndrome, pseudoxanthoma elasticum, hypomelanosis of Ito, Williams syndrome, cerebral dissecting and saccular aneurysms, sickle cell disease, β-thalassemia, Fanconi anemia, hereditary spherocytosis, LA, Sneddon syndrome, homocystinuria, oral contraceptives, factor XII deficiency, type I glycogenosis, reduced form of nicotinamide adenine dinucleotide phosphate (NADP)—coenzyme Q reductase deficiency, renal artery stenosis, Down syndrome, Apert syndrome, Graves' disease, coarctation of the aorta, Alagille syndrome, hyperphosphatasia, Schimke immuno-osseous dysplasia, primary oxalosis, pulmonary sarcoidosis, and Hirschsprung disease.

Moyamoya disease may cause TIAs, including hemodynamic paraparetic TIAs secondary to watershed paracentral lobule ischemia, headaches, seizures, movement disorders (chorea, hemidystonia, hemichoreoathetosis), mental deterioration, cerebral infarction, or intracranial hemorrhage. TIAs are often precipitated by crying, blowing, or hyperventilation.

Moyamoya disease has a bimodal age distribution, with peaks in the first and fourth decades of life. Childhood moyamoya is characterized by ischemic manifestations, whereas adult moyamoya disease presents with hemorrhagic manifestations. Diagnosis is based on a distinct arteriographic appearance as described by Suzuki's 6 angiographic stages: (1) stenosis of the carotid fork, (2) appearance of moyamoya vessels at the base of the brain, (3) intensification of moyamoya vessels, (4) minimization of moyamoya vessels, (5) reduction of moyamoya vessels, and (6) disappearance of moyamoya vessels (collaterals only from external carotid arteries) (Fig. 65.13). Moyamoya is characterized by progressive bilateral stenosis of the distal internal carotid arteries, extending to the proximal ACA and MCA, with development of an extensive collateral (parenchymal, leptomeningeal, and transdural) network at the base of the brain like a cloud or puff of smoke (moyamoya). Intracranial aneurysms, particularly located in the posterior circulation, may be present.

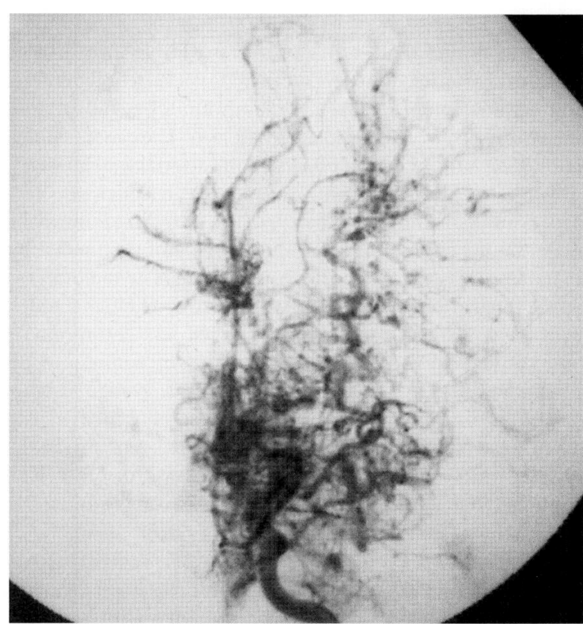

**Fig. 65.13** Left carotid angiogram (anteroposterior view) shows occlusion of the supraclinoid internal carotid artery and innumerable moyamoya vessels. *(Courtesy Vincent Mathews, MD.)*

The optimal treatment of ischemic moyamoya has not been determined. Platelet antiaggregants, vasodilators, calcium channel blockers, and corticosteroids have been used with variable results. Anticoagulants are not useful. Good results have been reported with superficial temporal artery to MCA anastomosis and other indirect or combined surgical revascularization procedures. No clear superior therapy to prevent rebleeding has been shown in the hemorrhagic type of moyamoya disease.

## Fibromuscular Dysplasia

FMD is a segmental, nonatheromatous, dysplastic, noninflammatory angiopathy affecting predominantly young and middle-aged women. Cervicocephalic FMD affects less than 1% of the population, occurs

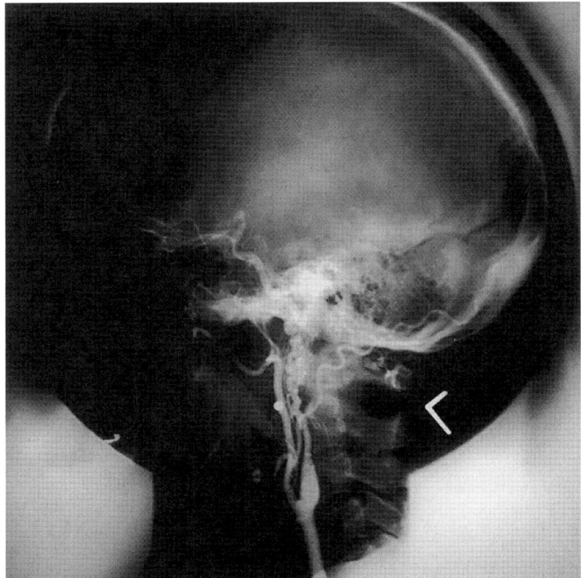

**Fig. 65.14** Lateral left carotid angiogram in a patient with fibromuscular dysplasia. Note "string of pearls" appearance at around the C2 level.

more often in Whites than in Blacks, and predominantly involves the cervical carotid arteries at the level of the C1–C2 vertebral bodies. FMD of the intracranial arteries is rare and mainly limited to the intrapetrosal internal carotid artery or carotid artery siphon. The cause is unknown. Immunological and estrogenic effects on the arterial wall may be causal mechanisms. An association with $\alpha_1$-antitrypsin deficiency has been reported. Four distinct histological types are recognized: intimal fibroplasia, medial hyperplasia, medial fibroplasia, and perimedial dysplasia. Medial fibroplasia is the most frequent form. The majority of cases involve the renal arteries, followed by the carotid and iliac arteries. The subclavian and vertebral arteries are affected less commonly. Some cases are familial. Most often, patients are asymptomatic or present with headaches, neck pain, carotidynia, tinnitus, vertigo, asymptomatic carotid bruits, transient retinal or cerebral ischemia, cerebral infarction, or subarachnoid hemorrhage. Cervicocephalic FMD may be associated with arterial dissection. Hypertensive patients may have concomitant renal FMD. Cerebral ischemia is usually related to the underlying arterial stenosis or arterial thromboembolism.

Cervicocephalic FMD may be diagnosed on the basis of MRA, CTA, or conventional catheter cerebral angiography. It is bilateral in approximately two-thirds of cases. The lesions of medial fibroplasia account for the characteristic "string of beads" angiographic appearance seen in approximately 90% of cases (Fig. 65.14).

The optimal treatment of symptomatic cervicocephalic FMD has not been determined. In view of the benign natural history of this condition, platelet antiaggregants are recommended. Surgical intervention with angioplasty and stenting, gradual arterial dilatation, resection and reconstruction, or interposition grafting is seldom warranted.

## Inflammatory Vasculopathies

Inflammatory vasculopathies can involve any size of vessel, including the precapillary arterioles and postcapillary venules. Many infectious and multisystem noninfectious inflammatory diseases cause cerebral vasculitis (see Box 65.4). Cerebral vasculitis is a consideration in young patients with ischemic or hemorrhagic stroke; patients with recurrent stroke; elderly patients with mental status or cognitive changes and leptomeningeal enhancement on imaging (Nouh et al. 2014); patients with stroke associated with encephalopathic features; and patients with stroke accompanied by fever, multifocal neurological events, mononeuritis multiplex, palpable purpura, or abnormal urinary sediment. Other manifestations of cerebral vasculitis include headaches, seizures, and cognitive deterioration. Laboratory studies typically show anemia of chronic disease, leukocytosis, and an elevated erythrocyte sedimentation rate. The diagnosis of vasculitis usually requires confirmation by arteriography or biopsy. Overall, these disorders have a poor prognosis, but corticosteroids and other immunosuppressive agents have improved survival (Biller and Grau, 2004).

## Infections and Stroke

Intracranial vasculitis and stroke can result from meningovascular syphilis; prodromal manifestations are common before stroke. The MCA territory is most commonly affected. Spinal cord infarction may result from meningomyelitis. Other neurological manifestations in patients with secondary syphilis include headaches, meningismus, mental status changes, and CN abnormalities. The cerebrospinal fluid (CSF) may show a modest lymphocytic pleocytosis, elevated protein content, and a positive Venereal Disease Research Laboratory (VDRL) test. Concurrent human immunodeficiency virus (HIV-1) infection can lead to rapid progression of early syphilis to neurosyphilis. Luetic aneurysms of the ascending aorta can extend to involve the great vessels. Treatment schedules for syphilis are listed in standard textbooks; patients with concurrent HIV-1 infection and meningovascular syphilis may require prolonged antibiotic treatment.

Worldwide, an estimated 1 billion people are infected with *Mycobacterium tuberculosis*. Neurotuberculosis affects predominantly the basilar meninges. Predisposing conditions include alcoholism, substance abuse, corticosteroid use, and HIV-1 infection. Strokes can result from tuberculous endarteritis. The exudative basilar inflammation entraps the CNs at the base of the brain, most frequently the third, fourth, and sixth CNs. The basilar arteriolitis most commonly involves penetrating branches of the ACA, MCA, and. There is usually a modest lymphocytic and mononuclear pleocytosis. The CSF protein is usually elevated, and the glucose level is depressed. In the early stages, a predominantly neutrophilic response may be noted. Smears of CSF demonstrate *M. tuberculosis* in 10%–20% of cases. Polymerase chain reaction testing of CSF for *M. tuberculosis* DNA may aid the diagnosis. Repeated CSF examinations increase the yield considerably.

Fungal arteritis may result in aneurysms, pseudoaneurysms, thrombus formation, and cerebral infarction. Complications of acute purulent meningitis include intracranial arteritis and thrombophlebitis of the major venous sinuses and cortical veins. Intracranial arterial stenoses have been associated with a complicated clinical course. Varicella zoster may cause a virus-induced necrotizing arteritis similar to granulomatous angiitis. Cerebral infarction is a complication of acquired immunodeficiency syndrome (AIDS) and may result from vasculitis, meningovascular syphilis, varicella-zoster virus vasculitis, opportunistic infections, infective endocarditis, aneurysmal dilation of major cerebral arteries, nonbacterial thrombotic endocarditis, aPL antibodies, or other hypercoagulable states, or from hyperlipidemia resulting from protease inhibitors and other factors such as HIV-1-related malignancy, cancer chemotherapy, and thrombotic thrombocytopenic purpura (TTP). Large-artery cerebrovascular occlusions have been found in association with meningoencephalitis caused by free-living amebae. Other infectious agents known to produce cerebral infarcts include *Mycoplasma pneumoniae, Aspergillus,* coxsackie 9 virus, California encephalitis virus, mumps paramyxovirus, hepatitis C virus, *Borrelia burgdorferi*, *Rickettsia typhi* group, cat-scratch disease, *Trichinella* infection, and the larval stage (cysticercus) of *Taenia solium*. Cerebrovascular involvement in neurocysticercosis is usually ischemic and is caused by chronic meningitis, arteritis, or endarteritis

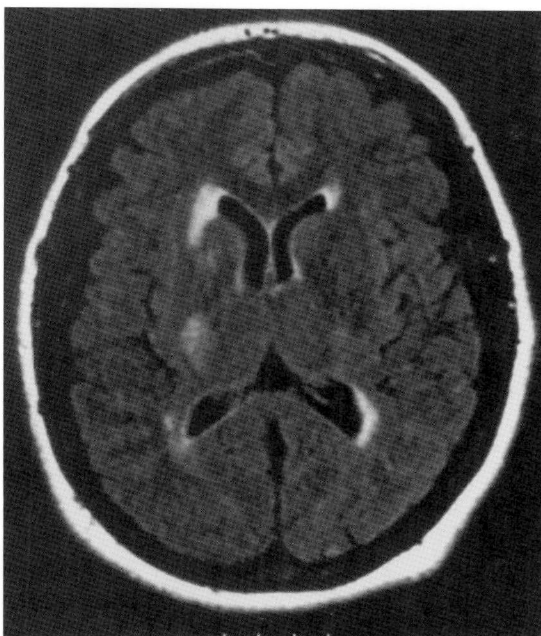

**Fig. 65.15** A 41-year-old woman with a history of cocaine abuse had acute onset of left-sided hemiplegia, left hemibody sensory deficit, and a left homonymous visual field deficit. Axial fluid-attenuated inversion recovery images of the brain demonstrate an area of infarction in the posterior limb of the right internal capsule in the distribution of the anterior choroidal artery territory. There is associated periventricular ischemia.

of small vessels. Unilateral or bilateral carotid artery occlusion can complicate necrotizing fasciitis of the parapharyngeal space. Infection with *C. pneumoniae* accelerates the process of atherosclerosis in animal studies; treatment with azithromycin has been shown to reduce the degree of atherosclerotic lesions in a rabbit model.

## Drug Abuse and Stroke

Ischemic stroke is a complication of illicit drug use and use of over-the-counter sympathomimetic drugs. Stroke mechanisms associated with the use of illicit drugs are multifactorial, including foreign-body embolization, vasculitis, vasospasm, acute onset of arterial hypertension or arterial hypotension, endothelial damage, accelerated atherosclerosis, hyper- or hypocoagulability, cardiac arrhythmias, embolism from an MI, or AIDS. The substances implicated most commonly are the amphetamines, cocaine, pentazocine (Talwin) in combination with Pyribenzamine ("Ts and blues"), phencyclidine, heroin, anabolic steroids, and glue sniffing. Ischemic or hemorrhagic strokes may follow within hours of cocaine use, whether the drug is smoked, snorted, or injected (Fig. 65.15) (see Chapter 87). The risk for intracerebral hemorrhage (ICH) led to removal from the American market of phenylpropanolamine. Ephedra, also called *ma-huang*, widely used in weight-loss products, has been associated with high blood pressure, heart attacks, and strokes. Stroke in young athletes may also be the result of anabolic-androgen steroid abuse and recombinant erythropoietin ("blood doping") administration.

## Stroke and Systemic Vasculitides

Ischemic stroke is also a complication of a variety of multisystem vasculitides. Stroke in patients with systemic lupus erythematosus (SLE) may be attributable to cardiogenic embolism (nonbacterial verrucous or Libman-Sacks endocarditis, which occurs in the ventricular surface of the mitral valve), aPL antibodies, underlying vasculopathy,

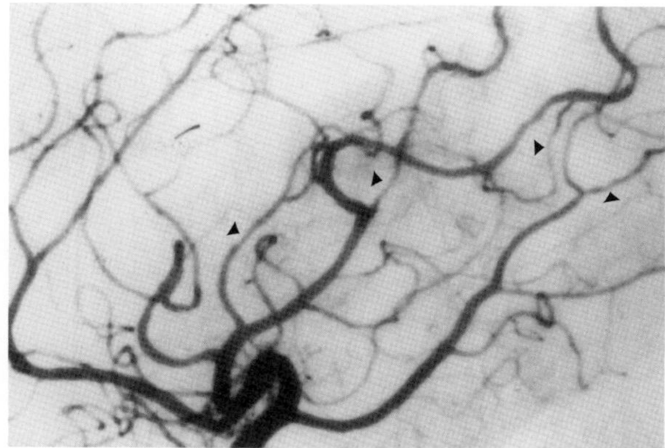

**Fig. 65.16** Lateral carotid angiogram demonstrates irregular beading appearance *(arrowheads)* of large and medium branches of the anterior, middle, and posterior cerebral arteries in a patient with systemic lupus erythematosus. *(Courtesy Vincent Mathews, MD.)*

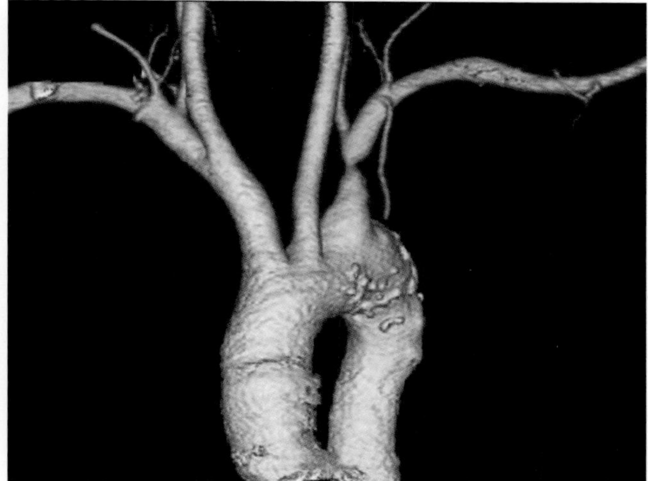

**Fig. 65.17** Computed tomographic angiogram demonstrating left subclavian stenosis in a 32-year-old woman with Takayasu arteritis.

nephrotic syndrome associated with lupus nephritis, or less often to an immune-mediated vasculitis (Fig. 65.16; see Chapter 58).

Behçet syndrome may involve vessels of any size. Venous thrombosis is more frequent than occlusive arterial compromise. Affected patients are mainly of Mediterranean or East Asian origin and may have a history of iritis, uveitis, and oral, genital, and mucocutaneous ulcerations. Cerebrovascular complications include strokes, carotid aneurysm formation, and cerebral venous thrombosis. Cogan syndrome is a rare condition characterized by nonsyphilitic interstitial keratitis, vestibular dysfunction, and deafness. Complications include aortic insufficiency and mesenteric ischemia. The angiitic form of sarcoidosis primarily affects the eyes, meninges, and cerebral arteries and veins. Kohlmeier-Degos disease, or malignant atrophic papulosis, is a multisystem occlusive vasculopathy characterized by cutaneous, gastrointestinal (GI), and neurological manifestations; it may be complicated by ischemic or hemorrhagic strokes. Cerebral vasculitis may also complicate the course of children with acute poststreptococcal glomerulonephritis. The multisystem vasculitides are described in more detail elsewhere in this book.

Takayasu arteritis is a chronic inflammatory arteriopathy of the aorta and its major branches, as well as the pulmonary artery (Fig. 65.17). The cause is unknown, but an immune mechanism is suspected. The disease,

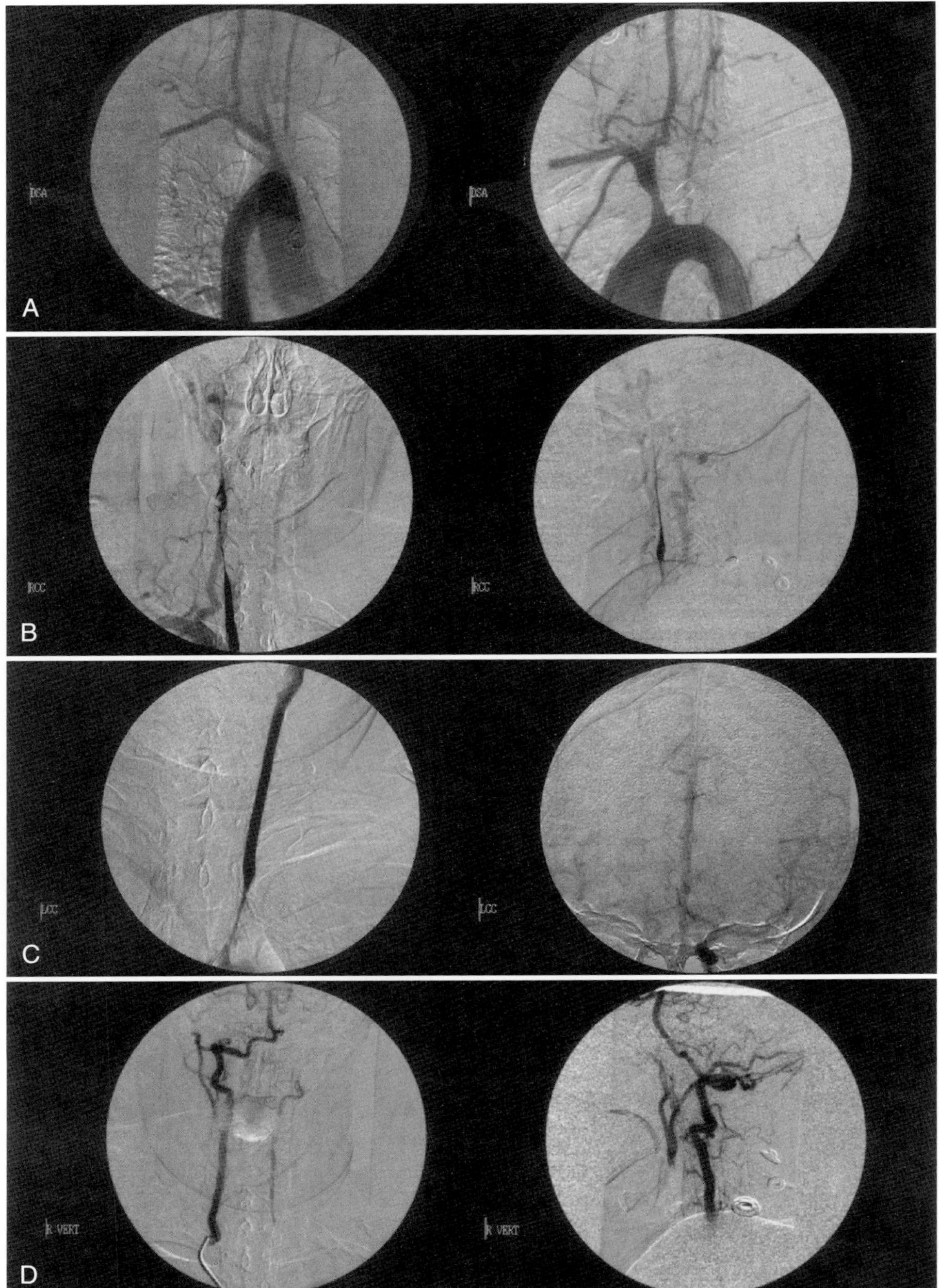


Fig. 65.18 A, Aortogram demonstrates a nonocclusive stenosis of the brachiocephalic artery. There is complete occlusion of the left subclavian artery. The left vertebra is absent or occluded. B, The right common carotid artery shows a long segment of critical stenosis extending from C3 to C5. C, There is also a very long stenosis of the left common carotid artery. D, A larger cervical right vertebral artery provides vigorous filling of the intracranial right internal carotid circulation.

prevalent in young women of Asian, Mexican, or Native American ancestry, develops insidiously, causing stenosis, occlusion, aneurysmal dilatation, or coarctation of the involved vessels. In the acute or "prepulseless" phase, nonspecific systemic manifestations are present. Patients have rashes, erythema nodosum, fever, myalgias, arthritis, pleuritis, carotidynia, and elevated erythrocyte sedimentation rate. Months or years later, the occlusive phase develops. Patients may have cervical bruits, absent carotid or radial pulses, asymmetrical blood pressure recordings, and arterial hypertension. Neurological symptoms result from CNS or retinal ischemia associated with stenosis or occlusion of the aortic arch and arch vessels, or arterial hypertension caused by aortic coarctation or renal artery stenosis. Visual disturbances are often bilateral. The diagnosis can be confirmed by MRA or CTA, but the most accurate assessment still requires aortography (Fig. 65.18).

Patients with active disease are treated with oral glucocorticoids; cyclophosphamide, azathioprine, or methotrexate may be needed in

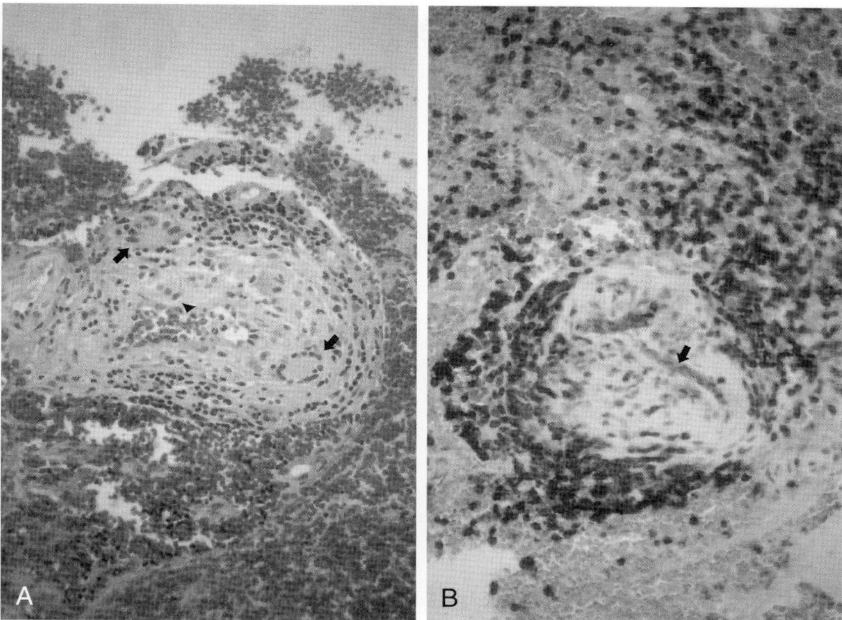


**Fig. 65.19** Cerebellum. **A,** Within an area of recent hemorrhage, there is a small blood vessel showing focal infiltration with lymphocytes and a couple of multinucleated giant cells *(arrows)*. Vessel lumen is marked with an *arrowhead* (hematoxylin and eosin, ×680). **B,** Same vessel as in **A**. Immunostain with CD3 demonstrates intense perivascular infiltration with T lymphocytes (×680).

special circumstances. Surgical treatment (angioplasty or bypass) of severely stenotic vessels may be required.

Cranial (giant cell or temporal) arteritis is a polysymptomatic systemic large-vessel arteritis with a predilection to involve carotid artery branches (see Chapter 102). Thromboangiitis obliterans, also known as *Buerger disease*, is a rare segmental, inflammatory, obliterative angiopathy of unknown cause. The condition involves small and medium arteries and veins. It is suspected in young men who smoke and have a history of superficial migratory thrombophlebitis presenting with distal limb ischemia accompanied by digital gangrene. The disorder is characterized by remissions and exacerbations. Cerebral involvement is uncommon. Strokes can result from isolated angiitis of the CNS, including amyloid-beta–related CNS angiits. Symptoms of large-vessel involvement include stroke-like presentations. Small-vessel involvement may be manifested as a mass lesion in the brain or multifocal encephalopathy (Fig. 65.19). The erythrocyte sedimentation rate is usually normal or minimally elevated.

## Migraine and Stroke

Migraine (see Chapters 20 and 102) affects women more often than men and may start during childhood or adolescence. Epidemiological studies suggest a nonrandom association of both headache and migraine with stroke, particularly among young women. The possible association between migraine headache and stroke was also evaluated by the Physician's Health Study; physicians reporting migraine had increased risks of subsequent total and ischemic stroke compared with those not reporting migraines (Buring et al., 1995). In the Women's Health Study, migraine with aura raised the stroke risk by 108% (95% CI, 30%–231%). Migraine without aura raised the stroke risk by approximately 25% (Kurth et al., 2005; Woodward, 2009). The risk of white-matter abnormalities on MRI is also increased, particularly among subjects with migraine with aura (Kruit et al., 2004). The risk of ICH is not increased.

The International Headache Society Classification and Diagnostic Criteria require that to establish a diagnosis of migrainous infarction, one or more migrainous aura symptoms must be present and not fully reversed within 7 days from onset, and must be associated with neuroimaging confirmation of ischemic infarction. This definition implies that a firm diagnosis of migraine with aura has been made in the past. Also, the clinical manifestations judged to be the result of a migrainous infarction must be those typical of previous attacks for that individual, and finally, other causes of infarction, including those related to migraine therapy, need to be excluded.

Headache accompanies a number of embolic or thrombotic causes of stroke, including cervicocephalic arterial dissections. Migraines also can be a prominent symptom in the aPL antibody syndrome (APAS). Symptomatic migraine attacks are more frequent than migraine-induced ischemic insults. The presence of headache with a stroke is therefore not sufficient to make the diagnosis of migraine as the cause of the patient's symptoms. Furthermore, patchy subcortical abnormalities on MRI in patients with migraine with aura should be interpreted with caution. Migrainous infarction remains a diagnosis of exclusion.

The pathogenesis of migrainous infarction is controversial. Cerebral infarctions complicating migraine are mostly cortical and involve the PCA distribution. The usual scenario is one of recurrent episodes of gradual buildup of unilateral throbbing headaches, associated with stereotyped visual phenomena occurring in both visual fields simultaneously, in one of which the vision loss becomes permanent. Migrainous infarctions have been subdivided as definite when all the International Headache Society criteria are fulfilled and possible when some but not all criteria are fulfilled. Patients with migrainous infarction are at increased risk for recurrent stroke.

*Cerebral autosomal dominant arteriopathy with subcortical infarcts and leukoencephalopathy* (CADASIL) is a familial microangiopathy characterized by migraine with aura, recurrent subcortical ischemic strokes starting in mid-adulthood, leading to pseudobulbar palsy, cognitive decline, subcortical dementia, and early white-matter hyperintensities on MRI (Fig 65.20). CADASIL is caused by simple missense mutations or small deletions in the *Notch 3* gene on chromosome 19q12 encoding a transmembrane receptor *Notch 3*. The *Notch 3* mutation

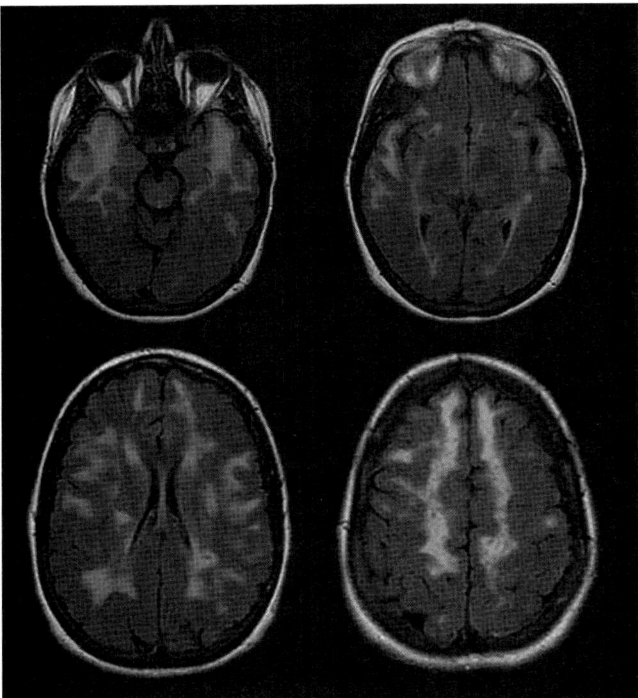

**Fig. 65.20** Fluid-attenuated inversion recovery magnetic resonance imaging sequences of a patient with cerebral autosomal dominant arteriopathy with subcortical infarcts and leukoencephalopathy.

has been thought to be one of the most common human mutations. Pathologically, there is a characteristic granular osmophilic material in arterial walls, including dermal arteries. A subtype of migraine known as *familial hemiplegic migraine* and characterized by transient weakness or frank paralysis during the aura has also been mapped close to the CADASIL locus. The acronym *CADASILM* (*c*erebral *a*utosomal *d*ominant *a*rteriopathy with *s*ubcortical *i*nfarcts, *l*eukoencephalopathy, and *m*igraine), refers to a subvariety of CADASIL characterized by the high frequency of migraine. A clinical trial of donepezil in CADASIL patients with subcortical vascular cognitive impairment showed no improvement in general cognition, but improvement in some executive functions such as processing speed and attention (Schneider, 2008).

## INHERITED AND MISCELLANEOUS DISORDERS

Homocystinuria, an inborn error of amino acid metabolism, is an unusual cause of stroke (Box 65.5). Three specific enzyme deficiencies responsible for homocystinuria have been identified: cystathionine-β-synthetase, homocysteine methyltransferase, and methylene tetrahydrofolate reductase. The accumulation of plasma homocysteine leads to endothelial injury and premature atherosclerosis. Patients may display a marfanoid habitus, malar flush, livedo reticularis, ectopia lentis, myopia, glaucoma, optic atrophy, psychiatric abnormalities, mental retardation, spasticity, seizures, osteoporosis, and a propensity for intracranial arterial or venous thrombosis. Death may result from pulmonary embolism, MI, or stroke. Hyperhomocysteinemia may be an independent risk factor for cerebrovascular disease, coronary artery disease, and peripheral arterial occlusive disease. Homocysteine levels can be reduced with folic acid, occasionally requiring the addition of vitamin $B_6$ and vitamin $B_{12}$, choline, betaine, estrogen, and acetylcysteine. However, reducing homocysteine levels with folic acid and B-complex vitamins has not been associated with decreased risk (Lonn et al., 2006; Toole et al., 2004).

### BOX 65.5 Inherited and Miscellaneous Disorders Causing Cerebral Infarction

Homocystinuria
Fabry disease
Marfan syndrome
Ehlers-Danlos syndrome
Pseudoxanthoma elasticum
Sneddon syndrome
Hereditary hemorrhagic telangiectasia
Neoplastic angioendotheliomatosis
Susac syndrome
Eales disease
Reversible cerebral segmental vasoconstriction syndrome
Hypereosinophilic syndrome
Cerebral amyloid angiopathy
Coils and kinks
Arterial dolichoectasia
Complications of coarctation of the aorta
Air, fat, amniotic fluid, bone marrow, and foreign particle embolism

Fabry disease is an X-linked disorder of glycosphingolipid metabolism characterized by deficient lysosomal α-galactosidase activity. Ceramide trihexosidase deposits in endothelial and smooth muscle cells. Patients have a painful peripheral neuropathy, renal disease, hypertension, cardiomegaly, autonomic dysfunction, and corneal opacifications. Characteristic dark red or blue lesions that do not blanch on pressure, called *angiokeratoma corporis diffusum*, are found between the umbilicus and knees. Stroke and MI are common. Female carriers may have mild disease or are asymptomatic.

Marfan syndrome is an autosomal dominant connective tissue disease associated with qualitative and quantitative defects of fibrillin. Histopathological studies of aortic segments show cystic medial necrosis. Patients may display arachnodactyly, extreme limb length, joint laxity, pectus excavatum or carinatum, subluxation of the lens, and aortic valvular insufficiency. Marfan syndrome is commonly associated with dilatation of the aortic root. Other cardiovascular abnormalities include aortic coarctation, mitral valve prolapse, and mitral annulus calcification with regurgitation. Progressive aortic root dilatation may lead to ascending aortic dissection, resulting in ischemia to the brain, spinal cord, or peripheral nerves. Saccular intracranial aneurysms or dissection of the carotid artery can occur. Annual echocardiographic studies are recommended. Patients should avoid contact sports.

Patients with Ehlers-Danlos syndrome (see Chapter 104), a common heritable connective tissue disorder, display hyperextensibility of the skin, hypermobile joints, and vascular fragility leading to a bleeding diathesis. Arterial complications such as dissections, arteriovenous fistulae, and aneurysms have been reported in association with Ehlers-Danlos syndrome types I, III, and IV, especially type IV. Other cardiovascular abnormalities in patients with type IV Ehlers-Danlos syndrome include ventricular and atrial septal defects, aortic insufficiency, bicuspid aortic valve, mitral valve prolapse, and papillary muscle dysfunction. Arteriography carries special risks and should be avoided if possible.

Patients with pseudoxanthoma elasticum, an inherited group of disorders of elastic tissue, often display loose skin and small, raised, orange-yellowish papules resembling "plucked chicken skin" in intertriginous areas. Patients with pseudoxanthoma elasticum have a higher risk for coronary artery disease and MI. These patients may also have arterial hypertension, angioid streaks of the retina, retinal hemorrhages, arterial occlusive disease, and arterial dissections. Women with pseudoxanthoma elasticum should avoid estrogens.

Sneddon syndrome consists of widespread livedo reticularis and ischemic cerebrovascular manifestations. A number of reports have documented a hereditary transmission and a link between Sneddon syndrome and aPL antibodies. An association with SLE is also described. However, the etiopathogenesis remains unknown, although an immune mechanism is suspected. Endothelial cells could be the primary target tissue. Antiendothelial cell antibodies may be present.

HHT is an autosomal dominant disorder. Ischemic stroke as a presenting manifestation of HHT disease has been reported infrequently. Paradoxical venous emboli passing through a pulmonary arteriovenous malformation can be the source of cerebral ischemia or abscess. Other potential causes leading to cerebral ischemia include air embolism and hyperviscosity secondary to polycythemia.

Neoplastic angioendotheliomatosis, also called *intravascular malignant lymphomatosis* or *angiotropic lymphoma*, is a rare disease characterized by multiple small- and large-vessel occlusions by neoplastic cell of lymphoid origin without an obvious primary tumor. Intravascular lymphomatosis has been reported to involve the skin, lungs, kidneys, adrenal glands, liver, pancreas, GI tract, ovary, prostate, testicles, heart, thyroid, and parathyroid glands. Bone marrow, spleen, and lymph nodes are usually spared. Simultaneous involvement of blood vessels throughout the body and compromise of different cerebral arterial territories is common. Patients may present with recurrent multifocal cerebral infarctions, dementia, or myelopathy. Diagnosis requires skin, liver, renal, or brain-leptomeningeal biopsy. Combination chemotherapy has been recommended. Autologous peripheral blood stem cell transplantation after chemotherapy may be useful.

Microangiopathy of the brain, retina, and inner ear (Susac syndrome), also known as *retinocochleocerebral vasculopathy*, is a very rare microcirculatory syndrome that affects mainly adult women (Susac, 2004). The syndrome is unrelated to arterial hypertension or diabetes and is characterized by arteriolar branch occlusions of the brain, retina, and inner ear, with resultant encephalopathy, vision loss, vestibular dysfunction, tinnitus, vertigo, and asymmetrical sensorineural hearing loss. CSF examination may be normal or show mild inflammatory response. MRI findings include multifocal white-matter hyperintensities with preferential involvement for the central fibers of the corpus callosum. Branch retinal artery occlusions may be seen on fluorescein angiography. Brain biopsy may show multifocal brain microinfarcts in both gray and white matter. Susac syndrome is due to an autoimmune endotheliopathy. Early treatment with intravenous (IV) immune globulin, plasmapheresis, and immunosuppression may be effective, but branch retinal artery occlusions and CNS infarctions may recur despite the treatment.

Eales disease, commonly reported in India and the Middle East, is a rare noninflammatory occlusive disease of the retinal vasculature characterized by repeated retinal and vitreous hemorrhages. The disorder affects mainly young men. Brain infarctions are rare.

Idiopathic reversible cerebral segmental vasoconstriction (RCVS) is a clinical angiographic syndrome characterized by recurrent sudden high-intensity headaches (Call-Fleming syndrome) and motor and sensory findings associated with reversible segmental arterial narrowing and dilatation. It has been associated with an expanding list of conditions including vasoconstrictive medication, sympathomimetic drug use, serotonergic medication, cannabis, pregnancy and the postpartum state, head trauma, and extreme hypertension among others. RCVS can be difficult to distinguish clinically and radiographically other arteriopathies. A proposed algorithm may help delineate those patients with RCVS (Rocha et al., 2019) with scores greater than 4 having a 99% specificity and 90% sensitivity for diagnosing RCVS and less than 3 with 100% specificity and 85% sensitivity for excluding RCVS.

The hypereosinophilic syndrome is a rare disorder caused by bone marrow overproduction of eosinophils that lodge in endothelial cells in the microcirculation primarily of heart, brain, kidney, lungs, GI tract, and skin. Neurological complications include emboli from involved endocardium and heart valves, and may also result from a hypercoagulable state with cerebral thromboses, and microcirculatory inflammation and occlusion by eosinophils. Cerebral infarction is a rare complication.

Cerebral amyloid angiopathy (CAA) occurs both sporadically or in rare instances as a hereditary disorder. It is characterized by the localized deposition of amyloid in the media and adventitia of small arteries and arterioles of the cerebral cortex and meninges in the elderly. CAA is more commonly associated with lobar hemorrhage than with ischemic stroke, but it has been associated with an increased frequency of cerebral infarction in patients with Alzheimer disease. Biopsy of the involved cortex and leptomeninges is the only definitive way to diagnose CAA. However, MRI evidence of superficial microbleeds or cortical siderosis can be supportive.

Redundant length of the cervical carotid artery causes coils and kinks and other forms of tortuosity. Occasionally associated with FMD, kinks and coils of the carotid artery are otherwise an infrequent cause of cerebral ischemia. Cerebral ischemia associated with kinking is due to a combination of flow reduction caused by obstruction, neck rotation, and distal embolization. Arterial kinking seldom affects the vertebrobasilar circulation, although there may be significant tortuosity of the vertebral or basilar arteries. Dolichoectasia, however, is an unusual vascular disease that causes enlargement and elongation of arteries, particularly the basilar artery. This arteriopathy causes a false aneurysm that leads to ischemic stroke, brainstem compression, cervicomedullary compression, CN palsies, cerebellar dysfunction, central sleep apnea, and hydrocephalus. The mechanisms of stroke are penetrating artery occlusion, basilar artery thrombosis, or embolism from the dolichoectatic artery.

Ischemic stroke and intracranial hemorrhage, the latter caused by arterial hypertension or ruptured intracranial aneurysm, are important complications of coarctation of the aorta. Spinal cord ischemia may also complicate surgery for aortic coarctation. Neurological complications also can result from aortic rupture, infective aortitis or endarteritis, associated aortic bicuspid valve, and dissection of the aorta proximal to the coarctation.

Atheromatous embolization (cholesterol emboli syndrome, blue toe syndrome, purple toe syndrome) may follow manipulation of an atherosclerotic aorta during catheterization or surgery. Clinical presentation may include TIAs, stroke, retinal embolism pancreatitis, renal failure, and livedo reticularis. Purple toes also may occur as a result of small cholesterol emboli lodging in the digital arteries. Pedal pulses are normal. Patients may have a low-grade fever, eosinophilia, anemia, elevated erythrocyte sedimentation rate, and elevated serum amylase. Anticoagulation may exacerbate further embolization, and its use should be discouraged.

Air embolism can be a cause of cerebral or retinal ischemia. It is a dreaded complication of surgical procedures, including intracranial operations in the sitting position; open heart surgery; surgery of the lungs, pleura, sinuses, neck, and axilla; hemodialysis; thoracocentesis; arteriography; central venous catheters; and scuba diving. Symptoms include seizures and multifocal neurological findings, such as cerebral edema, confusion, memory loss, and coma. CT scan may visualize the gaseous bubbles. Treatment includes prompt resuscitative measures, placement of the patient in the left lateral position with head down, and hyperbaric oxygen. Inotropic agents, pressors, anticonvulsants, and anti-edema agents may be indicated. Caisson disease can occur in persons who are scuba diving. Neurological features are due to multiple small nitrogen emboli that lead to ischemia of the brain and spinal cord; signs of spinal cord dysfunction are prominent. Hyperbaric oxygen therapy is the usual treatment.

Fat embolism to the brain complicates long-bone fractures, sickle cell disease, cardiopulmonary bypass, soft-tissue injuries, and blood transfusions (Morales-Vidal, 2019). This syndrome occurs suddenly, within hours to 3 or 4 days after injury, and is characterized by dyspnea, fever, tachycardia, tachypnea, cyanosis, cutaneous petechiae, and coagulopathy. Neurological manifestations are confusion, disorientation, delirium, hemiparesis, aphasia, and coma. Petechial hemorrhages may be apparent on funduscopy, conjunctivae, base of the neck, and axillary region. Vigorous respiratory supportive therapy is essential.

Amniotic fluid embolism is a rare catastrophic obstetrical complication caused by the entry of amniotic fluid into the maternal bloodstream during parturition. Vigorous supportive therapy with IV fluids and blood replacement to treat shock, respiratory distress syndrome, disseminated intravascular coagulation (DIC), and underlying fibrinolytic state are essential. Among other causes of emboli are large intracranial saccular aneurysms or extracranial false aneurysms of the internal carotid artery. Tumor emboli to the brain have been reported with osteosarcoma, atrial myxoma, and carcinoma of the lung, breast, pharynx, or esophagus. Talc, cornstarch, and other foreign particles injected as adulterants in illicit drugs can embolize to the brain or retina. Paradoxical embolism during bone marrow infusion is an infrequent complication.

## HYPERCOAGULABLE DISORDERS

Alterations in hemostasis are associated with an increased risk for cerebrovascular events, and may account for a considerable number of cryptogenic strokes (Box 65.6). These disorders account for 1% of all strokes and 2%–7% of ischemic strokes in young patients.

### BOX 65.6 Hypercoagulable States

**Primary Hypercoagulable States**

Antithrombin deficiency
Protein C deficiency
Protein S deficiency
Activated protein C resistance with or without factor V Leiden mutation
Prothrombin G20210 mutation
Dysfibrinogenemia
Hypoplasminogenemia
Abnormal plasminogen
Plasminogen activators deficiency
Antiphospholipid antibody syndrome (APAS)*

**Secondary Hypercoagulable States**

Malignancy
Pregnancy/puerperium
Oral contraceptive use
Ovarian hyperstimulation syndrome
Other hormonal treatments
Nephrotic syndrome
Polycythemia vera
Essential thrombocythemia
Paroxysmal nocturnal hemoglobinuria
Diabetes mellitus
Heparin-induced thrombocytopenia
Homocystinuria
Sickle cell disease (sickle cell anemia, sickle cell hemoglobin C)
Thrombotic thrombocytopenic purpura
Chemotherapeutic agents

* APAS may be primary or secondary.

### Primary Hypercoagulable States

Inherited thrombophilias especially affect the venous circulation. These disorders include AT deficiency, protein C and protein S deficiencies, APC resistance, fibrinogen abnormalities (dysfibrinogenemia), and abnormalities of fibrinolysis. Inherited thrombophilia should be suspected in patients with recurrent episodes of DVT, recurrent pulmonary emboli, family history of thrombotic events, unusual sites of venous (mesenteric, portal, or cerebral) or arterial thromboses, or in patients with thrombotic events occurring during childhood, adolescence, or early adulthood (deVeber et al., 2008). Approximately half of all thrombotic episodes occur spontaneously, although these patients are at greatest risk when exposed to additional risk factors such as pregnancy, surgery, trauma, or oral contraceptive therapy.

AT deficiency is inherited in an autosomal dominant fashion. There are three categories of inherited AT deficiency: classic or type I, characterized by decreased immunological and biological activity of AT; type II, characterized by low biological activity of AT but essentially normal immunological activity; and type III, characterized by normal AT activity in the absence of heparin but reduced activity in heparin-dependent assays. Acquired AT deficiency may follow acute thrombosis and DIC. It also has been associated with nephrotic syndrome, liver cirrhosis, eclampsia, various malignancies, estrogen or oral contraceptive use, L-asparaginase, tamoxifen, and heparin therapy. A normal AT activity level at the time of an acute thrombotic event is sufficient to exclude a primary deficiency. However, a low level of AT activity must be confirmed by repeat testing after resolution of the thrombotic episode and discontinuation of anticoagulant therapy. Confirmation of a low plasma level of AT activity on repeat testing is compatible with a primary deficiency and is an indication to investigate other family members. Thrombotic episodes associated with AT deficiency are treated acutely with heparin, with or without adjunctive AT concentrate. Prophylactic therapy in patients with recurrent thrombosis consists of long-term warfarin administration, keeping the therapeutic international normalized ratio [INR] range between 2.0 and 3.0.

Protein C deficiency is inherited in an autosomal dominant fashion. Homozygous protein C deficiency presents in infancy as purpura fulminans neonatalis. Heterozygotes are predisposed to recurrent thrombosis. Thrombotic manifestations are predominantly venous. Acquired protein C deficiency has been associated with the administration of L-asparaginase, warfarin therapy, liver disease, DIC, postoperative state, bone marrow transplantation, and the acute respiratory distress syndrome. Testing for immunological and functional assays of protein C should be performed after oral anticoagulation has been discontinued for at least a week. Heparin does not modify the levels of protein C. Warfarin-induced skin necrosis is a serious potential complication of protein C–deficient patients at the initiation of warfarin therapy; this syndrome typically occurs in association with large loading doses of warfarin. However, this deficiency is rare, and routine heparin administration prior to warfarin initiation is not mandatory unless there is clinical suspicion of protein C deficiency. In that case, the acute management of thrombosis associated with protein C deficiency consists of heparin. Long-term management requires warfarin.

Protein S deficiency also has an autosomal dominant mode of inheritance. Protein S exists in two plasma forms: approximately 40%

of the total protein S is functionally active or free, and the remaining is complexed to a binding protein. Homozygous protein S deficiency presents with venous thromboembolic disease. Heterozygotes are prone to recurrent thrombosis, including cerebral venous thrombosis. Acquired protein S deficiency occurs during pregnancy, in association with acute thromboembolic episodes, DIC, nephrotic syndrome, SLE, and with the administration of oral contraceptives, warfarin, and L-asparaginase. Immunological assays of total and free protein S and functional assay of protein S should be confirmed after resolution of the thrombotic episode and discontinuation of warfarin. Heparin therapy is effective in managing acute thrombotic events associated with protein S deficiency, whereas warfarin is advocated for patients with recurrent thromboembolism.

APC resistance and the prothrombin *PTG20210A* gene mutation are autosomal dominant and among the most common identifiable risk factors for venous thromboembolic disease, including cerebral venous thrombosis. However, their contribution to arterial ischemic stroke is less clear. APC resistance is 5–10 times more common than deficiencies of AT, protein C, or protein S. APC resistance is associated in most patients with a single point mutation in the factor V gene (factor V Leiden) that involves replacement of arginine 506 with glutamine 506 (Arg 506 Gln). Testing for APC resistance must be done after discontinuation of anticoagulants.

Fibrinogen abnormalities account for approximately 1% of all inherited thrombotic disorders. Fibrinogen cross-links platelets during thrombosis and is an important component of atherosclerotic plaques. High fibrinogen concentrations increase the risk for stroke and MI. Dysfibrinogenemia reflects a qualitative disorder in the fibrinogen molecule and may be associated with hemorrhagic or thrombotic episodes. Hereditary dysfibrinogenemia is inherited in an autosomal-dominant fashion. Decreased fibrinogen concentrations are associated with DIC, liver failure, snakebite, treatment with L-asparaginase, ancrod, fibrinolytic drugs, and valproate. Treatment consists of infusions of cryoprecipitate.

Hypoplasminogenemia, dysplasminogenemias, and defective release of plasminogen activators occur in families with recurrent thrombotic events. Cerebral venous thrombosis may occur. Prophylactic therapy in patients with recurrent thrombosis is lifelong anticoagulants.

LA, aCL antibodies, or anti-$\beta_2$-glycoprotein 1 antibodies, known collectively as *antiphospholipid antibodies*, have a pathogenetic role in arterial and venous thrombosis. Ischemic stroke is the most common arterial thrombotic event in patients with APAS. APAS associates the presence of aPL antibodies in high titers with recurrent arterial or venous thromboses, fetal loss, and livedo reticularis (Brey et al., 2001). Antiphospholipid antibodies are present in patients with SLE and related autoimmune disorders, Sneddon syndrome, acute and chronic infections (including HIV-1), neoplasias, inflammatory bowel disease, administration of certain drugs, early-onset severe preeclampsia, liver transplantation, and sporadically. A distinct group of patients has a primary APAS; its association with ischemic cerebrovascular disease is rare.

Antiphospholipid antibodies are associated with recurrent fetal loss, a prolongation of the activated partial thromboplastin time (aPTT) that does not correct on one-to-one mixing with normal plasma, thrombocytopenia, a false-positive VDRL test result, and livedo reticularis. They may also be associated with cerebral and ocular ischemia, cerebral venous thrombosis, migraine, vascular dementia, chorea, transverse myelopathy, MI, peripheral arterial thromboembolism, venous thrombosis, pulmonary embolism, and Degos disease. Multiple cerebral infarctions are common in patients with aPL antibodies; a subset of patients may present with vascular dementia (eFig. 65.21). Still another group may have an acute or progressive thrombotic ischemic encephalopathy. Pathological studies of cerebral arteries involved in association with aPL antibodies demonstrate the presence of a chronic thrombotic microangiopathy but no evidence of vasculitis. Patients with aPL antibodies have an increased frequency of mitral and aortic vegetations. There are findings resembling verrucous endocarditis (Libman-Sacks endocarditis). Left ventricular thrombus formation is a rare occurrence.

The diagnosis of APAS or Hughes syndrome requires high plasma LA titers (in the absence of other coagulopathies), moderately high aCL immunoglobulin G (IgG) (>40 IgG plasma level), or anti-$\beta_2$-glycoprotein 1 IgG antibodies in serum or plasma on at least two occasions at least 12 weeks apart, measured by a standardized enzyme-linked immunosorbent assay (ELISA). Patients with isolated immunoglobulin M (IgM) APS represent 14.3% of the APS population with an older age at diagnosis and strong association with stroke (Urbanski et al., 2018). Treatment for arterial thrombosis associated with aPL antibodies is not well established. In a prospective cohort study of a subgroup of patients with ischemic stroke in the Warfarin-Aspirin Recurrent Stroke Study trial, aspirin (325 mg) and warfarin (target INR 1.4–2.8) were equivalent for preventing recurrent strokes and venous thromboembolism (VTE) over a 2-year follow-up (Levine et al., 2004). To date, there is insufficient evidence to support the use of high-intensity warfarin (target INR >3.0) over moderate-intensity warfarin in patients who have recurrent VTE. Data are limited but also suggest that there is an increased frequency of recurrent thrombotic events in APL patients on DOACs as compared with warfarin (Martinelli et al., 2018). Because of its teratogenicity, warfarin should be avoided in the first trimester, and replaced in patients with APAS during pregnancy with low-molecular-weight heparin (LMWH) or unfractionated heparin (UFH). Pregnant patients without a history of stroke are often treated with prednisone, low-dose aspirin, or both.

## Secondary Hypercoagulable States

Strokes may complicate the clinical course of malignancies. In rare instances, stroke may be the initial manifestation of cancer. Cerebral infarction mostly complicates lymphomas, carcinomas, and solid tumors. Cerebral hemorrhages are more common with certain types of leukemia. Hypercoagulability is a common finding in patients with malignancy, especially myeloproliferative disorders, acute promyelocytic leukemia, brain tumors, and mucin-producing carcinomas of the pancreas, GI tract, and lung. Mucinous adenocarcinomas of the GI tract, lung, and ovary may produce infarcts from widespread cerebral arterial occlusions by mucin. The cause of the hypercoagulable state is often multifactorial. The pathophysiology may be due to a state of low-grade DIC and secondary fibrinolysis, but with the balance shifted toward clotting. Atherosclerosis is still the leading cause of infarction in patients with malignancy. Cerebral infarction in patients with malignancy also may be due to tumor emboli, bone marrow embolization, emboli originating from mural thrombi, or emboli arising from marantic vegetations associated with nonbacterial thrombotic endocarditis. Many patients with nonbacterial thrombotic endocarditis have associated DIC, which may cause capillary occlusion of multiple organs, especially the lungs, kidneys, GI tract, heart, and brain. Neurological manifestations produce a diffuse encephalopathy secondary to disseminated microinfarcts. Other patients with malignancy and cerebral infarction may have cerebral venous occlusive disease caused by thrombi, tumor invasion, or stroke associated with chemotherapy. In addition, cancer-enhanced atherothrombosis, neoplastic angioendotheliomatosis, arterial compression by tumor, occlusive vascular disease secondary to irradiation, and intercurrent angiitis may be responsible for cerebral infarction in some patients. Treatment consists of management of the underlying malignancy. Anticoagulants and platelet antiaggregants are used with variable success.

The postpartum period is a hypercoagulable state. Arterial thrombosis is more common during pregnancy, whereas venous thrombosis is more common during the puerperium (see Chapter 112).

Oral contraceptives may cause vascular intimal hyperplasia. They also may increase blood viscosity. There are decreased levels of protein S, AT activity, and plasminogen activator content in women taking oral contraceptives. There also may be an increase in the levels of fibrinogen, factor VII, and factor X. Oral contraceptive therapy may enhance arterial hypertension. Women taking oral contraceptives have an estimated ninefold increased risk for thrombotic stroke. This risk is increased by prolonged use, high estrogen dosage, cigarette smoking, concomitant diabetes, arterial hypertension, hyperlipidemia, and age older than 35 years. Current oral contraceptive users are at increased stroke risk; one study showed that oral contraceptives containing 30 μg of estrogen are associated with a one-third reduced risk compared with preparations containing 50 μg. The occurrence of intracranial venous thrombosis as a complication of oral contraceptives is well recognized. A patient on oral contraceptives occasionally presents with stroke secondary to paradoxical embolism associated with DVT.

Oral contraceptives probably should be avoided in women with arterial hypertension and in the first 2 weeks after delivery. Women older than 35 years who smoke cigarettes should consider a different contraceptive method. Women who smoke should not use oral contraceptives.

The ovarian hyperstimulation syndrome occurs in women after induction of ovulation with clomiphene, human menopausal gonadotropin, human follicle-stimulating hormone extracted from human pituitary, and human chorionic gonadotropin. Evidence of body-fluid shifts and hypercoagulability exist with this syndrome, contributing to thromboembolic events. Stroke is a rare consequence of severe ovarian hyperstimulation syndrome.

Thromboembolic events including cerebral infarction have occurred as a side effect of exogenous estrogen in male-to-female transgender persons. Likewise, TIAs and cerebral infarction may follow the administration of anabolic steroids for the treatment of hypogonadism and hypoplastic anemias and performance-enhancing use in athletes. Cerebral ischemia also has occurred following the use of human recombinant erythropoietin in the treatment of anemia for patients on hemodialysis.

The nephrotic syndrome may be accompanied by venous and arterial thromboses, including cerebral arterial and venous occlusive disease. The mechanism by which nephrotic syndrome causes hypercoagulability is multifactorial and includes elevated levels of fibrinogen; raised levels of factors V, VII, VIII, and X; thrombocytosis; enhanced platelet aggregation; and reduced levels of AT and protein S. A urinalysis is the initial clue to the diagnosis. The presence of severe proteinuria and a low serum albumin should prompt consideration of a hypercoagulable state. Treatment of thromboembolism associated with nephrotic syndrome consists of anticoagulants until remission of the renal condition.

Polycythemia vera and primary or essential thrombocythemia are typically disorders of middle-aged or elderly patients. Polycythemia vera is characterized by increased red blood cell mass and normal arterial oxygen saturation. Genomic studies have identified a mutation in the genetic sequence of a specific tyrosine kinase known as *Janus kinase* (JAK2). Patients have ruddy cyanosis, painful pruritus, hypertension, splenomegaly, elevated hemoglobin, high hematocrit value, thrombocytosis, leukocytosis, and elevated serum vitamin $B_{12}$ levels. Typically, the bone marrow is hypercellular. Secondary polycythemia may occur in association with cerebellar hemangioblastoma, hepatoma, hypernephroma, uterine fibroids, benign renal cysts, carbon monoxide exposure, and administration of androgens. CBF is reduced and cerebral hemorrhage and arterial or venous thrombosis can complicate the condition. The majority of the intracranial events are thrombotic in origin, the larger cerebral arteries being the most frequently involved. The stroke risk parallels the hemoglobin level. Headaches, dizziness, vertigo, tinnitus, visual disturbances, carotid and vertebrobasilar TIAs, chorea, and fluctuating cognitive impairment are well-recognized features of patients with polycythemia vera. Spinal cord infarction occurs rarely. Spinal cord and optic nerve syndromes may also be due to extramedullary hematopoiesis. Cautious lowering of the hematocrit is reasonable. Because of the potential risk for hemorrhagic intracranial complications, aspirin therapy should be used cautiously.

Cerebral thrombotic and hemorrhagic complications are common in primary or essential thrombocythemia. Patients may have splenomegaly, mucocutaneous hemorrhagic diathesis, persistent thrombocytosis (usually in excess of 1 million/mL), giant platelets, and bone marrow megakaryocyte hyperplasia. Frequent neurological complications include headaches, dizziness, amaurosis fugax, and TIAs. Cerebral arterial thrombosis caused by platelet-fibrin thrombi is a rare complication. Papilledema secondary to cerebral venous thrombosis may be a complication in patients whose platelet levels have not been controlled. Cerebral infarctions also have been reported in patients with thrombocythemia secondary to iron-deficiency anemia. Iron-deficiency anemia with or without thrombocytosis has been implicated as a cause of intraluminal thrombus of the carotid artery, intracranial venous thrombosis, and intracranial hemorrhage. Thrombocytosis is common after splenectomy but does not carry an increased thromboembolic risk. However, reactive thrombocytosis following cardiopulmonary bypass surgery may contribute to stroke in the late postoperative period. The role of rebound thrombocytosis in ischemic stroke among heavy alcohol drinkers is uncertain. Treatment of primary thrombocythemia includes hydroxyurea, plateletpheresis, recombinant interferon alfa (IFN-$\alpha$), and aspirin. Vigorous correction of anemia is indicated for those patients with thrombocytosis associated with iron-deficiency anemia.

Paroxysmal nocturnal hemoglobinuria is an acquired clonal stem-cell disorder characterized by severe hemolytic anemia and hemosiderinuria. Thrombosis of major cerebral veins or dural sinuses and portal vein thrombosis can occur and are the most frequent causes of death. Acute cerebral venous thrombotic episodes may be treated with thrombolytic agents, unless contraindicated, or anticoagulant therapy. Complement-lowering therapy with the monoclonal antibody eculizumab is recommended for secondary prevention and hematopoietic stem cell transplantation may be curative.

DM is a well-established stroke risk factor. DM associated with arterial hypertension or hyperlipidemia adds significantly to stroke risk. A variety of platelet, rheological, coagulation, and fibrinolytic abnormalities may play a role. Hemorheological alterations producing increased blood viscosity may include increased fibrinogen values, increased hematocrit, elevated factors V and VII, increased platelet aggregation, increased platelet adhesion, increased release of $\beta$-thromboglobulin, decreased red blood cell deformability, and decreased fibrinolytic activity.

Heparin-induced thrombocytopenia (HIT) can cause high morbidity and mortality from thrombotic complications. Heparin therapy may induce two types of thrombocytopenia. The most frequently observed is type I HIT, which is a mild and benign condition with platelet counts rarely less than 100,000/mL. This thrombocytopenia tends to occur early, within the first 48–72 hours after initiation of heparin treatment, and resolve spontaneously. Complications are rare. Type II HIT is a major, albeit infrequent (<3% with UFH and <1%

with LMWH) adverse effect of heparin therapy, with a delayed onset (5–15 days after heparin administration). An immune-mediated disorder characterized by increased levels of platelet-associated IgG and IgM, it increases the risk for venous and arterial thrombotic complications involving the brain, heart, and limbs. Fatalities are high, and hemorrhagic complications are rare. Unlike drug-induced immune TTP, petechiae are not seen in cases of type II HIT. Prevention is paramount, requiring reduction of heparin exposure to less than 5 days when possible, and platelet count monitoring during administration. Treatment requires immediate heparin discontinuation and initiation of recombinant hirudin or argatroban followed by oral anticoagulation for at least 3 months to prevent recurrence of thrombosis.

Patients with high plasma homocysteine levels have a greater likelihood of occlusive disease of the extracranial carotid arteries, cerebral arteries, and peripheral vascular and coronary beds when compared with the general population. Diagnosis of hyperhomocysteinemia may be made by demonstrating elevated basal plasma levels of homocysteine or raised levels after methionine loading. Reduction of homocysteine levels in plasma requires supplementation with folate and vitamins $B_6$ and $B_{12}$. However, the Vitamin Intervention for Stroke Prevention (VISP) study failed to show a benefit for vitamin B-complex supplementation for prevention of recurrent stroke, and a similar lack of benefit was noted for coronary heart disease (Lonn et al., 2006; Toole et al., 2004). The Vitamins to Prevent Stroke (VITATOPS) study showed no significant benefit of supplementation with folic acid and vitamins $B_6$ and $B_{12}$ for secondary stroke prevention (Vitatops Investigators, 2010). Homocystinuria is covered earlier in this chapter under Inherited and Miscellaneous Disorders.

### Sickle Cell Disease

Cerebrovascular disease is a major cause of morbidity and mortality in patients with sickle cell disease. Strokes in sickle cell anemia (hemoglobin SS [HbSS]) patients manifest as ischemic strokes in children and as intracerebral and subarachnoid hemorrhage in adults. The most common presentations are hemiparesis, seizures, language or visual impairments, and coma. Cognitive impairment may result from silent infarcts. Patients at greatest risk for stroke are those with HbSS severe anemia, higher reticulocyte counts, and lower hemoglobin F levels. Sickle cell disease leads to a hyperviscous condition within the microvasculature. At low oxygen tensions, erythrocytes containing hemoglobin S assume a sickle-like appearance. Sludge in small vessels occurs, resulting in microinfarctions in the affected organs. Although there is pathological evidence that microvascular occlusion and sludging caused by sickling does occur in the brain, the clinical and neurodiagnostic findings are consistent with a large-vessel arterial intimal hyperplasia with superimposed thrombosis affecting the major intracranial arteries. Ischemic stroke frequently involves the arterial border zones and adjacent deep white matter. Infarcts are more common in the ACA–MCA border zone. Sickle cell disease commonly causes a moyamoya syndrome. Sickle cell disease may be accompanied by thrombotic cerebral infarction, cerebral venous occlusive disease, or subarachnoid, intracerebral, or intraventricular hemorrhage. Delayed intracranial hemorrhage may follow cerebral infarction and has been described as a complication of bone marrow transplantation. Spinal cord infarction is rare. Neurological symptoms may be triggered by hypoxia, sepsis, dehydration, or acidosis.

The evaluation of the stroke patient with sickle cell anemia must be carefully individualized. Blood cell count, peripheral blood smear, hemoglobin electrophoresis, and sickling test are essential. Vascular imaging studies are valuable investigations in sickle cell patients. TCD ultrasound is useful in detecting the intracranial vasculopathy and may make it possible to detect patients at highest risk for cerebral infarction and to initiate preventive treatment. Maintenance of hemoglobin S below 30% is effective in reducing the stroke risk in children with sickle cell anemia. The Stroke Prevention Trial in Sickle Cell Anemia evaluated children with sickle cell anemia and no history of stroke (Adams et al., 1998). Children were screened for increased risk of stroke by TCD. The National Heart, Lung, and Blood Institute prematurely stopped the trial after 10 cerebral infarctions and 1 cerebral hemorrhage occurred among the standard care group, while only 1 ischemic stroke occurred among the transfused group. Since the publication of the STOP trial, additional data have pointed to the importance of the cerebral metabolic rates of oxygen utilization (a product of CBF, arterial oxygen content [Cao2], and oxygen extraction fraction [OEF]), as an important factor in the development of ischemia (Guilliams et al., 2019). Additional clinical trials identified patents who could be transitioned to hydroxyurea therapy from chronic transfusion therapy; the role of hydroxyurea as a primary stroke prevention strategy is also being explored worldwide (Guillams et al., 2019). For patients with severe SCD, stem cell replacement therapy may also be an option. Meticulous hydration, adequate oxygenation, and analgesia are necessary. Iron overload may be prevented by subcutaneous chelation with desferoxamine. If snoring is also identified in patients with sickle cell disease, a more aggressive approach to upper airway obstruction, including surgery, may be indicated.

### Thrombotic Thrombocytopenic Purpura

Thrombotic thrombocytopenic purpura (TTP) is a life-threatening, generalized microcirculatory condition of undetermined cause, characterized by fever, thrombocytopenia, microangiopathic hemolytic anemia, renal dysfunction, and fluctuating neurological signs. TTP is rare, with a reported incidence of 1 person per 1 million annually. Most cases are idiopathic, but TTP also may be caused by drug exposure or associated with pregnancy and the puerperium, connective tissue disorders, infective endocarditis, or neoplasms. There is widespread segmental hyaline microthrombi in the microvasculature. Neurological symptomatology is protean and may be fleeting, although stroke may occur. Patients frequently have headaches, visual disturbances, CN palsies, delirium, seizures, aphasia, paresis, and coma. Treatment is with infusions of fresh frozen plasma, plasmapheresis, corticosteroids, and platelet antiaggregants, singly or in combination. If plasma exchange fails, splenectomy combined with corticosteroids and IV vincristine may be used.

## INFARCTS OF UNDETERMINED CAUSE

Despite an extensive work-up, in a considerable percentage of persons with ischemic stroke, a causal factor cannot be determined. This percentage is possibly higher in patients younger than 45 years. Some of these ischemic strokes may result from asymptomatic paroxysmal AF; electrophysiological testing may be useful. More detailed investigation for thrombophilia may be warranted in selected patients. The recurrent stroke risk after stroke of undetermined cause appears to be less than that of other ischemic strokes types.

## ESSENTIAL INVESTIGATIONS

The diagnostic evaluation for all patients with TIAs or ischemic stroke includes complete blood cell count with differential white cell and platelet counts, prothrombin time (PT), aPTT, plasma glucose level, blood urea nitrogen, serum creatinine, lipid analyses, urinalysis, and 12-lead ECG. Glycated hemoglobin ($HbA_{1c}$) is measured in patients having or suspected of having DM. Chest roentgenography, laboratory tests for thrombophilia (Box 65.7), erythrocyte sedimentation rate, and luetic serology should be considered in appropriate circumstances.

**BOX 65.7 Specialized Laboratory Tests for Thrombophilia**

Antithrombin activity
Protein C
Protein S (total and free antigen levels)
Activated protein C resistance
Factor V Leiden
Prothrombin gene (G20210 A) mutation
Cardiolipin (IgG, IgM) antibodies
$\beta_2$-Glycoprotein 1 (IgG, IgM) antibodies
Lupus anticoagulant
Fibrinogen
Plasminogen
Plasminogen activator inhibitor
Plasmin functional activity
Factors V, VII, VIII, IX, X, XI, and XIII levels
Hemoglobin electrophoresis
Plasma homocysteine

## Neuroimaging

Initial emergent brain imaging is done in all patients, as it may detect hemorrhagic or mass lesions that can present as a TIA or evolving stroke. MRI is superior to computed tomography (CT) in cerebral ischemia but is not readily available for emergent use in many centers; it may be contraindicated in some patients, such as those with certain types of cardiac pacemakers. MRI is useful to delineate ischemic strokes, especially involving the brainstem or cerebellum, or lacunar strokes, because diffusion, perfusion, and gradient echo MR sequences can rapidly detect early ischemic and hemorrhagic lesions and also estimate tissue at risk (the "ischemic penumbra"). Approximately 10%–40% of patients with TIA symptoms have evidence of cerebral infarction on CT, while about 40%–60% of patients with TIA have evidence of ischemic injury on DW-MRI studies (Ay et al., 2002; Kidwell et al., 1999). Attention to early CT signs of ischemic stroke in the hemisphere, such as loss of gray/white-matter differentiation, sulcal effacement, effacement of the sylvian fissure, and obscuration of the lentiform nucleus, is critical. The intracranial large-vessel segments are occasionally hyperdense in the noncontrast CT (dense MCA sign, sylvian fissure dot sign, dense basilar artery) before the infarction becomes visible (Fig. 65.22). The dense MCA sign is indicative of a thrombotic or embolic occlusion of the MCA. It often predicts a large cortical infarct but is not always a poor prognostic indicator. MRA visualizes blood flow in the major cervical and cerebral arteries. The specificity and sensitivity of MRA is improved with gadolinium administration. The sensitivity of MRI in differentiating infarction or other lesions from normal tissue depends primarily on changes in tissue T1 and T2 relaxation times, which are related to tissue water content (Figs. 65.23 and 65.24). DW-MRI allows early detection of acute cerebral ischemia while also differentiating acute from chronic stroke. Within the first 24 hours, diffusion/perfusion mismatch may be present in as many as 70% of patients with ischemic stroke, complete ischemia in 10%–20% of patients, and a reperfusion pattern in 10%–15% of patients. A positive DW-MRI image with negative FLAIR (fluid-attenuated inversion recovery) image is now being used to identify patients potentially eligible for IV alteplase with an unknown time of stroke symptom onset (Thomalia et al., 2018).

Baseline changes on CT may also be used for patient selection for thrombolytic therapies via a quantitative scoring system that divides the MCA territory into 10 regions. This ASPECTS score has good predictive value for the risk of symptomatic ICH (sensitivity 0.9 and specificity 0.62, $P = .012$) and 3-month functional outcome (sensitivity 0.78 and specificity 0.96, $P < .001$) with good inter-rater reliability (kappa 0.71–0.89) (Barber et al., 2000).

CT perfusion imaging is a modality that is increasingly being used to evaluate patients with acute ischemic stroke and may increase the likelihood for early diagnosis of stroke when used in addition to acute imaging protocols of noncontrasted CT scan and CTA (Hopyan et al., 2010) (Fig. 65.25). CT perfusion imaging and CTA should be used selectively in stroke patients, because of the risks of increased radiation and contrast dye exposure (US Food and Drug Administration, 2010). Advanced multimodal imaging with CT- and MR-based perfusion protocols are increasingly being used to identify patients that may benefit from available acute treatment modalities in an expanded time window or when onset time is uncertain. New software techniques with high-speed automated computerized analysis, as utilized in recent mechanical thrombectomy trials, allow for rapid identification

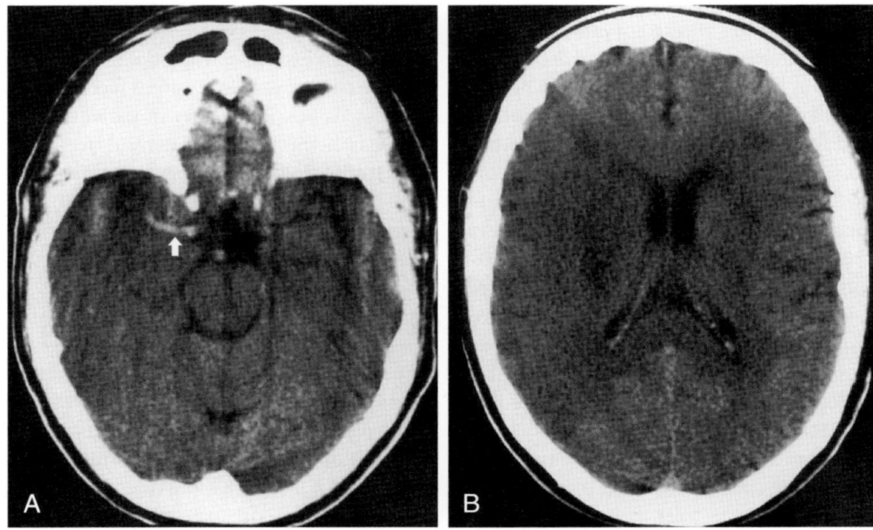


**Fig. 65.22** Nonenhanced axial computed tomographic scans show (**A**) a dense right middle cerebral artery (MCA) sign *(arrow)* on the M1 segment and (**B**) a complete right MCA territory infarction. *(Courtesy Vincent Mathews, MD.)*

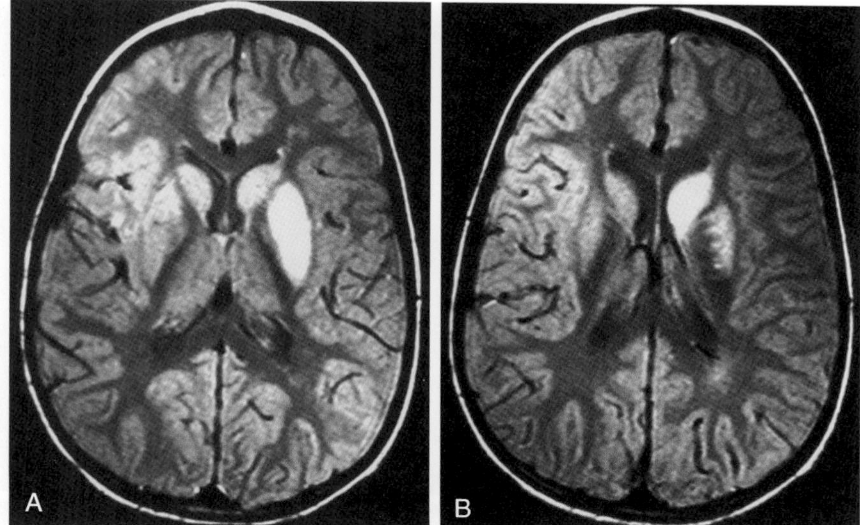


**Fig. 65.23** Axial proton density magnetic resonance imaging demonstrates areas of increased signal intensity involving the head of the left caudate nucleus and the left lenticular nucleus, consistent with infarction. The internal portion of the globus pallidus is spared (A–B).

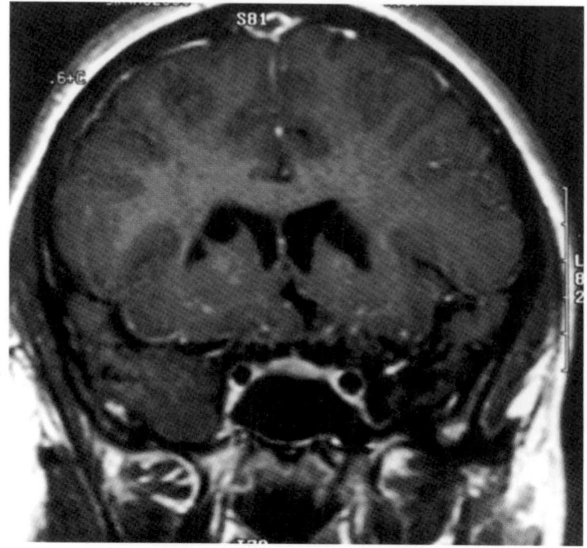

**Fig. 65.24** Coronal T1-weighted magnetic resonance imaging with contrast of a 14-year-old boy demonstrates bilateral recurrent artery of Heubner territory infarcts with involvement of the head of the caudate nucleus and anterior limb of the internal capsule. *(Courtesy Vincent Mathews, MD.)*

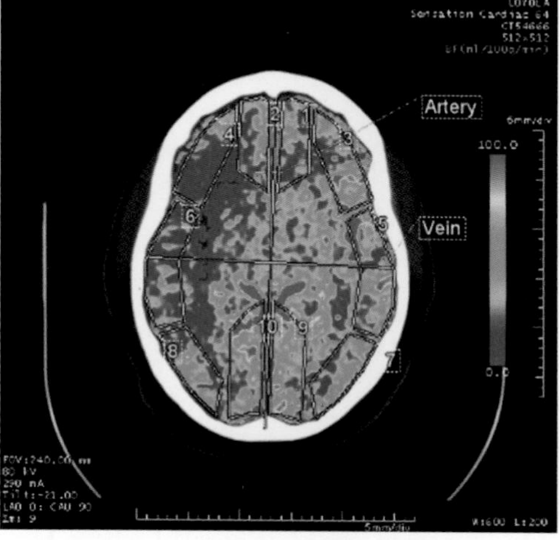


**Fig. 65.25** Example of a patient with prior strokes due to a middle cerebral artery proximal stenosis, with new left-sided weakness. There is a large area of computed tomography perfusion deficit as a result of new cerebral ischemia.

of CT or MR perfusion mismatch with report of estimated ischemic core volumes that, along with patient clinical factors, identify those patients who might gain benefit from stroke thrombolysis or mechanical thrombectomy (Campbell and Parsons, 2018; Thomalla et al., 2018; Fig. 65.26).

The emphasis in primary screening is on noninvasive testing, including Doppler imaging, B-mode scanning, duplex (combined B-mode and Doppler) scanning, and TCD imaging (see Chapter 41). In studies of duplex ultrasonography, sensitivity for detection of greater than 50% diameter carotid artery stenosis ranged from 87% to 96%, and specificity ranged from 81% to 96%. There are, however, practical limitations of the ultrasound techniques. Severe arterial stenosis or occlusion cannot be determined confidently by sonography. These methods also may fail to detect an intraluminal thrombus or a small atherosclerotic plaque, and some lesions are anatomically beyond the reach of the scanner. TCD assists in the evaluation of blood flow velocities and patency of the main intracranial arteries, hemodynamic reserve assessment, and identification of high-intensity transient microembolic signals. TCD is limited in that adequate signals are available in only 80% of patients, and the technique is highly operator dependent. The diagnostic evaluation of carotid plaque may now include new imaging modalities such as three-dimensional (3D) ultrasonography and TCD with microembolic detection for carotid plaque ulceration. Carotid plaque MRI is another useful modality for evaluation of carotid plaque morphology and stroke risk (Gupta et al., 2013; Treiman, 2015). Other additional techniques that can measure impairment of cerebrovascular reserve include positron emission tomography (PET), TCD with vasodilatory stimulus, CT perfusion, and MR perfusion. These techniques are being more frequently utilized to select those patients with asymptomatic carotid

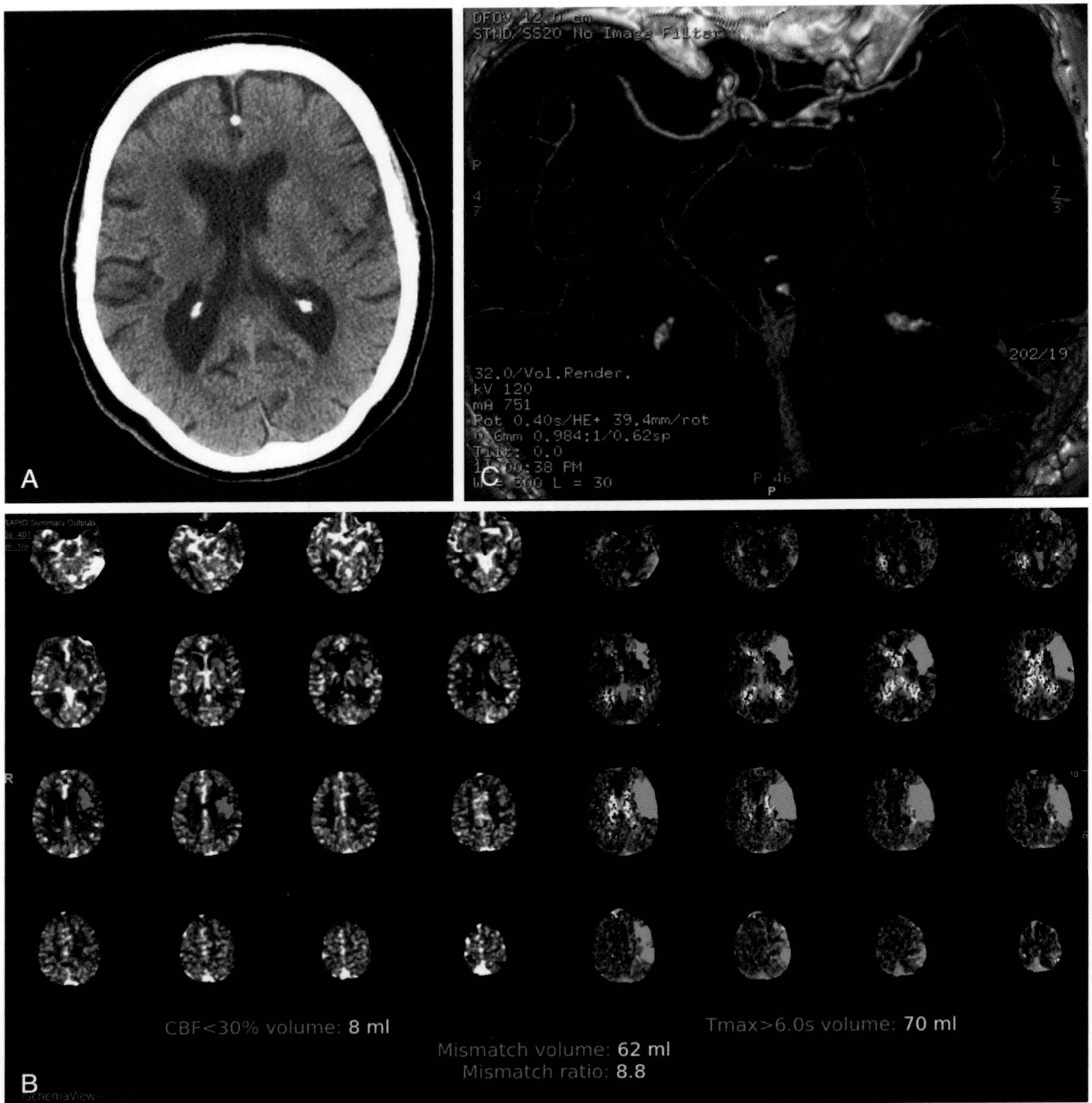


**Fig. 65.26** A 90-year-old woman with a prior history of MI, subarachnoid hemorrhage, and seizures, who presented with acute onset of aphasia and right hemiparesis, received IV alteplase within 2 hours of symptom onset. She was then transferred to a comprehensive stroke center for possible endovascular intervention. Head CT (non-contrast) with ASPECTS Score of 8 (**A**). CT Perfusion RAPID® study showed mismatch (**B**). She was found to have a superior M2 branch occlusion by CTA (**C**) (TICI 0). She had mechanical thrombectomy but her TICI score remained low (TICI 1).

artery stenosis, at greater stroke risk, who might then derive greater benefit from carotid artery revascularization (Gupta et al., 2013).

## Cardiac Evaluation of the Stroke Patient

Cardiac investigations to determine whether emboli have a cardiac source are advised in selected circumstances. Noninvasive cardiac imaging has expanded the ability to diagnose and assess a variety of cardiac conditions, many of which have been implicated as potential embolic causes. These techniques differ widely in the information they provide about the morphology, function, and metabolic status of the heart. Most institutions currently use two-dimensional (2D) echocardiography to detect left ventricular thrombus with injection of agitated saline or other contrast agents to screen for right-to-left cardiac shunts. A transthoracic or transesophageal approach can be used. The thrombus morphology predicts its embolic potential; left ventricular thrombi that have a protruding and mobile appearance on echocardiography are most likely to embolize. The sensitivity of TTE in detecting left ventricular thrombi varies from 77% to 92%, specificity varies from 84% to 94%, and predictive accuracy is 79% (Fig. 65.27).

Patients with AF are likely to develop atrial thrombi secondary to stasis of blood in the left atrium or left atrial appendage (LAA). Atrial thrombi are not always well visualized with TTE due to the distance between the LAA and chest wall. The LAA is often difficult to visualize with M-mode echocardiography. TEE remains the gold standard for identifying cardiac sources of emboli. TEE can also detect complex aortic plaques. TEE is used in selected individuals, particularly when TTE is technically inadequate for the evaluation of mitral and aortic prosthetic valves or vegetations, whenever there is a need for better visualization of the LAA or interatrial septum, or when a right-to-left shunt, left atrial spontaneous contrast, or aortic atherosclerosis is suspected. Two-phase 64-slice (or greater) cardiac CTA is also a useful noninvasive modality for detecting high-risk cardiac sources of embolism and differentiating

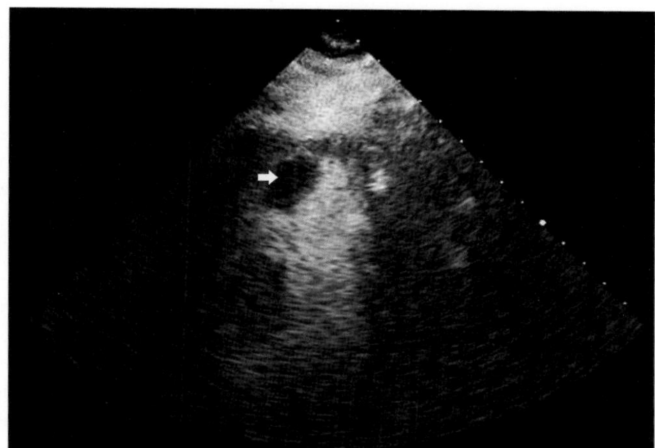

**Fig. 65.27** Contrast-enhanced transthoracic echocardiogram (two-chamber view) in a 62-year-old man with a left middle cerebral artery infarction showing a left ventricular apical thrombus *(arrow)*.

thrombus from circulatory stasis in stroke patients (Hur and Choi, 2017). Cardiac CT may detect intracardiac thrombi not seen on echocardiography with a sensitivity of 96% and specificity of 92%. It can also provide structural imaging of the LAA and guide selection of patients who might be eligible for LAA closure (Hur and Choi, 2017). Cardiac MRI may also improve identification of stroke etiology by detecting cardio-aortic embolic sources not otherwise seen on echocardiography, especially in patients with agnogenic stroke (Baher et al., 2014; Hur and Choi, 2017).

Routine cardiac telemetry in the acute stroke period may reveal unexpected paroxysmal disturbances of cardiac rhythm, often resulting in treatment modifications; it has become a crucial element of most acute stroke units. Prolonged arrhythmia monitoring beyond the acute hospital period may be useful in selected patients to detect paroxysmal AF. The 30-day Cardiac Event Monitor Belt for Recording Atrial Fibrillation after a Cerebral Ischemic Event (EMBRACE) study suggested that 30-day, noninvasive monitoring for AF in patients ≥ age 55, with a negative 24-hour cardiac monitor, was a cost-effective approach in identifying patients at risk for stroke recurrence, with 14-day monitoring as a reasonable alternative for lower-risk patients (Gladstone et al., 2014; Yong et al., 2016). The study randomized 572 patients with cryptogenic ischemic stroke or TIA within the prior 6 months to undergo either 30-day event-triggered non-implanted monitoring, or 24 hours of cardiac monitoring, with a primary outcome of the number of AF events with a duration of at least 30 seconds in the 90 days following randomization. A secondary outcome consisted of the number of AF events lasting 2.5 minutes or more. EMBRACE identified AF events in 16.1% of the prolonged monitoring group, compared with 3.2% in the control group ($P < .001$). AF events lasting 2.5 minutes or more occurred in 9.9% of the prolonged monitoring group and 2.5% of the control group ($P < .001$). The Cryptogenic Stroke and Underlying AF (CRYSTAL AF) study was an industry-sponsored randomized controlled trial to explore whether an insertable cardiac monitor was more effective than control in AF detection: 441 patients with no immediate detectable AF, with a miminimum of an initial 24 hours of ECG monitoring, were either randomized to device insertion, or control, with ECG monitoring in the control patients at the discretion of the sites (Sanna et al., 2014). AF was classified as an episode of irregular heart rhythm without detectable p waves, lasting more than 30 seconds, and the primary outcome was detection of an AF episode within 6 months. In the study, AF was detected in 8.9% of the device group versus 1.4% in the control group at 6 months (HR 6.4; 95% CI 1.9–21.7 ($P < .001$). The event rate rose to 12.4% in the device group and was 2% in the control group by 12 months. The median value for "the mean time in AF per day" was 4.3 minutes (interquartile range 0.7–34.5 minutes). The device was removed due to site infection or skin erosion in 2.4% of patients; 1.4% of patients had site infections, 1.4% had pain at the device site; and 1.9% had irrigation or inflammation at the device site. Of note, the median time to detection of an AF event was 41 days (interquartile range 14–84 days) in the device group and 32 days in the control group (interquartile range 2–73 days), suggesting that most AF events occur relatively early post-stroke. Also, the EMBRACE and CRYSTALAF studies used an AF event duration cutoff of 30 seconds, whereas other clinical trials only reported events of at least 5–6 minutes, duration, such that the cardioembolic risk (and associated benefit of anticoagulation ) of very short runs of AF remains less clear. Whether prolonged cardiac monitoring with an inserted cardiac monitor to detect possible AF events beyond 30 days is a cost-effective strategy is unknown at this time, but prolonged ambulatory monitoring for stroke of indeterminate cause, for which an embolic event is suspected, is a reasonable clinical approach.

## Cerebral Angiography

The gold standard for vascular imaging remains conventional catheter-based angiography. It can accurately determine the size and location of vascular lesions, detecting tandem arterial lesions and assessing the collateral circulation.

Cervicocerebral catheter-based angiography is not without complications, and its use is being challenged by the increasingly improving quality of MRA and CTA. A main disadvantage of MRA is that it overestimates the degree of stenosis related to disturbed signal from turbulent flow. Although the risks associated with cerebral angiography have been gradually decreasing, the risk for any complication is approximately 1%–5%, of which half are minor groin hematomas. The risk for permanent neurological disability is approximately 0.2%, and the risk for death has been estimated to be 0.05%. CTA has become another useful alternative for visualization of the intracranial and extracranial arteries and has replaced conventional catheter angiography for many patients.

Catheter-based conventional cerebral angiography is still indicated in several circumstances, particularly when the diagnosis remains uncertain. It remains the foundation for safe, successful cerebrovascular interventions including mechanical thrombectomy, and carotid angioplasty and stenting. When the evaluation fails to confirm the diagnosis, angiography may help differentiate between atherosclerotic cerebrovascular occlusive disease and nonatherosclerotic vasculopathies such as FMD, cervicocephalic arterial dissections, vasculitis, and moyamoya disease, as well as intracranial aneurysms or vascular malformations (Fig. 65.28).

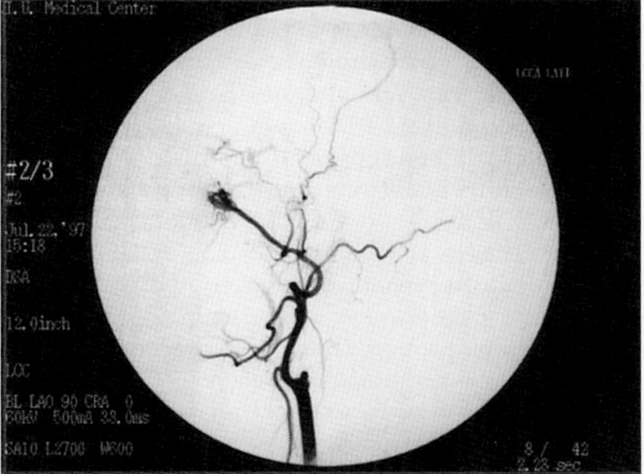


**Fig. 65.28** A 43-year-old woman with a history of hypertension, hypercholesterolemia, and tobacco use had right-sided hemiparesis. Cerebral angiogram demonstrates an occlusion of the left internal carotid artery just past the bifurcation. There is partial reconstitution via ethmoid collaterals.

Currently, angiography is seldom indicated when endarterectomy is planned; many physicians rely on CTA, MRA, and/or carotid ultrasound for preoperative assessment. Angiography may still be indicated when distinctions affecting treatment are unclear.

## PREVENTING STROKE RECURRENCE: MEDICAL THERAPY

At present, general measures including control of associated vascular risk factors, as well as the use of antithrombotic agents (platelet antiaggregants and anticoagulants), antihypertensive agents, and statin therapy, remain the mainstays of medical therapy.

### Platelet Antiaggregants

Evidence from several clinical studies favors the use of platelet antiaggregants as the first line of therapy in patients at high risk for stroke (Antithrombotic Trialists' Collaboration, 2002; Hankey, 2004). These agents are indicated for secondary prevention of stroke. Primary prevention studies do not support aspirin use for primary stroke prevention in low-risk, middle-aged people (Hebert et al., 2000). Aspirin (81 mg) every other day was effective in stroke primary prevention in older women (Ridker et al., 2005). Though aspirin did not offer a long-term protective effect among 372 asymptomatic patients with carotid bruits and greater than 50% carotid stenosis on duplex ultrasonography, many physicians continue its use in patients with carotid bruits or asymptomatic carotid stenosis; though reports regarding intraplaque hemorrhage caused by platelet antiaggregants are conflicting.

Aspirin, the oldest and most commonly used nonprescription drug in the world, is the standard medical therapy for preventing stroke in patients with transient cerebral ischemia and for reducing the risk for recurrent stroke and postoperative strokes after carotid endarterectomy (CEA). Aspirin is effective, inexpensive, and safe if started within 48 hours of acute ischemic stroke (Chinese Acute Stroke Trial, 1997; International Stroke Trial Collaborative Group, 1997). Meta-analyses have shown that aspirin reduces the combined relative risk for stroke, MI, and vascular death by approximately 25%. The optimal dose of aspirin remains uncertain. Higher doses confer more GI side effects. The recommended range of daily doses is between 50 and 325 mg of aspirin. There is a suggestion that aspirin is also effective in doses as low as 30 mg daily.

The mechanism of action of aspirin is the irreversible inhibition of platelet function by inactivation of cyclo-oxygenase (COX). Aspirin is a nonselective inhibitor of COX and is therefore able to inhibit both isoforms (COX-1 and COX-2). The antiaggregant effect is seen within 1 hour after administration. Aspirin is also anti-inflammatory, antioxidant, and may increase fibrinolytic activity up to 4 hours after administration. The main side effect of aspirin is gastric discomfort. GI hemorrhage occurs in 1%–5% of cases.

In the Aspirin in Carotid Endarterectomy (ACE) trial, 2849 patients who were scheduled for CEA were randomly assigned to compare the benefits of low-dose aspirin (81–325 mg daily) with high-dose aspirin (650 or 1300 mg daily). The primary endpoints in the ACE trial were stroke, MI, or death. At 3 months after surgery, the risk for stroke, MI, or death was 6.2% in the low-dose aspirin group, compared with 8.4% in the high-dose aspirin group. The difference was less apparent when only stroke or death was evaluated as the endpoint (Taylor et al., 1999). This was not a study of secondary stroke prevention, however, but a study of perioperative risk reduction in patients with asymptomatic or symptomatic carotid artery stenosis.

Ticlopidine and clopidogrel are structurally related thienopyridines that have antiplatelet effects.

*An extended version of this section is available online at http://expertconsult.inkling.com.* 

Ticlopidine reduces the relative risk for death or nonfatal stroke by 12% in comparison with aspirin. It has been supplanted by clopidogrel because of significant side effects of diarrhea, nausea, dyspepsia, and rash. Reversible neutropenia occurs in 2.4% of cases and is severe in 0.85%. Thrombocytopenia or TTP may also occur, with TTP risk related to ticlopidine among the highest reported.

*An extended version of this section is available online at http://expertconsult.inkling.com* 

The Clopidogrel versus Aspirin in Patients at Risk of Ischemic Events (CAPRIE) study assessed the relative efficacy of clopidogrel (75 mg daily) and aspirin (325 mg daily) in reducing the risk of ischemic stroke, MI, and vascular death in patients with previous ischemic stroke, MI, or symptomatic atherosclerotic peripheral arterial disease. The results of this study showed that clopidogrel was modestly more effective (8.7% RRR) than aspirin. Overall, the tolerability of clopidogrel was excellent, with no increased incidence of neutropenia, diarrhea, rash, and pruritus, and a lower incidence of GI hemorrhage and peptic, gastric, or duodenal ulcers when compared with aspirin.

Subsequent data from the Clopidogrel in Unstable Angina to Prevent Recurrent Events (CURE) study suggested that a combination of clopidogrel plus aspirin with doses ranging from 75 mg to 325 mg daily was superior to aspirin monotherapy (Yusuf et al., 2001) for patients with coronary artery disease. High-risk subgroups in the CAPRIE or CURE studies had greater benefit from clopidogrel, though the data should be interpreted with caution as it comes from a post hoc analysis. In CAPRIE, the benefit was seen in these subgroups; prior CABG, history of more than one prior ischemic event, involvement of multiple vascular beds (peripheral, coronary, or cerebrovascular), patients with hyperlipidemia, and/or diabetes. (Hirsch et al., 2004). Subsequently, the Management of Atherothrombosis with Clopidogrel in High-Risk Patients (MATCH) trial, comparing clopidogrel plus 75 mg of aspirin daily with clopidogrel monotherapy, showed a non-significant difference in benefit for combination therapy. The RRR for combination therapy in the MATCH trial was only 6.4% ($P = .244$) (Diener et al., 2004). Of great concern, combination therapy in the MATCH trial was associated with a 4.5% major and life-threatening bleeding events rate compared with 1.9% for clopidogrel monotherapy ($P < .0001$). A study of dual-antiplatelet therapy (DAPT) versus aspirin (325 mg daily) and aggressive blood pressure control versus conventional antihypertensive therapy in patients with MRI-proven small-vessel ischemic disease (SPS3) demonstrated no reduction in recurrent stroke for patients treated with the combination of aspirin and clopidogrel. DAPT patients experienced nearly twice the major hemorrhage risk and 52% higher all-cause mortality compared to those on aspirin alone (The SPS3 Investigators, 2012).

Early administration of DAPT within 12 hours after minor stroke or TIA appears to have some benefit. The POINT study enrolled 4881 patients with minor stroke (National Institutes of Health Stroke Scale [NIHSS] score <4 or TIA with ABCD2 score >3) at predominantly United States and European sites and randomized them to either clopidogrel 600 mg loading dose on day 1 followed by clopidogrel 75 mg and aspirin (50–325 mg daily) or aspirin alone with an endpoint of ischemic stroke, MI or vascular death at 90 days. DAPT was associated with a lower rate of ischemic events (5% for DAPT versus 6.5% for aspirin alone; HR 0.75 955 DI 0.59—0.95; $P = .02$), albeit with a higher risk of major hemorrhage (0.9% DAPT vs. 0.45 aspirin alone (HR 2.32 955 CI 1.10–4.87; $P = .02$). as compared with aspirin alone. Most events occurred in the first week after treatment initiation and were mainly ischemic strokes. The authors estimated there would be

15 ischemic events prevented and 5 major hemorrhages would occur following DAPT within those 90 days and the benefit of DAPT was concentrated within the first month. The CHANCE study enrolled 5170 patients at 114 Chinese study sites within 24 hours after minor stroke or high-risk TIA to DPAT with a 300 mg loading dose of clopidogrel plus aspirin 75 mg daily for the first 21 days following by clopidogrel 75 mg alone until day 90 or placebo plus aspirin 75 mg daily for 90 days. Stroke occurred in 8.2% of patients on DAPT and 11.7% of patients on aspirin alone (HR 0.68, 95% CI 0.57–0.81; $P < .001$) with moderate or severe hemorrhage occurring in 0.3% of the DAPT on aspirin only groups (Wang et al., 2013), Thus, DAPT is beneficial in the short term but, in the long run, the MATCH and SPS3 argument against DAPT long-term use remains appropriate.

Dipyridamole is a cyclic nucleotide phosphodiesterase inhibitor that increases the levels of cyclic adenosine monophosphate. The European Stroke Prevention Study 2 (ESPS-2), a multicenter randomized, double-blind, factorial, placebo-controlled trial, randomized patients with stroke or TIA within the previous 3 months to treatment with aspirin alone (25 mg twice a day), modified-release dipyridamole alone (200 mg twice a day), the two agents in combination, or placebo. The ESPS-2 investigators concluded that both low-dose aspirin and high-dose dipyridamole in a modified-release form alone were superior to placebo, and that the combination was significantly superior to each drug alone. Benefit was limited to stroke prevention in patients with prior stroke or TIA. There was little effect on fatal stroke and MI. The main side effects in the ESPS-2 study were headaches and GI distress with headache attributed to dipyridamole, and GI distress attributed to aspirin. The PRoFESS study, however, failed to show non-inferiority of extended-release dipyridamole plus low-dose aspirin compared with clopidogrel in recurrent stroke or a composite outcome of stroke, MI or death, and the rate of headache and hemorrhagic complications was higher in the aspirin plus dipyridamole group (Sacco et al., 2008). Cilostazol, another phosphodiesterase inhibitor, proved superior to aspirin in preventing recurrent strokes in patients with non-cardioembolic strokes (Shinohara, 2010).

## Oral Anticoagulants

Warfarin (4-hydroxycoumarin) inhibits the synthesis of factors II, VII, IX, and X, as well as proteins C and S. Oral anticoagulation with warfarin is indicated for primary and secondary prevention of stroke in patients with NVAF. Six randomized studies evaluated primary and secondary stroke prevention of stroke in the context of NVAF. Three of these studies also evaluated aspirin at daily doses of 75 mg, 300 mg, and 325 mg. These six studies demonstrated that the RRR for stroke was 68% with the use of warfarin (Koefoed et al., 1997). The RRR with aspirin therapy was 21% (18%–44%) (Atrial Fibrillation Investigators, 1997). Advancing age increases the risk for major hemorrhage in patients given warfarin for stroke prevention; patients older than 75 years are at greater risk for hemorrhagic complications. However, these older patients are at significantly greater risk for ischemic stroke compared to their risk for hemorrhage, and warfarin should still be considered for these patients. Therefore, NVAF patients at high risk for stroke should be treated with dose-adjusted warfarin (INR 2.0–3.0); INR values less than 2.0 and greater than 4.0 should be avoided. Patients younger than 65 years without other risk factors can be given aspirin, 325 mg/day ($CHA_2DS_2$-$VAS_C$ score 0–1). Low-intensity, fixed-dose warfarin plus aspirin is inadequate for stroke prevention in high-risk patients with NVAF. Warfarin plus antiplatelet therapy for AF is also not superior to warfarin alone, though combination therapy is sometimes used to treat AF patients who undergo stents. There is also no evidence that newer antiplatelet therapies are substitutes for warfarin. In those patients for whom the risk of bleeding complications of warfarin are unacceptably high, the combination of clopidogrel and low-dose aspirin (75–100 mg) was shown to be superior to aspirin monotherapy, though there was a slightly greater rate of bleeding complications with the combination therapy. At a median of 3.6 years of follow-up, major vascular events had occurred in 6.8% of patients receiving clopidogrel plus aspirin, compared with 7.6% of patients receiving aspirin monotherapy (RRR 0.89, 95% CI 0.81–0.98). Major bleeding occurred at a rate of 2% per year for patients receiving combination therapy and 1.3% in patients receiving aspirin alone (RR 1.57, 95% CI 1.29–1.92) (ACTIVE Investigators, 2009). Anticoagulation is also recommended for patients with AF and hyperthyroidism. Patients who cannot tolerate pharmacological cardioversion may benefit from electrophysiological or surgical procedures. However, cardioversion to sinus rhythm does not obviate the need for long-term anticoagulation (Sherman et al., 2005). Anticoagulant therapy has a protective effect against stroke following acute MI. To prevent arterial embolism, immediate anticoagulation with heparin is initiated, followed by oral anticoagulation for 6 months, following an anterior wall MI or an MI with apical wall motion abnormalities or left ventricular thrombus. Patients with mechanical prosthetic heart valves should receive lifelong therapy with warfarin to prolong the INR to a target of 3.5. Patients undergoing elective cardioversion for AF should receive anticoagulation for 3–4 weeks before cardioversion unless there was documented onset of AF less than 48 hours prior to cardioversion. Use of long-term anticoagulation in patients with left ventricular aneurysms and mural thrombi is not indicated because of the low risk for embolization. Prophylactic use of warfarin to a target INR 2.0–3.5 in patients with dilated cardiomyopathy in the Warfarin versus Aspirin in Reduced Cardiac Ejection Fraction study (WARCEF) did not show a reduction in the composite endpoint of ischemic stroke, ICH, or all-cause mortality compared to aspirin alone (325 mg daily) in the 2305 patients with low cardiac ejection fractions followed for up to 6 years. In the WARCEF study, however, there was a 48% reduction in the HR for ischemic stroke (95% CI 0.33–0.82; $P = .005$) in the warfarin-treated patients (Homma et al., 2012). Furthermore, there are no adequate data to support anticoagulation preferentially, as compared with antiplatelet therapy, in patients with a PFO or aortic arch atheroma–related stroke or TIA (Albers et al., 2004; Messe et al., 2004). For those patients with non-cardioembolic infarctions, the Warfarin Aspirin Recurrent Stroke Study (WARSS), a trial of 2206 patients randomized to warfarin (INR 1.4–2.8) or aspirin (325 mg daily), did not show additional benefit for warfarin in preventing recurrent ischemic stroke (Mohr et al., 2001). Additionally, while warfarin was previously thought to be beneficial for symptomatic intracranial atherosclerotic vascular disease, a randomized comparison of warfarin (INR 2.0–3.0) and high-dose aspirin (1300 mg daily) failed to show superiority of either therapy for the primary endpoint of stroke or vascular death (Chimowitz et al., 2005). The 2-year event rate was 22.1% for aspirin and 21.8% for warfarin, with $P = .83$. While there was a statistically nonsignificant ($P = .29$) benefit for warfarin (event rate 17.0%) versus aspirin (event rate 21.4%) for ischemic stroke, there was a statistically significant benefit for aspirin compared to warfarin for major bleeding (3.2% aspirin; 8.3% warfarin; $P = .01$) and nonsignificantly fewer vascular deaths (3.2% aspirin; 5.9% warfarin; $P = .16$). There was also a trend for aspirin superiority over warfarin in preventing subsequent MI, but the overall event rate was low, with a log-rank $P = .21$.

Factor Xa inhibitors and direct thrombin inhibitors are alternatives to warfarin in patients with NVAF. Dabigatran, a reversible oral thrombin inhibitor, at a dose of 110 mg was associated with rates of stroke and systemic embolism similar to those associated with warfarin, with lower rates of major hemorrhage (Connolly et al., 2009). Dabigatran at a dose of 150 mg was associated with lower rates of stroke and systemic embolism but similar rates of major hemorrhage compared with warfarin. The oral factor Xa inhibitor rivaroxaban (20 mg daily) was shown to be non-inferior to warfarin for stroke prevention and systemic embolism in 14,264 patients with NVAF. Stroke or systemic embolism rates were 1.7% per year for rivaroxaban-treated patients and 2.2% per year for warfarin-treated patients ($P < .001$ for non-inferiority). Major and nonmajor bleeding events were similar for both groups with slightly fewer intracranial (0.2% absolute reduction, $P = .02$) and fatal (0.3% absolute reduction, $P = .003$) hemorrhages in the rivaroxaban group (Patel et al., 2011). Another oral factor Xa antagonist, apixaban, (5 mg twice daily) was shown to significantly reduce stroke or systemic embolism compared to aspirin (HR 0.45, 95% CI 0.32–0.62; $P < .001$) in 5599 patients who were deemed unsuitable for warfarin, without significantly affecting rates of major bleeding, intracranial hemorrhage, or death (Connolly, 2011). Subsequently, apixaban (5 mg twice daily) was reported as being superior to warfarin (HR 0.79, 95% CI 0.66–0.95; $P < .01$) in 18,201 patients with AF and one or more additional stroke risk factors. The apixaban-treated group experienced significantly fewer major hemorrhages, hemorrhagic strokes, and death from all causes than the warfarin-treated group (Granger, 2011). Edoxaban, an oral factor Xa inhibitor, was compared to warfarin in a randomized controlled trial of 21,105 patients with AF and CHADS2 score of 2 or greater. Edoxaban 30 mg daily and 60 mg daily were reported to be non-inferior to warfarin (target INR 2–3) for preventing stroke or systemic embolism. A trend was seen for greater benefit in the group receiving the higher dose of edoxaban. Both doses of edoxaban were associated with fewer major bleeding events (Giugliano, 2013).

There are no data to support DOAC use above warfarin in stroke prevention for patients with mechanical heart valves. Additionally, DOACs are not associated with greater risk reduction, as compared with antiplatelet therapy, for patients with embolic strokes with unknown source (ESUS). The NAVIGATE-ESUS study of rivaroxaban 15 mg daily compared with aspirin 100 mg daily, for embolic stroke of undetermined source enrolled 7213 persons with a primary efficacy outcome of recurrent ischemic or hemorrhagic stroke or systemic embolism and a primary safety outcome of major bleeding. There was a median follow-up of 11 months but the study was terminated early due to an increased annualized bleeding risk (1.8% vs. 0.75; HR 1.07, 95% CI 1.68–4.39; $P < .001$) and no decrease in the primary outcome (5.1% vs. 4.8%; HR 2.72, 95% CI 0.87–1.33; $P = .52$) with rivaroxaban as compared with aspirin (Hart et al., 2018). The RESPECT-ESUS study randomized 5390 patients to dabigatran 2150 mg twice daily (110 mg twice daily for patients age 75 and older or patients with moderate renal impairment) or to aspirin 100 mg daily with a primary outcome of recurrent stroke and a primary safety outcome of major bleeding. There was a mean follow-up of 19 months with a stroke recurrence rate of 4.1% per year with dabigatran and 4.8% with aspirin (HR 0.85, $P = .01$). Major bleeding was similar in both arms of this study (1.7% for dabigatran and 1.4% for aspirin annually) (Diener et al., 2018).

### Alternatives to Anticoagulation

For AF patients in whom antithrombotic therapy is contraindicated, percutaneous closure of the LAA may be an alternative (Holmes et al., 2009). Multiple device options exist, with the choice contingent on patient cardiac anatomy and other factors, such as patient ability to undergo short-term anticoagulation in the case of the WATCHMAN device. The WATCHMAN device was associated in early studies with high periprocedural complication rates, but 5-year long-term follow-up of the two main WATCHMAN device clinical trials showed equivalence in terms of safety and efficacy compared with warfarin. Other percutaneous devices such as the LARIAT device and LAA plugs may be possible alternative options to the WATCHMAN device, as a reasonable consideration in patients for whom safety of oral anticoagulation is a concern (Patel et al., 2012; Reddy et al., 2017; Safavi-Naeni and Raskh, 2018). Moreover, a post hoc analysis of dronedarone, a novel antiarrhythmic drug, suggests a reduction of stroke risk by 34 % ($P = .027$) among patients with nonpermanent AF, in addition to standard therapy including antithrombotic agents (Rother and Laufs, 2010).

## TREATMENT OF ACUTE ISCHEMIC STROKE

Modern therapy for acute ischemic stroke is currently being approached in four different ways. First and most important are general measures aimed at preventing and treating complications. Second are reperfusion strategies directed at arterial recanalization. Third are cytoprotective strategies aimed at cellular and metabolic targets. The fourth approach targets inhibition of the inflammatory processes associated with cerebral ischemia. Eventually, combined therapy will be used for acute ischemic stroke treatment.

### Heparins and Heparinoids

UFH exerts its anticoagulant effect by binding to AT, whereas the anticoagulant effect of LMWH is primarily mediated through the inactivation of factor Xa. Randomized studies of UFH, LMWH, or heparinoids for acute ischemic stroke treatment continue to show no proven benefits in reducing stroke-related morbidity or mortality, early stroke recurrence, or stroke prognosis, except in the case of cerebral venous thrombosis. Time windows from stroke onset varied from 6 hours to 48 hours in these studies. LMWH or heparinoid therapy after acute ischemic stroke may decrease the occurrence of deep vein thrombosis compared to UFH (Sandercock et al., 2008).

Results are available from a randomized double-blind controlled trial of the LMWH nadroparin calcium. In this trial, 312 patients were randomized within 48 hours of stroke to receive either placebo or nadroparin calcium 4100 antifactor Xa IU subcutaneously once or twice daily. Treatment was continued for 10 days. After 10 days, all patients received aspirin, 100 mg/day. There was no difference between the groups at 3 months but, after 6 months, there was a significant dose-dependent reduction in the rate of poor outcome among the three study groups in favor of patients treated with nadroparin calcium twice daily, compared with those receiving treatment once daily or placebo (Kay et al., 1995). A second randomized double-blind study involving 750 patients in 120 centers (FISS bis) failed to confirm these initial observations.

The International Stroke Trial studied approximately 20,000 patients who were randomized within 48 hours of ischemic stroke onset to receive a fixed dose of 10,000 or 25,000 units of UFH subcutaneously daily (compared with no heparin). Treatment was continued for 14 days or hospital discharge, if shorter. There was no significant difference in rates of death or recurrent ischemic or hemorrhagic stroke at 2 weeks (11.7% with UFH and 12.0% without UFH). Patients receiving UFH had significantly fewer recurrent ischemic strokes at 2 weeks, but this was negated by a similar increase in hemorrhagic strokes (IST Collaborative Group, 1997).

Definite data regarding safety and efficacy of IV heparin for acute ischemic stroke or cardioembolic stroke are lacking, but to prevent recurrence, IV heparin is sometimes given to patients with small cardioembolic infarcts associated with intracardiac thrombi diagnosed by echocardiography. In a small trial performed by the Cerebral Embolism Study Group, 45 patients with acute cardioembolic stroke who presented within 48 hours of symptom onset were randomized to receive either early or delayed treatment. The early treatment group received an IV heparin bolus of 5000–10,000 units followed by a maintenance infusion for at least 96 hours before the patient was switched to warfarin. Patients in the control group received no heparin and were given platelet antiaggregants or warfarin 10 days post stroke. None of the 24 patients who received heparin experienced stroke recurrence or hemorrhage within the 96-hour treatment period. Of the 21 patients who received delayed anticoagulation, 2 experienced early recurrent embolic cerebral infarcts, 1 had a DVT, 2 had hemorrhagic transformations, and 3 died. The study suggested that heparin might be helpful, but the study was terminated prematurely. Heparin should not be used if a patient has a septic embolus or if CT shows a hemorrhagic or large infarction. When IV heparin is given, many physicians do not use an IV bolus and aim for a target aPTT of 55–75 seconds, or 1.5–2 times control.

IV UFH appears to be ineffective in patients with acute partial stable stroke. A large randomized study evaluated UFH in 225 patients with non-cardioembolic stroke. Patients who had progressing deficit in the first hour of observation were excluded from the study because of the prevailing belief at that time that stroke in evolution should be anticoagulated. There was no significant difference in stroke progression or death at 7 days. However, an Italian study of acute stroke patients suggested that heparin may be of benefit if given within 3 hours of symptom onset for nonlacunar stroke (Camerlingo et al., 2005).

Other LMWHs and heparinoids also remain unproven in acute ischemic stroke. The overall results of the TOAST study using danaparoid (a low-molecular-weight heparinoid) for patients with acute ischemic stroke treated within 24 hours of symptom onset showed no benefit for anticoagulation with this agent (TOAST Investigators, 1998). A subgroup post hoc analysis, however, of patients with more than 50% stenosis or ipsilateral occlusion of the internal carotid artery showed a favorable outcome for those patients given danaparoid as opposed to placebo at 7 days (53.8% favorable outcome for danaparoid versus 38% for placebo [$P = .023$]) and 3 months (68.3% favorable outcome for danaparoid versus 53.2% for placebo [$P = .021$]) (Adams et al., 1999). The current status of antithrombotic therapy of cerebral ischemia is shown in Table 65.5.

**TABLE 65.5 Current Status of Antithrombotic Therapy of Cerebral Ischemia**

| Therapy | Conclusion |
|---|---|
| Apixaban | Positive* |
| Aspirin | Positive |
| Dabigatran | Positive* |
| Edoxaban | Positive* |
| Clopidogrel | Positive |
| Ticlopidine | Positive |
| Slow-release dipyridamole and aspirin | Positive |
| Cilostazol | Positive |
| Rivaroxaban | Positive* |
| Sulfinpyrazone | Negative |
| Suloctidil | Negative |
| Glycoprotein IIb/IIIa receptor antagonists | Negative |
| Warfarin | Positive* |
| Warfarin | Negative† |
| Heparin | Negative |
| Fraxiparine | Negative |
| Dalteparin | Negative |
| Certoparin | Negative |
| Tinzaparin | Negative |
| Danaparoid | Negative |

*For primary and secondary prevention in patients with nonvalvular atrial fibrillation.

†No additional benefit in preventing recurrent ischemic stroke in patients with non-cardioembolic infarcts, including patients with high-grade symptomatic intracranial stenosis.

Though convincing statistical proof is still lacking, anecdotal evidence supports, at least for some clinicians, initiation of IV UFH to prevent stroke recurrence in several uncommon situations. These indications include cerebral infarction in the setting of inherited or acquired hypercoagulable states, intraluminal arterial thrombus, and extracranial cervicocephalic arterial dissections. Outcome of cerebral venous thrombosis is also improved with heparin therapy, with improvement beginning early in the course of therapy.

## Thrombolytic Therapy

If patients meet appropriate criteria, IV administration of alteplase, a recombinant tissue plasminogen activator (tPA), remains the only proven intervention for emergency management of acute ischemic stroke and the only approved therapy for acute ischemic stroke by the US Food and Drug Administration (FDA). A strong correlation has been shown between arterial recanalization and neurological improvement in acute cerebral ischemia. Understanding how baseline clinical, biological, and imaging variables impact outcome is critical for the subsequent management of patients with acute ischemic stroke and future acute stroke clinical trials design (Tomsick et al., 2010).

Intravenous thrombolytic therapy with alteplase is recommended within 4.5 hours from onset of ischemic symptoms, adhering to the eligibility criteria and therapeutic regimen provided by the National Institute of Neurological Disorders and Stroke (NINDS) and European Cooperative Acute Stroke Study III (ECASS III) (Hacke et al., 2008; NINDS rtPA Stroke Study Group, 1995). In addition to the 4.5-hour window for presentation, patients must have an unenhanced head CT scan that does not show hemorrhage and no other contraindications to the drug. The dose of alteplase is 0.9 mg/kg, with a maximum dose of 90 mg; 10% of the total dose is given as an initial bolus, and the rest is infused over 60 minutes.

Subsequent assessment of the NINDS tPA trial using a global statistic also demonstrated a sustained benefit of IV alteplase at 6 and 12 months after the intervention in patients treated within 3 hours after onset of ischemic stroke symptoms (Kwiatkowski et al., 1999). Reanalysis of the NINDS trial was performed, and a pooled analysis of the six major alteplase acute ischemic stroke trials was also published (Hacke et al., 2004; Ingall et al., 2004). The reanalysis confirmed the previously observed benefit for alteplase in the original NINDS rtPA study paper, despite apparent imbalances in baseline stroke severity; adjusted alteplase-to-placebo OR of a favorable outcome was 2.1 (95% CI, 1.5–2.9). The pooled analysis confirmed that earlier treatment of stroke patients is associated with a more favorable outcome. Based on the numbers needed to treat (NNT) ratio, for every 8 patients treated with alteplase, 1 patient has excellent or complete recovery, and for every 15 patients treated, 1 patient has a symptomatic intracranial hemorrhage. This ratio is similar to the findings for CEA for high-grade (>70%) symptomatic carotid stenosis (Schneck and Biller, 2005).

In the NINDS rtPA study, treatment did not lessen death rates or account for excess mortality. The frequency of symptomatic ICH was 10 times greater in patients given alteplase (6.4% in the treatment group compared with 0.6% in the placebo group). Most hemorrhages occurred within 36 hours of treatment. Thrombolytic-related intracranial hemorrhages are usually large-volume lobar bleeds, often multiple, with blood/fluid levels; intraventricular and subarachnoid extension is not uncommon. The rate of symptomatic intracranial hemorrhage in several phase IV series of alteplase in the community setting was similar to that seen in the NINDS trial (Albers et al., 2000; Chiu et al., 1998). Protocol violations have been associated with higher rates of symptomatic intracranial hemorrhages (Buchan et al., 2000; Katzan et al., 2000). Katzan and colleagues reported that in 1997–1998, fewer than 2% of all ischemic stroke patients received IV alteplase in Cleveland area hospitals. Close to 16% of those patients had a symptomatic intracranial hemorrhage, of which six were fatal. Overall, half the patients treated had deviations from national treatment guidelines. After initiation of a comprehensive stroke quality-improvement plan, however, alteplase administration rates went up dramatically, with the incidence of hemorrhage and other complications equal to that in the NINDS study (Katzan et al., 2003).

The benefits of treatment with IV alteplase also outweigh the risks among selected patients with acute ischemic stroke with symptom onset from 3 to 4.5 hours. Possible exceptions include patients older than age 80, patients with a combination of previous stroke and DM, patients on oral anticoagulants regardless of INR values, patients with NIHSS scores above 25, and patients with evidence of major infarct or head CT with compromise of more than one-third of the MCA territory (Hacke et al., 2008a). In ECASS 3, more patients had a favorable outcome (defined as a modified Rankin scale [mRS] of 0–1 at 3 months) with alteplase than with placebo (52% versus 45%). An expansion of the time window to 4.5 hours has been endorsed by the AHA/American Stroke Association (Del Zoppo et al., 2009) but as yet is not approved by the FDA. The time window for IV thrombolytic therapy may in the future be extended further. A recent clinical trial of MRI-guided thrombolysis for stroke with unknown time of onset suggested that patients with MR—DWI positive, FLAIR negative lesions showed a favorable outcome in the alteplase-treated group as compared with a placebo group (53.3% vs. 41.8%; $P = 0.02$) (Thomalla et al., 2018). Furthermore a recent trial using CT perfusion or MR diffusion/perfusion imaging found good functional outcome in patients treated with alteplase up to 9 hours after symptom onset (35% excellent outcome with alteplase vs 29% for placebo) with adjusted risk ratio of 1.44 (95% CI 1.01-2.06) with a P value of 0.042 (MA, 2019)).

Intravenous alteplase administration requires close adherence to protocol guidelines. Patient management following alteplase administration requires close neurological and blood pressure monitoring, as well as capabilities to handle potential hemorrhagic complications associated with thrombolytic therapy, by physicians experienced in the management of cerebrovascular disease. Centers that do not have these capabilities can still administer IV alteplase in partnership with tertiary care facilities by starting the drug and transferring the patient. Successful centers have treated up to 15%–20% of ischemic strokes with thrombolytic therapy, although nationally only a small percentage of patients are likely to be treated with thrombolytic therapies. Formal certification of primary stroke centers commenced in 2003. A model that mirrors the trauma system with primary and comprehensive designated stroke centers has evolved in the United States with the formal certification of comprehensive stroke centers in 2012 (Alberts et al., 2000, 2005).

Inclusion criteria for administration of alteplase in the NINDS rtPA trial were acute ischemic stroke with a clearly defined time of onset (<3 hours), neurological deficit measurable on the NIH Stroke Scale, and CT scan without evidence of intracranial hemorrhage. Patients who awoke from sleep had symptom onset defined as "when last seen awake and normal." Exclusion criteria for administration of alteplase were rapidly improving or isolated minor neurological deficits, seizure at the onset of stroke, prior intracranial hemorrhage, symptoms suggestive of subarachnoid hemorrhage, blood glucose less than 50 mg/dL (2.8 mmol/L) or greater than 400 mg/dL (22.2 mmol/L), GI or genitourinary bleeding within the 3 weeks before stroke, recent MI, current use of oral anticoagulants (PT >15 seconds or INR >1.7), a prolonged aPTT or use of heparin in the previous 48 hours, platelet count less than 100,000/mL, another stroke or serious head injury in the previous 3 months, major surgery within the previous 14 days, arterial puncture at a noncompressible site within the previous 7 days, or pretreatment SBP 185 mm Hg or above or DBP 110 mm Hg or above. Some of these original exclusion criteria were subsequently modified. In particular, seizure at onset of symptoms is considered an exclusion criterion only if residual impairments are postictal, and only blood glucose levels below 50 mg/dL are an exclusion, without an upper value as previously recommended (Jausch et al., 2013). More recently, recent MI, GI or genitourinary bleeding, and recent surgery have become relative contraindications and it may be reasonable to treat selected patients with these factors (Jauch, 2013).

The use of IV alteplase in the ATLANTIS trial was terminated early because of nonstatistical efficacy at interim analysis (Clark et al., 1999). Favorable outcome at 3 months was 42.3% for those treated with alteplase, versus 38.9% for those treated with placebo. Mortality at 3 months was 11.0% for alteplase-treated patients versus 6.9% for those patients receiving placebo. Symptomatic intracranial hemorrhage occurred in 7.0% of alteplase-treated patients. The Second European-Australasian Acute Stroke Study investigators assessed the safety and efficacy of IV alteplase (0.9 mg/kg of body weight) administered within 6 hours of ischemic stroke onset and failed to confirm a statistical benefit for alteplase; symptomatic intracranial hemorrhage occurred in 8.8% of alteplase-treated patients and in 3.4% of placebo-treated patients (Hacke et al., 2008b). An earlier study using a dose of alteplase of 1.1 mg/kg also failed to demonstrate therapeutic efficacy among 620 patients treated within 6 hours from ischemic stroke onset (Hacke et al., 1995). Favorable outcome at 3 months was 35.7% for those treated with alteplase versus 24.3% for those receiving placebo. Mortality at 3 months was 22.4% for alteplase-treated patients versus 15.8% for those treated with placebo (Clark et al., 1999).

The following seem to be predictors of favorable outcome with IV thrombolytic therapy with alteplase for acute ischemic stroke: treatment within 90 minutes of symptom onset, normal baseline CT scan, milder baseline stroke severity, no history of DM, normal pretreatment blood glucose level, and normal pretreatment blood pressure. The following seem to portend a less favorable outcome and/or increased risk for cerebral hemorrhage: extended area of low attenuation with mass effect or low attenuation on a third or more of the MCA territory on pretreatment CT scan; advanced age; prior head injury; DM; marked elevation of the blood pressure before, during, and after treatment; hypertension requiring post-randomization antihypertensive treatment; severe pretreatment neurological deficits; and protocol violations according to the NINDS study protocol (Hacke et al., 2004). Overall, for every 100 patients with acute ischemic stroke treated with IV alteplase in the 0- to 3-hour window, 32 patients benefit and 3 patients are harmed. For every 100 patients with acute ischemic stroke who are treated with IV alteplase in the 3- to 4.5-hour window, 16 patients benefit and 3 are harmed (Fig. 65.29).

While the various trials of alteplase did include patients with low NIHSS scores, patients without disabling deficits were not fluently enrolled. PRISMS was a randomized clinical trial of patients with NIHSS 0–5 with nondisabling clinical deficits and symptom onset

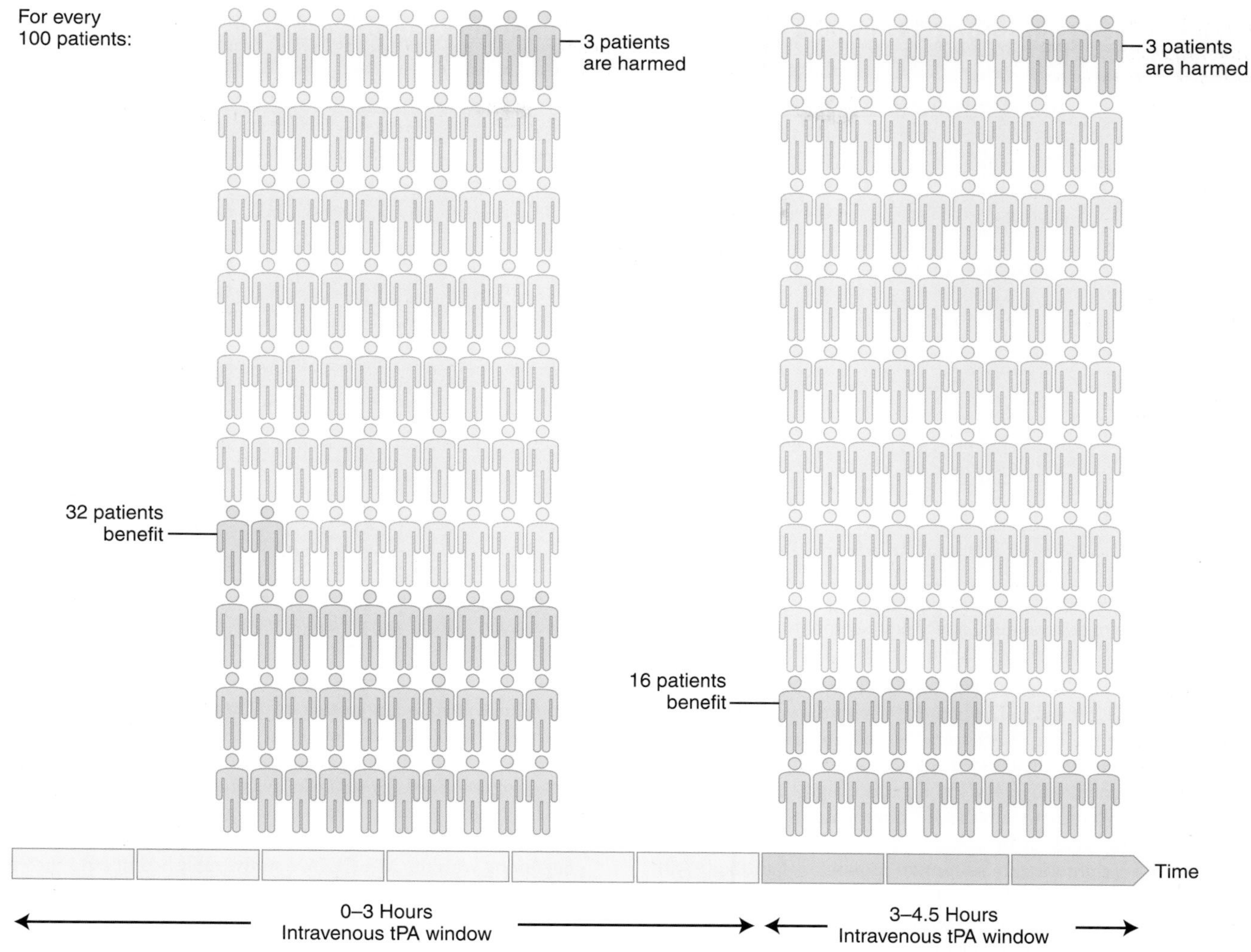


**Fig. 65.29** Risk/benefit ratio of IV tissue plasminogen activator (*tPA,* alteplase) for acute ischemic stroke in the 0- to 3-hour and 3- to 4.5-hour windows. (Created and designed by Gabriel A. Biller.)

within 3 hours of treatment. The study found that treatment with alteplase was not superior to aspirin (risk difference 1.1%, 95% CI 9.4% to 7.3%); 5 alteplase patients (3.2%) versus none of the aspirin-only patents had symptomatic ICH (risk difference 3.35, 95% CI 0.8–7.45). The study was terminated early, however, because of low enrollment. (Khatri et al., 2018).

The standard alteplase dose in the United States and Europe is 0.9 mg/kg. In Asian populations, however, studies have suggested that a lower dose of 0.6 mg/kg of alteplase may be equally effective. This recommendation is somewhat controversial. The Enhanced Control of Hypertension and Thrombolysis Stroke Study (ENCHANTED) found that patients with lower-dose alteplase failed to achieve non-inferiority in the primary outcome of death or disability, though there was less symptomatic ICH in the low-dose alteplase group. The current Chinese Stroke Association guidelines recommend full-dose IV alteplase, with lower-dose alteplase as a consideration for patients deemed at high risk of hemorrhage (Class IIb, Evidence level C) (Dong et al., 2017) In Japan, however, the lower alteplase dose of 0.6 mg/kg is recommended for acute stroke patients (Kern et al., 2013)

A number of other thrombolytic drugs have been investigated. Tenecteplase (TNK) is a thrombolytic agent with a longer half-life, improved fibrin specificity, and increased resistance to plasminogen activator inhibitor 1 (PAI-1) compared to alteplase (Haley et al., 2005). A small phase IIb dose-finding study of TNK in 75 patients randomized to TNK 0.1 mg/kg, TNK 0.25 mg/kg, or alteplase 0.9 mg/kg reported significantly favorable imaging and clinical outcomes for patients receiving the higher TNK dose without a significant impact on intracranial bleeding risk (Parsons et al., 2012). TNK before mechanical thrombectomy (0.25 mg/kg; maximum dose 25 mg) was associated with higher reperfusion rates and better functional outcome among patients eligible for mechanical thrombectomy, as compared with standard-dose alteplase (0.9 mg//kg; maximum dose 90 mg); 22% of tenecteplase and 10% of alteplase patients met the primary outcome of reperfusion in >50% of the involved ischemic territory or absence of retrievable thrombus at time of initial diagnostic angiogram (difference 12% with 95% CI 2–21; $P = 0.03$ for superiority) (Campbell et al., 2018)

Desmoteplase is a genetically engineered version of a clot-dissolving protein from vampire bats. The Desmoteplase in Acute Ischemic Stroke (DIAS) study and the Dose Escalation Study of Desmoteplase in Acute Ischemic Stroke (DEDAS) were randomized phase II clinical trials of patients who were enrolled within 3–9 hours of symptom onset using MRI criteria to identify those eligible for the trials on the basis of diffusion/perfusion mismatch. DEDAS demonstrated clinical improvement of up to 60% compared with placebo in patients who

**TABLE 65.6 Randomized Clinical Trials of Mechanical Thrombectomy for Acute Ischemic Stroke Within 12 Hours**

| | MR CLEAN | SWIFT PRIME | EXTEND-IA | ESCAPE | REVASCAT |
|---|---|---|---|---|---|
| Number of patients | 500 | 196 | 70 | 316 | 206 |
| IV tPA rate intervention vs. control | 87% vs. 91% | 100% vs. 100% | 100% vs. 100% | 73% vs. 79% | 68% vs. 77.7% |
| Imaging | CT/CTA | CT/CTA or MRA | CT/CTA/CTP | CT/multiphase CTA | CT/CTA MRDWI/MRA |
| Target vessels | ICA, M1, M2, A1, A2 | ICA, M1 | ICA, M1, M2 | ICA, M1, M2 | M1, ICA |
| NNT to achieve mRS 0–2 at 90 days | 7.4 | 4.3 | 3.2 | 4.2 | 6.4 |
| Median onset to groin puncture (minutes) | 260 | 252 | 210 | 185 | 269 |
| Treatment group sICH rate | 7.7% | 1% | 0% | 3.6% | 1.9% |
| Comments | | NIHSS improvement by 4.6 points at 27 hours | Lower mortality and improved 24h-NIHSS | | Sx onset to groin puncture delayed for CTA/MRA 30 minutes post IV tPA to exclude revascularized tPA patients |

*CT,* Computed tomography; *CTA,* computed tomography angiography; *ICA,* internal carotid artery; *IV tPA,* IV recombinant tissue plasminogen activator (alteplase); *M1,* middle cerebral artery first segment; *M2,* middle cerebral artery division; *MRA,* magnetic resonance angiography; *mRS,* modified Rankin scale; *NIHSS,* National Institutes of Health Stroke Scale; *NNT,* number needed to treat; *sICH,* symptomatic ICH.

received a dose of 125 mg/kg. The hemorrhage rate was relatively low, around 2% of patients. The DIAS study showed similar results (Hacke et al., 2005. The subsequent DIAS-2, DIAS-3, and DIAS-4 studies all failed to show a benefit above placebo for this drug, with DIAS-3 and DIAS-4 studying this drug within the 3–9 hour window after symptom onset (von Kummer et al., 2016).

Abciximab is a chimeric mouse/human monoclonal antibody with high binding for the platelet glycoprotein IIb/IIIa receptor. In a phase II safety study enrolling 400 patients within 6 hours of ischemic stroke, there was a low rate of symptomatic intracranial hemorrhage (3.6% of patients treated with drug [{7/195}] versus 1% for placebo [{2/199}]) (Abciximab Emergent Stroke Treatment Trial (AbESTT) Investigators, 2005). However, a subsequent phase III trial was stopped because of lack of benefit.

Argatroban is a direct IV thrombin inhibitor that was studied in a randomized double-blind placebo-controlled safety study of two doses in patients with acute stroke (<12 hours from symptom onset); there was no increase in hemorrhagic complications between low- and high-dose regimens. However, the study was not powered to assess efficacy of this agent (LaMonte et al., 2004). Argatroban has also been studied as an adjunct to both alteplase and mechanical endovascular thrombolysis to enhance vessel recanalization (Barreto et al., 2017). The Multi-arm Optimization of Stroke Thrombolysis (MOST) is a multicenter trial being initiated to determine if adding argatroban or eptifibatide results in better 90-day functional outcomes when used in conjunction with alteplase or mechanical thrombectomy (Adeoye et al., 2019; clincialtrials.gov).

Mechanical thrombectomy with newer catheter techniques has also been actively explored because of the hemorrhagic risks associated with various drugs. A number of devices have been tested for patients who are not within the time window or are not eligible for IV alteplase (e.g., recent surgery).

The MERCI coil retriever catheter was approved for retrieval of "cerebral clots" based on single-arm device studies. By 2013, a series of randomized clinical trials of endovascular mechanical thrombectomy trials were published, most prominently including the IMS-III trial that failed to show benefit of endovascular mechanical or pharmacological therapy above alteplase monotherapy. These trials are discussed in the Supplemental materials section.

*An extended version of this section is available online at http://expertconsult.inkling.com.* 

Beginning with the MR CLEAN study published in 2015, however, a number of thrombectomy trials have reported clinical benefits using newer-generation endovascular devices, including stent retrievers and newer aspiration devices (Berkehimer et al., 2015, Brocard et al., 2016; Campbell et al., 2015; Goyal et al., 2015; Jovin et al., 2015; Saver et al., 2015). The overall benefit in these trials for functional independence ranged from a NNT ratio of 3–7.5, which compares favorably with tPA alone in the 3–4.5 hour window (NNT of 5–13) (Saver et al., 2009), and in more severe patients (with MCA or distal ICA occlusions). Based on the clinical trials described below, the 2018 American Stroke Association guidelines recommend endovascular intervention for appropriately selected patients (Powers et al., 2018) (Table 65.6 and Box 65.8).

The Multicenter Randomized Clinical Trial of Endovascular Treatment for Acute Ischemic Stroke in the Netherlands (MR CLEAN) randomized 500 adult patients with ischemic stroke within 6 hours of onset, an NIHSS 2 or greater, and an established proximal vessel occlusion in the anterior circulation, to standard care including IV alteplase when appropriate or standard care plus endovascular treatment. Stent retrievers were employed in 81.5% of the endovascular group. Alteplase was given in 87% of patients randomized to endovascular therapy and 91% of control patients. The adjusted common OR for an improvement in the mRS at 90 days was 1.67 favoring intervention. At 90 days, mRS of 0–2 was achieved in 33% of the endovascular group compared to 19% of control patients. Mortality and serious adverse events, including symptomatic ICH, were similar between the groups (Berkhemer et al., 2015).

The Endovascular Treatment for Small Core and Anterior Circulation Proximal Occlusion with Emphasis on Minimizing CT to Recanalization Times (ESCAPE) trial was terminated after an interim analysis of the initial 315 randomized patients demonstrated efficacy. Eligible patients were 18 years or older with a disabling ischemic stroke

**BOX 65.8 Criteria for Intra-Arterial Thrombectomy Based on the 2018 AHA/ASA Guidelines Categorized by Evidence Class and Recommendation Grade**

1. Class Ia
   a. Pre-stroke mRS 0–1
   b. For eligible patients, receiving IV alteplase within 4.5 hours of symptom onset
   c. Occlusion of the iCA or proximal M1-MCA segment
   d. Age 18 or older
   e. NIHSS score ≥6
   f. ASPECTS score ≥6
   g. Time to groin puncture within 6 hours of symptom onset
   h. For selected patients within 6–16 hours of symptom onset with anterior circulation LVO who meet other eligibility criteria of the DAWN and DEFUSE-3 studies
2. Class IIa
   a. For selected patents who were last seen normal 16–24 hours from symptom onset with anterior LVO occlusion who meet the other criteria of the DAWN study
3. Class IIb
   a. Stent retrievers may be reasonable for M2 or M3 segments in patients for whom groin puncture is initiated within 6 hours
   b. Similarly, there may be benefit for select patients with occlusion of the ACA, PCA or vertebral and basilar arteries
   c. There may be benefit for selected patients with mRS >1, ASPECTS < or NIHSS <6 and ICA or M1 occlusions
   d. At the present time, stent retrievers are preferred to other endovascular devices

From Powers, W.J., Rabinstein, A.A., Ackerson, T., et al., 2018. The 2018 Guideline for the early management of patients with acute ischemic stroke: A guideline for healthcare professionals from the American Heart Association/American Stroke Association. Stroke 49, e46–e99. *ACA*, Anterior cerebral artery; *ICA*, internal carotid artery; *IV*, intravenous; *LVO*, large-vessel occlusion; *MCA*, middle cerebral artery; *mRS*, modified Rankin scale; *NIHSS*, National Institutes of Health Stroke Scale; *PCA*, posterior cerebral artery.

within 12 hours of onset. Additionally, patients had to have CT angiography evidence of proximal occlusion of the distal internal carotid artery, or M1 or M2 segment of the MCA, and good to moderate collateral filling by multiphase CT angiography. IV alteplase was used in 73% of patients in the intervention group and 79% of control patients. Only 15.5% of patients were randomized beyond 6 hours of onset. The median stroke onset to reperfusion was 241 minutes. The adjusted common OR for an improvement in mRS at 90 days was 3.1 in favor of intervention. A favorable outcome (mRS 0–2) at 90 days was achieved in 53% of patients in the interventional group compared to 29.3% of control patients. Mortality in the interventional group was half that of the control group and the symptomatic ICH rates were comparable (Goyal et al., 2015).

The Time for Thrombolysis in Emergency Neurological Deficits—Intra-Arterial (EXTEND-IA) trial was also halted early after the initial 70 patients had been randomized to either intervention (groin puncture within 6 hours of stroke onset) or standard care. Eligible patients had to have an ischemic stroke within 4.5 hours of onset, evidence of distal internal carotid artery or MCA stem occlusion, and received IV alteplase. Imaging eligibility requirements included an infarct core less than 70 mL and ischemic penumbra greater than 10 mL. Median time from stroke onset to initial recanalization was 248 minutes and reperfusion was achieved in 100% of the patients in the endovascular group compared to 37% of control patients ($P < .001$). By 24 hours, 80% of patients in the endovascular group had improved by 8 or more points on the NIHSS, compared to 37% in the control group ($P = .002$). Independent outcome (mRS 0–2) at 90 days was achieved in 71% of the endovascular treatment group and 40% of the control group ($P < .01$). There were no significant differences in mortality or symptomatic ICH between groups (Campbell et al., 2015).

The Solitaire FR With Intent For Primary Endovascular Treatment for Acute Ischemic Stroke (SWIFT PRIME) trial was also halted after 196 patients had been randomized. Patients 18–80 years old with NIHSS 8–29 and occlusion of the distal internal carotid artery or MCA stem were randomized to thrombectomy with a stent retriever (groin puncture within 6 hours of stroke onset) or control. Eligible patients had to present within 4.5 hours, and received IV alteplase. Functional independence (mRS 0–2) at 90 days was achieved in 60% of the intervention group and 36% of the control group ($P = .008$). Mean NIHSS at 27 hours was also significantly lower in the interventional group. Mortality, serious adverse events, and symptomatic ICH (ICH) rates were similar between the groups (see Table 65.6).

The Randomized Trial of Revascularization with Solitaire FR Device versus Best Medical Therapy in the Treatment of Acute Stroke Due to Anterior Circulation Large Vessel Occlusion Presenting within Eight Hours of Symptom Onset (REVASCAT) randomized 206 patients to receive medical therapy versus medical therapy with endovascular intervention with ICA or M1 occlusions (Jovin et al., 2015). Patients between ages 18 and 80 years were enrolled if they had a pre-stroke mRS of 0–1, NIHSS ≥ 6, and had an ASPECTS score of less than 7 by CT or DW-MRI ASPECTS score less than 6. After the first 100 patients were enrolled, the critiera were modified to include patients up to age 85 with an ASPECTS score greater than 8. The primary outcome was mRS at 90 days. The study was halted prematurely (original sample size of 690 patients) when the results of other stent-retriever thrombectomy trials were published. The study found that disability was decreased at 90 days across the mRS scale range (OR for 1 point improvement = 1.75, 95% CI 1.05–2.8) with higher rates of good outcome (mRS scores of 0–2) in the thrombectomy group (43.7%) versus the control group (28.2%) (OR 2.1, 95% CI 1.1–40). Symptomatic ICH rates were 1.9% in both groups and there were no significant differences in mortality rates between the groups. REVASCAT was unique among these stent-retriever mechanical thrombectomy trials because patients underwent vessel imaging with CTA or MRA 30 minutes after IV alteplase, and those without LVO were then excluded from the trial. The REVASCAT was also part of a nationwide Spanish registry of endovascular patients. In that registry, 540 patients underwent any type of endovascular treatment for acute stroke and 464 (86%) were treated at REVASCAT study hospitals; 111 of those patients met study criteria and only 8 study eligible patients were treated outside the REVASCAT protocol. Unlike some of the other studies, CT or MR perfusion imaging was not utilized as part of the REVASCAT patient selection strategy. The study did utilize the ASPECTS score, and retrospective central adjudicated imaging review demonstrated that 25% of enrolled patients had ASPECTS scores of ≤ 6 and 9% had M2 occlusions, which were exclusion criteria for intervention in the REVASCAT study. The enrollment of patients with possibly large infarcts (based on ASPECTS score), the longer time from symptom onset to groin puncture, and the decision to terminate the REVASCAT trial early, may also explain the lower treatment effect seen in this study compared to the other stent-retriever studies.

The DAWN trial reported results of mechanical thrombectomy for patients with large-vessel occlusion (LVO) of the proximal MCA or intracranial ICA who had been last seen well 6–24 hours prior to intervention; the DEFUSE-3 study reported similar results for patients last seen well 6–16 hours prior to intervention (Albers et al., 2018; Nogueira et al., 2018). In both trials, patients were enrolled if they had LVO on CT angiography and mismatch between infarct volume and clinical severity based on DW-MRI or perfusion CT measured using automated imaging software (RAPID; Campbell et al., 2018). Endovascular therapy was associated with a higher percentage of functionally independent patients, without an increase in serious adverse events. In the DEFUSE-3 study 45% of those who underwent thrombectomy versus 17% who did not undergo intervention ($P < .0010$) were functionally independent with mRS of 0–2. There was a similar result in the DAWN study, with functional independence at 90 days of 49% in the thrombectomy group versus 13% in the control group. In both studies, there was no increase in the rate of symptomatic ICH or death in the thrombectomy groups.

## Defibrinogenating and Hemorrheological Agents

Ancrod, an enzyme extracted from the venom of the Malayan pit viper, lowers fibrinogen and blood viscosity, inhibits erythrocyte aggregation, indirectly stimulates thrombolysis, and possibly causes local vasodilatation. It also has a weak anticoagulant effect at high dosages.

Its potential as a treatment for ischemic stroke was shown to be beneficial when initiated within 3 hours of stroke onset in the multicenter Stroke Treatment with Ancrod Trial (Sherman et al., 2000). The positive results of this study were not replicated in a subsequent study of IV ancrod within 6 hours after stroke onset (Levy and del Zoppo, 2009). Hemorheological therapy with isovolemic, hypovolemic, or hypervolemic hemodilution has been ineffective. A study of high-dose human albumin (2 g/kg 25% albumin) administered within 5 hours of ischemic stroke showed no benefit (90-day mRS 0 or 1) compared to an equivalent volume of isotonic saline (Ginsberg et al., 2013).

## Neuroprotective Agents

Despite widespread interest in neuroprotective drug therapy and positive results in experimental animals, no neuroprotective agent has been approved to date by the FDA for acute ischemic stroke (O'Collins et al., 2006).

More than 120 controlled clinical trials involving more than 21,000 subjects and investigating numerous neuroprotective interventions have yielded negative results. Unfortunately, very few of these studies included patients within the first 4–6 hours of ischemia. New agents (intrathecal agents, oxygenated fluorocarbon nutrient emulsions, α-amino-3-hydroxy-5-methyl-4-isoxazole propionic acid antagonists, potassium channel openers, minocycline, and high-dose statins) have been proposed. Intracellular adhesion molecules (ICAMs) are molecules to which leukocytes adhere and which facilitate migration of leukocytes through the endothelium. Some of these molecules are expressed in the cerebral vasculature during ischemia. Neutrophils in particular can contribute to tissue injury by obstructing capillaries and possibly by liberating cytotoxic products. Prevention of neutrophil adhesion by infusion of monoclonal antibodies directed at ICAMs improved neurological outcome in animal models of transient ischemia, but clinical trials yielded negative results. The sudden decrease in blood flow after ischemia provokes a cascade of events eventually leading to cell death. These events include the release of excitatory amino acids (EAAs) with secondary opening of ion channels, which leads to an increase in intracellular calcium concentration, activation of enzymes, and generation of free radicals. Several agents have been shown in vitro and in animal studies to interfere at various steps of this cascade, thus potentially protecting the cells from ischemia. Cerebro-selective calcium channel blockers such as nimodipine have been tested in acute stroke, but the benefits for patients with acute ischemic stroke remain unproven. Endogenous EAA neurotransmitters play a major role in the pathogenesis of cerebral ischemia. In animals, EAA antagonists reduce the size of an infarct after occlusion of a major artery. From preliminary studies, some of these compounds appear to be safe in humans, but their efficacy has not been demonstrated, and several clinical trials yielded negative results. Optimal protective regimens may necessitate blockading of both *N*-methyl-D-aspartate (NMDA) and non-NMDA receptors. Pre-hospital administration of magnesium, an NMDA antagonist, to patients with suspected stroke was reported to be safe but did not improve clinical outcomes in a randomized controlled trial (Saver, 2015). Free radicals produced during ischemia can degrade polyunsaturated lipids, which are building blocks of cellular membranes, by means of lipid peroxidation. The CNS appears particularly susceptible to free radical injury. The 21 aminosteroid compounds inhibit lipid peroxidation by scavenging free radicals. Tirilazad is one such compound that decreases damage secondary to global ischemia in experimental animal models, but its clinical application in the treatment of patients with ischemic stroke has not been established. Cerovive (NXY-059), a free-radical trapping agent, administered within 6 hours of symptom onset, was associated with improvement in primary outcome of disability post stroke ($P = .038$) by the mRS in the SAINT I study of 1722 patients (Lees et al., 2006). This randomized double-blind placebo-controlled study reported a favorable outcome regardless of stroke severity, with an OR of 1.2. The Barthel Index supported the primary mRS findings. However, no statistical difference of clinical deficits, as measured by the NIHSS scores, was seen in this trial. Safety of this drug was comparable with placebo, and there was also a suggestion of less intracranial hemorrhage in patients who received the study drug along with alteplase. A subsequent study showed no effect of treatment versus placebo in patients with acute ischemic stroke (Diener et al., 2008). Neurotrophins are factors known to promote cell growth in certain neuronal populations. Studies have shown that some of these factors given intraventricular route to animals during ischemia reduce infarct size. The mechanism of action is still unknown but could be related to interaction with EAAs. Calpains are cytosomal enzymes that are normally quiescent but become activated by increases in intracellular calcium concentration. These enzymes have many proteins as their targets, and thus their activation can cause considerable damage. In experimental models of stroke in animals, intra-arterial infusion of calpain inhibitors given after onset of ischemia significantly reduced infarct size compared with controls. The value of calpain inhibitors in humans has not been established. Treatments with gangliosides, barbiturates, prostacyclin, opiate antagonists, aminophylline, β-adrenergic receptor blockers, vasopressor therapy, naftidrofuryl, clomethiazole, inhibitors of leukocyte adhesion, fosphenytoin, lubeluzole, basic fibroblast growth factor, and citicoline have been ineffective.

## Hypothermia

Therapeutic hypothermia is a well-established neuroprotective strategy in the management of anoxic encephalopathy after cardiac arrest and perinatal asphyxia. Fever in stroke patients is associated with poor outcomes, and induced hypothermia may be neuroprotective in patients with acute cerebral ischemia. A number of hypothermic strategies are being investigated in acute ischemic stroke, and several small clinical trials have been performed, including the combination of caffeinol with hypothermia in patients with acute stroke given IV alteplase (Martin-Schild et al., 2009). While the validity of these hypothermia protocols is unproven, aggressive management of fever should be pursued in all acute stroke patients (Jausch et al., 2013). To date, however, induced hypothermia has no proven benefit for better outcome of acute ischemic stroke patients.

## Surgical Therapy

### Symptomatic Carotid Artery Stenosis

Stroke is often caused by atherosclerotic lesions of the carotid artery bifurcation; approximately 15% of ischemic strokes are due to extracranial internal carotid artery stenosis. Carotid atherosclerosis develops in areas of low vessel-wall shear stress, most commonly the carotid bulb. In addition to the degree of carotid artery stenosis, plaque structure has been postulated as a critical factor in defining stroke risk. Ulcers found during CEA have been associated with cerebral artery microemboli detected by TCD ultrasound. Echolucent carotid artery plaques may also be associated with an increased risk for stroke. CEA, by removing the atherosclerotic plaque, restores CBF, and reduces the risk for cerebral ischemia. Results from three major prospective contemporary studies provide compelling evidence of the benefit of CEA performed by experienced surgeons in improving the chance of stroke-free survival in high-risk symptomatic patients. Timely surgical intervention in selected patients with hemispheric TIAs, amaurosis fugax, or completed nondisabling carotid territory strokes within the previous 6 months, and with 70%–99% diameter-reducing carotid stenosis, can significantly reduce the risk for recurrent cerebral ischemia or death. Other factors that increase the risk for ipsilateral stroke are hemispheric (rather than retinal) site of ischemia, ulcerative nature of the stenosis, presence of contralateral carotid artery occlusion, and vascular risk factors. Benefits of CEA are similar for men and women for high-grade carotid stenosis, but the benefit is less certain for moderate-grade stenosis. Older age by itself should not be considered a contraindication for properly selected patients with symptomatic high-grade carotid artery stenosis, but there are no data supporting CEA for octogenarians.

The North American Symptomatic Carotid Endarterectomy Trial (NASCET) confirmed the effectiveness of CEA for preventing stroke in 659 symptomatic patients with TIAs or minor strokes with high-grade (70%–99%) diameter-reducing carotid artery stenosis. A uniform and strict technique measured carotid artery stenosis from an arteriogram. For different endpoints, absolute risk reductions in favor of surgery were 17.0% for ipsilateral stroke; 15.0% for all strokes; 16.5% for the combined outcomes of all strokes and death; 10.6% for major ipsilateral stroke; 9.4% for all major strokes; and 10.1% for major stroke and death. Longer-term outcome was also better for surgically treated patients despite an occluded contralateral carotid artery. The European Carotid Surgery Trial (ECST) also indicated the benefit from CEA compared with medical therapy in patients with mild carotid territory ischemic events associated with a diameter-reducing proximal internal carotid stenosis between 70% and 99%. The cumulative risk for any ipsilateral stroke at 3 years was 10.3% for the surgical group and 16.8% for the medical group. The ECST used different criteria than the NASCET for measurement of carotid artery stenosis on angiography.

A diameter-reducing carotid artery stenosis of 70%–99% by NASCET criteria is equivalent to a stenosis of 82%–99% by ECST methodology; likewise, a stenosis of 70%–99% by ECST criteria is equivalent to a stenosis of 50%–99% by NASCET criteria.

These methodological differences were more important with mild carotid artery stenosis. The Veterans Administration (VAH) Trial of Carotid Endarterectomy in Symptomatic Carotid Stenosis was terminated early because of the positive results of the NASCET and ECST. The VAH study also showed that CEA improved outcome in selected symptomatic patients with high-grade extracranial carotid artery stenosis. Among symptomatic patients with less than 30% stenosis, results from the ECST favor the use of medical therapy with platelet antiaggregants.

The utility of CEA for symptomatic patients with 30%–69% carotid artery stenosis has also been determined. Results were analyzed separately for those patients with 30%–49% and those with 50%–69% stenosis. Analysis from 1599 patients suggests that CEA is not indicated in most of these patients (European Carotid Surgery Trialists' Collaborative Group, 1996).

With a low surgical risk, CEA also provides modest benefit in symptomatic patients with carotid artery stenosis of 50%–69% (Barnett et al., 1998), especially among men with hemispheric ischemia who are not diabetic. CEA provides no benefit if the stenosis is less than 50% (50% by NASCET criteria is equal to 75% stenosis by ECST criteria).

Overall for patients with 70%–99% internal carotid artery stenosis, the absolute risk reduction with surgery, based on the 5-year risk of stroke combined data from NASCET, ECST, and VAH, was 15.6% with an RRR of 48%. This translates into a NNT of 6. Thus, 156 strokes could be prevented by 1000 carotid endarterectomies. For patients with 50%–69% stenosis, the absolute risk reduction is 7.8%, with an RRR of 28%. This translates into an NNT of 13. Thus, 78 strokes could be prevented by 1000 carotid endarterectomies. Conversely, for patients with a "string" sign, the absolute risk reduction was 0.1%; thus no strokes are prevented with carotid endarterectomies in this subgroup of patients. The benefit of CEA is highly dependent on surgical risk. Mortality and morbidity due to CEA are significantly lower for asymptomatic patients. The acceptable level of surgical risk varies with the indication for carotid artery surgery. Maximal acceptable limits of surgical risks for combined perioperative neurological morbidity and mortality are 3% for asymptomatic patients, 5% for patients with TIAs, 7% for patients with stroke, and 10% for patients with recurrent stenosis. A combined analysis of the NASCET and ECST also showed that men fared better than women, and patients in the seventh decade of life had equal or greater benefit compared to younger patients (Rothwell et al., 2004).

Whether selected patients should undergo CEA, on the basis of duplex scanning alone (without cerebral angiography) or duplex scanning complemented by MRA or CTA, remains controversial. However, early intervention following symptom onset is critical. Pooled data of the ECST and NASCET showed that time from the last symptomatic event to treatment is an important factor in modifying the benefit for CEA. As delays to CEA increased, there was a marked decline in CEA benefit. For patients with symptomatic stenosis of greater than 50% diameter, the NNT to prevent one stroke was 5 for those treated within 2 weeks of symptoms, compared to 125 for patients treated more than 12 weeks post-event (Rothwell et al., 2004).

Options for intervention are limited when the carotid artery is totally occluded. An estimated 61,000 first-ever strokes and 19,000 TIAs per year may be associated with carotid occlusion. However, as opposed to coronary artery occlusions, bypass of an occluded carotid artery has not been shown to be associated with better outcome. An early randomized study of medical therapy versus extracranial/intracranial (EC/IC) bypass surgery failed to show a benefit for surgery, and the procedure was largely abandoned in the ensuing decades, with exceptions for certain unique circumstances such as moyamoya disease. The original EC/IC bypass study was widely criticized, however, because of selection biases and failure to identify a subgroup with possible hemodynamic compromise that might be more likely to benefit from the procedure. The measurement of OEF by PET has allowed investigators to identify particular high-risk patients who might benefit from EC/IC bypass. These patients have been enrolled in the Carotid Occlusion Surgery Study (COSS) that screened patients with carotid occlusion for low OEF measured by PET; those patients were then randomized to best medical therapy or best medical therapy plus EC/IC bypass surgery. In spite of excellent graft patency, EC/IC bypass surgery was no better than best medical therapy in the secondary prevention of ischemic stroke in COSS (Powers et al., 2011).

## Asymptomatic Carotid Artery Stenosis

Asymptomatic carotid artery atherosclerosis is prevalent in the general population, especially in the elderly. Compared with symptomatic stenosis, asymptomatic carotid artery stenosis is associated with a relatively low risk for ipsilateral cerebral infarction. Clagett and colleagues followed only 57 asymptomatic patients with cervical bruits and abnormal ocular pneumoplethysmography; only 29 were truly randomized to aspirin therapy or CEA. More unfavorable outcomes were noted in those patients undergoing CEA, and the researchers concluded that most asymptomatic patients with cervical bruits and abnormal ocular pneumoplethysmography are appropriately managed without CEA. The Carotid Artery Surgery Asymptomatic Narrowing Operations versus Aspirin (CASANOVA) trial enrolled asymptomatic patients with 50%–90% carotid artery stenosis. Patients with greater than 90% carotid artery stenosis were excluded on the basis of presumed surgical benefit. Overall, the trial showed no difference between the medically and surgically treated groups. The Mayo Asymptomatic Carotid Endarterectomy Trial was terminated early because of higher rates of MI and TIA in the surgical group. Patients in the surgical group did not receive aspirin, probably explaining those results. The Veterans Affairs Asymptomatic Carotid Endarterectomy Trial evaluated 444 asymptomatic patients with angiographically proven carotid stenosis of 50%–99%. The study showed an RRR in the incidence of ipsilateral neurological events in favor of surgery when both TIA and stroke were included as composite endpoints. However, when ipsilateral stroke was considered alone, only a nonsignificant trend favoring surgery was noted. For the combined outcome of stroke and death, no significant differences were found between the two treatment arms. The Asymptomatic Carotid Atherosclerosis Study (ACAS) found that CEA combined with aspirin and risk factor reduction was superior to aspirin and risk factor reduction alone in preventing ipsilateral stroke in patients younger than 80 years who had greater than 60% asymptomatic carotid artery stenosis. The ACAS angiography methods were similar to those of the NASCET. All patients randomized to the surgical arm of the study had a catheter angiogram but it was not mandatory in the medically treated patients. The aggregate procedural morbidity and mortality of the ACAS participating surgeons were extremely low. Based on a 5-year projection, the ACAS showed that CEA reduced the absolute risk for stroke by 5.9% (which corresponds to an absolute risk reduction of only 1% per year), and the RRR for stroke and death of 53%. The surgical benefit incorporated a perioperative stroke and death rate of 2.3%, including a permanent arteriography complication rate of 1.2%. It is also important to note that all patients with 60%–99% stenosis were analyzed together in this study. Similar results have been reported from the Asymptomatic Carotid Surgery Trial (ACST), a European trial of highly selected patients with greater than 70% carotid artery stenosis (by ultrasound) and no prior history of cerebrovascular disease (Halliday et al., 2004). In the ACST, the 5-year stroke risk for surgery was 6.4% compared with 11.8% for medical therapy for the endpoints of fatal or nonfatal stroke, but the benefit was not substantiated for patients older than 75 years of age.

Based on the current guidelines, controversy still surrounds the selection of asymptomatic patients for CEA. Given the low risk for stroke for all deciles until 80%–89% carotid artery stenosis demonstrated by the European Carotid Artery Surgery Trialists (European Carotid Surgery Trialists' Collaborative Group, 1995), some experts recommend surgery only when the degree of stenosis is greater than 80%, provided that the operation is performed by an experienced surgeon with a complication rate (combined arteriography and surgical) of 3% or less. Additionally, current guidelines state that CEA for asymptomatic carotid artery disease is proven only for patients 40–75 years of age with very well-defined clinical characteristics, while women with either asymptomatic or moderate (50%–69%) symptomatic carotid artery disease seem to derive a less clear benefit from CEA as opposed to men (Chaturvedi et al., 2005). The CREST-2 study is a two-arm randomized trial of medical therapy versus carotid artery endarterectomy or medical therapy versus carotid artery stenting that may help further define the role of procedural interventions for asymptomatic carotid artery disease (Howard et al., 2017).

The value of impaired cerebral vasomotor reactivity using IV administration of acetazolamide as a predictor of stroke risk in patients with asymptomatic carotid artery stenosis is controversial. The necessity for widespread screening of patients with asymptomatic carotid artery stenosis is not supported by available data. Although concomitant CEA and CABG can be achieved with acceptably low operative risk, the risk is higher for combined procedures, and the best management for symptomatic patients with carotid stenosis and coexisting severe carotid and coronary artery disease is still unknown (Pullicino and Halperin, 2005). The risk for postoperative events related to carotid artery stenosis, compared with combined CEA (or stent) and surgery, seems to be low for asymptomatic carotid stenosis patients, and available data do not justify preoperative prophylactic CEA in patients requiring coronary angioplasty.

## Stenting of the Carotid Artery and Other Cervicocerebral Vessels

Carotid artery angioplasty and stenting (CAS) has emerged as an alternative treatment to CEA, particularly in patients with internal carotid artery stenosis in an anatomically high location in the neck, carotid artery restenosis following prior CEA, radiation-induced carotid artery stenosis, and among certain high-risk patients with serious medical comorbidities (Mas et al., 2006). There is strong evidence for the clinical efficacy of CEA compared to medical therapy, but only recently has there been evidence suggesting that CAS is a reasonable alternative to CEA (Fig. 65.30).

Early CAS trials did not show benefit as compared with CEA in reducing stroke or death related to carotid artery stenosis. The Stenting and Angioplasty with Protection in Patients at High Risk for Endarterectomy (SAPPHIRE) study reported that in high-risk patients who would have been ineligible for enrollment in NASCET or ACAS, CAS was not inferior to CEA (Yadav et al., 2004). Between August 2000 and July 2002, 747 patients were enrolled in the study, and 334 patients underwent randomization. Of the 413 patients who were not randomly assigned to treatment, 406 were entered into the stent registry, and 7 were entered into the surgical registry. The overall primary event rate of stroke, myocardial events, or death at 30 days in the randomized trial was high, with a cumulative 30-day event rate of 12.2% in the CAS arm and 20.1% in the CEA arm. The study conclusion was that CAS was not inferior to CEA, but there was no nonprocedural (medical) arm to serve as a baseline comparator.

Thereafter, two European studies, the Stent-Supported Percutaneous Angioplasty of the Carotid Artery versus Endarterectomy (SPACE) and the Endarterectomy versus Stenting in Patients with Symptomatic Severe Carotid Stenosis (EVA-3S) suggested that CAS was inferior to CEA. Arguments regarding the generalizability of these results, secondary to issues with study design and proceduralist capabilities, failed to resolve the debate regarding the relative merits of CEA versus CAS.

The Carotid Revascularization Endarterectomy versus Stenting Trial (CREST), a North American–based study, showed that among patients with either symptomatic or asymptomatic carotid artery stenosis, the risk of stroke, MI, or death did not differ statistically between those patients who underwent CEA or CAS (Brott et al., 2010). The overall 4-year rate was 7.2% for CAS and 6.8% for CEA. There was no difference by sex or symptomatic status, but older patients fared better

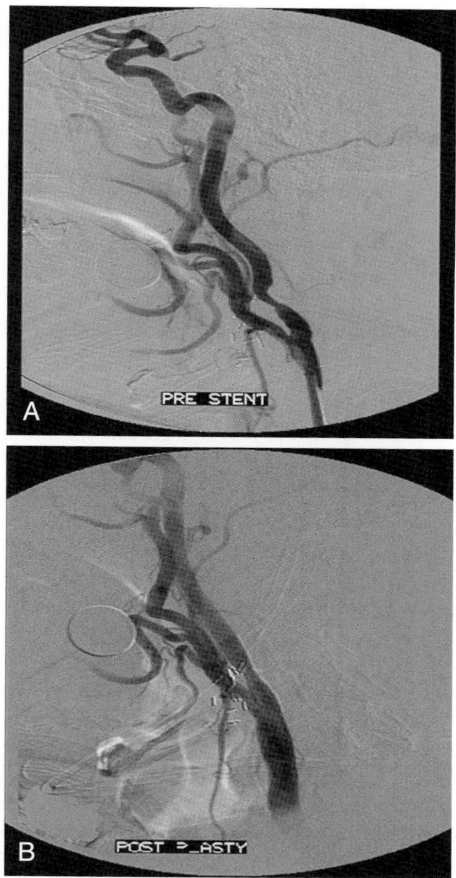


**Fig. 65.30** A 76-year-old man with 55% symptomatic right carotid artery stenosis presenting with decreased sensation on the left face, arm, and leg. **A**, The pre-stent cervical carotid artery. **B**, Same artery post-stent.

with CEA because of a lower stroke rate. Younger patients by contrast fared better with CAS as a result of a lower MI rate. Furthermore, there was a greater periprocedural stroke (CEA 2.3% versus CAS 4.3%; $P = .01$) or death rate in the CAS group (0.3% CEA versus 0.7% CAS; $P = .18$) and a greater MI (2.3% CEA versus 1.1% MI; $P = .03$) in the CEA group.

In contrast to CREST, the ICSS, a European study of 1713 patients with symptomatic carotid artery stenosis, reported a 30-day risk of stroke or death of 8.5% after CAS, versus 4.7% after CEA (HR 1.86, 95% CI 1.26–2.74; $P = .001$) (International Carotid Stent Study Investigators, 2010). In a substudy of 231 patients, there was a threefold excess risk of new ischemic lesions on DW-MRI in those patients who underwent CAS (Bonati et al., 2010). Furthermore, embolic protection devices did not protect CAS patients from developing new ischemic lesions. Thus, even though the CREST study suggests that CAS may be of benefit in selected patients when done by experienced proceduralists, the relative merit of CEA versus CAS remains a matter of considerable debate. CREST-2, described previously, may also give further perspective about stenting or surgery (as compared with medical therapy) in asymptomatic patients with high-grade carotid artery stenosis (Howard et al., 2017).

Stenting of intracranial arteries is still a procedure under development, though the frequency of ischemic stroke related to intracranial stenosis may be as high as that attributable to extracranial disease (Chimowitz et al., 1995). The procedure is not without risk, and compared to medical therapy, the rate of restenosis and other complications is not yet low enough to justify this procedure except in the context of clinical trials, although advocates have suggested that intracranial stenting is appropriate in cases with recurrent events despite aggressive medical therapy (Higashida et al., 2005). Two small single-arm studies have been published. In the Stenting of Symptomatic Atherosclerotic Lesions in the Vertebral or Intracranial Arteries (SSYLVIA) study, restenosis occurred in 12 of 37 (32.4%) intracranial cases and 6 of 14 (42%) extracranial vertebral artery stent cases; 39.1% of the restenosis cases were symptomatic (SSYLVIA Investigators, 2004), with a stroke rate of 4 in 55 (7.3%) within 6 months. In the Wingspan study, 45 patients underwent device placement for recurrent symptoms despite medical therapy (Higashida et al., 2005). Restenosis was low with this device, but the average stroke/death rate was 7.1% at 6 months (Fig. 65.31). The NINDS stopped enrollment early after 451 patients had been randomized in the Stenting versus Aggressive Medical Management for Preventing Recurrent Stroke in Intracranial Stenosis (SAMMPRIS) trial. Data indicated that aggressive medical management alone was superior to angioplasty combined with stenting in patients with symptomatic high-grade (equal or greater than 50%) intracranial arterial stenosis. Fourteen percent of patients in the angioplasty/stent arm experienced a stroke or died within the first 30 days of enrollment compared with 5.8% of patients treated with medical therapy alone (NINDS Clinical Alert, 2011).

## General Management of Acute Ischemic Stroke

Rapid diagnosis of stroke and initiation of treatment are important to maximize recovery, prevent recurrence of stroke, and prevent complications. Patients with a TIA or an acute stroke, regardless of severity, presenting within 72 hours of symptom onset should be admitted to the hospital for emergency evaluation and treatment,

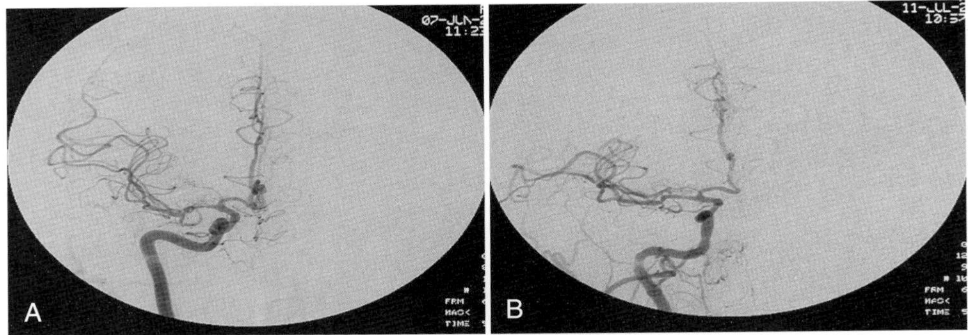


**Fig. 65.31** A 56-year-old man who had a transient ischemic attack and two ischemic strokes in the right middle cerebral artery (MCA) distribution. Because of recurrent strokes, despite optimal medical therapy in the context of a 65% to 70% focal stenosis of the M1 segment of the right MCA, the patient underwent placement of a Wingspan intracranial stent. **A**, The pre-stent proximal MCA stenosis. **B**, The immediate post-stent angiogram (note the wire in place following stent deployment).

preferably in a stroke unit or intensive care unit where close medical and nursing observation is available. Treatment of unselected acute stroke patients in specialized stroke units correlated with a lower mortality rate, reduced length of hospital stay, reduced frequency of discharge to a nursing home, and potentially reduced cost. Development of a stroke team is advantageous to expedite emergency care. Emergency care involves attention to the protection of the airway to avoid obstruction, hypoventilation, and aspiration. Pulse oximetry or arterial blood gases may be indicated. Supplemental oxygen and ventilatory assistance should be added if needed. Mild hypothermia protects the brain from ischemic injury; hyperthermia worsens ischemic outcome. Prevention of pulmonary complications is necessary in the bedridden patient or in the patient with impaired oropharyngeal function. The mortality rate from pneumonia is as high as 15%–25% in stroke patients. Aspiration was documented by video-fluoroscopic modified barium swallow examination in more than a third of patients with brainstem strokes, in one-fourth with bilateral hemispheric strokes, and one-tenth of patients with unilateral hemispheric strokes. If there is evidence of oropharyngeal dysfunction, it is important to place a temporary enteral feeding tube for administration of nutrition and enteral medication to minimize the risk for aspiration. Patients with oropharyngeal dysfunction, even if it appears to be mild, should receive nothing by mouth until evaluated by an experienced speech pathologist and until appropriate swallowing studies are completed. Frequent suctioning and maintenance of the head of bed greater than 30 degrees may help prevent aspiration of oral secretions.

The next step is assessment of the circulation. This involves evaluation of cardiac function and blood pressure. Because of the high frequency of cardiac dysfunction associated with stroke, cardiac monitoring is recommended for at least 48 hours after stroke. An immediate 12-lead ECG and troponin level should be obtained. Concomitant cerebral and myocardial ischemia can occur in approximately 3%–20% of cases. Ischemic stroke can be complicated by a variety of cardiac arrhythmias. If ischemic ECG changes occur or abnormal cardiac troponin levels are noted on admission, serial ECG and cardiac troponins are indicated. In patients with stroke, the blood pressure should be monitored frequently or even continuously for the first 48–72 hours. It is not unusual for the blood pressure to be transiently elevated after a stroke. Optimal arterial blood pressure post stroke appears to range from 160 to 200 mm Hg for SBPs and 70–110 mm Hg for DBPs (Castillo et al., 2004). Lower or higher arterial blood pressures were otherwise associated with an increased volume of stroke on CT scan 4–7 days post stroke. Following an acute event, the arterial blood pressure may return to pre-stroke levels within a few days. Whether transient elevations should be treated is controversial. It is important to not overtreat the blood pressure and cause hypotension. The most important objective is to maintain adequate CBF in the presence of impaired autoregulation. If urgent lowering of the blood pressure is indicated, IV labetalol can be given (e.g., 10 mg over 1–2 minutes, repeated or doubled every 10–20 minutes until the desired response has been achieved or a maximum dosage of 300 mg has been administered). Contraindications to the use of labetalol include congestive heart failure, asthma, second- or third-degree heart block, or cocaine use. Nicardipine may be a reasonable alternative IV agent. Therapy is usually initiated at 5 mg/h, and the infusion is titrated every 5–15 minutes by 2.5 mg/h to the desired rate, with a maximum dose of 15 mg/h. The use of immediate-release preparations of nifedipine, however, should be avoided because they lower the blood pressure in an unpredictable and sometimes dramatic fashion and have caused major cerebral infarcts. However, any blood pressure–lowering agent should be used with caution. The AHA guidelines suggest lowering the arterial blood pressure immediately post stroke only if the patient's blood pressure is above 220/130 mm Hg (Jausch et al., 2013) unless the patient is a candidate for thrombolytic therapy, in which case a target goal of less than 185/110 mm Hg is appropriate prior to thrombolysis. Pre-hospital acute treatment of elevated arterial hypertension does not appear to improve functional outcome (Right-2 Investigators, 2019). In patients presenting with acute ischemic stroke who are not candidates for thrombolytic therapy, the benefit of early treatment of arterial hypertension is uncertain within the first 48–72 hours (Whelton et al., 2017). For patients who received IV alteplase, a randomized study did not show a significant benefit as compared with prior guidelines for post-alteplase blood pressure management in the 72 hours post-thrombolysis, though perhaps with some non–statistically significant reduction in symptomatic ICH (Anderson et al., 2019).

Immediately after the patient's arrival in the emergency room, blood should be sent for appropriate studies, including a complete blood cell count, PT (INR), aPTT, and a general chemistry screen. A focused neurological examination should be performed to assess neurological stability and determine the extent of infarction. General signs that point toward a large infarction are forced eye deviation, hemiplegia, and altered consciousness. An NIHSS value of greater than 15 is another general indicator of a large infarction. Once stability of the airway, breathing, and circulation is determined and a focused neurological examination is performed to assess neurological stability, the patient should be sent immediately for emergent brain imaging with cranial CT scan without contrast or MRI. This can point the way to treat the patient with alteplase or to avoid antithrombotic therapies in patients with intracranial bleeds. CTA and/or CT perfusion studies may also be considered on an emergent basis for those patients who might be candidates for mechanical thrombectomy or alteplase in an extended time window.

Optimal target blood glucose levels in acute stroke patients remain largely unknown (Gray et al., 2004; Van den Berghe et al., 2006). The UK Glucose Insulin in Stroke Trial (GIST-UK) failed to demonstrate any clinical benefit of insulin-induced euglycemia (target glucose 72–126 mg/dL). Furthermore, mortality appeared to be higher among patients with the greatest glucose reduction (Gray et al., 2009). Moreover, in the Spectroscopic Evaluation of Lesion Evolution in Stroke: Trial of Insulin for Acute Lactic Acidosis (SELESTIAL), the infusion of glucose-potassium-insulin did not have a favorable impact on cerebral infarct growth (McCormick et al., 2010). Other studies, most recently including the Stroke Hyperglycemia Insulin Network Effort (SHINE) Trial, failed to show benefit for intensive glucose control immediately post stroke, with an increased risk of hypoglycemia compared with standard glucose control (Johnston et al., 2019). In the long term, however, pioglitazone may be of benefit for stroke patients without diabetes, who had insulin resistance, in preventing recurrent stroke or MI. There was also a lower risk of DM, albeit with significant risk of weight gain, edema, and fractures that might limit use of this drug in stroke patients (Kernan et al., 2016).

Attention should be directed not only to treating the stroke but also to preventing complications. A variety of neurological and medical complications can arise after a stroke. During the first week after an acute cerebral infarction, the most common cause of deterioration is development of brain edema. Brain edema begins to develop within the first several hours after an ischemic event and reaches its peak 72–120 hours after the stroke. Ischemic edema is initially cytotoxic and later vasogenic. Cytotoxic edema involves predominantly the gray matter, whereas vasogenic edema involves predominantly the white matter. Those at greatest risk for development of brain herniation due to edema are younger patients and those with large infarctions, often caused by large-artery occlusions. No specific pharmacological agent has been proven effective against ischemic cerebral edema. Corticosteroids are not indicated for acute ischemic stroke. Traditional treatment of increased intracranial pressure associated with acute ischemic stroke is shown in Box 65.9. In some circumstances of malignant cerebral edema associated with large MCA ischemic infarctions, hemicraniectomy and durotomy may be indicated (Gupta et al., 2004; Schneck et al., 2006; Vahedi et al., 2007a, 2007b) (Fig. 65.32). For cerebellar strokes with edema and herniation, posterior fossa decompression may be life saving (Fig. 65.33). Ventriculostomy may also be performed, but it carries the potential risk for upward herniation of the cerebellum.

### BOX 65.9 Medical Management Guidelines for Elevated Intracranial Pressure in Patients with Acute Ischemic Stroke

**Correction of Factors Exacerbating Increased Intracranial Pressure:**

Hypercarbia
Hypoxia
Hyperthermia
Acidosis
Hypotension
Hypovolemia

**Positional**

Avoidance of head and neck positions compressing jugular veins
Avoidance of flat supine position; elevation of head of bed 15 degrees

**Medical Therapy**

Endotracheal intubation and mechanical ventilation if Glasgow Coma Scale score ≤8
Hyperventilation to a $P_{CO_2}$ of 35 ± 3 mm Hg (if herniating)
Hyperosmolar therapy with mannitol or hypertonic saline.

**Fluid Management**

Maintenance of euvolemia with isotonic solutions using normal saline; avoidance of glucose-containing solutions because hyperglycemia is associated with worse prognosis for stroke; replacement of urinary losses with normal saline in patients receiving mannitol

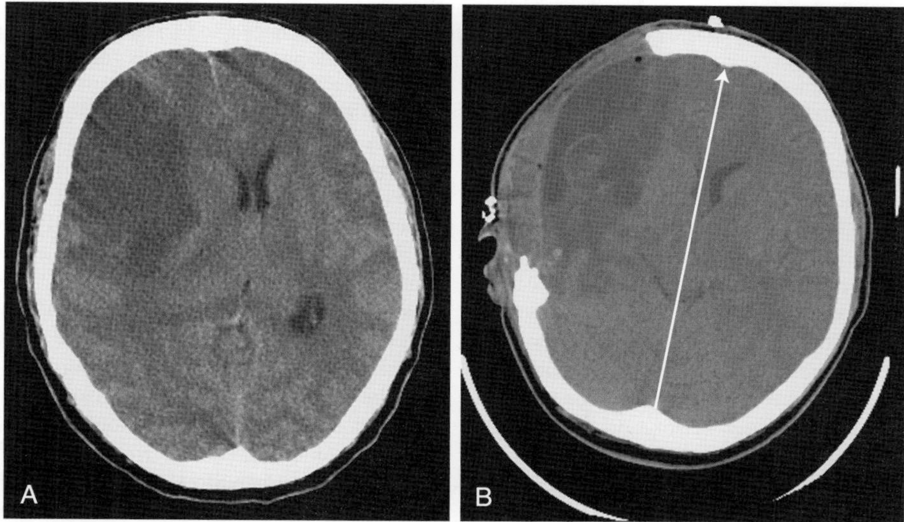


**Fig. 65.32** A 50-year-old man with right internal carotid artery occlusion who had acute onset of dysarthria, right gaze preference, left facial droop, left hemiplegia, and left hemianesthesia. He had a decline in the level of consciousness from admission and was taken to surgery 48 hours post stroke for large frontal-temporal-parietal-occipital craniotomy with temporal and frontal lobectomy and durotomy. **A,** Computed tomography (CT) scan showing a right frontal infarction with subfalcine herniation. **B,** CT scan 5 days following surgery showing outward swelling of the brain, with resolution of the right-to-left midline shift.

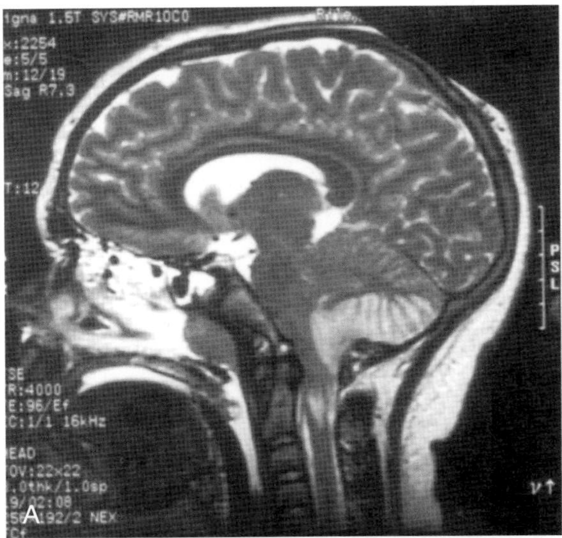


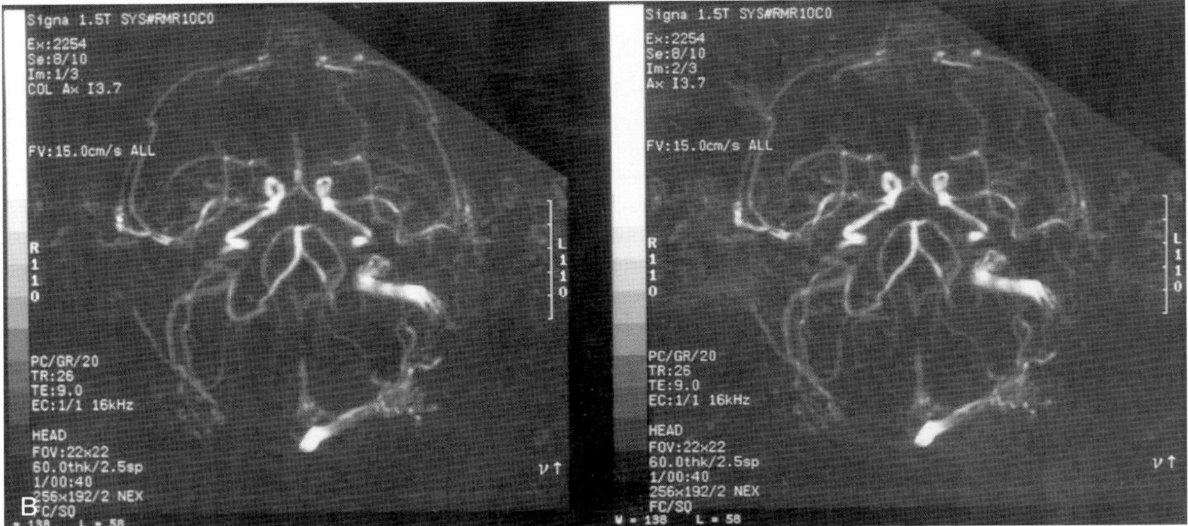


**Fig. 65.33** A 10-year-old girl with otomastoiditis was evaluated because of unresponsiveness. Magnetic resonance imaging shows areas of increased signal in the right cerebellum greater than the left cerebellum, consistent with infarctions. The cerebellar tonsils are herniated. **A**, Associated edema occurs in the superior cervical cord and inferior medulla. Phase-contrast magnetic resonance angiography images demonstrate lack of flow in the straight sinus and the right transverse sinus. Only a small amount of signal in the region of the right sigmoid and internal jugular vein is seen. **B**, Some arterial flow is represented in the examination.

In the second through the fourth weeks, pneumonia is the most common cause of non-neurological death. Many cases of pneumonia are caused by aspiration of food, saliva, or regurgitated gastric secretions, inert substances, or bacterial pathogens in saliva. Other potential complications include seizures, cardiac arrhythmias, MI, DVT, electrolyte disturbances, decubitus ulcers, and urosepsis. Cardiac dysfunction can manifest as ECG changes, arrhythmias, or myocardial ischemia.

Frequent neurological checks are essential for early recognition of neurological changes associated with herniation, recurrent or progressive stroke, or complications such as seizures. Seizures occur in a small percentage (<5%) of patients after an ischemic stroke. Antiseizure medications should be initiated if a seizure occurs.

DVT in a hemiparetic limb is common. The risk for VTE persists into the post-stroke period. If there are no contraindications, low-dose subcutaneous UFH at a dosage of 5000 units twice a day or LMWH is used. The Prevention of VTE after Acute Ischemic Stroke with LMWH (PREVAIL) study showed that enoxaparin (40 mg once daily) was superior to UFH in preventing VTE in patients with acute ischemic stroke but was associated with a small increase in extracranial hemorrhage rates (Kase et al., 2009). If heparin is contraindicated, intermittent pneumatic compression (IPC) of the lower extremities is recommended. Prophylactic doses of heparin can safely be given to patients receiving aspirin. The CLOTS 3 trial corroborated the effectiveness of IPC in reducing the risk of DVT in a wide variety of patients who were immobile following stroke (CLOTS (Clots in Legs OR sTockings after Stroke) Trials Collaboration, 2013).

The patient's nutritional status and fluid requirements should be assessed. Swallowing function should be assessed before intake of fluid or food is initiated. Patients who have significant oropharyngeal dysfunction require parenteral or tube feeding.

Although urinary incontinence is not uncommon in the acute phase of stroke, indwelling catheters should be avoided unless absolutely necessary and should be removed at the earliest possible time to avoid urosepsis. The chronic use of an indwelling catheter should be limited to patients with urinary retention that is refractory to other treatments. In the presence of an indwelling catheter, treatment of asymptomatic bacteriuria is usually not indicated. However, for significant clinical infections with pyuria and fever, treatment is recommended. Approximately 15% of patients develop pressure sores after a stroke. Steps to avoid this complication include frequent inspection of the skin, skin cleansing, frequent turning, use of special mattresses and protective dressings, maintaining adequate nutritional status, and trying to improve the patient's mobility early on. One of the most common causes of injury to the patient with a stroke is falling. Assessments of the risk for falling should be made at regular intervals during the acute hospitalization and also during the chronic rehabilitation phase. Reduction of postprandial SBP has been associated with a higher incidence of falls and syncope. Measures should be instituted to minimize the risk for falls (Divani et al., 2009). Shoulder subluxation can occur in hemiplegic patients. Chronic sequelae can be minimized if therapy is initiated before severe restriction of movement develops. Rehabilitation after stroke begins as soon as the diagnosis of stroke is established and any life-threatening neurological or medical complications have been stabilized (see Chapter 55). Patients are screened to evaluate whether they are candidates for rehabilitation. The criteria used to make this decision, including the stroke survivor's clinical and neurological status and social and environmental factors, are complex (Post-Stroke Rehabilitation Guideline Panel, 1995). The available evidence on the effectiveness of rehabilitation suggests that rehabilitation is beneficial to some patients, but the superiority of one type or the characteristics of patients most likely to benefit are not clear. Depressive symptoms are common after stroke, occurring in more than 25% of patients. Stroke patients should be screened for depression. Depression is more common following left hemispheric infarcts, especially in the frontal lobe, possibly caused by disruption of catecholamine pathways. Treatment with antidepressants is often successful in ameliorating symptoms.

## Cerebral Venous Thrombosis

Intracranial sinovenous occlusive disease is an infrequent condition (0.5%–1% of all strokes) with a variety of causes. The increasing recognition of this condition is probably due to an enhanced clinical awareness and the use of MRI. Intracranial venous thrombosis can be aseptic or septic. Septic intracranial venous thrombosis (resulting from skull osteomyelitis, suppurative infections of the inner ear, and erysipelas) is relatively infrequent in modern times and most often involves the cavernous sinus. Cavernous sinus thrombosis is typically a complication of a facial or orbital infection and often presents with proptosis, chemosis, and painful ophthalmoplegia. Septic lateral sinus thrombosis is an infrequent complication of otitis media or mastoiditis and often presents with headaches, fever, otalgia, vertigo, papilledema, and abducens nerve palsy (eFig. 65.34).

Aseptic intracranial venous thrombosis is divided into dural venous sinus thrombosis, DVT, and superficial or cortical vein thrombosis. The superior sagittal sinus is most frequently involved (Figs. 65.35 and 65.36). Causal factors are protean and the onset often insidious. The most common causal factors are listed in Box 65.10. However, in approximately 15%–20% of cases, no cause is found (Ferro et al., 2004). Although rare, cerebral venous thrombosis is a well-recognized disorder in children, with approximately half of cases occurring in neonates and young infants (deVeber et al., 2008).

Intracranial venous thrombosis may occur at any time from infancy to old age, but most reported modern cases have been in adult women in association with the puerperium. Onset of symptoms may be acute, subacute, or chronic. Cerebral venous infarction is the most serious consequence of cerebral venous thrombosis. Intracranial venous thrombosis should be considered a potential cause in patients with presumed idiopathic intracranial hypertension (pseudotumor cerebri) or unexplained hemorrhagic infarctions. Venous infarctions are often multifocal and bilateral, affecting both the gray matter and the subcortical white matter. Evidence of cerebral edema is unusual. Cerebral venous thrombosis may present without focal signs. Chief complaints are headaches, vomiting, transient visual obscurations, focal or generalized seizures, lethargy, or coma. Papilledema is common. There may be alternating focal deficits, hemiparesis or paraparesis, or other focal neurological deficits according to the location of the venous structure involved. Salient radiological features are the presence of low-density areas of infarction, hemorrhages, and small ventricles. There may be visualization of thrombus within the sinus on post-contrast images (empty delta sign) or direct visualization of the clot. The availability of MR venography makes it possible to diagnose early and atypical cases. MR venography is a reliable diagnostic tool and has replaced angiography for the diagnosis of cerebral venous thrombosis. Patients with intracranial venous occlusive disease should be screened for thrombophilia.

Accepted therapeutic measures include reduction of increased intracranial pressure, prophylactic seizure medications, and antibiotics in cases involving a septic causal factor. IV heparin or subcutaneous LMWH followed by warfarin for the treatment of intracranial venous thrombosis is also recommended (Stam et al., 2002). To date, there is no benefit of DOACs as compared with warfarin, although available studies are small and inconclusive. The efficacy of heparin has been shown even in patients who have evidence of intracranial hemorrhage by neuroimaging studies. In those instances or in patients failing to respond or who deteriorate despite anticoagulation, local infusion of thrombolytic agents and/or thrombectomy within the occluded intracranial venous sinus may be considered (Stam et al., 2008). Decompressive surgery may be required in selective instances (Crassard et al., 2010; Ferro et al., 2010).

*The complete references list is available online at http://expertconsult.inkling.com.*

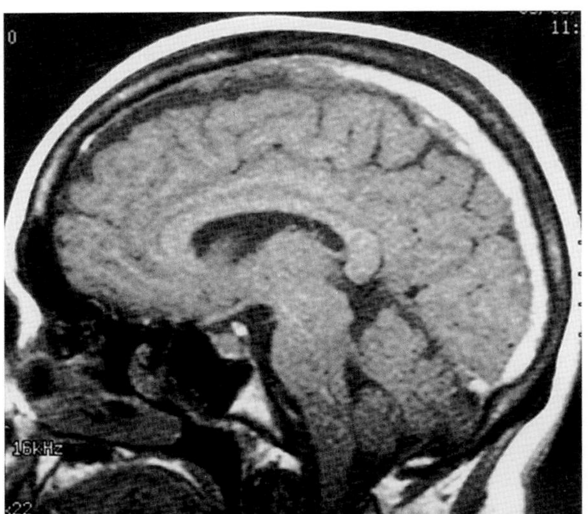


**Fig. 65.35** Unenhanced sagittal T1-weighted magnetic resonance imaging shows an area of increased signal and enlargement of the superior sagittal sinus throughout most of its course, consistent with superior sagittal sinus thrombosis. It also involves the region of the torcula.

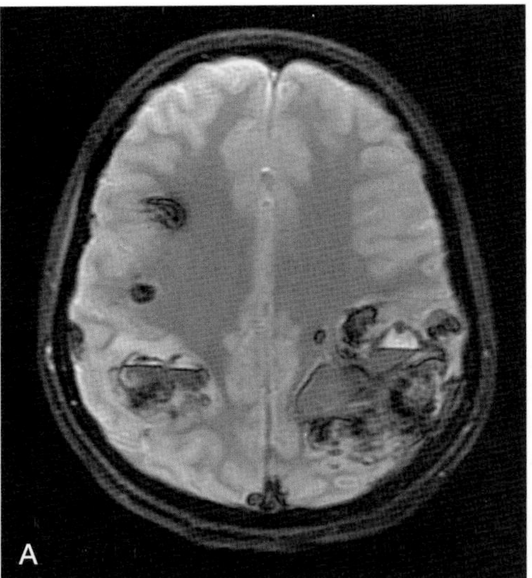


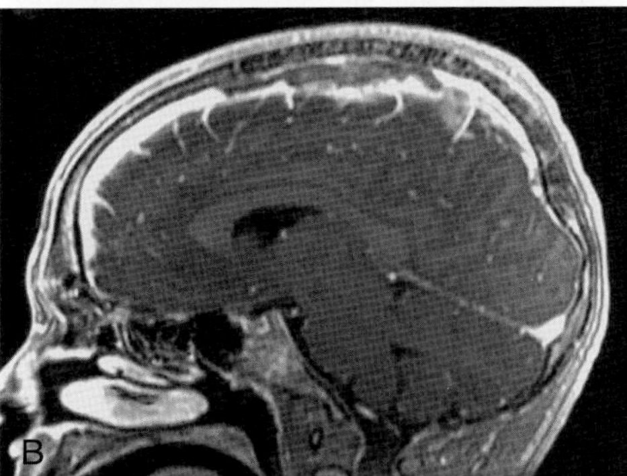


**Fig. 65.36** A 14-year-old boy with newly diagnosed acute lymphoblastic leukemia was on induction therapy that included L-asparaginase. He had a generalized seizure and postictal confusion. Head computed tomography showed bilateral hemorrhagic infarctions with fluid-fluid levels. Subsequent magnetic resonance imaging (MRI) showed a superior sagittal sinus thrombosis extending into cortical veins over the superior aspect of both parietal lobes, with associated early subacute hemorrhages in both parietal lobes. **A,** Gradient echo MRI demonstrating mixed and very irregular areas of intermediate and decreased T1 signal consistent with early subacute hemorrhage in both hemispheres. **B,** Venous phase MRI demonstrating proximal filling defects in the superior sagittal sinus and extending from the coronal to the lambdoid sutures, with possible filling defects extending into cortical veins near the midline in the high parietal regions bilaterally.

**BOX 65.10 Causes of Intracranial Sinovenous Occlusive Disease**

Facial/orbital/paranasal sinuses/middle ear infections
Trichinosis
Syphilis
Varicella-zoster virus infections
Human immunodeficiency virus infections
Sepsis
Pregnancy and puerperium
Carcinoma
Dehydration
Marasmus
L-Asparaginase therapy
Androgen therapy
Cisplatin and etoposide therapy
Epsilon-aminocaproic acid therapy
Medroxyprogesterone therapy
Cis-diamminedichloroplatinum (CDDP) and etoposide (VP-16) therapy
IV catheters, cardiac pacemakers
Polyarteritis nodosa
Systemic lupus erythematosus
Granulomatosis with polyangiitis
Behçet disease
Kohlmeier-Degos disease (malignant atrophic papulosis)
Osteopetrosis
Inflammatory bowel disease
Sarcoidosis
Osteoporosis
Congestive heart failure
Nephrotic syndrome
Budd-Chiari syndrome
Chronic lung disease
Diabetes mellitus
Cerebral arterial occlusions
Homocystinuria
Head injury
Paroxysmal nocturnal hemoglobinuria
Sickle cell disease and trait
Polycythemia vera
Essential thrombocythemia
Iron-deficiency anemia
Hypoplasminogenemia
Afibrinogenemia
Cryofibrinogenemia
Antiphospholipid antibody syndrome (APAS)
Disseminated intravascular coagulation
Antithrombin deficiency
Protein S deficiency
Protein C deficiency
Combined deficiencies (protein C, protein S, and antithrombin III)
Activated protein C resistance
Factor V Leiden mutation
Prothrombin G20210 mutation
Elevated factor VIII plasma levels
Heparin-induced thrombocytopenia
Maternal coagulopathy (twin transfusion reaction)
Familial histidine-rich glycoprotein deficiency
Arteriovenous malformations
Sturge-Weber syndrome
Neoplasm (meningioma, metastasis, glomus tumors)
Idiopathic

# 66

# Intracerebral Hemorrhage

*Ashkan Shoamanesh, Carlos S. Kase*

## OUTLINE



Intracerebral hemorrhage (ICH) accounts for approximately 10%–20% of strokes. Its clinical importance derives from its high frequency and 30-day mortality, which is close to 50%. The incidence of ICH has remained stable in the past 3 decades (van Asch et al., 2010), despite a gradually improved level of detection and treatment of hypertension, suggesting that ICH due to other mechanisms, such as anticoagulant use and cerebral amyloid angiopathy (CAA), has become more frequent (Flaherty et al., 2007). ICH continues to be a major public health problem, especially in populations at high risk such as young and middle-aged Blacks and Hispanics, in whom ICH occurs more frequently than in Whites; the medically indigent, who lack hypertension treatment; and the elderly on antithrombotic therapy. A growing body of evidence suggests that genetic factors such as possessing the ε2 and ε4 alleles of the apolipoprotein E gene play an important role in the occurrence of certain forms of ICH such as lobar hemorrhages (Greenberg et al., 2004).

The acute management of ICH entails treatment of elevated intracranial pressure (ICP), prompt blood pressure lowering, reversal of coagulopathies, and, less frequently, surgical hematoma evacuation. The hallmark of secondary ICH prevention is long-term blood pressure control and proper use of antithrombotic agents if needed for prevention of ischemic stroke. However, many treatment paradigms remain controversial and are under active investigation in randomized trials.

## MECHANISMS OF INTRACEREBRAL HEMORRHAGE

### Hypertension

The main cause of ICH is hypertension. The primary role of hypertension in ICH is supported by a high frequency (72%–81%) of history of hypertension, significantly higher blood pressure measurements at admission in comparison with patients with other stroke subtypes, high frequency of left ventricular hypertrophy, and over-representation of common genetic variants associated with hypertension (Falcone et al., 2012). Further support for the importance of hypertension in the pathogenesis of ICH is the steady increase in ICH incidence with advancing age, which is also associated with an increase in the prevalence of hypertension. Furthermore, mean systolic pressure increases steeply in the days leading to an ICH (Fischer et al., 2014).

The vascular lesion produced by chronic hypertension that leads to arterial rupture and ICH is probably lipohyalinosis of small intraparenchymal arteries. The role of microaneurysms of Charcot and Bouchard is uncertain, although their anatomical location at sites preferentially affected by ICH supports their causal importance. The nonhypertensive causes of ICH are listed in Box 66.1.

In one study of 188 patients with primary ICH (i.e., excluding patients with hemorrhage associated with ruptured arteriovenous malformations [AVMs], tumor, anticoagulant and thrombolytic therapy, and cocaine use), it was determined that the cause was hypertension in 72% of patients. Similarly, a multicenter international case-controlled study determined hypertension as the strongest risk factor for ICH, accounting for 56% of the population-attributable risk (PAR) (O'Donnell et al., 2016). Other modifiable risk factors for ICH included sedentary lifestyle (PAR 35%), unhealthy diet (25%), psychosocial stress (25%), central obesity (13%), current alcohol intake (10%), and smoking (4%). In total, these modifiable risk factors accounted for 87% of the PAR of global ICH, providing a significant opportunity to mitigate the global burden of ICH. It is recommended to target a long-term blood pressure of less than 130/80 mm Hg for the secondary prevention of ICH (Hemphill et al., 2015). Additionally, lifestyle modifications

**BOX 66.1 Nonhypertensive Causes of Intracerebral Hemorrhage**

Vascular malformations (saccular or mycotic aneurysms, arteriovenous malformations, cavernous angiomas)
Intracranial tumors
Bleeding disorders, anticoagulant and fibrinolytic treatment
Cerebral amyloid angiopathy
Granulomatous angiitis of the central nervous system and other vasculitides, such as polyarteritis nodosa
Sympathomimetic agents (including amphetamine and cocaine)
Hemorrhagic infarction
Head trauma
Miscellaneous: other vasculopathies (e.g., moyamoya disease, reversible cerebral vasoconstriction syndrome, cerebral autosomal dominant arteriopathy with subcortical infarcts and leukoencephalopathy [rarely]), and septic emboli/arteritis in the setting of infective endocarditis (all discussed elsewhere)

consisting of healthy diet, regular exercise, alcohol and smoking cessation, and stress management are likely to provide additional benefits.

## Vascular Malformations

Because a detailed discussion of intracranial aneurysms and AVMs is provided elsewhere (see Chapter 67), the analysis is limited here to the role of small vascular malformations in the pathogenesis of ICH. These lesions are often documented by magnetic resonance imaging (MRI), by pathological examination of specimens obtained at the time of surgical drainage of ICHs, or at autopsy. However, cerebral angiography also plays an important role in the diagnosis of these lesions.

ICHs caused by small AVMs or cavernous angiomas are frequently located in the subcortical white matter of the cerebral hemispheres. The clinical presentation of the ICH in this setting has a few distinctive characteristics: the hematoma is generally smaller, and symptoms develop more slowly than with hypertensive ICH; the presence of associated subarachnoid hemorrhage on computed tomography (CT) scan, although nonspecific, could suggest an aneurysm or AVM as the cause of a lobar ICH; and ICHs associated with small vascular malformations generally tend to occur in younger patients than those with hypertensive ICH, and have a female preponderance.

Cavernous angiomas are often recognized by MRI as a cause of ICH in the subcortical portions of the cerebral hemispheres and in the pons. This technique demonstrates a characteristic pattern on T2-weighted images, with a central nidus of irregular bright signal intensity mixed with mottled hypointensity (the "popcorn" pattern), surrounded by a peripheral hypointense ring corresponding to hemosiderin deposits (Fig. 66.1), reflecting previous episodes of blood leakage at the edges of the malformation. These lesions are predominantly supratentorial, favoring the temporal, frontal, and parietal lobes, whereas the less frequent infratentorial locations favor the pons. They are generally single lesions, but multiplicity is not rare, especially in patients with familial cavernous angiomas. Familial clustering is common among individuals of Mexican descent, in whom cavernous angiomas are inherited in an autosomal dominant pattern linked to a mutation in gene CCM1 in chromosome 7q (Gault et al., 2006). Cavernous angiomas manifest with seizures (27%–70%), ICH (10%–30%), or focal neurological deficits (29%–35%). ICH occurs in both the supratentorial and infratentorial varieties. A progressive course due to recurrent small hemorrhages within and around the malformation is occasionally seen in posterior fossa (especially pontine) lesions, and the deficits can evolve over protracted periods, at times suggesting a diagnosis of multiple sclerosis or a slowly growing brainstem tumor.

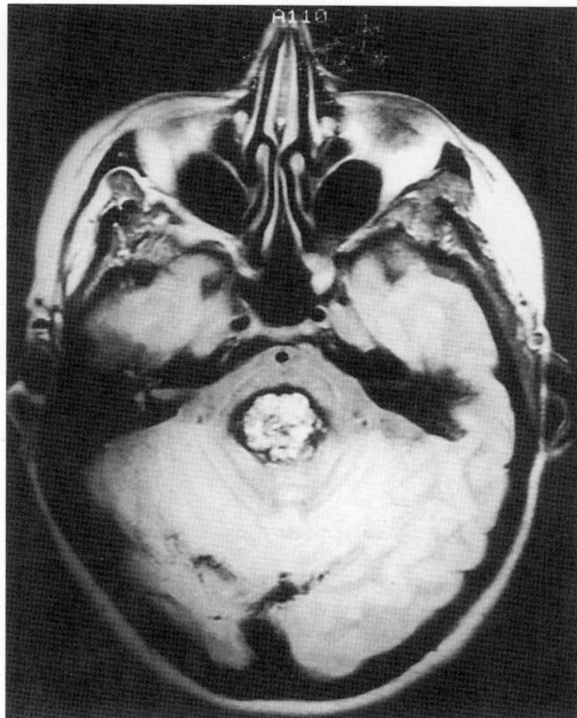

Fig. 66.1 Magnetic resonance imaging (proton density) of large cavernous angioma of the midpons in axial view, showing mixed-signal central nidus with peripheral hemosiderin ring.

A clinical profile thus can be suggested for cases of ICH due to small vascular malformations. These occur in generally young, predominantly female patients who present often with a syndrome of lobar ICH in which CT may document a superficial lobar hematoma with adjacent local subarachnoid hemorrhage, or MRI demonstrates the characteristic features of a small AVM or cavernous angioma. Lack of documentation of the vascular malformation on angiography is the rule—especially in the slow-flow cavernous angiomas—and definite diagnosis requires either MRI, delayed repeat angiography once the compressive forces of the hematoma have resolved, or the histological examination of a sample of the hematoma and its wall.

The overall annual rate of ICH in persons with cavernous angiomas is 0.15%–6%, with higher rates reported in persons initially manifesting with hemorrhage, particularly in the brainstem, and lower rates in incidental cases found on neuroimaging (Al-Shahi Salman et al., 2012; Flemming et al., 2012). The risk of recurrent hemorrhage is highest in the first 2 years following initial ICH and occurs more frequently in women.

## Intracranial Tumors

Bleeding into an underlying brain tumor is relatively rare in series of patients presenting with ICH, accounting for less than 10% of the cases. The tumor types most likely to lead to this rare complication are glioblastoma multiforme or metastases from melanoma, bronchogenic carcinoma, choriocarcinoma, or renal cell carcinoma (Fig. 66.2). The ICHs produced in this setting may have clinical and imaging characteristics that should suggest an underlying brain tumor, including: (1) the presence of papilledema on presentation,

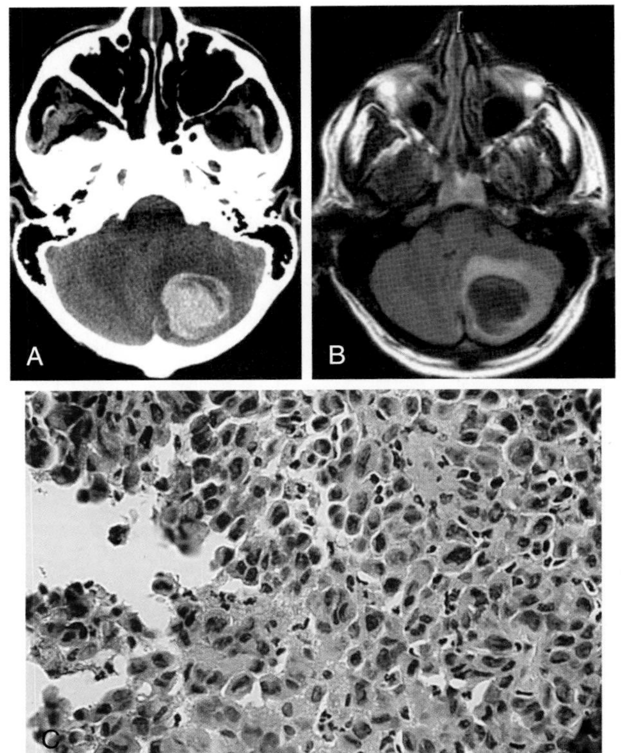


**Fig. 66.2** Computed tomography scan **(A)** and magnetic resonance imaging fluid-attenuated inversion recovery (FLAIR) sequence **(B)** of hemorrhage in left cerebellar hemisphere, showing moderate amount of surrounding edema in patient with history of lung cancer. **C,** Highly cellular pleomorphic metastatic tumor with multiple mitoses documented in biopsy of residual cavity after drainage of intracranial hemorrhage (H&E, ×20).

(2) the location of ICH in sites that are rarely affected in hypertensive ICH, such as the corpus callosum, which in turn is commonly involved in malignant gliomas (Fig. 66.3), (3) the presence of ICH in multiple sites simultaneously, (4) a CT scan characterized by a ring of high-density hemorrhage surrounding a low-density center in a noncontrast study, (5) enhancing nodules adjacent to the hemorrhage on contrast CT or MRI, and (6) a disproportionate amount of surrounding edema and mass effect associated with the acute hematoma. In these circumstances, a search for a primary or metastatic brain tumor should follow, and should include evaluation for systemic malignancy; if there is none, cerebral angiography and eventually craniotomy for biopsy of the wall of the hematoma cavity should be considered. Confirmation of the diagnosis of ICH secondary to malignant brain tumor carries a dismal prognosis, with a 30-day mortality rate in the 90% range.

## Bleeding Disorders, Anticoagulants, and Fibrinolytic Treatment

Inherent bleeding disorders due to abnormalities of coagulation are rare causes of ICH. Hemophilia caused by factor VIII deficiency leads to ICH in approximately 2.5% to 6.0% of patients, half with ICH and half with subdural hematomas. The majority of these hemorrhages occur in young patients, generally younger than age 18, and their mortality is high, about 10% for subdural hematomas and 65% for ICH. Immune-mediated thrombocytopenia, especially idiopathic thrombocytopenic purpura, is associated with life-threatening ICH in approximately 1% of patients. Bleeding occurs when the platelet count drops below 10,000/μL, and the hemorrhages may occur anywhere in the brain. Acute leukemia, especially the acute lymphocytic variety, is a common cause of ICH that favors the lobar white matter of the cerebral hemispheres. The occurrence of ICH frequently coincides with systemic bleeding, mostly mucocutaneous and gastrointestinal. These bleeding complications of acute lymphocytic leukemia are often accompanied by both thrombocytopenia (platelet counts of 50,000/μL or less) and rapidly increasing numbers of abnormal circulating leukocytes of 300,000/μL or more (blastic crisis). Acute promyelocytic leukemia, a variant of acute myelogenous leukemia, has a particular propensity to produce ICH secondary to disseminated intravascular coagulation.

Treatment with oral vitamin K antagonists (VKA) increases the risk of ICH by 2- to -4 fold compared with individuals with otherwise similar risk factors for ICH who are not receiving anticoagulants. Anticoagulant-related cases account for 9% to 14% of ICH (Pezzini et al., 2014). Potential risk factors for intracranial bleeding in patients receiving anticoagulants include advanced age, hypertension, East-Asian, Black and Latin American ethnicity, prior stroke or transient ischemic attack (TIA), anticoagulation with warfarin, concomitant antiplatelet use, head trauma, and excessive prolongation of the international normalized ratio (INR) (Hankey et al., 2014; Hart et al., 2012; Lopes et al., 2017). The last factor plays a major role in the pathogenesis of ICH in patients receiving VKAs. In the secondary stroke prevention trial SPIRIT (Stroke Prevention in Reversible Ischemia Trial), 651 patients assigned to warfarin treatment were maintained at an INR of 3.0–4.5, resulting in 24 instances of ICH (14 fatal), in comparison with 3 ICHs (1 fatal) in the group of 665 patients treated daily with 30 mg of aspirin (SPIRIT Study Group, 1997). These data further support the recommendation that oral anticoagulation in patients with cerebrovascular disease should aim at an INR of 2–3 to reduce the frequency of this complication. The presence of severe leukoaraiosis and cerebral microbleeds (CMBs) on neuroimaging are additional factors that independently increase the risk of ICH in patients on anticoagulation (Marti-Fabregas et al., 2019; Wilson et al., 2018 ). CMBs are characterized pathologically by small areas of previous bleeding, in the form of hemosiderin-laden macrophages, and often represent the presence of a bleeding-prone microangiopathy, most commonly hypertensive arteriopathy or CAA (Shoamanesh et al., 2011). However, as these imaging markers additionally increase the risk of ischemic events, the absolute rates of ischemic stroke far supersede that of ICH in ischemic stroke/TIA patients with CMBs, even in the setting of high microvascular burden or patterns consistent with CAA (Wilson et al., 2019) Current evidence would thus suggest that the presence, number, and/or distribution of CMBs should *not* be factored into decision making in ischemic stroke/TIA populations where anticoagulation has significant established benefit for stroke prevention (i.e., atrial fibrillation) (Shoamanesh et al., 2017, 2020).

Hemorrhages in the setting of VKA use have certain distinctive clinical characteristics: they tend to present with a slowly progressive course, at times over periods as long as 48–72 hours, in contrast with the usually more rapidly evolving presentation of hypertensive ICH; hematomas in patients receiving anticoagulants expand and reach volumes that are, on average, larger than those occurring in hypertensive ICH, in turn resulting in the higher mortality rate of approximately 65%; signs of systemic bleeding rarely accompany ICH in this setting. Anticoagulant-related ICH may represent bleeding from vessels different from those involved in ICH of hypertensive origin. Certain angiopathies with bleeding potential, such as CAA, may play a causal role in the ICHs that occur in patients treated with anticoagulants (Falcone et al., 2014). The available data largely pertain to oral anticoagulation with VKA. Direct

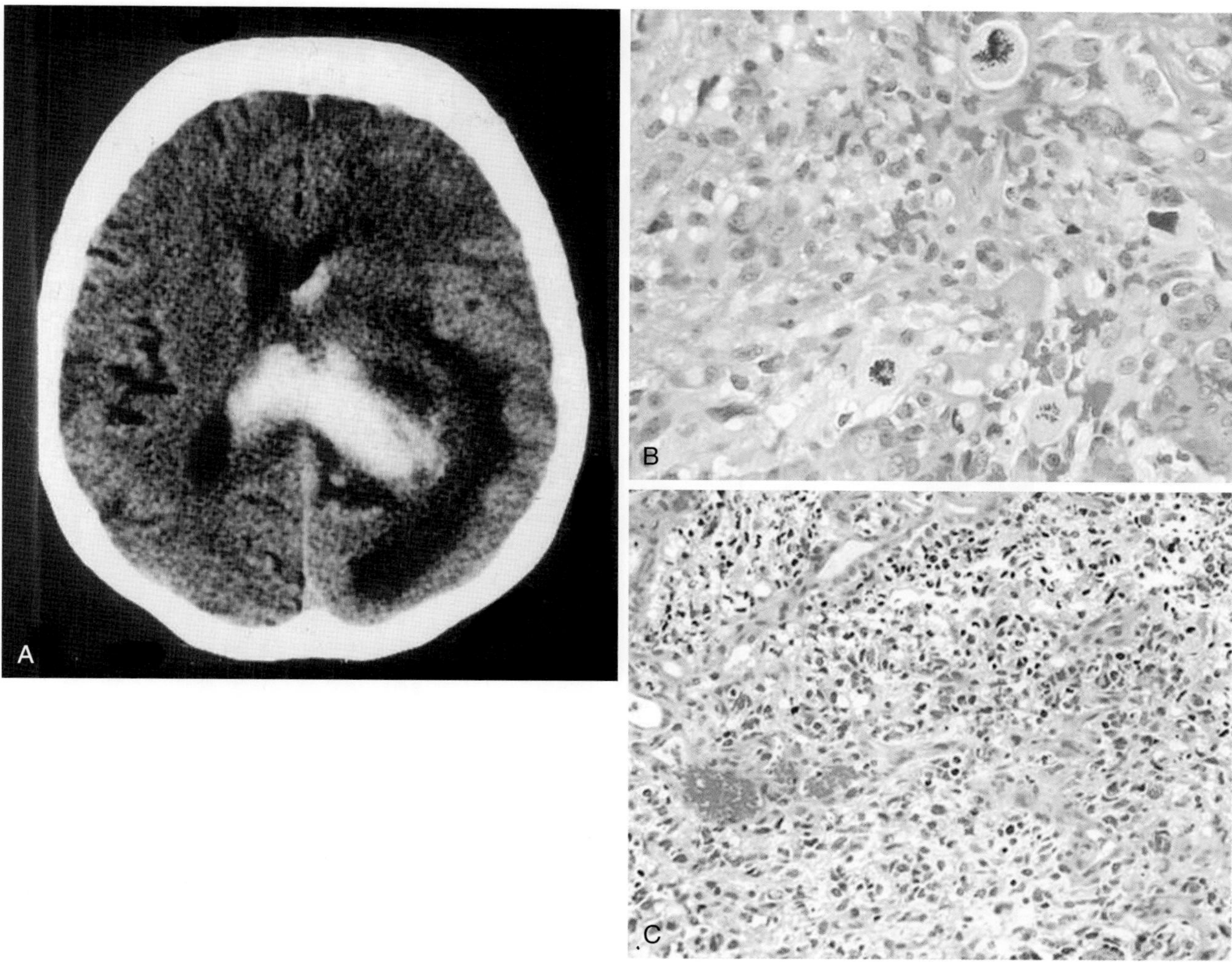

**Fig. 66.3** Noncontrast CT scan of acute hemorrhage into the deep white matter of the left parietal lobe with extension into the corpus callosum and across the midline **(A)**, due to glioblastoma multiforme with giant cells with atypical mitoses (B, H&E, x100), and high cellularity, pleomorphism, and endothelial proliferation (C, H&E, x20).

oral anticoagulants (DOACs; direct thrombin or factor Xa inhibitors) may have more favorable profiles. Randomized controlled trials have shown lower ICH rates amongst the DOACs in comparison to warfarin therapy in the management of nonvalvular atrial fibrillation. The specific targeting of the direct acting agents of a single factor within the coagulation cascade (factor Xa or IIa [thrombin]) that still allows for a robust hemostatic response to vessel rupture through tissue factor–factor VIIa complex mediated pathways, rather than the inhibition of four vitamin K-dependent factors (II, VII, IX, and X) by VKA, has been speculated to account for these differences. Although observational studies have additionally suggested smaller hematomas among DOAC-related ICH relative to warfarin-related ICH, mortality rates among DOAC-treated patients suffering an ICH have not differed from those occurring while on VKA in randomized trials. A comparison of VKA-related and DOAC-related ICH using an individual patient data meta-analysis from cohort studies documented lower admission National Institutes of Health Stroke Scale (NIHSS) scores and smaller baseline ICH volumes in patients on DOACs, but with similar hematoma expansion rates, in-hospital mortality, modified Rankin Scale (mRS) at discharge, and mRS at 30 days (Tsivgoulis et al., 2018). In addition, this study documented no differences in 30-day mortality rates for ICH patients on various DOACs, including dabigatran, rivaroxaban, and apixaban.

In addition to the anticoagulants, other substances with the potential for altering clot formation mechanisms are occasionally associated with ICH. These include drugs with fibrinolytic properties, such as streptokinase and tissue plasminogen activator (tPA). There is evidence to suggest that this complication of thrombolytic therapy may be favored by pre-existing vasculopathies with bleeding potential such as CAA. Recombinant tPA for the treatment of acute ischemic stroke was complicated by ICH in 6.4% of cases (NINDS rtPA Stroke Study Group, 1995), which is 10 times the rate found in the placebo group. Risk factors for ICH in this setting include a severe neurological deficit at presentation and documentation of hypodensity or mass effect on CT before treatment (NINDS tPA Stroke Study Group, 1997). Intra-arterial thrombolysis with pro-urokinase for middle cerebral artery occlusion leads to improved clinical outcomes but is associated with an 11% rate of early symptomatic ICH (Furlan et al., 1999). These hemorrhages occur at the site of the preceding cerebral infarct, are generally large (Fig. 66.4), and carry a dismal prognosis (Kase et al., 2001). Hyperglycemia at pretreatment baseline has been identified as a potential risk factor for ICH in patients treated with either intra-arterial prourokinase (Kase et al., 2001) or intravenous (IV) tPA (Poppe et al., 2009) for acute ischemic stroke. Additional risk factors for post-thrombolysis ICH include post-thrombolysis elevated blood pressure (Butcher et al., 2010), baseline dual antiplatelet therapy

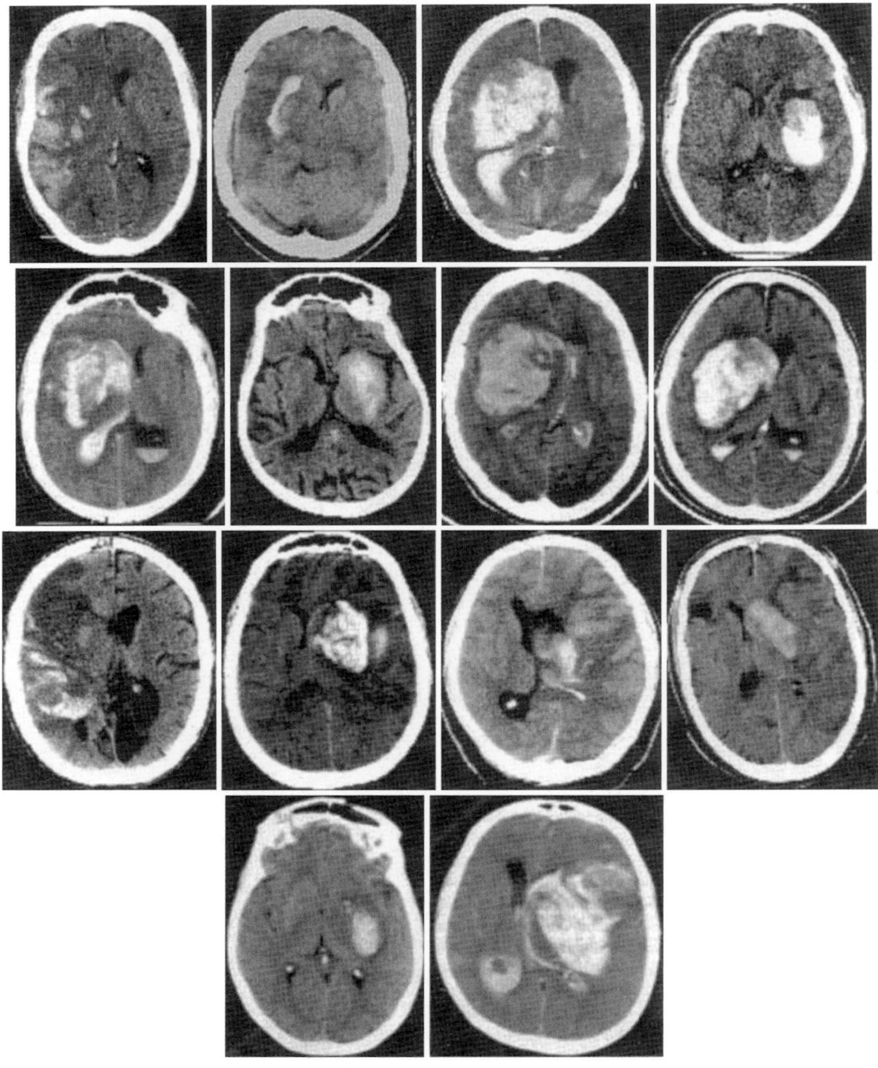

Controls

**Fig. 66.4** **Symptomatic Intracerebral Hemorrhages After Intra-Arterial Thrombolysis of Middle Cerebral Artery Occlusion with Prourokinase.** *(Reprinted with permission from Kase, C.S., Furlan, A.J., Wechsler, L.R., et al., 2001. Cerebral hemorrhage after intra-arterial thrombolysis for ischemic stroke: the PROACT II Trial. Neurology 57, 1603–1610.)*

with aspirin and clopidogrel (Diedler et al., 2010), and the presence of leukoaraiosis.

Another potential risk factor for ICH after thrombolysis is the presence of incidental CMBs, which can be easily detected with gradient echo or susceptibility-weighted MRI sequences (Fig. 66.5). Systematic reviews have suggested that individuals with CMBs are at higher risk of both intra-ischemic and remote post-thrombolysis ICH, particularly in patients with higher lesion burden (Shoamanesh et al., 2013). However, no firm recommendations can be given at present for using or withholding thrombolytics based solely on the presence of these often incidentally detected lesions.

The initiation or reintroduction of antithrombotic medications following ICH in patients with concomitant cardioembolic or vaso-occlusive diseases is controversial. The benefit of continued antiplatelet therapy following a spontaneous ICH was recently tested in the randomized multicenter RESTART trial (RESTART Collaboration, 2019), where randomization to antiplatelet therapy compared to no antithrombotic therapy did not increase the risk of recurrent ICH, and led to a 35% ($P$ = .025) relative risk reduction in the secondary composite outcome of nonfatal myocardial infarction, nonfatal stroke, and vascular death. Unexpectedly, there was a statistically nonsignificant trend for a reduction in recurrent ICH with antiplatelet therapy resumption (adjusted hazard ratio [aHR] 0.51 [95% confidence interval [CT] 0.25–1.03, $P$ = .06). Whether these provocative findings hint at novel mechanisms in our understanding of ICH pathophysiology, or are simply due to chance, remains uncertain. However, the RESTART results provide landmark data on the relative safety and net benefit of antiplatelet therapy in patients with ICH and concomitant vaso-occlusive diseases. Further reassurances are provided in the RESTART MRI subgroup analyses that did not demonstrate any treatment modification according to ICH location, or the presence and burden of MRI markers of cerebral small-vessel disease, including CMBs or cortical superficial siderosis.

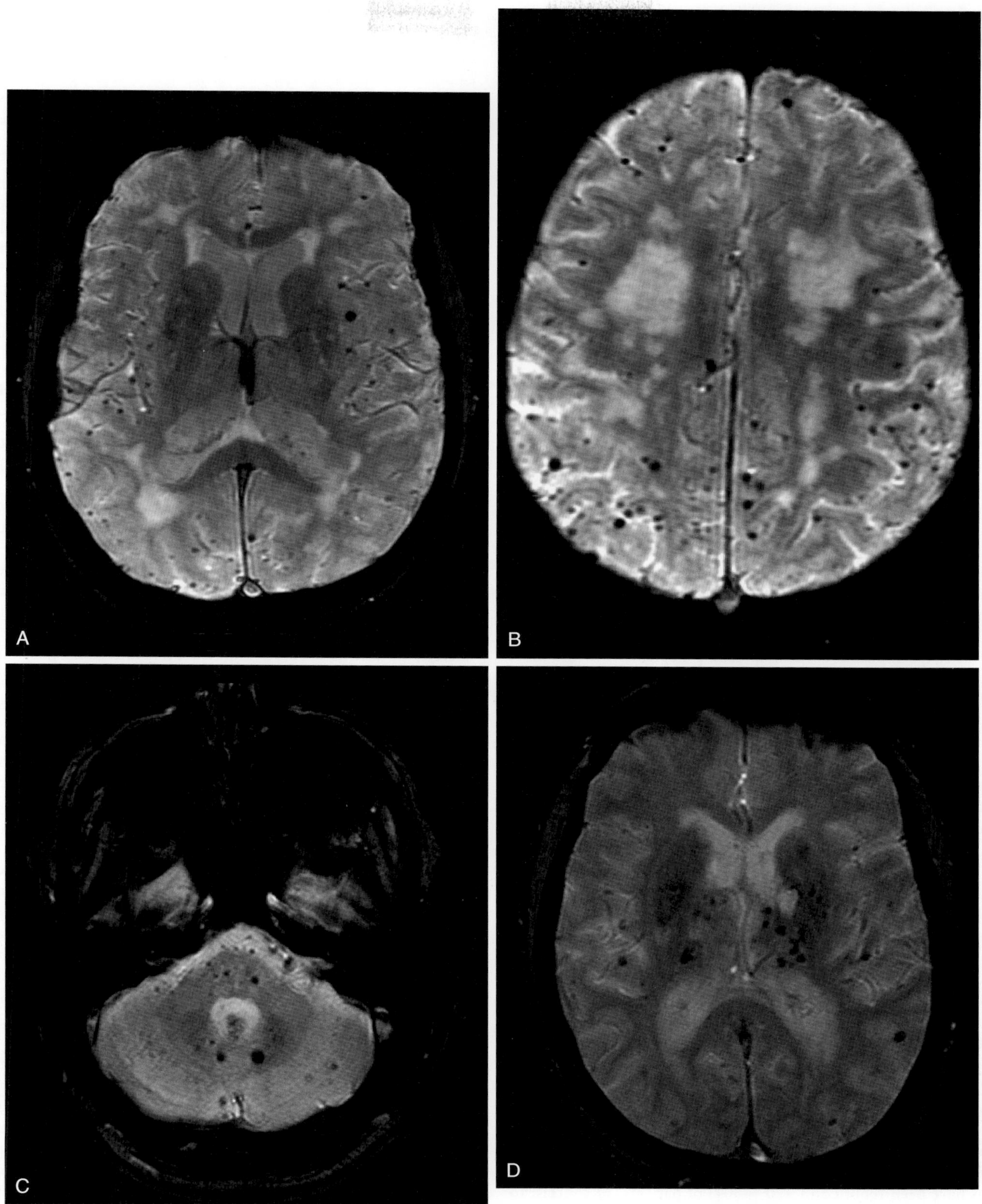


**Fig. 66.5** Magnetic resonance imaging T2* susceptibility-weighted sequence with multiple, strictly lobar, cerebral microbleeds (CMBs) in a subject with cerebral amyloid angiopathy (A and B), and multiple predominantly deep CMBs in a subject with hypertensive arteriopathy (C and D).

Similarly, multiple national observational registries have suggested continued benefit without an increased risk of ICH recurrence from oral anticoagulation in ICH survivors with atrial fibrillation (Biffi et al., 2017; Murthy et al., 2017). However, the likelihood of confounding by indication limits interpretation of these observational findings and several large randomized trials (including the global ENRICH-AF trial) are underway to confidently address this clinical dilemma.

## Cerebral Amyloid Angiopathy

CAA is characterized by selective deposition of β-amyloid in the walls of cerebral vessels, primarily small and medium-sized arteries of the cortex and leptomeninges. Because the frequency of CAA increases steadily with age, reaching 60% in unselected autopsies of individuals older than 90 years, it characteristically causes ICH in the elderly and is rarely documented before the age of 55 years. In addition, the superficial location of the affected vessels in the cortex and leptomeninges is responsible for a predominantly lobar location of ICH. The widespread character of the angiopathy is responsible for the observation of both recurrent and multiple simultaneous, predominantly lobar, hemorrhages in elderly patients. An additional characteristic of CAA is its association with histopathological features of Alzheimer disease. There is clinical and progressive dementia in 10% to 30% of patients with CAA and neuritic plaques in approximately 50% of cases. CAA may present with features other than ICH, such as episodes of transient focal neurological deficits, previously termed "amyloid spells."

Transient focal neurological episodes (TFNEs) are rarely disabling, but are rather a source of discomfort and concern for a proportion of CAA patients. The underlying pathophysiology of TFNEs is poorly understood, but experimental models, the semiology of TFNEs (Charidimou et al., 2012a), and lack of associated epileptiform activity, implicate cortical spreading depression as the most likely mechanism. As focal seizures could still potentially contribute to TFNEs in a subset of patients, a trial of an antiepileptic agent that is also effective for cortical spreading depression, such as topiramate, valproic acid, or gabapentin, can be attempted in patients with recurrent events. These episodes are often self-limited; treatment should be tapered off within 1–3 months following symptomatic control. Most often, the culprit lesion seems to be convexal subarachnoid hemorrhage or cortical superficial siderosis (Fig. 66.6; Charidimou et al., 2012a).

The histological lesion in CAA is deposition of Congo red–positive, birefringent amyloid material in the media and adventitia of small cortical and leptomeningeal arteries. The actual mechanism of rupture of an affected artery may be either a weakening of the wall or formation of microaneurysms at sites of amyloid deposition, particularly in advanced cases with fibrinoid necrosis and concentric splitting of the vessel with the characteristic "double-barrel" appearance. Other conditions may combine with CAA to produce rupture of affected vessels, including head trauma, neurosurgical procedures, hypertension, use of antithrombotic and fibrinolytic agents, and possibly statin treatment. The clinico-radiographic modified Boston Criteria (Table 66.1) are a validated useful tool to determine the probability of underlying CAA pathology in the absence of tissue biopsy (Linn et al., 2010). CAA-related ICH can often have overlying convexal subarachnoid hemorrhages, and overlying subdural hematomas have been reported in ~20%–30% of patients. In contrast to deep ICH resulting from hypertensive arteriopathy, which have an ICH recurrence rate of about 2% per annum, the recurrence rate of lobar ICH resulting from CAA is on the order of 5%–10% per annum. The presence of multiple strictly lobar CMBs, and cortical superficial siderosis in particular, can mark CAA patients who are at the highest risk of recurrent ICH.

CAA-related inflammation (and amyloid β-related angiitis) is a rare manifestation of CAA clinically characterized by the rapid onset of new headaches, seizures, cognitive decline/dementia, behavioral changes, and focal neurological deficits. It should be suspected in patients 40 years of age or older who present with these clinical signs and symptoms, and who have asymmetric subcortical white matter hyperintensities that extend to the U-fibers and multiple cortico-subcortical hemorrhagic lesions on MRI (macrobleeds, CMBs, and/or cortical superficial siderosis; Table 66.2; Auriel et al., 2016). The presenting clinical symptoms and asymmetric white matter lesions should not be attributable to an ICH or other cause. The clinical and radiographic findings are often completely reversible with immunosuppressive therapy. High-dose corticosteroid therapy with IV methylprednisolone 1 g daily for 3–5 days followed by a rapid oral prednisone taper is first-line treatment. Most cases of CAA-related inflammation are monophasic, but relapses have been reported in up to a third of patients (Kinnecom et al., 2007).

## Granulomatous Angiitis of the Central Nervous System and Other Vasculitides

Granulomatous angiitis of the CNS, also referred to as *isolated angiitis of the CNS*, is characterized by mononuclear inflammation with giant cell formation in the media and adventitia of small and medium-sized intracranial arteries and veins (see Chapter 70). An associated element of intimal hyperplasia leads frequently to cerebral infarcts and occasionally to ICH.

Among the vasculitides, the other variety that is known to present with ICH is polyarteritis nodosa. As opposed to granulomatous angiitis of the CNS, this form of necrotizing vasculitis depicts prominent signs of systemic involvement, including fever, malaise, weight loss, anemia, elevated erythrocyte sedimentation rate, and renal impairment with hypertension.

## Sympathomimetic Agents

Sympathomimetic agents can cause ICH after IV, oral, or intranasal use (see Chapter 86). The hemorrhages usually occur within minutes to a few hours after drug use, and the majority are located in the subcortical white matter of the cerebral hemispheres. In approximately half of reported cases, transient hypertension has been documented, as well as multifocal areas of spasm and dilatation ("beading") of intracranial arteries on angiography. Although the latter is frequently referred to as vasculitis or arteritis, histological proof is lacking, and this angiographic picture probably represents multifocal spasm secondary to the drug. The decongestant and appetite-suppressant phenylpropanolamine has been associated with ICH in young patients (median age in the early 30s), predominantly women (Kernan et al., 2000), usually without a history of hypertension but with acute hypertension on admission in a third of patients. Beading of intracranial arteries is frequent on angiography.

Cocaine (see Chapters 85 and 86) has become the most common sympathomimetic agent associated with ICH. Both ICH and subarachnoid hemorrhage can occur within short periods (generally minutes) of the use of both the alkaloid (free-base) form of cocaine and its precipitate form, known as *crack*. The ICHs favor the subcortical white matter but occasionally occur in the deep portions of the hemispheres (Fig. 66.7). There may be multiple simultaneous ICHs, both deep and superficial, the mechanism of which remains unknown. In some instances, the origin of the ICH can be traced to a coexistent AVM or aneurysm, whereas the remainder are probably associated with either cocaine-induced vasoconstriction followed by reperfusion, concomitant heavy alcohol intake, or (rarely) a drug-induced cerebral vasculitis.

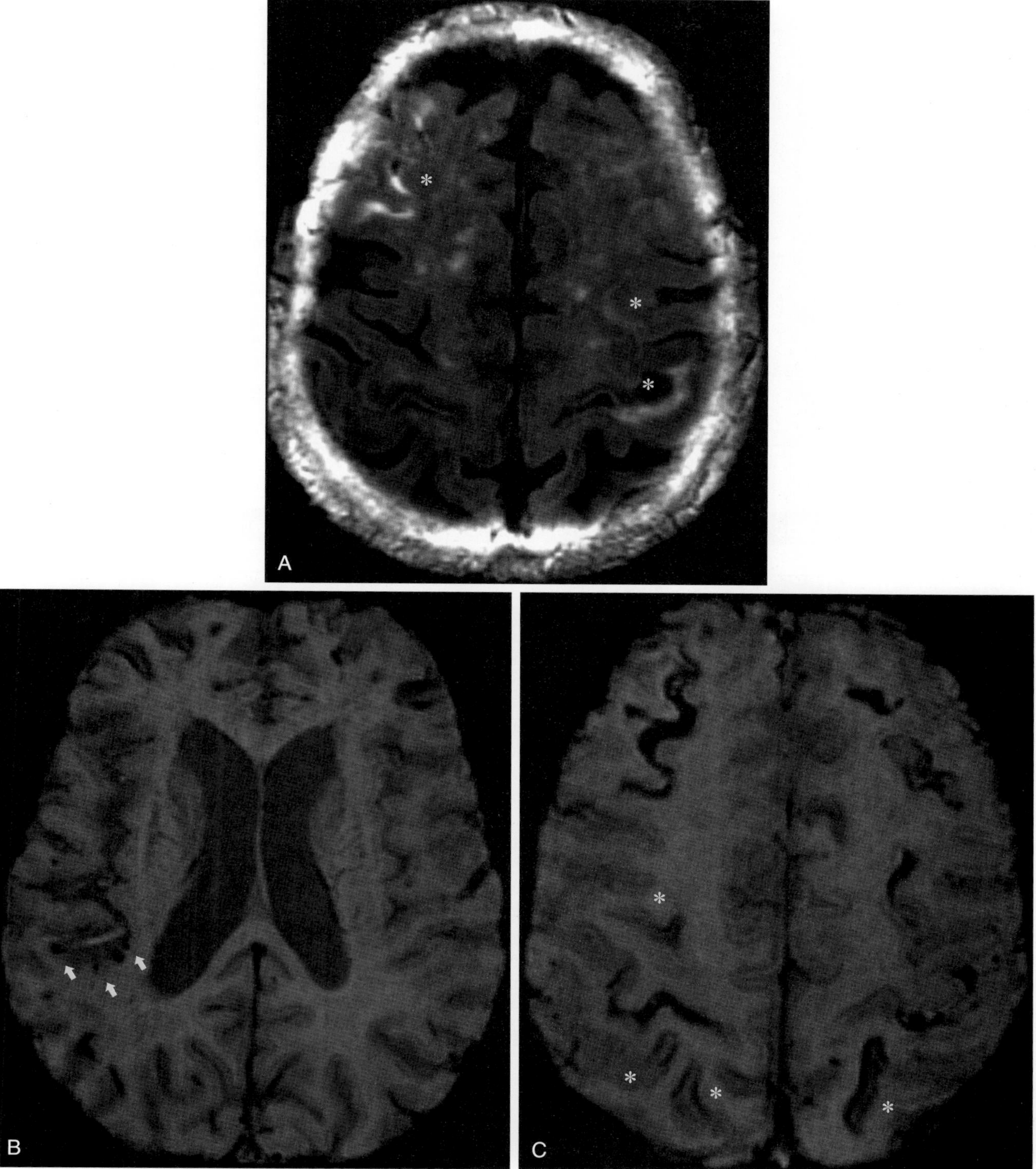


**Fig. 66.6 Magnetic Resonance Imaging in an 84-Year-Old Woman Presenting with Confusion and Word Finding Difficulty.** Fluid-attenuated inversion recovery (FLAIR) sequence (**A**) demonstrates bihemispheric convexal subarachnoid hemorrhage *(asterisks)* and susceptibility-weighted imaging (**B** and **C**) shows multiple cortical cerebral microbleeds (*arrows*, **B**), and areas of cortical superficial siderosis (*asterisks*, **C**) suggestive of prior occult convexal subarachnoid hemorrhage. This constellation of findings is highly suggestive of cerebral amyloid angiopathy.

**TABLE 66.1 Modified Boston Criteria for Cerebral Amyloid Angiopathy**

| Level of Certainty | Criteria (*Linn et al., 2010*) |
|---|---|
| Definitive CAA | Full postmortem examination demonstrating:<br>• Lobar, cortical, or subcortical hemorrhage<br>• Severe CAA vasculopathy<br>• Absence of other diagnostic lesion |
| Probable CAA with supporting pathology | Clinical data and pathological tissue (evacuated hematoma or cortical biopsy) demonstrating:<br>• Lobar, cortical, or subcortical hemorrhage<br>• Some degree of CAA in specimen<br>• Absence of other diagnostic lesion |
| Probable CAA | Clinical data and CT or MRI demonstrating:<br>• Age ≥55 years<br>• Multiple hemorrhages restricted to lobar, cortical, or corticosubcortical regions (cerebellar hemorrhage allowed) OR<br>• Single lobar, cortical, or corticosubcortical hemorrhage and focal or disseminated superficial siderosis<br>• Absence of other cause of hemorrhage or superficial siderosis |
| Possible CAA | Clinical data and CT or MRI demonstrating:<br>• Age ≥55 years<br>• Single lobar, cortical, or corticosubcortical hemorrhage OR<br>• Focal or disseminated superficial siderosis<br>• Absence of other cause of hemorrhage or superficial siderosis |

*CAA,* Cerebral amyloid angiopathy; *CT,* computed tomography; *MRI,* magnetic resonance imaging.

**TABLE 66.2 Diagnostic Criteria for Cerebral Amyloid Angiopathy-Related Inflammation**

| Level of Certainty | Criteria (*Auriel et al., 2016*) |
|---|---|
| Probable CAA-related inflammation | • Age ≥40 years<br>• Presence of ≥1 of the following clinical features: headache, decrease in consciousness, behavioral change, or focal neurological signs and seizures; the presentation is not directly attributable to an acute ICH<br>• MRI shows unifocal or multifocal WMH lesions (corticosubcortical or deep) that are asymmetric and extend to the immediately subcortical white matter; the asymmetry is not due to past ICH<br>• Presence of ≥1 of the following corticosubcortical hemorrhagic lesions: cerebral macrobleed, cerebral microbleed, or cortical superficial siderosis<br>• Absence of neoplastic, infectious, or other cause |
| Possible CAA-related inflammation | • Age ≥40 years<br>• Presence of ≥1 of the following clinical features: headache, decrease in consciousness, behavioral change, or focal neurological signs and seizures; the presentation is not directly attributable to an acute ICH<br>• MRI shows WMH lesions that extend to the immediately subcortical white matter<br>• Presence of ≥1 of the following corticosubcortical hemorrhagic lesions: cerebral macrobleed, cerebral microbleed, or cortical superficial siderosis<br>• Absence of neoplastic, infectious, or other cause |
| Ancillary findings (not included in the criteria) | CT angiography: Normal<br>• MRI post gadolinium: No enhancement or mild overlying leptomeningeal enhancement<br>• Cerebrospinal fluid: Can have mild pleocytosis or cytoalbuminologic dissociation, increased anti-Aβ autoantibodies and t- and p-τ, with decreased Aβ40 and Aβ42 levels<br>• APOE genotyping: APOE ε4 allele carried frequently |

*APOE,* apolipoprotein E; *CAA,* Cerebral amyloid angiopathy; *ICH,* intracerebral hemorrhage; *MRI,* magnetic resonance imaging; *WMH,* white matter hyperintensities.

## Hemorrhagic Infarction

Hemorrhagic infarction is pathologically and pathogenically different from ICH in that it results from restoration of blood flow to infarcted tissue that had previously ensued from arterial or venous occlusion (Alvarez-Sabin et al., 2013). As a result, its pathological aspect is one of multifocal petechial hemorrhagic staining of an area of the brain primarily affected by ischemic necrosis (i.e., infarction; Fig. 66.8). Hemorrhagic infarction characteristically occurs in the setting of cerebral embolism or, rarely, following restoration of cerebral perfusion to border-zone infarcts that had resulted from global hypoperfusion, such as in the case of cardiac arrest. Cerebral infarction secondary to venous occlusion (e.g., thrombosis of superior sagittal sinus or cortical veins) is also frequently hemorrhagic as a result of venous stasis in the necrotic area. In all these instances of hemorrhagic infarction, the bleeding namely reflects the mechanism of the infarct.

Clinical differences between hemorrhagic infarction and ICH usually permit their clear distinction (Table 66.3), but severe and confluent foci of hemorrhagic infarction may at times be difficult to distinguish from foci of primary ICH.

## Head Trauma

ICH caused by cerebral contusion characteristically occurs in the surface of the brain, because its mechanism is one of direct brain trauma against its bony covering at the time of an acceleration–deceleration head injury (see Chapter 62). This explains the sites of predilection for traumatic brain hemorrhages in the basal frontal, anterior temporal, and occipital areas, resulting from the *coup* and *contrecoup* mechanisms of injury. Thus, traumatic brain hemorrhages are frequently multiple.

# CLINICAL FEATURES OF INTRACEREBRAL HEMORRHAGE

The clinical presentation of ICH has two main elements: symptoms that reflect the effects of intracranial hypertension and those that are specific for the location of the hematoma. The general clinical manifestations of ICH related to ICP (headache, vomiting, and depressed level of consciousness) vary in their frequency at onset of ICH. The correlation of these symptoms (especially abnormal level of consciousness) with hematoma size applies to all anatomical varieties of ICH, which in turn relates directly to mortality.

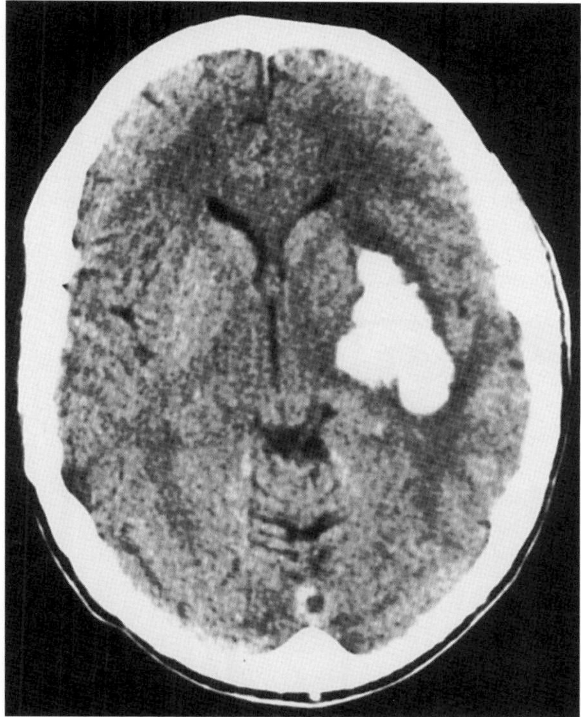

Fig. 66.7 Left Putaminal Hemorrhage After Use of Crack Cocaine. *(Courtesy of Susan S. Pansing, MD.)*

A characteristic of ICH at presentation is the frequent progression of focal neurological deficits over periods of hours. This early course reflects progressive enlargement of the hematoma (Fig. 66.9), which at times amounts to volume increments of more than 300% as measured by serial CT scans (Demchuk et al., 2012). Clinical features that predict hematoma growth include early time from symptom onset to baseline CT imaging, higher baseline ICH volumes, and antiplatelet and anticoagulant therapy (Al-Shahi Salman et al., 2018). The presence of small foci of contrast extravasation, referred to as the *spot sign*, during CT angiography (CTA) in patients with acute ICH is additionally predictive of hematoma enlargement (Goldstein et al., 2007; Wada et al., 2007). When CTA is performed within the first few hours post–ICH onset, the presence of the spot sign (Fig. 66.10) correlates with a frequency of hematoma enlargement in up to 77% of patients, compared to only 4%–22% in patients without the sign (Demchuk et al., 2012; Wada et al., 2007). Additionally, a number of noncontrast CT head markers of expansion are currently being actively investigated (Fig. 66.11).

MRI adds further precision to the diagnosis of ICH, especially in determining the time elapsed between onset and time of MRI examination. The type of signal intensity change depicted by T1- and T2-weighted MRI sequences can be correlated with the hyperacute, acute, subacute, and chronic stages of evolution of an intracerebral hematoma (Table 66.4). The increased use of acute/subacute MRI in ICH patients has led to the recognition of punctate DWI hyperintense lesions remote from the area of hematoma in about ~25% of patients. These are mainly ischemic lesions, yet a small fraction have the radiographic hallmarks of small hematomas captured in an extracellular methemoglobin stage of evolution (Shoamanesh et al., 2013). Although their pathophysiology is an area of active investigation, these lesions seem to be a manifestation of advanced underlying cerebral small-vessel disease, rather than indicative of proximal origin thromboembolism.

Physical examination findings that relate to the different anatomical locations of ICH are summarized in Table 66.5.

## Putaminal Hemorrhage

The most common variety of ICH, putaminal hemorrhage, represents approximately 35% of cases (Kase et al., 2011; eFig. 66.12). A wide 

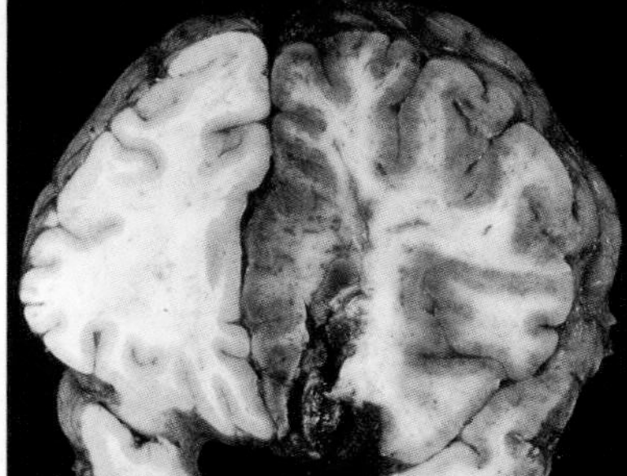


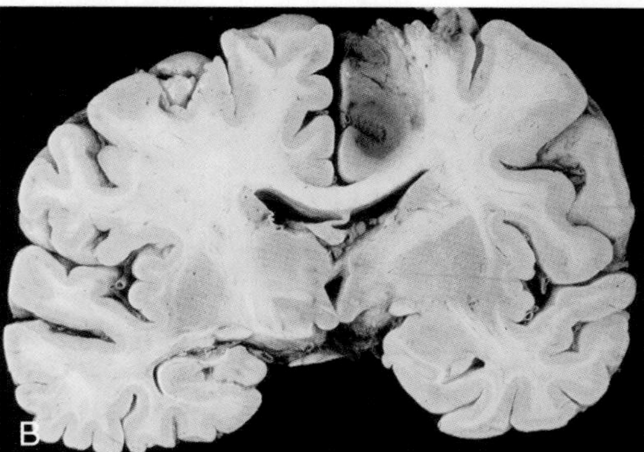


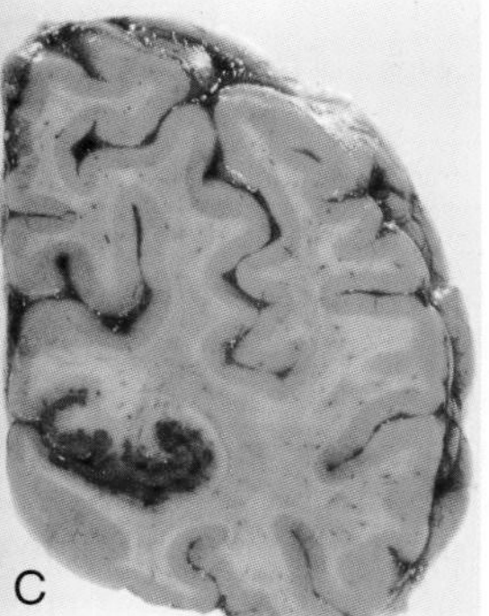


Fig. 66.8 A, Left hemispheric hemorrhagic infarction in the territory of the middle cerebral and anterior cerebral arteries as a result of intracranial internal carotid artery embolic occlusion. B, Left anterior cerebral artery distribution hemorrhagic infarction. C, Small hemorrhagic infarction in the left medial occipital (calcarine) cortex due to embolic occlusion of distal branch of the posterior cerebral artery.

**TABLE 66.3 Differences Between Intracerebral Hemorrhage and Hemorrhagic Infarction**

| | Intracerebral Hemorrhage | Hemorrhagic Infarction (Embolic) |
|---|---|---|
| **Clinical** | | |
| Onset of deficit | Sudden, followed by progression | Maximal from onset |
| Raised intracranial pressure | Prominent | Absent |
| Embolic source | No | Yes |
| **Computed Tomography** | | |
| High attenuation | Dense, homogeneous | Spotted, mottled |
| Mass effect | Prominent | Absent or mild |
| Location | Subcortical, deep (gray nuclei) | Cortex more than subcortical white matter |
| Distribution | Beyond arterial territories | Along branch distribution |
| Late enhancement | Ring-type | Gyral-type |
| Ventricular blood | Yes | No |
| **Magnetic Resonance Imaging*** | | |
| Hypointense blood (T2) | Homogeneous | Patchy, mottled |
| Hyperintense edema (T2) | Thin peripheral halo | Extensive, in vascular territory |
| **Angiogram/Magnetic Resonance Angiography** | | |
| Characteristics | Mass effect (avascular) | Branch occlusion |

*Magnetic resonance imaging (MRI) depicts the same features as computed tomography (CT) in regard to mass effect, location, distribution, late enhancement, and ventricular blood. This table lists only the features MRI adds to those of CT.

*Reprinted with permission from Kase, C.S., Mohr, J.P., Caplan, L.R., 2004. Intracerebral hemorrhage. In: Mohr, J.P., Choi, D.W., Grotta, J.C., et al. (Eds), Stroke: Pathophysiology, Diagnosis, and Management, fourth ed. Churchill Livingstone, Philadelphia.*

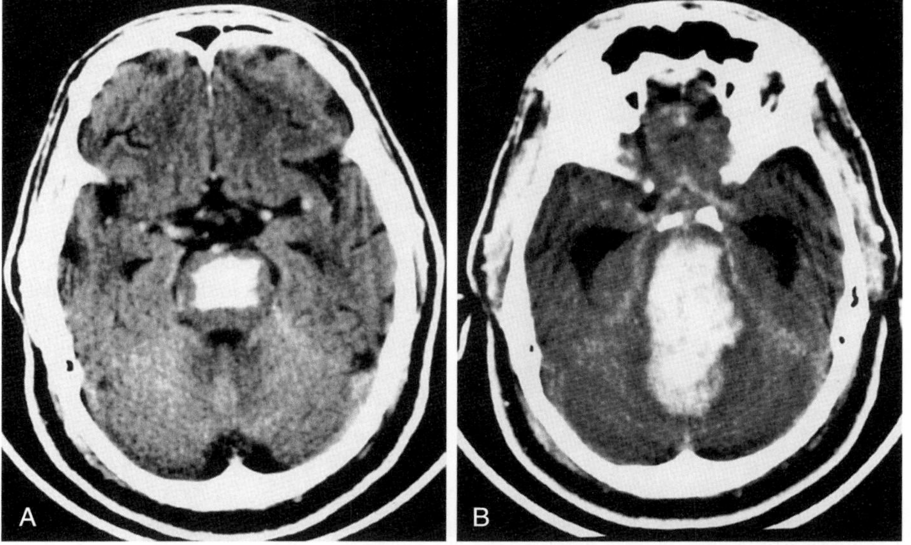


**Fig. 66.9** A, Basal-tegmental pontine hemorrhage at the time of admission. B, Massive enlargement of hemorrhage with extension into the fourth ventricle and hydrocephalus of temporal horns, 6 hours later.

spectrum of clinical severity relates to hematoma size, from minimally symptomatic cases presenting with pure motor hemiparesis or slight hemiparesis and dysarthria, to the extreme of coma with decerebrate rigidity in instances of massive hematomas with rupture into the ventricles. Modern CT series of putaminal hemorrhage document a mortality rate of 37%, in contrast to 65% to 75% from pre-CT data. This difference reflects the description of the full spectrum of hematoma size in recent reports, including smaller hematomas with benign outcomes, which were misdiagnosed as infarcts in the pre-CT era. Ventricular extension carries an invariably poor prognosis in putaminal hemorrhage.

## Caudate Hemorrhage

Caudate hemorrhage is a rare variety of ICH that accounts for only approximately 5% of cases (Kase et al., 2011; Fig. 66.13). It results from rupture of penetrating arteries from the anterior and middle cerebral arteries, and its most common cause is hypertension. Presentation is similar to that of subarachnoid hemorrhage in that the clinical picture is dominated by signs of intracranial hypertension and meningeal irritation, with focal neurological deficits (hemiparesis, horizontal gaze palsy, Horner syndrome) being minimal and transient or altogether absent. At times, the main manifestations of caudate ICH are neuropsychological deficits including

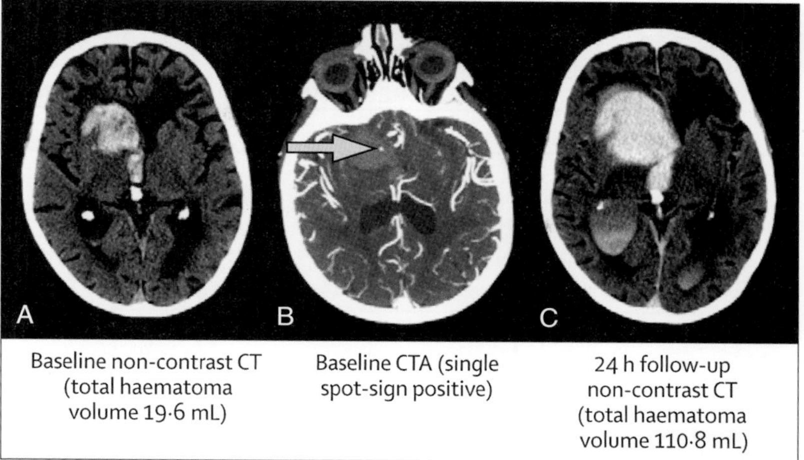


**Fig. 66.10 "Spot Sign" in Intracerebral Hemorrhage.** Baseline (**A**) and 24-hour (**C**) noncontrast computed tomography *(CT)* scans show expansion of a right caudate hemorrhage with ventricular extension. CT angiography *(CTA)* at baseline (**B**) shows an area of contrast extravasation ("spot sign") suggestive of ongoing bleeding *(arrow)*. *(From Demchuk, A.M., Dowlatshahi, D., Rodriguez-Luna, D., et al., 2012. Prediction of haematoma growth and outcome in patients with intracerebral haemorrhage using the CT-angiography spot sign (PREDICT): a prospective observational study. Lancet Neurol 11, 307–314.)*

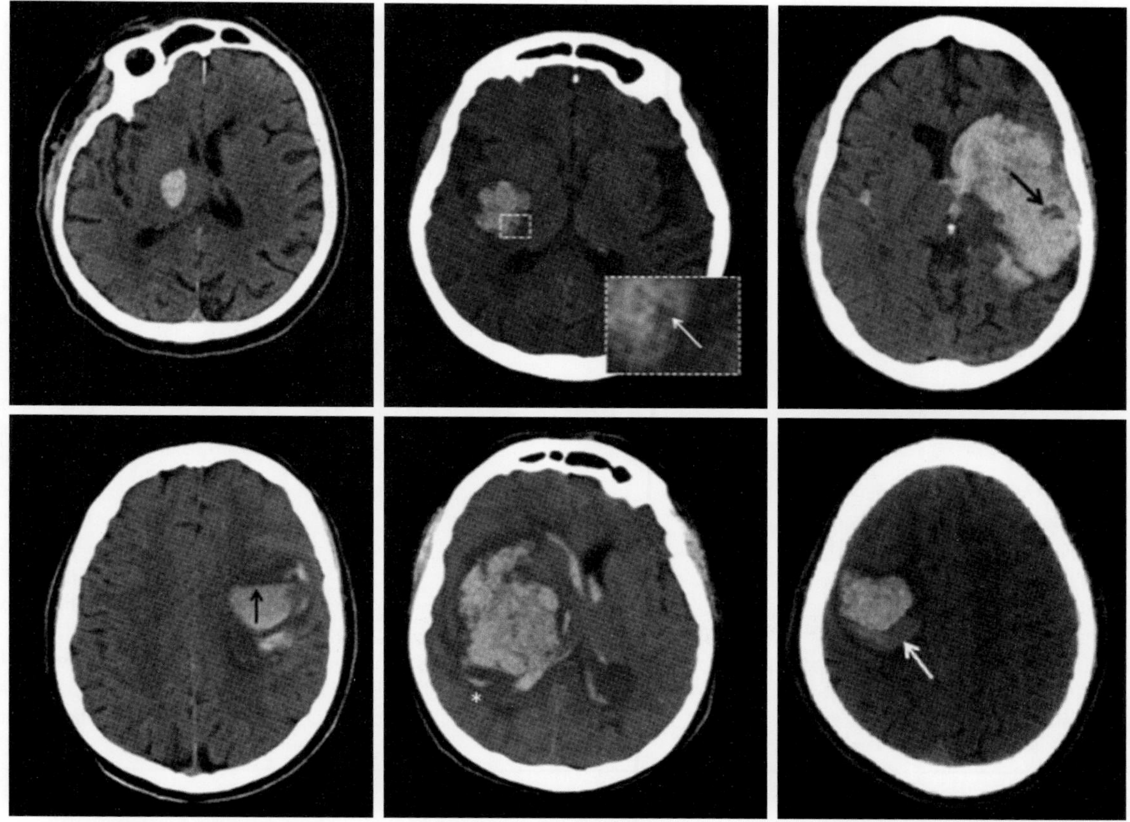

**Fig. 66.11 Noncontrast Computed Tomography (CT) Markers of Hematoma Expansion.** (**A**) Regular shape and homogeneous density*. (**B**) Irregular shape and homogenous density**. (**C**) Swirl sign *(black arrow)***. (**D**) Fluid level *(black arrow)***. (**E**) Satellite sign *(asterisk)***. (**F**) Blend sign *(white arrow)***. *No high risk features for expansion. **High risk features for expansion. *(Images courtesy of Drs. Andrea Morotti and Andreas Charidimou.)*

abulia, disorientation, and memory disturbances, occasionally accompanied by language disturbances (Kase, 2010). The main differential diagnosis of caudate ICH is ruptured anterior communicating artery aneurysm with bleeding through the septum pellucidum into the ventricular system. In this instance, CT shows blood in the interhemispheric fissure and in the lowermost frontal cuts, as opposed to the higher location of the unilateral clot in the head of one caudate nucleus in primary caudate ICH. Ventricular

**TABLE 66.4 Temporal Changes in Magnetic Resonance Imaging Features of Intracerebral Hemorrhage**

| Stage of Intracerebral Hemorrhage | MAGNETIC RESONANCE IMAGING SIGNAL INTENSITY | | |
|---|---|---|---|
| | Type of Hemoglobin | T1-Weighted | T2-Weighted |
| First hours | Oxyhemoglobin | Same or ↓ | ↑ |
| Hours to days | Deoxyhemoglobin | Same or ↓ | ↓↓ |
| First days | Methemoglobin, intracellular | ↑ | ↓ |
| Several days to months | Methemoglobin, extracellular | ↑↑ | ↑↑ |
| Several days to indefinitely | Ferritin/hemosiderin | Same or ↓ | ↓↓ |

*Same,* Equal signal with surrounding brain; ↓, hypointense to brain; ↑, hyperintense to brain; ↓↓, marked hypointensity; ↑↑, marked hyperintensity.

**TABLE 66.5 Clinical Features of Anatomical Forms of Intracerebral Hemorrhage**

| Type of Intracerebral Hemorrhage | Hemiplegia | Hemisensory Syndrome | Aphasia | Homonymous Visual Defects | Gaze Palsy: Horizontal | Gaze Palsy: Vertical | Brainstem Signs |
|---|---|---|---|---|---|---|---|
| Putaminal | Generally dense | Frequent | Global>motor>conduction | In large hematomas | Contralateral | No | No (only present with herniation) |
| Caudate | Absent or mild, transient | Absent | Transcortical motor (in dominant hemisphere hematomas) | No | Generally absent | No | No |
| Thalamic | Generally dense | Frequent, prominent | Occasional, thalamic variety | In large hematomas | Contralateral, occasionally ipsilateral | Yes, upward | Skew deviation, Horner syndrome, Parinaud syndrome |
| Lobar | Prominent in frontoparietal location | Prominent in frontoparietal location | In dominant temporoparietal location | In occipital hematomas | Contralateral in frontal hematomas | No | No (only present with herniation) |
| Cerebellar | Absent | Absent | No | No | Ipsilateral | No | Ipsilateral fifth through seventh nerve palsy, Horner syndrome |
| Pontine | Variable, usually bilateral | Variable, usually bilateral | No | No | Bilateral | No | Pinpoint reactive pupils, ocular "bobbing," decerebrate rigidity, respiratory rhythm abnormalities |
| Mesencephalic | Variable, usually present | Rare | No | No | No | Occasional, upward | Unilateral or bilateral third nerve palsy |
| Medullary | Generally absent | Occasional | No | No | No | No | Nystagmus, ataxia, hiccups, facial hypesthesia, dysarthria, dysphagia, 12th nerve palsy, Horner syndrome |
| Intraventricular | Generally absent | Rare | No | No | Occasional | Occasional | Rare (decerebrate rigidity) |

extension of the hemorrhage is a regular feature in caudate ICH, and hydrocephalus is usually present. Nevertheless, the outcome is generally good. The majority of patients recover without neurological sequelae, although at times neuropsychological deficits persist.

### Thalamic Hemorrhage

Thalamic hemorrhage represents 10% to 15% of ICH cases (Kase et al., 2011; eFig. 66.14).  Its onset tends to be more abrupt than that of putaminal hemorrhage, and slow progression of deficits is less common. These features may reflect early communication of the medially located hematoma with the third ventricle. The prognosis in thalamic hemorrhage relates to hematoma size and level of consciousness at presentation (Kase, 2010). Another reliable sign of poor prognosis in thalamic ICH is the presence of hydrocephalus, an occasional complication that can occur abruptly secondary to aqueductal obstruction by an intraventricular clot, with potential for a reversal of symptoms by ventriculostomy.

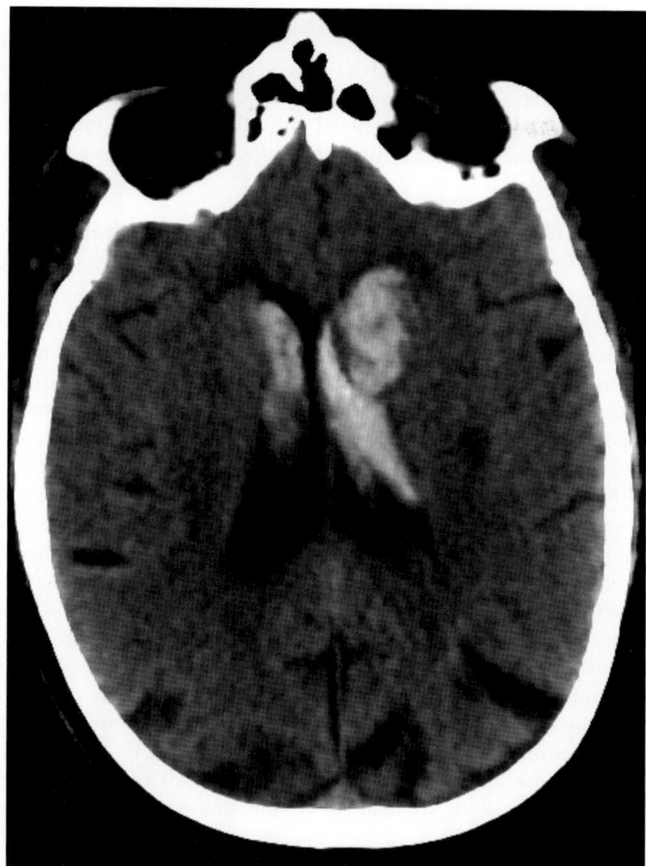

**Fig. 66.13** Left Caudate Hemorrhage with Extension into the Lateral Ventricles.

## Lobar Hemorrhage

Lobar hemorrhage is second to putaminal hemorrhage in frequency, accounting for approximately 25% of ICH cases (Kase et al., 2011; eFig. 66.15). Nonhypertensive mechanisms including AVMs, sympathomimetic agents (in young patients), and CAA (in elderly patients) are frequent causes. The peripheral (subcortical) location of these hematomas explains the lower frequency of coma at onset, as compared with the deep ganglionic forms of supratentorial ICH. Although seizures at the time of presentation of ICH are rare, they occur in as many as 28% of patients with lobar ICH. The clinical features reflect location: hemiparesis of upper limb predominance in frontal hematomas, sensorimotor deficit and hemianopia in parietal hemorrhages, fluent aphasia with relatively preserved repetition in dominant temporal hematomas, and homonymous hemianopia in occipital lobe hemorrhages. The mortality rate in individuals with lobar ICH is lower than in those with hematomas in other locations, and the long-term functional outcome may also be better.

## Cerebellar Hemorrhage

Cerebellar hemorrhage represents approximately 5% to 10% of ICH cases (Kase et al., 2011; eFig. 66.16). Its clinical presentation is characteristic, with abrupt onset of vertigo, headache, vomiting, and inability to stand and walk, but absence of hemiparesis or hemiplegia. The physical findings that allow its clinical diagnosis are the triad of appendicular ataxia, horizontal gaze palsy, and peripheral facial palsy, all ipsilateral to the hemorrhage.

The clinical course in cerebellar hemorrhage can be difficult to predict at onset. There is a notorious tendency for abrupt deterioration to coma and death after a period of clinical stability under hospital observation. This unpredictable course has stimulated a search for early clinical or CT signs that may separate patients with benign outcome from those who deteriorate clinically with the onset of brainstem compression and a high likelihood of mortality. These include clinical evidence of compromise of brainstem function, CT features of hydrocephalus, hematomas of 3 cm or more in diameter, and effacement of the quadrigeminal cistern.

## Pontine Hemorrhage

Pontine hemorrhage represents approximately 5% of ICH cases (Kase et al., 2011; Fig. 66.17). The massive bilateral basal-tegmental variety produces the classic picture of coma, quadriplegia, decerebrate posturing, horizontal ophthalmoplegia, ocular bobbing, pinpoint reactive pupils, abnormalities of respiratory rhythm, and preterminal hyperthermia. Since the introduction of CT and MRI, less severe forms of pontine hemorrhage that are compatible with survival are recognized. These hemorrhages are frequently located in the tegmentum, lateral to the midline, and thus produce syndromes of predominantly unilateral dorsal pontine involvement ("one-and-a-half" syndrome [see Chapter 21], internuclear ophthalmoplegia, fifth and seventh nerve palsies), with variable degrees of long-tract interruption. These hematomas result from rupture of distal tegmental branches of a long circumferential artery originating from the basilar trunk.

## Mesencephalic Hemorrhage

Mesencephalic hemorrhage is exceptionally rare (Kase et al., 2011). The causal mechanism was hypertension or ruptured AVM in half of the reported cases, the others being of undetermined cause. Occasional unilateral hematomas (eFig. 66.18) can present with ipsilateral third nerve palsy, cerebellar ataxia, and contralateral hemiparesis. Bilateral cases frequently have prominent tectal-tegmental signs, with bilateral ptosis, paralysis of upward gaze, and small pupils with light-near dissociation (see Chapter 21). Often patients survive without surgical treatment, but with persistent sequelae.

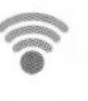

## Medullary Hemorrhage

Examples of pure primary ICH involving the medulla alone (eFig. 66.19) are rare, with most reported cases representing medullary extension of caudal pontine hematomas. The clinical presentation of primary medullary hemorrhage reflects the location of the lesion on one-half of the medulla, generally extending beyond the dorsolateral region, both medially (resulting in ipsilateral hypoglossal nerve palsy) and ventrally (resulting in contralateral hemiparesis). These two features distinguish most examples of medullary hemorrhage from the classical presentations of Wallenberg lateral medullary syndrome, caused by infarction rather than hemorrhage (see Chapter 21).

## Intraventricular Hemorrhage

Extension of hemorrhage into the ventricular system is a common feature of caudate and thalamic hemorrhages and of large putaminal and lobar hemorrhages. As a primary form not associated with a component of intraparenchymal bleeding, intraventricular hemorrhage is rare, accounting for only about 3% of ICHs. The site of origin of the hemorrhage is thought to be the vasculature of the subependymal region, and rarely the source can be identified in the choroid plexus.

The causes of intraventricular hemorrhage are similar to those of ICH elsewhere, including hypertension, aneurysm, AVM, coagulation disorders, cerebral tumors, cocaine use, and rare vasculopathies such as moyamoya disease. Those from aneurysm rupture are generally due to an anterior communicating artery aneurysm that ruptures in an upward direction, bleeding directly into one of the lateral ventricles;

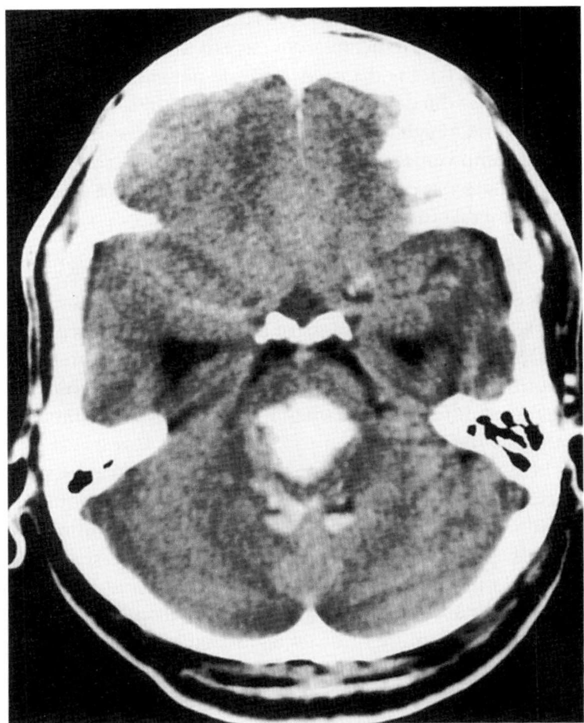

**Fig. 66.17** Large Tegmental-Basal Pontine Hemorrhage with Hydrocephalus of Temporal Horns.

in these instances, basal frontal subarachnoid hemorrhage and interhemispheric hemorrhage accompany the intraventricular hemorrhage and should always suggest a ruptured aneurysm. AVMs that cause purely intraventricular hemorrhage are generally small and located in the medial aspect of the basal ganglia or thalamus. Rarely, an intraventricular AVM or cavernous angioma may cause a primary intraventricular hemorrhage.

The clinical presentation of intraventricular hemorrhage is with acute onset of headache, nausea, vomiting, and decreased level of consciousness, with focal neurological deficits either minimal or altogether absent (Flint et al., 2008). This presentation is identical to that of subarachnoid hemorrhage from ruptured aneurysm or AVM. If focal deficits such as hemiparesis or ocular motor disturbances are prominent, the picture is not strictly that of a pure intraventricular hemorrhage but rather one of primary ICH with ventricular extension.

Intraventricular hemorrhage can be diagnosed reliably with CT and MRI, the latter being more sensitive in detecting a small component of subependymal intraparenchymal hemorrhage. Also, MRI can suggest a diagnosis of aneurysm, AVM, or cavernous angioma as the mechanism of hemorrhage. Even after extensive testing, the cause of many intraventricular hemorrhages remains unknown.

The prognosis of intraventricular hemorrhage is strongly dependent on the severity of the initial manifestation and its mechanism. Patients who are comatose as a result of the initial hemorrhage generally succumb, especially if they have early signs of brainstem involvement (ophthalmoparesis, loss of pupillary reflexes, decerebrate rigidity). Those who remain alert or obtunded without signs of parenchymal involvement tend to recover without neurological sequelae, although memory disturbances may be a relatively frequent residual deficit (Flint et al., 2008). Patients with the idiopathic form of intraventricular hemorrhage have the best prognosis.

## TREATMENT OF INTRACEREBRAL HEMORRHAGE

Issues related to treatment of ICH have been dominated by two main considerations: (1) the type and intensity of medical interventions required to improve the functional and vital prognosis and (2) the choice between medical and surgical therapy. These two issues are discussed separately.

### General Management of Intracerebral Hemorrhage

Because ICH is frequently associated with increased ICP, most of the therapies used in this setting are directed at lowering the ICP or preventing hematoma expansion, which occurs in 28%–38% of ICH presenting within 3 hours of symptom onset. Among the many medications and procedures available, a small group has come into customary use in most institutions, despite their value not being proven in properly controlled studies.

#### Initial Evaluation

On arrival in the emergency department, patients with ICH need to be immediately evaluated for stabilization of vital signs and airway protection. If the patient has a depressed level of consciousness and a Glasgow Coma Scale score of 8 or less, endotracheal intubation should follow. This is best performed with pretreatment with a short-acting IV agent as such as fentanyl (2-3 mcg/kg) to block the increases in ICP that result from tracheal stimulation.

Following emergent evaluation of vital signs and laboratory studies, clinical examination and CT are needed to establish the topography and size of the ICH, which determine the plan for further management. These decisions are made in conjunction with a neurosurgical consultant.

Laboratory testing in cases suggestive of ICH should include complete blood count for hematological disorders, a toxicology screen for sympathomimetic drug use, and serum glucose, as elevated levels have been associated with hematoma expansion and worse outcomes. Coagulation studies are essential, especially in instances of hemorrhage in patients receiving anticoagulants, those previously treated with thrombolytic agents, or patients with liver disease. It is important to establish the timing of the last anticoagulant dose in patients treated with DOACs or low-molecular-weight heparin in order to determine the need for OAC reversal strategies.

Anticoagulation-related coagulopathies should be treated emergently, because, if anticoagulation is not reversed, it can lead to progressive enlargement of the hematoma (see Hemostatic Therapy of Intracerebral Hemorrhage below).

#### General Measures for Prevention of Further Elevation of Intracranial Pressure

General measures include control of hypertension and treatment of seizures. The potential benefit of antihypertensive therapy is limited by the lack of present knowledge concerning optimal balance between adequate cerebral perfusion and control of ICP. The rapid lowering of blood pressure does not seem to have a significant effect on perihematomal cerebral perfusion in moderate-sized ICH (Butcher et al., 2013), nor does it seem to result in further neurological deterioration (Anderson et al., 2013; Qureshi et al., 2016). Pharmacological correction of severe hypertension (blood pressure >180/105 mm Hg) is recommended in the acute phases of ICH, with the goal being maintenance of normal cerebral perfusion pressure levels on the order of 50–70 mm Hg. Current evidence is unclear regarding whether further reduction of systolic blood pressure to less than 140 mm Hg improves clinical outcomes (Anderson et al., 2013; Qureshi et al., 2016). However, rapid reduction to below this target with the use of IV nicardipine in acute

ICH patients presenting with systolic blood pressures above 180 mm Hg has been shown to increase the risk of acute kidney injury (Qureshi et al., 2016). Most experts aim to keep the systolic blood pressure at various individual targets less than 160 mm Hg for the first 24–48 hours following ICH. Given the totality of current literature, a target of less than 140 mm Hg seems reasonable, where such a target would not result in greater than an 60 mm Hg absolute reduction in their presenting systolic blood pressure (i.e. presenting systolic blood pressures <200 mm Hg). The antihypertensive agent of choice in this setting is the IV beta- and alpha-blocking agent labetalol, often used in combination with loop diuretics. The use of the IV calcium channel blocker nicardipine is an equally appropriate choice in this setting in view of its lack of cerebral vasodilatory effect. These IV agents have the advantage of being rapidly effective and easy to titrate. Nitrovasodilators should be avoided where possible.

Seizures, a feature of the lobar rather than deep ganglionic varieties of ICH, typically occur at onset. EEG for the diagnosis of nonconvulsive status epilepticus should be considered in patients with depressed level of consciousness that is out of proportion to the size and location of ICH.

In patients who did not have early seizures, there is a negligible risk of late epilepsy. Thus the routine prophylactic use of anticonvulsants in patients with ICH is not justified. Early tonic-clonic convulsions need immediate control because they can contribute to increased ICP. The major anticonvulsants are of comparable value in this situation.

### Specific Treatment of Increased Intracranial Pressure

The mainstays of treatment of intracranial hypertension have been hyperventilation, osmotic diuretic therapy, and corticosteroids. Hyperventilation is most effective in rapidly lowering intracranial hypertension, usually within minutes of achieving levels of hypocapnia in the range of 25–30 mm Hg. IV mannitol (0.25–1 g/kg), a rapid and reliable way of lowering ICP, may be used along with hyperventilation in situations of neurological deterioration with impending herniation. Although dexamethasone is frequently given with the purpose of decreasing intracranial hypertension by reducing cerebral edema, it may be harmful and its use is not supported by data (Hemphill et al., 2015).

Intensive monitoring of ICP together with aggressive medical treatment of intracranial hypertension appears to improve the outcome of comatose patients with ICH. Failure to control raised ICP with these measures can be used as an objective indicator that surgical evacuation of the hematoma may be required, because persistently elevated ICP in these circumstances invariably results in progression to coma and death.

## Choice Between Medical and Surgical Therapy in Intracerebral Hemorrhage

A direct surgical approach is considered frequently in patients with superficial (lobar) hematomas of the cerebral hemispheres or with cerebellar hemorrhage, whereas patients with deep hemorrhages (caudate, thalamic, pontine, mesencephalic, and medullary in location) are rarely if ever surgical candidates. Putaminal hemorrhage occupies an intermediate position and is most controversial. Few scientific data are available to assist the clinician in this therapeutic choice.

Several randomized clinical trials compared surgical with nonsurgical treatment of ICH, and the results were generally inconclusive, mostly because of methodological issues. Mendelow and Associates (2005) reported the results of a prospective international multicenter clinical trial comparing surgical and nonsurgical treatment of ICH. The international STICH (Surgical Trial of Intracerebral Haemorrhage) randomized 1033 patients into each treatment arm, with the surgery for hematoma evacuation being performed within 4 days of ICH onset. The primary trial outcome, death or disability (measured with the extended Glasgow Outcome Scale) at 6 months, was virtually identical in the two groups: 74% in the surgical group and 76% in the nonsurgical group. Similarly, mortality at 6 months was 36% and 37%, respectively. Prespecified subgroup analyses showed no superiority of one treatment modality over the other, with the only exception being that hematomas located at a depth of less than 1 cm from the cortical surface fared better with surgical treatment. Based on this observation, the subsequent STICH II examined the benefit of initial conservative management versus surgical therapy within this particular subgroup and there were no significant differences found (Mendelow et al., 2013). Minimally invasive procedures for hematoma evacuation in patients with ICH are a promising alternative to craniotomy. In the MISTIE III trial, minimally invasive thrombolytic-assisted aspiration of large ICH did not improve functional outcomes compared with standard medical care, but did seem to lower mortality (Hanley et al., 2019). Exploratory analyses suggested functional gains in patients with greater extent of hematoma clot removal, but these findings need to be confirmed in future randomized trials.

In view of these data, most patients are currently treated nonsurgically, with the exception of those with lobar hemorrhage with progressive deterioration in the level of consciousness, and most instances of cerebellar hemorrhage. In addition, the presence of a lesion with potential for causing recurrence of ICH, such as an AVM, aneurysm, or cavernous angioma, is another indication for surgical therapy. Patients with putaminal and lobar ICH who undergo a steady decline in level of consciousness, with onset of coma, have a mortality of 100% with medical therapy. On the basis of this consideration, occasional patients with putaminal ICH are treated surgically, with a slight improvement in survival rates but without any demonstrated improvement in functional outcome. This raises a difficult ethical dilemma contrasting improved survival rates with poor quality of life in patients with massive basal ganglionic ICHs, in whom severe hemiplegia, hemisensory loss, and aphasia or hemi-inattention syndromes are the expected permanent sequelae.

The other group for whom surgery is frequently considered includes patients with cerebellar hemorrhage. Although a benign outcome without surgical evacuation is well documented in small cerebellar hemorrhages, the potential for sudden deterioration to coma and death, not infrequently after a clinically stable course under hospital observation, is well recognized. CT criteria for early selection of candidates for surgical therapy are large hematomas (diameter of 3 cm or more), presence of hydrocephalus, and obliteration of the quadrigeminal cistern (eFig. 66.20).  In addition to these CT features, early signs of pontine tegmental compression, such as ipsilateral gaze and facial palsy, and development of obtundation and extensor plantar responses, constitute indications for emergency surgical therapy, because otherwise the outcome is often fatal.

In addition to direct evacuation of a hematoma, there is the option of ventricular drainage for the relief of hydrocephalus and increased ICP in cases of cerebellar, thalamic, and caudate ICH. In cerebellar hemorrhage, massive hydrocephalus can be a major cause of clinical deterioration, and ventriculostomy may provide dramatic improvement, serving as a bridge to surgical evacuation rather than a substitute, since ventricular drainage does not diminish compression of the brainstem, and may exacerbate the potential for upward transtentorial cerebellar herniation due to decompression of the supratentorial ventricular system. Patients with thalamic hemorrhage occasionally show a dramatic reversal of ocular motor signs, coma, or both, after ventricular drainage. Patients with primary intraventricular hemorrhage and hydrocephalus benefit from ventricular drainage as well. Preliminary data suggest that ventricular drainage facilitated by local intraventricular instillation of tPA achieves a more rapid and efficient removal of the intraventricular blood, without an increase in the risk of rebleeding; this has yet to translate to proven improvements in functional outcomes, however.

## Hemostatic Therapy of Intracerebral Hemorrhage

Similar to the acute management of ischemic stroke, rapid emergent treatment is essential for hemostatic therapies to mitigate further hematoma growth and avoid neurological deterioration.

Patients with ICH in the setting of heparin anticoagulation should be treated with protamine sulfate, 1 mg per 100 units of heparin estimated in plasma, whereas those on warfarin should receive 5–25 mg of IV vitamin $K_1$ and, most important, IV prothrombin complex concentrate (PCC; 25–50 U/kg). The direct benefit of PCC over fresh frozen plasma in rapidly reversing abnormally prolonged INR in warfarin-related ICH was established in the INCH trial (Steiner et al., 2016). Fresh frozen plasma (10–20 mL/kg) can be used as a less favorable alternative where PCC is not available. As factor VIIa replaces only one of the four deficient vitamin K-dependent factors, anticoagulation may not be completely reversed in vivo despite rapid normalization of the INR, which is heavily dependent on factor VIIa activity. Accordingly, factor VIIa is currently not recommended for warfarin-related ICH (Hemphill et al., 2015).

Drug-specific antidotes are now available for DOAC-related ICH. IV idarucizumab 5 g (provided as two separate 2.5 g doses no more than 15 minutes apart) can rapidly and safely reverse the anticoagulant effect of dabigatran (Pollack et al., 2017). IV andexanet alfa (400 mg bolus followed by 480 mg infusion over 120 minutes or 800 mg bolus followed by 960 mg infusion over 120 minutes depending on the strength and last timing [more or less than 8 hours, respectively] of the factor Xa-inhibitor dose) reduces anti-factor Xa activity and is associated with high proportion of hemostatic efficacy in factor Xa-inhibitor (apixaban, edoxaban, and rivaroxaban) treated patients (Connolly et al., 2019). The ongoing ANNEXA-I trial will confirm whether these effects of andexanet alfa translate to meaningful improvements in clinical outcomes in intracranial hemorrhage patients. Limited data suggest that PCC (50 U/kg to maximum of 3000 U) may offer some benefit in reversing DOAC-related hemorrhage and can be considered where direct-acting reversal agents are unavailable (Schulman et al., 2018).

Platelet transfusions should be avoided in the case of antiplatelet-related ICH as they do not provide any benefit and may worsen outcomes (Baharoglu, et al. 2016). The use of platelet transfusions to reverse severe thrombocytopenia is still recommended, however. Instances of ICH after thrombolytic therapy are best treated with infusions of 10 units of cryoprecipitate (or fibrinogen concentrate equivalent where available) and 1 g of tranexamic acid.

The documented tendency of hematomas to enlarge after onset, even in the absence of inherent or drug-induced coagulopathies, have stimulated an interest in developing treatments aimed at mitigating this process. Mayer and colleagues (2005) tested the procoagulant agent, recombinant activated factor VII (rFVIIa), in 399 patients with ICH within 4 hours from symptom onset and documented a significant reduction in hematoma growth with three dosages of rFVIIa (40, 80, 160 μg/kg) in comparison with placebo. This was also associated with a significant trend in favor of rFVIIa when clinical outcomes and mortality were compared at 90 days. Thromboembolic complications were more frequent in the rFVIIa groups (7%) than in the placebo group (2%). These encouraging preliminary results were tested in the phase III FAST (rFVIIa in Acute Haemorrhagic Stroke Treatment) trial. This study compared rFVIIa in two dosages (20 and 80 μg/kg) with placebo in patients with ICH treated within 4 hours from onset. Although the subjects treated with 80 μg/kg of rFVIIa had a significantly smaller increase in hematoma volume at 24 hours post-treatment, this was not translated into clinical benefit: mortality and severe disability at 90 days occurred with essentially the same frequency in the three treatment groups (Mayer et al., 2008). In addition, the rate of arterial thromboembolic complications was significantly higher (10%) in the group that received rFVIIa at a dose of 80 μg/kg than in the group that received placebo (5%). Given the front-loaded nature of hematoma expansion, the NINDS-sponsored FASTEST trial will be further testing this agent in a targeted ICH subpopulation presenting within 2 hours of symptom onset to maximize its potential treatment effect.

The benefits of tranexamic acid in major trauma have increased interest in its potential benefits in spontaneous ICH. In the TICH-2 trial (Sprigg et al., 2018), the use of tranexamic acid (1 g bolus, followed by 1 g infused over 8 hours) was shown to be safe and seemed to reduce hematoma expansion and early deaths, but ultimately did not improve functional outcomes at 90 days in spontaneous ICH patients treated within 8 hours of symptom onset. Further trials are currently in preparation to validate and further explore these findings.

*The complete reference list is available online at https://expertconsult.inkling.com/.* 

# 67

# Intracranial Aneurysms and Subarachnoid Hemorrhage

*Viktor Szeder, Satoshi Tateshima, Reza Jahan, Jeffrey L. Saver, Gary R. Duckwiler*

## OUTLINE



An intracranial aneurysm is a cerebrovascular disorder in which weakness in the wall of a brain artery causes dilation or ballooning, which can grow and rupture over time. The term aneurysm originally comes from the Greek *aneurysma—ana* meaning "across" and *eurys* meaning "broad." Rupture of an intracranial aneurysm causes aneurysmal subarachnoid hemorrhage (aSAH), which accounts for 5%–10% of all strokes. aSAH causes greater morbidity and mortality than other stroke types. At least one-quarter of patients who are admitted to the hospital die, and half of the survivors have permanent neurological deficit. Two-thirds of aSAH survivors regain functional independence but half have cognitive impairments, half are dissatisfied with life, and only one-third resume the same work as before the rupture (Rinkel and Algra, 2011). Fortunately, there is a trend of improving outcomes in these patients thanks to early aneurysm repair, aggressive management of hydrocephalus and delayed cerebral ischemia (DCI), as well as better management of general medical complications. As there are an increasing number of neurointensivists and neurohospitalists as well as practicing vascular and general neurologists taking care of these patients, there is also a need to increase the exposure of neurology trainees to the management of aSAH.

Intracranial aneurysms are becoming more frequently detected, given the increased availability of advanced noninvasive diagnostic neurovascular imaging technologies such as computed tomographic angiography (CTA) and magnetic resonance angiography (MRA). Considering that intracranial aneurysm is a fairly common disease and is frequently discovered incidentally or presents symptomatically in young patients, at an age at which a disabling or fatal aSAH can jeopardize decades of otherwise healthy life, in-depth understanding of intracranial aneurysms and their complications is very important for modern comprehensive management of aSAH patients.

## EPIDEMIOLOGY

The annual incidence of aSAH varies across the world, ranging from 2 to 16 cases per 100,000, with the highest rate in Tbilisi, Georgia and the lowest in Dijon, France (Feigin et al., 2009). In the United States, an analysis of the Nationwide Inpatient Sample provided an annual estimate of 14.5 discharges for aSAH per 100,000 adults (Shea et al., 2007). However, up to 15% of patients with acute aSAH die before hospital admission, so the true incidence of aSAH might be even higher (Schievink et al., 1995 and Truelsen et al., 1998). aSAH is uncommon in children and increases with pediatric age. Resulting in an incidence from 0.18 to 2.0 per 100,000 (de Rooij et al., 2007 and Jordan et al., 2009). The average age of adult patients with aSAH is 55 years (Ingall et al., 2000; van Donkelaa et al, 2019). The incidence of aSAH is overall 1.2 times higher in women than in men. However, some evidence suggests an interaction of age and sex, with a higher incidence in younger men (25–45 years of age), women between 55 and 85 years of age, and men older than 85 (de Rooij et al., 2007).

The prevalence of unruptured aneurysms in the general adult population is estimated at 3.2% in imaging studies and 5% adults in autopsy series (Vlak et al., 2011). Fortunately, most intracranial aneurysms do not rupture during the lifetime of an individual. While most persons harbor a single aneurysm, multiple aneurysms are common, occurring in 10%–30% of patients in large clinical series (Juvela et al., 2000; Qureshi et al., 1998). Multiple aneurysms can be mirror aneurysms or located asymmetrically in different locations in the circle of Willis.

Aneurysms can appear sporadically or in family clusters, with familial aneurysms, defined as ≥2 first-degree relatives affected, accounting for between 7% and 20% of patients (Brown and Broderick, 2014; Ronkainen et al., 1997). Inheritance pattern is unclear. Leading possibilities are single-gene mutations with highly incomplete penetrance or multiple interacting genetic variations each with small effect size, and multiple intracranial aneurysms risk genes have been identified (Zhou, et al, 2018). Familial aneurysms tend to be located in the middle cerebral artery and rupture at a younger patient age (Ruigrok et al., 2004; Slot et al., 2019).

### Associated Conditions

Several hereditary and acquired conditions are associated with the formation of intracranial aneurysms and aSAH (Box 67.1). More generally, any congenital or acquired condition that produces vascular wall weakening and/or increased hemodynamic stress could result in the formation of intracranial aneurysms.

**BOX 67.1 Risk Factors and Associated Conditions for Intracranial Aneurysms**

Hypertension
Tobacco smoking
Autosomal dominant inherited polycystic kidney disease
Ehlers-Danlos syndrome, vascular type (formally called type IV)
Fibromuscular dysplasia
Coarctation of the aorta
Moyamoya syndrome
Pseudoxanthoma elasticum
$\alpha_1$-Antitrypsin deficiency
Systemic lupus erythematosus
Sickle cell anemia
Bacterial endocarditis
Fungal infection
Neurofibromatosis type 1
Tuberous sclerosis
Pheochromocytoma
Arteriovenous malformations
Anomalous carotid-vertebrobasilar anastomoses
Cocaine use

Approximately 5% of aneurysms are associated with connective tissue disorders, the most important being Ehlers-Danlos syndrome, vascular type (type IV), neurofibromatosis type 1, and autosomal dominant polycystic kidney disease (Hitchcock et al., 2017). Among all patients with polycystic kidney disease, approximately 8% harbor saccular aneurysms (Cagnazzo et al., 2017). The vascular type of Ehlers-Danlos syndrome, formally called *type IV*, has a defect of type-III collagen synthesis, which is a major component of distensible tissues such as vessels. A higher incidence of intracranial aneurysms in the cavernous segment of internal carotid artery (ICA) has been reported. The indication of arterial or venous puncture for catheter angiography in patients with Ehlers-Danlos syndrome should be carefully discussed because of increased vascular fragility and complications.

There are several known modifiable risk factors for aSAH, including—most prominently—hypertension, smoking, alcohol abuse, and the use of sympathomimetic drugs (e.g., cocaine). The role of elevated blood pressure in the formation of intracranial aneurysms has been supported by the association of aneurysms coarctation of the aorta, pheochromocytoma, and cocaine use—all conditions that can cause severe elevated blood pressure. Hypertension likely contributes to aneurysm formation and rupture via multiple mechanisms, including promoting wall injury and remodeling, and increasing radial force upon weakened wall segments. Active cigarette smoking is a risk factor for intracranial aneurysm formation (Inagawa, 2010) and may increase the risk of aneurysm rupture. American Heart Association/American Stroke Association guidelines recommend treatment of these risk factors to avert first or recurrent subarachnoid hemorrhage (Connolly et al., 2012). Interestingly, despite the increased success in the treatment of these factors, the incidence of aSAH has not changed in 35 years, though this may, in part, reflect improved detection counterbalancing mild actual incidence decline (Lovelock et al., 2010; Mackey et al., 2016).

## PATHOPHYSIOLOGY

Intracranial aneurysms are classified according to their morphology, size, pathogenesis, and anatomical location (Box 67.2). There are three morphological types of intracranial aneurysms: saccular, fusiform, and dissecting (Fig. 67.1).

**BOX 67.2 Classification of Intracranial Aneurysms**

**By Morphology**
Saccular
Fusiform
Dissecting

**By Pathogenesis**
Genetic
Hemodynamic (arteriovenous malformation, contralateral carotid ligation, etc.)
Infection (bacterial, fungal)
Trauma
Atherosclerosis
Neoplasm (primary or metastatic)
Radiation
Drug abuse
Connective tissue disorders
Vasculopathy
Miscellaneous conditions (moyamoya disease, etc.)

**By Size**
<3 mm (small)
3–6 mm (small)
7–12 mm (small-medium)
13–25 mm (large)
>25 mm (giant)

**By Location**

***Internal Carotid Artery***
1. Cavernous
2. Carotid cave
3. Paraclinoid
4. Ophthalmic
5. Superior hypophyseal
6. Posterior communicating
7. Anterior choroidal
8. Carotid bifurcation

***Anterior Cerebral Artery***
1. A1
2. Anterior communicating
3. A1–2
4. A2 and distal

***Middle Cerebral Artery***
1. M1
2. Bifurcation
3. M2 and distal

***Vertebral Artery***
1. PICA

***Basilar Artery***
1. Trunk
2. Fenestration
3. AICA
4. SCA
5. Basilar apex

***Posterior Cerebral Artery***
1. P1
2. P2 and distal

*AICA,* Anterior inferior cerebellar artery; *PICA,* Posterior inferior cerebellar artery; *SCA,* Superior cerebellar artery.

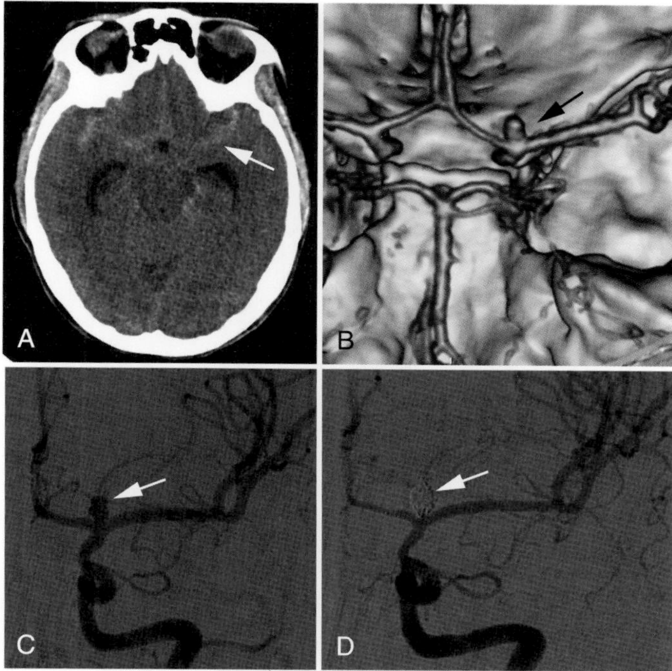


**Fig. 67.1 A 33-Year-Old Patient With Hunt and Hess Grade III Subarachnoid Hemorrhage.** **A,** Computed tomography (CT) scan shows an extensive subarachnoid hemorrhage *(white arrow)*, Fisher grade 3. **B,** Three-dimensional CT angiography demonstrates a saccular aneurysm *(black arrow)* arising from the left internal carotid artery terminus. **C,** Digital subtraction angiography, anteroposterior view, prior to endovascular treatment shows the aneurysm measuring 4.7 mm in height and 3.2 mm in width *(white arrow)*. **D,** After treatment, the aneurysm was completely obliterated using platinum coils *(white arrow)*.

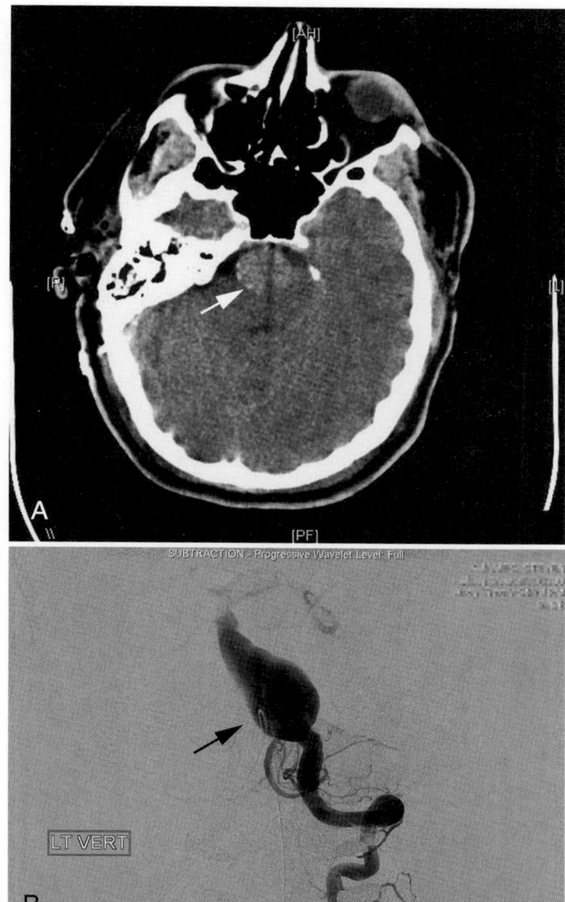


**Fig. 67.2 Patient Who Presented With Symptoms of Brainstem Mass Effect.** **A,** Computed tomography scan of brain shows an enlarged basilar artery *(white arrow)* in the basal cistern and severe mass effect on the belly of the pons. **B,** Digital subtraction angiography of the left vertebral artery shows a dolichoectasia involving the left vertebral artery and entire basilar trunk *(black arrow)*.

## Saccular Aneurysm

The most common morphological aneurysm type is *saccular aneurysms*, rounded, berry-like, outpouchings arising from first- and second-order branches in the circle of Willis (see Fig. 67.1). Saccular aneurysms may have narrow or wide openings (necks) leading into the aneurysm from the parent artery. They account for approximately 90% of intracranial aneurysms and are responsible for most of the morbidity and mortality from aSAH.

Intracranial arteries are structurally unique since they lack external elastic lamina, which in the anterior circulation disappears in the horizontal segment of the cavernous internal carotid arteries. Reduction and disappearance of the external elastic lamina and of elastic fibers in the tunica media also occurs in the vertebral arteries as they enter the skull. These structural alterations weaken the arterial walls making them less resistant to constant hemodynamic forces such as dynamic pressure, blood pressure, and shear stress. Although the etiology of intracranial saccular aneurysm formation involves multiple factors, a key pathogenetic step is degeneration of tunica media and internal elastic lamina at the branching sites of intracranial arteries in regions of chronic hemodynamic stress. In children with intracranial aneurysms, the abnormalities of tunica media and internal elastic lamina may be congenital rather than degenerative as in adults (Takemoto et al., 2014).

## Fusiform Aneurysm

A *fusiform aneurysm* is defined as a circumferential dilatation in a segment of an intracranial artery. Unlike a saccular aneurysm that has a single orifice (neck) through which blood passes into and out of the aneurysm cavity, a fusiform aneurysm does not have a defined orifice (neck). The inflow and outflow of fusiform aneurysms are longitudinally separate, which often makes surgical or interventional treatment of these aneurysms challenging. Fusiform aneurysms are often associated with atherosclerosis, which causes extensive damage to the tunica media and results in arterial stretching to all sides or elongation. Although infrequent, other diseases are known to cause vessel damage resulting in fusiform aneurysms. If an arterial fusiform dilatation is accompanied by a marked elongation and tortuosity, it is called a *dolichoectasia* (*dolichos*, long; *ectasia*, distended). Dolichoectatic fusiform aneurysms are often seen in the posterior circulation and can reach several centimeters in diameter (Fig. 67.2). Patients with dolichoectatic aneurysms characteristically present with mass effect on cranial nerves or brainstem compression, but also less frequently may present with subarachnoid hemorrhage or with ischemic stroke due to thrombosis in the dilated arterial segment or displacement and kinking of penetrating arteries (Lou and Caplan, 2010).

## Dissecting Aneurysm

A *dissecting aneurysm* is formed as a result of splitting or dissection of an arterial wall by blood entering or exiting through a tear. This may cause inward displacement of the vessel wall narrowing the lumen (stenosis) or outward displacement of the vessel wall (dissecting aneurysms). While

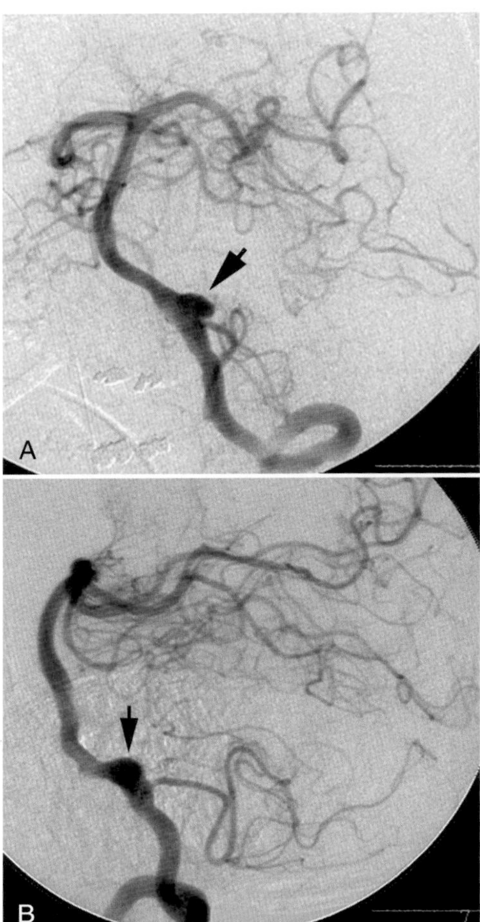


**Fig. 67.3 Digital Subtraction Angiograms of the Left Vertebral Artery.** Anteroposterior view (**A**) and lateral view (**B**) show a dissecting aneurysm *(short arrow)* just distal to the origin of the left posterior inferior cerebellar artery.

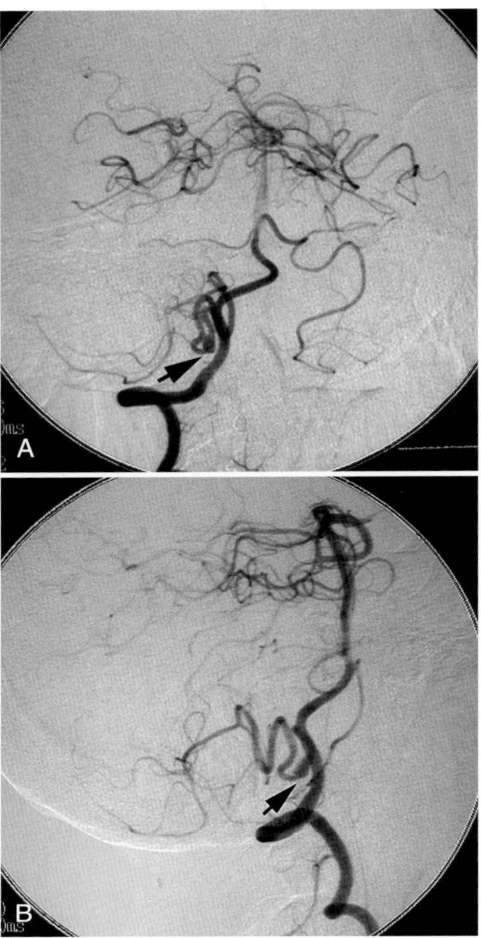


**Fig. 67.4 Patient With a Ruptured Dissecting Aneurysm of the Posterior Inferior Cerebellar Artery (PICA).** Digital subtraction angiograms of the right vertebral artery, anteroposterior view (**A**) and lateral view (**B**), show a small fusiform dilatation *(short arrow)* in the right PICA.

extracranial dissections typically cause intimal-media intramural hematomas with inward wall displacement and arterial narrowing (classic radiographic appearance of string-and-pear sign), intracranial dissections typically cause medial-adventitial intramural hematomas with outward wall displacing and saccular- or fusiform-like aneurysmal appearance (Fig. 67.3). Intracranial dissecting aneurysms often present with subarachnoid hemorrhage. In patients with severe SAH but no clear angiographic evidence of the source of the hemorrhage, very careful review of the angiograms should be conducted to search for a small dissecting aneurysm (Figs. 67.4 and 67.5). Intracranial dissections can occur spontaneously, but they are commonly associated with trauma or an underlying vasculopathy such as fibromuscular dysplasia. Minor trauma such as head turning, chiropractic manipulation, sneezing, or variety of sports activities may promote intracranial dissection or resultant dissecting aneurysm, with or without underlying vasculopathy (Smith et al., 2003).

## Mycotic Aneurysm

*Mycotic aneurysms* (infectious intracranial aneurysms) are rare infectious lesions that occur secondary to the spread of microbial infections to the arterial vessel wall, resulting in its weakening and aneurysmal dilatation. An early canine model of aortic infectious aneurysms experiments revealed first changes by the bacterial emboli in the adventitial layer and spread to involve media (Molinari et al., 1973). Aneurysmal enlargement occurs by the arterial pulsation against a weakened wall. Contiguous extension of an intracranial infectious focus could also weaken the arterial wall, causing mycotic aneurysm (Suwanwela et al., 1972). Further classification of these aneurysms includes septic embolic, contiguously infected, and cryptogenic. The most common cause is bacterial infections, with Streptococcus viridans being the most frequent. Fungal infections such as *Aspergillus* and *Candida* spp. are also common. Nevertheless, in about 13% of cases blood cultures could be negative.

Mycotic aneurysms are more prevalent in men and are reported across a wide range of age groups, with most patients being young to middle-aged adults (Alawieh et al., 2018). The average mortality significantly improved over the last two decades. However, the most common presentation of mycotic aneurysms (over 70%) is brain hemorrhage, with about half of the cases being SAH, leading to a potential mortality of up to 80% (Singla et al., 2016).

Ruptured mycotic aneurysms causing SAH require urgent treatment. Neuroendovascular intervention has been the preferred first-line therapy in the last decade, with significantly lower mortality, easier access to distal aneurysms, higher success in the treatment of multiple aneurysms, shorter delay to subsequent cardiac surgery, and lower risk of hemorrhage from anticoagulation compared with microsurgical craniotomies (Petr et al., 2016). The overall management also has to include targeted antimicrobial therapy and cardiac intervention in patients with infective endocarditis.

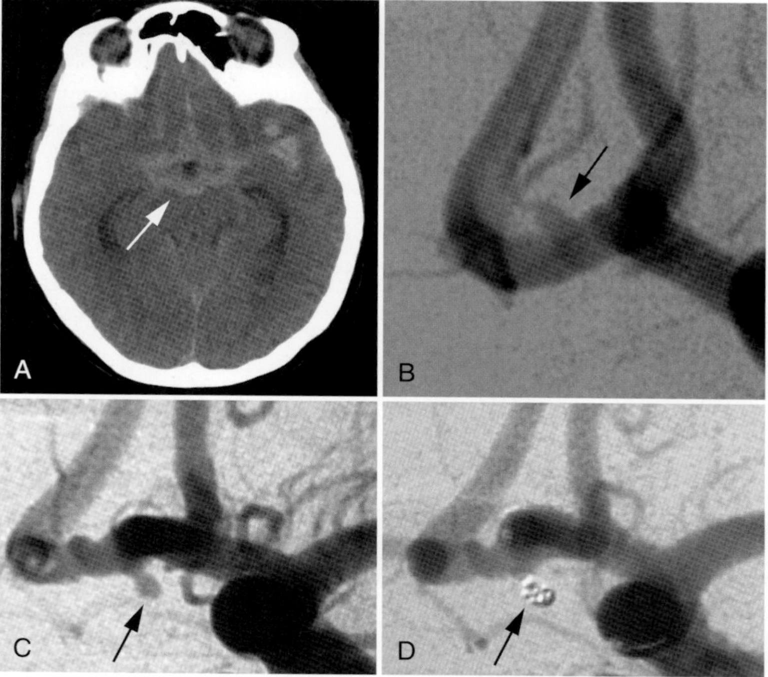


**Fig. 67.5** Patient With Hunt and Hess Grade I. **A,** Computed tomography (CT) of brain showed aneurysmal subarachnoid hemorrhage (aSAH) *(white arrow),* Fisher grade 4. **B,** At the time of admission digital subtraction angiography showed no clear evidence of an aneurysm in the anterior communicating artery (Acomm) region. There is an infundibulum *(arrow)* of an Acomm perforator pointing superiorly. **C,** Digital subtraction angiography at day 7 shows a small 2 mm aneurysm *(arrow)* pointing inferiorly. **D,** After treatment, the aneurysm was completely obliterated using 1 platinum coil *(arrow).*

## NATURAL HISTORY OF INTRACRANIAL ANEURYSMS

Several large, multicenter studies have delineated rates and predictors of growth and rupture of intracranial aneurysms. Understanding their natural history as well as the risks associated with their repair is mandatory for appropriate management. Several single center and retrospective observational studies suggested annual rupture rates between 1% and 6.5%, with increased rupture rates in women, older patients, symptomatic aneurysms, aneurysms in the posterior circulation, and those of a larger size greater than 10 mm (Juvela 2000, Morita 2005). However, annual rupture rates proved lower in multicenter and prospective studies (ISUIA Investigators, 1998, Wiebers et al., 2003).

The two influential, large, prospective multicenter studies were the International Study of Unruptured Intracranial Aneurysms (ISUIA) and the UCAS Japan study, both showing similar findings (Wiebers et al., 2003; UCAS Japan Investigators et al., 2012). The ISUIA study evaluated 4060 patients with unruptured intracranial saccular aneurysms in North America and Europe, and UCAS Japan assessed 5720 patients with unruptured intracranial saccular aneurysms in Japan. The ISUIA study's 4060 patients included 1692 who were treated medically, 1917 treated with open surgery (generally clipping), and 451 treated with endovascular procedures (generally coiling). Among the 1692 patients in the medically treated cohort, there were a total of 2686 aneurysms, and 1077 patients had no prior history of SAH (group 1), while 615 had a prior history of a SAH from another aneurysm (group 2). In the medically treated patients, over 5 years of follow-up, larger aneurysm size and posterior circulation location were the most important predictors of subsequent rupture. The 5-year cumulative risk of rupture for anterior circulation (Internal carotid artery [ICA], anterior cerebral artery (ACA), and middle cerebral artery [MCA]) aneurysms was 0% for less than 7 mm diameter, 2.6% for 7–12 mm diameter, 14.5% for 13–24 mm diameter, and 40% for ≥25 mm diameter. The risk of rupture for posterior circulation aneurysms was 2.5% for less than 7 mm, 14.5% for 7–12 mm, 18.4% for 13–24 mm, and 50% for ≥25 mm. For small aneurysms (<7 mm), patients with a prior aSAH had a higher cumulative risk of rupture (1.5% anterior circulation, 3.4% posterior circulation; Table 67.1). The Japanese study identified aneurysm morphology as an additional independent risk factor. Aneurysms with a daughter sac or multilobuations were also more likely to rupture (hazard ratio 1.63).

In the ISUIA study, among patients treated initially with interventional therapy, 30-day morbidity and mortality rates were 13.2% for open surgery and 9.1% for endovascular therapy. In the surgical group, predictors of poor outcome included age ≥50 years, aneurysm diameter ≥12 mm, posterior circulation location, previous ischemic cerebrovascular disease, and unruptured aneurysm presenting with symptoms. In the endovascular group, predictors of poor outcome were aneurysm diameter ≥12 mm and posterior circulation location, but age was not a predictor.

Both the ISUIA and UCAS Japan studies have limitations. As treatment was nonrandomized, there likely was some degree of selection bias, with lower-risk patients being allocated to medical therapy and higher-risk patients allocated to interventional treatment. Fusiform, saccular traumatic, and mycotic aneurysms were excluded from both the IUISA and UCAS Japan studies, so their long-term outcomes under different treatment approaches are less well characterized.

In addition to its baseline characteristics, subsequent growth of an unruptured intracranial aneurysm identifies lesions at increased risk of rupture potentially warranting interventional therapy. Serial imaging cohort studies have developed a scale predictive of subsequent aneurysm growth with eight component items: older patient age, MCA or

**TABLE 67.1 Five-Year Cumulative Hemorrhage Rates of Unruptured Aneurysms, by Site, Size, and Association With Other Ruptured Aneurysm***

| | <7 mm | <7 mm | 7–12 mm | 13–24 mm | >25 mm |
|---|---|---|---|---|---|
| | No Prior SAH | Prior SAH From Other Aneurysm | | | |
| Cavernous carotid artery | 0% | 0% | 0% | 3% | 6.4% |
| Anterior circulation | 0% | 1.5% | 2.6% | 14.5% | 40% |
| Posterior circulation | 2.5% | 3.4% | 14.5% | 18.4% | 50% |

*Anterior circulation includes anterior communicating artery, internal carotid artery other than cavernous carotid artery, and middle cerebral artery, but does not include posterior communicating artery.

†Posterior circulation includes vertebrobasilar artery posterior cerebral artery, and posterior communicating artery.

*Reported in International Study of Unruptured Intracranial Aneurysms Investigators, 2003 (Wiebers, D. O., Whisnant, J. P., Huston, J., 3rd, Meissner, I., Brown, R. D., Jr., Piepgras, D. G., et al. (2003). International study of unruptured intracranial aneurysms Investigators. Unruptured intracranial aneurysms: Natural history, clinical outcome, and risks of surgical and endovascular treatment.* Lancet, *362, 103–110).*

posterior circulation location, earlier subarachnoid hemorrhage from a different aneurysm, location in MCA or posterior circulation, older age, Japanese or Finnish population, larger size, and irregular shape of the aneurysm. On the resulting ELAPSS scale, 5-year growth risk ranges from under 9% to over 60% (Backes et al., 2017). A potential emerging imaging tool to identify unstable aneurysms at higher risk of growth and rupture is enhancement of the aneurysm wall after gadolinium on magnetic resonance imaging (MRI) (Lv et al. 2018; Edjlali et al., 2018).

A particular management challenge is patients with small aneurysms ≤7mm. These are by far the most numerous and least risky of unruptured aneurysms, but still account for an important fraction of subsequent subarachnoid hemorrhages. Additional studies are needed to improve identification of high-risk aneurysms in this small size range. In addition to irregular contour (including blebs and daughter sacs) identified in UCAS Japan, other aneurysm morphology indices may be helpful, including aspect ratio (i.e., ratio of aneurysm neck-to-dome length to aneurysm neck width) and height-to-width ratio, but firm evidence from adequately powered prospective studies using multivariable analyses is lacking (Kleinloog et al., 2018).

Management decisions for patients with unruptured aneurysms should be made on an individual basis, with careful consideration of life expectancy, estimated risks for hemorrhage, and estimated risks associated with interventional treatment (Harrigan and Deveikis, 2013; Thompson et al., 2015).

## IMAGING MODALITIES AND DIAGNOSIS

### Subarachnoid Hemorrhage

Brain noncontrast computed tomography (NCCT) is a highly sensitive imaging modality for diagnosis of aSAH (see Fig. 67.1, *A*). NCCT also provides other important information, including the presence of early hydrocephalus. The distribution of subarachnoid blood on NCCT suggests the location of the rupture site, and the extent of blood is a predictor of the probability of vasospasm and DCI (Box 67.3). In addition, CTA can directly visualize the aneurysm.

Compared with the gold standard of lumbar puncture, NCCT scan confirms a SAH with very high sensitivity, close to 100%, in the first 3 days (Cortnum et al., 2010). The sensitivity decreases moderately with time as the subarachnoid blood is metabolized and cleared. If there is a strong clinical suspicion for aneurysm rupture and a computed tomography (CT) scan fails to reveal a SAH, lumbar puncture should be performed. Cerebrospinal fluid (CSF) characteristics indicating a SAH are elevated red blood cell count and xanthochromia. Approximately 2 hours after the hemorrhage, xanthochromia becomes detectable and may last as long as several weeks. In a patient where there is clinical suspicion for SAH but negative NCCT and lumbar puncture, angiography should be used to search for a potential a SAH source.

**BOX 67.3 Computed Tomography Scan Classification of Subarachnoid Hemorrhage (Fisher Scale)**

Group 1: No blood detected

Group 2: Diffuse deposition or thin layer of blood, with all vertical layers of blood (interhemispheric fissure, insular cistern, ambient cistern) <1 mm thick

Group 3: Localized clots or vertical layers of blood 1 mm or greater in thickness

Group 4: Diffuse or no subarachnoid hemorrhage but with intraparenchymal or intraventricular clots

Multimodal MRI, including fluid-attenuated inversion recovery (FLAIR), proton density, and gradient echo (GRE) sequences, is becoming an important diagnostic tool to detect acute and chronic a SAH. FLAIR MRI sequences detect acute a SAH with equal sensitivity to NCCT. GRE MRI sequences can demonstrate subacute and chronic a SAH blood that is not apparent on CT (Kidwell and Wintermark, 2008) (Fig. 67.6).

For initial evaluation of, and screening for, unruptured intracranial aneurysms, either of the noninvasive angiographic imaging modalities, CTA and MRA, are preferred. Noncontrast time-of-flight MRA is the least-invasive modality to visualize the intracranial vasculature and is useful for screening but has lower sensitivity in detecting aneurysms with slow blood flow. Contrast-enhanced MRA and the use of higher strength, 3 tesla (3 T) provides very clear visualization of the intracranial vasculature. However, longer acquisition times and higher susceptibility to patient motion than CTA make it unsuitable as a first-line imaging modality in acute SAH. In some patients, CTA or MRA findings provide sufficient aneurysm characterization to guide management decision making. However, in some cases, four-vessel conventional catheter angiography (both two-dimensional [2D] and rotational three-dimensional [3D] angiography) is an important modality in the assessment of SAH. In a case of clear SAH with negative CTA, four-vessel conventional catheter angiography with 3D reconstruction is mandatory. If four-vessel angiography and/or CTA do not reveal any source of the hemorrhage, six-vessel angiography (including external carotid injections) should be performed to rule out rare causes of hemorrhage such as a dural fistula or venous pathology. Use of 3D rotating catheter angiography is also essential to delineate the clear relationship of a saccular aneurysm to its parent and daughter arteries (Fig. 67.7), as well as the details of the aneurysm morphology necessary for planning its treatment. Catheter angiography with carotid compression (Matas test and Alcock test) is used

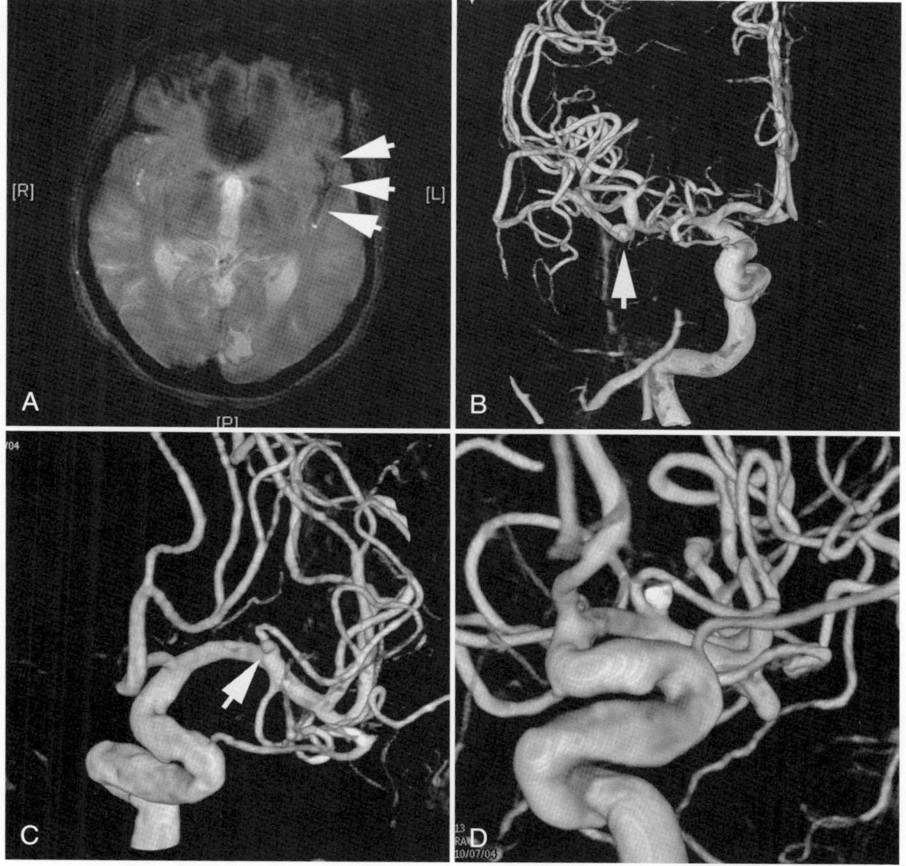


**Fig. 67.6 Patient with Bilateral Middle Cerebral Artery (MCA) Aneurysms and Subarachnoid Hemorrhage was Transferred to Our Hospital at Day 10.** Computed tomography was not helpful in determining the rupture site. However, gradient echo magnetic resonance imaging (**A**) shows blooming artifact centered in the left sylvian fissure *(arrows)* and aneurysm on the left was determined to be the rupture site. **B** and **C**, Digital subtraction three-dimensional angiography shows a small saccular aneurysm in the right MCA bifurcation (**B**, *arrow*), and smaller saccular aneurysm in the left MCA bifurcation (**C**, *arrow*). **D**, The left MCA aneurysm was completely embolized with platinum coils.

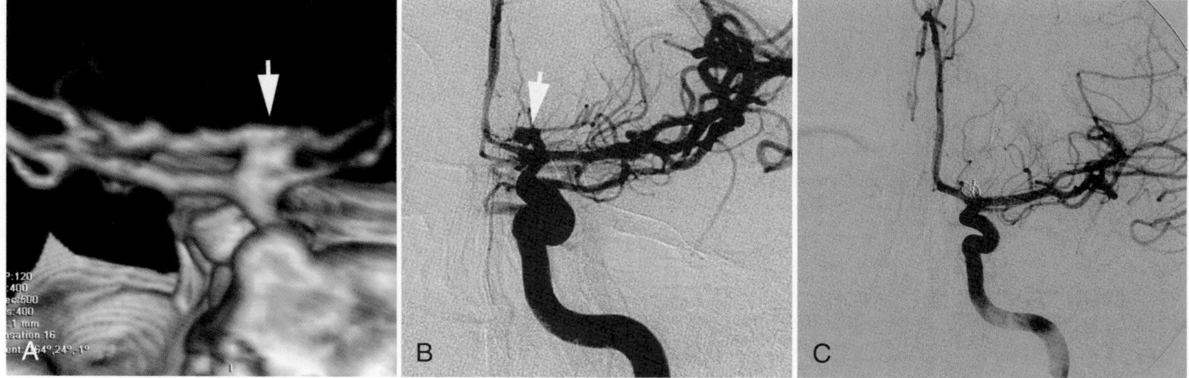


**Fig. 67.7 Patient With Hunt and Hess Grade 1 Subarachnoid Hemorrhage. A**, Computed tomographic angiography, posterior-anterior view, shows a small-domed, broad-necked aneurysm at the left internal carotid artery bifurcation *(arrow)*. Aneurysm shape was obscured by venous structures, and relationship of aneurysm dome and anterior cerebral artery was unclear, so digital subtraction catheter angiography was performed. **B**, Arterial phase of catheter angiography, anteroposterior view, shows a boot-shaped, very small-necked aneurysm with a clear separation of the left anterior cerebral artery from the aneurysm dome *(arrow)*. **C**, Owing to the small neck morphology seen on the catheter angiogram, endovascular embolization could be performed and the aneurysm was completely obliterated.

to visualize cross-flow via the anterior and posterior communicating arteries and is required if a parent artery occlusion must be considered as a treatment option.

Although the capability of separate acquisition of arterial, capillary, and venous phases as well as high spatial resolution are advantages of catheter angiography, it has intrinsic limitations. For instance, in order to choose an adequate treatment strategy for a partially thrombosed aneurysm, visualization of patent lumen by catheter angiography is not sufficient. A variety of 3D imaging methods with CTA, including volume rendering, maximal intensity projection, and axial, coronal, and sagittal 2D images, provide pertinent information including the true size of the aneurysm, the presence and degree of mural calcification, and the mass effect on surrounding structures.

In a patient with multiple aneurysms, identifying the rupture site requires thorough investigation, including the distribution of aSAH, clinical signs, and angiographic findings. CT or MR findings such as a focal parenchymal or cisternal hematoma adjacent to an aneurysm strongly suggest the rupture site. Aneurysmal wall enhancement with gadolinium on MRI additionally implicates an aneurysm as recently ruptured. A larger and irregularly shaped aneurysm is more likely to be the rupture site. Focal spasm is also a reliable sign but is relatively uncommon.

In approximately 10%–15% of patients with aSAH, no aneurysm or other source of hemorrhage can be detected. If the amount of aSAH is small and its distribution is anterior to the midbrain, without filling of the anterior interhemispheric fissure, extension to the lateral sylvian fissure, or presence of frank intraventricular hemorrhage, the diagnosis of perimesencephalic SAH may be established (Mensing et al., 2018). The prognosis is generally benign and the etiology may be spontaneous rupture of perimesencephalic veins. In a patient with an extensive SAH but negative angiography, repeating the imaging studies after a delay, including catheter angiography or CTA, is mandatory and can lead to the detection of small aneurysms in up to 14% of cases (see Fig. 67.5). The repeat study should be performed 1–2 weeks after the initial study, paying particular attention to identifying small dissecting aneurysms and pseudoaneurysms (false aneurysms with ruptured walls and a SAH but no enlargement of any layer of the vessel wall). CTA with intravenous administration of contrast is more sensitive in identifying very-slow-flowing lesions such as pseudoaneurysms.

## SYMPTOMS

Most aneurysms remain asymptomatic until the time of rupture. The typical symptom patients report with aneurysmal rupture is sudden onset of severe (thunderclap) headache described as "the worst headache of my life" in 80% of cases. This may be associated with other symptoms, such as nausea and/or vomiting, stiff neck, photophobia, brief loss of consciousness, or focal neurological deficits (including cranial nerve palsies). Aneurysms are a little more likely to rupture during physical exertion and during activities associated with a Valsalva maneuver (e.g., defecation/micturition, heavy lifting); most aneurysms rupture during regular daily activity (Matsuda et al., 2007).

A warning, sentinel headache, may precede aSAH in 10%–43% of patients (de Falco, 2004). Sentinel headaches increase the odds of early rebleeding after the first overt aSAH by 10-fold (Beck et al., 2006). The causes of sentinel headaches are likely several, including minor aneurysm rupture with a small degree of a SAH, hemorrhage into the wall of an aneurysm without complete rupture or a SAH, and expansion and stretching of an aneurysm wall.

Approximately 1 in 20 aSAH patients may be misdiagnosed during emergency department visits (Vermeulen and Schull, 2007), mostly due to mild and uncommon symptoms. Unfortunately, missed initial recognition of aSAH is associated with nearly a fourfold higher likelihood of death or disability at 1 year (Kowalski, 2004). A validated technique for identifying which headache patients should receive brain imaging and lumbar puncture to screen for SAH is the Ottawa Subarachnoid Hemorrhage Rule, which says definitive work-up is indicated in patients presenting with new severe nontraumatic headache reaching maximum intensity within 1 hour plus any one or more of the following six features: neck pain or stiffness, age greater than 40, loss of consciousness, onset during exertion, thunderclap (instant peak) onset, or reduced neck flexion on examination (Perry et al, 2017).

**TABLE 67.2 Most Commonly Used Clinical Grading Scales for Subarachnoid Hemorrhage**

**Hunt and Hess Scale**

Grade 0: Asymptomatic
Grade 1: Mild headache and mild nuchal rigidity, no neurological deficit
Grade 2: Moderate to severe headache but no neurological deficit other than cranial nerve palsy
Grade 3: Drowsy, confused, or mild focal deficit
Grade 4: Stupor, moderate to severe hemiparesis, and early decerebrate posturing
Grade 5: Deep comatose, decerebrate posturing

**WORLD FEDERATION OF NEUROLOGICAL SURGEONS SCALE**

| | Glasgow Coma Scale | Motor Deficit |
|---|---|---|
| Grade 0 | 15 | Absent |
| Grade 1 | 15 | Absent |
| Grade 2 | 13–14 | Absent |
| Grade 3 | 13–14 | Present |
| Grade 4 | 7–12 | Present or absent |
| Grade 5 | 3–6 | Present or absent |

Several formal grading scales using clinical variables are available to characterize presenting severity of SAH. The most widely used grading methods are summarized in Table 67.2. These methods are known to correlate with clinical outcomes.

A common presentation of intracranial aneurysms, especially of the ICA–posterior communicating artery segment, is with third cranial nerve palsy due to mass effect from aneurysm expansion or escaped blood. Unilateral ptosis, outward eye deviation, and a dilated pupil are the classic presentation of aneurysm-induced third-nerve palsy. These may be accompanied by retrobulbar pain. The ipsilateral pupil is often compromised by the mass effect from an expanded or ruptured aneurysm, since the nerve fibers controlling the pupils are located on the outer portion of the third nerve. In contrast, pupil-sparing third nerve palsies generally reflect lesions within the core of the third nerve, such as ischemia, and only very rarely arise from aneurysms or other sources of external compression (Fujiwara et al., 1989).

Basilar artery–superior cerebellar artery aneurysms can also present with third nerve palsies even if they are small in size. Other aneurysm–cranial nerve presentations include third-, fourth-, and sixth-nerve palsies from cavernous ICA aneurysms and optic nerve visual field defects from internal carotid–ophthalmic artery aneurysms. An important factor influencing the recovery of the cranial nerve palsy is the time interval between onset and intervention, with shorter intervals having a better prognosis. New or progressive mass effect from an aneurysm in the absence of a SAH indicates aneurysm growth and instability. Therefore, intracranial aneurysms, including cavernous aneurysms, presenting with mass effect should be considered for

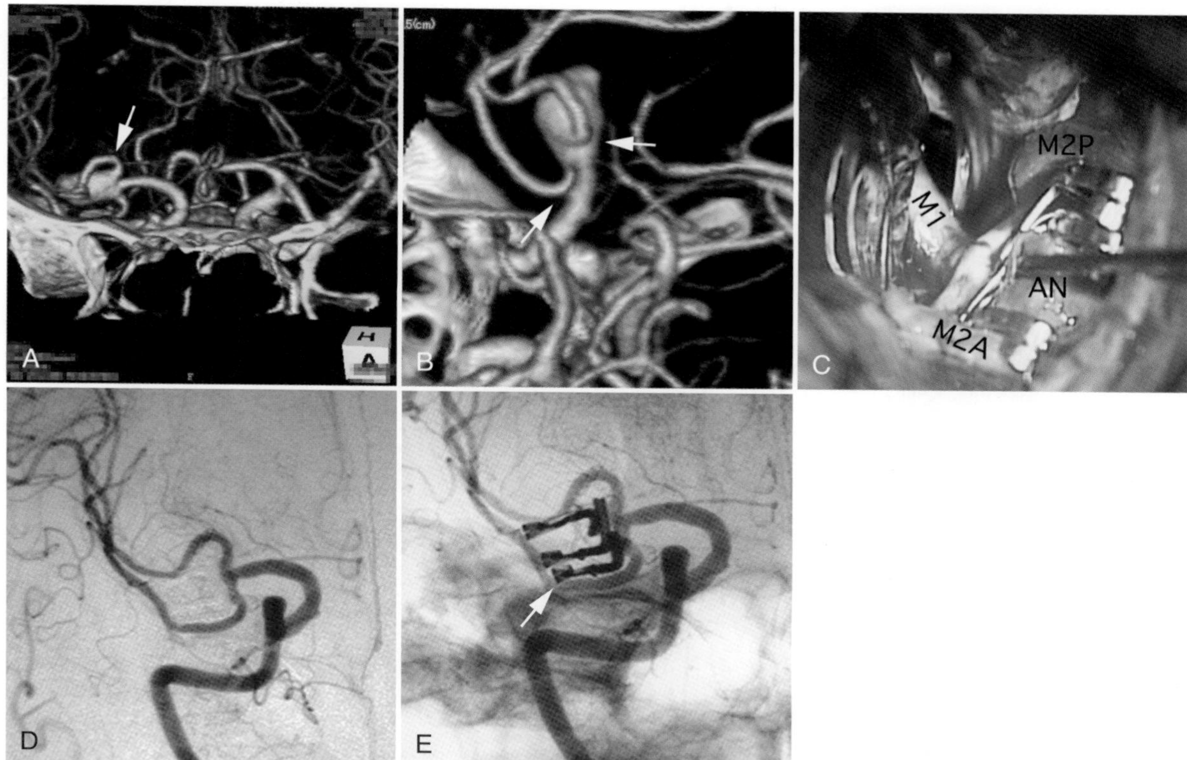


**Fig. 67.8 Patient With Hunt and Hess Grade 2, Fisher Group 3 Subarachnoid Hemorrhage. A,** Computed tomographic angiogram (CTA), anteroposterior view, shows a large saccular aneurysm *(arrow)* in the right middle cerebral artery (MCA) bifurcation. **B,** CTA, left inferior to right anterior view, shows both M2 branches are incorporated into aneurysm base *(arrows)*. **C,** Reconstructive surgical clipping was performed. *AN,* Aneurysm; *M1,* M1 segment; *M2A,* M2 segment anterior division; *M2P,* M2 segment posterior division. Follow-up catheter angiograms with subtraction (**D**) and without subtraction (**E**) show complete obliteration of the aneurysm by surgical clips *(arrow)*, with preservation of both MCA branches.

surgical or endovascular interventions to prevent catastrophic a SAH, as well as further cranial neuropathy and other mass effect symptoms.

## TREATMENT OF INCIDENTAL INTRACRANIAL ANEURYSMS

Management options of an incidentally discovered, unruptured aneurysm should be carefully considered and should be made on an individual basis, with consideration of life expectancy, estimated risk for hemorrhage, and estimated risks associated with treatment. Based on several risk factors for rupture, the PHASES score has been recently proposed to evaluate 5-year absolute risk of aneurysm rupture in individual patients, and takes into account risk factors of age, hypertension, history of a SAH from another aneurysm, size, location, and patient geographical region (Greving et al., 2014).

In individual patients, additional risk factors should be considered as well, such as known vascular fragility, family history, cigarette smoking, and other comorbidities. Cessation of cigarette smoking and adequate maintenance of normal blood pressure are the first steps in management, regardless of the overall treatment plan. Depending on the patient's clinical condition, aneurysm configuration, aneurysm size, vascular anatomy in the circle of Willis and proximal cervical vessels, the most suitable treatment modality should be selected for each patient.

### Open Surgical Treatment

A variety of surgical approaches have been developed for direct surgical clipping to close aneurysm necks, with each approach tailored to the specific anatomy and location of the intracranial aneurysm. Advances in the development of microsurgical techniques and research on microsurgical anatomy have improved the safety of surgical clipping procedures for aneurysms (Rice et al., 1990; Sano, 2010). A surgical clip is usually placed across the aneurysm neck, with preservation of the parent artery. Multiple surgical clips may be placed on an aneurysm that has branches so that the parent artery and the branches remain patent (Fig. 67.8). Surgical clipping is highly effective, with reported rates of complete aneurysm occlusion of 90%–95%. However, surgical clipping carries risks of procedural morbidity and mortality. In the ISUIA study, the risks of morbidity and mortality at 1 year were 9.8% and 2.3%, respectively (ISUIA Investigators, 1998; Wiebers et al., 2003). When a clip cannot be safely applied at the neck of an aneurysm, alternative modalities such as wrapping or trapping may be performed (Fig. 67.9). Surgical treatment of intracranial aneurysms of the posterior circulation, such as the upper basilar region, is associated with higher risks. Other known risk factors for surgery are advanced patient age, large or giant aneurysms, past history of ischemic cerebrovascular disease, and symptomatic aneurysms other than rupture.

### Endovascular Treatment

Endovascular treatment of intracranial aneurysms has evolved rapidly since the introduction of Guglielmi detachable coils (Guglielmi et al., 1991) and now is more common in the United States than surgical clipping. In the endovascular procedure, a microcatheter is placed in the dome of an aneurysm, and the aneurysm is tightly packed with a variety of coils to induce thrombosis (see Fig. 67.1, *C* and *D*). The success of endovascular treatment of intracranial aneurysms is less dependent on their location and more dependent on their anatomical

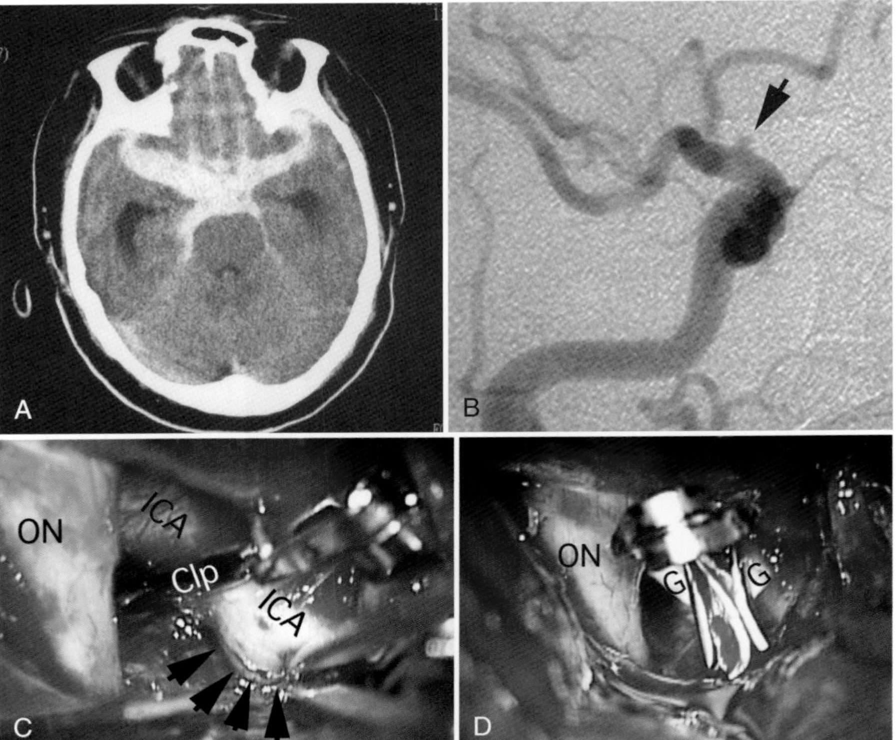


**Fig. 67.9 Patient With Hunt and Hess Grade 3 Subarachnoid Hemorrhage. A,** Computed tomography (CT) shows diffuse subarachnoid hemorrhage (Fisher grade 3) but slightly greater in the right sylvian cistern. Initial CT angiography and digital subtraction angiography failed to depict the site of rupture. **B,** Another digital subtraction angiography a week later shows a small outpouching in the anterior wall of the right internal carotid artery *(arrow)*. **C,** Intraoperative photo shows a laceration of the right internal carotid artery *(four arrows)* underneath a subadventitial pseudoaneurysm. **D,** The laceration was sutured with 11-0 Proline and subsequently wrapped with a Gore-Tex sheet and one L-shaped aneurysm clip. *Clp,* Temporary clip; *G,* Gore-Tex sheet; *ICA,* internal carotid artery; *ON,* optic nerve.

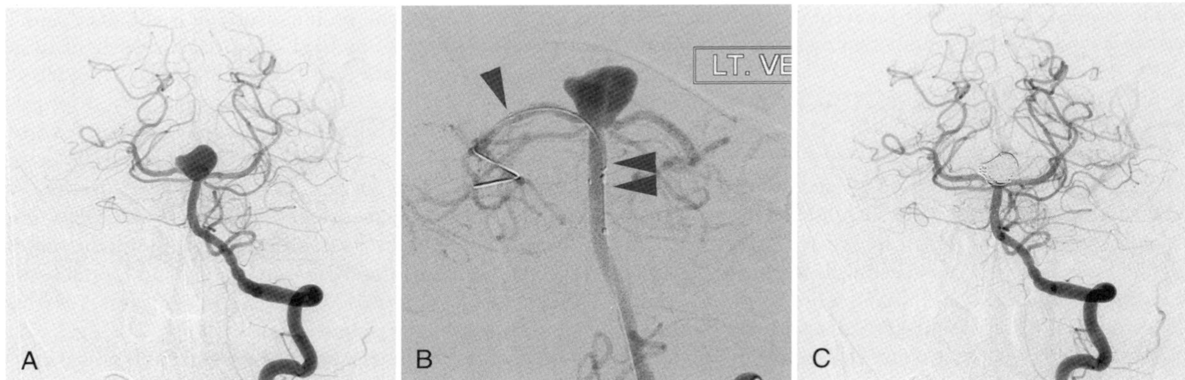


**Fig. 67.10 A,** Patient with an incidental basilar tip aneurysm. Aneurysm grew over a conservative follow-up period (10 to 18 mm in the largest dimension), and a decision was made to proceed with stent-assisted coil embolization. Aneurysm incorporates both posterior cerebral arteries. **B,** A 4 × 30 mm Neuroform stent was placed from the right posterior cerebral artery *(arrowhead)* down to the mid-basilar artery *(arrowheads)* over an exchange wire. Aneurysm was subsequently packed with platinum coils from two microcatheters placed in left and right sides. **C,** Postembolization angiogram shows complete obliteration of aneurysm, with preservation of blood flow to both posterior cerebral arteries.

configuration. Endovascular treatment is particularly beneficial in the treatment of aneurysms located at the upper basilar and paraclinoid regions, where the surgical exposure of aneurysm is challenging (Tateshima et al., 2000). Conversely, endovascular treatment of middle cerebral artery aneurysms raises more technical difficulty due to the high incidence of wide-necked configurations, whereas surgical treatment of middle cerebral artery aneurysms is less difficult than other sites because they are closer to the brain surface and are accessible with limited brain retraction (Suzuki et al., 2009). The introduction of complex-shaped coils, double microcatheter technique, adjunct technology (e.g., balloon or stent-assisted coiling) have improved the immediate and long-term occlusion success rate of endovascular treatment for fusiform or wide-necked aneurysms (Mocco et al., 2006; Piotin et al., 2009) (Fig. 67.10).

In the ISUIA multicenter cohort study, endovascular treatment resulted in less procedural morbidity and mortality than conventional surgical treatment (ISUIA Investigators, 1998; Wiebers et al., 2003). The 1-year morbidity was 6.4% and mortality 3.1%, despite the treatment of older patients, larger aneurysms, and more posterior circulation aneurysms. However, a limitation in the current endovascular treatment of intracranial aneurysms is aneurysm recanalization. It is highly unlikely that a completely coiled, small-necked, aneurysm will recanalize. Overall, unruptured aneurysms treated with coiling are successfully occluded 86.1% of the time based on postprocedure imaging, with recurrence in 24.4% and need for retreatment in 9.1% (Naggara et al., 2010).

More recently, endovascular techniques of flow diversion and flow disruption have been developed that permit treatment of aneurysms lacking a small enough neck to be addressed with simple coiling alone. Flow-diversion stent technology is used for large and wide-neck unruptured and aneurysm recurrence (Lylyk et al., 2009 and Wakhloo and Gounis, 2014). Placed at the wide aneurysm neck, the flow diverter redirects blood flow into the parent vessel, thus promoting stagnation of blood and thrombosis within the aneurysm. The aneurysmal thrombosis caused by the flow diverter develops over time, typically up to 6–12 months after treatment (Szikora et al., 2015). Flow diverters are typically self-expanding stents delivered with a microcatheter after dual antiplatelet therapy loading. The Pipeline embolization device (Medtronic Neurovascular, Irvine, CA) and Surpass (Stryker Neurovascular, Freemont, CA) were the first flow diverters clinically available (excluding clinical trials) in the United States. Flow disruption is an innovative endovascular approach, which involves placement of an intrasaccular device in order to modify the blood flow at the level of the neck and to induce aneurysmal thrombosis with a mechanism of action relatively similar to intravascular flow diversion. The WEB device (Woven EndoBridge, Sequent Medical, Aliso Viejo, CA) was the first available for clinical use in the United States.

With all endovascular treatment approaches, the issue of aneurysm recanalization remains, and early catheter angiography follow-up and long-term CTA or MRA imaging surveillance are indicated. Fig. 67.11 illustrates endovascular techniques that are currently used for treating intracranial aneurysms.

## MANAGEMENT OF SUBARACHNOID HEMORRHAGE

As soon as the diagnosis of aSAH is made, one should consider early transfer to a high-volume center (e.g., >35 aSAH cases per year) with experienced cerebrovascular surgeons, endovascular specialists, and multidisciplinary neurointensive care services (Connolly et al., 2012). Larger hospitals, with high case volumes, are associated with better outcomes and lower mortality rates, reflecting the importance of highly specialized and experienced care for aSAH (Andaluz et al., 2008; Cross et al., 2003; Johnston et al., 2000; Varelas et al., 2008). Institutions that used endovascular services had lower in-hospital mortality rates and a 9% reduction in risk for every 10% of cases treated. In addition, there was a 16% reduction in risk of in-hospital death at institutions that used interventional therapies, such as balloon angioplasty, to treat arterial vasospasm (Bardach et al., 2002).

An important first step in the management of aSAH is to assess the neurological condition and the source of the hemorrhage. The severity of aSAH is measured using widely accepted grading systems (see Table 67.2). A poor neurological condition may be due to direct damage to the brain tissue caused by the hemorrhage or acute hydrocephalus secondary to intraventricular blood or thick blood in the posterior fossa. Placement of a ventricular drainage catheter should be urgently considered to treat hydrocephalus. Intraparenchymal hematomas accompany 20% of aSAH, arising when the bleeding jet from the aneurysm penetrates the brain parenchyma, and can be the cause of the poor neurological condition.

Ruptured aneurysms are at extremely high risk for early re-rupture. Because rebleeding can cause devastating additional injury, re-rupture is a most feared event. Rebleeding rates within the first 24 hours are between 4% and 13.6% (Naidech et al., 2005; Ohkuma et al., 2001). The risk of re-rupture is maximal in the first 2–12 hours. Features associated with aneurysm rebleeding are longer time to aneurysm treatment, worse neurological status on admission, initial loss of consciousness, previous sentinel headaches, larger aneurysm size, and possibly systolic blood pressure greater than 160 mm Hg (Naidech et al., 2005; Ohkuma et al,, 2001).

Early ablative treatment of the ruptured aneurysm to reduce the risk of rebleeding is highly recommended. Until the aneurysm has been structurally addressed, medical therapies to deter rebleeding are pursued. Acute hypertension should be controlled: a decrease in systolic blood pressure to less than 160 mm Hg is reasonable. Titratable intravenous antihypertensives provide more adjustable blood pressure control, and nicardipine may exert smoother blood pressure control than labetalol or sodium nitroprusside. The benefit of antifibrinolytic therapy to prevent rebleeding during the interval before aneurysm occlusion is being investigated. It reduces rebleeding when there is a delay in aneurysm obliteration, but increases thromboembolic complications (Starke et al., 2008). It is reasonable in patients with an unavoidable delay in aneurysm obliterative treatment, a high risk of rebleeding, and no compelling medical contraindications, to use short-term (<72 hours) therapy with tranexamic acid or aminocaproic acid (Connolly et al., 2012).

### Endovascular and Surgical Treatment of Ruptured Aneurysms

Both endovascular and microsurgical approaches to occlude recently rupture aneurysms are continually undergoing technical advancement. The best approach for each individual patient should be determined by multidisciplinary team discussion, taking into account institutional expertise, grade of a SAH, overall clinical condition of the patient, aneurysm location, aneurysm size, age of the patient, and presence of parenchymal hematoma.

The only multicenter randomized trial comparing microsurgical and endovascular repair, the International Subarachnoid Aneurysm Trial (ISAT), enrolled patients with aSAH across 42 centers (Molyneaux et al., 2005). ISAT was a multicenter, prospective, randomized, controlled trial of endovascular coiling versus neurosurgical clipping in patients with ruptured cerebral aneurysms suitable for either therapeutic modality. A total of 9559 patients were assessed for eligibility and 2143 (22.4%) were randomized to coiling (1073) versus clipping (1070). The study was stopped early for overwhelming efficacy after a planned interim analysis found lower dependency or death (modified Rankin Scale 3–6) with coiling versus clipping, 23.7% versus 30.6%, $P = .0001$. Despite the slightly higher aneurysm recurrence or rebleeding risk in the coiling patients, long-term follow-up from ISAT has confirmed the superiority of coiling, with greater disability-free survival in the endovascular group at 10 years (Molyneux et al., 2015).

The results of ISAT do not apply to the whole aSAH population—they are only valid when a patient with a ruptured aneurysm qualifies for either treatment. In ISAT, the majority of patients (7416 out of 9559) were not enrolled. Among these, 2737 underwent endovascular treatment and 3615 surgical clipping. In ISAT there were more good-grade aSAH patients and fewer posterior circulation aneurysms than in large nonrandomized clinical series. This finding suggests that practitioners in the participating centers already favored endovascular treatment for poor-grade patients and posterior circulation aneurysms. The

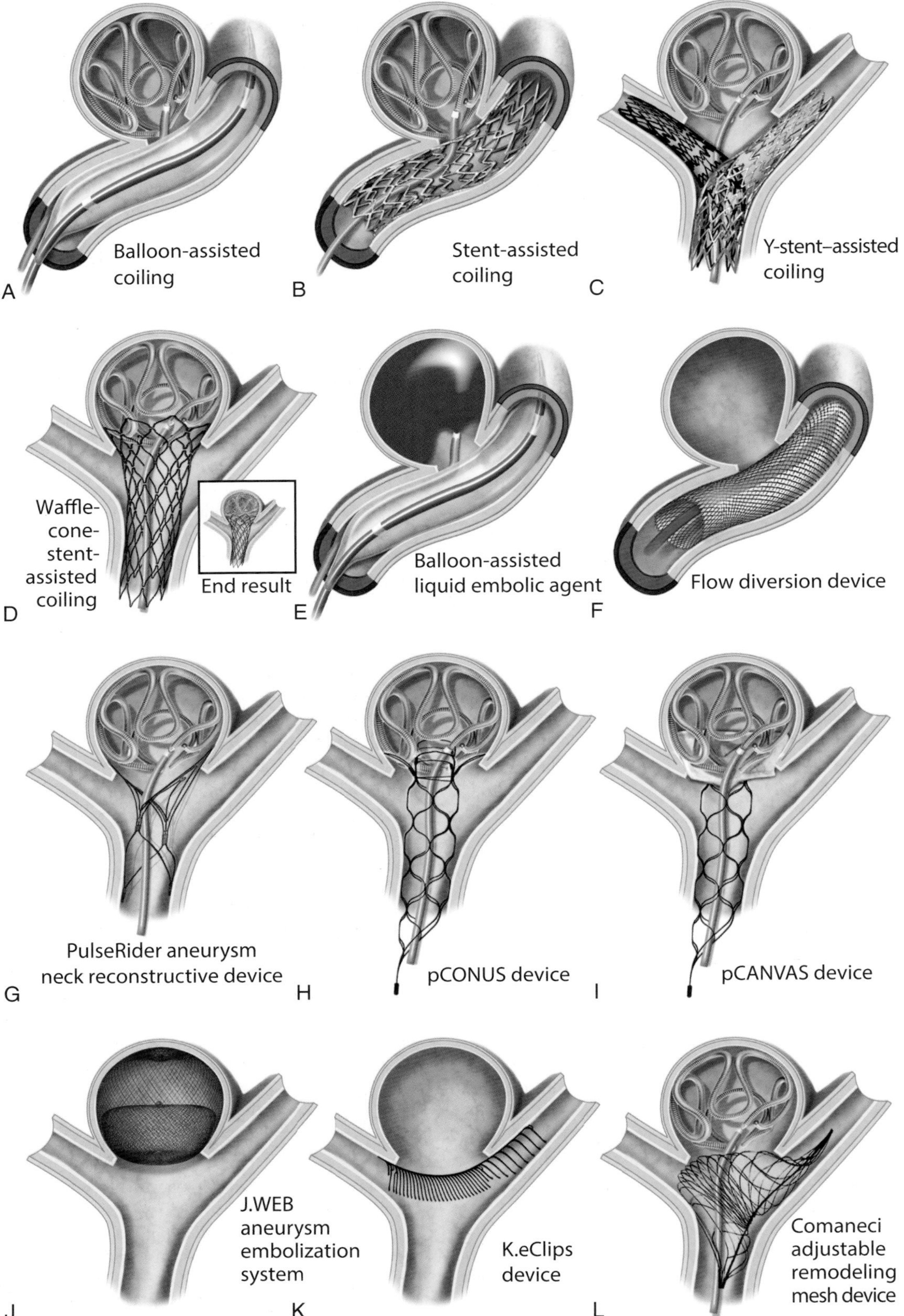


**Fig. 67.11** Endovascular Techniques Used in the Treatment of Intracranial Aneurysms. **A,** Balloon-assisted coiling; **B,** stent-assisted coiling; **C,** Y-stent–assisted coiling; **D,** waffle-cone-stent-assisted coiling, while coiling *(left)* and the end result *(right)*; **E,** balloon-assisted liquid embolic agent; **F,** flow diversion device; **G,** PulseRider aneurysm neck reconstruction device; **H** and **I,** pCONUS and pCANVAS bifurcation aneurysm implants; **J,** WEB aneurysm embolization system; **K,** eClips device; **L,** Comaneci adjustable remodeling mesh device. *(Adapted from* McPheeters, M. J., Vakharia, K., Munich, S. A., & Siddiqui, A. H. (2019). Wide-Necked Cerebral Artery Aneurysms: Where Do We Stand? *Endovascular Today, 18, 70-79.)*

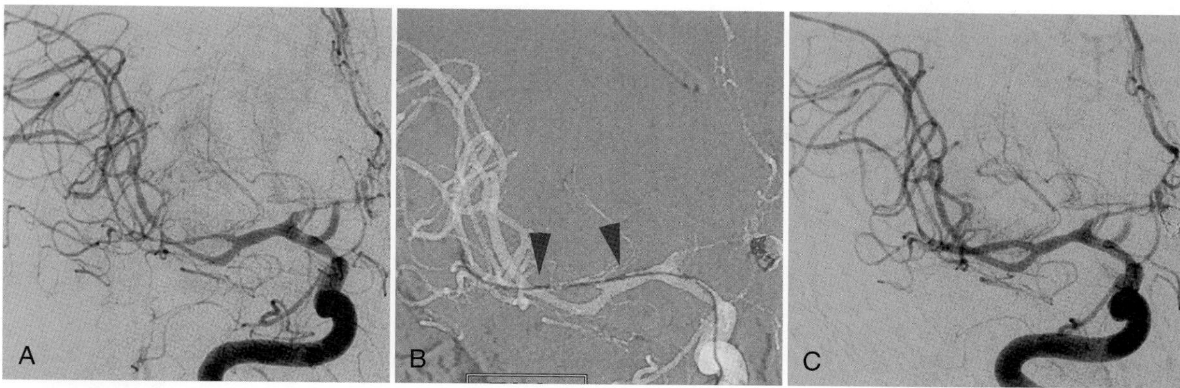


**Fig. 67.12 Patient With a Ruptured Anterior Communicating Artery, Day 9, Developed Left-Sided Weakness. A,** Right internal carotid artery angiogram shows severe vasospasm in the post-bifurcation M1 segment and M2 segment of the right middle cerebral artery, as well as in the A1 and A2 segments of the right anterior cerebral artery. Superselective papaverine infusion was performed in the M1, M2, and A1 segments. **B,** Subsequently, balloon angioplasty was performed in the post-bifurcation M1 segment *(arrowheads)*. **C,** Postendovascular intervention angiogram shows restoration of the caliber of the right middle cerebral artery and the distal anterior cerebral artery.

less invasive nature of endovascular coiling may be favorable for older-age patients and those with serious comorbid medical conditions (Gonzalez et al., 2010).

Despite continued evolution of endovascular techniques and positive results from ISAT, some ruptured aneurysms may not be best treated by endovascular methods. Newer endovascular techniques to treat wide-necked and complex-shaped aneurysms, such as flow-diverter stents and liquid embolic materials, require aggressive antiplatelet therapy due to their thrombogenic nature, rendering more suitable for unruptured than ruptured aneurysms. The term *coilable* in ISAT should be interpreted as suitable for primarily coiling or balloon-assisted coiling. For instance, middle cerebral artery bifurcation aneurysms often show complex wide-necked configurations with incorporation of important branches in the dome, so they are better clipped surgically. The decision between open surgery and endovascular treatment should be made on an individual basis with input from the patient and family members after clear explanations of both treatment modalities.

There has been a debate about whether the incidence of symptomatic vasospasm differs following surgical clipping or endovascular coiling. Theoretically, surgical clipping has an advantage in this regard because the clot (a presumed cause of vasospasm) surrounding the ruptured aneurysm can be removed. Nevertheless, several clinical studies have failed to demonstrate a difference in the incidence of symptomatic vasospasm between these two modalities (Dumont et al., 2010). Surgical manipulation, including the exposure of major arteries, the retraction of brain, and the disruption of 3D integrity of subarachnoid space, may have an offsetting effect promoting development of vasospasm. Based on current knowledge, the amount of subarachnoid blood is not a major determining factor in selecting the appropriate treatment modality for patients with ruptured aneurysms.

## Vasospasm and Delayed Cerebral Ischemia

*Cerebral vasospasm*—a delayed and sustained contraction of cerebral arteries—continues to be a leading cause of morbidity and mortality in patients with aSAH after aneurysm rupture (Fig. 67.12, *A*). Once blood leaks out of cerebral blood vessels, the blood or its breakdown products irritate the adjacent vessels and induce delayed vasospasm. Cerebral vasospasm may arise 3–20 days after SAH, most frequently 7–10 days after. If the arterial narrowing is sufficient to produce a critical reduction in cerebral blood flow, the result is *DCI*. Vasospasm is initiated, in part, by the release of oxyhemoglobin, one of the breakdown products of blood, and involves multifactorial mediators including free radicals, lipid peroxidation, and endothelin-1. Prolonged smooth-muscle contraction occurs in affected arteries. Vessel wall hypertrophy, fibrosis, degeneration, and inflammatory changes are also observed. Angiographic vasospasm occurs in as high as 70% of patients with aSAH and becomes clinically symptomatic in up to 30% (Romner and Reinstrup, 2001).

Close clinical and imaging monitoring in the neurointensive care unit for development plays a fundamental role in care of the aSAH patient after initial aneurysm occlusive treatment. New neurological signs or worsening of preexisting neurological deficits suggest potential symptomatic vasospasm. Serial transcranial Doppler (TCD) testing provides important presymptomatic screening and information regarding response to medical and interventional therapies. An elevation of blood-flow velocity suggests cerebral vasospasm.

Treatment of cerebral vasospasm and DCI is multimodal. Nimodipine is begun when a SAH is diagnosed and continued for 21 days. This calcium channel blocker protects against DCI by neuroprotective and potentially antivasospastic effects (Dorhout Mees et al., 2007; Pickard et al., 1989). Management of fluid and electrolyte balance is essential in the management of vasospasm. To optimize blood flow through both vasospastic arteries and collateral channels, hypotension and hypovolemia should be aggressively avoided. Mild induced hypertension may further augment cerebral blood flow but has the potential to provoke cardiopulmonary adverse effects (Gathier et al., 2008). Induced hypertension and hypervolemia have the potential to prevent or minimize DCI in patients with vasospasm by augmenting cerebral blood flow, both through vasospastic arteries and collateral vessels.

As neurointerventional technology has improved, endovascular treatment of cerebral vasospasm has become a therapeutic option. There are two types of endovascular treatment approaches: angioplasty using a microballoon and superselective injection of pharmacological vasodilators into the affected arteries (see Fig. 67.12). The effect of balloon angioplasty lasts longer than vasodilator injections and it is most useful in treating severe spasm in relatively proximal arteries (Boulouis et al., 2017). Superselective injection of vasodilators is most useful for distal spasm, and a variety of vasodilators (e.g., papaverine, verapamil, fasudil) have been used (Venkatraman et al., 2018). Large clinical series and small randomized trials suggest that endovascular treatment of vasospasm improves the angiographic appearance of vasospastic vessels and likely improves clinical outcome. However, endovascular interventions can be associated with major complications; therefore they should not be a first-line treatment option.

*The complete reference list is available online at https://expertconsult.inkling.com.* 

68

# Stroke in Children

*Meredith R. Golomb, José Biller*

## OUTLINE



## STROKE AND THE DEVELOPING CEREBROVASCULAR SYSTEM

Unlike adults, in most children with stroke, conditions such as diabetes and hypertension make little contribution to the etiology of stroke. Developmental, genetic, and environmental factors are the major contributors to cerebrovascular injury in children.

## EPIDEMIOLOGY

### Full-Term and Near-Term Neonates

Neonates appear to be at higher risk for stroke than older children. Asymptomatic subdural hemorrhage affects almost half of term neonates and can occur in infants delivered by both vaginal and cesarean delivery (Rooks et al., 2008). Symptomatic intracranial hemorrhage (ICH) affects 1 in 100 full-term neonates (Gradnitzer et al., 2002). Estimates place the rate of arterial ischemic stroke between 1 in 4000 neonates and 1 in 10,000 neonates (deVeber et al., 2017; Lynch and Nelson, 2001). Laugesaar et al. (2007) looked at all prospectively and retrospectively diagnosed perinatal stroke in Estonia and found a rate of 1 in 1587 live births. DeVeber and colleagues (2001) found a rate of 0.67 cases of cerebral venous thrombosis (CVT) per 100,000 children per year, with neonates making up 43% of cases; rates were not described in relation to the number of term births.

Chapter 110 discusses cerebral vascular injury in the premature neonate.

### The General Population of Children

Estimates of the incidence of all pediatric stroke in the United States and France have ranged from 2.6 to 13 cases per 100,000 children per year (Giroud et al., 1995), with some variation among studies on the inclusion of neonates, traumatic strokes, and meningitis and whether to use 16 or 18 as the cutoff age for pediatric stroke. A review of 17 years of data in the Greater Cincinnati Northern Kentucky Stroke Study found a stroke incidence of 4.4 per 100,000 per year (Lehman et al., 2018).

### High-Risk Subgroups

Certain subgroups of children are at high risk for stroke, with rates approaching or surpassing those in older adults. Medical conditions may place children at risk for ICH, ischemic stroke, or both.

Some types of central nervous system (CNS) vascular malformations (e.g., arteriovenous malformations, telangiectasias) are part of well-known neurocutaneous syndromes such as Sturge-Weber, Osler-Weber-Rendu, Louis-Bar syndrome, Wyburn-Mason syndrome, and Klippel-Trénaunay syndrome. Vascular malformations may present with ICH. A review of 70 cases of spontaneous intracranial hemorrhage seen over 30 months at a Chinese hospital found that 62.9% had arteriovenous malformation (Fig. 68.1), 5.7% had cavernous malformation, 2.9% had aneurysm, 2.9% had moyamoya vasculopathy, 2.9% had tumors, and 20% had unclear etiology (Liu et al, 2015). Cavernous malformations and aneurysms may be genetic and can present in childhood. Risk varies depending on the mutation involved (Denier et al., 2006). Brain aneurysms are rare in children and are often dysplastic. The carotid bifurcation is the most common site for pediatric intracranial aneurysms, followed by the posterior circulation. ICH may lead to vasospasm and resultant ischemic stroke, but this is less common in children than in adults (Menkes et al., 2000).

Children with bleeding disorders are at high risk for intracerebral hemorrhage. The US Centers for Disease Control and Prevention hemophilia surveillance project found ICH in 37 of 547 (7%) infants and children with hemophilia 2 years old or younger; 14 were delivery related (Kulkami et al., 2017). A 21-year retrospective and prospective and retrospective study of children and adolescents with severe hemophilia A or B seen at 33 hemophilia centers found that untreated patients had an ICH rate of 0.017 cases/patient-year, while full prophylaxis treatment lowered it to 0.00033 cases/patient-year (Andersson et al., 2017). Worldwide, the prevalence of sickle cell disease is highest in sub-Saharan Africa, the Caribbean, Saudi Arabia, India, Southern Turkey, and some parts of Brazil, Greece, and Sicily. Sickle cell disease affects approximately 100,000 Americans. Among African Americans, approximately 1 in 365 births have sickle cell disease, and 1 in 13 African Americans are born with sickle cell trait (Piel et al., 2013; Ware et al., 2017). Children with sickle cell anemia are at risk for ischemic stroke because sickling red blood cells may lead to thrombosis or endothelial injury and in some patients are associated with moyamoya syndrome (Pegelow, 2001; Pegelow et al., 2002; Fig. 68.2). Cerebral fat embolism may result as a complication of sickle cell crisis (vaso-occlusive crisis), causing bone marrow infarction. Cerebral fat embolism has a characteristic "starfield" pattern on magnetic resonance imaging (MRI) and may reach the brain by a patent foramen ovale (PFO; Dhakal et al., 2015; Gibbs et al., 2012). The rate of stroke in children with sickle cell anemia has dropped since the institution of transfusion therapy (see the later section Treatment). In California, the incidence of first stroke in children with sickle cell anemia dropped from 0.88 per 100 person-years to 0.17 per 100 person-years (Fullerton et al., 2004); however, approximately 30% of children aged 5–15 years old have silent infarcts (DeBaun et al., 2012). Children with sickle cell anemia may also develop aneurysms and resultant ICH, but this is more common in adults with sickle cell anemia (Pegelow, 2001; Yao et al., 2017).

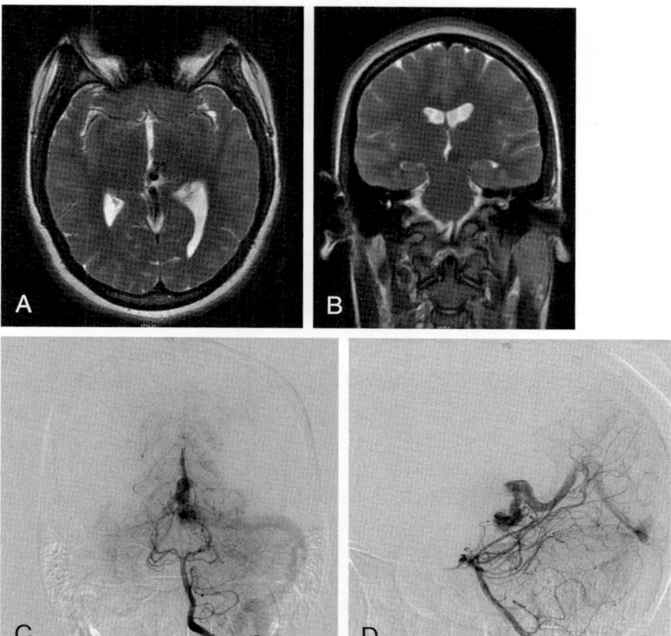


**Fig. 68.1** Axial **(A)** and coronal **(B)** T2-weighted magnetic resonance imaging and anteroposterior **(C)** and lateral **(D)** views of catheter cerebral angiography of a 17-year-old female with a left thalamic arteriovenous malformation (grade III Spetzler-Martin) fed from the posterior cerebral artery territories bilaterally. *AP,* antero-posterior; *PCA,* posterior cerebral artery; *T2,* Transverse relaxation time.

Children treated with mechanical circulatory support are at increased risk for both ICH and embolic ischemic stroke. The rates of infarction after extracorporeal membrane oxygenation (ECMO) vary dramatically among series, ranging from 0% to 28%; one study examined the brains of 44 patients who died while on ECMO and found evidence of focal ischemic infarct in 50% and ICH in 52%. A large study of 3517 cardiac surgery patients who received ECMO survivors found stroke in 12% (Werho et al, 2015). Stroke may occur in as many as 1 in 3 children treated with the Berlin Heart EXCOR ventricular assist device, but more intensive antiplatelet therapy may lower that risk (Rosenthal et al, 2017).

Children with complex congenital heart disease are at risk for cardioembolic stroke, thrombotic stroke, watershed infarcts from drops in perfusion pressure, and CVT (Fig. 68.3). The rates of stroke in children with complex congenital heart disease also vary among series, with some of the variation due to the severity of the malformation, the number of corrective surgeries required, anesthetic techniques during surgery, patient selection, and length of follow-up. A large Canadian study looked at 5526 children who underwent cardiac surgery and found a stroke rate of 5 per 1000 children (Domi et al., 2008). Data from the International Society for Heart and Lung Transplantation Registry revealed stroke in 3% of pediatric heart transplant patients (Morgan et al, 2016). The greatest risk for children with congenital heart disease occurs at the time of surgery or cardiac catheterization. One study found that 27% of children with stroke associated with cardiac disease had recurrent stroke. Mechanical heart valves, prothrombotic conditions, and infection at the time of first stroke all raised the risk of stroke recurrence (Rodan et al., 2012).

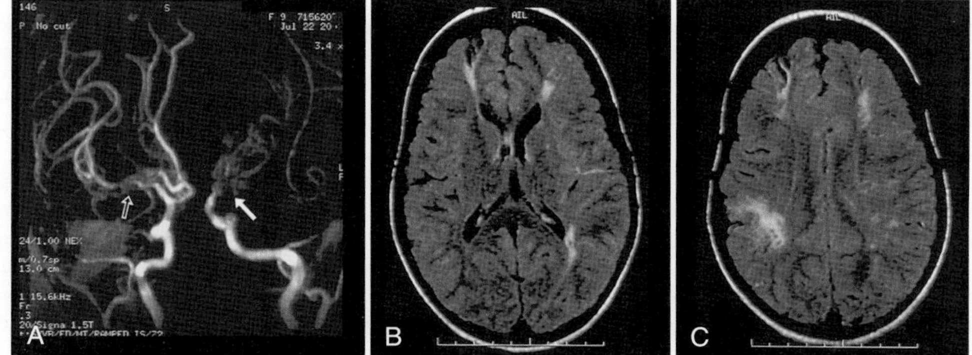


**Fig. 68.2** Magnetic resonance imaging (MRI) of a 10-year-old girl with sickle cell anemia. At age 5, she presented with a left hemiparesis. MRI then showed acute ischemia in the right middle cerebral artery (MCA) territory and chronic ischemic changes in the left cerebral hemisphere. Magnetic resonance angiography (MRA) showed stenoses in both anterior circulations. These stenoses progressed over time, and she was treated with pial synangiosis and burr holes. There was no clear progression of ischemic lesions. **A,** MRA demonstrates complete occlusion of the left M1 segment of the MCA *(solid arrow),* and severe stenosis of the M1 segment of the right MCA *(open arrow)* and both A1 segments of the anterior cerebral arteries. There are multiple small vessels at the stenotic sites consistent with moyamoya. There appears to be an anastomosis between the left superficial temporal branches and the distal left M1. **B, C,** Fast spin echo inversion recovery MRI demonstrates multiple old infarcts in the bilateral frontal and parieto-occipital regions and centrum semiovale.

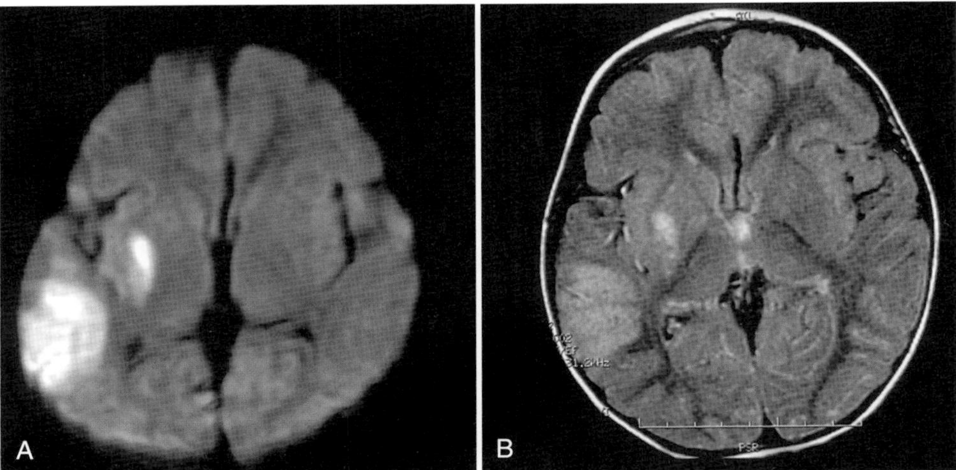


**Fig. 68.3** Magnetic resonance imaging (MRI) of a 3-year-old girl with a history of complex congenital heart disease. At age 10 months, she had a procedure to repair a double inlet left ventricle and left transposition of the great arteries. She presented with seizures and dysconjugate gaze 3 weeks later, and an acute right pontine infarct was diagnosed. Magnetic resonance angiography and catheter angiography demonstrated narrowing of the distal basilar artery and the right superior cerebellar artery. At age 3, she presented with acute left hemiparesis. Diffusion-weighted MRI (**A**) and fast spin echo inversion recovery MRI (**B**) demonstrate multiple infarctions in the right temporal lobe, inferior parietal region, and lentiform nucleus, consistent with cardioembolic stroke.

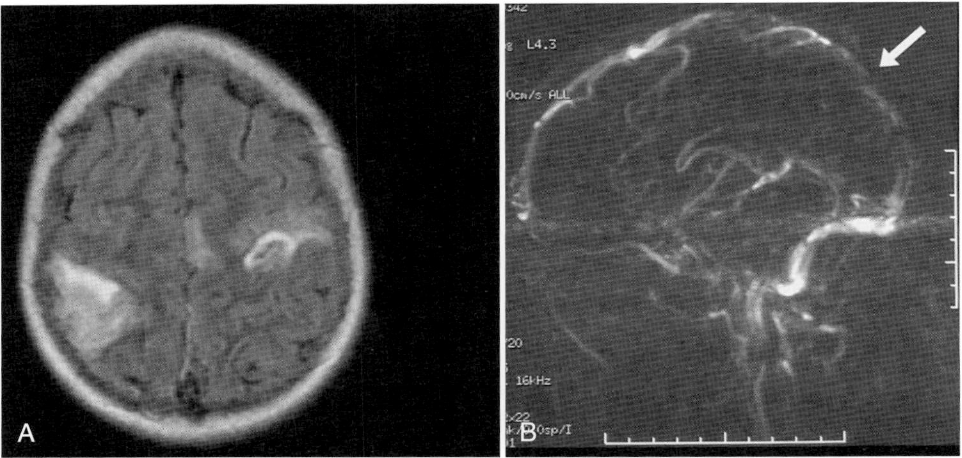


**Fig. 68.4** Magnetic resonance imaging (MRI) of an 8-year-old boy with leukemia who developed headaches and left-hand numbness during induction chemotherapy with L-asparaginase. **A**, Fast spin echo inversion recovery MRI demonstrates multifocal bilateral hemorrhagic infarctions. **B**, Magnetic resonance venogram demonstrates irregularity of the superior sagittal sinus consistent with thrombosis *(arrow)*.

Children with cancer are at risk for both ICH and ischemic infarction. ICH occurs secondary to thrombocytopenia from bone marrow suppression or bleeding within the tumors. Children with cancer may develop ischemic infarction or CVT due to leukostasis in the setting of leukemia; complications of chemotherapy such as L-asparaginase, which cause decreases in antithrombin, fibrinogen, and plasminogen; fungal or bacterial meningitis leading to arteritis; vasculopathy secondary to radiation; or complications of intracranial surgery (Fig. 68.4). Stroke affects approximately 1% of children with cancer, most commonly children with leukemia or brain tumors (Noje et al., 2013). One institutional study found that 4% of children treated with cranial and/or cervical radiation had stroke during the 10 years after radiation (Mueller et al., 2013).

Children with certain syndromes are predisposed to stroke, sometimes for multiple reasons. Children with Down syndrome have higher-than-average rates of leukemia, which in turn may lead to hemorrhagic stroke; moyamoya vasculopathy, which may lead to ischemic or hemorrhagic stroke; complex congenital heart disease, which may lead to cardioembolic stroke; and atlantoaxial instability and other abnormalities of the cervical spine, which increase the risk for vertebral artery dissection. Children with neurofibromatosis type 1 have higher-than-average rates of moyamoya and other occlusive vasculopathies that are sometimes but not always associated with radiation. Connective tissue disorders such as Marfan and Ehlers-Danlos syndromes and pseudoxanthoma elasticum may predispose to cervicocephalic arterial dissection or aneurysmal dilatation. Metabolic syndromes that damage the endothelium (e.g., homocystinuria, Fabry disease, familial hyperlipidemia) may predispose to vascular damage and thrombosis.

## PRESENTATIONS

Seizures are the most common manifestation of ICHs, arterial ischemic strokes, and CVT in term neonates. Seizures are a presenting sign for more than 65% of term neonates with ICH (Cole et al., 2017), at least 80% of term neonates with arterial ischemic stroke (deVeber et al., 2017; Volpe et al., 2001), and more than 50% of neonates with CVT (Berfelo et al., 2010; Fitzgerald et al., 2006). Other presenting signs include apnea, irritability, jitteriness, lethargy, and bulging fontanelle. The immature CNS may not demonstrate focal signs, and hemiparesis may not be apparent until a child is older than 6 months of age.

Children older than 6 months of age may present with seizures or focal signs similar to those seen in adult stroke, with hemiparesis, ataxia, or aphasia. Children younger than 1 year of age are more likely to present with seizures and altered mental status, whereas children older than 1 year of age are more likely to present with focal motor signs (Zimmer et al., 2007). Although severe headaches such as those in ICH often prompt parents to seek medical attention immediately, most children arrive at the emergency room more than 6 hours after the event (Gabis et al., 2002), and even in the emergency room, many children do not receive immediate cranial imaging (Surmava et al., 2019). Parents may not detect focal motor weakness in a young child who has not yet started to walk or aphasia in a young child who is just starting to speak. Parents may interpret the sudden onset of focal neurological signs as behavioral rather than neurological. It can be easier to detect focal neurological signs and symptoms in older children, but these are also often missed in the first minutes to hours, possibly because many parents and children do not realize children can have strokes. Some children may have no symptoms or only gradual onset of developmental delay. Although silent strokes are recognizable in the sickle cell population and several studies have screened for them, the rates of silent infarction in other cerebrovascular disorders are unclear because radiological investigations are lacking in the absence of clinical manifestations.

## ETIOLOGY

### Cardiac

Complex congenital heart disease may lead to thrombosis and ischemic stroke through several mechanisms. Abnormal cardiac anatomy or associated cardiac arrhythmias lead to abnormal flow and may predispose to the formation of intracardiac thrombi. Septal defects may lead to right-to-left shunts that allow venous thrombi to cross to the arterial side and cause cerebral infarction. Surgery and cardiac catheterization can disrupt the endothelium and lead to thrombosis. Cardiac surgery itself may lead to a temporary prothrombotic state (Heying et al., 2006; Petaja et al., 1996). An abnormal heart valve can serve as a nidus for bacterial or fungal vegetations that may cause cardioembolic stroke. Chronic hypoxemia in severe cases of congenital heart disease may lead to polycythemia, and the increased blood viscosity may promote thrombosis. Aortic coarctation may be complicated by infective endarteritis or ischemic or hemorrhagic strokes, including brain aneurysms. Based on autopsy findings, a PFO is found incidentally in 20%–35% of the general population. PFO is more common in patients with cryptogenic stroke than in the general population. Therapeutic options for patients with PFO include antiplatelet drugs, oral anticoagulants, percutaneous closure, or open heart procedures. Recent randomized clinical trials in adults support PFO closure among patients younger than 60 years with large PFOs and atrial septal aneurysms. However, there were potential biases due to unblinded referral decisions for endpoint and adjudications. There are no trials of PFO treatment in children (Mas et al., 2017; Saver et al., 2017; Sondergaard et al., 2017).

### Hematological

Any hematological disorder that disrupts coagulation can place a child at risk for hemorrhagic stroke. Newborns have lower levels of coagulation factors and have a drop in the vitamin K–dependent factors in the first days of life. Bleeding due to vitamin K deficiency was more common before intramuscular or oral administration to neonates became widespread; Cornelissen and colleagues (1996) found that administering vitamin K lowered the incidence of vitamin K deficiency bleeding from 7 to 1.1 per 100,000 births per year. However, late-onset vitamin K deficiency bleeding can occur in children with undiagnosed cholestatic jaundice who received oral vitamin K and are exclusively breastfed, because they cannot absorb the vitamin, and breast milk is low in vitamin K (Ijland et al., 2008). Schulte and colleagues (2014) reported a rise in late-presentation vitamin K deficiency bleeding in Tennessee because parents were refusing vitamin K, believing it was unnecessary or that the vitamin K injection included "toxins." Accidental ingestion or overdose of warfarin has the same effect as a vitamin K deficiency and may occur when a young child finds an older family member's medications. The most common congenital coagulation factor deficiencies are deficiencies of coagulation factor VIII (hemophilia A), coagulation factor IX (hemophilia B), and von Willebrand factor. ICH is the most common cause of death from bleeding in patients with hemophilia; the site of ICH can be epidural, subdural, or intraparenchymal. Spinal cord compression may result from spinal hematomas.

A deficiency or imbalance of factors involved in regulating coagulation may place the child at risk for thrombosis. Pediatric ischemic stroke has been associated with iron-deficiency anemia (Maguire et al., 2007), deficiencies of protein C, protein S, and antithrombin; activated protein C resistance due to the factor V Leiden mutation; the prothrombin gene 20210A mutation; the methylene tetrahydrofolate reductase (MTHFR) gene variants; the ATG haplotype of the protein Z gene (Nowak-Göttl et al., 2009); elevated lipoprotein (a); elevated antiphospholipid antibodies (Kenet et al., 2010) and lupus anticoagulant; elevated factor VIII levels; and low plasminogen or high fibrinogen. The importance of the plasminogen activator inhibitor promoter polymorphism (PAI-1) in childhood stroke is controversial. Temporary hematological abnormalities and resultant thrombosis may result from intercurrent illness; for example, idiopathic nephrotic syndrome is associated with decreased antithrombin levels and CVT and/or arterial thromboembolic events (Fluss et al., 2006). The role of prothrombotic factors in perinatal stroke is less clear. Although earlier studies have found a clear association, this has not been found in more recent work (Curtis et al., 2017).

Abnormalities of blood cells or blood cell concentration may place the child at risk for hemorrhagic or ischemic stroke. Stroke occurs in children with β thalassemia intermedia (βTI) and children with paroxysmal nocturnal hemoglobinuria. Low platelet count due to autoimmune thrombocytopenia or bone marrow suppression leads to hemorrhage. Anything that increases blood viscosity (e.g., sickled cells, polycythemia, chronic hypoxia) may predispose a child to arterial or venous infarct. Dehydration is associated with arterial strokes and CVT, possibly because it increases viscosity. Anemia has also been associated with arterial ischemic infarction and CVT, possibly due to alterations in hemodynamics or imbalances in thrombotic pathways.

Several authors have noted the presence of multiple prothrombotic abnormalities in some children with ischemic stroke (Kenet et al., 2010). The combination of MTHFR and endothelial nitric oxide synthase gene variants may raise stroke risk more than MTHFR alone (Djordjevic et al., 2009). Children with congenital heart disease or leukemia may be at higher risk for developing thrombotic complications during hospitalization if they also have a prothrombotic abnormality.

More recent work has identified multiple biomarkers associated with pediatric stroke. Inflammatory biomarkers such as C-reactive protein and myeloperoxidase are elevated in cardioembolic stroke, and serum amyloid A is elevated in arteriopathic stroke. Children who had progressive arteriopathy tended to have higher levels of C-reactive protein and serum amyloid A, suggesting these biomarkers might help to predict recurrent stroke (Fullerton et al, 2016).

## Trauma and Vascular Compression

Trauma is a risk factor for both ischemic and hemorrhagic stroke. Trauma can injure vessels directly, leading to hemorrhage from torn vessels, thrombosis in damaged intima, or traumatic pseudoaneurysm. Subdural hemorrhages, subarachnoid hemorrhages, and ischemic infarctions occur in head injury. Ascertaining the cause of the trauma is important; at one pediatric trauma center, the mortality rate for nonaccidental trauma was 9.7%, while the mortality rate for accidental trauma was 2.2% (Roaten et al., 2006). Most subdural hemorrhages in infants are due to abuse (Matschke et al., 2009). In older children and adults, low-admission Glasgow Coma Scale (GCS) score, low systolic blood pressure, brain herniation, and requirement for decompressive craniotomy are all predictors of posttraumatic cerebral infarction (Tian et al., 2008). Bony abnormalities of the vertebrae or abnormalities of vessel walls due to collagen-vascular disease or metabolic disease may predispose to cervicocephalic arterial dissection after mild trauma. Arterial dissection may be idiopathic in otherwise apparently normal children (Rafay et al., 2006). A prothrombotic state associated with trauma can promote thrombosis and worsen outcome; trauma patients who go into disseminated intravascular coagulation (DIC) have worse outcomes than those who do not. Trauma is the most common precipitant of hemorrhages in children with hemophilia. In neonates, compression of the sagittal sinus due to head position has been associated with cerebral sinovenous thrombosis; changing head position or minimizing compression with a specialized pillow may improve venous flow (Tan et al., 2013).

## Infection

The consequences of bacterial meningitis are DIC and vascular inflammation, and subsequent arterial or venous thrombosis and infarction. Other cerebrovascular complications of meningitis include vasculitis, vasospasm, intracranial aneurysm formation, and rarely subarachnoid hemorrhage. Group B streptococcal meningitis is an important cause of stroke in neonates and transmitted vertically from the mother or horizontally by nursery staff. During the first 2 months of life, infants are susceptible to bacteria found in maternal flora or in the local environment, including group B stretococci, gram-negative enteric bacilli, and *Listeria monocytogenes*. After 2 months of age, *Streptococcus pneumoniae* and *Neisseria meningitides* are the most common causes of bacterial meningitis. The institution of *Haemophilus influenzae* type b vaccination at 2 months of age has led to a dramatic drop in *H. influenzae*-b meningitis. In immunosuppressed patients such as those with cancer or acquired immunodeficiency syndrome (AIDS), *Aspergillus* species may lead to vasculitis and infarction. There are numerous possible causes of ischemic and hemorrhagic stroke in human immunodeficiency virus (HIV)/AIDS. Patients with AIDS may develop marantic endocarditis, arteriopathy of medium and small vessels, or aneurysms, and although the presumed cause for most cases is direct or secondary infection, the exact pathophysiology is not always clear. Highly active antiretroviral therapy for AIDS may result in dyslipidemia and may itself cause vascular injury and accelerated atherosclerosis (Mondal et al., 2004). Tuberculosis leads to meningitis in 1%–2% of cases, which may cause vasculitis and infarction (Starke, 1999). Several cases of stroke occurred in children with neurobrucellosis (Salih et al., 2006b). Lyme disease is a rare cause of infectious vasculitis and aneurysm formation. Varicella-zoster virus (VZV) may cause vasculitis by direct infection of the arterial wall or by a postinfectious inflammatory reaction that manifests weeks to months after the primary infection. Even minor recent infection has been identified as a risk factor for stroke and may act by inducing an inflammatory prothrombotic state or by causing vascular endothelial injury (Hills et al., 2014). In some cases, arteriopathy is associated with recent upper respiratory infection (Amlie-Lefond et al., 2009a). Asymptomatic herpes simplex type 1 infection has been associated with increased risk of vasculopathy and childhood stroke (Elkind et al., 2016). Children who are fully vaccinated may have lower risk than children who are not or who are incompletely vaccinated against routine childhood illnesses (Fullerton et al., 2015).

## Vascular Malformations/Vasculopathy/Migraine/ Anatomical Variation

As discussed previously, vascular malformations may present with intracerebral hemorrhage, and resulting vasospasm may lead to ischemic infarction (Fig. 68.5, *A-H*). Arterial abnormalities such as large-artery stenosis are common in otherwise healthy children with arterial ischemic stroke (Ganesan et al., 2003). At least 10% of hemorrhagic strokes and most subarachnoid hemorrhages in children are caused by ruptured aneurysms (Jordan et al., 2009).

One potential cause for stroke in pediatric patients is moyamoya disease. Moyamoya is a rare, chronic, progressive steno-occlusive intracranial vasculopathy involving the distal supraclinoid internal carotid artery and the proximal anterior artery and middle cerebral artery (MCA), and is associated with the formation of an abnormal vascular network at the base of the brain resembling a "puff of smoke" on angiography. The mechanism of the disease is still unknown. Moyamoya disease has a high prevalence in Japan, Korea, and China but has been reported worldwide (Han et al., 2012). There is a bimodal distribution, presenting most often in children (girls more common than boys) younger than 10–15 years and in adults in the third to fifth decades of life. Children usually present with recurrent transient ischemic attacks or strokes, headaches, seizures, or movement disorders. Adults may present with ICH, including subarachnoid hemorrhage, subependymal hemorrhage, or intraventricular hemorrhage (IVH). Some patients with moyamoya develop brain aneurysms. Many disorders have been associated with moyamoya disease (Table 68.1).

Fibromuscular dysplasia (FMD), a segmental, nonatherosclerotic, noninflammatory vascular disease of unknown pathophysiology, may result in arterial stenosis, vessel occlusion, aneurysm, and/or arterial dissection. FMD most commonly affects adult women and is rarely recognized in children with cerebral ischemia (DiFazio et al., 2000; Kirton et al., 2013; Zurin et al., 1997).

Primary angiitis of the central nervous system (PACNS) may occur in children and can be fatal if not treated with aggressive immune suppression. There are more frequently reported cases of less virulent vasculopathies in children, often occurring after varicella infection, which respond to aspirin alone and do not require immune suppression (Chabrier et al., 1998; Lanthier et al., 2001). Deficiency of adenosine deaminase type 2 (DADA2) may account for pediatric patients with intermittent fevers, diagnosed with polyarteritis nodosa–like disease, "lacunar" strokes, and systemic vasculopathy (Zhou et al., 2014). Stroke can result from vasculopathy outside the brain. Childhood stroke can be a first manifestation of Takayasu arteritis, an inflammatory large-vessel vasculitis that affects the aorta and its branches

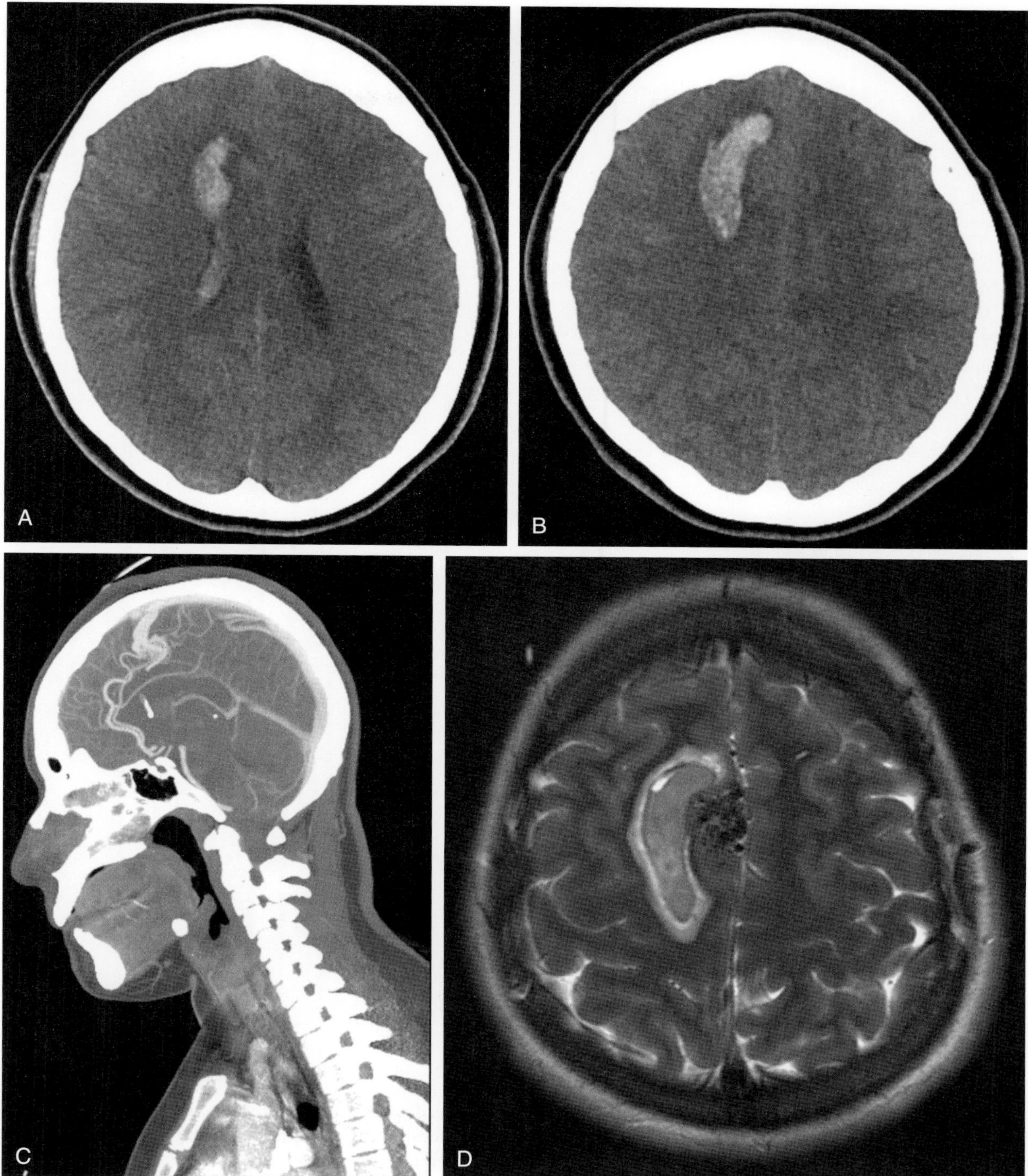

Fig. 68.5 A–H, A 15-year-old girl with right frontal intracranial hemorrhages secondary to a ruptured arteriovenous malformation (AVM), grade 1 Spetzler-Martin.

(Brunner et al., 2008). A growing body of literature exists examining the role of inflammatory factors in stroke in children and in adults.

Migraine is common in the pediatric populations, occurring in 3%–5% of young children and up to 18% of adolescents (Lewis et al., 2004). Although true migrainous infarctions are rare, migraine is associated with a twofold increased risk of ischemic stroke. The risk is more apparent for individuals who have migraine with aura, smokers, and women who use oral contraceptives (Shürks et al., 2009). Although migraine has been associated with childhood stroke in large studies (Gioia et al., 2012; Pezzini et al., 2014), a prospective study of 1008 children with migraine did not detect any clear infarcts (Mar et al., 2013).

Variations in vascular anatomy that are congenital or secondary to pathology may play a role in some strokes. Cerebral arterial tortuosity may predispose to dissection (Saba et al, 2015), and may be congenital in some cases or secondary to vasculopathy (Wei et al, 2016; Devela et al, 2018). One study found anatomical venous variants in 43% of children with sinovenous thrombosis (Kouzmitcheva et al, 2018).

## Drugs/Toxins

Abuse of illicit drugs is an important cause of ischemic and hemorrhagic strokes in young patients. Maternal use of cocaine may lead to vasospasm and cerebral infarction in the fetus, and use of cocaine by children

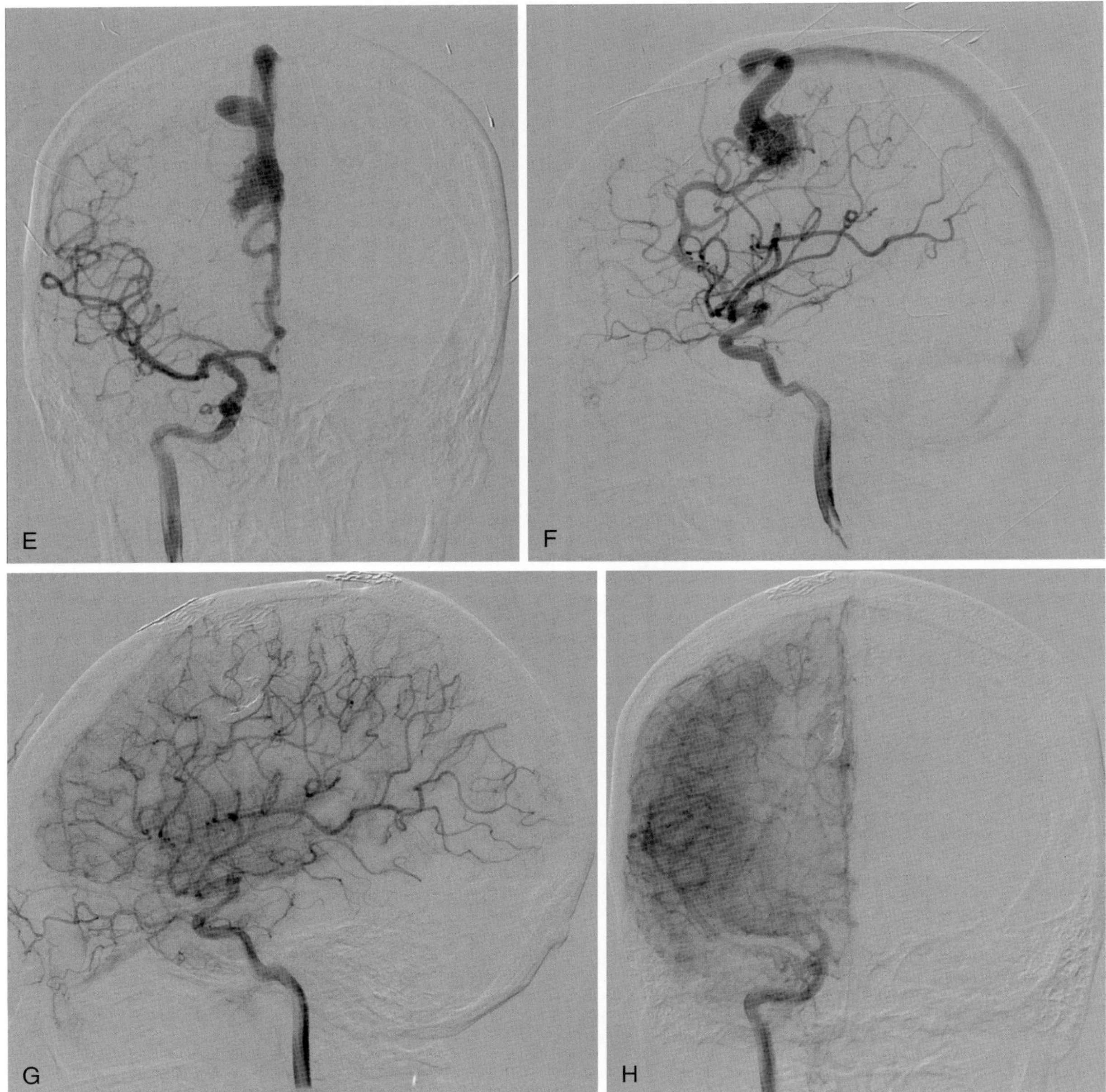


Fig. 68.5, cont'd

may lead to ICH or ischemic stroke. Other drugs such as amphetamines, which lead to sudden increases in blood pressure or vasospasm, also raise the risk of infarction. Ischemic stroke has been associated with both "natural" and "synthetic" ("Spice") marijuana use. Proposed mechanisms include cannabinoid-induced intracranial arteriopathy and/or cardiovascular effects such as arrhythmias (Barber et al., 2013; Freeman et al., 2013; Wolff et al., 2011). Accidental ingestion or overdose of medications used to treat thrombosis may lead to hemorrhage.

## Metabolic

The mitochondrial diseases may lead to metabolic strokes, particularly during times of metabolic stress. MRI can demonstrate infarction in nonvascular territories (Fig. 68.6). However, in rare cases, mitochondrial mutations have been associated with moyamoya vasculopathy (Longo et al., 2008; Papavasiliou et al., 2007).

Other metabolic diseases lead to cerebral infarction by contributing to thrombosis from arterial damage. Homocystinuria may lead to infarction, presumably through elevated homocysteine levels and subsequent vascular injury. The C677T MTHFR gene variant may be associated with childhood stroke, but it is not clear how large a role it plays; at least 10% of healthy children are homozygous for the MTHFR C677T (Gunther et al., 2000; Koch et al., 1999; Nowak-Göttl et al., 1999). Studies vary on the degree of associated risk, and carriers do not always have elevated homocysteine levels at the time of infarction. Fabry disease is an X-linked lysosomal storage disease that causes a deficiency of α-galactosidase and resultant accumulation of glycolipids in the endothelial wall. Male patients experience paresthesias of the hands and feet and cardiac abnormalities that can begin in childhood; hypohidrosis and renal dysfunction tend to occur later in the course of the disease (Ries et al., 2005). Both male and female heterozygotes are susceptible to cerebral thrombosis, possibly because of an increase in vasoreactivity in damaged vessels or endothelial and leukocyte activation. Males may be more severely

**TABLE 68.1 Disorders Associated with Moyamoya**

| | |
|---|---|
| Neonatal anoxia | Brain tumors |
| Head trauma | Parasellar tumors |
| Basilar meningitis | Wilms' tumor |
| Leptospirosis | Post-radiation vasculopathy |
| Tuberculosis | Atherosclerotic disease |
| Neurofibromatosis 1 | Hypertension |
| Tuberous sclerosis complex | Cerebral dissecting and saccular aneurysms |
| Sturge-Weber syndrome | Fibromuscular dysplasia |
| Phakomatosis pigmentovascularis type IIIB | Coarctation of the aorta |
| Pseudoxanthoma elasticum | Renal artery stenosis |
| Hypomelanosis of Ito | Arteriovenous malformations |
| Marfan syndrome | Cavernous malformations |
| Turner syndrome | Systemic lupus erythematosus |
| Williams syndrome | Sneddon syndrome |
| Noonan syndrome | Polyarteritis nodosa |
| Prader-Willi syndrome | Sjögren syndrome |
| Alagille syndrome | Sarcoidosis |
| Apert syndrome | Use of oral contraceptives |
| Down syndrome | Drug abuse (cocaine) |
| Sickle cell anemia | Homocystinuria |
| β-Thalassemia | Type I glycogenosis |
| Fanconi anemia | Osteogenesis imperfecta |
| Aplastic anemia | Glycogen storage disease |
| Hereditary spherocytosis | Hyperlipoproteinemia |
| Protein C deficiency | Primary oxalosis |
| Protein S deficiency | Hirschsprung disease |
| Antiphospholipid antibody syndrome (APAS) | Giant cervicofacial hemangiomas |
| Thrombotic thrombocytopenic purpura | Hyperthyroidism |
| Factor XII deficiency | Graves disease |

*Adapted from Houkin, K., Mikami, T., 2014. Moyamoya disease and moyamoya syndrome. In: J. E. Wanebo, N. Khan, J. M. Zabramski, R. F. Spetzler (Eds.), Moyamoya Disease: Diagnosis and Treatment. Thieme, New York.*

affected but rarely show cerebrovascular involvement before age 23 (Schiffmann, 2001). $\alpha_1$-Antitrypsin deficiency may lead to decreased structural integrity of the arterial wall by disrupting the balance of activity between proteases and antiproteases. $\alpha_1$-Antitrypsin deficiency has been associated with aneurysms and with vascular changes consistent with FMD. The hyperlipidemias can cause atherosclerotic vascular changes in children similar to those in older adults.

## Gender and Ethnicity

The role of gender in pediatric stroke has been controversial. One study found that both arterial ischemic stroke and sinovenous thrombosis are more common in boys, with male predominance particularly in cases of stroke caused by trauma-associated arterial dissection (Golomb et al., 2009). However, a recent population-based study in England did not find male gender to be a risk factor (Mallick et al., 2014). Higher testosterone levels have been associated with increased risk of stroke in boys (Normann et al., 2009).

Ethnicity is a risk factor for stroke. Black children appear to be at an increased risk for both ischemic and hemorrhagic stroke which cannot be fully explained by sickle cell disease. Asian ethnicity has been associated with stroke risk in the United Kingdom but not in the United States; differences in the ethnic makeup of the Asian populations between countries may explain some of the difference (Fullerton et al., 2003; Mallick et al., 2014). Multiple human leukocyte antigen (HLA) types have been associated with moyamoya disease in Asians (McCrea et al., 2019).

Gender and ethnicity may influence recovery from stroke. A study of mortality from childhood stroke in England and Wales from 1921 to 2000 found that boys had a higher mortality rate (Mallick et al., 2009). Black children have had higher stroke mortality than White children in the United States. This has been in part due to sickle cell anemia, and the disparity has decreased since the Stroke Prevention Trial in Sickle Cell Anemia (STOP) (Lehman et al., 2013).

## Genetic

Genome-wide association studies and whole-exome sequencing have led to the identification of genetic risk factors, but the function of the identified genes is not always clear. Mutations in the *CECR1* (cat eye syndrome chromosome region, candidate 1), which encode adenosine deaminase 2, have been associated with early stroke and vasculopathy.

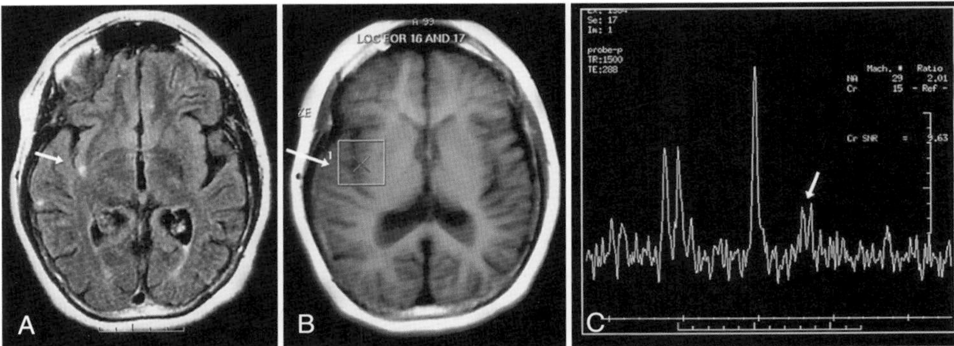


**Fig. 68.6** Magnetic resonance imaging (MRI) of an 18-year-old girl who presented at age 12 with headaches and went on to develop bilateral incoordination, decreased attention span, decline in school performance, and fatigability. **A,** Fluid spin echo inversion recovery MRI demonstrates multiple bilateral lesions in nonvascular territories. **B,** A section of the involved area is selected for evaluation using MR spectroscopy (MRS). **C,** MRS demonstrates a lactate doublet peak consistent with mitochondrial disease in an area of signal abnormality *(arrows)*.

Zebrafish and human studies suggest that adenosine deaminase 2 may function as a growth factor for endothelial cell development (Zhou et al., 2014). Mutations in genes such as alpha-actin (ACTA2) and myosin heavy chain 11 (MYH11) that can lead to smooth muscle dysfunction have been associated with dissection and vasculopathy that can affect children (McCrae et al, 2019). The AB collagen type IV alpha 1 and alpha 2 genes (*COL4A1* and *COL4A2*) code for a collagen which plays a role in the basement membranes of cerebral vasculature, and mutations can lead to vasculopathy and ischemic or hemorrhagic strokes starting in childhood (Jeanne et al., 2012; McCrea et al., 2019; Shah et al., 2010). Genetic variants in the plasma glutathione peroxidase gene *(GPX3),* which codes an enzyme which may modify fibrinogen, have been associated with pediatric ischemic stroke due to arteriopathy (Nowak-Göttl et al., 2011). A predisposition to pediatric stroke has been associated with four members of the ADAMTS gene family: *ADAMTS13, ADAMTS17, ADAMTS2,* and *ADAMTS12.* The currently best-understood of these genes, *ADAMTS13,* codes for von Willebrand factor–cleaving protease and leads to increased von Willebrand factor–induced endothelial platelet aggregation (Arning et al., 2012; Stoll et al., 2016).

## DIFFERENTIAL DIAGNOSIS

Children with stroke often present with seizures, and in the first few hours after a seizure, before cranial imaging, it can be difficult to determine whether a new hemiparesis is due to a temporary postictal Todd paresis or to infarction. Todd paresis usually does not last more than 24 hours, although in rare cases it may persist several days. Migraine may lead to infarction and permanent motor impairment, but hemiplegic migraine may lead to temporary motor impairment. A strong family history of hemiplegic migraine or documentation of a missense mutation of the *CACNA1A* calcium channel gene on chromosome 19p13 may help to differentiation (Terwindt et al., 2002), but variation exists in mutations among families (see Chapter 102). Alternating hemiplegia of childhood is a progressive neurodegenerative condition. The origin is generally unclear, although cerebrovascular factors and mitochondrial disease may be contributory. Neuroimaging studies usually do not demonstrate pathology. Edema, bleeding, or shifting of brain tumor may cause sudden onset of neurological signs. Encephalitis or meningoencephalitis may lead to sudden onset of focal neurological symptoms. Several metabolic diseases, including glutaric aciduria and carbohydrate-deficient glycoprotein syndrome (see Chapter 90), can present with stroke-like episodes, and serum and urine testing together with MRI help to make the diagnosis. Acute disseminated encephalomyelitis (ADEM), multiple sclerosis, vasculitis, and the vasculitic form of Hashimoto encephalopathy (Salpietro et al., 2014) are all causes of sudden onset of focal or multifocal neurological symptoms, and all may cause multiple T2 bright lesions on MRI.

## EVALUATION

### History and Physical

In the young patient, the history should include questions about delivery and the perinatal period, attainment of hand preference, and basic developmental milestones. Development of a hand preference before 1 year of age may be a sign of a mild hemiparesis in the nondominant hand, which could be due to a perinatal infarction. Any early hemorrhagic or ischemic infarction may lead to slowed development. Medical history should include questions about previous hemorrhages, abnormal bruising, petechiae, thromboses, and other medical conditions that may raise the risk of early stroke (e.g., complex congenital heart disease, renal failure, sickle cell anemia). Children with moyamoya usually present with recurrent transient ischemic attacks or cerebral infarction. Symptoms may be triggered by crying, physical exertion, or hyperventilation. Family history should include questions about abnormal bleeding in other family members, strokes or heart attacks before age 45, peripheral arteriopathy, or deep venous thrombosis. A history of multiple miscarriages may be suggestive of antiphospholipid antibody syndrome.

Physical examination should include examination of the face for signs of dysmorphic features suggestive of a genetic syndrome. Always assess head circumference. Early stroke may lead to macrocephaly due to hydrocephalus or to microcephaly due to tissue loss and poor brain growth from infarction. Examination of the skin should document signs of bruising or petechiae, livedo reticularis suggestive of Sneddon syndrome, systemic lupus erythematosus or other autoimmune disorders, café au lait spots suggestive of neurofibromatosis type 1, hypopigmented macules suggestive of tuberous sclerosis complex, excess skin laxity suggestive of a collagen disorder such as Ehlers-Danlos syndrome, cyanosis suggestive of heart failure and anoxia, and pallor suggestive of anemia. The head and neck should be auscultated for vascular bruits and the heart for murmurs and arrhythmias; peripheral pulses should be compared, and the abdomen should be auscultated for renal bruits suggestive of a systemic vascular disorder. Neurological examination should look for signs of focal abnormality, with the caveat that signs may not localize well in the very young child or may be difficult to assess in the frightened or uncooperative child (Table 68.2).

### Imaging Studies

Ultrasound (see Chapter 41) is useful in assessing IVH or periventricular leukomalacia in the premature infant or carotid flow in any child, but its sensitivity for detecting arterial stroke in the neonate is probably less than 50% (Golomb et al., 2001). Power Doppler ultrasound may be useful in detecting CVT in the neonate. Transcranial Doppler ultrasound is used to screen children with sickle cell anemia, and higher blood flow velocities are associated with higher stroke risk. Studies have suggested that this screening should begin in infancy (Telfer et al., 2007).

Cranial computed tomography (CT) (see Chapter 40) is better at assessing hemorrhage in the older child and ischemic stroke in the neonate and older child, but it may not detect arterial stroke until 24 hours or more after the event. CT angiography and venography (see Chapter 41) can image the cerebral vasculature.

MRI is the imaging tool of choice for most types of childhood stroke, and diffusion-weighted imaging (DWI) can detect brain ischemia within hours (see Chapter 40). DWI stays bright for approximately 2 weeks in the older child or adult but may "normalize" (pseudonormalization) within days in the neonate (Mader et al., 2002). Stroke imaging at any age should include DWI, T2, and fluid-attenuated inversion recovery (FLAIR) to detect areas of early infarction. Magnetic resonance angiography (MRA) may be helpful in diagnosing vasculitis and dissection involving larger vessels. In moyamoya, MRI typically demonstrates diminished flow voids in the distal ICAs, and proximal MCAs and ACAs, in addition to prominent collateral flow voids in the basal ganglia region (Fig. 68.7). Magnetic resonance spectroscopy (MRS) and single-photon emission CT (SPECT) demonstrate changes in regional blood flow and may be helpful in assessing patients with moyamoya disease and other sources of vasculopathy. MRS provides the earliest detection of ischemic lesions. Conventional angiography can clarify the structure of vascular malformations and is the most accurate method for detecting moyamoya, vasculitis, and dissection, but angiography may not always be possible in the acutely ill child. In patients suspected of moyamoya, six-vessel angiography remains the "gold standard" and should include selective injections of both ICAs, external carotid arteries, and vertebral arteries. Use all forms of neuroimaging in combination with other laboratory and physical findings because no one technique has perfect sensitivity or specificity for detecting vasculopathy. Continuous arterial spin labeling MRI has been used in research settings to study regional cerebral blood flow in persons with sickle cell anemia (Van den Tweel et al., 2009). Other newer forms of imaging such as functional MRI and diffusion-weighted tensor imaging are used in research settings and may provide insights into stroke evolution and recovery but are not widely available.

### Coagulation Work-up

The basic evaluation for prothrombotic disorders may include prothrombin time (PT) with international normalized ratio (INR) and activated partial thromboplastin time (aPTT) and a complete blood cell count, including platelets, protein C, protein S, and antithrombin levels, activated protein C resistance, plasminogen, fibrinogen, homocysteine, antiphospholipid antibody screen, lipoprotein (a), and a lipid panel. Genetic testing may include screening for the factor V Leiden mutation, the prothrombin 20210A gene, and the MTHFR gene variants. Some mutations are very common, and the ratio of symptomatic to nonsymptomatic carriers may be very high in some populations; more than 40% of healthy children in a European study were either homozygous or heterozygous for the C677T MTHFR variant (Koch et al., 1999). The frequency of different prothrombotic risk factors varies among populations (Salih et al., 2006a). Unfortunately, identifying asymptomatic carriers of prothrombotic genes might adversely affect later health, life, and disability insurance status (Golomb et al., 2005). Prothrombotic screening may not be warranted in otherwise healthy neonates with arterial ischemic stroke who do not have other areas of thrombosis (Curtis et al., 2017).

### Cardiac Evaluation

The basic cardiac evaluation may include electrocardiogram (ECG) with rhythm strip and a transthoracic echocardiogram with injection of agitated saline to screen for a PFO. If any suspicion exists for cardioembolic events and those two studies are unrevealing, perform transesophageal echocardiography and a Holter monitor study.

### Other Studies

Flexion and extension radiographs of the cervical spine may identify bony abnormalities predisposing to dissection. Electroencephalogram (EEG) may help to localize the lesion in children who present with seizures and is helpful for evaluating cerebral function in the unresponsive and possibly locked-in patient with a brainstem stroke (see Chapter 5). Visual evoked potentials and brainstem auditory evoked potentials may be particularly helpful in evaluating the very young or somnolent patient (see Chapter 35).

Serum and plasma studies may help to identify the cause of the stroke. Thrombocytopenia, deficiencies of factors I, VII, VIII, IX, and XIII, and deficiency of von Willebrand factor are all risk factors for ICH, whereas polycythemia, thrombocythemia, and anemia are all risk factors for ischemic stroke. Abnormalities in platelet count and fibrinogen may be markers for DIC, which may lead to thrombosis and ischemic stroke. Elevated serum lactate is a marker for mitochondrial disease, but not all patients with mitochondrial disease have elevated serum lactate; genetic tests may be required to confirm the diagnosis. Muscle biopsy may help to confirm mitochondrial disease (see Chapter 92). Serum studies for plasma α-galactosidase will identify Fabry disease. Serum ammonia, amino acids, and organic acids may help to identify metabolic disease such as hyperhomocysteinemia and mitochondrial diseases that can lead to stroke (Menkes, 2000).

## TREATMENT

### The Acute Period and Initiating Chronic Therapy

Children with ICH or hemorrhagic stroke require close observation in the first hours. Children with hemophilia need immediate factor replacement and may require blood transfusion. Children with large hematomas with significant mass effect may need surgery (Johnson, 2000). Any child presenting with unexplained or poorly explained ICH should also be evaluated for other sites of injury and possible child abuse.

Intravenous thrombolysis, intraarterial thrombolysis, and mechanical thrombectomy have been used in small numbers of children with good results, but there are no clear guidelines for use (Bigi et al, 2018.)

Some of these children were not treated in accordance with guidelines used for adults (Amlie-Lefond, 2009b; Ferriero et al., 2019; Roach et al., 2008). Few children present within the mandated 4.5 hours of ischemic stroke onset. Unfortunately, a National Institutes of Health (NIH)-funded dose-finding study of tissue plasminogen activator for

**TABLE 68.2 Physical Examination of the Child with Stroke**

| Finding | Possible Significance/Suggestive of |
|---|---|
| **Head Circumference** | |
| Macrocephaly | Hydrocephalus caused by IVH, SDH, SAH, or vascular malformation |
| Microcephaly | Failure of brain growth resulting from stroke or genetic disorder |
| **Eyes** | |
| ***External/Iris*** | |
| Epicanthal folds, Brushfield spots | Down syndrome |
| Horner syndrome | Carotid dissection (postganglionic)/vertebral dissection (central) |
| Pulsating exophthalmos | Carotid-cavernous fistula |
| Lens subluxation | Marfan syndrome, homocystinuria |
| Angioid streaks | Pseudoxanthoma elasticum |
| Xanthelasma on lids, corneal arcus | Hyperlipidemia |
| Corneal opacity | Fabry disease |
| ***Retina*** | |
| Papilledema | Increased ICP resulting from hydrocephalus, vascular malformation, or acute brain edema |
| Hemorrhages | Trauma (consider child abuse), bleeding diathesis, ruptured aneurysm, collagen disease, emboli |
| Vasculopathy | Systemic vasculitis |
| Angioid streaks | Pseudoxanthoma elasticum, Paget disease, sickle cell anemia |
| Angioma | Familial cavernous angiomatosis, von Hippel-Lindau disease |
| **Skin** | |
| Bruising | Bleeding diathesis (consider child abuse) |
| Petechiae | Platelet count low or dysfunction; DIC |
| Purpura | Henoch-Schönlein purpura |
| Pallor | Anemia |
| Erythema | Polycythemia |
| Cyanosis | Complex congenital heart disease, other cause of hypoxia |
| Skin necrosis | Meningococcemia |
| Café au lait spots | Neurofibromatosis type 1 |
| Hypopigmented macules, shagreen patches, facial angiofibromas | Tuberous sclerosis complex |
| Yellow papules | Pseudoxanthoma elasticum |
| Premature aging | Progeria |
| Malar rash | Systemic lupus erythematosus |
| Skin laxity | Ehlers-Danlos syndrome type IV |
| Telangiectasias | Osler-Weber-Rendu disease (hereditary hemorrhagic telangiectasia) |
| Oral/genital ulcers | Behçet disease |
| Angiokeratomas | Fabry disease |
| Lentigines in non–sun-exposed areas | Predisposition to dissection or to atrial myxoma, which may lead to cardioembolic stroke |
| Discoloration of fingers with cold: white, blue, then red | Raynaud phenomenon as sign of collagen disease or systemic lupus erythematosus |
| Livedo reticularis | Antiphospholipid syndrome, Sneddon syndrome, homocystinuria, systemic vasculitis, DADA2, cutis marmorata-telangiectatica congenita |
| Subcutaneous nodules on elbows, forehead, tendons | Rheumatic fever, systemic lupus erythematosus, rheumatoid arthritis |
| Erythematous macules that evolve to clear, fluid-filled vesicles | Acute varicella (chicken pox); shingles if in a dermatomal distribution |
| Multiple round, white, puckered scars | Past varicella infection |
| Needle tracks | IV drug addiction with risk for endocarditis and HIV |

Continued

**TABLE 68.2 Physical Examination of the Child with Stroke—cont'd**

| Finding | Possible Significance/Suggestive of |
|---|---|
| **Mouth** | |
| High, arched palate | Marfan syndrome |
| Petechial hemorrhages | Infective endocarditis |
| **Heart and Peripheral Pulses** | |
| Murmur | Complex congenital heart disease, valve abnormality |
| Decreased pulses | Takayasu arteritis |
| Increased pulses | Hypertension |
| ***Abdomen*** | |
| Hepatomegaly | Infection, cancer, liver failure |
| Bruit | Renal artery stenosis |
| **Back** | |
| Scoliosis, vertebral anomalies | Possible increased risk of dissection |
| **Hands** | |
| Long, tapering fingers | Marfan syndrome |
| Other anomalies of bones of hands | May be seen in association with congenital heart disease |
| Clubbing of fingers | Congenital heart disease |
| **Joints** | |
| Painful, restricted movement | Arthritis due to autoimmune disease, past bleeds (hemophilia) |
| Warm | Autoimmune disease, infection |
| **Overall Size** | |
| Tall | Marfan syndrome, homocystinuria |
| Short | Progeria, mitochondrial disease, dwarfism (risk of vertebral anomalies) |

*DADA2*, adenosine deaminase type 2; *DADA2*, Deficiency of Adenosine Deaminase 2; *DIC*, disseminated intravascular coagulation; *HIV*, human immunodeficiency virus; *ICP*, increased intracranial pressure; *IV*, intravenous; *IVH*, intraventricular hemorrhage; *SAH*, subarachnoid hemorrhage; *SDH*, subdural hematoma.

*Physical findings taken from Hurst, J.W., 1993. Cardiovascular Diagnosis: The Initial Examination. Mosby-Year Book, St. Louis. Information on lentigines from Neau, J.P., Rosolacci, T., Pin, J.C., et al., 1993. Cerebral infarction, cardiac myxoma and lentiginosis. Rev Neurol (Paris) 149, 289–291; and Schievink, W.I., Michels, V.V., Mokri, B., et al., 1995. Brief report: a familial syndrome of arterial dissections with lentiginosis. N Engl J Med 332, 576–579.*

acute pediatric stroke was closed because of difficulty enrolling patients (Rivkin et al., 2014). Thrombolytic therapy may not be helpful in neonates, who have lower levels of plasminogen than older children (Andrew et al., 2000).

No clear guidelines are available on the use of heparin (unfractionated or low-molecular-weight heparins) in pediatric arterial stroke and CVT patients either. Pilot studies and case series have described good results with heparin and low-molecular-weight heparins (deVeber et al., 1998; Massicotte et al., 1996). Large-scale studies with catheter-related noncranial thrombosis have shown good results (Andrew et al., 2000). Moharir et al. (2009) showed that neonates and children with sinovenous thrombosis who are not anticoagulated are at increased risk for thrombus propagation, which can be asymptomatic and lead to poor outcome. Other agents which either inhibit thrombin formation or account for direct thrombin inhibition may be required for patients with immune-mediated heparin-induced thrombocytopenia (Ahmed et al., 2007; Alsoufi et al., 2004; Neuhaus et al., 2000; Ranze et al., 1999; Risch et al., 2006).

In sickle cell anemia, exchange transfusion is the usual treatment for acute ischemic stroke (Menkes et al., 2000). The STOP demonstrated that, in children with vasculopathy shown by transcranial Doppler ultrasound screening, regular transfusions to keep the sickle hemoglobin (HbS) concentration at less than 30% reduced the risk of recurrent stroke by 92% (Adams, 2000). This trial has helped to decrease the disparity in stroke mortality between Black children and White children in the United States (Lehman et al., 2013). However, chronic transfusions carry the risk of infection and cause increases in serum ferritin (Files et al., 2002). Some children require treatment with deferoxamine chelation to prevent iron overload (Wayne et al., 2000). Stopping exchange transfusion therapy leads to increased vascular disease and stroke risk (Adams and Brambilla, 2005).

Attempts at treating and preventing metabolic stroke and cerebrovascular disease have been made by addressing the pathological defects in metabolic pathways, using coenzyme $Q_{10}$ and other antioxidant vitamins. L-Arginine improves endothelial dysfunction in children with MELAS (mitochondrial encephalopathy, lactic acidosis, and strokes) and may aid in treating the stroke-like episodes (Koga et al., 2006). Folate, vitamin $B_6$, and vitamin $B_{12}$ all play a role in homocysteine metabolism, which is impaired in homocystinuria and in carriers of the MTHFR C677T gene variant. Several different enzyme abnormalities may lead to homocystinuria, and

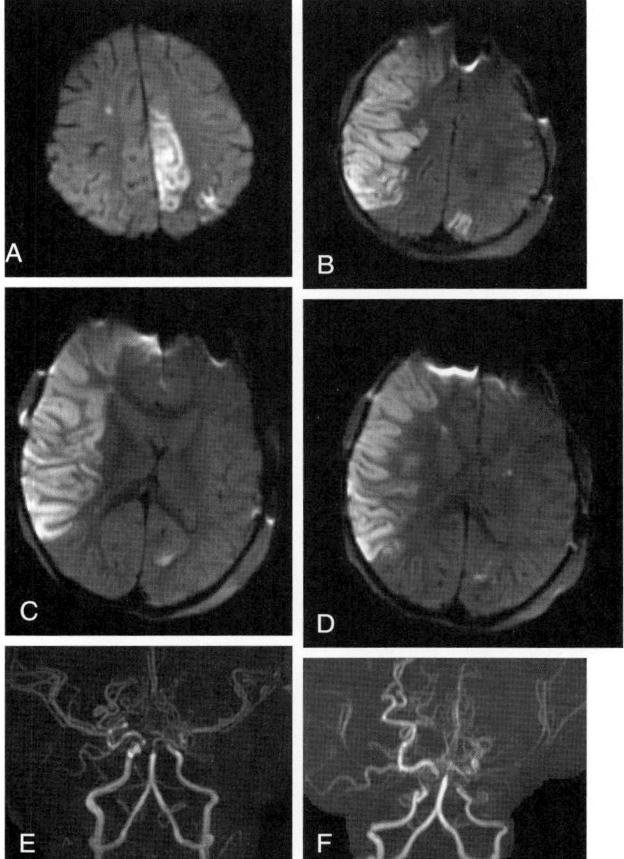

**Fig. 68.7** A 14-month-old girl with a history of complex partial seizures now develops a postictal right hemiparesis. **A–F,** Diffusion-weighted magnetic resonance imaging shows acute transcortical infarcts involving the right middle cerebral artery (MCA) territory, small segment of the left anterior cerebral artery territory, small segmental left posterior cerebral artery territory, and punctate left MCA territory. On magnetic resonance angiography, the intracranial arterial circulation demonstrates left supraclinoid carotid occlusion and reconstitution of left M1 and A1 segments via moyamoya-type collaterals. There was normal course and caliber of both cervical carotid and vertebral arteries. ACA, anterior cerebral artery; DWMRI, diffusion weighted magnetic resonance imaging; PCA, posterior cerebral artery.

the enzyme affected determines whether supplementation with folate, vitamin $B_6$, or vitamin $B_{12}$ is helpful (Menkes, 2000). Dietary supplementation with folate lowers serum homocysteine levels in adults with the MTHFR C677T gene variant (Thuillier et al., 1998) and may be helpful in children with it. Enzyme replacement with α-galactosidase decreases the symptoms of Fabry disease and normalizes cerebrovascular reactivity but does not remove the risk of recurrent stroke (Schiffmann et al., 2006).

Patients with protein C deficiency have been treated with protein C concentrate (Manco-Johnson et al., 2016; Minford et al., 2014). Antithrombin concentrate has been used to treat consumptive coagulopathy and severe antithrombin deficiency at the time of acute stroke or other thrombosis (Stockton et al., 2017), but it is not clear that it prevents thrombosis in leukemia patients treated with L-asparaginase (Ranta et al., 2013).

## Additional Issues in Chronic Therapy

Patients with hemophilia and severe bleeding may require prophylaxis with regular factor transfusions. Young or ataxic children may need to wear protective helmets until their balance improves.

Patients with genetic chronic thrombotic abnormalities such as protein C or S deficiency, or with antiphospholipid antibody syndrome, may require long-term care with low-molecular-weight heparin or warfarin (Andrew et al., 2000). However, for many patients, the best long-term therapy is not clear. Low-molecular-weight heparin may be used for 3–6 months after cervicocephalic arterial dissection or CVT (Andrew and deVeber, 1999), with an Insuflon patch to make administration tolerable. Warfarin or aspirin have been used for long-term therapy (Andrew et al., 2000). The Cervical Artery Dissection in Stroke Study (CADISS) in adults showed no differences in efficacy of antiplatelet and anticoagulant drugs at preventing stroke and death in patients with symptomatic cervical (carotid and vertebral) dissection. Of note, stroke recurrence was rare in both groups (CADISS Trial Investigators, 2015). Unfortunately, there are no trials on treatment of dissection in children. Families of children on warfarin need to be counseled about regulating vitamin K levels in the diet, bony changes, possible teratogenicity, and the risks of undertreatment or overtreatment. Families of children taking aspirin are generally concerned about Reye syndrome, but there are no reports in children taking aspirin for stroke prophylaxis (Roach, 2000). Strater and colleagues (2001) did a prospective follow-up study of 135 children with first onset of ischemic stroke. The children received prophylactic treatment with either low-dose low-molecular-weight heparin or aspirin and were followed for a median of 36 months. Low-dose low-molecular-weight heparin was not superior to aspirin in preventing stroke recurrence. For children with sickle cell anemia, chronic treatment with hydroxyurea can increase levels of fetal hemoglobin and decrease complications of sickle cell anemia, but careful monitoring is required for cytotoxicity and genotoxicity (Khayat et al., 2006). Bone marrow transplantation with allogeneic hematopoietic stem cell transplant may be an option for some children (Kassim et al., 2017; Vermylen, 2003; Ware et al., 2016). Surgery or interventional procedures play a role in treating some types of cerebrovascular disease. Indirect surgical revascularization procedures, such as encephaloduroarteriosynangiosis (EDAS), encephalomyosynangiosis (EMS), encephalomyoarteriosynangiosis (EMAS), pial synangiosis, multiple burr holes, craniotomy with inversion of the dura, omental transplantation, omental pedicle graft, and cervical sympathectomy, may be used to treat children with moyamoya disease. Direct revascularization procedures such as superficial temporal artery (STA) to MCA bypass are technically difficult to perform in children. Other surgical procedures such as clipping, coiling, radioablation, or removal may be useful in the treatment of aneurysms or malformations.

Socioeconomic status and social stressors may play a role in family compliance with therapy and patient outcome. A large multinational study of children with arterial ischemic stroke found that very low family income level was associated with worse outcome (Jordan et al., 2018).

## Other Issues

The risks that accompany pregnancy in adolescence are greater for young women with a history of hemorrhagic or ischemic stroke (see Chapter 112).

Oral contraceptives carry a very small risk for the general population but may carry more risk for women with prothrombotic disorders (Slooter et al., 2005). Oral contraceptive use raises the risk of both arterial thromboembolism and CVT. These issues require explicit discussion with patients and their families, preferably before adolescence, as some oral contraceptives are used to treat acne or menstrual disorders in young adolescent women.

## SUMMARY

Children with stroke are at risk for future cognitive impairment, motor impairment, and epilepsy. In full-term neonates, it is difficult to predict outcome based on initial cranial imaging, and it is unclear whether the side on which the infarcts occur affects language development. Evidence of degeneration of corticospinal tracts and resulting asymmetry in the midbrain on MRI performed during the second 6 months of life does predict hemiplegia. Approximately half of children with neonatal arterial ischemic stroke have feeding problems; when severe, feeding dysfunction can lead to aspiration and failure to thrive (Barkat-Masih et al., 2010). Children who present with signs of perinatal stroke after the perinatal period appear to have worse motor outcomes than children with perinatal stroke who present in the neonatal period (Lee et al., 2005). For these children, young age at presentation, fever at presentation, and right MCA infarction have been associated with poor outcome (Cnossen et al., 2010). Bilateral hemispheric lesions and low muscle tone of affected limbs at presentation have also been associated with poor outcome (Kim et al., 2009). Studies in both infants and older children show that larger and multiple infarcts are more likely to cause cognitive and motor impairment as well as epilepsy. Overall, the intelligence of children with stroke falls within the normal range, but some require extra help in school.

The prognosis for children with progressive cerebrovascular diseases is particularly problematic. Those children with severe forms of sickle cell disease or moyamoya disease who are not treated or who do not respond to therapy may develop significant cognitive and motor disabilities and epilepsy (Lagunju et al., 2013; Weinberg et al., 2011). More than 20% of children who survive childhood arterial ischemic stroke may have recurrent transitory ischemic attacks or stroke (Ganesan et al., 2002). Prothrombotic disorders and abnormalities on vascular imaging raise the risk of recurrence (Strater et al., 2002).

*The complete reference list is available online at https://expertconsult.inkling.com/.* 

69

# Spinal Cord Vascular Disease

*Michael J. Lyerly, Asim K. Bag, David S. Geldmacher*

OUTLINE



The spinal cord is subject to many of the same vascular diseases that involve the brain, but its unique anatomy and embryology render it susceptible to some syndromes that do not have intracranial counterparts. Although some vascular myelopathic processes have classic syndromic presentations, many may be more challenging to differentiate from other forms of myelopathy. Ischemic diseases of the spinal cord have been well characterized; however, the spinal cord may also be affected by vascular malformations and hemorrhagic processes that require prompt identification and management. A firm understanding of the vascular anatomy of the spinal cord is critical to understanding these disease processes.

## VASCULAR ANATOMY OF THE SPINAL CORD

Additional text available at http://expertconsult.inkling.com.

## SPINAL CORD INFARCTION

Paraplegia complicating aortic surgery was recognized as early as 1825, although it was not attributed to spinal cord ischemia until the 1880s. By the early twentieth century, cardiac embolism, atheromatous disease, and decompression sickness were also described as causes of paraplegia attributable to spinal cord ischemia. The actual prevalence of spinal cord infarction is unknown but is generally cited as representing 1%–2% of all central neurovascular events and 5%–8% of all acute myelopathies. The median age of presentation of all spinal cord infarction is 60 years, although this may vary based on the underlying pathophysiological process. The clinical presentation of spinal cord syndromes is presented in more detail in Chapter 27.

### Presentation and Initial Course

Similar to cerebral infarction, most patients present with sudden onset of neurological dysfunction that evolves over minutes to hours. In rare cases of spontaneous spinal cord infarction, transient symptoms referred to as "spinal transient ischemic attacks" have been reported. Symptoms depend on the vascular territory involved, with the ASA territory being most often affected. The ASA syndrome is characterized by loss of strength and pain/temperature sensation, with sparing of vibration/proprioception below the level of the infarction. This syndrome is most often bilateral but may be unilateral or incomplete, depending on the degree of collateral vessels. Autonomic dysfunction including hypotension, bowel/bladder dysfunction, or sexual dysfunction may also occur. The posterior spinal artery (PSA) syndrome is less common and typically presents with isolated loss of vibration and proprioception below the level of the lesion.

Weakness (89%–100%), sensory loss (89%–95%), back pain at onset (72%–82%), and urinary complaints requiring catheterization (75%) are the most common presenting symptoms of cord ischemia in multiple series (Kumral et al., 2011; Masson et al., 2004; Zalewski et al., 2019). Hyperacute onset is the clue to the diagnosis, with most patients reaching a nadir of their symptoms within 12 hours. The most common location to be affected is the mid-to-low thoracic spine. Lower cervical lesions are less common and upper thoracic spinal infarcts are rare. Cervical lesions may cause respiratory failure and quadriparesis. Pain and sensory changes occur first in most cases, followed by weakness within minutes or hours. More than 80% of back pain with spinal infarction follows a radicular pattern, but in cases of acute aortic disease, pain may have a more visceral character. Back pain typically occurs at the level of the infarction, which may assist with localization. Urinary retention is typical in the acute phase, but involuntary voiding or defecation may be associated with the onset of the ischemic insult.

The dominant clinical presentation depends on the vascular territory involved. ASA distribution infarction typically presents with weakness (ventral gray matter involvement), loss of pain and temperature sensation (spinothalamic tract involvement), and areflexia with bladder and bowel dysfunction. Asymmetry of these symptoms is not uncommon. Posterior spinal infarctions result in loss of proprioception and vibration sense, paresis, and sphincter dysfunction. Acute severe

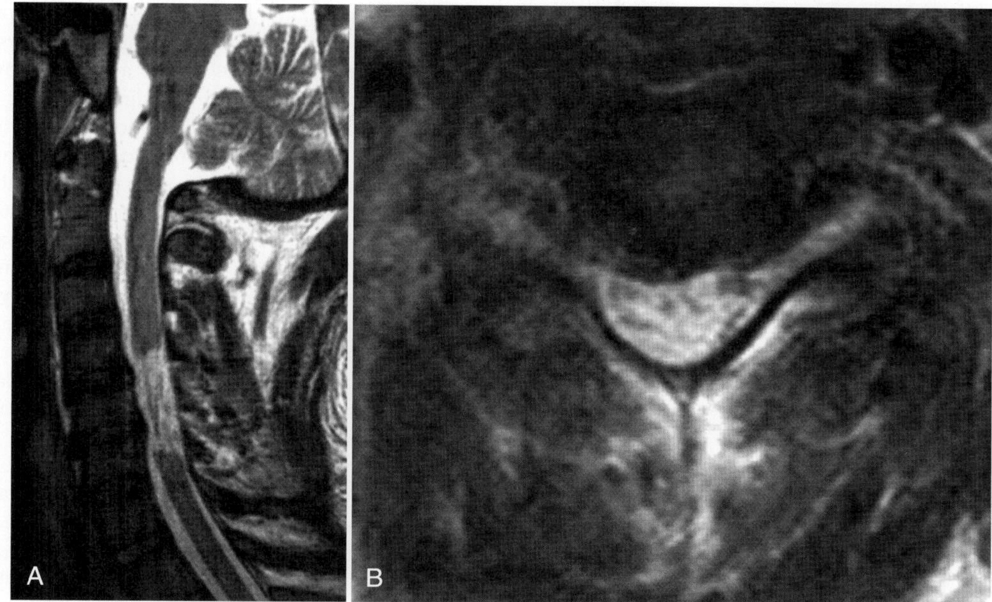


**Fig. 69.3 Subacute Infarction of the Cervical Cord.** A 32-year-old patient had presented with acute-onset quadriparesis and pain in the neck region. Over time, the patient regained function in his upper extremity but remained paraplegic. **A,** Sagittal T2-weighted image through the cervical spine and, **B,** axial T2-weighted image through the level of C5 vertebra were obtained 2 weeks after the initial presentation. Images demonstrate diffuse increased T2 signal involving almost the entire cross-sectional area of a segment of the spinal cord due to ischemic infarction.

hypotension and aortic surgery can present as bilateral sensory symptoms with preserved motor function (central infarction) or focal combined motor and sensory symptoms (complete transverse infarction).

## Examination Findings

Weakness most commonly affects both lower limbs. Examination typically reveals flaccid paresis acutely accompanied by diminished superficial and tendon reflexes below the level of the lesion. Preservation of strength and reflexes suggests PSA territory infarction. Upper motor neuron signs, including spasticity and hyperreflexia, may develop in the subsequent weeks. Sensory changes, when present, nearly always affect spinothalamic modalities. Isolated proprioceptive loss is rare. Hypotension may be present, suggesting autonomic involvement, and respiratory function may be compromised with cervical cord lesions.

## Investigations

Magnetic resonance imaging (MRI) is the diagnostic procedure of choice for detecting spinal cord ischemia, although the results can be normal in a minority of patients (19% in one series). Infarctions do not always fit perfectly with a vascular territory on imaging. In the acute phase, MRI may be negative on routine sequences. Therefore it is very important to incorporate diffusion-weighted imaging (DWI), preferably in both axial and sagittal planes, in patients with clinical suspicion of spinal cord infarction. Similar to brain infarction, DWI demonstrates diffusion restriction in the infarcted segment(s) of the spinal cord with increased signal matching low apparent diffusion coefficient value. Hyperintense signals on T2-weighted images initially appear between 2 hours to several days. Variable contrast enhancement can be seen in the subacute phase and may persist up to 3 weeks. Both T2-weighted images and contrast-enhanced T1-weighted images may demonstrate a double-dot ("owl's eyes") pattern if bilateral anterior horns are involved, an H-shaped pattern if the entire central gray matter is involved, or a more diffuse pattern if both gray and white matters are involved (Fig. 69.3). The diffuse pattern may be difficult to distinguish from venous congestion. When cord infarction results from compromise of a segmental artery, branches supplying the ipsilateral half of the vertebral body may also be affected. Vertebral body infarct is best detected on sagittal Short-TI Inversion Recovery (STIR) weighted images, usually appearing as a triangular area of increased signal near the end-plate and/or deep medullary portion of the vertebral body.

Other laboratory and radiographic studies are frequently nondiagnostic in noncompressive spinal cord ischemia; however, further testing may be necessary to rule out alternative diagnoses or determine the mechanism of infarction. Myelography is usually normal. Computed tomography angiography (CTA) or magnetic resonance angiography (MRA) may be useful for evaluating for vertebral or aortic dissection. If embolism is suspected, an echocardiogram may be performed as well as hypercoagulability studies. MRI of the brain may be useful if there is concern for an inflammatory etiology affecting other parts of the central nervous system (CNS). Cerebrospinal fluid (CSF) analysis will also help to evaluate for inflammatory or infectious processes but is frequently normal in spinal cord infarction. The most common CSF finding is an elevated protein; however, a pleocytosis may rarely be seen.

## Course and Prognosis

The course of spinal ischemic syndromes is variable. Although most patients reach maximum symptomatology within 12 hours, some have a longer course, possibly related to variations in collateralization of blood supply. Transient ischemic attacks with spinal cord symptoms have been reported to precede up to 10% of cord infarcts.

Rates of recovery vary widely among case series, which were collected by different methods; however, most patients demonstrate some degree of functional improvement. In a prospectively collected series, approximately half the patients had a favorable outcome, defined as the ability to walk with one assistive device (or none) and no need for urinary catheterization at the time of hospital discharge (Masson et al., 2004). Retrospective series also suggest that ambulation can be restored in approximately 50% of patients, although a

**BOX 69.1 Causes of Spinal Cord Ischemic Syndromes**

Local mechanical vascular compression
Regional hemodynamic compromise
Systemic hypotension
Occlusive vascular disease
Thromboembolism
Endovascular procedures
Fibrocartilaginous (intervertebral disk) embolism
Vasculitis
Arterial dissection
Thrombosis
Venous occlusion

quarter of patients remain wheelchair bound (Zalewski et al., 2019). The likelihood of recovery is higher when the deficits are less severe at presentation. Over a mean follow-up period of 4 years, more than 90% of patients with the mildest severity of deficit during the acute phase were able to walk independently or with assistive devices; in contrast, nearly one-third of more severely affected patients required a wheelchair (Nedeltchev et al., 2004). Poor outcome is predicted when proprioceptive loss, gait impairment, or urinary dysfunction were present at the onset. Female sex and advanced age have also been associated with a lower likelihood of recovery. Chronic pain can be a disabling consequence of cord ischemia, but it tends to occur only in individuals with spinothalamic sensory impairment early in the course. The duration of motor dysfunction is also useful in determining prognosis. Unless significant motor recovery occurs in the first 24 hours, the likelihood of major improvement is low. The case fatality rate ranges from 2% to 20%. Patients at highest risk are those with ischemia secondary to aortic dissection or those with ischemic injury to the high cervical cord.

## Causes of Spinal Cord Infarction

In recent series, the cause of spinal cord infarction could not be identified in up to 68% of cases. Patients with an idiopathic etiology frequently have traditional vascular risk factors, including hypertension, dyslipidemia, or tobacco abuse, suggesting that processes such as atherosclerosis may contribute to the pathogenesis. Among cases with identifiable causes, iatrogenic injury to the thoracoabdominal aorta during surgical repair is the most common etiology. Other common mechanisms can be divided into mechanical compression, diseases of the aorta or spinal arteries, systemic hypoperfusion, vascular malformations, and venous infarctions. Most infarcts associated with intrinsic spinal disease (e.g., chronic radicular pain, compression fractures) follow anterior or PSA patterns and occur at the level of the mechanical stresses in the spine. Mechanical triggering events are not associated with central or transverse infarct patterns. Systemic arterial disease was noted more frequently in patients with transverse patterns. Other typical causes of spinal ischemia are summarized in Box 69.1.

Aortic pathologies with regional hemodynamic compromise accounted for 30%–40% of cord infarcts in older case series. Complications of aortic surgery represented the largest proportion of those cases. Advanced age, prior cerebrovascular disease, intraoperative hypotension, prolonged clamping of the aorta above the renal arteries (e.g., for more than 20–30 minutes), and operative ligation of lower thoracic intercostal vessels are risk factors for cord ischemia and infarction. Open thoracoabdominal aortic aneurysm repairs are associated with up to a 10%–30% risk of significant neurological deficits. Although endovascular techniques appear to be safer, they do not completely eliminate the risk for spinal cord ischemia. Intraoperative interventions like distal aortic perfusion and CSF drainage may contribute to lower complication rates.

Atherosclerotic plaques in the aorta may overlie the origin of branches to the spinal cord and diminish their blood flow or be a source of embolism. As noted previously, many patients with spinal cord infarction have one or more vascular risk factors. Transesophageal echocardiography may identify such plaques in the descending aorta. Occlusive arterial disease may result in intermittent claudication of the spinal cord, manifested by activity-induced transient symptoms of myelopathy. Intermittent spinal claudication may respond positively to aortobifemoral bypass. Aortic dissection may also disrupt blood flow to the radicular arteries, particularly in the thoracic cord. This should be considered in a patient with symptoms concerning for spinal cord ischemia coupled with chest pain (particularly radiating to the back), abnormal pulses, or connective tissue diseases that may predispose to arterial dissections.

Systemic hypotension may also produce cord ischemia, but because other end-organ damage is common in such cases, including cerebral hypoxic-ischemic encephalopathy, this condition may be difficult to recognize and isolated spinal cord syndromes are infrequent. Transverse cord infarcts are associated with prolonged hypotension. Localized thoracic cord ischemia may result from disordered autoregulation following percutaneous radiofrequency spinal rhizotomy.

Radiotherapy produces myelopathy associated with occlusive changes in parenchymal spinal cord arterioles. The degree of myelopathy depends on the total radiation dose, dose per fraction, and the length of the irradiated segment of the cord.

Thromboembolism causes both acute and stepwise spinal cord dysfunction. Emboli may arise from the mitral valve in rheumatic heart disease, acute bacterial endocarditis, or an atrial myxoma. Myelopathy associated with decompression sickness (also known as *caisson disease*) results from circulating nitrogen bubbles that block small spinal arteries. Spinal cord ischemia also may complicate therapeutic renal or bronchial artery embolizations.

Fibrocartilaginous emboli from ruptured intervertebral disks are the cause of an ischemic syndrome unique to the spinal cord. Fragments of connective tissue material from the damaged disk are traumatically forced into bone marrow sinusoids by local fracture. The increased tissue pressure at the site of injury allows retrograde entry of emboli into the spinal vertebral plexus as well as into arterial channels, leading to cord infarction (Fig. 69.4). Approximately half of these events are purely arterial; the rest have mixed arterial and venous involvement. The anterior portion of the cervical cord is affected in up to 70% of such cases. Women are affected twice as often as men.

Vasculitic and thrombotic causes of spinal cord ischemia are well known. Before the antibiotic era, meningovascular syphilis was a common cause of ASA ischemic syndromes, and spinal meningitis continues to be occasionally associated with paraplegia of vascular origin. Systemic inflammatory conditions such as Crohn disease, polyarteritis nodosa, and giant cell arteritis may also lead to myelopathy. Sickle cell disease, intrathecal chemical irritants, angiographic contrast material, the postpartum state, and intravascular neoplastic invasion all predispose to thrombosis and spinal cord infarction.

Venous infarction without hemorrhage is clinically indistinguishable from the arterial ischemic syndromes. There may be an associated systemic thrombophlebitis that propagates into the spinal canal via the venous plexus. A subacute necrotizing myelitis (Foix-Alajouanine syndrome) causing stepwise spinal cord dysfunction occurs with extensive spinal cord thrombophlebitis in association with chronic obstructive pulmonary disease or a neoplasm (usually of the lung). This condition may also be the end-stage result of chronic venous hypertension and congestion resulting from dural venous fistula. Polycythemia rubra

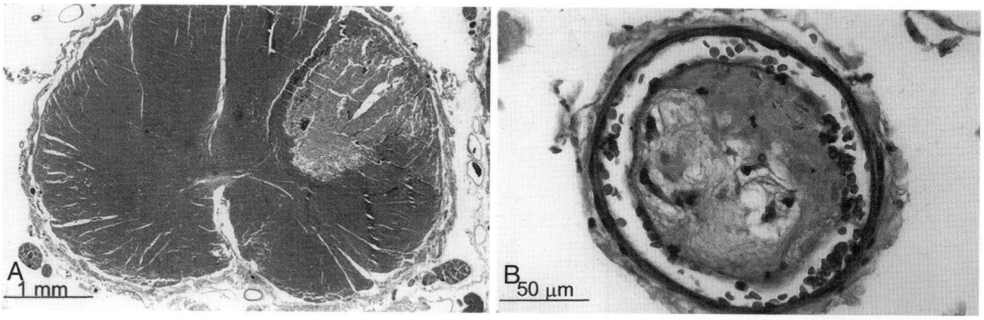

**Fig. 69.4** Pathological Sections From a 19-Year-Old Man Who Died After Cervical Fibrocartilaginous Embolism. **A,** Segmental infarction in the posterolateral cord. **B,** Intraluminal fibrocartilaginous material in the infarcted region. *(From Freyaldenhoven, T.E., Mrak, R.E., 2001. Fibrocartilaginous embolization. Neurology 56, 1354, with permission.)*

**BOX 69.2 Classification of Spinal Arteriovenous Malformations**

Type I: Dural arteriovenous fistula (AVF), subtypes IA (single feeding artery) and IB (multiple feeding arteries).

Type II: Intramedullary glomus-type arteriovenous malformation (AVM).

Type III: Intramedullary juvenile-type AVM, which is more extensive than a glomus-type AVM, frequently having an extramedullary component and sometimes an extradural component.

Type IV: Intradural extramedullary (perimedullary) AVF; subtypes IVA, IVB, and IVC correspond to lesions with progressively increased arteriovenous shunting, manifested as increased number, size, and tortuosity of feeding arteries.

vera can also lead to noninflammatory spinal venous thrombosis with subsequent cord ischemia.

### Treatment

The medical management of spinal cord ischemia focuses on supportive measures to minimize complications and on reducing risk for recurrence. Acute therapies have not been rigorously studied, but some protocols exist for specific situations. For patients with infarction secondary to aortic surgery, some authors advocate an algorithm for gradually increasing the mean arterial pressure with vasopressors and placing a lumbar drain (McGarvey et al., 2007). Although some improvement has been reported using this approach, more data are needed to evaluate the effectiveness of this algorithm. There are case reports of the use of thrombolytics, but the utility of this strategy is limited by the ability to make an accurate diagnosis of cord infarction within a suitable time window. There are no data to support the use of corticosteroids for spinal cord infarction, but this may be considered in cases where concern exists for an inflammatory myelopathy. Beyond the acute period, management consists of early bed rest and reversal of proximate causes such as hypovolemia or arrhythmias. Physical and occupational therapy are useful in promoting functional recovery.

Patients with cervical or high thoracic lesions should be monitored in an intensive care setting for potential life-threatening complications. These patients are at risk for developing autonomic dysreflexia or neurogenic shock including fluctuating blood pressures, pulmonary edema, and bradycardia. Blood pressure may require augmentation to avoid further extension of the cord infarction. High cervical lesions may also result in diaphragmatic and respiratory failure. Patients should be carefully monitored for pressure sores and given prophylaxis to avoid gastrointestinal ulceration and deep venous thrombosis. Many patients will also require urinary catheterization, which has the potential to lead to infection complications. Intermittent catheterization should be substituted for indwelling catheterization as early as possible.

## SPINAL ARTERIOVENOUS MALFORMATIONS

Spinal arteriovenous malformations (AVMs) are developmental or acquired abnormal direct communication of normal-sized to enlarged radiculomedullary arteries with enlarged tortuous radiculomedullary veins, without an intervening capillary network. Multiple classification schemes have been proposed for spinal AVM. A commonly accepted classification system (Anson and Spetzler, 1993) categorizes spinal AVM into four types (Box 69.2). Spinal vascular malformations not included in this radiological-pathological classification system include cavernous malformations, developmental venous anomalies (venous angiomas), telangiectasias, and epidural and paraspinal AVMs. Complex spinal cord vascular malformations such as metameric angiomatosis (Cobb syndrome) and disseminated angiodysplasia (Osler-Rendu-Weber syndrome) are also not included in this classification.

### Distribution and Prevalence

Spinal AVMs are rare and, consequently, do not have substantial epidemiological data. Dural arteriovenous fistula (AVF), the most common variety accounting for 80% of all spinal vascular malformations, has been reported to occur in five patients per million. The actual frequency of malformations could be higher because patients with small asymptomatic or misdiagnosed lesions may have been overlooked.

Spinal dural AVFs are identified most frequently between ages 30 and 70 (although classically reported in the 60s), and there is a 9:1 male predominance. Type II or IV malformations tend to occur in young adulthood. Type III malformations occur in childhood and typically have multiple feeding vessels that may extend into the vertebral bodies or paraspinal muscles (Fig 69.5). The predominant locations for these vascular malformations are the lower thoracic and lumbar spine regions. Spinal dural AVF usually drain to the dorsal surface of the cord and extend into the dural sleeve of the spinal nerve as it courses into the intervertebral foramen.

### Clinical Presentation and Course

Spinal vascular malformations, especially dural AVFs, are frequently misdiagnosed. The onset of symptoms can be acute or insidious, and the course may include remissions and relapses. The most common complaints at onset are pain, weakness, and sensory symptoms referable to the lower thoracic and lumbar regions. Later, bowel and bladder complaints may evolve. Triggering factors include trauma, exercise, pregnancy, or menstruation. Nonetheless, the interval between symptom onset and accurate diagnosis may be years. Severe locomotor

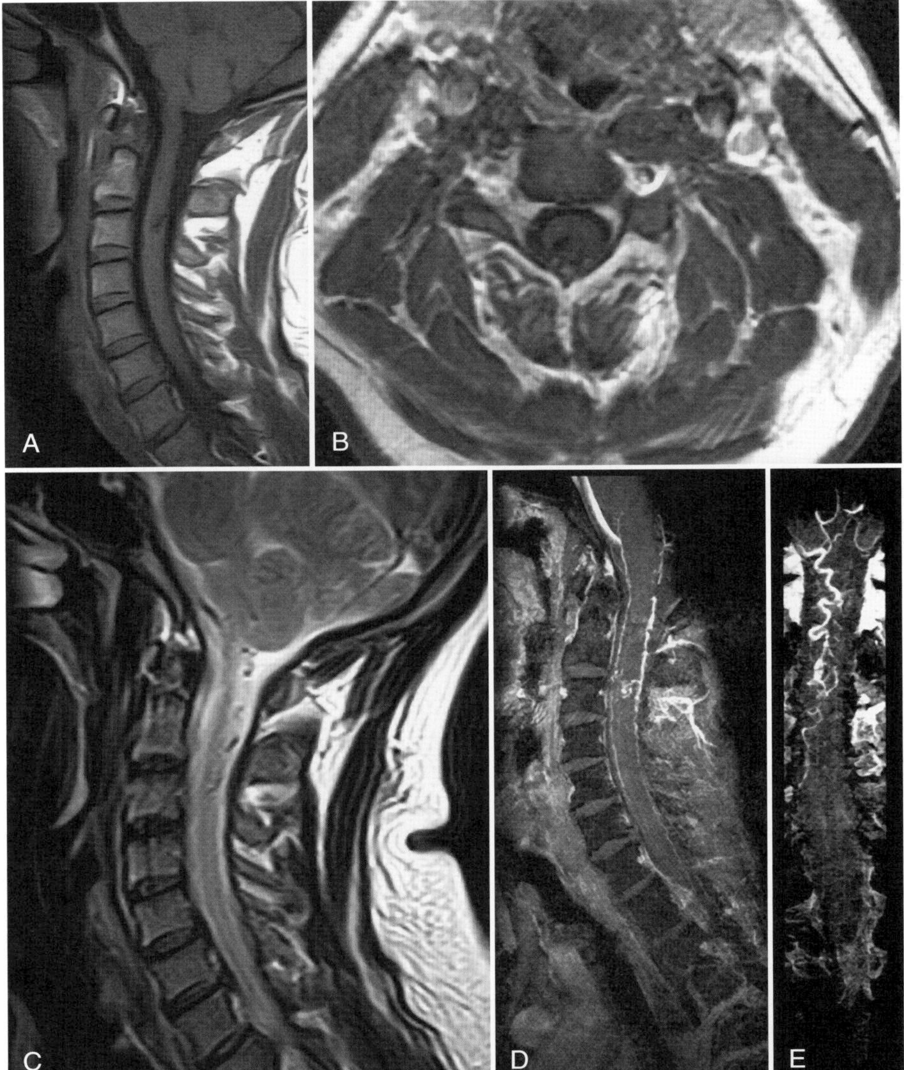


**Fig. 69.5 Magnetic Resonance Imaging and Contrast-Enhanced Three-Dimensional Magnetic Resonance Angiography (3D Mra) of a Cervical Intramedullary Glomus-Type Arteriovenous Malformation.** **A,** Precontrast T1-weighted sagittal image shows a focal hypointense intramedullary lesion at C3. The cord is not enlarged. **B,** Postcontrast T1-weighted axial image confirms the intramedullary location of the lesion. **C,** T2-weighted, fast spin-echo sagittal image shows serpentine flow voids posterior to the cervical cord from C1 to C3. Sagittal **(D)** and coronal **(E)** targeted magnetic resonance angiograms demonstrate the intramedullary nidus communicating with an enlarged posterior median vein. *(From Bowen, B.C., Saraf-Lavi, E., 2005. Magnetic resonance imaging and magnetic resonance angiography of spinal vascular lesions. In: Latchaw, R.E., Kucharczyk, J., Moseley, M.E. (Eds.), Imaging of the Nervous System: Diagnostic and Therapeutic Applications, vol. 2. Mosby, Philadelphia, pp. 1707–1722, with permission.)*

disability develops in approximately 20% by 6 months after onset of symptoms and in 50% by 3 years. Once leg weakness or gait difficulties emerge, they tend to progress rapidly.

The signs and symptoms of spinal vascular malformations are attributable to mass effect and ischemia. It is unusual for an unruptured spinal AVM to produce sufficient mass effect to cause spinal cord dysfunction. However, epidural, subdural, or intramedullary hemorrhage can arise from the malformation and produce spinal cord compression. Dural AVFs rarely produce hemorrhage and typically present as a slowly progressive myelopathy, which has been attributed to venous hypertension and intramedullary venous congestion that eventually can progress to infarction.

Pain may be local, radicular, diffuse, or any combination of these. Upper motor neuron weakness, lower motor neuron weakness, or both may occur. A spinal bruit is a highly specific (although uncommon) finding that is diagnostic of a spinal AVM. Exercise or Valsalva maneuver may exacerbate the symptoms by leading to an increase in venous congestion. Vascular malformations in the skin or paraspinal muscles are sometimes noted in conjunction with spinal AVMs. In cutaneomeningospinal angiomatosis (Cobb syndrome), a cutaneous angioma appears in the dermatome corresponding to the AVM's spinal segment. Foix-Alajouanine syndrome (see "Causes of Spinal Cord Infarction" earlier in this chapter) has been associated with end-stage dural AVF with thrombosis and venous infarction.

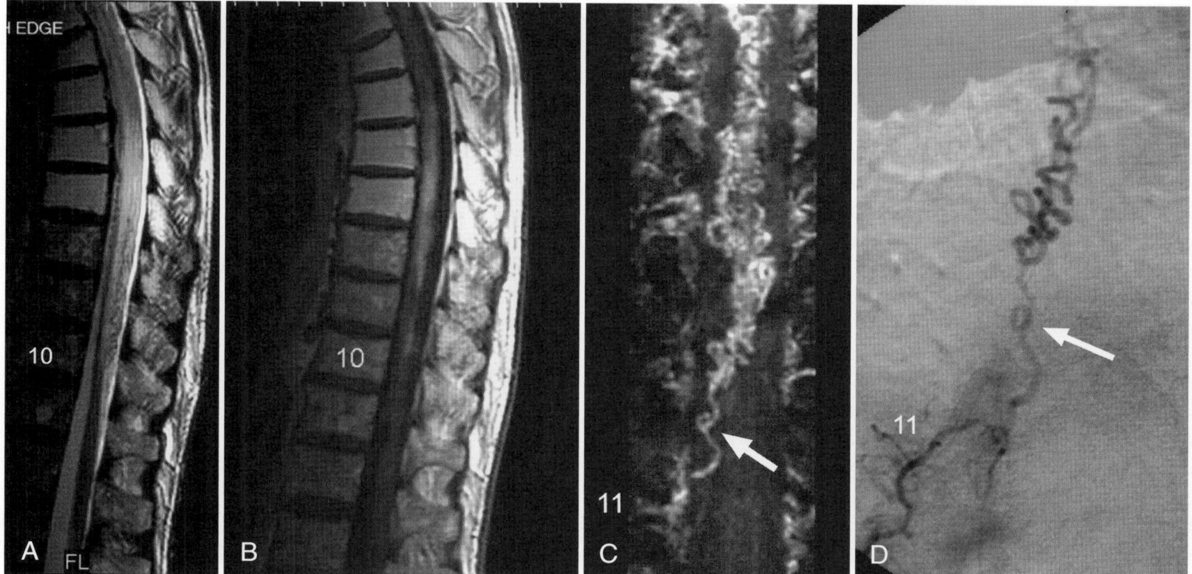


**Fig. 69.6 Magnetic Resonance Imaging (MRI) and Contrast-Enhanced Three-Dimensional Magnetic Resonance Angiography (3D Mra) of a Right T11 Dural Arteriovenous Fistula.** At the time of the MRI, this 68-year-old man had a 3-year history of progressive myelopathy. His symptoms began approximately 6 months after radiotherapy and surgical excision of a carcinoma of the right lung apex. His progressive neurological deficits were initially attributed to radiation myelitis of the upper thoracic cord. After surgical obliteration of the fistula, his symptoms improved. **A,** Fast spin-echo T2-weighted image shows hyperintense cord from T6 to T10 and serpentine flow voids, consistent with enlarged intradural vessels, posterior to the cord from T8 to T10. **B,** Postcontrast T1-weighted image shows hyperintense vertebral bodies from T4 to T7, as seen in **A** and consistent with radiation changes. There is patchy enhancement within the cord from T6 to T10. **C,** MRA (targeted to posterior half of the spinal canal) demonstrates an enlarged tortuous vessel *(arrow)* extending from the right T11 foramen to the posterior cord surface, where numerous convoluted vessels are seen. The right T11 vessel corresponds to the posterior medullary vein draining the fistula. **D,** Digital subtraction (catheter) angiogram (anteroposterior view) following injection of the right T11 posterior intercostal artery demonstrates a fistula in the region of the right neural foramen, with drainage into the canal via the medullary vein *(arrow)*. *(From Bowen, B.C., Pattany, P.M., 1999. Vascular anatomy and disorders of the lumbar spine and spinal cord. In: Ross, J. (Ed.), The Lumbar Spine. Magnetic Resonance Imaging Clinics of North America. Saunders, Philadelphia, pp. 555–571, with permission.)*

In some patients, the onset of symptoms is abrupt and may represent spinal hemorrhage. This is more commonly seen with type II malformations. Spinal hemorrhage usually has an abrupt onset and may be associated with the typical symptoms of subarachnoid hemorrhage (SAH), including headache, meningeal infection, and cord and nerve root damage.

Vascular malformations (AVMs and dural AVFs) may cause increased local venous pressure, decreased perfusion pressure, decreased tissue perfusion, and finally tissue ischemia. This explains the coexistence of deficits in more than a single arterial territory and the symptomatic improvement that results from ligation of feeding vessels. The sometimes confusing and widely varied presentation of spinal vascular malformations results in a large differential diagnosis that includes neoplasms, herniated disks, multiple sclerosis, intracranial SAH, subacute combined degeneration, meningovascular syphilis, and transverse myelitis (see Chapter 27).

## Investigations

MRI with and without MRA is the initial diagnostic test of choice. The definitive radiological procedure in the pretreatment evaluation of vascular malformations is selective spinal catheter digital subtraction angiography (DSA). Selective spinal angiography is tedious and typically requires injection of each segmental artery in the region being examined. DSA may be augmented by newer technologies such as flat-detector CT angiography (FD-CTA) or flat-panel catheter angiotomography (FPCA) that allow generation of multiplanar as well as three-dimensional (3D) images that accurately demonstrate the malformation and help treatment planning in addition to shortening the duration of the angiographic procedures. In cases of a single feeding vessel, the diagnosis is more straightforward. Type II and III malformations tend to have more complex vascular anatomy that can be more difficult to fully assess.

The characteristic MRI features of dural AVF (Fig. 69.6) are cord edema and dilated perimedullary vessels. T2-weighted images typically demonstrate swelling and increased cord signal that extends several segments due to venous hypertension. Abnormal T2 signal may be limited to the central "H-shaped" gray matter. A hypointense rim surrounding the cord on a T2-weighted sequence can be seen in some cases due to deoxygenated blood within the congested capillaries. Enhancement of the swelled cord is frequent and is due to venous engorgement. Prominent perimedullary vessels are best seen on sagittal T2-weighted images as serpiginous flow voids in the thecal sac posterior to the cord. If the AV shunting is very small, perimedullary vessels may not be visualized on any sequence or only on postcontrast images. If the AVM is not treated, the cord becomes atrophic with time.

Although the type of AVM cannot be differentiated, MRI can localize the AVM in relation to the spinal cord and dura and can distinguish high-flow versus low-flow AVM. The typical imaging appearance of spinal cord AVMs are conglomerate perimedullary or intramedullary blood vessels that appear as flow voids on T2-weighted sequences. Appearances of the vessels on T1-weighted sequences are variable and depend upon the velocity and direction of flow. Swelling of the cord with associated intramedullary T2 hyperintensity can also be seen as a result of venous hypertension. Contrast enhancement is also variable. Intramedullary hemorrhage can also occur that can further complicate the imaging appearance secondary to presence of blood products of different ages. SAH has also been described with spinal cord AVM.

Different MRA techniques have been used to diagnose and localize AV shunts. Although 2D and 3D phase contrast MRA was used initially, contrast-enhanced MRA techniques are more commonly used nowadays. Time-resolved contrast-enhanced MRA (TRCE-MRA) is a new technique that has better spatial resolution than older MRA techniques. In addition, TRCE-MRA provides dynamic information similar to that of DSA. Localization of the AVM with MRA can reduce duration, cost, morbidity, and mortality associated with spinal DSA. DSA remains the "gold standard" for evaluation of spinal dural AVF and can be complemented with FD-CTA and FPCA.

### Treatment

The treatment of spinal vascular malformations is by surgical resection and/or angiographically directed embolization of the malformation. Surgical approaches tend to have better rates of obliteration of the fistula, although some authors advocate attempting a less-invasive endovascular approach first. Endovascular approaches promote thrombosis and decrease blood flow through iatrogenic embolization but have the potential to cause additional infarction if the embolic material migrates. As the complexity of the malformation increases, the likelihood of achieving full obliteration of the lesion decreases and complications may occur more frequently. A sequential approach of embolization, followed by definitive surgical therapy, is common. Radioablation is also being explored for some lesions.

## SPINAL CAVERNOUS MALFORMATIONS

Spinal cavernous malformations (SCMs) are slow-flowing vascular malformations without arteriovenous shunting. Their exact frequency is not known, although they are estimated to represent 5% of spinal vascular malformations. SCMs preferentially affect women and may be seen in conjunction with intracranial cavernous malformations. They can be sporadic or familial. Multiple genetic mutations have been linked to SCM. Trauma and prior radiation are also associated with the development of SCMs. Typically, an SCM is an intramedullary lesion and can involve any segment of the spinal cord including the conus medullaris. SCMs are pathologically identical to intracranial cavernous malformations. Most commonly they are well-circumscribed lesions surrounded by hemosiderin-stained gliotic tissue. Constant presence of blood products suggests recurrent low-grade hemorrhage or episodic diapedesis into the lesion.

Clinical presentation of an SCM depends upon the size and location. Smaller SCMs can be asymptomatic. The usual age at presentation is in the fourth decade. Discrete episodic neurological deficit with variable recovery between episodes is the typical presentation. Acute presentation is typically due to hemorrhage within the lesion. Back pain frequently accompanies neurological symptoms. Gradual enlargement of the lesions can result in progressive myelopathy.

Characteristic MRI findings include heterogeneous (both high and low) signal intensity within the lesion on both T1- and T2-weighted sequences, resulting in a "popcorn"-like appearance surrounded by a hypointense rim on T2-weighted sequences. On a gradient echo sequence, the lesions demonstrate profound hypointensity due to blood products. Enhancement is not a typical feature. If the characteristic imaging findings are seen on MRI, angiographic evaluation is not necessary.

Management depends upon symptoms and the patient's age. No treatment is required for asymptomatic lesions. In symptomatic patients, surgical exploration and resection is the standard of care.

## SPINAL HEMORRHAGE

Subarachnoid, intramedullary, subdural, and epidural hemorrhage may affect the spine. The onset is usually sudden and painful and most commonly is related to trauma or vascular malformations.

### Subarachnoid Hemorrhage

Spinal SAH accounts for less than 1% of all SAHs. The most common cause is a spinal angioma, but these account for only approximately 10% of the total. Other associated conditions include trauma, coarctation of the aorta, rupture of a spinal artery, mycotic and other aneurysms of the spinal arteries, polyarteritis nodosa, spinal tumors, iatrogenic (lumbar puncture), blood dyscrasias, and therapeutic thrombolytics, and anticoagulants.

Clinical presentation of spinal SAH is characterized by the sudden onset of severe back pain, which localizes near the level of the hemorrhage. The pain typically becomes diffuse, and signs of meningeal irritation become prominent within minutes. Multiple radiculopathies and myelopathy may be present. Headache, cranial neuropathies, and a decreased level of consciousness are associated with diffusion of blood above the foramen magnum. The CSF is grossly bloody, and intracranial pressure is frequently elevated. Papilledema may be present.

Correct diagnosis requires a strong clinical suspicion. The evaluation of spinal SAH frequently follows negative radiological studies of the intracranial structures. History may reveal the initial severe back pain, traumatic injury, or prior anticoagulant use. Physical examination may reveal a spinal bruit, cutaneous angioma, sensory level, the stigmata of collagen vascular disease, or evidence suggesting septicemia. Radiological studies are discussed under "Spinal Arteriovenous Malformations" (see earlier discussion). Treatment is directed toward the underlying cause.

### Hematomyelia

Hematomyelia is intramedullary spinal hemorrhage that most often results from trauma. It may follow direct trauma to the spinal column or hyperextension injuries of the cervical spine. Spontaneous hematomyelia most often results from bleeding of a spinal vascular malformation, hemorrhage into a spinal tumor or syrinx, a bleeding diathesis, anticoagulant drug use, or venous infarction. The hemorrhage tends to disrupt spinal gray matter more than white matter. There are no recognized intraspinal counterparts to intracerebral hypertensive hemorrhage or amyloid angiopathy. Hematomyelia most commonly presents as spinal shock associated with the sudden onset of severe back pain, which is often radicular. Later, spasticity develops below the level of the lesion, with lower motor neuron signs occurring in the myotomes corresponding to the lesion.

MRI is the best imaging modality to detect intramedullary hemorrhage. CSF findings may be consistent with SAH. The initial treatment is supportive. Laminectomy and drainage of the hematoma, followed by resection of the tumor or vascular malformation, can be performed if neurological deficits are incomplete or progressive.

### Spinal Epidural and Subdural Hemorrhage

Spinal epidural hemorrhage (SEH) occurs more frequently than spinal subdural hemorrhage (SSH). SEH is more commonly observed in men and has a bimodal distribution, with peaks during childhood and the fifth and sixth decades of life. Cervical lesions are more common in childhood, whereas thoracic and lumbar lesions predominate in adults. Hemorrhages can be spontaneous but often occur following exertion or trauma. SEH is a complication of both lumbar puncture and epidural anesthesia and is more likely in anticoagulated patients. Other causes include blood dyscrasia, thrombocytopenia, neoplasms, trauma, and vascular malformations. Pregnancy also appears to increase risk for SEH.

SSH is most common in women. It may occur at any age but tends to predominate in the sixth decade. Most occur in the thoracic and lumbar regions. Hemorrhagic diatheses, including treatment with anticoagulants, blood dyscrasias, and thrombocytopenia, are the precipitating factors most commonly associated with SSH. Other factors include trauma, lumbar puncture, vascular malformation, and spinal surgery.

The clinical presentations of SEH and SSH are indistinguishable. The initial symptom is severe back pain at the level of the bleed. Myelopathy or cauda equina syndrome, with motor and sensory findings corresponding to the level of the lesion, develops over hours to days. The diagnosis should be suspected in patients with disorders of coagulation who have undergone recent lumbar puncture and develop back pain or signs of spinal cord or root dysfunction. Patients with a rapidly decreasing platelet count or less than 40,000 platelets/μL are at particular risk of developing SEH or SSH as a complication of lumbar puncture and should receive a platelet transfusion prior to the procedure. Clotting studies and a platelet count are important in the initial evaluation. In SEH and SSH, the CSF may be normal or xanthochromic and may contain increased protein.

MRI can delineate the size and location of the hematoma. In addition, gadolinium-enhanced MRI and MRA may show an underlying vascular malformation. In patients unable to tolerate MRI or where it is unavailable in the acute phase of the illness, myelography with computed tomography (CT) scanning provides an alternative. Myelography can reveal a partial filling defect or complete blockage to the flow of contrast material at the level of the lesion. However, the myelographic appearances of SEH and SSH may be indistinguishable.

Both SEH and SSH are surgical emergencies. Operative treatment is directed toward relief of local pressure and repair of any underlying defect. Laminectomy with evacuation of the clot should be performed as soon as possible to minimize the risk of permanent neurological dysfunction. The prognosis for recovery is better when the preoperative deficits are not severe; timing of surgery appears less important.

*The complete reference list is available online at https://expertconsult.inkling.com/.*

70

# Central Nervous System Vasculitis

*Olivia Groover, Fadi Nahab*

## OUTLINE



Central nervous system vasculitis (CNSV), alternatively termed primary angiitis of the central nervous system (PACNS) or granulomatous angiitis of the central nervous system, is a rare diagnosis with an estimated incidence rate of 2.4 cases per 1 million person years (Salvarani et al., 2007). The diagnosis can be challenging given the nonspecific presenting signs of headache, encephalopathy, and variable focal neurological signs. Here we outline some of the typical features and methods of distinguishing CNSV from mimics to create a framework for improving the diagnosis of this often discussed but rare disease.

## FEATURES AND DIAGNOSIS

### Clinical Features

Clinical symptoms are often nonspecific, can include headache (50%–60%), progressive cognitive difficulties (50%–70%), confusion, personality changes, and vision loss, and vary depending on the central nervous system (CNS) region affected. Ischemic strokes, intracranial hemorrhage, and subarachnoid hemorrhage can be seen but are less common than the aforementioned symptoms. Although fever, weight loss, rash, night sweats, arthritis, and peripheral neuropathy have been reported in a minority of patients with CNSV, systemic features should prompt a workup to rule out secondary vasculitis due to systemic cause (Limaye, 2018). The Calabrese diagnostic criteria include the presence of unexplained neurological deficits with evidence of either classic angiographic or histopathological features of angiitis within the CNS and no evidence of a systemic vasculitis or any other condition that could elicit the angiographic or pathological features (Calabrese and Hajj-Ali, 2013).

### Pathology

Features on histology have been subcategorized into granulomatous lymphocytic and necrotizing vasculitis (Salvarani et al., 2007; Limaye, 2018). Amyloid beta–related angiitis (ABRA) shares clinical and physiological characteristics but represents a separate disease entity (Salvarani et al., 2013).

Brain biopsy remains the "gold standard" of diagnosis for CNSV and is recommended to confirm diagnosis given the ongoing commitment for immunosuppressive therapy and potential side effects. Biopsy may also be helpful in making an alternate diagnosis (Miller et al., 2006).

### Laboratory

There are no specific laboratory data that can confirm CNSV. However, cerebrospinal fluid (CSF) analysis is helpful in differentiating noninflammatory vasculopathies from inflammatory vasculitides in cases where imaging shows findings concerning for vasculitis (Limaye, 2018). In a study of 101 patients with biopsy-proven CNSV, 96% had abnormal CSF showing either elevated protein or lymphocytic pleocytosis (Salvarani et al., 2007). Hence a normal CSF analysis effectively rules out CNSV. CSF analysis also assists with diagnosis of CNSV mimics, including infections such as neurosyphilis and varicella zoster (Bhattacharyya and Berkowitz, 2016).

### Imaging

#### Magnetic Resonance Imaging

Magnetic resonance imaging (MRI) of the brain is abnormal in more than 90% of cases (Birnbaum and Hellmann, 2009; Pipitone et al., 2008), making an alternate diagnosis more likely in the setting of a normal MRI. Diffusion-weighted imaging (DWI) sequences to identify recent ischemic lesions, fluid-attenuated inversion recovery (FLAIR) to establish chronicity, and precontrast and postcontrast T1 and T2 sequences are recommended to identify inflammatory lesions. The use of 3T MRI with T1 sequence after gadolinium administration in CNSV can also identify cerebral arterial wall enhancement, not seen in noninflammatory mimics. MR angiography (MRA) may identify abnormalities in large vessels found in CNSV mimics but has limited sensitivity to detect abnormalities in small vessels.

#### Computed Tomography

Although a computed tomography (CT) of the brain is less sensitive than MRI for detection of ischemic lesions in CNSV, CT angiography (CTA) may show abnormalities of sequential dilation and stenosis as seen in vasculitis. Because CTA has limited ability to show abnormalities of small vessels, it may be used as a screening test to identify large-vessel involvement prior to performing conventional angiography (Limaye, 2018).

### Digital Subtraction Angiography

Cerebral angiography may show the classical multifocal pattern of narrowing and dilatation referred to as "beads on a string"; however, this

TABLE 70.1 **Clinical Characteristics and Diagnostic Evaluation of Disorders That Mimic Primary Central Nervous System Vasculitis**

| Disease | Clinical Features | Diagnostic Testing | Diagnostic Results |
|---|---|---|---|
| Reversible cerebral vasoconstriction syndrome | Thunderclap headache, associated with vasoactive drugs including marijuana, amphetamines, and SSRIs. May occur during postpartum period | LP, MRA, CTA, or cerebral angiography | Spinal fluid has no pleiocytosis and normal protein level. Cerebral angiography may show normalization of artery spasm with intraarterial vasodilator |
| Intracranial atherosclerosis | Presence of risk factors including hypertension, diabetes, hyperlipidemia. More common in non-White race | MRA, CTA, testing for hyperlipidemia, diabetes | Larger intracranial vessels normally affected, atherosclerotic calcification can be seen on CTA |
| Radiation vasculopathy | History of radiation to the head | MRA, CTA, or angiography | Atherosclerotic stenosis advanced for age |
| Intravascular lymphoma | Systemic symptoms including skin involvement common, progressive dementia or focal signs | LP, brain biopsy required for definitive diagnosis, LDH | LP may show elevated protein with normal cell count, cytology normal, biopsy with malignant lymphoid cells |
| Amyloid beta–related angiitis (ABRA) | Possible cognitive impairment | LP, cerebral angiography, biopsy | LP with elevated protein, angiography typically normal, biopsy shows extensive amyloid B in vessel walls |
| Systemic vasculitis | Renal dysfunction, abdominal pain, pulmonary hemorrhage | Erythrocyte sedimentation rate (ESR), C-reactive protein (CRP), anti-nuclear antibodies (ANA), anti-neutrophil cytoplasmic antibodies (ANCA), cryoglobulins, hepatitis serology | Elevated ESR or CRP. Positive ANA or ANCA antibodies. Cryoglobulin may be present. Positive hepatitis serologies may be present |
| Varicella zoster vasculitis | May have history of shingles | LP | Positive CSF VZV PCR or elevated ratio of CSF:serum VZV IgG |
| Meningovascular syphilis | Evidence of tertiary syphilis, including tabes dorsalis | Treponemal antibody, LP | Positive serum treponemal antibody with inflammatory CSF and VDRL positive |
| Susac syndrome | Encephalopathy, branch retinal artery occlusion and hearing loss | MRI brain, retinal fluorescein angiography, audiogram, LP | Contrast-enhancing multifocal T2 hyperintensities on MRI during attacks typically involving corpus callosum, retinal fluorescein angiography with distal branch retinal artery occlusions, audiogram with sensorineural hearing loss, LP with elevated protein and mild pleiocytosis |

*ANA,* Anti-nuclear antibody; ANCA, Anti-neutrophil cytoplasmic antibody; CRP, C-reactive protein; *CSF,* Cerebrospinal fluid; *CTA,* CT angiography; *ESR,* Erythrocyte sedimentation rate; *LDH,* Lactate dehydrogenase; *LP,* Lumbar puncture; *MRA,* MR angiography; *MRI,* magnetic resonance imaging; *PCR,* polymerase chain reaction; *SSRI,* Selective serotonin reuptake inhibitor; *VDRL,* Venereal disease research laboratory; *VZV,* varicella-zoster virus.

pattern can be seen in mimics as well. In biopsy-proven CNSV, cerebral angiography had variable performance with abnormalities seen in 33%–87% of cases (Salvarani Medicine, 2015; de-Boysson H Arthritis Rheumatol, 2014).

## TREATMENT

There are no large prospective clinical trials to help guide treatment. However, high-dose glucocorticoids are widely accepted as the first-line treatment of choice. For biopsy-proven cases, cyclophosphamide may be used to achieve remission, after which transition to a steroid-sparing agent such as methotrexate, azathioprine, or mycophenolate is desirable. Newer agents such as rituximab or etanercept have also been used with some benefit (Salvarani 2013; Bhattacharyya and Berkowitz, 2016).

## MIMICS

Because of the significant difficulty in diagnosing CNSV, a knowledge of conditions which may masquerade as CNSV is important to successfully distinguish it from other conditions and avoid misdiagnosis, including unnecessary exposure to immunosuppressive therapy. Table 70.1 provides a list of mimics and differentiating features.

## CONCLUSIONS

Despite the challenges in diagnosing CNSV, a methodical and detailed approach can improve the accuracy of diagnosis.

*The complete reference list is available online at https://expertconsult.inkling.com/.* 

71

# Epidemiology of Brain Tumors

*Dominique S. Michaud*

## OUTLINE



Primary brain tumors are a diverse group of neoplasms arising from different cells of the central nervous system (CNS), including neuroepithelial tissue, the meninges, and cranial and spinal nerves. Within each of these cell types, tumors can exhibit distinct pathological characteristics, biological behavior, and clinical outcomes, leading to the complex classification of more than 100 different subtypes of brain tumors (Louis et al., 2007). Tumors originating from glial cells, known collectively as gliomas, are the most common malignant primary brain tumors (81%) and constitute 26% of all brain and CNS tumors; these tumors arise from astrocytes (astrocytomas), oligodendrocytes (oligodendrogliomas), or ependymal cells (ependymomas). Glioblastomas, the most aggressive type of brain tumors, account for approximately half of gliomas (47.7%), and astrocytomas (which includes glioblastomas) account for approximately three-quarters of all gliomas (75%; Ostrom et al., 2018). Meningiomas, which arise in the meninges, are also common brain tumors (37%), but unlike gliomas, more than 98% demonstrate nonmalignant behavior (Ostrom et al., 2018). In children (0–14 years), the most common brain tumors include pilocytic astrocytomas (17.5%), embryonal tumors (15.7%), and malignant gliomas (25.7%).

The etiology of brain tumors remains unknown despite substantial research conducted to identify the causes of brain tumors. Brain tumors are associated with a unique set of challenges for observational study designs (Box 71.1), hindering advances in identifying risk factors associated with this disease.

## CLASSIFICATION

The different cellular origins and behavioral characteristics of brain tumors contribute to the difficulty in achieving a single, widely accepted classification system. Historical attempts at developing a classification system for brain tumors date back to the 1830s. The most widely accepted classification for primary CNS tumors is the World Health Organization (WHO) system, developed in 1979 and subsequently revised in 1993, 2000, and 2007 (Kleihues et al., 2000; Louis et al., 2007). In this system, all CNS tumors are assigned different grades (I–IV) representing an estimate of malignancy. Molecular subclassification of specific primary CNS tumors has become routine in clinical practice, when feasible, as prognosis and clinical care are often driven by genetic characteristics. Future epidemiological studies will likely focus on specific molecular subtypes of brain tumors. Chapter 72 contains a comprehensive discussion of brain tumor classification.

## DESCRIPTIVE EPIDEMIOLOGY

### Incidence

The traditional source of descriptive data on brain tumors has been the Surveillance, Epidemiology, and End Results (SEER) program sponsored by the National Cancer Institute (NCI). The SEER 18 areas collect population-based cancer data on approximately 28%

## BOX 71.1 Challenges in Brain Tumor Epidemiology Studies

Uncommon form of cancer
Diversity of brain tumor types
Changing methods of ascertainment (clinical, radiography, histology, molecular characteristics)
Variable reliability of exposure assessment (cognitive impairment of subjects, remote exposures)

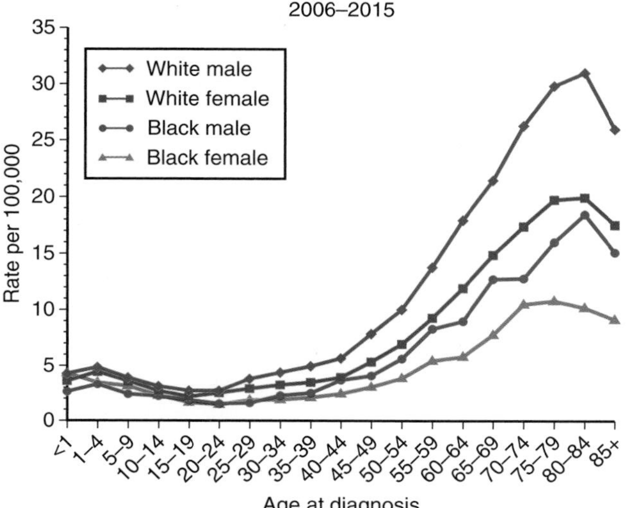


**Fig. 71.1** US age-specific incidence rates for malignant brain cancer and other nervous system cancer for 2006–2015, by race and sex. *(From Surveillance, Epidemiology, and End Results [SEER] 18 areas;*http://www.seer.cancer.gov)

of the US population to gauge national trends in cancer incidence and survival (National Cancer Institute, 2019). Until recently these data encompassed only malignant tumors; however, effective January 2004, all cancer surveillance registries are required to expand their primary brain tumor data collection to include tumors of benign or uncertain behavior (Benign Brain Tumor Cancer Registries Amendment Act; Public Law 107–260). The Central Brain Tumor Registry of the United States (CBTRUS) established in 1992 is the nation's largest population-based registry of primary brain and CNS tumors, compiling information from 50 population-based state cancer registries (Ostrom et al., 2018).

Incidence estimates differ according to the inclusion or exclusion of nonmalignant brain tumors. The American Cancer Society estimated the diagnosis of approximately 23,820 new cases of malignant primary CNS tumors in the United States in 2019 (American Cancer Society, 2019). For 2019, CBTRUS estimated approximately 26,170 new cases of malignant and 60,800 nonmalignant primary CNS tumors in the United States; approximately 5270 of these cases will be diagnosed in children (Ostrom et al., 2018). The annual incidence rate for malignant brain cancer for all races from 2011 to 2015 was 9 per 100,000 person-years in older adults (40+ years old) (Ostrom et al., 2018). The incidence of childhood primary malignant and nonmalignant brain and CNS tumors is 5.9 cases per 100,000 person-years (Ostrom et al., 2018; Fig. 71.1).

## Mortality and Prognostic Factors

Although primary malignant brain tumors account for only 2% of all cancers and are one-fifth as common as breast or lung cancer, they contribute to substantial morbidity, and prognosis is poor. The 5-year survival rate for primary malignant brain tumors (35% between 2008 and 2014) is the sixth lowest among all types of cancer (following pancreas, liver, lung, esophagus, and stomach, respectively) despite having increased over the past 30 years (from 23%; American Cancer Society, 2019). The 5-year survival rates vary substantially by histological subtypes: 81.6% for oligodendroglioma, 30% for anaplastic astrocytoma, and 5.6% for glioblastoma (Ostrom et al., 2018). Malignant CNS tumors will account for approximately 17,760 deaths in 2019 (American Cancer Society, 2019). Age-specific incidence rates from brain tumors among all races demonstrate gradual increases with each decade until age 55, after which the rate increases dramatically (see Fig. 71.1).

Young age and lower pathological grade are favorable prognostic factors for primary brain tumors (Ostrom et al., 2018). Less significant predictors of favorable prognosis include long duration of symptoms, absence of mental changes at the time of diagnosis, cerebellar location of the tumor, small preoperative tumor size, and completeness of surgical resection.

## Gender and Race

A slight male predominance exists in the incidence of malignant CNS tumors (7.5 per 100,000 person-years for men versus 5.4 per 100,000 person-years for women in 2010) (Ostrom et al., 2018). However, when assessing nonmalignant and malignant CNS tumor types together, the incidence rate in men is lower than in women (20.6 per 100,000 person-years for men versus 25.3 per 100,000 person-years for women; Ostrom et al., 2018). A partial explanation of this sex disparity is the predominance of meningiomas in women (11.5 per 100,000 person-years) compared with men (5.3 per 100,000 person-years; Ostrom et al., 2018).

Fig. 71.1 compares the age-adjusted incidence rates of malignant brain tumors among Whites and Blacks and by male and female. Compared with Blacks, Whites have a higher incidence of malignant brain tumors for both sexes; white males have an incidence rate of 8.5 per 100,000 person-years compared with black males at 4.8 per 100,000 person-years, whereas white females have an annual incidence rate of 6.0 per 100,000 person-years versus an annual incidence rate of 3.6 per 100,000 person-years among black females (Howlader et al., 2013). Mortality among Whites is higher (4.8 per 100,000 persons; 2011–2015) than among Blacks (2.6 per 100,000 persons; 2011–2015) (Howlader et al., 2013), and 5-year relative survival is lower among Whites (32%) than Blacks (39.5%) (Howlader et al., 2013). Incidence and mortality rates of malignant brain tumors among Asian Americans and Native Americans are lower than for either white or black Americans (Howlader et al., 2013).

## Temporal Trends

Increases in US incidence rates for malignant brain cancers that were observed between 1975 and 1985 (Fig. 71.2) have been largely attributed to improved diagnostic technology, increased use of noninvasive diagnostics, and changes in classification of tumors. An increase in brain tumor incidence in the late 1980s correlated with the use of computed tomography (CT) in the 1970s and magnetic resonance imaging (MRI) in the 1980s. In addition, in a study using CBTRUS data, increases in the incidence of most glioma subgroups were mirrored by decreases in the incidence of "not otherwise specified" (NOS) subgroups, suggesting that changes in classification and coding of brain tumors were likely responsible for some of the temporal trends (Jukich et al., 2001). However, the same study identified increases in the incidence of ependymomas and nerve sheath tumors, which were less likely to be artifacts of improvements in diagnosis.

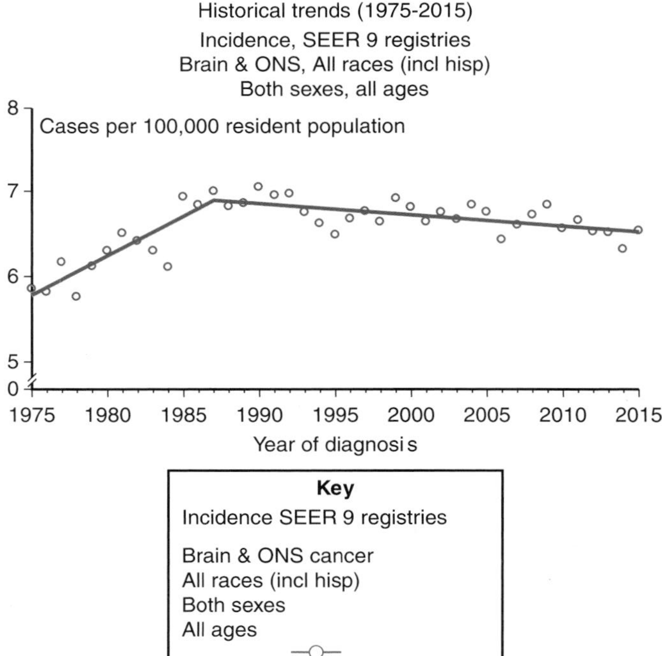


**Fig. 71.2** Age-adjusted incidence rates for invasive brain and other nervous system cancer in the United States between 1975 and 2015. Rates calculated using SEER* Stat. (*From* http://statecancerprofiles.cancer.gov). *ONS*, other nervous system cancer; *SEER*, surveillance, epidemiology, and end results.

Since 1987, age-adjusted incidence rates for malignant brain tumors decreased by 0.2% annually through 2015 (National Cancer Institute 2019; see Fig. 71.2); the decline occurred in both men and women and across different racial groups. A similar decline in incidence rates is observed with data representing all US states and territories (2008–2015; Ostrom et al. 2018).

## Geographical Trends and Migrant Studies

In general, brain cancer incidence is associated with level of economic development; concomitant differences in the availability of diagnostic technology (CT, MRI, neurosurgical technology), access to health care, and accuracy and completion rate of cancer diagnosis, and reporting, likely account for most of the observed disparities. However, variations in the incidence of primary malignant brain tumors within the United States are difficult to explain; Hawaii has the lowest rate (4.5 per 100,000 person-years), and Kentucky has the highest rate (8.18 per 100,000 person-years; Ostrom et al., 2018; Fig. 71.3).

In a study of Italians who migrated to Argentina, brain tumor mortality rates were lower among the migrants than in the country of origin (Roman, 1998). This suggests that environmental factors may influence the development of brain tumors. However, disparities in completeness of case ascertainment in the countries under study complicate the interpretation of this study.

## Primary Central Nervous System Lymphoma

The epidemiology of primary central nervous system lymphoma (PCNSL), a type of non-Hodgkin lymphoma, deserves special comment. A significant increase in the incidence of PCNSL occurred over the past few decades. This parallels a doubling of the incidence rate of systemic non-Hodgkin lymphoma over the past four decades. The incidence peaked in the early 1990s and subsequently declined. The primary factor behind the rising incidence is the acquired immunodeficiency syndrome (AIDS) epidemic. Two to six percent of individuals with AIDS develop PCNSL at some point in their disease course (Fine and Loeffler, 1999). The incidence of AIDS has decreased along with the rate of PCNSL since the beginning of the 1990s. However, AIDS does not fully account for the total increase in the incidence of PCNSL (Rubenstein et al., 2008). Recent studies suggest a continuing increased PCNSL incidence among non-AIDS populations (Haldorsen et al., 2007; Makino et al., 2006), particularly among men and women older than 65 years old (O'Neill et al., 2013).

# ANALYTICAL EPIDEMIOLOGY

## Study Designs

Analytical epidemiology involves identifying risk factors for particular diseases using the application of case-control or cohort study designs. The case-control study design has been the most commonly used in the search for brain tumor risk factors, due to low incidence rates. In a case-control study, the basis for subject classification is the presence (case) or absence (control) of the outcome of interest (e.g., brain tumor). An exposure of interest (e.g., head trauma) is then determined in a uniform manner for cases and controls. An odds ratio (OR) of disease for the exposed compared with the unexposed is generated. Case-control studies are most useful in the study of uncommon diseases (e.g., brain tumors) or those with a long period between the exposure of interest and the development of disease, but unfortunately, biases are common in these studies. In a cohort study, subject selection is from the population, and the presence or absence of an exposure is determined during recruitment when the subjects are free of disease. Participants are followed forward in time to ascertain the development of the outcome/disease of interest. Cohort studies are most useful when the outcome under study is common. Recent large cohort studies with long follow-up periods identified sufficient cases to examine lifestyle exposure in relation to brain tumor incidence.

## Methodological Challenges

Poor response rates in case-control studies can often lead to selection bias, and recall bias may be an especially important limitation in retrospective case-control studies of brain tumors. Individuals with brain tumors often have cognitive and language difficulties. Therefore reliable exposure assessments are difficult to achieve. To address this issue and to include patients who died of brain cancer before study recruitment, some case-control studies have used proxies (e.g., next of kin) to obtain information on the patient; unfortunately, this method is not accurate because proxies often misreport the patient's exposure. Another shortcoming of observational studies is the tendency to group all brain tumors together as one entity. Given brain tumor heterogeneity, this grouping may hide underlying associations unique to one subtype of tumor. Although exceptions exist, small effects and marked inconsistencies across studies characterize most exposures analyzed. This chapter provides a review of the major categories of exposure.

## Radiation

### Ionizing Radiation

Ionizing radiation exposure (e.g., radiation therapy or among atomic bomb survivors) is an established cause of certain types of brain tumors, especially meningiomas and nerve sheath tumors. The latency between irradiation and the development of brain tumors may be as short as 5 years but can also be many decades long. In a cohort study of 10,834 children treated with cranial radiation for tinea capitis in the 1950s (mean estimated radiation dose, 1.5 Gy), elevated risks were found for nerve sheath tumors (relative risk [RR] 18.8), meningiomas (RR 9.5), and malignant gliomas (RR 2.6; Ron et al., 1988).

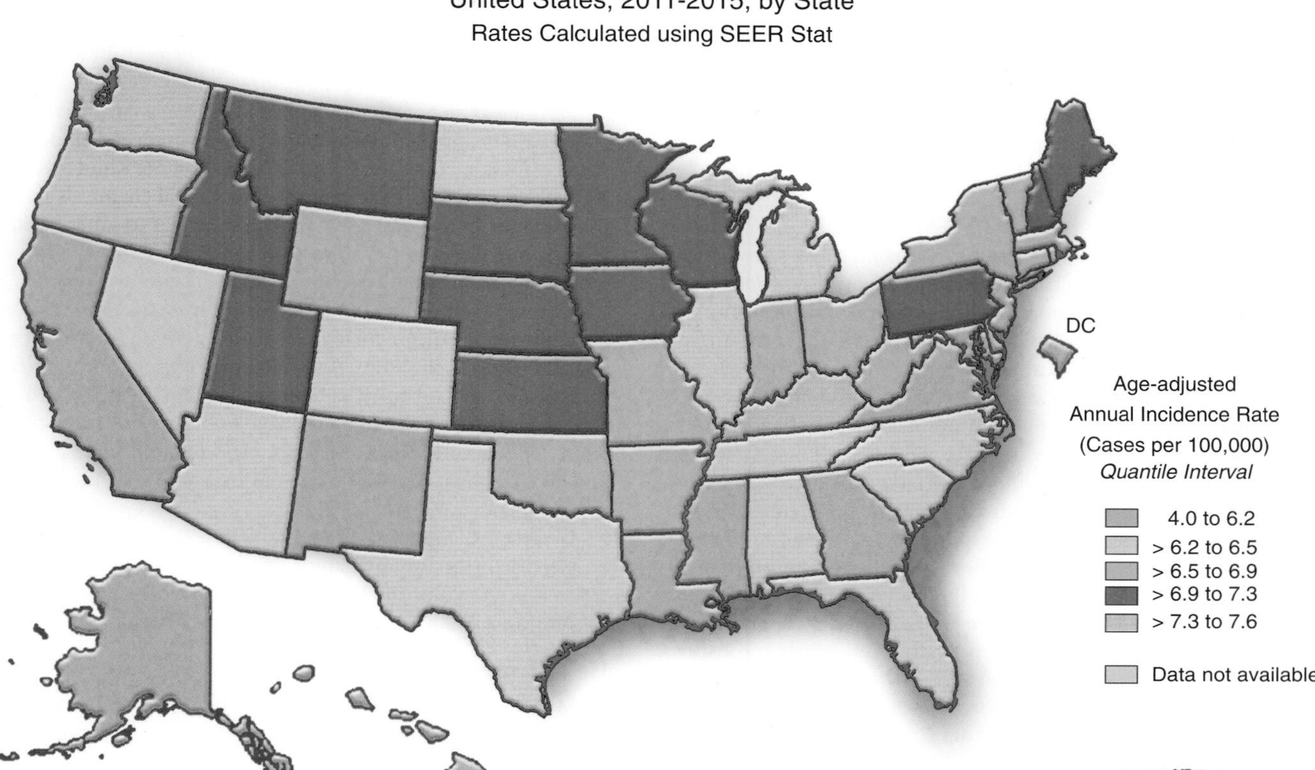


**Fig. 71.3** Age-adjusted incidence rates for malignant brain and other nervous system cancer in the United States for 2011–2015, by state. Rates calculated using SEER* Stat. (*From* http://statecancerprofiles.cancer.gov)

A strong dose-response relationship was observed, such that those who received an estimated dose of 2.5 Gy had RRs approaching 20 for all brain tumors. With an additional 16 years of follow-up, the RR for meningioma remained high (overall, RR 4.63; 95% confidence interval [CI] 2.43–9.12) and was elevated regardless of age at exposure or latency period (Sadetzki et al., 2005). In the same study, the highest risk of malignant glioma was observed among children who were exposed when they were less than 5 years old (RR 3.56; 95% CI 0.96–9.91). Reports of less dramatic but still significant elevations of risk for meningioma and nerve sheath tumors exist among individuals treated with variable doses of ionizing radiation for thymic enlargement, enlarged tonsils and adenoids, and thyroid and nasopharyngeal conditions. In a mutagen sensitivity assay, peripheral blood lymphocytes from glioma subjects were more prone to chromosomal damage when exposed to gamma radiation. In this study, mutagen sensitivity of lymphocytes was associated with an increased risk of glioma (OR 2.09; 95% CI 1.43–3.06; Bondy et al., 2001).

Radiation exposure from diagnostic x-rays is substantially lower than from therapeutic radiation; consequently, the association with brain tumors is not established. Prior to the introduction of fast-speed film in 1956, exposures were several orders of magnitude higher than those used nowadays. Therefore, despite some reports of positive associations between diagnostic x-rays and certain brain tumors (mostly meningioma), most of these included periods of exposure when diagnostic radiation levels were higher. In a recent study with detailed information on dental history, an elevated risk of meningioma was observed among individuals who reported six or more x-rays involving full-mouth series (OR 2.06; 95% CI, 1.03–4.17), but the associations were strongest among those who had frequent dental x-rays in years when doses were higher (Longstreth et al., 2004). In the same study, associations were not observed for bite-wings, lateral cephalometric, and panoramic radiographs. For gliomas, past and current studies consistently show no increase in risk with dental x-rays.

Overall, therapeutic ionizing radiation is an uncommon exposure and explains only a small proportion of brain tumors.

### Electromagnetic Field Radiation

Numerous studies examining low-frequency electromagnetic field (EMF) radiation and risk of brain cancer have yielded inconsistent results. Several observations cast doubt on the possibility that EMF exposure causes brain tumors; biological plausibility is not established, results of subsequent studies are conflicting, and bias and confounding played a role in earlier studies. Electrical workers have been the subject of several occupational cohort studies based on exposure to EMFs.

The possible role of EMFs as a cause of brain tumors is in question. Measuring magnetic field exposure is extremely challenging because there is great variability in field intensity, frequency, and temporal patterns. Earlier studies on this topic did not accurately measure EMF exposure. Some recent studies using accurate estimates of total EMF exposure show a slight increase in risk for brain tumors among workers with very high EMF exposures (Savitz and Loomis, 1995; Savitz et al., 2000), while others did not. Overall, the findings are insufficiently robust to establish causation, and, unfortunately, improvements in measurement assessment are unlikely to exceed those currently existing (Ahlbom et al., 2001).

### Radiofrequency and Cellular Telephone

Radiofrequency (RF) radiation exposures mainly involve microwave and radar equipment, as well as occupational exposures (sealers, plastic welders, amateur radio operators, medical personnel, and telecommunications workers). Cellular telephones are a source of RF radiation exposure and have received significant attention as a potential risk factor for brain tumors. Despite lack of strong biological plausibility, coverage in the popular media has caused public concern, and contradictory reports frequently appear in the news. In 2011 the International Agency for Research on Cancer (IARC) working group tasked to review the evidence on RF EMFs, including exposure from mobile phones, concluded that there was limited evidence that these exposures cause cancer in humans and experimental animals, and classified RF EMFs only as "possibly carcinogenic to humans (group 2B)." Results from numerous epidemiological studies conducted to examine the relationship between cell phone use and different brain tumor subtypes have been largely inconsistent (Christensen et al., 2004; Christensen et al., 2005; INTERPHONE Study Group, 2010; Inskip et al., 2001; Johansen et al., 2001; Lonn et al., 2005; Rothman et al., 1996; Schoemaker et al., 2005). The controversy stems from potential biases in these studies, including recall bias (especially with respect to side of use), selection bias (e.g., controls tend to be more educated and own phones), measurement error (e.g., reported phone usage does not correlate well with actual use determined from phone records), and brain tumor heterogeneity. Experts have been conflicted on this topic, with some concluding that the current epidemiological data do not support a causal association between cellular phones and brain tumors when examined critically (Ahlbom et al., 2009), whereas others have cautioned that only time will provide the answer because years of exposure to high levels of cell phone use are still relatively low (Saracci and Samet, 2010). It is worth noting that since this publication, incidence rates for primary brain tumors have been declining in the United States, despite continued increase in cellular phone use.

### Occupational Studies

Several occupational studies focusing on brain tumors in cohorts of workers who share common potentially harmful exposures report standardized incidence or mortality ratios using expected rates from the general population. Detection bias may occur because working adults with health insurance may be more likely to undergo diagnostic tests. This may lead to better ascertainment of brain tumors in the worker cohort as compared with the general population and potentially result in spurious associations. In general, data on occupational exposures and brain tumors are inconsistent. Small numbers of cases, imprecise methods of exposure assessment, potential confounding, and bias have complicated interpretation of many studies. Study validity is often questionable, and better exposure assessment using biological measures of exposure is mostly lacking.

Several observational studies have found that workers in "white collar" professions have higher rates of brain tumors (Brownson et al., 1990; Carozza et al., 2000). Some of these occupations, such as laboratory research and health professions, involve radiation or chemical exposures that support a biological plausibility for a causal relationship. Alternatively, detection bias may account for the excess risk in professionals because they are more likely to have health insurance and seek medical attention. However, higher rates of brain tumors among professionals in Sweden, where health care is free and available to all citizens, suggest that detection bias may not fully account for the observations (McLaughlin et al., 1987).

Farming as an occupation and residence on a farm have been associated with an elevated risk of brain tumors in several epidemiological studies (meta-analysis RR 1.30; 95% CI 1.09–1.56; Khuder et al., 1998). Agricultural workers have exposures to several chemicals in the form of pesticides, herbicides, and fungicides. Similar to other occupational studies, one limitation of studies on agricultural workers is the use of job classification as a proxy for nonspecific chemical exposures. Studies with more detail on individual exposure to pesticides and herbicides have not reported convincing associations with brain tumors (Ruder et al., 2009; Samanic et al., 2008). Reports of increased risks for brain tumors also exist for workers in the vinyl chloride, petrochemical, and rubber industries. Other studies have found an increased risk among aircraft pilots, firefighters, welders, glass manufacturers, tile makers, and metal cutters. However, these findings have been inconsistent over time (Samkange-Zeeb et al., 2010).

Despite the large number of studies in several occupational settings, an increased risk of brain tumor development based on occupational status is not established. The reported studies are characterized by significant design flaws and yielded conflicting results.

### Head Trauma

Head trauma is a potential risk factor for brain tumor development. The evidence is strongest for meningiomas and less convincing for gliomas (Wrensch et al., 2000). Anecdotal reports of brain tumors arising after head trauma date back to Harvey Cushing in 1922. Cushing reported the presence of a head scar or skull depression in 8% of meningioma patients. Experimental studies have also implicated physical trauma as a cocarcinogen. An excess risk of meningiomas in persons with a history of serious or repetitive head trauma has been observed in several case-control studies (Preston-Martin et al., 1989, 1998). Other studies have not confirmed an increased risk among children with head injuries (Gousias et al., 2009; Gurney et al., 1996).

Ionizing radiation may be a confounding factor in studies of head trauma and brain tumors. Individuals with a history of head trauma are more likely to have had skull x-rays. Recall bias is another factor complicating interpretation of case-control studies of head trauma and risk of brain tumors. Persons with brain tumors may be more likely to recall minor and major episodes of head injury compared with controls. One study reporting a positive association between head trauma and risk of brain tumors found no association when the definition of head trauma was restricted to episodes requiring medical attention. In a cohort study with an average of 8 years of follow-up, individuals hospitalized for head injury were not at higher risk for subsequent nonmalignant and malignant brain tumors after removing the first year of follow-up; detection bias was likely responsible for the higher risks observed in the first year (Inskip et al., 1998). No association was established between head trauma and brain tumor in a similar cohort with an average follow-up of 10 years (Nygren et al., 2001).

Acoustic neuroma (nerve sheath tumor of cranial nerve VIII) was associated with acoustic noise (trauma) of 10 years' duration in a case-control study (OR 2.2; 95% CI 1.12–4.67; Preston-Martin et al., 1989). A blinded review of job histories was the basis for noise exposure. In a study with a larger sample, a similarly elevated risk of acoustic neuroma was observed among individuals reporting loud noise exposure from any source (OR 1.55; 95% CI 1.04–2.30; Edwards et al., 2006). The association was stronger among individuals with exposure to loud noise from machines, power tools, or construction equipment (OR 1.79; 95% CI 1.11–2.89) or to loud music (OR 2.25; 95% CI 1.20–4.23; Edwards et al., 2006). Experimental studies of tissue destruction and repair following acoustic trauma support the biological plausibility of this association.

## *N*-Nitroso Compounds

*N*-Nitroso compounds (NOCs) are potent carcinogens in animal models. NOCs include nitrosamines, which require metabolic activation to a carcinogenic form, and nitrosamides, which do not require activation. It is well established that nitrosamines can form endogenously from foods treated with sodium nitrite and that certain foods such as bacon and beer contain preformed nitrosamines (Lijinsky, 1999). Although preformed nitrosamine levels in beer and nitrite levels have declined substantially since the 1980s, the small amounts of nitrosamines in food are nonetheless significant because of the possibility that humans are more sensitive to these carcinogens than laboratory rodents (Lijinsky, 1999). A long-standing hypothesis in the epidemiology of gliomas is that NOC exposure may increase risk. Transplacental exposure to ethylnitrosourea, a nitrosamide, results in formation of brain tumors including gliomas in rodents and primates. The addition of vitamin C to the diet prevents tumor formation in this model. Human NOC exposure divides equally between exogenous and endogenous sources. Nitrosamines in tobacco (mainly sidestream smoke), cosmetics, automobile interiors, and cured meats are the best-established exogenous (environmental) sources of NOC exposure. Other sources include rubber products (baby pacifiers, bottle nipples) and certain drugs including antihistamines, diuretics, oral hypoglycemic agents, antibiotics, tranquilizers, and narcotics. N-nitrosodiethanolamine, a carcinogen in animal models, occurs mainly as a contaminant in cosmetic products, soaps, shampoos, and hand lotions. Some environmental sources may contain both nitrosamines and nitrosamides. Endogenous formation of NOCs is a complex process that occurs in the stomach. This process is dependent upon the presence of NOC precursors (i.e., nitrates and nitrites), gastric pH, the presence of bacteria, and other physiological parameters.

Measurement of NOC exposure is difficult, given the many exogenous and endogenous sources. Thus misclassification of exposure is a major limitation for any study on this topic. However, because processed and cured meats are sources of NOC precursors and some preformed nitrosamines, dietary assessment may serve as a useful surrogate marker for NOC exposure.

Epidemiological support for NOC exposure as a risk factor for brain tumors comes mostly from studies of pediatric brain tumors and maternal diet. Several studies have assessed the association between maternal diet and childhood brain tumor risk (Dietrich et al., 2005). A meta-analysis determined that frequent intake of processed meats during pregnancy was associated with an elevated risk of childhood brain tumors (RR 1.68; 95% CI 1.30–2.17; Huncharek et al., 2003). However, the authors of this meta-analysis warn not to draw definitive conclusions, based on several study-design limitations such as recall bias and selection bias.

Case-control studies on dietary intakes of foods containing preformed nitrosamines or compounds that can be converted to nitrosamines yield inconsistent results. A few case-control studies reported strong positive associations (e.g., Blowers et al., 1997; Lee et al., 1997), but the potential for bias in these studies is high. Two large prospective cohort studies, with more than 300 incident cases of glioma in each study, examined meats and foods high in nitrites or nitrates; no increase in glioma risk was observed for meat, processed meats, nitrites from animal products, or nitrates (Dubrow et al., 2010; Michaud et al., 2009). Data from these two large studies, which are less prone to bias than case-control studies, provide little evidence for the NOC hypothesis, at least as it pertains to adult gliomas.

## Vitamins

Vitamins C and E inhibit nitrosation reactions in vivo, and intake of these vitamins can reduce the endogenous formation of NOC in the stomach. Epidemiological studies have demonstrated that consumption of vitamin C reduces the risk of gastric cancer (La Vecchia and Franceschi, 2000), a tumor for which NOC may be a risk factor (Neugut et al., 1996). Statistically significant inverse associations with dietary vitamin C or supplemental intake have been observed in a few case-control studies. Furthermore, no associations were observed in a large prospective cohort study examining intakes of vitamins C and E and a total antioxidant score and risk of glioma (Michaud et al., 2009). Currently, evidence does not support causation for vitamins and risk of glioma.

As with vitamin intake, findings on fruit and vegetable intake have been inconsistent. Inconsistent results for fruit, vegetable, and vitamin intakes are not surprising; in addition to the problems inherent in case-control designs, the initial design of several studies was not to test a dietary hypothesis. Consequently, most were limited in their ability to capture dietary exposures. Furthermore, the majority of studies on diet and gliomas have limited statistical power, making it difficult to draw conclusions from those findings. In a large prospective cohort study, fruit and vegetable intake, overall or within subgroups, was not associated with risk of glioma (Holick et al., 2007).

## Tobacco and Alcohol

The presence of nitrosamines in tobacco smoke has stimulated interest in tobacco exposure as a potential risk factor for primary brain tumors. Several case-control and cohort studies have assessed the relationship between cigarette smoking and the risk of adult glioma; few have reported any positive association with cigarette smoking. Overall, the 2004 Surgeon General's Report on the Health Consequences of Smoking concluded that "the evidence is suggestive of no causal relationship between smoking cigarettes and brain cancer in men and women" (US Department of Health and Human Services, 2004). Findings from studies of maternal smoking (active and passive) and risk of primary brain tumors in offspring have been inconsistent, but overall the data do not support an increase in brain tumor risk with maternal smoking (Norman et al., 1996).

Because beer and liquor contain nitrosamines, speculation that consumption of alcoholic beverages may increase the risk of brain tumors exists. However, no consistent association is demonstrable between consumption of different types of alcoholic beverages and the risk of gliomas or meningiomas in childhood (maternal consumption) or adulthood.

## Tea and Coffee

Several large prospective cohort studies have examined coffee and tea consumption in relation to risk of glioma. In a meta-analysis of six published studies on this topic (four cohort and two case-control studies), inverse associations were noted for tea (summary RR 0.88; 95% CI 0.69–1.12) and coffee plus tea (summary RR 0.75; 95% CI 0.54–1.05) when comparing highest with lowest categories of consumption (Malerba et al., 2013). Although the overall summary estimates were not statistically significant in the meta-analysis, several of the largest prospective studies reported significant inverse trends for at least one of these beverages (Dubrow et al., 2012; Holick et al., 2010; Michaud et al., 2010). An additional cohort study conducted in Japan, published after the meta-analysis was conducted, also reported inverse associations between coffee intake and brain cancer risk (for ≥3 cups/day vs. <4 cups/wk, HR 0.47, 95% CI 0.22–0.98 combined glioma and meningioma; HR 0.54, 95% CI 0.16–1.80 for glioma), but not for green tea (Ogawa et al., 2016).

## Infections, Allergies, and Immunity

The concern that simian virus 40 (SV40) may have human carcinogenic potential dates back to the early 1960s (Fraumeni et al., 1963). The detection of viruses and virus-like particles in brain tumor specimens resulted in speculation that viral infections could be involved in brain tumor development. Interest in SV40, a polyomavirus, was stimulated by animal studies documenting brain tumor development after intracerebral inoculation with SV40 and human studies in which SV40 was isolated from brain tumor tissue. Accidental contamination of administered poliomyelitis vaccine with SV40 occurred between 1955 and 1962. However, to date, numerous long-term follow-up studies of these vaccinated individuals have not revealed any increase in the risk of brain tumors (Engels, 2005). Other types of infections hypothesized to increase the risk of brain cancer have not been associated with glioma or have been associated with reduced risks of glioma. In one study (Schlehofer et al., 1999), subjects who reported a history of infectious diseases (e.g., colds, flu) had a 30% reduction in risk (RR 0.72; 95% CI 0.61–0.85) compared with those with no such history.

A possible protective role for antecedent infection with chickenpox (varicella-zoster virus [VZV]) has been reported in several case-control studies using self-report measures and serological measures of the antibodies to VZV (Wrensch et al., 1997, 2001, 2005; Amirian et al., 2016). In the largest case-control study, which included 4533 cases and 4171 controls, history of chickenpox was associated with a 21% decreased risk of glioma (OR 0.79; 95% CI, 0.65–0.96; Amirian et al., 2016). Furthermore, in a different case-control study, higher levels of immunoglobulin directed against VZV were associated with a 59% decreased risk of glioma (OR 0.41; 95% CI 0.24–0.70; Wrensch et al., 2005). Similar findings were observed in a prospective study using prediagnostic bloods; elevated antibodies to VZV were marginally associated with lower risk of glioma (OR = 0.68, 95% CI 0.41–1.13, fourth vs. first quartile; *P* for trend = .06), and no associations were observed for EBV, CMV, and adenovirus (Sjöström et al., 2011). In contrast, no associations were seen with three other herpesviruses (Epstein-Barr virus [EBV], cytomegalovirus [CMV], and herpes simplex virus; Wrensch et al., 2001, 2005).

The role of the immune response in the etiology of brain tumors has also been highlighted by findings that allergies such as asthma or eczema have been consistently linked to reduced risk of glioma. Although these associations may not have any direct clinical or preventive implications, it may shed some light on mechanisms and the role of the immune system in the pathogenesis of primary brain tumors. Several plausible biological mechanisms exist that could explain the role of allergies. Although complex, most relate to the immune system response and the tendency for individuals with allergies to mount a stronger type 2 response.

In a meta-analysis based on 3450 cases of glioma, a 39% decrease in risk of glioma was observed among those reporting any form of allergy (RR 0.61; 95% CI 0.55–0.67); the association was similar for asthma or eczema (Linos et al., 2007). The association is weaker for meningiomas. Two studies focused on allergies to specific exposures (e.g., medicine, foods) and reported inverse associations for most types of allergies (Brenner et al., 2002; Wiemels et al., 2002). In one of these studies (Brenner et al., 2002), self-report of any type of allergy was associated with a 33% reduction in the risk of glioma (OR 0.67), and the OR for individual allergies ranged from 0.23 (allergy to chemicals) to 0.97 (hay fever). In the other study (Wiemels et al., 2002), a dose-response relationship was observed between increasing numbers of specific allergens and risk of glioma, with an OR of 0.37 for five or more described allergens compared with none.

In a case-control study (Wiemels et al., 2004), measures of biological markers of allergies reduced the bias that arises from self-reporting in a case-control setting and increased the specificity of exposure assessment. Serum samples collected from 226 adult glioma cases and 289 age-gender-ethnicity frequency-matched controls measured immunoglobulin E (IgE), a clinical marker of atopic allergies. Compared with normal levels (<25 kU/L), individuals with elevated IgE levels (>100 kU/L) had an OR of 0.37 (95% CI 0.22–0.64), and individuals with intermediate IgE levels (25–100 kU/L) had an OR of 0.64 (95% CI 0.42–0.96) for glioma risk. Chemotherapy, radiation, surgery, and medication use (including nonsteroidal antiinflammatory drugs, allergy drugs, steroids, and antibiotics) did not affect IgE levels in cases or controls in this study. A similar finding was observable in a follow-up study on IgE levels and risk of glioma, although the association was weaker than in the first study, and drug treatment might have been a confounding factor (Wiemels et al., 2009).

The association between blood IgE levels and risk of glioma was recently examined in three large prospective studies (Calboli et al., 2011; Schlehofer et al., 2011; Schwartzbaum et al., 2012); given that measures were taken on prediagnostic blood, these studies were less prone to reverse causation (bias that arises when measured biomarkers are impacted by disease status). Calboli et al. (2011) observed a U-shaped (i.e., higher risk at low and high IgE plasma levels; lower risk in middle ranges of IgE levels) associated with IgE plasma levels and glioma risk, similar to the observed association in the earlier case-control study. In the European Prospective Investigation into Cancer and Nutrition (EPIC) cohort, the risk of glioma was inversely related to allergic sensitization (i.e., specific IgE level ≥0.35 kUA/L [kilo antibody units per liter], OR = 0.73; 95% CI 0.51–1.06) (Schlehofer et al., 2011). The third cohort study also reported a lower risk for glioma (OR 0.75, 95% CI 0.56–0.99, >100 kUA/L vs. ≤100 kUA/L); testing positive for total IgE at least 20 years before diagnosis was associated with an even greater risk reduction compared with testing negative (OR 0.54; 95% CI 0.30–0.99; Schwartzbaum et al., 2012). Combined, these studies provide additional support for the role of allergies in the etiology of glioma; however, the shape of the association with total IgE levels remains uncertain and suggests that the relation with innate immunity is likely very complex. The high degree of consistency in all reports, despite differences in study designs and geographical location of the study, suggests that an etiological basis for allergies and the related immune response may exist. Moreover, the fact that allergy was not a risk factor for meningioma in most studies (Brenner et al., 2002; Schlehofer et al., 1999) argues against bias as being responsible for the inverse association with glioma risk. Taken together, studies on infections and allergies suggest that the innate immune system plays an important role in glioma etiology. Further research should aim to elucidate specific components of the innate immune response that are critical to the development of glioma.

## Genetic Syndromes

Genetic syndromes that increase the risk of nervous system tumors cause approximately 1%–5% of brain tumors (Kleihues et al., 2000). Neurofibromatosis type 1 (NF1; see Chapter 99) occurs in 1 in 4000 newborns and is linked to a gene on chromosome 17. Approximately 5%–10% of persons with NF1 develop brain tumors, including malignant peripheral nerve sheath tumors, pilocytic astrocytomas of the optic nerve, and other astrocytomas. Neurofibromatosis type 2 (NF2) occurs in 1 in 40,000 newborns and has a corresponding link to a gene on chromosome 22. The presence of bilateral acoustic neuromas is the defining feature. Astrocytomas and other brain tumor types occur.

The Li-Fraumeni syndrome, an autosomal dominant condition, may involve a mutation in the tumor suppressor gene *TP53*, conferring an increased risk of soft-tissue sarcomas, osteosarcomas, breast cancer, and

TABLE 71.1 Genetic Syndromes Associated with Nervous System Tumors

| Syndrome | Chromosome or Gene | Inheritance | CNS Tumors |
|---|---|---|---|
| Neurofibromatosis type 1 (NF1) | 17q1 | Autosomal dominant | Pilocytic astrocytomas of the optic nerve, other gliomas, meningiomas, nerve sheath tumors |
| NF2 | 22q | Autosomal dominant | Nerve sheath tumors, glioma, meningioma |
| Li-Fraumeni syndrome | TP53 germline mutations | Autosomal dominant | Glioma, medulloblastoma, choroid plexus tumors, nerve sheath tumors, meningioma |
| Turcot syndrome | APC and *hMLH1/hPSM2* germline mutations | Autosomal dominant | Medulloblastoma |
| Gorlin syndrome | 9q22.3 microdeletions<br>*PTCH1* gene | Autosomal dominant | Medulloblastoma |
| Tuberous sclerosis | 9q32-34 | Autosomal dominant | Subependymal giant cell astrocytoma (SEGA) |
| Von Hippel-Lindau disease | 3p13-14<br>3p25-26 | Autosomal dominant | Hemangioblastoma |

*APC*, Adenomatous polyposis coli; *CNS*, central nervous system.

brain tumors. Approximately 12% of cancers in families with *TP53* germline mutations are brain tumors; astrocytomas are the predominant type (Kleihues et al., 1997). Turcot syndrome is associated with adenomatous polyps and increased risk of medulloblastoma and glioblastoma. Individuals with Gorlin syndrome (mutations in *PTCH1* gene) and Wilms tumor have an increased risk of medulloblastoma. Table 71.1 summarizes inherited syndromes associated with an increased risk of nervous system tumors.

Familial clustering of brain tumors is also recognized outside of these defined syndromes. The chance of having a family member with a brain tumor is twice as high in adult brain tumor patients (8%) as in controls (4%). This familial clustering is greater for children and certain histological types of brain tumors (medulloblastoma). Although genetic syndromes account for only a small fraction of brain tumors in the United States, further study of the affected genes may provide insight into the molecular pathogenesis of sporadic brain tumors.

## Genetic Susceptibility

Recently, researchers have focused on genetic factors of brain cancers with the increased availability of new technologies that allow rapid, effective, and affordable measurement of thousands of genetic variants. Genome-wide association studies (GWAS) involve the analysis of genetic variants in the whole genome and their relation to disease onset. Several GWAS have been conducted for glioma, providing new clues into possible genetic regions that may play a role in this disease. In one study, five susceptibility loci in genes TERT, CCDC26, CDKN2A/CDKN2B, RTEL1, and PHLDB1 were identified by genotyping 550K tagging single-nucleotide polymorphisms (SNPs) in a total of 2545 glioma cases and 2953 controls (Shete et al., 2009). In another study, the identification of two susceptibility loci (CDKN2B and RTEL1) was based on the analysis of 275,895 SNPs in 692 adult high-grade glioma cases and 174 controls (Wrensch et al., 2009). Strong replication of three regions (RTEL, TERT, and CDKN2B) was obtained in a GWAS analysis consisting primarily of cohort studies (Rajaraman et al., 2012). Consistent signals at 7p11.2 (EGFR) have also been reported in three studies (Rajaraman et al., 2012; Sanson et al., 2011; Wrensch et al., 2009). For meningiomas, two susceptibility loci have been identified (10p12.31 and 11p15.5; Claus et al. 2018), which are distinct from those identified for gliomas. Based on a genome-wide complex trait analysis that allows for evaluation of risk based on contribution of multiple SNPs simultaneously (vs. single-SNP analysis), it was estimated that 25% of glioma risk is inherited (i.e., due to variation in common genetic polymorphisms. genetic variation; Kinnersley et al. 2015).

Genetic polymorphisms in specific detoxification/metabolic enzymes have been implicated in the pathogenesis of certain cancers. The association between chemical carcinogens and brain tumors in experimental models raises the possibility that susceptibility may be related to genetic polymorphisms at loci encoding phase I cytochrome P450 (CYP450) and phase II glutathione *S*-transferase (GST) enzymes. Several potential neurocarcinogens (polycyclic aromatic hydrocarbons, nitrosoureas, and methyl halide) are substrates for these enzymes. Several case-control studies of brain tumors have assessed polymorphic enzymes (e.g., GSTT1, GSTM1, GSTP1, CYP2D6, NAT2, HRAS1) implicated in the activation or detoxification of potential neurocarcinogens; results from these studies are inconsistent. A meta-analysis of eight studies concluded that no evidence exists for an association between GST variants and risk of glioma (Lai et al., 2005). Other studies have been conducted on genetic polymorphisms involved in DNA repair, immune function, inflammation, and allergies; results from these studies need to be replicated.

## SUMMARY

Brain tumors are an uncommon but especially lethal form of cancer of unknown etiology. The only established environmental risk factor, ionizing radiation, accounts for only a small fraction of incident cases. Genetic predisposition exists in only a small percentage of cases through various familial syndromes. Similarly, genetic susceptibility plays a role in brain tumor etiology, and new findings have demonstrated that glioma is a polygenic disease and that common genetic variants may explain up to 25% of all glioma cases. Several factors complicate the study of brain tumors, including the large number of biological subtypes and low incidence compared with other cancers. Recent epidemiologic studies have unraveled new risk factors, namely a role for allergies and the immune response, and have provided a consensus on other risk factors that do not appear to be etiologically relevant, including exposure to nonionizing sources of radiation, meats and nitrosamines, and SV40. Future studies will likely provide a better understanding of the role of the immune response in risk of glioma and of genetic variability in immune pathways. Changes in reporting of meningiomas to cancer registries will also likely provide new opportunities to examine the etiology and recurrence of these benign tumors.

*The complete reference list is available online at https://expertconsult.inkling.com/.* 

# 72

# Pathology and Molecular Genetics

*Leomar Y. Ballester, Jason T. Huse*

## OUTLINE



## GENERAL PRINCIPLES OF NERVOUS SYSTEM TUMOR BIOLOGY

Tumors of the nervous system, like other human neoplasms, are dysregulated clonal proliferations that arise secondary to changes in cellular genetics and physiology. In many cases, alterations involving growth-promoting oncogenes, growth-checking tumor suppressors, and cell death genes are involved in brain tumorigenesis. However, recent work in brain tumors as well as other cancer types has expanded conventional notions of cancer-related genes, implicating chromatin-binding proteins and other regulators of cellular epigenetics in the oncogenic process (Plass et al., 2013). Some of the specific genes affected in human nervous system tumors are discussed with their respective tumor types later in this chapter. Because oncogenic transformation requires cell division, postmitotic cells, such as neurons, should not be susceptible to tumorigenic events. However, it remains possible that nervous system tumors arise when oncogenic changes occur in precursor cells rather than mature nervous system components. Such precursor cells reside in the brain into adult life (Vescovi et al., 2006).

While much progress has been made in recent years in characterizing the underlying genetics and epigenetics of brain tumors, precise etiological mechanisms remain unclear. To date, radiation and hereditary predisposition are the only clearly implicated factors in the genesis of nervous system tumors. See Chapter 71 for a discussion of ionizing radiation as a risk factor for specific types of brain tumors. Hereditary predisposition to brain tumors is rare and confined to specific syndromes (e.g., neurofibromatosis type 1 [NF1], neurofibromatosis type 2 [NF2], tuberous sclerosis, von Hippel–Lindau disease, Li-Fraumeni syndrome, Turcot syndrome, and Gorlin syndrome). These conditions highlight the critical roles played by specific genes in brain tumorigenesis. Tumors arising with these syndromes are discussed at multiple points within this chapter.

## NERVOUS SYSTEM TUMOR CLASSIFICATION

The foundation of the first comprehensive classification of nervous system tumors, formulated by Percival Bailey and Harvey Cushing in 1926, presumed parallels between embryological and neoplastic cells. In large part, this histogenetic model based on the presumed cell of origin still forms the basis for current nomenclature, although molecular factors are becoming increasingly important. In 1949, as a means of enhancing the clinical utility of tumor classification, Kernohan contributed a tumor grading system whose purpose was assessing patient prognosis. Russell and Rubinstein modified and updated the Bailey and Cushing system during the 1960s, 1970s, and 1980s. Further updates were incorporated into the World Health Organization (WHO) classification, first completed in 1979 and then revised in 1993, 2007, and most recently in 2016 (Louis et al., 2016). The WHO classification has become the system most widely used by neuropathologists today. The latest 2016 effort is the first to incorporate defining molecular features into specific diagnostic entities.

The WHO classification currently lists more than 100 types of nervous system tumors and their variants. This level of complexity may seem daunting at first, but consideration of key clinical and imaging characteristics typically narrows the differential diagnosis to only a few common possibilities (Table 72.1). Specific differential diagnoses vary substantially for supratentorial versus infratentorial, pediatric versus adult, and enhancing versus nonenhancing tumors.

Light microscopic examination of hematoxylin and eosin–stained sections is the basis of most classification and grading systems for nervous system tumors. The approach to nervous system neoplasia recapitulates that used to classify human tumors from all parts of the body; thus, many neuropathological terms derive from the discipline of general pathology. The fundamental concept of grading utilizes distinct histopathological features to stratify nervous system tumors on the basis of anticipated biological behavior. In the WHO scheme, grade I is equivalent to benign; II is low-grade malignant; III is intermediate-grade malignant, often associated with the term *anaplastic*; and IV is high-grade malignant. *Grading*, which depends on histological assessment, should not be confused with *tumor staging*, which depends on gross/radiographic characteristics and extent of tumor spread.

## Intraoperative Consultation

Intraoperative frozen sections are more difficult to interpret than fixed tissue sections, but their use has the advantage of speed, requiring only a few minutes to prepare. This technique is requested for several reasons, including simple curiosity and a desire to provide rapid feedback to patients and their families. However, the most important reasons for performing this technique are to ensure that the pathologist obtains a representative sample for permanent sections and to provide information that may alter the surgical procedure. For example, a neurosurgeon may opt to stop at a limited biopsy for a suspected lymphoma, aggressively resect for an ependymoma, or send additional material to the microbiology laboratory for an abscess. Because the process of tissue freezing produces significant cytological artifacts, another popular technique has been the preparation of touch imprints, or smears, from fresh tissue. Although underlying tissue architecture is lost, sample requirements are minimal, and cytological preservation is typically excellent. This may be critical for diagnoses based primarily on nuclear cytology, such as reactive gliosis versus low-grade diffuse glioma. It is

**TABLE 72.1 Common Central Nervous System Tumor Diagnoses by Location, Age, and Imaging Characteristics**

| Location | Child/Young Adult | Older Adult |
|---|---|---|
| Cerebral/supratentorial | Ganglioglioma (temporal lobe, cyst-MEN)<br>DNT (temporal lobe, intracortical nodules)<br>AT/RT (infant) | Grade II–III glioma (NE)<br>Glioblastoma (ring E, butterfly)<br>Metastases (gray/white junctions, E)<br>Lymphoma (periventricular, E) |
| Cerebellar/infratentorial | Pilocytic astrocytoma (cyst-MEN)<br>Medulloblastoma (vermis, E)<br>Ependymoma (fourth ventricle, E)<br>Choroid plexus papilloma (fourth ventricle)<br>AT/RT (infant) | Metastases (multiple, E)<br>Hemangioblastoma (cyst-MEN)<br>Choroid plexus papilloma (fourth ventricle) |
| Brainstem | Diffuse midline glioma<br>Pilocytic astrocytoma (dorsal brainstem) | Gliomatosis cerebri (multifocal) |
| Spinal cord (intra-axial) | Ependymoma<br>Pilocytic astrocytoma (cystic) | Ependymoma<br>Diffuse astrocytoma (ill-defined)<br>Paraganglioma (filum terminale) |
| Extra-axial/dural | Secondary lymphoma/leukemia | Meningioma<br>Metastases<br>Secondary lymphoma/leukemia |
| Intrasellar | Pituitary adenoma<br>Craniopharyngioma<br>Rathke cleft cyst | Pituitary adenoma<br>Rathke cleft cyst |
| Suprasellar/hypothalamic/optic pathway/ third ventricle | Germinoma/germ cell tumor<br>Craniopharyngioma<br>Pilocytic astrocytoma | Colloid cyst (third ventricle) |
| Pineal | Germinoma/germ cell tumor<br>Pineocytoma<br>Pineoblastoma<br>Pineal cyst | Pineocytoma<br>Pineal cyst |
| Thalamus | Pilocytic astrocytoma<br>Anaplastic astrocytoma/glioblastoma | Anaplastic astrocytoma/glioblastoma<br>Lymphoma |
| Cerebellopontine angle | Vestibular schwannoma (NF2) | Vestibular schwannoma<br>Meningioma |
| Lateral ventricle | Central neurocytoma<br>SEGA (tuberous sclerosis)<br>Choroid plexus papilloma<br>Choroid plexus carcinoma (infant) | Central neurocytoma<br>SEGA (tuberous sclerosis)<br>Choroid plexus papilloma<br>Subependymoma |
| Nerve root/paraspinal | Neurofibroma (NF1)<br>MPNST (NF1) | Schwannoma<br>Meningioma<br>Secondary lymphoma<br>Neurofibroma (NF1)<br>MPNST |

*AT/RT*, Atypical teratoid/rhabdoid tumor; *DNT*, dysembryoplastic neuroepithelial tumor; *E*, enhancing; *MEN*, mural enhancing nodule; *MPNST*, malignant peripheral nerve sheath tumor; *NE*, nonenhancing; *NF1*, neurofibromatosis type 1; *NF2*, neurofibromatosis type 2; *SEGA*, subependymal giant cell astrocytoma.

also important to realize that the frozen section technique results in substantial tissue loss and morphological artifacts in the thawed residual specimen. Therefore, it is best to omit its use in limited biopsies for which the surgical procedure will not be altered. In other words, it is imperative to save at least some optimally fixed nonfrozen tissue for final diagnosis on sections from paraffin-embedded material.

## Immunohistochemistry

Immunohistochemistry is an ancillary diagnostic technique for detecting protein expression within tumor cell nuclei, cytoplasm, and cell membranes. It is used most commonly to determine lines of cellular differentiation, proliferation indices, or the status of disease-defining molecular markers. Monoclonal antibody technology and recently improved antigen-retrieval methods have greatly expanded the versatility of this technique in routine formalin-fixed paraffin-embedded tissue, although a number of pitfalls remain, and considerable experience is necessary to make accurate determinations. Commercial antibodies vary greatly in terms of sensitivities, specificities, and clinical utilities. Most laboratories use the immunoperoxidase technique because staining is permanent and the reaction product is visible by conventional light microscopy. The application of several antibodies is usual for studying the more common CNS tumors:

*Lineage markers*: *Glial fibrillary acidic protein* (GFAP), an intermediate filament, remains the primary molecular marker used to designate glial cell lineage. Although it is commonly considered an astrocytic marker, it does not reliably distinguish astrocytic from oligodendroglial or ependymal ontogeny. Likewise, some degree of glial differentiation or GFAP expression may occur in choroid plexus tumors, medulloblastomas, gangliogliomas, and even some peripheral nerve sheath and cartilaginous tumors.

*Neurofilaments* are heteropolymers composed of three subunits with molecular weights of 68, 150, and 200 kD that are unique to neurons and their axonal processes. Normal neurons and mature neuronal tumors (e.g., gangliogliomas) stain for neurofilament protein, although primitive neuronal tumors, such as medulloblastoma, are often negative. Nevertheless, the staining of axons has great utility for highlighting a tumor's growth pattern. For example, discrete tumors such as metastases and ependymomas will push axon-bearing parenchyma to the side, whereas diffuse gliomas will contain entrapped neurofilament protein-positive axons within their substance. Another commonly utilized neuronal cell marker is *synaptophysin*, a 38-kD glycosylated polypeptide that is a component of presynaptic vesicle membranes. It is a relatively reliable marker of neuronal differentiation and is typically found even in the most primitive neuronal tumors, such as medulloblastoma. This marker, along with *chromogranin*, is also useful for highlighting normal and neoplastic ganglion cells, as well as neuroendocrine tumors such as pituitary adenomas, carcinoids, and paragangliomas. Lastly, *NeuN* (neuronal nuclear antigen), a protein marker of relatively mature neuronal differentiation, has the advantage of clearly marking tumor nuclei rather than surrounding neuropil, but it also clearly labels normal neurons.

*S100* protein expression is common to neuroectodermal cells, including melanocytes, glia, Schwann cells, chondrocytes, and the sustentacular cells in tumors such as paraganglioma, pheochromocytoma, and olfactory neuroblastoma. To a lesser extent, it also stains neuronal tumors and fibrous meningiomas. S100 protein is particularly useful for demonstrating Schwann cell differentiation in benign and malignant peripheral nerve sheath tumors. *Cytokeratins* are a class of intermediate filaments primarily expressed in epithelial cells. Antibodies against cytokeratin are commonly useful in the diagnosis of metastatic carcinomas but can also identify craniopharyngiomas, chordomas, and choroid plexus tumors. *Epithelial membrane antigen* (EMA) is a glycoprotein constituent of normal and neoplastic epithelial cells. In the central nervous system (CNS), EMA is a particularly useful marker for meningiomas, which unlike true epithelial tumors, display minimal to no cytokeratin expression in most cases.

***Cell proliferation markers***: The simplest and least expensive method for estimating cellular proliferation is the *mitotic index*, usually expressed as either the average or the maximal attainable count per 10 high-power fields (HPF). Difficulties in this type of proliferative assessment stem from pyknotic nuclei mimicking mitoses in poorly preserved specimens, variable field sizes among microscopes, and lack of uniform methods for counting. Underestimates of the proliferation index are common as well, given that the cells undergoing mitosis represent only a small fraction of cycling cells within a tumor.

Most proliferation antigens are nuclear constituents manifested during one or more proliferative phases in the cell cycle, allowing the recognition of cycling cells by routine immunohistochemistry. These markers are already valued in the diagnosis and management of brain tumors. The monoclonal antibody *Ki-67* (also known as *MIB-1*) binds to a human nuclear protein expressed during the cellular growth fraction (G1, S, G2, and M phases of the cell cycle). In most tumor types, the Ki-67 or MIB-1 labeling indices increase with degree of malignancy. *Phospho-histone H3* (pHH3) is a protein expressed exclusively during mitosis, and accordingly labels mitotically active cells, localizing to the spindle formation itself. Automated, computer-assisted algorithms to precisely quantify the extent of Ki-67 and/or pHH3 labeling further enhance the utility of both methodologies to accurately ascertain proliferative index.

***Disease-defining and disease-associated markers***: Several proteins directly involved in the pathogenesis of brain tumors are assessable by immunostaining. These include markers of diagnostic significance, such as IDH1 R132H, p53, ATRX, and BRAF V600E as well as markers reflecting the activation state of important oncogenic signaling networks, such as PTEN. Widespread use of markers like these has greatly facilitated the incorporation of molecular criteria into brain tumor diagnostics. Their precise application is discussed more extensively with associated tumor entities below.

## Molecular Diagnostics

As stated above, tumors arise when alterations occur in key molecular mechanisms governing cell growth, proliferation, differentiation, and cell death. The recent identification of many such alterations has greatly clarified the pathogenesis of brain tumors and led to significant revisions of the WHO classification scheme (Table 72.2). Relevant molecular abnormalities are detectable at the level of genomic DNA, messenger ribonucleic acid (mRNA), and protein. Some, such as large chromosomal translocations and/or deletions, can even be visualized cytogenetically as "signature" events. However, most abnormalities are undetectable by routine karyotyping and must be ascertained with molecular approaches. Focused assays based on loss of heterozygosity (LOH), fluorescence in situ hybridization (FISH), and quantitative polymerase chain reaction (PCR) enable the detection of specific biomarkers of interest (e.g., 1p/19q codeletion) at relatively low cost, as do immunohistochemical surrogates, which are available for IDH1 R132H, ATRX, BRAF V600E, and INI1, among others. However, the increasing requirement for more sophisticated disease stratification based on multiple biomarkers of interest has necessitated the development of multiplexed assays, which have now been adopted as clinical platforms in most large medical centers. These most notably include next-generation sequencing approaches that assess mutational profiles in hundreds of genes simultaneously (Wagle et al., 2012), RNA sequencing techniques to detect fusion transcripts (Maher et al., 2009), and array-based technology to determine global DNA copy number

**TABLE 72.2 Molecular Alterations in Primary Brain Tumors**

| | |
|---|---|
| Pilocytic astrocytoma | *KIAA1549-BRAF* fusion, BRAF p.V600E |
| Rosette-forming glioneuronal tumor | *PIK3CA* and *FGFR1* |
| Ganglioglioma | BRAF p.V600E, *KRAS*, FGFR1/FGFR2 |
| Pleomorphic xanthoastrocytoma | BRAF p.V600E |
| Low-grade diffuse astrocytoma | *IDH1/IDH2, ATRX, TP53* |
| Ependymoma | *C11orf95-RELA* fusion (supratentorial location) |
| Oligodendroglioma | *IDH1/IDH2, TERT* promoter, 1p deletion, 19q deletion |
| Glioblastoma (adults) | *EGFR, PTEN, CDKN2A, TERT* promoter, *NF1* |
| Glioblastoma (pediatric) | *H3F3A* (H3.3 p.K27M—diffuse midline glioma) |
| | (H3.3 p.G34R/V—hemispheric location) |
| ETMR | C19MC amplification |
| Craniopharyngioma | Adamantinomatous type—*CTNNB1* |
| | Papillary type—BRAF p.V600E |
| Primary CNS lymphoma | *MYD88 p.L265P* |

*CNS*, Central nervous system; *ETMR*, Embryonal Tumor with Multilayered Rosettes.

(Craig et al., 2012). Finally, recent work has demonstrated that global DNA methylation profiling effectively segregates primary neuroepithelial tumors by lineage and molecular features, designating previously unappreciated diagnostic categories (Capper et al., 2018). The importance of methylation profiling to routine brain tumor classification is likely to become evident in the next several years.

## PRIMARY NEUROEPITHELIAL TUMORS

Primary neuroepithelial tumors are nervous system neoplasms that arise from resident cells of origin within the CNS (i.e., glia, neurons, or their precursors).

### Infiltrating Gliomas

Gliomas constitute the largest group of neuroepithelial tumors from a clinical standpoint, and the term *diffuse glioma* encompasses all widely infiltrative glioma subtypes: astrocytomas and oligodendrogliomas (grade II to III), and glioblastoma (grade IV). While the histopathology and molecular foundations of these tumors vary, they are united by a shared tendency to widely infiltrate surrounding brain, a property that renders them incurable at present. Recent large-scale molecular profiling efforts have established striking biological distinctions between adult and pediatric gliomas, as well as between WHO grade II–III and WHO grade IV gliomas (see discussion in the sections that follow).

#### Infiltrating (Diffuse) Astrocytoma (WHO Grade II–III)

Diffuse astrocytoma is a slow-growing tumor with a median age at the time of diagnosis of 35 years. Radiographically, these tumors are ill-defined nonenhancing cerebral masses with a small proportion of diffuse astrocytomas occurring in the spinal cord, cerebellum, and brainstem. Microscopically, these tumors are characterized by hypercellularity, mild cellular pleomorphism, and a low mitotic count. Genetically, most diffuse astrocytomas exhibit a combination of mutations in the *IDH1, ATRX, TP53* genes (see below). This molecular signature is a strong prognostic indicator in diffuse gliomas. Astrocytomas with an *IDH1* or *IDH2* mutation have a better prognosis than *IDH1/IDH2*-wild-type astrocytomas. Moreover, the prognostic significance of *IDH1/IDH2* mutations in diffuse astrocytomas is superior to that based on histological features alone. As a result, the presence or absence of *IDH1/IDH2* mutations has been incorporated in the diagnosis of astrocytoma within the larger classification scheme for diffuse gliomas.

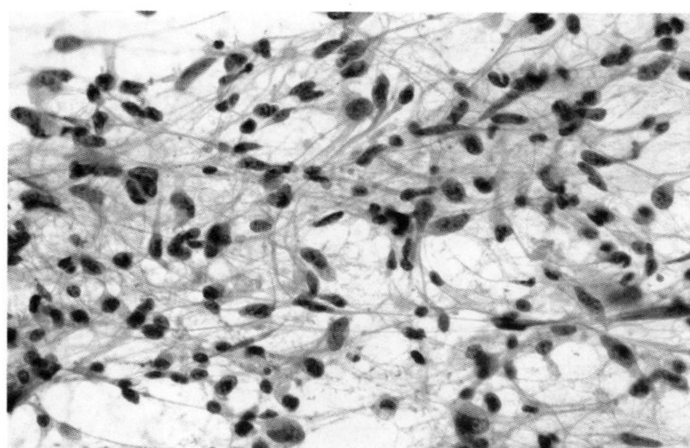

**Fig. 72.1 Diffuse Astrocytoma on an Intraoperative Smear.** Cytological preservation is superior to that of a typical frozen section, and cytoplasmic processes are easier to discern. The oval- to spindle-shaped hyperchromatic nuclei are typical of diffuse astrocytoma (hematoxylin-eosin stain, ×400).

Grossly, diffuse astrocytomas are poorly circumscribed tumors in which the CNS parenchyma variably expands, but the overall disruption of anatomy is minimal, although there can be significant edema and mass effect. Given its diffusely infiltrative nature and general lack of solid mass formation, large portions of the tumor may appear invisible to the naked (or radiographic) eye (i.e., microscopic disease). Also, this infiltrative growth pattern makes therapy a challenge because it has not been possible to address microscopic foci of disease adequately with focal treatments such as surgery and radiation. Particularly widespread infiltration involving multiple lobes and even the brainstem (gliomatosis cerebri) is rare and tends to have a poor prognosis regardless of histological grade.

While the morphology of diffuse astrocytoma varies, most are at least partially composed of irregular elongated hyperchromatic nuclei, either appearing "naked" in an otherwise fibrillary background or displaying discernible cytoplasmic processes (Fig. 72.1). GFAP immunostains highlight the latter, although this is neither absolutely sensitive nor specific, because (1) some astrocytomas harbor minimal quantities of GFAP-positive cytoplasm, (2) interpretation may be difficult owing to staining of nonneoplastic astrocytic elements or high background in general, and (3) other gliomas display GFAP immunoreactivity. Gemistocytic or "stuffed cell" architecture, characterized by strongly GFAP-positive cells with eccentric bellies of eosinophilic cytoplasm, may also be present to varying degrees. By definition, grade II astrocytomas lack significant mitotic activity, microvascular proliferation, and necrosis (see Glioblastoma [WHO Grade IV]). Ancillary staining for MIB-1 (Ki-67) generally reveals a low proliferative index as well.

The clinical presentation and radiographic features of anaplastic astrocytoma (WHO grade III) are similar to those of grade II astrocytoma, except that some cases show contrast enhancement on magnetic resonance imaging (MRI). Histologically, anaplastic astrocytomas are more cellular than grade II counterparts and display a greater degree of proliferation. The presence of mitotic figures primarily defines these tumors, as does a generally higher Ki-67 proliferative index on immunostains. Necrosis and microvascular proliferation are absent by definition.

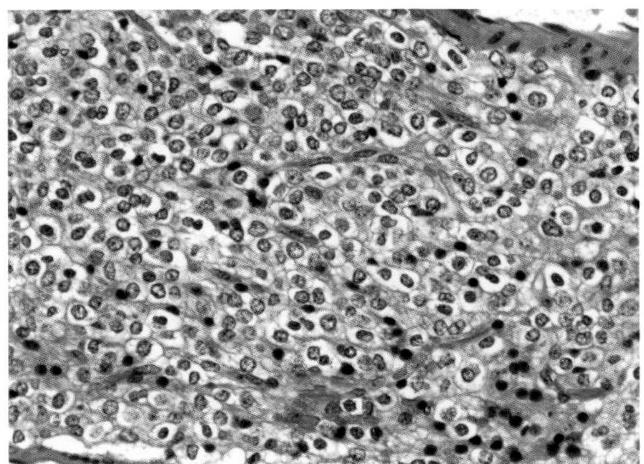

**Fig. 72.2 Oligodendroglioma.** Cells have uniform round nuclei with bland chromatin and a clear perinuclear halo, producing a "fried-egg" appearance. The rich, branching capillary network has been likened to chicken wire (hematoxylin-eosin stain, ×200).

## Oligodendroglioma, IDH-Mutant and 1p/19q Codeleted (WHO Grade II–III)

Oligodendrogliomas most commonly present as grade II tumors, occurring in young to middle-aged adults. Most are hemispheric masses, with the frontal lobe representing a favored location. On imaging studies, oligodendrogliomas are virtually indistinguishable from astrocytomas. However, gyriform calcifications are an uncommon but characteristic imaging feature. The prognosis for grade II oligodendrogliomas is significantly better than for astrocytomas, with average survival times of 10 years or more and improved chemosensitivity profiles. Oligodendrogliomas are defined by a specific molecular signature that includes a combination of *IDH1* or *IDH2* mutations and the codeletion of the 1p and 19q chromosomal regions (1p/19q codeletion). Accordingly, these genomic features are now included in the formal diagnosis of both WHO grade II and WHO grade III oligodendroglioma.

The classic microscopic features of oligodendroglioma include uniformly round nuclei, bland chromatin, clear perinuclear haloes imparting a "fried egg" appearance, and a rich branching capillary network reminiscent of "chicken wire" (Fig. 72.2). Less specific findings include cortical involvement, microcalcifications, mucin-rich microcystic spaces, and perineuronal satellitosis. Although helpful, the so-called fried-egg appearance is a formalin fixation artifact that is neither necessary for diagnosis nor encountered in frozen sections or rapidly fixed specimens. The morphological spectrum includes two strongly GFAP-positive cells: minigemistocytes (or microgemistocytes) and gliofibrillary oligodendrocytes. The former are gemistocyte-like cells with small bellies of eosinophilic cytoplasm, round bland nuclei resembling those of classic oligodendroglioma nuclei, and no cytoplasmic processes. The latter are histologically identical to classic oligodendroglioma cells but exhibit a thin perinuclear rim of GFAP immunoreactivity. Hypercellularity, numerous mitoses, and microvascular proliferation define anaplastic oligodendroglioma (grade III). Some oligodendrogliomas have regions that are histologically similar to diffuse astrocytoma, which caused significant diagnostic difficulty in the past. However, *IDH1* or *IDH2* mutations combined with 1p/19q codeletion represent defining molecular alterations for oligodendrogliomas, and the application of these biomarkers to routine clinical diagnosis has eliminated the diagnostic uncertainty associated with ambiguous and overlapping microscopic features.

## Oligoastrocytoma (WHO Grade II–III)

Previous editions of this book included a description of oligoastrocytomas. These tumors were characterized by the presence of microscopic features classically associated with both astrocytomas and oligodendrogliomas in the same lesion. However, the diagnosis of oligoastrocytoma demonstrated little agreement between pathologists and the incorporation of genetic alterations as defining features for brain tumor classification has led to the understanding that the vast majority of oligoastrocytomas can be classified as either astrocytomas or oligodendrogliomas based on highly recurrent molecular alterations.

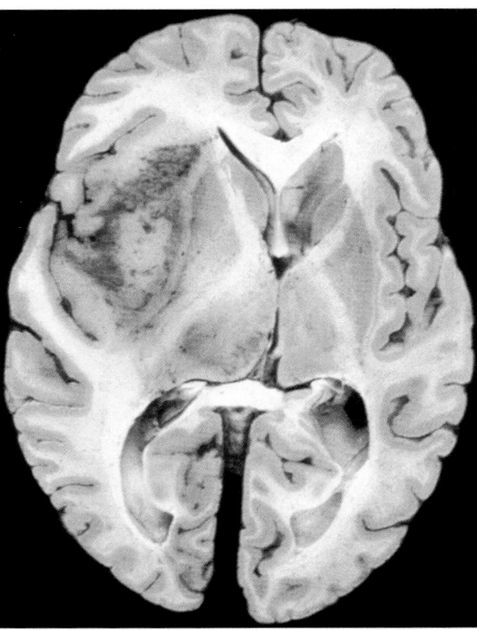

**Fig. 72.3 Glioblastoma (Cut in Axial Imaging Plane).** This patient's right hemispheric glioblastoma demonstrates central necrosis, a deceptively demarcated hyperemic rim (endothelial hyperplasia), and an infiltrative component that extends well beyond the grossly discernible margins (note expansion of right thalamus, with blurring of gray/white junctions).

## Glioblastoma (WHO Grade IV)

Glioblastoma (previously known as *glioblastoma multiforme*) is the most common malignant primary brain tumor in adults, accounting for approximately 80% of all infiltrating gliomas. The peak age at onset is 50–60 years. Unfortunately, several decades of basic and clinical research have had little impact on the clinical outcomes of glioblastoma, and average survival remains at approximately 1–1.5 years following radiation therapy and chemotherapy. Most glioblastomas arise de novo—primary glioblastomas—in a fully malignant state, while a minority emerges from lower-grade (WHO grade II or III) astrocytomas (secondary glioblastomas).

Glioblastoma most commonly occurs in the deep white matter, basal ganglia, or thalamus and is rarely found in the cerebellum or spinal cord. On imaging, these tumors typically present as an irregular ring of contrast enhancement, with a necrotic center, and significant edema. Gross and microscopic features are heterogeneous. Replacing the affected portion of the brain is a single mass that may grossly appear deceptively well circumscribed but microscopically infiltrates widely, often spreading to the opposite hemisphere via the corpus callosum (butterfly glioblastoma). Multifocal tumors may occur and, in some cases, they likely represent separate regions of malignant transformation within a widely disseminated astrocytoma. In advanced stages, the tumor may extend into the meninges or the ventricles. Seeding of the neuraxis as multiple implants on the brain or ventricular surfaces is an atypical growth pattern, and extracranial metastases are extremely rare. Glioblastomas exhibit a variegated appearance (Fig. 72.3) characterized by central yellow or white

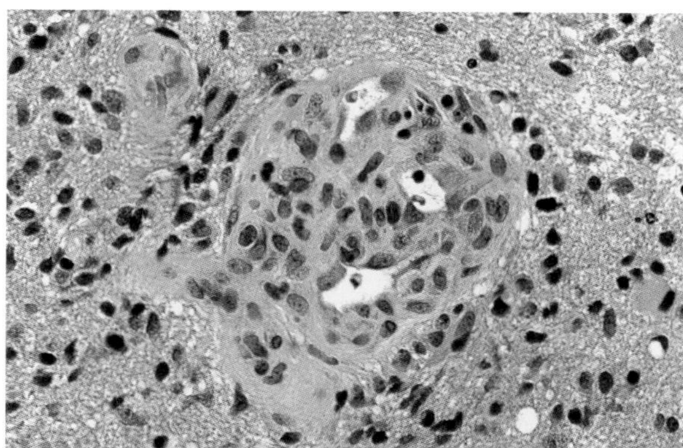

**Fig. 72.4 Glioblastoma.** Focus of endothelial hyperplasia with glomeruloid multilayered vessel (hematoxylin-eosin stain, ×400).

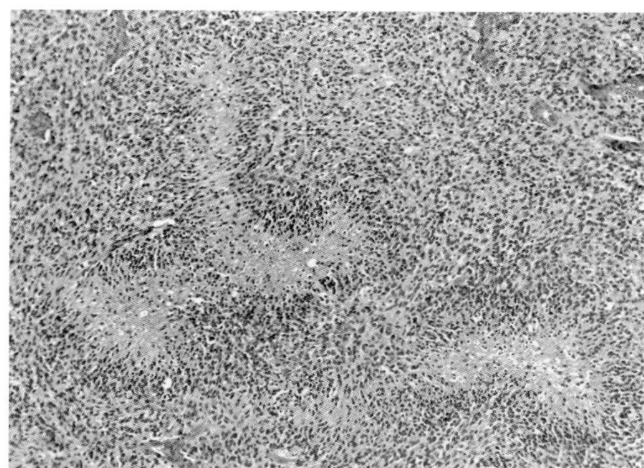

**Fig. 72.5 Glioblastoma.** Nuclear pseudopalisading surrounding foci of central necrosis (hematoxylin-eosin stain, ×100).

zones of necrosis and hemorrhage surrounded by a hyperemic ring (endothelial hyperplasia) and "edematous" brain with variable mixtures of vasogenic edema, gliosis, and tumor infiltrates. Microscopically characterizing glioblastomas are all the features of anaplastic astrocytoma plus endothelial hyperplasia or necrosis. Endothelial hyperplasia is defined as thickened or glomeruloid vessels with multilayering (Fig. 72.4), representing a form of tumor-induced angiogenesis. The necrosis is often associated with a characteristic serpiginous distribution and associated nuclear pseudopalisading (Fig. 72.5). Several histological variants exist, including giant cell glioblastoma, small-cell glioblastoma, and gliosarcoma. Characteristic of the latter is a sarcomatous element, currently felt to arise most likely from mesenchymal metaplasia within a glioblastoma. No significant clinical differences are identifiable in these variants when compared with conventional glioblastoma. However, some histological variants are associated with specific molecular alterations, which may have diagnostic or therapeutic relevance.

## Diffuse Midline Glioma (WHO Grade IV)

This recently defined disease entity includes midline infiltrating astrocytomas (thalamus, brainstem, and spinal cord) that occur in children and younger adults, including the majority of tumors previously designated "diffuse intrinsic pontine glioma" (DIPG). Histologically, these tumors frequently present with features of high-grade infiltrating astrocytomas or glioblastomas. However, traditional histological grading has been eliminated in the diagnosis of these tumors, given its poor correlation with tumor behavior. Diffuse midline gliomas are defined by the pathogenic *K27M* mutation involving genes encoding histone 3 monomers (H3-K27M; see below) and correspond to WHO grade IV, regardless of the presence/absence of histological features classically associated with grade IV tumors (i.e., increased mitotic activity, vascular proliferation, and necrosis). This represents the first example, in the WHO classification system for CNS tumors, of a molecular alteration replacing histological features as criteria for predicting tumor behavior. However, the diagnosis itself is predicated on the tumor in question being a diffusely infiltrating glioma arising in the midline, as very recent literature has identified H3-K27M mutations in other tumor types (e.g., pilocytic astrocytoma) characterized by less aggressive clinical course (Hochart et al., 2015; Orillac et al., 2016).

## Molecular Characteristics of Infiltrating Gliomas

As alluded to earlier, extensive molecular profiling has greatly clarified the molecular foundations of infiltrating glioma. In particular, a defined set of highly recurrent molecular alterations appear to transcend histopathological distinctions and have been incorporated into the diagnosis of more biologically uniform disease entities. The striking biological distinctions between primary glioblastoma and its lower-grade counterparts are most notably delineated by the presence or absence of point mutations in *IDH1/IDH2*, which occur in 70%–90% of astrocytomas and in 100% of oligodendrogliomas as currently defined (Yan et al., 2009). In this way, *IDH1/IDH2* mutations represent a defining molecular alteration segregating rapidly progressive infiltrating glioma from more indolent variants. Indeed, glioma patients with *IDH*-mutant tumors are younger and exhibit longer overall survival than those with *IDH*-wild-type tumors, with the latter distinction appearing to transcend conventional WHO grading. IDH proteins are metabolic enzymes that normally convert isocitrate to α-ketoglutarate as core components of the citric acid cycle. Glioma-associated *IDH* mutations alter enzymatic activity such that large amounts of the metabolite D-2-hydroxyglutarate (D-2-HG) are generated (Dang et al., 2009). While many of the downstream effects of D-2-HG accumulation remain unclear, it has been shown to dramatically alter cellular epigenomes and DNA methylation profiles. In particular, *IDH* mutation is sufficient to generate the so-called CpG island hypermethylator phenotype (G-CIMP) seen in *IDH*-mutant gliomas (Turcan et al., 2012).

Additional highly recurrent molecular alterations almost invariably co-occur with *IDH1/IDH2* mutations. By definition, oligodendrogliomas exhibit 1p/19q codeletion, which has been associated with both prolonged survival and a favorable response to cytotoxic therapy in both WHO grade III (Cairncross et al., 1998; Kaloshi et al., 2007) and WHO grade II variants (Kaloshi et al., 2007). Two of the likely tumor suppressors targeted by 1p/19q codeletion—*CIC* on chromosome 19q and *FUBP1* on chromosome 1p—were identified by high-throughput sequencing approaches (Bettegowda et al., 2011; Yip et al., 2012a, 2012b). Oligodendrogliomas also harbor activating mutations in the promoter region of the *TERT* gene, which encodes the catalytic core of the telomerase enzyme, in virtually all cases (Killela et al., 2013). In contrast to oligodendrogliomas, astrocytomas have long been associated with mutations in *TP53* and/or chromosome 17p losses (Louis, 2006). More recently, loss-of-function mutations in *ATRX* have also been identified in >70% of *IDH*-mutant tumors without 1p/19q codeletion (Jiao et al., 2012; Kannan et al., 2012). Therefore, the vast majority of *IDH*-mutant gliomas appear to harbor either 1p/19q codeletion and *TERT* mutation or *TP53* and *ATRX* mutations, with almost complete mutual exclusivity.

Early data indicate that 1p/19q-codeleted tumors are associated with longer overall survival than their *TP53/ATRX*-mutant counterparts, with both *IDH*-mutant variants exhibiting considerably better outcomes than *IDH*-wild-type gliomas (Brat et al., 2015; Jiao et al., 2012;

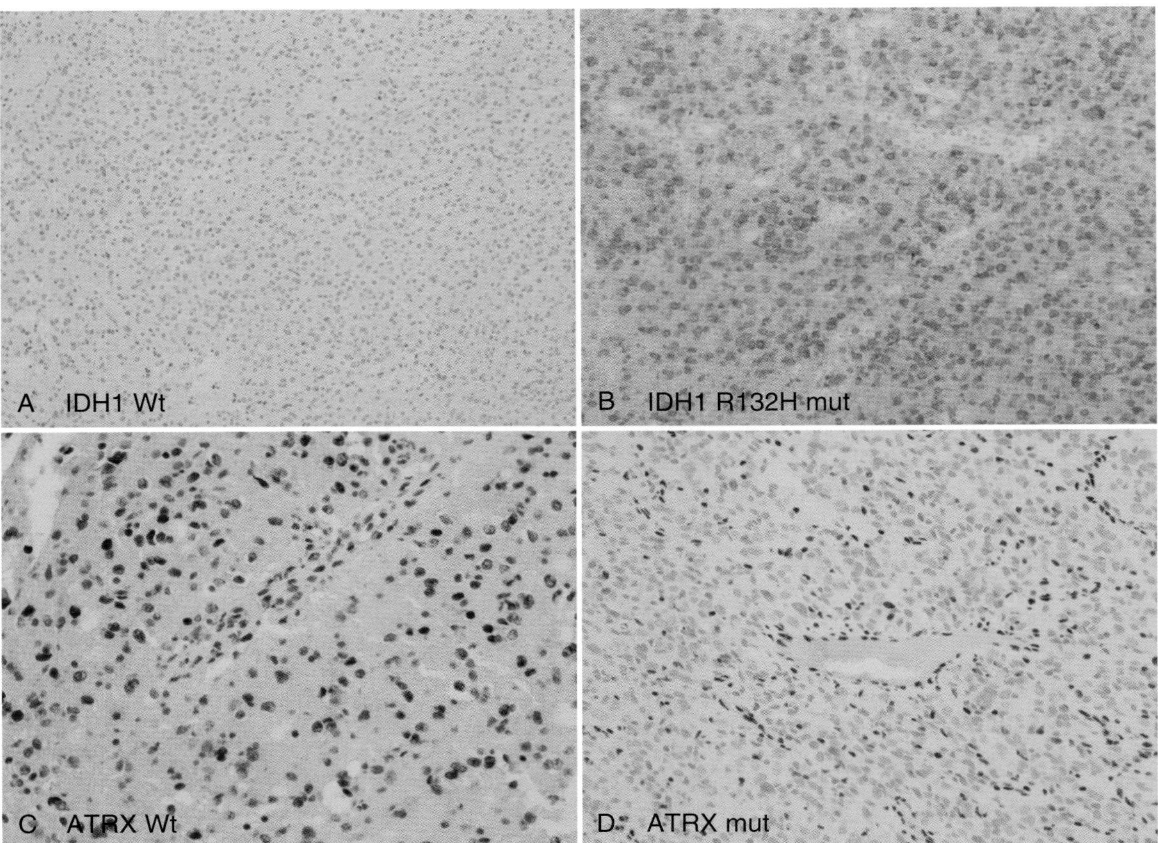


**Fig. 72.6** Immunohistochemical biomarkers for diffuse glioma. **A** and **B**, IDH1 R132H immunostaining in wild type (Wt; **A**; ×100) and mutant (mut; **B**; ×200) gliomas. **C** and **D**, ATRX immunostaining in wild type (Wt; **C**; ×200) and mutant (mut; **D**; ×200) gliomas.

Wiestler et al., 2013). Moreover, these distinctions appear to be more marked than those stratified by conventional histopathology alone. Thus, assessments of *IDH1/IDH2*, *TP53*, and *ATRX* mutations, along with 1p/19q codeletion, carry clinical relevance, and should be obtained whenever possible. Fortunately, rapid immunohistochemical assays exist for the detection of the most common *IDH* mutation (IDH1 p. R132H; Fig. 72.6, *A*), nuclear p53 accumulation (which frequently co-occurs with *IDH1/IDH2* mutation), and ATRX deficiency (see Fig. 72.6, *B*), and well-validated methodologies, most commonly FISH-based, are widely used for 1p/19q analysis.

Primary glioblastomas often harbor numerous cytogenetic and molecular genetic aberrations with frequent involvement of core components in the PI3K/MAPK, p16/CDK4/RB, and p53 signaling networks (Brennan et al., 2013). Promoter mutations in TERT, identical to those found in oligodendrogliomas, are also common (Killela et al., 2013). Mutations in *IDH1*, *IDH2*, and *ATRX* are rarely seen. Instead, 30%–40% of primary glioblastomas harbor *EGFR* amplifications, often with an associated constitutively activating mutation (Louis et al., 2001). *EGFR* amplifications are also particularly common (≈70%) in the small-cell histopathological variant of glioblastoma. Alterations of the p16/CDK4/RB pathway are nearly universal in glioblastoma, and many cases harbor chromosome 10 loss. Moreover, the *PTEN* gene on chromosome 10q23 is mutated in a subset of these. The list of additional glioblastoma-associated alterations is growing rapidly. Recent large-scale sequencing studies have shown that glioblastomas harbor somatic mutations of multiple genes (Brennan et al., 2013). These studies have confirmed the incidence of mutated and/or amplified genes such as *EGFR*, *PTEN*, *RB1*, and *PIK3CA* and showed higher prevalence for mutations in *TP53*, *NF1*, and *PIK3R1*, as well as new candidate genes involved in tumorigenesis.

Methylation of the *MGMT* gene promoter has emerged as a prognostic and predictive biomarker in glioblastoma. MGMT is a DNA repair enzyme, and promoter methylation leads to downregulation of expression, presumably reducing the capacity of tumor cells to correct DNA damage caused by cytotoxic chemotherapy. Patients whose tumors harbor MGMT promoter methylation demonstrate improved survival following treatment with the alkylating agent temozolomide (Hegi et al., 2005). Furthermore, resistance to alkylating chemotherapy in glioblastoma is associated with therapy-related inactivation of MSH6, a DNA mismatch repair enzyme, allowing increased mutagenesis and the emergence of a hypermutated phenotype (Cahill et al., 2007; Yip et al., 2009). Similar observations have been made recently for WHO grade II astrocytoma (Johnson et al., 2014).

Finally, recent sequencing studies have identified mutations in genes encoding for H3.3 core histone proteins—*H3F3A* and *HIST1H3B*—as highly recurrent in aggressive gliomas arising most often in the pediatric population (Schwartzentruber et al., 2012; Wu et al., 2012). Intriguingly, these mutations invariably involve amino acid residues either at or close to sites of post-translational modification in the histone tail known to impact associated gene expression, suggesting the potential for epigenomic consequences. Subsequent data have confirmed this conjecture, with H3.3-mutant tumors demonstrating unique gene methylation profiles and globally altered patterns of histone modification (Sturm et al., 2012). Additionally,

H3.3 mutations frequently co-occur with *ATRX* and *TP53* mutations, suggesting pathogenic parallels with adult gliomas. *TERT* mutations are uncommon. Striking correlations between tumor location and precise H3.3 mutation exist in these tumors. As described above, diffuse midline gliomas, are defined by the H3-K27M mutation; by contrast, hemispheric pediatric glioblastomas frequently (~30%) harbor the H3-G34R or H3-G34V mutations. A specific antibody targeting the H3-K27M mutant epitope has greatly facilitated the diagnosis of diffuse midline glioma (Fig. 72.7).

## Other Glial and Glioneuronal Tumors

A broad spectrum of glial and glioneuronal tumors impact pediatric and adult populations at lower rates than infiltrating gliomas. Many of these tumor variants are characterized by relatively indolent growth and discrete demarcation, although some can widely permeate surrounding brain. In general, clinical outcome associated with these tumors compares favorably to that seen in infiltrating gliomas. Molecular profiles are also distinct from those described above for astrocytomas, oligodendrogliomas, and glioblastomas, exhibiting high rates of abnormalities in *FGFR1/2*, *BRAF*, and other *MAPK* signaling pathway constituents. Finally, several of these morphologically diverse tumor types are strongly associated with seizure activity, and the broad designation "LEAT" (long-term epilepsy associated tumor) has been used to describe their functional intersection (Blumcke et al., 2014). While the precise classification of tumors within this group remains a work in progress, several entities are well established (see below).

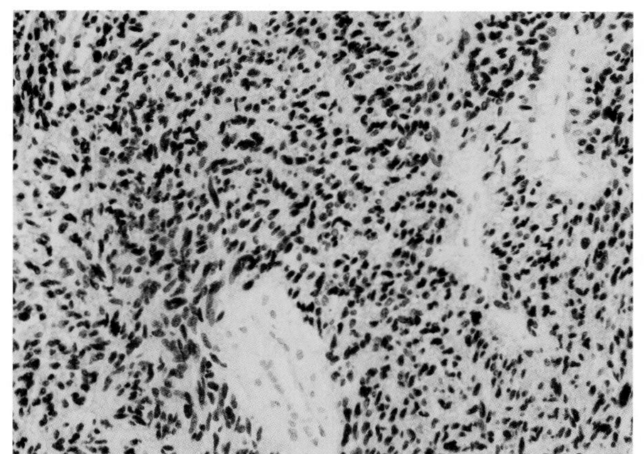

**Fig. 72.7** H3-K27M immunostaining in a mutant protein-expressing diffuse midline glioma (×200).

### Pilocytic Astrocytoma (WHO Grade I)

Usually, pilocytic astrocytomas are well-circumscribed tumors, both grossly and radiographically, although limited degrees of microscopic infiltration are not unusual. They arise in both children and adults, and are more common in the cerebellum, hypothalamus, third ventricle, optic nerve, spinal cord, and dorsal brainstem but may also involve the cerebrum. The adjective *juvenile* often added to pilocytic astrocytoma is misleading because most adult cases are histologically and clinically indistinguishable from their pediatric counterparts. Outcome depends on the surgical accessibility of the tumor but is usually excellent (80% 20-year survival), and many are curable with resection alone. Gross appearance varies somewhat with anatomical location. Cerebellar tumors, which are often hemispheric, are typically composed of a large fluid-filled cyst with an enhancing mural nodule. Hypothalamic and optic nerve tumors are usually solid. Optic nerve gliomas appear as a focal segmental nerve swelling. Both unilateral and bilateral optic nerve gliomas are particularly common in NF1 patients, a setting in which most tumors are indolent and do not progress to a point requiring surgical intervention.

The distinctive histological feature of pilocytic astrocytoma is a biphasic pattern with compact pilocytic areas interspersed with microcystic, spongy, or loose areas (Fig. 72.8). Dense portions contain piloid (hairlike) or bipolar astrocytes with long spindle-shaped processes. *Rosenthal fibers* are common. These are aggregates of intracellular astrocytic filaments, fusiform or corkscrew shaped, with a hyaline appearance (see Fig. 72.8, *A*). In addition, mulberry-shaped eosinophilic granular bodies (EGBs) also occur in most cases (see Fig. 72.8, *B*). Although not entirely specific, both Rosenthal fibers and EGBs are generally signs of an indolent process and represent important diagnostic clues that distinguish pilocytic astrocytoma from diffuse astrocytoma or glioblastoma. *NF1* gene inactivation occurs in NF1-associated pilocytic astrocytomas but is much less common in sporadic examples. Instead, most (~70%) pilocytic astrocytomas are characterized by a unique *KIAA1549:BRAF* fusion protein that serves as a constitutively active BRAF isoform (Jones et al., 2008). Additional *BRAF* fusion events and the known oncogenic *BRAF* p. V600E mutation are also found in lower percentages of tumors. Finally, mutations in *FGFR1* and *PTPN11*, along with *NTRK2* fusion genes, have been identified in small subsets of pilocytic astrocytoma (Jones et al., 2013).

Pilomyxoid astrocytoma is a variant of pilocytic astrocytoma that was historically associated with more aggressive behavior corresponding to WHO grade II. This tumor mainly affects children younger than 3 years of age and occurs predominantly in the hypothalamic region. The most recent WHO classification of CNS tumors in 2016 recommends not grading pilomyxoid astrocytomas. It is now believed that the more

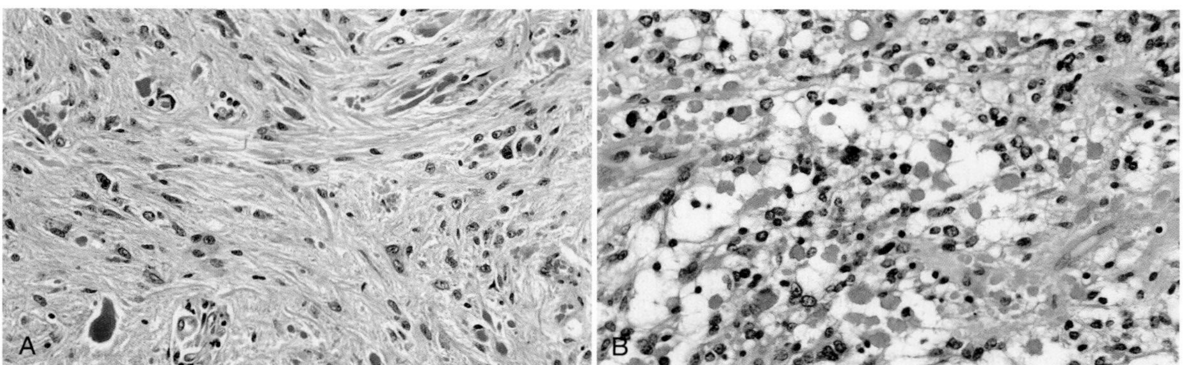


**Fig. 72.8 Pilocytic Astrocytoma.** Classic examples are biphasic with dense (**A**) and loose (**B**) regions. Helpful markers include bright red corkscrew-shaped Rosenthal fibers (**A**) and mulberry-shaped eosinophilic granular bodies (**B**) (hematoxylin-eosin stain, ×200).

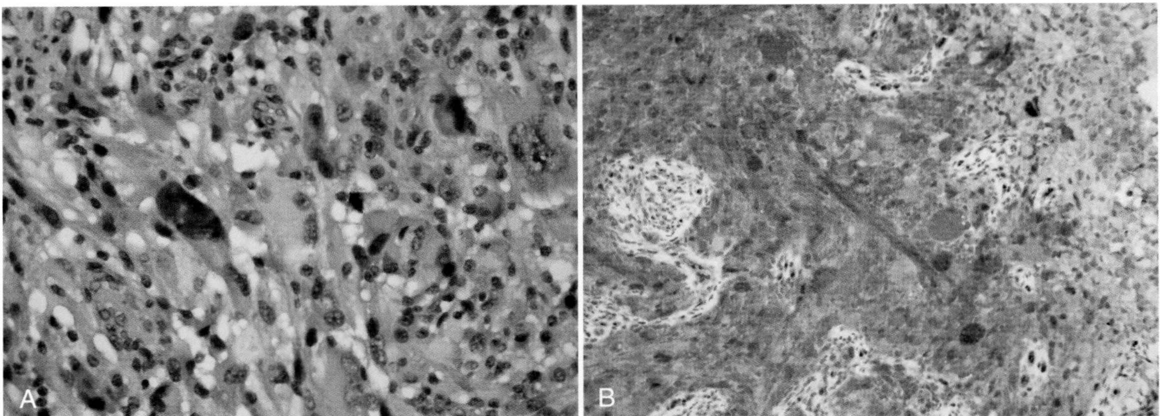


**Fig. 72.9** Pleomorphic Xanthoastrocytoma (PXA). **A,** Haphazardly arranged, bizarrely pleomorphic tumor cells with astrocytic features (hematoxylin-eosin stain, ×200). **B,** Positive immunostaining for BRAF V600E in a PXA (×200).

unfavorable course associated with pilomyxoid histology might reflect the limitations of obtaining complete surgical resection in the hypothalamic region rather than more inherently aggressive tumor biology. Pilomyxoid astrocytoma lacks a biphasic appearance and Rosenthal fibers but shows piloid cells, often with an angiocentric arrangement in a myxoid matrix. EGBs are often rare or absent.

### Pleomorphic Xanthoastrocytoma (WHO Grade II–III)

PXA is a rare and distinctive astrocytic neoplasm associated with a favorable prognosis and has often been misdiagnosed in the past as glioblastoma due to its marked cellular pleomorphism. The average age at diagnosis is 26 years, and a history of seizures often precedes diagnosis (Giannini et al., 1999). PXA usually involves the cerebral cortex and overlying meninges, and the preferred site is the temporal lobe. Histological features include hypercellularity and many atypical and pleomorphic tumor astrocytes (Fig. 72.9, *A*). Bizarre giant cells are present, but mitoses are unusual. Probably the most helpful pathological finding is that of EGBs, since these do not occur in glioblastomas. Despite its name, xanthomatous cells (lipidized astrocytes) with foamy lipid-filled cytoplasm only occur in approximately one-fourth of cases. PXA has a relatively favorable prognosis (WHO grade II), with postoperative survival averaging 81% at 5 years and 70% at 10 years. However, it is estimated that 15%–20% of these tumors undergo malignant transformation (WHO grade III) and are associated with an aggressive clinical course. When fully malignant, PXAs often acquire a discohesive cellular architecture, reminiscent of malignant epithelioid neoplasms like melanoma, and are often classified as "epithelioid glioblastoma." Recent studies have shown that *BRAF* p.V600E mutations occur in the majority of PXAs (see Fig. 72.9, *B*), whether WHO grade II or III, emphasizing the importance of the MAPK signaling pathway in the pathogenesis of these tumors (Schindler et al., 2011).

### Subependymal Giant Cell Astrocytoma (WHO Grade I)

Most subependymal giant cell astrocytomas (SEGAs) are associated with tuberous sclerosis, and the suggestion is that SEGA patients lacking other features of tuberous sclerosis have a *forme fruste* of this disorder. An elongated, sausage-like, or lobulated gross appearance is typical. Histologically identical smaller masses resembling candle gutterings (the drippings of tallow from a burning candle) on the wall of the lateral ventricle are common in tuberous sclerosis–associated cases. Hydrocephalus may result secondary to obstruction of the foramen of Monro.

The rich vascularity of the tumor gives the cut surfaces a red and beefy appearance. Calcification is almost invariable and is at times so extensive that the mass has the consistency of stone. SEGAs are moderately cellular, consisting of closely packed astrocytes with abundant cytoplasm. Tumor cells often sweep in fascicles or around blood vessels, analogous to the pseudorosettes in ependymomas. Some SEGAs may have a gemistocyte-like or spindled morphology.

Some tumor cells are clearly of astrocytic origin, and GFAP fills the cytoplasm. Other tumor cells resemble neurons having prominent nucleoli, and many have intermediate features with astrocytoma-like cytoplasm and neuronal-like nuclei. Positive immunohistochemical staining for neuronal markers further suggests neuronal differentiation. Tumor cells may stain with both neuronal and glial markers or with neither, explaining the preference of some neuropathologists for the term *subependymal giant cell tumor* rather than SEGA. These tumors are related to alterations in the *TSC1* (hamartin) and *TSC2* (tuberin) genes and thus involve aberrant signaling through downstream growth-regulatory pathways.

### Ganglioglioma/Gangliocytoma (WHO Grade I or III)

Most gangliogliomas occur before age 21 and comprise 4%–8% of all pediatric brain tumors. Gangliogliomas grow slowly and tend to show benign biological and clinical behavior. The most common site of involvement is the temporal lobe, and seizures are a typical presenting symptom. Other lobes of the cerebral hemispheres, cerebellum, and spinal cord are less often affected. Tumors are often cystic and well circumscribed, extending to the surface of the brain. Solid portions are firm, gray, and gritty due to calcium deposits that are evident on computed tomography (CT) scans.

Portions of the tumor resemble a low-grade astrocytoma, either pilocytic or fibrillary in nature. Unlike native entrapped neurons within an infiltrative glioma, some of the tumor ganglion cells have a dysmorphic appearance, as evidenced by their lack of polarity, clustering, cytoplasmic vacuolation, increased nuclear pleomorphism, or multinucleation (Fig. 72.10). Binucleate or multinucleate neurons are particularly helpful for diagnostic purposes when present. Otherwise, the most useful features to distinguish this tumor from diffuse gliomas include relative circumscription and eosinophilic granular bodies. Perivascular lymphocytic cuffing, microcystic spaces, and fibrosis with collagen deposition are other common findings. Rosenthal fibers are common, particularly at the edges of the lesion. Those without an obvious astrocytic component are sometimes referred to as *gangliocytoma*, although it is not yet clear that this distinction has any clinical relevance. The term *ganglion cell tumor* is less specific and incorporates both entities. Rare cases demonstrate signs of anaplasia (grade III), almost invariably in the glial component, but grading criteria and their predictive value have yet to be firmly established. GFAP expression is abundant in the astrocytic component, whereas the ganglion cell component expresses most markers of mature neurons such as synaptophysin, chromogranin, neurofilament, and NeuN. While the molecular basis of these tumors remains unclear, a significant minority has been shown to harbor *BRAF* V600E mutations (Schindler et al., 2011). Mutations in other genes involved in the MAPK pathway such as *KRAS, NF1*, and *FGFR1/FGFR2*, have also been associated with gangliogliomas. The recently described multinodular and vacuolating neuronal tumor (VNT) may represent a unique morphological variant of gangliocytoma, and is also characterized by mutations in genes encoding MAP kinase pathway effectors (e.g., *MAP2K1, BRAF*) (Huse et al., 2013; Pekmezci et al., 2018).

### Dysembryoplastic Neuroepithelial Tumor (WHO Grade I)

Dysembryoplastic neuroepithelial tumor (DNT) is a benign hamartomatous-like tumor with an excellent prognosis. DNTs occur throughout childhood and early adulthood, with a mean age at diagnosis of 9 years. These tumors are usually supratentorial and intracortical in location and are often associated with a long history of intractable seizures. The temporal lobe is the most common location for DNTs, although histologically similar tumors occur in rarer sites such as the basal ganglia, thalamus, lateral ventricle, septum pellucidum, and brainstem. DNTs are well-demarcated, multinodular, intracortical growths that may be associated with adjacent cortical dysplasia.

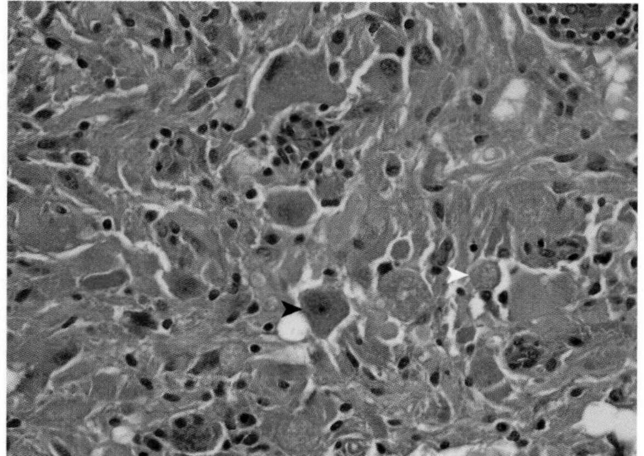

**Fig. 72.10 Ganglioglioma.** Abnormally clustered neoplastic ganglion cells *(black arrowhead)* admixed with eosinophilic granular bodies (*white arrowhead;* perivascular lymphocytic cuffing is also evident (*green arrowhead;* hematoxylin-eosin stain, ×200).

Histologically, there is a wide range of appearances, although the most characteristic features include patterned (i.e., with ribbons or arcades), mucin-rich, cortical nodules, and "floating neurons," the latter consisting of ganglion cells that appear to float within a lacune-like mucin-filled space (Fig. 72.11). The cytology of the tumor cells varies, although most resemble oligodendroglioma cells. In fact, on a small biopsy, it may be virtually impossible to distinguish these two entities, but the presence of diffuse cortical invasion on larger samples argues against a diagnosis of DNT. Moreover, unlike oligodendrogliomas, DNTs do not carry 1p/19q codeletion. Recent work indicates that DNTs are highly enriched for FGFR1 fusions and mutations at the molecular level (Qaddoumi et al., 2016).

### Rare Glioneuronal Tumors

*Papillary glioneuronal tumor* is possibly a ganglioglioma variant. These tumors are generally located in the cerebral hemispheres, particularly the temporal lobe, and have a characteristic pseudopapillary appearance conferred by single-layered cuboidal glial cells ensheathing fibrovascular cores with interpapillary aggregates of neurocytic and/or ganglioid cells. They correspond to WHO grade I.

*Rosette-forming glioneuronal tumor (RFGNT) of the fourth ventricle* is a very rare entity found in the posterior fossa, usually presenting with obstructive hydrocephalus. It is a biphasic tumor with a predominant glial component, often resembling pilocytic astrocytoma, and a neurocytic component comprising uniform cells forming neurocytic rosettes or perivascular pseudorosettes. Neurocytic rosettes surround a neuropil center that can be highlighted with antibodies against synaptophysin. RFGNTs frequently harbor mutations in *PIK3CA* and *FGFR1*, often concurrently in the same tumor (Kitamura et al., 2018). They correspond to WHO grade I.

## Ependymal Neoplasms

Ependymal neoplasms are thought to arise from specialized neuroepithelial cells lining the ventricular wall. Their neuraxial distribution, histopathological features, molecular characteristics, and biological behavior vary widely depending on precise disease variant.

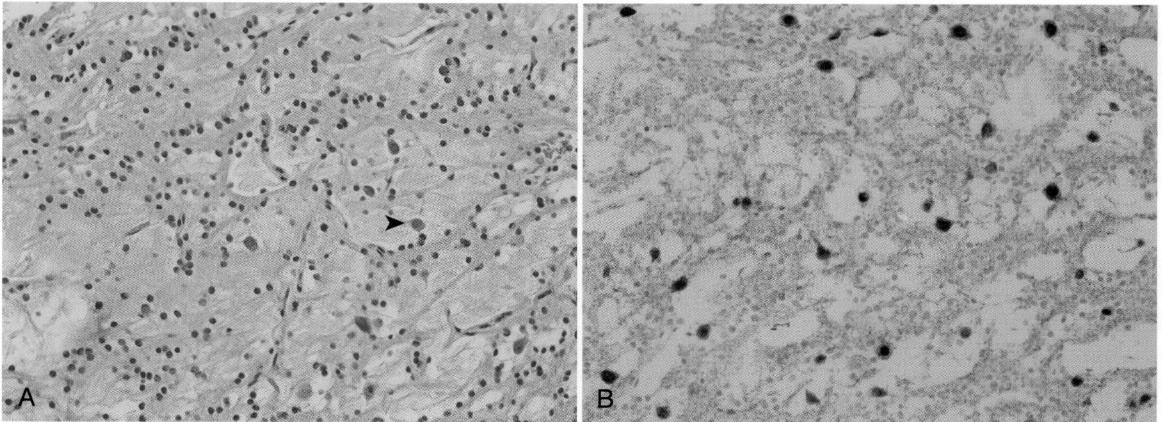


**Fig. 72.11 Dysembryoplastic Neuroepithelial Tumor.** Classic architecture consisting of oligodendroglioma-like cells arranged in mucin-filled spaces along with "floating neurons" (**A**; hematoxylin-eosin stain, ×200), the latter highlighted by NeuN immunostaining (**B**; ×200).

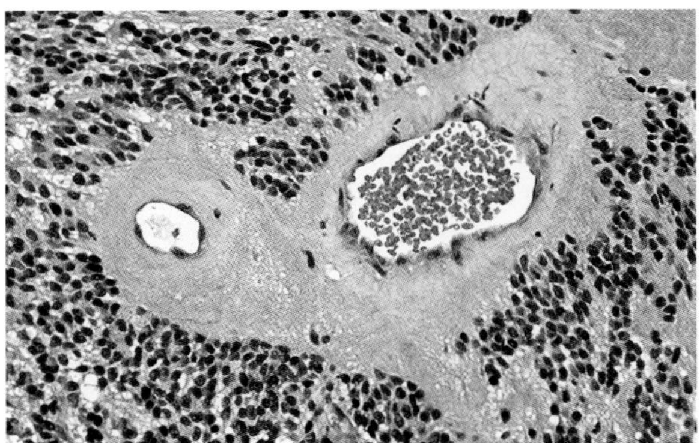

**Fig. 72.12 Ependymoma.** Perivascular pseudorosette characterized by a fibrillary-appearing perivascular nuclear-free zone (hematoxylin-eosin stain, ×200).

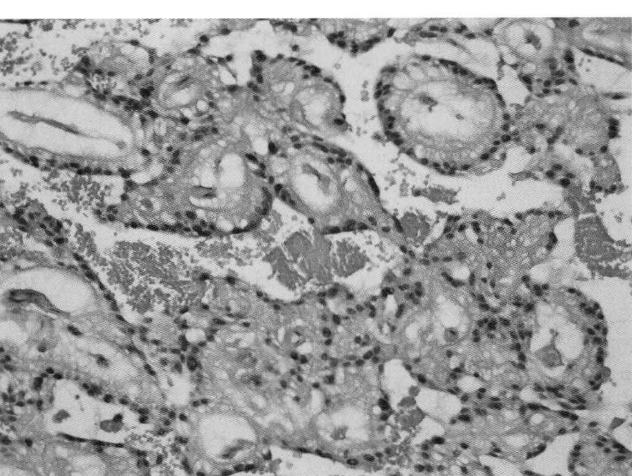

**Fig. 72.13 Myxopapillary Ependymoma.** Bland tumor cells arranged around blood vessels and myxoid material in a pseudopapillary architecture (hematoxylin-eosin stain, ×200).

## Ependymoma (WHO Grade II–III)

Ependymomas comprise 4% of all brain tumors and are the third most common CNS tumors in children. They may occur at any age but are most frequent in the first decade; patients younger than age 3 years have a significantly worse prognosis. Ninety percent of tumors are in the brain, with infratentorial sites twice as common a supratentorial sites, and 10% are in the spinal cord, often in adults. The typical infratentorial ependymoma occupies the fourth ventricle. Noncommunicating hydrocephalus develops when tumors are large enough to obstruct the flow of cerebrospinal fluid (CSF). On the other hand, these tumors may be periventricular or may not have any obvious association with native ependyma (e.g., spinal cord, cerebral hemispheres).

Ependymomas are usually well-circumscribed masses that tend to compress rather than infiltrate the adjacent parenchyma. As such, some cases may be surgically curable, and the extent of resection constitutes a much more important prognostic variable in ependymomas than in diffuse gliomas. Ependymomas in contact with CSF pathways may seed the subarachnoid space and generate drop metastases in approximately 5% of cases, a condition associated with a poor prognosis. The characteristic features of ependymomas are sheets of cells interrupted by perivascular pseudorosettes, nuclear free zones surrounding a central blood vessel (Fig. 72.12). True ependymal rosettes (i.e., containing a central lumen) and canals (i.e., slit-like structures resembling small ventricles) are even more specific but only occur in approximately 10% of cases.

Ependymoma is one of the few remaining tumors in which ultrastructural examination verifies the diagnosis in morphologically ambiguous cases. Electron microscopy shows a combined glial and epithelial-like appearance with intermediate filaments, microvilli, zipper-like intercellular junctions, intracellular lumina, cilia, and their basal attachments, known as *basal bodies* or *blepharoplasts*. Immunohistochemistry for GFAP may be particularly helpful in highlighting the thin processes radiating toward vessels in pseudorosettes, and dot-like cytoplasmic inclusions may be highlighted with EMA, CD99, and D2-40 immunostains, although none of these markers are entirely specific. Establishing the diagnosis of anaplastic ependymoma (grade III) requires hypercellularity, increased mitotic activity, and microvascular proliferation, although the clinical significance of these features remains controversial. In fact, histological grading of ependymomas may be abandoned altogether in future classification schemes, as disease outcomes appear to depend much more on molecular rather than morphological characteristics.

Ependymomas are often aneuploid, exhibiting a variety of complex, albeit nonspecific, alterations. Chromosome 22q deletions are among the most common, with associated *NF2* mutations primarily restricted to spinal ependymomas, a fact that fits with the spinal location of most ependymomas in NF2 patients (Singh et al., 2002). Other 22q tumor suppressors are likely, and the existence of many additional ependymoma-associated genes is expected. Multiple studies have shown that gene expression profiling delineates subgroups of ependymoma that also exhibit shared patterns of DNA copy number alterations, sites of origin (i.e., supratentorial, posterior fossa, or spinal ependymoma), and age of onset (Johnson et al., 2010; Witt et al., 2011). Recently, transcriptional signatures have been found to specify two distinct subgroups of posterior fossa ependymoma, further distinguished by their extent of genomic alterations, age of onset, and clinical performance. Interestingly, one of these subgroups, consisting of more aggressive tumors occurring in younger patients, appears to be entirely driven by epigenomic alterations that include widespread DNA hypermethylation (Mack et al., 2014). Additionally, a large percentage of supratentorial ependymomas in children have been found to harbor *C11orf95-RELA* fusions events, the presence of which is associated with unfavorable prognosis. *C11orf95-RELA* fusion activates oncogenic nuclear factor kappa B (NF-kB) signaling downstream, pointing to strategies for therapeutic intervention (Parker et al., 2014).

## Myxopapillary Ependymoma (WHO Grade II)

Myxopapillary ependymoma is a distinct variant that is virtually restricted to the filum terminale. These tumors may also occur in the presacral soft tissue. Myxopapillary ependymomas are more common in adults than in children, tend to be red because of their rich vascularity, and are sometimes frankly hemorrhagic and gelatinous in their gross appearance. Typically surrounding the tumor is a thin collagenous capsule. These tumors have a variable papillary architecture, with numerous hyalinized vessels surrounded by mucin and an outer layer of tumor cells (Fig. 72.13). Prognosis can be excellent, particularly when tumor is resected with its collagenous tumor capsule intact. Tumors taken out piecemeal with mucin spillage have a higher likelihood of subsequent recurrence with seeding of the spinal cord and significant associated morbidity. Soft-tissue myxopapillary ependymomas may metastasize to the lungs or other sites, despite their benign appearance. Other tumors that may present as cauda equina masses include meningiomas, schwannomas, metastatic lesions (from either hematogenous or CSF dissemination), and paragangliomas. *Paraganglioma* is a neuroendocrine neoplasm arising from the autonomic nervous system, rarely in the filum terminale but often in other systemic sites. Usually

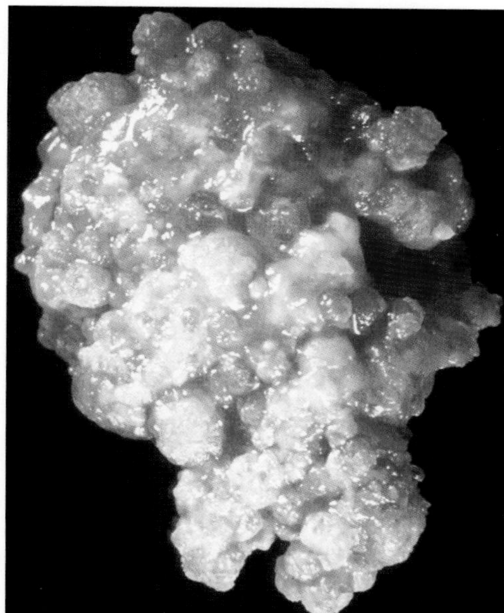

**Fig. 72.14 Choroid Plexus Papilloma.** Polypoid or cauliflower-like lesion with a nodular and partially calcified surface, taken from the fourth ventricle.

these tumors present in the cauda equina, with symptoms related to mass effect. Histologically they may mimic ependymoma and metastatic carcinoma but have a characteristic immunohistochemical profile (with chromogranin staining of the packed cells and S100 positivity of the surrounding sustentacular cells), permitting accurate distinction. Complete excision is usually curative.

### Subependymoma (WHO Grade I)

Subependymomas are slow-growing tumors often detected by MRI in the absence of clinical manifestations; 90% of subependymomas occur in adults, where they are small and incidental. Subependymomas appear as glistening, pearly white, lobulated, intraventricular protuberances, most often in the fourth ventricle. Large tumors may obstruct the ventricle and cause noncommunicating hydrocephalus. Clusters of bland rounded nuclei embedded in a fibrillary matrix with microcysts and foci of calcification characterize these tumors microscopically. The proliferative index is typically low. Rare cases contain foci of classic ependymoma; these are named *mixed ependymoma/subependymoma*. These cases are graded and treated according to the potentially more aggressive ependymoma component. The histogenesis of subependymomas is still a matter of debate, with candidates including subependymal glia, astrocytes, ependymal cells, or some mixture of these. Genetic changes are largely unknown.

## Choroid Plexus Tumors

The choroid plexus is a specialized secretory epithelium that grows in papillary structures within the ventricular system and whose main function appears to be the production of cerebrospinal fluid. Tumors involving the choroid plexus can be either benign or malignant.

### Choroid Plexus Papilloma (WHO Grade I)

Choroid plexus papillomas (CPPs) comprise approximately 0.5% of all intracranial tumors. As a rule, the location of these tumors is solely in the portion of the ventricular system that contains normal choroid plexus. Approximately half are in the fourth ventricle, often occupying the cerebellopontine angle, typically in adults. Tumors in the lateral ventricle are more common in children and may cause hydrocephalus by a combination of outflow obstruction and excess CSF production. The onset of symptoms is usually in the first decade and may occur at birth (i.e., congenital). In most cases, papillomas are surgically curable tumors.

CPPs have a pink or red, highly vascular, polypoid or cauliflower appearance, often with chalky calcifications (Fig. 72.14). Large tumors in the third or fourth ventricle may occlude or even distend the ventricle, causing noncommunicating hydrocephalus. Histologically, CPPs resemble normal choroid plexus in terms of a well-formed papillary structure with true fibrovascular cores and, in most cases, a single-layered epithelial covering. However, the lining of papillomas lacks the cobblestone-like appearance of normal choroid plexus and instead tends to form a uniform layer of tall cuboidal to columnar cells without intervening spaces. Calcifications and clear intracytoplasmic vacuoles are common. The mitotic index is low. Immunohistochemically, these tumors are consistently positive for cytokeratin, sometimes revealing a paranuclear ball-like pattern of staining. Immunoreactivity for transthyretin/prealbumin is also typical. A subset of CPP expresses GFAP focally; this reflects ependymal differentiation. The majority of CPP are well-differentiated neoplasms (WHO grade I).

### Choroid Plexus Carcinoma (WHO Grade III)

The diagnosis of choroid plexus carcinoma in adults is exceedingly rare and first requires exclusion of metastatic adenocarcinoma, most often from the lung. Carcinoma of the choroid plexus tends to arise in the lateral ventricle of infants and then invades the adjacent brain parenchyma and seeds throughout the subarachnoid spaces. Systemic metastases occur occasionally. The clinical course is generally quite aggressive, and mortality rates are high.

Histologically, choroid plexus carcinoma resembles high-grade papillary adenocarcinoma but does not secrete mucin, an important distinction from the majority of metastatic adenocarcinomas. Some cases have a small-cell appearance reminiscent of embryonal tumors like medulloblastoma or rhabdoid cells similar to those of atypical teratoid/rhabdoid tumor (AT/RT) (see below). The genetics of these high-grade malignancies remains unknown, although the possible involvement of the *INI1/SMARCB1* gene on 22q11.2 has been raised. However, it remains possible that reported tumors with such genetic changes are really AT/RT. Choroid plexus carcinomas are observed in Li-Fraumeni syndrome kindreds (Wolburg & Paulus, 2010). In addition, sporadic choroid plexus carcinomas lacking a germline *TP53* mutation may have a more favorable prognosis (Tabori et al., 2010).

## Neurocytic Tumors

These tumors are so-named due to their cellular constituents, which morphologically and immunohistochemically resemble small, mature neurons.

### Central Neurocytoma (WHO Grade II)

Central neurocytomas are slow-growing tumors located in the lateral or third ventricle near the foramen of Monro, frequently involving the septum pellucidum. Age at diagnosis is usually in the second or third decade. They are usually sharply demarcated, sometimes lobulated masses that fill the ventricular space without significant infiltration of the surrounding brain.

The main histological feature is a proliferation of uniformly round tumor cells that mimic oligodendroglioma (Fig. 72.15, *A*). Unlike oligodendrogliomas, these tumors often display *neurocytic rosettes*, exaggerated or irregular Homer Wright–like rosettes with central axon-rich neuropil. These rosettes are indistinguishable from the pineocytic rosettes encountered in pineocytoma, another tumor of small mature

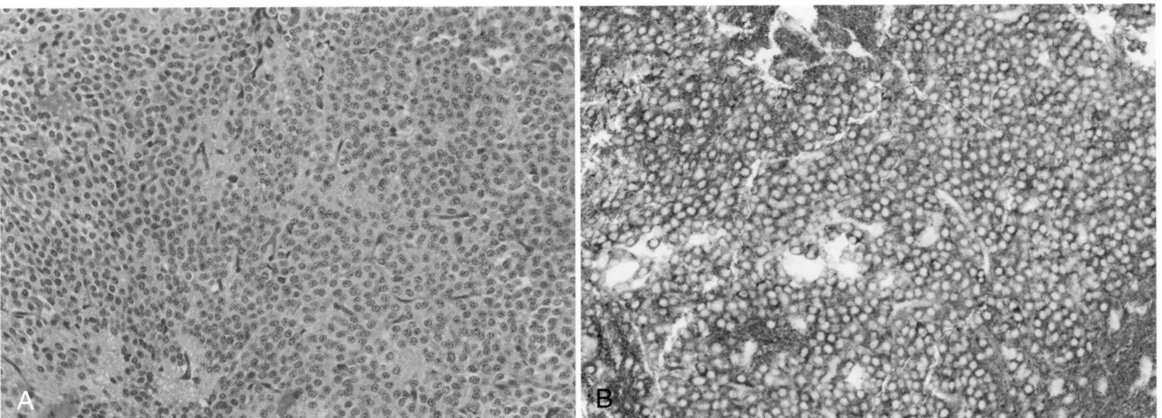

**Fig. 72.15 Central Neurocytoma. A,** Cellular neoplasm consisting of uniformly round tumor cells mimicking those of oligodendroglioma (hematoxylin-eosin stain, ×200). **B,** Immunostaining for synaptophysin is strongly positive (×200).

neurons, with similar cytological features to those of central neurocytomas. Ultrastructurally, their cytoplasm contains microtubules, synapses, and neurosecretory granules, belying their neuronal nature. Moreover, central neurocytomas are generally immunoreactive for the neuronal markers synaptophysin and NeuN (see Fig. 72.15, *B*). Central neurocytomas with elevated proliferative indices (e.g., >2%) and vascular hyperplasia tend to have a higher rate of recurrence and are sometimes referred to as *atypical neurocytomas*, although grading criteria have not been firmly established. Rare examples of extraventricular neurocytomas and liponeurocytomas (with fat metaplasia) occur in the cerebral hemispheres, cerebellum, and spinal cord, but it is yet to be determined whether these represent the same family of tumors. Extraventricular neurocytoma is now recognized as a similarly behaving counterpart to central neurocytoma. The WHO also recognizes the cerebellar liponeurocytoma as a distinct entity. The genetic alterations of neurocytoma are largely unknown; as expected, central neurocytomas do not harbor the 1p and 19q deletions seen in oligodendrogliomas.

## Embryonal Neoplasms

The term "embryonal" essentially refers to a "small round blue cell tumor" that in most cases shows evidence for primarily neuronal differentiation, albeit immature. Glial, mesenchymal, or melanotic elements may occur as well. Medulloblastoma represents the prototype embryonal neoplasm of the CNS. Other than medulloblastomas, embryonal tumors of the CNS are relatively uncommon and, as we shall see below, may only represent a relatively narrow spectrum of distinct disease entities.

### Medulloblastoma (WHO Grade IV)

The name *medulloblastoma* is misleading because it is doubtful that any cell identifiable as a medulloblast exists during histogenesis. Instead, medulloblastomas likely arise from either the external granular layer, the subependymal matrix cells of the fourth ventricle, or both. Much progress has been made in the treatment of medulloblastomas, with 5-year survival rates now as high as 70%–80%.

More than 50% of medulloblastomas occur in children younger than age 10. A second smaller frequency peak occurs between ages 18 and 25. Medulloblastoma, by definition, originates in the cerebellum. It is generally well defined, soft, friable, and focally necrotic. Medulloblastomas have a proclivity to invade the ventricle and disseminate along CSF pathways. Affirmation of their potential aggressiveness comes from rare reports of metastases to bone, lymph nodes, and other extracranial sites, and recent work in animal models supports the notion of hematogenous metastatic potential (Garzia et al., 2018).

Medulloblastomas consist of small immature cells with hyperchromatic round to carrot-shaped nuclei with minimal cytoplasm, as well as numerous mitoses and apoptotic bodies. These tumors typically display limited degrees of neuronal maturation, with neuropil formation, synaptophysin immunoreactivity, and occasional Homer Wright (neuroblastic) rosettes (Fig. 72.16, *A*). Established morphological variants of medulloblastoma include the *anaplastic/large-cell subtype,* which shows widespread cellular anaplasia and has an aggressive clinical course with a high frequency of metastasis (see Fig. 72.16, *B*). The *desmoplastic/nodular variant* is recognized by the presence of pale nodular areas representing foci of neuronal differentiation surrounded by proliferating cells with hyperchromatic nuclei (see Fig. 72.16, *C*). When strictly applied, nodular/desmoplastic features are associated with a better prognosis than "classic" medulloblastoma. Some evidence exists that the nodular or desmoplastic variant is encountered most frequently in adults, in the lateral cerebellar hemispheres, and in patients with Gorlin nevoid basal cell carcinoma syndrome (NBCCS) where there is loss of the tumor suppressor gene, *PTCH*, on chromosome 9q (see later discussion). The *extensively nodular variant* occurs in infants and features marked expansion of the pale areas described in desmoplastic medulloblastoma with elaboration of neuropil-like tissue. It is associated with much better survival than classic medulloblastoma (Eberhart et al., 2002).

Familial forms of medulloblastoma have provided important clues regarding the inherited and sporadic forms of the tumor. These include the patched (*PTCH*)/sonic hedgehog (*SHH*) signaling pathway implicated from studies of NBCCS and the APC/Wingless (WNT) pathway associated with a form of Turcot syndrome (polyposis coli and brain tumors). However, sporadic medulloblastoma appears to be a heterogeneous genetic tumor, with no single alteration accounting for the majority of cases. Comprehensive molecular profiling has greatly clarified the molecular composition of medulloblastoma, delineating molecularly stratified subgroups (Taylor et al., 2012), some of which now constitute *bone fide* diagnostic categories under the revised 2016 WHO classification scheme (Table 72.3). In particular, medulloblastomas characterized by activated WNT or SHH pathway signaling have been identified as distinct entities. WNT-activated medulloblastomas are driven by activating mutations in *CTNNB1* (β-catenin) in the vast majority of

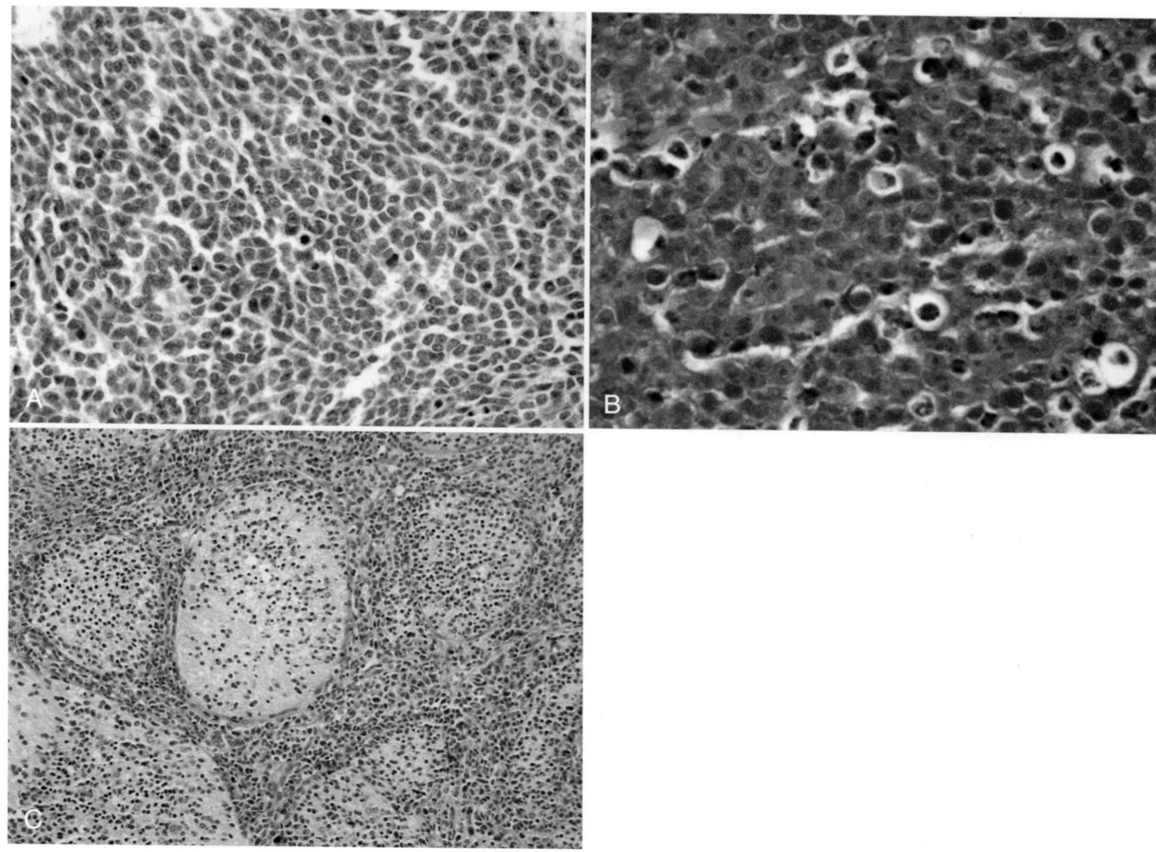

**Fig. 72.16 Medulloblastoma Morphological Variants. A,** Classic medulloblastoma composed of tightly packed, proliferative small round blue cells (hematoxylin-eosin stain, ×200). **B,** Large cell/anaplastic medulloblastoma featuring discohesive large anaplastic tumor cell nuclei and frequent apoptotic bodies (hematoxylin-eosin stain, ×200). **C,** Nodular/desmoplastic medulloblastoma exhibiting paucicellular and mitotically inert differentiating nodules (hematoxylin-eosin stain, ×100).

**TABLE 72.3 Molecular Alterations in Medulloblastomas**

| Medulloblastoma Subtype | Molecular Alterations |
|---|---|
| Medulloblastoma, WNT-activated | *CTNNB1* mutation, monosomy 6 |
| Medulloblastoma, SHH-activated | If *TP53* wild type; mutations in *PTCH1, SMO,* or *SUFU* |
| | If *TP53* mutant; amplification of *GLI2, MYCN,* or *SHH* |
| Medulloblastoma, non-WNT/non-SHH | *MYC* amplification |
| | Isochromosome 17q |

*SHH,* Sonic hedgehog.

cases, although those associated with Turcot syndrome feature loss-of-function mutations in *APC*. They are most common in children, although all age groups can be affected, and they tend to exhibit classical histopathology on microscopic examination. Importantly, WNT subgroup tumors are associated with the best prognosis of any medulloblastoma variant, with long-term survival exceeding 90%. SHH-activated tumors are driven by mutations in genes encoding a range of SHH pathway constituents, including *PTCH* (the gene most often associated with NBCCS), smoothened (*SMO*), and suppressor of fused (*SUFU*). *TP53* mutations also feature prominently in this tumor subgroup. Dichotomous age distribution, with high incidence in infancy and adults, but low incidence in children, characterizes the SHH-activated variant, which can also exhibit all histopathological patterns, including the vast majority of tumors with nodular/desmoplastic architecture. Prognosis is variable, and, in part, depends on the *TP53* mutational status.

Two additional, more loosely defined medulloblastoma subgroups, commonly known as subgroups 3 and 4, have been designated by global transcription and gene methylation profiling. Subgroup 3 tumors frequently overexpress MYC and a substantial minority harbor high-level amplification of the *MYC* locus. By contrast, subgroup 4 tumors exhibit the highest rates of isochromosome 17q, the most characteristic medulloblastoma-associated molecular aberration. Subgroup 4 tumors occur across a wide age range while subgroup 3 tumors tend to affect younger children and infants. Although histopathological patterns vary, subgroup 3 tumors are particularly enriched for large-cell/anaplastic architecture, with classic morphology accounting for the remainder of subgroup 3 and 4 medulloblastomas. Finally, subgroup 3 tumors, especially those harboring *MYC* amplification, are associated with poor prognosis, while outcomes for subgroup 4 tumors are more intermediate. Unlike WNT and SHH-activated counterparts, subgroup 3 and 4 medulloblastoma constitute heterogeneous collections tumors, each of which are characterized by variable pathogenic mechanisms. Recent work has emphatically confirmed this notion, and further studies in the near future are likely to identify additional distinct tumor variants within subgroups 3 and 4.

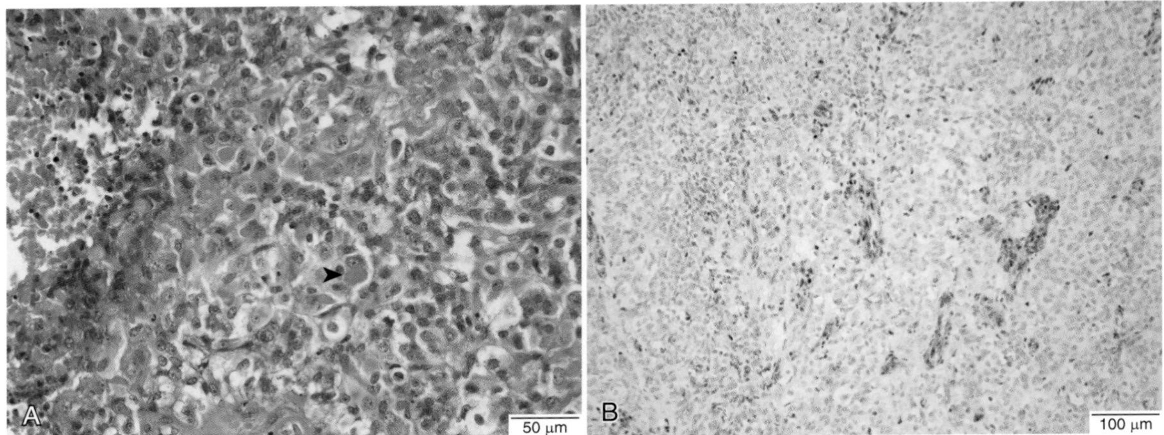


**Fig. 72.17 Atypical Teratoid/Rhabdoid Tumor. A,** High-grade, partially necrotic neoplasm composed of rhabdoid cells (black arrowhead (hematoxylin-eosin stain, ×200). **B,** Immunostaining shows loss of nuclear SMARCB1 in tumor cell nuclei with retention in associated vasculature (×100).

### Atypical Teratoid/Rhabdoid Tumor (WHO Grade IV)

AT/RT is an embryonal CNS neoplasm often misdiagnosed as medulloblastoma because of the prominence of small round blue cells in many cases. The name of this tumor derives from the fact that it may resemble either epithelial tumors (teratoid) or malignant rhabdoid tumors seen in the kidney, soft tissue, and other organ sites throughout the body. Mostly restricted to infants, AT/RT is one of the most aggressive human tumors. Average survival times are in the range of 6–8 months, and these tumors typically do not respond to conventional medulloblastoma-associated therapies. These dramatic biological differences make it critical to distinguish AT/RT from medulloblastoma.

Although small blue cells are common and may predominate in some cases, the defining histopathological feature of AT/RT is the *rhabdoid cell*, an enlarged cell featuring an eccentric oval to kidney-shaped nucleus with vesicular (open or clear) chromatin, as well as an eosinophilic rounded paranuclear inclusion (Fig. 72.17, *A*), often highlighted by immunostains for vimentin. Carcinoma-like and sarcoma-like foci are also evident in some cases. AT/RT represents a classic example of a *polyphenotypic tumor*, defined by coexpression of antigens normally associated with differing histogenetic lines (e.g., epithelial, mesenchymal, neuronal, glial). The list of potentially positive immunostains is long, but as opposed to medulloblastoma, the vast majority of AT/RTs express EMA, smooth muscle antigen (SMA), and vimentin. Despite the name *teratoid*, no relationship exists between these tumors and germ cell tumors; generally, they do not express germ cell markers.

Genetically, the majority of AT/RTs harbor monosomy 22 or 22q deletions coupled with mutations in the *INI1/SMARCB1* tumor suppressor gene, which leads to loss of expression of the *SMARCB1* gene product, a SWI/SNF family chromatin regulator. Germline mutations may occur in familial or disseminated forms of this disease. Loss-of-function mutations involving SMARCA4, another SWI/SNF family chromatin regulator, are also associated with AT/RT (Hasselblatt et al., 2011). Mutational inactivation of either *SMARCB1* or *SMARCA4* in AT/RT provides specific molecular markers for diagnosis, and monoclonal antibodies directed against the protein products of these genes have now found widespread implementation in clinical labs (see Fig. 72.17, *B*).

### Embryonal Tumor With Multilayered Rosettes (WHO Grade IV)

This newly described embryonal tumor represents an amalgamation of multiple rare diagnostic entities previously considered distinct, specifically ependymoblastoma, medulloepithelioma, and embryonal tumor with abundant neuropil and true rosettes (ETANTRs). Embryonal tumors with multilayered rosettes (ETMRs) primarily impact infants and young children, behave aggressively, and can occur in both supratentorial and infratentorial distributions. While precise histopathological features may vary, they are invariably composed of small round blue cells of embryonal morphology, organized into hypercellular clusters interspersed with relatively paucicellular, neuropil-rich regions. So-called multilayered or ependymoblastomatous rosettes, featuring pseudostratified, mitotically active tumor cells surrounding round or slit-like lumina, represent histopathological hallmarks. Molecularly, ETMRs are defined by a unique driver alteration involving amplification of a microRNA locus on chromosome 19q13.42 (Pfister et al., 2009). Demonstrating this event by FISH is diagnostic. ETMRs also selectively express the RNA-binding protein LIN28, which can be extremely helpful in designating this rare tumor variant from more common embryonal neoplasms (Korshunov et al., 2012).

### Central Nervous System Embryonal Tumor Not Otherwise Specified (NOS)

A heterogeneous group of aggressive small round blue cell tumors exhibiting histopathological similarities to medulloblastoma and other embryonal neoplasms, and arising in the supratentorium, have historically been grouped under the designation supratentorial primitive neuroectodermal tumor (PNET). Recent work, in particular global methylation profiling, has revealed that the majority of these neoplasms represent morphological variants of well-established disease entities, most notably glioblastoma and ependymoma (Sturm et al., 2016). These studies have also designated rare, but molecularly distinct, supratentorial embryonal variants within the larger histopathological pattern. According to the current WHO classification system, (Louis et al., 2016) these tumors are now classified as CNS embryonal tumors NOS. The diagnostic category PNET is no longer in use.

## Pineal Region Neoplasms

Pineal region tumors can arise from the pineal gland itself, or from rests of specialized cells in the immediate geographic vicinity that undergo selective transformation. Both are discussed below.

### Pineal Parenchymal Tumors

The pineal gland is an endocrine organ in the epithalamus that produces melatonin and is involved in the regulation of the circadian

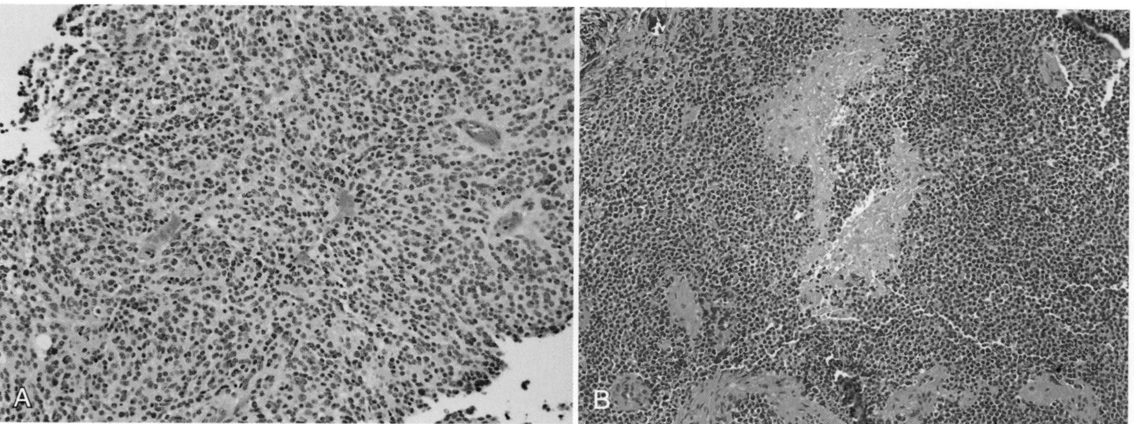


**Fig. 72.18 Pineal Parenchymal Tumors. A,** Pineal parenchymal tumor of intermediate differentiation showing cellular sheets of minimally proliferative tumor cells. **B,** Pineoblastoma exhibiting dense cellularity and foci of necrosis (hematoxylin-eosin stain, ×100).

rhythm. It is formed by clusters of pinealocytes with associated glial cells. Microcalcifications (also known as corpora arenacea) are common in the pineal gland, as is cystic degeneration, often an incidental finding on imaging or postmortem analysis. Tumors originating in the pineal gland are known as pineal parenchymal tumors and consist of three basic entities; pineocytoma (WHO grade I), pineal parenchymal tumor of intermediate differentiation (PPTID) (WHO grade II–III), and pineoblastoma (WHO grade IV).

Pineocytomas are slow-growing neoplasms with lobular architecture and characteristic pineocytomatous rosettes, which are formed by tumor cells arranged around an acellular central zone containing neuropil. Mitotic figures and/or necrosis are rare and should prompt consideration of PPTID or pineoblastoma. PPTID have intermediate features between pineocytomas and pineoblastomas. They are formed by sheets of tumor cells with minimal pleomorphism and minimal mitotic activity (Fig. 72.18, *A*). The pineocytomatous rosettes typically seen in pineocytomas are usually not present in PPTIDs. Pineoblastomas consist of cellular sheets characterized by marked pleomorphism, nuclear molding, numerous mitoses, apoptotic bodies, and necrosis (see Fig. 72.18, *B*). Histologically, pineoblastomas resemble other embryonal tumors, including medulloblastoma. The prognosis of pineoblastomas is poor. Similar to normal pinealocytes, pineal parenchymal tumors avidly express synaptophysin. Rare GFAP-expressing cells can be seen within the tumors, likely representing entrapped glial cells normally encountered in the pineal gland. A recent molecular analysis of pineoblastoma revealed heterogeneous genomic features with high rates of mutations in *DROSHA*, which encodes a microRNA processing enzyme, and duplications involving myomegalin (*PDE4DIP*), a gene involved in cardiac muscle contraction (Snuderl et al., 2018).

## Papillary Tumor of the Pineal Region

Another unusual neuroepithelial tumor that arises at this location is the papillary tumor of the pineal region (PTPR). Although it is thought to arise from specialized ependymocytes of the subcommissural organ, not from the pineal gland itself, we will include it in this section. PPTRs are very rare and have been reported in children and adults. Given their anatomical location, the tumors may cause hydrocephalus. On histology, PPTRs show papillary architecture with large cuboidal/columnar tumor cells growing along fibrovascular cores. The tumor cells express keratin and S100. Molecular studies have shown that PPTR frequently harbors mutations in *PTEN* and loss of chromosome 10 (Goschzik et al., 2014).

## Germ Cell Tumors

While not derived from neuroepithelial tissue per se, germ cell tumors are considered here due to their predilection for growth in the pineal region. Germ cell tumors of the nervous system are most common in children and are analogous to their counterparts in the gonads, retroperitoneum, and mediastinum. As indicated above, the pineal region is the most common site of involvement, followed by the suprasellar/hypothalamic region and the striatum. Germ cell tumors as a group grow rapidly, with a propensity to seed the subarachnoid space. CSF examination for both cytology and marker levels may be diagnostic. Elevations of placental-like alkaline phosphatase (PLAP) are most suggestive of germinoma, alpha fetoprotein (AFP) of yolk sac tumor, and beta human chorionic gonadotropin (β-hCG) of choriocarcinoma or a syncytiotrophoblastic element. For reasons not understood, pineal germ cell tumors are virtually restricted to boys; in some cases, the clinical and radiographical features are so typical that a biopsy is not necessary before therapy. Pure germinoma is most common and is virtually 100% curable because of its radiosensitivity. Mature teratoma is rarely pure, is slow growing and cystic, and typically does not respond well to chemotherapy or radiation. However, demarcation is often excellent, and surgical cure is possible. Most of the remaining cases of germ cell tumor consist of mixed tumors with various malignant elements, such as embryonal carcinoma, yolk sac tumor, choriocarcinoma, and immature teratoma. Such cases have a significantly worse prognosis, but survival rates have improved with modern multiagent chemotherapy regimens. In occasional cases that are successfully treated, the only viable element remaining on "recurrence" is mature teratoma.

Histologically, germinomas are identical to testicular seminoma and ovarian dysgerminoma, with two distinct cell populations (Fig. 72.19). The neoplastic element resembles primordial germ cells with abundant glycogen-rich clear cytoplasm and both PLAP and c-kit immunoreactivity. Immunoreactivity for the transcription factor OCT4 is a useful diagnostic marker for the neoplastic cells. The stroma is often rich in reactive lymphocytes, primarily T cells. Sarcoid-like granulomas are also quite common and may obscure the diagnosis in biopsies where the reactive response overshadows the tumor cells. Embryonal carcinoma resembles a poorly differentiated carcinoma. Endodermal sinus tumor (yolk sac tumor) forms loose papillary epithelial structures known as *Schiller-Duval bodies.* Combinations of mononucleated cytotrophoblasts and multinucleated syncytiotrophoblasts characterize choriocarcinoma. The tumor is highly vascular and particularly prone to hemorrhage. Teratomas differentiate into elements from all three germ layers,

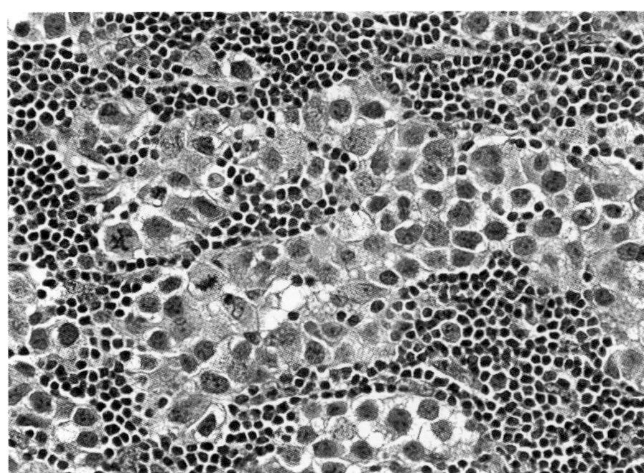

**Fig. 72.19 Pineal Germinoma.** The dual cellular population consists of numerous small reactive lymphocytes and large clear tumor cells, which resemble primordial germ cells (hematoxylin-eosin stain, ×400).

exhibiting mature components such as teeth, hair, muscle, cartilage, and bronchial wall. While arranged in a haphazard nonfunctional manner, these components are benign. Immature teratoma contains the same elements but has a fetal rather than mature appearance. Foci of immature brain with neural tube-like structures are particularly common.

Molecular analysis has shown frequent KIT, KRAS, and HRAS mutations in germinomas, with much lower rates in other types of germ cell tumors (Fukushima et al., 2014). These mutations appear to be mutually exclusive, firmly implicating RAS/MAPK signaling in germinoma pathogenesis while also pointing to viable strategies for the application of targeted therapeutics.

## Pituitary Neoplasms

The pituitary gland is located in a depression in the sphenoid bone called the sella turcica, and is divided into anterior (adenohypophysis), intermediate (pars intermedia), and posterior (neurohypophysis or pars nervosa) segments. Sellar tumors can originate from any of the aforementioned structures and will be discussed in more detail below. Although the adenohypophysis is an endocrine organ and not part of the CNS proper, given its anatomical location, lesions in this region often present with neurological symptoms due to mass effect, are surgically removed by neurosurgeons, and are examined histopathologically by neuropathologists: hence their inclusion herein.

### Pituitary Adenoma

Pituitary adenomas are the most common pituitary tumors and originate from the adenohypophysis. Clinical presentation is often associated with visual disturbances (e.g., bitemporal hemianopsia) due to compression of the optic chiasm, which lies directly above the sella turcica. Other frequent clinical presentations of pituitary adenomas are related to the systemic effects of hormonal excess resulting from the uncontrolled proliferation of a particular type of adenohypophyseal cell. Six hormones are secreted by the adenohypophysis—growth hormone (GH), adrenocorticotropic hormone (ACTH), prolactin, follicle-stimulating hormone (FSH), luteinizing hormone (LH), and thyroid-stimulating hormone (TSH)—any of which can be secreted by a given pituitary adenoma, both alone and in combinations (Table 72.4). Most adenomas are benign tumors confined to the sella turcica. However, macroadenomas, defined as >1 cm in greatest dimension, frequently extend outside of the sella, causing compression of the optic chiasm. Microadenomas are smaller than 1 cm; they usually present due to manifestation of hormonal excess, and more commonly secrete ACTH or GH.

**TABLE 72.4 Types of Pituitary Adenomas Based on Hormones Secreted**

| Adenoma Type | Hormones | Possible Clinical Manifestations |
|---|---|---|
| Somatotroph adenoma | Growth hormone | Gigantism, acromegaly |
| Mammosomatotroph | Growth hormone + prolactin | Gigantism or acromegaly along with galactorrhea or amenorrhea |
| Corticotroph adenoma | Adrenocorticotropic hormone | Cushing disease |
| Lactotroph adenoma* | Prolactin | Women: Reproductive or sexual dysfunction, galactorrhea, amenorrhea, ovulatory disorders<br>Men: erectile dysfunction, decreased libido |
| Gonadotroph adenoma | Follicle-stimulating hormone or luteinizing hormone | Most are clinically silent and usually present due to mass effect |
| Thyrotroph adenoma | Thyroid-stimulating hormone | Hyperthyroidism |
| Plurihormonal | Growth hormone, prolactin, thyroid-stimulating hormone, various hormonal combinations | Most are clinically silent |
| Null cell adenoma | No hormones | No symptoms of hormonal excess, usually present due to mass effect |

*Most common type of adenoma (~40% of cases).

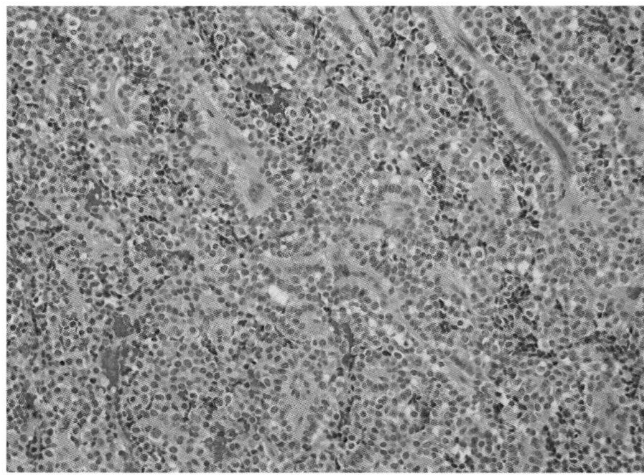

**Fig. 72.20 Pituitary Adenoma.** Neuroendocrine neoplasm growing in sheets and trabeculae. Proliferative activity is minimal (hematoxylin-eosin stain, ×200).

The adenohypophysis consists of acini of hormone-producing cells. These acini are surrounded by a connective tissue network, predominantly composed of collagen, that can be highlighted by reticulin histochemical staining. This normal acinar architecture and reticulin network are typically disrupted in pituitary adenomas, with neoplastic cells growing as trabeculae and/or unstructured sheets (Fig. 72.20). Microscopically, pituitary adenomas consist of relatively uniform tumor cells with neuroendocrine features, and frequently express chromogranin and synaptophysin. Mitotic activity and proliferation

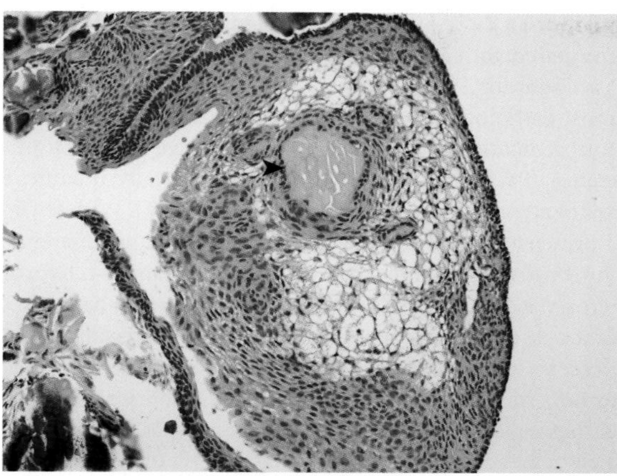

**Fig. 72.21 Craniopharyngioma, Adamantinomatous Type.** Modified squamous epithelium demonstrating central cobweb-like loosening (stellate reticulum) and peripheral palisading. A nodule of wet keratin is also present (*black arrowhead;* hematoxylin-eosin stain, ×200).

indices (e.g. Ki-67) are usually low, even in locally invasive adenomas. The designation of pituitary carcinoma is reserved for tumors that have metastasized to distant organs. Histopathological features have been found to correlate poorly with frankly malignant behavior in pituitary neoplasms. The treatment of pituitary adenomas usually consists of surgical resection, performed via a transsphenoidal approach. In some cases, prolactinomas (adenomas that secrete prolactin) are treated with dopamine receptor agonists (e.g., cabergoline), which reduce hormonal secretion.

### Parenchymal Tumors of the Neurohypophysis

The neurohypophysis is formed by glial cells (pituicytes) and axons derived from hypothalamic neurons that are involved in storing and secreting oxytocin and vasopressin. Three histologically distinct tumors arising from the neurohypophysis are pituicytoma, spindle cell oncocytoma, and granular cell tumor. All are rare, low-grade lesions with relatively good prognoses, and are non-functioning (i.e., do not cause hormonal excess). Therefore, clinical presentation is usually related to mass effect on adjacent structures.

Histologically, pituicytomas are composed of spindle- or stellate-shaped cells with round-oval-to-elongated nuclei. They exhibit a storiform architecture and a rich capillary network. Granular cell tumors usually arise in the pituitary stalk and present as a suprasellar (rather than intrasellar) lesions. Spindle cell oncocytomas show interwoven fascicles of spindle cells exhibiting abundant eosinophilic cytoplasm of granular (oncocytic) appearance. Ultrastructural examination shows that the tumor cell cytoplasm is rich in mitochondria. All three tumors express, as does the normal neurohypophysis, the thyroid transcription factor 1 (TTF1) and S100 protein. Expression of GFAP is variable and, in contrast to pituitary adenomas, these tumors do not express synaptophysin. It is still unclear if these tumors represent truly distinct entities or histological variants of the same neoplasm, partly because underlying genetic alterations are unknown. Treatment typically consists of surgery, although subtotal resection is associated with recurrence.

### Craniopharyngioma

Craniopharyngiomas comprise 2%–5% of CNS tumors. Most become symptomatic in the first two decades but can occur at any age. Craniopharyngiomas probably arise from cell rests of the Rathke pouch, an evagination of the primitive stomodeum. Craniopharyngiomas may be intrasellar or (more frequently) suprasellar in location, often involving the hypothalamus and the optic nerve or chiasm. The expanding mass causes hydrocephalus by encroaching on the third ventricle.

The advancing margins of the craniopharyngioma may appear deceptively sharp, but microscopic finger-like extensions into surrounding tissue are common. Both solid and cystic areas are intermingled. Cysts can become large and typically fill with a dark, viscous, cholesterol-rich fluid likened to motor oil. Irregularly shaped calcium deposits, varying in size from grains of sand to fine gravel, occur in approximately 75% of cases. The microscopic appearance is comparable to that of adamantinoma of the tibia and ameloblastoma of the jaw. Therefore, sometimes the classic craniopharyngioma is named *adamantinomatous craniopharyngioma.* The tumor demonstrates benign-appearing epithelium with central cobweb-like loosening (stellate reticulum) and peripheral palisading (Fig. 72.21). Squamoid foci may occur, and the pattern of keratinization with ghostlike nests of keratinocytes is called *wet keratin.* Wet keratin differs from the dry, flaky keratin of epidermoid and dermoid cysts and is unique to craniopharyngioma. Therefore, it is diagnostic on a biopsy, even without the presence of viable epithelium. A rare variant is the papillary craniopharyngioma, which often presents in the third ventricle of adults. A characteristic feature is a true nonkeratinizing squamous lining over fibrovascular cores. Goblet cells are another feature. It is uncertain whether this variant has a better prognosis.

Aberrant nuclear accumulation of β-catenin occurs in 94% of adamantinomatous craniopharyngiomas, indicating the likely pathogeneic importance of Wnt signaling in tumorigenesis. Recently, next-generation sequencing studies confirmed earlier work identifying high rates (92%) of *CTNNB1* (β-catenin) mutations in adamantinomatous craniopharyngiomas (Brastianos et al., 2014; Sekine et al., 2002). Interestingly, papillary craniopharyngiomas, which do not show nuclear translocation of β-catenin, demonstrate equally high rates (95%) of *BRAF* p V600E mutation (Brastianos et al., 2014). These findings point to fundamental biological distinctions between the different subtypes of craniopharyngioma while also providing molecular metrics to distinguish craniopharyngiomas from other sellar tumors in the event of a small, histologically indistinct biopsy.

## PRIMARY EXTRA-AXIAL NEOPLASMS

The most common extra-axial brain and spinal tumors are meningiomas, although hemangiopericytomas, sarcomas, lymphomas, metastatic tumors, schwannomas, and inflammatory masses also occur adjacent to the brain and spinal cord.

### Meningeal Neoplasms

These tumors arise from the soft-tissue coverings surrounding the brain and originate from either meningothelial or fibrous cellular constituents.

#### Meningioma (WHO Grade I)

Meningiomas comprise 20%–25% of all intracranial tumors. They are most prevalent after age 50. The female-to-male ratio is 2 : 1 in adults, nearly 10 : 1 in the spinal cord, and 1 : 1 in pediatric or malignant forms. Although most are benign (roughly 80%), a subset is aggressive with high-grade histology, high recurrence rates, or substantial morbidity and mortality. Even some histologically benign meningiomas are associated with disfigurement, neurological deficits, and major therapeutic challenges, particularly when located in sites at the skull base that preclude complete resection. Generally, extent of surgical resection and histological grade represent the most important prognostic variables.

The locations of meningiomas, in descending order of frequency, are the cerebral convexity, parasagittal region, sphenoid wing,

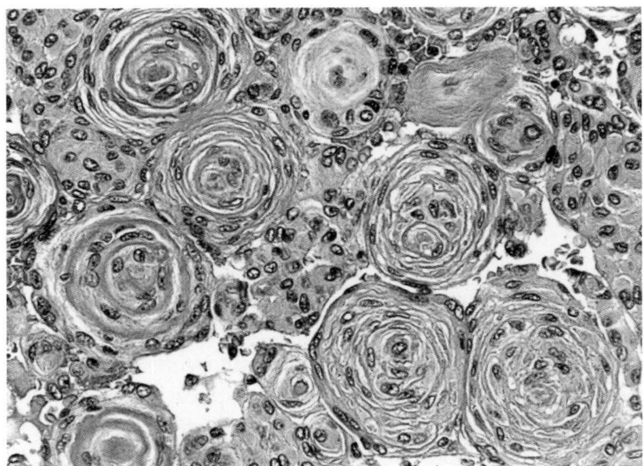

**Fig. 72.22 Meningioma.** Typical meningothelial nests and whorls with focal hyalinization, the first step in the formation of concentrically laminated calcifications, or psammoma bodies (hematoxylin-eosin stain, ×400).

parasellar region, and spinal canal. Posterior fossa and lateral ventricle locations are more common in children. Multiple meningiomas suggest the possibility of NF2, although forms not associated with NF2 also occur. Interestingly, a number of such cases show identical mutations in each meningioma arising from a single patient, suggesting that dural dissemination may account for multifocality, despite a histologically benign appearance.

Benign meningiomas are well-demarcated and compress rather than invade the adjacent brain or spinal cord. Nevertheless, bone and soft-tissue invasion may occur and is typically associated with hyperostosis. Notably, this type of invasion does not constitute evidence for malignancy, and those tumors that are grossly totally resected share the same excellent prognosis as those without invasion. *Meningioma en plaque* is a pattern of diffuse carpet-like tumor spread along the dural surface. Meningiomas are generally firm in consistency and often gritty because of the presence of sand-like calcifications, referred to as *psammoma bodies.*

Meningiomas are histologically heterogeneous. However, four rare variants are considered more aggressive by definition: clear cell (grade II), chordoid (grade II), papillary (grade III), and rhabdoid (grade III). The other nine subtypes are considered benign unless they fulfill additional criteria for atypical (grade II) or anaplastic (grade IIII) meningioma (see below). The majority of meningiomas have two basic histological patterns—meningothelial or fibroblastic—with the transitional variant having features of both. Meningothelial tumors are composed of arachnoidal epithelioid cells arranged in lobules, often with prominent whorls and psammoma bodies (Fig. 72.22), which represent laminated calcifications of degenerated meningothelial whorls. Fibroblastic meningiomas are distinguished by their spindled appearance, fascicular or storiform architecture, and abundant collagen deposition. The most helpful immunohistochemical marker suggesting meningothelial differentiation is EMA, which is detectable at least focally in the vast majority of meningiomas. Progesterone receptor immunopositivity is present in more than 50% of cases. While the pathogenic significance of this finding is unclear, meningiomas can enlarge dramatically with pregnancy and regress after delivery.

### Atypical Meningioma (WHO Grade II)

The intermediate-grade category of atypical meningioma defines a meningioma type that carries a considerable increased risk of recurrence, even after achieving gross total resection. These tumors are also associated with a slight but statistically significant increase in mortality when compared with age- and sex-matched controls. Atypical meningiomas account for 15%–20% of all meningiomas.

In most pathology series, mitotic or proliferative index is the most powerful predictor of outcome. Based on a large Mayo Clinic series, the presence of at least 4 mitoses/10 HPF, even focally, qualifies for the diagnosis of atypical meningioma (Perry et al., 1997). With fewer mitoses, the presence of at least three of five additional parameters (sheeting architecture, hypercellularity, macronucleoli, small-cell formation, and necrosis) also suffices. The issue of brain invasion has been debatable; although once considered the ultimate manifestation of malignancy, recent studies suggest that in the absence of frank anaplasia, these tumors have similar recurrence and mortality rates as those of atypical meningioma. Similar to mitotic counts, MIB-1 (Ki-67) labeling indices may be helpful for predicting the risk of recurrence, particularly in borderline atypical cases. Meningioma grade is also inversely proportional to progesterone receptor expression, so that, in general, fewer atypical meningiomas are progesterone receptor immunoreactive than their benign counterparts.

### Anaplastic Meningioma (WHO Grade III)

With the omission of brain invasion as a criterion for anaplastic meningioma, these tumors have become quite rare, accounting for no more than 1%–2% of all cases. Many of these tumors start as benign or atypical meningiomas and progress over time, although de novo presentations also occur. As a group, anaplastic meningiomas are highly aggressive, rapidly growing, and highly infiltrative, with a median survival of less than 2 years (Perry et al., 1997). Nevertheless, extent of resection remains important, and long-term survival is still possible in a subset of patients. Histologically, anaplastic meningiomas are defined by the presence of excessive mitotic activity (>20/10 HPF) and/or frank anaplasia with a carcinoma-like or sarcoma-like appearance. These tumors are highly cellular, with extensive sheeting, necrosis, and nuclear atypia. Often, lower-grade elements, more easily recognizable as meningioma, are present. For those lacking this feature, immunohistochemistry or electron microscopy is often necessary to exclude hemangiopericytoma or other tumors such as dural-based sarcoma, metastatic carcinoma, or melanoma. In most anaplastic meningiomas, the MIB-1 (Ki-67) labeling index is markedly elevated, and there is no discernible progesterone receptor expression.

### Molecular Features of Meningioma

Recent genomic profiling studies have confirmed earlier work indicating that the majority of meningiomas are associated with losses of chromosome 22 or portions thereof, with most of these tumors also harboring inactivating mutations in *NF2* (Brastianos et al., 2013; Clark et al., 2013). These findings correlate well with the fact that meningiomas are the second most common tumor type in NF2 patients. The remaining subset of meningiomas not characterized by NF2 loss exhibit either *TRAF7* or *SMO* mutations in a mutually exclusive pattern. Moreover, the majority of *TRAF7*-mutant meningiomas appear to harbor either *KLF4* or *AKT1* mutations, also in a mutually exclusive distribution. These findings provide unprecedented insights into meningioma biology, while also pointing to readily druggable targets in the case of *SMO*- and *AKT1*-mutant tumors.

While less is currently known about the molecular foundations of WHO grade II and III meningiomas, mutational profiling suggests that the majority of atypical variants fall into the NF2-deficient subgroup (Clark et al., 2013). Moreover, a growing number of cytogenetic alterations have been associated with malignant progression, though specific target genes remain unidentified. Anaplastic meningiomas appear to share the genetic features of lower-grade meningiomas but

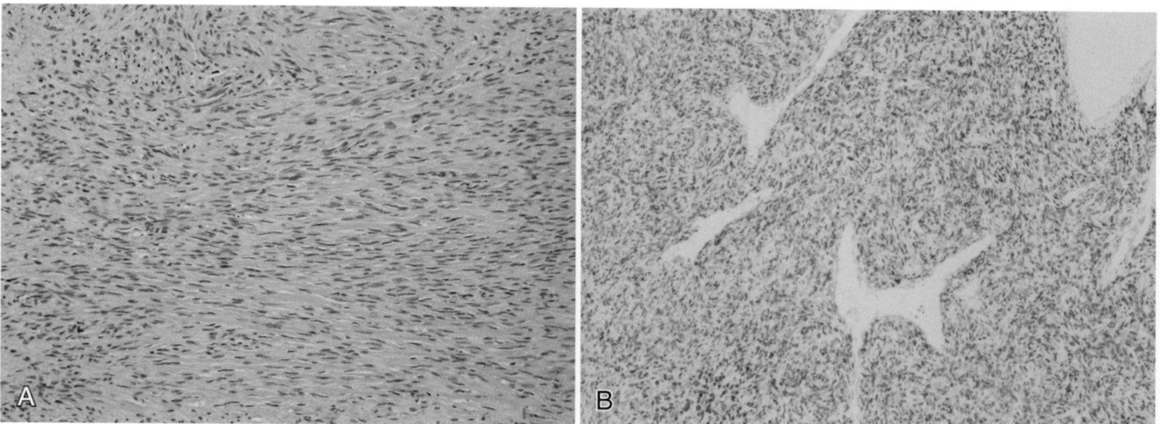


**Fig. 72.23 Solitary Fibrous Tumor. A,** Spindle cell tumor with exhibiting "patternless" pattern and extensive collagen band deposition (hematoxylin-eosin stain, ×200). **B,** Immunostaining for STAT6 is strongly positive in tumor cells (×100).

additionally harbor chromosome 17q gains/amplifications and 9p/p16 losses in many cases. Recent work has identified promoter mutations in *TERT* as a key prognostic indicator for meningiomas, designating aggressive behavior across WHO grades (Sahm et al., 2016).

### Hemangiopericytoma and Solitary Fibrous Tumor (WHO Grade II–III)

Hemangiopericytoma (HPC), once considered an angioblastic variant of meningioma, is now generally accepted to be a highly vascular dural-based sarcoma, analogous to those encountered in soft-tissue sites and of uncertain histogenesis. Solitary fibrous tumors (SFTs) were initially characterized as primary mesenchymal neoplasms of the pleura but have in recent years been described in many extrapleural sites including the meninges. Although still debated, it has been suggested that HPC and SFT may represent ends of the same biological spectrum. However, it is clear that tumors fulfilling criteria for HPC typically have high rates of local recurrence (60%–80%) and systemic metastasis (25%). In contrast, SFTs of the meninges generally behave in a more indolent fashion, one study demonstrating excellent local control through surgical resection alone (Tihan et al., 2003). Both tumors occur at all ages, peaking in the fourth to sixth decades. Unlike meningiomas, there is no female predilection, and there is no association with NF2 or any of the known meningioma-associated genetic alterations.

Histologically, HPC is a highly cellular reticulin-rich neoplasm with numerous branching (staghorn) thin-walled vessels, an architectural feature also shared by SFT (Fig. 72.23, *A*). HPCs are formed of densely packed hyperchromatic cells that are oval to spindled and display variable proliferative indices. Tumors with more than 5 mitoses/10 HPF or hemorrhage/necrosis are considered high grade (grade III), although even the low-grade (grade II) examples are considered malignant. Prototypic SFTs are less cellular tumors that have a so-called patternless pattern lacking characteristic architectural details. The tumors are composed of spindled cells with indistinct cell borders and finely dispersed chromatin, admixed with dense collagen bands.

Both SFT and HPC are EMA negative but positive for CD34, which is characteristically described as diffusely strong in SFT. Bcl2 is described as strongly staining cells in SFT, but HPC frequently also shows a positive signal. *NAB2–STAT6* gene fusion, which results in a chimeric protein that effectively targets the STAT6 carboxy-terminal transactivation domain to its downstream effector genes in the cell nucleus, was recently identified as a consistent driving alteration in SFTs and HPCs. This fusion event can be visualized easily by immunohistochemical positivity for STAT6 in tumor cell nuclei (Doyle et al., 2014; see Fig. 72.23, *B*).

## Nerve Sheath Tumors

Schwannomas and neurofibromas represent the most common peripheral nerve sheath tumors but may occur "centrally" when they arise from paraspinal nerve roots or cranial nerves. Multiple neurofibromas or schwannomas should suggest NF1 and NF2, respectively, particularly in younger individuals. Even the most cellular and mitotically active schwannoma virtually never undergoes malignant transformation, although plexiform and intraneural neurofibromas harbor a small but significant risk of this complication. Malignant peripheral nerve sheath tumor (MPNST) may therefore develop de novo or within a pre-existing tumor, most often a plexiform neurofibroma from an NF1 patient. The risk of developing MPNST is also increased in previously irradiated tissue (e.g., mediastinal radiation for Hodgkin lymphoma) in both NF1 and non-NF1 patients. Generally, MPNSTs occur in soft-tissue sites but may be seen more centrally owing to paraspinal localization. These sarcomas are usually high grade and have a dismal prognosis.

### Schwannoma (WHO Grade I)

The frequency of schwannomas peaks in the fourth and fifth decades. Most are located on the vestibular portion of the eighth cranial nerve. Other cranial nerves, particularly the trigeminal, are much less frequent sites of involvement. Bilateral vestibular schwannomas (acoustic neuroma) are diagnostic of NF2. Vestibular schwannomas erode the internal auditory meatus and occupy the cerebellopontine angle; with increasing size, the tumor mass may compress and deform the pons. Spinal schwannomas comprise about 30% of intraspinal tumors. Most arise from the dorsal roots, preferring sensory nerves like their cranial counterparts. Spinal schwannomas may extend through the dura or, in some cases, through the intervertebral foramen as a dumbbell-shaped mass that is partly within and partly outside the spinal canal.

As opposed to neurofibromas, schwannomas are pure Schwann cell proliferations, typically arranged in two architectural patterns. Cellular dense zones, known as *Antoni A areas*, contain spindle-shaped cells arranged in nuclear palisades, termed *Verocay bodies* (Fig. 72.24). *Antoni B areas* are myxoid and microcystic in appearance, with thin wavy cells and foci of collagenization highly reminiscent of

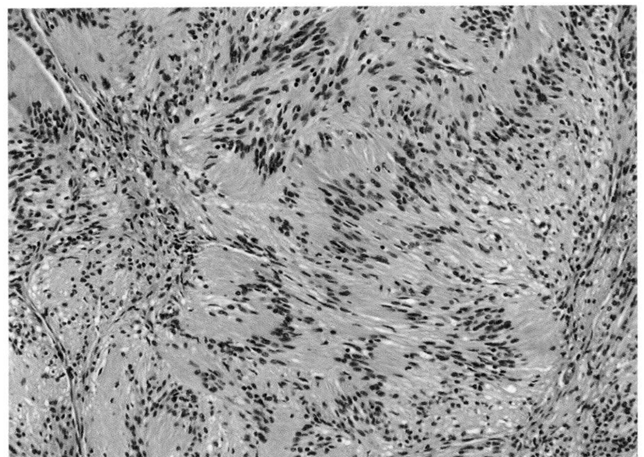

**Fig. 72.24 Schwannoma.** Spindle cell neoplasm arranged in nuclear palisades (Verocay bodies; hematoxylin-eosin stain, ×200).

neurofibromas. Degenerative changes are common and include hemorrhage, cystic breakdown, vascular hyalinization, and calcification. As opposed to neurofibromas, schwannomas typically have a discernible capsule and push the parent nerve aside rather than invading it. Immunohistochemical studies reveal strong and diffuse S100 immunoreactivity, diffuse collagen IV positivity, reflecting the rich network of Schwann cell-associated basement membranes, and a relative lack of neurofilament-positive entrapped axons.

The vast majority of both sporadic and familial (mostly NF2-associated) schwannomas are associated with loss of expression for the NF2 protein product, merlin or schwannomin (Stemmer-Rachamimov et al., 1997). *NF2* gene deletions and LOH are common, though other mechanisms may also be involved. Additionally, *INI1* expression is likely altered (Hulsebos et al., 2007). Indeed, INI1 immunohistochemistry shows a mosaic pattern of staining in tumors from familial and sporadic schwannomatosis patients, as well as in schwannomas from NF2 patients, contrasting with a strong uniform nuclear signal in sporadic tumors. These findings suggest a role for *INI1* in multiple schwannoma syndromes (Patil et al., 2008).

### Neurofibroma (WHO Grade I)

Neurofibromas are less commonly encountered centrally than schwannomas. Involvement of multiple spinal nerve roots is virtually pathognomonic of NF1. They more typically originate from nerve terminals in the dermis and from large nerve trunks such as the brachial plexus. Unlike the eccentric globular growth pattern of schwannomas, neurofibromas grow within the substance of a nerve, generating a fusiform intraneural mass. A plexiform ("bag of worms") growth pattern results from the involvement of multiple nerve fascicles and is virtually diagnostic of NF1. On gross inspection, neurofibromas are typically gray and gelatinous.

Histologically, bundles of cells with thin wavy nuclei suspend haphazardly in a myxoid or mucin-rich stroma. There are variable degrees of collagenization, depending on the age of the lesion, and the resulting hyaline silhouettes have been likened to "shredded carrots." As opposed to schwannomas, neurofibromas are a mixture of cell types that include not only Schwann cells but also fibroblasts, perineural-like cells, mast cells, and entrapped elements from the parent nerve. Most cases are hypocellular; therefore, foci of marked cellularity, increased cell size, and mitotic activity should raise concern for transformation to MPNST. Immunostains demonstrate patchy S100 and collagen IV expression because only a portion of the intratumoral cells are Schwann cells. Entrapped neurofilament-positive axons are usually present except in dermal neurofibromas. The MIB-1 (Ki-67) index is generally low, and p53 protein expression absent except in foci of transformation to MPNST.

Studies suggest that the Schwann cell is the neoplastic component within neurofibromas, with remaining cell types likely representing reactive or entrapped elements (Perry et al., 2001). Deletions of the *NF1* gene and losses of its protein product, neurofibromin, are detectable in a subset of both familial and sporadic neurofibromas.

### Hybrid Nerve Sheath Tumor (WHO Grade I)

Tumors exhibiting morphological and immunohistochemical features of both schwannoma and neurofibroma in segregated regions not infrequently arise in patients with NF1, NF2, and schwannomatosis. They have been associated with more frequent progression to MPNST.

## MISCELLANEOUS TUMORS

### Central Nervous System Lymphoma

CNS involvement by lymphoma may be either primary or secondary. Secondary CNS involvement occurs in 5%–29% of systemic non-Hodgkin lymphomas but is exceptional in Hodgkin disease. Systemic lymphomas tend to infiltrate the leptomeninges and spare the parenchyma. The epidural spinal space is a favored site, and spinal compression is a common complication. In contrast, primary CNS lymphoma (PCNSL), a type of extranodal non-Hodgkin lymphoma, typically presents deep in the brain parenchyma (e.g., periventricular) and usually spares the meninges, which may explain why the CSF cytological examination contains tumor cells in only a minority of patients. The incidence of CNS lymphoma increases in immunodeficient patients, including those with acquired immunodeficiency syndrome or organ transplant. Such cases are typically associated with Epstein-Barr virus (EBV), and CSF PCR studies take advantage of this common finding. Primary CNS lymphoma has also increased in the elderly immunocompetent population for poorly understood reasons. These cases are generally not associated with EBV. Survival without treatment is typically less than 1 year, but prolonged survivals with methotrexate-based chemotherapy regimens have been reported. Primary CNS lymphoma is unique in that approximately half are multifocal tumor masses that may disappear or regress after corticosteroid therapy, and they often recur in a completely different CNS site from that of the initial lesion.

Of non-HIV-associated PCNSL, 90% are diffuse large B-cell type, with the remaining 10% being poorly characterized low-grade lymphomas, Burkitt lymphomas, or T-cell lymphomas. These tumors show a distinctive angiocentric pattern in which malignant cells surround and invade blood vessels in concentric layers (Fig. 72.25). Reactive T cells are often numerous as well. Cases from immunosuppressed patients are characteristically necrotizing and EBV immunoreactive, whereas those from immunocompetent patients are not. Biopsies from patients treated preoperatively with corticosteroids are a common source of frustration and diagnostic difficulty for pathologists because the tumor cells often die, leaving behind a process that resembles either an inflammatory or demyelinating disorder. In such cases, an accurate diagnosis may await the time of recurrence. In addition, because sometimes cellularity is low in comparison to lymph node biopsies and the infiltrate typically mixed, wherein reactive T cells may outnumber tumor cells, flow cytometry is often less sensitive for establishing the diagnosis than routine histology and may waste a considerable amount of limited tissue.

Immunohistochemical expression of the germinal-center B-cell subgroup surrogate marker BCL-6 occurs at a lower frequency in primary CNS lymphoma than in nodal lymphoma and may be a favorable prognostic marker (Lin et al., 2006). The majority of CNS lymphomas

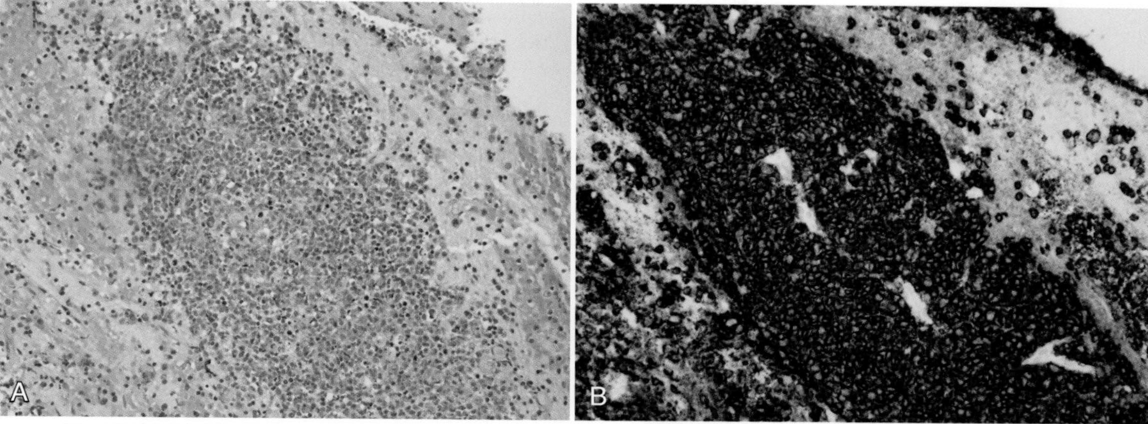


**Fig. 72.25 CNS Lymphoma. A,** Infiltrative angiocentric (aggregating around and within the vessel walls) neoplasm composed of immature lymphoid elements with a high nucleus-to-cytoplasm ratio, vesicular nuclei, and prominent nucleoli (hematoxylin-eosin stain, ×100). **B,** Immunostaining for the B-cell marker CD20 is strongly positive (×100). *CNS,* Central nervous system.

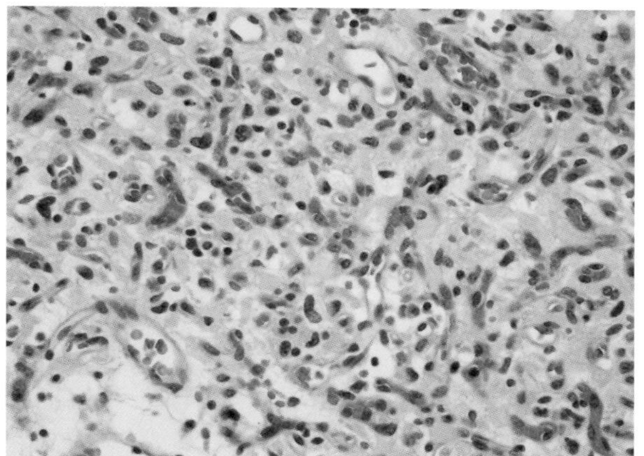

**Fig. 72.26 Hemangioblastoma.** Heterogeneous neoplasm featuring foamy stromal cells and a rich microvascular network.

harbor mutations in the *MYD88* gene. In particular, the *MYD88 p.L265P* mutation is the most common single genetic alteration in CNS lymphomas (Fukumura et al., 2016). Dysregulated *MYD88* signaling can be targeted with ibrutinib, a Bruton's tyrosine kinase (BTK) inhibitor (Grommes et al., 2017), and clinical trials are currently evaluating this potential therapeutic strategy. The *MYD88 p.L265P* mutation is a rare occurrence in other tumors, and thus, could serve as a specific diagnostic marker for CNS lymphomas.

## Hemangioblastoma (WHO Grade I)

Hemangioblastomas are benign vascular tumors of uncertain histogenesis. Approximately 10% of patients with hemangioblastoma have von Hippel–Lindau disease; the rest are sporadic. The age at diagnosis ranges from adolescence to the sixth decade, with the peak frequency at 40 years. Hemangioblastomas are more common in males. The tumor usually presents as a cyst with an enhancing mural nodule in the cerebellum and is the most common primary cerebellar neoplasm in adults. Hemangioblastomas are sometimes located in the retina, brainstem, spinal cord, or paraspinal nerve roots, sites more commonly involved in patients with von Hippel–Lindau disease.

Hemangioblastomas are cystic and sharply demarcated, often allowing complete surgical resection. Solid portions of the tumor are dark red because of a rich vascular supply, which predisposes to spontaneous hemorrhage. Histological examination shows abundant capillaries coursing throughout the tumor mass, though the actual neoplastic component is believed to be the foamy lipid-laden stromal cells residing amidst this rich vascular network (Fig. 72.26). These cells stain consistently with inhibin, S100 protein, neuron-specific enolase, and brachyury. Use of additional markers such as α-inhibin, D2-40, and EGFR immunohistochemistry may aid in the distinction between hemangioblastoma and potential mimics such as metastatic renal cell carcinoma, especially in the context of von Hippel–Lindau disease. Patchy GFAP expression occurs occasionally.

The *VHL* gene on 3p25–26 is a growth regulator that behaves as a classic tumor suppressor gene, with von Hippel–Lindau patients harboring a germline mutation ("first hit"). In these patients, it predisposes to a variety of tumors and malformative lesions, but the majority of the morbidity and mortality result from renal cell carcinomas, CNS hemangioblastomas, and, in a subset of patients, pheochromocytomas.

## Epidermoid and Dermoid Cysts

Presumably, epidermoid and dermoid cysts are implantation or sequestration cysts derived from misplaced ectoderm. These cysts may be congenital or acquired. The cause of the congenital type is inclusion of ectodermal tissue during embryonic closure of the neural groove or during coalescence of epithelial fusion lines in the cranium. Sequestration cysts accompany dysraphism, such as spina bifida, and may communicate with the skin surface through a sinus tract.

Epidermoid cysts occur in young adults and are usually found in the cerebellopontine angle or skull. Dermoid cysts are more common in children and tend to occur near the midline in the cerebellar vermis, parasellar or parapontine region, and spinal canal, especially in the lumbosacral region. A fibrous capsule that has a glistening white surface (like mother-of-pearl) envelops intact tumors called *pearly tumors.* The lining and contents of the epidermoid are composed of keratinizing squamous epithelium that may attenuate or focally stratify. The thin wisps of flaky intraluminal keratin are dry keratin, in contrast to the type seen in craniopharyngiomas. The adjacent collagenous wall often partially calcifies, producing a linear or speckled pattern in CT images. The inner layer of a dermoid cyst is also composed of squamous epithelium, but the presence of hair follicles and other skin appendages distinguishes dermoid cysts from epidermoid cysts. The cyst contents, once introduced into the meninges by spontaneous rupture or during surgery, can incite chemical meningitis.

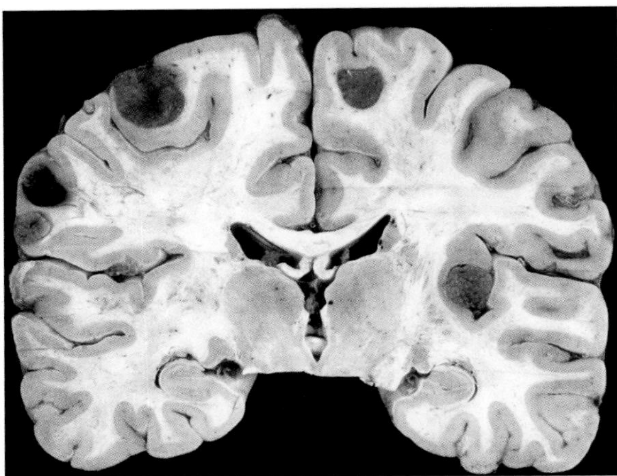

**Fig. 72.27 Metastatic Small-Cell Carcinoma.** Foci of well-demarcated tumor, primarily localized to corticomedullary junctions.

### Neuroenteric, Colloid, and Rathke Cleft Cysts

Cysts lined by cuboidal to columnar mucin-producing epithelial cells, resembling those of respiratory or enteric lining, may occur in several sites throughout the CNS. Such cysts are referred to as a *Rathke cleft cyst* in the sella, *colloid cyst* in the third ventricle, and *neuroenteric cyst* (or enterogenous, bronchogenic, or neuroepithelial cyst) when they occur in the anterior spinal region or rarely at intracranial sites. The origin of these cysts, thought to be developmental rather than neoplastic, is unknown. Although the presumed embryology may differ at these sites, the histological appearance is otherwise similar.

## METASTATIC TUMORS

Metastatic tumors of the nervous system are far more common than primary brain tumors. Most occur in middle-aged and older adults, with multiple CNS metastases commonly detected. Metastases often lodge in the corticomedullary junction. A zone of vasogenic edema customarily surrounds even small metastatic lesions.

The typical metastasis is round, sharply demarcated, with central necrosis or hemorrhage (Fig. 72.27). Spontaneous bleeding is characteristic of choriocarcinoma, melanoma, or renal carcinoma metastases. However, metastatic lung carcinoma is so much more common that it accounts for most hemorrhagic cases. In fact, lung carcinoma represents by far the most common primary tumor that metastasizes to the brain. Most other primary tumors metastasize to the lung before they gain access to the brain. Histological appearances are variable and recapitulate the morphology of the primary tumor in question. Most metastatic lesions are carcinomas or melanomas rather than sarcomas or lymphomas.

### Acknowledgments

Michael Jansen, Arie Perry, Reid R. Heffner, Jr., and David N. Louis were authors of this chapter in the previous edition.

*The complete reference list is available online at https://expertconsult.inkling.com/.* 

73

# Clinical Features of Brain Tumors and Complications of Their Treatment

Reena P. Thomas, Michael Iv

## OUTLINE



## CLINICAL FEATURES OF BRAIN TUMORS

### Overview of Symptoms

Patients with both primary and metastatic brain tumors can present with a variety of clinical symptoms and neurological signs. These manifestations are not specific for individual tumor subtypes or brain tumors, and symptoms can easily be mistaken for a number of other neurological conditions. In general, symptoms and signs are influenced by the underlying tumor's location, size, and growth rate. Some symptoms are focal, allowing clinical localization of the underlying tumor, while others are generalized and nonlocalizing. At the same time, it is important to note that brain tumor patients may have very few, if any, symptoms at the time of diagnosis.

Focal brain tumor symptoms are typically caused by tumor invasion into brain parenchyma, or by local compression from tumor, associated edema, or hemorrhage. In contrast, most generalized symptoms are the result of an increase in intracranial pressure that results from mass effect of the tumor, malignant edema, or hydrocephalus from cerebrospinal fluid (CSF) outflow obstruction. Brain tumors rarely cause constitutional symptoms associated with other advanced systemic cancers such as fevers, night sweats, anorexia, or weight loss. Symptoms produced by brain tumors are typically subacute and progressive, developing over days to weeks. However, because initial symptoms are often subtle, delayed recognition can make their eventual appearance seem acute. Obvious exceptions include symptoms from seizures, hemorrhages, and herniation, which can appear suddenly. Often even large brain tumors produce surprisingly few symptoms, which speaks to the nervous system's ability to accommodate gradual tumor growth. In fact, radiographic evidence of midline shift or herniation caused by a brain tumor may have minimal clinical consequences, in stark contrast to more acute neuropathology (Fig. 73.1). Unfortunately, as a result, even a seemingly normal neurological examination cannot completely rule out the presence of an underlying brain tumor.

Patient age can influence presentation, as in the case of elderly patients where cerebral atrophy may mitigate mass effect, or infants who may present with increasing head circumference. Patient comorbidities can also affect the recognition of brain tumor symptoms, as with headaches in a patient with a history of migraines or cognitive changes in the elderly. In the end, the presentation of a patient with a brain tumor can be quite variable, and there are no symptoms or signs specific to the diagnosis. Instead, a thorough history and neurological examination are required together with a high level of suspicion, particularly in at-risk populations such as those with a history of systemic cancer, prior brain radiation, or tumor predisposition syndromes. Understanding the ways in which brain tumors can present and some of the "red flags" to look for will help clinicians know when to suspect the diagnosis.

### Specific Symptoms and Signs

#### Focal Symptoms

***Focal motor symptoms.*** The frontal lobe is a common location for both primary and metastatic brain tumors, which frequently cause motor weakness in the contralateral face or limbs (Fig. 73.2). Weakness can result from tumors invading or compressing motor tracts in the cortex, subcortical white matter, internal capsule, or brainstem. Symptoms generally begin as subtle incoordination or loss of fine motor control and progress gradually, so that patients may not initially recognize weakness, though signs may be found on neurological examination. This gradual development of weakness is unlike the sudden weakness seen in stroke, though acute weakness can develop after a seizure or in the setting of intratumoral hemorrhage. Because hemorrhage is common, particularly in pilocytic astrocytoma, in high-grade glioma, and in metastases from melanoma and thyroid and renal cell carcinoma, it is important to obtain a 1- to 2-month follow-up magnetic resonance imaging (MRI) in any patient presenting with an otherwise unexplained intracranial hemorrhage (Li et al., 2013; Little et al., 1979).

Brain tumors rarely present with extrapyramidal motor manifestations, and though there are reports of patients with thalamic or basal ganglia tumors presenting with tremors or parkinsonism (Frosini et al., 2009; Grover, 2010), these symptoms rarely occur in isolation.

***Ataxia.*** Tumors of the cerebellum and brainstem tumors infiltrating the cerebellar peduncles can frequently produce symptoms and signs of ataxia. Cerebellar hemispheric tumors can cause ipsilateral limb ataxia, though many produce few symptoms. In contrast, involvement of the cerebellar vermis tends to be more symptomatic, producing truncal ataxia, often with nystagmus, scanning dysarthria, and ataxic gait. Less well localizing is a more general gait unsteadiness frequently experienced by brain tumor patients. This may be due to subtle limb weakness, disequilibrium, or sensory disturbances, and a detailed neurological examination is necessary to distinguish these causes from ataxia. In addition to symptoms of ataxia, large cerebellar tumors can cause CSF outflow obstruction (with symptoms of increased intracranial pressure) or compressed brainstem structures. Ataxia can, therefore, be an important initial clue to a tumor with the potential for acute neurological decline. Ataxia and associated symptoms from cerebellar tumors are much more common in children, where more than half of primary brain tumors arise in the posterior fossa (Pollack, 1994). In contrast to children, ataxia is relatively uncommon in adults, as fewer than 20% of adult brain tumors arise in the posterior fossa.

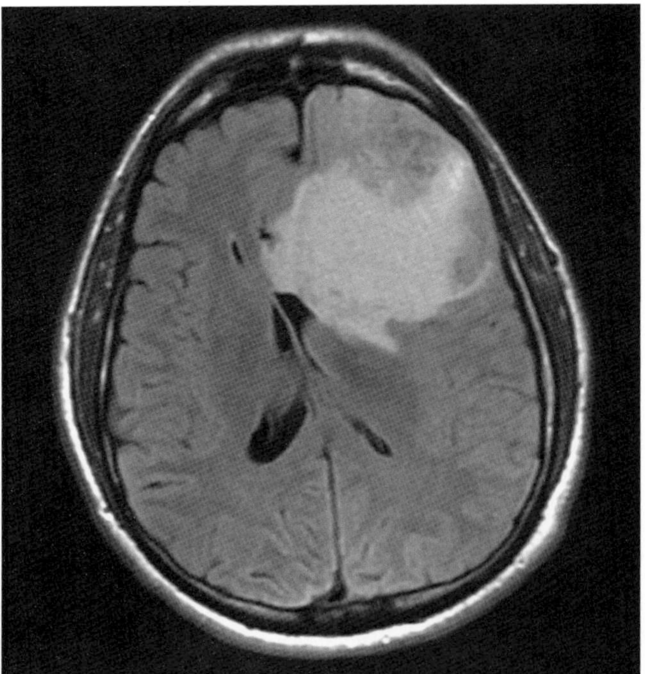

**Fig. 73.1** T2 FLAIR (fluid-attenuated inversion recovery) magnetic resonance image demonstrates a large left frontal glioblastoma causing subfalcine herniation and producing minimal symptoms in the form of a mild headache.

***Aphasia.*** Tumors involving the inferior frontal or superior temporal lobes of the dominant hemisphere frequently present with language difficulty. As with other brain tumor symptoms, language impairment is usually subtle at first and progresses gradually; however, sudden-onset aphasia can occur in the setting of a seizure and may be mistaken for a transient ischemic attack. Most brain tumor patients with aphasia have a mixture of expressive and receptive language impairments that defy simple classification. Given variable language localization between individuals and the reorganization that can occur in the vicinity of a brain tumor, the use of cortical stimulation mapping with awake craniotomy at the time of surgery can allow identification of areas essential for language in patients with mild language impairment (De Witt Hamer et al., 2012). This intraoperative technique can improve the extent of tumor resection while minimizing the risk of permanent language deficits.

***Visual problems.*** Brain tumors can cause a number of different visual symptoms depending on which portions of the visual pathway they involve. The somatotopic organization of vision often allows visual symptoms to reflect tumor location, though precise localization can require detailed testing and a cooperative patient. Tumors that affect the retina or the optic nerve anterior to the chiasm cause monocular visual symptoms ranging from scotoma to monocular blindness. Tumors that arise from the sella, most frequently including pituitary adenomas, craniopharyngiomas, and meningiomas, can compress the optic chiasm, classically causing a bitemporal hemianopsia. Post-chiasmatic tumors cause a homonymous hemianopsia, which becomes increasingly symmetric the more posteriorly the tumor is located. Parietal tumors can give rise to contralateral visual neglect, which can be difficult to distinguish from frequently co-occurring visual field loss. Particularly in the case of slow-growing tumors, the onset of visual field deficits can occur so gradually that patients may not seek medical attention for many months or years. Beyond vision loss itself, tumors involving the midbrain or pons, or directly compressing the third, fourth, or sixth cranial nerves, can impair coordinated eye movement, leading to double vision. Compression of the dorsal midbrain, most often by pineal tumors, can cause vertical gaze palsy, which, together with convergence-retraction nystagmus, light-near pupillary dissociation, and eyelid retraction, make up the Parinaud syndrome.

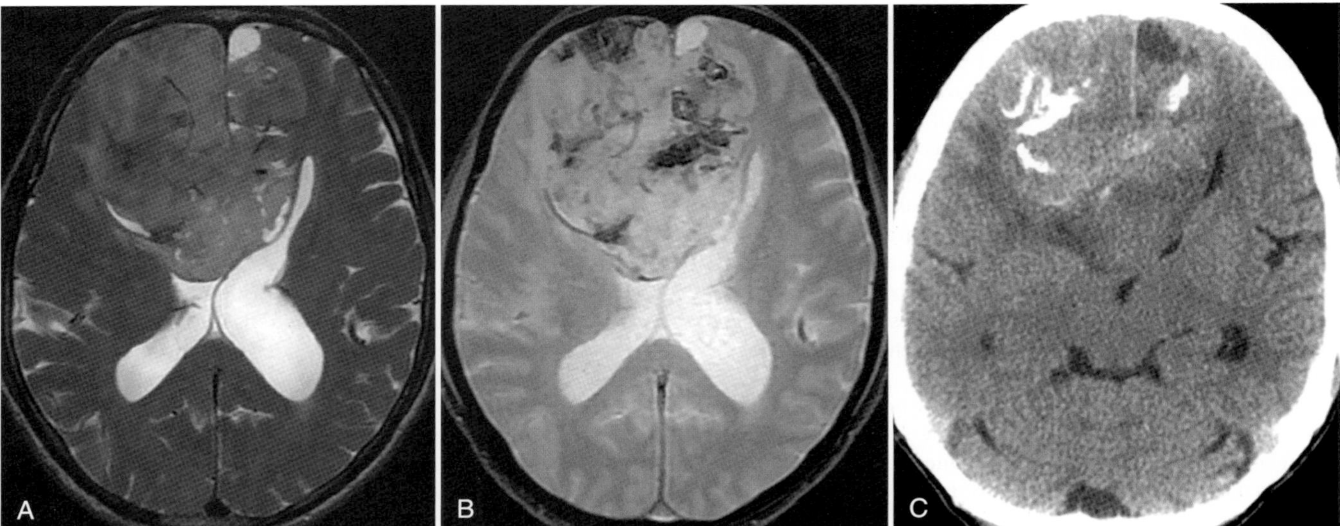


**Fig. 73.2** Large calcified anaplastic oligodendroglioma in the bilateral frontal lobes on axial T2-weighted **(A)** and gradient echo (GRE) **(B)** magnetic resonance images and non-contrast computed tomography image **(C)**.

A number of apparently focal visual signs can actually be falsely localizing manifestations of an increase in intracranial pressure (Lepore, 2002). Double vision can be caused by an increase in intracranial pressure causing sixth cranial nerve palsies; this false localizing sign is presumed to be due to traction of the nerve along its extended extracranial course. Pupillary dilatation followed by diplopia from a third cranial nerve palsy can be an ominous sign of uncal herniation. A contralateral hemiparesis is often seen, though ipsilateral hemiparesis can be a false localizing sign resulting from brainstem displacement and compression of the contralateral cerebral peduncle against the tentorium (Kernohan notch). Finally, increases in intracranial pressure are reflected at the optic nerve head, where signs of papilledema can manifest as decreased visual acuity and episodes of transient visual loss known as visual obscurations.

***Seizures.*** Seizures are a common brain tumor manifestation that can occur at initial presentation or anytime over the subsequent course of the disease. New onset or increasing frequency or severity of seizures can be a sign of underlying tumor progression and should prompt re-evaluation. The overall incidence of seizures varies with underlying tumor type and location. Tumors that involve the cerebral cortex are most likely to cause seizures, and temporal, frontal, and parietal lobe tumors are more commonly associated with seizures than those in the occipital lobe. In contrast, tumors in the deep gray nuclei, sella, and posterior fossa rarely cause seizures. Seizures are generally more common in primary brain tumors than in brain metastases, and slow-growing low-grade tumors cause seizures more frequently than high-grade tumors. Certain low-grade glial and glioneuronal tumors are particularly epileptogenic (Japp et al., 2013; van Breemen et al., 2007), including dysembryoplastic neuroepithelial tumors (where seizures occur in essentially 100% of patients), gangliogliomas (80%–90%), and low-grade oligodendrogliomas (90%) and astrocytomas (75%). Despite the high frequency of seizures in patients with brain tumors, prophylactic use of antiepileptic drugs (AEDs) in patients with no seizure history is currently not recommended, though AEDs are often used for 1–2 weeks postoperatively to decrease the risk of potentially devastating perioperative seizures.

Seizures resulting from brain tumors invariably originate focally, with initial seizure symptoms or lateralizing postictal signs often reflecting the location of the tumor. However, rapid secondary generalization can obscure initial symptoms, making it difficult to appreciate the seizure's partial onset. As a result, many seizures appear or are remembered as generalized and nonlocalizing. In the evaluation of brain tumor patients with loss of consciousness, it is important to also consider syncope and intracranial pressure waves alongside generalized seizures.

### Generalized Symptoms

***Headaches.*** Headaches are a common reason for neurological referral and although they occur at some point in 50%–70% of patients with brain tumors, most headaches without other neurological signs or symptoms are not associated with an underlying tumor (Forsyth and Posner, 1993; Goffaux and Fortin, 2010; Schankin et al., 2007; Suwanwela et al., 1994). Headaches are generally described by patients as bifrontal and tension-like, with constant, dull pressure, though they may mimic migraine, especially in patients with a prior history of migraine (Forsyth and Posner, 1993). *Classic brain tumor headaches* occur in the early morning with nausea and vomiting and improve over the course of the day; however, these symptoms only occur in 5%–17% of all brain tumor patients, 42% of whom have posterior fossa tumors (Forsyth and Posner, 1993; Schankin et al., 2007; Valentinis et al., 2010).

Headaches can be associated with signs of increased intracranial pressure, including nausea and vomiting and worsening with Valsalva maneuvers. Patients with infratentorial tumors can also develop occipital headaches. Schwannomas and posterior fossa meningiomas can occasionally present with trigeminal autonomic cephalalgias. Throbbing headaches and pulsatile pain can be seen in patients with pituitary adenomas and meningiomas (Gondim et al., 2009; Schankin et al., 2007). Episodic headaches and signs of plateau waves may occur in pedunculated tumors of the third ventricle, leading to intermittent obstruction of CSF flow precipitated by positional change. Headaches are more common in brain metastases and glioblastomas where most patients experience headache, while only 10% of patients with low-grade gliomas suffer from headaches. Factors that predispose brain tumor patients to headache include a prior history of headaches, location and size of the tumor, surrounding edema, mass effect, and midline shift (Schankin et al., 2007; Valentinis et al., 2010). A new-onset headache in an adult with no prior history of headaches or change in the quality, severity, or location of a pre-existing headache should be evaluated with detailed neurological examination and brain imaging.

***Nausea and vomiting.*** Nausea and vomiting can be generalized signs of increased intracranial pressure in patients with brain tumors, and are most common in tumors of the posterior fossa. Vomiting occurs as a result of stimulation of the chemotactic trigger zone in the area postrema near the floor of the fourth ventricle, which is sensitive to raised intracranial pressure. Alternatively, this region can be directly compressed by midline tumors of the posterior fossa such as medulloblastomas or ependymomas. Brainstem tumors involving tractus solitarius can also lead to vomiting in the absence of intracranial hypertension. Projectile vomiting is typically seen in children with posterior fossa tumors, and is rare in adults. Vomiting as seizure semiology is rare, but has been described in insular and mesiotemporal lobe tumors (Chen et al., 1999; Schauble et al., 2002).

***Syncope.*** Brain tumor patients can experience syncope or transient loss of consciousness and tone for a variety of reasons. Changes in position can trigger pressure waves and syncope in patients with elevated intracranial pressure. Syncope may also result from tumor involvement or compression of the brainstem. Third ventricular masses such as colloid cysts or pineal tumors most commonly seen in children can cause syncope or drop attacks due to intermittent obstruction of the cerebral aqueduct. Syncope may also be the result of hormone deficiency caused by pituitary tumors, or more commonly from adrenal insufficiency following rapid taper of long-standing corticosteroids. Syncope should be differentiated from generalized seizures, which are more frequent in this patient population and require distinct treatment with AEDs. Finally, cardiac rhythm abnormalities with or without seizures should be ruled out as a cause of syncope in brain tumor patients (van der Sluijs et al., 2004), particularly those with tumors affecting the insular cortex (Cole et al., 2013; Montenegro et al., 2011).

***Mental status and behavioral changes.*** Nonspecific mental status and cognitive changes are common in patients with brain tumors, though they may be subtle early in the course of the disease. Symptoms can include change in personality, irritability, disinhibition, lack of initiative, withdrawal, emotional lability, inattentiveness, apathy, somnolence, and lethargy. These symptoms can be seen in up to 34% of patients with brain tumors (Chang et al., 2005). Cognitive and behavioral symptoms are difficult to localize, though they often correlate with involvement of the corpus callosum, thalamus, or frontal lobes. Mental status change may alternatively be a sign of elevated intracranial pressure. Patients presenting with gradually progressive focal symptoms, such as aphasia (especially receptive aphasia), apraxia, agnosia, alexia, or abulia, may be perceived as having altered mental status or confusion, and a detailed neurological evaluation is important to differentiate these focal symptoms from mental status changes.

## COMPLICATIONS OF BRAIN TUMOR TREATMENT

Primary brain tumors are treated with a combination of surgery, radiation, and chemotherapy. This section discusses the neurological complications that can result from the treatment of primary brain tumors. A larger discussion of all potential side effects from brain tumor treatment or neurological complications from all anticancer therapy is beyond the scope of this chapter.

### Surgery

Surgical resection can improve brain tumor symptoms by relieving mass effect, by improving seizure control, and—depending on the tumor type—by reducing the risk of recurrence and by improving survival (Fig. 73.3). Most series have demonstrated perioperative mortality of 1.5%–3% with craniotomy (Chang et al., 2003; Fadul et al., 1988; Paek et al., 2005). Neurological complications from surgery may be the result of direct injury to the brain or arterial or venous infarction. Incidence ranges from 5% to 32%, with more recent series documenting lower incidence (Chang et al., 2003; Fadul et al., 1988; Gulati et al., 2011; Hoover et al., 2013; Sawaya et al., 1998). Regional complications may result from hemorrhage, CSF leak, or wound infection. There is an increased risk of impaired wound healing or wound dehiscence with multiple surgeries, radiation, or treatment with anti-angiogenic agents like bevacizumab (Barami and Fernandes, 2012). Postoperative seizures can occur in 1%–7.5% of patients after craniotomy (Chang et al., 2003; Hoover et al., 2013; Paek et al., 2005; Sawaya et al., 1998). Cerebellar mutism following midline posterior fossa surgery can be seen in up to 24% of children (Robertson et al., 2006).

In general, factors contributing to increased risk of neurological complications include age greater than 60 years, poor performance status, eloquent or deep location, and prior surgery or radiation

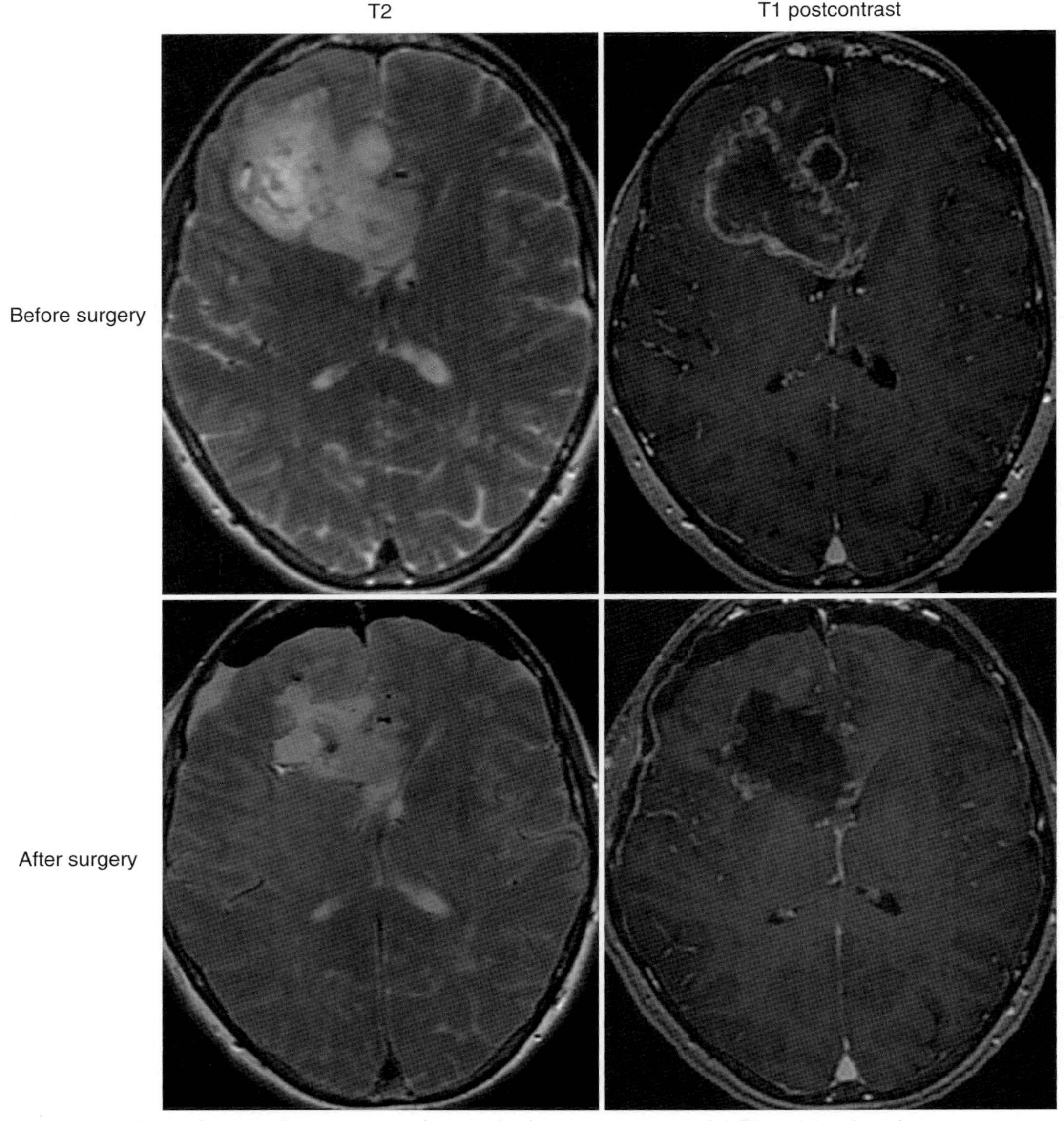


**Fig. 73.3** Right frontal glioblastoma before and after surgery on axial T2-weighted and postcontrast T1-weighted images.

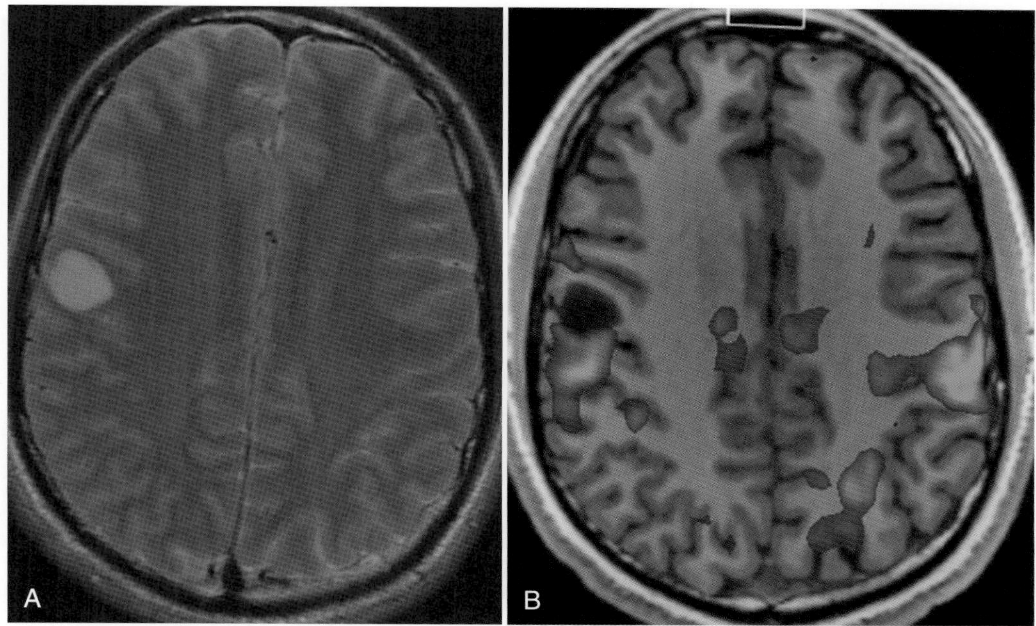

**Fig. 73.4 Right Lateral Frontal Lobe Dysembryoplastic Neuroepithelial Tumor. A,** Axial T2-weighted image shows a circumscribed and T2 bright mass in the right lateral frontal lobe. **B,** Following acquisition of task-based functional magnetic resonance imaging (specifically during movement of the tongue), there is motor activation along the posterior margin of the tumor.

(Chang et al., 2003; Fadul et al., 1988; Vorster and Barnett, 1998). One recent study has shown that the highest risk of neurological complications is between the first and second surgery (4.8% vs. 12.1%) and plateaus thereafter. In contrast, the risk of regional complications has been shown to increase with each surgery (6%–22% from 1 to ≥4 surgeries) (Hoover et al., 2013). Advances in neurosurgery, including neuronavigation, cortical mapping, intraoperative neuro-physiological monitoring, intraoperative MRI, functional MRI (Fig. 73.4), and awake craniotomy, have led to reduced risk of neurological complications.

## Radiation

Radiation is a standard treatment modality for patients with both primary and metastatic brain tumors (Fig. 73.5). Radiation damage to the brain can be acute (within days), early-delayed (1–6 months), and late-delayed (months to years) (Sheline et al., 1980; Soussain et al., 2009). Acute encephalopathy is related to raised intracranial pressure and presents as reversible headache, vomiting, focal signs, and fatigue. Early-delayed encephalopathy can present as neurological deterioration or somnolence. Patients with malignant glioma may demonstrate areas of contrast enhancement on MRI within a few months of concurrent chemoradiation with temozolomide. This *pseudoprogression* can be managed with corticosteroids (Brandsma et al., 2008), and should be differentiated from true disease progression that could necessitate a change in therapy. Late-delayed encephalopathy may be seen as radiation necrosis presenting with focal signs responding to corticosteroids, or atrophy with ventriculomegaly and leukoencephalopathy presenting as memory loss, gait ataxia, and incontinence, which may benefit from ventriculoperitoneal shunt placement (Thiessen and DeAngelis, 1998). The risk of leukoencephalopathy is higher with whole-brain radiation, old age, vascular risk factors, and combined chemoradiation. Neurocognitive decline can be seen in many patients after radiation and its treatment is difficult. A recent randomized trial

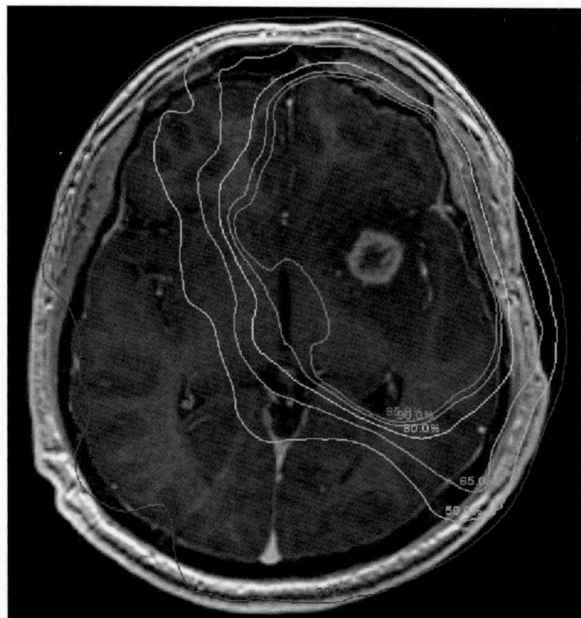

**Fig. 73.5** Radiation planning magnetic resonance image in a patient with a left frontal glioblastoma.

suggested that patients undergoing radiation who were treated with the *N*-methyl-D-aspartate (NMDA) receptor antagonist memantine had better cognitive function over time, although this was not statistically significant (Brown et al., 2013). Cranial neuropathies, including optic neuropathy, may develop as late complications. Radiation vasculopathy can occur years later and may lead to ischemic events such as stroke from intracranial vascular stenosis or hemorrhage from cavernomas. Stroke-like migraine attacks after radiation or SMART syndrome has been described (Black et al.,

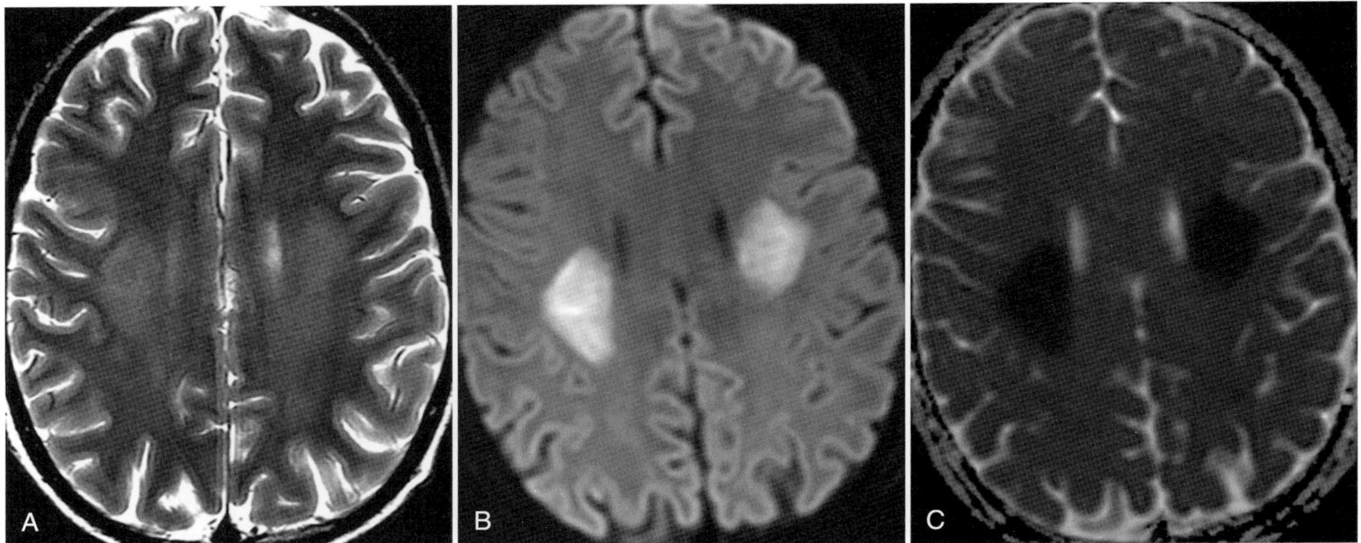

**Fig. 73.6 Acute Methotrexate Leukoencephalopathy. A,** Axial T2-weighted image showing symmetric bright signal intensity in the centrum semiovale. There is corresponding diffusion restriction—i.e., bright signal on diffusion-weighted **(B)** and dark signal on apparent diffusion coefficient **(C)** images—in the white matter, which is consistent with the acute phase of disease.

2006; Kerklaan et al., 2011). Other late complications include radiation-induced meningiomas, gliomas, sarcomas, and peripheral nerve sheath tumors.

## Chemotherapy and Biological Therapy

*Temozolomide* is an alkylating agent used in the initial treatment of glioblastoma, and is generally well tolerated with largely non-neurological side effects. Common neurologically relevant side effects include fatigue and thrombocytopenia, which can predispose to hemorrhage, including intracranial or intratumoral hemorrhage.

*Nitrosoureas* (*lomustine and carmustine*) typically do not cause neurotoxicity at the doses used for treatment of primary brain tumors. Higher-dose intravenous or intraarterial administration, especially in patients who have received prior radiation, can cause encephalopathy, seizures, and optic neuropathy. Carmustine biodegradable wafers are approved for placement directly into the tumor bed at the time of resection, but treatment can be complicated by local inflammation, infection, CSF leak, and seizures (Sabel and Giese, 2008).

*Procarbazine* (or PCV—procarbazine, CCNU (lomustine), vincristine) can cause encephalopathy and peripheral neuropathy.

*Vincristine* can cause a dose-limiting sensorimotor neuropathy, cranial neuropathy, and autonomic neuropathy. Risk factors include older age, dose, other neurotoxic drugs, and pre-existing neuropathy.

*Methotrexate* can cause acute or chronic neurotoxicity after oral, intravenous, or intrathecal use (Fig. 73.6). Acute encephalopathy can result from intrathecal or high-dose intravenous injection. Aseptic meningitis or myelopathy can also develop after intrathecal treatment. Chronic or diffuse leukoencephalopathy may appear months to years after treatment. There is a synergistic effect of cranial radiation (Correa et al., 2012).

*Bevacizumab* is a humanized monoclonal antibody against vascular endothelial growth factor, and is the only targeted therapy currently US Food and Drug Administration-approved for the treatment of glioblastoma. Neurological side effects include intracranial or intratumoral hemorrhage, ischemic events (including strokes/transient ischemic attacks), reversible posterior leukoencephalopathy syndrome (RPLS), and impaired wound healing following craniotomy (Clark et al., 2011; Fraum et al., 2011; Lou et al., 2011).

## Immunotherapy

There are many approved strategies to employ immune system–based therapies for cancer treatment, including immune checkpoint blockade and chimeric antigen receptor (CAR) T-cell therapy; however, immune-related adverse events (IRAEs) may occur as a result of treatment. Most commonly, the gastrointestinal tract, endocrine glands, skin, and liver may become affected; however, with increased use of these therapies, we are also seeing adverse events having a negative impact on the central nervous system. Clinical practice of how to effectively manage specific IRAEs remains variable, although the use of high-dose corticosteroids—including dexamethasone and methylprednisolone—remains a key aspect of clinical care for IRAE and immune effector cell–associated neurotoxicity syndrome (ICANS) (Postow et al., 2018; Neelapu et al., 2019).

*The complete reference list is available online at https://expertconsult.inkling.com/.* 

74

# Primary Nervous System Tumors in Adults

*Ashley Roque, Fred H. Hochberg, Joachim M. Baehring*

## OUTLINE



In the year 2019, approximately 86,970 cases of primary nervous system tumors are expected to occur in the United States (Ostrom et al., 2018). The World Health Organization (WHO) distinguishes between six groups of neoplasms. Meningeal tumors (mostly meningioma) and neuroepithelial tumors (astrocytic tumors including glioblastoma multiforme [GBM], oligodendrogliomas, and others) each account for about one-third of nervous system neoplasms. The remaining one-third is composed of tumors of the sellar region (pituitary adenoma, craniopharyngioma), tumors of peripheral nerves, lymphatic and hematopoietic tumors, and germ cell neoplasms.

Management of patients with primary brain tumors is an interdisciplinary effort that includes neurosurgeons, neurologists, radiation oncologists, medical oncologists, neuroradiologists, and neuropathologists. Neurologists are involved in the clinical diagnosis, treatment with chemotherapeutic agents or new medical strategies, and symptomatic therapy. Over the last 30 years, progress has been made in diagnostic procedures, monitoring of therapeutic efficacy, optimizing standard treatments for selected tumor subtypes, understanding the pathogenesis of primary brain tumors, and developing new treatment concepts. Surgical techniques have been refined and now allow the use of the operating microscope, intraoperative magnetic resonance imaging (MRI), preoperative mapping using functional MRI and fiber tractography, or intraoperative immunofluorescence technology. Surgery is curative for completely resectable meningioma and noninfiltrative gliomas. As surgery has become more precise, so has radiation therapy (RT). Conventional strategies provide cure for patients with germinomas. Highly focused external radiation strategies have improved local tumor control with reduced damage to contiguous normal brain. Chemotherapy improves survival and function of patients with lymphoma or glial brain tumors.

High-grade gliomas remain the biggest therapeutic challenge. Despite the provision of radiation therapy and chemotherapy as adjuvant treatment, fewer than 20% of patients with GBM are alive 2 years after diagnosis. Thus tertiary centers are consulted to provide experimental approaches to treat these patients.

Novel therapies must take into account issues specific to brain tumors. The blood–brain barrier (BBB) prevents access to the brain by hydrophilic chemotherapeutic agents and large molecules. Cells of brain tumors are uniquely able to resist chemotherapeutic agents by overexpressing membrane proteins that eliminate these drugs or by inducing enzymes to inactivate them. Even when drugs enter brain tumors, not all cells are sensitive. The hypoxic areas of tumors are in cell-cycle arrest and resistant to cell cycle–dependent agents or radiation. Other factors confounding therapy include corticosteroids that alter the BBB penetration of drugs, the host immunological reaction to the tumor, as well as the cytotoxic effects of chemotherapy.

This chapter reviews current therapeutic principles of brain tumors in adults and provides an approach to specific neoplasms.

## GENERAL ASPECTS

### Established Treatment Strategies

#### Surgery

Surgery, the primary modality of management for patients with brain masses, provides indispensable diagnostic information, alleviates mass effect, reduces seizure activity, and may offer cure.

No rational therapy can be administered without a histological diagnosis. Stereotactic biopsy uses targets acquired by computed tomography (CT) or MRI. A stereotactic frame or fiducial markers are placed on the patient's head assuring appropriate sampling and diagnosis in over 95% of patients. Functional MRI and diffusion-tensor imaging are performed to identify contiguous, eloquent areas of the brain and white matter tracts. The data is co-registered on three-dimensional MRI reconstructions from which biopsy coordinates are drawn. A probe is then passed through a small drill hole that retrieves cylindrical samples 1 cm in length and 1–2 mm in diameter. The procedure is safe and associated with less than a 2% risk of seizure, hemorrhage, or infection.

Some intracranial tumors can be cured by complete surgical resection (noninfiltrative gliomas, pituitary adenoma, meningioma). Less clear is the benefit of resecting the infiltrating diffuse astrocytoma or "partial" decompression of an aggressive tumor. Resection provides prolonged survival for oligodendrogliomas and most clinicians support "subtotal" resection in the setting of increased intracranial pressure; steroid-obligating mass effect, hemorrhage, or impending herniation; the presence of necrotic tumor cysts; and uncontrollable seizures. Often the decision to operate depends on preoperative MRI mapping of both gray and white matter functions. Aids to the surgeon also include tumor resection based on intraoperative MRI, intraoperative cortical stimulation mapping, and monitoring of somatosensory evoked potentials. It is often argued that surgery will reduce the burden of tumor prone to malignant degeneration, but this view is countered by the occurrence of infiltrates of tumor extending at distances from the main mass. The advocates of subtotal resection often cite the diminished likelihood of sampling error associated with stereotactic biopsy. Following operation, within 48 hours, a contrast-enhanced MRI is recommended as an objective measure of residual tumor. After 48 hours, perioperative changes occur in the brain and prevent accurate determination of residual tumor.

A device has been approved by the US Food and Drug Administration (FDA) for intraoperative MRI-guided laser interstitial thermocoagulation therapy (LITT) and is currently used for treatment of brain metastases, primary brain tumors, and radiation necrosis when conventional treatment strategies have been exhausted. The laser probe is passed through a small burr hole in the skull so that the high-intensity laser energy can be applied directly to brain tumor tissue (Torres-Reveron et al., 2013).

In 2017 the FDA approved the use of Gleolan (aminolevulinic acid hydrochloride or ALA HCl), a fluorescing agent, for use as an adjunct for visualization of malignant tissue during glioma surgery. ALA occurs endogenously as a metabolite that is formed in the mitochondria from succinyl co-enzyme A (succinyl coenzyme A) and glycine. Exogenous administration of ALA leads to accumulation of the ALA metabolite protoporphyrin IX (PpIX) in tumor cells, which causes violet-red fluorescence of the cells after excitation with a 405-nm-wavelength blue light. Three to four hours prior to induction of anesthesia, Gleolan is administered orally to the patient. Intraoperatively, the tumor is then visualized with a standard surgical operating microscope adapted with a "fluorescence mode," which is switched on to allow for real-time intraoperative guidance using the fluorescent properties of PpIX. Multiple studies have shown that ALA-induced tumor fluorescence extends beyond the area of gadolinium enhancement seen on preoperative MRI, allowing for maximal resection of infiltrative cells at the tumor margin (Hadjipanayis et al., 2015).

## Radiation Therapy

Radiation therapy is commonly provided to treat brain tumors. Some tumors, such as germinomas, can be cured and others are slowed in their progression. Survival is improved in many glial and nonglial tumors, and symptoms, including seizures, are reduced. Palliation is the goal for older adult patients or those with leptomeningeal tumor.

The target for radiation cell death is the DNA molecule. High-energy beams cause breaks in the DNA double strand either by ionization of the target atom or by production of free radicals. The effect of radiation depends on the dose applied, how often it is applied, and how much time is available for the target to repair the damage. Dividing cells are more susceptible to irradiation than are nondividing cells, especially during the M(mitotic) and $G_2$ phase of the cell cycle.

Photons are the most commonly used particles in the radiation therapy of brain tumors. Examples of nonphoton irradiation modalities (most of them only available in experimental facilities) include neutrons, protons, and heavy ions (carbon, argon, neon).

Radiation therapy is usually delivered by a linear accelerator (LINAC), which uses high-frequency electromagnetic waves to accelerate electrons to high energies. The electron beam is used directly for the treatment of superficial tumors or indirectly by producing x-ray beams for the treatment of deep-seated lesions. Shielding blocks are built for each patient to restrict the beam to the target volume. The size of the treatment field depends on the tumor type. For infiltrative tumors, such as malignant gliomas, therapy is provided to the volume of enhancement or $T_2$ abnormality on MRI and a margin of 1–3 cm. For noninfiltrative tumors, a narrower margin suffices. On the other hand, whole-brain radiation therapy (WBRT) is provided to treat multifocal infiltrating tumors seen in gliomatosis cerebri (GC) or the multiple masses of recurrent brain lymphoma. Strategies, mainly of experimental nature, to improve tumor cell kill and minimize damage to normal tissue include increasing the number of treatment fractions to two or more per day, the use of multiple fields, the use of radiosensitizing agents, or localized high-field strength sources.

The clinician should be aware of radiation therapy complications. Within 10 days of the start of irradiation, patients may become fatigued and experience altered appetite and sleep patterns resulting from brain edema. Six to 18 months after radiation, contrast-enhanced masses reflect radiation-induced white matter necrosis. Additional complications include pan–hypothalamic-pituitary dysfunction, elevated prolactin levels, impotence, or amenorrhea. Exposure to therapeutic doses of ionizing radiation increases the risk for secondary malignancies within the radiation field (4% in 10 years; Packer et al., 2013).

***Conventional fractionated radiotherapy.*** Conventional three-dimensional–conformal radiation therapy is provided in daily fractions of 1.8–2.0 Gy. The total dose seldom exceeds 60 Gy to avoid radiation necrosis, or damage to normal brain. "Hyperfractionation" protocols decrease the dose per fraction, but increase the number of fractions per day. With accelerated fractionation, the dose is applied over a shorter period by increasing the number of daily treatments. In theory, this reduces repopulation of tumor cells during irradiation. Fractionation strategies require immobilization devices such as bite blocks and thermoplastic molds that allow reproducible positioning of the patient with each treatment. The use of multiple radiation fields or three-dimensional conformal irradiation limits the exposure of overlying skin and normal brain tissue.

***Brachytherapy.*** In brachytherapy, radiation is delivered by implanting the irradiation source close to or into the target tissue. Interstitial therapy uses iridium-192 or iodine-125 seeds. Scalp infections have been described after therapy with high-activity brachytherapy seeds, and there is a 50% risk of the development of necrosis in the radiation site. Nearly half of patients require surgical removal of this tissue. Intratumoral positioning of miniature x-ray–generating devices or temporary intracavitary placement of a balloon catheter through which radionuclide can be administered are other forms of local radiation delivery. Survival outcomes using this technique have been variable. Given the technical complexity and potential for toxicity, the use of brachytherapy in the treatment of brain tumors is limited in current practice.

***Sensitization of tumor cells to ionizing radiation.*** Hypoxic tumor cells likely evade the lethal effect of irradiation. Rapidly growing tumors such as malignant gliomas contain a fraction of hypoxic cells that may represent one-third of the tumor burden. Fractionation of irradiation allows reoxygenation of tumor tissue during the resting intervals. Pharmacological strategies include nitroimidazoles such as metronidazole, misonidazole, or etanidazole, and the hypoxic cytotoxin tirapazamine. Oxygen delivery to the tumor can be increased by the application of hyperbaric oxygen or the provision of agents that alter the hemoglobin–oxygen dissociation curve (RSR13). Examples for nonhypoxic radiosensitizers are halogenated pyrimidines such as 5-bromodeoxy-uridine and hydroxyurea. Radiosensitization is also provided by certain chemotherapeutic agents (cisplatin or doxorubicin), the antitrypanosomal agent suramin, or the angiogenesis inhibitor thalidomide. Thus far, radiosensitizers have not shown to be of any benefit to brain tumor patients.

***Stereotactic radiosurgery techniques.*** Radiosurgery is the name given to single fractions of stereotactic radiosurgery (SRS) and multiple fractions of stereotactic radiation therapy (SRT). These techniques deliver large doses of radiation to well-circumscribed tumor sites while minimizing exposure to normal tissue. Three types of facilities are typically used. *LINAC radiosurgery* uses a modified LINAC to produce high-energy photon beams. Heavy charged particle beams such as helium or protons *(proton radiosurgery)* offer optimal physical characteristics for stereotactic applications. The beam penetration into tissue reflects the energy imparted to the particle and reaches relatively finite depths (Bragg peak). *Gamma knife* provides irradiation using 200 separate and collimated cobalt-60 sources in a hemispherical array aimed at the target. These radiosurgery techniques require some means of fixation of the patient's head in space. Devices include immobilization masks, rigid frames affixed to the patient's skull, or fitted mouthpieces. The acute complications of these therapies include cerebral edema and seizures. The major late complication is radiation necrosis manifested as early as 2–4 months after treatment, but maximal at 18 months.

A unique device equipped with a light-weight, high-energy radiation source is available for performing robotic frameless SRS (CyberKnife). The technique uses an image-to-image correlation algorithm for target localization and has been increasingly applied to neoplasms of brain, skull base, and spine. Other devices are available for frameless SRS (Novalis Tx).

### Chemotherapy

***Standard cytotoxic chemotherapy.*** Chemotherapy is provided to most patients with malignant brain tumors. Less commonly treated are nonresected low-grade but symptomatic tumors prior to or following radiation therapy. Chemotherapy is becoming increasingly important for patients with brain lymphoma or anaplastic oligodendroglial tumors (Table 74.1).

Alkylating agents are the major compounds used against brain tumors. Their antitumor effect is based on covalent binding of alkyl groups to DNA, which results in intra- and interstrand crosslinks. Gliomas resist these effects by reducing drug uptake, overexpression of cellular sulfhydryl groups, and elimination of alkylated nucleosides by the repair enzyme O-alkyl-guanine-alkyl-transferase (AGAT). Common toxicities of these agents include myelosuppression, nausea, and infertility. Secondary malignancies occur in 5%–10% of patients with a peak incidence 5–7 years after exposure.

The antifolates interfere with the synthesis of tetrahydrofolates, one-carbon carriers essential for synthesis of thymidylate and purines. *Methotrexate,* a potent inhibitor of dihydrofolate reductase (DHFR), is given by vein in gram-equivalent doses to achieve therapeutic concentrations within the brain, spinal fluid, nerve roots, and eye. This mandates the establishment of alkaline diuresis, because concentrations in urine can exceed the level of solubility, depending on urine pH. Drugs competing for excretion in the proximal tubule such as acetyl salicylic acid, penicillin G, or probenecid cannot be used concomitantly. *Pemetrexed* inhibits at least three enzymes involved in folate metabolism and DNA synthesis: thymidylate synthase, DHFR, and glycinamide ribonucleotide formyltransferase.

The deoxycytidine analogue cytosine arabinoside competitively inhibits DNA polymerase A. After incorporation into DNA, there is inhibition of chain elongation and template function.

Microtubular components of the mitotic spindle apparatus can be inhibited within tumor cells, with resulting reduction of cell division, intracellular transport, and secretion. The *vinca alkaloids* (vinblastine, vincristine), naturally found in *Catharanthus roseus,* inhibit polymerization of tubulin and the disassembly of microtubules, and thus produce cell-cycle arrest in metaphase. The *taxanes* (paclitaxel, docetaxel) disrupt microtubule dynamics by stabilization against depolymerization and enhancement of polymerization.

Platinum compounds form bifunctional bonds to DNA to produce intrastrand adducts linking two nucleotides. The cell repair of these links makes use of nucleotide excision-DNA repair. Defects in the DNA mismatch repair system may prevent recognition of platinum adducts and result in failure to initiate apoptosis.

Topoisomerase inhibitors catalyze the process of catenation and decatenation, the temporary uncoiling and unlinking of the DNA double strand. The topoisomerases bind to the free ends of the cut DNA molecule using a specific tyrosine residue. Topoisomerase I introduces single-strand breaks into the DNA molecule. Its inhibitors are derivatives of camptothecin (irinotecan, topotecan). Topoisomerase II catalyzes linking and unlinking by causing double strand breaks. Etoposide and teniposide, semisynthetic derivatives of podophyllotoxin, a substance found in mayapple extracts, inhibit the re-ligation of DNA from the cleavage complex.

Myeloablative doses of chemotherapy followed by autologous peripheral blood stem cell transplantation have failed to produce higher response rates in malignant gliomas when compared with conventional adjuvant chemotherapy (Finlay et al., 1996). Moreover, this approach is associated with considerable treatment-related morbidity and mortality, and thus has not found widespread use. Results of high-dose chemotherapy with peripheral blood stem cell rescue in patients with chemosensitive brain tumors like anaplastic oligodendroglioma or primary central nervous system lymphoma (PCNSL) are more promising (Abrey et al., 2006; DeFilipp et al., 2017).

***Delivery strategies.*** The BBB is the major anatomical obstacle for chemotherapy of primary brain tumors. It is composed of the endothelial cell layer of cerebral capillaries sealed by intercellular tight junctions, the vascular basal membrane, and astrocytic foot processes. Few studies have measured brain concentrations of systemically administered agents but delivery strategies developed to circumvent the barrier include the following: (1) Intrathecal administration of methotrexate, triethylenethiophosphoramide (thio-TEPA), or cytosine-arabinoside for leptomeningeal metastases. (2) Intracarotid infusion of hypertonic solutions (25% mannitol or 15% glycerol) to produce reversible opening of the BBB. This approach, selectively used in specialized centers, produces 1–2 hours of barrier lysis during which hydrophilic chemotherapeutic agents such as methotrexate or cyclophosphamide are provided. The technology obligates general anesthesia and serial angiographic procedures and is associated with toxicity, including seizures and transient encephalopathy. (3) Biodegradable polymers impregnated with bis-chloroethylnitrosourea (carmustine) (BCNU) increase local drug concentration without notable systemic toxicity. Dime-sized wafers of poly [bis (p-carboxyphenoxy)] propane and sebacic acid release the chemotherapeutic agent over 7–10 days into tumor surrounding the resection site. The polymer-based delivery strategy is associated with median survival improvements of 2 months in patients with malignant glioma (Westphal et al., 2003). Complications include infection, wound healing impairment, brain necrosis, and cerebrospinal fluid (CSF) leak.

## Novel Treatment Strategies

Various compounds interfering with pathways regulating cell growth have been developed for numerous cancer types. Cell growth control can be attacked at different levels: growth factors, growth factor receptors, intracellular signal transducers, nuclear transcription factors, and cell-cycle control proteins. Various strategies are available to interfere with proteins or the transcription/translation of their encoding genes at each level. Modified peptides or peptidomimetics, such as imatinib,

**TABLE 74.1 Cytotoxic Chemotherapeutic Agents, Applications in Neuro-Oncology, Associated Toxicities, and Unique Properties**

| | Neuro-Oncology Indications | Toxicity | Unique Drug Properties |
|---|---|---|---|
| **Alkylating Agents** | | | |
| ***Nitrogen Mustards*** | | | |
| Cyclophosphamide | Supratentorial PNET, esthesioneuroblastoma | Leukopenia, alopecia, hemorrhagic cystitis | Does not affect marrow stem cells, no cumulative myelotoxicity |
| Ifosfamide | MPNST, germ cell tumors | Leukopenia, alopecia, hemorrhagic cystitis | |
| thio-TEPA | Meningeal carcinomatosis (it); PCNSL (iv) | Myelosuppression | |
| ***Nitrosoureas*** | | | |
| BCNU | Malignant gliomas | Cumulative myelosuppression | Used also as local therapy (BCNU-impregnated wafers) |
| CCNU | Malignant gliomas | Cumulative myelosuppression | |
| ***Atypical Alkylating Agents*** | | | |
| Procarbazine | Anaplastic oligodendroglioma and other gliomas (as part of PCV); PCNSL | Extended interactions with foods and drugs that induce the microsomal cytochrome P450 oxidoreductase system; nausea, mild leukopenia, thrombocytopenia; hypersensitivity reactions; gonadotoxicity | |
| Temozolomide | Glioblastoma multiforme and other malignant gliomas | Lymphopenia, thrombocytopenia | Spontaneous conversion at physiological pH to active metabolite; excellent oral bioavailability; resistance is the result of MGMT-mediated repair of $O^6$-methylated guanine residues, defects in the cellular DNA mismatch repair system, and induction of poly (ADP-ribose) polymerase, a constituent of the nucleotide excision repair system |
| **Antifolates** | | | |
| Methotrexate | PCNSL, MPNST | Renal failure (from late excretion or precipitation of metabolites with low solubility), mucositis, hepatitis | Resistance results from altered transmembrane transport of the drug, decreased affinity of DHFR, or overexpression of the enzyme |
| Pemetrexed | In clinical trial for PCNSL | Myelosuppression | Administered by short infusion without need for alkaline diuresis |
| **Cytidine Analogs** | | | |
| Cytosine arabinoside | PCNSL (iv); meningeal NHL (it) | Myelotoxicity, gastrointestinal side effects, encephalopathy (after high-dose therapy in patients older than 40 years) | |
| **Antimicrotubule Agents** | | | |
| ***Vinca Alkaloids*** | | | |
| Vincristine | Anaplastic oligodendroglioma and other gliomas as part of PCV; PCNSL; medulloblastoma | Noncumulative autonomic neurotoxicity (constipation, paralytic ileus, dysuria, blood pressure instability); cumulative somatic peripheral neuropathy | Resistance based on overexpression of P-glycoprotein, a large transmembrane protein encoded by the *MDR1* gene that functions as a drug-pump transporting a variety of drugs from the intracellular to the extracellular compartment |
| Vinblastine | | | |
| ***Taxanes*** | | | |
| Paclitaxel | Intracerebral administration through convection-enhanced delivery for glioblastoma in clinical studies | | Poor penetration through blood–brain barrier |

Continued

**TABLE 74.1 Cytotoxic Chemotherapeutic Agents, Applications in Neuro-Oncology, Associated Toxicities, and Unique Properties—cont'd**

| | Neuro-Oncology Indications | Toxicity | Unique Drug Properties |
|---|---|---|---|
| **Compounds Based on Elemental Platinum** | | | |
| Cisplatin | Neuroblastoma, pineal parenchymal tumors, embryonal tumors, non-germinomatous germ cell tumors, recurrent malignant gliomas | Highly emetogenic; peripheral neuropathy, seizures, ototoxicity, renal toxicity, myelosuppression | |
| Carboplatin | | Myelosuppression | |
| **Topoisomerase Inhibitors** | | | |
| ***Topoisomerase I Inhibitors*** | | | |
| Irinotecan | Relapsed malignant glioma | Acute cholinergic syndrome, delayed diarrhea, myelosuppression, nausea, vomiting, and alopecia | |
| Topotecan | Second-line drug for methotrexate-resistant PCNSL | Leukopenia, thrombocytopenia | |
| ***Topoisomerase II Inhibitors*** | | | |
| Etoposide | PNET, ependymoma, pinealoma, embryonal tumors, nongerminomatous germ cell tumors, relapsed malignant gliomas, relapsed PCNSL; high-dose chemotherapy protocols followed by stem-cell rescue | Myelosuppression | Resistance based on adenosine triphosphate-dependent transporters such as P-glycoprotein and mutations within the topoisomerase gene |

*ADP,* Adenosine diphosphate; *ATP,* adenosine triphosphate; *BCNU,* Bis-chloroethylnitrosourea (carmustine); *CCNU,* cyclohexylchloroethylnitrosourea (lomustine); *DHFR,* dihydrofolate reductase; *MPNST,* malignant peripheral nerve sheath tumor; *PCNSL,* primary central nervous system lymphoma; *PCV,* procarbazine, lomustine, vincristine; *PNET,* primitive neuroectodermal tumor; *thio-TEPA,* triethylenethiophosphoramide; *it,* intrathecal; *iv* intravenous; *MGMT* methylguanine methyltransferase; *NHL* non-Hodgkin lymphoma; *MDR1* multidrug resistance 1.

are molecules designed to bind to the active sites of proteins such as the tyrosine kinase domain of growth factor receptors. Imatinib, a synthetic inhibitor of the tyrosine kinase receptors abl and c-kit, has been of value in the therapy of chronic myelogenous leukemia and gastrointestinal stromal tumors. This has inspired the use of similar agents to target analogous brain tumor pathways. Antisense oligonucleotides injected into tumors hybridize with transcripts of growth control genes and inhibit their translation. Ribozymes degrade transcripts with high specificity. Monoclonal antibodies directly target growth control proteins. Gene therapy may restore the function of mutated cell-cycle control proteins. A summary of new treatment strategies can be found in (Box 74.1).

Epidermal growth factor receptor (EGFR) is an attractive target as it is commonly overexpressed or mutated. However, monotherapy with agents targeting this receptor (gefitinib, erlotinib, and tyrphostin) has been disappointing (Rich et al., 2004). Molecular predictors of the rare responses have been identified (Mellinghoff et al., 2005). ABT-414, a drug–antibody conjugate that specifically targets tumor cells overexpressing EGFR, is currently being evaluated in clinical trials in newly diagnosed and recurrent disease (van Den Bent et al., 2017). Inhibition of platelet-derived growth factor receptor (PDGFR) with imatinib proved unsuccessful. Monotherapy failure of small molecule inhibitors has led to the development of compounds with a broader spectrum or "dual" inhibitors. AEE788 and vatalanib interfere with both EGFR- and vascular endothelial growth factor receptor (VEGFR) signal transduction. Lapitinib inhibits EGFR and ErbB2, two members of the ErbB family of transmembrane tyrosine kinase receptors. Many of these compounds have likewise failed to prolong survival in glioblastoma patients but clinical evaluation of combination regimens using growth factor receptor and downstream signal transduction inhibitors are still ongoing.

A variety of compounds were designed to block intracellular signal transduction such as phosphoinositide-3-kinase/protein kinase B (PI3K/Akt), protein kinase C (PKC), Ras, the mitogen activated protein kinase pathway Raf/MEK/ERK, and the NFκ-B pathway. These agents have been used as monotherapy and in combination with classical cytotoxic agents or growth factor receptor inhibitors. Inhibition of mTOR, a downstream constituent of the Pi3K/Akt pathway, has proven successful in the treatment of subependymal giant cell astrocytoma (SEGA; Franz et al., 2006). Large-scale genetic investigations have shown that several different glioma subtypes harbor mutations in the *BRAF* gene. Missense mutations of the V600E were identified in pleomorphic xanthoastrocytoma (PXA), ganglioglioma, pilocytic astrocytoma, and less frequently in glioblastoma. A fusion between the KIAA1549 and *BRAF* gene can be found in over 60% of pilocytic astrocytomas (Khater et al., 2018; Schindler et al., 2011). Targeted treatment with a BRAF inhibitor in combination with a MEK inhibitor has shown success in other malignancies including melanoma, thyroid carcinoma, hairy cell leukemia, and Erdheim- Chester disease. In gliomas, use of these agents has been reported with varying success in individual patients and small cohorts. Larger trials, mainly in pediatric populations, are underway. A combination of the BRAF inhibitor dabrafenib and the MEK inhibitor trametinib has demonstrated activity in papillary craniopharyngioma (Brastianos et al., 2016). Inhibition of the constitutively activated Nf-κB pathway using lenalidomide, pomalidomide, or ibrutinib has shown a promising effect on relapsed/

## BOX 74.1 Targeted Therapies for Intracranial Neoplasm

**Inhibition of Aberrant Receptor Signaling**

***EGFR Inhibitors***
Erlotinib
Afatinib
ABT-414

***PDGFR Inhibitors***
Imatinib
Tandutinib

***c-MET/HGF Inhibitors***
AMG102

***Glutamate Receptor Inhibitors***
Talampanel

***Small Molecule Inhibitors Targeting More Than One Growth-Promoting Pathway***
Lapatinib
Nintedanib
Vandetanib
Pazopanib

**Small Molecule Inhibitors of Intracellular Signal Transduction Pathways**

*Inhibition of the Phosphoinositide-3-Kinase/Protein Kinase B (PI3K/Akt) Pathway*
Sirolimus
Temsirolimus
Everolimus

***Inhibition of Protein Kinase C***
Enzastaurine

***Inhibition of Bruton Tyrosine Kinase***
Ibrutinib

***Inhibition of the Ras Signaling Pathway***
Farnesyltransferase inhibitors

***Inhibition of the raf/MEK/ERK Pathway***
Sorafenib
Vemurafenib
Dabrafenib
Trametinib
Selumetinib

***SRC- and SRC-Family Kinases***
Dasatinib

***Proteasome Inhibitors***
Bortezomib

***Histone Deacetylase Inhibitors***
Suberoylanilide hydroxamic acid (vorinostat)
Panobinostat

**Inhibitors of DNA Repair Mechanisms**
Veliparib, olaparib (inhibition of PARP)

**Inhibitors of Angiogenesis or Cell Invasion**

***Agents Targeting Endothelial Cell Migration or Integrin Expression***
Thalidomide
Pomalidomide
Cilengitide

***VEGF-/VEGF Receptor Antagonists***
Bevacizumab
Sunitinib
Cediranib

**Immunotherapies**
Immune checkpoint inhibitors
Nivolumab, pembrolizumab (anti-PD1 antibodies)
Atezolizumab (anti-PD-L1 antibody)
Targeting inhibitory cytokines
Galunisertib (TGF)

While many of these agents are approved by the Federal Drug Administration for various indications, most of them are considered experimental for brain tumor therapy at this point.

*EGFR,* Epidermal growth factor receptor; ERK, extracellular signal-regulated kinase; *HGF,* hepatocyte growth factor; MEK, mitogen-activated protein kinase kinase; MET mesenchymal-epithelial transition factor; *PARP,* poly (ADP-ribose) polymerase; *PD,* programmed death; *PDGFR,* platelet-derived growth factor receptor; raf, rapidly accelerated fibrosarcoma kinase; Ras rat sarcoma viral oncogene homologue; SRC, sarcoma viral proto-oncogene. *VEGF,* vascular endothelial growth factor; *TGF,* transforming growth factor;

refractory primary and secondary central nervous system (CNS) non-Hodgkin lymphoma in early phase trials.

Another therapeutic strategy targets intracellular protein degradation. The proteasome is a cellular protein degradation complex that recognizes and degrades polyubiquitinated substrates such as cell-cycle control proteins. Although a fairly nonspecific apparatus, the overall effect of some proteasome inhibitors such as bortezomib, a dipeptidyl boronic acid derivative, is the induction of apoptosis. The drug is approved for use in multiple myeloma but remains investigational for primary brain tumors.

Histone deacetylase (HDAC) inhibitors interfere with transcription. HDAC induces hyperacetylation of histones resulting in chromatin relaxation and transcriptional activation. The anticancer properties of various HDAC have been recognized and are likely the complex result of activation of differentiation programs, cell-cycle inhibition, and induction of apoptosis in cancer cells (Johnstone, 2002). HDAC inhibitors are of particular interest in the treatment of patients with midline gliomas (mostly children) as they often harbor mutations in the histone gene *H3.3K27M*. Less frequently, gliomas outside the midline may harbor mutations in *H3.3 G34R* or G34V (Schwartzentruber et al., 2012). Compounds such as phenylacetate, phenylbutyrate, or valproic acid display HDAC inhibiting properties but are unlikely to play a role as brain cancer therapeutics. Suberoylanilide hydroxamic acid (vorinostat), the fungal tetrapeptide depsipeptide, and panobinostat have been studied in early phase clinical trials and have not shown benefit in patients with glioma thus far (Galanis et al., 2018); Lee et al., 2015). However, several clinical trials using HDAC inhibitors in combination with various other treatment modalities in both adults and children with diffuse intrinsic pontine glioma are still ongoing. Infiltrative gliomas harbor mutations in isocitrate dehydrogenase (IDH)1 and IDH2, which encode two isoforms of IDH (Yan et al., 2009). Mutant IDH1/2 produce 2-hydroxyglutaric acid, a molecule that alters gene expression and appears to be promoting malignant degeneration by inhibiting histone- and DNA-modifying enzymes (Dang et al., 2009; Zhao et al., 2009). Inhibitors of these mutant enzymes may normalize gene expression and reverse malignant degeneration (Rohle et al., 2013). The use of IDH inhibitors and mutation-specific vaccines in low-grade and anaplastic gliomas is currently under clinical investigation.

The elucidation of the molecular pathways facilitating DNA repair have prompted new treatment strategies. Small molecular inhibitors of DNA repair are being tested as adjuvant therapy and in combination with radiation therapy in hope of inducing synergistic lethality. For example, poly (adenosine diphosphate [ADP]-ribose) polymerase (PARP) inhibitors (e.g., olaparib and veliparib) have been shown to disrupt the excision repair pathway in preclinical evaluations and are currently being tested in several phase I/II studies in gliomas. There is particular interest in their use with IDH mutant gliomas as evidence suggests that these mutations induce homologous recombination defects (Sulkowski et al., 2017). Agents targeting alternative repair pathways such as ataxia telangiectasia mutated (ATM) and ataxia telangiectasia and Rad3-related protein (ATR) signaling, nonhomologous end joining, and G2/M checkpoint (i.e., Wee1 inhibitor, AZD1775) are also in preclinical development or early phase trials in glioma (Bindra et al., 2017; Touat et al., 2017).

Inhibition of angiogenesis or cell invasion represents another approach to brain tumor therapy. Gliomas greater than a few millimeters in size stimulate new blood vessel formation. This induction is affected by promoters including VEGF (hypoxia-inducible endothelial cell mitogen, vascular permeability factor), basic fibroblast growth factor (bFGF), platelet-derived growth factor (PDGF), transforming growth factor (TGF), and tenascin. Endogenous inhibitors of angiogenesis include angiostatin, endostatin, thrombospondin, and heparin. Kinase insert domain receptor (KDR) and FMS-related tyrosine kinase 1 are receptors for VEGF. Bevacizumab, a humanized monoclonal antibody with murine complementarity-determining regions binding VEGF, is now approved for use in patients with relapsed glioblastoma. Several "small molecule" inhibitors of VEGFR are at various stages of development. Sunitinib is already in clinical use for advanced renal cell cancer. Early experience with cediranib in glioblastoma was promising (Batchelor et al., 2007) but a phase III study in patients with newly diagnosed disease failed to demonstrate survival benefit (Batchelor et al., 2013). Other potential therapies targeted to endothelial cells include thalidomide, interleukin (IL) 12, cyclooxygenase II inhibitors, and cilengitide, a cyclic pentapeptide inducing apoptosis of growing endothelial cells through inhibition of their $\alpha_V\beta_3$-integrin interaction with the matrix proteins vitronectin and tenascin.

Gene therapy of brain tumors encompasses a wide spectrum of various strategies. A comprehensive review of these approaches goes beyond the scope of this chapter and the interested reader is referred to excellent review articles (Kwiatkowska et al., 2013; Lam and Breakefield, 2001). Viral vectors create localized inflammation while expressing transgenes that activate cytokines and chemotherapies. Transfection efficiency depends on the agent and the mode of introduction. Cells are killed not only by transfection but also by the cellular reaction that damages adjacent tumor cells: the "bystander effect." The delivery of a therapeutic gene can be enhanced by improving the vector or delivering it through infusional clysis. Ligands or antibodies targeted at receptors expressed on tumor cells (EGFR, transferrin receptor, integrin receptor) can be incorporated into the capsid of adenoviral vectors. Tumor-specific expression systems make use of the human telomerase reverse transcriptase (hTERT) promoter. hTERT is the catalytic subunit of the telomerase ribonucleoprotein and is expressed in glioma cells but not in normal glia cells. Tumor selectivity can also be accomplished by using replication-conditional viral vectors, retroviruses, or placement of genes essential to virus replication under the control of promoters that are selectively active in gliomas (such as the nestin promoter). Currently used vector systems are either replication-defective or replication-conditional and include recombinant herpes simplex virus, adenovirus, retrovirus, and hybrid vectors. Gene therapy delivery involves stereotactic injection into the tumor or intraoperative insertion into the wall of the resection cavity, convection-enhanced delivery, intra-arterial or intraventricular application. Nonviral strategies have made use of naked DNA, polycationic polymers, and liposomes.

Therapies based on immune-mediated strategies aim to increase immune responses to the tumor. Whether primary brain tumors suppress immune reaction, are poorly recognized by the immune system, or are protected by the immunosuppressive effects of concurrent glucocorticoid administration is uncertain. Tumor vaccination makes use of immunogenic peptides, attenuated autologous tumor cells, or dendritic cells loaded with tumor antigens (Okada et al., 2011). These tumor antigens create an immune reaction enhanced by irradiation, transfection with cytokine genes, or transfection with major histocompatibility complex (MHC) class II genes. The antigen can be presented in subcutaneous tissues, after which cytotoxic T cells infiltrate the site of injection as well as the brain. A "one-fits-all" immunization strategy targeting a somatic mutant of EGFR (EGFRvIII) showed promising results in an early phase II trial; however, the phase III study was terminated early as it was felt to be unlikely to show a significant difference in survival (Elsamadicy et al., 2017).

There are various mechanisms by which gliomas evade recognition by the immune system. Potential mediators include inhibitory cytokines (TGF-β, prostaglandin E, IL-10), defective cytokine receptors on tumor-infiltrating T lymphocytes, and inhibitory molecules expressed on tumor cells, stromal cells, and immune cells. Strategies rendering glioblastoma cells immunogenic have included transfection with antisense TGF-β (Bogdahn et al., 2011) or decorin, a TGF-β–binding and TGF-β–inhibiting proteoglycan.

Cytokines can be linked to bacterial toxins as genetically engineered fusion proteins that enter the tumor cell via binding to selectively expressed receptors. A phase III clinical trial of cintredekin besudotox (IL-13 linked to pseudomonas exotoxin) administered intracerebrally through convection-enhanced delivery failed to demonstrate a survival benefit (Kunwar et al., 2010).

T-cell activation and tolerance are dependent upon interactions with antigen-presenting cells (APCs). T cells are activated when specific antigens on MHC molecules expressed by APCs are presented to the T-cell receptor. The T-cell response is modulated by numerous inhibitory and activating molecules on APCs: for example, B7.2 (binding to cytotoxic T-lymphocyte–associated antigen 4 [CTLA-4]) and B7-H1 (PD-L1, binding to programmed death 1 [PD-1]) (Zou and Chen, 2008). Cancer cells, stromal cells, and immune cells in the cancer microenvironment upregulate expression of inhibitory molecules, leading to tumor immune evasion. The immune checkpoint inhibitor ipilimumab, a fully human IgG1 monoclonal antibody blocking CTLA-4 and various antibodies blocking PD-1 or PD-L1, have recently been shown to have activity in a variety of cancers, including patients with CNS metastatic disease (Long et al., 2018; Topalian et al., 2012; Wolchok et al., 2013). Case reports have described a few patients with glioblastomas in the setting of hereditary DNA mismatch repair deficiency resulting in a hypermutated genome that achieved clinical and radiographic responses to immune checkpoint inhibition (Bouffet et al., 2016; Johanns et al., 2016). The first randomized prospective trial using immunotherapy in recurrent glioblastoma failed to show a significant difference between bevacizumab and nivolumab (published only in abstract form; Reardon et al., 2017). However, a recent study in a small cohort of patients with recurrent glioblastoma treated with pembrolizumab before and after surgical re-resection at recurrence showed that neoadjuvant PD-1 blockade led to improved overall survival (OS) compared with the adjuvant setting (Cloughesy et al., 2019). Further studies in recurrent disease that combine immunotherapy with re-irradiation are ongoing, as are trials using immunotherapy in newly diagnosed disease.

Antibodies alone or conjugated with toxins or radioactive isotopes (iodine-131, yttrium-90) can target epitopes on tumor cells (EGFR, neural cell adhesion molecule, tenascin). These approaches are hampered by insufficient delivery, lack of tumor specificity, and concerns regarding ventricular or subarachnoid exposure.

Oncolytic viruses are modified viruses that preferentially replicate in and destroy cancer cells. For example, ONYX-015 is a replication competent, E1B-attenuated adenovirus. E1B is a viral protein that binds and inactivates p53, a prerequisite for the virus' ability to replicate in its host cell, and lacking E1B can only replicate in TP53-deficient cells. Loss of TP53 function is an early event in the pathogenesis of gliomas and thus renders them susceptible to lytic infection with this attenuated virus (Chiocca et al., 2004). Clinical trials have proven safe but delivery systems have thus far proven insufficient. The search for viruses with enhanced tumor cell selectivity and killing is ongoing (Wollmann et al., 2010). The interested reader is referred to an excellent review (Wollmann et al., 2012).

New delivery strategies are designed to circumvent the BBB to treat malignant gliomas. Intraoperative injection of resection margins with various therapeutic agents (viral vectors, oncolytic viruses) does not depend on BBB permeability but is highly inefficient. Tissue penetration can be improved using convection-enhanced delivery. This technique requires intraoperative or stereotactic placement of infusion catheters in the wall of the resection cavity. Using microinfusion pumps, therapeutic agents are administered postoperatively over up to 96 hours. Exposure may be even further enhanced by packaging the therapeutic compound (cytotoxic chemotherapy agent, vector, antibody, etc.) into microspheres from which it is released over a modifiable period of time (Saltzman and Olbricht, 2002). Brain-penetrating polymeric nanoparticles loaded with drugs and optimized for intracranial convection-enhanced delivery have yielded promising results in terms of intracerebral distribution and survival in animal models (Zhou et al., 2013). Neuroprogenitor cells may deliver vectors or therapeutic genes to tumors. Animal experiments have shown that systemically administered neural stem cells home to brain tumors. Progenitor cells have been found within experimental brain tumors following injection into the contralateral cerebral hemisphere—an observation that may indicate the stem cells' ability to track down migratory brain tumor cells (Aboody et al., 2000).

## MANAGEMENT OF SPECIFIC BRAIN TUMORS

### Neuroepithelial Tumors

#### Astrocytic Tumors

##### *Noninfiltrative tumors*

**Pilocytic astrocytoma.** Composing 85% of infratentorial astrocytomas, most pilocytic astrocytomas are benign tumors located in the cerebellum and occur in the first and second decade (Burkhard et al., 2003). The remainder grow in the hypothalamus, the walls of the third ventricle, the optic pathway, and the brainstem. The tumor likely emerges from true astrocytes or subependymal precursors. Pilocytic astrocytoma, usually of the optic nerve, is the most common CNS tumor associated with neurofibromatosis type I. The tumor diagnosis is heralded by symptomatic obstructive hydrocephalus, headache, or hypothalamic/pituitary dysfunction. Posterior fossa signs include neck stiffness, head tilt, and incoordination. The masses enhance with gadolinium and appear in proximity to the ventricle or subarachnoid space. Cysts, focal hemorrhage, and calcification are described. Much of the tumor contains benign features: bipolar (piloid) cells with Rosenthal fibers in addition to microcysts surrounded by protoplasmic astrocytes and eosinophilic granular bodies. Three-quarters of patients receive surgical resection. For the unresectable case exhibiting progressive growth or symptoms refractory to treatment, involved field radiation therapy is given with a narrow margin. Chemotherapy can be used prior to irradiation or for tumor progression. The 25-year survival rate is between 50% and 94% following surgical resection. Malignant transformation of pilocytic astrocytoma is highly unusual.

**Pleomorphic xanthoastrocytoma.** PXA is a rare superficial cortical glioma (Fig. 74.1, *A*). Two-thirds of cases are diagnosed before age 25. Seizures anticipate diagnosis by 3 years. The masses are located in the temporal lobes and extend into the leptomeninges and Virchow-Robin spaces. PXAs are well demarcated from surrounding tissue and may contain cysts. The solid portion of the tumor usually enhances markedly on MR images with gadolinium. On unenhanced T1-weighted images it is hypo- to isointense. The pleomorphic cells vary in size and shape and include single and multinucleated giant cells. The large cells accumulate lipids—hence the term "xanthoastrocytoma." There is some uncertainty as to the true aggressive potential of the masses, as mitoses and necrosis are seen and malignant forms have been identified. Cells of origin are probably subpial astrocytes. Complete resection is feasible in most patients and radiation or chemotherapy is provided for aggressive or recurrent tumors. Two-thirds of PXAs carry mutation in *BRAF* (V600E), rendering them potentially susceptible to targeted therapy (Kaley et al., 2018; Schindler et al., 2011). The survival is more than 80% after 5 years and 70% after 10 years, with well-resected lesions faring the best (Giannini et al., 1999). Anaplastic transformation occurs in 15%–20% of patients for whom the natural history may be indistinguishable from that of glioblastoma.

**Subependymal giant cell astrocytoma.** SEGA occurs in patients with tuberous sclerosis and may be unique to that disease, although it is only reported in 6.1% of patients afflicted with this phakomatosis (Shepherd et al., 1991). Hydrocephalus emerges before the third decade as tumors in the wall of the lateral ventricles or in the interventricular foramen clog CSF outflow. Epilepsy of long-standing duration may change pattern. The well-circumscribed MRI masses rarely have hemorrhage or calcification but may show enhancement. The tumor cells stain with glial (GFAP) and neuronal (synaptophysin and neuron-specific enolase) markers and may be mixed with large cells which resemble gemistocytic astrocytes, elongated tumor cells, and giant multinucleated pyramidal cells. Surgery is curative and required when CSF flow is obstructed. Rapamycin and everolimus at standard immunosuppressive doses can induce regression of SEGA (Franz et al., 2006, 2013).

**Neuroepithelial tumors of unknown origin: chordoid glioma of the third ventricle.** Chordoid gliomas occur in the third ventricle of adult women (Brat et al., 1998). These tumors arise in the anterior third ventricular surface and commonly are diagnosed when CSF flow is obstructed or visual field deficits or signs of pituitary dysfunction arise. They commonly fill the third ventricle and obstruct the lateral ventricles. On MRI, chordoid glioma is characterized by homogeneous enhancement. Microscopically, tumors are composed of GFAP and vimentin-positive cells in a mucinous matrix. Some

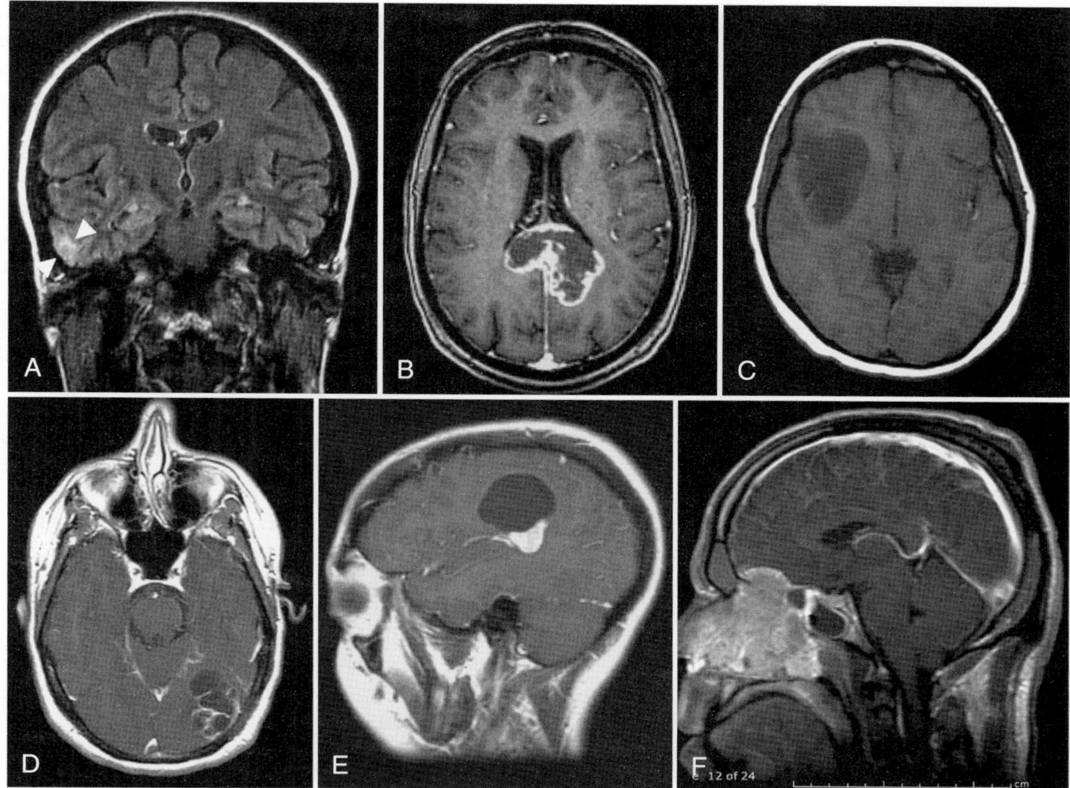


**Fig. 74.1 Neuroepithelial Tumors. A,** Pleomorphic xanthoastrocytoma. The tumor is seen on this fluid attenuated inversion recovery magnetic resonance image as an area of increased signal intensity in the right temporal lobe *(arrowheads)*. **B,** Glioblastoma multiforme. A rim-enhancing mass lesion is identified in the splenium of the corpus callosum (T1-weighted magnetic resonance imaging [MRI] with gadolinium). **C,** Oligoastrocytoma. The tumor in the right subinsular region has distinct margins on T1-weighted MRI, suggesting lack of deletion of chromosome 1p. **D,** Anaplastic ependymoma. T1-weighted MRI with gadolinium demonstrates a partially cystic, partially nodular tumor within the left temporo-occipital area. **E,** Ganglioglioma. This mass is composed of a large cyst and an enhancing nodule at its inferior margin (T1-weighted MRI with gadolinium). **F,** Esthesioneuroblastoma. The tumor occupies the entire nasal cavity and invades the neurocranium through the lamina cribrosa (T1-weighted MRI with gadolinium).

reports suggest that chordoid gliomas of the third ventricle arise from the lamina terminalis and perhaps from tanycytes in this region. Surgical resection is the treatment of choice but complete removal is often not possible due to location of the tumor and adherence to vital structures. This procedure has been aided by the use of endoscopic techniques or intraoperative MRI scanning. Adjuvant radiotherapy is used for tumors that progress after surgery. The excellent prognosis reflects the extent of surgical resection.

***Infiltrative low-grade astrocytomas.*** A tumor of young adulthood, symptoms appear either during the first or between the third and fourth decade. Representing fewer than 5% of brain tumors, there is a slight male predominance. Seizures herald the appearance of a lesion and a careful history often discloses symptoms of many years or decades. Commonly afflicted are the frontal and temporal lobe of the cerebral hemispheres where MRI studies reveal poorly demarcated hypointense T1- and hyperintense T2-weighted lesions that do not enhance after gadolinium administration. Surgically resected material contains one of three main subtypes: fibrillary, protoplasmic, and gemistocytic astrocytoma (in order of frequency). The cells appear cytologically benign but infiltrate surrounding brain tissue. Inactivation of *TP53* tumor suppressor gene, heterozygous point mutations of IDH1, and loss of chromosome 22p are common genetic alterations involved in formation of low-grade astrocytomas (Louis, 2006). The goal of surgery is tumor removal to the largest possible extent without risking the loss of neurological function. Surgery establishes a diagnosis. Symptoms are alleviated, including those associated with mass effect, hydrocephalus, hemorrhage, cyst formation, or seizure activity. Surgery reduces the cell pool at risk of malignant degeneration and removes potentially more aggressive foci within radiographically benign-appearing tumors. After surgery, treatment decisions are influenced by patient risk factors and molecular characteristics of the tumor. Favorable outcomes follow gross-total resection of tumors in young patients and patients with IDH1 or 2 mutations. In the majority of patients with lower-grade glioma who do not have an IDH mutation, clinical outcome and tumor behavior is similar to that of glioblastoma (Network, 2015). Additional unfavorable prognostic factors for survival are age over 40 years, a tumor diameter exceeding 6 cm, tumor crossing the midline, and presence of neurological deficit before surgery (Piepmeier et al., 1996; Pignatti et al., 2002). In patients with favorable risk factors, gross total resection can be followed by observation with further treatment reserved for progressive disease, uncontrollable seizures, or steroid dependence. In patients who undergo subtotal resection or have unfavorable risk factors, early postoperative therapy is generally indicated. Early radiation alone only prolongs recurrence-free survival (5.3 years) compared with the control group (3.4 years) but does not influence OS (median 7.4 years vs. 7.2

years; Van den Bent et al., 2005). Radiation dose escalation has no impact on survival (Karim et al., 1996). The radiation field includes the area of radiographically identifiable tumor (fluid attenuated inversion recovery [FLAIR] or T2 margin) and an additional margin of 1–2 cm. Recent long-term data from a large trial of high-risk low-grade glioma patients including both astrocytoma and oligodendroglioma (RTOG 9802) showed that the addition of procarbazine, lomustine, vincristine (PCV) chemotherapy to early radiation after resection improved OS almost twofold (13.3 years vs. 7.8 years; Buckner et al., 2016). In exploratory subgroup analyses, the effect was larger in those tumors categorized as oligodendroglioma and oligoastrocytoma. In clinical practice temozolomide has been widely used although no prospectively acquired data are available on its comparative efficacy. Off-label use in low-grade neoplasms follows treatment protocols established for malignant gliomas. Unfortunately, despite treatment, most patients eventually suffer anaplastic transformation of their tumor.

#### High-grade astrocytomas

**Anaplastic astrocytoma.** Anaplastic astrocytomas account for 5% of all primary brain tumors. Clinical presentation is similar to low-grade infiltrative gliomas, although neurological syndromes tend to evolve faster. MRI typically demonstrates heterogeneously enhancing lesions. Nonenhancing lesions are rarely anaplastic but the older the patient, the less reliable this feature is (Barker et al., 1997). Diffusion-weighted imaging can identify areas of increased cellularity within low-grade neoplasms and thus may be useful in identifying foci of early anaplastic transformation. After tumor resection, adjuvant therapy is required. Optimal treatment for these tumors remains an area of active debate. Long-term results of the NOA-04 trial, which included both anaplastic astrocytoma and oligodendroglioma, showed no difference in outcome when either irradiation or chemotherapy was used at initial diagnosis when followed by the other modality at the time of disease progression (Wick et al., 2016). With this approach, median time to treatment failure is 4.4–4.6 years. Interim results of a randomized controlled trial showed improved OS in patients treated with radiation and adjuvant temozolomide compared with patients treated without adjuvant temozolomide (radiation was given with or without concurrent temozolomide; van den Bent et al., 2017). Prognostically favorable are methylation of the methylguanine-methyltransferase (MGMT) promoter and somatic mutations in the *IDH1* gene. Carmustine-impregnated wafers are available for patients with newly diagnosed and relapsed disease (Brem et al., 1995; Westphal et al., 2003). Based on a population-based registry, the relative survival rate at 2 years is 46% and at 5 years, 30% (Ostrom et al., 2018).

**Glioblastoma multiforme.** GBM is the most common neuroepithelial tumor (50%) and the second most common primary nervous system tumor. Approximately 10,000 cases are diagnosed each year. Common clinical presentations are headache, seizures, or rapid progression of a focal neurological deficit. The deep-seated infiltrative masses can also cause cognitive difficulties or personality change. MRI identifies a single rim-enhancing lesion with central necrosis surrounded by vasogenic edema (see Fig. 74.1, *B*). "Multifocal" disease is characterized by the occurrence of more than one enhancing lesion—a misnomer as GBM by definition is a diffuse or multifocal disease. FLAIR sequences reveal areas of nonenhancing brain infiltration. Prior to evolution of the typical rim-enhancing appearance, diffusion-weighted images are useful in the diagnosis of these tumors. Gross total resection is recommended whenever feasible to reduce mass effect, improve quality of life, reduce the residual malignant cell pool to be targeted by adjuvant therapies, and extend survival. Biopsy for histological confirmation is offered to older adult patients with lesions in proximity to sensitive cortical areas or deep-seated locations. Radiation therapy doubles the median survival of patients with GBM (Walker et al., 1980). The treatment consists of fractionated external beam irradiation to a total dose of 55–60 Gy. Standard therapy combines irradiation with concomitant and adjuvant temozolomide. Given continuously at low dose (75 mg/m$^2$/day) during the 6 weeks of radiotherapy followed by six 4-week cycles (150–200 mg/m$^2$ on days 1–5), median OS is increased from 12.1 to 14.6 months with acceptable toxicity (Stupp et al., 2005). The efficacy of temozolomide is particularly pronounced in patients whose tumors exhibit MGMT promoter methylation (Hegi et al., 2005). In elderly patients, a shorter course of radiotherapy can be used alone or in combination with concurrent and adjuvant temozolomide (Malmström et al., 2012; Perry et al., 2017). Monotherapy with temozolomide represents an option for individuals with MGMT promoter methylation (Malmström et al., 2012). Two phase III double-blind placebo-controlled trials evaluated bevacizumab in combination with standard radiochemotherapy in patients with newly diagnosed GBM. The first study met its co-primary endpoint of improved progression-free survival (PFS); however, OS did not reach statistical significance (Chinot et al., 2014). In the second trial, no difference was found between arms for OS (median 16.1 months vs. 15.7 months, $P = .11$). PFS was extended for patients treated with bevacizumab but the prespecified significance criterion was not reached (7.3 months vs. 10.7 months, $P = .004$). Increased grade ≥3 toxicity was seen with bevacizumab. Risk subset analysis raised concern for worse outcome in patients with the best prognosis (MGMT promoter methylated, favorable gene profile; Gilbert et al., 2014).

In 2011, NovoTTF-100A, a medical device, was approved by the FDA for use in recurrent glioblastoma. The device delivers low-intensity alternating electrical fields via two pairs of transducer arrays worn on the scalp. The electrical field probably interferes with assembly of the mitotic spindle and cell. A phase III trial in which 695 GBM patients were randomized to receive adjuvant temozolomide alone or in combination with TTFs demonstrated statistically significant improvement in PFS (6.7 months vs. 4 months) and OS (20.9 months vs. 16.0 months) in the device group (Stupp et al., 2017). Biodegradable polymers impregnated with carmustine are available for intracavitary application after tumor removal (Brem et al., 1995).

At first tumor recurrence, patients are enrolled on a clinical trial or treated with bevacizumab. Bevacizumab was approved for this indication based on phase II trial data demonstrating a response rate of 28%–35% and a median duration of response of ~4 months (Friedman et al., 2009; Kreisl et al., 2009). The drug is frequently combined with cytotoxic agents, although evidence of superior outcome from this approach remains to be shown. Patients who have failed standard therapies and are not eligible for a clinical trial are provided nitrosoureas; platinum compounds (cisplatin, carboplatin); or combination therapy with ifosfamide, carboplatin, and etoposide. Small molecule inhibitors of EGFR and its signal transduction pathways may benefit a molecularly defined subset of patients (expression of the somatic mutant EGFRvIII and the tumor suppressor gene product PTEN; Mellinghoff et al., 2005). Patients with small, radiographically distinct areas of residual or recurrent tumor can be considered for stereotactic treatment. But this treatment fails for the same reason other localized therapies cannot contain these tumors—their diffusely infiltrative nature. The adverse effects of this aggressive approach include seizures, transient focal neurological deficits, and radiation-induced necrosis developing within 3–18 months (Shrieve et al., 1999). The prognosis of patients reflects age at diagnosis, performance status prior to treatment, MGMT promoter methylation status, and somatic *IDH1* mutation. Median survival of glioblastoma remains less than 1 year in population-based statistics (Ostrom et al., 2018). Concomitant radiochemotherapy results in a probability of survival of 27% at 2 years and 10% at 5 years (Stupp et al., 2009).

#### Others

**Gliomatosis cerebri.** GC is a glial neoplasm characterized predominantly by diffusely infiltrative growth involving at least three lobes of the brain. While the updated WHO classification no longer lists this entity, it remains a clinically useful category (Louis et al., 2016). Patients present with headache or other signs of increased intracranial pressure, seizures, or focal deficits. Symptom onset can be insidious or fulminant ("neoplastic encephalitis"). Surgery, limited to stereotactic or incisional biopsy, establishes the diagnosis. Histopathologically, the tumor cells are either astrocytic, oligodendroglial, or mixed. Involved field or whole-brain radiation is standard therapy, but provides only marginal benefit and, given the size of the irradiated field, is associated with substantial morbidity in the form of psychomotor decline. Thus chemotherapy is often used with agents including PCV or temozolomide. Observation may be justified as the infiltrative tumor may be slow growing.

**Diffuse midline glioma, H3 K27M-mutant,** represents a new category in the WHO classification system of nervous system tumors and was initially described in children (**Schwartzentruber et al.**, 2012). These tumors are found in spinal cord, thalamus, brainstem, cerebellum, hypothalamus, or pineal region. Patients tend to be younger than those with IDH and H3 wild-type neoplasms. Outcomes of standard therapy (radiation, alkylating chemotherapy) are equally poor (Kleinschmidt-DeMasters and Levy, 2018; Meyronet et al., 2017). Whether these tumors are amenable to targeted therapy awaits further study.

### Oligodendroglial Tumors

***Oligodendroglioma and oligoastrocytoma.*** Oligodendroglial tumors account for 4% of newly diagnosed neoplasms. Of note, in 2016, the WHO classification of nervous system tumors was updated to include both histopathological appearance as well as molecular features (*IDH* mutation and 1p/19q co-deletion). Classical oligodendrogliomas are molecularly defined by IDH1/2 mutations and whole- arm deletion of chromosome 1p and 19q. *IDH1*-mutant oligodendrogliomas lacking 1p/19q deletion are treated like astrocytic tumors and share their response rate and prognosis. The diagnosis of oligoastrocytoma no longer exists for tumors in which molecular information is available. Clinical presentation of these tumors mimics that of other infiltrative glial tumors. Gross total resection prolongs survival (see Fig. 74.1, *C*). Debulking is needed for symptoms of mass effect and hemorrhage. Similar to astrocytic low-grade tumors, need for postoperative therapy is generally based on extent of resection and patient risk factors. Asymptomatic patients who are less than 40 years old and undergo gross total resection are followed without immediate therapy after surgery. Benefit is achieved with adjuvant radiation therapy and chemotherapy at progression (Karim et al., 2002). Based on the RTOG 9802 trial, postoperative therapy at initial diagnosis is recommended to patients with high-risk low-grade oligodendrogliomas (>40 years of age or incomplete resection) and symptomatic individuals (refractory seizures). Radiation therapy followed by PCV results in improved both overall and progression-free survival as compared with radiation therapy alone. Given the excellent prognosis in this patient population, benefits have to be carefully weighed against possible adverse effects, especially with respect to cognitive performance. Therefore in the absence of clear guidance from clinical trials, patients with large, unresectable tumors involving the dominant hemisphere are often treated with a modified approach (postoperative chemotherapy, radiation at the time of tumor progression). Temozolomide is often used instead of PCV. Prospective comparative efficacy data are not available (Buckner et al., 2016; Lassman et al., 2011). The median survival time of patients with oligodendrogliomas exceeds 10 years (Ostrom et al., 2013). Key prognostic variables are age at diagnosis, extent of resection, and the provision of adjuvant therapy.

***Anaplastic oligodendroglioma.*** Anaplastic oligodendroglial tumors (AO) are outnumbered by their low-grade equivalents (2% of all newly diagnosed neoplasms). A multimodality approach is always required. Resection or, if not possible, biopsy are followed by radiation or chemotherapy. RT is given in 30 fractions to a cumulative dose of 55 to 60 Gy. The exquisite chemosensitivity of these tumors was discovered at the end of the 1980s and in the early 1990s (Cairncross et al., 1994). Patients with tumors harboring deletions of chromosome 1p and 19q (the result of an unbalanced translocation) live longer than those with non–co-deleted tumors irrespective of therapy, and the median survival of those with co-deleted tumors treated with PCV plus RT is twice that of patients receiving RT (14.7 years vs. 7.3 years; Cairncross et al., 2013). A European trial yielded similar results (van den Bent et al., 2013). A prospective trial suggested equivalence of outcome irrespective of which adjuvant treatment modality was used at initial diagnosis after a median follow-up of 9.5 years (Wick et al., 2016). Whether PCV is interchangeable with temozolomide or RT can be withheld until tumor progression after initial chemotherapy remains subject to clinical investigation. Alternative treatment strategies include BCNU, melphalan, or high-dose, myeloablative chemotherapy followed by peripheral stem cell rescue. However, the latter approach remains experimental in this disease setting (Abrey et al., 2003). 1p/19q intact AOs resemble anaplastic astrocytoma in terms of treatment response and prognosis and are treated accordingly (Pajtler et al., 2015; van den Bent et al., 2013).

### Ependymal Tumors

***Ependymoma and anaplastic ependymoma.*** Two percent of all nervous system tumors are of ependymal differentiation. Ependymomas occur along the neuraxis, usually in proximity to the ventricles or subarachnoid space. Intracranial ependymoma is more common in children (infratentorial more frequent than supratentorial), spinal ependymoma in adults. Ependymoma is the most common intramedullary spinal cord tumor in adults and is typically in proximity to the conus medullaris. In this location, most are of the myxopapillary subtype. Only a small fraction of ependymomas are high-grade (see Fig. 74.1, *D*). Grading of these tumors remains difficult and morphology based, resulting in inconsistent correlation with outcome. As such, recent research efforts have focused on establishing a molecular classification scheme. A large international genomic study of 500 samples from both adult and pediatric ependymomas identified nine clinically and molecularly distinct entities, which fall into three subgroups based on anatomical location (spinal column, posterior fossa, and supratentorial). There are two groups which portend a poorer prognosis: a supratentorial group harboring RELA fusion (ST-EPN-RELA) and a posterior fossa group called PF-EPN-A (Pajtler et al., 2015). There is not enough evidence for treatment recommendations based on subgrouping at this time, but this information is likely to be incorporated into clinical trials going forward. Based on their location, symptoms related to obstruction of CSF pathways and myelopathies are common. The vast majority of tumors avidly enhance after gadolinium administration. Complete surgical removal is indicated and may cure the patient with a low-grade ependymoma. Resection of myxopapillary tumors is technically difficult because the masses adhere to nerve roots and have indistinct surgical margins that separate them from normal tissue of the conus medullaris. Radiation therapy is beneficial to patients with residual symptomatic tumor after operation, at recurrence, or with aggressive histology (Chang et al., 2002). Whether patients after gross total resection benefit from adjuvant radiotherapy remains a matter of debate. Recently published EANO guidelines for ependymoma suggest adjuvant local radiotherapy for pediatric patients with intracranial grade II and III ependymomas irrespective of residual tumor volume. In spinal ependymomas, radiation is recommended only if tumors are incompletely resected (Rudà et al., 2017). Conformal radiotherapy for supratentorial tumors results in good disease control and excellent neurocognitive outcome (Merchant et al., 2004). Craniospinal irradiation (CSI) is only needed if leptomeningeal spread occurs. The benefits of prophylactic CSI for high-grade ependymoma are unclear. Local failure tends to herald leptomeningeal spread. Chemotherapy for ependymoma includes temozolomide; carboplatin; PCV; combination chemotherapy with cisplatin, lomustine, and vincristine; or alternating cycles of cisplatin/etoposide and cyclophosphamide/vincristine (Chamberlain, 2002; Rudà et al., 2015). It is only indicated when local therapies have failed.

***Subependymoma.*** Subependymomas are benign tumors in proximity to the ventricles (Ragel et al., 2006). Not uncommonly, their detection as calcific masses is incidental, and therapy is only indicated when symptoms ensue. Enhancement on MRI with gadolinium is variable. The fourth ventricle is the most common location, followed by the septum pellucidum and the lateral ventricles. The tumor is well demarcated and surgical removal is curative. Subtotally resected tumors should be followed with serial MRI studies. Symptomatic residual tumors and those that show progressive growth should be irradiated.

### Choroid Plexus Tumors

***Choroid plexus papilloma and carcinoma.*** Choroid plexus papillomas are tumors of childhood. In adults they account for only 0.2% of all intracranial neoplasms. The tumor is located in the fourth ventricle, the cerebellopontine angle, or the lateral ventricles. Patients most commonly present with deficits of the eighth cranial nerve, signs of cerebellar dysfunction, or overproduction of CSF. The masses enhance homogeneously after gadolinium administration. Total resection is accomplished in fewer than half of cases. Frequently the tumor is attached to lower cranial nerves potentially increasing morbidity of surgical intervention. There is no role for adjuvant treatment modalities at diagnosis because long-term survival follows even subtotal resection. At progression or recurrence, treatment with conventional external beam radiation or SRS is of benefit. Obstructive hydrocephalus, a frequent complication of choroid plexus papilloma, is relieved by tumor removal, and shunt procedures are only indicated in a few cases (Tacconi et al., 1996). Rarely are low-grade neoplasms complicated by leptomeningeal seeding.

Choroid plexus carcinoma in adults is the subject of case reports only. Adjuvant treatment after surgical removal includes irradiation and chemotherapy. Therapeutic efficacy has been shown for lomustine.

### Neuronal and Mixed Neuronal-Glial Tumors

***Ganglioglioma and gangliocytoma.*** Seizures are the most common manifestations. These tumors contain two cell populations: gangliocytes and mature glial elements derived from precursor cells that can differentiate into both elements (see Fig. 74.1, *E*). Enhancement pattern on MRI is variable. The slow growth of these tumors is reflected by intratumoral calcification. Gross total resection results in survival ranging from 7 to 17 years. Thus adjuvant irradiation is only provided to tumors that are incompletely resected or those with anaplastic progression. These have a worse prognosis with an OS of 3 years or less (Hakim et al., 1997). Chemotherapy regimens for the rare anaplastic tumors are identical to the ones used for high-grade gliomas. A subset of gangliogliomas harbor *BRAF* mutations and may respond to targeted therapy (Schindler et al., 2011).

***Central neurocytoma.*** Central neurocytoma, a neuronal tumor, occurs in young adults in proximity to the supratentorial ventricular system. Accounting for less than 1% of all primary brain tumors, the tumor arises from the fornix, septum pellucidum, or the walls of the lateral ventricles. Symptoms resulting from CSF flow obstruction commonly precede its discovery. Enhancement on postgadolinium MRI is variable. Intratumoral hemorrhage is rarely observed but can give rise to acute obstructive hydrocephalus. A benign growth, surgical removal is performed by operations through the corpus callosum or cortex with attendant memory and cognitive problems, which are transient. Fewer than 50% of patients experience cure; for the remainder there is bleeding or adherence of tumor to adjacent structures. However, long-term tumor control can be achieved with partial resection. Instances of anaplasia or dissemination along CSF pathways are rare. Thus radiation therapy is recommended for tumors with a high proliferative index or growth. For tumors smaller than 3 cm, SRS may be beneficial. Adjuvant chemotherapy benefits a minority of patients treated with a combination of cisplatin, etoposide, and cyclophosphamide. The 5-year survival rate exceeds 80% (Brandes et al., 2000; Schild et al., 1997).

### Pineal Parenchymal Tumors

Tumors of pineal origin include pineocytoma, pineal parenchymal tumors of intermediate grade, and pineoblastoma. The more malignant tumors are seen in younger patients; more than 90% of patients with pineoblastoma are younger than age 23, whereas in patients older than the age of 40 years, one-third of the masses are tumors of low or intermediate grade (Chang et al., 1995). Less than 150 cases are diagnosed each year. Compression of tectal structures results in upgaze inhibition, dissociation of pupillary response, and retractory nystagmus (Parinaud syndrome) or syndromes related to CSF flow obstruction. Tertiary neurosurgical hospitals advocate complete tumor resection. Radiation therapy to the pineal region and the craniospinal axis is provided to patients with high-grade neoplasms, residual tumor after surgery, and subarachnoid dissemination. Chemotherapy is used in the setting of pineoblastoma or parenchymal tumors that are disseminated at onset or at recurrence. Commonly, preirradiation chemotherapy reduces tumor size. As with other neuroblastic tumors, platinum-based compounds are used, usually in combination with etoposide, alkylating agents (cyclohexylchloroethylnitrosourea (lomustine) [CCNU], procarbazine, cyclophosphamide), or vincristine. Long-term responders are reported, but estimates of survival are based on literature reviews or small retrospective institutional series.

### Peripheral Neuroblastic Tumors

***Esthesioneuroblastoma.*** Typically discovered when the nasal passage is obstructed, esthesioneuroblastoma arises from the neuroepithelium of the upper nasal cavity. From there it invades the neurocranium through the cribriform plate, compresses the frontal lobes of the brain, and may infiltrate the brain parenchyma or subarachnoid spaces (see Fig. 74.1, *F*). A standardized therapeutic approach has not been established for this exceedingly rare tumor. A grading (Hyams) and staging system (Kadish) have been established that correlate with outcome. Frequently, gross total resection via a craniofacial approach is followed by adjuvant external beam radiation therapy unless the tumor is excised completely or is low grade (Eich et al., 2001). Because gratifying responses are seen with chemotherapy, patients with disseminated or recurrent disease and those with high-grade tumors are treated with combinations such as cisplatin-etoposide, cyclophosphamide-vincristine-doxorubicin, or alternating cycles of cisplatin-etoposide and cyclophosphamide-vincristine (McElroy Jr. et al., 1998). Advocates of radiation and chemotherapy prior to surgery cite decreased tumor burden and facilitation of gross total removal with decreased morbidity as benefits of this approach. Others recommend chemotherapy with cisplatin and etoposide after biopsy, followed by proton-photon irradiation and postradiation chemotherapy (Fitzek et al., 2002). Patients with low-grade tumors have PFS exceeding 10 years, in comparison with less than 3 years for those with more aggressive tumors. Not uncommon are late local recurrences or metastases to cervical lymph nodes. When the tumor invades through the dura into the subarachnoid space, intrathecal methotrexate, cytosine-arabinoside, or thio-TEPA may be used. Radiation is administered to symptomatic or nodular leptomeningeal recurrences.

### Embryonal Tumors

***Medulloblastoma.*** Medulloblastomas in adults are rare neoplasms (<1% of all primary brain tumors). The majority of patients present before 40 years of age with cerebellar syndromes, headache, or other signs of increased intracranial pressure. Unlike childhood tumors, these are prone to the cerebellar hemispheres, less commonly in contiguity with the fourth ventricle. As a result, dissemination into the CSF is seen in fewer than one-third of cases. In general, the natural history is less aggressive: extraneural metastases have been reported in fewer than 150 patients, and then most frequently to bone (Chan et al., 2000). On a molecular level, four tumor subgroups with distinct clinical, biological, and genetic profiles are currently identified: tumors with activated wingless pathway signaling; tumors with sonic hedgehog pathway activation; group 3 (MYC amplified); and group 4 tumors (Robinson et al., 2012). A recently published integrative deep-sequencing analysis of 125 tumor-normal pairs described the genomic complexity and heterogeneity underlying medulloblastoma, including several recurrent mutations in known medulloblastoma-related genes (*CTNNB1*, *PTCH1*, *MLL2*, *SMARCA4*), in genes not previously linked to this tumor (DDX3X, CTDNEP1, KDM6A, TBR1), and fusion genes (Jones et al., 2012). Multidisciplinary management is critical for the successful treatment of these tumors. Resection, CSI, and adjuvant chemotherapy results in 5-year survival rates of 65% (Brandes et al., 2003). Obstructive hydrocephalus is a frequent complication of medulloblastoma requiring at least transient external ventricular drainage. Third ventriculostomy or ventriculoperitoneal shunting is provided to symptomatic patients with occlusion of the fourth ventricle persisting after resection. Resection is followed by evaluation of CSF and lumbar spine for tumor spread, and CSI (CSI; posterior fossa 54 Gy, whole-brain 40 Gy, and spine 36 Gy; Abacioglu et al., 2002). Adult patients treated with proton beam CSI (p-CSI) lose less weight; experience less nausea, vomiting, and esophagitis; and have a smaller reduction in peripheral white blood cells, hemoglobin, and platelets than individuals treated with conventional CSI (Brown et al., 2013). Chemotherapy is considered a standard component of medulloblastoma management in children and likely also benefits adults, especially high-risk patients with significant residual tumor, brainstem infiltration, or leptomeningeal metastases. Commonly used drugs either prior to or following irradiation include cisplatin or carboplatin, cyclophosphamide, nitrosoureas, and etoposide. The Pediatric Oncology Group pioneered the preirradiation use of alternating cycles of cisplatin (single dose on day 1 or divided in five daily doses on days 1–5) and etoposide (daily on days 1–5) with cyclophosphamide (daily on days 1 and 2) and vincristine (1.5 mg/m$^2$ day 1; Duffner et al., 1993). The "Packer protocol," likewise designed for pediatric medulloblastoma, consists of weekly vincristine (1.5 mg/m$^2$) during CSI therapy and for 6 weeks thereafter followed by eight cycles (one cycle every 6–8 weeks) of cisplatin (75 mg/m$^2$) and CCNU (50 mg/m$^2$) on day 1 and vincristine (1.5 mg/m$^2$) given three times per cycle (Packer et al., 1994). The latter protocol appears to be considerably more toxic in adults than in children and dose reductions of all drugs are required in the vast majority of cases (Greenberg et al., 2001). Rational administration of these drugs in adults provides for their use before irradiation because CSI limits bone marrow reserve, whereas in children, benefit from preradiation chemotherapy could only be demonstrated in the youngest patients (<3 years). Radiation therapy should certainly not be delayed by extended periods of myelosuppression from chemotherapy. Whether to offer prophylactic chemotherapy along with reduced-dose CSI to low-risk patients is uncertain. Ultimately this issue will be addressed by formal study.

Treatment of tumor recurrence after multimodality therapy is difficult due to the patients' limited bone marrow reserve. Re-resection or SRS may be offered to selected patients. High-dose chemotherapy followed by stem cell rescue may benefit young patients. Preliminary data on temozolomide in relapsed medulloblastoma have been published in the pediatric literature. New insights into the molecular pathogenesis of medulloblastoma will hopefully soon result in the implementation of new therapeutic agents. Hedgehog pathway inhibitors (such as vismodegib) are subject to clinical investigation and have shown some activity in recurrent SHH mutant medulloblastoma in small phase II studies (Robinson et al., 2015; Rudin et al., 2009; Yauch et al., 2009; ).

***Other Embryonal Tumors.*** The term "primitive neuroectodermal tumors" was removed from the most recent WHO guideline (2016) and most of these tumors now fall into the category "CNS embryonal tumor not otherwise specified." This classification excludes tumors with C19MC amplification, the presence of which results in a diagnosis of embryonal tumor with multilayered rosettes (ETMR), C19MC altered (Louis et al., 2016). These tumors are rarer than medulloblastomas. The clinical syndrome consists of seizures, headache, or focal neurological symptoms. The masses display heterogeneous enhancement on postgadolium MRI. Surgical resection reduces the tumor burden. Postsurgical therapy has been similar to that for patients with high-risk medulloblastoma. Adjuvant therapy consists of fractionated external-beam radiation to the primary site and the craniospinal axis. However, because these masses are sensitive to chemotherapy, many centers have begun to treat high-risk patients with low-dose radiation in conjunction with chemotherapy. Drugs used include the PCV combination, cisplatin-etoposide alone, or alternating with cyclophosphamide-vincristine, and are frequently given prior to radiation. Survival may exceed 5 years, but many patients succumb to their disease within a few years. Treatment failure usually occurs locally. Well-delineated tumors with minimal residual after surgery have a favorable prognosis.

## Tumors of Cranial and Peripheral Nerves

### Schwannoma and Neurofibroma

Schwannomas and neurofibromas are benign tumors of the peripheral nerve sheath (PNST) and account for ~9% of tumors diagnosed each year. Nerve sheath tumors, while commonly found along large nerve trunks, have been described in almost any location in the body. Schwannomas have a predilection for head, neck, and flexor surfaces of the extremities. Intracranial schwannomas commonly arise from the sensory branches of cranial nerves such as the acoustic or trigeminal nerves. Naturally, the clinical spectrum varies widely and symptoms arise from loss of function of the affected nerve or mass effect on adjacent structures. PNSTs display homogeneous contrast enhancement. A rim-enhancing appearance reflects degenerative changes and should not be confused with a malignant neoplasm. Surgical removal is the treatment of choice for PNST and is curative. Schwannomas can be resected with resolution of symptoms and preservation of function in 90% of cases (Kim et al., 2005; Tiel and Kline, 2004). Spinal PNSTs can adhere to spinal cord or critical extradural structures such as the vertebral artery, rendering complete removal difficult. Transection of the dorsal rootlets rarely results in paresthesias; segmental loss of motor function results from sacrificing the anterior portion of nerve roots at the level of the upper and lower extremities (C5-T1, L3-S1) but is frequently only transient, suggesting that nerves afflicted by a nerve sheath tumor are not functional (Jinnai and Koyama, 2005).

Using an interfascicular approach and neurophysiological monitoring, gross total removal can also be accomplished in the majority of solitary neurofibromas, although these tumors are not encapsulated and intertwined with their parent and surrounding fascicles. Complete resection of plexiform neurofibroma is not possible without nerve damage but subtotal decompressive surgery may relieve pain. Image-guided frameless radiosurgery will likely have a role in treatment of symptomatic spinal tumors that cannot be resected. The MAP kinase inhibitor selumetinib has shown efficacy in a small cohort of children with plexiform neurofibroma in the setting of neurofibromatosis (Dombi et al., 2016).

Small and stable asymptomatic acoustic schwannomas are followed with serial MRI scans on an annual basis. Symptomatic tumors are treated with microsurgical resection or SRS. Surgical risks include postoperative CSF leak, facial and trigeminal neuropathy, and deafness. These risks are directly related to tumor size (Kaylie et al., 2001). The use of proton radiosurgery or fractionated SRT achieves tumor "control" without disappearance in over 90% of patients, with hearing complications in approximately 20%. The risk of hearing loss has been decreased by limiting the dose to 12 Gy (prescribed to the 50% isodose line). Bevacizumab therapy shrinks vestibular schwannomas and improves hearing in patients who have neurofibromatosis, type 2 (Plotkin et al., 2009). A volumetric and functional response was also described after lapatinib treatment (Karajannis et al., 2012). Complete surgical removal provides long-term local control or cure for the patient with schwannoma and nodular neurofibroma. Malignant degeneration for those tumors is rare. Outcome is less favorable in patients with neurofibromatosis. Transformation into a malignant nerve sheath tumor is more common in plexiform neurofibroma.

### Malignant Peripheral Nerve Sheath Tumor

Malignant peripheral nerve sheath tumor (MPNST) is a rare neoplasm of peripheral nerves, including cranial nerves. The neurological syndrome progresses faster than with low-grade PNSTs. Wide surgical excision is the treatment of choice. Average extent of resection depends on tumor location and ranges from 20% in paraspinal nerve root and plexus masses to nearly 100% in tumors of the distal extremities. Radiation therapy is provided for residual disease in the form of external beam radiation alone or in combination with brachytherapy (iridium-192) or intra-operative high-energy electron irradiation. Although amputation has been historically offered, these approaches have improved limb-sparing control. Twenty to forty percent of patients are treated with adjuvant chemotherapy at diagnosis (2-mercaptoethane sulfonate Na (MESNA), doxorubicin, ifosfamide, and dacarbazine, or single-drug regimens such as high-dose methotrexate). Chemotherapy does not have a role in the initial treatment of completely resected, localized MPNST.

Treatment failure in half the patients is local within 3 years, but late local recurrences at 25 years have been described. The median survival exceeds 2–5 years. Tumor size, extent of surgery, and age at diagnosis are predictors of survival (Baehring et al., 2003).

## Meningeal Tumors

### Meningioma

Meningiomas are the most common intracranial tumors (over one-third of newly diagnosed nervous system tumors; Fig. 74.2, *A*). Clinical manifestation and management depend on location, coexistent morbidities, and the patient's age (Chamberlain, 2001). Incidentally found asymptomatic meningiomas lacking mass effect or compression of a venous sinus can be followed conservatively with serial MRI evaluations. Many meningiomas will not grow over years, sparing older adult patients the need for craniotomy (Black et al., 1998). However, when seizures occur, tumors grow, or focal signs emerge, surgical resection can be curative, especially in meningiomas overlying the hemispheres. Technically more challenging are tumors invading dural venous sinuses, tumors arising from the dura overlying the medial portions of the sphenoid bone or other parts of the skull base, meningioma en plaque, posterior fossa meningiomas, and the rare intraventricular meningiomas. Complete surgical removal may not be possible in these situations and may be complicated by infection, CSF leakage, cerebral venous thrombosis, or cranial neuropathies. Less aggressive surgery in association with stereotactic radiation reduces treatment morbidity and may improve PFS (Villavicencio et al., 2001). At recurrence or tumor progression, conventional external beam irradiation or SRS is the major treatment option.

Atypical (6%) and malignant meningiomas (2%) account for a small fraction of all meningiomas, but these tumors recur in spite of surgical resection and irradiation. A recent study of genome-wide DNA methylation patterns identified six distinct methylation classes which were better predictors of recurrence and survival than WHO grades (Sahm et al., 2017). Although meningiomas express estrogen and progesterone receptors, clinical trials with tamoxifen or progesterone receptor antagonists such as mifepristone (RU-486) have been disappointing. Similarly, somatostatin analogs have failed to show clear benefit in recurrent meningioma even though most meningiomas express somatostatin receptors. Because meningiomas are highly vascular tumors, there has been recent interest in the incorporation of VEGF inhibitors into their treatment. Retrospective analyses and small cohort studies using VEGF inhibitors such as bevacizumab, vatalanib, and sunitinib have suggested disease stability with the use of these agents (Grimm et al., 2015; Nayak et al., 2012; Shih et al., 2016). Some authors have reported partial responses or stable disease in patients with recurrent or malignant meningioma who receive hydroxyurea, alpha interferon, or drug regimens such as cyclophosphamide/doxorubicin/vincristine, ifosfamide/mesna, or doxorubicin/dacarbazine. Recent insights in the molecular pathogenesis of meningioma may lead to novel targeted therapies. In more than half of meningiomas, inactivation of NF2 is identified (Brastianos et al., 2013; Clark et al., 2013). One-quarter of tumors harbor mutations in TRAF7, a proapoptotic E3 ubiquitin ligase, often accompanied by mutations in KLF4, a transcription factor, or AKT1. SMO mutations are identified in ~5% of non-NF2 mutant meningiomas. Non-NF2 meningiomas are nearly always benign. Tumors with mutant NF2 or chromosome 22 loss are more likely to be atypical. Molecular profile correlates with anatomical location and histological subtype. Tumors with NF2 mutations or chromosome 22 loss are predominantly found over the hemispheres and within the lateral skull base. The few meningiomas with SMO mutations localize to the medial anterior skull base. Secretory meningiomas carry both TRAF7 and KLF4 mutations (Clark et al., 2013). Trials with agents targeting these mutations are ongoing.

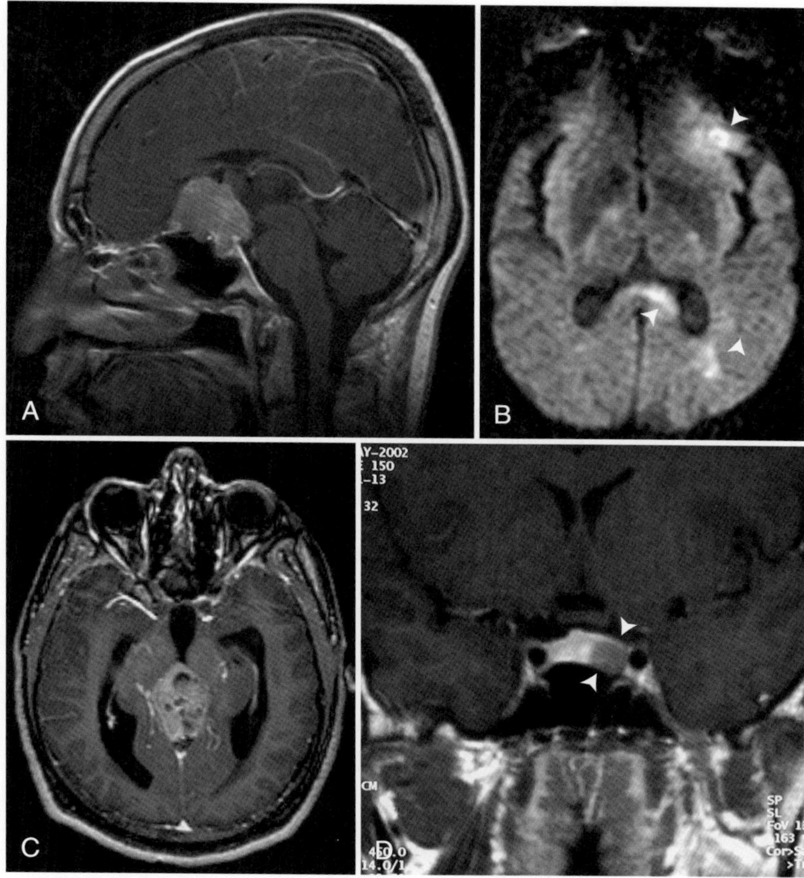

Fig. 74.2 Intracranial Neoplasms of Non-Neuroepithelial Origin. A, Meningioma of the planum sphenoidale. The homogeneously enhancing tumor invades the pituitary fossa and displaces the optic chiasm posteriorly and rostrally (T1-weighted magnetic resonance imaging [MRI] with gadolinium). B, Primary brain lymphoma. Highly cellular regions of this diffusely infiltrative neoplasm are seen as areas of increased signal intensity on this diffusion-weighted MRI. C, Germinoma. The homogeneously enhancing mass arises from the pineal region (T1-weighted MRI with gadolinium). D, Pituitary adenoma. The minimally enhancing tumor *(arrowheads)* can be seen in negative contrast to the surrounding cavernous sinus (T1-weighted MRI with gadolinium).

### Hemangiopericytoma/Solitary Fibrous Tumor

Intracranial hemangiopericytoma/solitary fibrous tumor is a rare meningeal neoplasm with a high rate of local recurrence and predisposition to metastases to bone and liver. Leptomeningeal spread has been described occurring beyond 5 years of diagnosis. Gross total resection emphasizes removal of surrounding normal dura or brain. Radiation therapy (fractionated to 48–60 Gy) reduces the local recurrence rate and prolongs PFS (Guthrie et al., 1989). Unfortunately, as with meningioma and schwannoma, tumor shrinkage cannot be expected until years after therapy.

At tumor recurrence, options include surgical resection, conventional external beam radiation, and SRS. Chemotherapy may benefit the patient with systemic metastases or local therapy-refractory disease (Galanis et al., 1998). Most protocols use doxorubicin in combination with cyclophosphamide, ifosfamide, cisplatin, or dacarbazine. Partial responses or stable disease for several months have been observed with these regimens. Anecdotal reports of successful therapy with alpha interferon 2A and small molecule inhibitors of VEGFR are available. Up to 90% of tumors recur locally or systemically within 9 years of initial manifestation. Extraneural recurrence is predictive of worsened prognosis. Median survival after first recurrence is between 4 and 5 years, but with aggressive management, long-term survival is possible.

## Neuraxis Tumors Derived from the Hematopoietic System

### Primary Central Nervous System Lymphoma

***Non-AIDS related disease.*** Approximately 1400 cases of PCNSL are diagnosed each year in the United States. The "chamaeleon" of modern clinical medicine, the disease presents with a wide variety of neurological syndromes. Common presentations are psychomotor decline and focal neurological symptoms. Diencephalic involvement results in disorders of sodium homeostasis, appetite control, and behavior. Neoplastic infiltrates have a predilection for ependymal or pial surfaces. Masses are homogeneously enhancing on post-gadolinium MRI. Tumor cellularity results in their hyperdense appearance on unenhanced CT scans and relative restriction of water diffusion visible on diffusion-weighted MRI. Diagnosis is established through stereotactic biopsy. Surgical resection is not indicated in the majority of cases. Methotrexate-based chemotherapy given in high doses (HDMTX; above 3.5 g/m$^2$) followed by leucovorin rescue has been shown to be the single most effective remission induction treatment for PCNSL. Its use, either alone or in combination before radiation therapy, has resulted in response rates of 70%–95% and survival durations in excess of 3 years (Hochberg et al., 2007). Methotrexate monotherapy is provided in 10–14 day intervals until complete radiographic remission is achieved followed by monthly consolidation treatments for 1 year (Batchelor et al., 2003). HDMTX seems to be well tolerated by the largely elderly patient population. The treatment produces no alopecia, minimal to modest myelotoxicity, and is compatible with normal cognitive function. Successfully used combination regimens include HDMTX, procarbazine, vincristine, cytarabine (Abrey et al., 2000); HDMTX, lomustine, procarbazine, methylprednisolone, and intrathecal chemotherapy with methotrexate and cytarabine (Hoang-Xuan et al., 2003); HDMTX with cyclophosphamide, ifosfamide, vincristine/vindesine, dexamethasone, cytarabine and intrathecal chemotherapy; or HDMTX with cytarabine, thio-TEPA, and rituximab (called the MATRix regimen) (Ferreri et al., 2017; Pels et al., 2003). Intra-arterial application of methotrexate preceded by mannitol-induced BBB disruption in combination with intravenous cyclophosphamide and etoposide is effective but requires monthly triple-vessel angiography and is associated with a high frequency of procedure-related, albeit reversible complications (Doolittle et al., 2000). Given its proven efficacy in systemic non-Hodgkin lymphoma, rituximab has been added to remission induction regimens for PCNSL, but its role remains to be defined. The administration of intrathecal or intraocular chemotherapy is of uncertain benefit. High-dose intravenous methotrexate results in cytotoxic drug levels within the CSF and in the vitreous body of the eyes. However, high tumor burden within CSF may be associated with methotrexate resistance and thus intrathecal chemotherapy may postpone the need for irradiation.

Historically, external beam irradiation was used for consolidation after chemotherapy (DeAngelis et al., 2002). When administered as part of the initial treatment protocol it seemed to result in a trend towards prolonged time to progression at the expense of earlier neurocognitive decline and without an increase in OS. Thus WBRT is now commonly deferred until the time of chemoresistant recurrence. More promising results have recently been reported combining chemotherapy with reduced-dose WBRT (23.4 Gy) for patients achieving complete remission after chemotherapy (Morris et al., 2013). Above doses of 35–45 Gy, escalation provides no survival benefit (Nelson et al., 1992).

Without consolidation therapy most patients relapse and systemic dissemination is encountered in up to 8%. At the time of recurrence, we and others have successfully used methotrexate even in prior recipients of this drug (Plotkin et al., 2004). Small clinical studies report responses at the time of relapse with the use of topotecan, rituximab (Batchelor et al., 2011), temozolomide, PCV, cytosine-arabinoside/etoposide, or pemetrexed (Zhang et al., 2013). Large-scale genomic investigations identified driver mutations in MYD88, CD79B, CARD11, and TNFAIP3 that constitutively activate the B-cell receptor (BCR) signaling axis. These discoveries have led to ongoing clinical trials using small molecule inhibitors targeting signal transduction pathways downstream of BCR, including NF-κB (Grommes et al., 2018). Ibrutinib, an inhibitor of Bruton tyrosine kinase, has shown activity in retrospective case studies as well as phase I clinical trials in patients with relapsed/refractory PCNSL (Chamoun et al., 2017; Grommes et al., 2017). Lenalidomide (Ghesquieres et al., 2019) and pomalidomide (Tun et al., 2018) have been studied in phase I and II studies and demonstrated promising efficacy. There are currently trials underway to evaluate use of immunotherapy (checkpoint blockade) in relapsed disease. Studies of CD19-targeting chimeric antigen receptor-T cell therapy for relapsed PCNSL are in preparation.

Addressing the high relapse rate in spite of successful remission induction, recent clinical studies have focused on intensification of consolidation regimens alone (Rubenstein et al., 2013) or combined with autologous stem cell transplantation (Kasenda et al., 2012). These studies have shown that high-dose chemotherapy followed by autologous stem cell transplant (using thio-TEPA, busulfan, and cyclophosphamide for myeloablation) results in favorable overall response rate (>90%) and progression-free survival (>74 months; DeFilipp et al., 2017; Illerhaus et al., 2016; Montemurro et al., 2006; Omuro et al., 2015; Soussain et al., 2008). As such this treatment is generally considered for consolidation in patients who are younger than 65 years, have good functional status, and achieved complete or near complete remission. Prospective randomized studies comparing various consolidation regimens are ongoing (clinicaltrials.gov, NCT01511562).

PCNSL is a highly aggressive tumor (see Fig. 74.2, *B*); left untreated, most patients succumb within 6 months. Unfavorable prognostic factors include older age (>60 years), low performance status, multiple brain lesions, evidence of leptomeningeal dissemination, lack of radiographic complete response to treatment, and elevated serum lactate dehydrogenase level (Ferreri et al., 2003). While in small series of patients treated at referral centers median survival of 3–5 years is reported, population-based registries document a survival rate of 54% at 1 year (Ostrom et al., 2018).

***AIDS-related primary central nervous system lymphoma.*** The introduction of highly active antiretroviral therapy (HAART) has not only reduced the incidence of brain lymphoma but also increased the number of patients eligible for systemic chemotherapy. Initiation of antiretroviral alone may facilitate remission induction of this EBV-driven disease. For remission induction, similar regimens are used as in the immunocompetent host. depending on patient's performance status and comorbidities.

## Germ Cell Tumors

Germ cell tumors of the CNS are rare adult tumors in the United States (<0.1% of primary brain tumors) occurring commonly in boys and young men before the age of 20 years. Incidence is considerably higher in East Asia. The most common germ cell tumor occurring within the CNS is germinoma. Less common are nongerminomatous germ cell tumors (teratoma, embryonal carcinoma, yolk sac tumor [endodermal sinus tumor], choriocarcinoma, and mixed germ cell tumors). The entire group has a proclivity for the sellar and suprasellar region, walls of the third ventricle, and the pineal gland. Accordingly, syndromes reflect pituitary or stalk dysfunction, or tectal compression. Surgical access is difficult and often limits intervention to biopsy or empiric radiation/chemotherapy. The latter approach is usually avoided, given the high incidence of mixed neoplasms. Treatment planning depends on careful analysis of resected tissue, often with evaluation of serum and CSF levels of β-human chorionic gonadotropin, α-fetoprotein, and placental alkaline phosphatase. The major determinants of outcome are local tumor control and histological subtype. Treatment schedules are still being optimized.

### Germinoma

Germinomas are infiltrative tumors with a tendency to subependymal and leptomeningeal spread (see Fig. 74.2, *C*). Traditionally, treatment included surgical resection or biopsy followed by CSI and a boost to the tumor bed resulting in high cure rates. It has been recognized that in patients with localized disease long-term survival can be achieved by extended focal irradiation including the third and lateral ventricles, the sella, and the pineal region (Matsutani et al., 1997). Thus CSI is now increasingly reserved for patients with cytopathological or radiographic evidence of leptomeningeal spread. Intracranial germinomas share with their extracranial counterparts sensitivity to platinum-based chemotherapy but relapses are common unless combined with radiotherapy (Allen et al., 1987; Balmaceda et al., 1996). The most commonly used protocols include cisplatin, etoposide, bleomycin, or cyclophosphamide. Long-term survivors of radiation are at risk of neuroendocrine morbidities reflecting dysfunction of the hypothalamic–pituitary axis. Preirradiation chemotherapy is given to high-risk patients to achieve complete responses and allows for radiation dose reduction (Matsutani et al., 1998; Sawamura et al., 1998). In a nonrandomized trial of patients with localized germinoma treated either with CSI or with chemotherapy (carboplatin/etoposide alternating with ifosfamide/etoposide) followed by localized irradiation, there was no difference in 5-year OS (95% ± 2% vs. 96% ± 3%). Five-year PFS was 97% ± 2% in the CSI group and 88% ± 4% in the combined modality group (Calaminus et al., 2013).

### Nongerminomatous Germ Cell Tumors

Gross total resection prolongs survival but is achieved in less than half the cases. Each of the nongerminomatous germ cell tumors (NGGCT) is approached differently (Schild et al., 1996). Mature or immature teratomas are operated on and then receive involved field radiation therapy with good control. If the teratoma has undergone transformation to malignancy, there is an increased risk of leptomeningeal metastases. This argues strongly for prophylactic whole-brain or craniospinal irradiation. Nonteratomatous, nongerminomatous germ cell tumors are provided adjuvant radiation therapy (above 50 Gy) and platinum-based polychemotherapy. The radiation therapy fields include the craniospinal axis followed by a "boost" to the tumor bed. These approaches are associated with complications of anterior pituitary dysfunction and intellectual decline—changes that have spurred the use of localized, lower doses or hyperfractionated radiation in the setting of polychemotherapy (carboplatin, etoposide; ifosfamide, cisplatin, etoposide; cisplatin, etoposide, cyclophosphamide, bleomycin/carboplatin, etoposide, and bleomycin [Kellie et al., 2004]; carboplatin, cyclophosphamide, etoposide). Recent results from the multicenter trial support the use of dose-intense chemotherapy followed by risk-adapted radiotherapy in nongerminomatous germ cell tumor (NGGCT). In this study 149 patients with NGGCT were treated with four courses of cisplatin/etoposide/ifosfamide followed by focal radiotherapy (54 Gy) in nonmetastatic patients and craniospinal RT (30 Gy) followed by 24 Gy boost in metastatic patients. Patients with localized malignant NGGCT demonstrated acceptable 5-year PFS and OS of 0.72 ± 0.04 and 0.82 ± 0.04, respectively. Patients with metastatic disease ($n$ = 33) demonstrated 5-year PFS and OS of 0.68 ± 0.09 and 0.75 ± 0.08, respectively (Calaminus et al., 2017). Prognosis for mature teratomas is excellent. On the other side, only 10%–15% of patients with embryonal carcinoma, yolk sac tumor (endodermal sinus tumor), or choriocarcinoma survive 3 years after diagnosis. Mixed germ cell tumors and immature teratomas fall in between these two extremes. High-dose chemotherapy followed by autologous stem cell transplantation is an option for salvage therapy (Modak et al., 2004).

## Tumors of the Sellar Region

### Craniopharyngioma

Craniopharyngioma is a tumor derived from Rathke's pouch epithelium, which may be present both within the sella turcica as well as other skull base locations. Less than 500 cases are diagnosed each year in adults. Masses may infiltrate the hypothalamus. Patients present with headache, visual field disturbances, or neuroendocrine dysfunction. Microsurgical resection via a subfrontal, pterional, or transsphenoidal approach is the primary treatment in symptomatic cases (Van Effenterre and Boch, 2002). External beam radiation therapy may extend PFS after incomplete resection, although long-term survival can be accomplished with surgery alone (Yasargil et al., 1990). Stereotactic radiation techniques have been successfully used. Intracavitary irradiation ($^{32}$P or $^{90}$Y; Hasegawa et al., 2004) or instillation of bleomycin is available for solitary cystic craniopharyngioma or cystic components of a mixed tumor following stereotactic aspiration of the cyst contents. Recent genomic evaluation has shown that nearly all papillary craniopharyngiomas (which are more common in adults) harbor mutations in BRAF p.Val600Glu and all adamantinomatous craniopharyngioma have mutations in CTNNB1 (Brastianos et al., 2014). This has led to successful use of targeted therapy with BRAF and MEK inhibitors in case reports and small case series of patients with papillary craniopharyngioma (Brastianos et al., 2016; Roque and Odia, 2017). A phase II study combining MEK/BRAF inhibition in these patients is now underway.

### Pituitary Adenoma

Pituitary adenoma is the third most common intracranial neoplasm (12.7% of newly diagnosed tumors). Clinical manifestation depends upon tumor size, hormone secretion by tumor cells, as well as compression of the normal gland and adjacent structures. Surgical resection is the treatment of choice for pituitary adenomas larger than 1 cm in diameter (Fig. 74.2, *D*), or those with compression of the optic chiasm, erosion of bone, or extension into the walls of the sella. The transsphenoidal approach (Hardy's procedure), preferable to the transcranial route (most often right pterional craniotomy), achieves gross total resection in one-third of patients. Improvement in microsurgical technique and imaging has reduced mortality to below 2%.

Radiation therapy is provided as primary treatment to older adult patients, those who are not surgical candidates, and following partial resection (Sasaki et al., 2000). Tumor shrinkage is seen only years after treatment. Adverse effects are infrequent and include necrosis of the adjacent portions of the temporal lobe, hearing loss, optic neuropathy, and radiation-induced sarcomas. Multiple field techniques and radiosurgery have reduced the incidence of these complications. The majority of patients treated with surgery and radiation require replacement of pituitary gland–dependent hormones. Local control rates are higher than 80% for patients with nonsecreting pituitary adenomas. Prognosis for secreting adenomas is slightly worse.

Dopamine agonists such as bromocriptine, cabergoline, quinagolide, and pergolide are effective in micro- as well as macroprolactinomas and lead to reduction in tumor size, improvement of symptoms, and normalization of prolactin levels (Vance, 2003).

*The complete reference list is available online at https://expertconsult.inkling.com/.* 

75

# Primary Nervous System Tumors in Infants and Children

*Vijay Ramaswamy, Sharon L. Gardner, Matthias A. Karajannis*

## OUTLINE



## PEDIATRIC PRIMARY NERVOUS SYSTEM TUMORS

Primary brain tumors account for nearly 20% of all malignancies during childhood and adolescence worldwide, with an age-standardized incidence rate of 28.2 per million persons (Steliarova-Foucher et al., 2017; Ward et al., 2014). These tumors are second only to leukemia in frequency among all childhood cancers and are the most common solid tumor in children (Steliarova-Foucher et al., 2017; Ward et al., 2014). The location, histological features, prognosis, and treatment of pediatric brain tumors are different from those of adult brain tumors and vary significantly according to age within the pediatric population (Table 75.1). The location of approximately 30% of primary brain tumors in children aged 0–14 years is the posterior fossa; however, supratentorial brain tumors are the most common location in adolescents and children younger than age 2 (Ostrom et al., 2015). Gliomas account for approximately half of pediatric central nervous system (CNS) tumors of which the majority are pilocytic astrocytomas (PAs) and other low-grade gliomas. In contrast to adult brain tumors, supratentorial high-grade astrocytomas (HGAs) represent only 6%–12% of all primary pediatric brain tumors, and diffuse intrinsic brainstem gliomas represent 10%. Embryonal tumors (14.5%), other gliomas (15%), ependymomas (6.5%), germ cell tumors (4.6%), and craniopharyngiomas (3%) account for most of the other types (Ostrom et al., 2015, 2018). Despite significant improvements in prognosis for many pediatric cancers over the past few decades, CNS malignancies remain a major cause of morbidity and mortality. However, the pace of both clinical and laboratory research has accelerated over the past decade, and classification and management of this diverse group of tumors is undergoing a transformation owing to a new understanding of brain tumor biology and genomics on a molecular level (Table 75.2).

## EMBRYONAL TUMORS

### Medulloblastoma

Medulloblastoma is a round blue cell tumor of the cerebellum and/or fourth ventricle, and is the most common malignant brain tumor of childhood. The World Health Organization (WHO) recognizes the medulloblastoma with five distinct molecular variants, termed subgroups: specifically, Wingless-activated (WNT), SHH-activated TP53 wild-type (SHH-TP53WT), SHH-activated TP53 mutant (SHH-TP53 mutant), and non-WNT/non-SHH comprising two provisional entities, Group 3 and Group 4 (Louis et al., 2016). The WHO also recognized histological variants defined as: large-cell medulloblastoma, anaplastic medulloblastoma, medulloblastoma with extensive nodularity, and desmoplastic/nodular medulloblastoma. Medulloblastoma represents approximately 65% of CNS embryonal tumors and 10% of all pediatric brain tumors. The incidence in males is twice that of females, and the median age at diagnosis is 5–7 years. Taken as a group, 80% of all CNS embryonal tumors are diagnosed before age 10. According to the incidence data generated by the National Cancer Institute's Surveillance, Epidemiology and End Results (SEER) registry and the CNS Tumors Diagnosed in the United States, the incidence of CNS embryonal tumors and medulloblastoma has remained fairly stable over the past 20 years (Linabery and Ross, 2008; Ostrom et al., 2015, 2018).

**TABLE 75.1 Pediatric Brain Tumors**

| Histology | Percent of All Tumors | Median Age | Rate* |
|---|---|---|---|
| Gliomas | 52.90 | 6 | 2.78 |
| *Pilocytic astrocytoma* | 17.60 | 7 | 0.93 |
| *Other low-grade glioma* | 14.30 | 6 | 0.75 |
| *High-grade glioma* | 11.10 | 7 | 0.59 |
| *Ependymal tumors* | 5.50 | 4 | 0.29 |
| *Other glioma* | 4.40 | 7 | 0.23 |
| Choroid plexus tumors | 2.30 | 1 | 0.12 |
| Tumors of the pineal region | 4.40 | 6.5 | 0.23 |
| Neuronal and mixed neuronal-glial tumors | 0.90 | 9 | 0.05 |
| Embryonal tumors | 15.00 | 4 | 0.79 |
| *Medulloblastoma* | 9.30 | 6 | 0.49 |
| *Primitive neuroectodermal tumor* | 2.20 | 3.5 | 0.12 |
| *Atypical teratoid/rhabdoid tumor* | 2.30 | 1 | 0.12 |
| *Other embryonal tumors* | 1.20 | 1 | 0.06 |
| Tumors of cranial and spinal nerves | 4.70 | 7 | 0.25 |
| Tumors of meninges | 2.90 | 9 | 0.15 |
| Lymphomas and hematopoietic neoplasms | 0.40 | 6 | 0.02 |
| Germ cell tumors | 3.70 | 9 | 0.19 |
| Tumors of the pituitary | 3.90 | 12 | 0.2 |
| Craniopharyngioma | 4.00 | 8 | 0.21 |
| Other/unclassified tumors | 4.90 | 9 | 0.26 |
| **TOTAL**[†] | **100.00** | **7** | **5.26** |

*Rates are per 100,000 and are age-adjusted to the 2000 US standard population.
[†]Refers to all brain tumors including histologies not presented in this table.
Average Annual Age-Adjusted Incidence Rates* for Brain and Central Nervous System Tumors (ages 0–14 years) by Major Histology Groupings, Histology, and Gender, CBTRUS Statistical Report: Alex's Lemonade Stand Foundation Infant and Childhood Primary Brain and Central Nervous System Tumors Diagnosed in the United States in 2007–2011 (http://www.cbtrus.org).

## Etiology

Although they are morphologically similar, integrated genomics have shown that medulloblastoma actually comprise four molecular variants, each with distinct signaling pathways that control brain development owing to different cells of origin (Hovestadt et al., 2019; Taylor et al., 2012; Vladoiu et al., 2019). These four molecular variants termed subgroups, are named WNT, SHH, Group 3 and Group 4 and have distinct demographics, genetics, and outcomes, and are now considered separate entities warranting dedicated approaches (Ramaswamy et al., 2016b). Approximately 10% of medulloblastoma patients have a germline predisposition, with highest incidence in children with SHH-activated medulloblastoma (Waszak et al., 2018).

The WNT tumors comprise 10%–15% of patients and are found most often in children and adults, occur equally in males and females, rarely metastasize, and are associated with an excellent prognosis (Kool et al., 2012; Ramaswamy et al., 2016b). They arise from the lower rhombic lip of the developing brainstem, and frequently invade the cerebellopontine angle (Gibson et al., 2010a; Perreault et al., 2014). The cytogenetic abnormality most commonly associated with this subgroup is monosomy of chromosome 6 and nearly all tumors have a somatic mutation the gene encoding beta-catenin *(CTNNB1)* (Cavalli et al., 2017; Northcott et al., 2017). These tumors almost always have nuclear immunohistochemical staining for beta-catenin, which signifies activation of the WNT pathway, although this marker should never be used in isolation due to the risk of false positives (Pietsch et al., 2014). Germline adenomatous polyposis coli *(APC)* mutations arise in 10% of WNT patients and are mutually exclusive from *CTNNB1* mutations. As such, all patients without a somatic mutation in *CTNNB1* require referral to a genetic counselor for germline testing for *APC* (Waszak et al., 2018). WNT tumors in patients under age 16 have an excellent prognosis across many studies, and currently several trials are ongoing evaluating de-escalation of radiotherapy (Ramaswamy et al., 2016b). The gold standard for diagnosis of a WNT-activated medulloblastoma is demonstration of an activating mutation in exon 3 of *CTNNB1*, with confirmation using a second method including immunohistochemistry, gene expression profiling, or DNA methylation profiling (Ramaswamy et al., 2016b).

Approximately 20%–25% of patients with medulloblastoma activation of the SHH pathway, where the majority have events such as mutations or amplifications, of which 20% are germline events (Cavalli et al., 2017; Northcott et al., 2017; Waszak et al., 2018). The SHH pathway is critically involved in the normal development of the cerebellum and SHH-activated medulloblastoma arise from the external granule layer of the cerebellum (Gibson et al., 2010b; Hovestadt et al., 2019; Vladoiu et al., 2019). Mutations in the SHH pathway can be either somatic or germline. The *PTCH* gene is the most commonly affected gene within this pathway, but mutations in other genes along this pathway including smoothened, fused, and suppressor of fused *(SUFU)* have also been identified (Northcott et al., 2017). Germline mutations in *PTCH* are associated with nevoid basal cell carcinoma syndrome, also known as *Gorlin syndrome*, and occur in 10%–15% of infants with SHH medulloblastoma with

**TABLE 75.2 Summary of the Common Genomic Alterations Across Pediatric Brain Tumors**

| Tumor Type | Molecular Subgroups | Main Genetic Alterations | Common Germline Predisposition |
|---|---|---|---|
| Medulloblastoma | WNT | SNV—*CTNNB1, TP53,* CNV—Monosomy 6 | Familial adenomatous polyposis |
| | SHH | SNV—*PTCH, SUFU, TP53, TERT, SMO* CNV—*GLI2, MYCN* | Gorlin syndrome, Li-Fraumeni syndrome |
| | Group 3 | CNV—*MYC* | |
| | Group 4 | CNV—*MYCN, CDK6,* SNV—*KDM6A* | |
| Embryonal tumors | ETMR | CNV—C19MC amplification, SNV - Dicer1 | |
| | Embryonal—NOS | CNV—FOXR2 fusions, MN1 rearrangements, BCOR alterations, CIC fusions | |
| ATRT | ATRT-MYC, ATRT-TYR, ATRT-SHH | *SMARCB1* deletions, mutation; SMARCA4 mutations | Rhabdoid predisposition syndrome |
| High-grade glioma | DIPG/DMG | Histone H3.1 and 3.3 K27M substitution (H3K27M) | |
| | Anaplastic astrocytoma/glioblastoma | SNV—Histone H3.1/3.3 G34V/R or K27M substitution, BRAF V600E, *IDH1*<br>CNV—*NTRK, ALK and MET* fusions<br>Hypermutation/mismatch repair deficiency | Constitutional mismatch repair deficiency (cMMRD), Li- Fraumeni syndrome |
| Low-grade glioma | Pilocytic astrocytoma | SNV—BRAF V600E<br>Germline—*NF1*<br>CNV—*KIAA1549-BRAF* fusion, FGFR-TACC fusions/duplication | Neurofibromatosis type 1 |
| | Diffuse astrocytoma | SNV—BRAFV600E, *FGFR1/2/3,* H3K27M, *IDH1*<br>CNV—*KIAA1549-BRAF, MYBL* fusions | |
| | Ganglioglioma/desmoplastic infantile astrocytoma | BRAF V600E mutations | |
| | Dysembryoplastic neuroepithelial tumor | *FGFR* mutations | |
| | Pleomorphic xanthoastrocytoma | SNV—BRAFV600E<br>CNV—*CDKN2A* deletion | |
| | Subependymal giant cell astrocytoma | *TSC1, TSC2* | Tuberous sclerosis |
| Ependymoma | PF-EPN-A | SNV—*EZHIP/CXorf67*<br>CNV—1q gain | |
| | PF-EPN-B | CNV—numerous arm level gains and losses | |
| | ST-EPN-RELA | Fusions of C11orf95-RelA, fusions on chromosome 11 | |
| | ST-EPN-YAP1 | Fusions of YAP1-MAMLD1 | |
| Craniopharyngioma | Adamantinomatous | *CTNNB1* mutations | |
| | Papillary | BRAF V600E | |

*ATRT,* Atypical/teratoid rhabdoid tumor; *CNV,* copy number variant; *CTNNB1,* beta-catenin; *DIPG/DMG,* diffuse intrinsic pontine glioma/diffuse midline glioma; *ETMR,* embryonal tumor with multilayered rosettes; *SNV,* somatic nucleotide variant.

an excellent prognosis (Garre et al., 2009; Waszak et al., 2018). This gene encodes for the protein that is the receptor of SHH. Gorlin syndrome is an autosomal dominant disorder characterized by the development of basal cell carcinomas, multiple bony cysts, and malignant tumors including medulloblastomas in young children. Germline *SUFU* mutations can result in a Gorlin-like syndrome and possibly portend a worse prognosis (Guerrini-Rousseau et al., 2018). SUFU is a suppressor of SHH signaling, downstream of PTCH and Smoothened. Older children (4–16 years) harbor germline mutations in the tumor suppressor *TP53* in 15%–20% of SHH-activated medulloblastomas, as part of the Li-Fraumeni syndrome (LFS). These patients have a very poor prognosis, and frequently have concurrent amplifications of *MYCN* and *GLI2*, with many somatic copy number changes observed, frequently harboring chromothripsis (chromosome shattering) (Rausch et al., 2012). All patients with SHH medulloblastoma should be referred to a geneticist for testing of germline (Ramaswamy et al., 2016b; Waszak et al., 2018).

SHH medulloblastoma are composed of four subtypes identified using integrated genomics, two observed in infants (SHHβ/SHH-I and SHHγ/SHH-II), one in the childhood age group (SHHα) and one adult group (SHHδ) (Cavalli et al., 2017). Infant SHH tumors are divided into two groups, whereby SHHβ/SHH-I have a frequent gain of chromosome 2p, *PTEN* loss, *SUFU* mutations, and a poor prognosis, whereas SHHγ/SHH-II have a blander genome and an excellent prognosis (Cavalli et al., 2017; Robinson et al., 2018). SHHα comprise the childhood age group, where *TP53* mutations (somatic or germline), *MYCN* amplification, *GLI2* amplification are common, and those with *TP53* mutations have a poor prognosis (Zhukova et al., 2013). SHHδ are primary adult-type medulloblastoma, and frequently harbor *TERT* promoter mutations and have an intermediate outcome (Kool et al., 2014; Remke et al., 2013) Nearly all desmoplastic, nodular medulloblastomas are found within the SHH subgroup, although only about 50% of SHH medulloblastomas have this histology, with the remaining tumors having either classic or large-cell anaplastic histology. Within adults, SHH comprise almost 70% of all medulloblastomas. Overall, metastasis at diagnosis is much less common in SHH tumors. At relapse SHH tumors recur in the surgical cavity in 50%–60% of cases (Ramaswamy et al., 2013; Zapotocky et al., 2018).

Group 3 tumors comprise approximately 25% of medulloblastoma and usually occur in children and infants, are rarely observed in adults, have a 3:1 male:female ratio, harbor classic or large-cell anaplastic histology, metastasize in up to 50%, and have a poor prognosis (Ramaswamy et al., 2016b). Postnatal cerebellar progenitor cells are candidate cells of origin for this subgroup (Hovestadt et al., 2019; Pei et al., 2012; Vladoiu et al., 2019). These tumors often have overexpression and amplification of the *MYC* oncogene, and activation of the *GFI* family of oncogenes (Northcott et al., 2014, 2017; Shih et al., 2014). Group 3 medulloblastomas recur almost exclusively with metastatic dissemination, particularly those children who are previously radiated (Ramaswamy et al., 2013). Germline predisposition is rare in Group 3; however, 1%–2% of patients have germline mutations in the Fanconi anemia/BRCA pathway, and should be suspected in those patients with significant treatment-related toxicity or suggestive family histories (Waszak et al., 2018).

Group 4 is the most common subgroup, and comprises 40%–45% of medulloblastomas in children aged between 4 and 16, and 10%–15% of adults (Taylor et al., 2012). There is a 3:1 male to female incidence, and between 30% and 35% of patients have metastasis at diagnosis. Group 4 medulloblastoma arises from the unipolar brush cells of the developing cerebellum, and transcriptionally have activation of glutaminergic pathways (Hovestadt et al., 2019; Vladoiu et al., 2019). Somatic nucleotide events in *KDM6A* have been observed to be a recurrent event in 10% of cases, with *MYCN* or *CDK6* amplifications observed in 15%–20% of cases. The most common cytogenetic aberration is isochromosome 17q, observed in almost 80%. Whole-chromosome loss of chromosome 11 or gain of chromosome 17 and 10p loss have been found to be associated with better survival within group 4 (Cavalli et al., 2017; Northcott et al., 2017; Shih et al., 2014). Additional heterogeneity has been observed within Groups 3 and 4, and the clinical relevance of this is currently being validated in prospective studies (Sharma et al., 2019). Group 4 medulloblastoma patients who have received radiotherapy recur almost exclusively with metastatic leptomeningeal dissemination, with the surgical cavity almost always devoid of tumor (Ramaswamy et al., 2013). In addition, late relapses are more frequently observed in Group 4, including after 5 years. Relapses in the surgical cavity in irradiated patients should prompt a suspicion for radiation-induced glioblastoma rather than medulloblastoma recurrence (Phi et al., 2018; Ramaswamy et al., 2013).

## Clinical Presentation

Many of the clinical manifestations of a medulloblastoma that arises in close proximity to the fourth ventricle are the result of increased intracranial pressure (ICP) due to obstructive hydrocephalus. Headache, vomiting, and ataxia are the most common initial symptoms and usually precede diagnosis by 2–8 weeks. Intractable nausea and vomiting occur frequently, characteristically in the morning. Personality changes, namely irritability, are an early feature, especially in infants, but may be difficult to recognize as a sign of a brain tumor. Other features that can lead to diagnosis include lethargy, diplopia, head tilt, and truncal ataxia. Interestingly, a longer time to diagnosis portends to an improved survival, which is related to a strong subgroup specificity (Ramaswamy et al., 2014).

Although contrast-enhanced magnetic resonance imaging (MRI) identifies leptomeningeal metastases in 20%–30% of children with medulloblastoma at the time of diagnosis, clinical manifestations are uncommon. Back pain and radicular pain indicate the rare complication of spinal dissemination. Less commonly, intratumoral hemorrhage may lead to acute onset of confusion, headache, and loss of consciousness. Among infants with posterior fossa tumors, diagnosis can be more challenging; thus, important features include changes in mood and personality as well as macrocephaly. Delay in achieving milestones or loss of previously achieved milestones and failure to thrive are characteristic.

## Diagnosis

A high level of clinical suspicion is critical to make an early diagnosis. Neuroimaging is usually the first step, with computed tomography (CT) scan of the brain frequently obtained in the acute setting. Contrast-enhanced cranial MRI provides definitive imaging of the tumor. Certain MRI features may help distinguish the various types of posterior fossa tumors (medulloblastoma, ependymoma, and PA) of childhood. Although no single radiological feature is pathognomonic of a medulloblastoma, certain common characteristics exist. On CT, a medulloblastoma is generally hyperdense and homogeneously enhancing, filling the fourth ventricle (Fig. 75.1, *A*). On contrast-enhanced cranial MRI, medulloblastomas are often isointense or hypointense to surrounding normal brain on T1-weighted images, with diffusion restriction observed in almost all tumors as a result of uniform hypercellularity (see Fig. 75.1, *B*). On T2-weighted images, medulloblastoma can appear to be hyperintense or more frequently can display mixed signal characteristics indicative of small intratumoral cysts, calcification, or small areas of hemorrhage (see Fig. 75.1, *C*). Because medulloblastoma typically arises in the roof of the fourth ventricle, a cleft of cerebrospinal fluid (CSF) beneath the tumor in the fourth ventricular canal helps distinguish this tumor from an ependymoma, which typically arises from the floor of the fourth ventricle. Ependymomas can fill the fourth ventricle and calcify more frequently than medulloblastomas. In addition, ependymomas often contain cysts, making their overall image appearance more heterogeneous. Because these tumors typically arise near the obex, ependymomas frequently extend out from the foramen of Magendie over the dorsal surface of the cervical spinal cord or through the foramen of Luschka. PAs typically arise in the cerebellar hemispheres and have the appearance of a cystic mass with an enhancing mural nodule. On T2-weighted MRI, these tumors often appear as areas of homogenous high signal intensity, with the fluid collections defining the less intense tissue components of the tumor (see Fig. 75.1, *D*). The four principal medulloblastoma subgroups have distinct imaging features, where SHH are almost always in the cerebellum, and Group 3 and 4 tumors occupy the fourth ventricle. Additionally, Group 4 tumors frequently do not enhance upon gadolinium administration, including non-enhancing metastasis. WNT tumors invade the lateral recess in 40%–50% of cases. Group 3 tumors avidly enhance upon gadolinium administration, and metastatic Group 3 tumors frequently have very small primaries. Thick bulky diffuse leptomeningeal metastasis is most commonly observed in Group 3 tumors (Zapotocky et al., 2018).

## Management

The first step in management after stabilization of the patient is surgery, which serves to decompress the posterior fossa and provide tissue for diagnostic purposes. In children in whom the diagnosis of medulloblastoma is suspected, a contrast-enhanced spinal MRI also should be obtained prior to surgery to assist in neurosurgical planning and staging. After imaging diagnosis, corticosteroids are frequently used to control increased ICP. If the child has unstable mental status or vital signs, emergency external ventricular drainage may be required before surgery. The goals of surgery are to control ICP, achieve a maximal safe surgical resection, establish a molecular diagnosis, and bank frozen tumor for molecular analysis prior to protocol therapy. Placement of a ventriculoperitoneal (VP)

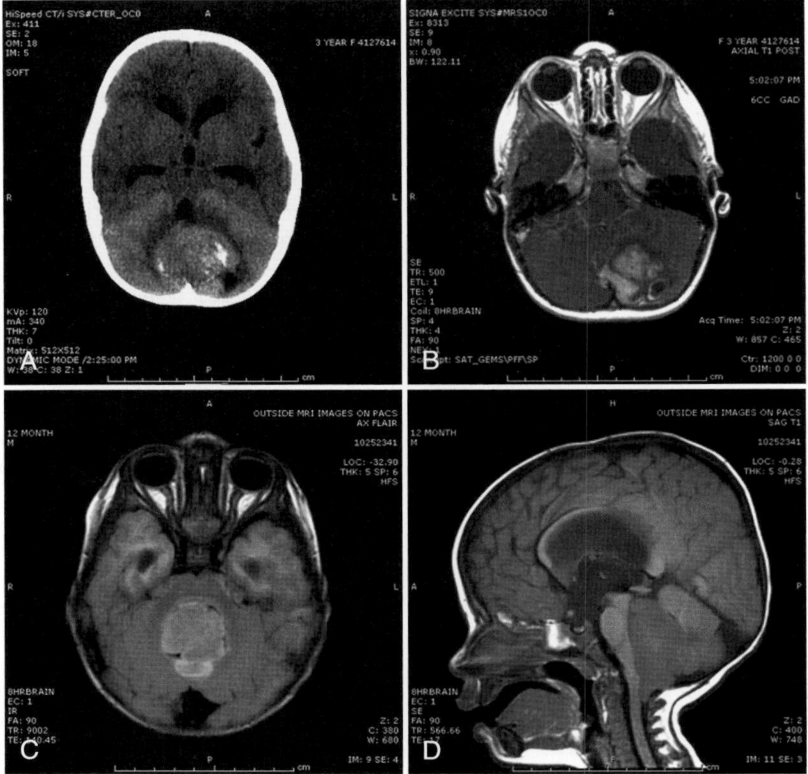


**Fig. 75.1** **A,** A 3-year-old girl presented with 3 weeks of worsening headaches that awakened her at night. A contrast-enhanced cranial computed tomography (CT) scan shows a large dense mass within the posterior fossa, containing internal calcifications. Surrounding edema can be seen. Compression of the quadrigeminal plate cistern and fourth ventricle led to obstructive hydrocephalus. **B,** Axial T1 postcontrast magnetic resonance image (MRI) of the same patient, showing heterogeneous enhancement of the lesion. MR spectroscopy showed a markedly depressed N-acetylaspartate (NAA) peak, with elevation of the choline peak consistent with high-grade tumor. Diffusion-weighted imaging showed restricted diffusion indicative of a highly cellular lesion. Resection of the mass showed it to be a medulloblastoma. **C,** A 13-month-old child presented with unsteady gait and vomiting over several days. MRI showed a large nonenhancing posterior fossa mass filling the fourth ventricle. Resection showed tumor consistent with ependymoma. Axial T2 fluid-attenuated inversion recovery (FLAIR) image shows T2 prolongation. **D,** Sagittal T1 image showing the ependymoma filling the fourth ventricle. The lesion extends out of the foramen of Magendie over the dorsal surface of the cervical spinal cord.

shunt before surgery is no longer commonly practiced but may be necessary after surgery. A lumbar puncture for CSF cytological evaluation should be performed 14–21 days after surgical resection to avoid false positivity. Potential complications of posterior fossa surgery include cerebellar mutism and aseptic meningitis. The posterior fossa syndrome (PFS), or cerebellar mutism, may occur in as many as 40% of children undergoing posterior fossa surgery (Gudrunardottir et al., 2016). The characteristics include reduced speech output or mutism, personality changes, hypotonia, ataxia, and reduced oral intake. Symptoms typically appear 1–2 days after surgery and may last for a few months, with varying degrees of recovery (Gudrunardottir et al., 2016).

Risk stratification is currently based on clinical staging and certain neuropathological features, although molecular observations are being incorporated into the next generation of clinical trials. Clinical staging follows the completion of perioperative brain and spine MRI and lumbar CSF cytological analysis. The M (metastasis) staging criteria include: M0, no metastases; M1, positive CSF cytology alone; M2, intracranial metastases; M3, spinal metastases; and M4, systemic metastases. The major determinants of clinical risk categorization are age at diagnosis, metastasis (M stage), primary tumor site, and volume of residual postoperative disease.

Patients are currently stratified into either standard-risk or high-risk prognostic groups. Standard-risk patients are those with medulloblastoma who are older than age 3–5 years at diagnosis, have residual tumor volume of less than 1.5 $cm^2$, have no evidence of metastasis (M0), and do not have anaplastic medulloblastoma. Children younger than age 3–5 are always at higher risk because they are frequently treated with radiation-sparing approaches, where the goal of therapy is delay and/or reduction of radiotherapy. In addition, patients with residual tumor volume greater than 1.5 $cm^2$, any metastatic disease, or large-cell/anaplastic medulloblastoma are at higher risk for recurrence. More recently, a molecular risk stratification is emerging which is helping to guide therapy, specifically, the division of patients into low, standard risk, high risk and very high risk. WNT patients under age 16 comprise low-risk patients. Metastatic and/or MYC amplified Group 3 and *TP53* mutant SHH-activated medulloblastoma comprise very-high risk patients, with survivals under 40% (Ramaswamy et al., 2016b).

Treatment of medulloblastoma is dependent on age, where infants are treated with radiation-sparing approaches, frequently at the expense of survival, due to the devastating side effects of craniospinal irradiation to the very young brain. The definition of "infant" is variable and depends on the cooperative group; historically, infants were defined as under 3 years old in North America, under 4 years old in International Society of Paediatric Oncology (SIOP) trials, and under 5 years old in France. Treatment of non-infants usually consists of surgery, radiation therapy, and chemotherapy. Maximal safe surgical resection is recommended for all patients, particularly those with non-metastatic disease, with the residual tumor being less than 1.5 cm$^2$. The current recommended therapy for standard-risk patients includes craniospinal irradiation (23.4 Gy) with a boost to the tumor bed to 55.8 Gy. Vincristine is commonly administered weekly with radiation therapy. Following radiation therapy, 4–8 cycles of cisplatin-based chemotherapy are administered, with either cisplatin, lomustine, and vincristine; or cisplatin, cyclophosphamide, and vincristine—both with similar survival. Those with metastatic dissemination or residual disease over 1.5 cm$^2$ are treated with 36–39 Gy of craniospinal irradiation with a boost to the tumor bed to 55.8 Gy, followed by 4–8 cycles of cisplatin, cyclophosphamide, and vincristine-based chemotherapy. In some cooperative groups, those with anaplastic and/or large-cell histology are treated on high-risk protocols; however, it is unclear if there is any benefit to this, particularly in WNT and Group 4 tumors. WNT patients are the subject of reductions in therapy, with the Children's Oncology Group (ACNS1422) and the European Society of Pediatric Oncology (PNET5) evaluating reductions to 18 Gy of craniospinal irradiation and the St. Jude group (SJMB12) evaluating reductions to 15 Gy for standard-risk patients. In Europe, the PNET5 trial allows WNT patients with metastatic disease or residual tumor to be treated with 23.4 Gy of craniospinal irradiation.

In addition to developing effective chemotherapy regimens with less toxicity, several groups are trying to decrease the toxicity associated with radiation therapy. The use of proton-beam radiation therapy as an alternative to high-energy x-rays (photons) has been studied and found to have the potential to limit late effects of radiation therapy by reducing the exposure of normal tissue to radiation (Durante et al., 2017). Proton radiation can spare adjacent critical structures such as the optic apparatus, cochlea, and hypothalamus as well as limit exposure to the trunk when they are not adjacent to tumor volume, potentially resulting in fewer long-term sequelae (Yock et al., 2016).

Infants are treated with radiation-sparing approaches post-surgery, where the treatment is highly dependent on both molecular subgroup and/or histology. In Europe the approach is to administer intraventricular methotrexate with induction chemotherapy, and in North America infants are treated with induction chemotherapy followed by 1–3 cycles of myeloablative chemotherapy with autologous stem cell transplant (Cohen et al., 2015; Lafay-Cousin et al., 2016; Rutkowski et al., 2005). Using this approach, patients with SHH medulloblastoma (or desmoplastic medulloblastoma) have excellent radiation-free survival of nearly 90%. Efforts to reduce therapy through omission of myeloablative chemotherapy or intraventricular methotrexate have resulted in dismal results for SHH medulloblastoma (Robinson et al., 2018). Group 3 infants have a poor prognosis without radiation, particularly those with metastatic disease and likely warrant new approaches. The role of focal radiation is not clear, and is likely of little to no benefit in Group 3 or 4 infants considering the metastatic pattern of relapse.

### Prognosis

Standard-risk medulloblastoma patients have a 5-year survival of approximately 80%; 5-year survival in high-risk medulloblastoma patients is approximately 50%–60% (Gajjar et al., 2006; Gandola et al., 2008; Jakacki et al., 2012; Lannering et al., 2012; Packer et al., 2006). Infants with SHH/desmoplastic histology can have radiation-free survival of close to 90% with intensive therapy, whereas Group 3 and 4 infants have dismal radiation-free survivals of less than 40% for non-metastatic disease, and less than 10% for metastatic disease (Lafay-Cousin et al., 2016; Pietsch et al., 2014; Robinson et al., 2018). The presence of CNS dissemination is the single most important factor that correlates with outcome, independent of subgroup (Jakacki et al., 2012; Ramaswamy et al., 2016b). Relapsed medulloblastoma in previously irradiated patients is associated with dismal survival rates of less than 10%, and although some approaches can provide extension of survival with good quality of life, these are essentially palliative (Pizer et al., 2011; Ramaswamy et al., 2013). Lifelong serial surveillance imaging is recommended in anticipation of radiation-induced secondary malignancies such as meningioma or high-grade glioma (Packer et al., 2013). Radiation therapy, particularly in young children, can also cause significant adverse late effects in cognitive development, growth, and endocrine function (Mulhern, 2005; Mulhern et al., 2004).

## Central Nervous System Embryonal Tumor and Embryonal Tumor with Multilayered Rosettes

Embryonal CNS tumors are the most common group of malignant brain tumors in children and include medulloblastomas, CNS embryonal tumors, embryonal tumor with multilayered rosettes (ETMR), and atypical teratoid/rhabdoid tumors (ATRT). There have been several changes to the categorization of embryonal tumors in the 2016 revised WHO classification of CNS tumors (Louis et al., 2016). A significant change from the 2007 WHO classification is the removal of the diagnosis 'CNS primitive neuroectodermal tumor (CNS-PNET)' and the inclusion of ETMR. CNS embryonal tumors are a diagnosis of exclusion, and morphologically are frequently mistaken for other supratentorial tumors, particularly high-grade gliomas. ATRT, ETMR, ependymoma, CNS sarcoma, and choroid plexus carcinoma must also be excluded. The remaining tumors formerly included in the diagnosis of CNS-PNET now comprise CNS neuroblastoma, CNS ganglioneuroblastoma, medulloepithelioma and CNS embryonal tumor not otherwise specified (NOS). Applying DNA methylation classification and unsupervised clustering, the majority of entities previously labeled CNS-PNET are reclassified as other entities. However, within the proportion of CNS embryonal tumors that do not reclassify, recurrent fusions and duplications of *FOXR2*, *BCOR*, *MN1*, and *CIC1* have been identified representing new brain tumor entities (Capper et al., 2018; Sturm et al., 2016). ETMR are divided into tumors harboring an amplicon at a microRNA (miRNA) cluster on chromosome 19, or with the morphological diagnosis without the amplicon. Pineoblastomas are embryonal tumors arising from the pineal gland, and frequently harbor recurrent homozygous deletion of DROSHA, the core nuclease that initiates miRNA processing in the nucleus (Snuderl et al., Nat Commun. 2018).

### Etiology

There is limited understanding of the etiology of CNS embryonal tumors, which have emerged as a highly heterogeneous group. A unifying molecular signature, including amplification of the C19MC oncogenic miRNA cluster and high LIN28 expression, has been found that encompasses several CNS embryonal tumor histological classes, including ETMR, medulloepithelioma, and CNS embryonal tumor NOS (Kleinman et al., 2014; Korshunov et al., 2014; Spence et al., 2014). These tumors have a very poor prognosis and tend to occur in children younger than 4 years old. Other markers for CNS embryonal tumors have not yet been defined, making further histopathological classification difficult. A major confounding issue to understanding the incidence and presentation of CNS embryonal tumors is that a significant proportion of these tumors are glioblastomas, resulting in difficulties in interpreting previous studies (Hwang et al., 2018).

Trilateral retinoblastoma is a well-recognized syndrome characterized by bilateral retinoblastomas occurring concurrently with a pineoblastoma with retinoblastic features. Although approximately half of the cases of trilateral retinoblastoma are associated with the familial form of retinoblastoma, one analysis indicates that most children with trilateral retinoblastoma have ordinary hereditary retinoblastoma that is complicated by trilateral disease by chance, thus dispelling the notion that trilateral retinoblastoma is caused by a different allele than that which causes ordinary retinoblastoma (de Jong et al., 2014).

Although earlier reports of supratentorial PNET have occurred in patients with the LFS (mutations in the *TP53* gene on chromosome 17), it is likely that these tumors represent misdiagnosed high-grade gliomas or glioblastomas, and molecularly defined cohorts are required to help elucidate this. Tumors previously described as PNET that are not reclassified as another entity after extensive molecular work-up, fall into one of four entities: CNS neuroblastoma with FOXR2 activation; CNS Ewing sarcoma family tumor with Capiciua transcriptional repressor (CIC) alteration; CNS high-grade neuroepithelial tumor with MN1 alteration; and CNS high-grade neuroepithelial tumor with Bcl6 co-repressor (BCOR) alteration. These entities require either DNA methylation analysis and/or RNA sequencing for diagnosis, and are the subject of ongoing studies (Capper et al., 2018; Sturm et al., 2016). The clinical implications and precise diagnosis of these groups is still emerging, and rendered challenging due to their rarity.

### Clinical Presentation

Similar to medulloblastoma, the presenting features of all CNS embryonal tumors are highly dependent on their location, including progressive headache, nausea, vomiting, seizures, and lethargy secondary to increased ICP. Children with pineoblastomas often present with dorsal midbrain compression (Parinaud syndrome) and obstructive hydrocephalus secondary to aqueductal occlusion.

### Treatment

CNS embryonal tumors, ETMR, and pineoblastomas have historically been stages and treated according to medulloblastoma protocols. Prognosis for tumors previously classified as supratentorial PNETs has been highly variable. ETMR usually arise in young infants, and carry a very poor prognosis, with survival less than 20%, despite aggressive therapies with upfront radiotherapy and high-dose chemotherapy with autologous stem cell transplant. The prognosis of CNS embryonal tumors and pineoblastoma are variable across studies. However, those with metastatic disease have much inferior survival compared with those with nonmetastatic disease, as do infants treated with radiation- sparing approaches. Future molecularly informed clinical trials are required to adequately determine optimal therapies for this heterogeneous group of patients.

## Atypical Teratoid/Rhabdoid Tumor

ATRT is a highly malignant tumor that was first recognized in the 1980s as a distinct entity (Biegel et al., 1989; Pomeroy et al., 2002). Rhabdoid tumors may arise anywhere in the body, but are most common in the kidney where they are referred to as malignant rhabdoid tumors and in the CNS where they are classified as ATRT. ATRTs can occur anywhere in the nervous system, and occur primarily supratentorially or in the posterior fossa, either in isolation or in association with germline predisposition, in other parts of the body such as the kidneys, or even with metachronous primary tumors. ATRT are defined by the loss of INI-1/BAF47, the protein encoded by the *SMARCB1* gene located on chromosome 22q, and is a germline event as part of the rhabdoid predisposition syndrome in 25%–35% of all cases.

Integrated genomic studies have revealed significant heterogeneity across ATRT, with at least three epigenetically defined subgroups. These groups—termed ATRT-SHH, ATRT-MYC, and ATRT-TYR—have distinct gene expression and DNA methylation patterns, distinct demographics, and genetics. The ATRT-SHH group is predominantly infratentorial with broad *SMARCB1* mutations, ATRT-TYR are composed of both infratentorial and supratentorial tumors with focal lesions in *SMARCB1*, and ATRT-MYC are composed of predominantly supratentorial tumors in older children (Johann et al., 2016; Torchia et al., 2016). The prognostic and therapeutic implications of these groups are currently unclear.

### Clinical Presentation

ATRTs are seen primarily in infants and young children, with a peak incidence between birth and age 3. ATRTs account for approximately 1%–2% of all childhood brain tumors, but these neoplasms represent nearly 10% of CNS tumors in infants (Ostrom et al., 2015). Children with ATRT often present with signs and symptoms consistent with the location of the primary tumor, similar to those with medulloblastoma or CNS embryonal tumor, including vomiting, loss of milestones, irritability, and increasing head circumference.

### Diagnosis

Owing to similar morphology, these tumors may be confused with medulloblastomas, CNS embryonal tumors, and choroid plexus carcinomas, and as such need to be considered in any young child presenting with a small-blue-cell tumor. The definitive diagnosis of ATRT is based on loss of immunoreactivity to INI1 and/or identification of a genetic lesion in the *SMARCB1* gene, which is present in almost all cases. There is a small, relatively poorly defined subset of molecularly defined ATRT lacking lesions in *SMARCB1*, but rather having inherited mutations in *SMARCA4*, with a poor prognosis (Hasselblatt et al., 2014). All patients diagnosed with ATRT should be referred to a geneticist for germline screening and counseling, and a surveillance protocol should be considered after completion of therapy (Foulkes et al., 2017).

### Management and Prognosis

Historically, ATRT have been treated as medulloblastoma with very poor survival, with the POG-9923/4 and CCG-9921 studies of conventional chemotherapy resulting in less than 10% survival. More recently, rhabdoid-specific multimodal therapy has been applied, with more favorable results, and the emergence of long-term survivors in upwards of 50% of patients. These treatments have included various combinations of aggressive surgery with complete resections and intensive chemotherapy, with and without irradiation, resulting in survivals of between 40% and 50% overall (Chi et al., 2009; Gardner et al., 2008; Lafay-Cousin et al., 2012; Seeringer et al., 2014). The Children's Oncology Group has recently completed a trial using multidrug chemotherapy with high-dose methotrexate, high-dose chemotherapy with autologous stem cell rescue, and radiation therapy, with promising results (Reddy et al., 2020). Germline predisposition is felt to have a worse survival; however, this is also unclear at the present time.

# ASTROCYTIC TUMORS

The spectrum of astrocytic tumors is broad and includes a wide range of glial neoplasms that differ in anatomical location, morphological features, degree of invasiveness, and clinical course. Grading of astrocytomas by the WHO is predictive of patient survival (Louis et al., 2016) (Box 75.1). Astrocytomas can be classified as low grade (WHO grade I and II) or high grade (WHO grade III and IV). Analogous to adult gliomas, the advent of molecular diagnostics has brought into question of the utility of WHO grading in isolation. However, currently, treatment protocols and clinical trials still rely on the distinction between low-grade and high-grade glioma. A crucial distinction between adult and pediatric low-grade gliomas are that pediatric low-grade gliomas rarely transform to higher-grade tumors, and in many instances eventually senesce, with the exception of a subset of *BRAF* mutant tumors harboring *CDKN2A* loss, and as such the approach and treatment should be commensurate with its natural history (Krishnatry et al., 2016; Mistry et al., 2015). The most

**BOX 75.1 WHO Classification and Grading of Low-Grade and High-Grade Glial and/or Neuronal Tumors**

| Astrocytic Tumors | Oligodendroglial and Oligoastrocytic Tumors | Neuronal and Mixed Neuronal-Glial Tumors |
|---|---|---|
| Pilocytic astrocytoma (I) | Oligodendroglioma (II) | Gangliocytoma (I) |
| Subependymal giant cell astrocytoma (II) | Anaplastic oligodendroglioma (III) | Ganglioglioma (I) |
| Pilomyxoid astrocytoma (II) | | Anaplastic ganglioglioma (III) |
| Diffuse astrocytoma (II) | | Desmoplastic infantile astrocytoma and ganglioglioma (I) |
| Pleomorphic xanthoastrocytoma (II) | | Dysembryoplastic neuroepithelial tumor (I) |
| Anaplastic astrocytoma (III) | | Central neurocytoma (II) |
| Glioblastoma (IV) | | |

*Adapted from Louis, D.N. Ohgaki, H. Wiestler, O.D., et al. (Eds.), 2016. WHO Classification of Tumors of the Central Nervous System, fourth ed. International Agency for Research on Cancer, Lyon, France.*

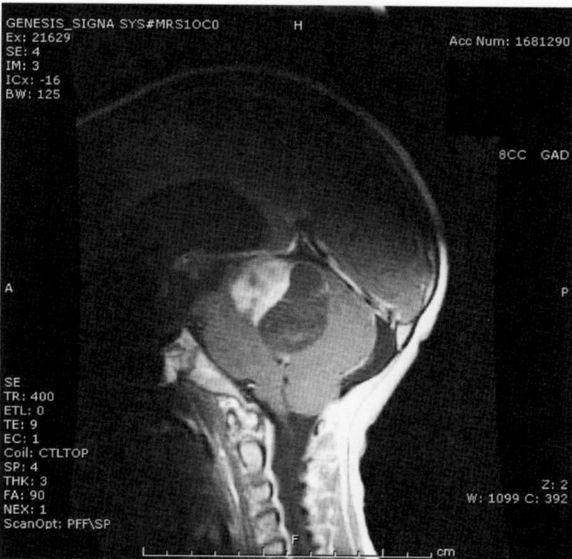


**Fig. 75.2** A 9-year-old boy who presented with a short history of headache and nausea. Contrast-enhanced cranial magnetic resonance imaging was obtained because of the severity of his headaches, which demonstrated an enhancing tumor with a solid portion in the anterior aspect of the posterior fossa, adjacent to the dorsal midbrain. A large cyst can be seen posterior to the solid mass. Resection revealed a pilocytic astrocytoma.

common pediatric subtypes recognized by the current WHO classification will be discussed.

## Pilocytic Astrocytoma

PAs are well-circumscribed, slow-growing tumors classified as WHO grade I (Louis et al., 2016). These tumors are the most common gliomas found in children and represent approximately 20% of all childhood brain tumors. PAs are typically diagnosed in the first two decades, with no clear gender predilection. Neurofibromatosis type 1 (NF1) is associated with an increased risk of PA (Evans et al., 2017). No other definite predisposing factors are known. Histologically, PAs consist of bipolar cells with long "fiber-like" processes: hence the name pilocytic. Other distinctive histological features of PAs include Rosenthal fibers, eosinophilic granular bodies, and microcysts. Constitutive activation of the mitogen-activated protein kinase (MAPK) signaling pathway through specific, recurrent gene fusions of BRAF and less commonly activating mutations (V600E) are by far the most common somatic events identified in PAs, as well as other pediatric low-grade astrocytomas (LGAs) (Jones et al., 2013; Pfister et al., 2008; Schindler et al., 2011; Zhang et al., 2013). This provides an opportunity for the development of molecular targeted therapies.

### Clinical Presentation

PAs can arise anywhere in the CNS, but most commonly occur in the cerebellum, optic pathways, hypothalamus, cerebral hemispheres, midbrain, and medulla. PAs of the spinal cord are less common. The spectrum of clinical manifestations depends on the structures involved and may include visual deficits, obstructive hydrocephalus, macrocephaly in younger patients, ataxia, endocrine dysfunction, focal neurological deficits, long-tract signs, cranial nerve dysfunction, and seizures if the tumor involves cortical structures. Cerebellar PAs usually present with symptoms indicative of increased ICP, such as headache, nausea, and vomiting. Brainstem PAs are usually dorsal and exophytic with obstructive hydrocephalus often the presenting feature. The diencephalic syndrome is unique to low-grade gliomas, usually juvenile PAs arising in infants in the hypothalamus or optic pathways, and consists of emaciation with normal linear growth, frequently accompanied by hyperemesis, hyperkinesis, and nystagmus (Fleischman et al., 2005; Kilday et al., 2014; Smith et al., 1965). Indeed, a hypothalamic glioma should be considered in young children presenting with failure to thrive without another apparent etiology.

### Diagnosis

A tissue diagnosis should be attempted in all children presenting with a suspected low-grade glioma and no clinical signs of neurofibromatosis type 1. The emergence of molecular diagnostics is significantly changing the diagnosis of low-grade gliomas, specifically the PA. Treatment and risk stratification now require the identification of specific alterations in BRAF, either tandem duplications with a fusion to KIAA1549, or, less frequently, point mutations at the V600E position. The history of illness is usually long; other signs of chronicity—such as bone remodeling, scoliosis, or hemihypotrophy—may be present, depending on the primary tumor location. The typical MRI appearance is a homogeneously enhancing mass with only minimal associated edema. Intratumoral cysts are common, depending on location—particularly in the cerebellum, where the typical appearance is one of a large cyst with mural nodule (Fig. 75.2). In approximately 5% of patients, PAs present with diffuse leptomeningeal dissemination, especially in infants and as such a baseline spinal MRI should be performed prior to initiation of therapy or surveillance (von Hornstein et al., 2011).

### Management

The mainstay of therapy for PAs is surgery. If feasible, gross total resection is "curative" even though residual microscopic disease always remains, and radiation or chemotherapy are typically not required. In situations where resection is not possible, tissue biopsy should be attempted to allow for an accurate molecular and histopathological diagnosis prior to initiation of therapy. Partial resections have little role in the treatment of PAs, with the exception of a symptomatic patient. Progressive or unresectable PAs, or those arising in infants or young children causing visual symptoms, may require adjuvant treatment.

Chemotherapy has an important role in the management of all progressive low-grade gliomas. The three most commonly used regimens are carboplatin/vincristine, TPCV (thioguanine, procarbazine, lomustine, and vincristine), and single-agent vinblastine monotherapy (Ater et al., 2012; Lassaletta et al., 2016b). Carboplatin/vincristine and TPCV regimens were compared in a randomized phase III trial by the Children's Oncology Group, and although TPCV was found to be moderately superior in regard to event-free survival, carboplatin/vincristine or vinblastine is considered the primary first-line therapy due to the poor safety profile of TPCV and increased risk of secondary malignancy (Ater et al., 2012). Historically, a substantial proportion of patients require multiple courses of chemotherapy, but eventually most low-grade gliomas stop progressing. The emergence of targeted agents in the form of MEK and/or BRAF inhibitors have emerged as powerful second-line options: specifically, BRAF/MEK inhibitors for BRAF V600E mutant tumors and MEK inhibition for BRAF fused tumors (Fangusaro et al., 2019; Jones et al., 2018). These agents have shown very impressive responses in early-phase clinical trials and randomized studies versus chemotherapy are currently ongoing through the Children's Oncology Group and the European Society of Pediatric Oncology. Because of concern for adverse effects, including neurocognitive and endocrine effects as well as secondary malignancies, early stroke, and the moyamoya syndrome, radiation therapy is usually deferred or omitted in children with low-grade gliomas, including those with multiple relapses (Krishnatry et al., 2016; Morris et al., 2009a; Mulhern et al., 2004). Radiation is a relative contraindication in children with NF-1 due to the very high risk of secondary high-grade gliomas and vasculopathies.

### Prognosis

The prognosis for resectable tumors is excellent, with 5-year recurrence-free survival of greater than 90% after gross total resection (Shaw and Wisoff, 2003). The most critical variable in the treatment of PAs is the anatomical location of the tumor. Complete resections are most difficult for tumors located in the brainstem, spinal cord, and hypothalamus. As such, the progression-free survival of children with centrally located tumors (e.g., optic chiasm, thalamus, hypothalamus) is reduced. The use of chemotherapy as initial treatment in patients with centrally located or unresectable tumors allows for the sparing or delay of radiation therapy until the child is less likely to suffer major developmental and neuropsychological sequelae. Ultimately, the quality of survival depends on multiple factors including tumor location, extent of tumor resection, timing of any radiation therapy, and side effects of surgery, chemotherapy, and radiation. Malignant transformation of PA and other LGAs in children is rare (Mistry et al., 2015). Targeted inhibitors v-Raf murine sarcoma viral oncogene homolog B (BRAF) and Mitogen-activated protein kinase kinase (MEK) now provide an option with a significant likelihood of tumor size reduction; however, the impact of these agents on long-term outcome and functional status is unknown.

## Optic Pathway Glioma

Optic pathway gliomas (OPGs) may be considered a subset of PAs, but their unique features and management requirements warrant a separate discussion. OPGs represent approximately 4%–6% of all primary pediatric brain tumors. These tumors may involve various parts of the optic pathway, such as the optic nerves, optic chiasm, optic tract, and optic radiations. The tumor may also infiltrate the adjacent hypothalamus and temporal lobes. Optic nerve gliomas are strongly associated with NF1, and NF1 patients represent about 50% of patients treated for OPG. Although approximately 20% of NF1 children scanned prospectively from birth will acquire MRI abnormalities suggestive of an anterior or posterior OPG, less than half of those will develop progressive neurological and radiological disease, and the occasional tumor may undergo spontaneous regression (Parsa et al., 2001). OPGs in NF1 patients have been suggested to have a more indolent course than those arising in patients without NF1 with improved progression-free survival compared with non-NF1 patients (Ater et al., 2012, 2016). Non-NF1 OPGs frequently harbor either *BRAF* fusions or *BRAF* mutations, similar to other low-grade gliomas of childhood (Lassaletta et al., 2017).

### Clinical Presentation

Most OPGs are LGAs, primarily PAs (WHO grade I) (Cummings et al., 2000). Although most OPGs are of lower histological grade, the clinical course of these tumors may be aggressive when the optic pathways and hypothalamus are invaded. Age is an important prognostic factor: children younger than 5 years of age experience a more aggressive course. Unilateral optic nerve gliomas present with the classic triad of vision loss, proptosis, and optic atrophy. Chiasmatic involvement may lead to unilateral or bilateral vision loss, optic tract involvement may lead to a visual-field deficit, and large dorsally exophytic or hypothalamic components of the tumor may lead to obstructive hydrocephalus. Further invasion into brain parenchyma may result in visual-field defects and hemiparesis. The diencephalic syndrome is unique to infant presentations of OPG and hypothalamic PA and presents with irritability, failure to thrive, nystagmus, visual loss, and hydrocephalus in the first or second year of life (Fleischman et al., 2005).

### Diagnosis and Management

The clinical diagnosis of an OPG should be suspected when a child presents with visual impairment associated with nystagmus and optic atrophy. It is very difficult to ascertain visual loss in younger children, but close behavioral observation during play may raise suspicion. Contrast-enhanced cranial or orbital MRI typically shows a solid, cystic, or solid and cystic tumor with enhancement (Fig. 75.3). MRI studies and clinical presentation may distinguish an OPG from other childhood tumors that arise in the suprasellar location, such as a germ cell tumor or craniopharyngioma. The unpredictable clinical course of patients with OPGs has led to controversy regarding the optimal management of these tumors. The clinical course, age of onset, severity of symptoms, size and extent of the tumor, and the presence of NF1 may all impact management decisions. Preservation of vision is paramount and the major indication for treatment, and although chemotherapy may cause stabilization or regression of the tumor on imaging studies the correlation with visual outcome is poor (Fisher et al., 2012; Silva et al., 2000). The emergence of targeted agents, specifically MEK and BRAF inhibitors, has the potential to significantly improve visual outcomes even in young children; however, the timing of their use is still not clear (Fangusaro et al., 2019; Lassaletta et al., 2016a). The chemotherapy regiments used for PA are also used for the treatment of OPG, most commonly carboplatin/vincristine and vinblastine monotherapy. Bevacizumab has shown the potential to significantly improve vision and can be considered in patients with progressive visual loss (Avery et al., 2014).

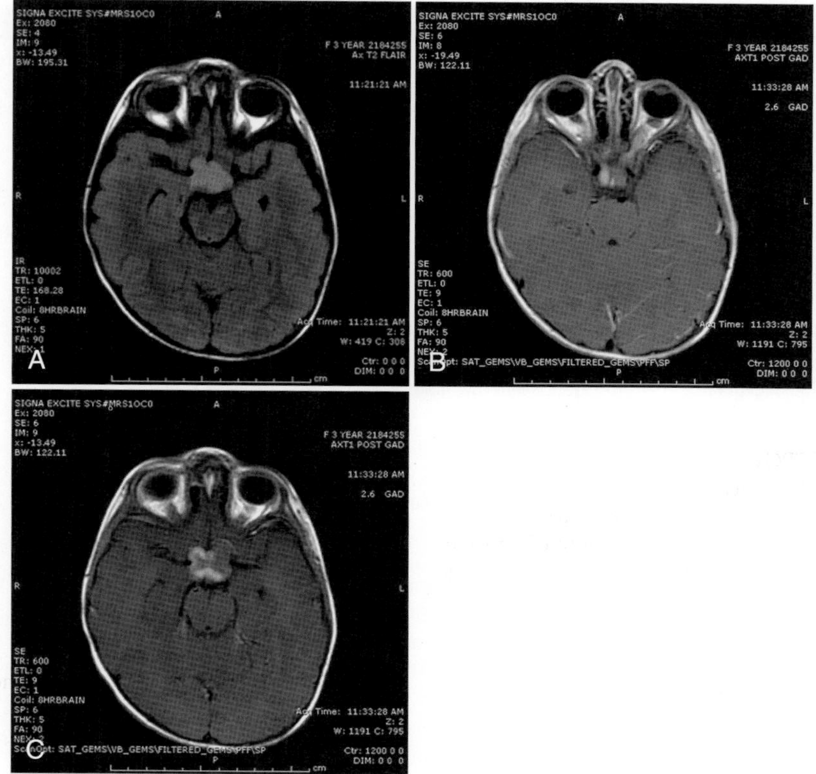


**Fig. 75.3** A 3½-year-old girl with a history of neurofibromatosis type 1 (NF1) who was seen after an ophthalmological evaluation revealed a left eye deviation and visual-field loss. **A,** Magnetic resonance imaging (MRI) reveals T2 prolongation in the optic chiasm. **B,** There is significant enlargement of the left optic nerve. **C,** Coronal T1 postgadolinium imaging shows the lesion to be contrast enhancing. The combined findings were highly suggestive of an optic pathway glioma.

### Prognosis

Although OPGs are histologically low-grade tumors, the location of these neoplasms often results in serious morbidity. The growth rate of OPGs often slows in older children and young adults. The most robust adverse prognostic factor across multiple studies has been age younger than 1 year at diagnosis, although some suggest that children with NF1 may have a longer progression-free survival (Opocher et al., 2006). Patients with OPGs associated with NF1 may remain stable for several years, and the indication for treatment is visual loss. Close observation and symptomatic management are appropriate for this subpopulation.

## Subependymal Giant Cell Astrocytoma

Subependymal giant cell astrocytomas (SEGAs) usually originate in the ependymal lining of the lateral ventricles and are associated almost exclusively with tuberous sclerosis (TS). Sporadic SEGAs are rare. TS is an autosomal dominant genetic syndrome caused by mutations in either *TSC1* (hamartin) or *TSC2* (tuberin), which are regulators of key cellular signaling pathways including the mammalian target of rapamycin (mTOR) pathway (Jozwiak et al., 2008).

### Clinical Presentation

Subependymal giant cell astrocytoma is sometimes the presenting feature of TS in patients without the typical physical stigmata of the syndrome. Although patients with TS typically have multiple periventricular SEGAs, the tumors that produce symptoms of hydrocephalus arise in close proximity to the foramina of Munro. Most patients with known TS have been followed with serial MRI scans, and newly identified SEGAs are typically removed in anticipation of more serious neurological syndromes such as headaches, altered sensorium, or weakness. These children may have other neurological symptoms such as seizures related to cortical tubers and cognitive deficiency.

### Diagnosis and Management

Contrast-enhanced cranial CT and MRI are essential for early and accurate diagnosis. Whereas the former is better for detecting small calcified lesions, MRI is superior to CT in identifying areas of gliosis, heterotopia, and SEGA, which gives the typical imaging appearance of candle dripping (Nabbout et al., 1999). SEGAs typically demonstrate diffuse contrast enhancement on both CT and MRI studies. Pharmacological inhibition of the mTOR signaling pathway with everolimus has been approved by the US Food and Drug Administration (FDA) and the European Medicine Agency (EMA) for the treatment of SEGA associated with TS (Franz et al., 2013, 2014; Krueger et al., 2010). SEGA may respond dramatically to mTOR inhibitors, but the tumors will recur once mTOR inhibition is terminated. Everolimus also improves seizure control in TS patients (Curatolo et al., 2018; Franz et al., 2018; French et al., 2016). The dramatic and sustained responses to mTOR inhibitors, along with the improvements in seizures, autism, and angiomyolipoma, has largely resulted in surgical intervention being displaced as a first-line approach, with surgery being reserved for those cases refractory to medical therapy.

**TABLE 75.3 Clinical Findings with Pediatric Brainstem Tumors**

| | Diffuse Tumors | Focal Tumors | Dorsally Exophytic Tumors | Cervicomedullary Tumors |
|---|---|---|---|---|
| Presenting symptoms | Progressive gait ataxia, weakness, and long-tract signs | Focal neurological signs and/or hydrocephalus (tectal gliomas) | Nausea and vomiting; long-tract signs are rare | Chronic nausea and vomiting |
| Cranial nerve (CN) involvement | Bilateral, asymmetrical; CN VI and VII most often | Unilateral; depends on location within the brainstem | Rare | Lower CNs (causing dysphonia, dysphagia) |
| Duration of symptoms prior to diagnosis | Short (≈6 wk) due to aggressive behavior of tumor | Longer duration; indolent course | Gradual course | Chronic course |
| Anatomical location | Almost always within the pons | Anywhere in the brainstem, but usually in the midbrain | Floor of the fourth ventricle | Cervicomedullary junction |
| Pathology | Often highgrade | Usually low-grade; solid or cystic | Usually lowgrade | Usually lowgrade |
| Imaging | Infiltrative lesion in the pons with rare enhancement | Occasional enhancement | Exophytic component strongly enhancing on CT and MRI | May show homogeneous or heterogeneous enhancement |
| Other signs/symptoms | Progressive gait ataxia; spastic quadriparesis | Contralateral hemiparesis | Early obstructive hydrocephalus, papilledema, ataxia, torticollis | Intractable neck pain; torticollis, hydrocephalus |
| Treatment | Palliative: radiation therapy (54 Gy); no clear role for chemotherapy | Surgery (depending on location); may need shunt<br>Radiation/chemotherapy if progressive or malignant component | Resection of exophytic component; re-resection for recurrence<br>Radiation therapy if malignant | Resection |
| Prognosis | Most die within 18 months | Relatively good course; can have long-term sequelae | Relatively good | Relatively good |

*CT,* Computed tomography; *MRI,* magnetic resonance imaging.

### Prognosis

SEGAs are typically low-grade tumors and, as such, gross total resection may be curative. However, multiple tumors may arise in some patients with TS. The overall prognosis for patients with TS is good, especially with the emergence of mTOR inhibition, despite increased susceptibility to other tumor types, including rhabdomyomas of the myocardium and angiomyolipoma of the kidney, liver, adrenals, and pancreas (Crino et al., 2006).

## Diffuse Astrocytoma

Diffuse astrocytomas (DAs, WHO grade II) are a common variant of LGA; they are composed primarily of fibrillary neoplastic astrocytes and are distinct from PAs. The most typical histological subtype is also termed fibrillary astrocytoma. DAs represent 12%–18% of all pediatric intracranial tumors. No gender predilection exists, and the peak age at diagnosis is 6–10 years. DAs may arise in any location within the CNS but are most commonly diagnosed in the frontal and temporal lobes. Brainstem and spinal cord are less common locations, and cerebellar DAs are rare. The spectrum of genetic abnormalities are similar to PAs, including BRAF fusions and BRAF V600E substitutions, and include mutations in the receptor tyrosine kinase *FGFR1*, as well as the transcription factors *MYB* and *MYBL1*, pointing to substantial biological heterogeneity among pediatric DAs (Ramkissoon et al., 2013; Zhang et al., 2013). Isocitrate dehydrogenase (IDH1/2) mutations are rare, but can arise in late adolescence (Yang et al., 2018). Midline DA, particularly the brainstem, thalamus, and multilobular (gliomatosis cerebri), can also harbor Histone 3 K27M, portending a very poor prognosis (Yang et al., 2018).

### Clinical Presentation

Initial symptoms vary, depending on the location of the tumor, and may exist for months to years before a definitive diagnosis (Table 75.3). DAs within the brainstem and thalamus harboring Histone 3 K27M have a different clinical course compared with DAs in other locations and will is discussed under "Diffuse Midline Glioma." Patients with medullary tumors may present with a long history of dysphagia, hoarseness, ataxia, and hemiparesis. Cervicomedullary tumors may cause medullary or upper cervical symptoms, such as neck discomfort, weakness, or numbness of the hands, and an asymmetrical quadriparesis. Patients with midbrain tumors such as a tectal glioma often present with signs and symptoms of increased ICP. Other symptoms include diplopia and hemiparesis.

### Diagnosis and Management

Most DAs appear isodense on CT scan, without significant contrast enhancement. The tumor is hypointense on T1-weighted and hyperintense on T2-weighted MRI, with minimal or no contrast enhancement with the exception of dorsally exophytic brainstem tumors (Fig. 75.4). The risk of malignant transformation appears to be much higher in adults with DA. Eighty percent of adult DAs harbor somatic mutations in the isocitrate dehydrogenase 1 *(IDH1)* gene (Sturm et al., 2012; Yan et al., 2009), which is rare in pediatric DAs. Management of children with DAs depends on the clinical prodrome and location of the primary tumor. Rapidly evolving clinical symptoms in the setting of a resectable tumor usually warrant prompt neurosurgical intervention. In patients with incidental diagnoses or lesions with a long history of indolent and mild symptoms, deferral of radical surgery is an option, with close MRI and clinical surveillance. If the tumor is surgically well accessible, some physicians and patients prefer a preemptive strategy with the hope of averting ultimate neoplastic transformation. Patients who show progressive neurological symptoms or MRI evidence of tumor growth require therapeutic intervention. The likelihood of gross total resection of a DA is low, especially when the tumor is located in an eloquent location such as the medulla. However, in patients with supratentorial

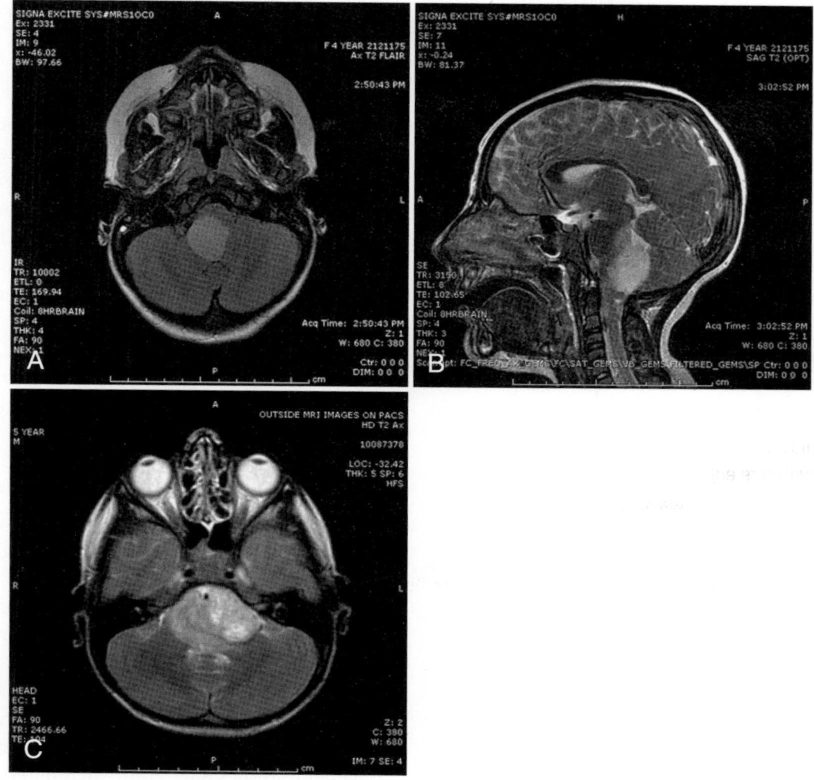


**Fig. 75.4** **A, B,** A 4-year-old girl with a several-week history of headache and a left cranial nerve VII palsy. Axial and sagittal magnetic resonance imaging (MRI) evaluation shows a dorsally exophytic mass in the medulla that is hyperintense on T2 fluid-attenuated inversion recovery (FLAIR) images. Biopsy showed the lesion to be consistent with a fibrillary (WHO grade II) astrocytoma. **C,** A 6-year-old boy with a several-week history of headache who subsequently developed right hand weakness along with a right-sided limp and ataxia. MRI demonstrates a diffusely infiltrating lesion of the pons that is hyperintense on T2-weighted images. Of note, the basilar artery is entirely surrounded by tumor. The lesion was noted to be strongly enhancing when contrast was administered. The radiological features of this tumor are consistent with a diffuse pontine glioma.

tumors, radical resection may confer a long symptom-free interval. Chemotherapy or radiation therapy is indicated when radical resection is not feasible or the tumor shows early signs of neoplastic transformation. Many DA harbor mutations and fusions in *BRAF* and less commonly *FGFR* mutations, and, as such, targeted agents such as BRAF and/or MEK inhibitors are an emerging treatment option. Although malignant transformation is rare, it can be observed in those tumors harboring BRAF mutations and histone 3 K27M mutations.

### Prognosis

Long-term survival is possible for children with supratentorial DAs despite most non-cortical tumors such as in the thalamus and brainstem not being amenable to surgical resection, with the notable exception of those with DMGs harboring histone 3 K27M mutations, in whom the prognosis is extremely poor.

## Diffuse Intrinsic Pontine Glioma/Diffuse Midline Glioma

DMG comprise malignant tumors of the thalamus and pons; they are termed diffuse intrinsic pontine glioma when they arise from the pons. Diffuse intrinsic pontine gliomas (DIPGs) represent up to 75% of all pediatric brainstem tumors and account for approximately 10% of all childhood brain tumors. Mean age at diagnosis is approximately 8 years, and there is no gender predilection (Hoffman et al., 2018). DMG/DIPG harbor K27M substitutions in histone 3.1 or 3.3 variants in over 80% of cases, and is a hallmark mutation, whereby the WHO classification terms them DMG H3 K27M-mutant (Mackay et al., 2017; Schwartzentruber et al., 2012). *ACVR1* mutations are observed in 20% of cases, and less commonly alterations in *PDGFR*, *EGFR*, *NTRK*, and *BRAF* are observed, usually in conjunction with histone 3.1 or 3.3 mutations (Buczkowicz et al., 2014b; Fontebasso et al., 2014; Jones and Baker, 2014; Khuong-Quang et al., 2012). Thalamic and pontine H3 K27M mutant tumors are histologically and biologically similar, and have similarly aggressive clinical behaviors (Castel et al., 2018; Mackay et al., 2017).

### Clinical Presentation

Most DIPG patients present with a relatively short (weeks to months) history of cranial nerve deficits, long-tract signs, and ataxia. A more protracted history may be seen in other brainstem tumors such as PAs. On MRI, DIPGs appear as infiltrative tumors within an enlarged pons (see Fig. 75.4). They are typically hypointense on T1-weighted imaging and hyperintense on T2-weighted imaging. Contrast enhancement is variable but usually absent to minimal at initial presentation. No specific imaging characteristics on conventional MRI at diagnosis are predictive of survival (Hargrave et al., 2008). Leptomeningeal spread may already be present at time of diagnosis, and MRI of the entire spine is therefore recommended initially as part of a staging work-up. Thalamic DMGs usually present with headaches, vomiting, and long-tract signs with an infiltrative appearance and enlarged thalamus on T2-weighted MRI.

### Diagnosis and Management

In patients with compatible history and MRI findings, the diagnosis of DIPG can be established without biopsy. In patients with a prolonged history, unusual neurological signs, or atypical MRI findings, diagnoses other than DIPG (e.g., PA) should be entertained and a biopsy strongly considered. Brainstem PAs usually display an anterior exophytic growth pattern. Embryonal tumors can occur in the brainstem, and diffusion imaging can help distinguish these, although biopsy is usually required to make this distinction. Demyelinating conditions may also resemble DIPG on imaging, and in addition to CSF analysis, diffusion tensor imaging fiber tracking has been suggested to aid in the diagnosis (Giussani et al., 2010). However, biopsies are frequently performed to determine the presence or absence of histone 3 K27M mutations in atypical cases, and to search for actionable targets such as *PDGFR* amplification, and *ACVR1* mutations. DIPG tissue samples obtained at initial diagnosis can usually be classified as WHO grade II–IV astrocytomas and carry no prognostic implications (Buczkowicz et al., 2014a). In contrast, specimens obtained from autopsies invariably show progression to glioblastomas (i.e., WHO grade IV astrocytomas), and genomic studies of DIPGs have revealed recurrent oncogenic alterations that share many similarities with pediatric supratentorial high-grade gliomas. Thalamic DMGs always require a biopsy for confirmation of diagnosis as the imaging and clinical presentation is not unique, and a wider range of genomic abnormalities are present in these tumors.

The standard treatment for DIPG/DMG consists of involved-field fractionated external beam radiotherapy at a dose of up to 59.4 Gy, and no chemoradiotherapy approach tested to date, including temozolomide, has proven superior to radiation therapy alone (Cohen et al., 2011). Re-irradiation can be considered at progression with a goal for extension of survival with acceptable quality of life (Tsang and Laperriere, 2019).

### Prognosis

Radiotherapy remains the mainstay of therapy and, although the majority of patients will initially respond on imaging and/or clinically, nearly all patients develop subsequent tumor progression, often with disseminated disease. Despite numerous attempts at improving survival with the addition of chemotherapy or biological modifiers, no therapy to date has resulted in significantly improved outcome compared to radiotherapy alone. Overall, the outcome for patients with DIPG/DMG remains dismal, with a median time to progression of approximately 6–9 months, median overall survival of less than 12 months, and only rare survivors beyond 2 years after initial diagnosis (Hoffman et al., 2018). DIPG remains one of the most frustrating entities in pediatric oncology, and novel treatment approaches are urgently needed.

## Pleomorphic Xanthoastrocytoma

Pleomorphic xanthoastrocytomas (PXAs) are uncommon cortical tumors that mainly occur in children, with a median age at diagnosis of 14 years.

### Clinical Presentation

PXAs are typically large and superficially located, especially in the temporal lobes. Seizures are the most common initial symptom. Contrast-enhanced MRI typically shows a large, enhancing tumor with occasional cystic components and calcification. On histopathological assessment, the proliferative indices are usually low, although necrosis, endothelial proliferation, and mitoses are observed in some patients. Consequently, PXAs may be confused with glioblastoma because of the presence of multinucleated cells and occasional foci of necrosis.

### Diagnosis and Management

PXA should be suspected in children presenting with new-onset seizures, focal deficits, and a large enhancing cortical mass on contrast-enhanced cranial MRI. The goal of surgery is to achieve a gross total resection, which is curative in the majority of patients (Rao et al., 2010). Adjuvant therapy should be deferred while the patient is monitored with serial MRI scans.

### Prognosis

The 5-year progression-free survival rate for patients with PXAs is better than 70%. However, the presence of mitoses, endothelial proliferation, or necrosis on the pathological specimen, although very rare, may significantly alter the clinical behavior and prognosis (Sugita et al., 2000). Patients with anaplastic PXA with malignant transformation have been reported, particularly those with *BRAF* mutations with concurrent *CDKN2A* homozygous deletion (Mistry et al., 2015). Up to two-thirds of PXAs harbor activating point mutations in the *BRAF* oncogene ($BRAF^{V600E}$) (Lassaletta et al., 2017), and targeted therapy with BRAF inhibitors was recently reported to have encouraging antitumor activity in patients with refractory PXA (Chamberlain, 2013; Nobre, 2020).

## Anaplastic Astrocytoma and Glioblastoma

Anaplastic astrocytoma (WHO grade III) and glioblastoma (formerly glioblastoma multiforme, WHO grade IV) are the most common high-grade astrocytomas (HGAs). The current WHO classification lists giant cell glioblastoma and gliosarcoma as histological subtypes. Overall, HGAs are much less common in children than in adults. Supratentorial HGAs represent only 6%–12% of all pediatric brain tumors, and diffuse intrinsic brainstem gliomas represent 10%. Most of these tumors arise in the cerebral hemispheres or within deeper midline structures such as the midbrain and pons. Recent genomic and epigenetic studies have confirmed that despite histological similarities, key biological differences exist between adult HGAs, pediatric HGAs, and diffuse intrinsic brainstem gliomas. Somatic mutations of the isocitrate dehydrogenase 1 and 2 genes (*IDH1*, *IDH2*) commonly seen in adult HGAs that evolved from lower-grade gliomas (i.e., secondary glioblastomas), are rarely seen in childhood HGAs (Sturm et al., 2012; Yan et al., 2009). In contrast, many pediatric tumors harbor unique oncogenic driver mutations in histone H3 leading to aberrant DNA methylation and gene expression (Sturm et al., 2012). This includes oncohistone mutations in histone H3 variants, particularly K27M substitutions in the midline and G34R/V substitutions in the cortex (Mackay et al., 2018; Schwartzentruber et al., 2012).

Several inheritable cancer predisposition syndromes have been found to be associated with HGAs. LFS, an autosomal-dominant condition caused by mutations in *TP53*, has been associated with gliomas of different grades, and somatic mutations in *TP53* are also common in pediatric HGAs in non-LFS patients (Schwartzentruber et al., 2012).

The autosomal-recessive constitutional mismatch repair deficiency syndrome (cMMRD) frequently presents with café-au-lait macules similar to NF1, resulting in occasional misdiagnosis. cMMRD is caused by germline biallelic (homozygous or compound heterozygous) mutations in one of the DNA mismatch repair (MMR) genes *MLH1*, *MSH2*, *MSH6*, and *PMS2*. Germline monoallelic mutations in MMR genes are found in hereditary nonpolyposis colon cancer, Lynch syndrome, and brain tumor polyposis syndrome type 1 (BTPS1 or Turcot type 1) (Bouffet et al., 2016; Shlien et al., 2015). Patients with cMMRD are predisposed to the development of HGAs and other brain tumors, as well as gastrointestinal and hematological cancers, typically within the first two decades of life.

### Clinical Presentation

The clinical manifestations of HGA depend on the anatomical location of the tumor as well as on the age of the patient. The clinical prodromes are usually short and rapidly evolving, with symptoms or signs of increased ICP or focal neurological dysfunction, although in some

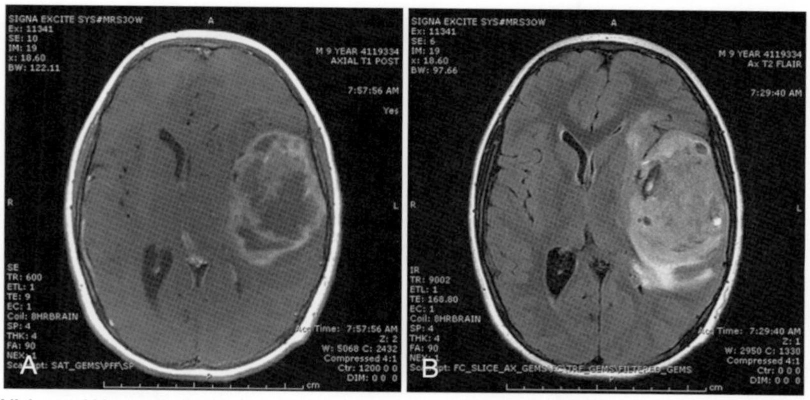

**Fig. 75.5 A 9-Year-Old Boy With a 1-Week History of Headache, Vomiting, and Increasing Somnolence.** He subsequently developed difficulties with word-finding and was seen in his local hospital, where a computed tomography scan showed a large left frontal mass with severe edema and midline shift. **A,** Magnetic resonance imaging shows a large (7 × 6 cm) left frontal lobe mass. T1-weighted image following the administration of contrast shows heterogeneous enhancement with hypointense areas consistent with intratumoral hemorrhage. **B,** Axial T2 fluid-attenuated inversion recovery (FLAIR) images show tumor-associated edema within the adjacent left frontal and parietal lobes. Resection of the lesion showed this lesion to be a glioblastoma (WHO grade IV).

patients, an HGA may arise in the setting of prolonged symptoms from an LGA (Tamber and Rutka, 2003).

### Diagnosis and Management

The basis for suspicion of HGA is the clinical presentation and the contrast-enhanced cranial MRI. The MRI features are a combination of diffuse non-enhancing signal abnormalities and focal enhancing solid lesions. Intratumoral cysts often correlate with spontaneous necrosis. The T2 signal is often more diffuse and is consistent with both infiltrative tumor and vasogenic tumor-associated edema (Fig. 75.5). Significant mass effect, hydrocephalus, and intratumoral hemorrhage may be present. Gross total resection is the initial treatment goal. This facilitates a more accurate diagnosis and makes subsequent radiation therapy tolerable. Unfortunately, the outcome for children with HGA remains poor. Single-agent temozolomide, when administered during and after radiotherapy, has been shown to significantly prolong both event-free and overall survival in adults with glioblastoma (Stupp et al., 2005); however, similar treatment strategies used in a single-arm pediatric trial did not improve outcome when compared with historical controls treated with other regimens (Cohen et al., 2011). Similar to DIPG, no chemoradiotherapy regimen has proven superior to radiation therapy alone in the treatment of pediatric HGAs. Exceptions to this are high-grade gliomas with MMR deficiency, usually in the context of cMMRD, which are ultra-hypermutant, and have been shown in some instances to have dramatic responses to immune checkpoint inhibition such as nivolumab (Bouffet et al., 2016). Moreover, a subset of pediatric high-grade gliomas have mutations in BRAF V600E (sometimes termed epithelioid glioblastoma), and may respond to BRAF inhibitors.

Pediatric high-grade gliomas frequently harbor fusion events, including *NTRK* fusions, which are highly actionable with available inhibitors, and should be evaluated in all cases. RNA sequencing either a panel or whole transcriptome analysis is emerging as a powerful tool in the evaluation and work-up of all pediatric high-grade gliomas (Jones et al., 2017; Mackay et al., 2017; Rogawski et al., 2017; Wu et al., 2014).

### Prognosis

Children with high-grade gliomas continue to have a poor prognosis, despite the use of multimodal therapy. Age younger than 3 years, radical resection, WHO grade III histology, and the presence of IDH1 mutations are favorable risk factors (Cohen et al., 2011). Patients with diffuse unresectable thalamic and pontine HGAs have the worst prognosis, particularly those harboring Histone 3 K27M mutations. Given the high prevalence of prognostically useful and/or therapeutically actionable genomic alterations in HGAs, including H3 K27M, IDH, NTRK, MET, ALK, BRAF as well as hypermutant MMR deficiency, comprehensive genomic testing of both tumor and germline is recommended for all pediatric HGA patients.

## NEURONAL AND MIXED NEURONAL-GLIAL TUMORS

The spectrum of neuronal and mixed neuronal-glial brain tumors represents several clinicopathological entities and includes tumors composed of mixed populations of cells of both glial and neuronal lineage. Similar to astrocytomas, neuronal and mixed neuronal-glial tumors can be classified as low-grade (WHO grade I and II) or high-grade (WHO grade III and IV), and the most relevant pediatric subtypes will be discussed.

### Ganglioglioma

These low-grade (WHO grade I) neuronal-glial tumors represent 4%–8% of primary brain tumors in children, and 80% occur in subjects younger than age 30. Constitutively activating mutations in the BRAF oncogene ($BRAF^{V600E}$) can be found in 18%–50% of these tumors with a minority harboring FGFR mutations (Schindler et al., 2011; Stone et al., 2018; Yang et al., 2018).

#### Clinical Presentation

Seizures are the initial manifestation in approximately 50% of ganglioglioma patients. Complex partial seizures are common because the typical tumor location is in the medial temporal lobe (Blumcke et al., 2017).

#### Diagnosis and Management

Contrast-enhanced cranial MRI often reveals a supratentorial cystic mass. The MRI appearance of these tumors is variable, but the lesion is frequently hypointense on T1-weighted sequences and hyperintense on T2-weighted images (Fig. 75.6, *A*). Contrast enhancement varies in intensity from marked to absent and may be nodular, solid, or circumferential. A large size and a supratentorial location characterize an infantile variant of ganglioglioma, desmoplastic infantile ganglioglioma, which frequently harbor

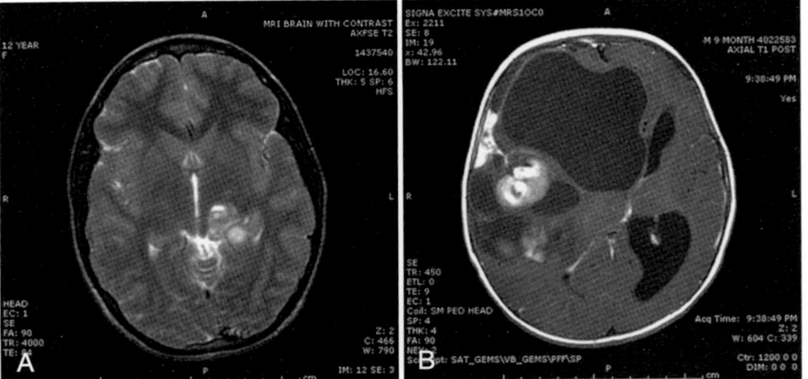


**Fig. 75.6** **A,** A 13-year-old girl with a several-month history of absence seizures. Contrast-enhanced cranial magnetic resonance imaging (MRI) demonstrated a lobulated lesion arising from the medial left temporal lobe extending and invading the left brainstem, the posterior left thalamic region, and the cingulate gyrus posterior to the splenium of the corpus callosum. Resection revealed the mass to be consistent with a ganglioglioma. Axial T2 fast-spin echo image shows T2 prolongation. **B,** A 9-month-old boy presented with a history of increasing irritability and increased head circumference. A contrast-enhanced MRI demonstrated a very large tumor consisting of both an enhancing solid component and multiple cystic components with surrounding edema, centered within the right frontal lobe. The mass caused subfalcine herniation and obstructed the third ventricle at the level of the foramen of Munro, resulting in marked hydrocephalus involving the lateral ventricles. MR spectroscopy demonstrated a markedly increased choline peak consistent with high cellularity. Resection revealed the mass to be consistent with a desmoplastic infantile ganglioglioma. Axial T1 postgadolinium contrast image shows the enhancing solid component with multiple cysts.

BRAF V600E mutations (see Fig. 75.6, *B*) (Bachli et al., 2003; Wang et al., 2018). Gross total resection is the treatment of choice for gangliogliomas. Unresectable or recurrent tumors may be treated with chemotherapy or targeted agents in the case of BRAF mutations (Lassaletta et al., 2016b).

### Prognosis

Gross total resection is often curative. Thus, location and extent of resection are the most important prognostic factors. In patients with recurrent or unresectable ganglioglioma, response to chemotherapy has been demonstrated. These tumors, when they harbor BRAF V600E mutations, may undergo malignant transformation over time, similar to a DA (WHO grade II) (Mistry et al., 2015). Similarly, desmoplastic infantile gangliogliomas, although often cured by resection, may undergo rapid progression and metastasis consistent with malignant transformation (Wang et al., 2018). The frequent constitutive activation of BRAF in these tumors, similar to PAs, provides the opportunity for molecular targeted therapies with small-molecule inhibitors, which are currently in early-phase clinical trials for children with brain tumors.

## Desmoplastic Infantile Astrocytoma or Ganglioglioma

Characteristic of desmoplastic infantile astrocytoma (DIA) or ganglioglioma (DIG) is their large size and superficial cortical location at presentation. These tumors may involve an entire hemisphere and are usually diagnosed in infants and children younger than age 2 years. The most common presentation consists of seizures, although progressive focal deficits may also be a first manifestation. The tumor is revealed by contrast enhancement on MRI and usually has a large cystic component. Histological features include collagenized regions with astrocytes and admixed small, primitive-appearing cells in nodular aggregates: hence the name *desmoplastic*. Regional leptomeningeal dissemination is common despite classification as a WHO grade I lesion. Nevertheless, patients with DIA often have a good prognosis if gross total resection can be achieved (Sugiyama et al., 2002). Similar to gangliogliomas, the BRAF$^{V600E}$ mutation can be found in a subset of DIAs/DIGs (Koelsche et al., 2014).

## Dysembryoplastic Neuroepithelial Tumor

### Background

Dysembryoplastic neuroepithelial tumors (DNETs) represent approximately 1% of all neuroepithelial brain tumors in patients younger than 20 years of age. DNETs are a common cause of tumor-related epilepsy, as two-thirds of DNETs are located in the temporal lobes, and 5%–15% of temporal lobe resections for intractable epilepsy show DNETs. These lesions are classified as WHO grade I tumors. Fibroblast growth factor receptor (FGFR) and BRAF V600E mutations are common in DNET and the emergence of BRAF inhibitors, clinically active FGFR inhibitors, and MEK inhibitors offers a potential treatment option in unresectable cases (Rivera et al., 2016).

### Clinical Presentation

Patients with these tumors typically present with a long history of complex partial seizures, which are often drug resistant. As such, the diagnosis of DNET is a consideration in children and young adults with either new-onset seizures or a long history of epilepsy. The average age of the onset of seizures is 9 years. The superficial cortical location of DNETs may account for the high risk of seizures.

### Diagnosis and Management

Contrast-enhanced cranial MRI shows absence of edema and only minimal if any enhancement (eFig. 75.7).  Pathological findings include a specific neuronal-glial element manifested by glial fibrillary acidic protein (GFAP)-negative oligodendroglia-like cells and neurons in a mucinous eosinophilic background that give the appearance of floating neurons. Because histopathological analysis shows oligodendrocytes, astrocytes, or both, the differential diagnosis often includes oligodendroglioma, mixed oligoastrocytoma, and ganglioglioma. DNETs typically do not grow or recur, so gross total resection is often curative of the tumor although seizures may recur even without tumor recurrence. Adjuvant chemotherapy and radiation therapy are not recommended.

### Prognosis

The stable behavior of DNETs over time results in an excellent prognosis after either gross total or partial resection (Sandberg et al., 2005).

## Central Neurocytoma

### Background

Central neurocytoma is a rare tumor of neuronal lineage that usually arises in a periventricular location. The diagnosis of a central neurocytoma should be a consideration in young patients with an intraventricular mass. Hydrocephalus may arise from obstruction of CSF flow at the level of the foramina of Munro (Schmidt et al., 2004). The molecular genetic underpinnings of this rare entity are currently unknown.

### Diagnosis and Management

Contrast-enhanced cranial MRI typically shows an isointense mass with minimal enhancement (eFig. 75.8). A tumor arising in the posterior third ventricular region may represent a pineocytoma, but a pineoblastoma must be excluded (Hirato and Nakazato, 2001). On pathological study, the presence of perinuclear halos on light microscopy may lead to a mistaken diagnosis of oligodendroglioma. Immunohistochemical staining with neuronal markers such as synaptophysin helps distinguish this tumor from an oligodendroglioma. Very rare atypical forms with mitoses, necrosis, and endothelial proliferation have been reported (Mackenzie, 2000; Soylemezoglu et al., 1997). Patients with a mitotic index greater than 3% have a worse prognosis (Rades et al., 2004). Gross total resection can be curative for central neurocytomas. Radiation and chemotherapy may be deferred in patients undergoing radical resections, but they should be monitored closely. This emphasizes the importance of differentiating central neurocytoma from oligodendroglioma, because the latter tumor may require adjuvant radiation and chemotherapy. Radiation therapy is a consideration only for atypical forms with a high mitotic index (>3%) and for recurrent unresectable tumors.

### Prognosis

The outcome in atypical central neurocytomas is difficult to predict accurately because of the rarity of the tumor. However, a meta-analysis has shown that lesions with a mitotic index less than 3% have a less than 15% risk of recurrence and a 95% 5-year overall survival, compared with 38% and 66%, respectively, for tumors with a mitotic index greater than 3% (Rades et al., 2004). Both chemotherapy and radiotherapy have been used in the recurrent setting and may produce prolonged disease stabilization and occasionally partial responses (Leenstra et al., 2007; Sharma et al., 2006). However, the role of adjuvant therapy after incomplete resection is not well defined.

# OTHER CENTRAL NERVOUS SYSTEM TUMORS

## Oligodendroglioma

Oligodendrogliomas are rare, accounting for less than 2% of pediatric brain tumors, and are diffusely infiltrative tumors. They are most commonly found in the cerebral cortex but may arise anywhere in the CNS. Depending on tumor location, most patients present with seizures or signs of raised ICP. Oligodendrogliomas are typically hypointense on T1-weighted MRI sequences and hyperintense on T2-weighted sequences. The tumor may appear partially contrast enhancing, cystic, hemorrhagic, and/or calcified. Histologically, the tumor cells resemble oligodendroglial cells. Oligodendrogliomas are graded as either WHO grade II or III(i.e., anaplastic oligodendroglioma [AO]). AO features frequent mitotic figures, nuclear atypia, microvascular proliferation, and occasional necrosis. Mixed tumors with both oligodendroglial and astrocytic components exist and are classified as oligoastrocytoma or anaplastic oligoastrocytoma. There is no specific immunohistochemical marker that unequivocally differentiates oligodendroglial from astrocytic tumors. Molecularly, oligodendroglial tumors are characterized by an unbalanced translocation of chromosomes 1 and 19, which results in a co-deletion of 1p and 19q. Several studies have established the 1p/19q co-deletion as a molecular signature for oligodendrogliomas in adults, although the prevalence in pediatric oligodendroglial tumors is rare (Kreiger et al., 2005; Raghavan et al., 2003). 1p/19q co-deleted oligodendrogliomas display a proneural gene expression signature (Cooper et al., 2010) and are associated with other favorable prognostic molecular features, including methylation of the MGMT promoter and somatic mutations of the *IDH* genes (Erdem-Eraslan et al., 2013). In addition, these tumors frequently harbor somatic mutations in *FUBP1*, located on 1p, and *CIC*, located on 19q (Bettegowda et al., 2011), although the mechanism of how these genetic alterations cooperate and contribute to tumorigenesis remains to be elucidated. The molecular features of pediatric oligodendrogliomas, which typically do not harbor 1p/19q co-deletions, are not currently defined.

### Management

Whenever feasible, gross total resection should be attempted. For residual, progressive, or recurrent tumors, optimal therapy in the pediatric population has not been established. Oligodendrogliomas are typically sensitive to chemotherapy and radiotherapy, and recent data indicate that a strong association with IDH mutational status exists (Cairncross et al., 2014). Based on adult experiences, chemotherapy such as PCV (procarbazine/CCNU/vincristine) and temozolomide have been used in pediatric patients in an attempt to delay radiotherapy. In adult studies, both chemotherapy and radiotherapy have been shown to prolong progression-free survival (Bromberg and van den Bent, 2009), but the optimal treatment sequence is subject to investigation in ongoing studies.

### Prognosis

In pediatric series, the most relevant prognostic factors for improved progression-free and overall survival were gross total resection and low tumor grade. For low-grade (i.e., non-anaplastic) oligodendrogliomas, 5-year progression-free survival and overall survival of 81% and 84%, respectively, have been reported (Peters et al., 2004). The 1p/19q co-deletion and IDH1/2 mutations, which have been associated with a favorable prognosis and sensitivity to chemotherapy in adult tumors, are rare in children and of unclear prognostic significance.

## Ependymoma

Ependymomas are glial tumors that arise from ependymal cells within the CNS. This tumor represents approximately 10% of all childhood intracranial neoplasms, constituting the third most common pediatric brain tumor after astrocytoma and medulloblastoma. Some 90% of pediatric ependymomas are intracranial, 75% of which arise in the posterior fossa. Most supratentorial ependymomas are located in the brain parenchyma away from the ependymal surface, in contrast to infratentorial ependymomas. Spinal cord ependymomas represent less than 10% of pediatric intramedullary spinal tumors, but more than 50% of intramedullary spinal tumors in adults. Although morphologically these tumors appear similar, supratentorial, posterior fossa, and spinal cord ependymoma are biologically completely different entities (Johnson et al., 2010; Taylor et al., 2005). A DNA methylation-based classifier divides ependymoma into nine distinct subgroups, three subgroups in each of the supratentorium, posterior fossa, and spinal cord (Pajtler et al., 2015, 2017). Supratentorial ependymoma are characterized by recurrent fusions on chromosome 11 involving either the nuclear factor kappa B (NF-κB) co-activator RelA fused to C11orf95 (ST-EPN-RELA), or recurrent fusions of *YAP1* and *MAML2* (ST-EPN-YAP) (Pajtler et al., 2015; Parker et al., 2014). Posterior fossa ependymoma can be subdivided into two distinct groups, termed PF-EPN-A or PF-EPN-B (Pajtler et al., 2015; Ramaswamy et al., 2016a; Witt et al., 2011). PF-EPN-A form the vast majority of young children, and are characterized by aggressive clinical behavior and a bland genome, with the exception of recurrent gains of chromosome 1q in 20% of cases, and either mutations (10%) or overexpression (90%) of the EZH2-binding protein EZHIP/CXorf67 (Hubner et al., 2019; Jain et al., 2019). PF-EPN-A are characterized by loss of histone H3 K27 trimethylation, and have a globally hypomethylated genome (Bayliss et al., 2016; Panwalkar et al., 2017). PF-EPN-B are more common in adolescents and adults, and are characterized by multiple chromosomal gains and losses, and retention of histone H3 K27 trimethylation. Significant heterogeneity exists across both PF-EPN-A and PF-EPN-B, with multiple subtypes identified within each group (Cavalli et al., 2018; Pajtler et al., 2018). A distinct subependymoma group, seen only in older adults exists in both posterior fossa and supratentorial ependymoma. Spinal ependymoma comprise three groups termed myxopapillary, classic, and subependymoma, with distinct epigenetic and gene expression profiles with distinct morphologies (Mack et al., 2015; Pajtler et al., 2017).

## Clinical Presentation

The presenting symptoms of infratentorial ependymomas relate to their origin from the ependymal tissue lining the fourth ventricle. Hydrocephalus results when the tumor fills the fourth ventricle, causing headache, irritability, nausea, vomiting, ataxia, and papilledema. A common sign of the tumor in infants is increased head circumference. Tumors that extend out one of the foramina of Luschka compromise lower cranial nerves and cause hoarseness and dysphagia. If the tumor extends through the foramen of Magendie, the patient may complain of neck discomfort and have torticollis. Spinal cord ependymomas are typically located in the cervical region. The most common presenting symptom is localized pain at the level of the lesion. The typical description of pain is that it is worse at night, presumably due to congestion of the spinal venous plexus in the recumbent position. The second most common symptom is radicular dysesthesias, and a late manifestation of this symptom is progressive spastic quadriparesis. Thoracic ependymomas are associated with scoliosis. Myxopapillary ependymomas of the conus medullaris and filum terminale may present with low back pain, radicular pain, saddle anesthesia, and sphincter dysfunction.

## Diagnosis

A typical MRI appearance of a fourth ventricular ependymoma is that of a homogeneously enhancing solid mass extending out one of the foramina of Luschka or the foramen of Magendie, with associated obstructive hydrocephalus (Fig. 75.9). Although there is no formal staging system for ependymomas, the WHO classification system recognizes three grades: grade I, subependymoma and myxopapillary ependymoma; grade II, classic ependymoma; and grade III, anaplastic ependymoma. This grading system is of limited utility due to extreme interobserver variability resulting in widely variable proportions of classic and anaplastic across different cooperative group studies (Ellison et al., 2011). Because ependymomas typically arise in the ependymal linings of ventricles, tumors may spread through the entire neuraxis. Evaluation of patients should include contrast-enhanced MRI scans of the brain and entire spinal cord. Cytological evaluation of the CSF is currently part of the metastatic work-up for patients at the time of initial presentation, albeit with a very low yield. The identification of fusions of C11orf95 to RelA allows for an

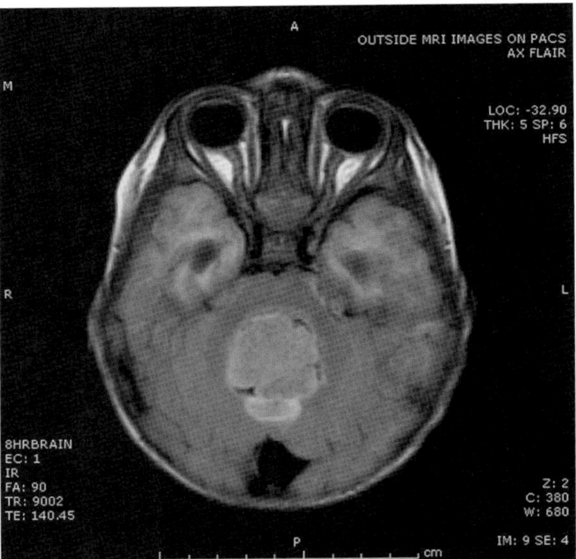


**Fig. 75.9** A 12-month-old boy who presented with a 1-week history of worsening balance, nausea, and vomiting. Brain magnetic resonance imaging showed a large fourth ventricle tumor (3 × 4 × 5 cm) extending out both foramina of Luschka, along with severe hydrocephalus. Biopsy showed a moderately cellular glial neoplasm with glial fibrillary acidic protein staining, visible mitoses, and an elevated proliferative index, consistent with an ependymoma (WHO grade II).

objective diagnostic and prognostic marker of supratentorial ependymoma. Immunoreactivity for L1CAM and CyclinD1 have been proposed as surrogates for RelA fusions; however, these markers can also be observed in high-grade glioma. A significant proportion of supratentorial ependymoma are misdiagnosed high-grade glioma or embryonal tumors and, as such, the presence of the RelA fusion should be evaluated in all cases. Posterior fossa ependymoma can be routinely divided into PF-EPN-A or PF-EPN-B using immunohistochemistry for H3K27me3, where the loss of H3K27me3 staining is highly suggestive of PF-EPN-A (Panwalkar P et al., 2017). PF-EPN-A harboring 1q gain are a very high-risk group and usually relapse quickly and with metastatic dissemination (Merchant et al., 2019).

## Management

The first line of treatment is surgery, with a goal of gross total resection, followed by postoperative conformal radiation. Technological advances, such as the operating microscope, the Cavitron ultrasonic aspirator, intraoperative ultrasound, MRI, and electrophysiological monitoring have reduced operative morbidity and allowed more complete tumor resection. Subtotal resections in both the posterior fossa and supratentorium carry a very poor prognosis, even with adjuvant radiotherapy, and second-look surgery and/or referral to more specialized centers should be considered in this event. Historically, the use of radiation in young children with ependymomas was avoided because the risks of cognitive, endocrine, and developmental side effects would be highest. Previous recommendations have been to reserve radiation for patients in whom a gross total resection was not possible or for patients with recurrent disease. However, the failure of adjuvant chemotherapy to delay radiation therapy for a significant time in younger patients with ependymomas of the fourth ventricle, as well as large cooperative group studies showing excellent survival for patients as young as 1 year old with complete resections and postoperative radiation has resulted in postoperative radiation being the standard of care

(Merchant et al., 2019). Long-term sequelae of conformal radiation in this age group has been shown to be manageable, and the advent of proton beam irradiation has the potential to further reduce long-term side effects (Merchant et al., 2005; Morris et al., 2009b; Mulhern et al., 2004; Zapotocky et al., 2019).

No clear role exists for adjuvant chemotherapy in the management of ependymomas (Bouffet and Foreman, 1999; Siffert and Allen, 1998). The Children's Oncology Group and the International Society for Pediatric Oncology are currently conducting studies with the primary aim of determining the role of maintenance chemotherapy. A secondary aim is to determine the survival of patients with supratentorial classic ependymoma treated with gross total resection alone.

Unfortunately, treatment options for children with recurrent ependymoma are quite limited; however, surgery and re-irradiation have been shown to significantly prolong survival (Tsang et al., 2018, 2019; Zapotocky et al., 2019).

### Prognosis

The most important prognostic factors for both infratentorial and supratentorial ependymoma are extent of surgical resection and postoperative radiotherapy. In PF-EPN-A tumors, 1q gain is a marker of poor prognosis even in those patients with complete surgical resections, and postoperative radiotherapy, with 5-year progression-free survival under 30% in this group. PF-EPN-A with balanced 1q status and a complete surgical resection have excellent 5-year progression-free survival approaching 80%. PF-EPN-B not only have excellent progression-free survival irrespective of 1q status but also benefit from complete surgical resections and radiation. Supratentorial ependymoma have survivals approaching 80% for those patients with complete resections and postoperative radiotherapy; however, up to 50% of patients with differentiated tumors can be cured without radiotherapy. Caution should be exerted with those supratentorial ependymomas that do not harbor a fusion of either RELA or YAP1, as a substantial portion of these patients are molecularly other entities such as high-grade glioma and embryonal tumors. Little is known regarding the optimal management of pediatric spinal cord ependymoma beyond the importance of complete surgical resections, specifically the role of postoperative radiotherapy.

## Germ Cell Tumors

Germ cell tumors are the most prevalent tumors of the pineal region and represent approximately 3%–5% of intracranial childhood malignances in the United States (Keene et al., 2007). These tumors are morphologically homologous to the germ cell tumors that arise in the gonads. The molecular pathogenesis of CNS germ cell tumors is not well understood; although similar to non-CNS germ cell tumors, somatic mutations in *KIT*, *mTOR*, and *RAS* can be found in a subset of intracranial germ cell tumors (Fukushima et al., 2014; Ichimura et al., 2016). Malignant germ cell tumors of the CNS are divided into two clinical categories reflecting relative sensitivities to cytotoxic therapies such as radiotherapy and chemotherapy: germinomas comprsie 60% of all CNS germ cell tumors and are the most sensitive; the second category comprises mixed malignant germ cell tumors (MMGCTs). MMGCTs (35%) include embryonal cell carcinoma, immature and mature teratomas, endodermal sinus tumor, choriocarcinoma, or combinations of the above (Robertson et al., 2014). Less than 5% of primary CNS germ cell tumors are mature or immature teratomas, which are primarily surgically controllable tumors.

The majority of germ cell tumors (95%) arise in midline CNS structures, with approximately 40% in the suprasellar/intrasellar region, 50% in the pineal region, and 5% involving both sites at diagnosis. Germinoma is the most common tumor arising in the pineal region; MMGCTs and germinomas arise with equal frequency in the suprasellar region.

Intracranial germ cell tumors present primarily in the second and third decades of life. Pineal region tumors are more common in males, whereas there is an equal sex distribution in the suprasellar region. The incidence of CNS germ cell tumors in Asian populations, such as in Korea and Japan, was thought to be higher than in other ethnic groups, but recent epidemiological studies question this disparity (McCarthy et al., 2012).

### Clinical Presentation

Patients diagnosed with suprasellar germ cell tumors may have an unusually long prodrome, often years in duration. The earliest symptoms—especially in patients with suprasellar primary tumors—include endocrine dysfunction (most frequently diabetes insipidus) with patients suffering from polyuria and polydipsia. Eventually other endocrine manifestations arise, such as growth impairment, precocious puberty, and hypothyroidism. Vision loss and symptoms of increased ICP are late manifestations when the tumor has either reached a large size or has spread in a periventricular distribution to the third and lateral ventricles. Patients with tumors arising in the pineal region usually present with a shorter prodrome consisting of symptoms of raised ICP; that is, headache, nausea, and vomiting due to obstructive hydrocephalus. Limitation of vertical gaze, convergence nystagmus, impaired pupillary reflexes, and double vision may be apparent on neurological examination, owing to compression of the midbrain tectum (Parinaud syndrome). Papilledema due to obstructive hydrocephalus is observed. Germ cell tumors can also cause precocious puberty when they release large concentrations of β-human chorionic gonadotropin (β-hCG) (Ogino et al., 2005).

### Diagnosis and Management

Contrast-enhanced cranial MRI is the most sensitive diagnostic modality when a primary CNS germ cell tumor is suspected. Pure germinomas are typically isointense on T1-weighted images and slightly hyperintense on T2-weighted images, with intense homogeneous contrast enhancement (Fig. 75.10). Intratumoral cysts or calcification may be present. MMGCTs (e.g., mixed germ cell tumors or teratomas) often have a more heterogeneous appearance due to a mixture of benign and malignant components. The specific type of pineal region tumor cannot be determined from the imaging appearance alone. Patients typically require histological or biochemical (tumor marker) confirmation of specific tumor histology at diagnosis for optimal management, because of the range of tumor types that arise in these areas. Histological confirmation may not be necessary in patients with elevated lumbar CSF concentrations of tumor markers (α-fetoprotein [AFP] or β-hCG) consistent with an MMGCT (Seregni et al., 2002). There is a strong association between the tumor marker profile in CSF and the types of MMGCT. Elevations of AFP occur with endodermal sinus tumor and embryonal carcinoma, whereas a high level (>2000 mIU/mL) of β-hCG alone is consistent with choriocarcinoma. Pure germinoma may have modest elevations of CSF β-hCG up to 100 mIU/mL. Elevations of lactate dehydrogenase isoenzymes and placental alkaline phosphatase are also detectable in CSF in germinoma patients.

Tumor markers are also useful in monitoring response to treatment and surveillance for early signs of recurrence. Approximately 60% of newly diagnosed germinoma patients will have normal β-hCG levels in both serum and CSF, and 35% of patients will have elevated lumbar CSF HCG levels only with normal serum values. Lumbar CSF values are usually 2–3 times higher than serum values (Allen et al., 2012). However,

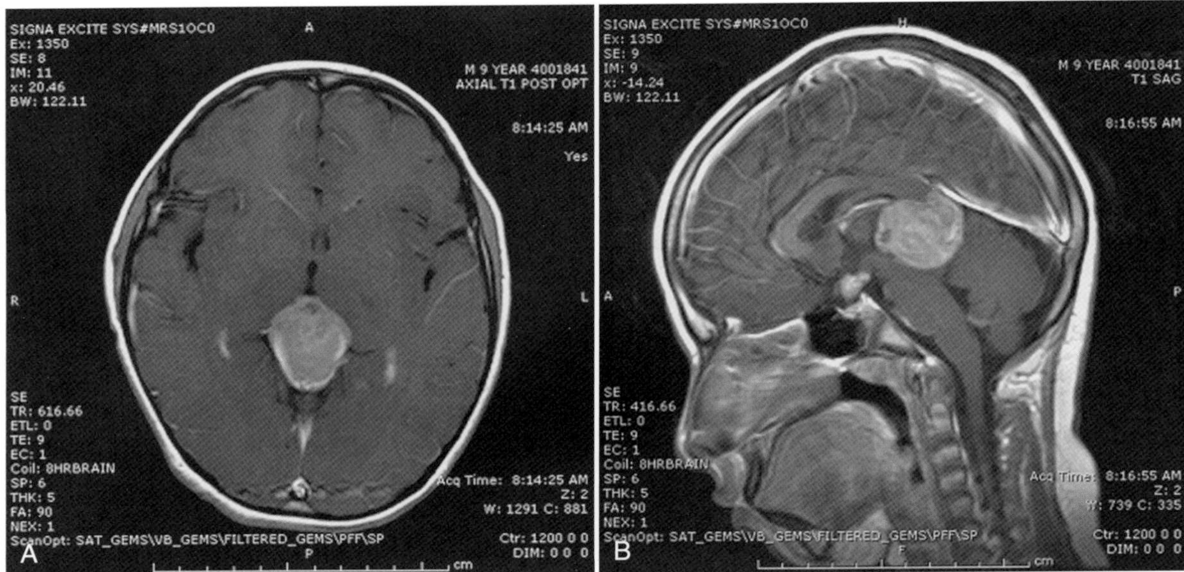


**Fig. 75.10** A 10-year-old boy who presented with an 18-month history of headache, fatigue, and diplopia. **A,** Contrast-enhanced cranial magnetic resonance imaging studies revealed a well-circumscribed, homogeneously enhancing pineal mass lesion measuring 3.6 × 2.9 × 3.0 cm. **B,** The mass was seen to extend anteriorly into the posterior aspect of the third ventricle and inferiorly into the midbrain, with compression of the tectum. A second homogeneously enhancing mass can be seen in the infundibular recess of the third ventricle, consistent with subarachnoid dissemination of disease. The patient underwent a biopsy that demonstrated that this lesion was a pure germinoma (no other mixed germ cell elements). Immunohistochemical analysis showed the tumor cells to be positive for placental alkaline phosphatase and PAS but negative for β-human chorionic gonadotropin and α-fetoprotein.

AFP values in the serum are usually comparable to those in lumbar CSF. Ventricular CSF is not an adequate substitute for lumbar CSF, since the ventricular tumor marker levels are usually lower than lumbar, and normative data are lacking. Furthermore, it is difficult to resample ventricular CSF following treatment (Legault and Allen, 2013).

Preoperative evaluation for patients with suspected CNS germ cell tumors should include contrast-enhanced cranial and spinal MRI, serum and CSF tumor markers (if lumbar puncture is safe to perform), CSF cytological analysis, and assessment of endocrine and visual function. Evaluation of the spine and CSF is necessary because germ cell tumors are capable of seeding the neuraxis via CSF. In cases of obstructive hydrocephalus, preoperative third ventriculostomy has the potential to eliminate the need for a VP shunt, which could carry a risk of infection as well as peritoneal dissemination of the tumor. The current neurosurgical management for pineal region tumors includes endoscopic or open biopsy for tissue diagnosis and/or possible resection, depending on the specific tumor type. For example, it is *not* prudent to incur the risks associated with radical resection of a pure germinoma, since the tumor is highly sensitive and curable with adjuvant therapy alone, but it *is* reasonable to radically resect an MMGCT if feasible, either at diagnosis or following adjuvant medical therapy if residual disease remains.

Radiation is frequently employed in the treatment of CNS germ cell tumors, with radiosensitivity determined by tumor histology. Germinomas are the most radiosensitive type, with 90% progression-free survival at 5 years, whereas MMGCTs have a 5-year survival rate of 30%–40% (Ogawa et al., 2004). However, multimodality therapy (chemotherapy and radiation therapy) is being used more commonly. Several treatment options exist regarding the management of intracranial germinomas. Radiation alone is usually administered in relatively high doses and large volumes (whole ventricular or craniospinal), even for localized disease. Although the 10-year survival ranges from 80% to 90% using this approach, children often suffer from the late consequences of radiation. Alternatively, the use of two to four courses of chemotherapy (carboplatin and etoposide) followed by whole ventricular radiation therapy appears to preserve the high survival statistics of higher-dose, larger-volume radiation only while minimizing long-term cognition (Calaminus et al., 2013, 2017). For MMGCTs, more aggressive chemotherapy and high-dose/large-volume radiation therapy are required to provide for a 5-year survival rate of greater than 70% (Kellie et al., 2004a, 2004b; Robertson et al., 2014).

### Prognosis

The prognosis for patients with pineal region tumors depends on histology. Their sensitivity to radiation and chemotherapy give germinomas an excellent prognosis. MMGCTs, on the other hand, tend to have a less favorable prognosis, but more recent treatment protocols that use combinations of chemotherapy and radiation have markedly improved outcome (Calaminus et al., 2017; Goldman et al., 2015). As CNS germinomas may recur late, patients should be imaged with brain and spine MRI at regular intervals for at least 10–15 years after diagnosis (Pruitt et al., 2015). Recurrent germ cell tumors may respond to salvage chemotherapy or additional radiation therapy.

## Craniopharyngioma

Craniopharyngiomas are the most common nonglial tumors in children and account for 3%–5% of all pediatric brain tumors. The peak age range for diagnosis of this tumor is 6–14 years. These are slow-growing tumors that arise in the sella and parasellar region, often extending into the parasellar cisterns and occasionally invading adjacent cortical and vascular structures. Although these tumors are histologically benign, compression of critical intracranial structures can lead to pituitary, hypothalamic, and optic dysfunction. As a result, these patients often have complicated medical courses and long-term sequelae.

## Clinical Presentation

The typical onset is insidious, and a 1- to 2-year history of slowly progressive symptoms is common; symptoms may include progressive vision loss, delay in sexual maturation, and tapering of growth velocity. Eventually, extension of the tumor dorsally in the third ventricle causes behavioral dysfunction and symptoms of raised ICP. More than 70% of children at the time of diagnosis present with growth hormone deficiency, obstructive hydrocephalus, short-term memory deficits, and psychomotor slowing. Craniopharyngiomas are divisible into adamantinomatous and papillary types. Adamantinomatous craniopharyngiomas are more common; they occur in children and young adults and typically have cystic and solid areas with calcifications. Papillary tumors, encountered almost exclusively in adults, are predominantly solid without calcification and are less infiltrative.

## Diagnosis and Management

The typical appearance on cranial MRI (Fig. 75.11, *A, B*) is a multicystic and solid enhancing suprasellar mass, which if large enough, results in hydrocephalus and forward displacement and stretching of the optic nerves and chiasm (Brunel et al., 2002). The cystic component is often bright on the T1 images prior to contrast. An important additional radiographic diagnostic sign is intratumoral calcifications on a nonenhanced CT scan (see Fig. 75.11, *C*).

Immunohistochemistry and sequencing studies have demonstrated *BRAF* V600E mutations in the majority of papillary craniopharyngiomas whereas mutations in *CTNNB1*, the gene encoding beta-catenin, have been found in the adamantinomatous subtype (Larkin et al., 2014). Although drugs targeting the beta-catenin pathway are still under development, there are currently drugs in clinical use targeting BRAF V600E.

Surgical removal of the tumor is an effective treatment for tumor control but unfortunately carries significant long-term morbidity and mortality in the form of profound hypothalamic dysfunction (Cohen et al., 2013; Elliott et al., 2010). In many centers, radical resection is still preferred, where transcranial or transsphenoidal surgical approaches are commonly used. Transsphenoidal resection is the preferred method for tumors in a subdiaphragmatic location and is associated with a lower incidence of postoperative diabetes insipidus (Elliott et al., 2011). Despite the surgical accessibility of many of these tumors, radical resection does not always guarantee recurrence-free survival. Moreover, aggressive resection can cause multiple hormonal deficiencies, visual-field and acuity deficits, and symptoms of hypothalamic injury, such as eating disorders, altered sleep/wake rhythms, memory impairment, and loss of impulse control. Another approach to craniopharyngioma combines incomplete surgical resection followed by radiation therapy in an attempt to preserve quality of life,

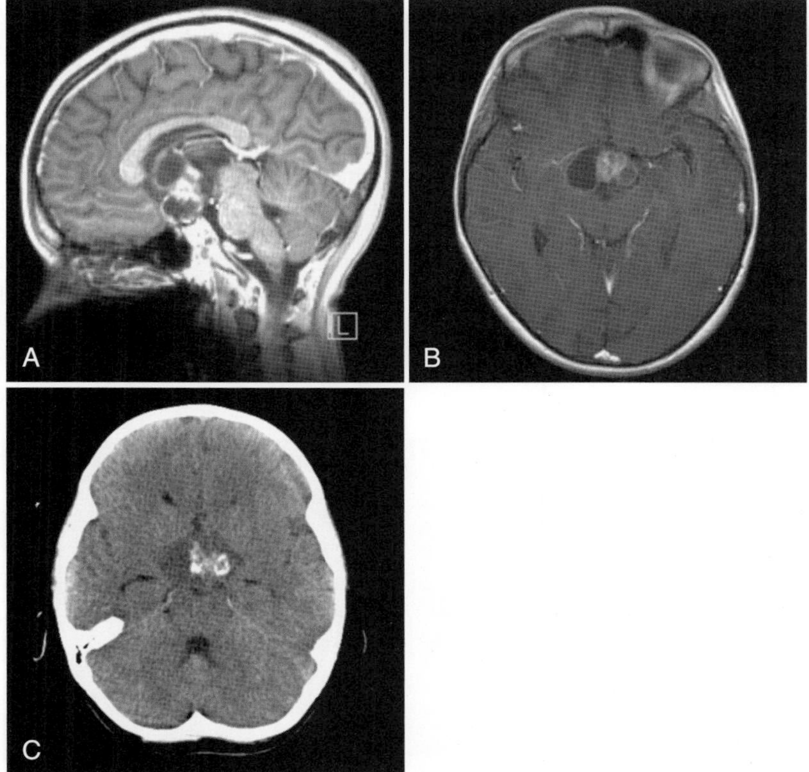


**Fig. 75.11** A 13-year-old girl who presented with a 1-year history of growth deceleration and delay of pubertal development followed by polyuria, nocturia, and polydipsia. **A, B,** Contrast-enhanced cranial magnetic resonance imaging demonstrated a contrast-enhancing, complex, solid and cystic suprasellar mass extending from the sella towards the third ventricle, with encroachment on the left foramen of Monro and displacement of the optic chiasm. **C,** Noncontrast cranial computed tomography revealed calcifications, as evidenced by hyperintense (bright) areas within the solid component of the tumor. Radiological findings were characteristic for a craniopharyngioma. Histopathological diagnosis after gross total resection showed craniopharyngioma, adamantinomatous subtype.

which is currently being evaluated by the German cooperative group (Marchal et al., 2005; Sainte-Rose et al., 2005). Long-term complications of radiation for craniopharyngiomas include cognitive and endocrine deficits, secondary malignancies, optic neuropathy, and vascular injury leading to moyamoya disease. A temporizing approach is the instillation of sclerosing agents such as interferon-alpha, 32P or bleomycin into the tumoral cysts although instillation of bleomycin carries the risk of severe neurotoxicity if the cyst has a leak into the CSF (Kim et al., 2007). Interferon has shown some encouraging results when the short acting or the pegylated form has been given subcutaneously, and more recently the administration of intracystic interferon has shown promise in delaying radiotherapy (Cavalheiro et al., 2010; Kilday et al., 2017). The optimal treatment for cystic craniopharyngioma is still evolving but quality of survival is of paramount importance in the approach.

### Prognosis

The most important factors that correlate with progression-free survival are extent of resection and administration of postoperative radiation. Recurrence occurs in 30% of cases after total resection and in 57% of cases after subtotal resection. The recurrence rate drops to 30% when radiation follows subtotal resection. Unfortunately, most long-term survivors experience significant morbidity related to panhypopituitarism, cognitive impairment, and obesity, and may have a shortened life expectancy from these sequelae (Cohen et al., 2013).

## Choroid Plexus Tumors

Choroid plexus tumors are rare tumors of neuroectodermal origin arising from the epithelium of the choroid plexus of the cerebral ventricles. Although tumors of the choroid plexus represent only 2%–4% of pediatric brain tumors, this group represents 10%–20% of tumors that develop in infancy. Three histological variants are described: choroid plexus papillomas (WHO grade I), atypical papillomas (WHO grade II), and choroid plexus carcinomas (WHO grade III) (Louis et al., 2016). Clear diagnostic criteria for atypical papillomas are not established; however, the presence of mitotic activity (≥2 mitoses per 10 high-power fields) is the sole histological feature independently associated with recurrence (Jeibmann et al., 2006). Choroid plexus papillomas outnumber choroid plexus carcinomas by a ratio of at least 5:1. Choroid plexus tumors are typically located in areas where choroid plexus tissue normally occurs. Most tumors arise from the lateral ventricles (50% of cases) and the fourth ventricle (40%). Choroid plexus carcinoma is associated with the LFS, in which patients have TP53 germline mutations (Merino et al., 2015).

### Clinical Presentation

Initial symptoms are usually secondary to increased ICP and hydrocephalus and include headaches, nausea, and vomiting. Other possible manifestations include lethargy, seizures, and failure to thrive. On physical examination, papilledema is often present. Infants may show irritability, lethargy, vomiting, a tense fontanelle, and macrocephaly with splayed sutures.

### Diagnosis and Management

The diagnosis is suspected when a large enhancing tumor in the lateral ventricle is visualized on contrast-enhanced cranial MRI (Fig. 75.12). Multilobular calcified contrast-enhancing intraventricular masses are characteristic of choroid plexus tumors. Preliminary molecular genetic studies of choroid plexus carcinomas have found several chromosomal losses more frequently in tumors in younger children (<36 months) and chromosomal gains in older patients (Merino et al., 2015). Multivariate analysis revealed that several of the chromosomal alterations were associated with survival. A substantial proportion of choroid plexus carcinomas are in the setting of LFS, and as such all patients should be referred for germline testing and genetic counseling.

The primary treatment objective for both low-grade and high-grade choroid plexus tumors is gross total resection (Lafay-Cousin and Strother, 2009; Sun et al., 2014). However, a major obstacle to surgical removal of choroid plexus tumors, particularly choroid plexus carcinomas, is the rich vascular network within these tumors. The choroid plexus receives its blood supply from the anterior and posterior choroidal arteries, branches of the internal carotid artery, and the posterior cerebral artery (Wolburg and Paulus, 2010). For patients who undergo gross total resection of their choroid plexus carcinomas, the role of adjuvant therapy is unclear. However, there does appear to be a role for neoadjuvant ifosfamide, carboplatin, etoposide (ICE) chemotherapy in patients with choroid plexus carcinomas followed by complete resection, which allows for reduction in blood loss and is compatible with excellent long-term survival (Schneider et al., 2015). The role of adjuvant radiation

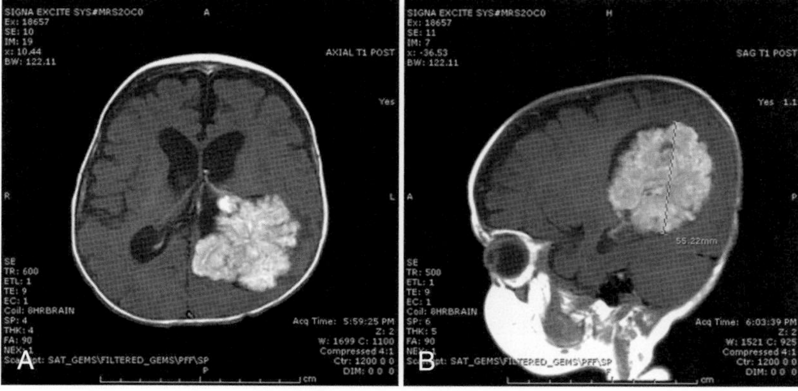


**Fig. 75.12** A 4-month-old boy who presented with irritability and macrocephaly. Contrast-enhanced cranial magnetic resonance imaging demonstrates a large, avidly enhancing heterogeneous mass centered in the trigone and body of the left lateral ventricle, consistent with a choroid plexus papilloma. Vascular flow voids are identified within the mass, which appears to demonstrate a frondlike papillary internal architecture. Branches of the left posterior choroidal arteries supply the lesion with prominent venous vascular structures draining into the internal cerebral veins at the foramen of Munro.

is controversial, particularly in light of a substantial proportion of choroid plexus carcinoma harboring germline *TP53* mutations. Radiation is reserved for older children, those who have had a subtotal resection, and those with malignant features within the tumor or dissemination of the tumor along the neuraxis.

### Prognosis

Gross total resection is often curative for choroid plexus papilloma. Although these benign tumors may disseminate into the CSF, such cases tend to be clinically asymptomatic. The prognosis is significantly worse for choroid plexus carcinomas, particularly those patients with p53 mutations (Gozali et al., 2012; Merino et al., 2015; Tabori et al., 2010). The latter tumors may produce nodular metastases along CSF pathways.

## TREATMENT-RELATED COMPLICATIONS IN INFANTS AND CHILDREN WITH PRIMARY NERVOUS SYSTEM TUMORS

The potential adverse effects of therapy should be considered by the physician before deciding on a particular modality of treatment for an infant or child with a tumor of the nervous system. It is often the profile of the potential late effects of one therapy versus another that determines which modality to apply. The particular importance of this concept in pediatric neuro-oncology is twofold. First, the developing nervous system is especially vulnerable to the toxic effects of chemotherapy and radiation compared with that of adults. Second, given that the chances for long-term survival are increasing for many children with brain tumors, the incidence of late effects is expected to increase as well.

### Surgery

Although radical resection is the objective of surgery for most types of brain tumors, local injury to eloquent neural tissue and postoperative complications, such as hemorrhage, infarcts, and infection, may result in additional neurological injury. Postoperative morbidity has been significantly reduced with the use of newer technology such as MRI-generated neuronavigation and stereotaxis, intraoperative microscopes, and safer techniques for resection (ultrasonic aspirator and laser). Nevertheless, there are several perplexing perioperative neurological syndromes that currently have defied understanding and prevention.

The cerebellar mutism or PFS has a wide range of expression and severity. The majority of patients develop diminished speech output within 24–48 hours of posterior fossa surgery, usually to resect a tumor that has presented with raised ICP. When severe, the mutism is often accompanied by emotional lability, profound hypotonia, dysphagia, and ataxia. Short-term interventions such as corticosteroids or VP shunts do not seem to have a beneficial role, but minor or major tranquilizers may mollify the severity of the behavioral effects. Improvement usually begins within several weeks, but there are often long-lasting if not permanent consequences including dysarthria, ataxia, emotional lability, and learning difficulties. Although PFS was once thought to be a fairly rare occurrence, with better methods of detection, signs of PFS may be found in as many as 40% of patients (Wells et al., 2010).

Aseptic meningitis syndrome often emerges within 1–2 weeks of surgery during a corticosteroid taper. It is thought to be related to the presence of blood and tissue contents mixing with CSF after surgery. Patients develope fever, increased nuchal rigidity, and signs of raised ICP. A pseudomeningocele may evolve, and if the ICP is not relieved, CSF leakage from the operative incision may ensue, leading to a septic meningitis. The simplest remedy is to rule out a septic meningitis by culturing the CSF, increasing the corticosteroid dose, and prolonging its taper (Carmel and Greif, 1993).

### Radiation Therapy

Radiation therapy may produce subacute and late effects on the CNS. Subacute effects include radiation somnolence syndrome (RSS) and Lhermitte sign (see later discussion). The RSS typically emerges within 1–2 months of initiating large-volume, high-dose cranial irradiation. Patients typically become lethargic and anorexic and may develop symptoms that recapitulate the symptoms at presentation of the initial tumor. RSS spontaneously resolves within 3 months in most cases, but occasionally low-dose corticosteroids are required to ameliorate the anorexia (Ryan, 2000). Lhermitte sign consists of a sensation of electric shocks traveling down the spine on neck flexion and usually arises within several months of cervicothoracic spinal radiation (Lewanski et al., 2000). It usually resolves spontaneously within months, without any apparent serious sequelae. Both of these syndromes are probably related to transient parenchymal edema induced by radiation therapy.

Long-term consequences of radiation therapy are becoming more apparent as survival rates increase; some of the more significant include endocrine effects, decrease in cognitive function, vascular effects, and secondary malignancies (Hoffman and Yock, 2009). Endocrine issues, including growth hormone and thyroid hormone deficiency, result from irradiation to the hypothalamus and pituitary glands (Heikens et al., 1998). Linear growth retardation may also result from irradiation to the spine. Neurocognitive studies in children with medulloblastoma treated with craniospinal irradiation have disclosed progressive loss of cognition and short-term memory and slower processing speeds (Mulhern et al., 2005). These deficits are more pronounced in children treated at a younger age and with higher doses of irradiation.

The use of concomitant or adjuvant chemotherapy may increase the acute and delayed neurotoxicity of CNS radiation therapy, or independently produce CNS injury. For example, a progressive leukoencephalopathy may emerge following administration of parenteral or intrathecal methotrexate, usually in the management of childhood acute lymphoid leukemia, and these effects are exacerbated by prior cranial radiation therapy (Mahoney et al., 1998). More severe hearing impairment may occur when cisplatin is used with whole-brain radiation therapy than when cisplatin is given alone (Walker et al., 1989). Pseudoprogression on MRI is more common following CNS radiation therapy when temozolomide and radiation therapy are given concomitantly than when radiation therapy is given alone (Brandsma et al., 2008; Clarke and Chang, 2009).

Radiation necrosis may occur after radiation delivery to the tumor and surrounding brain. The necrotic brain and tumor tissue can cause mass effect, edema, and contrast enhancement on MRI. This complication of radiation may be indistinguishable from progressive or recurrent tumor on conventional neuroimaging studies. In fact, cerebral radionecrosis can produce symptoms identical to those of an expanding tumor, including progressive focal neurological deficits, seizures, and increased ICP. Treatment of cerebral radionecrosis with corticosteroids may result in improvement of clinical symptoms and a reduction in contrast enhancement on CT or MRI studies. Bevacizumab, a monoclonal antibody against the vascular epidermal growth factor receptor (EGFR), decreases cerebrovascular permeability and confers some clinical benefit in adults with cerebral radionecrosis (Gonzalez et al., 2007); however, surgical debulking is often necessary to reduce mass effect and increased ICP. Involvement of small cerebral blood vessels may lead to ischemic strokes. For patients with suprasellar radiation doses exceeding 4000 cGy, progressive large artery stenosis and the development of multiple small collateral vessels may result in a moyamoya pattern of vascular abnormality, which, in turn, increases the risk for stroke or cerebral hemorrhage.

Secondary malignancies, including high-grade gliomas, atypical meningiomas (Santoro et al., 2002), and schwannomas, have been observed within the treatment field several years after the completion of radiation therapy. Patients with Turcot syndrome, Gorlin syndrome, and NF1 are more likely to develop a secondary malignant glioma after radiation therapy, compared with patients without these conditions (Stavrou et al., 2001). This provides additional rationale to defer radiation therapy (when possible) for low-grade gliomas.

As noted earlier in the chapter, in an effort to decrease radiation injury to normal tissues adjacent to a CNS target, protons rather than photons are being used with increasing frequency. Protons deposit their energy at the prescribed depth without the exit dose seen with photon radiation, owing to the Bragg peak effect (Hoffman and Yock, 2009). Although the number of children with CNS tumors treated with protons is still fairly small, the preliminary data—as well as models comparing proton and photon fields—suggest that this approach may result in similar tumor control with greater sparing of uninvolved normal tissue (MacDonald and Yock, 2010; Merchant et al., 2008).

### Chemotherapy

Bone marrow suppression is the most common hematological side effect of chemotherapy. Although this toxicity is usually reversible after suspension of chemotherapy, some patients develop prolonged cytopenias. These patients are at risk for recurrent and opportunistic infections due to neutropenia, hemorrhage due to thrombocytopenia, and fatigue, syncope, and cerebral and cardiac ischemia due to anemia. Secondary malignancies are also a potential late effect of chemotherapy. In children, acute myelogenous leukemia is the most common type of secondary malignancy induced by chemotherapy. Alkylating agents, platinum-based drugs, and etoposide are most commonly involved.

Peripheral neuropathy is a common late effect of several chemotherapies (Quasthoff and Hartung, 2002). Cisplatin and carboplatin mainly affect proprioception and spare pain and temperature sensation. The usual presenting symptoms are painful dysesthesias and tingling sensations in the toes and later in the fingers but sparing motor fibers. In contrast, vincristine produces a sensorimotor neuropathy. The first symptoms are usually tingling in the toes and fingers; loss of ankle jerk is typically the first objective sign. Continued use leads to areflexia and motor weakness involving the dorsiflexors of the feet (foot drop). Patients with preexisting neuropathies may become quadriparetic after treatment with vincristine. Cerebellar syndromes of acute onset may be seen with high-dose cytarabine and occasionally with 5-fluorouracil. These complications are usually reversible within 2 weeks, but severe irreversible damage to Purkinje cells may occur with chronic use of the drug (several months or if the drug is reintroduced) (Friedman and Shetty, 2001). Transverse myelopathy occurs with prolonged treatments with intrathecal methotrexate or cytarabine. The risk is higher when combined with spinal irradiation.

## SUMMARY

Pediatric brain tumors are more diverse in histology, location, and management than the spectrum of tumors that arise in adults. In contrast to the location of primary brain tumors in adults, posterior fossa tumors predominate in children. Pediatric brain tumors present with a variety of symptoms, usually involving nausea, vomiting, morning headaches, and changes in personality. Neurological deficits may not become evident until 1–2 months after the onset of symptoms. An accurate pathological and molecular diagnosis is critical for the management of pediatric brain tumors. Indeed, certain neoplasms have a benign course and a good prognosis after gross total resection, despite a malignant appearance on MRI and light microscopy (e.g., a PXA). Likewise, other tumors, such as a DNET or a central neurocytoma, may be mistaken for oligodendrogliomas. Because of the potentially severe side effects of adjuvant radiation and chemotherapy, these modalities should be reserved for malignant tumors or low-grade tumors that have demonstrated more aggressive behavior. Determining prognosis and managing pediatric brain tumors rely upon an assessment of various clinical, histopathological, and—more recently—molecular characterization of the tumor to more accurately assign a risk category and optimal therapy. Chemotherapy is assuming an increasingly important role in the management of many types of CNS tumors in children. Chemotherapy may not only improve survival but also permit deferral of, or the use of, less radiation therapy. The advent of integrated genomics has resulted in new targeted therapies that are currently being evaluated by cooperative groups, particularly in the realm of low- and high-grade gliomas. The majority of children with primary CNS tumors are managed in specialized pediatric oncology centers affiliated with clinical trials consortia that have access to pediatric subspecialists and a spectrum of support services and resources.

*The complete reference list is available online at https://expertconsult.inkling.com/.*

76

# Nervous System Metastases

*Ugonma Chukwueke, Robert Cavaliere, David Schiff, Patrick Wen, Kristin Huntoon*

## OUTLINE



## BRAIN METASTASES

### Epidemiology

Parenchymal brain metastases (BMs) are the most common direct neurological complication of systemic cancer. BMs are the most common intracranial tumor in adults, with 200,000–300,000 diagnosed annually in the United States (American Brain Tumor Association, 2016). In comparison, there are 35,000 new patients with primary brain tumors diagnosed each year in the United States. The precise incidence of BM is unknown and likely much higher, likely owing to improved tolerability and durability of systemic therapy and advances in imaging. Additionally, it is believed that up to 40% of adult patients with cancer are found to have undiagnosed BM at autopsy (Percy et al., 1970; Posner et al., 1978; Tsukada et al., 1983).

Any solid tumor may metastasize to the brain; however, the incidence of BM varies with the tumor type as well as molecular subtype. The most common primary tumors to metastasize to the brain include lung, breast, and melanoma (Barnholtz-Sloan et al., 2004). A population-based analysis of patients diagnosed with a primary lung, melanoma, renal, or colorectal cancer between 1973 and 2001 suggests that the true incidence percentages are lower than previously estimated (Barnholtz-Sloan et al., 2004). Overall, lung cancer accounts for up to 50% of all patients with BM, and breast cancer accounts for up to 20%. Melanoma, renal cell carcinoma, and gastrointestinal tumors each account for an additional 5%–10% of cases (Lassman and DeAngelis, 2003).

Given the advent of genomic characterization of solid tumors, the molecular subtype of the primary tumor may also influence the risk of development of BM. In breast cancer, the presence of human epidermal growth factor receptor 2 (HER2) amplification or hormone receptor (HR) negative and HER2-negative status have increased risk of development of BM (Martin et al., 2017; Sperduto et al., 2013). In non–small cell lung cancer (NSCLC), anaplastic lymphoma kinase (ALK)–rearranged tumors, the frequency of BM in this population may be up to 40%. In ALK-rearranged NSCLC, among patients who have received prior treatment with ALK tyrosine kinase inhibitors (TKIs), the incidence of BM is approximately 45%–70%.

Additionally, the blood–brain barrier prevents systemic therapeutic agents from entering the central nervous system (CNS), thereby creating a sanctuary for tumor cells. BM can arise anywhere in the brain, and the frequency of such tumors in various locations reflects the relative proportion of cerebral blood flow. Thus 80% of metastases arise in the supratentorial compartment. For unclear reasons, pelvic and gastrointestinal primary tumors are more likely to metastasize to the posterior fossa than to the supratentorial region (Delattre et al., 1988; Quattrochi et al., 2012).

Although most patients develop BM in the setting of known cancer, BM may be an initial manifestation of an underlying primary tumor in 10%–30% of cases (Drlicek et al., 2004). Less than one-fourth of such patients have clinical features suggesting location of the primary tumor. Nonetheless, 80% will eventually have the primary site of tumor identified during their lifetime. Lung cancer is the most common cause of BM presenting without a known primary, accounting for two-thirds of cases. Among lung tumor metastases, in patients with advanced NSCLC, approximately 20% have BM at the time of initial diagnosis (Arrieta et al., 2009; Hanna et al., 2015). A retrospective analysis of 176 patients with newly diagnosed brain masses concluded that chest computed tomography (CT) and brain magnetic resonance imaging (MRI), if used in concert as initial diagnostic studies, would have identified a biopsy site in 97%

of patients with a newly detected intracranial mass (Mavrakis et al., 2005). The high likelihood of a primary lung tumor and the fact that many patients with other primary tumors have lung metastases by the time they develop BM makes restricting initial radiological studies to the chest the more cost-effective approach. Because most BM are multiple, and most patients with BM have a known cancer, only 15% of solitary intracranial masses in patients not known to have cancer turn out to be metastatic tumors (Elder et al., 2019; Voorhies et al., 1980).

## Pathophysiology and Pathology

Parenchymal BM generally arise from hematogenous spread, typically through the arterial circulation directly or through the lymphatic system. Tumor emboli, like all emboli, tend to lodge at the gray/white junction because the caliber of blood vessels narrows at this site. These small emboli enlarge in a spherical fashion, eventually developing central necrosis as they outgrow their blood supply. They are usually associated with substantial surrounding vasogenic edema and well demarcated from the adjacent brain. The surrounding normally functioning brain tissue displaces, and herniation occurs if the displacement is not successfully treated. Metastases from certain primary tumors (squamous cell subtype of NSCLC, melanoma, choriocarcinoma, thyroid, and renal cell carcinoma) have a tendency for intratumoral hemorrhage. This may be attributable to a tendency for neovascularization or because they invade blood vessels.

The histopathology of BM usually closely resembles that of the underlying systemic tumor. BM may have a higher labeling index (percentage of cells going through the cell cycle) than the corresponding systemic tumor, suggesting that their growth rate is faster. Additionally, there is growing understanding that there may be genetic divergence between the primary tumor and BM, which provides an opportunity to investigate further the pathogenesis of BM and therapy.

## Clinical Presentations

BM may occur as long as 20 years after discovery of the primary tumor. Alternatively, BM may even antedate discovery of the underlying systemic cancer, as commonly occurs with lung cancer. Patients with specific subtypes of breast cancer and melanoma may enjoy years of apparent freedom from systemic cancer prior to discovery of cerebral metastasis (Henson and Urich, 1982). Conversely, the triple-negative breast cancers (TNBCs) often have a shorter period between initial diagnosis of primary disease and development of BM (Sperduto et al., 2013). The presenting features are usually progressive over days to weeks, although occasional patients present acutely with seizures or stroke-like syndrome in the setting of intratumoral hemorrhage. Half of patients complain of headache, and a third have mental status changes. Most headaches are indistinguishable from tension headache (Cavaliere, 2008). The "classic" brain tumor headache, which is worse in the mornings or awakens the patient from sleep, is uncommon, and its absence does not preclude the diagnosis of a brain tumor. Headache in the absence of other symptoms is more likely to be due to multiple metastases than a single metastasis. Over time, headache from brain metastasis becomes progressively more severe and may be accompanied by nausea, vomiting, and drowsiness. Unilateral weakness and gait disturbances are other common presenting complaints. Seizures are present at diagnosis in 18% of patients with BM (Cohen et al., 1988). Mental status changes and hemiparesis are the most common findings on neurological examination; each is present in approximately 60% of patients (Posner, 1995). Despite the frequent occurrence of increased intracranial pressure (ICP), papilledema is detectable in only 10% of patients.

## Differential Diagnosis

Several neurological conditions may mimic BM both clinically and radiographically. A primary brain tumor must be a consideration, especially in patients with a single brain mass. This is a particularly important consideration in patients with breast cancer and a dural-based tumor (Schoenberg et al., 1975). Abscess, demyelination, progressive multifocal leukoencephalopathy, cerebrovascular disease, and the effects of radiation or chemotherapy also simulate BM, both clinically and radiographically. Although the clinical syndrome and the neuroimaging studies usually provide a diagnosis, tissue sampling is often necessary for diagnosis or for symptomatic control of disease and to facilitate adjuvant therapy.

## Neuroimaging

Neuroimaging advances since the early 1970s have made the diagnosis of BM relatively straightforward in almost all cases. Noncontrast MRI is as sensitive as contrast-enhanced CT for detection of BM. Use of gadolinium-containing contrast agents dramatically improves the sensitivity of MRI, making it markedly superior to contrast-enhanced CT scanning (Fig. 76.1) (Yuh, et al., 1995).

In the pre-MRI era, approximately half of all patients were found to have a single brain metastasis, likely owing to the limits of detection of CT. It is now believed that solitary brain metastasis is relatively infrequent, and it is more common to have multiple BM. Approximately, 75% of patients with BM have multiple metastases when studied with MRI (Davis et al., 1991; Sze et al., 1990). Lung cancer and melanoma are somewhat more likely to produce multiple cerebral metastases, whereas renal cell, breast, and colon cancer tend to produce single metastases (Delattre et al., 1988). In addition to the number of BM (solitary vs. multiple), the size of the lesion also carries implications with regards to therapy, which will be discussed in subsequent sections on management.

## Management

### Supportive Care

Although other chapters address corticosteroids and antiepileptic drug (AED) usage, a few comments pertinent to their rational use in BM are appropriate. Corticosteroids improve symptoms associated with BM and should be considered for temporary symptomatic relief. One randomized controlled trial examined different doses in patients with BM. Patients with cerebral metastases and a Karnofsky Performance Score (KPS) (Table 76.1) less than or equal to 80 were randomized in two consecutive studies to 4 mg versus 16 mg and 8 mg versus 16 mg dexamethasone. All patients received standardized whole-brain radiotherapy (WBRT) after receiving dexamethasone for 1 week. At 1 week, patients treated with lower doses had similar outcomes to those treated with higher doses of dexamethasone. Patients treated with higher doses had increased toxicity at 1 month. The authors concluded that unless patients were in danger of herniation, 2 mg twice daily was an appropriate starting dose (Vecht et al., 1994). Although corticosteroids are part of the mainstay for management of peritumoral edema associated with BM, higher doses of corticosteroids are associated with increased toxicity (Table 76.2) (Arvold et al., 2018).

Approximately 20% of patients with BM present with seizures and require treatment with standard anticonvulsants. The use of prophylactic anticonvulsants in patients who have not had seizures is controversial. Fewer than 20% of these patients experience seizures later in the course of their illness, and this risk does not appear to be reduced with prophylactic anticonvulsants. A systematic review of the topic, specifically among patients with BM, concluded that the risk of seizure within 3 months was low (10%) and prophylaxis was not warranted (Mikkelsen et al., 2010). This agrees with other studies that evaluated prophylaxis in patients with all types of brain tumors (not limited to metastases) (Tremont-Lukats et al., 2008). Consequently, the American Academy of Neurology (AAN) has issued a practice parameter recommending against the prophylactic use of anticonvulsants in patients with brain tumors who have not had a seizure (Glantz et al., 2000). A more recent randomized study evaluated the role of phenytoin for 1 week in seizure-free patients following surgery to reduce the risk of seizure in the immediate postoperative period. The risk of seizure was in general low (8%) during this time and the use of prophylaxis did not alter the risk. Furthermore, toxicity was higher in the group that received phenytoin (Wu et al., 2013a,b). A subsequent study compared levetiracetam, a newer antiseizure agent, to phenytoin in patients undergoing craniotomy for resection of supratentorial tumor (Iuchi et al., 2015): 146 patients were randomized to either levetiracetam or phenytoin with primary endpoint of seizure and secondary endpoint of frequency of side effects. The incidence of seizure in the levetiracetam cohort was 1.4% compared to 15.1% with phenytoin. There were no treatment-related side effects with levetiracetam, where phenytoin was discontinued in five patients (Iuchi et al., 2015), indicating that levetiracetam is preferred to phenytoin. Potential exceptions to the AAN guideline include patients with metastases from melanoma (which may be more epileptogenic because of multiplicity or hemorrhage), tumors in motor cortex, or concomitant parenchymal and leptomeningeal disease

In contrast to seizure-free patients, those with seizures do require anticonvulsant therapy. Although efficacy is similar among the available anticonvulsants, differences in pharmacokinetic profile may influence which agent is used. Anticonvulsants metabolized by the P450 system interact with corticosteroids and many common antineoplastic therapies such as irinotecan and erlotinib. Consequently, the effectiveness of a given dosage of dexamethasone may be decreased, and tumor exposure to an antineoplastic agent may be reduced. Examples of enzyme-inducing anticonvulsants include phenytoin and carbamazepine. Alternatively, newer, nonenzyme-inducing agents such as levetiracetam and lacosamide do not interact with other medications administered concurrently. In addition, the side-effect profile of the more modern agents is more favorable, further supporting their use as first-line therapies.

### Radiation Therapy

While the goals of radiation therapy (RT) are to alleviate neurological deficits and provide disease control, whether or not RT prolongs survival or improves quality of life has yet to be demonstrated in a randomized clinical trial. The Quality of Life After Treatment for Brain Metastases (QUARTZ) study was a phase III, randomized non-inferiority trial in which patients with NSCLC BM were randomized 1:1 to either optimal supportive care (OSC) with dexamethasone and WBRT or OSC alone (Mulvenna et al., 2016). The primary outcome was quality-adjusted life years (QALYs), which was generated from OS

**TABLE 76.1 Karnofsky Performance Status**

| | |
|---|---|
| KPS 100 | Normal; no complaints, no evidence of disease |
| KPS 90 | Able to carry on normal activity; minor signs or symptoms of disease |
| KPS 80 | Normal activity with effort; some signs or symptoms of disease |
| KPS 70 | Cares for self; unable to carry on normal activity or do active work |
| KPS 60 | Requires occasional assistance but is able to care for most personal needs |
| KPS 50 | Requires considerable assistance and frequent medical care |
| KPS 40 | Disabled; requires special care and assistance |
| KPS 30 | Severely disabled; hospitalization is indicated, although death not imminent |
| KPS 20 | Very sick; hospitalization necessary, active support treatment necessary |
| KPS 10 | Moribund; fatal processes progressing rapidly |
| KPS 0 | Dead |

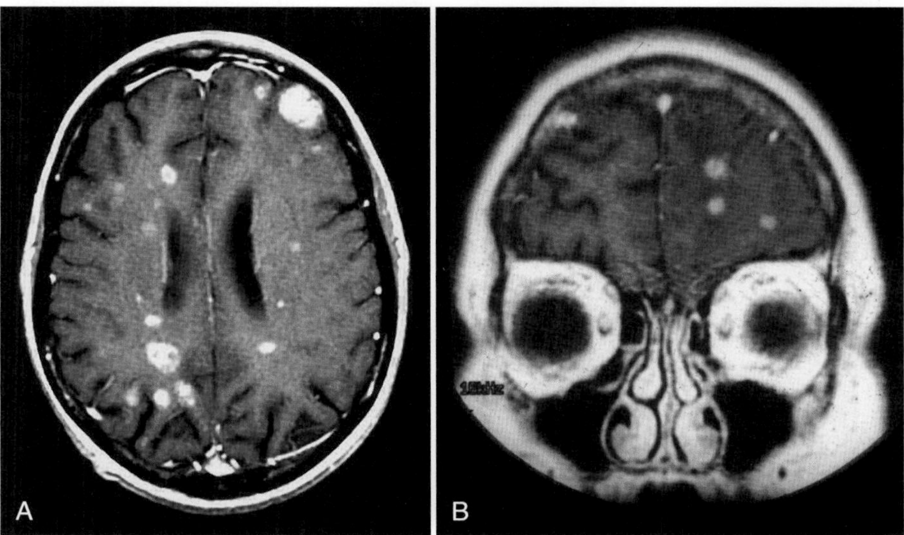


**Fig. 76.1** (A) Axial and (B) coronal T1-weighted, contrast-enhanced magnetic resonance image of the brain of a 58-year-old woman with breast cancer treated 1 year previously with whole-brain radiation therapy for brain metastases, who presents with multiple recurrent lesions. Treatment options are limited to chemotherapy or re-irradiation.

and patient-reported questionnaires. In this study, there was no difference in OS between the WBRT-treated and OSC-alone groups, with a difference in mean QALYs was 4.7 days, thus suggesting that WBRT did not provide an additional clinical benefit for patients in this group (Mulvenna et al., 2016).

For those patients treated with RT, the Radiation Therapy Oncology Group (RTOG) database has permitted the application of statistical techniques such as recursive partitioning analysis (RPA) to separate patients with BM treated with WBRT into different prognostic classes based on clinical features at presentation. Patients with BM can be divided into three classes. Class 1 consists of patients with a KPS greater than or equal to 70, age younger than 65 years, primary site of tumor resected or controlled with treatment, and no extracranial sites of metastatic tumor. Such patients have a median survival of 7.1 months. Class 3 is composed of all patients whose KPS is less than 70; the median survival in this group is only 2.3 months. Class 2 contains all patients who do not fall into classes 1 and 3; class 2 patients have a median survival of 4.2 months (Gaspar et al., 1997). Subsequent studies have validated these results (Gaspar et al., 2000). The limited number of patients with KPS less than 70 in the RTOG dataset precluded further analysis of this population.

**TABLE 76.2 Side Effects of Corticosteroids**

| Involved Organ System | Side Effect |
|---|---|
| Neurological/psychiatric | Insomnia |
| | Mood lability |
| | Anxiety/depression |
| | Psychosis |
| | Increased appetite |
| | Hiccups |
| | Tremor |
| Musculoskeletal | Proximal myopathy |
| | Osteoporosis |
| | Arthralgias |
| | Avascular necrosis |
| | Decreased growth/height (pediatric patients) |
| Gastrointestinal | Dyspepsia/gastritis |
| Hematological/immunlogical | Immunosuppression-related infections (oropharyngeal candidiasis, *Pneumocytis jiroveci* pneumonia) |
| Endocrine | Hyperglycemia |
| | Weight gain |
| | Cushingoid habitus |
| | Adrenal insufficiency (after discontinuation) |
| Cutaneous or vascular | Acne |
| | Striae |
| | Delayed wound healing |
| | Peripheral edema |
| Ocular | Visual blurring |
| | Cataract formation |

### Graded Prognostic Assessment

Survival following diagnosis of BM is dependent upon several factors, including primary tumor of origin. Given the limitations of existing prognostic indices at the time, the need for a reliable prognostic assessment for guidance of treatment led to the development of the graded prognostic assessment (GPA), which was found to be as prognostic as earlier prognostic measures and easier to use (Sperduto et al., 2008). The GPA is the sum of score (0, 0.5, and 1) for four factors, comprising age, KPS, extracranial metastases (none or present), and number of BM (1, 2–3, or >3) (Table 76.3). Subsequently, the diagnosis-specific GPA (DS-GPA) was proposed, incorporating both the primary diagnosis and criteria from RPA. Using data obtained from a retrospective analysis of 4259 patients with newly diagnosed BM, treated between 1985 and 2007, separate criteria were developed for patients with melanoma, lung, renal cell, breast, and gastrointestinal (GI) cancers. In this analysis, prognostic factors varied by diagnosis: in lung cancer, functional status, age, presence of extracranial disease, and number of BMs were significant, whereas only functional status was significant for breast and GI cancers (Table 76.4). Separate DS-GPAs are currently under investigation for specific cancers, including NSCLC with incorporation of molecular markers and melanoma (Sperduto et al., 2017a, 2017b).

***Radiation toxicity.*** With standard fractionation schemes, WBRT is tolerated well. Toxicity associated with radiation varies according to the duration of time following treatment: acute toxicity occurs during or within 6 weeks of completion of therapy, early-delayed appears up to 6 months from treatment completion, and late effects present at least 6 months after treatment. Acutely, patients may experience fatigue, alopecia, anorexia, nausea, and vomiting. Early-delayed effects may include fatigue, transient neurological worsening, or symptoms

**TABLE 76.3 Graded Prognostic Assessment for Brain Metastases from Solid Tumors**

| GPA of Newly Diagnosed BMs | Significant Prognostic Factors | GPA Scoring Criteria | | | | |
|---|---|---|---|---|---|---|
| NSCLC/SCLC | | 0 | 0.5 | 1 | — | — |
| | Age | >60 | 50–60 | <50 | — | — |
| | KPS | <70 | 70–80 | 90–100 | — | — |
| | ECM | Present | — | Absent | — | — |
| | No. of BMs | >3 | 2–3 | 1 | — | — |
| Melanoma/renal cell cancer | | 0 | 1 | 2 | — | — |
| | KPS | <70 | 70–80 | 90–100 | — | — |
| | No. of BMs | >3 | 2–3 | 1 | — | — |
| Breast/GI cancer | | 0 | 1 | 2 | 3 | 4 |
| | KPS | <70 | 70 | 80 | 90 | 100 |

*BM*, Brain metastases; *ECM*, Extracranial metastases; *GI*, gastrointestinal; *GPA*, graded prognostic assessment; *KPS*, Karnofsky Performance Score; *NSCLC*, non-small cell lung cancer; *SCLC*, small cell lung cancer.

related to pseudoprogression. Headache and nausea are generally alleviated with corticosteroids and antiemetics. In poor-prognosis patients, the acute side effects of WBRT must be considered, however, as they may have a significant impact on the quality of the remaining short predicted life span (Komosinska et al., 2010).

Long-term survivors of BM are at risk of suffering late complications of WBRT, of which neurocognitive effects are the most feared. Of WBRT recipients for BM, as many as 10%–30% develop cognitive impairment by 1 year if radiation doses per fraction exceed 300 cGy (Behin and Delattre, 2002). Symptoms commonly include poor short-term memory, abulia, gait unsteadiness, and urinary urgency. MRI frequently reveals extensive symmetrical periventricular white matter changes termed radiation leukoencephalopathy, ventriculomegaly, and sometimes cortical atrophy. The clinical picture may resemble normal-pressure hydrocephalus, but a positive durable response to ventriculoperitoneal shunt is rare (DeAngelis et al., 1989). Because the risk of this complication is greater with larger fraction sizes, radiation oncologists treat patients with good prognosis with 20 fractions of 200 cGy or similar regimens.

Neurocognitive decline in the setting of cancer is multifactorial, and establishing attribution is difficult. Progressive CNS disease, concurrent use of chemotherapy and other pharmacological agents (such as antiseizure medications), depression/anxiety, and neurological impairment, among other factors, may contribute. It is also recognized that patients with cancer may have cognitive impairment prior to any treatment or intervention. The true incidence of neurocognitive impairment from WBRT is unknown due to limitations of the available data to date. Many studies have relied on the Mini-Mental Status Examination (MMSE) assessment, which is not optimal given that these brief scales lack sensitivity and may not capture longitudinal decline in function when compared to formal neurocognitive testing (Phua et al., 2018). Comprehensive neurocognitive assessments that evaluate multiple cognitive domains provide more meaningful data but require expertise and are more expensive and labor intensive. Neurocognitive endpoints are increasingly being recognized as critical determinants of outcomes and are being used as primary measures of effectiveness in modern cerebral metastases studies. In contrast, overall survival is often used as a primary endpoint despite the fact that the majority of patients die of concurrent systemic disease. As neurocognitive toxicity related to cranial irradiation may present similarly to other neurodegenerative processes, an investigation of alternate or reversible etiologies should be undertaken.

Measures to mitigate the neurocognitive toxicity associated with WBRT have been under investigation. Neuroprotective strategies to date have included prophylactic use of memantine, an oral *N*-methyl-D-aspartate (NMDA) inhibitor, and use of hippocampal-sparing techniques during delivery of radiation. In a randomized, placebo-controlled study of 508 patients receiving WBRT, 256 patients received memantine starting 3 days prior to start of WBRT, which was continued for 6 months (Brown et al., 2013). Due to patient attrition, only 149 total patients were eligible for analysis, among which there was no difference in rate of memory decline between the two treatment groups, which was the primary endpoint. There was a trend toward delaying time to development of cognitive decline which favored the memantine-treated cohort; however, this was not statistically significant (Brown et al., 2013). In addition to memantine, donepezil, an anticholinergic typically used for mild to moderate Alzheimer's disease, has also been studied in this context, with modest benefit (Rapp et al., 2015, Shaw et al., 2006).

**TABLE 76.4 Recursive Partitioning Analysis of Prognostic Factors in Brain Metastases from Solid Tumors**

| | SCORE | | |
|---|---|---|---|
| | 0 | 0.5 | 1.0 |
| Age | >60 | 50–59 | <50 |
| KPS | <70 | 70–80 | 90–100 |
| No. of CNS metastases | >3 | 2–3 | 1 |
| Extracranial metastases | Present | — | None |

*CNS*, Central nervous system; *KPS*, Karnofsky Performance Score.

Hippocampal-avoidance radiation has been studied as well, given the role of the hippocampus in memory formation. A single-arm, phase II study of hippocampal-sparing was done in 113 patients with BM without involvement of the hippocampus. In comparison to historical controls, use of hippocampal avoidance was associated with lower rates of decline in recall in the 42 evaluable patients. In the subsequent phase III trial, the addition of memantine to hippocampal-avoidance WBRT led to reduction of risk of cognitive failure by 26%, in comparison to hippocampal-sparing WBRT alone. There were no differences noted in toxicity, progression-free survival (PFS), OS, or intracranial progression (Gondi et al., 2018).

***Prophylactic cranial irradiation.*** BMs are extremely common in small cell lung cancer (SCLC), being present in 10% of patients at diagnosis, increasing to 20% during therapy, and by some reports, up to 80% of patients with SCLC will have BM at autopsy (Jeyapalan and Henson, 2002; Nugent et al., 1979). At 2 years post-diagnosis, the cumulative risk of brain metastasis is 47% for patients with limited disease and 69% for those with extensive disease. Presumably the brain is a pharmacological sanctuary for microscopic tumor against systemic chemotherapy, which does not penetrate the intact blood–brain barrier. This has led to numerous trials designed to test whether prophylactic cranial irradiation (PCI) would decrease the incidence of brain relapse and improve survival in patients who achieved systemic CR in limited-staged SCLC (LS-SCLC, defined as disease confined to one hemithorax). A consistent finding was that PCI in LS-SCLC significantly decreased the risk of cerebral metastases. An often-cited meta-analysis of these studies indicated that PCI reduced the risk of subsequent brain metastasis (59% vs. 33% at 3 years) and modestly increased 3-year survival from 15.3% to 20.7% ($P = .01$) (Auperin et al., 1999). There was also suggestion of a dose response, although this was not confirmed in a recent randomized study in which patients were randomized to 25 or 36 Gy (Le Pechoux et al., 2009).

The role of PCI in patients with incomplete response to treatment or with extensive small-cell lung cancer remains unclear. The poor prognosis of these patients (median survival of 9 months) brings into question the utility of PCI. Slotman et al. randomized patients with extensive small-cell lung cancer that responded to treatment to observation or PCI. Patients treated with PCI had a cumulative risk of symptomatic BM of 14.6% compared to 40.4% among observation patients. Patients treated with PCI also had longer median overall survival (6.7 months vs. 5.4 months) with 1-year survival also favoring the PCI treated group (27% vs. 13%) (Slotman et al., 2007).

Although PCI appears to be well-tolerated, controversy still remains over whether the benefits of PCI outweigh its toxicities, particularly leukoencephalopathy. Two large prospective randomized trials of PCI did not document increased neuropsychological deficits among PCI recipients. Others argue that the small numbers of long-term survivors in these trials precluded accurate assessment of the risk of leukoencephalopathy, and that because PCI benefited only about a fourth of its recipients, it should not be considered standard therapy.

### Surgery

For several decades, neurosurgeons resected single BM in selected patients and argued that surgery produced better results than radiotherapy alone, particularly noting improvement in the percentage of long-term survivors. In 1990, a seminal randomized controlled trial verified the neurosurgeons' contention. In this study, eligible patients had a single surgically accessible metastasis identified by contrast CT or MRI scan. Patients with highly radiosensitive primary tumors were excluded. Enrolled patients were randomized to biopsy followed by WBRT (36 Gy in 12 fractions) versus resection and WBRT. Patients who underwent surgical resection of the metastasis followed by RT developed fewer local recurrences (20% vs. 52%) and significantly improved survival (40 weeks vs. 15 weeks) compared to those patients who received only a biopsy and RT. Patients who underwent surgical resection also had improved performance status and a reduced risk of dying as a result of neurological causes. Multivariate analysis showed that surgery and longer time between diagnosis of the primary tumor and the development of BM were associated with increased survival, whereas disseminated disease and increasing age were associated with decreased survival (Patchell et al., 1990). A significant prolongation in overall survival and improvement in quality of life among patients who underwent resection prior to whole-brain radiation was also noted in the randomized study by Vecht et al. (1993). The only patients who benefited from surgery, however, were those with stable extracranial disease. The results of these studies are in contrast to findings by Mintz et al. (1996) in their randomized study in which there was not survival benefit among patients with BM undergoing surgery. However, a higher proportion of patients in this study had active systemic disease, possibly influencing the results, as these were likely patients with poorer performance status. Thus, in patients with surgically accessible single BM and absent or controlled systemic cancer, surgical resection became the standard of care.

Alternatively, focal radiation to the surgical bed may reduce the risk of local recurrence, as patients with a solitary brain metastasis undergoing resection have 50%–60% risk of local recurrence over the following year (Kocher et al., 2011; Mahajan et al., 2017; Regine et al., 2002 ). Several retrospective studies examining the role of postoperative radiosurgery to the surgical bed found that focused radiation is efficacious in controlling local tumor growth and maintaining long-term quality of life (Jagannathan et al., 2009). Stereotactic radiosurgery (SRS) to the resection cavity has been a preferred approach for patients following resection of a solitary brain metastasis, thus improving local control and avoiding potential for neurocognitive side effects. In a randomized phase III trial of 194 patients with 1 resected brain metastasis and surgical cavity less than 5 cm, patients were randomized to either SRS or WBRT. At the time of follow-up, there was no difference in overall survival; however, cognitive decline was more frequent in the WBRT cohort (Brown et al., 2017). In a separate, randomized phase III trial comparing SRS to observation, 132 patients with BM (up to three treated with surgical resection) were randomized to either observation or SRS (Mahajan et al., 2017). Primary endpoint was local recurrence in the resection cavity: 72% of patients treated with SRS remained free from disease at 12 months in comparison to 43% of patients on observation (Mahajan et al., 2017).

### Multiple Metastases

Although the evidence presented in the previous section documents current concepts regarding treatment of solitary lesions, 50% of patients present with multiple BM. Autopsy studies indicate that 60%–85% of patients with BM have multiple lesions (Bindal et al., 1993). In the past, multiple brain lesions represented a relative contraindication to surgery due to the presumed poor survival of these patients. However, application of principles learned in studies regarding surgery for solitary lesions has yielded evidence suggesting that patients with multiple tumors may derive benefits from surgical resection similar to those of patients with solitary lesions. Currently, there is no level I evidence regarding the surgical treatment of patients with multiple BM (Siu et al., 2011). Some retrospective reviews have suggested a role for surgery in select patients, though the overall benefit of resection of a single symptomatic brain metastasis in the setting of multiple BM is unknown.

***Role of surgery in multiple metastases.*** One of the first large studies to review surgery for patients with multiple BM was Bindal et al. (1993), which retrospectively reviewed 56 patients with multiple BM. In group A, one or more lesions were not surgically removed, and in group B all lesions were resected. Patients in group B were compared to a cohort of patients with solitary lesions who underwent surgical resection matched by primary tumor, time from cancer diagnosis to brain metastasis, and status of systemic disease at the time of surgery (group C). Variables such as KPS, age, primary tumor, and systemic disease were similar between all three groups. All patients underwent postoperative WBRT. Median overall survival was 6 months for group A and 14 months for both group B and group C. Rates of surgical morbidity and mortality were similar between all groups, and a higher number of craniotomies per surgery was not associated with increased complication rate. Thus, surgery for resection of all lesions in patients with multiple tumors, up to 3 total, was determined to be as safe and effective as surgery for solitary tumors and provided significant survival benefit in patients amenable to surgical resection of all lesions.

Paek et al. (2005) retrospectively reviewed patients who underwent surgery for BM. Of 208 cases reviewed, 76 patients had multiple lesions and 17 of these underwent resection of two or more metastases. No differences in overall survival were seen when comparing patients with solitary metastases to those with two or three metastases. Evaluation of subgroups based on RPA class was performed. The authors concluded that surgical resection should be considered in patients with solitary and multiple BM, but that RPA class III solitary lesions and RPA class II multiple lesions may benefit more from SRS alone.

Based on available literature, surgical resection for patients with multiple metastases is indicated in a select group of patients. These patients have a low number of lesions (two or three) which are surgically accessible. Other favorable factors include stable systemic disease, high performance status, and age less than 65. However, patients who meet these criteria represent a relatively small subset of all patients who present with multiple metastases. Only approximately one-third of patients diagnosed with BM will be possible surgical candidates (Kalkanis et al., 2010).

Patients with a large number of BM are often not considered surgical candidates. In the retrospective reviews evaluating surgery in patients with multiple metastases (Bindal et al., 1993; Paek et al., 2005), most patients underwent one or two craniotomies to access one to three tumors. In general, better outcomes were observed in cases where all tumors were resected, and no patient had more than three craniotomies. However, certain clinical scenarios may warrant consideration for surgical intervention in these patients. For example, patients who present with poor or declining functional status in the setting of numerous BM may have a dominant lesion, or a specific lesion suspected of being the primary cause of the neurological decline. If the culprit lesion is removed, the patient's functional status may improve rapidly. Examples include lesions causing hydrocephalus or lesions with significant edema causing mass effect with midline shift and resulting altered mental status (Sunderland et al., 2016). Lesions affecting eloquent structures such as primary motor or speech areas may also cause significant neurological impairment either directly or indirectly, and surgical resection may allow significant rapid improvement in performance status. In these clinical settings, resection of a limited number of lesions thought to be directly responsible for neurological decline may allow for restoration of higher functional status and improved survival. However, as discussed in earlier section, the overall benefit of this approach has yet to be determined.

### Whole-Brain Radiotherapy in Multiple Metastases

Radiation has historically played an important role in the management of cerebral metastases. Its role, however, has evolved over the years as technology advanced. Consequently, several treatment paradigms have evolved. Central to the debate on cerebral metastases is balancing the toxicity of treatment against control of cerebral disease.

WBRT has long been a staple in the management of cerebral metastases. The rationale behind its use lies in the recognition of microscopic deposits seeding the brain in addition to macroscopic, visible disease. As such, it served to not only treat the visible disease but also prevent the development of new tumors. Consequently, neurological morbidity associated with progressive and new disease could be averted. The benefits of WBRT in patients with single metastatic deposits were first documented in the seminal randomized study by Patchell et al. (1998) in which patients who underwent a resection were randomized to radiation or observation. Although overall survival was identical between the two groups, the rate of local and distant control was better among treated patients. In addition, there was a significant reduction in neurological death.

Despite the apparent benefits of WBRT, long-term neurological toxicity remains a notable concern. This is particularly true as the number of long-term survivors increases. The exact incidence of neurocognitive impairment from WBRT is unknown. With neurocognitive testing, abnormalities can be seen in nearly half of patients after WBRT (Sun et al., 2011). Furthermore, treatments for the sequelae are limited. WBRT can be administered only once as the risks increase further with additional courses. As such, the routine use of WBRT in patients with limited disease limits future options in the event of CNS recurrence. Consequently, the routine use of WBRT was brought into question. With the evolution of stereotactic radiotherapeutic techniques, alternative treatment paradigms were developed. Specifically, treating macroscopic visible disease in select patients with a limited number of metastatic deposits (usually <4) and deferring WBRT became a common approach. However, the negative impact of CNS progression must be weighed against the disadvantages of early WBRT.

### Stereotactic Radiosurgery for Multiple Metastases

Like conventional surgery, SRS has emerged as a means of enhancing long-term local control of BM while also reducing risk of acute toxicity. SRS is a technique of external irradiation that uses multiple convergent beams to deliver a high single dose of radiation to a radiographically well-circumscribed treatment volume. SRS is generally administered either with a Gamma Knife apparatus or a modified linear accelerator. With either technique, the use of a stereotactic head frame secured to the head with screws and the radiation delivery system allow for great precision, with a rapid drop-off in radiation dose within millimeters of the target lesion, sparing normal brain the potentially deleterious consequences of high-dose radiation.

SRS offers several advantages to conventional surgery. SRS offers the potential of treating lesions in locations generally considered surgically inaccessible. Metastases in eloquent cortex, basal ganglia, thalamus, and even the brainstem can be treated with relatively low risk. In addition, multiple lesions can be treated with SRS simultaneously with significantly less risk. SRS is also more cost-effective than surgery and can be performed in an outpatient setting. A technical limitation of SRS, compared to conventional surgery, is the inability to treat metastases greater than 3.5 cm in median diameter due to excessive radiation toxicity. SRS has been frequently used to treat up to 4 BM; a greater number of lesions typically is treated with WBRT. SRS is sometimes associated with increased symptomatic edema, often necessitating treatment with corticosteroids and sometimes requiring surgical intervention. Surgery will alleviate mass effect quickly and allow for more rapid and complete discontinuation of corticosteroids.

Numerous single-institution experiences with radiosurgery for single or oligometastatic brain lesions have been published. In a review summarizing published series comprising more than 2000 patients treated over 8 years in the 1990s, Loeffler et al. (1999) found that SRS achieved permanent local control in more than 80% of patients, with complications in fewer than 10% (mainly radiation necrosis). Outcome appeared independent of the number of metastases treated. Median survival following SRS is approximately 9–10 months, very similar to surgical series. This raised the question of whether SRS can be performed in lieu of resection. An RTOG clinical trial has affirmed this hypothesis by randomizing patients with one to three BM to WBRT with or without SRS. Patients with a single brain metastasis had a significant survival benefit as well as improved performance status from the addition of SRS, as did patients younger than 50 and those in RPA class 1 (Andrews et al., 2004). Collectively, although the available data suggest similar efficacy of SRS and surgery, a randomized study comparing the two modalities has not been performed. Nonetheless, SRS may be an alternative to resection in select patients.

One consistent and remarkable finding across numerous SRS series is that metastases from highly radio-resistant tumors like melanoma and renal cell carcinoma, which respond very poorly to fractionated radiotherapy, respond virtually as well to SRS as tumors far more sensitive to conventional radiation. However, intracranial failure rates of highly radio-resistant tumors without WBRT were 25.8% and 48.3% at 3 and 6 months, respectively, according to a recent phase II trial conducted by the Eastern Cooperative Oncology Group. Therefore, delaying adjuvant WBRT may be appropriate for some subgroups of patients with radio-resistant tumors, but routine avoidance of WBRT should be approached judiciously (Manon et al., 2005).

Approximately 7% of metastases treated with SRS transiently increase in diameter on scan, reflecting a radiation reaction. According to an evidence-based review by the American Society for Therapeutic Radiation and Oncology (ASTRO), in selected patients with small (<4 cm) BM (up to three in number and four in one randomized trial), radiosurgery boost with WBRT improves local brain control compared to WBRT alone. Similarly, in patients with a single brain metastasis, radiosurgery boost following WBRT improves survival. In selected patients treated with radiosurgery alone for newly diagnosed BM, overall survival is not altered (Lutterbach et al., 2008). However, omission of upfront WBRT was associated with markedly poorer local and distant brain control (Tsao et al., 2005).

The relative effectiveness of radiosurgery versus surgery alone in patients with BM has never been ascertained. A retrospective review from the Mayo Clinic compared the efficacy of neurosurgery versus radiosurgery in local tumor control and patient survival in patients with solitary BM. There was no significant difference in patient survival ($P = .15$) between the 74 neurosurgery patients and the 23 radiosurgery patients. The 1-year survival rates for the neurosurgery and radiosurgery groups were 62% and 56%, respectively. There was a significant ($P = .020$) difference in local tumor control, but none of the radiosurgery group had local recurrence compared with 19 (58%) in the neurosurgery group (O'Neill et al., 2003). Although surgeons occasionally remove two or even three BM, surgery is generally restricted to single lesions, whereas multiple lesions generally present no problems for radiosurgery. Radiosurgery appears more cost-effective than surgery, although surgery alleviates symptoms of mass effect much more rapidly and reliably than SRS. In a single-institution retrospective review of 213 patients with large, previously treated BM (> 4 cm), 66 were treated with SRS alone and 157 were treated with surgical resection followed by SRS. The rate of local recurrence at 1 year was lower in the surgery and SRS group (20.5% vs. 36.7%); however, the rate of radiation necrosis was higher at 1 year (22.6% vs. 12.3%) (Prabhu et al., 2017). Phase III trials comparing these two modalities have been proposed, but no major multicenter study has yet been undertaken.

The role of WBRT following radiosurgery for BM is also uncertain. Two retrospective cohort studies have examined this issue. Pirzkall et al. (1998) compared outcomes in 158 patients treated with radiosurgery alone versus 78 receiving radiosurgery plus fractionated WBRT. All patients had three or fewer BM. The overall median survival was 5.5 months, with no difference between treatment groups. However, median survival in patients without extracranial tumor was increased in patients getting both forms of radiation (15.4 vs. 8.3 months, $P = .08$). A trend existed for superior local control in patients getting combined therapy. In a phase III EORTC trial of 359 patients with one to three BM treated with either SRS or surgical resection, 100 patients were randomized to observation and 99 to WBRT following SRS, while 79 patients were randomized to observation and 81 to WBRT following surgery. Although there was decreased intracranial relapse rate in the WBRT-treated group, there was no difference in overall survival between the observation group and WBRT (10.7 and 10.9 months) (Kocher et al., 2011).

### Fractionated Stereotactic Radiotherapy

Fractionated stereotactic radiotherapy (FSRT) is another radiotherapeutic modality that utilizes multiple beams that converge on a well-defined target. Similar to SRS, use of multiple beams reduces exposure to normal tissue by spreading out the dose as it passes through normal tissue before converging on the target lesion. In addition, the intensity of the individual beam can be modulated, allowing greater control of dose distribution. The increased conformality of the treatments allows for the delivery of a higher dose per fraction, which may have radiobiological advantages. FSRT does not require external fixation and can be done with a mask similar to conventional radiation. Fractionation requires multiple treatments, often single doses administered over 3–5 days. Treatment planning is more complex and requires more time. Compared to SRS, FSRT is not limited by the size of the lesion, so larger lesions can be treated. However, higher doses can still be delivered to target lesions. As such, it has emerged as another stereotactic option for patients with cerebral metastases. At this juncture, FSRT is not as well studied as SRS, although the available data suggest the efficacy and risk of the two modalities are similar (Fokas et al., 2012).

### Systemic Therapy

Although the mainstay of management for BM has been primarily surgery and RT, as discussed in previous sections of this chapter, systemic therapies have emerged as an attractive and, at times, first-line option for treatment of BM, specifically if synchronous with the diagnosis of extracranial disease. Advances in genomic characterization have led to improved understanding of the molecular underpinnings of solid tumors, thus paving the way for identification of important driver mutations and disease-modifying pathways which are being exploited for therapeutic benefit. While standard cytotoxic chemotherapy remains a significant component of treatment for some diseases, including some lung and gastrointestinal cancers, targeted therapies and immunotherapies are increasingly used for both solid tumors and BM.

***Epidermal growth factor receptor.*** Epidermal growth factor receptor (EGFR) is a member of the erbB family and is frequently overexpressed in NSCLC (Arteaga et al., 2002; Bunn et al., 2002). Mutations in EGFR are found in 15% of NSCLC patients and have been associated with adenocarcinoma histology, younger age at diagnosis, light or never smokers, women less than 35 years, and patients of Asian descent (Rosell et al., 2012). As the presence of EGFR confers sensitivity to EGR TKI, use of these agents, in patients with metastatic NSCLC harboring activating mutations in EGFR, is the standard of care (Soria et al., 2018).

Erlotinib is a first-generation EGFR TKI which was first shown to have activity against EGFR-mutated NSCLC BM. In a cohort of 17 patients treated with erlotinib, in the EGFR-mutated cohort, there was longer median time to progression (TTP) and higher objective response rate when compared to EGFR-wildtype patients. In a later phase II study of 48 patients with NSCLC BM, in the EGFR-mutated cohort, erlotinib was associated with longer median survival (PFS and OS) as well as a higher intracranial response rate (Wu et al., 2013a,b).

Osimertinib is a third-generation EGFR TKI which was initially used in EGFR-mutated NSCLC patients harboring T790M mutations, which may confer resistance to earlier generation EGFR TKIs (Wu et al., 2013a,b). It is also recognized for improved CNS penetration and response. In a phase III trial comparing osimertinib to chemotherapy (platinum and pemetrexed) in patients with NSCLC, among patients with BM, the osimertinib-treated cohort had longer median PFS (8.4 months vs. 4.2 months) (Mok et al., 2017).

***Anaplastic lymphoma kinase.*** In patients with NSCLC with fusion of ALK and echinoderm microtubule-like protein 4 (EML4), clinical characteristics are similar to that of EGFR: younger age, adenocarcinoma histology, female, and minimal smoking history. Alterations in ALK are present in 3%–7% of NSCLC and are mutually exclusive of other NSCLC-associated driver mutations, including EGFR and KRAS (Soda et al., 2007; Takahashi et al., 2010). Crizotinib is a first-generation ALK TKI which was prospectively investigated in patients with stable, previously treated BM (Costa et al., 2015). In patients treated with crizotinib, median PFS was 9 months, as compared to 4 months in the chemotherapy-treated arm. There are challenges, however, to broader use of crizotinib, including development of resistance. Additionally, a subset of patients who have been treated with crizotinib without history of BM often develop CNS disease as first site of relapse (Kim et al., 2017).

Alectinib and ceritinib are both second-generation ALK TKIs which have shown improved PFS and intracranial response rates in patients with ALK-rearranged NSCLC BM, in comparison to standard chemotherapy (Soria et al., 2017). In three separate phase III studies, alectinib, in comparison to crizotinib, demonstrated higher CNS penetration and delayed the risk of CNS progression in patients with baseline intracranial disease. Brigatinib is a third-generation ALK TKI which has also demonstrated improved intracranial response rates, particularly in patients with acquired resistance to the earlier-generation ALK TKIs (Kim et al., 2017). Similarly, lorlatinib is a dual ALK and ROS1 inhibitor which has gained use given its CNS penetration and ability to overcome ALK resistance. In a phase I study of lorlatinib in 54 patients with either ALK or ROS1-rearranged NSCLC, 39 patients had BM at baseline, 24 of which were evaluable (Shaw et al., 2017). Among the 19 patients with ALK-rearranged NSCLC BM, intracranial objective response was seen in 8 patients (Shaw et al., 2017). A subsequent phase II study, patients with either ALK or ROS1-rearranged NSCLC, were treated with lorlatinib one on six dose expansion cohorts based on prior exposure to earlier-generation ALK TKIs (Solomon et al., 2018). Among 30 patients in cohort 1 (ALK TKI-naïve), 8 patients had baseline CNS disease, of which 3 were measurable, and objective intracranial responses were observed in 2 patients. In cohorts 2–5, 133 of 198 patients who have been treated with at least one ALK TKI had baseline CNS disease. In the 81 evaluable patients, intracranial responses were observed in 51 patients and median duration of response was 14.5 months (Solomon et al., 2018).

***Human epidermal growth factor receptor 2.*** HER2 is overexpressed in up to 30% of breast cancer patients and is predictive of response to HER2-directed therapies, including trastuzumab, pertuzumab, ado-trastuzumab emtansine, and lapatinib (Lin et al., 2013; Ross et al., 2017; Tham et al., 2006). More important, these HER2-directed agents have demonstrated improved outcomes in HER2-positive CNS disease, including parenchymal and leptomeningeal disease (Dawood et al., 2010). In an observational study of factors determining outcomes in HER2-positive disease and BM, patients treated with trastuzumab had median OS of 11.6 months, versus 6.1 months in those who did not receive trastuzumab (Brufsky et al., 2011). Lapatinib is a small-molecule inhibitor that has been investigated for use in HER2-positive BM. In the LANDSCAPE trial, the combination of lapatinib and capecitabine was associated with longer overall survival rate at 6 months and prolonged time to intracranial disease progression in patients with untreated BM (Bachelot et al., 2013). Among 44 of 45 evaluable patients, 29 had objective CNS response (65.9%) and all patients had at least a partial response (Bachelot et al., 2013).

***Cyclin-dependent kinase.*** Whole-exome sequencing of 21 women with various HR and Her2 status revealed frequent alterations of the cyclin-dependent kinase (CDK) and PI3K pathways, which are frequently altered in breast cancer BM. Abemaciclib is an oral CDK inhibitor FDA-approved for initial treatment of postmenopausal women with HR-positive, HER2-negative breast cancer, as shown in the phase III study MONARCH 3. It has also now been used in the management of HR-positive, HER2-negative breast cancer BM.

***BRAF and mitogen-activated protein kinase.*** v-Raf murine sarcoma viral homolog (BRAF) is found in up to 50% of advanced melanoma patients, the majority of which are the result of a single substitution of valine to glutamate at codon 600 (V600E) (Berghoff et al., 2017). Vemurafenib and dabrafenib are BRAF inhibitors currently approved for treatment of melanoma BM. In comparison to dacarbazine, vemurafenib resulted in an intracranial response rate of 71% in patients with BM (Ramanujam et al., 2015). Similarly, in a phase II study of patients with untreated or previously treated BM, dabrafenib was associated with a higher intracranial response rate as well as improvement in OS and PFS (Long et al., 2011).

Mitogen-activated protein kinase (MEK) is downstream of BRAF in the MAP kinase pathway. Inhibitors of MEK are routinely used in combination with BRAF inhibitors in BRAF-mutated metastatic melanoma. Newer combinations of BRAF/MEK inhibition, including encorafenib and binimetinib, are currently under investigation in BM (Dummer et al., 2018)

***Immune checkpoint inhibition.*** Interleukin-2 (IL-2) was previously used for management of metastatic melanoma; however, significant toxicity has limited its use (Tawbi et al., 2018). Newer immune-based therapies have gained approval and are now widely used, specifically in metastatic melanoma and EGFR-wildtype NSCLC. The immune checkpoint inhibitors include nivolumab and pembrolizumab (anti-programmed death 1 or anti-PD-1) and ipilimumab (an anticytotoxic T-lymphocyte-associated protein 4 or CTLA-4). Nivolumab, either as monotherapy or in combination with ipilimumab has been associated with durable intracranial responses in melanoma BM (Long et al., 2018). In a phase II study comparing nivolumab monotherapy to nivolumab followed by combination of ipilimumab and nivolumab in patients with metastatic melanoma, there were higher rates of intracranial responses and a trend toward longer intracranial PFS in the combination therapy cohort (Tawbi et al., 2018).

## Management of Recurrent Brain Metastases

***Re-irradiation.*** Several case series have examined the safety and efficacy of administering a second course of fractionated WBRT to patients with recurrent or progressive BM. In general, this option is considered only for patients who had a good and relatively durable response to their prior course of WBRT and should only be considered in carefully selected patients in whom extracranial disease is stable and alternate CNS-directed treatment approaches are limited (unresectable disease). In a single-institution retrospective analysis of 17 patients who were re-treated with WBRT, median overall survival after re-irradiation was 5.2 months. In patients with stable extracranial disease, median survival time was 19.8 months versus 2.5 months in those with progressive disease (Son et al., 2012). Because survival in these circumstances is generally limited (median survival 4 months), clinical radiation-induced leukoencephalopathy is relatively uncommon (Wong et al., 1996). The interval between WBRT courses has yet to be established; however, most accept an interval of at least 4–6 months.

***Management of radiation necrosis.*** Necrosis is a common complication associated with RT, occurring in close to 10% of patients, up to several years following treatment (Kocher et al., 2011; Miller et al., 2016). The risk factors associated with development of necrosis include re-irradiation to the same lesion and the size of the lesion (Sneed et al., 2015). The increasing use of targeted therapies and immunotherapies has also been shown to increase the risk of radiation necrosis. Colaco et al. studied 180 patients who underwent SRS for BM who were subsequently treated with immunotherapy or cytotoxic or targeted therapy. Within the cohort, 21.7% of patients ultimately developed radiation necrosis; however, 37.5% of patients treated with immunotherapy versus 16.9% who received cytotoxic therapy were found to develop necrosis (Colaco et al., 2016).

Patients with radiation necrosis may be asymptomatic or may present with neurological symptoms related to perilesional edema. Corticosteroids may be used for initial management; however, if symptoms are refractory to steroids or intolerable side effects occur, surgical resection or use of bevacizumab may be appropriate. Bevacizumab is a monoclonal antibody against vascular endothelial growth factor (VEGF), which inhibits binding of the VEGF ligand to its receptor. Currently, bevacizumab is FDA-approved for treatment of multiple diseases including macular degeneration, metastatic colorectal cancer, ovarian cancer, and recurrent/progressive glioblastoma. In a randomized, double-blind study, 14 patients who had previously undergone radiation for head/neck carcinoma, meningioma, or glioma, with biopsy-proven radiation necrosis, were randomized to either bevacizumab or saline (Levin et al., 2011). The clinical status and volume of necrosis were assessed after 3 weeks of treatment. The patients in the bevacizumab-treated cohort all showed neurological improvement as well as radiographic response on postgadolinium images (Levin et al., 2011). Although the optimal dose and schedule of bevacizumab for radiation necrosis has yet to be established, treatment with 7.5 mg/kg of bevacizumab every 3 weeks has been accepted.

Surgical debulking may be considered for palliation and for diagnostic certainty in order to delay or avoid bevacizumab (McPherson et al., 2004). Laser interstitial thermal therapy (LITT) is also under investigation for treatment of symptomatic radiation necrosis, with the potential advantage of tissue acquisition for biopsy at the time of treatment (Eisele et al., 2015).

## METASTATIC EPIDURAL SPINAL CORD COMPRESSION

Spiller first described metastatic epidural spinal cord compression (MESCC) in 1925 as cancerous lesion metastasizing to the spine or epidural space, causing compression of the spinal cord (Spiller, 1925) (Box 76.1). If left untreated, the compression invariably can lead to paraplegia, which is the rationale of the emergent nature of its treatment. Thus, early diagnosis and swift appropriate treatment have resulted in preventing and in some instances reversing the condition in most patients (Abraham et al., 2008). MESCC was found to affect ~25,000 patients (Schiff, 2003); a frequency of 2%–3% was determined in a population-based study (Loblaw et al., 2003), and in autopsy study it was as high as 5% (Larsen et al., 1990). In 20% of patients, MESCC may herald the diagnosis of a malignancy (Savage et al. 2014; Schiff et al., 1997). The spine as a site for malignant growth of metastatic disease varies greatly; in one population-based study in Ontario it was concluded that there is a 40-fold variation in the cumulative incidence of MESCC among different types of cancer (Loblaw et al., 2003). Prostate, breast, and lung cancer accounted for 45%–61%; non-Hodgkin lymphoma (NHL), renal cell cancer, and multiple melanoma 5%–10%; and the remainder are due to colorectal cancer, sarcoma, and unknown primary tumors (Bach et al., 1990; Constans et al., 1983; Mut et al., 2005).

In children, however, MESCC are most commonly due to Ewing sarcoma, neuroblastoma, Hodgkin disease, and germ cell tumors (Tasdemiroglu et al., 1999). Approximately 20% of MESCC cases arise as the sole manifestation of cancer; this is particularly true of lung cancer (Schiff et al., 1997). The location on the spine of MESCC is thought to be a product of mass and blood flow; therefore, 15% occur in cervical spine, 60% in thoracic spine, and 25% in the lumbosacral spine (Bach et al., 1990; Constans et al., 1983).

### Pathophysiology and Pathology

Two main mechanisms account for metastatic cells reaching and seeding the epidural space and compressing the spinal cord. The less common route is the growth of a paravertebral tumor through an intervertebral foramen; this process accounts for 15% of MESCC and is associated with lymphomas and neuroblastomas. The vast majority, 85% of tumors (Gilbert et al., 1978), seed the vertebral body through hematogenous dissemination via arteries (Arguello et al., 1990) and the valveless low-pressure venous plexus of Batson (Coman and deLong, 1951). Slowly the tumor expands in size, spreading into the epidural space, secondarily causing spinal cord compression. Destruction of cortical bone may occur, causing vertebral body collapse, exacerbating spinal cord compression, and in some instances displaced bone fragments can protrude into the epidural space. The physical compression of the MESCC causes demyelination and axonal damage by secondary vascular compromise. In vivo animal studies demonstrated that acute anterior spinal cord compression resulted in occlusion of epidural venous plexus, causing breakdown on the blood–spinal cord barrier and ultimately vasogenic edema (Ushio et al., 1977). At this stage, steroids can have a possible effect; however, if not alleviated, the final stage of the compression is impaired arterial blood flow, causing ischemia and eventually infarction of the spinal cord.

**BOX 76.1 Differential Diagnosis of Epidural Spinal Cord Compression**

**Causes That Should Be Considered in Cancer Patients**

Vertebral metastases without ESCC
Intramedullary spinal cord metastases
Leptomeningeal metastases
Malignant plexopathy
Radiation myelopathy
Paraneoplastic myelopathy

**Benign Causes**

Osteoarthritis
Rheumatoid arthritis
Tophaceous gout
Spinal epidural abscess
Spinal epidural hematoma
Spinal epidural vascular malformation
Meningioma
Neurofibroma
Extramedullary hematopoiesis
Epidural lipomatosis
Sarcoidosis
Histiocytosis

*ESCC*, Epidural spinal cord compression.

### Clinical Presentation

The most common and earliest symptom for these patients is back pain, present in 83%–95% of patients at the time of diagnosis (Schiff, 2003). The time of diagnosis lags the symptoms of MESCC by 2 months (Schiff, 2003). The symptomology is usually indicative of tumor location: root pain and sensory loss are typically associated with lumbosacral tumors, whereas back pain associated with leg weakness is a hallmark of thoracic MESCC, where 60%–70% of MESCC arises. Additionally, back pain chronologically precedes motor weakness and later proceeds to sensory alterations. Several forms of pain can be experienced. Progressive localized pain, confined to the affected region, is usually the first symptom, and is thought to be due to the stretching of the periosteum as the lesion is growing and invading surrounding soft tissue. Radicular pain develops when there is further compression of nerve roots, unilateral in nature with cervical and lumbosacral MESCC and bilateral with thoracic MESCC. Patients describe worse pain at night, which is thought to cause distention of spinal epidural venous plexus, venous engorgement—these symptoms may not be due to direct nerve root compression from distended veins. Mechanical back pain is usually the result of vertebral body collapse and/or pathological fracture. Pain originates due to instability of the spine, which is amplified by any movement but can even be exacerbated by coughing. Lhermitte sign can be observed in patients with mechanical back pain in the cervical spine experiencing electrical sensations in the spine and extremities when their neck is flexed (Onimus et al., 1996).

The second most common symptom is motor weakness, ranging in reports from 60% to 85% at the time of diagnosis. Sadly, nearly two-thirds (50%–68%) of patients with MESCC are nonambulatory at the time of diagnosis (Bach et al., 1990; Constans et al., 1983; Gilbert et al., 1978; Helweg-Larsen and Sorensen, 1994). Weakness is most pronounced in thoracic spine MESCCs. Anatomically, this region of the spine is characterized by marked kyphosis, narrow canal, and limited vascular supply (Helweg-Larsen and Sorensen, 1994). Furthermore, due to delayed diagnosis of MESCC, nearly half of patients found with a MESCC are catheter dependent; thus, in patients with urinary retention, incontinence, and constipation, a high suspicion of MESCC should be present. Loss of sensation does occur in 50%–70% of patients with MESCC; the pattern typically is sensory loss distally to MESCC but can ascend with disease progression (Larsen et al., 1990; Mut et al., 2005). Occasionally, gait ataxia is observed due to spinocerebellar tract in the absence of pain or sensory aberrations (Cole and Patchell, 2008; Gilbert et al., 1978). Cauda equina syndrome may occur in patients in whom compressive lesions are present below the conus, characterized by radicular pain, asymmetric LE weakness, and dermatomal sensory loss.

## Differential Diagnosis

A wide differential diagnosis of MESCC should be explored, including neoplastic and non-neoplastic causes (Box 76.2). Spinal metastases not causing any cord compression can cause severe pain for patients appearing clinically similar to MESCC. Radiographically high-grade MESCC may not have signs of radiculopathy or myelopathy if the tumor and subsequent compression happened slowly. Intramedullary spinal cord metastases lesions should also be included but are much rarer. Leptomeningeal disease of the lower spine can cause cauda equina syndrome similarly to MESCCs. Both brachial and lumbosacral plexus neoplastic lesions should be considered as well in any weakness or sensory finding, but these typically are unilateral in nature (Fig. 76.2).

Paraneoplastic and radiation myelopathy can mimic MESCC. Radiation myelopathy generally develops 1–2 years after radiotherapy, presenting as numbness and asymmetrical dysfunction of the pyramidal tract, at times presenting as the Brown-Séquard syndrome. The risk increases with increasing dosages of RT, increased fraction size, and length or section of area irradiated. Paraneoplastic myelopathy should be included in the differential diagnosis, presenting as a painless myelopathy and frequently associated with encephalitis or secondary neuropathy.

Lastly, aberrations in the musculoskeletal system should be ruled out, especially osteoarthritis. MESCC can be distinguished from osteoarthritis by localization and frequency, as well as characterization of pain. MESCCs are much more common in the thoracic spine for reasons already discussed, whereas osteoarthritis is more common in the cervical and lumbosacral regions of the spine. Recumbency alleviates

### BOX 76.2 Differential Diagnosis of Leptomeningeal Metastases

**Neoplastic**
Parenchymal metastases
Dural metastases
Castleman disease

**Infections**
Bacterial/viral meningitis
Fungal infections, including *Cryptococcus*
Lyme disease
Neurocysticercosis
Tuberculosis

**Granulomatous Disorders**
Histiocytosis
Sarcoidosis
Granulomatosis with polyangiitis

**Inflammatory Disorders**
Multiple sclerosis
Paraneoplastic encephalomyelitis
Relapsing polychondritis
Rheumatoid nodules
Vasculitis (including granulomatous angiitis)

**Miscellaneous**
Enhancing meningeal blood vessels
Post–lumbar puncture changes (intracranial hypotension)

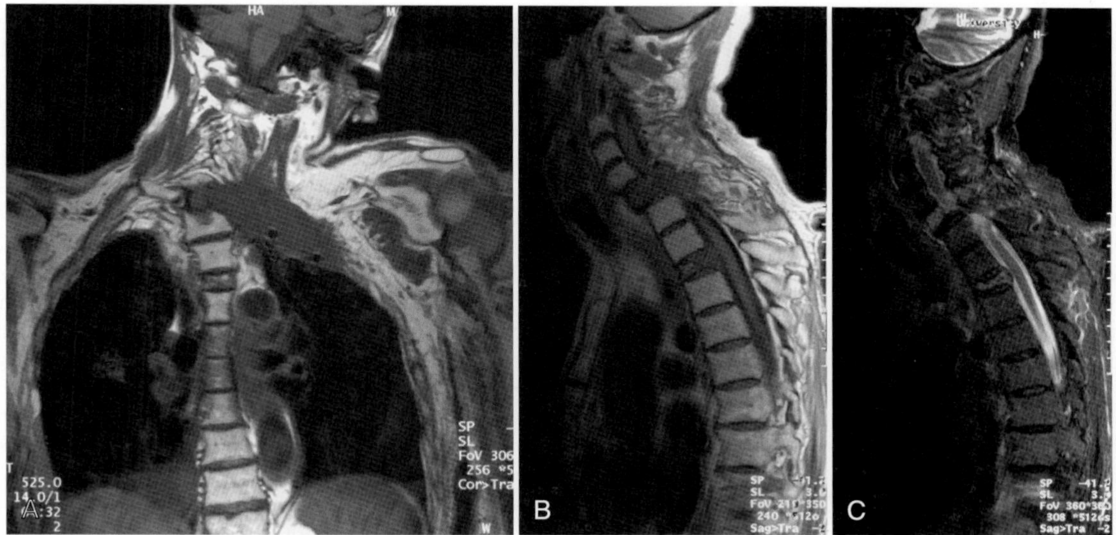


**Fig. 76.2** This 65-year-old woman with lung cancer presented with a left apical lung tumor and 3 months of distal left arm weakness and pain. She then developed distal right arm weakness consistent with C7, C8, and T1 polyradiculopathy. T1- and T2-weighted magnetic resonance imaging (MRI) scans demonstrate the apical mass extending into the neural foramina and vertebral bodies at C6 and C7, displacing the cord anteriorly and to the right. **A,** Coronal T1-weighted MRI showing left apical lung tumor extending into the neural foramina and vertebral bodies at C6 and C7. **B,** Sagittal T1-weighted MRI showing tumor infiltrating vertebral bodies at C6 and C7 and displacing the spinal cord. Also seen is a pathological compression fracture at T3, producing moderate canal stenosis. **C,** Sagittal T2-weighted MRI showing the same tumor infiltrating vertebral bodies at C6 and C7 and displacing the spinal cord. Also seen is a pathological compression fracture at T3, producing moderate canal stenosis.

benign causes of back pain, unlike MESCCs, which are exacerbated by this position. Other benign conditions include rheumatoid arthritis, tophaceous gout, benign tumors such as meningioma and neurofibromas, vascular malformations, epidural hematomas, extramedullary hematopoiesis, epidural lipomatosis, sarcoidosis, and histiocytosis.

## Neuroimaging

MRI is the imaging study with the highest sensitivity (93%) and specificity (97%) for MESCCs (Jarvik and Deyo, 2002) (see Fig. 76.2). Imaging is obtained noninvasively in one sitting and can demonstrate with one methodology the bone lesions, epidural, and intramedullary components as well as any leptomeningeal disease that may be associated. Likewise, with imaging not limited in space and scope the entire spine can be obtained, which is ideal as 30% of patients have more than one site of spinal cord compression (Mut et al., 2005). T1- and T2-weighted images can be used in screening for abnormalities in the bone and epidural space. Furthermore, administration of gadolinium may be helpful in delineating epidural tumor from leptomeningeal disease.

Prior to the advent of MRI, imaging for MESCC was dependent on CT scanning, myelography, or plain radiographs. The classical findings of plain films are pedicle thinning, widening of the neural foramina, compression fractures, osseous density changes, and soft-tissue paravertebral masses. Myelography is capable of demonstrating thecal sac compression; however, myelography images are dependent on flow and thus in the case of a complete block a second puncture rostral to the block may be necessary to the rostral edge of the epidural mass. Myelography is invasive and has the potential risk of precipitating a cerebral or spinal herniation syndrome, or subarachnoid block (Byrne, 1992); so it essentially has been replaced by MRI.

## Management

### Corticosteroids

First-line therapy for patients with MESCC is corticosteroids. Steroids are used for palliation and as a temporizing measure prior to initiation of definitive disease-directed therapy. The effectiveness of steroids in ameliorating neurological deficit was anecdotal as early as the 1960s and was confirmed in animal studies (Ushio et al., 1977). A randomized study compared high-dose steroids (96 mg bolus followed by 9 mg/day for 3 days with a 10-day taper before radiotherapy) to radiotherapy alone. Primary outcome revealed 3- and 6-month ambulation rates of 81% versus 63% and 59% versus 33%, respectively, in favor of steroid usage, which was statistically significant (Sorensen et al., 1994). Although the optimal dosing of steroids is variable, extrapolation of rodent modeling suggests 100 mg dexamethasone, followed by 24 mg 4 times daily, produces the maximum antiedema effect, specifically in patients with significant neurological deficit (Delattre et al., 1989). However, the toxicity of high-dose corticosteroids must be balanced against the potential benefits. A systematic review of literature to determine steroid dosing suggests an initial dose of dexamethasone 10 mg followed by 16 mg daily may be beneficial without increased risk of steroid-related toxicity (Kumar et al., 2017). Only one randomized study aimed to determine whether lower doses would still retain beneficial effects, that is, pain relief; they concluded that the use of lower doses while maintaining the high loading dose produced the same result (Vecht et al., 1989).

### Radiotherapy

Since the 1950s external beam radiation has been the standard treatment for MESCC. The evidence for radiotherapy lies in retrospective studies that show either preservation or improvement in function. Ideally, radiotherapy is most effective in treating radiosensitive lesions. Radiosensitive tumors include lymphoma, myeloma, and prostate; renal cell carcinoma and NSCLC are considered relatively radiosensitive. Ambulation was the primary outcome as in the steroid studies, and in general the ability to walk was preserved (Constans et al., 1983; Gilbert et al., 1978; Loblaw et al., 2003).

Despite the general consensus of the effectiveness of radiotherapy for MESCC, the optimal doses and regimen remain unclear. Radiation ports are designed based on diagnostic imaging and traditionally extend one vertebral level above and below the MESCC site and widen when paravertebral involvement is known. The determined radiation dosing is a compromise among tumor control, risk of radiation-induced myelopathy, and treatment duration based on the patient's condition. A multicenter study comparing 30 Gy over 10 fractions versus 40 Gy over 20 fractions demonstrated no statically significant difference in motor function or ambulatory scoring (Rades et al., 2004). Additionally, a retrospective study of over 1300 patients with five different radiation regimens ranging from 8 Gy to 40 Gy in 20 fractions all yielded similar results. The in-field recurrence rates were much lower in the protracted schedules (Rades et al., 2005). In a separate, non-inferior study, 233 patients with MESCC and poor survival were randomized to either short-course RT (4 Gy × 5 fractions) or longer-course RT (3 Gy × 10 fractions), with primary endpoint of improvement or stabilization of motor deficits at 1 month (Rades et al., 2016). At 1 month, improvement rates were 38.5% and 44% in the short-course and longer-course RT groups, respectively. PFS6 for the short-course group was 75% versus 81.8% in the longer-course RT with OS of 42.3% and 37.8%, respectively, suggesting that short-course RT was not significantly inferior to longer-course RT (Rades et al., 2016).

### Surgery

The role of surgery in the treatment of MESCC was controversial in the past but with advances its efficacy in selected patients has been established. Evidence of spinal instability is an absolute indication for surgical management. Prior to radiotherapy, decompressive laminectomy was the only surgical treatment. However, in several retrospective studies the results of laminectomy and radiotherapy did not differ from radiotherapy alone (Greenberg et al., 1980). This may be due to the fact that most MESCCs are located in the vertebral body, which is anterior to the spinal cord; thus, a laminectomy did not remove the tumor nor relieve any of the compression on the spinal cord associated with the MESCC. Additionally, the removal of the lamina and posterior elements further destabilized the spine.

In the 1980s, vertebral corpectomies were employed to treat patients afflicted with MESCCs. In this procedure the tumor in the vertebral body is removed by an anterior or lateral circumferential approach; decompression and reconstruction are achieved, providing immediate stabilization—meta-analysis has suggested that this surgery method is superior to radiotherapy alone (Klimo et al., 2005).

Several less-invasive surgical approaches have been introduced into the treatment paradigm for management of MESCC. Separation surgery (SS) has emerged in use, specifically in combination with spine stereotactic radiosurgery (SSRS). SS describes a posterolateral approach, which allows for stabilization and circumferential decompression of the thecal sac and nerve roots (Barzilai et al., 2018). Other techniques which have been employed include minimal access techniques combined with percutaneous screw instrumentation and cement augmentation for stabilization (Barzilai et al., 2018).

### Surgery with Radiation Therapy

To determine the role of surgery in the context of RT, a randomized clinical trial enrolled patients in RT only (30 Gy in 10 fractions in the first 24 hours) or surgery (first 24 hours) followed by RT (within 2 weeks of surgery). The primary outcome was ambulation; secondary outcomes included continence, time length of maintained strength, functional status, and survival. Ambulation rates were much higher in surgery with RT than in RT alone (84% vs. 57%) and patients were able to ambulate for longer periods of time (122 days vs. 13 days). Functional status and muscle strength were also maintained longer in the surgery with RT group than in those that received radiation alone. Survival was significantly longer in the surgery group as well (126 days vs. 100 days) (Patchell et al., 2005). This study showed surgery is superior, but the design of the study was for particular tumors and in select tumor types and presentation.

Recently, in surgical management of MESCC, there has been a trend toward hybrid therapy, in which SS is combined with SSRS. While the primary goal of surgery is for preservation of neurological function; in combination with SSRS, the aim is also to create a target for SSRS. In a retrospective study conducted by Laufer et al., adjuvant hypofractionated SSRS after surgery led to improved local progression rates of 5% (Laufer et al., 2013). Similar local control rates with SS followed by SSRS have been demonstrated in other studies (Moulding et al., 2010; Rock et al., 2006).

### Chemotherapy

Unlike with metastases to the brain, the blood–brain barrier is not a factor for MESCC; nevertheless, chemotherapy is rarely deployed in the acute management of MESCC, even if the metastasis involved is chemosensitive, as the response is too slow. However, the role of chemotherapy as adjunct therapy to RT is an area of growing interest (Wong et al., 1996).

## INTRAMEDULLARY SPINAL METASTASES

Spread of metastatic disease to the spine is rare but only 0.8%–3.5% of symptomatic metastases to the spine are intramedullary. Bronchogenic cancer is the most common, comprising 54%–85% of cases, with small-cell lung cancer accounting for the majority (47%) of these. Breast is the second most common (11%–13%), followed by renal cell carcinoma (4%–9%), melanoma (8%–9%), lymphoma (4%–5%), colorectal cancer (3%), thyroid (2%), ovarian (1%–2%), and other cancers. Several proposed mechanisms for the spread of metastatic disease to the spine are similar to that for the hematogenous spread of MESCC, venous plexus networks, and direct invasion, as approximately a quarter of the patients affected have leptomeningeal disease as well. Intramedullary spinal cord metastases can present in patients with progressive myelopathy (93%), a weak and sensory manifest of Brown-Séquard syndrome (22.5%), or pseudo or partial Brown-Séquard syndrome (22.5%). Lesions are detected on contrast-enhancing masses with large associated T2 signal abnormality due to edema produced on the surrounding spinal cord. More than half (57%) of patients with intramedullary spinal cord metastases have BM as well. The mainstay treatment of intramedullary spinal cord metastases is steroids and external beam radiation (Chi et al., 2006).

## SKULL AND DURAL METASTASES

### Skull Metastases

Metastases to the skull occur in approximately a quarter of patients with a known cancer history (Gloria-Cruz et al., 2000). Fortunately, these metastases are clinically silent, but in 8% of cases the presence of skull metastases is the first sign of cancer (Laigle-Donadey et al., 2005). In the case of prostate cancer, venous seeding appears to be the mechanism of hematogenous spread. In review of the literature, one study found that prostate cancer was the most common (38%), followed by breast cancer (20%), while all other pathologies (lung, renal, thyroid, and melanoma) constituted less than 10% (Laigle-Donadey et al., 2005). Renal cell and thyroid carcinoma may produce solitary calvarial metastasis. Rarely, extracranial tumors may extend centrally along cranial nerve branches and enter the skull foramina. Tumors with a predilection for perineural growth include squamous cell carcinoma of the nasopharynx, esthesioneuroblastoma, lymphoma, nerve sheath tumors, and skin cancer. While symptomatic patients may present with cranial neuropathy or craniofacial pain, several syndromes have been defined based on their location—parasellar and sellar syndromes were the most common (29%), followed by gasserian ganglion (6%) and jugular foramen syndrome (3%) (Laigle-Donadey et al., 2005).

Calvarial metastases are often asymptomatic. Occasionally they produce localized pain or a palpable mass. When metastases enlarge, they may cause focal neurological deficits or seizures. Rarely, calvarial metastases invade or compress cerebral venous sinuses, producing increased ICP and venous infarction.

Skull-base metastases often present with characteristic clinical features (Greenberg et al., 1981) (Table 76.5). The differential diagnosis includes leptomeningeal and parenchymal metastases, as well as benign conditions such as granulomatous or infectious diseases. Biopsy is a consideration if the diagnosis is inconclusive following clinical and radiological evaluation and CSF examination (to exclude leptomeningeal disease).

Calvarial metastases appear as irregular lucencies on skull radiographs. In 90% of patients, bony metastases are present elsewhere in the body. CT and MRI usually show lesions involving all three tables of the skull bone and provide information regarding the extent of intracranial extension and relation to venous sinuses (Jansen and Sillevis Smith, 2002). The differential diagnosis of multiple skull defects includes normal structures such as venous lakes, pacchionian granulations, and parietal foramina. Pathological conditions include Langerhans cell histiocytosis, hyperparathyroidism, osteomyelitis, and radiation necrosis. For single calvarial lesions, the differential diagnosis includes meningiomas (including primary intraosseous meningioma), hemangiomas, epidermoid cysts, leptomeningeal cysts (in children), Langerhans cell histiocytosis, Paget disease, postsurgical defect, and osteomyelitis (Jansen and Sillevis Smith, 2002). Radiological diagnosis of skull-base lesions tends to be more difficult. Contrast-enhanced MRI is the most useful diagnostic test, but CT scans with thin cuts through the skull base may help detect bony lesions.

**TABLE 76.5 Classification of Clinical Syndromes Caused by Skull-Base Metastasis**

| Site of Skull-Base Metastasis | Symptoms and Signs |
|---|---|
| Orbital | Local pain, proptosis, sensory loss ($V_1$), diplopia, decreased vision (late) |
| Parasellar/cavernous sinus | Unilateral frontal headache, oculomotor palsies (III, IV, VI), sensory loss ($V_1$) |
| Middle cranial fossa | Facial numbness or pain ($V_{2,3}$), sometimes abducens or facial nerve palsy (VI, VII) |
| Jugular foramen | Unilateral postauricular pain, hoarseness, dysphagia (IX, X), sternocleidomastoid or trapezius weakness (XI) |
| Occipital condyle | Unilateral occipital pain, stiff neck, unilateral tongue weakness (XII) |

*From Greenberg, H.S., Deck, M.D.F., Vikram, B., et al., 1981. Metastasis to the base of the skull: Clinical findings in 43 patients. Neurology 31, 530–537.*

Radiotherapy is the main form of therapy for skull metastases; in one study, overall symptomatic improvements of 86% were achieved with RT. The recommended dosage is 35 Gy in 14 fractions over 3 weeks. SRS has been utilized for primary skull-based metastases as well as in the treatment of postsurgical or postradiation residual or reoccurrence (Greenberg et al., 1981). Chemotherapy and immunotherapy may be of benefit for chemosensitive tumors, and hormonal therapy may benefit subsets of breast and prostate cancer patients. Occasionally, surgery may be required, based on location, functional status, and type of suspected primary since some tumor types are radio-resistant.

The prognosis of skull metastases depends on systemic tumor control as well as local factors including invasion of venous sinus or dura, leptomeninges, and brain parenchyma (Jansen and Sillevis Smith, 2002). In general, better outcomes are associated with starting treatment less than 1 month after diagnosis.

## LEPTOMENINGEAL METASTASES

Involvement of the leptomeninges (LM) by tumor is an increasingly common problem in patients with cancer and leads to significant morbidity and mortality (Kesari and Batchelor, 2003). Similar to parenchymal BM, the factors that have contributed to the increased incidence are a greater awareness of the condition among oncologists, improved diagnostic tests, and longer survival among patients with systemic malignancies due to tolerability of systemic and targeted therapies. Survival in this setting is usually short and averages 3–4 months (Jaeckle, 2006). Few randomized prospective trials of neoplastic meningitis have been conducted and standard therapeutic guidelines are still lacking at this time. Approaches to treatment are often guided by prognosis and the risk status of the individual patient. Previously defined prognostic factors have included female sex, history of intraparenchymal tumor, short duration of symptoms, and controlled systemic disease while negative prognosis was associated with age older than 55 years, increased CSF protein, hypoglycorrhachia, poor KPS, cranial nerve palsy, carcinomatous encephalopathy, concomitant bulky CNS metastases, poorly controlled systemic disease, and persistent CSF block (Gleissner and Chamberlain, 2006).

### Epidemiology

Approximately 5% of cancer patients have LM (Posner, 1995). The incidence varies with different tumor types. LM occurs in up to 8% of patients with solid tumors, 5%–29% of patients with NHL, and 11%–70% of leukemias (Kesari and Batchelor, 2003; Wen and Fine, 1997). Among solid tumors, adenocarcinomas have a particular propensity to metastasize to the leptomeninges. Among lung tumors, patients with SCLC have a greater tendency to develop LM than those with other lung cancer subtypes. In several large series, breast cancer accounted for 11%–64% of patients with LM, followed by lung cancer (14%–29%), melanoma (6%–18%), and GI cancers (4%–14%). Primary brain tumors, especially medulloblastoma and high-grade gliomas, also have a tendency for CSF spread. Some solid tumors (e.g., head and neck cancer, thyroid cancer, prostate cancer, carcinoid, bladder cancer) rarely seed the leptomeninges (Kesari and Batchelor, 2003; Wen and Fine, 1997).

LM associated with acute lymphoblastic leukemia (ALL) in children was previously common, but CNS prophylaxis has reduced the incidence from 66% to 5%. The incidence of LM in adults with ALL remains high despite similar prophylactic measures. Patients with acute myelogenous leukemia have a 5% risk of LM with CNS prophylaxis and 10% without it (Drappatz and Batchelor, 2007). LM is uncommon in patients with chronic myelogenous leukemia and hairy cell leukemia. Leptomeningeal involvement is present in up to 50% of patients with chronic lymphocytic leukemia at autopsy, although it is usually asymptomatic during life (Grossman and Moynihan, 1991). Seeding of the leptomeninges occurs in approximately 6% of patients with NHL. The highest risk occurs in those with diffuse, lymphoblastic, or Burkitt histology, or those who with involvement of the bone marrow, testes, or extranodal sites. Leptomeningeal disease is rare in patients with Hodgkin disease, mycosis fungoides, and multiple myeloma (Grossman and Moynihan, 1991).

### Pathogenesis

Tumor cells usually reach the leptomeninges by direct extension from a preexisting tumor in the brain parenchyma or epidural space or by hematogenous spread (Posner, 1995). Tumor cells may also spread along spinal nerve roots from a paraspinal mass or along cranial nerves from a head and neck tumor. Once tumor cells reach the leptomeninges, they spread along the surface of the brain, spinal cord, and nerve roots (Fig. 76.3). The flow of CSF carries exfoliated tumor cells to other parts of the neuroaxis, especially to the basal cisterns and cauda equina, where they tend to settle as a result of gravity and slow CSF flow.

The presence of tumor cells in the leptomeninges produces multifocal neurological dysfunction in several ways. Direct invasion of spinal and cranial nerves can cause demyelination and subsequent axonal degeneration of the nerves. Tumor cells may also grow along the Virchow-Robin spaces and directly invade the brain or spinal cord, producing symptoms of confusion and seizures (Wasserstrom, 1995). LM may also produce CNS dysfunction by causing hydrocephalus. Tumor cells can occlude the CSF outflow foramina of the fourth ventricle or impede the reabsorption of CSF through the arachnoid granulations, leading to hydrocephalus. Occasionally, ICP may increase without enlargement of the ventricles, and (rarely) herniation occurs. Tumor cells may interfere with the blood supply, decreasing cerebral blood flow and even producing transient ischemic attacks and strokes. Tumor cells may also directly compete with neurons for oxygen and essential metabolites such as glucose. This is the mechanism proposed

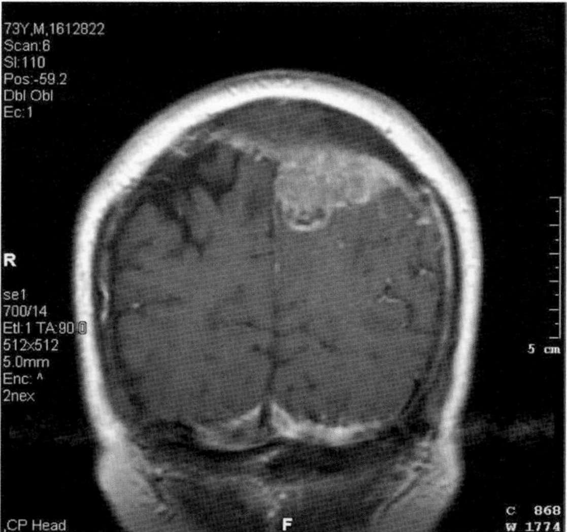


**Fig. 76.3** Gross appearance of tumor infiltrate in the subarachnoid space as evidenced by clouding of the leptomeninges. *(Courtesy Dr. Umberto De Girolami, Division of Neuropathology, Brigham and Women's Hospital.)*

for the weight gain seen in children with leukemic meningitis and infiltration of the hypothalamus (Posner, 1995).

## Clinical Features

LM is usually a late complication of systemic cancer, occurring 6 months to 3 years after the diagnosis of the primary tumor (Wasserstrom, 1995). In rare patients with breast carcinoma and melanoma, an interval of up to 10 years may exist between the diagnosis of the primary tumor and the leptomeningeal relapse. LM usually occurs in the setting of active disease outside the nervous system, although as systemic therapy improves, increasing numbers of patients are developing LM as the sole site of relapsed disease. In 5% of patients, leptomeningeal involvement is the initial presentation of a neoplasm (Posner, 1995).

The presentation of LM can be extremely variable and requires a high index of suspicion. Consider the diagnosis in any cancer patient, especially if there are symptoms and signs involving several different sites in the neuroaxis. Cerebral symptoms occur in up to 50% of patients (Kaplan et al., 1990; Wasserstrom, 1995). The most common are headaches, which can be nonspecific or have features suggestive of increased ICP. Other symptoms include nausea, vomiting, cognitive changes, and occasionally seizures. Focal cerebral symptoms such as hemiparesis, aphasia, or visual field deficits are relatively rare. Papilledema may occasionally be present in patients with hydrocephalus as evidence of increased ICP. This may be accompanied by dizziness or syncope which occurs with positional changes, suggestive of plateau waves or venous obstruction. Rarely, LM may produce a diencephalic syndrome, diabetes insipidus, central hypoventilation, cerebral infarction, and complex partial status epilepticus (Wen and Fine, 1997).

Some 30% of patients have cranial nerve symptoms, and 50% have cranial nerve signs. Involvement of the third, fourth, and sixth nerves is most common, followed by facial weakness, decreased hearing, and involvement of the optic, trigeminal, and hypoglossal nerves. Approximately 60% of patients have spinal symptoms, especially in the lumbosacral region, as a result of involvement of nerve roots. The most common symptoms are pain, weakness, and paresthesias. Sphincter dysfunction is less common. More than 70% of patients have signs of spinal cord dysfunction, including asymmetrical weakness, sensory loss, and depressed reflexes consistent with cauda equina syndrome.

## Diagnostic Tests

Table 76.6 summarizes the most useful tests for the diagnosis of LM.

### Cerebrospinal Fluid Examination

Examination of the CSF is the most important test for the diagnosis of LM. The finding of malignant cells in the CSF is the definitive diagnosis. However, the CSF is almost always abnormal even if the cytological examination result is negative. These most common findings include lymphocytic pleocytosis, elevated opening pressure, increased CSF protein, and a decreased glucose concentration (Kesari and Batchelor, 2003; Posner, 1995). It is worth noting that cytology may be negative in up to 20% of patients with LM—reasons for which are unknown but may be due to adherence of cells to the leptomeninges (Glantz et al., 1998a,b; Clarke et al., 2010). The opening pressure is elevated in approximately 50% of patients with LM as a result of tumor cells obstructing CSF outflow from the ventricles or interfering with CSF reabsorption by the arachnoid granulations. The CSF white blood cell count is elevated in more than 50% of patients with LM. This increase in cell count may range from a few cells to more than 1000. This is usually a lymphocytic pleocytosis, but occasionally polymorphonuclear cells are found. The elevated CSF protein in most patients is due to a combination of disruption of the blood–CSF barrier and exudation of serum protein into the CSF, and breakdown of tumor cells and lymphocytes. In most, the protein is moderately elevated, but levels in excess of 2 g/dL occur. Because normal levels of CSF protein are lower in the ventricle (10 mg/dL) than in the lumbar space (40–45 mg/dL), consider a CSF protein level of 15 mg/dL or greater from an Ommaya reservoir abnormal. In patients with leptomeningeal myeloma, CSF immunoglobulin (Ig)M may be elevated.

Low CSF glucose (hypoglycorrhachia) is present in approximately 30% of patients with LM (Wasserstrom, 1995). The precise cause of the low CSF glucose is unknown. Possible reasons include impaired carrier mediated transport of glucose across the blood–CSF barrier and increased utilization of glucose by tumor cells and reactive lymphocytes. The high rate of false-negative cytological findings may reflect the manner of spinal fluid collection and management. The sensitivity of cytology is dependent on the volume of CSF collected; thus a negative cytology in the setting of suspicious clinical presentation often merits repeat examination. Glantz et al. (1998a,b) in their unique prospective study of CSF collection among patients with suspected carcinomatosis meningitis reported a false-negative rate of a 3.5-mL sample of 32%, which decreased to 10% and 3% for 7.0- and 10.5-mL samples, respectively. Yet the mean CSF volume submitted to the cytology laboratory was 2.9 mL, with 97% of specimens less than 10.5 mL. In addition, the efficiency of processing collected CSF samples influenced outcomes. The false-negative rate after a 48-hour delay in processing the spinal fluid was 36%. The site from which CSF is collected, from the lumbar or cervical cistern or from the ventricles, may also influence the sensitivity of cytology. Several authors have noted a higher rate of positive cytological findings when collecting fluid from sites that approximate clinical or radiographic disease (Chamberlain et al., 2001; Glantz et al., 1998a,b). Repeat CSF analysis may further reduce false negatives when suspicion remains after a negative cytological study. In the often-cited study by Wasserstrom et al. (1982), cytological findings were positive in 54% at first lumbar puncture, which increased to 86% at the third sample. Other authors have reported similar findings in subsequent studies (Glantz et al., 1998a,b). Despite repeated samples, 8%–10% of patients with carcinomatosis meningitis have persistently negative cytology results.

When the CSF cytological examination result is negative, biochemical markers can sometimes be useful in assisting the diagnosis of LM

**TABLE 76.6 Diagnostic Tests for Leptomeningeal Metastases**

| Test | Measurement | Positive Findings |
|---|---|---|
| Lumbar puncture | Lymphocytic pleocytosis | >70% |
| | Elevated opening pressure | 50% |
| | Elevated protein | 75% |
| | Reduced glucose | 30%–40% |
| | Cytology after 1 LP | 50% |
| | Cytology after 3 LPs | 90% |
| | CSF markers | Variable |
| | Immunohistochemistry | Variable |
| | PCR | Variable |
| Brain MRI | Meningeal enhancement | >50% |
| | Enlarged ventricles | <50% |
| Spine MRI/myelogram | Subarachnoid masses | <25% |
| | Meningeal enhancement | >50% |

*CSF*, Cerebrospinal fluid; *LP*, lumbar puncture; *MRI*, magnetic resonance imaging; *PCR*, polymerase chain reaction.

and monitoring the response to therapy (Kesari and Batchelor, 2003; Wen and Fine, 1997). Table 76.7 lists some of the more commonly used markers. Although some of these markers are fairly specific, their lack of sensitivity often limits their usefulness. Occasionally, parenchymal metastases adjacent to leptomeningeal or ependymal surfaces falsely elevate the levels of biochemical markers in the CSF.

In some patients, immunocytochemistry can increase the sensitivity for detecting malignant cells. Monoclonal antibodies against surface markers on lymphocytes can be especially useful in distinguishing lymphoma cells (which are usually monoclonal B cells) from reactive T lymphocytes. However, because malignant lymphocytes can mix with reactive T cells, the presence of polyclonality does not exclude tumor. When the diagnosis of leptomeningeal lymphoma is difficult, the polymerase chain reaction (PCR) technique is useful for determining whether the Ig gene rearrangement is identical in all the lymphocytes, suggesting a neoplastic process (Thomas et al., 2000).

Rare cell capture technologies have been tested to identify circulating tumor cells (CTCs) in CSF for the diagnosis of leptomeningeal disease. Nayak et al., performed a pilot study of CSF samples from 60 patients, of which 51 patients with solid tumor and suspicion for leptomeningeal disease were ultimately analyzed. In addition to evaluation for presence of CTCs, imaging and cytology were also obtained. Fifteen patients were eventually found to have leptomeningeal disease and 16 patients were found to have CTCs (though one was false positive) (Nayak et al., 2013). A subsequent study of 95 patients with epithelial tumors and suspicion for leptomeningeal disease was performed; 30 patients were ultimately found to have positive cytology and CTCs were found in 43 patients. The presence of 1 CTC per 1 mL of CSF was identified as the diagnostic threshold, correlating with 93% sensitivity and 95% specificity (Lin et al., 2017).

## Neuroimaging

MRI is the most sensitive neuroimaging test for detecting LM. Meningeal enhancement is present in half of patients with LM. Also observed are small enhancing cortical nodules and communicating hydrocephalus from impaired CSF absorption. Rarely, focal LM may mimic a meningioma. Whenever possible, perform MRI before lumbar puncture as lumbar puncture occasionally results in intracranial hypotension and meningeal enhancement, which leads to an erroneous diagnosis of LM. Myelography shows thickening and nodularity of nerve roots in 25%–33% of patients with LM and may be helpful when MRI is not appropriate. Increasingly, the diagnosis of LM is established in patients with characteristic clinical and radiological findings, even if the CSF cytological examination result is negative (Freilich et al., 1995). Working groups, including RANO and the European Association of Neuro-Oncology/European Society of Medical Oncology (EANO-ESMO) have proposed criteria for response evaluation, which may aid in assessing disease activity in a standardized and systematic manner (Le Rhun et al., 2017).

## Diagnosis

The basis for the diagnosis of LM is the combination of characteristic clinical, radiological, and CSF features, and, ideally, positive CSF cytological findings. Other conditions causing subacute neurological deficits at multiple sites in the neuroaxis may mimic LM. These include parenchymal and epidural tumor deposits and subacute and chronic meningitides such as syphilis, sarcoidosis, Lyme disease, and fungal and tuberculous meningitis. Routine imaging, CSF studies, and positive cytology results usually distinguish other entities from LM (see Box 76.2). Specific serological tests are also useful. These include Lyme antibody titers; serum angiotensin-converting enzymes (sarcoidosis); fluorescent treponemal antibodies (syphilis); cryptococcal antigens; fungal cultures; and PCR for herpes simplex, varicella-zoster, and tuberculosis. A meningeal biopsy may be useful when the diagnosis remains in doubt.

## Treatment

Despite more than three decades of effort, the treatment options for LM remain limited. Reasons for the difficulty include (1) the need to treat the entire neuroaxis because of widespread dissemination of tumor cells throughout the subarachnoid space; (2) the close proximity of the tumor cells to neural structures; (3) the need to limit the administered doses of radiation and chemotherapy because of potential neurotoxicity; (4) the blood–CSF barrier, which limits access of many systemically administered drugs into the CSF; (5) the intrinsic resistance of many solid tumors; and (6) the routine presence of other sites of metastatic disease.

The goal of therapy is to improve or stabilize the patient's neurological status and prolong survival. Specific treatment depends on tumor type, site of the leptomeningeal tumor, and clinical condition of the patient. Without treatment, the median survival of patients with LM is 4–6 weeks. Death usually results from progressive neurological dysfunction. With treatment, median survival increases to 3–6 months. The response rate is 50%–60% for carcinomas and more than 80% for NHL (Wen and Fine, 1997). Although treatment often provides effective local control, LM usually occurs in the setting of systemic relapse, and most patients who survive beyond the first month (two-thirds of the total) eventually die of their systemic disease. For patients who are considered "good-risk", referring to favorable KPS,

**TABLE 76.7 Cerebrospinal Fluid Tumor Markers in Leptomeningeal Metastases**

| Marker | Tumor |
|---|---|
| **Relatively Specific** | |
| AFP | Teratocarcinoma, yolk sac tumor, ECC, endodermal sinus tumor |
| CA-125 | Ovarian cancer |
| CA-15-3 | Breast cancer |
| CA19-9 | Adenocarcinoma, biliary disease |
| Creatine kinase-1 (CK-1) | Small-cell lung cancer |
| hCG β-subunit (β-hCG) | Choriocarcinoma, ECC, germ cell tumor |
| 5-HIAA | Carcinoid |
| HPAP | Germinoma |
| IgM | Myeloma |
| Melanin | Melanoma |
| PSA | Prostate cancer |
| Tissue polypeptide antigen | Breast cancer |
| **Nonspecific** | |
| $\beta_2$-microglobulin | Lymphoma, infection, other tumors |
| β-glucuronidase | Nonspecific |
| CEA | Colon, ovarian, breast, bladder, lung |
| HMFG1 mAb | Nonspecific |
| LDH isoenzymes | Carcinoma, nonspecific |
| Telomerase | Nonspecific |
| VEGF | Nonspecific |

*AFP*, Alpha-fetoprotein; *CA*, carbohydrate antigen; *CEA*, carcinoembryonic antigen; *ECC*, embryonal cell carcinoma; *hCG*, human chorionic gonadotropin; *HIAA*, hydroxyindoleacetic acid; *HMFG*, human milk fat globule; *HPAP*, human placental alkaline phosphatase; *IgM*, immunoglobulin M; *LDH*, lactate dehydrogenase; *PSA*, prostate specific antigen; *VEGF*, vascular endothelial growth factor.

controlled systemic disease and minimal neurological symptom burden, treatment is often disease-directed: radiotherapy for treatment of bulky or symptomatic disease with consideration of systemic therapies which may have CNS penetration. "Poor-risk" patients are those with low KPS, high CNS symptom burden, and uncontrolled extracranial disease—in these instances, treatment is palliative.

Because tumor cells disseminate throughout the subarachnoid space, the entire neuroaxis requires treatment if therapy is to be effective. If only symptomatic sites are treated, early relapse is likely secondary to seeding from residual tumor cells in untreated areas of the leptomeninges. Currently, standard therapy for LM involves radiation to sites of symptomatic and bulky disease and regions of CSF flow interruption, intraventricular administration of chemotherapy via an Ommaya or Rickham reservoir, and optimal treatment of systemic disease (Box 76.3).

### Surgery

In general, LM is not a surgical condition. Surgery is limited to biopsy when diagnosis cannot be established via other methods. Patients who develop symptoms increased ICP which is inadequately controlled with dexamethasone, CSF diversion with placement of a ventriculoperitoneal shunt is recommended (Lamba et al., 2018; Omuro et al., 2005). A frequently cited concern of peritoneal spread of tumor appears to be less common than thought, perhaps owing to poor survival outcomes after diagnosis. Concurrent administration of intrathecal (IT) chemotherapy in a patient with a functioning shunt, however, remains problematic as it will shunt the chemotherapy out of the CNS. This makes it difficult to maintain therapeutic concentrations of chemotherapy within the spinal fluids. Strategies to resolve the issue involve the use of a programmable valve, allowing the shunt to be "shut off" if the patient can tolerate it (Lin et al., 2011).

### Radiation Therapy

RT is limited to symptomatic areas and sites of bulky disease where the penetration of IT drugs is limited. Although RT is more effective than chemotherapy in treating tumor cells in the Virchow-Robin spaces and nerve root sleeves, the use of craniospinal radiation to the entire neuroaxis is rare because of bone marrow suppression. This is of particular concern in patients with LM, because many have systemic metastases that require treatment with chemotherapy. In addition, adults tolerate craniospinal radiation poorly, often developing significant fatigues and encephalopathy which compromise quality of life. A commonly administered dose of radiation is approximately 30 Gy administered over 10 fractions; for poor-risk patients, a course of 20 Gy over 5 fractions is considered acceptable in order to maximize patient quality of life and minimize toxicity. When effective at restoring normal CSF circulation, radiation to sites of CSF flow obstruction may also improve outcome (Chamberlain and Kormanik, 1996). WBRT is also used in the setting of hydrocephalus, though CSF diversion with shunting is recommended for management of symptomatic hydrocephalus.

**BOX 76.3 Treatment of Leptomeningeal Metastases**

Radiation therapy to sites of symptomatic and bulky disease
Intrathecal chemotherapy:
- Methotrexate + leucovorin
- Thiotepa
- Cytarabine
- Liposomal cytarabine (DepoCyt)

Systemic chemotherapy (e.g., high-dose methotrexate)
Optimal treatment of systemic disease

### Intrathecal Chemotherapy

The administration of IT therapy is the delivery of chemotherapy directly into the CSF compartment, via repeated lumbar punctures or into the ventricles through an intraventricular cannula with a subcutaneous reservoir (Ommaya). Normal CSF circulation carries fluid preferentially out of the ventricles. Consequently, a uniform distribution of the drug may be achievable when injected into the ventricle rather than the lumbar cistern. This is particularly true of drugs with a short half-life (Glantz et al., 2010). In addition, it is less uncomfortable and avoids epidural and subdural leakage of the drug. In many patients with extensive LM, obstruction of CSF flow in the subarachnoid space decreases the effectiveness of IT chemotherapy and increases the likelihood of toxicity. In these patients, $^{111}$indium-DTPA CSF flow studies may be helpful in defining the CSF blocks (Mason et al., 1998). These blocks require treatment with RT and may influence outcome. Only a limited number of chemotherapeutic agents are available for IT administration, including methotrexate (MTX), cytarabine, and, infrequently, thiotepa (Kesari and Batchelor, 2003; Mason et al., 1998; Wen and Fine, 1997).

MTX is the most widely used drug and is administered both intrathecally and intravenously. It is an S-phase-specific antimetabolite and interferes with DNA synthesis by inhibiting dihydrofolate reductase. It is active against leukemia, lymphoma, breast cancer, and other solid tumors to a much lesser extent. The typical treatment is 10–12 mg twice weekly for 5–8 treatments, or until the CSF clears. Weekly and then monthly maintenance therapy follows. The most effective duration of treatment is unclear, but standard recommendations suggest treatment for at least 3–6 months, and perhaps indefinitely. MTX successfully clears malignant cells from the CSF in 20%–61% of cases (Glantz et al., 1998a,b). Therapeutic concentrations ($>10^{-6}$ molar) are attained in the CSF for 48 hours by administration of 12 mg of MTX. The MTX is gradually reabsorbed into the bloodstream by bulk flow, and transport via the choroid plexus results in a low systemic concentration (peak systemic concentration of $>10^{-7}$ molar), which may cause myelosuppression and mucositis. To reduce these systemic side effects, leucovorin (10 mg orally twice daily) should be administered for 3–4 days after administration of MTX. Complications of IT MTX include aseptic meningitis, leukoencephalopathy, mucositis, myelosuppression, encephalopathy, and opportunistic infections (Kesari and Batchelor, 2003).

Cytosine arabinoside (ara-C) is a synthetic pyrimidine nucleoside analog with activity against leukemias and lymphomas but not most solid tumors. The half-life of ara-C is very short in the serum but significantly longer in the CSF because of low levels of cytidine deaminase. The standard IT dose of ara-C is 50 mg twice a week. IT ara-C has relatively little systemic toxicity because of the rapid deamination of any drug reaching the systemic circulation. Neurological complications associated with IT ara-C include transverse myelopathy, aseptic meningitis, encephalopathy, headaches, and seizures (Kesari and Batchelor, 2003). A slow-release, liposomal formulation of cytarabine (DepoCyt) was approved for IT use in patients with lymphomatous meningitis (Glantz et al., 1999a, 1999b). An important advantage of this drug is that cytotoxic concentrations of cytarabine (>0.1 μg/mL) are maintained in the CSF for 2 weeks. In a randomized study of 28 patients with lymphomatous meningitis treated with either liposomal cytarabine (every 2 weeks) or ara-C (twice a week) for 1 month, the response rate in the liposomal cytarabine-treated patients was significantly higher than in the ara-C treated patients (71% vs. 15%) (Glantz et al., 1999b). Patients treated with liposomal cytarabine also had increased time to neurological progression and improvement in KPS compared with those treated with ara-C. A second phase III study compared the efficacy of DepoCyt to IT MTX in the treatment of LM from solid tumors. Cytarabine was slightly more effective with respect to cytological response (26% vs. 20%, *P* = .76) and median survival (105 days vs. 78 days, *P* = .15). Liposomal cytarabine treatment was significantly better in delaying the time to neurological progression (58 days vs. 30 days, *P* = .007) (Glantz et al., 1999a; Kesari and Batchelor, 2003). Arachnoiditis can occur in up to 60% of patients receiving liposomal cytarabine. As of 2017, liposomal cytarabine is no longer available for use in the United States.

Oral dexamethasone (4 mg twice daily for 5 days) reduces the frequency of arachnoiditis significantly.

Thiotepa (*N, N, N*-triethylenethiophosphoramide) is an alkylating agent with activity against a variety of tumors including leukemia and breast cancer. The dosage is 10 mg administered twice weekly. The rapid clearance of thiotepa from the CSF potentially limits its usefulness. However, in one randomized trial of IT chemotherapy in patients with LM, thiotepa was as effective as MTX and less toxic (Grossman and Moynihan, 1991).

Unlike combination chemotherapy for many systemic cancers, combinations of IT agents are not more effective than single agents and tend to be more toxic. More recently, IT administration of monoclonal antibodies in patients with selected tumors has been explored. The most common agents administered thus far are rituximab in CD20-positive lymphomas and trastuzumab in HER2-positive breast cancers. Large studies have not been performed to date, although small studies and case reports suggest that the treatment is well tolerated and may be effective (Figura et al., 2018). Optimal dosing has not been established. In addition, antibodies have been inconsistently given as single agents or in combination with other IT therapies (Perissinotti and Reeves, 2010; Zagouri et al., 2013). In patients with sensitive tumors this may be an effective approach although more study is needed.

### Systemic and Hormonal Therapy

The blood–brain barrier is often cited as an obstacle to the effective use of systemic chemotherapy for LM. However, it is accepted that the blood–brain barrier is "leaky" in the setting of CNS disease. This is evidenced by the enhancement present on MRI. Although not frequently evaluated in patients with tumors, the albumin CSF/serum quotient may characterize the extent of blood-derived proteins within the spinal fluid. This readily available test may be a tool to further assist clinicians in the management of LM and requires further testing (Reiber, 2003).

The interest in small-molecule tyrosine kinase is increasing in management of leptomeningeal disease, as in parenchymal BM. As discussed in prior sections, osimertinib, erlotinib and gefitinib are EGFR TKIs, while lapatinib targets HER2. Efficacy was initially noted in multiple published case reports that generated interest in additional investigations (Oliveira et al., 2011; Takenaka et al., 2011). Furthermore, pharmacokinetic studies have demonstrated that non-standard, more dose-dense schedules may further increase the ability of these agents to penetrate the CNS (Togashi et al., 2011). The early-generation EGFR TKIs gefitinib and erlotinib demonstrated either improvement in functional status or clinical and radiographic improvement following treatment, at both standard and high-dose regimens (Yi et al., 2009). In a phase I study of 20 patients with leptomeningeal disease from NSCLC, the third-generation EGFR TKI osimertinib showed radiographic and neurological improvement when used at high doses; similar activity has been shown at standard doses of osimertinib (Nanjo et al., 2018)

High-dose intravenous MTX achieves potentially cytotoxic CSF levels, and some evidence supports its utility in neoplastic meningitis. In one study, the treatment of patients with LM from solid tumors was with HD MTX with leucovorin rescue. Cytological clearing of CSF occurred in 13 of 16 patients, compared with 9 of 15 retrospective controls treated with IT MTX (Glantz et al., 1998a,b). High-dose systemic ara-C (3 g/m$^2$ every 12 hours) penetrates well into the CNS and is used sometimes in patients with leukemia or NHL who have both systemic and CNS disease. Recent data suggest that the 5-fluorouracil oral prodrug capecitabine may be useful in meningeal seeding from breast cancer (Ekenel et al., 2007; Rogers et al., 2004). A small study of showed durable responses in patients with leptomeningeal disease from lung and breast cancers treated with systemic HD-MTX (Tham et al., 2006; Vincent et al., 2013). Hormonal therapy may occasionally be of benefit in patients with LM due to hormone-sensitive tumors such as breast cancer and prostate cancer (Wen and Fine, 1997).

### Prognosis

Without treatment, patients with LM usually survive only 1–2 months, with occasional long-term survivals. The presence of encephalopathy in the setting of LM is associated with poor survival. In a cohort study of 40 patients, 20 had LM-related encephalopathy. Median survival in the group with encephalopathy was 10 weeks, compared to 24 weeks in the group without LM-associated encephalopathy (Chamberlain et al., 2004). Poor survival is also associated with CSF flow blocks in the setting of LM. Flow blocks culminate in nonuniform distribution of IT chemotherapy, which in turn creates regions of low and high concentrations of chemotherapy, resulting in tumor sanctuaries and increased toxicity, respectively. CSF flow blocks identified on CSF flow studies are often correctable with radiation. Uncorrectable flow blocks have been associated with significantly shorter survival (0.7 months) than in normal CSF flow (6.9 months) and abnormal but correctable flow blocks (13.0 months) (Glantz et al., 1995). Other prognostic factors include performance status, activity, and extent of systemic cancer, concomitant parenchymal metastases, and possibly histology. With treatment, the median survival increases to 3–6 months (Posner, 1995). Patients with NHL and breast cancer tend to respond better to treatment than those with other cancers, and the percentage of long-term survivors is increased. The 1-year survival rate for breast cancer is approximately 11%, whereas that for NHL is 6%–23%. In general, fixed neurological deficits such as cranial nerve palsies or paraplegia do not improve significantly with therapy, but encephalopathy may improve dramatically.

## PLEXUS METASTASES

### Brachial Plexopathy

The brachial plexus is the site of local metastasis or infiltration from adjacent tumors including lung cancer, breast cancer, and lymphoma. Local tumors of the nerve plexus may occur; however, this is less frequent. Anatomical upper and lower plexus lesions and panplexopathy are differentiated. Due to the vicinity of the lower brachial plexus to lymph nodes and apex of the lung, neoplasms of these origins are the most frequent presentation of neoplastic involvement (Jaeckle, 2004). Most common neoplastic plexus involvement is associated with lung cancer, breast cancer, and lymphoma. Less frequent causes include melanoma, sarcoma, unknown primaries, and laryngeal tumor. Infiltration via the supraclavicular lymph nodes resulting in damage of fibers from C5 and C6 nerve roots is rarely observed.

Axillary pain may be an indicator of upper thoracic root involvement. Likewise, depending on the topographical site of involvement, a radicular pain syndrome may also occur. Neurological signs such as motor, sensory, and autonomic may be involved but are much more delayed. Paresthesia is often perceived in the fourth and fifth digits.

Weakness caused by lower brachial plexus lesions affects the hand muscles, followed by weakness of the digit flexors. Damage to the sympathetic trunk causes Horner syndrome, which is a good indicator of prevertebral damage to the sympathetic trunk. The Pancoast tumor (superior pulmonary sulcus tumor or thoracic inlet tumor) (Pancoast, 1932) is usually caused by lung cancer at the apex of the lung but can also be caused by other tumors (Rao and Robins, 2001).

In patients with previous radiation, a differentiation between metastatic and radiation-induced plexopathy is required (Jaeckle, 2004, 2010; Mondrup et al., 1990). With new developments, the frequency of radiation brachial plexopathy is decreasing. Lymphoma can involve the brachial plexus in a variety of circumstances (Bokstein et al., 2005; Pietrangeli et al., 2000) and occurs usually as a late complication.

Enlarged lymph nodes can compress the brachial plexus and peripheral nerves, but also nerve infiltrations can be found. In lymphoma, secondary compression of the spinal cord can appear (Boes et al., 2008). In Hodgkin disease, brachial plexus infiltration occurs in 10%–15% of cases, more often affecting the upper brachial plexus (C5/C6). MRI is the best radiological method for exploring metastatic involvement of the brachial plexus and is superior to CT scan (Vargas et al., 2010a). MRI can show a mass adjacent to the plexus or metastatic infiltration and also cancer spread along nerve roots. A new technique such as magnetic resonance neurography (MRN) combines MRI with specially designed surface coils and allows visualization of the peripheral nerves (Zhou et al., 2004). This technique can detect both extraneural and intraneural lesions. MRI tractography of peripheral nerves is another promising investigation (Vargas et al., 2010b). Fluorodeoxyglucose–positron emission tomography (FDG–PET) is a good addition and its precision can be enhanced with an image fusion with CT or MRT scanning for anatomical localization. Rarely an open surgical exploration of the plexus is necessary. Ultrasound is a new and easily accessible tool for investigating the brachial plexus. Electrodiagnosis with electromyography (EMG) and nerve conduction velocity (NCV) is helpful for delineating the topographic aspects of the lesion as well as the electrical properties and function of the nerves and muscles (Boyaciyan et al., 1996). The complex distribution of peripheral nerves and muscles allows a topographical analysis and detection of denervation and reinnervation, which are suggestive of radiation damage.

The differential diagnosis of plexopathy in cancer patients includes epidural cord compression, neoplastic meningitis, primary plexus tumors, rarely paraneoplastic plexopathy, postinfectious plexopathy, and toxicity from intra-arterial chemotherapy. In patients with a history of radiotherapy, radiation-induced plexopathy may affect up to 5% of patients. Consequently, features that distinguish neoplastic plexopathy from radiation-induced brachial plexopathy can also be the result of postradiation subclavian artery occlusion, thrombosis of the axillary or subclavian vein, genetic susceptibility to develop nerve sheath tumors, and neuralgic amyotrophy (Lachance et al., 1991). Specific pain syndromes such as postmastectomy syndrome, which is typically a lesion of the intercostobrachial nerve, neuroma formation, post-thoracotomy syndrome, or phantom limb pain or stump pain must be excluded by clinical examination. Other differential diagnoses are malpositioning after interventions and neuralgic amyotrophy, and rarely a paraneoplastic cause has been suspected (Coppens et al., 2006). In patients with a history of radiotherapy, radiation-induced plexopathy may affect up to 5%. Consequently, features that distinguish neoplastic plexopathy from radiation-induced plexopathy have been subject to most reviews on brachial plexopathy. Distinction should be made between radiation-induced plexopathy and carcinomatous infiltration. Despite the fact that the distinction between radio-induced and tumor-related plexopathy has been given much deserved attention in previous textbooks, this can be a difficult issue. However, this distinction is of decreasing importance for two reasons: (1) RT treatment has improved over the past decades, and severe RT damage is infrequently seen; and (2) modern imaging, in particular MR, allows a distinction in many cases on imaging criteria. Additionally, fusion techniques (PET and MR or CT) allow the detection of neoplastic tissue.

As brachial plexus lesions are often a sign of advanced disease, surgical intervention is rarely indicated, although for Pancoast tumors and rare instances interventions have been described. Surgery is reserved for selected cases with neurological deficit (Lusk et al., 1987). Usually RT is the therapy of choice in neoplastic plexus involvement. RT with 3000–5000 cGy is more efficient on pain (Kori et al., 1981) than on motor and sensory deficits. Lymphedema, venous obstruction, and thromboses are late complications. Despite the improvement of RT techniques, it needs to be considered that RT of the brachial plexus can cause early, delayed, and late complications.

Early and early delayed complications occur within weeks or a few months and are attributed to conduction block (Soto, 2005). They are infrequently observed and can result in fibrosis of nerve and muscle (Wadd and Lucraft, 1998). Late complications are more frequent and must be distinguished from neoplastic recurrence (Lederman and Wilbourn, 1984). The mechanism is a radiation-induced vasculopathy, followed by radiation fibrosis (Fajardo and Berthrong, 1988). The median interval between RT and the onset of RT-induced late plexopathy ranges from 1 to 4 years or longer. The incidence of complications increases with the total radiation dose and dose per fraction (Johansson et al., 2002). Brachial plexus lesions during mantle field radiation have also been described (Wadd and Lucraft, 1998). Generally, new techniques reduce the number of side effects of RT (van Beek et al., 2008) and the extensive changes do not occur with new techniques. Medical therapies focus on the radiation-induced vascular lesions (Glantz et al., 1994). Pain relief must be obtained by pharmacological treatment focused on neuropathic pain. Opioids either orally or by spinal application are needed in severe pain cases. In tumor recurrence a repeated course of RT is also based on an individual decision. Chemotherapy and hormonal therapy (Bagley et al., 1978) can produce additional pain relief. Pain treatment is the most important feature for patients, either pharmacological or by local nerve blocks or other invasive techniques. In the older literature, even limb amputation for pain management has been described (Kori et al., 1981).

## Lumbosacral Plexopathy

As with brachial plexopathy, lumbosacral plexopathy is usually the result of direct invasion from the uterus, ovary, rectum, and prostate, or metastases to local lymph nodes or bone. Several cancers such as gynecological, gastrointestinal, prostate, lymphomas, and local sarcomas can invade either the lumbar or sacral plexus, usually as a late complication or recurrence. Lymphoma can also affect the sacral plexus, in particular diffuse large B-cell lymphoma, Burkitt, Hodgkin, and MALT type, and rarely T-cell lymphoma. Perineural spread via the pelvic plexus to the lumbosacral plexus has been described in prostate cancer with the use of high-resolution MRI and PET/CT (Hebert-Blouin et al., 2010; Ladha et al., 2006), and has been described in cervical cancer also. Locally invasive colorectal carcinoma is the most frequent cause of sacral plexus lesions. Pain is usually the most prominent symptom, radiating into the lumbar fossa, hip and buttocks, and legs. Pain is the dominating symptom, radiating to the buttocks and the posterior aspects of the thigh with symptomatic sensory loss, causalgia, and deafferentation. Numbness in the perianal region and also incontinence can occur. The involvement of sympathetic fibers causes the "hot and dry foot" syndrome (Dalmau et al., 1989). Several distinct pain syndromes with symptomatic sensory loss, causalgia, and deafferentation have been described in lower sacral and coccygeal plexus distribution (Caraceni and Portenoy, 1996).

Diagnostic methods are mostly dependent on CT, MR, and, increasingly, ultrasound. EMG/NCV techniques can help in localization and in the distinction between carcinomatous and radiation-induced plexopathy. Additionally, electrophysiological testing can help to determine the topography of involved structures. EMG can suggest findings relating to radiation plexopathy. Denervation of plexus-innervated muscles, absence of sensory nerve action potentials of the sural and fibular superficial nerve, and absence of paraspinal denervation are indicative of plexus lesions, but frequently definitive diagnosis of sacral plexus lesions cannot be made by electrophysiology alone. As in brachial plexus involvement, lumbar or sacral plexopathy is primarily treated with radiotherapy.

## PERIPHERAL NERVE METASTASES

Very rarely, mononeuropathies, mononeuropathy multiplex, and even a symmetrical polyneuropathy may result from direct nerve infiltration by tumor (Briemberg and Amato, 2003). Lymphomas and leukemias, particularly chronic lymphocytic leukemia, have been associated with peripheral neuropathy due to malignant infiltration of nerve. (Briemberg and Amato, 2003).

*The complete reference list is available online at https://expertconsult.inkling.com/.* 

77

# Neurological Manifestations of Human Immunodeficiency Virus Infection in Adults

Ashok Verma, Joseph R. Berger

## OUTLINE



## EPIDEMIOLOGY AND CURRENT TRENDS

Acquired immunodeficiency syndrome (AIDS) was first recognized in the United States in the summer of 1981 when unexplained occurrences of *Pneumocystis jirovecii* (formerly *carinii*) pneumonia and Kaposi sarcoma were reported in cohorts of previously healthy homosexual men in Los Angeles, New York, and San Francisco. Within months, the disease became recognized in intravenous drug users (IDUs) and soon thereafter in recipients of blood transfusion and blood products, including hemophiliacs. As the epidemiological pattern unfolded, it became clear that a microbe transmitted by sexual (homosexual and heterosexual) contact and through blood and blood products was the etiological agent of the epidemic. In 1983, human immunodeficiency virus type-1 (and later type-2, henceforth called HIV) was isolated and confirmed the following year as the causal agent of AIDS. In 1985, a sensitive enzyme-linked immunosorbent assay (ELISA) test was developed, which led to the recognition of the scope of HIV infection among cohorts of individuals in the United States and elsewhere. As the disease spread, seroprevalence studies revealed the enormity of the global pandemic, with AIDS cases reported from virtually every country.

Now, after three and a half decades of AIDS, this disease has become one of the greatest public health challenges globally. The HIV pandemic has resulted in an estimated 77.3 million infections worldwide and it has claimed the lives of 35.4 million persons (www.unaids.org). Although the trend in AIDS-related deaths and new HIV infection has declined in recent years, during the year 2017 alone, 1.8 million (compared to peak of 3.4 million in 2004) persons died from AIDS and 940,000 (compared to 1.9 million in 2004 and 1.4 million in 2010) were newly infected with HIV. At the end of 2017, an estimated 36.9 million (31.5 million adults, 1.8 million children younger than 15) were living with HIV disease (www.unaids.org). The latest epidemiological data indicate that globally the spread of HIV had peaked in the late 1990s, when yearly an estimated 3.5 million new infections occurred. In 2017, the estimated number of new infections was approximately 51% lower in adults than it was in late 1990s. However, the population of people living with HIV continues to rise, chiefly from the combined effects of continued high rates of new infections and the survival benefits of antiretroviral therapy.

HIV continues to disproportionately affect certain geographic regions (e.g., sub-Saharan Africa, Caribbean nations) and certain subpopulations (homosexual men, women in sub-Saharan Africa, intravenous drug abusers, and sex workers). East and Southern Africa is home to 6.2% of the world's population (440.2 million) but has 19.4 million people living with HIV, greater than 50% of the global total; Swaziland has the highest adult HIV prevalence in the world (27.2%), and HIV prevalence among sex workers varies between 50% and 70% in several countries in this region (www.unaids.org).

The staggering grim statistics of the worldwide HIV pandemic has been matched, however, by an explosion of information in the area of HIV virology, pathogenesis and treatment of HIV disease, treatment and prophylaxis of opportunistic diseases associated with HIV infection, and prevention of HIV infection. In the United States and other resource-rich countries, the incidence of AIDS and AIDS-related deaths has fallen by over 80% since 1995. This trend reflects reduced HIV infection rates since the mid-1980s and the use of highly effective combined active antiretroviral therapy (cART) early in the course of HIV infection. Perinatal HIV transmission from HIV-infected mothers has shown a dramatic decline (>95%) in the United States. This is attributable to several factors, including universal prenatal testing, antiretroviral prophylaxis, elective cesarean delivery, and avoidance of breastfeeding by infected mothers.

As the HIV epidemic has changed in recent years, new challenges have emerged. As more HIV-infected persons receive cART (50-fold increase in access to cART globally since 2001), the number of persons living with HIV is increasing, requiring that the prevention programs must be scaled up to prevent HIV transmission from those living with HIV infection to those at risk of infection. With no vaccine on the foreseeable horizon, stopping HIV transmission and halting AIDS-related deaths is the only practical strategy currently available to halt the AIDS epidemic.

## HUMAN IMMUNODEFICIENCY VIRUS GENOME, REPLICATION, AND MOLECULAR HETEROGENEITY OF HUMAN IMMUNODEFICIENCY VIRUS

HIV is an RNA virus belonging to the family of human retroviruses (Retroviridae) and the subfamily of lentiviruses. Electron microscopy shows that the HIV virion is an icosahedral structure. It contains numerous external spikes formed by the two major envelope proteins (gp120 and gp41) and one major core protein (p24). Like other retroviruses, HIV has genes that encode the structural and enzyme proteins of the virus: *env* encodes the surface glycoproteins, *gag* encodes the core protein, and *pol* and *integrase* encode for the enzymes responsible for reverse transcription and its integration into the nuclear genome. HIV also contains at least six other genes (*tat, rev, nef, vif, vpr,* and *vpu*), which encode for proteins involved in viral gene regulation and host cell modification to enhance viral growth. Several of these proteins play a role in the pathogenesis of HIV disease (see below). Flanking these genes are long terminal repeats that contain regulatory elements involved in gene expression. The major difference between the genomes of HIV-1 and HIV-2 is that HIV-2 lacks the *vpu* gene and has a *vpx* gene instead.

The replication cycle of HIV begins with high-affinity binding of the gp120 envelope protein to its receptor, the CD4 molecule, on the host cell surface (Greene and Peterlin, 2002). The CD4 molecule is a 55-kDa protein found predominantly on CD4+ helper-inducer lymphocytes (CD4+ T cells), but also on the surface of monocytes-macrophages and dendritic-Langerhans cells. After gp120 binds to the CD4 molecule, it undergoes a conformational change that facilitates its binding to a co-receptor (CCR5, CXCR4) (Xiao et al., 2000). These co-receptors belong to the family of transmembrane G protein-coupled cellular receptors, and the use of one or other of these receptors by the virus for entry into the cell determines the cellular tropism of the virus strain. Following surface attachment and fusion, the HIV genomic RNA is uncoated and internalized into the host cell. The subsequent steps in viral replication include activation of reverse transcriptase enzyme, reverse transcription of the genomic RNA into double-stranded DNA, and integration of DNA into the host cell chromosome through the action of another virally encoded enzyme—*integrase.* HIV integration into the nuclear DNA is not entirely random but is preferential for transcriptionally active genes and for some hotspots. This integrated provirus may remain latent (transcriptionally inactive) or it may manifest varying levels of gene expression, up to active production of the whole virus. Progression through the viral replication cycle is profoundly influenced by a variety of viral regulatory gene products and host factors (O'Brien and Moore, 2000).

Molecular analyses of various HIV isolates from a single person over time and from cohorts of patients reveal sequence variations over many parts of the viral genome. The degree of difference in coding sequences of the viral envelope genes, for example, can vary from a few percent to 50%. These sequence changes tend to cluster in hypervariable regions of the HIV genome. Single-base substitutions, insertions and deletions, recombinations, and gain or loss of glycosylation sites are involved in this phenomenon of genetic heterogeneity. The immune pressure and functional constraints on viral proteins (by antibodies, for example) and the use of retroviral therapy influence the level of variation in viral genes and protein products.

Detailed knowledge of the HIV agent is important for understanding the principles of HIV diagnostics and therapeutics. Diagnostic tests of HIV infection are based on host antibody response to viral proteins (ELISA), detection of major viral proteins (Western blot), or direct sequencing of viral genomic sites. The sensitivity and specificity of each of these tests differ. Likewise, each point in the replication cycle of HIV is a real or potential target for therapeutic intervention (see section on antiretroviral therapy). Study of viral genomic heterogeneity is also a powerful molecular tool to track viral trafficking worldwide and to understand drug resistance.

## NATURAL HISTORY OF HUMAN IMMUNODEFICIENCY VIRUS INFECTION AND NEURO-HUMAN IMMUNODEFICIENCY VIRUS DISEASE

The hallmark of HIV disease is the profound immunodeficiency resulting from a progressive loss or dysfunction of the subset of T lymphocytes referred to as helper or inducer T cells in conjunction with polyclonal immune activation (Fauci et al., 2018). The CD4+ T lymphocytes are phenotypically defined by the presence on their surface of the CD4 molecules that serve as the primary cellular receptor for HIV. A co-receptor (CCR5 or CXCR4, see previous section) must also be present together with CD4 for efficient fusion and entry of HIV into the target cells. CD4+ T cells are the initial and crucial natural activators in immune defense mechanisms. It is thus ironic that these helper/inducer CD4+ T cells are the cells most likely to bind to the virus, be infected, and themselves be destroyed. Whether direct infection and destruction, or activation-induced cell death, or a combination of these mechanisms is primarily responsible for progressive dysfunction and depletion of CD4+ T cells in vivo is unclear. But when the number of CD4+ T cells declines below a certain level, the person is at high risk of developing a variety of opportunistic diseases: chiefly the AIDS-defining infections and neoplasms. Some features of AIDS, such as neurological abnormalities (encephalopathy, dementia, polyneuropathy), cannot be explained entirely by the immunosuppressive effect of HIV, since they can arise before the development of severe immunological impairment.

The current Centers for Disease Control and Prevention (CDC) classification system of HIV-infected persons categorizes patients on

**TABLE 77.1 CDC Human Immunodeficiency Virus Infection Stages 1–3 Based on Specific CD4+ T cell Counts or CD4+ T cell Percentage of Total Lymphocytes**

| | AGE ON DATE OF CD4+ T CELL COUNT | | | | | |
|---|---|---|---|---|---|---|
| | ≤1 YEAR | | 1–5 YEARS | | 6 YEARS THROUGH ADULT | |
| Stage* | Cells/µL | % | Cells/µL | % | Cells/µL | % |
| 1 | ≥1500 | ≥34 | ≥1000 | ≥30 | ≥500 | ≥26 |
| 2 | 750–1499 | 26–33 | 500–999 | 22–29 | 200–499 | 14–25 |
| 3 | <750 | <26 | <500 | <22 | <200 | <14 |

*The stage is based primarily on the CD4+ T cell count; the CD4+ T cell count takes precedence over the CD4+ T cell percentage, and the percentage is considered only if the count is missing.

*Source: Morbidity and Mortality Weekly Report 63(Recommendations and Reports-03), 2014:1-10.*

the basis of clinical conditions associated with HIV infection and CD4+ T cell counts (Table 77.1). A confirmed HIV case can be classified in one of the five stages (0, 1, 2, 3, or unknown). Stage is 0 if the person was tested seronegative within previous 6 months of the first HIV infection diagnosis or until 6 months after diagnosis. Advanced HIV disease (AIDS) is classified as stage 3 if one or more specific opportunistic illness has been diagnosed. Otherwise, stage is determined by CD4+ T cell counts and immunological status. The stage is classified U (unknown) if none of these criteria apply (e.g., missing CD4+ T cell test results). The definition and staging criteria of AIDS are complex and comprehensive and were originally designed for surveillance purposes. The clinicians should not focus only on which stage is present, but instead should view HIV disease as a spectrum ranging from primary infection through asymptomatic stage to advanced disease.

The stage of systemic HIV infection influences both the risk and the nature of neurological disease as well as likely etiologies, and hence CD4+ T cell count provides critical information that helps guide the evaluation (Fig. 77.1). In early infection (corresponding to CD4+ T cell counts >500/μL) and in a setting of polyclonal immune activation, autoimmune disorders, such as inflammatory demyelinating neuropathies, may develop. During midstage infection (CD4+ T cell counts of 200–500/μL), primary HIV-related disorders, such as low-grade encephalitis or HIV-associated neurocognitive dysfunctions (HANDs), may become symptomatic, as may such infections as varicella-zoster virus (VZV) radiculitis (shingles). In advanced HIV infection (CD4+ T cell count <200/μL), the risk of dementia, myelopathy, and polyneuropathy increases further, and patients become increasingly vulnerable to major opportunistic infections (OIs), such as cerebral toxoplasmosis, progressive multifocal leukoencephalopathy (PML), and cryptococcal meningitis, as well as to neoplasms, in particular, such as primary central nervous system lymphoma (PCNSL).

It is important to appreciate that the pathogenic mechanisms of neuro-HIV disease are complex and varied, they are multifactorial and multiphasic, and they are different at different stages of the disease (Fauci et al., 2018; Malik and Eugenin, 2016; Patel and Spudich et al., 2018). Thus, it is essential to understand the typical clinical and immunological course of untreated HIV infection in order to fully appreciate the spectrum of HIV-associated neurological diseases.

There are a number of cardinal tenets of HIV-related neurological disease that need to be kept in mind in evaluating patients. First, neurological diseases are not infrequently the heralding manifestation of AIDS and may occur before HIV infection has been recognized. Second, HIV-related neurological disease may present in unusual fashions; common illnesses may present in atypical fashions. Third, despite upward of 36 years of experience with HIV/AIDS, new disorders attributed to the infection, including neurological illness, continue to be described (Fauci et al., 2018; Roh et al., 2013; Verma and Post 2013). Fourth, any part of the neuraxis may be affected by HIV infection. Fifth, the simultaneous presence of two or more HIV-related neurological disorders is frequently observed. Lastly, neurological disease occurring in the presence of HIV infection need not be related to the HIV infection or associated immunosuppression. Therefore, the clinician must have a high index of suspicion for HIV infection but not blindly attribute disease to the HIV infection.

## Primary Infection and Dissemination of Virus

HIV is transmitted by both homosexual and heterosexual contact; by sharing of contaminated needles in IDUs; by tainted blood and blood products; and from infected mothers to infants either intrapartum,

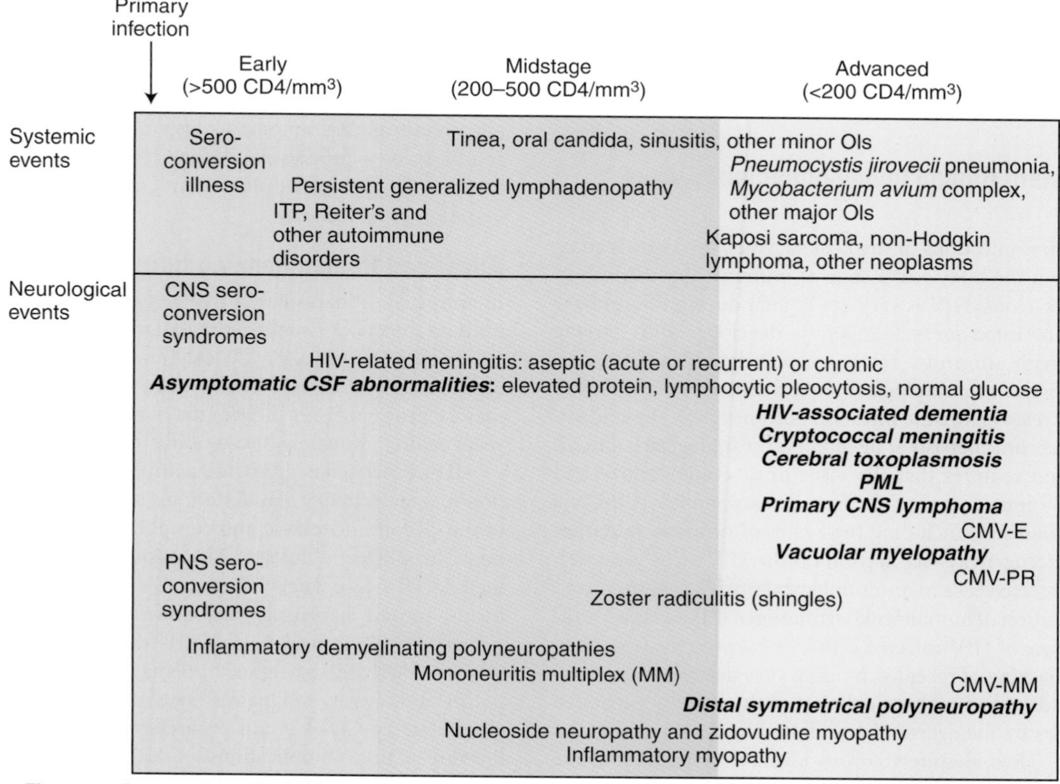


**Fig. 77.1 Systemic and Neurological Events in Human Immunodeficiency Virus (HIV) Infection.** Temporal sequence is approximate and indicates the increasing risk of systemic and neurological complications as HIV infection advances. *CMV-E,* Cytomegalovirus encephalitis; *CMV-PR,* CMV polyradiculitis; *CNS,* central nervous system; *CSF,* cerebrospinal fluid; *ITP,* idiopathic thrombocytopenic purpura; *OIs,* opportunistic infections; *PML,* progressive multifocal leukoencephalopathy; *PNS,* peripheral nervous system.

perinatally, or via breast milk (Hansasuta and Rowland-Jones, 2001). Virus that enters directly into the bloodstream via infected blood or blood products is trapped rapidly by the spleen and lymphoid tissue, whereas entry of virus through mucosal surface (sexual contact) requires mucosal dendritic cells or trafficking CD4+ T cells to first carry the virus to the regional lymphoid tissue. In either case, virus replication in CD4+ T cells intensifies (more rapidly with blood-borne infection) prior to development of the HIV-specific immune response, leading to a burst of viremia and rapid dissemination of the virus to other lymphoid organs, the brain, and other tissues. The initial viremic burst generally results in "acute HIV syndrome," and these individuals often have a high level of viremia, measured in millions of HIV RNA virions per milliliter, that lasts for several weeks. Virtually all patients develop initial viremia during primary infection, even though they may remain asymptomatic or not recall any clinical event. HIV infection of the brain is believed to occur within 2 weeks of the infection.

It is estimated that 50%–70% of individuals with HIV infection experience an acute clinical syndrome 1–6 weeks after the primary infection. The syndrome is typical of an acute viral syndrome and has been likened to acute infectious mononucleosis. Fever, erythematous or maculopapular rash, headache, nausea, anorexia, lethargy, arthralgia, sore throat, and lymphadenopathy occur in different combinations in this syndrome.

Neurological manifestations occur in as many as 10% of cases at the time of initial HIV infection. The neurological presentation frequently involves multiple parts of the nervous system, although one part is usually dominant. Meningitis, meningoencephalitis of varying severity, seizures, myelopathy, and cranial and peripheral neuropathies have all been linked to the primary HIV infection. Laboratory analysis at this stage (with or without neurological disease) reveals cerebrospinal fluid (CSF) abnormalities with mild mononuclear pleocytosis and moderate rise in protein. Imaging of the brain is usually normal, whereas the electroencephalogram (EEG) may be diffusely or focally slow in brain-symptomatic cases. In most cases, primary infection with or without the acute HIV syndrome is followed by a prolonged period of clinical latency.

## Chronic Persistent Human Immunodeficiency Virus Infection

In most human viral infections, if the host survives, the virus is completely cleared from the body and a state of immunity against subsequent infection develops. HIV is very rarely fatal during the primary infection. Chronic infection subsequently develops with varying degrees of virus replication in a setting of polyclonal immune activation and progressive immunological impairment over a median of approximately 10 years before the infection becomes clinically evident. Establishment of chronic persistent infection is the biological hallmark of HIV disease and requires that the virus must evade control and elimination by the immune system. The virus accomplishes this via a number of mechanisms, including high rates of genomic mutation and molecular heterogeneity (see section on the HIV virus genome), sequestration of infected cells in immunologically privileged sites (e.g., brain), downregulation of human leukocyte antigen (HLA) class I molecules on the surface of HIV-infected cells by viral proteins (e.g., *nef*), conformational masking of receptor-binding sites that fails to be neutralized by antibodies, and perhaps deletion of the initially expanded CD8+ T cell clones by the overwhelming initial burst of viremia and viral antigenemia. Thus, despite vigorous immune response and the marked downregulation of virus replication following primary HIV infection, HIV succeeds in establishing a state of chronic low-grade infection. Acute primary infection transitions to a relatively prolonged state of clinical latency. The level of steady-state plasma viremia (viral set point) in the latent phase probably determines the duration of this stage, or conversely, the rapidity of disease progression.

The half-life of a productively infected CD4+ T cell is approximately 1 day and that of a circulating virion is 30–60 minutes. Given the relatively steady level of plasma viremia and of infected cells in an individual, mathematical modeling indicates extremely large amounts of virus (over a billion or so copies) are produced and cleared from the circulation each day. Thus, clinical latency should not be confused with microbial latency. Vigorous virus replication, though with low-level viremia, is present during the period of clinical latency. Even the term "clinical latency" is misleading, because immunological progression of the HIV disease is generally relentless during this period.

Evidence indicates that the central nervous system (CNS) continues to harbor and mount a host reaction to the HIV throughout the asymptomatic or latent stage, yet without apparent immediate clinical sequelae (Spudich and Gonzalez-Scarano, 2012; Crossley and Brew, 2013; Saylor et al., 2016; Patel and Spudich, 2016). The CSF in patients with latent HIV infection generally shows abnormalities, including abnormal cell count, protein and immunoglobulin elevation, and local synthesis of anti-HIV antibodies within the CNS compartment; the intact virus can be recovered from the CSF. Pathological studies have shown evidence of inflammatory reactions in the CNS, with perivascular mononuclear cell infiltrations, although the HIV RNA burden, as measured by polymerase chain reaction (PCR) from CSF and brain samples, appears to be low at this stage. Neither overt nor subclinical cognitive or motor dysfunction appears to be common in the early latent stage. From a practical standpoint, the risk of cognitive decline in asymptomatic individuals is sufficiently small as to provide no basis for disability or disqualification from work based simply on HIV-positive status.

The length of the asymptomatic stage is determined by viral and host factors (Kinter et al., 2000; Xiao et al., 2000; Spudich and Gonzalez-Scarano, 2012; Fauci et al., 2018). Some patients, who are termed "long-term nonprogressors or elite controllers" show little if any decline in CD4+ T cell counts over many years. These patients generally have extremely low levels of HIV RNA. Certain other patients remain entirely asymptomatic despite the fact that their CD4+ T cell counts show a progressive decline to extremely low levels. In these patients, the appearance of a systemic or CNS OI may be the first manifestation of HIV disease.

## Advanced Human Immunodeficiency Virus Disease

In untreated or inadequately treated patients, after a variable period of primary infection, usually measured in years, the CD4+ T cell counts fall below a critical level (<200/μL) and patients become susceptible to opportunistic diseases. The depletion of CD4+ T cells continues and may be profound. Yet these patients may survive for months or even years before, ultimately, succumbing to OIs or neoplasia.

HIV-associated neurological complications in late-stage HIV infection include primary manifestations, secondary complications related to the OIs and neoplasia, and complications arising from antiretroviral or prophylactic therapy. The primary neurological complications include HIV-associated dementia (HAD) or its less severe HAND forms—minor neurocognitive disorder (MND) and asymptomatic neurocognitive impairment (ANI), vacuolar myelopathy (VM), and HIV-associated distal sensory polyneuropathy (DSP). Generally, the nature and severity of illnesses (systemic and neurological) that occur change as the CD4+ count progressively declines. The frequent and life-threatening complications of HIV infection typically occur in patients with a significant decline in CD4+ T cell counts below 100/μL. Although the causative agents of secondary infections are characteristically opportunistic organisms such as *Cryptococcus*, cytomegalovirus (CMV), and other microorganisms that do not ordinarily cause disease in the absence of a compromised immune system, they also include common bacterial and mycobacterial pathogens. Secondary complications (systemic and neurological) are of great importance because of their frequency and high mortality. Approximately 80% of deaths among AIDS patients are a direct result of an infection other than HIV.

## NEUROPATHOGENESIS OF HUMAN IMMUNODEFICIENCY VIRUS DISEASE

Neurons lack the conventional surface receptor for HIV binding and fusion, and therefore are not directly infected by the virus. The main cell types infected in the brain in vivo are those of the monocyte-macrophage lineage (Burdo et al., 2013). These include monocytes that have migrated into the brain from the peripheral blood, perivascular macrophages, and resident microglial cells. Although there have been reports of infrequent HIV infection of astrocytes, there is no convincing evidence that brain cells other than those of monocyte-macrophage lineage can be productively infected in vivo (Spudich and Gonzalez-Scarano, 2012). Nevertheless, in vivo infection of a neural cell line has been reported (Klein et al., 1999), and it appears that galactosylceramide on neuronal surface is an essential component of the HIV gp120 receptor and that antibodies to galactosylceramide inhibit the entry of HIV into the neural cell lines. Some studies have demonstrated that viral entry is due, in part, to the ability of virus-infected and immune-activated macrophages to induce adhesion molecules such as vascular adhesion molecule-1 (VCAM-1) on brain endothelium. Other studies have demonstrated that HIV gp120 enhances the expression of intercellular adhesion molecule-1 (ICAM-1) in glial cells; these effects may facilitate entry of HIV-infected cells into the CNS and may promote syncytia formation (Fig. 77.2).

The R5 (CCR5 co-receptor) virus strains which are macrophage-tropic preferentially gain access into the brain rather than R4 (CXCR4 co-receptor) strains. HIV-infected individuals who are heterozygous for CCR5-del.32 (co-receptor gene with 32-base deletion) appear to be relatively protected against the development of HIV encephalopathy, as compared with persons with homozygous wild-type CCR5 (Weiss et al., 1999). Host HLA, chemokine receptor (CCR5, CXR4), and innate immunity loci and certain HIV envelope sequences are also linked with the clinical manifestation of HANDs (Fauci et al., 2018; Saylor et al., 2016).

HIV-infected individuals may manifest white matter changes as well as neuronal loss (Saylor et al., 2016; Trentalange et al., 2020). Given the relative absence of evidence of HIV infection of neurons, it is unlikely that direct infection of these cells accounts for this cell loss. Rather, the HIV-mediated effects on brain tissue are thought to be due to a combination of indirect effects, either toxic or function-inhibitory of virus or viral antigens on neuronal cells and effects of a variety of neurotoxins released from the infiltrating monocytes, resident microglial cells, and astrocytes (Kamkwalala and Newhouse, 2017; Kovalevich and Langford, 2012; Levine et al., 2016; Scaravilli et al., 2007; Spudich and Gonzalez-Scarano, 2012; Saylor et al., 2016; Teodorof-Diedrich and Spencer, 2018). In this regard, it has been demonstrated that HIV-1 antigens—for example, *nef* and *tat* (viral core antigens)—can induce chemotaxis of leukocytes, including monocytes, into the CNS. Neurotoxins can be released from monocytes as a consequence of other HIV-associated infections or immune activation. Activated monocyte-derived neurotoxic factors have been reported to injure neurons via the *N*-methyl-D-aspartate (NMDA) receptor. Additionally, HIV gp120 shed by virus-infected monocytes, and a variety of cytokines, including tumor necrosis factor-alpha (TNF-α), interleukin (IL)-1, IL-6, interferon-α (IFN-α), and endothelin, can contribute directly or indirectly to the neurotoxic effects in HIV infection. Furthermore, infection or activation of monocyte lineage cells can result in increased production of eicosanoids, nitric oxide, and quinolinic acid, which may also contribute to the neurotoxicity.

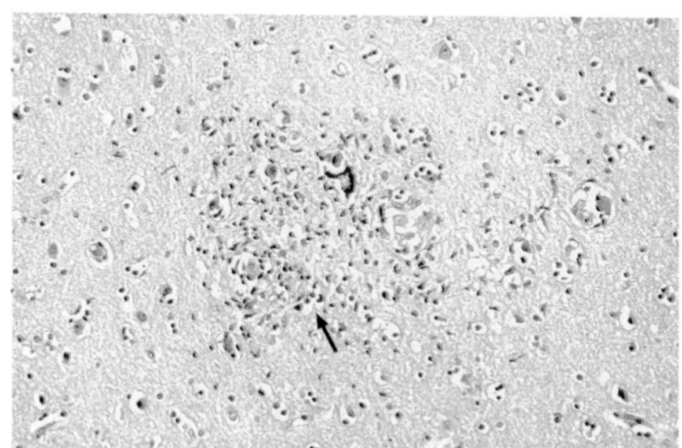

**Fig. 77.2 Human Immunodeficiency Virus Encephalitis.** Microglial nodule *(arrow)* containing multinucleated giant cells. (H&E, ×200.)

Older HIV-infected individuals (Kamkwalala and Newhouse, 2017; Saylor et al., 2016; Valcour, 2013; Yuen et al., 2017) and individuals with the E4 allele for apolipoprotein E (Corder et al., 1998; Saylor et al., 2016; Yuen et al., 2017) are reported to incur increased risk of HIV encephalitis and polyneuropathy. The fact that neuropsychiatric abnormalities may undergo remarkable and rapid improvement on the initiation of antiretroviral therapy, particularly in HIV-infected children, indicates that it is virus-driven, that the HIV or its products are involved in the neuropathogenesis of primary HIV neurological disorders, and that the dominant changes are either structural or functional at the synapses and dendritic spines, rather than indicative of neuronal death.

## ANTIRETROVIRAL THERAPY AND ITS EFFECT ON NEURO-HUMAN IMMUNODEFICIENCY VIRUS DISEASE

The dynamics of in vivo HIV production and turnover have been quantified using mathematical modeling in the setting of cART. Treatment with effective cART typically results in precipitous decline in the level of plasma viremia, often by well over 95% within a few weeks. The number of CD4+ T cells increases concurrently, suggesting that actively replicating virus is a major factor in CD4+ T cell depletion. Combination antiretroviral therapy therefore is the cornerstone of management of HIV infection. Suppression of HIV replication prolongs, as well as improves, the quality of life in patients with HIV infection.

Following the widespread use of cART in the United States from 1996, dramatic declines have been noted in the incidence of most AIDS-defining conditions, including neurological diseases (see earlier and following discussion). Successful cART with reconstitution of immune defense even has enabled some patients to discontinue secondary prophylaxis against CNS opportunistic pathogens, which had not been possible in the pre-cART era. It is recognized also that certain primary neurological diseases, in which the disease processes are driven by the HIV burden, can be prevented, delayed, or transformed into less severe forms by successful cART (Clifford, 2017; Sacktor et al., 2006; Saylor et al., 2016), although the evolution of drug-resistant viral strains may eventually limit the sustained benefits of antiretroviral therapy. It also appears that in the future, as patients survive longer and develop increasing drug-resistant HIV mutations to newer antiretroviral therapy, the incidence of neuro-HIV diseases may begin to actually rise again.

Treatment decisions must take into account the fact that one is dealing with chronic infection that can only be controlled; eradication of HIV infection has not yet been possible. Unfortunately, some of the most important questions related to the treatment of HIV disease lack definitive or straightforward answers. Among them are the questions of when cART should be started in an individual, what the best initial regimen is, when a given regimen should be changed, and what changes should be made once the decision to change is made. Notwithstanding these difficulties, the physician and patient must come to a mutually agreeable plan based on the best available data. Given the complexity of this field, decisions regarding antiretroviral therapy are best made in consultation with experts.

At present, the US Department of Health and Human Services Guidelines panel recommends everyone with HIV infection be treated with cART and the therapy be initiated as soon as possible after diagnosis. Therapy has been associated with a decrease in disease progression in patients at all stages of HIV infection and it leads to a decrease in the risk of transmission of infection. All pregnant women regardless of their stages of HIV disease should receive cART. In addition, one may wish to administer therapy to uninfected individuals immediately following a high-risk exposure; a 6-week course of cART therapy decreases risk of infection. Additionally, pre-exposure prophylaxis in individuals at high risk of HIV infection should be considered. For patients diagnosed with an OI and HIV infection at the same time, one may consider a 2- to 3-week delay in the initiation of cART during which time treatment is focused on the OI. This delay may decrease the severity of any subsequent immune reconstitution inflammatory syndrome (IRIS) by lowering the antigenic burden of the OI. However, for patients with advanced HIV infection (CD4+ <50/μm), cART should be initiated as soon as possible.

Currently licensed drugs for the treatment of HIV infection are summarized in Table 77.2. Fixed-dose combinations of many of these powerful drugs provide exciting new strategies for reducing pill burden, thus ensuring adherence and limiting the drug resistance (see Table 77.2).

Once the decision has been made to initiate therapy, the physician must decide which drugs to use as the first therapeutic regimen. Initial choice of drugs will determine the immediate response to therapy, and it will have implications regarding options for future therapeutic regimens. The goal of treatment is to achieve a viral load of less than 50 copies/μL within 4–6 months of initiation. The two options for initial therapy most commonly in use today involve a three- or four-drug regimen from two different antiretroviral classes (see Table 77.2). Recommendations regarding specific regimens are continuously evolving. In order to determine an optimal therapeutic regimen for initial therapy or for a patient on a failing regimen, one may attempt to measure antiretroviral drug susceptibility through genotyping or phenotyping of HIV quasispecies—to determine adequacy of dosing through measurement of drug levels. It is generally recommended that resistance testing be used in selecting initial therapy in settings where the risk of transmission of resistant virus is high and in determining new regimens for patients experiencing virological failure while on therapy.

For HIV-associated brain disease, drugs that exhibit good blood–brain barrier penetration should be preferred (see Table 77.2). Following the initiation of therapy, one should monitor virological (HIV RNA levels) and immunological (CD4+ T cell count) responses periodically. The HIV RNA levels in serum generally reflect viral levels in CSF, at least until late stages of the HIV disease. In terminal stages, the CNS compartment may harbor slightly different and divergent HIV strains, with different degrees of drug susceptibility (Crossley and Brew, 2013; Ellis et al., 2007; Spudich and Gonzalez-Scarano, 2012; Saylor et al., 2016). Maximal suppression of viral replication is the goal of therapy, not just to prevent the disease progression but also to prevent the appearance of drug-resistant HIV quasispecies. The principles of current therapy for HIV infection are well articulated in publications of the US Department of Health and Human Services (see updates at www.hivatis.org; www.nih.gov/phar/hiv-mgt).

As cART has become widely available and has prolonged the life of patients with AIDS, an increasingly observed rare manifestation has been noted characterized by a paradoxical clinical deterioration following therapy. Referred to as "the immune reconstitution inflammatory syndrome," it is defined as a paradoxical deterioration of the clinical status attributable to the recovery of the immune system. Although typically observed with OI, it may also occur as a response to noninfectious antigens. IRIS related to a known pre-existing infection or neoplasm is referred to as *paradoxical IRIS*, while IRIS associated with a previously undiagnosed condition is referred to as *unmasked IRIS*. IRIS has been described with a wide variety of systemic infections. In the CNS, IRIS has been well described with *Cryptococcus neoformans* infection, CMV retinitis, and PML, as well as other disorders. The term "immune reconstitution disease" is sometimes used to distinguish IRIS manifestations related to opportunistic diseases from IRIS manifestations related to autoimmune diseases. There is a suggestion that IRIS may attend primary HIV infection of the CNS. The symptoms mostly regress with continued cART, although a short course of high-dose parenteral corticosteroids has been suggested as effective in abrogating the response in some cases (Bahr et al., 2013; Roh et al., 2013).

## CLINICAL SPECTRUM OF NEURO-HUMAN IMMUNODEFICIENCY VIRUS DISEASE

The high prevalence and striking diversity of neurological disorders complicating AIDS were recognized early in the epidemic (Berger et al., 1987). Clinical description of neurological OIs and malignancies predominated in early reports, but it also became clear that AIDS was associated with distinct neurological syndromes, such as dementia and painful neuropathy, that appeared to result from the HIV itself. It also became recognized that the risk of neurological complications increased with the progression of the HIV infection and decline of the CD4+ T cell counts. Clinically apparent neurological disease develops in approximately one-half of HIV-infected patients. Neuropathological abnormalities are nearly universal in patients dying with AIDS, suggesting subclinical disease, underdiagnosis, or both, in many cases. Neurological disorders cause significant morbidity and mortality, and they may be the AIDS-defining illnesses in previously asymptomatic HIV disease or, occasionally, herald unrecognized HIV infection. Nervous system complications may directly threaten life, as well as impair a patient's ability to work or comply with complex cART regimens necessary to manage HIV disease optimally.

The neurological complications of HIV infection occur at all stages of the HIV disease (Simpson and Berger, 1996). Disorders of both the CNS and peripheral nervous system (PNS) can complicate HIV infection from the period after initial infection through the end stages of the severe immunosuppression. These neurological complications can be classified in a number of ways. A classification based on the underlying pathophysiology and HIV disease stages is summarized in Fig. 77.1. Box 77.1 presents classification based on neuroanatomical localization, following the classic proven methods of the neurologist. Clinicians must be aware that more than one site of neural axis can be involved in the same HIV-infected patient at the same time. Furthermore, the clinical deficits from one site may be masked by another lesion higher in the neuraxis; appropriate investigations may be necessary to delineate the complete

**TABLE 77.2 Currently Licensed and Most Commonly used Antiretroviral Drugs for Human Immunodeficiency Virus Infection**

| Drug | Dose | Toxicity | Remarks |
|---|---|---|---|
| **NRTIs** | | | |
| Abacavir (Ziagen) | 300 mg bid | Rash, GI, LA | Abacavir-resistant HIV strains are typically also resistant to Lamivudine, Didanosine, and Zalcitabine |
| Emtricitabine (FTC, Emtriva)* | 200 mg qd | Rash, GI | Generally well tolerated |
| Lamivudine (3Tc, Epivir)* | 150 mg bid | HA, GI, P, LA | May cause hepatic steatosis |
| Zidovudine (Retrovir)* | 300 mg bid | GI, HA, BM, rash | May cause myopathy, pancytopenia |
| **NtRTIs** | | | |
| Tenofovir alafenamide (Vemlidy) | 25 mg qd | GI, renal | Commonly used in combination therapy |
| Tenofovir disoproxil fumarate (Viread) | 300 mg qd | Renal, osteomalacia | Commonly used in combination therapy |
| **NNRTIs** | | | |
| Efavirenz (Sustiva)* | 600 mg qhs | Rash, liver, CNS | — |
| Etravirine (Intelence) | 200 mg bid | Rash, GI | Taken with food |
| Nevirapine (Viramune)* | 200 mg bid for 2 wk, then 200 mg bid or 400 mg extended release qd | Rash, liver | Close monitoring for initial 2 wk for rash and hepatitis |
| Rilpivirine (Edurant) | 25 mg qd | GI, liver, lipodystrophy | Mostly used in combination therapy |
| **PIs** | | | |
| Atazanavir (Reyataz) | 400 mg qd or 300 mg qd + Ritonavir 100 qd when given with Efavirenz | GI, metabolic changes | Mostly used in combination therapy |
| Darunavir (Prezista)* | 600 mg bid | Rash, liver, lipodystrophy | Mostly used in combination therapy |
| Ritonavir (Norvir) | 600 mg bid | GI, perioral paresthesia | Impairs metabolism of other PIs |
| **Entry Inhibitors** | | | |
| Enfuvirtide (Fuzeon)* | 90 mg SC bid | Local injection reaction, hypersensitivity | Increase incidence of bacterial pneumonia |
| Ibalizumab (Trogarzo) | Single-loading dose of 2000 mg followed by a maintenance dose of 800 mg q2 weekly | Rash, GI | Mostly used in combination therapy for multidrug-resistant HIV strains |
| Maraviroc (Selzentry) | 150–600 mg bid | Rash, fever, myalgia, cough | In combination therapy in adults infected with only CCR5-tropic HIV |
| **Integrase Inhibitors** | | | |
| Bictegravir (available only in combination therapy, Biktarvy)* | 25 mg qd | HA, GI | Available only in combination with Tenofovir alafenamide and Emtricitabine |
| Dolutegravir (Tivicay) | 50 mg qd in treatment-naïve and 50 mg bid in treatment-experienced cases | HA, hepatitis, CNS | Mostly used in combination therapy |
| Elvitegravir (available only in combination therapy, Stribild)* | 1 tablet qd | GI, HA, upper respiratory infection | Available only in combination with Cobicistat***, Tenofovir, and Emtricitabine |
| Raltegravir (Isentress)* | 400 mg bid | HA, GI, myopathy | Mostly used in combination therapy |
| **Combination Formulations** | | | |
| Atripla** | | Tenofovir disoproxil fumarate + Emtricitabine + Efavirenz | |
| Biktarvy** | | Tenofovir alafenamide + Emtricitabine + Bictegravir | |
| Combivir | | Zidovudine + Lamivudine | |
| Complera** | | Tenofovir disoproxil fumarate + Emtricitabine + Rilpivirine | |
| Descovy | | Tenofovir alafenamide + Emtricitabine | |
| Epzicom | | Abacavir + Lamivudine | |
| Genvoya** | | Tenofovir alafenamide + Emtricitabine + Elvitegravir + Cobicistat*** | |
| Kaletra | | Lopinavir + Ritonavir | |
| Odefsey** | | Tenofovir alafenamide + Emtricitabine + Rilpivirine | |

*Continued*

**TABLE 77.2 Currently Licensed and Most Commonly used Antiretroviral Drugs for Human Immunodeficiency Virus Infection—cont'd**

| Drug | Dose | Toxicity | Remarks |
|---|---|---|---|
| Prezcobix | | Darunavir + Cobicistat*** | |
| Stribild** | | Tenofovir disoproxil fumarate + Emtricitabine + Elvitegravir + Cobicistat*** | |
| Symfi** | | Tenofovir disoproxil fumarate + Lamivudine + Efavirenz (600 mg) | |
| Symfi Lo** | | Tenofovir disoproxil fumarate + Lamivudine + Efavirenz (400 mg) | |
| Triumeq** | | Abacavir + Lamivudine + Dolutegravir | |
| Trizivir | | Zidovudine + Lamivudine + Abacavir | |
| Truvada | | Tenofovir disoproxil fumarate + Emtricitabine | |

*Good CNS penetration.
**Complete, once-daily, single tablet regimens.
***Inhibits cytochrome CYP3A enzyme and enhances the levels of antiretroviral agents that are metabolized by this enzyme.
*BM,* Bone marrow suppression; *CNS,* central nervous system toxicity; *GI,* gastrointestinal toxicity; *HA,* headache; *HIV,* human immunodeficiency virus; *LA,* lactic acidosis; *NNRTIs,* nonnucleoside reverse transcriptase inhibitors; *NRTIs,* nucleoside reverse transcriptase inhibitors; *NtRTIs,* nucleotide reverse transcriptase inhibitors; *P,* pancreatitis; *PIs,* protease inhibitors.

**BOX 77.1 Major Human Immunodeficiency Virus-Associated Central Nervous System Disorders Classified by Neuroanatomical Localization**

**Meninges**
- Aseptic HIV meningitis
- Cryptococcal meningitis
- Tuberculous meningitis
- Syphilitic meningitis
- *Listeria monocytogenes* meningitis
- Lymphomatous meningitis (metastatic)

**Brain**

***Predominantly Nonfocal***
- HIV-associated neurocognitive disorders (HANDs)
  - HIV-associated dementia (HAD)
  - Mild neurocognitive disorder (MND)
  - Asymptomatic neurocognitive impairment (ANI)
- Toxoplasmic encephalitis
- Cytomegalovirus (CMV) encephalitis
- Aspergillus encephalitis
- Herpes encephalitis
- Metabolic encephalopathy (alone or concomitantly)

***Predominantly Focal***
- Cerebral toxoplasmosis
- Primary CNS lymphoma (PCNSL)
- Progressive multifocal leukoencephalopathy (PML)
- Cryptococcoma
- Tuberculoma
- Varicella-zoster virus (VZV) encephalitis
- Stroke

***Spinal Cord***
- Vacuolar myelopathy (VM)
- CMV myeloradiculopathy
- VZV myelitis
- Spinal epidural or intradural lymphoma (metastatic)
- Human T cell lymphocytotropic virus-1 (HTLV-1)-associated myelopathy

**Peripheral Nerves and Nerve Roots**

***Early Stages (Immune Dysregulation)***
- Acute inflammatory demyelinating polyradiculoneuropathy (AIDP)
- Chronic inflammatory demyelinating polyradiculoneuropathy (CIDP)
- Vasculitic neuropathy
- Brachial plexopathy
- Lumbosacral plexopathy
- Cranial mononeuropathy
- Multiple mononeuropathies

***Mid- and Late Stages (HIV-Replication Driven)***
- Distal sensory polyneuropathy
- Autonomic neuropathy

***Late Stages (Opportunistic Infection, Malignancy)***
- CMV polyradiculomyelitis
- Syphilitic polyradiculomyelitis
- Tuberculous polyradiculomyelitis
- Lymphomatous polyradiculopathy
- Zoster ganglionitis
- CMV mononeuritis multiplex
- Nutritional neuropathy (vitamin $B_{12}$, $B_6$)
- AIDS-cachexia neuropathy
- ALS-like motor neuronopathy

***All Stages (Toxic Neuropathy)***
- Nucleoside reverse transcriptase inhibitors (ddI, ddC, d 4 T)
- Other drugs (vincristine, isoniazid, ethambutol, thalidomide)

**Muscle**
- Polymyositis
- Pyomyositis
- Inclusion body myositis
- Toxic (zidovudine) myopathy
- AIDS-cachexia myopathy

**Treatment-Related Immune Reconstitution Inflammatory Syndrome (IRIS)**
- IRIS from cryptococcal CNS disease
- IRIS form of CMV retinitis
- IRIS forms of PML
- Other IRIS events

*ALS,* Amyotrophic lateral sclerosis; *CNS,* central nervous system; *ddC,* dideoxycytidine; *ddI,* didanosine; *d 4 T,* didehydrodeoxythymidine; *HIV,* human immunodeficiency virus.

clinical diagnosis. The clinician must be vigilant also for other common conditions that are not necessarily associated with the HIV or AIDS.

Experience in large HIV clinics indicates that the diagnosis of the neurological complications of HIV infection and AIDS is far from being an academic exercise. Rather, precise diagnosis is critical, and it frequently leads to specific therapy, with resultant reduction in morbidity and mortality, and in preservation of meaningful function and quality of life. Fig. 77.3 summarizes a diagnostic algorithm for CNS manifestations in HIV-infected patients.

## MAJOR HUMAN IMMUNODEFICIENCY VIRUS-ASSOCIATED NEUROLOGICAL SYNDROMES

### Diffuse Disorders of the Meninges and Brain

#### Aseptic Human Immunodeficiency Virus Meningitis

Diverse clinical forms of meningitis, without other evident cause, may develop during HIV infection. Although headache and meningeal irritation may accompany the initial seroconversion-related illness, chronic meningitis which is often subclinical, in less severe and protracted form, is more frequent in the later course of HIV infection. It occurs more commonly in patients experiencing progressive HIV disease, with decline in CD4+ T cell counts and clinical manifestations of HANDs. Isolated persistent headache is common in HIV-infected patients and it often occurs in the same setting as chronic aseptic meningitis.

Included among HIV-related meningitides is acute aseptic meningitis, which occasionally accompanies or follows the flu-like, febrile illness frequently associated with HIV seroconversion (see previous discussion). Preserved alertness and cognition accompanying headache and other symptoms of meningeal inflammation indicate HIV-associated meningitis. Seizures, encephalopathy, and additional signs and symptoms of parenchymal cerebral dysfunction suggest the presence of acute HIV-associated meningoencephalitis related to the HIV—a relatively rare seroconversion syndrome. The typical CSF profile consists of slightly elevated protein (<100 mg/dL) and mild lymphocytic pleocytosis (<25/μL), with normal glucose levels. Meningeal exposure to HIV can occur early in systemic infection, as inferred by recovery of HIV from CSF and evidence of intrathecal anti-HIV immunoglobulin G (IgG) synthesis. CSF pleocytosis of moderate degree is common in all stages of HIV infection and appears to correlate with CSF viral load, but not plasma viral levels (Spudich et al., 2005). The practical consequence of the CSF abnormalities routinely observed in HIV infection is that they can complicate interpretation of CSF obtained to diagnose other neurological disorders.

HIV-related meningitis is principally a diagnosis of exclusion, and hence evaluation for other causes of aseptic or chronic meningitis, such as parameningeal infection, other infections (syphilis, tuberculosis, listeriosis, fungal, etc.), lymphomatous or carcinomatous meningitis, other noninfectious causes (sarcoid, Behçet syndrome, etc.), or medications (nonsteroidal anti-inflammatory agents, intravenous immunoglobulin [IVIG], etc.) is usually undertaken. Patients thought to have acute HIV meningitis with an initially negative HIV test result require repeat testing in several months, because HIV antibodies may not be detectable in early infection. The prognosis in acute HIV meningitis is generally good and requires no specific therapy.

#### Human Immunodeficiency Virus-Associated Neurocognitive Disorders

HANDs, also called AIDS dementia complex (ADC) or HIV encephalitis, is characterized by cognitive, behavioral, and motor dysfunction, usually developing later in the course of infection (Clifford, 2017;

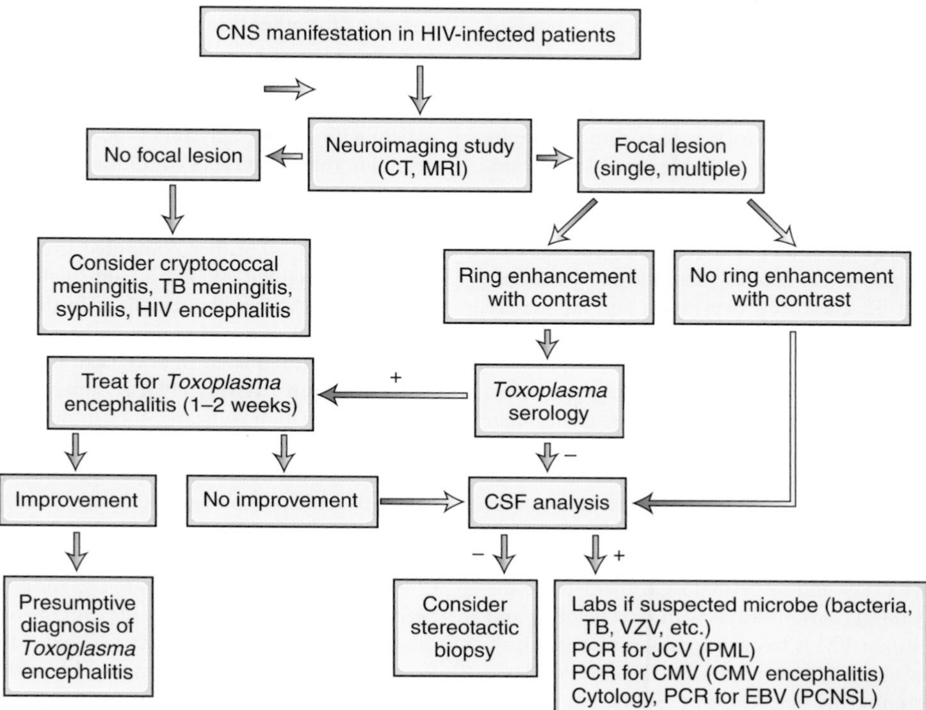


**Fig. 77.3 Diagnostic Algorithm for the Management of Human Immunodeficiency Virus (HIV) Disease with CNS Involvement.** +, Positive; –, negative; *CNS,* central nervous system; *CMV,* cytomegalovirus; *CSF,* cerebrospinal fluid; *CT,* computed tomography; *EBV,* Epstein-Barr virus; *JCV,* John Cunningham virus; *MRI,* magnetic resonance imaging; *PCNSL,* primary central nervous system lymphoma; *PCR,* polymerase chain reaction; *PML,* progressive multifocal leukoencephalopathy; *TB,* tubercular infection; *VZV,* varicella-zoster virus.

Spudich and Gonzalez-Scarano, 2012; Saylor et al., 2016). HAD and its less severe form, minor neurocognitive disorder (MND) and ANI, are the most common complications of untreated HIV disease. An alternative terminology, HIV-associated cognitive/motor complex, has also been proposed to encompass the full constellation of this syndrome. Characteristically, HAD and MND forms of HANDs manifest after patients have developed AIDS-defining systemic illnesses. However, a small number of patients present with HAD at a time when they do not yet fulfill formal diagnostic criteria of AIDS, although typically they show significant immunosuppression by laboratory criteria. Recognition of this early presentation was instrumental in the addition of HAD to the diagnostic criteria of AIDS. Later age, apoE4 allele, cardiovascular risk factors, and concurrent hepatitis C infections are linked to higher incidence of HAND (Clifford, 2017; Kamkwala and Newhouse 2017; Saylor et al., 2016; Yuen et al 2017). Smoldering IRIS mounted against compartmentalized HIV following brain-penetrant cART may cause encephalopathy (Apostolova et al., 2015; Roh et al., 2013).

### Clinical Features

ANI is the mildest form of HANDs and occurs in about 30% of individuals (Clifford, 2017; Saylor et al., 2016; Spudich and Gonzalez-Scarano, 2012). ANI is characterized by measurable neurocognitive impairment that is often unrecognized by the patient, or fails to impact function. ANI can be considered a presymptomatic form of HANDs; individuals with ANI are likely to go on to develop symptomatic cognitive dysfunction.

MND, the symptomatic form of neurological impairment of ANI, can be identified in about a quarter of HIV-positive persons. Early symptoms usually consist of difficulties with attention and concentration. Impaired executive function and cognitive slowing is often striking. Complex tasks become more difficult and take longer to complete, and forgetfulness and difficulty in concentration lead to missed appointments and the need to keep detailed lists outlining each day's plan. MND and HAD forms of HANDs are recognized early if patients require a high level of concentration and organization in their occupation or at home, because impaired performance becomes obvious in such situations. In many instances, an employee coworker, friend, or family member may be the first to notice subtle cognitive and personality changes as the patient begins to withdraw socially and appears apathetic and uncharacteristically quiet and forgetful. An agitated organic psychosis and dysphoria are rare as presenting or predominant aspects of this illness. Psychological depression and fatigue are not uncommon in HIV-infected individuals and require differentiation from early HANDs.

One major component of HAD syndrome is psychomotor dysfunction. Although cognitive dysfunction usually appears earlier than motor symptoms and continues to predominate, motor manifestations in the form of poor balance and incoordination may be an initial presentation. Fine and skilled hand movements are affected early, often resulting in a deterioration of handwriting. Gait incoordination may result in frequent tripping or falling or a need for extra caution in walking. The latter may impart a slow and somewhat rigid character to the gait. The appearance may mimic parkinsonism with slow pivoting and stooped posture. Concomitant VM is frequently observed at autopsy. Even if not symptomatic, motor abnormalities, such as hyperreflexia and positive Babinski sign, may be detected on examination early in the course of the disease.

Initially, formal mental status testing in ANI may be normal. As the disease progresses, however, patients begin to perform poorly on tasks requiring concentration and attention, such as digit and word reversals and serial sevens. Later, a large array of mental status tests become abnormal with advancing disease; multiple domains of cognitive function are affected. However, mental slowing continues to remain a prominent feature, and afflicted individuals often appear apathetic with poor insight, and even indifferent to their illness. Parallel to cognitive deterioration, ataxia, which at first affects only rapid turns or tandem gait, may become disabling. HIV-associated VM results in spastic lower extremity weakness, gait abnormalities, and sphincter dysfunction. Postural tremors are common, and on occasion, patients may exhibit choreiform movements and myoclonic jerks. Bowel and bladder disturbances are common in the later stages of the disease. In the end stage, patients become almost vegetative, lying in bed mute with vacant stare, unable to ambulate, and incontinent. Characteristically, the course is notable for the absence of focal or lateralizing neurological deficit, such as hemiparesis or aphasia. Their presence suggests another etiology for cognitive impairment.

### Neuropsychological Tests

Formal neuropsychological testing can be useful in diagnosis, management, and clinical monitoring of individual patients and in clinical research studies. Appropriately chosen neuropsychological tests that target the same cardinal cognitive dysfunction delineated by the AIDS-directed clinical assessment provide a formal, quantitative means of monitoring patients serially. These assessments focus chiefly on motor speed, concentration, and motor manipulation. However, the bedside neuropsychological tests (Power et al., 1995) have been developed to provide a quantitative scale of cognitive impairment in the same fashion as the Mini-Mental State Examination for Alzheimer disease. Neuropsychological test findings are not disease-specific and should always be interpreted in the clinical context. Neuropsychological tests do not substitute for the clinical neurological examination. Clinicians should be vigilant because some patients with MND perform within the population norms and some without HAD/MND perform poorly on testing for other reasons.

### Neuroimaging

Neuroimaging procedures are essential in evaluation of the AIDS patient with cognitive dysfunction. First, neuroimaging is particularly helpful in ruling out other conditions, such as PCNSL. Second, it often reveals abnormalities that are characteristic, although not pathognomonic, of HAD. Diffuse cerebral atrophy, generally greater centrally than cortically, on either computed tomography (CT) or magnetic resonance imaging (MRI), is an anticipated finding in HAD. In some patients, MRI shows abnormalities in the hemispheric white matter (Fig. 77.4) and, less commonly, in basal ganglia and thalamus, with patchy or diffusely abnormal signals, most apparent on fluid-attenuated inversion recovery (FLAIR) images (Trentalange et al., 2020). Results of metabolic imaging, such as diffusion tensor imaging (DTI), single-photon emission computed tomography (SPECT), and MR spectroscopy have also been reported, although their utility in clinical diagnosis remains uncertain.

### Cerebrospinal Fluid Analysis

CSF examination is used chiefly to exclude other diagnoses. The results need to be considered in the context of the nonspecific changes found in clinically normal HIV-infected individuals (discussed earlier). Routine examination of CSF in patients with HAND reveals nonspecific findings of mild mononuclear pleocytosis and mildly elevated protein in approximately 60% of the cases. Specialized CSF examination may also reveal abnormalities in immunoglobulin, including evidence of intrathecal IgG synthesis and the presence of oligoclonal bands, but because these abnormalities are also detected in patients who do not have HAD, their diagnostic utility is uncertain. HIV can be

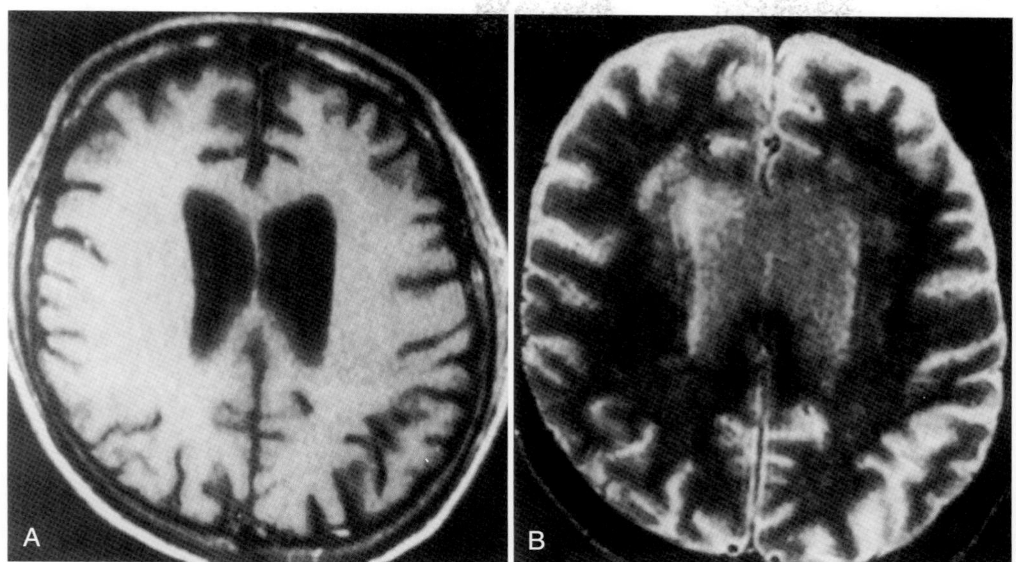


**Fig. 77.4 Human Immunodeficiency Virus-associated Dementia.** Gadolinium-enhanced (A) T1- and (B) T2-weighted magnetic resonance images obtained from a patient with acquired immunodeficiency syndrome and progressive cognitive impairment show marked cerebral atrophy and diffuse white-matter abnormalities.

isolated directly or HIV DNA can be amplified from the CSF sample by PCR, and HIV antigens can be detected in many of these patients, but these findings, too, are common in infected patients without neurological symptoms.

## Management

Accumulating evidence indicates that HAD can be treated and even prevented, at least to some extent, by antiretroviral therapy. Controlled studies have shown that cART improves neuropsychological performance in patients with HAD (Clifford, 2017; Sacktor et al., 2006; Saylor et al., 2016; Spudich and Gonzalez-Scarano, 2012). There has been at least an 80% decrease in HAD in developed countries since cART introduction in the late 1990s. With a growing list of HIV therapies in several classes of drugs (described previously) (see Table 77.2), many combination regimens are potentially available. It also appears that in the cART era, as the incidence of HAD has decreased, the milder forms of HAND (ANI and MND) have become more common (Clifford, 2017; Saylor et al., 2016).

For the successful management of HAD, cART should be designed to enhance the probability of a patient's adherence to the therapy. By the nature of the disorder, adherence to complicated treatment schemes is particularly difficult. Simpler regimens with the least number of drug side effects are important to enhance the adherence to therapy. For example, a once-daily dose of efavirenz is possible, and single-tablet combination formulations (see Table 77.2) may be better for patient compliance. Adherence may also be enhanced by the patient entering an assisted living facility with active support of family and close friends, and careful organization of medications (timers, pill boxes, etc.). A directly observed treatment is desirable in the later stages of HAND.

Although the data are scanty and controversial, selecting antiretroviral drugs that enter the CSF and brain optimally has been suggested to be advantageous in patients with HAD (Apostolova et al., 2015; Letendre et al., 2008). The relative CNS penetration of different antiretroviral drugs is summarized in Table 77.2. Effective cART outside the CNS compartment with rapid reduction of plasma HIV RNA copies also results in low viral copies in CNS and clinical neurological improvement (Clifford, 2017; Crossley and Brew, 2013; Spudich and Gonzalez-Scarano, 2012; Saylor et al., 2016). This indicates a dynamic exchange of virus between these two compartments. In patients with effective cART, HAD is now uncommon and has been replaced by milder forms of HANDs. Patients should be encouraged to participate in clinical trial research that may provide the patient the best available therapy and also assist future development of therapy. Treatment trials and a listing of health providers with expertise in this area may be accessed through the Neurological AIDS Research Consortium website at http://www.neuro.wustl.edu/narc.

## Cryptococcal Meningitis

Cryptococcal meningitis is covered in Chapter 79. Approximately 10% of patients with AIDS developed cryptococcal meningitis, a neurological OI caused by the encapsulated yeast *Cryptococcus neoformans* in the pre-cART era. Although the incidence has decreased with the widespread use of cART in resource-rich countries (Bicanic and Harrison, 2005; Crossley and Brew, 2013), cryptococcosis remains the most common cause of adult meningitis in Southern and East Africa, where it also remains the major cause of mortality. Cryptococcal meningitis is the initial AIDS-defining illness currently in ~2% of patients and generally occurs in patients with CD4+ T cell count less than 100/μL. It presents as headache, fever, stiff neck, and photophobia. However, meningeal symptoms and signs may be minimal or absent in over one-half of the cases, and the rather broad clinical spectrum includes failure to thrive, malaise, personality change, cognitive impairment, cranial neuropathy, altered mentation, and coma. Cranial CT or MRI, typically obtained to exclude focal cerebral disorders, sometimes reveals complications of cryptococcal meningitis, such as hydrocephalus, gelatinous pseudocysts, infarction, or cryptococcoma (Fig. 77.5). More commonly, neuroimaging reveals only cerebral atrophy related to the advanced HIV disease. Elevation of intracranial pressure (ICP) and hydrocephalus are common in cryptococcal meningitis. The CSF profile ranges from striking protein elevation, mononuclear pleocytosis, and hypoglycorrhachia to minimal abnormalities that overlap with those attributable to HIV infection alone. Fungal CSF culture is the gold standard, but incubation requires weeks before a positive result is obtained and it limits its clinical utility. India ink smear is helpful when positive but is too insensitive to exclude the diagnosis if negative.

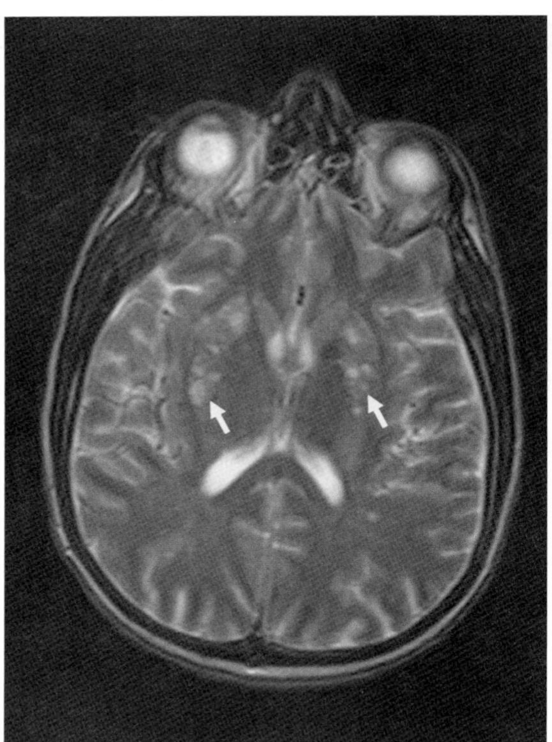

**Fig. 77.5 Cryptococcal Meningitis in Acquired Immunodeficiency Syndrome.** Axial T2-weighted magnetic resonance imaging showing multiple small gelatinous pseudocysts in basal ganglia *(arrows)*.

Fortunately, CSF cryptococcal antigen (CrAg) testing is a rapid, specific test with a sensitivity exceeding 90%. The rather diverse clinical presentations of cryptococcal meningitis may indicate that CrAg be performed routinely in patients with AIDS undergoing diagnostic CSF examination.

Similar to other CNS OIs in HIV-infected patients, the treatment for cryptococcal meningitis consists of an induction phase followed by maintenance therapy or secondary prophylaxis to prevent relapse (Table 77.3). A typical acute (induction) regimen consists of amphotericin B (0.5–0.7 mg/kg/day) with or without flucytosine (75–150 mg/kg/day) for 2–3 weeks. Renal insufficiency, hypokalemia, and hypomagnesemia may complicate amphotericin B therapy, and the hematological toxicity of flucytosine sometimes precludes its use in patients with AIDS, in whom pancytopenia is common. Patients who are doing well can be switched to fluconazole, 200 mg twice a day for 8–10 weeks, and then placed on maintenance therapy of 200 mg daily to prevent relapse. Although fluconazole therapy may be as effective as amphotericin B for acute therapy of cryptococcal meningitis, delayed CSF clearance of the fungus and a trend toward poorer outcomes among fluconazole-treated patients suggest this approach be reserved for patients with mild disease.

Poor prognostic features at presentation include impaired level of consciousness, increased ICP, CSF cell count less than 20 cells/μL, and CSF CrAg greater than 1:1024. Acute mortality in 10 weeks ranges from 10% to 25% in the developed world and up to 43% in resource-poor environments. Medical management with corticosteroids or acetazolamide and CSF drainage with repeated lumbar punctures or ventriculostomy can be used to lower ICP, although none of these interventions has been subjected to clinical trial. Optic nerve sheath fenestration has been suggested as an adjunct to these measures when increased ICP threatens vision. Without chronic suppressive therapy, relapse rates exceed 50%. As noted, first-line maintenance therapy is fluconazole, 200 mg daily; second-line agents include weekly amphotericin B or itraconazole. Secondary prophylaxis to prevent relapse after induction therapy should be continued at least until there is a sustained response in CD4+ T cell counts (i.e., >200 cells/μL for at least 6 months). In patients who escape early complications, long-term survival with cryptococcal meningitis is compatible with patients who tolerate and adhere to cART.

### Neurosyphilis

Neurosyphilis is covered in Chapter 79. Diagnosis and management of neurosyphilis in HIV-infected patients pose some complex challenges (Ahbeddou et al., 2018; Berger and Dean, 2014). Syphilis and HIV infection often coexist, as the disorders share risk factors. Moreover, both infections are characterized by diverse neurological syndromes affecting brain, meninges, spinal cord, and nerve roots. CNS invasion in early syphilis appears to occur at similar rates in patients with and without HIV infection. Individuals without HIV infection frequently clear *Treponema pallidum* from CSF even without antibiotic therapy (Berger and Dean, 2014). Whether the same is true in HIV-infected patients is less certain. Meningeal disorders characteristic of early neurosyphilis dominate case reports of HIV infection and neurosyphilis, perhaps implicating impaired CSF clearance of *T. pallidum* in HIV-infected patients, even with adequate therapy for early syphilis. Other clinical syndromes described in association with HIV infection include syphilitic eye disease, gumma, and myelopathy. Clinical experience indicates that co-infection with HIV and syphilis accelerates the development of meningovascular complications of the latter, often with early strokes (Ahbeddou et al., 2018).

Several factors complicate the diagnosis of neurosyphilis, particularly asymptomatic forms, in the setting of HIV infection. Individuals co-infected with HIV and *T. pallidum* may demonstrate unusual serological responses. When clinical suspicion of neurosyphilis is high and syphilis serology results are negative, repeat testing to exclude the prozone effect and darkfield examination or immunofluorescence staining of the lesion obtained by biopsy may be necessary (Berger, 1991; Berger and Levy, 1997). Assuming an atraumatic lumbar puncture, the CSF Venereal Disease Research Laboratory (VDRL) test is quite specific, but not particularly sensitive, for diagnosing neurosyphilis (Berger and Dean, 2014). Moreover, relying on CSF pleocytosis and protein elevation to make the diagnosis, as is done for HIV-negative individuals, is complicated by the high frequency of these CSF abnormalities caused by HIV infection alone. Importantly, a CSF pleocytosis is less common in HIV infection when CD4+ T cell counts are low. *Treponema*-specific tests in CSF are quite sensitive, but not specific, for neurosyphilis. Hence negative CSF fluorescent treponemal antibody or microhemagglutination *T. pallidum* generally excludes the diagnosis of neurosyphilis, but a positive result does not establish the diagnosis. HIV-infected patients with late latent syphilis or syphilis of unknown duration should undergo CSF examination before therapy, regardless of whether there are associated ophthalmic, vestibular, or neurological symptoms (Berger and Dean, 2014).

Regardless of HIV status, recommended treatment for neurosyphilis consists of a 10- to 14-day course of either aqueous crystalline penicillin G, 3–4 million units intravenously every 4 hours, or procaine penicillin, 2.4 million units intramuscularly daily, with or without oral probenecid, 500 mg four times a day. Because alternative agents, such as doxycycline and tetracycline, are of uncertain efficacy in neurosyphilis, desensitization should be considered in patients allergic to penicillin. The CDC recommends CSF examination every 6 months after therapy for all patients with neurosyphilis, regardless of HIV status, until pleocytosis, if initially present, resolves.

**TABLE 77.3 NIH/CDC/IDSA Guidelines for Therapy and Prevention of Select Human Immunodeficiency Virus-Associated Neurological Complications**

| Causal Organism/ Disorder | Therapy | Major Side Effects | Primary Prophylaxis |
|---|---|---|---|
| *Cryptococcus neoformans* (meningitis, meningoencephalitis, abscess) | *Induction*: amphotericin B (0.7 mg/kg/day IV) for 3 wk; adjust for renal status, + flucytocine (induction: 25 mg/kg/day PO) q6h for ×3 wk or fluconazole 400 mg/day PO ×3 wk, then 200 mg/day PO<br>*Maintenance*: fluconazole (200 mg qd) or amphotericin (0.6–1 mg/kg/wk IV) or itraconazole (200 mg/day)<br>Note: may stop if CD4+ T cell count ≥200/μL for ≥3 months | Renal toxicity, chills, hepatic toxicity (amphotericin B)<br>Bone marrow suppression (flucytosine)<br>Hepatotoxicity (fluconazole) | (If prior documented disease elsewhere and CD4+ T cell <100/μL)<br>Fluconazole 200 mg/day PO |
| *Toxoplasma gondii* (encephalitis, abscess) | *Induction*: sulfadiazine (induction: 1.5 g PO q6h ×6 wk; maintenance: 0.5 g PO qid) + pyrimethamine (200 mg PO 1 day, then 75 mg/day PO), + folinic acid 10 mg/day PO, or clindamycin (induction: 600 mg/day IV or PO qid; maintenance up to 450 mg PO qid)<br>*Maintenance*: pyrimethamine (25–50 mg/day) + sulfadiazine (0.5–1 g qid) + folinic acid (10 mg/day) PO<br>Note: may stop if CD4+ T cell count >200/μL for ≥3 months | Rash, bone marrow suppression, crystalluria (sulfadiazine)<br>Rash, leukopenia (pyrimethamine)<br>Rash, diarrhea, pseudomembranous colitis (clindamycin) | (If IgG antibody seropositive and CD4+ T cell <100/μL) trimethoprim/sulfamethoxazole DS PO 3× weekly, or trimethoprim/sulfamethoxazole SS PO qd, or atovaquone 1.5 g PO qd, or dapsone 50 mg PO qd + pyrimethamine 50 mg/wk PO, + folinic acid 25 mg/wk PO or dapsone 200 mg PO + pyrimethamine 75 mg PO + folinic acid 25 mg PO weekly |
| Cytomegalovirus (encephalitis, polyradiculomyelitis, mononeuropathy multiplex) | *Induction*: valganciclovir 900 mg PO bid or ganciclovir (induction: 5 mg/kg/day IV q8h ×2 wk; maintenance: 5 mg/kg/day IV 5 days/wk) ∓ foscarnet (induction: 60 mg/kg IV q8h ×2 wk, adjust for renal function; maintenance: 90 mg/kg/day IV) or cidofovir (5 mg/kg/wk IV) ×2 wk, then every 2 wk<br>Note: may stop if CD4+ T cell count >100/μL for ≥6 months and no evidence of active disease. Restart if prior retinitis and CD4+ T cells >100/μL | Bone marrow toxicity (ganciclovir)<br>Renal toxicity, hypocalcemia (foscarnet)<br>Renal failure, neutropenia, iritis, uveitis, ocular hypotony (cidofovir) | (If prior cytomegalovirus retinitis) ganciclovir 5 mg/kg/day IV 5 days/wk, or foscarnet 90–120 mg/kg/day IV, or cidofovir 5 mg/kg IV every other wk + probenecid |
| *Varicella zoster* (Shingles, zoster vasculitis) | acyclovir 800 mg PO 5× daily for 5–7 days or valacyclovir 1 g PO tid for 5–7 days | | Significant exposure to chickenpox or shingles in a patient with no history of immunization or prior exposure: varicella zoster immunoglobulin, IM, within 10 days of exposure |
| AIDP | IVIG 0.4 g/kg/day IV ×5 days | Flulike syndrome, renal failure, headache | — |
| CIDP | IVIG 0.4 g/kg/day IV ×5 days for relapse<br>prednisone 1 mg/kg/day until improvement, then titrate downward | Flulike syndrome, renal failure, headache (IVIG) | — |
| Polymyositis | prednisone 1 mg/kg/day PO until improvement, then titrate downward | GI, hypertension, weight gain, infection | — |

*AIDP*, Acute inflammatory demyelinating polyradiculoneuropathy; *CDC*, Centers for Disease Control and Prevention; *CIDP*, chronic inflammatory demyelinating polyradiculoneuropathy; *DS*, double strength; *GI*, gastrointestinal; *HIV*, human immunodeficiency virus; *IDSA*, Infectious Diseases Society of America; *IgG*, immunoglobulin G; *IVIG*, intravenous immunoglobulin; *NIH*, National Institutes of Health; *SS*, single strength.

### Cytomegalovirus Encephalitis and Ventriculoencephalitis

CMV is a B herpes virus with worldwide distribution; most adults have serological evidence of latent CMV infection. Clinically evident CMV encephalitis represented about 2% of all neurological complications in HIV patients in the pre-cART era. The incidence of CMV disease, including CNS infection, has decreased substantially in the cART era. Now an uncommon cause of global cerebral dysfunction in advanced AIDS (CD4+ T cell count <50/μL), CMV encephalitis and ventriculoencephalitis often cause death within weeks to months. Prior or active disseminated CMV disease, such as retinitis, esophagitis, or colitis, may provide important clues to the neurological diagnosis.

CMV encephalitis typically presents as a confusional state evolving over weeks and can resemble HAD. In addition to a course that is more subacute than chronic, focal cerebral signs, hyponatremia, and cranial

MRI showing periventricular enhancement are other factors that favor a diagnosis of CMV encephalitis over HAD. CSF abnormalities are typically nonspecific, and CMV PCR is positive in less than one-half of cases. Pathological findings include microglial nodules and cytomegalic cells in cortical and subcortical gray matter, thought to be consistent with hematogenous spread of CMV to brain. By contrast, CMV ventriculoencephalitis may reflect dissemination from CSF and presents more acutely than CMV encephalitis, often on a background of CMV retinitis or concurrently with polyradiculomyelopathy. Brainstem signs and neuroimaging studies revealing dilated ventricles also suggest the diagnosis. CSF abnormalities tend to be more striking than with CMV encephalitis, revealing elevated protein, polymorphonuclear or lymphocytic pleocytosis, and normal or low glucose levels. CMV viremia is quite common in late-stage AIDS, and hence viral detection in this setting by culture, antigen testing, or PCR from blood does not help establish the diagnosis of CMV-related neurological syndromes.

Four drugs are currently available for treating systemic CMV infection: ganciclovir, a guanosine nucleoside analog; valganciclovir (valyl ester of ganciclovir); foscarnet, a pyrophosphate analog; and cidofovir, a cytosine nucleoside analog. All have major limitations in AIDS patients because they are only virostatic, administration is inconvenient, and they have major side effects. Clinical trial data for the efficacy of ganciclovir, foscarnet, cidofovir, or combination therapy for CMV encephalitis and ventriculoencephalitis are lacking, though a trial of empiric therapy is probably appropriate given the poor prognosis (see Table 77.3). Effective cART and thereby successful restoration of the immune response against CMV is the most efficacious therapy to improve the dismal outcome in these patients.

### Other Meningitis and Meningoencephalitis Syndromes

Other causes of meningitis complicating HIV infection include other rare infections, neoplasms, and medications. Additional infectious causes of meningitis include bacteria (*Salmonella typhi, Pneumococcus pneumoniae, Mycobacterium tuberculosis, Nocardia asteroides, Listeria monocytogenes, Bartonella henselae*) and fungi (*Histoplasma capsulatum* and *Coccidioides immitis* in individuals who have lived in endemic regions, and *Candida albicans, Blastomyces dermatitidis*, and *Sporothrix schenckii*). Pyogenic meningitis can be complicated by subdural empyema that may require surgical drainage. Patients with AIDS are at increased risk for systemic lymphoma, which can cause lymphomatous meningitis. Medications are often overlooked as a cause of meningitis; implicated agents in common use for HIV infection include nonsteroidal anti-inflammatory drugs, trimethoprim/sulfamethoxazole (TMP/SMX), and IVIG.

## Focal Central Nervous System Disorders

Four disorders account for most HIV-related focal CNS dysfunction: cerebral toxoplasmosis, PCNSL, PML, and VM. The epidemiology of CNS OIs (toxoplasmosis, PML, PCNSL) associated with HIV infection has changed dramatically following the availability of cART since 1996. All of them are the disorders of advanced HIV infection, when CD4+ T cell counts are typically below 100/μL. Although they share focal hemispheric and, less commonly, brainstem and cerebellar or spinal cord symptoms as a prominent clinical feature, other aspects of the history, supplemented by neuroimaging studies, response to therapeutic trial, and occasionally brain biopsy, usually allow each to be diagnosed quickly and accurately (see Fig. 77.3).

### Cerebral Toxoplasmosis

CNS toxoplasmosis is described in Chapter 79. Toxoplasmic encephalitis (TE) was the most frequent CNS OI in AIDS in the pre-cART era; it occurred in 10% of patients or more, depending on the geographic origin. It is still very common in areas where cART is not used widely. Its incidence is significantly reduced in the post-cART era (Martin-Iguacel et al., 2017). Cerebral toxoplasmosis in AIDS almost always occurs from recrudescence of previously acquired infection and relates to the loss of the immune defenses that maintain *Toxoplasma gondii* in an inactive, encysted form. It is 10 times more common in patients with antibodies to the organism than in patients who are seronegative. It is generally a late complication of HIV infection and usually occurs in patients with CD4+ T cell counts lower than 100/μL.

The most common clinical presentation in TE is headache and focal neurological deficit with or without fever. Patients may present with seizure, hemiparesis, or aphasia as a manifestation of these focal lesions or with a picture more influenced by the accompanying cerebral edema characterized by confusion, mental torpor, and lethargy, which can progress to coma. Diagnosis is usually suspected on the basis of CT or MRI findings of multiple lesions in multiple locations, although in some cases only a single lesion is seen and, rarely, toxoplasmosis may present as a meningoencephalitis without any identifiable intraparenchymal lesions. The lesions have a predilection for the basal ganglia. Pathologically, these lesions generally exhibit inflammation and central necrosis and, as a result, demonstrate ring enhancement on contrast CT or MRI (Fig. 77.6). There is usually surrounding edema. In addition to toxoplasmosis, the differential diagnosis of multiple mass lesions in the HIV-infected patient includes PCNSL (see the following discussion) and, less commonly, tubercular, fungal, or bacterial abscesses. Resolution of lesions on anti-*Toxoplasma* therapy confirms the clinical diagnosis. The definitive diagnostic procedure is brain biopsy, but it carries morbidity and therefore is generally reserved for the patient who has failed 2 weeks of empirical anti-*Toxoplasma* therapy (see Fig. 77.3); however, open biopsy and decompression should be performed in the setting of impending brain herniation.

Standard therapy in TE is sulfadiazine (0.5–1.5 g by mouth every 6 hours) and pyrimethamine (200 mg loading day 1, then 75 mg by mouth every day). Folinic acid 10 mg/day is given to counteract pyrimethamine bone marrow toxicity. Clindamycin (600 mg intravenously or by mouth every day) can be substituted for sulfadiazine in sulfa-allergic patients. Long-term suppressive therapy is generally required, but doses may be tapered to pyrimethamine 25 mg/day and sulfadiazine 2 g/day. In patients who do not tolerate sulfa drugs, clindamycin (300–450 mg by mouth three or four times daily) can be substituted. Rarely, toxoplasmosis manifests as acute meningoencephalitis, variably accompanied by muscle involvement. In even the most unusual circumstance in which the diagnosis is made premortem, anti-*Toxoplasma* therapy may be lifesaving. Maintenance therapy should be continued for life in the absence of cART. Patients on cART with immune reconstitution, as measured by a sustained increase in CD4+ T cell counts above 200 cells/μL for at least 6 months, discontinuation of therapy may be accomplished safely.

Patients with CD4+ T cell counts below 100/μL and IgG antibodies to *Toxoplasma* should receive primary prophylaxis against toxoplasmosis (see Table 77.3). HIV-infected patients who are seronegative for *Toxoplasma* should be counseled about ways to minimize the risk of primary infection, including avoiding consumption of undercooked food and careful hand-washing after contact with soil or after changing the cat litter box.

### Progressive Multifocal Leukoencephalopathy

JC virus, named after the initials of the patient (John Cunningham) from whom it was first isolated, is a DNA-containing human papillomavirus—the causal agent for PML—which is an important opportunistic pathogen in patients with AIDS (Berger 2014; Berger et al., 2013; Berger and Mucke, 1988). Approximately 70%–90% of the adult population harbors antibodies to JC virus, indicative of prior infection in childhood or early adulthood, but less than 10% of healthy persons show any evidence of ongoing viral replication. PML is the only known complication of JC virus infection. It is a late manifestation of AIDS and is seen in approximately 4%–5% of patients with AIDS (Berger et al., 1987, 1998), Although its incidence seems to have decreased somewhat during the past several years, the decline has not been as marked as for other OIs.

PML is a demyelinating disease of the central nervous system that results from infection of oligodendrocytes with the JC virus (Berger and Khalili, 2011). The lesions of PML begin as small foci of demyelination in subcortical white matter, often in the parieto-occipital area, that eventually coalesce. The cerebellum, the brainstem, and, very rarely, the spinal cord can be involved in PML. Patients typically have a protracted course with focal neurological deficit, with or without changes in mental status. Visual field defects, hemiparesis, aphasia and other language disorders, sensory deficits, and ataxia may occur. MRI typically reveals multiple, nonenhancing white matter lesions that may coalesce and have a predilection for occipital or parietal lobes (Fig. 77.7); however, even in the era before the availability of antiretroviral therapy, contrast enhancement on MRI was observed in as many as 15% of patients (Berger et al., 1998). CSF is usually normal or shows nonspecific changes, but the viral DNA can be amplified from the CSF sample. CSF PCR for JC virus DNA coupled with the appropriate clinical findings and characteristic lesions of PML on MRI obviates the need for brain biopsy (Berger et al., 2013). In cases in which viral DNA is not detected in CSF, a brain biopsy is necessary to confirm the diagnosis. Brain biopsy reveals bizarre giant astrocytes with pleomorphic hyperchromatic nuclei, altered oligodendrocytes with enlarged nuclei that contain viral inclusions, and demyelination.

There is no specific therapy for PML despite anecdotal reports regarding cytosine arabinoside, cidofovir, mirtazapine, mefloquine, and other drugs. Mean survival in the pre-cART era was 2–4 months (Simpson and Berger, 1996); however, in the cART era, as many as 50% of patients experience median survival of 24 months and some surviving greater than 15 years. Factors influencing a favorable outcome include higher CD4+ T cell counts, low HIV viral load, undetectable JC virus in CSF following cART, and contrast-enhancing lesions at the time of diagnosis.

## Primary Central Nervous System Lymphoma

PCNSLs of B-cell origin are considered opportunistic neoplasms that complicate the course of AIDS in up to 5% of patients. The incidence of PCNSL in HIV-infected individuals dropped substantially following the introduction of cART in 1996, but now it appears to be cumulatively rising because of the increased longevity of HIV-infected persons, following the efficacy of both prophylactic and therapeutic measures against OIs and cART. Patients with PCNSL present with progressive focal or multifocal neurological deficits similar to those seen with toxoplasmosis and PML. Autopsy studies have revealed that PCNSL is virtually always multifocal, even when solitary lesions are seen on neuroimaging studies. The tempo of symptom evolution in PCNSL is generally slower than in toxoplasmosis and faster than in PML, with patients with PCNSL presenting several days or a few weeks after the onset of symptoms, which may include headache, hemiparesis, aphasia, ataxia, behavioral changes, and altered mentation. Lymphomatous meningitis or ocular involvement occurs in about 15% of cases. Systemic dissemination of PCNSL occurs in about 5% of patients, mainly in the final stages of the disease. Fever and constitutional symptoms are absent, except in patients with associated systemic infection.

The diagnosis of PCNSL is generally considered following review of neuroimaging in the appropriate clinical setting. MRI is more sensitive than CT scan, and characteristically shows one or more lesions. Lesion location is typically deep in the brain, adjacent to the lateral ventricles and often in white rather than gray matter; MRI may show characteristic subependymal extension (Fig. 77.8). In about 10% of patients, PCNSL is located in the posterior fossa. Mass effect may be present. Contrast enhancement may be irregular or peripheral and ring-like. Edema may be absent or minimal. CSF cytology is frequently unhelpful, although the presence of monoclonal B lymphocytes by flow cytometry, if demonstrated, indicates PCNSL. PCR amplification of

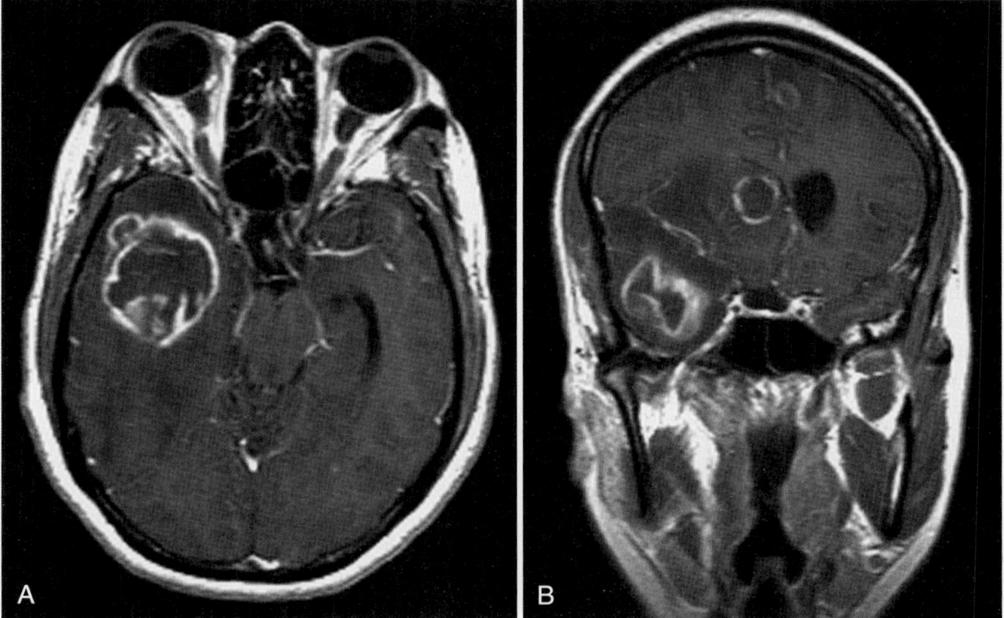


**Fig. 77.6 Cerebral Toxoplasmosis in Acquired Immunodeficiency Syndrome.** Postgadolinium axial **(A)** and coronal **(B)** T1-weighted magnetic resonance imaging showing multiple ring-enhancing lesions with mass effect.

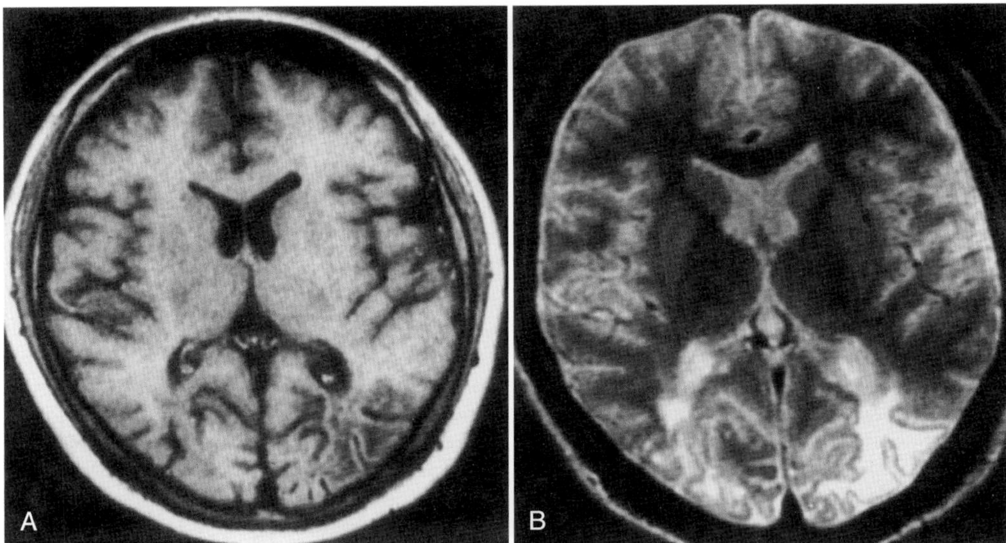


**Fig. 77.7 Progressive Multifocal Leukoencephalopathy.** (**A**) T1- and (**B**) T2-weighted cranial magnetic resonance images show bilateral lesions in occipital white matter, without mass effect.

Epstein-Barr virus DNA in CSF corroborates the diagnosis of PCNSL. The definitive diagnosis of PCNSL generally requires brain biopsy. Often, brain biopsy is undertaken after a therapeutic trial for cerebral toxoplasmosis. Uptake on thallium-201 SPECT may be useful in supporting the diagnosis of PCNSL and prompting early biopsy. The use of stereotactic biopsy techniques has increased the access to these tumors and reduced the morbidity of biopsy.

Before the cART era, the outcome of AIDS-associated PCNSL had been dismal, with median survival of approximately 2–3 months. The most important factors related to survival are the clinical condition of the patient, the CD4+ T cell count, and the absence of OIs. As with PML, the prognosis in PCNSL is improved by successful cART and immune reconstitution, and vigorous attempts to suppress HIV replication are recommended in all patients (Cingolani et al., 2005). Mass effect is treated by high-dose corticosteroid therapy. Palliative whole-brain irradiation therapy is recommended. The use of chemotherapy remains controversial outside a clinical research trial setting.

## Stroke

Cerebrovascular disease also causes focal brain dysfunction in HIV infection. A wide spectrum of cerebrovascular disorders has been associated with HIV infection (Dobbs et al., 2009). Ischemic and hemorrhagic strokes have been reported in up to 4% of clinical series and up to 34% of autopsy series (Pinto, 1996). HIV infection has been reported to cause carotid endothelial disease and atherosclerosis. HIV should be considered in the setting of stroke in young patients. Thrombocytopenia, coagulopathy related to liver disease or disseminated intravascular coagulation, PCNSL, metastatic Kaposi sarcoma, and rarely, toxoplasmosis may be associated with cerebral hemorrhage. Causes of ischemic stroke include an HIV cerebral vasculitis, co-infection with syphilis with early meningovascular strokes (see previous discussion), bacterial endocarditis, particularly in IDUs, as well as nonbacterial thrombotic endocarditis, vasculitis, and procoagulant states. VZV and tuberculous meningitis can cause infectious vasculitis, as can the angioinvasive fungi, *Aspergillus* and *Mucor*.

## Other Focal Central Nervous System Disorders

Numerous other infections have been reported to cause focal cerebral dysfunction in HIV-infected patients. Bacteremia from indwelling catheters needed to manage other aspects of HIV infection or from parenteral drug use predisposes to bacterial brain abscess (Fig. 77.9). Other bacterial causes of focal cerebral dysfunction include *M. tuberculosis* abscess, syphilitic gumma, *B. henselae*, and *N. asteroides*. Fungal causes of focal brain disease, in addition to the angioinvasive fungi discussed previously, include cryptococcoma, *B. dermatitidis*, and *H. capsulatum*. Among parasites, relevant diagnostic considerations in patients who have lived in or traveled through endemic areas are cysticercosis and intracerebral Chagas disease (*Trypanosoma cruzi*). Interestingly, although HIV infection does not appear to significantly increase the risk for *Herpes simplex* virus encephalitis, it may alter its clinical presentation. The long-term effect of the protease inhibitor–induced metabolic syndrome on atherosclerosis and stroke remains the topic of ongoing clinical research.

## Human Immunodeficiency Virus-Associated Myelopathy

Myelopathy is present in ~20% of patients with AIDS, often as part of HAND and DSP. Two main types of primary myelopathies are seen in patients with AIDS: VM and dorsal column sensory tractopathy. VM was the most common cause of spinal cord dysfunction in untreated patients with AIDS in the pre-cART era, apparent pathologically in ~25%–55% of AIDS autopsy series (Di Rocco and Simpson, 1998; McArthur et al., 2005; Petito et al., 1985). Affected patients develop gait difficulty, caused by spasticity, leg weakness, and impaired proprioception, often accompanied by sphincter dysfunction, evolving over several months. Back pain is not a prominent feature. Examination reveals spastic paraparesis with hyperreflexia and Babinski signs, unless concomitant neuropathy is severe. Sensation in the legs, particularly proprioception and vibratory sense, is usually impaired, but a clear discrete sensory level should suggest another etiology of the myelopathy. The arms are typically spared until VM is advanced. MRI may occasionally reveal cord atrophy, but usually is unremarkable. Pathological findings are most striking in the dorsolateral thoracic cord and include vacuolar changes in myelin sheaths with relative preservation of axons. Despite the clinical and pathological resemblance to combined systems degeneration, vitamin $B_{12}$ levels are typically normal in affected patients. HIV-induced release of neurotoxic cytokines or abnormalities in vitamin $B_{12}$ utilization may contribute to the development of VM. Spinal dorsal sensory tractopathy appears to be a milder form of VM.

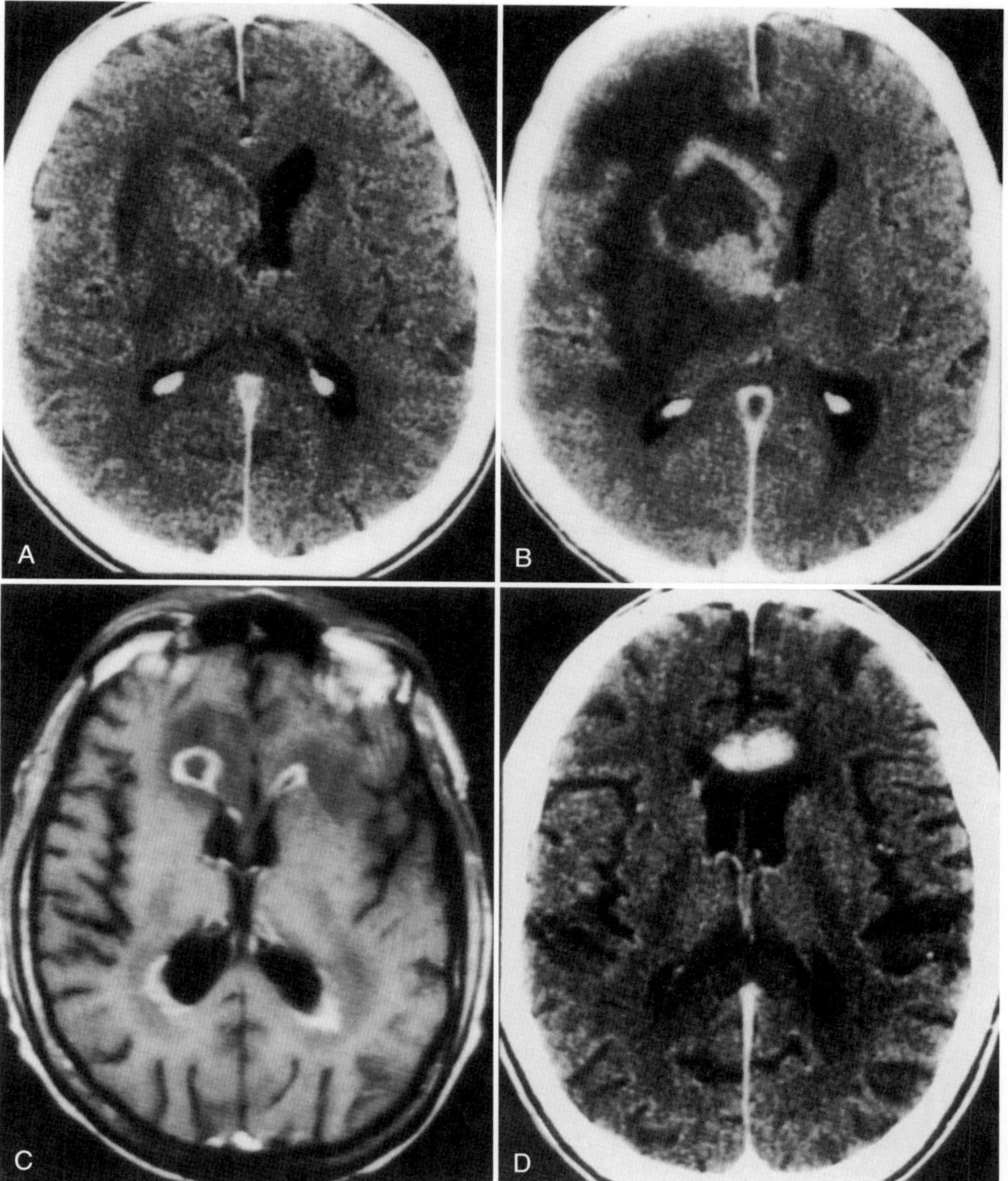


**Fig. 77.8 Primary Central Nervous System Lymphoma.** **A,** Contrast-enhanced computed tomography (CT) shows a solitary enhancing lesion adjacent to the right frontal horn, with edema and mass effect. **B,** Repeat contrast-enhanced CT after empirical anti-*Toxoplasma* therapy shows increased lesion size, enhancement, edema, and mass effect, consistent with lymphoma. Images from two additional patients show **(C)** involvement of subependymal regions in gadolinium-enhanced T1-weighted magnetic resonance imaging and **(D)** corpus callosum on contrast-enhanced CT.

Evidence that viral control can result in improved neurological function is not well documented in VM, but there are anecdotal reports, making the effort to control the infection important. Patients with myelopathy and paraplegia require considerable assistance, comparable to that of other spinal cord–injured patients. Care of the neurogenic bladder, bladder infection, management of limb spasticity, prevention of skin breakdown and decubiti, and assist devices to improve mobility are the issues that require individualized attention.

Numerous other infectious, neoplastic, and metabolic disorders occasionally cause myelopathy in patients with HIV infection, and they need to be differentiated from VM. Compared with VM, these disorders may progress more rapidly, often with associated back or radicular pain and the presence of a discrete sensory level over the trunk. CMV, VZV, herpes simplex virus type-2, and other pathogens may cause myelitis. Helpful diagnostic tests include spinal MRI, which may reveal cord swelling with intramedullary enhancement and T2 signal changes, and CSF PCR testing for viral DNA. Because HIV shares risk factors with human T cell lymphotropic virus I and II, co-infection with these retroviruses also may cause myelopathy in the HIV-infected patient.

## HUMAN IMMUNODEFICIENCY VIRUS-ASSOCIATED NEUROMUSCULAR DISORDERS

### Neuropathies

Peripheral neuropathies are common in HIV infection (Centner et al., 2013 Cornblath and Hoke, 2006; Schütz and Robinson-Papp, 2013; Verma, 2001;). Peripheral neuropathies complicate all stages of the HIV disease and cause considerable morbidity and disability

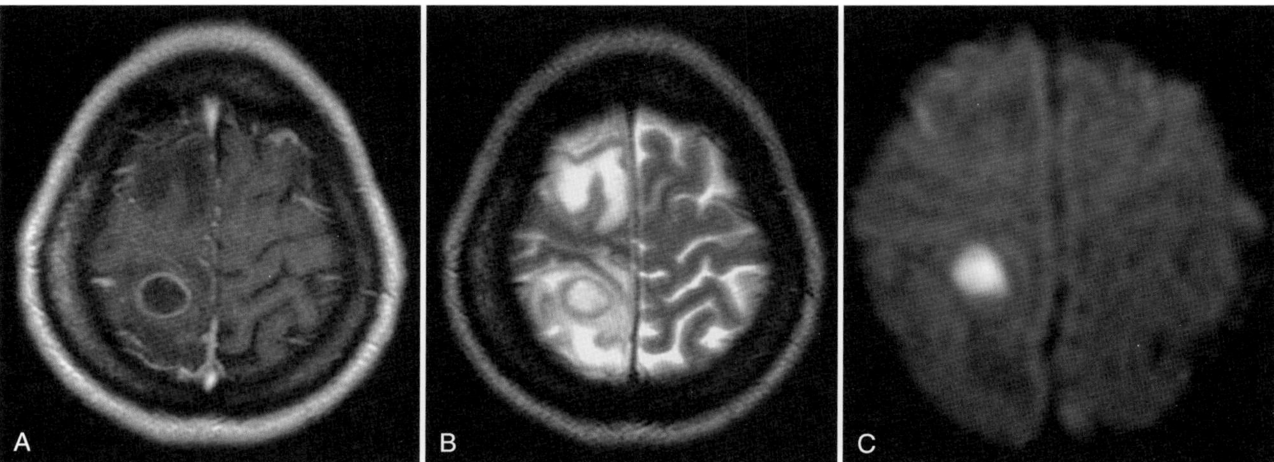


**Fig. 77.9 Pyogenic Brain Abscess in Acquired Immunodeficiency Syndrome.** Postgadolinium axial T1-weighted magnetic resonance image showing ring-enhancing lesion (**A**), with surrounding edema best seen in T2-weighted sequence (**B**) and with associated intralesional diffusion restriction (**C**).

in HIV-infected individuals and AIDS patients. Although symptomatic neuropathy occurs in approximately 15%–25% of HIV-infected patients overall, pathological evidence of peripheral nerve involvement is present in virtually all end-stage AIDS patients. There are five major clinical types of HIV-associated neuropathies that are regularly seen in large HIV clinics: DSP, acute and chronic inflammatory demyelinating polyradiculoneuropathies (AIDP and CIDP), CMV-associated polyradiculomyelopathy, and drugs-associated toxic neuropathies. Vasculitic neuropathy is less common, but often responds well to corticosteroid treatment (Bradley and Verma, 1996).

### Distal Sensory Polyneuropathy

Of the various peripheral nerve syndromes that complicate HIV infection, the most common is DSP, also called HIV-associated neuropathy or AIDS neuropathy. This axonal, predominantly sensory, length-dependent polyneuropathy develops in approximately one-third of patients with AIDS, becoming more prevalent as the CD4+ T cell count decreases. The 1-year incidence of DSP showed a steep decline in the post-cART compared with the pre-cART period. However, just like milder forms of HAND, the overall prevalence of DSP appears to be increasing as HIV-infected persons live longer with the disease (Centner et al., 2013; Schütz and Robinson-Papp, 2013).

Depressed or absent ankle jerks and mild pain, temperature, and vibratory sensory loss in the feet, with or without associated foot paresthesia and numbness, may be the only evidence of the disorder, and probably make up the more common clinical syndrome. Less frequently, severe burning pain and paresthesia develop in the feet, often disrupting sleep in a manner reminiscent of diabetic or nutritional sensory polyneuropathies. Symmetrical involvement is a characteristic clinical feature, and the hands are usually spared until the disorder is advanced. Even though DSP typically spares motor function and proprioception, walking may be impaired because of severe pain. The pathogenesis of DSP is not well understood; proposed mechanisms include toxicity to the dorsal root ganglion neurons from cytokine upregulation in advanced infection, as well as dorsal root ganglion toxicity of HIV, HIV antigens, and the effects of chronic, multisystemic illnesses.

The rather typical clinical features of DSP usually obviate the need for electromyography and nerve conduction studies. Exposures to neurotoxins, including ethanol, should be reviewed. Enquiry for neurotoxic antiretroviral drugs, in addition to isoniazid, pyridoxine, dapsone, metronidazole, and vincristine, and screening for vitamin $B_{12}$ deficiency and diabetes mellitus, are important.

Treatment goals in DSP include minimizing neurotoxic exposures, viral suppression by cART, and management of pain. Tricyclic antidepressants and anticonvulsants ameliorate neuropathic pain in DSP. When there is coexisting dementia or other cerebral disease, the anticholinergic effects of amitriptyline may be poorly tolerated. Using very low doses or switching to a less anticholinergic tricyclic antidepressant such as nortriptyline, plus addition of a selective serotonin reuptake inhibitor, may facilitate tolerance. With regard to anticonvulsants, the high rate of adverse reactions and drug interactions with carbamazepine in patients with AIDS limits its utility for the management of neuropathic pain. The favorable side-effect and drug-interaction profiles of gabapentin make it the treatment of choice for managing neuropathic pain in AIDS. Other useful treatments include nonsteroidal anti-inflammatory drugs, duloxetine, pregabalin, and transcutaneous electrical nerve stimulator units, but some patients may require chronic narcotic-analgesic therapy.

### Nucleoside Analog-Associated Toxic Neuropathy

A painful polyneuropathy that closely resembles DSP is the major dose-limiting toxicity of the nucleoside analog antiretroviral agents didanosine, zalcitabine, and stavudine (Centner et al., 2013; Cornblath and Hoke, 2006; Schütz and Robinson-Papp, 2013; Verma, 2001). Their exclusion in modern cART regimens has dramatically reduced the incidence of toxic polyneuropathy in the United States. Two clinical features can help distinguish nucleoside neuropathy from DSP. First, nucleoside neuropathy typically evolves over weeks following initiation of therapy, in contrast to DSP, which progresses over months or even years. Second, stopping the offending agent eventually leads to stabilization and regression of nucleoside neuropathy over several months, although coasting, in which symptoms worsen for several weeks before improvement, may complicate the evaluation of this strategy for diagnosis. Although preexisting DSP increases the risk for nucleoside neuropathy (Verma et al., 1999), many patients with DSP tolerate neurotoxic antiretrovirals, particularly if the dose is kept low. Other aspects of the evaluation and treatment are similar to those for DSP.

### Inflammatory Demyelinating Polyradiculoneuropathies

Less common than the DSP related to HIV or nucleoside antiretrovirals are the inflammatory demyelinating polyradiculoneuropathies, acute (AIDP), and chronic (CIDP) (Centner et al., 2013; Cornblath and Hoke, 2006; Schütz and Robinson-Papp, 2013). These disorders resemble the syndromes seen in individuals without HIV infection with regard to pathogenesis and most clinical features. The precise prevalence is unknown, but case series from the United States and Africa suggest that they more often develop during early HIV infection, sometimes around the time of seroconversion. AIDP or the Guillain-Barré syndrome typically presents as rapidly progressive ascending weakness with areflexia, variably accompanied by respiratory failure and dysautonomia. The Miller Fisher variant, in which cranial nerve dysfunction, areflexia, and ataxia are more prominent than limb or respiratory weakness, has also been described during HIV infection. In CIDP, neuropathic weakness and sensory loss occur in a more indolent or episodic manner than in AIDP. In both AIDP and CIDP, electrophysiological studies reveal slowed conduction, temporal dispersion of evoked response amplitudes, multifocal block, and prolonged F waves, indicating demyelination. In HIV-infected patients with inflammatory demyelinating polyradiculoneuropathy, the CSF often shows a lymphocytic pleocytosis (10–50 cells/μL) in addition to increased protein. Clinical experience suggests that intravenous immunoglobulin, plasmapheresis, and corticosteroids (only in CIDP) are beneficial.

### Lumbosacral Polyradiculomyelitis

Subacute lumbosacral polyradiculomyelitis with variable cord involvement is an uncommon HIV-related syndrome that results from a variety of infectious agents, most notably CMV. Clinical manifestations suggest a rapidly developing cauda equina syndrome, with leg weakness and later paralysis, sphincter dysfunction, sacral and leg paresthesias and sensory loss, and areflexia, typically evolving over several days (Centner et al., 2013). When such a syndrome develops in a patient with a CD4+ T cell count less than 50/μL, and CSF reveals marked polymorphonuclear pleocytosis, elevated protein, and low to normal glucose levels, CMV infection of the nerve roots, with subsequent inflammation and necrosis, is the likely cause. CMV PCR or branched DNA assay in CSF is a helpful confirmatory test, but treatment should not be delayed pending these results. Intravenous ganciclovir (see Table 77.3) can arrest and reverse the deficit in CMV polyradiculomyelitis, which is fatal without treatment. Polyradiculomyelitis caused by ganciclovir-resistant CMV has been reported and may respond to foscarnet, either alone or with cidofovir. Other causes of polyradiculomyelopathy in AIDS include tuberculosis, neurosyphilis, HSV type 2, and lymphomatous meningitis.

### Other Neuropathies and Neuronopathies

Mononeuritis multiplex (MM) is a relatively rare peripheral nerve syndrome of HIV infection that manifests clinically as multifocal, asymmetrical peripheral nerve lesions that may include cranial nerves. Acute seventh cranial nerve palsy is not uncommon in early HIV disease. When the MM syndrome develops in early or midstage HIV infection, it often responds well to corticosteroid therapy, though it may be self-limited, not requiring immunosuppressive therapy (Bradley and Verma, 1996). MM complicating advanced HIV infection, with CD4+ T cell count less than 50/μL, may be caused by CMV and responds to intravenous ganciclovir. An amyotrophic lateral sclerosis (ALS)-mimic syndrome (Moulignier et al., 2001; Verma and Berger, 2006) has also been reported in HIV disease.

## Myopathies

Myopathic symptoms in HIV-infected individuals can arise from toxic (zidovudine) or dysimmune (polymyositis) causes or from AIDS cachexia (muscle wasting syndrome) (Authier et al., 2005; Centner et al., 2013). In HIV-associated polymyositis, patients develop proximal weakness and, less commonly, myalgia, both of which are ascribed to a polyclonal hyperimmune response following HIV infection. On occasion it may occur with immune restoration following cART (Sellier et al., 2000). Serum creatine kinase is elevated in most cases, and electrophysiological studies often reveal myopathic motor units and increased insertional activity and spontaneous activity typical of an inflammatory myopathy. Muscle biopsy reveals fiber size variability, fiber necrosis and regeneration, and endomysial mononuclear infiltrates. Cytoplasmic bodies and nemaline rod bodies are other common histological features. HIV does not appear to directly infect muscle fibers, but rather induces them to express major histocompatibility complex I, triggering cell-mediated muscle fiber injury. Even so, inflammatory myopathy is among the few HIV-related neurological disorders that develop at any time during HIV infection. Despite the potential risks of corticosteroid therapy in the setting of HIV infection, such treatment is often well tolerated. Prednisone has helped in motor recovery and pain improvement in HIV-associated polymyositis. Starting with a dose of 1 mg/kg/day, the dose is titrated downward as strength improves. Inclusion body myositis also has been reported in association with HIV infection (Authier et al., 2005).

Zidovudine myopathy is a toxic mitochondrial disorder that presents with the insidious onset of proximal weakness and myalgia, making it difficult to distinguish this condition clinically from HIV-associated inflammatory myopathy (Centner et al., 2013). Though first described in patients taking zidovudine in doses of 1000 mg/day or more, zidovudine myopathy also develops on lower-dose regimens in cART regimen. Affected patients typically have taken zidovudine for at least 6 months. Serum creatine kinase may be normal or slightly elevated, and muscle biopsy shows histological features suggesting mitochondrial dysfunction, with no or scanty inflammation. Clinical response to a drug holiday or reduction in zidovudine dose often obviates the need for muscle biopsy.

Pyomyositis, a focal suppurative bacterial muscle infection, was more common in the tropics and rare in developed nations before the AIDS cART era. Blood cultures may reveal the causative organism, usually *Staphylococcus aureus* or, less commonly, *S. typhi* or other gram-negative bacilli. Empirical intravenous antibiotic therapy should be given to cover these pathogens. Surgical drainage may be required.

*The complete reference list is available online at https://expertconsult.inkling.com/.* 

78

# Viral Encephalitis and Meningitis

*John David Beckham, Marylou V. Solbrig, Kenneth L. Tyler*

## OUTLINE



Hundreds of viruses exhibit tropism for the central (CNS) and/or peripheral (PNS) nervous systems. In the case of some viruses, involvement of the CNS or PNS is the predominant feature of illness, whereas in others involvement of the nervous system is a rare complication of a more generalized illness. Viral infection of the nervous system can result in a myriad of clinical presentations occurring separately or in combinations including acute or chronic meningitis, encephalitis, myelitis, ganglionitis, and polyradiculitis. Viruses may also incite para- or post-infectious CNS inflammatory or autoimmune syndromes such as acute disseminated encephalomyelitis (ADEM) or encephalitis associated with autoantibodies (see Chapter 80). The neurological complications of human immunodeficiency virus (HIV) and human T-cell lymphotropic virus (HTLV) infections are discussed separately (see Chapter 77).

Table 78.1 lists the most common viral causes of nervous system disease in North America and the relative propensity of each virus to cause meningitis, encephalitis, post-infectious encephalomyelitis, or myelitis. Infections that occur in residents or travelers to areas outside the United States are listed in Table 78.2. In the United States, the most common viruses causing meningitis are enteroviruses (EVs), herpes simplex virus type 2 (HSV-2), and arboviruses. The most common identified viral causes of encephalitis are herpesviruses, notably HSV-1, and arboviruses. Even with the best diagnostic efforts, up to 70% of cases of suspected viral encephalitis remain of unknown etiology (Glaser et al., 2003, 2006; Kupila et al., 2006). However, cases of antibody-mediated autoimmune encephalitis are increasingly recognized as important causes of encephalitis and may represent a substantial portion of the unknown or unidentified encephalitis cases. In an analysis of patients < 30 years of age and enrolled in the California Encephalitis Project (CEP), anti-*N*-methyl-D-aspartate (NMDA)-receptor encephalitis was as common as viral encephalitis (Gable, 2012). Worldwide, there are tens of thousands of deaths from rabies each year (Warrell and Warrell, 2004), and in Asia, nearly 68,000 cases and 13,000–20,000 deaths from Japanese encephalitis virus (JEV; WHO, 2015). Since the original outbreak of West Nile virus (WNV) in 1999, the Centers for Disease Control (CDC) tracks reported cases of WNV disease in the United States https://www.cdc.gov/westnile/statsmaps/index.html From 1999 through 2018, there have been approximately 51,000 cases of WNV disease, including 24,000 cases of WNV neuroinvasive disease, and 2300 deaths.

Although the basic clinical features of most types of viral meningitis and encephalitis are generally similar, specific physical examination findings may help narrow the possible viral etiologies of nervous system disease (Tables 78.3 and 78.4). It is important to recognize that several nonviral diseases can mimic the clinical features of viral CNS infection (Table 78.5) (DeBiasi and Tyler, 2006a). The treatment, prophylaxis, and immunotherapy of specific viral infections are summarized later in the chapter.

## DEOXYRIBONUCLEIC ACID VIRUSES

### Herpesviruses

Multiple members of the herpesvirus family cause neurological disease in humans: HSV-1 and HSV-2, varicella-zoster virus (VZV), human cytomegalovirus (HCMV), Epstein-Barr virus (EBV), human herpesviruses (HHV-6, HHV-7, and HHV-8), and the simian ("monkey") herpes B virus.

#### Herpes Simplex Viruses Type 1 and 2

***Herpes simplex encephalitis.*** HSV-1 encephalitis is the most common identified cause of sporadic fatal encephalitis in the United States, accounting for approximately 10% of all cases of encephalitis and occurring with a frequency of about 2–4 cases per

TABLE 78.1 **Primary Causes of Viral Nervous System Infection in North America**

| Agent | | Meningitis | Encephalitis | Postinfectious Acute Disseminated Encephalomyelitis | Myelitis |
|---|---|---|---|---|---|
| Arboviruses (United States and Canada) | | | | | |
| Togaviruses | | | | | |
| Flavivirus | West Nile virus (WNV) | * | * * | | * * |
| | St. Louis encephalitis virus (SLE) | * | ** | | * * |
| | Powassan | | ** | | |
| Alphavirus | Eastern equine encephalitis (EEE) | * | *** | | |
| | Western equine encephalitis (WEE) | * | ** | | |
| | Venezuelan equine encephalitis (VEE) | * * | * | | |
| Reoviridae: orbivirus | Colorado tick fever | ** | * | | |
| Bunyavirus | California (La Crosse) | * | ** | | |
| | Jamestown Canyon | * | * | | |
| | Snowshoe hare | * | * | | |
| Herpes viruses | Herpes simples virus (HSV)-1 | * | ** | | * |
| | HSV-2 | ** | * | | ** |
| | Varicella-zoster virus (VZV) | * | ** | * | ** |
| | Human Cytomegalovirus (HCMV) | * | ** | | ** |
| | Epstein-Barr virus (EBV) | * | * | * | ** |
| | Human herpesvirus (HHV)-6 | * | ** | | * |
| | HHV-7 | * | | | |
| | HHV-8 | | * | | |
| | Herpes B virus | | *** | | ** |
| Lymphocytic choriomeningitis virus (LCMV) | | ** | * | | ** |
| Mumps virus | | ** | * | * | * |
| Human immunodeficiency virus (HIV) | | ** | * | | * |
| Rabies virus | | | *** | * | * |
| Measles virus | | | * | *** | * |
| Rubella virus | | | | * | * |
| Enteroviruses | | *** | * | | *** |
| Adenovirus | | * | ** | | |
| Vaccinia | | | | * | |
| Influenza | | | | * | * |
| Parainfluenza | | * | * | * | |
| Rotavirus | | * | * | | |
| Parvovirus B-19 | | * | * | | |
| Coronavirus | SARS-CoV2 | * | ** | ** | * |

*rare, **common, ***frequent clinical presentation of the indicated virus

1,000,000 population per year (Bradshaw and Venkatesan, 2016; Whitley, 2006). Early recognition is important because the efficacy of the antiviral drug acyclovir (ACV) in reducing morbidity and mortality decreases as neurological disease progresses (Sili et al., 2014; Erdem et al., 2015; Whitley et al., 1986). HSV-1 strains cause over 90% of cases of herpes simplex encephalitis (HSE) in adults, with the remainder due to HSV-2. Conversely, HSV-2 is a more common cause of meningitis and neonatal meningoencephalitis than HSV-1. Both HSV types 1 and 2 have been associated with myelitis.

Fever is present in about 75%–80% and headache in about 60%–70% of patients with brain biopsy or cerebral spinal fluid (CSF) polymerase chain reaction (PCR) proven HSE (Gnann and Whitley, 2017). Other common features include disorientation or altered consciousness (70%–90%), personality change (60%), focal or generalized seizures (55%), memory disturbance (35%), motor deficit (40%), and aphasia (40%–60%) (Domingues et al., 1997; Gnann and Whitley, 2017; Sili et al., 2014; Whitley, 2006; Whitley et al., 1986). Immunocompromised patients may have atypical clinical and MRI presentations including the absence of prodromal symptoms, fewer focal findings, and MRI abnormalities outside the "classical" frontotemporal areas (Tan et al., 2012). Atypical presentations may also occur in young children (Schleede et al., 2013).

It is important to recognize that no sets of signs or symptoms are pathognomonic of HSE, and multiple infectious and

**TABLE 78.2 Additional Causes of Viral Nervous System Infection Resulting from Foreign Exposures**

| Agent | | Geographical Distribution |
|---|---|---|
| Nipah virus | | Malaysia, Singapore, India, Bangladesh |
| Measles virus | | Europe, Middle East, Asia, Africa, the Pacific |
| Filovirus | Ebola | Rainforest Africa |
| | Marburg | |
| Mosquito-borne | Eastern equine | Caribbean and South America (plus United States) |
| | Venezuelan equine | Central and northern South America (plus United States) |
| | St. Louis | Caribbean, Central and northern South America (plus United States) |
| | Japanese B | Japan, China, Southeast Asia, India, parts of Northern Australia, western Pacific |
| | Kunjin | Australia |
| | Murray Valley | Australia and New Guinea |
| | West Nile | Africa and Middle East, parts of Europe (plus United States) |
| | Ilheus | South and Central America |
| | Rocio | Brazil |
| | Dengue | All tropical areas (plus United States) |
| | Zika | Caribbean, Central and South America, Southeast Asia, Pacific Island nations, Africa |
| | Yellow Fever | Sub-Saharan Africa, Central and South America |
| | Chikungunya | Africa, southern Asia, Oceania, Indian Ocean countries, Caribbean, Central and South America (plus United States) |
| Sand fly–borne | Toscana | Italy, Spain, Portugal, France |
| Tickborne complex | Far Eastern (formerly Russian spring-summer) | Eastern Russia and neighboring north Asian countries |
| | Siberian | Russia and neighboring Asian countries, Scandinavia |
| | Central European | Eastern and Central Europe, Scandinavia |
| | Kyasanur Forest | India |
| | Louping Ill | England, Scotland, and Northern Ireland |
| | Negishi | Japan |
| Bunyavirus | Tahyna | Czechoslovakia, Yugoslavia, Italy, southern France |
| | Inkoo | Finland |
| | Rift Valley | East Africa |
| Rhabdovirus | Rabies | Asia, Africa, South America, eastern Europe (plus United States) |
| Enterovirus | Poliovirus | Afghanistan, Pakistan, India, Nigeria (endemic) |
| Arenavirus | LCMV | All continents except Antarctica |
| | Lassa fever virus | West Africa |
| Orthopoxvirus | Monkeypox | Central and West Africa |

*LCMV*, Lymphocytic choriomeningitis virus.

inflammatory processes can mimic HSE (Whitley, 2006; Whitley et al., 1986). Definitive diagnosis of HSE is based on amplification of HSV DNA in CSF using an HSV-specific PCR assay or, less commonly, isolation of virus, or detection of viral antigen or viral nucleic acid from brain tissue at biopsy or autopsy (see later discussion).

Examination of CSF is a critical diagnostic test in suspected cases of HSE. CSF is usually under increased pressure, with a median lymphocytic pleocytosis of 25–150 white blood cells (WBC) per μL (range 0–1000). In early studies, over 95% of PCR or biopsy-proven cases of HSE have a CSF pleocytosis (Domingues et al., 1997; Whitley et al., 1986), although some more recent reports suggest normocellular CSF can occur in up to 26% of cases (Saraya et al., 2016), and this phenomenon may be more common in patients with HIV-infection or otherwise immunocompromised (Saraya et al., 2016). A recent retrospective multicenter review of pediatric HSE found that 16% of children with HSE had normal CSF glucose, protein, and cell counts (Schleede et al., 2013). HSE is often hemorrhagic, and both red blood cells and xanthochromia can be detected in CSF, although neither feature occurs with significantly greater frequency in HSE compared to other causes of focal encephalitis (Whitley et al., 1986). The presence of red cells in CSF may be associated with a worse prognosis (Poissy et al., 2012). CSF protein concentration is moderately elevated (65–85 mg/dL) in about 60%–70% of patients and glucose concentration is normal in the majority (75%–90%) patients (Sili et al., 2014; Gnann and Whitley, 2017). Autoantibodies, notably those against the NMDA receptor, may develop as a consequence of HSE in 30% of patients (Pruss et al., 2012). A retrospective study found that 30% of patients with PCR confirmed HSE had detectable serum NMDAR antibodies (Pruss et al., 2012). In adult HSE cases the presence of NMDAR antibodies has been associated with delayed recovery and resurgent symptoms suggesting disease relapse, that can respond to appropriate immunomodulatory therapies. In children, NMDAR antibodies may be associated with choreiform and other movement disorders (Armangue et al., 2015; Nosadini et al., 2017).

CSF PCR is the diagnostic assay of choice in HSE, as virus is cultured from CSF in less than 5% of cases. Amplification of HSV

**TABLE 78.3 Skin/Mucous Membrane Findings Suggesting Specific Viral Central Nervous System Diseases**

| Exanthem or Mucous Membrane Change | Viral Agent | Specific Changes |
|---|---|---|
| Vesicular eruption | Enterovirus (A71) | "Hand, foot, and mouth disease": Macules/papules/vesicles on palms, soles, buttocks |
| | Herpes simplex | Grouped small (3 mm) vesicles on an erythematous base |
| | Varicella-zoster virus | Zoster: Vesicles in dermatomal distribution |
| | | Primary VZV: Multiple vesicles, papules, pustules in various stages of eruption |
| Maculopapular eruption | Epstein-Barr virus | Diffuse maculopapular eruption following ampicillin treatment |
| | Measles | Diffuse maculopapular erythematous eruption beginning on face/chest and extending downward |
| | HHV-6 | Roseola: Diffuse maculopapular eruption following 4 days of high fever |
| | Colorado tick fever | Maculopapular rash in 50% |
| | LCMV | Occasionally occurs with lymphadenopathy |
| | WNV, ZIKV | Diffuse erythematous maculopapular rash on chest and arms |
| Erythema multiforme | (*Mycoplasma*) | Many types of rash |
| Confluent macular rash | Parvovirus | Confluent erythema over cheeks ("slapped cheeks") followed by lacy reticular rash over extremities (late) |
| Purpura | Parvovirus | Rare "stocking glove" syndrome: Purpuric lesions on distal extremities |
| Pharyngitis | Enterovirus | Herpangina: Vesicles on soft palate |
| | Adenovirus | Pharyngitis, conjunctivitis |
| Conjunctivitis | St. Louis encephalitis | Conjunctivitis |
| | ZIKV | Conjunctivitis |
| | Adenovirus | Conjunctivitis with pharyngitis (see above) |

*HHV-6*, Human herpesvirus type 6; *LCMV*, lymphocytic choriomeningitis virus; *VZV*, varicella-zoster virus; *WNV*, West Nile virus, *ZIKV*, Zika virus.

**TABLE 78.4 Other Specific Findings Associated with Viruses Causing Central Nervous System Disease**

| Finding | Viruses |
|---|---|
| Alopecia | LCMV |
| Arthritis | LCMV, parvovirus, Chikungunya |
| Biphasic illness | LCMV, Colorado tick fever |
| Lymphadenopathy | LCMV, mumps, HIV |
| Mastitis | Mumps |
| Mononucleosis | HCMV, EBV, CMV |
| Myelitis | WNV, St. Louis encephalitis virus, VZV, EBV, HSV-1, CMV, herpes B virus, LCMV, EV-D68, EV-A71 |
| Myocarditis/pericarditis | Enterovirus, (mumps, LCMV) |
| Orchitis/oophoritis | Mumps (LCMV, EBV) |
| Paresthesias | Colorado tick fever, LCMV, rabies |
| Parotitis | Mumps (LCMV) |
| Pneumonia | Influenza, parainfluenza, SARS-CoV2 |
| Retinitis | HCMV, WNV, ZIKV (congenital) |
| Tremors, myoclonus | Arbovirus (e.g., WNV), EV-A71 |
| Urinary retention | St. Louis encephalitis virus, VZV, HCMV, HSV, herpes B virus, LCMV (see myelitis causing viruses) |

*EBV*, Epstein-Barr virus; *EV*, Enterovirus, *HCMV*, human cytomegalovirus; *HSV*, herpes simplex virus type; *LCMV*, lymphocytic choriomeningitis virus; *VZV*, varicella-zoster virus; *WNV*, West Nile virus; *ZIKV*, Zika virus.

DNA from CSF by PCR testing has a sensitivity of 98% and specificity of 94%–99% for the diagnosis of HSE compared to brain biopsy (Gnann and Whitley, 2017; Lakeman and Whitley, 1995; Tebas et al., 1998) (Table 78.6). Surprisingly, CSF HSV genome copy number ("HSV viral load") is not a reliable predictor of outcome (Poissy et al., 2012). HSV CSF PCR results must be interpreted considering the pre-test probability that a patient has HSE (Bayesian decision analysis). For example, a negative HSV CSF PCR in a patient with a low (~5%) prior probability of HSE reduces the post-test likelihood of HSE to approximately 0.2%, whereas a negative PCR in a patient with a high (~60%) pre-test likelihood of HSE only reduces the post-test likelihood of HSE to around 6% (Tebas et al., 1998). CSF PCR remains a sensitive technique for the detection of HSE, even in patients who have received up to a week of ACV therapy (Lakeman and Whitley, 1995). Despite the high overall sensitivity of CSF HSV PCR, false-negative results have been reported, most notably in patients in whom CSF was obtained within the first 72 hours of illness onset (Weil et al., 2002). For this

**TABLE 78.5 Diseases That Can Masquerade as Viral Nervous System Disease**

| Etiology | Agent | Disease | Suggestive features |
|---|---|---|---|
| Infectious | Bacterial | Parameningeal focus (sinusitis, intracranial abscess) | Very mild pleocytosis, focal neurological exam |
| | | Partially treated bacterial meningitis | Prior antibiotic treatment |
| | | Lyme disease | Tick exposure, arthritis, appropriate geography, erythema migrans |
| | | Tuberculosis | Very high protein, hypoglycorrhachia |
| | | Leptospirosis | Conjunctival suffusion, jaundice |
| | | Syphilis (primary and tertiary) | Chronic |
| | | *Brucella* | Farm animal or unpasteurized milk exposure |
| | | Whipple disease | Gastrointestinal complaints |
| | | *Bartonella* (cat scratch disease) | Cat exposure, adenopathy |
| | | *Listeria* | Brainstem encephalitis |
| | | Typhoid fever | Exposure history, bradycardia |
| | Fungal | *Cryptococcus* | Usually immunocompromised patient (pt) |
| | | *Coccidioides* | Southwestern US exposure, pulmonary symptoms |
| | | *Histoplasma* | Pulmonary nodules |
| | | Blastomycosis | Midwest, pulmonary symptoms |
| | | *Candida* | Immunocompromised pt |
| | | *Nocardia* | Immunocompromised pt |
| | Parasitic | *Toxoplasma* | Retinitis, cat exposure |
| | | Cysticercosis | Calcified lesions |
| | | Amoebic | Fresh water: *Naegleria* |
| | | Malaria (*Plasmodium falciparum*) | Exposure history, cyclic fevers |
| | Rickettsial | Rocky Mountain spotted fever | Leukopenia, thrombocytopenia, hyponatremia, petechial rash |
| | | *Ehrlichia* | See above |
| | | *Coxiella burnetii* (Q fever) | Exposure to sheep, wildlife pulmonary disease |
| | *Mycoplasma* | | Precedent pulmonary symptoms |
| Parainfectious | Acute disseminated encephalomyelitis (ADEM) | | Characteristic MRI findings |
| Noninfectious | Anti-neuronal Antibodies, e.g., anti-NMDA receptor Abs | Autoimmune Encephalitis | Atypical psychiatric presentations or movement disorders and young age |
| | Connective tissue disorders | Systemic lupus erythematosus (SLE) | Malar rash, multisystem organ involvement |
| | | Sarcoidosis | Hilar adenopathy, erythema nodosum |
| | Uveomeningitic syndromes | Behçet disease | Genital/oral ulcers, uveitis |
| | Intracranial tumors and cysts | | Recurrent episodes, dermal sinus tract |
| | Drugs | NSAIDs, antibiotics, immunomodulators, anticonvulsants | Exposure history |
| | Intracranial or subarachnoid hemorrhage | | |
| | Encephalopathy | Toxic or metabolic, mitochondrial disorders, particularly MELAS | |

*MRI*, Magnetic resonance imaging; *NMDA*, N-methyl-D-aspartate; *NSAIDs*, nonsteroidal antiinflammatory drugs.

reason, caution should be used in stopping ACV therapy in patients with suspected HSE on the sole basis of a single negative CSF PCR test obtained within 72 hours of symptom onset, unless a suitable alternative diagnosis has been established.

When definitive diagnosis of HSE was dependent on brain biopsy, patients often had significantly depressed levels of consciousness and advanced neurological disease at the time of diagnosis. With routine use of HSV CSF PCR instead of brain biopsy for definitive diagnosis of HSE, patients are often identified at an earlier stage of illness, exhibit less depression of consciousness, and have improved response to therapy. Over 75% of cases with PCR-proven HSE had a Glasgow Coma Score (GCS) above 12 (Domingues et al., 1997), whereas only 30% of cases with biopsy-proven HSE had a GCS above 10 in the Collaborative Antiviral Study Group (CASG) trial of vidarabine versus ACV therapy (Whitley et al., 1986).

Magnetic resonance imaging (MRI) is significantly more sensitive than computed tomography (CT) and is the neuroimaging procedure of choice in patients with suspected HSE. Approximately 90% of patients with PCR-proven HSE will have MRI abnormalities involving the temporal lobes (Domingues et al., 1997; Raschilas et al., 2002; Silli et al., 2014) (Fig. 78.1). The electroencephalogram (EEG) may be abnormal early in the course of disease, demonstrating diffuse slowing, focal abnormalities in the temporal regions, or periodic lateralizing epileptiform discharges (PLEDs). EEG abnormalities involving the temporal lobes are seen in approximately 75% of patients with PCR-proven HSE (Domingues et al., 1997).

**TABLE 78.6 CSF PCR Diagnosis of Viral Nervous System Disease**

| Virus | Sensitivity | Specificity |
|---|---|---|
| Adenovirus | Unknown | |
| Dengue | Unknown | |
| Enterovirus | >95% (meningitis), <10% for AFM with EV-D68 or <25% with Neuroinvasive EV-A71 | >95% |
| Herpesviruses | | |
| HCMV | 100% in immunocompromised | High |
| | >60% in congenital CMV infection | High |
| EBV | 98.5% as tumor marker in HIV patients with Primary CNS lymphoma | Unknown |
| HSV-1 and -2 | >95% | >95% |
| HHV-6 | Unknown | Unknown |
| VZV | >95% | >95% |
| HIV | HIV RNA present at all stages | High |
| HTLV I and II | 75% | 98.5% |
| Influenza | Unknown but > culture | Unknown |
| Japanese encephalitis virus | Unknown (higher early) | High |
| JC virus | 50%–90% in PML, lower copy # in more immunocompetent pts | 98% |
| LCMV | Unknown | Unknown |
| Mumps | Unknown | High |
| Measles | Unknown | High |
| Parvovirus B-19 | 80% | Unknown |
| Rabies | 90% | High |
| WNV | 70% (higher early) | High |
| SARS-CoV2 | Unknown, likely low (Nasopharyngeal RT-PCR high acutely) | High |
| ZIKV | Unknown (congenital ZIKV syndrome) | High |

*AFM,* Acute flaccid myelitis; *CNS,* central nervous system; *CSF,* cerebral spinal fluid; *EBV,* Epstein-Barr virus; *HCMV,* human cytomegalovirus; *HHV,* human herpesvirus; *HSV,* herpes simplex virus; *HTLV,* human T-cell lymphotropic virus; *LCMV,* lymphocytic choriomeningitis virus; *PCR,* polymerase chain reaction; *PML,* progressive multifocal leukoencephalopathy; *VZV,* varicella-zoster virus; *WNV,* West Nile virus; *ZIKV,* Zika virus.

Brain biopsy is now only rarely performed for diagnosis of HSE. Biopsy is reserved for atypical cases in which the diagnosis remains in question and for those who respond poorly to treatment. Biopsy specimens from patients with HSE show hemorrhagic necrosis, HSV antigen in infected cells, and accumulations of viral particles forming acidophilic intranuclear inclusion bodies in neurons (Cowdry type A inclusions; Fig. 78.2).

Empirical therapy with ACV should be started immediately in acute cases of focal encephalitis of suspected viral etiology (Table 78.7). Delay in the institution of ACV therapy is surprisingly common and occurs more frequently in patients with other severe underlying diseases, chronic alcohol abuse, pleocytosis of less than 10 cells/μL, and delayed initial neuroimaging studies, as these factors may make clinicians less likely to consider HSE in the differential diagnosis (Poissy et al., 2009). Mortality in untreated cases of HSE is around 70%, but this is reduced to 19%–28% in patients treated with ACV (Whitley et al., 1986), and to less than 10% in more recent studies (Erdem et al., 2015; Sili et al., 2014). Morbidity due to HSV-1 encephalitis remains high even in patients receiving ACV, with only 37.5% of all patients surviving with no or only mild deficits (Whitley et al., 1986). In a more recent study 23% had no sequelae and 32% mild sequelae (Sili et al., 2014). However, in specific subpopulations of ACV-treated HSE patients, prognosis can be considerably better. For example, 50% (12/24) of patients in whom treatment with ACV was initiated when their GCS exceeded 6 survived with no or only minor sequelae, and more than 60% who were younger than age 30 and had a GCS above 6 survived with no or only minor sequelae (Whitley et al., 1986). Outcomes have been generally similar in cases of PCR-proven HSE treated with ACV, with 35%–56% of patients returning to normal functional status or having only mild disability or residual sequelae at 6 months follow-up (Domingues et al., 1997; Raschilas et al., 2002; Singh et al., 2016). Survival and prognosis are influenced by several factors including level of consciousness at initiation of therapy (e.g., GCS), patient age, and duration of disease before therapy (Erdem et al., 2015; Marton et al., 1996; Raschilas et al., 2002; Singh et al., 2016; Whitley et al., 1986). In the CASG trial, all (9/9) patients treated with ACV within 4 days of onset of fever, headache, and focal neurological deficits survived, whereas the mortality was 35% in those in whom ACV treatment was initiated when disease was more than 4 days old (Whitley et al., 1986). In another study, the recovery rate was 50% in patients treated within 5 days of illness onset (Marton et al., 1996). In a third study of PCR-proven HSE, 75% of patients with an ultimately favorable outcome had received ACV therapy within 2 days of hospital admission compared to only 30% of those with a poor outcome (Raschilas et al., 2002).

The standard adult dose of ACV for HSE is 10 mg/kg, given intravenously (IV) every 8 hours (20 mg/kg every 8 hours in neonates and children) for 14–21 days. Renal insufficiency is an infrequent, usually reversible side effect of ACV therapy and the risk is reduced by appropriate hydration. Neither higher doses of ACV nor prolonged therapy with oral valacyclovir after a standard intravenous course improved outcomes in adults (Gnann et al., 2015; Stahl et al., 2012). ACV dosing should be adjusted appropriately in patients with renal insufficiency. Periodic shortages of intravenous ACV and the cost of intravenous preparations in resource-poor countries have led some to suggest that oral valacyclovir may be an alternative when intravenous ACV is unavailable (Pouplin et al., 2011), but it is critical to emphasize that there are only isolated case reports and no comprehensive studies of the efficacy of oral drugs in HSE and this alternative should only be considered in

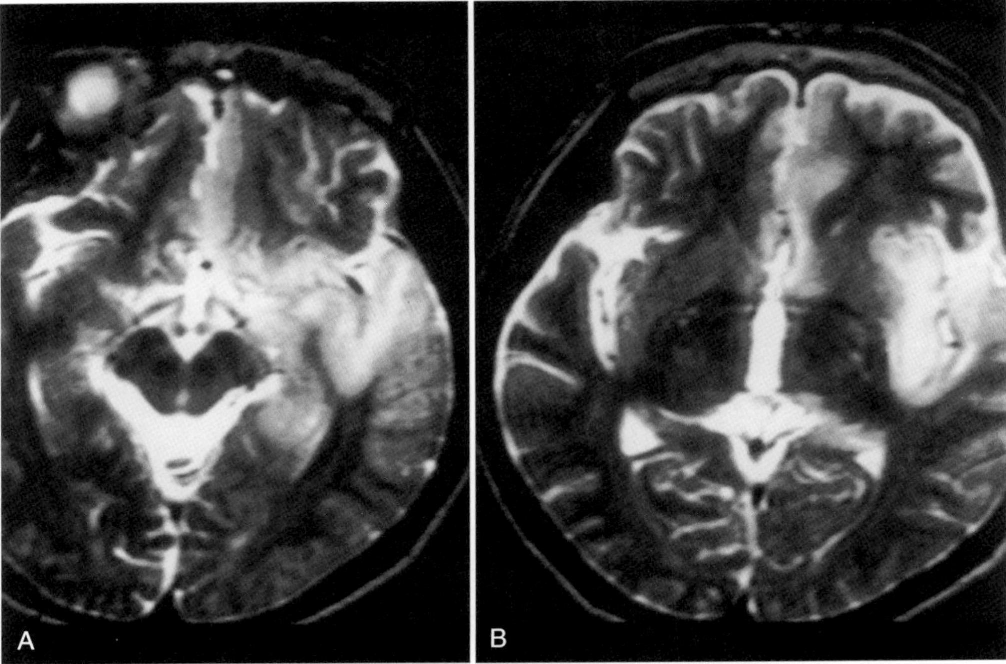


**Fig. 78.1 Herpes Simplex Encephalitis.** T2-weighted magnetic resonance image showing increased signal in left medial temporal lobe, inferior frontal lobe, and insular cortex. Sections at level of the midbrain (A) and thalamus and basal ganglia (B). (Courtesy J. Healy.)

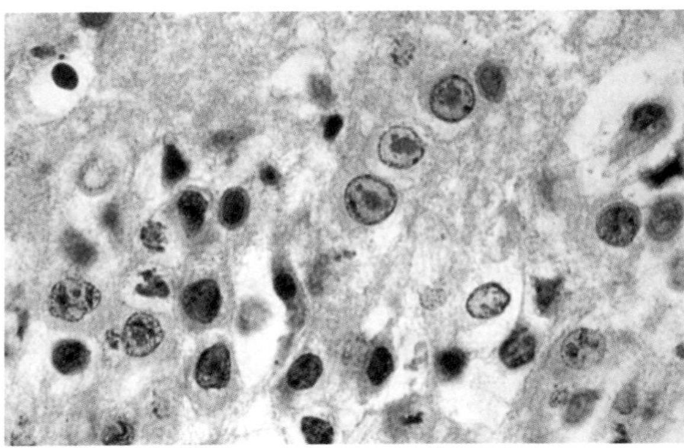

**Fig. 78.2 Hippocampal Granule Cell Neurons in Herpes Simplex 1 Encephalitis.** Many nuclei contain acidophilic Cowdry type A intranuclear inclusions, which are surrounded by halos and marginated nuclear chromatin. (Hematoxylin-eosin stain, ×350.) (Courtesy R. Kim.)

extraordinary circumstances or settings. When a specific shortage of intravenous formulations of ACV exists, ganciclovir can be used as an alternative. Retrospective studies have suggested that there may be some benefit in adding corticosteroids to ACV treatment (Kamei et al., 2006), although controlled clinical trials are needed before the role of steroid therapy as an adjunct to ACV can be definitively established. Cases of HSE due to ACV-resistant HSV strains have been reported predominantly in immunocompromised patients and in extraordinarily rare instances in immunocompetent individuals (<1%) who have never been exposed to antiviral drugs (Bergmann et al., 2017). Foscarnet (180 mg/kg IV daily given in two or three divided doses) is an alternative therapy for patients with suspected or proven ACV-resistant strains or with allergy to ACV (Bergmann et al., 2017; Schulte et al., 2010).

***Neonatal herpes simplex virus meningoencephalitis.*** In contradistinction to adults, in whom HSE is usually caused by HSV-1, HSV-2 is the most common causal agent of meningoencephalitis in neonates (although HSV-1 disease may also occur). Neonates who acquire HSV from the birth canal develop infection of the CNS in 50% of cases (Kimberlin, 2005). CNS disease occurs as either a component of an overwhelming sepsis-like disseminated disease with multiorgan involvement (in the first week of life) or as isolated CNS disease that usually presents later (weeks 2–10 of life), with or without accompanying vesicular skin, mucous membrane, or conjunctival lesions (skin, eye, mouth disease). The presence of vesicular skin or mucosal lesions in an infant of this age, even in the absence of fever or systemic symptoms, warrants immediate evaluation of CSF for HSV infection, because up to 30% of infants with presumed isolated skin, eye, and mouth disease are subsequently identified as having CNS involvement. Neonates with possible HSV disease should be treated empirically with IV ACV, 20 mg/kg, every 8 hours (Kimberlin et al., 2001). Treatment should be continued for 14 days in HSV-infected infants with isolated skin, eye, and mouth disease and 21 days in infants with sepsis or CNS involvement. Relapses of skin, eye, and mouth disease (with the potential for CNS involvement and subsequent neurological deficits) are common in the first year of life following neonatal HSV disease. A recent double-blind, placebo-controlled study found that a 6-month course of oral ACV (300 mg/meter sq. of body surface area 3× daily), after completion of the standard 14- to 21-day course of intravenous ACV, resulted in improved neurodevelopmental outcomes at 12 months after treatment compared to placebo and this has become standard of care (Kimberlin et al., 2011).

***Herpes simplex virus meningitis.*** HSV meningitis accounts for approximately 10% of acute viral meningitis in adults. In most series greater than 75% of those affected are women (Landry et al., 2009; Miller et al., 2013). At the time of their first episode of genital herpes (generally due to HSV-2), approximately 36% of women and 11% of men have symptoms of meningitis including fever, headache, and nuchal rigidity. In a review of the Mayo Clinic experience with HSV-2 meningitis all patients had headache and about half had fever, photophobia, and meningismus, and just over a quarter had nausea

TABLE 78.7 **Treatment and Prophylaxis of Viral Infections**

| Antiviral Class | Antiviral Agent | Dose | Indications | Toxicity or Cautions |
|---|---|---|---|---|
| Nucleoside analogs | Acyclovir | 10 mg/kg/dose (IV) q 8 h ×14–21 days | HSV encephalitis in adults | Renal impairment |
| | | 20 mg/kg/dose (IV) q 8 h ×21 days | Neonatal HSV encephalitis | |
| | | (IV) q 8 h ×21 days<br>10–12 mg/kg/dose in adults and up to 20 mg/kg/dose in infants) IV q 8 h ×21 days | VZV encephalitis in normal or immunocompromised patient (pt) | |
| | | 15 mg/kg/dose (IV) q 8 h ×21 days | Herpes B virus | |
| | | 800 mg (PO) 5×/day ×7 days | Dermatomal zoster or primary VZV in immunocompromised pt | Low solubility |
| | Famciclovir | 200 mg (PO) tid ×7 days | Dermatomal zoster or primary VZV in immunocompromised pt | Headache, nausea |
| | Valacyclovir | 1 g (PO) qid ×7 days | Dermatomal zoster or primary VZV in immunocompromised pt | Thrombotic thrombocytic purpura/hemolytic uremic syndrome in HIV patients |
| | Ganciclovir | 5 mg/kg (IV) q 12 h ×14–21 days | HCMV, herpes B virus | Bone marrow suppression |
| | Valganciclovir | 900 mg (PO) bid ×21 days (induction), then 900 mg (PO) daily (maintenance) | HCMV retinitis | Bone marrow suppression |
| | Ribavirin | 2 g (IV) ×1, then 1 g (IV) q 6 h ×4 days, then 0.5 g (IV) q 8 h ×6 days | Lassa fever | Hemolytic anemia |
| | | 20–35 mg/kg/day ×7 days | Measles virus | |
| | | 600 mg/day to 1400 mg/day (PO) divided in 2 doses | Hepatitis C | |
| | Cytarabine | 2 mg/kg (IV) ×5 days ×4 wk | PML | Bone marrow suppression |
| | Trifluridine | 1% ophthalmic solution | Herpetic keratoconjunctivitis | |
| Nucleotide analog | cidofovir | 5 mg/kg (IV) every 1–2 wk or 1 mg/kg (IV) 3×/wk for 3 wk | DNA viruses:<br>Severe AdV, monkeypox, resistant HCMV | nephrotoxicity |
| | Remdesevir (Gilead, EUA) | 200 mg IV x1 then 100mg IV q24h x 4-9d | Severe COVID-19 | |
| Pyrophosphate analog | Foscarnet | 90 mg/kg (IV) q 12 h ×14–21 days | Acyclovir-resistant HSV/VZV<br>Ganciclovir-resistant HCMV | Hypocalcemia, renal impairment |
| Neuraminidase inhibitors | Oseltamivir | 75 mg (PO) bid ×5 days | Influenza A and B | |
| | Zanamivir | 10 mg (inhalation) bid ×5 days | Influenza A and B | |
| Cytokine | Interferon alfa | 3 million U/day (SQ) | PML, acyclovir-resistant VZV, hepatitis C | Flulike side effects |
| | Pegylated interferon alfa-2b | 1.5 μg/kg/wk (SQ) | | |
| | | $10^5$–$10^6$ U/m$^2$ body surface (intrathecal) | SSPE | |
| Supplements | Vitamin A | 400,000 IU (IM) | Acute measles in vitamin A deficiency | |

*bid*, Twice daily; COVID-19, *COVID-19*, SARS-CoV2 Disease 2019; EUA, FDA Emergency Use Authorization; *HCMV*, cytomegalovirus; *HSV*, herpes simplex virus; *IM*, intramuscularly; *IV*, intravenously; *PML*, progressive multifocal leukoencephalopathy; *PO*, orally; *qid*, four times daily; *SQ*, subcutaneously; *SSPE*, subacute sclerosing panencephalitis; *tid*, three times daily; *VZV*, varicella-zoster virus.

or vomiting (Miller et al., 2013). Only ~13%–25% of patients have a history of genital herpes or active lesions (Landry et al., 2009; Miller et al., 2013; O'Sullivan et al., 2003). The CSF shows a lymphocytic pleocytosis with an average of ~500 cells/μL, an elevated protein (average ~150 mg/dL) and a normal glucose. Neuroimaging is normal in nearly 85% but may show meningeal enhancement in rare cases (Miller et al., 2013). Following an initial episode of HSV-2 meningitis, 20%–30% go on to develop recurrent episodes (Landry et al., 2009). A randomized double-blind controlled study failed to show any effect of long-term valacyclovir suppressive therapy (500 mg 2×/day) in reducing the frequency of recurrent episodes of meningitis (Aurelius et al., 2012). CSF viral cultures are invariably negative during recurrent episodes of meningitis, although the virus may be isolated during the first (primary) episode. Other neurological complications such as paresthesias, urinary retention, and transverse myelitis have been described with HSV-2 infections.

CSF PCR has identified HSV-2 as the primary etiological agent in patients with benign recurrent lymphocytic meningitis (Mollaret meningitis) (Shalabi and Whitley, 2006; Tedder et al., 1994). This syndrome may be associated with the presence in the CSF of large cells of monocyte-macrophage lineage (Mollaret cells).

Treatment of HSV-2 meningitis varies considerably across published series and no high-quality randomized controlled trials have been performed (Landry et al., 2009; Miller et al., 2013). A typical regimen is to use oral valacyclovir (500 mg 3×/day) for 7–10 days. Patients with more severe symptoms may benefit from an initial short course of intravenous ACV (e.g., 500 mg q8h ×3 days) followed by oral valacyclovir.

### Varicella-Zoster Virus

***Primary infection.*** At least 95% of the adult population has been infected with VZV, and the lifetime risk of developing shingles is 3%–5%. VZV can involve virtually every part of the CNS and PNS (Gilden, 2004; Gilden et al., 2000, 2005; Grahn and Studahl., 2015; Kennedy and Gershon, 2018; Kleinschmidt-DeMasters and Gilden, 2001). Primary VZV may produce meningitis or encephalitis in immunocompromised patients. An acute self-limited cerebellar ataxia occurs in about 1 in 4000 children (<15 years of age) during or immediately following primary VZV infection (chickenpox). Postinfectious encephalomyelitis follows an estimated 1 in 2500 cases of primary VZV infection.

Reactivation of herpes zoster can produce meningitis, myelitis, and encephalitis in older children and adults. Zoster "encephalitis" can occur in both immunocompetent and immunocompromised hosts and in adults typically results from reactivation of herpes zoster decades after an initial infection with varicella (chickenpox). It has been suggested that VZV encephalitis may be second only to that caused by HSV as a cause of sporadic encephalitis in adults, and may be the leading cause of sporadic encephalitis in children (Grahn and Studahl., 2015). VZV encephalitis is in fact a vasculopathy rather than a true encephalitis (Gilden, 2004; Gilden et al., 2000, 2005, 2009; Kennedy and Gershon, 2018; Kleinschmidt-DeMasters and Gilden, 2001; Nagel et al., 2017). In older (>60 years) immunocompetent adults, VZV vasculopathy (previously called *granulomatous arteritis*) typically presents with acute focal stroke-like deficits due to inflammatory involvement of large cerebral arteries, typically occurring in the trigeminal distribution. Most cases are monophasic, although rare cases follow a chronic or relapsing-remitting course (Gilden, 2004; Gilden et al., 2005; Gilden et al., 2009; Nagel et al., 2017). CSF shows a lymphocytic pleocytosis. MRI shows a large single infarct, most commonly in the carotid, middle, or anterior cerebral territory. At autopsy, viral particles, antigen, and DNA can be found in the involved artery. Diagnosis can be made by demonstration of VZV DNA in CSF by PCR or by demonstration of VZV immunoglobulin (Ig)M or intrathecal synthesis of VZV IgG in CSF.

In immunocompromised individuals, VZV reactivation produces a multifocal vasculopathy predominantly involving small and medium-sized arteries, resulting in a clinical syndrome of mental status changes, focal deficits, and a CSF mononuclear pleocytosis (Gilden, 2004; Gilden et al., 2005; Gilden et al., 2009; Nagel et al., 2017). The typical rash of zoster may be absent. Neuroimaging shows multifocal hemorrhagic and ischemic cortical and subcortical infarcts. Diagnosis can be established by VZV CSF PCR or by demonstration of CSF VZV IgM or intrathecal VZV-specific IgG antibody synthesis. While most cases of VZV encephalitis present as a vasculopathy on imaging, a recent case series of VZV encephalitis cases found that 14 of 20 patients had a nonvascular, nonspecific or normal neuroimaging result (DeBroucker et al., 2012).

VZV can also cause an aseptic meningitis in immunocompetent hosts even in the absence of a characteristic varicella (chickenpox) or zoster (shingles) rash (Kupila et al., 2006; Mogensen and Larsen, 2006). VZV accounts for up to 8% of viral meningitis cases, making it third in importance behind EVs and HSV-2 (Kupila et al., 2006).

VZV has recently been associated with giant cell arteritis (GCA). VZV antigen can be detected in up to 75% of temporal artery biopsy specimens from patients with associated evidence of GCA (Nagel et al., 2017). VZV antigen is also detected in a high percentage (64%) of biopsy specimens of temporal arteries taken for diagnosis of GCA even when histological evidence of GCA is not found. The incidence of VZV in "normal" temporal arteries is reported at 8%–22%. The significance of these findings and their implications for pathogenesis and potentially treatment remain to be established. Although the suggestion that GCA patients be treated with valacyclovir in combination with prednisone has been made (Nagel et al., 2017), no clinical trials of this strategy have been reported.

There are no controlled randomized clinical trials of antiviral therapy of CNS VZV infection. Intravenous ACV (10 mg/kg every 8 hours) for 7–10 days is generally recommended for treatment of immunocompromised children and adults with chickenpox. Patients with VZV CNS disease including vasculopathy receive IV ACV (10–20 mg/kg or 500 mg/m$^2$ every 8 hours) for a minimum of 7 (Gilden, 2004) to 14 (Steiner et al., 2005) days, combined with a steroid pulse for 3–5 days (e.g., prednisone 60–80 mg/day) (Gilden, 2004; Steiner et al., 2005). HIV-infected individuals with localized (non-disseminated) dermatomal zoster can be treated with oral famciclovir (500 mg 3× daily) or valacyclovir (1000 mg 3× daily) for 7–10 days.

***Herpes zoster.*** Following primary infection, VZV becomes latent in cells of the dorsal root ganglia. Reactivation of endogenous latent virus produces herpes zoster (shingles). The virus can reactivate after injury or trauma to the spine or nerve roots or in response to waning cell-mediated immunity to VZV caused by age or immunosuppression related to HIV infection, cancer, cytotoxic drugs, or systemic illness. Herpes zoster is frequently the first clinical presentation of underlying HIV infection and may present as protracted or multidermatomal disease. The incidence of shingles is up to 25-fold greater in HIV-infected individuals than in the general population. Following universal varicella vaccination for US children, concerns arose that decreases in exposure and boosting of immunity in older adults would result in increased rates of zoster. However, recent work shows that widespread childhood immunization against zoster did not seem to affect the incidence of herpes zoster from 1992 to 2010 (Hales et al., 2013).

Herpes zoster typically begins with pain and paresthesias in one or two adjacent spinal or cranial dermatomes (Gilden et al., 2000; Kennedy and Gershon, 2018). Pain is followed in 3–4 days by a painful pruritic vesicular eruption in the area supplied by the affected root. The eruption typically lasts 10–14 days. Eruption most commonly occurs in the lower thoracic dermatomes but also commonly involves the trigeminal distribution and the cervical or lumbosacral dermatomes. Involvement of the first division of the trigeminal ganglion produces ophthalmic zoster and may be associated with conjunctivitis, keratitis, anterior uveitis, or iridocyclitis. Fortunately, vision loss following herpes zoster ophthalmicus is rare. Involvement of the geniculate ganglion produces otic zoster, or the Ramsay Hunt syndrome—painful facial paresis accompanied by tympanic membrane and external auditory canal vesicular rash. Herpes zoster involving cervical and thoracic levels may be associated with myelitis, and in the lumbosacral region may be accompanied by bladder dysfunction or ileus. Complications of zoster include postherpetic neuralgia, segmental motor atrophy in the affected dermatome, meningitis, myelitis, large-vessel vasculitis (usually involving the carotid or its branches on the side of zoster ophthalmicus), and multifocal leukoencephalitis or encephalitis with generalized cerebral vasculopathy (Gilden, 2004; Gilden et al., 2000, 2005, 2009).

Risk factors for postherpetic neuralgia in patients with shingles include age older than 50 years and prodromal sensory symptoms. Treatments are directed toward lessening pain, reducing virus shedding, and shortening healing time. ACV (800 mg orally, 5× daily for 7 days), famciclovir (200 mg orally, 3× daily for 7 days), or valacyclovir (1 g orally, 4× daily for 7 days) accelerates cutaneous healing and decreases acute zoster pain if begun within 72 hours of onset of rash. Whether these agents significantly decrease the incidence, duration, or severity of postherpetic neuralgia is uncertain. In patients without contraindications, a short course of corticosteroids (e.g., 40 mg prednisolone/day, tapered over 3 weeks) may be added to antiviral therapy. Compared with ACV therapy alone, addition of corticosteroids has been shown to improve comfort levels (pain reduction during the acute phase) following herpes zoster, although its efficacy in reducing subsequent risk of postherpetic neuralgia remains uncertain. Currently, zoster vaccination is the primary approach to decreasing zoster incidence and the associated risk of developing post-herpetic neuralgia. A new vaccine ("Shingrix") containing VZV glycoprotein E and adjuvant has recently been licensed. In phase III trials the vaccine (IM ×2 doses 2 months apart) reduced the incidence rate of shingles from 9.1/1000 person-years to 0.3 per 1000 person years in individuals over the age of 50 followed for a median of ~3 years (Lal et al., 2015). Vaccine efficacy was estimated at between 96.6% and 97.9% for all age groups. The safety profile was excellent, although local injection site and systemic reactions (grade 3) were common (17%). This vaccine is now recommended for all adults over the age of 50 regardless of their prior VZV vaccination history or history of shingles. Because this is not a live attenuated vaccine it can also be used safely in immunocompromised individuals.

### Human Cytomegalovirus

HCMV is a ubiquitous virus that causes acute infections with a worldwide distribution resulting in seropositivity in the overwhelming majority of the population. The virus spreads from person to person through direct contact with bodily secretions. Like other herpesviruses, HCMV is never completely cleared from the host and remains latent for the life of the host with periods of persistent or sporadic shedding. Shed virus is an important source of virus transmission. As a rule, infection with HCMV in immunologically normal hosts is clinically silent but can occasionally cause self-limited, febrile, mononucleosis-like illness (Macarski et al., 2013). Severe HCMV disease is most commonly associated with congenital fetal infection or infection in immunocompromised hosts. When disease does occur, HCMV-related neurological complications include retinitis, encephalitis, polyradiculomyelopathy, neuropathy, and Guillain-Barré syndrome (Griffiths, 2004). In immunocompetent hosts, HCMV may rarely cause asymptomatic infection, a mononucleosis syndrome, aseptic meningitis, or the Guillain-Barré syndrome. HCMV encephalitis is rare in immunocompetent hosts beyond the neonatal period but is reported (Rafailidis et al., 2008). However, immunocompromised adults and developing fetuses are at high risk of developing CNS disease due to CMV. CMV infection of peripheral nerves, nerve roots, and spinal cord, particularly in patients with AIDS, causes ascending myeloradiculitis (Miller et al., 1996).

***Congenital human cytomegalovirus.*** HCMV infection is the most common human congenital infection and can cause severe injury to the infected fetus. Up to 75% of congenital HCMV infections are due to nonprimary maternal infection, implying that better screening procedures are needed to detect and prevent HCMV reactivation and fetal infection (Wang et al., 2011). A review of 15 studies published from 1970 to 2004 that screened newborns for HCMV reported that 12.7% of 117,986 newborns with congenital HCMV infection were symptomatic at birth (Dollard et al., 2007). The mortality for newborns with symptomatic disease is 10%–30%, and up to 90% of survivors will have neurological sequelae. The rate of sequelae in newborns with asymptomatic primary infection has been estimated at roughly 15% (Griffiths and McLaughlin, 2004), most commonly including microcephaly, poor feeding, lethargy, hypotonia, and seizures. In addition to congenital cases, there are cases that arise in the perinatal period as a consequence of passage through an infected birth canal or following breastfeeding. Persistent high levels of viral replication in the eye and brain of the developing fetus produce encephalitis, ependymitis, and retinitis, a pattern similar to that seen in patients with opportunistic HCMV infection in the setting of HIV infection. Pathologically, encephalitis occurs in a periventricular pattern and may cause polymicrogyria and hydrocephalus (Fig. 78.3). CT scans show characteristic periventricular calcifications in 20%–30% of children with symptomatic HCMV infection. Retinitis with optic atrophy is seen in about 15% of those affected and results in characteristic hyperpigmented retinal scars. As noted, 90% of survivors of congenital HCMV infection have residual neurological sequelae including psychomotor retardation, learning delays, mental retardation, seizures, optic atrophy and retinitis, and hearing loss. Mild or subclinical congenital infections may also manifest later in childhood as sensorineural deafness or developmental delay. Congenital human HCMV infection is the most common, nonheritable cause of hearing loss in the United States.

Diagnosis of congenital HCMV is made by identification of HCMV DNA using PCR testing of urine, saliva, or CSF during the immediate postnatal period. Because urinary excretion of HCMV can often persist during the first year of life, isolation of virus or viral DNA from urine may be useful in later diagnosis. HCMV inclusion-bearing cells may also be found in affected organs (Fig. 78.4) and in stained preparations of urinary sediment and saliva. Serological studies may be difficult to interpret owing to transplacental transfer of antibody from the mother. Although detection of virus-specific IgM antibodies has been used to diagnose congenital HCMV, direct detection of viral markers is more accurate and preferred.

In a study evaluating the efficacy of IV ganciclovir therapy (4–6 mg/kg every 12 hours for 6 weeks) in neonates with symptomatic congenital HCMV infection, 69% of treated children, compared to only 39% of untreated children, showed improvement in brainstem auditory evoked potentials. More significantly, none of the ganciclovir-treated children, compared to 42% of those not

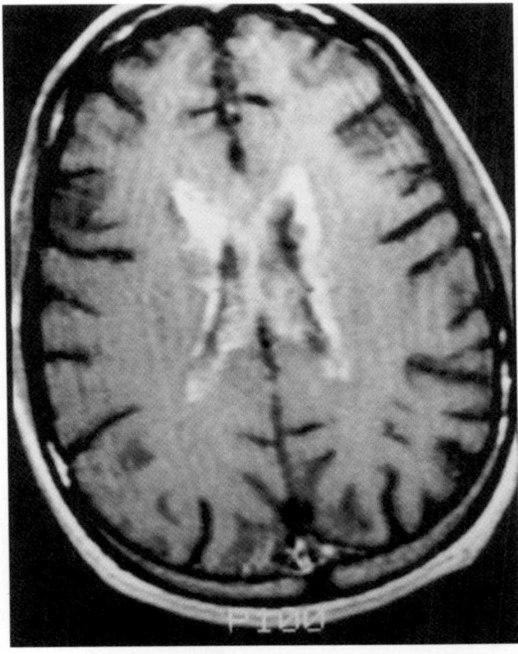

**Fig. 78.3 Human Cytomegalovirus Ventriculitis.** Axial gadolinium-enhanced T1-weighted magnetic resonance image showing contrast enhancement of ependyma of lateral ventricles. (Courtesy J. Healy.)

treated, showed worsening hearing loss over the initial 6 months post infection (Kimberlin et al., 2003; Whitley et al., 1997). In another study, 6 weeks of ganciclovir therapy in neonates with symptomatic congenital CMV infection involving the CMS led to fewer developmental delays at 6 and 12 months as compared to untreated infants (Oliver et al., 2009). While 6 weeks of therapy was beneficial, it was not known how long infants with congenital CNS HCMV disease should be treated. In a randomized, placebo-controlled study of 96 neonates, infants treated with valganciclovir (16 mg/kg, orally, twice daily) for 6 months were more likely to have normal hearing (73% vs. 57%) at 12- and 24-month follow-up and had improved neurodevelopmental scores when compared to infants treated with valganciclovir for 6 weeks and placebo for 4.5 months (Kimberlin et al., 2015). Thus, treating infants diagnosed with congenital HCMV infection for 6 months with valganciclovir may decrease the risk of hearing loss or neurodevelopmental abnormalities.

***Cytomegalovirus in immunocompromised adults.*** HCMV can cause neuroinvasive infections in immunocompromised patients with hematopoietic stem cell transplants, solid organ transplants (SOTs), or in patients with acquired immunodeficiency syndrome (AIDS) (Griffiths, 2004; Tselis and Lavi, 2000).

HCMV is an important pathogen following SOT and hematopoietic stem cell transplantation (HSCT). Risk factors for CNS disease in this group include delayed T-cell recovery, umbilical cord blood transplantation, graft versus host disease, and a history of recurrent HCMV viremia (Ariza-Heredia et al., 2014; Reddy et al., 2010). Antiviral prophylaxis for prevention of primary infection or recurrence is indicated when either or both donor (D+) and recipient (R+) are seropositive for HCMV. A phase 3, double-blind, randomized, placebo-controlled clinical trial recently showed that HSCT patients treated with letermovir prophylaxis (a new antiviral drug that inhibits the CMV-terminase complex) showed reductions in clinically significant CMV disease (37.5%) compared to the placebo group (60.6%) (Marty et al., 2017). Use of valganciclovir or ganciclovir is often limited in the HSCT patient population due to the associated myelosuppressive side effects of treatment, so the availability of a less myelosuppressive alternative (letermovir) that can be more widely employed may decrease the risk of CNS disease in this patient population. Prior to the availability of letermovir, a preemptive treatment strategy was used in HSCT patients instead, defined as prevention of development of disease when reactivation has occurred. Patients were monitored for CMV viremia and started on therapy with antiviral treatment to prevent clinical CMV disease and minimize the toxic effects of antiviral drugs to engrafted bone marrow.

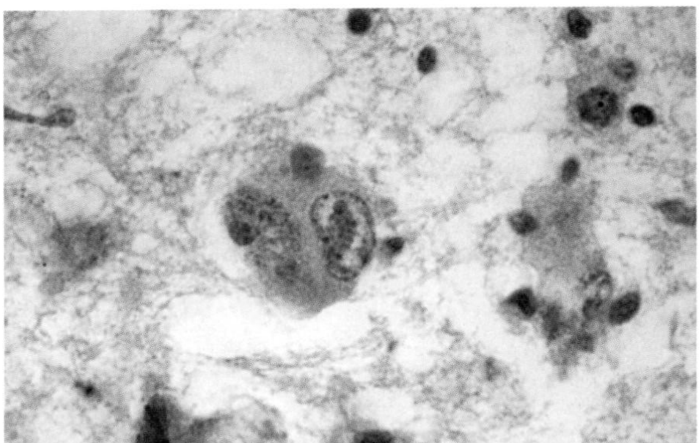

**Fig. 78.4 Ballooned Cell with Eccentric Nucleus in Human Cytomegalovirus Encephalitis.** An acidophilic Cowdry type A intranuclear inclusion body (with its surrounding halo) marginates nuclear chromatin. Cytoplasm also contains granular inclusion material. (Hematoxylin-eosin stain, ×350.) (Courtesy R. Kim.)

Despite recent advances, HCMV infection remains one of the most common complications affecting SOT patients. All patients undergoing SOT who are at risk for CMV disease receive universal prophylaxis, most commonly with valganciclovir starting within 10 days after transplantation and continuing for a period of 3–6 months.

HCMV encephalitis typically occurs in HIV+ patients with a CD4+ cell count of less than 50 cells/mm$^3$, although patients with counts below 100/mm$^3$ are at increased risk of developing HCMV viremia (Griffiths, 2004). In HIV patients with low CD4 counts in the era before highly active antiretroviral therapy (HAART), HCMV most commonly caused retinitis, esophagitis, and colitis and less commonly caused encephalitis, peripheral neuropathy, or polyradiculoneuritis. The increased use of HAART for the treatment of HIV has dramatically reduced the occurrence of HCMV viremia and disease.

HCMV encephalitis presents either as a microglial nodular encephalitis with acute onset of confusion and delirium, or as a more slowly progressive ventriculoencephalitis characterized by confusion and cranial nerve palsies. There is a broad pathological spectrum of HCMV infection of the brain, ranging from scattered microglial nodules to widespread necrotizing leukoencephalopathy or focal necrosis deep in the parenchyma.

Diagnosis of HCMV is largely dependent on quantitation of viral load in the blood using PCR and evidence of end organ disease or involvement consistent with HCMV infection. CSF HCMV PCR has a reported sensitivity of 82% and specificity of 99% in AIDS patients with CNS disease due to HCMV (Cinque et al., 1997). In immunosuppressed patients, a wide spectrum of neuroimaging results are reported, ranging from normal findings to detection of generalized atrophy, periventricular abnormalities, and focal discrete white-matter lesions. The most characteristic MRI finding is periventricular increased signal on T2-weighted images and ependymal enhancement following gadolinium administration on T1-weighted images. In advanced HIV disease, HCMV can manifest as polyradiculitis with diffuse enhancement of cauda equina nerve roots and is often associated with concurrent HCMV infection elsewhere in the body (Miller et al., 1996). Many patients with this syndrome have an almost pathognomonic CSF profile of neutrophilic pleocytosis with a low glucose concentration. The diagnosis is confirmed by PCR amplification of HCMV DNA in CSF.

Ganciclovir, foscarnet, and cidofovir all have efficacy against HCMV *in vitro* and in some clinical settings *in vivo*. In all immune suppressed patients, immune reconstitution following introduction of HAART or decreasing immune suppressing medications may help control HCMV replication and disease. General recommendations for immunocompromised patients, including those with AIDS, are for initial antiviral therapy with IV ganciclovir (5 mg/kg every 12 hours for 2–3 weeks), followed by maintenance dosing with either IV ganciclovir (5 mg/kg/day, 5 days/wk) or oral valganciclovir (900 mg daily) for at least an additional 4 weeks. For SOT patients, oral valganciclovir or intravenous ganciclovir treatment are associated with similar long-term outcomes based on the VICTOR study conducted in adult renal, liver, heart, and lung transplant recipients (Kotton et al., 2018). However, patients with severe or life-threatening HCMV disease were excluded from this study, so intravenous ganciclovir is still recommended for CNS disease in this population. A full discussion of CMV resistance and treatment is beyond the scope of this chapter. Briefly, foscarnet should be reserved for treatment of ganciclovir-resistant HCMV because of its nephrotoxicity and IV administration (Griffiths, 2004). Foscarnet dosage is 60 mg/kg IV, 3 times daily for 2–3 weeks for initial therapy, then 90–120 mg/kg IV daily for maintenance.

There are limited clinical data on the use of cidofovir for treatment of HCMV CNS disease (Table 78.8). In transplant cases, CNS disease is treated with IV ganciclovir, 5–7.5 mg/kg per dose 2 or 3 times daily with the addition of IV foscarnet 90 mg/kg twice daily for refractory cases (Ljungman, 2008).

### Epstein–Barr Virus

Primary EBV infection may be asymptomatic, present as a nonspecific febrile illness, or as the infectious mononucleosis syndrome with cervical lymphadenopathy, exudative pharyngitis, and splenomegaly. The pathogenesis of EBV-associated CNS disease remains uncertain because virus, viral antigen, or viral nucleic acid are only rarely isolated directly from CNS tissue in patients with encephalitis or myelitis, raising the possibility that at least some CNS manifestations may be post- or para-infectious immune-mediated phenomena. However, recent studies suggest that patients with EBV-associated neurological disease frequently have EBV DNA that can be amplified from CSF, and that this is frequently associated with amplifiable viral RNA consistent with lytic viral replication (Weinberg et al., 2002, 2005).

Nervous system disease occurs in 1%–7% of EBV infectious mononucleosis cases and can manifest as meningitis, encephalitis, acute hemiplegia, Alice in Wonderland syndrome, cerebellitis, cranial neuropathy, transverse myelitis, Guillain–Barré syndrome, or as small-fiber sensory or autonomic neuropathy syndromes (Doja et al., 2006; Tselis, 2014). The most common symptomatic EBV-associated CNS infection is meningitis. Cases of asymptomatic laboratory-defined meningitis probably vastly exceed symptomatic cases; up to 25% of patients with acute infectious mononucleosis may have a CSF pleocytosis despite the absence of signs or symptoms of meningitis. There are no unique features of EBV meningitis, although the presence of atypical lymphocytes in CSF may suggest the diagnosis. Diagnosis is typically made by amplification of EBV DNA by CSF PCR. In rare cases, EBV-specific IgM antibodies can be detected in CSF. Attempts to isolate virus from CSF are almost invariably negative. The presence of serum serologies indicative of recent primary infection supports the diagnosis (e.g., IgM antibodies against viral capsid antigen [VCA], presence of antibodies against early antigen [EA], but not Epstein-Barr nuclear antigen [EBNA]).

In rare cases, EBV is associated with frank encephalitis, presenting with altered consciousness including coma, seizures, and focal neurological signs and symptoms. Cases of EBV CNS disease may occur before, during, or after infectious mononucleosis or even in its absence. In one series of 21 cases of EBV encephalitis in children (Doja et al., 2006), only one patient had classic infectious mononucleosis; the remainder had a nonspecific prodrome that included fever (81%) and headache (66%). Seizures occurred in 48%, and 57% had EEGs with a diffusely slow background. CSF pleocytosis (81%) and MRI abnormalities (71%) were common. Mortality was 10%, with 80% neurologically normal at follow-up and an additional 10% having mild deficits. EBV encephalitis may mimic HSE, and in the CASG studies, EBV encephalitis accounted for about 8% of the HSV-negative cases of focal encephalitis in which an etiology was established. In a registry of childhood (ages 3–17) encephalitis cases at a large children's hospital, EBV accounted for 6% of total cases (Doja et al., 2006).

EBV myelitis can occur as an isolated syndrome or in association with meningoencephalitis. Most patients have CSF mononuclear pleocytosis and diagnosis is made by amplification of EBV DNA from CSF or by appropriate serological testing (see later discussion). Myelitis typically follows mononucleosis, although in some patients the symptoms of the initial infection may be mild or even absent. A variety of clinical forms have been reported and include transverse myelitis, myeloradiculitis, and a poliomyelitis-like syndrome of acute flaccid paralysis. MRI may show increased T2-weighted intramedullary signal or evidence of cord swelling. Nerve root enhancement has been reported in patients with myeloradiculitis. No controlled treatment trials are available, although isolated cases have been treated with IV ACV and ganciclovir with or without the addition of corticosteroids (Tyler, 2004).

Specific diagnosis of CNS EBV disease requires either amplification of EBV DNA from CSF or serological studies indicative of acute infection. In serum, the presence of EBV VCA IgM antibody is indicative of

**TABLE 78.8 Immunotherapy of Viral Infections**

| Immunotherapy Class | Immunotherapy | Dose or Route | Indications |
|---|---|---|---|
| Specific hyperimmune globulin | VZIG (varicella-zoster) | One vial (125 U) per 10 kg of body weight, intramuscularly (IM) | Postexposure prophylaxis in hypogammaglobulinemic patient (pt) |
| | RIG (rabies) | Human RIG, 20 IU/kg (inject as much as possible in area of wound and remainder IM at site distant from vaccine) | Postexposure prophylaxis |
| | Human cytomegalovirus hyperimmunoglobulin | Intravenous (IV) | Prophylaxis after bone marrow transplantation |
| | Central European encephalitis hyperimmunoglobulin | IM | Postexposure prophylaxis following multiple tick bites in endemic area |
| | Measles hyperimmunoglobulin | IV | Treatment of measles inclusion body encephalitis in immunocompromised pt |
| Polyvalent immune globulin | IVIG | IV | Treatment of chronic enterovirus meningoencephalitis in hypogammaglobulinemic pt |
| | IVIG | IV | Treatment of CNS parvovirus B19 infection |
| | IVIG | IV | Treatment of human T-cell leukemia virus I myelopathy |
| Monoclonal Antibody | Bamianivimab (Lily, EUA)<br>REGN10933/10987 Mab Cocktail (Regeneron, EUA) | IV | COVID-19 |
| Cytotoxic T cells | Epstein-Barr virus (EBV)-specific cytotoxic T lymphocytes | | Prophylaxis of EBV lymphoproliferative disease in bone marrow transplant recipients |
| Corticosteroids | Dexamethasone | PO/IV 6 mg/d x 10d | EUA for hospitalized COVID-19 pts |

*CNS*, Central nervous system; *EUA*, FDA Emergency Use Authorization; *IV*, intravenous; *IVIG*, intravenous immunoglobulin.
Live vaccines include yellow fever, measles, mumps, rubella, smallpox, polio, and varicella-zoster virus. Killed vaccines include polio, rabies, influenza, arboviruses (Japanese encephalitis, tickborne encephalitis, Kyasanur Forest, Rift Valley, eastern equine encephalitis, western equine encephalitis, and Venezuelan equine encephalitis). Soluble protein includes hepatitis B.

recently acquired active EBV infection. The presence of EBV VCA IgG antibody and antibody against EA in the absence of antibodies against EBNA antibodies is also indicative of recent infection. The presence of serum IgG VCA and EBNA antibodies indicates remote infection, and these antibodies persist for the lifetime of the infected individual.

CSF PCR for EBV is positive during the acute phase of illness in children with infectious mononucleosis and neurological complications such as transverse myelitis, meningoencephalitis, and aseptic meningitis. CSF PCR is negative in EBV-seropositive individuals in the absence of CNS infection. However, positive EBV PCR may be seen in patients with evidence of other viral or nonviral CNS infection, raising the possibility that these infections may trigger viral reactivation in the absence of EBV-associated disease. EBV has been one of the most frequent agents associated with dual-positive CSF PCR testing and may not always correlate clinically with the presence of CNS infection known to be caused by this virus (Weinberg et al., 2005).

There are no randomized controlled trials for any antiviral or immunosuppressive agent for the treatment of EBV-associated neurological disease. Supportive care is important, and death due to EBV neurological disease is uncommon. ACV inhibits EBV DNA polymerase *in vitro*, although viral production returns to normal levels after the drug is stopped, even after 11 months of therapy, because ACV does not affect the latent viral burden and latent virus can reactivate and replicate using host-dependent enzymes (Tselis, 2014). There are few studies supporting the use of ACV for EBV encephalitis, and the data supporting efficacy of other antivirals, including ganciclovir and foscarnet, are also limited. Treatment with intravenous immunoglobulin (IVIG) may improve EBV-associated small-fiber sensory or autonomic neuropathies if treatment begins during acute disease.

### Human Herpesvirus Type 6

HHV-6 was first isolated in 1986 from human peripheral blood mononuclear cells of patients with lymphoproliferative disorders. Two variants, HHV-6A and HHV-6B, are known. Primary infection with HHV-6 usually occurs during infancy, producing exanthem subitum (or roseola) or a syndrome of generalized lymphadenopathy. HHV-6 infects a broad range of cell types including T-cells, monocytes, dendritic cells, oligodendrocytes, microglia, and astrocytes. Primary HHV-6 infection may cause febrile seizures or acute meningoencephalitis in children. Cases of focal encephalitis in immunocompetent patients have been attributed to HHV-6, as has a syndrome of acute limbic encephalitis occurring in both SOT patients (post-transplant acute limbic encephalitis [PTALE]) and those receiving HSCT (Isaacson et al., 2005; McCullers et al., 1995; Mori et al., 2010; Seeley et al., 2007) (Fig. 78.5). MRI demonstrates symmetric hyperintensities in the medial temporal lobes. The role, if any, for HHV-6 in inducing medial temporal sclerosis temporal lobe epilepsy (Fotheringham et al., 2007) and as a co-factor in other neurological disorders including multiple sclerosis remains unproven.

There are no approved therapies for HHV-6 infection. HHV-6 isolates generally resemble HCMV in their *in vitro* susceptibility to antiviral drugs by exhibiting resistance to ACV and sensitivity to ganciclovir and foscarnet (Birnbaum et al., 2005; Seeley et al., 2007).

### Herpes B Virus (Cercopithecine Herpesvirus 1)

Additional text is available online at http://expertconsult.inkling.com. 

## Polyomaviruses (JC) and Progressive Multifocal Leukoencephalopathy

Progressive multifocal leukoencephalopathy (PML), a subacute demyelinating disease of the CNS, is a result of infection of oligodendrocytes by the polyomavirus, JC virus (JCV) (Brew et al., 2010; Koralnik, 2006). Specific criteria for establishing the diagnosis have been developed. Definitive diagnosis generally requires either neuropathological confirmation or the presence of consistent radiographic and clinical features with the associated demonstration of JCV DNA in CSF by PCR (Berger et al., 2013). Seroepidemiological studies indicate that asymptomatic primary infection with JCV occurs in childhood, and that by adult life roughly 55%–85% of the population is seropositive. Following primary infection, JCV becomes latent in sites including kidney, bone marrow, and tonsil. It is unclear whether CNS latency occurs. Reactivation in immunocompetent hosts usually takes the form of asymptomatic viruria. In the setting of impaired cell-mediated immunity, including immunosuppressive drug treatment, lymphoproliferative disorders, chronic infectious or inflammatory diseases such as tuberculosis and sarcoidosis, and most importantly AIDS, virus can reactivate to produce PML. In most modern series, over 80% of PML patients have underlying HIV infection. Treatment of patients with several immunomodulatory biologicals, as exemplified by natalizumab, has been linked to increased risk of developing PML (Brew et al., 2010; Clifford et al., 2010; Ho et al., 2017; Major, 2010; Tan et al.,

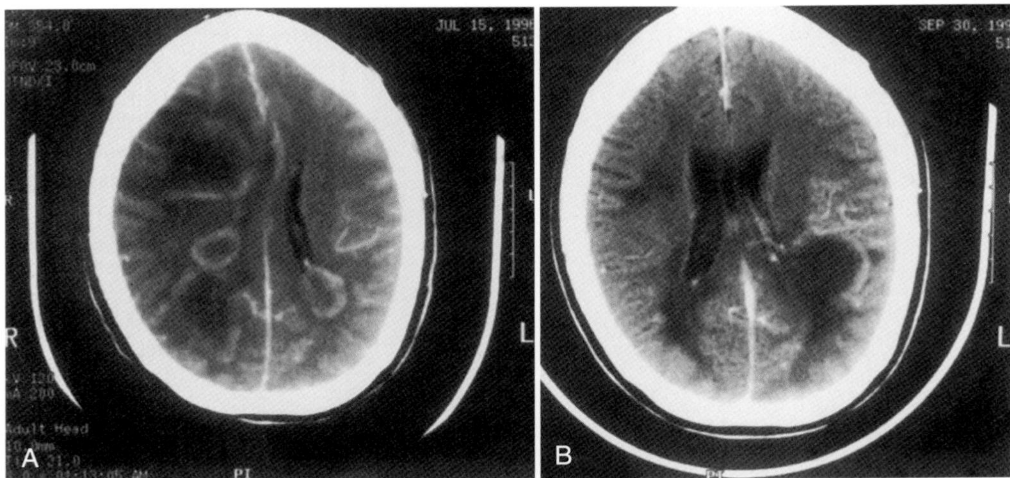


**Fig. 78.5 Concurrent Human Herpesvirus Type 6 and Human Immunodeficiency Virus Disease.** A) Contrast computed tomographic scan showing multiple ring-enhancing frontal, parietal, and occipital lesions. B) Second image shows parietal recurrence 3 months later. Pathology demonstrated perivascular lymphocytic infiltrates, demyelination, and axonal sparing. (Courtesy S. Busono.)

2010). The first reports involved patients treated for multiple sclerosis (2 cases) or Crohn disease (1 case) with natalizumab (Tysabri), a humanized monoclonal antibody that blocks lymphocyte binding to $\alpha_4$-integrin and inhibits trafficking into the CNS (Kleinschmidt-DeMasters and Tyler, 2005; Langer-Gould et al., 2005; Yousry et al., 2006). Over 750 cases of natalizumab-associated PML have now been reported (January, 2018), with a global risk of ~4.2/1000 treated patients. Key risk factors associated with increased risk of PML development include the presence of JC virus antibodies and higher values of the JCV Ab index, the use of prior immunosuppressive therapy (e.g., mitoxantrone, azathioprine, cyclophosphamide, methotrexate, mycophenolate mofetil), and the duration of natalizumab therapy (Bloomgren et al., 2012; Ho et al., 2017). Ninety-nine percent (205 of 207) of patients who developed natalizumab-associated PML were JCV seropositive at least 6 months before the onset of PML (Biogen Idec Safety data). The risk of developing PML among natalizumab-treated JCV seronegative individuals is ~0.07 PML case/1000 patients (95% CI 0.00–0.40). By contrast, in patients who are JCV seropositive but have not received prior immunosuppressive therapy the risk climbs as high as 1.7% (17/1000) in those who have received 72 months of therapy. In patients who are both JCV seropositive and have received prior immunosuppressive therapy, risk increases to 2.7% (27/1000) in those with 72 months of natalizumab exposure (see Bloomgren et al., 2012; Ho et al., 2017 and Biogen Idec Safety Data).

At least 124 cases of PML have been reported in patients receiving rituximab (Rituxan), an antibody directed against CD20 on B cells. The majority of cases occurred in patients being treated for non-Hodgkin lymphoma, although cases have also been reported in patients receiving rituximab for other diseases including systemic lupus erythematosus, rheumatoid arthritis, and autoimmune hemolytic anemia. Each of these diseases has been associated with PML in the absence of rituximab therapy, and patients were often receiving multiple immunosuppressive medications. A "disproportionality analysis" based on expected versus actual cases reported to the US Adverse Events Reporting System (AERS) suggested that immunosuppressive drugs associated with the highest risk of PML and their associated "reporting odds ratio" (ROR) included rituximab (ROR 73), Mycophenolate mofetil (ROR 23), natalizumab (ROR 22), azathioprine (ROR 22), cyclophosphamide (ROR 18), efalizumab (ROR16), methotrexate (ROR 9), tacrolimus (ROR9), and cyclosporine (ROR 6). The ROR was determined from estimates of number of reported cases and number of exposed individuals (Schmedt et al., 2012). In addition, three or four cases of PML have occurred in patients being treated for chronic plaque psoriasis with efalizumab (Raptiva), a monoclonal antibody directed against the CD11a lymphocyte antigen. The magnitude of the risk was estimated at approximately 1 in 400 treated patients and resulted in this drug being removed from the market.

The likely pathogenesis of PML includes reactivation from an extraneural primary site, dissemination of virus to the CNS through the bloodstream, and subsequent productive lytic infection of oligodendrocytes to induce demyelination (Brew et al., 2010; Koralnik, 2006). Infection of astrocytes is abortive, although resulting in striking and characteristic bizarre enlarged cells. Neuronal infection does not occur in classic PML but variant forms of JCV encephalitis and JCV cerebellar granule cell infection with distinct clinical presentations have been described (Koralnik, 2006). Rearrangements in the regulatory region of the viral genome appear to play a key role in neuropathogenesis insofar as viruses lacking these regulatory region rearrangements have not been isolated from PML brain specimens.

Onset of PML is subacute, with signs and symptoms of multifocal asymmetrical white-matter involvement. In non-AIDS-associated PML, early lesions tend to be in subcortical white matter of the occipital lobes, causing visual-field deficits or cortical blindness. Motor weakness, behavior changes, cognitive impairment, cerebellar ataxia, dysarthria, and sensory abnormalities also are seen, whereas headache, seizures, and extrapyramidal syndromes are rare. The disease progresses to dementia as the number of lesions increases.

CSF cell counts and protein levels are usually normal. Neuroimaging results help suggest the diagnosis. MRI studies show focal or multifocal lesions of subcortical white matter, sometimes involving the cerebellum, brainstem, and spinal cord, without mass effect or contrast enhancement. Fluid-attenuation inversion recovery (FLAIR) sequences, which remove CSF signals, are particularly good for demonstrating paraventricular disease (Fig. 78.6). White-matter lesions are larger and more confluent than those of multifocal leukoencephalitis of VZV. Patients with natalizumab-associated PML typically have large (>3 cm), subcortical, T2 and diffusion hyperintense and T1 hypointense lesions. The lesions have a sharp border on their cortical side and an ill-defined border at their white-matter side. In distinction to the experience with HIV-PML, ~40% of patients have some contrast enhancement on T1-weighted gadolinium-enhanced images (Yousry et al., 2012). Lack of CSF pleocytosis and an indolent course distinguish PML from ADEM. Brain biopsy definitively establishes the diagnosis by showing characteristic changes, including demyelination, bizarre astrocytes, and oligodendrocytes with enlarged nuclei that contain inclusion bodies, as well as viral particles and antigen or viral DNA (Berger et al., 2013). JCV has never been cultured from CSF, but JCV DNA may be detected in CSF using PCR amplification. Finding JCV DNA in CSF by PCR in the appropriate clinical setting with appropriate imaging abnormalities is also diagnostic of PML (Berger et al., 2013) and obviates the need for brain biopsy. Although the specificity of CSF PCR for JCV in the appropriate clinical setting approaches 100%, its sensitivity may be as low as 75%, reflecting variances in the amount of viral load in the CSF in different conditions. For example, 57% of Tysabri-associated PML cases were reported to have fewer than 500 copies of JCV DNA per mL, which is close to the sensitivity limit of some commercial assays (Clifford et al., 2010).

No specific therapy is available. Isolated reports of benefit from cytarabine were not confirmed in a randomized prospective clinical trial (Hall et al., 1998). Cidofovir was also found not to be of significant clinical benefit in HIV-associated PML in a prospective clinical trial (Marra et al., 2002). Interferon alfa has been reported to be of benefit in case reports but has not been tested in clinical trials. A study showing that JCV binds the 5HT receptor in cultured cells led to the use of mirtazapine, a serotonin receptor blocker, in patients with PML (Elphick et al., 2004). However, 12-month follow-up in patients with PML treated with mirtazapine showed no evidence of improved survival (Marzocchetti et al., 2009). A screen of chemical compounds found that mefloquine, a malarial drug, inhibits JCV replication (Brickelmaier et al., 2009). A multicenter clinical trial investigating the role of mefloquine treatment of JCV in PML patients did not show significant clinical benefit (clinicaltrials.gov identifier NCT00746941) (Clifford et al., 2013). A significant new development in therapeutics has been the use of virus-specific T-cells to treat cases of PML. This typically involves isolating T-cells from an HLA-matched donor, amplifying the JCV antigen-specific cytotoxic T lymphocyte (CTL) population, or the closely related BK-virus-specific CTLs by *ex-vivo* stimulation of these cells with JCV or BKV proteins or peptide mimics, and adoptive transfer of the amplified cells into a patient. No controlled clinical trials are yet available, although several small studies have shown clinical benefit or disease stabilization, and reduction in viral load in treated patients (Balduzzi et al., 2011; Muftuoglu et al., 2018). Until the effectiveness of adaptive T-cell therapy can be confirmed in controlled clinical trials, the most effective therapy for PML

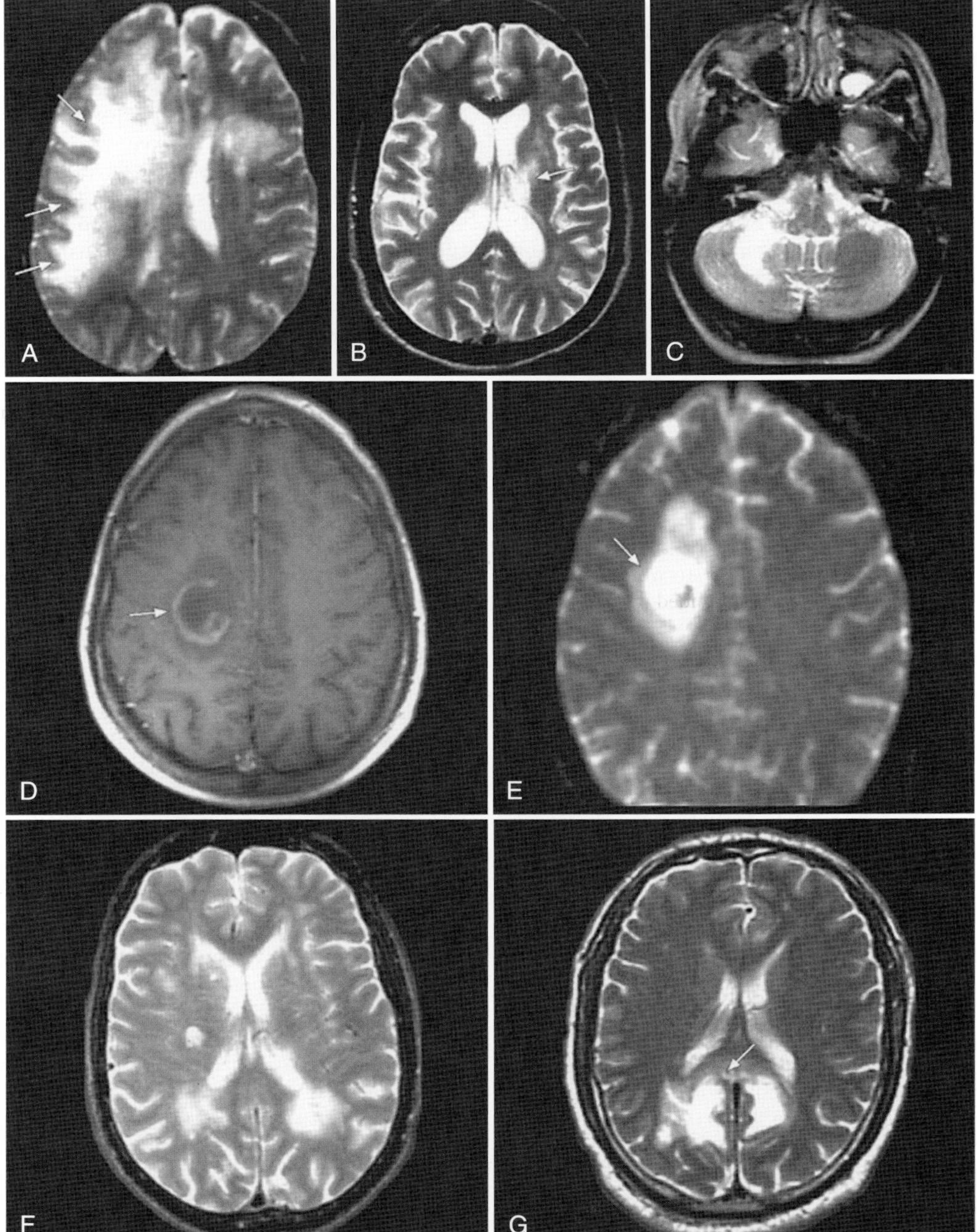


**Fig. 78.6 Progressive Multifocal Leukoencephalopathy Brain Magnetic Resonance Imaging Lesion Patterns. A,** Large, confluent, granular T2-weighted lesions *(arrows)*. **B,** Deep gray matter involvement *(arrow)*. **C,** Crescent-shaped cerebellar lesion. **D,** Gadolinium-enhancing lesions *(arrow)*. **E,** Tumefactive lesion *(arrow)*. **F,** Multiple sclerosis-like appearance. **G,** Transcallosal lesion *(arrow)*. All brain magnetic resonance images are axial T2-weighted except for **(D)**, which is an axial T1-weighted image acquired after the intravenous administration of gadolinium. (From Boster, A., Hreha, S., Berger, J.R., et al., 2009. Progressive multifocal leukoencephalopathy and relapsing-remitting multiple sclerosis: a comparative study. Arch Neurol 66, 593–599. Copyright © 2009 American Medical Association. All rights reserved.)

remains treatments which reverse any underlying immunosuppression. Unfortunately, immune reconstitution is often associated with an immune reconstitution inflammatory syndrome (IRIS) that causes paradoxical clinical and radiographic worsening as the host mounts an effective cellular immune response to the JC virus present in PML lesions. No controlled clinical trials of treatment of IRIS are currently available; however, cases are often treated with high-dose intravenous corticosteroids (Tan et al., 2011). A single intriguing case report describes successful use of the small-molecule CCR5 antagonist maraviroc rather than corticosteroids (Giacomini et al., 2014) to prevent development of IRIS in an HIV woman with natalizumab-associated PML. It was suggested maraviroc acted by inhibiting trafficking of CCR5+ immune-cell subsets into the CNS and preventing their immunopathological role in disease initiation.

### Adenovirus

Adenoviruses cause acute respiratory disease in children and adults in crowded settings such as military recruits, along with conjunctivitis, hemorrhagic cystitis, and gastroenteritis. The most common associated CNS diagnosis is febrile or afebrile seizure in children under 5 years. Meningoencephalitis or unilateral deafness coincident with nasopharyngeal infection are rare complications in normal hosts. Immunosuppression is a risk factor for encephalitis, with fatal meningoencephalitis reported in AIDS and bone marrow transplant patients and encephalomyeloradiculitis reported in an umbilical cord stem cell transplant recipient (Awosika et al., 2013). Clinical and histopathological features of adenovirus disease may resemble those of HCMV disease, such as adenovirus encephalitis and ependymitis in a child with AIDS (Anders et al., 1990). Diagnosis is by PCR or isolation of virus from extraneural sites, by serology, or by identification of virus or DNA in brain tissue or CSF. Adenovirus-infected neurons and glia have enlarged nuclei with amphophilic inclusions and a thin rim of cytoplasm, referred to as "smudge" cells. Diagnosis of adenoviral infection is complicated by the existence of 51 viral serotypes. Different serotypes have different tissue tropisms. Serotypes 1, 2, 3, 4, 5, 6, 7, 11, 12, 26, 31, 32, and 41 in mixture with 49 have been implicated in CNS infection (Huang et al., 2013). Cidofovir is used for severe adenovirus infections; viral clearance and patient survival is aided by lymphocyte reconstitution (Echavarria, 2008).

### Parvovirus

Acute infection with B19 parvovirus causes the febrile exanthematous illness, fifth disease (erythema infectiosum, or "slapped cheek rash") in childhood, transient aplastic crises (particularly in immunocompromised and sickle-cell patients), and small-joint arthritis in adults. Parvovirus B19 infections have been described as a potential trigger for various autoimmune disorders including necrotizing vasculitis resembling granulomatosis with polyarteritis in association with meningoencephalitis (Nolan et al., 2003). According to a systematic review of 129 cases of Parvovirus B19 (PVB19)-associated neurological disorders, 50 (39%) were diagnosed with encephalitis and only 14% were immunocompetent adults (Barah et al., 2014). Patients can develop neurological disease in the absence of systemic symptoms such as rash, anemia, and arthropathy (Jun et al., 2017). Neurological manifestations have included encephalitis, chorea, stroke, optic neuropathy abnormal pupillary reflexes, brachial plexitis, and autonomic, sensory, or motor neuropathies and recurrent paresthesias. In CNS disease, PVB19 DNA and less often IgM can be detected in CSF. IVIG speeds clearance of viremia in immunocompromised patients and rescues from rituximab-induced hypogammaglobulinemia and parvovirus infection. IVIG with or without steroids is increasingly used in all CNS disease cases (Douvoyiannis et al., 2009).

### Orthopoxviruses

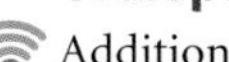
Additional text is available online at http://expertconsult.inkling.com.

Monkeypox has become the most important orthopoxvirus infection of humans worldwide due to population loss of vaccinial protection against smallpox in the smallpox post-eradication era. Early symptoms are fever and lymphadenopathy (a distinguishing feature), followed by a maculopapular rash that begins on the face and evolves through papular, vesicular, pustular, and umbilicated lesion stages. Face, palms, and soles are most commonly affected. Antipox antibodies in an ill unvaccinated individual support infection.

Since 2003, there had been no cases of human monkeypox outside Africa until two cases were diagnosed in the UK in 2018 in travelers from Nigeria. These were the first reports of travel-associated cases diagnosed outside Africa (Vaughan et al., 2018).

## RIBONUCLEIC ACID VIRUSES

### Poliovirus and Other Nonpolio Enteroviruses

The EV family comprises over 100 different serotypes within the Picornaviridae family. They can be subgrouped into the polioviruses, coxsackieviruses A and B, echoviruses, and the newer sequentially numbered EVs. Collectively, the EVs are the leading identified causes of viral meningitis, accounting for over 80% of cases in some series. Other severe neurological syndromes including encephalitis, brainstem encephalitis and acute anterior poliomyelitis are also associated with several of these agents.

#### Poliovirus

Poliovirus is transmitted by fecal-oral contact and, during epidemics, also by pharyngeal spread. Three antigenically distinct types of poliovirus have been defined. All can cause paralytic disease through destruction of motor neurons in the spinal cord and brainstem. In 2013, 404 cases of poliomyelitis were reported worldwide from eight countries. The majority of cases were due to serotype 1 viruses. Countries reporting cases included Somalia (193), Pakistan (93), Nigeria (53), Syria (24), Kenya (14), Afghanistan (14), Ethiopia (9), and Cameroon (4).

Clinically apparent infection with poliovirus results in aseptic meningitis (8% of cases) or paralytic illness (1% of all cases). A 7- to 14-day incubation period is followed by headache, fever, signs of meningeal irritation, drowsiness, and seizures in infants. Asymmetrical flaccid weakness of limbs, diaphragm, or cranial nerve-innervated muscles develops within days and progresses, on average, for 3–5 days. Cerebellitis, transverse myelitis, and facial paresis also have been reported.

Diagnosis, when based on the clinical picture and presence of CSF pleocytosis, is confirmed by serology, virus isolation, or PCR amplification of poliovirus RNA from CSF. In the CSF, polymorphonuclear cells predominate early, with a shift to lymphocytes after several days. CSF protein concentration is slightly elevated; levels of 100–300 mg/dL may accompany cases of severe paralysis.

Approximately one-quarter of polio patients develop an exacerbation of existing or new progressive lower motor neuron weakness 30–40 years after acute polio ("the post-polio syndrome"). Atrophy, fasciculations, and electromyographic evidence of active denervation are found in involved muscle groups. Diagnosis depends on the documentation of antecedent poliomyelitis and the exclusion of other new causes of lower motor neuron syndromes. Electrophysiology suggests that new weakness likely results from ongoing denervation that exceeds compensatory reinnervation. The exact cause of the syndrome remains uncertain; both immune-mediated processes and chronic persistent viral infection have been speculated to be potential triggers. No specific therapy has been shown to be of proven benefit, although patients may respond to a carefully designed program of physical therapy and the use of orthoses and assistive devices (Gonzalez et al., 2010).

Treatment of poliomyelitis is supportive, with particular attention to ventilatory assistance. Mortality from paralytic poliomyelitis is less than 10%, but bulbar forms have a poorer prognosis, and mortality may approach 50%.

There have been no cases of polio caused by wild-type viruses in the United States since 1979, and none in the Western Hemisphere since 1991. For this reason, the Advisory Committee on Immunization Practices recommended in 2000 that the inactivated (Salk, intramuscular) polio vaccine replace the live attenuated (Sabin, oral) vaccine in the United States for the entire primary immunization series in the first year of life, as well as the booster dose prior to school entry. In areas of the world in which poliovirus is still endemic, primary immunization is still carried out with trivalent live attenuated (Sabin, oral) vaccine, because the mucosal immunity conferred outweighs the small risk of reversion to virulence. Inactivated polio vaccine should always be used for vaccination of persons with immunodeficiency diseases, in whom the risk of vaccine-associated paralytic polio from the live attenuated vaccine strain is high. Vaccine-related cases of paralytic polio have included infants with unrecognized immunodeficiency who have received their first oral polio vaccine dose and immunocompromised patients who have been in contact with recipients of live attenuated oral polio vaccine.

### Nonpolio Enteroviruses

The nonpolio EVs may cause a wide spectrum of CNS and PNS disease, including aseptic meningitis, encephalitis, brainstem encephalitis, acute anterior poliomyelitis, acute cerebellar ataxia, peripheral and optic neuropathy, cranial polyneuritis, and epidemic myalgia. In neonates, encephalitis is generally part of an overwhelming sepsis-like illness with up to 10% mortality. Congenital CNS defects are associated with infection acquired *in utero*. Infection of hypogammaglobulinemic patients commonly leads to progressive meningoencephalitis. Certain strains have also been associated with an acute motor neuron disease in association with epidemic hemorrhagic conjunctivitis.

***Meningitis.*** Nonpolio EVs are the most common cause of viral meningitis in adult and pediatric populations (Kupila et al., 2006), with over 75,000 cases of EV meningitis in the United States each year. Spread of infection is by fecal-oral and (rarely) respiratory routes. Outbreaks tend to cluster in the late summer and early fall and may be associated with pharyngitis and gastrointestinal symptoms such as anorexia, vomiting, or diarrhea. Other associated findings are the exanthem of herpangina or the rash of hand, foot, and mouth disease (HFMD) (commonly associated with Coxsackievirus A16 and Enterovirus 71). Fortunately, EV meningitis occurring beyond the neonatal period in immunocompetent hosts is only rarely associated with severe disease or subsequent neurological deficits (Sawyer, 2002).

Meningitis caused by coxsackievirus produces CSF cell counts typically up to 250 WBC/μL with 10%–50% polymorphonuclear cells. Echovirus infections are associated with CSF pleocytosis from several hundred to greater than 1000 WBC/μL, 90% of which may be polymorphonucleocytes in the first 24 hours of infection. Amplification of EV RNA from CSF by reverse transcriptase (RT)-PCR has now replaced viral culture as the diagnostic procedure of choice for enteroviral CNS infections (Ramers et al., 2000). PCR primers and probes are directed against the 5′ non-translated region of the viral genome, which is highly conserved among almost all enteroviral strains. Currently available commercial enteroviral RT-PCR assays on CSF have better than 95% sensitivity and nearly 100% specificity for amplification of RNA from known strains of EV (Kost et al., 2007; Pillet et al., 2010).

***Meningoencephalitis.*** Although more commonly the etiological agent in aseptic meningitis, EVs may also cause encephalitis, particularly in immunodeficient patients with hypogammaglobulinemia and in neonates. Focal and generalized presentations of encephalitis have been reported. EV strain 70 has been implicated most frequently in instances of encephalitis. In neonates, meningoencephalitis is generally a component of an overwhelming sepsis-like illness with up to 10% mortality. Infection of hypogammaglobulinemic patients leads to a chronic and progressive meningoencephalitis; these patients should be treated with IVIG therapy.

***Enterovirus-68 associated acute flaccid myelitis.*** At least 400 cases of an acute poliomyelitis-like illness affecting predominantly (90%) children (median age 6 years) have been reported from over 40 states in the United States and over 16 foreign countries during the period 2014–2018 (Knoester et al., 2019; Messacar et al., 2016; Sejvar et al., 2016). The disease in the United States shows a biannual peak (cases increased in 2014, 2016, 2018) with a summer–fall seasonal predilection. Children present with a viral prodrome (>90%) with fever, upper respiratory and gastrointestinal symptoms followed several days later by the acute onset of an asymmetric flaccid paralysis. Limb weakness predominates in the upper extremities and is typically proximal greater than distal in distribution with associated decreased tone and hyporeflexia. Limb involvement can range from monoplegia to quadriplegia with respiratory impairment. Imaging studies show a multi-segmental T2 and FLAIR hyperintense abnormality involving predominantly the central gray matter and the anterior horns particularly. Cranial nerve abnormalities occur in about 30% of cases. Sensory abnormalities when present are typically mild and transient. The overwhelming majority have an associated CSF lymphocytic pleocytosis with normal or mildly elevated protein and normal glucose concentrations. The etiology of this syndrome remains controversial, as virus is not typically found in CSF specimens by RT-PCR and since fatality is rare, autopsy specimens from the acute phase have not been available for study. However, enteroviruses/rhinovirus group RT-PCRs are positive in about 50% of cases when obtained during the first few days after onset of illness. The most frequently isolated and typed EV has been EV-D68. Increasing evidence links EV-D68 as a major etiological factor in the recent spikes of acute flaccid myelitis (AFM) cases (Messacar et al., 2018), although isolated clusters of cases meeting the syndromic definition of AFM have also been linked to EV-A71. Patients with EV-D68-associated disease often have slow recovery and substantial residual weakness. No specific treatment of proven efficacy is currently available, although mouse models suggest that early administration of IVIG may ameliorate disease. Retrospective uncontrolled studies in children have not shown benefit for steroids, IVIG, or fluoxetine to date.

### Epidemic Conjunctivitis and Acute Motor Neuron Disease

EV type 70 is the etiological agent of a syndrome of conjunctivitis and an acute motor neuron disease. Epidemic acute hemorrhagic conjunctivitis first appeared in Ghana, West Africa, in 1969 and spread across Africa, Asia, and Europe in 1970 and 1971 to involve tens of millions of people. The eye disease was characterized by severe eye pain, photophobia, blurred vision, and varying degrees of subconjunctival hemorrhage. In a minority of patients, usually young men, a neurological (polio-like) phase developed 2 weeks after the conjunctivitis as acute asymmetrical hypotonic or flaccid weakness of the lower extremities. Isolated facial nerve palsy; upper limb weakness; radicular, myelopathic, dysautonomic syndromes; or multiple cranial neuropathies were also reported. Acute hemorrhagic conjunctivitis surfaced again in 1981 in many of the same countries, in French Polynesia, and in other Pacific Islands, was imported to the United States, and spread among household contacts. A similar disease caused by EV type 71 has occurred in Bulgaria and moved around the world. The other agent of epidemic hemorrhagic conjunctivitis, coxsackie A24, has not been associated with an acute motor neuron disease. These are highly contagious viruses for which there is no specific antiviral treatment, underscoring the importance of surveillance, public health measures, and sanitation in limiting disease.

### Enterovirus 71

EV71 was first isolated in the United States in 1969, and has been responsible for several massive outbreaks of herpangina and hand, foot, and mouth disease in Southeast Asia, likely totaling over 6 million cases (McMinn, 2014). One in 300 symptomatically infected patients develops severe disease, often involving the CNS. The most common neuroinvasive infections include a relatively benign aseptic meningitis, an AFM syndrome, and a severe brainstem encephalitis (rhombencephalitis) (Hu et al., 2015; Teoh et al., 2016). Brainstem encephalitis may be associated with neurogenic pulmonary edema which has been associated with sudden death. EV71 may also cause postinfectious immune-mediated syndromes including opsoclonus myoclonus, transverse myelitis, and Guillain-Barré syndrome. Hand, foot, and mouth disease signs and symptoms occur in about 40% of patients, and respiratory or GI symptoms in a similar number. Almost all patients are febrile. Diagnosis typically depends on identification of viral RNA in feces or rectal swabs (>90%) and less commonly in nasal or oropharyngeal swabs (50%–75%). CSF RT-PCR is only positive in a minority of cases (<25%) but when present is diagnostic of neuroinvasive disease. CSF shows a lymphocytic pleocytosis in the majority of cases, with a normal or mildly elevated protein and a normal glucose. MRI shows increased FLAIR and T2 signal in the dorsal pons and spinal cord and patients with AFM show multi-segmental spinal cord lesions involving the central gray matter. No specific therapy is available although patients with severe neurological illness have been treated with IVIG. Recently completed phase III trials with inactivated whole virus vaccines indicate that these are safe, immunogenic, and protective (Li et al., 2014; Zhu et al., 2014).

## Arboviruses

The term *arbovirus* (*ar*thropod-*bo*rne virus) is a general term for viruses transmitted to humans by mosquito and tick (arthropod) vectors. Arboviruses exist in nature in complex cycles involving birds and mammals that serve as viral reservoirs and amplifying hosts. When transmitted to humans, arboviruses can cause fever, headache, meningitis, encephalitis, and myelitis. Arboviruses comprise a group of over 500 RNA viruses, of which more than 100 are known to infect humans. Arboviruses are divided between four taxonomic families: Togaviridae (alphaviruses), Flaviviridae (flaviviruses), reoviruses, and bunyaviruses. Considered together, arboviruses represent the leading cause of encephalitis worldwide. Key features of arboviral infections occurring in North America are summarized in Table 78.9.

### West Nile Virus (Flavivirus)

WNV was already one of the world's most widely distributed arboviruses, present in many parts of Africa, West Asia, the Middle East, Eastern Europe, and Australia, when it emerged in North America in 1999. However, the emergence of WNV in 1999 was complicated by a marked increase in neuroinvasive infections compared to past WNV infections. In New York in 1999, a reported 59 people were hospitalized with encephalitis or meningitis in late summer, with seven resultant fatalities (Nash et al., 2001). WNV has subsequently become the most important cause of arboviral meningitis, encephalitis, and acute flaccid paralysis in the continental United States (Bode et al., 2006; Davis et al., 2006; DeBiasi and Tyler, 2006).

Transmission occurs overwhelmingly as the result of the bite of an infected mosquito; however, person-to-person transmission through organ transplantation, blood and blood product transfusion, and intrauterine spread can occur. WNV is maintained and amplified in an enzootic transmission cycle with *Culex* mosquitoes and passeriform birds, with occasional spillover transmission to horses or humans who serve as dead-end hosts (Weaver et al., 2010). Since its emergence in New York City in 1999, there have been approximately 51,000 cases of WNV disease, 24,000 cases of WNV neuroinvasive Infections, and 2300 deaths in the United States (https://www.cdc.gov/westnile/statemaps/cumMapsData.html). The epidemics of WNV in 2003 and 2012 were the largest outbreaks of neuroinvasive viral infections ever reported in the Western Hemisphere. The incidence of disease in the United States remains greatest in the central part of the country, where it can exceed 100 cases per million population per year in specific areas. Since 2009, WNV disease has increased throughout Europe as well with recent outbreaks throughout southern countries (Burki, 2018).

Approximately 80% of human WNV infections are asymptomatic. Following an incubation period of 3 to 14 days, around 20% of infected individuals develop a nonspecific febrile illness (West Nile fever [WNF]). Approximately one in 150 infected persons will develop encephalitis and/or meningitis (Davis et al., 2006; DeBiasi and Tyler, 2009). Older individuals (>50 years of age) are at increased risk of developing encephalitis, although meningitis and acute flaccid paralysis occur in middle-aged and younger individuals. Neurological disease is rare in infants and children but does occasionally occur. Clinical features suggestive of WNV CNS infection include the presence of movement disorders (e.g., tremor, myoclonus, parkinsonism) and severe weakness, often of a lower motor neuron type (flaccid tone, reduced or absent reflexes) (Bode et al.,

**TABLE 78.9 Details of North American Arboviruses**

| Agent | Geographical Distribution | Reservoir | Vector | Season | Group Affected | Mortality (Encephalitis) | Neurological Sequelae |
|---|---|---|---|---|---|---|---|
| Eastern equine | Atlantic and Gulf coasts, Great Lakes region | Birds | Mosquito | June–Aug | Children | 50%–70% | 80% (esp. young) |
| Western equine | Western United States and Canada | Birds and small mammals | Mosquito | June–Sept | Infants, adults >50 years | Adults: 3%–5% Infants: 10%–20% | Adults: 5% Infants: 50% |
| Venezuelan equine | Texas and Florida | Horses, small animals | Mosquito | Rainy season May–Sept | Adults | <1% | Rare |
| St. Louis | Throughout United States but greatest prevalence in Texas, Florida, and Ohio–Mississippi River Valley | Birds | Mosquito | June–Aug | Adults >50 years | 2%–20% | 25%–50% mild, < 10% severe |
| California (La Crosse) | Midwest and northeast United States, southern Canada | Chipmunk, squirrel, small mammals | Mosquito | June–Sept | Children | <1% | Rare |
| West Nile virus | Throughout United States | Birds | Mosquito | June–Oct | All ages, adults > 50 with severe disease | ≈10%–15% | Evolving data |
| Powassan | North-central United States, eastern Canada | Squirrel, porcupine, groundhog | Tick | Spring/summer | | Rare | 35% |
| Colorado tick fever | United States and Canadian Rocky Mountains | Chipmunk, squirrel, rodents | Tick | March–Sept | Children and adults | <1% | Rare |

2006; Davis et al., 2006; DeBiasi and Tyler, 2006). In many cases, weakness appears to result from injury to spinal cord motor neurons (a true "poliomyelitis"). In patients with weakness, electromyography (EMG) and nerve conduction velocity (NCV) studies are often consistent with injury to motor neurons and anterior roots, including reduced amplitudes of compound motor action potentials (CMAPs) with relatively preserved sensorineural action potentials (SNAPs). Evidence of denervation may be present on EMG studies after an appropriate interval. The case fatality among hospitalized patients, most of whom have encephalitis, is approximately 12%–14%.

Neuroimaging studies and CSF analysis may assist in the diagnosis. In contrast to HSE, about 50% of patients with WNV encephalitis have initially negative or normal imaging studies (Petropoulou et al., 2005). When abnormalities occur, they are best detected on FLAIR or diffusion-weighted images and typically involve the basal ganglia, thalamus, upper brainstem, and cerebellum. CSF evaluation invariably shows a pleocytosis (>95% of cases), with a mean of 225 cells/mm$^3$. Forty-five percent of meningitis and 37% of encephalitis patients have a neutrophil-predominant CSF pleocytosis (Tyler et al., 2006). The protein is typically elevated, and the glucose is almost invariably normal.

In immune competent individuals, WNV RNA viremia has often resolved by the time symptoms of disease develop and diagnosis is made by detection of IgM antibodies in CSF and/or IgM and IgG antibodies in serum. Since serum IgM antibodies do not cross the blood–brain barrier in significant amounts, the detection of WNV-specific IgM in CSF is evidence of both WNV infection and neuroinvasive disease. The prevalence of positive CSF IgM WNV antibodies increases as a function of time after infection at an approximate rate of 10%/day. As a result, by the first week after onset of illness, over 70% of patients are seropositive. Although IgM antibody responses against many viruses last only several months, there have been several reports of persisting serum and CSF WNV-specific IgM for a year or more following infection. CSF PCR is less sensitive than serological studies (70%) but virtually 100% specific. CSF PCR may be useful in diagnosis of WNV infection in immunocompromised patients who may fail to mount or have delayed WNV-specific antibody responses. WNV may be isolated from serum, blood, and CSF early in the febrile stage and from brain tissue. Because of potential cross-reactions with antibodies to other flaviviruses (yellow fever [YF], dengue virus (DENV) Japanese encephalitis antigen-complex members), care should be taken in interpreting positive serology test results in patients with potential exposure to other flaviviruses, or a history of yellow fever virus (YFV) or JEV vaccination.

There is no therapy with proven efficacy for WNV infection in humans, and treatment of WNV neuroinvasive disease is supportive. A randomized controlled, multicenter trial of high-titer anti-WNV IVIG (Omr-IgG-am) was conducted (NCT00069316) but results were not conclusive (Agrawal and Petersen, 2003). A phase II/III clinical trial to evaluate the safety and efficacy of a humanized monoclonal antibody (MGAWN1) for the treatment of WNV infection (clinicaltrials.gov identifier NCT00927953) was closed due to low enrollment. Although the titer of WNV-specific antibody in US lots of IVIG is increasing (Planitzer et al., 2007), its efficacy in treatment of WNV disease is unproven. Ribavirin did not show efficacy in uncontrolled clinical use, and no controlled trials demonstrate the efficacy of interferon alfa preparations in treatment of WNV infection (Chan-Tack and Forrest, 2005; Kalil et al., 2005). Three WNV vaccines have completed phase I human clinical trials for safety and immunogenicity but have not completed efficacy studies due to problems with enrollment. Two of these are chimeric vaccines in which genes encoding WNV structural protein envelopes are inserted into the backbone of attenuated yellow fever or dengue virus strains (see NCT00094718), and the third is a recombinant plasmid DNA vaccine (NCT00300417).

## St. Louis Encephalitis Virus (Flavivirus)

St. Louis encephalitis (SLE) virus is a cause of late summer encephalitis outbreaks in North America. Like WNV, SLE virus maintains an enzootic cycle between *Culex* species of mosquitoes and passeriform birds, with spillover transmission to dead-end hosts such as humans during late summer months. From 1999 to 2007, SLE virus caused 188 confirmed cases of neuroinvasive infection in the United States, with a peak in 2001–2003 paralleling that of the WNV epidemic (Reimann et al., 2008). In 2015–2016, there was a significant increase in SLE cases in the southwest United States localized to Arizona and California with 19 cases reported in 2015 (https://www.cdc.gov/sle/technical/epi.html).

Clinical symptoms of SLE virus infection are characterized by a febrile syndrome or neuroinvasive disease presenting with aseptic meningitis, encephalitis, or meningoencephalitis. Signs and symptoms of CNS infection progress over several days to a week. The incidence of encephalitis is higher in the elderly with a case fatality rate approaching 30%. Season, place of residence, exposure, and presence of similar cases in the community are important considerations in the diagnosis. CSF cell counts are generally less than 200 WBC/μL, with lymphocytic predominance, mildly elevated CSF protein, and normal CSF glucose. Although the virus may be isolated from serum or CSF, specific diagnosis usually relies on serological testing. IgM antibodies may be present in the CSF as early as day 3 of illness and are diagnostic.

No specific antiviral treatment exists for SLE. In an open-label study of interferon alfa-2b (Rahal et al., 2004), 13% of treated patients, compared to 65% of historical controls, had quadriplegia, quadriparesis, or respiratory insufficiency persist after the first week of hospitalization. At week 2, these endpoints were present in 7% of treated patients and 29% of historical controls. This study suggests that interferon alfa-2b might reduce the severity and duration of complications of SLE, although this interpretation must be viewed with extreme caution because of significant limitations in study design and methodology.

## Japanese Encephalitis Virus (Flavivirus)

JEV is the most common cause of mosquito-borne encephalitis in the world, with an estimated 67,900 annual cases, a 20%–30% case fatality ratio, and 30%–50% rate of neurological or psychiatric sequelae in survivors (Solomon, 2004; Solomon et al., 2003) (MMWR, 2013). One in 200 infections result in severe disease. The virus is widely distributed in Asia throughout Japan, China, Taiwan, Korea, the Far Eastern former Soviet Union, Southeast Asia, and India, with recent range expansion to Western Pacific islands and Northern Australia. JEV cycles between *Culex*, *Aedes*, or *Anopheles* species of mosquitoes, pigs, wading birds, and ducks, with Culex species the principal vectors throughout Asia. Lineage I and II strains of JEV are now endemic in Northern Australia owing to the presence of competent mosquito vectors and susceptible vertebrate hosts (Weaver and Reisen, 2010).

Following an incubation period of 6 to 16 days, patients present with a febrile headache syndrome, aseptic meningitis, or encephalitis. The encephalitic form is characterized by a 2- to 4-day viremic prodrome of headache, fever, nausea, vomiting, dizziness, drowsiness, and abdominal symptoms in children, progressing to meningoencephalitis with signs of cortical, subcortical, extrapyramidal, bulbar, cerebellar, and spinal cord involvement. Excitability or delirium, seizures, hyperthermia, expressionless facies, axial rigidity, limb tremors and other involuntary movements, erratic eye movements, cranial nerve palsies, ataxia, limb paresis including lower motor neuron-type weakness in the arms, and segmental sensory disturbance are reported. Prolonged fever, seizures, coma, respiratory complications, and high CNS virus load are all associated with a poorer prognosis. The case fatality rate is 30%–40%, and neurological sequelae include parkinsonism, seizure disorders, paresis, mental retardation, and psychiatric disorders.

JEV encephalitis is characterized by CSF pleocytosis, with 10–500 (rarely to 1000) WBC/μL and early polymorphonuclear predominance, elevated CSF protein (50–100 mg/dL), and areas of abnormal signal in thalamus and basal ganglia on MRI. The first-line rapid diagnostic assay recommended by WHO is JEV-specific IgM antibody capture enzyme-linked immunosorbent assay (ELISA), detecting IgM in serum or CSF. JEV-specific IgM antibodies can be measured in the CSF of most patients by 4 days after onset of symptoms and in serum by 7 days after onset.

The sensitivity of commercial IgM-ELISA assays in the CSF ranges from 65% to 69% with a specificity of 89%–100% (Moore et al., 2012). Plaque reduction neutralization test (PRNT) is the gold standard in flavivirus diagnosis, distinguishing between potentially cross-reacting antibodies of other flaviviruses. When PRNT is not available, a four-fold rise in IgG titer is confirmatory. Viral nucleic acid can be detected by RT-PCR in blood or CSF in early or acute phase infection. Like other flaviviruses, virus is expected to be detectable in the first few days of illness, at which time it is replaced by antibody. In JE cases, virus isolation from the blood is infrequent, but virus can be isolated from the CSF in up to a third of patients.

No specific therapy is available for JEV encephalitis. In a randomized double-blind trial, interferon alfa-2a (10 million units/m$^2$ daily ×7 days) treatment failed to reduce either mortality (≈20%) or the incidence of severe neurological sequelae (≈15%) (Solomon et al., 2003).

The most effective prevention is vaccination. The risk of developing encephalitis among travelers to endemic areas has been estimated to be between 1 in 5000 and 1 in 20,000 cases per week of travel, with the higher risks in rural areas. Japanese encephalitis vaccine used in the United States is the inactivated virus JE-VC vaccine. Originally licensed for people 17 years and older, in 2013 the recommendations were expanded to include children from 2 months of age. JE-VC primary immunization is two doses separated by 28 days, with the second dose at least a week before travel, followed by a single booster dose at 1 year. Revaccination is recommended at 3-year intervals (MMWR, 2010). Immunity is shorter with inactivated virus vaccines than with live attenuated vaccines.

## Zika Virus (Flavivirus)

Zika virus (ZIKV) is transmitted by Aedes species mosquitoes to cause a fever-rash-arthralgia syndrome. ZIKV is a member of the *Flaviviridae* family and the virus most closely related to dengue virus. ZIKV was first isolated from a rhesus monkey in Zika Forest, Uganda in 1947 and later found in other monkey species. The role of some animals as reservoir in the virus' ecology is not clear. Since 1947, there had been only sporadic human cases and seroprevalence studies concluding clinical disease was rare in man. That changed in 2007 when the first human outbreak was reported on Yap Island, Micronesia. Six years later, in 2013 in French Polynesia, ZIKV caused 28,000 cases and a 20-fold increase in incidence of Guillain-Barre Syndrome (GBS) cases. The first infections in the Americas were in Brazil and Columbia in 2015. A major outbreak followed, reaching most of South and Central America and Florida. There were hundreds of thousands of infections in adults and infants and alarming increases in GBS and microcephaly cases, prompting WHO to declare ZIKV a Public Health Emergency of International Concern from February to November, 2016. Maternal-fetal transmission, sexual transmission, breast milk infectivity, and risk of spread by blood transfusion were recognized. The large-scale outbreaks revealed severe neurological presentations previously unknown for Zika: brain malformations in children born of mothers infected during pregnancy, and Guillain-Barré-type syndromes in adults (De Brouker et al., 2017; Leonard et al., 2018; Reid et al., 2018).

Congenital Zika syndrome (CZS) is the result of vertical transmission from mother to fetus during pregnancy. Acquisition of infection in the first trimester poses the greatest risk. CZS features (by CDC criteria) are (1) severe microcephaly with partial collapse of the skull; (2) decreased brain tissue, with patterns of damage that include subcortical calcifications; (3) retinal injury including macular scarring and focal pigmentary retinal mottling; (4) congenital contractures, arthrogryposis; and (5) hypertonia shortly after birth. Recent reports indicate CZS can present with a spectrum of changes including post-natal or no microcephaly, hearing or visual loss, MRIs with cortical, callosal, and cerebellar malformations, or novel imaging abnormalities: multiple cranial nerve enhancement or chronic ischemic infarcts. Long-term management requires a comprehensive combination of developmental and psychosocial support systems (Reid et al., 2018).

In contrast to other Flaviviruses, the most frequent neurological presentations of ZIKV infection after the perinatal period are Guillain-Barré-type syndromes, not the encephalitis and myelitis complications dominant in WNV and JEV infections. Three different neurophysiology patterns—acute inflammatory demyelinating polyneuropathy (AIDP), acute motor axonal neuropathy (AMAN), and acute sensory motor axonal neuropathy (ASMAN) subtypes—have been identified. Their close temporal proximity to symptomatic Zika infection (6–7 days rather than the 2–4 weeks after infection for classic GBS) has raised the possibility of direct viral and/or parainfectious pathogenic mechanisms: acute ZIKV neurotropism boosted by a hyperimmune response, including active immunity against other arboviruses. Miller-Fisher variant, small-fiber or sensory neuronopathy cases have also been reported. No particular antiganglioside autoantibody markers to assist in diagnosis have been found (De Broecker et al., 2017; Munoz et al., 2017; Mehta et al., 2018b).

Presentations other than Guillain-Barré include: meningitis, encephalitis, radiculitis, or combinations; encephalopathy (reversible CNS symptoms with normal CSF and MRI studies) myelitis; ADEM with para- and post-infectious profiles; seizures; and myasthenia gravis. Patients may have dual infections with other co-distributed arboviruses, dengue or Chikungunya (alphavirus), and prior dengue may predispose to more severe Zika through antibody dependent enhancement (Parra et al., 2016; Brito et al., 2017; Munoz et al., 2017; Mehta et al., 2018b).

Zika is diagnosed by detection of ZIKV nucleic acid in serum, CSF, or urine by RT-PCR, or serological detection of anti-ZIKV IgM and ZIKV-specific neutralizing antibodies in serum or CSF (Leonhard et al., 2018). If the IgM result is positive or equivocal, because of poor specificity due to cross-reactivity with antibodies to other structurally similar viruses such as dengue, IgM testing is followed by PRNT available at specialized centers. ZIKV PRNT ≥10 and DENV PRNT <10 indicate a ZIKV infection, either current or prior infection (Reid et al., 2018). ZIKV-specific IgM in serum or CSF can be detected from about 4 days to 12 weeks after exposure. Although time between ZIKV onset and neurological complications may miss a narrow viremic window for ZIKV nucleic acid detection by PCR in serum or CSF, ZIKV RNA can be detected in urine up to 6 weeks to 3 months after symptom onset, and has been used to diagnose GBS associated with Zika (Roze et al., 2016). Because of CNS cases with dual infections, patients with acute neurological syndromes are investigated for Zika as well as cocirculating arboviruses, particularly Chikungunya and dengue (Mehta et al., 2018b, Leonhard et al., 2018).

Treatment of encephalitis is supportive. Treatment of GBS and myelitis include immunomodulatory therapy and supportive care, as per management guidelines and standards of care for these syndromes of other causes. Aspirin is not used because of a thrombocytopenia association with severe disease.

## California Serogroup of Viruses (Bunyaviruses)

The California (CAL) serogroup viruses are the second most common domestic arboviruses causing neuroinvasive disease/encephalitis in the United States after WNV, and cause approximately 80–100 cases per year. Members include La Crosse virus, Jamestown Canyon virus, and California encephalitis virus. These viruses are maintained in an enzootic cycle between (non-Culex) mosquito vectors and small mammals or deer hosts in a limited geographic range and spread to man by infected mosquito bite. Almost all recognized CAL serogroup viral disease, and encephalitic disease, is caused by La Crosse virus (LACV). La Crosse was found predominantly in the Midwestern United States, Wisconsin, Minnesota, and Ohio (McJunkin et al., 2001), but recent outbreaks of La Crosse virus demonstrate a shift in incidence to the Appalachian region, West Virginia, eastern Tennessee, and western North Carolina (Haddow et al., 2011). Jamestown Canyon virus (Michigan, New York), Snowshoe Hare virus (Alaska, Canada, and the northern United States), and California encephalitis virus are associated with viral meningitis or encephalitis.

The majority of La Crosse encephalitis cases occur in children under 16 years. Patients present with fever (>70%), headache (>70%), nausea and vomiting (>70%), disorientation and/or depressed consciousness (≈50%), and seizures (≈50%), including status epilepticus. Focal neurological signs including aphasia and hemiparesis mimic features of HSE. CSF has a lymphocytic pleocytosis and normal or elevated (30%) protein, and hyponatremia secondary to SIADH occurs in about 20%. LACV is difficult to isolate from clinical samples, and nearly all isolates and positive PCR results have come from CSF or brain tissue. Without a sensitive and non-invasive pathogen detection method, serology with detection of IgM antibody in serum or CSF, is the main method for early diagnosis. A fourfold rise in IgG provides confirmatory or retrospective diagnosis. Treatment is supportive. Ribavirin is not recommended due to problems with pharmacokinetics, toxicity, and CNS penetration (McJunkin et al., 2011). Fatalities are rare, 1%–3%, but children who recover may have seizures (10%), cognitive dysfunction (2%), weakness (<2%), or behavioral problems.

Other members of the California serogroup viruses causing meningitis or encephalitis, with their place of discovery are: California Encephalitis Virus, Kern County CA, which causes most disease in children; Jamestown Canyon Virus, Jamestown Canyon, CO, which affects mainly elderly persons and circulates in the northern United States; Snowshoe Hare Virus, in Montana; and Tahyna Virus, in central Europe, found in Tahyna, former Czechoslovakia.

## Equine Encephalitis Viruses (Alphaviruses)

Eastern equine encephalitis (EEE) virus, a summertime epizootic virus maintained between mosquito vectors and birds in the eastern United States, causes the most severe of US arboviral encephalitides, with an estimated mortality of 50%–70%, and neurological impairment in many survivors. Approximately seven cases are reported per year in the United States, with most cases in Atlantic and Gulf Coast states. Mosquitoes of Aedes, Coquillettidia, and Culex species are the principal vectors of disease transmission to man, with EEE virus-related horse or pheasant deaths often preceding human cases. However, rare cases have been associated with organ transplant (Pouch et al., 2019). Patients present with febrile headache, and progress rapidly to delirium and coma. Meningeal signs and excessive salivation are common CSF that contains 500–3000 WBC/μL, polymorphonuclear leukocyte predominance, and elevated protein concentration. The "parentheses sign," linear areas of T2/FLAIR hyperintensities in the external and internal capsules, with sparing of the lentiform nuclei, when present, distinguish EEE from other encephalitides (Babi et al., 2014; Nickerson et al., 2016; Berlin et al., 2017). Diagnosis is made by PCR detection of viral nucleic acid in serum or CSF, virus isolation from sera or CSF, detection of virus-specific IgM in serum or CSF, or the documentation of seroconversion and rise in antibody titer. At least three cases had good outcomes with steroids and IVIG supplementing supportive care that included ICP monitoring (Golomb et al., 2001; Wendell et al., 2013; Mukerji et al., 2016).

Western Equine Encephalitis virus, transmitted to people and horses by infected, mainly Culex tarsalis, mosquitoes, was responsible for 639 confirmed human cases in the United States from 1964–1997, in 21 Midwest and western states. Despite no recent US cases, WEE virus remains a cause of encephalitis in South America (Delfraro et al., 2011). Encephalitis has a fatality rate of 3%–7%.

Venezuelan equine encephalitis (VEE) virus occurs from Bolivia to Mexico, with occasional cases in Florida. VEE virus circulates in a permanent zoonotic cycle between Culex species mosquitoes and rodents, with epizootic cases in horses producing high viremias to infect a wide range of mosquitoes resulting in human cases. VEE virus causes a febrile illness with myalgias, progressing to encephalitis and coma in a small proportion of cases. Encephalitis has a fatality rate of about 1%. Epilepsy, paralysis, tremor, hallucinations, and emotional lability may persist as permanent sequelae in children, and occasional cases of residual epilepsy or tremor have been reported in adults. Because the clinical presentation of VEE infection may be febrile illness rather than primary encephalitis, the diagnosis may be missed unless recent travel in an area of disease activity in tropical America is taken into account. Both saliva and blood are infectious early in the disease. Diagnosis is by detection of viral nucleic acid or virus-specific antibodies in serum or CSF.

The live attenuated VEEV strain TC-83 is a licensed veterinary vaccine and the only strain available for protecting laboratory workers, military, or others in high-risk occupations (Leibovitch and Jacobson, 2016).

## Chikungunya Virus (Alphavirus)

Chikungunya virus (CHIKV) is an alphavirus, family Togaviridae belonging to the "new world" group of alphaviruses that includes Eastern, Western, and VEE viruses. CHIK is transmitted by Aedes species mosquitoes, the same vectors that transmit dengue and Zika, and occasionally from mother to child. After decades of low transmission starting in the 1960s, a divergent strain emerged in 2004 and CHIK became a major public health problem with explosive outbreaks and rapid global expansion. The first local US transmission of CHIK was in 2014 in Florida, Puerto Rico, and the US Virgin Islands. Like the flaviviruses dengue and Zika, CHIK causes a fever-rash-arthralgia syndrome and is associated with neurological complications. Differing from the flaviviruses, CHIK arthralgias often progress to chronic debilitating arthritis. Increasing reports of cocirculation and coinfection of these three arboviruses in the Americas present challenges in determining the underlying viral etiology in arbovirus-associated encephalitis and other neurological diseases (Mehta et al., 2018a). CHIK has been associated with antiganglioside antibodies.

An estimated 1 in 1000 CHIK cases develop neurological disease as: encephalitis, encephalopathy, myelitis, the full range of GBS variants, mixed central and peripheral syndromes, ADEM, inflammatory ocular disease, retinal detachment or hemorrhage, or branch retinal artery occlusion (Mehta et al., 2018a). Autoimmune or peripheral disease is more common in middle age, and CNS disease in the elderly (Cerny et al., 2017). Coinfection with dengue caused encephalitis, transverse myelitis, and unusual laminar cortical MRI patterns (Farias et al., 2018). Coinfection of CHIK plus Zika or dengue or both has caused myeloradiculitis, meningoencephalomyelitis, myelitis, GBS, and may be responsible for more severe disease (Mehta et al., 2018b). With the concurrent epidemics of dengue virus, ZIKV, and CHIKV in tropical areas where large proportions of the population are exposed to Aedes mosquitoes, these agents may be accounting for greater proportions of encephalitis cases in the future.

Neonatal disease is a consequence of transmission in the intrapartum period, with overt disease as: meningoencephalitis, sepsis, or white matter disease and extensive demyelination. Infection may not be obvious at birth but can cause neurocognitive development delay, found when neonates with suspected infection were followed for 2 years (Mehta et al., 2018a).

MRI may be normal or have nonspecific changes: increased T2 FLAIR signal of white matter, cortical, diencephalic, brainstem areas, restricted diffusion areas, hemorrhage, or medial temporal lobe abnormalities (Cerny et al., 2017; Doughty et al., 2017). Laboratory diagnosis is by detection of viral nucleic acid by RT-PCR in serum or CSF in the first few days of infection (urine and saliva may also be positive), or detection of anti-CHIKV IgM by ELISA in serum or CSF, which may be present as early as 2–3 days after infection, and persist for several months (Doughty et al., 2017). PRNT, a four-fold rise in CHIKV IgG in convalescent serum or demonstration of intrathecal IgG synthesis have also been used (Barr et al., 2018; Puccioni-Sohler et al., 2018).

There are no specific antivirals or vaccines. Ribavirin has been used in treatment of post-CHIK arthritis.

Mayaro virus, another alphavirus spread by Aedes mosquitoes, may be the new Chikungunya, as it expands across tropical forested areas of South America and the Caribbean. It produces symptoms that closely resemble CHIK: headache, fever, rash, severe and long-term arthralgias, and in endemic areas of Peru, has been reported with neurological complications.

### Colorado Tick Fever Virus (Coltivirus) and Banna Virus (Seadornavirus)

Colorado tick fever virus is a member of the family Reoviridae and the genus *Coltivirus* (Attoui et al., 2005). Ticks (e.g., *Dermacentor andersoni*) are the principal vectors of disease transmission, although rare human cases have been associated with blood transfusion and bone marrow transplants. The virus is found predominantly in the Rocky Mountain region of the United States and Canada, at altitudes of 4000–10,000 feet. Human infection is characterized by abrupt onset of fever, chills, retro-orbital pain, and myalgia (Attoui et al., 2005; Goodpasture et al., 1978). Up to 65% of cases have associated leukopenia and thrombocytopenia. Neurological manifestations of aseptic meningitis, meningoencephalitis, or encephalitis are more common in children. Patients with meningitis or encephalitis can have a lymphocytic CSF pleocytosis (up to 300 WBC/mm$^3$). Laboratory diagnosis is by detection of viral RNA or virus-specific IgM or neutralizing antibodies in serum. RT-PCR is the more sensitive test for early diagnosis because antibodies may not be present for 14–21 days after onset of symptoms. In specialty labs, diagnosis is also made based on isolation of virus from erythrocytes in blood, where it can persist for months. Treatment is supportive, and aspirin is avoided because of thrombocytopenia associated with infection. A related virus, Banna virus, belonging to the genus *Seadornavirus*, is transmitted by mosquitoes and has been isolated in cases of encephalitis in humans and animals, predominantly in China and Indonesia.

### Powassan Virus (Flavivirus)

Powassan virus (POWV), isolated from the brain of an encephalitic patient in Powassan, Ontario, Canada, is the only North American member of tickborne encephalitis (TBE) virus serogroup of flaviviruses. The virus, which cycles between ticks and small to medium-sized mammals or deer, is spread to man by tick bite.

POWV is the cause of sporadic encephalitis in Canada, the United States (mainly in northeastern and midwestern states), and Russia. In the US Great Lakes region, cases link to traditional lineage POWV, and in the Northeast to POWV lineage II (also known as deer tick virus). Since its discovery, there have been about 100 cases in the United States.

POWV infection is diagnosed by virus isolation, detection of IgM antibodies by ELISA with a confirmatory PRNT in serum, detection of IgM (ELISA) and PRNT in CSF with negative results for other causes of encephalitis, or four-fold rise in antibody titer in serum or CSF. Serological diagnosis is not genotype-specific, so the causal agent may be POW or DTV lineage. MRI show T2/FLAIR abnormalities most commonly in deep gray structures, but also affecting brainstem, cortex, or periventricular white matter (Piantadosi et al., 2016), evidence of hemorrhagic encephalitis with bilateral thalamic, frontal or temporal hemorrhages (Hermance and Thangamani, 2017), or images consistent with widespread necrotizing meningoencephalitis (Tavakoli et al., 2009).

Treatment is supportive. Use of IVIG was associated with good outcome in one patient and survival in a second patient (Piantadosi et al., 2016). POW encephalitis is fatal in 10%–15% of cases, or causes neurological sequelae in 50% of survivors (CDC, 2001; Ebel, 2010).

### Murray Valley Encephalitis Virus (Australian X Disease; Flavivirus)

Additional text is available online at http://expertconsult.inkling.com. 

### Tickborne Encephalitis Virus (Flavivirus)

Additional text is available online at http://expertconsult.inkling.com. 

### Rift Valley Fever Virus (Phlebovirus)

Additional text is available online at http://expertconsult.inkling.com. 

### Toscana Virus (Phlebovirus)

Toscana virus, a neurotropic arbovirus carried by sand flies, was first isolated in 1971. It has become the leading cause of summertime viral meningitis in Italy, accounting for 30%–50% of cases in some series (Charrel et al., 2005; Valassina et al., 2003). Additional human cases of meningitis were subsequently reported in many European countries including France, Spain, and Portugal (Charrel et al., 2005). Toscana virus is transmitted by *Phlebotomus* (sand fly) species, and dogs, cats, goats, sheep, and bats around the Mediterranean basin can be infected. In man, after an incubation period of a few days to 2 weeks, Toscana virus infection produces abrupt onset of either a self-limited febrile illness or various CNS syndromes: meningitis, encephalitis, or meningoencephalitis that may be severe and associated with coma and systemic disease (rash, adenopathy, hepatosplenomegaly, renal involvement, disseminated intravascular coagulation, and bleeding diathesis). Patients typically have headache (100%), fever (76%–97%), nausea and vomiting (67%–88%), and myalgia (18%). Diagnosis is by immunoenzymatic IgM testing of serum and CSF, or PCR detection of Toscana viral sequences in CSF (taken within 4 days of symptom onset) (Osborne et al., 2016). Virus can be isolated from CSF, plasma, or urine (Arden et al., 2017). Treatment is supportive. Other sand fly fever group viruses around the Mediterranean are associated with febrile illness (pappataci fever) (Osborne et al., 2016).

## Rabies

Rabies is a significant cause of encephalitis worldwide, with approximately 55,000 cases per year and nearly 100% mortality. Reservoirs of infection are bats, wild carnivores (skunks, foxes, raccoons, coyotes, wolves), and unimmunized dogs. In the United States, the bulk of human rabies cases are linked to bat exposures, often in the absence of a recognized or documented bite or scratch. Transmission can also occur following direct exposure (scratch or bite) from a reservoir species including skunks, fox, or racoon, as well as bats. Rare non-bite (aerosol) exposures, in the bat-inhabited Frio cave in Texas and in laboratory accidents, have also been documented. In 2004, four recipients of kidneys, a liver, and an arterial segment from an organ donor died within a month of transplantation from encephalitis characterized by rapid neurological deterioration, seizures, respiratory failure, and agitated delirium progressing to coma. The cause of illness was subsequently identified as rabies, and the donor was retrospectively found to have a history of a possible bat bite before he died of unrelated causes (subarachnoid hemorrhage) (Srinivasan et al., 2005). There were three more cases in 2005 in recipients of solid organs. A liver recipient with a history of vaccination 20 years earlier and the two corneal recipients survived (Maier et al., 2010). In Europe, a long incubation period transplant case was reported in 2013 (Vora et al., 2013).

The incubation period of rabies is usually from 1 to 3 months but may vary from 1 week to several years. A prodrome of headache, fever, paresthesias, and pain at the site of inoculation is followed by an acute neurological phase, then coma. Cases in which hyperactivity dominates have been called *furious* rabies. Characteristic neuropathological intraneuronal inclusions (Negri bodies; Fig. 78.7) and inflammatory changes are maximal in the brainstem and limbic system. A mainly mononuclear CSF pleocytosis is found in over half the cases during the first week of illness, and in 87% beyond the first week (Anderson et al., 1984), and MRI evidence of gray matter involvement: basal ganglia, thalamus, midbrain, and pontine nuclei, is described on FLAIR or T2-wieghted sequences (Jain et al., 2013). Up to 80% of patients may exhibit hydrophobia or aerophobia, spasms of pharyngeal and nuchal muscles lasting from 1 to 5 minutes, triggered by swallow attempts or tactile, auditory, visual, and olfactory stimuli. The spasms are thought to be an exaggerated respiratory tract protective reflex. As the disease progresses, spasms can increase in frequency and are accompanied by agitation, hallucinations, autonomic hyperactivity, and seizures. Body temperature may reach 105°F–107°F. Abnormal cranial nerve, motor, sensory examinations, tremor, myoclonus, local sensory symptoms, symptoms at the exposure site are more common with bat-acquired rabies (Udow et al., 2013). Paralytic, myelitic, or "dumb" rabies, accounting for 20% of patients, is characterized by paresthesias, weakness, and flaccid paralysis in the bitten extremity, progressing to quadriplegia.

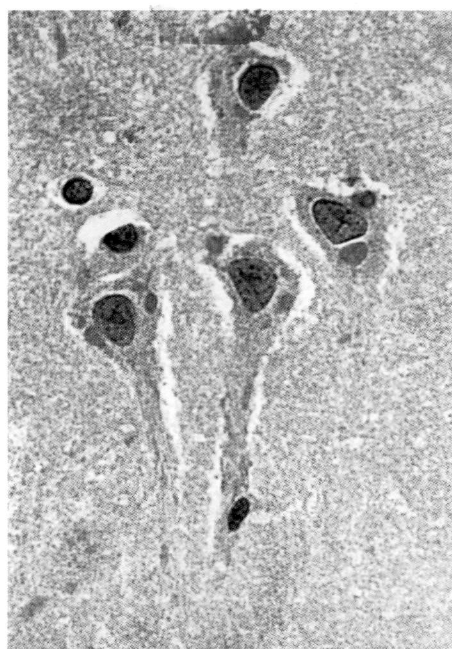

**Fig. 78.7 Hippocampal Neurons in Human Rabies Encephalitis.** Cytoplasm of these neurons bears one or more rounded or oval Negri inclusion bodies. (Hematoxylin-eosin stain, ×350.) (Courtesy R. Kim.)

The diagnosis of rabies should be considered in any patient, with or without a history of exposure, who has a clinical picture of agitated or paralytic encephalitic illness or acute flaccid paralysis without clinical brain involvement. When no history can be obtained, rabies should be included in the differential diagnosis of any encephalitis progressing rapidly to coma, particularly if the patient has been to an endemic area. Other differential diagnostic considerations include intoxications, postvaccinal encephalitis, tetanus (which has a shorter [<2-week] incubation period and normal spinal fluid), or rabies phobia (a hysterical response to an animal bite).

Examination of a skin biopsy from a hairy region of the posterior neck (nuchal biopsy) for the presence of rabies virus antigen by immunofluorescence, and RT-PCR testing of saliva are the most rapid methods of antemortem diagnosis. Corneal smears are rarely used because of low sensitivity. The presence of neutralizing antibodies in the serum and CSF of an unimmunized patient is diagnostic but these are not highly sensitive methods. Active disease produces high titers (>1:5000), which may be helpful for diagnosing acute rabies in previously immunized individuals. RT-PCR protocols for detection of viral sequences in saliva, skin biopsies, CSF, or brain specimens have been established (Wacharapluesadee and Hemachudha, 2001). The sensitivity for CSF is low, and this type of test is not usually needed for brain tissue.

Transdermal bites or scratches and mucous membrane contact with saliva from known reservoir animal species constitute exposure. In addition, any history of bat exposure, with or without recognized bite, should be considered a significant exposure. Superficial bat-inflicted wounds carry a high risk because of the ability of bat rabies variants to infect and multiply within epithelial cells and fibroblasts. Although CNS tissues are highly infectious, infectious rabies virus is only rarely isolated from CSF, and RT-PCR. Saliva should be considered infectious, and appropriate precautions taken. Postexposure treatment and prophylaxis of rabies includes wound care and the early initiation of rabies vaccine and antirabies immunoglobulin to nonimmune individuals (Rupprecht and Gibbons, 2004). Wounds should be cleansed with soap and water followed by povidone-iodine. Human diploid cell rabies vaccine (HDCV) or purified chick-embryo vaccine (PCEC) should be administered intramuscularly on days 0, 3, 7, and 14 into the deltoid or anterolateral thigh muscles (Rupprecht and Gibbons, 2004). Previously immunized individuals should be given booster doses of vaccine on days 0 and 3. Human rabies immunoglobulin (HRIG), 20 IU/kg, should be administered once as soon as possible after exposure (up to 7 days after the first dose of vaccine) at the beginning of prophylaxis to patients who have not been previously vaccinated. As much of the entire dose as possible should be administered in the area of the wound, and the remainder should be administered intramuscularly at a site distant from the vaccine administration. Because HRIG may partially suppress active production of antibody, the recommended dose should not be exceeded.

Local public health officials should be consulted before postexposure prophylaxis is started to avoid unnecessary vaccination and to assist in proper handling of the suspect animal if confinement or testing is appropriate. A dog or cat immunized within the previous 3 years is considered an unlikely source of infection but should be confined and observed for 10 days. Unimmunized dogs, cats, and ferrets can also be confined for 10 days. If ill, the animal should be euthanized and the brain examined at a regional health laboratory by IHC for rabies virus antigen. Therapy should be initiated if results are positive. Based on area health department data, wild animals belonging to known infected species should be considered rabid until laboratory test results are negative. Treatment can be stopped if the animal remains healthy for the 10-day observation period or if the euthanized animal is confirmed antigen negative.

Pre-exposure prophylaxis is available to veterinarians, animal handlers, laboratory workers, or travelers to endemic areas.

Recovery from rabies has been documented in only a few human cases worldwide. All but three had received rabies vaccinations before illness. One was the widely reported successful case of treatment of an adolescent patient with clinical rabies who did not receive antecedent postexposure prophylaxis (Willoughby et al., 2005). The patient was a 15-year-old girl who developed clinical rabies 1 month after a bat bite. She was treated with therapeutic ketamine/midazolam/phenobarbital coma, IV ribavirin (33 mg/kg load, then 16 mg/kg every 6 hours), enteral amantadine (200 mg/day), tetrahydrobiopterin, coenzQ10, and ascorbic acid, without active or passive immunization. It is unclear whether this patient's survival was related to any of the specific therapies used (Jackson, 2009); similar treatment of at least 26 other patients failed (Jackson, 2013).

Eight cases of rabies have followed corneal transplantation, and there have been several clusters of rabies virus transmission through solid organ or arterial segment transplantation in Texas, Florida, and Germany. The transmission of rabies virus through solid organ (kidney) transplantation in Germany differed from prior cases because of the long (18 months) incubation period in the recipient who developed rabies, and survival of three other recipients without pretransplant rabies vaccination (Vora et al., 2013). The low incidence of disease or suspicion has so far prevented mandatory donor testing. Transplant rabies is a complex issue. Pre-mortem testing never excludes rabies. Postmortem testing prior to transplantation is problematic because of logistical issues and organ wastage due to false positive results obtained in regular hospital but nonreference laboratories.

### Australian Bat Lyssavirus

Additional text is available online at http://expertconsult.inkling.com.

### Chandipura Virus "Encephalitis"

Additional text is available online at http://expertconsult.inkling.com.

### Measles

Measles, the most contagious virus yet known, is still an important cause of childhood mortality and blindness in developing countries, as well as in sporadic outbreaks in industrialized nations (Parker et al., 2006). Endemic measles was eliminated from the United States in 2000, but outbreaks associated with imported measles continue to occur and very recent outbreaks have been reported in low-vaccine-rate populations in the Pacific northwest and elsewhere. As long as measles remains endemic worldwide and subpopulations within the United States remain unvaccinated for religious or cultural reasons, there will be the risk of future outbreaks. From 2001 to 2016, 553 imported US cases of measles were reported with a median of 28 cases/year (Lee et al., 2018). 87% of cases were unvaccinated or had unknown vaccination status, and US residents accounted for 62% of imported measles cases following travel to countries in the Western pacific or European regions. Risk of measles importation was related to the incidence of measles and the volume of travel to the source country.

Measles causes four major CNS syndromes: acute encephalitis, postviral encephalomyelitis, measles inclusion body encephalitis, and subacute sclerosing panencephalitis (SSPE).

#### Acute Encephalitis and Postviral Encephalomyelitis

Fever, maculopapular rash, cough, coryza, and Koplik spots are characteristic of acute measles. CSF pleocytosis and generalized slowing on EEG may be documented in otherwise uncomplicated cases, but true encephalitis is rare. Keratitis and corneal ulceration accompany measles in children with preexisting malnutrition, particularly vitamin A deficiency. High-dose vitamin A supplementation, a single intramuscular dose of 400,000 IU for all ages, is recommended in regions with vitamin A deficiency or measles fatality rates greater than 1%. Postinfectious encephalomyelitis follows an estimated one in 1000 cases, usually within 2 weeks of the rash.

#### Measles Inclusion Body Encephalitis

Measles inclusion body encephalitis is a rapidly progressive dementing illness with behavior changes, myoclonus, refractory focal or generalized seizures, delirium, or coma developing 1–9 months after measles exposure in individuals with deficiencies in cell-mediated immunity. Patients are afebrile, and CSF analysis is normal. Measles virus is detected by PCR in brain or CSF. Treatment is supportive, plus reduction in immunosuppression if possible, and passive immunoglobulin therapy.

#### Subacute Sclerosing Panencephalitis

SSPE is a rare late complication of measles, caused by persistent nonproductive measles virus infection of neurons and glia in immunocompetent patients. The pathogenesis of SSPE is related to defective measles virus maturation in neural cells. Aberrant M (matrix) protein as well as other envelope proteins interfere with assembly and budding of infectious virus. The virus remains in intracellular form and spreads by cell-to-cell contact.

SSPE has an annual incidence from under 0.1 cases to 5 or 6 cases per million in unimmunized populations. In areas of high early-life measles attack rates, SSPE accounts for a portion of childhood neurodegenerative conditions. Children infected in the first 2 years of life are at greater risk, and case series consistently show SSPE to be more frequent in boys (male/female ratio 3:1). The median interval between acute measles infection and SSPE is 8 years, with a range from 2 to 12 years. The early stage is marked by behavioral or personality changes and declining school performance. Myoclonus, seizures, spasticity, choreoathetoid or ballistic movements, ataxia, and chorioretinitis can occur in the second stage of disease. Optic atrophy, quadriparesis, autonomic instability, akinetic mutism, and coma are seen in the final stage. The majority of cases follow a progressive downhill course to death within a few years (Garg, 2002).

At the time neurological symptoms occur, neurons and glia contain nuclear and cytoplasmic viral inclusion bodies (Fig. 78.8), and high titers of antimeasles antibody is found in both serum and CSF. The CSF/serum antibody ratio is consistent with high levels of intrathecal synthesis of measles antibody. CSF pleocytosis is absent, glucose is normal, and total protein is normal or elevated. Acute symptoms together with increased intracranial pressure are poor prognostic signs. The earliest MRI findings are high signal intensity on T2-weighted images of gray and subcortical white matter in posterior portions of the hemispheres. During the second stage of disease, the EEG shows a pattern of generalized slow-wave complexes with a regular periodicity (Fig. 78.9). The complexes may last up to 3 seconds and occur at regular intervals, between 4 and 14 seconds, against a background of depressed activity. Psychiatric illness presentations with alpha coma are also reported (Kartal et al., 2013).

There is no known effective therapy for SSPE. An estimated 30%–35% of patients have improved or stabilized after 1- or several 6-week treatments with intraventricular interferon alfa through an Ommaya reservoir (starting at 100,000 U/m$^2$ body surface area per day, with daily increments up to $10^6$ U/m$^2$/day over 5 hospital days, then $10^6$ U/m$^2$ twice a week for 6 months), combined with oral isoprinosine (inosiplex), 100 mg/kg/day to a maximum of 3 g/day taken orally in three divided doses for 6 months (Gascon, 2003; Gutierrez et al., 2010). Response to IV ribavirin in combination with intrathecal interferon alfa (Tomoda et al., 2001) and symptomatic improvement in myoclonus and encephalopathy with levetiracetam have been reported. The laboratory endpoint of treatment is eradication of detectable measles antigen from the CSF. Systemic (subcutaneous) interferon alfa in daily doses of up to 5 million units has been used with intrathecal interferon alfa to simultaneously treat the peripheral reservoirs of measles virus, lymphoid, and glandular tissue. Prolonged or repeated treatments carry the risks of meningitis, interferon alfa-induced encephalopathy, and interferon alfa upper and lower motor neuron toxicity. Spontaneous remissions are estimated at 5%.

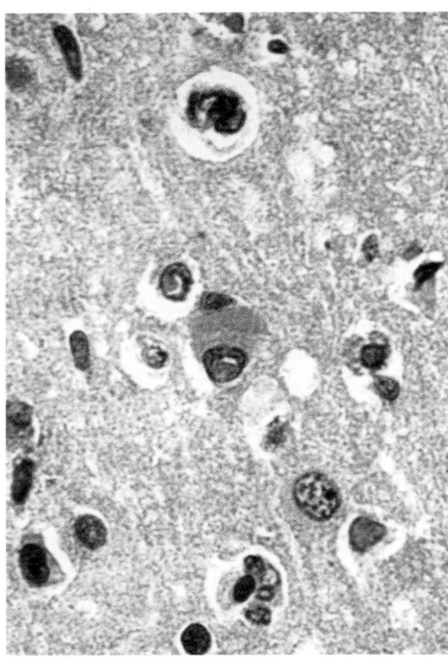

**Fig. 78.8 Cerebral Cortex in Subacute Sclerosing Panencephalitis.** A pyramidal neuron contains both a Cowdry-type A intranuclear inclusion and a cigar-shaped cytoplasmic inclusion. Cowdry A inclusions are also present in nuclei of several nearby glia cells. (Hematoxylin-eosin stain, ×350.) (Courtesy R. Kim.)

Immunization with attenuated live measles vaccine is recommended for infants between 12 and 15 months of age, with a second dose at age 4–6 years. Measles vaccine is one component of the combination quadrivalent measles, mumps, rubella, varicella (MMRV) vaccine and the trivalent measles, mumps, rubella (MMR) vaccine. Full recommendations of the Advisory Committee on Immunization Practices have been published (CDC, 2010b).

## Mumps

Mumps virus causes a mild childhood illness characterized by parotitis, but it has the capacity for widespread invasion of visceral organs, the vestibular labyrinths, and the CNS. In unimmunized populations, mumps is a common cause of aseptic meningitis and, less commonly, encephalitis. Before introduction of widespread vaccination in the United States, mumps virus was the leading cause of viral meningitis in the United States, with over 200,000 cases reported in 1964. Since the introduction of effective vaccination strategies, there has been a steady decrease in the incidence of mumps virus infection, with an all-time low of 231 US cases reported in 2001. The incidence of mumps meningitis and encephalitis varies with different epidemics, from less than 1% to 70%. Mumps meningitis may precede parotitis and can occur without salivary gland enlargement in 40%–50% of patients. In the remainder of cases, mumps meningitis or encephalitis develops approximately 5 days after the onset of parotitis. Postinfectious encephalomyelitis follows an estimated 1 in 6000 cases and develops 7–15 days after parotitis. Postinfectious encephalomyelitis may resemble ADEM with predominantly white-matter manifestations. Mumps virus-associated acute encephalopathy, an early, rapidly progressive coma, with raised intracranial pressure and prolonged convulsions, is a different syndrome, distinguished from meningoencephalitis by its acellular CSF, normal glucose and protein, but elevated CSF inflammatory cytokine profile in a pattern similar to that of influenza-associated encephalopathy (Watanabe et al., 2013). Outcomes vary from full recovery to death.

Seizures are estimated in 20%–30% of patients with CNS symptoms, but follow-up EEGs can be normal. Obtunded patients may

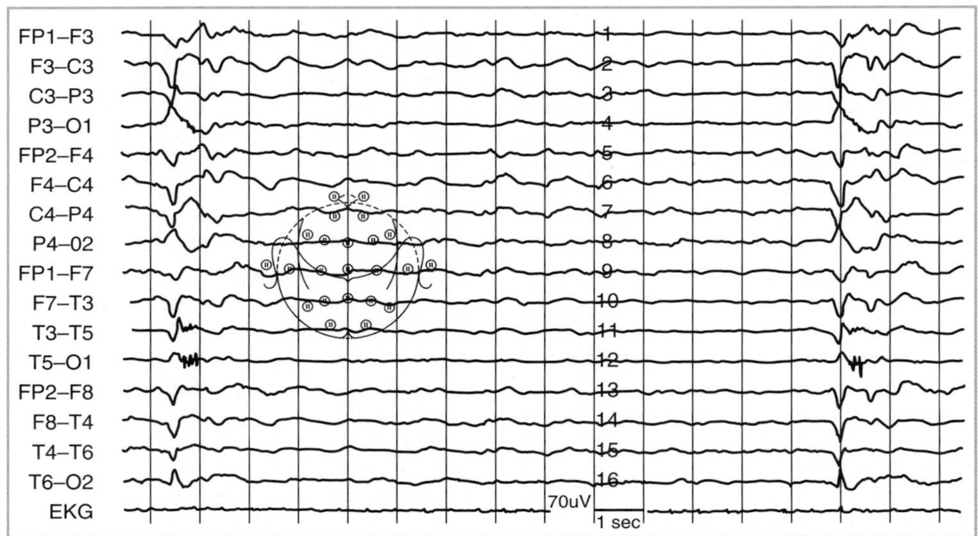


**Fig. 78.9** Electroencephalogram of a 23-year-old man with subacute sclerosing panencephalitis, showing generalized slow-wave co plexes occurring approximately every 12 seconds. (Courtesy K. Nudleman.)

have relatively mild EEG changes and recover with few sequelae. Complications include deafness from labyrinth membrane and sensory transducer damage, myelitis, or hydrocephalus following viral replication in choroidal and ependymal cells.

In mumps meningoencephalitis, there is a CSF pleocytosis of 25–500 WBC/μL with lymphocytic predominance, although higher counts may occur occasionally (as high as 3000 WBC/μL). CSF protein concentration is normal or moderately elevated and may include mumps-specific oligoclonal IgG; glucose concentration is depressed in 29% of cases. Diagnosis can be confirmed by serology with detection of anti-mumps-specific immunoglobulin M (IgM) during the acute phase (7–10 days after symptom onset). Alternatively, seroconversion or a four-fold increase in mumps IgG titers between acute and convalescent sera can support the diagnosis.

Mumps prevention is best achieved by vaccination with live attenuated virus at 12–15 months of age and an additional booster dose at 4–6 years of age; mumps vaccine is one component of the trivalent MMR or quadrivalent MMRV vaccine. Studies evaluating the use of the current MMR vaccine (containing Jeryl-Lynn strain) have not documented any association between vaccination and encephalitis, aseptic meningitis, or autism (Makela et al., 2002).

## Rubella

Rubella virus infection in childhood or adult life is usually a mild illness. Maculopapular rash, fever, and lymphadenopathy characterize clinically apparent infection. Acute encephalitis is rare, and may occur without rash (Guler et al., 2009). Postinfectious encephalomyelitis is estimated to complicate one of 6000 cases, with onset 1–6 days after the appearance of the rash.

Gestational rubella, especially infection acquired during the first trimester, has serious consequences for the fetus; 80% of children with a congenital rubella syndrome have some form of nervous system involvement. Signs in infancy include bulging fontanelle, lethargy, irritability, and abnormalities in muscle tone. CSF protein concentration is elevated, and the virus may be isolated from the CSF. Sequelae in survivors include mental retardation, microcephaly, sensorineural hearing loss, motor and posture abnormalities, cataracts, pigmentary retinopathy, and congenital heart disease. Congenital rubella syndrome has become rare in the United States since the institution of effective vaccination strategies in the 1960s (Reef et al., 2002).

A rare late-onset encephalitis may follow congenital rubella or natural childhood rubella ("progressive rubella panencephalitis"). There is a prolonged asymptomatic period followed by the onset of neurological deterioration during the second decade of life. Symptoms include behavioral changes, intellectual decline, ataxia, spasticity, and seizures. Although progressive rubella panencephalitis may exhibit some of the clinical features of SSPE, patients with progressive rubella panencephalitis tend to be older, have more protracted clinical courses, and lack generalized myoclonus or periodic burst-suppression EEG patterns. The typical course is one of progressive neurological decline leading to death within 8 years. Sera and CSF from affected children contain antirubella IgG antibodies and MRI may show diffuse brain atrophy. Since institution of widespread administration of live attenuated rubella virus vaccine to preschool children (as a component of the MMR vaccine), the incidence of rubella and rubella-associated ADEM has drastically declined. Postexposure vaccination is not recommended. A current discussion of the trivalent MMR vaccine for children is found in the Cochrane database (Demicheli et al., 2012).

One case of fatal encephalitis in a young adult male associated with a vaccine strain of rubella was reported after the 2008 measles/rubella (MR) vaccine immunization campaign in Brazil (Gualberto et al., 2013). RV isolated from brain tissue excluded a postinfectious diagnosis. RV encephalitis is usually diagnosed by rubella IgM antibodies in CSF and serum. However, this patient had received one dose of rubella vaccine previously, and instead showed elevated rubella IgG antibodies, a finding usually associated with secondary infection.

## Henipaviruses

Henipaviruses (Hendra virus [HeV] and Nipah virus [NiV]) are emerging zoonotic viruses associated with encephalitis in Australia and Southeast Asia.

### Hendra Virus

Additional text is available online at http://expertconsult.inkling.com. 

### Nipah Virus

NiV, closely related to HeV, was discovered in 1999 as the agent of an outbreak of encephalitis among pig farmers and others with close contacts to pigs in Malaysia and abattoir workers in Singapore. A major outbreak of mild disease in pigs but fatal encephalitic or respiratory diseases in humans from September 1998 to April 1999 resulted in 265 infected persons, 105 deaths, and the eventual destruction of 1.1 million pigs. There were no further Malaysian nor Singaporean cases. However, in 2001, annual outbreaks of Nipah encephalitis in Bangladesh and West Bengal, India began. As of 2015, there had been 13 Nipah annual outbreaks in Bangladesh, 261 laboratory-confirmed cases, and 199 deaths (Sharma et al., 2018). No evidence of transmission through pigs was found, but consumption of food, particularly raw date palm sap contaminated by fruit bats (flying foxes, Pteropus sp.), was a main source of infection (Luby, 2013). Ongoing transmission between humans is presumed via respiratory droplets. Like HeV, the natural reservoir is the fruit bat, and member species are found from the western Pacific to the eastern coast of Africa. Flying foxes were responsible for introduction to the Philippines in a 2014 outbreak of severe illness in horses and humans recognized as Nipah, with horse-to-human and human-to-human transmission (Ang et al., 2018).

NiV causes a wide spectrum of disease from mild to rapidly progressive encephalitis or respiratory illness, with 40% mortality in Malaysia, and 75%–94% mortality in Bangladesh (Sharma et al., 2018). Clinical signs and symptoms include fever, headache, myalgia, drowsiness, stupor, coma, and stroke (Goh et al., 2000). Diagnosis is by detection of anti-NiV IgM (which peaks on day 12 of illness) or IgG antibody in serum or CSF, detection of viral RNA by RT-PCR of serum, CSF, or urine, or virus isolation from blood, CSF, or respiratory secretions (Ahmad and Tan, 2014). Treatment is supportive.

Both NiV and HeV preferentially infect endothelial cells, causing a systemic vasculitis particularly of small arteries and capillaries of the brain. CSF can be normal or have a pleocytosis. In Malaysia, acute encephalitis patients had MRIs showing small disseminated discreet hyperintense lesions generally in subcortical and deep white matter, less often, in gray matter, consistent with focal areas of ischemia and microinfarctions. CNS hemorrhage may be present. Twenty-one percent of Malaysian survivors had neurological or neuropsychiatric sequelae.

Like HeV, NiV infection is also the cause of relapsed and late-onset encephalitis months to years after initial illness, with the longest interval 11 years. The syndrome is acute onset fever, headache, seizures, focal signs, and CSF pleocytosis with MRI evidence of areas of confluent cortical involvement rather than small discrete hyperintense areas of acute cases. Relapsed and late-onset NiV encephalitis are thought to be recurrent infection. Viral antigen is present but replication-competent NiV is not isolated from CNS. These syndromes have a lower mortality rate (18%) than acute Nipah encephalitis or pneumonia (Chong and Tan, 2003; Tan et al., 2002; Wilson, 2013; Ahmad and Tan, 2014).

## Influenza

Encephalitis, first recognized in association with the 1918 flu pandemic, is a rare complication of influenza, primarily described with influenza A and in children. The estimated incidence of neurological complications was 1.2/100,000 of symptomatic influenza cases in the 2009 A(H1N1) pandemic, and presented as seizures (57.1%), encephalopathy/encephalitis (37.7%), meningitis (3.9%), and Guillain-Barré syndrome (1.3%) in the United States. (Glaser et al., 2012). A national surveillance study of children and adults across the UK seen during the period when influenza A:H1N1 (2009) was the predominant subtype in circulation reported the most common presentations as encephalopathy and/or seizures in children, and added several rare syndromes: acute infantile encephalopathy predominantly affecting the frontal lobes, acute necrotizing encephalopathy (with imaging evidence of bilateral thalamic/basal ganglia/brainstem inflammation and edema), hemorrhagic shock and encephalopathy syndrome, and acute hemorrhagic leukoencephalopathy (Goenka et al., 2014).

Apparently, there has been no difference in the risk of encephalitis after seasonal influenza compared with the 2009 main pandemic wave. Influenza encephalitis in adults is more likely in unvaccinated patients, and neurological symptoms appear few days into an influenza-like illness (Piet et al., 2017). Focal encephalitis of brainstem, both thalami or small cortical areas, and white-matter disease including ADEM, PRES (posterior reversible encephalopathy syndrome), and reversible splenial lesion syndrome, have appeared in recent case reports. Myositis, myopathy, and Reye syndrome are other complications. Recurrence of an unusual encephalopathy in a child, for example, characterized by diffuse gray matter restricted diffusion during Influenza A infection, may signify an inborn error of metabolism (maple syrup urine disease in this case) (Szuch and Auriemma, 2018).

Laboratory diagnosis of influenza is by detection of viral RNA by RT-PCR or by culture from nasopharyngeal specimens or endotracheal aspirates. Rapid influenza diagnostic tests, antigen detection assays for respiratory samples or swabs have an estimated 50%–70% sensitivity. In CNS cases, CSF pleocytosis is rare, and viral RNA has not been amplified from CSF.

Treatment in the United States is with the neuraminidase inhibitors oral oseltamivir (Tamiflu), inhaled zanamivir (Relenza), or IV peramivir (Rapivab). Treatment of 2009 H1N1 and seasonal H3N2 viruses in adults is oral oseltamivir, 75 mg twice daily for 5 days, increased to 150 mg twice daily in severe cases; or zanamivir, 10 mg (25-mg inhalations) twice daily for 5 days, or peramivir 600 mg IV once (CDC, 2010c). The benefit of oseltamivir has not been demonstrated for influenza encephalitis (Piet et al., 2017), and oseltamivir has neuropsychiatric side effects. Add-ons to antiviral treatment, pulse steroids and IVIG, have been used in children with encephalopathy/encephalitis, ADEM, or ANE (Chen et al., 2018) and pulse steroids used in an adult with ANE had a good outcome (Alsolami and Shiley, 2017). Xofluza is a newly approved single dose oral inhibitor of polymerase acidic endonuclease for influenza.

An association between swine influenza vaccination and Guillain-Barré syndrome was reported in 1976–1977, but no increase in risk for Guillain–Barré syndrome associated with influenza vaccination was found when evaluated during the 1992–1993 and 1993–1994 flu seasons. GCA has been reported with influenza vaccination (Piyasirisilp and Hemachudha, 2002). Multivalent seasonal and 2009 H1N1 influenza vaccination are effective at preventing illness, and recommended starting from 6 months of age.

## Covid-19

The worldwide pandemic of coronavirus disease (COVID19)) caused by Severe Acute Respiratory Syndrome-coronavirus-2 (SARDCoV2) has as of mid-September 2020 been responsible for over 30 million disease cases and nearly 1 million fatalities. The United States has the world's highest case number (>7 million cases) as well as the most recorded deaths (>200,000). Severe illness and death generally result from respiratory complications of SARSCoV2 infection, notably acute respiratory distress syndrome (ARDS), however, the neurological manifestations of COVID19 are an important source of morbidity and mortality (see Ellul et al., 2020; Iadecola et al., 2020; Koralnik & Tyler, 2020; Pezzini A & Padovani, 2020 for review). The exact frequency of neurological complications of COVID19 remain to be determined but appear to be common, especially in hospitalized and more severely ill patients. In a review of over 200 hospitalized patients with COVID19 in Wuhan China, 36% of cases had neurological signs and symptoms (Mao et al, 2020). In another study of patients hospitalized with COVID19-associated ARDS, 84% had neurological signs (Helms et al., 2020).

The major neurological manifestations of COVID19 can be broadly categorized into: (1) those reflecting the effects of systemic illness on the CNS, (2) direct viral invasion of the CNS including encephalitis, and (3) post-infectious presumably immune-mediated syndromes (Koralnik & Tyler, 2020).

The most common effect on the CNS of systemic COVID19 is the development of encephalopathy. This is typically characterized by altered mental status, agitation, and in some cases, a dysexecutive syndrome. It is seen most commonly in severely ill patients often with multi-organ system impairment that can include respiratory failure and hypoxemia, hepatic dysfunction, renal failure, and cardiac or hemodynamic impairment. Many patients have associated co-morbidities including diabetes and hypertension. Patients are often older and male, as these demographic factors are linked to risk of more severe disease. Patients frequently have very elevated markers of inflammation (e.g., HS-CRP, ESR, ferritin) and signs of systemic coagulopathy (e.g., elevated d-dimer). CSF examination is typically normal or may show a mild protein elevation. Virus is not detected in CSF by RT-PCR. The EEG shows either diffuse or anteriorly predominant slowing. MRI may be normal but, in more severe cases, can show diffuse white matter changes, and juxtacortical and callosal petechial micro-hemorrhages (Radmanesh et. al, 2020). It remains to be seen whether aspects of this syndrome are unique for COVID19 or merely reflect the severity and type of organ system dysfunction including the severe hypoxemia and need for prolonged mechanical ventilation.

Patients with COVID19 may develop or even present with acute cerebrovascular disease. Ischemic large vessel strokes, at times in multiple vascular territories, appear to be the most common manifestation, followed in order of decreasing frequency by intracerebral hemorrhage, venous infarctions, and, possibly, vasculitis. The frequency has been reported at between 1-6% in hospitalized patients with the higher percentages seen in more critically ill cases. The group at highest risk appears to be older and more severely ill patients. These individuals frequently have associated vascular disease risk factors including hypertension, diabetes, smoking, dyslipidemia and heart disease. Strokes often occur 1-3 weeks following the onset of COVID19 symptoms. The mechanism is likely due to thrombosis secondary to the associated hyper-coagulable state, and patients may have evidence of thrombosis in multiple organs including the lungs in addition to the CNS. In some reports there has been a high incidence of pro-thrombotic autoantibodies including lupus anticoagulant, anticardiolipin and anti-beta2-glycoprotein-1 antibodies (Beyrouti et al., 2020).

Not all patients with COVID19-associated strokes are older individuals with associated vascular risk factors. Stroke can also be the presenting manifestation of COVID19 in younger adults (Oxley, et al., 2020). These patients often do not have significant risk factors for stroke and may have only mild or even absent respiratory symptoms of COVID19. Like their older counterparts, the strokes frequently involve large vessel territories and patients often have elevated inflammatory markers and evidence of a pro-thrombotic state. Because SARSCoV2 can infect endothelial cells in the cerebral circulation, it has been suggested that endothelial injury may be another contributing factor to COVID-associated strokes, both in younger individuals and the elderly.

In contrast to neurological events that reflect the systemic disease process induced by SARSCoV2, there is also increasing evidence that the virus can be neuroinvasive and neurotropic. There have now been several reports in which patients develop focal neurological signs and symptoms with associated MRI abnormalities, a CSF lymphocytic pleocytosis, and a positive CSF RT-PCR for SARSCoV2 (Moriguichi, et al., 2020; Duong et al., 2020; Huang et al., 2020). In some cases, viral nucleic acid has been detected by RT-PCR in brain tissue when CSF RT-PCR studies have been negative (Paniz-Mondolfi et al., 2020). Coronavirus-like virion particles have also been described after electron microscopy in endothelial cells and neurons (Paniz-Mondolfi, et al., 2020). There are also reports of detection of SARSCoV2 neutralizing antibodies in CSF of patients and detection of viral antigen in cortical neurons by immunohistochemistry (Song et al., 2020).

Although cases of encephalitis due to direct viral infection have been documented, in a larger group of patients with encephalitis (e.g., focal neurological signs and symptoms, CSF pleocytosis, MRI abnormalities), CSF RT-PCR for SARSCoV2 has been negative. It is possible that this may reflect a lack of sensitivity of the CSF RT-PCR for detection of CNS virus, as at least one reported case had a negative CSF RT-PCR but a positive brain tissue RT-PCR (Paniz-Mondolfi et al., 2020). Some cases of encephalitis may also potentially result from the hyper-inflammatory state ("cytokine storm") or even development of autoantibodies as both elevated CSF pro-inflammatory cytokine and chemokine levels and autoantibodies (NMDAR antibody) have been reported in isolated cases.

In addition to the acute neurological manifestations resulting from effects of infection of the CNS or direct viral invasion, a large number of post-infectious immune mediated syndromes have been associated with COVID19. The most commonly reported post-infectious syndrome is Guillain-Barre Syndrome (GBS). Toscano and colleagues reported five such cases that occurred 5-10 days after CIOVID19 symptom onset (Toscano et al., 2020). The clinical manifestations included areflexia, flaccid paralysis and in some patients bifacial weakness and respiratory failure. Nerve conduction studies were consistent with the axonal form of GBS in three patients and the demyelinating form in two. CSF was normo-cellular and had a negative SARSCoV2 RT-PCR in all patients, with elevated CSF protein in three (albuminocytological dissociation). Although careful epidemiological studies have not yet been performed the large number of reports of GBS in close temporal association with COVID19 make it seem likely that there is a causal association, but the magnitude of the risk remains to be determined.

In addition to GBS and its variants, there have also been several reports of clinical, radiographic, and neuropathological findings consistent with a COVID19-associated acute disseminated encephalomyelitis (ADEM) (Reichard et al., 2020). In some cases the imaging or neuropathology has also shown associated microhemorrhages in addition to demyelination. Several case reports of acute necrotizing encephalopathy (ANE) following COVID19 have also appeared (Poyiadji et. al., 2020). Patients with ANE typically present with rapid deterioration in mental status with seizures and hyper-reflexia. MRI shows a striking pattern of bilateral medial thalamic signal intensity, at times with involvement of the insula, basal ganglia and brainstem. The mechanism of this syndrome remains uncertain, but it has been associated previously with other respiratory infections including influenza.

Some types of COVID19 associated neurological signs and symptoms currently have an uncertain pathogenesis. Loss, reduction, or perturbations of taste and/or smell have been commonly reported in many COVID19 patients. In one European study olfactory dysfunction was reported in 86% of examined cases (80% with anosmia, 20% with hyposmia). (Lechien et al., 2020). The mechanism remains unclear, as olfactory neurons lack the human ACE2 receptor for SARSCoV2, making their infection and injury unlikely. Infection of nasal epithelial cells with associated dysfunction of the interspersed neurons may be a more likely mechanism. 67-73% of cases in one series recovered within 8 days of onset, also arguing against neuronal injury which would have been expected to induce more long-lasting dysfunction. Muscle injury characterized by pain and elevated muscle enzymes have been reported in 10% of hospitalized patients and up to 20% of those with more severe disease (Mao et al., 2020) but the mechanism remains unclear.

Treatment of COVID19 associated neurological manifestations generally parallels those utilized for the underlying disease process in non-COVID19 settings. For example, patients with acute strokes have been treated with clot retrieval and clot lysis or anti-coagulant therapy. GBS cases have received plasmapheresis or intravenous immunoglobulin, and patients with ADEM-like syndromes corticosteroids. It remains to be determined whether these therapies are as efficacious in COVID-19 associated disease as in other settings, or whether specific modifications or preferential treatments should be made in COVID19 patients. Recent studies of patients with more severe COVID19 have suggested beneficial effects of corticosteroids and remdesevir but have failed to show a significant benefit for chloroquine or hydroxychloroquine. Large scale studies of the use of convalescent plasma are also underway, but no randomized controlled data on efficacy are yet available. A trial of an anti-SARSCoV2 humanized monoclonal antibody cocktail has also shown promising results in initial early phase studies, with larger advanced phase trials planned. It remains to be seen whether these treatments have specific roles in COVID19-associated neurological disease settings. Obviously, disease prevention strategies would result in associated reduction in risk of neurological disease. Several vaccine candidates have now advanced to Phase III trials, with efficacy data expected to be available for some trials before the end of 2020.

## Arenaviruses

Arenaviruses are rodent-borne viruses, with human infection usually occurring through exposure to rodent excreta. An estimated 5% of house mice in the United States carry lymphocytic choriomeningitis virus (LCMV). Person-to-person transmission has occurred as maternal-fetal transmission or solid-organ transplantation for LCMV, or contact with blood or body fluids for the other arenaviruses. The arenaviruses of neurological consequence are LCMV, Lassa fever, and Argentine hemorrhagic fever viruses.

LCMV causes CNS disease that varies from meningitis to severe encephalomyelitis. Although usually causing aseptic meningitis, 5%–34% of serologically confirmed LCMV CNS cases have been diagnosed as encephalitis. CSF cell counts in excess of the 10–500 WBC/μL range usually seen in viral meningitis may be present with LCMV. Ascending or transverse myelitis, bulbar syndromes, parkinsonism, sensorineural hearing loss, and hydrocephalus as sequelae of ependymitis or ventriculitis have been reported. LCMV infection of the fetus has produced hydrocephalus, diffuse parenchymal disease, mental retardation, chorioretinitis, and congenital microcephaly. The incidence of congenital LCMV is unknown (Bonthius, 2012).

Four times in the past decade in the United States, and a fifth time worldwide, groups of solid-organ transplant recipients have developed severe LCMV disease, characterized by encephalopathy, coagulopathy, thrombocytopenia, fever, and leukocytosis. Outcomes varied. A single survivor out of the first three clusters (10 cases) had received ribavirin and reduction of immunosuppression. Two of four recipients in the fourth cluster survived without specific antiviral treatment (MacNeil et al., 2012).

Argentine hemorrhagic fever has been associated with an acute encephalitic syndrome with tremor, seizures and coma, acute- and convalescent-phase ataxia, and a late neurological syndrome of cerebellar ataxia, oculomotor disorder and cranial nerve palsies after immune plasma treatment.

Lassa fever, a West African viral hemorrhagic fever with high mortality (20%–55% of hospitalized cases), is a multisystem disease with fever, pharyngitis, hemorrhage, hepatic involvement, and shock, plus neurological syndromes in 40% of hospitalized patients. One-third of all patients with Lassa fever develop hearing impairments, two-thirds of whom are left with significant sensorineural hearing loss. Encephalitis with seizures, depressed consciousness, amnesic syndromes, dystonia or tremor, convalescent ataxic syndromes, and neuropsychiatric sequelae have been described. Imported cases are seen in Europe, North America, Asia, and Australia. The first report of a secondary case following import to a non-endemic country was in Germany in 2016 (Ehlkes et al., 2017).

Arenavirus diagnosis is by RT-PCR of acute serum or CSF, serology, or viral culture in specialized labs. IgM antibody to LCMV is present in serum, CSF, or both during acute meningitis. CSF may be positive for Lassa fever virus by RT-PCR in encephalitis/encephalopathy cases and rarely, virus has been cultured from CSF. Lassa fever is treated with IV ribavirin administered as a 2-g loading dose, followed by 1 g every 6 hours for 4 days, then 0.5 g three times daily for 6 additional days or per manufacturers protocol. WHO presented a similar regimen in 2004: loading dose 17 mg/kg (max 1 g per dose) or 30 mg/kg (max 2 g) if treatment were delayed, followed by 17 mg/kg IV (max 1 g per dose) every 6 hours for 4 days, followed by 8 mg/kg IV (max 500 mg per dose) every 8 hours for 6 days (WHO 2004). Oral ribavirin is available through the CDC (Atlanta, Georgia) for the prophylaxis of contacts. Year 2017 was the first time the broad-spectrum antiviral favipiravir, licensed for influenza in Japan, was added to ribavirin for treating Lassa fever (as oral favipiravir 2000-mg loading dose followed by 1200 mg twice daily for 4 days (De Clercq, 2012) (Raabe et al., 2017).

## Other Hemorrhagic Fever Viruses

### Arboviral Agents of Hemorrhagic Fevers

***Dengue (Flavivirus).*** For size of epidemics, with an estimated 400 million people infected each year, and severity of disease, dengue fever and dengue hemorrhagic fever are the most important arthropod-borne viral diseases of humans. Dengue virus, having lost its requirement for enzootic amplification, cycles between humans and mosquitoes and causes extensive epidemics in tropical urban centers. *Aedes aegypti*, the most important vector, is a mosquito that has evolved to live in proximity to humans and breeds well in manufactured throwaway containers holding stagnant water. The expansion of *A. aegypti* throughout the Americas and the inadvertent import of another competent vector, *Aedes albopictus*, to the United States and Brazil from Asia have established dengue on all continents with tropical and subtropical areas. Dengue fever outbreaks in the United States since 2001 have been in Hawaii (2001), Brownsville, Texas (2005) and south Florida (2009–2011). Today, one in six tourists returning from the tropics is likely infected with dengue (Solbrig and Perng, 2015).

Dengue fever is a fever-rash-arthralgia syndrome with a 2- to 7-day incubation period. Dengue hemorrhagic fever is the severe form of disease, occurring in persons (usually children) previously sensitized by infection with a heterologous dengue serotype through antibody-dependent enhancement.

Neurological complications range from 0.5% to 18%. Dengue, as pure (self-limited, classic) dengue fever or dengue hemorrhagic fever, causes meningitis, meningoencephalitis, bitemporal encephalitis, thalamic, basal ganglia, or corpus callosum lesions, rhombencephalitis, hemorrhagic encephalitis, opsoclonus-myoclonus, cerebellitis, myelitis, acute polyradiculoneuritis, CN palsy, ADEM, retinochoroiditis, retinal vasculopathy, subdural hematoma, ischemic or hemorrhagic stroke, encephalopathy, cerebral edema, Reye syndrome, cortical laminar necrosis, or reversible splenial lesions (Solomon et al., 2000; Sreedharan et al., 2011; Wasay et al., 2008; Yeo et al., 2005; Borawake et al., 2011; Kamble et al., 2007). Peripheral syndromes associated with dengue are: Guillain-Barré, acute motor sensory axonal neuropathy, brachial plexitis, mononeuritis multiplex, hypokalemic quadriparesis or plegia, diaphragmatic paralysis, and myositis (Jha and Ansari 2010; Sharma et al., 2011). Convalescent or recurring immune-mediated syndromes include Miller-Fisher variant Guillain-Barré (Carod-Artal et al., 2013; Puccioni-Sohler et al., 2013), and neuromyelitis optica (NMO)-like illnesses: aquaporin-4 negative neuromyelitis optica spectrum disorders. Single case reports of steroid-responsive syndromes are: an optic-spinal syndrome in a child of Japanese ancestry (deSouza et al., 2006) and brainstem and transverse myelitis associated with persistent DENV infection (Puccioni-Sohler et al., 2017).

Diagnosis is by virus isolation, RT-PCR of serum in the early viremic stages, or serology, CNS cases may have laboratory evidence of DENV in CSF by viral isolation, RT-PCR, NS1 Ag, or IgM detection. CSF usually contains few (<30) or no WBCs. Care is supportive, and salicylates are contraindicated because of the risk of hemorrhagic exacerbation and Reye syndrome. Numbers of severe or complicated CNS cases may increase due to expansion of other arboviruses, such as Chikungunya and Zika, associated with neurological disease in the same geographic areas. Of the flaviviruses, ZIKV is most closely related to the 4 serotypes of DENV. The similarity presents problems for diagnosis, and has implications for disease augmentation or possibly mitigation, from antibody cross-reactivity.

A universal vaccine that includes all four serotypes of dengue, Sanofi Pasteur (CYD-TDV) (Dengvaxia) vaccine, is licensed with an indication for use in individuals aged 9 years and older. There are certain qualifications for use, described in WHO publications (Imai and Ferguson, 2018; WHO 2018).

***Yellow fever (Flavivirus).*** YF is a viral disease in tropical South America and sub-Saharan Africa, principally affecting humans and nonhuman primates and spread by the bite of infected mosquitoes. The risk of YF returning to the Americas to produce large urban epidemics has increased, owing to large numbers of susceptible people and successful expansion of the host range of the mosquito vector, *A. aegypti*. The 17D vaccines have been widely accepted as one of the safest vaccines in use. Vaccination with YF 17D strain, a live attenuated viral vaccine developed by the WHO, has been associated with rare encephalitis cases in infants (within 30 days of immunization). Viscerotropic adverse events, multisystem illnesses, and death following YF vaccination have been reported, and because of the risk of encephalitis, the vaccine is contraindicated for infants younger than 6 months of age. WHO advises vaccination for all individuals greater than 9 months living in countries or areas at risk, except pregnant women and breastfeeding mothers, and vaccination of at-risk laboratory personnel (Staples et al., 2010; Thomas et al., 2011). The World Health Assembly adopted the recommendation to remove the 10-year booster dose requirement from International Health Regulations by June 2016 (World Health Organization, 2014).

Pharmacovigilance databases provide estimates of YF vaccine-associated neurological disease ranging from 0 to 7.8 cases per million vaccinated, with the highest rate in people over 60 years of age. Illness is 1–30 days after vaccination with meningoencephalitis, ADE, Guillain-Barré, myelitis, bulbar or Bell's palsy and detection of YFV-specific IgM antibodies in CSF (Pires-Marczeski et al., 2011). A French vaccine produced from infected mouse brains associated with a 1% incidence of postvaccinal encephalitis is no longer manufactured.

***Filoviruses.*** Additional text is available online at http://expertconsult.inkling.com.

***Filoviruses.*** Ebola and Marburg viruses, members of the family Filoviridae and genus Ebolavirus or Marburgvirus, cause severe or fatal viral hemorrhagic fever in humans and nonhuman primates. Species of Ebolavirus pathogenic for man are Zaire ebolavirus, Sudan ebolavirus, Tai Forest ebolavirus, and Bundibugyo ebolavirus.

Spread of filovirus infections is by direct contact with infected animals, close contact with another case through body fluid contact, or in the case of Ebola, sexual contact with a recovered patient up to months after hospital discharge. Natural reservoirs for Ebola and Marburg viruses are fruit and insectivorous bats (Leroy et al., 2005; Mari Saez et al., 2015). Both viruses are characterized by highly efficient replication in liver, spleen, lymph nodes, gastrointestinal tract, and lung, leading to fulminating hemorrhagic fever with shock and high mortality.

Filovirus disease, as Marburg Disease, was first recognized in Marburg Germany in 1967 in laboratory workers who had handled monkey blood, tissues, or cell cultures from African green (vervet) monkeys from Uganda. Neuropathy, restless legs, psychosis, amnesia, depression, and fatigue (Martini 1971) were found in survivors, and live virus was recovered from the anterior chamber of the eye of a uveitis patient 2 months after recovery (Gear et al., 1975).

The geographic range of known Ebola human cases has included most of the African rain forest. The severe Ebola epidemic of West Africa (2013–2016) caused by Zaire-Ebolavirus was thought to start with a single zoonotic transmission event from an insectivorous bat to a 2-year-old boy. Human-to-human transmission followed (Mari Saez et al., 2015).

Prior to the 2013–2016 West Africa epidemic, with its 28,616 cases and 11,310 deaths, there had been 2317 human clinical infections and 1671 confirmed deaths caused by Ebola-Zaire and Ebola-Sudan since Ebola viruses (EBOV) were first identified in 1976 in the 2 countries.

EBOV can infect the CNS during acute infection causing encephalitis or behavior changes, associated with +CSF EBOV RT-PCR (Sagui et al., 2015; de Greslan et al., 2016); delirium, myoclonus, eye movement changes, and multiple foci of small lesions in white matter and around the fourth ventricle on MRI (Chertow et al., 2016); a delayed encephalitis (day 14–40 of illness) with +CSF and negative serum EBOV PCR (Howlett et al., 2016); and late Ebola relapse causing meningoencephalitis and radiculitis with infectious virus in CSF 9 months after initial treatment and recovery (Jacobs et al., 2016).

"Post-Ebola syndromes," the spectrum of diseases in survivors, include headache, long-term neurological and psychiatric sequelae, and visual and hearing losses (Howlett et al., 2018). Visual changes are from uveitis or a novel retinal lesion of pale peripapillary lesions that may represent spread of virus along retinal ganglion cell axons (Steptoe et al., 2017). Viral persistence in CNS, eye, semen, and urine cause public health concern.

Rapid diagnostic testing of blood using RT-PCR nucleic acid amplification tests are deployed through portable labs to health centers in an outbreak. Between 2014 and 2016, patients in the United States and Europe were treated with: ZMapp, a cocktail of three humanized monoclonal antibodies against EBOV glycoprotein; Gilead's GS-5734, a nucleoside inhibitor; favipiravir; brincidofovir; TKM-Ebola small interfering RNA; and passive immune therapy (blood or plasma from convalescent patients). The US Food and Drug Association and drug manufacturers have up-to-date information on availability and use of new therapies. Merck's recombinant vesicular stomatitis virus (rVSV) ebola virus vaccine (ZEBOV) vaccine, which halted the spread of Ebola in Guinea, was offered to international responders, local health care personnel, and contacts of Ebola patients in the Democratic Republic of Congo's 2018 Ebola epidemic prior to licensing.

## Hepatitis Viruses

The viral causes of hepatitis are hepatitis A, B, C, D (delta), and E viruses. Hepatitis B has been associated with vasculitis, cryoglobulinemia, polyarteritis nodosa, and myelitis, and post-vaccination ADEM with hepatitis B vaccination. Hepatitis C virus (HCV), causing chronic infection and complex immune responses in patients, has the potential to cause neurological illness both by direct infection (Wilkinson et al., 2009) and by immune-mediated and enhanced autoimmune responses. Extrahepatic manifestations of HCV are stroke (accelerated atherosclerotic or inflammatory vascular disease with or without cryoglobulins and antiphospholipid antibodies), encephalitis, immune-mediated demyelinating disease, myelitis, NMO antibody disease, neuropsychiatric disorders, cranial and peripheral nerve disorders (associated with cryoglobulin, vasculitic, or gammaglobulin diseases), and polymyositis (McCarthy and Ortega, 2012). Ribavirin plus interferon-alfa and direct-acting antivirals, telaprevir or boceprevir, treat liver and renal disease. Complications of interferon alfa treatment include exacerbation of autoimmunity, manifest as neuromuscular, CNS demyelinating, and neuropsychiatric disorders. Depression, a common complication of treatment with interferon alfa, is treated with selective serotonin reuptake inhiitor (SSRI). Plasma exchange may benefit patients whose neuropathy is worsened by interferon alfa. Intracerebral hemorrhage is a complication of combination therapy (standard or pegylated interferon alfa-2b and ribavirin) in patients with chronic hepatitis C who may or may not have additional risk factors such as hypertension and diabetes (Nishiofuku et al., 2006). HCV/HIV co-infections may adversely affect performance on neurocognitive tests compared to HIV alone (Winston et al., 2010), particularly if both infections are untreated or poorly controlled (Ryan et al., 2004). Alternatively, HCV infection may not impact performance of patients with virologically controlled HIV infection (Clifford et al., 2009).

*The complete reference list is available online at https://expertconsult.inkling.com/.*

# Bacterial, Fungal, and Parasitic Diseases of the Nervous System

*Nicolaas C. Anderson, Anita A. Koshy, Karen L. Roos*

## OUTLINE



Prior to the modern antimicrobial era, non-viral infections of the central nervous system (CNS) were almost universally fatal. The diagnosis and treatment of CNS infections have improved significantly with advancements made in spinal fluid diagnostic tests, neuroimaging, antimicrobial therapy, and neurosurgical techniques. Despite these advancements, diagnosing CNS infections can be difficult, and a delay in diagnosis and treatment can lead to increased morbidity and mortality. Thus, it is important to quickly recognize when CNS infections are high on the differential diagnosis.

When considering an infectious cause of a CNS disorder, it is important to know predisposing conditions for infection, including geographic residence, travel history, occupational and recreational activities, recent sinus or middle ear infections, chronic medical illnesses, vaccination history, and the patient's immune status. In general, the immunocompromised will be susceptible to the same organisms as the immunocompetent but will also be susceptible to organisms that are rarely or never seen in the immunocompetent host. In addition, clinical manifestations in immunocompromised patients may be subtle or even absent as they may not generate a brisk immune response to the pathogen. Thus, the differential must always be broader and the bar lower for starting empirical treatment in these patients. The immune status of a patient is particularly important when considering fungal and parasitic diseases.

## BACTERIAL INFECTIONS OF THE CENTRAL NERVOUS SYSTEM

Bacteria are prokaryotic organisms that colonize all human mucosal and skin surfaces. Only rarely are bacteria pathogenic. The pathogenic bacteria that cause CNS infections can be acquired in a variety of ways, including simple colonization via oral and nasal secretions that becomes invasive *(Streptococcus pneumoniae, Neisseria meningitidis)*, via contaminated food *(Listeria monocytogenes)*, as a complication of a systemic infection, from a neurosurgical procedure, or via a contiguous focus of infection (skin, sinuses, or middle ear infections). Most pathogenic bacteria have virulence factors that partially explain why they cause disease, but various host factors (low immunoglobulin levels, impaired T-cell immunity, complement deficiencies) also play a role.

### Meningitis

#### Etiology

Bacterial meningitis can be divided into acute bacterial meningitis and chronic meningitis. *S. pneumoniae* and *N. meningitidis* are the most common causes of community-acquired acute bacterial meningitis. In mastoiditis-associated meningitis, sinusitis, or otitis media, anaerobes often play a role. *S. pneumoniae* and *N. meningitidis* colonize the nasopharyngeal mucosa, which provides a route of entry for these bacteria. *L. monocytogenes* is usually acquired via contaminated food.

Historically, children had the highest incidence of meningitis. However, with the development of an extremely effective *Haemophilus influenzae* type b (Hib) vaccine, adults now have the highest incidence of meningitis in developed countries. The *S. pneumoniae* vaccine has also decreased the incidence of meningitis in children by decreasing the incidence of otitis media (Thigpen et al., 2011). Though an absolute increase in the number of cases of *H. influenzae* non-b and *S. pneumoniae* serotypes not in the vaccine ("replacement phenomena") has been seen, this increase in absolute number is small (Bender et al., 2010). The incidence of meningitis due to *N. meningitidis* has decreased with the tetravalent (serogroups A, C, W-135, and Y) meningococcal glycoconjugate vaccine, but the vaccine does not provide lasting immunity and does not include one of the major serotypes, serotype B. Vaccination against serogroup B is a separate vaccine, the MenB vaccine (MMWR, 2017), and has become part of the required vaccination schedule for students matriculating at most American universities. *L. monocytogenes* accounts for approximately 8% of acute bacterial meningitis cases and is an uncommon cause of meningitis in healthy children and adults. The most common predisposing factors for *L. monocytogenes* meningitis are age older than 50, diabetes, chronic illness, malignancy, and immunosuppressive therapy or an immunosuppressed state.

Subacute or chronic meningitis is caused by a more diverse group of organisms, and more typically by fungi than bacteria, with the exception of *Mycobacterium tuberculosis*. Given its endemicity around the world, *M. tuberculosis* is the leading cause of chronic

**TABLE 79.1 Bacterial Meningeal Pathogens and Their Diagnostic Tests**

| Organism | Blood | Cerebrospinal Fluid |
|---|---|---|
| *Streptococcus pneumoniae* | Culture | Gram stain: gram-positive diplococci in pairs<br>Culture<br>Meningitis/encephalitis panel |
| *Listeria monocytogenes* | Culture | Gram stain: gram-positive rods<br>Culture<br>Meningitis/encephalitis panel |
| *Neisseria meningitides* | Culture | Gram stain: gram-negative diplococcus<br>Culture |
| *Haemophilus influenzae* type b | Culture | Gram stain: gram-negative coccobacillus<br>Culture<br>Meningitis/encephalitis panel |
| *Mycobacterium tuberculosis* | | 20–30 mL for AFB stain and culture; PCR |
| *Treponema pallidum* | RPR/VDRL; MHA-TPA; FTA-ABS; TPPA | VDRL (nontraumatic tap) |
| *Coxiella burnetii* | Acute and convalescent serologies | |
| *Brucella* spp. | Culture: acute and convalescent serologies | Gram stain: gram-negative coccobacillus<br>Culture |
| *Borrelia* spp. | ELISA→if equivocal or +, then IgG and IgM WB (follow CDC guidelines for + WB) | Antibody index: anti-*Borrelia* IgG in CSF/anti-*Borrelia* IgG in serum to total IgG in CSF/total IgG in serum |
| *Leptospira* spp. | Acute and convalescent serologies (MAT only done in reference labs, ELISA and lateral flow dipstick less sensitive and specific)<br>Culture: special media; may need to keep for 8–12 wk | Culture: Special media, fastidious |

*AFB,* Acid-fast bacilli; *CDC,* Centers for Disease Control and Prevention; *CSF,* cerebrospinal fluid; *ELISA,* enzyme-linked immunosorbent assay; *FTA-ABS,* fluorescent treponemal antibody absorbed; *Ig,* immunoglobulin; *MAT,* microscopic agglutination test; *MHA-TPA,* microhemagglutination assay–*Treponema* antibody absorption test; *PCR,* polymerase chain reaction; *RPR,* rapid plasma reagin test; *TPPA, Treponema pallidum* particle agglutination; *VDRL,* Venereal Disease Research Laboratory test; *WB,* Western blot test.

bacterial meningitis worldwide. At the present time, *Treponema pallidum*, the causative agent of neurosyphilis, typically causes a meningitis or a meningovasculitis and less often tabes dorsalis or dementia. Other bacterial etiological agents of chronic meningitis include nontuberculous mycobacteria, *Coxiella burnetii*, *Brucella* spp., *Leptospira* spp., *Francisella tularensis*, *Actinomyces* spp., *Ehrlichia chaffeensis*, and *Anaplasma phagocytophilum*.

Table 79.1 lists the most common bacterial causes of acute or chronic meningitis and diagnostic tests for identifying different organisms.

## Clinical Presentation

The classic symptoms of acute bacterial meningitis are fever, headache, meningismus, and a progressive decrease in the level of consciousness. In a study that evaluated the symptoms in 666 episodes of meningitis in adults, headache was the most common complaint (87%), followed by neck stiffness (83%), fever (77%), and altered mental status (69%). While no single symptom is particularly sensitive or specific, 95% of the patients had two of the four symptoms and only 1% had none. A petechial rash can be present, especially when *N. meningitidis* is the causative agent, although *S. pneumoniae* can produce a similar rash (van de Beek et al., 2004). In immunocompromised patients, fever and meningismus may not be present.

Chronic bacterial meningitis presents more subtly than acute meningitis and is defined as symptoms of meningeal inflammation lasting longer than 4 weeks. Symptoms of chronic bacterial meningitis include insidious new headache with or without mild neck stiffness, low-grade fever, and night sweats. Often, it is not until the patient presents with a focal neurological finding, such as cranial nerve palsies, that the syndrome is recognized.

Neurosyphilis typically presents with signs and symptoms of meningitis (meningeal signs, cranial nerve palsies) or meningovasculitis (focal neurological deficits/stroke).

## Diagnosis

The diagnosis of acute bacterial meningitis depends on recognizing the clinical picture as one consistent with acute meningitis and performing a lumbar puncture (LP) to evaluate for meningeal inflammation and bacteria. Brain imaging prior to LP is recommended in patients with any of the following: altered level of consciousness, focal neurological deficits, new-onset seizures, papilledema (or other signs of increased intracranial pressure), or an immunocompromised state. The utility of imaging is twofold: (1) to evaluate for focal mass lesions and edema that put the patient at risk for uncal herniation, and (2) to find those diseases that might mimic acute bacterial meningitis but in fact are quite distinct (bacterial abscess, tumor). The imaging modality to use in such patients is computed tomography (CT), which can be done quickly and is sensitive enough to rule out lesions that predispose patients to herniation. Non-contrast imaging may show no abnormality while postcontrast images will often show diffuse meningeal enhancement. If head imaging before LP is appropriate, and acute bacterial meningitis is high in the differential, obtaining blood cultures and beginning empirical antibiotics before the patient is sent for imaging is essential. Starting empirical antibiotics quickly is critical because there is burgeoning evidence that delays in initiating antibiotic treatment for bacterial meningitis lead to increased morbidity and mortality (Auburtin et al., 2006; Proulx et al., 2005). If antibiotics are not initiated prior to imaging, it is also clear that imaging prior to LP significantly delays the time to antibiotics (Proulx et al., 2005).

The gold standard for the diagnosis of bacterial meningitis is identification of the meningeal pathogen on Gram stain and/or culture of

TABLE 79.2 **Empiric and Specific Antibiotics for Bacterial Infections of the Central Nervous System**

| Disease Entity | Organisms | Antibiotics |
|---|---|---|
| Acute bacterial meningitis: | | |
| Age <50 and no risk factors for *Listeria* | *Streptococcus pneumoniae, Neisseria meningitidis* | Vancomycin + ceftriaxone *or* cefotaxime *or* cefepime |
| Age >50 and/or risk factors for *Listeria* | As above + *Listeria monocytogenes* | As above + ampicillin |
| Sinusitis, mastoiditis, or otitis predisposing cause of meningitis | As above (depending on age and risk factors) + anaerobes | As above (depending on age and risk factors) + metronidazole |
| Brain abscess | *Staphylococcus aureus*, aerobic and anaerobic streptococci, oral and gastrointestinal flora (including *Bacteroides* spp.) | Vancomycin + ceftriaxone *or* cefotaxime *or* cefepime+ metronidazole |
| | *Nocardia* | Trimethoprim-sulfamethoxazole |
| Spinal epidural abscess (SEA) | *Staphylococcal* spp., *Streptococcal* spp., enteric gram-negative bacilli | Vancomycin + ceftriaxone *or* cefotaxime *or* cefepime |
| Chronic meningitis or SEA | *Mycobacterium tuberculosis* (high suspicion) | Four-drug therapy (isoniazid, rifampin, ethambutol, pyrazinamide) |
| Neurosyphilis | *Treponema pallidum* | Intravenous aqueous crystalline penicillin G |

cerebrospinal fluid (CSF). Cultures may take 48–72 hours to be positive. The organism may also be cultured from blood. Newer diagnostic techniques include polymerase chain reaction (PCR) assays; the Meningitis/Encephalitis panel has the advantage of both being sensitive and having a rapid turnaround rate (Liesman et al., 2018). The Meningitis/Encephalitis panel can detect the DNA of 14 pathogens, 6 of which are bacteria. The bacteria included in this panel are *S. pneumoniae, N. meningitidis, H. influenzae, L. monocytogenes, Escherichia coli and Streptococcus agalactiae.* The advantage to PCR-based diagnostics is rapid turnaround, but the disadvantages are that these tests are not routinely available, and antibiotic sensitivity data, which are essential, can only be obtained from culture. Thus, in many hospitals, Gram stain and culture remain the best tools for diagnosing bacterial meningitis.

The CSF cell count, and protein and glucose concentrations, can be helpful in differentiating bacterial meningitis from viral meningitis. In general, the classic CSF abnormalities in bacterial meningitis are pleocytosis with a predominance of neutrophils, mild to moderate increase in protein concentration, and decreased glucose concentration (or low CSF/serum glucose ratio, usually ≤0.3.) The classic CSF abnormalities in viral meningitis are a pleocytosis with a lymphocytic predominance, normal to mild elevation in protein concentration, and normal glucose concentration and CSF/serum glucose ratio.

The diagnosis of chronic infectious meningitis is much more complicated and has a broad differential whose specific etiology will often require extensive testing. LP is important in documenting meningeal inflammation, although if there are clinical signs or symptoms consistent with increased intracranial pressure, neuroimaging should be done prior to LP. To identify the cause of chronic meningitis, repeat high-volume CSF cultures or testing may be necessary. In addition, obtaining CSF from a site close to abnormalities on neuroimaging, including cervical punctures, may increase yield. These same principles hold true for accurately diagnosing *carcinomatous meningitis*, which can be clinically indistinguishable from chronic bacterial meningitis. Neoplastic leptomeningeal metastasis is discussed at length in Chapter 76.

Magnetic resonance imaging (MRI) with and without contrast is the neuroimaging study of choice because of increased sensitivity compared to CT and the decreased urgency to start empirical treatment and obtain CSF for diagnostic studies. Depending on the CSF abnormalities, certain etiologies may be more or less likely. For example, a mononuclear predominance with a mildly decreased glucose concentration and increased protein concentration suggests tuberculous meningitis, while a CSF pleocytosis with a mononuclear predominance and a normal glucose concentration and either a normal or mildly elevated protein concentration is more consistent with neurosyphilis. To distinguish between these two possibilities, send serum and CSF tests for syphilis (see Table 79.1) and high-volume CSF acid-fast bacilli smear, culture, and PCR for *M. tuberculosis.*

The diagnosis of neurosyphilis is based on either a positive CSF Venereal Disease Research Laboratory (VDRL) test or a combination of a CSF pleocytosis with an elevated protein concentration in a patient with symptoms suggestive of neurosyphilis and a positive serological test (rapid plasma reagin [RPR], VDRL, fluorescent treponemal antibody–absorbed [FTA-ABS], or *Treponema pallidum* particle agglutination [TPPA]).

### Management

Bacterial meningitis is treated initially with empirical antibiotics, which can be narrowed once the specific organism and its antibiotic sensitivities have been determined. Choosing the appropriate empirical regimen depends on the likely organism, which is dependent upon the patient's age and risk factors. Table 79.2 identifies which antibiotics should be used for specific patient populations, and Table 79.3 lists the recommended CNS dosing for these antibiotics. Antibiotic therapy is modified when the antimicrobial sensitivity tests results are available.

Early treatment with dexamethasone before or with the first dose of antibiotics has been shown to improve outcomes in patients with bacterial meningitis. In 2002, a landmark prospective double-blinded, placebo-controlled randomized study showed that adjunctive dexamethasone at the time of initiation of empirical antibiotics significantly improved the overall mortality and morbidity of those with bacterial meningitis. Subgroup analysis showed that all mortality and morbidity benefits were derived from the group that had *S. pneumoniae* meningitis (de Gans et al., 2002). This was followed by evidence that the nationwide implementation of dexamethasone for pneumococcal meningitis led to a decline in fatality rates (Brouwer et al., 2010). Thus, the current recommendations are to initiate dexamethasone just before or with the administration of empirical antibiotics. A favorable trend for reduced rates of death and hearing loss has been demonstrated for dexamethasone therapy in patients with meningococcal meningitis (Heckenberg et al., 2012). Based on animal model data, there was concern that the addition of steroids to empirical antibiotics would decrease the CSF concentration of vancomycin, leading to undertreatment of penicillin-resistant *S. pneumoniae* meningitis, an issue not addressed by the 2002 study, as all of their isolates were penicillin-sensitive. A study in 2007 prospectively evaluated the CSF vancomycin concentration in patients with suspected *S. pneumoniae* meningitis who were placed on empirical antibiotics and dexamethasone. Over half of this group had penicillin-resistant *S. pneumoniae*, and all had CSF vancomycin concentrations at least fourfold higher than the minimum inhibitory concentration (MIC) of the cultured organism. On repeat LP, none of the patients had positive *S. pneumoniae* cultures, and the CSF vancomycin levels were proportional to the serum vancomycin levels (Ricard et al., 2007). Thus, it appears that concurrent administration of dexamethasone does not decrease vancomycin CSF penetration in a clinically significant manner and that in these patients, serum vancomycin levels are similarly related to the CSF concentration, as in patients without concomitant dexamethasone.

The management of chronic bacterial meningitis is highly dependent on the organism isolated. Antibiotics are important in all cases, but the appropriate antibiotic(s), length of therapy, and adjunctive use of corticosteroids are all dependent upon the etiology.

## Brain Abscess

Brain abscess has become much less frequent in the post-antibiotic era where otitis media rarely goes untreated or becomes a chronic process. Though fewer abscesses occur now, contiguous infections still make up a considerable proportion of the group; while neurosurgical procedures and trauma also account for a significant proportion of cases. Other risk factors include bacterial endocarditis, diabetes, immunosuppression (alcohol, immunosuppressive drugs), and vascular abnormalities (congenital heart disease, hereditary hemorrhagic telangiectasia). The most commonly isolated bacteria are related to the source of infection and include aerobic and anaerobic streptococci, staphylococci, *Bacteroides* spp., Enterobacteriaceae, and anaerobic organisms. In endemic areas or in patients who have moved from endemic areas, tuberculomas and cysticercosis are also in the differential diagnosis. In immunocompromised patients, *Nocardia* spp. and *Rhodococcus equi* become possible etiologies, especially in those with a concomitant lung infection.

**TABLE 79.3 Central Nervous System Dosages for Commonly Used Antibiotics**

| Drug | Dose (Adult, Assuming a Normal Creatinine Clearance) |
|---|---|
| Vancomycin | 40–60 mg/kg/day, divided into q 8-12 h dosing |
| Ceftriaxone | 2 g, q 12 h |
| Cefepime | 2 g, q 8 h |
| Cefotaxime | 2 g, q 4–6 h |
| Ampicillin | 2 g, q 4 h |
| Metronidazole | 500 mg, q 6 h |
| Aqueous penicillin G | 18–24 million U/day |

### Clinical Presentation

Most patients with brain abscess will present with the signs and symptoms of a space-occupying lesion, such as headache. They may also present with confusion, alterations in consciousness, seizure, or focal neurological deficits. Fever occurs in fewer than half of patients with brain abscess (Carpenter et al., 2007) and should not be used to exclude brain abscess from the differential diagnosis. As in any space-occupying lesion, progressive nausea and vomiting can be seen as the mass expands and intracranial pressure increases. There are no signs or symptoms that definitively exclude or prove bacterial brain abscess in a patient presenting with a space-occupying lesion.

### Diagnosis

CNS imaging has highly improved the ability to diagnose bacterial brain abscesses and thus decreased mortality from 20%-50% to less than 20% in most modern series (Seydoux and Francioli, 1992). Every patient with a suspected brain abscess needs timely contrast-enhanced brain imaging. As seen in Fig. 79.1, the contrast imaging will often show a ring-enhancing mass. Although blood cultures are usually negative, positive cultures, which occur most often in the setting of hematogenous dissemination, can be helpful. Predisposing factors such as otitis media or sinusitis can suggest the likely etiology, but definitive diagnosis requires either a culture from another source (e.g., sputum in disseminated tuberculosis) or directly from the abscess itself. Given the improvements in neurosurgical techniques, including stereotactic aspiration, the ability to treat and definitively diagnose the etiological agent of the abscess has greatly improved. If the patient is stable from a hemodynamic and neurological standpoint, and stereotactic

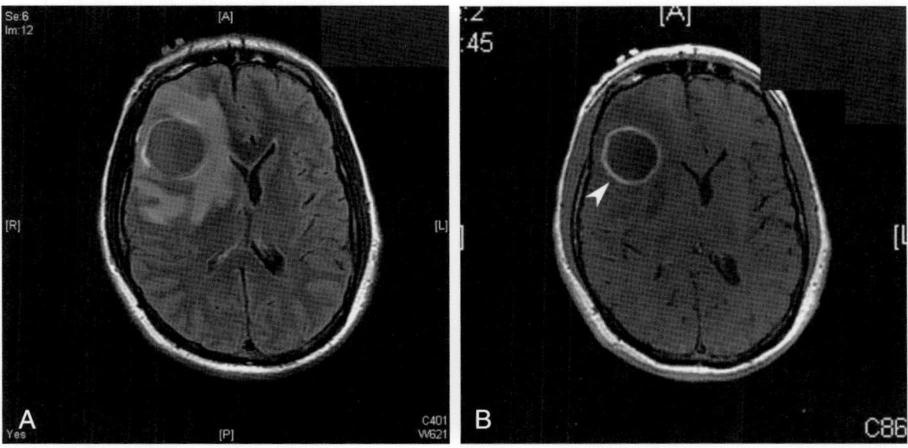


**Fig. 79.1** Magnetic resonance imaging of a 47-year-old man with a new, progressive headache starting 1 week after infected tooth extraction. **A,** Fluid-attenuated inversion recovery (FLAIR) image showing the central hypodense lesion with surrounding edema. **B,** T1 image after gadolinium administration, which shows a thick rim of contrast enhancement around the lesion *(white arrowhead). (Courtesy Dr. Anita Koshy, Stanford University.)*

aspiration and cultures can be obtained quickly (within 24–48 hours of presentation), empirical antibiotics should be avoided until after abscess cultures have been obtained. The pathogen is preliminarily identified at the time of stereotactic aspiration by Gram stain, and culture is obtained for definitive identification and antimicrobial sensitivity testing.

Notably, LP plays no role in the diagnosis of brain abscess. LP has the potential to lead to brain herniation if the abscess is large, culturing the causative bacteria from CSF is uncommon, and there is nothing specific about the CSF profile that will suggest or confirm bacterial brain abscess (Seydoux and Francioli, 1992).

### Management

Currently, CT-guided stereotactic aspiration of the abscess in combination with antibiotics is the standard of care. While there are reports of patients surviving with antibiotic treatment alone (typically if the abscess is very small, very deep, or there are multiple abscesses), generally both antibiotics and surgical aspiration are recommended. Aspiration offers the opportunity for both diagnosis and decreasing the size of the abscess, allowing for quicker resolution. Patients with small abscesses (<2.5 cm diameter), those who are poor surgical candidates, and those who have abscesses in deep brain structures can be treated with medical management alone, although with improved surgical technique, even some deep brain structures can be drained (Wait et al., 2009).

The usual empirical antibiotics are those that have good CNS penetration and cover both aerobes and anaerobes. Thus, a third-generation cephalosporin in combination with metronidazole is often used. Vancomycin is added if there is concern that the organism is a *Staphylococcus* species. If the aspirated material or blood cultures yield an organism(s), empirical antibiotics are modified accordingly. The duration of intravenous antimicrobial therapy is usually 6–8 weeks, and some experts recommend continued oral therapy beyond this period. Imaging follow-up is recommended to assess response to treatment.

## Spinal Epidural Abscess

### Etiology

Spinal epidural abscesses (SEAs) are increasingly common due to the increasing number of diabetics, a major predisposing condition. *Staphylococcus aureus* is the most commonly isolated organism (~50%–60% of the isolated organisms in any series), with *Streptococcus* spp., coagulase-negative staphylococci, and enteric gram-negative rods making up the remainder of the nontuberculous SEA (Curry et al., 2005; Davis et al., 2004; Reihsaus et al., 2000; Soehle and Wallenfang, 2002). In areas with endemic tuberculosis or in patients who have recently emigrated from endemic areas, *M. tuberculosis* as a cause of SEA associated with vertebral osteomyelitis should be high on the differential diagnosis.

The development of SEA can occur from direct spread (i.e., psoas abscess, vertebral osteomyelitis) or from hematogenous spread from a distant site. The cervical spine is less frequently involved than the thoracic or lumbar spine, which may be related to the extent of the epidural space and the venous drainage of the thoracic and lumbar spine (Reihsaus et al., 2000).

### Clinical Presentation

SEA is a progressive disease that usually begins with new-onset back pain or localized tenderness and progresses to radicular pain and ultimately to neurological deficits, including bowel and bladder dysfunction. The classic triad of SEA is back pain or localized tenderness, fever, and progressive neurological deficits localized to the spinal cord. Similar to bacterial meningitis, this triad is highly specific but has low sensitivity, especially early in the disease course (Davis et al., 2004; Reihsaus et al., 2000). In most studies, back pain is a presenting feature in 60%–70% of patients, and "fever" is present in 50%–60%, although it is not always clear if this is a reported or documented fever. In addition, as one study noted, patients with back pain often use anti-inflammatory medications, which have antipyretic effects, making the presence of a fever even less likely in these patients (Davis et al., 2004).

When trying to determine whether a patient with new-onset back pain should be imaged to rule out SEA, one should assess the patient for the known risk factors for SEA. The most common risk factors are diabetes mellitus, intravenous drug use, alcohol abuse, immunocompromised state (including immunosuppressive drugs, acquired immunodeficiency syndrome (AIDS), cancer patients), spinal surgery/procedure, trauma (spinal or extraspinal), and extraspinal infections (furunculosis/cellulitis, psoas abscess, etc.). Which risk factor is most highly related to SEA depends on the study and likely reflects the different populations studied (Davis et al., 2004; Pradilla et al., 2009; Reihsaus et al., 2000). In every study there are a small number of patients without any risk factors, but in general, most patients have at least one of the previously listed risk factors (Davis et al., 2004; Reihsaus et al., 2000). In addition, while SEA can be located anywhere along the spinal axis, up to a third of patients will present with thoracic pain. As the thoracic spine is an unusual place to develop mechanical back pain, new-onset thoracic back pain should make one consider SEA sooner rather than later.

### Diagnosis

Diagnosing SEA is difficult because the vast majority of patients with back pain (>99%) will not have SEA. Thus, in this group of patients, choosing whom to further evaluate, especially early on when the patient has no neurological deficits and may not have fever, is extremely difficult. Using risk factors, fever, and location of pain can help narrow the number of patients sent to neuroimaging. One provocative retrospective study suggested that using risk factors to evaluate which patients were at high risk for an SEA had a sensitivity of 98% and a negative predictive value of 99%. Yet, given the high incidence of risk factors and back pain compared to SEA, 50 patients would need further evaluation to catch a single case of SEA (Davis et al., 2004). Clearly, better biomarkers for SEA are needed. The erythrocyte sedimentation rate (ESR) may be the one laboratory test that has a role in helping to narrow the patients for evaluation, as the majority of patients with SEA have an ESR greater than 20 mm/h (Davis et al., 2004; Reihsaus et al., 2000). As with the risk factor assessment, the sensitivity of this test will be very good, but the specificity will be poor. Ultimately, determining whether a patient is at high risk for SEA requires the physician to integrate risk factors, the neurological examination, and limited laboratory data.

Once a patient is felt to be at risk for SEA, MRI with gadolinium is the standard of care. MRI has the capability to evaluate the bones and discs for signs of infection (osteomyelitis and discitis) as well as to look for the presence and extent of an epidural abscess. Fig. 79.2 demonstrates a ventral epidural abscess with associated discitis. In patients who cannot undergo MRI, CT myelogram is the next best choice. SEA is a neurological emergency because limited evidence suggests that the outcome is better if patients are treated before the onset of neurological deficits or if neurological deficits have only been present for a short time period (<48–72 hours) (Khanna et al., 1996; Reihsaus et al., 2000). This assumes the deficits are from cord compression and not ischemia.

The full diagnostic work-up for SEA includes blood cultures and an ESR, which is useful to follow for patients with associated osteomyelitis. LP is contraindicated, as the procedure offers little help with

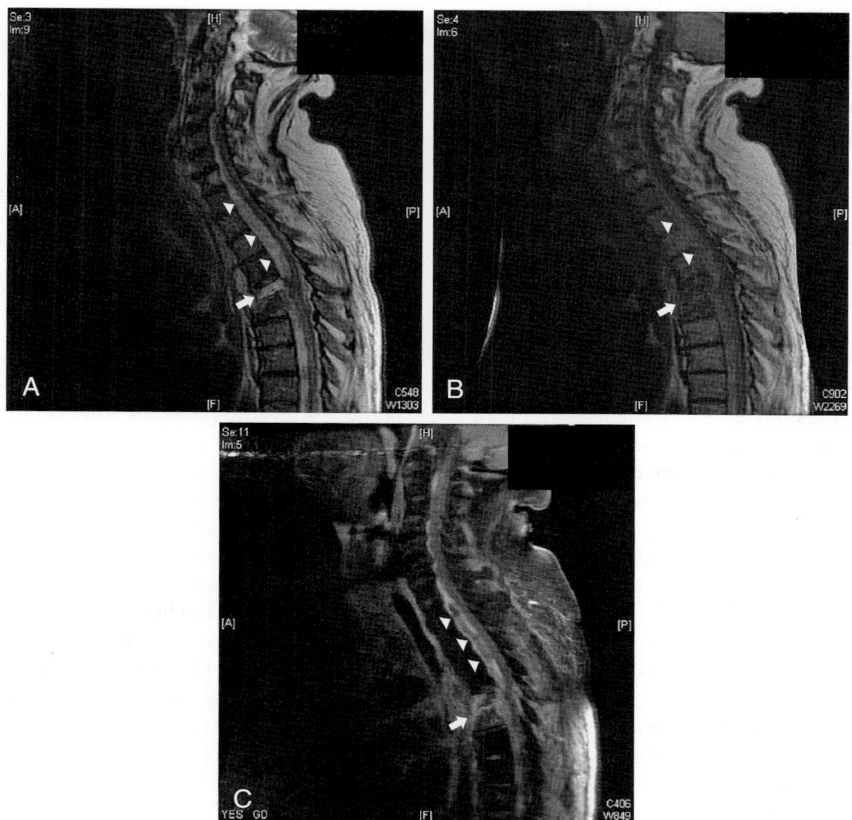

**Fig. 79.2** A 66-year-old woman who presented with fevers and four-limb weakness. **A,** T2-weighted sagittal image showing discitis *(arrow)* and extensive ventral epidural abscess *(arrowheads)* with spinal cord displacement and compression. **B,** T1-weighted sagittal image without contrast also shows discitis and abscess, as well as abnormal vertebral body signal secondary to osteomyelitis. **C,** T1-weighted sagittal image post contrast showing the rim-enhancing epidural abscess *(arrowheads)* and discitis and vertebral osteomyelitis *(arrow)*. *(Courtesy Dr. Nancy Fischbein, Stanford University.)*

diagnosis or culturing the organism and has the risk of seeding the meninges or subarachnoid space.

### Management

There are no randomized controlled trials to evaluate the efficacy of medical management with or without surgical treatment. The current standard of care is to employ both surgical (aspiration or evacuation of the abscess) and medical management (antibiotics). While there have been reports of patients doing equally well with medical management alone (Tang et al., 2002), there are similar reports showing that patients treated with surgery as well as antibiotics have better outcomes than those who only receive medical management (Curry et al., 2005). In addition, the reasons for choosing medical management alone are usually the lack of neurological deficits or poor surgical candidates—baseline differences that undoubtedly impact outcomes. Thus, at this time, the management of SEA relies on both surgical and medical management, with the appropriateness of medical management alone being reserved for a small group of well-defined patients who will have excellent follow-up.

Empirical antibiotics for suspected or confirmed SEA must cover *S. aureus*, streptococci, coagulase-negative staphylococci, and enteric gram-negative bacilli. If *M. tuberculosis* is highly suspected, four-drug therapy should be initiated until the etiological agent is identified. Once the organism is isolated from the blood or the abscess itself, antibiotics can be modified. Please see Table 79.2 for suggested empirical antibiotics. The length of intravenous antibiotic treatment is not well defined, but usually 6–8 weeks is recommended, with some clinicians preferring to switch to oral medications for further treatment. *M. tuberculosis* vertebral osteomyelitis with or without associated epidural abscess is treated for 6–9 months (American Thoracic Society/Center for Disease Control/Infectious Disease Society of America, 2003).

Follow-up MRIs to guide decisions about treatment failure is a common practice, but clinical evidence to support this approach is limited. Two studies have addressed the utility of follow-up MRIs for SEA/vertebral osteomyelitis. While both studies were small, neither found that routine follow-up MRIs were cost-effective predictors for clinical outcomes. Thus, both studies recommended not obtaining routine follow-up studies (Carragee, 1997; Kowalski et al., 2006) but rather limiting follow-up imaging to those patients who are clinically worse (Kowalski et al., 2006).

## FUNGAL INFECTIONS OF THE CENTRAL NERVOUS SYSTEM

Fungi are eukaryotic organisms that do not have organelles for movement (such as flagella) and generally develop from spores. Fungi range from mushrooms to bread mold, but only a small group is pathogenic in humans, with a subset causing CNS infection. While immunocompromised patients are at higher risk for fungal infections, some fungi, such as dimorphic fungi, are found frequently in immunocompetent patients as well. Immunocompetent patients can also develop CNS disease as a complication of neurosurgery, craniofacial surgeries, or IV drug use.

Finally, it is important to recognize that "immunocompromised" hosts include the traditional patients (e.g., high-dose steroids, organ transplant, human immunodeficiency virus (HIV)/AIDS) as well as those patients on newer immunomodulatory drugs (e.g., fingolimod, tumor necrosis factor [TNF] inhibitors) and patients with rare underlying immune defects (e.g., chronic granulomatous disease) (Schwartz et al., 2018). In all patients, the most frequent CNS manifestations of fungal infections are meningitis and brain abscesses, though other manifestations such as strokes, vasculitis, and SEA can also be seen.

## Meningitis

### Etiology

Unlike the common bacteria that cause meningitis, which are generally ubiquitous, fungi that cause meningitis are either widely prevalent (*Cryptococcus* spp., *Aspergillus* spp., *Pseudallescheria boydii/Scedosporium* spp.) or have restricted geographic regions (*Coccidioides* spp., *Blastomyces dermatitidis*, *Histoplasma capsulatum*) (Schwartz et al., 2018). In general, endemic fungi and *Cryptococcus* spp. cause meningitis more often than fungi such as *Aspergillus*, zygomycetes, or *P. boydii*. Like most invasive fungal disease, fungal meningitis more commonly occurs in the immunocompromised, though *Coccidioides* spp. and *Cryptococcus gattii* routinely cause disease in the immunocompetent. In addition, *Aspergillus* spp. can rarely cause a pure meningeal syndrome, which occurs more often in the immunocompetent (Antinori et al., 2013). Thus, understanding the exposure history (e.g., geographic regions) and the immune state of the patient is critical to determining which fungus is the most likely causative organism. Finally, awareness of ongoing outbreaks is essential, as highlighted by the 2012 multistate outbreak of predominantly *Exserohilum rostratum* parameningeal and meningeal infections linked to epidural injection of contaminated methylprednisolone acetate (MPA) (McCotter et al., 2015).

### Clinical Presentation

The clinical presentation of fungal meningitis is similar to bacterial meningitis except that the time course is usually subacute to chronic rather than acute, and the patients are more commonly immunocompromised. Fever as a presenting sign can vary by organism as well as immune state. In 71 cases of CNS coccidioidomycosis in which less than half were immunocompromised, 77% of the patients presented with headache, but only 28% presented with fever (Drake and Adam, 2009). Conversely, in patients with cryptococcal (HIV+ or −) and *Aspergillus* meningitis, fever is often present (Antinori, 2013; Antinori et al., 2013). Altered mental status is also relatively common in fungal meningitis, which may be a direct result of the infectious process or secondary to complications, such as hydrocephalus or vasculitis.

### Diagnosis

In general, the CSF profile of fungal meningitis resembles that of *M. tuberculosis* meningitis, with a mononuclear pleocytosis and an elevated protein concentration, though in *Aspergillus* meningitis, most of the literature-described cases had a neutrophil predominance (>60%) in the CSF regardless of immune status (immunocompromised 14/20 and immunocompetent 25/37) (Antinori et al., 2013). Additionally, in both *Coccidioides* and *Blastomyces* meningitis, a minority of patients will also present with a CSF neutrophil predominance (Bariola et al., 2010; Drake and Adams, 2009). The CSF glucose concentration in fungal meningitis is moderately decreased, while in tuberculous meningitis, the CSF glucose concentration is only mildly decreased. Imaging studies often show basilar meningitis with contrast enhancement or unexplained hydrocephalus. Determining the exact fungal etiology is highly dependent on the suspected fungal species. CSF fungal smears (India ink) may demonstrate the organism but isolating the organism by culture is preferred. While *Candida* spp. readily grow in culture, many of the fungi rarely produce positive CSF cultures. In general, CSF fungal cultures require high volumes (10–30 mL) and may require up to 3 weeks to grow. Thus, identifying the agent often occurs through antibody and/or antigen detection or rarely through meningeal biopsy. For *Cryptococcus* spp., rapid cryptococcal antigen testing (lateral flow assay or latex agglutination assay) from the CSF is recommended (WHO, 2018). For *Coccidioides immitis*, serum and CSF should be tested for coccidioidal antibodies and antigen (Kassis et al., 2015; Galgiani et al., 2016). For *H. capsulatum*, a CSF *Histoplasma* polysaccharide antigen test is the test of choice, though a recent report suggests that antigen detection, in combination with detection of anti-*Histoplasma* antibodies, especially via a more sensitive enzyme immunoassay (EIA), significantly improves the diagnostic sensitivity (Bloch et al., 2018; Wheat et al., 2018). CNS involvement with *Blastomycosis* is uncommon (Bariola et al., 2010), making it difficult to determine the best diagnostic algorithm, but tests for *Blastomycosis* antigen and antibody detection are available. The dimorphic fungi can produce cross-reactive antibodies, and a recent report highlights that cryptococcal antibodies can also cause cross-reactivity to the dimorphic fungal EIAs (Bahr et al., 2019), so confirmational antigen testing or culture is important. The utility of tests for fungal components such as β-glucan (all except *Mucor* and *Cryptococcus*) and galactomannan (*Aspergillus* spp.) on CSF have shown mixed results, which appear to vary by fungal etiology (Chong et al., 2016; Myint et al., 2018). Though relatively rarely done now, in certain cases meningeal biopsies may be of use. Biopsies and CSF should be sent for culture and/or PCR as well as histopathology (Brown et al., 2015). The next horizon for diagnostic testing in high-resource countries is likely broad-spectrum pathogen detection using PCR targeted at rRNA (18s and 28s rRNA for fungi) or next-generation sequencing (RNA or DNA depending on the platform), which should identify any microbe. While proof-of-principle findings are encouraging (Wagner et al., 2018; Wilson et al., 2018), rigorous prospective data on the yield, turnaround time, and cost-effectiveness of these techniques remain limited.

### Management

Compared to bacterial meningitis, fungal meningitis is more indolent and thus requires longer courses of therapy. There are very comprehensive guidelines written by the Infectious Diseases Society for America (IDSA) for the following fungi that cause meningitis: *B. dermatitidis*, *Coccidioides* spp., *Aspergillus* spp., *Candida* spp., *H. capsulatum*, and *Sporothrix schenckii*. The World Health Organization (WHO) has recently released guidelines for cryptococcal disease in HIV$^+$ patients, while the older IDSA guidelines for cryptococcal disease in non-HIV$^+$ patients remains informative. These guidelines are written by experts in the field, are updated as necessary, and the recommendations are graded by level of evidence. In general, management will consist of several phases: induction, consolidation, and maintenance. The agents used and the length of each phase depends on the specific pathogen and the patient population. Table 79.4 summarizes recommended treatment as determined by the fungus identified or suspected.

Increased intracranial pressure is another factor that requires attention in fungal infections. It often develops secondary to hydrocephalus caused by CSF flow obstruction at the level of the third or fourth ventricle and may require a shunt. A ventriculostomy is typically inserted and converted to a ventriculoperitoneal shunt after the infection has been treated.

Currently corticosteroids are not routinely indicated for fungal meningitis though corticosteroids may be required in patients with

**TABLE 79.4 Suggested Treatment for Specific Fungal Diseases of the Central Nervous System**

| Infection | Treatment |
|---|---|
| Aspergillosis | Primary: voriconazole. Alternative primary in select patients: liposomal amphotericin B, isavuconazole<br>Secondary/salvage therapies: amphotericin B lipid complex, caspofungin, micafungin, posaconazole, or itraconazole; primary combination therapy (azole + echinocandin) not recommended except in severe disease<br>Consider surgical resection if possible; no role for adjunct steroids |
| Zygomycosis | Aggressive surgical débridement<br>Standard or lipid-formulation amphotericin<br>Some experts advocate addition of echinocandin or posaconazole. |
| Cryptococcosis: | |
| HIV patients | Induction: liposomal amphotericin B + flucytosine x 2 weeks (can use amphotericin B or ABLC); lower/middile income countries: amphotericin B + flucytosine ×1 wk, followed by 1 wk of fluconazole (1200 mg/day, adult)<br>Alternate induction: fluconazole (400-1200 mg/day, adult) + flucytosine ×2 wk<br>Consolidation: oral fluconazole 800 mg/day ×8 wk (minimum)<br>Maintenance/secondary prophylaxis: oral fluconazole 200 mg/day<br>Corticosteroids: not recommended during induction<br>Antiretroviral therapy (ART) initiation: defer for 4–6 wk from start of antifungal treatment |
| Organ transplant patients | Induction: lipid-formulation amphotericin + flucytosine ×2 wk (minimum)<br>Consolidation: oral fluconazole 400–800 mg/day ×8 wk<br>Maintenance: oral fluconazole 200–400 mg ×6–12 mo |
| Immunocompetent patients | Induction: amphotericin B/lipid-formulation amphotericin + flucytosine ×4 wk<br>Consolidation: oral fluconazole 400–800 mg/day ×8 wk<br>Maintenance: oral fluconazole 200–400 mg ×6–12 mo |
| Increased intracranial pressure (ICP) (any group) | If ICP ≥ 25 cm $H_2O$ and symptomatic, then remove cerebrospinal fluid (CSF) via lumbar puncture (LP) to closing pressure of ≤20 cm $H_2O$ or ≤50% of opening pressure (OP) if OP very high<br>Persistence/recurrence of signs or symptoms of elevated ICP defines frequency of therapeutic LP. For persistent symptoms, recheck and treat OP daily until symptoms abate or ICP stable ×2 days |
| Coccidioidomycosis | Oral fluconazole; itraconazole also okay<br>Salvage: intrathecal amphotericin B ± oral azole<br>Recommendation after CSF normalized is lifelong azole therapy<br>Increased ICP: if ≥25 cm $H_2O$, follow *Cryptococcus* guidelines. Continue daily LPs for at least 4 days or until OP stable <25 cm $H_2O$. High likelihood of requiring permanent shunting |
| Blastomycosis | Induction: intravenous liposomal or standard amphotericin ×4–6 wk<br>Consolidation/maintenance: oral azole therapy (fluconazole, itraconazole, or voriconazole*) »>12 mo and resolution of CSF abnormalities. |
| Histoplasmosis | Induction: intravenous lipid-formulation amphotericin ×4–6 wk<br>Consolidation/maintenance: itraconazole ≥12 mo and resolution of CSF abnormalities including *Histoplasma* antigen.<br>If relapse or CSF does not normalize, patient may need life-long therapy |
| Sporotrichosis | Induction: intravenous lipid-formulation amphotericin ×4–6 wk<br>Consolidation/maintenance: itraconazole 200 mg bid ≥12 mo and resolution of CSF abnormalities. |
| Candidiasis | Induction: intravenous lipid-formulation amphotericin ± flucytosine for several weeks<br>Consolidation/maintenance: fluconazole 400–800 mg until CSF and radiological abnormalities resolve. If possible, remove any associated central nervous system devices.<br>For ventricular devices that cannot be removed: amphotericin B should be administered through the device |

*Voriconazole is generally the azole of choice given its high CSF penetration and effectiveness against *Blastomycosis.* Standard dosing: amphotericin B = 0.7-1 mg/kg/day IV; liposomal amphotericin B = 3-4 mg/kg/day IV; amphotericin B lipid complex (ABLD) = 5 mg/kg/day IV; Flucytosine 25 mg/kg po qid.
*From Chapman et al. (2008), DHHS (2016), Galgiani et al. (2016), Kauffman et al. (2007), Pappas et al. (2016), Perfect et al. (2010), Patterson et al. (2016), Wheat et al. (2007), WHO (2018).*

immune reconstitution inflammatory syndrome (IRIS), most often associated with cryptococcal meningitis. Additionally, some experts advocate using corticosteroids for *Coccidioides*-associated CNS vasculitis (Galgiani et al., 2016).

## Brain Abscess

### Etiology

In general, fungal brain abscesses are found in immunocompromised organ transplant patients, hematological malignancy patients, and AIDS patients, with *Candida* and *Aspergillus* spp. topping the list of etiologies (Leventakos et al., 2010), though a review of *Aspergillus* cases suggested that ~20%–30% of patients with CNS involvement had no associated immunosuppression (Kourkoumpetis et al., 2012). Candidal abscesses are usually secondary to disseminated disease. *Aspergillus* involvement may be secondary to hematogenous dissemination from invasive pulmonary disease or due to direct extension from the paranasal sinuses. Zygomycetes (*Rhizopus* spp., *Mucor*) generally involve the CNS by direct extension from paranasal sinuses, though a recent report highlights that isolated cerebral mucomycosis can occur through IV drug use (Kerezoudis et al., 2019). This disease occurs in classically immunosuppressed patients, though diabetes mellitus is the most commonly cited risk factor. While the *Scedosporium* spp. complex was previously considered a rare cause of brain abscess associated with near-drownings or trauma, this group of fungi are now being recognized as important opportunistic pathogens in a range of immunocompromised patients (Seidel et al., 2019). *Cladophialophora bantiana*, a dematiaceous fungus, is a rare but potentially increasing cause of fungal brain abscesses in both immunocompromised and immunocompetent patients. *C. bantiana* brain abscesses have been reported from many countries, though most reported cases have come from India (Chakrabarti et al., 2016; Kantarcioglu et al., 2017). Finally, the fungi mentioned in the preceding section can also be associated with isolated brain abscesses but are more commonly associated with meningitis or meningoencephalitis. In general, these infections are extremely difficult to treat, often because they occur in the most immunosuppressed patients, and thus carry a high mortality rate.

### Clinical Presentation

As with most brain abscesses, these patients present with focal neurological signs or symptoms and may or may not have fever. Headache is a common symptom, and other signs will be dependent upon the size and location of the abscess. Given its ability to invade blood vessels and cause thrombosis, *Aspergillus* infections can present with strokes. As with fungal meningitis, the immunocompromised state of many of these patients often means they have very little manifestation of disease until they are morbid.

### Diagnosis

Diagnosis depends upon a high degree of clinical suspicion in the correct clinical context. Brain contrast imaging with MRI or CT is the preferred evaluation technique. Determining the etiology of the lesion will depend on concomitant risk factors and previous or ongoing infection in extra-CNS organs. A brain biopsy with cultures and/or molecular studies may be required. If fungal disease is on the differential, histopathology should not be the only mechanism for definitive identification of the organism, as many fungi can look like *Aspergillus* on brain biopsy. Thus, confirmatory tests such as culture or PCR should be done.

### Management

The suspected organism determines the definitive antimicrobial agent used, but azoles and a lipid formulation of amphotericin B are the most common agents. Table 79.4 provides a summary of recommended treatments for suspected or isolated fungi. It is important to recognize the Achilles heels of the different antifungal agents. For example, voriconazole is the drug of choice for treating CNS aspergillosis, but is not effective against Zygomycetes. Thus, in a patient with sinus disease and infectious extension into the brain, until a final diagnosis is determined, empirical treatment with amphotericin is appropriate. Very limited data suggest that, compared to medical therapy alone, neurosurgical debridement improves outcomes for *C. bantiana* abscesses and *Aspergillus* abscesses or sinusitis with extension into the CNS (Chakrabarti et al., 2016; Kourkoumpetis et al., 2012). In neither case do the data control for how patients were selected for neurosurgical intervention, which by itself may explain the difference in outcomes. Despite new antifungal agents with more potency against fungi, the mortality of CNS fungal abscesses remains high.

## PARASITIC INFECTIONS OF THE CENTRAL NERVOUS SYSTEM

Parasites are a group of organisms that obtain the resources required for their survival and proliferation from a host organism at the host's expense. Parasitic infections of the CNS are uncommon, but should be considered in the setting of specific environmental, food, or animal exposures. The relevant parasites can be broadly categorized as protozoa (single-celled) or helminths (worms). Parasitic infections of the CNS can cause focal lesions, meningitis, encephalitis, or a combination of these.

### Acute Meningitis

#### Etiology and Clinical Presentation

The presentation of acute parasitic meningitis is similar to that of other infections, such as bacteria and viruses. Typical symptoms are meningeal signs, headache, seizure, and encephalopathy.

Primary amebic meningoencephalitis (PAM) is caused by *Naegleria fowleri*, a free-living ameba. This disease has a clinical presentation similar to that of acute bacterial meningitis, with symptoms of fever, headache, nuchal rigidity, seizures, and a progressive decrease in the level of consciousness. It should be suspected when there has been recent exposure to untreated fresh water, such as swimming in a lake. *Naegleria* invades the CNS along the olfactory nerve. PAM is almost always fatal.

Unlike *Naegleria*, *Angiostrongylus cantonensis* causes eosinophilic meningitis, which is defined as 10 or more eosinophils/microliter of CSF or a CSF eosinophilia of 10% or greater (Lo Re and Gluckman, 2003). This parasite should be considered in those with exposure to snails and slugs. The differential diagnosis for eosinophilic pleocytosis should include coccidioidomycosis, neurocysticercosis, tuberculosis, sarcoidosis, and others (Greenlee and Carroll, 1997).

#### Diagnosis

Table 79.5 provides specific diagnostic tests for the common parasites that cause acute meningitis.

#### Management

Table 79.5 lists the recommended treatment for acute meningitis based on the parasite.

### Chronic Meningitis and Encephalitis

#### Etiology and Clinical Presentation

Granulomatous amebic encephalitis (GAE) is most commonly (>99%) caused by *Acanthamoeba* spp. and *Balamuthia mandrillaris*, which are free-living amebas. GAE most often occurs in immunocompromised patients; however, *Balamuthia* GAE can also occur in immunocompetent individuals. The presentation usually resembles chronic meningitis, but can also resemble tumor, abscess, and other neurological conditions; therefore, a biopsy is typically required for specific diagnosis (Durack, 1997). Typical symptoms include headache, low-grade fever, and focal neurological deficits. Progression usually occurs over a 2- to 8-week period before eventual death.

Cerebral malaria is an encephalopathy that is caused by *Plasmodium falciparum* and leads to coma. The diagnosis should be considered in individuals living in or traveling to endemic areas, which involve most of the tropical and subtropical latitudes, including sub-Saharan Africa, Southeast Asia, Central America, and South America. Children less than 5 years of age who live in endemic areas and nonimmune travelers to endemic areas are at highest risk for cerebral malaria (Cegielski and Warrell, 1997). Treatment with IV medications, such as artesunate, is preferred over the older oral treatment with quinine (WHO, 2015).

African sleeping sickness or African trypanosomiasis is caused by *Trypanosoma brucei*, a parasite that uses the tsetse fly as a vector and leads to progressive encephalopathy and death. For further details please see Chapter 101 on sleep disorders.

Trichinosis is caused by *Trichinella spiralis* and can be acquired by eating undercooked pork that contains *Trichinella* cysts (larvae migrate

**TABLE 79.5 Parasites of the Central Nervous System**

| Organism (Disease) | Symptoms | History/At-risk Population | Diagnosis/Testing | Treatment |
|---|---|---|---|---|
| *Naegleria fowleri* (primary amebic meningoencephalitis), free-living ameba | Acute meningoencephalitis similar to bacterial meningitis, fever, headache, nuchal rigidity, seizure, encephalitis | Young, healthy individuals with exposure to untreated fresh water (e.g., swimming in a lake) | CSF profile consistent with acute bacterial meningitis; however, Gram stain will be negative, CSF wet prep (motile trophozoites), PCR offered by the CDC | High-dose IV amphotericin with possible addition of azoles, rifampin, or miltefosine |
| *Acanthamoeba* species (granulomatous amebic encephalitis [GAE], *Acanthamoeba* keratitis), free-living ameba | Chronic insidious meningitis, headache, low-grade fever, focal neurological symptoms | Immunocompromised > immunocompetent | Contrast MRI/CT (focal lesions), CSF profile consistent with aseptic meningitis, biopsy, PCR offered by the CDC | Combination of pentamidine, an azole, a sulfonamide, flucytosine, and miltefosine |
| *Balamuthia mandrillaris* (GAE), free-living ameba | Chronic insidious meningitis, headache, low-grade fever, focal neurological symptoms | Immunocompetent > immunocompromised | Contrast MRI/CT (focal lesions), CSF profile consistent with aseptic meningitis, biopsy, PCR offered by the CDC, utility of serology is unclear | Combination of pentamidine, flucytosine, a sulfonamide, albendazole, an azole, a macrolide, amphotericin, and/or miltefosine |
| *Plasmodium falciparum* (cerebral malaria), protozoan | Fever, encephalopathy, seizure | Travel to endemic regions (sub-Saharan Africa, South Asia, Southeast Asia, Central America, South America) | Thick and thin blood smears with Giemsa stain, ELISA, PCR | First line: IV artesunate. Alternative: IV quinine |
| *Taenia solium* (neurocysticercosis), helminth | Headaches, seizures, hydrocephalus, focal neurological symptoms | Worldwide, exposure to individuals with cysticercosis, ingestion of undercooked pork | Contrast MRI/CT (cystic lesion with scolex), direct visualization or parasites by fundoscopic examination, serum EITB, CSF ELISA for anticysticercal antibodies | Albendazole, praziquantel, and steroids |
| *Entamoeba histolytica* (cerebral amebiasis), free-living ameba | Focal neurological symptoms, headache, seizure, meningeal signs, fever, weight loss, abdominal pain, diarrhea | Travel to endemic regions (Mexico, Latin America, Southeast Asia, Africa), recent intestinal amebiasis | Clinical, contrast MRI/CT, presence of liver abscess, serology | Metronidazole and paramomycin |
| *Toxoplasma gondii* (toxoplasmosis), protozoan | Focal neurological symptoms, headache, change in mental status, change in personality | Immunocompromised | Contrast MRI/CT (diffuse enhancement or ring-enhancing lesions), serology, CSF PCR | Pyrimethamine plus sulfadiazine |

*CDC,* Centers for Disease Control and Prevention; *CSF,* cerebrospinal fluid; *EITB,* enzyme-linked immunoelectrotransfer blot; *ELISA,* enzyme-linked immunosorbent assay; *IV,* intravenous; *MRI/CT,* magnetic resonance imaging/computed tomography; *PCR,* polymerase chain reaction.

and encyst in muscle). Initial symptoms often include myalgias and fever, followed by meningeal signs and encephalitis. Diagnosis is made clinically; however, testing that can be helpful includes brain imaging, serology, muscle biopsy, and CSF studies.

Other uncommon causes of parasitic meningitis or encephalitis include *Gnathostoma spinigerum* (Asia, especially Southeast Asia, dogs and cats, eating raw fish), *Strongyloides stercoralis* (Far East, exposure to soil, can cause bacterial meningitis), *Toxocara* genus (worldwide, dogs and cats), and *Schistosoma* spp. (*S. japonicum* in Japan, China, Southeast Asia; *S. mansoni* in Africa, Southwest Asia, Caribbean, South America; *S. haematobium* in Africa and Southwest Asia, exposure to freshwater). There are case reports of other parasitic causes of meningitis and encephalitis but these are too rare to be discussed here.

### Diagnosis

The various parasitic infections that cause chronic meningitis and encephalitis have specific diagnostic tests based on the individual organism. Table 79.5 provides specific diagnostic tests corresponding to common organisms.

### Management

The treatment of chronic meningitis and encephalitis caused by parasitic CNS infections should be tailored to the specific organism. Table 79.5 lists specific agents targeting the most common organisms.

## Focal Lesions

### Etiology and Clinical Presentation

Patients with focal lesions caused by parasites will present with symptoms similar to those of other space-occupying lesions. Common symptoms are focal neurological symptoms, headache, seizures, nausea, vomiting, or papilledema (obstructive hydrocephalus). Focal CNS lesions caused by parasites can occur in immunocompetent or immunocompromised patients.

The most common parasitic infection causing focal lesions in the CNS is neurocysticercosis, caused by the intestinal tapeworm *Taenia solium*. Humans are the definitive hosts, although both humans and pigs can also function as intermediate hosts. *T. solium* infection was previously associated with ingestion of undercooked pork but is now more commonly thought to spread from human to human. An individual can be infected with the tapeworm (cysticercosis) via the gastrointestinal

TABLE 79.6 **Diagnostic Criteria for Neurocysticercosis**

| Categories of Criteria | Criteria |
|---|---|
| Absolute | Histological demonstration of the parasite from biopsy of a brain or spinal cord lesion |
| | Cystic lesions showing the scolex on CT or MRI |
| | Direct visualization of subretinal parasites by fundoscopic examination |
| **Neuroimaging criteria:** | |
| Major | Cystic lesions without a scolex |
| | Enhancing lesions |
| | Multilobulated cystic lesions in the subarachnoid space |
| | Typical parenchymal brain calcifications |
| Confirmative | Resolution of cystic lesions after cysticidal drug therapy |
| | Spontaneous resolution of single small enhancing lesions |
| | Migration of ventricular cysts on sequential neuroimaging studies |
| Minor | Obstructive hydrocephalus |
| | Abnormal enhancement of basal leptomeninges |
| **Clinical/exposure criteria:** | |
| Major | Detection of specific anticysticercal antibodies or cysticercal antigens |
| | Cysticercosis outside the CNS |
| | Evidence of a household contact with *Taenia solium* infection |
| Minor | Clinical manifestations suggestive of neurocysticercosis |
| | Individuals coming from or living in an area where cysticercosis is endemic |

| Diagnostic certainty | Criteria |
|---|---|
| Definitive | One absolute criterion |
| | Two major neuroimaging criteria and any clinical/exposure criteria |
| | One major neuroimaging criterion, one confirmative neuroimaging criterion, and any clinical/exposure criteria |
| | One major neuroimaging criterion, two clinical/exposure criteria (including at least one major clinical/exposure criterion), and the exclusion of other pathologies producing similar neuroimaging findings |
| Probable | One major neuroimaging criterion and any two clinical/exposure criteria |
| | One minor neuroimaging criterion and one major clinical/exposure criterion |

*CNS,* Central nervous system; *CT,* computed tomography; *MRI,* magnetic resonance imaging.
*Adapted from Del Brutto, O.H., Nash, T.E., White Jr., A.C., et al., 2017. Revised diagnostic criteria for neurocysticercosis. J. Neurol Sci. 372, 202–210.*

tract, after which this individual can autoinfect himself or infect others. In autoinfection, the ingested eggs hatch in the small intestine, after which the parasite migrates through the mucosal layers into the vascular circulation, allowing spread to various tissues, especially the CNS and eyes. Initially, edema forms around the parasite. Over months, a cyst forms around the organism. The organism will eventually die and the cyst degrades to leave a calcified nodule (Cameron and Durack, 1997). Patients can present at any time during this progression, although most commonly they present after a cyst has formed.

Cerebral amebiasis is a condition that often produces multiple brain abscesses in individuals who have had an intestinal infection with *Entamoeba histolytica*. The brain lesions, which consist of hemorrhagic necrotic tissue, are almost always associated with hepatic abscesses, and are often concomitantly associated with abdominal pain and weight loss (Durack, 1997).

*Toxoplasma gondii* is one of the most common human parasites with up to one-third of the human population latently infected. Humans most commonly become infected through ingestion of contaminated food or water, or congenital transmission. Rarely, blood transfusion and organ transplantation have resulted in infection (Halonen and Weiss, 2013). In immunocompetent individuals, acute infection is usually asymptomatic, but can rarely produce a mono-like illness or present as acute chorioretinitis. These acute manifestations appear to occur more commonly in South America than in North America and Europe and are thought to be secondary to the genotypic diversity of *Toxoplasma* strains found in South America (Pfaff et al., 2014). Chronic infection of the CNS, skeletal muscle, and heart is asymptomatic in immunocompetent persons, but in immunocompromised patients, such as those with HIV/AIDS and bone marrow transplant patients, the parasite can reactivate and cause cerebral toxoplasmosis, or toxoplasmic encephalitis (TE). TE presents most often as focal ring-enhancing CNS lesions, especially in AIDS patients, but can also present as a diffusely infiltrating process in areas such as the basal ganglia, which is more common in bone marrow transplant patients. Clinical presentation includes focal neurological symptoms, headache, or changes in mental status or personality.

Rare parasitic causes of focal CNS lesions include *T. spiralis* (worldwide, pigs and bears), *Taenia* genus (*T. multiceps* in Europe, Africa, and Brazil; *T. serialis* in Canada and the United States; *T. brauni* and *T. glomerata* in Africa, dogs), *Echinococcus* genus (*E. granulosus*, *E. multilocularis*, *E. vogeli*, *E. oligarthrus*, worldwide, dogs and sheep), and *Spirometra* genus (*S. mansonoides* in the Western Hemisphere; *S. ranarum*, *S. mansoni*, and *S. erinacei* in the Far East, dogs and cats).

## Diagnosis

Determining the etiology of the lesions will depend on the particular overall clinical picture. Imaging studies, such as contrast MRI or CT, are useful in establishing the presence of focal CNS lesions, and in some cases, can be helpful in defining the etiology of the lesions. Neurocysticercosis can be diagnosed to different degrees of certainty using the recently revised diagnostic criteria (Table 79.6; Del Brutto et al., 2017). Table 79.5 provides specific diagnostic tests corresponding to common organisms.

**TABLE 79.7 Treatment for Neurocysticercosis**

| Form | Subgroup | Recommendation |
|---|---|---|
| **Parenchymal Neurocysticercosis** | | |
| Viable (live cysts) or enhancing lesions (degenerating cysts) | 1–2 cysts | Antiparasitic treatment (albendazole monotherapy) with steroids |
| | >2 cysts | Antiparasitic treatment (albendazole and praziquantel) with steroids |
| Calcified cysticerci | Any number | No antiparasitic treatment |
| Encephalitis (with diffuse cerebral edema) | | No antiparasitic treatment, use steroids |
| **Extraparenchymal Neurocysticercosis** | | |
| Intraventricular | Surgical removal feasible | Lateral or third ventricle: neuroendoscopic removal<br>Fourth ventricle: neuroendoscopic or microsurgical removal based on experience of surgeon<br>No medical therapy if removal successful |
| | Removal not feasible | Ventricular shunt followed by antiparasitic treatment with steroids (antiparasitic treatment can precipitate hydrocephalus) |
| Subarachnoid | | Ventricular shunt first if there is hydrocephalus, followed by antiparasitic treatment (prolonged course of albendazole, or albendazole and praziquantel) |
| Hydrocephalus with no visible cysts on neuroimaging | | Ventricular shunt, no antiparasitic treatment |
| Spinal cysticercosis, intra- or extramedullary | | Surgical removal or antiparasitic treatment with steroids (individualized based on circumstances) |
| Ocular cysticercosis | | Surgical resection of cysts |

*Adapted from Garcia, H.H., Evans, C.A., Nash, T.E., et al., 2002. Current consensus guidelines for treatment of neurocysticercosis. Clin. Microbiol. Rev. 15, 747–756; and White Jr., A.C., Coyle, C.M., Rajshekhar, V., et al., 2018. Diagnosis and treatment of neurocysticercosis: 2017 Clinical Practice Guidelines by the Infectious Diseases Society of America (IDSA) and the American Society of Tropical Medicine and Hygiene (ASTMH). Clin. Infect. Dis. 66 (8), e49–e75.*

### Management

The treatment of focal parasitic CNS infections should be tailored to the specific organism. For specific agents targeting the most common organisms, see Table 79.5. Table 79.7 outlines recommendations adapted from consensus guidelines (Garcia et al., 2002) and clinical practice guidelines (White et al., 2018) for the treatment of neurocysticercosis. Other associated conditions should be managed as needed (e.g., antiepileptic drugs for seizure and surgical intervention for symptomatic obstructive hydrocephalus).

### Prevention

The prevention of most parasitic diseases relies on access to clean water, soap, education about good hygiene (e.g., handwashing before eating or when preparing food), and eating well-cooked food. For malaria, global prevention includes early detection and treatment of disease, insecticide-impregnated bed-nets, and controlling environmental breeding areas (NVBDCP, 2009). For travelers to endemic areas, including expats who are returning to visit friends and family, antimicrobial prophylaxis is the best mechanism for preventing malaria.

## SUMMARY

Bacterial, fungal, and parasitic infections of the CNS are important diseases generally associated with decreasing mortality over the past century as a result of advancements in antimicrobial therapy, improved imaging, and enhanced neurosurgical techniques. Although infectious diseases have continued to expand as pathogenic organisms find new niches and the number of immunosuppressed patients increases, our ability to diagnose and treat these infections will likely continue to improve as well.

*The complete reference list is available online at https://expertconsult.inkling.com/.* 

80

# Multiple Sclerosis and Other Inflammatory Demyelinating Diseases of the Central Nervous System

*Michelle T. Fabian, Stephen C. Krieger, Fred D. Lublin*

## OUTLINE



Diseases affecting central nervous system (CNS) myelin can be classified on the basis of whether a primary biochemical abnormality of myelin exists *(dysmyelinating)* or whether some other process damages the myelin or oligodendroglial cell *(demyelinating)*. Demyelinating diseases in which normal myelin is disrupted include autoimmune, infectious, toxic and metabolic, and vascular processes. Dysmyelinating diseases in which a primary abnormality of the formation of myelin exists include several hereditary disorders. Infectious demyelinating disease (progressive multifocal leukoencephalopathy [PML]), toxic and metabolic demyelinating diseases, and vascular demyelinating disease (Binswanger disease) are discussed elsewhere. The present chapter concentrates on multiple sclerosis (MS) and other inflammatory demyelinating diseases of myelin as well as other CNS diseases that are presumably immune mediated (Box 80.1).

**BOX 80.1 Diseases of Myelin**

**Autoimmune**
Acute disseminated encephalomyelitis
Acute hemorrhagic leukoencephalopathy
Multiple sclerosis

**Infectious**
Progressive multifocal leukoencephalopathy

**Toxic/Metabolic**
Carbon monoxide poisoning
Vitamin $B_{12}$ deficiency
Mercury intoxication (Minamata disease)
Alcohol/tobacco amblyopia
Central pontine myelinolysis
Marchiafava-Bignami syndrome
Hypoxia
Radiation

**Vascular**
Binswanger disease

**Hereditary Disorders of Myelin Metabolism**
Adrenoleukodystrophy
Metachromatic leukodystrophy
Krabbe disease
Alexander disease
Canavan-van Bogaert-Bertrand disease
Pelizaeus-Merzbacher disease
Phenylketonuria

## CHARACTERISTIC CLINICAL SYMPTOMS AND PHYSICAL FINDINGS IN MULTIPLE SCLEROSIS

MS is classically described as principally a demyelinating disorder that affects multiple white matter tracts within the CNS. The variability of MS in clinical presentation is well known. This heterogeneity includes age of onset, mode of initial manifestation, frequency, severity and sequelae of relapses, extent of progression, and cumulative deficit over time, as will be discussed across this chapter. The clinical features reflect the widespread distribution of CNS injury, and we will begin with an overview of the signs and symptoms of this disease, referable to characteristic demyelinating localizations: optic neuritis (ON), brainstem, and spinal cord.

## CRANIAL NERVE DYSFUNCTION

### Impairment of Visual Pathways

ON, inflammation at any point of the optic nerve, is common at some point in the course of patients with relapsing MS, and frequently it may be the presenting symptom. The optic nerve is the most commonly affected site of the visual pathway. It usually manifests as an acute or subacute unilateral syndrome characterized by pain in the eye that is accentuated by ocular movements, followed by a variable degree of visual loss affecting mainly central vision and sometimes decreased color vision as well. Patients with ON often have a relative afferent pupillary defect (Marcus Gunn pupil) and most have a normal fundoscopic exam; papillitis is rarely seen. Mapping of visual fields reveals a central or cecocentral scotoma (central scotoma involving the physiological blind spot). After an attack of acute ON, 90% of patients regain normal vision, typically over a period of 2–6 months.

It is important to note that bilateral, simultaneous ON is rare in MS, and its occurrence may suggest another diagnosis such as Leber hereditary optic neuropathy, toxic optic neuropathy, neuromyelitis optica, or anti-MOG antibody associated ON. In bilateral ON in MS cases, the impairment usually begins asymmetrically and is more severe in one eye.

### Impairment of Ocular Motor Pathways

Impairment of individual ocular motor nerves is infrequent in MS but may occur in isolation or as part of a brainstem syndrome. When present, the involved nerves are, in decreasing order of frequency, cranial nerves VI, III, and (rarely) IV.

Brainstem syndromes in MS causing eye movement abnormalities are frequently those that reflect lesions of vestibulo-ocular connections and internuclear connections. Nystagmus is a common finding in MS. One form of nystagmus particularly characteristic of MS is *acquired pendular nystagmus*, in which there are rapid small-amplitude pendular oscillations of the eyes in the primary position. Patients frequently complain of *oscillopsia* (subjective oscillation of objects in the field of vision). This type of nystagmus is most often bilateral, but can also be unilateral and may be seen as consequent of an optic neuropathy, or because of involvement in the cerebellum or dorsal pontine tegmentum (Brazis et al., 2011).

Internuclear ophthalmoplegia (INO), defined as abnormal horizontal ocular movements with lost or impaired adduction and horizontal nystagmus of the abducting eye, is secondary to a lesion of the medial longitudinal fasciculus on the side of diminished adduction. Convergence is preserved. When present bilaterally, it is usually coupled with vertical nystagmus on upward gaze. Often a patient with an INO does not complain of a visual disturbance and it is instead recognized first by the examiner. Ocular pursuit movements are frequently saccadic rather than smooth. In the appropriate epidemiological context, the identification of an INO is highly suggestive of MS and should prompt a work-up for this diagnosis.

### Impairment of Other Cranial Nerves

Impairment of facial sensation—subjective or objective—is a relatively common finding in MS and may occur in isolation or as part of a hemisensory syndrome. The occurrence of trigeminal neuralgia in a young adult may prompt a work-up for MS, yet is an uncommon presenting symptom and, if it occurs, it is typically later in the course. *Facial myokymia*, a fine, undulating wavelike facial twitching, and hemifacial spasm can be caused by MS, but other causes of a focal brainstem lesion must be excluded (Mehanna and Jankovic, 2013). Unilateral facial paresis can occur. Complete hearing loss, usually unilateral, is an infrequent complaint. Isolated dysfunction of taste sensation is rare but has been well characterized with localization to the brainstem (McGraw et al., 2012). Malfunction of the lower cranial nerves is usually of the upper motor neuron type (pseudobulbar syndrome) and a rather late finding in MS. Vertigo is a reported symptom in 30%–50% of patients with MS and is commonly associated with dysfunction of adjacent brainstem or cranial nerves.

### Impairment of Cerebellar Pathways

Cerebellar pathway impairment, due to a lesion or lesions in the posterior fossa, results in gait imbalance, difficulty performing coordinated actions with the arms, and slurred speech. Examination reveals the usual features of cerebellar dysfunction. Ocular findings of nystagmus, ocular dysmetria, and frequent refixation saccades suggesting cerebellar or cerebellovestibular connection dysfunction are common. Speech can be either scanning or explosive in character. Dysmetria, decomposition of complex movements, and hypotonia are most often observed in the upper extremities. An intention tremor in the limbs and titubation of the head may be seen. Walking is impaired by ataxia. In severe cases, even with full strength, there is inability to use the arms because of a violent intention tremor and inability to stand. Such profound impairment of cerebellar function is rarely the permanent residua of acute relapse, and instead is typically a manifestation of progressive MS.

### Impairment of Sensory Pathways

Spinal cord white-matter lesions are common in MS, and as such, sensory manifestations are a frequent initial feature of MS and are present in almost every patient at some time during the course of disease. The sensory features can reflect spinothalamic, posterior column, or dorsal root entry zone lesions. The sensory symptoms are commonly described as numbness, tingling, pins and needles, tightness, coldness, itching, or a feeling of swelling of limbs or trunk. Radicular sensations, unilateral or bilateral, can be present, and a bandlike abdominal sensation may be described, euphemistically described as "the MS hug."

The most frequent sensory abnormalities on clinical examination are varying degrees of impairment of vibration and joint position sense, decrease of pain and light touch in a distal distribution in the four extremities, and patchy areas of reduced pain and light touch perception in the limbs and trunk. A bilateral sensory level, frequently ascending in character, is a more frequent finding than a hemisensory spinal cord (Brown-Séquard) syndrome.

The deafferented "useless" hand is a characteristic but uncommon feature, consisting of an impairment of function secondary to a pronounced alteration of proprioception, without loss of power. A lesion of the relevant root entry zones or posterior columns in the spinal cord may be responsible in such cases.

### Impairment of Motor Pathways

Corticospinal tract dysfunction is common in MS, and can occur in the setting of acute relapse or progressive disease. Weakness as a result of a relapse, typically due to a partial myelitis affecting motor pathways, can involve one or all limbs, although a devastating relapse resulting in permanent inability to walk is exceedingly rare. More commonly, sustained motor weakness can be either partial, as the residual of a relapse, or worsen gradually as a result of progressive disease. Paraparesis, or paraplegia with a lower extremity preponderance, occurs more frequently than significant weakness in the upper extremities (Giovannoni et al., 2017). A hemiparesis sparing the face is also common. Most patients with weakness develop spasticity to some degree. This can manifest as a feeling of muscle tightness, cramping, and stiffness with walking. In advanced cases of paralysis and severe spasticity, joint contractures may occur. The physical findings include an increased spastic tone, usually more marked in the legs than in the arms. The deep tendon reflexes of the affected limbs are exaggerated, sustained clonus may be elicited, and extensor plantar responses are observed. Occasionally, reduced reflexes reflect hypotonia due to cerebellar pathway lesions. Amyotrophy, when observed, most frequently affects the small muscles of the hand; lesions of the motor root exit zones may produce muscle denervation secondary to axon loss.

### Impairment of Bladder, Bowel, and Sexual Functions

The extent of sphincter and sexual dysfunction is typically the consequence of MS-related myelopathy, and often parallels the degree of motor impairment in the lower extremities. The most common complaint related to urinary bladder dysfunction is initially urgency, usually the result of uninhibited detrusor contraction, reflecting a suprasegmental lesion. As the disease progresses, urinary incontinence due to urgency becomes more frequent. With involvement of sacral segments of the spinal cord, symptoms of bladder hypoactivity may evolve (e.g., decreased urinary flow, interrupted micturition, incomplete bladder emptying). An atonic dilated bladder that empties by overflow results from loss of perception of bladder fullness and is usually associated with urethral as well as anal and genital hypoesthesia, and sensory deficits in the sacral dermatomes. A dyssynergic voluntary sphincter that interrupts bladder emptying will lead to frequent, small-volume urinations combined with a large postvoid residual. Urinary tract infections are common in MS, especially in women, and may present in atypical patterns without hallmark pain due to concomitant interruption of ascending nociceptive signal in the spinal cord.

Constipation is very common and is generally due to a combination of factors: spinal cord involvement, decreased general mobility, dietary issues, and the tendency of some patients to restrict their fluid intake in a misguided attempt to decrease urinary urgency and incontinence. Almost all patients with paraplegia require special measures to maintain regular bowel movements. Bowel urgency can also be a troubling symptom for patients.

Sexual dysfunction, although frequently overlooked, occurs in 40%–80% of patients with MS (Schairer et al., 2014). Men experience various degrees of erectile dysfunction, often trouble maintaining erection, whereas inability to ejaculate is less common. Sexual dysfunction in women manifests as inability to orgasm and decreased libido. Sexual dysfunction can be the result of multiple problems, including the direct effects of lesions on the motor, sensory, and autonomic pathways within the spinal cord as well as psychological factors that affect libido: depression, self-image, self-esteem, and fear of rejection by the sexual partner. Mechanical difficulties created by spasticity, paraparesis, and incontinence may further aggravate the problem.

## PATHOPHYSIOLOGY

The symptoms and signs of MS are the result of the pathological process that occurs in the CNS. In early relapsing disease, new lesion formation is responsible for acute symptom development. In the natural history of the disease state, a progressive phenotype develops in most; axonal loss then results in the gradual accumulation of neurological deficit.

### Changes in Axonal Conduction with Demyelination

A comparison of the physiological properties of normally myelinated axons and demyelinated axons provides insight into the disease process. Compacted myelin is the lipid-rich plasma membrane of oligodendrocytes that provides insulation for electrical impulses traveling along axons. Myelinated axons propagate nerve impulses rapidly in a saltatory fashion, with a high safety factor for transmission (five to seven times above threshold). Current is induced by the opening of voltage-gated $Na^+$ channels found at the nodes of Ranvier. The resultant $Na^+$ influx creates a current that then moves toward the next node of Ranvier, as current cannot flow outward in myelinated internodal segments (Fig. 80.1). $K^+$ channel opening terminates current flow and leads to repolarization. Several types of $K^+$ channels exist in the axon. Fast $K^+$ channels sensitive to 4-aminopyridine are located in internodal axonal membrane and contribute to repolarization of demyelinated axons. Slow $K^+$ channels are found at the nodes of Ranvier and have a role in modulating repetitive firing. The $Na^+/K^+$-adenosine triphosphatase (ATPase) in the axon membrane restores ionic balance after high-frequency firing.

Demyelination interrupts current flow by removing the insulator of internodal axon current flow. After a relapse, remyelination occurs with recovery of clinical function to some degree in most cases. Transient worsening of function reflects a drop below the safety threshold for conduction because of physiological changes involving the partially demyelinated axon. This explains the characteristic Uhthoff phenomenon, a temporary worsening of previous symptoms with increased body temperature. To contrast, persistent neurological deficit happens in areas that have been less completely myelinated. In those regions, severe conduction block remains or severe axonal destruction has taken place.

## Formation of the Multiple Sclerosis Lesion

Although debated, it is generally thought that activation of myelin-specific T cells in the periphery precede the formation of an MS lesion, as opposed to a CNS location as the origin of attack. The trigger for each relapse is generally unknown, though some relapses may occur after immune system activation secondary to a viral infection, or in the postpartum setting. One of the earliest features of acute MS lesion formation is the interruption of the blood-brain barrier (BBB). The BBB normally functions to regulate protein transport and ion concentration, and to block pathogens and immune cells from CNS entry. It is composed of a thick membrane of glycocalyx, non-fenestrated endothelial cells, a vascular basement membrane, the glia limitans, and astrocytic end-feet. The endothelial cells of the BBB are connected through tight junctions (Varatharaj and Galea, 2017).

During a relapse, activated CD4 T cells are likely the first to enter the CNS, bringing a plethora of immune cells behind. Grossly, the pathological hallmark of MS is the cerebral or spinal plaque, which consists of a discrete region of demyelination with relative preservation of axons, although spectroscopic and pathological studies suggest some axonal loss may be an integral part of the disease process. Examination of the brain in MS often reveals atrophy and ventricular dilatation. Plaques may be visible on the surface of the spinal cord on inspection. The cut surface of the brain reveals the plaques, which when active, appear whitish yellow or pink with somewhat indistinct borders. Older plaques appear translucent with a blue-gray discoloration and sharply demarcated margins. Individual lesions are generally small (1–2 cm) but may become confluent, generating large plaques. Plaques develop in a perivenular distribution and are seen most frequently in the periventricular white-matter, brainstem, and spinal cord (Figs. 80.2 and 80.3), a finding confirmed with magnetic resonance imaging (MRI) studies. However, large numbers of small plaques, often detected only by microscopy, are found in cortical regions affecting intracortical myelinated fibers. Histological examination of active plaques has revealed abnormal infiltration of lymphocytes, monocytes, and macrophages, with occasional plasma cells around a central vein. The process then propagates radially (Gaitán et al., 2011) and myelin

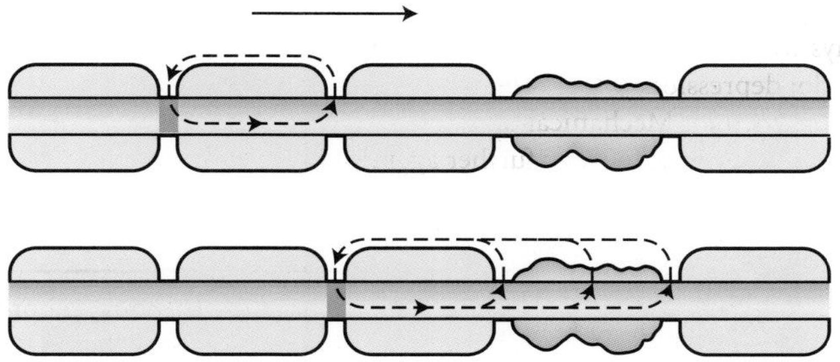

**Fig. 80.1** Schematic diagram of impulse conduction in normal *(upper)* and demyelinated *(lower)* regions of a nerve fiber. *Solid arrow* indicates the direction of impulse conduction; *red area* indicates the region occupied by the impulse. Current flow is indicated by *broken arrows*. In normally myelinated regions *(upper)*, the high resistance, low capacitance directs the majority of action current to the next node of Ranvier. In contrast, in demyelinated regions *(lower)*, action current is short-circuited through the damaged myelin sheath or denuded regions of the axon, so further propagation of the action potential is blocked. (*Reprinted with permission from Waxman, S.G., 1982. Membranes, myelin, and the pathophysiology of multiple sclerosis. N Engl J Med 306, 1529–1533.*)

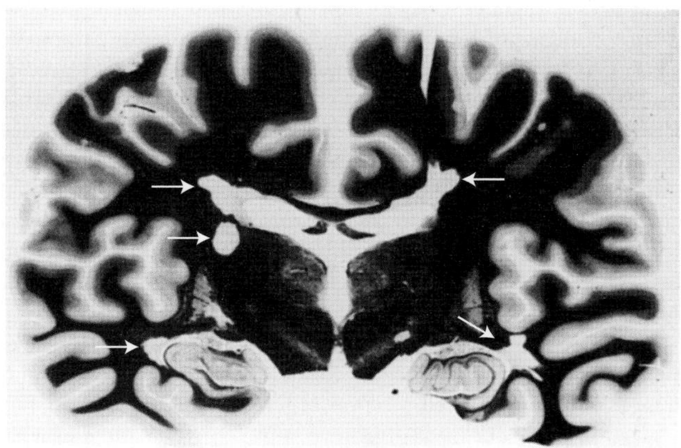

**Fig. 80.2** Coronal section of brain showing large plaques adjacent to lateral ventricles and temporal horns. A plaque is also seen in the left internal capsule *(arrows)* (Heidenhain myelin stain). (*Courtesy Dr. S. Carpenter.*)

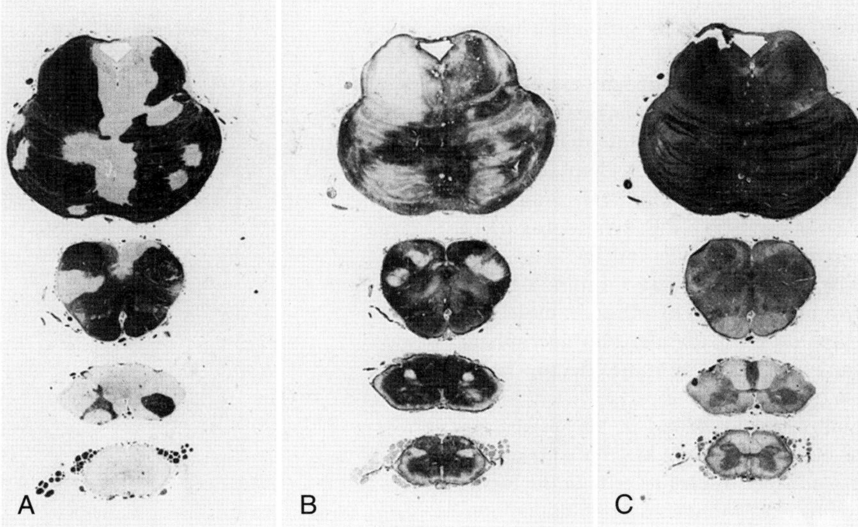


**Fig. 80.3** Brainstem and spinal cord sections from patient with multiple sclerosis stained with Heidenhain myelin stain (**A**), Holzer stain for gliosis (**B**), and Bodian stain for axons (**C**). Note mirror image of myelin and Holzer stains in the pons. Also note dramatic demyelination of sacral cord with preserved myelin in nerve roots (A, *bottom*). (*Courtesy Dr. S. Carpenter.*)

is disrupted, resulting in myelin debris found in clumps and within lipid-laden "foamy" macrophages. Reactive astrocytes are prominent in plaques. Immunohistochemical studies have found increased levels of cytokines in active plaques, indicative of ongoing immunoreactivity.

Oligodendroglia numbers are reduced proportionate to myelin loss in the plaque center, whereas at the plaque edge, oligodendroglia are preserved or even increased, suggesting an attempt at remyelination. Remyelination may involve either oligodendrocytes that previously produced myelin or maturation of progenitor cells. Such remyelination may explain the clinical finding of slow and delayed recovery from an acute attack, whereas rapid clinical recovery presumably reflects the resolution of edema, inflammation, and removal of toxic factors associated with acute plaques in which myelin destruction is minimal. Pathological studies demonstrate that the extent of remyelination can be quite extensive, even in patients with progressive disease (Patrikios et al., 2006).

Data derived from biopsy as well as autopsy material (Lucchinetti et al., 2000) have emphasized the heterogeneity of the MS lesion. These investigators have described four distinct pathological patterns. Some lesions appear to be chiefly inflammatory (types I and II), with retention of active oligodendrocytes derived from identifiable precursor cells and evidence of remyelination. The most common pathological pattern seen (type II) had inflammatory infiltrates and deposition of complement and immunoglobulin (Ig)G. In other patients, extensive destruction of oligodendrocytes, little replacement, and closer resemblance to a viral or toxic cell apoptosis or necrosis was found (types III and IV). All active lesions from an individual patient were of the same type. A follow-up to this study reported that patients with repeat biopsies continued to exhibit the same pathological subtype over time (Metz et al., 2014). The specific target of the immune-mediated injury in MS remains undetermined.

Lymphocytes in the lesion are specifically sensitized to myelin antigens. Reports vary with regard to the extent of restriction and the precise profile of the T-cell receptor repertoire of CNS T cells. T-cell sensitization could occur via direct exposure to myelin antigens within the CNS or within cervical lymph nodes, a site to which CNS antigens are transported through draining, or via exposure to exogenous agents sharing antigenic determinants with myelin, termed molecular mimicry. Microglial cells, endothelial cells, and astrocytes can be induced to express major histocompatibility complex (MHC) antigens and function as antigen-presenting cells, thus potentially promoting myelin antigen interaction with immune-mediating cells.

Activated T cells and the microglia-macrophages can contribute to tissue injury via non-antigen-restricted mechanisms. Each of these cell types releases an array of soluble factors that can contribute to tissue injury, including oligodendroglia. Cytokines characteristic of T cells include interleukin 2 (IL-2), interferon gamma (IFN-γ), and tumor necrosis factor β (TNF-β; lymphotoxin). A shift toward $T_H1$ cells expressing IFN-γ, TNF, and IL-2 and away from $T_H2$ cells is characteristic. Many of these immunologically active substances can result in upregulation of adhesion molecules that can promote or facilitate nonspecific lymphocyte-macrophage migration to the site of immune injury and immune effector–target cell interactions.

B cells and immunoglobulins are also found in MS lesions. To date, no specific antibody has been identified in MS, but anti-myelin antibodies have been shown to enhance disease severity in the experimental allergic encephalomyelitis (EAE) model, suggesting that both cellular and humoral mechanisms may be needed for full expression of immune injury. Furthermore, the marked effect of B-cell depleting therapies such as rituximab and ocrelizumab allude to their critical role in the pathogenic process.

Chronic inactive plaques are hypocellular and show astrocytic proliferation with denuded axons and an absence of oligodendroglia (Figs. 80.4 and 80.5). Axonal loss also may be noted to a variable extent. Microglia and macrophages are scattered throughout the lesion. The edge of chronic plaques may still exhibit hypercellularity, suggesting continued disease activity.

In progressive MS, ongoing low-grade demyelination is found at the borders of plaques, and this may explain the slow expansion of plaques and occurrence of more diffuse inflammation leading to progressive loss of function (Kutzelnigg et al., 2005; Prineas et al., 2001).

Recent pathological studies have focused on the gray matter in MS and have found a lesion load within the cortex and deep gray structures. The nature of the intracortical plaques differs from those seen in white matter because there is less inflammation but considerable reactive microgliosis (Bo et al., 2003).

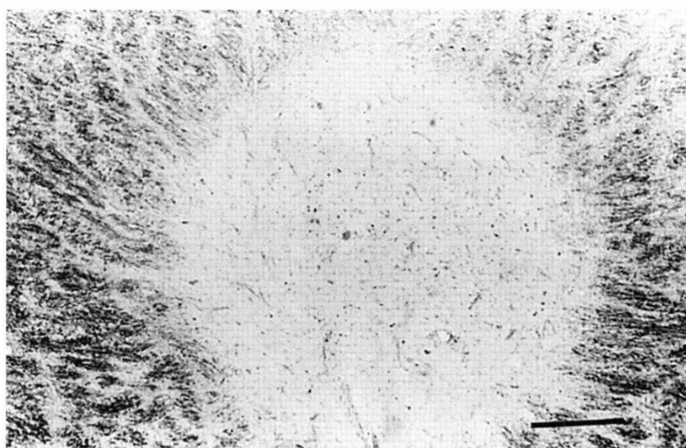

**Fig. 80.4** Punched-out appearance of an old multiple sclerosis plaque surrounded by regions with varying amounts of myelin preservation (periodic acid-Schiff luxol fast blue; bar = 100 μm). (*Courtesy Dr. S. Carpenter.*)

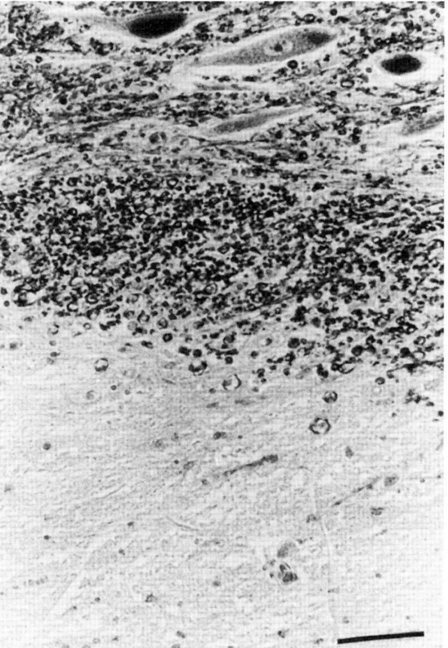

**Fig. 80.5** Plaque edge of an old plaque with a sharply demarcated zone of demyelination and normal myelin above (periodic acid-Schiff luxol fast blue; bar = 50 μm). (*Courtesy Dr. S. Carpenter.*)

## ETIOLOGY

### Autoimmunity

Low levels of autoreactive T cells and B cells are present in normal individuals. Presumably they have escaped from clonal deletion during the process of immune development and are now tolerant of their antigens. Autoimmunity develops when these cells lose tolerance and a complex process of immune reactivity in target tissues begins. One potential way tolerance can be broken is by means of molecular mimicry between self-antigens and foreign antigens—for example, viral components. Several viral and bacterial peptides share structural similarities with important proteins of myelin, and a few of them are able to activate specific T-cell clones derived from patients with MS. Another way tolerance can be broken is by CNS infection that causes tissue damage and antigen release into the peripheral circulation, where corresponding autoreactive T cells may be encountered.

Myelin basic protein (MBP) has long been considered one of the primary candidates for an autoimmune attack. T cells that respond to MBP are found in the peripheral blood in both normal persons and those with MS, possibly at higher levels in MS patients with active disease. MBP, which accounts for 30% of the protein of myelin, can be an antigen for EAE, the primary animal model of MS.

Several other myelin proteins are also candidates for an autoimmune attack. Proteolipid protein accounts for 50% of CNS myelin protein and is an integral membrane protein of the myelin leaflets. Myelin-associated glycoprotein, myelin oligodendrocyte glycoprotein, and cyclic nucleotide phosphodiesterase are proteins that each account for a few percent of myelin. Myelin oligodendrocyte glycoprotein and cyclic nucleotide phosphodiesterase are not found in peripheral nerve myelin and are therefore of special interest.

Although the possibility of pure autoimmunity as the causal mechanism for MS exists, the issue is not proven. The evidence for MS being a dysimmune condition is more compelling; with alterations in the immune cell repertoire and activation state both in blood and cerebrospinal fluid (CSF) of MS patients compared to others (Conlon et al., 1999; Hafler et al., 2005).

### Genetics

MS is a genetically complex disease. Compared to the general population, a higher frequency of familial occurrence of MS suggests a strong but non-Mendelian inheritance of susceptibility. Twin studies established the importance of genetic factors: the concordance rate for a clinical diagnosis of MS in female monozygotic twins is about 30%, whereas in dizygotic twins it is 2%–5% (Ebers et al., 1995; Willer et al., 2003). The risk is highest for siblings: 3%–5%, or 30–50 times the background risk for this same population. Adoptive relatives, when raised from infancy with the patients with MS, are no more likely to develop MS than the general population.

MS is associated with both MHC and human leukocyte antigen (HLA) class I A3 and B7 antigens. The class II polymorphisms, Dw2 and DR2, also show strong association, and specifically the HLA DRB1*1501 allele (Oksenberg et al., 2004). Additional HLA alleles that carry protective as well as detrimental effects with regard to MS susceptibility have been identified. HLA-A*02, for example, has a protective effect relative to MS susceptibility. Additional MS susceptibility loci outside of the MHC have been described. Specifically, the loci coding for IL-7 receptor and IL-2 receptor are strongly linked with MS susceptibility (Zuvich et al., 2010). IL-7 and IL-2 receptor signaling is critical for the differentiation of $CD4^-$ $CD8^-$ thymocytes and has a role in survival of $CD4^+$ $CD8^+$ cells after positive selection. This may be important not only in MS predisposition but also in disease course and outcome.

In recent years, multiple genome-wide association studies (GWAS) have been performed, allowing for the analysis of a larger number of genetic variants that individually have a small, but still significant, impact on MS risk. Greater than 230 genetic variants have been identified through these studies, yet combined they account for only 20% of the heritability risk. Recently, an important study analyzed 32,367 MS cases and 36,012 controls and found 4 novel gene variants that independently contribute an additional 5% risk (International Multiple Sclerosis Genetics Consortium: chris.cotsapas@yale.edu & International Multiple Sclerosis Genetics Consortium, 2018). Although there have been clear advancements in this area of study, current knowledge of MS genetics has not enabled the creation of reliable diagnostic or prognostic tools for use in the clinic.

### Infection

A possible role for microbial infection in the causation of MS has been a matter of ongoing debate for decades. However, beyond speculation, little direct evidence supports the concept. Specific efforts to recover a known viral genome have been fruitless. Despite this, in recent decades pathogens such as human herpesvirus 6 (HHV6), Epstein-Barr virus (EBV), and *Chlamydia pneumoniae* have been the focus of interest as potential triggers for MS.

Perhaps the most compelling argument has been made for a possible role for EBV in MS pathogenesis. Although EBV is extremely common in the population, with a prevalence between 90% and 95%, multiple studies have shown seroprevalence to be greater than 99%, though importantly not 100%, in MS patients. Furthermore, history of infectious mononucleosis, as opposed to the more common asymptomatic EBV infection, seems to further predispose to risk for MS (Handel et al., 2010). Potential mechanisms invoking EBV in the development of MS include an inappropriate autoreactive immune response as the result of molecular mimicry or a more direct role of the EBV virus promoting persistent inflammation in the CNS (Pakpoor et al., 2013).

### Vitamin D

Although there is no definitive evidence for vitamin D deficiency as a causative factor in the pathogenesis of MS, low levels of vitamin D have now been associated with an increased risk for MS in many different studies. Early epidemiological studies in MS noted an increasing prevalence of MS in populations at increasing distances from the equator. This led to the hypothesis that decreasing levels of vitamin D, related to lower levels of sun exposure, could explain this phenomenon. Cohort studies supported this theory, as vitamin D supplementation was inversely related to the risk for MS in two groups of nurses (Munger et al., 2004), and similarly, the highest serum levels of 25-hydroxy vitamin D correlated to the lowest risk for MS and vice versa in a group of 7 million US military recruits (Munger et al., 2006). Multiple studies since have also shown this association. Furthermore, the correlation between low serum vitamin D levels and an increased risk for continued MS disease activity has been made both radiologically (Mowry et al., 2012) and with data from a clinical trial cohort (Ascherio et al., 2014). The SOLAR trial is the largest completed trial to date of vitamin D supplementation in MS. This 48-week, double-blind placebo-controlled trial of high-dose (14,000 IU daily) vitamin $D_3$ as an add-on to 44-μg scIFN β-1a did not find a difference in disease activity free status or in relapse rate between the groups (Smolders, 2016). Thus, despite many indications of the role of vitamin D in MS, it remains to be seen if supplementing an MS patient can alter the disease course.

### Smoking

The association between smoking and an increased risk for MS has been established with evidence from multiple case control studies.

Smoking increases the risk of developing MS and the risk of conversion from CIS to clinically definite MS (CDMS; van der Vuurst de Vries et al., 2018). There is also evidence, albeit weaker, that smokers have a more severe course than nonsmokers (Manouchehrinia et al., 2013). Smoking is thought to be a direct neurotoxin, but also may bring about immunomodulatory changes that promote inflammation (Goodin, 2014).

### Diet and the Microbiome

Although several studies have linked MS and childhood obesity (Hedstrom et al., 2014; Munger et al., 2013), there are no specific dietary factors that are known to provoke or ameliorate the MS course. However, there is a plethora of ongoing research in this area. Likewise, the human microbiome is also a topic of interest in relation to the risk of getting MS, as well as to its impact on the MS course. Thus far, researchers have been able to show that both adult and pediatric patients with MS do have a different microbiome signature than people without (Chen et al., 2016, Tremlett et al., 2016). Furthermore, treatment with MS disease-modifying therapies (DMTs) also has been shown to impact the composition of the microbiome (Katz Sand et al., 2019). However, further work needs to be done to understand the complexities of the relationship between the microbiome and MS.

## EPIDEMIOLOGY

### Age of Onset

Most studies agree that the mean and median age of onset in relapsing forms of MS is age 29–32. The peak age of onset is approximately 5 years earlier for women than for men. Primary progressive multiple sclerosis (PPMS) has a mean age of onset of 35–39 years. It is well recognized that the onset of MS can occur well outside of these ranges; 5% of cases of MS have their onset before age 18. Most of these cases occur in adolescence, but a small percentage have an onset in the first decade of life (Fig. 80.6). Patients may also present with first symptoms after age 50, in 3%–12% of incident cases (Tremlett et al., 2006).

### Sex Distribution

Similar to most other autoimmune conditions, MS affects more women than men. During the 20th century the female: male ratio of incident relapsing MS cases has increased in most geographic locations (Westerlind et al., 2014). Although some have hypothesized that this is due to ascertainment bias (milder cases in females discovered through increased use of MRI and more sensitive diagnostic criteria), most agree that changes in childbearing patterns and epigenetic and environmental factors also likely contribute to this trend (Miller et al., 2014). The female: male ratio in relapsing-remitting MS in most countries is 2–3:1, although interestingly it has remained steady at 1:1 in PPMS (Kalancik et al., 2013).

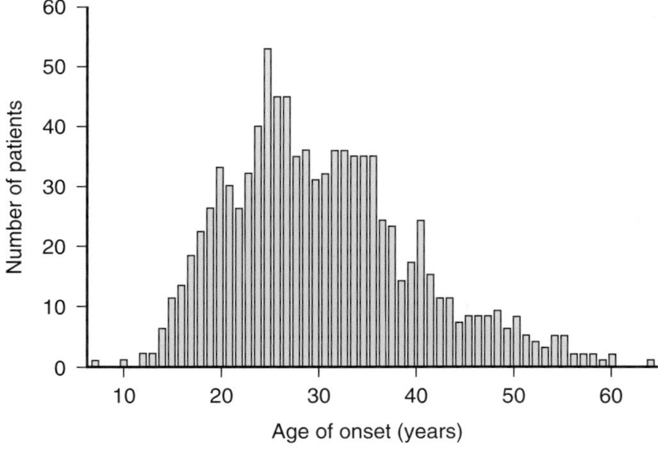


**Fig. 80.6** Age at onset of symptoms of multiple sclerosis in 940 patients followed at the Multiple Sclerosis Clinic of the Montreal Neurological Institute. Mean age of onset is 30.6 years, median is 27 years, and peak incidence is 25 years.

### Geographical Distribution

Hundreds of prevalence surveys have been carried out, serving as the basis for the delineation of geographical risk for MS depicted in Fig. 80.7. Worldwide, it is estimated that in 2016 2.2 million people had MS, which is 10.4% more cases than in 1990 (GBD 2016 Multiple Sclerosis Collaborators et al., 2019). High-frequency areas of the world include all of Europe (including Russia), southern Canada, the northern United States, New Zealand, and the southeastern portion of Australia. In many of these areas, the prevalence is far greater than 100 cases per 100,000. The largest increase in MS prevalence has been in Canada where there has been an 82% upsurge in the last 25 years. The number of cases of MS in the United States was estimated by the National MS Society in 2002 to be approximately 400,000 persons, yet more recent 2017 estimates are greater than 900,000 (Wallin et al., 2019). The rise in numbers is likely due to a combination of factors, including more sensitive criteria for diagnosis and increased survival.

One possible conclusion, as mentioned above, regarding geographical differences in prevalence is that MS is a location-related illness with a latitude gradient. However, this risk is clearly modulated genetics, as notable exceptions exist. Japan, situated at the same latitude as areas of high prevalence in Europe, is a low-risk area. Second-generation Japanese in the United States retain their parents' low risk of MS. The White population of South Africa, with medium prevalence of MS, is surrounded by a Black population in whom the disease is very uncommon. Native North Americans, especially of pure Amerindian background, have a very low prevalence but are surrounded by a White population with a medium or high risk for MS. People of Asian, African, or Native American origin have the lowest risk.

Migration data have often been used to support the view that an environmental agent is involved in the pathogenesis of MS. The data indicate that persons migrating from an area of high risk to an area of low risk after the age of puberty carry their former high risk with them. With migration during childhood, the risk seems to be that of the new area to which the person has migrated.

### Mortality

Most studies of MS and mortality have shown that MS shortens life span, on average, by a period of 7–14 years (Lunde et al., 2017, Scalfari et al., 2013). Death due to a catastrophic MS relapse is extraordinarily uncommon. Although MS is listed as the primary cause of death on an MS patient's death certificate approximately 50% of the time (Leray et al., 2015), more typically an infection or other complication of progressive MS is the actual cause. Cardiovascular disease, accidents, and suicide seem to be represented in a higher proportion in the MS population.

The evidence suggests that the increased rate of death in patients with MS does seem to be declining relative to that of the general population. In Denmark, an exceptionally complete survey of the country found the median survival after diagnosis for men was 28 years and for women 33 years, compared with matched population death rates of 37 and 42 years, respectively. The 10-year excess mortality was reduced by 50% in recent decades, even before the introduction of DMTs (Bronnum-Hansen et al., 2004). This trend seems to have continued

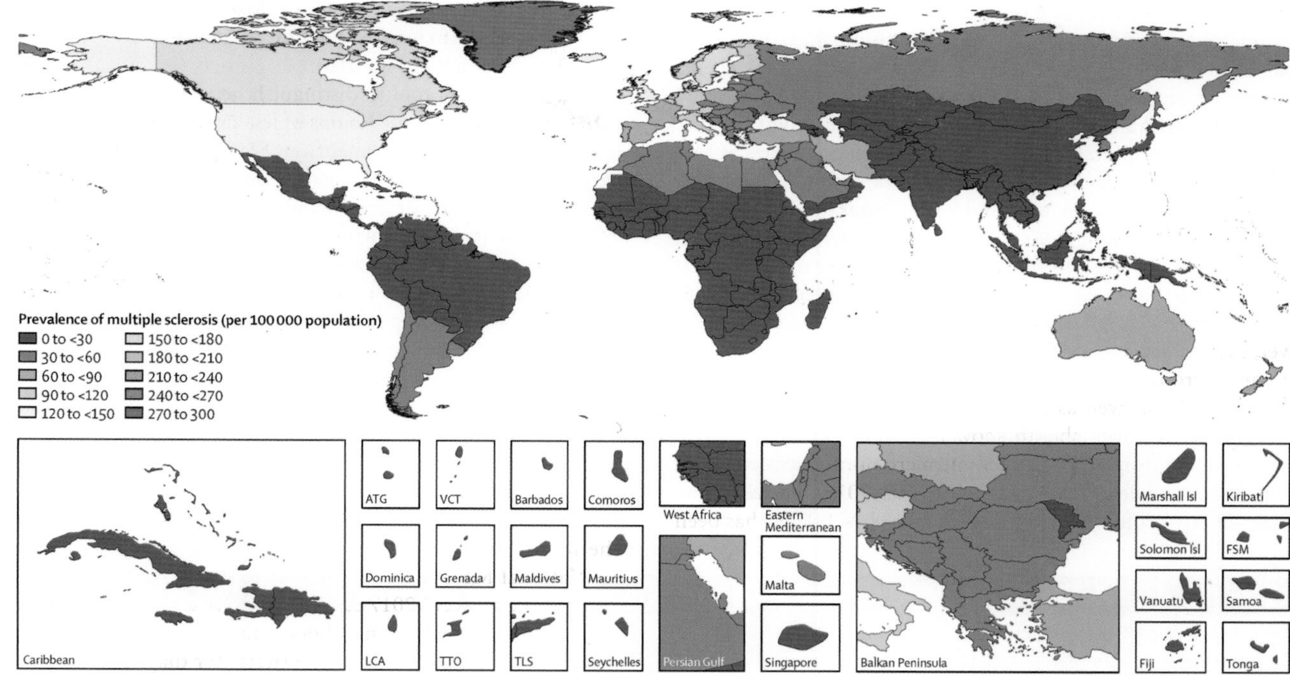


**Fig. 80.7** Worldwide distribution of multiple sclerosis as of 2016. (*From GBD 2016 Multiple Sclerosis Collaborators., 2019. Global, regional, and national burden of multiple sclerosis 1990–2016: a systematic analysis for the Global Burden of Disease Study 2016. Lancet Neurol. 18(3), 269–285.*)

in the post-DMT era. In another important study, a 21-year follow-up that included 98.4% of the patients enrolled in the pivotal IFN-β-1b trial, the risk for death in patients initially randomized to IFN-β-1b 250 μg was found to be decreased, with a hazard ratio (HR) of 0.53 versus those initially on placebo (Goodin et al., 2012), thus suggesting that early initiation of DMT might further alter mortality outcomes. These findings were replicated in a case-control study where greater than 3 years of IFN-β reduced the chance for death by 32% in a cohort composed of Canadian and French patients (Kingwell, 2019).

## DIAGNOSIS

### Diagnostic Criteria

In a condition such as MS, where a diagnosis proven by biopsy is rare and undesirable in almost all cases, formulating criteria that produce an accurate diagnosis through other means is of crucial import. There have been multiple sets of diagnostic criteria utilized over the years, in an effort to assist the clinician in making the correct diagnosis as well as to allow the researcher to identify those appropriate for studies. The common thread among all MS diagnostic criteria has been the requirement for symptoms and signs that are disseminated in time and space (more than one episode involving more than one area of the CNS).

Before 2001, the accepted criteria allowed for the diagnosis of MS based on clinical features alone—namely, history and physical examination—with support for the diagnosis gained by the use of CSF analysis, evoked potentials, and neuroimaging. In the Poser criteria, used from 1983 to 2001, a patient must have had two clinical attacks with evidence to support this on examination in order to be diagnosed with CDMS.

#### The McDonald Criteria

In 2001, McDonald and colleagues initiated the modern era of MS diagnosis by proposing diagnostic criteria that permitted activity on follow-up MRIs to substitute for a second clinical attack in order to meet dissemination in space (DIS) and dissemination in time (DIT). These criteria maintained an acceptable level of diagnostic sensitivity and specificity despite less rigorous clinical requirements. Importantly, incorporating subclinical activity on MRI into the criteria allowed for the diagnosis of MS to be made sooner, instead of waiting for additional clinical episodes as diagnostic confirmation.

The McDonald criteria were most recently revised in 2017 (Thompson et al., 2018) (Table 80.1). This version aimed to refine the earlier iterations, with only minor changes made. Like the previous 2010 criteria, at least one characteristic demyelinating episode is required in order to diagnosis relapsing-remitting multiple sclerosis (RRMS). DIS is satisfied if MRI reveals ≥f1 lesion in two out of four typical locations: periventricular, cortical/juxtacortical, infratentorial, and spinal cord. Here, the most important change is that cortical lesions were added as a typical lesion location interchangeable for a juxtacortical lesion. For the DIT criteria, the requirement is met when there is simultaneous presence of gadolinium-enhancing and nonenhancing lesions at any time, or a new T2 or T1 gadolinium-enhancing lesion on a follow-up MRI scan. To contrast, the 2010 criteria mandated that symptomatic lesions in the brainstem and spinal cord could not be used to support DIS or DIT.

One key addition to the 2017 criteria is the use of lumbar puncture to confirm a diagnosis. For patients with only one clinical event that meets DIS criteria, positive oligoclonal bands (OCBs) in the CSF now can substitute for DIT. This decision was made based on multiple studies that show that positive bands are an independent risk factor for further clinical activity (Thompson et al., 2018). Additionally, the panel maintained that the clinician should ascertain disease phenotype at diagnosis, and should periodically reassess.

### Diagnostic Studies

#### Magnetic Resonance Imaging

MRI is the preferred imaging modality for both making the diagnosis of MS and longitudinal follow-up of patients. MRI is based on relaxation properties of water in tissues and is sensitive to T2 (transverse) and T1 (longitudinal) relaxation rates of protons. Gadolinium (Gd) diethylenetriamine penta-acetic acid (DTPA) is a paramagnetic contrast agent. It crosses the disrupted BBB, indicating increased vascular permeability in association with inflammation. Gd enhancement is best seen on spin-echo T1-weighted imaging. These fundamental properties of MR image acquisition provide a sensitive measure of pathology; areas of brain inflammation, demyelination, and loss of axons can be especially well seen with this technique. Virtually all patients with MS have T2 and fluid-attenuated inversion recovery (FLAIR) abnormalities. New lesions occur 9–10 times more often than new clinical attacks in RRMS.

Characteristic cerebral lesions, or plaques, are focal and discrete, have an ovoid appearance, and are oriented perpendicularly to the plane of the lateral ventricles. These are classically referred to as Dawson's fingers and are thought to represent perivenular inflammation, seen pathologically in MS plaques. Additionally, lesions are characteristically located in the deep white matter and the centrum semiovale, as well as in cortical and deep gray-matter structures. Juxtacortical lesions affecting U-fibers are often seen in MS. Posterior optic radiation lesions are also frequently present. Posterior fossa lesions are commonly present in the cerebellum, middle cerebral peduncles, and in areas adjacent to the fourth ventricle (Fig. 80.8).

MRI is a helpful tool to distinguish between acute, subacute, and chronic MS lesions. Acute lesions of less than 12 weeks duration often show Gd contrast enhancement on T1-weighted sequences, indicating inflammation and BBB disruption. Enhancement patterns can appear as incomplete or, less commonly, complete rings, or as patchy or homogeneously enhancing lesions (Fig. 80.9). Ring-enhancing lesions are associated with significant tissue destruction (Minneboo et al., 2005). They may also be associated with a bright signal on diffusion-weighted imaging (DWI). Contrast-enhancing lesions are most often associated with a bright T2 or FLAIR signal, denoting an acute MS lesion. Acute MS lesions tend to be larger in size, with less well-defined margins. Infrequently, acute T2 bright lesions can disappear on subsequent scans, indicating reversible tissue inflammation and edema. At times, acute MS lesions may show an associated dark signal on T1 noncontrast scan (acute T1 lesion), consistent with edema and demyelination. Subacute MS plaques may no longer show contrast

**TABLE 80.1 McDonald Criteria for the Diagnosis of Multiple Sclerosis (MS)**

2017 revised McDonald MS diagnostic criteria*

Diagnosis of MS requires elimination of more likely diagnoses and demonstration of dissemination of lesions in space (DIS) and time (DIT)

| Clinical (Attacks) | Lesions | Additional Criteria to Make DX |
|---|---|---|
| 2 or more | Objective clinical evidence of ≥2 lesions or objective clinical evidence of 1 lesion with reasonable historical evidence of a prior attack | None. Clinical evidence alone will suffice; additional evidence desirable but must be consistent with MS |
| 2 or more | Objective clinical evidence of 1 lesion | DIS; OR await further clinical attack implicating a different CNS site |
| 1 | Objective clinical evidence of ≥2 lesions | DIT; OR await a second clinical attack OR demonstration of CSF-specific oligoclonal bands |
| 1 | Objective clinical evidence of 1 lesion | DIS; OR await further clinical attack implicating a different CNS site AND DIT; OR demonstrations of CSF-specific oligoclonal bands OR await a second clinical attack |
| 0 (progression from onset) | | One year of disease progression (retrospective or prospective) AND at least two of: DIS in the brain based on ≥1 T2 lesion in periventricular, cortical/juxtacortical or infratentorial regions; DIS in the spinal cord based on ≥2 T2 lesions; positive CSF |

*Thompson, A, Banwell, B, Barkoff, F., 2018. Diagnosis of multiple sclerosis: 2017 revisions of the McDonald Criteria. Lancet Neurol. 17(2), 162–173.*

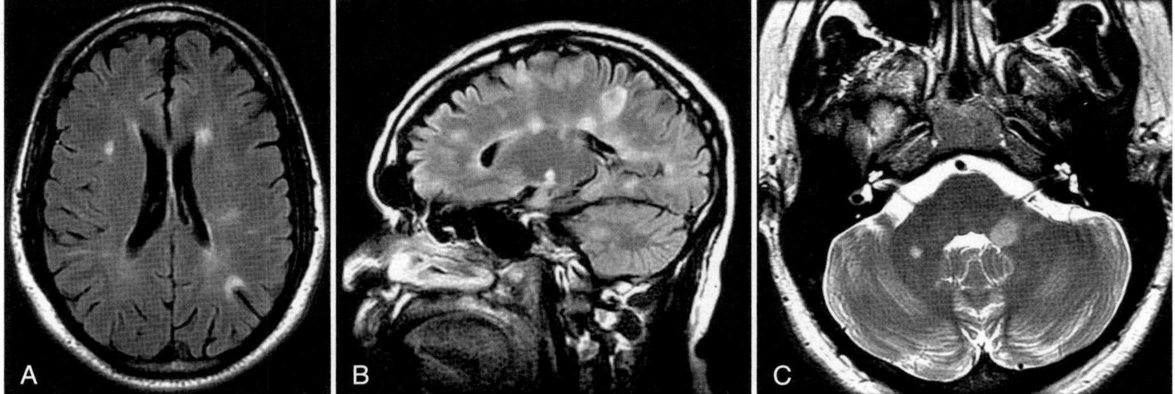


**Fig. 80.8 Typical Magnetic Resonance Imaging Appearance of Multiple Sclerosis Lesions in Brain. A,** Axial view with presence of both periventricular (PV) and juxtacortical lesions. **B,** Sagittal view with classic Dawson's finger appearance of PV lesions. Also present are juxtacortical and posterior fossa lesions. **C,** Axial view of posterior fossa lesions. T2 images are often best for viewing infratentorial lesions.

enhancement but may continue to show bright DWI abnormality. Chronic MS plaques appear hyperintense on T2 or FLAIR sequences, are usually smaller, and have sharper margins. Persistent and profound T1 hypointensity (also known as a "black hole") usually reflects irreversible tissue damage such as axonal loss and permanent demyelination (Neema et al., 2007; Fig. 80.10).

### High-Field Strength Magnetic Resonance Imaging

High (3 T) and ultra-high (7 T) MRI scanners greatly improve sensitivity for detecting T2 and Gd-enhancing lesions. Cerebral lesion volume also increases with higher field strength (Bachmann et al., 2006; Sicotte et al., 2003), and cortical lesions are easier to detect. Moreover, more patients fulfill the diagnostic criteria for MS when studied with 3 T or higher MRI because of improved lesion detection in both supra- and infratentorial compartments (Bakshi et al., 2008; Sicotte et al., 2003).

### Brain Atrophy

Progressive MS-related cerebral atrophy has been documented with various MRI techniques for over a decade. The rate of atrophy is estimated to be between 0.6% and 1.35% per year (Bermel and Bakshi, 2006). Semi-automated (atlas-based) and fully automated (voxel-based) segmentation tools are used in imaging research and clinical trials to assess loss of cerebral volume in MS. The brain parenchymal fraction (BPF), defined as the ratio of brain parenchymal volume to the total volume within the brain surface contour, is used to measure whole brain atrophy (Rudick et al., 1999). In clinical practice, cerebral volume loss is immediately apparent through progressive enlargement of CSF spaces including lateral ventricles and subarachnoid spaces (gyri and sulci) seen on conventional MRI. Gray matter is affected by atrophy more profoundly than white matter, and deep gray-matter nuclei are even more susceptible. Higher rates of atrophy

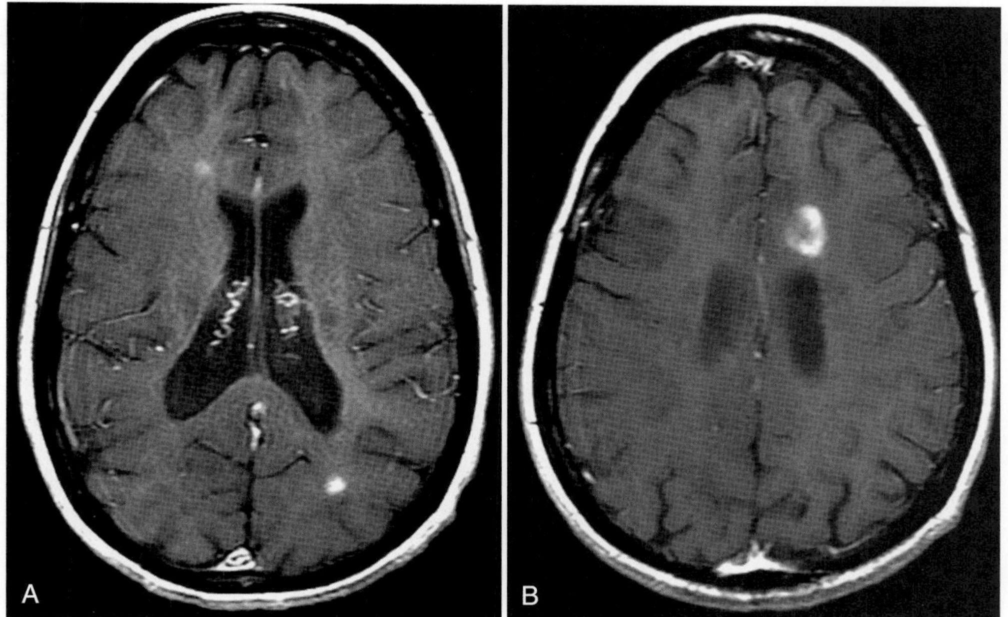


**Fig. 80.9** Common Enhancement Patterns in the Brain. A, Homogeneous uptake of contrast. B, Open-ring pattern, specific for demyelinating lesions.

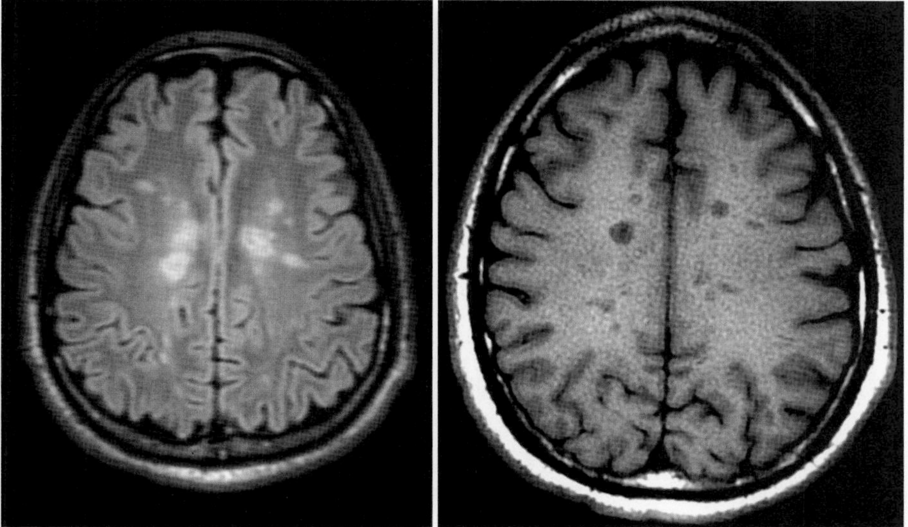

**Fig. 80.10** Axial fluid-attenuated inversion recovery (FLAIR) magnetic resonance imaging with corresponding T1 image showing evidence of black holes, areas believed to represent permanent tissue destruction and atrophy.

have been correlated with progressive disease and have become a target in clinical trials, functioning as a surrogate marker for progression itself (University of California, San Francisco MS-EPIC Team et al., 2019). While cerebral tissue loss in MS is an important factor, the ability to reliably measure it in a clinical setting remains suboptimal. Confounding factors include effects of aging, osmotic agents, and even anti-inflammatory treatments—all of which can decrease cerebral water content and result in a skewed finding of atrophy progression (Fig. 80.11).

***Spinal cord imaging.*** Over 90% of MS patients have spinal cord lesions at some point in their disease course, and 30% of patients presenting with CIS other than transverse myelitis have (asymptomatic) disease in the spinal cord (Dalton et al., 2003). They typically involve fewer than two contiguous segments of the spinal cord and are asymmetric (Fig. 80.12). Spinal cord lesions can be in the form of discrete isolated plaques or manifest as more confluent affected areas, especially in SPMS or PPMS patients. It is less common to have T1 hypointensities in the spinal cord. Lesions in the spinal cord produce neurological symptoms with a greater frequency than those in the brain, and cord atrophy has a strong correlation with neurological disability (Lukas, 2013).

## Cerebrospinal Fluid Analysis

CSF findings alone neither make nor exclude the diagnosis of MS. However, CSF analysis remains important in atypical clinical syndromes, atypical or nondiagnostic MRI findings, or unusual clinical manifestations such as a course of progressive neurological impairment without history of relapses. CSF does not show any gross abnormalities in MS; it is clear, colorless, and has a normal opening pressure. Cell counts are typically normal but may be slightly elevated in 15%–20% of patients. The predominant cells are T lymphocytes. Significant pleocytosis with greater than 50 white blood cells should raise suspicion of another etiology. Determining the presence of OCBs is the most important diagnostic test. These bands represent excess antibody produced by one or more clones of plasma cells. The pattern of banding remains relatively stable in an individual patient throughout the course of the disease. However, 10%–20% of patients with confirmed CDMS do not have OCBs at any given point in time. Presence of OCBs in a patient with CIS independently confers a higher rate of conversion to CDMS (Ferraro et al., 2013), and thus substitutes for DIT in the 2017 McDonald criteria. MBP in the CSF is a marker of tissue damage and has been used as a measure of CNS myelin breakdown. The levels of the protein may be quite increased in MS patients, but the specificity

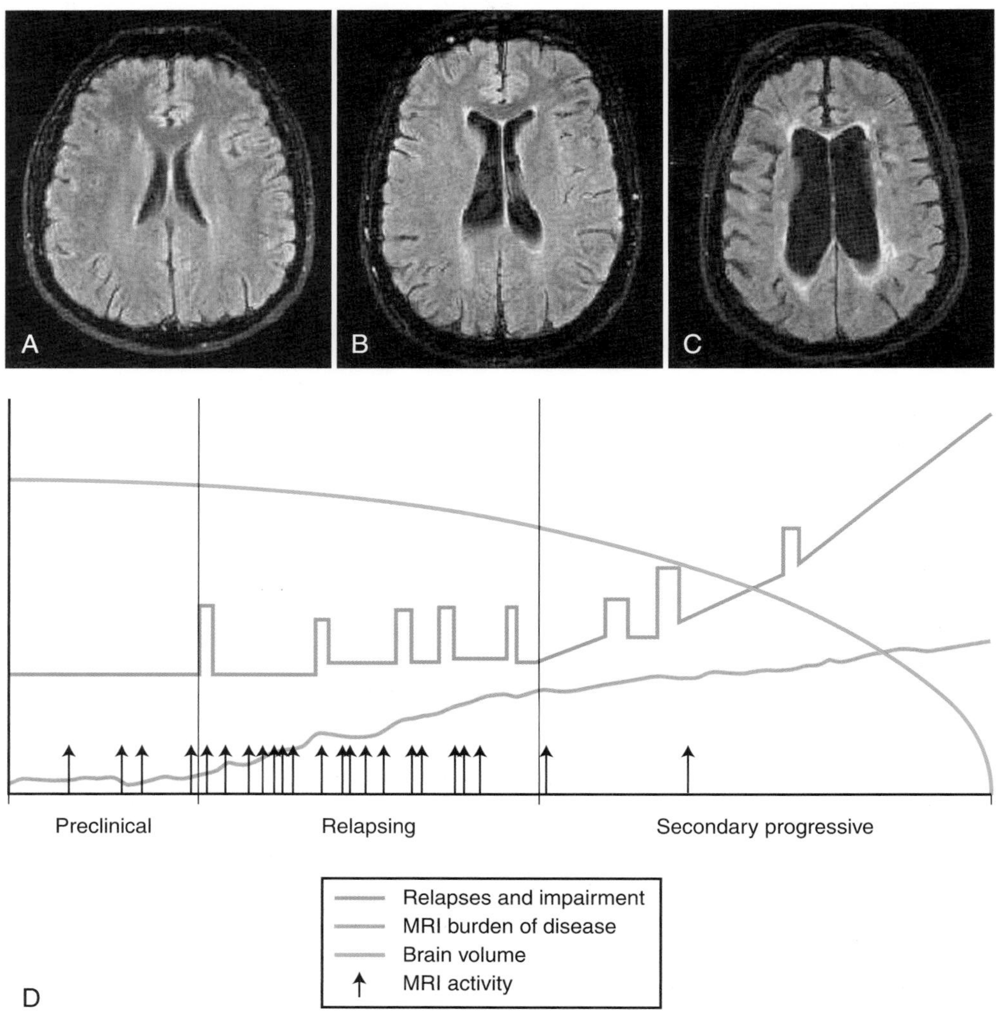


**Fig. 80.11** Changes in magnetic resonance imaging (*MRI*) scans with duration of disease. **A–C,** Comparison of three scans from patients with different disease duration, indicating the appearance of atrophy and ventricular dilation with time. **D,** As brain atrophy appears, it is common to observe that the number of gadolinium-enhancing lesions declines.

of these findings is not known and thus it is not recommended for use in diagnosis. An abnormality in CSF IgG production (as measured by the IgG index, or as a percentage of total protein or albumin) is found in over 90% of patients with confirmed MS (Table 80.2).

### Optic Coherence Tomography

Optic coherence tomography (OCT) can measure the retinal nerve fiber layer (RNFL) using a process analogous to ultrasound imaging, with light instead of sound. The RNFL is devoid of myelin and contains axons that converge to form the optic nerve. OCT can be used to noninvasively quantify axonal damage following an ON event. There is a correlation between optic nerve atrophy and RNFL thinning, suggesting that OCT may be useful in clinical trials aiming at neuroprotection. Despite the important information that OCT may provide, it is not used in the diagnosis of MS at this point in time.

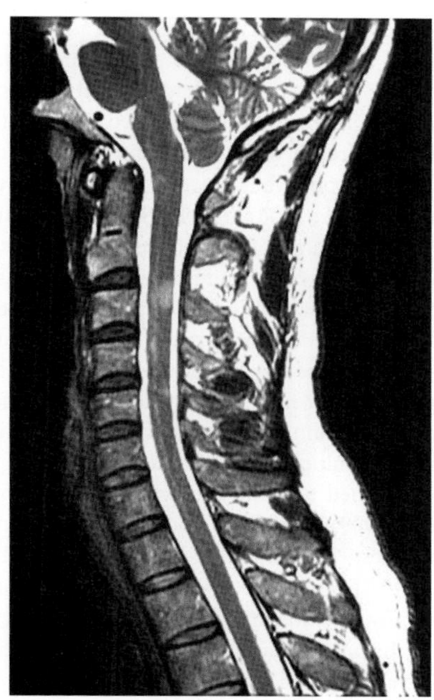

**Fig. 80.12** Sagittal, T2-weighted image of spinal cord with multiple, characteristic cord lesions.

### Evoked Potentials

Evoked potentials (EPs) are CNS electrical events generated by peripheral stimulation of a sensory organ and are useful to determine abnormal function that may be clinically unapparent. Detecting a subclinical lesion at a site remote from the region of clinical dysfunction supports the multifocal disease portion of the diagnostic criteria for MS. The three most commonly used EPs are visual evoked potentials (VEPs), somatosensory evoked potentials (SSEPs), and brainstem auditory-evoked responses (BAER). In a review of the role of EPs in MS, only VEPs were thought to be useful to determine increased risk for MS (Gronseth and Ashman, 2000). Using pattern shift VEPs, abnormalities (P100 wave prolongation) are detected in over 90% of patients with a history of ON, even in a setting of complete restoration of vision (Table 80.3). Although VEPs may be abnormal in many MS patients, they have not been used in the McDonald criteria. Furthermore, the use of MRI has supplanted their utility in most cases and thus VEPs are not routinely included as a part of the diagnostic work-up.

## Differential Diagnosis

In a person of typical age for onset of MS with two or more clinically distinct episodes of CNS dysfunction with at least partial resolution, there is little in the way of a differential diagnosis. In this case, doing testing beyond MRI and basic laboratory tests rarely, if ever, leads to an alternate diagnosis. However, the differential broadens with atypical presentations, monophasic episodes, or progressive deficits (Box 80.2). A monophasic illness with symptoms attributable to one site of the CNS creates a large differential diagnosis that includes neoplasms, vascular events, and infections. Appropriate imaging studies may help clarify the situation, depending on the site of involvement and clinical progression.

Great care must be taken in those with progressive CNS dysfunction to exclude treatable etiologies (e.g., vitamin $B_{12}$ deficiency, compressive spinal cord lesions, arteriovenous malformations, cavernous angiomas, Arnold-Chiari malformation), infectious causes (syphilis, human T-cell lymphotropic virus type 1 [HTLV-1], human immunodeficiency virus [HIV]), and hereditary disorders (adult metachromatic leukodystrophy, adrenomyeloneuropathy, spinocerebellar disorders, CADASIL).

A common diagnostic error is to misinterpret multiple hyperintense lesions on MRI as equivalent to MS. A few white-matter lesions on T2-weighted MRI scans are not infrequent, particularly in the elderly or migraineurs, but do not indicate a diagnosis of MS. CNS vasculitides such as systemic lupus erythematosus (SLE), Sjögren disease,

**TABLE 80.2 Cerebrospinal Fluid Abnormalities in Multiple Sclerosis**

| | Albumin | IgG/TP | IgG/Albumin | IgG Index | Oligoclonal Banding of Ig |
|---|---|---|---|---|---|
| Clinically definite multiple sclerosis | 23% | 67% | 60%–73% | 70%–90% | 85%–95% |
| Normal controls | 3% | — | 36% | 3% | 7%* |

*IgG/TP*, Immunoglobulin G value/total protein.
*Other neurological disease.

**TABLE 80.3 Comparison of Sensitivity of Laboratory Testing in Multiple Sclerosis**

| | VER | BAER | SSEP | OCB | MRI |
|---|---|---|---|---|---|
| Clinically definite multiple sclerosis | 80%–85%* | 50%–65% | 65%–80% | 85%–95% | 90%–97% |

*BAER*, Brainstem auditory evoked response; *MRI*, magnetic resonance imaging; *OCB*, oligoclonal band; *SSEP*, somatosensory evoked potential; *VER*, visual evoked response.
*Numbers show the percentage of patients with abnormal study results.

polyarteritis nodosa, syphilis, retroviral diseases, and Behçet disease may all produce multifocal lesions with or without a relapsing-remitting course. SLE can present as a recurrent neurological syndrome before the systemic manifestations of this disease declare themselves. Behçet disease is characterized by buccogenital ulcerations in addition to the multifocal neurological findings. CNS sarcoidosis can be mistaken for MS with multifocal neurological and MRI lesions. An MS-like phenotype associated with mitochondrial gene defects has been described.

More important than features characteristic for MS are features that should prompt the clinician to reconsider the diagnosis of MS—red flags indicating that another diagnosis is more likely (see Miller et al., 2008 for a complete discussion on this topic). Some features that should alert the clinician to the possibility of other diseases include (1) family history of neurological disease, (2) a well-demarcated spinal level in the absence of disease above the foramen magnum, (3) prominent back pain that persists, (4) symptoms and signs that can be attributed to one anatomical site, (5) patients who are older than age 60 or younger than age 15 at onset, and (6) progressive disease.

### Multiple Sclerosis Misdiagnosis

Despite significant gains made in accurate diagnosis of MS over the years through more sensitive and specific criteria, misdiagnosis of MS remains a significant issue. This problem has been highlighted by a number of recent articles (Kaisey et al., 2019, Solomon et al., 2016) that reported that a relatively high proportion of patients referred to MS centers with a diagnosis of MS were subsequently given alternate diagnoses. The clinician must remain vigilant with every patient in order to accurately diagnosis MS, or to exclude it as a possibility.

#### BOX 80.2 Differential Diagnosis in Multiple Sclerosis

**Inflammatory Diseases**
Granulomatous angiitis
Systemic lupus erythematosus
Sjögren disease
Behçet disease
Polyarteritis nodosa
Paraneoplastic encephalomyelopathies
Acute disseminated encephalomyelitis, postinfectious encephalomyelitis
Neuromyelitis optica
MOG antibody-associated disease

**Infectious Diseases**
Neuroborreliosis
Human T-cell lymphotropic virus type 1 infection*
Human immunodeficiency virus infection
Progressive multifocal leukoencephalopathy*
Neurosyphilis*

**Granulomatous Diseases**
Sarcoidosis
Granulomatosis with polyangiitis (formerly, Wegener's granulomatosis)
Lymphomatoid granulomatosis

**Diseases of Myelin**
Metachromatic leukodystrophy (juvenile and adult)*
Adrenomyeloleukodystrophy*

**Miscellaneous**
Spinocerebellar disorders*
Arnold-Chiari malformation
Vitamin $B_{12}$ deficiency*
Optic neuritis
Cerebellitis
Brainstem encephalitis

* Indicates disorders that are predominantly important to differentiate in the setting of progressive disease.

## CLINICAL COURSE AND PROGNOSIS

### Measures of Disability

MS clinical course is characterized by both relapsing and progressive contributions to the accumulation of disability. The most commonly used index for characterizing MS disability, the Kurtzke Expanded Disability Status Scale (EDSS), uses numbers ranging from 0 for normal examination and function to 10 for death caused by MS. This scale is nonlinear, with great emphasis on ambulation capabilities with scores above 4. Most MS populations have bimodal distributions of EDSS scores, with peaks at values of 1 and 6 (ambulation with unilateral assistance). In a cohort of patients followed for 25 years (in the pretreatment era), the following data emerged: 80% of the patients had reached the progressive phase by 25 years, 15% had died, 65% had reached EDSS 6 (requiring aids for walking), and 50% reached EDSS 6 within 16 years of onset. More recent studies suggest a somewhat slower course of progression (Pittock et al., 2004; Tremlett et al., 2006). The EDSS, although universally used in clinical trials, has a number of limitations. Even with special training and examiner blinding, interrater and intrarater variations in scoring are common. EDSS scores of 4 and higher depend almost entirely on the ability to walk; developing dementia, vision loss, and weakness of hands may pass undetected by the scoring once one reaches these levels. An obvious implication of these facts is that other outcome measures should be used as well, and that minor changes in EDSS score alone should not be overinterpreted. The Multiple Sclerosis Functional Composite (MSFC) is a clinical tool designed to avoid the problems encountered with the EDSS (Cutter et al., 1999). The MSFC consists of three parts: paced auditory serial addition test (PASAT), nine-hole peg test (9HPT), and timed 25-foot walk (T25FW). These three measures take into account cognition, upper-extremity function, and lower-extremity function. A *z*-score is obtained for each measure, and a combined *z*-score is then derived. The MSFC has been validated in several clinical trials. Additional measures including patient reported outcomes and quality-of-life indices have been developed and validated in MS populations.

### Clinical Phenotypes (RRMS, SPMS, PPMS)

Approximately 80%–90% of MS cases begin as a relapsing disease characterized by acute neurological events referable to focal inflammatory lesions. MS relapses are defined as the acute or subacute onset of clinical dysfunction, usually reaching its peak in days to several weeks, followed by a remission during which the symptoms and signs usually resolve partially or completely. The minimum duration for a relapse has been arbitrarily established at 24 hours. Clinical symptoms of shorter duration are less likely to represent what is considered a true relapse (i.e., new lesion formation or extension of previous lesion size). Worsening of previous clinical dysfunction can occur concurrently with fever, infection, physical activity, or metabolic upset and last for hours to a day or more and is referred to as *pseudo-relapse*. Summaries of many studies provide an average figure of 0.4–0.6 relapses per year in patients in the relapsing-remitting phase of the illness, though this varies widely across individuals. In general, relapses are more frequent during the first years of the disease and tend to wane in later years, at which point it is more common for worsening to occur via a progressive course.

A standardization of terms used to describe the pattern and course of the illness was introduced in 1996 (Lublin and Reingold, 1996) and revised in 2013. The current classification identifies three main clinical course phenotypes:

1. RRMS: Clearly defined relapses with full recovery or with sequelae and residual deficit on recovery. The periods between disease relapses are characterized by a lack of disease progression.
2. SPMS: Initial relapsing-remitting disease course followed by progression with or without occasional relapses, minor remissions, and plateaus.
3. PPMS: Disease progression from onset, with occasional plateaus and temporary minor improvements allowed.

The 2013 revisions to the clinical courses advise sub-categorizing the clinical course by whether there is evidence of activity and, in progressive forms of the illness, whether there is evidence of ongoing progression. Both characterizations should be qualified by a time frame. Activity is defined as either the occurrence of an acute relapse or new MRI changes defined as a new or, unequivocally, an enlarging T2 lesion or a gadolinium-enhancing lesion. Thus a patient with RRMS who has had a relapse or new MRI lesion over the past year would be characterized as *RRMS with activity*. Patients with PPMS or SPMS are further sub-categorized as *progressing* or *not progressing* over a defined period of time. Thus a progressive patient might be active or inactive and progressive or not progressing over the defined period of time (Lublin et al., 2014). PPMS remains a distinct clinical phenotype, although it is recognized that disease activity as seen on MRI can occur even in the absence of a history of relapses. Besides being able to more accurately describe a patient's course, the new categorizations differ from previous in that progressive relapsing MS would be categorized as progressive with disease activity instead of being a separate disease classification (Fig. 80.13, *A*, *B*).

The topographical model of MS was proposed as a unified depiction of MS clinical course across the spectrum of relapsing and progressive forms of the disease (Krieger et al., 2016). This conceptual model blurs the distinctions between phenotypic categories and animates dynamic periods of transition across them, taking into account that in practice there can be a long period of diagnostic uncertainty as patients transition from RRMS to SPMS (Katz Sand et al., 2014) and a precise moment of "conversion to SPMS" can rarely be identified.

In the topographical model the CNS is visualized as a pool with increasing levels of depth, where the depth of the water corresponds with the degree of functional reserve, or compensatory ability, intrinsic to these different regions of the CNS (Fig. 80.14). Thus the spinal cord and optic nerves—the simplest, most linear structures commonly affected by MS lesions—have the least redundancy and capacity for organizational plasticity, while the cerebral hemispheres possess the greatest such structural and functional resilience (Laitman et al., 2018). In the topographical model, lesions rise as focal peaks emerging from the base of the pool; those that cross the surface of the water—the clinical threshold—cause demonstrable signs and symptoms of an MS relapse. Disease activity in the shallow end—spinal cord and optic nerves—is predisposed to causing the hallmark clinical relapses of MS: symptoms referable to partial myelitis and ON.

It is hypothesized that the accelerated loss of brain volume in MS yields a loss of the compensatory mechanisms that constitute neurological reserve, and that MS progression may become clinically apparent after reserve is depleted. The topographical model depicts this, in that as time passes and functional reserve (the water level) declines, progression clinically recapitulates a patient's prior relapse symptoms and unmasks previously clinically silent lesions, incrementally manifesting above the clinical threshold of a patient's underlying disease topography (Laitman et al., 2018). This recapitulation hypothesis is based on the observation that the clinical signs and symptoms of a patient's progression manifest as a permanent, incremental recapitulation of prior relapse symptoms and a cumulative unmasking of previously clinically silent lesions.

In addition to the heterogeneity of clinical course as encapsulated in the distinct phenotypes and the topographical model, the disease is also notably heterogeneous in severity and prognosis. Two extremes of disease severity have been described: *benign MS* is disease in which the patient remains fully functional in all neurological systems 15 years after the disease onset, and *malignant MS* is disease with a rapid progressive course leading to significant disability in multiple neurological systems or death in a relatively short time after disease onset. These terms should be used judiciously as MS is an unpredictable condition that is difficult to characterize in broad terms, particularly for individual patients.

## Radiographically Isolated Syndrome

The diagnostic entity of *radiographically isolated syndrome* (RIS) addresses the category of asymptomatic patients who have MRI-detected anomalies highly suggestive of MS. Typically, these patients get an MRI for a completely unrelated reason, such as an accident or a headache syndrome. A multi-center, retrospective study found that the risk for a clinical event in a group of RIS patients was 34% within 5 years of the

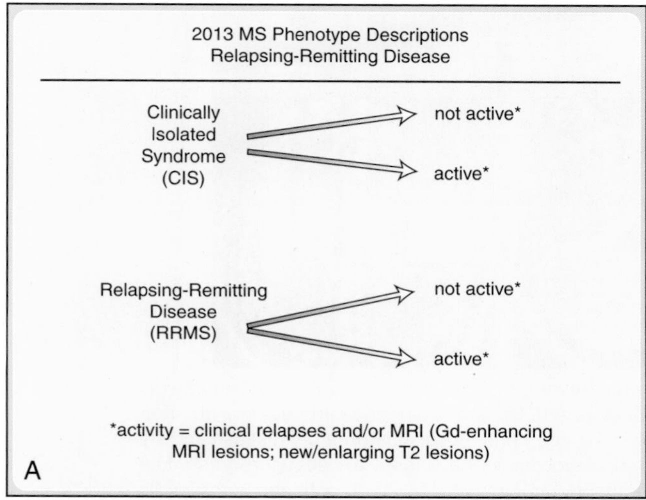


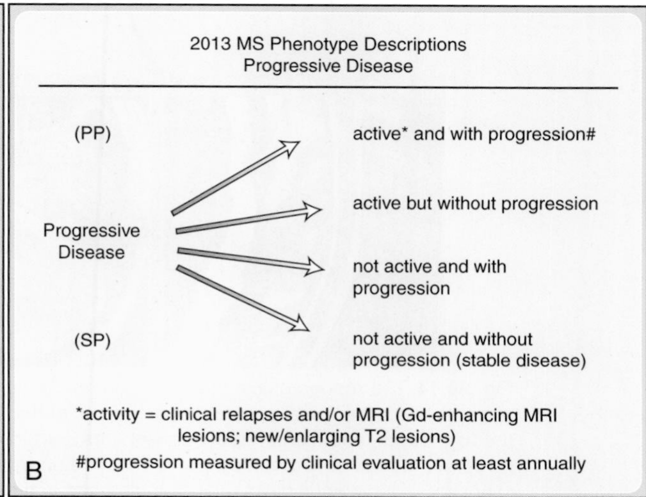


**Fig. 80.13** A and B, The 2013 clinical courses of multiple sclerosis. *Gd*, Gadolinium; *MRI*, magnetic resonance imaging; *MS*, multiple sclerosis. *(Courtesy F. Lublin.)*

first brain MRI (Okuda et al., 2014). RIS patients with enhancing lesions and spinal cord lesions have a higher risk for conversion. It is important to recall that without a characteristic clinical syndrome suggestive of demyelinating disease, patients with RIS cannot be formally diagnosed with MS according to the McDonald criteria. The question of which RIS patients, if any, should be started empirically on DMTs remains unanswered and is currently under study.

### Clinically Isolated Syndrome

Although many more patients with a first clinical demyelinating event are now immediately given a diagnosis of MS based on the clinical history and an MRI that meets the current McDonald criteria, there still exist those patients who present with an event that is clinically consistent with MS and accompanied by typical multifocal white-matter lesions on MRI, yet the MRI does not meet criteria for DIS and time. This situation is referred to as the *clinically isolated syndrome* (CIS). In the long-term study by Brex et al. (2002) that followed patients with initial demyelinating episodes for up to 14 years, in practical terms no diagnoses were encountered other than MS or suspected MS. Multiple clinical trials have been completed which show favorable outcomes in reduction of recurrent MRI and clinical activity for CIS patients who begin DMTs.

## FACTORS INFLUENCING CLINICAL COURSE

### Predictive Value of Magnetic Resonance Imaging in Conversion to Clinically Definite Multiple Sclerosis

Studies suggest that MRI may provide some prediction of the risk of conversion to CDMS based on the presence and number of T2 lesions within 1–5 years following CIS. Increasingly higher numbers of T2 lesions result in greater likelihood of conversion to CDMS and higher disability scores at 5 years. Two long-term follow-up studies of 10–14 years show that most patients with CIS and MRI abnormalities will develop CDMS (70%–80%), while only 20% of patients with normal cerebral MRI scans will be diagnosed with MS over this time period (Beck et al., 2003; Brex et al., 2002; O'Riordan et al., 1998). These data in part have led to the 2010 and 2017 revisions to the McDonald criteria, allowing for an earlier diagnosis of MS in CIS cases meeting DIS on MRI.

### Prognosis Based on Patient Characteristics

Although great individual variability exists with regard to disease prognosis, a variety of factors have been identified as possible prognostic indicators:

- Sex: MS may follow a less severe course in women than in men.
- Age at onset: Average is 29–32 years. Onset at an early age is a favorable factor, whereas onset at a later age carries a less-favorable prognosis. RRMS is more common in younger patients, and PPMS and SPMS are more common in the older age group. Data are lacking as to whether prognosis differs as a function of age in patients with similar patterns of disease.
- Initial disease course: Relapsing form of the disease is associated with a better prognosis than progressive disease. A high rate of relapses early in the illness and a short first interval between attacks may correlate with shorter time to reach EDSS 6.
- Initial manifestations: Among initial symptoms, impairment of sensory pathways or ON has been found in several studies to be a

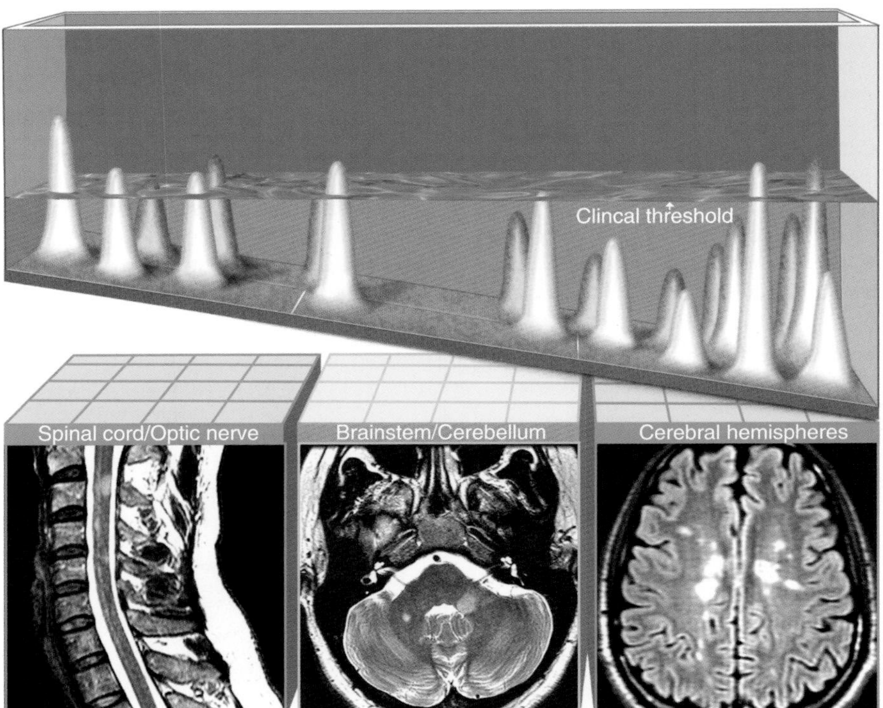


**Fig. 80.14** The topographical model visualizes the central nervous system as a pool with increasing levels of depth, with the spinal cord and optic nerves at the shallow end, the brainstem and cerebellum with intermediate depth, and the cerebral hemispheres comprising the deep end. Focal inflammatory disease activity is represented as topographical peaks that rise up from the pool base. The single view shown represents a snapshot of a patient's disease at a single point in time; the water is translucent, with both above-threshold clinical signs and subthreshold lesions shown. The combined volume of above-threshold topographical peaks corresponds with the degree of accumulated disability, unmasked as functional reserve declines.

favorable prognostic feature, whereas pyramidal and, particularly, brainstem and cerebellar symptoms carry a poor prognosis.

In general, when considering disability as measured by the EDSS (which prioritizes ambulatory function), patients with mild disease (EDSS score 0-3) 5 years after diagnosis only uncommonly progress to severe disease (EDSS score 6) by 10 years (7.5% of patients) and 15 years (11.5% of patients). It remains difficult to effectively prognosticate at the individual level, and clinical, imaging, and laboratory biomarkers for disease severity such as neurofilament light chain (NfL) are still being investigated (Siller et al., 2019).

### Effect of Exogenous Factors on Clinical Course

The role of a variety of exogenous factors either influencing the development of MS or inducing disease exacerbations has been examined using epidemiological techniques. Relapses may occur with higher frequency in MS patients who have suffered recently from viral infections, and a high number of such infections are followed by acute attacks. Controversy exists about co-occurrence of stressful events and exacerbation of MS, though in the authors' view stress may commonly worsen existent MS symptoms without inciting a new focal inflammatory event. Trauma appears not to be implicated in disease induction or relapse. Performance of neurological diagnostic procedures such as myelography and lumbar puncture has not been linked to aggravation of the MS, nor has administration of local or general anesthetics or surgery. There is no established link between acellular (non-live virus) vaccinations and disease exacerbations, and there are no convincing data to support withholding immunizations—for example, for influenza or hepatitis. However, caution should be used in the administration of live, attenuated vaccines, such as yellow fever, as an increased risk for relapse may exist.

### Pregnancy in Multiple Sclerosis

MS preferentially affects women of childbearing age. Pregnancy is recognized to induce changes in the maternal immune system, including both immunosuppression on a local level and a heightened state of immunocompetence on a global level. Several retrospective studies reported an overall increase in relapse rate during the postpartum period and a lower relapse rate during pregnancy itself (Weinshenker et al., 1989). Pregnancy in Multiple Sclerosis (PRIMS) was a seminal prospective study of 254 women (269 pregnancies) regarding MS and pregnancy. Subjects were followed for 2 years after delivery (Confavreux et al., 1998; Vukusic et al., 2004; Vukusic and Confavreux, 2006). In the cohort, a pre-pregnancy rate of 0.7 relapses per year decreased to 0.2 per year in the third trimester. The relapse rate increased to 1.2 per year in the first 3 months postpartum. However, 72% of women did not experience any relapses during the study period. An increased relapse rate in the year before pregnancy, an increased relapse rate during pregnancy, and a higher EDSS score at the beginning of pregnancy correlated significantly with occurrence of a postpartum relapse. Epidural anesthesia and breastfeeding were not predictive of a subsequent relapse or disability progression. More recent studies have suggested a protective benefit to exclusive breastfeeding in the postpartum period (Hellwig et al., 2015). There are no contraindications to cesarean section or vaginal delivery in MS patients.

A prospective 5-year study compared the rate of progression in disability between childless women, women who had onset of MS after childbirth, and women who had onset before or during their pregnancy (Stenager et al., 1994). The rates of disability increased most rapidly in nulliparous women. Another study retrospectively examined childbirth's effects on disability progression in 330 women with MS (D'hooghe et al., 2010). Women who gave birth after MS onset reached EDSS scores of 6 significantly later in the disease course than those who did not (median time to progression, 13–15 years vs. 22–23 years). Overall, there is no compelling evidence of adverse effects of pregnancy on MS progression. However, potential risks of prolonged MS therapy discontinuation, level of baseline neurological disability, and other factors need to be taken into consideration when counseling patients on family planning.

Although MS is not known to affect fertility, in patients who require assisted reproductive technologies (ART) for other fertility issues there is evidence through multiple case series that ART utilizing a gonadotropin-releasing hormone agonist (GnRH agonist) can increase the risk for MS relapse, especially in the case of an unsuccessful trial (Bove et al, 2020; Correale et al., 2012).

Another related issue is whether the disease has any effects on pregnancy outcomes, risk of malformations, fetal birth weight, or duration of pregnancy. Some groups report no increased risk in incidence of pregnancy and labor and delivery–related adverse events in MS patients (Mueller et al., 2002). Other reports indicate higher rates of operative deliveries and induced labor as well as greater numbers of neonates with low birth weight or being small for gestational age (Dahl et al., 2005). Kelly and colleagues evaluated obstetric outcomes in women with MS, epilepsy, or pregestational diabetes mellitus (DM) and in healthy controls. MS patients had a 30% higher risk for cesarean delivery and 70% higher rate of intrauterine growth restriction (IUGR) than healthy women. There were no long-term adverse pediatric outcomes (Kelly et al., 2009).

## VARIANTS OF MULTIPLE SCLEROSIS

### Tumefactive Multiple Sclerosis

Rarely, patients present with a large (>2 cm), acute demyelinating lesion in one hemisphere, the brainstem, or even the spinal cord (Fig. 80.15), known as tumefactive MS. A tumefactive lesion may be the cause of the initial presentation, or may occur as part of a relapsing MS course. In a series of 54 Turkish patients, the tumefactive lesion was the initial event in 54% of cases and occurred in RRMS patients in 46% of cases (Altintas et al., 2012). Depending on the size of the lesion, there may be prominent mass effect with compression of the lateral ventricle and shift across the midline. Clinical presentation in such patients is variable, ranging from mild to severe, and is at times

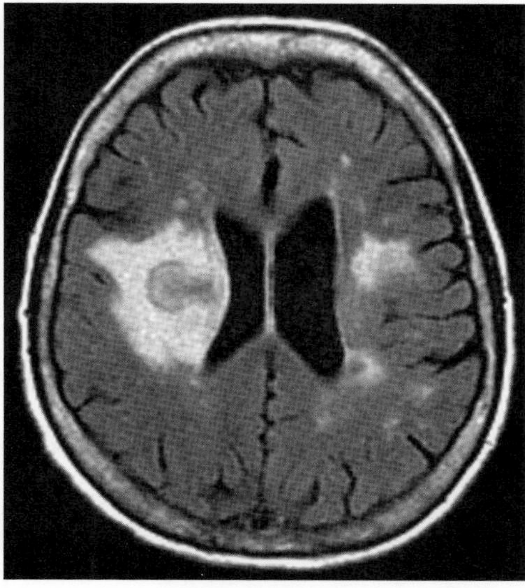

**Fig. 80.15** A tumefactive lesion in the setting of other, more typical multiple sclerosis lesions. Note the vasogenic edema and mass effect on the ipsilateral ventricle.

atypical for MS and more reflective of a space-occupying lesion, with symptoms including encephalopathy, seizure, hemiparesis, neglect, or other cortical syndromes. Important diagnostic clues toward a demyelinating etiology include typical location for an MS lesion, presence of other more characteristic MS lesions, an incomplete ring of enhancement (classically open toward the gray matter), and peripheral restriction on DWI (Hardy and Chataway, 2013). Ultimately, biopsy may be necessary to establish the correct diagnosis.

In terms of prognosis, in another large series of 168 patients with a biopsy-proven tumefactive lesion, after a median follow-up time of 4.8 years 70% developed MS, 9% were called probable MS, and only 14% were still free of a second event. Furthermore, in a comparison to a MS cohort matched for disease duration, disability seemed to be similar in the tumefactive MS group (Luchinetti et al., 2008).

### Marburg Variant

Marburg variant MS refers to an exceptionally uncommon form of MS with a relentless, fulminant course. Classically, the presentation is multifocal and may include encephalopathy, motor and sensory deficits, seizures, and aphasia. Imaging shows many bilateral, large, acute lesions that may all enhance (Fig. 80.16). There may be prominent subcortical and brainstem involvement. Pathology reveals confluent, destructive lesions consistent with demyelination and with relative preservation of axons (Letournel et al., 2008). Untreated, the prognosis is extremely poor, and death may occur within 1 year of symptom onset. Thus, aggressive treatment with steroids, plasma exchange (PLEX), and/or immunosuppressive therapy should be given immediately when the condition is recognized (Cappello and Mancardi, 2004).

### Baló Concentric Sclerosis

Baló concentric sclerosis is often thought of as an MS variant, though it is possible that it represents a separate demyelinating syndrome (Hardy et al., 2016). The characteristic pathological findings are alternating rings of myelin preservation or remyelination and myelin loss, consistent with demyelination. On MRI, Baló lesions appear as concentric rings or a whorled appearance on T2-weighted and contrast-enhanced T1-weighted images (Fig. 80.17) (Karaarslan et al., 2001). Symptomatically, patients may present similar to a typical MS relapse; however, symptoms may also reflect the fact that these lesions are space occupying in nature and may include headache, cognitive difficulty, behavioral changes, muteness, urinary incontinence, seizures, aphasia, and hemiparesis (Hardy and Miller, 2014). Before the advent of MRI, it was thought that Baló disease was a universally lethal condition, presumably because all cases were recognized only at autopsy. However, multiple series have been published that show this not to be the case, and patients may have a good recovery and long-term prognosis that is similar to those with RRMS.

## TREATMENT AND MANAGEMENT

Since the introduction of IFN-β-1b in the early 1990s, MS has morphed from being a virtually untreatable disease to arguably the most dynamic area of new treatment methodologies and applied research in all of neurology (Krieger, 2011).

Nine distinct agents have been approved by the US Food and Drug Administration (FDA) that are capable of modifying the disease course in RRMS. The existing medications are, however, only partially effective in preventing MS relapses, and have a limited impact on the accrual of disability. Modifying the course of progressive forms of the disease remains a major unmet need.

Treatment of the MS patient should be directed toward these fundamental goals:

- Treating acute relapses to shorten their duration and limit their residual effects
- Disease modification to reduce the frequency of relapses and prevent the accrual of disability
- Relief or modification of symptoms.
- Supporting family and patient, alleviating social and economic effects, and advocating for the disabled.

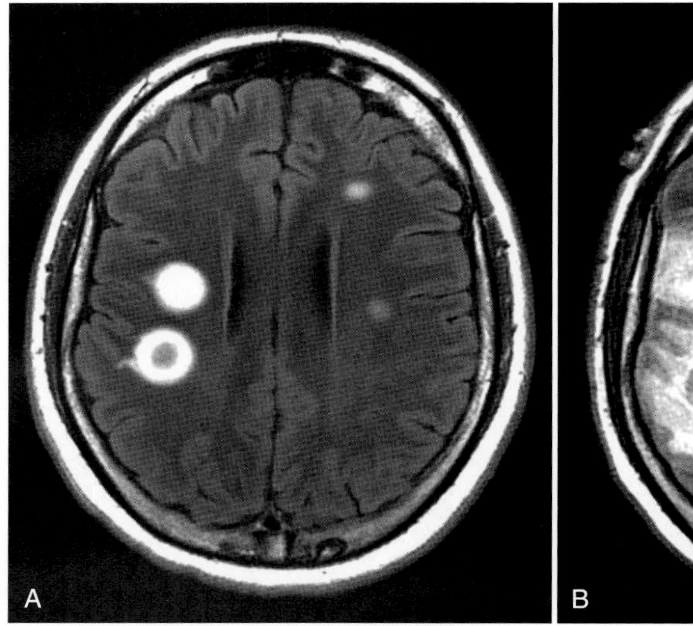


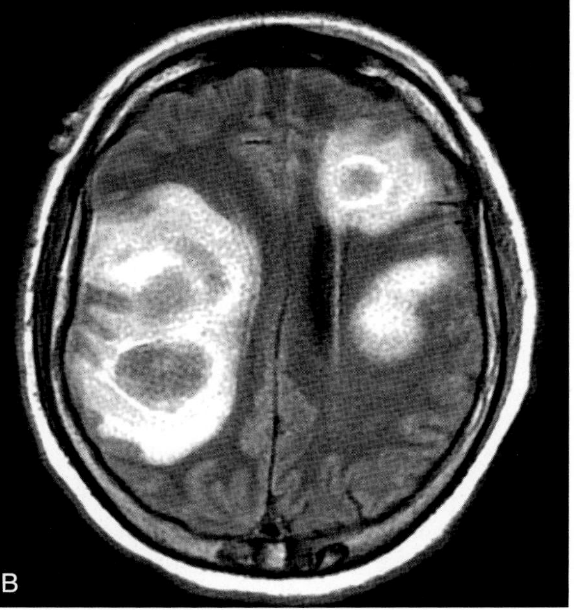


**Fig. 80.16** Marburg variant multiple sclerosis in a 29-year-old male. **A,** Brain magnetic resonance imaging (MRI) at onset of symptoms. Patient presented with altered mental status and dysarthria as well as focal motor deficits. **B,** Brain MRI 1 month later. Despite aggressive immunosuppression, the patient died within 1 year of disease onset.

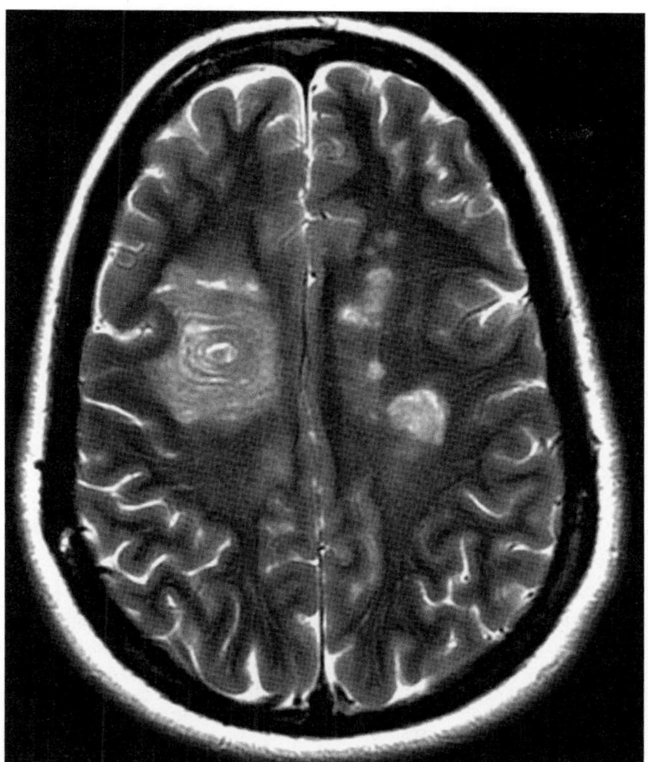

**Fig. 80.17** Baló concentric sclerosis. Note the alternating rings of demyelinated and, presumably, normal tissue.

## Treatment of Acute Attacks

High-dosage corticosteroids are considered most effective for the management of acute relapses of MS. Numerous studies have found that this treatment is associated with a faster recovery rate, though the final recovery from a relapse is thought to be independent from steroid. Thus, indications for treatment of a relapse include functionally disabling symptoms with objective evidence of neurological impairment or those that result in pain, yet mild sensory attacks may not be treated. Treatment with short courses of intravenous (IV) methylprednisolone, typically 1000 mg daily for 3–5 days, with or without a short prednisone taper, has commonly been used. The 1992 Optic Neuritis Treatment Trial demonstrated that patients treated with oral prednisone alone were more likely to suffer recurrent episodes of ON compared with those treated with IV methylprednisolone followed by oral prednisone. Furthermore, definite MS developed in 7.5% of the IV methylprednisolone group, 14.7% of the oral prednisone group, and 16.7% of the placebo group over a 2-year period. Development of disability, even when the diagnosis of MS had been made, was very rare, reemphasizing the need for follow-up periods of decades and the sometimes benign nature of MS presenting with ON. These data support the use of high-dose IV methylprednisolone for acute MS attacks, and do not support the use of low-dose oral steroid regimens for this purpose (Beck et al., 1992). High-dose IV methylprednisolone is accompanied by relatively few side effects in most patients, although psychiatric changes (insomnia, anxiety, mania), gastrointestinal disturbances, fluid retention, and hyperglycemia may occur, and an increased predilection for infections, fractures, or avascular necrosis of the femoral head has been observed. The immunological mechanisms of high-dose corticosteroids include reduction of $CD4^+$ cells and decrease in cytokine release from lymphocytes, including TNF, IFN-$\gamma$, and decreased MHC complex class II expression. Corticosteroids have been shown to decrease IgG synthesis in the CNS. Intravenous methylprednisolone may decrease the entry of cells into the brain by stabilizing the BBB.

In 2015 a randomized, double-blind study was done in 199 MS patients in acute relapse that showed that high-dose oral methylprednisolone (1000 mg daily × 3 days) was not inferior to the equivalent IV dose of methylprednisolone in regard to improvement in disability scores 1 month after steroid administration (Le Page et al., 2015). Side effects and adverse events were similar in both groups, except for a higher rate of insomnia in those on oral treatment. Based on this study, high-dose oral steroids provide another option for relapse treatment.

For refractory or steroid-nonresponsive relapses, adrenocorticotropic hormone (ACTH) and plasmapheresis are additional treatment strategies. Placebo-controlled studies (Rose et al., 1970) have demonstrated the ability of ACTH to hasten recovery in MS relapses, and there is a commercially available form for this indication given by subcutaneous injection. Accelerated recovery from acute MS relapses with ACTH may be due to its effects on both corticosteroid and the melanocortin pathways. Updated evidence-based guidelines from the American Academy of Neurology (AAN) characterized plasma exchange as "probably effective" for the management of corticosteroid-resistant acute relapses of relapsing forms of MS based on the strength of a study by Weinshenker (2001). Plasma exchange typically requires inpatient hospitalization, and adverse events resulting from the procedure include heparin-associated thrombocytopenia, anemia, and hypotension.

## Treatment Strategies and Goals of Therapy

Much controversy has arisen since the introduction of the approved medications for RRMS as to how best to choose and utilize them in practice. The diverse array of disease-modifying agents makes MS one of the more unique neurological diseases. As a general rule, all patients with active relapsing forms of MS should be receiving one of the immunomodulatory agents indefinitely. Numerous clinical trials of initiating these agents at the time of the CIS have demonstrated with remarkable consistency the benefit of early treatment at preventing conversion to clinically definite or McDonald criteria MS, the prevention of subsequent relapses or new MRI lesions, and the prevention of accumulated disability.

The availability of newer, highly efficacious DMTs has made it possible for clinicians to aim for much better disease control than in previous times. In recent years, the goal of MS disease control has been more sharply defined as no evidence of disease activity (NEDA). A patient meets NEDA when there is no evidence for new or enlarging MRI lesions, no new clinical relapse, and no evidence upon examination of disease progression over time (Banwell et al., 2013). NEDA-4 also includes no evidence for brain atrophy above and beyond the normal physiological rate. Although NEDA is a worthy treatment goal (Giovannoni et al., 2018a) it may not be achievable over the long term for most patients who, despite DMT treatment, may still have ongoing, subclinical activity. Furthermore, it has not been definitively established that those that have minimal evidence for disease activity (MEDA) have a worse prognosis than those that are NEDA (Río et al., 2018).

Most experts do agree that a patient should be switched to a different DMT if they have had a clinical relapse after the drug would be expected to be fully effective, as relapses on DMT portends a poorer long-term outcome (Jokubaitis et al., 2016). However, the decision to switch DMTs based on MRI activity alone is more debatable. In certain circumstances, brain MRI may be particularly helpful. MRI scans can be evaluated and compared at baseline and within 6–12 months after the initiation of a DMT. If a patient has two or more active lesions, modifying the DMT should be considered as this confers a risk of suboptimal clinical response to therapy (Rio et al., 2009). An MRI scan can be done after a relapse to evaluate the number of new lesions. Unfortunately, general agreement about the definition of treatment failure does not currently exist, though a lower tolerance for breakthrough disease activity certainly exists now compared to previous times.

## Disease-Modifying Therapy

Variability of signs and symptoms, in both type and timing, is the hallmark of MS. The disease confers a considerable degree of randomness in terms of frequency and severity of relapses, and in the extent and onset of gradual development of disability. The profound individual clinical variability poses challenges at all levels of MS management—diagnosis, prognosis, clinical trial design, and particularly DMT decisions for an individual patient (Krieger et al., 2009).

For some patients, MS is a disease with one or two acute relapses, with no further evidence of disease activity. In others, it is a chronic relapsing or progressive disease wherein neurological disability accumulates. Treatment of MS, as with other diseases, is based on the results of prospective well-controlled clinical trials. Most of these trials have been designed to establish efficacy in RRMS but have not followed patients in controlled fashion for longer than 2 or 3 years, and have provided only limited insight as to the long-term results of treatment. Long-term placebo-controlled trials are not ethically possible once effective therapies are established. Patients in clinical practice may differ markedly from those who have been treated in clinical trials, yet therapeutic decisions must be made, and these trials provide best evidence. Despite the evidence for efficacy in clinical trials, inter-individual treatment response to these agents is heterogeneous (Aktas et al., 2010), and it is as yet not possible to prospectively identify likely responders or nonresponders to a given treatment modality. The following section will provide an overview of available DMTs, followed by a discussion of treatment strategy.

### Injectable Agents

***Interferons.*** The first medicine for use in RRMS was approved by the FDA in 1993. It was a recombinant IFN-β-1b, which was shown in a double-blind placebo-controlled trial of 372 patients to decrease the frequency of relapses by 34% after 2 years. Treatment had an additional effect on decreasing MRI T2 lesion burden (an increase in lesion volume of 3.6% compared with 30.2% in the placebo group over 5 years). No significant change in disease progression occurred over 5 years. The mechanism of action of IFN-β-1b may relate to antiproliferative effects, cytokine changes, effects at the BBB, and alterations of T-cell subsets.

A second double-blind placebo-controlled study in 301 patients with relapsing-remitting disease investigated the efficacy of weekly intramuscular (IM) injections of 30 μg of IFN-β-1a, a glycosylated recombinant IFN-β (Jacobs et al., 1996). Over 2 years, the annual exacerbation rate decreased by 29%. MRI data revealed significantly decreased T2 lesion volume and number of enhancing lesions over the 2 years of the study. There was also a 37% reduction in progression of neurological disability in the treatment group.

Another randomized double-blind placebo-controlled study of IFN-β-1a in higher doses was conducted in Europe and Canada (Ebers, 1998). This involved 560 patients with relapsing-remitting disease given subcutaneous IFN-β-1a. Patients were randomized to placebo, 22 μg, or 44 μg of IFN-β-1a three times a week for 2 years. There was a 27% reduction in the relapse rate in the group receiving 66 μg/week and a 33% reduction in the group receiving 132 μg/week. There was also a significant reduction in disability. The MRI lesion burden showed a decrease of 1.2% in the group receiving 66 μg/week, a decrease of 3.8% in the group receiving 132 μg/week, and an increase of 10.9% in the group receiving a placebo. Based on these data and a comparison trial of weekly IM IFN-β-1a versus the thrice-weekly 44 μg subcutaneous dose (Panitch et al., 2002), the latter was approved by the FDA in March 2002.

Side-effect profile is similar between all IFNs and includes influenza-like symptoms, which usually diminish over weeks to months and can be well managed by nonsteroidal anti-inflammatory drugs. Local reactions at the injection site are common. Elevated liver enzymes, leukopenia, and anemia can occur, and blood monitoring is recommended every 3–6 months. Depression has been associated with IFN therapy and mood should be monitored. Furthermore, a variable number of patients develop neutralizing antibodies against IFNs that may reduce the clinical efficacy of the drug.

***Glatiramer acetate.*** Glatiramer acetate (GA) is a synthetic polypeptide administered by daily subcutaneous injection. In a large double-blind trial in RRMS involving 251 randomized patients (Johnson et al., 1995), the patients receiving GA had a 29% reduction in the relapse rate over 2 years. Extension data show that over 140 weeks, 41% of patients receiving placebo experienced worsening of their disability by 1.5 EDSS steps or greater, whereas only 21.6% of GA-treated patients had worsening (Johnson et al., 1998). There were also modest MRI effects, with an observed decrease in new T2 lesion load, enhancing lesions, and T1 hypointense lesions (T1 black holes). The mechanism by which GA may work in humans is unknown but may relate to interference with antigen presentation and induction of regulatory cells ($T_H2$) that traffic to the CNS and induce bystander suppression of immune responses.

In 2014, a new dosing strategy for GA was approved by the FDA, based on the 40 mg subcutaneous (SC) injections given TIW as studied in the GALA trial (Khan et al., 2013). In this trial, a 34% reduction was seen in annualized relapse rate between GA 40 mg TIW and placebo, which satisfied the primary endpoint for the trial. Secondary outcomes including T2 lesion formation and T1 gadolinium-enhancing lesions were also reduced by 35% and 45%, respectively. These data were roughly congruent with those seen in the pivotal trials of GA 2 decades earlier.

Side effects included local injection site reactions and lipoatrophy with cutaneous indentations at the injection sites after prolonged use. Transient systemic postinjection reactions may be seen, characterized by chest pain, flushing, dyspnea, palpitations, and anxiety. No laboratory monitoring is necessary.

***Comparison between interferon and glatiramer acetate.*** The REGARD study examined the effects of high-dose IFN against GA in RRMS patients (Mikol et al., 2008). The study had an open-label, randomized, multicenter, comparative, assessor-blinded design and enrolled close to 800 subjects. There was no difference between the two agents in reaching the primary endpoint, which was time to the first relapse. There was also no difference in the annualized relapse rate. The BEYOND study was designed to compare a 500-μg IFN-β-1b subcutaneous injection treatment every other day with the currently approved 250 μg Betaseron subcutaneous treatment every other day, to assess in a double-blinded manner whether efficacy can be further improved while maintaining safety and tolerability. Treatment with GA as an active comparator arm examined the difference between the MS treatments, IFN-β-1b and GA, in a rater-blinded manner (Comi et al., 2009). No significant difference in risk for relapses was found between the treatment arms. BECOME examined IFN-β-1b versus GA in MS with triple-dose Gd and 3 T MRI endpoints in this investigator-initiated randomized prospective rater-blinded trial to directly compare these two agents in the treatment of MS (Cadavid et al., 2009). No difference in MRI or clinical outcomes was observed between the drugs. Therefore, there is no clear evidence of superior efficacy between GA and high-dose IFN in multiple head-to-head trials, and these agents are generally thought to be equivalent.

### Infusion Therapies

***Natalizumab.*** Natalizumab is a monoclonal antibody directed against the adhesion molecule $\alpha_4$-integrin. Blocking this molecule inhibits trafficking of lymphocytes from the blood into the CNS. Two well-designed trials led to FDA approval of this agent. In a placebo-controlled clinical trial (AFFIRM), natalizumab reduced relapse rate by 68% and progression of disability by 42% over 2 years (Polman et al., 2006). MRI metrics were similarly affected. In a second study (SENTINEL), significant improvements in both clinical and MRI outcomes were seen when subjects who had had an exacerbation while on IFN-β-1a once weekly were treated concomitantly with natalizumab (an add-on study), as compared to those who received a placebo add-on (Rudick et al., 2006). During the studies, the safety profile was quite good; however, during the extension phase, two cases of PML occurred in subjects receiving both natalizumab and IFN (Kleinschmidt-DeMasters and Tyler, 2005; Langer-Gould et al., 2005). A third case of PML occurred in a subject who had received natalizumab in a Crohn disease study. This led to withdrawal of natalizumab from the market until July 2006, when it was reintroduced with a risk management program to try to better determine the risks of this agent and monitor its use. Enrollment in a TOUCH (Tysabri Outreach: Unified Commitment to Health) prescribing program is mandatory for those patients who are receiving natalizumab. This program is designed to monitor monthly for new neurological symptoms that may be concerning for PML. Over 800 cases of natalizumab-related PML have been identified as of mid-2019.

Data published in 2012 allow for the risk of natalizumab-associated PML to be estimated with increased precision and these data have stood constant since. Three risk factors for PML have since been identified that allow for the stratification of individual patients by relative risk of PML. Positive status with respect to anti-JC virus antibodies, prior use of immunosuppressants, and increased duration of natalizumab treatment are associated with distinct increased levels of PML risk in natalizumab-treated patients with MS (Bloomgren et al., 2012).

Among the risk factors, the JCV Ab has emerged as the crucial predictor of risk for development of PML. Approximately 50%–60% of adults are seropositive for the JC Ab. Patients who test JCV Ab negative have a less than 1:10,000 risk of developing PML; JC-negative patients are however at an annual risk for seroconversion of approximately 2%–3% per year. As such, the current recommendations are to re-test JCV Ab status every 6 months in seronegative patients on natalizumab therapy. JC-positive patients should be counseled regarding risk stratification and treatment decisions as the cumulative exposure to natalizumab increases. Patients who are JC positive have a PML risk of approximately 1:200 after 2 years of natalizumab treatment; this rises to 1:150 after 4 years. These data have significant implications regarding patient selection for natalizumab therapy, as well as for the ongoing decision to keep JC Ab-positive patients on natalizumab for prolonged duration (Sorenson, 2012).

***Alemtuzumab.*** Alemtuzumab is a recombinant humanized monoclonal antibody that has been used in the treatment of B-cell chronic lymphocytic leukemia. It targets CD52, a glycoprotein expressed mainly by B and T lymphocytes, though also by various other components of the immune system such as dendritic cells, monocytes/macrophages, natural killer cells, and some granulocytes (Hu et al., 2009). Administration of alemtuzumab by IV infusion causes widespread and sustained depletion of lymphocytes, followed first by slow repopulation of B cells and eventually of T cells. Several studies have suggested a "sparing" of T cells with a regulatory phenotype, thus inducing a durable regulatory "resetting" of the immune system that may contribute to alemtuzumab's effect in MS (Cox et al., 2005). Unlike other MS therapies, this agent has a durable mechanism of action, and is dosed intravenously for 5 or 3 consecutive days only once yearly.

CARE-MS I was a multicenter, rater-blind phase III trial that randomized treatment-naïve RRMS patients to alemtuzumab (12 mg/day for 5 days by IV infusion followed by a second 3-day infusion 1 year later) or IFN-β-1a (44 μg subcutaneous three times per week) and followed them over 2 years (Cohen et al., 2012). Treatment with alemtuzumab resulted in a 55% reduction in relapse rate compared to IFN (adjusted risk ratio [AR] 0.18 vs. 0.39, $P < .0001$), satisfying one of the study's primary endpoints. However, there was no significant difference in the other primary endpoint, 6-month confirmed disability progression measured by EDSS. As for MRI endpoints, the number of new GEL, new T2 lesions, and new T1 lesions were all significantly reduced in the alemtuzumab group. CARE-MS II, a second phase III, rater-blind, active-comparator trial, randomized RRMS patients who had experienced at least one relapse while on some DMT to either alemtuzumab or IFN-β-1a (both administered as in CARE-MS I) (Coles et al., 2012). In this study, evaluating patients with more active and treatment-refractory MS, both co-primary outcomes were satisfied: alemtuzumab demonstrated a 49% reduction in relapse rate ($P < .0001$) and a 42% reduction in disability progression measured by EDSS ($P = .0084$).

Several safety concerns were raised by the above studies, particularly an increased risk of infection and emergent autoimmune diseases in patients treated with alemtuzumab. All three studies showed a modest increase in the incidence of infections, though there have been no treatment-related fatalities reported in the phase III studies. Approximately 18% and 16% of alemtuzumab patients developed an autoimmune thyroid disorder and 0.8% and 1% developed immune thrombocytopenic purpura (ITP) in CARE-MS I and II, respectively. Of note in the two phase III studies, these adverse events were anticipated, detected by monitoring, and appropriately managed.

***Ocrelizumab.*** Ocrelizumab was approved by the FDA in 2017 for relapsing-remitting MS. Many would argue that its approval has made the most dramatic impact on the ability of the practitioner to effectively treat even the most aggressive cases of RRMS with a safe and tolerable therapy. Notably, it is the only treatment that has also been FDA-approved for PPMS (see below). Ocrelizumab is a humanized monoclonal antibody aimed at CD20, a cell surface antigen specific to pre-B cells, memory B cells, and mature B cells. Administration of ocrelizumab produces profound and sustained depletion of B cells. Importantly, plasma cells are spared, which allows for preservation of humoral immunity (Hauser et al., 2017). Ocrelizumab is almost identical to rituximab, a chimeric mouse/human anti-CD20 antibody. Early trials using rituximab showed potent efficacy in treating patients with active MS (Hauser et al., 2008, Naismith et al., 2010). Based on these results, phase III trials in RRMS and PPMS were conducted with ocrelizumab, an analogous but humanized antibody.

OPERA I and OPERA II were identical trials that were carried out in over 1650 RRMS patients (Hauser et al., 2017). These trials were both 96-week randomized, placebo-controlled trials of ocrelizumab (300 mg IV once, repeated in 2 weeks and then 600 mg IV q24 weeks) against an active comparator, IFN-β-1a (44 μg SC, three times a week). Both trials found marked efficacy of ocrelizumab over IFN with an ARR difference of 0.16 vs. 0.29 (47% absolute decrease, $P < .001$) and a difference in mean number of new T1-enhancing lesion per MRI of 0.02 vs. 0.29 (94%–95% reduction, $P < .001$). These results were coupled with a favorable side-effect profile. Infusion reactions consisting mainly of rash, itching, and throat irritation were reported in 34.3% of patients on ocrelizumab. No fatal infusion reactions were reported. Overall infections were slightly higher in the ocrelizumab group (56.9% vs. 54.3%). The main infections reported were sinusitis, bronchitis, and urinary tract infection. Herpes infections of mild to moderate severity were also more common in those on ocrelizumab (5.9% vs. 3.4%). Surprisingly, serious infection was reported to be slightly higher in the IFN group. Although infrequent cases of PML in patients on rituximab have occurred, PML has not been reported in patients on ocrelizumab, except a few case reports of so called "carry-over" PML. In these cases, the patient was previously on either natalizumab or fingolimod, switched to ocrelizumab and subsequently diagnosed with the infection (Genentech, 2019). Thus, unlike natalizumab, the treatment is not limited by a patient's JC antibody status. Furthermore, the benefit of ocrelizumab was maintained across different demographics and levels of disease activity (Turner et al., 2019). Based on these results, ocrelizumab has become a widely used DMT for RRMS patients.

### Oral Therapies

***Fingolimod.*** Fingolimod (Gilenya) is a compound with structural similarity to sphingosine-1-phosphate (S1P). It was initially investigated to prevent renal allograft rejection and primarily acts to sequester circulating lymphocytes into secondary lymphoid organs. Fingolimod causes reduction of $CD3^+$, $CD4^+$, $CD8^+$, $CD45RA^+$ (naive T cells), $CD45RO^+$ (memory T cells), and $CD19^+$ cells but has no effect on lymphocyte induction, proliferation, or memory function. FREEDOMS was a 24-month, randomized, double-blind, placebo-controlled, parallel-group multicenter study to investigate fingolimod 1.25 mg versus 0.5 mg versus placebo on the annualized relapse rate (primary endpoint) and EDSS and MRI progression (secondary endpoints) over 24 months (Kappos et al., 2010). There was 60% reduction in annualized relapse rate and significant decrease in disability progression and MRI lesions. No improved efficacy was reported at the higher dose of fingolimod. TRANSFORMS compared daily fingolimod 0.5 mg against weekly IM IFN 30 μg. Superior efficacy was seen in the fingolimod group with annualized relapse rate reduction and the MRI metrics of disease activity and progression. Adverse events observed in these trials included bradycardia, herpesvirus infections, basal cell skin cancer, macular edema, and pulmonary function test abnormalities.

Safety monitoring for fingolimod includes baseline blood tests including pre-screening for varicella-zoster virus (VZV) immunity, ophthalmological evaluation to screen for macular edema, and electrocardiographic (ECG) testing to rule out cardiac conduction abnormalities. Fingolimod should not be prescribed to patients with a recent myocardial infarction, unstable angina, stroke, transient ischemic attack, decompensated heart failure requiring hospitalization, a history or presence of Mobitz type II second- or third-degree atrioventricular block, baseline QTc interval ≥ 500 ms, or treatment with class Ia or class III anti-arrhythmic drugs (Gilenya, 2012).

***Siponimod.*** Siponimod was approved in 2019 by the FDA for the treatment of CIS and relapsing-remitting MS. The pivotal trial for siponimod, EXPAND, was conducted in secondary progressive MS patients. It is discussed below in the section on DMT use in progressive MS.

***Teriflunomide.*** Teriflunomide (Aubagio) is a metabolite of leflunomide (Arava) that is approved for treatment of rheumatoid arthritis. This agent reversibly inhibits the mitochondrial enzyme dihydroorotate dehydrogenase, which provides the rate-limiting step in de novo pyrimidine synthesis, a crucial pathway for proliferating lymphocytes. Teriflunomide therefore selectively targets blasting rather than quiescent lymphocytes. This agent became the second oral agent approved for RRMS in 2012 after several successful phase III trials.

TEMSO was a multicenter double-blind trial that randomized 1088 patients with relapsing forms of MS to placebo or 7- or 14-mg doses of oral teriflunomide daily for 108 weeks (O'Connor et al., 2011). The study met its primary endpoint with significant reduction in ARR, from 0.54 in the placebo group to 0.37 in both teriflunomide groups, corresponding to relative risk reduction of 31.2% and 31.5% for the 7- and 14-mg doses of teriflunomide, respectively ($P <$ .001). The key secondary endpoint, reduction in confirmed disability progression as defined by sustained increase in EDSS over 12 weeks, was met at the 14-mg dose (20.2% vs. 27.3%; $P = .03$). The key MRI endpoint, change in total lesion volume, was also met by both doses, with the higher dose of teriflunomide demonstrating somewhat more robust efficacy than the lower. There was no statistically significant difference in serious adverse events, or adverse events requiring discontinuation of the study drug. Adverse events that were more common with teriflunomide include diarrhea, nausea, and hair thinning, which only very rarely resulted in discontinuation of the study drug. Those receiving teriflunomide were more likely to have mildly elevated alanine aminotransferase levels, but no case of severe hepatic dysfunction was seen.

A second randomized, double-blind, placebo-controlled phase III study (TOWER) (Confavreux et al., 2014) also demonstrated lower annualized relapse rates with teriflunomide 7 mg/day (0.39, $P = .0183$) and teriflunomide 14 mg/day (0.32, $P = .001$) compared with placebo (0.50) in 1169 patients with relapsing MS. Similar to results seen in the TEMSO trial, only the teriflunomide 14 mg/day dose significantly decreased the risk of sustained accumulation of disability (relative HR reduction 32%, $P = .0442$). A third phase III study, TENERE (Vermersch et al., 2014), was performed in 324 patients with relapsing MS, and compared the same two doses of teriflunomide with injectable IFN-β-1a (44 μg) (Rebif). The primary composite endpoint, time to failure as defined by first occurrence of a confirmed relapse or permanent treatment discontinuation for any cause, did not differ between the three treatment groups. The annualized relapse rates did not significantly differ between teriflunomide 14 mg/day (0.26) and IFN-β-1a (44 μg) (0.22, $P = .6$). When considering treatment initiation with teriflunomide, patients should be screened for latent tuberculosis and women of childbearing potential should undergo pregnancy testing. Liver function tests should be obtained monthly during the first 6 months of treatment, and intermittently thereafter.

***Dimethyl fumarate (BG-12).*** An oral fumaric acid ester (Fumaderm) was previously shown to be effective in patients with psoriasis and various formulations of fumaric acid esters have been in use for this disease in Germany for many years (Katz Sand and Krieger, 2012). Dimethyl fumarate is rapidly metabolized to its main active metabolite, monomethylfumarate. The mechanism of action in MS is still under investigation; however, it seems that at least some of the drug's activity is related to monomethylfumarate's release of the transcription factor Nrf-2, which ultimately leads to a decrease in several inflammatory cytokines, chemokines, and adhesion molecules (Gold et al., 2012b). Work in animal models suggests BG-12 may have neuroprotective properties, with positive effects on the preservation of oligodendrocytes, myelin, and axons through the reduction of oxidative stress (Linker et al., 2011).

Dimethyl fumarate has had positive outcomes in two phase III trials, leading to its FDA approval in 2013. DEFINE (Gold et al., 2012a) was a multicenter, double-blind trial of dimethyl fumarate 240 mg twice daily (BID), and three times daily (TID) versus placebo for 2 years. The study met its primary endpoint with a 49% (BID) and 50% (TID) reduction in the proportion of patients who relapsed during the study period ($P < .0001$). The annualized relapse rate at 2 years was 0.36 for placebo, 0.17 for dimethyl fumarate 240 mg BID, and 0.19 for dimethyl fumarate 240 mg TID, corresponding to a relative reduction by dimethyl fumarate of 53% and 48%, respectively ($P < .001$ for either dose). Risk of 12-week disability progression was reduced by 38% with dimethyl fumarate BID ($P < .01$) and 34% with dimethyl fumarate TID ($P < .05$).

CONFIRM (Fox et al., 2012) was also a multicenter, double-blind trial comparing the same two doses of dimethyl fumarate with placebo and daily subcutaneous injection of GA for 2 years. The study met its primary endpoint with reduction in ARR of 44% for dimethyl fumarate BID ($P < .0001$) and 51% for dimethyl fumarate TID ($P < .0001$) compared to placebo, while glatiramer reduced ARR by 29% compared to placebo. The study was not designed to test for superiority or noninferiority of dimethyl fumarate versus GA. There was no statistically significant difference in the remaining clinical endpoint, 12-week confirmed disability progression, possibly due to the unexpectedly low rate of progression in the placebo group.

The incidence of serious adverse events and events leading to drug discontinuation was similar in all groups in both trials. There were neither opportunistic infections nor treatment-related fatalities in either phase III trial. Flushing and gastrointestinal adverse effects (nausea, abdominal pain, diarrhea) were more common with dimethyl fumarate than with placebo. Because of the partially transient nature of these adverse effects, patient education and close monitoring is important, particularly during the first weeks of treatment, to ensure treatment tolerability and adherence. Because dimethyl fumarate may cause lymphopenia, a complete blood count should be obtained prior to treatment and repeated as suggested by the prescribing information.

***Cladribine.*** Cladribine is a purine nucleoside analogue that primarily interferes with DNA synthesis in B and T cells with less impact on innate immunity (Cree et al., 2019). Previous indications include the treatment of multiple forms of leukemia and lymphoma. Cladribine is dosed 4–5 days of the first month based on weight, with this cycle repeated 4 weeks later. In year 2, the cycle is repeated. Redosing after the second cycle is not advised for at least another 2 years.

CLARITY was a study published in 2010 that enrolled 1330 patients in a 1:1:1 fashion to 3.5 mg/kg of cladribine, 5.25 mg/kg, or placebo (Giovannoni et al., 2010). The study found that cladribine decreased the rate of relapse compared to placebo (ARR 0.14 and 0.15 vs. 0.33 ($P < .001$) and decreased MRI activity as well. A second study, ORACLE, was conducted in patients with CIS. Cladribine decreased the risk for a second MS relapse by 67% versus placebo. Although Russia and Australia approved cladribine for use in 2010, both the EMA and the FDA delayed approval with concern over risk. A total of 867 of the original CLARITY patients were enrolled in the CLARITY Extension study. This study showed sustained effect for up to 4 years in the majority of patients treated with cladribine and provided additional information on tolerability and risk (Giovannoni et al., 2018b). Overall, the side effects reported in the trials were minimal. Lymphopenia was the most commonly reported adverse event, with sustained, severe lymphopenia occurring very rarely. Malignancy was also reported in 1.4% of patients in the study. Infections were increased over placebo, though they were typically mild. The data from the Extension study ultimately resulted in EMA approval in 2017 and FDA approval in 2019.

### Treatment of Progressive Disease

A number of clinical trials have investigated treatments for progressive MS. Since the last edition of this chapter, there are have been 2 DMTs that have shown efficacy in progressive MS in phase II I clinical trials: ocrelizumab in PPMS and siponimod in SPMS.

Most past clinical trials in progressive MS have used chemotherapeutic agents. These all have the disadvantage of producing generalized immunosuppression and have considerable potential systemic toxicity. In addition, the toxic and long-term residual effects of these agents tend to limit or preclude chronic or repetitive dosing, further restricting their usefulness.

The most successful historical trial for progressing patients was performed in Europe using the chemotherapeutic agent mitoxantrone (Novantrone), which produced a reduction in the progression of disability and a considerable decrease in relapse rate in patients with worsening RRMS, PPMS, and SPMS over a 2-year period (Hartung et al., 2002). Improvement in MRI measures of disease was also demonstrated. At 3 years, an appreciable benefit was still evident, even though the dosing had been stopped at 2 years. The agent has dose-related cardiac toxicity that limits lifetime dosing to 140 mg/m$^2$. Other side effects include nausea, alopecia, and neutropenia. Secondary leukemias have been uncommonly reported, though this combined risk profile has significantly limited the use of mitoxantrone in MS in recent years.

A number of studies of cyclophosphamide treatment of progressive MS have been conducted, with some suggesting a benefit and others not. Comparison between trials is always hazardous, and various induction protocols have been used, some with the addition of steroids or plasmapheresis. Nevertheless, many anecdotal reports of success led to use of this agent in rapidly progressive cases.

IFN-β-1b has been used in two studies of SPMS. The first was a European multicenter controlled trial of IFN-β-1b in 718 patients with SPMS treated with either IFN-β-1b, 8 MIU subcutaneously every other day, or placebo. The study was planned for 3 years but was stopped after enrollees had completed 2 years because an interim analysis demonstrated efficacy (Kappos, 1998). Analysis of this study revealed that patients treated with IFN-β-1b had significant delays in progression of disability. On average, this delay amounted to 9–12 months. A second study of IFN-β-1b was performed in North America. In this study, SPMS patients were treated with placebo, IFN-β-1b, 8 MIU every other day, or IFN-β-1b 5 MIU/m$^2$ every other day (this group had an average dose of 9.6 MIU). As opposed to the European study, in this study no effect on the primary outcome assessment of reduction in time to worsening disability was found (Kappos et al., 2004). Further analysis of these two studies suggested that the marked difference in their outcomes might relate in part to differences in the degree of MS disease activity between the groups. Although the entrance criteria were very similar, the actual groups differed in several ways (Kappos et al., 2004). This highlights the difficulty in trying to compare results across studies, even those that attempt to evaluate the same problem with the same type of subject.

Ocrelizumab became the first FDA-approved DMT for use in PPMS in 2017 after a successful trial, ORATORIO. ORATORIO randomized 732 PPMS patients 2:1, ocrelizumab:placebo. Key inclusion criteria were age less than 55 years old, presence of elevated IgG index or OCBs in CSF, and an EDSS between 3.0 and 6.5. ORATORIO found that ocrelizumab-treated patients had a 30% less chance for sustained 24-week disability progression compared to patients on placebo ($P = .04$). The side-effect and risk profiles were similar to the RRMS trials (Montalban, 2017). Furthermore, the rate of brain atrophy was less in treated patients. ORATORIO was designed after a failed trial of rituximab in PPMS, OLYMPUS, suggested that younger patients with enhancing lesions on baseline MRI did benefit from rituximab. Extension studies have showed continued benefit of those treated earlier with ocrelizumab versus placebo.

Siponimod was approved for the treatment of SPMS with activity in 2019. Siponimod targets the S1P1 and S1P5 receptors, similar to fingolimod, though notably it has less specificity for the S1P3 receptor, and thus bradycardia during first-day dosing is less of a concern. Siponimod was tested in the EXPAND trial, a study of 1600 patients with SPMS. Siponimod reduced 6-month sustained disability progression 24% versus placebo and decreased ARR and new lesion formation as all. Despite subanalyses that showed that patients who had evidence for inflammatory disease activity in the 2 years leading up to the study received the most benefit, statistical analysis also found that much of the benefit of siponimod was unrelated to this effect (Cree et al., 2019). This implies that there may be a neuroprotective effect of siponimod in addition to the known anti-inflammatory mechanism.

In summary, there is now a treatment option for patients with PPMS and an additional treatment option for patients with SPMS. It is likely that younger patients with progressive MS with evidence for ongoing disease activity will benefit more from the currently available treatments versus those with a purely progressive phenotype. Although there have been significant advancements made in the treatment of progressive MS, further work needs to be done to provide treatments that prevent neurodegeneration and repair previous neurological injury.

## CLINICAL SYMPTOMS AND SYMPTOM MANAGEMENT

Symptom recognition and management is an essential component of MS care, and necessarily evolves over the course of the disease. Symptom management also goes beyond the pharmacological treatment of individual symptoms; it represents an opportunity to reassess polypharmacy, increase safety (such as minimizing risk of urinary infections and hospitalizations), prevent injury (such as due to falls), reduce social isolation and promote satisfying personal relationships, enable self-sufficiency with activities of daily living, and relieve caregiver burden when possible. The AAN published a Multiple Sclerosis Quality Measurement Set in 2015, and the majority of it included measures directly pertaining to symptom management: fall risk, bladder infection, physical activity, fatigue, cognitive impairment, depression screening, depression outcomes, and overall quality of life (Rae-Grant et al., 2015).

### Gait and Ambulatory Dysfunction

Loss of mobility is an important symptom of MS, a major concern for patients diagnosed with this condition and a significant contributor to quality of life. Physical rehabilitation, bracing, and assistive devices all can confer an improvement in mobility for appropriate MS patients. Minimizing fall risk is an essential goal of mobility management. Physical and occupational therapy are important components of comprehensive care and can be employed early in disease course to maximize compensatory strategies and optimize energy utilization to help preserve function and limit fatigue.

The first medication designed to engender functional improvement in MS patients, the oral medication dalfampridine was approved in 2010 (Krieger, 2011). Dalfampridine is a potassium channel blocker that has been hypothesized to restore conduction in demyelinated axons and potentiate synaptic transmission via voltage-dependent potassium channel blockade (Judge et al., 2006). In a series of clinical trials, dalfampridine (sustained-release fampridine) was studied with a primary outcome measure based on changes in walking speed as measured by the timed 25-feet walk (T25FW). In several trials, approximately 35% of patients receiving dalfampridine were timed-walk responders compared with 8% of those given placebo (Goodman et al., 2008, 2009). While modest, this improvement was associated with a reduction of patients' reported ambulatory disability, indicating a clinically meaningful therapeutic benefit for this subset of MS patients.

Dalfampridine is unique among MS agents in having an indication specifically for improving walking (as opposed to reducing relapses or delaying disability). Unlike the immunomodulator treatments for relapse prevention in MS, the efficacy of which can only be assessed in groups of patients, the symptomatic effects of BID oral dalfampridine are rapid and reversible, which makes it possible to detect response in individuals (Goodman et al., 2008). The medication is contraindicated in patients with a history of seizure.

### Fatigue

Fatigue is very common, though not universal, and is usually described as physical exhaustion unrelated to the amount of activity performed. Fatigue occurs in as many as 78% of patients and often interferes with daily activities. The degree of fatigue correlates poorly with the overall severity of disease or the presence of any symptom or sign. In contrast to the situation with cognitive deficits, no MRI findings correlate with fatigue. Fatigue may often be reported in association with an attack and persist long after resolution of other neurological symptoms.

The initial treatment approach to fatigue in MS should include an evaluation of sleep habits, including consideration of treating insomnia, anxiety, depression, nocturia, spasticity, and pain, all of which can undermine sleep integrity and contribute to fatigue. For primary MS fatigue, amantadine (Symmetrel), 100 mg BID, has relatively few side effects and is well tolerated by most patients. Caution must be used in patients with renal insufficiency or seizure disorders. Studies have reported an efficacy rate of 40%.

Modafinil (Provigil) is a wakefulness-promoting agent approved for use in narcolepsy that is chemically and pharmacologically distinct from CNS stimulants, although the precise mechanism of action is unknown. A single-blind crossover study suggested improvement, but a double-blind placebo-controlled parallel group study failed to demonstrate a benefit. Oral dosage starts at 100 mg in the morning and can be increased up to 400 mg/day. Armodafinil is a related vigilance-promoting agent that can be utilized. Some patients also may respond to methylphenidate (Ritalin), 10–60 mg/day in 2–3 divided doses, or to other stimulants such as atomoxetine. In addition to treating the depressive symptoms associated with MS, selective serotonin reuptake inhibitors (SSRIs), especially those with activating properties, have been used to treat fatigue. Bupropion may also alleviate fatigue at times, even in the absence of overt depression. The drug should be avoided in patients with a history of seizures.

### Cognitive Impairment

Cognitive involvement in MS was documented as early as 1877 by Charcot. He observed that patients with "multilocular sclerosis" are slow to form conceptions, have "marked enfeeblement of the memory, and blunting of intellectual and emotional faculties." However, the subsequent era of research in MS focused primarily on physical disability. There was a paucity of rigorous studies, with a focus on cognition. In 1981, Kurtzke reported that only 5% of patients with MS suffered from cognitive impairment. The Kurtzke EDSS focused primarily on somatic disability measures. A decade later, data from formal neuropsychological studies indicated that cognitive involvement has been underreported in MS (Rao et al., 1991). Neuropsychological test results have shown that 34%–65% of patients with MS have some degree of cognitive impairment (Nocentini et al., 2006).

Cognitive abnormalities affect patients across the disease spectrum and involve all MS subtypes. Some 49%–53.7% of CIS and early RRMS patients show significant impairment in one or more cognitive domains that impacts their quality of life (Achiron and Barak, 2003; Glanz et al., 2007). A longitudinal study reported 29% of early PPMS patients (within 5 years from disease onset) as cognitively impaired (Penny et al., 2010; Ukkonen et al., 2009). It is increasingly recognized that low physical disability can coexist with significant cognitive disease.

In general, the most frequently reported abnormalities are with working memory, attention, and speed of information processing. Patients complain of memory loss, difficulties at work or with interpersonal relations, inability to multitask, and "mental fog and fatigue." Comorbid depression, anxiety disorders, and emotional lability may further affect cognitive performance. Mild to moderate abnormalities are usually not apparent during a routine office visit, and simple screening tools for cognitive dysfunction such as the Symbol Digit Modalities Test (SDMT) offer increased sensitivity to MS-related cognitive dysfunction (Benedict et al., 2017). Longer neuropsychological testing batteries are designed to assess cognitive impairment in MS patients and are used primarily in research trials. The Brief Repeatable Battery of Neuropsychological Tests (BRB-N) (Rao et al., 1991) and Minimal Assessment of Cognitive Function in Multiple Sclerosis (MACFIMS) (Benedict et al., 2002) are the most widely used cognitive batteries for MS assessment.

Treatment of cognitive impairment in MS is challenging. There are limited data on the effectiveness of DMTs at preventing the development of cognitive dysfunction. A trial of IM IFN-β-1a showed a 47% reduction in cognitive decline on PASAT testing over 2 years of follow-up (Fischer et al., 2000). A subsequent randomized study of 469 patients showed that treatment with higher versus lower doses of SC IFN-β-1a was predictive of lower cognitive impairment at 3 years of follow-up (Patti et al., 2010).

Pharmacological therapy focuses on treatment of underlying disease as well as symptomatic manifestations of declining mental function, such as difficulties with attention, memory, and fatigue. There is no convincing evidence that cholinesterase inhibitors improve memory in MS patients. A small study assessed the effects of donepezil on SPMS patients who were residents in a nursing home, documenting improvement in several cognitive domains after 8 weeks of therapy (Greene et al., 2000). There are additional anecdotal reports of efficacy in small numbers of subjects, though these agents are not widely employed in MS. Modafinil may also improve focused attention. It has a favorable safety profile and can be used for symptomatic management of MS patients with severe fatigue and decreased focus. There is some evidence that treatment with l-amphetamine is associated with improved learning and memory in cognitively impaired MS patients (Benedict et al., 2008; Morrow et al., 2009).

Appropriate management of superimposed or comorbid psychiatric disease (notably depression and/or anxiety) often improves cognitive performance. Cognitive-behavioral therapy, family and individual counseling, strategies to improve day-to-day function, physical and occupational therapy evaluations, and necessary job modifications and accommodations can be of great help to MS patients suffering from cognitive decline.

## Mood and Affective Disorders

Cross-sectional studies have shown some degree of affective disturbance in a significant number of patients with MS (Goldman Consensus Group, 2005). The AAN quality measure set recommends screening for depression and assessing depression as two separate components of comprehensive MS care. Depression is the most common manifestation and may in part be due to the burden of having to cope with an unpredictable and chronic disease. However, it is more prevalent in MS than in other chronic diseases, suggesting a disease-related component as well. The lifetime risk of major depression in patients with MS is up to 50% (Sadovnick et al., 1996). Patients taking multiple medications are prone to depression, and the side-effect profile of the IFN-β medications includes depression. Some data indicate a comorbid association between bipolar illness and MS. Suicide rates are higher in patients with MS than in the general population or when compared to patients with other chronic illnesses (Bronnum-Hansen et al., 2005). Frontal or subcortical white-matter disease may also be a contributory causative factor.

Depression in MS is a treatable condition, irrespective of whether it is considered a symptom or a comorbidity. SSRIs are the medications of choice for depressive symptoms in patients with MS, and any of the other medications in this class may be used. More stimulating SSRIs may help to address concurrent fatigue; Serotonin and norepinephrine reuptake inhibitors (SNRIs) such as duloxetine are also potentially effective for depression in MS, and may have benefit for MS-related pain in patients with both symptoms. Amitriptyline is a second-line choice because of its anticholinergic side effects. However, anticholinergic properties may also be helpful to patients with symptoms of bladder spasticity or chronic pain.

Euphoria, formerly considered to be common in MS, is actually infrequent and is usually associated with moderate or severe cognitive impairment and greater disease burden on MRI. However, emotional "dyscontrol," also known as *pseudobulbar affect*, is quite common, and patients with this condition may oscillate frequently between expressing sad and happy states, at times without clear precipitants and in situations not congruent with the emotional expression. Dextromethorphan with quinidine has been shown to be effective for MS patients with pseudobulbar affect (PBA) (Pioro et al., 2010).

## Spasticity

Spasticity slows voluntary movement, impairs balance and gait, and may cause painful flexor or extensor spasms. Rehabilitation interventions like stretching, Pilates, yoga, and functional electrical stimulation, along with weight-bearing exercises, and pool/aquatic therapy are important nonpharmacological management approaches.

Baclofen is a $\gamma$-aminobutyric acid (GABA) agonist that can effectively relieve spasms and has modest effects in improving performance. Daily divided doses of 20–120 mg and occasionally more are used. Too large a dose may produce drowsiness or hypotonicity that may aggravate weakness, especially in those individuals who require a degree of spasticity to stand and transfer. Intrathecal baclofen via an implanted pump can be effective against spasticity in suitable patients. Its effectiveness has been demonstrated in several controlled trials, and the side effects are few.

Tizanidine (Zanaflex), a centrally active $\alpha_2$-noradrenergic agonist, may be used alone or in combination with baclofen because the mechanism of action is different. The medication should be gradually increased, starting with 2 mg at bedtime. The side effects are similar to those seen with baclofen; however, a blind prospective trial in patients with MS showed that tizanidine relieved spasticity without adversely affecting strength.

Benzodiazepines contribute to the control of spasticity, although sedation and possible drug dependency are limiting factors, and these agents can worsen cognition and ataxia, and potentially increase the risk of falls.

Botulinum toxin type A (Botox) injections into spastic or contracted muscles may also be effective in cases with more focal or localized spasticity.

## Tremor

Tremor is one of the most disabling and difficult-to-treat symptoms in MS. Appendicular tremors are usually seen in action or intention and may limit activities of daily living. Weighted wrist bracelets and specially adapted utensils are nonpharmaceutical options. Most attempts at pharmacological amelioration of tremor are minimally successful. Anticonvulsants have been tried with little success. Carbamazepine (Tegretol) in divided doses up to 800 mg/day has been used. Gabapentin (Neurontin) in daily divided doses up to 3600 mg has shown some benefit, and anecdotal reports of a benefit with topiramate (Topamax) have been noted. Primidone (Mysoline), 125–250 mg BID or TID, may be tried. Dizziness, somnolence, and nausea are the primary side effects.

Clonazepam (Klonopin), 0.5–2 mg one to four times daily, may be mildly effective. i 20–40 mg BID or TID, is another option, and may help with an anxiety or underlying essential tremor component than be medication responsive. Caution must be exercised in patients with concomitant cardiac, circulatory, or respiratory disorders.

Surgical thalamotomy or deep brain stimulation may be used in patients with refractory tremors.

### Bladder Dysfunction

Symptomatic bladder dysfunction occurs at some time during the course of MS in 50%–80% of patients. Recurrent urinary tract infections should alert the practitioner to the need for a urological evaluation, if this has not been done previously. The severity of bladder symptoms is unrelated to the duration of the disease but often parallels the severity of other myelopathic symptoms. Differentiating between bladder spasticity (urinary frequency, urgency, incontinence) and hypotonia (urinary hesitancy, retention, and overflow incontinence) is important before initiating therapy, because different therapies are employed for each condition. Initial steps in managing bladder dysfunction include fluid management, timed voiding, and the use of a bedside commode. Anticholinergic medications are often used for patients with a hyperreflexic bladder without outlet obstruction. Oxybutynin (Ditropan) is often a first-line medication because it is available generically at relatively low cost and has been very extensively used. Dosage usually ranges from 2.5 to 5 mg one to three times daily. An extended-release formulation is available. Other medications with similar action include tolterodine (Detrol), trospium (Sanctura), darifenacin (Enablex), and solifenacin (VESIcare).

Desmopressin is also effective for hyperreflexic bladder without outlet obstruction, especially when taken at bedtime. Doses of 20–40 mg daily are suggested. Adverse effects include nausea, flushing, and headache. Detrusor hyperreflexia with outlet obstruction may respond to Credé maneuvers, antispasticity medications, or anticholinergics in combination with α-sympathetic blocking agents such as terazosin hydrochloride (Hytrin). Adverse effects include tachycardia, dizziness, syncope, headache, and asthenia. Botulinum toxin injection to the bladder musculature may be helpful in medication-refractory hyperreflexic bladder. Intermittent catheterization, often self-performed, may be very helpful for patients with retention. Occasionally, chronic indwelling catheterization may be required. Surgical correction, such as augmentation of bladder capacity with an exteriorized loop of bowel, is another alternative for appropriate patients, when other measures have failed.

### Sexual Dysfunction

Studies suggest that 45%–74% of women with MS experience sexual dysfunction. These symptoms have been associated with depression, bowel dysfunction, fatigue, spasticity, and pelvic floor weakness. Referral for urogynecological evaluation and consideration of pelvic floor exercises, lubricants, stimulator devices, and therapeutic techniques may be of value. Erectile dysfunction in men is common, especially in patients with spinal cord involvement. Adverse effects of medication or psychological issues may also be associated with sexual dysfunction.

Sildenafil and multiple similar medications have supplanted older approaches to erectile dysfunction in men. Caution should be taken in patients with cardiovascular disease and concomitant cardiac medications. In both women and men with MS, consequent effects of sexual dysfunction involve social isolation, depression, anger, guilt, spousal burden, and self-image, which can be addressed through counseling and sexual therapy.

### Transient and Paroxysmal Symptoms Particularly Characteristic of MS

Clinical features that are characteristic, though not pathognomonic of MS include bilateral INO, the Lhermitte sign, paroxysmal episodes, and the Uhthoff phenomenon (Table 80.4). Lhermitte sign is the brief occurrence of an electrical sensation down the spine and/or into the limbs, usually provoked by flexion of the neck. It is experienced commonly in MS patients with spinal cord disease, but other spinal cord pathologies may also cause the same symptomatology. Paroxysmal episodes refer to brief, stereotyped attacks of motor or sensory phenomena such as diplopia, focal paresthesia, trigeminal neuralgia and other paroxysmal pain syndromes, ataxia, dysarthria, and tonic spasms, including hemifacial spasm and dystonia (Mehanna and Jankovic, 2013). They may be triggered by a specific movement or stimulus, but frequently there is no identifiable inciting factor. They do not always occur as the result of a new disease activity, but may occur as a consequence of a pre-existing lesion.

Anticonvulsants have been used for their membrane-stabilizing properties in their usual or lower doses with some benefit at decreasing the frequency and intensity of paroxysmal symptoms. Carbamazepine is perhaps the most widely utilized, particularly extended-release formulations. Benzodiazepines also have been effective in some patients. Baclofen, acetazolamide, and bromocriptine have been cited as potentially beneficial for these paroxysmal symptoms. A new onset of a "flurry" of paroxysmal symptoms may be considered an MS relapse, and a course of high-dose IV steroids as described in the section on treatment of acute attacks may be employed.

Heat sensitivity is a well-known occurrence in MS. Specifically, *Uhthoff phenomenon* describes the recurrence or worsening of a focal MS deficit (i.e., visual blurring) due to decreased conduction through demyelinated fibers at higher body temperatures. Similarly, recrudescence of prior symptoms in the setting of a febrile illness such as urinary tract infection, often termed a *pseudoexacerbation*, is a consequence of the same process and needs to be distinguished from a true new relapse before steroids are utilized.

## OTHER INFLAMMATORY DEMYELINATING DISEASES OF THE CENTRAL NERVOUS SYSTEM

### Acute Disseminated Encephalomyelitis

*Acute disseminated encephalomyelitis* (ADEM) is a demyelinating syndrome that often occurs in association with an immunization or vaccination (postvaccination ADEM) or systemic viral infection (parainfectious ADEM), but may also occur without any known trigger. This disorder is almost always monophasic. Recurrent cases have been reported, but this occurs rarely and distinction from MS or other CNS demyelinating disorders is unclear.

**TABLE 80.4 Characteristic Clinical Features of Multiple Sclerosis**

| Clinical Features Suggestive of Multiple Sclerosis |
|---|
| Onset between ages 15 and 50 |
| Involvement of multiple areas of the central nervous system |
| Optic neuritis |
| Lhermitte sign |
| Internuclear ophthalmoplegia |
| Fatigue |
| Worsening with elevated body temperature |

### Postvaccination Acute Disseminated Encephalomyelitis

The occurrence of "neuroparalytic accidents" as a consequence of the Pasteur rabies vaccine prepared from spinal cords of rabbits inoculated with fixed rabies virus was recorded soon after introduction of the treatment. Similar neurological complications were associated with the Jenner vaccine used for smallpox prevention. Reports have associated ADEM with other vaccines including pertussis, rubella, diphtheria, and measles. The association of the swine influenza vaccine with ADEM has been the subject of medicolegal controversy. ADEM is not known to be clearly associated with any vaccine currently used in the United States. ADEM developing after drug administration has been reported with sulfonamides and para-aminosalicylic acid/streptomycin.

### Parainfectious Acute Disseminated Encephalomyelitis

Descriptions of cerebral and cerebellar abnormalities after measles appeared in the mid- to late 19th century. The overall experience suggests that neurological sequelae complicate 1 in 400 to 1 in 1000 cases of measles infection, and that patients do not develop peripheral nerve damage, nor do relapses occur. Less compelling associations with ADEM have been made with a wide array of viral and bacterial infections including rubella, mumps, herpes zoster, herpes simplex, influenza, EBV, coxsackievirus, *Borrelia burgdorferi*, *Mycoplasma*, and *Leptospira*.

### Clinical Features

Cases of acute encephalomyelitis occurring in a setting without a recent known infection or vaccination or with only nonspecific viral symptoms are difficult to diagnose with certainty and distinguish from episodes of MS. An initial attack of MS is considerably more common than ADEM. Cases occurring in children at an extremely young age are perhaps the most readily delineated.

The hallmark clinical feature of ADEM is the development of a focal or multifocal neurological disorder following exposure to virus or receipt of vaccine. In some but not all cases, a prodromal phase of several days of fever, malaise, and myalgia occurs. Onset of the CNS disorder is usually rapid (abrupt or up to several hours), with peak dysfunction within several days. Initial features include encephalopathy ranging from lethargy to coma, seizures, and focal and multifocal signs reflecting cerebral, brainstem, and spinal cord involvement. Clinically, fever, encephalopathy, and multifocal presentation can be most helpful in distinguishing ADEM from the first episode of MS. Other reported findings include movement disorders and ataxia.

Recovery can begin within days; complete resolution is occasionally noted within a few days but more often evolves over the course of weeks or months. Poor prognosis is correlated with severity and abruptness of onset of the clinical syndrome. Measles virus-associated ADEM may carry a worse prognosis than vaccine-associated disease.

### Laboratory and Radiological Features

The usual CSF findings are normal opening pressure, little or modest increase in cell count (<100 cells/mL), and a moderate increase in protein. Cases with high cell counts, including some polymorphonuclear cells and high protein values, occur. The high counts usually return to normal within a few days. OCBs occur less commonly than in MS.

Radiologically, an important feature of ADEM is that the great majority of the T2 lesions enhance, suggesting they were of recent onset, consistent with a monophasic illness (Fig. 80.18). Unlike MS, in ADEM, after several weeks, lesions show at least partial resolution without the appearance of new lesions.

Pathologically, ADEM lesions display perivascular inflammation and surrounding demyelination within the CNS. Vessel necrosis is frequently observed. The demyelinating aspect may be minimal or widespread, with coalescence of the multiple lesions. Some meningeal reaction may also be apparent.

The diagnosis of ADEM can usually be made with confidence in the setting of a clear-cut antecedent event strongly associated with the disorder, such as measles infection or vaccination. The occurrence of an acute focal or multifocal CNS syndrome subsequent to a nonspecific viral illness creates a wider differential diagnosis. Apart from the first episode of MS, CNS vasculitis, embolic disease, direct infection, and granulomatous disease should be considered.

## Acute Hemorrhagic Leukoencephalitis

Acute hemorrhagic leukoencephalitis is a rare entity that represents a hyperacute form of ADEM. The most frequent antecedent history is that of an upper respiratory infection. The clinical manifestations

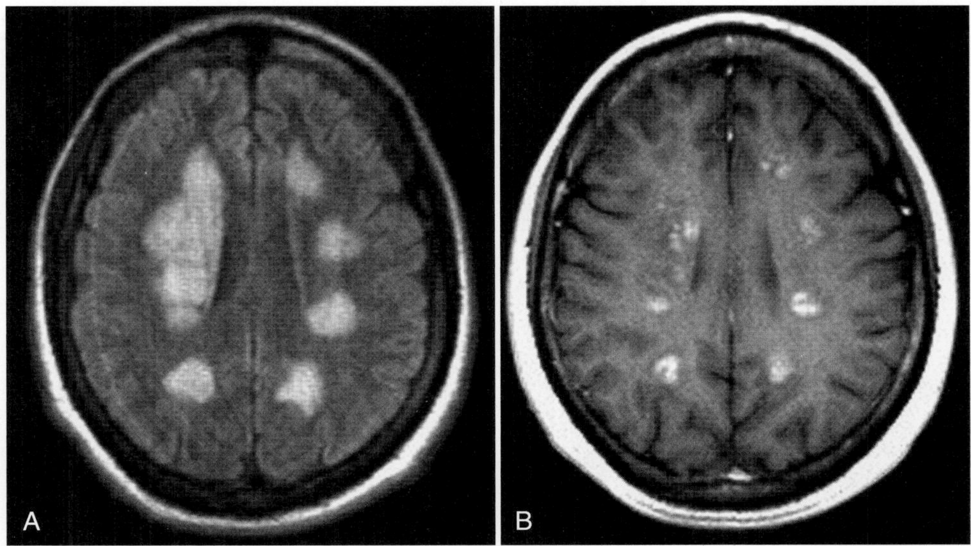


**Fig. 80.18** Acute disseminated encephalomyelitis in a 20-year-old male. **A,** Fluid-attenuated inversion recovery (FLAIR) images. **B,** Corresponding postcontrast images showing enhancement of all lesions. The patient presented with encephalopathy, headache, and a dense left hemiplegia. Two years later he had developed no further symptoms or magnetic resonance imaging lesions, but a left hemiparesis was still present.

mimic ADEM but are more abrupt and more severe. MRI usually shows large, confluent FLAIR bright lesions with petechial hemorrhages. Pathology shows necrotizing vasculitis involving venules and capillaries and features perivascular accumulations of polymorphonuclear cells and red blood cells.

### Treatment

The current favored therapy for ADEM is high-dose corticosteroids, although no controlled clinical studies have been conducted. Plasmapheresis and immunosuppressants, such as cyclophosphamide, have been used in refractory cases.

## Neuromyelitis Optica

Eugene Devic coined the phrase "neuromyelitis optica" (NMO) in the late 1800s to describe a devastating demyelinating syndrome characterized by ON and myelitis, either simultaneously or in sequential relapses. Despite Devic's and others' belief that NMO was a unique disease entity, until 2004 many considered NMO to be a severe variant of MS. In 2004, the aquaporin-4 antibody was identified in a majority of patients with the clinical syndrome of NMO, while at the same time showing a high specificity (Lennon et al., 2004), thus confirming long-standing suspicions that NMO is a different disease entirely than MS.

The target of the NMO antibody is the aquaporin-4 (AQP4), a transmembrane protein which facilitates water transport in the CNS. AQP4 is heavily expressed at astrocytic foot processes at the BBB. The NMO lesion is a result of compliment activation at the site of the AQP4 protein, leading to a distinctive "rim and rosette" pattern of immune complexes in the NMO lesion (Luchinetti et al., 2002). The result is astrocyte death and tissue necrosis in both gray and white matter. Although T cells, B cells, and macrophages are important in NMO pathophysiology similar to MS, in NMO, neutrophils and eosinophils also contribute to tissue damage (Jacob et al., 2013).

Epidemiologically, NMO patients differ significantly from MS patients. NMO is a much rarer condition, with an overall prevalence thought to be approximately 2–4/100,000 in most populations (Flanagan et al., 2016; Houzen et al., 2017). The female to male ratio is even more disparate in NMO versus MS at 9:1. The age of onset is older (median age 40 years vs. 28 years). There is a non-Caucasian predominance in the NMO population, with patients of Hispanic and African descent being commonly affected (Mata and Lolli, 2011). The course of NMO also differs from that of MS. Although NMO patients are much less likely to transition to a progressive course, the disability accumulated from NMO relapses tends to be more severe; patients more commonly have a deficit of total blindness or paralysis from NMO attacks, something that is uncommon in MS patients.

Classically, NMO patients have relapses consisting of ON, myelitis, or area postrema syndrome. ON in NMO is typically severe, more likely to be bilateral, and the recovery may not be as complete. Spinal cord relapses, another hallmark of NMO, are often a longitudinally extensive myelitis (LETM), defined as a spinal cord lesion that is contiguous and greater than three vertebral segments but may be many more, often extending from the cervical junction throughout the cervical and thoracic cord (Fig. 80.19). Myelitides in NMO may involve motor, sensory, and/or bowel and bladder functions. Although classically NMO was defined as a condition that spared the brain itself, it is now well recognized that NMO lesions can also cause brainstem and cerebral symptoms. Brainstem symptoms may include intractable nausea and vomiting and hiccupping (also known as the area postrema syndrome, the presenting symptom in up to 10% of NMO patients), double vision, dysphagia, and respiratory compromise. Cerebral symptoms may include motor or sensory deficits and encephalopathies.

The key diagnostic test in NMO is the NMO antibody. Depending on the assay employed, sensitivity ranges from 70% to 80%, with specificity close to 100% (Wingerchuk et al., 2015). Patients with NMO often have positive antibodies for other conditions such as Sjögren syndrome or lupus. If they have clinical symptoms suggestive of these other conditions as well, it is likely that there are two coexisting autoimmune syndromes. The reverse scenario, a patient with another rheumatological condition displaying seropositivity for the NMO antibody, is rare. CSF shows OCB positivity in only 10% of cases. Commonly there can be a mild elevation in CSF white blood cell (WBC) count and protein.

The currently accepted diagnostic criteria for NMO spectrum disorders (NMOSD) from Wingerchuk et al., (2015) requires that a patient with AQP4 IgG have a history of a core clinical syndrome (ON, myelitis, area postrema syndrome, brainstem syndrome, narcolepsy or other acute diencephalic syndrome, or symptomatic cerebral syndrome with typical NMOSD lesions) along with a positive anti-AQP4-IgG test and exclusion of other causes. The requirements for a diagnosis of NMOSD

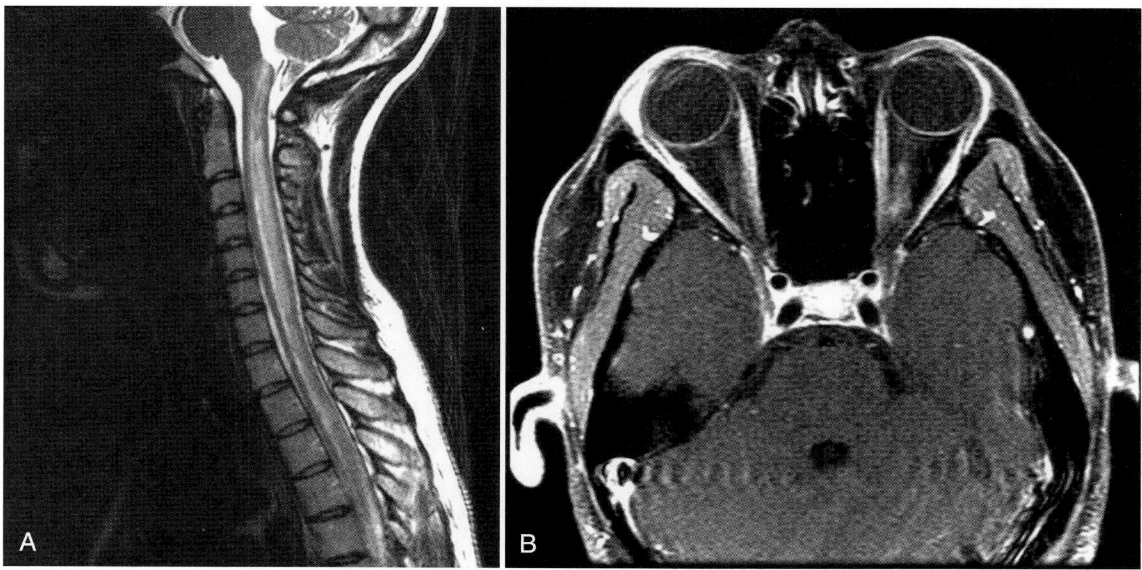


**Fig. 80.19** Neuromyelitis optica in a 30-year-old female of Caribbean origin. **A,** Longitudinally extensive cervical spine lesion. **B,** Avid enhancement of left optic nerve.

for seronegative cases are more rigorous in order to maintain diagnostic accuracy (Table 80.5).

One important subset of AQP4-seronegative NMOSD patients are those patients that are now known to test positive for myelin oligodendrocyte glycoprotein (MOG) antibody. Transient seropositivity of MOG antibody has been associated with a monophasic course versus those with a persistently high titer who had a higher risk for relapsing disease (Hennes et al., 2017; Hyun et al., 2017). As with NMO, MOG antibody-associated disorders include ON, myelitis, and brainstem syndromes, though there are subtle differences between the conditions. MOG antibody disease is more common in males than in NMO. ADEM is a common presenting feature. The ON in MOG antibody-associated disease often presents with disc edema, involves a long section of the optic nerve, and is bilateral (Chen et al., 2018). Myelitis is often lower in the spinal cord than in AQP4-positive patients and may be longitudinally extensive or involve only a short segment (Weber et al., 2018). The area postrema syndrome is less common. Overall, the prognosis for MOG antibody-associated disorders appears to be better than for AQP4-IgG disorder. Patients are less likely to have severe neurological deficits after a relapse and more likely to maintain function, though bowel/bladder/erectile dysfunction may be permanent in MOG antibody disease patients (Jurynczyk et al., 2017).

The approach to treatment in NMOSD and MOG antibody disease is currently almost identical and contains three parts: treatment of relapse, prevention of relapse, and treatment of chronic symptoms. Treatment of an NMOSD attack should be prompt and aggressive, as it may influence the neurological outcome. Typically, high-dose IV methylprednisolone is given for a period of 5 days followed by a prednisone taper. Depending on treatment response, plasmapheresis or IVIG may be used for relapses with incomplete recovery after steroid. Early plasmapheresis is encouraged for those patients with serious deficit or those that do not respond initially to steroid, and treatment of subsequent attacks may be treated with plasmapheresis as a first line, as it has been shown to bring about a better outcome when used earlier in the course (Kleiter et al., 2016). Historically, azathioprine, mycophenolate mofetil, rituximab, mitoxantrone, and cyclophosphamide have all been used as preventive treatments in NMO (Kimbrough et al., 2012). Recently, three randomized, controlled studies to assess efficacy of disease-modifying treatments in NMO have been completed. Eculizumab, a complement inhibitor, showed a 94% reduction risk for new relapses when it was added on to a patient's previous immunosuppressive regimen versus patients who were given placebo and continued their previous DMT treatment. It is now FDA-approved for the treatment of NMOSD. Satralizumab and inebilizumab both showed marked reduction in new NMOSD relapse versus the comparison group as well (Collongues et al., 2019). Importantly, multiple disease-modifying agents commonly in MS, including IFNs and natalizumab, are suspected to worsen the disease course in NMO. This makes early and accurate diagnosis that much more critical.

## Site-Restricted Forms of Demyelinating Disorders

### Transverse Myelitis

*Acute transverse myelitis* is defined as the development of isolated spinal cord dysfunction over hours or days in patients in whom no evidence of a compressive or vascular lesion exists. Further categorization can

**TABLE 80.5 Diagnostic Criteria for NMOSD with AQP4 IgG**

**Diagnostic Criteria for NMOSD *with* AQP4 IgG**

- At least one core clinical characteristic
- Positive test for AQP4 IgG using best available assay
- Exclusion of other alternative diagnosis

**Diagnostic Criteria for NMO *without* AQP4-IgG or NMOSD *with unknown* AQP4-IgG status**

- At least two core clinical characteristics occurring as a result of one or more clinical attacks and meeting all of the following requirements:
  - a. At least one core clinical characteristic must be optic neuritis, acute myelitis with longitudinally extensive transverse myelitis, or area postrema syndrome
  - b. Dissemination in space (2 or more different core clinical characteristics)
  - c. Fulfillment of additional MRI requirements, as applicable
- Negative tests for AQP4 IgG using best-available method or unavailable
- Exclusion of alternative diagnoses

**Core Clinical Characteristics**

- Optic neuritis
- Acute myelitis
- Area postrema syndrome: episode of otherwise unexplained hiccups or nausea and vomiting
- Acute brainstem syndrome
- Symptomatic narcolepsy or acute diencephalic clinical syndrome with NMOSD-typical diencephalic MRI lesions
- Symptomatic cerebral syndrome with NMOSD-typical brain lesions

**Additional MRI Requirements for NMOSD *without* AQP4-IgG and NMOSD *with unknown* AQP4-IgG Status**

- Acute optic neuritis: requires brain MRI showing (a) normal findings or only nonspecific white-matter lesions, OR (b) optic nerve MRI with T2-hyperintense lesion or T1-weighted gadolinium-enhancing lesion extending over more than half optic nerve length or involving optic chiasm
- Acute myelitis: requires associated intramedullary MRI lesion extending over ≥c3 contiguous segments of focal spinal cord atrophy in patients with history compatible with acute myelitis
- Area postrema syndrome: requires associated dorsal medulla/areas postrema lesions
- Acute brainstem syndrome: requires associated periependymal brainstem lesions

*AQP4*, Aquaporin-4; *IgG*, immunoglobulin G; *MRI*, magnetic resonance imaging; *NMO*, neuromyelitis optica; *NMOSD*, neuromyelitis optica syndrome disorder.

*Adapted from Wingerchuk, D.M., Banwell, B., Bennett, J.L., et al., 2015. International consensus diagnostic criteria for neuromyelitis optica spectrum disorders. Neurology 85(2), 177–189.*

be made into acute complete transverse myelitis (ACTM), idiopathic inflammation of the spinal cord causing symmetrical and moderate or severe loss of function relative to a distinct spinal cord level and acute partial transverse myelitis (APTM), asymmetric involvement or partial involvement of the spinal cord (Scott, 2007).

In the absence of a brain MRI that is characteristic, ACTM rarely evolves into MS and is typically a monophasic event. Conversely, APTM is a precursor to MS in 50%–90% of patients who have two or more typical MS lesions on cerebral imaging and 20%–30% in those with negative brain MRIs (Scott, 2007). Acute transverse myelitis is also known to occur on a background of systemic vasculitis. NMO antibody and a complete rheumatological panel should be tested. Positivity of OCBs may help in differentiating between idiopathic cases and either MS or NMO, as they are rarely present without an underlying cause. Similarly, an elevation in CSF white count and CSF viral testing may be associated with an infectious or parainfectious etiology (Scott et al., 2011).

## Isolated Optic Neuritis

The clinical features of ON are described earlier in the chapter. The issue remains whether some cases of isolated ON represent formes frustes of ADEM. In this regard, cases of ON occurring after childhood exanthemas would represent the best example of parainfectious ON. Cases have been reported following measles, rubella, mumps, and varicella. Most patients had bilateral optic nerve involvement; additional neurological abnormalities occurred in only a minority of patients. The young age of the patients further suggests that these events are not the initial manifestations of MS. The prognosis for recovery of vision is good in most cases, perhaps less so in post-varicella cases.

## Chronic Relapsing Inflammatory Optic Neuropathy

Chronic relapsing inflammatory optic neuropathy (CRION), first described in 2003, is a condition characterized by relapsing ON without known involvement in other areas of the CNS. Presentations of this condition vary and include a unilateral relapsing ON, sequential relapses of both optic nerves, and simultaneous, bilateral ON. Characteristic features used to make a diagnosis include history of ON with at least one relapse, objective loss of visual function, NMO IgG negative, contrast enhancement of the affected optic nerve on MRI, and often there is a response to steroid treatment followed by relapse with dose reduction or discontinuation (Petzold and Plant, 2014). The differential diagnosis for CRION includes NMOSD, MOG-associated ON, SLE, sarcoidosis, and atypical MS presentation.

*The complete reference list is available online at https://expertconsult.inkling.com/.*

81

# Paraneoplastic Disorders of the Nervous System

Myrna R. Rosenfeld, Josep Dalmau

## OUTLINE



## PATHOGENESIS

Paraneoplastic neurological syndromes (PNSs) are a heterogeneous group of disorders that are immune mediated (Table 81.1). It is postulated that the expression of neuronal proteins (called onconeuronal proteins) by a tumor provokes an immune response that is misdirected against the nervous system. This hypothesis is supported by the detection in the serum and cerebrospinal fluid (CSF) of anti-neuronal antibodies that react with antigens expressed by the tumor and the nervous system (Dalmau et al., 2008; Darnell et al., 2003). Antibodies that target intracellular antigens (e.g., anti-Hu, Ri, Ma2) are most commonly associated with PNS of the central nervous system (CNS). The detection of one of these antibodies is highly predictive of the presence of a cancer (Table 81.2). The PNSs associated with antibodies to intracellular antigens are likely mediated by cytotoxic T-cell responses that produce irreversible neuronal cell death, explaining why many PNSs are not reversible. Since the T cells appear to be directed against the same antigens as the antibodies, the antibodies and the T cells likely play cooperating roles in the pathogenesis of the PNSs that have yet to be defined (Blachere et al., 2014). Other antibodies, in particular those that target antigens on the neuronal cell surface (e.g., acetylcholine receptor [AChR] or γ-aminobutyric acid type B receptor [GABAbR]) occur with specific neurological syndromes regardless of the presence or absence of cancer. These antibodies are pathogenic and act by binding to and altering the function of the target antigens (Dalmau et al., 2018; Ruff et al., 2018). Cytotoxic T-cell mechanisms are not involved and the antibody effects are reversible. Thus these disorders often respond to treatment of the associated cancer (when paraneoplastic) and B-cell or antibody depleting strategies.

## GENERAL DIAGNOSTIC APPROACH

The specificity of paraneoplastic anti-neuronal antibodies for PNSs or some types of cancer makes them useful diagnostic tools (see Table 81.2). In approximately 65% of patients with PNS, the neurological symptoms precede the tumor diagnosis (Giometto et al., 2010). Therefore in the right clinical context the detection of a paraneoplastic antibody in the serum or CSF helps to diagnose the PNS and focus the search for the neoplasm (Graus et al., 2004). Most paraneoplastic neuronal antibodies can also be detected, usually at low titers, in the serum of a variable proportion of patients with cancer but without PNS (Monstad et al., 2009). Therefore, if the detected antibody does not correspond with the antibody that usually associates with the neurological syndrome, other causes for the neurological dysfunction should be considered. Similarly, if the detected cancer is not the histological type typically found in association with the antibody (e.g., anti-Yo with lung cancer rather than breast or ovarian cancer), a second neoplasm should be suspected. A search for another neoplasm is required if the tumor cells do not express the target antigen of the paraneoplastic antibody (Graus et al., 2001). Clinical experience suggests that detection of paraneoplastic antibodies in CSF confirms that the neurological disorder is paraneoplastic.

The diagnosis of PNS can be made to different degrees of certainty by taking into consideration the type of syndrome, detection of a tumor, and presence or absence of paraneoplastic antibodies (Graus et al., 2004). The diagnosis of PNS is relatively straightforward for patients who develop symptoms of a well-defined syndrome that is typically associated with cancer. Patient age is important because symptoms that associate with paraneoplastic mechanisms in adults (e.g., subacute cerebellar dysfunction) are less typical of paraneoplasia in children. Conversely, the development of opsoclonus in children is often paraneoplastic, but in adults is less suggestive of a paraneoplastic cause. In these settings, the detection of an antibody known to be associated with PNS or cancer is practically confirmatory of paraneoplasia. If a cancer is not discovered, the presence of an occult neoplasm is assumed unless proven otherwise. Body [$^{18}$F]- fluorodeoxyglucose-positron emission tomography (FDG-PET) scans can detect tumors that escape detection by other standard imaging methods (Garcia Vicente et al., 2017;

**TABLE 81.1 Paraneoplastic Neurological Syndromes**

| Syndromes Affecting the Central Nervous System |
|---|
| Cerebellar degeneration |
| Encephalomyelitis* |
| Limbic and brainstem encephalitis |
| Opsoclonus-myoclonus |
| Stiff-person spectrum disorders |
| Necrotizing myelopathy† |
| Motor neuron syndromes† (ALS; subacute motor neuronopathy; upper motor neuron dysfunction) |
| **Syndromes Affecting the Visual System** |
| Retinopathy |
| Optic neuritis |
| Uveitis (usually in association with encephalomyelitis) |
| Bilateral diffuse uveal melanocytic proliferation |
| **Syndromes Affecting the Peripheral Nervous System** |
| Sensory neuronopathy |
| Vasculitis of the nerve and muscle |
| Subacute and chronic sensorimotor peripheral neuropathy |
| Sensorimotor neuropathies associated with plasma cell dyscrasias and B-cell lymphoma |
| Autonomic neuropathy† |
| Brachial neuritis† |
| Acute polyradiculoneuropathy (Guillain-Barré syndrome) |
| Peripheral nerve hyperexcitability |
| **Syndromes Affecting the Neuromuscular Junction and Muscle** |
| Lambert-Eaton myasthenic syndrome |
| Myasthenia gravis |
| Dermatomyositis |
| Necrotizing autoimmune myopathy |

*ALS,* Amyotrophic lateral sclerosis.
*Includes focal cortical encephalitis, cerebellar dysfunction, and myelitis.
†Not discussed further in this chapter.

**TABLE 81.2 Paraneoplastic Anti-neuronal Antibodies, Associated Syndromes, and Cancers***

| Antibody | Syndrome | Associated Cancers |
|---|---|---|
| Anti-Hu (ANNA1) | Focal encephalitis, PEM, PCD, PSN, autonomic dysfunction | SCLC, other |
| Anti-Yo (PCA1) | PCD | Gynecological, breast |
| Anti-Ri (ANNA2) | PCD, opsoclonus-myoclonus | Breast, gynecological, SCLC |
| Anti-Tr | PCD | Hodgkin lymphoma |
| Anti-CV2/CRMP5 | PEM, PCD, peripheral neuropathy chorea, uveitis | SCLC, other |
| Anti-Ma proteins† | Limbic, diencephalic, brainstem encephalitis, PCD | Germ cell tumors of testis, other solid tumors |
| Anti-VGCC‡ | LEMS, PCD | SCLC |
| Anti-AChR‡ | MG | Thymoma |
| Anti-amphiphysin | Stiff-person syndrome, PEM | Breast |
| Anti-recoverin or against other retinal proteins | Retinopathy | SCLC |
| Anti-bipolar cells of the retina | Retinopathy | Melanoma |

*Does not include antibodies against extracellular neuronal antigens, which associate with the autoimmune encephalitis syndromes; these syndromes may occur with or without cancer and are not discussed in this chapter.
†Patients with antibodies to Ma2 are usually men with testicular cancer. Patients with additional antibodies to other Ma proteins are men or women with a variety of solid tumors.
‡These antibodies are markers for the neurological disorder and can occur in patients with or without cancer. These neurological disorders (MG, LEMS) frequently associate with specific cancers and cancer screenings are recommended in all patients with these diagnoses.
*AChR,* Acetylcholine receptor; *LEMS,* Lambert-Eaton myasthenic syndrome; *MG,* myasthenia gravis; *PCD,* paraneoplastic cerebellar degeneration; *PEM,* paraneoplastic encephalomyelitis; *PSN,* paraneoplastic sensory neuronopathy; *SCLC,* small-cell lung cancer; *VGCC,* voltage-gated calcium channels.

Sundermann et al., 2017). Although almost any type of neoplasm can cause PNS, the tumors more frequently involved are small-cell lung cancer (SCLC); cancers of the breast and ovary; thymoma, neuroblastoma, and plasma cell tumors. The development of PNS frequently heralds tumor recurrence in patients with a history of cancer or those who have recently gone into tumor remission.

The diagnosis of PNS is more difficult in patients who develop less characteristic symptoms (e.g., brainstem dysfunction, myelopathy), especially if no antibodies are found in the serum or CSF. Most PNSs have an acute or subacute onset compared with noninflammatory neurodegenerative disorders that are chronically progressive. If the patient is known to have cancer, the possibility of metastases and nonmetastatic neurological complications of cancer (side effects of treatment, metabolic encephalopathy, infection, or cerebrovascular disorders resulting from coagulopathy) should be considered before the diagnosis of PNS. Novel immunotherapeutic treatment strategies such as chimeric antigen receptor (CAR) T cells and immune checkpoint inhibitors can produce a wide variety of immune-related neurological complications, including CAR T-cell–related encephalopathy caused by cytokine-release syndrome (Neelapu et al., 2018), or immune-related adverse events caused by immune checkpoint blockade. In fact, there is evidence that immune checkpoint blockade can favor the development of PNS, which may be associated with classic paraneoplastic neuronal antibodies targeting intracellular antigens or antibodies against neuronal cell surface antigens (Graus and Dalmau, 2019).

Neuroimaging, in particular magnetic resonance imaging (MRI), helps to exclude some of these complications. Brain FDG-PET in the early stages of some PNS of the CNS may show hypermetabolism in the involved regions even when MRI is normal, and may be indicative of early inflammatory changes (Basu and Alavi, 2008; Ances et al., 2005). The CSF profile in patients with PNS of the CNS often suggests an inflammatory process: pleocytosis, increased protein concentration, intrathecal synthesis of immunoglobulin (Ig)G, and oligoclonal bands (Psimaras et al., 2010).

## SPECIFIC PARANEOPLASTIC NEUROLOGICAL SYNDROMES AND THEIR TREATMENT

### Paraneoplastic Cerebellar Degeneration

Paraneoplastic cerebellar degeneration (PCD) is characterized by the rapid development of severe pancerebellar dysfunction, including truncal and appendicular ataxia, dysarthria, and downbeat nystagmus. Frequently the symptoms of cerebellar dysfunction are preceded by dizziness and vertigo, suggesting peripheral vestibular dysfunction. In adults, the subacute onset of PCD differentiates it from chronic degenerative diseases of the cerebellum. A subset of patients with SCLC develops PCD associated with Lambert-Eaton myasthenic syndrome (LEMS), often before the tumor is diagnosed (Mason et al., 1997). In some cases LEMS may be overlooked unless it occurs prior to the onset of PCD. The tumors more frequently associated with PCD are SCLC, breast and ovarian tumors, and Hodgkin lymphoma (Shams'ili et al., 2003). Anti-Yo (PCA1) is the most frequent antibody found in PCD and is usually associated with breast or gynecological tumors (Peterson et al., 1992). Anti-Yo antibodies have been identified in a few male patients with PCD and cancer of the salivary gland, lung, and esophagus. Some patients with predominant truncal ataxia, opsoclonus, and other ocular movement abnormalities may harbor an antibody called anti-Ri. In such cases, the tumor is usually a breast carcinoma or, less frequently, gynecological cancer, bladder cancer, or SCLC (Luque et al., 1991). These patients may also develop dementia, peripheral neuropathy, axial rigidity, myoclonus, brainstem encephalitis, and laryngeal spasms (Pittock et al., 2010).

In patients with SCLC the development of PCD may be the presenting symptom of paraneoplastic encephalomyelitis (PEM) in which case other areas of the nervous system become involved and anti-Hu or anti-CV2/CRMP5 antibodies are usually identified (Fig. 81.1). Patients with symptoms restricted to cerebellar dysfunction and negative anti-Hu antibodies often harbor voltage-gated calcium channel (VGCC) antibodies (Graus et al., 2002). Patients with PCD associated with Hodgkin disease develop Tr antibodies (Graus et al., 1997); these antibodies are directed against Delta/Notch-like epidermal growth factor-related receptor (DNER). The neurological disorder may develop before or after the diagnosis of the lymphoma, sometimes heralding tumor recurrence. Sox1 antibodies are found in about 50% of patients with PCD and SCLC but are not found when PCD is associated with other cancers (Sabater et al., 2013).

Antibodies reported in isolated cases or small series of patients with acute to subacute onset ataxia and cancer have been shown to target protein kinase Cγ (PKCγ), carbonic anhydrase related protein 8 (CARPVIII), or tripartite motif-containing (TRIM) protein 9 or TRIM protein 67 (Bataller et al., 2004; Do et al., 2019; Hoftberger et al., 2013). These antibodies should be considered in patients for whom there is a strong suspicion of PCD and who do not have any of the more common PNS-associated antibodies.

Several single case reports describe patients with PCD who improved after treatment of the tumor, plasma exchange, intravenous immunoglobulin (IVIG), rituximab, or immunosuppression with cyclophosphamide or corticosteroids (Blaes et al., 1999; Shams'ili et al., 2006). However, due to early, irreversible neuronal loss most patients with PCD do not improve with any of these treatments (Vedeler et al., 2006) (see Fig. 81.1).

### Paraneoplastic Encephalomyelitis

Patients with PEM develop features of dysfunction at different levels of the neuraxis (Dalmau et al., 1992; Graus et al., 2001; Sillevis et al., 2002). Many patients will develop a sensory neuronopathy (see paraneoplastic sensory neuronopathy [PSN]) and cerebellar dysfunction:

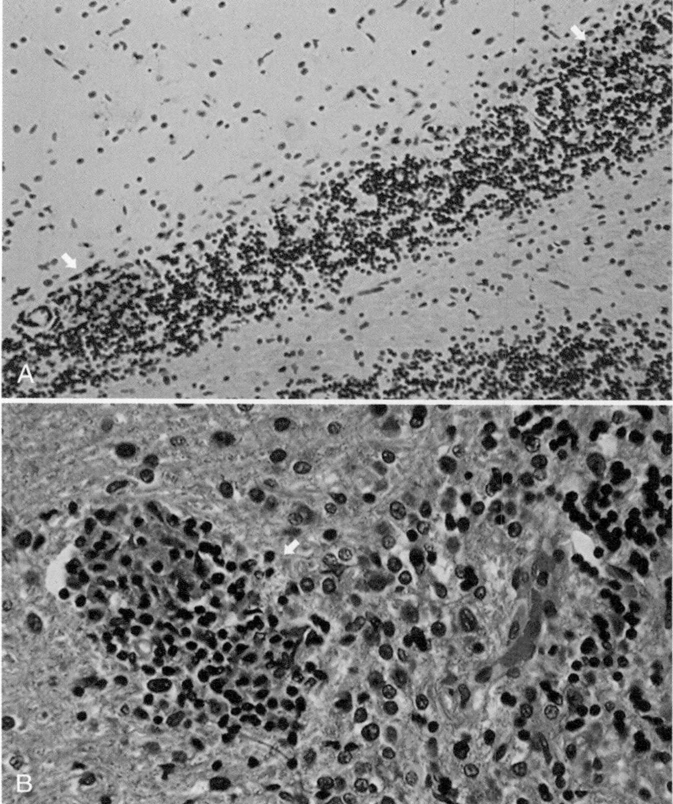


**Fig. 81.1** A, Extensive loss of Purkinje cells in a patient with a subacute cerebellar syndrome in the context of encephalomyelitis and anti-Hu antibodies. The *arrows* showing clusters of CD3 T cells in Purkinje cell layer. **B,** A higher magnification of the Purkinje cell layer shows a neuronophagic nodule of T lymphocytes that are probably destroying a Purkinje cell. A: (A, ×100, immunostained for CD3 and counterstained with haematoxylin B: × 400 haematoxylin-eosin. (*Reprinted with permission from* Dalmau et al., 2008.)

gait ataxia, in particular. Limbic and/or brainstem encephalopathy (see limbic and brainstem encephalitis) occur in up to one-third of patients with PEM. Lower motor neuron involvement secondary to myelitis occurs in approximately 20%; the presence of symptoms affecting other areas of the neuraxis and MRI findings help to rule out pure motor neuron disorders (Flanagan et al., 2011). Approximately one-fourth of patients with PEM develop autonomic nervous system dysfunction, including postural hypotension, gastroparesis and intestinal dysmotility, sweating abnormalities, neurogenic bladder, and erectile dysfunction. Cardiac dysrhythmias or respiratory failure are frequent causes of death.

PEM, with or without PSN, can be associated with almost any tumor, but in the majority of patients the underlying tumor is lung carcinoma, particularly SCLC (Graus et al., 2001). Patients with PEM/PSN and SCLC often have anti-Hu antibodies, and at a much lower frequency, anti-CV2/CRMP5 antibodies, or both. CV2/CRMP5 antibodies occur more frequently in the context of PEM with chorea, uveitis, or peripheral neuropathy that is different from PSN (Dubey et al., 2018; Vernino et al., 2002). Anti-CV2/CRMP5 antibodies are also associated with thymoma and other cancers (Benyahia et al., 1999).

In general, PEM is poorly responsive to treatment, although there are reports showing symptom stabilization or improvement with prompt treatment of the tumor and immunotherapy (Sillevis et al., 2002; Vernino et al., 2004).

## Limbic and Brainstem Encephalitis

Patients with limbic encephalitis have memory deficits with relative preservation of other cognitive functions. The memory deficits may be masked by concurrent confusion, depression, agitation, and anxiety. Complex partial seizures are also common. Brainstem encephalitis is characterized by oscillopsia, diplopia, dysarthria, dysphagia, gaze abnormalities, and sometimes subacute hearing loss.

Limbic encephalitis is one of the few PNSs in which neuroimaging can suggest the diagnosis. Typical MRI findings include unilateral or bilateral mesial temporal lobe abnormalities best seen on T2-weighted and fluid-attenuated inversion recovery (FLAIR) images (Gultekin et al., 2000; Ances et al., 2005). The temporal-limbic regions may be hypointense on T1-weighted sequences and rarely enhance with contrast.

Limbic and brainstem encephalitis occur in both paraneoplastic and non-paraneoplastic settings. The cancers most commonly associated are SCLC, testicular germ-cell tumors, teratoma (usually of the ovary), thymoma, and Hodgkin lymphoma (Gultekin et al., 2000).

The immune responses in limbic and brainstem encephalitis are classified according to the location of the target antigen; intracellular or on the neuronal cell surface. The main intracellular antigens are Hu, Ma2, and less commonly CV2/CRMP5. In patients with Hu antibodies, limbic encephalitis usually develops as part of a more widespread disorder such as PEM (Dalmau et al., 1992). Most of these patients have SCLC (Alamowitch et al., 1997).

Men younger than 45 years of age with symptoms of limbic, hypothalamic, and brainstem dysfunction are likely to have antibodies against Ma proteins and an underlying germ cell tumor of the testis (Dalmau et al., 1999). Ma antibodies are also encountered in older patients with similar neurological symptoms and other cancers (Dalmau et al., 2004). In contrast to patients with Hu antibodies, in whom the lower brainstem is predominantly affected and symptoms progress in an upward direction, patients with Ma antibodies often present with an upper brainstem syndrome with vertical gaze palsy or hypokinesis, and symptoms progress in a downward direction (Saiz et al., 2009).

Limbic or brainstem encephalitis associated with CV2/CRMP5 antibodies usually form part of a syndrome that may include cerebellar ataxia, chorea, uveitis, optic neuritis, or sensorimotor neuropathy (Honnorat et al., 1997). CV2/CRMP5 antibodies can co-occur with Hu antibodies, in which case patients almost always have multifocal deficits or PEM.

Limbic encephalitis is a frequent manifestation of autoimmune encephalitis syndromes that are associated with antibodies to neuronal cell surface or synaptic proteins such as AMPA or GABAb receptors, LGI1 and Caspr2 proteins. These disorders are discussed further in the chapter on autoimmune encephalopathies with antibodies to cell surface antigens.

In general, limbic and brainstem encephalitis associated with antibodies targeting intracellular antigens show limited response to treatment of the tumor or immunotherapy. About one-third of patients with syndromes associated with antibodies against Ma proteins show neurological improvement after treatment of the tumor (usually a testicular germ-cell neoplasm) and immunotherapy (Dalmau et al., 2004).

## Paraneoplastic Opsoclonus-Myoclonus

Opsoclonus-myoclonus consists of spontaneous, arrhythmic, large-amplitude conjugate saccades occurring in all directions of gaze that are associated with myoclonus of the head, trunk, or extremities. In children, paraneoplastic opsoclonus-myoclonus usually has a subacute onset with staggering and falling, suggesting the diagnosis of acute cerebellitis; these symptoms are followed by body jerks, drooling, refusal to walk or sit, ataxia, opsoclonus, hypotonia, irritability, and sleep disturbances (Russo et al., 1997; Tate et al., 2005). In adults, symptoms range from opsoclonus with mild truncal ataxia to a more severe syndrome characterized by opsoclonus, myoclonus, ataxia, and encephalopathy that can lead to stupor and death (Bataller et al., 2001).

In children, opsoclonus-myoclonus is usually a manifestation of neuroblastoma, although similar neurological symptoms may result from viral infections. The neurological symptoms precede the tumor diagnosis in 50% of patients. Children with neuroblastoma and opsoclonus have a better tumor prognosis than those without opsoclonus (Tate et al., 2005). In adults several underlying tumors have been reported, but the most common are SCLC and cancers of the breast and ovary.

Studies have shown the presence of autoimmune responses against a variety of neuronal antigens but no clinically relevant opsoclonus-specific antibodies have been identified (Bataller et al., 2003; Armangue et al., 2016). Patients with breast and gynecological cancers usually harbor anti-Ri (ANNA2) antibodies (Luque et al., 1991). These patients often have additional brainstem and cerebellar dysfunction. Some adult patients, in particular those with SCLC, have anti-Hu or glycine receptor antibodies while 5% of children with neuroblastoma have anti-Hu antibodies (Armangue et al., 2016; Dalmau et al., 1995).

In children, the ocular and motor symptoms may resolve spontaneously or after immunotherapy and treatment of the tumor, if applicable (Bell et al., 2008; Pranzatelli et al., 2018). However, most children are left with cognitive and behavioral abnormalities and language and psychomotor deficits (Catsman-Berrevoets et al., 2009). Sleep disturbance may respond to trazodone (Pranzatelli et al., 2005). Paraneoplastic opsoclonus-myoclonus in adults may respond to immunosuppression and IVIG; spontaneous remissions rarely occur. Patients whose tumors are treated promptly have a better neurological outcome than those whose tumors are not treated (Bataller et al., 2001). In the latter group, the disorder often progresses to severe encephalopathy and death.

## Stiff-Person Spectrum Disorders

These disorders share core features of muscle stiffness, spasms, and heightened stimulus sensitivity, but have distinct phenotypes. Stiff-person spectrum disorders (SPSDs) include stiff-person syndrome (SPS), progressive encephalomyelitis with rigidity and myoclonus (PERM), and stiff-limb syndrome (SLS). In some patients SPS or SLS can also overlap with other syndromes such as ataxia, epilepsy, or encephalitis (Malter et al., 2010; Saiz et al., 2008). In a series of 121 patients with SPSD, the median age was 51 years with a female predominance (62% of the cases) (Martinez-Hernandez et al., 2016).

SPS is characterized by stiffness and rigidity of the axial musculature with superimposed spasms. Muscle stiffness primarily affects the lower trunk and legs, but it can extend to the arms, shoulders, and neck. Muscle spasms are usually precipitated by emotional upset and auditory or somesthetic stimuli. Electrophysiological studies show continuous activity of motor units innervating the stiffened muscles that improves after treatment with diazepam. The rigidity disappears during sleep and after local or general anesthesia (Espay and Chen, 2006). In SLS one or more limbs are affected with distal rigidity and abnormal posturing of the hands or feet (Saiz et al., 1998) whereas PERM can also associate with cerebellar, brainstem, or autonomic dysfunction (Meinck and Thompson, 2002).

Multiple auto-antigenic targets have been described. The most common are glutamic acid decarboxylase (GAD) and the α-subunit of the glycine receptor (αGlyR). About one-third of patients are seronegative or rarely have other antibodies (e.g., amphiphysin, GABAaR,

DPPX) (Martinez-Hernandez et al., 2016). Antibodies to GAD are more frequent in patients with SPS or with overlapping syndromes, while antibodies to αGlyR are more often associated with PERM (Carvajal-Gonzalez et al., 2014). The type of antibody and severity of symptoms—but not the syndrome—appear to correlate with outcome; αGlyR antibodies associate with better outcome compared with GAD antibodies or being seronegative, the latter 2 groups having similar outcomes (Martinez-Hernandez et al., 2016).

The majority of SPSDs are not paraneoplastic except for those associated with amphiphysin antibodies, which usually occur with breast cancer (Pittock et al., 2005); for αGlyR antibodies the frequency of an underlying malignancy is about 10%–20% (Carvajal-Gonzalez et al., 2014). Patients with SPSD or αGlyR antibodies are more responsive to immunotherapy than those who do not harbor antibodies or who have antibodies against GAD or amphiphysin (Martinez-Hernandez et al., 2016).

Treatment of the tumor, corticosteroids, and IVIG may improve paraneoplastic SPS; the usefulness of IVIG has been demonstrated in patients with non-paraneoplastic SPS (Dalakas et al., 2001). GABA-enhancing agents, such as benzodiazepines, gabapentin, or baclofen among others, provide symptomatic relief.

## Paraneoplastic Sensory Neuronopathy

PSN is characterized by progressive sensory loss that may involve limbs, trunk, and face, and sometimes sensorineural hearing loss. Painful dysesthesias are common. At onset, symptoms are usually asymmetrical and can be confused with radiculopathy or polyneuropathy. All modalities of sensation are eventually affected, and, with progression, the sensory deficits result in sensory ataxia, gait difficulty, and pseudoathetoid movements. In the majority of cases the clinical picture progresses rapidly over a few weeks, although about 10% of cases have a chronic, less severe course (Graus et al., 1994). PSN may develop alone or more commonly in association with PEM (Dalmau et al., 1992; Graus et al., 2001). Neurological dysfunction precedes the cancer diagnosis in two-thirds of patients. Typically, nerve conduction studies show small-amplitude or absent sensory nerve action potentials (SNAPs), although motor nerve and F-wave studies are usually normal. These findings are consistent with the pathological involvement of the neurons of the dorsal root ganglia, but some patients also have electrophysiological evidence of axonal and demyelinating neuropathy (Camdessanche et al., 2002; Oh et al., 2005). The CSF often shows an increased protein level with pleocytosis, oligoclonal bands, and intrathecal synthesis of IgG. For patients with no known cancer, PSN should be suspected when sensory symptoms develop subacutely and asymmetrically, and involve the trunk and cranial nerves, particularly if the patient is a smoker. One study comparing the clinical features of sensory neuronopathies due to a variety of causes found that paraneoplastic cases more often had subacute onset, were older (> 60 years) men, and there was early pain and frequent involvement of the arms (Camdessanche et al., 2012).

Approximately 80% of patients with PSN have cancer of the lung, usually SCLC, but virtually any type of neoplasm may be found. The anti-Hu antibody is almost always detected in the serum of patients with PSN and SCLC but is rarely present in PSN associated with other tumors (Molinuevo JL et al., 1998; Honnorat et al., 2009). A few patients with PSN have been reported with antibodies to amphiphysin or CV2/CRMP5 (Saiz et al., 1999; Antoine et al., 2001). Patients with CV2/CRMP5 antibodies often have motor involvement and evidence of axonal and demyelinating features on electrophysiological studies (Antoine et al., 2001); in these patients the symptom presentation can also be asymmetrical and associated with pain (Dubey et al., 2018).

Studies of patients with SCLC and anti-Hu-associated PSN and PEM indicate that neurological symptoms in patients whose tumors completely responded to therapy were more likely to stabilize or improve, as compared with those with untreated tumors or tumors that did not respond to therapy (Graus et al., 2001; Sillevis et al., 2002). In some patients, prompt treatment with corticosteroids may partially improve sensory deficits. The effects of IVIG, cyclophosphamide, or rituximab are uncertain although there are case reports of responses (Shams'ili et al., 2006; Giometto et al., 2012).

## Vasculitis of the Nerve

Vasculitis of the nerve usually occurs in older men. It can present as a painful symmetric or asymmetric, subacute, sensorimotor polyneuropathy (Oh, 1997). Electrophysiological findings are compatible with multifocal neuropathy or diffuse axonal sensorimotor neuropathy (Zivkovic et al., 2007). The erythrocyte sedimentation rate and the CSF protein concentration are elevated. Nerve and muscle histology shows intramural and perivascular inflammatory infiltrates composed of $CD8^+$ T cells (Vincent et al., 2007). The most common tumor association is with SCLC. Less frequently found are lymphoma, cancer of the colon, kidney, bile duct, stomach, and prostate (Oh, 1997). The disorder has no specific serological markers of paraneoplasia, although patients with SCLC may have anti-Hu antibodies. The vasculitis often responds to treatment with steroids, cyclophosphamide, or both (Oh, 1997).

## Subacute and Chronic Peripheral Neuropathies

A mild peripheral neuropathy is common in patients with cancer, especially in the advanced stages of the disease. The cause is multifactorial and includes metabolic and nutritional deficits and toxicity from chemotherapy. Paraneoplastic sensorimotor neuropathy may develop before or after the diagnosis of cancer. The onset may be subacute or acute, with symmetric, distal paresthesias, occasionally associated with pain. The course is usually progressive. with late development of weakness. A relapsing and remitting course suggests chronic inflammatory demyelinating polyneuropathy (CIDP) (Antoine et al., 1999). The tumors most commonly associated are lung and breast cancers; anti-neuronal antibodies are usually absent, but some patients with lung cancer or thymoma harbor CV2/CRMP5 antibodies (Antoine et al., 2001). Patients with electrophysiological signs of demyelination may improve with steroids or IVIG (Antoine et al., 1999).

The use of immune checkpoint inhibitors may result in several types of immune-related adverse effects, including acute or subacute inflammatory neuropathies, and Guillain-Barré syndrome (GBS); differentiation from paraneoplastic syndromes can be challenging (Graus and Dalmau, 2019.)

## Peripheral Neuropathy Associated with Plasma Cell Dyscrasias and B-Cell Lymphoma

Several malignancies of plasma cells and lymphocytes are associated with neuropathy and include multiple myeloma, Waldenström macroglobulinemia, POEMS syndrome, Castleman disease, and B-cell lymphoma. A sensorimotor neuropathy may develop in patients with multiple myeloma that is similar to those seen in other advanced cancers. If the myeloma is complicated by amyloidosis, the neuropathic symptoms often include autonomic dysfunction and lancinating and burning dysesthesias. In both cases, treatment of the myeloma does not affect the neurological symptoms.

Patients with Waldenström macroglobulinemia can develop a symmetrical, demyelinating, sensorimotor neuropathy predominantly involving large sensory fibers, especially those for vibration sense, often resulting in gait disturbance. Patients whose IgM paraprotein reacts with myelin-associated glycoprotein tend to have sensorimotor axonal loss and demyelination while patients with IgM targeting sulfatide have sensory axonal loss (Levine et al., 2006). The neuropathy may respond to treatment directed at the Waldenström macroglobulinemia including plasma exchange, IVIG, rituximab, chlorambucil, cyclophosphamide, or fludarabine (Latov, 2000; Weide et al., 2000).

POEMS syndrome stands for *p*olyneuropathy, *o*rganomegaly, *e*ndocrinopathy, *M* protein, and *s*kin changes. This syndrome may result from sclerotic myeloma or Castleman disease, among others. While not all features must be present for the diagnosis to be made, peripheral neuropathy is one of the mandatory criteria for a POEMS diagnosis (Dispenzieri, 2012). The neuropathy is typically a subacute or chronic demyelinating, symmetric, ascending sensorimotor neuropathy. This presentation and the fact that there can be CSF albumin-cytologic dissociation often leads to an initial diagnosis of CIDP (Isose et al., 2011). A series comparing patients with POEMS and CIDP showed that patients with POEMS were significantly more likely to have muscle atrophy, distal muscle weakness, and severe leg pain (Nasu et al., 2012). Electrophysiological studies demonstrate that the neuropathy of POEMS has more marked features of axonal loss with greater reductions in compound muscle action potential (CMAP) and SNAP amplitudes, compared to CIDP, among other differentiating features (Mauermann et al., 2012).

Treatment of the plasma cell dyscrasia can result in improvement of the neuropathy and includes high-dose alkylator chemotherapy with peripheral blood stem cell transplant or low-dose alkylator chemotherapy with corticosteroids (Dispenzieri, 2014). The use of gabapentin, pregabalin, amitriptyline, and related medications may help if the neuropathy is associated with pain (Dispenzieri, 2012).

Castleman disease (also called angiofollicular lymph node hyperplasia) is a lymphoproliferative disorder that can present with unicentric or multicentric disease. About one-third of patients with multicentric Castleman disease also fulfill criteria for POEMS syndrome (Dispenzieri et al., 2012). However, compared with POEMS, the neuropathy in Castleman disease tends to be less severe and mostly sensory (Naddaf et al., 2016). Treatment is aimed at the underlying lymphoproliferative disorder and may include resection or radiation for unicentric disease and immunotherapy with or without corticosteroids for multicentric disease (Mitsos et al., 2018; van Rhee et al., 2018).

An acute to subacute paraneoplastic polyradiculoneuropathy clinically identical to GBS appears to occur at a higher frequency in patients with cancer (Vigliani et al., 2004). The neoplasm most commonly implicated is Hodgkin lymphoma but other cancers including solid tumors have been reported. In some patients, GBS may be the first manifestation of tumor recurrence. Treatment is the same as for the noncancer-related form and consists of plasma exchange and IVIG. There is some evidence suggesting that patients with cancer-associated GBS have worse neurological outcome compared to patients with GBS without cancer (Vigliani et al., 2004). In a patient with cancer the differential diagnosis of GBS should include leptomeningeal carcinomatosis or neurolymphomatosis. These cases tend to have asymmetric involvement, are often associated with pain, and do not evolve acutely. The use of immune checkpoint inhibitors may also lead to adverse effects resembling GBS. These adverse effects often respond to immunotherapy and discontinuation of the immune checkpoint inhibitor (Graus and Dalmau, 2019).

## Lambert-Eaton Myasthenic Syndrome

The onset of LEMS symptoms is usually progressive over weeks or months. In most patients the symptoms develop before the tumor diagnosis has been made. Clinical features include fatigue, proximal muscle weakness, and paresthesias with involvement of the legs as the most common initial symptom (Wirtz et al., 2002). Over time the weakness spreads proximally to distally (Titulaer et al., 2011a). Almost 80% of patients have autonomic dysfunction that includes dry mouth, erectile dysfunction, and blurry vision. Cranial nerve dysfunction may produce diplopia, ptosis, or dysphagia. Neurological examination shows proximal weakness, occurring in the legs more than the arms, and absent or depressed tendon reflexes, which may potentiate after a brief muscle contraction. Strength may improve after brief exercise, but continued exercise increases weakness. The diagnosis is based on electrophysiological studies. Nerve conduction studies show small-amplitude CMAPs. At slow rates of repetitive nerve stimulation (2–5 Hz), a decremental response of greater than 10% is obtained. At fast rates of repetitive nerve stimulation (20 Hz or greater) or after maximal voluntary muscle contraction, facilitation occurs and an incremental response of at least 100% is seen. LEMS can develop in association with other paraneoplastic syndromes such as PCD and PEM (Mason et al., 1997). Recurrence of LEMS after remission often heralds tumor recurrence.

Approximately 60% of patients with LEMS have an underlying neoplasm, usually SCLC or rarely other tumors such as lymphoma. The non-paraneoplastic cases often have slower symptom presentation and associate with other autoimmune conditions such as thyroiditis and insulin-dependent diabetes mellitus, among others (Wirtz et al., 2002). The presence of LEMS in a patient with SCLC is associated with improved tumor survival (Maddison et al., 1999). The Dutch-English LEMS Tumor Association Prediction (DELTA-P) score can be used to predict patients with a high risk of an associated SCLC (Titulaer et al., 2011b). Aggressive tumor screening should be carried out as soon as the LEMS diagnosis is confirmed. In one study, 91% of SCLCs were detected within 3 months of LEMS onset and 96% within 1 year (Titulaer et al., 2008).

The majority of patients with LEMS have serum antibodies against P/Q type VGCCs (Motomura et al., 1997). The antibodies interfere with the quantal release of acetylcholine at the presynaptic neuromuscular junction, resulting in failure of neuromuscular transmission. Antibodies to P/Q type VGCCs also occur in a subset of patients with SCLC and paraneoplastic PCD (with or without LEMS). There is a mouse model showing that cisternal injection of these antibodies produces cerebellar dysfunction (Martin-Garcia et al., 2013). When LEMS develops in association with PEM, patients often have anti-Hu antibodies. Detection of Sox1 antibodies in patients with LEMS predicts the presence of SCLC and may be used to follow those LEMS patients with no evidence of cancer at the initial evaluation (Sabater et al., 2008). In about 10% of patients with LEMS no autoantibodies are detected. The clinical phenotype and electrophysiological features of seronegative patients are similar to the seropositive cases except for a lower incidence of SCLC (Nakao et al., 2002).

Most patients with cancer improve neurologically with combined treatment of their cancer and therapy for LEMS. The latter includes medication to increase the release of acetylcholine (3,4-diaminopyridine). and immunomodulation, resulting in improvement of muscle strength and mean resting CMAP amplitude in most patients. The use of 3,4-diaminopyridine results in moderate to marked neurological improvement in 80% of patients (Keogh et al., 2011; McEvoy et al., 1989). Plasma exchange and IVIG are useful for treating severe weakness; strength improves within days or weeks, but the benefits are transient (Bain PG et al., 1996). Long-term immunosuppression with prednisone or azathioprine should be considered if symptoms continue despite the use of 3,4-diaminopyridine. Several reports have demonstrated responses to rituximab in patients who did not respond to other treatments (Maddison et al., 2011).

## Myasthenia Gravis

Myasthenia gravis (MG) is a postsynaptic disorder of neuromuscular transmission. The main features are weakness and fatigability of skeletal muscles that improves with rest and worsens with activity (Gilhus, 2016). Ptosis and diplopia occur in most patients, and symptoms remain localized to the extraocular and eyelid muscles in 15% of patients. In the rest, weakness becomes generalized and can impair respiration to the extent that mechanical ventilation is necessary. Tendon reflexes and sensation are normal.

A thymic epithelial tumor (thymoma or thymic carcinoma) is found in 10% of patients with MG, and one-third of patients with thymoma develop MG. In a few instances, MG has been reported in association with other tumors, including thyroid gland tumors, SCLC, breast cancer, and lymphoma.

Antibodies to AChR are found in 80%–90% of patients with generalized MG, and in 50% of those with ocular MG. A small percent of AChR-negative patients have antibodies to muscle-specific tyrosine kinase (MusK). Compared to patients with AChR antibodies, those with MusK antibodies have more prominent facial and bulbar involvement and more severe muscle weakness (Gilhus, 2016). Antibodies to lipoprotein receptor-related protein 4 (LRP4) are found in 1%–3% of all patients; the presence of these antibodies associates with mild to moderate symptoms. Thymoma-related MG almost invariably associates with AChR antibodies, but not anti-MusK or LRP4 antibodies. Patients with thymoma often have additional antibodies against skeletal muscle proteins such as titin and ryanodine (Romi et al., 2005).

Treatment strategies for MG include symptomatic treatment (e.g., acetylcholinesterase inhibitors) immunomodulation (e.g., plasma exchange, IVIG), immunosuppression (e.g., steroids, azathioprine, methotrexate, and others) and treatment of the tumor if found (Skeie et al., 2010).

## Dermatomyositis

Dermatomyositis and polymyositis are immune-mediated inflammatory diseases of muscle. An association exists between cancer and dermatomyositis in adults (Yang et al., 2015), but an association with malignancy is less clear for polymyositis, with cohort studies reporting conflicting results (Chen et al., 2010; Antiochos et al., 2009). The symptoms of paraneoplastic dermatomyositis are the same as those in patients without cancer. The typical neurological presentation is the subacute onset of proximal muscle weakness. Neck flexors and pharyngeal and respiratory muscles are commonly involved and may lead to dysphagia and aspiration. Facial weakness and dysarthria can occur but are uncommon. Cutaneous changes include periorbital purplish discoloration (heliotrope rash), edema and erythematous lesions over the knuckles (Gottron papules), and an erythematous macular rash on the face, neck and chest, shoulders and upper back. Tendon reflexes and sensation are normal. Serum creatine kinase concentrations are often elevated, although normal levels are occasionally found, even in patients with profound muscle weakness. Electromyography (EMG) shows increased spontaneous activity (fibrillations, positive sharp waves, and complex repetitive discharges), and short-duration, low-amplitude polyphasic motor unit action potentials on voluntary activation. Muscle histology shows inflammatory infiltrates ($CD4^+$ T cells predominate in dermatomyositis and $CD8^+$ T cells in polymyositis) and muscle necrosis; the presence of perifascicular atrophy is characteristic of dermatomyositis, but is only found in about half of patients (Dalakas, 2002).

About 10%–15% of adults with dermatomyositis develop a malignancy, usually within 2–3 years of presentation (Yang et al., 2015). Juvenile-onset dermatomyositis is not cancer-associated. Many histological types of cancers have been reported in association with dermatomyositis. The most common are hematological and lymphatic cancers (e.g., lymphoma, leukemia, multiple myeloma) followed by breast, lung, ovarian, and gastrointestinal malignancies. Risk factors for malignancy include older age, male gender, necrotic skin ulcerations, and rapid onset of symptoms.

About 60%–70% of patients have a dermatomyositis-specific antibody. These include antibodies to Mi-2, melanoma differentiation-associated protein 5 (MDA5), transcriptional intermediary factor 1 (TIF1), and nuclear matrix protein 2 (NXP-2). The presence of antibodies to TIF1 or NXP-2, are predictive of an increased risk of malignancy (Fiorentino et al., 2013; Trallero-Araguas et al., 2012).

In some patients, muscle and dermatological symptoms improve coincidently with treatment of the tumor. No studies are available on the efficacy of immunosuppressants in cancer-associated dermatomyositis, but it seems reasonable to use strategies similar to those used in non-paraneoplastic dermatomyositis (corticosteroids, methotrexate, azathioprine, mycophenolate mofetil, IVIG) (McGrath et al., 2018). Rituximab has been considered effective in some patients but its efficacy in general remains unclear (Nalotto et al., 2013).

## Necrotizing Autoimmune Myopathy

This disorder is characterized by the acute to subacute onset of severe, progressive, and symmetric proximal muscle weakness (Allenbach et al., 2013). Neck weakness, dysphagia, and dyspnea are common. Serum creatine kinase concentrations are markedly elevated and electrophysiological studies demonstrate myopathic findings. Muscle histology shows severe necrotic changes and fiber regeneration with minimal or no inflammatory infiltrates. The disorder can be paraneoplastic and also occurs in association with connective tissue disease, exposure to statin medication, and after treatment with immune checkpoint inhibitors.

Antibodies associated with the disorder include anti-3-hydroxy-3-methylglutaryl-coenzyme A reductase (HMGCR) and anti-signal recognition particle (SRP). Compared to patients with HMGCR antibodies or seronegative cases, patients with SRP antibodies have a more severe and refractory disease course. Necrotizing autoimmune myopathy has been reported in association with a variety of solid tumors including carcinomas of the gastrointestinal tract, lung, and ovary (Kassardjian et al., 2015). Cancer occurs more often in patients with HMGCR antibodies and seronegative cases compared with patients with SRP antibodies (Allenbach et al., 2016).

No large clinical trials are available to direct treatment strategies. Recent recommendations include the upfront use of corticosteroids and methotrexate (Allenbach et al., 2018). Other agents such as azathioprine, mycophenolate, tacrolimus, cyclosporine, or cyclophosphamide can substitute for methotrexate, with no data supporting increased benefit of one over the other (Kassardjian et al., 2015). Relapses can occur, often when immunotherapy is tapered or discontinued (Kassardjian et al., 2015). For paraneoplastic cases, tumor treatment is important. Statin-induced necrotizing myopathy may be responsive to IVIG; the efficacy of IVIG in idiopathic or paraneoplastic forms has not been clarified.

## Paraneoplastic Visual Syndromes

Paraneoplastic involvement of the visual system may affect the retina, and less frequently, the uvea and optic nerves (Thirkill, 2005; Ko et al., 2008). Because paraneoplastic visual syndromes are rare, the more important considerations are metastatic infiltration of the optic nerves, toxic effects of chemotherapy or radiation therapy, and severe anemia. The symptoms of cancer-associated retinopathy (CAR) are photosensitivity, progressive loss of visual acuity and color perception, central or ring scotomas, and night blindness. Attenuation of photopic and scotopic responses is recorded on the electroretinogram

(ERG). Funduscopic examination is frequently normal, or may show nonspecific optic disc pallor and arteriolar narrowing. When one eye is affected, the other becomes symptomatic within days or weeks. Imaging studies and evaluation of the CSF are not revealing.

Melanoma-associated retinopathy (MAR) affects patients with metastatic cutaneous melanoma (Boeck et al., 1997). Patients typically present with the acute onset of night blindness and shimmering, flickering, or pulsating photopsias. Symptoms often progress to complete visual loss. The ERG typically demonstrates reduction in the b-wave amplitude.

Paraneoplastic optic neuritis is very uncommon, and, although it may develop in isolation, it is usually associated with PEM. The onset is subacute with painless, bilateral visual loss. Papilledema may be present.

Bilateral diffuse uveal melanocytic proliferation is a rare syndrome that has largely been described in patients with advanced cancers who develop rapid and severe vision loss due to accumulation of uveal tract melanocytes leading to retinal detachment (Gass et al., 2003). Funduscopic examination is often initially normal but eventually shows multiple round or oval pigmented and nonpigmented patches. Fluorescein angiography reveals multifocal hyperfluorescence corresponding with these patches. The underlying mechanism of the melanocytic proliferation has not been elucidated.

SCLC is the tumor most commonly associated with CAR. Optic neuritis has been described with SCLC and non-SCLC, as well as with other solid tumors. Bilateral diffuse uveal melanocytic proliferation has most commonly been described with gynecological cancers in women and lung cancers in men.

In patients with CAR the antibody most frequently identified is against recoverin, a retinal-specific calcium-binding protein. However, an increasing number of retinal proteins have been found to be antigenic targets in both paraneoplastic and non-paraneoplastic retinopathy, including tubby-like protein 1 (TULP1), α-enolase, the photoreceptor-specific nuclear receptor, carbonic anhydrase, and arrestin, among others (Adamus et al., 2004). Anti-enolase antibodies predominantly associate with central cone abnormalities and may also occur without a cancer association (Adamus et al., 2004). Patients with MAR typically have antibodies that react with the bipolar cells of the retina. Anti-CV2/CRMP5 antibodies are reported in some patients with PEM, uveitis, and optic neuritis.

Although the paraneoplastic retinopathies rarely improve, responses to tumor treatment, corticosteroids, plasma exchange, IVIG and rituximab have been reported (Ferreyra et al., 2009; Or et al., 2013).

*The complete reference list is available online at https://expertconsult.inkling.com/.* 

# Autoimmune Encephalitis with Antibodies to Cell Surface Antigens

Myrna R. Rosenfeld, Josep Dalmau

## OUTLINE



Autoimmune encephalitis with antibodies to neuronal cell surface/synaptic antigens (further referred to as autoimmune encephalitis) are a group of neuropsychiatric disorders (Table 82.1) in which the antibodies produce neuronal dysfunction by direct interaction with their target antigen (Dalmau et al., 2017, 2018). These disorders can occur with and without a cancer association and while they affect individuals of all ages, some syndromes preferentially affect young adults and children (Armangue et al., 2012; Wells et al., 2018). The antibody effects are reversible and although the process of recovery can be prolonged, patients with autoimmune encephalitis often have full or substantial recovery after immunotherapy. Autoimmune encephalitis syndromes are therefore different from the classical paraneoplastic encephalitis that are always cancer associated and in which the associated antibodies target intracellular neuronal proteins but do not directly mediate the neuronal dysfunction. Rather in the classical paraneoplastic encephalitis, T-cell mechanisms appear to play a predominant role and the neuronal effects are often irreversible (Dalmau et al., 2017, 2018).

Patients with autoimmune encephalitis develop complex neuropsychiatric symptoms including memory loss, changes in behavior or cognition, psychosis, seizures, and movement disorders. At presentation one or a few of these symptoms may predominate and can mislead the diagnosis until additional symptoms develop over days or weeks. Patients may initially be diagnosed with idiopathic encephalitis, likely viral but with negative viral studies. Autoimmune encephalitis should be included in the differential diagnosis of any patient, especially if young, with a rapidly progressive encephalopathy of unclear origin. For some disorders such as anti-*N*-methyl-D-aspartate receptor (NMDAR) encephalitis, patients may initially be given a primary psychiatric diagnosis, and the accompanying signs and symptoms such as abnormal movements or fever erroneously ascribed to the use of antipsychotic medication (Kayser et al., 2013; Lejuste et al., 2016). Some patients with autoimmune encephalitis, especially those with NMDAR antibodies, experience a viral-like prodrome including lethargy, headache, upper respiratory symptoms, nausea, diarrhea, among others (Titulaer et al., 2013). In some but not all cases supporting findings such as inflammatory signs in cerebrospinal fluid (CSF) or the presence of oligoclonal bands can be useful. Abnormalities on magnetic resonance imaging (MRI) fluid-attenuated inversion recovery (FLAIR) sequences are more commonly seen in some syndromes than others, as discussed below. Any immunological type of autoimmune encephalitis can have a relapsing course and therefore the diagnosis of these disorders should be considered in a patient with a past history of encephalitis or relapsing encephalopathy.

The diagnosis of autoimmune encephalitis is confirmed by the presence of specific neuronal cell surface/synaptic antibodies in serum and CSF. While some laboratories state that evaluation of serum is sufficient, this is incorrect and CSF should always be included in the initial evaluation. A study of patients with anti-NMDAR encephalitis demonstrated that depending on how the testing was performed, up to 13% of CSF positive cases had no antibodies detectable in serum, and thus the diagnosis would have been missed (Gresa-Arribas et al., 2016). Institution of treatment should not be delayed until the results of antibody testing are available as this can negatively affect the outcome. Guidelines for the diagnosis of autoimmune encephalitis based on standard neurological assessment and routinely available laboratory testing are available (Graus et al., 2016). Based on the level of evidence, therapy should be initiated promptly and then adjusted when antibody results become available.

The immunological trigger of autoimmune encephalitis is varied and, in many cases, is yet to be established. In some patients, the presence of a systemic tumor that expresses the target neuronal/synaptic proteins appears to be important. About 25% of patients with herpes simplex viral encephalitis develop autoimmune encephalitis after recovery from the viral infection (Armangue et al., 2018). Specific human leukocyte antigen (HLA) associations have been reported for anti-LGI1 encephalitis, anti-CASPR2 encephalitis, and anti-IgLON5 disease (Sabater et al., 2016; van Sonderen et al., 2017). There are some patients in whom autoimmune encephalitis overlaps with demyelinating disorders (Titulaer et al., 2014); whether there is a relationship between the two syndromes is not yet clear.

TABLE 82.1 **Autoimmune Encephalitis with Antibodies to Cell Surface Antigens**

| Antigen Target | Syndrome | Other Associations | Responses to Immunotherapies |
|---|---|---|---|
| NMDA receptor | Psychiatric symptoms, seizures, memory deficits, decreased level of consciousness, dyskinesias, seizures, and autonomic disturbances | Predominantly affects young adults, teenagers, and children with an age-related association with ovarian teratoma | Almost 80% of cases have full or substantial recoveries. Improvement occurs slowly and can continue for over 18 months |
| $GABA_B$ receptor | Limbic encephalitis with prominent seizures | Median age 62 years. About 50% of the patients have an associated cancer (SCLC or other neuroendocrine tumor). Frequent coexisting autoimmunities | Patients can have full or partial recovery, but this is dependent on tumor control |
| AMPA receptor | Limbic encephalitis with prominent psychiatric symptoms | Predominantly affects middle-aged women; about 70% with an associated cancer (breast, thymus, lung) | About 70% improve with therapy, but neurological relapses without tumor recurrence are frequent and lead to cumulative disability |
| LGI1 | Limbic encephalitis. About 60% develop hyponatremia, and less often REM behavior disorder. About 30%–40% patients faciobrachial dystonic seizures that precede the limbic encephalitis. | Median age 60 years (men > women). Less than 10% have an underlying tumor (usually thymoma) | Almost 80% have recovery but are often left with residual memory or cognitive deficits |
| CASPR2 | Morvan syndrome, limbic encephalitis, neuropathic pain, peripheral nerve hyperexcitability | Frequent coexisting autoimmunities | About 70% have full or substantial recovery |
| $GABA_A$ receptor | Rapidly progressive, severe encephalopathy with refractory seizures | Extensive MRI FLAIR/T2 cortical-subcortical abnormalities. Frequent coexisting autoimmunities (TPO, GAD antibodies) | Half of patients have good response to immunotherapy, but patients may die from medical complications during status |
| DPPX | Agitation, paranoia, hallucinations, tremor, myoclonus, and/or seizures. Less often cerebellar signs, hyperekplexia, or PERM-like syndrome. Symptoms are usually preceded by severe diarrhea | Protracted course with relapses when immunotherapy is reduced | Partial but meaningful improvement |
| mGluR5 | Encephalitis, no specific syndrome | Hodgkin lymphoma or no tumor | Full recovery |
| mGluR1 | Cerebellar ataxia | No tumor or rarely lymphoma | May respond to immunotherapy |
| Dopamine receptor 2 | Infrequent cases of basal ganglia encephalitis, Sydenham chorea | No tumor association | Improvement or full recovery with early immunotherapy |
| Neurexin 3α | Encephalopathy with seizures | No tumor association | May partially respond to immunotherapy |
| IgLON5 | Encephalopathy with REM and non-REM parasomnias, obstructive sleep apnea, stridor preceded by or concurrent with gait dysfunction, chorea, and cognitive decline | Usually chronic and slowly progressive, less often rapidly progressive | Largely unresponsive to immunotherapy. Patients usually have sudden death during wakefulness |

*AMPA,* Alpha-amino-3-hydroxy-5-methyl-4-isoxazolepropionic acid receptor; *CASPR2,* contactin-associated protein-like 2; *DPPX,* dipeptidyl-peptidase-like protein 6; *FLAIR,* fluid attenuated inversion recovery; *$GABA_A$,* Gamma-aminobutyric acid-A; *$GABA_B$,* Gamma-aminobutyric acid-B; *GAD,* glutamic acid decarboxylase; *IGLON5,* immunoglobulin-like cell adhesion molecule 5; *LGI1,* leucine-rich glioma-inactivated protein-1; *mGluR5,* metabotropic glutamate receptor 5; *mGluR1,* metabotropic glutamate receptor 1; *MRI,* magnetic resonance imaging; *NMDA, N*-methyl-D-aspartate; *PERM,* progressive encephalomyelitis with rigidity and myoclonus; *REM,* rapid eye movement. *SCLC,* small-cell lung cancer; *TPO,* thyroid peroxidase.

## SPECIFIC SYNDROMES

### Anti-NMDAR Encephalitis

Anti-NMDAR encephalitis is the most frequent antibody-associated encephalitis and the second most common cause of immune-mediated encephalitis after acute disseminated encephalomyelitis (ADEM) (Granerod et al., 2010). It is most common in young women and children who represent about 80% of patients but can also affect men and older individuals. The syndrome is highly characteristic and usually occurs as a multistage process. Patients develop acute psychiatric symptoms, seizures, memory deficits, decreased level of consciousness, and dyskinesias (orofacial, limb, and trunk) (Dalmau et al., 2008; Titulaer et al., 2013). Autonomic instability is common, and, in some patients, it results in central hypoventilation, often requiring weeks of mechanical ventilation. Many adults are initially evaluated by psychiatry services. Patients or their families should be questioned about a viral-like prodrome that can elevate the suspicion for an autoimmune process. Children are often brought to medical attention due to mood and behavioral change at times with new-onset seizures, movement disorders, insomnia, or reduction of speech. Partial syndromes with predominant psychiatric symptoms or abnormal movements, and less severe phenotypes can occur, although almost all patients eventually develop several elements of the syndrome (Kayser et al., 2013;Titulaer et al., 2013). Atypical symptoms, such as cerebellar ataxia or hemiparesis, can occur and are more common in children than in adults. Approximately 40% of female patients over 18 years have uni- or bilateral ovarian teratomas compared to less than 9% of girls under 14 years of age. Younger children and men only rarely have tumors. Isolated cases with other tumor types—including teratoma of the mediastinum, small-cell lung cancer (SCLC), Hodgkin lymphoma, neuroblastoma, breast cancer, and germ-cell tumor of the testis—have been reported (Titulaer et al., 2013).

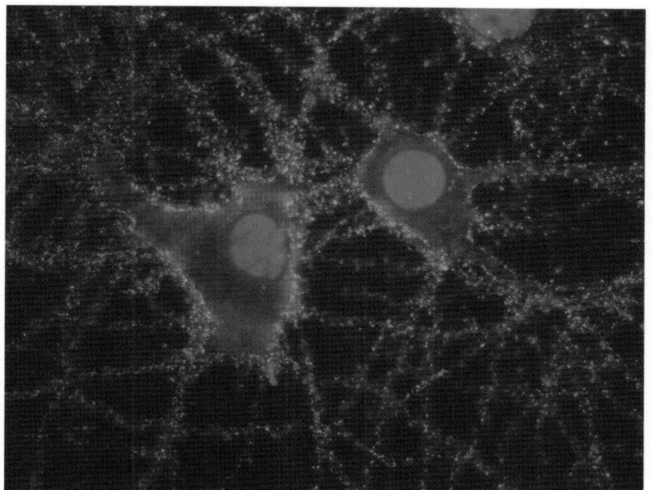

**Fig. 82.1** Antibodies to GluN1 subunit of the NMDA receptor in a patient with anti-NMDAR encephalitis. Live rat hippocampal neurons incubated with the patient's CSF are immunolabeled with antibodies against cell surface antigens; subsequent characterization demonstrated that the antigen is the GluN1 subunit of the NMDA receptor. *CSF*, Cerebrospinal fluid; *NMDA*, *N*-methyl-D-aspartate; *NMDAR*, *N*-methyl-D-aspartate receptor.

In almost 80% of patients the CSF shows lymphocytic pleocytosis and, less commonly, increased proteins and/or oligoclonal bands. About 35% of the patients have increased signal on MRI FLAIR/T2 sequences and less often, faint or transient contrast enhancement of the cerebral cortex, overlaying meninges, basal ganglia, or brainstem. The electroencephalogram (EEG) is abnormal in 95% of cases and usually shows focal or generalized slow or disorganized activity without epileptic discharges that may overlap with electrographic seizures (Sonderen et al., 2018). About 10%–30% of patients have a unique EEG pattern called extreme delta brush due to its similarity to the delta brush pattern seen in neonatal EEG (Schmitt et al., 2012). This pattern may be associated with prolonged illness and the finding of extreme delta brush in a patient with an undiagnosed encephalopathy should raise consideration for anti-NMDAR encephalitis.

Diagnosis of the disorder is confirmed by demonstration of NMDAR antibodies in CSF and serum (Fig. 82.1). As noted above, testing of CSF should be done for all initial evaluations (Gresa-Arribas et al., 2014). The antibodies are immunoglobulin G (IgG) subtype and target the GluN1 (previously called NR1) subunit of the NMDAR. These antibodies are highly specific for anti-NMDAR encephalitis and are different from other less nonspecific and unrelated immunoglobulin M (IgM) and immunoglobulin A (IgA) anti-NMDA antibodies, or IgG antibodies that target other NMDAR subunits such as the GluN2 (Hara et al., 2018). The pathogenicity of the antibodies has been shown in vitro and in vivo animal models. These studies show that the antibody binding to the NMDAR results in a reversible internalization of NMDARs that associates with a reduction of NMDAR-mediated currents (Hughes et al., 2010; Planaguma et al., 2015)

## Anti-GABA$_B$ Receptor Encephalitis

Anti-gamma-aminobutyric acid B receptor (GABA$_B$R) encephalitis similarly affects men and women and more than half have an associated tumor, almost always a SCLC (Boronat et al., 2011). When the disorder is cancer-related, the onset of the encephalitis usually precedes the cancer diagnosis. The median age of patients in one study was 62 years, with older patients more likely to have cancer. The presenting features are almost always those of typical limbic encephalitis with memory loss, confusion, and prominent seizures (Hoftberger et al., 2013; Jeffery et al., 2013). Rare cases presenting with ataxia or opsoclonus-myoclonus have been reported, but in these cases the syndrome progresses to include limbic encephalitis (Hoftberger et al., 2013). Most seizures appear to have a temporal-lobe onset with secondary generalization, while some patients have status epilepticus or subclinical seizures demonstrated on EEG.

The brain MRI is abnormal is almost two-thirds of the patients, showing unilateral or bilateral medial temporal lobe FLAIR/T2 signal, which is consistent with limbic encephalitis. As in other autoimmune encephalitis, the CSF can show lymphocytic pleocytosis.

In addition to the presence of GABA$_B$R antibodies, these patients may have other autoantibodies (e.g., TPO, ANA, GAD65) reflecting a tendency to autoimmunity or the presence of an underlying cancer (e.g., Sox1, amphiphysin, and/or Ri antibodies). In contrast to NMDAR antibodies, patient GABA$_B$R antibodies act as selective GABA$_B$R antagonists without causing receptor internalization (Dalmau et al., 2017).

Patients who receive immunotherapy together with tumor control often have full or substantial recoveries, including cases where treatment is delayed by several months. A previously healthy 3-year-old child developed GABA$_B$R and GABA$_A$R antibodies with opsoclonus, limb and trunk ataxia, and seizures; he died as a result of sepsis while receiving intensive care support (Kruer et al., 2014; Petit-Pedrol et al., 2014).

## Anti-AMPA Receptor Encephalitis

Anti-alpha-amino-3-hydroxy-5-methyl-4-isoxazolepropionic acid receptor (AMPAR) encephalitis predominantly affects middle-aged women (median age 62 years). Just over half the patients present with subacute (<8 weeks) symptoms of limbic encephalitis including confusion, disorientation, and memory loss (Hoftberger et al., 2015; Lai et al., 2009). Other patients present with limbic dysfunction in association with multifocal or diffuse encephalopathy. Unusual presentations (psychosis, motor dysfunction) have also been reported (Graus et al., 2010; Hoftberger et al., 2015). Seizures have been reported in under half of cases. About 60% of the patients have an underlying tumor, most often in the lung, breast, or thymus. The antibodies target the GluA1/2 subunits of the AMPAR. The binding of patient antibodies to the AMPAR results in receptor internalization; compensatory changes include insertion of GluA1 homomers in the synapses, increasing synaptic excitability (Haselmann et al., 2018).

The brain MRI usually shows abnormal FLAIR signal involving the medial temporal lobes, rarely with transient signal changes in other areas. The CSF often reveals lymphocytic pleocytosis. In one reported series, half of the patients had a history of, or concurrent findings of, systemic autoimmunity such as insulin-dependent diabetes with glutamic acid decarboxylase (GAD) antibodies, hypothyroidism, or Raynaud syndrome (Lai et al., 2009). As in GABA$_B$R encephalitis, the presence of additional paraneoplastic immune responses related to cytotoxic T-cell mechanisms is associated with worse outcome (Hoftberger et al., 2015).

The majority of patients respond to immunotherapy; however, approximately half have relapses. Those with relapses usually respond to treatment, but these responses are often partial, resulting in cumulative memory or behavioral deficits. It is unclear if chronic immunosuppression has a role in preventing or reducing the risk of relapses.

## Anti-LGI1 Limbic Encephalitis

Anti-leucine-rich glioma-inactivated 1 (LGI1) encephalitis predominantly occurs in older men (median age 60 years; men > women) who develop memory loss, confusion, and temporal lobe seizures. About

60% of patients also develop hyponatremia and less often rapid eye movement (REM) sleep behavior disorders, which can be additional clues in formulating the differential diagnoses (Lai et al., 2010). About 30%–40% of patients develop brief tonic or myoclonic-like seizures (also called faciobrachial dystonic seizures) (Irani et al., 2011). In a few cases patients develop additional symptoms of peripheral nerve hyperexcitability (PNH) (Morvan syndrome). The rapidly progressive memory disturbance along with myoclonic-like movements can lead to the suspicion of rapid onset dementia such as Creutzfeldt-Jakob disease. In one study, about 15% of patients presented with rapidly progressive cognitive deficits with no clear evidence of encephalitis (Arino et al., 2016). The disorder is usually not cancer associated, and less than 10% of patients have an underlying neoplasm, usually a thymoma. The MRI often shows findings typical of limbic encephalitis, although seizures can result in similar abnormalities, confounding interpretation. The CSF is usually normal, although mild inflammatory changes or oligoclonal bands may be present; despite normal routine CSF studies, the antibodies are almost always detectable in both serum and CSF.

Patients' antibodies target LGI1, a secreted neuronal protein that interacts with pre- and postsynaptic epilepsy-related proteins (Fukata et al., 2006). The antibodies cause a decrease of Kv1.1 and AMPAR altering pre- and postsynaptic signaling and resulting in neuronal hyperexcitability (Petit-Pedrol et al., 2018). Mutations in LGI1 are linked to the human disorder, autosomal dominant lateral temporal lobe epilepsy (also called autosomal dominant partial epilepsy with auditory features) (Gu et al., 2002; Kalachikov et al., 2002).

About 80% of patients have substantial responses to immunotherapy although many are left with deficits that prevent them from returning to work. Relapses occur in about 27%–35% of the patients (Arino et al., 2016; van Sonderen et al., 2016b).

## Anti-CASPR2 Associated Encephalitis

Patients with contactin-associated protein-like 2 (CASPR2) antibodies often develop symptoms involving both the central nervous system (e.g., encephalopathy, cerebellar dysfunction, hallucinations, seizures, insomnia, autonomic dysfunction) and peripheral nervous system (PNH, neuropathy, allodynia) (Irani et al., 2012; Lancaster et al., 2011a; van Sonderen et al., 2016a). The combination of the indicated CNS symptoms and PNH is called Morvan syndrome. Rare cases of isolated limbic encephalitis or PNH have been reported. Patients may have other coexisting immune-mediated disorders such as myasthenia gravis with anti-acetylcholine (AChR) or muscle-specific kinase (MuSK) antibodies (Fleisher et al., 2013). Anti-CASPR2 associated encephalitis is usually not cancer related, and those patients with a tumor (most commonly thymoma) are more likely to have Morvan syndrome as opposed to isolated central or PNH symptoms.

In contrast to most of the autoimmune encephalitis (LGI1, DPPX, and IgLON5 are other exceptions), antibodies to CASPR2 are primarily of the IgG4 isotype. Studies suggest that patient CASPR2 antibodies interfere with the normal clustering of VGKCs at juxtaparanodes, resulting in hyperexcitability of peripheral nerves (Patterson et al., 2018).

## Anti-GABA$_A$ Receptor Encephalitis

The median age of patients with this syndrome is 40 years, but it may occur in children and adolescents. Patients develop a progressive, severe encephalopathy that in 90% of cases includes refractory seizures with frequent status epilepticus. Other symptoms include cognitive impairment, altered behavior, decreased consciousness, and movement disorders (Petit-Pedrol et al., 2014; Spatola et al., 2017). Over half of the patients have CSF abnormalities, including pleocytosis, increased proteins, and/or oligoclonal bands. In contrast to other autoimmune encephalitis in which the brain MRI is either normal or shows predominant involvement of the limbic system, almost all patients have extensive MRI abnormalities on FLAIR/T2 imaging with multifocal cortical-subcortical involvement without contrast enhancement (Fig. 82.2). Almost one-third have an associated tumor (mostly thymoma). More than half of the patients have partial or complete response to immunotherapy despite the severity of the illness and the seizures. Deaths that have been reported were attributed to status epilepticus or complications such as sepsis.

Most patients also have coexisting autoimmunity including antibodies to GAD or thyroid peroxidase (TPO), raising the question of whether some patients with severe seizures attributed to GAD65 antibodies may in fact have other more disease-relevant antibodies such as GABA$_A$R. The findings may also provide an explanation for some encephalitis attributed to TPO antibodies (erroneously considered Hashimoto encephalitis). The disorder can be triggered by viral encephalitis (herpes simplex virus 1 or human herpesvirus 6), and these patients usually have coexisting anti-NMDAR antibodies.

Patients' have antibodies that target the gamma aminobutyric acid A receptor (GABA$_A$R). These antibodies produce a relocation of the receptor from synaptic to extrasynaptic sites, leading to neuronal hyperexcitability and supporting a pathogenic role (Petit-Pedrol et al., 2014).

## Anti-DPPX Encephalitis

Patients with encephalitis associated with antibodies to dipeptidyl-peptidase-like protein6 (DPPX) develop severe prodromal weight loss or diarrhea followed by the development of prominent neuropsychiatric symptoms, CNS hyperexcitability (e.g., agitation, hallucinations, myoclonus, tremor, seizures, hyperekplexia), and/or cerebellar or brainstem dysfunction (Boronat et al., 2013; Hara et al., 2017; Tobin et al., 2014).The weight loss and severe diarrhea occur, on average, 4 months before the onset of neurological symptoms and can result in extensive evaluations for a primary gastrointestinal disorder. The triad of weight loss, cognitive dysfunction, and symptoms of CNS hyperexcitability should raise the suspicion for anti-DPPX encephalitis. The encephalitis is chronic and progresses over months (median 8 months to disease peak). The CSF can show pleocytosis or oligoclonal bands but can be normal. The MRI is usually nonspecific. Tumor associations are unusual but do occur (mostly B-cell neoplasms). Some patients develop a syndrome resembling progressive encephalomyelitis with rigidity and myoclonus (PERM) or present with hyperekplexia (Balint et al., 2014; Hara et al., 2017). The prodromal gastrointestinal symptoms, severe loss of weight, and/or prominent cognitive or mental alterations helps to distinguish DPPX encephalitis from PERM. Patients often respond to immunotherapy with relapses mainly occurring in the setting of reduced immunotherapy.

All patients have a combination of IgG1 and IgGg4 anti-DPPX antibodies. These antibodies produce a reversible decrease of the density of DPPX receptor clusters as well as the associated Kv4.2 potassium channels (Hara et al., 2017). The myenteric plexus is enriched in DPPX receptors and this may explain the prominent gastrointestinal symptoms.

## Anti-mGluR5 Encephalitis

Anti-mGluR5 antibodies were initially described in two patients with limbic encephalitis and Hodgkin lymphoma (Ophelia syndrome) (Lancaster et al., 2011b). An evaluation of additional patients showed that most have a viral-like prodrome followed by the development of a complex neuropsychiatric syndrome with prominent psychiatric and cognitive dysfunction, movement disorders, sleep dysfunction, and/or seizures (Spatola et al., 2018). There is CSF pleocytosis in almost all cases and, less commonly, oligoclonal bands. In approximately half of the

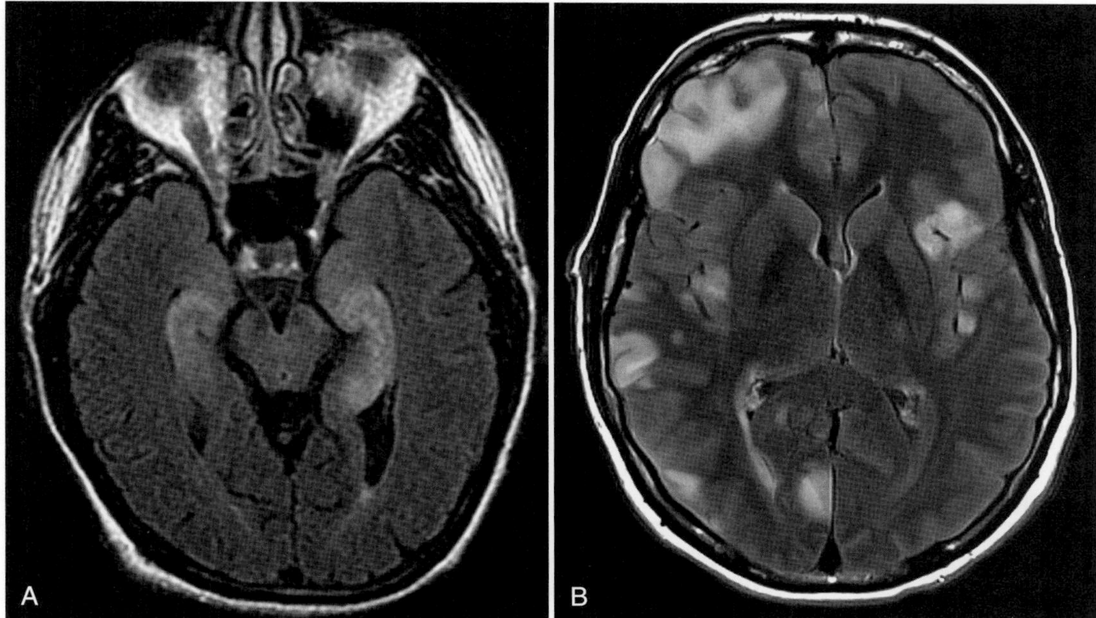


**Fig. 82.2** A, Brain MRI of a patient with limbic encephalitis and antibodies against LGI1, showing typical increased FLAIR signal involving the medial temporal lobes. Similar findings occur in greater than 50% of patients with AMPA or $GABA_B$ receptor antibodies, and less frequently in patients with CASPR2 antibodies. B, Brain MRI of a patient with $GABA_A$ receptor antibodies showing FLAIR abnormalities involving multiple cortical and subcortical regions. These abnormalities occur in 80% of patients with this disorder; diffusion weighted imaging rarely show restricted diffusion. These multifocal abnormalities appear and disappear in an asynchronous manner, are highly suggestive of $GABA_A$ receptor encephalitis, and do not occur in patients with other types of antibody-mediated encephalitis. *AMPA*, alpha-amino-3-hydroxy-5-methyl-4-isoxazolepropionic acid; *CASPR2*, contactin-associated protein-like 2; *FLAIR*, fluid-attenuated inversion recovery; *$GABA_A$*, gamma-aminobutyric acid A; *$GABA_B$*, gamma-aminobutyric acid B; *LGI1*, leucine-rich glioma inactivated 1; *MRI*, magnetic resonance imaging. (*Reprinted with permission from Lancaster et al., Neurology 2011;77(2):179–189 and Spatola et al., Neurology 2017;88(11):1012–1020.*)

patients, the MRI showed FLAIR abnormalities in limbic or extralimbic regions. There was a tumor association in about half of the cases (most commonly Hodgkin lymphoma, and one patient reported with SCLC). Patients can respond to immunotherapy and tumor treatment when appropriate, but can have relapses.

## Anti-mGluR1 Cerebellar Dysfunction

Cerebellar ataxia in association with antibodies to the mGluR1 receptor was initially described in two patients with a history of Hodgkin disease (Sillevis et al., 2000). Since then a few additional patients have been reported but other than one patient with a T-cell lymphoma, the disorder was not cancer related (Lopez-Chiriboga et al., 2016). All patients developed cerebellar ataxia, and rarely cognitive changes, psychiatric symptoms, and/or seizures. Some patients responded to early administration of immunotherapy. Injection of patient antibodies to the subarachnoid space near the cerebellum resulted in progressive ataxia, suggesting a direct pathogenic role of the antibodies in the disorder (Sillevis et al., 2000).

## Anti-Dopamine Receptor Encephalitis

A very rare number of patients, mostly children with basal ganglia encephalitis, Sydenham chorea, or Tourette syndrome have been reported to have antibodies to the dopamine-2 receptor (Dale et al., 2012). There is preliminary evidence that the antibodies have pathogenic effects. These antibodies have also been found in some patients with autoimmune encephalitis, which developed after a herpes simplex viral infection. Most of these patients have concurrent antibodies to NMDAR. Patients can have full recovery with early immunotherapy (Dale et al., 2012).

## Anti-neurexin 3α Encephalitis

This disorder was initially described in five patients (median age 44 years) who presented with prodromal fever, headache, or gastrointestinal symptoms followed by the onset of confusion, seizures, and a decreased level of consciousness (Gresa-Arribas et al., 2016). Two of the patients developed facial dyskinesias suggestive of anti-NMDAR encephalitis (anti-NMDAR antibodies were absent). The MRI was normal in four patients, and in one showed medial temporal lobe FLAIR abnormality. Three patients had partial recovery after immunotherapy; however, two patients died—one death was related to refractory seizures and brain edema and the other to sepsis. Studies in cultured neurons showed that the patient antibodies decrease receptor cluster density as well as the number of synapses (Gresa-Arribas et al., 2016).

## Anti-IgLON5 Disease

Patients with this disease develop a characteristic sleep disorder before or concurrently with the onset of bulbar symptoms, gait abnormalities, chorea, oculomotor problems and, less commonly, cognitive decline (Sabater et al., 2014). The sleep disorder includes REM and non-REM sleep disturbances characterized by abnormal movements and behaviors that predominate in the early hours of sleep. In some patients the disorder is progressive over years while in other patients the course is rapidly progressive and may result in death within months of symptom onset. The disorder is poorly responsive to treatment.

Video polysomnography demonstrates undifferentiated non-REM sleep or poorly structured non-REM stage N2, along with REM parasomnias and sleep breathing dysfunction, including obstructive sleep apnea and stridor. The brain MRI, EEG, CSF studies, and electromyography are usually normal. In the patients who were studied, the CSF hypocretin levels were normal. Autopsy studies of six patients showed neuronal loss and gliosis associated with an atypical tauopathy mainly involving the tegmentum of the brainstem and the hypothalamus. There was no glial pathology, grains, or globular glial inclusions that would allow classification of these cases within any of the presently known tauopathies (Gelpi et al., 2016).

All patients have antibodies targeting immunoglobulin-like cell adhesion molecule 5 (IgLON5), a member of the IgLON family, which is part of the immunoglobulin superfamily of cell adhesion molecules. The antibodies are predominantly of the IgG4 subclass, and there is a strong association with the HLA-DRB1*10.01 allele (Gaig et al., 2017). The IgLON proteins appear to play a role in neuronal pathfinding and synaptic formation although the exact function of IgLON5 is unknown.

## GENERAL TREATMENT RECOMMENDATIONS

The optimal management of these disorders is still being elucidated, and current recommendations are largely derived from the experience with anti-NMDAR encephalitis (Titulaer et al., 2013). Based on data that demonstrate a pathogenic role of the antibodies, treatments are focused on antibody depletion and immunosuppression. In tumor-associated cases, the first step in management should be its identification and treatment. Patients with anti-NMDAR or AMPAR encephalitis, whose tumors were not removed, had less frequent recoveries and an increased risk of relapses compared to those whose tumors were treated. While it is not known if this applies to other disorders it strongly supports early tumor treatment when appropriate (Titulaer et al., 2013).

Despite the severity of many patients' symptoms, the majority of patients respond to treatment. Recovery can be slow and some disorders have a tendency to relapse. Corticosteroids and/or intravenous immunoglobulin (IVIG) or plasma exchange are considered first-line therapies and should be considered in all patients. There are no data to support the use of IVIG over plasma exchange, although the poor medical condition and autonomic instability of some patients may favor the use of IVIG. For patients who do not show early improvement with these therapies or who are severely affected, rituximab and/or cyclophosphamide should be considered and are increasingly being used upfront (Nosadini et al., 2015). The use of rituximab appears to reduce the risk of relapses and there is evidence it is effective for IgG4 antibody-mediated diseases (Huijbers et al., 2015), supporting its early or upfront use.

*The complete reference list is available online at https://expertconsult.inkling.com/.* 

83

# Anoxic-Ischemic Encephalopathy

Jennifer E. Fugate, Eelco F.M. Wijdicks

## OUTLINE



When the heart stops and cerebral blood flow is interrupted during a cardiac arrest, patients lose consciousness and may remain comatose after resumption of circulation. Such a global injury to the brain is understandably profound, and more than 70% of patients die or remain comatose 24 hours after cardiopulmonary resuscitation (CPR) (Rogove et al., 1995; Zandbergen et al., 2006). Anoxia describes the complete lack of oxygen delivery (e.g., complete cessation of blood flow during cardiac arrest), whereas hypoxia describes what may occur during times of decreased oxygen delivery, but with some degree of continued blood flow. Hypoxic-ischemic brain injury—albeit less well defined and less clearly understood than anoxic-ischemic injury—can occur in patients with respiratory arrest or severe hypoxemia (e.g., asphyxia).

Approximately 100,000 patients a year in the United States are admitted to intensive care units with anoxic-ischemic brain injury after CPR (Peberdy et al., 2003). Although the pathophysiology of brain injury caused by cardiac arrest is reasonably well understood, less is known about neuroprotection. For nearly two decades, there was enthusiasm that induced hypothermia could not only improve survival rates but also improve neurological outcomes (Broccard, 2006), but these beliefs have been challenged (Nielsen et al., 2013). This chapter critically evaluates the current knowledge of anoxic-ischemic brain injury. Studies have reported tools for predicting outcomes, and guidelines for prediction of poor outcome have been developed by the American Academy of Neurology (Wijdicks et al., 2006). The accuracy of these predictors after the use of therapeutic hypothermia or targeted temperature management (TTM) is a subject of ongoing research.

## PATHOPHYSIOLOGICAL CONCEPTS

One of the more vital questions for scientists and clinicians is whether there is a specific period during resuscitation in which interventions can modify the degree of anoxic-ischemic brain injury and improve clinical outcomes. Is the damage to the brain permanent and present at ictus, or are there processes at work that could potentially be influenced and modulated? Several clinical facts are important. First, with cardiac arrest, whether due to asystole or ventricular fibrillation, there is no measurable flow to the brain. Moreover, even with standard CPR techniques, only one-third of the pre-arrest cerebral blood flow can be attained (Maramattom and Wijdicks, 2005). In addition, the shockable rhythms (ventricular tachycardia and ventricular fibrillation) have a better outcome than nonshockable rhythms such as asystole, pulseless electrical activity, and bradyarrhythmias, reflected by restoration of adequate cerebral blood flow when ejection fraction of the ventricle improves (Callans, 2004). Secondly, there might be a critical time period after which CPR may fail to restore neuronal function. This time interval is poorly defined, but we know that the neuronal oxygen stores are depleted within 20 seconds of cardiac arrest, and cerebral necrosis occurs as a result of ischemia. There is some uncertainty about whether hypoxemia alone could produce necrosis, and, although it can cause damage (preferentially in the striatum), necrosis is rarely seen even in patients with arterial $Pao_2$ values less than 20 mm Hg.

After 2–4 minutes of anoxia, several biochemical mechanisms that result in irreversible neuronal damage may become operative (Fig. 83.1). Selective neuronal vulnerability to this type of injury involves areas in the CA-1 sector of the hippocampus, the thalami, the neocortex, and the cerebellar Purkinje cells (Fig. 83.2). Necrosis of the cortex involves layers three, four, and five and is pathologically known as *laminar necrosis*. The vulnerability of these areas may be explained by the presence of receptors for excitatory neurotransmitters or the high metabolic demands of these neurons. An important question is whether necrosis or apoptosis occurs. The cell death cascade that involves several modulatory and degradation signals has been documented in global cerebral ischemia, but whether these processes can be effectively manipulated remains unclear (Ogawa et al., 2007). A caspase inhibitor did not affect neurological outcome after 6 minutes of cardiopulmonary arrest in rats (Teschendorf et al., 2001).

Another mechanism of neuronal and glial damage is excitatory brain injury. Glutamate efflux due to ischemic injury increases intracellular calcium concentration, which results in neuronal injury. The excess release of calcium leads to other processes that include activation of catabolic enzymes and endonucleases. Glutamate excitotoxicity has remained the major hypothesis to explain this type of neuronal injury and was made more probable after the documentation of neuroprotection with *N*-methyl-D-aspartate (NMDA) or α-amino-3-hydroxy-5-methyl-4-isoxazolepropionic acid (AMPA) receptor antagonists.

In addition, research interest in anoxic brain injury has pointed toward a phenomenon called *no reflow*. This concept is based on the premise that after resumption of circulation, there are major microcirculatory reperfusion deficits. Coagulation may occur within these reperfusion zones, with intravascular fibrin formation and

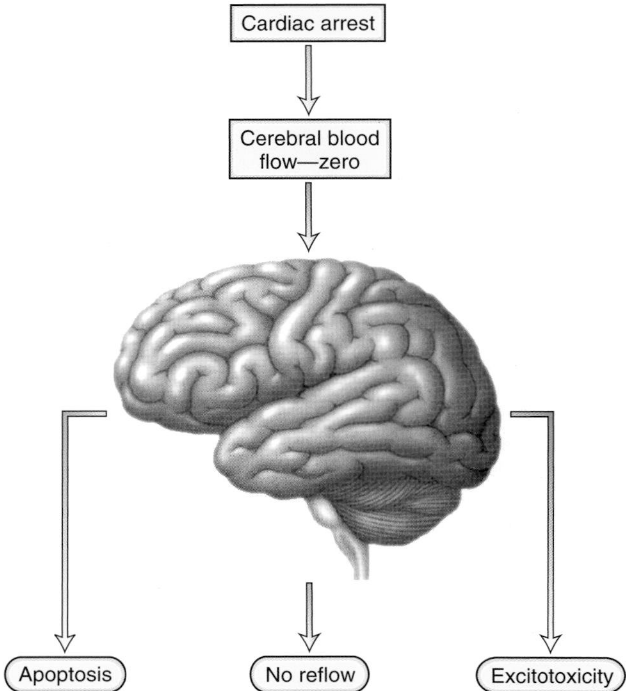


**Fig. 83.1** Mechanisms of Brain Injury after Cardiac Arrest.

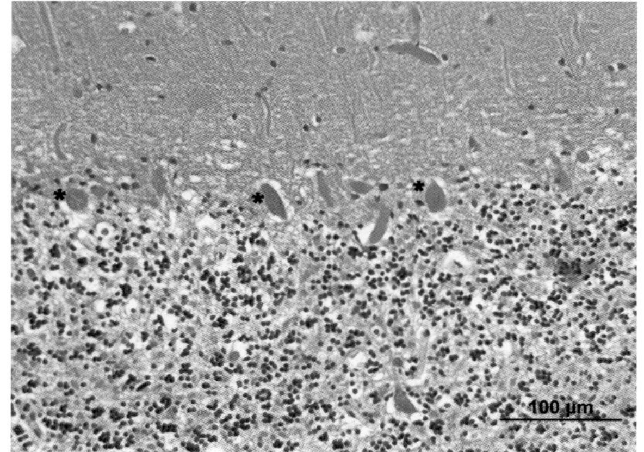


**Fig. 83.2** Purkinje Cell Loss after Cardiac Arrest (*Asterisks* Point to a Few Surviving Cells).

microthrombosis. This concept has served as a basis for experimental studies using recombinant tissue-type plasminogen activator (tPA) (Echeverry et al., 2010; Haile et al., 2012). Despite our understanding of the pathophysiology of anoxic-ischemic injury based on careful animal experiments, the clinical reality of neuroprotection is discouraging. Clinical trials using barbiturates or calcium channel antagonists have been unsuccessful (Maramattom and Wijdicks, 2005). Induced hypothermia, which inhibits apoptosis and reduces free radical formation and excitatory neurotransmitters, was considered to be the only potentially beneficial intervention (Bernard et al., 2002; HACA Study Group, 2002), but even this has come into question and strict normothermia may be just as beneficial (Nielsen et al., 2013). Patients who are comatose after CPR unfortunately often have a devastating outcome. Improvement of outcome might come from very early intervention and administration of neuroprotective agents at the onset of resuscitation, rather than when a patient enters the hospital.

## CLINICAL EXAMINATION

Early awakening after CPR, clinical signs of localizing pain stimuli, and following commands are generally considered positive. However, the current literature provides no criteria on which a good long-term outcome can be reliably predicted. Most studies that have concentrated on the examination of the patient assume a poor outcome.

Clinical neurological examination follows a standard procedure, with examination of brainstem reflexes, motor response to pain, specific attention to myoclonus, and spontaneous or elicited eye movements. Because the brainstem is far more resilient to anoxic-ischemic injury than the cortex, brainstem reflexes, including the pupillary reflex to light, are often normal. Absent pupil responses can be caused by a high dose of intravenous atropine used during resuscitation, although a pupil response might still be found when examined under the magnifying glass. Fixed, dilated pupils presenting 6 hours after resuscitation are a sign of poor prognosis, but this is rarely present in isolation and is usually an indication that the rest of the brainstem has also been involved in the anoxic-ischemic injury. The eye examination may provide useful supporting evidence of anoxic injury (Wijdicks, 2002). Sustained upward gaze is often indicative of a significant global bihemispheric injury that may include the thalamus. A proposed mechanism explaining this phenomenon is a complete disinhibition of the vestibulo-ocular reflexes from the cerebellar flocculus (Nakada et al., 1984). Although forced upgaze is usually associated with poor outcomes, it is still compatible with survival in approximately 12%–15% of cases (Fugate et al., 2010). In some patients, downward gaze can be elicited using rapid head shaking or attempting to elicit a vestibular ocular response (Johkura et al., 2004). Other eye abnormalities, including ping-pong gaze or periodic lateral gaze deviations, have not been specifically examined for their prognostic value (Diesing and Wijdicks, 2004). Continuous blinking is often a common finding in comatose patients, although its anatomical substrate is unknown.

An important clinical sign is *myoclonus status epilepticus*, defined as continuous and vigorous jerking movements involving facial muscles, limbs, and abdominal muscles (Thomke et al., 2005; Young et al., 2005). These jerks can often be elicited or aggravated by touch or hand clap and may also involve the diaphragm, which complicates ventilation. Myoclonus status epilepticus has classically been considered an agonal phenomenon indicating an almost invariably poor prognosis, although exceptional cases have been reported (Greer, 2013). This sustained, diffuse, vigorous myoclonus should not be confused with occasional myoclonic jerks. The majority of these patients have a malignant burst-suppression pattern on electroencephalogram (EEG) and do not survive. In others, EEG may show a continuous background with polyspikes concordant with myoclonic jerks, and, in these cases, favorable outcome is possible (Elmer et al., 2016). Myoclonus status epilepticus must be distinguished from myoclonus due to intoxication or hepatic encephalopathy and from generalized tonic-clonic seizures. Convulsive status epilepticus is uncommon, as is nonconvulsive status epilepticus (NCSE).

The motor response to pain should be classified and described as absent to pain, extensor response, pathological flexion response, withdrawal to pain, or localization. Lack of motor response to nail-bed compression at the initial assessment does not necessarily predict poor outcome. It may represent the "man-in-the-barrel" syndrome that occurs after bilateral border-zone infarction in the anterior and middle cerebral watershed regions. Involvement in this territory will result in prolonged weakness of the arms, with normal findings in the lower limbs. The outcome in these patients is often better than that for other patients with ischemic-anoxic injury.

**TABLE 83.1 Clinical Syndromes after Post–Anoxic-Ischemic Encephalopathy**

| Clinical Syndrome | Mechanism | Outcome |
|---|---|---|
| "Man-in-the-barrel" syndrome | Bilateral watershed infarcts | Uncertain, may improve substantially |
| Parkinsonism | Infarcts in the striatum | Improvement possible |
| Action myoclonus | Cerebellar infarcts | In awake patients, could improve with medication |

**TABLE 83.2 Sedative and Analgesic Medications**

| Agent | Elimination Half-Life (h) |
|---|---|
| Morphine | 1.5–4 |
| Fentanyl | 2–5 |
| Alfentanil | 1.5–3.5 |
| Midazolam | 1–4 |
| Lorazepam | 10–20 |
| Propofol | 2 |

The outcomes for patients in coma range from death, including brain death, to persistent vegetative state (see Chapters 5 and 6), to awakening with disabilities ranging from the minimally conscious state (see Chapter 6) to complete recovery (see Chapter 55).

Awakening from coma can be protracted and prolonged, although the vast majority of patients who will awaken will do so within the first few days, provided they are not kept sedated. In our series of patients, 94 of 101 patients with post–anoxic-ischemic injury awoke within 3 days after cardiac arrest and induced hypothermia did not seem to directly influence this (Fugate et al., 2011). However, awakening can occur even 3 months after onset, although rarely without a severe deficit such as an amnesic syndrome or other neurological findings (Table 83.1).

The neurological examination can be confounded by an additional systemic injury associated with CPR. Several patients may have an associated acute renal failure or liver injury. In addition, medications may have been administered to counter pain or to facilitate mechanical ventilation. Often patients have been treated with fentanyl and lorazepam, both of which have long elimination half-lives (Table 83.2). The use of therapeutic hypothermia (TH) or targeted temperature management (TTM) may further prolong medication effects, as hepatic metabolism and renal clearance are decreased, which may cause an enhanced and prolonged effect of medications (Polderman, 2009).

## MANAGEMENT

The optimal management of anoxic-ischemic injury is unclear, and little guidance is available from clinical trials. The initial management of a comatose patient requires intubation and mechanical ventilation. Optimal hemodynamic goals are not well established. A mean arterial pressure of 65–80 mm Hg is a common goal and often requires norepinephrine, with or without inotropes, in addition to fluid resuscitation (Hassager et al., 2018). Blood pressure, clearance of lactate, and adequate urine output are important measures of the initial resuscitative efforts. Patients with severe cardiogenic shock may require more advanced interventions such as intraaortic balloon pumps or extracorporeal membrane oxygenation. Prevention of hyperglycemia that may reduce regional cerebral blood flow is advised. This includes the avoidance of dextrose-containing solutions and use of insulin drips to

**BOX 83.1 Temperature Control Protocol for Out-of-Hospital Cardiopulmonary Arrest**

Sedate patient prior if paralysis is initiated:

Midazolam, initial dose 0.01–0.05 mg/kg intravenously (IV), then 0.02 mg/kg/h IV, titrate up to 0.1 mg/kg/h IV

*or*

Propofol, 5 mcg/kg/min, titrated by 5 mcg/kg/min IV every 5 min to a goal of 30–50 mcg/kg/min as tolerated by the blood pressure

*or*

Fentanyl, 0.7–10 mcg/kg/h IV as tolerated by the blood pressure

Paralysis:

Atracurium, 0.2–0.5 mg/kg bolus, followed by an infusion of 11–13 mcg/kg/min

*or*

Vecuronium 0.1 mg/kg bolus, then 1 mcg/kg/min; titrate paralysis to a 1–2/4 train-of-four every hour to suppress shivering

Lacri-Lube to eyes

Target temperature control with cooling device

Place bladder catheter to monitor temperature

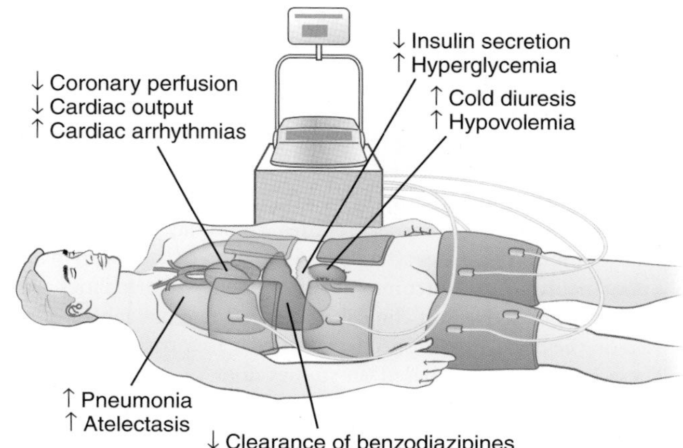


**Fig. 83.3** Potential Systemic Effects of Induced Hypothermia.

maintain a normoglycemic state. The practice of induced hypothermia in post–cardiac arrest management became widespread after the publication of two influential trials in 2002 (Bernard et al., 2002; HACA Study Group, 2002). These early trials found improved survival, but details on the neurological condition of the patients were insufficient (Maramattom and Wijdicks, 2005). The beneficial effect of cooling has been challenged by two more recent clinical trials. One showed that prehospital cooling did not improve outcomes, and the other—the TTM trial—found no benefit in targeting 33°C compared with 36°C (Kim et al., 2014; Nielsen et al., 2013). The results of the latter study raise the possibility that it is the avoidance of hyperthermia—and not the induction of moderate hypothermia—that may confer the neuroprotective effect. An ongoing clinical trial (TTM 2) aims to answer that hypothesis.

A cooling protocol for out-of-hospital cardiopulmonary arrest is shown in Box 83.1. This requires reduction in core temperature with ice packs, rapid infusion of cold intravenous fluids, and the use of external cooling devices or endovascular cooling systems (Holzer et al., 2006). Temperature management is initiated within 2–3 hours to reduce core temperatures to 32°C–36°C and is maintained for 24 hours, followed by gradual rewarming. Sedation and neuromuscular blockade are needed to control shivering. Major potential systemic complications may include pneumonia, cardiac arrhythmias, pancreatitis, and hyperglycemia, particularly in those cooled to 32°C–34°C (Fig. 83.3). The benefit of

**BOX 83.2 Concerns When Evaluating Patients Treated with Cooling Protocols**

Potentially confounded neurological examination because hypothermia necessitates sedatives, neuromuscular blockers, and analgesics:
- Motor response and corneal reflexes may not be reliable as early as day 3
- Pupil examination maintains prognostic reliability

Decreased metabolism and clearance of sedative and analgesic medications related to hypothermia effects and kidney/liver injury
Metabolic abnormalities and systemic shock
Nonconvulsive seizures are not uncommon and require electroencephalogram for detection

hypothermia has not been established in patients after in-hospital CPR or in those with initial cardiac rhythms other than ventricular fibrillation.

## PREDICTING PROGNOSIS

In the prehypothermia era, the assessment of prognosis was summarized in practice guidelines commissioned by the Quality Standard Subcommittee of the American Academy of Neurology (Wijdicks et al., 2006). This extensive literature review found that the circumstances surrounding CPR were not predictive of outcome. Several clinical features were highly predictive. The presence of myoclonus status epilepticus within the first 24 hours in patients with circulatory arrest, absence of pupillary responses within day 1–3 after cardiopulmonary arrest, absence of corneal reflexes within day 1–3, and absent or extensor motor responses after day 3 were all associated with invariably poor neurological outcome. Eye movement abnormalities were insufficiently predictive, but clinical studies in these patients have not focused on the prediction of specific eye motor abnormalities.

These guidelines were based on studies done prior to the routine use of TTM, and the reliability of predictors in this setting has been an area of great interest and investigation. Neurologists need to consider key factors when prognosticating for patients treated with cooling protocols (Box 83.2). A suggested algorithm for estimating neurological prognosis is shown in Fig. 83.4. Brainstem reflexes are crucial in the clinical evaluation of comatose patients after cardiac arrest. Because the brainstem is relatively resistant to anoxic-ischemic injury, the absence of pupil or corneal reflexes indicates a severe and often widespread injury that also involves much of the cortex. In a meta-analysis of 10 studies of prognostication after mild therapeutic hypothermia (TH), the pupil response was tested in 566 patients at 72 hours. The absence of pupillary light reactivity remained a reliable predictor of poor outcome with a false-positive rate (FPR) of 0.004 (confidence interval [CI] 0.001–0.03) (Kamps et al., 2013). In contrast, after TH, the absence of corneal reflexes at 72 hours did not remain as reliable in outcome prediction with an FPR of 0.02 (CI 0.002–0.13).

The reliability of the motor response at 72 hours after TH protocol has also been questioned (Al Thenayan et al., 2008; Rossetti et al., 2010). Although it is still associated with outcome, an absent or extensor motor response at 72 hours after cardiac arrest after TH appears less reliable than in studies done in the pre-TH era (Rossetti et al., 2010). In a meta-analysis, the motor response at 72 hours in 811 patients treated with TH had an unacceptably high FPR of 0.21 (CI 0.08–0.43) (Kamps et al., 2013). Patients treated with TH are more likely to receive sedation than those not treated with TH, and in studies with a "normothermia" comparison group, the motor response in patients sedated in that group also can be unreliable (Fugate et al., 2010; Samaniego et al.,

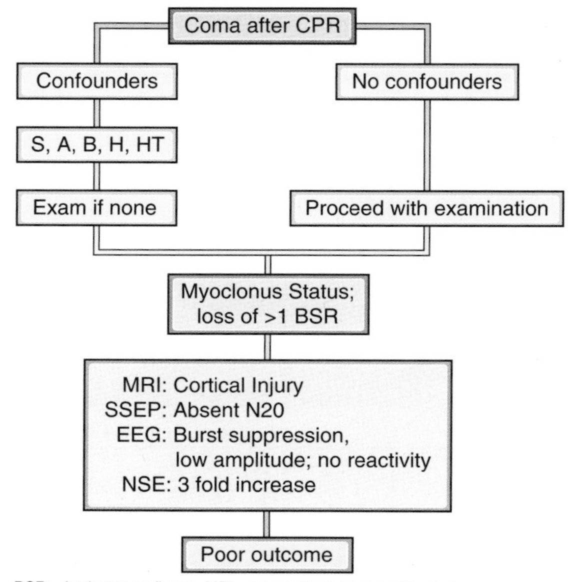


BSR = brainstem reflexes, MRI = magnetic resonance imaging, SSEP = somatosensory evoked potentials, EEG = electroencephalography NSE = neurospecific enolase, S = sedatives, A = analgesics, B = neuromuscular junction blockers, H = hypothermia

**Fig. 83.4**

2011). Thus it is crucial to ensure that there are no residual effects of sedative or analgesic medications used when assessing motor responses in patients who remain comatose after cardiac arrest.

## LABORATORY AND ELECTROPHYSIOLOGICAL TESTING

As a complement to the clinical examination, several widely used tests are EEG, neuroimaging (computed tomography [CT] or magnetic resonance imaging [MRI]), evoked potentials, and serum biomarkers. However, an evidence-based review of all laboratory tests found that many have insufficient prognosticating value (Wijdicks et al., 2006). These tests can be useful adjuncts in the estimation of neurological prognosis but should not be interpreted or used for decision making in isolation. The approach to estimating neurological prognosis in comatose survivors of cardiac arrest should be multifaceted: a combination of the neurological examination, results of tests, and the overall clinical context.

EEG has been used since the 1950s to aid in prognostication. "Highly malignant" patterns defined by the American Neurophysiological Society include suppressed background, suppressed background with continuous periodic discharges, and burst suppression These predict a poor outcome with 50% sensitivity and 100% specificity. A continuous background with preserved background reactivity is considered "benign" and has a positive predictive value of about 80% for good outcomes (Rossetti et al., 2017).

Continuous electroencephalography (cEEG) monitoring after cardiac arrest has become more widely applied as it has become recognized that nonconvulsive seizures and NCSE can occur (Abend et al., 2009; Al Thenayan et al., 2010; Legriel et al., 2009; Rundgren et al., 2006). Electrographic seizures have been found in 9%–33% of patients (Cloostermans et al., 2012; Crepeau et al., 2013; Knight et al., 2013; Mani et al., 2012; Rittenberger et al., 2012; Sadaka et al., 2014) and NCSE in 2%–12% (Crepeau et al., 2013; Legriel et al., 2009; Rittenberger et al., 2012) who are monitored during cooling protocols. Although continuous EEG (cEEG) monitoring increases the detection of epileptiform activity, it has not been shown that earlier detection and treatment of seizures in this setting changes outcomes. The labor and resources needed for cEEG are substantial, and the added value and yield of cEEG compared with "spot" EEGs in this population are not clear (Alvarez et al., 2013; Crepeau et al., 2014; Fatuzzo et al., 2018).

Also of interest are somatosensory evoked potentials (SSEPs) (Madl and Holzer, 2004). SSEPs are not influenced by drugs, temperature, or acute metabolic derangements and thus are a useful adjunct for prognostication (Chen et al., 1996). SSEP requires stimulation of the median nerve that then results in a potential at the brachial plexus, cervical spinal cord, and finally bilateral cortex potentials (N20). For SSEPs to be reliable, the cervical spine potential must be recognized, and this could be of potential concern in patients with injury involving the cervical spinal cord. The bilateral absence of cortical potentials (N20 component) is nearly 100% specific in predicting unfavorable outcomes when performed between 1 and 3 days after cardiac arrest (Wijdicks et al., 2006). However, the presence of N20 cortical responses—the much more common finding—is less useful because they have very low sensitivity to predict outcomes. Evidence indicates that absent N20 responses during mild hypothermia after resuscitation maintains accuracy in predicting a poor neurological outcome (Bouwes et al., 2009; Rossetti et al., 2010). In a meta-analysis including 492 TH-treated postarrest patients with bilaterally absent cortical responses on SSEPs, the FPR was 0.007 (CI 0.001–0.047), which is comparable with that in patients not treated with TH (Kamps et al., 2013).

Serum biomarkers have also been used in prognostication. Most studies of biomarkers in comatose survivors of cardiac arrest have examined serum neuron-specific enolase (NSE) and S100. NSE is a gamma isomer of enolase that is located in neurons, and S100 (Bottiger et al., 2001; Tiainen et al., 2003; Wang et al., 2004) is a calcium-binding astroglial protein. The usefulness of these biomarkers in prognostication may be more limited than the electrophysiological testing because none of these studies are automated, long lab turn-around times may be impractical, and standardization may not be optimal. In studies done prior to the routine use of hypothermia, only NSE predicted outcomes well, with a level greater than 33 μg/L at days 1–3 being associated with poor outcome. However, TH may have an effect on the metabolism and clearance of these biomarkers, clouding their prognostic value. Results of studies on the predictive value of NSE during or after cooling protocols are conflicting, with some finding that NSE levels maintain prognostic accuracy (Oksanen et al., 2009; Rundgren et al., 2009) and others finding the prognostic value to be reduced (Fugate et al., 2010; Steffen et al., 2010). With a cutoff value of 33 μg/L, FPRs have been reported as high as 22%–29% after TH protocols (Fugate et al., 2010; Samaniego et al., 2011) and one study found an NSE level as high as 79 μg/L is needed to achieve an FPR of 0% for predicting unfavorable outcomes (Steffen et al., 2010). In a large study of 686 TTM-treated patients (1823 NSE samples), NSE values of 61, 46, and 35, at 24, 28, and 72 hours, respectively, corresponded to an FPR less than 5% (Stammet et al., 2015). Differences in laboratory assays have made comparisons difficult, and there is not a strict threshold level of NSE that can be recommended for use in prognostication after cardiac arrest after hypothermia until there is further research and standardization of laboratory assays.

Tau protein, an indicator of axonal injury, is another promising serum biomarker. In patients from the TTM trial, a tau protein threshold of 11.2 ng/L at 72 hours after arrest had a 98% specificity and 66% sensitivity to predict poor neurological outcomes (Mattsson et al., 2017). It may be more accurate than NSE (area under the ROC curve 0.91 vs. 0.86), but it is not currently widely available.

## NEUROIMAGING

The use of neuroimaging is growing as an adjunct to estimating neurological prognosis in comatose survivors of cardiac arrest, despite a lack of high-quality evidence (Hahn et al., 2014). CT imaging performed early is often normal and cannot determine the severity of anoxic-ischemic injury. After 3–5 days in severe cases, global brain edema may be visualized. Several studies have found that the disappearance of the gray/white junction on noncontrast head CT has been associated with poor outcomes and failure to awaken (Inamasu et al., 2010; Torbey et al., 2000). Findings should be interpreted cautiously because much of the literature is limited to retrospective case series and the timing of CT has ranged from minutes to nearly 3 weeks after the insult. Still, a more recent study based on the TTM trial cohort showed that edema on brain CT detected qualitatively predicts poor neurological outcome with 97.4% specificity and 14.4% sensitivity within 24 hours of cardiac arrest (Moseby-Knappe et al., 2017).

Imaging with MRI holds promise as an adjunct to prognosis in comatose patients after cardiopulmonary arrest (Wijman et al., 2009), but there are currently insufficient data to systematically guide prognostication with MRI. Diffusion-weighted imaging (DWI) is particularly sensitive to ischemia, and apparent diffusion coefficient (ADC) values can provide a quantitative measure of injury. Current literature is limited by heterogeneity of MRI timing and patient selection bias. MRI parameters associated with poor outcome include widespread and persistent cortical DWI abnormalities (Barrett et al., 2007; Wijdicks et al., 2001), the combination of cortical and deep gray matter DWI/fluid-attenuated inversion recovery (FLAIR) abnormalities (Greer et al., 2011; Mlynash et al., 2010), and severe global ADC reduction (Wijman et al., 2009; Wu et al., 2009). Still, 20%–50% of patients with good outcomes have DWI abnormalities on MRI (Choi et al., 2010; Greer et al, 2012; Roine et al., 1993), and some patients have poor outcomes despite a normal MRI (Fig. 83.5). Thus decisions on continuing medical care or withdrawal of life-sustaining treatments should not be made on the basis of MRI findings alone, and larger prospective studies with standardized imaging are needed. Some practical limitations that could impact the widespread use of MRI in this population include the difficult nature of transporting patients who may be too hemodynamically unstable to move to the MR suite.

The assessment of prognosis in comatose survivors of CPR is important in clinical practice. It allows discussion about the level of care, whether the patient would have wanted another resuscitative effort, or whether medical care should be escalated. In many cases the family will decide to withdraw support. However, with all of these prognosticating studies, there continues to be a concern about prognostication error. Prognostication is difficult in patients who have received sedative drugs, despite examination beyond drug elimination half-life, and in patients who have had a cardiorespiratory arrest in the setting of drug overdose. In these patients, one should be prudent in making a definitive assessment.

In conclusion, anoxic-ischemic injury to the brain is damaging at ictus and often leads to prolonged coma, and in many patients a persistent unconsciousness can be anticipated if care is not withdrawn. The continuous care of comatose patients after cardiopulmonary arrest results in a major burden to the healthcare system, and family members should be adequately informed about the chances of recovery. There is some indication that treatments are on the horizon, but for now, early resumption of circulation is the best guarantee for awakening.

*The complete reference list is available online at https://expertconsult.inkling.com/.*

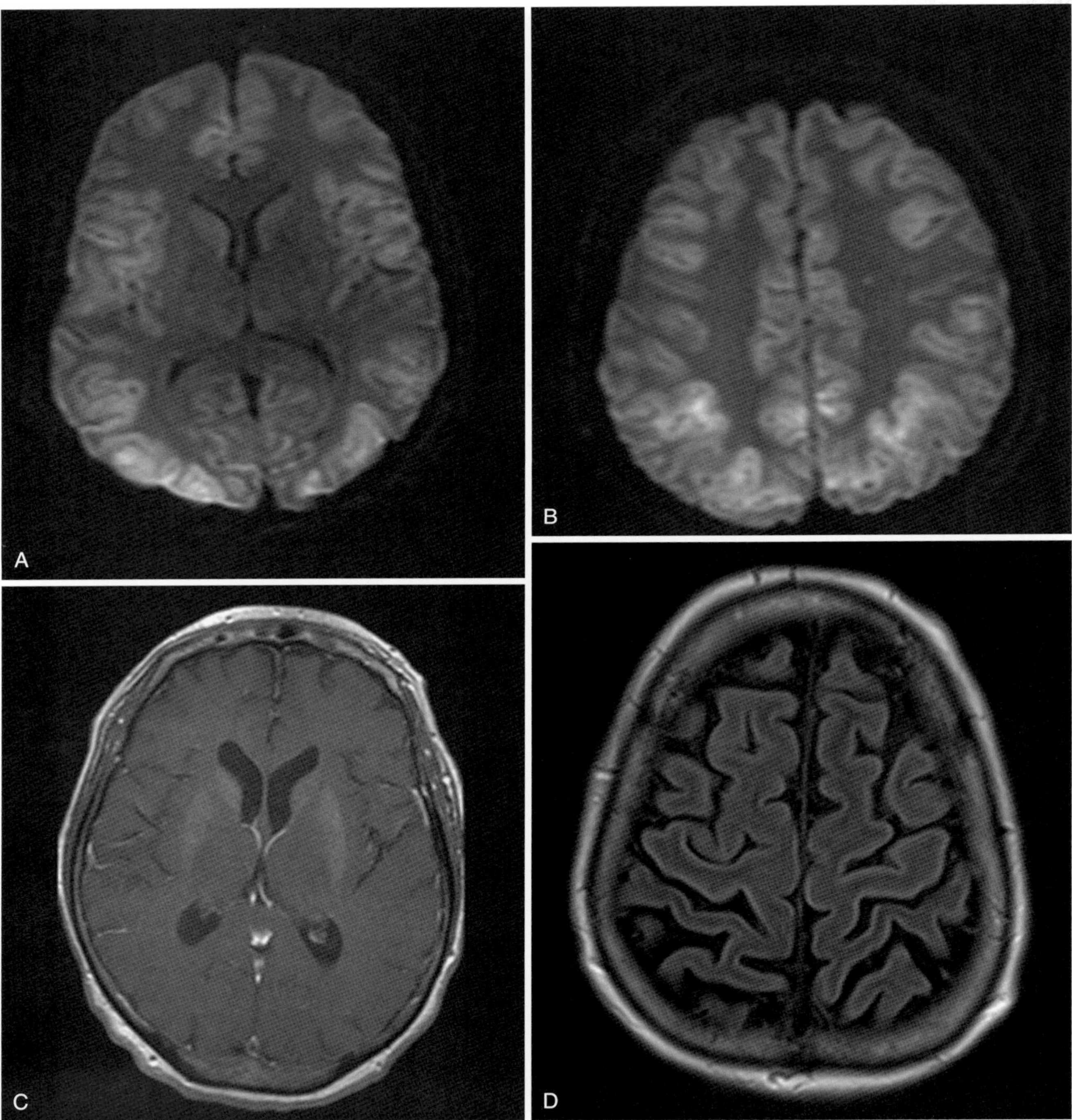

**Fig. 83.5** Diffusion-weighted magnetic resonance imaging (MRI) in anoxic-ischemic injury show diffuse cortical hyperintensities indicative of cortical injury, likely laminar necrosis (**A**, **B**). In a different patient, T1 post-gadolinium MRI shows contrast enhancement in the basal ganglia (**C**) and T2 hyperintensity involving the cortex (**D**), indicative of some anoxic injury despite clinical awakening. Noncontrast head computed tomography shows diffuse cerebral edema, loss of gray-white differentiation

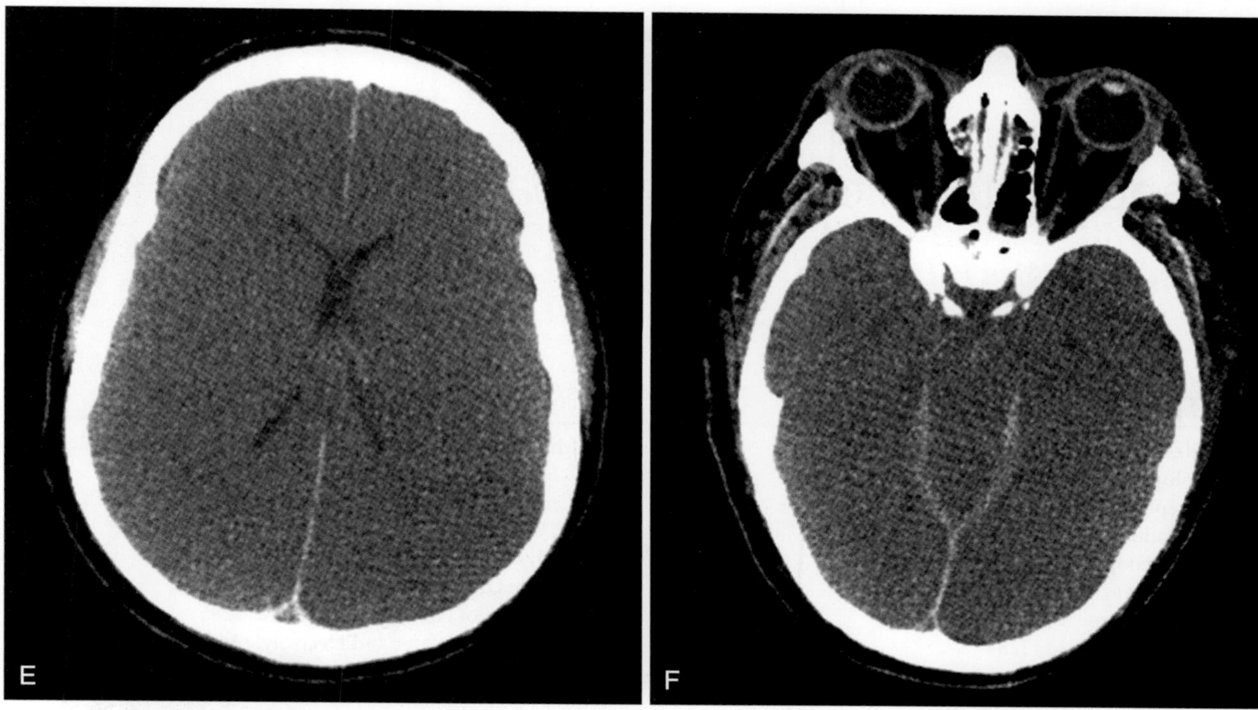


**Fig. 83.5 cont'd** (E), and "pseudosubarachnoid hemorrhage" (F) in a patient who did not survive.

84

# Toxic and Metabolic Encephalopathies

*Karin Weissenborn, Alan H. Lockwood*

## OUTLINE



Toxic and metabolic encephalopathies are a group of neurological disorders characterized by an altered mental status—that is, a *delirium*, defined as a disturbance of consciousness characterized by a reduced ability to focus, sustain, or shift attention that cannot be accounted for by preexisting or evolving dementia and that is caused by the direct physiological consequences of a general medical condition (see Chapter 4). Fluctuation of the signs and symptoms of the delirium over relatively short time periods is typical. Although the brain is isolated from the rest of the body by the blood-brain barrier, the nervous system is often affected severely by organ failure that may lead to the build-up of toxic substances normally removed from the body. This is encountered in patients with hepatic and renal failure. Damage to homeostatic mechanisms affecting the internal milieu of the brain, such as the abnormalities of electrolyte and water metabolism also affects brain function. In some cases, a deficiency of a critical substrate such as glucose is the precipitating factor. Frequently, the history and physical examination provide information that defines the affected organ system. In other cases, the cause is evident only after laboratory data are examined.

## CLINICAL MANIFESTATIONS

Encephalopathy that develops insidiously may be difficult to detect. The slowness with which abnormalities evolve and replace normal cerebral functions makes it difficult for patients and families to recognize deficits. When examining patients with diseases of organs that are commonly associated with encephalopathy, neurologists should include encephalopathy in the differential diagnosis.

Mental status abnormalities are always present and may range from subtle abnormalities, detected by neuropsychological testing, to deep coma. The level and content of consciousness reflect involvement of the reticular activating system and the cerebral cortex. Deficits in selective attention and the ability to process information underlie many metabolic encephalopathies and affect performance on many tasks. These deficits are manifested as disorders of orientation, cognition, memory, affect, perception, judgment, and the ability to concentrate on a specific task. Evidence from studies of patients with cirrhosis suggests that metabolic encephalopathies are the result of a multifocal subcortical and cortical disorder rather than uniform involvement of all brain regions. Abnormalities of psychomotor function may also be present. Among patients with coma of unknown cause, nearly two-thirds ultimately are found to have a metabolic cause. A complete discussion of coma is found in Chapter 5.

The neuro-ophthalmological examination is extremely important in differentiating patients with metabolic disorders from those with structural lesions. The pupillary light reflex and vestibular responses are almost always present, even in patients in deep coma. However, it is common for these reflexes to be blunted. Exceptions include severe hypoxia, ingestion of large amounts of atropine or scopolamine, and deep barbiturate coma, which is usually associated with circulatory collapse and an isoelectric electroencephalogram (EEG). The pupils are usually slightly smaller than normal and may be somewhat irregular. The eyes may be aligned normally in patients with mild encephalopathy. With more severe encephalopathy, dysconjugate roving movements are common. Other cranial nerve abnormalities may be present but are less useful in formulating a differential diagnosis. Motor system abnormalities, particularly slight increases in tone, are common. Other signs and symptoms of metabolic disorders may include spasticity with extensor plantar signs and extrapyramidal as well as cerebellar signs (in patients with liver disease), multifocal myoclonus (in patients with uremia), cramps (in patients with electrolyte disorders), Trousseau sign (in patients with hypocalcemia), tremors, and weakness.

Asterixis, a sudden loss of postural tone, is common. To elicit this sign, the patient should extend the arms and elbows while dorsiflexing the wrists and spreading the fingers. Small lateral movements of the fingers may be the earliest manifestation. More characteristically, there is a sudden flexion of the wrist with rapid resumption of the extended position, the so-called flapping tremor. Asterixis also may be evident during forced extrusion of the tongue, forced eye closure, or at the knee in prone patients asked to sustain flexion of the knee. Electrophysiological studies have shown that the onset of the lapse of posture is associated with complete electrical silence in the tested muscle. This sign, once thought to be pathognomonic of hepatic encephalopathy (HE), occurs in a variety of conditions including uremia, other metabolic encephalopathies, and drug intoxication. Asterixis may also be present in patients with structural brain lesions, especially thalamic lesions.

Generalized seizures occur in patients with water intoxication, hypoxia, uremia, and hypoglycemia, but only rarely as a manifestation of chronic liver failure. Seizures in patients with liver failure are generally due to alcohol or other drug withdrawal, or cerebral edema associated with acute liver failure (ALF). Focal seizures, including epilepsia partialis continua, may be seen in patients with hyperglycemia, and multifocal myoclonic seizures may occur in patients with uremia. Myoclonic status epilepticus may complicate hypoxic brain injury (see Chapter 83).

## TOXIC ENCEPHALOPATHIES

### Hepatic Encephalopathy

Cirrhosis of the liver affects an estimated 5.5 million adults in the United States. In 2011, over 33,000 Americans died as the result of chronic liver disease (Tsochatzis et al., 2014). Among the poor, the incidence of cirrhosis may be as much as 10 times higher than the national average and accounts for almost 20% of their excess mortality. As patients with chronic liver disease enter the terminal phases of their illness, HE becomes an increasingly important cause of morbidity and mortality. In this portion of the chapter, the term *hepatic encephalopathy* will be used to differentiate this condition from disorders associated with ALF, discussed in the next section. About 20,000 patients per year were hospitalized in the United States between 2005 and 2009 after developing HE (Stepanova et al., 2012). It is important to stress that minimal HE—the mildest form of HE, which interferes with the patients' daily living ability but usually does not result in seeking medical care—is far more common, affecting about half of all patients with cirrhosis. Minimal HE can be diagnosed using neuropsychological tests, EEG, or critical flicker frequency (CFF), for example, but is commonly overlooked.

A World Gastroenterological Association consensus statement seeks to minimize the substantial confusion in the literature and in clinical practice concerning the diagnosis of HE by using a multiaxial approach (Ferenci et al., 2002). The initial categorization addresses the presence of hepatocellular disease and portacaval shunting. Patients with acute liver disease or fulminating hepatic failure, a disorder occurring in patients with previously normal livers who exhibit neurological signs within 8 weeks of developing liver disease, form the first group (type A HE). A second group consists of a small number of patients who are free of hepatocellular disease but have portacaval shunting of blood (type B HE). The largest number of patients have hepatocellular disease with shunts (type C HE). Further subdivisions address temporal aspects—whether HE is episodic, chronic progressive, or persistent. Causal considerations are then applied to separate patients with precipitated HE from those with recurrent and idiopathic encephalopathy, and to identify the severity of the syndrome. The features that differentiate patients with ALF from those with the much more common portal systemic encephalopathy are shown in Table 84.1.

Rating the severity of HE is complex but essential for evaluating the results of the treatment of individual patients and for evaluating potential treatments in the research setting. The so-called West Haven criteria supplemented by an evaluation of asterixis was used in the large multicenter trial that led to the approval of rifaximin for the treatment of HE. Both scales are ordinal. The West Haven Scale is scored as the following: 0, no personality or behavioral abnormality detected; 1, trivial lack of awareness, euphoria, or anxiety, shortened attention span, or impairment of the ability to add or subtract; 2, lethargy, disorientation with respect to time, obvious personality change or inappropriate behavior; 3, somnolence or semistupor, responsiveness to verbal stimuli with confusion or gross disorientation; 4, coma. Asterixis is graded as follows: 0, no tremors; 1, few flapping tremors; 2, occasional flapping tremors; 3, frequent flapping tremors; 4, almost continuous flapping tremors.

**TABLE 84.1 Features Distinguishing Acute Liver Failure from Chronic Hepatic Encephalopathy or Portal Systemic Encephalopathy**

| Feature | Acute Liver Failure | Portal Systemic Encephalopathy |
|---|---|---|
| **History** | | |
| Onset | Usually acute | Varies; may be insidious or subacute |
| Mental state | Mania may evolve to deep coma | Blunted consciousness |
| Precipitating factor | Viral infection or hepatotoxin | Gastrointestinal hemorrhage, exogenous protein, drugs, uremia, infection |
| History of liver disease | No | Usually yes |
| **Symptoms** | | |
| Nausea, vomiting | Common | Unusual |
| Abdominal pain | Common | Unusual |
| **Signs** | | |
| Liver | Small, soft, tender | Usually large, firm, no pain |
| Nutritional state | Normal | Cachectic |
| Collateral circulation | Absent | May be present |
| Ascites | Absent | May be present |
| **Laboratory Test** | | |
| Transaminases | Very high | Normal or slightly high |
| Coagulopathy | Present | Often present |

Recently, a subdivision into "covert" and "overt" HE has been recommended (Vilstrup et al., 2014). Patients with grade 2–4 according to the West Haven Scale thereby are included in the "overt HE" group, while those with grade 1 according to the West Haven Scale and those with only psychometric or neurophysiological but no clinical signs of HE are included in the "covert HE" group. The decision to combine grade 1 HE and minimal HE to "covert HE" originates from the observation of a significant inter-rater variability in diagnosing grade 1 HE but is still controversial.

An episode of HE may be precipitated by one or more factors, some of which are iatrogenic. In one series, the use of sedatives accounted for almost 25% of all cases. A gastrointestinal (GI) hemorrhage was the next most common event (18%), followed by drug-induced azotemia and other causes of azotemia (15% each). Excessive dietary protein accounted for 10% of episodes; hypokalemia, constipation, infections, and other causes accounted for the remaining cases. As liver disease progresses, patients appear to become more susceptible to the effects of precipitants. This phenomenon has been referred to as *toxin hypersensitivity*. A transjugular intrahepatic portosystemic shunt (TIPSS), an endovascular procedure developed to treat intractable severe ascites, predisposes a patient to the development of encephalopathy, particularly among the elderly. TIPSS is more effective than large-volume paracentesis but does not prolong survival. TIPSS-related encephalopathy often responds to conventional treatment. Refractory cases may require endovascular treatment with coils to block a portion of the shunted blood.

### Laboratory Evaluations

The diagnosis of HE is based on the signs and symptoms of cerebral dysfunction in a setting of hepatic failure. Usually, standard laboratory test results, including serum bilirubin and hepatic enzymes, are abnormal. Products of normal hepatic function, including serum albumin and clotting factors, often are low, leading to elevation of the international normalized ratio (INR). Measurements of the arterial ammonia level may be helpful in diagnosing HE, but an ammonia level within the normal range does not exclude HE.

Several consensus conferences sponsored by the International Society for Hepatic Encephalopathy and Nitrogen Metabolism have made recommendations concerning the use of electrophysiological and neuropsychological tests to evaluate patients with HE (Guerit et al., 2009; Randolph et al., 2009). The favored electrophysiological tests are those that are responsive to cortical function and include event-related potentials (ERPs) such as P300 tests and the EEG. Bursts of moderate- to high-amplitude (100–300 μV), low-frequency (1.5–2.5 Hz) waves with predominance in the frontal derivations are the most characteristic EEG abnormality in patients with severe HE. But even patients without clinical signs of HE may show a reduction of the mean dominant frequency. Recently EEG was used to investigate functional cortical connectivity in patients with liver cirrhosis and an alteration was shown as well in patients with normal cognitive function compared to controls (Olesen et al., 2019). Abnormal ERPs may also be found in patients with minimal encephalopathy. Auditory P300 potential recordings, in which the subject is asked to discriminate between a rare and a common tone, showed prolonged latencies in patients with overt encephalopathy (including HE grade 1) and in some of the patients without clinical evidence of HE, indicating minimal encephalopathy. The need of more sophisticated equipment for the P300 assessment than for the EEG assessment has precluded broad use of this method for clinical purposes.

Neuropsychological tests are useful for diagnosing minimal HE and for follow-up of patients with low-grade HE (grades mHE–grade II HE). Domains to be evaluated include attention, visuoconstructional ability, and motor speed and accuracy.

Up to 60% of all patients with cirrhosis with no overt evidence of encephalopathy exhibit significant abnormalities when given a battery of neuropsychological tests. Tests of attention, concentration, visuospatial perception, and motor speed and accuracy are the most likely to be abnormal (Schomerus and Hamster, 1998). The Portosystematic Encephalopathy (PSE) Syndrome Test—a test battery consisting of the Number Connection Tests A and B, serial dotting, line tracing, and the Digit Symbol Test—has been recommended for evaluating patients who may have HE (Randolph et al., 2009; Weissenborn et al., 2001). This battery is sensitive and relatively specific for the disorder, compared with other metabolic encephalopathies.

Besides EEG and neuropsychological tests, occasionally the analysis of the CFF is used for diagnosing HE and follow-up (Vilstrup et al., 2014).

Subclinical cognitive impairment of patients with cirrhosis, particularly attention deficits and impairment in the visuospatial sphere, may be severe enough to interfere with the safe operation of an automobile or other dangerous equipment. A study comparing patients with minimal encephalopathy with nonencephalopathic patients with cirrhosis and a third group with GI disease found that those with minimal encephalopathy performed the worst during an on-the-road driving test. Specific problems centered on handling, adaptation to road conditions, and accident avoidance. Language functions are usually normal. These data, combined with other studies showing that the quality of life is affected by these abnormalities, suggest that neuropsychological tests should be used more extensively for routine evaluation of all patients with cirrhosis, particularly those without overt evidence of HE.

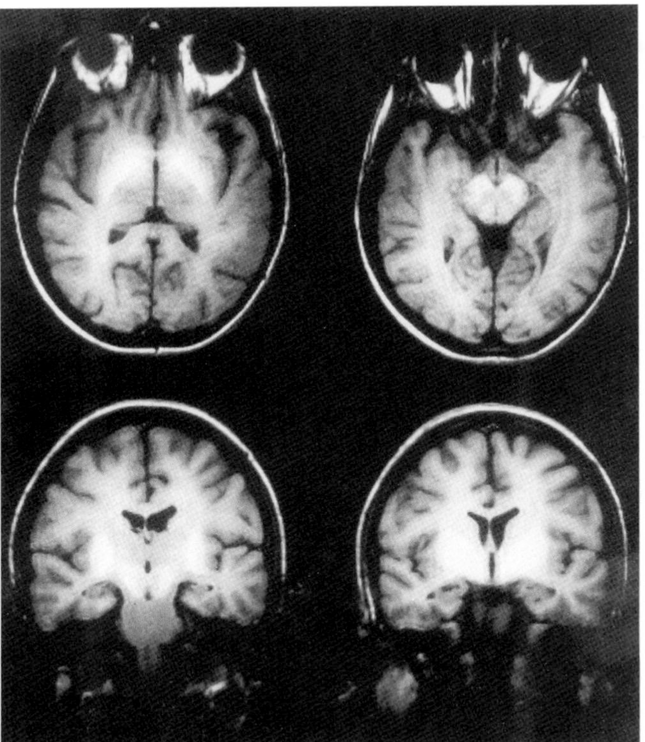

**Fig. 84.1** T1-weighted magnetic resonance images from a patient with cirrhosis of the liver. Note high signal in basal ganglia, cerebral peduncles, and substantia nigra.

Although the diagnosis of HE is typically made on the basis of clinical criteria, neuroimaging techniques are commonly employed to exclude structural lesions. Magnetic resonance imaging (MRI) and spectroscopic (MRS) studies have revealed new insights into the pathophysiology of HE (Lockwood et al., 1997). On T1-weighted images, it is common to find abnormally high signals arising in the pallidum. These are seen as whiter-than-normal areas in this portion of the brain, as shown in Fig. 84.1. In addition to these more obvious abnormalities, a systematic analysis of MR images shows that the T1 signal abnormality is widespread and found in the limbic and extrapyramidal systems, and generally throughout the white matter. A generalized shortening of the T2 signal also occurs. These abnormalities have been linked to an increase in the cerebral manganese content. The abnormalities become more prominent with time and regress after successful liver transplantation. The unexpected finding of high T1 signals in the pallidum should suggest the possibility of liver cirrhosis.

Proton MRS techniques also have been applied to the study of patients with cirrhosis and are available in many centers. In the absence of absolute measures that are referable to concentrations, the signal of specific compounds has often been referenced to creatine and expressed as a compound-to-creatine ratio in the past. Irrespective of the use of a quantitative or semi-quantitative approach, there is general agreement among studies that an increase in the intensity of the signal occurs at approximately 2.5 ppm; this is attributed to glutamine plus glutamate (Glx). With high-field-strength magnets, this peak can be resolved into its components; the increase is attributed to glutamine, as expected on the basis of animal investigations. Glx increase is accompanied by a decrease in my-oinositol and choline signals, whereas *N*-acetylaspartate resonances (a neuronal marker) are consistently normal. Correlations between the glutamine concentration, generally considered to be a reflection of exposure of the brain to ammonia, and the severity of the encephalopathy, have led some to propose that MR spectroscopy may be useful in the diagnosis of HE. However, the data currently available are controversial.

Neuroimaging is useful in the diagnosis of coexisting structural lesions of the brain, such as subdural hematomas or other evidence of cerebral trauma, or complications of alcohol abuse or thiamine deficiency, or both, such as midline cerebellar atrophy, third ventricle dilatation, mamillary body atrophy, or high-signal-strength lesions in the periventricular area on T2 fluid-attenuated inversion recovery (FLAIR) images.

It must be emphasized that none of the methods described in this section delivers findings that are specific for HE. Thus, a diagnosis of HE can be made only after exclusion of other possible causes of cerebral dysfunction.

## Pathophysiology

The pathophysiological basis for the development of HE is still not completely known. However, treatment strategies for the disorder are all founded on theoretical pathophysiological mechanisms. A number of hypotheses have been advanced to explain the development of the disorder. Suspected factors include hyperammonemia, altered amino acids and neurotransmitters—especially those related to the γ-aminobutyric acid (GABA)–benzodiazepine complex—mercaptans, short-chain fatty acids, and manganese deposition in the brain. An interaction between hyperammonemia and a systemic pro-inflammatory status is now considered a major cause of HE (Cabrera-Pastor et al., 2019).

## Cerebral Blood Flow and Glucose Metabolism

Whole-brain measurements of cerebral blood flow (CBF) and metabolism are normal in patients with grade 0–1 HE. Reductions occur in more severely affected patients. Sophisticated statistical techniques designed to analyze images have made it possible to identify specific brain regions in which glucose metabolism is abnormal in patients with low-grade encephalopathy and abnormal neuropsychological test scores (Lockwood et al., 2002). These positron emission tomography (PET) data show clearly that minimal forms of HE are caused by the selective impairment of specific neural systems rather than by global cerebral dysfunction. Reductions occur in the cingulate gyrus, an important element in the attentional system of the brain, and in frontal and parietal association cortices. These PET data are in accord with cortical localizations based on the results of neuropsychological tests. Fig. 84.2 shows the results of correlation analyses between scores on selected neuropsychological tests and sites of reduced cerebral glucose metabolism.

## Role of Ammonia

HE is linked to hyperammonemia. Patients with encephalopathy have elevated blood ammonia levels that correlate to a degree with the severity of the encephalopathy. Metabolic products formed from ammonia—most notably glutamine and its transamination product, α-ketoglutaramic acid—also are present in excess in cerebrospinal fluid (CSF) in patients with liver disease. Treatment strategies that lower blood ammonia levels are the cornerstone of therapy.

Tracer studies performed with [$^{13}$N]-ammonia have helped clarify the role of this toxin in the pathophysiology of HE. Ammonia and other toxins are formed in the GI tract and carried to the liver by the hepatic portal vein, where detoxification reactions take place. Portal systemic shunts cause ammonia to bypass the liver and enter the system circulation, where it is transported to the various organs as determined by their blood flow. The liver is the most important organ for the detoxification of ammonia. However, in patients with portacaval shunting of blood, because of the formation of varices, TIPS, or other surgically created shunts, skeletal muscle becomes more important as the fraction of blood bypassing the liver increases. Under the most extreme conditions, muscle becomes the most important organ for ammonia detoxification. It is partly for this reason that nutritional therapy for patients should be designed to prevent development of a catabolic state and muscle wasting.

Ammonia is always extracted by the brain as arterial blood passes through the cerebral capillaries. When ammonia enters the brain, metabolic trapping reactions convert free ammonia into metabolites (Fig. 84.3). The adenosine triphosphate (ATP)–catalyzed glutamine synthetase reaction is the most important of these reactions. The blood-brain barrier is approximately 200 times more permeable to uncharged ammonia gas ($NH_3$) than it is to the ammonium ion ($NH_4^+$); however, because the ionic form is much more abundant than the gas at physiological pH values, substantial amounts of both species appear to cross the blood-brain barrier. Because of this permeability difference and because ammonia is a weak base, relatively small changes in the pH of blood relative to the brain have a significant effect on brain ammonia extraction. As blood becomes more alkalotic, more ammonia is present as the gas and cerebral ammonia extraction increases; however, the role this has in the production of HE is not known. The permeability surface-area (PS) product of the blood-brain barrier may be affected by prolonged liver disease. However, the experimental data about this change are in conflict: one study reported an increase in the PS product, others reported no change (Ahl et al., 2004; Dam et al., 2013; Goldbecker et al., 2010; Keiding et al., 2006; Lockwood et al., 1991).

## Other Pathophysiological Mechanisms

***Astrocyte swelling and the role of concomitant disorders.*** Although there is a strong correlation between the plasma ammonia level and the grade of HE, there is also substantial overlap in ammonia levels by grade of HE, indicating that other factors besides hyperammonemia must play a role in the development of HE. An increase in ammonia detoxification in the brain is associated with an increase of glutamine concentrations within astrocytes and cell swelling. Initially, glutamine is counterbalanced by the release of cellular osmolytes such as myo-inositol to avert cell swelling. If the cells are depleted of myo-inositol, cell swelling can be induced with small amounts of ammonia. Astrocyte swelling may be induced also by inflammatory cytokines, hyponatremia, or benzodiazepines. This is of special interest since HE episodes are frequently precipitated by infection, electrolyte dysbalance, or the application of sedative drugs. Overall, the vulnerability of the brain against these precipitating factors increases with decreasing concentration of intracellular myo-inositol.

Astrocyte swelling is considered a key factor in the pathogenesis of HE (Häussinger and Sies, 2013). It has been shown to trigger multiple alterations of astrocyte function and gene expression. Astrocyte swelling induces the formation of reactive oxygen species and nitrogen oxide. Ammonia has been shown to induce the mitochondrial permeability transition (mPT) probably mediated by oxidative stress. Induction of the mPT leads to a collapse of the mitochondrial inner membrane potential, swelling of the mitochondrial matrix, defective oxidative phosphorylation, cessation of ATP synthesis, and finally the generation of reactive oxygen species. Thus, induction of the mPT is part of the vicious circle of oxidative/nitrosative stress and astrocytic dysfunction (Norenberg et al., 2009). Oxidative stress is closely related

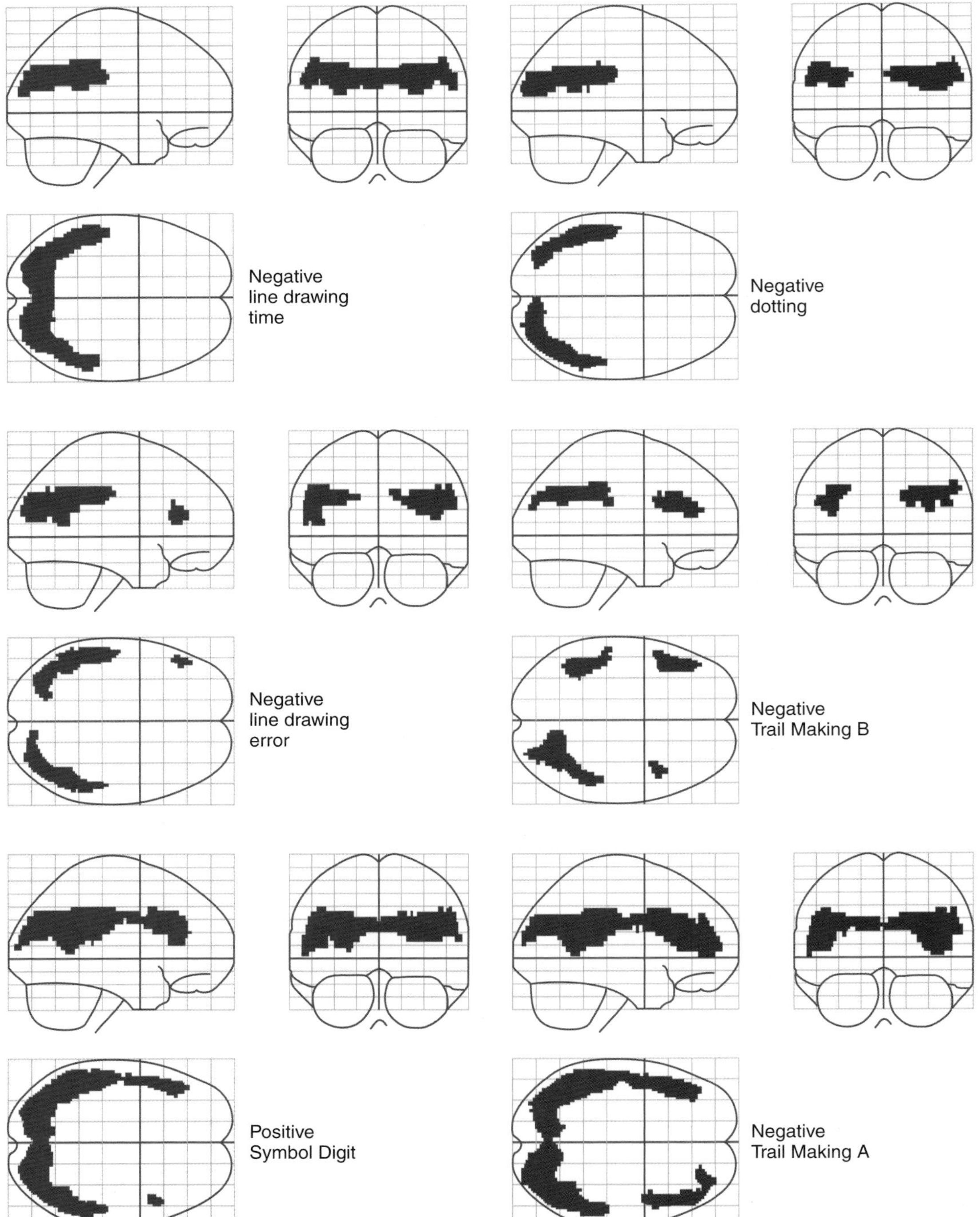


**Fig. 84.2** Correlations between performance in the various subtests of the PSE Syndrome Test, as measured by age-corrected z scores, and cerebral glucose metabolism, as measured by fluorodeoxyglucose-positron emission tomography metabolism. Only those subjects able to complete the test are included in the analyses. The statistical parametric mapping Z image projections show significant correlations with bilateral parietal associative cortex, with increasing correlations with frontal regions. *(Used with permission from Lockwood, A.H., Weissenborn, K., Bokemeyer, M., et al., 2002. Correlations between cerebral glucose metabolism and neuropsychological test performance in nonalcoholic cirrhotics. Metab Brain Dis 17, 29–40.)*

to astrocytic senescence; it has recently been suggested that this plays an important role in the pathophysiology of HE (Görg et al., 2018).

***Abnormalities of neurotransmission.*** Since the early 1970s, a variety of hypotheses have suggested that HE is caused by disordered neurotransmission. Although early hypotheses related to putative false neurotransmitters were disproved, there is still effort in this direction.

As a result of the false neurotransmitter hypothesis, it was shown that the ratio of plasma amino acids (valine + leucine + isoleucine) to (phenylalanine + tyrosine) was abnormal in encephalopathic patients, leading to the development of branched chain amino acid (BCAA) solutions designed to normalize this ratio, which are now commercially available. A meta-analysis of studies analyzing the effects of

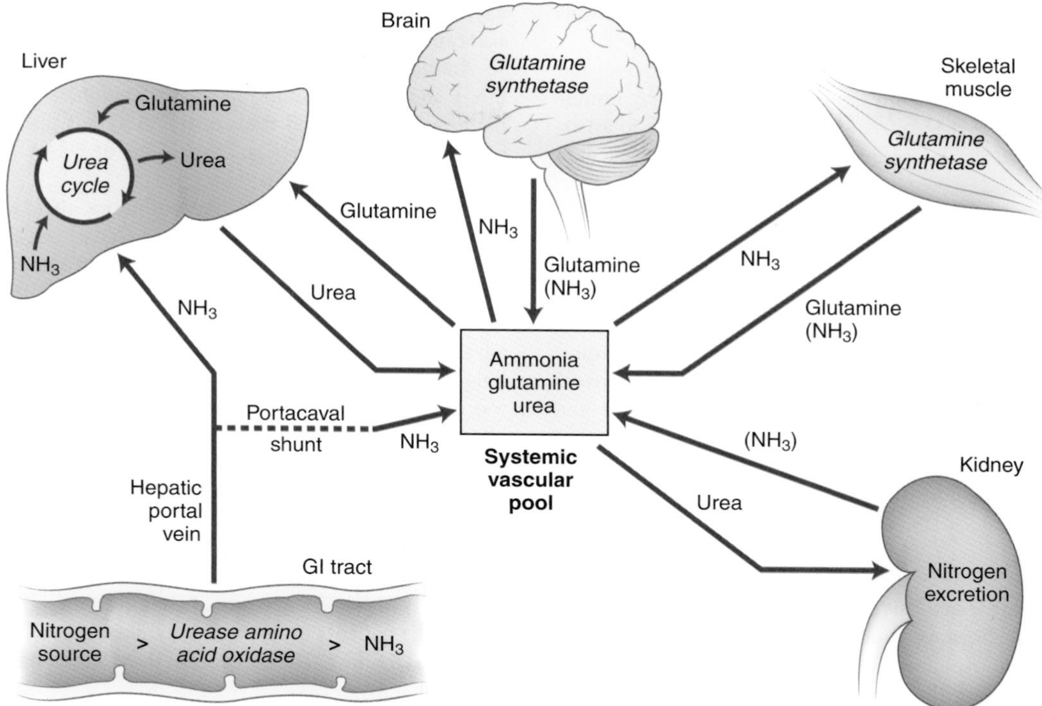


**Fig. 84.3 Human Ammonia Metabolism.** The brain becomes more sensitive to ammonia as time progresses. The reasons for this are largely unknown. In addition, ammonia may cause anorexia by stimulating hypothalamic centers, leading to reductions in muscle mass and an impaired ability of muscle to detoxify ammonia. *GI*, Gastrointestinal. *(Adapted from Lockwood, A.H., McDonald, J.M., Reiman, R.E., et al., 1979. The dynamics of ammonia metabolism in man: effects of liver disease and hyperammonemia. J Clin Invest 63, 449–460.)*

oral or intravenous application of BCAA came to the conclusion that BCAAs have a beneficial effect upon HE, but not upon mortality in patients with liver cirrhosis (Gluud et al., 2017). Substantial effort has been focused on potential abnormalities of the GABA–benzodiazepine complex. Initial attention was directed at GABA itself. However, early reports that GABA concentrations were elevated in patients with encephalopathy have been disproved. Still, a number of anecdotal reports have described dramatic improvements in patients after they were given flumazenil—a benzodiazepine antagonist; very low concentrations of benzodiazepines and their metabolites may be found in blood and CSF of patients with encephalopathy. In controlled studies, patients given flumazenil are more likely to improve than those given placebo. It is unclear whether benzodiazepine displacement is the mechanism because these patients do not usually have clinically significant blood levels of benzodiazepines.

More recent theories have linked the presence of increased expression of peripheral types of benzodiazepine receptors (currently called translocator protein [TSPO]) to HE. These receptors are found on mitochondrial membranes and are implicated in intermediary metabolism and neurosteroid synthesis. Hyperammonemia causes an increase in TSPO and thereby stimulates the production of neurosteroids such as allopregnanolone, which activates GABA and benzodiazepine receptor sites of the GABA-A receptor, resulting in an increase in GABA-ergic tone in the brain.

In addition, there are significant alterations in cerebral serotonin and dopamine metabolism and a reduction in postsynaptic glutamate receptors of the *N*-methyl-D-aspartate type. Thus, there is a substantial interest in the potential role of neurotransmitters in the pathogenesis of HE. As of yet, there is no unifying hypothesis and no rational therapeutic approach based on altering neurotransmission.

***Manganese.*** Blood manganese levels are increased in patients with liver cirrhosis due to an impairment of biliary manganese excretion. Manganese deposition within the brain increases, with predominance in the basal ganglia. These manganese deposits are considered to cause the brain MRI signal alterations in patients with liver cirrhosis. Manganese potentiates the toxic effects of ammonia. Moreover, manganese deposition per se results in neuronal loss, Alzheimer type II astrocytosis, alteration of dopaminergic neurotransmission, and expression of the "peripheral-type" benzodiazepine receptor (TSPO) mentioned earlier (Butterworth, 2010).

## Neuropathology

The Alzheimer type II astrocyte is the neuropathological hallmark of hepatic coma. An account of the original descriptions of this change was provided in translation by Adams and Foley in 1953. In this report, they presented their own findings concerning this astrocyte change in the cerebral cortex and the lenticular, lateral thalamic, dentate, and red nuclei, offering the tentative proposal that the severity of these changes might be correlated with the length of coma. The cause of the astrocyte change was established by studies that reproduced the clinical and pathological characteristics of HE in primates by continuous infusions of ammonia. In studies of rats with portacaval shunts, astrocyte changes become evident after the fifth week. Before coma develops, astrocytic protoplasm increases and endoplasmic reticulum and mitochondria proliferate, suggesting that these are metabolically activated cells. After the production of coma, the more typical signs of the Alzheimer type II change became evident as mitochondrial and nuclear degeneration appeared. Norenberg (1987) suggested that HE is an astrocytic disease, although oligodendroglial cells are affected as well. More recent evidence from his laboratory has shown that ammonia affects a wide variety of astrocytic functions and aquaporin-4.

The neuropathological–neurochemical link between astrocytes and the production of hyperammonemic coma is strengthened by immunohistochemical studies that localized glutamine synthetase to astrocytes and their end-feet. Similar findings for glutamate dehydrogenase have been described.

Long-standing or recurrent HE may lead to the degenerative changes in the brain characteristic of non-Wilson hepatocerebral degeneration. Brains of these patients have polymicrocavitary degenerative changes in layers five and six of the cortex, underlying white matter, basal ganglia, and cerebellum. Intranuclear inclusions that test positive by periodic acid–Schiff are also seen, as are abnormalities in tracts of the spinal cord. More recent histopathological studies showed lymphocyte infiltration in the meninges, microglia activation in the molecular layer, and loss of Purkinje and granular neurons of the cerebellum, already in patients with steatohepatitis grade 1, and increasing glial activation and neuronal loss with progression of the liver disease to cirrhosis (Balzano et al., 2018).

### Treatment

Ideally, the management of cirrhosis should involve a cooperative effort between hepatologists, surgeons, neurologists, and psychologists, with additional input from nurses and dieticians. Practice guidelines published by the European and the American Association for the Study of the Liver (EASL/AASL) recommend a four-pronged approach to management of HE: (1) provision of supportive care, (2) identification and treatment of precipitating factors, (3) search for and treatment of concomitant causes of encephalopathy, and (4) commencement of empirical HE treatment (Vilstrup et al., 2014).

Initial diagnostic and therapeutic efforts should be directed at the identification and mitigation of precipitating factors, and at reducing the nitrogenous load arising from the GI tract. This is accomplished by a brief withdrawal of protein from the diet and the administration of cleansing enemas, followed by the use of lactulose. Antibiotics such as rifaximin, metronidazole, or neomycin may be used as an alternative or add-on to lactulose. Rifaximin has the advantage of showing no systemic side effects (Bass et al., 2010). Oral BCAAs were shown to improve both overt and minimal HE, and thus are a possible add-on therapy if a patient does not respond to conventional therapy. After the acute phase of HE, patients should receive the maximum amount of protein that is tolerated. Prolonged periods of protein restriction should be avoided. Protein is required for the regeneration of hepatocytes and prevention of a catabolic state and muscle wasting.

In patients without overt encephalopathy, diagnostic efforts should be directed toward identifying patients with minimal encephalopathy and monitoring the effects of treatment. Patients with minimal encephalopathy have a diminished quality of life and benefit from therapy, typically lactulose. Follow-up testing is needed to monitor treatment.

***Lactulose.*** Lactulose is a mainstay for the treatment of both acute and chronic forms of HE. It has been used for the treatment of overt HE for decades despite sparse data from randomized placebo-controlled trials. According to a recent Cochrane review, lactulose has a beneficial effect on minimal and overt HE and also may prevent recurrence of HE (Gluud et al., 2016). Lactulose is a synthetic disaccharide metabolized by colonic bacteria to produce acid, and causes an osmotic diarrhea. The effect of lactulose is attributable to its role as a substrate in bacterial metabolism, leading to an assimilation of ammonia by bacteria or reducing deamination of nitrogenous compounds. It is probably the single most important agent in the treatment of acute and chronic encephalopathy. The usual dose of lactulose is 20–30 g, 3 or 4 times a day, or an amount sufficient to produce 2 or 3 stools per day. Lactulose also can be given as an enema.

***Amino acids.*** BCAAs improve skeletal muscular protein synthesis and thereby ammonia detoxification. A meta-analysis of 16 randomized controlled trials of BCAA versus placebo, diet, lactulose or neomycin showed a significant effect of BCAA upon minimal and overt HE (Gluud et al., 2017).

***Antibiotics.*** Nonabsorbable antibiotics such as neomycin were among the initial treatments for HE but have been abandoned because of their nephrotoxicity and ototoxicity. In 2010, the US Food and Drug Administration (FDA) approved the use of oral rifaximin, 550 mg, twice daily "to reduce risk for recurrence of overt HE in patients with advanced liver disease." This nonabsorbable antibiotic had a relatively long history of use for the treatment of traveler's diarrhea. Its efficacy was shown in a multicenter randomized, placebo-controlled, double-blind clinical trial involving 299 patients who were in remission after sustaining at least two episodes of HE (Bass et al., 2010). A breakthrough episode of HE occurred in 22.1% of the patients in the rifaximin group and in 45.9% of the patients in the placebo group, yielding a hazard ratio of 0.42 (95% confidence interval [CI] 0.28–0.64; $P < .001$). There was also a significant reduction in a secondary endpoint, the probability of rehospitalization. It is important to note that more than 90% of the patients in this trial were already receiving and continued to receive lactulose. Thus, rifaximin should be considered as a valuable add-on therapy.

### Complications and Prognosis

Although studies done over 2 decades ago demonstrated that patients with hepatic coma were more likely to survive with minimal residua, this disorder still carries a substantial risk of death. Transplant-free survival at 1 year is less than 50% after an initial episode and less than 25% at 3 years. To aid in the selection of patients for transplantation, a simple rating system or MELD (Model for End-stage Liver Disease) score has been developed and validated to predict mortality. HE has no effect in the selection of patients for transplantation. The MELD score is based on bilirubin, serum creatinine, and the INR. The higher the MELD score, the worse the prognosis. Currently the use of the MELD score is controversial. While the mortality on the waiting list for liver transplantation decreased since introduction of the MELD score as a means for organ allocation, the mortality after transplantation continuously increased.

The incidence of HE is probably underestimated, mainly because neurologists are not usually the primary physicians of these patients, and early subtle signs of cerebral dysfunction may be missed. It is important to establish the diagnosis of HE promptly and proceed with vigorous treatment. HE was considered completely reversible in the past. There is, however, increasing evidence that the recovery may remain incomplete (Bolzano et al., 2018; Campagna et al., 2014). Prolonged or repeated episodes risk transforming this reversible condition into non-Wilson hepatocerebral degeneration, a severe disease with fixed or progressive neurological deficits including dementia, dysarthria, gait ataxia with intention tremor, choreoathetosis, and—most frequently—parkinsonism (Tryc et al., 2013). Other patients may develop evidence of spinal cord damage, usually manifested by a spastic paraplegia. This complication may be a part of the spectrum of hepatocerebral degeneration. Differentiating correctly between early myelopathy or hepatocerebral degeneration and the motor abnormalities that characterize reversible encephalopathy may not always be possible in a first visit but can be done with follow-up examinations.

Patients with HE may develop toxin hypersensitivity, wherein previously innocuous levels of toxins cause symptoms. This concept implies that there may be a steadily increasing risk for developing permanent neurological damage as toxin hypersensitivity evolves.

## Acute Liver Failure

ALF is usually the result of massive necrosis of hepatocytes and is defined as a syndrome in which the signs of encephalopathy develop within up to 3 months after the onset of the symptoms of liver disease in a patient with a previously normal liver. Modern classifications differentiate between hyperacute (HE within 1 week), acute (HE within 4 weeks), and subacute courses (HE develops between 1 and 3 months after the onset of the liver disease). Hyperacute, acute, and subacute ALF differ in regard to etiology and prognosis (Bernal, 2017; Bernal and Wendon, 2013). HE in patients with ALF and HE in patients with cirrhosis share many symptoms. However, due to the different time course and extent of the metabolic alterations, there are some significant differences. In contrast to patients with cirrhosis, patients with ALF frequently develop irritability, agitation, seizures, and brain edema, whereas extrapyramidal and cerebellar symptoms, which are frequent in patients with cirrhosis, are lacking in ALF. In patients with ALF, blood ammonia levels may rise extremely, and have been shown to correlate with intracranial pressure (ICP), severity of clinical presentation, and death by brain herniation (Bernal et al., 2007; Bernal and Wendon, 2013). Recently, it was shown that persistent hyperammonemia above 122 μmol/L for 3 days is accompanied with increased risk of developing brain edema, seizures, and death. Brain edema is present in 25%–35% of patients with grade 3 HE and in 65%–75% of those with grade 4 HE in ALF. According to a retrospective analysis from King's College, London, the percentage of patients with intracranial hypertension significantly decreased between 1973 and 2008 from 76% to 20% (Bernal et al., 2013). Nevertheless, brain edema is one of the leading causes of mortality in ALF, while both diagnosis and treatment are difficult. The diagnosis is impeded by the fact that the patients are intubated and mechanically ventilated, and thus a clinical neurological assessment is impossible. Repeated brain imaging is not feasible. In addition, there is no strong correlation between ICP and CCT results. Therefore, occasionally continuous monitoring of ICP is recommended, but is not without controversy, since these patients with altered hemostasis may develop intracranial hemorrhages. In a series of 324 patients with acute hepatic failure, 28% underwent ICP monitoring. In a subset of these, 10.3% had radiographic evidence of an intracranial hemorrhage, half of which were incidental findings (Vaquero et al., 2005).

Basic treatment of patients with ALF aims to reduce plasma ammonia levels and systemic cytokine levels, and to hold plasma sodium levels within the normal range. Therefore, patients are treated prophylactically with antibiotics as well as early renal support. Of note, lactulose has not shown a significant effect in ALF, neither with regard to plasma ammonia levels nor with survival. Brain edema is treated with mannitol infusion given either every 6 hours (1 g mannitol/kg body weight) or in patients with ICP monitoring as a response to ICP increases above 20–25 mm Hg. A precondition is that serum osmolality is less than 320 mOsm/L and patients have not yet developed acute renal dysfunction. Based on clinical observations, moderate hypothermia (32°C–34°C) has been recommended to reduce ICP in patients with uncontrolled intracranial hypertension who are awaiting emergency liver transplantation. However, a randomized, controlled, multicenter study has not confirmed these observations (Bernal et al., 2016). Besides supportive care, the quick identification of those patients who will need liver transplantation is important. Risk factors considered for this decision are the grade of encephalopathy and coagulopathy, age, bilirubin and creatinine plasma levels, and pH. Substantial research efforts have been devoted to the development of artificial livers or cell-based perfusion systems designed to remove toxins from circulating blood. But none of the systems has shown significant effect on survival (Bernal and Wendon, 2013; Lee, 2012; Shawcross and Wendon, 2012). In contrast, a recent multicenter study showed a significant effect of therapeutic plasma exchange upon liver transplant–free survival (Larsen et al., 2016).

ALF has been described as "metabolic chaos" because of coexisting acid-base, renal, electrolyte, cardiac, and hematological abnormalities, usually culminating in GI bleeding, ascites, sepsis, and often death. Due to continuous improvement in intensive care management and emergency liver transplantation, mortality of ALF decreased from about 80% in the 1970s to currently about 30%–40%.

## Uremic Encephalopathy

Neurological disorders in patients with renal failure may present more problems for the neurologist than are found in patients with failure of other organ systems. This is primarily because of the complexity of the clinical status of many of these patients. Many of the disorders that lead to the development of renal failure (e.g., hypertension, systemic lupus erythematosus, diabetes mellitus) are frequently associated with disorders of the nervous system that are independent of a patient's renal function. Thus it may be difficult to determine whether new neurological problems are caused by the primary disease or by the secondary effects of uremia. Similarly, it is frequently difficult to determine whether neurological problems are the consequence of the progression of renal disease and progressive azotemia, the treatment of renal failure by measures such as dialysis and its associated dysequilibrium and dementia syndromes, or a complication of transplantation and immunosuppression. With increasing numbers of renal transplants and improved treatment designed to prevent rejection, it is likely that the complexity of these issues will continue to increase. For these reasons, good cooperation and communication between neurologists and the nephrologists and transplant teams who care for these patients are important.

Uremic encephalopathy is considered to be caused by uremic toxins, in particular guanidino compounds, that accumulate due to renal dysfunction. These compounds interfere with both glutamatergic and GABA-ergic neurotransmission, finally leading to an enhanced excitability. In addition, disturbance of the dopaminergic neurotransmission has been observed in experimental animals (uremic rats) and was related to impairment of motor activity. Secondary hyperparathyroidism is suggested as leading to increased neuronal calcium levels and neuroexcitation. Experimental studies have shown a doubling of the brain calcium content and serum parathyroid hormone levels within days of the onset of acute renal failure. EEG slowing correlates with elevations in the plasma content of the N-terminal fragment of parathyroid hormone. Treatment with 1,25-dihydroxyvitamin D leads to improvements in the EEG and reductions in N-terminal fragment parathyroid hormone concentrations. Alteration of the blood-brain barrier due to uremia as well as systemic inflammation that accompanies renal failure facilitates access of toxins to the brain (Jabbari and Vaziri, 2018).

Clinical symptoms range from emotional alterations, especially depression, and slight attention and memory deficits to severe alterations of consciousness and cognition, including (mostly agitated) confusion, psychosis, seizures, and coma. Slight neuropsychiatric symptoms are present in about 30% of patients on dialysis therapy. The advanced grades of uremic encephalopathy with confusion or coma are currently predominantly observed in patients in whom a decision has been made not to start dialysis. Action tremor, asterixis, and myoclonus, as well as hyperreflexia, are characteristic features of uremic encephalopathy. Occasionally, choreatic movements have been described. Both asterixis and myoclonus may be provoked by several drugs such as opioids, antiepileptic drugs, phenothiazines, or metoclopramide in patients with impaired renal function due to increased plasma levels.

The diagnosis of uremic encephalopathy is made in the presence of the characteristic symptoms in a patient with severe renal dysfunction after exclusion of other possible causes. The diagnosis is proven if symptoms disappear with successful renal replacement therapy. EEG, CSF, and brain imaging produce unspecific results. The EEG shows a generalized slowing with excess theta and delta activity. Sometimes bilateral spike-wave complexes are found. EEG correlates with clinical findings: with progression of encephalopathy, EEG becomes slower, but normalizes with successful therapy. CSF is often abnormal, and shows increased protein levels (<1 g/L) and a slight pleocytosis (<25 cells/mL). In contrast to patients with liver cirrhosis, in patients with renal dysfunction brain imaging is completely unspecific, showing just a decrease in brain volume.

Uremic encephalopathy can successfully be treated by the initiation of renal replacement therapy. Symptoms usually regress within days or weeks after the initiation of dialysis, but mild symptoms may persist. Successful renal transplantation results in resolution of symptoms within days.

Cognitive dysfunction in patients with end-stage renal disease has several possible causes in addition to the accumulation of uremic toxins; these include chronic renal anemia, hyperparathyroidism, or obstructive sleep apnea (here, independent of a patient's weight!). Improvement of cognitive function can be achieved by increasing a patient's hemoglobin level to about 11–12 mg/dL or treatment of obstructive sleep apnea by using continuous positive airway pressure ventilation, similar to treatment of obstructive sleep apnea in obese patients (Brouns and DeDeyn, 2004; Seifter and Samuels, 2011).

## Twitch-Convulsive Syndrome

The twitch convulsive syndrome was first described by Victor and Adams in 1977. They observed patients with end-stage renal function who showed varying degrees of muscle twitching and fasciculations, arrhythmic tremors, random and asynchronous jerking of the limbs, myoclonus, asterixis, and seizures. The motor symptoms were associated with various degrees of mental dysfunction: some were mentally unaltered, others showed a delirium. Guadino compounds are considered to play a major role in the development of these symptoms. Recently, dexmedetomidine substantially improved the clinical symptoms in a patient with twitch-convulsive syndrome. Dose reduction led to a rapid increase of symptoms (Nomoto et al., 2011).

## Restless Leg Syndrome

With a prevalence of about 68%, restless leg syndrome (RLS) is a frequent attendant phenomenon of renal failure. It is characterized by a need to move the legs, is worsened by periods of inactivity, and can be relieved by walking or stretching. Thus, patients suffer especially during the night. RLS is considered to result from a decrease in dopaminergic modulation of intracortical excitability. Iron deficiency plays a major role in the development of RLS since iron is a cofactor for the enzyme tyrosine hydroxylase, the rate-limiting step in the biosynthesis of dopamine. Accordingly, treatment includes the application of dopamine receptor agonists, L-dopa combined with dopa decarboxylase inhibitors, and the adjustment of any iron deficit. These treatments are often combined with the application of benzodiazepines, opioids, or gabapentin. RLS often persists after the initiation of dialysis therapy, but resolves after kidney transplantation (Seifter and Samuels, 2011).

## Wernicke Encephalopathy

Another possible cause of encephalopathy in hemodialysis patients is thiamine deficiency due to poor intake caused by decreased appetite and increased loss of this water-soluble vitamin in the dialysis procedure. The significance of thiamine deficiency in patients with renal replacement therapy who develop brain dysfunction became evident in a study that showed a 33% prevalence of thiamine deficiency in 30 dialysis patients who presented with clinical symptoms of encephalopathy (Hung et al., 2001).

## Mild Cognitive Impairment/Dementia in Chronic Renal Disease

Several studies provide evidence that patients with chronic renal disease (CRD) develop cognitive dysfunction from mild impairment to frank dementia (Bugnicourt et al., 2013; Elias et al., 2013; Tryc et al., 2011). Since CRD is more frequent with increasing age, most of the studies have been performed in older populations, thus raising the question as to which part of cognitive deterioration is due to CRD and which to age. Considering only studies in patients aged less than 65 years, however, a recent review did show a close correlation between the grade of CRD and the extent of cognitive dysfunction that was independent of age-related changes (Brodski et al., 2019).

The frequency of dementia in patients of old age undergoing dialysis therapy has been estimated as about 4%, with predominance of multi-infarct dementia. Multi-infarct dementia is about 7 times more frequent in dialysis patients than in the general elderly population.

Neuropsychological studies showed alterations especially of attention, concentration, and memory, even in some patients who appeared normal in a clinical examination. Among 374 dialysis patients, 55 years of age or older, who were tested in the domains of memory, executive function, and language, only 12.7% were normal. Almost 14% had mild impairment, 36.1% had moderate impairment, and 37.3% had severe impairment (Murray et al., 2006). ERP studies applying an oddball experiment showed, as in patients with HE, an increase in P300 latency and a decrease in P300 amplitude in patients with chronic kidney disease but no clinical symptoms of brain dysfunction compared to controls. The pathophysiology is multifactorial: uremic toxins, hypertension, microangiopathic lesions, anemia, hyperparathyroidism, and others may play a role.

## Central Nervous System Symptoms Associated with Dialysis Therapy

### Dialysis Dysequilibrium Syndrome

Dialysis dysequilibrium syndrome is especially observed after the initiation of renal replacement therapy. Rapid normalization of electrolytes, urea, and creatinine result in water influx into brain cells because the intracellular osmolyte levels cannot be normalized as fast as the intravascular levels. As a consequence, cerebral edema evolves and presents with headache, nausea, vomiting, confusion, and seizures. The diagnosis of dialysis dysequilibrium syndrome can be made only by exclusion of other possible causes of brain dysfunction. Of special interest are hypertensive encephalopathy (or posterior reversible encephalopathy syndrome [PRES]) and intracranial bleeding as a complication of hypertension and anticoagulation with hemodialysis. Dialysis dysequilibrium syndrome responds to a decrease of dialysis length to 2–3 hours, daily dialysis, and reduced dialysis efficacy (Seifter and Samuels, 2011).

## Dialysis Encephalopathy

Dialysis encephalopathy has been observed, especially with the use of aluminum-containing dialysate and aluminum-based phosphate binders to treat hyperphosphatemia, and thus has been referred to the neurotoxicity of aluminum. Most cases were observed in the 1970s. Dialysis encephalopathy is currently reported only sporadically. Clinical features are dysarthria, aphasia, apraxia, myoclonus, seizures, and cognitive decline.

## METABOLIC DISTURBANCES

### Disorders of Glucose Metabolism

Under normal conditions, glucose is the exclusive fuel for the brain, which unlike other organs such as the liver and skeletal muscle, is able to store only trivial quantities of glucose as glycogen. Because brain glucose concentrations are normally low (i.e., ≈25% of the plasma concentration) and the cerebral metabolic rate for glucose is high, the brain is highly vulnerable to interruptions in the supply of glucose. Hyperglycemia is tolerated by the brain better than hypoglycemia, but it also produces neurological symptoms, largely due to osmotic effects.

#### Physiology

**Glucose homeostasis.** After food is ingested, blood glucose levels begin to climb, which, in concert with a number of complex factors, leads to the release of insulin from the pancreas. Insulin has the combined effects of suppressing hepatic glucose production and fostering the storage of glucose, particularly as glycogen in the liver. After carbohydrate absorption is complete, homeostasis is maintained by hepatic glycogenolysis. The liver normally contains sufficient glycogen stores to maintain the blood glucose concentration at 80–90 mg/dL for 24–36 hours. After this time, gluconeogenesis becomes the principal mechanism for maintaining adequate plasma glucose levels. Alanine and glutamine are the amino acids that, along with lactate and pyruvate, are the most important glucose precursors. Initially, most gluconeogenesis takes place in the liver, but with extended starvation, the kidney begins to produce glucose, accounting for roughly half of the glucose produced. Approximately half of the glucose produced in the postabsorptive state is metabolized by the brain. Because the metabolic processes of glucose homeostasis, including insulin release, glycogen breakdown, and gluconeogenesis, are complex and involve the pancreas, liver, and other organs, it is not surprising that an extensive list of conditions may manifest as hypoglycemia.

**Cerebral glucose metabolism.** Under normal conditions, with a mean CBF of 50 mL/100 g of brain per minute and a glucose concentration of approximately 5 mmol/L, large amounts of glucose are presented to the brain at all times. As blood traverses the cerebral capillary bed, approximately 10% of the glucose is transported across the blood-brain barrier by a glucose transporter enzyme (GLUT1) that exhibits Michaelis–Menten kinetics. GLUT1 further facilitates the glucose uptake into glial cells while the neuronal glucose uptake is mediated by the glucose transporter 3 (GLUT3), which has a higher transport rate than GLUT1 (Mergenthaler et al., 2013). The local glucose utilization rate is driven by functional activity that allows imaging of the cerebral glucose utilization via PET using an $^{18}$F-labeled glucose analog, fluorodeoxyglucose (FDG), to visualize brain regions with increased or decreased neuronal activity.

#### Clinical Aspects of Hypoglycemia

Diagnosing hypoglycemia on the basis of clinical symptoms is fraught with hazards. Although the majority of symptoms are attributable to nervous system dysfunction, they are extremely varied, nonspecific, and not always present even when blood glucose levels are very low. Because of the close link between the symptoms of hypoglycemia and the brain, some authors use the term *neuroglycopenia* to refer to *symptomatic hypoglycemia*. There are three syndromes: acute, subacute, and chronic.

The acute syndrome most commonly develops as the result of the action of insulin preparations or oral antihyperglycemics and begins with vague symptoms of malaise, feeling detached from the environment, restlessness associated with hunger, nervousness that may lead to panic, sweating, and ataxia. Patients may recognize these symptoms. The symptoms respond quickly to oral or parenteral glucose. An EEG performed during this period may reveal nonspecific abnormalities. Attacks may proceed rapidly to generalized seizures and coma, with the attendant risk of permanent brain injury. These patients may arrive in the emergency department in a coma with no history. Of note, hypoglycemia may also mimic stroke, with an acute-onset focal neurological deficit including hemiparesis or aphasia.

The subacute syndrome is the most common form and occurs in the fasting state. Most of the symptoms listed for the acute syndrome are absent. In their place is a slowing of thought processes and a gradual blunting of consciousness with a retention of awareness, although amnesia for the episode is common. The diagnosis may be difficult to establish until the possibility of hypoglycemia is considered or routine testing uncovers the abnormality. Hypothermia is encountered frequently in this form of the disorder, and unexplained low body temperatures always should be followed by a blood glucose measurement.

Chronic hypoglycemia is rare and, if confirmed, suggests a probable insulin-secreting tumor or obsessively good control by a diabetic. This syndrome is characterized by insidious changes in personality, memory, and behavior that may be misconstrued as dementia. Unlike those of the acute and subacute forms of hypoglycemia, these symptoms are not relieved by administering glucose, suggesting the presence of neuronal injury. Clinical improvement after removal of the source of the exogenous insulin is gradual, extending over periods as long as a year.

Diabetics may develop hypoglycemia without being aware of the usual warning symptoms, a condition known as *hypoglycemia unawareness*, which may occur in a complete or partial form in up to 17% of all episodes in patients with type 1 diabetes. The underlying mechanisms appear to be related to the occurrence of prior episodes of hypoglycemia, altered neuroendocrine responses that regulate blood glucose levels, and central nervous system dysfunction that may interfere with symptom detection and analysis. This is supported by studies that show that patients with the syndrome exhibit a reduction in β-adrenergic sensitivity. In these patients, the glucose concentration needed to initiate counter-regulatory hormonal response was lower than normal. Imaging studies using FDG and PET to measure neuronal activity in the subthalamic area, a site implicated as a glucose sensor, showed an abnormal response in patients with symptoms of hypoglycemia unawareness (McCrimmon, 2012).

The presence of the unawareness syndrome poses a special challenge for these patients, their caregivers, and colleagues. Precautions should be taken to minimize the chance that a patient with the syndrome might have a prolonged and unrecognized period of hypoglycemia that could result in permanent injury to the brain; the patient should not be allowed to drive, make critical decisions, and the like while in an impaired state.

Because of the complexity of glucose homeostasis, the causes of hypoglycemia are many and varied, and a detailed discussion is beyond the scope of this chapter. In general, most authors present a physiological classification as shown in Box 84.1.

Drugs are an important cause of hypoglycemia. In some cases, the effect of a drug may be potentiated by a restriction of food intake. Age-varying causes have been found and should aid in the diagnosis of the disorder. Sulfonylureas and oral hypoglycemics dominate in the age group 50 years and older. Alcohol predominates between the ages of 30 and 50 years. Of note, beta-blockade was a factor in masking the symptoms of developing hypoglycemia. The use of beta-blockers in patients receiving insulin or oral hypoglycemic agents therefore should be avoided. A number of risk factors have been recognized that predispose to the development of hypoglycemia. These include (in addition to diabetes) decreased caloric intake (usually related to severity of some illness or disruption of dietary routines), uremia, liver disease, infection, shock, pregnancy, neoplasia, and burns.

Hypoglycemia is associated with a substantial morbidity. A study of 600 patients with diabetes showed that the frequency of severe hypoglycemia was 1.60 episodes per patient per year and that it occurred twice as

**BOX 84.1 Causes of Hypoglycemia**

**Postprandial Hypoglycemia (Reactive)**
Postoperative rapid gastric emptying (alimentary hyperinsulinism)
Fructose intolerance
Galactosemia
Leucine intolerance
Idiopathic

**Fasting Hypoglycemia**
Overuse of glucose
Elevated insulin levels
Exogenous insulin (therapeutic, factitious)
Oral hypoglycemic (therapeutic, factitious)
Islet cell disorders (adenoma, nesidioblastosis, cancer)
Excessive islet cell function (prediabetes, obesity)
Antibodies to endogenous insulin
Normal to low insulin levels
Ketotic hypoglycemia
Hypermetabolic state (sepsis)
Rare extrapancreatic tumors
Carnitine deficiency

**Underproduction of Glucose**
Hormone deficiencies (growth hormone, glucagon, hypoadrenalism)
Enzyme disorders
Glycogen metabolism (glycogen phosphorylase, glycogen synthetase)
Hexose metabolism (glucose-6-phosphatase, fructose-1,6-biphosphatase)
Glycolysis, Krebs cycle (phosphoenolpyruvate carboxykinase, pyruvate carboxylase, malate dehydrogenase)
Alcohol and probably other drugs
Liver disease (cirrhosis, fulminant hepatic failure)
Severe malnutrition

often in patients with the type 1 form of the disorder. The risk of severe hypoglycemia episodes increases with the duration of the disease. Among patients with severe episodes of hypoglycemia, injuries and convulsions occurred at rates of 0.04 and 0.02 episodes per patient per year, respectively. Five patients had automobile accidents caused by hypoglycemia. But, in general, patients with diabetes are not more prone to automobile accidents than subjects without diabetes. Patients with episodes of severe hypoglycemia were more likely to have had prior severe episodes, were on insulin longer, and had lower hemoglobin $A_{1c}$ concentrations. A southern California medical examiner found 123 deaths caused by hypoglycemia in a series of 54,850 autopsies. According to data from the Diabetes Control and Complications Trial (DCCT) more than half of the hypoglycemia episodes occur during the night (Diabetes Control and Complications Trial Research Group, 1997). Recently the dead-in-bed syndrome—a term used to describe the sudden unexplained deaths of young people with type 1 diabetes—could be related to hypoglycemia-related autonomic failure.

Hypoglycemia is a medical emergency, and this diagnosis should be considered among virtually all patients with an altered mental status of unknown cause. Most of these patients should be treated with parenteral glucose after adequate blood samples are obtained for laboratory testing. It is prudent to draw extra blood so that insulin, C-peptide, and hemoglobin $A_{1c}$ levels can be measured if indicated by the patient's subsequent course. These measures are particularly important in patients with obscure histories and in whom factitious hypoglycemia may be present.

## Clinical Aspects of Hyperglycemia

Although there are many causes of hyperglycemia, diabetic ketoacidosis (DKA), nonketotic hyperosmolar coma, and iatrogenic factors such as parenteral hyperalimentation are the most important. DKA is a relatively common disorder, predominantly affecting patients with type 1 diabetes. It is frequently precipitated by an infectious process in a patient who has been otherwise stable, develops over several days, and is heralded by polyuria and polydipsia caused by the osmotic diuresis produced by glucosuria. These symptoms are followed by anorexia, nausea, disorientation, and coma. On physical examination, sustained hyperventilation is common, especially in patients with severe acidosis. The diagnosis is frequently suspected on the basis of clinical findings, but laboratory data including the plasma glucose, arterial blood gases, electrolytes, and an appropriate test for ketone bodies are essential for confirming the diagnosis and management.

In contrast, nonketotic hyperosmolar coma—currently also called hyperosmolar hyperglycemic state—is a feature of type 2 diabetes and is thus encountered in older patients, commonly as the first manifestation of the disease. This syndrome evolves more slowly than DKA, and the period of polyuria is more prolonged, leading to much more severe dehydration. Because glucose is a less effective dipsogen than other solutes, water-seeking behavior is not as strong in this group of patients as it is in patients with hypernatremic hyperosmolality, thus promoting the development of dehydration. The disorder's signs and symptoms are those of hyperosmolality, hypovolemia, and cerebral dysfunction, with epileptic seizures occurring in some individuals. Precipitating factors include infection, gastroenteritis, pancreatitis, and occasionally, treatment with glucocorticoids or phenytoin. Because many total parenteral nutrition protocols use solutions with high glucose contents, hyperglycemia is a potential complication of their use.

DKA is an insulin-deficient state, and insulin is the cornerstone of therapy. In the absence of insulin, peripheral glucose uptake and glycogen formation are reduced, and glycogenolysis and lipolysis are accelerated, leading to the formation of acidic ketone bodies and hyperglycemia. When plasma glucose levels exceed the renal threshold (usually approximately 180 mg/dL), glucosuria and a forced osmotic diuresis ensue. The treatment of DKA is designed to reverse these pathophysiological abnormalities and consists of administering insulin to enhance glucose uptake, enhance glycogen formation by noncerebral tissues, and reduce the rate of ketone body formation occurring during low-insulin, high-glucagon states that promote the entry of fatty acids into mitochondria, where they are converted to ketones. Usually a bolus of 0.1 U insulin/kg bodyweight (BW) is applied followed by a continuous infusion of 0.1 U/kg BW/h until blood glucose levels are below 200 mg/dL. Thereafter the insulin rate may be decreased (minimum 0.5 U/h) but should be adjusted to maintain a plasma glucose level of 150–200 mg/dL until ketoacidosis is resolved. Intravenous insulin application must not be stopped before normalization of the anion gap (Echouffo-Tcheugui and Garg, 2017). Acidosis (pH $< 7.0$) should be treated with 50–100 mmol sodium bicarbonate. Replacing fluid and electrolytes is also required, as is treatment of precipitating factors. It is important to remember that overly vigorous treatment with rapid restoration of plasma osmolality to normal levels can lead to the development of cerebral edema (see Complications of Treatment, next section) (Nyenwe and Kitabchi, 2011).

Neurologists may become involved in the diagnosis and management of nonketotic hyperosmolar coma when a patient is brought to the emergency department with unexplained coma or seizures. Alterations of consciousness, seizures, and focal neurological deficits are more frequent in patients with nonketotic hyperosmolar coma than in those with DKA. Neurologists should be aware that stroke might accompany a nonketotic hyperosmolar coma, either as a complication due to the procoagulant status or as precipitant. Two characteristic, though rare, complications of the nonketotic hyperosmolar state are epilepsia partialis continua (Kojewnikow's syndrome) and hemichorea.

Because hyperosmolality and the associated hypovolemia are usually much more severe in this condition than in DKA, maintaining an adequate blood pressure and cardiac output are the first priorities in treatment. One liter of normal saline per hour should be given during the first 3 hours to restore blood volume and to begin to reduce plasma osmolality. If serum sodium levels are above 150 mmol/L, 1–2 L 0.45% saline solution should be given, followed thereafter by 5% glucose solution. Glucose 5% should be used as soon as the blood glucose levels are lower than 11.2 mmol/L. Insulin therapy follows the same rules as in DKA, while the insulin infusion rate can be decreased in patients with hyperosmolar coma when plasma glucose is lower than 300 mg/dL. Blood glucose levels should not decrease more than 100 mg/dL/h; the optimum would be 50 mg/dL/h. In addition, blood glucose levels should be maintained between 10 and 15 mmol/L for the first 24 hours after initiation of treatment. If serum potassium levels are 3.5–5.5 mmol/L, 20 mmol potassium chloride should be added to every liter of the infusion, and 40 mmol if serum levels are below 3.5 mmol/L. Recent Joint British Diabetes Societies guidelines even recommend initiation of hyperglycemic hyperosmolar status treatment with fluid replacement, exclusively, while low-dose intravenous insulin (0.05 units/kg/h) is advocated only if significant ketonemia (3-hydroxybutyrate >1 mmol/L) or ketonuria (>2+) is seen at presentation or if plasma glucose is falling at a rate of less than 5 mmol/h (90 mg/dL) despite adequate fluid replacement (Gouveia and Chowdhury, 2013).

The patients may require intensive monitoring with arterial and central venous catheters to monitor the circulatory system status and avoid inducing a volume overload. The exact mechanisms leading to the development of the syndrome, particularly the absence of ketosis, are not fully explained.

### Complications of Treatment

Although treatment of DKA has improved, the mortality rate is still appreciable. Among adults, the mortality rate of DKA is estimated as about 1%. However, DKA remains a leading cause of mortality in children and young adults with type 1 diabetes. The majority of patients who succumb do so because of cardiovascular collapse or from complications of the precipitating factor. A small number of patients die unexpectedly when laboratory and clinical indicators all show initial improvement.

Clinically, patients with DKA who die experience rapid neurological then cardiovascular deterioration. Postmortem examinations of the brain show lesions similar to those seen in acute asphyxia, including capillary dilation with perivascular and pericellular edema. Death is heralded by a rapid evolution of signs and symptoms indicating an increase in ICP. About half of patients die during the initial episode of DKA. The rate and degree to which the plasma glucose level is lowered is not a major risk factor for death.

Some degree of cerebral edema attends the treatment of most patients with DKA, occasionally to the high level of 600 mm $H_2O$ CSF pressure, as shown in Fig. 84.4.

The data suggest that at least mild clinically silent cerebral swelling may be much more common than is realized in cases of DKA. Rare unknown factors appear to trigger a malignant increase in ICP in a small number of patients. Published experience suggests that if this diagnosis is made, prompt aggressive treatment of cerebral edema is indicated, preferably using ICP monitoring as a guide to therapy. Nevertheless, the associated mortality rate is high.

The estimated mortality rate in patients with nonketotic hyperosmolar coma, ranging between 5% and 20%, is much higher than that of DKA. This difference is partially due to affected patients being older and with comorbid conditions that contribute to volume depletion more often than those with DKA. Available evidence suggests that hyperglycemic emergencies are associated with an inflammatory and procoagulant state, which both contribute to an increased risk of thrombotic complications. Thus, heparin should be administered subcutaneously for prophylaxis of thrombosis.

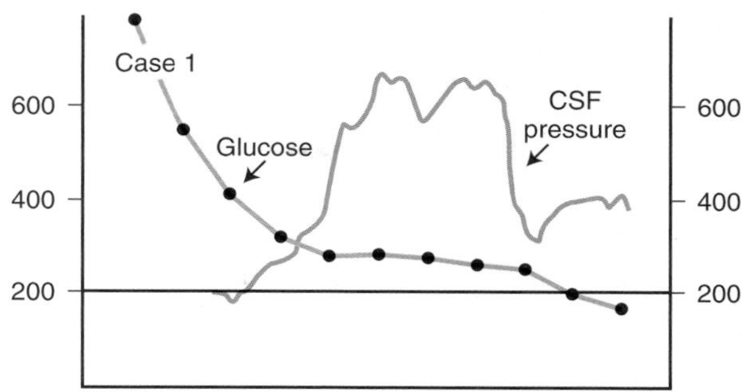


**Fig. 84.4 Blood Glucose and Intracranial Pressure During Treatment of Diabetic Ketoacidosis.** The untreated hyperosmolar state leads to the intracerebral accumulation of idiogenic osmoles. As blood glucose and osmolality levels decrease during treatment, free water enters the brain more rapidly than idiogenic osmoles are shed, leading to an increase in intracranial pressure from the swollen brain. This mechanism presumably operates in all cases in which hyperosmolality is corrected rapidly. *CSF,* Cerebrospinal fluid. *(Reprinted with permission from Clements, R.S. Jr., Blumenthal, S.A., Morrison, A.D., et al., 1971. Increased cerebrospinal fluid pressure during treatment of diabetic ketoses. Lancet 2, 671–675.)*

## Disorders of Water and Electrolyte Metabolism

Patients with abnormalities of water and electrolyte metabolism frequently exhibit signs and symptoms of cerebral dysfunction. Typically these patients have altered states of consciousness or epileptic seizures that herald the onset of the abnormality. The vulnerability of the nervous system to abnormalities of water and electrolyte balance arises from changes in brain volume, especially the brain swelling that may be associated with water intoxication. The role played by electrolytes is also important in maintaining transmembrane potentials, neurotransmission, and a variety of metabolic reactions. Although most clinicians are aware of the importance of water and electrolyte disturbances as a cause of brain dysfunction, the importance of the brain in the control of water and electrolytes is less well appreciated. Excellent reviews of these disorders have been written by Adrogué and Madias (2000a, 2000b, 2012, 2014).

### Disordered Osmolality

***Osmotic homeostasis.*** Serum osmolality, and hence whole-body osmolality, are regulated by complex neuroendocrine and renal interactions that control thirst and water and electrolyte balance. When serum osmolality increases, the brain loses volume; when osmolality falls, the brain swells. Events related to water loss are illustrated in Fig. 84.5. The brain has little protection in terms of volume changes when osmotic stress is acute. Examples of acute osmotic stress may be found in patients with heatstroke, inadvertent solute ingestion (particularly in infants), massive ingestion of water (which may be psychogenic), hemodialysis, and diabetics with nonketotic coma. Recent reports also suggest that excessive water consumption occurs in some marathon runners, leading to acute water intoxication. When osmotic stress is applied more slowly over a longer period, the predicted volume changes are smaller than would be expected. The mechanisms that underlie these protective adaptations are not known completely but involve the gain of amino acids in the case of the hyperosmolar state and the loss of potassium in the hypo-osmolar state. Experimental studies have failed to identify all of the osmotically active particles that must exist in the brain after a given osmotic stress is applied. These unidentified molecules are called *idiogenic osmoles.*

***Hypo-osmolality and hyponatremia.*** Hypo-osmolality is almost always associated with hyponatremia. The diagnosis usually is made by

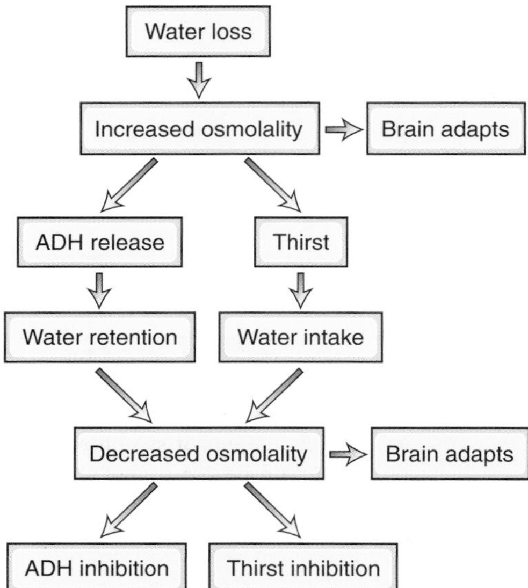


**Fig. 84.5 Water Balance and the Brain.** A reduction in water (or an increase in water loss or solute gain) stimulates thirst and vasopressin release, leading to increased water conservation and intake, which in turn reduces vasopressin levels and ends thirst. Excessive water intake or excessive water loss leads to hypo-osmolality or hyperosmolality and the loss or gain of osmotically active particles in the brain, respectively. Excessively rapid treatment of these conditions may lead to the development of neurological symptoms. *ADH*, Antidiuretic hormone.

laboratory testing. Conditions associated with hyponatremia are shown in Box 84.2. When hyponatremia is encountered, a measurement of serum osmolality should be performed to differentiate true from pseudo hypo-osmolality, which may be encountered in patients with lipidemic serum or in neurological patients treated with mannitol.

Elevated osmolality may be encountered in patients with hyponatremia due to elevated urea or ethanol concentrations who are subject to the same risks as patients with hyponatremia associated with reduced osmolality.

A large and diverse group of neurological conditions is associated with hyponatremia as a result of syndrome of inappropriate antidiuretic hormone secretion (SIADH), as shown in Box 84.3. SIADH is characterized by hyponatremia in the face of normal or increased blood volume, normal renal function, and the absence of factors that normally operate to produce antidiuretic hormone (ADH) release. The syndrome may be relatively asymptomatic, in which case water restriction is the treatment of choice. In more severe cases, hypertonic saline combined with a diuretic may be required. Overly zealous treatment may produce central pontine myelinolysis (see the upcoming section, Therapy). Chronic syndromes have been treated successfully with a variety of drugs including the tetracycline demeclocycline, which interferes with the action of ADH on the renal tubules.

Great care must be taken when considering the diagnosis of SIADH in patients with subarachnoid hemorrhage. Patients with subarachnoid hemorrhage, hyponatremia, and reduced blood volume may not have true SIADH. In these patients, fluid restriction may lead to further volume reduction and cerebral infarcts during the period of the highest risk for vasospasm. The mechanisms underlying this phenomenon are unclear but may be related to the complexity of the peptidergic neurotransmitter systems in the vicinity of the third ventricle and to the possibility that they are damaged by the ruptured aneurysm. Damage is especially likely with an aneurysm on the anterior communicating artery.

Hyponatremia occurs in approximately 1% of patients with recent surgical procedures. Because the symptoms are frequently mild or

## BOX 84.2 Causes of Hyponatremia

**Combined Water and Sodium Depletion (Hypovolemia)**

***Renal Loss***

Primary renal disease
Osmotic diuresis (glucose, mannitol)
Adrenal insufficiency

***Nonrenal Loss***

Gastrointestinal (diarrhea, suction, vomiting)
Transcutaneous (sweating, burns)
Sequestration (ascites, peritonitis)

***Hyponatremia without Water Loss***

Edema with water and sodium retention
Dilutional (iatrogenic, psychogenic)
Sick cell syndrome
Hyperosmotic (hyperglycemia or mannitol administration)
Syndrome of inappropriate antidiuretic hormone secretion
Artifact (laboratory error, hyperlipidemia)

attributed to the surgery itself, this diagnosis may be missed. Typically, these patients seem to do well in the immediate postoperative period and then develop symptoms and signs of encephalopathy. Men and postmenopausal women are less likely to develop postoperative hyponatremia than women who are still menstruating. Complications such as respiratory arrest are particularly likely to occur more frequently in menstruating women than in men or menopausal women. Thus, it is important to be particularly vigilant when evaluating younger women with postoperative encephalopathy.

***Clinical features.*** The signs and symptoms of deranged osmolality depend on the severity of the disturbance and the length of time elapsed between onset and clinical presentation. Often these syndromes are of insidious onset. Typical complaints are nonspecific and include malaise, nausea, and lethargy, leading to obtundation and coma. Headache due to brain swelling, and epileptic seizures may be encountered in patients with hyponatremia, especially in patients with an acute alteration of serum sodium levels, as for example in patients with psychosis, Ecstasy use, or in patients with postoperative intravenous fluid application. Although serum sodium levels below 120 mmol/L are considered serious, patients who develop this level of hyponatremia as a side effect of diuretics or antiepileptic treatment over a long period of time may present with only minor, if any, symptoms. Minor symptoms include dizziness, cognitive dysfunction, gait disturbances, and falls. Since, in these chronic states of hyponatremia, the brain can counteract cell swelling by release of endogenous osmolytes, severe symptoms often occur only after serum sodium levels have decreased below 110 mmol/L. However, patients in whom serum sodium levels decrease within a short time interval due to an acute overload of total body water are prone to develop brain edema, alterations of consciousness, and seizures. Children and young women are particularly vulnerable to hyponatremic brain damage. Of note, brain adaptation to low serum sodium levels increases the risk of osmotic demyelination after rapid resolution of hyponatremia. Symptoms of the osmotic demyelination syndrome (ODS) occur several days after successful treatment of hyponatremic encephalopathy. Characteristic are seizures, behavioral disturbances, swallowing dysfunction, dysarthria, paralysis, or movement disorders. Cerebral MRI may show demyelination in the pons or symmetrically extra-pontine in the white matter. The extent of MRI lesions, however, does not correlate with the severity of clinical symptoms.

**BOX 84.3 Causes of the Syndrome of Inappropriate Antidiuretic Hormone Secretion**

**Malignant Neoplasms**
Small cell carcinoma of lung
Pancreatic tumors
Thymoma
Mesothelioma
Lymphoma (lymphosarcoma, reticulum cell sarcoma, Hodgkin disease)
Bladder, ureter, prostate tumors
Duodenal tumors
Ewing sarcoma

**Central Nervous System Disorders**
Infections (meningitis, encephalitis, abscess, Rocky Mountain spotted fever)
Trauma
Subarachnoid hemorrhage
Infarction
Guillain-Barré syndrome
Acute intermittent porphyria
Hydrocephalus
Neonatal hypoxia
Shy-Drager syndrome
Delirium tremens
Systemic lupus erythematosus

**Drugs**
Vasopressin
Oxytocin
Vinca alkaloids
Thiazides
Chlorpropamide
Phenothiazines
Carbamazepine
Clofibrate
Nicotine
Monoamine oxidase inhibitors
Tricyclic antidepressants
Cyclophosphamide
Narcotics

**Pulmonary Diseases**
Tuberculosis
Other pneumonias
Abscess or cavity
Empyema
Cystic fibrosis
Obstructive airway disease
Pneumothorax
Asthma
Positive pressure ventilation

**Miscellaneous Causes**
Hypothyroidism
Acute psychosis
Postoperative state
Idiopathic

Of note, rapid correction of hyponatremia is not the only known cause of pontine myelinolysis (ODS). Other possible causes include hypernatremia, severe hyperglycemia, malignancy, hyperammonemia, or alterations of serum potassium levels. Patients after liver transplant seem especially at risk to develop ODS.

***Therapy.*** Current European and US guidelines recommend slow correction of hyponatremia in patients who developed the electrolyte imbalance in an interval of more than 48 hours, but a more rapid correction in case of acute water intoxication. In acute hyponatremia a rapid correction by about 4–6 mmol/L is considered both effective in regard to counteracting osmotic brain swelling and safe in regard to the risk of osmotic demyelination. Fortunately, both death from cerebral edema as well as osmotic demyelination are rare complications of hyponatremia. However, the risk increases with extremely low serum sodium levels. Fifty percent of rapidly corrected patients develop osmotic demyelination if their serum sodium levels at baseline were lower than 105 mmol/L. The preferred therapy for hyponatremia might be water restriction and discontinuing diuretics if patients show only slight if any symptoms.

The recommendations for treatment of symptomatic hyponatremia differ slightly between the European and the US guidelines. The former differentiate between severely and moderately symptomatic cases and recommend infusion of two 150-mL boluses of 3% saline, measuring serum sodium levels in between for severely symptomatic hyponatremia, and repeating this treatment until the serum sodium level has increased by 5 mmol/L. In case of moderately severe symptoms a single 150-mL infusion of 3% saline is recommended. The US experts recommend an infusion of 100 mL of 3% saline up to 3 times if needed in case of severe symptoms such as seizures and coma and in case of acute water intoxication. In patients with mild to moderate symptoms, 3% saline at 0.5–2 mL/kg per hour to correct by 4–6 mmol/L is recommended. Caution is recommended in patients with hypovolemic hyponatremia. Correction of hypovolemia may induce brisk water diuresis and then lead to rapid sodium correction. The limits for sodium level correction are 10 mmol/L within the first 24 hours, and 8 mmol/L/day thereafter in the European guidelines while the American guidelines set a daily 4–6 mmol/L goal and a limit of 8 mmol/L per day for patients with high risk to develop ODS, and a daily correction goal of 4–8 mmol/L for those with low risk

In patients with euvolemic or hypervolemic hyponatremia, vaptans, which antagonize the effect of vasopressin, thereby promoting aquaresis, can be administered.

Sodium replacement cannot be done without considering potassium levels. Replacement of 1 mmol/L potassium affects serum sodium levels as much as 1 mEq of retained sodium.

The effect of a given infusate on the serum sodium concentration can be estimated from the formula $\Delta Na^+$ in serum = $[Na^+ + K^+]$ in infusion—$[Na^+]$ in serum/total body water +1, where total body water is calculated as fraction of body weight. This fraction is 0.6 in children, 0.55 in men, and 0.5 in women. In case of substantial ongoing fluid loss, it is recommended to combine this formula with the so-called fluid loss formula (see Adrogué and Madias, 2012). In case of severe symptomatic hyponatremia, continuous monitoring of vital signs and repeated measurement (every 2 hours) of the electrolyte levels are mandatory. Overcorrection of the serum sodium level should be treated by prompt administration of 5% glucose solution.

***Hyperosmolality.*** Hyperosmolality is less common than hypo-osmolality but may manifest with similar symptoms or evidence of intracranial bleeding caused by the tearing of veins that bridge the space between the brain and dural sinuses. Usually, hyperosmolality is diagnosed by laboratory findings of an elevated serum sodium level or, perhaps more commonly, hyperglycemia in diabetics. The syndrome frequently is caused by dehydration (especially in hot climates), by uncontrolled diabetes with or without ketosis, and (less frequently) by central lesions that reset the osmotically sensitive regions of the brain. As with hypo-osmolality, cautious correction of the defect is important. Replacement should be given orally if possible. Treatment is based on the answers to two questions: What is the water deficit?

How rapidly should it be corrected? The deficit can be computed for adults from the equation deficit = current body water ($Na^+/140 - 1$). Current body water can be estimated as ranging from 50% to 60% of the lean body weight. A safety factor of 10% has been suggested; therefore, current body water should be taken as about 45% of the lean body weight. Thus, a 70-kg person with a sodium concentration of 160 mEq/L would require about 4.5 L of free water.

Chronic hyperosmolality is associated with relative brain volume preservation as a result of the production of idiogenic osmoles, as described earlier. Administering free water at a rate that exceeds the rate at which the brain is able to rid itself of idiogenic osmoles is associated with the development of paradoxical brain edema that occurs at a time when serum glucose and electrolyte concentrations are normalized. This is illustrated by the data in Fig. 84.4, in which the CSF pressure was measured continuously as hyperglycemia due to diabetes mellitus was corrected. The increase in ICP is undoubtedly caused by adapted brain cells imbibing free water as serum osmolality decreases in response to therapy. If patients undergoing treatment for hyperosmolar states develop new neurological signs, including altered consciousness and seizures, the diagnosis of brain swelling should be considered. Mannitol treatment to restore osmolality to the prior elevated level may be required to prevent death due to brain swelling.

To avoid the production of brain edema, seizures, and other complications, the rate of correction should not exceed 0.5 mmol/L in any given hour, and no more than 10 mmol/L/day.

## Disorders of Calcium Metabolism

Hypercalcemia and hypocalcemia both have diverse causes associated with disordered parathyroid gland function and a variety of other conditions. In normal circumstances, approximately half of the total serum calcium is bound to proteins, mainly albumin, and half is in the ionized form, the only form in which it is active. When there is doubt about the $Ca^{2+}$ concentration, as in patients with hypoalbuminemia, direct measurement of $Ca^{2+}$ with ion-sensitive electrodes may be required.

Hypercalcemia is associated with hyperparathyroidism, granulomatous diseases (especially sarcoidosis), treatment with drugs including thiazide diuretics, vitamin D, calcium itself, tumors that have metastasized to bone, and thyroid disease. Many cases are idiopathic.

The symptoms and signs of hypercalcemia may be protean. Severe hypercalcemia affects the brain directly, causing coma in extreme cases. In this group of patients, metastatic tumors are common, especially multiple myeloma and tumors of the breast and lung. Cancer patients seem to be particularly vulnerable to developing hypercalcemia after a change in therapy. Less severe hypercalcemia may cause altered consciousness, with a pseudodementia syndrome and weakness. GI, renal, and cardiovascular abnormalities also may be present.

Severe hypercalcemia is life threatening. Initial treatment consists of a forced diuresis using saline and diuretics. Because the volumes of saline that are required may be large, a central venous or Swan-Ganz catheter may be needed to monitor therapy. Once the initial phase of treatment is accomplished, further management is determined by the cause of the hypercalcemia.

Hypocalcemia usually is associated with hypoparathyroidism. The neurological symptoms are attributable to the enhanced excitability of the nervous system. Symptoms include paresthesias around the mouth and fingers, cramps caused by tetanic muscle contraction, and in more extreme cases, epileptic seizures. In more chronic hypocalcemia, headache secondary to increased ICP may occur, and extrapyramidal signs and symptoms such as chorea or parkinsonism may be encountered. These patients may have calcification of the basal ganglia, evident on computed tomography of the brain. The physical examination should include attempts to elicit Chvostek and Trousseau signs. Cataracts and papilledema may be seen.

Severe hypocalcemia should be treated with infusions of calcium to treat or prevent epileptic seizures or laryngeal spasms, both of which are life-threatening but unusual complications. Chronic therapy usually involves administration of calcium and vitamin D. Care must be taken to avoid hypercalcemia and hypercalciuria. Consultation with an endocrinologist is prudent, but continued neurological care may be necessary, especially in patients with extrapyramidal syndromes, who may require specific treatment.

## Disorders of Magnesium Metabolism

Hypermagnesemia is an unusual condition because of the ease with which normal kidneys act to preserve magnesium homeostasis. Hypermagnesemia is most commonly due to infusions given to treat blood pressure and nervous system dysfunction in patients with eclampsia. Care must be observed in administering magnesium to patients with renal failure. This group of patients is the most vulnerable and the most likely to develop hypermagnesemia because the kidneys' homeostatic function is impaired. Hypocalcemia potentiates the effects of excess magnesium. Severe hypermagnesemia is life threatening, and concentrations in excess of 10 mEq/L must be treated. Discontinuation of magnesium preparations usually suffices. When cardiac arrhythmias are present or circulatory collapse is possible, calcium must be infused, especially when hypocalcemia is present.

Isolated hypomagnesemia is unusual. Magnesium deficiency usually occurs in patients with deficiencies of other electrolytes. Hypomagnesemia may result from a diet deficient in magnesium, including prolonged parenteral alimentation with insufficient or no magnesium replacement, malabsorption, and alcoholism. Excess magnesium loss from the GI tract or the kidneys may also lead to calcium deficiency. Magnesium deficiency is usually part of a complex electrolyte imbalance, and accurate diagnosis and management of all aspects of the state are necessary to ensure recovery.

Pure magnesium deficiency has been produced experimentally and is expressed primarily through secondary reductions in serum calcium levels despite adequate dietary calcium intake. Ultimately, anorexia, nausea, a positive Trousseau sign, weakness, lethargy, and tremor develop but are rapidly abolished by magnesium repletion. Balance studies indicate that magnesium deficiency causes a positive sodium and calcium balance and a negative potassium balance. Magnesium is necessary for proper mobilization and homeostasis of calcium and the intracellular retention of potassium. Some of the effects of magnesium depletion are secondary to abnormalities of potassium and calcium metabolism.

## Disorders of Manganese Metabolism

Manganese poisoning occurs primarily in manganese ore miners and causes parkinsonism. As presented in the Hepatic Encephalopathy section, there is increasing evidence that accumulation of this metal in the brain causes hyperintensities on T1-weighted MRI and may be associated with disorders of dopaminergic neurotransmission.

*The complete reference list is available online at https://expertconsult.inkling.com/.* 

85

# Deficiency Diseases of the Nervous System

Yuen T. So

## OUTLINE



Malnutrition causes a wide spectrum of neurological disorders (Table 85.1). Despite socioeconomic advances, nutritional deficiency diseases such as kwashiorkor and marasmus are still endemic in many underdeveloped countries. The problem in Western countries is usually the result of dietary insufficiency from chronic alcoholism or malabsorption due to gastrointestinal (GI) diseases. Bariatric surgery has become an important risk factor of malabsorption due to its increased use in the treatment of obesity.

Individual vitamin requirements are influenced by many factors. The daily need for thiamine and nicotinic acid, important compounds in energy metabolism, increases proportionally with increasing caloric intake and energy need. For example, symptoms of thiamine deficiency may occur in at-risk patients during periods of vigorous exercise and high carbohydrate intake. Other factors such as growth, infection, and pregnancy may also worsen deficiency states.

## COBALAMIN (VITAMIN $B_{12}$)

The terms *vitamin $B_{12}$* and *cobalamin* are used interchangeably in the literature. Cobalamins are abundant in meat, fish, dairy, and other animal byproducts. Vegetables generally contain only trace amounts of cobalamin (Watanabe, 2014). Although only 1 μg/day of cobalamin is needed, strict vegetarians are at risk and may rarely develop clinically significant deficiency. Intestinal absorption of cobalamin requires the presence of intrinsic factor, a binding protein secreted by gastric parietal cells. Cobalamin binds to intrinsic factor, and the complex is transported to the ileum where it is absorbed into the circulation. A small amount of free cobalamin, about 1%–5%, is also absorbed through the entire intestine without intrinsic factor. Once absorbed, cobalamin binds to a transport protein, transcobalamin, for delivery to tissues. As much as 90% of total body cobalamin is stored in the liver. Even when vitamin absorption is severely impaired, many years are needed to deplete the body store. A clinical relapse in pernicious anemia after interrupting cobalamin therapy takes an average of 5 years to be recognized.

Two biochemical reactions depend on cobalamin. One involves methylmalonic acid as precursor in the conversion of methylmalonyl coenzyme A (methylmalonyl-CoA) to succinyl-CoA. The importance of this to the nervous system is unclear. The other is a folate-dependent reaction in which the methyl group of methyltetrahydrofolate is transferred to homocysteine to yield methionine and tetrahydrofolate. The reaction depends on the enzyme methionine synthase, which uses cobalamin as a cofactor. Methionine is converted to *S*-adenosylmethionine (SAM), which is used for methylation reactions in the nervous system.

### Causes of Deficiency

The classic disease pernicious anemia is caused by defective intrinsic factor production by parietal cells, leading to malabsorption. These patients may have demonstrable circulating antibodies to parietal cells or lymphocytic infiltrations of the gastric mucosa, suggesting an

**TABLE 85.1 Neurological Manifestations in Deficiency Diseases**

| Neurological Manifestations | Associated Nutritional Deficiencies |
|---|---|
| Dementia, encephalopathy | Vitamin $B_{12}$, nicotinic acid, thiamine, folate |
| Seizures | Pyridoxine |
| Myelopathy | Vitamin $B_{12}$, vitamin E, folate, copper |
| Myopathy | Vitamin D, vitamin E |
| Peripheral neuropathy | Thiamine, vitamin $B_{12}$, vitamin E, and many others |
| Optic neuropathy | Thiamine, vitamin $B_{12}$, and many others |

underlying autoimmune disorder. A more common cause of malabsorption is food-cobalamin malabsorption (Dali-Youcef and Andres, 2009). Under some clinical settings, the normal digestive process fails to release cobalamin from food or intestinal transport protein. Cobalamin remains bound and cannot be absorbed even in the presence of available intrinsic factors. Predisposing factors include atrophic gastritis and hypochlorhydria, and malabsorption may be seen with *Helicobacter pylori* infection, gastrectomy or other gastric surgeries, intestinal bacterial overgrowth, and prolonged use of $H_2$ antagonists, proton pump inhibitors, or biguanides (e.g., metformin). Patients with human immunodeficiency virus (HIV) are often observed to have a low serum cobalamin level, usually with normal homocysteine and methylmalonic acid. The significance of this association is unknown.

Nitrous oxide, a commonly used anesthetic gas, may cause a clinical syndrome of myeloneuropathy indistinguishable from that of cobalamin deficiency. It interferes with the cobalamin-dependent conversion of homocysteine to methionine. Prolonged exposure is necessary to produce neurological symptoms in normal individuals and is primarily seen in individuals who abuse the gas for its euphoric properties (Keddie et al., 2018). By contrast, patients who are already deficient in cobalamin may experience neurological deficits after only brief exposures during routine general anesthesia with nitrous oxide. Symptoms appear subacutely after surgery and resolve quickly with cobalamin treatment (Singer et al., 2008).

## Clinical Features

The onset of symptoms is insidious, with paresthesias in the hands or feet experienced by most patients. Weakness and unsteadiness of gait are the next most frequent complaints. Lhermitte sign may be present. Mental slowing, depression, confusion, delusions, and hallucinations are common, and occasionally patients present with only cognitive or psychiatric symptoms.

On examination, signs of both peripheral nerve and spinal cord involvement may be present, although either can be affected first or disproportionately. Loss of vibration or joint position sense in the legs is common. If impaired position sense is severe, a Romberg sign may be present. Motor impairment, if present, results from pyramidal tract dysfunction and is most severe in the legs, ranging from mild clumsiness and hyperreflexia to spastic paraplegia and extensor plantar responses. Tendon reflexes are variably affected depending on the degree of pyramidal and peripheral nerve involvement. Visual impairment is occasionally present and may antedate other manifestations of vitamin deficiency. Ophthalmological examination may reveal bilateral visual loss, optic atrophy, and centrocecal scotomata. Brainstem or cerebellar signs, chorea, autonomic insufficiency, or even reversible coma may rarely occur.

## Laboratory Studies

Serum assays of vitamin $B_{12}$ and cobalamin-dependent metabolites provide direct measures of cobalamin homeostasis, although there are important limitations. Blood cobalamins are bound to two transport

**BOX 85.1 Causes of Elevated Serum Levels of Homocysteine and Methylmalonic Acid**

**Elevated Methylmalonic Acid**
Cobalamin deficiency
Renal insufficiency
Inherited metabolic disorders
Hypovolemia

**Elevated Homocysteine**
Cobalamin deficiency
Folate deficiency
Pyridoxine deficiency
Renal insufficiency
Hypothyroidism
Psoriasis
Inherited metabolic disorders
Hypovolemia

proteins, transcobalamin and haptocorrin. The cobalamin bound to transcobalamin, known as *holotranscobalamin*, is the fraction that is available to tissues, although it accounts for only 10%–30% of the serum level measured by standard laboratory methods. Serum levels are influenced by conditions that affect the concentrations of these transport proteins. Myeloproliferative and hepatic disorders may raise the concentration of haptocorrin and cause a falsely normal serum level. A misleadingly high serum level also may result from the presence of an abnormal cobalamin-binding protein. In contrast, pregnancy and contraceptives may give falsely low measurements in the absence of deficiency. Folate deficiency also causes a falsely low cobalamin serum level that corrects after folate replacement. These confounding factors diminish the sensitivity and specificity of the commonly used assay of total serum cobalamin in the diagnosis of deficiency state. Although measurement of holotranscobalamin is better in theory, available data suggest that its diagnostic sensitivity is approximately equivalent or only modestly better than that of total serum cobalamin, and its specificity is uncertain (Oberley and Yang, 2013).

Homocysteine and methylmalonic acid are precursors of cobalamin-dependent biochemical reactions. The concentrations of these metabolites increase during cobalamin deficiency. Measurement of these metabolites is especially useful when the serum cobalamin concentration is in the low range of normal, between 200 and 350 pg/mL, and in patients with suspected nitrous oxide abuse who may have normal serum cobalamin levels. Homocysteine level should be measured either at fasting or after an oral methionine load. The blood sample should be refrigerated immediately after collection because the level increases if whole blood is left at room temperature for several hours. Elevated levels of homocysteine and methylmalonic acid are not specific for cobalamin deficiency, as there are many other causes of increase in these metabolites (Box 85.1).

In patients with autoimmune gastritis and intrinsic factor deficiency, antibodies against parietal cell and intrinsic factor may be elevated. Anti-parietal cell antibodies are nonspecific and are present in other autoimmune endocrinopathies as well as occasional normal individuals. Anti-intrinsic factor antibodies are less sensitive (50%–70%) but are specific for pernicious anemia. Elevated serum gastrin level is a marker of atrophic gastritis and hypochlorhydria and is a sensitive (up to 90%) but nonspecific indicator of pernicious anemia.

The classic hematological manifestation of pernicious anemia is a macrocytic anemia. Erythrocyte or bone marrow macrocytosis or hypersegmentation of polymorphonuclear cells may be present

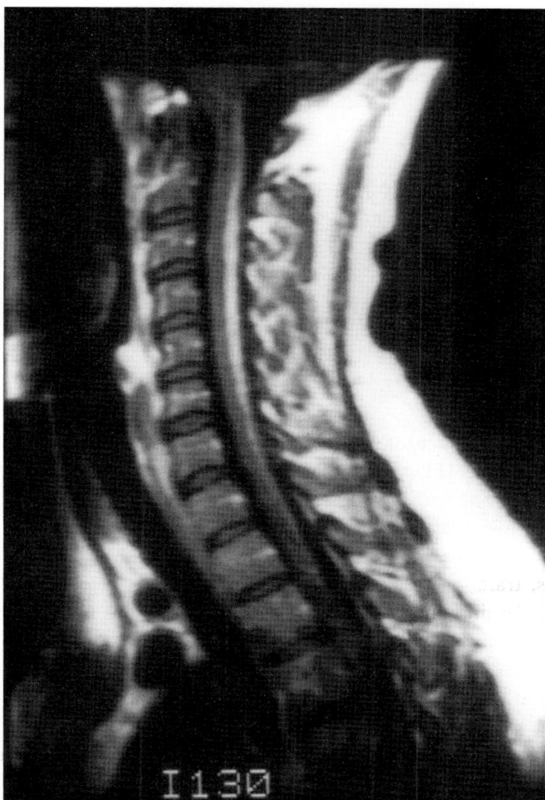


**Fig. 85.1 Vitamin $B_{12}$ Deficiency Myelopathy.** Gadolinium-enhanced, T1-weighted cervical and upper thoracic magnetic resonance image showing marked enhancement of posterior cord of a 30-year-old African American woman wheelchair-bound due to an 18-month history of progressive myelopathy; vitamin $B_{12}$ level, 60 pg/mL. *(Courtesy Dr. R. Laureno.)*

without anemia. Hematological abnormalities may be absent at the time of neurological presentation and are thus insufficiently sensitive for use in diagnosis.

Because most patients present with clinical features suggesting a myelopathy or encephalopathy, imaging studies are necessary to exclude structural causes. Results of magnetic resonance imaging (MRI) may be normal, or T2-signal abnormalities may be seen in the lateral or posterior columns in patients with subacute combined degeneration (Kumar and Singh, 2009) (Fig. 85.1). Both gadolinium enhancement and spinal cord swelling have been described. Patients with encephalopathy or dementia often have multiple foci of T2 signal abnormalities in the deep white matter that may become confluent with disease progression. Diffusion tensor imaging (DTI) may be more sensitive in revealing brain changes that correlate with cognitive dysfunction (Gupta et al., 2014). Nonspecific abnormalities of electroencephalography, as well as visual and somatosensory evoked responses, are present in many patients with neurological abnormalities. Nerve conduction studies show small or absent rural nerve sensory potentials in approximately half of patients, providing evidence for an axonal polyneuropathy.

## Pathology

The term *subacute combined degeneration of the spinal cord* describes the pathological process seen in this disorder. Microscopically, spongiform changes and foci of myelin and axon destruction are seen in the white matter of the spinal cord. The most severely affected regions are the posterior columns at the cervical and upper thoracic levels (Fig. 85.2). Pathological changes also are seen commonly in the lateral columns, whereas the anterior columns are involved in only a small number of the advanced cases. The pathological findings of the peripheral nervous system are those of axonal degeneration, but in some cases there is evidence of demyelination. Involvement of the optic nerve and cerebral white matter also occurs.

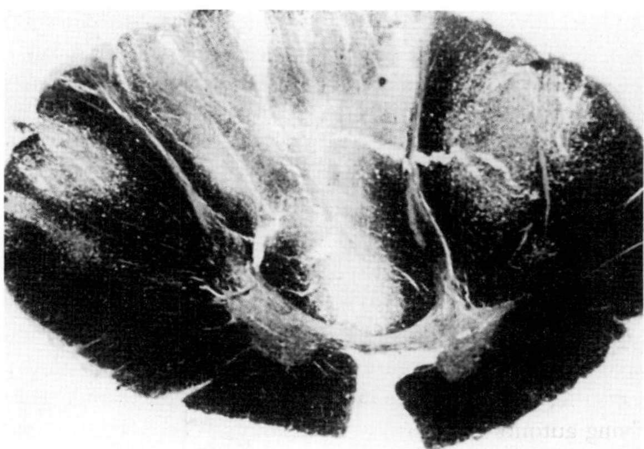

**Fig. 85.2 Subacute Combined Degeneration of the Spinal Cord in Vitamin $B_{12}$ Deficiency.** Demyelination and loss of axons are more widespread in posterior than in lateral columns (Weigert stain). *(Courtesy Dr. Michael F. Gonzales.)*

## Treatment

Recommendations for treatment of cobalamin deficiency vary widely. A typical regimen uses intramuscular daily injections of 1000 µg for the first week, followed by weekly 1000 µg injections for 1 month, and monthly injections thereafter. These parenteral doses provide quantities considerably higher than the body requirement. There is no evidence that overdosing can speed neurological recovery, but high doses of cobalamin appear to be safe. Oral supplementation at 1000 µg daily has also been used with some success, even in patients with suspected malabsorption, although close monitoring is necessary to ensure adequacy of treatment.

With proper treatment, serum levels of homocysteine and methylmalonic acid return to normal in about 2 weeks. Neurological improvement is more delayed and may be incomplete. Most of the symptomatic improvement occurs during the first 6–12 months of therapy. The need for early diagnosis and treatment is underscored by the observation that remission correlates inversely with the time lapse between onset of symptoms and initiation of therapy.

# FOLATE DEFICIENCY AND HOMOCYSTEINE

Folate deficiency may produce the same neurological deficits as those seen in cobalamin deficiency because of its central role in the biosynthesis of methionine, SAM, and tetrahydrofolate (see the previous section Cobalamin [Vitamin $B_{12}$]). Overt neurological manifestations are rare in folate deficiency, probably owing to alternative cellular mechanisms that are available to preserve SAM levels in times of folate scarcity.

## Causes of Deficiency

Absorption of folate occurs in the jejunum and to a lesser extent the ileum. Chronic alcoholism is an important cause of folate deficiency. Folate deficiency also may complicate small-bowel disease (e.g., sprue, Crohn disease, ulcerative colitis). Other populations at risk are pregnant women and patients receiving anticonvulsant drugs that interfere with folate metabolism. Sulfasalazine, methotrexate, triamterene, and oral contraceptives also can cause folate deficiency. Intrathecal methotrexate, in particular, causes a leukoencephalopathy associated with marked elevation of homocysteine levels in the cerebrospinal fluid (CSF).

### Clinical Features

The majority of patients with laboratory evidence of folate deficiency do not have overt neurological findings. The classic syndrome of folate deficiency is similar to subacute combined degeneration seen in cobalamin deficiency. Presenting symptoms are limb paresthesias, weakness, and gait unsteadiness. These patients have megaloblastic anemia, impaired position and vibration sense, pyramidal signs, and possibly dementia. Chronic folate deficiency may result in mild cognitive impairment or increased stroke risk in adults. Although low folate level is present in many elderly asymptomatic people, the prevalence seems to be higher in the psychiatric and Alzheimer disease populations. Moreover, a low folate level appears to correlate with depression and cognitive impairment. Even in healthy older adults, a low folate level is associated with subtle deficits in neuropsychological test performance. Chronic folate deficiency during pregnancy leads to an increased frequency of neural tube defects in babies.

Serum homocysteine is an important surrogate marker for folate metabolism, although there are other causes of elevated homocysteine levels (see Box 85.1). Hyperhomocysteinemia is a risk factor for vascular diseases and venous thrombosis. For cerebrovascular disease, the association is strongest for multi-infarct dementia and white-matter microangiopathy. Even a modestly increased serum level in the range of 15–20 mmol/L engenders a recognizable increase in vascular risk. A meta-analysis of randomized control trials suggests a modest 10% reduction in stroke and 4% reduction in cardiovascular risk with long-term folate supplementation (0.5–15 mg/day, mean duration 3.2 years) (Li et al., 2016).

Clinical observations in two inborn errors of metabolism reinforce our understanding of the role of homocysteine in neurological diseases. Hereditary deficiency of cystathionine β-synthase leads to hyperhomocysteinemia and hyperhomocysteinuria. The homozygous form presents with markedly elevated homocysteine levels, mental retardation, premature atherosclerosis, and seizures. Heterozygous individuals have milder elevations of homocysteine and also have increased risk of vascular disease. A much more common condition is a C-to-T substitution at codon 677 in the gene coding for N5, N10-methylenetetrahydrofolate reductase (MTHFR). Some 5%–10% of the White population are homozygotes for this C677T mutation. These individuals have mildly elevated homocysteine levels and increased risk of vascular disease.

### Laboratory Studies

Plasma and erythrocyte folate levels may be measured directly. Erythrocyte level is generally more reliable than plasma level because it is less affected by short-term fluctuation in intake. Serum homocysteine is increased in folate deficiency. Its measurement is discussed in Laboratory Studies under the previous section, Cobalamin (Vitamin $B_{12}$).

### Treatment

In patients with documented folate deficiency, the initial dose is usually 1 mg of folate several times per day, followed by a maintenance dose of 1 mg/day. For acutely ill patients, parenteral doses of 1–5 mg may be given. Even with oral doses as high as 15 mg/day, there is no report of toxicity. In women of childbearing potential with epilepsy, daily folate supplementation of 0.4 mg or more is recommended as prophylaxis against neural tube defects. Since 1998, in an attempt to lower the incidence of neural tube defects, the US Food and Drug Administration (FDA) has mandated fortification of grain products with folate. The fortification translates to an increased daily intake of 0.1–0.2 mg in a typical adult.

**BOX 85.2 Causes of Vitamin E Deficiency**

Gastrointestinal diseases
Biliary atresia, chronic cholestasis
Intestinal resection
Crohn disease
Pancreatic insufficiency (e.g., cystic fibrosis)
Blind loop syndrome and bacterial overgrowth
Bowel irradiation
Celiac disease
Other causes of steatorrhea
Hereditary diseases: abetalipoproteinemia, hypobetalipoproteinemia, Anderson disease, α-tocopherol transfer protein mutation

## VITAMIN E

*Vitamin E* refers to a group of tocopherols and tocotrienols, of which α-tocopherol is the most important. It is a free-radical scavenger and an antioxidant and has attracted attention for its potential in the prevention and treatment of a wide range of diseases. Unfortunately, the value of vitamin E for these indications has yet to be proven. We limit discussion here to the neurological manifestations of vitamin E deficiency.

Like other fat-soluble compounds, vitamin E depends on the presence of pancreatic esterases and bile salts for its solubilization and absorption in the intestinal lumen. Neurological symptoms of deficiency occur most commonly in patients with fat malabsorption (Box 85.2). A reduced bile salt pool may be caused either by reduced hepatic excretion, as in congenital cholestasis, or by interruption of the enterohepatic reabsorption of bile, as in patients with extensive small-bowel resection. Pancreatic insufficiency contributes to malabsorption. Another setting is cystic fibrosis.

A number of rare familial disorders lead to chronic diarrhea, abnormal blood lipid profile, and malabsorption of fat and fat-soluble vitamins. In addition to vitamin E deficiency, these patients also have deficiency of vitamins A and D. Abetalipoproteinemia or Bassen-Kornzweig syndrome is an autosomal recessive disorder due to mutation in the microsomal triglyceride transfer protein (MTP) gene. This results in impaired absorption of fat and fat-soluble vitamins (Zamel et al., 2008). In addition to a neurological syndrome similar to that seen in other vitamin E-deficient states, spiky red blood cells (acanthocytes) and retinal pigment changes are characteristic. Two other disorders are also characterized by chronic fat malabsorption and vitamin E deficiency. SAR1B gene mutation leads to chylomicron retention disease or Anderson disease. Familial hypobetalipoproteinemia presents with variable degrees of malabsorption and symptoms, and about 50% are due to mutation in the APOB gene (Peretti et al., 2010).

Another rare syndrome of ataxia with isolated vitamin E deficiency (AVED) occurs in patients without GI disease or generalized fat malabsorption. Mutations in the α-tocopherol transfer protein gene (TTPA) on chromosome 8q are responsible (El Euch-Fayache et al., 2014; Mariotti et al., 2004). This condition is inherited in an autosomal recessive manner. The defect appears to be impaired incorporation of the vitamin into hepatic lipoproteins that are necessary for delivery to tissues.

### Clinical Features

Clinical symptoms typically do not begin until many years of malabsorption deplete the vitamin reserves. This takes 15–20 years in adults, but clinical onset as early as age 1–2 years may occur in children because of their small vitamin reserves. The usual presenting symptoms are weakness or gait unsteadiness. Neurological examination reveals a syndrome of spinocerebellar degeneration accompanied by peripheral nerve involvement. Some patients are diagnosed erroneously with Friedreich ataxia. The most consistent abnormalities are limb ataxia, areflexia, and loss of vibration and position sense. Cutaneous sensation usually is spared or affected to a lesser degree. About half of patients have nystagmus, ptosis, or partial external ophthalmoplegia. Mild to moderate proximal weakness is common, and some patients may have a myopathy. The pattern of weakness may also be diffuse or predominantly distal. Babinski sign may be present.

### Laboratory Studies

The diagnosis is not difficult when the appropriate neurological syndrome and a low serum vitamin E level are both present. Serum level should be interpreted in light of the clinical findings. Some patients with low levels do not have demonstrable neurological deficits. Moreover, plasma vitamin E is largely incorporated into chylomicrons and is highly dependent on the concentrations of total plasma lipids, cholesterol, and very low-density lipoproteins.

Other laboratory abnormalities, despite their nonspecific nature, help clarify the diagnosis. Stool fat is increased in many patients, and serum carotene concentration is often abnormally low, both reflecting a generalized state of fat malabsorption. CSF should be normal. Nerve conduction studies usually reveal a sensory polyneuropathy, although motor conduction abnormality and features of a demyelinating neuropathy have been reported rarely (Puri et al., 2005). Somatosensory and visual evoked responses are frequently abnormal, and there may be high signal lesions in the posterior columns on T2-weighted MRI.

### Treatment

The recommended daily requirement of vitamin E in normal adults is 10 mg (equivalent to 10 IU) of DL-α-tocopherol acetate, a commonly available form of the vitamin. A wide range of doses has been used, from 200 mg/day to 100 mg/kg/day. Improvement, or at least stabilization, of neurological status is possible, even in those patients with hereditary diseases (El Euch-Fayache et al., 2014; Peretti et al., 2010), although there is no consensus on the optimal therapeutic dosage. A reasonable approach is to begin therapy with an oral preparation of water-miscible tocopherol at a dose of 200–600 mg/day. The clinical picture and serum level should be followed; if no improvement occurs, higher oral dosages or even parenteral administration should be tried. Supplementation of bile salts may be of value in those patients with intestinal malabsorption.

## PELLAGRA (NICOTINIC ACID DEFICIENCY)

Nicotinic acid or vitamin $B_3$ is converted in the body to two important coenzymes in carbohydrate metabolism: nicotinamide adenine dinucleotide (NAD) and nicotinamide adenine dinucleotide phosphate (NADP). *Niacin*, another term for nicotinic acid, was introduced to avoid confusion with the alkaloid nicotine. Dietary deficiency of nicotinic acid produces pellagra (from the Italian *pelle agra*, meaning "rough skin"). Pellagra classically occurs in populations who consume primarily corn. Corn lacks nicotinic acid as well as tryptophan, a precursor that can be converted in the body to nicotinic acid. In underdeveloped countries, pellagra is still a common health problem. Even in the United States, pellagra was endemic until around 1940 in the South and in alcoholic populations. The disease is now rare due to the widespread consumption of bread enriched with niacin. In addition to cases still encountered in alcoholics, there are case reports of individuals with malabsorption from GI diseases or concurrent use of medications that interfere with the production of niacin from tryptophan, such as isoniazid, azathioprine, and some chemotherapy agents (Li et al., 2016).

Pellagra affects three organ systems in the body: the GI tract, skin, and nervous system (hence the mnemonic of "three Ds": diarrhea, dermatitis, and dementia). The chief GI symptoms are anorexia, diarrhea, stomatitis, and abdominal discomfort. Skin changes range from erythema to a reddish-brown hyperkeratotic rash distributed over much of the body, with the face, chest, and dorsal surfaces of the hands and feet being most involved.

The neurological syndrome of pellagra is not well defined. Reported cases, especially of patients with alcoholic pellagra, frequently are confounded by other coexisting central nervous system disorders such as Wernicke encephalopathy. The primary early symptoms are neuropsychiatric (e.g., irritability, apathy, depressed mood, inattentiveness, memory loss) and may progress to stupor or coma. In addition to the confusional state, spasticity, Babinski sign, gegenhalten, and startle myoclonus may be prominent on neurological examination. Nonendemic pellagra occurs rarely in patients with alcoholism or malabsorption secondary to GI disease. The diagnosis of nonendemic pellagra can be made only on clinical grounds because there is no available method to make a blood niacin level determination, and this diagnosis may be difficult because diarrhea and dermatological changes are often absent. The condition is likely under-recognized and mistaken for other causes of encephalopathy. A postmortem study found pathological features suggestive of pellagra encephalopathy in 5 of 59 patients with suspected Creutzfeldt-Jakob disease (Kapas et al., 2012).

The recommended daily allowance for nicotinic acid is 6.6 mg/1000 kcal dietary intake. Oral nicotinic acid in doses of 50 mg several times a day is usually sufficient to treat symptomatic patients. Alternatively, parenteral doses of 25 mg can be given 2–3 times a day. Nicotinamide has similar therapeutic efficacy in pellagra, but it does not have the vasodilatory and cholesterol-lowering activities of niacin.

## VITAMIN $B_6$ (PYRIDOXINE)

Although the term *pyridoxine* often is used synonymously with vitamin $B_6$, two other naturally occurring compounds—pyridoxal and pyridoxamine—possess similar biological activities. All three compounds are converted to pyridoxal-5'-phosphate (PLP), an important cofactor for glucose, lipids, and amino acid metabolism as well as neurotransmitter synthesis.

In the early 1950s, physicians in the United States encountered cases of an unusual seizure disorder in infants at the age of several weeks to a few months. These seizures were difficult to control with the usual anticonvulsants. In contrast, the response was dramatic when vitamin $B_6$ was given. It eventually became clear that the symptomatic infants were fed a commercial formula that contained approximately one-third the vitamin $B_6$ found in other infant formulas. The cause was then traced to a manufacturing process that reduced the pyridoxine content.

Even with better awareness of the problem, sporadic cases of infantile seizures from dietary vitamin $B_6$ deficiency still occur, most commonly as a result of breastfeeding by malnourished mothers from poor socioeconomic backgrounds or in underdeveloped countries. The typical patients have a normal birth history and are entirely healthy until the development of hyperirritability and an exaggerated auditory startle. Recurrent convulsions often occur abruptly, as may status epilepticus. Once the dietary insufficiency is corrected, patients become free of seizures and develop normally.

Another rare form of pyridoxine-responsive seizure occurs in infants with inborn errors in PLP metabolism. Mutations in several genes have been implicated. The current list includes ALDH7A1, ALDH4A1, PNPO, TNSALP, PLPBP, and PLPHP, and will likely continue to expand with advances in our understanding of this group of diseases (Johnstone et al., 2019; Pearl and Gospe, 2014; Wilson et al., 2019). In these children, seizures appear during the neonatal period. The seizures typically respond poorly to anticonvulsants. Long-term administration of large amounts of pyridoxine or PLP is needed to control seizures and to minimize adverse effects on cognitive development.

Although adults are more tolerant of vitamin $B_6$ deficiency, a high prevalence of low serum level is present in women and elderly populations (Morris et al., 2008), people with malabsorptive predisposition such as bariatric surgery, and renal failure patients with high loss of vitamins through dialysis. Medications such as isoniazid, hydralazine, penicillamine, and L-dopa/carbidopa intestinal gel have also been linked to pyridoxine deficiency (Loens et al., 2017). Chronic vitamin $B_6$ deficiency probably causes a subacute sensory or sensorimotor neuropathy (Ghavanini, 2014). This is best described in patients receiving isoniazid. Sensory symptoms appear first in the distal feet. Burning pain may be disabling. Examination may show impaired sensation, distal weakness, and depressed tendon reflexes. In patients taking isoniazid, pyridoxine supplementation of 50 mg/day prevents the development of neuropathy, although a lower dose likely suffices. Acute overdose of isoniazid may rarely lead to coma, metabolic acidosis, and seizures, and pyridoxine provides a specific antidote.

Indiscriminate use of pyridoxine supplements may be harmful. The recommended daily allowance of vitamin $B_6$ is approximately 2 mg. High doses of pyridoxine (1000 mg/day or more) can reliably cause a sensory neuropathy within a few months (Berger et al., 1992). Patients ingesting a high dose for a prolonged period have been described as developing sensory ataxia with impaired sensation, areflexia, and Romberg sign. Many years of taking doses as low as 200 mg/day of pyridoxine have been associated with a mild predominantly sensory polyneuropathy, although a safety threshold for chronic lower-dose usage has not been established. In general, it is prudent to limit the daily dosage to 50 mg or less for the therapeutic use of pyridoxine.

## THIAMINE

Thiamine is synonymous with vitamin $B_1$. It is a water-soluble vitamin that plays a crucial role in the metabolism of carbohydrates, amino acids, and lipids. It is absorbed in the jejunum and ileum by active transport as well as passive diffusion. Thiamine is mostly stored in the liver. A continuous dietary supply is necessary as only a small amount is stored. Demand for thiamine increases with high glucose intake and during periods of high metabolic demands such as pregnancy and many systemic illnesses. The minimum daily requirement of thiamine is 0.3 mg/1000 kcal dietary intake in normal subjects, but the requirement is higher during pregnancy and old age. For therapeutic purposes, a target of 50–100 mg/day is often used.

Diagnosis of thiamine deficiency is based on the appearance of appropriate clinical features in the setting of either nutritional deficiency or high metabolic demands. Thiamine levels in serum and urine may be decreased, although the levels do not reliably reflect tissue concentrations. Erythrocyte transketolase activity level is dependent on thiamine and provides an assay of functional status. Pyruvate accumulates during thiamine deficiency, and elevated serum level provides additional confirmation. A blood sample should be drawn before initiation of treatment because these laboratory abnormalities normalize quickly.

### Thiamine Deficiency Neuropathy (Beriberi)

*Beriberi* literally means extreme weakness. It is caused by thiamine deficiency and affects the heart and peripheral nerves, producing congestive cardiomyopathy, sensorimotor polyneuropathy, or both. The classical *wet* and *dry* forms refer to the presence or absence of edema. The neuropathy generally develops over weeks or months. Affected patients complain of paresthesias or pain in the feet. Walking becomes difficult. The most common neurological finding is distal sensory loss. Weakness appears first in the finger and wrist extensors and the ankle dorsiflexors. Ankle stretch reflexes are lost in most patients. When cardiac dysfunction is present, patients also experience tachycardia, palpitations, dyspnea, fatigue, and ankle edema.

Electrodiagnostic studies show an axonal neuropathy with reduced amplitude of sensory or motor responses, normal or mildly reduced conduction velocity, and neuropathic changes on electromyography. Lumbar puncture sometimes shows a mildly elevated opening pressure, a finding probably related to the presence of congestive heart failure. Findings of CSF examination are otherwise unremarkable. If cardiac impairment is present, electrocardiographic or other cardiac abnormalities may be seen.

Thiamine, 100 mg, may be given intravenously (IV) in the acute stage, especially if there is doubt about adequate GI absorption. Long-term treatment consists of a balanced diet with oral supplements of thiamine and other vitamins. Gradual return of sensory and motor function can be expected after thiamine replenishment. In severe cases, improvement may take many months and may be incomplete.

### Infantile Beriberi

An acute syndrome of thiamine deficiency in infants occurs in the rice-eating populations of Asia, most frequently in breastfed infants younger than 1 year of age. Thiamine is often deficient in breast milk from mothers who eat primarily polished rice. Although the disorder is called *infantile beriberi*, it bears little resemblance to the adult form. Acute cardiac symptoms are common, often preceded by a prodrome of anorexia, vomiting, deficient weight gain, and restlessness. Dyspnea, cyanosis, and signs of heart failure follow and can lead rapidly to death. Arytenoid edema and recurrent laryngeal neuropathy may give rise to hoarseness, dysphonia, and eventually aphonia. Early signs of coughing and choking may be mistaken for respiratory tract infections. Central nervous system manifestations include drowsiness, ophthalmoplegia, and convulsions. These symptoms often begin abruptly and carry a grave prognosis. If given promptly, parenteral administration of 5–20 mg of thiamine can be lifesaving.

## WERNICKE-KORSAKOFF SYNDROME

In 1881, Carl Wernicke described a syndrome of mental confusion, ophthalmoplegia, and gait ataxia in three patients, two of whom were alcoholics. At autopsy, multiple small hemorrhages were seen in the periventricular gray matter, primarily around the aqueduct and the third and fourth ventricles. Shortly after Wernicke's original treatise, Korsakoff, a Russian psychiatrist, described an amnesia syndrome in 20 alcoholic men. At the time, neither Wernicke nor Korsakoff recognized the relationship between the encephalopathy and impaired memory. The clinical connection and the pathological similarity between the two conditions were not appreciated until 10 years later by other investigators. Korsakoff syndrome and Wernicke encephalopathy do not represent separate diseases but are different stages of one disease process (Wernicke-Korsakoff syndrome). Korsakoff syndrome typically follows Wernicke encephalopathy, emerging as ocular symptoms and encephalopathy subside.

**BOX 85.3 Associated Conditions in Nonalcoholic Patients with Wernicke Encephalopathy**

Hyperemesis of pregnancy
Systemic malignancy
Gastrointestinal surgery (e.g., bariatric surgery)
Hemodialysis or peritoneal dialysis
Prolonged intravenous feeding
Refeeding after prolonged fasting or starvation
Anorexia nervosa
Dieting
Acquired immunodeficiency syndrome

Wernicke encephalopathy is due to thiamine deficiency. The most common clinical setting for this disorder is chronic alcoholism. However, a large number of cases occur in other conditions, with the only prerequisite being a poor nutritional state, from inadequate intake, malabsorption, or increased metabolic requirement (Box 85.3). Wernicke encephalopathy may be precipitated acutely in at-risk patients by IV glucose administration or carbohydrate loading.

The classic triad in Wernicke encephalopathy is the combination of confusion, ophthalmoplegia, and gait ataxia, although all three elements are seen in fewer than half of all patients. In a retrospective study of 468 patients in Spain, the triad was present in only 39% of alcoholic and 29% of nonalcoholic patients (Chamorro et al., 2017). The Caine criteria was often used for its higher sensitivity in diagnosis of Wernicke encephalopathy (Caine et al., 1997). It requires only two of the following four features: dietary deficiency, oculomotor abnormalities, cerebellar ataxia, and confusion. Eighty-five percent of autopsy-confirmed cases of Wernicke encephalopathy met the Caine criteria, although the specificity is likely low.

Confusion is the most common symptom and develops over days or weeks. This is characterized by inattention, apathy, disorientation, and memory loss. Stupor or coma is rare. Gait ataxia is likely a result of cerebellar abnormality, neuropathy, and vestibular dysfunction. On examination, truncal ataxia is common, but limb ataxia is not—findings similar to those seen in alcoholic cerebellar degeneration. Ophthalmoplegia, when present, commonly involves both lateral recti, either in isolation or together with palsies of other extraocular muscles. Patients may have horizontal nystagmus on lateral gaze, and many also have vertical nystagmus on upgaze. Sluggish reaction to light, light-near dissociation, and other pupillary abnormalities are sometimes seen. The clinical findings reflect the localization of pathological abnormalities in this disease—namely, the prominent symmetrical involvement of periventricular structures at the level of the third and fourth ventricles. Lesions of the nuclei of cranial nerves III, VI, and VIII are responsible for the eye findings. Other frequent findings include hypothermia and postural hypotension, reflecting involvement of hypothalamic and brainstem autonomic pathways.

The Korsakoff syndrome follows repeated bouts of encephalopathy or an inadequately treated acute encephalopathy. As the acute encephalopathy subsides, it becomes obvious that the patient has an amnestic disorder. The memory impairment is out of proportion to other cognitive dysfunction and consists of both anterograde and retrograde amnesia. Affected patients have severe difficulty establishing new memories, always coupled with a limited ability to recall events that antedate the onset of illness by several years. Most patients are disoriented as to place and time. Alertness, attention, social behavior, and most other aspects of cognitive functioning are relatively preserved. Confabulation can be a prominent feature, especially in the early stages, although it

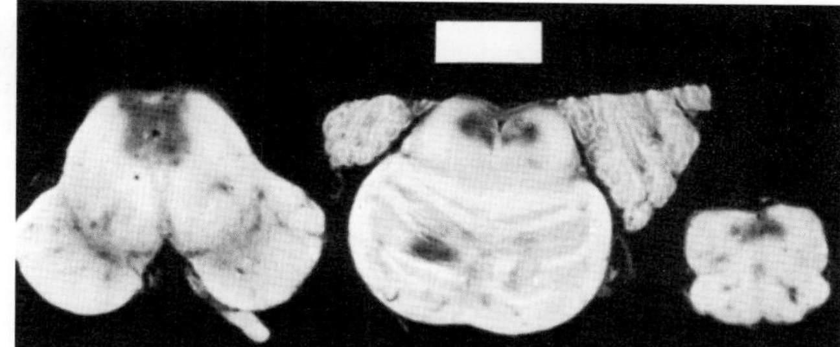

**Fig. 85.3 Acute Wernicke Disease.** Hemorrhagic areas are seen adjacent to the fourth ventricle and aqueduct in the *(from right to left)* medulla, pons, and midbrain. *(Courtesy Dr. Michael F. Gonzales.)*

may be absent in some patients. The memory disorder reflects the predilection of the lesions for the diencephalon and temporal lobes. Injury to these regions, regardless of cause (e.g., infarction, trauma, tumors, herpes encephalitis), can produce a syndrome indistinguishable from the amnesia syndrome seen in alcoholic patients.

## Laboratory Studies

Brain MRI is helpful in acute Wernicke encephalopathy. MRI typically shows signal abnormalities on T2-weighted fluid-attenuated inversion recovery (FLAIR) and diffusion-weighted images, symmetrically distributed around the periaqueductal regions, tectal plates, medial thalami, and bilateral mammillary bodies. Other regions such as the cerebellar vermis, pons, medulla, dentate nuclei, cranial nerve nuclei, and basal ganglia are at times affected. Some lesions may show contrast enhancement. Petechial hemorrhages may be seen on T2-weighted images using susceptibility-weighted imaging (SWI) (Hattingen et al., 2016). There are differences in the distribution of lesions between alcoholic and nonalcoholic patients, but there is a considerable overlap between the two groups (Zuccoli et al., 2009). Brain computed tomography (CT) may be used when MRI is unavailable but is much less sensitive in demonstrating abnormalities. MRI signal abnormalities typically resolve completely with prompt treatment, but shrunken mammillary bodies may be seen as a late residual finding. The CSF is either normal or shows a mild elevation in protein. Serum thiamine level and erythrocyte transketolase activity may be depressed, and there may be an elevation of serum pyruvate.

## Pathology

The pathological process depends on the age of the lesions. Macroscopically, varying degrees of congestion, petechial hemorrhages, shrinkage, and discoloration are present (Fig. 85.3). Glial proliferation and myelin pallor characterize the more chronic lesions. The regions affected are the same as those observed to be involved on MRI. The frequency of Wernicke encephalopathy as estimated from autopsy studies is approximately 0.8%–2.8%, a figure far greater than that expected from clinical studies. Only 20% of the autopsy cases in one series were diagnosed during life. This is unfortunate because Wernicke encephalopathy is preventable and treatable. The under-recognition may result from an overemphasis on alcoholism as a cause (see Box 85.4) or a misconception that all three elements of the clinical triad are needed for a diagnosis. Wernicke encephalopathy occurring under other settings may be mistaken for encephalopathy of uremia, dialysis, sepsis, or other systemic diseases.

## Treatment

Wernicke encephalopathy should be suspected in all patients with encephalopathy and at risk for nutritional deficiency (see Box 85.3) (Galvin et al., 2010). Treatment should not be delayed while waiting for laboratory confirmation of thiamine deficiency. Intravenous thiamine is safe, inexpensive, and effective in the treatment of Wernicke encephalopathy. Patients suspected of having the disorder should receive thiamine *before* administration of glucose to avoid precipitation of symptom worsening. A dose of 500 mg should be given IV in the acute stage, followed by 100 mg 3 times daily during the first week. Parenteral administration is preferable over oral supplements because intestinal absorption is unreliable in debilitated and alcoholic patients.

If left untreated, Wernicke encephalopathy is progressive. The mortality, even with thiamine treatment, was 10%–20% in the early studies. With treatment, the majority of ocular signs resolve within hours, although a fine horizontal nystagmus persists in approximately 60% of patients. The gait disturbance resolves slowly, and in over one-third of the cases, gait may be abnormal even months after treatment. As the global confusional state recedes, some patients are left with the Korsakoff syndrome. The treatment of Korsakoff syndrome is usually limited to social support. Many patients require at least some form of supervision, either at home or in a chronic care facility. There are anecdotal reports of success treating the memory loss with acetylcholinesterase inhibitors or memantine, but controlled studies in small numbers of patients did not show a consistent benefit (Luykx et al., 2008).

## OTHER DISEASES ASSOCIATED WITH ALCOHOLISM

The diverse neurological consequences of alcohol abuse have been recognized for centuries. Alcohol is a potent central nervous system depressant. It facilitates the inhibitory neurotransmitter γ-aminobutyric acid (GABA) and inhibits the excitation induced by *N*-methyl-D-aspartate (NMDA). It also has effects on the opioid, dopamine, and serotonin systems in the brain. Sustained heavy consumption of alcohol leads to dependency and increased tolerance, along with reduced sensitivity to GABA and increased sensitivity to NMDA. These alcohol abusers are also at risk for the development of withdrawal symptoms after cessation of alcohol consumption.

In addition to the increased susceptibility to withdrawal symptoms, dietary deficiency is common in alcohol abusers. Alcohol contains so-called empty calories because it does not provide significant amounts of protein and vitamins. A gram of pure ethanol contains 7 calories. A person who drinks a pint of 86-proof liquor daily consumes well over 1000 calories a day, approximately half of the daily caloric requirement. The alcohol consumption inevitably results in reduced intake of other foods. The problem is compounded further by malabsorption and abnormal metabolism of vitamins, both of which are common in alcoholics.

Despite the increased risk of malnutrition, only Wernicke-Korsakoff syndrome and rare cases of pellagra in alcoholics are clearly linked to nutritional deficiency. The pathogenesis of other neurological disorders is less clear (Box 85.4), though many have postulated a direct toxic effect of alcohol on both the central and peripheral nervous systems. For instance, neuropathy sometimes develops in alcohol abusers with normal nutritional status. The pattern of nerve fiber loss in these patients appears to be different from that in beriberi neuropathy from thiamine deficiency, thus suggesting a different pathological mechanism (Koike et al., 2003).

**BOX 85.4 Neurological Complications Associated with Alcohol Abuse**

**Nutritional Deficiency**
Wernicke encephalopathy
Korsakoff syndrome
Pellagra

**Direct Effects of Alcohol**
Acute intoxication
Fetal alcohol syndrome

**Abnormalities of Serum Electrolytes and Osmolality**
Central pontine myelinolysis

**Alcohol Withdrawal**
Withdrawal seizures
Alcoholic hallucinosis
Delirium tremens

**Diseases of Uncertain Pathogenesis**
Alcoholic neuropathy
Alcoholic myopathy
Amblyopia
Cerebellar degeneration
Marchiafava-Bignami disease

### Alcohol-Withdrawal Syndromes

Alcohol-withdrawal syndrome typically occurs in patients with a long history of sustained alcohol use. Symptoms appear 4–12 hours after the last consumption of alcohol. The initial symptoms are insomnia, anxiety, tremulousness, palpitations, and diaphoresis. It is not uncommon for symptoms to appear even when there is a significant alcohol level in the blood. Mild cases of alcohol withdrawal are self-limiting, with symptoms peaking and resolving within 72 hours. Moderate to severe cases require urgent medical attention, as they are often complicated by withdrawal seizures, alcoholic hallucinosis, and delirium tremens.

Alcohol-withdrawal seizures are generalized clonic-tonic convulsions that usually occur between 12 and 48 hours from the last drink, though shorter or longer time intervals are possible. Most patients have either a single seizure or seizures occurring in a brief flurry. Status epilepticus is rare in isolated alcohol withdrawal, though alcohol withdrawal frequently complicates seizure disorders from other causes. The occurrence of status epilepticus or the presence of ominous features such as focal seizures or focal deficits in the postictal state should prompt an investigation into other structural, metabolic, or infectious causes. Although most alcohol-withdrawal seizures are self-limiting, recurrent or prolonged seizures require treatment. Benzodiazepines or phenobarbital are preferred over phenytoin, which is ineffective in withdrawal seizures.

With or without seizures, the initial symptoms of alcohol withdrawal may further progress to altered mentation. Visual and sometimes auditory and tactile hallucinations (alcoholic hallucinosis) often occur in the first 2 days after the last drink. They are then followed by delirium and agitation, accompanied by tachycardia, hypertension, fever, or diaphoresis (delirium tremens). Fluid and electrolyte disturbances often accompany delirium tremens. Hypovolemia, hypokalemia, hypomagnesemia, and hypophosphatemia are common and should be promptly treated if present. Other secondary complications may include cardiac failure, dysrhythmia, rhabdomyolysis, alcoholic pancreatitis, hepatitis, and pneumonia.

Benzodiazepines and supportive care are the mainstays in the treatment of a severe alcohol-withdrawal state. A fast-acting benzodiazepine such as diazepam, lorazepam, or oxazepam should be given via the IV route. They are effective in controlling the agitation and sympathetic hyperactivity as well as any withdrawal seizures. This should be accompanied by aggressive support with IV fluids, nutritional supplementation (see the earlier section Wernicke-Korsakoff Syndrome), treatment of coexisting complications, and close monitoring of vital signs, fluid status, and electrolytes. Less-proven agents such as β-adrenergic antagonists, clonidine, and carbamazepine may also be used as adjunctive measures in controlling alcohol-withdrawal symptoms. The improvement of treatment has reduced the mortality rate of delirium tremens from over 30% at the beginning of the 20th century to the current rate of no more than 5%.

## Alcoholic Neuropathy

Neuropathy is the most frequent neurological complication of alcoholism. Depending on the method of ascertainment, it may be diagnosed in 10%–75% of alcoholic patients. Most affected patients are between age 40 and 60, and, in essentially all cases, there is a history of chronic and heavy alcohol intake for many years.

### Clinical Features

Alcoholic neuropathy is a mixed sensory and motor disorder that affects large- and small-diameter nerve fibers to varying degrees (Zambelis et al., 2005). Symptom onset is insidious, beginning in the feet and progressing proximally and symmetrically. Paresthesia is the most common presenting complaint. Many patients also complain of pain, either an aching discomfort in the calves or a burning sensation over the soles. Dysesthesia may be so severe that a light touch or gentle rubbing over the skin is intensely unpleasant. Interestingly, pain is more often a problem in those with milder neuropathy. On examination, both deep and superficial sensations are affected. Ankle tendon reflexes and sometimes knee reflexes are lost. Weakness and wasting are limited to the distal feet in mild cases but can involve the distal upper extremities in more severe cases. Rarely there may be vagus or recurrent laryngeal nerve involvement, with prominent hoarseness and weakness of voice. Both alcohol neurotoxicity and thiamine deficiency likely play important roles in alcoholic neuropathy. One study (Koike et al., 2003) suggests that pure alcoholic neuropathy without thiamine deficiency is more likely to be painful and has less motor involvement than that associated with concomitant thiamine deficiency.

Other manifestations of chronic alcoholism are often evident. Liver cirrhosis, hepatic encephalopathy, Wernicke-Korsakoff syndrome, alcoholic cerebellar degeneration, and alcohol-withdrawal symptoms all occur frequently at the time of evaluation. Trophic skin changes in the form of hyperpigmentation, edema, ulcers, and cellulitis in the distal part of the feet are sometimes encountered. There may be radiological suggestions of a distal neuropathic arthropathy (Charcot forefeet, acrodystrophic neuropathy), with phalangeal atrophy, bony resorption, and subluxation of small joints in the feet. Repeated trauma and infections to insensitive parts of the feet are probably responsible. This syndrome is prevalent in the south of France and Spain, where the term *Thevenard syndrome* is applied.

### Laboratory Studies and Pathology

The pathology of alcoholic neuropathy is predominantly axonal loss. Nerve conduction studies show reduced amplitude of sensory nerve responses, with normal or mildly reduced conduction velocities. Electromyography may reveal signs of denervation and reinnervation in distal muscles of the lower extremities. Axonal degeneration of both myelinated and unmyelinated fibers is present on sural nerve biopsy. In some patients, autonomic dysfunction may be demonstrated by abnormalities in heart rate variation to deep breathing, Valsalva maneuver, and postural change.

### Treatment

It is prudent to treat most affected patients with abstinence from alcohol, supplemental multivitamins, and a balanced diet. Even under ideal conditions, recovery is slow and incomplete.

## Tobacco–Alcohol or Nutritional Amblyopia

Tobacco–alcohol amblyopia is a syndrome of vision loss caused by a selective lesion of the optic nerves. In Western countries, most affected patients are chronic and severe alcoholics, often with a history of poor dietary intake or marked weight loss. Vision loss occurs insidiously and painlessly, progressing in both eyes over a period of several weeks. The most common deficits are impaired visual acuity and the presence of central or centrocecal scotomata. Even in severely affected subjects, the optic discs may show only mild pallor. The commonly used term *tobacco–alcohol amblyopia* is likely incorrect, as neither agent has been proven to be directly responsible. The disease is probably identical to the nutritional amblyopia seen in prisoners of war and malnourished individuals who have no access to either alcohol or tobacco. Moreover, treatment with a combination of an adequate diet and B vitamins, despite the continuation of drinking and smoking, results in visual recovery. Dietary deficiencies of vitamin $B_{12}$, thiamine, folate, and riboflavin, all of which have been linked to optic neuropathy, may individually or together be responsible.

## Marchiafava-Bignami Disease

In 1903, Marchiafava and Bignami, two Italian pathologists, described a syndrome of selective demyelination of the corpus callosum in alcoholic Italians who indulged in large quantities of red wine. The disease seems to affect primarily severe and chronic alcoholics in their middle or late adult life, with a peak incidence between ages 40 and 60. It is not restricted to any one ethnic group, and consumption of red wine is not an invariable feature. With the widespread use of MRI, there has been an increase in recognition of this previously rare disorder. A few cases have also been reported in nonalcoholics.

The neurological presentation is variable. The most common are an acute confusional state or a dementing syndrome. Patients may present with a variable combination of psychomotor slowing, behavioral changes, incontinence, dysarthria, and spasticity. Seizures, hemiparesis, and coma are sometimes seen. Pathologically, there is selective involvement of the central portion of the corpus callosum; the dorsal and ventral regions are spared or affected to a lesser degree. There also may be symmetrical involvement of other white-matter tracts. MRI is valuable and shows increased T2 and FLAIR signals along with restricted diffusion in the body of the corpus callosum, sometimes with extension into the genu or the splenium (Menegon et al., 2005). Abnormalities may also be seen in the subcortical white matter and cerebellar peduncles. Thinning of the corpus callosum is seen commonly in alcoholics without symptoms of Marchiafava-Bignami disease. It is unclear what causes the overt disease in susceptible individuals.

Treatment of Marchiafava-Bignami disease should be directed at supportive care, nutritional supplements, and rehabilitation from alcoholism. In those patients who recovered, it is not clear whether improvement was a result of nutritional supplementation or merely a reflection of the disease's natural history.

## Alcoholic Cerebellar Degeneration

Alcoholic cerebellar degeneration is likely the most common of the acquired degenerations of the cerebellum. Men are affected more frequently than women, and the incidence peaks in the middle decades of life. Alcohol abuse is long-standing in all patients, and alcoholic polyneuropathy accompanies most of them. The clinical syndrome is usually quite stereotyped. The presentation is a progressive unsteadiness in walking that evolves over weeks or months. Less commonly, a mild gait difficulty may be present for some time, only to worsen suddenly during binge drinking or an intercurrent illness. On examination, the most prominent finding is a truncal ataxia, demonstrated by a wide-based gait and difficulty with tandem walking. Limb ataxia, if present, is much milder than the truncal ataxia and more severe in the legs than in the arms. In contrast to Wernicke encephalopathy, nystagmus and ocular dysmetria are uncommon. Dysarthria, tremor, and hypotonia are rare findings.

The pathogenesis of cerebellar degeneration is unknown, though both nutritional deficiency and direct toxicity of alcohol may play a role. The pathological changes consist of selective atrophy of the anterior and superior parts of the cerebellar vermis, with the cerebellar hemispheres involved to a lesser extent. Cell loss involves all neuronal types in the cerebellum, although Purkinje cells are the most severely affected. A mild secondary loss of neurons is common in the deep cerebellar nuclei and the inferior olivary nuclei. In some patients, concomitant pathological changes of Wernicke encephalopathy may be present. Abstinence is the main treatment and can lead to a partial but incomplete improvement. With abstinence from alcohol and nutritional supplements, improvement in cerebellar symptoms occurs slowly but is often incomplete.

## VITAMIN A

Dietary deficiency of vitamin A is uncommon in Europe and the United States. Deficiency may occur rarely in fat malabsorption syndromes such as sprue, biliary atresia, and cystic fibrosis. A few cases have occurred in infants put on nondairy formula free of vitamin A. The earliest sign of deficiency is reduced ability to see in dim light. Retinol, an aldehyde form of vitamin A, binds with the protein, opsin, to form rhodopsin, which is responsible for vision at low light level. Xerosis, or keratinization, of the conjunctiva and cornea often accompanies night blindness. Some patients have the characteristic Bitot spots, which are white foam-like spots appearing at the side of the cornea. These eye findings are caused by metaplasia of epithelial cells and, if severe, can lead to permanent blindness. Rarely, infants may manifest a syndrome of raised intracranial pressure, bulging fontanelles, and lethargy.

Patients with signs of vitamin A toxicity or overdose are also likely to see a neurologist. The classic syndrome of toxicity is that of pseudotumor cerebri with headache, papilledema, nausea, and vomiting. The skin is often dry and pruritic, and patients may complain of generalized joint or bone pain. Especially in children, joint swelling and hyperostoses are often evident on roentgenography. Chronic daily consumption of more than 25,000 IU may produce toxicity, although most reported patients consumed much higher doses over a shorter period of time. Unusual foods, such as polar bear liver and halibut liver, contain high concentrations of vitamin A and have caused acute toxicity. Serum retinol level is useful in the diagnosis. The generally accepted lower limit of normal is 20 mg/dL, whereas concentrations in excess of 100 mg/dL are suggestive of toxicity.

## VITAMIN D

Vitamin D is important for bone and calcium metabolism. Deficiency may be caused by a diversity of systemic conditions including dietary insufficiency, malabsorption, inadequate sunlight exposure, immobility, anticonvulsant use, hypophosphatemia, and hyperparathyroidism. The recommended laboratory assay is the serum level of 25-hydroxyvitamin D (25[OH]D). The optimal 25(OH)D level is unsettled, although most favor a serum level between 20 and 40 ng/mL for ideal bone health. A recent surge in interest in the role of vitamin D in neurological disorders arose from three lines of observation. First, a large portion of the elderly population may be deficient in vitamin D, most likely from a combination of inadequate dietary intake, decreased exposure to sunlight, and decreased vitamin D skin production with aging. Second, vitamin D has potentially diverse effects in the nervous system through its action on inflammatory cytokines, neurotrophins, and calcium-binding proteins. Third, low levels of 25(OH)D have been associated with a number of neurological diseases including multiple sclerosis, Parkinson disease, stroke, and cognitive decline (Miller, 2010). On the other hand, an observed association does not prove causation. Whether vitamin D supplementation has any beneficial impact in central nervous system diseases remains to be seen (McLaughlin et al., 2018).

The best-documented neurological syndrome attributable to overt vitamin D deficiency is a myopathy characterized by proximal weakness (Al-Said et al., 2009). Progressive weakness develops over many months. Weakness leads to difficulty in going up stairs and rising from a chair. When severe, some patients are wheelchair dependent. Diffuse bone pain, muscle pain, or back pain is common. Stretch reflexes and sensation are normal. Some patients may already have a diagnosis of osteomalacia. Serum creatine kinase level is usually normal or only mildly elevated. Serum alkaline phosphatase is abnormally high, and calcium and phosphorus may be normal or mildly decreased. Electromyography typically shows short-duration low-amplitude and polyphasic motor unit potentials without spontaneous activities; these features are similar to those of other metabolic myopathies. Nonspecific type II muscle fiber atrophy is seen on biopsy.

Oral supplementation of vitamin D is recommended in patients with low serum 25(OH)D levels. There are various effective regimens. Cholecalciferol, vitamin $D_3$, appears slightly more effective than ergocalciferol, vitamin $D_2$, although both are suitable. One approach in severely depleted patients (<12 ng/mL) is to employ weekly oral supplementation of 50,000 IU ($D_2$ or $D_3$) for 6 weeks, followed by 800–1000 IU daily afterwards. Less-depleted patients may be treated with daily oral doses of 800–1000 IU. In patients with myopathy from vitamin D deficiency, prompt improvement occurs after supplementation (Al-Said et al., 2009; Mokta et al., 2017). Pain usually subsides first, and laboratory abnormalities return to normal after a short period of repletion. Satisfactory recovery of muscle weakness follows over subsequent months.

The role of vitamin D deficiency in other causes of muscle pain is less clear in light of the high prevalence of low serum 25(OH)D levels in otherwise asymptomatic subjects. There is some suggestion that patients with statin-related myalgia and low serum vitamin D level may improve their statin tolerance after vitamin D supplementation (Riche et al., 2016). Regardless, it is prudent to check serum 25(OH)D level in patients with proximal weakness or muscle pain, as vitamin D deficiency is an easily amendable condition.

## MISCELLANEOUS DEFICIENCY DISEASES

### Complications after Bariatric Surgery

In the United States, surgery is increasingly used to treat obesity. The devised surgical strategies involve some combination of gastroplasty or gastric bypass, and they share the common goals of limiting food absorption and inducing early satiety. These patients are at great risk for development of deficiency in multiple micronutrients (especially B vitamins and folate, and less commonly vitamin E, vitamin D, vitamin A, and trace elements such as copper). Aside from compressive neuropathies that can result from a dramatic weight loss, clinically significant malabsorption and vitamin deficiency syndromes are common. The estimated frequency of these neurological disorders varies widely. An early retrospective study of 500 patients reported that 4.6% had neurological complications 3–20 months after surgery (Abarbanel et al., 1987).

The most commonly reported neurological complication is peripheral neuropathy. A retrospective study of 435 patients found 16% with peripheral neuropathy (Thaisetthawatkul et al., 2004). Most of these patients have a sensorimotor polyneuropathy. Mononeuropathies and plexopathies are less frequent. Wernicke encephalopathy is the most common central nervous system disorder. Uncommon complications include vitamin A-deficiency retinopathy, optic neuropathy, myelopathy, and myopathy (Koffman et al., 2006). Some patients may not become symptomatic until many years after surgery. All patients should have long-term medical follow-up, dietary counseling, and periodic laboratory evaluations. They should all take dietary supplements on an indefinite basis. Supplements should include multivitamins with additional oral vitamin $B_{12}$ supplement, iron, calcium, and the essential trace elements.

## Acute Nutritional Neuropathy

While the majority of neuropathies due to nutritional deficiencies are chronic in nature, a diffuse axonal neuropathy may rarely present in an acute or subacute manner (Hamel and Logigian, 2018; Thaisetthawatkul et al., 2004). This occurs typically in the setting of alcoholism, bariatric surgery, or anorexia. The neurological disease is accompanied by weight loss, vomiting, or diarrhea. Patients present with progressive, length-dependent sensory loss and areflexia, gait ataxia, and sometimes lower limb weakness. Nerve conduction study shows an axonal sensorimotor polyneuropathy. The condition may be distinguished from axonal Guillain-Barré syndrome by its slower onset over many days or a few weeks, absence of cranial nerve involvement, lack of antecedent infection, and occurrence in the setting of severe nutritional derangement. This condition is likely an extension of the acute beriberi syndrome seen in thiamine deficiency. In the reported patients, thiamine level, if measured before supplementation, was low, and there was also deficiency of other vitamins such as pyridoxine (Hamel and Logigian, 2018).

## Copper Deficiency

Deficiency of copper classically leads to a myelopathy or myeloneuropathy characterized by sensory ataxia and gait difficulty (Jaiser and Winston, 2010). The syndrome may be difficult to distinguish from the subacute combined degeneration of vitamin $B_{12}$ deficiency. Common symptoms are lower-limb paresthesias and gait difficulty. The syndrome is characterized by sensory loss and sensory ataxia. Examination shows prominent proprioceptive impairment, less severe sensory loss to other modalities, brisk reflexes, and variable presence of Babinski sign (Kumar, 2006). Diminished ankle reflex and evidence of axonal loss on nerve conduction studies, indicating the presence of a sensorimotor polyneuropathy, are common. Other observers have described unusual clinical features such as cognitive dysfunction, optic neuropathy, sensory ganglionopathy, and asymmetrical weakness from a lower motor neuron syndrome.

Finding a low serum copper level, along with low serum ceruloplasmin and low urinary copper excretion, helps to establish the diagnosis of copper deficiency. There may be associated hematological abnormalities such as anemia (microcytic, normocytic, or macrocytic) and neutropenia. Abnormal T2 signals on MRI may be seen along the posterior column of the spinal cord. Interpretation of copper and ceruloplasmin levels may be complicated. Ceruloplasmin is the chief carrier protein for copper, and its serum level generally parallels that of copper. Ceruloplasmin is also an acute-phase reactant, and its concentration increases in pregnancy, liver disease, and various infectious and inflammatory disorders. Thus, serum copper level in a deficiency state may be falsely normal under some conditions. Low levels of ceruloplasmin and low serum copper are seen in Wilson disease (see Chapter 95). In such patients, urinary copper excretion is typically elevated (>100 μg over 24 hours).

The most common cause is impaired absorption of dietary copper after gastric surgeries, including bariatric surgery. GI disorders predisposing to malabsorption, such as sprue, celiac disease, and bacterial overgrowth, are also risk factors. Excessive dietary consumption of zinc and iron may impair the absorption of copper. Some cases have been reported in the setting of parenteral zinc overload from renal dialysis. Menkes disease is a form of congenital copper deficiency and is due to an inherited disorder of intestinal copper absorption. Clioquinol, an antibiotic with the property of being a copper-zinc chelator, may rarely be responsible. Even in cases of malabsorption, dietary supplementation of 2–6 mg of copper salt per day is usually sufficient to reverse a deficiency state. Intravenous infusion may be used if needed. Replenishment appears to halt progression of disease but with little neurological improvement (Jaiser and Winston, 2010; Kelkar et al., 2008).

## Protein-Calorie Malnutrition

Millions of infants and children in underdeveloped countries suffer from varying degrees of protein and calorie deficiencies and manifest two interrelated syndromes: marasmus and kwashiorkor. Marasmus is primarily a result of caloric insufficiency and is characterized by extreme emaciation and growth failure in early infancy. These infants usually have never been breastfed or were weaned before 1 year of age. Kwashiorkor is seen most commonly in children weaned between 2 and 3 years of age, and its primary underlying cause is protein deficiency. The signs of kwashiorkor are edema, ascites, hepatomegaly, sparse hair, and skin depigmentation.

The earliest and most consistent neurological signs in these children are apathy to the environment and extreme irritability. Weakness, generalized muscle wasting, hypotonia, and hyporeflexia occur frequently. Cognitive deficits may be permanent despite improvement in nutrition. It is difficult to separate the effects of malnutrition from those of socioeconomic deprivation, but comparison studies in siblings show persistent impairment of intelligence attributable to malnutrition. Autopsy and imaging studies show the brain to be slightly atrophic, and neuronal development is less mature. A mild encephalopathy, usually no more than transient drowsiness, sometimes occurs during the first week of dietary treatment. Occasionally, children develop asterixis or coma or even die as a result of their treatment. Other children manifest a transient syndrome of rigidity, coarse tremors, myoclonus, and exaggerated tendon reflexes during the first few weeks of recovery from malnutrition.

*The complete reference list is available online at https://expertconsult.inkling.com/.* 

86

# Effects of Toxins and Physical Agents on the Nervous System

*Michael J. Aminoff, Yuen T. So*

## OUTLINE



Neurotoxic disorders are occurring increasingly as a result of occupational or environmental exposure and often go unrecognized. Exposure to neurotoxins may lead to dysfunction of any part of the central, peripheral, or autonomic nervous system and the neuromuscular apparatus. Neurotoxic disorders are recognized readily if a close temporal relationship exists between clinical onset and prior exposure to an agent, especially one known to be neurotoxic. Known neurotoxins produce stereotypical neurological disturbances that generally cease to progress soon after exposure is discontinued and ultimately improve to a variable extent. Recognition of a neurotoxic disorder may be difficult, however, when exposure is chronic or symptoms are nonspecific. The problem is compounded when the exposure history is unclear. Diagnosis may also be clouded by concerns about other confounding factors, such as other drugs, illnesses, and possible litigation. Patients often attribute symptoms of an idiopathic disorder to an exposure when no other cause can be found.

Single case reports that an agent is neurotoxic are unreliable, especially when the neurological symptoms are frequent in the general population. Epidemiological studies may be helpful in establishing a neurotoxic basis for symptoms. However, many of the published studies are inadequate because of methodological problems such as the selection of appropriate control subjects. Recognition of a neurotoxic basis for neurobehavioral disorders, for example, requires matching of exposed subjects and unexposed controls for many factors including age; gender; race; premorbid cognitive ability; educational, social, and cultural background; and alcohol, recreational drug, and medication use. Laboratory test results are often unhelpful in confirming that the neurological syndrome is caused by a specific agent, either because the putative neurotoxin cannot be measured in body tissues or because the interval since exposure makes such measurements meaningless.

The part of the central, peripheral, or autonomic nervous system and the neuromuscular apparatus damaged by exposure to neurotoxins depends on the responsible agent. The pathophysiological basis of neurotoxicity is often unknown. In considering the possibility of a neurotoxic disorder, it is important to obtain a detailed account of the exposure, including details of the duration and severity, and any protective measures taken, if applicable. Then it must be determined whether any of these agents are known to be neurotoxic and whether symptoms are compatible with the known toxicity of the suspected compound. Many neurotoxins can produce clinical disorders that resemble other known metabolic, nutritional, or degenerative neurological disorders, and it is therefore important to consider these and any other relevant disease processes in the differential diagnosis. In recognizing new neurotoxic disorders, a clustering of cases is often important, but this may not be evident until patients are referred for specialist evaluation.

Neurotoxins cause diffuse rather than focal or lateralized neurological dysfunction. The neurological disorder is typically monophasic. Depending on the neurotoxin, and on the duration and level of exposure, it most commonly takes the form of an acute or chronic encephalopathy or a peripheral neuropathy. Although progression may occur for several weeks after exposure has been discontinued ("coasting"), it is eventually arrested, and improvement may then follow, depending on the severity of the original disorder. Prolonged or progressive deterioration long after exposure has been discontinued, or the development of neurological symptoms months to years after exposure, suggests that a neurotoxic disorder is not responsible.

Any discussion of developmental neurotoxicity (i.e., the adverse effects of industrial chemicals on the development of the brain and behavior) is beyond the scope of the present chapter.

## OCCUPATIONAL EXPOSURE TO ORGANIC CHEMICALS

### Acrylamide

Acrylamide polymers are used as flocculators and are constituents of certain adhesives and products such as cardboard or molded parts. They also are used as grouting agents for mines and tunnels, a solution of the monomer being pumped into the ground where polymerization is allowed to occur. The monomer is neurotoxic, and exposure may occur during its manufacture or in the polymerization process. Most cases of acrylamide toxicity occur by inhalation or cutaneous absorption. Acrylamide can be formed by cooking various carbohydrate-rich foods at high temperatures, but consumption is unlikely to be sufficient for neurotoxicity. The acrylamide is distributed widely throughout the body and is excreted primarily through the kidneys. The mechanism responsible for its neurotoxicity is unknown, but it has been related to an inhibitory effect on presynaptic function (LoPachin and Gavin, 2012), by damage to the nerve terminal involving membrane fusion mechanisms and tubulovesicular alterations (Pennisi et al., 2013), and to abnormalities of kinesin-based fast axonal transport. Axonal swellings due to accumulations of neurofilaments relate to impaired retrograde axonal transport.

Clinical manifestations of acrylamide toxicity depend on the severity of exposure. Acute high-dose exposure results in confusion, hallucinations, reduced attention span, drowsiness, and other encephalopathic changes. A peripheral neuropathy of variable severity may occur after acute high-dose or prolonged low-level exposure. The neuropathy is a length-dependent axonopathy involving both sensory and motor fibers. Hyperhidrosis and dermatitis may develop before the neuropathy is evident clinically in those with repeated skin exposure. Ataxia from cerebellar dysfunction also occurs and relates to degeneration of afferent and efferent cerebellar fibers and Purkinje cells. Neurological examination reveals distal sensorimotor deficits and early loss of all tendon reflexes rather than simply the Achilles reflex, which is usually affected first in most length-dependent neuropathies. Autonomic abnormalities other than hyperhidrosis are uncommon. Gait and limb ataxia are usually greater than can be accounted for by the sensory loss. With discontinuation of exposure, the neuropathy "coasts," arrests, and may then slowly reverse, but residual neurological deficits are common. These consist particularly of spasticity and cerebellar ataxia; the peripheral neuropathy usually remits because regeneration occurs in the peripheral nervous system. No specific treatment exists but recovery may occur if further exposure is prevented. Studies in rats have shown that administration of FK506 to increase Hsp-70 expression may exert a neuroprotective effect and have therefore suggested that compounds eliciting a heat shock response may be useful for treating the neuropathy in humans (Gold et al., 2004).

Electrodiagnostic studies provide evidence of an axonal sensorimotor polyneuropathy. Workers exposed to acrylamide may be monitored electrophysiologically by recording sensory nerve action potentials, which are attenuated early in the course of the disorder, or by measuring the vibration threshold. Histopathological studies show accumulation of neurofilaments in axons, especially distally, and distal degeneration of peripheral and central axons. The large myelinated axons are involved first. The affected central pathways include the ascending sensory fibers in the posterior columns, the spinocerebellar tracts, and the descending corticospinal pathways. Involvement of postganglionic sympathetic efferent nerve fibers accounts for the sudomotor dysfunction. Measurement of hemoglobin–acrylamide adducts may be useful in predicting the development of peripheral neuropathy.

### Allyl Chloride

Allyl chloride is used for manufacturing epoxy resins, certain insecticides, and polyacrylonitrile. Exposure leads to a mixed sensorimotor distal axonopathy. Cessation of exposure is followed by recovery of variable degree. Intra-axonal accumulation of neurofilaments occurs multifocally before axonal degeneration in animals exposed to this compound. Similar changes may also occur in the posterolateral columns of the spinal cord.

### Carbon Disulfide

Carbon disulfide is used as a solvent or soil fumigant, in perfume production, in certain varnishes and insecticides, in the cold vulcanization of rubber, and in manufacturing viscose rayon and cellophane films. Toxicity occurs primarily from inhalation or ingestion but also may occur transdermally. The pathogenetic mechanism is uncertain but may involve an essential metal-chelating effect of carbon disulfide metabolites, direct inhibition of certain enzymes, or the release of free radicals following cleavage of the carbon–sulfur bond. Most reported cases have been from Europe and Japan.

Acute inhalation of concentrations exceeding 300–400 ppm leads to an encephalopathy, with symptoms that vary from mild behavioral disturbances to drowsiness and, ultimately, to respiratory failure. Behavioral disturbances may include explosive behavior, mood swings, mania or depression, confusion, and other psychiatric disturbances. Long-term exposure to concentrations between 40 and 50 ppm may produce similar disturbances. Minor affective or cognitive disturbances may be revealed only by neuropsychological testing.

Long-term exposure to carbon disulfide may lead also to extrapyramidal (parkinsonian) or pyramidal deficits, impaired vision, absent pupillary and corneal reflexes, optic neuropathy, and a characteristic retinopathy. A small-vessel vasculopathy may be responsible (Huang, 2004). Neuroimaging may reveal cortical—especially frontal—atrophy, as well as lesions in the globus pallidus and putamen. Computed tomography (CT) angiography and perfusion studies have revealed decreased cerebral blood flow in total brain parenchyma and basal ganglia, decreased cerebral blood volume in the basal ganglia, and a prolonged mean transit time in the total brain parenchyma and the territories of the internal carotid artery, basal ganglia, and occipital lobe. Such findings have been held to support the presence of a microangiopathy (Chuang et al., 2007).

A clinical or subclinical polyneuropathy develops after exposure to levels of 100–150 ppm for several months or to lesser levels for longer periods and is characterized histologically by axonal loss, focal axonal swellings, and neurofilamentary accumulations. Clinically there is stocking-glove impairment of all sensory modalities together with distal weakness and absent ankle reflexes. The concurrence of neuropathy and parkinsonism should suggest the possibility of carbon disulfide intoxication.

No specific treatment exists other than the avoidance of further exposure. Recovery from the peripheral neuropathy generally follows the discontinuation of exposure, but some central deficits may persist.

## Carbon Monoxide

Occupational exposure to carbon monoxide occurs mainly in miners, gas workers, and garage employees. Other modes of exposure include poorly ventilated home heating systems, stoves, and suicide attempts. The neurotoxic effects of carbon monoxide relate to intracellular hypoxia. Carbon monoxide binds to hemoglobin with high affinity to form carboxyhemoglobin; it also limits the dissociation of oxyhemoglobin and binds to various enzymes. Acute toxicity leads to headache, disturbances of consciousness, and a variety of other behavioral changes. Motor abnormalities include the development of pyramidal and extrapyramidal deficits. Seizures may occur, and focal cortical deficits sometimes develop. Treatment involves prevention of further exposure to carbon monoxide and administration of pure or hyperbaric oxygen. New therapies aimed at the inflammatory effects and oxidative stress induced by carbon monoxide poisoning or helping remove carbon monoxide from the body, as with porphyrin complexes or modified globin proteins, are under study (Rose et al., 2017).

Neurological deterioration may occur several weeks after partial or apparently full recovery from the acute effects of carbon monoxide exposure, with recurrence of motor and behavioral abnormalities. The degree of recovery from this delayed deterioration is variable; full or near-full recovery occurs in some instances, but other patients lapse into a persistent vegetative state or severe parkinsonism. Neuroimaging may show lesions in the periventricular white matter, globus pallidus, and elsewhere. There may be diffuse brain atrophy.

Pathological examination shows hypoxic and ischemic damage in the cerebral cortex as well as in the hippocampus, cerebellar cortex, and basal ganglia. Lesions are also present diffusely in the cerebral white matter. The delayed deterioration has been related to a diffuse subcortical leukoencephalopathy, but its pathogenesis is uncertain.

## Ethylene Oxide

Ethylene oxide is used to sterilize heat-sensitive medical equipment and as an alkylating agent in industrial chemical synthesis. A by-product, ethylene chlorohydrin, is highly toxic. Operators of sterilization equipment should wear protective ventilatory apparatus to prevent occupational exposure. Acute exposure to high levels produces headache, nausea, and a severe, reversible encephalopathy, with seizures and disturbances of consciousness. Respiration may be impaired. Treatment is supportive. Long-term exposure to ethylene oxide or ethylene chlorohydrin—as can occur, for example, in operating-room nurses and sterilizer workers—may lead to a peripheral sensorimotor axonopathy and mild cognitive changes. Recovery generally follows the cessation of exposure. Neuropathy may be produced in rats by exposure to ethylene oxide, and the residual ethylene oxide in sterilized dialysis tubing may contribute to the polyneuropathy occurring in patients undergoing chronic hemodialysis.

## Hexacarbon Solvents

The hexacarbon solvents n-hexane and methyl-n-butyl ketone are both metabolized to 2,5-hexanedione, which is responsible in large part for their neurotoxicity. This neurotoxicity is potentiated by methyl ethyl ketone, which is used in paints, lacquers, printer's ink, and certain glues. n-Hexane is used as a solvent in paints, lacquers, and printing inks and is used especially in the rubber industry and in certain glues. Workers involved in the manufacturing of footwear, laminating processes, and cabinetry, especially in confined, unventilated spaces, may be exposed to excessive concentrations of these substances. Methyl-n-butyl ketone is used in the manufacture of vinyl and acrylic coatings and adhesives and in the printing industry. Exposure to either of these chemicals by inhalation or skin contact leads to a progressive distal sensorimotor axonal polyneuropathy; partial conduction block may also occur. Optic neuropathy or maculopathy and facial numbness also have followed n-hexane exposure. The neuropathy is related to a disturbance of axonal transport, and histopathological studies reveal giant multifocal axonal swelling and accumulation of axonal neurofilaments, with distal degeneration in peripheral and central axons. Myelin retraction and focal demyelination are found at the giant axonal swellings.

Acute inhalation exposure may produce feelings of euphoria associated with hallucinations, headache, unsteadiness, and mild narcosis. This has led to the inhalation of certain glues for recreational purposes, which causes pleasurable feelings of euphoria in the short term but may lead to a progressive, predominantly motor neuropathy and symptoms of dysautonomia after high-dose exposure and a more insidious sensorimotor polyneuropathy following chronic use.

Electrophysiological findings include increased distal motor latency and marked slowing of maximal motor conduction velocity, as well as small or absent sensory nerve action potentials and electromyographic (EMG) signs of denervation in affected muscles. The conduction slowing relates to demyelinating changes and is unusual in other toxic neuropathies. A reduction in the size of sensory nerve action potentials may occur in the absence of clinical or other electrophysiological evidence of nerve involvement. Central involvement may result in abnormalities of sensory evoked potentials. The cerebrospinal fluid (CSF) is usually normal, but a mildly elevated protein concentration is sometimes found.

Despite cessation of exposure, progression of the neurological deficit may continue for several weeks or, rarely, months (coasting) before the downhill course is arrested and recovery begins. Clinical and electrophysiological recovery of the peripheral neuropathy may take several years and may not be complete when involvement is severe (Little and Albers, 2015). As the polyneuropathy resolves, previously masked signs of central dysfunction, such as spasticity, may become evident.

## Methyl Bromide

Methyl bromide has been used as a refrigerant, insecticide, fumigant, and fire extinguisher, but its use has been banned in many countries because of its ozone-depleting properties. Its high volatility may lead to work-area concentrations sufficient to cause neurotoxicity from inhalation. Following acute high-level exposure, an interval of several hours or more may elapse before the onset of symptoms. Because methyl bromide is odorless and colorless, subjects may not even be aware that exposure has occurred, so chloropicrin, a conjunctival and mucosal irritant, is commonly added to methyl bromide to warn of inhalation exposure. Acute methyl bromide intoxication leads to an encephalopathy with convulsions, delirium, hyperpyrexia, coma, pulmonary edema, and death. Acute exposure to lower concentrations may result in conspicuous mental changes, including confusion, psychosis or affective disturbances, headache, nausea, dysarthria, tremulousness, myoclonus, ataxia, visual disturbances, and seizures. The electroencephalogram (EEG) may show frontally predominant slow waves or polyspike-wave complexes, while magnetic resonance imaging (MRI) reveals involvement of the dentate nucleus, brainstem, and splenium of the corpus callosum (De Souza et al., 2013).

Long-term, low-level exposure may lead to a polyneuropathy in the absence of systemic symptoms. Distal paresthesias are followed by sensory and motor deficits, loss of tendon reflexes, and an ataxic gait. Visual disturbances, optic atrophy, and upper motor neuron deficits may occur also. Calf tenderness is sometimes conspicuous. The CSF is unremarkable. Electrodiagnostic study results reveal both sensory and motor involvement. Gradual improvement occurs with cessation of exposure.

The basis of the neurotoxicity is uncertain but methyl phosphates formed in cells may contribute to its neuron-specific toxicity via cholinesterase inhibition (Bulathsinghala and Shaw, 2014). Treatment is symptomatic and supportive. Hemodialysis may help in removing bromide from the blood. Chelating agents are of uncertain utility.

## Organochlorine Pesticides

The organochlorine pesticides include aldrin, dieldrin, and lindane, as well as the once-popular insecticide dichlorodiphenyl-trichloroethane, commonly called *DDT*. Exposure is typically through inhalation or ingestion. Tremor, convulsions, and coma may follow acute high-level exposure, but the effects of chronic low-level exposure are uncertain. Chlordecone, which belongs to this group, may produce a neurological disorder characterized by "nervousness," tremor, clumsiness of the hands, gait ataxia, slurred speech, and opsoclonus. Minor cognitive changes, memory loss, and benign intracranial hypertension may occur. The signs may reverse over months or longer. The pathophysiology of the disorder has not been established.

The risk of developing Parkinson disease (PD) is reportedly increased by exposure to organochlorine insecticides but the involved mechanisms are unclear (Costa, 2015).

## Organophosphates

Organophosphates are used mainly as pesticides and herbicides but are also used as petroleum additives, lubricants, antioxidants, flame retardants, and plastic modifiers. Most cases of organophosphate toxicity result from exposure in an agricultural setting, not only among those mixing or spraying the pesticide or herbicide but also among workers returning prematurely to sprayed fields. Absorption may occur through the skin, by inhalation, or through the gastrointestinal tract. Organophosphates inhibit acetylcholinesterase by phosphorylation, with resultant acute cholinergic symptoms, with both central and neuromuscular manifestations. Symptoms include nausea, salivation, lacrimation, headache, weakness, and bronchospasm in mild instances and bradycardia, tremor, chest pain, diarrhea, pulmonary edema, cyanosis, convulsions, and even coma in more severe cases. Death may result from respiratory or heart failure. Treatment involves intravenous (IV) administration of pralidoxime (1 g) together with atropine (1 mg) given subcutaneously every 30 minutes until sweating and salivation are controlled. Pralidoxime accelerates reactivation of the inhibited acetylcholinesterase, and atropine is effective in counteracting muscarinic effects, although it has no effect on the nicotinic effects, such as neuromuscular cholinergic blockade with weakness or respiratory depression. It is important to ensure adequate ventilatory support before atropine is given. The dose of pralidoxime can be repeated if no obvious benefit occurs, but in refractory cases, it may need to be given by IV infusion, the dose being titrated against clinical response. Cardiac and respiratory function must be supported and seizures controlled pharmacologically. Functional recovery may take approximately 1 week, although acetylcholinesterase levels take longer to reach normal levels. Measurement of paraoxonase status may be worthwhile as a biomarker of susceptibility to acute organophosphate toxicity; this liver and serum enzyme hydrolyzes a number of organophosphate compounds and may have a role in modulating their toxicity (Costa et al., 2005).

Carbamate insecticides also inhibit cholinesterases but have a shorter duration of action than organophosphate compounds. The symptoms of toxicity are similar to those described for organophosphates but are generally milder. Treatment with atropine is usually sufficient.

Certain organophosphates cause a delayed polyneuropathy that occurs approximately 2–3 weeks after acute exposure even in the absence of cholinergic toxicity. In the past, contamination of illicit alcohol with tri-ortho cresyl phosphate ("Jake") led to large numbers of such cases. There is no evidence that peripheral nerve dysfunction follows prolonged low-level exposure to organophosphates (Vale and Lotti, 2015). Paresthesias in the feet and cramps in the calf muscles are followed by progressive weakness that typically begins distally in the limbs and then spreads to involve more proximal muscles. The maximal deficit usually develops within 2 weeks. Quadriplegia occurs in severe cases. Although sensory complaints are typically inconspicuous, clinical examination shows sensory deficits. The Achilles reflex is typically lost, and other tendon reflexes may be depressed also; however, in some instances, evidence of central involvement is manifested by brisk tendon reflexes. Cranial nerve function is typically spared. With time, there may be improvement in the peripheral neuropathy, but upper motor neuron involvement then becomes unmasked and often determines the prognosis for functional recovery. There is no specific treatment to arrest progression or hasten recovery. Electrodiagnostic studies reveal an axonopathy with partial denervation of affected muscles and small compound muscle action potentials but normal or only minimally reduced maximal motor conduction velocity.

The delayed syndrome follows exposure only to certain organophosphates, such as tri-ortho cresyl phosphate, leptophos, trichlorfon, and mipafox. The neurological disturbance relates in some way to phosphorylation and inhibition of the enzyme, neuropathy target esterase (NTE), which is present in essentially all neurons and has an uncertain role in the nervous system (Lotti and Moretto, 2005). In addition, "aging" of the inhibited NTE (loss of a group attached to the phosphorus, leaving a negatively charged phosphoryl group attached to the protein) must occur for the neuropathy to develop. The precise cause of the neuropathy is uncertain, however, as is the role of NTE in axonal degeneration. No specific treatment exists to prevent the occurrence of neuropathy following exposure, but the measurement of lymphocyte NTE has been used to monitor occupational exposure and predict the occurrence of neuropathy. Moreover, the ability of any particular organophosphate to inhibit NTE in hens may predict its neurotoxicity in humans.

Three other syndromes related to organophosphate exposure require brief comment. The *intermediate syndrome* occurs in the interval between the acute cholinergic crisis and the development of delayed neuropathy, typically becoming manifest within 4 days of exposure and resolving in 2–3 weeks (Abdollahi and Karami-Mohajeri, 2012). It reflects excessive cholinergic stimulation of nicotinic receptors and is characterized clinically by respiratory and bulbar symptoms as well as proximal limb weakness. Symptoms relate to the severity of poisoning and to prolonged inhibition of acetylcholinesterase activity but not to the development of delayed neuropathy. The syndrome of *dipper's flu* refers to the development of transient symptoms such as headache, rhinitis, pharyngitis, myalgia, and other flulike symptoms in farmers exposed to organophosphate sheep dips. Vague sensory complaints (but no objective abnormalities on sensory threshold tests) may also occur (Pilkington et al., 2001). Whether these complaints relate to mild organophosphate toxicity is uncertain. Similarly uncertain is whether *chronic effects* (persisting behavioral and neurological dysfunction) may occur in the absence of acute toxicity or follow acute exposure to organophosphates as a result of the respiratory and cardiac complications that sometimes occur (Vale and Lotti, 2015). A meta-analysis of well-designed studies, however, did find an association between low-level exposure and impaired neurobehavioral function (Ross et al., 2013). Evaluation of reports is hampered by incomplete documentation and the variety of agents to which exposure has often occurred. Carefully controlled studies may clarify this issue in the future.

## Pyrethroids

Pyrethroids are synthetic insecticides that affect voltage-sensitive sodium channels. Their neurotoxicity in mammals may also relate to their effect on sodium channels but voltage-gated calcium and chloride channels have been implicated as alternative or secondary sites of action for certain pyrethroids (Soderlund, 2012). Occupational or residential exposure is increasing, is mainly through the skin but may also occur through inhalation, and has led to paresthesias that have been attributed to repetitive activity in sensory fibers as a result of abnormal prolongation of the sodium current during membrane excitation. The paresthesias affect the face most commonly and are exacerbated by sensory stimulation such as scratching; they typically resolve within a day. Local application of a cool cloth or of a cream containing vitamin E may help relieve the sensory complaints. Treatment is otherwise purely supportive. Coma and convulsions may result if substantial amounts of pyrethroids are ingested, however, necessitating urgent hospitalization.

In laboratory animals, two syndromes relating to neurotoxicity have been described, but these are poorly defined in humans. The first syndrome (type I) is characterized by reflex hyperexcitability and fine tremor, whereas the second (type II) consists of choreoathetosis, salivation, and seizures.

## Pyriminil

Exposure to pyriminil (Vacor), a rodenticide, has led to severe autonomic dysfunction accompanied by a usually milder sensorimotor axonopathy following its ingestion. The mechanism by which this develops is unclear, but it may relate to an impairment of fast anterograde axonal transport. Acute diabetes mellitus also results from necrosis of the beta islet cells of the pancreas.

## Solvent Mixtures

In the 1970s, a number of reports from Scandinavia suggested that house painters, in particular, developed an irreversible disturbance of cognitive function that related to long-term exposure to mixtures of organic solvents. Many studies of exposed workers since then have documented the occurrence of cognitive symptoms (impaired memory, difficulty in concentration, poor attention span), affective complaints, and changes in personality, with impaired motivation and ease of fatigue. The symptoms are generally nonspecific in nature. The neurological examination is typically normal or reveals minor nonspecific abnormalities, as do neuroimaging and electrophysiological tests. However, other studies (including cases previously diagnosed with the disorder) have failed to validate the earlier reports, which, in many instances, were methodologically flawed. Furthermore, workers performing the same basic tasks in different companies have highly variable levels of solvent exposure, and solvent mixtures vary in different occupational settings, complicating the interpretation of published studies. Because of these factors and the nonspecific character of symptoms, the existence of so-called painter's (or chronic solvent) encephalopathy in those exposed to low levels of organic solvents for a prolonged period has been questioned. Nevertheless, the World Health Organization has published diagnostic criteria for this syndrome, later refined by a commission of the European Union and by others (Sainio, 2015; van Valen et al., 2018), and it is accepted as an occupational disease by the International Labour Organization.

Certain neurodegenerative diseases, including Parkinson and Alzheimer diseases, have been related to occupational exposure to organic solvents in some but not other studies. Difficulties in interpreting individual studies relate to methodological factors such as the manner in which exposure is estimated, varying diagnostic criteria, and the presence of confounding risk factors. Certain neurodegenerative disorders are not homogeneous but consist of a heterogeneous group of conditions with a similar clinical phenotype, complicating still further the interpretation of different epidemiological studies concerning their possible association with solvent exposure.

## Styrene

Styrene is used for manufacturing reinforced plastic and certain resins. Occupational exposure occurs by the dermal or inhalation routes and is typically associated with exposure to a variety of other chemicals, thereby making it difficult to define the syndrome that occurs from styrene exposure itself. Exposure (inhalation or dermal) occurs particularly among those working in industries manufacturing or using styrene, those exposed to automobile exhaust or cigarette smoke, and those using photocopiers. Styrene may also be ingested in drinking water or certain foods. Further details and allowable limits are provided by the Agency for Toxic Substances and Disease Registry (2007). Acute exposure to high concentrations of styrene has led to cognitive, behavioral, and attentional disturbances. Less clear are the consequences of exposure to chronic low levels of styrene. Abnormalities in psychomotor performance have been reported, but there is little compelling evidence of persisting neurological sequelae in this circumstance. Visual abnormalities (impaired color vision and reduced contrast sensitivity) also occur.

## Toluene

Toluene is used in a variety of occupational settings. It is a solvent for paints and glues and is used to synthesize benzene, nitrotoluene, and other compounds. Exposure, usually by inhalation or transdermally, occurs in glue-sniffers and among workers laying linoleum, spraying paint, and working in the printing industry, particularly in poorly ventilated locations. Chronic high exposure may lead to cognitive disturbances and to central neurological deficits with upper motor neuron, cerebellar, brainstem, and cranial nerve signs and tremor (Filley et al., 2004). An optic neuropathy may occur, as may ocular dysmetria and opsoclonus. Disturbances of memory and attention characterize the cognitive abnormalities, and subjects may exhibit a flattened affect. The cerebellar dysfunction, which may be permanent, may lead to dysarthria, action tremor, gait ataxia, and occasionally downbeat nystagmus (Manto, 2012). MRI shows cerebral atrophy and diffuse abnormalities of the cerebral white matter; symmetrical lesions may be present in the basal ganglia and thalamus and the cingulate gyri. Thalamotomy may ameliorate the tremor if it is severe. Lower levels of exposure lead to minor neurobehavioral disturbances.

## Trichloroethylene

Trichloroethylene is an industrial solvent and degreaser that is used in dry cleaning and the manufacture of rubber. It also has anesthetic properties. Recreational abuse has occurred because it may induce feelings of euphoria. Acute low-level exposure may lead to headache and nausea but claims that an encephalopathy follows chronic low-level exposure are unsubstantiated. Higher levels of exposure lead to dysfunction of the trigeminal nerve, with progressive impairment of sensation that starts in the snout area and then spreads outward. This has been particularly associated with rebreathing anesthetic circuits where the trichloroethylene is heated by the carbon dioxide absorbent. With increasing exposure, facial and buccal numbness is followed by weakness of the muscles of mastication and facial expression. Ptosis, extraocular palsies, vocal cord paralysis, and dysphagia may occur also, as may signs of parkinsonism (Gash et al., 2008; Goldman et al., 2012) or an encephalopathy, but the occurrence of a peripheral neuropathy is uncertain. The clinical deficit relates to neuronal loss in the cranial nerve nuclei and nigrostriatal dopaminergic system and degeneration in related tracts. Upon discontinuation of exposure, the clinical deficit generally resolves, sometimes over 1–2 years, but occasional patients are left with residual facial numbness or dysphagia.

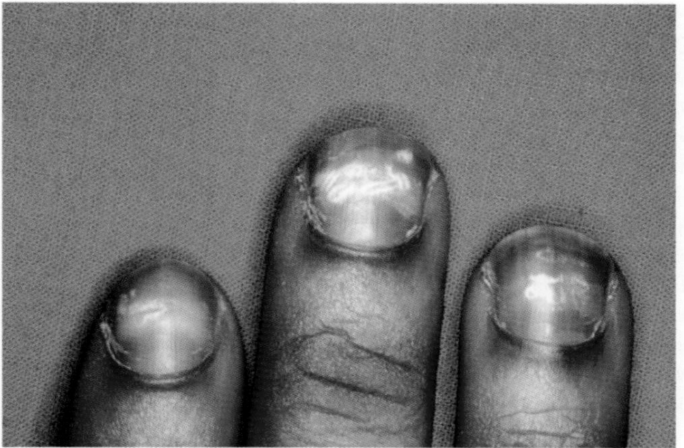

**Fig. 86.1 Mees Lines in Arsenic Neuropathy.** *(From Johnston, R., 2012. Weedon's Skin Pathology Essentials, first ed. Churchill Livingstone, Elsevier.)*

## OCCUPATIONAL EXPOSURE TO METALS

### Aluminum

Aluminum exposure is responsible for dialysis encephalopathy, which is characterized by speech disturbances, cognitive decline, seizures, and myoclonus. Some reports suggest that workers exposed to aluminum dust or aluminum-containing welding fumes may develop depression and mild cognitive dysfunction, but whether this relates to the occupational exposure is unclear; individual studies are difficult to interpret because of methodological and other issues. A role for aluminum in the pathogenesis of Alzheimer disease is disputed (Virk, 2015; Wang, 2016).

### Arsenic

Arsenic poisoning can result from ingestion of the trivalent arsenite in murder or suicide attempts. Large numbers of persons in areas of India, Pakistan, and certain other countries are chronically poisoned from naturally occurring arsenic in groundwater. Traditional Chinese and Tibetan medicinal herbal preparations may contain arsenic sulfide and mercury and are a source of chronic poisoning. Uncommon sources of accidental exposure include burning preservative-impregnated wood and storing food in antique copper kettles. Exposure to inorganic arsenic occurs in workers involved in smelting copper and lead ores.

With acute or subacute exposure, nausea, vomiting, abdominal pain, diarrhea, hypotension, tachycardia, and vasomotor collapse occur and may lead to death. Obtundation is common, and an acute confusional state may develop. Arsenic neuropathy takes the form of a distal axonopathy, although a demyelinating neuropathy is found soon after acute exposure. The neuropathy usually develops within 2–3 weeks of acute or subacute exposure, although the latent period may be as long as 1–2 months. Symptoms may worsen over a few weeks despite lack of further exposure, but they eventually stabilize. With low-dose chronic exposure, the latent period is more difficult to determine. In either circumstance, systemic symptoms are also conspicuous. With chronic exposure, similar but less severe gastrointestinal disturbances develop, as may skin changes such as melanosis, keratoses, and malignancies. Mees lines are white transverse striations of the nails (striate leukonychia) that appear 3–6 weeks after exposure (Fig. 86.1). As a nonspecific manifestation of nail matrix injury, Mees lines can be seen in a number of other conditions, including thallium poisoning, chemotherapy, and a variety of systemic disorders.

The neuropathy involves both large- and small-diameter fibers. Initial symptoms are typically of distal painful dysesthesias and are followed by distal weakness. Proprioceptive loss may be severe, leading to marked ataxia. The severity of weakness depends on the extent of exposure. The respiratory muscles are sometimes affected, and the disorder may simulate Guillain-Barré syndrome both clinically and electrophysiologically. Electrodiagnostic studies may initially suggest a demyelinating polyradiculoneuropathy, but the changes of an axonal neuropathy subsequently develop. Arsenic levels in hair, nail clippings, or urine may be increased, especially in cases of chronic exposure.

Detection of arsenic in urine is diagnostically useful within 6 weeks of a single large-dose exposure or during ongoing low-level exposure. Total inorganic arsenic urinary excretion should be measured over 24 hours. Methods are available in reference laboratories for distinguishing between inorganic (toxic) and organic (seafood-derived) arsenic compounds. Arsenic bound to keratin can be detected in hair or nails months to years after exposure. Pubic hair is preferable to scalp hair for examination because it is less liable to environmental contamination. Levels exceeding 10 μg/g of tissue are abnormal. Other abnormal laboratory features include aplastic anemia with pancytopenia and moderate CSF protein elevation. Nerve conduction studies in chronic arsenic neuropathy reflect the changes of distal axonopathy with low-amplitude or unelicitable sensory and motor evoked responses and preserved conduction velocities. EMG typically shows denervation in distal extremity muscles. In the subacute stages, however, some electrophysiological features such as partial motor conduction block, absent F responses, and slowing of motor conduction velocities are suggestive of demyelinating polyradiculoneuropathy. Progressive slowing of motor conduction velocities sufficient to invoke consideration of segmental demyelination has been reported in the first 3 months after massive exposure. Biopsies of peripheral nerves show axonal degeneration in chronic cases. Arsenite compounds react with protein sulfhydryl groups, interfere with formation of coenzyme A and several steps in glycolysis, and are potent uncouplers of oxidative phosphorylation. These biochemical reactions are responsible for the impaired neuronal energy metabolism, which in turn results in distal axonal degeneration.

Chelation therapy with water-soluble derivatives of dimercaprol (DMSA or DMPS) is effective in controlling the systemic effects of acute arsenic poisoning and may prevent the development of neuropathy if it is started within hours of ingestion. There is little evidence that chelation in the later stages of arsenic neuropathy promotes clinical recovery. The neuropathy itself often improves gradually over the course of many months, but depending on the severity of the deficit when exposure is discontinued, a substantial residual neurological deficit is common.

## Lead

Occupational exposure to lead occurs in workers in smelting factories and metal foundries and those involved in demolition, ship breaking, manufacturing of batteries or paint pigments, and construction or repair of storage tanks. Occupational exposure also occurs in the manufacture of ammunition, bearings, pipes, solder, and cables. Nonindustrial sources of lead poisoning are home-distilled whiskey, Asian folk remedies, earthenware pottery, indoor firing ranges, and retained bullets. Lead has been used to artificially increase the weight of illicit marijuana and has then been inhaled with it (Busse et al., 2008). Artificial turf may also pose an exposure threat to unhealthy levels of lead: the lead is released in dust that may be ingested or inhaled, but whether there is a sufficient amount to cause neurotoxicity is unclear. Lead neuropathy reached epidemic proportions at the end of the 19th century because of uncontrolled occupational exposure but now is rare because of strict industrial regulations. Exposure also may result from ingestion of old lead-containing paint in children with pica and consumption of illicit spirits by adults. Absorption is commonly by ingestion or inhalation but occasionally occurs through the skin.

The toxic effects of inorganic lead salts on the nervous system commonly differ with age, producing acute encephalopathy in children and polyneuropathy in adults. Children typically develop an acute gastrointestinal illness followed by behavioral changes, confusion, drowsiness, reduced alertness, focal or generalized seizures, and (in severe cases) coma with intracranial hypertension. At autopsy, the brain is swollen, with vascular congestion, perivascular exudates, edema of the white matter, and scattered areas of neuronal loss and gliosis. In adults, an encephalopathy is less common, but behavioral and cognitive changes are sometimes noted. In adults, lead produces a predominantly motor neuropathy, sometimes accompanied by gastrointestinal disturbances and a microcytic, hypochromic anemia. The neuropathy is manifest primarily by a bilateral wrist drop sometimes accompanied by bilateral footdrop or by more generalized weakness that may be associated with distal atrophy and fasciculations. Sensory complaints are usually minor and overshadowed by the motor deficit when the neuropathy develops subacutely following relatively brief exposure to high lead concentrations, but they are more conspicuous when the neuropathy develops after many years of exposure. The tendon reflexes may be diminished or absent. Older reports describe a painless motor neuropathy with few or no sensory abnormalities and distinct patterns of weakness affecting wrist extensors, finger extensors, and intrinsic hand muscles. Preserved reflexes, fasciculations, and profound muscle atrophy may simulate amyotrophic lateral sclerosis. A rare sign of lead exposure is a blue line at the gingival margin in patients with poor oral hygiene. Hypochromic microcytic anemia with basophilic stippling of the red cells, hyperuricemia, and azotemia should stimulate a search for lead exposure. Prognosis for recovery from the neuropathy is good when the neuropathy is predominantly motor and evolves subacutely, but it is less favorable when the neuropathy is motorsensory in type and more chronic in nature.

Lead intoxication is confirmed by elevated blood and urine lead levels. Blood levels exceeding 70 μg/100 mL are considered harmful, but even levels greater than 40 μg/100 mL have been correlated with minor nerve conduction abnormalities. Subjects should be removed from further occupational exposure if a single blood lead concentration exceeds 30 μg/100 mL or if two successive blood lead concentrations measured over a 4-week interval equal or exceed 20 μg/100 mL (Kosnett et al., 2007). Discontinuation of lead exposure should be considered when exposure control measures over an extended period do not reduce blood lead concentrations to less than 10 μg/dL or if selected medical conditions exist that increase the risk of continued exposure. It has been recommended that medical surveillance should include quarterly blood lead measurements for individuals with blood lead concentrations between 10 and 19 μg/dL and semiannual measurements when sustained blood lead concentrations are less than 10 μg/dL (Kosnett et al., 2007).

Lead inhibits erythrocyte δ-aminolevulinic acid dehydratase and other enzymatic steps in the biosynthetic pathway of porphyrins. Consequently, increased red cell protoporphyrin levels emerge together with increased urinary excretion of δ-aminolevulinic acid and coproporphyrin. Excess body lead burden, confirming past exposure, can be documented by increased urinary lead excretion after a provocative chelation challenge with calcium ethylenediaminetetraacetic acid. Only a few electrophysiological studies have been reported in patients with overt lead neuropathy. These investigations indicate a distal axonopathy affecting both motor and sensory fibers. These observations corroborate changes of axonal degeneration seen in human nerve biopsies. Contrary to the findings in humans, lead produces segmental demyelination in animals.

The biochemical mechanisms leading to neurotoxicity remain unknown but may include oxidative stress, disruption of calcium-dependent cell signaling, inhibition of nitric oxide synthase, and changes in glutamatergic signaling (Caito and Aschner, 2015). Lead encephalopathy is managed supportively, but corticosteroids are given to treat cerebral edema. Chelating agents (dimercaprol or 2,3-dimercaptopropane sulfonate) are also prescribed for patients with symptoms of lead toxicity (Kosnett et al., 2007). No specific treatment exists for lead neuropathy other than prevention of further exposure to lead. Chelation therapy does not hasten recovery. It is continued until a steady-state level of lead excretion is reached. With large lead stores in bone, chelation may be followed by movement of lead back into the blood and soft tissues, and thus by a rebound increase in blood lead level after an initial decline. Chelation therapy should not be used as attempted prophylaxis against rising blood levels in workers with continuing lead exposure.

## Manganese

Manganese miners may develop neurotoxicity following inhalation for prolonged periods (months or years) of dust containing manganese. Headache, behavioral changes, and cognitive disturbances ("manganese madness") are followed by the development of motor symptoms such as dystonia, parkinsonism, retropulsion, and a characteristic gait called *cock-walk*, manifested by walking on the toes with elbows flexed and the spine erect. There is usually no tremor, and the motor deficits rarely improve with L-dopa therapy. MRI may show changes in the globus pallidus, and this may be helpful in distinguishing manganese-induced parkinsonism from classic PD. Any relationship between welding and the development of PD itself is disputed.

Manganese intoxication has been reported in miners, smelters, welders, and workers involved in the manufacture of dry batteries, after chronic accidental ingestion of potassium permanganate, and from incorrect concentration of manganese in parenteral nutrition. Manganese toxicity also may occur with chronic liver disease and long-term parenteral nutrition.

Manganese intoxication may be associated with abnormal MRI (abnormal signal hyperintensity in the globus pallidus and substantia nigra on T1-weighted images). In contrast to PD, fluorodopa positron emission tomography (PET) studies are usually normal in patients with manganese-induced parkinsonism, and raclopride ($D_2$ receptor) binding is only slightly reduced in the caudate and normal in the putamen. Neuronal loss occurs in the globus pallidus and substantia nigra pars reticularis, as well as in the subthalamic nucleus and striatum. There is little response to L-dopa of the extrapyramidal syndrome, which may progress over several years. Myoclonic jerking may occur, sometimes without extrapyramidal accompaniments.

Chelation therapy is of uncertain benefit in patients with manganese toxicity, although claims of improvement in parkinsonism among small series of manganese-exposed subjects have been made.

## Mercury

The neurotoxic effects of elemental mercury (mercury vapor), inorganic salts, and short-chain alkyl-mercury compounds predominantly involve the central nervous system (CNS) and dorsal root ganglion sensory neurons. Inorganic mercury toxicity may result from inhalation during industrial exposure, as in thermometer and battery factories, mercury processing plants, and electronic applications factories. In the past, exposure occurred particularly in the hat-making industry. No evidence exists that the mercury contained in dental amalgam imposes any significant health hazard. The extent to which mercury exposure accounts for differences in health and cognitive function between dentists and control subjects is unclear. Clinical consequences of exposure include cutaneous erythema, hyperhidrosis, anemia, proteinuria, glycosuria, personality changes, intention tremor ("hatter's shakes"), and muscle weakness. The personality changes ("mad as a hatter") consist of irritability, euphoria, anxiety, emotional lability, insomnia, and disturbances of attention with drowsiness, confusion, and ultimately stupor. A variety of other central neurological deficits may occur but are more conspicuous in patients with organic mercury poisoning. A few cases presenting with peripheral neuropathy or a predominantly motor neuronopathy resembling amyotrophic lateral sclerosis have been described in association with intense exposure to elemental mercury vapors.

The effects of methyl mercury (organic mercury) poisoning have come to be widely recognized since the outbreak that occurred in Minamata Bay (Japan) in the 1950s, when industrial waste discharged into the bay led to a contamination of fish that were then consumed by humans. Outbreaks have also occurred following the use of methyl mercury as a fungicide, because intoxication occurs if treated seed intended for planting is eaten instead. Methyl and ethyl mercury compounds have been used as fungicides in agriculture and in the paper industry. Methyl mercury and elemental mercury are potent neurotoxins that cause neuronal degeneration in the cerebellar granular layer, calcarine cortex, and dorsal root ganglion neurons. The mechanisms involved in methyl mercury toxicity may include increased oxidative stress; inhibition of proteins involved in calcium homeostasis, glutamate transport, and $\gamma$-aminobutyric acid (GABA) synthesis; and alterations in several cell signaling pathways (Caito and Aschner, 2015).

The characteristic features of chronic methyl mercury poisoning are sensory disturbances, constriction of visual fields, progressive ataxia, tremor, and cognitive impairment. Electrophysiological studies have shown that these symptoms relate to central dysfunction. Sensory disturbances result from dysfunction of sensory cortex or dorsal root ganglia rather than peripheral nerves, and the visual complaints also relate to cortical involvement. Pathological studies reveal neuronal loss in the cerebral cortex, including the parietal and occipital regions, as well as in the cerebellum. The diagnosis of elemental or inorganic mercury intoxication usually can be confirmed by assaying mercury in urine. Monitoring blood levels is recommended for suspected organic mercury poisoning.

Chelating agents increase urinary excretion of mercury, but the evidence is incomplete that chelation increases the rate or extent of recovery.

## Tellurium

Tellurium is used in the manufacture of various alloys, the production of rubber, the manufacture of thermoelectric devices, and the coloring of glass, ceramics, and metalware. Inhalation of volatile tellurium compounds may lead to headache, drowsiness, a metallic taste, hypohidrosis, rashes and skin discoloration, and a curious odor resembling garlic on the breath. Recovery generally occurs spontaneously.

## Thallium

Thallium has been used until recently as a rodenticide and insecticide. It has also been used as a depilatory and in various industrial contexts. It is absorbed through the skin and also by ingestion or inhalation. Thallium exposure causes mitochondrial damage and impairs energy production. It leads to increased oxidative stress, changes in the physical properties of cell membranes, and the activation of antioxidant mechanisms (Osorio-Rico et al., 2017). There are changes in antiapoptotic and proapoptotic proteins, cytochrome c, and caspases (Osorio-Rico et al., 2017). The toxic effects of thallium have been related to the binding of sulfhydryl groups or displacement of potassium ions from biological membranes.

Thallium salts cause severe neuropathy and CNS degeneration that has led to their discontinued use as rodenticides and depilatories. Most intoxications result from accidental ingestion, attempted suicide, or homicide. After consumption of massive doses, vomiting, diarrhea, or both occur within hours. Neuropathic symptoms, heralded by limb pain and severe distal paresthesia, are followed by progressive limb weakness within 7 days. Cranial nerves, including optic nerves, may be involved. Ptosis is common. In severe cases, ataxia, chorea, confusion, and coma, as well as ventilatory and cardiac failure, may ensue. Alopecia, which appears 2–4 weeks after exposure, provides only retrospective evidence of acute intoxication. A chronic progressive, mainly sensory neuropathy develops in patients with chronic low-level exposure. In this form, hair loss is a helpful clue.

Electrocardiographic findings of sinus tachycardia, U waves, and T-wave changes of the type seen in potassium depletion are related to the interaction of thallium and potassium ions. Electrophysiological findings are characteristic of distal axonal degeneration. Autopsy study results confirm a distal axonopathy of peripheral and cranial nerves. Studies in animals show an accumulation of swollen mitochondria in distal axons before wallerian degeneration of nerve fibers. The diagnosis is confirmed by the demonstration of thallium in urine or bodily tissues. High levels are found in CNS gray matter and myocardium.

With acute ingestion, gastric lavage and cathartics are given to remove unabsorbed thallium from the gastrointestinal tract. Oral potassium ferric ferrocyanide (Prussian blue), which blocks intestinal absorption, together with IV potassium chloride, forced diuresis, and hemodialysis, has been used successfully in acute thallium intoxication.

## Tin

Although ingested inorganic tin usually produces little or no systemic or neurological complications, organic tin compounds used in various industrial processes have definite neurotoxicity. Intoxication with trimethyl tin leads to multifocal central dysfunction with conspicuous behavioral disturbances, emotional lability, confusion, disorientation, cognitive disturbances, sleep dysfunction, headaches, and visual disturbances. Triethyl tin may lead to severe cerebral edema with headache, papilledema, and behavioral abnormalities that generally resolve some weeks after discontinuation of exposure.

# EFFECTS OF IONIZING RADIATION

Electromagnetic and particulate radiation may lead to cell damage and death. Radiation therapy affects the nervous system by causing damage to cells (particularly their nuclei) in the exposed regions; these cells include neurons, glia, and the blood vessels supplying neural structures. As a late carcinogenic effect, radiation therapy may also produce tumors, particularly sarcomas, that lead to neurological deficits. Neurological injury is proportional to both the total dose and the daily fraction of radiation received. The combination of radiation therapy with chemotherapy may increase the risk of radiation damage. Preclinical studies are investigating whether certain growth factors or metalloporphyrin antioxidants can prevent damage or hasten the recovery of neural structures from radiation injury (Pearlstein et al., 2010). Neurological deficits may also arise as a secondary consequence of radiation (e.g., from vertebral osteoradionecrosis), leading to pain or compression of the spinal cord or nerve roots.

### Encephalopathy

Radiation encephalopathy is best considered according to its time of onset after exposure (Grimm and DeAngelis, 2008).

*Acute radiation encephalopathy* occurs within a few days of exposure and is characterized by headache, nausea, and a change in mental status. It may be related to increased intracranial pressure from breakdown of the blood–brain barrier due to the immediate effects of the energy dispersal in the nervous tissue. It typically occurs after exposure of a large brain volume to more than 3 Gy. Treatment with high-dose corticosteroids usually provides relief.

*Early delayed radiation encephalopathy* is probably caused by demyelination and occurs between 2 weeks and 4 months after irradiation. Headache and drowsiness are features, as is an enhancement of previous focal neurological deficits. Symptoms resolve after several weeks without specific treatment. A brainstem encephalopathy that manifests as ataxia, nystagmus, diplopia, and dysarthria also may develop if the brainstem was included in the irradiated field. Spontaneous recovery over a few weeks is usual, but the disorder sometimes progresses to obtundation, coma, or death.

*Delayed radiation encephalopathy* occurs several months or longer after cranial irradiation, particularly when doses exceed 35 Gy. It may be characterized by diffuse cerebral injury (atrophy) or focal neurological deficits. Slowness of executive function may occur, and there may be marked alterations of frontal functions such as in attention, judgment, and insight. Some patients develop a progressive disabling disorder with cognitive and affective disturbances and a disorder of gait approximately 6–18 months after whole-brain irradiation. Verbal and spatial memory become impaired, as does problem-solving ability. Cognitive deficits increase with time, leading to dementia. Such a disturbance may occur more commonly in elderly patients after irradiation. Pathological examination in some instances has shown demyelinating lesions. Radiation-induced late effects have been attributed to dynamic interactions between multiple cell types within the brain, including glial cells, neurons, and endothelial cells, and include inflammatory responses, radiation-induced neuronal loss, vascular changes, and changes in neuronal function, particularly synaptic plasticity (Greene-Schloesser et al., 2013). The precise mechanisms involved are unclear. Bevacizumab, a monoclonal antibody that inhibits vascular endothelial growth factor A, may help in some instances. Therapeutic strategies to prevent these disorders are focusing experimentally on stem cell or drug-based anti-inflammatory therapies (including blockade of the renin–angiotensin system; Greene-Schloesser et al., 2013).

### Myelopathy

A myelopathy may result from irradiation involving the spinal cord. Transient radiation myelopathy usually occurs within the first year or so after incidental spinal cord irradiation in patients treated for lymphoma and neck and thoracic neoplasms. Paresthesias and the Lhermitte phenomenon characterize the syndrome, which is self-limiting and probably relates to demyelination of the posterior columns. A delayed severe radiation myelopathy may occur 1 or more years after the completion of radiotherapy, especially with total doses exceeding 60 Gy to the spinal cord. The size of individual treatment fractions is also important, but it is unclear whether concomitant chemotherapy influences the risk. Patients present with a focal spinal cord deficit that progresses over weeks or months to paraplegia or quadriplegia. This may simulate a compressive myelopathy or paraneoplastic subacute necrotizing myelopathy, but the changes on MRI are usually those of a focal increased T2-weighted myelomalacia with cord atrophy in the originally irradiated field. The CSF is usually normal, although the protein concentration is sometimes elevated. Corticosteroids may lead to temporary improvement or slow progression, but no specific treatment exists. Anecdotal reports of benefits from hyperbaric oxygen are not supported by more detailed studies. The utility of bevacizumab is being studied. The disorder is caused by necrosis and atrophy of the cord, with an associated vasculopathy. Occasional patients develop sudden back pain and leg weakness several years after irradiation, with MRI revealing hematomyelia; symptoms usually improve with time.

Inadvertent spinal cord or cauda equina involvement, usually by irradiation directed at the para-aortic nodes, sometimes leads to a focal lower-limb lower motor neuron syndrome. The neurological deficit may progress over several months or years but eventually stabilizes, leaving a flaccid asymmetrical paraparesis. Recovery does not occur.

### Plexopathy

A radiation-induced plexopathy may rarely occur soon after radiation treatment for neoplasms, particularly of the breast and pelvis, and must be distinguished from direct neoplastic involvement of the plexus (Dropcho, 2010). Paresthesias, weakness, and atrophy typify the disorder, which tends to plateau after progressing for several months. The plexopathy may develop 1–3 years or longer after irradiation that involves the brachial or lumbosacral plexus. In this regard, doses of radiation exceeding 60 Gy, use of large daily fractions, involvement of the upper part of the brachial plexus, lymphedema, induration of the supraclavicular fossa, and the presence of myokymic discharges on EMG all favor a radiation-induced plexopathy. Although radiation plexopathy is often painless, a point favoring this diagnosis rather than direct infiltration by neoplasm, pain is conspicuous in some patients. Symptoms progress at a variable rate. The plexopathy is associated with small-vessel damage (endarteritis obliterans) and fibrosis around the nerve trunks.

## EFFECTS OF NONIONIZING RADIATION

Nonionizing radiation that strikes matter is transformed to heat, which may lead to tissue damage. Ultraviolet radiation is produced by the sun, incandescent and fluorescent light sources, welding torches, electrical arc furnaces, and germicidal lamps. Ultraviolet radiation is absorbed primarily by proteins and nucleic acids. Susceptibility to it is increased by certain drugs such as chlorpromazine and tolbutamide and by certain plant substances such as materials from figs, lemon and lime rinds, celery, and parsnips, which contain furocoumarins and psoralens. Short-term exposure to ultraviolet light can damage the retina and optic nerve fibers. A severe central scotoma may result from macular injury. Prevention requires the use of goggles and face masks in work environments where exposure to high-intensity ultraviolet radiation is likely to occur.

Infrared radiation is found in various industrial settings or where lasers or arc lamps are used, with a range of wavelengths between microwaves and visible light. By heating the eyes, infrared radiation can cause cataracts, cornea damage, and retina burns. Protection is afforded by wearing filters or reflective coatings.

Exposures to laser radiation can also induce ocular damage. This is particularly a problem when the wavelength of the laser beam is not in the visible portion of the electromagnetic spectrum, because the patient may not be aware of the exposure. Protection may be provided by safety goggles for those known to be at risk.

Microwaves have frequencies ranging from 1 to 300 GHz. Exposure to modulated electromagnetic energy in this frequency range can cause the perception of audible noises or actual speech within the head. This has been suggested as the cause for the symptoms developed by certain US diplomats in Cuba and China in 2017.

Concern has been raised that occupational or environmental exposure to high-voltage electric power lines may lead to neurological damage from exposure to high-intensity electromagnetic fields. However, the effects of such exposure are uncertain and require further study.

Nonionizing radiation at the radiofrequency used by cellular telephones has been reported to cause brain tumors or accelerate their growth (Hardell et al., 2013; Morgan et al., 2015), but the evidence is conflicting, and a clear theoretical basis for such an association with brain tumors is lacking. Most safety standards for exposure to radiofrequency radiations relate to the avoidance of harmful heating or electrostimulatory effects. There are case reports of burning sensations or dull aches of the face or head on the side that the telephone is used. Radiofrequency radiations have also been associated with dysesthesias, generally without objective neurophysiological evidence of peripheral nerve damage (Westerman and Hocking, 2004). The basis of such symptoms is unclear.

High-intensity noise in the acute setting may lead to tinnitus, vertigo, pain in the ear, and hearing impairment. Chronic exposure to high-intensity noise of any frequency leads to focal cochlear damage and impaired hearing.

## ELECTRIC CURRENT AND LIGHTNING

Electrical injuries (whether from manufactured or naturally occurring sources) are common. Their severity depends on the strength and duration of the current and the path in which it flows. Electricity travels along the shortest path to ground. Its passage through humans can often be determined by identifying entry and exit burn wounds. When its path involves the nervous system, direct neurological damage is likely among survivors. With the passage of the current through tissues, heat is produced, which is responsible at least in part for any damage, but nonthermal mechanisms may also contribute (Winkelman, 2014). In addition, neurological damage may result from circulatory arrest or trauma related to falling or a shock pressure wave.

A large current that passes through the head leads to immediate unconsciousness, sometimes associated with ventricular fibrillation and respiratory arrest. Confusion, disorientation, seizures, and transient focal deficits are common in survivors, but recovery generally occurs within a few days. Some survivors develop a cerebral infarct after several days or weeks, attributed to thrombotic occlusion of cerebral blood vessels. Residual memory and other cognitive disturbances are also common. Weaker currents lead only to headaches or other mild symptoms for a brief period.

When the path of the current involves the spinal cord, a transverse myelopathy may occur immediately or within 7 days or so, and may progress for several days. The disorder eventually stabilizes, after which partial or full recovery occurs in many instances (Lakshminarayanan et al., 2009). Upper and lower motor neuron deficits and sensory disturbances are common, but the sphincters are often spared. Unlike traumatic myelopathy, pain is not a feature. Autopsy studies show demyelination of long tracts, loss of anterior horn cells, and areas of necrosis in the spinal cord.

Segmental muscle atrophy may occur within a few days or weeks of electrical injury of the spinal cord. Whether this relates to focal neuronal damage or has an ischemic basis is uncertain. The current pathway is typically across the cervical cord from one arm to the other, and the resulting muscle atrophy in the arms may be accompanied by an upper motor neuron deficit in the legs. Sensory disturbances (in upper or lower limbs) and sphincter dysfunction also occur. Occasional reports have suggested the occurrence of a progressive disorder simulating amyotrophic lateral sclerosis after electrical injury.

Peripheral or cranial nerve injury in the region of an electrical burn is often reversible, except when high-tension current is responsible and when the damage is severe, in which case thermal coagulation necrosis is likely. Care must be taken to distinguish such neuropathies from compartment or entrapment neuropathies, which are suggested by severe pain and a delay between injury and development of the neuropathy. Compartment syndromes develop because of muscle swelling and necrosis, and entrapment syndromes because of swelling of tissues in confined anatomical spaces. Immediate decompression of the compartment is indicated in these cases.

For uncertain reasons, occasional patients have developed hemorrhagic or thrombotic stroke after electrical injuries. Venous sinus thrombosis has also been described. Suggested mechanisms include coagulation necrosis of part of the vascular wall, with aneurysmal distention and rupture or intramural thrombosis. Intense vasospasm, acute hypertension, intramural dissections, or transient circulatory arrest may also contribute.

Trauma resulting from the electrical injury (e.g., falls) may lead to intracranial hemorrhage, subdurally, epidurally, or in the subarachnoid space. Long-term consequences of electrical injuries include neuropsychological symptoms such as fatigue, impaired concentration, irritability and emotional lability, and posttraumatic stress disorder (Ritenour et al., 2008).

## VIBRATION

Exposure to vibrating tools such as pneumatic drills has been associated with both focal peripheral nerve injuries such as carpal tunnel syndrome and vascular abnormalities such as Raynaud phenomenon (Sauni et al., 2009). The mechanism of production is uncertain but presumably reflects focal damage to nerve fibers. The designation of *hand-arm vibration syndrome* has been applied to a combination of vascular, neurological, and musculoskeletal symptoms and signs that may occur in those using handheld vibrating tools such as drills and jackhammers. There may be blanched, discolored, swollen, or painful fingers; paresthesias or weakness of the fingers; pain and tenderness of the forearm; and loss of manual dexterity (Weir and Lander, 2005). The pathophysiological basis of the syndrome is poorly understood, and treatment involves the avoidance of exposure to cold or vibrating tools.

## HYPERTHERMIA

Exposure to high external temperatures may lead to heat stress disorders. Heat stroke, the most severe condition, sometimes has an exertional basis, and disturbances of thermoregulatory sweating may be contributory. Classic heat stroke occurs, especially in older persons, with chronic disorders such as diabetes or obesity and in hypermetabolic states such as thyrotoxicosis. Anticholinergic or diuretic drugs and dehydration predispose to heat stroke because they impair sweating and thereby limit heat dissipation.

Hyperthermia leads to thirst, fatigue, nausea, weakness, and muscle cramps and eventually to confusion, delirium, obtundation, or coma, but coma can develop without any prodrome. Seizures are frequent, focal neurological deficits are sometimes present, and papilledema may occur. With recovery, symptoms and signs generally clear completely, but cognitive changes or focal neurological deficits may persist. Cataracts have been attributed to dehydration. Cardiac output is reduced, pulmonary edema may occur, and adult respiratory distress syndrome is sometimes conspicuous.

Other systemic manifestations include a respiratory alkalosis and often a metabolic acidosis, hypokalemia or hyperkalemia, hypoglycemia, other electrolyte disturbances, and various coagulopathies. Rhabdomyolysis is common, and acute renal failure may occur in exertional heat stroke.

The prognosis depends on the severity of hyperthermia and its duration before the initiation of treatment. With proper management, the mortality rate is probably about 5%. Treatment involves control of the body temperature by cooling, rehydration of the patient, correction of the underlying cause of the hyperthermia, and prevention of complications. When excessive muscle activity is responsible, neuromuscular blockade may be necessary.

In the malignant hyperthermia syndrome, the responsible anesthetic agent is discontinued, the patient is vigorously cooled, oxygenation is ensured, and IV dantrolene is administered. In the neuroleptic malignant syndrome, the responsible neuroleptic and other psychotropic agents should be stopped and the patient should be treated supportively; fever is reduced with cooling blankets, cardiorespiratory function is maintained, and agitation is controlled with benzodiazepines.

Among other conditions predisposing to hyperthermia are thyrotoxicosis and pheochromocytoma. Thyrotoxic crisis is treated with thyroid-blocking drugs. Patients with pheochromocytoma are treated with α-adrenergic antagonists.

Cooling is achieved by evaporation or direct external cooling, as by immersion of the patient in cold water. The skin should be massaged vigorously to counteract the cutaneous vasoconstriction that results from external cooling and impedes heat removal from the core. Antipyretic agents are unhelpful. Hypotension is treated by fluid administration rather than vasoconstrictor agents, which should be avoided if possible. High doses of mannitol and use of diuretics may be required to promote urinary output. Electrolyte and glucose abnormalities also require treatment.

Patients who received 915-MHz hyperthermia treatment together with ionizing radiation for superficial cancers and developed nonspecific burning, tingling, and numbness in the territory of an adjacent nerve have been described (Westerman and Hocking, 2004). Once the symptoms developed, they occurred with the application of power without any time lag and ceased as soon as power was removed, suggesting that they were not a thermal effect. Dysesthesias have also been reported after accidental exposures in faulty microwave ovens (Westerman and Hocking, 2004). The precise neurophysiological basis for such symptoms has not been elucidated.

## HYPOTHERMIA

A core temperature below 35°C may occur in very young or elderly persons with environmental exposure, coma, hypothyroidism, malnutrition, severe dermatological disorders (due to excessive heat loss and inability to regulate cutaneous vasoconstriction), and alcoholism. Alcohol promotes heat loss by vasodilation and may directly lead to coma or predispose impaired individuals to trauma, with resultant environmental exposure to cold. Hypothermia also occurs in persons exposed to low temperatures in the working environment, such as divers, skiers, and cold-room workers.

The usual compensatory mechanism for cooling is shivering, but this fails at body temperatures below 30°C or so. As the temperature declines, respiratory requirements diminish, cardiac output falls, and significant hypotension and cardiac arrhythmias ultimately develop. Neurologically, there is increasing confusion, psychomotor retardation, and obtundation until consciousness is eventually lost. The tendon reflexes are reduced and muscle tone increases, but extensor plantar responses are not usually found. The EEG slows and ultimately shows a burst suppression pattern or becomes isoelectric with increasing hypothermia. At core temperatures below 32°C, the appearance of brain death may be simulated clinically and electroencephalographically, but complete recovery may follow appropriate treatment. Management involves the slow rewarming of patients and preventing complications such as aspiration pneumonia and metabolic acidosis. Hypotension may occur from dehydration but can usually be managed by fluid replacement. Plasma electrolyte concentrations must be monitored closely, especially because of the risk of developing cardiac arrhythmias. With recovery, there are usually no long-term sequelae.

Nerve damage may occur as a consequence of the tissues becoming frozen by the cold (frostbite). This involves the extremities and is usually irreversible.

## BURNS

Following common usage, the term *thermal burn* refers to a burn caused by direct contact with heat or flames. Patients with severe burns may have associated disorders such as anoxic encephalopathy from carbon monoxide poisoning, head injury, or respiratory dysfunction from smoke inhalation. Central neurological disorders may occur later during hospitalization and are secondary to various systemic complications. Metabolic encephalopathies may relate to anoxia, liver or kidney failure, and hyponatremia, and central pontine myelinolysis may occur also. Infections (meningitis or cerebral microabscesses) are common, especially in the second or third week after the burn. Vascular complications, including multiple strokes, may result from septic infarction, disseminated intravascular coagulation, venous thrombosis, hypotension, or intracranial hemorrhage. Imaging studies are therefore important in clarifying the underlying disorder.

Peripheral complications of burns are also important. Nerves may be damaged directly by heat, leading to coagulation necrosis from which recovery is unlikely. A compartment syndrome may arise from massive swelling of tissues and mandates urgent decompressive surgery. In other instances, neuropathies result from compression, angulation, or stretching due to incorrectly applied dressings or improper positioning of the patient. A critical illness polyneuropathy and myopathy is now well recognized in patients with multiorgan failure and sepsis, including patients with burns, and is discussed in Chapters 106–109.

## NEUROTOXINS OF ANIMALS AND INSECTS

Neurotoxins of animals, insects, plants, and fungi are of great scientific interest. Many of them serve as important tools used by neuroscientists to probe the workings of the nervous system. One of the oldest and best-known examples is curare, a plant toxin that was used in Claude Bernard's classical experiments on neuromuscular transmission. α-Bungarotoxin from the venom of the banded krait is a competitive blocker of the acetylcholine receptor that has been invaluable in studies of the neuromuscular junction.

Venoms are used by animals or insects to defend against predators and to immobilize prey. Each contains a wide range of incompletely characterized enzymes that may include metalloproteinases, phospholipases, acetylcholinesterases, collagenases, phosphodiesterases, and others. The composition varies not only from species to species but also according to season and geographical region, so the clinical effects of venomous injuries are highly variable. In addition to their effects on the nervous system, most venoms possess hemorrhagic, necrotic, inflammatory, and coagulopathic properties, and are capable of inducing tissue necrosis and systemic cardiovascular collapse. Despite their biological potency, death from venoms is uncommon in developed countries. The rarity is in part a result of the healthy respect most people have for snakes, spiders, and scorpions. Moreover, most injuries result in a small amount of envenomation that is usually below lethal dosage. Mortality is more likely in children and the elderly.

## Snakes

More than 5 million snakebites occur worldwide per year, with half of them venomous, resulting in about 400,000 amputations and up to 138,000 deaths. About 6800 cases with fewer than 10 deaths are reported in the United States each year (Langley, 2008). In contrast, cases are far more common in Africa, Asia, and Latin America, with mortality and morbidity particularly high in impoverished rural communities (Gutierrez et al., 2017; Williams et al., 2010).

The majority of venomous snakebites are inflicted by snakes from the families Viperidae (true vipers and pit vipers) and Elapidae. Pit vipers (Crotalinae), so named because of an identifiable heat-sensing foramen, or "pit," between each eye and nostril, include rattlesnakes (genera *Crotalus* and *Sistrurus*), fer-de-lances or lanceheads (*Bothrops*), and bushmasters (*Lachesis*). Moccasins (*Agkistrodon*), including cottonmouths and copperheads, account for up to half of pit viper envenomations in the United States. The true vipers (Viperinae) include the puff adder, rhinoceros-horned viper and Gaboon viper (*Bitis*), and Russell viper (*Daboia russelii*), and are important venomous snakes worldwide. Important venomous snakes of the Elapidae family include cobras, mambas, kraits, coral snakes, and sea snakes.

Low-molecular-weight polypeptides in snake venoms have neurological activities on both pre- and postsynaptic elements of the neuromuscular junction. Some toxins may be directly myotoxic, resulting in rhabdomyolysis and compartment syndromes. Just as important are the diverse systemic effects that affect platelets, endothelial cells, coagulation cascade, and other organs. As many as 25% to 50% of venomous snakebites are "dry" and do not result in envenomation. When envenomation occurs, signs and symptoms vary and depend on the venom composition of the local snakes. Bites by the same species may cause primarily neuromuscular paralysis in one region and coagulopathy and hemorrhage in another area. In general, snakes from the family Viperidae induce mostly coagulopathies, bleeding, and local tissue damage, while the family Elapidae are more likely to produce neuromuscular toxicity.

Patients typically present with local pain, swelling, and erythema after a snakebite. Early indications of envenomation include tender regional lymph nodes, nausea, and a metallic, rubbery, or minty taste in the mouth. Systemic symptoms appear over the ensuing 12–24 hours and consist of a variable combination of perioral or limb paresthesias, muscle fasciculations, weakness, hypotension, and shock. Ptosis, oculomotor palsies, dysphagia, diffuse weakness, areflexia, and respiratory suppression may develop. If weakness is present, the pattern generally resembles myasthenia gravis, with predilection for the neck flexors, ocular, bulbar, and proximal limb and respiratory muscles. Clinical outcome principally depends on the availability and sophistication of emergency medical care.

Initial laboratory evaluation should include complete blood cell and platelet counts, coagulation panel, fibrinogen, fibrin split products, serum chemistries, creatine kinase, and urinalysis. In patients with weakness, nerve conduction studies with repetitive stimulation may reveal a pattern of either pre- or postsynaptic blockade. The observed changes consist of reduced amplitude of compound muscle action potentials, decremental response to low-frequency repetitive stimulation, and postexercise and posttetanic facilitation. Treatment includes calming and supportive measures. Even in the absence of life-threatening symptoms, a patient should be monitored for at least 6–12 hours if bitten by a venomous snake. Antivenom immunoglobulin is the only effective antidote. If available for the specific snake responsible for envenomation, antivenom should be administered as soon as possible (Gutierrez et al., 2017; Warrell, 2010). Patients should be monitored closely for anaphylactic and infusion reactions to antivenom. Additional supportive measures to counter organ and circulatory failure are equally important. In survivors of snakebites, the main source of disability is local tissue necrosis, which may lead to disfigurement or limb amputation.

## Spiders

Of the commonly encountered spiders, few produce significant symptoms in humans. The female widow spider (*Latrodectus* sp.) is the most important to the neurologist. Of the approximately 2600 widow bites reported annually in the United States, 13 had major health consequences, and no fatality occurred (Langley, 2008). Black widow spider (*Latrodectus mactans*) venom contains α-latrotoxin, a potent neurotoxin capable of inducing release and blocking reuptake of neurotransmitter at presynaptic cholinergic, noradrenergic, and aminergic nerve endings. Venom of *Phoneutria* banana spiders from South America and *Atrax* funnel-web spiders from Australia also causes neurotoxicity. Another clinically important spider, the brown recluse spider (*Loxosceles reclusa*), is responsible for local tissue damage and systemic symptoms that rarely may include disseminated intravascular coagulation, hemolysis, shock, and multisystem failure.

Although the latrotoxins found in widow spider venom are more potent than the neurotoxins found in snake venom, most spider bites lead to only a small volume of envenomation. Children are most vulnerable, although symptoms are usually minor (Glatstein et al., 2018). Sometimes a characteristic erythematous ring surrounding a paler center ("target" or "halo" lesion) develops around the site of the spider bite. In the rare instances with sufficient envenomation, pain and involuntary muscle spasms spread from the bite site and appear in abdominal muscles and distant limb musculature (so-called latrodectism). Symptoms may appear as early as 30–60 minutes, and spread to distant muscles, usually by 3–4 hours. Tachycardia, hypertension, piloerection, and diaphoresis may be present. Other associated symptoms include priapism, salivation, bronchospasm, and bronchorrhea. Serum creatine kinase may be elevated. In very rare instances, respiratory failure can result from diaphragmatic muscle involvement. Treatment begins with careful monitoring of vital signs and intensive care support if necessary. Benzodiazepines and opioids are used to control spasmodic effects and pain. Muscle spasms may also be treated with slow infusion of calcium gluconate or methocarbamol. Antivenom may be beneficial, but there are no vigorous clinical trial data.

## Scorpions

Of the approximately 1400 scorpion species, about 25 are of neurological importance with venom that may be deadly to humans. Scorpion envenomation is second only to snakebites as a public health problem in the tropics and North Africa. In Mexico alone, 100,000–200,000 scorpion bites occur annually, resulting in 400–1000 fatalities. In the United States, approximately 17,000 scorpion bites are reported annually, with the majority from Arizona, followed by Texas, Nevada, and Southern California (Kang, 2017). The Arizona bark scorpion (*Centruroides sculpturatus*) is of particular concern because of its neurotoxic venom. The venoms contain a wide range of polypeptides with molecular targets at the voltage-gated sodium and potassium channels. Small children are especially prone to developing neurological complications, and as many as 80% of bites are symptomatic.

Presenting symptoms are highly variable, from local pain to serious systemic complications. Paresthesias are common and usually experienced around the site of the bite but also may be felt diffusely. Autonomic symptoms of sympathetic excess (tachycardia, hypertension, and hyperthermia) are often present, but parasympathetic symptoms including the SLUD syndrome (salivation, lacrimation, urination, and defecation) may be present as well. Muscle fasciculations, spasms, limb flailing, dysconjugate roving or rotary ocular movements, dysphagia, and other cranial nerve signs are sometimes seen. With severe envenomation, encephalopathy may result from direct CNS toxicity or secondary to uncontrolled hypertension. Symptom control, cardiovascular and respiratory support, and antivenom administration are the mainstays of treatment. *Centruroides* scorpion antivenom appeared to be effective in a small, randomized control trial in children with neurotoxicity (Boyer et al., 2009). Efficacy was reaffirmed when a subsequent larger treated cohort was compared to historical controls (Boyer et al., 2013).

### Tick Paralysis

Tick paralysis is caused by envenomation during tick bites. The vast majority of reported cases occur during the spring-summer breeding seasons in Australia and North America. *Ixodes* species are largely responsible in Australia, and *Dermacentor* are in America. Most cases in North America appear in the Pacific Northwest and Rocky Mountains, and only a few in the eastern United States (Diaz, 2015). Paralysis is due to inoculation of a toxin during the tick bite. Continuing attachment of the tick for 1 or more days is necessary before clinical symptoms appear. In most cases, the tick is eventually found on the scalp and neck, or around the ear. Other areas where a tick may go undetected for days are the ear and nose canals and the genital areas. Children are the most likely victims. Girls outnumber boys in the United States, perhaps because a tick is harder to find in longer hair.

The clinical presentation of tick paralysis often mimics Guillain–Barré syndrome. Weakness typically starts in the legs and spreads to the arms and eventually to the bulbar and respiratory muscles. Gait ataxia or limb incoordination may be the first sign in young children. Examination shows limb weakness (most prominent in the legs), hypoactive or unobtainable stretch reflexes, and normal or mildly impaired sensation. Respiratory muscle weakness, if present, manifests as rapid shallow breathing and diminished forced vital capacity. Mechanical ventilation was necessary in 11% of US cases and 3% of Australian cases (Diaz, 2015). There are reports of atypical presentations such as cranial neuropathy, encephalopathy, autonomic dysfunction, and brachial plexopathy.

Electrodiagnostic findings are likely to be nonspecific during the acute phase of the disease, although only limited data are available. Low-amplitude compound muscle action potentials may be the only abnormality (Vedanarayanan et al., 2002). Motor nerve conduction velocities, sensory nerve conduction studies, and repetitive nerve stimulation are typically normal. There is a case report of unilateral conduction block at the lower trunk of the brachial plexus from a tick bite in the ipsilateral axilla (Krishnan et al., 2009). CSF is usually normal. The key to diagnosis is to find the culpable tick by careful inspection of the patient's skin. The tick can then be removed, leading to clinical improvement that may start within a few hours and complete in 1–2 days.

## NEUROTOXINS OF PLANTS AND FUNGI

Pharmacologically active agents are present in thousands of plants and fungal species. Although fatal poisoning is rare, many of the commonly encountered species are capable of inducing serious neurological symptoms. Toxicity occurs in several circumstances. Approximately 75% of cases occur in children younger than age 6 as a result of accidental ingestion. Adult poisoning may happen when toxic plants or mushrooms are mistaken for edible species. Another category arises with intentional consumption by those seeking drug-induced mood effects from plants such as Jimson weed.

Plant identification is difficult and should be left to a trained botanist or mycologist. Common names of plants are inadequate, and botanical names should be used whenever possible. Even without a definitive identification, the history of ingestion and recognition of a characteristic syndrome are often sufficient for a tentative diagnosis. Initial treatment is usually empirical, consisting of gastric lavage or catharsis and supportive measures. With the exception of anticholinergic poisoning, there are few specific antidotes.

A comprehensive review of the numerous botanical toxins is impossible. Table 86.1 lists several major categories and the commonly associated plants in each category. Omitted are plants that do not have direct toxicity on the nervous system, such as those containing cardiac glycosides, coumarin, oxalates, taxines, andromedotoxin, colchicine, and phytotoxins. Secondary neurological disturbances may result from these toxins because some can cause electrolyte abnormalities, cardiovascular dysfunction, or coagulopathy.

### Jimson Weed

Jimson weed (*Datura stramonium*), first grown by early settlers in Jamestown from seeds brought from England, was initially used to treat asthma. The plant is now found throughout the United States. Intoxication primarily occurs among young people who intentionally ingest the plant for its psychic effects. The chief active ingredient is the alkaloid hyoscyamine, with lesser amounts of atropine and scopolamine. Symptoms of anticholinergic toxicity appear within 30–60 minutes after ingestion and often continue for 24–48 hours because of delayed gastric motility. The clinical picture can include hyperthermia, delirium, hallucinations, seizures, and coma. Autonomic disturbances such as mydriasis, cycloplegia, tachycardia, dry mouth, and urinary retention are often present. Treatment includes gastrointestinal decontamination with or without the induction of emesis. Supportive measures and symptom relief should be provided, but physostigmine should be reserved for severe or life-threatening intoxications.

### Poison Hemlock

The dangers of ingesting poison hemlock (*Conium maculata*) have been known since ancient times. This was reportedly the method used to execute Socrates. The Old Testament describes rhabdomyolysis in Israelites who ate quail fed on hemlock (coturnism). The highest concentration of toxin is in the root of this plant that may be mistaken for wild carrots. Alkaloid toxins structurally similar to nicotine initially cause CNS activation and general autonomic stimulation. In severe cases, a depressant phase may then ensue, presumably secondary to acetylcholine receptor depolarization blockade. Death is usually secondary to respiratory paralysis.

### Water Hemlock

Water hemlock (*Cicuta maculata*) is a highly toxic plant found primarily in wet, swampy areas and is sometimes mistakenly ingested as wild parsnips or artichokes. Although related to poison hemlock, its clinical toxidrome is quite different. The principal toxin, the long-chain aliphatic alcohol cicutoxin, is a highly potent noncompetitive GABA receptor antagonist (Uwai et al., 2000). Symptoms consist of initial gastrointestinal effects (abdominal pain, salivation, and diarrhea) followed by generalized convulsions, obtundation, and coma. Mortality

**TABLE 86.1 Neurotoxicity of Plants**

| Principal Toxins | Plants (Representative Examples) | Main Clinical Features |
|---|---|---|
| Tropane (belladonna) alkaloids | Jimson weed (*Datura stramonium*); deadly nightshade (belladonna, *Atropa belladonna*); matrimony vine (*Lycium halimifolium*); henbane (*Hyoscyamus niger*); mandrake (*Mandragora officinarum*); jasmine (*Cestrum* spp.) | Mydriasis, cycloplegia, tachycardia, dry mouth, hyperpyrexia, delirium, hallucinations, seizures, coma |
| Solanine alkaloids | Woody nightshade (bittersweet, *Solanum dulcamara*); black nightshade (*S. nigrum*); Jerusalem cherry (*S. pseudocapsicum*); wild tomato (*S. gracile*); leaves and roots of the common potato (*S. tuberosum*) | As above |
| Nicotine-like alkaloids (e.g., cytisine) | Tobacco (*Nicotiana* spp.); golden chain (*Laburnum anagyroides*); mescal bean (*Sophora* spp.); Scotch broom (*Cytisus* spp.); poison hemlock (*Conium maculatum*) | Variable sympathetic and parasympathetic hyperactivity, hypotension, drowsiness, weakness, hallucinations, seizures |
| Cicutoxin | Water hemlock (*Cicuta maculata*) | Diarrhea, abdominal pain, salivation, seizures, coma |
| Triterpene | Chinaberry (*Melia azedarach*) | Confusion, ataxia, dizziness, stupor, paralysis, seizures |
| Anthracenones | Buckthorn (*Karwinskia humboldtiana*) | Ascending paralysis; polyneuropathy |
| Excitatory amino acid agonists | Chickling pea and others (*Lathyrus* spp.); cycad (*Cycas rumphii*); false sago palm (*Cycas circinalis*) | Possible chronic myelopathy with spasticity and motor neuron degeneration |

is secondary to refractory status epilepticus; seizures are treated with standard protocols.

### Peyote

Peyote (*Lophophora williamsii*) is a small cactus native to the southwestern United States and Mexico, but it can be cultivated anywhere. The principal agent is mescaline, which has actions similar to those of the hallucinogenic indoles. A peyote button, the top portion of the cactus, contains about 45 mg of mescaline; approximately six to nine buttons are sufficient to be hallucinogenic. Dizziness, drowsiness, ataxia, paresthesias, sympathomimetic symptoms, nausea, and vomiting are frequent accompanying clinical features. Ingestions are rarely life threatening.

### Morning Glory

The active agents in morning glory (*Ipomoea tricolor*) seeds are various amides of lysergic acid. The seeds are consumed for purposes of drug abuse. The neuropsychological effects are similar to those of lysergic acid diethylamide (LSD) and consist of hallucinations, anxiety, mood changes, depersonalization, and drowsiness. Acute clinical effects may also include mydriasis, nausea, vomiting, and diarrhea.

### Medicinal Herbs

Treatment of illness with herbal remedies, either purchased over the counter at health food stores or procured from practitioners of traditional medicine, may lead to undesired toxicity. The labels, if present, may not fully represent the myriad of compounds contained within. Potentially harmful ingredients may be included as contaminants or intentionally added to increase a desired effect. Contamination of products with *Atropa belladonna* (deadly nightshade), *Datura* spp., and *Mandragora officinarum* (mandrake) have been reported. Common herbal preparations such as kava-kava (*Piper methysticum*) and St. John's wort (*Hypericum perforatum*) have neurotoxic potential, particularly if combined with other herbal or standard pharmaceuticals. Mayapple (*Podophyllum peltatum*), widely used in Chinese herbal medicine, is potentially neurotoxic.

### Excitatory Amino Acids

Various *Lathyrus* species, including *Lathyrus sativus* (chickling pea), Lathyrus *clymenum* (Spanish vetch), and Lathyrus *cicera* (flat-podded pea), are responsible for lathyrism. These hardy plants are an important part of the diet of people in India, Africa, China, and some parts of Europe. Epidemics of lathyrism often coincide with periods of famine or war, probably a result of excessive dietary dependency on these legumes. The putative toxin is β-*N*-oxalylamino-L-alanine (L-BOAA), an amino acid with potent agonist activity at the (RS)-α-amino-3-hydroxy-5-methyl-4-isoxazolepropionic acid (AMPA) subclass of glutamate receptors. L-BOAA is capable of inducing lathyrism in several animal models. Clinically affected patients present with subacute or insidious onset of upper motor neuron signs and gait instability. Muscle aching and paresthesias may be present, but the sensory examination is largely normal. Cognition and cerebellar functions are spared. Partial recovery after discontinuation of *Lathyrus* intake is possible, but interestingly, there are reports of deterioration without further exposure many years later.

Another excitatory amino acid, β-methylamino-L-alanine (BMAA), is found in cycad seeds, a dietary staple of the Chamorro people of Guam. When given in sufficient quantity, BMAA can induce neurotoxicity in primates. An unusually high incidence of amyotrophic lateral sclerosis, parkinsonism, and dementia was observed in the Chamorros around the Second World War, and it has been postulated that BMAA may play an etiological role (Bradley and Mash, 2009). A causal relationship in humans, however, is difficult to prove.

### Mushroom Poisoning

Of the more than 5000 varieties of mushrooms, approximately 100 are known to be toxic to humans. Accidental poisoning is common because poisonous mushrooms often closely resemble edible varieties. Aside from accidental ingestion, mushrooms such as *Psilocybe* spp., *Panaeolus*, *Amanita muscaria*, and *Amanita pantherina* are popular among drug users for their psychoactive effects. The common mushrooms associated with neurological morbidity are listed in Table 86.2.

Supportive care and decontamination are the mainstays of treatment. This can be further supplemented by specific treatments such as infusion of pyridoxine (gyromitrin poisoning), atropine (muscarine poisoning), or physostigmine (ibotenic acid and muscimol poisoning) as needed.

## MARINE NEUROTOXINS

Descriptions of marine food poisoning date back to ancient times. A carving on the tomb of the Egyptian Pharaoh Ti (*c.* 2700 BC) depicts the toxic danger of the puffer fish. Ciguatera intoxication was known during the T'ang Dynasty (618–907 AD) in China. It was later described by early Spanish explorers and in the journals of Captain Cook's expedition in 1774 (Doherty, 2005). George Vancouver recognized

**TABLE 86.2 Poisonous Mushrooms**

| Principal Toxins | Mushrooms (Representative Examples) | Mode of Action | Time of Onset/Main Clinical Features |
|---|---|---|---|
| Monomethylhydrazines (gyromitrin) | *Gyromitra* spp. ("false morels") | Functional pyridoxine deficiency; GABA deficiency (through decreased GAD activity) | 6–10 h: GI symptoms, hemolysis; seizures respond to pyridoxine |
| Coprine | *Coprinus atramentarius* ("inky cap") and other Coprinaceae | Inhibition of aldehyde dehydrogenase (disulfiram-like) | 20–120 min: Flushing, palpitations, and headache after alcohol ingestion |
| Muscarine | *Clitocybe* and *Inocybe* genera | Cholinergic agonist | 15–120 min: Cholinergic hyperactivity |
| Isoxazoles (muscimol, ibotenic acid) | *Amanita muscaria* ("fly agaric"), *A. gemmata, A. pantherina* ("the panther"), *A. cothurnata* | GABA receptor agonist; glutamate receptor agonist; anticholinergic | 30–90 min: Ethanol-like intoxication; euphoria, hallucinations, dysarthria, ataxia, myoclonic jerks, seizures, and coma |
| Indoles (psilocybin, psilocin) | *Psilocybe caerulipes, Psilocybe cubensis, Panaeolus foenisecii, Gymnophilus spectabilis, Psathyrella foenisecii* | Structural analog of serotonin (5-HT); actions resemble LSD | 30–60 min: Euphoria, hallucinations, mydriasis, tachycardia, seizures (in children) |

*GI*, Gastrointestinal; *GABA*, γ-aminobutyric acid; *GAD*, glutamic acid decarboxylase; *5-HT*, 5-hydroxytryptamine; *LSD*, lysergic acid diethylamide.

paralytic shellfish poisoning (PSP) in the Pacific Northwest toward the end of the 18th century.

Most marine toxins originate from microorganisms, typically unicellular flagellated algae (dinoflagellates). The proliferation of toxin-producing algae depends on environmental and seasonal factors. During periods of intense algal proliferation ("blooms"), high concentrations of toxins accumulate in fish or shellfish, which then act as transvectors for human disease. Outbreaks may also lead to widespread mortality of fish, shellfish, or marine mammals. One of the algal blooms familiar to residents of the United States is the so-called red tide, which refers to the reddish-brown discoloration of seawater.

All the common marine toxins are colorless, tasteless, and odorless. They are often stable to heat, acid, and normal food preparation procedures, making them particularly dangerous to unsuspecting consumers. Many of these toxins affect the $Na^+$ channels in peripheral nerves, causing disorders that range from mild sensory symptoms to life-threatening weakness. The diagnosis depends on a history of ingestion and recognition of the appropriate clinical features. Whenever possible, the contaminated food should be retrieved and tested, as assays for many toxins are available.

## Ciguatera Fish Poisoning

The ciguatera toxins are produced by algae that thrive in the tropical or subtropical coral reef ecosystem, mainly in the Indo-Pacific and the Caribbean waters between latitudes 35°N and 35°S. The algae are consumed by small herbivorous fish that in turn are eaten by carnivorous ones. As a result, predatory fish such as barracuda, eel, sea bass, grouper, red snapper, and amberjack are likely to be more toxic, although practically any reef fish eaten in significant quantity can cause ciguatera. Outbreaks can also occur in residents of temperate areas after a return from travel or from consumption of imported fish. The prevalence of ciguatera ranges from 0.1% in residents of large continents to 50% or more in those living in South Pacific and Caribbean islands (Dickey and Plakas, 2010).

A number of toxins are responsible for ciguatera, including ciguatoxins and maitotoxin. Ciguatoxins are a group of lipid-soluble molecules that act on tetrodotoxin-sensitive voltage-gated $Na^+$ channels in nerve and muscle, leading to increased $Na^+$ permeability at rest and membrane depolarization. Maitotoxin is the most potent nonproteinaceous toxin known. It is a water-soluble compound that increases $Ca^{2+}$ influx through voltage-independent $Na^+$ channels. Gambierol and palytoxin have also been implicated in ciguatera poisoning.

Symptoms are typically dose-dependent, with more severe poisonings occurring after consumption of the toxin-rich head, liver, and viscera of contaminated fish. Abdominal pain, nausea, vomiting, and diarrhea first appear within hours of ingestion. Bradycardia and hypotension may accompany the initial acute symptoms. Neurological symptoms then follow (Lewis, 2006). Patients develop centrifugal spread of paresthesias, involving the oral cavity, pharynx, limbs, trunk, genitalia, and perineum. Particularly characteristic is cold allodynia and a paradoxical temperature reversal when cold is perceived as burning, tingling, or unbearably hot. Less frequently, warm is perceived as cold. Headache, weakness, fatigue, arthralgia, myalgia, metallic taste, and pruritus are common. Symptoms may be worsened by alcohol consumption, exercise, sexual intercourse, or diets. Some patients are referred to psychiatrists by clinicians unfamiliar with the disease.

Cold allodynia in the distal limbs is a common finding on neurological examination (Schnorf et al., 2002). Some patients have findings of a mild sensory neuropathy. Weakness is generally not present, though rare cases of polymyositis have been reported. Most neurological symptoms remit in approximately 1 week, although some degree of paresthesias, asthenia, weakness, and headache may persist for months to years. Ciguatera can be rarely life threatening, with serious complications such as seizure, coma, and respiratory failure (Chan, 2016).

Diagnosis is based on a history of ingestion and the characteristic gastrointestinal, cardiovascular, and neurological disturbances. Clustering of cases in people who consumed the same fish helps with the diagnosis, though there is variation in individual susceptibility. An assay for ciguatoxins in fish is commercially available. Nerve conduction studies may show slowing of both sensory and motor conduction velocities, with prolongation of the absolute refractory, relative refractory, and supernormal periods. Although the chief neurological symptoms are attributable to the peripheral nerves, brain MRI may show reversible white-matter abnormalities (diffusion-weighted imaging [DWI] hyperintensity and apparent diffusion coefficient [ADC] reduction) in the corpus callosum, pyramidal tracts, and cerebellar peduncles (Yalachkov et al., 2019).

Gastric lavage may be beneficial if the patient presents soon after ingestion. Intravenous mannitol (20%; 1 g/kg at 500 mL/h) has been used for treatment of acute ciguatera poisoning. The mechanism of action is postulated to be reduction of edema in Schwann cells. The efficacy of mannitol is supported only by uncontrolled case series that report dramatic neurological improvement, especially if mannitol is given soon after symptom onset. One small controlled trial in 50 patients found no difference in outcome between mannitol and saline placebo (Schnorf et al., 2002), although many of the patients were treated over 24 hours after symptom onset. Supportive care during acute disease may include fluid replacement, control of bradycardia, and symptomatic treatment of anxiety, headache, and pain. Calcium gluconate, anticonvulsants, and corticosteroids have been tried with varying results. The chronic symptoms of ciguatera poisoning are difficult to treat. Gabapentin, pregabalin, amitriptyline, or other tricyclic antidepressants may provide partial relief of neuropathic pain.

## Puffer Fish Poisoning

Tetrodotoxin (TTX) is the causative agent in puffer fish poisoning. Puffer fish (family Tetraodontidae) have a worldwide distribution in both fresh and salt waters but are most commonly found in Japan and China. Other sources of TTX include the ocean sunfish, toadfish, parrotfish, Australian blue-ringed octopus, gastropod mollusk, horseshoe crab (eggs), atelopid frogs (skin), newts (genus *Taricha*), and some salamanders. Imported dried puffer fish has also been reported as a source of poisoning. TTX concentrations are especially high in the skin, liver, roe, and gonads, and relatively low in the muscles. *Fugu* refers to a preparation of puffer fish in Japan that is considered a delicacy. Specially trained and certified fugu chefs fillet the fish in such a way to avoid contamination by the deadly viscera. Despite these precautions, fugu poisoning accounts for approximately half of the fatal food poisonings in Japan, with up to 50 deaths each year.

Tetrodotoxin is a heat-stable, water-soluble small molecule that selectively blocks voltage-gated $Na^+$ channels in excitable membranes. It interferes with the inward (excitatory) flow of $Na^+$ current that occurs during an action potential, blocks impulse conduction in somatic and autonomic nerve fibers, reduces the excitability of skeletal and cardiac muscles, and has profound effects on vasomotor tone and central mechanisms involved in respiration. A dose of 1–2 mg of purified TTX can be lethal. Toxicity has been documented with the consumption of as little as 1.4 ounces (39.69 g) of fugu.

Lip, tongue, and distal limb paresthesias appear within minutes to about 2 hours of ingestion. Nausea, vomiting, diarrhea, and abdominal pain are common. Perioral paresthesias and progressive ascending weakness are apparent in moderately severe cases. Dysphonia, dysphagia, hypoventilation, bradycardia, and hypotension develop in severe intoxications. Coma and seizures may be seen. Fatality rates are high in severely affected individuals due to respiratory insufficiency, cardiac dysfunction, and hypotension (Chowdhury et al., 2007).

Diagnosis may be made on the basis of the patient's ingestion history and clinical features on presentation. Liquid chromatography may detect TTX in serum or urine. Electrophysiological tests of nerve excitability sometimes show a characteristic elevation in electrical threshold (Kiernan et al., 2005). There may be mild to moderate slowing of nerve conduction velocities, especially in the sensory nerves and in the more severely affected patients (Liu et al., 2011).

Treatment is supportive. Gastric lavage and charcoal are indicated if presentation is early. Neostigmine has been used with anecdotal success. Patients who survive the acute period of intoxication (approximately the first 24 hours) often recover without neurological sequelae.

## Shellfish Poisoning

Three neurological syndromes result from consumption of shellfish contaminated by toxins: PSP, neurotoxic shellfish poisoning (NSP), and amnestic shellfish poisoning (ASP; James et al., 2010). All of them are primarily associated with the ingestion of bivalve mollusks (clams, mussels, scallops, oysters)—filter feeders that can accumulate toxic microalgae. Rarely, poisoning is seen after consumption of other seafood such as predator crabs that may have eaten contaminated shellfish. Outbreaks are more frequent during the summer months, especially during periods of red tides, but they may occur in any month and in the absence of red tides. Shellfish may remain toxic for several weeks after the bloom subsides.

### Paralytic Shellfish Poisoning

PSP occurs in the United States along the coasts of New England, the Pacific Northwest, and Alaska. It is the most common and most severe of the shellfish intoxications. Mortality rates range from 1% to 12%, with higher rates in areas without advanced life support capabilities. Children appear to be more sensitive than adults. Saxitoxin (STX) is a heat-stable toxin that binds reversibly to voltage-gated $Na^+$ channels in nerve and muscle membrane. Its action is similar to tetrodotoxin. Symptoms usually appear within 30 minutes to 3 hours of ingestion. Paresthesias develop and initially involve the perioral areas, oral cavity, face, and neck. These symptoms spread to the limbs and trunk in severe cases. Other manifestations may include dysarthria, dysphagia, headache, gait ataxia, limb incoordination, ophthalmoplegia, and pupillary abnormality. Despite the name of this syndrome, muscle paralysis does not develop in every patient. If present, weakness may involve muscles of the face, jaw, swallowing, respiration, and the upper and lower limbs. Respiratory paralysis appears within 2–12 hours and is the primary cause of death in PSP. Spontaneous recovery begins after 12 hours and is usually complete within a few days. Weakness, however, may persist for weeks. There is no antidote, and treatment is supportive.

Initial diagnosis depends largely on recognizing the history and clinical features. Nerve conduction studies may show reduced amplitude of the sensory and motor-evoked responses and prolonged latencies with slowed nerve conduction velocities. Unlike acute demyelinating neuropathies in which electrophysiological abnormalities lag behind clinical findings, the electrophysiological abnormalities in PSP are most prominent at symptom onset and improve over a few days as clinical symptoms resolve. STX may be detected by high-performance liquid chromatography (HPLC) or enzyme-linked immunosorbent assay (ELISA). A mouse bioassay is commonly employed to monitor commercial shellfish production in many parts of the world. A mouse unit is the minimum amount needed to produce the death of a mouse in 15 minutes. The lethal dose for humans is approximately 5000–20,000 mouse units.

### Neurotoxic Shellfish Poisoning

NSP is more restricted geographically than PSP and is found primarily in the Gulf of Mexico, the Caribbean Sea, and the waters around New Zealand (Watkins et al., 2008). The responsible toxins are *brevetoxins* that cause activation of voltage-gated $Na^+$ channels, leading to nerve membrane depolarization and spontaneous action potential firing. These toxins are probably more toxic to wildlife than humans, as red tides from blooms of *Gymnodinium breve* are typically associated with massive fish, invertebrate, and seabird kills. Clinical presentation is characterized by the simultaneous onset of gastrointestinal and neurological symptoms within minutes to hours after ingestion. Nausea, vomiting, and diarrhea are common. Numbness and tingling appear around the mouth and face, as well as the extremities. Some patients may develop slurred speech, ataxia, headache, and limb weakness. Reversal of hot and cold sensation, similar to that in ciguatera poisoning, has been reported. No human deaths have been associated with NSP. The toxin may be detected by HPLC, radioimmunoassay (RIA), or ELISA are also available. There is also a mouse bioassay.

### Amnestic Shellfish Poisoning

*Amnestic shellfish poisoning* (ASP) was first described in 1987 in Canadians who ate blue mussels harvested off the Prince Edward Island coast (Pulido, 2008). Gastrointestinal symptoms were followed by cognitive dysfunction and headache. The putative toxin is domoic acid, which has since been found in mussels, clams, and other shellfish in many coastal regions worldwide. Domoic acid is an analog of kainic acid and acts as a potent excitatory neurotransmitter. Neurological disease results from its excitotoxic actions, especially on the limbic system. Symptoms appear within a few hours of ingestion, with diarrhea, vomiting, or abdominal cramps. Roughly half of patients experience headaches, and approximately 25% have memory loss, disorientation, mutism, seizures, myoclonus, or coma. Two patients were reported to have a unique alternating hemiparesis and complete external ophthalmoplegia. Gradual improvement occurs over a 3-month period. Those with residual deficits often have anterograde amnesia with relative preservation of intellect and other higher cortical functions. Some patients develop temporal lobe epilepsy. In the only reported outbreak, the mortality rate was 3%, all occurring in elderly patients. Autopsy revealed neuronal loss in the amygdala and hippocampus. Treatment is primarily symptomatic. Diagnosis may be established by the identification of domoic acid with HPLC. A surveillance program is now routine in high-risk regions of the United States and Canada to monitor commercial shellfish operations.

Low levels of domoic acid are persistent in some shellfish year-round. In a study of Native Americans in the Pacific Northwest, a high level of consumption of razor clams appeared to negatively impact everyday memory (Grattan, 2018). Further studies are needed to clarify the clinical significance of repeated low-level exposure to domoic acid.

*The complete reference list is available online at https://expertconsult.inkling.com.* 

87

# Effects of Drug Abuse on the Nervous System

John C.M. Brust

## OUTLINE



Drug dependence is of two types. *Psychic dependence* (addiction) refers to craving and drug-seeking behavior. *Physical dependence* refers to an adaptive state in which abrupt cessation of drug use results in somatic withdrawal symptoms. *Tolerance* refers to the need for increasing doses of a drug to produce a desired effect or to avoid withdrawal. *Abuse* refers to the perception that use of a drug, or the manner in which it is used, whether licit or illicit, is harmful.

Worldwide, numerous drugs, licit and illicit, are used recreationally, resulting in different patterns of intoxication and withdrawal. Symptoms and signs can be confusing. Polydrug users might experience intoxication from one agent while simultaneously withdrawing from another (Brust, 2004).

In 2016, a national epidemiological survey of American adults reported a 9.9% lifetime prevalence of DSM-5 drug use disorder (not including ethanol or tobacco) (Grant, 2016).

## DRUGS OF DEPENDENCE

### Opioids

Opioids include agonists, antagonists, and mixed agonist–antagonists (Box 87.1). In the past, the opioid most often used recreationally was heroin (diacetylmorphine), which is classified by the US Drug Enforcement Agency (DEA) as Schedule I (high potential for abuse, no accepted medical use).

Beginning in the 1990s, the United States and other countries experienced a steady rise in the use of prescription opioids to treat chronic noncancer pain (Han et al., 2017; Volkow et al., 2018). There soon emerged an epidemic of recreational use of these products (Walsh and Babalonis, 2017; Vadivelu et al., 2018), which in turn was followed by an epidemic of illicit opioid use, including heroin, fentanyl, and "designer opioids" (principally fentanyl analogs and novel synthetic opioids) (Frisoni et al., 2018; Karila et al., 2019). These agents are often taken with other drugs, including cocaine, benzodiazepines, and ethanol. Of 72,306 drug overdose deaths in the United States during 2017, 84% were opioid-related (Seth et al., 2018; CDC Wonder, 2018).

Desomorphine, a designer opioid, has become increasingly popular in Eastern Europe. Termed "crocodile" for the green-black skin lesions found on parenteral users, the drug is made by cooking crushed codeine pills with household hydrocarbons such as gasoline or paint thinner. Vascular damage causes gangrene and multiorgan failure, and average life expectancy in users is estimated at 2 years (Gahr et al., 2012). Since 2013, undocumented reports of crocodile use in North America have appeared (Grund et al., 2013).

Kratom, obtained from a Southeast Asian tree, contains mitragynine, which has opioid-like as well as serotonergic and noradrenergic effects. Usually smoked, Kratom produces stimulatory effects at low doses and opioid effects at higher doses (Rosenbaum et al., 2012). Fatal overdose has been reported (Gershman et al., 2019).

At desired levels of intoxication, opioid agonists produce drowsy euphoria, analgesia, cough suppression, miosis, and often a variety of other symptoms and signs (Box 87.2). Taken parenterally or smoked, heroin produces a "rush," a brief ecstatic feeling followed by euphoria and either "nodding" or garrulous hyperactivity.

Heroin overdose causes coma, respiratory depression, and pinpoint but reactive pupils; hypotension, if present, is usually secondary to hypoventilation. Treatment of overdose, including naloxone and ventilator support, depends on the degree of respiratory depression (Box 87.3). Fentanyl, fentanyl analogs, and novel synthetic opioids, some of which are thousands of times more potent than morphine, require larger and often repeated doses of naloxone to reverse respiratory depression. In response to the opioid epidemic, naloxone is now available over the counter as a nasal spray or an auto-injector.

Opioid agonist withdrawal produces a characteristic syndrome (Box 87.4). Seizures and delirium are not features, and their presence mandates identification of another cause (e.g., cocaine overdose or ethanol withdrawal). Craving is intense and is not explained by the unpleasantness of the somatic symptoms. Opioid withdrawal in adults is seldom life-threatening and can usually be prevented or treated with methadone 20 mg taken once or twice daily. With morphine or heroin, withdrawal symptoms usually appear several hours after the last dose,

**BOX 87.1 Commonly Used Opioids**

**Agonist**
Camphorated tincture of opium (paregoric)
Morphine
Meperidine (Demerol)
Methadone
Fentanyl
Hydromorphone (Dilaudid)
Oxycodone
Hydrocodone
Propoxyphene (Darvon)
Heroin

**Antagonist**
Naloxone (Narcan)
Naltrexone

**Mixed Agonist–Antagonist**
Pentazocine (Talwin)
Butorphanol (Stadol)
Buprenorphine (Buprenex)

**BOX 87.2 Acute Effects of Opioid Agonists**

"Rush"
Euphoria or dysphoria
Drowsiness, "nodding"
Analgesia
Nausea, vomiting
Miosis
Dryness of the mouth
Sweating
Pruritus
Cough suppression
Respiratory depression
Hypothermia
Postural hypotension
Constipation
Biliary tract spasm
Urinary retention

**BOX 87.3 Treatment of Opioid Overdose**

Respiratory support
If hypotension does not respond promptly to ventilation, IV fluids (pressors rarely needed)
Consider prophylactic intubation
If respiratory depression, naloxone, 2 mg IV, IM, or SC, and then 2–4 mg repeated as needed up to 20 mg. If no respiratory depression, naloxone 0.4–0.8 mg IV, IM, or SC, and if no response, 2 mg repeated as needed
Hospitalization and close observation, with additional naloxone as needed
Consider additional drug overdose, e.g., alcohol or cocaine

peak at 24–72 hours, and last a week or two. With methadone, symptoms appear at 12–24 hours and can last several weeks.

In newborns, untreated opioid withdrawal is severe, protracted, and often fatal. Seizures and myoclonus are described but can be difficult to tell from jitteriness. Treatment is with titrated doses of methadone or paregoric. Phenobarbital can be added for intractable seizures or if additional drug withdrawal is suspected.

**BOX 87.4 Symptoms and Signs of Opioid Withdrawal**

Drug craving
Anxiety, irritability
Lacrimation
Rhinorrhea
Yawning
Sweating
Mydriasis
Myalgia, muscle spasms
Piloerection
Anorexia, nausea, vomiting
Diarrhea
Abdominal cramps
Productive coughing
Hot flashes
Fever
Tachycardia
Tachypnea
Hypertension
Erection, orgasm

**BOX 87.5 Commonly Used Psychostimulants**

Dextroamphetamine
Methamphetamine
Ephedrine
Pseudoephedrine
Methylphenidate (Ritalin)
Pemoline (Cylert)
Phenmetrazine (Preludin)
Phentermine
3, 4-Methylenedioxymethamphetamine (MDMA, "Ecstasy")
Cocaine
Cathinone, methcathinone

Opioid dependence is treated pharmacologically with maintenance doses of methadone or buprenorphine (Hser et al., 2013; Mattick et al., 2014). Treatment failure is most often attributable to inadequate dosage. Despite US Food and Drug Administration (FDA) approval, oral treatment with the opioid antagonist naltrexone has limited usefulness in treating opioid dependence (O'Connor and Fiellin, 2000; Walley, Wakerman, and Eng, 2019). Proposed alternative therapies include injectable extended-release naltrexone (Krupitsky et al., 2013), slow-release oral morphine (Ferri et al., 2013), injectable heroin (Byford et al., 2013), acupuncture (Cui et al., 2013), and deep brain stimulation (Kuhn et al., 2013). Treatment with the West African hallucinogenic alkaloid ibogaine has been associated with sudden cardiac death (Jalal et al., 2013).

## Psychostimulants

Psychostimulants comprise a large number of licit and illicit drugs that include cocaine and amphetamine-like agents (Box 87.5).

Cocaine is an alkaloid present in the South American plant *Erythroxylon coca.* Unlike other psychostimulants, cocaine is also a local anesthetic. As a street drug, cocaine hydrochloride is sniffed or

## BOX 87.6 Acute Toxic Effects of Cocaine and Amphetamine-Like Psychostimulants

**Psychiatric**

Anxiety, insomnia, paranoia, agitation, violence, depression, suicide, hallucinations, psychosis

**Neurological**

Dizziness, syncope, vertigo, mydriasis, headache, paresthesias, tremor, stereotypy, bruxism, chorea, dystonia, myoclonus, seizures, coma, ischemic or hemorrhagic stroke

**Cardiopulmonary**

Chest pain, dyspnea, palpitations, sweating, pulmonary edema, cardiac arrhythmia, myocardial infarction, cardiac arrest

**Other**

Nasal congestion, nausea, vomiting, abdominal pain, fever, chills, myalgia, rhabdomyolysis, myoglobinuria

## BOX 87.7 Treatment of Psychostimulant Overdose

Sedation with intravenous benzodiazepine
Oxygen
Sodium bicarbonate for acidosis
Anticonvulsants
Antihypertensives (nitroprusside or α-adrenergic blockers; avoid β-adrenergic blockers)
Ventilatory support
Blood pressure support
Cardiac monitoring and treatment of cardiac arrhythmia
Treatment of hyperthermia
For rhabdomyolysis: vigorous hydration, sodium bicarbonate

injected. An alkaloidal preparation ("crack") is smoked, thereby avoiding complications of parenteral use and allowing sustained administration of very large doses. Methamphetamine ("speed," "crystal meth") is easily manufactured from commercially available pseudoephedrine. In the United States it is especially popular in midwestern and rural areas. Methamphetamine can be taken orally, sniffed, injected, or, as "ice," smoked. During 2010 it was estimated that worldwide 17.9 million people were dependent on amphetamine-like psychostimulants and 6.7 million on cocaine (Degenhardt et al., 2014).

Intended effects of cocaine and methamphetamine include alert euphoria with increased motor activity and endurance. Taken parenterally or smoked, they produce a rush distinguishable from that of opioids. With repeated use there is stereotypic activity progressing to bruxism and dyskinesias and paranoia progressing to frank hallucinatory psychosis.

Cocaine or methamphetamine overdose causes psychiatric, cardiopulmonary, and neurological symptoms, which can progress to shock, coma, and death (Box 87.6). Malignant hyperthermia and disseminated intravascular coagulation occur. Treatment includes sedation, cooling, anticonvulsants, antihypertensives, and cardiac monitoring (Box 87.7).

Withdrawal from these agents produces fatigue, hunger, craving, and depression. Objective signs are few, but depression can be suicidal.

The phenylalkylamine 3,4-methylenedioxymethamphetamine (MDMA, "Ecstasy"), popular on college campuses, appears to combine the psychostimulant properties of amphetamine-related agents and the hallucinogenic properties of drugs such as D-lysergic acid diethylamide (LSD). Many analogs of MDMA are marketed for oral use. At low doses, MDMA reportedly facilitates communication and empathy. Undesired effects include anxiety, tremor, muscle tightness, sweating, profuse salivation, blurred vision, and ataxia. As with methamphetamine, overdose causes hypertensive crisis, hyperthermia, tachyarrhythmia, psychosis, delirium, seizures, and rhabdomyolysis. Treatment is similar to that for psychostimulant toxicity.

Khat, a shrub indigenous to East Africa and the Arabian Peninsula, contains an amphetamine-like compound, cathinone, and the plant's leaves are chewed for their stimulant effects. During the past decade "designer" analogs of cathinone have become popular recreational drugs in Europe and North America. Purchased through the Internet as "legal highs" and collectively marketed as "bath salts," dozens of compounds are available, including methcathinone (ephedrone), mephedrone, methylone, and methylenedioxypyrovalerone (MDPV) (Angoa-Perez et al., 2017; Benzer et al., 2013; Glennon, 2014; Iverson et al., 2014; Miotto et al., 2013; Rech et al., 2015; Valente et al., 2014). Overdose is similar to what is encountered with methamphetamine. Numerous fatalities have been reported (Karila et al., 2019).

In addition to cathinone derivative, a wide array of novel designer psychostimulants have appeared on European and North American markets. Chemically characterized as aminoindanes, piperazines, and pipradrol, these agents have varying degrees of noradrenergic, dopaminergic, and serotonergic activity, and some are used as MDMA substitutes in products sold as Ecstasy (Iverson et al., 2014; Rosenbaum et al., 2012; Simmler et al., 2014).

Phenylpropanolamine, an amphetamine-like compound, was present in decongestants and diet pills and also available on the Internet as a "legal high" until a case-control study demonstrated it carried a risk for stroke. It was withdrawn from the US market in 2000 (Kernan et al., 2000).

Dietary supplements containing ephedra alkaloids ("ma huang") were available in "health food" stores until stroke and seizure risk led to their withdrawal in 2003 (Haller and Benowitz, 2000).

Despite clinical trials involving dozens of agents, an effective pharmacotherapy for psychostimulant dependence does not exist. Studies have involved dopamine, serotonin, opioid agonists and antagonists (Bidlack, 2014), GABAergic agents (modify effects of γ-aminobutyric acid [GABA]), glutamate inhibitors (Li et al., 2013a), sigma receptor ligands (Matsumoto et al., 2014), calcium channel blockers, ketamine (Dakwar et al., 2014), glial modulators (Beardsley and Hauser, 2014), bupropion (Carroll et al., 2014), guanfacine (Fox and Sinha, 2014), metyrapone (Goeders et al., 2014), salvinorin A analogs (Kivell et al., 2014), *N*-acetylcysteine (Berk et al., 2013; Corbit et al., 2014), orexin antagonists (Merlo Pich and Melotto, 2014), and deep brain stimulation (Yadid et al., 2013).

## Sedatives

Sedative drugs include barbiturates, benzodiazepines, and miscellaneous products (Chen et al., 2011) (Boxes 86.8–86.10). Intended effects and overdose resemble ethanol intoxication, but respiratory depression is much less with benzodiazepines than with barbiturates. Treatment of overdose includes ventilator support. For severe benzodiazepine poisoning, a specific antagonist flumazenil can reverse coma, but its action is brief and it can trigger seizures. As with ethanol, sedative withdrawal causes tremor, seizures, or delirium tremens; treatment can require intensive care and very high-titrated doses of a benzodiazepine.

"Designer benzodiazepines" began appearing early in the 21st century, and it is estimated that worldwide over 3000 such compounds have been synthesized. Biological half-lives of these agents vary widely, and they are difficult to detect using standard assays (Carpenter et al., 2019; Moosman and Auwarter, 2018).

**BOX 87.8 Commonly Used Barbiturates**

**Long-Acting**
Phenobarbital
Barbital
Primidone

**Intermediate-Acting**
Amobarbital
Butalbital (only in mixtures, e.g., Fioricet)

**Short-Acting**
Pentobarbital
Secobarbital

**Ultra-Short-Acting**
Methohexital
Thiopental

**BOX 87.9 Commonly Used Benzodiazepines**

**Marketed as Tranquilizers**
Alprazolam
Clorazepate
Chlordiazepoxide
Diazepam
Lorazepam
Oxazepam

**Marketed as Hypnotics**
Flurazepam
Temazepam
Triazolam

**Marketed as Anticonvulsants**
Clonazepam

**Marketed for Anesthesia Induction and for Treatment of Status Epilepticus**
Midazolam

**BOX 87.10 Miscellaneous Sedatives**

Buspirone
Chloral hydrate
Paraldehyde
Diphenhydramine
Ethchlorvynol
Glutethimide
Hydroxyzine
Meprobamate
Methaqualone (no longer produced in the United States)
Zolpidem (Ambien, Stilnox, Niotal)
Zaleplon (Sonata)
γ-Hydroxybutyric acid (Xyrem)

γ-Hydroxybutyric acid (GHB) and its precursors, γ-butyrolactone and 1,4-butanediol, are GABAergic sedatives. Classified as Schedule III, GHB is approved in the United States for treating narcolepsy. Notorious as "date-rape" drugs, these agents produce ethanol-like intoxication and withdrawal symptoms.

**BOX 87.11 Acute Effects of Marijuana**

Relaxation, euphoria, jocularity
Jitteriness, anxiety, paranoia, panic
Depersonalization, subjective time-slowing
Dizziness, sensation of floating
Impaired coordination and balance
Impaired memory and judgment
Conjunctival injection, decreased salivation
Urinary frequency
Tachycardia
Systolic hypertension and postural hypotension
Bradycardia, hypotension
Increased appetite and thirst
Decreased intraocular pressure
Analgesia
Auditory and visual illusions or hallucinations
Psychosis

## Marijuana

Consisting of leaves and flowers of the hemp plant *Cannabis sativa*, marijuana is usually smoked but can be eaten. The plant contains more than 60 cannabinoid compounds, of which δ-9-tetrahydrocannabinol (δ-9-THC) is the principal psychoactive ingredient. Hashish, prepared from resin covering the leaves, has a much higher concentration of δ-9-THC.

In the United States, pure δ-9-THC (dronabinol) and a close analog (nabilone) are FDA-approved for anorexia and chemotherapy-induced nausea but not for neurological disease (Koppel et al., 2014). A nonpsychoactive cannabinoid, cannabidiol (CBD), is FDA-approved for treating seizures in patients with Dravet or Lennox-Gastaut syndrome (Gaston and Szaflarski, 2018). A 2014 systematic review from the American Academy of Neurology found evidence for efficacy of oral cannabis extracts containing combinations of δ-9-THC and CBD in treating spasticity, central pain, painful spasms, and urinary frequency in patients with multiple sclerosis. Evidence of benefit in a variety of other neurological conditions was lacking, as was evidence of benefit from smoked marijuana in any neurological disorder (Bowen and McRae Clark, 2018; Koppel et al., 2014; Torres-Moreno et al., 2018; Rice and Cameron, 2018). Nonetheless, as of 2018, 30 states and Washington, DC had approved the use of marijuana or cannabinoid compounds for a variety of disorders, most with little or no evidence of efficacy, and putting users in violation of federal law.

The discovery of cannabinoid receptors with endogenous ligands in the brain led to the pharmaceutical development of synthetic receptor agonists. A number of these soon became popular recreational agents, marketed as "Spice" and "K2" (Brust, 2013; Seely et al., 2012). Up to 200 times more potent than δ-9-THC, dozens of these compounds, with ever-changing formulations, are available through the Internet. "K2" products are currently the second most popular illicit drug (after marijuana) among US high school students (Johnson et al., 2011).

Smoked marijuana produces dreamy euphoria, often with jocularity and disinhibition, plus an array of somatic symptoms (Box 87.11). Sometimes there is dysphoria or panic. Incoordination and impaired judgment increase the risk of traffic accidents, and because δ-9-THC is taken up by fat and slowly released, subtle effects on cognition can last more than 24 hours. High doses cause auditory or visual hallucinations, confusion, and psychosis, but fatal overdose has not been documented. Withdrawal symptoms are usually mild, with headache, jitteriness, sleep difficulty, and anorexia, but psychic dependence can be marked. The lifetime dependence risk of marijuana users is 9% but doubles for those who use it before age 17 (Bostwick, 2012; Kilmer, 2017; Volkow et al., 2014).

Synthetic cannabinoids ("K2," "Spice") frequently produce serious adverse effects, including psychosis, hallucinations, self-mutilation, cardiac arrhythmia, myocardial infarction, vertigo, hypertension, protracted vomiting, convulsive seizures, acute kidney injury, stroke, and death (Adams et al., 2017; Armenian et al., 2017a; Branchoff et al., 2018; Cooper, 2016; Courts et al., 2016; Fattore, 2016; Langford and Bolton, 2018; Mills et al., 2015; Paul et al., 2018; Riederer et al., 2016; Tait et al., 2016). Similarly, withdrawal symptoms are more severe than with marijuana, and dependence liability is greater (Nacca et al., 2013). Synthetic cannabinoids are not identified in toxicology screens, and there is no antidote for overdose.

### Hallucinogens

Dozens of hallucinogenic plants are used ritualistically and recreationally around the world. In the United States, the most popular hallucinogenic agents are the phenylalkylamine mescaline from peyote cactus, the indolealkylamines psilocin and psilocybin from different mushroom species, dimethyltryptamine (DMT) in ayahuasca, and the synthetic ergot LSD (Graddy et al, 2018; Feng et al, 2017; Nichols, 2016). Increasingly popular is the herb *Salvia divinorum*, which contains the kappa opioid receptor agonist salvinorin A (Pourmand et al., 2018; Ranganathan et al., 2012; Rech et al., 2015; Rosenbaum et al., 2012). Numerous designer hallucinogens are available, with such street names as "Fly" and "Bromodragonfly" (Hill and Thomas, 2011). "2C drugs" are phenylethylamines with hallucinogenic properties (Weaver et al., 2015).

Acute effects are perceptual (visual distortions or hallucinations, often formed and elaborately beautiful), psychological (depersonalization or altered mood), and somatic (dizziness, paresthesias, or tremor). Some users experience paranoia or panic, and some have "flashbacks," a spontaneous recurrence of symptoms in the absence of drug use. High doses can cause seizures or stupor but fatalities are usually attributable to accidents or suicide. Treatment of overdose usually requires no more than calm reassurance. Withdrawal symptoms do not occur.

### Inhalants

Recreational inhalant use is a worldwide phenomenon, especially popular among children and adolescents. A wide variety of products containing different volatile compounds are available (Table 87.1).

Despite chemical diversity, intended effects are similar to ethanol intoxication; symptoms usually last only 30 minutes or so, leading to repeated use over many hours. Overdose can cause respiratory depression, hallucinations, psychosis, seizures, and coma; death has resulted from cardiac arrhythmia, accidents, aspiration of vomitus, and asphyxiation during sniffing from plastic bags. Treatment consists of respiratory and cardiac monitoring. There is no predictable withdrawal syndrome other than craving.

### Phencyclidine

Developed as an anesthetic, phencyclidine (PCP) was withdrawn because it caused psychosis. As a recreational drug (PCP, "angel dust"), it is easily manufactured by kitchen chemists and usually smoked. Also used recreationally are the related agents ketamine and dextromethorphan (Majlesi et al., 2011). Among a variety of PCP analogs, methoxetamine has a much longer duration of action than ketamine (Corazza et al., 2012).

**TABLE 87.1 Inhalants**

| Products | Contents |
|---|---|
| Aerosols | Fluorinated hydrocarbons, propane, isobutane |
| Cleaning fluids, furniture polish | Chlorinated hydrocarbons, naphtha |
| Glues, cements | Toluene, acetone, benzene, trichloroethylene, *n*-hexane, xylene |
| Paints, enamels, paint thinners | Toluene, methylene chloride, aliphatic acetates |
| Lighter fluid | Aliphatic and aromatic hydrocarbons |
| Fire extinguishing agents | Bromochlorodifluoromethane |
| Natural gas | Methane, ethane, propane, butane |
| Petroleum | Many aliphatic and aromatic hydrocarbons |
| Anesthetics | Nitrous oxide, diethyl ether, halothane, chloroform, trichloroethylene |
| "Room odorizers" | Amyl, butyl, and isobutyl nitrite |

Low doses of PCP produce relaxation and euphoria, but sometimes dysphoria predominates, and with higher doses symptoms progress to agitation, violent behavior, hallucinations, psychosis, myoclonus, seizures, coma, respiratory depression, and shock. Unlike psychostimulants, PCP reproduces both positive and negative symptoms of schizophrenia, including catatonia. Treatment includes a calm environment, benzodiazepine sedation, and restraints as needed. Psychic dependence occurs but withdrawal symptoms are usually limited to nervousness and tremor.

### Anticholinergics

Worldwide, a number of plants contain atropine and scopolamine. In North America, *Datura stramonium* ("jimson weed") grows abundantly, and ingestion of its seeds (or, less often, leaves and roots) is popular among adolescents. Less often used recreationally are antiparkinsonian anticholinergics and the tricyclic antidepressant amitriptyline. The result is a predictable intoxication that includes delirium, fever, and dilated unreactive pupils. Treatment includes physostigmine, gastric lavage, and, if necessary, anticonvulsants. Neuroleptics, which have anticholinergic properties, are contraindicated, and sedatives should be used cautiously. There is no withdrawal syndrome.

## NEUROLOGICAL COMPLICATIONS

### Trauma

Drug intoxication can result in trauma; for example, driving accidents with marijuana, acts of violence with psychostimulants, or self-mutilation with hallucinogens. Among users of illicit drugs, trauma is most often related to the illegal activities necessary to distribute and procure them.

### Infection

Parenteral drug abusers are subject to local and systemic infections that affect the nervous system. Hepatitis can result in encephalopathy or hemorrhagic stroke. Cellulitis and pyogenic myositis can lead to peripheral nerve damage, vertebral osteomyelitis with radiculopathy or myelopathy, and meningoencephalitis. Tetanus affecting injectors is often severe. Botulism can originate at injection sites or, in cocaine snorters, in paranasal sinuses. Endocarditis, bacterial or fungal, can cause meningitis, brain abscess, infarction, and septic ("mycotic") aneurysm.

Drug injection is a major risk factor for human immunodeficiency virus (HIV) infection, and acquired immunodeficiency syndrome (AIDS) in this population is associated with the same neurological complications that affect nondrug users. Especially notable are syphilis and tuberculosis, including drug-resistant forms. Promiscuity and associated sexually transmitted diseases put nonparenteral cocaine users at increased risk for AIDS (DesJarlais et al., 2014; Centers for Disease Control and Prevention, 2018).

Progressive myelopathy occurs in parenteral drug users infected with either human T-cell lymphotropic virus (HTLV) I HTLV II.

During 2009–10, 199 cases of anthrax, many fatal, were reported in Europe as a result of contaminated heroin (Hanczaruk et al., 2014).

## Seizures

Some drugs cause seizures as a toxic effect. With amphetamine-like psychostimulants seizures are usually accompanied by other symptoms of intoxication such as fever, hypertension, or delirium. With cocaine, seizures are more likely to occur in the absence of obvious overdose. Cocaine-related seizures have a "kindling" effect—repeated use progressively reduces seizure threshold.

Opioids lower seizure threshold, but seizures in someone with heroin overdose mandate search for an alternative cause such as concomitant cocaine intoxication or ethanol withdrawal. Meperidine more often causes seizures or myoclonus, attributable to its metabolite normeperidine.

Like ethanol, sedative drugs, including barbiturates, benzodiazepines, and GHB, cause seizures as a withdrawal phenomenon.

A case-control study found that marijuana use was protective against the development of incident seizures (Ng et al., 1990). In animals the nonpsychoactive cannabinoid CBD is anticonvulsant. Its efficacy in treating human epilepsy is uncertain.

## Stroke

Illicit drug users often smoke tobacco or abuse ethanol, increasing their risk for ischemic or hemorrhagic stroke. Parenteral drug abusers are additionally at risk for stroke related to endocarditis, hepatitis, and AIDS. Heroin nephropathy carries risk for stroke.

Heroin users are at risk for ischemic stroke in the absence of systemic disease or other stroke risk factors; an immunological mechanism has been proposed (Brust, 2011). Magnetic resonance imaging (MRI) studies in heroin users found reduced perfusion in anterior cingulate cortex, medial prefrontal cortex, and insula (Denier et al., 2013a). Pulse wave analysis revealed "advanced vascular stiffness and ageing" among opioid-dependent subjects compared with controls (Reece and Hulse, 2014).

With amphetamine-like psychostimulants (including MDMA) hemorrhagic stroke has occurred in the setting of overdose, often with severe hyperthermia. Ischemic stroke attributed to large- and small-vessel vasculitis is also described in amphetamine/methamphetamine users, although the diagnosis of vasculitis has often been based on angiographic "beading," a nonspecific sign.

Over 600 cases of stroke have been reported in cocaine users, roughly half ischemic and half hemorrhagic (Brust, 2011), and epidemiological data confirm that cocaine is a significant stroke risk factor (Westover et al., 2007). Cerebral vasculitis is rare in cocaine users, in whom hemorrhagic stroke is probably most often caused by hypertensive surges (often with an underlying saccular aneurysm or vascular malformation). Ischemic stroke is most often associated with direct cerebrovascular constriction. Cocaine affects platelets and other coagulation factors, and some of its metabolites are pharmacologically active, plausibly accounting for strokes occurring hours or even days after use.

Anecdotal reports describe stroke temporally associated with marijuana smoking in young people without other vascular risk factors (Wolff et al., 2013). Marijuana users are also at risk for myocardial infarction and Buerger-like peripheral vascular disease. A population-based study of hospitalized patients reported an adjusted odds ratio of 1.76 for marijuana exposure and ischemic stroke (Westover et al., 2007). Another population survey, adjusting for covariates, found that subjects who used marijuana at least weekly had 4.7 times the rate of stroke compared with nonusers (Hemachrandra et al., 2016). Proposed mechanisms for stroke include postural hypotension with impaired autoregulation, cardioembolism, and reversible cerebral vasoconstriction syndrome. Of 48 consecutive young people with acute ischemic stroke, marijuana use was associated with "multiple intracranial stenosis" in 10 (Wolff et al., 2011).

A number of reports describe ischemic stroke in synthetic cannabinoid users (Bernson-Leung, 2014; Brust, 2013; Freemen et al., 2013; Khan et al., 2018; Pacher et al., 2018; Rose et al., 2015; Takematsu et al., 2014). A review of 98 cases of cannabinoid-related stroke (87% ischemic, 8% hemorrhagic) identified 85 following marijuana use and 13 following synthetic cannabinoid use (Wolff and Jouvanis, 2017).

LSD and PCP are vasoconstrictive, and ischemic and hemorrhagic strokes have followed use (Brust, 2011).

## Cognitive Effects

Chronically altered mentation in drug users might be related to ethanol, infection (e.g., AIDS dementia), malnutrition, or trauma. Determining whether the drugs themselves cause lasting cognitive or behavioral abnormality has been difficult; intoxication or withdrawal effects can persist for uncertain durations, and baseline cognitive performance prior to drug use is seldom available.

A meta-analysis of studies addressing "neuropsychological consequences of chronic opioid use" (including prescription analgesics and methadone maintenance therapy) identified significant impairments in verbal working memory, verbal fluency, and "cognitive impulsivity," but the authors stressed methodological problems in the studies reviewed (Baldacchino et al., 2012). Structural and functional imaging studies have demonstrated reduced cerebral gray-matter density and decreased white-matter fractional anisotropy in heroin users (Bora et al., 2012; Denier et al., 2013a, 2013b; Goldstein and Volkow, 2011; Guihua et al., 2013; Li et al., 2013a, 2013b; Qiu et al., 2013a, 2013b; Wang et al., 2012, 2013; Yuan et al., 2009; Wollman et al., 2015). Abnormal connectivity patterns are described in both heroin users (Liu et al., 2009) and recreational users of oxycodone and hydrocodone (Upadhyay et al., 2010).

In animals and humans, dextroamphetamine damages dopaminergic nerve terminals, methamphetamine damages both dopaminergic and serotonergic nerve terminals, and MDMA damages serotonin nerve terminals. The effects are partially reversible, but regeneration can lead to aberrant pathways. Abnormal cognition and behavior, as well as functional MRI abnormalities, are described in methamphetamine and MDMA users (Murphy et al., 2009). In a study of MDMA, subjects were matched on neuropsychological testing and functional imaging prior to taking up drug use and re-examined after 12–36 months. Those who had used MDMA during that interval, even in small doses, had decreased verbal memory and abnormal fractional anisotropy in the thalamus, globus pallidus, and cerebral white matter (deWin et al., 2008). Serotonin transporter binding was decreased in the cerebral cortex of abstinent MDMA users who, although "grossly behaviorally normal," demonstrated abnormalities on trials of attention, memory, and executive function (Kish et al., 2010).

Cocaine is not neurotoxic to axon terminals, but cognitive impairment is described. High doses of cocaine decrease hippocampal neurogenesis and impair working memory in rats (Sudai et al., 2011). Lasting cognitive impairment and structural alterations in frontostriatal systems are described in heavy cocaine users (Ersche et al., 2011; Lucantonio et al., 2012; Tau et al., 2014). Cocaine-treated rats demonstrate abnormal dendritic spines on neurons in the nucleus accumbens, and in both rodents and humans, diffusion tensor imaging shows abnormal fractional anisotropy in cerebral white matter (Moeller et al., 2007; Narayana et al., 2009; Shen et al., 2009; Wang et al., 2013). Rhesus monkeys self-administering cocaine developed abnormal central nervous system (CNS) myelin composition (Smith et al., 2014). Reduced resting state functional connectivity between amygdala and prefrontal cortex predicted relapse in abstinent cocaine addicts (McHugh et al., 2014). Reduced frontal gray matter volume and increased striatal volume are described in users of either cocaine or amphetamine (Crunelle et al., 2014; Ide et al., 2014; Mackey and Paulus, 2013; Moreno-Lopez et al., 2012). In rodents, cocaine alters *N*-methyl-D-aspartate (NMDA) receptor subunit composition and redistributes the assembled protein at the synapse (Ortinski, 2014).

A meta-analysis of neuroimaging studies in "stimulant-dependent individuals" found consistent reduction of prefrontal gray matter," which was plausibly linked to impaired "self-regulation and self-awareness." Direction of causality, however, remained open to question (Ersche et al., 2013).

A review of studies describing the long-term cognitive effects of cocaine concluded, "The current evidence does not support the view that cocaine use is associated with broad cognitive deficits" (Frazer et al., 2018). Another review during the same period concluded, "Long-term effects of cocaine show a wide array of deteriorated cognitive function" (Sprunk et al., 2018).

Clinical, imaging, and animal studies provide persuasive evidence that marijuana and synthetic cannabinoid use, especially during adolescence, causes lasting behavioral and cognitive alteration (Batalla et al., 2013; Battistella et al., 2014; Broyd et al., 2016; Brust, 2012; Bolla et al., 2002; Cohen and Weinstein, 2018; Davidson et al., 2017; Gilman et al., 2014; Greydenus et al., 2013; Hall, 2015; Pujol et al., 2014; Steel et al., 2014; Volkow et al., 2014). In the New Zealand Dunedin cohort study, which followed individuals from birth to age 38 years, heavy marijuana use by adolescents and young adults was associated with neuropsychological decline across multiple domains of functioning. The most persistent users had an average IQ drop of eight points from childhood to adulthood, and impairment was still evident after cessation for a year or more (Meier et al., 2012).

Functional imaging during testing of executive function found abnormal patterns of activation after several weeks of abstinence from marijuana (Bolla et al., 2005; Eldreth et al., 2004). Diffusion-weighted MRI and connectivity mapping identified microstructural alterations affecting axonal pathways in long-term marijuana users (Pujol et al., 2014). Volume reductions in brain regions rich in CB1 receptors have also been observed (Battistella et al., 2014; Gilman et al., 2014). Animal studies have reproduced such findings (Steel et al., 2014; Verrico et al., 2014).

Epidemiological studies offer compelling evidence that marijuana is a significant risk factor for schizophrenia (Le Bec et al., 2009; van Winkel and Kuepper, 2014).

Sedative drugs cause reversible dementia in the elderly and delayed learning in small children.

Controversial is whether psychostimulants predispose to depression or whether PCP predisposes to schizophrenia.

Leukoencephalopathy and dementia are described in toluene sniffers. Lead encephalopathy is described in gasoline sniffers.

## Fetal Effects

Adverse effects of in utero exposure to drugs are difficult to disentangle from inadequate prenatal care, concomitant ethanol or tobacco, malnutrition, and home environment.

Fetal exposure to prescription opioids is associated with decreased gestational size, respiratory distress, and, later, cognitive impairment (Broussard et al., 2011).

In utero exposure to methamphetamine is significantly associated with restricted fetal growth, depressed arousal in neonates, and in older children, lower verbal memory, spatial memory, working memory, attention, and visual-motor integration. Lasting metabolic and structural changes affect frontostriatal circuitry (Roussotte et al., 2011; Thompson et al., 2009).

A 10-year prospective study controlling for such confounders as additional drugs and environmental influences concluded that first trimester exposure to cocaine conferred risk for reduced height, weight, and head circumference and for lower sociability and increased withdrawn behavior (Richardson et al., 2013). A systematic review of 27 studies concluded that prenatal cocaine exposure "increases the risk for small but significantly less favorable adolescent functioning," including behavior, language, and memory. Eight studies reported morphological abnormalities of brain structure (Buckingham-Howes et al., 2013). A meta-analysis of studies of newborns exposed to cocaine found "clear evidence that crack cocaine contributes to adverse perinatal outcome," including reduced head circumference (dos Santos et al., 2018). A review of "congenital cocaine syndrome" concluded, "...maternal cocaine use during pregnancy...is associated with a host of neurological and developmental abnormalities in the offspring," including microcephaly, perinatal cerebral infarction, brain abnormalities on MR diffusion tensor imaging, and lower volumes of cortical grey matter (Todd et al., 2018).

Human and animal studies offer evidence that in utero exposure to marijuana carries risk for later cognitive impairment (Dinieri and Hurd, 2012; Gilbert et al., 2016; Richardson et al., 2016). Long-term cohort studies have demonstrated impaired performance on tasks of attention and visual memory as well as greater impulsivity and smaller head size, persisting into adolescence (Fried et al., 2002, 2003; Richardson et al., 2002). In animals, prenatal exposure disrupts cortical development by interfering with cytoskeletal dynamics critical for axonal connectivity between neurons (Tortoriello et al., 2014). A literature review concluded that although marijuana use is not teratogenic in the sense of causing morphological abnormalities, it does have negative long-term effects on executive functioning (Grant, 2018).

Organic solvents are teratogenic in animals.

## Miscellaneous Effects

Guillain-Barré polyneuropathy and brachial or lumbosacral plexopathy, probably immunological in origin, are described in heroin users. Severe axonal sensorimotor polyneuropathy affects sniffers of glue containing *n*-hexane.

Rhabdomyolysis, myoglobinuria, and renal failure have followed use of heroin, psychostimulants, and PCP (as well as ethanol) (Adrish et al., 2014).

Myeloneuropathy indistinguishable from cobalamin deficiency and combined systems disease affects sniffers of nitrous oxide. Vitamin $B_{12}$ levels are often normal. The mechanism is inactivation of the cobalamin-dependent enzyme methionine synthetase.

Severe irreversible parkinsonism affected Californians exposed to 1-methyl-4-phenyl-1,2,3,6-tetrahydropyridine (MPTP), an unintended by-product in the manufacture of a synthetic meperidine-like opioid.

"Chasing the dragon" consists of heating heroin mixture on metal foil and inhaling the fumes. Such practice is associated with dementia, ataxia, dystonia, quadriparesis, blindness, and death as a result of a spongiform leukoencephalopathy most often affecting the posterior cerebrum and internal capsule. The responsible toxin has never been identified (Cordova et al., 2014; Alambyan et al., 2018). A similar spongiform encephalopathy has infrequently been reported from intravenous heroin (Pirompanich and Chankrachang, 2015). Refractory hydrocephalus is also described in dragon chasers (Bui et al., 2015).

Irreversible extrapyramidal symptoms, including bradykinesia and dystonia, are described in users of methcathinone, a result of exposure to potassium permanganate used in preparing the drug (Steppins et al., 2014).

Blindness occurred in a heroin user whose preparation contained large quantities of quinine.

Cocaine users develop extrapyramidal symptoms progressing from repetitive stereotypic behavior ("punding") to choreoathetosis and dystonia. Cocaine can precipitate or aggravate symptoms of Tourette syndrome (Brust, 2010).

Marijuana inhibits follicle-stimulating and luteinizing hormones, causing reversible erectile dysfunction in men and menstrual irregularity in women.

Toluene sniffers develop cerebellar white-matter lesions and ataxia.

Sensorineural hearing loss has followed overdose with either heroin or methadone (Aulet et al., 2014; Saifan et al., 2013).

Hallucinogen users not only experience flashbacks but also the visual phenomena—geometric shapes, objects in the peripheral field, flashes of color, enhanced color sensitivity, trailing and stroboscopic perception of moving objects, after images, halos, and macro/micropsia—can persist for years ("hallucinogen-persisting perception disorder") (Hermle et al., 2012).

US cocaine samples are frequently adulterated with the immunomodulatory drug levamisole, which has an amphetamine-like metabolite and causes leukopenia and vasculitis (Baptiste et al., 2015; Le Graff et al., 2016). An associated leukoencephalopathy has been described in a number of cocaine users (Cascio and Jun, 2018).

The vitamin K anticoagulant brodifacoum, present in rodenticides, is a common adulterant in preparations of synthetic cannabinoids. Coagulopathy and spontaneous intracranial hemorrhage have been reported (Kelkar et al., 2018).

*The complete reference list is available online at https://expertconsult.inkling.com/.* 

88

# Brain Edema and Disorders of Cerebrospinal Fluid Circulation

*Gary A. Rosenberg*

## OUTLINE



## BRAIN EDEMA AND DISORDERS OF CEREBROSPINAL FLUID CIRCULATION

Increased intracranial pressure (ICP) and cerebral edema are life-threatening complications of shifts in water between cells and tissue that are final common pathways of injury in many neurological disorders. Separation of brain fluids from blood is maintained by a complex series of interfaces between the blood and brain tissues with the major one referred to as the neurovascular unit (NVU). The cerebrospinal fluid (CSF) is continuously formed mainly at the choroid plexus and absorbed at the arachnoid granulations. The interstitial fluid (ISF) bathes the brain cells delivering nutrients and removing waste. Early investigators realizing that the brain lacked a true lymphatic drainage system recognized that the ISF functioned as the lymphatic system and that the CSF and ISF were a continuous fluid. In 1925, Cushing and Weed named this the "third circulation" elevating it to the level of blood and lymph fluid. In 1885, Ehrlich injected blue dye into the bloodstream of mice. The dye stained all of the animals' organs blue—except their brains. In a follow-up experiment in 1913, one of Ehrlich's students injected the same dye directly into the brains of mice. This time, the brains turned blue, whereas the other organs did not. From these early studies the concept of a blood–brain barrier (BBB) emerged. It is now well established that at all the interfaces between the blood and brain tissues there are specialized proteins that form tight junctions. In addition to the tight junctions, the NVU has carrier molecules and electrolyte pumps to preserve the fluid balance, provide nutrients, and remove waste materials from metabolism (Iadecola et al., 2007).

Cellular membranes preserve the compartmental structure with water in extracellular and intracellular spaces. When shifts in water from one compartment to another occur under pathological conditions, swelling in the various compartments leads to increased ICP. If the increased water is blocked from exiting the ventricles, hydrocephalus results with transependymal flow of water into the periventricular white matter, resulting in interstitial edema. Loss of energy stores results in cell swelling due to failure of the membrane pumps, which is called cytotoxic edema. Damage to blood vessels leads to leakage of fluid, which expands extracellular space with intact cell membranes, leading to vasogenic edema (Higashida et al., 2011; Simard et al., 2007).

Hypoxia/ischemia and brain trauma initiate a series of molecular events that ultimately lead to cell death. Several molecules play key roles in the injury cascade: aquaporin forms pores in membranes that facilitate passive water movement; hypoxia inducible factor-1α (HIF-1α) is another key molecule that plays a key role in brain injury and repair by activating a cassette of inflammatory and repair-promoting genes (Agre et al., 2003; Semenza, 2014). Cytokines, proteases, and free radicals amplify the tissue damage. Advances in magnetic resonance imaging (MRI) have improved the diagnosis of CSF disorders and brain edema. Although we understand the underlying molecular processes involved in edema formation and have better ways of observing its evolution, treatment of brain edema remains a major challenge.

Brain edema represents a serious, often life-threatening consequence of many common brain disorders, including stroke, trauma, tumors, and infection. Early anatomists realized that the bony skull provided a rigid case that prevented expansion of the contents inside the skull and that such an expansion causes increases in ICP. Herniation

**TABLE 88.1 Causes of Increased Intracranial Pressure**

| Site of Increased Intracranial Pressure | Diseases |
|---|---|
| Increased tissue volume | Tumor, abscess |
| Increased blood volume | Hypercapnia, hypoxia, venous sinus occlusion |
| Cytotoxic edema | Ischemia, trauma, toxins, metabolic diseases |
| Vasogenic edema | Infections, brain tumors, hyperosmolar states, inflammation |
| Interstitial edema | Hydrocephalus with transependymal flow |

of brain tissues at several sites occurs when there is an increase in any of the three main brain compartments: brain tissue, blood, or CSF. Brain tumors and space-occupying infections damage cells because the mass distorts the surrounding tissues by compressing vital regions of the brain. Cell injury that occurs in cerebral ischemia, hypoglycemia, and some metabolic disorders causes tissue damage via cell swelling or breakdown of the BBB. It is important to appreciate the physiology of brain fluids as a basis for understanding the pathological changes encountered in clinical practice.

The human nervous system has evolved mechanisms to provide a stable microenvironment for the normal functioning of neurons and other cells. The electrolyte and protein contents of the brain fluids are normally kept within a constant range, which differs greatly from the systemic circulation of blood and lymph. The key to maintaining this privileged environment is a series of interfaces at each of the sites of potential brain and blood interaction. Interfaces formed by endothelial cells, choroid plexuses, ependymal cells, and arachnoid have tight-junction proteins that restrict the transport of nonlipid soluble substances and large protein molecules. In the major site formed by the endothelial cells, other components are important, including astrocytes, pericytes, and the basal lamina. Energy is expended at these interfaces to preserve this balance, and functions that are unique to the brain have evolved to provide for a constant delivery of oxygen and glucose to brain cells as well as the removal of metabolic products.

CSF fills the cerebral ventricles and subarachnoid spaces around the brain and spinal cord, serving along with the fluid between the cells, ISF, as a lymph-like fluid for brain tissue. ISF circulates between cells, draining into the CSF in the ventricle and subarachnoid space. Water moves into the extracellular space along osmotic gradients created at the capillary abluminal surface by the exchange of three sodium molecules for two molecules of potassium through the action of the sodium/potassium-triphosphatase ($Na^+/K^+$-ATPase) pump. Once within the ventricles, CSF/ISF circulates through the foramina of Magendie and Luschka to return to the systemic circulation at the sagittal sinus by way of one-way valves at the arachnoid granulations.

Examination of the CSF by lumbar puncture (LP) can provide unique information, aiding diagnosis and patient management. Increased ICP can only be determined by measurements made during removal of CSF; this information is critical in the diagnosis of raised CSF pressure in idiopathic intracranial hypertension (IIH). Studies of cells and proteins in the CSF provide information about infection and inflammation. Cancer cells can be detected and antibodies to infectious agents identified. When the BBB is disrupted, increased blood-derived proteins, mainly albumin that is produced in the liver, move into the CSF. Albumin levels in the blood are in the range of 3–5 g/dL, and in the CSF they are normally 15–60 mg/dL. CSF is critical in diagnosis of brain infection, such as meningitis, and in selection of appropriate treatment. Detection of cells in the CSF aids in the diagnosis of neuroinflammation. Detection of proteins in the CSF is important in the diagnosis of multiple sclerosis (MS): there are increased levels of myelin basic protein along with immunoglobulin (Ig)G endogenous production, which is expressed as an IgG index that is formed by dividing CSF albumin into IgG. When it is elevated, it suggests the IgG is formed in the brain rather than transported into the CSF across a damaged BBB. Patients with Alzheimer disease have low levels of amyloid-$\beta_{1\text{-}42}$ ($A\beta_{1\text{-}42}$), and elevated levels of phosphorylated tau. The ratio of $A\beta_{1\text{-}42}/A\beta_{1\text{-}40}$ is more accurate in identifying Alzheimer's disease (AD) patients (Janelidze et al., 2016). Thus, LP to obtain CSF is one of the most cost-effective procedures in daily clinical practice, and when done correctly, it can provide critical diagnostic information that is only available from CSF.

The recognition that the total volume of fluid and tissue contained within the skull of an adult is constant is called the *Monro–Kellie doctrine*, named after two early anatomists. Changes in volume of blood, CSF, or brain compartments produce compensatory changes in the others, with a resultant increase in CSF pressure. When CSF outflow pathways are blocked, enlargement of the ventricles or hydrocephalus follows, resulting in a buildup of pressure in the ventricles that forces the CSF to move transependymally into the periventricular white matter (Rosenberg et al., 1983). Masses enlarge the tissue space and compress CSF and blood spaces. When the compensatory mechanisms are overwhelmed, ICP increases and herniation of brain tissue occurs. Disruption of the blood vessels leads to vasogenic edema that moves through the more compliant extracellular space of the white matter. HIF-1$\alpha$ is another novel molecule that plays a key role in brain injury and repair matter. Finally, an increase in blood volume, as seen in hypercapnia and hypoxia, increases the ICP (Table 88.1).

## BLOOD–BRAIN INTERFACES

### Cerebral Blood Vessels and the Neurovascular Unit

The large surface area of capillary endothelial cells forms the major interface between the blood and brain. Other, less-extensive, interface surfaces include choroid plexuses and arachnoid granulations (Table 88.2). At each of the BBB interfaces, high-resistance junctions between cells, which make the surface into an epithelial-like structure, restrict transport. The epithelial sheets impede nonlipid-soluble substances, charged substances, or large molecules, whereas lipid-soluble substances, such as anesthetic gases and narcotics, pass easily through the cells. Water has an anomalous structure that allows it to pass rapidly through endothelial cells but with slight restrictions (Raichle et al., 1974).

ISF surrounds brain cells. It is formed by capillaries via an active transport mechanism. It is similar in composition to CSF and circulates. This lymph-like ISF fluid is formed by cerebral blood vessels, which have electrolyte pumps that make fluid in a fashion similar to that of the epithelial cells. Flowing around cells, ISF brings nutrients such as glucose and oxygen to neurons and astrocytes and removes the products of metabolism. ISF is absorbed either into the blood via terminal capillaries and venules or into CSF for eventual absorption through the arachnoid granulations (Fig. 88.1). CSF from the subarachnoid space moves rapidly into the brain along paravascular routes surrounding penetrating cerebral arteries, exchanging with ISF and facilitating the clearance of interstitial solutes, which may be driven by arterial pulsation (Iliff et al., 2013). Measurements of movement of ISF

**TABLE 88.2 Characteristic Features of the Blood–Brain Interfaces**

| Interface | Tight-Junction Location | Functional Aspects |
|---|---|---|
| Blood–CSF | Choroid plexus cell | Active secretion of CSF via ATPase and carbonic anhydrase |
| CSF–blood | Arachnoid membrane | Arachnoid granulations absorb CSF by one-way valve mechanism |
| Blood–brain | Capillary endothelial cell | Active transport of ISF via ATPase; increased mitochondria and glucose transporters in capillary endothelial cells |

*ATPase*, Adenosine triphosphatase; *CSF*, cerebrospinal fluid; *ISF*, interstitial fluid.

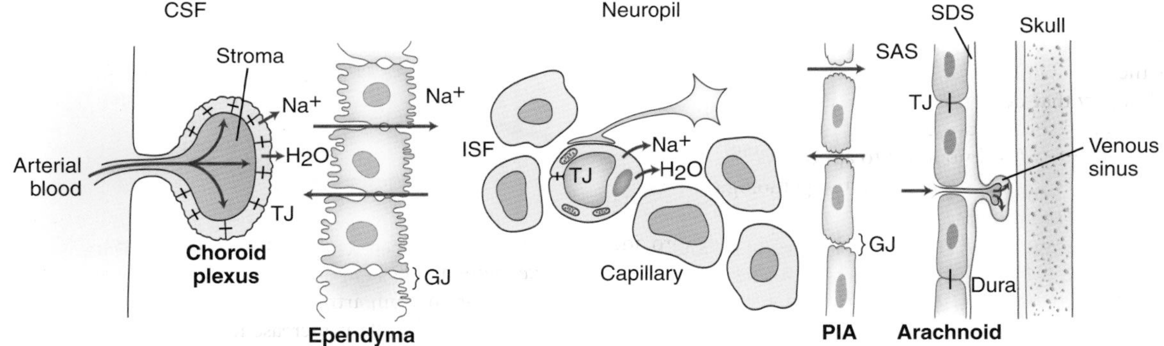


**Fig. 88.1 Illustration of the Third Circulation.** Cerebrospinal fluid *(CSF)* is formed by the choroid plexuses in the ventricles, and interstitial fluid *(ISF)* is formed by cerebral capillaries. At both sites, the action of the $Na^+/K^+$-ATPase pump creates the osmotic gradient that pulls water from the blood. Tight junctions *(TJ)* are found at each site of blood–brain interface. This includes the apical surface of the choroid plexus epithelial cells, the cerebral endothelial cells, and the arachnoid. Substances move between the brain and CSF across the gap junctions *(GJ)* on ependymal and pial surfaces. *SAS,* Subarachnoid space; PIA, pia mater; SDS, subdural space.

made with MRI indicate that inspiration facilitates the flow of ISF by its effect on the veins. Studies in mice have shown an influence of arterial pulse pressure on the movement of ISF into and out of the brain, but these studies need to be replicated in higher mammals.

Brain extracellular space comprises 15%–20% of the total brain volume. Complex carbohydrates are found in the extracellular space, including hyaluronic acid, chondroitin sulfate, and heparan sulfate. Hyaluronic acid forms large water domains. These large extracellular matrix glycoproteins impede cell movement. After an injury, astrocytes secrete an extracellular molecule, hyaluron, which impedes movement of fluids in the extracellular space, slowing tissue repair. Treatment with hyaluronidase reduces hyaluron and improves regrowth of injured fibers (Back et al., 2005).

Proteases are secreted during development, angiogenesis, and neurogenesis to clear a path for the growing cells, similar to the secretion of proteases by spreading cancer cells (Yong et al., 2001). Rather than a unitary endothelial BBB, transport between blood and brain is modulated by neurons, astrocytes, pericytes, and endothelial cells, forming an NVU. On the abluminal surface of the endothelial cells is a basal lamina composed of type IV collagen, fibronectin, heparan sulfate, laminin, and entactin. Entactin connects type IV collagen and laminin to add a structural element to the capillary. Fibronectin from the cells joins the basal lamina to the endothelium. Basal lamina provides structure through type IV collagen, charge barriers by heparan sulfate, and binding sites on the laminin and fibronectin molecules. Pericytes are embedded in the basal lamina; they are a combination of smooth muscle and macrophage. Pericytes are important in preserving the BBB. Loss of pericytes occurs in a number of neurodegenerative diseases (Bell et al., 2010). Astrocyte foot processes form a layer that surrounds the basal lamina. Glia limitans is found at the pial surface and at the interface between astrocytes and blood vessels (Owens et al., 2008; Fig. 88.2).

Cerebral blood vessels have very low permeability and high electrical resistance, making them more similar to epithelial cells than systemic capillaries, which are passive structures with low electrical resistance and fenestrations that permit passage of large protein molecules. In addition, cerebral blood vessels have highly selective molecular transport properties. During development, cerebral blood vessels acquire the characteristics that distinguish them from systemic capillaries. Astrocytes are critical in this differentiation process, which involves interactions between blood vessels and astrocytes. The critical nature of the astrocytes in this process was shown in transplantation studies involving chicken and quail cells, which can be separated histologically. Quail brain grafts from 3-day-old quails transplanted into the coelomic cavity of chick embryos become vascularized by chick endothelial cells and form a competent BBB. On the other hand, when avascular embryonic quail coelomic grafts are transplanted into embryonic chick brain, chick endothelial cells form leaky capillaries and venules (Stewart et al., 1981). Astrocytes are critical in the differentiation process (Janzer et al., 1987).

At the interface between the systemic circulation and brain cells there are specialized proteins that form the poorly permeable vessels. Tight-junction proteins have been isolated and cloned, permitting immunocytochemical studies of their location in the endothelial cells. Zona occludins tether the tight-junction proteins to actin within the endothelial cells; occludin and claudin form the actual tight junctions within the endothelial clefts. Occludin attaches to the zona occludins, while claudins attach to occludin and protrude into the clefts between cells. The extracellular tails of claudins from adjacent cells self-assemble to form the tight junctions that are "zip-locked" together (Hawkins et al., 2005). During an ischemic injury, the tight junction proteins are degraded, contributing to the disruption of the BBB (Yang et al., 2018).

Tight junctions between the endothelial cells create the unique membrane properties of the cerebral capillaries by greatly increasing

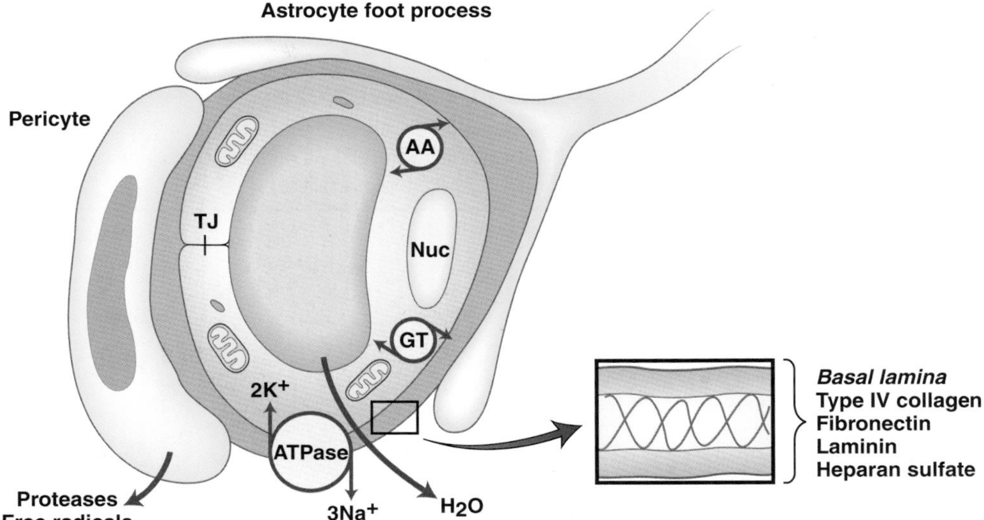


**Fig. 88.2 The Cerebral Capillary Is a Fluid-Secreting, Epithelial-Like Cell with a High Metabolic Rate.** The $Na^+/K^+$-ATPase pump on the apical surface forms cerebrospinal fluid. Tight junctions *(TJ)* between the endothelial cells maintain the electrical resistance. A large number of mitochondria are seen in the capillary. Amino acid and glucose transporters are present. Around the cell is a basal lamina composed of type IV collagen, laminin, fibronectin, and heparan sulfate. Astrocytic end-feet surround cells. Pericytes, which are embedded in the basal lamina, are macrophage-like cells that have macrophage and smooth-muscle functions in the perivascular space.

## BOX 88.1 Unique Features of Cerebral Capillaries

- Tight junctions create high electrical resistance
- Adenosine triphosphatase pumps on abluminal surfaces form interstitial fluid
- Increased numbers of mitochondria for high-energy needs
- Glucose transporters and amino acid carriers
- Basal lamina contributes to the barrier
- Pericytes act as perivascular macrophages
- Astrocytes maintain the tight junctions

electrical resistance, blocking transport of nonlipid-soluble substances (Box 88.1).

Brain tissue has a very high demand for glucose and essential amino acids, which can be met by specialized molecules that transport glucose and amino acids across the BBB. Glucose transporters are densely distributed in the capillaries. At low levels of blood glucose, the carrier proteins function at full capacity to meet metabolic needs, but at higher levels of blood glucose, the carriers are saturated, and transport is dominated by diffusion rather than active transport (Vannucci et al., 1997). High concentrations of one isoform, GLUT1, are found on cerebral blood vessels. GLUT3 is found on neurons and GLUT5 in microglia. GLUT2 is found predominantly in the liver, intestine, kidney, and pancreas. Amino acid transporters carry essential amino acids into the brain. Competition for the amino acid transporters can lead to a deficiency state; serotonin uptake is decreased in patients with phenylketonuria, which competes for the transporter.

Steady-state levels of brain electrolytes are preserved by transport mechanisms at the BBB. Potassium is maintained at a constant level in the CSF and brain by the BBB. This prevents fluctuations of electrolyte levels in the blood from influencing brain levels. Calcium is similarly regulated. Glutamate, which is an excitotoxin, is excluded from the brain. Highly lipid-soluble gases such as carbon dioxide and oxygen are rapidly exchanged across the capillary. Anesthetic gases are effective because they readily cross the BBB and enter the brain.

The presence of the BBB creates a major impediment for the transport of drugs into the brain. For example, penicillin is restricted from entry into the brain; high doses are needed to achieve therapeutic brain levels. Newer generations of antibiotics, such as the cephalosporins, penetrate more readily, making them better agents for treatment of brain infections. Chemotherapy of brain tumors has been hampered by the poor lipid solubility of most agents; to overcome this impediment, chemotherapeutic agents can be injected intrathecally or into catheters implanted into the ventricles, with injection bulbs buried beneath the scalp. Drugs of addiction are often modified to allow them to more readily cross the BBB. For example, heroin, which is derived from morphine, has increased lipid solubility, which enhances its transport into the brain. Similarly, other addictive substances, such as nicotine and alcohol, are highly lipid soluble and easily transported into brain.

Different rates for equilibration of various substances between blood and brain can cause paradoxical clinical situations. For example, to compensate for a metabolic acidosis, bicarbonate levels fall in both the blood and the brain. Metabolic acidosis is balanced by a respiratory alkalosis due to lowering of carbon dioxide by hyperventilation, which compensates for the acidosis; carbon dioxide is reduced in both the blood and CSF compartments, since it readily crosses the BBB, while bicarbonate is much more slowly exchanged between the two compartments. This adjustment results in a stable, albeit pathological, situation. However, when the metabolic acidosis is corrected by intravenous infusion of bicarbonate, there is a rapid adjustment of $Pco_2$ as the hyperventilation stops and $CO_2$ builds up. Bicarbonate adjusts very slowly because of the limited transport across the BBB, and the $CO_2$ entering the brain causes a further fall in brain pH. This dangerous situation continues until the bicarbonate levels in the brain rise. Although treatment is necessary to correct the metabolic acidosis, patients may become worse due to brain acidosis if treatment is too rapid (Posner et al., 1967).

## Production of Cerebrospinal Fluid and Interstitial Fluid

Production of brain fluids comes from multiple sources including the choroid plexuses within the ventricles, the electrolyte pumps on the abluminal surface of the cerebral capillaries, and metabolism. The main source is the choroid plexuses, which form an important interface between CSF and blood. Choroid plexuses protrude into the cerebral ventricles; they are covered with a specialized type of ependymal cell that has tight junctions on the apical surface.

Choroid plexus capillaries are fenestrated. Substances from the blood can cross into the stroma next to the ependymal cells. They are blocked from entering the CSF by tight junctions that form at the apical surface of the ependymal cells. Choroid plexus ependymal cells are enriched with mitochondria, Golgi complexes, and endoplasmic reticulum—suggesting a high rate of metabolic activity—and are covered with microvilli that increase their surface area.

In humans, the volume of CSF in the ventricles and around the spinal cord is approximately 140 mL, with a rate of CSF production of 0.35 mL/min or about 500 mL/day, which explains why obstruction of CSF leads rapidly to life-threatening hydrocephalus. CSF production occurs at both choroidal and extrachoroidal sites, and estimates of the proportion of CSF from each site vary, depending on the species and the method of measurement. Removal of the choroid plexus in nonhuman primates only reduces CSF production by 40%, leaving 60% presumably from extrachoroidal production (Milhorat, 1969).

Higher levels of sodium, chloride, and magnesium and lower levels of potassium, calcium, bicarbonate, and glucose are found in CSF than are expected from a plasma ultrafiltrate, which suggests that the CSF is actively secreted. An ATPase pump on the apical surface of the choroidal cells secretes three sodium ions in exchange for two potassium ions; osmotic water follows the increased sodium gradient. Carbonic anhydrase converts carbon dioxide and water into bicarbonate, which is removed along with chloride to balance the sodium charge. Production of CSF continues even when the ICP is high. Only acetazolamide, which inhibits carbonic anhydrase, can be used for the long-term reduction in CSF production. Experimentally, hypothermia, hypocarbia, hypoxia, and hyperosmolality have been shown to reduce production, but these are not practical to use for other than short periods. Osmotic agents such as mannitol and glycerol increase serum osmolality, lowering CSF production temporarily by about 50%. Agents that interfere with $Na^+/K^+$-ATPase reduce CSF production. Digitalis has an effect on the rate of CSF production, but ouabain, which is a more effective agent experimentally, is too toxic for use in patients. Recently, hypertonic saline has been shown to reduce CSF pressure; some of this effect may be due to a reduction in CSF production, but the mechanism of action remains to be clarified.

Capillaries, which have $Na^+/K^+$-ATPase on the abluminal surface, are a source of extrachoroidal ISF production. Gray matter has a dense neuropil that impedes the flow of water, whereas white matter, being more regularly arranged, is a conduit for normal bulk flow of ISF as well as a route for movement of edema under pathological conditions. Normally the flow of ISF in the white matter is toward the ventricle, where it mixes with the CSF from the choroid plexus to be eventually drained across the arachnoid granulations that protrude into the sagittal sinus.

## Water Molecules: Basis for Magnetic Resonance Imaging

Water molecules have a magnetic moment that allows them to be aligned in a magnetic field. Such a field is created in a magnetic resonance scanner. Because brain tissue is 80% water, and water dipoles can be aligned by manipulating the magnetic fields, they can be made to resonate and the resonance signals from water protons can be detected by MRI; since water is the most abundant source of protons in the brain, water protons dominate the signals.

MRI can detect water diffusion by the use of appropriate pulse sequences. The complex diffusion signals are obtained mainly from intracellular water, with some contribution from extracellular water. Water diffusion between cells in the extracellular space occurs normally. When there is cellular swelling and the extracellular space is compressed, the diffusion of water slows, and the apparent diffusion coefficient (ADC) shows a loss of signal, which appears black on the image. The diffusion-weighted image (DWI) has a bright signal. Because the DWI may show T2 shine-through that will be misinterpreted as restricted diffusion, both a darkened ADC and a bright DWI should be seen in the region of the infarct. In cerebral ischemia, the DWI is abnormal within minutes after the onset of the ischemia, making this an excellent diagnostic test for the presence of acute cerebral ischemia.

Diffusion tensor imaging (DTI) reveals the patterns of white-matter tracts in three dimensions. Taking advantage of the directional flow of water protons along white matter, diffusion is measured in three planes, and the separate pathways for water movement between the fibers are traced. In patients with white-matter pathology, such as in vascular cognitive impairment and MS, injury patterns in the white matter can be revealed by DTI (Maillard et al., 2013).

Contrast agents are important in determining injury to the BBB. Iodine-containing contrast agents are used in computed tomography (CT) scanning because they are radiopaque. When injected intravenously, contrast agents show the site of injury to the blood vessels by the appearance of the contrast agent on the scan. Iodine-containing contrast agents can cause anaphylactic reactions, however, particularly in individuals with allergy to shellfish. Contrast agents used in MRI studies are safer and more sensitive, making them the agents of choice. Gadolinium-containing compounds are used in MRI because they produce a paramagnetic effect. When they leak from the vessels into tissue, they cause a rapid relaxation of the protons that can be seen on T1-weighted images as a hyperintensity, compared to the pre-contrast scan. There is some retention of gadolinium in the brain, but the significance of this finding is uncertain. However, it has led to more cautious use of gadolinium.

## Anatomical Sites of Central Nervous System Infection

The terminology used to describe various types of central nervous system (CNS) infections is anatomically based (Table 88.3). An infection limited to the subarachnoid space, with inflammation of the meninges, is called *meningitis*. Meningeal signs of headache, stiff neck, and photophobia are present without focal findings that would indicate spread into the parenchyma. When the infection spreads contiguously from the subarachnoid space through the pial surface or along Virchow-Robin spaces, crossing gap junctions, the brain parenchyma is infected, and the term *meningoencephalitis* is used. In addition to meningeal signs, there are focal findings and possibly impaired consciousness and seizures. An infection in the brain tissue that is most likely to spread via blood begins as a loose collection of invading cells referred to as a *cerebritis*; walling off of the infected brain tissue leads to an *abscess*. Finally, the term *encephalitis* is used to describe a more diffuse brain infection in both the gray and white matter, which is usually indicative of a viral infection. Occasionally the infection spreads in a potential space beneath the dura but outside the arachnoid; *subdural empyema* describes a life-threatening collection of pus over the brain surface that has often spread from an infected sinus through the venous plexus of the ethmoid or sphenoid sinuses into the subdural space. The presence of a subdural empyema should be suspected in a patient with sinus infection, fever, seizures, focal findings, and altered consciousness. Diagnosis of meningitis can be done by examination of CSF for signs of infection such as increased white blood cells or protein. Infections

**TABLE 88.3 Terms Used to Describe Different Sites of Inflammation in the Central Nervous System**

| Infection | Symptoms | Site of Inflammation |
|---|---|---|
| Meningitis | Fever, stiffness, photophobia, headache | Cells confined to subarachnoid space (SAS) |
| Meningoencephalitis | Meningeal symptoms with focal findings | SAS and brain inflammation |
| Encephalitis | Headache, seizures, altered mental state | Multiple sites of cellular response in brain tissue |
| Cerebritis/abscess | Fever, seizures, focal findings | Cerebritis, early collection of inflammatory cells around vessels; abscess is the walled-off stage |
| Subdural empyema | Fever, seizures, coma | Diffuse collection of pus over the surface of the brain between the dura and arachnoid |

that invade the brain are best diagnosed with MRI, which can readily demonstrate a meningoencephalitis, cerebritis, abscess, or encephalitis. Use of contrast agents increases the potential of reaching a correct diagnosis based on site of infection. Subdural empyema is the most difficult condition to diagnose because it may only be a thin layer of pus on the surface of the brain and be obscured by the skull. Diagnosis can be missed on LP or CT, and MRI is more sensitive.

## Gap Junctions on Ependymal and Pial Surfaces

Lining the cerebral ventricles (other than over the choroid plexus) is a layer of ciliated ependymal cells connected by gap junctions. Pial cells lining the surface of the brain, which form the limiting glial membrane, the glial limitans, also have gap junctions. Fluid, electrolytes, and large protein molecules move through the gap junctions, allowing exchange between the CSF and ISF. Intrathecal administration of antibiotics and chemotherapeutic agents has been used to bypass the BBB.

Blood vessels penetrate the brain from the surface. As they enter the brain, they are invested with pia mater. The space between the penetrating blood vessels and the brain, prior to the point where only brain tissue surrounds the vessels, is called the *Virchow-Robin space.* After injection of substances intrathecally, the large proteins in the CSF space penetrate into the brain from the surface via the Virchow-Robin spaces. These perivascular routes may be involved in the spread of infection into the brain from the subarachnoid space in meningitis.

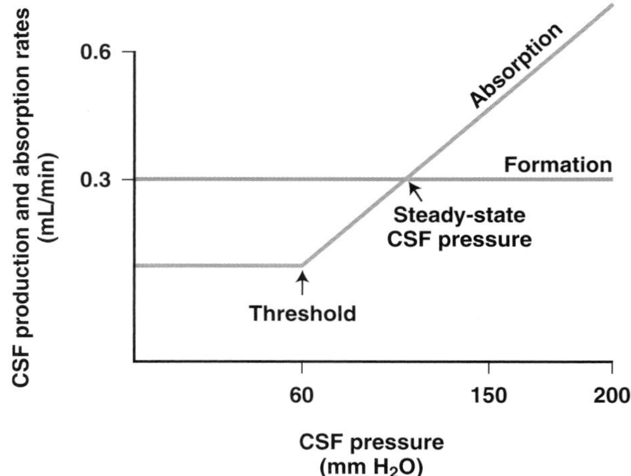


**Fig. 88.3 Schematic Drawing of the Relationship of Cerebrospinal Fluid Formation and Absorption to Pressure.** Cerebrospinal fluid *(CSF)* is formed at a constant rate of 0.35 mL/min. Absorption begins above a threshold value that varies from person to person. Once CSF absorption begins, it is linear, as seen in a one-way valve. When formation rate equals absorption rate, the steady-state CSF pressure is determined. *(Modified with permission from Cutler, R.W., Page, L., Galicich, J., et al., 1968. Formation and absorption of cerebrospinal fluid in man. Brain 91, 707–720.)*

## Arachnoid Granulations and Absorption of Cerebrospinal Fluid

Arachnoid granulations (pacchionian granulations) are the major sites for the drainage of CSF into the blood. They protrude through the dura into the superior sagittal sinus and act as one-way valves. As CSF pressure increases, more fluid is absorbed. When CSF pressure falls below a threshold value, the absorption of CSF ceases (Fig. 88.3). In this way, CSF pressure is maintained at a constant level, with the rate of CSF production as one determining factor.

Although channels are seen in the arachnoid granulations, actual valves are absent. Tissue appears to collapse around the channel as the pressure falls, and the channels enlarge as pressure rises. Resistance to outflow across the arachnoid granulations leads to CSF pressure elevation. Substances can clog outflow channels and increase resistance to CSF absorption. Blood cells are trapped in the arachnoid villi, and subarachnoid hemorrhage causes a transient increase in CSF pressure and can occasionally lead to hydrocephalus. Similarly, white blood cells and increased protein from meningitis can block the arachnoid granulations and increase CSF pressure.

## Cerebrospinal Fluid Pressure

Measurement of CSF pressure is a critical part of the LP. Pressures should be measured with the patient in the lateral recumbent position, and a narrow-bore spinal needle should be used to minimize CSF leakage. Performing the LP with the patient in the sitting position, although easier for the physician, eliminates the possibility of obtaining an accurate CSF pressure. Whenever CSF pressure is a critical piece of information, such as in the diagnosis of IIH, the sitting position should not be used.

The opening CSF pressure is measured with a manometer attached to the needle. Normal CSF pressure ranges from 80 to 180 mm $H_2O$ but may go as high as 200 mm $H_2O$ in obese patients or those who are not relaxed. Three components contribute to the measured pressure: volume of blood within the cranial cavity, amount of CSF, and the brain tissue. The CSF pressure recorded by the manometer represents the venous pressure transmitted from the right side of the heart through the venous sinuses. Small fluctuations from the cardiac systolic pulse and larger fluctuations from respirations can be seen in the column of fluid in the manometer. Pulsations in the manometer represent the fluctuations in the thin-walled veins. Arteries have thick elastic walls that dampen the pulsations from arteries. Deep respirations cause wide fluctuations in the CSF pressure, whereas changes in arterial pressure are barely visible. As ICP rises, tissue compliance falls and reserve capacity of the intracranial contents is lost. When tissue compliance is lost, small changes in fluid volume may lead to large increases in ICP.

Patients with increased ICP can be continuously monitored with indwelling catheters in the ventricles or with a pressure sensor implanted over the dura. Both procedures are invasive and only used in critically ill patients. Pathological elevations in ICP cause plateau waves that increase in steps to 50 mm Hg, where they persist for up to 20 minutes before returning to baseline. Treatment of patients with raised ICP can be monitored at the bedside with pressure monitors. Monitoring is used to gauge response to osmotic agents and to determine the severity of head injury. Despite use of intracranial monitoring in patients with severe brain injury, clinical utility has not been shown.

### Composition of the Cerebrospinal Fluid

CSF resembles water; the protein content is low and no more than five lymphocytes and no neutrophils should be present. Glucose values are two-thirds of those in blood. Some IgG is produced in the brain, but in the absence of an inflammatory disease (e.g., MS), amounts should be very small. The IgG index can be used to determine the source of CSF IgG. While meningitis is the major disease diagnosed exclusively by detection of cells in the CSF, other neurological diseases result in abnormal levels of proteins. Acute MS attacks cause an increase in myelin basic protein, which represents breakdown of myelin; oligoclonal bands suggest a longer disease course (Noseworthy et al., 2000). The ratio of IgG to albumin in both the blood and brain is calculated according to the formula (CSF IgG × serum albumin)/(serum IgG × CSF albumin). Dividing the ratio in the brain by that in the blood indicates whether the IgG comes from the blood across a leaky BBB, in which case the ratio is low, or whether the source of IgG is the brain, in which case the IgG index is elevated. An IgG index above 0.6 generally indicates intrathecal IgG synthesis.

Cells in the CSF provide an important indication of the underlying pathology. Bacterial infection typically leads to an increase in polymorphonuclear leukocytes; viruses cause a lymphocytosis. Large numbers of red blood cells in the CSF suggests a subarachnoid hemorrhage, which is confirmed by the presence of xanthochromia due to breakdown of blood products. In some forms of encephalitis, such as herpes encephalitis, there may be red blood cells in the CSF. Vasculitis can increase white blood cell numbers, as can an acute attack of MS. The presence of more than 50 cells increases the likelihood of vasculitis over MS. Parameningeal infections may not cause an increase in white blood cells but will increase CSF protein. CSF can aid in the diagnosis of neurodegenerative diseases.

## BRAIN EDEMA

### Molecular Cascade in Injury

Cerebral edema, which is the end result of many neurological diseases, is classified into cytotoxic or cellular swelling, ionic or extracellular edema that occurs in the presence of an intact BBB, vasogenic or vascular leakage, and interstitial edema, when the fluid accumulates in the interstitial spaces as occurs in hydrocephalus. Disruption of the BBB leads to vasogenic edema, which expands the extracellular space. Vasogenic edema moves more readily in between the linearly arranged fibers that form the white matter. The gray matter restricts water movement because of the dense mat-like nature of the neuropil, while the more loosely connected fiber tracts can be separated to allow edema fluid to flow. Cytotoxic edema, which results from pathological processes that damage cell membranes, constricts the extracellular spaces, constraining movement of fluid between the cells. Because of the lack of cell damage in vasogenic edema, once the damage to the blood vessel resolves, there may be a return to normal in the edematous tissue. This is generally not the case in cytotoxic edema, which is due to direct injury to cells. The resolution of interstitial edema from hydrocephalus is variable; some resolution may occur once the pressure in the expanded cerebral ventricle is reduced by insertion of a ventriculoperitoneal shunt.

Cellular and blood vessel damage follows activation of an injury cascade. The cascade begins with depletion of energy and glutamate release into the extracellular space (Fig. 88.4). This occurs during a hypoxic, ischemic, or traumatic injury and causes cytotoxic damage. Release into the extracellular space of excessive amounts of the excitatory neurotransmitter glutamate opens calcium channels on cell membranes, allowing extracellular calcium to enter the cells. Because one calcium ion is exchanged for three sodium ions, the removal of excess calcium from the cell, which requires an intact cellular membrane, causes a buildup of sodium within the cell, creating an osmotic gradient that pulls water into the cell. While the cell membrane is intact, the increase in water causes dysfunction but not necessarily permanent damage. If the blood vessels are intact, this stage has been referred to as ionic edema (Simard et al., 2017).

Accumulation of calcium ions within the cell activates intracellular cytotoxic processes, leading to cell death. An inflammatory response is initiated by the formation of immediate early genes (e.g., *c-fos* and *c-jun*) and cytokines, chemokines, and other intermediary substances. Microglial cells are activated and release free radicals and proteases, which contribute to the attack on cell membranes and capillaries. Irreversible damage to the cell occurs when the integrity of the membrane is lost. *Free radicals* are pluripotential substances produced in the ischemic brain and after traumatic injury. The arachidonic acid cascade produces reactive oxygen species such as superoxide ion, hydrogen peroxide, and hydroxyl ion. Release of fatty acids (e.g., arachidonic acid) provides a supply of damaging molecules. Superoxide dismutase-1 and catalase are the major enzymes that catalyze the breakdown of reactive oxygen species. Other defenses include glutathione, ascorbic acid, vitamin E, and iron chelators such as the 21-amino steroids. The role of oxygen radicals has been extensively studied. Transgenic mice that overexpress the superoxide dismutase-1 gene have smaller ischemic lesions than controls (Jung et al., 2009).

Nitric oxide (NO) is another source of free radicals, which have both positive and negative effects. NO synthetase (NOS) has three forms: neuronal NOS (nNOS), endothelial NOS (eNOS), and inducible or immunological NOS (iNOS). Macrophages and activated microglial cells form NO through the action of iNOS in response to ischemia, injury, and inflammatory stimuli. NO acts as both a normal vasodilator of blood vessels, by release of cyclic guanosine monophosphate in smooth muscle, and as a toxic compound under pathological conditions through the action of peroxynitrite anions ($ONOO^-$), which are formed from the reaction of NO with superoxide anions (Endres et al., 2004).

Manipulation of the *NOS* gene has helped reveal the action of the enzyme. nNOS produces toxic free radicals early in ischemic injury. Deletion of the *nNOS* gene in transgenic mice results in smaller infarcts from middle cerebral artery occlusion. On the other hand, eNOS causes vasodilatation and increases cerebral blood flow. Removing the *eNOS* genes leads to increased infarct size. Inflammation induces iNOS, which enhances injury and reaches a maximum at 24 hours (Iadecola, 1997).

### Neuroinflammation and Vasogenic Edema

Vasogenic edema occurs when there is damage to the cells of the NVU and subsequent disruption of the BBB. Protein and blood products enter brain tissue, increasing the oncotic pressure in the brain and exposing brain cells to toxic products from the blood. Opening of the BBB could occur by loosening of tight junctions, development of pinocytotic vesicles in the endothelial cell, or an alteration in the

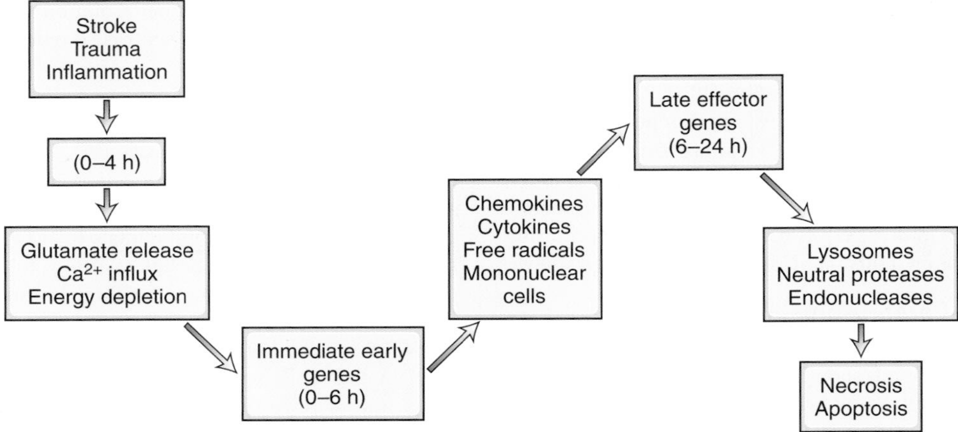


**Fig. 88.4 Mechanisms of Ischemic-Hypoxic Injury Leading to Cell Swelling and Death.** Chart shows the time course of early events involving glutamate release, immediate early gene production, and energy failure. This leads to changes in electrolytes and initiation of the inflammatory response. Cytokines continue the damage, which results in opening of the blood–brain barrier. Chemokines attract white blood cells to the injury site, where they release free radicals and proteases and enhance the injury. Finally, the proteases attack structural components, leading to membrane damage and cell death.

basal lamina surrounding the capillaries. Tight junctions in the endothelial cells are the first line of protection. Proteases and free radicals are the major substances that attack the capillaries (Candelario-Jalil et al., 2009). The layer of basal lamina around the capillary, containing type IV collagen, fibronectin, and laminin, is degraded by proteases. The proteases involved include the serine proteases, plasminogen activators/plasmin system, and matrix metalloproteinases (MMPs) (Cunningham et al., 2005). Free radicals activate the proteases and attack the membranes directly. Brain cells and infiltrating leukocytes are the sources of proteases and free radicals. Neutrophils contain prepackaged gelatinase B (MMP-9), which is released in an activated form at the injury site.

Extracellular matrix undergoes remodeling by the action of MMPs during development and repair. The MMPs are a gene family of over 24 enzymes that are expressed constitutively during normal remodeling but are induced in an injury. MMPs are expressed in a latent form that requires activation. Constitutively expressed MMP-2 is normally expressed by astrocytic foot processes around cerebral blood vessels, where it modulates the permeability of the BBB. Membrane-type MMP (MT-MMP) is membrane bound and forms a trimolecular complex with tissue inhibitor to metalloproteinases 2 (TIMP-2) to activate MMP-2. This configuration keeps the action of MMP-2 close to the membrane where it can gradually remodel the extracellular matrix around the blood vessel (Liechti et al., 2014). Synaptic remodeling is an important feature of learning. MMP-9 is involved in the formation of the neural nets as part of the synapse formation. Treatment with MMP inhibitors blocks this critical process and impedes learning. The dual function of proteases, such as the MMPs, in perpetuating injury and facilitating repair illustrates the important concept that the beneficial effects of drugs in the early phases of injury is offset by the detrimental effects of blocking proteases during the repair process.

Bacterial meningitis initiates an inflammatory response in the meninges caused by the invading organisms and by the secondary release of cytokines and chemokines. The secondary inflammatory response may aggravate the infection. Cytokines, including tumor necrosis factor (TNF)-α and interleukin (IL)-6, are elevated in the CSF of patients with bacterial meningitis and contribute to the secondary tissue damage. MMPs are increased in bacterial meningitis, and MMP inhibitors (e.g., doxycycline) block the damage secondary to infection (Lietchti et al., 2014). Steroids suppress the expression of MMPs and other inflammatory mediators. In children, treatment of bacterial meningitis with steroids along with the antibiotic reduces secondary injury. Use of steroids in adults with bacterial meningitis is more controversial. Doxycycline, a tetracycline derivative, suppresses MMP-9 expression and has a beneficial effect in reducing inflammation in meningitis when combined with another antibiotic (Meli et al., 2006).

## Cytotoxic Brain Edema

Stroke, trauma, and toxins induce cytotoxic edema. After a stroke, brain water increases rapidly owing to energy failure and loss of adenosine triphosphate (ATP). Cytotoxic edema begins soon after the onset of ischemia as shown by DWI, reaching a maximum between 24 and 72 hours, when the danger of brain herniation is greatest (Fig. 88.5). The initial cellular swelling due to an increase in water is the result of the accumulation of ions in the intracellular and extracellular spaces. This is referred to as ionic edema since the BBB remains intact. As the energy failure progresses there is further deterioration of the cell, threatening cell death. The next stage is the damage to the blood vessels, resulting in vasogenic edema, which occurs at multiple times depending on the cause of the injury. In brain trauma, there is an early opening of the BBB along with extensive damage to the brain tissue, and a mixture of cytotoxic and vasogenic edema leads to severe brain edema in the early stages after injury. Ischemic injuries with permanent occlusion of a blood vessel decrease blood flow to the vessel territory, and unless collateral vessels take over, there is infarction of the ischemic tissue. Greater damage occurs in transient ischemia, because the restoration of blood flow returns oxygen and white blood cells to the region, enhancing the damage. Reperfusion injury particularly damages the capillary, with disruption of the BBB seen in two phases: an early opening after several hours and a more disruptive secondary opening after several days (Kuroiwa et al., 1985). The initial opening, which is transient, is related to the activation of MMP-2, which is constitutively expressed and normally found in the latent form. Opening of the tight junctions is seen transiently after the onset of reperfusion, where disruption of tight-junction proteins is observed. A second, more disruptive, phase of injury to the capillary begins around 24–48 hours after the onset of reperfusion. This is related to activation of MMP-3 and MMP-9, along with cyclooxygenase-2, which are induced

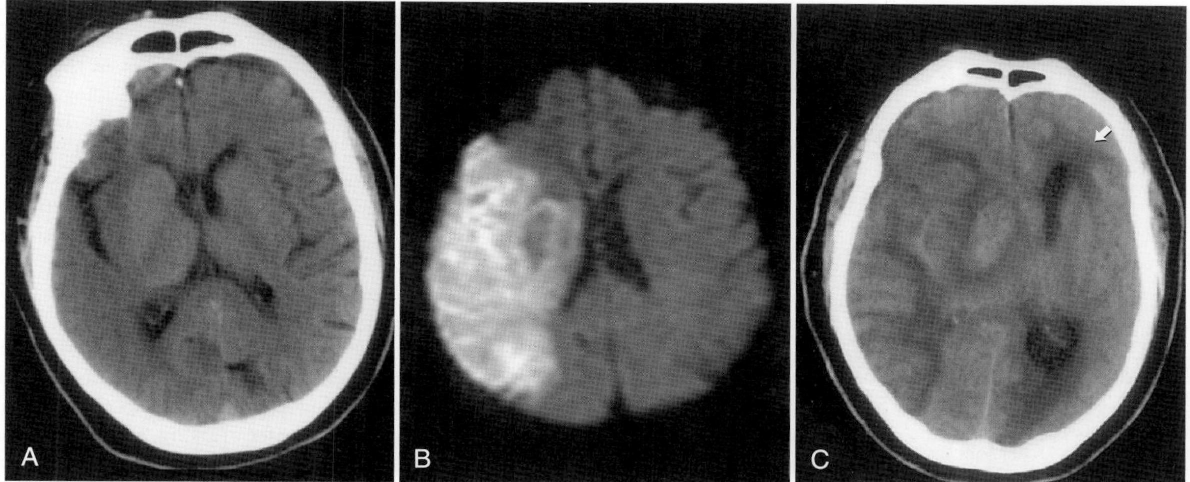


**Fig. 88.5 Patient with Cytotoxic Edema Secondary to a Large Middle Cerebral Artery Infarction. A,** Computed tomography (CT) shows early stages of infarction, with loss of definition of the insular stripe, an early sign of infarction. **B,** Diffusion-weighted image later that day shows restricted diffusion in region of infarct. **C,** One week after admission, CT shows mass effect and herniation, with hydrocephalus on contralateral side *(arrow)* due to obstruction of foramen of Monro.

from several cell types including microglia/macrophages during the amplification phase of the secondary inflammatory response. Emboli are more likely to lead to reperfusion injury than thrombosis because the breaking up of the clot can restore blood flow to a previously ischemic region. When that occurs, the risk of hemorrhage is increased (Fig. 88.6).

Cerebrovascular diseases are the major cause of brain edema in the adult because of the high incidence of cerebral ischemia in the elderly, but other causes include acute hepatic failure, osmotic changes, exposure to toxins, and high altitude. In acute hepatic failure, cerebral edema may cause death. Patients with hepatic failure are often young and have an acute cause for liver failure. They may have overdosed on a drug that is toxic to the liver, such as acetaminophen, or they may have infectious hepatitis. Long-standing liver disease with cirrhosis and hepatic encephalopathy shows changes of astrocytes in the brain, but it is generally not complicated by cerebral edema (Norenberg et al., 2005). Reye syndrome, which is seen primarily in children after an influenza infection (particularly when they are treated with aspirin), has a high incidence of brain swelling. Parents are warned not to use aspirin for childhood fevers, and since warnings appeared and use of aspirin declined, the number of patients with Reye syndrome has decreased.

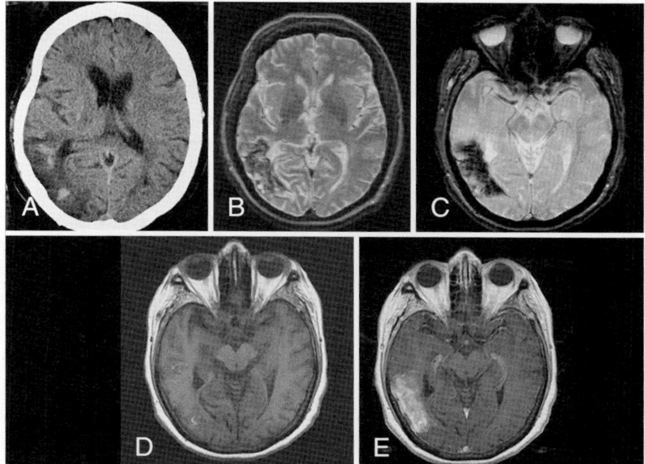


**Fig. 88.6 Hemorrhagic Transformation and Enhancement of an Infarct.** Patient presented with left-sided weakness of uncertain duration but probably less than 12 hours. Computed tomography (CT) without intravenous (IV) contrast **(A)** shows a posterior right temporo-occipital, cortically based area of low attenuation with smaller areas of higher attenuation. Magnetic resonance imaging (MRI) was performed the following day. The greater sensitivity of MRI for hemorrhage is illustrated by the areas of low T2 signal intensity on an axial spin-echo image **(B)** and even more prominently on a gradient-echo image **(C)**. Follow-up CT showed very little change; difference is due primarily to differences in imaging technique and sensitivity, not further hemorrhage. Minimal foci of T1 hyperintensity are present before IV contrast administration **(D)**. After gadolinium administration **E**, extensive enhancement within the area of infarct indicates breakdown of the blood–brain barrier.

## Effect of Blood Pressure and Osmolality Changes on Brain Edema

Cerebral blood flow is tightly regulated in the waking state to ensure adequate flow to the brain. Loss of autoregulation occurs at both the lower and upper extremes of blood pressure, with resulting syncope and hypertensive encephalopathy, respectively. The normal level of autoregulation varies greatly between patients, depending on age, prior diseases such as hypertension and diabetes, and years of treatment for hypertension. The hypertensive blood vessel undergoes changes over a long period of time with the lumen becoming narrower and the outer wall thickening. This results in a noncompliant vessel that restricts blood flow and responds slowly to an increase in metabolic need (Rigsby et al., 2011). When a young patient with average blood pressures in the 100/60 range has an increase to 160/110, there may be hypertensive crisis, whereas in an older individual with long-standing hypertension, a blood pressure of 160/110 would most likely have no adverse effects. When an individual with chronic hypertension has a stroke, the blood pressure may increase to 200/120 without producing a hypertensive crisis. In fact, lowering the blood pressure too rapidly may worsen the ischemia; a gradual reduction in blood pressure is safer. Therefore, it is critical to understand the normal range for the individual before deciding to treat.

Rapid elevation of blood pressure causes hypertensive encephalopathy. In experimental animals, hyperemia is present, suggesting

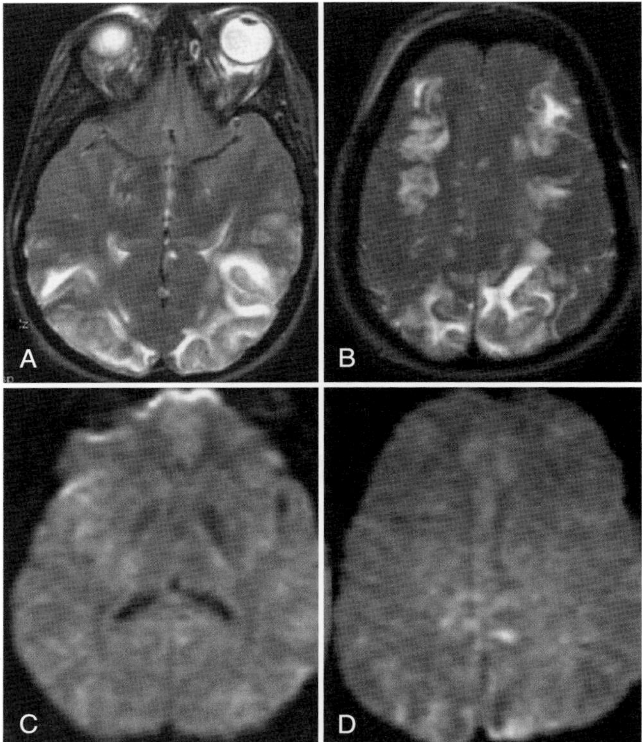


**Fig. 88.7 Patient with Hypertensive Encephalopathy Secondary to Eclampsia, with the HELLP (Hemolysis, Elevated Liver Enzymes, and Low Platelets) Syndrome. A,** T2-weighted magnetic resonance imaging shows extensive cerebral edema in posterior white-matter regions, with less involvement of the gray matter. **B,** A higher level of the same scan sequence as in **A,** showing some frontal lobe involvement. **C and D,** Diffusion-weighted images (DWIs), with only one small area of involvement. The lack of DWI changes is consistent with this being a vasogenic type of edema, and the patient had a good recovery without residual effects.

that the blood vessels are dilated and have increased permeability. Confusion, focal findings, seizures with papilledema, and increased CSF protein are present in some patients with hypertensive encephalopathy. MRI shows vasogenic edema, primarily in the posterior white matter of the brain (Fig. 88.7), a condition referred to by some as *reversible posterior leukoencephalopathy syndrome.* Common causes of rapid elevations of blood pressure are acute kidney disease, particularly in children with lupus erythematosus or pyelonephritis, and in eclampsia. Changes may be transient, and complete recovery is possible if treatment is instituted before hemorrhage or infarction occurs. A characteristic pattern of vasogenic edema without cytotoxic edema is present on MRI: there is extensive edema seen in the white matter, generally in the posterior regions, but spread in frontal regions can be seen, and an absence of DWI lesions indicating this is only vasogenic edema without tissue ischemia. Absence of signs of ischemia, such as a normal DWI in the face of marked white-matter edema, supports a good prognosis for recovery (Covarrubias et al., 2002). Rapid reduction in blood pressure is necessary. The reason for involvement of the posterior circulation is uncertain. Eclamptic patients have visual disturbances due to involvement of the occipital lobes; rarely is this a life-threatening condition, but when death occurs, on postmortem examination, petechial hemorrhages may be seen in the occipital lobes, explaining the visual symptoms.

Another cause of cerebral edema is a rapid change in serum osmolality. For example, rapid reduction of plasma glucose and sodium puts patients treated for diabetic ketoacidosis at risk for edema secondary to water shifts into the brain (Bohn and Daneman, 2002). Long-standing hyperosmolality leads to solute accumulation in the brain to compensate for hyperosmolar plasma levels. These idiogenic osmoles are thought to include taurine and other amino acids. During treatment of diabetic ketoacidosis, blood osmolality is reduced, and water moves into brain along the osmotic gradient, resulting in cerebral edema. Rapid reduction of serum hyperosmolality, as in diabetic ketoacidosis, should be avoided to prevent brain edema due to the residual idiogenic osmoles (Edge et al., 2001). Dialysis dysequilibrium also may be due to an osmotic imbalance that results from urea buildup in brain tissue.

Rapid correction of chronic serum hyponatremia can cause central pontine myelinolysis (Murase et al. 2006). In this syndrome, patients have very low sodium, usually less than 120 mEq/L, secondary to a variety of causes including inappropriate secretion of antidiuretic hormone (ADH), excessive water drinking, anorexia nervosa, alcohol withdrawal, meningitis, and subarachnoid hemorrhage. When there is inappropriate secretion of ADH, serum osmolality is low in the face of high urine osmolality. Treatment involves water restriction. In other patients, there is a salt-wasting syndrome that is treated by careful salt replacement. Low serum sodium can develop over an extended time period and be remarkably well tolerated. Shifts of water during treatment can result in central pontine myelinolysis due to damage to the myelinated tracts, particularly in the brainstem, but extrapontine myelinolysis may also be present.

## Edema in Venous Occlusion and Intracerebral Hemorrhage

Occlusion of the venous sinuses draining the brain can cause increased ICP and venous hemorrhagic infarction. When the superior sagittal sinus is involved, there may be hemorrhagic infarction in both hemispheres (Fig. 88.8). Dehydration and hypercoagulable states are often found in such patients. Early symptoms may be subtle, with headache due to vessel occlusion or increased ICP. However, as infarction develops, other symptoms such as seizures develop, leading to hemorrhagic conversion of the infarction, herniation, and death. A CT scan is usually unhelpful, and MRI may have subtle findings. Diagnosis can be made with an MR venogram showing the occluded veins. Partial occlusions resulting in increased ICP are underdiagnosed. Patients may recanalize the thrombosed superior sagittal sinus and have an excellent outcome (Fig. 88.9). Although still controversial, most studies suggest that anticoagulation of the patient with sagittal sinus thrombosis is indicated even when there is hemorrhage into the brain.

Intracerebral hemorrhage (ICH) causes brain edema around the hemorrhagic mass. This edema is both cytotoxic (direct damage to cells) and vasogenic (inflammatory response induced by toxic blood products). Growth of hematoma was observed after 24 hours in 38% of patients who were imaged within 3 hours of hemorrhage onset and again within 24 hours (Brott et al., 1997). Determining the cause of the ICH is generally difficult because the origin of the intracranial bleeding is obscured by the tissue destruction following the bleed and cellular necrosis. In primary ICH, a vessel ruptures, releasing blood into the brain. Secondary hemorrhagic transformation can occur in an area of infarction, particularly when the ischemic region is large. Generally, the hemorrhagic transformation is found 24–72 hours after the insult. Primary ICH most commonly occurs in the region of the basal ganglia, where the lenticulostriate arteries are subjected to hypertensive changes. The pons and cerebellum are less common sites (Fig. 88.10). Accumulation of blood causes both mass effect on the surrounding tissues and release of toxic blood products into adjacent tissues. Mass effect can lead to herniation. Blood contains coagulation cascade enzymes such as thrombin and plasmin, which are pluripotential

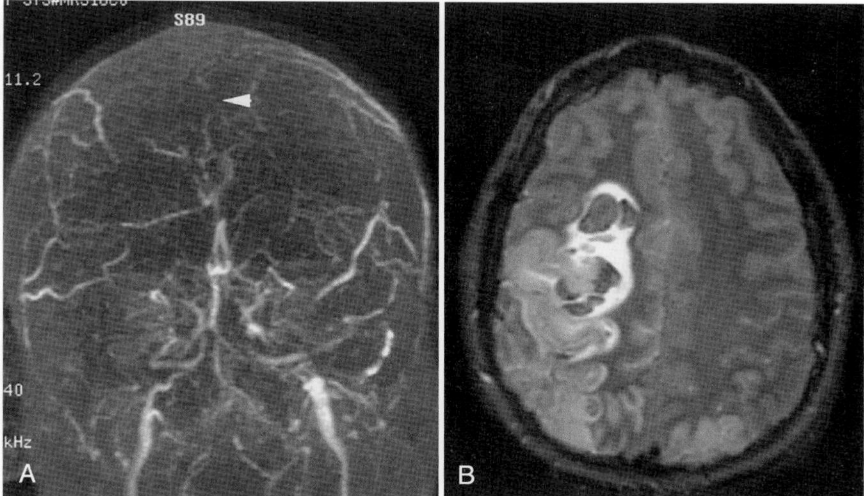


**Fig. 88.8 Sagittal Sinus Occlusion in a 17-Year-Old with Severe Dehydration. A,** Magnetic resonance venogram shows absence of sagittal sinus on coronal view *(arrowhead)*. **B,** T2-weighted image shows extensive venous hemorrhagic infarction.

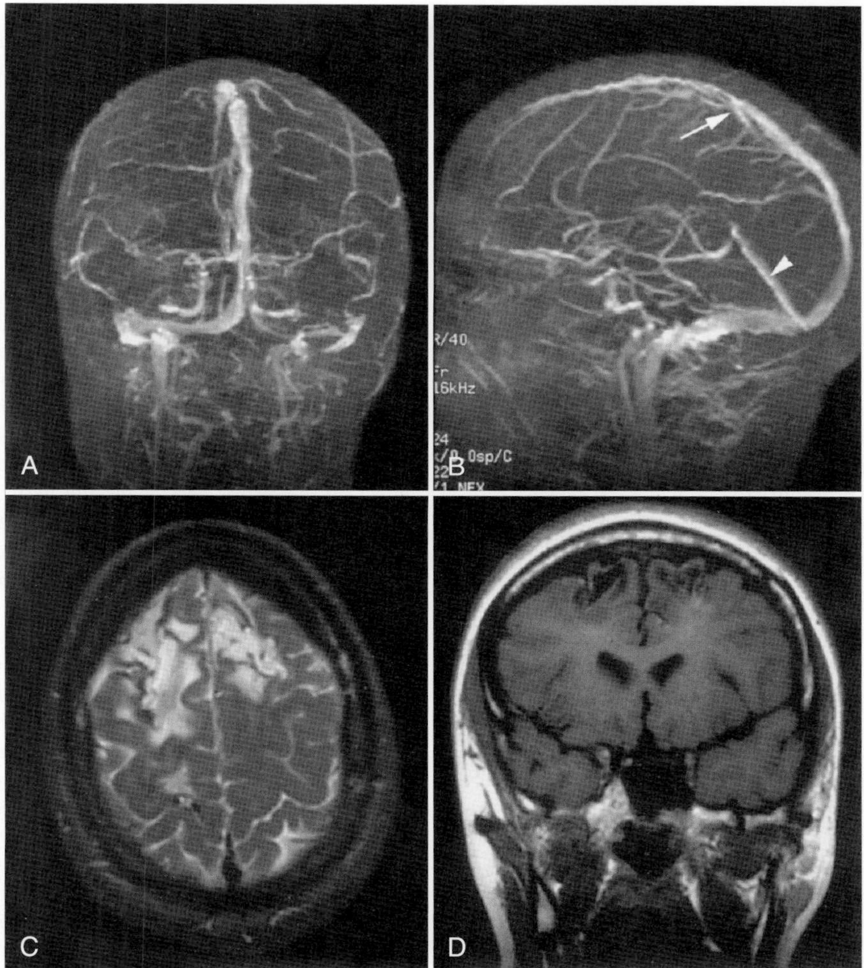


**Fig. 88.9 Patient with Sagittal Sinus Occlusion That Developed After Pregnancy.** Images shown were obtained several months after the event and demonstrate ability to recover. At illness onset, there was papilledema and increased intracranial pressure. **A,** Sagittal sinus is intact in this coronal view from a magnetic resonance (MR) venogram. **B,** Lateral view from venogram, showing flow in sagittal sinus *(arrow)* and straight sinus *(arrowhead)*. **C,** Region of prior venous infarction is shown on axial T2-weighted MR image. **D,** Same region as in **C** on the coronal T1-weighted image.

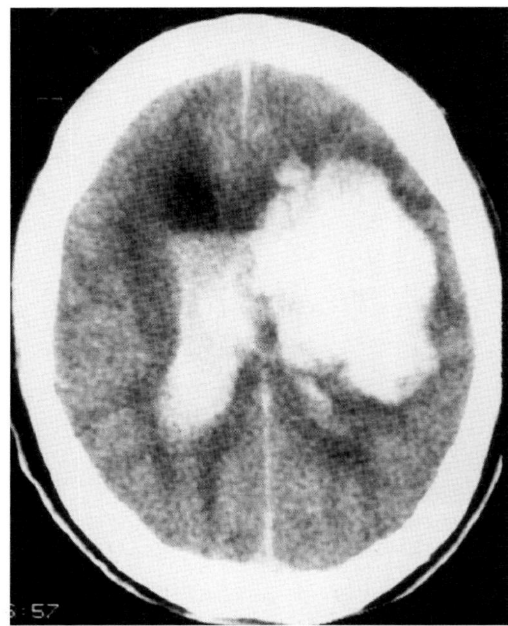

**Fig. 88.10 Computed Tomography Scan Shows Intracerebral Hemorrhage with Rupture into the Ventricle.** Contralateral ventricle is dilated as the result of compression of cerebrospinal fluid outflow.

molecules that can damage cells both directly by their toxic effects and indirectly by activation of other proteases. In experimental animals, injection of thrombin into the brain produces a focal increase in brain water content (Xi et al., 2006). In addition to proteases, free radicals are thought to be involved in hemorrhagic injury, but evidence of free radical involvement is indirect and comes from studies showing that free radical scavengers and spin trap agents reduce bleeding and improve function in experimental models of ICH (Peeling et al., 1998).

Many studies have been carried out to assess treatment of ICH. Two recent large clinical trials of surgical removal of the deep and lobar hematomas (STICH I) and of lobar hematomas only (ISTITCH II) failed to show a beneficial effect from surgery (Mendelow et al., 2013). A minimally invasive procedure to remove the blood via a catheter with the aid of thrombolysis is under evaluation but has not been proven to be effective (Hanley et al., 2017).

## High-Altitude Cerebral Edema

High-altitude cerebral edema (HACE) occurs when the concentration of oxygen, which is normally maintained at 21%, is markedly reduced. As the altitude increases and the atmospheric pressure is reduced, the amount of oxygen is also reduced, reaching dangerously low levels when climbing the highest mountains. Acute reductions in oxygen cause a constellation of cerebral symptoms that includes, initially, headache, ataxia, and short-term memory impairment, and can progress to life-threatening cerebral edema with papilledema, coma, and death. Two major mechanisms are thought to be involved in HACE: (1) hypoxia may increase cerebral blood flow, leading to an increase in intravascular pressure and vasogenic edema; and (2) disruption of the $Na^+/K^+$-ATPase pump due to the hypoxic conditions could lead to cytotoxic edema (Wilson et al., 2009). Both the vasogenic and the cytotoxic edema raise the intracranial pressure and impede venous outflow, adding another possible factor. Reduced oxygen content of the air leads to a compensatory hyperventilation, lowering the partial pressures of both oxygen and carbon dioxide. Since hypoxia causes vasodilatation and hypocapnia vasoconstriction, the combined effects initially balance each other. However, extreme exertion at altitude leads to levels of hypocapnia that produce vasoconstriction, reducing blood flow to the brain, which may reach ischemic levels. One study found that breathing into a bag to increase the concentration of $CO_2$ could relieve high-altitude symptoms (Harvey et al., 1988). Persistent impairment in memory has been reported in mountain climbers who have climbed to over 8000 m without supplemental oxygen (Regard et al., 1989). In nine patients with HACE after mountain climbing or skiing, MRI in seven of them demonstrated increased T2 signal in the splenium, with additional involvement in the centrum semiovale (Hackett et al., 1998). These abnormalities resolved in the four patients who had a repeat MRI; all seven patients recovered. Prophylactic treatment with the carbonic anhydrase inhibitor acetazolamide is beneficial for prevention of the initial symptoms of acute mountain sickness. Steroids may be used in individuals who are unable to tolerate acetazolamide: steroids probably act in altitude sickness by decreasing the release of cytokines and preserving the integrity of the BBB. Patients with HACE need to be transported as quickly as possible to lower altitudes.

## Treatment of Brain Edema

Treatment of brain edema has lagged behind the advances in understanding the mechanisms producing the edema. Reduction of volume in one of the three compartments may be helpful. Blood volume can be reduced with hyperventilation, which lowers carbon dioxide. However, excessive hyperventilation can cause vasoconstriction and ischemia. Reduction of CSF volume can be done mechanically by placing a drainage catheter into one of the ventricles. This can be difficult when cerebral edema has compressed the ventricular system. Intraventricular drainage is mainly used in patients with head injuries or acute hydrocephalus or is done post-surgically. Agents that reduce the production of CSF (e.g., acetazolamide, diuretics) may be used but are of marginal benefit.

For many years, osmotic therapy has been the treatment of choice for temporarily lowering ICP. Initially, urea was used, but the small molecule entered the brain, causing rebound edema. Current osmotic treatment is done primarily with mannitol, which reduces brain volume, lowers CSF production, and improves cerebral blood flow. Osmotherapy with low-dose mannitol infused over several days lowers ICP. Earlier studies employed 3 g/kg of mannitol, which had a drastic effect on the serum electrolytes and permitted only one or two doses to be given. More recently, it was found that low doses of mannitol (0.25–1 g/kg) are as effective as higher doses, without less effect on electrolytes. Lower doses raise serum osmolality only slightly, suggesting that mannitol has several mechanisms of action. The effect of the small change in osmolality is to reduce brain tissue volume; this effect is more prominent in the noninfarcted than the infarcted hemisphere. Other effects are that mannitol reduces CSF and ISF secretion by 50%, which may contribute to its action. Some investigators have proposed that mannitol hyperosmolality alters the rheological properties of blood, whereas others have noted an antioxidant effect. Prolonged administration of mannitol results in an electrolyte imbalance that may override its benefit and that must be carefully monitored. Although mannitol has been used to treat edema in acute stroke, its efficacy has not been proven. More recently, hypertonic saline has been advocated for use in treatment of cerebral edema (Fink, 2012).

Corticosteroids lower ICP primarily in vasogenic edema because of their beneficial effect on blood vessel permeability. However, they have been less effective in cytotoxic edema, and are contraindicated in the treatment of edema secondary to stroke or hemorrhage. In fact, systemic complications of corticosteroids can worsen the patient's condition when used to treat ICH. Edema surrounding brain tumors, particularly metastatic brain tumors, responds dramatically to treatment with high doses of dexamethasone; this corticosteroid rapidly closes the BBB. Hence, it is important to obtain contrast-enhanced MRI or CT scans before treatment with corticosteroids. Otherwise, enhancement of the lesion may be missed. High doses of corticosteroids have been shown to be effective in brain edema secondary to inflammation in MS; the steroids act by closing the BBB, which can be seen on contrast-enhanced MRI (Rosenberg et al., 1996). Inflammatory lesions such as those that occur in acute attacks of MS respond well to high-dose methylprednisolone. Treatment with 1 g/day of methylprednisolone for 3–5 days reduces the inflammatory changes in the blood vessels during an acute exacerbation. Dramatic reduction in enhancement on MRI may be seen after treatment. However, the effect is lost after several months.

## IDIOPATHIC INTRACRANIAL HYPERTENSION

Before the advent of CT or MRI scanners, the complaint of headache and the finding of papilledema raised the suspicion of hydrocephalus or tumor. When tests were negative for either of these conditions, confusing names for the syndrome were invented, which have led to the use of inappropriate terms for this syndrome. It was first noted that otitis media was at times associated with papilledema that was suspected to be due to hydrocephalus, leading to the pre-imaging term *otitic hydrocephalus*. During the era of pneumoencephalography, which was done to show distortion of the ventricles to diagnose hydrocephalus or tumors, the term *pseudotumor cerebri* was invented to describe patients with papilledema who had neither. More recently, the syndrome has been called *benign intracranial hypertension*, but when blindness occurs it cannot be considered benign. None of these terms are satisfactory, and the descriptive term IIH is preferred, although, through common usage, *pseudotumor cerebri* has persisted in the literature.

### Clinical Features

Patients with IIH have a constellation of symptoms that includes headaches, transient visual obscurations, pulsatile tinnitus, diplopia, and sustained visual loss. Headache is the most frequent symptom; it is the presenting symptom in most patients and is an important reason for searching for papilledema in all headache patients. The pain characteristically wakes the patient from sleep in the early morning hours. Sudden movements such as coughing aggravate the headache. Headaches may be present for months before a diagnosis is made. Some patients complain of dizziness. Transient obscuration of vision occurs when changing position from sitting to standing. Visual fields show an enlarged blind spot due to the encroachment of the swollen optic nerve head. Prolonged papilledema may lead to sector scotomas and, rarely, vision loss when the swollen disc encroaches on the region of the macula. It is important to differentiate papillitis due to inflammation from papilledema due to increased CSF pressure. In the former, vision loss is prominent early in the course and the pupillary response is abnormal, whereas with papilledema, the vision is preserved until the late stages when the swollen disc encroaches on the macula. Dysfunction of one or both sixth cranial nerves may occur as an effect of shifts of cerebral tissue. Because the sixth cranial nerve is remote from the site of the process producing intracranial hypertension, the cranial neuropathy is a false localizing sign. The sixth nerve has a long course as it travels to the eye. Before entering the eye socket, it makes a 90-degree turn and goes through the canal of Dorello at the tip of the temporal bone. It is possibly at this site that compression of the abducens nerve could occur (Nathan et al., 1974).

Diagnosis requires ruling out other causes of increased ICP. All patients require a CT or MRI scan to look for hydrocephalus and mass lesions. After a mass lesion is ruled out, LP is needed, with careful attention to accurately measuring the CSF pressure, which must be elevated by definition. Characteristic CSF findings include normal or low protein, normal glucose, no cells, and elevated CSF pressure. The upper limit for normal CSF pressure is 180 mm $H_2O$. Most IIH patients will have readings above 200 mm $H_2O$, with pressures at times exceeding 500 mm $H_2O$. Measurement of CSF pressure should be done with the patient's legs extended and neck straight. As noted earlier, pressures taken with the patient in the sitting position are inaccurate. Movements of the fluid column with respiration should be seen to confirm proper placement of the needle. It is important to obtain an accurate pressure reading at the time of the initial LP, since measurements of pressure in subsequent LPs may be falsely reduced by damage to the dura and the loss of fluid during the initial puncture. Occasionally, CSF leaks into the epidural space and forms a false pocket; subsequent attempts at LP may sample this space rather than the actual CSF space.

IIH occurs more frequently in women than in men. Obesity and menstrual irregularities, with excessive premenstrual weight gain, are often present. Because many illnesses may be associated with increased ICP, a search for an underlying cause is essential before the diagnosis of IIH is made by exclusion of other causes.

MRI has rekindled interest in conditions that cause occlusions of the venous sinuses. When the sinuses draining blood from the brain are obstructed, absorption of CSF is reduced, causing the pressure of the CSF to increase. MR venography (MRV) is better for showing thrombosis of the sinuses than conventional MRI. The role of venous sinus obstruction in raising ICP, although important to rule out, is uncommon. When venous sinus obstruction is found as the cause, a hypercoagulable work-up is important.

Obesity is often found in women with IIH. Endocrine abnormalities have been extensively investigated in both obese and nonobese subjects, but none have been identified. Drugs associated with the syndrome include tetracycline-type antibiotics, nalidixic acid, nitrofurantoin, sulfonamides, and trimethoprim-sulfamethoxazole (Box 88.2). Paradoxically, the withdrawal of corticosteroids used to treat increased ICP can cause an increase in ICP. Large doses of vitamin A, which are used in the treatment of various skin conditions, may cause the syndrome. Hypercapnia leads to retention of carbon dioxide and increase in blood volume. Sleep apnea and lung diseases may cause headaches and papilledema due to this mechanism. Less frequent causes include Guillain–Barré syndrome, in which increased CSF protein clogs the arachnoid villa, leading to an increase in ICP. Similarly, a cellular response in meningitis may increase CSF pressure by blocking outflow pathways. Uremic patients have an increased incidence of papilledema with IIH. Renal failure patients have increased levels of vitamin A, use

**BOX 88.2 Drugs Frequently Associated with Idiopathic Intracranial Hypertension**

Minocycline
Isotretinoin
Nalidixic acid
Tetracycline
Trimethoprim-sulfamethoxazole
Cimetidine
Prednisolone
Methylprednisolone
Tamoxifen
Beclomethasone

*From Schutta, H.S., Corbett, J.J., 1997. Intracranial hypertension syndromes. In: Joynt, R.J., Griggs, R.C. (Eds.), Clinical Neurology, twelfth edition. Lippincott, Philadelphia, pp. 1–57.*

corticosteroids, and take cyclosporine, which have all been linked to IIH.

Other less well-substantiated causes of elevated CSF pressure include obstruction to venous outflow. Venous pressure measurement has shown high pressure in the superior sagittal sinus and proximal transverse sinuses, with a drop in venous pressure distal to the transverse sinus. In patients without a documented structural defect in the venous sinuses, increased right atrial filling pressure that was transmitted to the venous sinuses has been shown (Karahalios et al., 1996). Whether the high venous pressure and imaging evidence of venous narrowing is the cause or the result of the increased ICP is controversial.

### Treatment

Treatment involves reducing ICP. Acetazolamide is an inhibitor of carbonic anhydrase that lowers CSF production and pressure. It is given in a dose of 1–2 g/day. Electrolytes must be monitored to look for metabolic acidosis. Distal paresthesias are reported to occur in up to 25% of patients. The hyperosmolar agent glycerol (0.25–1 g/kg, two or three times daily) was advocated at one time but is no longer indicated; the increased blood sugar caused weight gain in a group of patients that are often obese. Corticosteroids reduce increased ICP, but the pressure may increase when they are tapered. In patients with rapidly progressive visual loss, corticosteroids can be given in high doses for several days before a more definitive treatment is started.

Drug effects are often transient, and when the syndrome does not resolve spontaneously, other treatments are needed. Although the relationship of obesity to IIH is uncertain, loss of weight can lead to resolution of the syndrome, and some patients have undergone bariatric surgery to control the obesity, but controlled studies of this procedure are lacking.

Visual fields should be measured and the size of the blind spot plotted. Swelling of the optic disc causes the enlarged blind spot. When papilledema spreads into the region of the macula, visual acuity falls, and, in extreme cases, blindness may occur. Although most patients with IIH retain normal vision, a small percentage of patients develop impairment of vision. When vision is threatened and drugs and LPs fail to lower CSF pressure, surgical intervention is necessary.

Lumboperitoneal shunting has a high initial success rate, but subsequent shunt failure is common. Fenestration of the optic nerve sheath to drain CSF into the orbital region reduces the ICP, and some consider it the treatment method of choice in medically refractory patients. Stereotactic insertion of ventriculoperitoneal shunts is now possible and provides better long-term patency than lumboperitoneal shunts. In obese patients with IIH, weight loss is an important adjunct treatment, and some authors argue that it is as important as acetazolamide.

Patients with fulminant IIH are rare but require urgent treatment with acetazolamide, high-dose steroids, and optic nerve fenestration or ventriculoperitoneal shunting. In one study from two institutions, a total of 16 patients were studied, all of who were women between the ages of 14 and 39 years. All were obese with mean CSF pressures of 541 mm $H_2O$. All had surgical treatment, which reduced headaches and vomiting, but 50% remained legally blind, showing the serious nature of this form of the illness (Thambisetty et al., 2007).

Patients with venous sinus occlusion as the suspected cause of increased ICP have had intravascular stents placed to improve flow. In a series of 12 patients with refractory IIH who had venous pressure gradients, stenting the transverse sinus stenosis improved 7, but the natural history of the illness is that most improve over time (Higgins et al., 2002). Although placement of a stent is less invasive than placement of an intraventriculoperitoneal shunt, there are sparse data on which to base a treatment strategy. There are no controlled studies of the efficacy and long-term consequences of placing venous stents in this population of younger patients. Most reports of stenting are anecdotal and endovascular procedure should be considered experimental until controlled studies are done (Mollan et al., 2018).

### Brain Edema in Idiopathic Intracranial Hypertension

Two MRI studies showed edema in the white matter in patients with IIH; there was an increase in white-matter water signal of a heavily T2-weighted imaging sequence obtained at 1.5 T (Gideon et al., 1995). Another study compared diffusion maps of the ADC in 12 patients fulfilling conventional diagnostic criteria for IIH and in 12 healthy volunteers. They reported a significantly larger ADC within subcortical white matter in the patient group than in the control group, without significant differences within cortical gray matter, the basal nuclei, the internal capsule, or the corpus callosum. In addition, four of seven patients with increased ADC in subcortical white matter also had increased ADC within gray matter (Moser et al., 1988). Another group measured mean diffusivity of water and the proton longitudinal relaxation time in 10 patients with IIH and 10 age-, sex-, and weight-matched controls. They failed to find significant differences in DWI and T1 values between patient and control groups in any of the brain regions investigated, concluding that IIH is not associated with abnormalities of convective transependymal water flow leading to diffuse brain edema (Bastin et al., 2003). Thus, based on the results of MRI studies, there is no consensus as to the presence of brain edema.

## HYDROCEPHALUS

Hydrocephalus is a pressure-dependent enlargement of the cerebral ventricles due to obstruction of drainage of the CSF. Mainly occurring in infants and the elderly, ventricular enlargement rarely causes diagnostic problems, because detection of enlarged ventricles has been greatly aided by CT and MRI. However, determining the underlying cause is still difficult, particularly in the elderly where separation of ventricular enlargement due to hydrocephalus from that due to loss of brain tissue can be challenging. In early life, obstruction of ventricular outflow often occurs in the cerebral aqueduct that opens into the fourth ventricle, leading to noncommunicating hydrocephalus. In the elderly, the site of obstruction is drainage from the subarachnoid space; when resistance to drainage of the CSF occurs outside the ventricles, it is referred to as *communicating hydrocephalus*.

Hydrocephalus in the adult may be acute and life threatening, as when a cerebellar infarct or hemorrhage obstructs CSF outflow from the ventricles, and ventricular enlargement is rapid. Or it may be insidious and slowly produce symptoms, with normal pressure measured at the lumbar sac when the symptoms are finally diagnosed. Although CSF pressure may be normal at the time of discovery, most likely there was a period of increased pressure when ventricular enlargement initially began.

### Hydrocephalus in Children

In children younger than 2 years of age, enlargement of the ventricles produces an increase in head circumference because the skull sutures are still open. Children with head growth that is more rapid than expected for their age are suspected of having hydrocephalus and are imaged early in the course, preventing the large heads and lower-extremity spasticity that once occurred as part of the childhood form of hydrocephalus.

The cause of hydrocephalus in newborns is often an infection in utero that causes scarring and closure of the cerebral aqueduct, with subsequent obstruction to the outflow of CSF. Infection in the meninges can cause scarring over the channels connecting the CSF in the ventricles with that in the subarachnoid space. Closure of the foramina

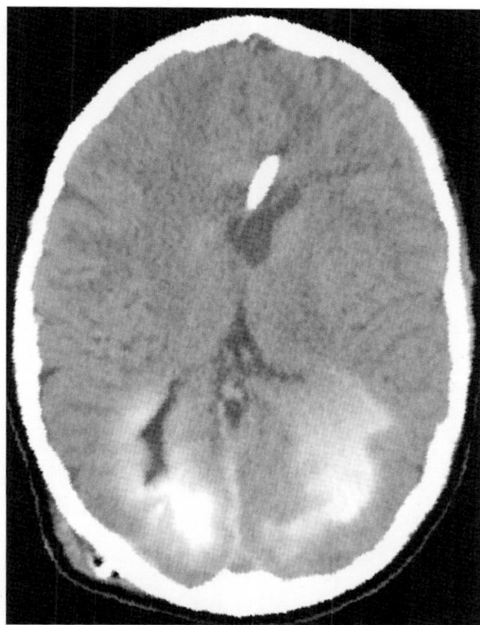

**Fig. 88.11 Transependymal Flow.** Computed tomography scan performed several hours after a small amount of contrast material was infused through a ventricular shunt catheter to evaluate communication shows that dependent contrast in the lateral ventricles has diffused into the surrounding brain through the ependyma.

of Magendie and Luschka leads to noncommunicating hydrocephalus. Obstruction of CSF circulation may result in increased CSF pressure as the cerebral ventricles enlarge, but once that has occurred compensatory drainage mechanisms may lower the CSF pressure, as is often the case in the adult with idiopathic normal-pressure hydrocephalus (NPH).

Acute noncommunicating hydrocephalus develops rapidly, reaching 80% of maximal ventricular enlargement within 6 hours owing to the continued production of CSF despite the increased pressure. A slower phase of enlargement follows the initial rapid expansion, and ventricular enlargement plus continual production of CSF causes fluid accumulation in the periventricular white-matter interstitial space, producing interstitial brain edema. When the hydrocephalus stabilizes and enters a chronic phase, CSF pressure may decrease, resulting in normal-pressure recordings on random measurements, although long-term monitoring reveals intermittent increases in ICP.

Long-standing hydrocephalus may cause atrophy in the white matter surrounding the ventricles but rarely affects the gray matter. When the rate of ventricular enlargement stabilizes in patients with incomplete ventricular obstruction, CSF production is balanced by transependymal absorption (Fig. 88.11). Occasionally a patient escapes detection of hydrocephalus in early life, and an enlarged head is the only sign of an underlying problem. Many years may elapse before the hydrocephalus manifests symptoms, and they may decompensate after many years of stability.

Hydrocephalus in children is often due to a structural abnormality such as a Chiari I or II malformation, aqueductal stenosis due to intrauterine infection, or other congenital causes such as anoxic injury, intraventricular hemorrhage, and bacterial meningitis. When the sutures are open and some expansion of the skull may be possible, the only sign of increased ICP may be bulging of the anterior fontanelle along with thinning of the skull and separation of the sutures. If the diagnosis is delayed, abnormal eye movements and optic atrophy may develop. Spasticity of the lower limbs may be observed at any stage. Acute enlargement of the ventricles is associated with nausea and vomiting.

During the neonatal and early childhood period, irritability is a common symptom of hydrocephalus. The child feeds poorly, appears fretful, and may be lethargic. In the older child, headache may be a complaint. Vomiting due to increased ICP may be present in the morning. Remote effects of the increased pressure may affect the sixth cranial nerves on one or both sides, leading to the complaint of diplopia in the older child. The enlarged ventricles affect gait. A wide-based ataxic gait due to the stretching of the white-matter tracts from the frontal leg regions around the ventricles may be present.

Premature infants weighing less than 1500 g at birth have a high risk of intraventricular hemorrhage, and approximately 25% of these infants develop progressive ventricular enlargement, as shown by CT, MRI, or ultrasound (Mazzola et al., 2014). Ventricular size in the neonate may be followed at the bedside with B-mode ultrasound through the open fontanelle. Long-term, follow-up studies of children with intraventricular hemorrhage due to prematurity show that 5% require shunting for hydrocephalus. The survivors of a large germinal plate hemorrhage often have multiple disabilities. Angiogenic factors play a role in the development of the hemorrhages (Ballabh et al., 2007).

Once the sutures are closed, which generally occurs by the age of 3, hydrocephalus causes signs of increased ICP rather than head enlargement. Meningitis, aqueductal stenosis, Chiari malformations, and mass lesions may be the cause of hydrocephalus in these young children. Tumors originating from the cerebellum and brainstem produce acute symptomatology, including headaches, vomiting, diplopia, visual blurring, and ataxia. Symptoms are due to the acute hydrocephalus secondary to obstruction of the cerebral aqueduct and to pressure on brainstem structures.

Examination shows papilledema, possible sixth cranial nerve palsy, and spasticity of the lower limbs. When the hydrocephalus is more long-standing, endocrine dysfunction may occur, involving short stature, menstrual irregularities, and diabetes insipidus. Excessively rapid growth of the head is the hallmark of hydrocephalus in the child before closure of the sutures. Charts are available to plot head growth and compare it with standardized curves for normal children. Bulging of the anterior fontanelle is found even with the child relaxed and upright. After 1 year, the firmness of the fontanelle cannot be used, because the sutures have closed. Other findings include the "cracked-pot" sound on percussion of the skull (McEwen sign), engorged scalp veins, and abnormalities of eye movements. As spasticity develops, the deep tendon reflexes are increased.

Treatment involves shunting CSF from the ventricles to drain fluid into another body cavity. The shunted CSF is generally drained into the peritoneal cavity. Complications of shunt placement include malfunction and shunt infection. Revisions of the shunt as the child grows are frequently necessary.

## Adult-Onset Hydrocephalus

In the adult, symptoms of acute hydrocephalus include headaches, papilledema, diplopia, and mental status changes. Sudden death may occur with severe increases in pressure. Although rare, hydrocephalus can cause an akinetic mutism due to pressure on the structures around the third ventricle. Other symptoms include temporal lobe seizures, CSF rhinorrhea, endocrine dysfunction (e.g., amenorrhea, polydipsia, polyuria), and obesity, which suggest third ventricle dysfunction. Gait disturbances are reported in patients with aqueductal stenosis, but hyperreflexia with Babinski sign is infrequent.

The causes of adult-onset hydrocephalus are similar to those in children, but the frequencies differ. As in children, acute obstruction of the ventricles in adults results in rapidly progressive hydrocephalus with symptoms of raised ICP. Adults are more likely than children to present with an acute blockage of CSF flow by intraventricular masses, such as a colloid cyst of the third ventricle, an ependymoma of the fourth ventricle, or the intraventricular racemose form of cysticercosis. Masses obstructing CSF outflow cause sudden headaches, ataxia, and loss of consciousness. Diagnosis may be difficult in patients with colloid cysts when the symptoms are intermittent because of the ball-valve effect of the mass.

Cerebellar hemorrhage and cerebellar infarction with edema cause an acute hydrocephalus by compressing the brainstem, occluding the cerebral aqueduct and fourth ventricle outflow pathways, and causing noncommunicating hydrocephalus and acute elevation in intraventricular pressure. Patients with cerebellar hemorrhage usually have a history of hypertension. Increasing drowsiness and difficulty walking often follow the acute onset of headache. Hemiparesis and brainstem findings evolve after the ataxia, providing a clue that the origin of the problem is in the posterior fossa. The expanding hemorrhagic mass in the posterior fossa, if it is encroaching on the brainstem, requires urgent neurosurgical attention, with placement of a ventricular catheter to decompress the lateral and third ventricles, followed by posterior fossa craniectomy to remove the mass and reduce pressure on the brainstem (Adams et al., 1965). In patients with cerebellar infarction, the progression is generally slower, since the maximum swelling takes place in 24–48 hours, but the consequences of the enlarging posterior fossa mass are the same as with hemorrhage, and surgery may be necessary to remove the necrotic tissues and restore normal CSF flow. CT is helpful to show enlargement of the ventricle, but MRI is better for imaging the cerebellar infarction (Fig. 88.12).

Treatment of adult hydrocephalus involves an operation to insert a tube to shunt CSF from the ventricles to the peritoneal cavity. These devices have one-way valves that respond to pressure. In an emergency, hydrocephalic ventricles can be assessed readily owing to the increase in their size. Shunt malfunction may cause abrupt decompensation. Symptoms of acute increased ICP from a shunt malfunction resemble those seen with onset of the hydrocephalic process.

Adult-onset hydrocephalus that is communicating may be due to a tumor in the basal cisterns, subarachnoid bleeding, or infection or inflammation of the meninges. In the pre-antibiotic era, syphilis, tuberculosis, and fungal infections were a common cause of hydrocephalus due to chronic obstruction of subarachnoid pathways. CSF cultures are indicated in the elderly patient with enlarged ventricles, and searching for other sources of infection in lungs and other organs may be helpful in establishing the type of infection.

## Normal-Pressure Hydrocephalus

Chronic hydrocephalus in the adult can produce symptoms of gait disturbance, incontinence, and memory loss, with or without symptoms and signs of raised ICP including headache, papilledema, and false localizing signs. Causes of chronic hydrocephalus include post–subarachnoid hemorrhage, chronic meningeal infections (e.g., fungal, tuberculosis, syphilis), and slow-growing tumors blocking the CSF pathways.

*Normal-pressure hydrocephalus* is a term commonly used to describe chronic communicating adult-onset hydrocephalus. Typically, patients with NPH have the triad of mental impairment, gait disturbance, and incontinence. NPH can develop secondary to trauma, infection, or subarachnoid hemorrhage, but in about one-third of patients no etiology is found. Enlarged ventricles are seen on CT, and MRI shows both the enlarged ventricles and the transependymal CSF absorption. By definition, LP generally reveals a normal or minimally elevated CSF pressure. *Normal pressure* is an unfortunate term, because patients who have undergone long-term monitoring with this syndrome have intermittently elevated pressures, often during the night.

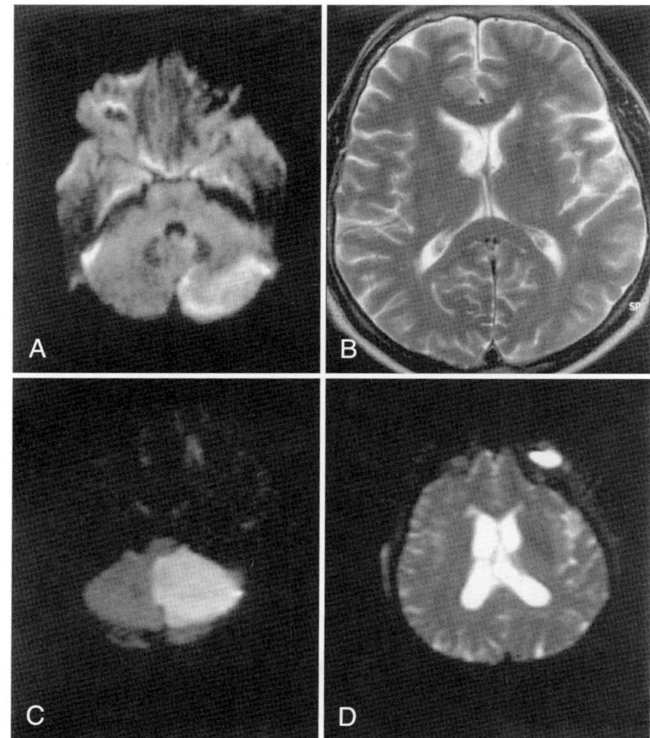


**Fig. 88.12 Cerebellar Infarct with Secondary Hydrocephalus. A,** Initial diffusion-weighted image with cerebellar infarct in the territory of the left posterior inferior cerebellar artery. **B,** Initial axial T2-weighted magnetic resonance imaging shows normal ventricular size. **C,** Diffusion-weighted image 3 days later, showing swelling of the infarction in the cerebellum. **D,** Echo-planar T2 axial image shows enlargement of the ventricles prior to surgery for hydrocephalus.

The presenting symptoms may be related to gait or mental function. When gait is the presenting factor, the prognosis for treatment is better. NPH causes an apraxic gait, which is an inability to lift the legs, as if they were stuck to the floor. Motor strength is intact, reflexes are usually normal or slightly increased, and Babinski signs are absent. In some patients, attempts to elicit a Babinski sign will result in a grasp response of the toes, suggestive of frontal lobe damage. Patients may be misdiagnosed as having Parkinson disease, because the gait disorder is similar in the two syndromes, suggesting that the etiology of the problem in the hydrocephalic patient lies in the basal ganglia. Because many of these patients also have hypertension, and some have small or large strokes, such patients may have other neurological findings including spasticity and hyperreflexia with Babinski signs.

NPH leads to a reduction in intellect, which at times may be subtle. The dementia is of the subcortical type and involves slowing of verbal and motor responses, with preservation of cortical functions such as language and spatial resolution. Neuropsychological testing quantifies the decline in intellect and the degree of dementia. Patients are apathetic and appear depressed. Incontinence of urine may occur, particularly in patients with prominent gait disturbance. In the early stages of the illness, presumably as the ventricles are undergoing enlargement, patients can experience drop attacks or brief loss of consciousness. Headache and papilledema are generally not part of the syndrome.

Diagnosis of adult-onset hydrocephalus and selection of patients for placement of a ventriculoperitoneal shunt has been difficult. Many of these patients have hypertensive vascular disease with lacunar infarcts. Features of Parkinson disease were noted in earlier reports of the

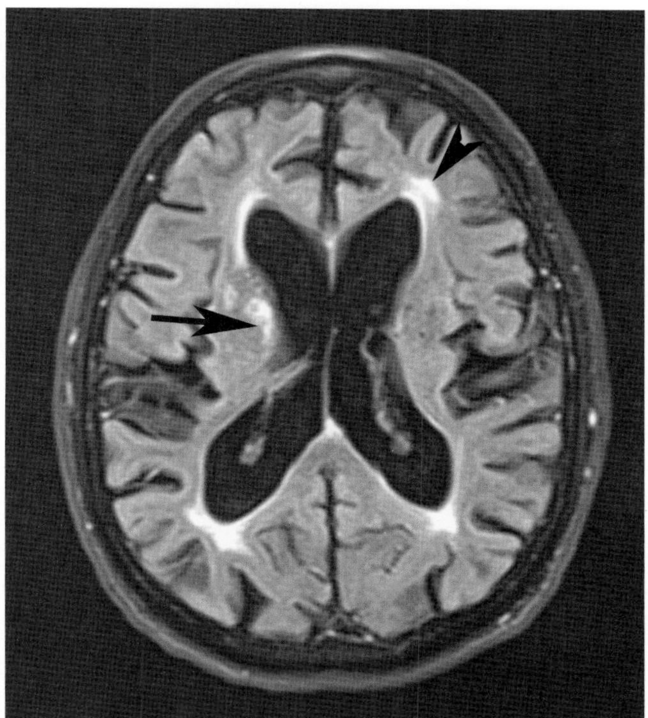

**Fig. 88.13 Magnetic Resonance Imaging of a Patient with Possible Normal-Pressure Hydrocephalus Who Had Extensive Vascular Disease with White-Matter Changes and Suspected Transependymal Absorption of Cerebrospinal Fluid (CSF).** He had a large-volume lumbar puncture to remove CSF, but failed to show improvement, and did not have a shunt placed. There is evidence of a stroke in the basal ganglia *(arrow)*, and of transependymal flow of CSF *(arrowhead)*. He had features of Parkinson disease and responded to treatment with Sinemet. This patient illustrates the overlap of normal-pressure hydrocephalus with chronic microvascular disease, lacunar strokes, and Parkinson disease. Such patients may not benefit from shunting.

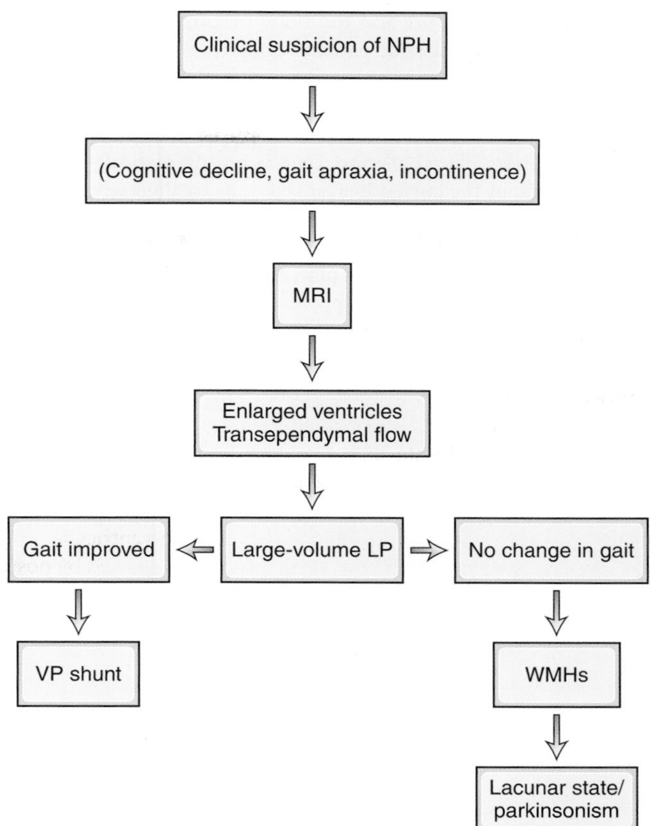


**Fig. 88.14 An Algorithm for Selection of Patients for Ventriculoperitoneal (VP) Shunt.** Patients with the clinical triad undergo FLAIR MRI. If communicating hydrocephalus is found without excessive atrophy and with transependymal absorption, then a large volume of cerebrospinal fluid is removed and the changes in the gait observed over several days. In those with improvement in gait, a VP shunt is done. Patients with white-matter changes in the deep white matter probably have lacunar state. Those with white matter changes compatible with microvascular disease most likely have lacunar state or parkinsonism. *FLAIR*, Fluid-attenuated inversion recovery; *LP*, lumbar puncture; *MRI*, magnetic resonance imaging; *NPH*, normal-pressure hydrocephalus; WMHs, white matter hyperintensities.

syndrome, and it is now recommended that all patients with Parkinson disease have scans to rule out hydrocephalus. CT and MRI have aided in separating Parkinson disease, lacunar state, and NPH, although NPH may occasionally coexist with these diseases (Fig. 88.13). Patients diagnosed with vascular diseases, such as lacunar state or subcortical arteriosclerotic encephalopathy (Binswanger disease) along with the hydrocephalus, respond poorly to shunting, and, if there is a positive response, it may be transient as the underlying disease progresses (Tullberg et al., 2002). LP with 20–40 mL removed often improves the gait, leading some investigators to use response to the removal of CSF as a diagnostic test for placement of a lumbar peritoneal shunt. Placing a lumbar catheter for continuous drainage improves diagnostic accuracy. Finally, although not used routinely, radionuclide cisternography may be helpful. The selection of patients for shunting requires a combination of clinical findings and diagnostic test results; no test can predict whether a patient should undergo an operation (Fig. 88.14). Drainage of CSF may involve the lymphatics of the brain, which are also called the glymphatics. Intrathecal injection of gadobutrol, a gadolinium contrast agent that can be imaged with T1-weighted MRI, can aid in visualizing pathways of CSF removal. There was reduced clearance of the contrast agent from the subarachnoid space and accumulation in the Sylvian fissure (Ringstad et al., 2017). A high incidence of vascular risk factors was found in patients with NPH, suggesting that it is a form of vascular dementia (Israelsson et al., 2017).

Neuroimaging in patients with NPH has shown an enlargement of the temporal horns of the lateral ventricle, with a disproportionate amount of cortical atrophy to that anticipated for the age of the patient. This is in contrast to patients with hydrocephalus ex vacuo due to a degenerative disease, such as Alzheimer disease, in which there is atrophy of the cerebral gyri and enlargement of both the sulci and ventricles. Another useful finding on proton-density MRI is the presence of presumed transependymal fluid in the frontal and occipital periventricular regions. Quantitative cisternography with single-photon emission CT has been successfully used to predict the results of a shunt. Other proposed diagnostic methods, including measuring the rate of absorption of CSF by infusion of saline or artificial CSF into the thecal sac, clinical improvement after CSF removal, or the prolonged monitoring of ICP, have been used with some success to select patients for surgery. Decreased cerebral blood flow has been reported in NPH; regional cerebral blood flow is reduced in both cortical and subcortical regions. Patients who show clinical improvement with shunting have a concomitant increase in cerebral blood flow. Removal of CSF may result in an increase in cerebral blood flow in patients in whom NPH is likely to respond to shunt therapy.

After the initial report and the hope of curing many people of dementia, a large number of patients underwent placement of ventriculoperitoneal shunts. As the number of patients who showed no improvement with shunts grew and the complication rates of placing a shunt in an elderly patient became evident, the rate of diagnosis and number of shunts placed at most centers has dramatically declined. However, none of the currently available tests by themselves identify the patients who will benefit from shunting. Most helpful is a combination of clinical signs and judiciously chosen laboratory tests.

Various success rates for shunt placement have been reported; some reports describe improvement in approximately 80% of treated patients, while others report lower rates. In the early days of treatment of NPH patients with shunts, a high rate of shunt failure occurred, with complications of shunting being a major problem. Serious complications occurred in as many as one-fourth of the patients, including infection and subdural hematomas. More recently, the rates of correct diagnosis and complication-free treatments have improved, but the definitive diagnostic test and complication-free treatment remain elusive goals. Clearly, more information is needed to aid in the diagnosis and management of patients with this potentially treatable syndrome.

## Acknowledgments

The neuroradiological illustrations were generously provided by Blaine Hart, MD, Department of Radiology (Neuroradiology), University of New Mexico Health Sciences Center.

*The complete reference list is available online at https://expertconsult.inkling.com.* 

89

# Developmental Disorders of the Nervous System

Harvey B. Sarnat, Laura Flores-Sarnat

## OUTLINE



## EMBRYOLOGICAL AND FETAL DEVELOPMENT OF THE NERVOUS SYSTEM

Neuroembryology integrated with molecular genetics provides the key to understanding congenital malformations of the nervous system. Modern neuroembryology or ontogenesis encompasses not only classical descriptive morphogenesis but also the molecular genetic programming of development and the immunocytochemical demonstration of maturation of neuronal and glial proteins in individual cells and sequences of neurotransmitter biosynthesis, synapse formation, and myelination. Neuroimaging and electrocerebral maturation, as determined by electroencephalogram (EEG) in preterm infants, contribute other aspects of ontogenesis of normal and abnormal brain formation that are particularly relevant to clinical neurology. *Maturation* refers to both growth, a measure of physical characteristics over time, and development, the acquisition of metabolic functions, reflexes, sensory awareness, motor skills, language, and intellect. *Molecular development*, by contrast with molecular biology, refers to the maturation of cellular function by changes in molecular structures such as the phosphorylation of neurofilaments. In neurons, it also includes the development of an energy production system that actively maintains a resting membrane potential, the synthesis of secretory molecules as neurotransmitters, and the formation of membrane receptors. Membrane receptors respond to various transmitters at synapses, to a variety of trophic and adhesion molecules, and during development to substances that attract or repel growing axons in their intermediate and final trajectories. *Molecular biology* is the basis of linking a DNA sequence to a specific gene and a particular locus on a specific chromosome, and ultimately making a correlation with normal function and a particular disease.

Table 89.1 shows known genetic loci and mutations in human central nervous system (CNS) malformations. In most cases, mutations affect the genetic programming of the spatial and temporal sequences of developmental processes. Molecular genetic data are rapidly becoming available because of intense interest in this key to understanding neuroembryology in general and neural induction in particular. Other aspects of current investigative interest include the roles of neurotropic factors, hormones, ion channels, and neurotransmitter systems in fetal brain development. Genetic manipulation in animals has created many genetic models of human cerebral malformations. These contribute greatly to our understanding of human dysgeneses and provide insights into the pathogenesis of epilepsy and other functional results of dysgeneses.

Maturation progresses in a predictable sequence with precise timing. Insults that adversely affect maturation influence events occurring at a particular time. Some are brief (e.g., a single exposure to a toxin),

**TABLE 89.1 Genetic Loci of Known Human Mutations in Central Nervous System Malformations**

| Malformation | Inheritance | Locus | Symbol: Gene or Transcription Product |
|---|---|---|---|
| Agenesis anterior commissure; hypoplasia corpus callosum | | | PAX6 |
| Agenesis corpus callosum with neuropathy | AR | | SLC12A6 for transporter protein |
| Aicardi-Goutières syndrome | AR | | CC3 ribonuclease H2 subunits |
| Cerebellar hypoplasia | XR | Xq12 | OPHN1 |
| Cerebellar hypoplasia, Hutterite dysequilibrium | AR | | VLDLR |
| Cerebrohepatorenal syndrome (Zellweger)* | AR | Xq22.3-q23 | DCX |
| Coffin-Lowry syndrome | XR | Xp22.2 | RSK2 |
| Congenital muscular dystrophy with cerebral/cerebellar dysplasia | AR | | FKRP (fukutin) |
| Dandy-Walker malformation | AD | 2q36.1 | |
| Hemimegalencephaly[†] | AR | Xq28 | L1-CAM AKT3; somatic mutation |
| Hemimegalencephaly, isolated (sporadic) | | | |
| Hemimegalencephaly associated with epildermal nevus or especially proteus syndrome | | | AKT1; somatic mutation |
| Holoprosencephaly[‡] | AD, AR | 7q36-qter | SHH |
| Holoprosencephaly | AR; sporadic | 13q32 | ZIC2 |
| Holoprosencephaly | AR; sporadic | 2q21 | SIX3 |
| Holoprosencephaly | AD, sporadic | 18p11.3 | TGIF |
| Holoprosencephaly | AR; sporadic | q22.3 | PTCH (SHH receptor) |
| Holoprosencephaly | AR; sporadic | 10q11.2 | DKK (head inducer) |
| Holoprosencephaly | AR; sporadic | | Dhcr7 (SHH-related) |
| Joubert syndrome (JBTS1) | AR | 9q34.3 | ? |
| Joubert syndrome (JBTS2) | AR | 11p11.2-q12.3 | ? |
| Joubert syndrome (JBTS3) | AR | 6q23 | AHI1; jouberin |
| Joubert syndrome with nephronophthisis | AR | ? | NPHP1 |
| Kallmann syndrome* | XR | Xp22.3 | KAL1;EMX2 |
| Lissencephaly I (isolated and Miller-Dieker syndrome) | AR | 17p13.3 | LIS1 |
| Lissencephaly II with cerebellar hypoplasia | AR | 7q22 | RELN |
| Lissencephaly II, muscle-eye-brain disease | AR | 1p32 | POMGnT1 |
| Lissencephaly II, Walker-Warburg syndrome | AR | | POMGnT1 |
| Lissencephaly II, Fukuyama muscular dystrophy | AR | | fukutin |
| Lissencephaly with genital anomalies | XR | | ARX |
| Meckel-Grüber syndrome | AR | | MKS3; meckelin |
| Microcephaly, primary | AR | 1pq25-q32 | MCPH5 |
| Midbrain agenesis and cerebellar hypoplasia | ?AR; sporadic | 7q36 | EN2 |
| Periventricular nodular heterotopia | XD | Xq28 | FLN-A |
| Periventricular nodular heterotopia | AD | ? | ? |
| Periventricular nodular heterotopia and posterior pituitary ectopia | AR | | HESX1 |
| Pituitary aplasia, ectopia (neurohypophysis) | AR | | HESX1 |
| Pituitary aplasia (adenohypophysis) | | | Pitx2 |
| Pontocerebellar hypoplasia, nondyskinetic | AR | 7q11-21 | ? |
| Rett syndrome | XD | Xq28 | MECP2 |
| Sacral agenesis[§] | AD | 7q36.1-qter<br>1q41-q42.1 | SHH<br>HLXB9 |
| Schizencephaly | AR | Unknown | |
| Septo-optic-pituitary dysplasia | AR; sporadic | 3p21.1-p21.2 | HESX1, PAX3 |
| Sotos syndrome (megalencephaly) | AD, AR, sporadic | 5q35 | NSD1 |
| Subcortical laminar heterotopia (band heterotopia) | XD | Xq22.3-q23 | DCX |
| Tuberous sclerosis | AD | 9q34.3,<br>16p13.3 | TSC1; hamartin<br>TSC2; tuberin |
| X-linked hydrocephalus (X-linked aqueductal stenosis and pachygyria) | XR | Xq28 | L1-CAM |

*The DCX (doublecortin) mutation is primary in subcortical laminar heterotopia but also is described in Zellweger syndrome, though it is likely only a secondary defect in this lysosomal disease associated with major neuroblast migratory defects; DCX is localized on the X chromosome, and Zellweger syndrome is an autosomal recessive trait. DCX also is a secondary genetic defect in Kallmann syndrome (anosmia due to agenesis or defective migration of olfactory bulb neurons and hypogonadotropic hypogonadism, the hypothalamic secretory cells having the same origin as the olfactory neurons).

**TABLE 89.1 Genetic Loci of Known Human Mutations in Central Nervous System Malformations—cont'd**

†The role of L1-CAM in hemimegalencephaly is not certain and is more likely a secondary defect and not the primary genetic mutation.
‡Holoprosencephaly is associated with many chromosomal defects in addition to those listed here, but the gene products associated with the others have not yet been identified. Only 20% of genetically studied cases have one of the six genetic mutations demonstrated.
§Sacral agenesis (AD form) maps to the same locus at 7q36 as one form of holoprosencephaly and also is associated with defective SHH expression, the same genetic defect expressed at opposite ends of the neural tube. Both sacral agenesis and holoprosencephaly also occur with a high incidence in infants born to mothers with diabetes mellitus. Agenesis of more than two vertebral bodies is generally associated with dysplasia of the spinal cord in that region during fetal development: fusion of ventral horns; deformed central canal with heterotopic ependyma, consistent with defective neural induction. A second gene with a locus at 1q41-q42.1 is also identified as another cause of autosomal dominantly transmitted sacral agenesis.
*AD*, Autosomal dominant; *AR*, autosomal recessive; *CAM*, cell adhesion molecule; *OPHN1*, oligophrenin-1; *RELN*, Reelin; *SHH*, Sonic hedgehog; *TGIF*, TG-interacting factor; *XD*, X-linked dominant; *XR*, X-linked recessive.

whereas others act over many weeks or throughout gestation (e.g., congenital infections, maternal diabetes mellitus, and genetic or chromosomal defects). Even brief insults may have profound influences on later development by interfering with processes essential to initiate the next stage of development. Often this makes the timing of an adverse event difficult. Timing of onset of mutated genetic expression or of embryonic or fetal exposure to a teratogenic exogenous toxin is one of the most important determinants of the nature and extent of cerebral malformations (Sarnat, 2018a; Sarnat and Flores-Sarnat, 2017).

The anatomical and physiological correlates of neurological maturation reflect the growth and development of the individual neuron and its synaptic relations with other neurons. The mature neuron is a secretory cell with an electrically polarized membrane. Though endocrine and exocrine cells are secretory and muscle cells possess excitable membranes, only neurons embrace both functions. Some epithelial cells are adherent to neighboring cells forming a sheet of epithelium or glandular villi, and have weakly polarized membranes, but they are not excitable. The precursors of neurons are neither secretory nor excitable. The cytological maturation of neurons is an aspect of ontogenesis that is as important as is their spatial relations with other cells, both for future function and for the pathogenesis of some functional neurological disorders of infancy such as neonatal seizures (Sarnat, 2013, 2015; Sarnat and Flores-Sarnat, 2014).

Neuroblasts are postmitotic neuroepithelial cells committed to neuronal lineage. These cells have not yet achieved all functions of mature neurons such as membrane polarity, secretion, and synaptic relations with other neurons, and often they are still migratory. Use of the term *blast* is different for neural development than for hematopoieses, in which blast cells are still in the mitotic cycle or may even be neoplastic. The events of neural maturation after initial induction and formation of the neural tube are each predictive of specific types of malformation of the brain and of later abnormal neurological function. These are (1) neurulation or formation of the neural tube, (2) mitotic proliferation of neuroblasts, (3) programmed death of excess neuroblasts, (4) neuroblast migration, (5) growth of axons and dendrites, (6) electrical polarity of the cell membrane and the energy pump to maintain a resting membrane potential, (7) synaptogenesis, (8) biosynthesis of neurotransmitters, and (9) myelination of axons.

Malformations of the nervous system are unique. No two individual cases are identical, even when categorized as the same anatomical malformation, such as alobar holoprosencephaly (HPE), syndromic or isolated agenesis of the corpus callosum, and types 1 and 2 lissencephaly. Functional expression of anatomically similar cases also may vary widely. For example, two cases of HPE with nearly identical imaging findings and similar histological patterns of cortical architecture and subcortical heterotopia at autopsy may differ in that one infant may have epilepsy refractory to pharmacological control, whereas the other may have no clinical seizures at all. The difference may be at the level of synaptic organization and the relative maturation of afferent input and neuronal maturation (Sarnat and Born, 1999; Sarnat et al., 2010). A discussion of the critical sequence of events in neural maturation follows.

## NEURULATION

*Neurulation* refers to the formation and closure of the neural tube. The formation of the neural tube from the neural plate starts with the establishment of the axis in the neural plate. The three early axes—longitudinal, horizontal, and vertical—persist during life and correspond to the basic body plan of all vertebrates (Sarnat and Flores-Sarnat, 2001b). Gastrulation occurs at 16 days' gestation in the human; the Henson node and primitive streak establish bilateral symmetry as the basic body plan and the three axes of the body, as well as of the future neural tube. A flat neural plate is formed around the primitive streak and is the earliest differentiation of a neuroepithelium. The lateral margins of this neuroepithelial neural plate contain the precursors of neural crest cells. Shortly thereafter, grooving and bending of the neural plate occurs in the rostrocaudal axis. Subsequent closure of the lateral margins of the folding neural placode ensues in the dorsal midline to form the neural tube. To accomplish closure, intercellular filaments interdigit cells of the two sides to form a veil at midline closure points and the neuropores. At this time, the neural crest separates bilaterally at the two fusing lips of the closing neural tube, and its cells migrate along predetermined pathways to form the peripheral nervous system including autonomic ganglion cells and their axons and Schwann cells, chromaffin tissue, melanocytes, adipocytes, blood vessels, and various other cells derived from all three of the traditional germ layers: ectoderm, mesoderm, and endoderm. Because of the pervasiveness of neural crest derivatives and the expression of the same genes in all germ layers, Hall has proposed that the neural crest be regarded as a fourth germ layer with status equal to the other three (Hall, 2009). Neural crest cells terminally differentiate only after reaching their final destination. The inhibitory function of versican, a chondroitin sulfate proteoglycan, is an important factor of the extracellular matrix for neural crest cell migration (Dutt et al., 2006).

The process just described is *primary neurulation*. Another process, *secondary neurulation*, occurs in the most caudal regions of the spinal cord and is limited to the lower sacral region, the part of the incipient spinal cord that formed caudal to the posterior neuropore, which is not at the extreme posterior end of the neural placode. During secondary neurulation, rather than the ependyma forming from the dorsal surface of the placode, which then becomes folded, a central canal grows rostrally from the posterior end of the solid cylinder of neural tissue within its core. It may or may not reach the central canal of primary neurulation more rostrally, and often in the midgestational or earlier fetus in particular, a transverse section through the lower sacral spinal cord reveals two ependymal-lined central canals, both in the vertical axis and one above the other. This is a normal condition, by contrast with two central canals side-by-side in the horizontal axis, at any level of the spinal cord, which represents duplication from the overexpression of a dorsalizing gene in the vertical axis of the neural tube and is found in some malformations.

Following neurulation, an associated process begins: segmentation of the neural tube and its compartmental division into neuromeres (called rhombomeres in the hindbrain). Segmentation of the neural tube is one of three independent segmentation processes in the vertebrate body, the others being the branchial arches and the somites (Graham et al., 2014).

### Disorders of Neurulation (1–4 Weeks' Gestation)

Incomplete or defective formation of the neural tube from the neural placode is the most common type of CNS malformation in the human. Anencephaly and meningomyelocele are the most frequent forms.

Anencephaly (aprosencephaly with open cranium) is a failure of the anterior neuropore to close at 24 days' gestation, or perhaps to remain closed. The lamina terminalis and its derivatives fail to form, and most forebrain structures do not develop. Structures derived from the ventral part of the lamina terminalis, the basal telencephalic nuclei, may form imperfectly. Because the deficient forebrain neuroectoderm does not induce development of the overlying mesoderm, the cranium, meninges, and scalp do not close in the sagittal midline, exposing the remaining brain tissue to the surrounding amniotic fluid throughout gestation. The original induction failure, however, is probably that of mesodermal tissue on neuroectoderm, and is due to a defective rostral end of the notochord. Failure of craniofacial induction by the neural tube, mediated through the prosencephalic and mesencephalic neural crest, is another major pathogenetic factor (Sarnat and Flores-Sarnat, 2005).

The small nodule of residual telencephalic tissue called the *area cerebrovasculosa* consists of haphazardly oriented mature and immature neurons, glial cells, and nerve fibers. Perfusing this neural matrix is an extensive proliferation of small, thin-walled vascular channels, so concentrated in places as to resemble a cavernous hemangioma. This abnormal vasculature, particularly prominent at the surface of the telencephalic nodule, is probably the result of a necrotizing and resorptive process. Cephaloceles (encephalocele, exencephaly) are less serious defects than those found in anencephaly. A *cephalocele* is a mass of neural tissue protruded through a developmental defect in the cranium. The cerebral tissue in the cephalocele sac is usually extremely hamartomatous without recognized architecture. It may include heterotopia from an unexpected site. Zones of infarction, hemorrhage, calcifications, and extensive proliferations of thin-walled vascular channels are common, approaching the disorganized tissue of the area cerebrovasculosa of anencephaly. The remaining intracranial brain is often dysplastic as well. The ventricular system may be partially incorporated into the cephalocele sac.

*Meningomyelocele* (spinal dysraphism, rachischisis, spina bifida cystica) involves the caudal end of the neural tube and results from the posterior neuropore not closing at 28 days prenatally. The hypothesis that meningomyelocele and atelencephaly are due to increased pressure and volume of fluid within the primordial ventricular system of the developing neural tube, which causes rupture at one end and prevents reclosure, has not been widely embraced. Formation of the choroid plexuses has not yet occurred at the time of neural tube closure, and embryological evidence of hydrocephalus at that stage in experimental animals is lacking. Although many mechanical theories have been proposed and several teratogenic drugs, hypervitaminosis A, and genetic models are able to produce neural tube defects and hydrocephalus in experimental animals, none explains the pathogenesis of faulty neurulation in humans.

## MITOTIC PROLIFERATION OF NEUROBLASTS (NEURONOGENESIS)

After formation of the neural tube, proliferation of neuroepithelial cells in the ventricular zone associated with mitoses at the ventricular surface generates neurons and glial cells. The rate of division is greatest during the early first trimester in the spinal cord and brainstem and during the late first and early second trimester in the forebrain. Within the ventricular zone of the human fetal telencephalon, only 33 mitotic cycles provide the total number of neurons required for the mature human cerebral cortex (10 cycles in rodents), because of an exponential increase (Caviness et al., 1981). Most mitotic activity in the neuroepithelium occurs at the ventricular surface, and the orientation of the mitotic spindle determines the subsequent immediate fate of the daughter cells. If the cleavage plane is perpendicular to the ventricular surface, the two daughter cells become equal neuroepithelial cells preparing for further mitosis. If, however, the cleavage is parallel to the ventricular surface, the two daughter cells are unequal (asymmetrical cleavage). In that case, the one at the ventricular surface becomes another neuroepithelial cell, whereas the one away from the ventricular surface separates from its ventricular attachment and becomes a postmitotic neuroblast ready to migrate to the cortical plate. Furthermore, the products of two genes that determine cell fate, called *numb and notch*, are on different sides of the neuroepithelial cell. Therefore, with symmetrical cleavages, both daughter cells receive the same amount of each, but. With asymmetrical cleavage, the cells receive unequal ratios of each, which also influences their subsequent development (Mione et al., 1997). The orientation of the mitotic spindle requires *centractin*. The mitotic spindle, the strands of which are microtubules, is linked to the plasma membrane during the splitting of the cytoplasm (cytokinesis) by a protein complex called *centralspindlin* (Lekomtsev et al., 2012).

Active mitoses cease well before the time of birth in most parts of the human nervous system, but a few sites retain a potential for postnatal mitoses of neuroblasts. One recognized site is the periventricular region of the cerebral hemispheres (Kendler and Golden, 1996). Another is the external granular layer of the cerebellar cortex, where occasional mitoses persist until 1 year of age. Postnatal regeneration of these neurons after destruction of most by irradiation or cytotoxic drugs occurs in animals and may occur in humans as well. Primary olfactory receptor neurons also retain a potential for regeneration. In fact, if a constant turnover of these neurons in the olfactory epithelium did not occur throughout life, the individual would become anosmic after a few upper respiratory infections, which transiently denude the intranasal epithelium.

Neuronogenesis also involves the biosynthesis of cell-specific proteins. Many of these are detectable in the germinal matrix as evidence of early commitment of cells not only to a neuronal lineage but also to a fate as a specific type of neuron. The previously held concept that germinal matrix cells were uniformly undifferentiated postmitotic neuroepithelial cells was incorrect. But a population of "stem cells" with mitotic potential also is present in the subventricular zone and just beneath the hippocampal dentate gyrus (Johansson et al., 1999). These have generated considerable interest because of a potential for regeneration of the damaged adult brain and because they may be induced to mature as neurons (Schuldiner et al., 2001). Transplanted stem cells have an increased risk of neoplastic transformation, however (Dlouhy et al., 2014). Cultures of stem cells not only can generate neurons but also may even generate a poorly formed miniature cortex or whole brain (Lancaster et al., 2013; van den Ameele et al., 2014).

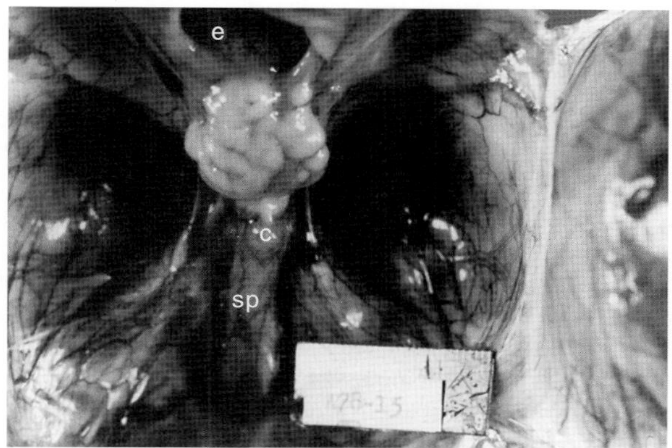


**Fig. 89.1 Severe Cerebral Hypoplasia.** The brain of this full-term neonate weighed only 12.6 g (normal mean is 350 g), although the cranium was closed and mainly filled with fluid. The dysplastic architecture of the telencephalon, including dysplastic cerebellar tissue, extended into a frontal encephalocele *(e)* and was not that of a neural tube defect or fetal infarction. The spinal cord *(sp)* is well formed except for the absence of descending tracts. The cerebellum *(c)* is small but normally laminated. This brain probably represents lack of neuronal proliferation. Note the well-formed fossae at the base of the skull, despite the absence of cerebral development. *(Reproduced with permission from Sarnat, H.B., de Mello, D.E., Blair, J.D., et al., 1982. Heterotopic growth of dysplastic cerebellum in frontal encephalocele in an infant of a diabetic mother. Can J Neurol Sci. 9, 31–35.)*

### Disorders of Neuronogenesis

Destructive processes may destroy so many neuroblasts that regeneration of the full complement of cells is impossible. This happens when the insult persists for a long time or is repetitive, destroying each subsequent generation of dividing cells. Inadequate mitotic proliferation of neuroblasts results in hypoplasia of the brain (Fig. 89.1). Such brains are small and grossly malformed, either because of a direct effect on neuroblast migration or by destruction of the glial cells with radial processes that guide migrating nerve cells. The entire brain may be affected, or portions may be selectively involved. Cerebellar hypoplasia often is a selective interference with proliferation of the external granular layer. In some cases, cerebral hypoplasia and microcephaly are the result of precocious development of the ependyma before all mitotic cycles of the neuroepithelium are complete, because ependymal differentiation arrests mitotic activity at the ventricular surface. The mutation of a gene that programs neuronogenesis may be another explanation for generating insufficient neuroepithelial cells. In somatic mutations that give rise to hamartomatous malformations of the brain, such as hemimegalencephaly and tuberous sclerosis, the genetic program for neuronal lineage, differentiation, and cellular growth is altered such that proliferation may be deficient and those neuroblasts that do form are dysmorphic, often megalocytic, and do not function normally, including becoming epileptogenic.

## PROGRAMMED CELL DEATH (APOPTOSIS)

Normal mitotic proliferation produces excessive neuroblasts in every part of the nervous system. Reduction of this abundance by 30%–50% is by a programmed process of cell death, or apoptosis, until achieving the definitive number of immature neurons. The factors that arrest the process of apoptosis in the fetus are multiple and are in part genetically determined. Cells that do not match with targets are more vulnerable to degeneration than those that achieve synaptic contact with other cells. Endocrine hormones and neuropeptides modulate apoptosis. Some homeotic genes such as *c-fos* are important in the regulation of apoptosis in the nervous system, and other suppressor genes stop the expression of apoptotic genes. Caspase-3 is a key mediator of apoptosis, a protease activated as early as neural tube formation; it also is active in many neurodegenerative diseases (D'Amelio et al., 2012). During apoptosis, cells break up into membrane-bound fragments, a process regulated by the protein pannexin-1, which has its own membrane channels; it can be deregulated by quinolone antibiotics (Poon et al., 2014).

Two phases of apoptosis are distinguished. One involves as-yet undifferentiated neuroepithelial cells or neuroblasts with incomplete differentiation; the other phase involves fully differentiated neurons of the fetal brain. The first phase begins during embryonic life and may extend to midgestation in some parts of the brain (e.g., periventricular telencephalic neuroepithelium) until ependyma differentiates at the ventricular surface. The second phase may be ongoing throughout life, as occurs in primary olfactory neurons of the nasal mucosa, and in the olfactory bulb and hippocampus, closely associated with a reservoir of stem cell progenitors.

In addition to cellular apoptosis, mitochondria within cells also undergo a similar autophagy (mitophagy), largely mediated by the genes *Parkin* and *PINK1*, mutations of which explain some hereditary neurodegenerative diseases (Scarffe et al., 2014).

### Disorders of Programmed Cell Death

Spinal muscular atrophy (see Chapter 98) is an example of a human disease caused by apoptosis not stopping at the proper time. In this disorder, continued loss of spinal motor neurons (SMNs) after the normal deletion of surplus embryonic neuroblasts expresses itself as a progressive denervating process. Genetic factors are crucial in determining the arrest of cell death, which accounts for the hereditary character of spinal muscular atrophy. The SMN defective gene at the chromosome 5q13.1 locus has now been isolated and is normally responsible for arresting apoptosis in motor neuroblasts (Roy et al., 1995).

Other neurodegenerative diseases of fetal life and infancy are more widespread within the CNS, rather than limited to one type of neuron such as the motor neuron. The characteristic feature is also progressive neuronal loss that is apoptotic rather than necrotic in character: No inflammatory or glial reaction occurs, and the features of the DNA degradation differ from ischemic necrosis. An example is pontocerebellar hypoplasia, a group of progressive degenerative diseases that begin prenatally and continue postnatally (Barth et al., 1995). Despite the name, they involve much more than the cerebellar system. These diseases are associated with extensive cerebral cortical and basal ganglionic abnormalities even in motor neurons, which cause a clinical presentation at birth resembling spinal muscular atrophy. This autosomal recessive group of diseases, all genetically distinct from olivopontocerebellar atrophy, exemplifies a semantic difficulty. If an atrophic process begins before development is complete, it results in both hypoplasia and superimposed atrophy. In the CNS, glial cells also undergo apoptosis. Glial necrosis intimately links to the interhemispheric passage of commissural fibers in the corpus callosum. In a murine model of callosal agenesis, glial cells that do not degenerate act as a barrier to crossing axons and prevent the corpus callosum from forming.

## NEUROBLAST MIGRATION

No neurons of the mature human brain occupy their site of generation from the neuroepithelium. They migrate to their mature site to establish the proper synaptic connections with appropriate neighboring neurons and send their axons in short or long trajectories to targets. The *subependymal germinal matrix* (Fig. 89.2) is the subventricular zone of the embryonic concentric layers and consists of postmitotic premigratory neuroblasts and glioblasts. In general, the movement of maturing nerve cells is centrifugal, radiating toward the surface of the brain. The cerebellar cortex is exceptional in that external granule cells first spread over the surface of the cerebellum and then migrate into the folia. Migration of neuroblasts begins at about 6 weeks' gestation in the human cerebrum and is not completed until at least 34 weeks of fetal life, although the majority of germinal matrix cells after midgestation are glioblasts. Glioblasts continue to migrate until early in the postnatal period. Within the brainstem, neuroblast migration is complete by 2 months' gestation. Cerebellar external granule cells continue migrating throughout the first year of life.

Neuroblast migration permits a three-dimensional spatial relationship to develop between neurons, which facilitates the formation of complex synaptic circuits. The timing and sequence of successive waves of migrating neuroblasts are precise. In the cerebral cortex, immature nerve cells reach the pial surface and then form deeper layers as more recent arrivals replace their position at the surface. Neurons forming the most superficial layers of neocortex are thus the last to have migrated, although in the three-layered hippocampus, the most superficial neurons represent the earliest migratory wave. Three major groups of molecules control neuroblast migration (Gressens, 2006): (1) molecules of the cytoskeleton that determine the initiation (filamin-A and ADP-ribosylation factor GEF2) and ongoing progression (doublecortin and LIS1) of neuroblast movement; (2) signaling molecules involved in lamination, including reelin and other proteins not yet associated with human diseases; and (3) molecules modulating glycosylation that provide stop signals to migrating neuroblasts (e.g., POMT1 [protein *O*-mannosyl-transferase], involved in Walker-Warburg syndrome; POMGnT1 [protein *O*-mannose β-1,2-*N*-acetylglucosaminyltransferase], involved in muscle-eye-brain disease; and fukutin, involved in Fukuyama muscular dystrophy).

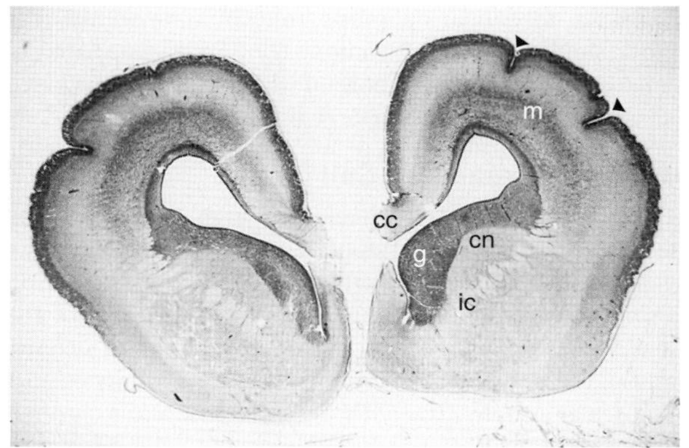


**Fig. 89.2** Coronal section of forebrain of 16-week normal fetus, showing extensive subependymal germinal matrix *(g)* of neuroblasts and glial precursors that have not yet migrated. The surface of the brain is just beginning to develop sulci *(arrowheads)*. Migrating neuroblasts *(m)* are seen in the subcortical white matter. The corpus callosum *(cc)* is artifactually ruptured, and the two hemispheres should be closely approximated. (Hematoxylin-eosin stain.) *cn*, Caudate nucleus; *ic*, anterior limb of internal capsule.

The laminated arrangement of the mammalian cerebral cortex requires a large cortical surface area to accommodate increasing numbers of migrating neuroblasts and glioblasts. Initially the cortical plate shows no histological layering, a process beginning at about midgestation, but rather has an immature columnar architecture. The lamination is superimposed upon this columnar pattern, but columnar architecture is still seen postnatally, particularly at the crowns of gyri and the depths of sulci. Even before histological lamination is evident, ribonucleic acid (RNA) probes for specific neuronal identities can already detect future organization of the cortical plate (Hevner, 2007). Convolutions provide this large surface area without incurring a concomitant increase in cerebral volume. The formation of gyri and sulci is thus a direct result of migration (Fig. 89.3). Most gyri form in the second half of gestation, which is a period of predominant gliogenesis and glial cell migration. Therefore, the proliferation of glia in the cortex and subcortical white matter may be more important than neuroblast migrations in the formation of convolutions, but the growth of dendrites and synaptogenesis also may influence gyration by contributing mass to the neuropil.

## Major Mechanisms of Neuroblast Migration: Radial Glial Fiber Guides and Tangential Migration along Axons

The majority of neuroblasts arriving at the cortical plate do so by means of radial glial guides from the subventricular zone. A second route, tangential migration, uses axons as the guides for the migratory

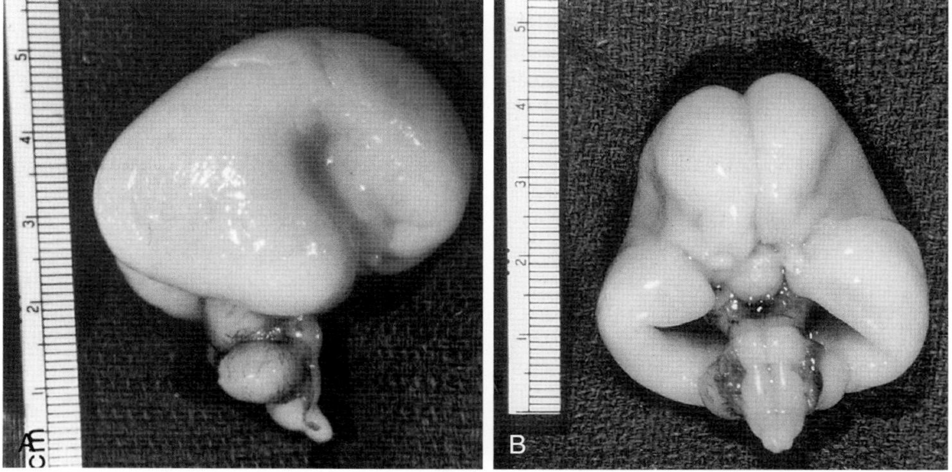


**Fig. 89.3** Lateral (**A**) and ventral (**B**) views of a normal brain of a 16-week fetus. Primary fissures (e.g., sylvian, calcarine) are formed early in gestation, but primary sulci, such as the central and parieto-occipital, form at midgestation, and secondary and tertiary sulci and gyri develop after 22 weeks. At midgestation the surface of the cortex is essentially smooth.

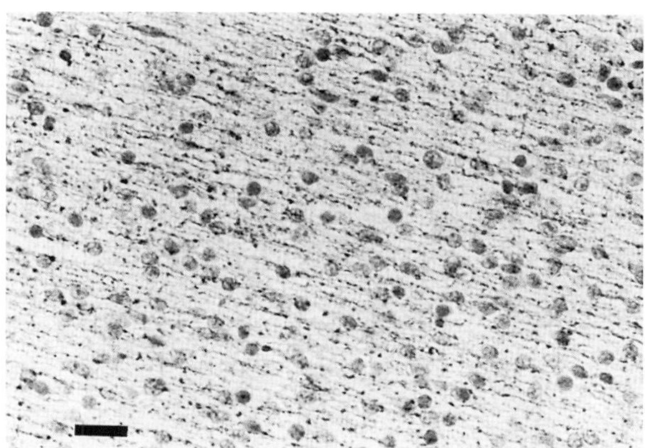

**Fig. 89.4** Radial glial fibers extending from subependymal region *(right)* toward cerebral cortex *(left)*, guiding migrating neuroblasts in a 16-week fetus. (Glial fibrillary acidic protein reaction. Bar = 10 μm.)

neuroblasts. The genetically determined programming of neuroblast migration begins when cells are still undifferentiated neuroepithelial cells and even before all their mitotic cycles are complete. Neuroepithelial cells express the gene products of the lissencephaly gene (*LIS1*), as do ependymal cells and Cajal-Retzius cells of the molecular layer of cerebral cortex. The expression of this gene is defective in type 1 lissencephaly (Miller-Dieker syndrome), a severe disorder of neuroblast migration (Clark et al., 1997). An understanding of its function in migration is incomplete. The guidance of most neurons of the forebrain to their predetermined site from the germinal matrix (embryonic subventricular zone) is by long radiating fibers of specialized fetal astrocytes (Fig. 89.4). The elongated processes of these glial cells span the entire wall of the fetal cerebral hemisphere; their cell bodies are in the periventricular region, and their terminal endfeet are on the limiting pial membrane at the surface of the brain (see Fig. 89.4). Radial glial cells are the first astroglial cells of the human nervous system converted into a mature fibrillary astrocyte of the subcortical white matter; some are still present at birth. Mature astrocytes are present throughout the CNS by 15 weeks' gestation, and gliogenesis continues throughout fetal and postnatal life. Several types of glial cells are recognizable between 20 and 36 weeks' gestation.

Facilitating the mechanical process of neuroblasts gliding along a radial glial fiber are several specialized proteins at the radial glial fiber surface membrane or extracellular space. An example is astrotactin, secreted by the neuroblast (Zheng et al., 1996). Glial cells and neural cell adhesion molecules also facilitate gliding (Jouet and Kenwrick, 1995). These adhesion molecules must be deactivated when the migratory neuroblast reaches the neural plate so that the next arriving neuroblast on the same radial glial fiber can bypass the first to establish the inside-out arrangement of the cortical plate, with the earliest migratory waves forming the deep layers and the last arrivals forming the superficial layers. Fetal ependymal cells have radiating processes that resemble those of the radial glial cell but do not extend beyond the germinal matrix and secrete molecules in the extracellular matrix. Some adhesion molecules are present in the extracellular matrix (Thomas et al., 1996). These molecules serve as lubricants, as adhesion molecules between the membranes of the neuroblast and the radial glial fiber, and as nutritive and growth factors. They stimulate cell movement. Deficient molecules lead to defective migration. For example, the abnormality of the L1 adhesion molecule is the defective genetic program in X-linked hydrocephalus accompanied by polymicrogyria and pachygyria. Other inhibitory cell adhesion molecules also are essential for detachment of neuroblasts from radial glia (Anton et al., 1996).

The process of transformation of radial glial cells into astrocytes and ependymal cells begins during the first half of gestation and completes postnatally. During midgestation when neuronal migration is at a peak, many radial glial cells remain attached to the ventricular and pial surfaces, increasing in length and curving with the expansion and convolution of the cerebral wall. From 28 weeks' gestation to 6 years of age, astrocytes of the frontal lobe shift from the periventricular to the subcortical region. The centrifugal movement of this band of normal gliosis marks the end of neuronal migration in the cerebral mantle. Ependyma does not completely line the lateral ventricles until 22 weeks' gestation. Studies of messenger RNA (mRNA) in individual glioblasts indicate that these immature glial precursors already exhibit differences related to their final differentiation (Rao et al., 2016).

Radial glial cells also act as resident stem cells in the fetal brain. In the presence of injury, such as a cortical microinfarct, radial glia are capable of differentiating as neurons to replace those that were lost. Radial glia express nestin and other primitive proteins found only in cells of multipotential lineage or that participate in early developmental processes, such as floor-plate ependymal cells.

In addition to the radial migration to the cerebral cortex, tangential migration also occurs, but the number of neuroblasts is far smaller (Rakic, 1995; Takano et al., 2004). These migrations perpendicular to the radial fibers probably use axons rather than glial processes as guides for migratory neuroblasts. This explains why not all cells in a given region of cortex are from the same clone or vertical column. Most of the tangentially migrating neuroblasts in the cerebral cortical plate are generated in the fetal ganglionic eminence, a deep telencephalic structure of the germinal matrix that gives origin to basal ganglionic neurons and to the γ-aminobutyric acid (GABA)-ergic inhibitory interneurons of the cerebral cortex. These neurons in the cortex from tangential migration have some unique metabolic features and distinctive immunoreactivities in tissue section for antibodies against soluble calcium-binding molecules, such as calretinin and parvalbumin (Sarnat, 2013; Takano et al., 2004; Ulfig, 2002). Calretinin-reactive inhibitory interneurons in the cerebral cortex comprise about 12% of total neurons and are a subset of total neurons arriving at the cortical plate by tangential migration, which represent about 20% of total cortical neurons. These also include a population of disinhibitory interneurons that suppress the activity of inhibitory interneurons (Pi et al., 2013).

Tangential migrations occur in the brainstem and olfactory bulb as well as in the cerebrum. The subpial region is another site of neuroblast migration that does not use radial glial cells. Calretinin-reactive neurons are in the cerebellum as well as the cerebral cortex (Yew et al., 1997), particularly Purkinje cells, basket cells, and neurons of the dentate and inferior olivary nuclei of the cerebellar system, but not those of the pontine nuclei, which similarly originated in the rhombic lip of His.

## Disorders of Neuroblast Migration

Nearly all malformations of the brain are a direct result of faulty neuroblast migration, or at least involve a secondary impairment of migration. Imperfect cortical lamination, abnormal gyral development, subcortical heterotopia, and other focal dysplasias relate to some factor that interferes with neuronal migration, whether vascular, traumatic, metabolic, or infectious. The most severe migratory defects occur in early gestation (8–15 weeks), often associated with even earlier events in the gross formation of the neural tube and cerebral vesicles. Heterotopia of brainstem nuclei also occurs. Later defects of migration are expressed as disorders of cortical lamination or gyration such as lissencephaly, pachygyria, and cerebellar dysplasias. Insults during the third trimester cause subtle or focal abnormalities of cerebral architecture that may express in infancy or childhood as epilepsy.

Most disturbances of neuroblast migration involve arrested migration before the journey is complete. These disorders are divisible into three anatomical phases, depending on where the migratory arrest occurred. An example of neuroblasts never having begun migration from the periventricular region is periventricular nodular heterotopia, an X-linked genetic disorder due to defective expression of the gene, filamin-A (*FLNA*). Subcortical laminar heterotopia results when neuroblasts begin migration but arrest in the subcortical white matter before reaching the cortical plate. This is another X-linked recessive trait but is due to a different gene called *doublecortin* (*DCX*). The term *double cortex* is sometimes used, but this name is incorrect because unlike a true cortex, the subcortical heterotopia lacks lamination. If the neuroblasts reach the cortical plate but lack correct lamination, accompanying this abnormal architecture of the cortical plate are abnormalities of gyration such as lissencephaly or pachygyria. Several different genes, including *LIS1* and reelin (*RLN*), are important in cortical plate organization (Curran and D'Arcangelo, 1998) and mutated in malformations of the terminal phase of neuroblast migration.

*Lissencephaly* is a condition of a smooth cerebral cortex without convolutions. Normally at midgestation, the brain is essentially smooth; the interhemispheric, sylvian, and calcarine fissures are the only ones formed. Gyri and sulci develop between 20 and 36 weeks' gestation, and the mature pattern of gyration is evident at term, although some parts of the cerebral cortex (e.g., frontal lobes) are still relatively small. In lissencephaly type 1 (Miller-Dieker syndrome), the cerebral cortex remains smooth. Lesser degrees of this gross morphological defect exist, with a few excessively wide gyri (pachygyria) or multiple excessively small gyri (polymicrogyria). The histopathological pattern is that of a four-layer cortex in which the outermost layer (1) is the molecular layer, as in normal six-layered neocortex. Layer 2 corresponds to layers 2 through 6 of normal neocortex, layer 3 is cell-sparse as a persistent fetal subplate zone, and layer 4 consists of incompletely migrated neurons in the subcortical intermediate zone. In lissencephaly type 2 (Walker-Warburg syndrome), poorly laminated cortex with disorganized and disoriented neurons is seen histologically, and the gross appearance of the cerebrum is one of a smooth brain or a few poorly formed sulci (Fig. 89.5). The term *cobblestone* refers to the aspect of the surface, with multiple shallow furrows not corresponding to normal sulci. The cerebral mantle may be thin, suggesting a disturbance of cell proliferation as well as of neuroblast migration. Malformations of the brainstem and cerebellum often are present as well (see Fig. 89.5). Lissencephaly type 1 and type 2 (Walker-Warburg syndrome, Fukuyama muscular dystrophy, muscle-eye-brain disease of Santavuori) are genetic diseases. *LIS1* was the first gene discovered in the lissencephalies, but many more have now been identified (Fry et al. 2014). Lissencephaly also results from nongenetic disturbances of neuroepithelial proliferation or neuroblast migration, including destructive encephaloclastic processes such as congenital infections during fetal life. More recently it has been recognized that the lissencephalies, including those resulting from mutations in *LIS1, DCX,* and *ARX* genes, are disturbances not only in radial migration but also involve tangentially migrating neuroblasts (Marcorelles et al., 2010).

Other abnormal patterns of gross gyration of the cerebral cortex occur secondary to neuroblast migratory disorders. *Pachygyria* signifies abnormally large, poorly formed gyri and may be present in some regions of cerebral cortex, with lissencephaly in other regions. *Polymicrogyria* refers to excessively numerous and abnormally small gyri that similarly may coexist with pachygyria. The small gyri often show fusion of adjacent molecular zones and other gaps in the pial membrane and leptomeninges that also result in overmigration (Squier and Jansen, 2014). However, polymicrogyria does not necessarily always denote a primary migratory disorder of genetic origin.

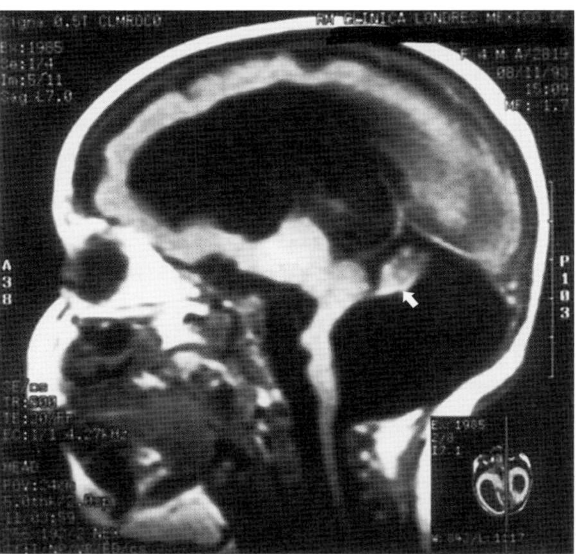

**Fig. 89.5** Sagittal T1-weighted magnetic resonance image of a 10-month-old girl with lissencephaly type 2 and Dandy-Walker malformation. The cerebral mantle is thin, and the lateral ventricles are greatly enlarged. A few abnormal shallow fissures at the cerebral surface may indicate abortive gyration or pachygyria. The cerebellum is severely hypoplastic (*arrow* indicates anterior vermis), and the posterior fossa contains a large fluid-filled cyst. The brainstem also is hypoplastic, and the basis pontis is nearly absent. A differential diagnosis of this image is pontocerebellar hypoplasia, but the high position of the torcula indicates a Dandy-Walker malformation.

Small, poorly formed gyri may occur in zones of fetal ischemia, and they regularly surround porencephalic cysts due to middle cerebral artery occlusion in fetal life.

In the cerebral hemisphere, most germinal matrix cells become neurons during the first half of gestation, and most form glia during the second half of gestation. Nonetheless, a small number of germinal matrix cells are neuronal precursors, migrating into the cerebral cortex in late gestation. Because the migration of the external granular layer in the cerebellar cortex is incomplete until 1 year of age, a potential for acquired insults to interfere with late migrations persists throughout the perinatal period. Anatomical lesions such as periventricular leukomalacia, intracerebral hemorrhages and abscesses, hydrocephalus, and traumatic injuries may disrupt the delicate radial glial guide fibers and prevent normal migration even though the migrating cell itself may escape the focal destructive lesion. Damaged radial glial cells tend to retract their processes from the pial surface. The migrating neuron travels only as far as its retracted glial fibers carry it. If this fiber retracts into the subcortical white matter, the neuroblast stops there and matures, becoming an isolated heterotopic nodule composed of several nerve cells that were migrating at the same time in the same place. In these nodules, neurons of various cortical types differentiate without laminar organization and with haphazard orientations of their processes, but a few extrinsic axons may prevent total synaptic isolation of the nodule. Interference with the glial guide fibers in the cerebral cortex itself results in neurons either not reaching the pial surface or not being able to reverse direction and then descending to a deeper layer. The consequence is imperfect cortical lamination, which interferes with the development of synaptic circuits. These disturbances of late neuroblast migration do not produce the gross malformations of early gestation and may be undetectable by imaging techniques. They may account for many neurological sequelae after the perinatal period, including seizures, perceptual disorders, impairment of gross or fine motor function, learning disabilities, and intellectual disability.

In sum, either defective genetic programming or acquired lesions in the fetal brain that destroy or interrupt radial glial fibers may cause disorders of neuroblast migration. Cells may not migrate at all and become mature neurons in the periventricular region, as occurs in X-linked periventricular nodular heterotopia (Eksioglu et al., 1996) and in some cases of congenital cytomegalovirus infection. Cells may become arrested along their course as heterotopic neurons in deep subcortical white matter, as occurs in many genetic syndromes of lissencephaly-pachygyria and in many metabolic diseases including cerebrohepatorenal (Zellweger) syndrome and many aminoacidurias and organic acidurias. The same aberration may occur in acquired insults to the radial glial cell during ontogenesis. Cells may overmigrate beyond the limits of the pial membrane into the meninges as ectopic neurons, either singly or in clusters known as *marginal glioneuronal heterotopia*, or brain warts. Rarely, herniation of the germinal matrix into the lateral ventricle may occur through gaps in the ependyma; those cells mature as neurons, forming a non-neoplastic intraventricular mass that may or may not obstruct cerebrospinal fluid (CSF) flow. Whether disoriented radial glial fibers actually guide neuroblasts to an intraventricular site or neuroblasts are physically pushed in a direction of less resistance is uncertain.

### Architecture of the Cortical Plate

The first wave of radial migration brings subventricular neuroblasts to the middle of the marginal zone at 7 weeks' gestation. These initial cells forming the cortical plate separate the marginal zone into a superficial molecular layer that includes the Cajal-Retzius neurons, and the deeper subplate zone, a transitory lamina that has disappeared by about 34 weeks. More than 90% of radial migration of neuroblasts is complete by 16 weeks' gestation, and most of the remaining immature cells of the periventricular germinal matrix yet to migrate will become glioblasts. After reaching the cortical plate, migratory neuroblasts must detach from their radial glial fiber by losing the adhesion molecule that has held it in place, so that the next migratory neuroblast may pass to a more superficial position in the mature cortex, an inside-out arrangement described by Rakic (1972, 2002) so that the deepest cortical layers are from the earliest migratory waves and layer 2 neurons are the last wave.

The histological architecture of the cortical plate in the first half of gestation is radial microcolumnar. Synaptic layers between neurons also are initially radial. Horizontal lamination is superimposed, beginning at about 22 weeks' gestation, and becomes the dominant architecture of the mature cortex. If neuroblasts cannot detach from their radial glial fiber, a disorganized cortical plate results (Anton et al., 1996). Another mechanism of cortical dysplasia is a maturational arrest with persistence of radial architecture. This pattern is seen in some metabolic diseases such as methylmalonic acidemia, in some chromosomopathies such as DiGeorge syndrome (22q11.1 deletion), and in focal cortical dysplasias type 1 (Sarnat and Flores-Sarnat, 2013a). Such maturational arrest is epileptogenic, but fetuses of less than 26 weeks cannot have seizures generated in the cortex because cortical synapses are too few. Despite the change from radial to horizontal histological layering, metabolic cell markers show specific neuronal types already positioned before this transition (Hevner, 2007). Genetic patterning of specific areas is programmed in part by the thalamocortical projections (O'Leary et al., 2007).

The U-fiber layer beneath the cortex and following the gyral contours consists of short association axons of layer 6 neurons that connect different parts of the same gyrus and immediately adjacent gyri, but do not provide commissural fibers or descending projections to subcortical structures. U-fibers generally myelinate later than the deep white matter, except those lining primary fissures and major sulci such as the Rolandic and parieto-occipital. The U-fiber layer does not begin to form until midgestation, when gyration and sulcation of the cortex is initiated. The U-fiber layer beneath focal cortical dysplasias contains excessive neuronal dispersion from layer 6 and elaborate synaptic plexi formed from and between these displaced neurons (Sarnat et al., 2018).

**BOX 89.1 Fissures of the Developing Brain**

**Forebrain Fissures**

Interhemispheric (4.5 weeks)
Choroidal (5 weeks)
Optic/ocular (5 weeks)
Hippocampal (6 weeks)
Sylvian (8–9 weeks)
Calcarine (10–12 weeks)
There also are more than 30 sulci in the mature cerebral cortex

**Hindbrain and Cerebellar Fissures**

Sagittal intercollicular (10 weeks)
Transverse intercollicular (10–11 weeks)
Longitudinal paravermal
Transverse cerebellar fissures:
- Primary (anterior/posterior lobes)
- Posterolateral (flocculonodular lobe)
- Posterior superior
- Horizontal
- Prepyramidal

Sagittal basilar pontine
Sagittal interpyramidal

## FISSURES AND SULCI OF CORTICAL STRUCTURES

Fissures and sulci are grooves that form in laminated cortices, principally cerebral and cerebellar. Such folding accomplishes a need for an enlarging surface area without a concomitant increase in tissue volume as development proceeds. Without gyration of the cerebral cortex and foliation of the cerebellar cortex, the brain would be so large and voluminous at birth that neither the neonate nor the mother would survive delivery. Fissures and sulci both result from mechanical forces during fetal growth, but they differ in that fissures form from external forces and sulci form from internal forces imposed by the increased volume of neuronal cytoplasm and the formation of neuropil, the processes of neurons and glial cells (Sarnat and Flores-Sarnat, 2013c). The ventricular system acts as another external force, surrounded by but outside of the brain parenchyma. Whereas fissures generally form earlier and often are deeper than sulci, these are not the most important differences. Box 89.1 lists the various fissures of the brain, and Fig. 89.6 is a drawing of the development of the human telencephalic flexure, which becomes, after closure of the operculum, the sylvian fissure. It should be noted that the ventral bending of the primitive oval-shaped telencephalic hemisphere results in the original posterior pole becoming the temporal—not the occipital—lobe, and that the lateral ventricle bends with the brain. The occipital horn of the lateral ventricle is a more recent diverticulum of the original simple ventricle and, as such, remains the most variable part of the ventricular system, symmetrical in only 25% of normal individuals. Cerebellar folia are the equivalent of cerebral cortical gyri. A temporally and spatially precise sequence of the development of fissures, sulci, and cerebellar folia is genetically programmed and enables the neuroradiologist and neuropathologist

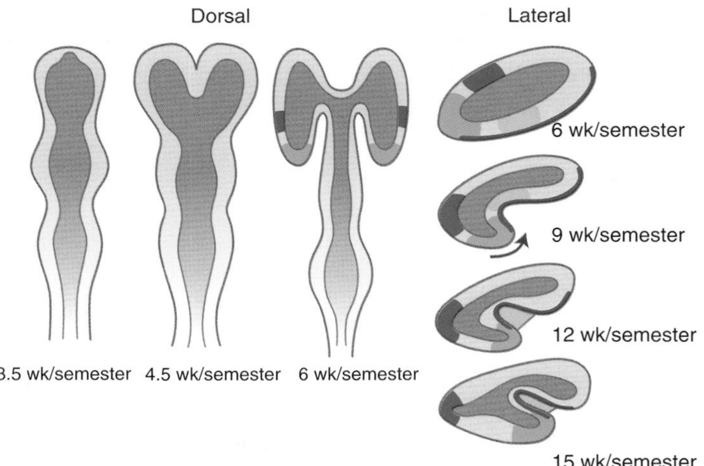


**Fig. 89.6** The Telencephalic Flexure that Forms the Sylvian Fissure.

to also assess maturational delay of this aspect of ontogenesis. The gestational age of a premature infant may be determined to within a 2-week period or less from the convolutional pattern of the brain.

### Disorders of Fissures and Sulci

The telencephalic sylvian fissures fail to form in HPE and form abnormally in many major malformations of the brain, including lissencephalies, schizencephaly, and severe cerebral hypoplasias. Abnormal gyration is a regular feature of many neuroblast migratory disorders, including lissencephaly, pachygyria, and polymicrogyria, and also in alobar and semilobar HPE (Sarnat et al., 2013c). Accurate diagnosis by neuroimaging thus not only is available postnatally but also by prenatal fetal magnetic resonance imaging (MRI), even though microscopic details of cortical lamination and organization are below the resolution of these techniques.

## GROWTH OF AXONS AND DENDRITES

During the course of neuroblast migration, neurons remain largely undifferentiated cells, and the embryonic cerebral cortex at midgestation consists of vertical columns of tightly packed cells between radial blood vessels and extensive extracellular spaces. Cytodifferentiation begins with a proliferation of organelles, mainly endoplasmic reticulum and mitochondria in the cytoplasm, and clumping of condensed nuclear chromatin at the inner margin of the nuclear membrane. Rough endoplasmic reticulum becomes swollen, and ribosomes proliferate.

The outgrowth of the axon always precedes the development of dendrites, and the axon forms connections before the differentiation of dendrites begins. Ramón y Cajal first noted the projection of the axon toward its destination and named this growing process the *cone d'accroissement* (growth cone). The tropic factors that guide the growth cone to its specific terminal synapse, whether chemical, endocrine, or electrotaxic, have been a focus of controversy for many years. However, we now know that diffusible molecules secreted along their pathway by the processes of fetal ependymal cells and perhaps some glial cells guide growth cones during their long trajectories. Some molecules (e.g., brain-derived neurotropic growth factor, netrin, S-100β protein) attract growing axons, whereas others (e.g., the glycosaminoglycan keratan sulfate—not to be confused with another very different protein, keratin) strongly repel them and thus prevent aberrant decussations and other deviations.

The proteoglycan keratan sulfate has been known since 1990 to be an important molecule in the dorsal median septum of the spinal cord that prevents rostrally growing dorsal column axons from crossing the midline before their intended destinations in the nuclei gracilis and cuneatus at the caudal medulla oblongata; aberrant decussation would confuse the brain about laterality of sensory stimuli (Snow et al., 1990). Keratan sulfate is selective, however, repelling excitatory glutamatergic axons while facilitating inhibitory GABAergic axons. The great majority of dorsal root ganglion neurons that project axons into the dorsal columns are glutamatergic, by contrast with spinothalamic fibers that mainly are GABAergic; ascending axons of the nuclei gracilis and cuneatus to the thalamus also are GABAergic. Another repulsive factor for guidance of olfactory axons away from septal receptors is a secreted protein called *Slit*, which is the ligand for the *Slit* receptor *Robo* (Brose et al., 1999; Li et al., 1999; Rothberg et al., 1990). Commissural axons also are enabled to cross the ventral median septum of the spinal cord that repulses longitudinal axons growing rostrally or caudally in the longitudinal axis of the neural tube and early fetal spinal cord (Bovolenta and Dodd, 1990)

Keratan sulfate also occurs in the forebrain and is strongly expressed in early fetal life in the thalamus and globus pallidus, later appearing in the molecular zone and later diffusely in the cortical plate, finally becoming more localized in the deep cortical laminae and the U-fiber layer, where it impedes the penetration of axons from deep white-matter heterotopia so that they cannot integrate into cortical synaptic circuitry and epileptic networks (Sarnat, 2019). Granulofilamentous keratan sulfate also binds to neuronal somatic membranes, but not to dendritic spines, explaining why axosomatic synapses are inhibitory and axodendritic synapses are excitatory (Sarnat, 2019). An additional function of keratan sulfate in the brain, where is it secreted by astrocytes into the intercellular matrix, is to surround axonal fascicles so that axons can neither enter nor exit the fascicles except at programmed places. Both large and long fascicles, such as the corticospinal tract, and short fascicles, such as the coarse local axonal bundles within the globus pallidus and similar but smaller "pencil fibers of Wilson" within the corpus striatum, are insulated (Sarnat, 2019). Keratan sulfate also has a wider distribution in the body in organs other than the CNS. It is strongly expressed in cornea, cartilage, bone, synovium, connective tissues, and other sites (Caterson and Melrose, 2018; Pomin, 2015, 2018). It may explain why cartilage is not penetrated by nerves except at designated foramina.

Matrix proteins such as laminin and fibronectin also provide a substrate for axonal guidance. Cell-to-cell attractions operate as the axon approaches its final target. Despite the long delay between the migration of an immature nerve cell and the beginning of dendritic growth, the branching of dendrites eventually accounts for more than 90% of the synaptic surface of the mature neuron. The pattern of dendritic ramification is specific for each type of neuron. Spines form on the dendrites as short protrusions with expanded tips, providing sites of synaptic membrane differentiation. The Golgi method of impregnation of neurons and their processes with heavy metals such as silver or mercury, used for more than a century, continues to be one of the most useful methods for demonstrating dendritic arborizations. Among the many contributions of this technique to the study of the nervous system, beginning with the elegant pioneering work of Ramón y Cajal, none has surpassed its demonstration of the sequence of normal dendritic branching in the human fetus. Newer immunocytochemical techniques for demonstrating dendrites also are now available, such as microtubule-associated protein 2. These techniques are applicable to human tissue resected surgically, as in the surgical treatment of epilepsy, and to the tissue secured at autopsy.

### Disorders of Neurite Growth

If a neuron disorients during migration and faces the wrong direction in its final site, its axon is capable of reorienting itself as much as 180 degrees after emerging from the neuronal cell body. Dendrites, by contrast, conform strictly to the orientation of the cell body and do not change their axis. The dendritic tree growth stunts if axodendritic synapses are not established. Because so much dendritic differentiation and growth occurs during the last third of gestation and the first months of the postnatal period, the preterm infant is particularly vulnerable to noxious influences that interfere with maturation of dendrites. Extraordinarily long dendrites of dentate granule cells and prominent basal dendrites of pyramidal cells occur in full-term infants on life-support systems. Retardation of neuronal maturation in terms of dendrite development and spine morphology occurs more frequently in premature infants, compared with term infants of the same conceptional age, possibly as a result of asphyxia. Infants with fetal alcohol syndrome also have a reduced number and abnormal geometry of dendritic spines of cortical neurons.

Traditional histological examination of the brains of intellectually disabled children often shows remarkably few alterations to account for their profound intellectual deficit. The study of dendritic morphology by the Golgi technique has revealed striking abnormalities in some of these cases. The best documentation of these alterations occurs in chromosomal diseases such as trisomy 13 and Down syndrome. Long, thin, tortuous dendritic spines and the absence of small stubby spines are a common finding. Children with unclassified intellectual disability but normal chromosomal numbers and morphology also show defects in the number, length, and spatial arrangement of dendrites and synapses. Abnormalities of cerebellar Purkinje cell dendrites occur in cerebellar dysplasias and hypoplasias. They consist of cactus-like thickenings and loss of branchlet spines. Abnormal development of the dendritic tree is also a common finding in many metabolic encephalopathies, including Krabbe disease and other leukodystrophies, Menkes kinky hair disease, gangliosidoses, ceroid lipofuscinosis, and Sanfilippo syndrome. Among genetically determined cerebral dysgeneses, reports of aberrations in the structure and number of dendrites and spines exist in cerebrohepatorenal (Zellweger) syndrome and in tuberous sclerosis.

## ELECTRICAL POLARITY OF THE CELL MEMBRANE

The development of membrane excitability is one of the important markers of neuronal maturation, but knowledge is incomplete about the exact timing and duration of this development. Membrane polarity establishes before synaptogenesis and before the synthesis of neurotransmitters begins. Because the maintenance of a resting membrane potential requires considerable energy expenditure to fuel the sodium-potassium pump, the undifferentiated neuroblast would be incapable of maintaining such a dynamic condition as a resting membrane potential. The development of ion channels within the neural membrane is another important factor in the maturation of excitable membranes and the maintenance of resting membrane potentials.

### Disorders of Membrane Polarity

Epileptic phenomena are largely due to inappropriate membrane depolarizations. They represent a complex interaction of excitatory and inhibitory synapses that modulate the resting membrane potential, metabolic alterations, and many unknown factors that also contribute to the discharge threshold of neural membranes. Cerebral malformations are often associated with seizures because of abnormal synaptic circuitry, and the role of abnormal resting membrane potentials in development is largely speculative at this time. Electrolyte imbalances in the serum certainly influence the depolarization threshold, and hypothalamic disturbances may alter endocrine function and electrolyte balance. Finally, abnormal membrane receptors and ion channels in the neuronal plasma membrane are the result of many recently discovered genes associated with specific types of epilepsy and may or may not have a histopathologically abnormal phenotype.

## SYNAPTOGENESIS

Synapse formation follows the development of dendritic spines and polarization of the cell membrane. The relation of synaptogenesis to neuroblast migration differs in different parts of the nervous system. In the cerebral cortex, synaptogenesis always follows neuroblast migration. In the cerebellar cortex, however, the external granule cells develop axonal processes that become the long parallel fibers of the molecular layer and make synaptic contact with Purkinje cell dendrites before migrating through the molecular and Purkinje cell layer to their mature internal position within the folium. Synaptophysin immunoreactivity is a useful marker for studying normal and abnormal synaptogenesis in the fetus and newborn. Throughout the brain, the precisely programmed sequence of synaptogenesis can be identified in sections of fetal brain of various gestational ages (Sarnat et al., 2010, 2013a, 2013b, 2013c).

Afferent nerve fibers reach the neocortex early, before lamination occurs in the cortical plate. The first synapses are axodendritic and occur both external to and beneath the cortical plate in the future layers I and VI, which contain the first neurons that have migrated.

An excessive number of synapses form on each neuron, with subsequent elimination of those that are not required. Outside the CNS, muscle fibers also begin their relation with the nervous system by receiving multiple sources of innervation from multiple motor neurons, later retaining only one. Transitory synapses also form at sites on neurons where they no longer exist in the mature condition. The SMNs of newborn kittens display prominent synapses on their initial axonal segment, where they never occur in adult cats. Somatic spines are an important synaptic site on the embryonic Purkinje cell, but these spines and their synapses disappear as the dendritic tree develops. A structure/function correlation is possible in the developing visual cortex. In preterm infants of 24 to 25 weeks' gestation, the visual evoked potentials (VEPs) recorded at the occiput exhibit initial long-latency negativity, but by 28 weeks' gestation, a small positive wave precedes this negativity. The change in this initial component of the VEP corresponds to dendritic arborization and the formation of dendritic spines that occurs at that time.

The EEG of the premature infant follows a predictable and time-linked progression in maturation. The EEG reflects synaptogenesis more closely than any other feature of cerebral maturation and thereby provides a noninvasive and clinically useful measure of neurological maturation in the preterm infant. Fetal EEG may even detect neurological disease and seizures in utero.

### Disorders of Synaptogenesis

Because the formation of dendritic spines and the formation of synapses are so closely related, the same spectrum of diseases already discussed is equally appropriate for consideration in this section. In preterm infants, who are generally unwell even if they do not have specific neurological disease, the rate of maturation of the EEG is often slow, which may reflect an impairment of synapse formation. Chronic hypoxemia particularly delays neurological maturation, including synapse formation. Deletions of δ-catenin, a neuron-specific catenin implicated in adhesion and dendritic branching, lead to severe synaptic dysfunction and correlate with the severity of intellectual disability in cri du chat syndrome (Israely et al., 2004). Delayed synaptogenesis occurs in many chromosomopathies and genetic diseases involving the fetal brain, as well as in many inborn metabolic diseases. Precocious synaptogenesis also can occur, as demonstrated in fetal HPE in the cerebral cortex and the retina of the cyclopean eye (Sarnat and Flores-Sarnat, 2013b; Sarnat et al., 2014). Precocious synapse formation is not advantageous because it is out of synchrony with other simultaneous processes of neuronal maturation and may lead to early development of epileptic circuitry and severe infantile epilepsies.

## BIOSYNTHESIS OF NEUROTRANSMITTERS

The basis for synthesis of neurotransmitters and neuromodulating chemicals is the secretory character of the neuron, without which synaptic transmission is impossible. Several types of substances serve as transmitters: (1) acetylcholine (ACh); (2) monoamines, including dopamine, norepinephrine, epinephrine, and serotonin; (3) neuropeptides, including substance P, somatostatin, and opioid-containing peptide chains such as the enkephalins; and (4) simple amino acids, including glutamic acid, aspartic acid, GABA, and glycine. Some transmitters are characteristically inhibitory (e.g., glycine, GABA, and ACh in the CNS). Each neuronal type produces a characteristic transmitter—motor neurons produce ACh, cerebellar Purkinje cells produce GABA, and granule cells produce glutamic acid in the adult. Neuropeptides may coexist with other types of transmitters in some neurons.

In some parts of the brain, transitory fetal transmitters may appear during development and then disappear. Substance P and somatostatin are present in the fetal cerebellum at midgestation, but these neuropeptides are never found in the mature cerebellum. In the cerebral cortex of the frontal lobe, the pattern of laminar distribution of cholinergic muscarinic receptors in the mature brain is the inverse of that in the fetus. The functions of these transitory transmitter systems are unknown. Some serve as tropic molecules rather than transmitters in early development. Even amino acid transmitters such as GABA may serve mainly a tropic function at an early stage in development. In situ hybridization and immunocytochemical techniques demonstrate neurotransmitters in neurons of the developing brain of experimental animals and may be applicable to human tissue under some circumstances (Dupuy and Houser, 1997). The ontogeny of neurotransmitter systems depends not only on the mechanisms of synthesis of chemical transmitters but also on the development of highly specific receptors of these chemical signals and their ability to modify excitability of neuronal membranes and trigger action potentials after the recognition of specific molecules (Rho and Storey, 2001; Simeone et al., 2003).

### Disorders of Neurotransmitter Synthesis

Ischemic and hypoxic insults impair RNA transcription and result in arrest of the synthesis of secretory products. Many of the clinical neurological deficits observed in asphyxiated neonates are probably the result of neurotransmitter depletion and functional synaptic block. Some amino acid neurotransmitters, by contrast, are neurotoxic when released in large quantities. The excitatory amino acids glutamic acid and aspartic acid induce transsynaptic degeneration when released in this way (as might occur with hypoxic stresses) and may be a major source of irreversible brain damage in asphyxiated neonates.

Developmental disorders due to inborn errors of metabolism that block the chemical pathway of transmitter synthesis may occur, but they are probably incompatible with survival if they interfere with synthesis of a major transmitter such as ACh, monoamines, or an essential peptide. Many defects in the metabolic pathways of particular amino acids are associated with intellectual disability, epilepsy, spastic diplegia, and other chronic neurological handicaps. Phenylketonuria (a disorder of phenylalanine metabolism) and maple syrup urine disease (a disorder of the metabolism of the branched-chain amino acids leucine, isoleucine, and valine) are well-documented examples. However, it is not certain whether absence of the product of the deficient enzyme, or toxicity of high levels of precursors upstream from the enzyme deficiency, is the principal insult to the nervous system.

## MYELINATION

Myelin insulates individual axons and provides greatly increased speed of conduction. It is not essential in all nerves, and many autonomic fibers of the peripheral nervous system remain unmyelinated throughout life. Conduction velocity in central pathways is important in coordinating time-related impulses from different centers that converge on a distant target and in ensuring that action potentials are not lost by synaptic block. The basis of nervous system functions is the temporal summation of impulses to relay messages across synapses.

Myelination of pathways in the CNS occurs in a predictable spatial and temporal sequence. Some tracts myelinate as early as 14 weeks' gestation and complete their myelination cycle in a few weeks. Examples include the spinal roots, medial longitudinal fasciculus, dorsal columns of the spinal cord, and most cranial nerves. Between 22 and 24 weeks' gestation, myelination progresses in the olivary and cerebellar connections, the ansa lenticularis of the globus pallidus, the sensory trigeminal nerve, the auditory pathways, and the acoustic nerve, as well as the trapezoid body, lateral lemniscus, and brachium of the inferior colliculus. By contrast, the optic nerve and the geniculocalcarine tract (i.e., optic radiations) do not begin to acquire myelin until near term. Some pathways are late in myelinating and have myelination cycles measured in years. The corpus callosum begins myelinating at 4 months postnatally and is not complete until mid-adolescence. Some ipsilateral association fibers connecting the frontal with the temporal and parietal lobes do not achieve full myelination until about 32 years of age.

Myelination can now be accurately measured in specific central pathways by using T2-weighted MRI sequences, but the time at which myelination can be detected is somewhat later than with traditional myelin stains of brain tissue sections, such as Luxol fast blue. Newer neuropathological methods using gallocyanin and immunoreactivity to myelin basic protein may detect myelination even earlier than the traditional stains. Electron microscopy remains the most sensitive method of demonstrating the earliest myelination in tissue sections.

### Disorders of Myelination

Many metabolic diseases impede the rate of myelination. Hypothyroidism is a classic example. Menkes kinky hair disease, a disorder of copper absorption and metabolism, is another example. Many aminoacidurias, including phenylketonuria, are also associated with delayed myelination. The neuropathological findings in cerebrohepatorenal (Zellweger) syndrome include disorders of neuroblast migration and myelination. Some leukodystrophies (e.g., Krabbe disease, perinatal sudanophilic leukodystrophy) express defective myelination in fetal life.

Chronic hypoxia in premature infants is probably the most common cause of delayed myelination and contributes to the delay found in clinical neurological maturation. Myelination depends on fatty acids supplied by the maternal and infant diet; nutritional deficiencies during gestation or in postnatal life may result in delayed myelination and be clinically expressed as developmental delay. Unlike disorders of neuronal migration, delay in myelination is reversible. Removing the insult may allow myelination to catch up to reach the appropriate level of maturity.

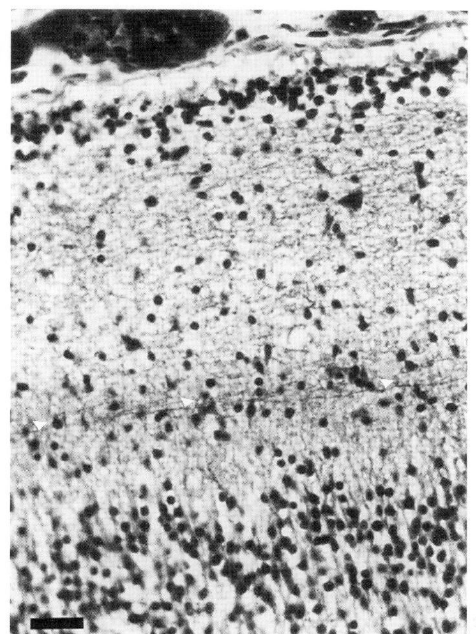

**Fig. 89.7** Silver stain of molecular layer of motor cortex in a 20-week fetus. The long fibers *(arrowheads)* extending parallel to the surface of the brain are axons of Cajal-Retzius neurons. (Bielschowsky stain. Bar = 10 μm.)

## CAJAL-RETZIUS NEURONS AND SUBPLATE NEURONS OF THE FETAL BRAIN

Cajal-Retzius cells are large, mature, stellate neurons in the marginal (outermost) zone of the fetal cerebral cortex. They are the first cells to appear at the surface of the embryonic cerebrum, preceding the first wave of radial migration from the subventricular zone and forming a plexus in the marginal (later the molecular) zone. They migrate to the surface from the ganglionic eminence, the source of GABAergic inhibitory interneurons that will later arrive at the cortical plate by tangential migration (Sarnat and Flores-Sarnat, 2002). The first afferent processes to enter the marginal layer are dendrites of pyramidal cells of layer VI; synapses between Cajal-Retzius and pyramidal neurons of layer VI form the first intrinsic cortical circuits (Marín-Padilla, 1998). They eventually have synaptic contacts with cortical neurons in all layers.

Cajal-Retzius cells contain acetylcholinesterase and oxidative enzymes and secrete GABA and probably ACh as neurotransmitters. Their long axons extend parallel to the surface of the brain, plunging short branches into layer II (Fig. 89.7). Cajal-Retzius neurons are sparse by term but persist even in the adult, though their function after maturity is uncertain. They strongly express the transcription product of the *LIS1* gene, which is defective in X-linked hydrocephalus associated with polymicrogyria and defective neuroblast migration. Cajal-Retzius neurons also strongly express spastic diplegia, *RLN*, another gene essential for radial neuroblast migration and organization of the cortical plate (Clark et al., 1997; Sarnat and Flores-Sarnat, 2002). This is the only specific disease involving Cajal-Retzius neurons.

The subplate zone is a transitory layer of neurons in early development that will regress at midgestation and eventually disappear, its neurons being incorporated into the deep layers of the cortical plate. The subplate zone also is essential for organization of the cortical plate and, in preterm infants, can contribute to subcortical white-matter injury (Pogledic et al., 2014).

The fetal cerebral cortex has a subpial or external granular layer that histologically resembles that of the cerebellum but is of quite a different character. Cells of the cerebral cortex rise in columns from the germinal matrix of the hippocampus to form a thin layer on the surface of the archicortex at 12 weeks' gestation. They rapidly spread over the neocortex in a predictable sequence to cover the entire convexity by the 16th to 18th week, with the layer reaching the greatest thickness by 22 weeks' gestation. Subsequent involution of the external granular layer results from migration of these cells into the cerebral cortex, where they can no longer be distinguished. Only remnants of this once prominent layer persist at term, confined to the inferior temporal and orbital surfaces. These surfaces are the last sites from which they finally disappear from the neocortex, although a few may persist over the paleocortex even into adult life. Their fate within the cerebral cortex is unknown, but speculation is that they mature into glial cells, because they lack ultrastructural features of neurons, and they stain immunocytochemically for glial fibrillary acidic protein but not for vimentin. The subpial granular layer of the cerebral hemispheres is partially or totally absent in most cases of HPE, even at the gestational period when it is normally most prominent; this absence may contribute to the marginal glioneural heterotopia found in the meningeal spaces and superficial cortical layers. The layer of the subpial granule cells may serve as a barrier to reverse the direction of migration in neuroblasts reaching the surface. In the Fukuyama type of congenital muscular dystrophy associated with cerebral cortical dysplasia, a heterotopic layer of stellate glial cells forms at the surface of the cerebral cortex, into which migrating neurons accumulate as they reach the surface, rather than reversing direction and entering deeper layers of the cortex.

## ETIOLOGY OF CENTRAL NERVOUS SYSTEM MALFORMATIONS

The causes of cerebral malformations generally fall into one of two categories. The first category is genetic and chromosomal disease in which programming of cerebral development is defective. This genetic category also includes many inborn metabolic diseases in which cerebral dysgenesis may be due to biochemical insults during development, rather than (or in addition to) primary errors in molecular genetic codes for neural programming. The second category is epigenetic and includes all induced malformations in which a teratogenic influence acts at a particular time in ontogenesis; the malformation depends on the timing of the insult in relation to brain development at that moment. The timing may be brief, as with a single exposure to a toxic drug, a dose of radiation, or a traumatic injury of the fetal brain. It may be repeated two or more times or may be prolonged and involve the fetus at several stages of development. Examples of the latter include certain congenital infections such as toxoplasmosis and cytomegalovirus infection, which may be active throughout most of gestation, even into the postnatal period. Genetic factors are the most frequent causes of malformations during the first half of gestation. Environmental factors are more important in late gestation and may cause disturbances of late neuroblast migrations, particularly in premature infants. In some cases, no definite inductive factor is identifiable despite intensive clinical investigations during life and meticulous postmortem studies. Fetal alcohol syndrome in which the fetus is exposed to maternal alcohol intake results in a small brain with delayed synaptogenesis and other maturational features. The vascular development of the fetal and neonatal brain is impaired by alcohol and contributes to deficient growth and chronic ischemia (Jégou et al., 2012).

### Ischemic Encephalopathy in the Fetus

Among the environmental factors that may interfere with the developmental process in utero or postnatally, either briefly or more chronically, none is more important as a cause of morbidity than ischemic encephalopathy. Circulatory insufficiency or, less often, hypoxemia may interfere with migrations by causing infarction, which interrupts glial guide fibers. After birth, hypoxia is more frequent than pure ischemia as a cause of encephalopathy.

Ischemia also affects the fetal cerebrum by producing watershed infarcts between zones of arterial supply because of the fetus's poorer collateral circulation compared with that of the mature brain. Thin-walled vessels radiate perpendicular to the surface of the brain. The precursors of these radial vessels originate from leptomeningeal arteries and are evident at 15 weeks' gestation in the human embryo; horizontal branches appear in deep cortical layers at 20 weeks' gestation and increase to supply the superficial cortex by 27 weeks' gestation. The capillary network of the cortex proliferates mainly in the postnatal period as radial arterioles decrease in number. Severe ischemia of the immature brain may result in cuffs of surviving nerve cells surrounding the radial arterioles, with vertical columns of necrotic tissue between these zones related to immaturity of the vascular bed. Alternating radial zones of viable cerebral tissue and infarcted tissue thus occur in the cerebral cortex. Infarcts not only destroy maturing nerve cells that have already completed their migration but also interfere with continuing and future migrations into those regions. The zones of infarction eventually become gliotic and disrupt the geometric architecture of the cortex.

The existence of fetal watershed zones of the cortical vascular bed is important in the pathogenesis of *ulegyria*, an atrophy of gyri that grossly resembles polymicrogyria. Focal areas of cortical atrophy and gliotic scarring occur after perinatal ischemic or hypoxic encephalopathy. The four-layered cortex of polymicrogyria is quite a different lesion from ulegyria, resulting from a primary disturbance of neuroblast migration. Some authors question this interpretation, however, and provide evidence of postmigratory laminar necrosis of the cortex. The distribution of polymicrogyria is frequently in vascular territories of fetal brain and often forms a rim surrounding a porencephalic cyst in the territory of the middle cerebral artery. Multicystic encephalomalacia and hydranencephaly are end-stage sequelae of massive cerebral infarction in the developing brain. Watershed zones also exist in the brainstem between the territories supplied by paramedian penetrating short and long circumferential arteries, which originate from the basilar artery. Transitory hypoperfusion in the basilar artery in fetal life may produce watershed infarcts in the tegmentum of the pons and medulla oblongata. This is a probable pathogenesis of Möbius syndrome and probably also of "failure of central respiratory drive" in neonates with hypoventilation not due to pulmonary or neuromuscular disorders (Sarnat, 2004b). The cause is involvement of the tractus solitarius, which receives afferents from chemoreceptors such as the carotid body and provides efferent axons to motor neurons that innervate the diaphragm and intercostal muscles.

Mitochondria are the energy-generating organelles of all cells (except mature erythrocytes) and produce enzymes essential for cellular respiration. In mitochondrial diseases of early infancy, mitochondria of endothelial cells are more severely altered in muscle and brain than surrounding myofibers and neural cells, unlike the reverse involvement in adults (Sarnat et al., 2012a). In infants suffering hypoxic/ischemic insults, who do not have primary mitochondrial disease, their endothelial mitochondria may also be impaired and contribute to ischemic lesions of the brain.

## MOLECULAR GENETIC CLASSIFICATION OF MALFORMATIONS OF THE NERVOUS SYSTEM

Classification is a fundamental human thought process, allowing us to organize data in a systematic manner and understand relations. The traditional basis for classification of CNS malformations is descriptive morphogenesis. New insights into the molecular genetic programming of neural development require the integrations of this information with the anatomical criteria (Sarnat and Flores-Sarnat, 2001b, 2004; Simeone, 2002). For example, lissencephaly and HPE are two important malformations, each formerly thought to be distinctive. It is now recognized that many different genetic defects cause each; hence they are end stages of ontogenetic errors with diverse causes (see following discussion). A pure genetic classification to replace anatomical criteria, by contrast, would not be useful to clinicians, radiologists, or pathologists, and would be incomplete because many genetic mutations remain unknown. A compromise that addresses the deficiencies of both pure anatomical and pure genetic schemes of classification is one based on patterns of genetic expression in which the precise genetic mutation may or may not be known but is stated while preserving anatomical criteria (Sarnat and Flores-Sarnat, 2001b; Sarnat and Menkes, 2000). The upregulation or downregulation of a dorsalizing or ventralizing gene may be recognizable by its anatomical effect on neural tube development, even if the precise gene is unknown.

The traditional categories of CNS development that allow categories of ontogenetic processes, such as neuronogenesis, neuroblast migration, and synaptogenesis, and their disturbances in malformations, may be preserved in the proposed new scheme of classification. They are supplemented by new categories such as "disturbances of cellular lineage" (e.g., tuberous sclerosis; hemimegalencephaly) and disorders of embryonic neuromeric segmentation (e.g., absence of the midbrain and upper pons; absence of the basal ganglia; Chiari malformations). Some genes specify particular types of cellular differentiation and may change the cell type at different stages of development (Marquardt and Pfaff, 2001). One of the most important concepts in the integrated morphological-molecular-genetic scheme is the gradients of genetic expression (Sarnat and Flores-Sarnat, 2001b). The gradients are those of the axes of the neural tube: dorsoventral and ventrodorsal, rostrocaudal and sometimes caudorostral, and mediolateral. Nearly all genes have gradients of expression, with stronger expression in some regions and gradually lesser influence more distally. For example, if the rostrocaudal gradient in HPE extends as far as the midbrain, mesencephalic neural crest migration is impaired, and midfacial hypoplasia results, regardless of the severity of the forebrain malformation (see following discussion). Some authors attempt to develop schemes of regional classification for malformations (e.g., limited to the cerebral cortex for use in genetic epilepsies). All classifications should consider the entire CNS, however, because the rostrocaudal gradients of genetic expression may cause important subcortical defects, and indeed some seizure disorders may even originate in subcortical structures. The upregulation and downregulation of genes also is sometimes easier to understand in the anatomically simpler structures of the brainstem and spinal cord, allowing extrapolation to more complex forebrain structures.

A simple chronological listing of genes in the order from those that are initially expressed in the embryo is not feasible because most genes express at several different stages of development. Genes subserve different functions at each stage, initially as organizer genes for the basic architecture of the neural tube such as axes, cephalization, dorsal and ventral surfaces, and segmentation. These same genes later express as regulator genes for the differentiation and maintenance of particular cellular identities and functions.

Focal cortical dysplasias are a special group because in general they are highly epileptogenic and often refractory to medical treatment, requiring surgical excision. An international consortium of neuropathologists established by the International League Against Epilepsy (ILAE) defined and standardized diagnostic criteria and terminology for the focal cortical dysplasias. A scheme was thus published and is widely accepted, yet still has the flexibility to undergo present and future modifications as more data and new concepts emerge (Blümcke et al., 2011). After years of additional experience by the ILAE Consortium on Neuropathology, recommendations for revision of the original 2011 scheme were published (Najm et al. 2018). One major distinction is altered cortical architecture with disoriented and displaced but normal neurons, and those dysplasias that additionally involve cytological abnormalities of the neurons themselves. These abnormalities of growth and morphogenesis of some clones of neurons and glial cells in postzygotic somatic mutations are related to the mammalian target of rapamycin (mTOR) signaling pathway (Lindhurst et al. 2011; Mühlebner et al. 2019; Xu et al. 2019). Other pathways integrating with mTOR include the *PI3K* and *AKT* gene families that are the genetic etiology of many neurocutaneous syndromes, particularly epidermal nevus syndrome, including Proteus and CLOVES that also involves progressive overgrowth in the extremities, viscera and in the brain as hemimegalencephaly (Flores-Sarnat, 2013, 2016).

An additional factor in the pathogenesis of mTOR pathway disorders, particularly in tuberous sclerosis complex, is the expression of inflammatory markers in fetal brain (Prabowo et al., 2013; Sarnat and Scantlebury, 2017). The role of inflammation since fetal life in such genetic diseases has been little studied and much new data are anticipated.

## CLINICAL EXPRESSION OF SELECTED MALFORMATIONS OF THE NERVOUS SYSTEM

Table 89.2 summarizes the clinical features of major malformations of the brain.

### Disorders of Symmetry and Cellular Lineage

#### Hemimegalencephaly

Hemimegalencephaly is one of the most enigmatic cerebral malformations, because it is a severe dysgenesis limited to one cerebral hemisphere or, less commonly, includes the ipsilateral cerebellar hemisphere and brainstem (total hemimegalencephaly). Though traditionally regarded as another disorder of neuroblast migration, this feature is probably only secondary to involvement of radial glial cells and perhaps the neuroblasts themselves, and the primary process is a disturbance of cellular lineage and also involvement of genes of symmetry expressed as early as gastrulation (Flores-Sarnat, 2002a, 2003, 2008). Individual neural cells exhibit both glial and neuronal proteins and have abnormal growth and morphology. Some cases of hemimegalencephaly are isolated, but others are particularly associated with neurocutaneous syndromes: epidermal nevus syndrome and Klippel-Trénaunay syndrome (Flores-Sarnat, 2006). Neurological clinical features and neuropathological findings are virtually identical in isolated and associated forms. Partial epilepsy is the principal clinical feature in severe and moderate forms, often refractory to medical treatment and abolished only by hemispherectomy or other surgical resections. In epidermal nevus syndrome, 38% of patients have hemimegalencephaly and 77% have epilepsy, infantile spasms being the most frequent form (Flores-Sarnat, 2016). Other less constant features include variable intellectual disability and contralateral motor deficit. Mild as well as severe forms occur. Associated forms additionally include the features of the particular syndrome, such as lipomatosis of the ipsilateral face in epidermal nevus syndrome and Proteus syndrome (Flores-Sarnat, 2013). Hamartomatous brain malformations, such as tuberous sclerosis and hemimegalencephaly as isolated or neurocutaneous-associated forms, are now known to be somatic mutations, which explains patchy involvement of skin and brain and multisystemic involvement in many cases (Lee et al., 2012; Poduri et al., 2012). Hemimegalencephaly is a mutation in the *AKT3* gene, and the mTOR pathway is activated as it is in tuberous sclerosis. In addition, abnormal phosphorylated tau is upregulated in both disorders. Tau is a microtubule-associated protein and microtubules in early development are essential in establishing neuronal polarity, growth, differentiation, synapse formation and other cytological features (Sarnat et al., 2012b; Sarnat and Flores-Sarnat, 2015).

Hemimegalencephaly and focal cortical dysplasia type 2 are a spectrum of the same disorder. The difference between the extent of the focal malformation with dysplastic neurons is the timing of onset of mutated genetic expression in the 33 mitotic cycles of periventricular primitive neuroepithelium (Sarnat, 2018; Sarnat and Flores-Sarnat, 2017a,b). This neuroembryological evidence is confirmed by genetic evidence with the same conclusion (D'Gama et al., 2015, 2017; Lee et al., 2012).

### Disorders of Neurulation (1–4 Weeks' Gestation)

Incomplete or defective formation of the neural tube from the neural placode is the most common type of malformation of the human CNS. Anencephaly has an incidence of 1 per 1000 live births; meningomyelocele is almost as frequent. Geographical and ethnic differences occur among various populations in the world. Nonetheless, it is a medical problem and human tragedy of much greater proportions because the majority of infants affected with defects of the posterior neural tube survive with major neurological handicaps. The causes of these disorders in the first month of gestation are usually not evident, despite intensive epidemiological, genetic, dietary, and toxicological surveys.

#### Anencephaly (Aprosencephaly With Open Cranium)

Anencephaly is a failure of the closing of the anterior neuropore at 24 days' gestation. Death in utero occurs in approximately 7% of anencephalic pregnancies, 34% of such babies are premature, and 53% at term. Stillbirth, presumably resulting from intrapartum death, occurs in 20% of these deliveries. In one study of 211 pregnancies, 72% (153) of anencephalic offspring were liveborn; of those, 67% (103) died within 24 hours, but six survived 6 or more days (maximum 28 days) (Jaquier et al., 2006). The prenatal diagnosis of anencephaly is by examination of amniotic fluid for elevation of $\alpha$-fetoprotein, and confirmation is by sonographic imaging as early as 12 weeks' gestation. The face may show a midline hypoplasia, similar to HPE (see following section on HPE), probably because the rostrocaudal gradient of a defective genetic expression extends to the midbrain and interferes with mesencephalic neural crest migration (Sarnat and Flores-Sarnat, 2001a).

#### Cephalocele (Encephalocele; Exencephaly)

Most encephaloceles are parietal or occipital (Fig. 89.8) and contain supratentorial tissue, cerebellar tissue, or both. Frontal encephaloceles are less common in North America and Europe but are the most frequent variety in Thailand, Vietnam, and surrounding countries. They usually include olfactory tissue. Cases of encephaloceles related to Agent Orange (containing the herbicides 2,4-dichlorophenoxyacetic

**TABLE 89.2 Summary of Clinical Features of Major Malformations of the Brain**

| | Microcephaly | Cephalo- cele | Dysmorphic facies | Hydrocephalus | Epilepsy | Visual Impairment | Intellectual Disability | Hypotonia | Spasticity | Ataxia | Myopathy | Endocr- inopathy |
|---|---|---|---|---|---|---|---|---|---|---|---|---|
| Holoprosencephaly, lobar, semilobar* | +++ | ++ | +++ | + | ++ | + | ++++ | +++ | + | ++ | 0 | ++ |
| Holoprosencephaly, lobar, middle interhemispheric variant* | + | 0 | + | ++ | ++ | 0 | +++ | ++ | + | + | 0 | + |
| Septo-optic-pituitary dysplasia | + | 0 | + | + | ++ | +++ | +++ | ++ | + | + | 0 | +++ |
| Callosal agenesis, complete or partial | 0 | 0 | ++ | + | +++ | + | +++ | + | + | 0 | 0 | + |
| Callosal agenesis, Aicardi syndrome | ++ | 0 | ++ | + | ++++ | ++ | +++ | +++ | ++ | + | 0 | 0 |
| Callosal agenesis lipoma | 0 | 0 | + | + | ++++ | 0 | + | ++ | 0 | 0 | 0 | 0 |
| Colpocephaly, primary | ++ | 0 | ++ | 0 | ++ | ++ | ++ | ++ | + | 0 | 0 | 0 |
| Lissencephaly type 1 (Miller-Dieker syndrome) | + | 0 | ++++ | 0 | +++ | + | ++++ | +++ | + | ++ | 0 | + |
| Lissencephaly type 2 | +++ | ++ | ++++ | ++ | +++ | +++ | ++++ | +++ | ++ | ++ | ++++ | ++ |
| (Walker-Warburg syndrome) | ++ | 0 | ++ | + | +++ | ++ | ++++ | + | +++ | + | 0 | 0 |
| Pachygyria (Fukuyama muscular dystrophy) | +++ | 0 | ++ | 0 | +++ | + | ++++ | ++++ | 0 | ++ | ++++ | + |
| Cerebrohepatorenal disease (Zellweger syndrome) | ++ | 0 | ++++ | + | ++++ | ++ | ++++ | ++++ | 0 | 0 | ++ | + |
| Tuberous sclerosis | + | 0 | ++++ | ++ | ++++ | + | ++++ | ++ | ++ | + | 0 | + |
| Hemimegalencephaly[†] | 0 | 0 | ++ | + | +++ | ++ | ++++ | + | ++ | 0 | 0 | + |
| Chiari malformations | + | + | 0 | ++++ | + | 0 | ++++ | 0 | +++ | + | 0 | 0 |
| Dandy-Walker malformation | 0 | + | 0 | +++ | + | 0 | +++ | +++ | ++ | +++ | 0 | 0 |
| Aqueductal stenosis/ atresia | 0 | 0 | + | ++++ | + | 0 | ++ | + | ++ | + | 0 | 0 |
| Cerebellar hypoplasias | 0 | 0 | 0 | 0 | + | 0 | ++ | ++++ | 0 | ++++ | 0 | 0 |

0, <5% of patients; +, 5%–25%; ++, 26%–50%; +++, 51%–75%; ++++, >75% of patients involved.
*In holoprosencephaly, anatomical varieties do not correspond to genetic defect and correlate poorly with midfacial hypoplasia.
[†]Normal face in isolated form, cutaneous or subcutaneous signs in associated forms. Most are unilateral findings.

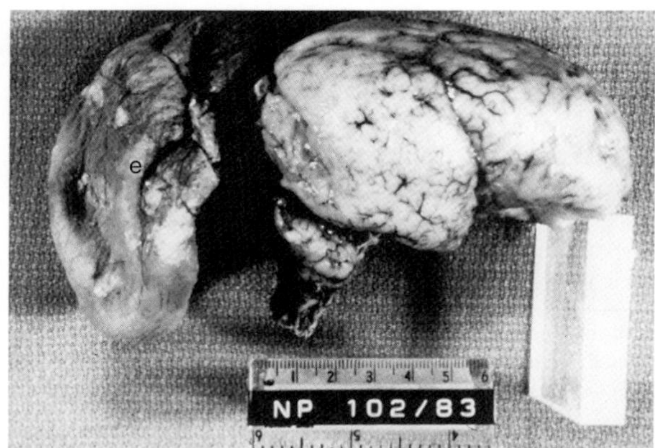


**Fig. 89.8** Lateral view of the brain of a term neonate with Meckel-Grüber syndrome. This dysplasia is a large occipital encephalocele *(e)* and lissencephaly. The brain is smooth and shows only a sylvian fissure and a few shallow abnormal sulci near the vertex. The encephalocele contains disorganized neural tissue, angiomatous malformations, focal hemorrhages, and zones of infarction.

acid [2,4-D] and 2,4,5-trichlorophenoxyacetic acid [2,4,5-T]), which was used in the Vietnam War, are still reportedly observed in Cambodia.

Skin may completely cover the encephalocele, or thin, distorted meningeal membranes may be exposed. When the ventricular system also is herniated into the encephalocele sac, hydrocephalus develops. Leaking CSF rapidly leads to infection. Some encephaloceles, particularly those of the occipital midline, may become so large that they exceed the size of the infant's head. Nasopharyngeal encephaloceles are rare but may be a source of meningitis from CSF leak through the nose. Malformations of the visceral organs often coexist with encephaloceles, and other congenital anomalies of the eyes and face, cleft palate, and polydactyly are also common. The entire brain may be severely hypoplastic (see Fig. 89.1).

Frontal and nasal encephaloceles protrude though bony foramina that normally close in the fetus: the fonticulus frontalis in the case of frontal (forehead midline) encephaloceles and the foramen cecum in the case of intranasal encephaloceles. Nasal encephaloceles might be confused clinically with nasal polyps, and CSF leak in the nose may be confused with benign nasal secretions. Both of these foramina fail to close because of defective prosencephalic neural crest tissue, which migrates from the dorsal part of the lamina terminalis as a vertical sheet of cells in the frontal midline.

Neurological handicaps may be severe because even if the herniated tissue within the encephalocele is small and easily excised, concomitant intracranial malformations of the brain often result in epilepsy, intellectual disability, and motor impairment. Cortical blindness often occurs in the case of occipital encephaloceles. The treatment of choice of small encephaloceles is surgical excision and closure of overlying cutaneous defects. Seizures and hydrocephalus are common but treatable complications.

## Meningomyelocele (Spinal Dysraphism, Spina Bifida Cystica)

The basis of classification of spina bifida syndromes is on either the bony vertebral deformity or the neurological lesion and associated clinical deficit. No deficits are associated with spina bifida occulta without herniation of tissue or mild spina bifida cystica with herniation of meninges alone. Deficits from herniation of nerve roots include motor, sensory, and autonomic neuropathy (meningomyelocele). Extensive defects occur with herniation of the parenchyma of the spinal cord (myelodysplasia). Most lesions are lumbosacral in location, but meningomyelocele also may occur in the thoracic or even the cervical region, usually as an extension rostrally of lumbosacral lesions. The level of involvement determines much of the clinical deficit. Type II Chiari malformation is consistently present, and aqueductal stenosis coexists in 50% of cases. Hydrocephalus is a common complication involving most patients with meningomyelocele; it causes neurological deficit.

The treatment of meningomyelocele is controversial and enters the arena of medical ethics. Surgical closure of small defects in the neonatal period is the rule. Large defects associated with complete paraplegia and flaccid neurogenic bladder, often accompanied by hydronephrosis, severe hydrocephalus, and other cerebral malformations, are associated with poor quality of life. A decision not to treat such infants or not to prolong survival poses a moral question addressed by the physicians in consultation with parents, hospital ethics committees, and other individuals the parents may identify. The most important immediate complications of large meningomyeloceles are hydrocephalus and infection from leaking CSF. Long-term complications include chronic urinary tract infections, decubiti, hydrocephalus, paraplegia, and other neurological deficits. Intellectual disability is common but may be mild.

### BOX 89.2 Causes of Congenital Aqueductal Stenosis

**Genetic or Presumed Genetic Causes**

Holoprosencephaly
Chiari II malformation
X-linked hydrocephalus with aqueductal stenosis and pachygyria
Autosomal recessive hydrocephalus with aqueductal stenosis
Mutation of dorsalizing gene in vertical axis of neural tube
Agenesis of mesencephalic and metencephalic neuromeres
Primary defective ependymal and choroid plexus epithelia (?)

**Acquired Causes in Utero**

Intraventricular hemorrhage with thrombus in aqueduct
Congenital infections (e.g., cytomegalovirus infection, mumps)
Ependymitis/ventriculitis with gliosis around and within aqueduct
Chronic arachnoiditis
Hydranencephaly
Aqueductal membrane across lumen
Amnion rupture sequence
Aneurysms, venous angiomas, and other vascular malformations
Cystic dilatation of perivascular Virchow-Robin spaces in midbrain
Tumors of aqueduct (e.g., ependymoma, astrocytoma, glioneuronal hamartoma, neuroepithelial tumor of subcommissural organ)
Tumors that compress the midbrain tectum from above (e.g., pineal tumors and cysts, arachnoidal cysts, lipomas)

## Congenital Aqueductal Stenosis

Another aspect for consideration in the category of disorders of neurulation is the downregulation of genes in the vertical axis of the neural tube. In the case of the ventrodorsal gradient due to defective sonic hedgehog (SHH) expression, sacral agenesis with dysplastic spinal cord at the levels of the deficient vertebrae (and notochord) is the best example. Downregulation in the dorsoventral gradient of several genes or gene families, including *ZIC2, SHH* in the forebrain, *BMP,* and *PAX,* may result in HPE (see following section on HPE) or may cause defective development of the dorsomedial septum of the midbrain with aqueductal stenosis (Sarnat and Flores-Sarnat, 2001a). Box 89.2 lists the various causes of congenital aqueductal stenosis (Sarnat and Flores-Sarnat, 2001a).

TABLE 89.3 **Best Documented Genetic Mutations in Holoprosencephaly**

| Chromosomal Locus | Defective Gene | Vertical Gradient Effect |
|---|---|---|
| 2p21 | *SIX3* | Dorsoventral |
| 7q36 | *SHH* | Ventrodorsal (spinal cord, hindbrain), dorsoventral (midbrain, forebrain)* |
| 13q32 | *ZIC2* | Dorsoventral |
| 18q11.3 | *TGIF* | Ventrodorsal |
| 9q22.3 | *PTCH* | Ventrodorsal |
| 10q11.2 | *DKK* | Ventrodorsal |

*Although *SHH* is a powerful ventralizing gene in the embryonic spinal cord and hindbrain, recent evidence indicates that at the level of the midbrain and most rostral regions of the neural tube, it changes its gradient and becomes dorsalizing in the vertical axis.

*Data from Blaess, S., Corrales, J.D., Joyner, A.L., 2006. Sonic hedgehog regulates Gli activator and repressor functions with spatial and temporal precision in the mid/hindbrain region. Development 133, 1799–1809.*

## Midline Malformations of the Forebrain (4–8 Weeks' Gestation)

Several developmental malformations of the prosencephalon relate embryologically to failure of the lamina terminalis to differentiate into telencephalic structures. The *lamina terminalis* is the rostral membrane of the primitive neural tube that forms with closure of the anterior neuropore. The expression of such disorders is mainly as midline defects, not only because of its location in the midline but also because of impaired lateral growth of the cerebral hemispheres due to deficient or abnormal cellular migration centrifugally to form the cerebral cortex. The series of midline prosencephalic malformations relates to the embryological time of the beginning of each and includes alobar, semilobar, and lobar HPE, arhinencephaly, septo-optic dysplasia, colpocephaly, and agenesis of the corpus callosum.

The lamina terminalis, after differentiating the forebrain structures, becomes the anterior wall of the third ventricle in the mature brain. It extends between the optic chiasm ventrally and the rostrum of the corpus callosum dorsally. Some authors contend that a defective cephalic notochord induces midline forebrain defects. Understanding of the complex embryological relationship of neuroectoderm and mesoderm in early ontogenesis is incomplete.

### Holoprosencephaly

HPE is a malformation in which the two cerebral hemispheres appear fused in the midline but is really a failure of cleavage in the midsagittal plane of the embryonic cerebral vesicle at 33 days' gestation and thus a paramedian hypoplasia of the forebrain (Fallet-Bianco, 2018). HPE has a frequency of one in 16,000 live births but one in 250 spontaneously aborted fetuses in the first trimester; hence it is among the most common of the major cerebral malformations.

Traditionally, HPE was a single malformation with three variants: alobar, semilobar, lobar. A fourth was added later: the middle interhemispheric variant (Hahn and Pinter, 2002; Simon et al., 2002). Another variant recently described is septopreoptic HPE, demonstrated as noncleavage restricted to the preoptic and septal region by MRI in seven patients (Hahn et al., 2010); we have now recognized two additional cases (unpublished). Recent molecular genetic data redefine HPE as a common end-stage malformation with six known different genetic mutations demonstrated in various cases (Golden, 1998; Table 89.3). Other chromosomal defects (in loci 3p26, 4,5, 6, 14q13, 14q21.1-q21.2, 20, 21q22.3) are known in which the specific genetic mutation is not yet identified. All six known defective genes together account for only about 20% of cases, so many more gene defects remain undiscovered. Furthermore, each of the traditional anatomical variants of HPE is demonstrable in each of the six known genetic forms, signifying that these merely represent degrees of severity without etiological implication. A defect in the *ZIC2* gene is associated with chromosome 13q deletions, and HPE is frequent in infants with trisomy 13 (Brown et al., 1998). One of the most studied of the genetic mutations is the strong ventralizing gene, *SHH*; lack of expression of this gene in the prechordal mesoderm ventral to the rostral end of the neural tube results in no neural induction (Roessler et al., 1996). Abnormal *SHH* expression also may be altered in metabolic diseases with impaired cholesterol synthesis and high serum levels of the cholesterol precursor molecule7-dehydrocholesterol, as in the Smith-Lemli-Opitz syndrome associated with HPE (Kelley et al., 1996).

After chromosomal defects, the most common association of HPE is maternal diabetes mellitus; sacral agenesis is another common malformation in infants of diabetic mothers. Both involve downregulation of SHH. A defect at the same chromosome 7p36.2 locus associated with an autosomal dominant form of HPE also affects SHH at the posterior, rather than the anterior, end of the neural tube and results in sacral agenesis (Lynch et al., 1995). Disturbed insulin metabolism may affect SHH in programming the neural tube.

Olfactory bulbs and tubercles differentiate at 41 days, a few days after forebrain cleavage, but olfactory agenesis usually accompanies all but the mildest forms of HPE; therefore, the term *arhinencephaly*, often used interchangeably, is incorrect. Callosal agenesis also is a uniform feature except in the mildest forms, and the cerebral mantle shows gross disorganization with multiple heterotopia, poorly laminated cortical gray matter, and heterotopic neurons and glial cells in the overlying meninges. Extensions of germinal matrix into the lateral ventricles through gaps in the ependyma are common. Thus, although HPE can be dated to about 33 days' gestation at onset, the pathological process extends throughout most of fetal life.

Five different anatomical variants of HPE reflect different degrees of abnormal cerebral architecture. Characteristic of alobar HPE is a brain with a single midline telencephalic ventricle rather than paired lateral ventricles and continuity of the cerebral cortex across the midline frontally. The roof of the monoventricle balloons into a dorsal cyst. The corpus striatum and thalamus of the two sides are uncleaved, and the third ventricle may obliterate with rudiments of ependymal rosettes in its place. In semilobar HPE, an incomplete interhemispheric fissure forms posteriorly, and the occipital lobes, including the occipital horns of the ventricular system, may approach a normal configuration despite noncleavage of the frontal lobes across the midline. Lobar HPE is a less severe dysgenesis; the hemispheres form well but are in continuity through a band of cortex at the frontal pole or the orbital surface, and the indusium griseum and cingulate gyri overlying the corpus callosum are in continuity. The corpus callosum incompletely forms but is not totally absent, as in alobar and semilobar HPE. The middle interhemispheric variant consists of hypoplasia of the middle part of the corpus callosum and associated structures of the medial side of the hemispheres. The most recently recognized and rarest form of HPE, demonstrated by MRI, is the septo-preoptic, which seems transitional between this malformation and septo-optic-pituitary dysplasia (Hahn et al. 2010).

In the more severe forms of HPE, the optic nerves are hypoplastic or fused to enter a single median eye. Midline cerebellar defects, absent pyramidal tracts, and malformed brainstem structures accompany the more severe forms of this malformation. Meningeal heterotopia or marginal glioneuronal nodules commonly result from overmigration, perhaps associated with hypoplasia or absence of the transitory external granular glial layer of Brun of the fetal brain in HPE.

The diagnosis of HPE often occurs at the time of delivery, because 93% of patients exhibit midline facial dysplasias. Midfacial hypoplasia is present in most patients with HPE, but others have a normal face. The facial dysmorphism ranges from mild hypotelorism and vomer bones to severe forms including cebocephaly with a single naris, severe hypotelorism and absence of the premaxilla and vomer bones to produce a midline cleft lip and palate, or cyclopia with a midline proboscis dorsal to the single median eye. This eye, resulting from fusion of the two lateral halves of the incipient globes, is associated with a persistent long hyaloids canal containing a hyaloids artery that normally regresses at 7 weeks' gestation; precocious synapse formation is seen around ganglion cells of the retina (Sarnat et al., 2014). The severity of the facial dysmorphism does not correlate as well with the anatomical variant as originally expressed in the often-cited statement "the face predicts the brain." Midfacial hypoplasia does correlate, however, with the rostrocaudal extent of the defective genetic expression. If the gradient extends to the embryonic mesencephalic neuromere and causes hypoplasia of the midbrain, neural crest formation and migration are affected (Sarnat and Flores-Sarnat, 2001a). The mesencephalic neural crest is the most rostral origin of neural crest, and this tissue forms not only peripheral neural structures such as the ciliary ganglion but also most of the membranous bones of the face, globe of the eye (except the retina and choroid), and much of the facial connective tissue.

The various forms of HPE are well demonstrated by most imaging techniques (Fig. 89.9), including prenatal ultrasound. The imaging features of each anatomical variant are distinctive (Hahn and Pinter, 2002) and correspond well to the gross neuropathological findings (Golden, 1998). The anterior cerebral artery is usually a single azygous vessel coursing just beneath the inner table of the skull, a pathognomonic finding. The sagittal sinuses, deformed or replaced by a network of large abnormal veins, resemble the early embryonic pattern of venous drainage.

The EEG in HPE shows multifocal spikes that often evolve into hypsarrhythmia. In the neonatal period, the characteristic feature of the waking EEG is almost continuous high-voltage alpha-theta monorhythmic activity, becoming discontinuous in sleep. VEPs also are abnormal or altogether absent. The characteristic clinical course of HPE is severe developmental delay and a mixed pattern of seizures that often are refractory to antiepileptic drugs. The presence or absence of seizures does not correlate with the anatomical severity or variant of the defective forebrain and correlates poorly with the genetic mutation (Hahn and Pinter, 2002). A better correlation may be with the degree of mediolateral extension of genetic expression in disrupting the histological architecture of the cortex, or it may relate to an abnormal sequence of maturation of axosomatic (inhibitory) and axodendritic (excitatory) synapses in relation to the maturation of the neuron innervated by these axonal terminations (Sarnat and Flores-Sarnat, 2001a). Some patients develop hydrocephalus that requires a ventriculoperitoneal shunt. This condition is paradoxically more common in the less severe anatomical forms of the malformation. In the severe alobar form, a "dorsal cyst" occupies the entire posterior one-half to two-thirds of the intracranial space and, occasionally, even protrudes through the anterior fontanelle as a unique encephalocele that may be larger than the rest of the head. No other type of encephalocele occurs at the anterior fontanelle. The dorsal cyst seems to originate from a dilated suprapineal recess of the third ventricle and later is a dorsal membrane that includes the roof of the forebrain, extending from the hippocampi (Sarnat and Flores-Sarnat, 2001a).

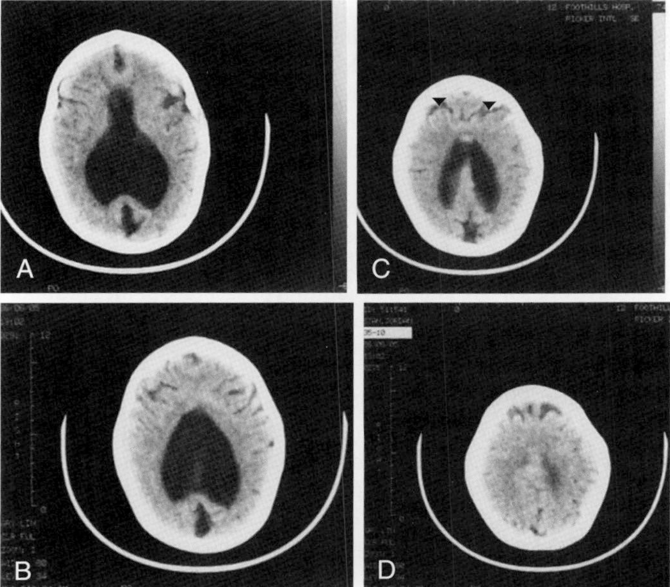

**Fig. 89.9** (A-D) Unenhanced computed tomographic scan of a 6-year-old boy with semilobar holoprosencephaly. The lateral ventricles are fused, particularly frontally, but show some division into two occipital horns. A deep abnormal sulcus is seen across the fused frontal lobes *(arrowheads)*. This is one of several radiological variants of holoprosencephaly.

Endocrine dysfunction may be present, associated with hypothalamic or pituitary involvement, and vasopressin-sensitive diabetes insipidus occurs in about 86% of cases, other hypothalamic–pituitary dysfunction being much less frequent (Plawner et al., 2002). The basis of this specific involvement of the paraventricular and supraoptic hypothalamic nuclei may be hypoplasia in some cases in which the midline hypoplasia involves the diencephalon as well as the forebrain (most patients), but it also occurs in some children without hypothalamic noncleavage. One hypothesis is that the primary gene defect suppresses expression of the gene orthopedia (*OTP*). *OTP* and downstream genes such as *SIM1* and *BRN2* are essential for terminal differentiation of neuroendocrine cells of these hypothalamic nuclei (Sarnat and Flores-Sarnat, 2001a).

The treatment of HPE symptoms entails treating the complications (e.g., seizures, hydrocephalus, endocrine disturbances). Educational potential and needs depend on the degree of intellectual, speech, and visual impairments.

### Isolated Arhinencephaly and Kallmann Syndrome

Absence of olfactory bulbs, tracts, and tubercles commonly accompanies extensive malformations such as HPE and septo-optic dysplasia but may occur with callosal agenesis or as an isolated cerebral anomaly. *Kallmann syndrome* is an X-linked autosomal dominant condition limited to males, in which anosmia secondary to arhinencephaly without other forebrain malformations is associated with lack of secretion of gonadotropic hormones. The defective gene is *KAL1* at the chromosome Xp22.3 locus. Also implicated is the *EMX2* gene, though schizencephaly does not occur with Kallmann syndrome (Taylor et al., 1999). Olfactory reflexes may be elicited in the neonate consistently after 32 weeks' gestation and provide a useful supplement to the neurological examination of newborns suspected of cerebral dysgenesis.

The olfactory bulb develops in a unique manner and also is unique in being the only special sensory system to not project efferent axons to the thalamus, because the deep granular cell core of the olfactory bulb that extends into the olfactory tract is its own thalamic equivalent (Sarnat and Flores-Sarnat, 2017b). Many abnormalities of olfactory bulb development are known in addition to agenesis. Some are abnormal lamination and fusion of the bulbs of the two sides (Sarnat and Flores-Sarnat, 2017a, 2017b).

## Septo-Optic-Pituitary Dysplasia

De Mosier first recognized the association of a rudimentary or absent septum pellucidum with hypoplasia of the optic nerves and chiasm in 1956. Underdevelopment of the corpus callosum and anterior commissure and detachment of the fornix from the ventral surface of the corpus callosum are additional features. Patients with this combination of anomalies overlap others with semilobar HPE, and some many children with septo-optic-pitutary dysplasia have hypoplasia of the olfactory bulbs arhinencephaly as well, though olfactory perception is not totally abolished (Sarnat and Flores-Sarnat, 2017a, 2017b).

Disturbances of the hypothalamic–pituitary axis often occur in septo-optic dysplasia, ranging from isolated growth hormone deficiency to panhypopituitarism and deficient secretion of antidiuretic hormone. Hypothalamic hamartomas, gliosis, and the absence of some hypothalamic nuclei may be associated with a histologically normal pituitary. Absence of the neurohypophysis is demonstrable postmortem in some cases.

Midline cerebellar defects and hydrocephalus occur inconsistently in septo-optic dysplasia. One cerebellar lesion, called *rhombencephalosynapsis* is aplasia of the vermis and midline fusion of the cerebellar hemispheres and of the dentate nuclei, probably the downregulation of a dorsalizing gene at the level of rhombomere 1 (Sarnat, 2000).

Clinical manifestations relate mainly to the endocrine deficiencies and vision impairment. Ataxia may be compensable if the cerebellar vermis is mildly involved. Seizures are uncommon. Intellectual development usually is normal. Hypertelorism is not a constant finding. Chromosome analysis is invariably normal. The gene *HEXS1* is is defective in at least some cases (Dattani et al., 1998). No reports of familial cases exist. However, a high incidence of teenage pregnancy and drug abuse in early gestation occurs in mothers of affected infants. Septo-optic-pituitary dysplasia has occurred in an infant of a diabetic mother.

## Rhombomeric Deletions and Ectopic Genetic Expression

Rare patients with absence of certain parts of the brain appear in the literature. Only recently, by understanding the families of genes responsible for neural tube segmentation (e.g., *HOX, WNT, PAX*), have these conditions been understood at the level of molecular embryology. Agenesis of the midbrain and upper pons (metencephalon) with cerebellar hypoplasia are attributable to the *EN2* gene, which produces an almost identical malformation in the knockout mouse model (Sarnat et al., 2002). *EN1* and *WNT1* genes also are essential for development of the mesencephalic and rhombomere 1, but the animal models of these genetic defects produce total agenesis of the cerebellum. *SHH* also regulates the temporal and spatial precision of the midbrain–hindbrain junction, mediated through *Gli* activator (Blaess et al., 2006). Absence of the corpus striatum might be due to mutation of the *EMX1* gene, which is essential in the programming of the basal telencephalon but not the cerebral cortex (Sarnat and Flores-Sarnat, 2001a). The Chiari malformations, particularly type II, were incompletely explained by mechanical theories of pathogenesis, but a molecular genetic hypothesis of ectopic expression provides a more complete and reasonable explanation (see the online section Chiari Malformation at http://expertconsult.inkling.com) (Sarnat and Flores-Sarnat, 2001b, 2004).  Despite documentation of many of these genetic malformations in experimental animal models, definitive confirmation in humans has not occurred.

## Agenesis of the Corpus Callosum

A commissural plate differentiates within the lamina terminalis at day 39 of embryonic life. The plate acts as a bridge for axonal passage and provides a preformed glial pathway to guide decussating growth cones of commissural axons. Microcystic degeneration in the commissural plate and physiological death of astrocytes precedes the interhemispheric projection of the first axons. The earliest callosal axons appear at 74 days in the human embryo, the genu and the splenium are recognizable at 84 days, and the adult morphology is achieved by 115 days.

The pathogenesis of callosal agenesis relates to the commissural plate; if this plate is not available to guide axons across, the corpus callosum does not develop. Failure of physiological degeneration of a portion of the plate results in a glial barrier to axonal passage and the disappearance or deflection of primordial callosal fibers posteriorly to another destination within their hemisphere of origin (bundle of Probst). Other destinations of callosal axons that are unable to cross the midline at their expected site include passage into the anterior commissure, which can become enlarged as much as four times its normal volume by the addition of these axons; aberrant sites of crossing of individual fibers not forming large bundles; and, occasionally, callosal axons descending within the internal capsule with the corticospinal tract as far as the spinal cord, where their termination and function remain unknown (Sarnat, 2008). The anterior commissure also passes through the embryonic lamina terminalis, more ventrally than the corpus callosum; its earliest pioneer axons traverse the midline 3 weeks earlier than those of the corpus callosum, at about 7–8 weeks' gestation (Cho et al., 2013). Tridimensional diffusion tensor imaging (tractography) now enables assessment of white-matter connectivity prenatally, including corpus callosal fibers that are unable to cross the midline normally at the commissural plate, in second and third trimester fetuses (Kasprian et al., 2013).

Agenesis of the corpus callosum is a common malformation, having a 2.3% prevalence in computed tomography (CT) scans in North America and 7%–9% prevalence in Japan. Most cases are isolated malformations, but callosal agenesis is an additional feature of many other prosencephalic dysplasias; it also occurs with aplasia of the cerebellar vermis and anomalous pyramidal tract. Simple callosal agenesis may involve the entire commissure or may be partial, usually affecting only the posterior fibers. Hypoplasia or partial agenesis of the commissure is much more common than total agenesis. In callosal agenesis, the anterior and hippocampal commissures are always well formed or large.

A rare genetic form of callosal agenesis is associated with defective neural crest migration causing aganglionic megacolon (Hirschsprung disease). The cause is a defective human gene, Smad-interacting protein 1 (*SMAD1*), at the chromosome 2q22-q23 locus (Cacheux et al., 2001). In the absence of a corpus callosum, the lateral ventricles displace laterally, and the third ventricle rises between them (Fig. 89.10). Often the ventricles dilate mildly, but intraventricular pressure is normal. The anomaly may be demonstrable by most imaging techniques. The varying degrees of partial callosal agenesis produce several radiographic variants.

Clinical symptoms of callosal agenesis may be minimal and unrecognized in children of normal intelligence. Detailed neurological

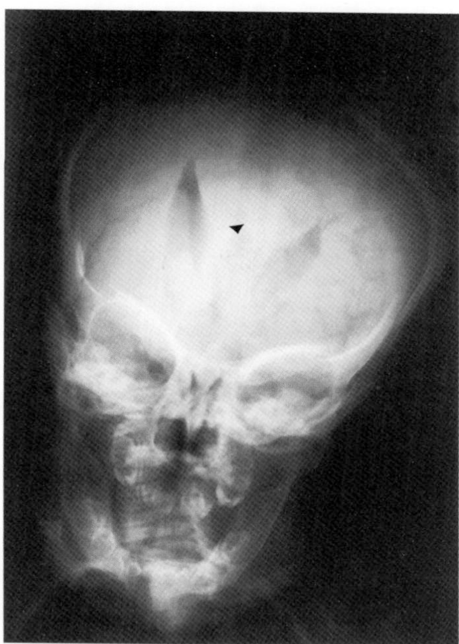

**Fig. 89.10** Pneumoencephalogram (from the preimaging period) of an 18-month-old boy with agenesis of the corpus callosum associated with an interhemispheric arachnoidal cyst *(arrowhead)*, a complication of some cases of callosal agenesis. The lateral ventricles are widely separated from the medial side of each hemisphere by the bundle of Probst; the third ventricle rises between them. The brainstem, cerebellum, and cerebral cortical convolutions appear normal. The patient has intellectual disability and epilepsy.

examination discloses deficits in the interhemispheric transfer of perceptual information for verbal expression. Intellectual disability or learning disabilities occur in some cases. Epilepsy is common, particularly in patients diagnosed early in life. Seizures may relate more to minor focal cortical dysplasias than to the callosal agenesis itself. Hypertelorism is present in many and often is associated with exotropia and inability to converge.

The EEG characteristically shows interhemispheric asynchrony or poor organization, with or without multifocal spikes, but is not specific enough to establish the diagnosis. Asynchronous sleep spindles after 18 months of age are a good clue to the diagnosis. Several hereditary forms of callosal agenesis occur besides its occurrence as an additional anomaly in some cases of tuberous sclerosis and other genetic syndromes. Andermann syndrome is an autosomal recessive syndrome of callosal agenesis, mental deficiency, and peripheral neuropathy. Aicardi syndrome consists of agenesis of the corpus callosum, chorioretinal lacunae, vertebral anomalies, intellectual disability, and myoclonic epilepsy. This disorder is found almost exclusively in girls and is thought to be X-linked dominant (Xp22) and generally lethal in the male fetus. The EEG shows a typically asymmetrical asynchronous burst-suppression pattern. Neuropathological findings in Aicardi syndrome include a variety of minor dysplasias in addition to agenesis of the corpus callosum and anterior commissure, and nonlaminated polymicrogyric cortex with abnormally oriented neurons. Callosal agenesis is a common component in many chromosomal disorders, particularly trisomies 8, 11, and 13. Interhemispheric lipoma replacing part of the corpus callosum is associated with a high incidence of epilepsy.

### Colpocephaly

Colpocephaly is a selective dilatation of the occipital horns, *not* due to increased intraventricular pressure but rather due to loss of white matter. Colpocephaly occurs in three conditions:

1. It appears as a primary malformation, histologically associated with poorly laminated striate cortex, subcortical heterotopia, and defective ependymal lining of the occipital horns.
2. It is common in many cases of agenesis of the corpus callosum because of absence of the splenium and hypoplasia of white matter.
3. It may be the acquired result of periventricular leukomalacia, especially in premature infants, because of loss of periventricular white matter in the posterior half of the cerebral hemispheres.

Clinical findings are usually those of intellectual disability, spastic diplegia, epilepsy, and vision loss, but it does not always cause complete blindness. CT in the neonatal period or early infancy demonstrates most cases. Isotope cisternography shows normal CSF dynamics in most. Colpocephaly is associated with several syndromes and systemic disorders including cerebrohepatorenal (Zellweger) disease, hemimegalencephaly, and several chromosomal disorders. The EEG in colpocephaly ranges from normal in mild cases to near-hypsarrhythmia in infants who develop myoclonic epilepsy. Bilateral posterior slowing of low voltage with occipital spikes is common. Colpocephaly also develops late in fetal life because of infarction and cystic degeneration of the deep white matter of the posterior third of the cerebral hemispheres, rather than as a developmental disorder of neuroblast migration. It is often confused with hydrocephalus.

## Disorders of Early Neuroblast Migration (8–20 Weeks' Gestation)

### Lissencephaly (Agyria, Sometimes With Pachygyria)

Lissencephaly is a failure of development of convolutions in the cerebral cortex because of defective neuroblast migration. The cortex remains smooth, as in the embryonic brain (see Fig. 89.8). The migrations of the cerebellum and the brainstem also usually are involved, but the thalamus and basal ganglia form properly. Structural and metabolic abnormalities of the fetal ependyma may be supplementary factors in disturbing the normal development of radial glial cells.

The cytoarchitecture of the neocortex in lissencephaly takes one of two forms. In the first, a four-layered sequence develops. The outermost layer is a widened molecular zone; layer 2 contains neurons corresponding to those of normal laminae III, V, and VI; layer 3 is cell-sparse; and layer 4 contains heterotopic neurons that have migrated incompletely. Decreased brain size leads to microcephaly with widened ventricles, representing a fetal stage rather than pressure from hydrocephalus, and an uncovered sylvian fossa representing lack of operculation. The second form of cortical architectural abnormality in lissencephaly is disorganized clusters of neurons with haphazard orientation, forming no definite layers or predictable pattern. Type 2 lissencephaly is associated with several closely related genetic syndromes: Walker-Warburg syndrome, Fukuyama muscular dystrophy, muscle-eye-brain disease of Santavuori, and Meckel-Grüber syndrome, the latter often associated with posterior encephalocele (see Fig. 89.8).

Additional text available at http://expertconsult.inkling.com. 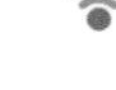

## Disturbances of Late Neuroblast Migration (after 20 Weeks' Gestation)

Additional text available at http://expertconsult.inkling.com. 

## Disorders of Cerebellar Development (32 Days' Gestation to 1 Year Postnatally)

Additional text available at http://expertconsult.inkling.com. 

*The complete reference list is available online at https://expertconsult.inkling.com.* 

90

# Autism and Other Neurodevelopmental Disabilities

*Reet Sidhu, D. David O'Banion, Christine Hall*

## OUTLINE



## AUTISM SPECTRUM DISORDERS

### Diagnostic Criteria

Autism spectrum disorder (ASD) is a neurodevelopmental disorder characterized by impairments in two areas: (1) deficits in social communication and social interactions; and (2) restricted and repetitive patterns of behavior, interests, and activities (APA, 2013a). With the revised *Diagnostic and Statistical Manual of Mental Disorders,* 5th edition (DSM-5), ASD now subsumes what were previously separate diagnostic categories of autistic disorder (also referred to as classic autism or early infantile autism), pervasive developmental disorder–not otherwise specified (PDD-NOS), and Asperger syndrome. The changes are based on research results which, thus far, have failed to document either PDD-NOS or Asperger syndrome as separate biological entities. The prior diagnostic manual also included deficits in language expression as a criterion, but this is no longer the case as not all children with ASD have language disorders. However, pragmatic language skills are incorporated into the social domain as all individuals with ASD have deficits in this domain of language. Under the DSM-5, diagnosis of ASD requires an individual to exhibit three deficits in social communication and at least two symptoms in the category of restricted range of activities/repetitive behaviors. Within the second category, a new symptom is included: hyper- or hyporeactivity to sensory input or unusual interests in sensory aspects of the environment. Deficits in social communication and interactions include those in social reciprocity, nonverbal communication, and skills in developing, maintaining, and understanding social relationships. Symptoms must be present in early development but need not be shown until social demands exceed the individual's capacity. Furthermore, DSM-5 specifies three levels of severity (mild, moderate, severe) rated separately for social communication and restricted, repetitive behaviors, based on what level of support the individual requires. In addition to the diagnosis, individuals are also described in terms of any known genetic cause (e.g., fragile X syndrome [FXS], Rett syndrome), level of language and intellectual disability (ID), and presence of medical conditions such as seizures, psychiatric disorders (e.g., anxiety, depression), and/or gastrointestinal disorders. (See Box 90.1 and Table 90.1 for DSM-5 criteria for ASD.) The range of disabilities seen among children on the spectrum cannot be overemphasized.

### Epidemiology

There has been a significant increase in the prevalence of ASD in the United States, particularly since the late 1990s. In the 1990s, the estimated frequency was about 1 per 1000 for autism and 2 per 1000 for ASD (Williams et al., 2006), while, more recently, the estimated prevalence is much higher. The Autism and Developmental Disabilities Monitoring Network (2018), which identifies ASD through screening and review of health and education records that document behaviors associated with ASD in 11 sites in the United States, most recently reported a prevalence rate of 16.8 per 1000 (1 in 59) among 8 year olds, with prevalence estimates varying from 5.7 to 21.9 per 1000 in the different sites. Non-Hispanic White children were approximately 7% more likely to be identified with ASD than non-Hispanic Black children and 22% more than Hispanic children. ASDs are four times more likely in males than in females.

Whether there has been an actual increase in ASD prevalence or if the apparent increase is due to other factors is still under investigation. Factors such as increased awareness among parents and professionals (Fombonne, 2009), broadening of the diagnosis with emphasis on the spectrum aspect of the disorder, including mildly affected individuals (Shattuck, 2006; Wing and Potter, 2002), change in referral patterns, and using the diagnosis as a basis for intervention services (Blumberg et al., 2013; Idring et al., 2014; Shieve et al., 2011) may account for an apparent increase in prevalence rates. Both advanced maternal and paternal age may play a role in increasing the frequency of autism (Durkin et al., 2008). The theory that the measles, mumps, rubella (MMR) vaccine plays any role in the increase has been completely discredited (Marshall et al., 2015, Maglione et al., 2014).

The prevalence of ASD in siblings of children with ASD ranges from 2% to 18% (Lauritesen et al., 2005; Ozonoff et al., 2011; Schaefer and Mendelsohn, 2013). The high concordance in monozygotic twins (Rosenberg et al., 2009), the increased risk for recurrence in siblings (≈5%–10%), a broader autistic phenotype in families with an autistic proband,

## BOX 90.1 DSM-5 Criteria for an Autistic Spectrum Disorder

A. Persistent deficits in social communication and social interaction across multiple contexts, as manifested by the following, currently or by history (examples are illustrative, not exhaustive, see text):

1. Deficits in social-emotional reciprocity, ranging, for example, from abnormal social approach and failure of normal back-and-forth conversation; to reduced sharing of interests, emotions, or affect; to failure to initiate or respond to social interactions.
2. Deficits in nonverbal communicative behaviors used for social interaction, ranging, for example, from poorly integrated verbal and nonverbal communication; to abnormalities in eye contact and body language or deficits in understanding and use of gestures; to a total lack of facial expressions and nonverbal communication.
3. Deficits in developing, maintaining, and understanding relationships, ranging, for example, from difficulties adjusting behavior to suit various social contexts; to difficulties in sharing imaginative play or in making friends; to absence of interest in peers.

   Specify current severity:

   Severity is based on social communication impairments and restricted repetitive patterns of behavior (see Table 90.8).

B. Restricted, repetitive patterns of behavior, interests, or activities, as manifested by at least two of the following, currently or by history (examples are illustrative, not exhaustive; see text):

1. Stereotyped or repetitive motor movements, use of objects, or speech (e.g., simple motor stereotypies, lining up toys or flipping objects, echolalia, idiosyncratic phrases).
2. Insistence on sameness, inflexible adherence to routines, or ritualized patterns or verbal nonverbal behavior (e.g., extreme distress at small changes, difficulties with transitions, rigid thinking patterns, greeting rituals, need to take same route or eat food every day).
3. Highly restricted, fixated interests that are abnormal in intensity or focus (e.g., strong attachment to or preoccupation with unusual objects, excessively circumscribed or perseverative interest).
4. Hyper- or hyporeactivity to sensory input or unusual interests in sensory aspects of the environment (e.g., apparent indifference to pain/temperature, adverse response to specific sounds or textures, excessive smelling or touching of objects, visual fascination with lights or movement).

   Specify current severity:

   Severity is based on social communication impairments and restricted, repetitive patterns of behavior (see Table 90.8).

C. Symptoms must be present in the early developmental period (but may not become fully manifest until social demands exceed limited capacities, or may be masked by learned strategies in later life).

D. Symptoms cause clinically significant impairment in social, occupational, or other important areas of current functioning.

E. These disturbances are not better explained by intellectual disability (intellectual developmental disorder) or global developmental delay. Intellectual disability and autism spectrum disorder frequently co-occur; to make comorbid diagnoses of autism spectrum disorder and intellectual disability, social communication should be below that expected for general developmental level.

Note: Individuals with a well-established DSM-5 diagnosis of autistic disorder, Asperger disorder, or pervasive developmental disorder not otherwise specified should be given the diagnosis of autism spectrum disorder. Individuals who have marked deficits in social communication, but whose symptoms do not otherwise meet criteria for autism spectrum disorder, should be evaluated for social (pragmatic) communication disorder.

Specify if:

With or without accompanying intellectual impairment

With or without accompanying language impairment

Associated with a known medical or genetic condition or environmental factor

Associated with another neurodevelopmental, mental, or behavioral disorder

With catatonia

*Reprinted with permission from the Diagnostic and Statistical Manual of Mental Disorders, Fifth Edition (© 2013). American Psychiatric Association.*

## TABLE 90.1 Severity Levels for Autism Spectrum Disorder

| Severity Level | Social Communication | Restricted, Repetitive Behaviors |
|---|---|---|
| Level 3 "Requiring very substantial support" | Severe deficits in verbal and nonverbal social communication skills cause severe impairments in functioning, very limited initiation of social interactions, and minimal response to social overtures from others. For example, a person with few words of intelligible speech who rarely initiates interaction and, when he or she does, makes unusual approaches to meet needs only and responds to only very direct social approaches | Inflexibility of behavior, extreme difficulty coping with change, or other restricted/repetitive behaviors markedly interfere with functioning in all spheres. Great distress/difficulty changing focus or action |
| Level 2 "Requiring substantial support" | Marked deficits in verbal and nonverbal social communication skills; social impairments apparent even with supports in place; limited initiation of social interactions; and reduced or abnormal responses to social overtures from others. For example, a person who speaks simple sentences, whose interaction is limited to narrow special interests, and who has markedly odd nonverbal communication | Inflexibility of behavior, difficulty coping with change, or other restricted/repetitive behaviors appear frequently enough to be obvious to the casual observer and interfere with functioning in a variety of contexts. Distress and/or difficulty changing focus or action |
| Level 1 "Requiring support" | Without supports in place, deficits in social communication cause noticeable impairments. Difficulty initiating social interactions, and clear examples of atypical or unsuccessful response to social overtures of others. May appear to have decreased interest in social interactions. For example, a person who is able to speak in full sentences and engages in communication but whose to-and-fro conversation with others fails, and whose attempts to make friends are odd and typically unsuccessful | Inflexibility of behavior causes significant interference with functioning in one or more contexts. Difficulty switching between activities. Problems of organization and planning hamper independence |

*Reprinted with permission from the Diagnostic and Statistical Manual of Mental Disorders, Fifth Edition, (© 2013). American Psychiatric Association.*

which includes anxiety and mood as well as social style and obsessive characteristics (Daniels et al., 2008), and the association with a number of genetic disorders support a hereditary basis in many cases (Gillberg, 2010).

Developmental regression or loss of previously established skills during the first 1–3 years of life has been estimated as occurring in approximately one-third of children with ASD at an average age of 1.78 years (Barger et al., 2013). A meta-analysis of studies on the prevalence of developmental regression in children with ASD found that rates differed based on type of regression measured. Studies focusing on language regression (e.g., loss of words) were estimated as occurring in 25%; those on both language and social regression (e.g., play skills, joint attention, response to name) in 38%; mixed regression (including cognitive and/or motor skills) in 33%; and unspecified regression in 39%. Similarly, regression prevalence differed based on sampling methods, with population-based studies showing a prevalence rate of 22%; clinic-based prevalence at 34%; and parent survey-based prevalence as 41% (Barger et al., 2013). While most studies on regression in autism have relied on retrospective parent reports, recently there has been a shift towards prospective studies that focus on infants who are at genetically high risk for autism. These studies have tracked early-appearing social behaviors such as shared affect, social interest, gaze to face and eyes, and response to name. In a review of these prospective studies, Ozonoff and Iosif (2019) found evidence that most children with autism had a period of relatively typical development followed by decline in social behaviors starting at about 9 months. In some studies, as many as 80% of infants with ASD demonstrated this early regression in social behaviors (Jones et al., 2014; Ozonoff et al., 2018b; Pearson et al., 2018).

While ASD cannot be reliably diagnosed until 18 months of age, there is evidence that ASD can be detected as early as 12 months old based on early social behaviors, including looking at people, use of gestures, response to name, and repetitive motor actions (Osterling et al., 2002). An eye-tracking study found that typical eye gaze is present but declines in 2- to 6-month-old children who are later diagnosed with ASD (Johnson and Klin, 2013).

## Clinical Features

The intelligence quotient (IQ) is not one of the defining criteria for an ASD diagnosis (Matson and Shoemaker, 2009). The Autism and Developmental Disabilities Monitoring Network (2018) found that 31% of children with ASD have an ID (IQ < 70), 25% are in the borderline range (IQ 71–85), and 44% have IQ scores in the average to above average range (i.e., IQ > 85). Normal range IQ is a positive prognostic sign. Having a higher verbal IQ at 2–3 years of age appears to predict better outcome, particularly if intervention is delivered early (Anderson et al., 2014) Long-term prognosis also correlates with acquisition of language skills. An estimated one-third of people with autism are nonverbal, and those with verbal language often demonstrate significant difficulties with prosody and pragmatic language (Rapin and Tuchman, 2006; Tager-Flusberg et al., 2009). Individuals with conversational language by age 5–6 do significantly better than children with little or no language. Early joint attention (the ability to draw another person's attention to an object of interest through the use of eye gaze and gestures, such as pointing), as well as vocal and motor imitation skills, was more impaired in children who did not develop language by age 5 (but had relatively strong nonverbal cognitive skills) than in children who did develop language by 5 years (Thurm et al., 2007).

The dominant feature of ASD is a difference in a child's social communication and interaction. Typically developing children show a natural proclivity to learn from the social world, and they seek out social input spontaneously and frequently starting in the first weeks of life. By contrast, children with ASD tend to be more drawn to interaction with the physical world (Klin et al., 2002) and are less likely to show interest in interacting with others. They tend to have difficulty attending to others, interpreting the social intent of others, and sharing enjoyment. In toddlers and preschoolers, social deficits include reduced eye contact, reduced enjoyment in social games, lack of joint attention, and lack of interest in other children. Because of these social vulnerabilities, they struggle to learn appropriate social communication strategies including verbal speech as well as nonverbal communication strategies such as gestures and body language. They also tend to struggle to engage in age-appropriate functional and pretend play with others. As children with ASD progress through school, they can struggle with forming friendships, engaging appropriately in back-and-forth conversation, appropriate body language, and knowing how to initiate and respond to interactions with their peers appropriately.

A restricted range of behaviors, interests, and activities is another hallmark feature of autism. Many children with ASD demonstrate stereotypic motor behaviors such as hand flapping, tensing and shaking, toe walking, or spinning. In addition, they may use language in repetitive or idiosyncratic ways such as echoing statements made by others or heard on television, or repeating certain sounds/words/phrases over and over again. They may also like spinning, dropping, or lining up objects, or opening and closing doors. Second, children with ASD often are highly dependent on routines or rituals and have significant difficulty with change or transitions. Third, children with autism may be overly focused on a particular topic, object, or area of interest. For example, a child may be fixated on trains, super heroes, bunnies, the constitutional convention, or air conditioning units. Finally, children with ASD often demonstrate differences in how they respond to sensory input. They may seek out sensory input in unusual ways such as smelling or licking objects, or rubbing items on their face. In other instances, they may be highly sensitive to sensory input such as loud noises, textures, or crowded environments.

### Evaluation

The clinical history and observations of the child are the basis for the diagnosis of an ASD. Research indicates that ASDs may be identified as young as 18 months of age or younger. By age 2 years, it is expected that a qualified professional can reliably make the diagnosis. The American Academy of Pediatrics recommends screening all children at well-child visits at 18 months and at 24 months of age (Johnson et al., 2007). A number of questionnaires and observation measures are available to screen for ASDs. Probably the most commonly used is the Modified Checklist for Autism in Toddlers–Revised (M-CHAT-R), which is a parent-completed questionnaire designed to identify children at risk for autism in the general population.

There are a number of tools used to assess ASDs, but experts believe that no single tool should be used to make a diagnosis. The Autism Diagnostic Observation Schedule-2 (ADOS-2) is considered the "gold standard" in diagnosing ASD. It consists of a semi-structured, standardized assessment of social interaction, play, and imaginative use of material for individuals suspected of having ASDs from 12 months old to adults. The ADOS often is used in conjunction with the Autism Diagnostic Interview–Revised (ADI-R), a clinical diagnostic interview for diagnosing autism in children and adults with mental ages of 18 months and above that focuses on assessing reciprocal social interactions, communication, and language; and restricted and repetitive, stereotyped interests and behaviors. Both the ADOS and ADI-R are time consuming and the ADOS requires special training to administer and score. Other well-known assessments include the Childhood Autism Rating Scale–Second Edition (CARS-2) that is appropriate for children over age 2 and draws from observations on different areas of behavior associated with ASDs. Several rating scales, such as the Social Responsiveness Scale (SRS-2) and the Social Communication Questionnaire (ScQ) can be helpful for eliciting information from parents and teachers.

The standard neurological examination is generally normal, although children with ASDs are often clumsy and have mild hypotonia.

Macrocephaly occurs in about one-third of children with autism and generally becomes apparent around the age of 1–3 years. The fact that macrocephaly is not present at birth suggests there is an increased rate of brain growth in the first years of life that diminishes and may become subnormal in later childhood; macrocephaly in adults with autism is less common than in children with ASD (Sacco et al., 2007). Skin examination requires careful attention, given high co-occurrence with tuberous sclerosis (Gillberg, 2010). Dysmorphology examination should be performed to facilitate the diagnosis of genetic syndromes (e.g., FXS, velocardiofacial syndrome, and Smith-Magenis syndrome). Hearing impairment should be excluded by a formal audiology assessment. Electroencephalogram (EEG), including a sleep record or overnight video-EEG monitoring, is appropriate when seizures occur or if developmental regression has occurred (see the Epilepsy section).

There are multiple neurometabolic causes of ASD, many of which are not usually associated with any dysmorphology. Primary inborn errors of metabolism in simple (e.g., nonsyndromic) autism are a rare occurrence. Treatable conditions include PKU (phenylketonuria), hyperammonemia/urea cycle defects, and creatine synthesis/creatine transporter defects. Other conditions include purine and pyrimidine abnormalities, Smith-Lemli-Opitz syndrome, and lysosomal storage disorders. Primary mitochondrial disease and ASD is a subject of much debate. Some investigators report a significant incidence of mitochondrial DNA changes or functional disturbances in children with ASD but whether these are the primary cause of ASD remains to be defined. The extent of the evaluation for an underlying metabolic disorder depends on clinical suspicion and the relevance to family counseling. Box 90.2 lists some disorders that can be associated with an ASD phenotype.

## Medical Comorbidities

Medical comorbidities frequently occur in ASD, including epilepsy, gastrointestinal dysfunction, sleep disorders, and psychiatric conditions (e.g., anxiety, depression, obsessive-compulsive disorder [OCD]). It is important to consider medical causes for any change in behavior, especially in those individuals who are nonverbal or with limited language capability. Examples of such medical conditions include, but are not limited to, the following: pain (due to migraine headaches, ear infection, fractures, etc.), gastrointestinal disorders (e.g., gastroesophageal reflux disorder [GERD], constipation), gastrourinary conditions (e.g., urinary tract infection [UTI]), hormonal imbalance/endocrine dysfunction (e.g., menstruation), and sleep disturbance (e.g., sleep apnea).

## Epilepsy

The association of epilepsy with autism provided one of the first clues to suggest that autism was a neurodevelopmental disorder of brain function. It is now well established that individuals with ASD have a higher risk of epilepsy than the general population. Epilepsy is commonly reported to occur in approximately one-third of individuals with ASD but the exact prevalence is unknown, with reports in the literature ranging from 5% to 46% (Spence and Schneider, 2009). Variation in estimates is likely related to multiple factors such as sample ascertainment, degree of ID, age, gender, and type of ASD (simple/nonsyndromic vs. complex/syndromic). ID and motor impairments (e.g., cerebral palsy) have been identified most commonly as significant risk factors for epilepsy in ASD, with higher rates in those with more severe cognitive impairments (Amiet et al., 2008; Hara, 2007; Parmeggiani, Barcia, Posar, & et al, 2010a, 2010b, Viscidi et al., 2013). Age of onset of epilepsy in ASD has generally been thought to occur in two peaks, one in early childhood (<5 years) and the other in adolescence (10–15 years) (Kawasaki et al., 2010, Parmeggiani et al., 2010a, 2010b). However, the peak, before age 5 years, includes those children with ASD secondary to infantile spasms (frequently as part of tuberous sclerosis) and other epileptic encephalopathies. A community-based study of ASD in children with epilepsy has found that only 5%–15% of children with epilepsy have autism (Berg et al., 2011).

Given the prevalence of epilepsy in autism, it is important to consider the possibility of seizures when evaluating an individual with autism, but currently there is inadequate evidence to recommend EEG in all individuals with autism (Filipek et al., 2000; Johnson et al., 2007; Kagan-Kushnir et al., 2005). Although all seizure types are present in ASD, the most commonly observed are complex partial seizures (85%) and generalized tonic-clonic seizures (7%). Absence and myoclonic seizures occur less commonly (1%–4%) (Yasuhara, 2010).

ASD can occur in the context of other comorbid medical conditions. Some of the most widely recognized syndromes associated with ASD and epilepsy include tuberous sclerosis, FXS, MECP2-related disorders (Rett syndrome), Angelman syndrome, and 15q duplication

### BOX 90.2 Double Syndromes: Medical Disorders Associated With Autistic Spectrum Disorder Phenotypes

**Genetic and Metabolic Disorders**

Angelman
CHARGE association
Cohen
de Lange
DiGeorge (22q11 deletions)
Fragile X
Hypomelanosis of Ito
Joubert
Lujan-Fryns
Moebius sequence
Neurofibromatosis
Noonan
Oculoauriculovertebral spectrum (including Goldenhar)
Partial monosomy 1p36
Partial tetrasomy 15
Prader-Willi
PTEN
Rett complex
Sex chromosome aneuploidies
Sotos
Smith-Magenis
Timothy
Tuberous sclerosis
Williams

**Metabolic Disorders**

Adenylosuccinate lyase deficiency
Cerebral folate deficiency
Cystathionine β-synthase deficiency
Dihydropyrimidinase deficiency
Disorders of creatine transport or metabolism
Ehlers-Danlos syndrome
Homocysteine
Marfan syndrome
Mitochondrial disorders
Mucopolysaccharidosis, including Sanfilippo
Smith-Lemli-Opitz syndrome
Succinic semialdehyde dehydrogenase deficiency
Urea cycle disorders

*Modified from Gillberg, C., 2010. Double syndromes: autism associated with genetic, medical and metabolic disorders. In: Nass, R.D., Frank, Y. (Eds.), Cognitive and Behavioral Manifestations of Pediatric Diseases. Oxford University Press, New York, pp. 100–110.*

syndrome. A targeted physical examination should consider other risk factors for epilepsy including head circumference (microcephaly), dysmorphisms, skin lesions (tuberous sclerosis, neurofibromatosis type 1 [NF-1]), and focal neurological findings. It is crucial to assess for medical comorbidities which may mimic seizures, including sleep disorders, GERD, and other gastrointestinal disorders, and psychiatric disorders including attention-deficit/hyperactivity disorder (ADHD).

Epileptiform EEG abnormalities are frequently seen in children with ASD, with or without epilepsy. Interictal epileptiform discharges (IEDs) are detected in approximately 20% of ASD children without epilepsy and 80% of ASD children with epilepsy on routine EEG (Chez et al., 2006; Hara 2007; Hughes and Melyn, 2005). Since these background or epileptiform EEG abnormalities can occur in ASD individuals without a clinical history of seizures, they are not to be considered evidence for epilepsy. The significance of these abnormalities, especially in the absence of clinical seizures, is quite unclear. At the present time, there are no data to support the use of antiepileptic drugs or epilepsy surgery in the treatment of these abnormalities in the absence of clinical seizures (Tuchman, 2004). The relationship of autistic regression to epilepsy and epileptiform EEG abnormalities is unclear. Findings in the literature are inconsistent with some studies reporting higher rates of epilepsy in children with ASD and regression, and others showing no relationship (Chez et al., 2006; Hrdlicka et al., 2004; McVicar et al., 2005; Tuchman and Rapin, 1997). However, language regression is a hallmark of Landau-Kleffner syndrome (LKS), a rare childhood-onset epileptic encephalopathy in which loss of previously acquired language skills occurs in the context of an epileptiform EEG activated in sleep. Electrical status epilepticus (ESES) during slow-wave sleep is the electroencephalographic pattern seen in LKS. The degree of overlap between LKS, ESES, and autistic regression with epileptiform EEG is currently poorly understood, although it is known that this ESES is rarely seen in children with a more global autistic regression (Galanopoulou et al., 2002; Tuchman and Rapin, 2002). At the current time, there are no data to support the use of LKS- or ESES-specific treatment regimens in those with more classic autistic regression and epileptiform EEG without clinical seizures.

## Etiology

***Genetics.*** ASDs are clinically and etiologically heterogeneous. Twin and family studies provide evidence for ASD as a highly genetic disorder with heritability estimates of 85%–92%. A recent large multinational population-based cohort study, which included more than 2 million individuals from five countries, estimated the heritability of ASD to be approximately 80% (Bai et al., 2019). With routine use of chromosomal microarray (CMA) and more recently whole-exome and genome sequencing, a genetic correlate can be identified in 30%–40% of children with ASD (Schaefer and Mendelsohn, 2013). Having an etiological diagnosis offers clinicians the opportunity to provide better guidance regarding recurrence risks, as well as prognostic information, and obviates the need for additional medical or neurodiagnostic testing. Furthermore, a specific diagnosis can alert clinicians to be aware of other comorbidities associated with certain genetic syndromes to provide more personalized care.

Known genetic causes of ASD include cytogenetically visible chromosomal abnormalities (5%), copy number variants (CNVs) (e.g., submicroscopic deletions and duplications) (10%–20%), and single-gene disorders in which neurological findings are associated with ASD (5%–10%). CMA has replaced high-resolution chromosomes as the initial test of choice to evaluate children with ASD. CMA has identified clinically relevant de novo genetic imbalances in 7%–20% of individuals with autism of unknown cause. As CMA will not detect balanced translocations or low-level mosaicism, a karyotype should be done when there is a family history of multiple miscarriages or there is high suspicion of mosaic aneuploidy.

The most frequent chromosome abnormality found in 1%–3% of individuals with ASD is maternally derived 15q11q13 duplication (Hogart et al., 2010). Aneuploidies are also found in ASD: 21 (Down syndrome), X (Turner syndrome, Klinefelter syndrome, XXX syndrome), and Y (XYY syndrome) (Devlin and Scherer, 2012).

Monogenic syndromes are found in 5%–10% of individuals with ASD. The most common is FXS, which is found in 1.5%–3%, and is caused by mutations in the *FMR1* gene. Tuberous sclerosis (*TSC1* and *TSC2* genes) occurs in about 1% of patients diagnosed with ASD. Mutations in the MECP2 protein (methyl CpG-binding protein 2) are known to cause Rett syndrome and are found in 1% of females with ASD. Mutations in the *PTEN* gene are found in ASD with macrocephaly (occipital frontal head circumference [OFD] > 3 standard deviations [3 SD] above the mean). Other single gene disorders associated with ASD include neurofibromatosis, type 1 (*NF1* gene), Duchene muscular dystrophy (*DMD* gene), and Timothy syndrome (*CACNA1C* gene) (Wisniowiecka and Nowakowska, 2019).

The most common autism-related CNVs are 16p11.2 microdeletions and microduplications that are identified in about 1% of individuals with ASD. Individuals with deletions have commonly been found to have macrocephaly versus those with duplications often have microcephaly. Other recurrent CNVs found in ASD include 1q21.1, 15q13.3, 17p11.2, 22q11.2, 16p13.1, and microduplication of 7q11.23 (Wisniowiecka and Nowakowska, 2019).

Mutations in genes encoding synaptic adhesion molecules like neuroligin, neurexin, contactin-associated protein (CNTNAP), and cell-adhesion molecule 1 (CADM1) suggest that impaired synaptic function underlies ASDs (Miller et al., 2005). However, knockout mouse models of these mutations do not show the full range of autistic symptoms. This could mean that gain of function as well as loss of function arising from these mutations is required for the full ASD picture. Endoplasmic reticulum stress due to these mutations may cause a trafficking disorder of synaptic receptors like gamma-aminobutyric acid B (GABAB) receptors, resulting in impaired synaptic function and signal transduction. This theory provides for epigenetic factors playing a role as well (Momoi et al., 2010). Genes encoding postsynaptic scaffold proteins (SHANK2 and SHAN3) and ion channel proteins (CACNA1A, CACNA1H, SCN1A, SCN2A) also have been implicated in ASD (Montiero and Feng 2017, Daghsni et al., 2018).

***Neuropathology.*** Based on the core symptoms of autism, neuropathological abnormalities would be anticipated and are found in regions important to social function (frontal lobe, superior temporal cortex, parietal cortex, and amygdala), language function (language cortex), and repetitive behaviors and stereotypies (orbital frontal cortex and caudate) (Amaral et al., 2008; Bauman and Kemper, 2005; Casanova and Trippe, 2009; Casanova et al., 2006; Herbert et al., 2002, 2005; Pardo and Eberhart, 2007; Schumann et al., 2010; Vargas et al., 2005). Functional imaging studies demonstrate that neural systems related to social functioning, such as emotional face recognition, are abnormal (Corbett et al., 2009). Abnormalities of mirror neurons are also seen when subjects imitate and observe emotions (Rizzolatti and Fabbri-Destro, 2010).

ASDs are now considered disorders of the development of the connectivity of the neurons of the cerebral cortex, which results in disturbances in the highly specialized connections that provide for uniquely human abilities. The occurrence of mutations in genes that act on molecular signaling pathways involved in the development and maintenance of neuronal and synaptic connections has reinforced the centrality of disruption of cortical connectivity in ASD (Konopka et al., 2012; Parikshak et al., 2013; Pinto et al., 2014; Scott-Van Zeeland et al., 2010).

Studies of brain structure have implicated multiple events in the prenatal and postnatal brain development, particularly neuronal organizational events. A recent study supports a prenatal onset of ASD, occurring during the second and third trimester of pregnancy. Courchesne and colleagues found focal patches of abnormal laminar cytoarchitecture and cortical disorganization of neurons, but not glia, in the prefrontal and temporal cortical tissue from 10 of 11 children with autism and from 1 of 11 unaffected children, supporting a probable dysregulation of layer formation and layer-specific neuronal differentiation prenatally (Stoner et al., 2014).

Increased total brain volume, primarily due to increased white matter, is the most frequently replicated imaging finding (Verhoeven et al., 2010). Very young children with autism (18 months to 4 years) have a 5%–10% increase in brain volume, especially in the frontal lobe compared to controls, which parallels the increasing head circumference during this period. A recent study suggests that changes in brain growth rate between the ages of 6 and 12 months may predict changes in the brain that occur between the ages of 12 and 24 months and correspond with the development of ASD symptoms (Hazlett, 2017).

In contrast to other white-matter structures, both volume and density of the corpus callosum are reduced (Hardan et al., 2008; Minshew, 2009), perhaps resulting in decreased interhemispheric communication (Williams and Minshew, 2007). Imaging studies also highlight the dissociation between white-matter tract overgrowth and gray-matter dendritic and synaptic underdevelopment. Spectroscopy studies suggest that the gray matter is abnormal and dendritic arborization and synaptosome density reduced. Some investigators speculate that gray-matter abnormalities trigger the white-matter overgrowth (Williams and Minshew, 2007).

The white-matter abnormalities result in abnormality of connectivity. At the cytoarchitectonic level, minicolumns that determine connectivity are abnormal, especially in the dorsolateral prefrontal cortex (Casanova et al., 2006). As a result, and well delineated on diffusion tensor (DT) imaging (Keller et al., 2007; Sundaram et al., 2008), short-range connectivity is increased, and long-range connectivity is decreased (Williams and Casanova, 2010). The hyperconnected local networks may become partially isolated and acquire novel functional properties. By contrast, the decrease in long-range connections could explain the problems with top-down control and integration (Williams and Casanova, 2010). A recent study of toddlers, ages 1–4 years, with ASD found axonal overconnectivity in frontal lobes with growth pathology thought to be due to neuron excess. This is thought to lead to underfunctional connectivity and resultant impairments in social communication (Solso et al., 2016).

Given that the brain mechanisms causing ASD are largely at the level of connections among neurons and are not detectable on gross structural neuroimaging, imaging is not considered a routine part of the evaluation of individuals with ASD.

### Management

Both behavioral and educational interventions target the core symptoms of ASDs. Usually, children with ASD require a combination of therapies and interventions to address their individual groups of symptoms. It is recommended that children receive educational intervention as soon as they are suspected of having ASD, with services being provided a minimum of 25 hours a week on a yearly basis. Preschool children with ASDs should receive special education preschool or a home-based behavioral modification program (Handelman and Harris, 2002). Intensive behavioral interventions, such as applied behavior analysis (ABA), based on the work of Lovaas (1987) use multiple prompting paradigms, reinforcement schedules, and imitation and modeling. Another type of intervention, the Treatment and Education of Autistic and Related Communication-Handicapped Children (TEACCH) method, uses structured teaching to help improve skills, with the therapist functioning as a generalist in treating the whole child. Developmental and relationship-based models, such as the Developmental Individual Difference, Relationship approach (DIR or Floortime), focus on teaching skills, such as social communication and interpersonal skills. The Early Start Denver Model (ESDM) is considered an integrative approach, as it uses a combination of intensive ABA and developmental and relationship-based intervention and includes parents as therapists. Parental involvement is considered an important part of the treatment program and parent-mediated treatment may result in better parent–child interaction and reduced severity of ASD symptoms than in children in nonmediated groups (Oono et al., 2013).

A variety of other interventions are used to target specific areas of development (e.g., social skills groups, video modeling, occupational therapy). Table 90.2 lists medications that have been helpful in some children.

### Prognosis

Based on current outcome data, children who receive early intensive behavioral intervention can show significant improvement in the core features of autism including social communication, emotional/behavioral regulation, as well as in IQ and adaptive behavior (Zwaigenbaum et al., 2015; Howelen et al.; Reichow et al.). Findings suggest that best prognosis is associated with normal IQ, intensive intervention before age 3, and intervention that includes active involvement of families or caregivers (Zwaigenbaum et al., 2015, Granpeesheh, 2009). Some Swedish studies, conducted before the introduction of early identification and intervention, demonstrated poor outcomes for many adults with ASD. In a prospective study, Billstedt et al. (2005) followed 120 individuals diagnosed in childhood and reevaluated them at ages 17 and 40 with regard to employment, higher education, independent living, and peer relationships. Outcomes were generally poor in 78% of cases, and only 4 of 120 individuals were living independently. Better outcomes were associated with childhood IQ level and existence of communicative phrase speech at age 6. Cederlund et al. (2008) found that approximately two-thirds of adults with autism showed poor social adjustment (limited independence in social relations). Even though higher-functioning individuals with autism (including those previously diagnosed as Asperger syndrome) had the best outcome, only 15%–30% had fair to good outcomes, and only 5%–15% became competitively employed, led independent lives, married, and raised families. Psychiatric problems were common in this group. Probably, some "odd" adults go undiagnosed in childhood and adolescence, thus increasing the proportion of those with ASD who ultimately function in the mainstream. Some are highly productive and original in their work (Billstedt et al., 2007; Seltzer et al., 2003).

## INTELLECTUAL DISABILITY

### Clinical Features

ID, also known as intellectual developmental disorder, requires limitations in both intellectual ability and deficits in adaptive skills, as expressed in conceptual, social, and practical adaptive skills, relative to the child's age, experience, and environment. Specifically, the diagnosis requires that the following criteria are met: (1) Deficits in intellectual functioning (i.e., reasoning, abstract thinking, learning, both experiential and academic) that must be confirmed through both clinical evaluation and individualized, standardized IQ testing; (2) limitations in adaptive functioning that result in failure in meeting developmental

**TABLE 90.2 Medications for Autism Spectrum Disorders**

| | |
|---|---|
| Hyperactivity and inattention | Psychostimulants (methylphenidate; dextroamphetamine);<br>α-agonists (clonidine, Tenex, Intuniv, Kapvay) |
| Obsessive-compulsive behaviors and anxiety | Selective serotonin reuptake inhibitors: fluoxetine (Prozac), sertraline (Zoloft), paroxetine (Paxil), fluvoxamine (Luvox), citalopram (Celexa)<br>Anxiolytics: buspirone (BuSpar)<br>Tricyclics: clomipramine (Anafranil) |
| Aggressive and impulsive behaviors | Atypical neuroleptics: risperidone (Risperdal), olanzapine (Zyprexa), ziprasidone (Geodon), aripiprazole (Abilify)<br>α-agonists: clonidine (Catapres), guanfacine (Tenex), Intuniv, Kapvay<br>Beta-blockers: propranolol (Inderal)<br>Mood stabilizers: carbamazepine (Tegretol), divalproex sodium (Depakote), gabapentin (Neurontin), topiramate (Topamax), lithium (Lithium) |
| Tics/stereotypies | Clonidine, Tenex, clonazepam (Klonopin), pimozide (Orap), haloperidol (Haldol), risperidone (Risperdal), baclofen (Lioresal), deep brain stimulation |
| Self-mutilation | Naloxone (Narcan), propranolol, fluoxetine, clomipramine, lithium |
| Psychosis | Neuroleptics: haloperidol, risperidone, olanzapine, ziprasidone |
| Seizures | Depakote, Lamictal, Trileptal, Tegretol, Topamax |

*Modified from Soorya, L., Kiarashi, J., Hollander, E., 2008. Psychopharmacologic interventions for repetitive behaviors in autism spectrum disorders. Child Adolesc Psychiatr Clin N Am 17, 753–771.*

and social standards for personal independence and social responsibility; and (3) onset of intellectual and adaptive deficits occurs during the developmental period. Moreover, the level and severity of ID (mild, moderate, severe, and profound) is defined on the basis of adaptive skills rather than the IQ score. The definition links the severity of ID to the degree of community support required to achieve optimal independence (Katz and Lazcano-Ponce, 2008). Mild ID indicates the need for intermittent support; moderate ID for limited support; severe ID for extensive support; and profound ID for pervasive support. Although both intellectual and adaptive functioning are pertinent in defining ID, impairment of adaptive function is more likely to be the presenting feature than low IQ; however, it is expected that there is an association between intellectual functioning and adaptive skills.

The term *global developmental delay* (GDD) is used to describe children under the age of 5 years with significant delays in developmental milestones in several areas of functioning (APA, 2013b). GDD can be diagnosed using a standardized test, which shows performance at least 2 SD below the mean in at least two developmental domains: motor, speech and language, cognition, personal-social, and/or adaptive (daily living). The diagnosis of ID is not used for children under 5 years old since IQ scores are not reliable until after 5 years and because some children with a GDD diagnosis will not meet criteria for ID as they get older.

The IQ definition of ID uses 100 as the mean and 15 as the SD. An IQ score of 65–75 (≈2 SD below the mean, with a variation of ±5 points) is the demarcation point. Previously, children with an IQ of 55–69 were considered mild ID, those with an IQ of 40–54, as moderate ID; those with an IQ of 25–39, severe ID; and those with an IQ under 25, profound ID.

The prevalence of ID varies due to differences in diagnostic approach, population characteristics, and study design. In the general population, it is considered to be 1% when ID is defined as deficits in both adaptive and intellectual functioning (Harris, 2006; Maulik et al., 2011; Szymanski and King, 1999). The prevalence of intellectual deficits only (IQ < 75), based on IQ score alone, is 3% (Szymanski and King, 1999). Mild ID represents the majority (85%), but roughly 0.4% of the general population is severely intellectually disabled. As a rule, those with severe ID are more likely to have a definable biological cause, whereas those with mild ID tend to come from socially disadvantaged backgrounds and often have a family history of borderline intellectual function or mild ID (Kaufman et al., 2010; Stromme and Magnus, 2000). The prevalence of GDD (in children under 5 years) is estimated at 1%–3% (Shevell et al., 2003). The ratio of boys to girls with ID, especially mild ID, is 1.4:1. Male excess is present in ASD with ID, syndromic X-linked ID (S-XLID) (associated with a specific phenotype), and nonsyndromic X-linked ID (NS-XLID). About 15% of males with ID have X-linked intellectual disability (XLID) (Stevenson and Schwartz, 2009). About 25% of all males with severe ID have XLID, and almost 50% of all cases of mild ID are due to XLID (Partington et al., 2000; Ropers and Hamel, 2005). The recurrence of ID in families with one previous child with severe ID is reported to be between 3% and 9% (CDC, 2009).

## Diagnosis and Etiology

The diagnosis of ID now includes a measure of both intellectual functioning and adaptive skills. The most commonly used tests of IQ are the Wechsler Scales and the Stanford-Binet tests; however, other tests are used to assess intellectual ability, several of which are measures of nonverbal intelligence. Clinical interview with the individual and a collateral contact who knows the individual well can help assess adaptive functioning, as can standardized measures of adaptive behaviors. The most commonly used standardized measure is the Vineland Adaptive Behavior Scale-II (VABS-2), which assesses and provides a general adaptive behavior composite score. A valid determination of ID (intellectual and adaptive abilities) also considers differences in language and culture, as well as in communication, motor, sensory, and behavioral factors.

Children with ID often have neurological and psychiatric comorbidities. Epidemiological studies suggest that as many as one-fifth of them have epilepsy by the age of 10 years (Airaksinen et al., 2000). The probability of developing epilepsy is fivefold greater for children with severe ID (35%) than for those with mild ID (7%). Cerebral palsy (CP) coexists in 6%–8% of the mildly ID and as many as 30% of the severely ID. Microcephaly occurs in one-fifth of XLID syndromes. Macrocephaly also occurs secondary to increased brain volume or hydrocephalus. Children with GDD and ID are at risk for physical disabilities. Impaired vision occurs in 15%–50% and impaired hearing in about 20%. An increased prevalence of psychopathology and maladaptive behavior occurs in children with ID. Table 90.3 details specific cognitive and behavioral problems in several common genetically defined ID syndromes, along with the possible neuropathological basis of these disorders.

Etiology is ultimately determined in anywhere from 10% to 81% of children with GDD/ID. Evaluation of ID should be sequential;

**TABLE 90.3 Cognitive and Behavioral Problems in Several Genetically Defined Intellectual Disability Syndromes**

| Syndrome | IQ | Language | Spatial Skills | Executive | Social Skills | Neuropathology |
|---|---|---|---|---|---|---|
| Down trisomy 21 | Range 30–70, usually moderate, dementia in adulthood | Good vocabulary and conversation, weaker grammar, impaired verbal short-term memory | Commensurate with IQ | Perseverative, impulsive | Often relative strength, but autism reported | Reduced gray-matter volumes, especially with infantile spasms |
| Williams deletion 7q11 | Mild to moderate | Expressive language and conversation a strength, grammar preserved, loquacious | Weak visuospatial and global processing, face recognition spared | Inattentive, distractible, impersistent | Social perception spared (facial emotional expression), social cognition impaired, overly social, musical | Reduced volume with overall preservation of gray matter, except for right occipital lobe, abnormal cerebellar metabolism |
| Prader-Willi deletion 15q11–q13 | Mean 70, range profound MR to average | Oromotor dysfunction | Visuospatial strength, jigsaw puzzles a special interest | Obsessive, skin picking, paternal imprinting in uniparental disomy increases likelihood of autism | Internalizing, externalizing problems and ADHD can interfere with social functioning<br>Aggressive behavior maximal in young adults, psychosis occasional with maternal uniparental disomy | Hypothalamic dysfunction, bifrontal, thalamus, internal capsule, splenium of the corpus callosum abnormal |
| Fragile X males 1/2000B 6000 | Moderate to severe, decline after puberty, fully methylated patients have more decline, academics decline over time | Poor articulation, cluttering, verbal dyspraxia, weak word finding, poor pragmatics and conversational skills | Sporadic weakness of visual-motor skills | Weak attention, planning, shifting sets | Strength in adaptive functioning until puberty, normal recognition of facial emotions, autistic features common | 10% seizures, loss of expression of FMRP maximal in hippocampus, cerebellum, cortex and nucleus basalis magnocellularis, decreased cerebellum, superior temporal gyrus, enlarged thalamus and caudate, hippocampal volume reflected in cognitive functioning |
| Fragile X females | Normal to mild to moderate | Generally intact | Visuospatial and nonverbal memory problems | Relatively weak, ADHD, poor cognitive flexibility and working memory | Very shy, anxious | |
| VCF 22q11 haplo-insufficiency (reduced gene dosage) | Borderline to mild MR | Speak in single words despite their ability to converse, but verbal skills stronger than nonverbal | Impairments in visuoperceptual ability, NVLD | Weak problem solving, planning, abstraction, ADHD | Poor social interactions, anxiety, increased prevalence of psychosis/schizophrenia | Decreased gyrification, reduced volume bilaterally in the occipital parietal lobes, larger right caudate nucleus, reduced cerebellar gray matter, reduced white matter in frontal lobe, cerebellum, internal capsule; correlates with psychiatric problems |

*Continued*

**TABLE 90.3 Cognitive and Behavioral Problems in Several Genetically Defined Intellectual Disability Syndromes—cont'd**

| Syndrome | IQ | Language | Spatial Skills | Executive | Social Skills | Neuropathology |
|---|---|---|---|---|---|---|
| Rett syndrome mutations in the X-linked gene encoding methyl-CpG-binding protein 2* | Appear to develop normally until 6–18 months, deteriorating to severe retardation | Gradually lose speech and purposeful hand use | Stereotypical hand movements | | Autistic-like behavior | Progressive microcephaly, seizures |

*ADHD*, Attention-deficit/hyperactivity disorder; *FMRP*, fragile X mental retardation protein; *IQ*, intelligence quotient; *MR*, mental retardation; *NVLD*, nonverbal learning disability; *VCFS*, velo-cardio-facial syndrome.
*Prevalence is 1–3 per 10,000 live births.
*Data from Adegbola, A.A., Gonzales, M.L., Chess, A., et al., 2009. A novel hypomorphic MECPs point mutation is associated with a neuropsychiatric phenotype. Hum Genet 124 (6), 615–623; Campbell, L., Daly, E., Toal, F., et al., 2006. Brain and behaviour in children with 22q11.2 deletion syndrome: a volumetric and voxel-based morphometry MRI study. Brain 129, 1218–1228; Hooper, S.R., Hammer, J., Roberts, J.E., 2010. Down syndrome. In: Nass, R.D., Franks, Y. (Eds.), Cognitive and Behavior Abnormalities of Pediatric Diseases. Oxford University Press, New York, pp. 159–169; Mastergeorge, A., Au, J., Hagerman, R., 2010. Fragile X: a family of disorders. In: Nass, R., Frank, Y. (Eds.), Cognitive and Behavioral Abnormalities of Pediatric Diseases. Oxford University Press, New York, pp. 170–187; Renieri, A., Mari, F., Mencarelli, M.A., et al., 2009. Diagnostic criteria for the Zappella variant of Rett syndrome (the preserved speech variant). Brain Dev 31, 208–216; Robertson, L., Hall, S.E., Jacoby, P., et al., 2006. The association between behavior and genotype in Rett syndrome using the Australian Rett Syndrome Database. Am J Med Genet B Neuropsychiatr Genet 141B, 177–183; Zarcone, J., Welsh, S.S., 2010. Prader-Willi syndrome. In: Nass, R.D., Franks, Y. (Eds.), Cognitive and Behavior Abnormalities of Pediatric Diseases. Oxford University Press, New York, pp. 213–230.*

key elements include the medical, family, and developmental histories, dysmorphology and neurological examinations, and appropriate laboratory and neuroimaging tests (Moeschler and Shevell, 2006; Shevell et al., 2003). The latter can include careful metabolic evaluation together with neuroimaging studies, EEG, cytogenetic studies, and genetic and ophthalmological consultations as appropriate (Mao and Pevsner, 2005; Shevell et al., 2003). Auditory and visual function must be determined, since these are common comorbidities. If a child was born in a locale without universal newborn screening, consider a screening metabolic evaluation that includes a capillary blood gas, serum lactate and ammonia levels, serum amino acids and urine organic acids, and thyroid function studies. An EEG is appropriate when the history suggests possible seizures, paroxysmal behaviors, or an underlying epilepsy syndrome. Neuroimaging is recommended as part of the diagnostic evaluation of a child with GDD (Level B; class III evidence, AAN 2003 Practice Parameter for GDD). Computed tomography (CT) contributes to the etiological diagnosis of GDD in approximately 30% of children. Magnetic resonance imaging (MRI) is more sensitive than CT, with abnormalities found in 48.6%–65.5% of children with global delay (Level C; class III evidence, AAN 2003 Practice Parameter for GDD). The chance of detecting an abnormality increases if physical abnormalities, particularly CP, are present (AAN 2003 Practice Parameter for GDD).

Environmental factors play a role in the causation of ID. Nongenetic prenatal causes of ID include congenital infections; environmental toxins, such as lead, mercury, hydantoin, alcohol, and valproate; iron deficiency; and radiation exposure, especially between 9 and 15 weeks' gestation. Smoking during pregnancy is associated with more than a 50% increase in the prevalence of ID. Perinatal conditions that may lead to ID include very preterm birth, hypoxia, stroke, trauma, and intracranial hemorrhage. Postnatal and acquired causes of ID include head trauma, hypoxia, central nervous system (CNS) hemorrhage, psychosocial deprivation, malnutrition, CNS malignancy, acquired hypothyroidism, and environmental toxins.

Inherited metabolic diseases are responsible for 1%–5% of unspecified ID, with a yield of between 0.2% and 4.6%, depending on the presence of clinical indicators and the range of testing performed (Michelson et al., 2011). ID is rarely a unique symptom in inborn errors of metabolism. Table 90.4 lists some of the metabolic disorders that cause isolated ID, some of which are potentially treatable.

Genetic defects are important causes of ID. Approximately 25%–50% of identified cases are genetic in origin. Genetic etiologies include cytogenic abnormalities, CNVs, for example, submicroscopic deletions/duplications/rearrangements, and single-gene disorders. Recent years have seen important progress in identifying the genes involved in ID. To date, 450 genes have been implicated in ID, with 400 attributed to syndromic ID and 50 to nonsyndromic ID.

Despite the advancements in genetic testing, only a few specific well-characterized single-gene disorders with a recognizable clinical phenotype (e.g., FMR1-fragile X and MECP2-Rett syndrome) are routinely tested for during the diagnostic process (Sherr et al., 2013). The diagnostic evaluation should focus on clues for a genetic versus acquired etiology for ID. If a family history of consanguinity exists or a close family member (sibling, aunt/uncle, or first cousin) is known to have GDD/ID, testing specific to the known disorder should be performed. A history of pregnancy losses/stillbirths, postnatal deaths of prior offspring, or birth defects should raise suspicion for a genetic etiology (Srour and Shevell, 2014). Observed dysmorphic features may prompt specific testing for such entities as Down syndrome, FXS, Rett syndrome, Prader-Willi/Angelman, or congenital hypothyroidism (Jones, 2006).

Increasingly sophisticated genetic testing is becoming more readily available. The AAN 2011 Evidence Report for genetic and metabolic testing on children with GDD/ID found that CMA testing is abnormal on average in 7.8% of subjects with GDD/ID and in 10.6% of those with syndromic features. Karyotype studies are abnormal in at least 4% of subjects with GDD/ID and in 18.6% of those with syndromic features. Mutations in X-linked genes may explain up to 10% of all cases of GDD/ID. *FMR1* testing has a combined yield of at least 2% in males and females with mild GDD/ID. MECP2 mutations are found in 1.5% of girls with moderate/severe GDD/ID and in less than 0.5% of males with GDD/ID (Michelson et al., 2011). CMA has emerged as the most commonly ordered initial diagnostic test in individuals with unexplained GDD/ID. A 2010 consensus

TABLE 90.4 **Metabolic Disorders Associated With Intellectual Disability**

| Disorder | Intellectual Disability | Expressive Speech Disturbances | Psychiatric Disturbances | Epilepsy | Cerebellar Involvement | Brain MRI | Other Signs | Diagnostic Tests |
|---|---|---|---|---|---|---|---|---|
| Creatine transporter deficiency | Mild to moderate | Severe | Autistic-like behavior | 50% of cases, in general, good response to conventional therapy | No | Usually normal (low or absent creatine peak in spectroscopy) | Hypotonia, slight pyramidal signs, dysmorphy, often short statured | High creatine/creatinine in urine; low creatine peak in MRS; fibroblast creatine incorporation; mutations SLC6A8 |
| 4-Hydroxybutyric aciduria | Mild to moderate | Severe | Autistic-like, attention deficit, hyperactivity, anxiety, obsessive-compulsive disorder, aggression | 50% of cases; some patients may be resistant to conventional therapy, others demonstrate EEG abnormalities without seizures | Nonprogressive ataxia, cerebellar atrophy (not constant) | 40% of cases involving cerebellum, subcortical white matter, and/or pallidum | Hypotonia, movement disorders, sleep disturbances | 4-Hydroxybutyric acid in urine; SSDH activity in fibroblasts; SSDH mutations |
| Adenylosuccinate lyase deficiency | Moderate to severe | Moderate | Autistic-like | 80% of cases, often resistant to therapy | May be present (nonprogressive ataxia, cerebellar atrophy) | Not specific; cerebellar atrophy and white-matter high intensity may be present | Nonspecific dysmorphic features | SAICAR and S-Ado in urine; ADLS activity and mutations |
| Sanfilippo B | Mild to severe | Mild | Hyperactivity, aggressiveness | Not frequent | May appear in later stages | Similar to Sanfilippo A | Mildly coarse facies and abundant thick hair in childhood and adolescence, which sometimes normalizes late in adulthood | GAGs: heparin sulfate |

*EEG*, Encephalogram; *GAGs*, glycosaminoglycans; *MRS*, magnetic resonance spectroscopy.
*From García-Cazorla, A., Wolf, N.I., Serrano, M., et al., 2009. Mental retardation and inborn errors of metabolism. J Inherit Metab Dis 32, 597–608.*

statement indicated that CMA should be used instead of karyotyping as the first-line cytogenetic diagnostic test for individuals with GDD/ID, ASD, or multiple congenital anomalies (Miller et al., 2010). Advancements in technology have allowed genome-wide analyses to move into clinical practice. Whole-exome sequencing (WES) or whole[-genome sequencing (WGS) are such techniques that potentially can identify a causative mutation in an individual with GDD/ID for whom conventional testing (CMA or karyotype) has been unrevealing. This type of testing is not without its limitations and challenges (Flore and Milunsky, 2012).

## Management

Available evidence demonstrates the benefits of early intervention through a variety of programs, at least with respect to short-term outcomes, and suggests that early diagnosis of a child with global delay may improve long-term outcome (Shevell et al., 2003). The management of children with ID focuses on finding the appropriate educational setting for children with mild ID, vocational training for those with moderate ID, and determining home or institutional placement for those with severe and profound ID.

Advances in genetic diagnosis have had immediate benefits for families, allowing for carrier testing, genetic counseling, prenatal diagnosis, and preimplantation genetic diagnosis. Some of the gene discoveries have also pointed to potential strategies for treatment, for example, FXS. In a recent study, Jaffrey and colleagues studied stem cells from donated human embryos that have a genetic mutation resembling that in FXS (Colak et al., 2014). They found a malfunction in fragile X cells in which messenger RNA sticks to mutated DNA segments during early cell development, thereby blocking the gene's expression and, as a result, preventing the cell from producing a protein critical to the transmission of signals between neurons. The malfunction appears to occur suddenly before the end of the first trimester in humans and after 50 days in cultured stem cells. A drug compound was used to bind to the fragile X gene's RNA before the malfunction occurs, allowing the gene to continue producing the critical brain protein. This represents a potential prevention or treatment strategy for FXS (Colak et al., 2014).

## LEARNING DISABILITY

Learning disability (LD) occurs in 5%–15% of school-aged children and is characterized by persistent difficulties learning academic skills in reading, writing, or mathematics. Most educational institutions abide by the Individuals with Disabilities Education Act (IDEA, 2004), which subsumes all of these learning problems under the general category of *Learning Disabled.* The IDEA (2004) states that "a specific learning disability means a disorder in one or more of the basic psychological processes involved in understanding or in using language, spoken or written, that may manifest itself in the imperfect ability to listen, think, speak, read, write, spell or do mathematical calculations" (CFR 300.8, 10).

### Dyslexia

#### Clinical Features

The best-studied and probably the most common learning disability (LD) is dyslexia. It occurs in as many as 10% of school-aged children and in 80% of LDs. Males are more often affected. *Developmental dyslexia* is marked by reading achievement that falls substantially below that expected given the individual's chronological age, measured intelligence, and age-appropriate education (ICD-10). As with other LDs, major neurological abnormalities are not present, but minor abnormalities (soft signs) may be detected (Denckla, 1985) (Tables 90.5 and 90.6). Major sensory functions must be normal and the child must have been in a social and educational environment conducive to learning to read. It should be noted that the nomenclature in the DSM-5 uses the term Specific Learning Disorder with Impairment in Reading and describes dyslexia as an alternative term used to refer to difficulties with word recognition, decoding, or spelling (APA, 2013a).

#### Diagnosis and Etiology

Most school systems abide by the IDEA (2004), which uses the Response to Intervention (RTI) model for the identification of dyslexia and other learning disorders. This model emphasizes evidence-based practices for monitoring progress, screening, and offering intervention for struggling readers (Fletcher and Vaughn, 2009). While this method is useful for providing early intervention, the RTI model does not explain why a child is having reading difficulties or rule out differential diagnoses. Thus, children with early reading problems should have a formal neuropsychological evaluation to examine their pattern of strengths and weaknesses and to exclude comorbid problems (e.g., ADHD) that might affect treatment. Deficits in phonological awareness frequently underlie reading difficulties and persist even into adolescence (Shaywitz et al., 1999) and adulthood. Measures that assess phonological functioning (e.g., segmenting words [say *cowboy* without the *boy*, say *smack* without the *m*], word and nonword blending, sound matching of first and last syllables) best differentiate dyslexic from normal readers. The *double-deficit hypothesis* of developmental dyslexia proposes that deficits in phonological processing and naming speed represent independent sources of dysfunction in dyslexia (Vukovic and Siegel, 2006). Although phonological processing issues appear to be the primary and/or most common cause of dyslexia, neuropsychological studies have identified other deficit clusters in dyslexics. For example, Crews et al. (2009) identified three dyslexia subtypes: (1) no language or memory deficit, (2) global language and memory deficit, and (3) global memory deficit. Few children fail to read because of visual perceptual difficulties or extraocular motility problems. However, processing by the lateral geniculate magnocellular system (important for monitoring motion, stereopsis, spatial localization, depth, and figure-ground perception) may not appropriately modify the information received from the fast parvocellular system (crucial for color perception, object recognition, and high-resolution form perception) (Amitay et al., 2002; Angélique et al., 2002).

**TABLE 90.5 Common Soft Signs Associated With Learning Disabilities**

| | |
|---|---|
| Cranial nerves | Head turns with eyes |
| | Mouth opens when eyes open |
| | Difficulty with grimace |
| Motor | Excess upper-extremity posturing on stressed gait |
| | Excess overflow during finger tapping and sequencing |
| | Unsustained one-foot stand |
| | Difficulty with hopping |
| | Excess choreiform movements with arms extended |
| Cerebellar | Dysrhythmic rapid alternating movements |
| | Excess overflow during rapid alternating movements |
| | Ballistic finger-nose-finger test |
| | Difficulty with tandem gait |
| Sensory | Extinction on double simultaneous stimuli |
| | Poor finger localization |
| DTR | Minor reflex asymmetries |

*DTR*, Deep tendon reflexes.
*Modified from Denckla, M.B., 1985. Revised neurological examination for subtle signs. Pharmacol Bull 21, 773–789.*

**TABLE 90.6 Natural History of Soft Signs**

| Neurological System Affected | Soft Sign | Age of Appearance or Disappearance |
|---|---|---|
| Cranial nerves | Head does not move with eyes | 6–7 years |
| | Sticks tongue out for 10 s | 6–7 years |
| Motor | Toe-heel walk | 3 years |
| | Heel walk without associated movements | 5 years |
| | Hop 10 times | 5 years |
| | Hops indefinitely | 7 years |
| | One-foot stand for 30 s | 7 years |
| | No longer drifts up and down with pronated and supinated arms | 3–4 years |
| | Rigid tripod | 5 years |
| | Dynamic tripod | 7–8 years |
| | Choreiform movements | 7–10 years |
| | Athetoid movements | 2–4 years |
| Cerebellar | Tandem | 6 years |
| | No overflow during rapid alternating movements | 7–8 years |
| Sensory | Stereognosis, graphesthesia | 6 years |
| | No longer extinguishes on double simultaneous stimulation | 8 years |

The standard neurological examination is normal. Routine imaging is normal and unnecessary, except perhaps in children with atypical features (Box 90.3).

Dyslexia has a significant genetic component with heritability estimated at 54%–84% (Astrom et al., 2007; DeFries et al., 1987; Scerri and Schulte-Korne, 2010). Dyslexia-susceptibility-1-candidate-1 (*DYX1C1*) was the first gene reported to be associated with dyslexia, possibly with

**BOX 90.3 Atypical Features in Dyslexia**

Female gender
Left-handed without family history
Strongly left-handed, early declaration
Dyslexic without family history
No history of developmental language problems
Large discrepancy between verbal and spatial skills
Neurological abnormalities or seizures

a memory-deficit dyslexia phenotype (Dahdouh et al., 2009). Numerous candidate dyslexia susceptibility genes have subsequently been identified from cytogenic, linkage, association, and biological studies (e.g., DYX1C1 at DYX1, KIAA0319 and DCDC2 at DYX2, MRPL19, and C20RF3 close to DYX3, ROBO1 at DYX5, and KIAA0319L at DYX8), including several that affect neuronal migration (Anthoni et al., 2007; Cope et al., 2005; Hannula-Jouppi et al., 2005; Harold et al., 2006; Meng et al., 2005; Paracchini et al., 2006; Schumacher et al., 2006; Taipale et al., 2003).

Pathological studies suggest that those with dyslexia have both atypical planum temporale asymmetries and areas of cortical dysplasia, reflecting abnormal neuronal migration, particularly in the left hemisphere (Galaburda et al., 2006). Structural imaging demonstrates that in about two-thirds of normal adults, the left planum temporale is larger than the right, but by contrast, only 25% of dyslexics have this same left/right planum asymmetry (Eckert and Leonard, 2000). Dyslexics with atypical asymmetry tend to have more severe language and/or reading deficits. In a group of children with dyslexia with or without ADHD, the presence of an extra sulcus in the left pars triangularis was associated with poor expressive language ability. In those with adequate expressive language functioning, left pars triangularis length related to phonological awareness, phonological short-term memory, and rapid automatic naming (RAN). Right pars triangularis length related to RAN and semantic processing (Kibby et al., 2009). Evidence of decreased gray matter has been found not only in the left temporal lobe and bilaterally in the temporoparietooccipital juncture but also in the frontal lobe, caudate, and thalamus (Brown et al., 2001).

Interhemispheric transfer of information may be abnormal in dyslexia (Beaton et al., 2006). Structural differences of the corpus callosum exist in normal versus dyslexic readers. Theoretically, the splenium is critical because it contains axons linking the planum temporale and angular gyrus.

Functional imaging studies demonstrate that fluent reading requires functional integrity of three left hemisphere regions—an inferior frontal region and two posterior systems (a temporal-parietal system and a ventral occipital-temporal system). Developmentally, the temporal-parietal system predominates initially and is required for learning to integrate the printed word with its phonological and semantic features. The occipital-temporal system constitutes a late-developing rapid sight word identification system that underlies word recognition in skilled readers. Disruption of both posterior systems may occur in developmental dyslexia. In contrast to normal readers, dyslexics may rely on left and right inferior frontal and right posterior regions (Blau et al., 2010; Pugh et al., 2000). Thus, they make inefficient use of the posterior system. Functional imaging also implicates the cerebellum, an area that other studies suggest is crucial for language functioning (Fulbright et al., 1999). Positron emission tomography (PET) studies have shown reduced activation within the left insula (Paulesu et al., 1996) and within temporal, parietal, and occipital left hemisphere regions (McCrory et al., 2005).

Connectivity abnormalities in dyslexics occur in two areas associated with working memory. Within a "phonological" left-lateralized prefrontal network, increased functional connectivity occurs in left prefrontal and inferior parietal regions. Within an "executive" bilateral frontoparietal network, dyslexics showed a decreased connectivity pattern in bilateral dorsolateral prefrontal and posterior parietal regions and increased connectivity in the left angular gyrus, left hippocampal cortex, and right thalamus (Wolf et al., 2010). Abnormalities of very short-range connectivity (e.g., angular gyrus, striate cortex), in association with larger gyri, may explain reading difficulties (Casanova et al., 2010; Silani et al., 2005).

In a study using diffusion tensor imaging (DTI), positive correlations were found with three tests of reading ability (word reading, decoding, and reading fluency) in the bilateral white matter, particularly in the frontal lobes but also involving the thalamus, and temporoparietal regions (Lebel et al., 2013).

### Management

Although dyslexia does not disappear, most children with early reading problems learn to read at average to above-average levels if they are diagnosed by the age of 8–9 years (third to fourth grade) and evidence-based reading instruction is provided. Children diagnosed later, even if remediated, are likely to continue to have reading problems. Three out of four children with reading problems at the end of third grade are still having trouble in seventh grade. In the Connecticut Longitudinal Study, dyslexic children (diagnosed after the third grade) never caught up to average or superior high school readers (Shaywitz et al., 1999). Early identification and provision of evidence-based reading instruction, systematic, phonetic, and multisensory approaches such as the Orton Gillingham or Wilson method can reduce the percentage of children reading below grade level in fourth grade from 37% to 6% (Bakker, 2006). However, large population studies suggest that some degree of reading disability persists into adulthood in most, and occupational attainment is lower in some (Undheim, 2009). The magnitude of phonological impairment alone does not appear to fully predict reading outcome. Phonological deficits appear to interact with other cognitive factors, such as nonverbal IQ and linguistic skills, particularly syntactic processing in determining long-term outcome (Peterson et al., 2009; Wiseheart et al., 2009).

*Compensated readers*, who are accurate but not fluent, demonstrate a relative underactivation in posterior neural systems for reading located in left parietotemporal and occipitotemporal regions. *Persistently poor readers*, who are both not fluent and less accurate, activate posterior reading systems but engage them differently from nonimpaired readers; they rely more on memory-based rather than analytic word identification strategies (Shaywitz et al., 2003). The majority of high-risk responder children benefit from systematic reading instruction and develop adequate reading abilities with successful recruitment of temporoparietal and visual association areas for reading (Simos et al., 2005). In another study correlating outcome with anatomy, 8- to 10-year-old poor readers had significantly lower fractional anisotropy (FA) in the left anterior centrum semiovale than good readers; 100 hours of intensive remedial instruction resulted in improved decoding ability and increased FA, consistent with enhanced myelination (Keller and Just, 2009). Although vision problems can interfere with reading, they are not the cause of dyslexia. Eye exercises, behavioral vision therapy, and special tinted filters or lenses are not effective treatments for dyslexia (American Academy of Pediatrics, 2009).

## Dyscalculia

### Clinical Features

Developmental dyscalculia (DD) can involve any or all aspects of mathematics, from difficulties representing and manipulating numeric information nonverbally, to learning and remembering arithmetic facts, to executing arithmetic procedures. The prevalence of dyscalculia is approximately 6%–14% (Shalev, 2007). A developmental Gerstmann syndrome (right/left disorientation, finger agnosia, dysgraphia, dyscalculia, and sometimes, constructional apraxia) occurs in as many as 2% of school-aged children. The mean IQ of children with dyscalculia is generally normal; one-fourth show symptoms of ADHD and approximately one-fifth are dyslexic. As with dyslexia, the DSM-5 uses the nomenclature Specific Learning Disorder with impairment in mathematics to refer to problems with number sense, calculation or math reasoning (APA, 2013a).

### Evaluation and Etiology

Comprehensive neuropsychological evaluations are recommended in individuals suspected of having dyscalculia. Children with neuropsychological signs of both left and right hemisphere dysfunction can have dyscalculia. Both groups have similar problems on arithmetic batteries, but those with left hemisphere dysfunction seem to perform significantly worse in addition, subtraction, complex multiplication, and division and also make more visuospatial errors (Shalev and Gross-Tsur, 2001). Imaging studies show that parietal and frontal abnormalities predominate. Children with DD have been shown to have weaker brain activation in the intraparietal sulcus (IPS) and inferior frontal gyrus of both hemispheres for approximate calculation than typically achieving children (Kucian et al., 2006). Evidence of parietal dysfunction (Grafman and Romero, 2001; Price et al., 2007) and reduced gray-matter volumes in frontal and parietal areas (Rotzer et al., 2008) are also reported in DD. Deficits in parietal and frontal lobe function in children with DD relate to poor spatial working memory (Rotzer et al., 2009). Several studies implicate deficit in working memory, a factor associated with DD (Camos, 2008).

### Management

Math remediation is appropriate for the child with isolated difficulties or with mathematics difficulties in combination with other learning difficulties.

## Disorder of Written Communication

In addition to reading and mathematics disorders, the DSM-5 Specific Learning Disorder classification includes a specifier for disorder of written expression. This is coded as “Specific Learning Disorder with Impairment in Written Expression” (DSM-5; American Psychiatric Association, 2013). The IDEA (2004) also identifies written expression as one of the eight areas of eligibility under the category of Specific Learning Disability. Under both classification systems, a disorder in written expression can include a variety of problems in writing, including difficulty expressing oneself in writing, spelling difficulties, and poor handwriting. Thus, the etiology and clinical presentation of writing disabilities is heterogeneous and most individuals who have difficulties in written expression also have other learning or behavioral difficulties, including dyslexia, motor coordination disorder/dysgraphia, language disorders, or ADHD. Katusic et al. (2009) found that 75% of children with written language disorders also had problems with reading, and Berninger and May 2011 found that writing disability is associated with dysgraphia, dyslexia, and/or oral language impairments.

## Developmental Coordination Disorder

### Diagnosis

Developmental coordination disorder (DCD) refers to problems with motor coordination that (1) are substantially below expectations for the individual’s age and opportunity for skill learning and use, (2) interfere with activities of daily living appropriate for age, and (3) negatively affect academic achievement, prevocational and vocational activities, and social integration. DCD is not better explained by other conditions, such as ID, visual impairment, neurological conditions, such as cerebral palsy, neuromuscular disease, or neurodegenerative disorders, vertigo, ASD, or ADHD (APA, 2013a; see Box 90.4).

A wide range of motoric difficulties are often considered synonymous with DCDs, including clumsiness, mild gross motor delay, decreased dexterity, visual motor problems, motor learning difficulty, dysgraphia, dyspraxia, and even adventitious movements (Blank et al., 2012; Mcnab et al., 2001). Generally, children with DCD are competent in the basic developmental motor skills such as walking, but it is in everyday activities such as tying shoe laces, buttoning a coat, riding a bike, or writing homework assignments where the greatest impact of the disorder is apparent (Box 90.5). Approximately 5% of school-aged children have DCD, with prevalence estimated to be three to four times greater in males (Kirby et al., 2014). Neither socioeconomic status nor education level is a factor.

A diagnosis of DCD is typically made at school age and is rarely made in children under age 5 years (Blondis, 1999), although delayed achievement of early motor milestones, problems with sucking or swallowing in infancy, persistent drooling (after 2½ years old), toe walking, or wide-based gait after 14 months may be associated with later DCD (Summers et al., 2008; Taft and Barowsky, 1989). Longitudinal studies suggest that the frequency of DCD changes with age (Hadders-Algra, 2002; Hadders-Algra et al., 2004). DCD does not necessarily resolve and continues into adolescence and adulthood (Losse et al., 1991). The presence of early neurological symptoms increases the frequency. In that respect, it is not surprising that children born prematurely (<32 weeks, gestation) and at a low birth weight (<1500 g), both appropriate for gestational age (AGA) and small for gestational age (SGA), are significantly more likely to have higher prevalence of DCD (Edwards et al., 2011; Faebo et al., 2013).

**BOX 90.4 Developmental Coordination Disorder, DSM-5 Diagnostic Criteria**

A. The acquisition and execution of coordinated motor skills is substantially below that expected given the individual’s chronological age and opportunity for skill learning and use. Difficulties are manifested as clumsiness (e.g., dropping or bumping into objects) as well as slowness and inaccuracy of performance of motor skills (e.g., catching an object, using scissors or cutlery, handwriting, riding a bike, or participating in sports).
B. The motor skills deficit in Criterion A significantly and persistently interferes with activities of daily living appropriate to chronological age (e.g., self-care and self-maintenance) and impacts academic/school productivity, prevocational and vocational activities, leisure, and play.
C. Onset of symptoms is in the early developmental period.
D. The motor skills deficits are not better explained by intellectual disability (intellectual developmental disorder) or visual impairment and are not attributable to a neurological condition affecting movement (e.g., cerebral palsy, muscular dystrophy, degenerative disorder).

*Reprinted with permission from the Diagnostic and Statistical Manual of Mental Disorders, Fifth Edition, (© 2013). American Psychiatric Association.*

**BOX 90.5 Development of Pencil Grip**

Ulnar/vertical—1.5–3 years
Radial—acceptable until 3.5 years
Tripod (static)—50% by 3 years, 80% by 4 years
Tripod (dynamic)—5–6 years

### Comorbid Conditions

DCDs often co-occur with ADHD (Pitcher et al., 2003), ASDs (Green et al., 2009), developmental language disorders, and dyslexia (Smits-Engelsman et al., 2003; Zwicker et al., 2009), in addition to other childhood-onset epilepsy syndromes (e.g., benign epilepsy of childhood with centrotemporal spikes [BECTS]) (Scabar et al., 2006). Anomalous dominance/handedness may also co-occur with DCDs, as approximately half of children with DCD are left-handed or ambidextrous in comparison to 10%–15% in the general population. Strong left-handedness, particularly when established before 1 year of age, should raise concerns that handedness is pathological (reflects left hemisphere dysfunction) (Cairney et al., 2008; Goez and Zelnik 2008; Hiscock and Chapieski, 2004).

### Evaluation and Etiology

A diagnosis of DCD should be made through a combination of history taking and standardized tests of gross and fine motor functioning (Kirby et al., 2014). The most commonly used standardized tests are the Bruininks-Oseretsky Test of Motor Proficiency (Bruininks and Bruininks, 2005) and the Movement Assessment Battery for Children (MABC-2) (Henderson et al., 2007). There are several clinical indicators that should prompt more emergent referral to a pediatric neurologist in order to rule out other neurological conditions (Kirby et al., 2014; see Box 90.6).

**BOX 90.6 Clinical Indicators Prompting Emergent Referral to Child Neurologist When Evaluating a Clumsy Child**

- Recent history of head injury or trauma
- History of deterioration of motor skills
- History of headaches, eye pain, blurred vision
- Gait abnormalities (ataxic, wide-based, prolonged toe walking)
- Increased muscle tone, fluctuating tone, or significant hypertonia
- Asymmetric muscle tone or strength
- Dysarthria, swallowing or feeding difficulties
- Gower's sign—difficulty rising to a standing position

*With permission from Kirby, A., Sugden, D., Purcell, C., 2014. Diagnosing developmental coordination disorders. Arch Dis Child 99(3), 292–296.*

Geuze (2005) suggests that DCDs are characterized by poor postural control (hypotonia or hypertonia, poor distal control, static and dynamic balance), difficulty in motor learning (learning new skills, movement planning, adaptation to change, automatization), and poor sensorimotor coordination (coordination within/between limbs; sequencing of movement; use of feedback, timing, anticipation, strategic planning). An evaluation for *dyspraxia* (the inability to perform learned skilled movement despite the motor abilities to do so) is probably required for a comprehensive assessment, as is a neurological examination for soft signs (Denckla, 1985). Dysgraphia, for example, is a common problem for children with DCDs, which can occur for many reasons. It can result from a primary/isolated disorder or exist as a symptom of visuomotor difficulties, dexterity deficits, or dyspraxia (part of a generalized deficit or a material-specific deficit). It can also occur along with dyslexia as a higher-order cognitive disorder (Table 90.7).

The neural substrate of DCD is not well characterized. There are very few studies of neuroimaging in children with DCD, with limited evidence pointing toward involvement of multiple brain areas (Peters et al., 2013). Poor postural control is a hallmark of DCD (O'Hare and Khalid, 2002). Theoretically, the cerebellum, parietal lobe, and basal ganglia could each/all be involved in DCD (Zwicker et al., 2009). The soft neurological signs seen in children with DCD (e.g., dysmetria, dysdiadochokinesia, impaired timing) all suggest cerebellar involvement (Ivry, 2003; Lundy-Ekman et al., 1991). Parietal lobe involvement could underlie the visuospatial problems as well as the imagery problems that characterize DCD (Wilson, 2004; Box 90.7; see also Box 90.8).

### Management

Children with significant DCDs may benefit from process-oriented occupational therapy, motor imagery intervention, and perceptual motor training (Wilson et al., 2002). A recent meta-analysis by Fereguson et al. (2013) supported *task-oriented therapies* and did not recommend *process-oriented* approaches for improving motor performance in DCD. Computers can facilitate output for those with poor graphomotor skills. Sometimes difficulties are sufficient to require taping of lectures and access to a scribe. Extended time is often required in the classroom setting and for test taking. Physical activity and therapy are priorities (Zwicker et al., 2009).

**TABLE 90.7 Natural History of Developmental Coordination Disorders**

| Age at Evaluation | Abnormal Neonatal Course, % With DCD | Normal Neonatal Course, % With DCD | Mechanisms |
|---|---|---|---|
| 4 years | 10% | 7% | Interval complications could induce DCDs in normal children and hamper recovery in those with neonatal problems |
| 9 years | Mild DCD, 25%; severe DCD, 35% | 20% | Emergence of dysfunction in circuits not previously used |
| DCD mild, <2 symptoms* | Mild neonatal problems, 15%; definite neonatal problems, 15% | 15% | DCDs mild and severe, differ in degree of associated cognitive and behavior problems |
| DCD 2, >2 symptoms* | Mild neonatal problems, 10%; definite neonatal problems, 18% | 5% | |
| 12 years | 49% | 22% | DCDs can develop even after a long silent interval |
| 14 years | 28% | 6% | Puberty causes a dramatic decrease in DCDs |

*DCD*, Developmental coordination disorder.

*Developmental coordination difficulties considered: (1) posture and muscle tone, (2) reflex abnormalities, (3) choreiform movements, (4) coordination and balance problems (most often related to preterm birth), (5) fine manipulative ability (most often related to neonatal difficulties).

*Modified from Hadders-Algra, M., 2002. Two distinct forms of minor neurological dysfunction: perspectives emerging from a review of data of the Groningen Perinatal Project. Dev Med Child Neurol 44, 561–571.*

**BOX 90.7 Signs of Visuospatial Learning Disabilities**

1. Can the child easily memorize material such as names, information, and poems?
2. Is the child able to make use of the available space when drawing?
3. Can the child use tools such as scissors, set square, or ruler that require independent and coordinated use of both hands?
4. Does the child understand spoken commands or texts that involve space relationships?
5. Is the child able to execute complex everyday movements such as tying shoelaces?
6. Does the child show good understanding of spatial relationships in calculation; can he or she write numbers in a column correctly?
7. Does the child have good spatial orientation abilities?
8. Is the child good at drawing?
9. Can the child easily interact with friends?
10. Has the child reached a good linguistic learning level for his or her age?
11. Has the child reached a good mathematical learning level for his or her age?
12. Is the child competent in learning contexts that rely on visuospatial skills?
13. Is the child distracted easily?
14. Is the child often restless or hyperactive?
15. Is the child a good observer of the environment in which he or she lives?
16. Does the child demonstrate an interest in new objects, and can he or she deal with them?
17. Does the child show good overall cognitive potential?
18. Does the child have a poor sociocultural background?

**BOX 90.8 Draw a Person: Expectations at Different Ages**

Humpty Dumpty or better, 50% at 3 years, 80% at 3.5 years
Intermediate man or better, 50% at 4 years, 80% at 4.5 years
Mature man, 50% at 4.5 years
10-part person at 5.5 years
14 parts at 6.5 years
18 parts at 7.5 years
22 parts at 8.5 years
26 points at 9.5 years
30 parts at 10.5 years
42 parts at 13.5 years

## ATTENTION-DEFICIT/HYPERACTIVITY DISORDER

### Clinical Features

ADHD is a disorder that begins in childhood with symptoms of hyperactivity, impulsivity, and/or inattention. Box 90.9 delineates the specific DSM-5 criteria for diagnosis. For children under 17 years of age, the DSM-5 diagnosis requires six or more symptoms of hyperactivity and impulsivity and six or more symptoms of inattention. For individuals 17 years and older, five or more symptoms of hyperactivity and impulsivity and five or more symptoms of inattention are required. Depending on the predominance of symptoms, ADHD can be considered to be one of the three subtypes: predominantly inattentive; predominantly hyperactive-impulsive; and combined type. Symptoms of hyperactivity/impulsivity and inattention must occur often; be present in more than one setting, such as school or work and home; persist for at least 6 months; be present before age 12 years; impair academic, social, or occupational functioning; and be excessive for the developmental level of the child. Furthermore, ADHD is classified as mild (few or no symptoms in excess of those necessary to make the diagnosis and no more than minor impairments in social or occupational function); moderate (symptoms or functional impairment between "mild" and "severe"); and severe (many symptoms in excess of those that are required to make the diagnosis, several symptoms that are particularly severe, or symptoms that result in marked impairment in social or occupational functioning).

The reported prevalence of ADHD in school-aged children in the United States is 9.4% (Danielson et al., 2018) and worldwide ranges vary, with the pooled estimated prevalence at 7.2% (Thomas et al., 2015). The DSM-5 conservatively estimates the prevalence of ADHD as about 5% of children and 2.5% of adults in most cultures. However, data from the National Survey of Children's Health (NSCH), a national, cross-sectional online/mail survey reported in 2016 that the prevalence remained similar to the 2011 survey. However, the prevalence from the 2007 to 2011 surveys was increasing remarkably, and now that the NSCH will be conducted annually the prevalence will be followed closely for future deviations. ADHD occurs approximately twice as often in males (Visser et al., 2014), but when affected, females are more likely to present primarily with inattentive features. Although complete recovery from ADHD was previously thought to be the rule, ADHD is considered a chronic condition (Subcommittee on Attention-Deficit/Hyperactivity Disorder & Management, 2011) and persists into adulthood in 60%–70% of people diagnosed with ADHD in childhood (Kessler et al., 2005). ADHD occurs and can be diagnosed in the toddler (although the false-positive rate is relatively high). Box 90.10 lists symptoms, which, in addition to DSM-5 criteria, may suggest ADHD in preschoolers. Hyperactive and impulsive symptoms typically are apparent and are more reliably recognized by the time a child reaches 4 years old and increase during the next 3–4 years, peaking at 7–8 years old. By adolescence, hyperactivity symptoms are less discernible, although symptoms of impulsivity and feelings of restlessness persist. Symptoms of overt inattention may not seem obvious until the child is 8–9 years old, but ability to complete tasks due to distractibility is present early.

### Evaluation and Etiology

History is the primary basis of ADHD diagnosis. Since symptoms must be present in at least two settings and interfere with functioning in at least one setting, multiple informants are helpful for the diagnosis. In addition to an interview, questionnaires for parents, teachers, and the child or adolescent him/herself are useful for making the diagnosis. Given the high rate of ADHD comorbidities (e.g., anxiety and mood disorders, oppositional defiant disorder, conduct disorders), both narrow-band questionnaires that specifically assess for ADHD and broad-band questionnaires that assess not only for ADHD but also for other psychiatric comorbidities should be used (Nass, 2006). The traditional neurological examination is generally normal, although soft signs are common (e.g., synkinesis during repetitive finger tapping and sequencing tasks). Neuropsychological testing is not absolutely necessary unless comorbid learning issues are suspected. The neuropsychological profile usually reveals a normal IQ, but low scores are common on the Wechsler IQ subtests that demand attention or rapid processing (e.g., digit span, coding, arithmetic, symbol search) and intra-test scatter often is found, reflecting variability in attention. Executive frontal lobe functioning—the ability to initiate, inhibit, sustain, and shift attention, working memory, and organizational skills—is often impaired (Crosbie et al., 2007). Measures of spatial working memory, stop task response suppression, continuous performance tasks (CPT), Stroop naming speed, and mazes score have been found to correlate most highly with a clinical ADHD diagnosis. CPTs like the Testing of Variables of Attention Deficit (TOVA) or the Conners

## BOX 90.9 Criteria for Diagnosis of Attention-Deficit/Hyperactivity Disorder

People with ADHD show a persistent pattern of inattention and/or hyperactivity-impulsivity that interferes with functioning or development:

1. Inattention: Six or more symptoms of inattention for children up to age 16, or five or more for adolescents 17 and older and adults; symptoms of inattention have been present for at least 6 months, and they are inappropriate for developmental level:
   - Often fails to give close attention to details or makes careless mistakes in schoolwork, at work, or with other activities.
   - Often has trouble holding attention on tasks or play activities.
   - Often does not seem to listen when spoken to directly.
   - Often does not follow through on instructions and fails to finish schoolwork, chores, or duties in the workplace (e.g., loses focus, side-tracked).
   - Often has trouble organizing tasks and activities.
   - Often avoids, dislikes, or is reluctant to do tasks that require mental effort over a long period of time (such as schoolwork or homework).
   - Often loses things necessary for tasks and activities (e.g., school materials, pencils, books, tools, wallets, keys, paperwork, eyeglasses, mobile telephones).
   - Is often easily distracted.
   - Is often forgetful in daily activities.
2. Hyperactivity and impulsivity: Six or more symptoms of hyperactivity-impulsivity for children up to age 16, or five or more for adolescents 17 and older and adults; symptoms of hyperactivity-impulsivity have been present for at least 6 months to an extent that is disruptive and inappropriate for the person's developmental level:
   - Often fidgets with or taps hands or feet, or squirms in seat.
   - Often leaves seat in situations when remaining seated is expected.
   - Often runs about or climbs in situations where it is not appropriate (adolescents or adults may be limited to feeling restless).
   - Often unable to play or take part in leisure activities quietly.
   - Is often "on the go" acting as if "driven by a motor."
   - Often talks excessively.
   - Often blurts out an answer before a question has been completed.
   - Often has trouble waiting his/her turn.
   - Often interrupts or intrudes on others (e.g., butts into conversations or games).

In addition, the following conditions must be met:

- Several inattentive or hyperactive-impulsive symptoms were present before age 12 years.
- Several symptoms are present in two or more settings (e.g., at home, school or work; with friends or relatives; in other activities).
- There is clear evidence that the symptoms interfere with, or reduce the quality of, social, school, or work functioning.
- The symptoms do not happen only during the course of schizophrenia or another psychotic disorder. The symptoms are not better explained by another mental disorder (e.g., mood disorder, anxiety disorder, dissociative disorder, or a personality disorder).

Based on the types of symptoms, three kinds (presentations) of ADHD can occur:

*Combined presentation*: if enough symptoms of both criteria inattention and hyperactivity-impulsivity were present for the past 6 months.

*Predominantly inattentive presentation*: if enough symptoms of inattention, but not hyperactivity-impulsivity, were present for the past 6 months.

*Predominantly hyperactive-impulsive presentation*: if enough symptoms of hyperactivity-impulsivity but not inattention were present for the past 6 months.

Because symptoms can change over time, the presentation may change over time as well.

*Reprinted with permission from the Diagnostic and Statistical Manual of Mental Disorders, Fifth Edition, (© 2013). American Psychiatric Association.*

## BOX 90.10 Signs of Preschool Attention-Deficit/Hyperactivity Disorder (Nuances in Addition to DSM-5 Core Symptoms)

High activity
Poor persistence and follow through
Problems staying with the class in group activities
Weak behavior modulation for age
Poor social interactions, over-eager physical play
Silliness unusual for age
Impulsiveness in physical play
  Requires constant supervision in tasks *and* play
  Anxiousness/difficult behavior when required to wait
  Toileting accidents due to forgetfulness
  Inappropriate behavior

Continuous Performance Test are not useful as isolated diagnostic measures because of the high rate of both false-positive and false-negative results.

Overall, neuropsychological deficits are consistent with dysfunction of the basal ganglia–frontal circuits. However, these neuropsychological test abnormalities do not really explain the cognitive neurobiology of ADHD: hence the search for endophenotypes (Castellanos and Tannock, 2002; Konrad et al., 2010; Sonuga-Barke, 2010). Some candidates for core deficits of ADHD include failure of inhibitory control, dysregulation of brain systems mediating reward and response cost, and deficits in arousal, activation, and effortful control. Better delineation of endophenotypes not only would enhance understanding of the disorder but also would increase the power of genetic research to identify susceptibility genes (Crosbie et al., 2007).

Several medical causes of ADHD exist (Box 90.11). The pediatric neurologist should take particular note of its high frequency of co-occurrence in infants who were born preterm (about 20%) and its relatively high frequency in patients with epilepsy, for example, which is as high as 30% in children with BECTS (Tovia et al., 2011).

ADHD has a substantial genetic component (Larsson et al., 2013). Reported heritability of ADHD ranges from 0.70 to 0.88 in twins. Approximately one-fourth of the first-degree relatives of a child proband with ADHD also has or had ADHD. ADHD co-occurs with other neurobehavioral disorders such as Tourette syndrome, obsessive-compulsive disorder, anxiety, and learning disabilities, raising the question of possible shared susceptibility genes. An increasing number of studies have attempted to elucidate specific genes involved in ADHD and the genetic impact on ADHD biology (Banaschewski et al., 2010). The identification of the exact genes is still unknown and a recent meta-analysis of genome-wide association studies has been unrevealing (Neale et al., 2010). Many different environmental factors have been reportedly associated with ADHD but it is difficult to identify which are definitely causal. Pre- and perinatal factors, environmental toxins, dietary factors, and psychosocial adversity have all been implicated, with the most reliable associations being with low birth weight/prematurity and exposure to maternal smoking in utero (Thapar et al., 2013). Given variability in heritability and phenotypic expression, it is likely that environmental influences play a role in concert with genetic factors.

Dopamine appears to be the primary neurotransmitter involved in ADHD (Cools, 2008; Solanto, 2002). Hence, genetic studies have focused on candidate genes involved in dopaminergic transmission (dopamine transporter and dopamine receptors genes). The dopamine $D_4$ receptor (DRD4) has been the most well studied and is prevalent in the basal ganglia–frontal networks implicated in the pathophysiology of ADHD (Albayrak et al., 2008). Data suggest that the genotype may even influence the physiological response to medication in ADHD (Gilbert et al., 2006).

While not clinically indicated, most research structural imaging studies reveal abnormalities in frontal and striatal regions (Cubillo et al., 2012), but imaging research in ADHD has blossomed in the past several decades and has broadly implicated executive function networks (Fig. 90.1). For an excellent review see Bush (2009). Children with ADHD show relative cortical thinning in regions important for attentional control, most prominently in the medial and superior prefrontal and precentral regions (Shaw et al., 2006). Children with a worse outcome have "fixed" thinning of the left medial prefrontal cortex, which may compromise the anterior attentional network and encumber clinical improvement. Right parietal cortex thickness normalization in patients with a better outcome may represent compensatory cortical change (Shaw et al., 2006). Cortical volume, surface area, and folding throughout the cerebral cortex appear to be decreased, suggesting the disorder begins prenatally and affects neurogenesis (Wolosin et al., 2009). Variations in corpus callosum have been observed between ADHD subjects and controls, but these may be impacted by gender differences (Hutchinson et al., 2018). DTI studies point to altered structural connectivity in white-matter tracts linking areas previously implicated in the pathophysiology of ADHD.

**BOX 90.11 Possible Environmental Causes/Contributors to Attention-Deficit/Hyperactivity Disorder**

Chronic illness: allergy, asthma, celiac disease, sleep disorders
Endocrine: thyrotoxicosis, hypothyroidism, generalized resistance to thyroid hormone
Epilepsy
Genetic disorders: Turner syndrome, fragile X syndrome
Infectious disease: otitis media, human immunodeficiency virus
Metabolic disorders: phenylketonuria
Prematurity
Psychosocial adversity
Toxins, pre- and postnatal: maternal smoking, drugs, alcohol; lead, mercury
Trauma: concussion, closed head injury

*From Mill, J., Petronis, A., 2008. Pre- and peri-natal environmental risks for attention-deficit hyperactivity disorder (ADHD): the potential role of epigenetic processes in mediating susceptibility. J Child Psychol Psychiatry 49, 1020–1030; Nass, R., 2006. Evaluation and assessment issues in the diagnosis of attention deficit hyperactivity disorder. Semin Pediatr Neurol 12, 200–216; Nass, R.D., Frank, Y. (Eds.), 2010. Cognitive and Behavioral Abnormalities of Pediatric Diseases, Oxford University Press, New York.*

Functional neuroimaging studies have assessed the degree of brain activation associated with various neuropsychological tasks implicated in ADHD and executive function (Rubia, 2018). Results are varied, and promises of biomarker identification in single-subject prediction are thus far unmet due to bias, methodology, and sampling (Arbabshirani et al., 2017; Pulini et al., 2019). In many studies, the ADHD and control subjects do equally well on the experimental task. Thus, activation differences indicate group differences in the neural systems used to accomplish the task. Results of most of these studies are consistent with the structural studies locating abnormalities of brain activation in patients with ADHD in fronto-basal ganglia-cerebellar circuits (Biederman and Faraone, 2005; Biederman et al., 2006; MTA Cooperative Group, 2004). Functional connectivity during "default mode" (Raichle et al., 2001) when individuals are in a task-free condition, also has been studied. Fair et al. (2010) showed that children with ADHD had dysfunctional connectivity in the default-mode network (brain regions that are active when an individual is not focused on the outside world and is in a state of wakeful

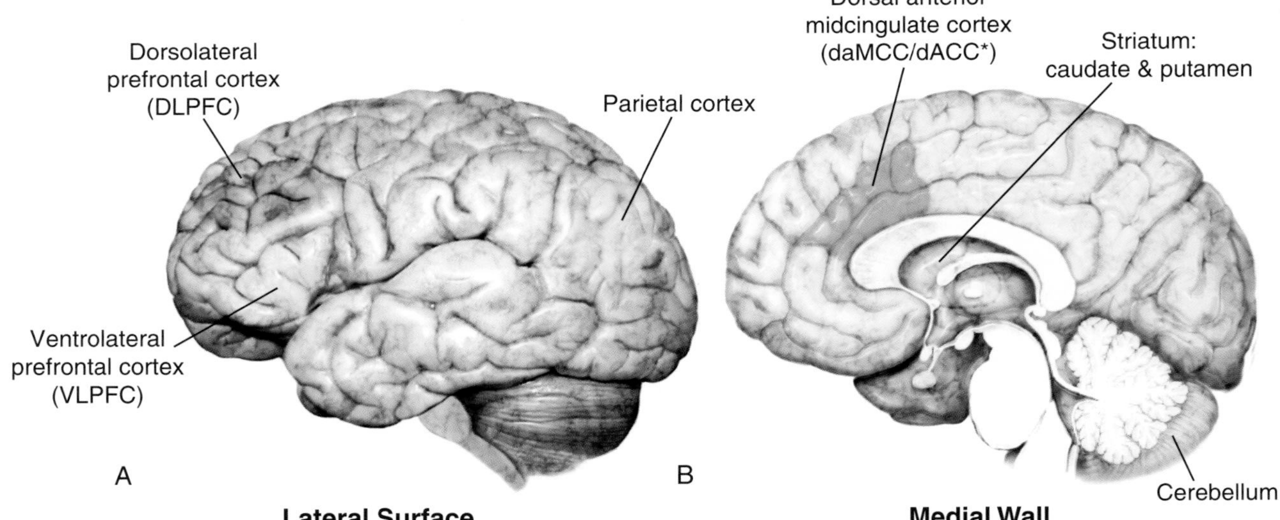


**Fig. 90.1** Brain Structures Implicated in Attention-Deficit/Hyperactivity Disorder *(ADHD).* Interacting neural regions have been implicated in ADHD. In particular, the dorsal anterior midcingulate cortex *(daMCC)*, dorsolateral prefrontal cortex *(DLPFC)*, ventrolateral prefrontal cortex *(VLPFC)*, parietal cortex, striatum, and cerebellum—all key elements of cognitive/attention networks—have also been found to display functional abnormalities in multiple studies of ADHD. *(From Attention-Deficit/Hyperactivity Disorder and Attention Networks from Bush 2010 (Bush, 2009))*

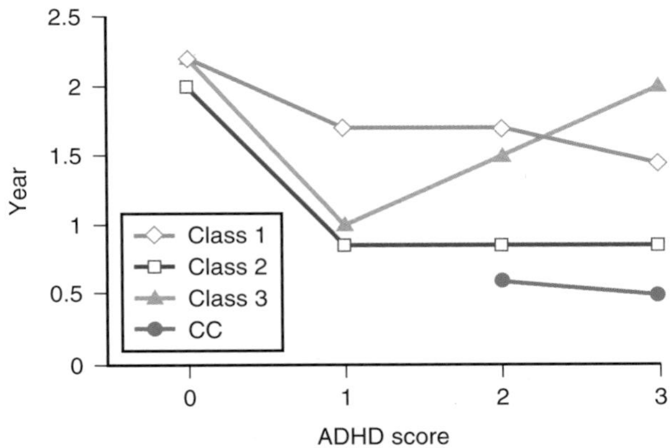


**Fig. 90.2** MTA Study Outcome of Co-Occurring Disorders in Children. *ADHD,* Attention-deficit/hyperactivity disorder. (*Data from MTA Cooperative Group, 1999. Arch Gen Pysch 54, 1088.*)

**TABLE 90.8 Pharmacological Treatment of Attention-Deficit/Hyperactivity Disorder**

| | |
|---|---|
| Stimulants | Methylphenidate (Ritalin, Focalin, Concerta, Daytrana), dextroamphetamine (Dexedrine, Adderall, Vyvanse) |
| α-Agonists | Clonidine (Catapres), guanfacine (Tenex), Intuniv |
| Antidepressants | SSRIs; tricyclic antidepressants; bupropion (Wellbutrin); trazodone; SSNRIs (venlafaxine [Effexor], duloxetine [Cymbalta]); MAOIs (selegiline [Deprenyl]) |
| Antimanic | Lithium carbonate (Lithium) |
| Mood stabilizers | Carbamazepine (Tegretol), divalproex sodium (Depakote), gabapentin (Neurontin), topiramate (Topamax) |
| Beta-blockers | Propranolol (Inderal), atenolol (Tenormin) |
| Anxiolytics | Buspirone (BuSpar); clonazepam (Klonopin), SSRIs |
| Atypical neuroleptics | Risperidone (Risperdal, Zyprexa) and others |
| Nonstimulants | Atomoxetine (Strattera), modafinil (Provigil) |

*MAOI,* Monoamine oxidase inhibitor; *SSNRI,* selective serotonin and norepinephrine reuptake inhibitor; *SSRI,* selective serotonin reuptake inhibitor. *Data from Biederman, J., Faraone, V., 2005. ADHD. Lancet 366, 237–245.; Dopheide, J.A., Pliszka, S.R., 2009. Attention-deficit-hyperactivity disorder: an update. Pharmacotherapy 29(6), 66–79; Swanson, J.M., Greenhill, L.L., Lopez, F.A., et al., 2006. Modafinil film-coated tablets in children and adolescents with attention-deficit/hyperactivity disorder: results of a randomized, double-blind, placebo-controlled, fixed-dose study followed by abrupt discontinuation. J Clin Psychiatry 67, 137–147.*

rest), compared with children without ADHD. Functional MRI has also been used to investigate the effects on ADHD drugs on neural functioning. Rubia et al. (2009, 2011a, 2011b) have shown that methylphenidate normalizes abnormal brain activation and connectivity. A recent qualitative review supports these findings (Spencer et al., 2013).

## Management

Medication, in particular psychostimulants, is the mainstay of treatment (Greenhill et al., 2002) (Table 90.8). The National Institutes of Health (NIH) sponsored Multimodal Treatment Study of ADHD (MTA) (The MTA Cooperative Group, 1999) has shown the effectiveness of stimulants both behaviorally and by neuropsychological testing, and the effectiveness is greater than behavioral modification alone (Biederman et al., 2006; Epstein et al., 2006). Approximately 75% of children initially respond to stimulants. During the initial 14 months of the MTA study, children randomized to intensive behavioral management rather than stimulants did not do as well with respect to the core symptoms of ADHD (inattention, hyperactivity, impulsivity) as those receiving stimulants, demonstrating that medication is critical to managing ADHD. Those children who had comorbid issues, such as anxiety or oppositional behavior, did best with both medication and behavioral management. Some longitudinal data from the MTA study suggest that the effectiveness of medication may decrease over time (Molina et al., 2009). The initial trajectory in treatment is prognostic, and adolescent impairments remain. Three subgroups that did not correspond to the initial treatment groups were identified at year 3. Group 1 had gradual improvement over time, with increasing and significant benefit from medication use at 3 years out (34% of the sample). Group 2 had a larger initial improvement that was maintained over time (52% of the sample). Group 3 returned to baseline symptoms after initial benefit (14% of the sample) (Fig. 90.2). So, although the same treatment benefits were not present at year 3, most of the children were doing well nonetheless. Intensive medication management may only make a persistent long-term difference if continued with the same intensity as during the MTA's initial 14-month study period. In contrast, starting or adding medication at a less-than-optimal intensity and/or too late in a child's ADHD clinical course, particularly if a child's behavior is deteriorating, may not only be ineffective, but also (if not carefully examined in data analysis) even make medication appear to be associated with worse outcomes. Some children may eventually be able to stop medication, perhaps just because of early intensive treatment. Medication alone and combined therapy (medication and behavioral management) did decrease the number of ADHD children who developed oppositional defiant disorder at the 3-year follow-up (Molina et al., 2009).

Stimulant benefits occur on initiation of treatment as do side effects, and dose response is expected for both. Limitations to persistence in treatment include not only the side effects (e.g., emotional lability, daytime appetite suppression, sleep dysregulation) but also the practice and policy barriers to obtaining refills. Guidelines for ADHD treatment include combinations of stimulant use and evidence-based behavior therapy (Subcommittee on Attention-Deficit/Hyperactivity Disorder & Management, 2011), and best practices in ADHD for the specialist should not be limited to pharmacology (Fig. 90.3). Many different formulations of the stimulants exist, with differing duration of action (Table 90.9). No stimulant has a buildup period, and titrations can be made to clinical effect in weekly increments with good communication between providers and caregivers. Neither epilepsy, tics, or Tourette syndrome is a contraindication to stimulant use in ADHD, although they may affect medication choices (Pliszka et al., 2006). Comorbid mood or anxiety disorders also affect their use (Brown, 2000; Pliszka et al., 2006). In addition to stimulants, other medications can be used to treat ADHD. Atomoxetine (i.e., Strattera) is a nonstimulant treatment with acceptable treatment effect size but different side-effect profile. Adjunct therapy with the α-agonists (clonidine, guanfacine) is common, though a common practice of initiating treatment with these medications is not recommended. Tricyclics, selective serotonin reuptake inhibitors, serotonin-norepinephrine reuptake inhibitors, bupropion, and modafinil have all been used, generally in those who failed to respond to stimulants (see Table 90.8).

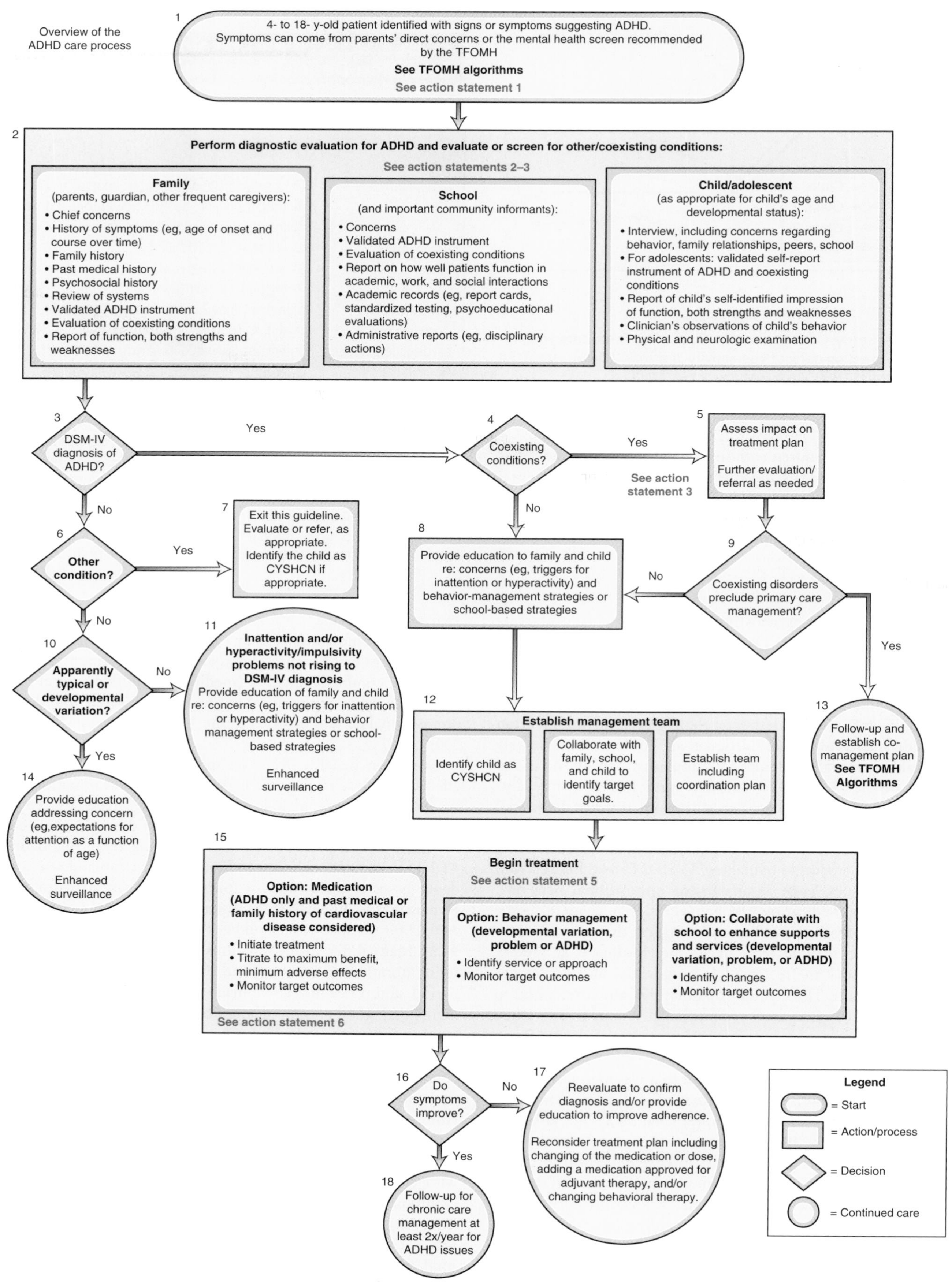


**Fig. 90.3** Attention-Deficit/Hyperactivity Disorder *(ADHD)* Diagnosis and Treatment Algorithm. (*From Wolraich, M., Brown, L., Brown, R. T., et al. (2011, November). ADHD: Clinical practice guideline for the diagnosis, evaluation, and treatment of attention-deficit/hyperactivity disorder in children and adolescents. Pediatrics. https://doi.org/10.1542/peds.2011-2654.*)

TABLE 90.9 **Duration and Preparation of Stimulants**

| Medication | Brand | Initial Titration Dose | Frequency | Time to Initial Effect | Duration, hours | Maximum Dose | Available Doses |
|---|---|---|---|---|---|---|---|
| Mixed amphetamine salts | Adderall[a] | 2.5–5.0 mg | QD-BID | 20–60 min | 6 | 40 mg | 5.0-, 7.5-, 10.0-, 12.5-, 15.0-, 20.0-, and 30.0-mg tablets |
| | Adderall XR[a] | 5 mg | QD | 20–60 min | 10 | 40 mg | 5-, 10-, 15-, 20-, 25-, and 30-mg capsules |
| Dextroamphetamine | Dexedrine[a]/ Dextrostat | 2.5 mg | BIO-TIO | 20–60 min | 4–6 | 40 mg | 5- and 10-mg (Dextrostat only) tablets |
| | Dexedrine Spansule[a] | 5 mg | QD-BID | ≥60 min | ≥6 | 40 mg | 5-, 10-, and 15-mg capsules |
| Lisdexamfetamine | Vyvanse | 20 mg | QD | 60 min | 10–12 | 70 mg | 20-, 30-, 40-, 50-, 60-, and 70-mg capsules |
| Methylphenidate | Concerta | 18 mg | QD | 20–60 min | 12 | 54 mg (<13 years); 72 mg (≥13 years) | 18-, 27-, 36-, and 54-mg capsules |
| | Methyl ER | 10 mg | QD | 20–60 min | 8 | 60 mg | 10- and 20-mg tablets |
| | Methylin | 5 mg | BID-TID | 20–60 min | 3–5 | 60 mg | 5-, 10-, and 20-mg tablets and liquid and chewable forms |
| | Daytrana | 10 mg[b] | Apply for 9 h | 60 min | 11–12 | 30 mg | 10-, 15-, 20-, and 30-mg patches |
| | Ritalin[a] | 5 mg | BID-TID | 20–60 min | 3–5 | 60 mg | 5-, 10-, and 20-mg tablets |
| | Ritalin LA | 20 mg | QD | 20–60 min | 6–8 | 60 mg | 20-, 30-, and 40-mg capsules |
| | Ritalin SR[a] | 20 mg | QD-BID | 1–3 h | 2–6 | 60 mg | 20-mg capsules |
| | Metadate CD | 20 mg | QD | 20–60 min | 6–8 | 60 mg | 10-, 20-, 30-, 40-, 50-, and 60-mg capsules |
| Dexmethylphenidate | Focalin[a] | 2.5 mg | BID | 20–60 min | 3–5 | 20 mg | 2.5-, 5.0-, and 10.0-mg tablets |
| | Focalin XR | 5 mg | QD | 20–60 min | 8–12 | 30 mg | 5-, 10-, 15-, and 20-mg capsules |
| Atomoxetine | Strattera | 0.5 mg/kg/day, then increase to 1.2 mg/kg/day; 40 mg/day for adults and children at > 154 lb, up to 100 mg/ct | QD-BID | 1–2 weeks | At least 10–12 h | 1.4 mg/kg | 10-, 18-, 25-, 40-, 60-, 80-, and 100-mg capsules |
| Extended-release guanfacine | Intuniv | 1 mg/ct | QD | 1–2 weeks | At least 10–12 h | 4 mg/ct | 1-, 2-, 3-, and 4-mg tablets |
| Extended-release clonidine | Kapvay | 0.1 mg/ct | QD-BID | 1–2 weeks | At least 10–12 h | 0.4 mg/ct | 0.1- and 0.2-mg tablets |

[a]Available in a generic form.
[b]Dosages for the dermal patch are not equivalent to those of the oral preparations.*BID*, Twice daily; *TID*, three times daily; *QD*, indicates daily.
*Subcommittee on Attention-Deficit/Hyperactivity Disorder, S. C. on Q. I., & Management., 2011. ADHD: Clinical Practice Guideline for the Diagnosis, Evaluation, and Treatment of Attention-Deficit/Hyperactivity Disorder in Children and Adolescents. Pediatrics, 128(5), 1007–1022. https://doi.org/10.1542/peds.2011-2654*

In addition to medication, treatment should focus on parent skills training, educational accommodations (504 plans: preferential seating, extended time/separate testing site for testing, organizational supports), cognitive behavioral therapy, social skills training, and behavioral modification. Behavioral modification requires setting goals, defining progress, and determining the incentives. The specialist treating ADHD should be prepared to link families to these services for maximum gain and potential reduction of secondary disability. Evidence is emerging in therapeutic devices and alternative approaches to stimulant treatment, especially as they pertain to the challenges facing the maturing population with ADHD (Christiansen et al., 2019).

*The complete reference list is available online at https://expertconsult.inkling.com/.* 

91

# Inborn Errors of Metabolism and the Nervous System

*Phillip L. Pearl, Melissa L. DiBacco, K. Michael Gibson*

## OUTLINE



The concept of inborn errors of metabolism (IEM) was introduced by Sir Archibald Garrod in the 1908 Croonian Lectures, and further developed in his Huxley Lecture presented at Charing Cross Hospital in London (Garrod, 1927). IEM constitute a heterogeneous group of disorders resulting from abnormalities in the synthesis, transport, and turnover of dietary and cellular components. Although individually uncommon, IEM collectively represent a significant cause of morbidity and mortality. In aggregate, approximately 1 in 1000 individuals is born with an IEM. Recent advances in expanded newborn screening (NBS) for IEM have allowed earlier identification and decreased sequelae associated with acute decompensation.

Defects of intermediary metabolic pathways induce disease through either accumulation of a toxic metabolite, depletion of a metabolic by-product, or impaired inter- or intracellular transport. When an enzyme deficiency blocks normal catabolic routes, the diversion of metabolism to alternative pathways may disrupt cellular integrity. Deficient enzyme activity may arise from (1) mutations in the primary gene sequence for the protein, with loss of activity; (2) abnormal processing (i.e., defects of post-translational modification); (3) mistaken intracellular localization; (4) mutation resulting in superactivity of enzyme function; and (5) "gain-of-function" mutations. Metabolic defects may also result from defects of a noncatalytic cofactor, structural, or transport protein.

Most IEM are multiorgan disorders that usually impact the nervous system. The clinical course can be acute, subacute, or chronic. Disorders characterized by intoxication or energy depletion usually manifest acutely as altered mental status, often associated with seizures, hypotonia, ataxia, or myopathy. Vomiting and peripheral organ dysfunction (cardiac, hepatic, renal, pancreatic) are other clinical features of acute intoxication. Some IEM follow an insidious course characterized by developmental delay or intellectual deficiency, behavioral problems, sensory–motor impairment, or dementia. In terms of pathophysiology, it is advantageous to categorize IEM into one of three diagnostic groups: (1) disorders involving complex molecules (e.g., lysosomal storage disorders [LSDs]), peroxisomal diseases, congenital defects of glycosylation (CDG), defects of cholesterol synthesis); (2) disorders involving "small molecules" (e.g., amino and organic acidurias, hyperammonemias, lactic acidemias, disorders of vitamins, metal ions); and (3) disorders associated with disruption of cellular energy metabolism (e.g., mitochondrial respiratory-chain defects, disorders of carbohydrate metabolism, disorders of ). Metabolic defects involving complex molecules are generally progressive and unrelated to food intake, whereas those involving small molecules and cellular energy metabolism may be temporally correlated with food intake or metabolic status (e.g., immunization, postsurgical stress, anabolic vs. catabolic status).

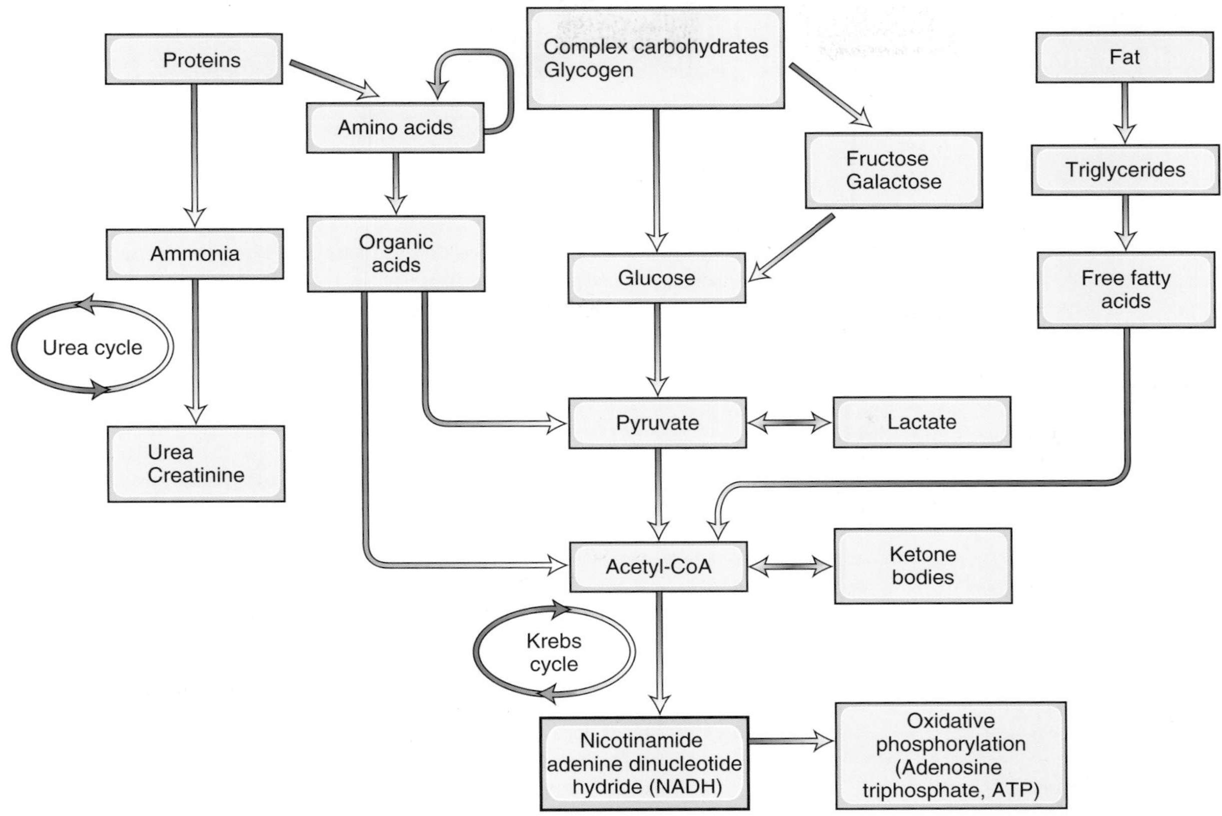


**Fig. 91.1** Overview of Metabolic Pathways. ATP, Adenosine triphosphate; NADH, reduced nicotinamide adenine dinucleotide.

Most often, the inheritance of IEM is autosomal recessive, and the heritable trait results in the deficiency of an enzyme or its cofactor. Autosomal-recessive inheritance often accounts for the absence of a family history when the sibship size is small. A smaller number of IEM are transmitted as autosomal-dominant traits (e.g., acute intermittent porphyria [AIP], familial hypercholesterolemia), as X-linked traits (e.g., Fabry disease, Hunter syndrome, Lesch-Nyhan syndrome, ornithine transcarbamylase deficiency), or segregate in a matrilineal fashion (e.g., mitochondrial DNA defects), the latter requiring a sufficient heteroplasmic burden of mutant mitochondria to enable disease expression.

Early diagnosis is important for treatment intervention, genetic counseling, and family support. A major goal of NBS is to reduce the functional impairment of affected probands, and this has been the greatest advance made through the expansion of NBS for the ~30 disorders on the current list of screened IEM. In addition, most families are unaware of their a priori risk, and early diagnosis of an affected proband facilitates the potential for prenatal diagnosis in future pregnancies. Therapeutic advances in recent years are considerable, especially in the realm of LSDs and ERT (enzyme-replacement therapy) and early diagnosis provides for optimal outcomes. Furthermore, treatment of secondary disabilities (e.g., seizures, sensory impairments, behavioral problems) positively impacts quality of life.

This chapter provides an overview of the major IEM (Fig. 91.1), except for the mitochondrial disorders. Most neurologists are neither metabolic specialists nor biochemical geneticists and are not expected to be knowledgeable concerning the details of all biochemical pathways. This chapter describes those IEM that prominently associate with nervous system dysfunction. A partial listing of IEM associated with key clinical presentations is shown in eTable 91.1. For more comprehensive coverage, the reader may consult several recently published books (Blau et al., 2014; Hoffman et al., 2010; Sarafoglu et al., 2009; Saudubray et al., 2012).

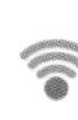

## GENERAL CONSIDERATIONS

### Diagnostic Approach

Clinical features, family history, and baseline testing help focus the diagnostic approach. In the setting of acute illness with neurological signs and symptoms, an IEM should be considered, in parallel with more common disorders, even in the face of a noninformative family history. Examine the blood and urine of patients with acute neurological deterioration or even static encephalopathy for signs of acidosis, ketosis, hypoglycemia, and hyperammonemia (Table 91.2 and eTable 91.3). The caveat is that absence of abnormalities of blood pH, base deficit, blood sugar or ammonia do not necessarily rule out an IEM (e.g., succinic semialdehyde dehydrogenase [SSADH] deficiency) (Kim et al., 2011). Moreover, consider screening tests for abnormalities of amino or organic acid metabolism, and be aware that abnormal metabolites may not be present during stable periods or in samples obtained after the acute illness has resolved. Certain static or progressive encephalopathies require analysis of cerebrospinal fluid (CSF; Opladen and Hoffmann, 2014) (Table 91.4). While CSF examination is time-honored and standard in neurological evaluations, it bears emphasis that hypoglycorrhachia for the diagnosis of glucose transporter 1 (GLUT1) deficiency requires a lumbar puncture, and diagnosis mandates initiation of the ketogenic diet along with carnitine supplementation in the classic neonatal presentation (Wang et al., 2019). There is a differential diagnosis to hypoglycorrhachia, including bacterial and tuberculous meningitis, meningocarcinomatosis, subarachnoid hemorrhage, peripheral

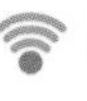

**TABLE 91.2 Commonly Requested Primary/Secondary Tests for the Evaluation of a Patient Suspected for an Inborn Error of Metabolism***

| Tests | Clinical Utility |
|---|---|
| Blood gas, anion gap | Urea cycle defects, organic and amino acidurias, fatty acid oxidation disorders, selected glycogen storage disorders, ketone synthesis/utilization defects, OXPHOS defects |
| Ammonia | Urea cycle defects, organic and amino acidurias, fatty acid oxidation defects, hyperinsulinemia-hyperammonemia (HIHA) syndrome |
| Glucose | Organic and amino acidurias, fatty acid oxidation defects, glycogen storage disorders, ketone synthesis/utilization disorders, OXPHOS defects |
| Lactate† | Selected glycogen storage disorders, defects of gluconeogenesis, fatty acid oxidation (often in conjunction with hypoglycemia); OXPHOS defects |
| Urinary ketones | Organic acidurias, fatty acid oxidation defects, selected glycogen storage disorders, ketone utilization/synthesis disorders, selected amino acidurias (predominantly MSUD); gluconeogenic disorders, OXPHOS defects; ability to distinguish hypo- and hyperketotic disorder (especially pertinent to hypoglycemic disorders) |
| Uric acid | Organic and amino acidurias, fatty acid oxidation defects, glycogen storage disorders, ketone synthesis/utilization disorders, OXPHOS defects; disorders of purine and pyrimidine metabolism |
| Creatine kinase | Disorders of fatty acid oxidation, selected glycogen storage disorders, OXPHOS defects |
| Reducing substances (urine) | Disorders of carbohydrate metabolite (primarily galactosemia) |
| Insulin levels (with ketones and/or free fatty acids) | Useful in the differential diagnosis of the hypoglycemic patient; comparisons between the ratio of free fatty acids/ketone bodies, in conjunction with glucose and ketone bodies, assist in differentiating hypo- and hyperketotic disorders. |
| Amino acid analysis (sera/plasma) | Amino acidurias, selected organic acidurias, defects in gluconeogenesis, urea cycle disorders |
| Organic acid analysis (urine) | Organic and amino acidurias, urea cycle defects, fatty acid oxidation disorders, selected glycogen storage disorders, ketone synthesis/utilization defects, defects in gluconeogenesis, OXPHOS defects (urinary orotic acid can also be beneficial in the differential diagnosis of urea cycle defects) |
| Acylcarnitine profile (sera/plasma/bloodspot) | Organic acidurias, defects of fatty acid oxidation, limited utility in differential diagnosis of ketone utilization/synthesis defects |
| Congenital disorders of glycosylation | Isoelectric focusing of serum transferrin (possible to miss selected disorders); isoelectric focusing of serum apolipoprotein C-III; analysis of lipid-linked oligosaccharides; glycan structural analysis (usually MALDI-TOF, or combined with capillary electrophoresis); mutation analyses and/or whole exome sequence analysis |

*MALDI-TOF*, Matrix-assisted laser desorption/ionization-time of flight mass spectrometry; *MSUD*, maple syrup urine disease; *OXPHOS*, disorders of oxidative phosphorylation.

*The above list only represents a brief overview of primary and secondary tests to pursue. Depending upon outcomes (or specific clinical features), more detailed analyses may be warranted, potentially including purine and pyrimidine analyses (urine), neurotransmitter evaluation (cerebrospinal fluid), lipoprotein profile, cholesterol-related metabolites (often in the context of dysmorphia), creatine, polyols, bile acids, very-long chain fatty acids (VLCFA, peroxisomal disease, in conjunction with phytanic acid), and potentially Nuclear magnetic resonance (NMR) spectroscopy.

†Presence or absence of hypoglycemia can be a useful aid to differential diagnosis of disorders that lead to lactic acidemia.

*Adapted from Grünewald, S., Davison, J., Martinelli, D., Duran, M., Dionisi-Vici, C., 2014. Emergency diagnostic procedures and emergency treatment. In Blau, N., Duran, M., Gibson, K. M., Dionisi-Vici, C. (Eds.), Physician's Guide to the Diagnosis, Treatment, and Follow-Up of Inherited Metabolic Diseases. Springer, New York, pp. 709–719.*

hypoglycemia, and, in some cases, status epilepticus and mitochondrial disorders. The phenotypic spectrum of GLUT1 deficiency is considerable, from neonatal seizures to later exertional dyskinesias, as well as myoclonic-atonic seizures and early-onset generalized absence seizures (Fig. 91.2).

Neurological deterioration is a characteristic feature of acute intoxication disorders (e.g., certain aminoacidopathies, organic acidurias, and the urea cycle disorders). However, with the revolution of NBS, many patients are identified prior to a potential acute decompensation episode. Abnormal urine odor may be present in diseases associated with the excretion of volatile metabolites (keto-acids [maple syrup] in maple syrup urine disease [MSUD]; sweaty feet in isovaleric acidemia [IVA]; and glutaric acidemia type II). Isolated seizures may be the initial features of vitamin-responsive disorders (e.g., defects of pyridoxine [vitamin $B_6$] and folinic acid metabolism, biotinidase deficiency, and biotin-responsive multiple carboxylase deficiency [MCD]), and are a prominent feature in glycine encephalopathy, sulfite oxidase (SO) deficiency, and formation of the molybdenum cofactor complex. Congenital lactic acidosis and central hypotonia are features of abnormalities of pyruvate metabolism and the Krebs cycle (De Meirleir, 2013; Pithukpakorn, 2005). Recurrent hypoglycemia, in the face of pronounced organomegaly, typically occurs in the glycogen storage disorders (GSDs) affecting the liver and in defects of fatty acid oxidation (FAO; consequent to overutilization) (Spiekerkoetter and Mayatepek, 2010); these diseases are also frequently associated with signs of cardiac involvement (cardiomyopathy, arrhythmias). In the mitochondrial FAO defects, urinary ketone concentrations are pathologically low (associated with the inability to metabolize fatty acids of variable chain length). Analysis of plasma acylcarnitines, and the profile of urinary acylglycines, is helpful in the differential diagnoses of the FAOs (Spiekerkoetter and Mayatepek, 2010). Renal tubular acidosis associated with bicarbonate wasting can be encountered in pyruvate carboxylase (PC) deficiency, methylmalonic

**TABLE 91.4 Selected Cerebrospinal Fluid Abnormalities in Disorders of Monoamine Neurotransmitter Metabolism and Tetrahydrobiopterin Synthesis**

| | LEVELS IN CEREBROSPINAL FLUID | | | | | | | |
|---|---|---|---|---|---|---|---|---|
| **Disorder** | **Neopterin** | **Sepiapterin** | **Biopterin** | **5-HTP** | **HVA** | **5-HIAA** | **3-OMD** | **MHPG** |
| Dopamine β-hydroxylase deficiency | | | | | | N | ↑ | ↓↓ |
| Tyrosine hydroxylase deficiency | | | | | ↓↓ | N | n | ↓ |
| Aromatic-L-amino acid decarboxylase deficiency | | | | ↑↑ | ↓↓ | ↓↓ | ↑↑↑ | |
| Monoamine oxidase A deficiency | | | | | ↓ | ↓ | n | ↓ |
| Dopamine transporter deficiency | | | | | ↑ | N | | |
| Dopamine-serotonin vesicular transport defect | | | | | n | N | | |
| Guanosine triphosphate (GTP) cyclohydrolase deficiency | ↓↓ | | ↓↓ | | ↓↓ | ↓ | | |
| 6-Pyruvoyl-tetrahydropterin synthase (6-PTPS) deficiency | ↑↑↑ | | ↓↓↓ | | ↓↓ | ↓↓ | | |
| Dihydropteridine reductase deficiency | n | | n-↑ | | ↓↓ | ↓↓ | | |
| Pterin-4-α-carbinolamine dehydratase deficiency (primapterinuria) | ↑-↑↑ | | | | | | | |
| Dopa-responsive dystonia (Segawa disease) | ↓ | | ↓ | | ↓ | ↓-n | | |
| Sepiapterin reductase deficiency | n | ↑↑ | ↑ | | ↓↓↓ | ↓↓↓ | | |

*3-OMD*, 3-ortho-methyldopa (derived from L-dopa); *5-HIAA*, 5-hydroxyindoleacetic acid (derived from serotonin); *5-HTP*, 5-hydroxytryptophan; *HVA*, homovanillic acid (derived from dopamine); *MHPG*, 3-methoxy-4-hydroxyphenylglycol (norepinephrine metabolite).

*Adapted from Opladen, T., Hoffmann, G.F., 2014, Neurotransmitter disorders, in addition to Blau, N., van Spronsen, F.J., 2014, Disorders of phenylalanine and tetrahydrobiopterin metabolism, both in. In: Blau, N., Duran, M., Gibson, K.M., Dionisi-Vici, C. (Eds.), Physician's Guide to the Diagnosis, Treatment, and Follow-Up of Inherited Metabolic Diseases. Springer, New York, pp. 515–528 and 3–22.*

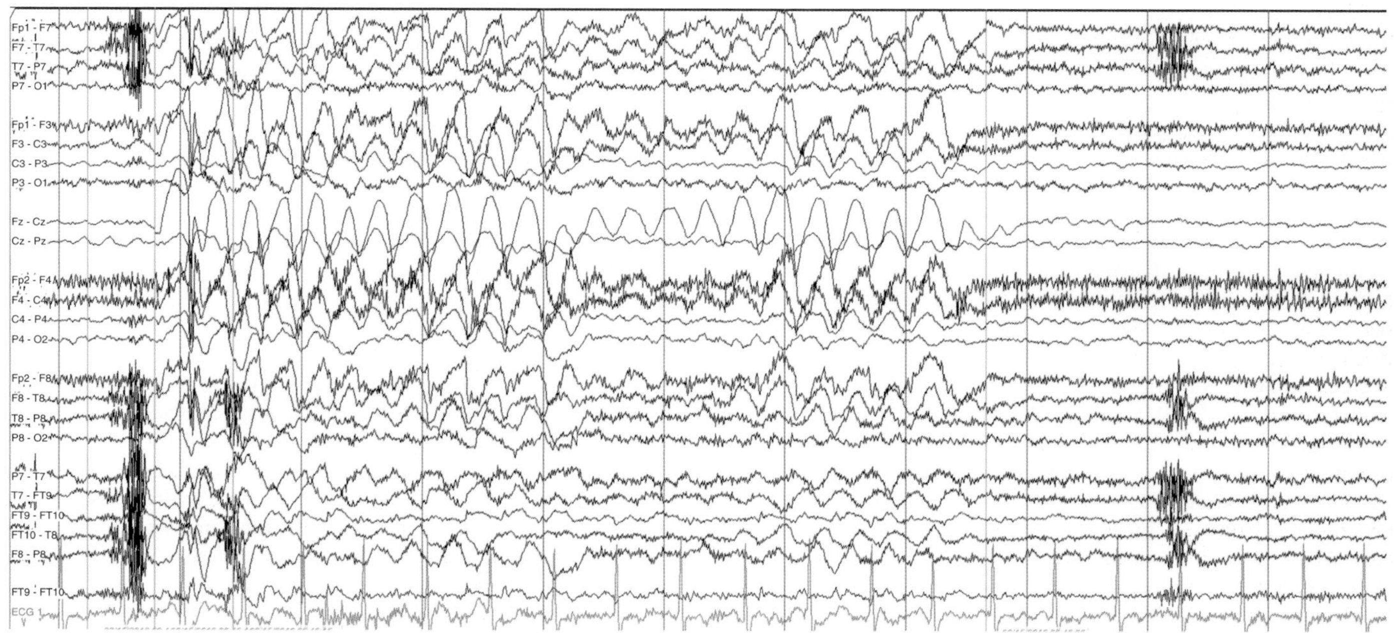

**Fig. 91.2** Electroencephalogram (EEG) in 2-year-old boy presenting with absence seizures at only 23 months of age. High voltage generalized 3–4 Hz paroxysmal slow waves superimposed upon a normal background accompany staring spells. Subsequent evaluation confirmed glucose transporter 1 deficiency. HFF 70 Hz, LFF 1 Hz, time base 30 mm/s. Note sensitivity is 30 mcV/mm.

acidemia (MMA), carnitine palmitoyltransferase I (CPT-I) deficiency, and cystinosis.

Ophthalmological examination often provides important insight into the diagnosis of IEM. Vertical supranuclear ophthalmoplegia occurs in Niemann-Pick type C disease, and saccadic initiation failure and defective optokinetic nystagmus may be observed in Gaucher disease type III. Kayser-Fleisher rings (orange or greenish deposits around the limbus of the cornea due to copper deposition within the Descemet basement membrane of the cornea) are strongly suggestive of Wilson disease (eTable 91.5). Hepatosplenomegaly and other signs of storage (e.g., coarse facies, nonimmune hydrops fetalis, dysostosis multiplex, kyphoscoliosis) occur within the broad spectrum of lysosomal disorders, especially the mucopolysaccharidoses. Liver dysfunction or hepatomegaly (or both) usually manifests in disorders of carbohydrate metabolism (e.g., galactosemia, hereditary fructose intolerance [HFI], GSD [particularly Pompe disease, or GSD type II]), bile acid synthesis defects, tyrosinemia, and CDG. Inability to synthesize and mobilize bile acids (and conjugates) can also result in extensive cholestatic disease (Lemonde et al., 2003). Unconjugated hyperbilirubinemia associated with liver dysfunction or hemolysis in infancy may lead to permanent brain damage due to kernicterus, a major concern in the Crigler-Najjar disorder (Erlinger et al., 2014).

Cardiomyopathy, both dilated and hypertrophic, may develop in IEM associated with infiltrative (storage) disorders and deficits of energy metabolism. The presence of hepatomegaly and other signs of systemic involvement (e.g., cataracts, coarse facies, renal disease, dysostosis multiplex) may suggest storage disorders of mucopolysaccharide mobilization.

Some disorders may have both a young and a later age of onset, or follow an atypical course. Allelic mutations with partial enzyme activity, or organ-specific expression, may underlie these presentations. Examples include acid maltase deficiency (muscle weakness and respiratory problems without cardiomyopathy), FAO deficits (myoglobinuria and rhabdomyolysis post-exercise) (Spiekerkoetter and Mayatepek, 2010), X-linked adrenomyeloneuropathy (spastic paraparesis associated with spinal cord and peripheral nerve demyelination), glycogen brancher enzyme deficiency (adult polyglucosan body disease with progressive motor neuron disease, sensory loss, neurogenic bladder, and dementia), and AIP (abdominal pain, psychosis). The myopathy associated with statin use may suggest that the use of these drugs in disorders of FAO is contraindicated (Isackson et al., 2011).

Assessment of the L-carnitine profile (total and esterified carnitine levels in plasma) may be useful when suspecting a primary or secondary carnitine deficiency, as well as defects of fat oxidation and organic acidurias. Carnitine plays an essential role in the transfer of long-chain fatty acids across the inner mitochondrial membrane, in the detoxification of acyl moieties, and in the maintenance of free coenzyme A (CoA) levels. Primary carnitine deficiency (due to defects in the *OCTN2* gene associated with defective carnitine transport) leads to cardiac and skeletal muscle disease. Secondary carnitine deficiency occurs in several IEM and is often responsive to oral L-carnitine supplementation that enhances detoxification of accumulated acyl-CoA species and excretion of toxic organic acid species as acylcarnitine analogues.

Tandem mass spectrometry (TMS) analysis of blood spots on filter paper is an effective means of screening for some defects of amino and organic acid metabolism, and FAO defects, among

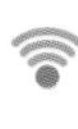

others (Pasquali et al., 2006) (eTable 91.6). The massive expansion of NBS using TMS has taken advantage of the numerous acylcarnitine analogues associated with multiple disorders, which affords specific identification of disease patterns (Greene and Matern, 2014). Methods for screening of LSDs by TMS have also been recently introduced (Liao et al., 2014; Matern, 2008; Ombrone et al., 2013).

Histological examination of appropriate tissue samples can provide important insights into the nature of the storage materials found in certain IEM (e.g., lysosomal disorders) (Bali et al., 2012; Warren and Alroy, 2000). When performing a skin biopsy, it is advisable to obtain samples for microscopic examination in addition to tissue culture. These cultured cells are useful as source material for subsequent biochemical or molecular (genetic) testing. For disorders of amino and organic acids, skin fibroblasts allow confirmatory diagnosis by enzymatic assays. Many laboratories certified to provide clinical biochemical genetic testing are moving away from complex enzymology for diagnostic confirmation, primarily related to expense, complexity, and poor cost recovery issues with insurance. The gold standard for diagnoses has more recently turned to molecular genetic testing (Zschocke and Janssen, 2008), and the latter has been considerably expanded to deep-genomic and whole exome sequencing (WES) (Alavi et al., 2013; Kevelam et al., 2013; Rosenthal et al., 2013). Biopsy of various tissues (liver, heart, and muscle) is necessary for diagnosis of selected diseases (e.g., glycogen storage, disorders of oxidative phosphorylation). Lastly, microscopic examination of scalp hair can provide important diagnostic information, such as Menkes syndrome (pili torti) (Cosimo et al., 2011; Smith et al. 2005).

Careful attention to sample requirements and shipping and handling considerations is key for optimal testing outcomes. Clinical information is required to receive guidance in both testing interpretation and patient evaluation. In cases with an established diagnosis, detailed information may be obtained from several websites, including Gene Reviews (https://www.ncbi/nlm/nih/gov), Online Mendelian Inheritance in Man (OMIM, <http://www.ncbi.nlm.nih.gov/OMIM>), GeneClinics (<http://www.geneclinics.org>), the National Organization for Rare Disorders (NORD, <http://www.rarediseases.org>), the Online Metabolic and Molecular Bases of Inherited Disease (<ommbid.mhmedical.com>), the Society for Inherited Metabolic Disorders (<http://www.simd.org>), and the Society for the Study of Inborn Errors of Metabolism (<http://www.ssiem.org>). Several patient advocacy support groups provide information about community resources and ongoing clinical trials (e.g., the National PKU Alliance [<http://www.npkua.org>], the Organic Acidemia Association [<http://www.oaanews.org>], the MSUD Family Support Group [<http://www.msud-support.org>], the SSADH Foundation [<http://www.ssadh.net>], and many others).

## Mutation Analysis

Molecular genetic techniques offer an alternative means for the diagnostic confirmation of IEM, especially in those instances in which a biochemical or enzymatic diagnostic test is unavailable or requires invasive approaches. This is particularly true for diseases with a *founder effect*—common mutations in which one or a few alleles account for a significant proportion of cases (e.g., Finnish and Jewish "heritage" diseases). In diseases with a known causal mutation, testing of other family members permits accurate carrier identification, but significant ethical considerations arise and certified genetic counselors should be involved. DNA testing for prenatal diagnosis provides rapid diagnosis in relation to the use of chorionic villi or amniocytes which do not require cell culture. Molecular diagnostic analyses are not completely foolproof, and several caveats exist. For example, when two mutant alleles are identified in an autosomal-recessive disorder, are they on the same chromosome or different chromosomes (e.g., *cis* or *trans*)? Studies in parental samples usually help to clarify this issue. Additionally, is the disease predicted from the identified alleles 100% penetrant (e.g., the penetrance of a disease-causing mutation is the proportion of individuals with the mutation who exhibit clinical symptoms)? Caution should always be applied in assignment of causality, particularly for novel mutations or sequence alterations for which functional impacts have not been established (Geneletti et al., 2011).

Examples of disorders for which DNA testing has proven useful include medium-chain acyl-CoA dehydrogenase (MCAD) deficiency (Gregersen et al., 2004; Leal et al., 2014), Gaucher disease (Sidransky, 2012), and classical MSUD in the old-order Amish (Jain et al., 2013). Among patients with MCAD deficiency of northwestern European descent, ~80% are homozygous for a single missense mutation (A985G), and 17% carry this mutation in combination with another less common allelic alteration. This finding has improved the reliability of MCAD carrier identification and diagnosis, particularly for siblings who may be affected but asymptomatic at the time of family screening. Certain metabolic disorders (e.g., Tay-Sachs disease, Gaucher disease, Niemann-Pick disease type A, and Canavan disease) have an increased prevalence among individuals of Ashkenazi Jewish ancestry (i.e., of Central and Eastern European descent). A limited number of "common" mutations in this population cause the disease, which facilitates targeted screening for appropriate genetic counseling prior to marriage and conception. A number of scanning and screening methodologies exist for molecular genetic analyses in DNA, including polymerase chain reaction (PCR) amplification, discontinuous gradient gel electrophoresis (DGGE), restriction digestion analyses (in which a putative allelic alteration either induces a new restriction site or removes a preexisting site), and dot-blot analyses (using radiolabeled or chemiluminescent-labeled oligonucleotides to bind to a DNA region harboring the mutation). Nonetheless, direct sequencing remains the gold standard (Zschocke and Janssen, 2008). More recent DNA sequencing methods have expanded the molecular diagnostic menu, including multiplex ligation-dependent probe amplification (MLPA) and WES (Vozzi et al., 2013; Zheng et al., 2013).

## Special Considerations

Generally, mutations in IEM associate with loss of function, but there are instances in which mutations can result in gain of function, as well as superactivity of enzyme function that can be deleterious. For example, heterozygous somatic mutations in the isocitrate dehydrogenase isozyme 2 that disable the enzyme to catalyze its normal reaction (isocitrate conversion to 2-oxoglutarate) confer a new function: namely, conversion of 2-oxoglutarate to D-2-hydroxyglutarate (Kranendijk et al., 2010). Alternatively, specific mutations in the phosphoribosyl pyrophosphate synthetase isoform 1 (PRPP synthetase 1) result in superactivity of the enzyme and the induction of a severe form of hyperuricemia and gout (Chen et al., 2013; Moran et al., 2012).

## Inborn Errors of Metabolism Associated with Hearing Abnormalities

A number of IEM manifest with hearing dysfunction (eTable 91.7). For example, sensorineural deafness is a prominent finding in the LSDs, peroxisomal and mitochondrial diseases, and the congenital disorders of glycosylation (CDG) (Morava et al., 2012; Rafique et al., 2013; Sarig et al., 2013). Recurrent otitis media in the mucopolysaccharidoses reflects the storage pathophysiology associated with glycosaminoglycan accumulation (Brands et al., 2013), while conductive deafness may be prominently associated with CDG and the pyrimidine biosynthetic disorders, the latter including dihydroorotate dehydrogenase deficiency (Beck et al., 2013; Jaeken, 2011; Morava et al., 2012). It may be prudent, therefore, for the clinician confronted with idiopathic deafness or hearing loss to consider an IEM in the differential diagnosis.

## Inborn Errors of Metabolism Associated with Abnormal Brain Development and Encephaloclastic Lesions

Several IEM disrupt the normal sequence of brain development and lead to multiple anomalies, including agenesis or dysgenesis of the corpus callosum, neuronal migration defects, and dysmyelination (Braverman et al., 2013; Hennekam, 2005; Jeng et al., 2001; Lee et al., 2013; Nissenkorn et al., 2001) (Table 91.8; eTables 91.9–91.13). Cystic necrosis of white matter, with or without basal ganglia involvement, occurs in deficiencies of pyruvate dehydrogenase (PDH), PC, and molybdenum cofactor. Nonsyndromic congenital microcephaly has been associated with maternal PKU, phosphoglycerate dehydrogenase deficiency (a serine biosynthetic disorder), and 2-ketoglutaric aciduria (associated with Amish lethal microcephaly). Multiple mechanisms have been proposed to explain abnormal brain development and encephaloclastic lesions (such as porencephalic cysts) in IEM, including production of a toxic or energy-deficient intrauterine milieu, modification of the content and function of membranes, and disturbance of the normal expression of intrauterine genes responsible for neurulation and neuronal migration (Prasad et al., 2009).

## Neuroimaging

Magnetic resonance imaging (MRI) is widely employed to obtain brain anatomical data in patients with static and progressive encephalopathy. Advanced imaging techniques such as MR spectroscopy (MRS) and diffusion-weighted imaging (DWI) provide additional insights into brain biochemistry and cell viability, and may highlight diagnostic criteria (Cheon et al., 2002; Faerber and Poussaint, 2002; Kanekar and Byler, 2013; Kaye, 2001; Stence et al., 2013). For example, MRI shows great utility in the diagnosis of pantothenate kinase-associated neurodegeneration (PKAN) associated with brain iron accumulation, in relation to the characteristic "eye-of-the-tiger" pattern that is observed (Diaz, 2013). MRS and DWI represent quantitative techniques that may prove useful in assessing disease severity and potential response to treatment. MRS may even afford a diagnostic pattern: that is, increased gamma-aminobutyrate (GABA) peak in GABA-transaminase deficiency (Tsuji et al., 2010).

White-matter signal abnormalities suggestive of leukodystrophy can be found in several IEM, including Krabbe disease, metachromatic leukodystrophy (MLD), X-linked adrenoleukodystrophy (ALD), and Canavan disease. In addition to signal hyperintensities noted on T2-weighted imaging, selected features may provide additional diagnostic clues. For example, enlarged perivascular spaces or small cysts are characteristic of the mucopolysaccharidoses and Lowe syndrome. Gray-matter lesions may be found in Zellweger syndrome and other peroxisomal disorders. In glutaric aciduria type 1, imaging may show selective frontotemporal atrophy, especially involving subcortical white matter, accompanied by prominent extra-axial CSF collections and widening of the sylvian fissure with poor opercularization ("bat wing" appearance) (Nunes et al., 2013; Oguz et al. 2005). The presence of hyperintense lesions in the subcortical cerebral white matter, basal ganglia, and dentate nuclei, together with cerebellar atrophy, is strongly suggestive of L-2-hydroxyglutaric aciduria (Isikay, 2014; Steenweg et al., 2009). The latter is of interest in comparison to patients with combined D/L-2-hydroxyglutaric aciduria and isolated D-2-hydroxyglutaric aciduria, in which the phenotype features developmental delay, hypotonia, epilepsy, and cardiomyopathy without extensive imaging abnormalities (Muhlhausen et al., 2014).

**TABLE 91.8 Developmental Brain Malformations Associated with Inborn Errors of Metabolism***

| Abnormality | Associated Inborn Errors of Metabolism |
| --- | --- |
| Agenesis, corpus callosum | CHILD syndrome; glycine encephalopathy; pyridoxine-dependent epilepsy; pyruvate dehydrogenase complex (PDH) E1α, E1β, and E3 deficiencies; combined oxidative phosphorylation defect 2 (combined with dysmorphism and fatal lactic acidosis); S-adenosylmethionine (SAM) hydrolase deficiency; Smith-Lemli-Optiz (SLO) syndrome; chondrodysplasia punctate 2 (male); desmosterolosis; 3-hydroxyisobutyryl-CoA deacylase deficiency; congenital disorders of glycosylation (CDG) |
| Atrophy, corpus callosum | Hyperprolinemia; mucolipidosis II; pyrroline-5″-carboxylate synthetase deficiency |
| Atrophy, cerebellum | CDG; succinic semialdehyde dehydrogenase (SSADH) deficiency |
| Atrophy, cerebrum | CDG; cerebral folate deficiency; maple syrup urine disease; 3-methylcrotonyl-CoA carboxylase deficiency; 3-methylglutaconyl-CoA hydratase deficiency (type I methylglutaconic aciduria); Costeff syndrome; 3-methylglutaconic acidurias (idiopathic forms); 3-hydroxy-3-methylglutaryl-CoA (HMG-CoA) lyase deficiency; 3-phosphoglycerate dehydrogenase deficiency; propionic acidemia; methylmalonic acidemia; molybdenum cofactor deficiency; cobalamin disorders; coenzyme $Q_{10}$ deficiency; CDG; SSADH deficiency; dihydropyrimidine dehydrogenase deficiency; deoxyguanosine kinase deficiency; mucolipidosis II, III |
| Atrophy, combined cerebrum and cerebellum | CDG; sulfite oxidase deficiency; MEGDEL syndrome; folate receptor (FOLRI) deficiency; combined saposin deficiency; neuronal ceroid lipofuscinosis (Batten disease); SLC33A1 deficiency with low plasma copper and ceruloplasmin; SSADH |
| Atrophy, frontotemporal | 2-Methyl-3-hydroxybutyryl-CoA dehydrogenase (MHBD) deficiency; malonic aciduria |
| Atrophy, striatal | Glutaric aciduria type I (GA-I) |
| Cerebral infarction | Fabry disease; 3-hydroxy-3-methylglutaryl-CoA (HMG-CoA) lyase deficiency; oxidative-phosphorylation (OXPHOS) disorders (e.g., MELAS) |
| Cerebral white matter lesions | 3-Phosphoglycerate dehydrogenase deficiency; L-2-hydroxyglutaric aciduria; Zellweger syndrome; ribose-5′-phosphate isomerase deficiency; SSADH deficiency |
| Dysplasia, cerebellum | CDG; glutaric acidemia II; Menkes disease; Refsum (infantile) disease; Pyruvate dehydrogenase complex (PDHC) deficiency; peroxisomal diseases (neonatal pseudo-ALD, bifunctional enzyme deficiency); respiratory chain enzyme deficiency; SLO syndrome; Zellweger syndrome |
| Holoprosencephaly | SLO syndrome |
| Hypopmyelination | SAM hydrolase deficiency; serine deficiency disorders; AGC1 deficiency (global cerebral hypomyelination); folate receptor-α deficiency; mucolipidosis II; multiple sulfatase deficiency; SLC33A1 deficiency with low plasma copper and ceruloplasmin |
| Hypoplasia, pons | SAM hydrolase deficiency |
| Hypoplasia, unilateral | CHILD syndrome |
| Hypoplasia, temporal | GA-I; |
| Hypoplasia, cerebellar | CDG; cerebral folate deficiency; glutamine synthetase deficiency; neonatal mitochondrial encephalocardiomyopathy; SAM hydrolase deficiency; adenylosuccinate lyase deficiency; |
| Hypoplasia, cerebellar vermis | CDG; phosphoserine aminotransferase deficiency; phosphoserine phosphatase deficiency |
| Lissencephaly/pachygyria | 3-OH-isobutyric aciduria; bifunctional enzyme deficiency, CDG; desmosterolosis; fumarase Pyruvate dehydrogenase complex (PDHC) deficiency; glutaric acidemia 2; glycine encephalopathy; PDHC deficiency; SLO syndrome; Zellweger syndrome |

*The listing is necessarily incomplete but meant to demonstrate notable patterns of reported findings in selected IEM.

*ALD*, Adrenoleukodystrophy; *CoA*, coenzyme A; *IEM*, inborn errors of metabolism; *MELAS*, mitochondrial encephalopathy, lactic acidosis, and stroke-like episodes.

*Adapted from all chapters in Blau, N., Duran, M., Gibson, K.M., Dionisi-Vici, C. (Eds.), 2014, Physician's Guide to the Diagnosis, Treatment, and Follow-Up of Inherited Metabolic Diseases. Springer, New York.*

The creatine deficiency syndromes, featuring significant developmental delays, hypotonia, and extrapyramidal movement abnormalities, include guanidinoacetate methyltransferase (GAMT), arginine: glycine amidinotransferase (AGAT), and creatine transporter deficiencies. All feature cerebral creatine deficiency detected through MRS (Stockler et al., 2007). A secondary disruption in creatine levels is observed in ornithine aminotransferase (OAT) deficiency, in which the brain creatine : phosphocreatine ratio is decreased. Brain MRS reveals elevated levels of *N*-acetylaspartate (NAA) in patients with Canavan disease, whereas patients with mitochondrial defects and defects of gluconeogenesis may show elevated brain lactate. In MLD, MRS reveals decreased NAA and increased choline and myoinositol, compatible with axonal loss, dysmyelination, and gliosis.

## Imminent Death Prior to Diagnosis in a Child with a Suspected Inborn Error of Metabolism

A metabolic autopsy is recommended when a patient develops acute fatal metabolic decompensation, and in cases of sudden and unexpected death (Ernst et al., 2006; Lee et al., 2010; Olpin, 2004). A correct diagnosis facilitates appropriate counseling and prenatal diagnosis for subsequent pregnancies. Blood and bile (obtained by direct puncture of the gall bladder) specimens should be collected, spotted on filter paper (two circles for each, about 25 μL), and dried prior to storage. Plasma should be separated from whole blood and frozen, as should urine. A portion of liver tissue should be obtained, rinsed with phosphate buffered saline (PBS), and deep frozen without preservative at −80°C. A skin sample should be obtained under sterile technique (use alcohol and not iodine, which interferes with cell growth), and stored at room temperature in tissue culture medium. When suspecting a storage disorder, obtain a small snip of skin and place it in glutaraldehyde for subsequent electron microscopic studies. Excellent guidelines exist for the metabolic autopsy (<http://www.sudc.org/Portals/0/medical/Mayo_Metabolic_Protocol_2009.pdf>).

## Management Considerations Following Diagnosis

The appropriate management of IEM depends upon the particular metabolic and/or molecular derangement. Therapeutic strategies may include one or more of the following approaches: (1) substrate

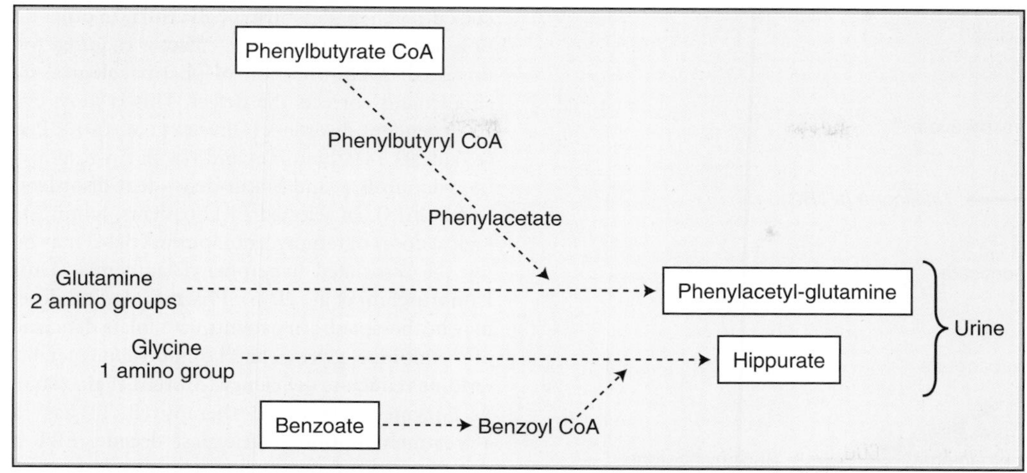


**Fig. 91.3** Alternative Pathways to Reduce Accumulation of Ammonia. *CoA,* Coenzyme A.

reduction by dietary manipulation or precursor synthesis inhibition; (2) removal (or enhanced clearance) of the toxic metabolite(s); (3) replenishment of depleted metabolites or cofactor supplementation (or both), (4) enzyme (replacement or enhancement via chaperone intervention) therapy; and (5) cell or organ replacement (e.g., bone marrow, liver, heart, or kidney transplantation, hepatocyte transplantation) (Chakrapani and Wraith, 2002; Leonard and McKiernan, 2004; Vogel et al., 2014; Wilcken, 2003). Gene therapy is rapidly progressing, with trials recruiting or completed in aromatic amino acid decarboxylase (AADC) deficiency, MLD, Tay-Sachs, Pompe, and Fabry diseases (<http://www.clinicaltrials.gov>). Gene therapeutic approaches are accepted interventions in severe combined immunodeficiency (SCID) and adenosine deaminase deficiency. Numerous gene therapy protocols are active in a number of murine models of IEM, including PKU, Canavan disease, L-AADC deficiency, and others (Ahmed et al., 2013; Koeberl and Kishnani, 2009; Lee et al., 2014; Viecelli et al., 2014). Liver repopulation (hepatocyte transplant) is feasible, but challenges with early engraftment and long-term expansion remain, and this approach is predominantly useful for instances of liver failure and bridging to eventual liver transplant (Vogel et al., 2014). Chaperone-mediated therapy for IEM associated with residual enzyme activity is under active examination, especially the utility of cofactors such as sapropterin (tetrahydrobiopterin) in helping to rescue misfolded proteins and enhance enzyme activity in phenylalanine hydroxylase and other proteins (Gregersen et al., 2001; Pastores and Sathe, 2006; Sarkissian et al., 2012; Underhaug et al., 2012). Drug repurposing is gaining increasing interest, such as use of the compound NTBC (see later; employed in patients with tyrosinemia type I) for possible intervention in PKU to increase brain dopamine (Harding et al., 2014), or the utility of phenylbutyrate (employed in urea cycle disorders to regulate blood ammonia) to alter the regulation of branched-chain ketoacid dehydrogenase in MSUD (NCT01529060; <http://www.clinicaltrials.gov>). The potential to transplant stem cells with directed differentiation potential remains a very active avenue of research (Desnick, 2004; Grompe, 2002; Kawashita et al., 2005; Lund, 2013; Sokal et al., 2014).

Each patient requires an individualized approach, and some disorders require more than one management option. For patients with IEM, generally the "team" approach is necessary, with collaboration between medical geneticist, the biochemical genetics laboratory, genetic counselor, and other specialties as needed. The clinical response to most treatment plans may vary, and residual disturbances are common. Patients may remain at risk for metabolic decompensation when stressed (infection, trauma, surgery, vaccination). Reducing energy expenditure and promoting anabolism are immediate management goals in almost all instances. Emergency measures may prevent further deterioration, but most options are nutritionally incomplete, and extension beyond 48 hours without dietary review is often not prudent. In most situations, provision of symptomatic treatment may necessitate the need for specialized care units with expertise in the specific disease.

Special diets require attention to caloric requirements and balanced nutrition; this is particularly true for minerals and supplements, trace metals, and other parameters. Diseases managed with dietary restriction include phenylketonuria (PKU), MSUD, and homocystinuria. Nonetheless, despite excellent metabolic control, patients with PKU and MSUD may still manifest long-term neurocognitive deficits (Hood et al., 2014; Muelly et al., 2013). Other disorders, such as serine, glutamine, and proline biosynthesis disorders, benefit from recognition and supplementation (de Koning, 2013; van der Crabben et al., 2013). Multiple clinical studies suggest that treatment of PKU patients with sapropterin (a cofactor of phenylalanine hydroxylase) provides better disease control and increases dietary phenylalanine tolerance for selected patients, allowing relaxation of dietary phenylalanine restriction (Blau et al., 2009; Camp et al., 2014; Vockley et al., 2014). In classic Refsum disease, reduction in dietary phytanate results in significant attenuation of the biochemical and clinical phenotype.

Selected IEM require alternative dietary sources. Medium-chain triglycerides may be administered as a lipid source to patients with very-long-chain acyl-CoA dehydrogenase (VLCAD) and long-chain acyl-CoA dehydrogenase (LCHAD) deficiencies. In Smith-Lemli-Opitz syndrome (SLOS) (7-dehydrocholesterol reductase deficiency), the use of cholesterol supplementation improves somatic parameters and may benefit neurodevelopmental status, although clinical response is variable. In the GSDs, carbohydrate supplementation (usually in the form of cornstarch) prevents hypoglycemia and suppresses secondary metabolic derangement, such as hyperlipidemia and hyperuricemia. In the disorders of the urea cycle, arginine or citrulline supplementation can prime the cycle via replenishment of intermediates not synthesized secondarily to the metabolic block.

When dietary manipulation fails to correct the accumulation of toxic metabolites, the primary clinical approach is to utilize methods to enhance their excretion or detoxification. For example, in patients with hyperammonemia, sodium benzoate and sodium phenylbutyrate may be orally supplemented, which conjugate with glycine and glutamine, respectively, to facilitate nitrogen excretion (Fig. 91.3). Clinical care must be taken to monitor sodium intake with these supplements,

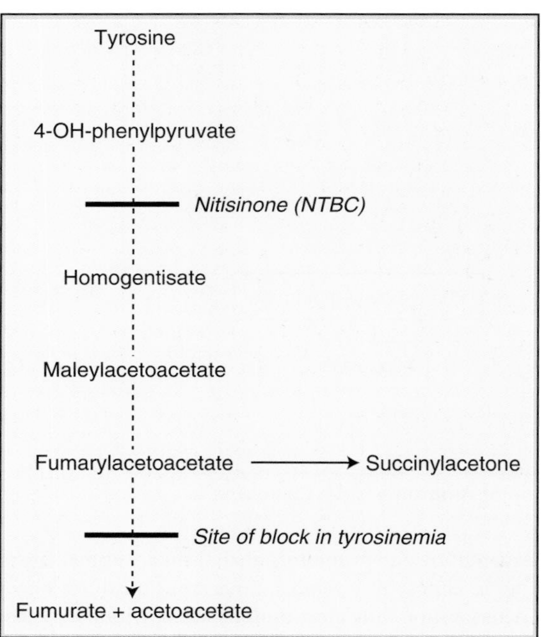


**Fig. 91.4** Substrate Reduction Therapy. *NTBC,* 2-Nitro-4-trifluoro-methylbenzoyl-1,3-cyclohexanedione.

however. In IVA, treatment with oral glycine results in enhanced conjugation and excretion of isovalerylglycine. Administration of cysteamine to patients with cystinosis promotes the formation of cysteine, which is subsequently excreted. Cysteamine has also been piloted in the treatment of neuronal ceroid lipofuscinosis (Gavin et al., 2013). Carnitine supplementation given to patients with organic acidemia prevents carnitine deficiency secondary to the excretion of acylcarnitine species, while simultaneously repleting intracellular concentrations of CoA. During acute metabolic decompensation, dialysis and hemofiltration facilitate the rapid clearance of toxic metabolites. These techniques are already a part of the treatment of multiple IEM, especially the urea cycle disorders and the ensuant hyperammonemia encountered with decompensation (Daschner and Schaefer, 2002; Tsai et al., 2014). In X-linked ALD, administration of glycerol trioleate and trierucate (Lorenzo's oil) to asymptomatic patients may modify the disease course and progression (Moraes, 2013; Moser et al., 2005). A large number of novel therapeutic strategies for IEM employ substrate synthesis inhibitors to block the production of toxic metabolites (Fig. 91.4). An excellent example is the use of NTBC (2-nitro-4-trifluoro-methylbenzoyl-1,3-cyclohexanedione) in tyrosinemia type I (fumarylacetoacetate hydrolase deficiency), a defect in the distal tyrosine metabolic pathway. Via blockade of an early step of tyrosine metabolism, NTBC administration prohibits the production of cytotoxic succinylacetone and fumarylacetoacetate, which are associated with the development of hepatocellular carcinoma. For tyrosinemia type I, NTBC is a life-saving intervention (Larochelle et al., 2012). Miglustat, an iminosugar that inhibits glycosphingolipid biosynthesis in a reversible fashion, has shown clinical utility (improved peripheral organ and hematological parameters) in a variety of glycosphingolipid storage disorders, including Gaucher disease and Niemann-Pick C disease (Lyseng-Williamson, 2014; Pastores and Barnett, 2005; Patterson et al., 2007). It has also been piloted in Tay-Sachs and Sandhoff diseases, cystic fibrosis, and GM2 gangliosidosis.

Replenishing depleted substrates may significantly correct the underlying defect in some IEM. In carnitine transport defects, L-carnitine supplementation can resolve cardiomyopathy and prevent further episodes of hypoketotic hypoglycemia. In other disorders, the production or binding affinity of a cofactor required for enzyme function is impaired. Administration of pharmacological doses of the required supplement corrects the defect. This is most evident in the vitamin $B_6$-dependent disorders (Oliveira et al., 2013; Pearl and Gospe, 2014) (eTable 91.14), thiamine- and riboflavin-responsive defects, as well as the vitamin $B_{12}$- and biotin-dependent disorders (Plecko et al., 2014; Sedel, 2013). In selected PKU patients, administration of pharmacological doses of tetrahydrobiopterin (BH4) may be beneficial in reducing the associated hyperphenylalaninemia (Humphrey et al., 2011; Lambruschini et al., 2005). Pharmacological doses of tetrahydrofolate may be therapeutic in patients with folate deficiency, selected disorders of methionine, glycine, and homocysteine metabolism, and dihydropteridine reductase deficiency (Moretti et al., 2005).

Enzyme replacement therapy (ERT) has rapidly expanded as a treatment option in the past decade. ERT has been piloted in the majority of the mucopolysaccharidoses, Gaucher, Fabry, and Niemann-Pick diseases, and others (Boudes, 2013; Mahmud, 2014; Pastores and Barnett, 2005; Pastores and Gupta, 2013). The utility of ERT relies on the presence of the appropriate sugar residues on the exogenously administered enzyme that can target it to, and facilitate the intake into, the appropriate cell organelle (e.g., usually the lysosome). Enzymes produced in culture or in batch processes are purified and administered via regular intravenous infusions of the recombinant protein. While benefits are substantial in relation to peripheral organ function and hematological parameters, neurological complications (if present) are generally nonresponsive due to the inability of recombinant proteins to cross the blood-brain barrier (BBB). Moreover, the annual cost of replacement therapy is substantial. A valuable adjunct to ERT, bone marrow transplant (BMT) and hematopoietic stem cell transplantation (HSCT) have been performed in patients with LSD for more than 25 years (Lund, 2013). The primary goal of these approaches is to provide enzyme-replete cells. The advantage of BMT/HSCT is the capacity to impact brain function, and to potentially slow neurodegenerative outcomes. Challenges with both approaches remain, however, including donor limitation issues, procedural risks, long-term immunosuppression, and graft-versus-host disease (GVHD) (Mitchell et al., 2013). Storage disorders characterized by rapid neurodegeneration, such as Hunter and Sanfilippo syndromes, were previously felt to be poor candidates for either protocol, but emerging data indicate that neurodegeneration may be slowed in these disorders employing HSCT (Annibali et al., 2013; de Ruijter et al., 2011).

Organ transplantation is a concomitant therapy for several IEM, including those with a significant hepatic phenotype. The latter include Crigler-Najjar syndrome, the hyperoxalurias, ornithine transcarbamylase deficiency, and classical MSUD (primarily for patients carrying the classical Amish allele) (Dhawan et al., 2005; Inderbitzin et al., 2005; Mazariegos et al., 2012; McLaughlin et al., 2013; Vogel et al., 2014). Concomitant single-organ failure is seen in many IEM, including end-stage renal insufficiency in Fabry disease, cystinosis, and methylmalonic aciduria. Domino liver transplantation continues to gain traction in the clinic. In the latter, the diseased organ (e.g., MSUD liver) is transplanted to an individual with end-stage hepatic failure who is a very low candidate on the transplant list (Badell et al., 2013), generating a chimeric individual with regard to enzyme function.

Symptomatic treatment remains a vital component of patient care. Indeed, several palliative measures improve quality of life and reduce the incidence and severity of disease-related complications. For instance, corticosteroid and mineralocorticoid replacement are essential in patients with ALD and adrenal insufficiency, while supplementation with L-dopa improves motor function in patients with tyrosine hydroxylase (TH) deficiency. D-Deamino-arginine-vasopressin (DDAVP) reduces the tendency for abnormal bleeding during surgery of patients with GSD type 1A (von Gierke disease), while granulocyte colony-stimulating factor (G-CSF) administered to patients with GSD IB and neutropenia minimizes the risk of recurrent bacterial infection and gastrointestinal tract ulceration. Additionally, patients with certain metabolic disorders necessitate special considerations for anesthesia and surgery. For instance, upper airway obstructive disease in patients with mucopolysaccharidosis may lead to problems during induction and extubation. Hypoglycemia must be avoided in patients with FAO defects, GSD, and disorders of gluconeogenesis, which may require careful planning in terms of the time the procedure is undertaken and maintenance of euglycemia throughout, employing intravenous administration of 10% glucose.

Finally, the importance of effective genetic counseling must be reinforced, for both the patient and the family coping with the affected patient. Since the majority of IEM are autosomal-recessive disorders, prenatal diagnosis is available for most disorders, employing either metabolite, enzymatic, or, more commonly, molecular-based diagnostics. Parents of children with IEM display higher scores on a stress index, lower scores on adaptive behavior scales, and greater anxiety concerning their child's future and that of their composite family (Weber et al., 2012).

## Adolescent with an Inborn Error of Metabolism and Transition to Adulthood

Because of earlier diagnosis and intervention, many affected children with IEM have achieved longer survival. This is in large part due to the evaluation of NBS noted earlier, which has often provided diagnoses within the first week, thereby obviating major episodes of acute decompensation in the neonatal period due to an absence of diagnosis. In most instances, the provision of early patient care has been by pediatricians and metabolic specialists. Most physicians caring for adults are not prepared to assume the care of these patients as they grow older, and the services of well-trained medical geneticists are needed in these instances. Familiarity with the natural history of the disease, offered by the medical geneticist and the biochemical genetics laboratory, may lead to anticipatory guidance and appropriate monitoring, with early intervention at the first sign of trouble (Camp et al., 2014; Enns and Packman, 2002; Packman et al., 2012; Papetti et al., 2013; Walterfang et al., 2013) (see Chapter 56 for further discussion of care transition). Several examples illustrate this. Hepatic adenomas, which may become malignant, develop in the second and third decade of life in patients with GSD IA, while patients with tyrosinemia are also at risk for hepatocellular carcinoma. Other late complications include acute and chronic recurrent pancreatitis, which occurs in association with the hyperlipidemias, porphyrias, and organic acid disorders (Baertling et al., 2013; Rafique, 2013; Simon et al., 2001; Stefanutti et al., 2013). Cholelithiasis is a common occurrence in patients with MLD and Gaucher disease, and in disorders of bile formation and biliary transport. Thromboembolism causes morbidity in homocystinuria and methylenetetrahydrofolate reductase (MTHFR) deficiency. Cardiomyopathy and retinopathy may complicate LCHAD and other selected disorders of fat oxidation. Renal insufficiency or failure may develop in patients with cystinosis, Fabry disease, GSD I, and MMA. Metabolic stroke with bilateral globus pallidus abnormalities and extrapyramidal signs may be associated with metabolic decompensation in MMA.

As most IEM affect multiple systems, the involvement of a multidisciplinary team with central coordination by a primary physician is essential, and the roles of the medical geneticist and counselor remain critical. Patients and family members usually appreciate being included in the decision-making process. These moments of interaction provide an opportunity to assess the family's understanding of the disease and its management as well as their coping mechanisms, and provide a guideline for the need of additional counseling and guidance. Efforts must be directed to ensuring that the patient reaches his or her maximum potential, and educational programs must be adapted to the appropriate developmental level and cognitive capacity to minimize frustration and associated behavioral problems. It is important to prepare for increasing handicap, and to take appropriate steps to facilitate individual performance during activities of daily living, since self-care, communication skills, and mobility issues will likely require special and individualized attention. Quality-of-life surveys are emerging in the rare-disease community for both the patient and the caregiver (Bose et al., 2019).

All individuals become increasingly self-conscious of their body image during puberty. It is critical that caregivers enhance self-esteem in adolescents who feel stigmatized by their physical appearance, especially in instances in which facial dysmorphic features and skeletal deformities are involved. Dysarthria impedes communication, and disturbances of bowel and bladder continence undermine self-confidence and social interaction. Some disorders are associated with delayed puberty (GSD IA, galactosemia, and CDG), or premature ovarian failure (hypergonadotropic hypogonadism). Osteoporosis is often underrecognized as an associated condition of IEM. This most often occurs in disorders causing poor mobility due to cognitive or neuromuscular impairment, or those IEM characterized by chronic acidosis and renal insufficiency. When dietary regimens are required for disease control, be aware that the nature of adolescence may lead to nonconformity and a state of "rebellion." Peer pressure may lead to noncompliance, and the patient must understand the potential implications of the disease, his or her role in management, and long-term outcomes. An engaged family support group is fundamental to this process. Pregnancy is a critical time, requiring measures to ensure a good maternal-fetal outcome (Preece and Green, 2002). This is especially reflected in the maternal PKU syndrome, for which pregnant PKU patients who maintain inadequate control of their phenylalanine levels are at heightened risk of delivering a fetus with microcephaly, developmental delays, and heart defects (Grange et al., 2014). Nonetheless, early diagnosis and excellent long-term management have led to successful pregnancies in many IEM, including MMA, homocystinuria, propionic acidemia, and glutaric aciduria type I, among others (Langendonk et al., 2012). Clearly, the role of pre-pregnancy counseling and interim management of risks pertinent to each disorder require close attention (Lamb et al., 2013; Sechi et al., 2013; Singh et al., 2013).

Selected IEM have particular requirements and concerns. For example, women with homocystinuria may have an increased risk for spontaneous abortion and preeclampsia. Pregnancy may exacerbate the cutaneous lesions of porphyria cutanea tarda during the first trimester. Women who are carriers of ornithine transcarbamoylase (OTC) deficiency may develop a hyperammonemic encephalopathy during the postpartum period, and postpartum metabolic decompensation also occurs in MSUD. Lysinuric protein intolerance (LPI) is associated with increased risk of anemia, toxemia, and intrauterine growth retardation during pregnancy, and bleeding complications during delivery. Attention to maternal protein intake and control of hyperammonemia and other problems during pregnancy are essential (Tanner et al., 2006; Unal et al., 2013).

Psychiatric symptoms are primary features of some disorders or may develop secondary to metabolic decompensation (Gray et al., 2000). For example, there is a growing association between the presentation of autism spectrum and the neurological sequelae of many IEM (Ghaziuddin and Al-Owain 2013; Schulze, 2013; Spilioti et al., 2013).

Behavioral changes (e.g., agitation, delirium) occur in individuals with X-linked ALD, late-onset GM2 gangliosidosis, MLD, urea cycle defects, and porphyria. Cognitive and behavioral problems also occur in children with PKU, especially in those who are not compliant with dietary restriction. Neuropsychiatric findings, such as OCD, PDD, ADD, and attention-deficit/hyperactivity disorder (ADHD), are prominent in numerous IEM, especially in SSADH deficiency and disorders of monoamine metabolism, involving the metabolism of dopamine and serotonin. Children subjected to BMT are at risk for neuropsychological complications secondary to chemotherapy and irradiation.

### Animal Models of Human Inborn Errors of Metabolism

Several spontaneous animal models of human IEM exist, but successful breeding is uncommon. For example, Sly syndrome has been found to occur in a breed of beagle, while the Watanabe heritable hyperlipidemic rabbit (WHHL), the Gunn rat, and the Long Evans Cinnamon (LEC) rat models have been instrumental in defining the pathophysiology of hypercholesterolemia, Crigler-Najjar syndrome, and Wilson disease (Vogel et al., 2014). The literature is abundant with IEM occurring in selected canine strains, particularly relevant to the dog due to the tendency for inbreeding and drift to enhanced expression of rare, autosomal-recessive variants (Fieten et al., 2012). The seminal work by Capecchi and colleagues on homologous recombination in the mouse led to the genesis of knockout mice for the characterization of disease, especially the IEM (Capecchi, 2008). Valuable murine knockouts have been developed in a plethora of IEM, including MSUD, PKU, tyrosinemia type I, SSADH deficiency, and many of the mucopolysaccharidoses and LSDs (Hamman et al., 2005; Kim et al., 2011; Skvorak et al., 2013; Wu et al., 2011). Currently available animal models have proven useful in defining the pathophysiology of many IEM and in the preclinical testing of various drugs. In some cases, these investigations have provided the rationale for further clinical trials in humans (Vogel et al. 2013). Although similarities may exist between knockout mice and the corresponding human IEM, species-specific differences in disease expression result from alternative pathways of substrate processing. These considerations highlight the need for caution in carrying over observations made in animal models to humans.

## DISORDERS INVOLVING COMPLEX MOLECULES

The metabolism of complex molecules in lysosomes and peroxisomes involves different biochemical pathways from those responsible for the processing of dietary constituents. This highlights why dietary manipulation, efforts at enhanced product clearance, and vitamin or cofactor supplementation are not effective treatments for LSDs.  eTables 91.15–91.17 provide an overview of the classification and genetic and phenotypic findings of the major LSDs. LSDs involve tissues and organs that develop normally but later malfunction. In contrast, the expression of early-onset peroxisomal disorders often associates with severe developmental malformation.

### Lysosomal Storage Disorders

The lysosome is a membrane-bounded intracytoplasmic vacuole that contains enzymes required for the degradation of complex lipids, proteins, and nucleotides. Its acidic milieu (pH 5.4) is required for optimal activity of multiple endogenous hydrolytic enzymes and their cofactors and activators. The estimated combined incidence of LSDs is 1 in 5000–8000.

Clinically the LSDs represent a heterogeneous group of disorders involving multiple organ systems. The clinical features reflect the cellular sites of substrate storage and associated organ dysfunction. There is incomplete understanding of disease pathogenesis, but there is increasing evidence for various mechanisms such as aberrant inflammation, induction of apoptosis, enhanced oxidative damage, and defects of autophagy having a contributory role (Ballabio and Gieselmann, 2009; Maejima et al., 2013).

In rapidly progressive forms, the onset of clinical features begins in the neonatorum or early infancy. With later-onset forms, the initial features are delayed until adolescence or adult life, and the course can vary from acute to chronic. Acute and subacute courses are usually associated with primary central nervous system (CNS) involvement, developmental delay, and intellectual deficiency.

Unlike the small-molecule diseases, the characteristic clinical features of LSDs are either a subacute or chronic encephalopathy. Myoclonic seizures occur in fucosidosis, Gaucher disease types II and III, GM2 gangliosidosis, Schindler disease (α-*N*-acetylgalactosaminidase deficiency), and sialidosis type 1. Some LSDs do not have primary CNS involvement (e.g., Fabry disease, Gaucher disease type I, MPS I [Scheie syndrome], MPS IV [Morquio syndrome], mild MPS VI [Maroteaux-Lamy syndrome], and Niemann-Pick disease type B).

Defects in the enzyme cofactor/activator required for complete substrate hydrolysis, rather than a primary enzyme defect, result in rare variants of sphingolipid storage disorders. Two categories of sphingolipid activators exist. One represents the GM2 activator and the other a group of four molecules (saposin A, B, C, and D) derived via proteolytic cleavage of a common precursor, prosaposin. Deficiency of the GM2 activator results in the AB variant of GM2 gangliosidosis. Saposin B activates arylsulfatase A, deficiency of which gives rise to a variant of MLD. Saposin C activates glucocerebrosidase and β-galactocerebrosidase. The clinical picture of deficiency of the latter is that of an atypical form of Gaucher disease because of its clinical overlap with the type III variant (subacute neuronopathic Gaucher disease). Disorders resulting from cofactor deficiencies often result in enzymatic activities in vitro that are within normal limits when using a synthetic (artificial) substrate. Accordingly, routine biochemical testing will likely fail to make the diagnosis, underscoring the absolute need for a board-certified clinical biochemical genetics laboratory being involved in the laboratory testing. Molecular analysis may reveal the presence of mutations in the relevant genes.

The transmission of all LSDs is autosomal recessive, except for Danon disease, Fabry disease, and Hunter syndrome (MPS-II), representing X-linked recessive traits. As noted earlier, interpretation of certain enzyme assay results (e.g., arylsulfatase activity, galactocerebrosidase) must be cautiously interpreted, because low values may be obtained in the presence of pseudo-deficiencies (Lorioli et al., 2014). Diagnostic confirmation is also available by molecular (DNA) testing. Prenatal diagnosis is possible for almost all LSDs. Preimplantation genetic diagnosis may also be possible (Tomi et al., 2006).

Neufeld and colleagues showed that exchanging the growth media surrounding fibroblasts with different disease gene mutations for mucopolysaccharidoses (MPS I [Hurler] and MPS II [Hunter] diseases] led to the clearance of intracellular storage material (Neufeld and Muenzer 2001; <http://www.ommbid.com>). The metabolic cross-correction correlated with the secretion of the functional enzyme from one cell line, followed by intracellular uptake by the deficient cells (e.g., complementation). These studies provided the rationale for treatment of the LSD by ERT, which has undergone an explosion as a therapeutic mechanism (see earlier; Anderson et al., 2014), as well as additional exploratory therapeutic strategies such as substrate synthesis inhibitors, chaperone-mediated agents (Fig. 91.5), neuronal stem cell transplantation, and gene therapy (Ferla et al., 2014; Sands and Davidson, 2006). The first ERT for a LSD was approved in 1991 for Gaucher disease; currently ERTs are approved to treat Gaucher, Fabry, and Pompe diseases, and MPS I, II, and IV (Lachmann, 2019). Additional gene therapy studies utilizing viral vectors are underway to

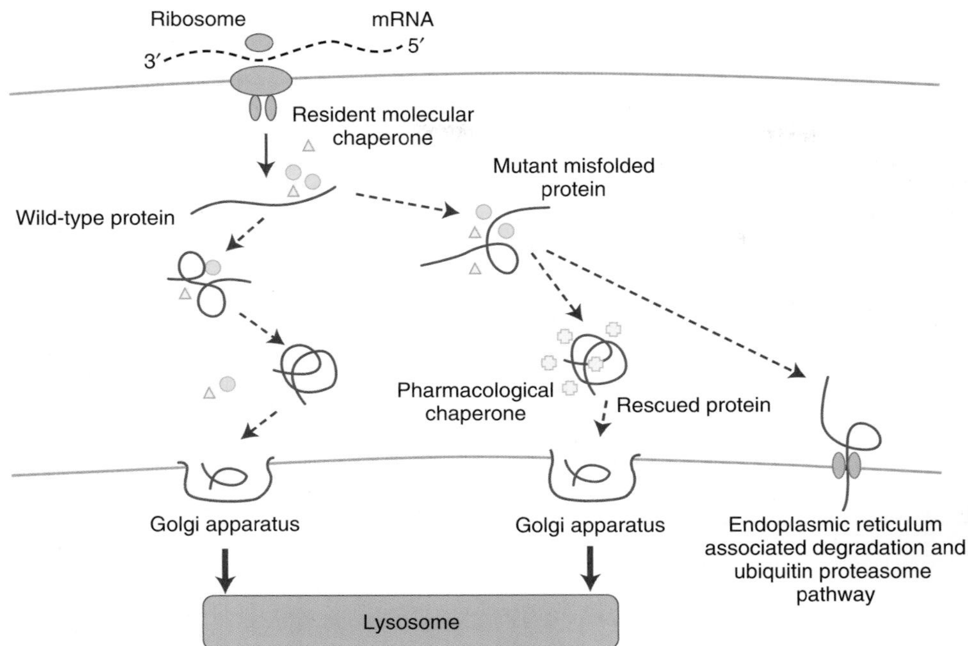


**Fig. 91.5** Chaperone-Mediated Enzyme Enhancement Therapy.

overcome limitations of the approved ERTs (Ohasi, 2019). HSCT is effective for MLD when implemented early. To overcome the limitation of needing to find a donor match as well as GVHD with HSCT, lentiviral-mediated gene therapy trials are in progress.

## Neuronal Ceroid Lipofuscinoses

The neuronal ceroid lipofuscinoses (NCLs) are neurodegenerative diseases of childhood and adulthood associated with lysosomal accumulation of autofluorescent material (Hollak and Wijburg, 2014). Cumulative incidence of the NCLs is ~1:20.000, and contains approximately 13 known disorders. Cardinal clinical manifestations include developmental regression, movement disorders, myoclonic epilepsy, progressive loss of vision, behavioral disturbance, and a progressive course of cognitive decline resulting in dementia.

The primary site of neuropathology is the grey matter, associated with brain atrophy, decerebration, and premature death. Five clinical syndromes are categorized by age of onset, including congenital, infantile, late-infantile, juvenile, and adult forms associated with multiple genetic lesions (see eTable 91.16). The majority of NCLs are inherited as autosomal-recessive traits, although one subtype of the adult disorders is an autosomal dominant.

Food and Drug Administration (FDA) approval of human recombinant ERT, tripeptidyl peptidase 1 (cerliponase alfa), for CLN2 type Batten disease, as an intraventricular infusion, was the first therapeutic breakthrough for these heretofore untreatable progressive myoclonic epilepsies (Schulz et al., 2018). This leads to prolonged survival and improvement in neurological morbidity, although not reversal of vision loss. A pre-clinical study focusing on CLN6 disease shows promising results for use of an adeno-associated viral vector for gene therapy delivered as an intraventricular single dose in mice and an intrathecal single dose in a nonhuman primate, improving motor function, learning deficits, and survival (Cain et al., 2019).

## Peroxisomal Disorders

The peroxisome is an organelle involved in β-oxidation of very-long-chain fatty acids (VLCFAs), the synthesis of plasmalogen (an ether lipid) and bile acids, and oxidation of pipecolic, phytanic, and dicarboxylic acids (Engelen et al., 2012; Fidaleo, 2010). The classification of peroxisomal disorders is generally by the presence of single or multiple enzyme deficiencies (see eTable 91.15). The combined incidence is ~1:25,000. The internalization of most peroxisomal matrix proteins occurs via one of two targeting sequences in a unique system enabling the importation of oligomerized proteins through a specific shuttle involving a receptor and its cargo. Defects of these cellular mechanisms (involving peroxins encoded by *PEX* genes) lead to disruption of peroxisomal metabolic functions (Engelen et al., 2012; Oglesbee, 2005). Peroxisomal disorders primarily transmit in an autosomal-recessive pattern of inheritance, with the exception of X-linked ALD, the most prevalent clinical type (incidence ~1:17,000). While boys are affected with the progressive leukodystrophy (vide infra), female carriers are at high risk for adult-onset slowly progressive myelopathy, and a small percentage develop adrenal insufficiency (Engelen et al., 2014; Huffnagel et al, 2019).

The phenotype of the peroxisomal disorders includes craniofacial abnormalities, encephalopathy, neuronal migration and brain cortical defects, limb malformations, ocular abnormalities, and hepatic and intestinal dysfunction. In the late-onset types, the features are nonspecific and include behavioral changes and deterioration of intellectual function. Demyelination occurs in X-linked ALD, visual and hearing deficits in Refsum disease, and peripheral neuropathy with gait abnormality in Refsum disease and the atypical peroxisomal biogenesis defects. In ALD patients, the onset of MRI abnormalities may be evident up to 12 months prior to onset of neurological symptoms. BMT is generally well tolerated and slows to stops disease progress, with optimal outcomes when administered at an early stage of cerebral disease (Awaya et al., 2011; Gassas et al., 2011; Rockenbach et al., 2012). In May 2018, the FDA approved gene therapy mediated by a lentiviral vector for cerebral-type ALD after a phase 2/3 study of 17 patients showed safety and efficacy (Eichler et al., 2017). Replacement therapy with adrenal corticosteroids is required for all patients with ALD and impaired adrenal function.

The demonstration of elevated plasma VLCFA concentrations enables screening for peroxisomal disorders. Plasma VLCFA levels are normal in rhizomelic chondrodysplasia punctata (RCDP), the latter associated with impaired erythrocyte plasmalogen synthesis. Increased phytanic acid occurs in Refsum disease and RCDP. Since the majority of genes identified in these disorders have been identified (see eTable 91.15), the majority of pre- and postnatal studies are undertaken through molecular genetic analyses for individuals having anomalous VLCFA and phytanic acid findings. In general, treatment options for the Zellweger spectrum disorders are limited and results are conflicting. There are reservations about the ketogenic diet because of the possibility of increasing VLCFAs and phytanic acid. Docosahexaenoic acid, cholic acid, and supplementation of plasmalogens have been attempted with mixed results (Klouwer et al., 2015). Studies utilizing patient-derived fibroblasts to test suitable pharmacological components are ongoing (MacLean et al., 2019).

## DISORDERS INVOLVING SMALL MOLECULES

Disorders of intermediary metabolism often result in the accumulation of compounds that cause acute progressive neurological disorders. The term *defects of small molecules* is used because the compounds that accumulate proximal to the metabolic block are typically elevated in blood and/or CSF and often excreted in the urine. Detection in blood, CSF, or urine facilitates diagnosis. Conversely, as noted earlier, the disorders of serine and creatine biosynthesis result in low levels of these intermediates. Serial measurements monitor the effectiveness of disease intervention and progression. Treatment often requires elimination of the accumulating toxic species, supplementation with missing end-products or intermediates, and use of dietary restriction or the provision of vitamins or cofactors. During episodes of acute decompensation, metabolic homeostasis may be rapidly achieved by exchange transfusion or preferably by peritoneal or hemodialysis. Continuous control of many small molecule disorders (primarily the organic acidurias) necessitates the use of compounds that bind with accumulated intermediates and facilitate alternative pathways of clearance (e.g., glycine, L-carnitine, benzoate, among others). Included in this group of small molecules are the aminoacidopathies, organic acidemias, and urea cycle defects.

### Disorders of Amino and Organic Acid Metabolism

*Aminoacidopathies* result from abnormalities in the catabolism of amino acids, whereas *organic acidemias* are distinguished by their involvement of CoA-activated intermediates. The main clinical feature of these conditions is a symptom-free interval followed by an acute catastrophic event (e.g., vomiting, lethargy, coma, metabolic acidosis, hyperammonemia, hypoglycemia), although the expansion of NBS has prevented many such events due to anticipatory monitoring (Ogier de Baulny and Saudubray, 2002). These metabolic disorders can lead to progressive developmental regression. Typifying MSUD is an acute encephalopathy without hyperammonemia or significant metabolic acidosis, failure to thrive, and mild to moderate psychomotor slowing. Although dysmorphic features suggest organelle pathologies, disorders of organic acid metabolism (i.e., mevalonic aciduria, glutaric aciduria type II [GA-II], among others) often present with severe malformations. A specific diagnosis relies on the disease-specific pattern of abnormalities displayed on the amino and organic acid screening profile, and by detection of the relevant acylcarnitine compounds in plasma. The usual treatment of these disorders is by dietary restriction, elimination of toxic compounds, and adjunctive treatments using specific cofactor or vitamin supplements and carnitine as indicated.

#### Hyperammonemia

Blood ammonia is derived from protein catabolism and as a metabolic by-product of bacterial reactions in the gastrointestinal tract. Ammonia is neurotoxic and promotes excessive glutamine production in the cytosol of astrocytes through its action on glutamine synthetase. It can promote cellular swelling and brain edema by its osmotic effect. Blood ammonia concentrations are elevated by primary defects of the urea cycle (urea cycle disorders, UCD) or secondarily in disorders of amino and organic acid metabolism. In the organic acidemias, intramitochondrial accumulation of acyl-CoA esters decreases the synthesis of *N*-acetylglutamate, the natural activator of carbamyl phosphate (CP) synthetase that primes the urea cycle. Assessment of the plasma amino acid and ammonia levels and analysis of the urine organic acid profile establish the diagnosis. Elevated plasma glutamine levels are common to all the UCDs. Measurement of orotic acid levels in urine is useful in the differential diagnosis. Elevated ammonia enhances orotic acid production in liver through shunting of CP to the cytoplasm from the mitochondria (where the urea cycle is housed). CP is eventually converted to orotic acid, and from that to the pyrimidine triphosphates, cytidine triphosphate and thymidine triphosphate. UCDs are inherited as autosomal-recessive traits except for OTC deficiency (the most common form of UCD), which is an X-linked trait. In addition to protein restriction and alternative pathway therapy, maintenance of arginine and ornithine levels is an important consideration to maintain urea cycle function.

The clinical features of the UCDs are variable; newborns may exhibit rapidly progressive neurological deterioration, with irritability or lethargy, seizures, coma, and respiratory arrest (Haberle et al., 2012; Singh et al., 2005; Steiner and Cederbaum, 2001). Transitory hyperammonemia of the newborn (THAN) must also be considered. Compared with neonates affected with UCD, those with THAN have a significantly lower birth weight for gestational age and chest radiographic findings are usually abnormal. Treatment of newborns with a UCD may be by exchange transfusion and preferably by peritoneal dialysis or continuous arteriovenous hemofiltration as required. Most THAN survivors have normal neurological and developmental examinations later on and do not experience recurrent episodes of hyperammonemia.

Clinical manifestations of later-onset UCDs include developmental delay, behavioral problems, hepatomegaly, and gastrointestinal symptoms. Morbidity may be high (Bachmann, 2005; Ibarra-Gonzalez et al., 2010; Nassogne et al., 2005). Affected children and adults may show confusion, irritability, and cyclic vomiting, with deterioration in mental status during metabolic stress. Among the UCDs, the unique clinical characteristics of arginase deficiency are postneonatal onset of spastic diplegia, dystonia, ataxia, and seizures (Fig. 91.6) (Haberle et al., 2012).

Two disorders of amino acid metabolism, LPI and hyperammonemia-hyperornithinemia-homocitrullinemia (HHH syndrome), are associated with hyperammonemic encephalopathy. The initial features of LPI are growth impairment, hepatic and renal dysfunction, and hematological and pulmonary abnormalities. The primary defect resides in dibasic amino acid transport that leads to an increased urinary excretion of arginine, ornithine, and lysine. LPI is secondary to a functional disorder of the urea cycle. HHH syndrome, caused by mutations in the gene encoding the mitochondrial ornithine transporter, is associated with an elevation of plasma ornithine and increased urinary excretion of homocitrulline (a derivative of lysine and carbomyl phosphate) (Ersoy Tunali et al., 2014; Korman et al., 2004) The clinical features include protein intolerance, vomiting, seizures, and developmental delay. Ornithine administration improves urea cycle function by providing the required precursor for sequential metabolic steps

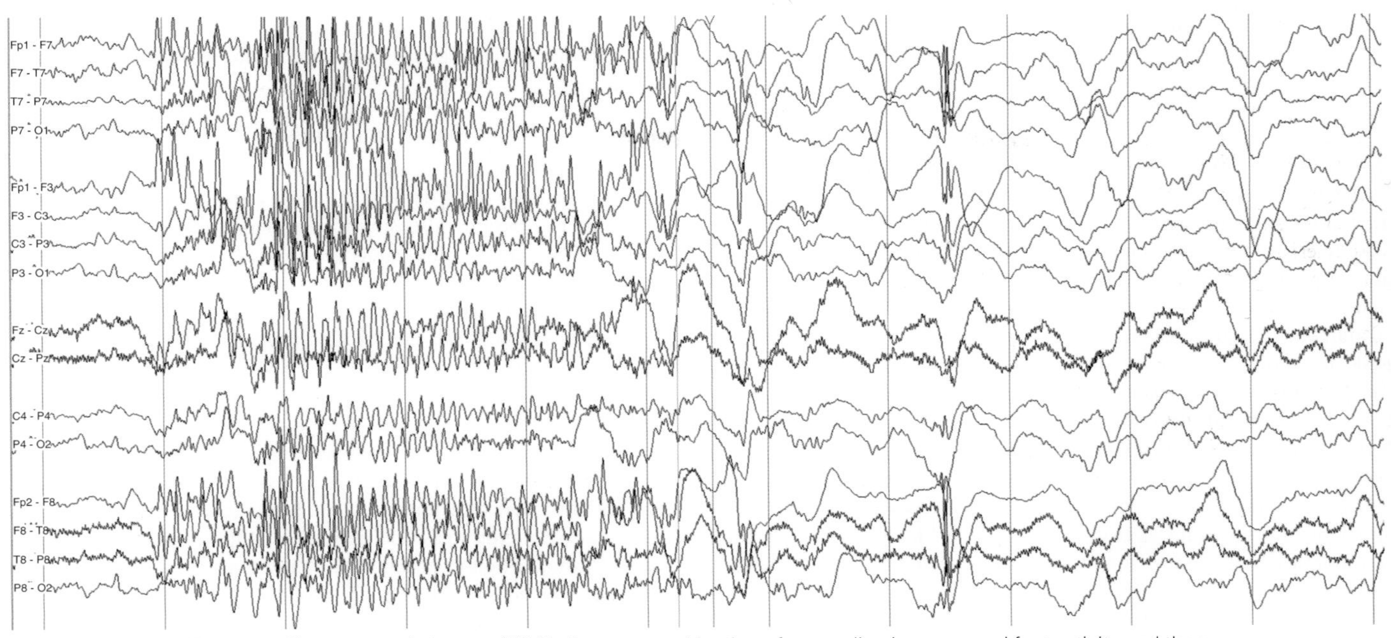


**Fig. 91.6** Electroencephalogram (EEG) shows a combination of generalized paroxysmal fast activity and then slow spike-wave in a 20-year-old patient with urea cycle disorder arginase deficiency, presenting with status epilepticus at 3 years of age. HFF 70 Hz, LFF 1 Hz, sensitivity 7 mcV/mm, time base 30 mm/s.

(Kim et al., 2012; Summar, 2001). Progressive spastic paraparesis is a late complication.

Two additional disorders prominently associated with hyperammonemia are the hyperinsulinism-hyperammonemia (HIHA) syndrome and citrin deficiency. HIHA is a form of congenital hyperinsulinism caused by missense mutations in glutamate dehydrogenase (GLUD1). Inherited mutations lead to a gain in enzyme function. The phenotype includes recurrent hypoglycemia, which responds well to diazoxide treatment and/or protein restriction (Kelly and Stanley, 2008; Plaitakis et al., 2013). Citrin deficiency includes both adult-onset type II citrullinemia (CTLN2) and neonatal intrahepatic cholestasis (NICCD), both associated with mutations in the *SLC25A13* gene that encodes citrin. Adult patients with CTLN2 suffer from recurring neuropsychiatric symptoms associated with hyperammonemia, including disorientation, delirium, seizures, and coma. Patients with NICCD show multiple metabolic abnormalities: aminoacidemias with an increased threonine/serine ratio, galactosemia, hypoproteinemia, cholestasis, and fatty liver (Kimura et al., 2010; Zhang et al., 2014). Conventional therapeutic procedures for hyperammonemia are counterproductive and result in suppression of ureagenesis (Fukushima et al., 2010; Song et al., 2013). Low-carbohydrate coupled with high-protein/fat diets are beneficial, and liver transplantation may optimize outcome in some patients.

## Disorders of Energy Metabolism

The energy requirements of cellular metabolism derive from carbohydrates in the nourished state and glycogen and fat stores during fasting. Cellular energy is stored in the form of adenosine triphosphate (ATP) and creatine phosphate, generated in the cytoplasmic and mitochondrial compartments from glucose and FAO. Hormones primarily mediate the relevant metabolic pathways. Tissues with high aerobic metabolic rates, such as the brain, skeletal muscle, and cardiac muscle, are most vulnerable to IEM involving energy metabolism.

Various clinical presentations suggest an underlying defect of energy metabolism (Rahman, 2012; Sedel, 2013; Sim et al., 2002; Vockley and Whiteman, 2002). In the amino and organic acidemias, deficiency in gluconeogenic substrates occurs accompanied by limited availability of free CoA for mitochondrial FAO, which compromises energy metabolism. Acute or recurrent exercise intolerance and myoglobinuria, with or without cramps, are features of the glycogen and FAO disorders. An inability to perform sudden intense exercise suggests a problem with glycogenolysis or glycolysis, while inability to perform at a sustained level suggests an FAO defect. Progressive neuromuscular weakness and hypotonia are features of the glycogenoses (acid maltase, debrancher enzyme, and brancher enzyme deficiencies), FAO defects (involving carnitine uptake and carnitine acylcarnitine translocase defects), and mitochondrial disorders (cytochrome oxidase deficiency). Acute or chronic weakness occurs in VLCAD or LCAD, short-chain L-3-hydroxyacyl-CoA dehydrogenase, and trifunctional protein deficiencies. Avoidance of fasting is key in the management of disorders of carbohydrate metabolism (glycogenolysis), FAO, and ketogenesis. In some cases, nasogastric or gastrostomy tube feedings are required to maintain caloric requirements.

### Glycogen Storage Diseases

Enzyme defects of glycogen degradation/substrate utilization cause the GSDs. The GSDs are generally identified by a number reflecting the historical sequence of their first clinical characterization. There are also several subtypes of each disorder which reflect the first description of that subgroup. For instance, Pompe disease is the eponymous designation for GSD type II, an LSD. Hepatomegaly and hypoglycemia characterize the GSD resulting from liver enzyme defects. Cramps on exertion and progressive weakness characterize the GSD resulting from muscle enzyme defects (e.g., McArdle disease caused by muscle glycogen phosphorylase deficiency, also associated with rhabdomyolysis and myoglobinuria) (DiMauro and Lamperti, 2001; Oldfors and DiMauro, 2013; Scarlato and Comi, 2002; Witting et al., 2014) The majority of GSDs transmit in an autosomal-recessive fashion, except for the X-linked deficiencies of GSD type IIb (LAMP2 deficiency) and the phosphoglycerate kinase (PGK) deficiencies (GSD IX, either muscle or liver specific). GSD IX manifests with hemolytic anemia, seizures, intellectual deficiency, and exercise intolerance, with myoglobinuria.

### Disorders of Glycolysis and Gluconeogenesis

Deficiency of glycolytic enzyme in muscle can associate with myopathy and hemolytic anemia (Berardo et al., 2010; Naini et al., 2009). Characteristic disorders include PGK, phosphoglycerate mutase, and α-enolase deficiencies, all of which are inherited as autosomal-recessive traits with the exception of X-linked PGK deficiency (Chiarelli et al., 2012; Salameh et al., 2013). Neurological morbidity in PGK deficiency encompasses intellectual deficiency, behavioral abnormalities, and seizures. Defects of gluconeogenesis result in recurrent combined hypoglycemia and lactic acidosis, with or without ketosis. Neurodegenerative features occur in PC and phosphoenolpyruvate carboxykinase (PEPCK) deficiencies. In the severe neonatal form of PC deficiency, there is congenital lactic acidosis along with citrullinemia and hyperammonemia. Citrullinemia can be highly suggestive, the result of the absent conversion of pyruvate to oxaloacetate, which leads to lowered aspartic acid (transamination product of oxaloacetate). Aspartate is a co-reactant in the condensation of citrulline to form argininosuccinic acid in the urea cycle. The integrity of glycogenolysis and gluconeogenesis can be examined with the glucagon stimulation test. In patients with glycogenosis type I (von Gierke disease), the glucose curve following glucagon administration (0.5 g intramuscularly) is usually flat, or there may be a decline associated with an increase in lactate and alanine levels.

### Fatty Acid Oxidation Defects

The oxidation of fatty acids involves four components: the carnitine cycle, mitochondrial β-oxidation, electron transfer, and the synthesis of ketone bodies (KB). Some tissues use fatty acids and KB as alternative energy sources to spare glucose consumption. Before undergoing β-oxidation, free fatty acids activate to the corresponding acyl-CoA thioesters. In contrast to muscle, the brain cannot fully oxidize fatty acids but can use KB synthesized by the liver. The different acyl-CoA dehydrogenases utilize electron-transferring flavoprotein (ETF) as a final electron acceptor. Early-onset FAO defects manifest episodic hypoketotic and hypoglycemic crises, and periods of metabolic decompensation during prolonged fasting, operations, or infections (Mak et al., 2013; Olpin, 2005; Spiekerkoetter and Mayatepek, 2010). Deficiency of mitochondrial trifunctional protein (MTP) and CPT II may present in the neonatal period as an acute fulminant illness. Congenital anomalies are observed in disorders involving ETF, ETF-CoQ oxidoreductase, and multiple acyl-CoA dehydrogenase deficiency (GA-II, or MADD). In GA-II, affected neonates can present with facial dysmorphism, muscular defects of the abdominal wall, hypospadias (in males), and cystic renal lesions. Rhabdomyolysis, cardiomyopathy, and skeletal muscle weakness comprise the phenotype of chronic late-onset cases of FAO defects. The initial acute-onset metabolic crisis in MCAD deficiency, the most common FAO defect, may have a high morbidity, but expanded NBS has substantially limited this outcome.

An intriguing advance has been the development of triheptanoin (C7 oil), an anaplerotic agent metabolized through the medium-chain component of FAO (Borges and Sonnewald, 2012). Anaplerotic trihepatonoin, an odd-chain-number fatty acid, generates a 3-carbon moiety upon completion of β-oxidation, which is converted to succinyl-CoA and replenishes the Kreb cycle (e.g., anaplerosis). The use of triheptanoin is under clinical investigation in a number of disorders, including FAO, GLUT-1 deficiency, and GSDs. Clinical trials in subjects with long-chain FAO disorders are demonstrating improved cardiac parameters during rest and exercise (Gillingham et al 2017), and in cardiac function in patients with cardiomyopathy (Vockley et al 2016).

### Disorders of Ketogenesis and Ketolysis

Excess acetyl-CoA, a by-product of FAO, is converted in hepatic tissue to the primary KB, 3-hydroxybutyrate and acetoacetate, which are transported to peripheral tissues for further metabolism. Ketone utilization by the brain spares glucose for use by other tissues, such as erythrocytes, the latter unable to meet their energy requirements from nonglucose substrates. In liver, condensation of acetyl-CoA occurs sequentially through the enzymes thiolase, 3-hydroxy-3-methylglutaryl-CoA (HMG-CoA) synthase, and HMG-CoA lyase. The latter is the final enzyme of L-leucine metabolism, making this amino acid a "ketogenic" amino acid.

The primary disorders of ketogenesis and ketolysis are rare, and include synthetic disorders (HMG-CoA synthase and lyase deficiencies) and disorders of ketone utilization, including 3-oxothiolase deficiency (also β-ketothiolase deficiency, on the L-isoleucine catabolic pathway) in addition to succinyl-CoA:3-ketoacid transferase (SCOT) deficiency (Fukao et al., 2014). Synthetic disorders prominently feature hypoketotic hypoglycemia (as expected for defects limiting KB formation). When unchecked, 3-oxothiolase deficiency features a prominent ketoacidosis, and is responsive to intravenous glucose. SCOT deficiency manifests permanent, unrelenting ketosis, a highly suggestive marker. SCOT may not be reliably diagnosed by NBS.

## OTHER SUBCLASSIFICATIONS OF INBORN ERRORS OF METABOLISM

### Disorders of Cholesterol and Lipoprotein Metabolism

Defects in the proximal portion of the cholesterol biosynthetic pathway are rare, including mevalonic aciduria and hyper IgD syndrome (HIDS; Tricaroico et al., 2013). Both phenotypes associate with deficiency of mevalonate kinase (MVK), the enzyme proximal to HMG-CoA reductase and first committed step in cholesterol synthesis. Urinary excretion of mevalonate is substantial in mevalonic aciduria and considerably lower in HIDS. The former prominently features neurological sequelae, such as ataxia, psychomotor slowing, and brain malformations associated with atrophy of the cerebellar hemispheres and vermis, as well as hepatomegaly. HIDS patients form a component of the periodic fever disorders, often prominently associated with skin rash (van der Hilst et al., 2008).

The remaining IEM on the cholesterol pathway are distal to the branch point at farnesyl diphosphate at which the sterol pathway branches to multiple intermediates, including isoprenoids (ubiquinone, dolichol) and several other intermediates critical in cell function. The best known of these disorders is the SLOS, a disorder characterized by multiple malformations, growth and psychomotor slowing, and behavioral disturbances (Porter, 2008; Yu and Patel, 2005). SLOS associates with mutations in dehydrocholesterol reductase (DHCR). The remaining disorders in cholesterol synthesis are quite rare, but all present with some form of unilateral (or bilateral) skin lesions (rash, psoriasis, etc.) or skeletal lesions (limb shortening, chondrodysplasia punctate, etc.) (Krakowiak, 2003). The phenotype of patients with desmosterolosis includes structural brain abnormalities, and variably, microcephaly, renal dysfunction, rhizomelic shortness, and large joint contractures (Schaaf et al., 2011). There is a related disorder of sterol-C4-methyl oxidase deficiency affecting the cholesterol synthesis pathway, with developmental impairment, microcephaly, congenital cataracts, arthralgias, and variable degrees of psoriatic dermatitis (Frisso et al., 2017; He et al., 2011). For the majority of these disorders, cholesterol supplementation may provide limited benefits, and intervention with statins is being increasingly considered (Svoboda et al., 2012). Although not a disorder in the synthetic pathway, autosomal-recessively inherited cerebrotendinous xanthomatosis (CTX) associates with mutations in the sterol 27-hydroxylase gene. The primary feature is the formation of xanthomatous lesions in the brain and tendons (Kulkarni et al., 2014; Luyckx et al., 2014; Moghadasian, 2004). Biochemical findings include elevated plasma and bile cholestanol levels (Samenuk and Koffman, 2001).

Disorders of lipoprotein metabolism are often referred to as dyslipidemias, or dyslipoproteinemias. The transport of lipids in plasma is on lipoproteins (consisting of a hydrophobic core of triglycerides and cholesterol esters, wrapped in an amphiphilic coating of apolipoproteins, phospholipids, and unesterified cholesterol). Diseases associated with abnormal lipid absorption and metabolism can result in depleted fat-soluble vitamins (A, D, E, and K). Biochemical diagnosis is obtained via identification of abnormal levels of the corresponding lipoprotein involved (e.g., LDL [low-density lipoprotein], HDL [high-density lipoprotein], or TG [triglyceride]), alone or in combination. The classic disorder is familial hypercholesterolemia, featuring defects in the LDL receptor. Abetalipoproteinemia and hypobetalipoproteinemia are disorders of reduced LDL cholesterol metabolism. In abetalipoproteinemia (Bassen-Kornzweig syndrome), plasma apolipoprotein B (apoB) levels are undetectable, and total cholesterol levels are low (usually <50 mg/dL). Patients manifest fat malabsorption and neurological disturbances, retinitis pigmentosa, and anemia with acanthocytosis, a consequence of reduced erythrocyte membrane fluidity. Acanthocytosis also occurs in vitamin E deficiency and neuroacanthocytosis (Rampoldi et al., 2002).

Hypobetalipoproteinemia, due to mutations in the *apoB* gene, causes a clinical syndrome similar to Friedreich ataxia (ataxia and peripheral neuropathy). Most patients have low LDL cholesterol concentrations (usually <60 mg/dL). Vitamin supplements (A and E) have a beneficial influence on the neurological and ocular symptoms (Lee and Hegele, 2014). Tangier disease is a rare autosomal-recessive disorder caused by mutations in the cell membrane protein ABCA1, which normally mediates the secretion of excess cholesterol from cells into the HDL metabolic pathway. Characteristic of Tangier disease is severe deficiency of HDL and tissue storage of cholesterol esters. Clinical features include enlarged, orange-yellow tonsils (filled with foam cells representing deposits of β-carotene cholesterol esters), splenomegaly, and a relapsing sensorimotor neuropathy (Pichit et al., 2010; Puntoni et al., 2014). Familial lecithin-cholesterol acyl transferase (LCAT) deficiency (also termed fish-eye disease in heterozygous inheritance) manifests impressive HDL deficiency and corneal opacifications (Dimick et al., 2014).

## Disorders of Metals (Copper, Zinc, Iron)

Copper and zinc are essential trace elements required for proper function of numerous metalloenzymes (Fuchs et al., 2012). Both are absorbed in the intestine through the function of specific transporters. Wilson disease is a recessive IEM of copper transport associated with mutations in the ATPase *ATP7B* (Davies et al., 2008). Excessive copper accumulates in liver and brain, resulting in liver failure and neurological features including tremor, loss of fine motor control, poor coordination, rigid dystonia, dysarthria, and swallowing difficulties (Kitzberger et al., 2005). Diagnostic findings include the presence of Kayser-Fleischer rings, increased urine copper excretion, low serum ceruloplasmin, increased liver tissue copper content, and basal ganglia degeneration as evident on MRI. Liver transplantation is associated with increased survival and reversal of the underlying copper defect with clinical improvement. Treatment includes lifelong supplementation with chelation therapy (penicillamine or trientine hydrochloride) and zinc. Menkes disease is an X-linked trait associated with mutations in the copper transporter, ATP7A, resulting in functional copper deficiency and low levels of serum copper and ceruloplasmin (Daniel et al., 2004). Progressive neurodegeneration, seizures, and marked connective tissue abnormalities, including the characteristic twisted hair (pili corti), with early lethality are characteristic of Menkes disease. Neuropathological findings include neovascularization and extreme reduplication of the cerebral arteries, in conjunction with cystic medial vessel wall degeneration, bilateral cerebellar hypoplasia and heterotopias, and focal cortical dysplasias. Daily intravenous copper histidine administration restores serum copper and ceruloplasmin levels and leads to favorable clinical results when started prior to neurodegeneration. Occipital horn syndrome is an allelic variant of Menkes syndrome with a milder phenotype, including abnormal skin and joint laxity. MEDNIK (mental deficiency, enteropathy, deafness, neuropathy, ichthyosis, keratodermia) syndrome associates with mutations in *AP1S1*, encoding the small subunit of the adaptor protein-1 (AP1) complex. Deficiency results in low serum copper and ceruloplasmin, associated with intestinal obstruction, ichthyosis, and intellectual deficiency (Martinelli et al., 2013).

Neurodegeneration with brain iron accumulation (NBIA) is a heterogeneous group of disorders that most prominently share accumulation of brain iron, principally in the basal ganglia, and movement disorders of childhood (Kurian and Hayflick, 2013). The two major types are PKAN and PLA2G6-associated neurodegeneration (PLAN), although there are additional disorders (mitochondrial membrane protein-associated neurodegeneration or MPAN, beta-propeller protein-associated neurodegeneration or BPAN, CoA synthase protein-associated neurodegeneration or CoPAN, fatty acid hydroxylase-associated neurodegeneration or FAHN, and others). Disorders of zinc and manganese homeostasis may also be associated with neurodegeneration (Ferreira and Gahl, 2017).

## Disorders of Polyol Metabolism, Including Galactose and Fructose

Polyols are alcoholic compounds containing multiple hydroxyl groups. Disorders in this group include IEM involving galactose and fructose. Disorders in the pentose phosphate pathway (PPP) have also been described (Kruger et al., 2011). Galactosemia is the most common disorder of galactose metabolism, and the most severe. The primary pathophysiology resides in the peripheral organs (liver, kidney, ovaries). Nonetheless, neurological complications are present, including movement disorders and motor, cognitive, and psychiatric impairment (Ridel et al., 2005; Rubio-Agusti et al., 2013). The extent to which galactose derivatives (galactose-1-phosphate, and the polyol galactitol) contribute to pathophysiology remains unknown, although the association of cataract formation has been linked to galactitol accumulation. Treatment of galactosemia centers on removal of galactose from the diet, but this sugar is prevalent in many foodstuffs and dietary restriction of intake remains a significant challenge. Detection on NBS and implementation of dietary restriction in the first week of life leads to a more favorable outcome in galactosemia. A less favorable outcome is associated with a homozygous c.563A>G (p.Gln188Arg) mutation, GALT enzyme activity less than 1%, and strict galactose restriction based on a recent international natural history study (Rubio-Gozalbo et al., 2019). Four disorders associated with fructose metabolism include fructokinase deficiency, fructose-1-phosphate aldolase deficiency (HFI), fructose-1,6-biphosphatase deficiency (FBP), and D-glyceric acidemia. Most symptoms in these disorders occur in peripheral tissues (liver) with the ingestion of fructose; FBP is a disorder of gluconeogenesis as well. The phenotype of D-glyceric acidemia, caused by deficiency of glycerate 2-kinase, is variable from healthy to a severe phenotype; however, if symptomatic, the presentation may be a progressive encephalopathy with microcephaly, seizures, and early fatality (Dimer et al., 2015).

## Disorders Associated with Vitamin Metabolism

Vitamin-dependent disorders involve primarily vitamin $B_6$, $B_{12}$, biotin, thiamine, and riboflavin. Pyridoxine-dependent epilepsy has been explained by antiquitin deficiency: that is, alpha-aminoadipic semialdehyde dehydrogenase of the lysine degradation pathway leading to accumulation of pipecolic acid and sequestration of pyridoxine from the nervous system (Plecko et al., 2014). There are a range of pyridoxine-responsive neurological phenotypes, although not all pyridoxine-responsive epilepsies are explained. A related disorder is pyridox(am)ine-5′-phosphate oxidase deficiency, with inability to convert pyridoxine to the biologically active form of pyridoxal-5-phosphate (P5P) and thus necessitating vitamin $B_6$ in the form of P5P. Type II hyperprolinemia (pyrroline-5-carboxylate dehydrogenase deficiency), congenital hypophosphatasia, tissue nonspecific alkaline phosphatase deficiency, and deficiency of the *PROSC* gene are also associated with pyridoxine dependency. In addition, CSF P5P levels may be decreased in patients with nonspecific diagnostic findings, and attributable to active epileptic encephalopathies (Goyal et al., 2013).

Cerebral folate deficiency is a transportopathy related to deficiency of the FOLR1 transporter. As with GLUT1 deficiency, peripheral measurements may be nondiagnostic and lumbar puncture is needed for biochemical confirmation. In this case, CSF requires quantification of the 5-methyltetrahydrofolate (MTHF) level. There is a differential diagnosis, to low CSF 5-MTHF levels, including disorders of folate absorption, but also a potassium channelopathy and medication effects, including valproate. Folinic acid (leucovorin) has BBB penetrability and is the mainstay of treatment for cerebral folate deficiency.

Approximately 15 disorders associated with vitamin $B_{12}$ (cobalamin) have been described (Baumgartner, 2013). This finding is of interest since cobalamin is only required for two intracellular reactions: methylation of homocysteine to methionine and conversion of methylmalonyl-CoA to succinyl-CoA. Most cobalamin-related disorders relate to hereditary anomalies in absorption, transport, and processing of cobalamin into the appropriate cofactor format. The biochemical hallmarks of these disorders are accumulation of methylmalonic acid and homocysteine, and the primary clinical features include varying degrees of hematological and neurological abnormalities. Disorders of biotin metabolism include holocarboxylase synthetase and biotinidase deficiencies, both of which respond to pharmacological dosages of biotin, although vision and sensorineural hearing loss persist once established. In the absence of intervention, both disorders feature a phenotype of ataxia, developmental delay, and seizures, often associated with a striking alopecia totalis and skin rash.

Thiamine is converted intracellularly to its main cofactor, thiamine pyrophosphate, the latter a cofactor in multiple intracellular reactions. Thiamine-responsive megaloblastic anemia (TRMA), due to mutations in the thiamine transporter *SLC19A2,* features progressive deafness, diabetes mellitus, and optic neuropathy (Sedel, 2013). Mutations in *SLC19A3* are linked to thiamine-responsive basal ganglia disease, recurrent seizures, and episodes of severe Leigh-like encephalopathy. A later-onset bilateral striatal necrosis disorder, associated with progressive peripheral neuropathy, is linked to mutations in *SLC25A19* (also referred to as mitochondrial thiamine pyrophosphate carrier deficiency, or Amish microcephaly).

Deficiency of molybdenum cofactor (MoCD) associates with neonatal seizures, progressive neurodegeneration, and diffuse cavitary leukomalacia, although therapy has been introduced using cyclic pyranopterin monophosphate (cPMP) (Hitzert et al., 2012). Deficiency of SO, one of four molybdenum cofactor–dependent enzymes, is believed to underlie the majority of this pathophysiology. Loss of SO function results in accumulation of neurotoxic sulfite, which may alter *N*-methyl-D-aspartate (NMDA) receptors and additionally sulfur-containing intermediates.

## Congenital Disorders of Glycosylation

The fastest-growing group of inborn metabolic errors is the CDG, with at least 150 types identified (eTable 91.18). Cardinal clinical features are shown in eTable 91.18, and span all organ systems (Fig. 91.7) (Chang et al., 2018, Freeze et al., 2014). CDGs are the result of defective glycosylation of glycoconjugates (e.g., glycoproteins, glycolipids, glycosylphosphatidylinositol anchors). Minimally, there are 4 subgroups: (1) defects in protein *N*-glycosylation; (2) defects in protein O-glycosylation; (3) disorders involving glycolipid and glycosylphosphatidylinositol anchor glycosylation; and (4) disorders involving multiple glycosylation pathways. It has been suggested that CDGs should be considered in any idiopathic multisystem syndromic patient, or single-tissue disorder, not adequately explained through the identification of another disorder (Wolfe and Krasnewich, 2013). Nonetheless, some 60%–70% of CDG patients present with some form of intellectual disability. Therapeutic options are limited, and largely supportive and symptomatic. Targeted therapies are available for MPI-CDG, SLC35C1-CDG, PIGM-CDG, and PGM1-CDG. Oral mannose use in mannose phosphate isomerase deficiency (MPI-CDG) has been successful (Wolfe and Krasnewich, 2013). Many clinical trials and pre-clinical trials are underway for other CDG, including utilizing mannose-1-phosphare substrate replacement therapy for PMM2-CDG (formerly congenital disorder of glycosylation type 1a), and *N*-acetylmannosamine in *GNE*-CDG (formerly hereditary inclusion body myopathy). Therapies utilizing simple sugars to improve hypoglycosylation are also ongoing. In PGM1-CDG, TMEM165-CDG, and SLC39A8-CDG galactose has demonstrated improvement in coagulopathy and endocrinopathy. Manganese has also shown improvement in SLC39A8-CDG. Sodium butyrate may be beneficial for seizure remission in CAD-CDG and PIGM-CDG. In PIGA-CDG the use of the ketogenic diet has demonstrated decrease in seizure frequency in some cases (Chang et al., 2018). Estimates indicate that 1%–2% of the human genome is actively involved in the process of glycosylation (involving the cytosol, ER, and Golgi of the cell), demonstrating the ubiquitous role for protein glycosylation and impact of this group of disorders (Losfeld et al., 2014).

## Disorders of Purine and Pyrimidine Metabolism

Purines and pyrimidines are essential cellular components involved in energy transfer and the metabolism of nucleic acids. Defects of purine and pyrimidine metabolism can result from disruption of biosynthetic, catabolic, and salvage pathways. Consider these disorders in patients presenting with psychomotor delay and behavioral problems, abnormalities of muscle tone, extrapyramidal features, and seizures (Jurecka, 2009). Nonetheless, they can include renal, musculoskeletal, immunological, and hematological manifestations. Due to the relative insolubility of many of the hydroxylated purines/pyrimidines, cholelithiasis, nephrolithiasis, hyperuricemia, hypouricemia, and gout are associated features (Kelley and Andersson, 2014; Peters et al., 2004; Weidensee et al., 2011).

Transmission of Lesch-Nyhan syndrome is X-linked recessive. Hypoxanthine guanine phosphoribosyl transferase (HGPRT), required in the purine salvage pathway, is deficient, causing hyperuricemia. Clinical features include chorea and athetosis, dysarthria, hyperreflexia, hypertonia, cognitive impairment, and behavioral

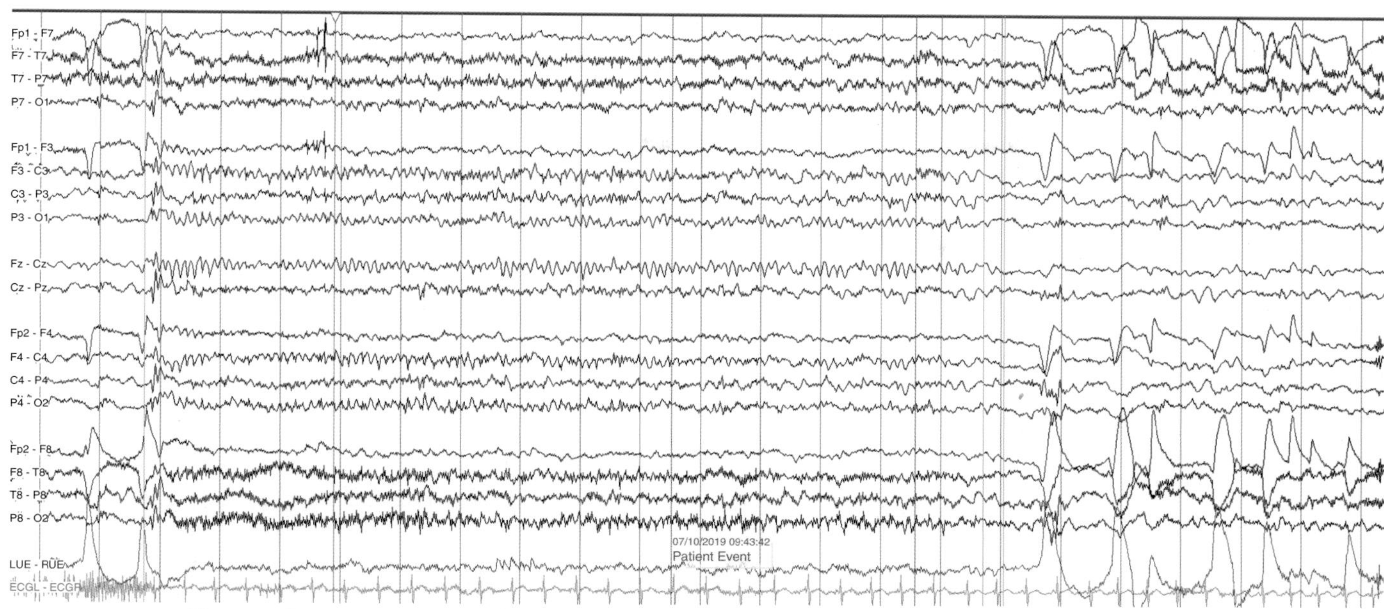


**Fig. 91.7** Electroencephalogram during tonic seizure in 2-year-old boy with congenital defects of glycosylation 1N (SLC39A8, related to Mn transporter) shows bilateral fast (beta) activity over the parasagittal regions bilaterally with abrupt onset and offset, followed by recurrent eye movement artifact, as corroborated with the left upper eye (LUE) - right upper eye (RUE) extraoculograph leads. HFF 70 Hz, LFF 1 Hz, sensitivity 10 mcV/mm, timebase reduced to 15 mm/s to capture entire 14-seconds seizure on the slide.

disturbances (including impulsive self-mutilation) (Schretlen et al., 2001). Reduced dopamine concentrations in the basal ganglia and CSF may account for some of the neurological features. Adenylosuccinate lyase deficiency is an autosomal-recessive trait in which de novo purine and adenosine monophosphate (AMP) synthesis are defective. The unique metabolites succinyl-aminoimidazole carboxamide riboside (SAICAR) and adenylosuccinate accumulate in cells and are detectable in urine. Severe developmental impairment including autism spectrum, seizures, and growth deficiency are characteristic (Salerno and Crifo, 2004).

Dihydropyrimidine dehydrogenase deficiency, a defect of pyrimidine metabolism, features developmental delay, autistic-like behavior, and seizures. It is associated with increased urinary excretion of thymine and uracil (van Kuilenburg et al., 2004). Deficiencies of two other enzymes involved in pyrimidine catabolism, dihydropyrimidinase and β-ureidopropionase, exist (Nyhan, 2005). These disorders have been associated with severe toxicity in patients with cancer, following the administration of the chemotherapeutic agent 5-fluorouracil. Autistic features are also a component of the phenotype of dihydropyrimidinase deficiency. Treatment remains supportive.

## Porphyrias

Porphyrias represent disorders in the metabolism of heme, and the accompanying neurotoxicity associates with accumulation of porphyrins and/or porphyrin precursors. The porphyrias can be divided into two classes, encompassing acute and non-acute disorders (Stolzel et al., 2010). Disorders in the former include AIP, variegate porphyria (VP), hereditary coproporphyria (HCP), and aminolevulinic acid dehydratase deficiency porphyria (ALADP). For these disorders, therapeutic strategies generally encompass intravenous glucose administration, electrolyte correction, and heme arginate. Symptoms can be triggered by administration of various antiseizure medicines, e.g., phenobarbital, and other 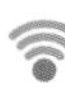 centrally acting agents (eTable 91.19). The non-acute disorders include porphyria cutanea tarda, erythropoietic protoporphyria, and congenital erythropoietic porphyria (Stolzel et al., 2010; Tracy and Dyck, 2014).

The heme synthetic pathway normally occurs in bone marrow (85%) or liver. Consider a diagnosis of porphyria in patients with unexplained neuropsychiatric signs, visceral (gastrointestinal and hepatic) symptoms, or cutaneous photosensitivity (Dombeck and Satonik, 2005; Seager et al., 2014; Stolzel et al., 2010). Cutaneous manifestations are prominent in HCP and VP, but the neurovisceral disturbances may be indistinguishable from those of AIP (Bonnot et al., 2014). Acute peripheral neuropathy and encephalopathy may develop in patients with AIP (Pischik and Kauppinen, 2009). Acute porphyric neuropathy is predominantly a motor disorder and is associated with a history of abdominal pain and dysautonomia, CNS involvement, and mild hepatopathy. Acute encephalopathy manifests as a combination of psychiatric symptoms and seizures. Porphyrias with neurological features have either a constant or an intermittent excretion of ALA and porphobilinogen. A recent pilot study of 17 patients described a decrease in mitochondrial oxygen consumption rates in peripheral blood mononuclear cells in patients with acute porphyria (including AIP and HCP), suggesting a deficit in mitochondrial function with reduction in electron transport and ATP production (Dixon et al., 2019). A phase 1 trial of givosiran (RNA interference agent that inhibits hepatic ALAS1 synthesis) recently concluded that subjects randomized to the monthly injection group resulted in reduced ALAS1 mRNA levels, reduced levels of the neurotoxic intermediates delta ALA and porphobilinogen to a near-normal range, and a lower neurovisceral attack rate (Sardh et al., 2019).

## Neurotransmitter Inborn Errors of Metabolism

Mammalian neurotransmitters are divisible into several groups: inhibitory (GABA, glycine), excitatory (aspartate, glutamate), cholinergic (acetylcholine), monoaminergic (epinephrine, norepinephrine, dopamine, and serotonin), and purinergic (adenosine, AMP, ADP, ATP). IEM associated with disrupted neurotransmitter metabolism include deficient synthesis, release, breakdown, transport, or reuptake. In addition, defects of receptors and failure of signaling pathways of glial cells may lead to disease. Clinical features vary from mild to severe and include psychomotor slowing, developmental

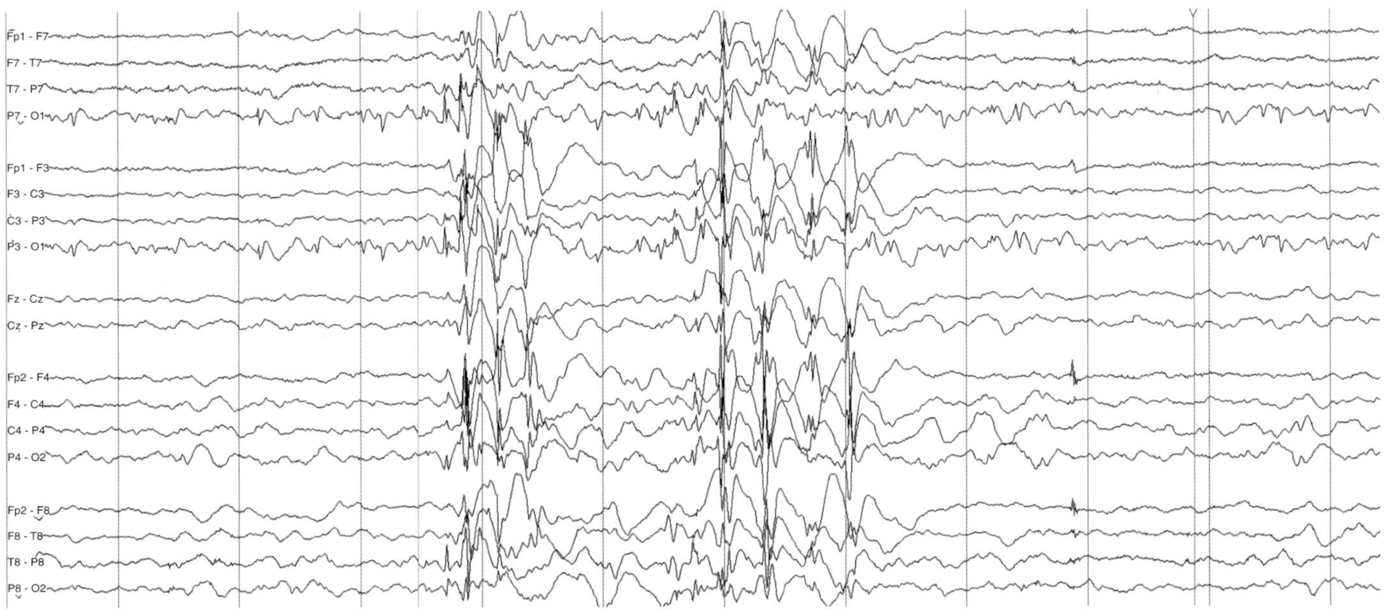


**Fig. 91.8** Electroencephalogram (EEG) in 10-year-old girl with Dihydropteridine reductase (DHPR) deficiency shows active generalized and multifocal spike and polyspike and wave discharges. Note highly active left occipital focus. HFF 70 Hz, LFF 1 Hz, sensitivity 20 mcV/mm, timebase 30 mm/s.

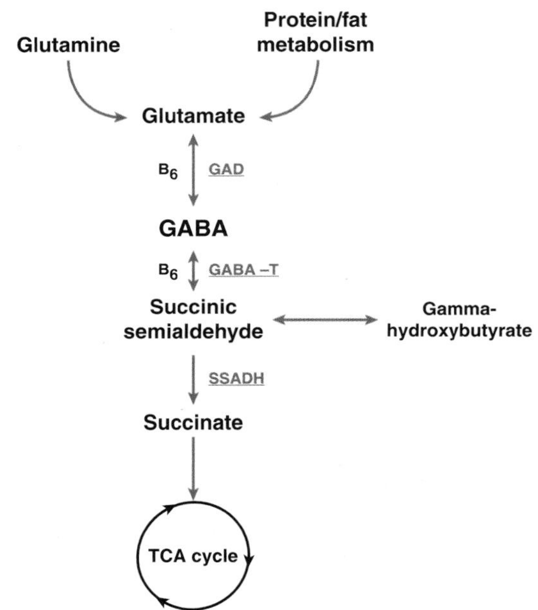


**Fig. 91.9** Gamma-Aminobutyrate (GABA) Metabolism Pathway. *GABA-T*, GABA transaminase; *GAD*, glutamic acid decarboxylase; *SSADH*, succinic semialdehyde dehydrogenase; *TCA*, tricarboxylic acid cycle.

delay, oculogyric crises, central and peripheral hypotonia, hypo- or hyperkinesia, mixed pyramidal and extrapyramidal motor disorders, epilepsy, and ataxia (Opladen et al., 2012; Pearl et al., 2004). Analysis of neurotransmitters and related metabolites in CSF can be critically important, and the inclusion of pterin/biopterin measurements helps to differentiate primary monoamine synthesis disorders: that is, AADC or TH deficiency, from defects in tetrahydrobiopterin (BH4) metabolism, a necessary cofactor for phenylalanine hydroxylation (Fig. 91.8; see Table 91.4).

There are two described disorders of GABA metabolism (Fig. 91.9). Succinic semialdehyde dehydrogenase (SSADH) deficiency disrupts the normal metabolism of GABA, resulting in the accumulation of gamma-hydroxybutyrate (GHB), a neuromodulator. The phenotype of SSADH deficiency comprises intellectual disability with disproportionate deficit in expressive language, hypotonia, ataxia, and epilepsy (Kim et al., 2011; Vogel et al., 2013). Prevalent neuropsychiatric morbidity includes OCD and ADHD, which can be debilitating especially in adulthood (DiBacco et al., 2018). Of interest, about half of the patients develop epilepsy, and there appears to be a risk for SUDEP (sudden unexplained death in epilepsy patients) in as high as 10%–15% of the adult cohort with otherwise normal or nearly normal life expectancy (Lapalme-Remis et al., 2015). Metabolic abnormalities are recapitulated in the murine model (Gupta et al. 2002, 2004), which manifests an evolving seizure disorder encompassing absence, tonic-clonic, and eventual lethal status epilepticus (Buzzi et al., 2006; Cortez et al., 2004; Wu et al., 2006). Of interest, vigabatrin (VGB; irreversible inhibitor of GABA-transaminase) has been broadly employed, with favorable outcomes in some, but not all, patients (Vogel et al., 2013). The use of VGB is rational, in relation to lowering of GHB, yet this gain may well be offset by further GABA elevation, and long-term VGB intervention is associated with visual-field impairments. Rescue studies in the murine model have led to clinical trials of taurine and an experimental GABAB receptor antagonist in patients (Pearl et al., 2014). GABA-transaminase has been described in about 15 cases worldwide. Initial reports described a severe neonatal- or infantile-onset epileptic encephalopathy and mortality within the first 2 years of life (Tsuji et al., 2010). Recently, expanding phenotypes emerged with evidence of survival into adulthood (Hegde et al., 2019). Experimental treatment with flumazenil, a GABA-A benzodiazepine receptor antagonist, may represent a therapeutic strategy (Koenig et al., 2017).

Several disorders of monoamine metabolism are known, primarily altering the production of dopamine and serotonin (Marecos et al.,

2014). TH deficiency involves the first committed step in dopamine, epinephrine, and norepinephrine formation. The clinical presentation of the infantile onset form includes a progressive hypokinetic-rigidity syndrome with dystonia and a more severe presentation with severe encephalopathy in the newborn period (Opladen et al., 2012). Aromatic L-amino acid decarboxylase (AADC) deficiency causes a deficiency of both serotonin and catecholamines, leading to a subacute encephalopathy. Autonomic dysfunction leads to ptosis, hypotension, gastric and intestinal dysmotility, and poor temperature regulation. Therapy for TH usually centers on bypass of the metabolic block with levodopa/carbidopa and dopamine agonists, whereas AADC patients also may receive MAO inhibitors, anticholinergics, and SSRIs in combination with pyridoxine and folinic acid. Preliminary work shows progress utilizing adeno-associated viral-mediated gene therapy in murine and clinical trials (Tseng et al., 2019; Kojima et al., 2019).

The conversion of dopamine to norepinephrine is catalyzed by dopamine β-hydroxylase (DBH), and deficiency results in primary autonomic failure, as expected. In the newborn period, muscular hypotonia, hypothermia, and hypoglycemia accompany hypotension, delayed eye opening, and ptosis (Marecos et al., 2014). Males with X-linked monoamine oxidase (MAO) deficiency manifest mild intellectual deficiency, stereotypical hand movements, and behavioral problems highlighted by aggressive outbursts (Opladen et al., 2012). Only a few specialized laboratories in the world are skilled in accurate, sensitive, and quantitative measures of monoamine metabolites in CSF. Age-matched reference ranges and special collection systems for CSF (to avoid auto-oxidation of reactive intermediates) must be employed (Hyland, 2008).

## Disorders of Glycine and Serine Metabolism

The primary disorder of glycine metabolism is glycine encephalopathy (GE; previously called non-ketotic hyperglycinemia), a disorder of the mitochondrial glycine cleavage system (Hennermann et al., 2012; Toone et al., 2002). The latter is a tetramer of four subunits; the predominance of mutations associate with the P (pyridoxal-containing) protein. Glycine is a simple amino acid that functions as a neurotransmitter with dual excitatory (cortical) and inhibitory (spinal cord and brainstem) effects. The clinically characteristic GE is a neonatal encephalopathy with lethargy, hypotonia, myoclonic seizures, apnea, burst-suppression pattern on electroencephalogram (EEG), and elevated plasma and CSF: plasma glycine. Neuropathological examination has revealed spongiform white-matter degeneration. Treatment is with dextromethorphan (as an NMDA receptor blocker) and ketamine to inhibit receptor excitation. Valproate should be avoided in GE. Prognosis is poor with early onset and in the presence of cerebral dysgenesis. Additional clinical variants have been described, including an infantile presentation after age 6 months with focal seizures or hypsarrhythmia; a childhood variant with mild intellectual deficiency, delirium, chorea, and vertical gaze palsies; and a late-onset pattern in adults with progressive spastic diplegia and optic atrophy (Dinopoulos et al., 2005; Terek et al., 2012).

L-serine is a precursor of several metabolic intermediates, including nucleotides, phospholipids, sphingolipids, and ceramides, and is necessary for myelin formation (de Koning, 2006). Disorders resulting in serine deficiency are caused by deficiency in one of three serine biosynthetic enzymes (de Koning, 2013; van der Crabben et al., 2013) (Fig. 91.10). Serine deficiency disorders present a neurological phenotype with psychomotor slowing, microcephaly, and seizures in newborns and children, and often a progressive polyneuropathy in adults. Prompt identification is critical in order to supplement with L-serine. Normal outcome is possible with early intervention, including prenatal administration (de Koning et al, 2004).

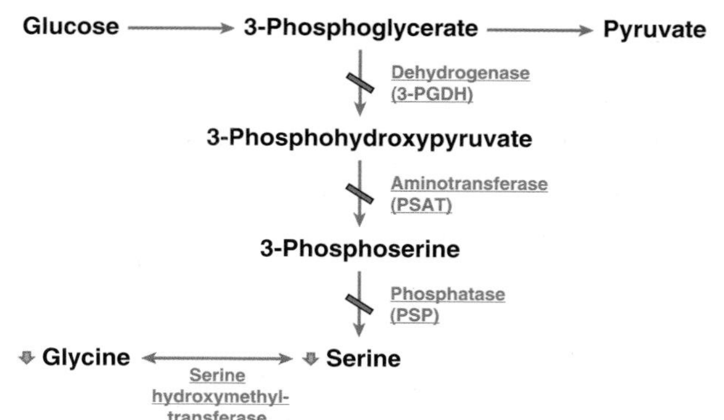


**Fig. 91.10** Serine Synthesis Pathway and Sites of Enzymatic Defects. *3-PGDH,* 3-phosphoglycerate dehydrogenase; *PSAT,* 3-phosphoserine aminotransferase; *PSP,* 3-phosphoserine phosphatase.

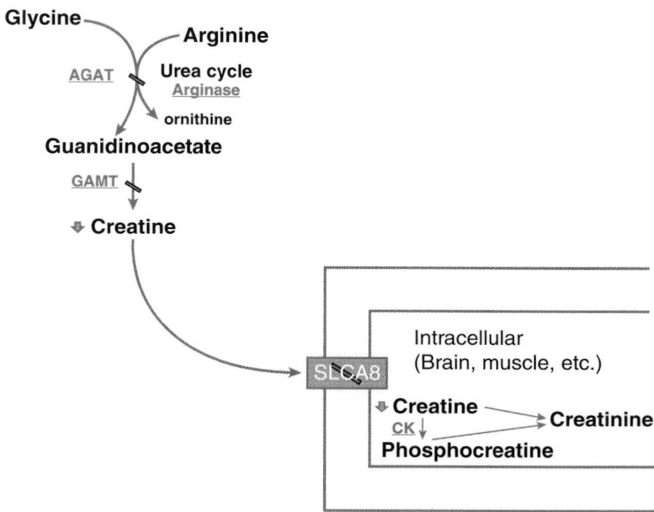


**Fig. 91.11** Creatine Synthesis and Transport Pathway. *AGAT,* Arginine:glycine aminotransferase; *CK,* creatine kinase; *GAMT,* guanidinoacetate methyltransferase; *SLCA8,* creatine transporter.

## Creatine Deficiency Syndromes

Creatine and phosphocreatine play essential roles in energy storage and transmission. Primary creatine deficiency can result from defects in one of two synthetic enzymes: arginine:glycine amidinotransferase (AGAT) and GAMT (Fig. 91.11). Although the brain can generate creatine, the majority of creatine is taken up from the circulation via a sodium/chloride-dependent transporter, SLC6A8, the so-called creatine transporter (Mercimek-Mahmutoglu et al., 2014; van de Kamp et al., 2013). The primary organ affected in the creatine deficiency syndromes is the brain, and this is readily documented with proton magnetic resonance spectroscopy which reveals absent or significantly decreased creatine (phosphate) (Dezortova et al., 2008; Stockler et al., 2007). Cardinal clinical findings in these disorders include intellectual disability, speech delay, autistic behavior, and variably degrees of epilepsy, from fever-associated seizures to medically refractory mixed seizures. Additional features variably include hypotonia and an extrapyramidal movement disorder. Supplementation with creatine is beneficial in the synthetic disorders of AGAT and GAMT (Stockler et al., 2007). Measurement of guanidinoacetate in body fluids enables discrimination of GAMT (high GAA concentration) and AGAT (low GAA) deficiencies from creatine transporter deficiency (normal GAA concentration). Multiple pre-clinical trials in a mice model are underway, one utilizing 4-phenylbutyrate to correct misfolding of the transporter in creatine transporter deficiency syndrome (El-Kasaby et al., 2019).

## CONCLUSION

Inherited disorders of metabolism may affect the central and peripheral nervous systems in a multitude of ways, and organizing the disorders into those of small-molecule, intermediary metabolism in contrast to large or complex molecular metabolism, as well as by principal organelle involved, is a helpful way to logically address them. Diagnosis requires a combination of clinical, electrophysiological, imaging, and laboratory analyses, including metabolic screening of peripheral fluids, especially CSF, and increasing utilization of phenotype-specific gene panels and WES. Treatment modalities traditionally have been substrate reduction, toxin removal, and replenishment of depleted nutrients or cofactors. While NBS and mutation analysis were initially transformational in the field diagnostically, currently next-generation sequencing and the advent of increasing use of ERT and gene therapy are ushering in a new transformational wave.

### Acknowledgment

This chapter, updated from the prior edition, was originally a revised version of the chapter by G.M. Pastores in the sixth edition.

*The complete reference list is available online at https://expertconsult.inkling.com/.* 

# 92

# Neurodegenerative Disease Processes

*Roger A. Barker, Kirsten M. Scott*

## OUTLINE



Neurodegenerative disorders of the central nervous system (CNS) are characterized by the loss of specific populations of neural cells, the pattern and distribution of which shape the clinical presentation of the patient. This has led to the standard way in which these disorders are diagnosed: namely, the clinical phenotype of motor impairment (tremor, rigidity, and hypokinesia) in Parkinson disease (PD) with a loss of nigral dopaminergic neurons, amyotrophic lateral sclerosis (ALS) with the loss of motor neurons, and so on (Table 92.1). These cellular losses are typically also defined by the accumulation of an abnormal protein that usually gives rise to an inclusion (e.g., α-synuclein–containing Lewy bodies (LBs) in PD or hyperphosphorylated tau neurofibrillary tangles in progressive supranuclear palsy [PSP]). This has led to calls to reclassify neurodegenerative disorders by the proteinopathy that characterizes them—α-synucleinopathies, tauopathies, etc. (see Table 92.1). Although this latter approach has much to merit it, especially when one comes to study disease pathogenesis, many clinicians would argue that they cannot see the pathology of cell inclusions (although this may change with the advent of new positron emission tomography [PET] ligands for these protein aggregates), only the clinical phenotype. Therefore most patients are still diagnosed using clinical criteria which predict a pathology and a therapeutic approach. In all cases this therapy serves to treat symptoms. There is an urgent unmet need to identify disease-modifying therapies for these disorders as the world's population ages and we face a burgeoning burden of age-related neurodegenerative diseases.

In this chapter we discuss some of the mechanisms underlying the loss of cells in neurodegenerative disorders and how this may shape future therapies.

However, before discussing this in more detail, it is worth making a few general points about neurodegenerative disorders of the CNS:

- Similar clinical presentations can have different disease causes: for example, idiopathic PD can initially look just like the parkinsonian form of multiple system atrophy (MSA); many cases of what look like corticobasal degeneration (CBD) end up having a pathological diagnosis of PSP or Alzheimer disease (AD) (Ouchi et al., 2014). This poses a challenge for the selection of patients for clinical trials who may not respond to a treatment because they do not have the target pathology (rather than the drug lacking efficacy).
- Similar pathological states can have different clinical presentations: for example, tauopathies presenting as PSP and CBD (Murray et al., 2014) or c9orf72 presenting as frontotemporal dementia (FTD) or ALS (Balendra and Isaacs, 2018)
- Many patients dying of specific diseases have a mixed pathology at postmortem, especially in the more elderly population (e.g., AD with amyloid plaques, tau tangles, along with vascular disease and α-synuclein deposition). Indeed there is even some suggestion that one pathology may trigger another: for example, AD in patients presenting initially with a cerebral amyloid angiopathy (Cupino and Zabel, 2013) or tau driving additional degeneration alongside α-synuclein pathology (Moussaud et al., 2014).
- All primary neurodegenerative disorders of the CNS have a glial response which may contribute to the disease state; for example, ALS may be driven by neurotoxic signals and/or abnormal glutamate handling by astrocytes (Pirooznia et al., 2014). In this respect, diseases that were once thought of as being more glial in nature—such as multiple sclerosis (MS)—are now being reclassified as neurodegenerative, given that this defines the disease in the secondary progressive phase after the initial inflammatory events (Coles et al., 2006).
- All neurodegenerative disorders generate an immune/inflammatory/microglial response, which again may be an integral part of the disease process; for example, in Huntington disease (HD) there are changes in the circulating immune cells that experimentally alter the disease course of HD in transgenic animals (reviewed in Soulet and Cicchetti, 2011).
- It is also increasingly being recognized that traditional single disease entities may have different "disease subtypes" within them; for example, in PD there is evidence to show that some patients develop dementia earlier than others, which is driven by certain genetic variants in tau and the glucocerebrosidase (GBA) gene, as well as possibly inflammation (Williams-Gray et al., 2009, 2016; Winder-Rhodes et al., 2013). As such, these diseases, despite superficially looking the same, may have different pathogenic pathways, or at least a similar pathogenic process with different kinetics. This disease heterogeneity is present across all neurodegenerative disorders and is an additional challenge for the design of clinical trials around disease modification.
- Over the past 25 years many Mendelian forms of classical neurodegenerative diseases of the CNS have been described (e.g., AD and PD). These monogenic forms of disease have been very helpful in identifying pathways of disease, especially through the generation of cell and animal models of disease (Levine et al., 2004). However, while instructive, understanding the basis of these disorders does not necessarily mean that the same processes occur in the commoner sporadic forms of disease, although in some cases genes linked to familial forms of the disease

**TABLE 92.1 Major Neurodegenerative Disorders of the Central Nervous System and Their Associated Protein Pathology**

**The Major Neurodegenerative Disorders of the CNS**

- Alzheimer disease (AD)
- Frontotemporal dementia (familial and sporadic) (FTD)
- Parkinson disease ± dementia (PD/PDD)
- Dementia with Lewy bodies (DLB)
- Multiple system atrophy (MSA)
- Progressive supranuclear palsy (PSP)
- Corticobasal degeneration (CBD)
- Huntington disease (HD)
- Spinocerebellar ataxias (SCAs)
- Motor neuron disease including amyotrophic lateral sclerosis (ALS)
- Vascular dementia including inherited conditions such as CADASIL
- Traumatic brain encephalopathy
- Multiple sclerosis (MS)
- Prion disease
- Human immunodeficiency virus (HIV)-associated neurocognitive disorder
- Inherited metabolic diseases of the CNS

**The Major Neurodegenerative Disorders of the CNS as Defined by Their Protein Pathology**

| | |
|---|---|
| Amyloid | • AD |
| Tau | • AD |
| | • PSP |
| | • FTD and especially FTD linked to chromosome 17 |
| | • CBD |
| | • Pick disease |
| | • Dementia pugilistica |
| | • Argyrophilic grain disease |
| α-Synuclein | • PD/PDD |
| | • MSA |
| | • DLB |
| Other | • TDP-43: ALS; some types of FTD |
| | • Mutant huntingtin, HD |
| | • Others in ALS include FUS; SOD 1; C9ORF72; OTN; UBQLN2 |
| | • Ataxins in various different types of autosomal dominant spinocerebellar ataxias |

*CADASIL*, Cerebral autosomal dominant arteriopathy with subcortical infarcts and leukoencephalopathy; *CNS*, central nervous system; *FUS*, fused in sarcoma protein; *OTN*, optineurin; *SOD1*, superoxide dismutase; *TDP-43*, TAR DNA-binding protein 43; *UBQLN2*, ubiquilin 2.

have also emerged from a genome wide association study (GWAS) (e.g., LRRK2 in PD) (Simón-Sánchez et al., 2009). For example, patients with Parkin mutations present with parkinsonism and have a pathology that affects protein degradation within the cell, but the few patients who have come to postmortem do not appear to have classical LB pathology, the hallmark of idiopathic PD (Doherty et al., 2013). As such, these patients do not have the same disease and thus the same fundamental disease process as that which underlies sporadic PD. In other words, many rare genetic forms of common sporadic disorders are instructive only up to a point.

- Finally it is currently recognized that many neurodegenerative disorders of the CNS may not have a pathology that is solely cell autonomous (i.e., driven only by an intrinsic problem within the neuron affected by the disease process). Rather, all disorders (even solely genetic disorders such as HD) have a noncell autonomous aspect to them that includes not only the glial/inflammatory component discussed earlier but also the possible spreading of pathogenic protein strains from one cell to another in a prion-like fashion (e.g., tauopathies, α-synuclein in PD, and certain forms of ALS) (Guo and Lee, 2014).

It is important to remember these major points when one comes to try and understand the relative role of different pathogenic pathways in neurodegenerative disorders of the CNS, because it is all too easy to study one isolated pathway as the only pathway to cell loss in these conditions. The reality is that many pathways are involved and that there is a significant degree of overlap between seemingly different disorders. Therefore we will briefly summarize all the pathways linked to cellular dysfunction and death in these disorders, highlighting commonalities as well as differences and how this may ultimately impact on new therapeutic approaches for these disorders. In the end, it is likely that successful therapeutic strategies will target a number of these pathways together rather than focusing on one, because this has so far proven unsuccessful (e.g., Jensen and Barker, 2019).

## WHERE DO NEURODEGENERATIVE DISORDERS BEGIN?

This seems to be a redundant question because clinicians can easily recognize a patient presenting with motor neuron disease or PD. However, in nearly all cases by the time the patient presents clinically they have already lost substantial numbers of neural cells and the disease process is well underway and may have passed a point at which the process can be reversed because the cells underlying the core aspects of the disease have been long lost; for example, in PD it is estimated that up to 50% of the nigral DA cells and up to 80% of the dopaminergic innervation to the striatum are lost by the time the patient presents with motor abnormalities (Lees et al., 2009). Therefore this tells us a number of things:

1. The disease process begins well ahead of clinical presentation.
2. The disease process may well originate outside the population of cells that determines the initial clinical expression.
3. The disease process may not begin in the nerve cell body but in other cellular compartments, such as the nerve terminals.

The recognition that disease processes begin well ahead of their overt clinical presentation has primarily come from studies looking at monogenic forms of neurodegeneration, such as HD and certain forms of AD (presenilin families, etc.) (Cash et al., 2013). In these studies, abnormalities in brain structure, typically using longitudinal magnetic resonance imaging (MRI), have been seen many years ahead of the patient presenting. Of course, when such abnormalities are detected decades ahead of clinical presentation, questions arise as to whether one is truly picking up the earliest pathology or a developmental state secondary to possessing the abnormal gene and its product (Dean et al., 2014). This early pathology often remains silent in terms of obvious clinical features, although it can in some cases be revealed using complex and specific motor or cognitive tests (e.g., in HD looking at emotional processing) (Labuschagne et al., 2013). This shows not only the degree of redundancy that exists in the adult CNS but also its compensatory capacity, which could be exploited therapeutically if we better understood it.

Nevertheless, at some point the patient presents, but by this stage the disease process is well established. Thus, if we are to truly stop or slow down the disease, it may be that searching for these early markers is likely to be most effective, to then intervene and slow down the pathology before the whole range of downstream processes have been activated. There is currently much interest in trying to identify such states: for example, prodromal PD; the form of mild cognitive impairment that truly evolves to AD; and the earliest reliable measure of change in premanifest HD patients (Barker and Mason, 2014; Bondi et al., 2005; Postuma et al., 2015; Stout et al., 2012; Tabrizi et al., 2009, 2011, 2012, 2013).

Knowing where the disease starts in terms of the temporal loss of cells is not straightforward, and this is perhaps best illustrated in PD. In PD, the patients present when there is extensive loss of nigral dopaminergic cells, but at this stage there is also extensive additional brainstem pathology as well as abnormalities in the olfactory bulb and even outside the CNS with involvement of the enteric nervous system and gut (Derkinderen et al., 2011; Shannon et al., 2012). The recognition of this by Braak and colleagues, using α-synuclein immunostaining to define the pathology, has led to the concept that PD may originate in the gut and olfactory system (possibly in response to some environmental insult in genetically susceptible people) with spread into the CNS (Del Tredici et al., 2002). As such nigral pathology occurs at a relatively advanced stage of the disease process, this in turn has contributed to the idea that in PD, α-synuclein acts in a prion-like fashion, seeding pathology as it spreads caudally (Guo and Lee, 2014; see later discussion).

Thus most neurodegenerative disorders are thought to start years ahead of clinical presentation and with a pathology not initially found in the cells classically defined as lying at the heart of the condition. Furthermore, it is now thought by many that the disease process itself may target the axon and synapse more than the cell body in the early stages of disease, which would help to explain why there can be a discordance between neurological deficits and overt cell loss, especially in transgenic models of human diseases. So, for example, in α-synuclein transgenic models of PD, the earliest changes relate to dopamine release in the striatum resulting from synaptic dysfunction (Spinelli et al., 2014). This then leads to synaptic terminal loss with axonal transport defects and a dying back of the axon toward the cell body, which atrophies before eventually being lost. This would account for the greater terminal loss of dopaminergic fibers than nigral cell body loss in the early stages of PD. In addition, this may also help to explain why therapies targeting the cell bodies may not necessarily be clinically successful not only in PD but in a range of diseases that affect neurons with long projecting axons and multiple synaptic targets.

## MECHANISMS OF CELL LOSS IN NEURODEGENERATION

Cells can die in disease through programmed cell death, be it apoptosis or necroptosis (Duprez et al., 2009; Galluzzi et al., 2012), or even phagoptosis (Brown and Neher, 2012), or through nonprogrammed processes such as necrosis, of which there are various different forms. Indeed more recently a form of programmed necrosis has been described, although the details of this lie beyond the scope of this review. For many years it has been thought that the only form of cell death in neurodegenerative disorders was an apoptotic one, and although this may be true in part, it is increasingly being recognized that the disease process induces a range of cell death processes (Jellinger, 2001), a point we will come back to later.

As to the mechanisms by which cells are induced to die, a number have been proposed that can broadly be thought of as being cell autonomous (i.e., triggered by an intrinsic disease process such as the production of mutant huntingtin in the case of HD; reviewed in Ross and Tabrizi, 2011) or noncell autonomous (e.g., the production of neurotoxic molecules by astrocytes in ALS) (Pirooznia et al., 2014). In both cases the disease process typically starts with the formation of an abnormal protein species (e.g., oligomeric α-synuclein), which then interferes with a whole range of intracellular processes that ultimately cause the cell to become dysfunctional and then die (Fig. 92.1). The processes that dominate in any one disease vary, but nevertheless they are probably all involved to some degree and as such may be amenable to therapies which could be used across all neurodegenerative disorders. In addition, all disorders have a noncell autonomous aspect to them, which again varies as a function of the disease state and the location of pathology.

The main pathogenic mechanism starts in most cases with the production of an abnormal protein species, which either can be defined by the underlying gene causing the condition (e.g., SOD 1 in some cases of familial ALS; mutant huntingtin in HD; ataxin in autosomal dominant spinocerebellar ataxias) or occurs through some poorly understood process (e.g., α-synuclein in sporadic PD; tau in PSP). In either case the abnormal protein undergoes some form of conformational change, which then leads to formation of oligomers and then protofibrils (Goedert et al., 2013). Downstream of the oligomers, fibrils are formed which finally aggregate into inclusion bodies that are used to define the pathology of the neurodegenerative disease (Peden and Ironside, 2012). Whether the oligomeric species, the protofibrils, or the aggregates are the most toxic forms of the protein is still a matter of debate (Winklhofer et al., 2008), because oligomers are entities in flux and there is no good way of detecting them in intact tissue. The mechanisms by which the toxic species instigate death pathways are also not clear, but major problems in several intracellular organelles, such as the mitochondria, and the ubiquitin-proteosomal and lysosomal degradation pathways, are implicated (see later discussion). Therapeutically, the aggregation cascade has led many to develop agents that block the production of the toxic protein species. This is clearly difficult in sporadic disease where the identity of the pathological protein strain is not known but is obviously more feasible in monogenic forms of disease where interfering with the production of the mutant protein (while not significantly reducing the production of the wild-type protein) can be done using strategies such as small interfering RNAs (siRNAs) or oligosense antinucleotides (OSAs) (Chandra et al., 2014). These therapies have entered the clinical arena for some childhood forms of ALS as well as HD (Jensen and Barker, 2019).

The production of toxic protein species results in perturbations to the normal physiology of the neuron and the network of cells it forms and is located within, and by so doing precipitates a disease state. The nature of these different perturbations is listed as follows, along with some of the therapeutic strategies that could be used to treat them:

- *Transcriptional dysregulation.* This is best described in diseases such as HD, where the abnormal gene product leads to transcriptional dysregulation in the early stages of the disease process (Moumne et al., 2013). As such, the cell undergoes a global change in its transcriptional profile, and this includes a number of key receptor/intracellular systems which in turn can then lead to cellular dysfunction and death. Most recently this has been described in those cases of ALS and FTD caused by an expansion of a repeated six-nucleotide sequence in the noncoding region of the c9orf72 gene (Woollacott and Mead, 2014). Although the optimal treatment in these conditions would be to silence the mutant gene with its expansion, an alternative approach, at least in the case of HD, has been the use of histone deacetylase inhibitors, which alter the global conformation of DNA but also target many other cellular processes. These have shown some success in slowing down the disease process in animal models (Jia et al., 2012), and although their precise mechanism of action is not known, they are now entering clinical trials (HDSA, 2015).
- *Mitochondrial dysfunction leading to oxidative stress and free radical production.* One of the earliest theories of neurodegeneration was that cells were lost as a result of mitochondrial dysfunction,

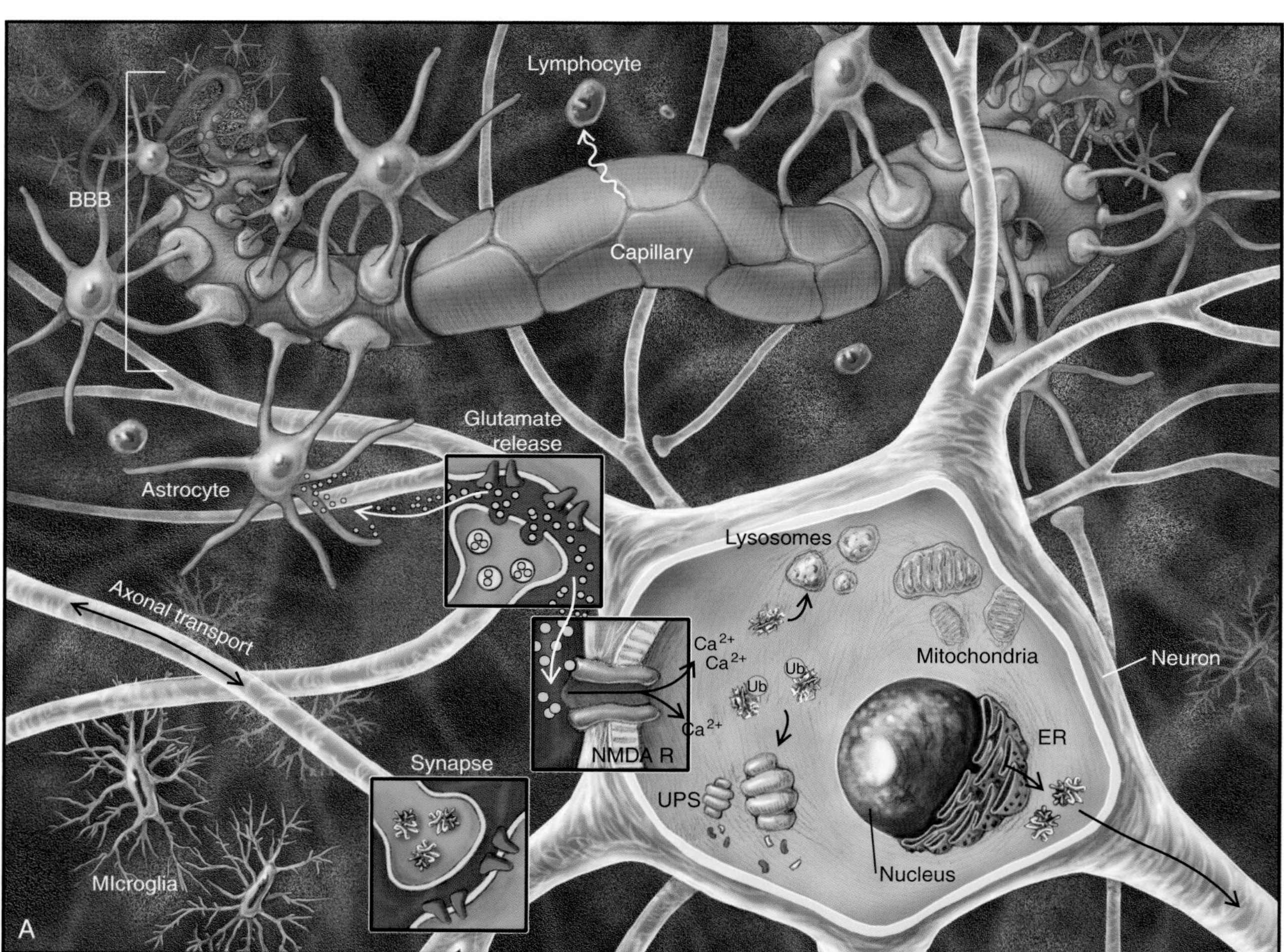


**Fig. 92.1** (A) Schematic figure of the normal brain. The intact blood-brain barrier *(BBB)* allows some circulating lymphocytes to enter the central nervous system (CNS), where they perform a surveillance role. In addition, there is evidence that the CNS has a lymphatic system of sorts (so called G-lymphatics), which also increases the crosstalk between the immune system and CNS pathology/homeostasis (Louveau et al., 2018). The neurons communicate via synapses, with any excess synaptic glutamate release being buffered by the neighboring astrocytes. The activation of *N-methyl*-D-aspartate receptor *(NMDA R)* by glutamate leads to a calcium influx that is buffered by intracellular mechanisms such as calcium-binding proteins and endoplasmic reticulum *(ER)*/mitochondria. The production of proteins within the neurons is tightly regulated, and abnormal proteins are removed by the ubiquitin proteasome system *(UPS)* and via the lysosomes through a process of autophagy. This involves chaperone proteins.

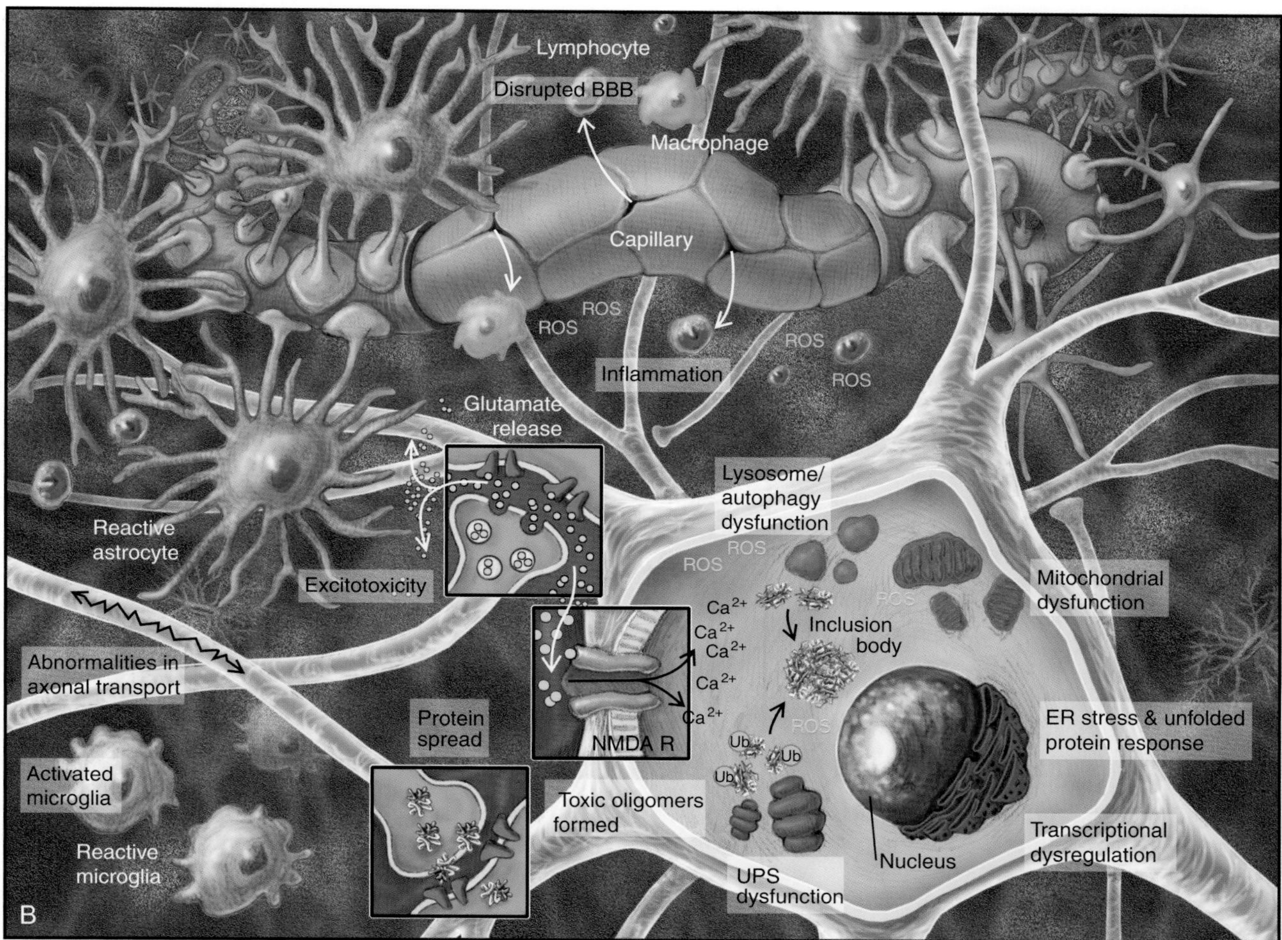


**Fig. 92.1—cont'd** (B) Schematic figure of the brain in neurodegenerative disorders. Under these conditions a number of linked pathways interact to cause neuronal dysfunction and then death. These include: (i) excitotoxicity due to reduced glutamate uptake by glial cells or increased release leading to excessive calcium influx and the production of reactive oxygen species *(ROS)*; (ii) the production of abnormal proteins or a change in the conformation of the protein leads to the formation of toxic oligomers or protofibrils, which (iii) may also be passed into the neuron transsynaptically from afferent neurons containing that protein. The abnormal form or strain of the protein then forms the toxic species which have a number of effects, including (iv) transcriptional dysregulation along with (v) ER stress that can also provoke an unfolded protein response which can ultimately lead to apoptosis. In addition, (vi) abnormalities in mitochondrial function occur through a variety of routes including direct interactions with the toxic protein species, and all of this is exacerbated by problems in protein clearance mechanisms linked to the (vii) UPS and autophagic systems. Superimposed on this is (viii) an inflammatory response that may be secondary or primary, and the elements that contribute to it include abnormalities in the BBB with increased migration of inflammatory cells into the CNS along with changes in the meningeal lymphatics, activation of microglia by the extracellular secretion of the toxic protein, and the loss of neurons themselves. All of these processes can affect (ix) axonal transport, which can also be primarily targeted in some forms of neurodegenerative disorders. As a result of this cascade of events, the neuron becomes dysfunctional and then is lost by one of several processes, typically programmed cell death (apoptosis), although in some cases the neurons either die through necrosis or are directly phagocytosed by microglia (phagoptosis).

leading to oxidative stress and the production of free radicals (Beal, 2005). This theory gained early support from the finding that some cases of familial ALS were due to SOD 1 mutations. This theory has waned in popularity (Dupuis, 2014) but is still considered by many to be an important player in the pathogenic cascade, although most would recognize that there are other processes involving mitochondria, such as fusion/fission and mitophagy, that may also be critical (Federico et al., 2012; Osellame and Duchen, 2014; see later discussion). Nevertheless, the idea that some of the cell death has a free radical basis has led to many trials using free radical scavengers and agents designed to reduce oxidative stress. This includes trials of vitamin E in PD and coenzyme $Q_{10}$ in PD and HD. To date, none of these trials have shown long-term benefits (e.g., see The Parkinson Study Group QE3 Investigators et al., 2014), and in reality the production of damaging free radicals lies downstream of many more significant events in most neurodegenerative disorders.

- *Mitophagy and abnormalities of mitochondria dynamics.* Mitochondria in cells are not static organelles but are in a dynamic equilibrium between dividing (fission) and fusing (fusion) as well as being removed through a selective autophagic pathway (mitophagy). The molecular signals underlying the dynamic interplay between these states are only now being understood, but in essence mitochondrial fission enables the neurons to shuttle mitochondria to nerve processes as well as to the mitophagy pathways in the case of abnormal mitochondria displaying bioenergetic failure. Fusion, on the other hand, protects against the dominant expression of mitochondrial mutations and may also help to maintain adenosine triphosphate (ATP) in cases of great cellular demand (Youle and van der Bliek, 2012). Of late there has been great interest in the possibility that this dynamic interplay may go awry in disease states and by so doing compromise the intracellular energetics of the cell, leading to its demise (Campello et al., 2014; Itoh et al., 2013). This has been studied in most detail in some of the genetic forms of PD: namely, those linked with gene products known to have a mitochondrial site of interaction (PINK 1, DJ 1, and Parkin) (de Vries and Przedborski, 2013). Currently this approach is being looked at in a trial in PD by Edison Pharmaceuticals (https://clinicaltrials.gov/ct2/show/NCT01923584).

- *Ubiquitin-proteasomal and autophagic dysfunction.* The production of abnormal proteins is an ongoing problem for any metabolically active cell, and this includes neurons. As such, the cell has powerful mechanisms for ridding the cell of abnormal or damaged proteins. One involves ubiquitylation and the shuttling of the protein to the proteasome system (ubiquitin proteasome system [UPS]), where it is broken down and removed (Lee et al., 2013). This process relies heavily on chaperone proteins. An alternative pathway involves directing the abnormal protein to lysosomes, where they are hydrolyzed and removed (so-called autophagy). There are several different forms of autophagy, some of which also rely on chaperone proteins. Loss of activity in these networks can lead to accumulation of aberrant protein, and in addition these proteins may then further inhibit the process in a positive feedback fashion. The extent to which abnormalities in these pathways are primarily or secondarily affected in neurodegenerative disorders is debated, but, regardless, they still offer an attractive therapeutic target (Boland et al., 2018). As a result, much work has gone into finding agents that could upregulate autophagy and by so doing enhance protein clearance within the cell, including the removal of aberrant pathogenic protein species such as mutant huntingtin in HD. This has led to early clinical trials with drugs such as rapamycin, an activator of autophagy, which have been shown to work well in a range of animal models of neurodegenerative diseases linked to intracellular protein accumulation and inclusion body formation. However, chronic use of a general mammalian target of rapamycin (mTOR) inhibitor is not without its problems (Aso & Ferrer, 2013), and so safer alternatives have been trialed such as rilmenidine (Underwood et al., 2017).
- *Endoplasmic reticulum stress and the unfolded protein response (UPR).* Of late there has been a great deal of interest in the role of the endoplasmic reticulum in disease pathogenesis and the effect of accumulated protein species within it, which in turn can activate the UPR. This evolutionary conserved response leads to the cell halting protein translation (and by so doing stopping the production of the aberrant protein) as well as the production of chaperone proteins that mediate protein folding and degradation. This system has obvious advantages to the cell in the short term but in the long term causes cell stasis and apoptosis (Jager et al., 2012). Recently there have been attempts to modulate this system and by so doing rescue cells affected by the neurodegenerative disease process; this has been most intensely studied in prion diseases. This has involved a number of small molecules that either activate or inhibit critical phosphatases known to regulate aspects of this pathway's activity (Moreno et al., 2012; Tsaytler et al., 2011) as well as drug repurposing studies (Halliday et al., 2017).
- *Synaptic trafficking abnormalities.* As already stated, it is currently recognized that many neurodegenerative disorders begin at the nerve terminal with a dying-back process eventually involving the cell body. This, in part, may relate to local protein accumulation as well as a global neuronal energy failure, given the metabolic activity of this part of the neuron. As a result there is early synaptic dysfunction which leads not only to abnormalities of synaptic transmission (giving symptoms in the absence of cell loss) but also impairments in endosomal-exosomal trafficking and protein aggregation.
- *Excitotoxicity.* In this situation there is an excessive influx of glutamate (whether from other afferent neurons or disordered glial uptake of glutamate), and this leads to a calcium influx which in turn overwhelms the intracellular calcium buffering system, which then triggers a whole series of downstream events including free radical production, oxidative stress, and loss of mitochondrial function (Cali et al., 2012; Lau and Tymianski, 2010), as well as triggering apoptosis. This is perhaps best studied in ALS and HD, and as a result much effort has been devoted to finding agents that block glutamate receptors (e.g., *N*-methyl-D-aspartate [NMDA] antagonists) or their action and calcium influx (e.g., calcium channel blockers). To date, none has been shown to be of value, although there is a lot of interest in calcium channel blockers and PD (e.g., there has been a recent trial of isradipine in the United States that reported negative results in 2020) https://clinicaltrials.gov/ct2/show/NCT02168842 because the vulnerable nigral neurons express specific calcium channels. In these neurons there is also a link between calcium influx and α-synuclein, which may help to explain why these neurons in particular are selectively targeted in PD and may also help to explain the anecdotal data from some epidemiological studies that calcium channel blockers protect against PD (Sulzer and Surmeier, 2012).
- *Abnormalities of axonal transport.* One of the fundamental ways in which cells maintain their integrity is through anterograde and retrograde axonal transport, where essential signaling molecules are exchanged between the cell body and its nuclear machinery and the nerve processes and their synaptic communication. In some disorders there is thought to be a major pathology in this pathway which leads to slowed axonal transport, which in turn deprives aspects of the cell of vital signals as well as the local accumulation of certain products within the axon, which can further disrupt the transport system. This is well studied in certain diseases where the cells affected have especially long axonal projections such as occurs in hereditary spastic paraparesis (HSP), PD, and ALS (Hinckelmann et al., 2013). The disruption of axonal transport is also thought to be important in the tauopathies, where alterations in the ratio of 3–4 repeat tau isoforms (which in the normal brain is 1:1) changes the ability of this protein to stabilize microtubules and maintain normal axonal transport (Brunden et al., 2014). Treating such deficits is difficult, but there has been great interest in using small molecules to stabilize tau and by so doing improve axonal transport and neuronal integrity and survival (Brunden et al., 2014).
- *Inflammation and immune-mediated processes of neuronal loss.* This is best seen in conditions in which there is a clear primary immune response as is seen in MS and related neuroinflammatory conditions, as well as in paraneoplastic and autoimmune disorders of the CNS. In these conditions an immune response targets a neural compartment and causes dysfunction and then secondary cell death—in the case of MS this targets the oligodendrocytes, leading to secondary axonal loss; in paraneoplastic conditions it targets neuronal antigens,

leading to their death, although in many cases a direct pathogenic link between the paraneoplastic antibody and disease state has not been proven (Graus and Dalmau, 2012). In all cases the treatment is designed to stop the inflammation using a range of immune modulatory drugs or, in the case of paraneoplastic syndromes, removing the underlying tumor that is driving the aberrant immune response. Although these conditions have not traditionally been regarded as being neurodegenerative, there is increasing recognition that this is a major part of their pathology if the disease process is allowed to progress unchecked. In addition, many primary neurodegenerative disorders have been postulated to have either a primary autoimmune component (e.g., calcium channel antibodies in ALS; Zhao et al., 2013) or a secondary inflammatory process driven by components of the pathologically diseased neural network. This involves activated microglia, which can be broadly divided into M1 and M2, with one type promoting repair and the other mediating cell toxicity (Benarroch, 2013), although it is also fair to say that the true heterogeneity of this cell type is only now being properly addressed (Böttcher et al., 2019). Thus simply stopping microglial activation, with drugs such as minocycline, may not necessarily be a good thing. Indeed more recently there has been evidence suggesting that these microglia interact with astrocytes to drive pathology and that this may represent an alternative therapeutic target (Liddelow et al., 2017; Yun et al., 2018).

In addition, there is evidence for peripheral immune involvement, involving both the innate and adaptive immune responses, as well as data from GWAS, which have thrown up loci linked to immune/inflammatory functions (Chang et al., 2017). As a result there are increasing efforts to develop antiinflammatory agents that can get into the CNS, and/or agents that by affecting peripheral immune cells can have CNS effects (Kaushik and Basu, 2013). In HD, where the mutant huntingtin changes peripheral immune function, selectively targeting this compartment can affect the CNS pathology (Soulet and Cicchetti, 2011). In PD there are emerging data showing that the immune system is important in the risk and progression of this disorder (Racette et al., 2018) and that the pathology of tauopathies involves complement activation (reviewed in Davies and Spires-Jones, 2018). In ALS, trials are ongoing of a number of immunomodulatory agents, with no evidence as yet of clear efficacy (Khalid et al., 2017). Peripheral immune cells in the CNS lymphatics may also play a role in clearance of toxic protein species with mouse models, showing worsening of Alzheimer pathology when CNS lymphatics are blocked and improvement when they are expanded following administration of vascular endothelial related protein C. This suggests that facilitation of immune-mediated clearance via the meningeal lymphatics may also be a promising therapeutic strategy (Da Mesquita et al., 2018).

- *Protein spread and the prion hypothesis of neurodegeneration.* This theory has become very popular of late and builds on the model first described in prion disorders of the CNS such as Creutzfeldt-Jakob (CJD) disease. In this condition the primary problem is thought to involve the normal prion protein (PrPc) undergoing a conformational change to a virulent form of the protein (PrPsc). This occurs either through infection with PrPsc (in the case of kuru or mad cow disease) or sporadically by chance. The PrPsc so produced then templates the normal PrPc into the abnormal form and by so doing catalyzes the disease process, such that once it has started the disease is self-propagating, which helps to explain its generally explosive onset and course. More recently it has been proposed that similar events underlie other sporadic CNS disorders characterized by protein pathologies such as PD, tauopathies, and ALS (Goedert et al., 2010; Polymenidou and Cleveland, 2011). In these cases it is postulated that the underlying native protein—α-synuclein in the case of PD, tau in the case of tauopathies—undergoes a conformational change to form a toxic strain, possibly in response to an environmental factor or by chance, as occurs in most cases of CJD. This abnormal strain of protein can then template the normal protein to convert it into a new toxic species and so the process continues, with the abnormal protein also being passed from cell to cell, possibly through exosomes (Guo and Lee, 2014). Although controversial, there has been a recent tranche of data in support of this in animal studies, which in turn has led to new therapeutic approaches attempting to remove the protein as it passes through the extracellular compartment from cell to cell—an approach that in particular has lent itself to immunization therapies which are now entering clinical trials (see, e.g., Golde et al., 2013; Jankovic, 2019; Jankovic et al., 2018; Mandler et al., 2014; Schenk et al., 2017).
- *Astrocyte dysfunction.* The astrocytes of the CNS are important in maintaining homeostasis by the removal of excess neurotransmitters, calcium, and potassium—this they do by forming a syncytium, which serves to support the neurons embedded within them. There has always been interest in the possibility that abnormalities in astrocyte function may disturb the local homeostatic environment and by so doing lead to neuronal compromise and death. This is perhaps best illustrated in ALS where abnormalities in glutamate transport have been reported, with the result that glutamate levels accumulate locally and by so doing cause local motor neuronal death through excitotoxicity (see earlier discussion; Pirooznia et al., 2014). This has led to attempts to modulate ALS not only by blocking glutamate and its effects (e.g., riluzole) but also by targeting the astrocytes which are thought to be primarily abnormal in ALS. Indeed, there is increasing evidence for this, using in vitro modeling systems involving induced pluripotent stem cell (iPS) cells as well as animal models where transplants of astrocytes have rescued motor neurons in transgenic ALS mice (Lepore et al., 2008; Pirooznia et al., 2014) as well as more mechanistic studies looking at the role of microRNAs is this crosstalk (Ferraiuolo and Shaw, 2018). In addition there have been recent studies in HD showing that astrocyte abnormalities exist and drive part of the clinical phenotype, at least in mouse models of disease (Benraiss et al., 2016).
- *Disturbances of sleep.* There has recently been interest in the idea that sleep has a vital function not only in maintaining synaptic homeostasis and allowing memory consolidation but also in the removal of extracellular proteins. This has perhaps best been seen in an animal model of AD, where it was shown that in sleep there were changes in extracellular fluid flow within the brain that altered the clearance of amyloid in a transgenic model of AD (Xie et al., 2013). More recently, similar results have been shown in sleep-deprived humans, where cerebrospinal fluid tau is increased compared with controls (potentiating the pathology in the corresponding mouse model) (Holth et al., 2019). If correct, then this opens up a new therapeutic approach, especially as it is well known that sleep/wake abnormalities are common in these chronic neurodegenerative disorders of the CNS and may in part be driving aspects of the pathology (Hasting and Goedert, 2013).

## CONCLUSION

The loss of neurons in chronic neurodegenerative disorders of the CNS can occur through many different routes, and this occurs in almost all diseases, albeit with one route being more dominant than others. Although this makes it difficult to unravel the exact series of events leading to neuronal dysfunction and death, it does offer the hope that the treatment of one condition will have implications for all neurodegenerative disorders. However, understanding when the pathological cascade begins and where in the cell will be critical in future therapeutic interventions: treating the disease as early as possible offers the best hope of slowing it down or even stopping it. Indeed there is now a growing realization that neurodegenerative disorders of the CNS are not just diseases of neurons but have an astrocyte, microglial, and inflammatory aspect to them, and this may even extend to the vasculature and more global CNS processes such as sleep homeostasis.

In this chapter we have tried to summarize new concepts in neurodegenerative diseases in terms of how they can be better classified and understood at the pathogenic level. With this comes a better understanding of the therapies of tomorrow, which will be designed to try and slow down or even stop the disease process in a series of conditions that will become only more common as the population ages and lives longer.

*The complete reference list is available online at https://expertconsult.inkling.com.* 

## ACKNOWLEDGMENTS

We thank Dr. Aviva Tolkovsky for her critical review of the original manuscript and Dr. Janelle Drouin-Ouellet for her help with the figure.

93

# Mitochondrial Disorders

*Chris Turner, Robert D.S. Pitceathly, Anthony H.V. Schapira*

## OUTLINE



The bacterial hypothesis of the origin of mitochondria suggests that approximately 1–2 billion years ago, alpha-purple bacteria were incorporated into evolving eukaryotic cells. During evolution, these bacteria transferred many of their essential genes to the nuclear chromosomes. Mitochondria still have many remnants of their bacterial origin, such as the use of *N*-formylmethionyl-tRNA (transfer ribonucleic acid) as the initiator of protein synthesis.

Our current knowledge of mitochondrial genetics began with evidence of cytoplasmic genetic inheritance (rho factor in yeast) in the 1940s. Two decades later, mitochondrial deoxyribonucleic acid (mtDNA) was first recognized in chick cells and shortly thereafter in yeast, establishing the identity of the rho factor with mtDNA. In 1951, Denis Leigh first described the striking neuropathology resembling Wernicke encephalopathy in a child who had died of a neurological disease that now bears his name, *Leigh syndrome*. In 1959, following astute bedside clinical observations made in a single patient with nonthyroidal hypermetabolism, Rolf Luft deciphered biochemical abnormalities involving a defect in oxidative phosphorylation (OXPHOS) and described a rare neurological condition that we now call *Luft disease*. In the 1960s, morphological abnormalities of mitochondria were recognized by electron microscopy and special stains (Gomori trichrome and its modification) in newly characterized muscle diseases. In the early 1970s, abnormalities in respiratory chain function were associated with disorders mainly involving the central nervous system (CNS) and muscle. In the following year, the first examples of myopathies due to isolated deficiencies of muscle carnitine and carnitine palmitoyltransferase (CPT) were reported. These clinical discoveries were the starting point for a rapid expansion in the field of mitochondrial pathophysiology. By 1981, the complete sequence of human mtDNA was elucidated.

In 1988 a major breakthrough in our understanding of mitochondrial disorders occurred with the report of the association of sporadic human encephalomyopathies with large deletions of mtDNA (Holt et al., 1988) and of Leber hereditary optic neuropathy (LHON) with a point mutation at nucleotide pair (np) 11778 in the mtDNA (Wallace et al., 1988). More than 250 pathogenic point mutations of the mtDNA, large-scale mtDNA deletions, and rearrangements have been subsequently reported (MITOMAP [2019]: A Human Mitochondrial Genome Database. http://www.mitomap.org, 2019). More than 85% of mitochondrial proteins are encoded by the nuclear DNA (nDNA), with at least 300 nuclear genes linked to mitochondrial disease (Rahman, 2018). However, given that approximately 1500 mitochondrial proteins are nuclear-encoded (Calvo, 2016), it is highly probable that many unknown mitochondrial disorders due to nDNA defects still exist. The delineation of human mtDNA variation and genetics has also provided startling new insights into the evolution and migration of human populations (Wallace, 1995). Mitochondria may also play an important role in neurodegenerative diseases and the aging process (Schapira, 2008, 2012; Turner and Schapira, 2010).

The diseases included under the term *mitochondrial disorders* are so diverse and involve so many parts of the nervous system and other organs that the whole spectrum cannot be easily addressed in any one chapter. Therefore the disorders related to intermediate metabolism and mitochondrial Krebs cycle are discussed with inborn errors of metabolism in Chapter 91. The syndrome that combines epilepsy and ragged-red muscle fibers (myoclonic epilepsy and ragged-red fibers [MERRF]) is discussed in Chapters 48 and 100. The syndrome of progressive external ophthalmoplegia (PEO) is discussed with other abnormalities of eye movement (Chapter 17), and LHON with other causes of vision loss (Chapter 16). This chapter overviews the principles of mitochondrial genetics and pathophysiology. It also provides a summary of the clinical features and management of patients with mitochondrial disorders and a brief review of those neurodegenerative diseases where mitochondrial dysfunction is best characterized (Schapira, 2012).

## GENETICS OF MITOCHONDRIAL DISORDERS

MtDNA is a 16,569-np double-stranded, closed, circular molecule located within the matrix of the double-membrane mitochondrion. Each human cell contains a dynamic network of mitochondria and hundreds of mtDNA molecules. Human mtDNA encodes 13 of the 89 subunits of the mitochondrial respiratory chain, as well as the small (12S) and large (16S) ribosomal RNAs (rRNAs) and 22 tRNAs necessary for intramitochondrial protein synthesis (Fig. 93.1, *A*).

The mtDNA is replicated and transcribed by using an origin and promoter for each of the two DNA strands, the G-rich heavy (H) strand and the C-rich light (L) strand. The H- and L-strand replication origins (OH and OL; see Fig. 93.1, *A*) are relatively distant within the molecule, but the H- and L-strand promoters (PH and PL) are closely spaced and located adjacent to OH in the approximately 1000-np noncoding control region. This region also encompasses the D-loop, which is formed by replication initiation events from the OH. Research involving evolution of mammalian species and origin and migration of humans on earth has focused on the variation in a small hypervariable noncoding region within the D-loop. The replication mechanism of mtDNA may be more complex than originally suggested, in that the mtDNA can also replicate by the extension of both leading and lagging strands, a process resembling nDNA replication (Holt et al., 2000).

The respiratory chain (see Fig. 93.1, *B*) is located within the mitochondrial inner membrane and is composed of five multimeric enzyme complexes whose genes are dispersed between the mtDNA and nDNA. Complex I (nicotinamide adenine dinucleotide [NADH]–ubiquinone oxidoreductase) accepts electrons from the reduced form of NADH, whereas complex II (succinate–ubiquinone oxidoreductase) collects electrons from succinate. Both NADH and succinate are the products of the Krebs cycle. Enzyme complexes I and II transfer electrons to coenzyme $Q_{10}$ ($CoQ_{10}$). From $CoQ_{10}$, the electrons flow through complex III (ubiquinone–cytochrome *c* oxidoreductase) to cytochrome *c*, then to complex IV (cytochrome *c* oxidase), and finally to oxygen to yield water. The electron transfer is coupled to proton ($H^+$) pumping by complexes I, III, and IV from the matrix to the intermembrane space, creating an electrochemical gradient across the inner membrane. This electrochemical gradient is used by complex V (adenosine triphosphate [ATP] synthase) as a source of energy to condense adenosine diphosphate (ADP) and inorganic phosphate (Pi) to synthesize ATP. ATP and ADP are then exchanged across the mitochondrial membrane by the adenine nucleotide translocator (ANT).

Complex I comprises approximately 46 subunits, 7 of which (ND-1, -2, -3, -4, -4L, -5, and -6) are encoded by the mtDNA; complex II has 4 subunits, none from the mtDNA; complex III includes 11 subunits, 1 (cytochrome *b*) from the mtDNA; complex IV contains 13 subunits, 3 (COX-1, -2, and -3) from the mtDNA; and complex V contains 13 subunits, 2 (ATPase-6 and -8) from the mtDNA. The remaining subunits of complexes I, III, IV, and V; the entire complex II; the two small electron carriers, $CoQ_{10}$ and cytochrome *c*, and ANT are encoded by the nDNA. The mitochondrial rRNA and tRNA genes provide the structural RNAs for mitochondrial protein synthesis (i.e., for the expression of 13 mtDNA-encoded polypeptides). The majority of mitochondrial respiratory chain proteins are encoded by the nDNA in the cytosol. A complex mitochondrial importation process therefore enables the cytosolically synthesized nuclear-encoded mitochondrial respiratory chain subunits to be coassembled with mtDNA-encoded counterparts in the inner mitochondrial membrane. There are more than 1000 other nuclear genes which express mitochondrial proteins that are important for mitochondrial function.

Mitochondrial diseases therefore can arise from defects in the mtDNA (sporadic or maternal inheritance, see following section) or nDNA (sporadic or Mendelian inheritance). nDNA-related mitochondrial disorders result from defects involving nDNA-encoded mitochondrial polypeptides, including respiratory chain complexes, respiratory chain assembly, mtDNA maintenance, protein import, lipid dynamics, and biosynthesis of $CoQ_{10}$. Table 93.1 summarizes a simplified clinical and genetic classification of mitochondrial diseases.

### Maternal Inheritance of Mitochondrial DNA

Patients inherit mtDNA from their mothers, and therefore the mode of transmission of mtDNA, including pathogenic mtDNA mutations, follows maternal line inheritance. A single case report has demonstrated paternal transmission of an mtDNA mutation (Schwartz and Vissing, 2002), although there is emerging evidence that biparental inheritance of mtDNA occurs in exceptional circumstances (Luo, 2018). *Maternal inheritance* implies maternal transmission of mtDNA to all offspring but subsequent transmission only by females. Thus a disease expressed in all children of both sexes of an affected individual, without evidence of paternal inheritance, strongly suggests an mtDNA point mutation. However, exceptions to this general rule are encountered in clinical practice. First, a de novo point mutation in the mtDNA of the maternal germ cell line will not necessarily be transmitted to all children. Second, for unknown reasons, mtDNA mutations involving large-scale deletions, rearrangements, and point mutations in some protein-coding genes may occur sporadically and be due to mutations arising in the oocyte. Bottleneck expression of an mtDNA mutation may be enhanced in the fetus. Multiple deletions and depletion of mtDNA are autosomally transmitted, because they are the consequence of mutations in nuclear-encoded factors involved in mtDNA metabolism or replication. Third, maternal inheritance may not always be clinically evident because of extreme variability of clinical expression among family members due to heteroplasmy and the threshold effect (described in the following section).

### Heteroplasmy and Mitotic Segregation of Mitochondrial DNA

Each cell contains thousands of mtDNA copies in a network of cytoplasmic mitochondria. MtDNA is constantly undergoing replication, fission, and fusion even in terminally differentiated cells. When all mtDNA molecules are identical, the mtDNA is *homoplasmic*. If pathogenic mtDNA mutations exist with normal (wild-type) mtDNA, then there are two populations of mtDNA in the system, and this is *heteroplasmy*. The severity of the phenotypic effects of the mtDNA mutations in heteroplasmic cells is determined by the proportion of the wild-type and mutant mtDNA. Neutral polymorphic sites (nonpathogenic mutations) of mtDNA are generally homoplasmic, whereas pathogenic mutations are mostly, but not invariably, heteroplasmic.

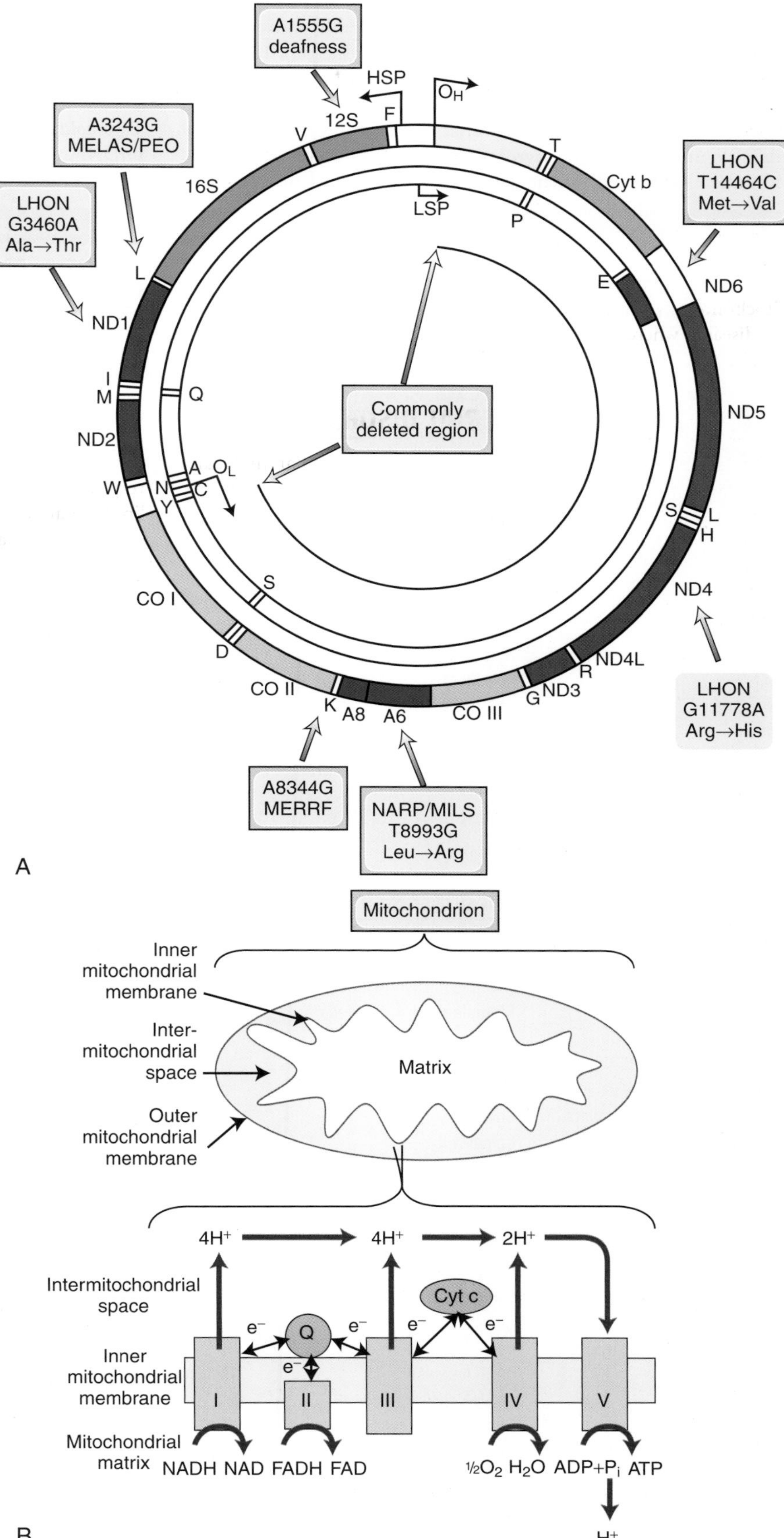


**Fig. 93.1** A, Human mitochondrial DNA (mtDNA) map. The mtDNA encompasses 16,569 np, with numbering starting at OH and proceeding counterclockwise around the circular map. Each gene is identified by shading, and the transfer RNA gene is identified by the letter of its cognate amino acid. Mutation sites of common mitochondrial diseases are indicated. B, Schematic representation of the mitochondrial respiratory chain located in the inner mitochondrial membrane. Electrons are transferred from complexes I and II to complex III via the mobile lipid carrier, coenzyme $Q_{10}$ ($CoQ_{10}$ [ubiquinone]). Electrons are then transferred to complex IV through the protein mobile carrier, cytochrome *c* (Cyt *c*). Electrons are finally transferred to molecular oxygen by complex IV. Three of the respiratory complexes (I, III, and IV) have a proton pumping mechanism coupled to the electron transfer. Pumping of protons to the intermembrane space generates a membrane potential and a proton gradient that flows back through complex V. The flow of protons through complex V enables ATP synthesis. *ATP*, Adenosine triphosphate; *HSP*, heavy strand promoter; *LHON*, Leber hereditary optic neuropathy; *LSP*, light strand promoter; *MELAS*, mitochondrial encephalomyopathy with lactic acidosis and stroke-like episodes; *MERRF*, myoclonic epilepsy with ragged-red fibers; *MILS*, maternally inherited Leigh syndrome; *NADH*, nicotinamide adenine dinucleotide; *NARP*, neuropathy, ataxia, and retinitis pigmentosa; *PEO*, progressive external ophthalmoplegia.

Heteroplasmy may occur at the level of the cell or at the level of the individual mitochondrion (intramitochondrial heteroplasmy). At cell division, mitochondria and mtDNA are randomly partitioned to be carried into the two daughter cells (mitotic segregation). Therefore mtDNA mutation is typically represented in a variable proportion of mitochondrial genomes, with the consequence that cells, tissues, and the whole individual would harbor variable proportions of mutant and wild-type mtDNA. Mitotic segregation explains how certain patients with mtDNA-related disorders may present with one manifestation at an early age and shift to another as they grow older as the proportions of heteroplasmy change with time in different tissues. For a disease to manifest in a tissue, the proportion of mutant mtDNA must be greater than the threshold level.

### Threshold Effect of Mitochondrial DNA Mutations

*Threshold effect* denotes the minimal critical number of mutated mtDNA molecules that would cause mitochondrial dysfunction in one or more tissues or organ systems. Variable somatic load of mtDNA

**TABLE 93.1 Major Gene Mutations in Mitochondrial Disorders**

| DEFECTS OF MITOCHONDRIAL DNA | | | |
|---|---|---|---|
| **Disease/Syndrome** | **Main Mutation** | **Gene Location** | **Mode of Inheritance** |
| PEO/multisystem with PEO | | Single large deletion | Sporadic |
| | | Deletion/duplication | Sporadic |
| | nt-A3243G | $tRNA^{Leu(UUR)}$ | Maternal |
| | nt-C3256T | $tRNA^{Leu(UUR)}$ | Maternal |
| KSS | | Single large deletion | Sporadic |
| | | Large tandem duplication | Sporadic |
| Pearson syndrome/KSS | | Single large deletion | Sporadic |
| MELAS | nt-A3243G | $tRNA^{Leu(UUR)}$ | Maternal |
| | nt-T3271C | $tRNA^{Leu(UUR)}$ | Maternal |
| MERRF | nt-A8344G | $tRNA^{Lys}$ | Maternal |
| Myopathy | | Single large deletion | Sporadic |
| | nt-A3243G | $tRNA^{Leu(UUR)}$ | Maternal |
| | nt-G15762A | Cytochrome *b* | Sporadic |
| MiMyCa | nt-C3254G | $tRNA^{Leu(UUR)}$ | Maternal |
| NARP/MILS | nt-T8993G | ATPase 6 | Maternal |
| LHON | nt-G3460A | ND1 | Maternal |
| | nt-G11778A | ND4 | Maternal |
| | nt-T14484C | ND6 | Maternal |
| Diabetes, optic atrophy, deafness | | Single large deletion | Sporadic |
| Tubulopathy, diabetes, ataxia | | Large tandem duplication | Maternal |
| Sideroblastic anemia | nt-T6721C | COX-I | Sporadic |
| **DEFECTS IN NUCLEAR DNA AFFECTING MITOCHONDRIAL DNA OR ENZYME COMPLEXES** | | | |
| **Disease/Syndrome** | **mtDNA/Enzyme Defect** | **Nuclear Gene/Locus** | **Mode of Inheritance** |
| PEO | Multiple mtDNA deletions | PEO1(Twinkle), ANT1, POLG1 and 2, SLC25A4 | Autosomal dominant/recessive |
| MNGIE | Multiple mtDNA deletions | ECGF1 | Autosomal recessive |
| Leigh syndrome | Complex IV | SURF1 | Autosomal recessive |
| | Complex I | NDUFS4, 6, 7, 8, NDUFV2 | Autosomal recessive |
| Leukodystrophy/myoclonus | Complex I | NDUFV1 | Autosomal recessive |
| Encephalopathy/cardiomyopathy | Complex I | NDUFV2 | Autosomal recessive |
| Leigh syndrome | Complex II | SDH | Autosomal recessive |
| GRACILE syndrome | Complex III | BCS1L | Autosomal recessive |
| Leigh syndrome | Complex IV | SCO1, COX10, COX15, RPPRC | Autosomal recessive |
| Encephalomyopathy/cardiomyopathy | Complex IV | SCO2 | Autosomal recessive |
| Encephalopathy, tubulopathy | Complex IV | COX10 | Autosomal recessive |
| Hypertrophic cardiomyopathy | Complex IV | COX15 | Autosomal recessive |
| Encephalopathy | Complex V | ATPAF2, ATP5E | Autosomal recessive |
| Encephalopathy, hepatopathy | mtDNA depletion | DGUOK, SUCLA2 | Autosomal recessive |
| Infantile myopathy | mtDNA depletion | Thymidine kinase 2 | Autosomal recessive |
| Alpers syndrome | mtDNA depletion | POLG | Autosomal recessive |
| CMT2 | Mitochondrial dynamics | MFN2, MT-ATP6 | Autosomal dominant, maternal |
| Optic atrophy, deafness, neuropathy | Mitochondrial dynamics | OPA1 | Autosomal dominant |
| Ataxia, Leigh syndrome, hepatorenal failure. | Coenzyme $Q_{10}$ function | Coenzyme $Q_{10}$ biosynthesis protein | Autosomal recessive |

**TABLE 93.1 Major Gene Mutations in Mitochondrial Disorders—cont'd**

| Disease/Syndrome | mtDNA/Enzyme Defect | Nuclear Gene/Locus | Mode of Inheritance |
|---|---|---|---|
| X-linked ataxia/sideroblastic anemia | Iron exporter | ABCB7 | X-linked |
| Friedreich ataxia | Iron storage protein | Frataxin | Autosomal recessive |
| Hereditary spastic paraplegia | Metalloprotease | Paraplegin | Autosomal recessive |
| Parkinsonism | Oxidant-sensing protein | DJ1 | Autosomal recessive |
| Parkinsonism | Respiratory chain function, mtDNA, maintenance, mitophagy | PTEN-induced kinase 1 | Autosomal recessive |
| Juvenile parkinsonism | Mitophagy | Parkin | Autosomal recessive |

*ABCB7*, ATP-binding cassette sub-family B member 7; *ANT1*, Adenine nucleotide translocator; *CMT2*, type 2 form of Charcot-Marie-Tooth disease; *COX*, cytochrome *c* oxidase; *ECGF1*, endothelial cell growth factor 1 (thymidine phosphorylase); *GRACILE*, growth retardation, amino aciduria, cholestasis, iron overload, lactic acidosis, and early death; *KSS*, Kearns-Sayre syndrome; *LHON*, Leber hereditary optic neuropathy; *MELAS*, mitochondrial encephalomyopathy, lactic acidosis and stroke-like episodes; *MERRF*, myoclonic epilepsy with ragged-red fibers; *MFN2*, mitofusin 2; *MILS*, maternally inherited Leigh syndrome; *MiMyCa*, mitochondrial myopathy and cardiomyopathy; *MNGIE*, myoneurogastrointestinal encephalopathy; *mtDNA*, mitochondrial DNA; *NARP*, neuropathy, ataxia, and retinitis pigmentosa; *NUDFS* and *NUDFV*, complex I components; *PEO*, progressive external ophthalmoplegia; *POLG*, DNA polymerase gamma; *PTEN*, phosphatase and tensin homolog; *SCO1* and *SCO2*, mitochondrial copper proteins; *SURF*, cytochrome *c* oxidase assembly protein; *Twinkle*, mtDNA helicase.

*Adapted from Servidei, S., 2003. Mitochondrial encephalomyopathies: gene mutation. Neuromuscul Disord 13, 109–114; DiMauro, S., Hirano, M., 2005. Mitochondrial encephalomyopathies: an update. Neuromuscul Disord 15, 276–286; and Rahman, S., Hanna, M., 2009. Diagnosis and therapy in neuromuscular disorders: diagnosis and new treatments in mitochondrial diseases. J Neurol Neurosurg Psychiatry 80, 943–953.*

mutation in different tissues and organ systems, or *skewed heteroplasmy*, is a universal finding in heteroplasmic states. It often changes over time, particularly in postmitotic cells such as neurons, and it increases with age. This in part explains the age-dependent penetration of many mitochondrial clinical phenotypes and age-related variability in their clinical features. The mtDNA mutation load needed for clinical expression is typically high and in the range of 70%–90% for both point mutations and deletions. The mutation threshold effect is believed to be affected by the oxidative metabolic requirement of a particular tissue. For example, the threshold effect may manifest itself at lower concentrations of mutated mtDNA in tissues that are inherently dependent on high oxidative metabolism, such as brain, eye, myocardium, and skeletal muscle.

Examples of threshold effect and mitotic segregation include patients with mitochondrial encephalomyopathy with lactic acidosis and stroke-like episodes (MELAS) who may present with only episodic headache in childhood but with stroke-like episodes and neurological deficits as they age and the pathogenic mutations accumulate in brain and cerebral vasculature. Infants with Pearson syndrome (a hematopoietic disease) may survive their disease because the proportion of mtDNA with deletions may decrease as bone marrow cells with heavy mutation loads are selected against. Following this process of outgrowing the hematopoietic disease in childhood, individuals with Pearson syndrome may later develop a different clinical phenotype such as Kearns-Sayre syndrome (KSS) as the mutation accumulates in their postmitotic neurons and muscle fibers.

## PATHOPHYSIOLOGY OF MITOCHONDRIAL DISORDERS

Mitochondria have several functions in maintaining cellular homeostasis, such as transient storage of intracellular calcium, fatty acid oxidation, the Krebs cycle, and iron metabolism (Kasahara and Scorrano, 2014; McBride et al., 2006; Schapira, 2006). Mitochondria also have a key role in the regulation of apoptosis (Chandel, 2014; Wang, 2001; Xiong et al., 2014). One of the most important roles of mitochondria is to catalyze the phosphorylation of the majority of cellular ADP to ATP. ATP is generated by oxidation of intermediates such as NADH and reduced flavin adenine dinucleotide (FADH2) via the process of OXPHOS within mitochondria by the respiratory chain enzymes. Several intermediary metabolic pathways from carbohydrates, fatty acids, and amino acids converge in mitochondria at the level of acetyl coenzyme A (acetyl CoA) for the final conversion of the fuel into ATP. Pyruvate is the terminal product of anaerobic glycolysis and is transported across the inner mitochondrial membrane to the mitochondrial matrix where it is converted to acetyl CoA. The transportation of pyruvate is coupled with the influx of hydrogen ions down their electrochemical gradient across the inner mitochondrial membrane. Pyruvate can also be generated during the catabolism of the amino acids alanine, serine, glycine, and cysteine. Transport of free fatty acids across the mitochondrial membrane requires two enzymes (CPTs I and II), a carrier molecule (L-carnitine), and a translocase (carnitine-acylcarnitine translocase). Fatty acids are also metabolized into acetyl CoA. Acetyl CoA enters the Krebs cycle, where three molecules of NADH and one molecule of $FADH_2$ are produced from each acetyl CoA. Molecules of NADH and $FADH_2$ donate electrons to the electron transport chain (NADH to complex I and succinate to FAD in complex II). The functional unit comprising the electron transport chain (complex I–IV) and complex V (ATP synthase) constitutes the OXPHOS system (see Fig. 93.1, *B*).

Lactic acid is the end product of glycolytic anaerobic metabolism and acts as a reservoir for excess pyruvate. Physiological states such as exercise may cause transient lactic acidosis. Pathological *lactic acidosis* occurs during anoxia/ischemia, in metabolic failure from liver disease and diabetes mellitus (secondary lactic acidosis), and in defects of OXPHOS (primary lactic acidosis) such as mitochondrial disorders. The blood lactate-to-pyruvate ratio reflects the NADH to $NAD^+$ ratio, or *redox state*, and is useful in the diagnosis of primary lactic acidosis. Defects in pyruvate dehydrogenase (PDH), which catalyzes the conversion of pyruvate to acetyl CoA with the conversion of $NAD^+$ to NADH, are associated with a low redox state (due to increased $NAD^+$), and usually produce elevated levels of lactate and pyruvate with normal or slightly low lactate/pyruvate ratios (<20). OXPHOS defects often cause a high redox state (due to increased NADH accumulation) and generally produce a high lactate/pyruvate ratio (>20) as NADH and pyruvate are converted to lactate by lactate dehydrogenase.

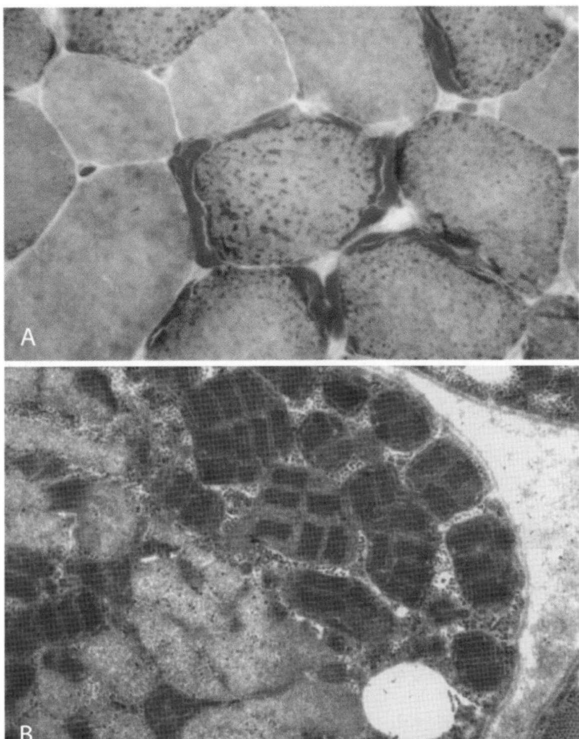


**Fig. 93.2** A, Modified Gomori trichrome section of a biopsy showing ragged-red muscle fibers. Increased mitochondrial staining in the subsarcolemmal and intermyofibrillar regions of the muscle fibers imparts the ragged-red appearance. B, Mitochondrial myopathy. Electron micrograph of a part of the muscle fiber showing mitochondrial proliferation; many mitochondria contain typical "parking lot" paracrystalline inclusions.

Neurons, myocardial and skeletal muscle, liver, and renal tissues are highly dependent on oxidative metabolism and are most commonly involved in mitochondrial diseases. Neurons especially require high levels of ATP production to maintain ion homeostasis following controlled flux of ions across the cell membrane during electrical signaling. Within the brain, the high metabolic activity of the basal ganglia makes them vulnerable to oxidative metabolic defects. Necrosis of the basal ganglia and brainstem is an early feature of Leigh syndrome and is common in other mitochondrial cytopathies.

In skeletal muscle, some fibers are severely involved and others may appear normal on histological analysis. With more severe involvement, the combination of patchy myofibrillar degeneration along with mitochondrial proliferation gives rise to the so-called ragged-red appearance of fibers on modified Gomori trichrome staining (Fig. 93.2, *A*). Defective OXPHOS may result in compensatory mitochondrial proliferation, particularly in type I and IIA muscle fibers. Ultrastructural analysis can demonstrate abnormal mitochondrial morphology such as intramitochondrial paracrystalline inclusions (see Fig. 93.2, *B*). Patients with mitochondrial disorders can show a wide range of symptoms, including any combination of developmental delay, short stature, small muscle bulk, seizures, vision loss, hearing impairment, peripheral neuropathy, autonomic nervous system difficulties, gastrointestinal dysfunction, endocrine problems, hematopoietic disease, and failure to thrive (Box 93.1). The presentation of a particular mitochondrial disorder can be variable, even among affected individuals in the same family. Conversely, more than one pathogenic mutation can give rise to similar clinical phenotypes.

## BOX 93.1 Clinical Features in Mitochondrial Diseases

**Central Nervous System Abnormalities**
Cognition dysfunction
Seizures
Myoclonus
Migrainous headache
Stroke-like episode
Ataxia
Dystonia
Parkinsonism
Visual impairment
Sensorineural deafness
Spinal muscular atrophy

**Peripheral Nervous System Abnormalities**
Sensorimotor polyneuropathy
Autonomic polyneuropathy

**Myopathy**
Progressive external ophthalmoplegia
Proximal limb myopathy
Exercise intolerance, myalgia, and fatigue
Rhabdomyolysis, myoglobinuria

**Cardiomyopathy**
Hypertrophic cardiomyopathy
Dilated cardiomyopathy
Cardiac conduction defects

**Liver Dysfunction**
Hepatic steatosis
Liver failure

**Renal Dysfunction**
Renal tubular acidosis
Fanconi syndrome
Myoglobinuric renal failure

**Gastrointestinal Disturbance**
Gastroparesis
Intestinal pseudo-obstruction
Constipation, diarrhea
Pancreatitis

**Endocrine Dysfunction**
Diabetes mellitus
Hypothalamic hypogonadism
Hypothyroidism
Hypoparathyroidism
Hypoadrenalism

**Miscellaneous**
Failure to thrive
Developmental delay or regression
Short stature
Cataracts
Anemia
Pancytopenia
Lipomas

## APPROACH TO THE DIAGNOSIS OF MITOCHONDRIAL DISORDERS

The complex inheritance patterns and clinical heterogeneity of mitochondrial diseases often result in incorrect or delayed diagnosis of the affected individuals. This delay can result in increased morbidity or mortality. For example, patients with specific metabolic defects such as β-oxidation of fatty acids can benefit from appropriate manipulations of diet and physical activity. $CoQ_{10}$ (ubiquinone) and L-carnitine replacements are often effective in rare metabolic disorders of $CoQ_{10}$ and primary systemic carnitine deficiencies. Failure to make a precise genetic diagnosis and, in turn, the lack of appropriate genetic counseling, can lead to the subsequent birth of affected children in unsuspecting families. Leigh syndrome is a good example in that the phenotype can vary among members of the same family and can be inherited in the maternal line (mtDNA-related mutations) or in Mendelian (autosomal or sex-linked) inheritance patterns.

A detailed clinical history and examination in conjunction with experienced interpretation of a battery of complex laboratory results are often required to make an accurate diagnosis. This process is often best carried out in a specialist mitochondrial clinic and subsequently discussed at a multidisciplinary meeting involving neurologists, pediatricians, geneticists, pathologists, and biochemists. Diagnostic criteria for mitochondrial disorders have previously been proposed (Bernier et al., 2002; Morava et al., 2006; Thorburn et al., 2004). However, the usefulness of categorizing patients as having "possible" mitochondrial disease has recently been questioned (Parikh et al., 2019).

Although the overall clinical spectrum of mitochondrial disorders is broad, recognized patterns of clinical presentations, clinical signs, and investigations have emerged. A detailed extended family history is essential in deciphering subtle clues suggesting a maternal line of inheritance. Any patient with unexplained multisystem problems, particularly affecting the nervous system, skeletal muscle, liver, kidney, and heart, may have mitochondrial disease. Rare presentations can be of mitochondrial origin, such as stroke-like episodes with MELAS, chronic ophthalmoplegia in KSS, and a movement disorder in children or young adults with Leigh syndrome. Patients and families often report a history of periods of severe fatigue with intercurrent illnesses, trauma, or surgery. Affected individuals may develop exacerbations, such as an increase in seizures, or new symptoms, such as an episode of lactic acidosis, during a seemingly minor illness. The patient may develop a permanent neurological deficit following these physiological stressors.

### Laboratory Findings

The mitochondrial metabolic test battery includes serum creatine kinase (CK), lactate and pyruvate, plasma and urine acylcarnitines, blood and urine amino acids, urine organic acids, and cerebrospinal fluid (CSF) lactate and pyruvate (if the CNS is involved). The lactate/pyruvate ratio may differentiate disorders of the OXPHOS system in comparison to more proximal metabolic defects such as PDH deficiency. However, normal values for the lactate and lactate/pyruvate ratio in a patient do not exclude mitochondrial disease; mtDNA-related diseases are generally associated with normal or only mildly elevated resting blood lactate levels but often with a significant rise with exercise. Serum CK is usually normal or mildly elevated in patients with mitochondrial myopathies. Blood levels of free carnitine are often decreased in mtDNA-related disorders, with a relative increase in acylcarnitine levels. The interpretation of test results of free and total carnitine, blood and urine amino acids, and urine organic acids is discussed in Chapter 91.

A controlled muscle exercise test may offer a useful noninvasive tool to investigate muscle oxidative metabolism. Lactate level, oxygen extraction from hemoglobin (near-infrared spectroscopy), and the ratio of phosphocreatine (PCr) to Pi ($^{31}P$ magnetic resonance spectroscopy [MRS]) have been measured in muscle at rest and during exercise and recovery. In patients with mitochondrial dysfunction, PCr:Pi ratios are lower than normal at rest, decrease excessively during exercise, and return to baseline values more slowly than normal controls. However, normative PCr:Pi values overlap with those in patients with mitochondrial disorders, and this test is not suitable for infants and young children because it requires a high degree of patient cooperation.

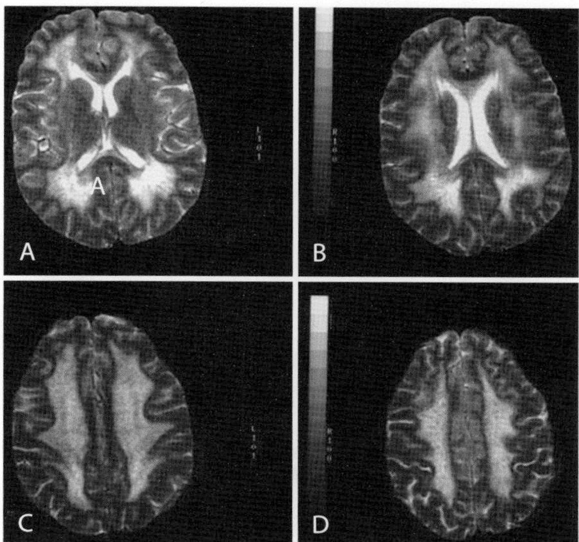

**Fig. 93.3 Mitochondrial Neurogastrointestinal Syndrome.** T2-weighted axial magnetic resonance images showing diffuse white-matter signal changes in cerebral hemispheres (A-D).

### Neuro-Ophthalmology

The four most common neuro-ophthalmological mitochondrial disorders are LHON, PEO, pigmentary retinopathy, and retrochiasmal visual loss. Standard flash electroretinograms are typically normal in LHON. Visual evoked responses are predictably abnormal in patients with visual loss. KSS is a subset of PEO associated with ataxia, cognitive dysfunction, cardiac conduction defects, and elevated protein in CSF. The most common pigmentary retinopathy appearance in mtDNA-related diseases is that of "salt-and-pepper" retinopathy that typically becomes more prominent with advancing age. Macular involvement and vascular attenuation are common in pigmentary retinopathy. Fluorescein angiography in LHON reveals vasculopathy without leakage, whereas rod-and-cone–specific electroretinography may help to confirm subtle changes of pigmentary retinopathy. Disruption of retrochiasmal visual pathways, generally due to stroke-like episodes, causes homonymous hemianopic defects or cortical blindness in patients with MELAS.

### Neuroradiology

The use of neuroimaging, especially brain magnetic resonance imaging (MRI), has greatly facilitated the detection of CNS involvement in mitochondrial disorders. Brain atrophy is common in children with mitochondrial disease. Developmental delay and basal ganglia calcification are common in KSS and MELAS, and diffuse signal abnormalities of the white matter are characteristic of KSS and myoneurogastrointestinal encephalopathy (MNGIE) (Fig. 93.3). The diagnosis of MELAS can be aided by the clinical association of stroke-like episodes with radiological lesions that do not conform to the anatomical territories of blood vessels and predominantly involve cortical gray matter (Fig. 93.4). The initial or predominant lesions in MELAS are

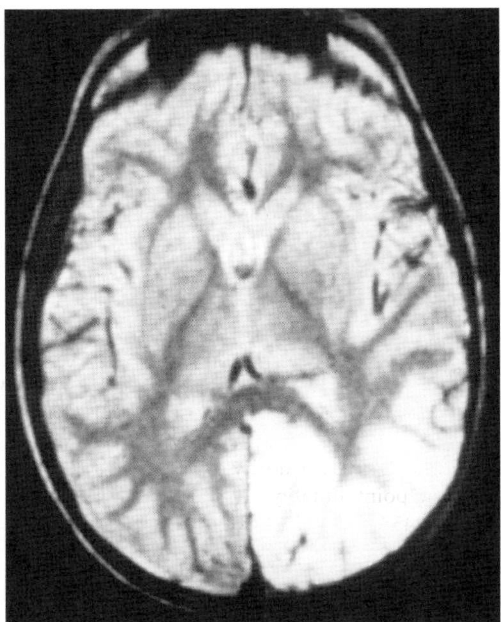

**Fig. 93.4** Mitochondrial encephalomyopathy, lactic acidosis, and stroke-like episodes syndrome (MELAS). Proton density axial magnetic resonance image showing ischemic lesions in the left occipital and posterior parietal regions (note predominantly cerebral cortical lesions).

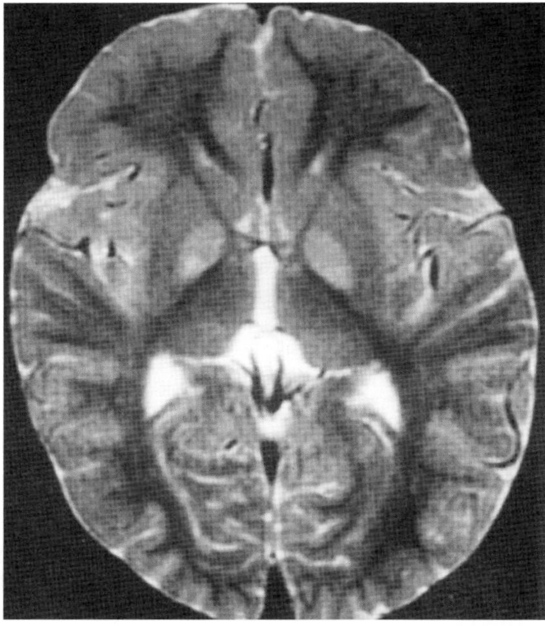

**Fig. 93.5 Leigh Syndrome.** T2-weighted magnetic resonance image showing symmetrical signal changes in the globus pallidus and putamen.

characteristically in the parietal-occipital region, and new lesions generally appear with acute illness and elevated CSF lactate levels. Leigh syndrome characteristically shows bilateral hyperintense signals on T2-weighted and fluid-attenuated inversion recovery (FLAIR) MRIs in the putamen, globus pallidus (Fig. 93.5), and thalamus.

Extraocular muscle T2 signal is elevated in chronic progressive external ophthalmoplegia (CPEO) and correlates negatively with ocular movements, thus providing a potential quantitative measure of disease severity (Pitceathly et al., 2016). $^{1}$H-MRS often detects lactate accumulation in the CSF and in specific areas of the brain, whereas positron emission tomography (PET), which measures metabolic flux, has identified several metabolic abnormalities in mitochondrial disease patients using radioisotopically labeled metabolites relevant to the study of bioenergetics.

## Muscle Biopsy

An open muscle biopsy under local anesthesia provides material for histochemistry, ultrastructural studies, biochemistry, myoblast culture, and molecular genetic studies.

### Histochemistry

Many of the histopathological abnormalities found in muscle biopsies from patients with mitochondrial diseases are nonspecific and include excessive variability of muscle fiber size, fiber type–specific atrophy, scattered myofibrillar necrosis and regeneration, and intermyofibrillar lipid or glycogen accumulation. Mild peripheral nerve involvement is common in mitochondrial diseases, and the muscle biopsy may reveal evidence of partial denervation. Oxidative enzyme staining may show core targetoid fibers and fiber type grouping.

The hallmark feature in mitochondrial diseases is the *ragged-red fiber* (RRF) (see Fig. 93.2, *A*). In frozen sections stained with modified Gomori trichrome, subsarcolemmal and intermyofibrillar accumulation of mitochondria appear as bright red masses on at least three sides of the fiber, against the background of the blue myofibrils. These abnormal accumulations represent a compensatory proliferation of mitochondria, some of which are ultrastructurally normal and others dystrophic (see Fig. 93.2, *B*). The same fibers stain intensely blue with the histochemical reaction for succinate dehydrogenase (SDH), an OXPHOS enzyme encoded entirely by the nDNA. SDH staining is more sensitive than the modified Gomori trichrome in detecting mitochondrial proliferation. NADH-tetrazolium reductase (NADH-TR) stains mitochondria-rich fibers even more intensely, but the enzyme reaction is less specific than SDH for mitochondria. RRFs are seen in most patients with mtDNA defects and in some patients with nDNA mutations, but RRFs are neither a universal feature in mitochondrial disorders, nor are they specific for primary mitochondrial diseases. RRFs can occur in other neuromuscular diseases such as inflammatory myopathies or inclusion body myositis, as well as in normal aging. They also occur in the toxic myopathy caused by the drug zidovudine, where the underlying pathogenesis is drug-induced damage of the mtDNA. Mitochondrial proliferation in the smooth muscle of intramuscular vessels results in strongly SDH-reactive vessels in MELAS. The histochemical stain for cytochrome oxidase (COX) activity may be helpful. COX or complex IV of the mitochondrial respiratory chain has 13 subunits; three—COX I, II, and III—are encoded in mtDNA, and the others are encoded in the nuclear genome. COX may be absent in myofibers from patients with defects of mtDNA, mitochondrial transcription and translation, or assembly of complex IV. RRFs which are COX negative suggest impaired mitochondrial protein synthesis in the face of mitochondrial proliferation and are typically seen in mtDNA deletions. In the combined COX-SDH histochemical stain, COX-negative fibers with normal or high concentrations of SDH stain blue against a background of normal brown fibers that have both COX and SDH. Single-fiber polymerase chain reaction (PCR) from these fibers (RRF/SDH rich and COX negative) shows higher levels of mutated mtDNA molecules, suggesting that these mutations are deleterious. Discordance between RRF status and COX activity is not uncommon in muscle fibers in mitochondrial diseases. In patients with mutations in mtDNA protein-coding genes and defects in complex IV, RRF and many non-RRFs are COX negative or deficient, whereas in patients with defects of complex I or III and tRNA mtDNA point mutations, many RRFs with normal COX activity may be seen. SCO2 and SURF1 nDNA mutations, which cause complex IV deficiency, are generally associated with diffuse COX deficiency but without RRFs. The absence of either RRFs or COX-negative fibers does not rule out mitochondrial disease. For instance, patients with neuropathy, ataxia, and retinitis pigmentosa–maternally inherited Leigh syndrome (NARP-MILS) or LHON do not have RRF or COX-negative fibers.

### Electron Microscopy

Electron microscopy of muscle biopsy specimens from patients with mitochondrial diseases may reveal subsarcolemmal and intermyofibrillar proliferation of mitochondria and the presence of abnormal mitochondria in muscle fibers. Enlarged, elongated, irregular, and dumbbell-shaped mitochondria with hypoplastic and dystrophic cristae and paracrystalline inclusions (see Fig. 93.2, *B*) may be seen in a patient's muscle biopsy with a diagnosis of mitochondrial disease. However, they are nonspecific and can be present in other neuromuscular disorders. Significant intermyofibrillar mitochondrial proliferation should be detectable by light microscopy in the modified Gomori trichrome, NADH-TR, and SDH stains. Isolated focal collections of mitochondria in the subsarcolemmal space or near the A–I junction in muscle fiber can be normal and should not be mistaken for pathological accumulation.

### Biochemistry

In specialized mitochondrial laboratories, expertise for biochemical analysis of OXPHOS enzymes in muscle, cultured skin fibroblasts, and peripheral blood lymphocytes can be performed. Muscle tissue is generally preferred for biochemical analysis because it has high oxidative metabolism, and it is more often affected in mitochondrial diseases. Biochemical analysis can be performed in fresh or frozen muscle tissue. The advantage of fresh muscle is that functionally intact mitochondria can be isolated for polarographic analysis, but the disadvantage is that the patient must travel to the site of the study laboratory. Frozen muscle sample can be stored and shipped to specialized laboratories for biochemical analysis of the OXPHOS enzymes in the muscle homogenate. The activities of specific respiratory complexes should be compared with the activity of an unrelated nuclear encoded mitochondrial enzyme such as citrate synthase to compensate for mitochondrial mass in the sample.

Isolated defects of complex I, III, or IV, each of which incorporates subunits encoded by mtDNA and nDNA, can occur in sporadic, Mendelian, or maternal line mutations. Combined defects of complexes I, III, and IV suggest either a single large deletion or tRNA mutations in mtDNA, or an nDNA defect that secondarily alters mtDNA (multiple mtDNA deletions, mtDNA depletion). The activities of specific respiratory complexes may be abnormal even when the muscle histochemistry is normal, especially in children.

The combined defect of complexes II/III when assayed together as succinate cytochrome *c* reductase with normal activities of the individual complexes suggests a possible diagnosis of $CoQ_{10}$ deficiency. The combined complex II+III assay requires endogenous $CoQ_{10}$, whereas the individual complex II and complex III assays are independent of $CoQ_{10}$. $CoQ_{10}$ levels can be determined by high-performance liquid chromatography (HPLC) in muscle and peripheral blood mononuclear cells.

### Blue Native Polyacrylamide Gel Electrophoresis

One of the most powerful tools to appear in the past few years for the analysis of the OXPHOS complexes is the resolution of the individual fully assembled complexes in blue native polyacrylamide gel electrophoresis (BN-PAGE). By using mild detergents, the OXPHOS complexes normally remain intact in the electrophoretic field, but they begin separating from each other if components of the OXPHOS are abnormal (Ugalde et al., 2004). The complexes and their components can be detected by direct staining of proteins, enzyme activity, or antibodies.

### DNA-Based Diagnosis

A large number of mtDNA and nDNA mutations are currently known to cause mitochondrial disorders, and their number (especially nDNA gene mutations) has continued to rise in recent years (Rahman, 2018). Further details about mtDNA mutations can be found in the MITOMAP database (http://www.mitomap.org). If a patient has a clearly defined clinical syndrome such as MELAS, MERRF, LHON, or NARP, the most common mutations associated with the syndrome can be initially screened in blood (see Table 93.1). Genetic tests for mutations at positions 3243, 8344, and 8993 are widely available in diagnostic laboratories. The majority of LHON cases will have one of the three common point mutations at positions 11778, 14484, or 3460. The level of np-3243A>G in blood declines with age and may become undetectable after the age of 30.

However, especially in adult mitochondrial disease, lymphocyte DNA may be normal, and skeletal muscle will have to be analyzed, such as in sporadic patients with isolated PEO. This is particularly true for mtDNA deletions and mtDNA depletion syndromes. The entire mitochondrial genome can be sequenced for a pathogenic mutation if there is a strong suspicion of a mitochondrial disease.

Advances in molecular diagnostics in the past decade, specifically high-throughput sequencing technology, have led to an exponential rise in known and novel disease-causing nuclear mitochondrial gene mutations. Although mutations in nuclear-encoded protein subunits of the mitochondrial respiratory chain enzymes occur, most nDNA mutations reported occur in gene products that regulate the assembly of OXPHOS complexes or control of mtDNA replication. The majority of nDNA mitochondrial disorders present with neonatal or early-childhood onset. Mutations in the nuclear gene encoding the catalytic subunit of the mtDNA polymerase gamma (POLG) have been described as presenting with a variety of phenotypes in childhood and adulthood (see later discussion). Nuclear gene tests can be performed from the DNA sample isolated from the peripheral lymphocytes.

Fig. 93.6 demonstrates an algorithm for the DNA diagnosis of a patient with suspected mitochondrial disease.

## MITOCHONDRIAL CLINICAL SYNDROMES

Numerous distinct mitochondrial clinical syndromes are reported. However, as increasing numbers of genetically confirmed patients are characterized, previously underrecognized clinical manifestations have emerged. These include upper and lower gastrointestinal involvement (Kaufmann et al. 2009, Kornblum et al. 2001, Nesbitt et al. 2013, Pitceathly et al. 2012) and sudden unexplained death (Ng et al. 2016), in addition to new genotypes linked to established syndromes and expanding phenotypic spectrums caused by known genes (Chinnery, 2015).

### Progressive External Ophthalmoplegia and Kearns-Sayre Syndrome

Clinically isolated PEO with progressive ptosis is a common manifestation of mitochondrial disease. Onset is often before 20 years of age or after 50. There is a slow evolution of symmetrical extraocular muscle weakness, and diplopia is uncommon. Ptosis progresses over time and often needs treatment such as eyelid props or eyelid surgery. A sporadic single clonal deletion of mtDNA is the most common genetic

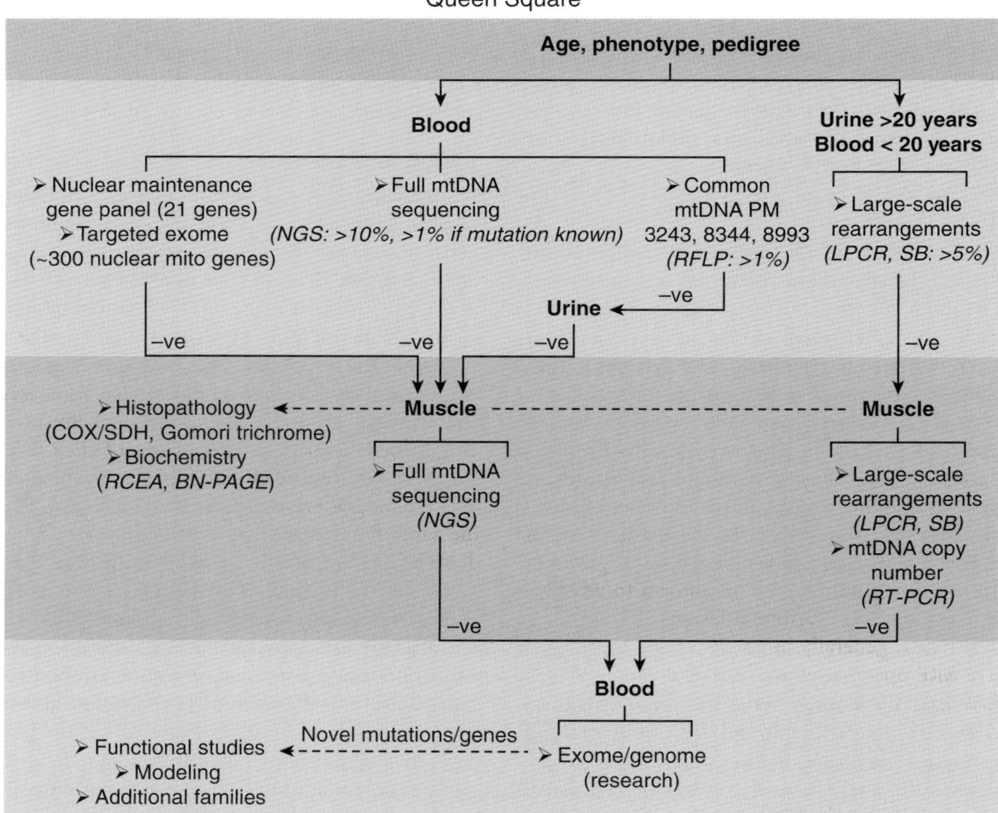


**Fig. 93.6** Queen Square Mitochondrial Disease Investigation Pathway. (1) Mitochondrial DNA *(mtDNA)* deletion screen can be performed on blood from patients younger than 20 years of age. (2) Perform respiratory chain enzyme assays even if histochemistry normal if strong clinical suspicion. (3) Sequence mtDNA even if respiratory chain enzyme assays normal if strong clinical suspicion. *BN-PAGE*, Blue native polyacrylamide gel electrophoresis; *COX*, cytochrome *c* oxidase; *LPCR*, long-range polymerase chain reaction; *NGS*, next-generation sequencing; *PM*, point mutation *RCEA*, respiratory chain enzyme analysis; *RFLP*, restriction fragment length polymorphism; *RRF*, ragged-red fiber; *RT-PCR*, real-time polymerase chain reaction; *SB*, Southern blot; *SDH*, succinate dehydrogenase. Italicized, laboratory techniques.

defect in patients with PEO, although point mutations in tRNA genes (e.g., A3243G mutation) and a duplication of mtDNA have also been reported.

Autosomal dominant or recessive PEO due to defects in nuclear genes involved in mtDNA maintenance results in multiple mtDNA deletions. It tends to present in adulthood and may be associated with multisystem involvement such as neuropathy, ataxia, tremor, parkinsonism, depression, cataracts, pigmentary retinopathy, deafness, rhabdomyolysis, and hypogonadism. Mutation in *POLG1* is one of the more common nuclear genes to cause this syndrome.

KSS is defined by the triad of PEO and onset before age 20, with at least one of the following: pigmentary retinopathy, cerebellar ataxia, heart block, and/or elevated CSF protein (>100 mg/dL). Patients often have a progressive limb myopathy and frequently require a pacemaker for atrioventricular block. Many patients with KSS have delayed motor milestones, are small of stature, and have cognitive impairment. Some clinical features of MELAS and MERRF may overlap with KSS. The clinical course in KSS is progressive, and many patients with CNS or cardiac complications die in the third or fourth decade. Nearly all cases of KSS are sporadic and usually caused by a single large clonal mtDNA deletion that arises in the mother's oocyte.

## Mitochondrial Myopathies without Progressive External Ophthalmoplegia

The clinical spectrum of isolated mitochondrial myopathy varies from mild nondisabling proximal limb weakness to severe infantile myopathy with lactic acidosis and death by 1 year. Exercise intolerance is common. Some of these cases present in adult life, but careful questioning usually elicits a history of lifelong exercise intolerance. A sporadic form of myopathy related to somatic mutations in the cytochrome *b* gene of mtDNA is associated with progressive exercise intolerance and weakness and, in some cases, attacks of rhabdomyolysis (Andreu et al., 1999). Less frequently, sporadic patients with exercise intolerance have been found to have mtDNA mutations in genes encoding subunits of complexes I or IV (DiMauro and Hirano, 2005). Some patients with mitochondrial myopathy without PEO will develop progressive PEO in later life, and others may have overlapping deficits with MERRF and MELAS.

## Mitochondrial Peripheral Neuropathy

Patients with complex mtDNA-associated mitochondrial phenotypes involving the CNS (e.g., MERRF, MELAS) often have a mild axonal sensorimotor neuropathy that may be subclinical. A peripheral neuropathy can be the dominant clinical feature in some patients. Mutations in the mitofusin 2 *(MFN2)* gene, which encodes a protein that influences mitochondrial dynamics, is a cause of Charcot-Marie-Tooth disease. Some families with *MFN2* mutations have additional clinical features, including optic atrophy (Züchner et al., 2006). Mutations in *POLG* can cause a prominent large-fiber sensory neuropathy with significant proprioceptive loss in the SANDO (sensory ataxic neuropathy dysarthria and ophthalmoplegia) syndrome. Axonal motor and sensorimotor polyneuropathy may also be a feature of dominant optic atrophy caused by mutations in the *OPA1* gene encoding a mitochondrial dynamin-like protein and *MT-ATP6* mutations, encoding the ATP6 subunit of the mitochondrial ATP synthase (Pitceathly et al., 2012).

## Mitochondrial Encephalomyopathy, Lactic Acidosis, and Stroke-Like Episodes

MELAS is a maternally inherited encephalomyopathy clinically characterized by short stature, stroke-like episodes, migrainous headaches, vomiting, seizures, and lactic acidosis. The stroke-like deficits are sometimes transient but can be permanent and cause progressive encephalopathy with dementia. Ataxia, deafness, muscle weakness, cardiomyopathy, and diabetes are common as the disease progresses.

A typical radiological feature is that the stroke involves the cerebral cortex, spares the white matter (see Fig. 93.4), mostly affects the parietal and occipital cortices, and does not conform to vascular territories. Neuroimaging may show additional lesions that have no clinical correlates. The onset is generally in childhood or early adult life. Most patients have RRF on muscle biopsy. Approximately 80% of patients with MELAS have an A-to-G point mutation at np-3243 ($tRNA^{Leu[UUR]}$ gene, *MT-TL1*). Another point mutation at np-3271 of the $tRNA^{Leu(UUR)}$ gene accounts for 10% of cases of MELAS.

## Myoclonic Epilepsy with Ragged-Red Fiber Myopathy

MERRF is a maternally inherited encephalomyopathy characterized by myoclonus, epilepsy, cerebellar ataxia, and myopathy with RRF. Onset is usually in childhood or early adulthood. The syndrome begins with stimulus-sensitive myoclonic epilepsy in childhood, which may be photosensitive. Worsening ataxia and mental retardation are seen in later childhood. Patients may also develop cardiomyopathy, short stature, deafness, optic atrophy, PEO, cutaneous lipomas, and neuropathy. Overlapping clinical features of MERRF and MELAS can occur in the same patient or among different members of the same family (Verma et al., 1996). The clinical course in MERRF is variable, but it is typically progressive.

Approximately 80% of MERRF cases have a point mutation at np-8344 of the $tRNA^{Lys}$ gene (*MT-TK2*). As with other mtDNA mutations, the time of onset and severity of the disease have been related to the quantitative burden of mutant mtDNA.

## Mitochondrial Neurogastrointestinal Encephalomyopathy

MNGIE is an autosomal recessive disease with secondary alterations of mtDNA. There is typically a combination of ptosis, PEO, severe gastrointestinal dysmotility leading to episodes of pseudo-obstruction and cachexia, peripheral neuropathy, leukoencephalopathy on brain MRI (see Fig. 93.3), and evidence of mitochondrial dysfunction (e.g., lactic acidosis or RRF in muscle biopsy) (Hirano et al., 2004). Onset is usually in the late teens, and most patients die before age 40. MNGIE is caused by mutations in the gene encoding thymidine phosphorylase. The disease can be diagnosed by blood tests demonstrating loss of thymidine phosphorylase activity or elevation of plasma thymidine and deoxyuridine.

## Neuropathy, Ataxia, Retinitis Pigmentosa Syndrome

NARP syndrome is a relatively rare disorder due to a point mutation at np-8993 of the mitochondrial ATPase-6 gene encoding subunit 6 of complex V, giving rise to two maternally inherited and clinically related phenotypes even within the same family: NARP and MILS. Other point mutations in the same gene have been reported with the NARP and MILS. The severity of the syndrome corresponds to the mutant mtDNA load in the tissues. A mutation load greater than 90% of mtDNA tends to cause the more severe phenotype of MILS.

## Subacute Necrotizing Encephalomyelopathy (Leigh Syndrome)

Leigh syndrome is a familial or sporadic mitochondrial disorder characterized by psychomotor regression and lesions in the basal ganglia and brainstem (see Fig. 93.5). Some cases display a maternal inheritance, such as mtDNA np-8993 and np-8344 mutations (MILS). Others follow an autosomal (pyruvate carboxylase, *SURF1* gene mutations with COX deficiency, complex I deficiencies) or sex-linked (*PDH E1* gene mutations) pattern of inheritance. More than 50% of cases present in the first year of life, usually before 6 months of age. Late-onset varieties with a greater degree of clinical heterogeneity are also reported. The precise clinical boundaries of Leigh syndrome have not been defined; there is clinical heterogeneity even among members of the same family. Leigh syndrome and congenital lactic acidosis are described further in Chapter 91.

## Leber Hereditary Optic Neuropathy

Patients with LHON usually present with a subacute bilaterally sequential and isolated optic neuropathy. LHON is expressed predominantly in males of the maternal lineage, and the greater susceptibility of males to vision loss in LHON remains unexplained. The age of onset is typically between 15 and 35 years, and the vision loss is painless, central, and usually occurs in one eye weeks or months before involvement of the other eye. Fundoscopic abnormalities may be seen in patients with LHON and in their asymptomatic relatives. During the acute phase of vision loss, there may be hyperemia of the optic nerve head, dilatation and tortuosity of peripapillary vessels, circumpapillary telangiectasia, nerve-fiber edema, and focal hemorrhage. Vision loss in LHON affects central or centrocecal fields and is usually permanent. A minority of patients show objective improvement, sometimes to a dramatic degree. Three primary point mutations at mtDNA np-11778 (69%), np-14484 (14%), and np-3460, all within coding regions for complex I subunits, account for 80%–95% of cases of LHON worldwide. These mutations are found in blood and are often homoplasmic. Patients with np-14484T>C have a better chance of some visual recovery. Some families have additional members with associated cardiac conduction abnormalities, especially preexcitation syndromes. There may also be a movement disorder such as dystonia or other mild neurological or skeletal abnormalities. Occasionally LHON is associated with an MS-like illness.

## Sensorineural Deafness

Sensorineural hearing loss (SNHL) is a feature of many mitochondrial diseases and commonly occurs in MELAS, maternally inherited diabetes and deafness (MIDD), MERRF, or KSS. The presence of SNHL in a patient with a complex multisystem phenotype suggests a possible mitochondrial disease. SNHL may also occur in isolation. The np-1555A>G mitochondrial mutation (which confers sensitivity to aminoglycoside-induced deafness and may cause nonsyndromic deafness) is present in 1 in 500 of the general population. Mutations in the tRNA gene for serine (*UCN*) may also cause isolated deafness. SNHL is also a feature of some nuclear-encoded mitochondrial disorders such as dominant optic atrophy associated with *OPA1* mutations.

## Mitochondrial DNA Depletion Syndrome

Mitochondrial DNA depletion syndrome (MDDS) is an autosomal recessive disorder caused by a quantitative reduction in the amount of mtDNA. A myopathic and a hepatocerebral form have been described.

Both forms are usually fatal in childhood, although patients with Navajo neurohepatopathy may survive into their late teens. MDDS may be caused by recessive defects of the mtDNA replication machinery (*POLG* or *PEO1*) or from defects of maintaining the deoxyribonucleoside triphosphate pool necessary for mtDNA replication.

## MANAGEMENT OF MITOCHONDRIAL DISEASES

### Treatment of Associated Complications

Treatment of mitochondrial disease is mainly symptomatic (but see later for treatment options that can be beneficial in mitochondrial diseases in specific scenarios), empirical, and often palliative (DiMauro and Mancuso, 2007; Pitceathly and McFarland, 2014). Patients and families with confirmed mitochondrial disease require management and support in a multidisciplinary clinical team setting. This is often coordinated by a neurologist with close links to a range of different disciplines such as rehabilitation medicine, physiotherapy, occupational therapy, cardiology, endocrinology, ophthalmology, audiology, and speech therapy. There is usually no specific treatment for most mitochondrial disorders, and therefore monitoring and treatment of complications arising from the disease are vital for improving quality of life and reducing morbidity.

#### Hearing and Vision

Hearing aids and, in severe cases, cochlear implantation are especially important to improve hearing in patients who have coexistent visual impairment from optic atrophy, pigmentary retinopathy, or cortical visual loss. Ptosis can be helped with eyelid props and surgery. Cataracts should be excluded as a cause of visual impairment.

#### Seizures

MELAS, MERRF, and Leigh syndrome are typically associated with seizures. Sodium valproate has been shown to inhibit mitochondrial OXPHOS and may cause clinical worsening, including precipitation of fatal hepatic failure in some cases of Alpers syndrome caused by *POLG* mutations. The treatment of myoclonus can be problematic, and many patients require several anticonvulsants, including piracetam, levetiracetam, and/or clonazepam.

#### Movement Disorders

Dystonia is often seen in Leigh syndrome, and treatment with anticholinergics may occasionally be helpful. Intramuscular electromyography (EMG)-guided botulinum toxin can be helpful for severe focal dystonia.

#### Diabetes

Oral hypoglycemics and/or comparatively low doses of insulin are often sufficient to treat diabetes. Metformin should be avoided because of the risk of lactic acidosis. One study suggested that long-term $CoQ_{10}$ administration prevented the progressive insulin secretory defect, exercise intolerance, and hearing loss in MIDD patients (Suzuki et al., 1998).

#### Respiratory

The combination of diaphragmatic and axial skeletal muscle weakness, with aspiration from bulbar weakness, can precipitate acute respiratory failure. Functional vital capacity (FVC) monitoring in patients with significant myopathy is important. Patients with bulbar weakness are also at risk of developing obstructive sleep apnea. CNS mitochondrial disease, especially Leigh syndrome, may cause central hypoventilation. A sleep study is mandatory if nocturnal hypoventilation is suspected, and noninvasive nocturnal ventilation can improve patients' quality of life.

#### Gastrointestinal

Gastrointestinal symptoms are common in patients with mitochondrial disease. These include swallowing difficulties, failure to thrive in children, weight loss/cachexia, constipation, pseudo-obstruction, nausea, and vomiting. Bulbar weakness can be compounded by cerebellar incoordination to cause severe dysphagia, especially in KSS and Leigh syndrome. Patients therefore require monitoring by speech and language therapy supplemented by videofluoroscopy assessment. The requirement for a percutaneous endoscopic gastrostomy (PEG) should be considered if there is a high probability of aspiration pneumonia. Weight loss can be dramatic, especially in the MNGIE syndrome, when it may be accompanied by recurrent pseudo-obstruction.

#### Heart

Cardiac screening is important in patients with mitochondrial disease. Tachyarrhythmia and bradyarrhythmia may require insertion of a permanent pacemaker or implantable cardiac defibrillator, especially in KSS and some cases of PEO. Preexcitation syndromes such as Wolff-Parkinson-White may cause supraventricular tachycardias in patients with np-3243A>G cardiomyopathy and in some patients with LHON. Progressive left ventricular hypertrophy may be a particular feature in patients with the np-3243A>G and np-8344A>G mutations and may progress to left ventricular failure due to cardiomyopathy. Cardiac problems should ideally be referred to a cardiologist with a specialist interest in inherited cardiac muscle disease, where patients can be monitored with echocardiography and electrocardiography and treated with agents such as angiotensin-converting enzyme inhibitors.

### Genetic Counseling, Prenatal Diagnosis, and Reproductive Options

If a nuclear gene mutation is identified, genetic counseling and prenatal diagnosis can be offered to the patient. Primary mtDNA mutations present in the male will not be transmitted. If an mtDNA mutation is identified in a woman with mitochondrial disease, it is more difficult to provide accurate genetic counseling advice. Most large-scale deletions of mtDNA are sporadic, and the risk of transmission is relatively low. Some mtDNA point mutations are also sporadic. For heteroplasmic mtDNA point mutations, the factors that determine the amount of a particular point mutation that will be transmitted to offspring are poorly understood. Although a heteroplasmic point mutation will be transmitted in the maternal line, because of the genetic bottleneck for mtDNA (where only a small number of mtDNA molecules in the mother are passed on to the next generation), large shifts in the proportion of mutant from mother to offspring may occur. It is therefore not possible to offer women who harbor heteroplasmic disease-causing point mutations accurate advice regarding the risk of transmission.

The offspring of a patient with a homoplasmic point mutation such as in LHON will be homoplasmic for the mutation, but they may not all develop the disease. Unknown non-mtDNA factors may be important in determining disease expression. At present, a number of reproductive choices exist for patients with mitochondrial disease harboring both mitochondrial and nuclear gene mutations. These include ovum donation (for mtDNA mutations) and preimplantation genetic diagnosis (for both mtDNA and nDNA mutations). Mitochondrial donation, which involves oocyte manipulation techniques aimed at replacing maternal mutant mtDNA with healthy donor mtDNA, has also recently been licensed in the United Kingdom for patients with mtDNA mutations. Individuals at risk of inheriting an mtDNA mutation may request predictive genetic testing. If they have any symptoms suggestive of mitochondrial phenotype, diagnostic genetic testing is appropriate.

### Pharmacological Approaches

There are certain treatment options that can be beneficial in mitochondrial disease for specific indications. These include $CoQ_{10}$ in disorders that impair $CoQ_{10}$ biosynthesis (Quinzii et al., 2007), allogeneic bone marrow transplantation in MNGIE (Halter et al., 2015), and riboflavin supplementation in adults with riboflavin transporter disorders (Foley et al., 2014). Despite a Cochrane review of treatments for mitochondrial disorders identifying more than 1300 reports using numerous strategies aimed at improving mitochondrial function, the majority were open-label studies comprising small patient cohorts. Of the 30 randomized trials, no treatment showed a significant benefit on a clinically meaningful endpoint (Kerr, 2013; Pfeffer et al., 2012). It is therefore likely that vitamins and cofactors traditionally used in mitochondrial disease do not confer a major therapeutic benefit. However, a number of promising new approaches are currently being evaluated at the preclinical and early clinical phase with the hope that these will ultimately be licensed for clinical use, particularly given increasing interest from industry in developing treatments for rare diseases (Pitceathly et al. 2020 a more detailed review of emerging therapies for mitochondrial disorders).

### Coenzyme $Q_{10}$ Deficiency

$CoQ_{10}$ is a lipophilic mobile electron carrier and antioxidant located in the inner mitochondrial membrane. Disorders of $CoQ_{10}$ biosynthesis are clinically heterogeneous. Presentations include recurrent rhabdomyolysis with seizures, multisystem disorder of infancy with prominent nephropathy, ataxia with or without seizures, Leigh syndrome, and pure myopathy. These disorders respond well to $CoQ_{10}$ supplementation if treatment is started early, but very large doses may be necessary because of poor uptake into the mitochondrion. The results of randomized controlled trials using $CoQ_{10}$ in other mitochondrial disorders have yielded conflicting results. Many specialists recommend $CoQ_{10}$ to all patients with a proven diagnosis of mitochondrial disease up to 200 mg 3 times daily in adults.

### Other Pharmacological Approaches

Although a number of pharmacological agents have been studied in mitochondrial disease, a Cochrane systematic review concluded that there was insufficient evidence to recommend any standard treatment (Pfeffer et al., 2012). There are anecdotal reports of benefit of various agents (e.g., riboflavin, succinate, L-carnitine, α-lipoic acid, creatine [Tarnopolsky et al., 1997], and vitamins C, E, and K), but the clinical heterogeneity and unpredictable natural history of mitochondrial disease, with a frequently relapsing-remitting course, makes interpretation of the effectiveness of any given agent in a single individual difficult. The few randomized double-blind clinical trials that have been performed yielded inconclusive or conflicting results. Novel pharmacological approaches have emerged which are aimed at stimulating mitochondrial biogenesis via the transcriptional coactivator PGC-1α. Drugs that may stimulate this pathway include bezafibrate and resveratrol, and these have demonstrated protective properties in animal models of Parkinson disease (Khan et al., 2010), Huntington disease (Ho et al., 2010; Maher et al., 2011), Alzheimer disease (Anekonda and Reddy, 2006), and other diseases including a mouse model of mitochondrial myopathy (Wenz et al., 2008). Finally, idebenone, a CoQ analog, has been approved by the European Medicines Agency to treat LHON, and an international consensus statement established the indication in patients with acute, subacute, or dynamic clinical course but did not recommended the treatment for chronic patients (Carelli et al. 2017).

### Removal or Neutralization of Toxic Metabolites

The pathophysiological mechanism of MNGIE syndrome (thymidine phosphorylase deficiency) is considered to result from an imbalance of intramitochondrial nucleosides, leading to stalling of the mtDNA replication apparatus. A rationale for treatment is thus to restore intramitochondrial nucleoside balance by removing accumulated nucleosides. In one study, renal dialysis was used to remove accumulated plasma thymidine and deoxyuridine in patients with MNGIE, but these metabolites reaccumulated within 24 hours of dialysis. Diuretics have also been used to increase renal excretion of thymidine and deoxyuridine but without success. Bicarbonate may be used to correct acute or chronic lactic acidosis. Dichloroacetate (DCA) is an inhibitor of PDH and thus maintains PDH in its active (phosphorylated) state, resulting in reduced lactate production. DCA can be effective in lowering lactate levels in acute acidotic states. A double-blind placebo-controlled trial aimed to investigate the efficacy of DCA in the MELAS syndrome but had to be terminated prematurely because of reversible peripheral nerve toxicity (Kaufmann et al., 2006).

### Enzyme and Metabolite Replacement

#### Thymidine Phosphorylase Replacement Therapy

A number of strategies have been used to replace thymidine phosphorylase activity in patients with MNGIE. Replacement by repeated platelet or encapsulated red cell transfusions has been shown to produce transient benefit. Allogeneic stem cell transplantation has proven to be the most successful method of restoring thymidine phosphorylase activity in MNGIE patients but is associated with a high level of mortality, possibly due to the advanced clinical state of the patients (Halter et al., 2011). More recently, allogeneic bone marrow transplantation has been shown to restore thymidine phosphorylase enzyme function in patients with MNGIE and improve clinical manifestations in the long term; thus it should be considered for selected patients with an optimal donor (Halter et al. 2015).

### L-Arginine Therapy in MELAS

The precise mechanisms leading to stroke-like episodes in MELAS have not been determined. Dehydration, fasting, sepsis, and seizures are all likely to contribute, thus emphasizing the importance of adequate hydration, electrolyte and acid-base balance, nutritional support, antibiotics, and anticonvulsants. A possible role of L-arginine therapy has been reported based on the possibility that impaired vasodilation might be a factor in the acute setting. The effects of administering L-arginine, a nitric oxide precursor, were assessed in patients with acute MELAS stroke-like episodes. The authors suggested that oral administration within 30 minutes of a stroke significantly decreased frequency and severity of stroke-like episodes. In a further study, the same group found that 2 years of supplementation with oral L-arginine improved endothelial function to control levels and normalized plasma levels of L-arginine in patients. It was suggested that L-arginine therapy improved endothelial dysfunction and may have potential in the prevention and treatment of stroke-like episodes in MELAS.

### Folate Deficiency

Low CSF folate levels were first reported in KSS 25 years ago. More recently, rapid clinical response to folinic acid was reported in an 8-year-old boy with an mtDNA deletion associated with cerebral folate deficiency and leukoencephalopathy. It seems likely that the folate deficiency is secondary in KSS; at present, the prevalence of CSF folate deficiency in patients with mitochondrial disorders is not known. If central folate deficiency is suspected, CSF must be analyzed because blood folate levels do not accurately reflect CNS folate status. Treatment with folinic acid rather than folate is necessary because the latter does not cross the blood–brain barrier.

### Carnitine Deficiency

Primary systemic carnitine deficiency generally shows dramatic response to replacement therapy (up to 200 mg/kg daily in 2–4 divided doses in adults; maximum 3 g per day). Early replacement therapy may prevent the neurological deficits.

## Gene Therapy

### Resistance Exercise Training to Shift mtDNA Genotype

The proportion of mutant mtDNA in muscle correlates with the degree of reduction in oxidative capacity. Recently there has been increasing interest in the role of exercise therapy to improve muscle respiratory chain oxidative capacity by potentially reducing mutant mtDNA load—a process known as *gene shifting*. Certain mtDNA mutations such as deletions and some tRNA point mutations are present in high levels in mature skeletal muscle, but for reasons that remain unclear, they are absent from the muscle satellite cell population, which harbors only wild-type mtDNA. Previous experimental work demonstrated that activation of satellite cells has the potential to introduce wild-type mtDNA into mature skeletal muscle, thereby lowering the proportion of mutant mtDNA and reversing the respiratory chain defect. Certain types of exercise protocols have the potential to induce satellite cell activation and promote entry of wild-type mtDNA into mature muscle. Endurance training has been demonstrated to improve aerobic capacity (Taivassalo et al., 2006) and OXPHOS capacity and exercise tolerance (Jeppesen et al., 2009) in patients with mitochondrial myopathy. A 12-week progressive overload leg resistance exercise training protocol has demonstrated increased muscle strength and improved muscle oxidative capacity, although there was no measurable reduction in deleted mtDNA (Murphy et al., 2008) and exercise has been accompanied by an increase in mutant mtDNA load in one study (Taivassalo et al., 2001).

### Other Gene Therapy Approaches for mtDNA Mutations

An allotropic expression strategy used a mitochondrial targeting sequence added to an *ATP6* gene, recoded using the nuclear rather than the mitochondrial genetic code, to rescue the NARP phenotype in a cell-culture model. Cell growth was restored, and ATP synthesis improved. More recently, a similar approach was used in a rat model of LHON with an *ND4* mutation. Other approaches have attempted to introduce cytosolic tRNAs into the mitochondrion, eliminate mutant mtDNAs using restriction enzymes targeted to the mitochondrion, reduce deleted mtDNA molecules in cultured cells by growing under ketogenic conditions, and shift heteroplasmy with zinc finger nucleases that bind to mutant mtDNA molecules, leading to their selective degradation. A range of techniques for manipulating mtDNA and their products is in the early stages of development (Kyriakouli et al., 2008).

A novel strategy involves the exchange of maternal mtDNA with that of a healthy donor (Craven et al., 2010). This technique requires in vitro fertilization with the parent ovum and sperm, removal of the pronucleus from the resulting zygote, and fusion into an enucleated donor oocyte (cytoplast). The reconstituted zygote can then be implanted into the mother's uterus for development. Inevitably, this process requires the molecular diagnosis to have been made in the host woman (and excluded in the donor) and is an important potential therapy for female mutation carriers (Tachibana et al., 2013).

# MITOCHONDRIAL DYSFUNCTION IN NEURODEGENERATIVE DISEASE

## Mitochondrial Dysfunction and Parkinson Disease

Mitochondrial dysfunction is now established as an important component of the etiology and pathogenesis of PD (Schapira et al., 2014). Detailed analysis using laser capture of dopaminergic neurons from parkinsonian brains has demonstrated a greater proportion of deleted mtDNA than that in age-matched controls. Mutations in the nuclear genes *parkin*, *PINK1*, and *DJ1* encoding the corresponding mitochondrial proteins cause autosomal recessive PD. *Parkin* mutations predominantly cause parkinsonism in patients younger than 30 years. Mitochondrial dysfunction and increased oxidative stress have been described in parkin-deficient *Drosophila*, mouse models, and peripheral tissues in patients with *parkin*-mutation-positive PD. Parkin is a ubiquitin E3 ligase and regulates expression of PGC1α through interaction with parkin-interacting substrate protein, which represses expression of PGC1α and nuclear respiratory factor 1. Both parkin and PINK1 proteins control mitochondrial turnover via autophagic destruction (mitophagy) of impaired mitochondria. Mutations in *parkin* or *PINK1* impair mitophagy, causing the accumulation of defective mitochondria. This process can be reversed by upregulation of parkin or PINK1 proteins and the removal of defective mitochondria. The demonstration of abnormal expression of autophagy proteins in the brain of patients with Parkinson disease has further drawn attention to the importance of degradation pathways to the pathogenesis of the disease. The upregulation of the translation inhibitor 4E-BP counteracts the effects of *PINK1* or *parkin* mutants in *Drosophila,* and rapamycin, a drug that activates 4E-BP and autophagy, is also protective in these mutants.

Mutations in *DJ1* are a rare cause of familial PD. *DJ1*-knockout mice demonstrate downregulated mitochondrial uncoupling proteins 4 and 5, impaired calcium-induced uncoupling, and increased oxidant damage. DJ1 may have a protective role in the reduction of protein misfolding and aggregation which may be a result of oxidative stress and can reduce α-synuclein aggregation. Genetic causes of Parkinson disease, other than those encoding mitochondrial proteins, can also affect mitochondrial function. α-Synuclein is a major component of Lewy bodies and neurites present in the brains of patients with Parkinson disease. Point mutations or multiplications of the α-synuclein gene cause familial PD. α-Synuclein is predominantly cytosolic, but a fraction has been identified in mitochondria and has been noted to interact directly with mitochondrial membranes, including at the neuronal synapse, and to inhibit complex I in a dose-dependent manner that shows regional expression of the protein. In addition to genetic causes, several environmental factors have been associated with both mitochondrial dysfunction and PD or parkinsonism, including a range of mitochondrial complex I inhibitors that are toxic to dopaminergic neurons.

## Mitochondrial Dysfunction and Alzheimer Disease

Apart from age, important risk factors for Alzheimer disease include apolipoprotein ε4 status and mutations of amyloid precursor protein or presenilin. Abnormalities of mitochondrial structure or function, or mtDNA defects in the brain and other tissues, of patients with Alzheimer disease have been described (Picone et al., 2014). The presence and relevance of these findings have remained controversial, and the data derived have not always been reproducible. Polymorphism of the *TOMM40* gene (2 kilobases away from the *APOE 4* gene on chromosome 19) has been described as an important risk factor for Alzheimer disease and its age of onset. TOMM40 protein forms part of a pore in the outer mitochondrial membrane and is involved in the transportation of cytoplasmic proteins into the mitochondrion. Amyloid precursor protein accumulates in this pore. Presenilins 1 and 2 and γ-secretase are associated with the mitochondria-associated membrane, a connection site between the endoplasmic reticulum and the mitochondrion that is dependent on mitofusin 2 function. Mitochondria-associated membranes contain acyl-CoA cholesterol acyltransferase—an important enzyme in cholesterol metabolism that is needed for the formation of amyloid β, which in turn can localize to mitochondria. Impaired mitochondria-associated membrane function may affect intracellular calcium homoeostasis and be relevant to calcium dysregulation by the endoplasmic reticulum and abnormal neuronal calcium handling detected in Alzheimer disease models and patients. Triple-transgenic mice expressing amyloid and tangle pathology similar to that noted in Alzheimer disease had pronounced mitochondrial abnormalities, such as reduced OXPHOS, decreased activities of complexes I and IV, lowered mitochondrial membrane potential, and increased free-radical generation. The potential contribution of mitochondria to Alzheimer disease continues to develop into a pivotal role in the downstream biochemical events that affect intracellular bioenergetics and homoeostasis.

## Mitochondrial Dysfunction and Huntington Disease

Huntington disease is caused by an unstable CAG triplet repeat expansion in exon 1 of the *huntingtin* gene. Mitochondrial defects have been described in patients with Huntington disease in vivo, in postmortem brain and muscle, and in cell and animal models of the disease (Schapira et al., 2014). The mitochondrial defects in Huntington disease are associated with abnormalities of calcium handling, increased susceptibility to calcium-induced opening of the mitochondrial permeability pore, and reduced respiration. Mutant huntingtin protein associates with mitochondrial membranes, can impair axonal trafficking of mitochondria, and can reduce synaptic ATP concentrations. Mutant huntingtin protein interacts with, and increases the sensitivity of, the inositol-1,4,5-trisphosphate receptor at the mitochondria-associated membrane and contributes to calcium dysregulation in Huntington disease. Mutant huntingtin protein also sensitizes cells to free radical–mediated damage, reduces ATP production and mitochondrial fusion, and induces increased fragmentation. These changes were prevented by overexpression of mitofusin 2. The role of mitochondrial quality control is further supported by the finding that the calcineurin-mediated dephosphorylation of dynamin-like protein 1 is increased in cells of patients with Huntington disease and leads to increases in mitochondrial translocation, promotion of fragmentation, and an increased cell susceptibility to apoptosis. Mutant huntingtin protein has an important role in transcription regulation, and the expression of a range of mitochondrial proteins is modified in Huntington disease striatal neurons, including the downregulation of COX subunit 2, mitofusin 1, mitochondrial transcription factor A, and PGC1α. This correlates with disease severity and increased expression of dynamin-like protein 1. The regulation of PGC1α by mutant huntingtin protein is of particular interest because of the potential to manipulate the expression of this molecule with drugs. Mutant huntingtin protein binds to the PGC1α promoter and blocks transcription of target genes in Huntington disease models and patient muscle. In view of the important regulatory role for PGC1α in mitochondrial biogenesis, this process might contribute to the mitochondrial dysfunction seen in Huntington disease, including impaired defense against free radicals.

## Other Neurodegenerative Diseases

Mitochondrial dysfunction has been identified in several other neurodegenerative diseases. Secondary abnormalities of mitochondrial morphology and function have been recorded in amyotrophic lateral sclerosis (Palomo and Manfredi, 2014), whereas in other disorders the causative gene mutation involves a mitochondrial protein (see Table 93.1)—for example, Friedreich ataxia and hereditary spastic paraplegia. Mutations in the *MFN2* gene are a common cause of autosomal dominant Charcot-Marie-Tooth type 2 disease, an early-onset axonal sensorimotor neuropathy. A proportion of patients have additional abnormalities, such as optic atrophy or deafness. Mutations of *OPA1* cause autosomal dominant optic atrophy, but the phenotype can include peripheral neuropathy, deafness, ataxia, and ophthalmoplegia with multiple mtDNA deletions. The part that both mitofusin 2 and optic atrophy protein 1 play in fission–fusion might at least partly explain both the pathophysiology of neuronal-axonal dysfunction and the overlapping phenotypes of mutations affecting these proteins, although an additional role in mtDNA maintenance cannot be excluded.

*The complete reference list is available online at https://expertconsult.inkling.com/.* 

94

# Prion Diseases

*Boon Lead Tee MD, Michael D. Geschwind MD PhD FAAN*

OUTLINE



Prion (pronounced *pree-ahn*) diseases (PrDs) are a group of uniformly fatal neurodegenerative diseases caused by the transformation of an endogenous protein, PrP (prion-related protein), into an abnormal conformation (misfolded protein) called the *prion*. The term *prion* is derived from the term *proteinaceous infectious particle* and was named by Stanley Prusiner, who discovered prions (Prusiner, 1998). For many years, prion diseases were mistakenly thought to be due to "slow viruses," in part owing to the transmissibility of the diseases and the long incubation period between exposure and symptom onset (Brown et al., 1986b; Gajdusek, 1977). Research by Prusiner and others, however, determined that the infectious agent did not contain nucleic acid, a component of viruses. Furthermore, treating prion-contaminated material with methods that inactivated viruses and other microorganisms did not prevent these diseases from being experimentally transmitted; yet methods that denatured or destroyed proteins prevented transmission, strongly supporting the theory that the causative agent was a protein (Gajdusek, 1977; Prusiner, 1982). The identification of the gene-encoding human PrP (Oesch et al., 1985), *PRNP*, and mutations of this gene in patients with familial prion disease (Goldgaber et al., 1989; Hsiao et al., 1989) further helped support the prion hypothesis. In 1997, Prusiner received the Nobel Prize in Physiology or Medicine for his work on identifying the prion (Prusiner, 1998). Through animal models, identification of prion gene mutations causing prion disease in humans, and in vitro production of prions with transmissibility, it essentially has been proven that the prion protein is necessary and sufficient to cause prion disease (Pritzkow et al., 2018; Prusiner, 2013). Although PrDs occur in animals and humans, this chapter focus on human PrDs, discussing animal prion diseases only relevant to human disease.

## HUMAN PRION DISEASES

### Introduction

Perhaps one reason many find PrDs so fascinating is that they are unique in medicine because they can occur in three ways in humans: spontaneously (sporadic), genetically, and through transmission (acquired) (Prusiner, 1998). Approximately 85% of human prion diseases are sporadic, 15% are genetic, and fewer than 1% are acquired (e.g., iatrogenic) (Begue et al., 2011; Klug et al., 2013; Nozaki et al., 2010; Prusiner, 1998). Sporadic prion disease, or sporadic Jakob-Creutzfeldt disease (sJCD), is thought to occur spontaneously. Genetic prion diseases (gPrD) are due to a mutation in *PRNP* and historically have been classified into three forms based on clinical and pathological features: familial JCD (fJCD), Gerstmann-Sträussler-Scheinker disease (GSS), and fatal familial insomnia (FFI). As noted in the gPrD section, however, this classification is somewhat antiquated. Although acquired (infectious) prion diseases are the least common form of human prion disease, they are perhaps the most notorious, in part owing to their occurrence through inadvertent transmission of prions from animals to humans and from human to human. Because the genetic and acquired forms of human prion disease are less common, they will be discussed in less detail in this chapter than the much more common form, sJCD.

### Epidemiology

The incidence of human prion diseases is about 1–1.5 per million per year in most developed countries, with some variability from year to year and between countries (Begue et al., 2011; Holman et al., 2010; Jansen et al., 2012; Klug et al., 2013; Litzroth et al., 2015; Maddox et al., 2020; Nozaki et al., 2010). Thus, annually there are about 6,000 human prion cases worldwide, including about 400–500 in the United States (Holman et al., 2010; Maddox et al., 2010). The incidence of cases can vary from year to year, particularly in countries with smaller populations in which a small fluctuation in cases can have a big impact on incidence (http://www.eurocjd.ed.ac.uk/surveillance%20data%201.html; Begue et al., 2011; Ladogana et al., 2005; Litzroth, Cras, De Vil & Quoilin, 2015; Nozaki et al., 2010; Ruegger et al., 2009). The peak age of onset of sJCD occurs around a unimodal, relatively narrow peak of about 68 years (Brown et al., 1994; Collins et al., 2006; Holman et al., 2010). Because sJCD tends to occur within a relatively narrow age range, a person's lifetime risk of dying from sJCD is estimated to be about 1 in 5000–10,000, much higher than the incidence (which is across all age groups) of 1 in a million (Maddox et al., 2020; Minikel et al., 2016).

## History of Creutzfeldt-Jakob Disease Nomenclature

The history of the nomenclature for JCD is quite interesting. In 1921 and 1923, Alfons Jakob published four papers describing five unusual cases of rapidly progressive dementia. He stated that his cases were nearly identical to a case described earlier by his professor Hans Creutzfeldt in 1920. This disease was referred to for many decades as *Jakob's disease* or *Jakob-Creutzfeldt disease* until Clarence J. Gibbs, a prominent researcher in the field, started using the term *Creutzfeldt-Jakob disease (CJD)* because the acronym was closer to his own initials (Gibbs, 1992). It turns out that the cases Jakob described were very different than Creutzfeldt's case, and that only two of Jakob's five cases actually had the disease that we now call JCD or CJD (prion disease), whereas Creutzfeldt's case did not (Katscher, 1998). Therefore, the name for prion disease should be *Jakob's disease* or possibly *Jakob-Creutzfeldt disease*. Unfortunately many continue to use the term CJD, either for historical reasons or because the term *JC disease* (JCD) can be easily confused with progressive multifocal leukoencephalopathy (PML) caused by the JC virus. In this chapter, we will use the more historically accurate terms *Jakob-Creutzfeldt disease* and *JCD*. Prion diseases also have been historically called *transmissible spongiform encephalopathies* (TSEs) due to two properties common to many prion diseases: transmissibility and, on neuropathology, spongioform changes. We will not use the older term TSE because some gPrDs might not be transmissible (Weissmann & Flechsig, 2003) and not all human prion diseases have spongiform changes (now called *vacuolation* due to fluid-filled vesicles in the dendrites) on pathology (Budka et al., 1995; Kretzschmar et al., 1996).

## What Are Prions?

Before further discussion, it is important to understand what a prion is. Just as the nomenclature for human prion diseases is complicated, unfortunately so is the terminology for the biology of prions. The normal prion protein (PrP) is referred to as *PrP^C^*, in which the *C* stands for the normal cellular form. Prion proteins, $PrP^C$, can be transformed into prions, an abnormal, "infectious" form of PrP often called either $PrP^{Sc}$ or $PrP^{Res}$ (*Sc* refers to the abnormally shaped PrP found in scrapie—the prion disease of sheep and goats—and *Res* refers to the fact that prion being partially resistant to digestion by proteases (enzymes that digest proteins). In this chapter we use the term $PrP^{Sc}$.

$PrP^C$ and $PrP^{Sc}$ essentially have identical amino acid sequences (except in gPrD; see later) but different three-dimensional structures, with the former mainly consisting of α-helical structure with little or no β-sheet structure and the latter mainly having β-sheet structure (Baldwin et al., 1994; Sarnataro et al., 2017), possibly stacked as a solenoid (Wille & Requena, 2018). Prions are characterized by the intrinsic ability of their structures to act as a template and convert the normal physiological $PrP^C$ into the pathological disease-causing form, $PrP^{Sc}$. Per the current prion model, when $PrP^C$ comes in contact with $PrP^{Sc}$, $PrP^C$ changes shape into that of $PrP^{Sc}$. Thus, $PrP^{Sc}$ acts as a template for the misfolding of $PrP^C$ into $PrP^{Sc}$. It is believed that it is the accumulation of prions, $PrP^{Sc}$, in the brain that leads to nerve cell injury and death (Prusiner, 1998, 2013), although some data suggest that it is the transformation of $PrP^C$ into $PrP^{Sc}$, and not the accumulation of $PrP^{Sc}$, that causes neuronal injury and subsequent disease (Mallucci et al., 2007). Sporadic JCD can present quite variably despite all cases having

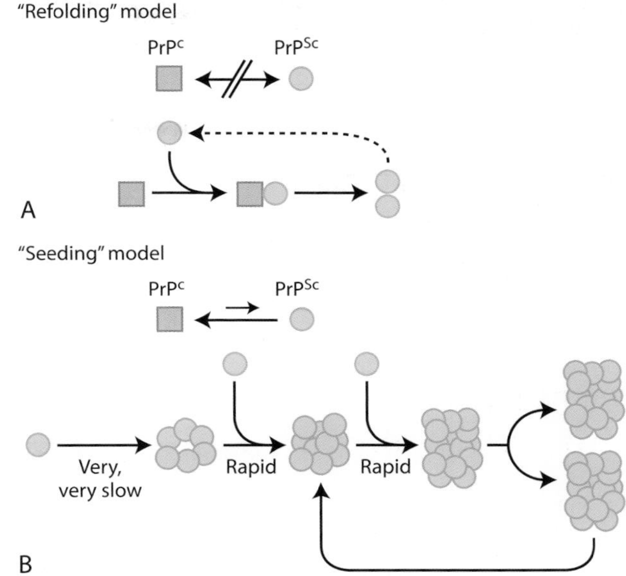


**Fig. 94.1** Models for the conformational conversion of cellular prion protein *($PrP^C$)* to scrapie prion protein *($PrP^{Sc}$)*. **A,** The refolding model. Conformational change is kinetically controlled, a high-activation energy barrier preventing spontaneous conversion at detectable rates. Interaction with exogenously introduced $PrP^{Sc}$ causes $PrP^C$ to undergo an induced conformational change to yield $PrP^{Sc}$. This reaction could be facilitated by an enzyme or chaperone. In the case of certain mutations in $PrP^C$, spontaneous conversion to $PrP^{Sc}$ might occur as a rare event, explaining why familial Creutzfeldt-Jakob disease (JCD) or Gerstmann-Sträussler-Scheinker disease arise spontaneously, albeit late in life. Sporadic JCD might come about when an extremely rare event (occurring in about one in a million individuals per year) leads to spontaneous conversion of $PrP^C$ to $PrP^{Sc}$. **B,** The seeding model. $PrP^C$ *(purple rectangles)* and $PrP^{Sc}$ (or a $PrP^{Sc}$-like molecule, *Orange circles*) are in equilibrium, with $PrP^C$ strongly favored. $PrP^{Sc}$ is stabilized only when it adds onto a crystal-like seed or aggregate of $PrP^{Sc}$ *(green circles)*. Seed formation is rare, but once a seed is present, monomer addition ensues rapidly. To explain exponential conversion rates, aggregates must be continuously fragmented, generating increasing surfaces for accretion. *(From Weissmann, C., Enari, M., Klöhn, P.C., et al., 2002. Transmission of prions. Proc. Natl. Acad. Sci. USA 99(16), 378–316, 383.)*

$PrP^{Sc}$ with an identical amino acid sequence; one reason for this is that there are different strains of $PrP^{Sc}$, each with slightly different biological and physicochemical properties. Such prion strain diversity contributes clinicopathologically to variabilities in tissue tropism, host affinity, and clinical presentations (Bartz, 2016; Morales, 2017; Safar et al., 1998).

Although it is not known how prions spread throughout the brain, at least two models have been proposed: a refolding model and a seeding model, which are not mutually exclusive (Fig. 94.1). Importantly, mice that are devoid of $PrP^C$ can neither be infected with nor replicate prions (Bueler et al., 1993; Katamine et al., 1998; Prusiner, 1998). Furthermore, when an explant of neuronal tissue overexpressing $PrP^C$ is explanted into a $PrP^C$ knockout mouse and inoculated with prions, the explant shows extensive $PrP^{Sc}$ accumulation and neurodegeneration, but host brain tissue shows no toxicity despite containing $PrP^{Sc}$ derived from the graft (Brandner et al., 1996a, 1996b; Weissmann et al., 1996). These studies provide strong evidence that $PrP^C$ is necessary for prion disease. Furthermore, propagation capacity of different prion strains is shown to be partly related to surrounding cellular cofactors (Fernandez-Borges et al., 2018).

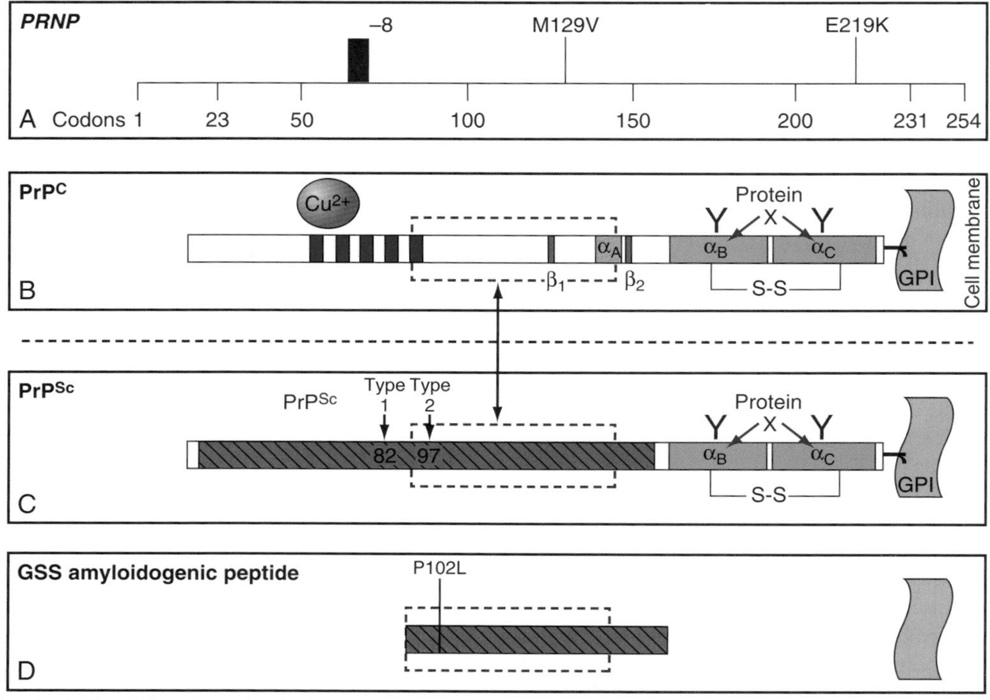


**Fig. 94.2 The Prion Protein. A,** The prion protein gene *(PRNP)* is located on the short arm of the human chromosome 20. Nonpathogenic polymorphism includes deletion of one of the octarepeat segments, methionine-valine polymorphism at the 129 position, and glutamine-lysine polymorphism at position 219. **B,** Post-translational modification truncates the cellular prion protein *(PrP^C)* at positions 23 and 231 and glycosylates (Y) at positions 181 and 197. The glycosylphosphatidylinositol *(GPI)* attached to serine at position 231 anchors the C-terminus to the cellular membrane. The intracellular N-terminus contains five octarepeat segments, P(Q/H)GGG(G/-)WGQ *(blue blocks)*, that can bind copper ions. The central part of the protein contains one short α-helical segment (α-helix A encompassing residues 144–157 *[green block]*), flanked by two short β-strands *(red blocks)*, β1(129–131) and β2(161–163). The secondary structure of the C-terminus is dominated by two long α-helical domains: α-helix B (residues 172–193) and α-helix C (residues 200–227), which are connected by a disulfide bond. The blue arrows indicate binding sites of the protein X within α-helices B and C. The dashed frame marks a segment between positions 90 and 150, which is crucial for the binding of PrP^C to scrapie prion protein *(PrP^Sc)*. **C,** PrP^Sc has increased β-sheet content (red dashed block). **D,** Unlike PrP^Sc, which is anchored to the membrane, Gerstmann-Sträussler-Scheinker *(GSS)* amyloidogenic peptides are truncated and excreted into the cellular space, where they aggregate and fibrillize into GSS amyloid deposits. This example is an 8-kD PrP fragment associated with the most common GSS/P102L mutation. A synthetic form of this peptide (90–150 residues), exposed to acetonitrile treatment to increase β-sheet content, is the only synthetically generated peptide that when injected intracerebrally into P102L-transgenic mice is able to induce the GSS disease. (*From Sadowski, M., Verma, A., Wisniewski, T., 2008. Infection of the nervous system: prion diseases. In: Bradley, W., Daroff, R., Fenichel, G., et al. (Eds.), Neurology in Clinical Practice, fifth ed. Butterworth-Heinemann, Philadelphia.*)

## Function of PrP^C

The function of PrP^C is still not entirely known (Castle & Gill, 2017; Gill & Castle, 2018; Wulf et al., 2017). It is evolutionary conserved, so it probably plays an important role in neuronal development and function (Kanaani et al., 2005). In humans, it is encoded by *PRNP*, located on the short arm of chromosome 20 (Basler et al., 1986; Oesch et al., 1985). PrP^C protein typically consists of a highly conserved central hydrophobic segment (HD) and a C-terminal hydrophobic region that is commonly attached to the outer cell membrane by a glycosylphosphatidylinositol (GPI) anchor and an amino terminal flexible tail (Borchelt et al., 1992, 1993; Sarnataro et al., 2017; Tarboulos et al., 1992) (Figs. 94.2 and 94.3). PrP^C is primarily membrane bound and resides primarily on nerve cell membranes and on other cells in the body, including lymphocytes. Mice that have had both copies of the open reading frame (ORF) of their PrP gene, *Prnp*, deleted (PrP$^{-/-}$) have a normal lifespan and appearance (Bueler et al., 1992; Manson et al., 1994). Furthermore, conditional knockout mice, in which the gene is not removed until after the mouse has already developed, also appear normal and unaffected by gene removal (Legname, 2017). Although the mice essentially were clinically asymptomatic, deeper phenotyping revealed several abnormalities, as discussed below.

PrP^C binds to many proteins and cellular constituents. Animal and cell models have suggested a variety of possible functions of PrP^C, including cell signaling, adhesion, proliferation, differentiation, and growth (Castle & Gill, 2017; Didonna, 2013; Gill & Castle, 2018; Wulf et al., 2017). Studies with various *Prnp* knockout mice models of mixed genetic backgrounds found they develop peripheral nerve demyelination (Nishida et al., 1999); have increased susceptibility to ischemic brain injury (Spudich et al., 2005; Weise et al., 2006); altered sleep and circadian rhythm (Nuvolone et al., 2016; Tobler et al., 1997); altered

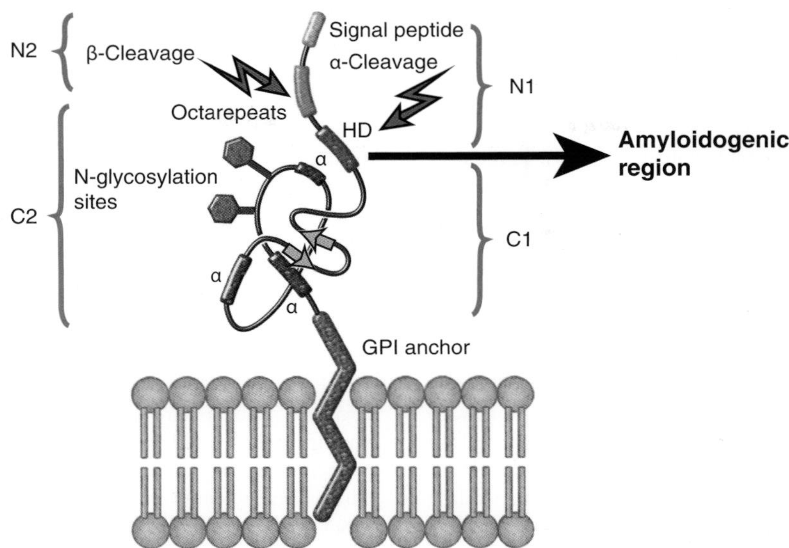


**Fig. 94.3 Schematic of Prion Protein (PrP$^C$) Attached to Cell Membrane.** This figure shows an outline of the structure of the cellular prion protein, including posttranslational modifications and representation of PrP$^C$ cleavages. A secretory signal peptide resides at the extreme N-terminus. Hydrophobic segment *(HD)* defines the hydrophobic region; α indicates alpha-helix and the arrows β-sheets; hexagons define N-glycosylation; the glycosylphosphatidylinositol *(GPI)* anchors PrP to the cell membranes. α-Cleavage acts in the HD generating N1 and C1 fragments, whereas β-cleavage acts in the octarepeat region generating N2 and C2. (*From Sarnataro, D., Pepe, A., Zurzolo, C., et al., 2017. Cell biology of prion protein. Prog. Mol. Biol. Transl. Sci. 150, 57–82, Figure 2.*)

hippocampal neuropathology and physiology, including deficits in hippocampal-dependent spatial learning and hippocampal synaptic plasticity (Colling et al., 1997; Criado et al., 2005); and olfactory dysfunction (Le Pichon et al., 2009). The octarepeat peptide regions of PrP$^C$ have even been implicated in playing an involved role in multidrug resistance of gastric cancer cells (Wang et al., 2012). There also have been several studies suggesting PrP$^C$ binds β-amyloid (Aβ), a major protein in Alzheimer disease (AD), and might play a role in the pathogenesis of AD (Kudo et al., 2013; Gunther & Strittmatter, 2010). Some studies in mice suggest that PrP$^C$ mediates the toxic effects of Aβ oligomers and might be necessary for memory deficits to occur in AD (Gimbel et al., 2010; Nygaard & Strittmatter, 2009). In fact, in one study infusion of anti-PrP$^C$ antibodies ameliorated cognitive deficits in an AD mouse model (Chung et al., 2010). This possible role of PrP$^C$ in binding to Aβ and causing dysfunction in AD is still controversial, however. In one study, with human APP (J20) crossed onto a PrP$^C$-deficient background still had the neurological impairment that was present in the J20 mice, suggesting PrP$^C$ might not be a major mediator of Aβ-induced impairment (Cisse et al., 2011).

For reasons that were unclear at the time, many phenotypes identified in certain *Prnp* knockout mice were not reproducible in knockout mice with different genetic backgrounds, resulting in confusion regarding the physiological role of PrP$^C$ in transgenic knockout mice models (*Prnp -/-*) (Wulf et al., 2017). One possible reason is that some reported findings were caused by knocking out genes adjacent to *Prnp* rather than *Prnp* itself; this is because the experiments were done with mice of mixed genetic backgrounds, which may harbor variable *Prnp*-flanking genes that can lead to poorly controlled Mendelian segregation of these polymorphic alleles. This led to systematic genetic confounds and in some cases incorrect conclusions regarding the function of PrP$^C$, such as the inhibition of macrophage phagocytosis (Aguzzi et al., 2013; Castle & Gill, 2017; Nuvolone et al., 2013; Striebel et al., 2013a, 2013b; Weissmann & Flechsig, 2003; Wulf et al., 2017). Using *Prnp* knockout mice with pure genetic backgrounds that do not possess flanking genes (Manson et al., 1994; Nuvolone et al., 2016), investigators found few of the prior putative phenotypes reported in *Prnp* knockout mice of impure genetic backgrounds (Castle & Gill, 2017; Wulf et al., 2017). Thus, genotype-phenotype relationships in impure mice strains need to be interpreted with caution and earlier experiments investigating the role of PrP$^C$ with impure mice models need to be replicated with *Prnp* mice with pure genetic backgrounds (Castle & Gill, 2017; Manson et al., 1994; Wulf et al., 2017). Phenotypes that remain in *Prnp* knockout mice with pure genetic background include chronic demyelinating peripheral neuropathy, suggesting a role for PrP$^C$ in myelin maintenance (Nuvolone et al., 2013), altered circadian rhythm and sleep pattern (Tobler et al., 1996), and altered synaptic plasticity (Wulf et al., 2017). Given the findings from *Prnp* mice with pure backgrounds, it seems that PrP$^C$ interacts with other membrane proteins, can regulate transport and regulation of these proteins, can modulate their functionality, and can even signal distinct biological pathways via its N-terminal tail cleavage products and scavenge Aβ amyloid aggregates (Wulf et al., 2017).

## Prion Protein Pathogenicity

Prion disease is generally regarded as a gain of function disease for at least two reasons: (1) deletion or reduction (e.g., hemizygous) of *Prnp* in mice results in mice that are normal or largely asymptomatic; and (2) the prion protein expression level in mice models is directly associated with the rate of disease progression (Fischer et al., 1996; Minikel et al., 2016; Weissmann & Flechsig, 2003; Wulf et al., 2017). Nevertheless, some of the roles for PrP$^C$ suggest that dysfunction in prion diseases might be due not only to pathogenicity of misfolded PrP$^C$ into prions but also to loss of normal function of PrP$^C$ (Castle & Gill, 2017).

Post-translational modification of prion protein and the GPI anchor may play a role in the pathogenesis of prion diseases. Different proteolytic processing of the prion protein generates protein fragments that have variable functions. For instance, the hydrophobic domain (HD) region in $PrP^C$ (amino acid 106–126) (see Fig. 94.3) is considered to have amyloidogenic properties (Tagliavini et al., 1993). In the normal state, α-cleavage occurs in this region, causing a loss of the amyloidogenic tendency and generating both a tethered C terminal protein (C1), which helps maintain myelin integrity, and a free N terminal fragment (N1), which has anti-apoptotic activity. In contrast, β-cleavage, which occurs more frequently in prion disease, generates a membrane-bound C terminal protein (C2) that retains the amyloidogenic core, and a free N terminal fragment (N2), the latter of which is speculated to have antioxidant instead of anti-apoptotic properties. It is believed that a higher-stress environment favors β-cleavage that tends to reduce oxidative stress but promote prion aggregation (Guillot-Sestier et al., 2009; Linsenmeier et al., 2017; Sarnataro et al., 2017). When $Prnp^{-/-}$ transgenic mice that retain the region encoding the C1 protein (i.e., less amyloidogenic) were inoculated with prions, they remained asymptomatic and showed resistance to protease-resistant PrP accumulation (Westergard et al., 2011). As aforementioned, these studies involved transgenic mice with mixed genetic backgrounds and further study replications using pure genetic mice models is warranted. Regarding the role of the GPI anchor attaching $PrP^C$ to the cell membrane, anchorless transgenic mice, which encode $PrP^C$ without the GPI anchor, remained asymptomatic when inoculated with $PrP^{Sc}$ but still showed diffuse amyloid $PrP^{Sc}$ plaques in the brain (Chesebro et al., 2005). Another version of anchorless transgenic mice, however, had spontaneous late-onset neurological symptoms and GSS-like pathology (i.e., amyloid plaques) (Stohr et al., 2011). The former anchorless $PrP^C$ study suggests that $PrP^{Sc}$ deposition alone might not be sufficient to cause neurotoxicity, but both studies suggest the GPI anchor might be involved in prion disease pathophysiology.

## CLINICAL ASPECTS OF HUMAN PRION DISEASES

### Sporadic Prion Disease

As noted above, nomenclature in prion diseases can be confusing, with the terms JCD or CJD used to refer to just sporadic JCD or to all human prion diseases interchangeably. To reduce confusion in this chapter, we refer to all human prion diseases as prion disease (PrD), whereas sJCD will be used to refer only to sporadic JCD. The rarity of sJCD and the fact that its incidence is similar (~1–1.5/million) in most countries with appropriate surveillance suggest that it is unlikely to be due to an environmental cause and likely arises as a rare stochastic event in otherwise healthy persons, possibly through the spontaneous transformation of the prion protein $PrP^C$ into $PrP^{Sc}$ or through a somatic mutation that results in the formation of a prion protein that is more susceptible to changing into $PrP^{Sc}$ (Alzualde et al., 2010; Will et al., 1998; see Watts et al., 2006, for a discussion on possible origins of sJCD).

Sporadic JCD is typically a very rapid disease with a median survival of about 4.5–6 (range 1–130) months (Collins et al., 2006; Parchi et al., 1999b) and mean survival of about 8±11 months (Brown et al., 1994). About 85% of patients die within 1 year from onset of symptoms (Collins et al., 2006), and ~ 50%–60% die in less than 5–6 months (Brown et al., 1994; Collins et al., 2006). The median age of onset is 60–67 years old, with a range from 12 to 95 (Brown et al., 1994; Collins et al., 2006; Parchi et al., 1999b) (Table 94.1). Occurrence of sJCD at young (20s–40s) (Belay et al., 2001; Martindale et al., 2003; Murray et al., 2008) or old (>80) ages is uncommon (Collins et al., 2006). Patients younger than 20 years of age are extremely rare, although a few have occurred, including a 13-year-old in the United States (Blase et al., 2014) and an unpublished case of a 12-year-old girl with sJCD in Spain (biopsy-proven with no *PRNP* mutation; M. Geschwind, personal communication). Sporadic JCD individuals with younger age of onset were reported to have longer survival and higher tendency to present with non-cognitive features including affective disorder, behavioral change, or sleep illnesses (Appleby et al., 2007; Corato et al., 2006).

Symptoms of sJCD vary widely but typically include cognitive changes (dementia), behavioral and personality changes, difficulties with movement and coordination, visual symptoms, and constitutional symptoms (Appleby et al., 2009; Brown et al., 1986a; Rabinovici et al., 2006). Cognitive problems are often among the first symptoms in sJCD and typically include mild confusion, memory loss, and difficulty concentrating, organizing, or planning. Motor manifestations of sJCD include extrapyramidal symptoms (bradykinesia, dystonia, tremor), cerebellar symptoms (gait or limb ataxia), and later in the disease, myoclonus (sudden jerking movements). Whereas the cognitive and motor symptoms are often obvious, other common early symptoms may be subtle. These include behavioral or psychiatric symptoms (i.e., irritability, anxiety, depression, or other changes in personality) and constitutional symptoms (i.e., fatigue, malaise, headache, dry cough, lightheadedness, vertigo, etc.). Visual symptoms typically present as blurred or double vision, cortical blindness, or other perceptual problems; they are due to problems with processing of visual information in the brain and not due to retinal or cranial nerve abnormalities. Other symptoms such as aphasia, neglect, or apraxia (inability to do learned movements) due to cortical dysfunction might also occur and can be presenting features. Sensory symptoms such as numbness, tingling, and/or pain are less well-recognized symptoms and are probably under-reported, given the magnitude of the other symptoms in sJCD (Brown et al., 1994; Lomen-Hoerth, 2010; Rabinovici et al., 2006; Will, 2004). sJCD can sometimes be classified based on the initial presenting symptoms (within the first few weeks of onset), into cognitive, Heidenhain (visual presentation), affective (mood disorders presentation), classic (cognitive symptoms and ataxia), and Brownell-Oppenheimer (ataxia presentation) variants, with cognitive and cerebellar symptoms being the most common initial presentations (Appleby et al., 2009; Rabinovici et al., 2006; Tsuji & Kuroiwa, 1983; Will et al., 2004). Each of these sJCD variants can have distinctive disease courses as well as electroencephalogram (EEG) and magnetic resonance imaging (MRI) findings (Appleby et al., 2009; Meissner et al., 2009). Classic and visual variants often progress most rapidly with the shortest survival time. Affective variants tend to have a younger age of onset and longest disease duration. In contrast, Oppenheimer-Brownell variants usually have an older onset age and lack presence of periodic sharp-wave complexes on EEG or basal ganglia hyperintensity on brain MRI (Appleby et al., 2009). Clinical symptomatology and course appear to vary, in part, based on the molecular classification of sJCD based on the prion type and a *PRNP* polymorphism (see later discussion) (Parchi et al., 1999b). Sporadic JCD usually progresses rapidly over weeks to months from the first obvious symptoms to death. The end stage is usually an akinetic-mute state (no purposeful movement and not speaking) (Brown et al., 1994). Most patients with prion disease die from aspiration pneumonia.

Typical neuropathological features of sJCD include neuronal loss, gliosis (proliferation of astrocytes), vacuolation (i.e., spongiform changes), and deposition of $PrP^{Sc}$; except for $PrP^{Sc}$ deposition, the other features are found in many other neurodegenerative and other neurological conditions and are not specific for JCD

(Kretzschmar et al., 1996) (Fig. 94.4). PrP$^{Sc}$ deposition followed by mild vacuolation (spongiform change), and gliosis are early features of prion diseases (Bouzamondo-Bernstein et al., 2004; Iwasaki et al., 2014), with later more severe vacuolation, gliosis, and neuronal loss (Iwasaki et al., 2014). Some pathologists are of the opinion that the term *vacuolation* is the more appropriate term to describe the spongiform changes, as these are not holes but rather fluid-filled vesicles formed in distal dendrites near synapses (Bouzamondo-Bernstein et al., 2004). Clinical and other features of several prion diseases are summarized in Table 94.1.

**TABLE 94.1 Major Characteristics of Major Types of Human Prion Diseases**

| Characteristic | sJCD | vJCD | fJCD | iJCD | FFI | GSS | Kuru |
|---|---|---|---|---|---|---|---|
| Average age at onset (years) | 67 | 28 | Variable among kindreds, 23–55 | All ages | 50 | 40 | All ages |
| Average duration of disease (months) | 8 | 14 | Variable among kindreds, 8–96 | 12 | 18 | 60 Variable among kindreds, 60–240 | 11 |
| Average incubation periods (range) | N/A | 17 years (12–23 years); blood transfusion, 7 years (6.5–8 years) | N/A | Neurosurgical, 18 months (12–28); dura graft, 6 years (1.5–23 years); hGH, 5 years (4–36 years) | N/A | N/A | 12 years (5–50 years) |
| Most prominent early signs | Cognitive and/or behavioral dysfunction | Psychiatric abnormalities, sensory symptoms (later dementia, ataxia, and other motor symptoms) | Cognitive and/or behavioral dysfunction | Cognitive dysfunction, ataxia | Insomnia, autonomic instability | Ataxia, tremor, extrapyramidal symptoms | Ataxia, tremor |
| Cerebellar dysfunction (%) | >40 | 97 | >40 | >40 | No | 100 in P102L mutation, less common in most other mutations | 100 |
| DWI/FLAIR MRI positive | Yes, >92% | Yes, pulvinar sign | Yes for most mutations | Variable; some positive in deep nuclei or cerebellum | Unclear | Variable; most negative | N/A |
| PSWCs on EEG | Yes, 65% | No (rarely at end stage) | Yes | Yes | No | No | N/A |
| Amyloidosis | Sparse plaques in 5%–10% | Severe in all cases | Sporadically seen | Sporadically seen | No | Very severe | 75% of cases |
| Presence of PrP$^{Sc}$ in the lymphoreticular system | No | Yes | No | Yes | No | No | Unlikely |

*DWI*, diffusion-weighted imaging; *EEG*, Electroencephalogram; *fJCD*, familial Creutzfeldt-Jakob disease; *FFI*, familial fatal insomnia; *FLAIR*, fluid-attenuated inversion recovery; *hGH*, human growth hormone; *iJCD*, iatrogenic Creutzfeldt-Jakob disease; *GSS*, Gerstmann-Sträussler-Scheinker; *mo*, months; *N/A*, not available or not applicable; PrP$^{Sc}$, scrapie prion protein; *PSWCs*, periodic sharp wave complexes; *sJCD*, sporadic Creutzfeldt-Jakob disease; *vJCD*, variant Creutzfeldt-Jakob disease; *yrs*, years.

*Modified from Sadowski M, Verma A, Wisniewski T. Infections of the nervous system. Chapter 59G. Prion diseases. In: Bradley WG, Daroff RB, Fenichel GM, Jankovic J,editors. Neurology in Clinical Practice. 5th ed. Newton, MA: Butterworth-Heinmann; 2008. p. 1566-82; and from these other references: Brandner, S., Whitfield, J., Boone, K., Puwa, A., O'Malley, C., Linehan, J.M., et al., 2008. Central and peripheral pathology of kuru: pathological analysis of a recent case and comparison with other forms of human prion disease. Philos. Trans. R. Soc. Lond. B, Biol. Sci. 363 (1510), 3755–3763; Brown, P., Brandel, J.P., Preece, M., Sato, T., 2006. Iatrogenic Creutzfeldt-Jakob disease: the waning of an era. Neurology 67 (3), 389–393. Brown, P., Gibbs, C.J., Jr., Rodgers-Johnson, P., Asher, D.M., Sulima, M.P., Bacote, A., et al., 1994. Human spongiform encephalopathy: the National Institutes of Health series of 300 cases of experimentally transmitted disease. Ann. Neurol. 35 (5), 513–529. Brown, P., Preece, M., Brandel, J.P., Sato, T., McShane, L., Zerr, I., et al., 2000. Iatrogenic Creutzfeldt-Jakob disease at the millennium. Neurology 55 (8), 1075–1081; Collie, D.A., Summers, D.M., Sellar, R.J., Ironside, J.W., Cooper, S., Zeidler, M., et al., 2003. Diagnosing variant Creutzfeldt-Jakob disease with the pulvinar sign: MR imaging findings in 86 neuropathologically confirmed cases. AJNR Am. J. Neuroradiol. 24 (8), 1560–1569; Collinge, J., Whitfield, J., McKintosh, E., Beck, J., Mead, S., Thomas, D.J., et al., 2006. Kuru in the 21st century—an acquired human prion disease with very long incubation periods. Lancet 367 (9528), 2068–2074; Heath, C.A., Cooper, S.A., Murray, K., Lowman, A., Henry, C., Macleod, M.A., et al., 2011. Diagnosing variant Creutzfeldt-Jakob disease: a retrospective analysis of the first 150 cases in the UK. J. Neurol. Neurosurg. Psychiatry 82 (6), 646–651; Huillard d'Aignaux, J.N., Cousens, S.N., Maccario, J., Costagliola, D., Alpers, M.P., Smith, P.G., et al., 2002. The incubation period of kuru. Epidemiology 13 (4), 402–408; Kong, Q., Surewicz, W.K., Petersen, R.B., Zou, W., Chen, S.G., Gambetti, P., et al., 2004. Inherited prion diseases. In: Prusiner, S.B., (Ed.), Prion Biology and Diseases, second ed. Cold Spring Harbor Laboratory Press, Cold Spring Harbor, pp. 673–775; Lewis, A.M., Yu, M., DeArmond, S.J., Dillon, W.P., Miller, B.L., Geschwind, M.D., 2006. Human growth hormone-related iatrogenic Creutzfeldt-Jakob disease with abnormal imaging. Arch. Neurol. 63 (2), 288–290; Parchi, P., Giese, A., Capellari, S., Brown, P., Schulz-Schaeffer, W., Windl, O., et al., 1999. Classification of sporadic Creutzfeldt-Jakob disease based on molecular and phenotypic analysis of 300 subjects. Ann. Neurol. 46 (2), 224–233; Valleron, A.J., Boelle, P.Y., Will, R., Cesbron, J.Y., 2001. Estimation of epidemic size and incubation time based on age characteristics of vCJD in the United Kingdom. Science 294 (5547), 1726–1728; Vitali, P., Maccagnano, E., Caverzasi, E., Henry, R.G., Haman, A., Torres-Chae, C., et al., 2011. Diffusion-weighted MRI hyperintensity patterns differentiate CJD from other rapid dementias. Neurology 76 (20), 1711–1719; Will, R.G. 2003. Acquired prion disease: iatrogenic CJD, variant CJD, kuru. Br. Med. Bull. 66, 255–265.*

### Molecular Classification of Jakob-Creutzfeldt Disease

Sporadic JCD has historically been divided into approximately six major molecular subtypes based on the genetic polymorphism at codon 129 in *PRNP* (MM, MV, or VV; Table 94.2) (Parchi et al., 1999b) (also see later discussion and Figs. 94.2 and 94.7) and the molecular weight of protease-resistant fragment of $PrP^{Sc}$ (type 1 or 2). When $PrP^{Sc}$ is extracted from brain tissue, and partially digested with proteinase, depending on the conformation of $PrP^{Sc}$, cleavage can occur at either of two sites (codon 82 or 97; see Fig. 94.2) resulting in, either a longer 21-kD (type 1) or a shorter 19-kD (type 2) peptide fragment is found when run on a Western blot. This classification, to some extent, separates sJCD cases based on their clinicopathological features into the six subtypes: MM1/MV1, VV2, MV2, MM2-thalamic, MM2-cortical, and VV1. MM1 and MV1 present clinicopathologically very similarly and are often, therefore, grouped together. They comprise the most common forms (~70%, the vast majority of which are MM1) and usually present as classic sJCD with rapidly progressive dementia and a duration of just a few months. VV2 (~16%) typically starts with ataxia, and has dementia later in the course, as well as a short disease duration. The remaining four types—MV2 (9%), MM2-thalamic (2%), MM2-cortical (2%), and VV1 (1%)— have median durations of about 1–1.5 years. MV2 presents similarly to VV2 with ataxia but has focal amyloid "kuru" plaques in the cerebellum. MM2-thalamic presents often with insomnia, followed later by ataxia and dementia, with most pathology confined to the thalamus and inferior olives and very little vacuolation; some researchers in the prion field call this form *sporadic fatal insomnia* (sFI), as it has some overlapping pathology with the genetic prion disease FFI (Parchi et al., 1999a), but this is simply the MM2-thalamic variant of sJCD (Parchi et al., 1999b). MM2-cortical patients have progressive dementia with large confluent vacuoles in all cortical layers with prolonged median duration of 15.7 months. VV1 patients also typically present with progressive dementia but have severe cortical and striatal pathology with sparing of the brainstem nuclei and cerebellum. Unlike MM2-cortical, sJCD VV1 patients generally do not have large confluent vacuoles but

**TABLE 94.2 Distribution of PRNP Codon 129 Polymorphism in Normal Population and Several Human Prion Diseases**

| | MV (%) | MM (%) | VV (%) |
|---|---|---|---|
| Normal population | 51 | 37 | 12 |
| sJCD | 12–17 | ~66–72 | 17 |
| iJCD | 20 | 57 | 23 |
| vJCD* | <1 | >99 | 0 |

**All but two clinical cases of vJCD have been MM; one probable and one definite vJCD case were codon 129 MV, and some subclinical cases with vJCD prions in the lymphoreticular system have been identified (see text). iJCD, Iatrogenic Creutzfeldt-Jakob disease; sJCD, sporadic Creutzfeldt-Jakob disease; vJCD, variant Creutzfeldt-Jakob disease. Data from Brown, P., Preece, M., Brandel, J.P., Sato, T., McShane, L., Zerr, I., et al., 2000. Iatrogenic Creutzfeldt-Jakob disease at the millennium. Neurology 55 (8), 1075–1081; Collins, S.J., Sanchez-Juan, P., Masters, C.L., Klug, G.M., van Duijn, C., Poleggi, A., et al., 2006. Determinants of diagnostic investigation sensitivities across the clinical spectrum of sporadic Creutzfeldt-Jakob disease. Brain 129(Pt 9), 2278–2287; Garske, T., Ghani, A.C., 2010. Uncertainty in the tail of the variant creutzfeldt-Jakob disease epidemic in the UK. PLoS One 5 (12), e15626; Knight, R., 2017. Infectious and sporadic prion diseases. Prog. Mol. Biol. Transl. Sci. 150, 293–318; Parchi, P., Giese, A., Capellari, S., Brown, P., Schulz-Schaeffer, W., Windl, O., et al., 1999. Classification of sporadic Creutzfeldt-Jakob disease based on molecular and phenotypic analysis of 300 subjects. Ann. Neurol. 46 (2), 224–233; Peden, A., McCardle, L., Head, M.W., Love, S., Ward, H.J., Cousens, S.N., et al., 2010. Variant CJD infection in the spleen of a neurologically asymptomatic UK adult patient with haemophilia. Haemophilia 16 (2), 296–304.*

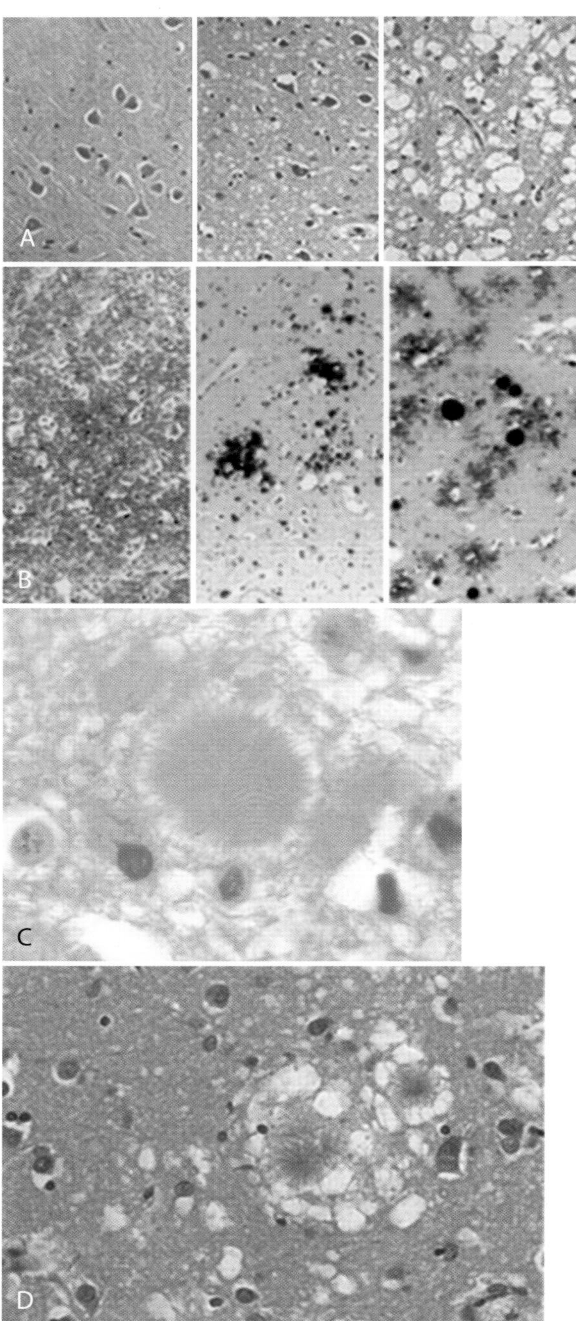


**Fig. 94.4 Neuropathology of Prion Disease. A,** In sporadic Creutzfeldt-Jakob disease (sJCD), some brain areas may have no (hippocampal end plate, *left*), mild (subiculum, *middle*), or severe (temporal cortex, *right*) spongiform change (hematoxylin and eosin [H & E] stain). **B,** Cortical sections immunostained for $PrP^{Sc}$ in sJCD: synaptic *(left)*, patchy/perivacuolar *(middle)*, or plaque-type *(right)* patterns of $PrP^{Sc}$ deposition. **C,** Large kuru-type plaque (H & E stain). **D,** Typical "florid" plaques in variant JCD (H & E stain). (*Modified from Budka, H., 2003. Neuropathology of prion diseases. Br Med Bull. 66, 121–130. Copyright © 2003 Oxford University Press.*)

TABLE 94.3 **Several Commonly Used Diagnostic Criteria for Probable sJCD**

| | 1998 WHO Revised Criteria (Geschwind et al., 2007; WHO, 1998) | 2007 UCSF Criteria (Geschwind et al., 2007; Young et al., 2005) | 2009 European Consortium | 2017 European Consortium (Hermann et al., 2018; UK National CJD Research & Surveillance Unit [NCJDRSU], 2017) |
|---|---|---|---|---|
| I. Clinical Features | Progressive dementia with two of the following:<br>• Myoclonus<br>• Visual or cerebellar disturbance<br>• Pyramidal/extrapyramidal signs<br>• Akinetic mutism | Rapidly progressive dementia with two of the following:<br>• Myoclonus<br>• Visual disturbance<br>• Cerebellar signs<br>• Pyramidal/ extrapyramidal signs<br>• Akinetic mutism<br>• Focal cortical signal (e.g.: neglect, aphasia, acalculia, apraxia) | Progressive dementia with two of the following:<br>• Myoclonus<br>• Visual or cerebellar disturbance<br>• Pyramidal or extrapyramidal signs<br>• Akinetic mutism | Rapidly progressive cognitive impairment with two of the following:<br>• Myoclonus<br>• Visual or cerebellar disturbance<br>• Pyramidal or extrapyramidal signs<br>• Akinetic mutism |
| II. Diagnostic Test | Typical EEG*<br>OR<br>• Elevated CSF protein 14-3-3 (with total disease duration < 2 years) | • Typical EEG*OR<br>• Typical MRI† | • Typical EEG*OR<br>• Elevated CSF protein 14–3-3 (with total disease duration <2 years)<br>OR<br>• Typical MRI‡ | • Typical EEG*OR<br>• Typical MRI†OR<br>• Elevated CSF protein 14–3-3<br>OR<br>• Positive RT-QuIC in CSF or other tissues in setting of any progressive neurological condition |
| III. Other | • Routine investigations should not suggest an alternative diagnosis | • Routine investigations should not suggest an alternative diagnosis | • Routine investigations should not suggest an alternative diagnosis | |

*Typical EEG: Periodic sharp waves complexes

†Typical MRI for University of California, San Francisco (UCSF) MRI criteria initially required diffusion-weighted imaging (DWI) brighter than fluid-attenuated inversion recovery (FLAIR) hyperintensity in the cingulate, striatum and/or > 1 neocortical gyrus, ideally with sparing of the precentral gyrus and apparent diffusion coefficient map supporting restricted diffusion. (See Table 1 in Vitali et al., 2011.) UCSF MRI criteria were updated in 2017 (See Table 2 in Staffaroni et al., 2017.)

‡Typical MRI for European criteria: High signal abnormalities in caudate nuclear and putamen or at least two cortical regions (temporal-parietal-occipital, but not frontal, cingulate, insular or hippocampal) either on DWI or FLAIR MRI.

*Reproduced permission from Tee, B.L., Longoria Ibarrola, E.M., Geschwind, M.D., et al., 2018. Prion disease. Neurol Clin. 36 (4):865–897.*

have faint synaptic $PrP^{Sc}$ staining (Parchi et al., 1999b). Complicating matters is the fact that anywhere from six (Collins et al., 2006) to as high as 50% (Polymenidou et al., 2005) of sJCD cases have both type 1 and 2 prions (Puoti et al., 1999). The clinicopathological presentation of each patient with mixed types appears to depend in part on the relative ratio of these prion types (Collins et al., 2006; Polymenidou et al., 2005; Puoti et al., 2012).

As shown in Table 94.2, heterozygosity at codon 129 in the prion gene *PRNP* is somewhat protective against prion disease. Additionally, a study from the UK Medical Research Council Prion Unit suggested that codon 129 alone affects rate of decline in sJCD independent of prion typing, with homozygosity (MM or VV) associated with faster decline than codon 129 heterozygosity (Thompson et al., 2013).

## DIAGNOSIS OF CREUTZFELDT-JAKOB DISEASE

Several criteria exist for the diagnosis of sJCD. Unfortunately, most patients will only fulfill existing criteria at later stages of the disease (Paterson et al., 2012), because most criteria are designed for epidemiological purposes, to ensure that all deceased, non-pathologically proven cases have a sufficient non-pathological diagnosis (Brandel, et al., 2000; WHO, 1998; Zerr et al., 2009). Thus, most epidemiological criteria designed for JCD surveillance do not allow diagnosis at early disease stages and are not very helpful when evaluating a patient early in the disease course. Criteria generally categorize patients by level of diagnostic certainty into definite, probable, and possible. *Definite criteria* require pathological evidence of the presence of $PrP^{Sc}$ in brain tissue (by biopsy or autopsy) (Budka, 2003; Kretzschmar et al., 1996). *Probable criteria* usually require a positive ancillary diagnostic test (e.g., EEG, cerebrospinal fluid [CSF] marker, or brain MRI) in addition to certain symptoms. Several *probable criteria* are shown in Table 94.3. The most commonly used *probable criteria* are based on the World Health Organization (WHO) Revised Criteria (1998) and require dementia plus at least two of four clinical signs or symptoms, and positive ancillary test (Geschwind, 2015; WHO, 1998; Zerr et al., 2009). Pyramidal findings are motor abnormalities on neurological exam (e.g., hyperreflexia, focal weakness, extensor response). Extrapyramidal findings in sJCD typically include rigidity, slowed movement (bradykinesia), tremor, or dystonia, typically due to problems in the basal ganglia or its connections. Myoclonus is sudden quick jerking of a limb or the trunk that can be spontaneous or stimulus induced, often by loud noise. *Akinetic mutism* describes patients who are without purposeful movement and mute; this typically and it occurs at the very end stage of the disease. WHO 1998 *possible JCD criteria* are the same as for *probable criteria* but do not require the ancillary testing (WHO, 1998). Many patients will not meet WHO revised criteria for probable sJCD until late in the disease course (Hermann et al., 2018). Criteria utilizing brain MRI were proposed in 2007 (Geschwind, 2015;

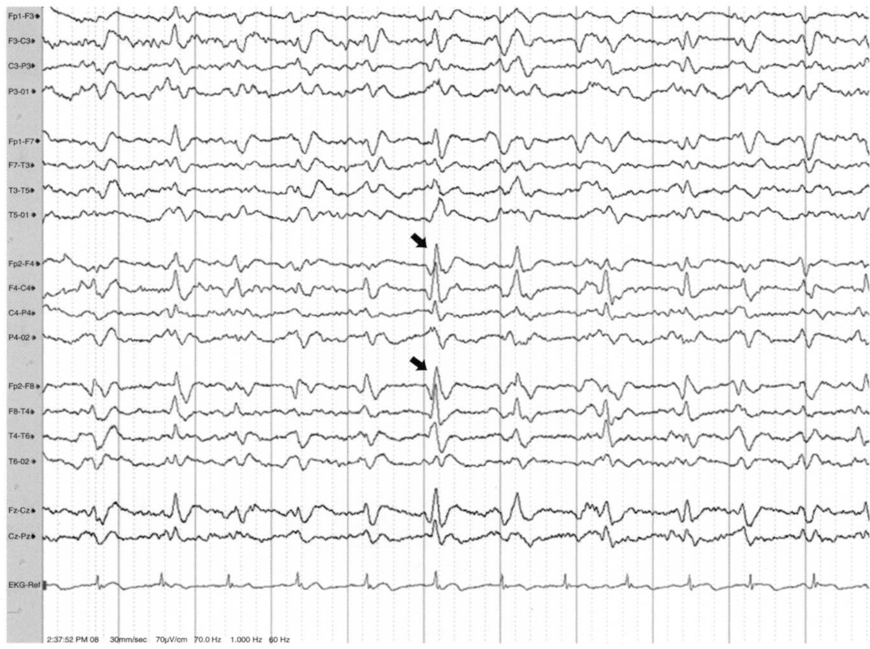


**Fig. 94.5** A typical electroencephalogram in a sporadic Creutzfeldt-Jakob disease patient, with diffuse slowing and 1-Hz periodic sharp wave complexes *(black arrows)*.

Geschwind et al., 2007), and, in 2009, modified European sJCD criteria also allowed inclusion of brain MRI (see later discussion) (Zerr et al., 2009) (see Table 94.3). To increase the diagnostic accuracy, especially at the early stages of sJCD, explicit details of MRI criteria (discussed in detail in next section) have been proposed and continue to be updated (Staffaroni et al., 2017; Vitali et al., 2011; Zerr et al., 2009). The German prion surveillance group recently proposed to ammend research diagnostic criteria to allow diagnosis of probable sJCD with either (1) progressive cognitive impairment or (2) one of the cardinal sJCD symptoms and a positive real-time quaking-induced conversion assay (RT-QuIC; see next section). Compared with WHO diagnostic criteria, this diagnostic criterion increased the sensitivity level of premorbid diagnosis from 74% to 97% among 65 definite sJCD individuals (Hermann et al., 2018). Thus, the more prion specific biomarkers such as RT-QuIC were incorporated into the 2009 and 2017 European sJCD criteria (see Table 94.3).

## Diagnostic Tests for Sporadic Jakob-Creutzfeldt Disease

A typical EEG in sJCD has sharp or triphasic waves (periodic sharp wave complexes, or PSWCs) occurring about once every second (Fig. 94.5); this EEG finding, however, is found in only about two-thirds of sJCD patients, typically only after serial EEGs and often not until later stages of the illness (Steinhoff et al., 2004; Zerr et al., 2000). The presence of PSWCs is very dependent on molecular classification; for example, they are found in 73% of MM1 and 53% of MV1 cases, but in only 12%–18% of MV2, VV2, and VV1/2 cases (Collins et al., 2006; Zerr et al., 2000). These EEG findings are relatively specific, but PSWCs are sometimes seen in other conditions including AD, Lewy body disease, toxic-metabolic and anoxic encephalopathies, PML, Hashimoto encephalopathy (Seipelt et al., 1999; Tschampa et al., 2001), and even voltage-gated potassium channel complex associated encephalopathy (Savard et al., 2016).

The first CSF biomarker for sJCD diagnosis, the 14-3-3 protein, was proposed in 1996, but the clinical utility of this and other biomarkers is controversial, in part because of varying degrees of sensitivity and specificity reported. The 14-3-3 protein was one of the first CSF proteins touted as a diagnostic marker for JCD, but its utility is controversial (Chapman et al., 2000; Forner et al., 2015; Geschwind et al., 2003), particularly as it is elevated in many non-prion neurological conditions (Foutz et al., 2017; Satoh et al., 1999).

This test is usually a Western blot that is read subjectively, or at best semiquantitatively, as positive, negative, or inconclusive. We believe that enzyme-linked immunosorbent assay (ELISA) tests, which provide quantitative values, are notoriously unreliable in the United States, although they have been reported to be very reliable in some other countries, including Germany (Hermann et al., 2018). The range of sensitivities in studies with 50 or more sJCD subjects vary from 51% to 95% (Castellani et al., 2004; Chohan et al., 2010; Collins et al., 2006; Forner et al., 2015; Hamlin et al., 2012; Ladogana et al., 2009; Sanchez-Juan et al., 2006; Zerr et al., 1998, 2000). Two larger European studies have found this protein to have a sensitivity and specificity of about 85%; the control patients, however, are probably not sufficiently characterized in some of these studies (Table 94.4) (Collins et al., 2006; Sanchez-Juan et al., 2006). Data from the US National Prion Disease Pathology Surveillance Center (NPDPSC) on 420 pathology-confirmed sJCD and non-prion cases in the United States found the sensitivity and specificity of the 14-3-3 Western blot to be only 74% and 56%, respectively (Hamlin et al., 2012). By restricting controls to pathology-proven cases, however, many studies exclude non-prion cases with clinical phenotypes that mimic JCD and often have elevated 14-3-3, but who eventually recover; these cases often include patients with strokes, seizures, autoimmune encephalopathies, and other conditions. Many dementia experts consider the 14-3-3 protein merely a marker of rapid neuronal injury that has poor specificity for sJCD (Chapman et al., 2000; Foutz et al., 2017; Geschwind et al., 2003; Hamlin et al., 2012; Satoh et al., 1999).

Other potential sJCD CSF biomarkers include total-tau (t-tau), neuron-specific enolase (NSE), and the astrocytic protein S100β (Hamlin et al., 2012). The sensitivity and specificity of these biomarkers for sJCD vary greatly among studies. One large multicenter European study examined four CSF biomarkers: 14-3-3, t-tau, NSE, and S100β. As not

**TABLE 94.4 Calculated Sensitivities and Specificities of Various Biomarkers in sJCD Based on Literature Review**

| | SENSITIVITY *(n)* | | |
|---|---|---|---|
| | **Definite** | **Definite + Probable**[§] | **Specificity** *(n)* |
| **EEG*** | **59.6% (2473)** | **59.7% (2488)**[¶] | **83.8% (99)** |
| **CSF Biomarkers** | | | |
| 14-3-3 protein (WB) | 86.7% (2675) | 86.3% (4266) | 88.1% (2209) |
| 14-3-3 protein (ELISA) | 80% (55) | 89.6% (201) | 84.2% (183) |
| Total tau | 85.8% (618) | 85.9% (1489) | 86.5% (1642) |
| NSE | 81% (42) | 74.5% (644) | 93.5% (186) |
| S100B | 75.8% (442) | 79.7% (1058) | 85.7% (1293) |
| RT-QuIC | 90.1% (455) | 88.9% (468) | 99.6% (498) |
| **Nasal Mucosa**[†] | | | |
| RT-QuIC | 97.9% (97) | 97.3% (111) | 100% (116) |
| Brain MRI DWI[‡] | 98.2% (57) | 94% (184) | 93.8% (195) |

For this table, we combined results from several papers to ascertain the sensitivities and specificities of various biomarkers in sJCD using published literature.

*Typical EEG findings: Periodic sharp waves complexes.

[†]Includes both olfactory mucosa brush and swab.

[‡]Only included literature based on DWI, not just T2 or FLAIR sequences.

[§]Unclear whether possible sJCD were included in Sanchez-Juan et al. (2006).

[¶]Levy et al. (1986) was published prior to WHO diagnostic criteria, 15 cases were clinically diagnosed without autopsy.

*CSF*, Cerebrospinal fluid; *DWI*, diffusion-weighted imaging; *EEG*, electroencephalography; *ELISA*, enzyme-linked immunosorbent assay; *MRI*, magnetic resonance imaging; *NSE*, neuron-specific enolase; *RT-QuIC*, real-time quaking-induced conversion; *S100B*, S100 calcium-binding protein B; *WB*, Western blot.

References for each category were as follows:

EEG: Collins et al., 2006; Levy et al., 1986; Steinhoff et al., 2004; Zerr et al., 2000.

14-3-3 protein (WB): Beaudry et al., 1999; Collins et al., 2000, 2006; Hamlin et al., 2012; Hsich et al., 1996; Kenney et al., 2000; Sanchez-Juan et al., 2006; Van Everbroek et al., 2003; Zerr et al., 1998, 2000; Baldeiras et al., 2009; Castellani et al., 2004; Chohan et al., 2010; Forner et al., 2015; Geschwind et al., 2003.

14-3-3 protein (ELISA): Geschwind et al., 2003; Kenney et al. 2000; Matsui et al., 2011.

Total Tau: Baldeiras et al., 2009; Chohan et al., 2010; Coulthart et al., 2011; Hamlin et al., 2012; Sanchez-Juan etal., 2006; Van EverBroek et al., 2003.

NSE: Beaudry et al., 1999; Sanchez-Juan et al., 2006; Pocchiari et al., 2000.

S100B: Beaudry et al., 1999; Sanchez-Juan et al., 2006; Baldeiras et al., 2009; Chohan et al., 2010; Coulthart et al., 2011.

RT-Quic: Atarashi et al., 2011; Bongianni et al., 2017; Foutz et al., 2017; McGuire et al., 2012, 2016; Orru et al., 2014, 2015; Sano et al., 2013.

Brain MRI: Forner et al., 2015; Shiga et al., 2004; Tian et al., 2010; Young et al., 2005

all patients were tested for all four biomarkers, nor were they necessarily tested using the same samples, this study did not allow proper comparison of these biomarkers. Nevertheless, they found the sensitivity and specificity of the 14-3-3 to be 85% and 84%, t-tau (cutoff > 1300 pg/mL) 86% and 88%, NSE 73% and 95%, and S100β 82% and 76%, respectively (Sanchez-Juan et al., 2006). A Canadian study, with 126 pathology-proven sJCD and 843 probable non-JCD cases, found CSF t-tau to be better than 14-3-3 and S100β (Coulthart et al., 2011). A study at our center similarly found CSF t-tau to be a better diagnostic marker than either 14-3-3 or NSE (Forner et al., 2015). The sensitivity and specificity of these CSF biomarkers in other forms of prion disease such as variant JCD and gPrD are usually much lower than for sJCD (Foutz et al., 2017; Hamlin et al., 2012; Sanchez-Juan et al., 2006). The ratio between T-tau and phosphorylated tau (T-tau/P-tau) also has been assessed as a diagnostic tool for sJCD, with reported sensitivities ranging from 63% to 94% and specificities ranging from 92% to 97% (Forner et al., 2015). Additional biomarkers, such as CSF and serum glial fibrillary acidic protein (GFAP) and serum neurofilament light chain (NfL), are also being evaluated for diagnosis and prognosis of prion diseases but are not yet in clinical practice. Given the nonspecificity of elevated NfL, it is unlikely to be used as a diagnostic marker but appears to show great potential as a prognostic marker in symptomatic prion disease (Kovacs et al., 2017; Staffaroni et al., 2019; Steinacker et al., 2016; Thompson et al., 2018; van Eijket al., 2010). Total-tau might be the best CSF non-prion diagnostic biomarker protein for sJCD, but it still is not close to the diagnostic utility of brain MRI (Forner et al., 2015; Shiga et al., 2004).

Most of the above biomarkers are not testing for prions, $PrP^{Sc}$, but are markers of rapid neuronal injury and can be elevated in various acute or rapidly progressive neurological disorders (Geschwind, 2015, 2016; Lattanzio et al., 2017). The relatively new RT-QuIC test enables detection of prions by amplifying them. It works by first mixing the sample to be tested for prions with a substrate containing $PrP^{C}$ (usually either recombinantly-derived or from healthy rodent brain). Then, by continuous shaking, $PrP^{Sc}$ in samples are brought into contact with $PrP^{C}$, allowing conversion into $PrP^{Sc}$, which aggregates into amyloid fibrils. These amyloid fibrils will fluoresce when thioflavin T is added. The fluorescent signal can be read on an automated plate reader (Atarashi et al., 2011; McGuire et al., 2012, 2016). Currently, this technique is used to detect prions in several human tissues, including brain, CSF, olfactory mucosa, skin biopsies, all layers of the eye, and even extra-ocular muscle (Orru et al., 2017, 2018), but does not work with blood or blood-contaminated CSF (Cramm et al., 2016; Shi et al., 2013). The sensitivity of RT-QuIC in sJCD CSF varies greatly in the literature, but is most commonly reported to be about 85%. In our University of California, San Francisco (UCSF) sJCD cohort, sensitivity was only around 60%, with testing being performed at two independent laboratories (unpublished data). In contrast, the specificity of RT-QuIC is very high, with many studies reporting 98% or higher (Atarashi et al., 2011; Bongianni et al., 2017; Foutz et al., 2017; Franceschini et al., 2017; Lattanzio et al., 2017; McGuire et al., 2016). Thus, in our opinion, a negative test does not exclude disease, but a positive test in the appropriate clinical context has great diagnostic value.

MRI has been shown to be highly sensitive and specific (91%–96%) for diagnosing sJCD (Shiga et al., 2004; Vitali et al., 2011; Young et al., 2005). The first MRI abnormalities reported in JCD were basal ganglia hyperintensities on T2-weighted sequences (Gertz et al., 1988; Rother et al., 1992). Later, cortical gyral hyperintensities (Urbach et al., 1998) were identified, and found to be more evident on fluid-attenuated inversion recovery (FLAIR) than T2-weighted sequences, and most evident on diffusion-weighted imaging (DWI) sequences. These cortical hyperintensities are commonly referred to as *cortical ribboning*. DWI has higher sensitivity than FLAIR (Fujita et al., 2012; Vitali et al., 2011). Whenever JCD is suspected, a brain MRI that includes diffusion sequences (e.g., DWI, ADC, and, if possible, exponential ADC [eADC]) should be obtained (Staffaroni et al., 2017). Some typical MRI features on FLAIR, DWI, and ADC sequences in sJCD and vJCD are shown in Fig. 94.6. Unfortunately, many radiologists, even at academic centers, are still not familiar with the findings indicative of prion disease, and a majority of sJCD MRIs are misread (Carswell et al., 2012; Geschwind et al., 2010). Several MRI criteria for sJCD diagnosis have been proposed and modified or improved over the years (Staffaroni et al., 2017). MRI (particularly DWI and FLAIR sequences) was first included in sJCD diagnostic criteria (UCSF sJCD diagnostic criteria) in 2007 (Geschwind et al., 2007; Young et al., 2005). MRI was subsequently incorporated into European sJCD criteria in 2009 (Zerr et al., 2009) (see Table 94.3). We believe that these European criteria are a step forward but have several limitations. First, many patients in the study did not have DWI MRI sequences, and the criteria allow for FLAIR hyperintensities alone without requiring diffusion abnormalities. This is a problem because FLAIR abnormalities in prion disease are more difficult to detect and less specific than diffusion abnormalities for sJCD. For example, deep nuclei hyperintensities on T2-weighted/FLAIR sequences can be seen in many conditions other than JCD, including metabolic and autoimmune conditions (Rosenbloom et al., 2015; Vernino et al., 2002; Vitali et al., 2008a, 2008b). Second, T2/FLAIR or DWI hyperintensities in the frontal and insular cortices, cingulate, and hippocampus were excluded in European 2009 criteria because of the high levels of artifact found in these regions that resulted in many false positives. We have found, however, that these artifacts, which are usually due to CSF–brain interface, can often be avoided by acquiring MRIs in multiple planes (e.g., axial and coronal), using an attenuation diffusion coefficient (ADC) map to confirm the presence of restricted diffusion, and improving image quality using various proprietary methods, such as readout segmentation of long variable echo trains (RESOLVE) (Staffaroni et al., 2017). Unfortunately, the European 2009 MRI criteria neither require the use of DWI nor include the ADC map sequences to confirm true restricted diffusion. This is important because the DWI sequence is a combination of both T2 and diffusion, so a T2 shine-through effect can make certain regions appear bright on DWI despite normal diffusion. Especially when the deep gray nuclei (basal ganglia and/or thalamus) are involved in sJCD, the ADC map typically is hypointense and shows reduced levels of diffusion (Staffaroni et al., 2017; Vitali et al., 2011). Evidence suggests that the reduced diffusion on MRI in JCD is from restricted flow of water molecules inside vacuoles in the dendritic tree (Geschwind et al., 2009; Manners et al., 2009).

Basic laboratory studies such as complete blood cell count (CBC), chemistry, liver function tests, erythrocyte sedimentation rate (ESR), antinuclear antibody (ANA), and so forth, are generally unremarkable in sJCD. CSF is typically normal with a mildly elevated protein (typically $< 100$ mg/dL). CSF shows normal red blood cells (RBCs) and white blood cells (WBCs). Pleocytosis ($>10$ WBCs), an elevated immunoglobulin (Ig)G index, or the presence of oligoclonal bands is unusual in sJCD and should lead to considering other conditions, particularly infectious or autoimmune disorders. As noted earlier, an EEG that is "typical" or classic for JCD has PSWCs (see Fig. 94.5), but often there is just slowing on EEG in sJCD.

*Variably protease-sensitive proteinopathy* (vPSPr) is a recently described, although very rare, form of sJCD (Head et al., 2013; Puoti et al., 2012; Zou et al., 2010). One hallmark of prion diseases has been that part of $PrP^{Sc}$ is resistant to proteases, but the degree of protease sensitivity of $PrP^{Sc}$ is strain dependent (Safar et al., 1998). In vPSPr, the vast majority of patients' $PrP^{Sc}$ is protease sensitive, so standard immunohistochemical techniques that depend on identifying the protease-resistant core of $PrP^{Sc}$ for diagnosis are insufficient (hence, the term "variably protease-sensitive"). Another key feature of vPSPr has been that when $PrP^{Sc}$ is detected on Western blot, there is no diglycosylated $PrP^{Sc}$ band, only the mono- and unglycosylated band, and there are also some smaller bands for a total of five bands (Xiao et al., 2013). The United States National Prion Disease Pathology Surveillance Center (US NPDPSC) and United Kingdom National JCD Surveillance and Research Unit (UK NCJCDSRU) estimated the prevalence of vPSPrs to be 0.7% and 1.7% respectively, among all sporadic PrDs (Notari et al., 2018; UK National CJD Research & Surveillance Unit (NCJDRSU), 2018). As of 2018, about 37 cases of vPSPr have been reported in the literature (Notari et al., 2018), although there are likely many more cases. The distribution of codon 129 genotype in vPSPr differs substantially from that of sJCDs, with ~65% being VV, 24% MV, and 11% MM (Notari et al., 2018). The codon 129 genotype also appears to affect the clinical presentation, age of onset, and the electrophoretic profile on Western blot. Many of these cases presented with psychiatric symptoms, speech/language problems, and frontal lobe dysfunction (Puoti et al., 2012). Unlike other sporadic prion diseases, most had negative ancillary tests (MRIs, EEGs, and CSF 14-3-3), making diagnosis more challenging. Although their mean age was commensurate with classic sJCD (late 60s), their mean disease duration was much longer, at about 2.5 years (Gambeti et al., 2011; Head et al., 2013; Notari et al., 2018; Zou et al., 2010). As the awareness of the disease rises, the spectrum of presentation continues to widen, including reports of vPSPr presenting as amyotrophic lateral sclerosis (ALS)/frontotemporal dementia (FTD) spectrum disorder (Cannon et al.,

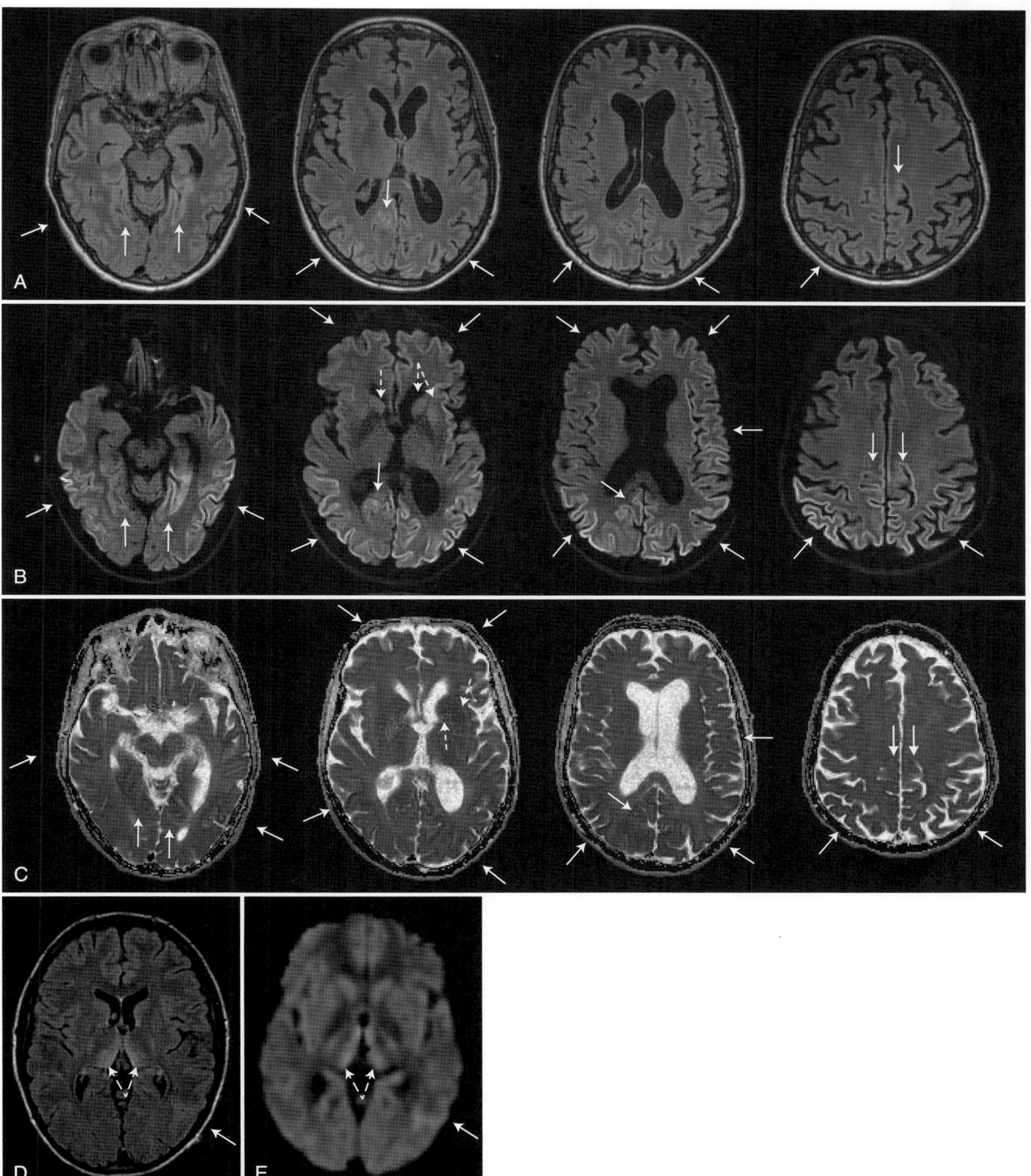


**Fig. 94.6** Brain magnetic resonance images (MRIs) in sporadic Jakob-Creutzfeldt disease (sJCD) and variant Jakob-Creutzfeldt disease (vJCD). Brain MRI in 59-year-old woman with sJCD showing both cortical *(solid arrows)* and subcortical *(dashed arrows)* abnormalities on fluid-attenuated inversion recovery (FLAIR) **(A)**, diffusion-weighted imaging (DWI) **(B)**, and apparent diffusion coefficient (ADC) **(C)** sequences in sporadic Jakob-Creutzfeldt disease (sJCD). This MRI shows a common pattern in sJCD, including cortical gyral ("cortical ribboning"; *solid arrows*) and deep nuclei *(dashed arrows)* hyperintensities on FLAIR and DWI sequences and corresponding hypointensity on ADC sequences. The DWI hyperintensities with corresponding ADC hypointensity confirm that there is restricted diffusion of water molecules, which is found in more than 95% of sJCD cases. Note that as seen in most brain MRIs in prion disease when restricted diffusion is present, the hyperintensities are much more evident on DWI than on FLAIR sequences. Brain MRI in a 20-year-old woman with variant JCD (vJCD) showing, on FLAIR **(D)** and DWI **(E)** sequences, hyperintensity of bilateral thalamic hyperintensity in the mesial pars (mainly dorsomedian nucleus) and posterior pars (pulvinar) of the thalamus, sometimes called the double hockey stick sign, which can be seen in many prion diseases. Importantly, this MRI also shows the pulvinar sign, in which the posterior thalamus (pulvinar; dashed *arrow*) is more hyperintense than the anterior putamen; this sign has much higher specificity for vJCD compared to other forms of prion disease. (D and E)

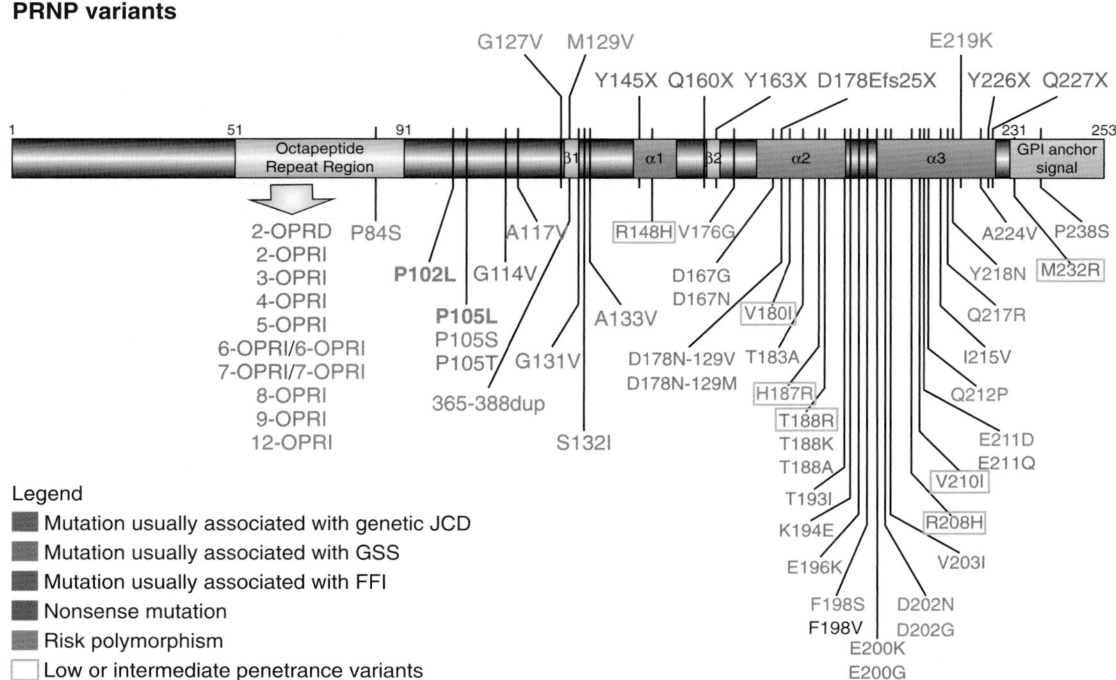


**Fig. 94.7 Schematic of Prion Protein Gene *(PRNP)* Disease-Associated Variants.** Mutations are color coded based on clinicopathological classification as genetic Jakob-Creutzfeldt disease *(JCD)*, Gerstmann-Sträussler-Scheinker *(GSS)*, fatal familial insomnia *(FFI)*, or nonsense mutations. *PRNP* mutations present in the UCSF cohort are in bold. Most mutations are shown below the gene schematic; nonsense mutations and polymorphisms associated with prion disease risk are above the gene schematic. Low or intermediate penetrance variants are based on Minikel et al. (2016) (not all low/intermediate penetrance variants are shown). For the F198V mutation, the clinical presentation was not classifiable as genetic JCD, GSS, or FFI, and neuropathology was not reported (Zheng et al., 2008). Variants that are probably benign (largely based on Minikel et al., 2016) are not included (e.g., G54S, P39L, E196A, R208C) (Beck et al., 2010; Minikel et al., 2016). *OPRD,* Octapeptide repeat deletion; *OPRI,* octapeptide repeat insertion. (*Reproduced with permission from Takada, L.T., Kim, M.O., Cleveland, R.W., Wong, K., Forner, S.A., Gala, II, et al., 2017. Genetic prion disease: Experience of a rapidly progressive dementia center in the United States and a review of the literature. Am. J. Med. Genet. B Neuropsychiatr. Genet. 174 [1]:36–69.*)

2014; Ghoshal et al., 2014; Vicente-Pascual et al., 2018). Such atypical features and varied presentations can make these cases difficult to diagnose.

## Genetic Prion Disease

Background on genetic prion disease Genetic forms of prion disease (gPrD) are caused by autosomal dominant pathogenic variants (i.e., mutations) in the human PrP gene, *PRNP*. More than 60 *PRNP* variants, mostly point mutations but some stop codons, insertions, and deletions, have been reported, but several of these are of low penetrance (e.g., less than 1%) and some are likely non-pathogenic (Kim et al., 2018; Minikel et al., 2016). Most *PRNP* variants considered as mutations are essentially 100% (i.e., fully) penetrant, meaning that a person with a mutation is virtually guaranteed to develop prion disease if they live a normal lifespan (Kim et al., 2018; Mead, 2006; Takada et al., 2017, 2018). Diagnosis of gPrD is made by identification of a pathogenic variant in *PRNP*. For a variant to be considered pathogenic, it should fulfill published guidelines for considering a variant to be causal for a disease (MacArthur et al., 2014; Richards et al., 2015) (Fig. 94.7 and Fig. 94.2). Based on a study combining data from nine prion disease surveillance centers, 85% of gPrDs are attributed to five mutations—E200K, V210I, V180I, P102L, D178N; with the first three presenting as JCD, P102L presenting as GSS and D178N as either CJD or FFI (Kim et al., 2018; Minikel et al., 2016; Takada et al., 2017). Several *PRNP* variants reported to be mutations in some literature, such as V210I, V180I, and M232R, have higher than expected prevalence in the general population and most carriers lack a family history of prion or other neurodegenerative disease. The penetrance of these three variants is estimated to be 10%, 1%, and 0.1%, respectively (Kim et al., 2018; Minikel et al., 2016; Takada et al., 2017). It usually is easiest to test for *PRNP* from blood (or saliva) while a patient is still alive; alternatively, in some countries, JCD surveillance centers can extract DNA from frozen brain autopsy tissue and sequence *PRNP* in order to identify variants (Kim et al., 2018). gPrDs are sometimes referred to as *familial*, but this term can be a misnomer because a family history is not always present or known. In a large European study, 47% of patients ultimately shown to have a *PRNP* variant causing gPrD did not have positive family history of dementia or prion disease. It is possible that this was because relatives were misdiagnosed or there was reduced penetrance of the *PRNP* variant or, less likely, that they were de novo mutations (Kovacs et al., 2005).

Although gPrDs historically were divided according to their clinical and pathological characteristics into familial JCD (fJCD), GSS, and FFI, this classification was developed prior to the discovery of *PRNP*. It is clear that several *PRNP* mutations such as H187R, the octapeptide insertion (OPRI) mutations, octapeptide deletion, and stop codon mutations do not fit into one of these three historical categories (Kim et al., 2018). Most *PRNP* mutations are associated with fJCD, more than a dozen are associated with GSS, and only the D178N *PRNP* mutation (usually with codon 129 cis methionine) results in FFI. Most forms of fJCD usually present clinically and pathologically as an RPD similarly to sJCD. GSS usually presents as a more slowly progressive ataxic, parkinsonian disorder often with dementia somewhat later in the course. FFI usually begins with dysautonomia and insomnia; motor and cognitive dysfunction usually appear later in the disease course. These are described in greater detail below. Many cases with *PRNP* mutations that can present as either fJCD or GSS, such as many of the OPRI mutations (discussed below), have features that blend these two phenotypes. Most *PRNP* mutations result in a younger age of onset (typically 40s–60s) than sJCD (Kim et al., 2018; Mead, 2006). Typically, however, there is great variability in clinical presentation and disease course within a *PRNP* mutation; in fact, even within a gPrD family, there can be great clinical variability (Takada et al., 2017, 2018; Webb et al., 2008).

Several *PRNP* polymorphisms have been identified that affect one's risk for developing non-genetic forms of prion disease and may also affect the way genetic and non-genetic PrD present. The most important polymorphism is at codon 129, which can be either a methionine (M) or valine (V) see Figs. 94.2 and 94.7 and Table 94.2). Although many older studies suggest that codon 129 can affect the age of onset in many gPrD mutations, a very comprehensive study suggests that codon 129 does not have this effect (Minikel et al., 2016), but it often affects the rate of disease progression as shown in sJCD (Mead et al., 2016).

Regarding how *PRNP* variants lead to gPrD, it is presumed that a mutation results in a protein $PrP^{MUT}$ that is more susceptible to misfolding and changing conformation into the abnormally shaped, disease-causing form, $PrP^{Sc}$ (see above discussions for more about prion proteins $PrP^{C}$ and $PrP^{Sc}$) (van der Kamp & Daggett, 2010). Presumably the nascent $PrP^{MUT}$ maintains a normal conformation for most of a patient's life and does not begin transforming shape into $PrP^{Sc}$ until a patient gets older, which is why the disease usually does not occur until adulthood. Alternatively, and possibly more likely, some transformation of $PrP^{MUT}$ into $PrP^{Sc}$ occurs throughout life, with small amounts of $PrP^{Sc}$ being removed by normal cellular protein degradation pathways but, due to the aging process, the cellular pathways for clearing out misfolded proteins do not work as efficiently. The increasing accumulation of $PrP^{Sc}$ causes transformation of nascent $PrP^{MUT}$ and $PrP^{C}$ (from the normal *PRNP* allele) into $PrP^{Sc}$ in an exponential manner, resulting in disease (Kim et al., 2018; Kong et al., 2004; Prusiner, 1998) (see Fig. 94.1).

## Familial Jakob-Creutzfeldt Disease

More than 20 *PRNP* missense variants (P105T, G114V, R148H, D178N (with codon 129 cis V) V180I, T183A, T188A, T188K, T188R, T193I, K194E, E196A, E196K, E200K, E200G, V203I, R208H, V210I, E211Q, I215V, A224V, M232R, and P238S), an insertion, and octapeptide repeat insertions (OPRI) with four or fewer 24-base-pair repeats typically present as fJCD (although often there is a great phenotypic variability in OPRI variants). Most of these patients present similarly to sJCD, often with overlapping clinical, MRI, and EEG findings. The E200K variant, causing an fJCD presentation, is the most common pathogenic *PRNP* variant worldwide (Kim et al., 2018; Kong et al., 2004; Mead, 2006). Several other reported *PRNP* variants are shown above the PrP gene in Fig. 94.7.

## Gerstmann–Sträussler–Scheinker Disease

Gerstmann-Sträussler-Scheinker disease was first reported by Dimitz in 1913 (Dimitz, 1913), followed shortly after by Gerstmann in 1928 and 1936 (Gerstmann, 1928; Gerstmann et al., 1936). They described a dominantly inherited neurological illness that occurred in members of an Austrian family that presented initially with cerebellar ataxia followed by gait difficulty, speech and swallowing problems, nystagmus, pathological reflexes, and behavioral and cognitive changes (Dimitz, 1913; Gerstmann, 1928; Gerstmann et al., 1936). In 1980, Schlote et al. first introduced the name Gerstmann-Sträussler-Scheinker disease (GSS) based on the author names of early literature (Schlote et al., 1980). Subsequent neuropathological studies showed presence of prion amyloidosis, in which prions often form large uni- or multicentric prion amyloid plaques in the brain parenchyma and/or have a prion cerebral amyloid angiopathy (CAA), with or without coexisting spongiform changes (Schlote et al., 1980; Seitelberger, 1962, 1981). These large prion amyloid plaques were initially called "kuru plaques" and considered a nearly pathognomonic neuropathology feature that separates GSS from most other prion diseases. Nonetheless, these plaques are also seen in a minority of sJCD cases, albeit more sparsely (see Fig. 94.4) (Parchi et al., 1990b; Wadsworth et al., 2006), and differ from the florid plaques of variant JCD (Sikorska et al., 2008) (see later discussion and Fig. 94.4). As the common pathological feature is PrP amyloid deposition, some experts adopted the umbrella term "dominantly inherited PrP cerebral amyloidosis" to describe various clinical syndromes that have autosomal dominant *PRNP* mutations and PrP amyloid plaques in the brain (Ghetti et al., 2018). Typically, these patients present as GSS clinical syndrome, which is commonly described as subacute progressive ataxia, parkinsonism, and behavioral changes, followed by cognitive impairment at the later stages, similar to that described by Gerstmann et al. (Ghetti et al., 2018). Some patients with dominantly inherited PrP cerebral amyloidosis, however, can present with psychosis and cognitive decline or even syndromes mimicking Alzheimer disease (AD) or FTD. The age of clinical symptom onset ranges widely, from the teens to the seventies (Ghetti et al., 2018).

In 1989, three *PRNP* variants P102L (Hsiao et al., 1989) and two ORF insertions (Collinge et al., 1989; Owen et al., 1989) were identified in three families with GSS. Since then, at least 24 *PRNP* mutations have been shown to cause dominantly inherited PrP cerebral amyloidosis, including 19 missense mutations (P84S, P102L, P105L, P105S, P105T, A117V, G131V, S132I, A133V, R136S, V176G, H187R, F198S, D202N, E211D, Q212P, Q217R, Y218N, and M232T), at least five stop codon mutations (Y145X, Q160X, Y163X, Y226X, and Q227X; see below) and several OPRIs (see Fig. 94.7) (Ghetti et al., 2018; Jansen et al., 2010, 2011; Kim et al., 2018; Kong et al., 2004). OPRI mutations with a higher number of repeats typically present as GSS, but there are many exceptions and considerable phenotypic variability within and between OPRI mutations and even within OPRI families (OPRIs discussed in more detail below) (Giovagnoli et al., 2008; Kim et al., 2018; Kong et al., 2004; Mead et al., 2006). Although stop codon mutations are prion amyloidoses and have some overlapping features with GSS, they are distinct and, thus, are discussed in a separate section below. Most reports suggest that the *PRNP* codon 129 polymorphism modifies the clinical phenotype and neuropathological features of dominantly inherited PrP cerebral amyloidosis, which make it important to consider codon 129 genotype in combination with *PRNP* mutations (Collinge, 2001; Dlouhy et al., 1992; Furukawa et al., 1995; Ghetti et al., 2018). Most dominant inherited PrP cerebral amyloidosis have longer disease duration than sJCD or many other gPrDs, ranging from a few months to 15 years or more (Kim et al., 2018). Thus, these patients sometimes are incorrectly diagnosed with other neurodegenerative conditions, such as multiple system atrophy (MSA), spinocerebellar ataxias, idiopathic PD, AD, or even Huntington disease (see Table 94.1) (Collinge et al., 1992; Kim et al., 2018). Less commonly, patients with mutations typically associated with GSS can have an fJCD-like presentation (similar to typical sJCD), with a rapidly progressive course leading to death within a few months from onset (Liberski, 2012). GSS generally has a distinct neuropathology from most other prion diseases, with large $PrP^{Sc}$ amyloid plaques called *kuru plaques*. These plaques also are seen in a minority of sJCD cases, albeit more sparsely (see Fig. 94.4) (Parchi et al., 1999b; Wadsworth et al., 2006), but differ from the florid plaques of variant JCD (Sikorska et al., 2008) (see later discussion and Fig. 94.4). The amyloid deposits seen in GSS contain fragments of $PrP^{Sc}$ (see Fig. 94.2). Because of the large deposits of prion amyloid in GSS, it might be possible to detect these pathological changes noninvasively prior to clinical onset through the use of amyloid-binding agents such as 2-(1-(6-[(2-[$^{18}$F] fluoroethyl) (methyl) amino]-2-naphthyl) ethylidene) malononitrile ([$^{18}$F]FDDNP) and PET scans (Kepe et al., 2010).

### Fatal Familial Insomnia

FFI usually starts with progressively worsening insomnia and dysautonomia. Autonomic symptoms often include tachycardia, hyperhidrosis, and hyperpyrexia. Progressive insomnia is often accompanied by disruption of circadian rhythm and is eventually associated with hallucinations. Importantly, insomnia is not unique to FFI; many other prion diseases, including sJCD, also can have early and/or prominent insomnia. Cognitive and motor deficits typically develop later in the disease course. FFI is caused by a single *PRNP* missense variant, D178N, usually with codon 129 M on the same chromosome (cis) (see Fig. 94.7). Persons with D178N but cis codon 129 V usually present with fJCD, not FFI. Age of onset is similar to sJCD, but most FFI patients survive slightly longer, about 18 months. Although brain MRI, including diffusion imaging, is usually normal, fluorodeoxyglucose (FDG)-PET imaging reveals thalamic and cingulate hypometabolism, often even before disease onset (Cortelli et al., 2006). Neuropathology of FFI includes profound thalamic gliosis and neuronal loss causing atrophy. Involvement of regions outside of the thalamus is greater in FFI with codon 129 MV than with MM (Budka, 2003; Cortelli et al., 2006, 2007).

## Octopeptide Repeat Insertions

The prion protein is normally composed of 253 amino acids. In the N-terminal domain, there is an unstable repeat region consisting of a nonapeptide repeat (Pro-Gln-Gly-Gly-Gly-Gly-Trp-Gly-Gln), termed R1, followed by four nearly identical octapeptide repeats (Pro-His-Gly-Gly-Gly-Trp-Gly-Gln). Some of the octapeptide repeats, however, have slightly different nucleotide sequences, and thus are termed R2, R3, and R4 to differentiate them (Hansen et al., 2011). Insertions of two or more octapeptides (OPRIs) and a deletion of two octapeptides (OPRD) have been associated with gPrD (Capellari et al., 2002; Kim et al., 2018; Takada et al., 2017). Two functional studies suggest that OPRIs, unlike other *PRNP* pathogenic variants, do not necessarily lead to protein conformational change, but rather result in $PrP^{C}$ that is more protease resistant and prone to aggregation, which in turn facilitates the formation of $PrP^{Sc}$ (Moore et al., 2006; Priola & Chesebro, 1998). Literature suggests that individuals with one to four additional OPRIs often present clinically as sJCD and tend to have a mid-late adulthood age of onset and short clinical course. In contrast, individuals with five to seven OPRIs first manifest symptoms around their early to mid-adulthood with more variable presentations and lengthier disease course (Croes et al., 2004; Kim et al., 2018). Those with eight or more additional octapeptide repeats more commonly manifest as a GSS phenotype (Gambetti et al., 2003). As with many other gPrDs, particularly those causing GSS or other slower forms of PrD, OPRIs rarely show typical sJCD findings on EEG, MRI, or CSF surrogate biomarkers (e.g., 14-3-3, NSE and total tau) (Kim et al., 2018; Takada et al., 2017).

### *PRNP* Nonsense Mutations

Pathogenic *PRNP* nonsense variants (stop codons) are very rare, and only a few families have been reported. Reported pathogenic nonsense variants (stop codons) occur at the C terminal of $PrP^{C}$ at codon 145 or higher and cause premature translational cessation, resulting in a truncated protein (Guerreiro et al., 2014; Minikel et al., 2016). Nonsense variants tend to present quite differently than other *PRNP* mutations. They often have relatively early onset (20s–50s) with long disease durations, ranging from 1 year to more than 3 decades. Early cognitive impairment and personality changes are common, and patients with nonsense variants can have phenotypes resembling AD or FTD. Other common early features include chronic diarrhea, other gastrointestinal upset, dysautonomia, and/or sensory neuropathy (Fong et al., 2017; Ghetti et al., 1996; Jayadev et al., 2011; Kim et al., 2018; Mead et al., 2013; Takada et al., 2017). It is not known if these stop codon variants are fully penetrant, but there have been cases in which parent carriers of symptomatic children are asymptomatic (Fong et al., 2017). Based on the available limited data, codon 129 in PRNP does not appear to play a role in age of onset (Kim et al., 2018). Interestingly, on autopsy, most of the reported cases were found to have $PrP^{Sc}$-amyloid plaques, $PrP^{Sc}$ amyloid angiopathy, and tau containing neurofibrillary tangles (Finckh et al., 2000a, 2000b; Ghetti et al., 1996; Jansen et al., 2010; Mead et al., 2013; Owen et al., 1989), suggesting a link between prionopathies and tauopathies.

### Conclusions Regarding gPrD

Confirmation of a known pathogenic *PRNP* variant in a patient with neurological symptoms consistent with the known presentation of a known clinical syndrome (e.g., fJCD, GSS, or FFI) generally is sufficient for diagnosis of gPrD. Pathology of gPrDs can aid in the diagnosis, but pathology alone often is insufficient for ascertaining that the diagnosis is definitively of a genetic etiology. GSS and FFI have rather distinct pathologies, but testing for a *PRNP* mutation after appropriate genetic counseling is important, particularly because many gPrD cases do not have a clearly positive family history and/or appear clinically similar to sJCD (Goldman et al., 2004).

## Acquired Prion Disease

### Background on Acquired Prion Diseases

Acquired forms of prion disease occur because of the transmissibility of prions (Brown et al., 1994). Although considered infectious, prion diseases are not as easy to transmit as many other infectious diseases such as respiratory-transmitted pathogens (e.g., certain viruses or *Mycobacterium tuberculosis*) or through exposure to bodily fluids (e.g., human immunodeficiency virus [HIV] and hepatitis). A relatively large amount of prions (probably several thousand proteins) are necessary to transmit prion disease. Thus, human prion diseases are not contagious; physical contact and even intimacy are not known to transmit prions between persons. Acquired prion diseases include kuru (now essentially extinct but at one time occurring among the Fore tribe in Papua New Guinea as a result of endocannibalism), iatrogenic JCD (iJCD), and the highly publicized variant JCD (vJCD), occurring primarily in the United Kingdom and France and caused by consumption of beef contaminated with bovine spongiform encephalopathy (BSE, or mad cow disease) (Collinge et al., 2006; Will, 2003; Will et al., 2000). Kuru, one of the first identified forms of transmitted human prion disease, is a neurodegenerative disease of the Fore ethnic group of the central highlands of Papua New Guinea. In the Fore language, *kuru* means "to shake or tremble." It was transmitted through a practice in which deceased relatives were honored by ritualized endocannibalism. Although it is not known how this disease began, it was presumably through cannibalism of a person with sJCD. Because women and children consumed the less-desirable tissues, including brain and spinal cord, which contained higher levels of prions, they were more likely than adult males to contract prion disease (Gajdusek et al., 1996). The disease was essentially eliminated with the cessation of ritual cannibalism several decades ago; rare cases have occurred recently, however, suggesting an incubation period as long as 50 years or more (Collinge et al., 2006), particularly in those who are heterozygous at codon 129 in *PRNP*. The fact that heterozygotes have longer incubation periods could suggest a similar phenomenon might occur with vJCD (see later discussion). Genetic risk factors, and more recently protective alleles, have been identified in the Fore population (Mead et al., 2009).

### Iatrogenic PrD

Approximately 400 cases of iJCD have occurred from the use of cadaveric-derived human pituitary hormones, dura mater grafts, corneal transplants, reuse of cleaned and sterilized EEG depth electrodes implanted directly into the brain, other neurosurgical equipment, and blood transfusion (Aarsland et al., 2005; Brown et al., 2000, 2006, 2012; Tullo et al., 2006; Will, 2003) (Table 94.5). Because the prion is a protein, not a virus or bacterium, it is not susceptible to typical decontamination methods that would inactivate such microorganisms (see Prion Decontamination) (Bellinger-Kawahara et al., 1987a, 1987b; Prusiner, 1998). This difficulty in inactivating prions has, in part, led to transmission of prion disease between patients. Most of the pituitary-derived (mostly human grown hormone and some gonadotrophin) cases occurred from contaminated batches in France, the United Kingdom, and the United States. As of 2012, 226 cases related to human growth hormone and four cases from gonadotrophins had been reported (Brown et al., 2012), but cases with long incubation periods continue to develop from exposures decades ago (Maddox et al., 2020). These patients typically present with a cerebellar dysfunction (Appleby et al., 2013; Brown et al., 2012). Methods have since been instituted to prevent prion transmission through such hormones (Brown et al., 2006). In the United States, pituitary hormone recipient patients exposed to JCD were informed of their potential risk for developing prion disease, whereas this was not always the case in other countries. As of 2012, the incubation period was estimated to be a mean of 17 years, which varies between countries, with a range of 5–42 years (Brown et al., 2012).

As of 2013, 228 cases of iJCD have been linked to exposure to contaminated batches of dura mater (mostly Lyodura brand), with a majority (154 as of 2017) of cases occurring in Japan (Ae et al., 2018; Brown et al., 2012). These exposures stopped after 1987, the year when a sodium hydroxide disinfection step was added to the processing protocol (Brown et al., 2000; Brown et al., 2006; Brown et al., 2012). New cases from remote past exposure continue to be

**TABLE 94.5 Iatrogenic Jakob-Creutzfeldt Disease Cases Through July 2017**

| Transmission Source | Case Number | Countries Reported Cases | Mean Incubation Period in Years (Range) | Clinical Signs | References |
|---|---|---|---|---|---|
| Growth hormone | 238 | Majority in France, United Kingdom and United States | 17 (5–24) | Cerebellar | Bonda et al. (2016), Brown et al. (2013), UK National CJD Surveillance Unit (2018) |
| Gonadotrophins hormone | 4 | Australia | 13.5 (12–16) | Cerebellar | Cochius et al, (1990, 1992), Healy and Evans (1993) |
| Dura mater grafts | 238 | Japan, France, Germany, Spain, United Kingdom, Australia, Canada, Italy, and United States in descending order | 12 (1.3–30) | Cerebellar, visual, dementia | Bonda et al. (2016), Centers Disease Control (CDC, 1987) |
| Corneal transplant | 2 | United States, Germany | 15.75 (1.5–30) | Dementia, cerebellar | Hammersmith et al. (2004), Heckmann et al. (1997), Maddox et al. (2008) |
| Neurosurgical instruments | 4 | United Kingdom and France | 1.6 (1.4–2.2) | Visual, dementia, cerebellar | el Hachimi et al. (1997), Will and Matthews (1982) |
| Brain depth electrodes | 2 | Switzerland | 1.5 (1.3–1.7) | Dementia, cerebellar | Bonda et al. (2016), Brown et al. (2000) |
| Packed red blood cells | 3* | United Kingdom | 7.53 (6.5–8.3) | Psychiatric, sensory, dementia, cerebellar | Llewelyn et al. (2004), Peden et al. (2004), Wroe et al. (2006) |

*This does not include the two asymptomatic vJCD cases (Brown et al., 2000; Collins et al., 2006; Garske and Ghani, 2010; Knight, 2010, 2017; Parchi et al., 1999; Peden et al., 2004, 2010).

*Data adapted from Brown, P., Brandel, J.P., Sato, T., Nakamura, Y., MacKenzie, J., Will, R.G., et al., 2012. Iatrogenic Creutzfeldt-Jakob disease, final assessment. Emerg. Infect. Dis. 18 (6), 901–907. https://doi.org/10.3201/eid1806.120116 and Bonda, D.J., Manjila, S., Mehndiratta, P., Khan, F., Miller, B.R., Onwuzulike, K., et al., 2016. Human prion diseases: surgical lessons learned from iatrogenic prion transmission. Neurosurg. Focus. 41 (1), E10. https://doi.org/10.3171/2016.5.FOCUS15126; Table published with permission from Tee, B.L., Longoria Ibarrola, E.M., Geschwind, M.D., et al., 2018. Prion disease. Neurol. Clin. 36 (4), 865–897.*

identified worldwide, however (Iwasaki et al., 2018; Van Iseghem et al., 2019). Symptoms typically include dementia with cerebellar and visual dysfunction. The mean incubation period is about 12 years, with a range of 1.3 to at least 30 years (Ae et al., 2018; Brown et al., 2012; Van Iseghem et al., 2019).

Six iJCD cases have been linked to neurosurgical procedures (including two EEG depth electrodes) and at least two to corneal implants (Brown et al., 2012). A few other cases might have occurred through neurosurgical or other surgical procedures, but in such cases it is often difficult to determine whether a case is iatrogenic or sporadic (Brown et al., 2006). Although it appears that the number of iJCD cases is declining, prion contamination still occurs, despite World Health Organization (WHO) and other recommended practices for managing potential prion-contaminated tissues, leaving patients at risk for iJCD.

Improved identification of prion disease should help prevent future iJCD cases, but cases will likely be missed by screening, and, thus, strict application of efficient decontamination procedures is still critical to prevent transmission. Unfortunately, the true risk of iJCD is still unknown; many of the decontamination procedures tested were based on models using animal prions, which appear easier to decontaminate than human prions (Peretz et al., 2006). Rather than trying to decontaminate neurosurgical equipment used during surgery on potential or suspected prion subjects, some medical centers dispose of all such equipment through incineration rather than take the risk of reusing it (UCSF Medical Center, 2012). The most recently identified form of iJCD has been the transmission of vJCD through blood products (Ironside, 2012) (see next section).

### Variant Jakob-Creutzfeldt Disease

Perhaps the most notorious form human PrD is variant JCD, first identified in 1995 (Will et al., 1996). There is strong epidemiological and experimental evidence that it is caused by inadvertent ingestion of beef contaminated with BSE (mad cow disease) or, in a few cases, blood or blood product transfusion from asymptomatic carriers of vJCD (Diack et al., 2014; Ironside, 2012; Knight, 2017; Zou et al., 2008). It is believed that BSE occurred through the practice of feeding scrapie-infected sheep products to cattle (Bruce et al., 1997; Scott et al., 1999; Wilesmith et al., 1988). In general, vJCD differs from sJCD in several ways. Patients with vJCD generally are much younger, with a median age of around 27 (range 12–74) and almost all cases have occurred in persons younger than age 50. The mean disease duration is longer, about 14.5 months, versus about 7 months for sJCD. As of 2017, 231 cases had been identified worldwide (Knight, 2017). Although psychiatric symptoms often occur early in sJCD (Rabinovici et al., 2006; Wall et al., 2005), in vJCD profound psychiatric symptoms are often the initial symptoms for several months before obvious neurological symptoms begin. A relatively unique symptom in vJCD is persistent painful paresthesias in various parts of the body. The EEG only rarely shows the classic PSWCs and then only at the end stage of disease (Binelli et al., 2006). Brain MRI often shows the "pulvinar sign," in which the pulvinar (posterior thalamus) is brighter than the anterior putamen on T2-weighted or DWI MRI (Collie et al., 2003) (see Fig. 94.6); this finding is rare in other human prion diseases (Haik et al., 2002; Martindale et al., 2003; Petzold et al., 2004; Zeidler et al., 2000). Diagnostic criteria for probable vJCD are shown in Table 94.6 (Heath et al., 2010). Although several features of vJCD overlap those of sJCD, vJCD's younger age of onset, MRI findings, prominent early psychiatric features, persistent painful sensory symptoms, and movement disorder such as chorea might help differentiate these conditions.

Definitive diagnosis of vJCD is based on neuropathological evidence of the variant form of $PrP^{Sc}$ in brain biopsy or autopsy. Because vJCD is typically acquired peripherally, $PrP^{Sc}$ can be found in the lymphoreticular system, including tonsillar tissue (Will, 2004). Brain pathology of vJCD typically shows abundant $PrP^{Sc}$ deposition; multiple fibrillary PrP plaques surrounded by a halo of spongiform vacuoles, often referred to as "florid" plaques; other PrP plaques; and amorphous pericellular and perivascular PrP deposits, which are especially prominent in the cerebellar molecular layer. The florid plaques are called such because they have the appearance of a flower with a dense center and surrounding ring of vacuoles, and are considered pathognomonic for vJCD (Budka, 2003) (see Fig. 94.4). The Western blot characteristics of vJCD $PrP^{Sc}$ also differ from those seen in other forms of prion disease; in vJCD, they are called type 2B, which have a 19-kD unglycosylated (lower) band and a prominent diglycosylated (upper) band (Ironside, 2012; Will, 2004; Will et al., 2000).

As of July 1, 2019, 228 probable or definite cases of vJCD had been documented, almost all in the United Kingdom (U.K.) (UK National CJD Research & Surveillance Unit, 2019). France has the

**TABLE 94.6 Current Diagnostic Criteria for Variant Creutzfeldt-Jakob Disease**

| |
|---|
| Definite: IA and neuropathological confirmation of vJCD* |
| Probable: I and 4/5 of II and IIIA and IIIB; or I and IV |
| Possible: I and 4/5 of II and IIIA |
| I |
| Progressive neuropsychiatric disorder |
| Duration of illness > 6 months |
| Routine investigations do not suggest an alternative diagnosis |
| No history of potential iatrogenic exposure |
| No evidence of a familial form of TSE |
| II |
| Early psychiatric features† |
| Persistent painful sensory symptoms‡ |
| Ataxia |
| Myoclonus or chorea or dystonia |
| Dementia |
| III |
| EEG does not show the typical appearance of sporadic JCD§ in the early stages of illness |
| Bilateral pulvinar high signal on MRI scan |
| IV |
| Positive tonsil biopsy¶ |

*Spongiform change and extensive prion protein deposition with florid plaques throughout the cerebrum and cerebellum.
†Depression, anxiety, apathy, withdrawal, delusions.
‡Includes frank pain and/or dysesthesias.
§The typical appearance of the EEG in sporadic JCD consists of generalized triphasic periodic complexes at approximately 1 per second. These may occasionally be seen in the late stages of vJCD.
¶Tonsil biopsy is not recommended routinely nor in cases with EEG appearances typical of sporadic JCD but may be useful in suspect cases in which the clinical features are compatible with vJCD and MRI does not show bilateral pulvinar high signal.
*EEG*, Electroencephalography; *MRI*, magnetic resonance imaging; *TSE*, transmissible spongiform encephalopathy; *vJCD*, variant Jakob-Creutzfeldt disease.
*Modified from Heath, C.A., Cooper, S.A., Murray, K., Lowman, A., Henry, C., MacLeod, M.A., Will, R.G., 2010. Validation of diagnostic criteria for variant Creutzfeldt-Jakob disease. Ann. Neurol. 67 (6), 761–770.*

second highest number of vJCD cases ($n = 27$), which probably have the same origin as those in the U.K. (Brandel et al., 2009). No cases of vJCD are thought to have been acquired in the Western Hemisphere; the six vJCD cases identified in North America—four patients in the United States and two in Canada are believed to have acquired it elsewhere (Coulthart et al., 2016; Maheshwari et al., 2015; UK National CJD Research & Surveillance Unit, 2019). Three of the North American cases were born and raised in the Saudi Arabia and are believed to have been exposed to BSE-contaminated beef there (Coulthart et al., 2016). The peak of the vJCD epidemic was in 2000, although it is not known whether other peaks will occur, particularly in persons with different genetic susceptibility to vJCD or iatrogenically through blood products (Andrews, 2010). A few studies have assessed the presence of latent vJCD in the UK and found it to be much higher than expected. In the first large study, researchers found vJCD prions by immunostaining in 3 of 11,246 appendix samples collected from 1995 to 2000, for an incidence of about one in 4,000. Another similar study, the National Anonymous Tonsil Archive, found one positive sample among a subset of 9,160 tested (de Marco et al., 2010; Garske & Ghani, 2010). A larger and more definitive follow-up study analyzing 32,441 anonymized appendix samples found an incidence of about 1 in 2000, double the previous estimate. About half of these positive appendix cases were homozygous for valine or heterozygotes at codon 129 in *PRNP*, unlike most affected vJCD cases who are methionine homozygous (Gill et al., 2013). Thus, it is estimated that as many as 1 in 2000 persons in the UK population are asymptomatic carriers with vJCD prions in their lymphoreticular system (subclinically infected). For these carriers, it is not clear if they will ever develop vJCD or if and when they will be infectious and passing it on to others, such as through medical/surgical procedures or blood products (Salmon, 2013). As of 2019, four patients had acquired vJCD infection through non-leukodepleted (WBCs removed) blood transfusions received before 1999; three patients (all codon 129 MM) had probable or definite vJCD, with incubation periods of about 6–8.5 years (Health Protection Agency, 2007; Llewelyn et al., 2004; Wroe et al., 2006). The fourth patient (heterozygous, MV, at codon 129) died from non-neurological causes five years after receiving a contaminated blood transfusion but at autopsy was found to have prions in his lymphoreticular system (Peden et al., 2004). Lastly, a 73-year-old male patient with hemophilia and no history of neurological disease, who was heterozygous (methionine/valine) at codon 129 and had received more than 9000 units of factor VIII concentrate prepared from plasma pools known to include donations from a vJCD-infected donor, was found at autopsy to have vJCD prions in his spleen (Peden et al., 2010). It is not known whether these latter two pre-clinical patients would have ever developed vJCD through spread to the brain or would have simply survived as carriers and possible reservoirs for vJCD (Garske & Ghani, 2010). A graph of presumed vJCD cases in the U.K. is shown in Fig. 94.8. As Fig. 94.8 shows, the number of cases has been very low over the past several years—at five or fewer per year, with the last death UK in 2016, in the U.K. There is great concern that, however, future cases of vJCD might occur iatrogenically through transfusion of blood products or because many exposed persons, particularly with codon 129 MV or VV polymorphism, might have longer incubation times. These asymptomatic carriers of vJCD might pose the greatest risk for spread of vJCD through transfusion of blood products or invasive procedures. Of great concern is that infected asymptomatic vJCD donors, who eventually became symptomatic, had transmitted the disease about 1.5–3.5 years before they became symptomatic (Health Protection Agency, 2007).

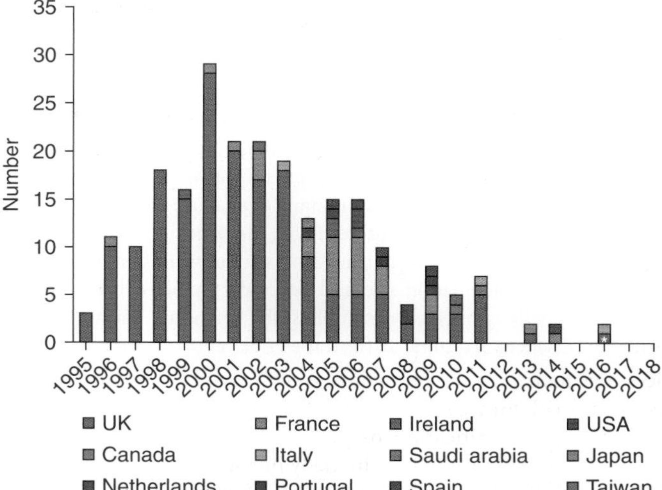


**Fig. 94.8** Incidence of Death Due To Variant Creutzfeldt-Jakob Disease *(vCJD)* Worldwide Between the Years 1995 and 2018. vCJD cases ($n = 231$) are color coded by the countries that diagnosed and reported cases. Not all cases contracted disease in the same country in which they were diagnosed and/or died (see text). (*Courtesy National CJD Surveillance Unit, Edinburgh,* UK.) Note, vCJD = vJCD.

## Prion Properties of Other Neurodegenerative Diseases

Numerous neurodegenerative diseases—including Alzheimer disease (AD), MSA, Parkinson disease (PD), dementia with Lewy bodies (DLB), FTD, ALS, and Huntington disease (HD)—have been described to exhibit prion-like features (Krejciova et al., 2019; Scheckel & Aguzzi, 2018). This is because the pathogenic proteins of these neurodegenerative diseases—specifically Aβ-amyloid, tau, synuclein, TDP 43, and huntingtin—tend to exist in the form of aggregated oligomeric or polymeric proteins that are folded into β-sheet structure and stacked into amyloid fibrils (Annus et al., 2016; Prusiner, 1998). As in prion diseases, these amyloid-like misfolded proteins are resistant to proteolysis, aggregate in the brain, and spread in a predictable pattern (Braak et al., 2003, 2006; Brettschneider et al., 2013), which is why these neurodegenerative diseases are sometimes referred as protein misfolding diseases (Knowles et al., 2014).

The idea that other neurodegenerative diseases might spread in the brain in a manner similar to prions was further supported when it was shown that α-synuclein pathology was found at autopsy in the healthy fetal graft tissue implanted into brains of patients with PD 11–16 years after dopaminergic neuron transplantation (Kordower et al, 2008a, 2008b). Since then, many in vitro and in vivo studies noted the presence of seeding properties and transcellular spreading abilities in Aβ amyloid, tau, synuclein, TDP 43, and huntingtin proteins (Clavaguera et al, 2013a. 2013b; Frost & Diamond, 2009, 2010; Frost et al., 2009a, 2009b; Hansen et al., 2011; Hasegawa et al., 2017; Holmes et al., 2013; Jeon et al., 2016; Jucker & Walker, 2013; Lasagna-Reeves et al., 2012; Luk et al., 2012; Luks et al., 2009; Masnata et al., 2019; Munch et al., 2011; Olsson et al., 2018; Sanders et al., 2014; Watts et al., 2013). For example, when inoculated intracerebrally and intraperitoneally with brain extracts from Alzheimer disease individuals, transgenic mice that express human amyloid precursor protein showed premature deposition of amyloid plaques and presence of CAA pathology (Eisele et al., 2009, 2010; Kane et al., 2000; Meyer-Luehmann et al., 2006). Injection of human AD brain homogenates into the dentate gyrus of mice successfully induced the aggregation of wild-type murine tau (Audouard et al., 2016). Furthermore, transgenic mice that harbor human α-synuclein transgene developed MSA symptoms and somewhat similar pathology when inoculated intracerebrally with brain homogenates of MSA patients (Prusiner et al., 2015; Watts et al., 2013). When studies re-examined brains of hGH iCJD cases in both UK and US cohorts, they found higher than expected frequency of vascular and gray matter amyloid β pathology. Given the young age of these cases, this caused concern of peripheral transmission of amyloid β pathology (Cali et al., 2018; Jaunmuktane et al., 2015; Jucker & Walker, 2015; Tousseyn et al., 2015). Interestingly, the depositions of these proteins in several of the above transmission studies were first found to be adjacent to the inoculation site and gradually involved brain regions that are axonally connected, resembling the spreading nature of prion proteins (Eisele et al., 2009, 2010; Kane et al., 2000; Meyer-Luehmann et al., 2006).

Despite possessing the molecular features of seeding, templating, misfolding, and transcellular spreading similar to prion protein, these protein aggregates have yet to be found to show any direct evidence of infectivity between hosts; thus, in the opinion of some, separating themselves from $PrP^{Sc}$. Various terms have been used to describe these other neurodegenerative diseases that display templated misfolding of proteins spreading in the brain, including "prionoid," "prion-like," and even simply considering them all prion diseases (Aoyagi et al., 2019; Prusiner, 2012; Scheckel & Aguzzi, 2018). There are a few arguments used to support the terminology "prion" diseases for all of these prion-like disorders. First, despite the definition of "prion" includes the term "infectious," fewer than 1% of classic PrP prion disease cases are actually infectious, in that they occurred through transmission; more than 99% are sporadic or genetic (Prusiner, 1998). Second, when first identified, viruses were referred to by many different terms because of the great diversity of shapes, sizes, and other characteristics; yet now, the term "viruses" applies to many small infectious agents that replicate only inside the living cells of an organism. Nevertheless, many in the field do not wish to call other prion-like neurodegenerative diseases "prion" diseases because of the implication that they are as infectious or transmissible as PrP prion diseases, which, among other issues, might make it difficult for patients to get standard invasive medical procedures due to infection control concerns. The debate on this nomenclature continues.

### Prion Decontamination

Decontamination of prions requires methods that will denature proteins, as prions resist normal inactivation methods used to kill viruses and bacteria. Typical methods for reducing the load of or inactivating prions include prolonged moist autoclaving at higher-than-normal temperatures and pressure, with or without denaturing agents (many of which are caustic). Unfortunately, recommended methods for prion decontamination that include very high temperatures with steam and caustic denaturing agents often damage equipment and instrumentation. WHO guidelines state the preferred method is steam sterilization for at least 30 minutes at 132°C in a gravity-displacement sterilizer. If a pre-vacuum sterilizer is used, they note that 18 minutes at 134°C is also effective. Another option is 1N sodium hydroxide or 2% sodium hypochlorite for 1 hour, with 134°C autoclaving for at least 18 minutes. Non-fragile items may be immersed in 1N sodium hydroxide, a caustic solution, for 1 hour at room temperature and then steam-sterilized for 30 minutes at 121°C (Condello et al., 2018; WHO, 2006). Unfortunately, most of the literature on prion infection control is based on non-human prions and using prion-infected brain homogenate, both of which have critical shortcomings. Certain strains of prions, including human prions, are much more difficult to denature than many prions (e.g., mouse or hamster) that have been tested in decontamination experiments. Furthermore, many disinfection studies used prion-infected brain homogenate, which is much easier to decontaminate than using small stainless steel wires incubated overnight in prion-infected brain homogenate, which also more closely approximates prions binding to steel surgical equipment. The steel-wire method is an important model because prions bind readily to metal and, thus, become more difficult to remove and denature (Condello et al., 2018; Peretz et al., 2006). Because of the risk of transmission to subsequent patients, when financially feasible, some hospitals dispose of neurosurgical and other surgical equipment potentially exposed to prions (usually by incineration) rather than attempting to decontaminate the equipment for future patient use. Particularly for instruments of intricate design or for which the complete removal of protein cannot be assured, single-use instruments are recommended when possible. Research into improved methods of decontamination of prions is ongoing (Condello et al., 2018; Ward et al., 2018).

### Animal Prion Diseases

The first known animal prion disease, scrapie, which occurs in sheep and goats, was first described more than 150 years ago. This disease was so named because the sick animals would scrape their skin by rubbing against fences or other objects, probably because of itching. Owing to a phenomenon called the *species barrier*, scrapie is not directly transmissible to humans. Species barriers prevent or reduce transmission of prions from one species to another, and animal models of prion disease support the idea that scrapie prions do not directly pass to humans (Igel-Egalon et al., 2018). Furthermore, there appear to be no differences in the incidence of human prion disease between countries that have little or no scrapie and those where scrapie is endemic.

Unfortunately, in the mid-1980s an outbreak of BSE occurred in the United Kingdom because scrapie-contaminated material was being fed to cattle (Houston & Andreoletti, 2018). Cattle with BSE develop an ataxic illness, weight loss, behavioral changes, and other neurological symptoms progressing to death. More than 280,000 cattle suffered from BSE. Initially, cases were only identified in the United Kingdom, but eventually cases were identified in other countries as well. When cases were identified, entire herds were killed to prevent the disease from spreading further. Fortunately, through proper epidemiological control, including feed bans and cessation of various feeding practices, the incidence of BSE has dropped dramatically now, with only a few, if any, cases occurring each year, some of which might be sporadic cases. Tragically, even though scrapie prions do not pass directly to humans, they were able to overcome the species barrier with humans by passing through cattle. Ingestion of BSE prions unfortunately led to vJCD in the United Kingdom and several other countries (see earlier discussion). The temporal relationship between the BSE epidemic and the rise of vJCD, coupled with data in mice showing the similarity between these conditions, are strong evidence for the link between these two diseases (Bruce et al., 1997; Houston & Andreoletti, 2018; Scott et al., 1999). As of December, 31, 2016, 24 isolated cases of BSE had been reported in North America (three in the United States and 21 in Canada) (Fig. 94.9) (World Organisation for Animal Health—OiE, 2019). Thus, it does not appear that there has been another outbreak, although it is possible that some cases are still getting into the food supply, as not all cattle are being inspected in most countries.

Chronic wasting disease (CWD) is a prion disease of mule deer, white-tailed deer, elk, and, more recently, moose. The first clinical cases were recognized in the late 1960s in Colorado, United States,

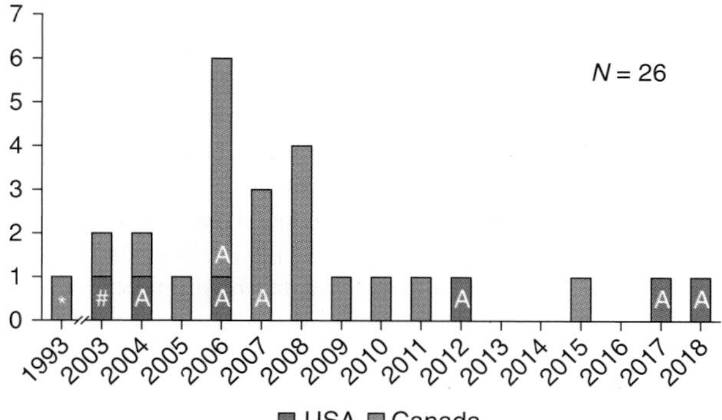


**Fig. 94.9 Bovine Spongiform Encephalopathy (BSE) in North America.** This figure illustrates the 26 BSE cases identified in North America, from 1993 through August 2018, of which 7 were atypical BSE cases and 19 were classic BSE cases. The only classic BSE case identified in the United States was imported from Canada. *(Courtesy Centers for Disease Control and Prevention. Available at: https://www.cdc.gov/prions/bse/bse-north-america.html.)*

but it was not recognized as a prion disease until 1980. Clinical features of the disease include weight loss, behavioral changes such as depression, and isolation from the herd. Some other features might also include hypersalivation, polydipsia/polyuria, and ataxia. The disease primarily has been reported in the United States and Canada, with the highest concentrations occurring in the Central Mountain region of the United States, especially Colorado and Montana, as well as the Canadian provinces of Saskatchewan and Alberta (Sigurdson, 2008; Williams, 2005). It has also been identified in South Korea, Finland, and Norway (Sigurdson et al., 2018). A map showing the distribution of CWD in North America is in Fig. 94.10. Most concerning aspect of CWD is its ease of horizontal transmission between cervids, which might be due, in part, to the fact that CWD appears to be transmissible through blood, urine, and saliva (Haley et al., 2009). This feature makes it very difficult to prevent spread of the disease in free-ranging cervid populations (Williams, 2005). It still is not clear whether CWD can spread to humans or whether there is a species barrier, but there has been no reported increase in human prion cases in states with the highest

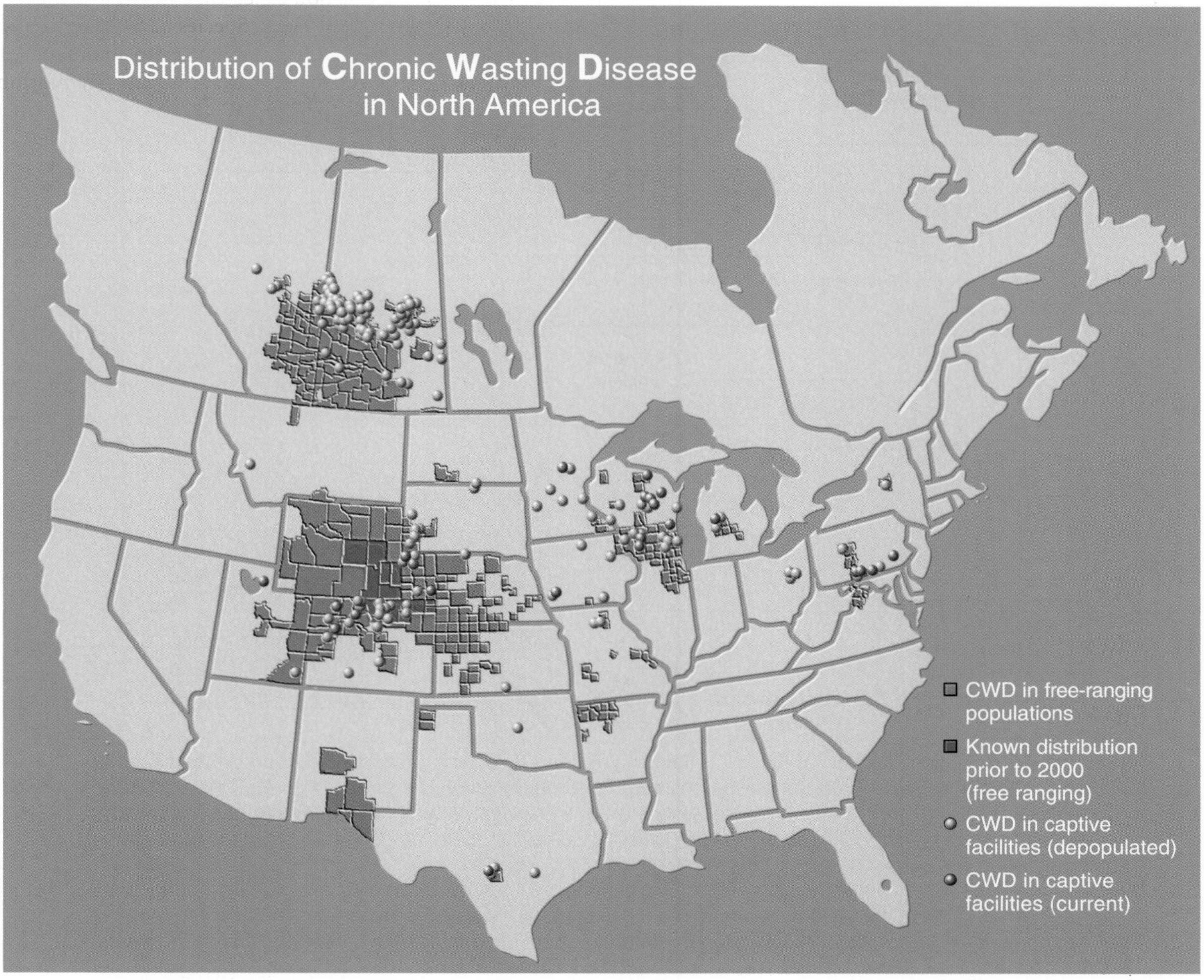

**Fig. 94.10 Distribution of Chronic Wasting Disease *(CWD)* in North America.** Figure shows the reported distribution of chronic wasting disease in North America as of April 1, 2018. (*Courtesy Bryan Richards, US Geological Service (USGS) National Wildlife Health Center. Public domain; https://www.usgs.gov/media/images/distribution-chronic-wasting-disease-north-america-april-2018.*)

rates of CWD (Sigurdson et al., 2009). Although it has been shown that CWD prions from brains on infected animals can be transmitted to squirrel monkeys by oral or intracerebral inoculation, at least two studies suggest they could not be transmitted to cymologous monkeys, which are closer genetically to humans than squirrel monkeys (Race et al., 2018). Of particular concern, an as-yet unpublished collaboration between Canadian and French scientists, presented at an international prion meeting, suggested that feeding some macaques meat from CWD animals resulted in transmission. To date, there have been no human cases of prion disease linked to CWD, although the Centers for Disease Control and Prevention (CDC) in the US is actively surveilling for new forms of human prion disease that might be linked to CWD.

## TREATMENT OF HUMAN PRION DISEASES

Currently, there is no known cure for human prion diseases; all cases are uniformly fatal. Some potential mechanisms for treating prion diseases are shown in Fig. 94.11. This include removing or reducing the endogenous substrate $PrP^C$, blocking the interaction of $PrP^C$ with $PrP^{Sc}$, removing $PrP^{Sc}$, and blocking its toxicity (Korth & Peters, 2006). Several medicines have been used to treat human prion disease, but only oral flupirtine, quinacrine, and doxycycline have been tested in randomized double-blinded placebo-controlled trials, and none were effective in prolonging survival in symptomatic patients (Geschwind, 2014; Geschwind et al., 2013; Haik et al., 2014; Korth & Peters, 2006; Stewart et al., 2008). Despite doxycycline not showing benefit in symptomatic patients (Haik et al., 2014), it is being tested in a decade-long, double-blinded study with 25 at-risk members (10 carriers and 15 non-carriers) of a single large Italian family with FFI to assess if it can delay onset in D178N/129M mutation carriers compared with historical controls; the study should be completed by 2023 (Forloni et al., 2015). Intraventricular pentosan polysulfate has been used on a compassionate basis in the United Kingdom, Japan, and a few other countries, but observational data suggest that it does not improve function. The fact that four of the five treated cases in the UK had significantly longer survival than untreated cases might suggest that the drug can prolong survival; it does not, however, appear to affect neuropathological damage or improve function (Newman et al., 2014). An antibody against $PrP^C$, PRN100, is being infused intravenously as an experimental treatment by the UK National Health Service to treat only UK patients with symptomatic prion disease. The first patient, with sJCD, began treatment in October 2018. The goal of this antibody is to block the contact of $PrP^{Sc}$ with $PrP^C$ and, thereby, prevent propagation of prions. As of May 2019, five patients had begun treatment, but the results have

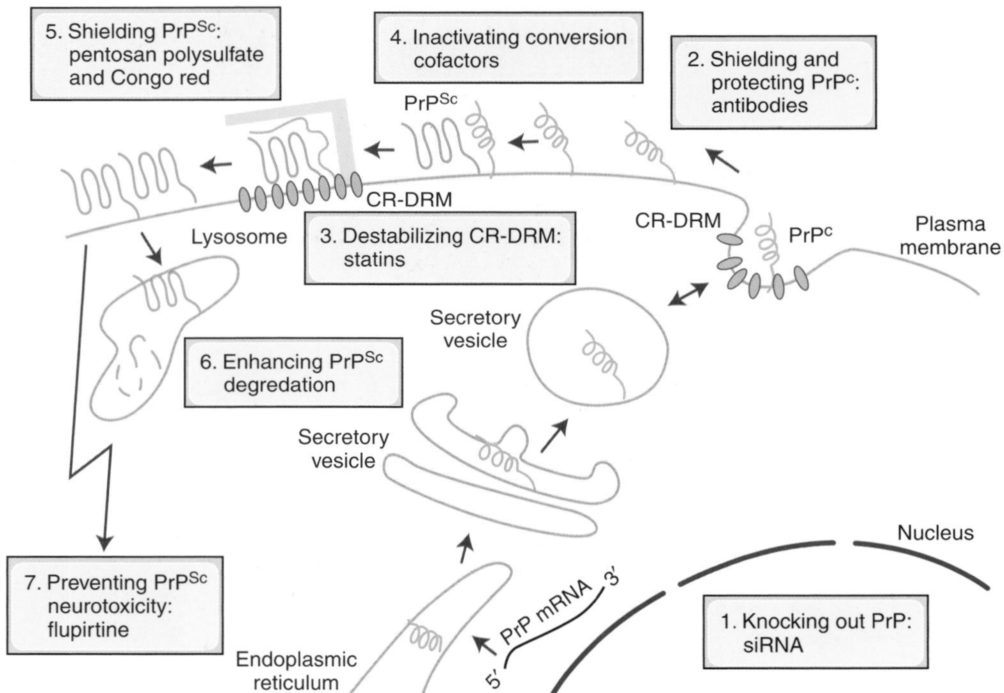


**Fig. 94.11** Schematic drawing of the life of the prion protein *(PrP)* inside the cell, its conversion to infectious prions, and cell biology-based possibilities of treatment intervention. The cellular PrP *($PrP^C$)* is *light blue*, and the scrapie PrP *($PrP^{Sc}$)* is *orange*. *Blue-filled ovals* within the plasma membrane are cholesterol-rich, detergent-resistant membrane domains *(CR-DRMs)*. The *light blue bar* represents a hypothesized conversion-assisting cofactor, sometimes referred to as protein X. For a more detailed explanation, see Korth and Peters (2006). *mRNA*, Messenger ribonucleic acid; *siRNA*, small interfering ribonucleic acid. Of note, for Step 2, attempts to treat human prion disease with antibodies targeting $PrP^C$ began in London under the Medical Research Council in October 2018 with five symptomatic patients treated with unreported results as of May 2019. Although not shown in this figure, as an addition to Step 1, as of 2019, antisense oligonucleotides (ASOs) are currently being used in clinical practice to treat spinal muscular atrophy (SMA), are being used in treatment trials for Huntington disease, and are actively being studied in animal models of prion disease. (*Modified from Korth, C., Peters, P.J., 2006. Emerging pharmacotherapies for Creutzfeldt-Jakob disease. Arch. Neurol. 63 [4], 497–501.*)

not been reported (Dyer, 2018; Klohn et al., 2012; Medical Research Council Prion Unit, 2019).

Several laboratories around the world are actively screening drug libraries and using medicinal chemistry to identify and develop anti-prion therapies (Lasmezas & Gabizon, 2018). One of the most promising potential treatments for PrDs is antisense oligonucleotides (ASOs), which are already being used for clinical treatment of spinobulbar muscular atrophy (SMA) in children (Finkel et al., 2017; Mercuri et al., 2018) and in trials for ALS and HD (Kordasiewicz et al., 2012; Ly & Miller, 2018; Rinaldi & Wood, 2017; Tabrizi et al., 2019a, 2019b). The goal of ASOs is to prevent specific proteins from being made; this is done by designing ASOs that bind to the mRNA of interest. When this occurs, the normally single-stranded mRNA becomes double-stranded, which the cell recognizes and degrades, preventing the protein of interest from being translated. ASOs can result in significant knock-down of brain mRNA, in ranges of about 15%–75% in animal models (Kordasiewicz et al., 2012; Rinaldi & Wood, 2017). When inoculated with prions, mice hemizygous for *Prnp* have significantly longer survival than wild-type mice (Bueler et al., 1994). This suggests that lowering $PrP^C$ might prolong survival of symptomatic disease as well as delay onset of pre-symptomatic or at-risk persons (i.e., *PRNP* mutation carriers or those exposed to prions via blood, surgery, or other methods). Supporting the notion that reduced levels of $PrP^C$ would be tolerated in humans is a large genomic data study that reported three individuals who remained healthy despite being hemizygous for *PRNP* (Minikel et al., 2016), suggesting that partial reduction of *PRNP* gene dosage can be tolerable. Treatment trials in HD have already demonstrated that intrathecally-delivered ASOs can reduce the level of mutant huntingtin protein in the CSF up to 42% (Tabrizi et al., 2019b). Although it is not yet known how much decrease of huntingtin level is occurring in the brain tissue of these patients with HD, this data is encouraging for the treatment of other proteinopathies, such as prion disease.

### Management of Prion Diseases

In the absence of any curative treatments, management of prion diseases involves treating symptoms as they arise and comfort care. Insofar as there are no approved drugs in any countries for treatment of prion disease, all medications are used off-label for symptomatic treatment. There are no data supporting the use of any medications, including those approved for certain dementias, such as AD and PD. At our center, we have managed hundreds of patients with prion disease and have empirically found certain medications to be helpful. For example, we commonly use selective serotonin reuptake inhibitors (SSRIs), such as escitalopram, to treat depression, anxiety, and mild agitation; atypical antipsychotics (particularly quetiapine as it is less likely to cause parkinsonism) to treat agitation and psychosis; and levetiracetam, clonazepam, or valproic acid to treat myoclonus. One study suggested valproic acid increases $PrP^C$ and $PrP^{Sc}$ in vitro but had no effect in an in vivo mouse model (Shaked et al., 2000), so one might consider avoiding use of this medicine when disease-modifying treatments become available. We, and others, have published recommendations on the care and ethical issues regarding managing patients with prion disease (Appleby & Yobs, 2018; Bechtel & Geschwind, 2013).

## DIFFERENTIAL DIAGNOSIS

Other conditions such as AD, Lewy body disease, Hashimoto encephalopathy, and hepatic encephalopathy rarely also have an EEG with PSWCs, typical of sJCD (Geschwind, 2016; Savard et al., 2016). Other rapidly progressive disorders to consider that might present similarly to JCD include paraneoplastic or other autoimmune limbic encephalopathies (Graus et al., 2016; Rosenbloom et al., 2009; Vernino et al., 2007), cancers (particularly lymphoma, either within or outside the nervous system), central nervous system vasculitis, metabolic or toxic disorders (e.g., bismuth intoxication, hepatic encephalopathy, electrolyte imbalance, etc.) (Geschwind, 2016; Rosenbloom et al., 2015), and atypical presentations of more common neurodegenerative conditions such as AD, Lewy body disease, and corticobasal degeneration (Drummond et al., 2017; Geschwind, 2016; Schmidt et al., 2012; Tartaglia et al., 2012).

*The complete reference list is available online at https://expertconsult.inkling.com/.* 

95

# Alzheimer Disease and Other Dementias

*Ronald C. Peterson, Jonathan Graff-Radford*

## OUTLINE



## NORMAL AGING AND MILD COGNITIVE IMPAIRMENT

### Normal Aging

A cognitive continuum exists from normal aging through mild cognitive impairment (MCI) to dementia. This continuum is better understood when realizing that it occurs on a background of some degree of cognitive decline with aging. While the theoretical ideal is to age without cognitive change, typically cognitive function declines over time. Research has provided normative data on cognitively normal individuals at each decade of life, but this approach has been criticized because these studies likely include individuals who subsequently develop cognitive impairment. Research on normal aging using biomarkers for both Alzheimer disease (AD) and non-AD related pathologies will hopefully improve these methodological issues. Despite the aforementioned limitations, a brief review of cognitive change with age is important.

Before age 60, a consistent pattern of cognitive change with age occurs. General knowledge and vocabulary are stable or improve while problem solving, speed of processing and reasoning decline (Salthouse, 2012).

Age-related decline occurs primarily in cognitive speed, working memory, and encoding (Hedden and Gabrieli, 2004). The pattern on neuropsychological testing associated with normal aging includes a decline in learning and acquisition performance with delayed recall relatively preserved (Petersen et al., 1992). Recognition performance also is preserved with age. Age-related cognitive decline is heterogeneous as a substantial minority may show minimal decline (Benton et al., 1981). Cognitive reserve refers to different capacities for the brain to maintain cognitive functioning in setting of brain pathology or injury (Stern et al., 2018).

Age-related cognitive decline is associated with different neuroanatomical changes compared to cognitive decline from AD. Loss of synaptic density occurs as a function of age independent of Alzheimer pathology (Masliah et al., 1993). While AD is characterized by early damage of the entorhinal cortex and relative preservation of the dentate, age-associated medial temporal lobe changes occur in the dentate with preservation of the entorhinal cortex (Small et al., 2011). Brain volume normally declines with age but at a significantly slower rate than AD patients. In addition to the hippocampus, which declines in volume by 1%–2% a year in normal aging (Du et al., 2006), the prefrontal cortex also undergoes an age-related decrease in volume (Raz et al., 2005).

## Preclinical Stage of Dementia

Many studies have shown the pathophysiological processes leading to dementia can begin decades prior to cognitive symptoms. An evolving understanding of the preclinical stages of dementia has resulted in significantly increased interest in targeting it as a possible therapeutic time window. In the preclinical phase of dominantly inherited AD, cerebrospinal fluid (CSF) amyloid beta 42 (Aβ42) decreases 25 years before expected symptom onset (Bateman et al., 2012). Recent studies have revealed that in the general population the sequence of biomarkers leading to dementia is more diverse than dominantly inherited AD. In addition to cognitively normal individuals with biomarkers compatible with preclinical AD, the Mayo Clinic Study of Aging identified a group of patients with evidence of neurodegeneration on fluorodeoxyglucose positron emission tomography (FDG-PET) or magnetic resonance imaging (MRI), but without cerebral amyloid deposition. This group, termed suspected non-Alzheimer pathophysiology (sNAP) did not have imaging evidence consistent with cerebrovascular disease or synucleinopathy as the cause of brain injury (Jack et al., 2012; Knopman et al., 2012b). In general, these sNAP patients have a lower risk of becoming symptomatic after 5 years compared to patients with amyloid or amyloid plus neurodegeneration related biomarkers (Vos et al., 2013). In synuclein-related neurodegenerative disorders, autonomic symptoms, rapid eye movement (REM) sleep behavior disorder, and anosmia can predate cognitive and motor symptoms by many years. Ioflupane dopamine transporter scanning appears to be a promising biomarker in these conditions (Boeve, 2013). Preclinical stages of frontotemporal dementia (FTD) have not been studied as much as AD. The available biomarker data will be reviewed subsequently in this chapter. The 2011 National Institute on Aging (NIA) (Sperling et al., 2011) preclinical AD criteria are summarized in Table 95.1 (Knopman et al., 2013; Vos et al., 2013).

## Mild Cognitive Impairment

MCI refers to an in-between state of normal cognitive aging and dementia. In MCI, cognitive change is greater than expected for age but independence in the community and activities of daily living are preserved (Petersen, 2004; Petersen et al., 2009). On average, MCI patients perform 1–1.5 standard deviations below matched normative data. In 2018, the American Academy of Neurology published evidence-based guidelines on the concept of MCI, documenting the prevalence of MCI to be 6.7% at 60–64 years, 8.4% between ages 65 and 69, 10.1% between ages 70 and 74, 14.8% between ages 75 and 79, and 25.8% for ages 80–84. The rate of progression from MCI to dementia was between 9% and 20% per year depending on the specific nature of the population (Petersen et al., 2018).

In 2004, Petersen published criteria for MCI (Table 95.2; Petersen, 2004). These criteria, proposed at the Key Symposium in Stockholm (Winblad et al., 2004), emphasized the concept as a syndrome between

**TABLE 95.1 National Institute on Aging Criteria for Preclinical Alzheimer Disease (AD)**

| Diagnostic Category | | Amyloid Beta (Positron Emission Tomography or Cerebrospinal Fluid) | Neuronal Injury* | Cognitive Change | % of diagnostic category (Knopman et al., 2013) | 5-Year Risk of Dementia (Vos et al., 2013) |
|---|---|---|---|---|---|---|
| Normal AD biomarkers | Stage 0 (normal AD biomarkers) | – | – | – | 43% | 2% |
| Preclinical AD | Stage 1 (asymptomatic amyloidosis) | + | – | – | 16% | 11% |
| | Stage 2 (amyloidosis plus evidence of neural degeneration) | + | + | – | 12% | 26% |
| | Stage 3 (amyloidosis, neurodegeneration, subtle cognitive change) | + | + | + | 3% | 56% |
| | sNAP† (neurodegeneration, no amyloidosis) | – | + | – | 23% | 5% |

*Biomarkers of neuronal injury include increased cerebrospinal fluid (CSF) tau, hippocampal atrophy, and abnormal fluorodeoxyglucose positron emission tomography (FDG-PET) metabolism.
†Suspected non-Alzheimer pathway, not part of 2011 NIA criteria.
*Data based on studies by Knopman, D.S., Jack, C.R., Jr., Wiste, H.J., Weigand, S.D., Vemuri, P., Lowe, V.J., et al., 2013. Brain injury biomarkers are not dependent on beta-amyloid in normal elderly. Ann. Neurol. 3, 472–480; and Vos, S.J., Xiong, C., Visser, P.J., Jasielec, M.S., Hassenstab, J., Grant, E.A., et al., 2013. Preclinical Alzheimer's disease and its outcome: a longitudinal cohort study. Lancet Neurol. 2, 957–965.*

normal aging and dementia. Diagnosing MCI is the initial step, followed by a determination of etiology of the syndrome.

In 2011, the NIA and the Alzheimer Association published guidelines for the diagnosis of MCI due to AD (Albert et al., 2011). More recently, the Diagnostic and Statistical Manual of Mental Disorders-5 (DSM-5) described an analogous concept of "mild neurocognitive disorder." A comparison of the recent MCI criteria is presented in Fig. 95.1 (Albert et al., 2011; Petersen et al., 2014). The American Academy of Neurology published guidelines recommending clinicians assess patients for MCI (Petersen et al., 2018).

**TABLE 95.2 Mild Cognitive Impairment Criteria**

| aMCI | naMCI |
|---|---|
| Cognitive decline with intact ADLs, often corroborated by an informant | Cognitive decline with intact ADLs, often corroborated by an informant |
| Memory impairment | Nonmemory cognitive impairment (language, attention, executive function, visual-spatial) |
| Multidomain aMCI if other domains involved | Multidomain naMCI if more than one other nonmemory domain involved |

*ADL*, Activity of daily living; *aMCI*, mild cognitive impairment—amnestic; *naMCI*, mild cognitive impairment—nonamnestic.

The concept of MCI is important because it identifies persons who are at great risk of developing dementia. While the annual risk of developing dementia in the elderly general population is approximately 1%–2%, MCI patients seen in the clinic setting have a 10%–15% annual risk. In population-based studies of MCI the annual risk of developing dementia is slightly lower at 5%–10% (Farias et al., 2009; Petersen et al., 2010; Roberts et al., 2014). The prevalence of MCI in subjects age 70–89 is approximately 16% (Petersen et al., 2010). Identifying MCI patients allows for monitoring of progression, provides opportunity for appropriate counseling, and offers a possible therapeutic window for intervention in the future.

Several biomarkers predict the risk of converting from MCI to dementia. On structural MRI, MCI patients with hippocampal volumes on the 25th percentile are 2–3 times more likely to convert to

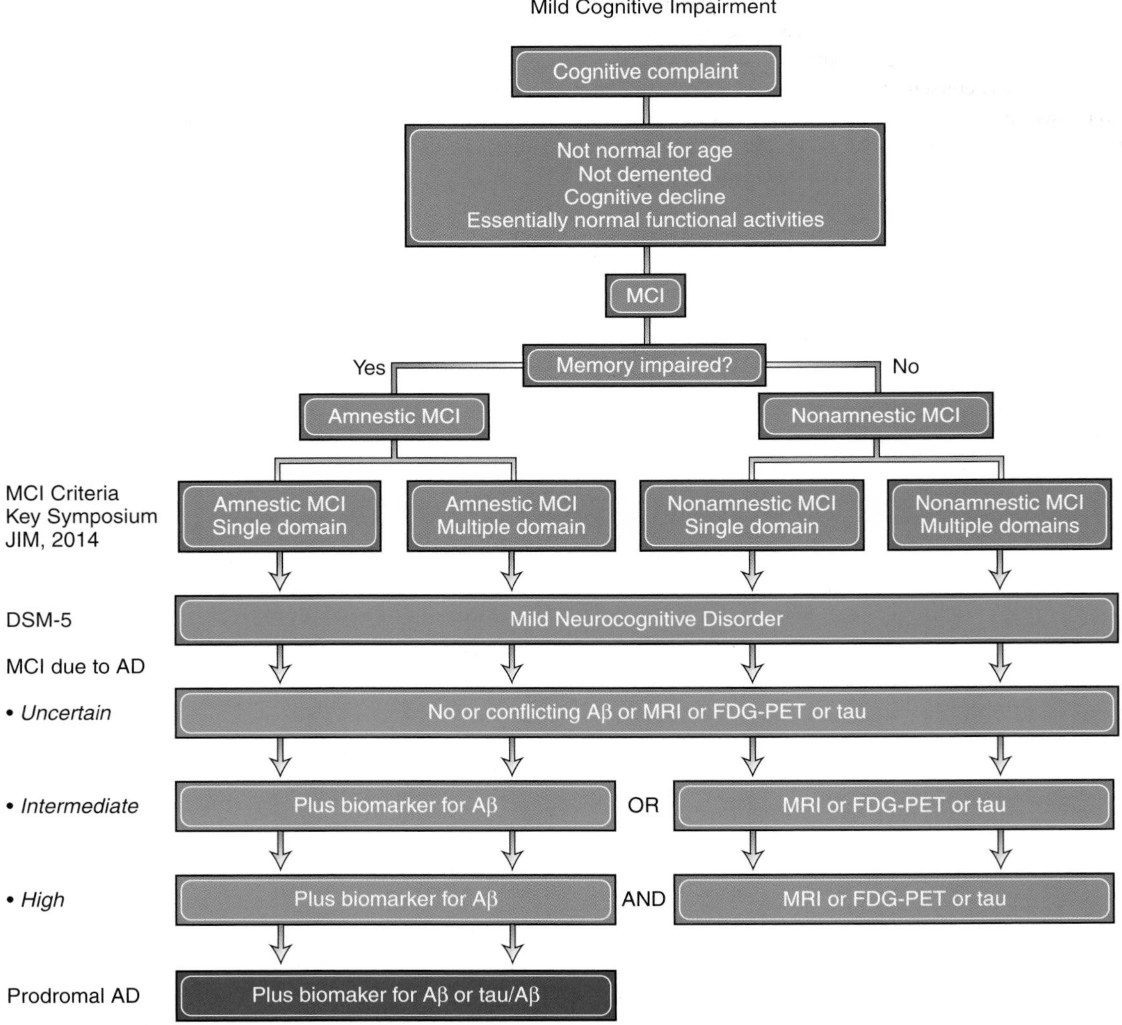


**Fig. 95.1 Comparison of Recent Criteria for Mild Cognitive Impairment *(MCI)*.** The criteria outlined in blue were proposed at the Key Symposium. Other criteria include those of the fifth edition of the Diagnostic and Statistical Manual of Mental Disorders *(DSM-5)* and MCI due to Alzheimer disease *(AD)* (Albert et al., 2011). *Aβ*, Amyloid beta; *FDG-PET*, fluorodeoxyglucose positron emission tomography; *MRI*, magnetic resonance imaging. (*Reproduced from Petersen, R.C., Caracciolo, B., Brayne, C., Gauthier, S., Jelic, V., Fratiglioni, L., 2014. Mild cognitive impairment: a concept in evolution. J. Intern. Med. 275, 214–228 with permission from Journal of Internal Medicine.*)

dementia compared to MCI patients with hippocampal volumes on the 75th percentile (Jack et al., 2010). In CSF, low Aβ 42 and high total tau (t-tau) and phospho tau (p-tau) levels are associated with progression in MCI patients (Mattsson et al., 2009). Other risk factors for conversion include APOE ε4 allele (Petersen et al., 1995, 2005), temporal-parietal hypometabolism on FDG-PET (Chetelat et al., 2003), and amyloid deposition on Aβ PET imaging (Wolk et al., 2009). One criticism of the MCI concept is that a proportion of patients diagnosed with MCI revert to normal. Interestingly, recent longitudinal studies demonstrated that those patients who fluctuate between normal cognition and mild cognitive impairment have a significantly higher risk of developing dementia over time. Therefore, a diagnosis of MCI even with reversion to normal has prognostic value (Lopez, 2013; Roberts et al., 2014). This fluctuation is analogous to labile hypertension and glucose intolerance with respect to the ultimate development of hypertension or diabetes mellitus.

Subtyping MCI into amnestic and nonamnestic categories also has predictive value. Amnestic MCI (aMCI), which is more common, refers to memory impairment often noticed by family and even the patient but with intact cognitive skills in other domains (language, executive function, visual-spatial) and preservation of functional capacity. In contrast, nonamnestic MCI (naMCI) patients have declines in nonmemory cognitive domains such as language, executive function, and visual-spatial skills. The vast majority of aMCI patients progress to AD dementia (Petersen et al., 2005). Those with naMCI may progress to dementia with Lewy bodies (DLB) but can also progress to FTD, vascular dementia, and even AD dementia (Ferman et al., 2013b; Molano et al., 2010).

### Subjective Cognitive Impairment

While restricted insight into memory loss has been a distinguishing feature of individuals with cognitive impairment, recent studies have demonstrated that patients with cognitive complaints, good insight, and normal cognitive testing called subjective cognitive decline (SCD) are three times more likely than controls to develop MCI with AD-related biomarkers (Jessen et al., 2010; van Harten et al., 2018). SCI has been associated with elevated levels of tau regionally in the entorhinal cortex and global elevation of Aβ (Buckley et al., 2017).

## DEMENTIA

Dementia is an encompassing syndromic term for a decline in cognitive abilities of sufficient severity to interfere with function during daily activities (i.e., shopping, paying bills, cooking, driving, etc.). The term dementia does not imply an underlying etiology, although neurodegenerative diseases represent the most common causes. The decline from a prior higher level of functioning must be present in order to distinguish dementia from a developmental cognitive disorder. The cognitive deficit cannot be due to delirium or altered sensorium, which can be distinguished by the presence of marked fluctuations and acute-to-subacute temporal pattern, although dementia patients are more susceptible to delirium than the general population. The practice guideline on dementia from the American Academy of Neurology (AAN) recommended use of the DSM-IIIR dementia criteria (which were subsequently updated to the DSM-5 criteria). The DSM-5 criteria use the term major neurocognitive disorder to approximate dementia.

### Dementia Epidemiology

An estimated 35.6 million worldwide were living with dementia in 2010, with a prediction the number would double approximately every

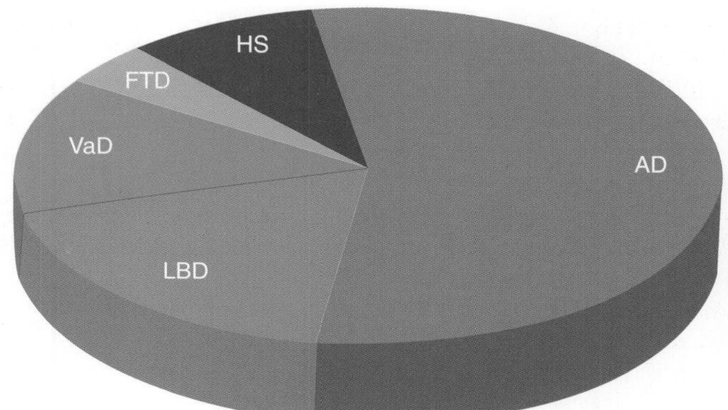


**Fig. 95.2 Frequency of Different Pathologies in State of Florida Brain Bank.** *AD,* Alzheimer disease; *LBD,* Lewy body disease; *VaD,* vascular dementia; *HS,* hippocampal sclerosis; *FTD,* frontotemporal dementia. (*Based on data from Barker, W.W., Luis, C.A., Kashuba, A., Luis, M., Harwood, D.G., Loewenstein, D., et al., 2002. Relative frequencies of Alzheimer disease, Lewy body, vascular and frontotemporal dementia, and hippocampal sclerosis in the State of Florida Brain Bank. Alzheimer Dis. Assoc. Disord. 16, 203–212.*)

20 years (Prince et al., 2013). In the United States, the estimated prevalence of dementia among those 71 and older using an in-home visit is 13.9%. A sharp increase in dementia prevalence occurs with age (Plassman et al., 2007).

However, data from the Rotterdam study indicate the incidence of dementia may be declining (Schrijvers et al., 2012). This has been replicated in the UK (Matthews et al., 2013) and Rochester, MN (Rocca et al., 2011). One possible explanation is that this decrease is related to improved treatment of vascular risk factors.

Dementia can result from numerous causes, including brain injury (cerebrovascular disease or trauma) or infectious and metabolic diseases, but the most common causes are neurodegenerative diseases. Fig. 95.2 represents frequency of the predominant pathologies in a large dementia brain bank (Barker et al., 2002). However, it is clear that while each patient has a predominant pathology, the majority of patients have multiple pathologies at autopsy. In fact, only 30% had AD pathology without other pathologies. Similarly, in the Rush Memory and Aging Project, over 50% of autopsied subjects with dementia had multiple pathological diagnoses (Schneider et al., 2007).

In a longitudinal clinicpathological study of aging, AD was the most common underlying pathology (65%) but occurred without other pathologies rarely (9%). On an individual level, AD pathology accounted for approximately 50% of cognitive decline on average, highlighting the importance of pathological heterogeneity in age-related cognitive decline (Boyle et al., 2018). In fact, even among patients diagnosed with AD-dementia, multiple pathologies are the rule rather than the exception (Schneider et al., 2007, 2009). With age, amyloid accumulation plateaus (Jack et al., 2017), tau, TAR DNA-binding protein 43 (TDP-43), and cerebrovascular pathologies continue to accumulate (Josephs et al., 2014; Schneider et al., 2007, 2009).

### Diagnostic Approach

In 2001, the AAN published evidence-based guidelines for the diagnosis of dementia (Knopman et al., 2001).

#### History

The history is the most important component of the dementia diagnosis. Ideally, the history should be taken from not only the patient but also an individual who knows the patient well as lack of awareness

TABLE 95.3 **Key Parts of the History**

| Cognitive Symptoms | Motor Symptoms | Autonomic Symptoms | Sleep | Behavioral |
|---|---|---|---|---|
| Impaired recent memory (repetitive questions/statements, forgets appointments, loses items easily) | Presence of tremor or myoclonus | Bowel/bladder symptoms | Presence of REM sleep behavior disorder | Change in personality, socially inappropriate behavior |
| Language difficulty (trouble understanding others, trouble getting words out, trouble finding words, uses incorrect words) | Trouble swallowing/ slurred speech | Presence of orthostasis | Excessive daytime sleepiness | Loss of empathy/interest in hobbies, family |
| Visual spatial difficulty (getting lost more easily, trouble reading, difficulty recognizing familiar people) | Change in gait/falls | Sexual dysfunction (erectile dysfunction) | Evidence of sleep apnea (snoring, stopped breathing during sleep) | Compulsive behaviors, change in dietary preference |
| Executive/attentional dysfunction (poor judgment, difficulty problem solving, difficulty maintaining focus, trouble with calculations) | Muscle cramps atrophy, fasciculations | Change in sweating | Evidence of stridor | Disheveled, decreased interest in hygiene |

*REM,* Rapid eye movement.

of impairment commonly accompanies dementia. This individual can provide invaluable information regarding impairment in activities of daily living (ADLs). Other key elements of the history include identifying the presenting symptom, mode of onset, duration of symptoms, and rate of progression. Neurodegenerative causes of dementia typically present with an insidious onset and slow rate of progression, while the sudden onset of symptoms should raise suspicion for stroke, medication effect, infection, autoimmune process, or psychosocial stressors. Patients may have a subacute onset over weeks or months. The dementias presenting with this course will be discussed in Chapter 94. Thorough evaluation of patients referred for cognitive symptoms to a memory clinic can identify a potentially reversible or partially reversible disorder in up to 9% of cases (Clarfield, 2003) and a treatable coexisting disorder in up to 23% (Hejl et al., 2002). Several key components of the dementia history are reviewed in Table 95.3. Background information such as age, level of education, occupation, social stressors, and cultural background can influence the presentation of dementia and should be taken into consideration. As a general framework, when an older patient presents with a progressive amnestic disorder with subsequent decline in other cognitive domains, AD dementia is the most common diagnosis. Alternatively, if the initial presentation is one of a change in language, personality, or behavior with relatively spared memory, FTD is the most likely consideration. The presence of parkinsonism, hallucinations, fluctuations, and REM sleep behavior disorder with dementia are most suggestive of DLB. Vascular cognitive impairment (VCI) (Corriveau et al., 2016) can be temporally related to a stroke or develop gradually with prominent cognitive slowing and executive dysfunction with cerebral small-vessel white matter disease. Often vascular disease occurs together with other causes of dementia as a comorbid component of the clinical picture. In the setting of subacute dementia, consider Creutzfeldt-Jakob disease, autoimmune dementia, and their differential diagnosis.

***Medical history.*** The past medical history can provide clues to the diagnosis or identify contributors to the cognitive decline. A careful head injury history is important because significant head trauma is a risk factor for dementia (Guo et al., 2000). Repeated head injuries may suggest chronic traumatic encephalopathy (CTE) such as can occur in contact sports or the military (McKee et al., 2013). Histories of stroke, hypertension, diabetes, high cholesterol, atrial fibrillation, smoking, or other vascular risk factors are important clues to vascular disease contributing to dementia. A history of cancer or autoimmune disease in the setting of a subacute cognitive decline may point to a paraneoplastic disorder or autoimmune dementia. A history of seizures, meningitis, or encephalitis, chemotherapy, brain radiation, sleep apnea, and other sleep disorders, depression and other psychiatric illness, and medication use may all be informative.

***Family history.*** Knowledge about genetic causes and risk factors has rapidly increased in the last few decades. Thus a careful family history is essential. Identify not only first degree relatives but other relatives with dementia. It is also important to ask about Parkinson disease, amyotrophic lateral sclerosis (ALS), and psychiatric disease. Patients with one phenotype may have relatives with another. For example, one patient may have FTD and a relative may have ALS from the same gene mutation.

***Medications.*** A thorough review of medications is essential as medication side effects exacerbate an underlying cognitive impairment or even mimic a dementia. A temporal association or worsening with starting a medication should be taken seriously and prompt consideration of a medication taper. While numerous medications are associated with cognitive side effects, the most common include anticholinergic agents (often present in medications for incontinence or antihistamines), benzodiazepines, zolpidem and other sedatives, opioids, and muscle relaxants. Table 95.4 is a partial list of medications that can be associated with cognitive symptoms.

***Neuropsychiatric history.*** A thorough neuropsychiatric history provides important information by identifying potentially treatable symptoms and narrowing the differential diagnosis. According to the AAN guidelines, depression should be screened for in all dementia patients because it occurs frequently and is treatable (Knopman et al., 2001). While depression can mimic dementia, depression is also a risk factor for and occurs frequently with AD and DLB (Boot et al., 2013; Ownby et al., 2006). Traditional teaching suggested that patients with dementia have consistent memory deficits and executive dysfunction of which they are unaware or minimize, while depressed patients are more likely to complain about cognitive impairment and perform variably on cognitive testing due to attention deficits and poor effort on testing (although in practice, distinguishing the two is difficult due to the significant overlap). However, more recent work on the MCI stage of dementia due to AD has demonstrated that early neuropsychiatric features such as apathy, agitation, and dysphoria may be presenting features of a neurodegenerative process (Geda et al., 2014). Important neuropsychiatric symptoms to review include change in mood (depression, mania), change in personality, and presence of delusions, obsessive behaviors, or hallucinations. The presence of certain neuropsychiatric features may narrow the differential diagnosis. For example, personality changes in behavioral variant FTD

**TABLE 95.4 Partial List of Medications Which Can Cause Cognitive Impairment**

| | | |
|---|---|---|
| **Sleep aids, cold medications, and antihistamines with an anticholinergic component:**<br>Diphenhydramine Acetaminophen/Dextromethorphan/Doxylamine succinate, Ibuprofen/Diphenhydramine | **Anticonvulsants**<br>Lamotrigine<br>Phenobarbital<br>Phenytoin<br>Levetiracetam<br>Topiramate<br>Zonisamide | **Anticholinergics**<br>Benztropine<br>Meclizine<br>Scopolamine |
| **Antihypertensives**<br>Beta-blockers | **Anticholinergics**<br>Tolterodine<br>Oxybutynin | **Muscle relaxants**<br>Baclofen |
| **Antidepressants**<br>Amitriptyline (anticholinergic property)<br>Imipramine (anticholinergic property) | **Antipsychotics**<br>Quetiapine<br>Olanzapine<br>Risperidone<br>Aripiprazole | **Cardiac**<br>Digoxin |
| **Opiates**<br>Oxycodone<br>Morphine<br>Hydrocodone<br>Fentanyl<br>Propoxyphene<br>Methadone | **Hypnotics**<br>Zolpidem<br>Eszopiclone | **Immunosuppressants**<br>Tacrolimus<br>Cyclosporine |
| **Benzodiazepines**<br>Alprazolam<br>Clonazepam<br>Lorazepam<br>Diazepam<br>Temazepam | **Antibiotics**<br>Metronidazole<br>Cefepime | **Mood stabilizer**<br>Lithium |

(bvFTD) or hallucinations or delusions in DLB. The Neuropsychiatric Inventory (NPI) can be used to screen for common neuropsychiatric manifestations of dementia (Cummings, 1997).

### Cognitive Assessment

Many useful cognitive screening instruments have been developed. Common well validated instruments include the Mini-Mental State Exam (MMSE) (Folstein et al., 1975), the Blessed Orientation Memory Concentration Test (Katzman et al., 1983), the Kokmen Short Test of Mental Status (STMS) (Kokmen et al., 1991), and the Montreal Cognitive Assessment (MOCA) (Nasreddine et al., 2005). Detailed cognitive testing by a neuropsychologist can be very helpful. The neuropsychologist provides an in-depth cognitive evaluation by administering a standardized battery of tests. These tests evaluate important cognitive domains such as attention and concentration, memory, language, visuospatial abilities, and executive function. They also gauge the psychiatric contributions to the clinical picture. Patients with different dementias have different strengths and weaknesses on these tests. The pattern of performance helps determine if the person is impaired, the severity of impairment, and the likely brain areas that are damaged. Neuropsychology can also be helpful in following a patient's progression over time.

### General Neurological Examination

A general neurological exam is a key part of the evaluation of dementia. While the general neurological exam is typically normal in early AD, abnormalities on exam may indicate other neurodegenerative processes. The presence of parkinsonism may suggest DLB or another parkinsonian dementia. Focal findings on exam such as asymmetric reflexes or other lateralizing signs may suggest a vascular component to the dementia. A coexisting peripheral neuropathy may suggest a metabolic disturbance. Fasciculations can be seen in patients with suspected FTD to suggesting coexisting motor neuron disease. A language screening exam and testing for apraxia should also be performed. The presence of a gait abnormality may indicate normal pressure hydrocephalus (NPH), parkinsonism, or vascular disease.

### Laboratory Evaluation

The AAN practice parameter recommends routine assessment for vitamin $B_{12}$ deficiency and thyroid hormone abnormalities because these conditions are common, and can affect cognitive function. Treatment of vitamin $B_{12}$ deficiency and hypothyroidism may not completely reverse cognitive symptoms, but recognition of these conditions is important. Other routine lab tests include a complete blood cell count, electrolyte panel, glucose, liver function tests, and creatinine. Screening for syphilis should be done based on clinical suspicion (Knopman et al., 2001). Special circumstances, including age less than 65 years, seizures, rapidly progressive dementia, history of cancer or autoimmune disease, suspicion of central nervous system (CNS) infection, constitutional symptoms, history of drug abuse or immunosuppression, systemic infection, suspicion of vasculitis, or other atypical features, can guide further laboratory evaluation, including CSF examination. In neurodegenerative disease, the cell count, protein, and glucose concentrations in the CSF are within normal limits and specific markers of AD pathology; for example, Aβ42 total and phospho-tau, may be useful.

The AAN practice parameter recommends against electroencephalogram (EEG) in the standard evaluation of dementia (Knopman et al., 2001). However, EEG may be very useful in a patient with a history of seizures, assessment of rapidly progressive dementia, a history of spells, or suspicion of transient epileptic amnesia (Butler et al., 2007).

### Neuroimaging

Structural neuroimaging modalities including computed tomography (CT) and MRI can identify potentially treatable causes of dementia including subdural hematoma, hydrocephalus, and intracranial neoplasm. The AAN practice parameter paper recommends screening with either CT or MRI to identify these conditions (Knopman et al., 2001). In a study evaluating the usefulness of the AAN dementia guidelines, 3% of dementia patients had a surgically treatable finding on neuroimaging (NPH, subdural hematoma, neoplasm). Neuroimaging changed management in 15% of cases and clinical diagnoses in 19%–28% (Chui and Zhang, 1997). In the recent "Imaging Dementia-Evidence for Amyloid" Scanning (IDEAS) study, the use of amyloid PET among Medicare beneficiaries with cognitive impairment of unclear etiology led to a change in diagnosis and clinical management in a significant proportion of the participants (Rabinovici et al., 2019).

### DSM-5

Recently, the DSM-5 was released, updating the prior criteria for dementia. DSM-5 introduces the terms "mild neurocognitive disorder," which is similar to MCI, and "major neurocognitive disorder," which is analogous to dementia. Major neurocognitive disorder represents a significant cognitive decline in at least one cognitive domain that interferes with daily function that is recognized by the individual, informant, or clinician and documented by neuropsychological testing. Mild neurocognitive disorder represents a cognitive decline which does not impair daily activities (American Psychiatric Association, 2013). DSM-5 recommends a two-tiered approach: (1) syndrome characterization as outlined above and (2) an etiological determination.

## ALZHEIMER DISEASE

### Background

In 1906 Alois Alzheimer, a German psychiatrist, reported the case of a woman in her 50s with paranoia and memory loss followed by aphasia whom he evaluated in a psychiatric unit. She eventually lost the ability to perform motor tasks. At autopsy, gross inspection revealed an atrophied brain with vascular changes. Microscopic sections prepared with Bielschowsky stain revealed the hallmark AD inclusions which would later be known as amyloid plaques and neurofibrillary tangles (NFTs). Although the patient had early onset of symptoms, Alzheimer's case summarizes many of the key clinical features of AD dementia.

### Definition of Alzheimer Disease Over Time

In 1984, the National Institute on Neurological and Communicative Disorders and Stroke and the Alzheimer's Disease and Related Disorders Association criteria were created conceptualizing Alzheimer disease as a clinicopathological entity for over 30 years (McKhann et al., 1984a). With advancing technology allowing in vivo detection of amyloid with PET and CSF as well as measurement of neurodegeneration, in 2011 revised AD criteria were proposed by the National Institute on Aging-Alzheimer's Association. Individuals were characterized by their clinical state (normal, MCI, and dementia) with biomarkers of amyloid and neurodegeneration providing the likelihood that their clinical state was due to Alzheimer disease. For example, if amyloid and neurodegeneration biomarkers were present in conjunction with the clinical syndrome of dementia, the diagnosis of dementia due to AD with high likelihood could be made (McKhann et al., 2011). But the diagnoses of MCI and dementia due to AD were still clinical-pathological conditions.

More recently, tau PET imaging and improvement in CSF assays has allowed detection of both hallmark AD proteins in vivo. This advance of being able to detect both amyloid and tau in conjunction with data from clinical trials, which suggested that almost a quarter of individuals enrolled in a trial targeting amyloid were considered amyloid negative (Siemers et al., 2016), led to a new research framework proposing that AD should be defined biologically by the presence of both amyloid and tau either with biomarkers during life or pathologically with a separation of the clinical syndrome from the disease definition. The advantages of this framework include the ability to classify individuals earlier in the disease process, prevention of individuals with an amnestic dementia being misclassified as AD dementia if they have an alternative pathology, and the ability for individuals with an atypical phenotype (nonamnestic) to be classified as AD. In this research framework, each individual would be characterized by 3 biomarker groupings: (1) β-amyloid deposition, (2) pathological tau, and (3) neurodegeneration [AT(N)]. In this research framework, neuritic plaques may be identified by decreased CSF Aβ42 or amyloid PET positivity and neurofibrillary tangles identified by a positive tau PET or elevated phospho-tau protein in the CSF (Jack et al., 2018a). The presence of an amyloid biomarker alone without tau would be referred to as Alzheimer pathological change and the absence of amyloid as non-Alzheimer pathological change. The authors cautioned that this framework is for research at this point in time and should not be used in routine clinical practice. This framework provides a universal terminology to allow comparison between research studies, avoiding misclassification and potential erroneous enrollment in randomized clinical trials of individuals with an amnestic dementia syndrome not due to Alzheimer pathology such as hippocampal sclerosis (Botha et al., 2018a). A cognitive staging scheme can be applied to an individual's biomarker status (Jack et al., 2018a). This history of Alzheimer disease definition was reviewed in the 2018 Wartenberg lecture (Petersen, 2018). Table 95.5 provides proposed cognitive stages applied to the new AD biomarker framework.

### Alzheimer Epidemiology

#### Prevalence

According to the Alzheimer's Association in 2018, 5.7 million Americans have AD dementia (2018) which represents 70% of dementia in the United States (not autopsy confirmed) (Plassman et al., 2007). The prevalence of Alzheimer dementia increases with age from 3% of people between the ages of 65 and 74 to 32% of people age 85 and older (Alzheimer's disease facts and figures 2018). While MCI is more common in men, the prevalence of AD dementia is higher in women. This in part can be explained by a longer life span in women than men. The lifetime risk of developing Alzheimer dementia from the age of 45 is approximately 10% for men and 20% for women (Alzheimer's disease facts and figures 2018). By 2060, the prevalence will increase to an estimated 15 million individuals in the United States (Brookmeyer et al., 2018).

#### Incidence

Age is the most important risk factor for AD dementia. The incidence of AD dementia increases with age: 2 new cases per 1000 for individuals age 65 to 74, 11 new cases per 1000 people age 75 to 84, and 37 new cases per 1000 people age 85 and older (Alzheimer's disease facts and figures 2018).

#### Societal Cost and Future Projections

Anticipated increases in cost to society for AD dementia are notsustainable. The total payments in 2018 for all individuals with dementia are estimated to be $277 billion (Alzheimer's disease facts and figures

**TABLE 95.5 Cognitive Stage**

| | Cognitively Unimpaired | Mild Cognitive Impairment (MCI) | Dementia |
|---|---|---|---|
| A⁻T⁻(N)⁻ | Normal Alzheimer disease (AD) biomarkers, cognitively unimpaired | Normal AD biomarkers with MCI | Normal AD biomarkers with dementia |
| A⁺T⁻ (N) | Preclinical Alzheimer pathological change | Alzheimer pathological change with MCI | Alzheimer pathological change with dementia |
| A⁺T⁺ (N)⁻<br>A⁺T⁺ (N)⁺ | Preclinical Alzheimer disease | Alzheimer disease with MCI (Prodromal AD) | Alzheimer disease with dementia |
| A⁺T⁻ (N)⁺ | Alzheimer and concomitant suspected non-Alzheimer pathological change, cognitively unimpaired | Alzheimer and concomitant suspected non-Alzheimer pathological change with MCI | Alzheimer and concomitant suspected non-Alzheimer pathological change with dementia |
| A⁻T⁺ (N)⁻<br>A⁻T⁻ (N)⁺<br>A⁻T⁺ (N)⁺ | Non-Alzheimer pathological change, cognitively unimpaired | Non-Alzheimer pathological change with MCI | Non-Alzheimer pathological change with dementia |

*A*, Amyloid status; *T*, tau status; *N*, neurodegeneration status.
*Adapted from Jack, C.R., Jr., Bennett, D.A., Blennow, K., Carrillo, M.C., Dunn, B., Haeberlein, S.B., et al., 2018a. NIA-AA Research Framework: toward a biological definition of Alzheimer's disease. Alzheimers Dement. 4, 535–562.*

2018). The Alzheimer Association estimates that by 2050 annual costs for AD dementia will reach approximately $1.2 trillion (Thies and Bleiler, 2013). Therefore, the burden on society will continue to be enormous unless a prevention or treatment is developed. The Health and Retirement Study has reported that AD is the costliest chronic disease in the United States exceeding those of cancer and heart disease (Hurd et al., 2013).

## Risk Factors

In addition to age and female gender, many other risk factors for AD dementia have been reported.

***Hypertension.*** After controlling for confounders, systolic blood pressure (>160 mm Hg) and elevated cholesterol increase risk for AD dementia later in life (Kivipelto et al., 2001). In the Honolulu-Asia Aging Study, the use of beta-blockers for hypertension was associated with less cognitive decline, especially among diabetics (Gelber et al., 2013). In the Ginkgo Evaluation of Memory Study, the use of a diuretic blood pressure medication, angiotensin-1 receptor blocker, or angiotensin-converting enzyme inhibitor was associated with reduced risk of AD dementia in those with normal cognition at baseline (Yasar et al., 2013). The relationship between hypertension and dementia is complicated. Counterintuitively, some studies have shown that low blood pressure is more commonly seen in demented patients than high blood pressure (Guo et al., 1996). A parsimonious explanation of this apparent discrepancy is that the association between hypertension and cognitive decline is age dependent. Mid-life hypertension and late-life hypotension are associated with AD dementia (Qiu et al., 2005). The relative risk of mid-life hypertension and dementia is 1.61 and it has been estimated that decreasing the prevalence of mid-life hypertension by 10% could result in a worldwide decrease of 160,000 AD dementia cases (Barnes and Yaffe, 2011). The recent SPRINT-MIND trial demonstrated that treating systolic blood pressure to a goal of less than 120 mm Hg compared to a goal of less than 140 mm Hg reduced the risk of mild cognitive impairment by approximately 19%, but the study did not meet its primary endpoint of showing a reduction in the risk of dementia (Williamson et al., 2019).

***Diabetes and elevated glucose.*** Type 2 diabetes is associated with hyperinsulinemia. Both insulin and Aβ are substrates for insulin-degrading enzyme. Therefore, hyperinsulinemia may result in accumulation of Aβ through competing with Aβ for insulin-degrading enzyme (Qiu and Folstein, 2006). However, at autopsy, type 2 diabetes is associated with vascular brain disease not increased AD pathology (Arvanitakis et al., 2006). Nonetheless, a meta-analysis estimated the relative risk of dementia related to diabetes was 1.39 (Lu et al., 2009). It has been estimated that a 10% decrease in diabetes prevalence may decrease the number of worldwide dementia cases by 81,000. Recently, a study has demonstrated that elevated glucose in the absence of diabetes also increases the risk of dementia (Crane et al., 2013).

***Head injury.*** A meta-analysis of 15 case-control studies demonstrated an increased risk of AD dementia with prior head injury in men (Fleminger et al., 2003). The mechanism is unclear, but after severe head injury, levels of Aβ42 in the CSF decrease, which also occurs in preclinical AD (Franz et al., 2003). The presence of the APOE4 allele may confer a higher risk of dementia after head injury (Koponen et al., 2004). In a population-based study, MCI subjects but not normal control subjects with history of head trauma had elevated brain Aβ deposition (Mielke et al., 2014).

***Sleep.*** The glymphatic system of the brain allows clearance of waste products. In mice, it has been shown that during sleep there is an increase in the interstitial space allowing for increased rate of clearance of β-amyloid (Xie et al., 2013b). Emerging evidence suggests that impaired sleep may alter β-amyloid dynamics in humans (Lucey et al., 2018; Shokri-Kojori et al., 2018). This is an active area of ongoing research.

***Others.*** Other risk factors associated with an increased risk of AD include smoking (Anstey et al., 2007), cerebrovascular disease (Pendlebury and Rothwell, 2009), anemia (Hong et al., 2013), and obesity (Profenno et al., 2010).

## Protective Factors

***Education/leisure activities/early-life cognitive abilities.*** In 1990, a study performed in Shanghai demonstrated an association between a lower educational attainment and dementia risk (Zhang et al., 1990). Subsequently, several other studies have demonstrated an association between low educational attainment and increased dementia risk (Qiu et al., 2001; Stern et al., 1994).

In addition to education, participation in certain leisure activities, including reading, dancing, playing board games, and playing musical instruments, is associated with a decreased dementia risk (Verghese et al., 2003).

These studies and others have led to the development of the cognitive reserve hypothesis. Which attempts to explain why those with certain life experiences, including higher educational attainment and increased leisure activity participation, are more resistant to neurodegenerative changes (Stern, 2012).

Early-life cognitive abilities also may play an important role in dementia risk. In the nun study, autobiographical essays from nuns at a mean age of 22 were evaluated for idea density and grammatical complexity. Those with low idea density and grammatical complexity had lower cognitive scores later in life, and, in a small sample of nuns who came to autopsy, those with low early-life linguistic ability had AD pathology while those with linguistic talent did not have AD pathology (Snowdon et al., 1996). Similarly in 1932, participants in the 1921 Scottish birth cohort took a test of intelligence at age 11. Lower mental ability at age 11 was associated with an increased risk of dementia (Whalley et al., 2000).

***Exercise.*** A Cochrane review of 11 studies of exercise in elderly non-demented participants concluded that exercise enhanced cognitive function (Angevaren et al., 2008). In addition, Yaffe and colleagues (Yaffe et al., 2001) reported that women with higher baseline levels of self-reported physical activity were less likely to decline cognitively. Similar findings were found in the nurses' health study (Weuve et al., 2004) and a population-based study (Geda et al., 2010). In addition to epidemiological studies, a single-blind prospective study of physical activity intervention in participants with subjective cognitive impairment but not dementia demonstrated modest but significant improvement in cognition at 18 months follow-up (Lautenschlager et al., 2008). The mechanism of how exercise can improve cognition is unclear, but exercise and improvement in aerobic fitness correlate with increased hippocampal volumes (Erickson et al., 2011). Even in autosomal dominant AD, self-reported exercise of greater than 150 minutes per week was associated with lower amyloid load compared to those who exercised less than 150 minutes per week (Brown et al., 2017).

***Diet.*** In a nested case-control study from the Cardiovascular Health Study, consumption of 1–6 alcoholic beverages per week was associated with decreased odds of dementia relative to abstinence (Mukamal et al., 2003). In contrast, heavy drinking (>3/day) was not associated with a lower AD dementia risk (Luchsinger et al., 2004). In fact, it is well described that alcoholic patients can develop dementia for multifactorial reasons. Korsakoff syndrome related to thiamine deficiency is primarily an amnestic disorder. Other neuropsychological features of alcoholics with dementia include impaired letter fluency, fine motor control, and delayed recall with relative preservation of recognition (Saxton et al., 2000).

Dietary fat intake has been associated with AD dementia risk. While intake of saturated fats and *trans*-unsaturated fats is associated with a higher risk, intake of unsaturated, unhydrogenated fats may be protective against AD dementia (Morris et al., 2003a, 2003b). Weekly fish consumption and increased intake of omega-3 fatty acid may also be associated with decreased AD dementia risk. Similarly, adherence to the Mediterranean diet, which recommends fish intake, is associated with decreased risk of AD and decreased risk of converting from MCI to AD dementia (Scarmeas et al., 2006, 2009). Cognitive outcome data from a clinical trial in which a Mediterranean diet was compared to a control diet demonstrated that a Mediterranean diet supplemented with olive oil or nuts was associated with better cognition than a control diet (Livingston et al., 2017).

## Alzheimer Clinical Features

AD dementia survival is shorter than predicted based on US population estimates, with a median survival from diagnosis of 4.2 years for men and 5.7 years for women (Larson et al., 2004).

### Early Presentation

Typical AD dementia initially presents with an episodic memory impairment reflecting the selective vulnerability of the medial temporal lobe to AD pathology. Episodic memory relates to our ability to remember information specific to a time and place when that memory was formed (e.g., "What did you eat for dinner? What did you do on a trip?"). Recent episodic memory is particularly impaired in early AD.

### Pattern of Progression

While episodic memory is the hallmark of early AD, subsequent cognitive decline is heterogeneous as the pathology spreads to the association cortices. While individual presentations vary significantly, Feldman and Woodward have described the typical symptom progression in AD dementia: Mild AD (recent memory impairment, repetitive questions, loss of interest in hobbies, anomia, impaired instrumental ADLs), moderate AD (aphasia, executive dysfunction, impaired basic ADLs), severe AD (agitation, complete loss of independence, sleep disturbance) (Feldman and Woodward, 2005).

### Common Clinical Features

Semantic memory dysfunction can be an early feature of AD but occurs after episodic memory involvement. Semantic memory is factual knowledge not linked to time or space context. Examples include naming or recalling animals, objects and tools, or landmarks. The preservation of semantic memory in a subset of early AD cases indicates that transentorhinal dysfunction is inadequate to disrupt semantic memory, which likely requires extension of pathology into the temporal neocortex (Hodges and Patterson, 1995). A category fluency test (asking the subject to generate as many items as possible from a given category such as fruits, animals, or vegetables) is commonly used as a brief test of semantic knowledge. This not only tests the ability to remember the names of objects but the ability to search one's mind for a category of objects. This test is often impaired early in the course of the disease and also tests executive function.

Executive function (planning, organization, problem solving, set switching) decline occurs in mild AD (Greene et al., 1995). The executive dysfunction in AD dementia is mild until later in the disease course compared to bvFTD.

Language disturbance often occurs in the mild-moderate stage of AD dementia. Initial complaints often include word-finding difficulty. In time, other features of aphasia may develop, and in the late states, language output can be limited.

Decline in visuospatial skills is common, often manifesting early with the complaint of becoming lost or being disorientated in unfamiliar places.

Apraxia often occurs later in the course of typical AD, although it may be an early feature in atypical AD.

Strikingly, several abilities are preserved until very late in the development of AD dementia. For example, AD dementia patients have preserved motor learning (procedural) (Eslinger and Damasio, 1986), motor, and sensory skills.

A useful way to think of the clinical picture of AD dementia is to look at the pattern of both deficits and strengths the patient exhibits. Patients with AD dementia have episodic memory loss and develop anomia, executive dysfunction, and visuospatial difficulty in the setting of preserved ability to walk, see, hear, and feel. AD dementia is also characterized by the juxtaposition of "knowing how" (procedural memory) and "not knowing what" (declarative memory). The clinical picture of deficits and preserved abilities is explained by the anatomical distribution of the NFT pathology. Arnold et al. (1991) demonstrated that tangle burden is greatest in the medial temporal lobe but spares the primary sensory and motor cortices until very late in the course, which is why AD dementia patients can see, hear, and move but not remember. Early AD is characterized by an isolated memory impairment resulting from significant pathology in the entorhinal cortex and hippocampus, which serves to disconnect the medial temporal lobe from other cortices. The spread of pathology to other association cortices results in accumulation of other symptoms: semantic memory involvement from spread to the anterior temporal lobes, executive dysfunction from spread to the frontal lobes, and visual-spatial dysfunction from spread to the occipitotemporal lobes. In contrast, the primary motor and sensory cortices are only affected late in the course. The preserved basal ganglia and cerebellum are involved in the procedural/motor learning (or knowing how).

## Atypical Alzheimer Disease

Occasionally, AD can present with focal cortical syndromes without memory loss initially. The three most commonly described atypical presentations are posterior cortical atrophy (PCA), logopenic aphasia (LPA), and frontal variant of AD.

### Posterior Cortical Atrophy

In 1988, Benson used the term posterior cortical atrophy to describe five cases with progressive dementia involving visual-spatial function, alexia, and partial Balint and Gerstmann syndromes with relatively preserved memory (Benson et al., 1988). Later, autopsy series of PCA revealed Alzheimer pathology as the most common underlying etiology. While AD is the most common pathology, other pathologies in clinically diagnosed PCA cases include corticobasal degeneration and prion disease. PCA patients are often initially referred to optometry or ophthalmology for difficulty seeing, which may manifest as driving impairment or trouble reading. Not uncommonly, PCA patients undergo procedures such as cataract removal without significant benefit, or alternatively, they may be told there is nothing wrong with their eyes prior to definitive diagnosis. The mean age of onset of PCA is approximately 60 (Tang-Wai et al., 2004). Compared to typical AD, insight is preserved (Mendez et al., 2002). In a large series of 40 PCA cases, complete or partial Balint syndrome (optic ataxia, oculomotor apraxia, simultanagnosia) was present at diagnosis in 88% of patients, complete or partial Gerstmann (left-right confusion, finger agnosia, agraphia, acalculia) was present in 62%, and visual field loss was present in 48%. Simultanagnosia is characterized by only being able to see one object at a time while viewing a scene. Ishihara plates used to assess color perception and complex scenes are good screening tools for the presence of simultanagnosia. Other important signs and symptoms include ideomotor apraxia, alexia, prosopagnosia, hemineglect (sensory or visual), achromatopsia, and dressing apraxia (Tang-Wai et al., 2004). PCA is associated with the APOE ε4 allele (Carrasquillo et al., 2014). Structural MRI reveals parieto-occipital atrophy and FDG-PET demonstrates associated parieto-occipital hypometabolism (Figs. 95.3 and 95.4, respectively). The distribution of amyloid is similar between PCA and typical AD (Rosenbloom et al., 2011). In contrast, PCA patients have significantly more tau deposition in the occipital lobe compared to typical AD (see Fig. 95.4), corresponding to their clinical symptoms (Hof et al., 1990). Adaptive equipment for the blind or those with low sight can be helpful. No randomized controlled trial supports the use of any drug therapies in PCA, although acetylcholinesterase inhibitors are commonly used since the most common underlying pathology is AD. Recent consensus criteria (Table 95.6) for the diagnosis of PCA have been published emphasizing PCA as a clinicoradiological syndrome (Crutch et al., 2017). The new classification recognizes that PCA can present in a "pure" form or overlap with other degenerative diseases such as corticobasal syndrome.

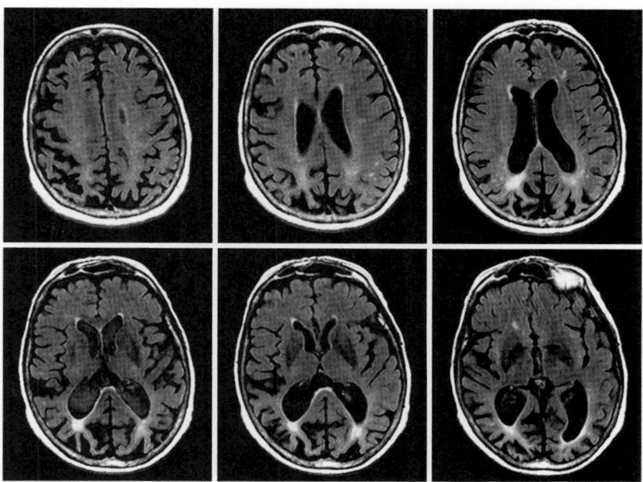

**Fig. 95.3** T2 fluid-attenuated inversion recovery magnetic resonance imaging scans in a patient with posterior cortical atrophy revealing significant parietal and occipital atrophy.

### Logopenic Primary Progressive Aphasia

LPA is one of the primary progressive aphasias. The distinguishing features of LPA include impaired naming, repetition, and word retrieval with phonological errors. Motor speech and grammar are spared. Gorno-Tempini et al. (2008) have suggested impairment in the phonological loop, which stores and rehearses verbal memory as the basis of the clinical presentation. In a study by Mesulam et al. (2008), 64% of logopenic patients had AD pathology at autopsy, and these patients had greater tangle burden in the left hemisphere language areas and fewer tangles in the entorhinal cortex when compared to typical AD pathology. In a large multicenter study, amyloid pathology was present in 86% of those with LPA compared to 20% of those with nonfluent/agrammatic PPA and 16% of those with semantic variant PPA (Bergeron et al., 2018). Phonological errors may be the strongest predictor of underlying AD pathology (Leyton et al., 2014). Structural MRI reveals left temporal-parietal atrophy. FDG-PET scans reveal temporal-parietal hypometabolism and tau PET demonstrates left greater than right temporal and parietal tau deposition (Fig. 95.5, *A* and *B*).

### Behavioral/Frontal or Dysexecutive Variant Alzheimer Disease

Rarely, patients with pathologically confirmed AD present with early impairment on tests of frontal lobe function including verbal fluency and Trails A. These patients may have behavioral and personality changes similar to patients with FTD. However, those with behavioral presentation of AD develop apathy as the most common behavioral feature, in contrast to hyperorality and perseverative/compulsive behaviors seen more commonly in bvFTD (Ossenkoppele et al., 2015). Interestingly, the NFT burden in these patients is increased in the frontal lobes (Johnson et al., 1999).

### Others

Other focal presentations with underlying AD pathology include corticobasal syndrome and, rarely, progressive agrammatic aphasia or semantic variant primary progressive aphasia, which are typically due to FTLD pathology (Alladi et al., 2007).

## Neuropsychiatric Features of Alzheimer Disease Dementia

In a study using the Neuropsychiatric Inventory in AD, apathy (72%) was the most common neuropsychiatric symptom, followed by

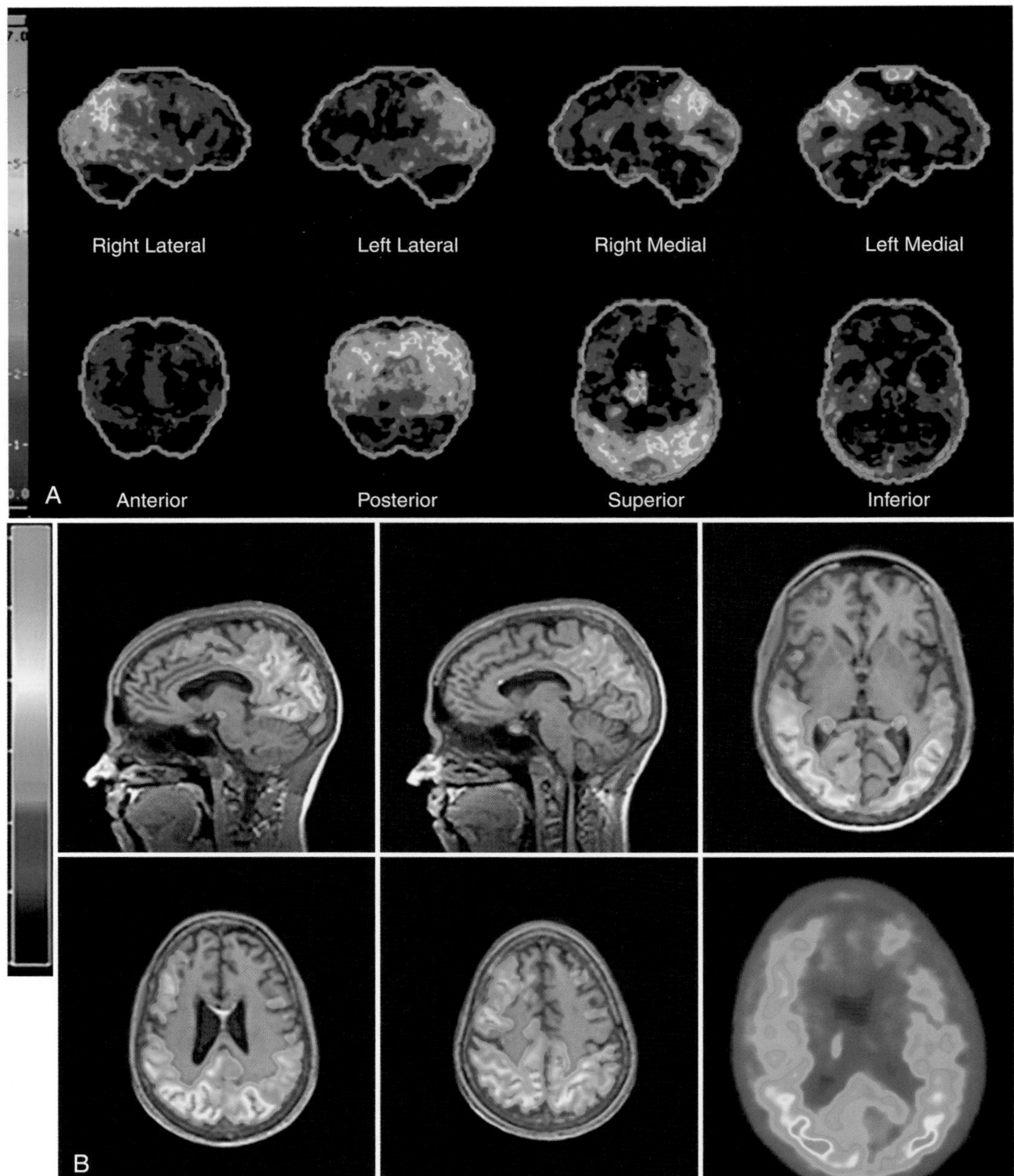


**Fig. 95.4** A, *Top row:* Fluorodeoxyglucose-positron emission tomography (PET) statistical stereotactic surface projection map (Cortex ID) in patient with posterior cortical atrophy demonstrating marked left greater than right occipital-parietal hypometabolism. B, *Bottom rows:* Tau PET in posterior cortical atrophy demonstrating posterior tau deposition.

agitation (60%) and anxiety (48%) (Mega et al., 1996). Identification of delusions is important because it often precedes physically aggressive behavior (Gilley et al., 1997). Common delusions in AD include paranoia and infidelity. Identification of neuropsychiatric features is important because these symptoms result in significant caregiver burden and can be targeted for treatment (Kaufer et al., 1998).

## Diagnostic Criteria

For many years, the most commonly used criteria for the diagnosis of AD were the National Institute of Aging and Stroke–Alzheimer's Disease and Related Disorders Association criteria (McKhann et al., 1984b). However, over the ensuing years, it became apparent that the pathophysiological underpinning of AD began many years before the symptoms of dementia presented themselves. Therefore, in 2011, the National Institute on Aging–Alzheimer's Association (NIA–AA) published revised criteria for the AD process. In this exercise, a distinction was drawn between the clinical symptoms of AD and the underlying pathophysiology. That is, prior to this point, AD was defined as a clinical–pathological entity, but that caused confusion in the field (Petersen, 2018). Therefore, the NIA–AA research criteria characterized the AD clinical spectrum in three phases: dementia, MCI, and preclinical. The dementia due to AD phase was quite similar to what had been defined in 1984 but was made more specific and suggested that biomarkers for AD may be useful in the future when they are validated. The new criteria, however, also recognized a

**TABLE 95.6 Posterior Cortical Atrophy Syndrome**

**Clinical Features**
Insidious onset
Gradual progression
Prominent early disturbance of visual ± other posterior cognitive functions

**Cognitive Features**
**At least three of the following must be present as early or presenting features:**
Space perception deficit
Simultanagnosia
Object perception deficit
Constructional dyspraxia
Environmental agnosia
Oculomotor apraxia
Dressing apraxia
Optic ataxia
Alexia
Left/right disorientation
Acalculia
Limb apraxia (not limb-kinetic)
Apperceptive prosopagnosia
Agraphia
Homonymous visual field defect
Finger agnosia
**All of the following must be evident:**
Relatively spared anterograde memory function
Relatively spared speech and nonvisual language functions
Relatively spared executive functions
Relatively spared behavior and personality
**Neuroimaging:**
Predominant occipito-parietal or occipito-temporal atrophy on magnetic resonance imaging/hypometabolism on positron emission tomography/hypoperfusion single-photon emission computed tomography

*Adapted from Crutch, S.J., Schott, J.M., Rabinovici, G.D., Murray, M., Snowden, J.S., van der Flier, W.M., et al., 2017. Consensus classification of posterior cortical atrophy. Alzheimers Dement. 13, 870–884..*

milder symptomatic stage of the AD process which was termed MCI due to AD (Albert et al., 2011). This stage recognized the growing literature on MCI that had been generated in the previous decade, documenting the existence of a clinical phase of the disease by which people may be mildly impaired from a cognitive perspective, usually with a memory disorder, but were otherwise intact in other cognitive domains and were functionally intact (Petersen et al., 2018). The most novel phase of the disease process was termed preclinical AD. In this phase, subjects were cognitively and functionally normal but harbored the underlying pathophysiological features of AD, such as amyloid deposition. This phase of the disease was meant to generate research on the preclinical aspects of the disease process to allow intervention when disease-modifying therapies become available. Subsequent research has demonstrated that these research criteria are reasonably accurate and data regarding the validation of the biomarkers are accumulating (Jack et al., 2012; Landau et al., 2012). The role of biomarkers has been documented using both neuroimaging and cerebrospinal fluid measures (Jack et al., 2012; Vos et al., 2013). Recent work has revealed a group of preclinical subjects without the typical AD biomarker profile (i.e., no evidence of Aβ deposition on PET or in the CSF) but evidence of neurodegeneration by FDG-PET or MRI, termed suspected non-Alzheimer disease pathophysiology or sNAP given the absence of Aβ deposition (Knopman et al., 2012b). A similar condition, sNAP MCI has been described (Knopman et al., 2013). Fig. 95.6 compares the newest research diagnostic criteria for AD (Dubois et al., 2014; McKhann et al., 2011) and reports the NIA–AA criteria, including the 2018 proposed research framework, which divorces the pathology from the clinical stage. This proposed framework is a significant departure from the 1984 and 2011 proposals since AD could only be called a disease if there was biomarker or autopsy evidence for the presence of amyloid (neuritic plaques) and tau (neurofibrillary tangles) independent of clinical state. One implication of this proposal is that a clinically unimpaired person could be labeled as having AD if there was biomarker evidence for amyloid and tau. Fig. 95.1 reports the NIA–AA criteria for MCI due to AD. The International Working Group has also incorporated biomarkers into updated criteria in 2007 (Dubois et al., 2007) and 2014 (Dubois et al., 2014).

## Neuropsychology in Alzheimer Disease Dementia

Neuropsychology provides a more detailed understanding of cognitive constructs, thereby allowing identification of what cognitive functions are deficient or preserved. The pattern of neuropsychometric testing abnormalities can assist in predicting underlying anatomy and in the differential diagnosis of dementia. Testing is particularly helpful early in the course. Neuropsychology uses well-developed standards based on normative data that improve clinical utility and predictive value. The NIA workgroup consensus criteria of MCI due to AD (Albert et al., 2011) recommend episodic memory evaluation to assist in predicting those with MCI at high risk of converting to AD dementia. Memory testing alone is insufficient, and simple bedside testing cognitive screens can be insensitive to early changes of neurodegeneration. The preservation versus impairment in memory subcomponent testing allows for differentiation among disorders. In brief, learning or encoding refers to the transfer of to-be-learned material from short-term sensory stores into consolidated traces in recent memory involving numerous integrated networks. Free recall pertains to the retrieval of that material without any cues or aids and recognition refers to the identification of the material from among several candidates. A classical memory test such as a verbal memory test consists of reading a list of words over multiple trials. An improvement in encoding over the learning trials (i.e., an increase in number of correct words per trial) is found in normal learning. An individual with an encoding problem may demonstrate a flat learning curve (i.e., the same number of words per trial). Despite the flat learning curve, an encoding problem might lead to preserved free recall and recognition of words with cues. A retrieval deficit is manifest when the person is unable to perform free recall of the material but is able to recall the items when retrieval cues are given. For example, if the person remembers the word "sweater" and is unable to free recall it but can recall it when cued, "It is an item of clothing," then the person was demonstrating a retrieval failure since the word was encoded but not recalled without cues. With a retention or consolidation problem, the individual generally encodes normally with improvement in number of words learned over trials, but with delayed recall has significant difficulty recalling words and does not benefit from recognition cuing. Encoding problems may correspond to attentional deficits or a failure of medial temporal lobe structures such as the hippocampus to facilitate consolidation of the material. This pattern of poor learning and consolidation is commonly seen in AD. In contrast, a relatively pure retrieval problem would be more characteristic of parkinsonian disorders, vascular cognitive impairment, or other disorders not involving the medial temporal lobe. Other neuropsychometric tests can provide discriminating information. For example, category and letter fluency tests may also provide useful diagnostic pattern in AD. Typically, fluency for semantic categories (e.g., fruits, vegetables, and animals) is impaired relative to letter fluency performance (e.g., words beginning with a certain letter). This discrepancy in verbal fluency performance

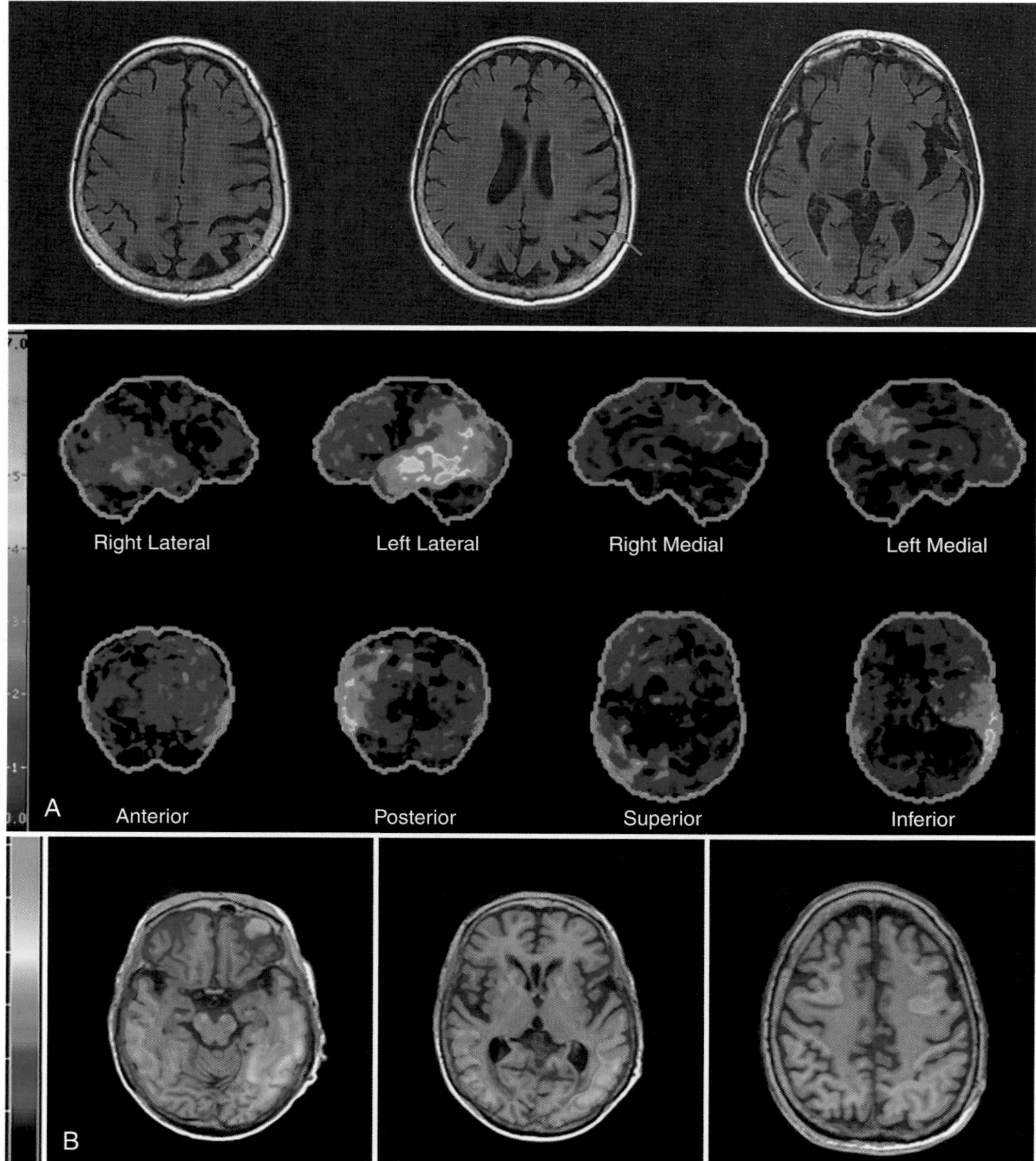


**Fig. 95.5** **A,** *Top row:* T2 fluid-attenuated inversion recovery magnetic resonance imaging scans in a patient with logopenic primary progressive aphasia revealing significant left parietal and temporal atrophy *(red arrows). Bottom row:* Fluorodeoxyglucose-positron emission tomography (PET) statistical stereotactic surface projection map (Cortex ID) in patient with logopenic aphasia demonstrating left temporal-parietal hypometabolism. **B,** Tau PET in logopenic primary progressive aphasia demonstrating left greater than right temporal and parietal tau deposition.

tends to reflect temporal lobe involvement in AD pathology and the relative preservation of subcortical circuitry. Confrontation naming of common objects is also impaired in early AD. Executive function tasks may also be impaired in early AD as evidenced by tasks requiring set-shifting and sequencing, including Trail Making Test Part B (Albert, 1996). Tests of visual spatial function including figure copying can also be impaired early in AD spectrum disorders.

## Biomarkers in Alzheimer Disease

### Cerebrospinal Fluid Biomarkers

The combination of reduction in the CSF Aβ42 and elevation in the CSF tau protein has a sensitivity of 85% and specificity of 86% for the diagnosis of AD dementia (Hulstaert et al., 1999). More recent studies using Aβ42 and tau or phosphorylated tau suggest these biomarkers can improve diagnosis in difficult cases and predict conversion from MCI to AD dementia (Hansson et al., 2006; Mattsson et al., 2009; Shaw et al., 2009). The current research framework includes elevated phosphorylated tau as evidence of pathological tau accumulation while the less specific total tau is used as a neurodegenerative biomarker (Jack et al., 2018a). While these biomarkers can provide important information, normal CSF Aβ42 and tau have been reported in autopsy-proven AD dementia patients (Brunnstrom et al., 2010). Recent data suggest that novel CSF markers, for example, neurofilament light protein, may be good index of neurodegeneration (Mielke et al., 2019).

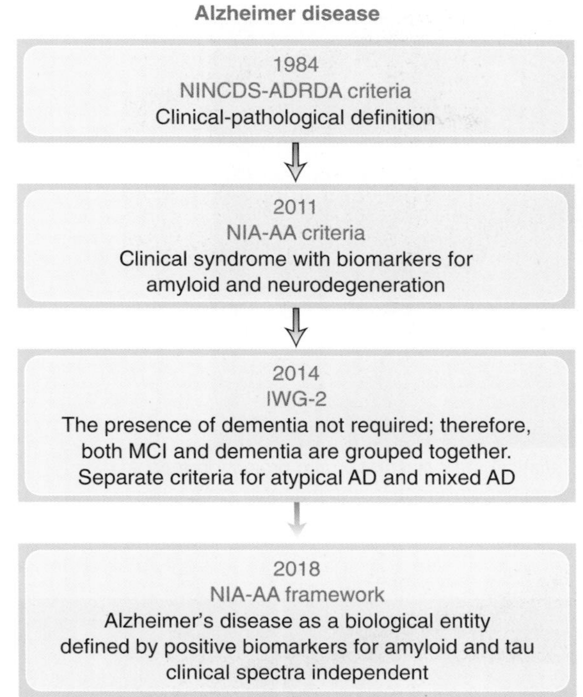


**Fig. 95.6** Timeline of Criteria and Research Frameworks for Alzheimer Disease *(AD)*. The International Working Group 2 *(IWG-2)* (Dubois et al., 2014) criteria do not require the presence of dementia: therefore, both mild cognitive impairment *(MCI)* and dementia are grouped together. IWG-2 includes separate criteria for atypical AD and mixed AD. The National Institute on Aging and the Alzheimer Association *(NIA-AA)* criteria (McKhann et al., 2011): Dementia due to AD criteria is separated into three subgroups, uncertain, intermediate, and high, representing the likelihood that the dementia syndrome is due to underlying AD pathology. Amnestic presentation refers to decline in learning and recall. Nonamnestic presentation refers to decline in language, visuospatial function, or executive function. Both sets of criteria include exclusionary criteria such as the presence of other types of dementia or systemic medical issues that better account for cognitive decline. In the 2018 research framework, the AD is defined purely on biological grounds requiring the presence of an amyloid and tau biomarker separate from clinical status.

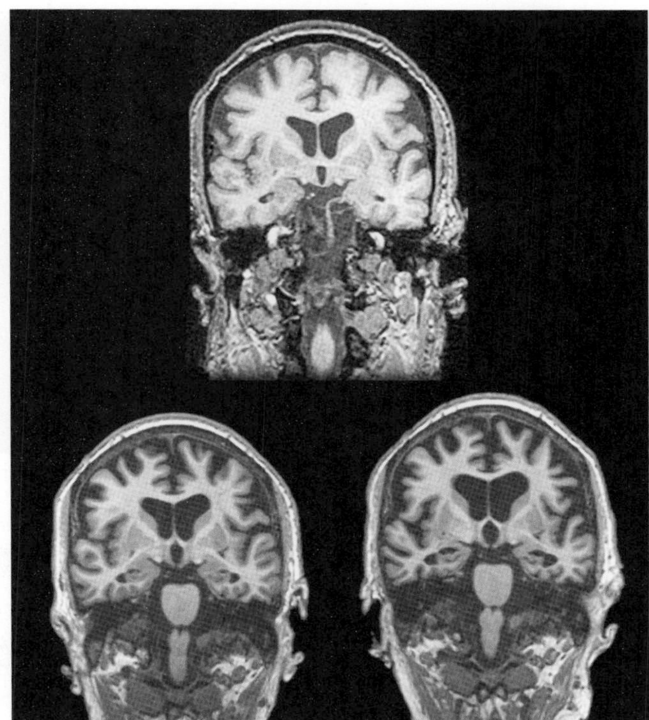

**Fig. 95.7** Longitudinal coronal T1 magnetic resonance imaging in a patient that progressed from normal cognition to amnestic mild cognitive impairment (aMCI) to dementia due to Alzheimer disease (AD). Note progressive hippocampal and cortical atrophy. *Top image:* Normal cognition age 75. *Bottom left image:* aMCI age 81. *Bottom right image:* Dementia due to AD age 86.

## Neuroimaging Biomarkers

Various neuroimaging biomarkers are sensitive to different stages and markers of AD.

***Structural imaging.*** The AAN practice parameter recommends that a neuroimaging examination, either CT or MRI, be performed at the time of the initial dementia assessment (Knopman et al., 2001). While this recommendation was primarily suggested to exclude reversible and treatable causes of dementias, MRI provides much higher resolution than CT and has proven very useful in the differential diagnosis of dementia and as a biomarker of neurodegeneration in AD dementia. Medial temporal lobe atrophy of the hippocampus and entorhinal cortex with concomitant dilatation of the temporal horns is an early characteristic of AD dementia (Fig. 95.7) and can predict conversion from normal cognition to MCI and MCI to AD dementia (Jack et al., 2000). Reduction in hippocampal volumes correlates with NFT pathology at autopsy and cognitive decline (Jack et al., 2002). In aMCI, atrophy is limited to the medial temporal lobe structures while with AD onset, atrophy spreads to the lateral temporal and parietal cortices. This change corresponds with Braak staging, which is why structural MRI serves as a biomarker of neurodegeneration (Braak and Braak, 1991).

The utility of volumetric measurements of the entorhinal cortex, while promising, is controversial. Although medial temporal lobe structures become atrophic in early AD and correlate with episodic memory performance, later in the disease atrophy rates are greater in the temporal, parietal, and frontal cortices and are associated with deterioration in other cognitive domains including language, praxis, and visuospatial (Frisoni et al., 2010). Medial temporal lobe atrophy is not specific for AD and can be seen in other degenerative and vascular processes. In particular neurodegenerative hippocampal sclerosis of aging can have a similar imaging appearance to Alzheimer dementia (Botha et al., 2018b). During the dementia stage, significant global atrophy occurs typically most significantly in a temporal-parietal distribution with coinciding ventriculomegaly.

The presence of white matter hyperintensities observed by FLAIR or T2 MRI also appears to contribute to cognitive impairment in AD (Provenzano et al., 2013).

***Cerebral amyloid angiopathy.*** Hypointense signal on MRI gradient-echo sequences represents hemosiderin deposition reflective of cerebral microbleeds. Newer techniques, such as susceptibility-weighted imaging, are more sensitive for these findings. In the Alzheimer's Disease Neuroimaging Initiative (ADNI) cohort, cerebral microbleeds were present in approximately 33% of cases and increased with Aβ load as measured by amyloid PET (Kantarci et al., 2013). When cerebral microbleeds occur in a lobar distribution in elderly patients, they often represent cerebral amyloid angiopathy (CAA). In a population-based study, β-amyloid load on PET was associated with lobar but not with deep cerebral microbleeds (Graff-Radford et al., 2019). Identification of coexisting CAA and AD has clinical importance because patients with AD and CAA have worse cognition

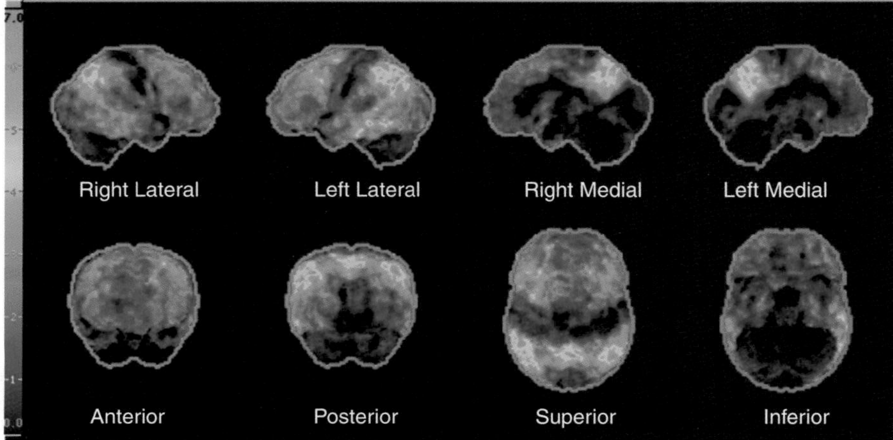


**Fig. 95.8** Fluorodeoxyglucose-positron emission tomography statistical stereotactic surface projection map (Cortex ID) showing marked hypometabolism involving the temporal-parietal junction and posterior cingulate gyri which is relatively symmetric. Relative preservation of the frontal and occipital lobes consistent with Alzheimer disease dementia.

and higher mean tangle and plaque rates than patients with just AD changes alone (Arvanitakis et al., 2011; Pfeifer et al., 2002). Specific cognitive correlates of CAA include decreased perceptual speed and episodic memory (Arvanitakis et al., 2011). CAA preferentially involves the occipital lobe.

***Functional imaging.*** Functional brain imaging using single-photon emission computed tomography (SPECT) and FDG-PET can suggest disease specific patterns. While functional imaging studies have not been endorsed by criteria for MCI or AD due to dementia (Albert et al., 2011; McKhann et al., 2011), their value is recognized in selected cases. Especially when the structural imaging scan is not informative, functional imaging modalities may provide additional useful information (Reiman et al., 1996; Sanchez-Juan et al., 2014).

Decreased blood flow in a temporal-parietal distribution seen on SPECT correlates with hypometabolism seen on FDG-PET and is suggestive of AD.

In aMCI, hypometabolism is primarily in the hippocampus and posterior cingulate. In AD dementia, the hypometabolism includes these regions as well as the temporal-parietal regions (Mosconi et al., 2008). Recent studies have indicated that FDG-PET can be used as an aid in the diagnosis of AD dementia, in particular in differentiating AD from FTD (Foster et al., 2007; Rabinovici et al., 2011), which has led to the Centers for Medicare and Medicaid Services approving reimbursement for evaluating this differential diagnosis. Several studies have validated the use of FDG-PET as a biomarker in AD, resulting in its inclusion as a biomarker in the most recent AD criteria (McKhann et al., 2011). In MCI ADNI participants, FDG-PET predicted conversion to AD dementia (Landau et al., 2010). Of particular interest, FDG-PET in cognitive normal homozygous carriers for APOE ε4 demonstrates hypometabolism in the posterior in the cingulate, temporal, and parietal cortices (Reiman et al., 1996). Fig. 95.8 demonstrates an FDG-PET in a patient with typical AD dementia.

***Amyloid imaging.*** The development of Pittsburgh Compound B (PiB) has allowed measurement of amyloid burden in living subjects (Klunk et al., 2004). While not currently recommended for routine clinical use, this imaging modality is already being used in clinical trials for identifying preclinical AD, MCI due to AD, and monitoring effectiveness of amyloid-targeted therapies. Appropriate-use criteria have been published which make recommendations regarding the clinical setting in which amyloid PET could be considered (Johnson et al., 2013). The deposition of amyloid as measured by PiB-PET occurs primarily in the frontal and temporal-parietal regions (see Fig. 95.9 for examples of PiB-PET imaging). Since its discovery, numerous studies have demonstrated possible clinical utilities. PiB-PET outperformed FDG-PET in discriminating FTD from AD (Rabinovici et al., 2011). PiB binding cross-sectionally correlates with cognitive function (Jack et al., 2008). Longitudinally, however, once, symptomatic, the deposition of β-amyloid plateaus demonstrating that PiB utility may be greatest in the preclinical stages (Engler et al., 2006).

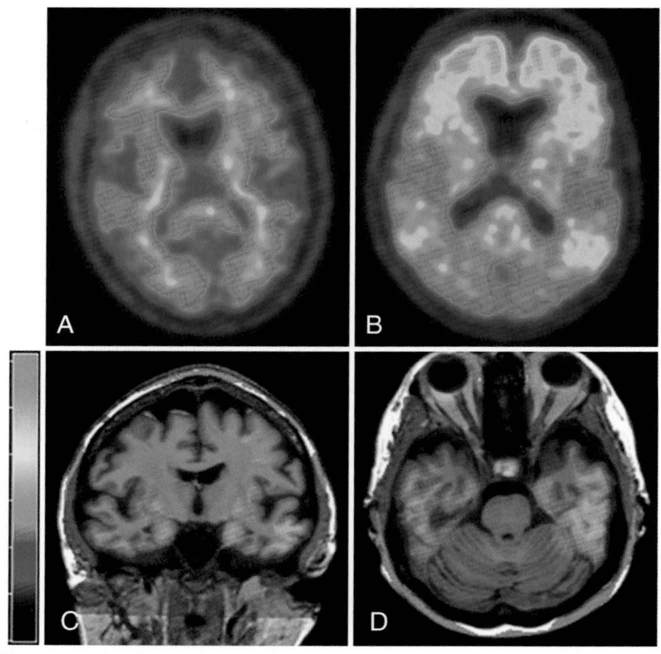


**Fig. 95.9 Top Row: Amyloid Pittsburgh Compound B (PiB)-Positron Emission Tomography Imaging. A,** PiB retention is not present. **B,** Significant PiB retention. **Bottom Row: Tau PET in Typical amnestic AD. C,** Coronal view of Tau signal in medial temporal lobe. **D,** Axial view of Tau PET signal in the bilateral temporal lobes *(Courtesy Dr. Val Lowe.)*

In a population-based study of cognitively normal individuals over age 70, approximately one-third have significant β-amyloid load (Kantarci et al., 2012b). The prevalence of a positive amyloid PET scan among cognitively unimpaired individuals in the general population increased from 2.7% in individuals between ages 50 and 59 years to 41% in those individuals between ages 80 and 89 years (Roberts et al., 2018). The high rate of amyloid-positive scans in the cognitively normal population along with the absence of any disease-modifying therapy would suggest amyloid imaging in cognitively normal elderly individuals should be reserved for research purposes until disease-modifying therapy is available.

Several F-18 analog amyloid tracers have been developed and approved for clinical use by the Food and Drug Administration (FDA) florbetapir, flutemetamol, and florbetaben. The F-18 agents provide comparable results to PiB imaging, but a longer half-life allows for transportation to clinical centers. Florbetapir performs well compared to autopsy confirmation (Clark et al., 2011). In the ADNI study, Aβ deposition, as measured with florbetapir, correlated with cognitive decline in cognitive normal and MCI participants. In the cognitive normal group this decline sometimes occurred in the absence of FDG abnormality (Landau et al., 2012). Multiple studies have demonstrated the prognostic importance of amyloid PET. The incident risk of developing mild cognitive impairment increased greater than twofold among cognitively unimpaired individuals who were amyloid PET positive compared to those who were amyloid PET negative (Roberts et al., 2018).

***Task-free functional magnetic resonance imaging.*** Functional MRI (fMRI) measures the blood-oxygen-level dependent (BOLD) signal, essentially relying on the fact that neuronal activation in a region produces associated increases in blood flow to that same region. Dementia caused by neurodegeneration is caused by the disruption of specific, large-scale neural networks (Seeley et al., 2009). fMRI is one technique to study these neural networks. The default mode network (DMN) refers to connected regions of brain that are active when an individual is at rest or not focused on the external environment (Raichle et al., 2001). In AD, the DMN is selectively targeted. The core regions of the brain activated in this default state include the medial prefrontal cortex, inferior parietal lobule, posterior cingulate gyrus, hippocampal formation, and lateral temporal cortex. These changes on fMRI occur early in the disease process. In cognitively normal APOE ε4 subjects, there is a decrease in connectivity relative to controls (Machulda et al., 2011). These changes occur in the absence of brain amyloidosis, as measured by amyloid PET and Aβ42 levels in the CSF (Sheline et al., 2010). Therefore, fMRI changes may be a very early marker of the pathophysiology of AD. While current use of fMRI in dementia is limited to research, it has provided substantial knowledge about degenerative disease and is actively being investigated as a biomarker.

***Tau imaging.*** Recently, several tau imaging tracers have been developed The FDA approved Tauvid (flortaucipir F18) for patients being evaluated for AD. Since tau comprises the other hallmark of the AD pathological process, neurofibrillary tangles, the ability to image it in vivo would be extremely useful. Tau is also implicated in a variety of other disorders and the ability to characterize this protein would be advantageous in diagnosis and following putative treatments.

The presence of tau PET signal in the inferior temporal cortex is closely linked to clinical symptoms (Johnson et al., 2016). Tau PET reliably distinguishes AD dementia from non-AD dementias (Ossenkoppele et al., 2018). Since flortaucipir binds to AD-type tau (3R,4R), it is not surprising that tau-PET levels in the temporal pole of tau mutation (microtubule-associated protein tau [MAPT]) cases were lower than in AD dementia cases, with the exception of tau mutation cases, whose MAPT mutation occurs outside of exon 10 (V337M and R406W) and, therefore, develop AD-like tau and have tau-PET signal close to the AD dementia levels (Jones et al., 2018a). Many issues exist regarding these tracers, such as specificity for tau and various tau isoforms, but it is a promising technique. For example, in semantic variant primary progressive aphasia, which is most often associated with TAR DNA-binding protein (TDP)-43-positive inclusions, tau-PET signal has been seen in areas of atrophy, possibly reflecting off-target binding (Josephs et al., 2018; Makaretz et al., 2018). Tau PET has allowed investigation into how patterns develop with age. In cognitively unimpaired individuals in the preclinical stage of AD, in addition to the expected medial temporal tau involvement, tau is present in extra-medial temporal regions and extra-temporal regions arguing against a region-region spread of tau pathology that has been previously proposed (Lowe et al., 2018) (see Fig. 95.9 bottom row for examples of tau-PET imaging).

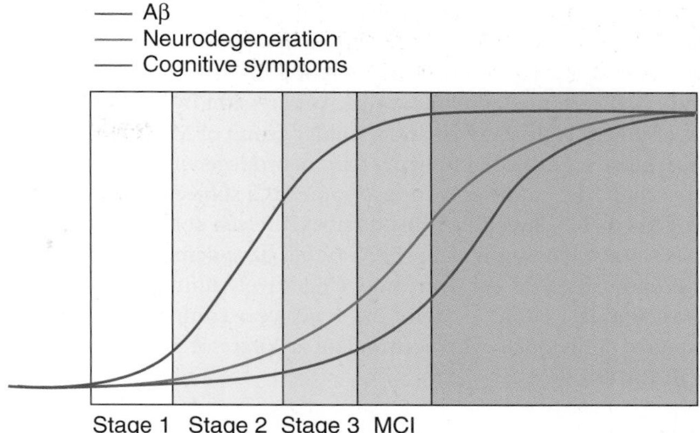


**Fig. 95.10** Hypothetical model for the sequence of biomarkers and pathological events in the development of Alzheimer disease. *Aβ,* Amyloid beta; *MCI,* mild cognitive impairment. (*Modified with permission from Jack, C.R. Jr., Knopman, D.S., Jagust, W.J., et al., 2010. Hypothetical model of dynamic biomarkers of the Alzheimer's pathological cascade. Lancet Neurol. 9, 119–128.*)

## Longitudinal Tracking of Biomarkers

The advent of biomarkers for tracking the progression of AD has vastly increased our knowledge about its temporal progression and will play a key role in clinical trial design and execution. Several key biomarker studies in conjunction with data of unselected autopsies published over a short period of time have provided evidence that the pathophysiological processes underlying AD start decades before cognitive decline. This knowledge has shifted the focus of disease therapies to the presymptomatic or early symptomatic phases of the disease. One influential hypothetical model for the sequence of these biomarkers was first proposed by Cliff Jack in 2010 (Jack et al., 2010) and revised in 2013 (Jack and Holtzman, 2013). This model represents the pathophysiological processes underlying AD, and is summarized in Fig. 95.10. The Dominantly Inherited Alzheimer Network (DIAN) study has provided important information regarding the timing of biomarkers in autosomal dominant AD largely consistent with the model described above (Bateman et al., 2012). This sequence can be summarized by the following: CSF Aβ42 declines over two decades before clinical symptoms; Aβ-PET abnormalities begin about 15 years before symptoms; brain volume loss and increased CSF tau also occur 15 years before symptoms; FDG-PET abnormalities occur 10 years before symptoms (Bateman et al., 2012).

While this sequence is predictable for dominantly inherited AD, the Mayo Clinic Study of Aging has demonstrated that a substantial proportion of cognitively normal subjects have neurodegeneration biomarkers but not amyloid biomarkers, as was noted earlier in this chapter (Jack et al., 2012; Knopman et al., 2012a). In preclinical AD, 42% of incident Aβ-PET positive cases also have positive neurodegeneration biomarkers first. This suggests that at least two biomarker profile pathways to preclinical AD exist, and some of the cases labeled sNAP are on the AD pathway but with a different biomarker progression (Jack et al., 2013). In the same framework, progression in MCI to dementia has also been characterized and a similar group of MCI sNAP subjects have been identified, implying that neurodegenerative pathologies other than AD may be operating in some MCI subjects, and while most progress to AD dementia, some do not (Petersen et al., 2013).

Recently, longitudinal tau-PET studies have demonstrated the rate of accumulation of tau over time. Cognitively unimpaired individuals accumulate tau at a rate of 0.5% per year compared to cognitive impaired individuals who accumulate at a rate of 3% per year (Jack et al., 2018b).

## Genetics

### Alzheimer Genetics

In a large twin study from Sweden based on 392 pairs of twins, the genetic component of AD was estimated to be 58%–79% (Gatz et al., 2006). Family history of AD can provide important risk information. The lifetime risk of AD dementia in first-degree relatives is approximately 39% and this risk increases to 54% by age 80 if both parents have AD dementia (Lautenschlager et al., 1996).

### Early-Onset Genes

Three rare, early-onset, fully penetrant gene mutations have been described to cause Alzheimer dementia. While mutations in these genes are rare, studying them has been instrumental in our understanding of AD. All three increase brain Aβ levels and form an important part of the amyloid hypothesis for AD (discussed later). This provided the basis for several animal models and biomarker development including development of CSF and PET Aβ.

***Amyloid precursor protein chromosome 21.*** Mutations in amyloid precursor protein (APP) were the first mutation to be described to cause AD. Chromosome 21 became a chromosome of interest for AD, since patients with trisomy 21 (Down syndrome) develop AD pathology after age 40. Investigators looked at the brains of patients with AD dementia and Down syndrome and found Aβ in both. Since Aβ is the product of APP (located on chromosome 21), APP became a candidate gene (Glenner and Wong, 1984; Goate et al., 1991; Goldgaber et al., 1987; St George-Hyslop et al., 1987). All APP mutations that cause AD change the Aβ42 to Aβ40 ratio. Recently, certain mutations in APP have been described to be protective against AD (Jonsson et al., 2012) by decreasing the production of Aβ. The mean age of onset for APP mutation families is approximately 50. In addition to early age of onset, the clinical presentation of APP mutations carriers may be distinguished from sporadic AD by the presence of myoclonus, seizures, early dyscalculia, cerebral white matter changes, and even corticospinal tract signs (Rossor et al., 1993).

***Presenilin 1 chromosome 14.*** The majority of early-onset familial AD cases are mapped to chromosome 14 (Rossor et al., 1993). In 1995, mutations on chromosome 14 were found in PSEN1 in autosomal dominant AD families (Sherrington et al., 1995). Interestingly, presenilin is part of the γ secretase complex that cleaves APP (Wolfe et al., 1999). Clinical features of PSEN1 families can include significant aphasia in addition to myoclonus and seizures (Lampe et al., 1994).

***Presenilin 2 chromosome 1.*** PSEN2 was discovered shortly thereafter (Rogaev et al., 1995). PSEN 2 mutations are the rarest of the autosomal dominant mutations. PSEN2 is part of the γ secretase complex that cleaves APP. Most of these individuals are descendants of families from the Volga River region of Russia. Similar to the other familial early-onset mutations, PSEN2 families have a higher rate of seizures than in sporadic AD (Jayadev et al., 2010).

### Late-Onset Genes

Apolipoprotein E (APOE) is the most important genetic risk factor for late-onset AD (Corder et al., 1993). APOE has three isoforms (E4 associated with high risk, E3 associated with neutral risk, and E2 which is protective). About 20% of all late-onset AD is thought to be related to APOE ε4 (Slooter et al., 1998). APOE ε4 affects AD risk and age of onset in a dose-dependent way; for example, E4 homozygotes have a mean age of onset of 68 with a lifetime AD risk of 91%; in E4 heterozygotes, the mean age of onset is 76 with a 47% lifetime risk (Liu et al., 2013). In contrast, E4 noncarriers have a mean age of onset of 84 with an approximately 20% lifetime frequency (Corder et al., 1993; Liu et al., 2013).

Trem2 variants have recently been identified as rare risk variants for AD dementia (Guerreiro et al., 2013b). The odds ratio is similar to APOE ε4 but it is rare, which is why it was not seen in previous genome-wide association studies. Its population-attributable risk is lower than APOE ε4 due to its lower frequency.

Many other risk loci have been associated with AD risk, but their overall impact is thought to be small. These include CD33 molecule, ATP-binding cassette, subfamily A, member 7 (ABCA7), sortilin-related receptor L (SORL1), clusterin (CLU), phosphatidylinositol binding clathrin assembly protein (PICALM), as well as many others (Guerreiro et al., 2013a).

### Genetic Testing

Genetic testing for APP, PSEN1, PSEN2, and APOE is commercially available in Clinical Laboratory Improvement Amendments (CLIA) laboratories. Routine genetic testing is not recommended by the practice parameter of the AAN, but if patients have testing, genetic counseling prior to testing is essential. Testing may have significant implications for patients and families in terms of family planning, financial costs, and risk of depression. Genetic testing currently does not change treatment of the patient but may provide opportunities to participate in research studies such as DIAN.

## Alzheimer Pathophysiology

All three early-onset AD genes (APP, PSEN1, PSEN2) play a role in Aβ metabolism which has provided the foundation for the amyloid hypothesis of AD. The basic hypothesis is that abnormal Aβ metabolism altering the Aβ42/Aβ40 ratio in the brain causes Aβ oligomer formation and aggregation to form fibrils, which form the amyloid plaque. This oligomer formation and aggregation results in a cascade of events, including tau protein tangle formation, increased inflammatory response, and oxidative injury, to cause neurotoxicity and neurodegeneration. More recent work has focused on the pathogenicity of soluble Aβ oligomers with converging basic scientific evidence that they play a major role in neurotoxicity. For example, human Aβ oligomers injected into the hippocampus of rats inhibit long-term potentiation (Walsh et al., 2002) and result in synaptic dysfunction which impairs memory formation (Walsh et al., 2002).

Aβ is derived from APP through proteolytic processing. Aβ is produced normally in the body but under normal circumstances it is removed efficiently by a number of mechanisms. These include breakdown by extracellular proteases, such as insulin-degrading enzyme, and receptor-mediated endocytosis followed by lysosomal degradation and drainage through the cerebral vasculature and into the CSF via the glymphatic system (Xie et al., 2013a).

### Amyloid Hypothesis

The amyloid hypothesis proposes that AD can result from too much Aβ production or a change in ratio with more Aβ42 than Aβ40 produced, or impaired clearance of Aβ. Understanding APP processing is central to the amyloid hypothesis (Hardy and Higgins, 1992).

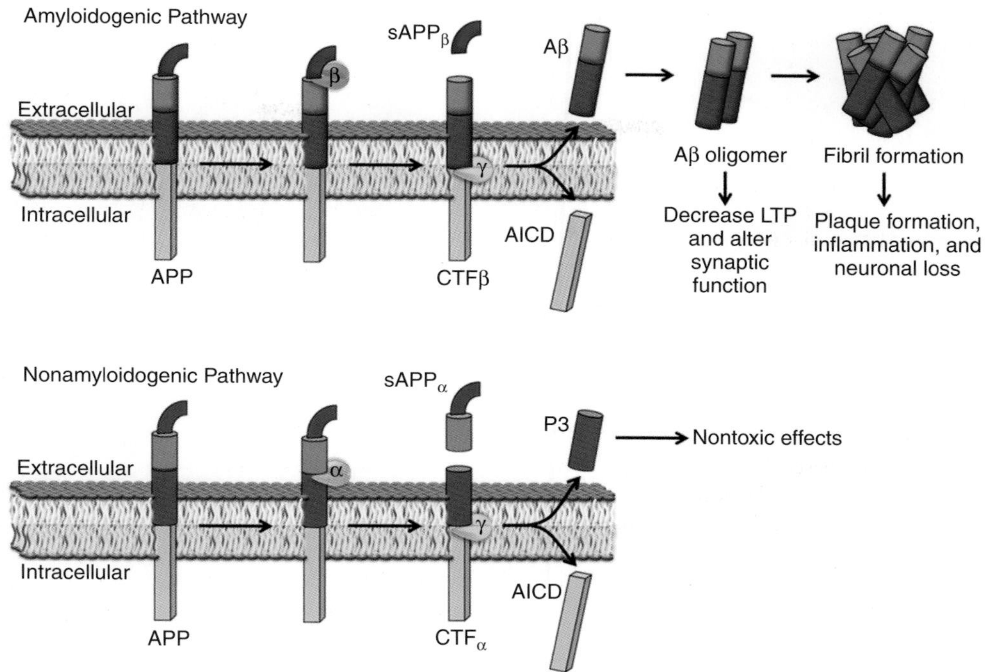


**Fig. 95.11** Amyloid Precursor Protein Processing. *Aβ,* Amyloid Beta; *AICD,* APP intracellular domain; *APP,* amyloid precursor protein; *sAPPα,* soluble APP α.

APP is a type 1 protein with the amino terminal in the extracellular space. APP is cleaved by three enzymes (α, β, and γ secretase) (Selkoe and Schenk, 2003) and can undergo processing either through the amyloidogenic pathway (γ and β secretases) which produces Aβ, or the nonamyloidogenic pathway (α secretase) (Fig. 95.11).

In the amyloidogenic pathway, APP is first cleaved by β secretase. This cleavage produces a β C-terminal fragment, which stays on the membrane and soluble APP Aβ. This β C-terminal fragment is then cleaved by γ secretase in the transmembrane region producing APP intracellular domain (AICD) and Aβ peptide, which is then released into extracellular space. PSEN 1 and 2 are part of the γ secretase complex (Iwatsubo, 2004). Other components of the γ secretase complex include nicastrin, APH-1. This aforementioned cleavage occurs by sequential events eventually producing β-amyloid fragments, either Aβ1-42 (about 10%) or Aβ1-40 (about 90%). Aβ can aggregate and these aggregates may form oligomers which may be toxic. Aβ1-42 has a greater tendency to aggregate and is found in greater concentration in plaques, while Aβ1-40 is the predominant form in vascular amyloid deposits.

In the nonamyloidogenic pathway, APP cleavage is mediated by α secretase. This cleavage is in the middle of the β-amyloid peptide above the surface of the membrane, thereby preventing the formation of Aβ. This cleavage generates soluble APP α (sAPPα) and α C-terminal fragments, which can also undergo cleavage by γ secretase, producing a nontoxic peptide called P3.

APOE functions primarily in the transport of lipids/cholesterol from astrocytes to neurons. The presence of the APOE ε4 allele is associated with decreased CSF Aβ42 and increased brain Aβ burden seen on Aβ (Morris et al., 2010). Despite these biomarker changes, the mechanisms of E4 leading to AD are numerous and include both Aβ-related and Aβ-unrelated mechanisms. Aβ-dependent mechanisms include interfering with cerebral Aβ clearance and promoting Aβ aggregation. Aβ-independent mechanisms include promoting abnormal lipid transport, thereby altering synaptic plasticity and the inflammatory response (Liu et al., 2013).

Accumulating evidence suggests that a common mechanism across neurodegenerative diseases may include the trans-synaptic spread of tau and other misfolded proteins to anatomically connected regions in a prion-like manner where the protein is released and taken up by the anatomically related neuron (Walker et al., 2013).

Recent efforts have been made to investigate how large-scale neural networks may be involved in the pathophysiology of AD and other neurodegenerative disorders. It has long been known that systems of connected neurons are selectively vulnerable to neurodegenerative disease, but the pathophysiology behind this association is debated. In contrast to disease models that emphasize the molecular misfolding of proteins spreading within connected systems, complex systems models emphasize the causal role of dynamic functional activity within brain systems interacting with molecular physiology (Jones et al., 2016).

## Alzheimer Pathology

Alzheimer disease is defined by two pathological findings: extracellular plaques composed primarily of amyloid and intraneuronal neurofibrillary tangles composed primarily of hyperphosphorylated tau. Both involve abnormal conformational changes in proteins. Proteolytic events are critical in APP processing that leads to Aβ. In neurofibrillary pathology, phosphorylation of tau is a critical event.

Macroscopically, AD is characterized by diffuse brain atrophy including significantly decreased weight at autopsy. Some areas are preferentially affected, including multimodal association areas, while others, like primary motor, somatosensory, auditory, and visual cortices, are relatively spared. The limbic areas including hippocampi and cingulate gyrus are severely affected. Substantia nigra (unlike in parkinsonian disorders) is relatively spared while locus coeruleus is severely affected. Work from Braak looking at autopsies of young adults suggests the earliest place neurofibrillary tangle pathology occurs is in the locus ceruleus, with tangles occurring in the third or fourth decades without involvement of tangles in the limbic areas or the presence of amyloid plaques (Braak et al., 2011). Fig. 95.12 summarizes typical examples of Alzheimer pathology.

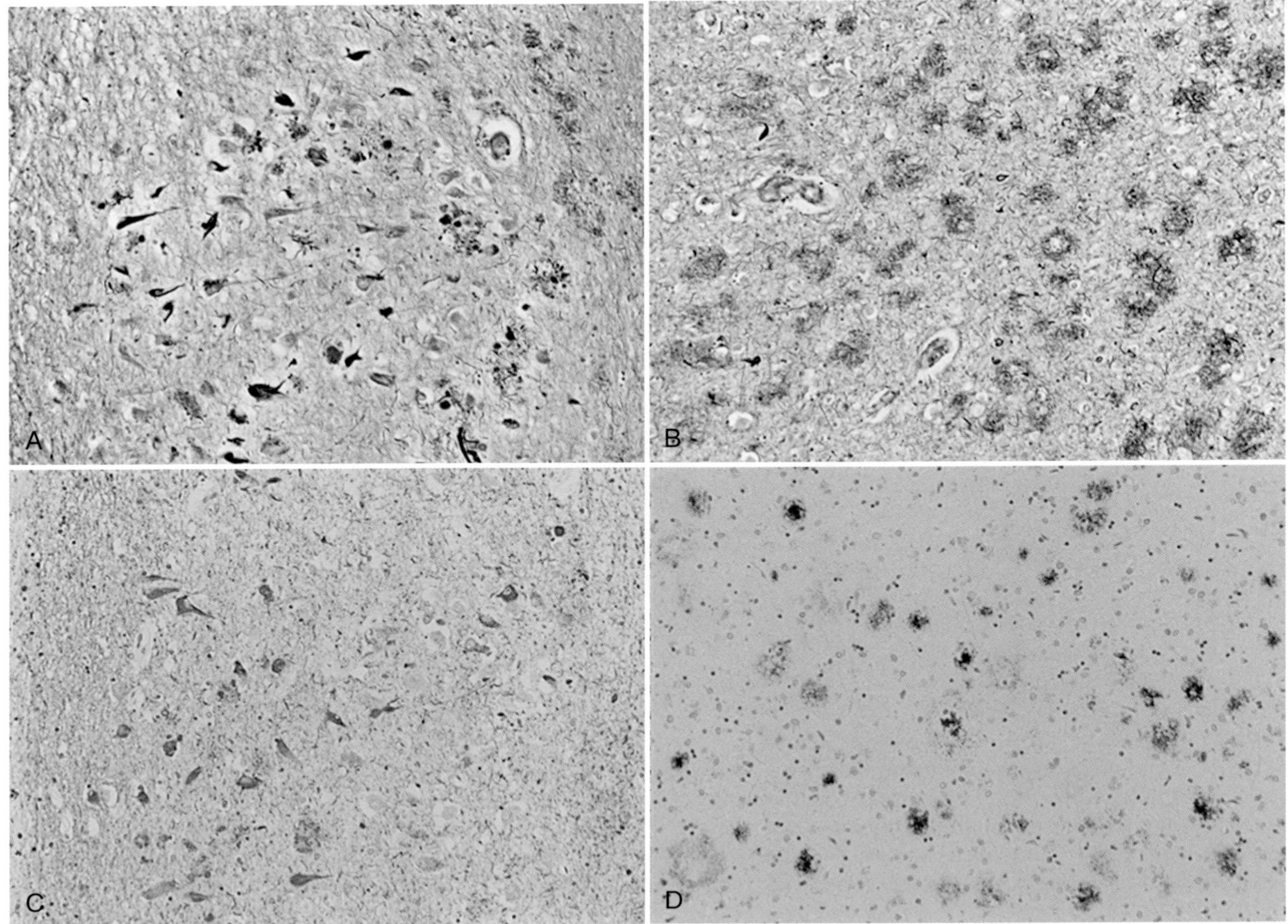

**Fig. 95.12 Alzheimer Disease Pathology.** Bielschowsky stain of CA1 of the hippocampus (**A**) and temporal cortex (**B**) demonstrating neurofibrillary tangles and amyloid plaques. **C**, Tau stain of CA1 of the hippocampus demonstrating neurofibrillary tangles. **D**, Aβ stain of the parietal cortex demonstrating plaques. (*Courtesy Dr. Joseph Parisi.*)

## Amyloid Plaques

Aβ deposition in the brain occurs in a sequential manner starting in the cortex, followed sequentially by the hippocampus, basal ganglia, thalamus, and basal forebrain before in the final stages reaching the brainstem and cerebellum (Thal et al., 2002). Plaques are complicated heterogeneous lesions composed of extracellular protein deposits and certain cellular components. Aβ derived from APP is the sine qua non of plaques, which are in turn the defining pathological finding in AD. Despite the strong association of Aβ with plaques, in reality plaques contain many other components. Other associated components of the plaque include APOE, alpha-1 antitrypsin, complement factors, and immunoglobulins. Plaques can be divided into diffuse (Aβ mainly) and neuritic plaques (includes damaged tau containing axons and dendrites, i.e., neurites). Cell components seen in plaques include neurites, microglia, and astrocytes. The typical neuritic plaque has a dense core of Aβ and less compact rim consisting of neurites, microglia, and astrogliosis at the periphery. Diffuse plaques have less diagnostic specificity and can be seen in a variety of different disorders. They contain Aβ but do not stain with tau-containing neurites and are not associated with synaptic loss, reactive astrocytes, or microglia.

## Neurofibrillary Tangles

The major component of the NFT is tau within neurons and their cell processes. First, pretangles form in the neuron cytoplasm, often concentrated around the membrane. Then, tau is organized into fibrils as NFTs. When the cell dies, the tangle may be situated extracellularly. Normal tau is a microtubule-associated protein and is not visible within the brain. In NFTs, tau has become hyperphosphorylated and abnormally conformed. This tau can be detected with immunostains that bind abnormally conformed tau. Braak and Braak (1991) have described a fairly predictable spread of NFT pathology through the brain occurring in six stages which can be reduced to three, consisting of transentorhinal (stages I, II), limbic (III, IV), and isocortical (V, VI) stages. Braak staging has recently been modified to include brainstem regions preceding medial temporal involvement (Braak et al., 2011).

Several other associated pathological findings may be seen with AD. CAA, often present in leptomeningeal vessels, capillaries, small arterioles, and middle-sized arteries, is seen in over 80% of AD cases. In contrast to cerebral plaques consisting primarily of Aβ42, CAA's major component is Aβ40. Granulovacuolar bodies, typically found in the hippocampus, are small dense granules within the vacuole and can be labeled with acid phosphatase, tubulin, ubiquitin, and neurofilament. Hirano bodies (eosinophilic rod bodies), also typically found in the hippocampus, are often in neuronal processes and contain actin and actin-binding proteins. The significance of granulovacuolar bodies and Hirano bodies is incompletely understood.

### Clinicopathological Correlations

Numerous studies have shown that dementia duration and severity correlate better with NFTs compared to amyloid plaques (Arriagada et al., 1992; Grober et al., 1999).

### Cholinergic Loss

Studies of subjects with advanced AD demonstrated depleted cholinergic neurons in the basal forebrain. This finding served as the basis for the cholinergic hypothesis, which postulated that memory loss in AD was caused by a cholinergic deficit. This hypothesis led to the development and approval of acetylcholinesterase inhibitors for AD. In one study (DeKosky et al., 2002), the loss of choline acetyltransferase (ChAT) and cholinergic neurons did not occur until late in the AD course.

### Neuropathological Criteria

The pathological criteria for AD are based not only on the presence of the pathological lesions but also the severity and location of the lesions. Original criteria (Khachaturian, 1985) were only plaque based and included all types of plaques. In 1991, modifications were then made by the Consortium to Establish a Registry for Alzheimer Disease (CERAD) (Mirra et al., 1991). These criteria emphasized the importance of neuritic plaques over diffuse plaques but lacked specificity because NFTs were not included. In 1997, the NIA and the Reagan Institute criteria were developed which included both neurofibrillary pathology and neuritic plaques and included probability statements (low, intermediate, or high likelihood AD) based on Braak stage and severity of plaques (none, sparse, moderate, or frequent). Most recently, the 2012 criteria incorporated evaluation of coexisting pathologies and the recognition that AD pathological changes can occur without cognitive decline (Montine et al., 2012).

The separation of the clinical symptoms from the pathological features of AD was an important advancement for the field. Alzheimer disease is no longer considered a "clinical-pathological" entity; rather there are two continua, clinical and pathophysiological.

### TAR DNA-Binding Protein 43

TDP 43 deposition was originally thought to be specific for frontotemporal lobar degeneration. Recent studies, however, have shown that TDP-43 pathology occurs in AD and may play an important role in neurodegeneration and clinical features (Josephs et al., 2014; Wilson et al., 2013).

### Alzheimer Pathology in Aging and Mild Cognitive Impairment

Plaques can be found in cognitively normal individuals. This has been termed "pathological aging," although there is significant evidence that these individuals may have preclinical AD (Dickson et al., 1992). The plaques seen in "pathological aging," unlike neuritic AD plaques, lack tau immunoreactivity. NFTs can also be seen with aging but are typically restricted to the medial temporal lobe and brainstem in cognitively normal individuals. In addition, cognitively normal individuals with tau in the entorhinal cortex will have neurons surrounding the tau, in contrast to AD where tau will be associated with significant neuronal loss. Not surprisingly, autopsies of patients with MCI typically fall in a transition pathological state between aging and AD dementia, most commonly Braak stage II or III (Petersen et al., 2006).

### Hippocampal-Sparing Alzheimer Disease

While progression of tangles from the medial temporal to association cortex is typical, there is a subgroup of individuals with a high burden of cortical tau pathology with relative sparing of the hippocampus. This is termed hippocampal-sparing AD. Despite the difference in tau pathology between sites, the amyloid burden is similar. Hippocampal sparing occurs in approximately 10% of cases (Murray et al., 2011). It occurs more often in men and is an early-onset disease with a more aggressive course. These patients are often clinically diagnosed with frontotemporal dementia, posterior cortical atrophy, or logopenic aphasia.

## Treatment

### Acetylcholinesterase Inhibitors

Acetylcholinesterase inhibitors (AChEIs) are recommended by AAN practice parameter for the treatment of dementia (Doody et al., 2001). The mechanism of action of AChEIs is to improve cholinergic functioning in the brains of patients with AD by increasing the concentration of acetylcholine through inhibition of acetylcholinesterase.

Tacrine was the first AChEI approved for use in AD but was limited by four times a day dosing and strict hepatic function monitoring requirements due to a risk of toxicity. These limitations in combination with the development of newer drugs resulted in its disappearance from the market place.

Donepezil, a reversible AChEI that can be administered with a single daily dose and does not require laboratory monitoring, was the next AChEI approved by the FDA. Donepezil is initiated at 5 mg per day for 28 days and if tolerated can be increased to 10 mg daily. Initial donepezil studies were 12–24 weeks in duration and demonstrated improvement on neuropsychological testing and clinician evaluation (Burns et al., 1999; Rogers and Friedhoff, 1996; Rogers et al., 1998). Double-blind placebo-controlled trials of up to 1 year demonstrated sustained medication benefit (Winblad et al., 2001). Common side effects include vivid dreaming, diarrhea, and nausea. Education to patients and caregivers about cholinergic mediated gastrointestinal side effects which often attenuate with time can lead to improved drug compliance. Giving the medication in the morning instead of the evening may decrease the vivid dreams. While not common, serious side effects may include provoking bradycardia and heart block in patients with cardiac conduction disorders. Recently, a 23-mg preparation of donepezil became available with inconclusive results as to its effectiveness (Doody et al., 2012).

Rivastigmine is another AChEI with FDA approval. Rivastigmine is initiated at 1.5 mg twice daily, which can be increased by 1.5 mg twice daily every 2 weeks to a maximum of 6 mg twice daily. The side effects of rivastigmine mirror those of donepezil, although gastrointestinal side effects may be more common (Rosler et al., 1999). Rivastigmine has been formulated in a patch form and has demonstrated similar efficacy with decreased side effects (Winblad et al., 2007).

Galantamine is a reversible AChEI. Galantamine is dosed twice daily, and should be titrated over 4 weeks. Dosing is initiated at 4 mg twice daily, with increases every 2 weeks to 8 mg twice daily and eventually 12 mg twice daily if tolerated. Galantamine is available in a sustained release formulation. The side-effect profile is similar to donepezil and rivastigmine; however, the FDA recommends caution when using galantamine for MCI due to concerns about an increase in cardiac-related deaths in clinical trials evaluating its use in MCI.

### *N*-Methyl-D-Aspartate Receptor Antagonist

Memantine is an *N*-methyl-D-aspartate (NMDA) receptor antagonist. It also blocks the 5-hydroxytryptamine-3 receptor. Memantine was approved by the FDA for the treatment of moderate to severe AD and can be used in conjunction with AChEIs (Tariot et al., 2004) or on its own (Reisberg et al., 2003). Side effects are rare, although confusion and dizziness have been reported.

### Vitamin E

In a large double-blind, randomized, placebo-controlled, multicenter trial, high-dose vitamin E (2000 IU a day) and selegiline delayed the progression of moderate AD to severe AD dementia. In contrast, high-dose vitamin E failed to delay progression of MCI to AD dementia (Petersen et al., 2005). This negative trial in concert with a meta-analysis which suggested an increase in all-cause mortality with high-dose vitamin E (Miller et al., 2005) resulted in a decreased enthusiasm for vitamin E in AD dementia. More recently, a large double-blind, placebo-controlled, randomized trial involving patients with mild-to-moderate AD dementia demonstrated less decline with high-dose vitamin E in the primary outcome of the Alzheimer's Disease Cooperative Study/Activities of Daily Living, which translated to a delay in progression of about 19% per year without an increase in mortality (Dysken et al., 2014). Further research into the safety of high-dose vitamin E in a dementia population will be needed before it can be recommended routinely.

### Estrogen Replacement Therapy

Epidemiological evidence has recognized that postmenopausal women who take estrogen replacement may be at decreased risk of AD. Randomized controlled trials showed no effect of estrogen on AD risk (Henderson et al., 2000; Mulnard et al., 2000), but there are issues pertaining to the time in life the estrogen was administered, e.g., around menopause or later in life.

### Antiinflammatory Medications

Converging basic science and epidemiological data suggested that antiinflammatory therapy may decrease the risk of developing AD. Clinical studies using prednisone (Aisen et al., 2000) and nonsteroidal antiinflammatory drugs (NSAIDs) (Aisen et al., 2003) have been negative.

### Treatment of Noncognitive Symptoms in Alzheimer Disease

Noncognitive side symptoms of AD play a major role in caregiver burden. Medical conditions such as urinary tract infections can present with confusion or agitation in dementia patients and should be excluded prior to considering other therapies. If possible, nonpharmacological treatment is preferred over pharmacological intervention to minimize undesirable side effects. Simple nonpharmacological approaches to neuropsychiatric problems include avoiding prior triggers, limiting changes to the environment, regular exercise, and shifting attention. Other techniques include aromatherapy and music therapy. "Sun-downing," the phenomenon of increased confusion or agitation late in the day, can be particularly problematic. This can occur in the hospital, in the nursing home, or at home. Nonpharmacological interventions during waking hours include maximizing patient activity, exposing the patient to light, and discouraging daytime napping. Prior to sleep, extra noise should be minimized.

Depression commonly accompanies AD. Selective serotonin reuptake inhibitors (SSRIs) are preferable to tricyclic antidepressants because the anticholinergic side effects of tricyclics can exacerbate cognitive decline. Agitation, psychosis, and aggressive behavior are also commonly seen in AD. Traditionally, these behaviors were treated with atypical antipsychotics (risperidone, olanzapine, quetiapine), which have a better side-effect profile than typical antipsychotics such as haloperidol. In 2006, a double-blind, placebo-controlled trial of atypical antipsychotics in Alzheimer patients demonstrated no significant difference in Clinical Global Impression of Change at 12 weeks, although patients in the placebo group stopped medication due to lack of efficacy more than those on olanzapine or quetiapine (Schneider et al., 2006). In addition to the limited effectiveness in randomized clinical trials, these medications are not approved by the FDA for behavioral disturbance in dementia and have been associated with increased mortality in dementia patients. In a meta-analysis of randomized placebo-controlled trials, the use of atypical antipsychotics in dementia was associated with an odds ratio of 1.54 for increased mortality (Schneider et al., 2005). The FDA has issued a black box warning for the use of these medications in dementia. After informing the patient and families of the increased risk of death, there is a minority of dementia patients in whom the benefits may outweigh the risks. In these cases, antipsychotics should be used at the lowest effective dose for the shortest period of time necessary. The Citalopram for Agitation in Alzheimer Disease Study demonstrated that the SSRI citalopram given at 30 mg daily improved agitation in AD dementia patients compared to placebo but was associated with prolonged QTc, which led the authors to conclude that it could not be routinely recommended for the treatment of agitation (Porsteinsson et al., 2014).

## Patient Safety

### Driving

In 2010, the AAN published a practice parameter on the evaluation and management of driving in dementia patients. This practice parameter reports that useful indicators of impaired driving performance include a Clinical Dementia Rating Scale (CDR) of 0.5 or above, MMSE score of ≤ 24, caregiving rating driving safety as unsafe, recent history of crashes or traffic violation, or aggressive or impulsive personalities (Iverson et al., 2010). Patients with MCI or mild dementia and no other risk factors for impaired driving may benefit from a driving-risk management strategy that includes regular roadside driving tests, while those with dementia and several risk factors for impaired driving should surrender driving privilege (Iverson et al., 2010).

### Medication Supervision

Given the cognitive impairment, medication errors are common when demented patients manage their own medications. The caregiver and patient should be educated to develop an organized system to prevent any medication errors.

### Other Safety Issues

Dementia patients with a propensity to wander can obtain an identity bracelet through the Alzheimer Association. The safety of the home living situation should be reviewed with the patient and caregiver, including support system need for adaptive equipment at home. While patients may live at home with a spouse for many years, assisted living and nursing homes may need to be considered based on level of care needed, behavioral disturbance, and caregiver burden. During the early stages of cognitive impairment, the healthcare provider should advise the patient to designate a healthcare durable power of attorney. Also, the healthcare provider should recommend the family help oversee finances to minimize errors and prevent any exploitation.

### The Future Treatment of Alzheimer Disease

To date, there have been no medications found definitely to modify the course of disease in AD. A wide array of studies, including those directed at inflammation, hormonal therapy, homocysteine, direct immunization against Aβ, passive immunization against Aβ, β, and γ secretase inhibitors, and those directed against tau, have been negative. There are ongoing anti amyloid and anti-tau medications still being studied. However, with all of the present failures, researchers have proposed that doctors may have to intervene earlier to modify AD. The biomarker studies in AD may provide such an opportunity. Biomarker studies indicate that AD pathogenesis starts many years before the symptoms occur. At this time, secondary prevention studies are beginning in this pre-symptomatic window. Ongoing studies include the Anti-Amyloid in Asymptomatic Alzheimer Disease (*A4*) study, the DIAN study, the Alzheimer's Prevention Initiative studies on the Columbian autosomal dominant kindred, and the APOE ε4 study as well. The A4 study is a 3-year, double-blind study evaluating solanezumab in cognitively normal persons who are florbetapir positive. The DIAN study is evaluating solanezumab and gantenerumab versus placebo in unaffected carriers of dominantly inherited gene mutation.

***Amyloid trials.*** After early negative trials with amyloid therapy, it was felt that two possible reasons for failure were that participants were enrolled based on clinical diagnosis rather than biomarker status and that the amyloid intervention may have taken place too late in the disease course. The EXPEDITION 3 trial of solanezumab in mild cognitive impairment or dementia in individuals with a positive Aβ biomarker did not reach its primary endpoint of cognitive improvement even though it restricted its criteria to individuals with early disease and required biomarker positivity for entry (Honig et al., 2018). Verubecestat, a β-secretase inhibitor, was tested in mild-to-moderate Alzheimer dementia and reduced CSF Aβ42 and amyloid PET levels. Verubecestat did not reduce cognitive decline, and the treated groups had a greater decline in hippocampal volume compared to placebo (Egan et al., 2018).

Two Aβ antibodies have demonstrated efficacy in lowering brain amyloid but whether they can influence cognitive decline remains to be seen (Sevigny et al., 2016). A recent trial using one of these Aβ antibodies, aducanumab, was prematurely stopped due to lack of efficacy in participants with MCI due to AD and mild AD dementia but subsequent analysis of the full data set reignited interest in Aducanumab and it continues to be investigated.

Some have viewed these results as indicating that Aβ-based therapies should be tried earlier in the disease course while others have taken these negative trials as impetus to try other non-Aβ-based therapeutic approaches.

## NEURODEGENERATIVE DEMENTIAS ASSOCIATED WITH PARKINSONISM

The neurodegenerative dementias associated with parkinsonism can be classified based on the molecular pathology found at autopsy:

- Synucleinopathies, which consist of DLB, Parkinson disease dementia (PDD), and multisystem atrophy (MSA); and
- Tauopathies, which consist of corticobasal degeneration (CBD), Guam dementia Parkinson complex, chronic traumatic encephalopathy (CTE), progressive supranuclear palsy (PSP), and familial FTD with parkinsonism.

Table 95.7 summarizes key clinical features of parkinsonian syndromes.

**TABLE 95.7 Clinical Features of Selected Parkinsonian Dementias**

| Subtype | Key Clinical Findings |
|---|---|
| Dementia with Lewy bodies | Fluctuations/hypersomnolence<br>Parkinsonism<br>Visual hallucinations<br>REM sleep behavior disorder |
| Progressive supranuclear palsy | Supranuclear gaze palsy<br>Axial rigidity<br>Gait disorder/frequent falls<br>Bulbar symptoms |
| Corticobasal syndrome | Asymmetric apraxia, dystonia, myoclonus<br>Cortical sensory findings, alien hand/limb<br>Rigidity |
| MSA-C/P | Ataxia, parkinsonism, long tract signs, autonomic dysfunction |

*MSA-C/P*, Multiple system atrophy—cerebellar/parkinsonian type; *REM*, rapid eye movement.

### Synucleinopathies

#### Dementia With Lewy Bodies

In 1961, Okazaki described two male patients with dementia who were admitted to the hospital and subsequently died and went to autopsy. One of the patients had been hallucinating for over 1 year. Autopsy of both patients revealed Lewy bodies in the cerebral cortex, brainstem, and spinal cord. Okazaki recognized the clinical presentation with distinctive pathological findings represented a unique disease entity (Okazaki et al., 1961). Lewy bodies are difficult to recognize with standard histological sections. Immunohistochemistry with ubiquitin in the 1980s led to a greater recognition of the disorder. A major breakthrough occurred in 1997, when mutations in alpha-synuclein were shown to be a cause of autosomal dominant Parkinson disease (Polymeropoulos et al., 1997). The same year it was shown that Lewy bodies were immunoreactive for alpha-synuclein (Spillantini et al., 1997), significantly improving recognition of Lewy bodies, leading to improved understanding of the clinical characteristics associated with Lewy body pathology.

***Prodromal dementia with Lewy bodies.*** Prior to cognitive decline, DLB patients often experience several clinical symptoms common to disorders with underlying synuclein pathology. DLB patients may variably report loss of smell, autonomic dysfunction, and REM sleep behavior disorder (RBD) prior to the onset of cognitive symptoms. In a series of patients with RBD who subsequently developed DLB, the mean age of onset of RBD was 61.5 while the age of cognitive decline was 68.1 (Boeve et al., 1998). More recently it has been reported that RBD can precede other symptoms of synucleinopathies by 50 years (Claassen et al., 2010), or can occur after cognitive decline has started. Similar to RBD, autonomic symptoms can precede DLB by many years (Kaufmann et al., 2004).

***Mild cognitive impairment due to dementia with Lewy bodies.*** In a large series of MCI patients, those with naMCI were much more likely to develop DLB, with over 80% having either attention or visual-spatial dysfunction (Ferman et al., 2013b). In an autopsy series of MCI patients with underlying DLB or AD pathology, MCI-DLB patients were distinguished from MCI-AD patients by the presence of more parkinsonism, hallucinations or episodes of delirium, and relatively preserved memory testing (Jicha et al., 2010).

***Epidemiology.*** DLB is the second most common cause of degenerative dementia. In autopsy series, DLB accounts for approximately 20% of dementia cases. Similarly, DLB accounted for approximately 20% of patients referred for dementia to specialty clinics in Norway (Aarsland et al., 2008).

The population-based incidence of DLB in France was estimated at 112 per 100,000 person-years (Perez et al., 2010).

The majority of DLB patients are male (around 70%) with average age of onset of approximately 72.5 years old (Boot et al., 2013). Compared to AD, DLB patients are more likely to have a history of depression and a positive family history of Parkinson disease (Boot et al., 2013). The prognosis is different between DLB and AD. DLB patients have a shorter survival compared to AD patients (Williams et al., 2006) and are admitted to nursing homes 2 years earlier in the disease course (Rongve et al., 2014).

***Clinical features.*** Consortium consensus criteria for the diagnosis DLB were published in 2005 and updated in 2017 (McKeith

**TABLE 95.8 Consensus Diagnostic Criteria for Dementia With Lewy Bodies**

| Symptom/Sign | Cardinal Manifestations | Frequency |
|---|---|---|
| Dementia (required criteria) | Attentional, frontal-executive, and visuospatial deficits, often worse than in AD dementia; episodic memory relatively better than in AD dementia | 100% |
| **Probable DLB** | | |
| (a) Presence of 2 or more core clinical features (with or without indicative biomarker) | | |
| (b) One core clinical feature plus at least one indicative biomarker | | |
| **Possible DLB** | | |
| (a) Presence of 1 core clinical feature (no indicative biomarker) | | |
| (b) Presence of 1 or more indicative biomarkers but no core clinical features | | |
| **Core Features** | | |
| Fluctuating cognition | Variable timing of altered level of attention or arousal; distinct from sundowning | 60%–89% |
| Visual hallucinations | Recurrent; typically involve animate subjects; variable degree of insight | 50%–75% |
| Parkinsonian motor signs | Spontaneous; rigidity and bradykinesia most common; action tremor more common than resting tremor | 50%–90% |
| REM sleep behavior disorder | Loss of atonia during REM sleep; individuals appear to act out dreams; may be combative or violent | 25%–76% |
| **Indicative Biomarkers** | | |
| 1. Reduced dopamine transporter uptake (SPECT or PET) | | |
| 2. Low uptake iodine-123-MIBG myocardial scintigraphy | | |
| 3. Confirmation of REM sleep without atonia on polysomnography | | |
| **Supportive Clinical Features** | | |
| 1. Neuroleptic sensitivity | | |
| 2. Postural instability | | |
| 3. Repeated falls | | |
| 4. Syncope | | |
| 5. Autonomic dysfunction | | |
| 6. Excessive daytime sleepiness | | |
| 7. Hyposmia | | |
| 8. Hallucinations (non-auditory) | | |
| 9. Delusions | | |
| 10. Apathy, anxiety, and depression | | |
| **Supportive Biomarkers** | | |
| 1. Preservation of medial temporal lobe volume on CT/MRI | | |
| 2. Generalized low uptake on SPECT/PET perfusion/metabolism scan with reduced occipital activity and/or the cingulate island sign on FDG-PET imaging | | |
| 3. Prominent posterior slow-wave activity on EEG with periodic fluctuations in the pre-alpha/theta range | | |

*CT*, Computed tomography; *EEG*, electroencephalogram; *FDG*, fluorodeoxyglucose; *MIBG*, metaiodobenzylguanidine; *MRI*, magnetic resonance imaging; *PET*, positron emission tomography; *REM*, rapid eye movement; *SPECT*, single-photon emission computed tomography.

*Modified from McKeith I.G., Boeve, B.F., Dickson, D.W., Halliday, G., Taylor, J.P., Weintraub, D., et al., 2017. Diagnosis and management of dementia with Lewy bodies: Fourth consensus report of the DLB Consortium. Neurology. 89, 88–100.,*

et al., 2005, 2017; Table 95.8). The major change was elevation of RBD to a core clinical feature. The cardinal features of DLB can present in any order but typically RBD precedes cognitive changes followed shortly thereafter by parkinsonism and hallucinations (Fields et al., 2011). DLB patients are also notably susceptible to delirium, which frequently occurs if they are hospitalized. DLB can rarely present as a rapidly progressive dementia (Fields et al., 2011).

***Parkinsonism.*** Parkinsonism is present in approximately 50% of DLB patients at diagnosis, but up to 25% in autopsy series do not develop parkinsonism (McKeith et al., 2004). The absence of parkinsonism is one of the major reasons for misdiagnosis (McKeith et al., 2000). Parkinsonian features of DLB tend to be symmetrical with action tremor greater than rest tremor. Parkinsonian features more severe in DLB than Parkinson disease (PD) include difficulty getting up from a chair, gait difficulty, impaired facial expression, and rigidity (Aarsland et al., 2001). While DLB patients respond to L-dopa therapy, the proportion that does not respond to L-dopa is higher than in PD patients (Bonelli et al., 2004).

***Cognitive fluctuations.*** Fluctuations have been reported to occur in up to 89% of DLB patients (Del Ser et al., 2000; McKeith et al., 2004). Cognitive fluctuations in DLB resemble delirium but do not have any provoking cause. Fluctuations are difficult to characterize and several fluctuations scales have been developed. Fluctuations in DLB can lead to variable performance on cognitive tests. Despite the difficulty in quantifying them, fluctuations can distinguish DLB from AD. One study found that the presence of at least 3 of 4 characteristic fluctuation features (staring into space, disorganized speech, drowsiness, and napping during the day despite getting adequate sleep) occurred in 63% of DLB patients, 12% of AD patients, and 0.5% of normal elderly persons, but asking specifically if the patient fluctuates did not distinguish DLB from AD (Ferman et al., 2004). Another fluctuations battery found the following four features distinguished DLB from

PDD, vascular dementia, and AD, with sensitivity ranging from 78.6% to 80.3% and specificity ranging from 73.9% to 79.3%:

1. Significant differences in daytime functioning;
2. Somnolence;
3. Drowsiness; and
4. Daytime altered levels of consciousness (Lee et al., 2014).

***Hallucinations.*** Hallucinations in DLB are often detailed, vivid visual images of people and animals. Children and insects are also common themes. Hallucinations tend to cluster in the evening, and patient insight is variable. Hallucinations occur in 63% of autopsy-confirmed DLB patients and are much more likely to be due to DLB when they occur in the first 5 years of the dementia (Ferman et al., 2013a).

***Rapid eye movement sleep behavior disorder.*** RBD refers to loss of the normal REM sleep with atonia. RBD can be screened for by asking "Does the patient act out his or her dreams while sleeping?" Polysomnogram is the gold standard for diagnosing RBD. In an autopsy series of patients with RBD, 141 of 172 had Lewy body disease of any kind (DLB, PDD, or PD) while 19 of 172 had MSA, demonstrating the relationship between synuclein pathology and the presence of RBD (Boeve et al., 2013). In autopsy-confirmed DLB patients, approximately 76% have RBD (Ferman et al., 2011). Patients who have DLB with RBD differ from those without RBD. DLB with RBD patients are more likely to be male, have earlier parkinsonism and hallucinations, and lower Braak tangle staging than those without RBD (Dugger et al., 2012). RBD improves the diagnosis of DLB. The odds ratio of DLB compared to other causes of dementia improves from 2 to 6 when RBD is added to visual hallucinations, parkinsonism, and fluctuations (Ferman et al., 2011). Other sleep disorders are often comorbid, including obstructive sleep apnea and periodic limb movements of sleep.

***Neuroleptic sensitivity.*** DLB patients experience greater neuroleptic sensitivity than AD patients. Of DLB patients who receive dopamine-blocking antipsychotics (e.g., haloperidol and risperidone), approximately 80% will experience an adverse reaction, with 50% experiencing a severe reaction (McKeith et al., 1992). Symptoms include worsening motor symptoms, confusion, and agitation.

***Autonomic dysfunction.*** Autonomic symptoms are common in DLB. The most common symptoms are orthostatic hypotension, urinary incontinence, and erectile dysfunction (Thaisetthawatkul et al., 2004).

***Other neuropsychiatric symptoms.*** Delusions occur in approximately 70% of DLB patients, with 40% developing misidentification syndromes (Ballard et al., 1999). Depression, anxiety, and apathy are also frequently seen.

***Falls.*** Falls are more common in DLB than AD. Falls may be related to a combination of parkinsonism and autonomic symptoms.

***Neuropsychology.*** The neuropsychological profile is helpful in distinguishing DLB from AD. Compared to AD dementia patients, DLB patients perform worse on tests of visual spatial ability (Mori et al., 2000) and attention but better on tests of naming and verbal memory (Ferman et al., 1999).

***Laboratory studies.*** No proven blood or CSF tests for DLB exist, although serum and CSF biomarkers are actively under development.

***Genetics.*** The genetics of DLB remain obscure. Genes implicated in PD and AD are also implicated in DLB and PDD. In a Belgian kindred with familial DLB, chromosome 2q35-q36 was mapped as the region of interest (Meeus et al., 2010). Duplications in the α-synuclein *(SNCA)* gene (Kasuga et al., 2010) and mutations in the leucine-rich repeat kinase 2 *(LRRK2)* gene on chromosome 12 also cause DLB (Qing et al., 2009). In a multicenter study, glucocerebrosidase *(GBA1)* mutations were associated with DLB with an odds ratio of 8.28 (Nalls et al., 2013). *GBA1* carriers had an earlier age of onset and worse parkinsonism. In all likelihood, there are multiple genes involved, with most undiscovered.

***Neuroimaging in dementia with Lewy bodies.*** The pathological overlap of AD and DLB results in significant overlap of the imaging biomarkers. A multimodal imaging approach (MRI, PiB-PET, FDG-PET) is additive in its ability to distinguish AD from DLB (Kantarci et al., 2012c).

**Structural magnetic resonance imaging.** Compared to AD, DLB patients have relatively preserved hippocampal volumes and less global atrophy although there is significant overlap. In DLB patients, lower hippocampal volumes correlate with higher Braak tangle stage (Kantarci et al., 2012a), indicating greater coexisting AD pathology. The posterior mesopontine region is also significantly smaller in DLB compared to AD (Kantarci et al., 2012a; Whitwell et al., 2007). The presence of hippocampal atrophy among DLB patients is associated with a shorter survival time compared to DLB patients with normal hippocampal volumes (Graff-Radford et al., 2016).

**Amyloid imaging in dementia with Lewy bodies.** Approximately 50%–80% of DLB patients are amyloid-positive on PiB-PET scans although at lower levels than AD patients and the pattern of deposition is similar to AD (Edison et al., 2008; Kantarci et al., 2012c). Therefore, amyloid PET should not be used to distinguish DLB from AD.

**Fluorodeoxyglucose positron emission tomography in dementia with Lewy bodies.** The FDG-PET pattern of DLB is very characteristic, involving parietal-occipital hypometabolism. In an autopsy-confirmed series, occipital hypometabolism distinguished DLB from AD dementia with a sensitivity of 90% and specificity of 87% (Minoshima et al., 2001), but it is important to understand that cases of atypical AD and late AD may show significant occipital hypometabolism. Since occipital hypometabolism does not occur in all cases, this limits its clinical utility. More recently, the relative preservation of the posterior cingulate metabolism relative to the precuneus and cuneus metabolism, termed the "cingulate island," has been shown to have the highest specificity in distinguishing DLB from AD (Graff-Radford et al., 2014; Lim et al., 2009).

Fig. 95.13 demonstrates imaging features of DLB.

**Dopamine transporter (DaT) scan.** Dopamine transporter imaging with [$^{123}$I]-FP-CIT SPECT differentiates DLB from other dementias with 78% sensitivity and 90% specificity (McKeith et al., 2007). In DLB patients, there is significantly decreased nigrostriatal uptake compared to AD, particularly in the putamen. The 4th consortium criteria for DLB recognized reduced dopamine transporter uptake in basal ganglia demonstrated by SPECT or PET as an indicative biomarker of the diagnosis of DLB (McKeith et al., 2017). Fig. 95.13 demonstrates a dopamine transporter scan in DLB. In an autopsy series, approximately 10% of patients with LBD pathology had a normal dopamine transporter scan with [$^{123}$I]-FP-CIT SPECT (Thomas et al., 2017).

**Myocardial iodine-131-meta-iodobenzylguanidine.** Myocardial iodine-131-meta-iodobenzylguanidine (MIBG) imaging can also help distinguish DLB from other dementias and is considered an indicative biomarker in the DLB criteria (McKeith et al., 2017; Yoshita et al., 2006). MIBG imaging measures postganglionic sympathetic cardiac innervation, which is reduced in DLB compared to AD.

***Pathology.*** α-Synuclein is the primary protein in Lewy bodies. The presence of Lewy bodies and Lewy neurites in limbic and cortical regions distinguishes DLB from PD, where Lewy bodies are limited to the brainstem. Lewy bodies in the cortex are more difficult to identify. In 2003, Braak proposed a staging scheme for synuclein pathology where the earliest region involved was the dorsal motor nucleus of the medulla followed by the pons, midbrain (nigra), basal forebrain, and then cortical

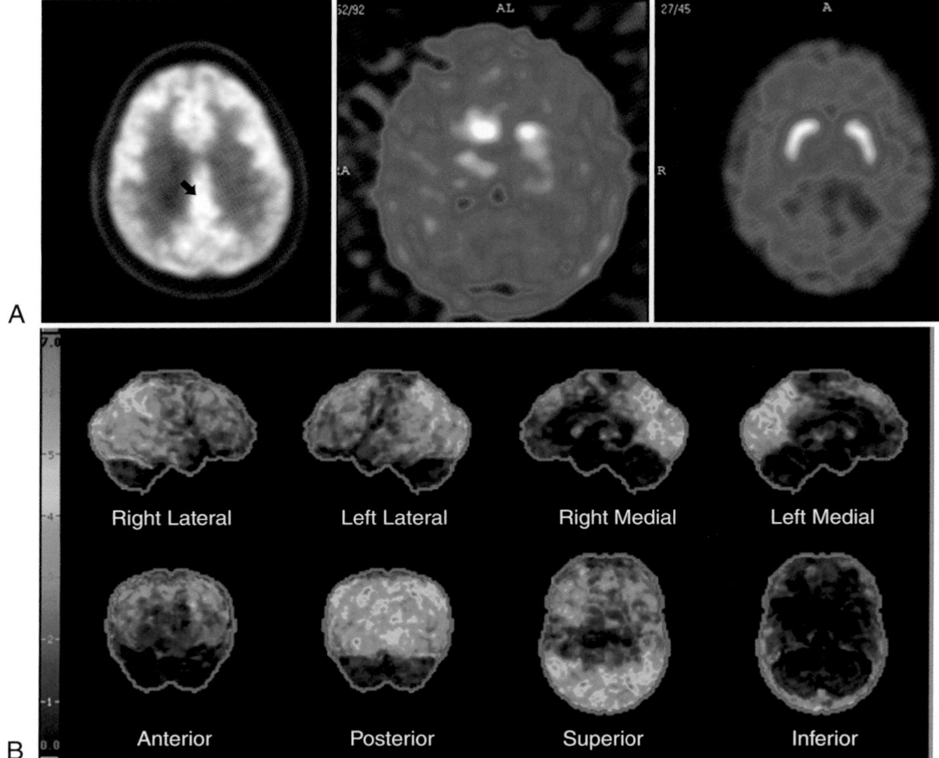


**Fig. 95.13** A, *Left:* Fluorodeoxyglucose positron emission tomography (FDG-PET) in dementia with Lewy bodies (DLB) patient demonstrating relative preservation of posterior cingulate *(arrow)* (e.g., cingulate island sign). *Middle:* Dopamine transporter single-photon emission computed tomography (DaT-SPECT) imaging with iodine-123-ioflupane in patient with DLB. There is markedly decreased striatal accumulation bilaterally, left greater than right. *Right:* Normal dopamine transporter imaging. **B,** FDG-PET statistical stereotactic surface projection map (Cortex ID) showing occipital hypometabolism in a DLB patient. (*DaT imaging courtesy Dr. Bradley Boeve.*)

areas, particularly frontal and temporal. Another early region involved is the olfactory bulb. Synuclein is also present in the striatum of DLB patients, although this was not included in Braak's staging scheme. Synuclein pathology in the spinal cord affects the intermediolateral cell column and less often Onuf's nucleus. There is significant pathological overlap between AD and DLB. The majority of DLB patients have amyloid plaques at autopsy. Most of the plaques in DLB tend to be diffuse without associated tau neuritic pathology. Interestingly, plaques may increase Lewy body density, suggesting a possible interaction between amyloid and synuclein. In the consortium criteria for DLB, the relative amount of Lewy body pathology to AD pathology is taken into account to determine the likelihood of the patient presenting with a clinical syndrome of DLB. Fig. 95.14 summarizes the pathological features of DLB.

***Treatment.*** A systematic approach to DLB patients aids in maximizing function. Cognitive symptoms, motor symptoms (parkinsonism, falls), neuropsychiatric symptoms, autonomic symptoms, and sleep disorders should all be addressed. Discontinuing medications which can exacerbate cognitive or motor symptoms is an important part of the management of DLB patients. These medications include those with anticholinergica properties, antipsychotic medications with antidopaminergic properties, and benzodiazepines.

***Cognitive symptoms***

Acetylcholinesterase inhibitor drugs. Compared to AD, DLB patients have a greater loss of cholinergic function. The loss of cholinergic function with comparatively intact structural integrity has provided the rationale to suggest that DLB patients may respond better to AChEIs than AD dementia patients. In 2000, a double-blind, randomized, controlled multicenter trial demonstrated that DLB subjects receiving rivastigmine improved significantly in neuropsychiatric features and a four-item DLB-specific subset of the NPI composed of delusions, hallucinations, apathy, and depression subscales (McKeith et al., 2007). In another randomized, double-blind, placebo controlled trial, donepezil 5 or 10 mg improved MMSE scores, caregiver burden, and behavioral symptoms in DLB patients relative to placebo (Mori et al., 2012a).

DLB patients without imaging markers of coexisting AD pathology (hippocampal atrophy, PiB-PET positivity) are more likely to improve with AChEIs compared to those with imaging markers of AD pathology (Graff-Radford et al., 2012).

### Parkinsonism

***Dopaminergic therapy.*** Parkinsonism in DLB is L-dopa responsive, although less so than PD. To minimize the risk of inducing or exacerbating neuropsychiatric symptoms such as hallucinations, L-dopa/carbidopa should be introduced at a low dose and titrated slowly. Many medications may exacerbate various symptoms of DLB and should be avoided where possible. Specifically, dopamine agonists are more likely to exacerbate hallucinations and behavioral disorders. Selegiline may also exacerbate psychosis, and anticholinergics such as benztropine and trihexyphenidyl can cause confusion.

Neuropsychiatric features. Depression and anxiety can be treated with SSRIs. As previously noted, it is important to avoid anticholinergic agents when selecting an antidepressant.

Hallucinations and delusions that do not bother the patient may not require treatment. First-line therapy for hallucinations and delusions in DLB should be AChEIs, which have been shown to improve delusions and hallucinations (McKeith et al., 2000c).

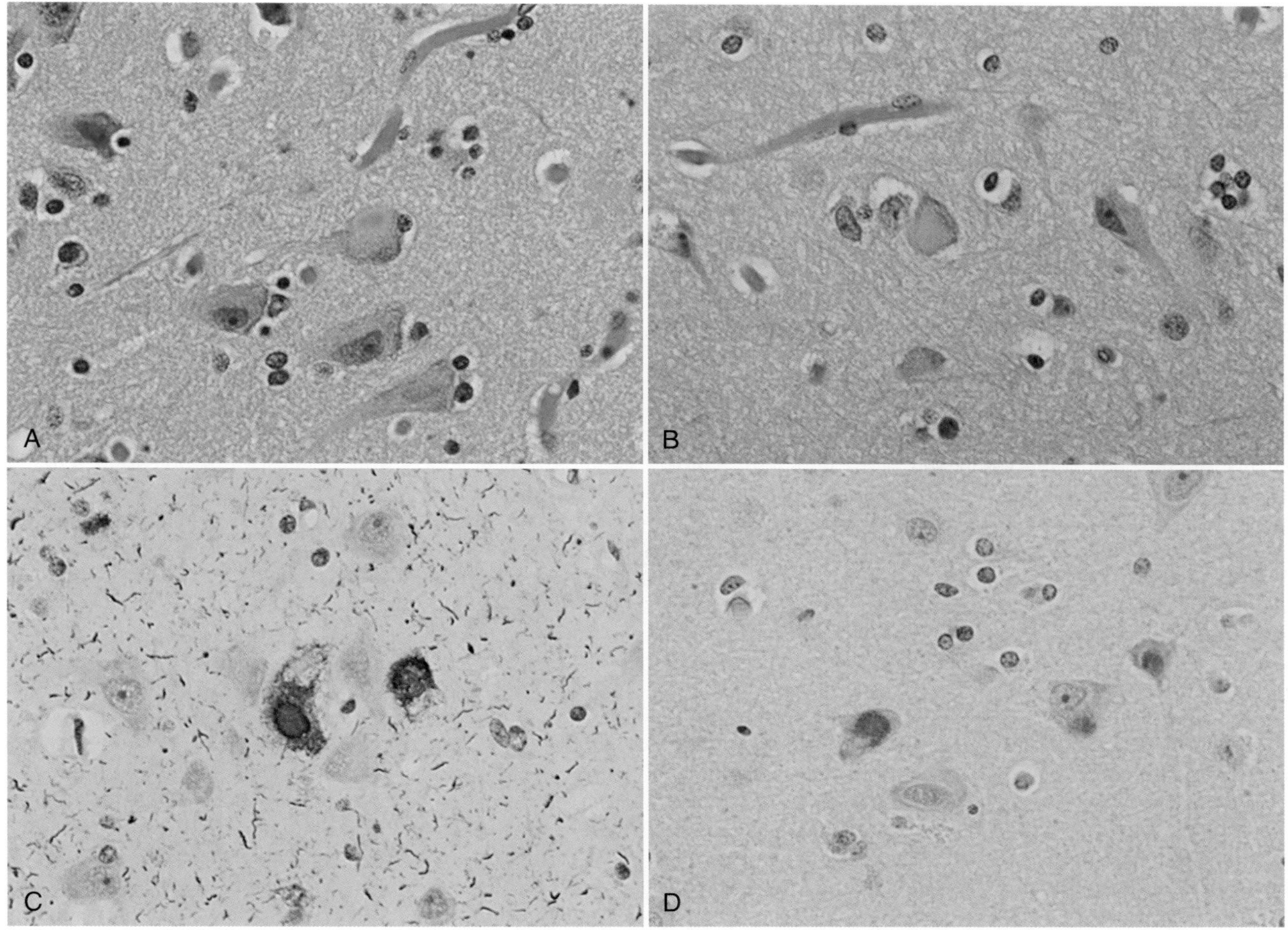


**Fig. 95.14** Dementia With Lewy Bodies Pathology. Hematoxylin and eosin (H&E) stain of anterior cingulate cortex (A) and temporal cortex (B) demonstrating Lewy bodies. Alpha-synuclein stain of anterior cingulate cortex (C) and temporal cortex (D) demonstrating Lewy bodies. (*Courtesy Dr. Joseph Parisi.*)

Typical antipsychotics are contraindicated in DLB due to severe sensitivity and association with increased mortality. Atypical antipsychotics (risperidone, olanzapine, and quetiapine) are associated with increased mortality in dementia and their use should be avoided if possible (Schneider et al., 2005). Pimavanserin was approved to treat Parkinson psychosis by the FDA and has not been approved for use in DLB. It also carries a black box warning that elderly patients with dementia treated with antipsychotics are at increased risk of death.

When the benefits of antipsychotics are felt to outweigh the risks, quetiapine and clozapine are often used to minimize the risk of worsening parkinsonism. The use of clozapine is limited because of the risk of agranulocytosis requiring routine blood monitoring. Antipsychotics should be used at the lowest effective dose for the shortest interval necessary, due to side effects.

**Autonomic symptoms.** Since autonomic symptoms vary significantly among patients, an individualized approach is necessary. Constipation can be treated by increasing water and fiber intake initially followed by over-the-counter therapies such as psyllium powder and rarely prescription therapies. Orthostasis can initially be treated by lifestyle modifications and limiting drugs that lower blood pressure. As dysautonomia worsens, pharmacological interventions with midodrine or fludrocortisone may become necessary. In appropriate patients, erectile dysfunction can be managed with phosphodiesterase inhibitors.

**Sleep disorders.** RBD is the most common sleep disorder in DLB, but other sleep disorders are common and can be treated. Therefore, patients should be screened for sleep apnea because treatment can improve daytime alertness. Treatment of RBD should be individualized to see if the patient is at risk of harming themselves or their bed partner. Nonpharmacological treatments include removal of sharp objects from around the bed, creating barriers between bed partners, or even bed alarms. Melatonin can improve RBD and is well tolerated. Clonazepam is often used as a second-line option at low doses, but this should be monitored carefully as benzodiazepines are typically avoided in dementia and may increase fall risk.

## Parkinson Disease Dementia

PDD is distinguished from DLB by the presence of parkinsonism preceding cognitive decline for at least 1 year. About 80% of PD patients will develop dementia (Aarsland and Kurz, 2010). The clinical features of PDD are otherwise similar to DLB and some authorities have questioned whether they are distinct entities or different presentations of the spectrum of Lewy body diseases.

There are some pathological differences between PDD and DLB. For example, PDD patients have greater substantia nigra neuronal loss.

In addition to treatment of motor symptoms, a recent multicenter placebo-controlled study of the AChEI rivastigmine in PDD showed an improvement in cognitive, neuropsychiatric, and functional features, leading to FDA approval (Emre et al., 2004). An MCI stage of PDD is recognized, and similar criteria to MCI due to AD have been suggested (Litvan et al., 2012).

## Multiple System Atrophy

Multiple system atrophy was known as striatonigral degeneration, olivopontocerebellar atrophy (OPCA), and Shy-Drager syndrome. Current consensus criteria (Gilman et al., 2008) recognize two types of MSA: MSA-P (L-dopa nonresponsive parkinsonism) and MSA-C (cerebellar ataxia). Approximately 58% of European patients with MSA have MSA-P (Geser et al., 2006) while MSA-C is more common in the Japanese population (84%) (Yabe et al., 2006). Mean age of onset is 54 (Ben-Shlomo et al., 1997) with mean survival from symptom onset of 5.7 years (Bjornsdottir et al., 2013). The average annual incidence rate of MSA is 3 per 100,000 person-years (Bower et al., 1997). The prevalence is estimated at 4.4 cases per 100,000 (Schrag et al., 1999).

Patients with pure autonomic failure may evolve into MSA. A prospective study of pure autonomic failure found that about one-third of patients later met clinical criteria for a synucleinopathy, including MSA within 4 years of follow-up (Kaufmann et al., 2017).

Clinical characteristics include autonomic dysfunction with any combination of parkinsonism and/or ataxia. Autonomic symptoms may manifest as cardiovascular in the form of orthostatic hypotension, urogenital or gastrointestinal dysfunction. Erectile dysfunction is common among male MSA patients. RBD is strongly associated with MSA, reflecting the underlying synuclein pathology. In MSA-C, ataxia progresses faster than in other degenerative ataxias (Klockgether et al., 1998). The parkinsonism in MSA-P typically lacks the classic rest tremor and L-dopa responsiveness seen in PD and progresses more rapidly than in PD (Seppi et al., 2005). Other key symptoms associated with MSA include pyramidal signs, stridor, dysarthria, oculomotor dysfunction, pseudobulbar affect, myoclonus, orofacial dystonia, and dysphagia (Gilman et al., 2008). Significant cognitive deficits at diagnosis are rare in MSA. In the 2nd consensus statement on the diagnosis of multiple system atrophy, the presence of dementia was considered a red flag against the diagnosis of MSA (Gilman et al., 2008), although in one clinical series, dementia was diagnosed in 10 of 58 MSA patients with 3 of 58 presenting with cognitive symptoms (Kitayama et al., 2009). Neuropsychological testing can often detect executive deficits and slowed processing speed. Common neuropsychiatric symptoms include depression and anxiety.

***Evaluation.*** Autonomic dysfunction can be detected by supine and standing blood pressure, with the drop of 30 mm Hg systolic or 15 mm Hg diastolic required in order to meet diagnostic criteria for probable MSA. Autonomic reflex screen testing may demonstrate the orthostatic blood pressure drop and other signs of adrenergic or cardiovagal failure. Thermoregulatory sweat testing demonstrates anhidrosis in a central pattern. Elevated postvoid residual volumes are often seen in patients with urological symptoms.

***Neuroimaging.*** The imaging features differ between the types of MSA. In MSA-C, atrophy of the pons, cerebellum, or middle cerebellar peduncles is characteristic. On T2-weighted MRI, hyperintensity can be seen in the pons ("hot cross bun sign"), middle cerebellar peduncles, and cerebellum. Putaminal abnormalities are more commonly seen in MSA-P with T2-hyperintensity of the lateral putaminal rim or hypointensity of the posterior putamen.

FDG-PET findings in MSA include hypometabolism of the basal ganglia and cerebellum (Eckert et al., 2005).

***Genetics.*** Recently, mutations in CoQ2 were shown to be associated with MSA in Japanese cases (2013), but this mutation was not confirmed in other populations.

***Pathology.*** The gross pathology of MSA-P demonstrates degeneration of the putamen and lateral substantia nigra. The hallmark lesion of MSA is glial cytoplasmic inclusions that consist of filamentous inclusions of synuclein in oligodendroglia. These can be located in the cortex, subcortical areas, cerebellum, spinal cord, and dorsal root ganglia.

***Treatment.*** Treatment is symptomatic, with autonomic dysfunction being most disabling. Early in the course, lifestyle modifications can be effective, including increasing salt and fluid intake, sleeping with the head of the bed elevated, learning physical maneuvers, and wearing compression garments. Later, pharmacological intervention may become necessary with fludrocortisone, midodrine, pyridostigmine, or droxidopa often providing a measure of symptomatic relief although they may cause supine hypertension. Raising the head of the bed can help mitigate the supine hypertension. A subset of MSA-P patients may respond to L-dopa, but the benefit is often transient and limited, with treatment exacerbating orthostatic hypotension. Physical and occupational therapy can be helpful with gait instability and safety evaluation. Referral to a sleep medicine specialist for evaluation of respiratory stridor should be considered as stridor carries a poor prognosis (Silber and Levine, 2000). Dysphagia should also be monitored.

## Tauopathies

### Corticobasal Degeneration/Corticobasal Syndrome

In the 1960s, Rebeiz reported three patients with an asymmetrical akinetic rigid syndrome and apraxia with unique pathological features which was called corticodentatonigral degeneration with neuronal achromasia (Rebeiz et al., 1968). Later the name changed to corticobasal ganglionic degeneration or corticobasal degeneration. The clinical syndrome of progressive asymmetric rigidity and apraxia became synonymous with corticobasal degeneration. Subsequent autopsy series revealed patients with this characteristic clinical syndrome had heterogeneous pathology including CBD, PSP pathology, AD pathology, or Creutzfeldt-Jakob disease (CJD) (Boeve et al., 1999). Currently, corticobasal syndrome (CBS) refers to a clinical syndrome characterized by asymmetric rigidity, apraxia, and alien limb phenomenon variably associated with cortical sensory loss, myoclonus, dystonia, and parkinsonism. This syndrome can be caused by several pathologies. The term CBD refers to the distinct pathological entity which can present with a variety of clinical syndromes. While CBD is the most common pathological substrate of CBS, this pathology only accounts for approximately 50% of cases of CBS (Boeve et al., 2003). In the most recent criteria for the diagnosis of CBD, four clinical phenotypes are recognized (corticobasal syndrome, frontal behavioral-spatial syndrome, nonfluent/agrammatic variant of PPA, and PSP-syndrome) (Armstrong et al., 2013). The mean age of symptom onset is approximately 64 years, with average disease duration of 6.6 years (Armstrong et al., 2013). CBS has an incidence rate per year of approximately 0.02 cases per 100,000 persons (Winter et al., 2010).

The key features of CBS are a progressive, asymmetric apraxia and rigidity. Cortical features variably associated with CBS include cortical sensory loss, alien limb syndrome, mirror movements, cognitive impairment, and myoclonus. Motor features associated with CBS include bradykinesia, dystonia, tremor, and poor L-dopa response. Additionally, the hand can form a characteristic fist. Common neuropsychiatric features include depression, disinhibition, and obsessive-compulsive features. Capgras and hallucinations are quite rare in CBS relative to other neurodegenerative diseases (Geda et al., 2007). Most patients with underlying CBD pathology present with cognitive or behavioral symptoms, with a significant portion presenting as bvFTD (Lee et al., 2011b).

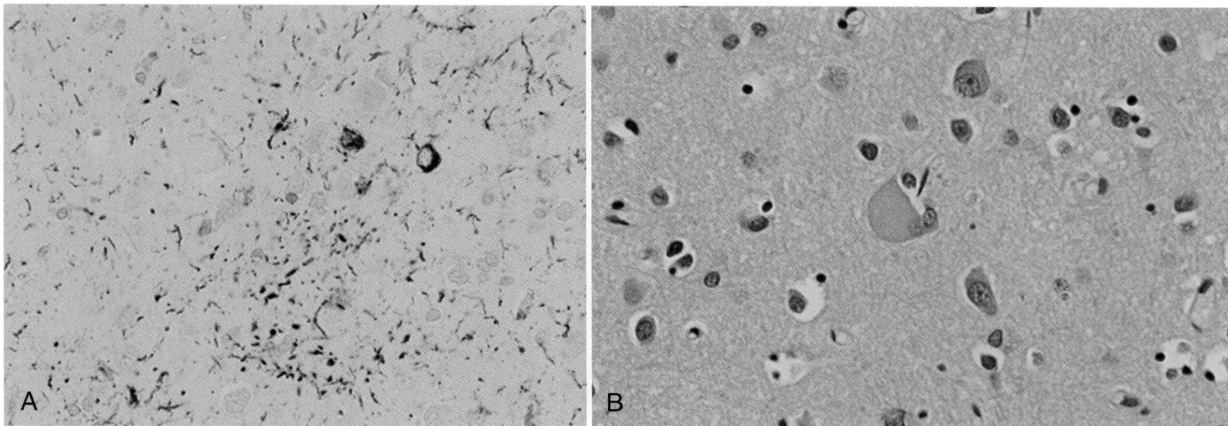

**Fig. 95.15 Corticobasal Degeneration Pathology. A,** Tau-positive astrocytic plaque with pleomorphic neuronal inclusions and neurites with tau staining. **B,** Balloon neuron on hematoxylin and eosin (H&E). (*Images courtesy Dr. Joseph Parisi.*)

Neuropsychological testing demonstrates prominent deficits in executive functions, language, and visual-spatial functions, with relative sparing of episodic memory at presentation (Murray et al., 2007).

Structural MRI in CBS often shows asymmetrical frontoparietal atrophy corresponding to the side contralateral to the affected limb. FDG-PET imaging demonstrates focal asymmetric hypometabolism in the posterior frontal, anterior parietal region.

***Pathology.*** The gross pathology of CBD includes atrophy of the superior frontal gyrus, thinning of the corpus callosum, and loss of pigment of the substantia nigra. CBD is a four-repeat (four microtubule-binding domains) tauopathy. The pathology in CBD occurs in both the cortex and white matter. Tau accumulates in certain regions including cortex, basal ganglia, basal nucleus of Meynert, thalamus, and brainstem (Dickson et al., 2002). Rebeiz described swollen achromatic neurons, now known as ballooned neurons, which are present in CBD but not specific (Rebeiz et al., 1968). The hallmark of CBD is the astrocytic plaque. These plaques are tau positive without amyloid. Research criteria for the pathological diagnosis of CBD also include tau-reactive gray- and white matter threadlike lesions (Dickson et al., 2002). Fig. 95.15 summarizes the key pathology of CBD. The clinical presentation is determined by the distribution of tau. In autopsy-proven CBD patients, tau deposition in the motor and somatosensory cortex was associated with a CBS presentation while tau deposition in limbic regions and the hindbrain was associated with PSP syndrome (Kouri et al., 2011).

The tau genotype consists of two haplotypes, H1 and H2. In typical populations approximately 60% are homozygous for H1/H1, but in PSP and CBD over 80% are H1/H1, indicating that being H1 is a risk factor for CBD (Houlden et al., 2001). Interestingly, some *MAPT* gene mutations can cause CBD pathology.

***Treatment.*** No disease-modifying therapy is available for CBD/CBS; therefore, treatment is symptomatic. A minority of patients will have a modest response of rigidity and bradykinesia to dopaminergic therapy. If myoclonus is problematic, clonazepam, levetiracetam, and gabapentin can be considered. Physical and occupational therapy are important to prevent falls, provide adaptive equipment, and maximize function with appropriate exercises.

## Progressive Supranuclear Palsy

The nomenclature of PSP is confusing. PSP syndrome (PSP-S) refers to the classical clinical presentation, while PSP pathology refers to pathological substrate. The classical clinical presentation of PSP-S is characterized by unexplained falls, symmetric predominantly axial rigidity, bradykinesia, poor L-dopa responsiveness, and impaired vertical gaze, especially downgaze. This typical presentation is also called Richardson syndrome. Other clinical features include eyelid apraxia, dysphagia, abnormal neck posturing, pseudobulbar affect, long tract signs, and impaired saccadic pursuits. Five clinical presentations associated with PSP pathology have been described:

1. PSP-S (described above).
2. PSP-parkinsonism (characterized by limb and axial rigidity, tremor, L-dopa responsiveness).
3. PSP-pure akinesia with gait freezing (early gait disorder with subsequent freezing, early micrographia, phonation difficulties, lack of L-dopa response, or early eye movement abnormalities).
4. PSP-corticobasal syndrome (CBS as previously described).
5. PSP-progressive nonfluent aphasia/apraxia of speech (language and/or speech disorder characterized by agrammatism and/or speech apraxia) (Williams and Lees, 2009).

In 2017, new criteria for PSP were published by the Movement Disorder Society recognizing four functional domains (ocular motor dysfunction, postural instability, akinesia, and cognitive dysfunction) which can predict PSP. Patients can be categorized as probable, possible, or suggestive of PSP based on degree of certainty (Hoglinger et al., 2017).

Neuropsychiatric features of PSP-S include prominent apathy, disinhibition, depression, and anxiety (Litvan et al., 1996). Bradyphrenia can be prominent and PSP can mimic bvFTD. The annual incidence rate of PSP-S is 5.3 per 100,000 person-years (Bower et al., 1997). The prevalence is approximately 6.4 per 100,000 (Schrag et al., 1999).

The disease duration is approximately 7 years. Most patients die from complications related to dysphagia. Neuropsychological profile includes prominent executive dysfunction. Language and speech difficulties can be present or even dominate the clinical presentation.

Structural MRI demonstrates midbrain atrophy and has been called the "hummingbird sign" (Kato et al., 2003). A small midbrain to pons ratio may also predict PSP (Massey et al., 2013). Enlargement of the third ventricle is also described in PSP. The FDG-PET scan reveals frontal-subcortical hypometabolism. Midbrain hypometabolism is also described and has been called the "pimple sign" (Botha et al., 2014).

Of patients clinically diagnosed with PSP-S, 76% will have PSP at autopsy, with CBD, MSA, and DLB accounting for most of the other pathologies (Josephs and Dickson, 2003). PSP-S caused by CBD differs from PSP-S caused by PSP pathology. PSP-S with underlying CBD

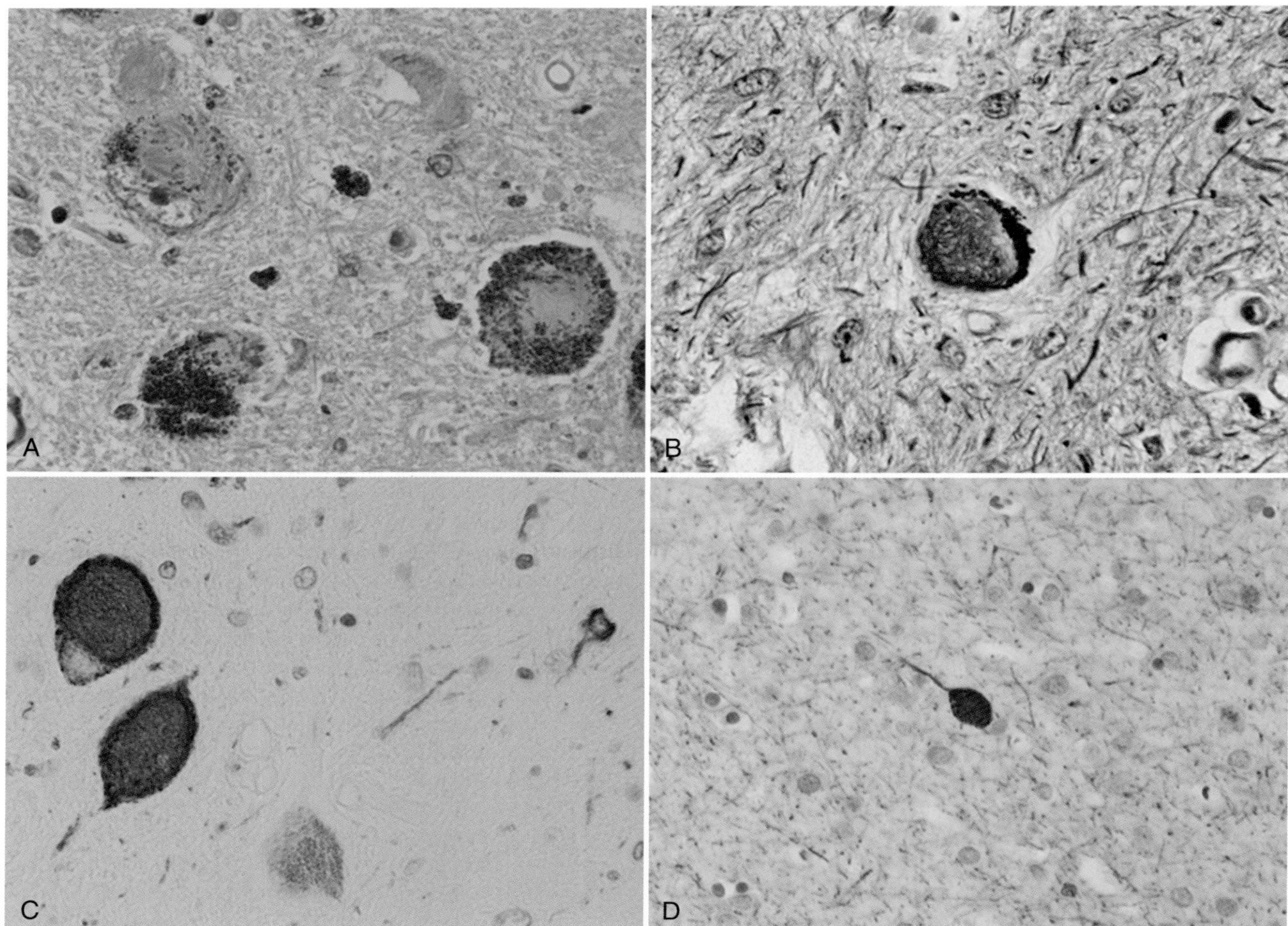


**Fig. 95.16 Progressive Supranuclear Palsy Pathology.** **A,** Hematoxylin and eosin (H&E) stain demonstrating globose neurofibrillary tangle. **B,** Bielschowsky stain demonstrating globose neurofibrillary tangle. **C,** Tau stain demonstrating globose neurofibrillary tangle. **D,** Neurofilament stain demonstrating ballooned neuron. *(Courtesy Dr. Joseph Parisi.)*

pathology is more associated with cognitive behavioral dysfunction and tends to have less subthalamic nucleus neuronal loss but more neuronal loss in the medial aspect of the substantia nigra and degeneration of the anterior part of the corpus callosum (Kouri et al., 2011).

Gross pathological findings with PSP pathology include midbrain, superior cerebellar peduncle, and subthalamic nucleus atrophy. PSP is a four-repeat tauopathy characterized by globose tangles in the globus pallidus, substantia nigra, and subthalamic nucleus. The pathology also affects motor cortex, striatum, pontine nuclei, inferior olive, and dentate nucleus. Tufted astrocytes are also present. The neuronal loss in PSP correlates with NFTs rather than the astrocytic pathology. Fig. 95.16 summarizes the key pathological features of PSP.

No disease-modifying treatment is available for PSP. Subgroups of PSP (PSP-parkinsonism) patients respond to L-dopa therapy. SSRIs can be used for depression, anxiety, and pseudobulbar affect.

## FRONTOTEMPORAL DEMENTIAS

In 1892, Arnold Pick described a patient with progressive aphasia associated with frontal and temporal lobar atrophy. This was the first description of FTD. In 1911, Alois Alzheimer described the pathological hallmark of this disorder, a rounded inclusion now called a Pick body (Alzheimer, 1911). Only later was it recognized that only a small proportion of FTD cases have Pick bodies at autopsy. In 1982, Mesulam reported six patients with "slowly progressive aphasia," and later introduced the term primary progressive aphasia (PPA) (Mesulam, 1982, 1987). Brun and Gustafson in Sweden (Gustafson et al., 1990) and Neary and Snowden in the UK (Neary et al., 1988) termed the group of disorders "frontal lobe dementia of the non-Alzheimer type," and "dementia of the frontal type," respectively.

### Nomenclature

FTD is an encompassing term that refers to a group of clinical syndromes that are characterized by degeneration of the frontal and temporal lobes, while frontotemporal lobar degeneration (FTLD) is an encompassing term for the spectrum of pathologies associated with FTD.

### Diagnostic Criteria

In 1998, consensus criteria were published that recognized three clinical variants of FTD that correlate with FTLD pathologically: FTD, progressive nonfluent aphasia (PNFA), and semantic dementia (Neary et al., 1998). More recently updated criteria have been proposed to further characterize FTD variants including bvFTD (Rascovsky et al.,

2011) and the PPA variants (Gorno-Tempini et al., 2011). Currently, three clinical variants of FTD are recognized: bvFTD, semantic dementia or semantic variant PPA (svPPA), and PNFA.

### Frontotemporal Dementia Epidemiology

In a UK-based study of dementia patients aged 45 to 64, the prevalence of FTD and AD was the same (15 per 100,000) (Ratnavalli et al., 2002). In a population-based study in Rochester, MN, the incidence rates (number of new cases per 100,000 person-years) of FTD were 2.2 for ages 40–49, 3.3 for ages 50–59, and 8.9 for ages 60–69 (Knopman et al., 2004). While FTD is an early onset dementia, 30% of FTD patients are estimated to be over the age of 65 (Knopman and Roberts, 2011). Median survival from symptom onset among FTD patients is approximately 6 years but FTD with motor neuron disease (FTD-MND) patients have a significantly shorter survival of approximately 3 years (Hodges et al., 2003).

### Behavioral Variant Frontotemporal Dementia

#### Clinical Presentation

The characteristic clinical features of bvFTD include a change in personality and behavior such as disinhibition, and executive dysfunction such as poor planning, loss of judgment, difficulty with organization and loss of insight. In bvFTD, patients exhibit social isolation, peculiar affiliations, antisocial behavior, compulsions, and drug or alcohol abuse. A change in dietary preference, particularly an increased interest in sweets, may occur, although indiscriminate overeating can also occur. Other features include apathy, decreased pain response, utilization behaviors, and obsessive compulsive and perseverative behaviors. Patients often lack empathy and insight. They may show little concern for friends or family members. Language deficits occur but are not the presenting feature. The most recent criteria for bvFTD are listed in Table 95.9A (Rascovsky et al., 2011). Differentiating features are summarized in Table 95.9B.

Parkinsonian features are often mild. Motor neuron disease more commonly occurs with bvFTD than PPA. Early in the disease course neuropsychological testing can be completely normal. Typically, neuropsychological testing demonstrates less episodic memory impairment than patients with semantic dementia or dementia due to AD (Hodges et al., 1999). Executive function deficits are characteristic but may be absent. Semantic memory is spared in bvFTD relative to semantic variant PPA and AD dementia (Rogers et al., 2006).

Hodges described a disorder he termed bvFTD phenocopy describing patients who met bvFTD criteria but had no major imaging findings of FTD and remained clinically stable over time. This disorder may represent lifelong personality quirks and unusual behaviors or, alternatively, a subset may represent a slowly progressive bvFTD secondary to a C9ORF72 mutation (Khan et al., 2012).

#### Primary Progressive Aphasias

The primary progressive aphasias refer to a group of disorders where neurodegeneration targets the language network. Two variants of PPA are under the FTD umbrella: PNFA and semantic dementia or svPPA. The logopenic variant is most frequently caused by AD pathology and is not considered a type of FTD. Criteria were published for the classification of the PPA variants (Gorno-Tempini et al., 2011).

***Nonfluent/agrammatic variant primary progressive aphasia.*** Agrammatic primary progressive aphasia is characterized by nonfluent, hesitant speech. Agrammatism occurs and is characterized by telegraphic speech, misuse of pronouns, and errors in sentence construction. Word and object knowledge is relatively spared. Early in the course, agrammatism may only be evident in writing samples. The Northwestern Anagram Test which focuses on grammar can be considered to aid in the diagnosis (Weintraub et al., 2009). Apraxia of speech often co-occurs and accounts for some of the appearance of nonfluency. Comprehension for complex sentences can be impaired. Behavioral symptoms often co-occur but are not the presenting feature. Over time, patients often develop a parkinsonian syndrome.

***Semantic variant primary progressive aphasia.*** svPPA is a fluent aphasia characterized by a prominent anomia with loss of single word meaning. Nouns are particularly difficult to comprehend. Patients will replace a specific word with a more general word such as "it" for "telephone." In most patients repetition is relatively spared, and grammar remains intact. The commonest age range of presentation in svPPA is between 66 and 70 years of age (Hodges and Patterson, 2007). Surface dyslexia occurs in svPPA, where irregularly pronounced words such as "colonel" and "pint" are pronounced phonetically. svPPA patients also may develop loss of visual object meaning and prosopagnosia (difficulty recognizing familiar faces) when the right temporal lobe is more affected than the left. Testing for prosopagnosia can be accomplished by showing pictures of famous celebrities and asking the patient to identify the famous face (Tiger Woods) among distractor (non-famous) faces. To test person knowledge, a follow-up question of asking who, in fact, Tiger Woods is can also be helpful. A svPPA patient may not know he is a golfer or in professional sports. Over time, svPPA patients commonly develop coexisting behavioral issues which overlap with bvFTD. svPPA patients are more likely to develop food fads and seek social attention, while bvFTD patients are more likely to overeat and become withdrawn (Snowden et al., 2001). Additionally, patients with svPPA tend not to have parkinsonism, a family history of dementia, or associated motor neuron disease. Some patients present with nonverbal semantic deficits, typically right greater than left temporal involvement, do not meet root criteria for PPA, and the term semantic dementia may continue to be most appropriate.

#### Amnestic Syndromes

Occasionally, elderly patients with FTLD pathology can present with an amnestic syndrome resembling AD.

## HIPPOCAMPAL SCLEROSIS OF AGING

Hippocampal sclerosis refers to loss of neurons and gliosis in the subiculum and CA1 of the hippocampus which is accompanied with TDP-43 pathology. Patients present typically over the age of 75 with a progressive amnestic course (Pao et al., 2011). In the elderly, hippocampal sclerosis is seen in approximately 13% of autopsy cases. It may occur as a co-pathology with AD or in isolation (Nag et al., 2015). While clinical features of hippocampal sclerosis and AD dementia overlap, the presence of focal medial temporal and posterior cingulate hypometabolism is a promising biomarker to distinguish hippocampal sclerosis from AD dementia (Botha et al., 2018).

### Argyrophilic Grain Disease

Argyrophilic grain (AG) disease is a 4-repeat tauopathy. Patients with AG may have an unusually long course of aMCI (Petersen et al., 2006) or present with an FTD syndrome.

#### Frontotemporal Dementia With Motor Neuron Disease

FTD-MND represents approximately 10%–15% of FTDs. Identification of MND in FTD patients is important because of the decreased survival compared to FTD patients (<3 years). BvFTD with MND is associated with a longer survival time compared to a language-dominant FTD-MND phenotype. Traditional teaching reported spared cognition in ALS patients, but recent studies have shown that cognitive impairment and subtle executive dysfunction is common in ALS (Phukan et al., 2007).

**TABLE 95.9A International Consensus Criteria for Behavioral Variant FTD**

I. Neurodegenerative disease. The following symptom must be present to meet criteria for bvFTD:
  A. Shows progressive deterioration of behavior and/or cognition by observation or history (as provided by a knowledgeable informant).

II. Possible bvFTD, Three of the following behavioral/cognitive symptoms (A–F) must be present to meet criteria. Ascertainment requires that symptoms be persistent or recurrent, rather than single or rare events.
  A. Early behavioral disinhibition (one of the following symptoms [A.1–A.3] must be present):
    A.1. Socially inappropriate behavior
    A.2. Loss of manners or decorum
    A.3. Impulsive, rash, or careless actions
  B. Early apathy or inertia (one of the following symptoms [B.1–B.2] must be present):
    B.1. Apathy
    B.2. Inertia
  C. Early loss of sympathy or empathy (one of the following symptoms [C.1–C.2] must be present):
    C.1. Diminished response to other people's needs and feelings
    C.2. Diminished social interest, interrelatedness, or personal warmth
  D. Early perseverative, stereotyped, or compulsive/ritualistic behavior (one of the following symptoms [D.1–D.3] must be present):
    D.1. Simple repetitive movements
    D.2. Complex, compulsive, or ritualistic behaviors
    D.3. Stereotypy of speech
  E. Hyperorality and dietary changes (one of the following symptoms [E.1–E.3] must be present):
    E.1. Altered food preferences
    E.2. Binge eating, increased consumption of alcohol or cigarettes
    E.3. Oral exploration or consumption of inedible objects
  F. Neuropsychological profile: executive/generation deficits with relative sparing of memory and visuospatial functions (all of the following symptoms [F.1–F.3] must be present):
    F.1. Deficits in executive tasks
    F.2. Relative sparing of episodic memory
    F.3. Relative sparing of visuospatial skills

III. Probable bvFTD All of the following symptoms (A–C) must be present to meet criteria:
  A. Meets criteria for possible bvFTD
  B. Exhibits significant functional decline (by caregiver report or as evidenced by Clinical Dementia Rating Scale or Functional Activities Questionnaire scores)
  C. Imaging results consistent with bvFTD (one of the following [C.1–C.2] must be present):
    C.1. Frontal and/or anterior temporal atrophy on MRI or CT
    C.2. Frontal and/or anterior temporal hypoperfusion or hypometabolism on PET or single-photon emission computed tomography

IV. Behavioral variant FTD with definite FTLD pathology. Criterion A and either criterion B or C must be present to meet criteria:
  Meets criteria for possible or probable bvFTD
  Histopathological evidence of FTLD on biopsy or at postmortem
  Presence of a known pathogenic mutation

V. Exclusionary criteria for bvFTD. Criteria A and B must be answered negatively for any bvFTD diagnosis. Criterion C can be positive for possible bvFTD but must be negative for probable bvFTD.
  A. Pattern of deficits is better accounted for by other non-degenerative nervous system or medical disorders
  B. Behavioral disturbance is better accounted for by a psychiatric diagnosis
  C. Biomarkers strongly indicative of Alzheimer disease or other neurodegenerative process.

*Reprinted with permission from Rascovsky, K., Hodges, J.R., Knopman, D., et al., 2011. Sensitivity of Revised Diagnostic Criteria for the Behavioural Variant of Frontotemporal Dementia. Brain. 134(Pt 9):2456–77.*

**TABLE 95.9B Features of Frontotemporal Dementia Subtypes**

| FTD type | BvFTD | SvPPA | Agrammatic/nonfluent PPA |
|---|---|---|---|
| % of FTD cases | 50 | 25 | 25 |
| Most common underlying pathology | Tau-related or TDP-43 | TDP type C | Tau-related |
| Typical anatomy | Insula, amygdala, orbitofrontal, anterior cingulate cortex | L. anterior temporal | L. inferior frontal gyrus |

### Expanded Frontotemporal Dementia Syndromes

Features of bvFTD and PPA are recognized in a subgroup of patients with progressive apraxia of speech, CBS or PSP-S. Therefore, these disorders are considered in the differential of FTD-related disorders (Boeve et al., 2003; Josephs, 2008). While CBS and PSP-S have unique features, there is significant clinical overlap including associated frontal lobe dysfunction on neuropsychometric testing.

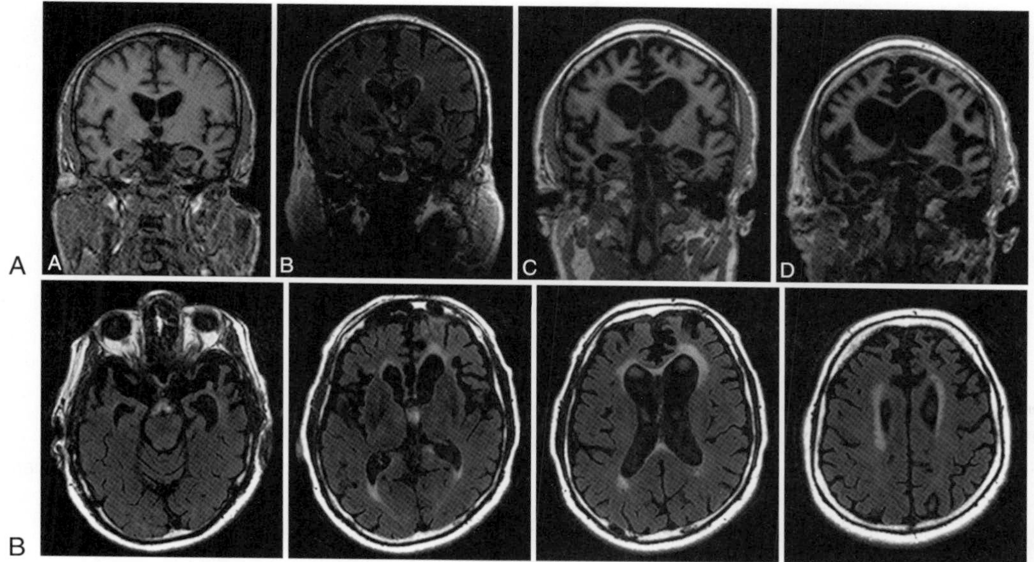


**Fig. 95.17** A, Longitudinal serial coronal magnetic resonance imaging (MRI) in patient with bvFTD demonstrating increasing frontal and temporal atrophy. *A,* 1 year of symptoms; *B,* 3 years of symptoms; *C,* 7 years of symptoms; *D,* 9 years of symptoms. B, T2 fluid-attenuated inversion recovery MRI in same patient 7 years after symptom onset. *bvFTD,* Behavioral variant frontotemporal dementia. (*Courtesy Bradley Boeve.*)

Progressive apraxia of speech is a disorder of motor speech planning. It can occur with agrammatism or on its own. When it occurs in isolation, it is called primary progressive apraxia of speech (PPAOS) (Josephs et al., 2012). The speech is characterized by slow rate, sound distortions, distorted substitutions, and trial-and-error articulatory movements. The anatomical correlate of PPAOS is atrophy/hypometabolism of the lateral premotor area and supplementary motor cortices. When apraxia of speech occurs with or without agrammatism, the pathology is most often tau (Josephs et al., 2006).

## Neuroimaging

### Structural Magnetic Resonance Imaging

Structural MRI and functional imaging studies provide complementary information in the diagnosis of FTD. In bvFTD, atrophy occurs in the anterior cingulate cortex, anterior insula, striatum, amygdala, hypothalamus, and thalamus comprising the salience network regardless of underlying pathological substrate (Perry et al., 2017; Rosen et al., 2002).

In svPPA, the left anterior temporal pole is the region of greatest atrophy (Mummery et al., 2000). Other regions that can be involved include the orbitofrontal region, insula, anterior cingulate right anterior temporal lobe, and hippocampus (Rosen et al., 2002). Agrammatic PPA is associated with left inferior frontal atrophy (Gorno-Tempini et al., 2004). When apraxia of speech is present, atrophy is predominantly in the superior premotor and supplementary motor regions (Josephs et al., 2013). Furthermore, in patients with progressive apraxia of speech, agrammatic PPA, or both, tests of apraxia of speech correlate with premotor volume while tests of aphasia correlate with regions of the left hemisphere language network including Broca's area (Whitwell et al., 2013). Fig. 95.17 provides an example of longitudinal change on MRI in a patient with bvFTD. Fig. 95.18 shows an MRI in a patient with svPPA.

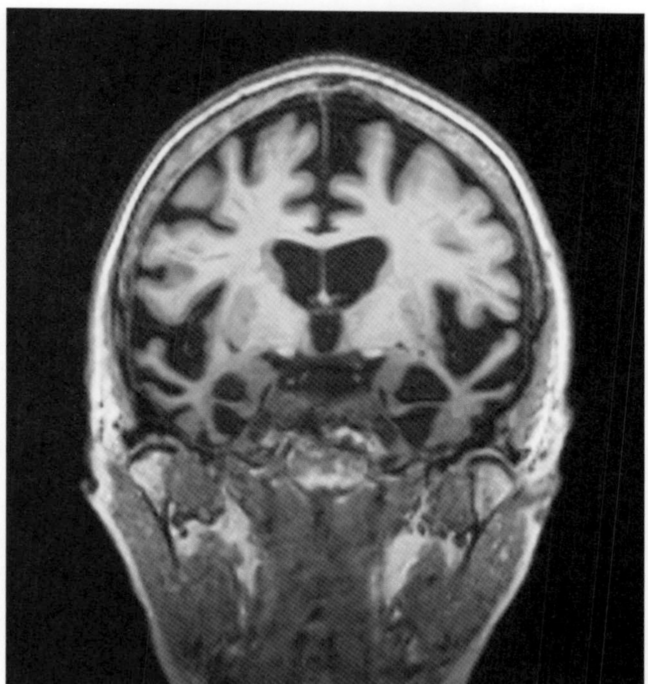

**Fig. 95.18** T1 coronal magnetic resonance imaging in patient with semantic variant primary progressive aphasia (svPPA) demonstrating asymmetric temporal atrophy and dilation of the collateral sulcus.

### Functional Imaging

FDG-PET has been shown to improve accuracy of diagnosis in autopsy-confirmed FTD patients (Foster et al., 2007). BvFTD is characterized by bilateral frontal-temporal hypometabolism. Agrammatic PPA is associated with the left posterior inferior frontal lobe hypometabolism. svPPA is associated with left anterior temporal hypometabolism. PPAOS is characterized by a focal hypometabolism in the supplementary motor area and superior premotor cortex. Figs. 95.19–95.21 show PET scans for subjects with svPPA, nonfluent/agrammatic aphasia, and PPAOS.

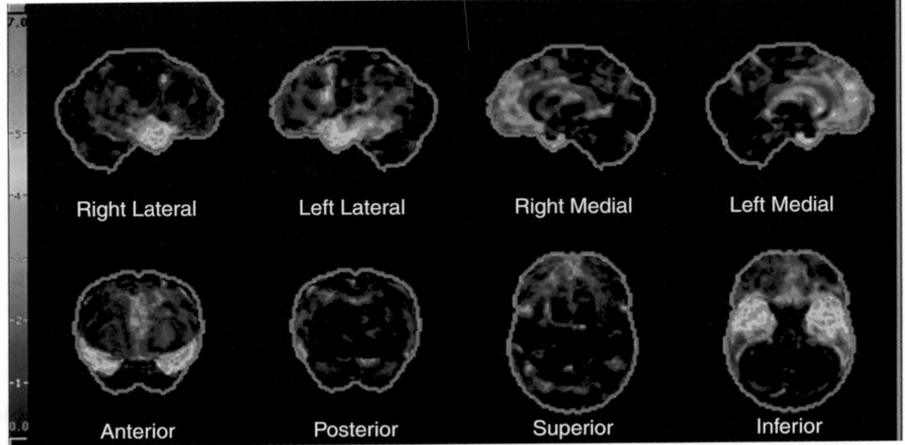


**Fig. 95.19** Fluorodeoxyglucose-positron emission tomography statistical stereotactic surface projection map (Cortex ID) in a semantic variant primary progressive aphasia (svPPA) patient.

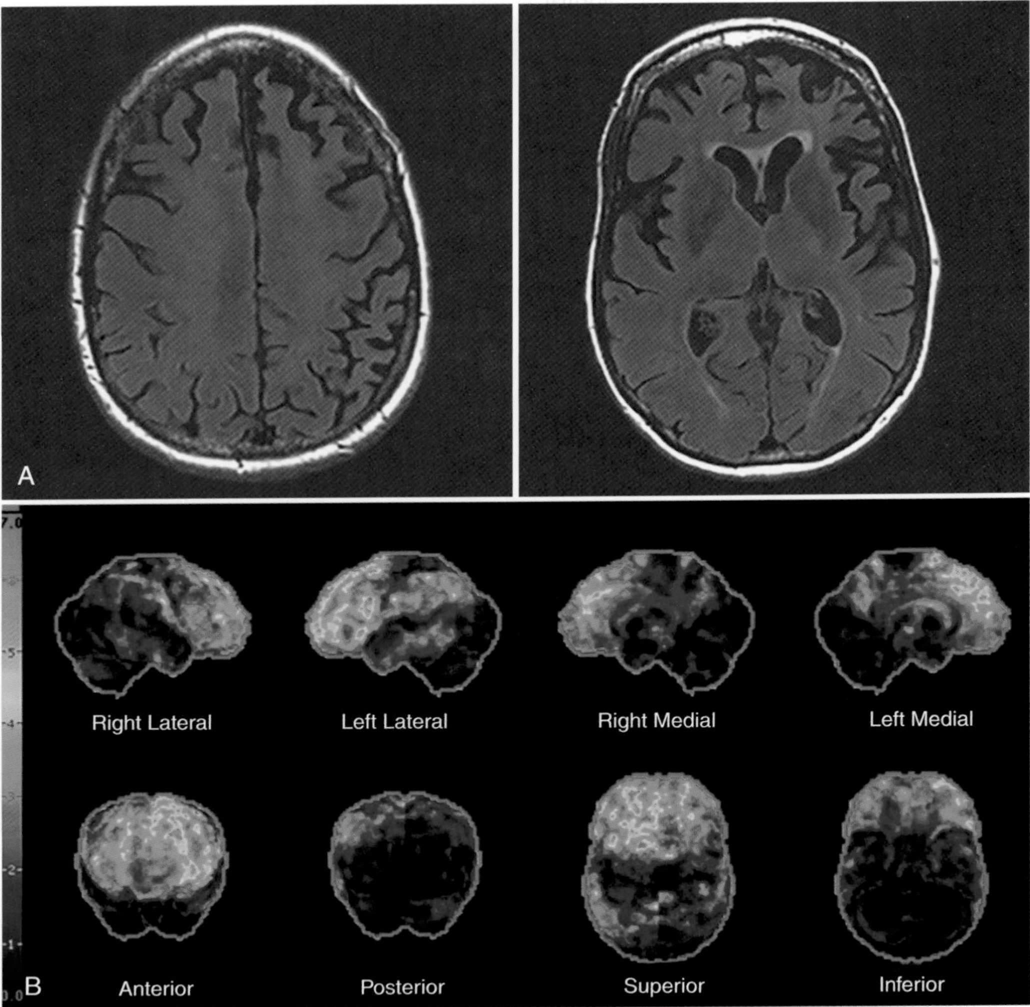


**Fig. 95.20** A, *Top row:* Axial magnetic resonance imaging brain in agrammatic aphasia demonstrating left inferior frontal atrophy. B, *Bottom row:* Fluorodeoxyglucose-positron emission tomography statistical stereotactic surface projection map (Cortex ID) in patient with progressive agrammatic aphasia showing hypometabolism in the left greater than right frontal lobe. Notice greatest area of hypometabolism near Broca's area.

### PiB-PET

PiB-PET has also proven useful in discriminating FTD from AD. PiB-PET is more sensitive than FDG-PET on both visual interpretation and quantitative measures while FDG-PET is more specific only quantitatively (Rabinovici et al., 2011).

### Tau-PET

[$^{18}$F]-AV-1451 (flortaucipir) was developed to bind to AD-type tau which is a mix of 3 microtubule-binding domain repeats (3R-tau) and 4R-tau. FTD syndromes due to 3R-tau such as Pick's pathology or 4R-tau such PSP or CBD pathology, therefore, do not bind the current tau PET ligand well. In FTD cases secondary to *MAPT* mutations whether the tau PET will be positive depends on where the mutation occurs. Inclusion of exon 10 in transcripts determines if 3 or 4R-tau is produced. *MAPT* mutations outside of exon 10 (V337M and R406W) produce AD-like tau (mixed 3R/4R), and, therefore, have tau-PET signal close to the AD dementia levels. Mutations inside exon 10 have lower levels of tau-PET SUVR than AD dementia participants (Jones et al., 2018b).

### Laboratory Evaluation

In the FTD spectrum disorders serum and CSF studies are normal. Active investigation for the role of serum and CSF biomarkers in predicting pathology for FTD subtypes is underway. Progranulin serum levels have shown promise in discriminating those with and without progranulin mutations (Finch et al., 2009). Some studies have demonstrated plasma TDP-43 and CSF TDP-43 may predict TDP-43 pathology although more research is needed to confirm these findings (Foulds et al., 2008; Steinacker et al., 2008).

## Genetics

A positive family history occurs in approximately 40% of FTD cases. Several genes associated with FTD have been described. The three major genes include *MAPT*, which account for approximately 5%–10% of FTD cases (10%–20% of familial cases), progranulin which accounts for 10% of FTD cases, and chromosome 9 open reading frame 72 (C9ORF72) which accounts for approximately 15% (25% of familial cases) of FTD cases. These genes are dominantly inherited. Several other genes have been implicated in FTD, including charged multivesicular body protein 2B (CHMP2B) on chromosome 3 (Skibinski et al., 2005) and valosin-containing protein (VCP) mutations on chromosome 9 (Watts et al., 2004). Mutations in VCP cause a syndrome of inclusion body myopathy, Paget disease of bone, and frontotemporal dementia. TAR DNA-binding protein 43 mutations have been reported in patients with FTD with or without MND (Benajiba et al., 2009; Borroni et al., 2009). Less common genes associated with FTD include *TBK1*, *TIA1*, and *FUS*.

### Frontotemporal Dementia and Parkinsonism Linked to Chromosome 17

Frontotemporal dementia and parkinsonism linked to chromosome 17 (FTD-P 17) refers to mutations in either MAPT or progranulin.

***Microtubule-associated protein tau mutations.*** The first FTD gene discovery was *MAPT* mutations as a cause of behavioral and personality changes associated with parkinsonism (FTD-P 17) (Hutton et al., 1998). Clinical phenotypes vary and can include FTD, PSP-S, and CBS. Despite this discovery, a group of families with FTD linked to chromosome 17 without *MAPT* mutations or tau pathology remained uncharacterized. Mutations in these remaining families were later linked to progranulin. For *MAPT* mutations, median age of onset is 45 while the median survival is 7 years. Anteromedial temporal atrophy is characteristic on MRI (Fig. 95.22; Whitwell et al., 2009).

***Progranulin mutations.*** In 2006, two groups demonstrated that these remaining chromosome 17 FTD families have mutations in the *PGRN* gene (Baker et al., 2006; Cruts et al., 2006). Plasma progranulin levels can be used as a diagnostic test to determine when a *PGRN* mutation is present (Finch et al., 2009). Low plasma progranulin levels are detected in both symptomatic and asymptomatic individuals with *PGRN* gene mutations. Significant clinical variability exists between individuals with the same *PGRN* mutation, indicating other genetic and environmental factors play an important role in the clinical phenotype (Rademakers et al., 2007). The clinical presentations include bvFTD, PPA, AD dementia phenotype, and CBS. The median age of onset is approximately 59, with median survival of 6 years (Boeve et al., 2012). Neuroimaging reveals asymmetric frontal-parietal and posterior temporal atrophy (Fig. 95.23; Boeve et al., 2012; Whitwell et al., 2012).

### Chromosome 9 Open Reading Frame 72

Most recently a noncoding repeat expansion in C9ORF72 was found in FTD and ALS patients (DeJesus-Hernandez et al., 2011). In healthy individuals 2–23 copies of GGGGCC repeat are present. In contrast, in FTD/ALS families hundreds to thousands of copies exist. This is the most common cause of familial FTD/ALS. It also accounts

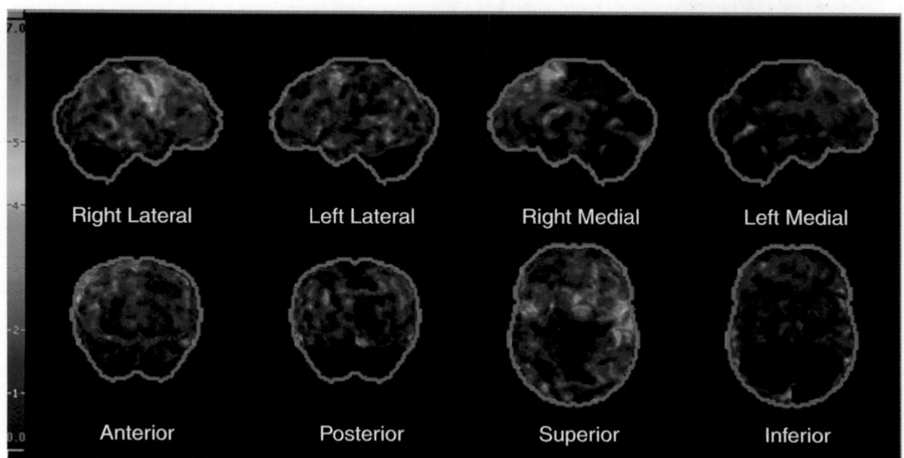


**Fig. 95.21** Fluorodeoxyglucose-positron emission tomography statistical stereotactic surface projection map (Cortex ID) showing hypometabolism in right premotor cortex and right supplementary motor area in a patient with primary progressive apraxia of speech (PPAOS).

for approximately 6% of sporadic FTD and approximately 25% of familial FTD (Majounie et al., 2012). While most patients present with FTD or ALS, approximately 30% have FTD-MND. BvFTD is the most common FTD presentation. The clinical phenotype can vary widely, including parkinsonism and psychosis. C9ORF72 mutations have been seen in clinically diagnosed AD, PD, and CBS. Recently, C9ORF72 mutations were shown to be the most common cause of Huntington disease phenocopy (Hensman Moss et al., 2014). Repeat length does not predict phenotype between FTD-MND, ALS, or FTD (van Blitterswijk et al., 2013). Median age (range) of onset is 52, with median survival of 5 years (Boeve et al., 2012). Neuroimaging reveals fairly symmetric bilateral frontotemporal atrophy (Fig. 95.24; Boeve et al., 2012). FDG-PET in a C9ORF72 patient is demonstrated in Fig. 95.25.

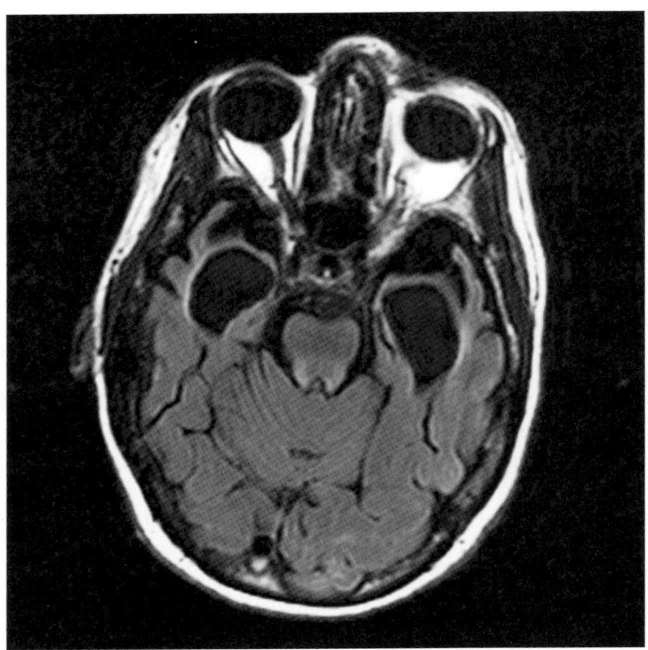

**Fig. 95.22** T2 fluid-attenuated inversion recovery magnetic resonance imaging in frontotemporal dementia patient with microtubule-associated protein tau (MAPT) mutation with characteristic bitemporal atrophy. (*Courtesy Dr. Bradley Boeve.*)

## Pathology

Gross findings include significant frontal and temporal lobar atrophy. Pathological diagnoses of FTLD are based on the major deposited protein in the brain. Three major proteins are associated with FTLD: the microtubule-associated protein tau (FTLD-tau) (approximately 40%), the TAR DNA-binding protein of 43 kD (FTLD-TDP) (approximately 50%), and the fused-in-sarcoma protein (FTLD-FUS) (approximately 9%). Approximately 1% remains uncharacterized.

FTLD-tau consists of PSP pathology, CBD, argyrophilic grain disease (4R tauopathies), globular glial tauopathy, and Pick disease (3R tauopathy). *MAPT* mutations are always associated with tau pathology. Pick disease is the prototype 3R tauopathy. Pick disease accounts for less than 5% of all FTLDs. The gross atrophy of Pick disease has been described as knife edge-like. Pick bodies, circumscribed tau positive inclusions, are the hallmark pathology of Pick disease. Pick disease has less neuritic pathology than other tauopathies. The Gallyas silver stain can distinguish Pick disease from other tauopathies. The inclusions are negative for the Gallyas silver stain and a 4R tau stain. Other pathological findings in Pick disease include "ballooned neurons." CBD and PSP pathology were previously discussed. Characteristic pathology is demonstrated in Fig. 95.26. Globular glial tauopathy is characterized by globular tau-reactive oligodendroglial and astrocytic inclusions.

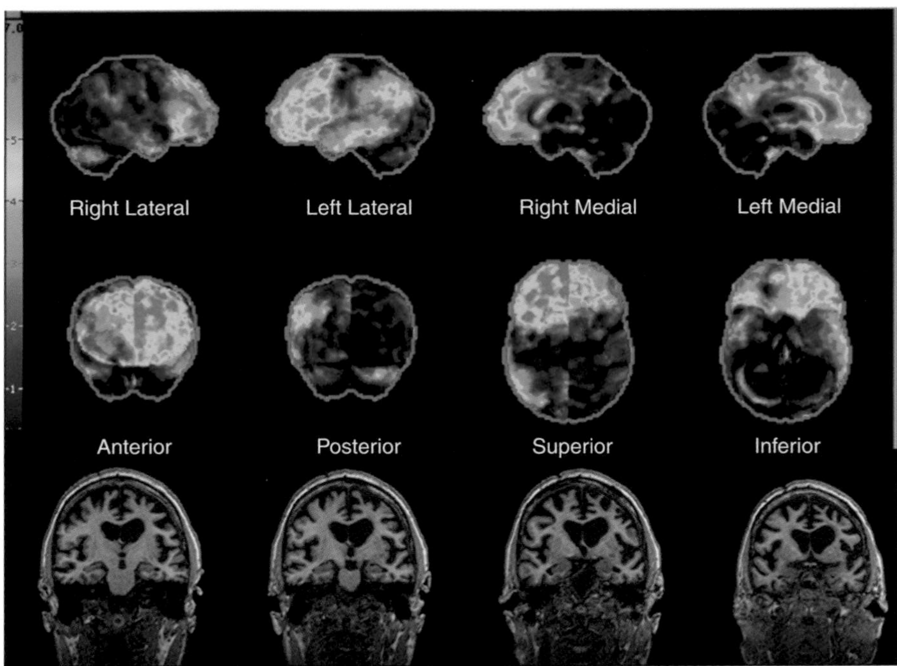


**Fig. 95.23** *Top 2 rows*: Fluorodeoxyglucose-positron emission tomography statistical stereotactic surface projection map (Cortex ID) in a primary progressive aphasia patient with progranulin mutation showing asymmetric left greater than right hypometabolism. *Bottom row*: Corresponding coronal T1 magnetic resonance imagings in bottom row. Notice asymmetric atrophy and ventricular dilation. (*Courtesy Dr. Bradley Boeve.*)

FTLD-TDP can be subdivided into types A, B, C, D, and E. Type A is associated with neuronal inclusions, intranuclear inclusions, and dystrophic neurites. Progranulin mutations are associated with FTLD-TDP-type A. Type B is associated with neuronal cytoplasmic inclusions. C9ORF72 mutations are associated with FTLD-TDP-type B, less likely A, C. C9ORF72 mutation cases also have characteristic cerebellar inclusions. FTLD-TDP-type B is also associated with FTD-MND. Type C is associated predominantly with neurites and characteristic Pick body–like neuronal inclusions. Semantic dementia is associated with TDP type C. VCP mutations are associated with FTLD-TDP type D pathology with abundant intraneuronal inclusions. TDP type E was recently described in association with a rapidly progressive FTD phenotype. Type E was characterized by granulofilamentous neuronal inclusions, abundant grains, and oligodendroglial inclusions (Lee et al., 2017).

FTLD-FUS is divided into three rare forms of FTLD: neurofilament inclusion disease, basophilic inclusion disease, and atypical FTLD with ubiquitin-only immunoreactive changes (aFTLD-U). All three are immunoreactive to FUS. Neurofilament inclusion disease (Josephs et al., 2003) is a rare cause of FTD that can also be associated with MND and parkinsonism. The pathology is characterized by neuronal and intranuclear inclusions that are immunoreactive to neurofilament and alpha-internexin (Uchikado et al., 2005). Basophilic inclusion disease is pathologically characterized by basophilic inclusions on hematoxylin and eosin (H&E) that are not immunoreactive to intermediate filaments. aFTLD-U does not have inclusions on H&E.

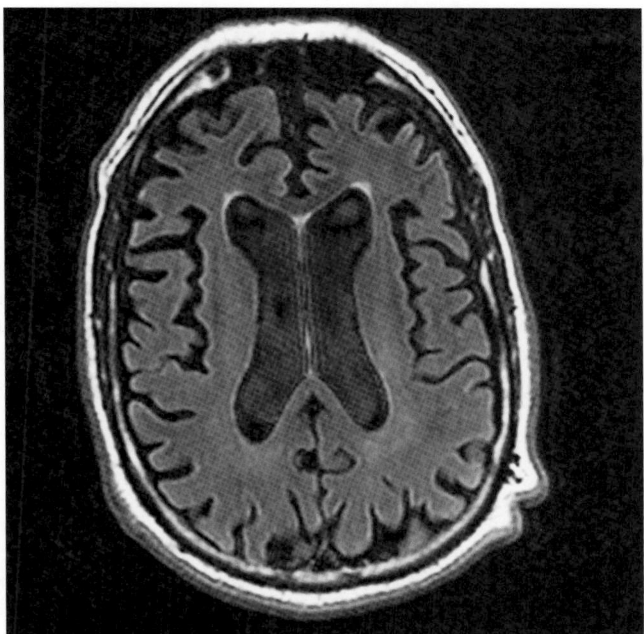

**Fig. 95.24** Axial T2 fluid-attenuated inversion recovery magnetic resonance imaging in a frontotemporal dementia patient demonstrating symmetric atrophy pattern in a patient with chromosome 9 open reading frame 72 mutation.

## Clinicopathological Correlations

bvFTD is associated most commonly with TDP (usually type A; ~40%) or tau pathology (~40%), with FUS pathology less likely (~10%). When bvFTD occurs in tauopathies, the underlying pathologies are in order of frequency: Pick disease (PiD), CBD, PSP, and argyrophilic grain disease (AGD) (Josephs et al., 2011). Agrammatic PPA is associated most commonly with tau (70%) (Josephs et al., 2011) pathology, especially if apraxia of speech is present (Josephs et al., 2006). CBS and PSP-S are also most commonly associated with tau pathology, although familial CBS has been associated with progranulin mutations (Josephs et al., 2011). FTD-MND is almost always associated with TDP pathology. svPPA is most commonly associated with TDP pathology (TDP-type C; 83%), although when it is caused by tau pathology Pick disease is most likely (Josephs et al., 2011).

Pick disease can present with bvFTD, PPA, or CBS (Boeve et al., 1999; Piguet et al., 2011). Although Pick disease is typically sporadic, familial cases can have a tau mutation. Globular glial tauopathies have a range of clinical presentations, including bvFTD, semantic variant PPA, PSP-S, CBS, and motor neuron disease.

Patients with FTLD-FUS tend to have a young age of onset (mean 41), stereotypies, hypersexuality, and hyperphagia. Striatal atrophy is a characteristic imaging feature (Josephs et al., 2010; Urwin et al., 2010).

## Pathophysiology

***TAR DNA-binding protein 43.*** TDP-43 normally resides in the nucleus of the cell. In neurodegenerative disease, TDP-43 relocalizes to the cytoplasm, forms inclusions, becomes cleaved,

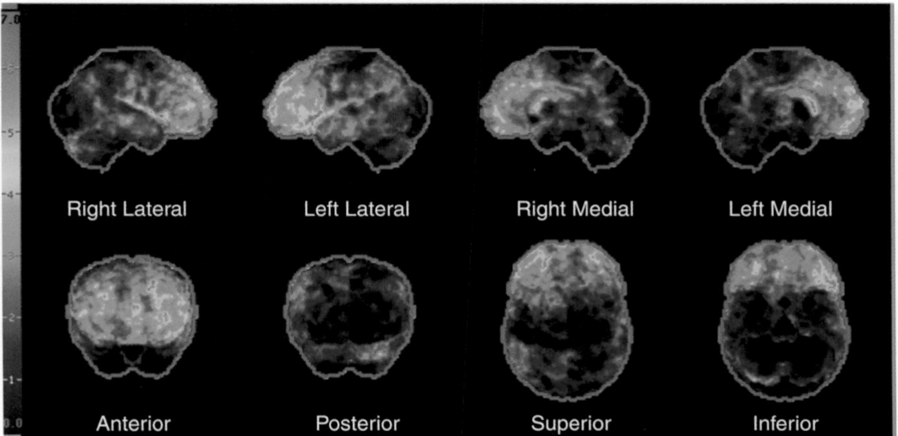


**Fig. 95.25** Fluorodeoxyglucose-positron emission tomography statistical stereotactic surface projection map (Cortex ID) in a patient with chromosome 9 open reading frame 72 mutation demonstrating bifrontal hypometabolism.

hyperphosphorylated, and aggregates. TDP-43 has numerous functions in the cell and how it is related to neurodegeneration is incompletely understood. Functions of TDP-43 include RNA metabolism, including transcription, splicing, and transport of RNA.

***Microtubule-associated protein tau.*** The tau protein promotes microtubule stabilization and assembly. Hyperphosphorylation of tau leads to microtubule destabilization under pathological conditions. The tau protein undergoes differential splicing. Inclusion of exon 10 in splicing of tau results in four microtubule-binding domains (4R), while exclusion of exon 10 results in 3 binding domains (3R). In normal adults, there is a 1:1 ratio of 4 and 3 binding domains. Most tau mutations cluster around the microtubule-binding domain. Mutations in tau disrupt the binding of tau to the microtubule and enhance tau aggregation or interfere with splicing, resulting in excessive exon 10 inclusion, increasing 4R/3R tau ratio (Rademakers and Hutton, 2007).

***Progranulin.*** The progranulin protein is a precursor protein that is cleaved into granulins. Progranulin functions as a growth factor with antiinflammatory properties. Granulins may serve as inflammatory mediators. Progranulin is expressed in neurons and glia. Neuronal progranulin regulates synaptic function and has neuroprotective and neurotrophic properties. All mutations in progranulin cause a reduction in progranulin levels (haploinsufficiency) which may cause a loss of trophic support and neuronal loss. The mechanism by which progranulin mutations result in TDP pathology is unknown, although in cells, suppression of progranulin leads to a caspase activation which leads to TDP-43 accumulation (Zhang et al., 2007). Patients with progranulin mutation carriers or svPPA patients have an increased prevalence of associated autoimmune disease and elevated levels of TNF-alpha, further implicating a relationship between inflammation and FTD associated with progranulin (Miller et al., 2013).

***Chromosome 9 open reading frame 72.*** The mechanism of how hexanucleotide expansions in C9ORF72 cause disease is under active investigation. Upon expansion in the noncoding region, a decrease in C9ORF72 mRNA occurs, resulting in haploinsufficiency. A decrease in expression of the mRNA transcript may occur through epigenetic events such as DNA and histone methylation, resulting in less protein (Belzil et al., 2013). In addition to haploinsufficiency as a mechanism of disease, the hexanucleotide repeat undergoes transcription, resulting in RNA. This RNA can form nuclear foci which bind and sequester RNA-binding proteins and prevent them from binding their RNA targets. This process can interrupt splicing. Alternatively, the RNA can undergo C9 repeat associated non-ATG translation (C9RAN) where the repeat sequences make proteins that normally do not exist (Zu et al., 2011). This results in different polypeptides, depending on the reading frames. An antibody that recognizes all of these polypeptides was created. All stained brains of C9ORF72 patients had these polypeptide inclusions (Gendron et al., 2013). It is possible that these C9RAN proteins inclusions are toxic although further research is required.

***TMEM106B.*** Genome-wide association studies (GWAS) in FTLD-TDP patients demonstrated an association with TMEM106B, which is an uncharacterized transmembrane protein (Van Deerlin et al., 2010). More recently, it was shown that TMEM106B single nucleotide polymorphisms may protect against developing FTD in progranulin mutation carriers by affecting progranulin levels (Finch et al., 2011). The protective variant results in less TMEM106B protein. A TMEM106B variant also protects against FTD but not ALS in C9ORF72 mutation carriers (van Blitterswijk et al., 2014).

### Frontotemporal Dementia Treatment

There are no FDA-approved medications for the treatment of FTD. While a meta-analysis has suggested benefit for the use of SSRIs in FTD to improve behavioral symptoms, most of the studies included were small and uncontrolled (Huey et al., 2006). Since the FDA has issued a warning that antipsychotic drugs increase risk of death in dementia patients, such agents must be used with caution. Nonpharmacological interventions including home safety evaluation and removal of weapons from the home are important. Family education about the disease and caregiver support groups can be helpful. Patients with PPA may benefit from evaluation and treatment by speech language pathologists to help with communication strategies.

## VASCULAR DEMENTIA (VASCULAR COGNITIVE IMPAIRMENT)

### History

Our understanding of the interaction among vascular disease, neurodegeneration, and cognition has evolved over time. Binswanger described "encephalitis subcorticalis chronica progressiva" as characterized by dementia, stroke, and white matter disease, which Alzheimer demonstrated was secondary to arteriolosclerosis of long perforating arteries. For many decades, narrowing of the arteries was thought to be the most common cause of dementia and doctors and patients attributed dementia to "hardening of the arteries." Hachinski introduced the term multi-infarct dementia (MiD), emphasizing prior clinical strokes with

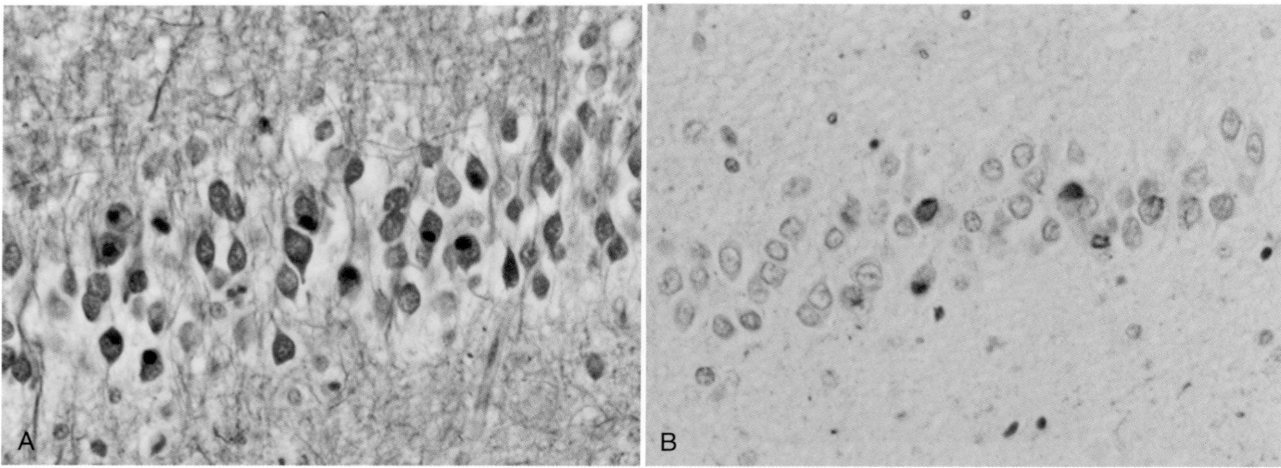


**Fig. 95.26 Pick Disease Pathology. A,** Bielschowsky stain showing Pick bodies in fascia dentate. **B,** Tau stain demonstrating Pick bodies in fascia dentate. (*Courtesy Dr. Joseph Parisi.*)

focal neurological signs and symptoms and "stepwise" cognitive decline (Hachinski et al., 1974). With advances in neuroimaging, investigators appreciated that multi-infarct was a small part of a wider spectrum of vascular diseases resulting in cognitive impairment. The term vascular cognitive impairment (VCI) was introduced to encompass all forms of cognitive impairment related to vascular disease including milder forms of cognitive impairment not meeting criteria for dementia and those with mixed pathology (O'Brien et al., 2003). Both multi-infarct dementia and vascular dementia (VaD) are now subgroups of VCI.

## Diagnostic Criteria

The American Heart Association and American Stroke Association (AHA-ASA) released a statement defining the term VCI (Table 95.10; Gorelick et al., 2011), but for many years the National Institute of

**TABLE 95.10 Vascular Cognitive Impairment**

| | |
|---|---|
| 1. The term VCI characterizes all forms of cognitive deficits from VaD to MCI of vascular origin.<br>2. These criteria cannot be used for subjects who have an active diagnosis of drug or alcohol abuse/dependence. Subjects must be free of any type of substance for at least 3 months.<br>3. These criteria cannot be used for subjects with delirium. | |
| Dementia | 1. The diagnosis of dementia should be based on a decline in cognitive function from a prior baseline and a deficit in performance in two or more cognitive domains that are of sufficient severity to affect activities of daily living.<br>2. The diagnosis of dementia must be based on cognitive testing, and four cognitive domains should be assessed: executive/attention, memory, language, and visuospatial functions.<br>3. The deficits in activities of daily living are independent of the motor/sensory sequelae of the vascular event. |
| Probable VaD | 1. There is cognitive impairment and imaging evidence of cerebrovascular disease and<br>a. There is a clear temporal relationship between a vascular event (e.g., clinical stroke) and onset of cognitive deficits, or<br>b. There is a clear relationship in the severity and pattern of cognitive impairment and the presence of diffuse, subcortical cerebrovascular disease pathology.<br>2. There is no history of gradually progressive cognitive deficits before or after the stroke that suggests the presence of a nonvascular neurodegenerative disorder. |
| Possible VaD | There is cognitive impairment and imaging evidence of cerebrovascular disease but<br>1. There is no clear relationship (temporal, severity, or cognitive pattern) between the vascular disease (e.g., silent infarcts, subcortical small-vessel disease) and the cognitive impairment.<br>2. There is insufficient information for the diagnosis of VaD (e.g., clinical symptoms suggest the presence of vascular disease, but no CT/MRI studies are available).<br>3. Severity of aphasia precludes proper cognitive assessment. However, patients with documented evidence of normal cognitive function (e.g., annual cognitive evaluations) before the clinical event that caused aphasia could be classified as having probable VaD.<br>4. There is evidence of other neurodegenerative diseases or conditions in addition to cerebrovascular disease that may affect cognition, such as<br>a. A history of other neurodegenerative disorders (e.g., Parkinson disease, progressive supranuclear palsy, dementia with Lewy bodies);<br>b. The presence of Alzheimer disease biology is confirmed by biomarkers (e.g., PET, CSF, amyloid ligands) or genetic studies (e.g., PS1 mutation); or<br>c. A history of active cancer or psychiatric or metabolic disorders that may affect cognitive function. |
| VaMCI | 1. VaMCI includes the four subtypes proposed for the classification of MCI: amnestic, amnestic plus other domains, nonamnestic single domain, and nonamnestic multiple domain.<br>2. The classification of VaMCI must be based on cognitive testing, and a minimum of four cognitive domains should be assessed: executive/attention, memory, language, and visuospatial functions. The classification should be based on an assumption of decline in cognitive function from a prior baseline and impairment in at least one cognitive domain.<br>3. Instrumental activities of daily living could be normal or mildly impaired, independent of the presence of motor/sensory symptoms. |
| Probable VaMCI | 1. There is cognitive impairment and imaging evidence of cerebrovascular disease and<br>a. There is a clear temporal relationship between a vascular event (e.g., clinical stroke) and onset of cognitive deficits, or<br>b. There is a clear relationship in the severity and pattern of cognitive impairment and the presence of diffuse, subcortical cerebrovascular disease pathology.<br>2. There is no history of gradually progressive cognitive deficits before or after the stroke that suggests the presence of a nonvascular neurodegenerative disorder. |
| Possible VaMCI | There is cognitive impairment and imaging evidence of cerebrovascular disease but<br>1. There is no clear relationship (temporal, severity, or cognitive pattern) between the vascular disease (e.g., silent infarcts, subcortical small-vessel disease) and onset of cognitive deficits.<br>2. There is insufficient information for the diagnosis of VaMCI (e.g., clinical symptoms suggest the presence of vascular disease, but no CT/MRI studies are available).<br>3. Severity of aphasia precludes proper cognitive assessment. However, patients with documented evidence of normal cognitive function (e.g., annual cognitive evaluations) before the clinical event that caused aphasia could be classified as having probable VaMCI.<br>4. There is evidence of other neurodegenerative diseases or conditions in addition to cerebrovascular disease that may affect cognition, such as<br>a. A history of other neurodegenerative disorders (e.g., Parkinson disease, progressive supranuclear palsy, dementia with Lewy bodies);<br>b. The presence of Alzheimer disease biology is confirmed by biomarkers (e.g., PET, CSF, amyloid ligands) or genetic studies (e.g., PS1 mutation); or<br>c. A history of active cancer or psychiatric or metabolic disorders that may affect cognitive function. |
| Unstable VaMCI | Subjects with the diagnosis of probable or possible VaMCI whose symptoms revert to normal should be classified as having "unstable VaMCI." |

*VaD,* Vascular dementia; *VaMCI,* vascular mild cognitive impairment; *VCI,* vascular cognitive impairment.

*Reprinted with permission from Gorelick, P., Scuteri, A., Black, S.E., et al., 2011, Vascular contributions to cognitive impairment and dementia: a statement for healthcare professionals from the American Heart Association/American Stroke Association. Stroke 42, 2672–2713.*

Neurological Disorders and Stroke and the Association Internationale pour la Recherche et l'Enseignementen Neurosciences (NINDS-AIREN) criteria were used for VaD (Roman et al., 1993). The NINDS-AIREN criteria rely heavily on symptomatic cerebrovascular disease including history of stroke, imaging of stroke, and focal exam findings consistent with stroke. These criteria have been shown to be specific, but not sensitive, overlooking infarcts that were clinically silent. In fact, the clinical diagnosis of "probable VaD" compared to subsequent pathological confirmation was 20% (Gold et al., 2002).

## Epidemiology

In the population-based Rotterdam study with a mean follow-up of 5.7 years using the conservative NINDS-AIREN criteria, the incidence of vascular dementia was 0.1 per 1000 person-years in those aged 60–64 years. The incidence increased with age to 7.0 per 1000 person-years in those aged 90–94 years, with a higher risk of VaD in men (Ruitenberg et al., 2001). In a Rochester, MN population-based study, approximately 13% of autopsy dementia cases were due to pure vascular dementia and 12% had significant vascular and AD pathology, making vascular disease an important component in at least 25% of dementia cases (Knopman et al., 2003). In a PiB-PET study (Lee et al., 2011a), amyloid imaging was used in 45 patients with subcortical vascular dementia. Approximately two-thirds of cases were negative for amyloid deposition, indicating the pure VaD phenotype can be appreciated antemortem.

## Vascular Risk Factors

Interestingly, stroke and Alzheimer dementia share many risk factors including diabetes, hypertension, and metabolic syndrome.

## Subtypes

Numerous subtypes of VCI have been proposed, including multi-infarct dementia, subcortical ischemic vascular dementia, dementia related to strategic strokes, perfusion-related dementia, hemorrhagic stroke-related dementia, dementia associated with arteriopathies, and mixed dementia (O'Brien et al., 2003).

## Clinical Presentation

Due to the heterogeneous causes of VCI, there is no typical clinical presentation. The severity, temporal course, and associated features vary widely. VaD patients with large territory stroke may have focal signs on exam (upper motor neuron pattern weakness, hemianopsia, sensory loss), while those with cerebral small-vessel disease may present with gait disturbance and cognitive slowing. Mixed AD and VaD patients may present with an amnestic syndrome indistinguishable from typical AD. In one large study that used NINDS-AIREN criteria, patients with large-vessel disease defined as those with strategic or territorial infarcts were compared to those with small-vessel disease defined as those with lacunar strokes and white matter hyperintensity (Staekenborg et al., 2008). A pattern emerged with small-vessel patients manifesting bulbar findings and parkinsonism, while large-vessel patients had more lateralizing language, motor, and sensory findings. The common clinical presentation associations with small- and large-vessel presentations may be useful in subtyping VCI, with the caveat that many patients have coexisting large-vessel and small-vessel disease.

## Large-Vessel Stroke

### Strategic Infarcts

Targeted strokes can present with memory loss. The amnesia can be distinguished from the episodic memory loss associated with AD dementia disease by the sudden onset. The posterior cerebral artery provides the blood supply to the posterior medial aspect of the hippocampus. Infarction of the bilateral posterior cerebral arteries may result in an amnestic syndrome (Benson et al., 1974), although isolated left posterior cerebral artery infarctions can produce amnesia as well. Common coexisting deficits include visual field cuts. The concept of strategic lesions is highlighted by thalamic infarction where a small infarction involving both hippocampal and amygdala pathways causes significant amnesia, but when the lesion involves only one pathway the memory impairment is quite mild (Cipolotti et al., 2008; Graff-Radford et al., 1990). Basal forebrain injury most commonly secondary to aneurysm rupture can manifest with amnesia associated with personality change (Damasio et al., 1985). Other strategically located infarcts mentioned in the NINDS-AIREN criteria include those involving the angular gyrus and anterior cerebral artery territory (Roman et al., 1993). Caudate infarcts may produce a syndrome similar to behavioral variant FTD but with a sudden onset resulting from interrupting the connectivity between the caudate and the frontal lobe (Graff-Radford et al., 2017).

### Multi-Infarct Dementia

MiD reflects traditional thinking that patients with multiple cortical strokes develop dementia with an abrupt onset and stepwise deterioration. These patients have focal neurological signs on exam such as hemiparesis.

### Dementia After Stroke

In the Canadian Study of Health and Aging, which sampled 9008 community-based individuals and 1255 institutionalized individuals over the age of 65, incident stroke increased the risk of converting from cognitively normal to dementia with a hazard ratio of 2.3. Stroke prevalence was 6 times higher in those with cognitive impairment relative to normal, and approximately two-thirds of stroke survivors had cognitive impairment or dementia in contrast to 21% of stroke-free individuals (Jin et al., 2006). In a population-based study, the incidence of dementia after stroke was 9 times greater than expected, and dementia risk remained double the control population even if there was no dementia the first year after stroke (Kokmen et al., 1996). The subtype of stroke may be important. In the Secondary Prevention of Small Subcortical Strokes trial, 47% of subjects had MCI even in the absence of physical disabilities related to the stroke. Therefore, the presence of a single stroke serves as a biomarker for more extensive cerebrovascular disease (Jacova et al., 2012). Approximately 20% of the population over the age of 65 has silent infarctions. In those with normal cognition at baseline and silent infarction, the risk of dementia is increased significantly (Vermeer et al., 2003). In a meta-analysis of poststroke dementia including population- and hospital-based studies, approximately 10% of patients have dementia prior to first stroke, 10% develop dementia shortly after first stroke, and about 33% develop dementia with recurrent stroke (Pendlebury and Rothwell, 2009). Risk factors for dementia after stroke include age, diabetes, severity of stroke, and white matter hyperintensity (Cordoliani-Mackowiak et al., 2003).

## Cerebral Small-Vessel Disease

### White Matter Hyperintensity

White matter hyperintensity, sometimes called leukoaraiosis, was initially thought to be of indeterminate significance but is increasingly recognized as detrimental. In the Cardiac Health Study, white matter hyperintensity was associated with lower cognitive and lower extremity function (Longstreth et al., 1996). The underlying causes of white matter hyperintensity are numerous, including arteriolosclerosis (vascular risk factor related), amyloid angiopathy, genetic (Fabry disease, etc.), inflammatory or immune (vasculitides, etc.), venous, and others (postradiation, etc.) (Pantoni, 2010). The Framingham study demonstrated, in younger persons (mean age 53), when dementia and CAA are less common, that atherosclerosis risk factors, particularly hypertension, are strongly related to cerebral white matter changes (Jeerakathil et al., 2004). Hypertension was also a risk factor for white matter hyperintensity in the Cardiac Health Study (Longstreth et al., 1996). Also in the Framingham study, white matter hyperintensity volume was associated with incident diagnosis of mild cognitive impairment (Debette et al., 2010). Specific cognitive functions associated with increasing white matter disease burden include executive dysfunction and episodic memory impairment (Maillard et al., 2012). White matter hyperintensity has also been associated with a decline in gait (Baezner et al., 2008), progression to disability (Inzitari et al., 2009), decreased cognitive speed (Valdes Hernandez Mdel et al., 2013), and incident depression (Firbank et al., 2012).

### Lacunar Stroke

Highlighting the overlap between vascular pathologies, white matter hyperintensity is associated with lacunar stroke, but both are independently associated with cognition (van der Flier et al., 2005). Incident lacunes predict decline in executive functions and psychomotor speed (Jokinen et al., 2011). Not surprisingly, the location of lacunes appears to play an important role in cognitive outcomes, with thalamic and putamen lacunes being worse than capsular, caudate, and white matter lacunes (Benisty et al., 2009). In the Secondary Prevention of Small Subcortical Strokes study, 47% of participants met criteria for MCI (36% amnestic, 37% amnestic multidomain, 28% nonamnestic) (Jacova et al., 2012).

### Cerebral Amyloid Angiopathy

CAA is very common. In the Religious Orders Study, 85% of subjects had CAA and approximately 25% of demented patients had severe CAA (Arvanitakis et al., 2011). The presence of significant CAA was associated with decreased perceptual speed and episodic memory, while mild CAA did not correlate to cognitive measures. In the Honolulu-Asia Aging Study, the presence of both CAA and AD at autopsy predicted worse cognitive scores than AD alone (Pfeifer et al., 2002). Amyloid angiopathy correlates with extent of white matter hyperintensity on MRI (Gurol et al., 2013). Lobar cerebral microbleeds in the elderly detected on gradient echo or susceptibility weighted MRI sequences can be used to identify CAA during life.

### Microinfarcts

Microinfarcts contribute to dementia as much as macroscopic infarcts (Troncoso et al., 2008). In an autopsy study, the population attributable risk of dementia for microinfarcts was 33% (Sonnen et al., 2007). In the Honolulu-Asia Aging Study (White, 2009), in autopsied demented or impaired subjects microvascular infarcts were the sole or dominant lesion in approximately 33% of subjects while AD pathology was the sole or dominant lesion in 18% of cases. Microinfarcts are not visible on MRI, but the presence of macroinfarcts, white matter hyperintensity, and hemorrhages correlates with presence of microinfarcts (Longstreth et al., 2009). Recently, it was estimated that identifying one or two microinfarcts on nine routine pathological specimens indicates a maximum-likelihood estimate of 552 to 1104 microinfarcts (Westover et al., 2013). A recent imaging pathology study demonstrated microinfarcts increase rate of brain atrophy independent of AD pathology on MRI, and this primarily occurs in a watershed distribution (Raman et al., 2014). Microinfarcts are associated with decreasing blood pressure, suggesting the pathophysiology of microinfarcts requires further investigation (Graff-Radford et al., 1989).

### Mixed Pathology

Mixed pathology is probably the most important subgroup of VCI. In a recent autopsy series, most demented patients had multiple pathologies at autopsy and the most common pathological diagnosis was AD with vascular pathology occurring in 38% of patients (Schneider et al., 2007). The coexistence of vascular pathology modifies clinical expression of dementia when AD pathology is present. The presence of coexisting cerebrovascular disease with AD requires a lower AD pathology burden to develop dementia (Nagy et al., 1997). In the nun study, at autopsy those with Alzheimer pathology and lacunar stroke were 20 times more likely to be demented during life (Snowdon et al., 1997). In the Baltimore Longitudinal Study of Aging Autopsy Program, the interaction between cerebrovascular disease and AD pathology in causing dementia was also assessed. In subjects with a limited degree of AD pathology, the average number of macroscopic infarcts in demented patients was 2.2, but those with an isolated infarct were not demented (Troncoso et al., 2008). Despite the interaction between cerebrovascular disease and AD pathology, an ADNI study reported that atherosclerosis risk factors and white matter changes were not related to Alzheimer-related biomarkers (CSF Aβ42, hippocampal atrophy, and cognitive tests with memory components) (Lo and Jagust, 2012). Similarly, the leukoaraiosis and disability in the elderly study (LADIS) demonstrated that t-tau, p-tau, and the different Aβ markers did not differ between groups of mild, moderate, and severe white matter hyperintensity (Jonsson et al., 2010).

### CADASIL

Cerebral autosomal dominant arteriopathy with subcortical infarcts and leukoencephalopathy (CADASIL) is a genetic cerebral small-vessel disease caused by mutations in the *NOTCH3* gene on chromosome 19. *NOTCH3* codes for a transmembrane receptor located on vascular smooth muscle cells. In Scotland, the prevalence has been estimated to be 1.98 per 100,000 adults (Razvi et al., 2005). Clinical features include migraine headaches, stroke, and dementia. The pattern of cognitive deficits on neuropsychometric testing includes impaired cognitive speed, executive function, and attention (Peters et al., 2005). Neuropsychiatric symptoms are common. MRI reveals significant white matter hyperintensity and ischemic lesions, particularly in subcortical regions. Involvement of the anterior temporal pole and external capsule are characteristic. Microhemorrhage also variably occurs.

## Neuropsychological Testing

Given the numerous presentations of VCI, no single neuropsychological profile exists. Nonetheless, a pattern emerges when studying groups of VCI patients. In an analysis of 27 prior studies, one study found that frontal executive function was more impaired in VaD relative to AD dementia and verbal memory scores were relatively preserved (Looi and Sachdev, 1999). In autopsy-proven AD, memory impairment is consistently worse than executive function, while in autopsy-proven VaD the findings are more variable, although the majority of patients perform poorly on tests of executive function (Reed et al., 2007). Compared to AD dementia patients, VCI patients have more difficulty with tasks of cognitive speed (Mendez et al., 1997). In a study of 170 patients with stroke or transient ischemic attack (TIA), those with cognitive impairment performed worse on tasks of abstraction, mental flexibility, and processing speed relative to those without cognitive impairment (Sachdev et al., 2004).

## Treatment

Treatment and prevention of vascular dementia should focus on identifying and managing hypertension, diabetes mellitus, atrial fibrillation, and hyperlipidemia. Although aggressive treatment of vascular risk factors is logical to prevent and slow progression of those on the trajectory to VCI, few prospective trials exist. In the double-blind placebo-controlled Systolic Hypertension in Europe trial, non-demented subjects age 60 and older with a baseline systolic blood pressure over 160 mm Hg were randomized to aggressive blood pressure treatment or placebo to determine whether blood pressure management could decrease the incidence of dementia. In the active treatment group at 2 years, blood pressure was decreased by 8.3 mm Hg on average and the incidence of dementia was reduced from 7.7 to 3.8 cases per 1000 patient-years (Forette et al., 1998). In the Perindopril Protection against Recurrent Stroke Study, which was a randomized, double-blind, placebo-controlled trial investigating antihypertensive treatment in patients with prior stroke or TIA, cognitive decline occurred in 9.1% of patients on treatment and in 11.0% on placebo (Tzourio et al., 2003). In the SPRINT-MIND trial, treating systolic blood pressure to a goal of less than 120 mm Hg compared to a goal of less than 140 mm Hg reduced the development of mild cognitive impairment at 1 year (Group, 2019).

### Symptomatic Treatment

AChEIs improve cognitive function to a small degree in patients with VCI (Birks and Craig, 2013; Malouf and Birks, 2004) but are not FDA approved for this indication. Since most patients have mixed vascular and Alzheimer pathology, it is reasonable to investigate AChEIs in this population.

Neuropsychiatric symptoms such as depression and pseudobulbar affect can respond to SSRIs. Dextromethorphan/quinidine has recently been approved by the FDA for treatment of pseudobulbar affect.

## NORMAL PRESSURE HYDROCEPHALUS

NPH refers to enlarged ventricles disproportionate to the degree of cortical atrophy on neuroimaging in patients with a normal opening pressure on lumbar puncture. Non-communicating hydrocephalus refers to a condition in which an obstruction of the CSF occurs within the ventricular system. The causes of NPH are heterogeneous. One cause of NPH is impaired absorption of CSF at the arachnoid granulations. NPH can be idiopathic or secondary to prior history of subarachnoid hemorrhage, meningitis, or other conditions that cause inflammation of the arachnoid granulations. Also, a significant minority (10%–20%) of NPH patients have increased head circumference, indicating that a subgroup of NPH patients may have congenital hydrocephalus that becomes symptomatic later in life (Krefft et al., 2004; Wilson and Williams, 2007). Hypertension may also be a risk factor (Graff-Radford and Godersky, 1987; Graff-Radford et al., 2013; Krauss et al., 1996). NPH is a rare disease. One Norwegian study estimated the prevalence of NPH to be around 21.9/100,000 and the incidence to be around 5.5/100,000 (Brean and Eide, 2008). A more recent population-based study in Sweden found the prevalence of probable idiopathic NPH was 0.2% in those aged 70–79 years and 5.9% in those aged 80 years and older, suggesting that the disorder may be more common than previously thought (Jaraj et al., 2014).

While the classical clinical triad of NPH is gait disturbance, urinary incontinence, and progressive cognitive impairment, many patients may have only one or two of these symptoms and still improve with shunt surgery. However, the core symptom is gait disturbance and shunting patients with hydrocephalus and cognitive impairment alone rarely results in improvement (Petersen et al., 1985). The symptoms are thought to arise from disturbance of white matter pathways subserving frontal lobe function.

### Gait Disturbance

Gait disturbance is an early feature in NPH and is sometimes referred to as an apraxic or magnetic gait. This can be misleading because it is neither pathognomonic nor typical. The typical gait is slow with a wide base and small steps, and turns using multiple steps (piecemeal). There is no mask-like face, hand tremor, arm rigidity, or impaired fine finger movements as in typical Parkinson disease. Postural instability and falls are common in NPH. The gait disorder is the feature most responsive to treatment.

### Cognitive Disorder

Stretching of the frontal white matter pathways results in a cognitive profile characterized by frontal-executive dysfunction, including cognitive slowing, impaired abstract thinking, and impaired set-shifting. Improvement in cognition is difficult to predict with shunting, but the presence of anomia has been associated with less benefit from surgery (Graff-Radford et al., 1989). The reason is that anomia is a marker of cortical dementia and indicates the patient may have comorbid neurodegenerative disease. In fact, at the average age of shunting, which is about 75, over 30% of normal persons have AD pathology as measured by PiB-PET (Knopman et al., 2013).

### Urinary Incontinence

Urinary urgency may occur very early, while later in the disease course incontinence is accompanied by a lack of distress.

### Assessing Comorbidities

Despite this clinical triad, the diagnosis of NPH remains challenging because the features of NPH are very common in the elderly population. Among non-demented patients aged 75–85, gait abnormalities occur in approximately 20% and are related to development of dementia (Verghese et al., 2002). Similarly, at age 60 the prevalence of incontinence is 17% in men and 31% in women (Anger et al., 2006). Therefore, careful evaluation of comorbidities and other diagnoses must be made prior to diagnosing NPH. Some possible comorbidities to investigate which can confound the evaluation of NPH by causing cognitive dysfunction or gait disturbance include the presence of arthritis, peripheral neuropathy, cervical spondylosis, vestibular dysfunction, medication use, and visual dysfunction. It is particularly important to look for parkinsonian disorders which can be associated with enlarged ventricles. To avoid shunting unnecessarily, some have advocated a L-dopa challenge to distinguish PD from NPH (Morishita et al., 2010).

### Neuroimaging

The hallmark neuroimaging feature is ventricular enlargement out of proportion to atrophy. When atrophy is proportionate to ventricular enlargement, the term ex vacuo hydrocephalus is used. The Evans index is used to assess ventriculomegaly. The Evans index is defined as the maximal diameter of the frontal horns to the largest width of the inner tables of the cranium with a ratio of greater than 0.30 considered consistent with ventriculomegaly (Mori et al., 2012b). Transependymal flow occurs and may be the result of extravasation of CSF into the white matter. This finding appears as white matter hyperintensity capping of the ventricles, but can be mistaken for periventricular white matter hyperintensities. Increased flow rate of aqueductal CSF through the third ventricle (Dixon et al., 2002) and radionucleotide cisternography (Vanneste et al., 1992) are probably not helpful in predicting shunt responsiveness. Recently, the MRI imaging finding of disproportionately enlarged subarachnoid space hydrocephalus (DESH) was reported. DESH is defined as the presence of a "tight" convexity in conjunction with enlarged sylvian fissure and associated hydrocephalus (Mori et al., 2012b). One important radiological finding is dilation of sulci. These enlarged sulci are indicative of a CSF dynamics disorder and are sometimes mistaken for focal atrophy.

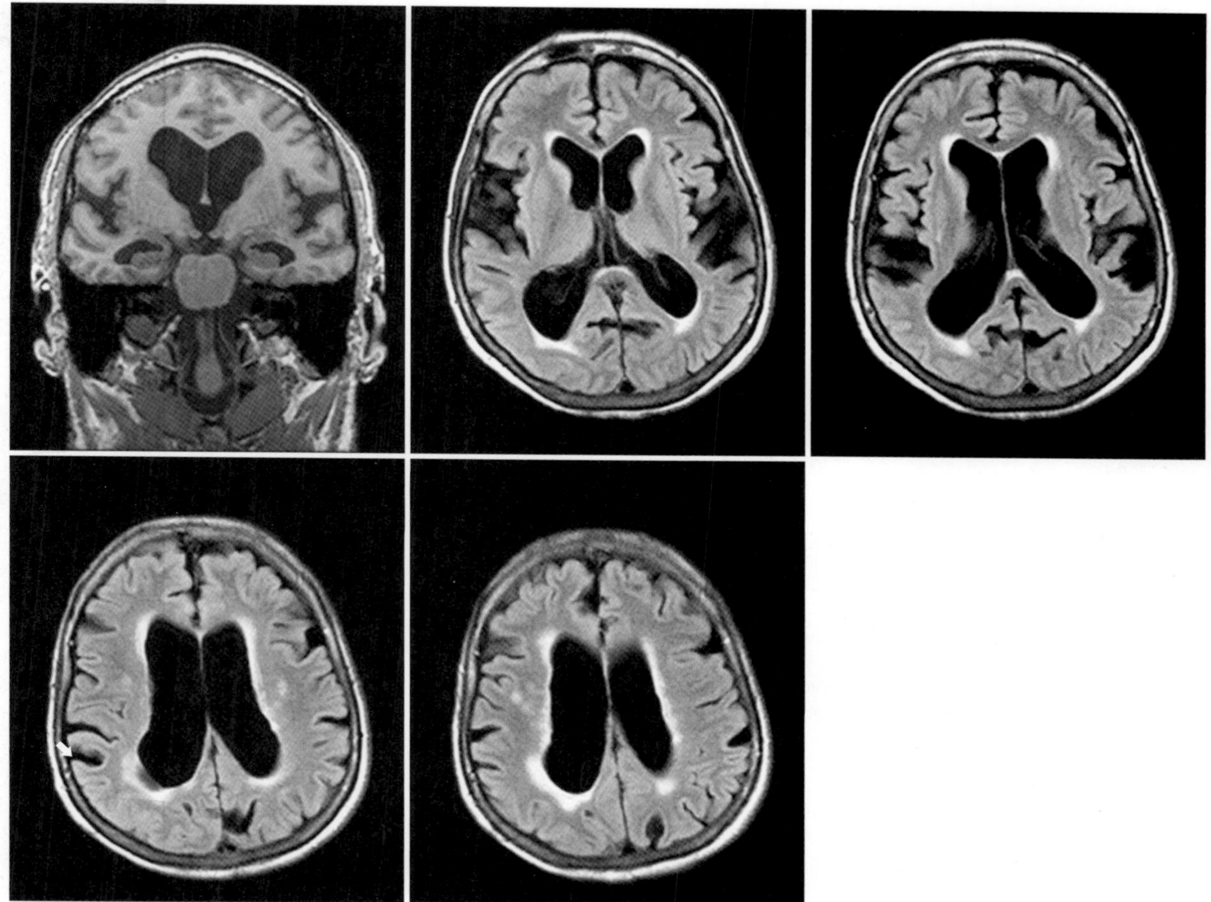

**Fig. 95.27** *Top row:* Left image reveals enlargement of the sylvian fissures and crowding at the apex consistent with disproportionately enlarged subarachnoid space hydrocephalus. Middle and right images demonstrate ventricular enlargement and transependymal flow seen in normal pressure hydrocephalus (NPH). *Bottom row:* Entrapped sulci seen in NPH *(white arrow)*.

Other helpful features to distinguish NPH from AD dementia include an enlarged anterior cingulate sulcus (Adachi et al., 2006) and narrow precuneus sulci (Ishii et al., 2008).

Fig. 95.27 demonstrates many of the hallmark imaging findings in NPH.

## Confirmatory Diagnostic Tests

Since shunting procedures are invasive and associated with possible serious complications, additional diagnostic tests are recommended prior to shunt placement. The best test to see if a shunt will work is a temporary shunt. This can be done with either a high-volume lumbar puncture or external CSF drainage over 1–3 days. The most common approach is a large-volume (30–50cc) lumbar tap test where gait is tested before and within 30 minutes of the tap. Improved gait after CSF has been removed constitutes a positive result and predicts a better response to shunting (Wikkelso et al., 1986). Most studies have shown that this test has a high positive predictive value but lower negative predictive value (Kahlon et al., 2002), indicating some patients who might benefit from shunting are missed with only the tap test. A more invasive method is placement of a temporary catheter in the lumbar CSF space and drainage of CSF at 10 cc per hour for a period of 1–3 days. This test is reported to be more sensitive than the lumbar puncture test but has a small risk of infection. Other tests that have been used include intracranial pressure monitoring (Graff-Radford et al., 1989) and CSF infusion tests (Boon et al., 1997).

## Biomarkers

The CSF biomarker profile of NPH is low CSF Aβ42 but normal CSF t-tau and p-tau similar to controls. Thus the features are in keeping with AD (low Aβ42) but also in keeping with normals (normal t-tau and p-tau). Therefore, CSF biomarkers may not be useful in distinguishing NPH from NPH plus comorbid AD (Kapaki et al., 2007).

## Biopsy Studies

Many NPH patients have AD pathology found through biopsies or autopsies. In a study of 56 probable NPH patients in their mid-70s who underwent cortical biopsies during shunt surgery, approximately 40% had AD pathology, and patients with a greater amount of amyloid plaque and NFT deposition had more cognitive dysfunction (Golomb et al., 2000). Gait improved regardless of biopsy findings. The number with AD pathology is similar to what would be expected in that age group. In a population-based study of cognitively normal individuals with a median age of 78 years, approximately 32% had amyloid deposition as measured by PiB-PET (Knopman et al., 2013).

**TABLE 95.11 Japanese Diagnostic Criteria of Idiopathic Normal Pressure Hydrocephalus**

**Possible iNPH (Meets All Five of the Following)**

1. Individuals who develop symptoms in their 60s or older.
2. More than one of the clinical triad (cognitive impairment, urinary incontinence, gait disturbance).
3. Ventricular dilation (Evans index > 0.3).
4. Above-mentioned symptoms cannot be completely explained by other neurological or non-neurological disease.
5. Preceding diseases possibly causing ventricular dilation are not obvious, including subarachnoid hemorrhage, meningitis, head injury, congenital hydrocephalus, and aqueductal stenosis.

**Possible iNPH Supportive Features**

(a) Small stride, shuffle, instability during walking, and increased instability with turning.
(b) Symptoms progress slowly; however, sometimes an undulating course, including temporal discontinuation of development and exacerbation, is observed.
(c) Gait disorder is the most prevalent feature, followed by cognitive impairment and urinary incontinence.
(d) Cognitive impairment is detected on cognitive tests.
(e) Sylvian fissures and basal cisterns are usually enlarged.
(f) Other neurological diseases such as Parkinson disease, Alzheimer disease, and cerebrovascular disease may coexist; however, all such diseases should be mild.
(g) Periventricular changes are not essential.
(h) Measurement of CSF is useful for differentiation from other dementias.

| Probable iNPH (Meets All of the Following Three Features) | Definite iNPH |
|---|---|
| 1. Meets criteria for possible iNPH.<br>2. CSF pressure <200 mm $H_2O$ and normal CSF content.<br>3. One of the following three investigational features:<br>(1) Neuroimaging of narrowing of the sulci and subarachnoid spaces over the high convexity/midline surface (DESH) in the presence of a gait disturbance<br>(2) Improvement of symptoms after CSF tap test<br>(3) Improvement of symptoms after CSF drainage test. | Improvement of symptoms after the shunt procedure |

*CSF,* Cerebrospinal fluid; *DESH,* disproportionately enlarged subarachnoid space hydrocephalus; *iNPH,* idiopathic normal pressure hydrocephalus.
*Reprinted with permission from Mori, E., Ishikawa, M., Kato, T., et al. 2012. Guidelines for management of idiopathic normal pressure hydrocephalus: second edition. Neurol. Med. Chir. 52, 775–809.*

### Diagnostic Criteria

Recently, the Japanese Society of Normal Pressure Hydrocephalus published updated guidelines for the diagnosis of NPH (Mori et al., 2012b; Table 95.11).

## CHRONIC TRAUMATIC ENCEPHALOPATHY/POST-TRAUMATIC DEMENTIA

An article in JAMA in 1928 described the concept of "punch drunk" in which boxers who received significant head injury later became cognitively impaired (Martland, 1928). "Punch drunk" was also known as dementia pugilistica. MacDonald Critchley later introduced the term CTE. Although CTE has received much attention in the literature recently, little is known about the pathogenesis. The clinical and radiological presentations associated with head trauma are variable. While the disorder is most often associated with athletes or military veterans who experience head injury, anyone who experiences head injury can develop symptoms. Cavum septum pellucidum can occur but is not universal. The mechanism is thought to be related to repetitive acceleration-deceleration of the head during concussion or more mild head injuries. While some patients have atrophy or hemorrhage on neuroimaging, the majority demonstrate normal imaging findings. The clinical presentation appears to have two distinct presentations that are age dependent. In a series of 36 individuals with autopsy-confirmed CTE, those presenting at a young age had a behavioral mood disorder characterized by violent behavior, aggression, and depression, while those presenting at an older age presented with cognitive decline (memory, executive, attention) (Stern et al., 2013). Currently CTE can only be definitely diagnosed at autopsy. Research criteria have been proposed for a clinical syndrome termed "traumatic encephalopathy syndrome" (Montenigro et al., 2014), but these criteria will require validation before they can be adopted into clinical practice.

The pathology of CTE is a tauopathy. CTE typically starts as foci in the frontal cortex and then spreads to other regions including limbic structures (McKee et al., 2013). The tau characteristically is perivascular and patchy. The most severe pathology is located at the bottom of sulci. CTE has also been associated with motor neuron disease and TDP-43 pathology (McKee et al., 2010). APOE ε4 is thought to be a risk factor for dementia in those with head injury. Among former NFL players, a neurodegenerative cause of death was approximately three times greater than controls (Lehman et al., 2012).

## OTHER CAUSES

Countless causes of dementia have been reported in the literature because it is a syndromic term. Partial lists of important subtypes of non-degenerative dementia are listed in Box 95.1.

### Autoimmune or Paraneoplastic Dementia

Clinical features of autoimmune dementia include a subacute course, personal or family history of autoimmunity or cancer, and myoclonus. Limbic encephalitis is one form of paraneoplastic/autoimmune disorder that can cause a dementia. Predictors of responsiveness to immunotherapy include subacute onset, fluctuating course, tremor, shorter delay to treatment, seropositivity for certain autoantibodies, pleocytosis in the CSF, and elevated CSF protein (>100 mg/dL) (Flanagan et al., 2010). Autoimmune dementias must be kept in the differential diagnosis of rapidly progressive dementias because they

**BOX 95.1 Partial List of Non-Degenerative Dementias**

**Vascular**
Vasculitis (primary or secondary)
Chronic subdural hematoma

**Infectious Causes**
Syphilis
Chronic meningitis
CJD and other prion disease
Whipple
PML
Sequelae of herpes encephalitis
HIV/AIDS-associated dementia
Neuro brucellosis
CNS tuberculosis
Parasitic infections (e.g., cysticercosis)
Lyme disease
Subacute sclerosing panencephalitis

**Toxic/Metabolic Causes**
Hypothyroidism
Liver disease
Kidney disease
Vitamin $B_{12}$ deficiency
Thiamine deficiency
Vitamin E deficiency
Marchiafava-Bignami disease
Deficiency of nicotinic acid (pellagra)
Heavy metal toxicity
Parathyroid hormone dysfunction
Adrenal and pituitary disorders
Carbon monoxide poisoning
Drugs (see prior table for list of drugs that can affect cognition)

**Structural Causes**
Primary or metastatic neoplasm
Hydrocephalus

**Immune/Inflammatory**
Autoimmune dementia
Multiple sclerosis
Sarcoidosis
Collagen vascular diseases (e.g., systemic lupus erythematosus, Sjögren syndrome)
Behçet

**Neoplastic**
Slow-growing neoplasm (e.g., meningioma, pituitary tumors)
Gliomatosis cerebri
Radiation effect
Paraneoplastic syndromes
Lymphoma

**Psychiatric**
Depression

**Inherited Disorders**
Leukodystrophies (e.g., metachromatic leukodystrophy, adrenoleukodystrophy)
Krabbe disease
Storage disorders: Gaucher disease, Niemann-Pick disease, cerebrotendinous xanthomatosis, and polysaccharidoses, neuronal ceroid lipofuscinoses
Wilson disease

*AIDS*, acquired immunodeficiency syndrome; *CJD*, Creutzfeldt-Jakob disease; *CNS*, central nervous system; *HIV*, human immunodeficiency; *PML*, progressive multifocal leukoencephalopathy.

can mimic CJD and cause an elevated 14-3-3 protein in the CSF, as well as demonstrate cortical diffusion-weighted imaging abnormalities on MRI (called cortical ribboning) (Geschwind et al., 2008b). In addition to autoimmune dementias associated with specific autoantibodies, patients with autoimmune conditions such as systemic lupus erythematosus (SLE) or Sjögren syndrome can present with cognitive decline. Neuropsychiatric symptoms occur in up to 90% of SLE patients, with cognitive dysfunction (approximately 80%) and mood disorder (43%) being quite common (Ainiala et al., 2001). Sjögren syndrome can be associated with a vasculitis and meningoencephalitis. Dementia and more subtle cognitive dysfunction may also occur.

## Other Non-Degenerative Dementias

### Rapidly Progressive Dementias

Rapidly progressive dementias typically present over weeks to months, but may still be considered up to 1–2 years after symptom onset (Paterson et al., 2012). A thorough work-up is important to identify treatable causes before they are irreversible. At the University of California-San Francisco, which is the referral center for rapidly progressive dementia, of 178 rapidly progressive dementia cases, approximately 75% of cases were prion disorders, 14.6% neurodegenerative diseases, and 8.4% autoimmune in etiology (Geschwind et al., 2008a). Four cases were infectious with viral encephalitis and three were cancer-associated encephalopathies without paraneoplastic antibodies. At the Mayo Clinic, the most common neurodegenerative diseases causing rapidly progressive dementia include FTD-MND, 4R tauopathy, and DLB (Josephs et al., 2009). In a retrospective review of brain biopsies referred to the US National Prion Disease Pathology Surveillance Center for rapidly progressive dementia, 71 out of 1106 had a potentially treatable condition (26 immune related, 25 neoplastic related, 14 infectious, and 6 metabolic [most commonly Wernicke]) (Chitravas et al., 2011). Chapter 94 reviews this subject in more detail. A partial list of causes of rapidly progressive dementia is listed in Box 95.2.

## YOUNG-ONSET DEMENTIA

Young-onset dementia has a wide differential diagnosis. Definitions vary but typically age of onset before 45 is used to distinguish it from early-onset dementia. At the Mayo Clinic, the most common causes were neurodegenerative (31.1%), autoimmune or inflammatory (21.3%), and metabolic (10.6%), with a substantial proportion remaining unknown (18.7%). Among the neurodegenerative diseases FTD and Huntington disease were most common (Kelley et al., 2008). When the age range is extended to 65, AD dementia becomes the most common neurodegenerative cause (Janssen et al., 2003). Given the number of potentially treatable etiologies, young-onset dementia requires a thorough work-up. The nine most common causes in the papers from Kelley et al. 2008 and Harvey et al. 2003 are listed in Table 95.12.

**BOX 95.2 Partial Differential Diagnoses of Rapidly Progressive Dementias**

Prion diseases
Autoimmune/paraneoplastic disorders
Infections: Viral encephalitis, Whipple disease, fungal meningitis, human immunodeficiency virus-related, Lyme disease, syphilis, tuberculosis
Neurodegenerative diseases presenting with rapid time course
Central nervous system (CNS) vasculitis and other vasculopathies (e.g., Susac syndrome, Abeta-related angiitis)
Neurosarcoidosis
Neoplastic: CNS lymphoma, gliomatosis, metastatic disease
Toxic/metabolic conditions: Vitamin $B_1$ (thiamine) deficiency, vitamin $B_{12}$ deficiency, alcohol related, uremia, hepatic failure, drug toxicity (e.g., lithium, methotrexate)
Wilson disease
Nonconvulsive status epilepticus
Subdural hematoma
Primary or secondary hydrocephalus

## Future Directions

It has become apparent in recent years that the most common neuropathology underlying cognitive changes in aging is multifactorial. As has been discussed above, age is the primary risk factor for virtually all of the degenerative and vascular diseases. In the early-onset cases, 65 years and younger, a single or a few pathological entities are more common, but when a person is older, most individuals will have a combination of contributing pathologies present, including amyloid, tau, alpha-synuclein, TDP-43, and vascular disease. The proportion of each of these will vary in each person and there are likely many factors contributing to this combination, genetic and lifestyle among them. A challenge for the field lies in our ability to identify these factors in life as early as possible with the goal of prevention. Biomarkers have taken on a huge role in this regard and progress is being made.

As is depicted in Fig. 95.28, ideally we would like to identify a biomarker for each pathological entity and develop therapies for each component (Petersen et al., 2018). This would result in combination therapy for each person tailored to that person's unique biomarker profile. If these therapies were shown to be preventive, early intervention would be the key. Due to the personal, societal, and economic burden of these diseases, attempts at prevention or delaying onset and slowing progression are essential. If a biomarker's proof of concept could be demonstrated with imaging and CSF measures, extension to involve blood-based biomarkers would be a major step forward. Ultimately, one could imagine a person having a blood panel drawn that would give the person and the physician a profile of biomarkers for a variety of neurodegenerative and vascular processes to direct individual therapy programs. While actual prevention may not be feasible, a delay and slowing of the underlying processes would produce huge benefits. A great deal of research is underway pursuing this approach.

*The complete reference list is available online at https://expertconsult.inkling.com.* 

**TABLE 95.12 Young-Onset Dementia**

| Nine Most Common Causes of Dementia (Ages 17–45) According to Kelley et al. (2008) | Nine Most Common Causes of Dementia (Ages 30–65) According to Harvey et al. (2003) |
|---|---|
| Frontotemporal dementia | Alzheimer dementia |
| Huntington disease | Vascular dementia |
| Multiple sclerosis | Frontotemporal dementia |
| Autoimmune encephalopathy (dementia) | Alcohol-related dementia |
| Neuropsychiatric lupus | Dementia with Lewy Bodies |
| Mitochondrial disease | Huntington disease |
| Storage disease | Multiple sclerosis |
| Prion disease | Dementia due to Down syndrome |
| Vasculitis | CBD/prion disease/Parkinson dementia |

*CBD,* corticobasal degeneration.

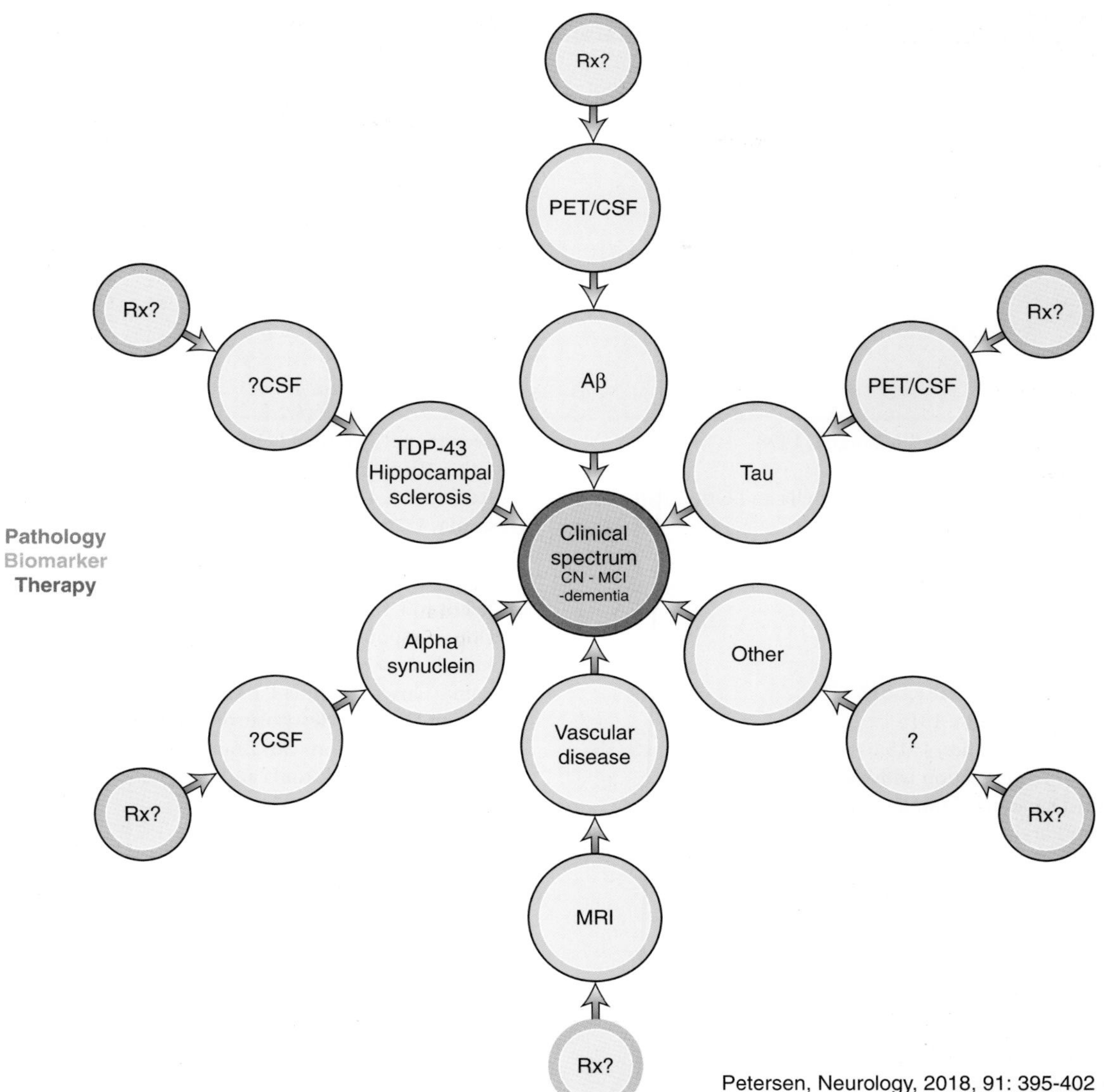


**Fig. 95.28** Clinical spectrum of cognitively unimpaired–mild cognitive impairment–dementia with its multiple potential etiologies. The contribution of Alzheimer disease (AD) is expressed by β-amyloid (Aβ) and tau. However, the other protein abnormalities, including TDP-43 and β-synuclein, as well as vascular disease may also contribute to cognitive impairment. Biomarkers for TDP-43, alpha-synuclein and other are under development. Treatments may be developed for each pathological entity.

96

# Parkinson Disease and Other Movement Disorders

*Joseph Jankovic*

## OUTLINE



## MOVEMENT DISORDERS AND THE BASAL GANGLIA

Neurologists often equate movement disorders with disease or dysfunction of the basal ganglia, so no review of movement disorders would be complete without a discussion of these subcortical structures and their connections. In some movement disorders such as parkinsonism, chorea, and ballism, the link to the basal ganglia is supported by clinicopathological, biochemical, functional neuroimaging, and electrophysiological data, whereas in other movement disorders such as tremor, dystonia, and tics, dysfunction of the basal ganglia is implied but not proven. Clinicopathological studies relate the signs of Parkinson disease (PD) to deficient dopaminergic neurotransmission in the striatum consequent to the death of dopaminergic neurons in the substantia nigra pars compacta (SNc). Choreic movements in Huntington disease (HD) are linked to the death of medium spiny neurons in the caudate and putamen. Hemiballism (HB) is typically associated with structural lesions in the contralateral subthalamic nucleus (STN) or its afferent or efferent connections. Changes in basal ganglia neurotransmission are well described in many movement disorders, and deepening understanding of basal ganglia neurotransmission has yielded promising symptomatic therapies in many such conditions.

Functional neuroimaging studies with specific radiopharmaceutical agents demonstrate abnormal function of basal ganglia structures, and intraoperative electrophysiology studies demonstrate abnormalities in neuronal firing rates and patterns, particularly in the STN and globus pallidus (GP) of patients with PD, dystonia, chorea, and other movement disorders. Animal models including the 1-methyl-4-phenyl-1,2,3,6-tetrahydropyridine (MPTP) model of PD, excitotoxic and transgenic models of HD, and the STN lesion model of HB confirm the central role of disordered basal ganglia function in these conditions. In other movement disorders such as dystonia, the link with basal ganglia function is more complex. For example, although secondary dystonias may result from structural lesions in the contralateral putamen, other sites of pathology include the thalamus, rostral brainstem, and cerebellum. Functional neuroimaging studies in patients with dystonia show abnormal activation of the lenticular nucleus, but neuroimaging and physiological studies provide support for additional involvement of the cortex, brainstem, and cerebellum. In other movement disorders such as essential tremor (ET), restless legs syndrome (RLS), stiff person syndrome (SPS), hemifacial spasm (HFS), spinal myoclonus, and painful legs–moving toes syndrome (PLMTS), the dysfunction appears to lie outside the basal ganglia, such as in the brainstem, cerebellum, spinal cord, or even in the peripheral nervous system.

## Basal Ganglia Anatomy

There is no clear consensus on which structures should be included in the basal ganglia. For the purposes of this discussion, we consider those structures in the striatopallidal circuits involved in modulation of the thalamocortical projection: the caudate nucleus, the putamen, the external segment of the GP (GPe), and the internal segment of the GP (GPi). In addition, the SNc, the substantia nigra pars reticulata (SNr), and the STN are included in the basal ganglia (Ellens et al., 2013). The substantia nigra (SN), a melanin-containing (pigmented) nucleus, normally contains about 500,000 dopaminergic neurons. Several transcriptional regulators, including Nurr1, Lmx1a, Lmx1b, Msx1, and Pitx3, are responsible for the development and maintenance of midbrain dopaminergic neurons (Le et al., 2009).

The *caudate nucleus* is a curved structure that traverses the deep hemisphere at the lateral edge of each lateral ventricle. Its diameter is largest at its head, tapering to a small tail. It is continuous with the putamen at the head and tail. The caudate and putamen together are called the *striatum*, and they form the major target for projections from the cerebral cortex and the SN. The putamen and the GP together form a wedge-shaped structure called the *lenticular nucleus*. The GP is divided into two parts, the GPe and the GPi. The GPi is structurally and functionally homologous with the SNr. The SNr and SNc extend the length of the midbrain ventral to the red nucleus and dorsal to the cerebral peduncles. The STN is a small lens-shaped structure at the border between the cerebrum and the brainstem. The basal ganglia and its relation to the thalamus and overlying cortex are illustrated in Fig. 96.1.

## Functional Organization of the Basal Ganglia and Other Pathways

Afferent projections to the striatum arise from nearly all areas of the cerebral cortex, the intralaminar nuclei of the thalamus, mesencephalic SN, and from the brainstem locus coeruleus and raphe nuclei. There is also a projection from the cerebral cortex to the STN (Eisenstein et al., 2014). The major efferent projections are from the GPi and SNr to the thalamus and brainstem nuclei such as the pedunculopontine nucleus (PPN). The GPi and SNr project to ventral anterior and ventrolateral thalamic nuclei. The GPi also projects to the centromedian thalamic nuclei, and the SNr projects to the mediodorsal thalamic nuclei and superior colliculi. The ventral anterior and ventrolateral thalamic nuclei then project to the motor and premotor cortex. Throughout, these projections are somatotopically organized (Rodriguez-Oroz et al., 2009).

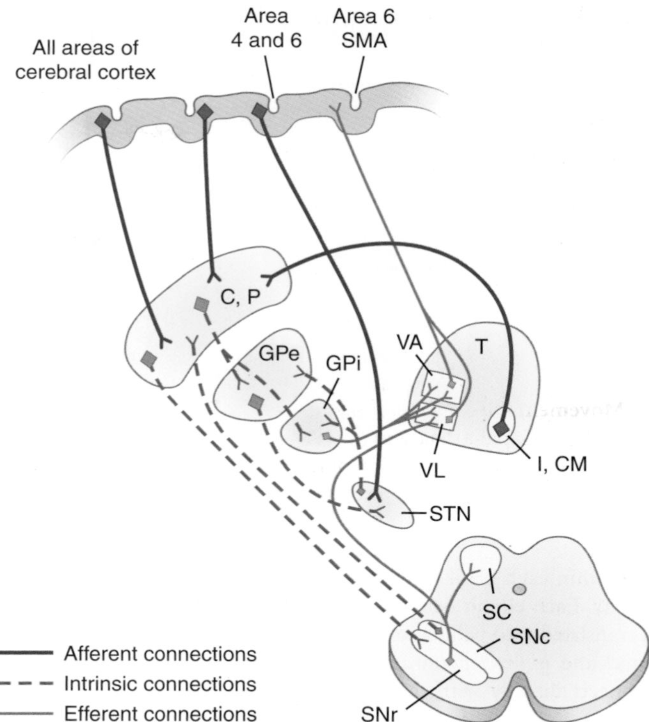


**Fig. 96.1** Schematic drawing of interconnections between the basal ganglia and its afferent and efferent connections. *CM*, Centromedian nucleus of thalamus; *C,P*, caudate, putamen (striatum); *GPe*, lateral (external) globus pallidus; *GPi*, medial (internal) globus pallidus; *SC*, superior colliculus; *SMA*, supplementary motor area; *STN*, subthalamic nucleus; *SNc*, substantia nigra pars compacta; *SNr*, substantia nigra pars reticulata; *T*, thalamus; *VA*, ventral anterior; *VL*, ventrolateral.

The basal ganglia has dense internuclear connections (see Fig. 96.1). Five parallel and separate closed circuits through the basal ganglia have been proposed. These are the motor, oculomotor, dorsolateral prefrontal, lateral orbitofrontal, and limbic loops (Rodriguez-Oroz et al., 2009). It is now generally accepted that these loops form three major divisions—sensorimotor, associative, and limbic—that are related to motor, cognitive, and emotional functions, respectively (Table 96.1). The functions of the sensorimotor striatum are subserved mainly by the putamen, which derives its afferent cortical inputs from both motor cortices. Sensorimotor pathways are somatotopically organized, and the pathway ultimately terminates in the premotor and primary motor cortices and the supplementary motor area (SMA). Cognitive functions are largely mediated by the associative striatum, particularly the dorsal caudate nucleus, which receives afferent input from the homolateral frontal, parietal, temporal, and occipital cortices. Projections from this pathway ultimately terminate in the prefrontal cortex. The limbic striatum subserves emotional and motivational functions. Its input derives from the cingulate, temporal, and orbitofrontal cortices, the hippocampus, and the amygdala. It mainly comprises the ventral striatum, with ultimate projections to the anterior cingulate and medial orbitofrontal cortices (Rodriguez-Oroz et al., 2009). Whether these divisions are interconnected or organized in parallel remains a topic of debate.

TABLE 96.1 **Divisions of the Striatum**

| | ORIGIN OF STRIATAL | | TERMINATION OF BASAL | |
|---|---|---|---|---|
| **Division** | **Afferents** | **Striatal Nucleus** | **Ganglia Efferents** | **Function** |
| Sensorimotor | Motor cortex | Putamen | Premotor cortex<br>Primary motor cortex<br>Supplementary motor area | Movement |
| Associative | Frontal cortex<br>Parietal cortex<br>Temporal cortex<br>Occipital cortex | Dorsal caudate | Prefrontal cortex | Cognition |
| Limbic | Hippocampus<br>Amygdala<br>Cingulate cortex<br>Temporal cortex<br>Orbitofrontal cortex | Ventral striatum | Anterior cingulated cortex<br>Medial orbitofrontal cortex | Emotion<br>Motivation |

Within each basal ganglia circuit lies an additional level of complexity. Each circuit contains two pathways by which striatal activity is translated into pallidal output. These two pathways are named the *direct* and *indirect pathways*, depending on whether striatal outflow connects directly with the GPi or first traverses the GPe and STN before terminating in the GPi. The direct and indirect pathways have opposite effects on outflow neurons of the GPi and SNr (Fig. 96.2, *A*).

In the motor direct pathway, excitatory neurons from the cerebral cortex synapse on putaminal neurons, which in turn send inhibitory projections to the GPi and its homolog, the SNr. The GPi/SNr sends an inhibitory outflow to the thalamus (see Fig. 96.2, *B*). Activity in the direct pathway disinhibits the thalamus, facilitating the excitatory thalamocortical pathway and enhancing activity in its target, the motor cortices. Thus, the direct pathway constitutes part of an excitatory cortical-cortical circuit that likely functions to maintain ongoing motor activity. In the indirect pathway, excitatory axons from the cerebral cortex synapse on putaminal neurons. These neurons send inhibitory projections to the GPe, and the GPe sends an inhibitory projection to the STN. The net effect of these projections is disinhibition of the STN. The STN in turn has an excitatory projection to the GPi (see Fig. 96.2, *C*). Activity in the indirect pathway thus excites the GPi/SNr, which in turn inhibits the thalamocortical pathway. Thus, the net effect of increased activity in the indirect pathway is cortical inhibition. There is growing appreciation of the importance of direct connection from the cortex to the STN, the so-called hyperdirect pathway, and to the thalamus (Coude et al., 2018).

The striatum also receives robust afferent input from the SNc. This projection from the SNc, an important modifier of striatal activity, facilitates activity in the direct pathway, mediated via $D_1$ dopamine receptors, and inhibits activity in the indirect pathway via $D_2$ dopamine receptors (see Fig. 96.2, *A*).

Disorders of the basal ganglia result in prominent motor dysfunction, though not generally in frank weakness. The absence of direct primary or secondary sensory input and lack of a major descending pathway below the level of the brainstem suggest that the basal ganglia moderates rather than controls movement. The direct pathway is important in initiation and maintenance of movement, and the indirect pathway apparently plays a role in the suppression of extraneous movement. From this model of basal ganglia connectivity, hypotheses about the motor function of the basal ganglia have been proposed. One hypothesis is that the relative activities of the direct and indirect pathways serve to balance the facilitation and inhibition of the same population of thalamocortical neurons, thus controlling the scale of movement. A second hypothesis proposes that direct pathway-mediated facilitation and indirect pathway-mediated inhibition of different populations of thalamocortical neurons serve to focus movement in an organization reminiscent of center-surround inhibition. These hypotheses relate activity in the direct and indirect pathways mainly to rates of firing in the STN and GPi. Thus, death of neurons in the SNc, as in nigrostriatal degeneration associated with PD, decreases activity in the direct pathway and increases activity in the indirect pathway. These changes cause an increased rate of firing of subthalamic and GPi neurons, with excessive inhibition of thalamocortical pathways, and produce the behavioral manifestations of bradykinesia in PD (Fig. 96.3, *A*).

On the other hand, predominant loss of indirect pathway neurons, as in HD, interferes with suppression of involuntary movements. Choreic involuntary movements are the usual result (see Fig. 96.3, *B*). Direct electrophysiological recordings of the STN and GP during stereotactic functional neurosurgical procedures confirm that the GPi and STN are overly active in patients with PD. The activity of these nuclei returns toward normal with effective pharmacotherapy, and chorea is associated with lower firing rates of neurons in these nuclei. Unfortunately, this model does not completely explain some important features of movement disorders. For example, bradykinesia and chorea coexist in HD and in patients with PD treated with levodopa (LD). Thalamic lesions that might be expected to worsen parkinsonism by reducing excitatory thalamocortical activity do not do so. Pallidal lesions that might be expected to worsen chorea by decreasing inhibition of thalamocortical pathways instead are dramatically effective at reducing chorea. The model is even more problematic when applied to dystonia. It has been suggested that in dystonia there is overactivity of both the direct and indirect pathways. Yet, intraoperative recordings in dystonia have shown low rates and abnormal patterns of neuronal firing in the GPi. A simple change in firing rate of the STN or GPi is thus insufficient to explain the underlying physiology of dystonia. It is likely that disordered patterns and synchrony of pallidal firing, as well as changes in sensorimotor integration and the control of spinal and brainstem reflexes, are important. These factors are under investigation, but current models remain useful for understanding the rationale of pharmacological and ablative surgical procedures for certain movement disorders.

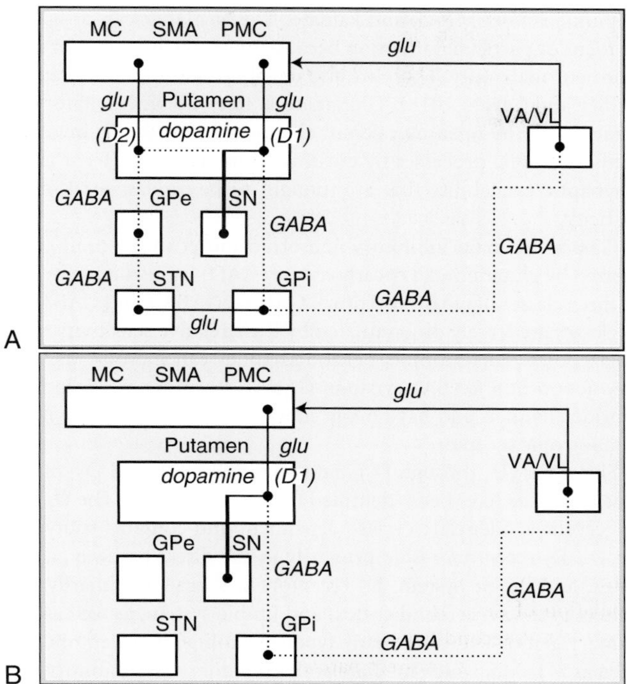


**Fig. 96.2** Schematic drawing of internuclear connections of basal ganglia, including **(A)** direct and indirect pathways and **(B)** direct pathway. (See Fig. 96.3 for depiction of indirect pathway.) Excitatory pathways in *solid lines*, inhibitory pathways in *dotted lines*. $D_1$, Dopamine $D_1$ receptor; $D_2$, dopamine $D_2$ receptor; *GABA*, γ-aminobutyric acid; *glu*, glutamate; *GPe*, external segment of the globus pallidus; *GPi*, internal segment of the globus pallidus; *MC*, motor cortex; *PMC*, premotor cortex; *SMA*, supplementary motor area; *SN*, substantia nigra; *STN*, subthalamic nucleus; *VA/VL*, ventral anterior/ventrolateral thalamic nuclei.

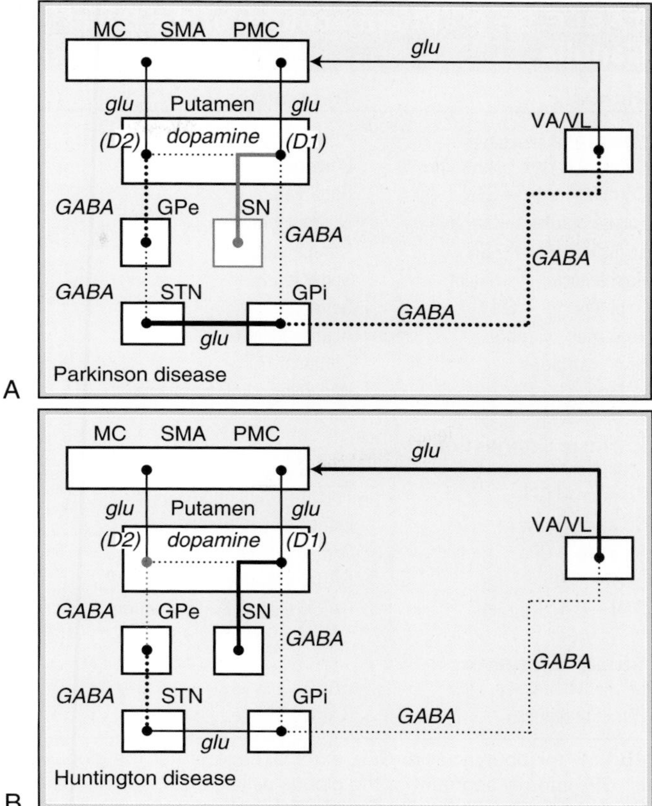


**Fig. 96.3** Schematic drawing of functional activities in the direct and indirect pathways in Parkinson disease (PD) and Huntington disease (HD). **A**, In PD, reduced dopaminergic facilitation of direct pathway and inhibition of indirect pathway due to death of dopaminergic neurons causes increased firing and increased inhibition of thalamocortical pathways, producing bradykinesia. **B**, In HD, loss of striatal neurons leads to reduced activity in indirect pathway, causing reduced inhibition of thalamocortical pathways, with production of excessive or involuntary movements. (See Fig. 96.2 for explanations to abbreviations.) $D_1$, Dopamine $D_1$ receptor; $D_2$, dopamine $D_2$ receptor; *GABA*, γ-aminobutyric acid; *glu*, glutamate; *GPe*, external segment of the globus pallidus; *GPi*, internal segment of the globus pallidus; *MC*, motor cortex; *PMC*, premotor cortex; *SMA*, supplementary motor area; *SN*, substantia nigra; *STN*, subthalamic nucleus; *VA/VL*, ventral anterior/ventrolateral thalamic nuclei.

Although much of the emphasis has been on GPi and SNr efferents to the thalamocortical system, there is growing evidence that descending pathways, particularly to the zona incerta and PPN, are important in movement disorders. The PPN appears to play a role in locomotion, muscle tone, and akinesia. A number of other pathways also seem particularly relevant to myoclonus, including a corticolemniscal-thalamocortical circuit and a spinobulbar-spinal circuit that primarily involves the spinoreticular tracts, nucleus reticularis gigantocellularis of the medullary reticular formation, and the reticulospinal tracts. The *Guillain-Mollaret triangle* is a network connecting the red nucleus, dentate nucleus, and inferior olive, which has been implicated in palatal myoclonus (PM) (also known as *palatal tremor*) and myorhythmia (Baizabal-Carvallo et al., 2015). The propriospinal pathways and segmental spinospinal loops are important in the genesis of propriospinal and spinal segmental myoclonus, respectively.

It is beyond the scope of this chapter to review all the brain structures involved in motor control, but there has been considerable recent interest in the lateral habenula, located above the posterior thalamus. The lateral part of the habenula has an inhibitory influence on the SNc, but its exact role in various movement disorders is unknown, although it has been implicated in some mood disorders (Yang et al., 2018). Another structure that has received some interest, particularly as it relates to ET, is zona incerta. This nucleus appears to be an extension of the reticular nucleus of the thalamus, situated between the thalamus and the fields of Forel, with its fiber tracts conveying the pallidal output to the thalamus. Chiefly inhibitory (GABAergic), the zona incerta may act to synchronize activity generated by the basal ganglia and cerebellum. Indeed, there is a growing body of evidence of communication between the cerebellum and basal ganglia involving γ-aminobutyric acid (GABA) and other neurotransmitters (Bostan and Strick, 2018).

## Biochemistry

Our understanding of basal ganglia neurotransmitters and pharmacology is growing rapidly. In addition to dopamine, there are many other neurotransmitters that play a role in motor and nonmotor functions (Stayte and Vissel, 2014; Klein et al., 2014). Along with this growth is an expanding spectrum of practical applications for pathology, neuroimaging, and therapeutics. For example, catecholamine and amino acid neurotransmitters coexist with peptides. This co-localization may allow histopathological differentiation among medium spiny striatal projection neurons that secrete γ-aminobutyric acid (GABAergic neurons), further elucidating the specific nature and progress of striatal

**TABLE 96.2 Pharmacology of the Basal Ganglia**

| Pathway | Transmitter |
|---|---|
| **Striatal Afferents** | |
| Cerebral cortex → striatum | Glutamate |
| Cerebral cortex → STN | Glutamate |
| Locus coeruleus → striatum | Norepinephrine |
| Locus coeruleus → SN | Norepinephrine |
| Raphe nuclei → striatum | Serotonin |
| Raphe nuclei → SN | Serotonin |
| Thalamus → striatum | Acetylcholine? |
| SNc → striatum | Glutamate? |
| | Dopamine, cholecystokinin |
| **Intrinsic Connections** | |
| Striatal interneurons | GABA, acetylcholine |
| Striatum → GPi | Somatostatin, neuropeptide Y |
| Striatum → SNr | Nitric acid, calretinin |
| Striatum → GPe | GABA, substance P |
| GPe → STN | GABA, dynorphin, substance P |
| STN → GPi, SNr, GPe | GABA, enkephalin, glutamate |
| **Striatal Efferents** | |
| GPi → thalamus | GABA |
| SNr → thalamus | GABA |

*GABA*, γ-Aminobutyric acid; *GPe*, external segment of the globus pallidus; *GPi*, internal segment of the globus pallidus; *SN*, substantia nigra; *SNc*, substantia nigra pars compacta; *SNr*, substantia nigra pars reticulata; *STN*, subthalamic nucleus.

neurodegeneration. Neuroimaging technology has been aided by the development of radiopharmaceutical ligands with such discrete targets as the dopamine transporter on the presynaptic dopamine neuron and subpopulations of dopamine receptors on the postsynaptic neuron. The pharmaceutical industry is searching for ways to provide better-targeted and more physiological stimulation of neurotransmitter receptors and is expanding its investigations from the primary targets themselves to approaches that may modify responsiveness of the primary targets.

The major neurotransmitters of the basal ganglia are outlined in Table 96.2 (see also Fig. 96.2). Most excitatory synapses of the basal ganglia and its connections—including those from the cerebral cortex to the striatum, the STN to the GPi, and the thalamocortical projections—use glutamate. Projections from the striatum to the GPe and GPi, from the GPe to the STN, and from the GPi to the thalamus are inhibitory and employ GABA. Medium spiny GABAergic neurons in the direct pathway co-localize substance P and dynorphin. GABAergic neurons in the indirect pathway co-localize enkephalin. Dopamine is the major neurotransmitter in the nigrostriatal dopamine system; it has excitatory or inhibitory actions depending on the properties of the stimulated receptor. Acetylcholine is found in large aspiny striatal interneurons and the PPN. Norepinephrine, important in the autonomic nervous system, is most concentrated in the lateral tegmentum and locus coeruleus. Serotonin is found in the dorsal raphe nucleus of the brainstem, hippocampus, cerebellum, and spinal cord.

For each of these neurotransmitters, multiple types of receptors may exist. Glutamate is active at a number of types of ligand-gated ion channel receptors named for their selective agonists: *N*-methyl-D-aspartate (NMDA), α-amino-3-hydroxy-5-methyl-4-isoxazole propionic acid (AMPA), and kainate. The NMDA receptor has been the focus of particular attention because of its potential role in excitotoxic neuronal injury. There are also metabotropic glutamate receptors (Reiner and Levitz, 2018). Glutamate is not only an excitatory neurotransmitter by opening calcium channels, but it is also involved in many metabolic processes by creating short- and long-term changes in synaptic excitability that are thought to be fundamental in brain plasticity.

GABA, the main inhibitory neurotransmitter in the brain, is synthesized by glutamic acid decarboxylase (GAD) from glutamate. There are three classes of GABA receptors, $GABA_A$, $GABA_B$, and GABAc. The subclasses are largely differentiated by their relative sensitivity to benzodiazepines. For example, benzodiazepines can increase the inhibitory action of a $GABA_A$ synapse. $GABA_A$ receptors are ligand-gated chloride channels and have many subtypes. The $GABA_B$ receptor is a metabotropic receptor.

Five types ($D_1$ through $D_5$) and two families ($D_1$ and $D_2$) of dopamine receptors have been identified (Klein et al., 2019). The $D_1$ family of receptor is adenylate cyclase dependent and contains subtypes $D_1$ and $D_5$. $D_1$ receptors reside primarily in the direct pathway, cerebral cortex, and limbic system. $D_2$ receptors are located primarily in the indirect pathway, cerebral cortex, and limbic system, as well as in the pituitary gland. There are many types of cholinergic receptors, designated as M1–M5, which mediate both excitatory and inhibitory effects (Liu and Su, 2018). Most striatal cholinergic receptors are muscarinic. In the norepinephrine system, there are two primary receptor systems, α and β. There are many distinct receptor subtypes of serotonin receptors, including G protein–coupled receptors in the 5-HT1, 5-HT2, 5-HT4, 5-HT5, 5-HT6, and 5-HT7 families and the 5-HT3-type ligand-gated ion channels. Adenosine $A_{2A}$ receptors are co-localized with striatal dopamine $D_2$ receptors on GABAergic medium spiny neurons, which project via the indirect striatopallidal pathway to the GPe. Drugs targeting specific subpopulations of receptors are in use or under development for movement disorders, but there remains a knowledge deficit about the relative clinical utility of specific receptor agonists and antagonists.

There is a growing interest in the tetrahydrocannabinol and the cannabinoid system but its role in motor control or various movement disorders is still not well understood, although there is evidence that the cannabinoids modulate dopaminergic effects (Bloomfield et al., 2016; Covey et al., 2017; Kluger et al., 2015). CB1 receptor is the principal receptor in the central nervous system (CNS), particularly abundant in the basal ganglia (Davis et al., 2018). $TRVP_1$ (transient receptor potential vanilloid type1) receptors also respond to cannabinoids. The main endogenous ligands for the CB1 receptor are anandamide and 2-arachidonoylglycerol (2-AG).

## MECHANISMS OF NEURODEGENERATION

Many of the neurodegenerative movement disorders share the property of neuronal damage caused by the accumulation of aggregation-prone proteins that have toxic effects (Table 96.3). For a protein to function normally, it must be properly synthesized and folded into its normal three-dimensional structure. Nascent proteins are aided in folding by molecular chaperones. Proteins that are not properly folded, are otherwise damaged, or are beyond their useful lives are degraded by the ubiquitin-dependent proteasome protein degradation system (Atkin and Paulson, 2014). In the ubiquitin-dependent proteasome system, proteins are first labeled for degradation by attachment of a polyubiquitin chain (Fig. 96.4). This three-step process involves activation, conjugation, and ligation steps catalyzed by three types of enzymes—E1,

**TABLE 96.3 Toxic Proteins and Neurodegenerative Movement Disorders**

| α-Synuclein | Tau | Polyglutamine Tract |
|---|---|---|
| Parkinson disease | Four-repeat tau | Huntington disease |
| Diffuse Lewy body disease | Progressive supranuclear palsy | Spinocerebellar ataxias |
| Multiple system atrophy | Corticobasal degeneration | Dentatorubral-pallidoluysian atrophy |
| | Frontotemporal dementia with parkinsonism (chromosome 17) | |
| | Parkinsonism dementia complex of Guam | |
| | Postencephalitic parkinsonism | |

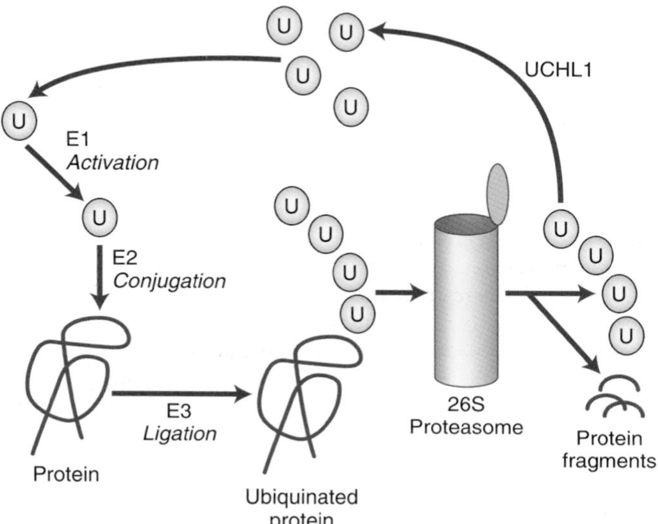


**Fig. 96.4 Ubiquitin-Dependent Proteasome Proteolysis.** Once a protein is tagged for degradation, it is tagged with a polyubiquitin chain, a three-step process involving first activation, then conjugation, then ligation. Ubiquitinated protein enters 26S proteasome, where it is degraded into protein fragments, and polyubiquitin chain is degraded back to monomeric ubiquitin. *E*, Enzyme; *U*, ubiquitin; *UCHL1*, ubiquitin carboxy-terminal hydrolase 1.

E2, and E3, respectively. Polyubiquitinated protein enters the 26S proteasome, a cylindrical complex of peptidases. The end products of proteasome action are protein fragments and polyubiquitin. The polyubiquitin is then degraded and recycled to the cellular ubiquitin pool, a process requiring enzymatic action by ubiquitin carboxy-terminal hydrolase 1.

The cascade of pathogenic events linking abnormal protein aggregation to cell death is the subject of intense investigation. Although aggregates are the most striking physical change in surviving cells, the actual role of the aggregate remains a mystery. Indeed, many now believe that the formation of aggregates may be a protective mechanism sequestering the wayward protein from vulnerable cell processes (Espay et al., 2019). Nevertheless, there are now many clinical trials designed to suppress α-synuclein as a potential disease-modifying strategy (Jankovic, 2019).

Misfolded proteins may produce the most mischief as they form protofibrils. A number of mechanisms have been described. In some cases, these are specifically related to the type of protein, but in many other cases, they are nonspecific mechanisms shared by all the misfolded protein diseases. There is growing evidence that preformed fibrils generated from full-length and truncated recombinant α-synuclein enter neurons, probably by endocytosis, and act as "seeds" that induce recruitment of soluble endogenous α-synuclein into insoluble

**BOX 96.1 Mechanisms of Neurodegeneration Related to Misfolded Protein Stress**

- Loss of protein function
- Interaction of the mutant protein with the wild-type protein
- Interaction with other proteins, including transcription factors
- Caspase activation
- Apoptosis
- Suppression of proteasome function
- Interference with mitochondrial function
- Oxidative stress
- Microglial activation

Lewy body–like inclusions, resulting in progressive prion-like spread of neurodegeneration (Recasens et al., 2014). Some potential mechanisms of neurodegeneration related to misfolded protein stress are listed in Box 96.1. The mutant protein may be unable to perform a vital function or may interfere with the function of the wild-type protein. Mutant protein, protofibrils, or aggregates might interfere with other proteins. Interference with transcription factors may be particularly important in this regard. Mutant proteins may activate caspases or in other ways activate the apoptotic cascade. They may interfere with intracellular transport or other vital processes. They may suppress activity of the proteasome, enhancing protein aggregation. They may interfere with mitochondrial function, making cells more vulnerable to excitotoxicity. In addition to the ubiquitin-proteasome system, lysosomes play an important role in degrading intracellular proteins by a process termed *autophagy* (Chu, 2019). When the function of the ubiquitin proteasome system is not sufficient to clear the accumulating cellular proteins, the autophagy lysosome pathway becomes the other important route for degradation of aggregated/misfolded proteins as well as sick or abnormal mitochondria. Indeed, mitophagy is an increasingly recognized mechanism for removing sick mitochondria and maintaining cellular health (Wang et al., 2019). Accumulation of iron, increased oxidative stress, and microglial activation have also been thought to play important roles in the pathogenesis of various neurodegenerative disorders (Dusek et al., 2012).

Many neurodegenerative movement disorders can be linked to abnormal synthesis, folding, or degradation of specific proteins or protein families and the notion that progression of neurodegenerative disease is mediated via seeding of misfolded proteins has extended to a broad range of mutated proteins, including α-synuclein, tau, huntingtin, SOD-1, and TDP-43. The synucleinopathies include PD, Lewy body disease (LBD), and multiple system atrophy (MSA). The tauopathies include progressive supranuclear palsy (PSP), corticobasal degeneration (CBD), familial frontotemporal dementia (FTD) with parkinsonism (FTDP), postencephalitic parkinsonism (PEP), post-traumatic parkinsonism, and amyotrophic lateral sclerosis (ALS)-PD of Guam. The polyQ disorders include HD, dentatorubral-pallidoluysian atrophy (DRPLA), and many spinocerebellar ataxias (Ling et al., 2010; Williams and Lees, 2009).

Within the CNS, certain neuronal populations seem selectively vulnerable to the various pathogenic mechanisms of cell death. This preferential degeneration of specific neuronal populations ultimately determines the phenotype of the disorder. Better understanding of the various pathogenic cellular mechanisms and selective vulnerability may lead to neuroprotective therapeutic strategies that favorably modify the natural course of the neurodegenerative disease.

## PARKINSONIAN DISORDERS

### Parkinson Disease

In his monograph, *The Shaking Palsy* (1817), James Parkinson identified the hallmark features of the illness through descriptions of cases observed in the streets of London as well as in his own patients (Obeso et al., 2017). Over time, *Parkinson disease* or *idiopathic PD* has replaced the original term *paralysis agitans* as the name for the clinical syndrome of asymmetrical parkinsonism, usually with rest tremor, in association with the specific pathological findings of depigmentation of the SN due to loss of melanin-laden dopaminergic neurons containing eosinophilic cytoplasmic inclusions (Lewy bodies) (see Chapter 24). Dopamine deficiency in parkinsonian brain was described by Hornykiewicz in 1959, a discovery that ultimately led to highly effective pharmacotherapy with LD and direct-acting dopamine agonists (DAs). Recently, genetic forms of parkinsonism that are clinically indistinguishable from PD have been linked to mutations in several genes (Rousseaux et al., 2017). The discovery of different genetic forms of parkinsonism with variable penetrance has led to the current concept of PD as a syndrome with genetic and environmental etiologies, but, overall, gene mutations are a rare cause of parkinsonism, particularly in those patients with late-onset disease (Deng et al., 2018; Trinh and Farrer, 2013) (Chapter 24).

#### Epidemiology

In community-based series, PD accounted for more than 80% of all parkinsonism, with a prevalence of approximately 360 per 100,000 and an incidence of 18 per 100,000 per year (de Lau and Breteler, 2006). PD is an age-related disease, showing a gradual increase in prevalence beginning after age 50, with a steep increase in prevalence after age 60. Disease before 30 years of age is rare and often suggests a hereditary form of parkinsonism. Prevalence rates in the United States are higher than those in Africa and China, but the role of race remains unclear. Within the United States, race-specific prevalence rates vary, with some studies suggesting a similar prevalence among Whites and Blacks. Unfortunately, Blacks make up only a small fraction of most specialty clinic populations and thus are underrepresented in clinic-based studies and clinical trials. One study showed the world's highest prevalence of PD may be among the Amish in the US Northeast—nearly 6% of those 60 years of age or older, more than three times the reported 1%–2% prevalence for the rest of the country (Racette et al., 2009).

***Clinical features.*** Typically, the onset and progression of PD are gradual. We have developed a screening tool that can be used to detect early symptoms of PD (York et al., 2020). The most common presentation is with rest tremor in one hand, often associated with decreased arm swing and shoulder pain (Ha and Jankovic, 2012; Jankovic, 2008). Although 4–5 Hz rest tremor is considered the typical tremor of PD, the more troublesome tremor experienced by patients with PD is postural tremor, either re-emergent tremor occurring after a latency of a few seconds following the assumption of position of outstretched arms, or the postural tremor of PD (Jankovic, 2016a).

**TABLE 96.4 Hoehn and Yahr Stage**

| Stage | Disease state |
|---|---|
| **Original Scale** | |
| I | Unilateral involvement only, minimal or no functional impairment |
| II | Bilateral or midline involvement, without impairment of balance |
| III | First sign of impaired righting reflex, mild to moderate disability |
| IV | Fully developed, severely disabling disease; patient still able to walk and stand unassisted |
| V | Confinement to bed or wheelchair unless aided |
| **Modified Scale** | |
| 0 | No signs of disease |
| 1 | Unilateral disease |
| 1.5 | Unilateral plus axial involvement |
| 2.0 | Bilateral disease without impairment of balance |
| 2.5 | Mild bilateral disease with recovery on pull test |
| 3.0 | Mild to moderate bilateral disease, some postural instability, physically independent |
| 4.0 | Severe disability, still able to walk or stand unassisted |
| 5.0 | Wheelchair bound or bedridden unless aided |

In contrast to the rest and re-emergent tremor which may be related to dopamine deficiency, the PD action-postural tremor appears to correlate with serotonergic deficiency (Jankovic, 2018a). Bradykinesia and rigidity are often detectable on the symptomatic side (Loane et al., 2013), and midline signs such as reduced facial expression or mild contralateral bradykinesia and rigidity may already be present. The presentation may be delayed if bradykinesia is the earliest symptom, particularly when the onset is on the nondominant side. The disorder usually remains asymmetrical throughout much of its course. With progression of the illness, generalized bradykinesia may cause difficulty arising from a chair or turning in bed. Patients typically develop stooped posture and in some cases the flexion of the trunk can become quite severe, the so-called camptocormia (see Videos 96.1 and 96.2) (Wijemanne and Jankovic, 2019). Some patients may also develop deformities in the hands and feet which can resemble arthritis, the so-called "striatal deformities" (see Video 96.3) (Wijemanne and Jankovic, 2019). The gait and balance are progressively affected, and falls may occur. Sudden arrests in movement, also called *freezing* or *motor blocks*, soon follow, first with gait initiation, turning and traversing narrow or crowded environments, and then during walking (see Video 96.4). Bulbar functions deteriorate, impairing communication and nutrition. The tremor-dominant form of PD generally has a more favorable clinical course than PD dominated by gait disorder and postural instability (Thenganatt and Jankovic, 2014a).

The Unified Parkinson's Disease Rating Scale (UPDRS) has been used to quantitate the various motor symptoms and signs of PD and to chart the course of the disease. This traditional scale, now known as the *Movement Disorder Society (MDS)-UPDRS*, has been revised to clarify some ambiguities in the original version and to capture early motor and also nonmotor symptoms associated with PD (http://www.movement-disorders.org). The *Hoehn and Yahr* staging, first described before effective dopaminergic treatment became available, outlines the milestones in progression of the illness from mild unilateral symptoms through the end-stage nonambulatory state. A modified version of the Hoehn and Yahr stage is commonly used in contemporary clinical trials (Table 96.4).

Nonmotor symptoms are increasingly recognized as a major cause of disability in PD and contribute prominently to declining quality of life, particularly in the more advanced stages of the disease (Marinus et al., 2018). Autonomic symptoms include reduced gastrointestinal transit time with postprandial bloating and constipation, urinary frequency and urgency (sometimes with urge incontinence), impotence, disordered sweating, and orthostatic hypotension. Cognitive and behavioral changes are also very common. Attention and concentration wane. Executive dysfunction with diminished working memory, planning, and organization is common. Global dementia occurs in approximately 30% of patients, increasing in frequency with the age of the patient. Those with prominent early executive dysfunction and more severe motor signs seem particularly at risk. Anxiety, depression, and other mood disorders are common in PD. Sleep disturbance is nearly universal in PD and is multifactorial.

Disordered sleep onset and maintenance lead to fragmentation of nocturnal sleep. A variety of motor movements including RLS and periodic leg movements of sleep may be seen, and many patients have rapid eye movement (REM) sleep behavior disorder (RBD) with active motor movements during REM sleep. The following question was found to have 94% sensitivity and 87% specificity in detecting RBD: "Have you ever been told, or suspected yourself, that you seem to 'act out your dreams' while asleep (for example, punching, flailing your arms in the air, making running movements, etc.)?" (Postuma et al., 2012). Some patients with PD have sleep apnea. Vivid dreams and nightmares are very common, particularly in treated patients. Sleep disorders in PD variably relate to the pathological changes of the disease itself, arousals due to immobility, comorbid primary sleep disorders, and side effects of antiparkinsonian medications. Many patients with PD are excessively sleepy during the day, sometimes with serious consequences such as unintended sleep episodes while driving. In most cases, this excessive daytime drowsiness is related to dopaminergic drugs. Fatigue is a common and complex symptom of PD. The differentiation of fatigue from excessive daytime sleepiness, depression, apathy, and other conditions can be difficult, and there is not yet a useful body of literature on its assessment and treatment.

Clinicopathological studies have found that the clinical variable that best predicts the typical pathological changes of PD, in the absence of other diagnoses known to cause parkinsonism, is an asymmetrical illness with rest tremor along with rigidity or bradykinesia and marked improvement with LD, motor fluctuations, dyskinesias, and hyposmia (Adler et al., 2014). Misdiagnosed cases generally are found to have MSA, PSP, or subcortical vascular disease. When making the diagnosis of early PD, the clinician should be aware of a number of red flags (Box 96.2) (see Chapter 24). Cognitive impairment within the first year should raise the possibility of Alzheimer disease (AD), dementia with Lewy bodies (DLB), corticobasal syndrome (CBS), PSP, or FTDP. Symmetrical or prominent midline or bulbar signs suggest MSA or PSP. Early gait disorder with falls points to the diagnosis of PSP or to subcortical vascular disease. Dependence on a wheelchair within 5 years of onset is suggestive of PSP or MSA. Early orthostatic hypotension or incontinence points to the autonomic dysfunction of MSA. Severe sleep apnea, inspiratory stridor, or involuntary sighing also suggests MSA. Apraxia, alien limb, or cortical sensory loss is typically seen in CBS.

Routine laboratory studies are not helpful in the diagnosis of PD, and their use should be reserved for patients with atypical features. There is a growing interest in serums and cerebrospinal fluid (CSF) biomarkers that may differentiate between PD and atypical parkinsonism. In this regard, several studies have found that neurofilament light chain (NFL) protein levels have been found elevated in the serum and CSF of patients with atypical parkinsonism but not in PD (Marques et al., 2019). When genetic causes (see below) are suspected, testing for specific PD-related monogenic mutations or by whole-exome or whole-genome sequencing may be indicated when coupled with appropriate genetic counseling (Sokol et al., 2017).

**BOX 96.2 "Red Flags" Suggesting a Diagnosis Other Than Parkinson Disease**

Early or prominent dementia
Symmetrical signs
Bulbar dysfunction
Early gait disorder
Falls within the first year
Wheelchair dependence within 5 years
Early autonomic failure
Sleep apnea
Inspiratory stridor
Apraxia
Alien limb
Cortical sensory loss

Neuroimaging studies such as computed tomography (CT) and magnetic resonance imaging (MRI) are usually not very helpful in making a diagnosis of PD, because they are generally normal or show only incidental abnormalities. Sometimes neuroimaging abnormalities can be useful in suggesting alternative diagnoses such as PSP or MSA (see below). The radiopharmaceutical 6-[$^{18}$F]-fluorodopa (F-dopa) is taken up by dopaminergic neurons in the SN and metabolized to 6-[$^{18}$F]-fluorodopamine. Positron emission tomography (PET) scans using this radiopharmaceutical agent show reduced F-dopa uptake in dopaminergic nerve terminals in the putamen and caudate proportional to the severity of degeneration in the ipsilateral SN and symptoms in the contralateral hemibody (Fig. 96.5). Although these tests are used in PD research, they are not readily clinically available at this time. Single-photon emission CT (SPECT) with radioligand that labels the dopamine transporter on nerve terminals in the striatum (DaTscan) is a very helpful tool in differentiating PD from ET, drug-induced parkinsonism (DIP), or functional (psychogenic) parkinsonism (Isaacson et al., 2017; Jankovic, 2011). Since most atypical parkinsonian disorders have striatal dopaminergic denervation, DaTscan is not helpful in differentiating these disorders from PD. Routine electrophysiological testing is not helpful in the diagnosis of PD.

## Pathology

The most striking pathological changes in PD occur in the SNc. The SN appears pale to the naked eye. Microscopic changes include neuronal loss, gliosis, and the presence of extracellular pigment. Surviving neurons may show characteristic cytoplasmic inclusions (Fig. 96.6). These inclusions, called *Lewy bodies*, have a dense eosinophilic core and a pale halo (except for those located in the cortex) (Jellinger, 2012). They contain hyperphosphorylated neurofilament proteins, lipids, iron, ubiquitin, and α-synuclein. Pigmented nuclei elsewhere in the brainstem, including the locus coeruleus, dorsal motor nucleus of the vagus, and others, may also show Lewy bodies and characteristic degenerative changes. The substantia innominata and intermediolateral cell column in the spinal cord also are affected. Patients with PD and dementia show more diffuse Lewy body pathology or comorbid AD. Even the myenteric intestinal and cardiac plexus of patients with PD may contain Lewy bodies, showing that PD is not just a CNS disease.

A staging system introduced by Braak (Goedert et al., 2013) has been developed to characterize the progression of neuropathological changes associated with PD. According to Braak staging, during the presymptomatic stages (1 and 2), the PD-related inclusion body pathology remains confined to the medulla oblongata and olfactory

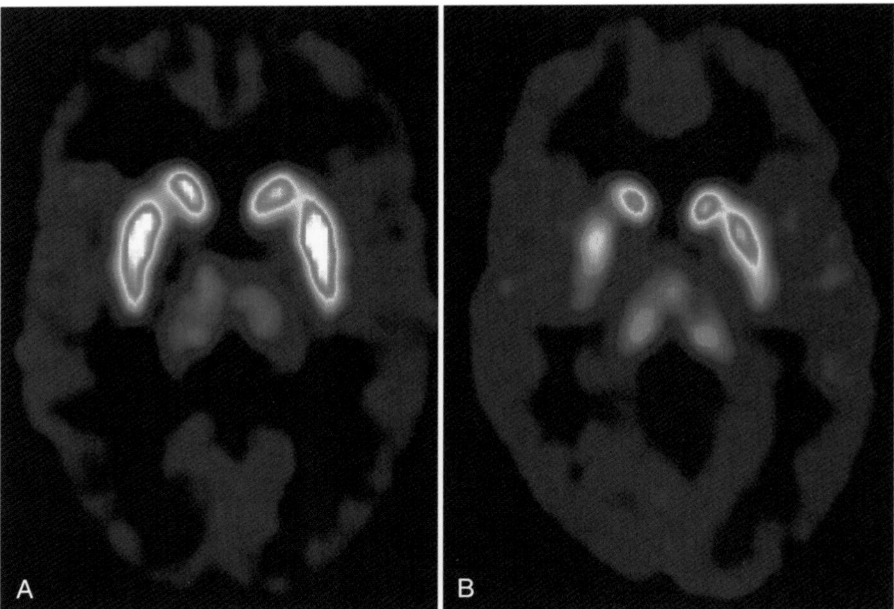


**Fig. 96.5** Positron emission tomography scan with [$^{11}$C]RTI-32, which labels the presynaptic dopamine transporter in a normal control **(A)** and a subject with early Parkinson disease (PD) **(B)**. There is asymmetrically reduced uptake in PD, indicating asymmetrical loss of presynaptic dopaminergic neurons. *(Courtesy Mark Guttman, MD.)*

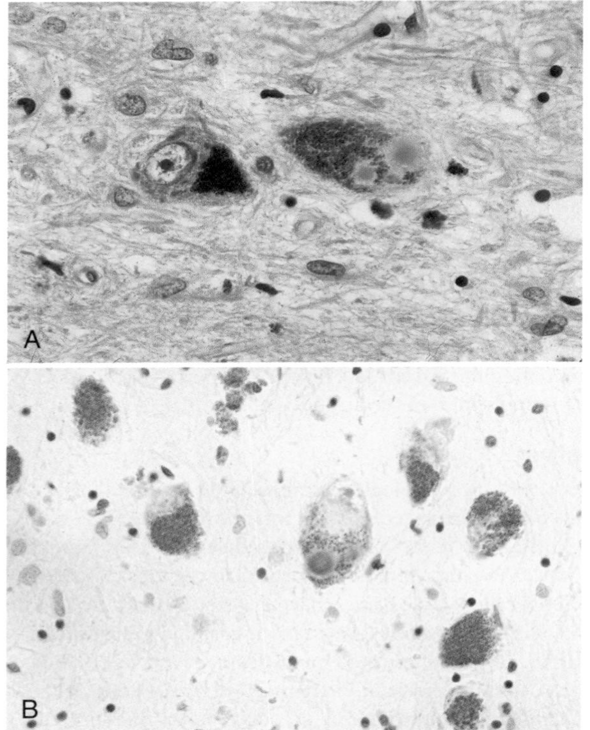


**Fig. 96.6 Brainstem Lewy Bodies. A,** Hematoxylin and eosin-stained section of substantia nigra with a pigmented neuron containing two Lewy bodies. Each is an eosinophilic cytoplasmic inclusion with a halo, displacing neuromelanin. **B,** α-Synuclein-immunostained Lewy body in a neuron of the substantia nigra; α-synuclein protein is stained *red* in this preparation. *(Courtesy Elizabeth Cochran, MD.)*

bulb. In stages 3 and 4, the SN and other nuclear grays of the midbrain and basal forebrain are the focus of initially subtle and then severe changes, and the illness reaches its symptomatic phase. In the end stages (5 and 6), the pathological process encroaches upon the telencephalic cortex. Although the Braak hypothesis is supported by early olfactory, sleep, and autonomic involvement in patients with PD, the staging proposal has been challenged for many reasons and inconsistencies, such as absence of cell counts to correlate with the described synuclein pathology, absence of immunohistochemistry to identify neuronal types, absence of observed asymmetry in the pathological findings that would correlate with the well-recognized asymmetry of clinical findings, absence of bulbar symptoms as early features of PD, and the observation that brain synucleinopathy consistent with Braak stages 4 and 6 has been found in individuals without any neurological signs. Although the Braak hypothesis and the central role of α-synuclein in the pathogenesis of PD have been challenged (Espay et al., 2019) these concepts provide a useful framework for understanding the progression of neurodegeneration in PD.

## Etiology

Studies of large numbers of patients with PD have suggested that PD is a multifactorial illness with likely genetic and environmental determinants (Rousseaux et al., 2017; Jankovic and Tan, 2020). Twin studies suggest that heredity plays a relatively small role in the population at large, but the hereditary component is greater if one twin has disease onset at younger than age 50. Moreover, PET studies of twins suggest that most monozygotic twins of patients with PD show subclinical declines in dopamine innervation, strengthening the evidence for a significant hereditary contribution irrespective of age at onset.

Although the majority of cases of PD appear to be sporadic, it is becoming increasingly evident that genetic factors play an important role in the pathogenesis of PD, particularly if onset is earlier than age 50 (see Chapter 24). Some 20%–25% of patients have at least one first-degree relative with PD, and first-degree relatives are two to three times as likely as relatives of controls to develop PD. The most cogent evidence for genetic contribution to the pathogenesis of PD has been provided by reports of large multicase kindreds with dominantly inherited autopsy-proven PD. A genome scan in the Contursi kindred of Greek-Italian origin found a genetic marker on chromosome 4q21-q23 linked to the PD phenotype. Subsequent studies identified at least three different mutations in the α-synuclein gene (SNCA), the first monogenetic form of PD, designated PARK1 (see Table 24.1). In addition to the typical PD features, this family exhibited dementia, severe central hypoventilation, orthostatic hypotension, prominent myoclonus, urinary incontinence, and pathological involvement of the brainstem pigmented nuclei, hippocampus, and temporal neocortex. Later, the application of quantitative real-time PCR amplification of the *SNCA* gene showed that some families with a PD phenotype, originally designated as PARK4, had duplication and triplication of the gene, with marked increase in the amount of α-synuclein protein. Thus, an overexpression of α-synuclein may lead to neurodegenerative disease, with features overlapping with PD, DLB, and MSA. Based on screening, the entire coding region of the gene in a large number of PD patients shows that mutation in the *SNCA* gene is a rare cause of PD.

Discovery of a linkage between an autosomal recessive, young-onset, LD-responsive form of PD to a locus on chromosome 6q25.2-27 led to subsequent identification of numerous mutations in the gene called *parkin* (PARK2). This 500-kb, 12-exon gene encodes a 465-amino acid protein with E3 ubiquitin-ligase activity through interaction with the ubiquitin-conjugating enzyme UbcH7 (E2). Associated with the Golgi complex, the parkin protein has also been thought to be involved in vesicular transport. Parkin strongly binds to a variety of proteins and microtubules, a disruption of which in patients with parkin mutations affects vesicular transport and may contribute to the nigrostriatal degeneration. Whereas normal parkin is involved in ubiquitination and subsequent degradation of certain proteins by proteasomes, mutated parkin protein loses this activity and thus may lead to an accumulation of proteins, causing a selective neural cell death without formation of Lewy bodies. In addition to typical PD features, patients with PARK2 exhibit a variety of atypical features such as hyperreflexia, dystonia, leg tremor, autonomic dysfunction, sensory axonal peripheral neuropathy, marked sleep benefit, LD-induced dyskinesias, psychosis, and other behavioral and psychiatric problems. Although PARK2 has been identified in patients with late age at onset, up to half of patients with onset of PD before age 40 years have *parkin* mutations.

A growing number of novel genes have been implicated in the pathogenesis of PD (Deng et al., 2018; Trinh and Farrer, 2013) (see Chapter 24). In addition to α-synuclein (*SNCA* gene), there are many other monogenetic causes of PD (see Table 24.1) (Deng et al., 2018) Mutations in the PTEN-induced putative kinase 1 *(PINK1)* gene on chromosome 1p36 were identified in autosomal recessive families with early-onset parkinsonism (PARK6). The *PINK1* gene codes for a putative serine-threonine kinase located in the mitochondria, thus providing further support for the role of oxidative stress in the pathogenesis of PD. The mean age at onset is in the fourth decade, and the course is quite benign, associated with LD-induced dyskinesias. These clinical features are similar to those of another autosomal recessive form of PD (PARK7) localized to the same chromosomal region in the *DJ-1* gene. Besides slow progression and good, prolonged response to LD, patients with a *DJ-1* mutation may exhibit blepharospasm, leg dystonia, anxiety, and parkinsonism-dementia-ALS complex. In contrast to *parkin* mutations that may account for up to 50% of young-onset PD, the *DJ-1* mutations account for approximately 1% of all young-onset PD cases.

Another locus mapped to 12p11.23-q13.11 (PARK8) was initially identified in a Japanese family with typical PD inherited in an autosomal dominant pattern with incomplete penetrance and has been subsequently found to be the most common form of familial adult-onset PD (Marras et al., 2016). The course of the disease is relatively benign, usually presenting with unilateral hand or leg tremor without cognitive deficit; the patients respond well to LD. Other clinical phenotypes have included parkinsonism with dementia, hallucinations, dysautonomia, amyotrophy, or both and otherwise typical ET. Autopsy studies demonstrate variable pathology, ranging from Lewy body and tau neurofibrillary tangle pathology to no pathological changes. The gene responsible for PARK8 on 12p11.2-q13.1, called *LRRK2* (leucine-rich repeat kinase 2), belongs to the ROCO protein family and includes a protein kinase domain of the MAPKKK class and several other major functional domains. The gene product, a protein called *dardarin* (from Basque word *dardara*, meaning "tremor"), is a novel protein that probably functions as a cytoplasmic kinase involved in phosphorylation of proteins such as α-synuclein and tau. LRRK2 is closely associated with a variety of membrane and vesicular structures, membrane-bound organelles, and microtubules, suggesting its role in vesicular transport and membrane and protein turnover, including the lysosomal degradation pathway. This mutation has been found to be particularly frequent in PD patients of North African origin and in Ashkenazi Jewish patients (Inzelber et al., 2014). The penetrance is quite variable, and many elderly individuals have the mutation but no signs of PD have been reported.

It is beyond the scope of this chapter to discuss all the various genetic causes of PD but the reader is referred to Chapter 24 and other reviews on this topic (Deng et al., 2018). The variable penetrance and growing number of causative and susceptibility genes, coupled with a growing number of commercially available DNA tests, has obvious implications for genetic counseling (Sokol et al., 2017).

Evidence for environmental causes of PD comes primarily from two sources: the fortuitous discovery of parkinsonism in parenteral drug users exposed to the contaminant MPTP and epidemiological associations of sporadic PD or other parkinsonisms with certain lifestyle or occupational exposures. The discovery that a handful of drug addicts had developed a severe LD-responsive form of parkinsonism following parenteral administration of a meperidine analog contaminated with the mitochondrial protoxin MPTP suggested that environmental toxins might cause PD. The discovery of MPTP-induced parkinsonism in humans was a sentinel event in our understanding of the disease because it pointed to a class of environmental toxins that might be important in sporadic disease. Although MPTP spawned the development of reproducible models of disease in many kinds of animals, its role in human disease is limited to the cluster of cases in drug addicts and a few others. Intriguing studies have confirmed that certain pesticides (e.g., paraquat, rotenone) can reproduce the pathology of PD in animals, but their role in human disease remains undefined.

Epidemiological studies suggest that exposure to environmental metals or organic toxins may be associated with an increased risk of PD or an earlier age at onset. Case-controlled studies have suggested that the risk of PD is increased in persons who have worked in the agricultural industry, have been exposed to pesticides, or have sustained significant head injury. Whether exposure to welding predisposes to earlier onset of PD, possibly as a result of manganese poisoning, is controversial (Jankovic, 2005). On the other hand, the risk of PD seems lower in those with a high dietary intake of antioxidant-rich foods, as well as caffeine drinkers and those who have smoked cigarettes. Although PD and cancer are two distinct diseases that result from either degeneration or over-proliferation, respectively, several recent studies have provided evidence that while PD provides some type of biological protection against most types of cancers, the disease confers increased risk for other cancers such as melanoma. The relationship between PD and melanoma is being explored, but the higher frequency of melanoma does not appear to be due to LD. It is possible that high concentrations of α-synuclein in the skin of patients with PD may increase their risk of melanoma by inhibiting tyrosine hydroxylase, an enzyme involved in dopamine and melanin biosynthesis or by some other mechanism (Pan et al., 2012).

### Treatment

Before discussing specific treatment strategies for PD, it is important to recognize that the quantitative assessment of clinical symptoms and progression of the course is an essential component of any therapeutic trial (Jankovic, 2008; Jankovic and Tan, 2020 Jankovic and Tan, 2020). In addition to sensitive clinical rating scales (e.g., MDS-UPDRS), reliable diagnostic, presymptomatic, and progression biomarkers are needed (Marek et al., 2018; Wu et al., 2011).

***Neuroprotective or disease-modifying therapies for Parkinson disease.*** A preclinical period lasting years, its slow progression rate, and our increasing understanding of disease etiopathogenesis make PD an ideal candidate for neuroprotective therapeutic strategies. However, double-blind placebo-controlled trials designed to explore therapies that may have favorable disease-modifying effects and slow disease progression have been thus far disappointing. The first "neuroprotective" trial, DATATOP (Deprenyl and Tocopherol Antioxidative Therapy of Parkinsonism), randomized patients with early PD to treatment with placebo, tocopherol, selegiline (deprenyl), or both, using the time until the patients needed potent symptomatic dopaminergic therapy, LD, as a proxy endpoint for disease progression. The selective monoamine oxidase (MAO-B) inhibitor, selegiline, successfully delayed this endpoint, but interpretation of the study was contaminated by the drug's mild symptomatic antiparkinsonian and antidepressant properties, as well as the potential effects of its amphetamine metabolites. Although disease-modifying effects of selegiline have been suggested by some clinical trials, further studies are needed before it can be concluded that selegiline is neuroprotective in PD. Another MAO-B inhibitor, rasagiline, has been shown to have modest symptomatic benefit (Jankovic et al., 2014), but its effects on disease progression are also still being debated. In a randomized multicenter, double-blind, placebo-controlled, parallel-group study prospectively examining rasagiline's potential disease-modifying effects (ADAGIO [Attenuation of Disease Progression with Azilect Given Once-Daily]), delayed-start design was used to assess the potential disease-modifying effects of rasagiline (Olanow et al., 2009). A total of 1176 patients with early untreated PD (mean time from diagnosis, 4.5 months) from 129 centers in 14 countries were randomized into 4 treatment groups (either 1 or 2 mg/day, early-start versus delayed-start treatment, 9 months each). Early-start treatment consisted of 72 weeks of rasagiline (either 1 or 2 mg once daily), and delayed-start treatment consisted of 36 weeks of placebo followed by 36 weeks of rasagiline (either 1 or 2 mg once daily [active treatment phase]). The primary analyses of the trial were based on change in total UPDRS score and included slope superiority of rasagiline over placebo in the placebo-controlled phase, change from baseline to week 72, and noninferiority of early-start versus delayed-start slopes during weeks 48 through 72 of the active phase. The 1-mg dose group met all three endpoints, but there was no observable benefit with the higher 2-mg dose, although when analyzing the upper quartile group, the 2-mg dose group met all the primary endpoints. Some possible explanations for the seemingly confusing outcome include early symptomatic treatment helping some compensatory mechanism, cumulative symptomatic effect, and other possibilities.

Development of neuroprotective strategies has been challenging, partly because of lack of reliable and sensitive biomarkers of progression (Jankovic and Sherer, 2014; Jankovic and Tan, 2020). Animal models are essential in preclinical testing of potential symptomatic and neuroprotective therapies (Le et al., 2014). One of the most exciting developments of potential neuroprotective or disease-modifying therapies is the use of α-synuclein monoclonal antibodies to reduce α-synuclein formation and rescue dying neurons (Savitt and Jankovic, 2019a; Tran et al., 2014).

***Symptomatic treatment of Parkinson disease.*** Many types of medications are available for symptomatic treatment of PD: anticholinergics, amantadine, LD, MAO inhibitors (MAOIs), catechol-O-methyltransferase inhibitors (COMTIs), and DAs (Jankovic et al., 2014; Obeso et al., 2017). Anticholinergics such as trihexyphenidyl and benztropine antagonize the effects of acetylcholine at muscarinic receptors postsynaptic to striatal interneurons. They reduce tremor and rigidity but have no effects on bradykinesia. Toxicity relates to antagonism of acetylcholine at central receptors, causing confusion, and peripheral receptors, causing blurred vision, dry mouth, constipation, and urine retention. Although amantadine has been available for nearly 4 decades (it was originally marketed as an anti-influenza, antiviral agent), its antiparkinsonian mechanisms have been poorly understood. It has been thought to stimulate release of endogenous dopamine stores, block reuptake of dopamine from the synaptic cleft, and have anticholinergic properties. However, amantadine has been found to have antiglutamatergic properties and as such is the only antiparkinsonian drug that improves LD-induced dyskinesia. Extended release formulation of amantadine has been found to improve not only dyskinesia but also motor fluctuations (Pahwa et al., 2017).

Combining LD with carbidopa, an aromatic acid decarboxylase inhibitor that prevents its peripheral metabolism, markedly reduces its peripheral adverse effects, particularly nausea. The global antiparkinsonian efficacy of LD is so dramatic and predictable that a positive therapeutic response is used to define the disease itself. Adverse effects of LD include nausea and vomiting, orthostatic hypotension, sedation, confusion, sleep disturbance, alterations of dream phenomena, hallucinations, and dyskinesias (see Video 96.6). Many studies have concluded that DAs such as pramipexole, ropinirole, and rotigotine, when introduced early in the course of PD treatment, may delay LD-related complications such as motor fluctuations and dyskinesias. But evidence is lacking to support the hypothesis that early introduction of DAs slows progression of the disease or even improves long-term quality of life (Espay and Lang, 2017). The PROUD study (Pramipexole on Underlying Disease), which assessed early versus delayed pramipexole treatment in early PD, involved 535 untreated PD patients who were randomized to double-blind placebo or pramipexole (1.5 mg/day) for 6–9 months and continued with pramipexole for up to 15 months. The researchers found no difference in UPDRS (−0.4 UPDRS units) or PDQ-39 scores in the 411 patients who completed the 15-month study, but at the end of the placebo-controlled phase, the difference in adjusted means was −4.8 UPDRS units (95% confidence interval [CT], −6.3, −3.2; $P < .0001$), and there was a significant difference in PDQ-39 ($P = .0001$), both in favor of pramipexole (Schapira et al., 2010). Furthermore, many studies have shown that LD is more effective than DAs in reducing motor symptoms in early as well as advanced stages of PD (PD MED Collaborative Group, 2014). In a pragmatic, open-label, randomized trial involving 1620 patients with a newly diagnosed PD randomized to receive a DA ($N = 632$), a monoamine oxidase inhibitor ($N = 460$), or LD ($N = 528$), after median follow-up of 3 years there was a slightly better (1.8 points) PDQ-39 mobility score with LD than with the other two treatments (PD MED Collaborative Group, 2014). Although the study suggested small but persistent benefits when PD patients were initially treated with LD compared with LD-sparing therapy, the study did not adequately address whether patients with young-onset PD should be treated differently than those with late-onset PD. Despite the findings from the PD MED study, most parkinsonologists would probably still employ LD-sparing strategy in patients with young-onset PD.

Because of various adverse effects related to their ergot structure, particularly fibroproliferative lesions of heart valves, lung, and other tissues, bromocriptine, pergolide, and cabergoline have been discontinued from clinical use. Apomorphine, a nonergoline DA, is water soluble and lipophilic and is therefore suitable for intravenous, subcutaneous, sublingual, intranasal, or transdermal administration. Apomorphine is available as an acute intermittent subcutaneous injection, as a rapid rescue from hypomobility off episodes (end-of-dose wearing off and unpredictable on/off episodes) associated with advanced PD. DAs cause side effects similar to those of LD, although orthostatic hypotension, sleepiness, and hallucinations are more common or severe. Continuous apomorphine infusion has been found to meaningfully reduce off time in PD patients who experience troublesome motor fluctuations (Katzenschlager et al., 2018).

One major concern with DAs is the relatively high frequency of a variety of behavioral problems that include pathological gambling, compulsive shopping and eating, hypersexuality, and other impulse-control disorders (ICD) (Zhang et al., 2019). Patients with PD who experience ICD seem to have a variety of associated psychiatric symptoms, such as psychoticism, interpersonal sensitivity, obsessive-compulsive symptoms, and depression (Jaakkola et al., 2014) and seem to be prone to dopamine dysregulation syndrome, an addictive behavior and excessive use of dopaminergic medication (Warren et al., 2017).

Selegiline and rasagiline block MAO-B-dependent dopamine degradation and have modest effects in potentiating the action of LD. These drugs are now used very infrequently, but some clinicians prescribe these MAO-B inhibitors as the initial pharmacological agents in newly diagnosed patients in an attempt to delay LD therapy. This approach is in part supported by the ADAGIO study (Olanow et al., 2009). COMTIs (entacapone and tolcapone) block peripheral degradation of peripheral LD and central degradation of LD and dopamine (tolcapone), increasing central LD and dopamine levels. Hepatotoxicity associated with tolcapone has limited its use. Triple-combination therapy containing LD, carbidopa, and entacapone is available for patients with moderately advanced PD. The primary role of COMTIs is to prolong the effects of LD, so they are useful as adjunctive drugs for patients who experience LD-related motor fluctuations. Besides increasing LD-related dyskinesias, COMTIs may cause nausea, postural hypotension, diarrhea, and orange discoloration of urine, but they are generally well tolerated. There is no evidence that COMTIs prevent or delay the onset of LD-related motor complications. Symptomatic pharmacological treatment should begin when the patient is noticing functional, occupational, or social disability related to PD symptoms. Prospective studies have suggested that approximately 70% of patients with PD will require symptomatic therapy within 2 years of disease onset. Less potent therapies such as selegiline, rasagiline, amantadine, and DAs may be useful for initial therapy, particularly in patients with young-onset PD, but LD should be used when more potent therapy is indicated or in patients with late-onset disease. The argument that LD might be toxic to dopaminergic neurons is based on (1) the recognition that dopamine metabolites increase oxidative stress and (2) the observation that LD is toxic to cultures of mesencephalic neurons in vivo. There is, however, no in vivo evidence from animal or human studies that LD accelerates disease progression, and it is difficult to reconcile the potential of dopamine toxicity with the obvious fact that the drug prolongs life in patients with PD. A 9-month study called the *Earlier versus Later* L-DOPA (ELLDOPA) trial compared different doses of LD with placebo and found no evidence of LD toxicity (Jankovic and Poewe, 2012). Nevertheless, as a result of "LD phobia," many patients and physicians still unnecessarily delay LD therapy in patients who would clearly benefit from symptomatic relief (Espay and Jankovic, 2017).

Clinical experience with LD treatment of PD indicates that there is a progressive increase in the prevalence of drug-related motor fluctuations (wearing off, dyskinesia) over time, and that about half of patients experience wearing off, and a third experience dyskinesias within 2 years after initiation of LD therapy. Wearing off results from loss of DA storage in the striatum as a result of loss of nigrostriatal terminals. Experiments in animal models relate the development of dyskinesia to changes in striatal glutamate receptor sensitivity consequent to pulsatile stimulation of striatal dopamine receptors. Continuous dopamine receptor stimulation with LD or with long-acting DAs prevents or reverses this phenomenon.

In eliciting a description of the patient's response to medication, it is important to understand the severity of symptoms in the morning on arising and the latency, magnitude, and duration of benefit from each dose of LD. Information about the onset of motor and nonmotor symptoms during wearing off as well as the phenomenology, timing, and distribution of dyskinesia. The usefulness of historical information may be augmented by careful patient education on symptom recognition and the development of a shared vocabulary. Completing motor diaries (Fig. 96.7) helps both the patient and the treating physician recognize patterns of motor response and adjust the medications accordingly.

*Wearing off* is the most common type of motor fluctuation. It refers to the return of parkinsonian symptoms following the previous dose in advance of the next scheduled antiparkinsonian dose. *On/off* is the unpredictable reappearance of parkinsonism at a time when central levels of antiparkinsonian drugs are expected to be within the target therapeutic range. *Delayed on* is a prolongation of the time required for the central antiparkinsonian drug effect to appear. *Dose failure* is a complete failure to develop a favorable response to an incremental dopaminergic dose. This may be related to protein intake which interferes with the transport of LD across the intestinal wall as a result of competition for facilitated transport by large amounts of neutral amino acids. A variety of dyskinesias can further complicate the response to LD. *Peak-dose dyskinesias* are usually choreiform or stereotypical movements, such as head bobbing movement of the head or choreic movements of limbs and trunk, present at the peak of the therapeutic response. *Off-period dystonia* usually appears in the more severely affected foot in the morning before the first daily doses, sometimes reappearing during wearing off. *Diphasic dyskinesias* are usually large-amplitude dyskinetic movements of the lower body during the time of increasing and decreasing LD levels.

Armed with a few basic principles and a commonsense approach, the clinician can usually smooth out fluctuations for most patients with appropriate selection of drugs and dose (Jankovic and Poewe, 2012) (Figs. 96.8 and 96.9). Delay to onset of therapeutic benefit can be hastened by taking the medication on an empty stomach (if tolerated without nausea), avoiding or reducing protein intake, or by crushing the LD tablet and mixing it with a carbonated beverage. The duration of benefit increases when the individual dose is increased or dopamine metabolism is blocked with an MAO-B or COMTIs. This, however, may increase the risk of dyskinesia and the patient may do better on smaller, more frequent LD doses. Thus fractionation of LD dose is usually the initial strategy in an attempt to smooth out fluctuations and prevent wearing off symptoms.

In addition to the fluctuating response, some patients, particularly those with advanced disease, may acquire LD-resistant motor symptoms such as freezing, progressive gait dysfunction, dysarthria and dysphagia, and recurrent falling due to loss of balance and postural instability. Other features of advanced illness (cognitive impairment, autonomic dysfunction, psychiatric complications) may limit the types and dosage of tolerated medications. *Freezing*, sudden immobility of the feet while walking, often with falls, may be seen in either the off or the on period. Although off-period freezing may improve with optimization of medications, on-period freezing is usually resistant to pharmacological treatment. Physical therapy, including strategies that

| Time | Medication | Meal | Asleep | Off | On | Dyskinesia |
|---|---|---|---|---|---|---|
| Midnight – 1:00 A | | | X | | | |
| 1:00 – 2:00 A | | | X | | | |
| 2:00 – 3:00 A | | | X | | | |
| 3:00 – 4:00 A | | | X | | | |
| 4:00 – 5:00 A | | | X | | | |
| 5:00 – 6:00 A | | | | X | | |
| 6:00 – 7:00 A | 1 Sinemet<br>½ Mirapex | X | | X | | |
| 7:00 – 8:00 A | | | | | X | |
| 8:00 – 9:00 A | | | | | X | X |
| 9:00 – 10:00 A | | | | X | | |
| 10:00 – 11:00 A | | | | X | | |
| 11:00 – noon | 1 Sinemet<br>½ Mirapex | X | | X | | |
| 1:00 – 2:00 P | | | | X | | |
| 2:00 – 3:00 P | | | | | X | X |
| 3:00 – 4:00 P | 1 Sinemet | | | X | | |
| 4:00 – 5:00 P | | | | | X | |
| 5:00 – 6:00 P | | X | | | X | X |
| 6:00 – 7:00 P | | | | | X | |
| 7:00 – 8:00 P | ½ Sinemet | | | X | | |
| 8:00 – 9:00 P | | | | | X | X |
| 9:00 – 10:00 P | | | | | X | X |
| 10:00 – 11:00 P | | | | X | | |
| 11:00 – midnight | | X | | | | |

**Fig. 96.7 Sample Diary in Parkinson Disease.** For each hour, the patient indicates whether and which antiparkinsonian drugs he or she has taken, then places a mark to indicate motor state for most of the hour.

utilize sensory cues, such as stepping over a horizontal laser beam, may be helpful. Dysarthria and dysphagia are often treated by speech therapists, although documentation of improvement from these techniques is scant.

Cognitive impairment increases mainly with the age of the patient and with disease severity. Preliminary reports suggest that cholinesterase inhibitors might be useful in PD-associated dementia, but these studies require confirmation in carefully controlled trials. Orthostatic hypotension can be managed conservatively with salt supplementation, fludrocortisone, midodrine, and droxidopa for orthostatic hypotension (Kaufmann et al., 2014). Urological medications may improve bladder dysfunction, and dietary changes along with medications such as linaclotide and lubiprostone may improve constipation. Hallucinations occur in approximately 30% of treated patients; a loss of insight that the visions are not real or the appearance of psychotic thinking signals a particularly disabling complication. Hallucinations often improve with atypical antipsychotics such as quetiapine and clozapine. Also, pimavanserin, a non-dopaminergic and selective serotonin inverse agonist with high affinity at the 5-HT2A receptor has been found to be effective in the treatment of psychosis and hallucinations related to dopaminergic therapy (Cummings et al., 2014).

Cholinesterase inhibitors, in addition to improving cognitive function, may reduce hallucinations in some patients. Sleep disorders may respond to hypnosedatives, tricyclic antidepressants, mirtazapine, trazodone, quetiapine, or nighttime dopaminergic therapy. Excessive daytime sleepiness may respond to methylphenidate, modafinil, or armodafinil.

***Surgical treatment of Parkinson disease.*** Despite optimal medical therapy, many patients with moderate to advanced disease have a poor quality of life because of fluctuating response, troublesome dyskinesia, or LD-unresponsive symptoms. Palliative surgical approaches such as stereotactic destruction of physiologically defined overactive brain nuclei (thalamotomy, pallidotomy) have been replaced by deep brain stimulation (DBS) using implanted pulse generators. The

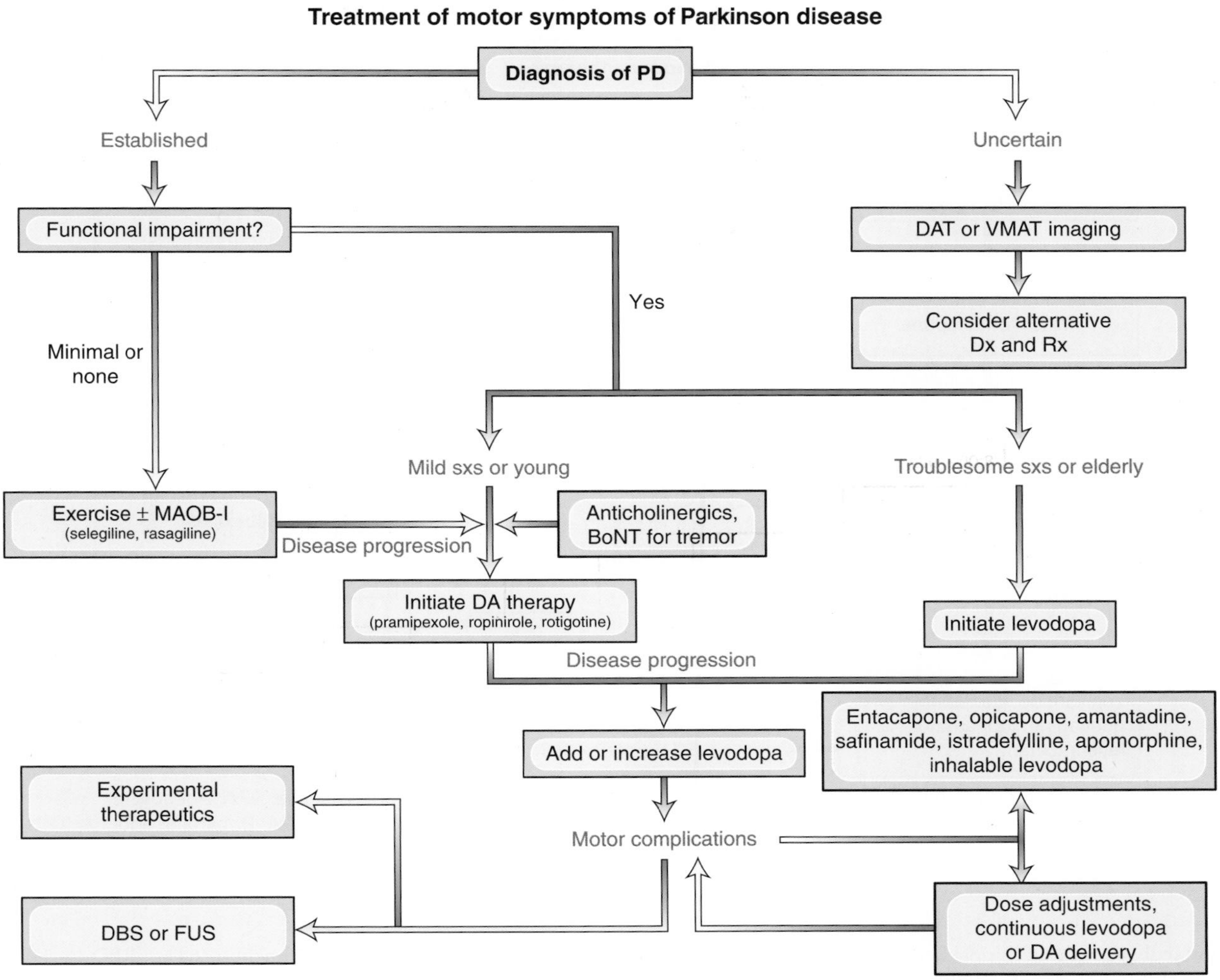

**Fig. 96.8 Treatment of Motor Symptoms of Parkinson Disease.** Algorithm for the treatment of Parkinson disease *(PD). BoNT* = botulinum neurotoxin; *DA,* Dopamine agonist; *DAT,* dopamine transporter; *DBS,* deep brain stimulation; *Dx,* diagnosis; *FUS,* focused ultrasound; *MAOB-1,*monoamine oxidase inhibitor type 1; *MAOI,* monoamine oxidase inhibitor; *Rx,* treatment; *VMAT2,* vesicular monoamine transporter 2.

chief advantage of DBS over ablative lesioning is that the stimulation parameters can be customized to the needs of the patient to optimize the benefits. With improvements in technology the outcomes of DBS will likely continue to improve (Okun, 2019).

Thalamic DBS is most frequently used to control high-amplitude tremor (either PD or ET), but STN or GPi are the most frequent targets for DBS treatment of patients with PD with disabling LD-related complications. To address the question whether optimal medical therapy or DBS provides more robust improvement, 255 patients at seven Veterans Affairs and six university hospitals were enrolled in a randomized controlled trial designed to compare the effects of DBS (STN, $n = 60$; or GPi, $n = 61$) and "best medical therapy" ($n = 134$) after 6 months of treatment (Weaver et al., 2009). Patients treated with DBS gained a mean of 4.6 hours/day of on time without troubling dyskinesia, compared to 0 hours/day for patients who received best medical therapy ($P < .001$). Furthermore, motor function improved by 5 or more points on the motor UPDRS in 71% of DBS and 32% of medical therapy patients. This was accompanied by improvements in the majority of PD-related HRQOL (health-related quality of life) measures and only minimal decrement in neurocognitive testing. The overall risk of experiencing a serious adverse event, however, was 3.8 times higher in the DBS than in the medical therapy group (40% vs. 11%). In a follow-up analysis of the Veterans Affairs Cooperative Studies Program outcomes, STN and GPi DBS were analyzed after 24 months in 299 patients, and there were no differences in mean changes in the motor (Part III) UPDRS between the two targets (Follett et al., 2010). Patients undergoing STN required a lower dose of DAs than those undergoing pallidal stimulation ($P = .02$), and visuomotor processing speed declined more after STN than after GPi stimulation ($P = .03$). On the other hand, there was worsening of depression after STN DBS, but mood improved after GPi DBS ($P = .02$). Slightly more than half of the patients experienced serious adverse events, but there was no difference in the frequency of these events between the two groups. Based on these and other studies, there is emerging evidence that GPi DBS may be particularly suitable for patients who may have troublesome dyskinesias as well as mild cognitive or behavioral impairment, whereas bilateral STN DBS may be the surgical choice for patients who are cognitively intact but in whom reduction in LD dosage is the primary goal. While DBS is a proven effective therapeutic strategy, its success depends on the appropriate selection of patients and the experience and skill of the stereotactic surgeon in order to optimize the results and minimize complications. Advances in DBS technology, such as the use of adaptive stimulation, improving connectivity, directional stimulation (Pollo et al., 2014), and searching for new targets,

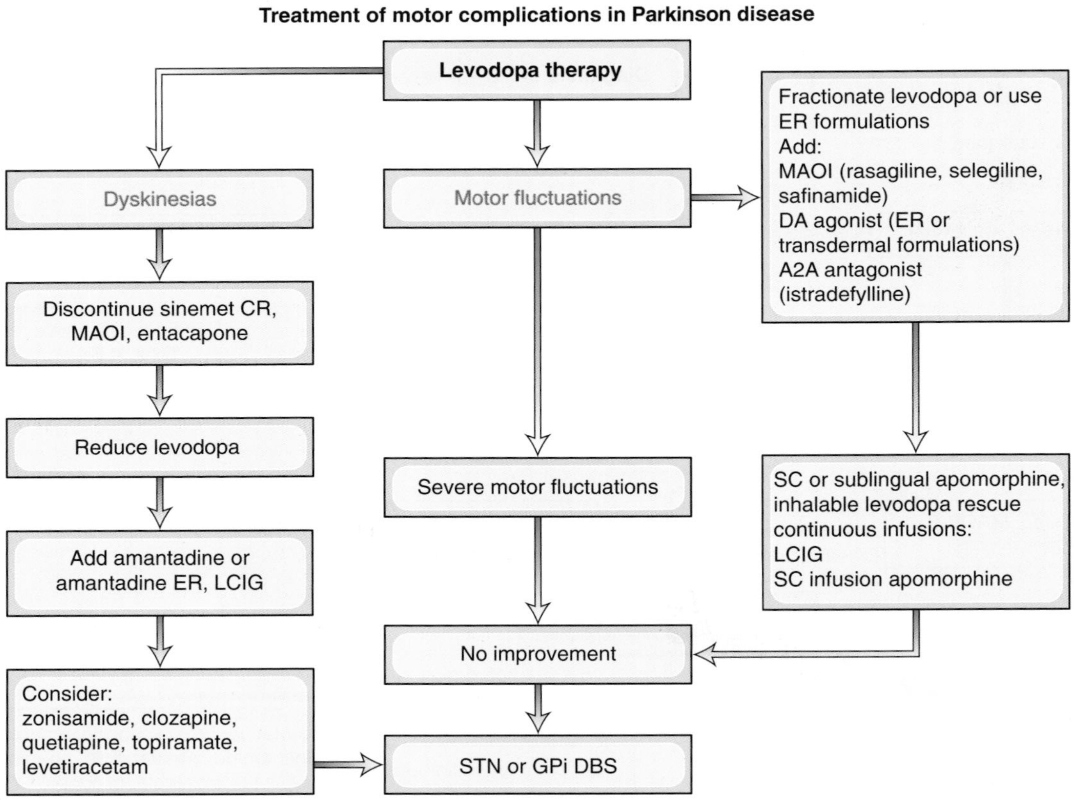

**Treatment of motor complications in Parkinson disease**

Levodopa therapy

Dyskinesias

Discontinue sinemet CR, MAOI, entacapone

Reduce levodopa

Add amantadine or amantadine ER, LCIG

Consider: zonisamide, clozapine, quetiapine, topiramate, levetiracetam

Motor fluctuations

Fractionate levodopa or use ER formulations
Add:
MAOI (rasagiline, selegiline, safinamide)
DA agonist (ER or transdermal formulations)
A2A antagonist (istradefylline)

Severe motor fluctuations

SC or sublingual apomorphine, inhalable levodopa rescue continuous infusions:
LCIG
SC infusion apomorphine

No improvement

STN or GPi DBS

**Fig. 96.9** Treatment of Levodopa-Related Motor Complications in Parkinson Disease. A2A, Adenosine A2A receptor; *COMTI*, catechol-o-methyl-transferase inhibitor; *CR*, Controlled release; *DA*, Dopamine agonist; *DBS*, deep brain stimulation; *ER*, extended release; *GPi*, globus pallidus interna; *LCIG*, levodopa-carbidopa infusion gel; *MAOI*, monoamine oxidase inhibitor; *SC*, subcutaneous; *STN*, subthalamic nucleus.

will undoubtedly provide additional benefits from this procedure and reduce complications (Baizabal-Carvallo et al., 2012). It should be noted that there is a trend toward recommending DBS earlier in the course of PD (Charles et al., 2014).

Unilateral focused ultrasound lesioning of the STN or thalamus (in tremor-dominant forms of PD) has been found to be beneficial in some patients, particularly if the symptoms are markedly asymmetric (Bond et al., 2017; Martínez-Fernández et al., 2018). Finally, spinal cord stimulation is increasingly being explored in patients with PD who are most troubled by their gait disorder (Samotus et al., 2018).

## Multiple System Atrophy

MSA is a neurodegenerative disorder manifested by dysautonomia and various combinations of parkinsonism and ataxia (Krismer and Wenning, 2017; Stamelou et al., 2013). Originally referred to as *Shy-Drager syndrome*, MSA is subdivided into two major categories according to the predominant clinical manifestation. *Predominantly parkinsonian MSA* (MSA-P) replaces the term *striatonigral degeneration. Cerebellar MSA* (MSA-C) replaces the now obsolete term *olivopontocerebellar atrophy*.

MSA is considerably less common than PD, with a prevalence of 4–5 per 100,000, compared to 360 per 100,000 for PD. This sporadic neurodegenerative disorder with a mean age at onset of 54 years may be difficult to differentiate from PD, particularly in the early stages. The most common signs of dysautonomia in pathologically confirmed cases are bladder dysfunction (89%), particularly urinary incontinence (44%) and urinary retention (26%), bowel dysfunction (77%), particularly constipation (46%) and fecal incontinence (27%), orthostatic hypotension (75%), sexual dysfunction (64%), RBD (54%), sweating dysfunction (40%), sleep apnea (37%), and nocturnal stridor (30%) (Iodice et al., 2012). In contrast to PD, MSA-P usually presents with symmetrical parkinsonism, often without tremor, with early instability and falls. Most patients become wheelchair bound within 5 years after onset (see Video 96.12).

Several clinical studies have addressed differentiating between MSA-P and parkinsonism, and a collection of "red flags" has been generated and recently validated as having high diagnostic specificity (Stefanova et al., 2009). The red flags were grouped into six categories: (1) early instability, (2) rapid progression, (3) abnormal postures (includes Pisa syndrome, disproportionate anterocollis, and/or contractures of hands or feet) (Fig. 96.10), (4) bulbar dysfunction (includes severe dysphonia, dysarthria, and/or dysphagia), (5) respiratory dysfunction (includes diurnal or nocturnal inspiratory stridor and/or inspiratory sighs) (Mehanna and Jankovic, 2010), and (6) emotional incontinence (includes inappropriate crying and/or laughing). They proposed that a combination of two out of these six red-flag categories be used as additional criteria for the diagnosis of probable MSA-P. Other characteristic features of MSA include early hypokinetic dysarthria, distal myoclonus, and cold hands and feet with bluish discoloration of the distal extremities. MSA patients also have more autonomic symptoms at baseline and more progression to global anhidrosis than patients with PD (Iodice et al., 2012). The autonomic symptoms (particularly sexual dysfunction) and RBD may precede the onset of motor symptoms by years or even decades. About 10% of patients originally diagnosed with pure autonomic failure eventually transition to MSA (Singer et al., 2017). Patients with MSA-C have parkinsonism with

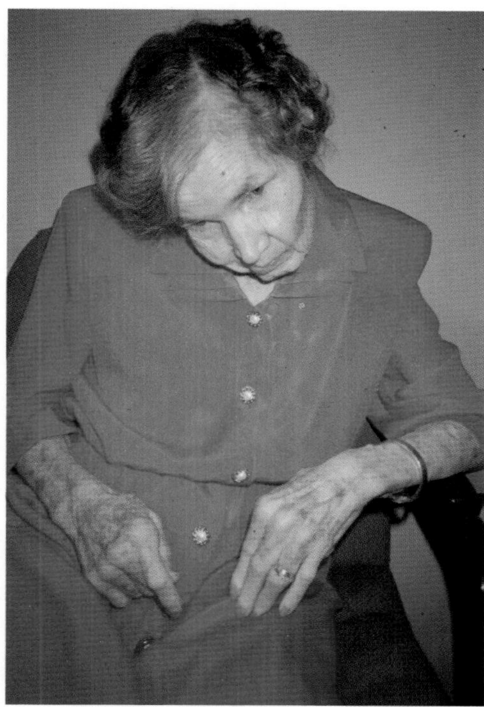

**Fig. 96.10** Patient with multiple system atrophy showing anterocollis and Pisa sign.

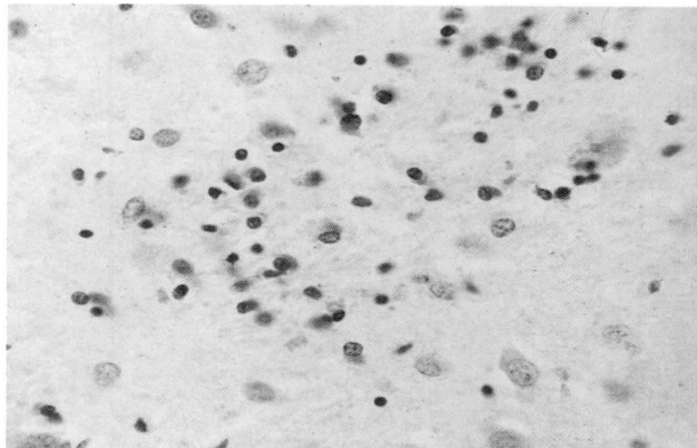

**Fig. 96.11** Glial cytoplasmic inclusions in basal ganglia, immunostained with α-synuclein—typical of multiple system atrophy. *(Courtesy Elizabeth Cochran, MD.)*

prominent cerebellar signs, especially wide-based ataxic gait. Although there may be a positive response to LD, this is generally relatively short lived and often associated with facial and oromandibular dyskinesia. In a prospective study of 141 patients with moderately severe MSA (mean age at symptom onset 56.2± 8.4 years) who had a median survival of 9.8 years (95% CI 8.1–11.4), shorter survival was suggested by the parkinsonian variant of MSA and incomplete bladder emptying, and shorter symptom duration at baseline and absent LD response predicted rapid progression (Wenning et al., 2013).

Clinical tests of autonomic dysfunction may be helpful in diagnosis or treatment (Mostile and Jankovic, 2010). Testing of cardiovascular reflexes such as heart rate variability at rest and during forced respiration, as well as blood pressure changes during head-up tilt, may help establish a clinical diagnosis of MSA. A lack of responsiveness of growth hormone to clonidine challenges and denervation on rectal sphincter electromyography (EMG) are also characteristic findings. T2-weighted MRI brain scans may show a hyperintense rim at the lateral edge of the dorsolateral putamen, with decreased signal within the putamen. Cruciform hyperintensity within the pons, the so-called hot-cross-bun sign, may also be a helpful marker (Brooks et al., 2009). PET scan with [11C]PMP that images subcortical acetyl cholinesterase (AChE) activity was significantly more decreased in MSA-P and PSP than in PD, possibly reflecting greater impairment in the pontine cholinergic group (PPN); this may account for the greater gait disturbances in the early stages of these two disorders compared to PD (Gilman et al., 2010). There is a need for development of highly specific and sensitive biomarkers that support the diagnosis and track the progression of the disease. In this regard, NFL protein levels have been found elevated in the serum and CSF of patients with MSA but not in PD but this does not differentiate between MSA and other forms of atypical parkinsonism (Marques et al., 2019).

At autopsy, MSA brains show neuronal loss and gliosis in the striatum, SN, locus coeruleus, inferior olive, pontine nuclei, Purkinje cells, intermediolateral cell column, and the Onuf nucleus in the sacral spinal cord. Glial cytoplasmic inclusions containing α-synuclein (Fig. 96.11) are the most characteristic histological features linking the different types of MSA. Neuron-to-oligodendrocyte transfer of α-synuclein by prion-like spread, leading to oligodendroglial and myelin dysfunction associated with chronic neuroinflammation, has been suggested to lead to the MSA pattern of neurodegeneration (Jellinger, 2014). There is a severe depletion of cholinergic neurons in the PPN and laterodorsal tegmental nucleus. The etiology of MSA remains unknown, but genetic factors do not seem to play an important role.

Treatment of MSA is difficult (Castro et al., 2017; Stamelou et al., 2013). There are no specific interventions, and symptomatic therapies provide only partial relief of disability. Parkinsonism may respond to LD, particularly early in the disease course, but the results are not dramatic or sustained. DAs are not helpful and may be poorly tolerated because of orthostatic hypotension. There is no effective treatment for the cerebellar signs. Orthostatic hypotension may improve with nonpharmacological measures such as liberal salt and water intake, compression stockings, and sleeping with the head up, but most patients require pharmacotherapy with fludrocortisone, midodrine, droxidopa, or other agents (Kaufmann et al., 2014). Treatment of orthostatic hypotension often worsens supine hypertension. Even in the best hands, MSA has a poor prognosis, with a mean survival of 7–9 years.

## Progressive Supranuclear Palsy

First described in 1964 by Steele, Richardson, and Olszewski as a progressive illness characterized by vertical supranuclear ophthalmoplegia, axial rigidity, pseudobulbar palsy, and mild dementia, PSP has evolved into a broad spectrum of syndromes with different pathological substrates (Boxer et al., 2017; Höglinger et al., 2017; Stamelou et al., 2013). In addition to the classic Richardson syndrome, other subtypes include PSP-parkinsonism (with features suggestive of PD), pure akinesia with gait freezing, CBS, non-fluent variant primary progressive aphasia, behavioral variant FTD, and PSP presenting with cerebellar ataxia (Boxer et al., 2017). In addition, based on four core clinical features of PSP (oculomotor dysfunction, postural instability, akinesia, and cognitive dysfunction) other variants of PSP have been described. These include PSP with predominant ocular motor dysfunction (PSP-OM), with predominant postural instability (PSP-PI), with predominant parkinsonism (PSP-P), with predominant frontal presentation (PSP-F), with progressive gait freezing (PSP-PGF), with predominant corticobasal syndrome (PSP-CBS), with predominant speech and language disorder (PSP-SL), with predominant ataxia (PSP-C), and with predominant primary lateral sclerosis (PSP-PLS) (Boxer et al., 2017; Höglinger et al., 2017).

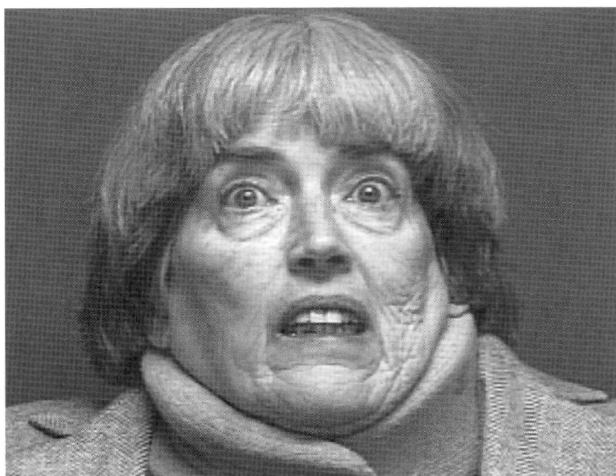

**Fig. 96.12** Typical facial expression of a patient with progressive supranuclear palsy, illustrating worried or surprised appearance, with furrowed brow and fixed expression of lower face.

After vascular parkinsonism (Mehanna and Jankovic, 2013), which can also have PSP-like features, PSP represents the third most common cause of parkinsonism, but it is still a relatively rare disease, with prevalence estimates ranging from 1.39 to 6.4 per 100,000. Men are affected more often than women.

The diagnosis of PSP is made based on clinical criteria (Höglinger et al., 2017; Stamelou et al., 2013). PSP typically begins with a gait disorder and falling in the sixth to seventh decades of life. Patients develop an akinetic rigid state with symmetrical signs and prominent axial rigidity. In contrast to the flexed posture of patients with PD, those with PSP may have an extended trunk or retrocolic neck posture. A characteristic facial appearance features a wide-eyed stare, furrowing of the forehead with frowning expression ("procerus sign"), and deepening of other facial creases, allowing experienced clinicians to make an instant diagnosis (Fig. 96.12; see also Videos 96.7–96.11). Pseudobulbar palsy with dysarthria and dysphagia lend the patient a characteristic dysarthria with spasticity, hypokinesia, and ataxia and often "silent" aspiration. Frontal lobe features are common. There is striking executive dysfunction early in the disease course; concrete thought, difficulty shifting set, decreased verbal fluency, and personality changes such as impulsivity and poor judgment are nearly universal. One of the characteristic, although not specific signs of PSP is the applause sign, which is manifested by persistence of applauding by the patient beyond the number of claps performed by the examiner. This is highly correlated with impairments in executive, visuospatial, and language function as well as measures of disease severity (Schönecker et al., 2019). A progressive apathetic state ensues, but true dementia may not be prominent until the advanced stages of the disease. The presence of square wave jerks should suggest the diagnosis of PSP, although this neuro-ophthalmological sign may also be observed, but much less frequently, in other parkinsonian disorders (Waln and Jankovic, 2018). Abnormal vertical saccades, best demonstrated by examination for opticokinetic nystagmus, compared to horizontal saccades, is one of the earliest ophthalmological signs of PSP. Typically, the vertical saccades are more impaired when the opticokinetic tape moves in an upward rather than downward direction. Electro-oculographic recordings in PSP show decreased amplitude and normal latency of horizontal saccadic eye movements. Although considered a clinical hallmark of PSP, supranuclear vertical gaze palsy may not appear until later in the disease course, and some patients may never develop gaze palsy. Another neuro-ophthalmological sign in PSP is blepharospasm with or without apraxia of eyelid opening (Waln and Jankovic, 2018).

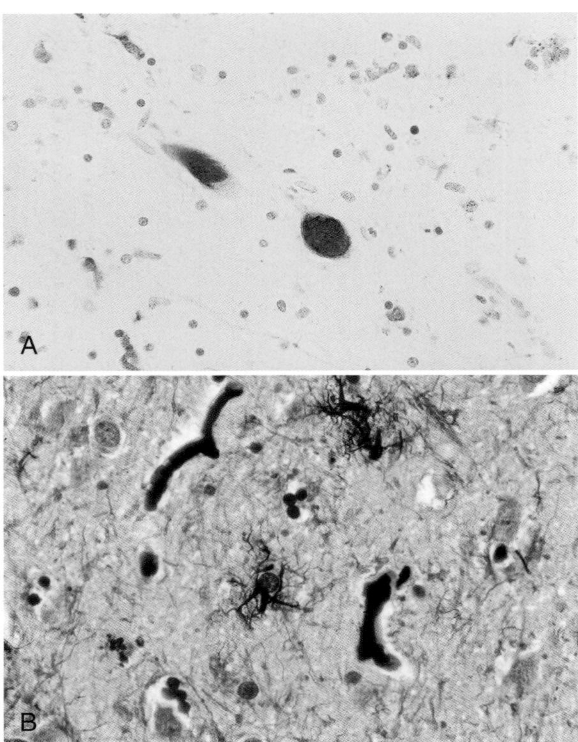


**Fig. 96.13** Globose neurofibrillary tangle and tufted astrocytes in progressive supranuclear palsy (PSP). **A,** Tau-immunostained globose neurofibrillary tangles in neurons of globus pallidus. **B,** Gallyas silver-stained tufted astrocytes in globus pallidus of patient with PSP.

In contrast to PD, patients with PSP tend to have a more broad-based gait with knee extension, and instead of turning en bloc they tend to pivot on their toes and sometimes even cross their legs, which contributes to frequent falls (Jankovic, 2015a). Atypical presentations are often seen, especially pure akinesia manifested by severe motor blocks while walking (freezing). PSP is rapidly progressive; by the fourth year of illness, half of patients need assistance for walking and have troublesome dysarthria and visual symptoms. Dysphagia becomes prominent shortly thereafter.

There are no diagnostic tests for PSP, but elevated serum and CSF levels of NFL have been found in patients with PSP compared to those with PD (Marques et al., 2019). Although not diagnostic, NFL can serve as a possible biomarker. Typical MRI signs of PSP include midbrain atrophy, increased signal in the midbrain and GP, atrophy or increased signal in the red nucleus, third ventricle dilation, and atrophy of the frontal or temporal lobes. On the midsagittal view of the MRI, as a result of atrophy of the rostral midbrain tegmentum, the most rostral midbrain, the midbrain tegmentum, the pontine base, and the cerebellum appear to correspond to the bill, head, body, and wing, respectively, of a hummingbird or a penguin.

At autopsy, the midbrain in PSP is atrophied, and the sylvian aqueduct is dilated. The SN is depigmented and appears orange and shrunken. The locus coeruleus may also show some depigmentation, but this is less prominent than in idiopathic PD. Other structures may also show atrophy, most notably the frontal lobe, STN, and superior cerebellar peduncle. Histopathologically, the degenerative process involves mainly the basal ganglia, diencephalons, and brainstem. Pathological findings include neuronal loss, gliosis, neurofibrillary tangles, and granulovacuolar degeneration in neurons of the brainstem. There are tufted astrocytes in the motor cortex and the striatum, and the typical neuronal lesion is the globose neurofibrillary tangle, made up of hyperphosphorylated four-repeat tau protein filaments (Fig. 96.13).

On the basis of an analysis of 103 pathologically confirmed consecutive cases of PSP, PSP was divided into two categories: *Richardson syndrome*, characterized by the typical features described in the original report, and *PSP-P*, in which the clinical features overlap with PD and the course is more benign (Williams and Lees, 2009). The latter group, representing about a quarter of all patients with PSP, has less tau pathology than the classic Richardson syndrome. The mean 4R-tau/3R-tau ratio of the isoform composition of insoluble tangle-tau isolated from the pons was significantly higher in Richardson syndrome (2.84) than in PSP-P syndrome (1.63).

PSP almost always occurs sporadically, yet an increasing number of familial cases suggests a genetic etiology in some cases. Pedigrees with apparent dominant and recessive inheritance have been described. Affected families may show phenotypical heterogeneity, with some affected persons showing dementia, dystonia, gait disorder, or tics. Mutations in the tau gene have been reported in patients with a familial PSP-like illness, but these have been quite rare, and mutations are not believed responsible for most PSP cases. However, patients with PSP are homozygous for a common haplotype that contains a normally occurring polymorphism in the tau intron immediately preceding exon 10. There is growing support for the notion of altered regulation of tau gene expression in PSP. Genetic polymorphisms are increasingly being identified, some of which might increase risk for PSP via effects on tau. No toxic, viral, or other environmental risk factors have been described.

Dopaminergic agents, particularly LD, may provide temporary improvement in bradykinesia in approximately 40% of patients, but LD usually does not improve dysarthria, gait, or balance problems. No other drug has been shown to provide any meaningful improvement in symptoms of PSP. A randomized placebo-controlled trial of donepezil showed modest cognitive improvements but poor tolerability. Amitriptyline may be helpful in improving pseudobulbar affect and emotional incontinence. Botulinum toxin injections may be useful to treat blepharospasm or retrocolic neck posture in PSP. The prognosis of PSP is poor, with serious impact on quality of life and a median duration of survival of approximately 8 years. It is possible that future strategies targeting toxic tau, currently investigated in other tauopathies, may also exert disease-modifying effects in PSP.

## Corticobasal Degeneration

In 1967, Rebeiz and colleagues described three patients with akinetic rigidity, apraxia, dystonia, tremor, and aphasia, who at autopsy had pale achromatic ballooned neurons similar to those seen in Pick disease. The condition was named *corticodentatonigral degeneration with neuronal achromasia* in 1989 but has since become known simply as *corticobasal degeneration*. Although CBD generally brings to mind a particular motor syndrome of asymmetrical rigidity, apraxia, and cortical sensory dysfunction, its underlying pathological features may be seen in other clinical syndromes including PSP, progressive aphasia, and FTDP. One study based on 35 cases from the Queen Square Brain Bank, in which there were 21 clinically diagnosed cases of CBS and 19 pathologically diagnosed with CBD, was designed to address the clinical and pathological overlap between CBD and PSP (Ling et al., 2010). Of 19 pathologically confirmed CBD cases, only five had been diagnosed correctly in life (sensitivity =26.3%). All had a unilateral presentation, a clumsy useless limb, limb apraxia, and myoclonus; four had cortical sensory impairment and focal limb dystonia, and three had an alien limb. Eight cases of CBD had been clinically diagnosed as PSP, all of whom had vertical supranuclear palsy, and seven had falls within the first 2 years. Of 21 cases with CBS, only five had CBD (positive predictive value = 23.8%); six others had PSP pathology, five had AD, and the remaining five had other non-tau pathologies. Forty-two percent of CBD cases presented clinically with a PSP phenotype, and 29% of CBS cases had underlying PSP pathology. The authors suggested the CBD-Richardson syndrome for the overlap cases and concluded that CBD "is a discrete clinico-pathological entity but with a broader clinical spectrum than was originally proposed" (Ling et al., 2010).

CBD is one of the least common and most asymmetrical forms of atypical parkinsonism (Stamelou et al., 2013). The mean age at onset is 60–64 years. In its most recognizable form, it is predominantly a motor disease, but its presentation is clinically heterogeneous. In addition to parkinsonism with strikingly asymmetrical rigidity, CBD patients often exhibit asymmetrical dystonia, myoclonus, apraxia, alien limb, and cortical sensory loss. They may also present with primary progressive aphasia and may evolve into global dementia (see Videos 96.13–96.16) (Lee et al., 2011).

Patients with CBS have asymmetrical and often focal cortical atrophy on MRI, with widening of the sylvian and interhemispheric fissures and dilation of frontal, parietal, and temporal sulci (Josephs, 2017). Fluorodeoxyglucose PET scans show asymmetrical hypometabolism in the thalamus and motor cortex. SPECT scans show marked asymmetry of cortical blood flow.

At autopsy, patients with a clinical syndrome consistent with CBD have gross brain atrophy. Typical microscopic changes are tau-positive neuronal and glial lesions, especially gray and white matter astrocytic plaques and threadlike lesions, and neuronal loss in the cortex and SN. The inclusions are formed of hyperphosphorylated four-repeat tau. Overlap with other conditions including AD, PSP, PD, FTDP, and hippocampal sclerosis is common (Ling et al., 2010).

As with other tauopathies, the etiology of CBD is unknown. There are no familial forms of the illness, and no mutations in the tau gene have been identified. There is clinical and pathological overlap with other tauopathies, and patients with CBD share a similar tau haplotype with patients with PSP.

There is no treatment for the degenerative process. Parkinsonian features do not seem to respond to LD or other dopaminergic drugs. Benzodiazepines, particularly clonazepam, may help myoclonus. Botulinum toxin injections may improve focal dystonia early in the disease and help relieve pain and facilitate care in advanced disease. The prognosis is poor, with a reported median survival after onset of about 7 years.

## Dementia with Lewy Bodies

DLB is the second most prevalent degenerative dementia after AD. In one study, among 542 incident cases of parkinsonism, 64 had DLB and 46 had PD dementia (PDD); the pathology was consistent with the clinical diagnosis in 24 of 31 patients (77.4%) who underwent autopsy (Savica et al., 2013). DLB is a progressive dementia characterized especially by fluctuating cognitive impairment, prominent disruption of attention and visuospatial abilities, visual hallucinations, and parkinsonism (see Video 96.5). RBD and depression are also very common. These behavioral symptoms are typically present at least 1 year prior to the onset of motor (parkinsonian) features (McKeith et al., 2017). Patients with DLB are extremely sensitive to dopamine receptor antagonists and experience severe parkinsonism when treated with neuroleptics.

Characteristic pathological changes include cortical and brainstem (SN) Lewy bodies. Spongiform changes, neurofibrillary tangles, and dystrophic Lewy neuritis may also be seen, and overlap with AD is considerable. Treatment of DLB is difficult but medications used in the treatment of both PD and dementia are often employed here. Although antiparkinsonian agents are used to treat parkinsonian signs, the degree of sensitivity of parkinsonian signs to dopaminergic therapy has not been well defined. Psychiatric and behavioral symptoms may improve with atypical antipsychotics, and cholinesterase inhibitors such as rivastigmine may improve delusions and hallucinations.

*PD dementia* is defined as cognitive impairment that includes cognitive and motor slowing, executive dysfunction, and impaired memory retrieval. The relationship of PDD to AD and other dementing disorders such as DLB has not yet been well defined. Although some investigators suggest that clear clinicopathological separation is possible between the three disorders, the differences in neuropathological and neurochemical characteristics suggest that there is a continuum.

## Frontotemporal Degeneration with Parkinsonism

Frontotemporal degeneration is a group of disorders characterized by behavioral changes and neuropsychological evidence of frontal lobe dysfunction. They include PSP, CBD, Pick disease, pallidopontonigral degeneration, disinhibition-dementia-parkinsonism-amyotrophy, familial multiple system tauopathy with presenile dementia, familial subcortical gliosis, FTD, FTD with ALS, FTD with inclusion body myopathy, and FTDP-17. In up to 60% of patients with FTD, there is a positive family history. Genetic loci on chromosomes 17 (FTDP-17), 9 (FTD with ALS; FTD with inclusion body myositis), and 3 (FTD) have been described. The prototype of FTDP is an inherited parkinsonism-dementia disorder, initially described as *Wilhelmsen-Lynch disease* (disinhibition-dementia-parkinsonism-amyotrophy complex) and subsequently found to be due to mutations in the tau gene on chromosome 17q21. Although tau mutations account for many of these diseases, similar phenotypes have been attributed to mutations in other genes such as p97 (also known as *valosin-containing protein*) on chromosome 9p21-p12, CHMP2B (charged multivesicular body protein 2B) on the pericentromeric region of chromosome 3, and progranulin (PGRN) on chromosome 17q21 (1.5 Mb centromeric of tau). Plasma and CSF levels of progranulin have been found to be reduced nearly fourfold in affected and unaffected subjects with PGRN mutations, and low (75% reduction) plasma progranulin levels may be used as a screening tool for PGRN mutations.

There is considerable phenotypical, genotypical, and pathological heterogeneity in FTDP (Spillantini and Goedert, 2013). The disorder most often begins in the 50s or 60s with personality and behavioral changes that include disinhibition and aggressiveness as well as frontal executive dysfunction. Other common signs include social misconduct, stereotyped verbalizations, impaired recent memory, and parkinsonism. Some families present with early parkinsonism. Many mutations have been reported in the tau gene. They comprise mainly three groups: mutations in the coding region for a microtubule-binding domain, resulting in a dysfunctional protein; mutations outside the microtubule-binding domains; and mutations that alter the ratio of three- to four-repeat tau isoforms. Pathological findings include tau-positive neuronal and glial inclusions distributed variably throughout the brain. In patients with prominent parkinsonism, there is severe neuronal loss in the SN. The response of parkinsonism to symptomatic treatment is not known. The prognosis is poor, with death occurring within 10 years.

## Parkinsonism-Dementia Complex of Guam

A high incidence of an ALS-like illness among the Chamorros, indigenous people of Guam, was noticed more than 50 years ago. In the same population, a smaller number of people had a syndrome of parkinsonism with dementia, the parkinsonism-dementia complex (PDC). Some had both motor neuron disease and PDC. Early in its course, PDC appears variably like PD, atypical parkinsonism, or PSP; however, in the end stages, it most resembles PSP. Familial aggregation of cases has been noted, but prior attempts to elucidate a hereditary basis to the illness proved fruitless. A similar constellation of ALS and PDC has been reported on the Kii peninsula of Japan.

Pathologically, the disorder is characterized by neuronal degeneration and abundant neurofibrillary tangles in the brain and spinal cord. A recent reanalysis of a patient registry suggests that both the spouses and the offspring of persons with PDC have a significantly higher risk of themselves developing ALS-PDC, suggesting both environmental and genetic risk factors. The critical age for exposure to the environmental factor was adolescence or early adulthood. Despite extensive analysis of the diet and other environmental factors, the etiology of PDC of Guam remains unknown, although neurotoxic damage from the cycad nut has been implicated.

## Guadeloupean Parkinsonism

A form of atypical parkinsonism has been described in the French West Indies. The so-called Guadeloupean parkinsonism shows clinical features of LD-unresponsive parkinsonism, postural instability with early falls, and pseudobulbar palsy. More than 25% of these patients have a phenotype like that of PSP. The etiology of this form of parkinsonism is unknown, but exposure to dietary or other environmental toxins is suspected. The disease may be associated with the use of indigenous plants (*Annona muricata* [synonyms: soursop, corossol, guanabana, graviola, and sweetsop]) that contain the mitochondrial complex I and dopaminergic neuronal toxins, reticuline and coreximine.

## Vascular Parkinsonism

After PD, vascular parkinsonism is the second most common form of parkinsonism encountered in movement disorders clinics, accounting for 8% of all parkinsonian patients (Mehanna and Jankovic, 2013). Vascular changes on imaging studies are common, but the cause and effect are not always clearly established. Among stroke patients, parkinsonism is more common in patients with lacunar stroke. Adult-onset diabetes, chronic hypertension, and hyperlipidemia seem to be the most common risk factors associated with vascular parkinsonism (De Pablo-Fernandez et al., 2018). Vascular parkinsonism usually presents as "lower body parkinsonism" with a broad-based shuffling gait and prominent start and terminal hesitation, as well as freezing (see Videos 96.17 and 96.18). Postural instability and a history of falls are common. Many patients have dementia and corticospinal findings of incontinence. In a systematic review of 25 articles, patients with vascular parkinsonism were older, had a shorter duration of illness, presented with symmetrical gait difficulties, were less responsive to LD, and were more prone to postural instability, falls, and dementia (Kalra et al., 2010). Pyramidal signs, pseudobulbar palsy, and incontinence were more common in vascular parkinsonism, but tremor was not a main feature. Structural neuroimaging was abnormal in 90%–100% of vascular cases, compared to 12%–43% of PD cases. In contrast to PD, there is usually no abnormality in presynaptic striatal dopamine transporters as measured by SPECT in vascular parkinsonism.

The pathology includes subcortical vascular disease with preservation of dopaminergic cells in the SN. There is a growing body of evidence that microstructural changes of normal-appearing white matter are common in the brains of patients with vascular parkinsonism (Salsone et al., 2019; van Veluw et al., 2017).

The symptoms of vascular parkinsonism are unlikely to show a significant response to LD, but a therapeutic trial is worth pursuing because as many as half of patients improve. Physical therapy may also be useful.

### Bilateral Striatopallidodentate Calcification (Fahr Disease)

Calcification of the basal ganglia has many causes. It is an incidental finding in up to 1% of all CT brain scans. Basal ganglia calcifications can also be seen in infectious, metabolic, and genetic disorders affecting this brain region. There are familial and sporadic forms. When symptoms occur, they usually begin in adulthood between age 30 and 60 years. Cognitive dysfunction, seizures, cerebellar signs, dysarthria, pyramidal signs, psychiatric illness, gait disorder, and sensory impairment are common. About half of symptomatic patients have movement disorders. Among these, parkinsonism and chorea are most common. Fewer than 10% of patients have tremor, dystonia, athetosis, or orofacial dyskinesia. The presence of symptoms correlates with the amount of calcification. Calcification is most often seen in the GP but may also occur in the caudate, putamen, dentate, thalamus, and cerebral white matter, as well as internal capsules. Calcium is deposited in the perivascular extracellular space. Dominant and recessive inheritance patterns with many different gene mutations have been described (Deng et al., 2015). There is no specific treatment other than symptomatic management.

### Postencephalitic Parkinsonism

Between 1916 and 1927, a worldwide epidemic of encephalitis lethargica killed approximately 250,000 persons and left an additional 250,000 with chronic disability. These survivors of the acute illness developed parkinsonism, usually within 10 years of the infection. PEP resembles PD, although more prominent behavioral and sleep abnormalities occur early in the disease course, extraocular movements are often abnormal, and oculogyric crises are common. Other common movement disorders include chorea, dystonia, tics, and myoclonus. Pyramidal tract signs are common. The pathological appearance of PEP includes degeneration of SN neurons, with neurofibrillary tangles in surviving neurons. Although the etiology is presumed to be a virus, none has ever been identified. There have been no subsequent epidemics of encephalitis lethargica, although sporadic cases of PEP are occasionally reported. The symptoms of PEP tend to be responsive to LD, but behavioral complications such as hallucinations and delusions are common, limiting therapy.

### Drug-Induced Parkinsonism

Dopamine receptor-blocking drugs reproduce the major clinical features of PD, although signs are usually symmetrical, and the tremor is more often present during posture holding than at rest (Savitt and Jankovic, 2018; Ward and Citrome, 2018). The most common causes of DIP are the typical neuroleptic antipsychotic drugs, antidopaminergic antiemetics, and drugs that deplete presynaptic nerve terminals of dopamine, such as reserpine, tetrabenazine, deutetrabenazine, and valbenazine. Despite the marketing efforts by the drug manufacturers to minimize the risk of tardive dyskinesia (TD) with the atypical (third-generation) neuroleptics, all these drugs have been reported to cause TD. Among the newer, or atypical, antipsychotics, the relative propensity to cause DIP is as follows: risperidone = ziprasidone > olanzapine > quetiapine > clozapine. This ranking reflects their respective affinity for the $D_2$ receptor. A number of other drugs have been associated with DIP: aripiprazole and other new atypical neuroleptics (Peña et al., 2011), selective serotonin reuptake inhibitors, lithium, phenytoin, methyldopa, valproic acid, and the calcium channel antagonists flunarizine and cinnarizine, which are not marketed in the United States. DIP generally appears subacutely after weeks to months of therapy. Although it is reversible, DIP may resolve very slowly over a period of up to 6 months, and symptomatic treatment with anticholinergics, amantadine, or LD may be required. Occasionally, parkinsonism does not resolve, suggesting that the offending drug likely has unmasked an underlying parkinsonism. The use of antipsychotic medications is a strong predictor of subsequent PD and patients taking neuroleptics may be five times more likely to begin antiparkinsonian medications than nonusers. In some cases of DIP when the offending dopamine receptor blocking drug is discontinued TD may emerge (Savitt and Jankovic, 2018).

### Toxin-Induced Parkinsonism

In 1982, a number of young California drug addicts developed acute and severe parkinsonism after intravenous injection of a synthetic heroin contaminated by MPTP. Subsequent study showed that the offending toxin was the metabolic product of MPTP produced by monoamine oxidase, 1-methyl-4-phenyl-propionoxypiperidine (MPP+). Postmortem examination in patients 10 years after the original exposure showed severe loss of SN neurons without Lewy body formation. Interestingly, despite the 10-year interval between exposure to the toxin and death, there was evidence of an active neurodegenerative process that included extracellular melanin and active neuronophagia. This suggests that intracellular mechanisms may promote neurodegeneration after a distant environmental insult. MPTP-induced parkinsonism is responsive to LD, but the response is complicated by early development of motor fluctuations and dyskinesias, which may become severe, and psychiatric complications such as hallucinations. Cognitive function usually remains intact.

Acute carbon monoxide poisoning is associated with parkinsonism. MRI scans show high-intensity white-matter lesions and necrosis of the GP bilaterally. Cognitive signs including decreased short-term memory, attention, and concentration are common. Patients with neurological sequelae of carbon monoxide intoxication may experience gradual clinical and radiological improvement over months to years.

Manganese toxicity is associated with LD-unresponsive symmetrical parkinsonism with dystonic features such as oculogyric crisis. The disorder may progress for years after cessation of exposure (Jankovic, 2005). Striatal MRI T2-weighted hyperintensity may be present during the acute phase of poisoning. F-dopa PET scans in subjects with manganism show normal presynaptic dopamine function, suggesting postsynaptic pathology. The fungicide maneb (manganese ethylene-bis-dithiocarbamate) has also been shown to induce a toxic parkinsonism.

## TREMOR

### Physiological Tremor

A fine tremor of the outstretched limbs is a universal finding. Physiological tremor appears to originate in the heartbeat, mechanical properties of the limbs, firing of motoneurons, and synchronization of spindle feedback. Its frequency ranges from 7 to 12 Hz. It is usually not noticeable except with electrophysiological recording, but its amplitude is accentuated by fatigue, anxiety, fear, excitement, stimulant use, and medical conditions such as hyperthyroidism (Box 96.3).

### Essential Tremor

#### Epidemiology and Clinical Features

ET is one of the most common movement disorders. In population-based studies, the prevalence increases steadily with age,

**BOX 96.3 Physiological Classification of Tremor**

**Mechanical Oscillations**
Physiological tremor

**Oscillations Based on Reflexes**
Neuropathic tremor

**Oscillations Due to Central Neuronal Pacemakers**
Palatal tremor
Essential tremor
Orthostatic tremor
Parkinsonian rest tremor
Holmes tremor

**Oscillations Due to Disturbances in Feed-Forward/ Feedback Loops**
Cerebellar tremor
Holmes tremor

occurring in up to 10% of patients older than 60 years of age. Meta-analysis of epidemiological studies has found the prevalence of ET to range between 0.01% and 20.5%, but the pooled prevalence is 0.9% (Louis and Ferreira, 2010). In its purest form, ET is a monosymptomatic illness characterized by gradually increasing-amplitude postural and kinetic tremor of the forearms and hands (with or without involvement of other body parts) in the absence of endogenous or exogenous triggers or other neurological signs. In clinic-based series, as many as 50% of patients exhibiting ET do not conform to this clinical picture, suggesting substantial heterogeneity and an overlap in some cases with dystonia and parkinsonism (Fekete and Jankovic, 2011). The clinical definition of ET is problematic because there are no pathological, biochemical, genetic, or other established and validated diagnostic criteria. The Movement Disorders Society issued a "consensus statement" on classification of tremors (Bhatia et al., 2018). It defined ET as isolated tremor syndrome of bilateral upper limb action tremor at least 3 years' duration with or without tremor in other locations (e.g., head, voice, or lower limbs), absence of other neurological signs, such as dystonia, ataxia, or parkinsonism. They acknowledged that patients frequently have a family history, of tremors and small doses of alcohol may improve the tremor, but they felt that these clinical features are not consistent enough to be included in the definition of ET. They also introduced the term "ET-Plus," a new tentatively and uncertainly defined entity characterized by the presence of additional neurological signs other than action tremor. This has engendered much controversy, and many believe that ET-Plus is more common than ET.

There seems to be a bimodal distribution for age at onset, peaking in the 2nd and 6th decade of life. The typical patient becomes aware of a barely perceptible postural or action tremor, usually in the distal arms and hands. The head and lower limbs are less commonly affected. Head tremor (titubation) is milder than limb tremor and is predominantly of a side-to-side, "no-no" type. Head tremor is often associated with cervical dystonia and some patients with head tremor merely have dystonic tremor as a manifestation of their cervical dystonia without associated ET (Merola et al., 2019). Tremor of the face, trunk, and voice may also be present in patients with ET. The kinetic tremor is typically higher in amplitude than the postural tremor (Fig. 96.14). In contrast to PD where the handwriting is small, the handwriting in patients with ET is tremulous.

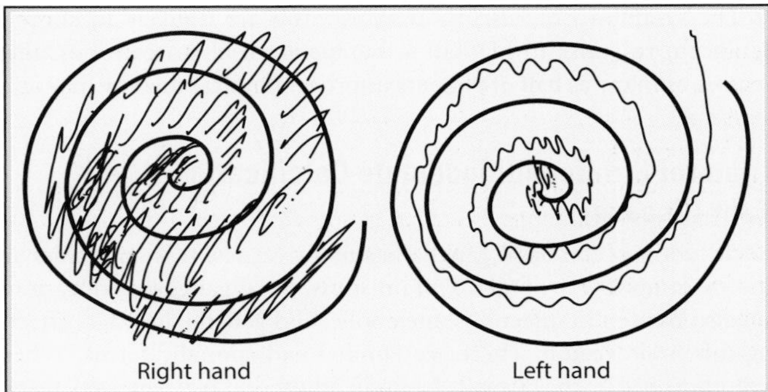

**Fig. 96.14** Writing sample from a man with asymmetrical postural and action tremor of essential tremor.

A striking improvement after ingestion of a small amount of ethanol is seen in 50% of patients and may be helpful in diagnosis (Mostile and Jankovic, 2010). Over time, the tremor worsens, causing increasing functional disability. Only a fraction of affected persons seek medical attention, and there is often a long latency from onset to presentation for care. At the time of diagnosis, nearly all patients with ET have significant social, functional, or occupational disability, and as many as 25% must make occupational adjustments as a result of tremor-related disability. ET is thought to be a monosymptomatic illness without changes in cognition, strength, coordination, or muscle tone, and the results of the neurological examination are usually normal. However, detailed studies of patients with ET have demonstrated frontostriatal cognitive deficits, changes in tandem gait, and other (albeit subtle) evidence of cerebellar dysfunction. The worsening of ET over time likely relates to two phenomena. First, the frequency of tremor in ET decreases over time, and its amplitude increases. This results from decreased attenuation of lower-frequency tremor secondary to age-related changes in the mechanical properties of limbs and muscle. A second possible contributor is true progression of the underlying disorder. According to recent studies, the severity of ET relates to disease duration independent of aging and age-related changes in mechanical properties of the muscles and limbs.

The diagnosis of ET is made by history and physical examination. A tremor rating scale known as *The Essential Tremor Rating Assessment Scale* (TETRAS) has been developed by the Tremor Research Group to assess ET and has been found to correlate well with quantitative assessments using the kinesia system (Mostile et al., 2010).

## Etiology

As many as two-thirds of patients give a positive family history of tremor, and first-degree relatives of patients with ET are 5–10 times more likely to have ET than first-degree relatives of control subjects. Direct questioning or examination of first-degree relatives increases the yield of family history to as high as 96%. In some families, pedigree analysis suggests ET is an autosomal dominant trait, with virtually complete penetrance by age 50 years. Twin studies suggest both hereditary and environmental factors are important in disease expression. Hereditary ET is genetically heterogeneous, with several described loci including ETM1 (FET1) on chromosome 3, ETM2 on chromosome 2, a $D_3$ receptor gene (DRD3) localized on 3q13.3, and a locus on chromosome 6p23 (Kuhlenbäumer et al., 2014). One study involving a North American population demonstrated a significant association between a LINGO1 variant and ET, but further studies are needed before this association can be confirmed (Deng et al., 2019).

The mechanism of disease production in these genetic disorders remains unknown, and no consistent pathological structural changes have been found in postmortem brain or nervous tissue, although cerebellar degeneration and Lewy bodies have been found in a few autopsied brains (Fekete and Jankovic, 2011; Louis et al., 2013). A number of lines of evidence point to cerebellar dysfunction in ET; abnormal tandem gait is one example. The tremor may resolve following ipsilateral cerebellar lesions. Motor control studies show evidence of abnormal production of ballistic movements in a pattern that suggests abnormalities in cerebellar timing. PET scans have shown evidence of bilaterally increased cerebellar activity at rest and during tremor. The demonstration of reduced *N*-acetyl-L-aspartate (NAA) relative to total creatine in the cerebellar cortex by magnetic resonance spectroscopy (MRS) suggests that the cerebellar disorder may be degenerative.

### Treatment

Patients with mild ET whose main source of disability is tremor during meals and whose tremors respond to ethanol often benefit from a cocktail before meals. The two most commonly used pharmacological treatments are β-adrenergic blockers and primidone. Placebo-controlled studies have shown that β-adrenergic blockers (e.g., 120–320 mg of propranolol per day) reduce tremor amplitude in 40%–50% of patients. Common side effects of these beta-blocker drugs include bradycardia, fatigue, nausea, diarrhea, rash, impotence, and depression. Beta-blockers are contraindicated in patients with congestive heart failure, asthma, third-degree atrioventricular block, and diabetes. Primidone improves ET about 50% in short-term controlled trials and has been suggested to be more effective for head tremor than other agents. Because of the risk of acute side effects such as vertigo, nausea, and unsteadiness, primidone is usually started at a dose of 25 mg at bedtime and then titrated as tolerated to its effective dose range of 50–350 mg daily. It can be given as a single nighttime dose or in divided-dose increments. Long-term primidone therapy is usually well tolerated. Propranolol and primidone combination therapy may be more effective than either agent alone. A double-blind placebo-controlled study of topiramate found that this antiepileptic drug may reduce ET. Other drugs such as alprazolam, gabapentin, pregabalin, clonazepam, acetazolamide, and nimodipine may also provide benefit in some patients with ET. Botulinum toxin injection in the wrist flexors in patients with prominent hand tremor and into cervical muscles in patients with head tremor provided a meaningful reduction in the amplitude of the tremor for about 3–4 months after each injection (Mittal et al., 2019a; Niemann and Jankovic, 2018). The pipeline of experimental therapeutics is beginning to expand and includes various tremor suppression devices, peripheral nerve stimulation and drugs that modulate GABA type A receptors and calcium-activated potassium channels, and Cav3 T-type calcium channel blockers.

Thalamic DBS has been reported to suppress contralateral tremor as much as 75% in up to 90% of cases, and bilateral stimulation can be performed safely with long-lasting benefits, although dysarthria and gait and balance problems may occur, particularly with bilateral stimulation (see Video 96.19) (Baizabal-Carvallo et al., 2014). Adverse effects are relatively rare and may include intracranial hematoma, postoperative seizures, dysarthria, paresthesia, dysequilibrium, headaches, dyspraxia, and word-finding difficulty. Problems with the stimulator itself are relatively uncommon but include lead fracture or migration and failure of the impulse generator. Reoperation may be necessary to correct device-related adverse effects. DBS should be considered for cognitively intact, otherwise healthy patients with disabling medication-resistant tremor. Unilateral focused ultrasound thalamotomy was evaluated in 27 patients with troublesome ET, who were randomized (2:1) to compare this with sham procedures (Bond et al., 2017). Using the Clinical Rating Scale for Tremor (CRST) as the primary endpoint along with several secondary outcomes the on-medication median tremor scores improved 62% after active treatment and 22% after sham procedures ($P = .04$).

### Primary Writing Tremor

Primary writing tremor is a rare condition characterized by a 4- to 7-Hz tremor in the hand while assuming a writing posture or during the writing task itself. Most patients are men. About one-third have a positive family history of writing tremor, and a similar number give a history of improvement after ethanol ingestion. Surface EMG shows isolated extensor tremor, alternating tremor in flexors and extensors, or co-contraction of flexors and extensors. Writing tremor may be difficult to distinguish clinically from ET and from task-specific or writing dystonia. Primary writing tremor is not usually associated with the phenomenon of overflow, typically seen in dystonia, and electrophysiological studies suggest it is distinct from both conditions. Accelerometry suggests that the primary writing tremor reflects the normal rhythmic movement of writing, but the amplitude of the movements is enhanced. The tremor may respond to β-adrenergic blockade or primidone or anticholinergic medications, but botulinum toxin injections provide the most benefit. Thalamic DBS has also been reported effective in some cases.

### Orthostatic Tremor

Orthostatic tremor consists of a high-frequency (14–18 Hz) isometric tremor in the legs during standing (see Video 96.21) (Yaltho and Ondo, 2014). Patients may not be aware of the tremor but complain of unsteadiness and vibration or discomfort in the legs that are relieved by leaning against a stationary object, by walking, or by sitting down. Leaning on the arms may precipitate a similar frequency tremor in the arms, and a tremor of the closed jaw has also been reported. Orthostatic tremor may be visible or palpable and can be confirmed by the appearance on EMG of high-frequency tremor when standing. Unlike parkinsonian tremors and ETs, orthostatic tremor shows significant side-to-side coherence, suggesting a central generator. PET scans have shown increased resting cerebellar activity similar to that seen in ET. A recent study has suggested that coherent high-frequency tremor in the legs may be a normal response to perceived unsteadiness when standing still, and that orthostatic tremor may be an exaggeration of this response. Clonazepam is thought to be the most effective pharmacological treatment, although there are reports of benefit from LD and gabapentin.

### Neuropathic Tremor

Tremors associated with neuropathy are usually postural and kinetic tremors with a frequency between 3 and 6 cycles per second. Demyelinating neuropathies have a particular association with tremor. The diagnosis is made when a typical tremor affects a person with neuropathy in the absence of other tremorgenic neurological disorders. The pathophysiology of neuropathic tremor is believed to be disordered feedback control related to abnormal peripheral sensory input. Some patients develop tremor after a peripheral injury, sometimes associated with abnormal posture as well as reflex sympathetic dystrophy or complex regional pain syndrome. The mechanism of this peripherally induced movement disorder is not understood. Pharmacological treatment is usually disappointing, but some patients respond to beta-blockers or clonazepam.

### Cerebellar Tremor

The tremor typically associated with cerebellar disease is a slow tremor that is absent during rest but appears and progressively increases in amplitude with movement, particularly with fine adjustments required for a precise movement. Sitting or standing unsupported may induce a tremor of the trunk and head (titubation). A variant of cerebellar outflow tremor is known as *Holmes tremor*, or *rubral tremor* (Raina et al., 2016). This tremor is present during rest, posture holding, and action. At rest, it is slower and less rhythmic than parkinsonian rest tremor. Holmes tremor results from acquired structural lesions in the ipsilateral cerebellar dentate nucleus and superior cerebellar peduncle. The usual causes are multiple sclerosis, stroke, and head injury. Pharmacological treatment of Holmes tremor is difficult, although some patients respond to LD. Thalamotomy or thalamic DBS may be useful in some cases (Oliveria et al., 2017) (see Video 96.20).

### Hereditary Geniospasm (Chin Tremor)

Hereditary geniospasm is characterized by involuntary vertical movement of the tip of the chin with quivering and mouth movements. Geniospasm may be spontaneous or stress induced. Trembling becomes apparent in infancy or early life. Trembling episodes last minutes. The attacks become somewhat less frequent with age. The disorder is genetically heterogeneous, with linkage to chromosome 9q13-21 in some but not all families. Geniospasm has been suggested to be a form of hereditary essential myoclonus (EM).

### Fragile X Premutation

Male carriers of the fragile X premutation have been found to have a neurodegenerative syndrome characterized by the onset after age 50 years of kinetic tremor, gait ataxia, executive cognitive dysfunction, parkinsonism, dysautonomia, erectile dysfunction, and peripheral neuropathy (Hagerman and Hagerman, 2013). Daughters of the patients often have ovarian failure. Bilateral cerebellar hyperintensities have been reported on T2-weighted MRI studies in some cases. Overexpression and CNS toxicity of the fragile X mental retardation 1 gene (FMR1) messenger ribonucleic acid (mRNA) has been thought to cause this fragile X-associated tremor/ataxia syndrome (FXTAS).

There are other, more unusual tremors that physicians should be able to recognize but their discussion is beyond the scope of this chapter (Ure et al., 2016). Functional (psychogenic) tremors are discussed below.

## CHOREA

### Huntington Disease

The first complete description of HD is attributed to George Huntington in 1872. He accurately reported the salient clinical features of the disease, its pattern of transmission from parent to child, and its dismal prognosis. HD is a highly penetrant autosomal dominant disease characterized by a progressive movement disorder associated with psychiatric and cognitive decline, culminating in a terminal state of dementia and immobility (Testa and Jankovic, 2019).

#### Epidemiology

Prevalence figures for HD vary depending on the geographical area, but the best estimate is 10 per 100,000. The disorder is reported in all races, although it is much more common in Scotland and Venezuela and less common in Finland, China, Japan, and Black South Africans. HD usually begins between the ages of 30 and 55 years, although it has been reported to begin as early as age 2 and as late as age 92. Approximately 5% of cases begin in patients younger than 21 years; the juvenile phenotype differs from the adult phenotype, and patients are often misdiagnosed. HD is a progressive degenerative disease that affects movement, behavior, and cognitive function.

#### Clinical Features

When clinical illness begins, it does so gradually, and it is best to define a "zone" rather than a time of onset. Patients with HD may present with motor signs, particularly chorea (about 60%), with behavioral signs (about 15%), or with both motor and behavioral signs (about 25%). Patients themselves may be unaware or unconcerned about early cognitive and motor changes. Concerned family members often bring them to medical attention. A change in the ability to generate saccadic eye movements and their speed is often the earliest sign. Eventually, a blink or head thrust may be required to initiate saccadic eye movements. The motor disorder usually begins with clumsiness and fidgetiness that evolves into chorea. The presence and severity of chorea vary markedly from person to person and over time. Some patients, particularly in early stages of the disease, are able to camouflage their chorea by incorporating the involuntary movements into seemingly volitional gestures such as touching their face or adjusting glasses (parakinesia). Chorea may not be recognized initially by family members or other observers. In addition to chorea, patients with HD have bradykinesia and motor impersistence, with difficulty sustaining ongoing movement. They may be unable to maintain forced eye closure, hold the mouth open, or protrude the tongue for long periods. With advancing disease, there is progression of bradykinesia, and dystonic movements appear. The chorea may become somewhat less prominent or may continue to worsen. The gait disorder of HD is complex, irregular, and dance-like, produced by a combination of chorea, parkinsonism, lapses in tone of antigravity muscles, and ataxia. The walking patient with HD resembles a marionette, lurching, swaying, dipping, and bobbing. Tandem walking becomes difficult, then impossible. Ultimately, progressive bradykinesia and intractable falls lead to the wheelchair- or bed-bound state. Dysarthria and dysphagia progressively impair communication and nutrition. Most patients spend the last several years of their lives in nursing home settings and die of complications such as pneumonia and head injury. Mean survival is 17 years, but the natural history varies and is influenced by genetic and environmental factors. Generally, patients with onset at a younger age have the largest number of CAG repeats and tend to progress more rapidly than patients with onset at an older age. The juvenile HD differs from the adult phenotype, with prominent parkinsonism and dystonia, even early in the course, and with myoclonus, seizures, and cognitive decline.

Behavioral changes contribute mightily to disability in HD; 98% of patients show one or more behavioral symptoms. The most common changes in early disease are irritability, anxiety, and mood disturbance. Irritability may be accompanied by verbal or physical aggression. Patients with HD often have a low threshold for anger and react to minimal provocation with an explosive response. Depressed mood is very common; 30% of patients meet criteria for major depressive disorder. Mania and hypomania are seen less commonly than depression. The risk of suicide is increased as much as sixfold over the general population. Unmarried and childless persons living alone, those who are depressed, and those with a family history of suicide are particularly at risk for suicide. Fear of the disease leads to an increased risk of suicide, even in first-degree relatives of affected individuals who are at autopsy found not to have inherited the mutant gene. Psychosis is rare and may be difficult to treat. Obsessive-compulsive disorder has been reported but can be difficult to differentiate from frontal lobe personality with perseveration. Apathy increases in concert with disease severity and is a nearly universal feature of advanced disease. Behavioral and psychiatric disorders may predate the onset of overt HD by as long as a decade, reflecting early pathological changes in the nonmotor areas of the striatum. Because some behavioral signs may be episodic and respond to pharmacotherapy, their severity does not progress in a linear fashion with cognitive and motor changes. Behavioral signs seem to improve in the terminal stages of the illness, but ascertainment may be hindered by the severe physical disability of such patients.

Cognitive changes are universal in HD. The dementia of HD fits the description of subcortical dementia, with disordered attention, concentration, motivation, insight, judgment, and problem solving rather than traditional cortical signs such as aphasia and apraxia. Executive dysfunction renders affected persons unable to work, drive, and manage family finances relatively early in the disease course, but prominent global dementia occurs later.

The diagnosis of HD in a patient with a typical clinical picture and a confirmed family history is straightforward. Unfortunately, the family history may be vague or it may be negative because of competitive mortality, misdiagnosis, denial, inaccurate parental information, or obfuscation. In addition, there is a small but definite new mutation rate as expansion occurs with transmission of a premutation. Although there is a broad differential diagnosis of chorea, there are few alternative causes of the fully developed syndrome. When the clinical suspicion of HD is high, the most cost-effective diagnostic procedure is genetic testing.

The direct DNA test for the CAG repeat expansion in the *huntingtin (HTT)* gene, formerly called *IT15*, which codes for the huntingtin (HTT) protein is highly sensitive and specific. A repeat CAG expansion length of 37 and longer is considered pathogenic, resulting in motor, cognitive, and neuropsychiatric manifestations of HD. CAG repeat lengths between 27 and 36 are considered to be intermediate in range, with some risk of expansion into the disease range during meiosis and manifested by typical HD in subsequent generations. Traditionally, these intermediate CAG repeat lengths have not been associated with clinical disease, but there has been a growing number of reports of patients with clinical (and neuropathological) evidence of HD who possess CAG repeats in the intermediate range (Savitt and Jankovic, 2019b).

The availability of the HD genetic test makes possible the identification of mutant gene carriers long before they become symptomatic. However, because of concerns about the potential for occupational, insurance, and social discrimination and the lack of neuroprotective treatment interventions, only a minority of eligible at-risk subjects pursue testing. This, however, may change as potential disease-modifying therapies are being developed (see below). Those who pursue testing do so either to help with reproductive choices or because their uncertainty about the future is unbearable. Women are more likely to request presymptomatic testing than men at equal risk. Although prenatal testing is also available, relatively few prenatal tests have been performed. Interested researchers working in concert with lay organizations have outlined principles that guide clinicians in the preparation of potential gene carriers for predictive genetic testing. These guidelines discourage genetic testing in asymptomatic minors and recommend genetic and psychological counseling before and after testing (Migliore et al., 2019). One obvious concern is the risk that once given a positive genetic test result, the patient may have a major depression or other psychopathology or may attempt suicide. When carefully managed, presymptomatic test programs are safe. In studies of life events after gene-carrier detection, less than 1% of patients have a potentially severe adverse outcome such as attempted or completed suicide or hospitalization for psychiatric illness. Adverse outcomes may be seen in patients whose predictive test suggests they are not gene carriers, the "survivor guilt" phenomenon. Depressive symptoms in such patients tend to become apparent several months after the testing process is completed. A premorbid history of depression increases the risk of an adverse outcome of testing irrespective of test results, confirming the need for careful screening and counseling in genetic testing programs.

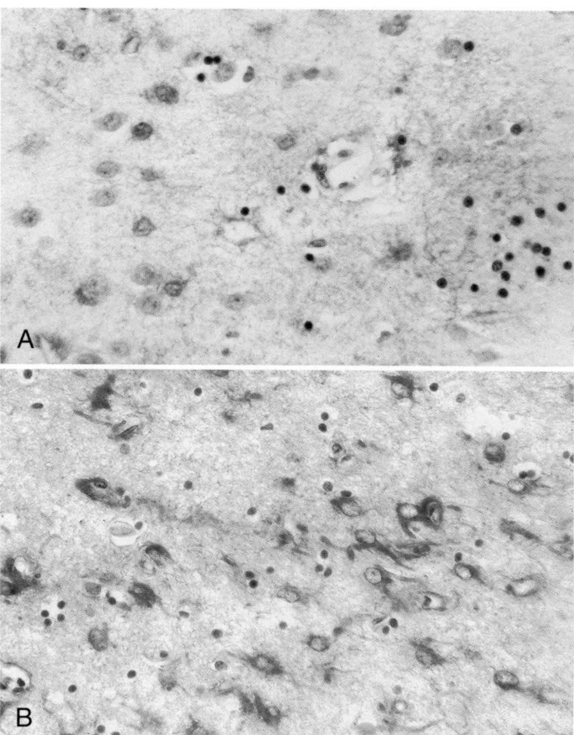


**Fig. 96.15 Pathology of Huntington Disease. A,** Glial fibrillary acidic protein immunostain of caudate nucleus of normal brain. **B,** Glial fibrillary acidic protein immunostain of caudate nucleus of patient with Huntington chorea. Note decreased neuronal density and marked reactive astrocytosis compared to normal brain. *(Courtesy Elizabeth Cochran, MD.)*

Neuroimaging studies can show generalized or preferential striatal atrophy, but these findings are not specific for the disorder. Although volumetric analysis of the striatum shows declining volume even in presymptomatic gene carriers, many obviously symptomatic patients do not have clinically apparent striatal atrophy. Somatosensory evoked potentials are abnormal in 94% of patients with HD, and abnormalities correlate with clinical signs of the illness. However, the usefulness of these and other electrophysiological studies for diagnosis or measuring illness progression remains unproven.

## Pathology

The pathology of HD includes prominent neuronal loss and gliosis in the caudate nucleus and putamen, along with regional and more diffuse atrophy (Fig. 96.15). At autopsy, HD brains show about 20% loss of brain weight, suggesting that the degenerative process is not confined to striatal tissues. Large cortical neurons in layer VI are also involved, as are neurons in the thalamus, SNr, superior olive, lateral tuberal nucleus of the hypothalamus, and deep cerebellar nuclei. Within the striatum, GABAergic medium spiny neurons bear the brunt of the degenerative process. Early, there is preferential loss of GABAergic neurons that co-localize enkephalin, dynorphin, and substance P. These neurons are thought to predominate in the indirect pathway, accounting for difficulties suppressing adventitious movement early in the disease course. With disease progression, all GABAergic medium spiny neurons are affected, including those in the direct pathway, explaining the emergence of parkinsonism in later disease. Juvenile-onset disease, more severe from the beginning, resembles late-stage HD with degeneration of GABAergic neurons in both pathways.

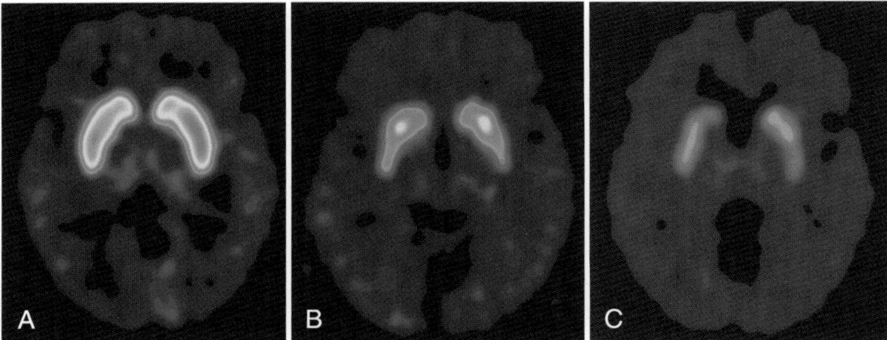


**Fig. 96.16** [$^{11}$C]-Raclopride positron emission tomography scans of **(A)** normal control subject, **(B)** asymptomatic carrier of Huntington disease (HD) gene, and **(C)** person with symptomatic HD, showing progressive loss of $D_2$-receptor-bearing striatal neurons.

## Pathogenesis

HD is a dominantly inherited condition caused by an unstable expanded CAG trinucleotide repeat in exon 1 of the *huntingtin (HTT)* gene on the tip of the short arm of chromosome 4, which codes for HTT (Testa and Jankovic, 2019). Because repeat instability of this mutation is much more common in spermatogenesis than in oogenesis, the offspring of men may have substantially greater CAG repeat lengths than their fathers. This feature accounts for the phenomenon of anticipation in HD. There is a well-documented inverse correlation between the CAG repeat length and the age at disease onset. The extreme manifestation of this relationship is the association of juvenile-onset illness with repeat lengths of 60 or greater and onset within the first decade with repeat lengths of 80 or greater. Approximately 5% of patients present before age 21 years; in nearly all cases of juvenile-onset disease, the mutant allele is inherited from the father. Likewise, very late disease presentations often are associated with repeat lengths between 36 and 41. The correlation between repeat length and age at onset is driven by a very tight relationship of these two factors at the two ends of the mutation spectrum. The repeat length, however, accounts for only about 50%–70% of the variance in age at disease onset, suggesting that other genetic or environmental factors are important. For this reason, the CAG repeat length is not a particularly useful tool for making predictions about disease onset, severity, or progression in individual patients.

HD is a true dominant condition. Homozygotes do not have an earlier onset or more severe form of the illness, suggesting the disorder results from a toxic effect of the mutant protein, a so-called gain of function (Cubo et al., 2019). The HD gene controls the synthesis of HTT, a widely expressed protein of uncertain function. HTT is a cytoplasmic protein, but ubiquitinated, mutant, proteolytic *N*-terminal huntingtin fragments form protein aggregates in the cytoplasm and nucleus of neurons. Mutant HTT interacts with a number of HTT-associated proteins and when it misfolds it can become more toxic. A number of lines of evidence point to impaired mitochondrial function in HD, including abnormalities in complex I, II, III, and IV in caudate nuclei of affected brains. PET studies show reductions in striatal glucose metabolism and loss of dopamine $D_2$ receptor-bearing neurons in the striatum (Fig. 96.16), and increased brain lactate levels. Systemic administration of the mitochondrial toxin 3-nitropropionic acid models the disease in animals. Intrastriatal administration of the excitotoxins kainate and quinolinic acid also reproduces the striatal lesions of HD. One theory that ties these animal models together is that of *indirect excitotoxicity*. Mitochondrial energy failure increases the vulnerability of the cell to excitotoxic injury because the resulting change in cell membrane potential results in loss of the magnesium ion from the NMDA receptor-associated ion channel, allowing ligand-associated depolarization of the postsynaptic receptor and excitotoxic-mediated damage. HTT may also interfere with the function of postsynaptic density protein 95, a scaffolding protein associated with NMDA and kainate receptors, rendering these glutamate receptors hypersensitive. Mutant HTT also interferes with gene transcription, leading to an alteration in cell phenotype and disrupting many cell functions. Mutant HTT may block the normal function of HTT to upregulate brain-derived neurotrophic factor. Mutant HTT likely also triggers apoptotic cell death, but its full effect on cellular function, interaction with other proteins, and how these actions lead to neurodegeneration in HD have not yet been fully elucidated.

## Treatment

As in all other neurodegenerative disorders, no treatment is yet proven to favorably influence disease progression (Schapira et al., 2014). As with other forms of neurodegeneration, many potential types of interventions might prove useful: blocking transcription of the mutant gene, enhancing chaperone function, interfering with association and aggregation of the protein, improving cell bioenergetics and mitochondrial integrity, and interfering with the triggers and ultimate steps in the process of apoptosis. Clinical trials of antioxidants designed to slow down the progression of the disease have been disappointing. One large-scale study assessed the potential neuroprotective effects of the mitochondrial complex 1 booster coenzyme $Q_{10}$ (600 mg/day), or the antiexcitotoxic agent remacemide (600 mg/day), on the decline of the total functional capacity score over 30 months. The study demonstrated a trend toward slowing the decline in this measure of disability in the coenzyme $Q_{10}$ treatment arm, but this did not achieve statistical significance. A number of other potential strategies have shown promise in transgenic disease models, although they have not been studied in human safety and efficacy trials. These include the caspase inhibitor minocycline, as well as creatine, lithium, ethyl eicosapentaenoic acid, cystamine, bile acids, and inhibitors of transglutaminase. As with other neurodegenerative diseases, there is no standard method for determining disease severity or its rate of change over time. Studies relying on clinical rating scales, such as the Unified HD Rating Scale, must be quite large and adequately powered to detect the disease-modifying effect.

One intriguing discovery in HD is that, in transgenic models, turning off the HD gene not only stops progression of the experimental illness but also reverses pathological findings, including aggregates, and is associated with clinical improvement. Apparently, continued production of the mutant protein is required for maintenance of cell dysfunction and ultimately for cell death. This argues for a period of cellular dysfunction before death and raises the possibility that neuroprotection might have the potential to at least partially reverse extant clinical features of the disease. In this regard, an antisense oligonucleotide designed to inhibit HTT messenger RNA and thereby reduce concentrations of mutant HTT has been tested in a randomized, double-blind, multiple-ascending-dose, phase 1-2a trial involving 46 patients with HD (Tabrizi et al., 2019). The intrathecal administration of 4 doses, 1 month apart, showed up to 38% reduction in the concentration of mutant HTT in CSF without any serious adverse effects. A confirmatory phase 3 trial, involving 660 patients, followed for up to 2 years is currently under way.

Treatment of HD begins with an assessment of the nature of the patient's complaints. Patients with chorea are often unaware of or untroubled by their involuntary movements (Jankovic and Roos, 2014). Although typical neuroleptics represent the conventional approach to chorea, they have been shown not to improve function in HD and are not used as much as in the past (Frank and Jankovic, 2010). Preliminary study suggests that the glutamate antagonist, amantadine, may improve chorea in HD and is well tolerated in doses up to 400 mg. Tetrabenazine and deutetrabenazine, inhibitors of the vesicular monoamine transporter 2 (VMAT2), that act by presynaptically depleting dopamine, have been approved by the US Food and Drug Administration (FDA) for the treatment of chorea associated with HD. Although similar to typical neuroleptics, these drugs may cause drowsiness, parkinsonism, depression, and akathisia; in contrast to the dopamine receptor blocking drugs, they do not cause TD (Bashir and Jankovic, 2018a). Some patients with prominent bradykinesia improve with dopaminergic therapy. Selective serotonin reuptake inhibitors seem to improve irritability, aggression, depression, and obsessive-compulsive symptoms. Irritability may respond to carbamazepine and some of the newer antiepileptic drugs. Quetiapine, an atypical antipsychotic with minimal risk for parkinsonism or TD, has been reported to be useful in patients with irritability and aggression.

## Dentatorubral-Pallidoluysian Atrophy

*Dentatorubral-pallidoluysian atrophy* is an inherited neurodegenerative disease that appears to be rare outside Japan but has been found to be relatively common in North Carolina: hence the alternative term *Haw River syndrome*. Typical symptoms of DRPLA include chorea, ataxia, myoclonic epilepsy, dystonia, parkinsonism, psychosis, and dementia. Onset is usually in the 20s, with death about 20 years later. Anticipation occurs with paternal transmission of the gene. The pathology of DRPLA includes degeneration of the dentate and red nuclei, the GP, and the STN. Neurodegeneration may also be found in the cerebral white matter, putamen, medulla oblongata, and spinal cord. Neuronal nuclear inclusions stain for ubiquitin and atrophin-1. There is also evidence for aberrant phosphorylation of the DRPLA protein complex and the nuclear membrane. DRPLA is associated with an expansion of CAG trinucleotide repeat in a gene on chromosome 12. In this region of the genome, the normal trinucleotide repeat length is 7–23. In DRPLA, the CAG repeat length is between 49 and 75. Because of the polyglutamine stretch in the mutant protein, neurodegeneration likely relates to interactions between the protein, other cellular components, and cellular proteins. The Haw River syndrome, described in a multigenerational African American family, is caused by the same repeat expansion as DRPLA. Clinical differences include lack of myoclonic epilepsy and the presence of subcortical white-matter demyelination, basal ganglia calcifications, and neuroaxonal dystrophy. No information is available about the treatment of DRPLA, but as in HD, the clinician should be guided by the nature and severity of symptoms.

## Neuroacanthocytosis and McLeod Syndrome

The term *acanthocyte* is derived from the Greek word for "thorn." Acanthocytes are contracted erythrocytes with unevenly distributed thorny projections, often with terminal bulbs. Acanthocytes are seen in peripheral blood smears in patients with three neurological syndromes: abetalipoproteinemia, neuroacanthocytosis, and McLeod syndrome (Walker et al., 2006). A broad spectrum of movement disorders is seen in neuroacanthocytosis and McLeod syndrome.

All forms of neuroacanthocytosis are rare disorders. Autosomal recessive neuroacanthocytosis is characterized by onset at around age 35 years of a progressive syndrome that includes a movement disorder and behavioral and cognitive changes. The movement disorder predominantly consists of chorea, dystonia, and tics; parkinsonism may occur in more advanced stages. There is also prominent orofacial dystonia with dystonic tongue protrusion interfering with eating. In addition, many patients exhibit lip and tongue biting and prominent dysarthria and dysphagia. Behavioral changes resemble those seen in HD: anxiety, depression, obsessive-compulsive disorder, and emotional lability. Subcortical dementia is a late feature. Seizures develop in approximately 50% of patients. There may be myopathy or axonal neuropathy, and the creatine kinase level is elevated. In patients with neuroacanthocytosis, acanthocytes usually make up 5%–20% of peripheral blood erythrocytes. Autopsy changes include atrophy of the caudate, putamen, GP, and SN, with marked neuronal loss and gliosis. The cerebral cortex is relatively spared. Mutations in the CHAC gene (recently renamed *VPS13A*) on chromosome 9 that lead to the production of chorein, a truncated protein of unknown function, have been found in this syndrome. Homologous proteins in animals seem important in intracellular trafficking.

McLeod syndrome is an X-linked recessive disorder linked to a number of mutations in the *XK* gene, a gene for the Kell group of erythrocyte membrane glycoprotein antigens on the X chromosome (Roulis et al., 2018). McLeod syndrome usually begins around age 50 and has a slowly progressive course. The most common clinical feature is an axonal peripheral neuropathy. Some patients have evidence of myopathy as well, and all have elevations in serum creatine kinase level. The CNS illness is characterized by limb chorea. Oral movements and lip and tongue biting are less common than in neuroacanthocytosis. Facial tics are common, and some patients have dystonia. Seizures may be seen. Subcortical dementia and behavioral changes occur later in the disease course in approximately 50% of patients. Cardiomyopathy and hemolytic anemia are other common manifestations. Neuroimaging studies may show caudate atrophy with secondarily enlarged lateral ventricles. Increased T2-weighted signals in the lateral putamen may be seen on MRI scans. Pathological changes include intense caudate atrophy, loss of small cells, and gliosis in the dorsolateral putamen, with less severe changes in the GP. Milder changes may be present in the thalamus, SN, and anterior horns of the spinal cord. Neurons in the cerebral cortex, STN, and cerebellum are spared. The reported mutations in the *XK* gene result in absence or truncation of the protein product. *Kell* is an endothelin processing enzyme. Endothelins are important in proliferation and development of neural crest–derived cells and are thought to be important in neurotransmitter release in dopaminergic neurons. No information is available about treatment of neuroacanthocytosis, but the physician should be guided by the clinical manifestations.

## Sydenham Chorea and Other Autoimmune Choreas

Sydenham chorea (SC), one of the major manifestations of rheumatic fever, typically appears months after the initial streptococcal infection (Baizabal-Carvallo and Jankovic, 2012). Because of the widespread availability of antistreptococcal therapy, SC is now extremely rare in developed countries. It is a disorder of children, mainly girls, between ages 5 and 15, with a mean age at onset of 8.4 years. The chorea begins insidiously, but progresses over a period of weeks, and it generally resolves within about 6 months. Choreic movements are usually generalized, but asymmetric and hemichorea may also be seen. Behavioral accompaniments such as restlessness, irritability, and obsessive-compulsive traits are common. It is a self-limited disorder, usually lasting up to 6 months. Approximately 20% of cases recur, but multiple recurrences are rare. Mild enlargement of the basal ganglia may be seen on MRI brain scan. Pathologically, SC is characterized by inflammation of the cortex and basal ganglia. Anti–basal ganglia antibodies can be detected by enzyme-linked immunosorbent assay and Western immunoblot. The mechanism of basal ganglia damage is likely molecular mimicry, with cross-reaction between antibodies directed against streptococcal and striatal antigens. Because it is often self-limited, the decision to treat SC depends on the magnitude of each patient's disability. A recent comparative trial suggested that valproic acid is the most effective treatment, followed by carbamazepine and haloperidol. The typical neuroleptics, such as haloperidol, however, are now rarely used in the treatment of chorea and instead VMAT2 inhibitors, such as tetrabenazine, deutetrabenazine, and valbenazine are now considered the drugs of choice (Bashir and Jankovic, 2018b). Because SC tends to be self-limited, periodic attempts should be made to wean from therapy. Intravenous methylprednisolone followed by oral prednisone may be useful in refractory cases. Later in life, people who have survived SC may have a recrudescence of chorea in the presence of hormonal stresses like pregnancy (chorea gravidarum) or estrogen treatment.

Besides SC, there are many other autoimmune choreas, including systemic lupus erythematosus and paraneoplastic choreas (Baizabal-Carvallo and Jankovic, 2012; Baizabal-Carvallo et al., 2013) and NMDAR encephalitis (Baizabal-Carvallo and Jankovic, 2018).

## Other Choreic Disorders

There are many causes of chorea but here we will focus only on the more common ones or those in which understanding of pathogenesis has improved. A condition previously referred to as benign hereditary chorea has been re-defined with the discovery of its genetic cause. Inherited as an autosomal-dominant disorder, this disorder has been linked to mutations in the *NKX2-1* (previously called *TITF1*) gene coding for a transcription essential for the organogenesis of the brain, lung, and thyroid. Since all three of these sites are affected, the condition has also been referred to as "BLT syndrome." Initially defined as a nonprogressive syndrome of inherited childhood-onset chorea with a good outcome in the absence of an underlying degenerative disease, the phenotype has been expanded markedly as new cases with mutations of the NKX2-1 gene are being reported (Patel and Jankovic, 2014). Chorea is present from early childhood, usually from the first decade of life, but a variety of other movement disorders and nonmotor features have been described. These include hypotonia in early infancy, delayed walking ability, dystonia, myoclonus, and tics as well as a variety of behavioral and cognitive features including attention-deficit/hyperactivity disorder. Because of the heterogeneity of clinical features, the term NKX2-1 disease has been suggested for this disorder.

Mutations in the adenylate cyclase 5 *(ADCY5)* gene have been associated with a variety of movement and behavioral disorders, including episodic and fluctuating chorea, dystonia, myoclonus, cognitive decline, delayed motor and speech milestones, hypotonia, ataxia, unexplained falls, and myopathy-like facial appearance (Carecchio et al., 2017). The disorder is frequently misdiagnosed as dyskinetic cerebral palsy (Monbaliu et al., 2017). A homozygous loss-of-function mutation in the *PDE2A* gene has been associated with early-onset hereditary chorea (Salpietro et al., 2018).

## Ballism

*Ballism* is usually a high-amplitude proximal ballistic flinging movement (see Chapter 24, Box 24.5) that most commonly affects the limbs on one side of the body (HB), but involvement in both legs (paraballism) or both sides of the body (biballism) is also possible. Ballism overlaps with choreas, and both movements may coexist. Acute-onset ballism often evolves into and is replaced by chorea. Animal models with lesions in the STN result in a mixture of choreic and ballistic movements. The development of ballism varies with the underlying etiology. HB related to stroke appears suddenly or emerges more slowly in a recovering plegic limb. Approximately 20% of cases relate to structural lesions within the contralateral STN and in 20% of cases no lesion can be demonstrated by MRI. In other cases, the lesion is usually found in the afferent or efferent projections of the STN. Rarely, other etiologies, even ipsilateral to the movement, have been described. Although the underlying lesion is usually cerebrovascular disease in the elderly and infectious or inflammatory disease in younger patients, any type of structural lesion, appropriately placed, can produce the characteristic movement. Metabolic disorders such as nonketotic hyperglycemia and drug exposure may also cause HB (Box 96.4). The mechanism of ballism is not well understood but loss of STN excitation of the GPi results in a loss of inhibitory drive to the thalamus, giving rise to excessive

### BOX 96.4 Etiology of Hemiballism

**Structural Lesions**

***Cerebrovascular Disease***

Infarction
Transient ischemic attack
Hemorrhage
Arteriovenous malformation
Subarachnoid hemorrhage
Subclavian steal syndrome

***Infection***

Syphilis
Tuberculoma
Toxoplasmosis
Acquired immunodeficiency syndrome
Influenza A

***Tumor***

Pituitary microadenoma
Metastasis

***Immune-Mediated***

Systemic lupus erythematosus
Sydenham chorea
Behçet disease
Scleroderma

***Other***

Static encephalopathy
Head injury
Demyelinating disease
Thalamotomy
Heredodegenerative disease

**Metabolic**

Nonketotic hyperosmolar hyperglycemia

**Drug-Induced**

Phenytoin and other anticonvulsants
Oral contraceptives
Neuroleptics (tardive)

motor activity which may be represented clinically by the ballistic movements. Low firing frequency of the STN has been confirmed in a few cases, using intraoperative recording.

Long-term prognosis and outcome closely relate to the underlying etiology. Movements often regress or become more choreic over several months, but they can be quite exhausting or disabling when present, and treatment is usually only indicated acutely and in patients whose movements do not resolve spontaneously. Although the rarity of the condition has precluded controlled clinical trials, there is ample evidence from case series and reports that dopamine antagonists and dopamine depleters (VMAT2 inhibitors) effectively decrease choreic movements. Beneficial results have also been obtained using gabapentin and valproic acid.

## DYSTONIA

### Childhood-Onset Generalized Primary Dystonia

#### Epidemiology and Clinical Features

Dystonia is a disorder dominated by sustained muscle contractions, which often cause twisting and repetitive movements or abnormal postures (Albanese et al., 2013; Balint et al., 2018) (see also Chapter 24). Generalized dystonia is quite rare, with an estimated prevalence of approximately 1.4 per 100,000. Most cases of primary generalized dystonia that begin in childhood have DYT-*TOR1A* dystonia, caused by a mutation in the torsin A gene (TOR1A) on chromosome 9q32-34 (Dauer, 2014; Marras et al., 2016) (see also Chapter 24). Also referred to as *Oppenheim dystonia* and previously called *dystonia musculorum deformans*, DYT1 is an autosomal dominant disorder with relatively low penetrance. DYT1 dystonia is one of several movement disorders particularly common in persons of Ashkenazi Jewish descent (Inzelberg et al., 2014). The reported prevalence of DYT1 dystonia is as high as 20–30 per 100,000. Half of patients are affected by age 9, and onset in patients older than 40 years of age is extremely rare. The earliest symptom is usually an action-induced dystonia in the leg or arm. Onset in the cervical, facial, laryngeal, or pharyngeal region is rare. In approximately 70% of patients, dystonic movements spread to the trunk and other limbs, and the condition generalizes over about 5 years. Patients with earlier onset and onset in the leg are more likely to develop generalized dystonia than those presenting later or with arm dystonia. Generalized dystonia produces severe disability, and most patients with this severe form of the illness are nonambulatory. Even in generalized disease, however, laryngeal and pharyngeal dystonia remains rare. The diagnosis of childhood-onset primary generalized dystonia is made clinically in a patient with onset before age 26 of limb dystonia, with subsequent spread; absence of other movement disorders, with the exception of tremor; normal intellect and neurological examination; and absence of a pronounced response to LD (see also Chapter 24).

Routine laboratory and neuroimaging studies do not contribute to the diagnosis. Simultaneous recording of EMG activity from antagonist muscles often reveals simultaneous contraction of antagonistic muscles and spread or overflow of activity to muscles not involved in the intended action. Such studies are not required for the diagnosis. DNA testing is available for DYT1 dystonia, but the low penetrance of the disease limits the usefulness of this test for prenatal or presymptomatic diagnosis.

#### Pathology

Pathological studies in childhood-onset primary generalized dystonia are limited. Although traditionally thought not to be associated with pathological changes, brains from genetically confirmed DYT1 dystonia patients showed perinuclear inclusion bodies in the midbrain reticular formation and periaqueductal gray matter of the PPN, cuneiform nucleus, and griseum centrale mesencephali. These inclusions stained positive for ubiquitin, torsin A, and the nuclear envelope protein lamin A/C. In addition, tau/ubiquitin-immunoreactive aggregates were found in the SNc and locus coeruleus. If confirmed by other studies, these findings support the notion that DYT1 dystonia is associated with impaired protein handling, particularly in brainstem nuclei such as the PPN.

#### Pathogenesis

The low penetrance of DYT1 dystonia, combined with variable expression that may range from an asymptomatic state to severe life-threatening dystonia (dystonic storm), may obscure its hereditary nature in many families. The disorder is genetically homogeneous in Ashkenazi Jews, 90% of whom are found to have the DYT1 mutation (Inzelberg et al., 2014). Non-Jewish patients are genetically more heterogeneous. The DYT1 mutation is a GAG deletion in the TOR1A gene on chromosome 9, with an estimated frequency of 1 per 2000 to 1 per 6000 in Ashkenazi Jews and about 1 per 20,000 to1 per 30,000 in non-Jewish populations. The high prevalence of DYT1 in Ashkenazi Jews is related to a founder mutation estimated to have originated about 350 years ago in Lithuania or Byelorussia and the subsequent large increase in the population from a limited number of ancestors.

The pathogenesis of generalized dystonia remains poorly understood, but progress is being made in unraveling the cellular and molecular mechanism of the genetic forms of dystonia (Dauer, 2014). Torsin A is a protein of unknown function that is homologous to the adenosine triphosphatases and heat-shock proteins. Its structure suggests a role in endoplasmic reticulum function, intracellular trafficking, or vesicular release. Mutant torsin A may interfere with these functions or may contribute to misfolded protein stress. Besides DYT1 there are many other genetic and non-genetic causes of dystonia (see Table 24.6A and 24.6B and Box 24.3).

There is experimental, clinical, neuroimaging, and electrophysiological evidence of dysfunction at the cortical, subcortical, brainstem, cerebellar, and spinal levels. Although sensation in patients with dystonia is normal, it has been suggested that there is disordered sensory function as suggested by the presence of alleviating maneuvers (see Chapter 24), a characteristic feature of dystonia (Patel et al., 2014). Deep brain recordings support abnormally low firing rates in the GPi, with an abnormal pattern of firing as well. During sustained dystonia, metabolic activity in the midbrain, cerebellum, and thalamus is increased. Functional neuroimaging of the dopamine system suggests decreased dopamine neurotransmission in the striatum, but decreased striatal dopamine has not been confirmed in postmortem tissue. Because dystonia may respond to pallidal lesions or stimulation, a central role of the GPi has been proposed. It is likely, however, that the pathophysiology of dystonia involves many factors that include changes in the rate and pattern of neuronal firing, the degree of synchronization of firing, and aberrant focusing of sensory input. There is no diagnostic test for dystonia, although simultaneous EMG recording of agonist and antagonist muscles may show inappropriate co-contraction. But this is not required for diagnosis of dystonia.

#### Treatment

Rather limited information is available on the medical treatment of childhood-onset primary generalized dystonia. Apart from an obvious neurotransmitter deficiency or excess, there is no compelling rationale for the use of any particular pharmacotherapy, and no drug has been found to be universally effective for symptom control (Balint et al., 2018; Jankovic, 2009a; Thenganatt and Jankovic, 2014b). In the absence of genetic confirmation of the DYT1 mutation, a trial of

LD should be considered in all patients with childhood-onset dystonia because up to 10% will have dopa-responsive dystonia (DYT5a) (Wijemanne and Jankovic, 2015). In patients younger than 20 years of age, some 50% will respond well to high-dose anticholinergic therapy. The response rate is better in patients treated within 5 years of onset. Baclofen, clonazepam, benzodiazepines, and dopamine-depleting medications may be useful in some patients. The treatment of childhood-onset primary generalized dystonia is a trial-and-error process. Treatment should be initiated with very small doses, and the dose should be increased slowly and gradually. Botulinum toxin injections may be considered to treat one or a few particularly problematic body areas in patients with generalized dystonia. Chronic intrathecal baclofen has been reported to help some patients with dystonia, especially those with concomitant spasticity.

Thalamotomy has been replaced by GPi or STN DBS as the treatment of choice for disabling medically intractable generalized or segmental dystonia. Long-term studies have established the sustained efficacy of DBS in patients with dystonia (Panov et al., 2013). Advances in DBS techniques and in defining the appropriate targets have resulted in improved outcomes in patients with dystonia treated with DBS (Cheung et al., 2014; Meoni et al., 2017; Ostrem et al., 2017).

## Adult-Onset Primary Focal and Segmental Dystonia

### Epidemiology and Clinical Features

A community-based postal survey of primary dystonia suggested the prevalence of adult-onset primary focal or segmental dystonia was 12.9 per 100,000. Cervical dystonia and blepharospasm were most commonly represented. The focal and segmental primary dystonias generally begin in adulthood with dystonic movements in the hand and arm, neck, or face. When spread occurs, the ultimate distribution tends to maintain a segmental pattern. Cervical dystonia is the most frequently diagnosed form of focal dystonia, accounting for about half of focal dystonia cases. Patients with cervical dystonia present with neck pain, difficulty maintaining a normal head position, and sometimes tremor. Dystonic tremor, which may be present not only in patients with cervical dystonia but also in those with limb dystonia, is usually an irregular oscillatory movement that stops when the patient is allowed to place the head or limb in the position of the dystonic pulling—the *null point*. There is a directional preponderance to dystonia movements that is usually maintained throughout the course of the disease. Alleviating maneuvers (also referred to as "sensory tricks") are often discovered and used by the patients to ameliorate the dystonia (see Chapter 24) and include resting the head against a wall or high-backed chair or touching the chin or back of the head lightly with one hand. Spontaneous remissions may be seen in as many as 20% of patients, although recurrence is common.

*Blepharospasm* is one of the most common forms of focal dystonia. Symptoms of blepharospasm are often preceded by photosensitivity and a gritty or otherwise abnormal sensation in the eye. Increased blinking may follow, or frank spasms of eyelid closure may begin. Symptoms of blepharospasm are typically worse with driving, reading, or watching television and when exposed to bright light, wind, or stress. Many patients notice improvement in their blepharospasm when they talk or sing and when they place a finger on the eye orbit (alleviating maneuver). Blepharospasm is often accompanied by oromandibular dystonia (cranial dystonia), or the latter may occur in isolation. Oromandibular dystonia typically causes involuntary jaw opening or closure (with trismus and bruxism), tongue protrusion, dysarthria, and dysphagia. Because the actions of eating and speaking activate the dystonia, these tasks are particularly affected. Alleviating maneuvers used by patients with oromandibular dystonia include touching the face or inserting an object such as a pencil into the mouth. Vocal cord involvement with adductor or abductor spasmodic dysphonia affects phonation, resulting in a harsh and strangled or breathy voice, respectively. Whispering and singing are often relatively unaffected in such patients. The occupational or task-specific dystonias are those that arise in the context of repetitive or skilled use of a body part. The most common task-specific dystonia is writer's cramp, in which action dystonia of the arm and hand develop during writing. Musicians, hair stylists, court reporters, and others who work repetitively with the hands may find these specific skills similarly affected. Players of wind instruments may develop embouchure dystonia, with difficulty maintaining the proper mouth and lip posture. Occasionally an adult patient presents with a pure truncal dystonia with flexion, extension, or lateral bending. As noted before, truncal dystonia is a typical manifestation of tardive dystonia. Isolated foot dystonia in an adult may be the initial manifestation of isolated dystonia although it is more commonly the initial presentation of an underlying neurodegenerative disorder, PD, or other form of parkinsonism, or SPS (see below). Some patients may become initially aware of their foot or leg dystonia while running, the so-called runner's dystonia, another example of task-specific dystonia (Wu and Jankovic, 2006). The diagnosis of adult-onset primary focal or segmental dystonia is made clinically. Neuroimaging studies are useful if an underlying cause is suspected but are generally normal.

### Pathogenesis

Besides generalized dystonia, many studies have suggested that focal and segmental dystonia might also have a genetic basis (Albanese et al., 2013; Balint et al., 2018; Dauer, 2014). Approximately 25% of adult-onset focal or segmental dystonia patients have a positive family history of dystonia, which would be consistent with an autosomal dominant condition with low penetrance (see also Chapter 24).

The pathogenesis of adult-onset primary focal or segmental dystonia is unclear, but similar mechanisms to childhood-onset primary generalized dystonia are proposed. Studies suggest that there is reduced intracortical inhibition in dystonia, believed related to impaired cortical and striatal GABA levels. Several lines of evidence suggest that abnormal central somatosensory processing may lead to insufficient sensorimotor integration in dystonia. PET scans suggest an abnormal pattern of regional glucose metabolism with hypermetabolism of the basal ganglia, cerebellum, and SMA.

### Treatment

Medical treatment of adult-onset primary focal and segmental dystonia is difficult and employs those agents typically used in generalized dystonia. Adults are less able to tolerate effective doses of these agents, so the response to therapy is somewhat more disappointing than that seen in children. Botulinum toxin injections, on the other hand, are very helpful in the treatment of focal and segmental dystonia (Jankovic, 2017). Botulinum toxin injections have been proven effective in the treatment of blepharospasm and other facial dystonias, as well as cervical dystonia (Mittal et al., 2019b; Simpson et al., 2016). Clinical experience suggests they are also useful in the treatment of oromandibular, laryngeal, truncal, and limb dystonia. Overall, more than 75% of treated patients report moderate to marked improvement in dystonic pain or posture. The procedure is generally well tolerated, with weakness of injected muscles or occasionally neighboring muscles the most often reported side effect. Botulinum toxin injections have a relatively brief duration of action, requiring repeated injections every 3–6 months. Secondary resistance occurs in some chronically treated patients, especially those injected frequently with higher doses of the toxin (Jankovic, 2018b).

Patients who fail to respond to botulinum toxin injections may be offered surgical interventions. Blepharospasm can be treated by orbital myectomy, although this procedure is now rarely needed as botulinum toxin provides adequate relief in most patients. Likewise, cervical rhizotomy or myectomy are rarely performed, even in patients with cervical dystonia who are resistant to botulinum toxin therapy. Pallidal or STN DBS has been tried with good results in some patients with refractory cranial-cervical dystonia, but this procedure is most frequently used in patients with generalized dystonia (Meoni et al., 2017; Ostrem et al., 2017).

## X-linked Dystonia-Parkinsonism (Lubag)

DYT/PARK-*TAF1* (DYT3), or Lubag, is an X-linked condition with progressive dystonia and parkinsonism affecting Filipino adult men descended from maternal lines from the Panay Island (Marras et al., 2016). In addition to dystonia and parkinsonism, patients may manifest tremor, chorea, and myoclonus. The phenotypical heterogeneity is evident in colorful descriptions of the disorder in the local dialect. *Lubag* means "intermittent," and *wa'eg* "sustained twisting or posturing," suggesting the predominantly dystonic form of the illness. Sudsud refers to shuffling gait, suggesting the parkinsonian form of the illness. Lubag affects men in the fourth or fifth decades, although much earlier-onset cases have been described. Symptoms predominantly relate to dystonia, although parkinsonism is present in more than 30% of patients. A nearly pure parkinsonian phenotype is thought to predict a more benign prognosis.

PET studies have shown both postsynaptic and presynaptic dopaminergic changes. Some brains of patients with this dystonia-parkinsonism syndrome have been found to have a mosaic pattern of striatal gliosis. In some patients, parkinsonian symptoms are LD-responsive, although there are reports that LD worsens symptoms in some predominantly dystonic patients.

## Dopa-Responsive Dystonia

Dopa-responsive dystonia (DRD) is an uncommon condition with a prevalence of 0.5–1 per 1,000,000. Girls are preferentially affected. DRD is a childhood-onset generalized dystonia with a dramatic, sustained, and uncomplicated response to low doses of LD. The disorder begins in the first decade of life, usually with an action leg dystonia. The condition then progresses to the fully formed illness that ranges in severity from mild focal to disabling generalized dystonia associated with marked gait difficulty and postural instability with a positive pull test. Early-onset cases may be mistakenly diagnosed as cerebral palsy. The most characteristic historical feature is prominent diurnal fluctuation, although this is present in only 50% of the cases. Affected patients may be almost normal in the morning, becoming progressively more disabled over the course of the day, with peak disability due to generalized dystonia and parkinsonism late in the evening. DRD is usually dominantly inherited with incomplete penetrance (DYT5a). DYT5 results from mutations in the guanosine triphosphate cyclohydrolase 1 *(GCH1)* gene on chromosome 14 (Wijemanne and Jankovic, 2015). Over 100 different mutations of the gene have been identified, and therefore commercially available DNA testing identifies only the most common mutations. Guanosine triphosphate cyclohydrolase 1 is an enzyme involved in the synthesis of tetrahydrobiopterin, a cofactor for tyrosine hydroxylase, the rate-limiting enzyme in the synthesis of LD. Other mutations affecting enzymes involved in tetrahydrobiopterin synthesis, such as tyrosine hydroxylase (DYT5b), have also been implicated in DRD. The DYT5b form of DRD is recessively inherited. Patients with DRD have low levels of tyrosine hydroxylase and therefore low levels of dopamine but F-dopa PET and postmortem studies confirm normal numbers of dopaminergic neurons. DRD responds very well to low doses of LD (100–300 mg daily). Patients with DRD do not typically develop the motor fluctuations and dyskinesias associated with chronic LD therapy in PD. DAs and anticholinergic drugs may also be useful.

Another childhood-onset dystonia related to deficient dopaminergic neurotransmission is aromatic acid decarboxylase deficiency. This disorder is recessively inherited. Dystonia, parkinsonism, oculogyric crises, autonomic symptoms, and progressive neurological impairment begin in childhood. There are deficiencies in central biogenic amines including dopamine, norepinephrine, epinephrine, and serotonin. Because the enzyme deficiency is distal to LD in the dopamine synthetic pathway, the symptoms are not LD responsive. However, direct-acting DAs and MAOIs may be useful.

## Myoclonus Dystonia (DYT11)

In myoclonus dystonia (MD), dystonia is the predominant symptom, but myoclonus in body parts not necessarily affected by dystonia is also present. Some patients have pure myoclonus. Symptoms usually begin before the teenage years and predominantly affect the head, arms, and upper body. The involuntary movements may be exquisitely sensitive to ethanol. Psychiatric features including affective disorder, obsessive-compulsive disorder, substance abuse, anxiety, phobic or panic disorders, and psychosis have been described. Cognitive decline has also been reported. No other neurological deficits are seen, and the course is usually benign. The pathology is unknown. A number of heterozygous mutations in the ε-sarcoglycan gene on chromosome 7 have been reported in families with MD. Another dystonic disorder associated with myoclonus is DYT-*KCTD17* (DYT26), an autosomal dominant disorder of childhood or adult onset, manifested by myoclonus and cranial-cervical dystonia. MD responds poorly to medical therapy, but beneficial responses to clonazepam, valproic acid, and trihexyphenidyl have been reported. Thalamic stimulation may also be beneficial.

## Rapid-Onset Dystonia Parkinsonism (DYT12)

Rapid-onset dystonia parkinsonism (RDP), DYT/PARK-*ATP1A3* (DYT12), is a very rare disorder in which signs of parkinsonism and upper-body dystonia develop subacutely (Heinzen et al., 2014). Onset ranges from childhood to adulthood. Dystonia preferentially affects bulbar muscles and progresses over a period of days to weeks but then remains stable. Although sporadic cases have been reported, most cases belong to a small number of families showing dominant inheritance with incomplete penetrance. A genetic locus on chromosome 19 has been discovered. Low levels of homovanillic acid have been detected in the spinal fluid, but PET scans using presynaptic markers fail to demonstrate a loss of dopaminergic neurons. There is no evidence of neurodegeneration, and symptoms do not improve with administration of LD. Mutations in the $Na^+/K^+$-ATPase $\alpha_3$ gene, *ATP1A3*, on chromosome 19q13 were found to be associated with RDP (see also Chapter 24).

## Wilson Disease (Hepatolenticular Degeneration)

### Clinical Features

Wilson disease (WD) is a rare, autosomal recessive, heredodegenerative disorder thought to affect 1–2 per 100,000 persons (Dusek et al., 2015; Hedera, 2019). The WD gene, termed *ATP7B*, on the long arm of chromosome 13 encodes copper-transporting P-type ATPase. Over 600 mutations have been identified and most patients carry at least two mutations. Because of the biallelic mutations in the *ATP7B* gene there is a loss of function of copper transporter ATPase, which results in an impaired excretion of copper into the bile and subsequent accumulation of copper in the liver and brain. Excessive copper not incorporated into copper-binding protein, ceruloplasmin, leads to cytotoxic effects in hepatic and central nervous tissues. Many patients present in childhood with symptoms and signs of liver disease ranging from cirrhosis to fulminant liver failure associated with progressive accumulation of copper. Once cirrhosis has developed, extrahepatic copper deposits begin to form, especially in the brain, eyes, and kidneys. Some patients present with hemolytic anemia, hypersplenism, or renal failure. Nearly half of all patients with WD present with CNS symptoms and signs. Neurological signs usually present during adolescence or early adulthood, but presentations up to age 51 have been reported. Neurological presentations include parkinsonism, postural and kinetic tremor, ataxia, titubation, chorea, seizures, dysarthria, and dystonia (see Video 96.22). A fixed stare with a smiling expression *(risus sardonicus)* and drooling are classic features of the illness but are not seen in all cases. Dystonia is a common sign, present in about a third of patients at presentation. Dystonia may be focal, segmental, or generalized. Dementia, if present, is mild, but psychiatric symptoms are common and may be quite disabling. Mood and personality disorders, behavioral changes, and psychosis are reported. In the presence of neurological signs, ophthalmological examination that includes slit-lamp examination essentially always demonstrates copper deposition in the Descemet membrane (*Kayser-Fleischer rings*; see Chapter 24, Fig. 24.1). Many patients with WD also have sunflower cataracts (Waln and Jankovic, 2018).

Laboratory studies often show abnormalities in hepatic enzymes, aminoaciduria, low uric acid, and demineralization of bone. MRI scan usually shows decreased signal intensity (hypodensity) in the striatum and superior colliculi and increased signal intensity in the midbrain tegmentum (except for red nucleus) and in the lateral SNr, giving the appearance of "face of the giant panda" on T2-weighted images. Low serum ceruloplasmin, elevated 24-hour copper excretion, and the presence of Kayser-Fleischer rings are useful in making the diagnosis, but confirmation by demonstrating elevated hepatic copper is occasionally required in ambiguous cases.

### Pathology

Gross inspection of the brain often reveals cerebral atrophy and shrunken discolored putamen and GP. Microscopically, WD brains show both preferential striatal and generalized neuronal loss. There is diffuse gliosis with Alzheimer types I and II astrocytes, as well as Opalski cells, cells of microglial origin.

### Pathogenesis

The mutated *ATP7B* gene on chromosome 13 regulates a copper-transporting adenosine triphosphatase. Although the neurological disorder clearly relates to harmful effects of intracellular copper, the precise mechanisms of cell dysfunction and death are not well understood.

### Treatment

The goal of treatment of WD is to reduce the body burden of copper and to prevent its reaccumulation (Aggarwal and Bhatt, 2018). Traditionally, acute chelation began with D-penicillamine, but more recent treatment strategies stress somewhat less toxic therapies such as trientine and zinc or ammonium tetrathiomolybdate. The effectiveness of initial de-coppering is monitored by serially measuring urine copper excretion and plasma copper levels. Although there may be an acute deterioration associated with the mobilization of copper stores, most patients improve over time. Long-term therapy must be maintained, usually with trientine and zinc. D-Penicillamine is associated with a number of systemic toxicities including dermatopathy, neuromuscular junction disorders, thrombocytopenia, and Goodpasture syndrome. Ammonium tetrathiomolybdate (WTX101), which offers potential advantages over zinc, penicillamine, and trientine in that it blocks copper absorption and forms complexes with copper in the blood, is emerging as the most effective and safest treatment of WD, but this drug is still considered experimental. Asymptomatic siblings should be tested for the disease because timely treatment prevents the illness. Orthotopic liver transplantation is curative but has been used largely in patients with fulminant hepatic failure who have not yet developed significant neurological signs. The response of neurological symptoms to liver transplantation is not completely understood.

## Neurodegeneration with Brain Iron Accumulation

Neurodegeneration with brain iron accumulation (NBIA), formerly known as *Hallervorden-Spatz disease*, includes pantothenate kinase-associated neurodegeneration (PKAN) and a variety of other genetic neurodegenerative disorders associated with accumulation of iron in the brain, particularly the basal ganglia (Dusek et al., 2012; Hayflick et al., 2018). PKAN is an autosomal recessive neurodegenerative disorder presenting in childhood with the insidious onset of dystonia and gait disorder. Rigidity, dysarthria, spasticity, dementia, retinitis pigmentosa, and optic atrophy develop and progress relentlessly until death in early childhood. T2-weighted MRI brain scans show areas of reduced attenuation in the GP surrounding an area of hyperintensity, the *eye of the tiger sign* (McNeill et al., 2008).

Autopsy studies show a brown discoloration of the GPi and SNr, reflecting pathological accumulation of iron. Microscopic changes include neuronal loss, gliosis, loss of myelinated fibers, and axonal swellings (spheroids). Families with typical PKAN have mutations in the pantothenate kinase gene (PANK2) on chromosome 20. Pantothenate kinase is an important regulatory enzyme in coenzyme A synthesis. Aceruloplasminemia, characterized by anemia, iron overload, diabetes, and neurodegeneration caused by homozygous mutation of the ceruloplasmin gene, may be associated with dystonia and akinetic-rigid syndrome. The four subtypes of NBIA—PKAN, neuroferritinopathy, infantile neuroaxonal dystrophy (INAD), and aceruloplasminemia—can be differentiated by gradient echo (T2*) and fast-spin echo (FSE) MRI (McNeill et al., 2008). Another subtype of NBIA, PLA2G6-associated neurodegeneration (PLAN), is manifested by early childhood-onset axial hypotonia, spasticity, bulbar dysfunction, ataxia, and dystonia. Previously diagnosed as INAD, NBIA2, or Karak syndrome, PLAN may also present as adult-onset LD-responsive dystonia-parkinsonism without iron on brain imaging. The *PLA2G6* gene on chromosome 22q13.1 encodes a calcium-independent phospholipase A2 enzyme that catalyzes the hydrolysis of glycerophospholipids. Iron chelation with deferiprone and fosmetpantotenate, a phosphopantothenic acid prodrug which aims to replenish phosphopantothenic acid have been reported to result in regression of symptoms after several months of treatment. Another form of NBIA, mitochondrial membrane protein-associated neurodegeneration (MPAN). may present as juvenile-onset LD-responsive parkinsonism as well as progressive dystonia-parkinsonism, optic atrophy, and axonal motor neuronopathy (Gregory et al., 2019).

## Post-traumatic Dystonia and Peripherally Induced Movement Disorders

Dystonia resulting from central trauma most often presents as hemidystonia, but cervical, segmental, or axial dystonia can also be seen as sequelae of brain or spinal cord trauma. Most cases of post-traumatic dystonia occurred in children or adolescents who have survived severe head injury. Often the dystonia emerges as a traumatic hemiparesis and later improves or resolves. There may be a latent period between the trauma and development of the dystonia from 1 day to 6 years, followed by slow progression of dystonic symptoms. Younger patients tend to have longer latencies than those who are older at the time of the head injury. Focal lesions in the caudate, putamen, or thalamus contralateral to the affected side are usually found on neuroimaging studies. Lesions of the mesencephalon or dentatothalamic pathways have also been found. The prognosis of this form of post-traumatic dystonia is poor, with a low rate of spontaneous improvement. Most cases are refractory to medical therapy, although some may respond to anticholinergic drugs. Botulinum toxin injections may be helpful in the treatment of focal or segmental dystonia. DBS may also provide some benefit, although the magnitude of response is much less than that seen in patients with primary dystonia.

Although still somewhat controversial, there is growing evidence that dystonia may also occur after peripheral injury (Jankovic, 2009b). For example, oromandibular dystonia may follow dental surgery or facial and jaw trauma. Indeed edentulous dyskinesia, usually an orolingual stereotypy or dystonia occurring after loss of teeth, may be considered a classic example of peripherally induced movement disorder. Limb dystonia has also been reported to occur after peripheral trauma, often in the context of a work- or sports-related injury, especially after immobilization as a result of casting (Pirio Richardson et al., 2017). Peripherally induced dystonia tends to manifest with a fixed rather than mobile dystonia and may be associated with complex regional pain syndrome, also known as causalgia or reflex sympathetic dystrophy (Jankovic, 2009b; van Rooijen et al., 2011). The response of this condition to medical or other therapies is disappointing.

## Paroxysmal Movement Disorders

Paroxysmal movement disorders consist of intermittent movements that are now classified both clinically and genetically (Erro and Bhatia, 2019; Waln and Jankovic, 2015) (see also Chapter 24).

Paroxysmal kinesigenic dyskinesia (PKD) is a disorder of childhood onset characterized by attacks of involuntary movements that include prominent dystonia, chorea, and other hyperkinesias. Because the attacks are often not witnessed and therefore appropriate phenomenological categorization is not possible, the less specific term, *paroxysmal dyskinesia*, is preferred. Boys make up 80% of cases. There is often a family history. Patients typically recount that episodes are triggered by rapid movement, often in response to an unexpected stimulus such as the telephone ringing. There may be a premonitory sensation in an affected limb, such as limb paresthesia before the onset of the abnormal involuntary movement. The movements may be unilateral or bilateral. The spells last less than 1 minute and occur up to 100 times daily. There is a tendency for spells to decrease in adulthood. Diagnosis depends on careful history taking; because the examination usually shows no abnormalities, typical spells may not be elicited in the examination setting, and neuroimaging and electrophysiological studies are usually normal.

Paroxysmal nonkinesigenic dyskinesia (PNKD) usually begins in infancy and affects boys more than girls. The spells of PNKD occur less often but are more prolonged than those in PKD. Their frequency ranges from several episodes a month to several episodes a day, and their duration is generally between 10 minutes and several hours. They are not precipitated by action but may be triggered by ethanol, caffeine, fatigue, or stress. Unlike PKD, PNKD does not show a dramatic response to anticonvulsants. Some patients respond to clonazepam, other benzodiazepines, carbamazepine, gabapentin, anticholinergics, LD, acetazolamide, and neuroleptics. Mutations in many genes, such as *PRRT2*, *MR-1*, *SCL2A1*, *SLC16A2*, *GLUT1*, *KNCMA1*, *SCN8*, *ECHS1*, *CACNA1A*, *ADCY5*, and *ATP1A3* have been identified to cause paroxysmal dyskinesia (Erro and Bhatia, 2019).

Secondary paroxysmal dyskinesia has been thought to be quite rare (Waln and Jankovic, 2015). However, in one series, 26% of paroxysmal dyskinesia cases occurred in the context of another nervous system disease. Underlying etiologies include cerebrovascular disease, trauma, infection, and metabolic encephalopathy. The clinical manifestations of secondary paroxysmal dyskinesia are heterogeneous. Some are kinesigenic and some are not. Some are associated with premonitory sensations; others have no warning signs. Treatment of the underlying cause may improve the dyskinesia.

# TICS

## Tourette Syndrome

### Clinical Features

The most common cause of childhood-onset tics is Tourette syndrome (TS), a complex neurological disorder, manifested not only by motor and phonic tics but also by many behavioral comorbidities, particularly attention-deficit and obsessive-compulsive disorders (Robertson et al., 2017; Thenganatt and Jankovic, 2016). The diagnosis of TS rests entirely on the history and physical examination. There is no diagnostic test for TS, but according to the *Diagnostic and Statistical Manual of Mental Disorders*, 5th Edition (DSM-5) (American Psychiatric Association, 2013) the following are criteria for the diagnosis of TS (refer to Box 24.8 for full DSM-5 diagnostic criteria):

A. Both multiple motor and one or more vocal tics are present at some time during the illness, although not necessarily concurrently.
B. The tics may wax or wane in frequency but have persisted for more than 1 year since first tic onset.
C. Onset is before age 18 years.
D. The disturbance is not attributable to the physiological effects of a substance (e.g., cocaine) or a general medical condition (e.g., HD, postviral encephalitis).

Prevalence estimates for TS vary from 10 to 700 per 100,000, depending on the population studied and the study methods used. Meta-analysis of 21 studies yielded a prevalence of TS at 0.52% (Scharf et al., 2015). Although the prevalence of tics is greater among children in special schools and those with disorders in the autism spectrum, the vast majority of patients with TS have normal intelligence.

Typical early signs of TS are motor tics, including eye blinks, facial grimacing, head jerks, shoulder shrugs, and a variety of limb and trunk movements (see Chapter 24). Phonic tics include sniffing, throat clearing, grunting, whistling, chirping, and words—including verbal obscenities *(coprolalia)* and obscene gestures *(copropraxia)*. Over time, the tics wax and wane, and new tics emerge as other tics resolve. Tics may be simple or complex and can resemble any voluntary or involuntary movement. Tics are often preceded by regional or generalized premonitory feelings, such as an urge to move, increased tension, a compulsive need to move or make sound, and other sensations. These premonitory phenomena differentiate tics from other jerk-like movements such as myoclonus and chorea and highlight the sensory aspects of movement disorders (Patel et al., 2014). Symptoms tend to increase throughout childhood, typically peaking just prior to puberty and spontaneously subsiding after the age of 18 years.

Behavioral changes are very common in TS, especially attention-deficit/hyperactivity disorder, obsessive-compulsive disorder, impulse control disorders, and a variety of conduct disorders. In one study involving 1374 patients with TS, 72.1% met the criteria for attention-deficit/hyperactivity disorder, obsessive-compulsive disorder (Hirschtritt et al., 2015).

### Pathogenesis

Although TS is clearly a biological genetic disorder, no causative gene or genes have been identified, although several susceptibility genes have been found through various genetic techniques, including genome-wide association studies (Deng et al., 2012; Yu et al., 2015). Possible reasons for the absence of reported causative genes include lack of specific diagnostic criteria, clinical and genetic heterogeneity, and bilineal transmission (inherited from both parents).

Because there is a robust response to dopamine receptor–blocking medications, altered central neurotransmission has been proposed to underlie TS. PET studies, however, have failed to provide evidence of dopaminergic hyperactivity in TS. One PET study, using [$^{11}$C]-flumazenil, and structural MRI provided evidence of decreased binding of GABAA receptors in TS patients bilaterally in the ventral striatum, GP, thalamus, amygdala, and right insula and increased binding in the bilateral SN, left periaqueductal gray, right posterior cingulate cortex, and bilateral cerebellum (Lerner et al., 2012). This suggests that the GABAergic system plays an important role in TS and provides evidence that TS represents a "disinhibition" disorder.

Adult-onset tics usually represent recurrences of childhood tics or may be present in the setting of cocaine use or with exposure to other CNS stimulants, dopamine receptor blockers (tardive tics), and in association with neuroacanthocytosis. Rarely, movement disorders resembling tics may be of psychogenic (functional) origin (Baizabal-Carvallo and Jankovic, 2014).

## Treatment

Treatment of TS must be individualized and should be reserved for patients who are experiencing interference from tics in the educational, social, or family spheres (Billnitzer and Jankovic, 2020) (Fig. 96.17). Disabling tics are most effectively suppressed by dopamine-receptor blocking drugs such as fluphenazine (Wijemanne et al., 2014), and dopamine-depleting drugs such as tetrabenazine, deutetrabenazine, and valbenazine (Jankovic, 2016b, 2020). But many other drugs have been reported to be effective in treating tics, such as cannabinoids, nicotine, ondansetron, and ecopipam, a $D_1$ receptor antagonist (Gilbert and Jankovic, 2014; Jankovic, 2015c). Obsessive-compulsive disorder responds to selective serotonin reuptake inhibitors. Comorbid ADHD can be safely treated with clonidine, methylphenidate, and other CNS stimulants. Guanfacine and clonidine have been found useful in patients with TS and impulse-control problems. Patients with disabling tics (with or without obsessive-compulsive disorder) may benefit from DBS of the thalamus or GPi (Martinez-Ramirez et al., 2018; Viswanathan et al., 2012). The American Academy of Neurology Practice Guideline made 46 recommendations regarding the assessment and management of TS, including treatment options such as Comprehensive Behavioral Intervention for Tics, antidopaminergic and other medications, botulinum toxin injections for focal motor and phonic tics, and DBS (Pringsheim et al., 2019).

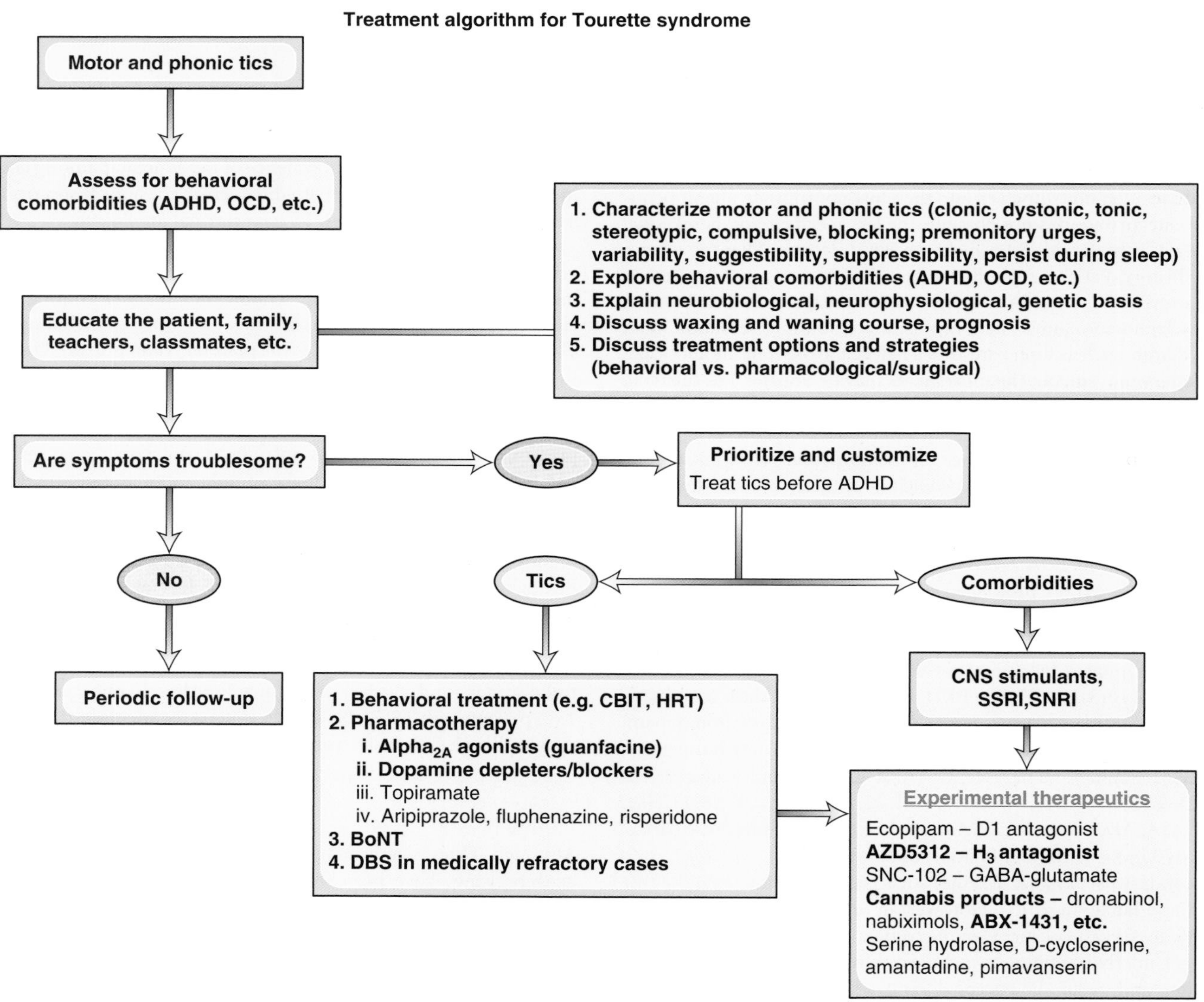


**Fig. 96.17** Treatment Algorithm for Tourette Syndrome. *ADHD.* attention deficit hyperactivity disorder; *CBIT,* comprehensive behavioral intervention for tics; *CNS,* Central nervous system; *DBS,* deep brain stimulation; *GABA,* γ-aminobutyric acid; *HRT,* habit reversal training; *OCD,* obsessive compulsive disorder; *SNc,* substantia nigra pars compacta; *SNRI,* selective noradrenergic reuptake inhibitor; SSRI, selective serotonin reuptake inhibitor.

## MYOCLONUS

### Essential Myoclonus

EM is diagnosed when myoclonus is present as an isolated neurological sign or is accompanied only by tremor or dystonia. EM can be sporadic or inherited. Dominantly inherited EM usually presents before age 20. EM is usually multifocal with upper body predominance. Although spontaneous jerks are seen, they are exacerbated by action. Alcohol may dramatically suppress the myoclonus. Sporadic forms of this illness are also described. Myoclonus-dystonia and EM are allelic disorders linked to the ε-sarcoglycan gene on chromosome 7. Besides DYT-*SGCE* (DYT11), other genetic forms of myoclonus-dystonia include *GCH1* (DYT5a), DYT/PARK-*TH* (DYT5b), DYT-*KCTD17* (DYT26) (see Chapter 24).

### Posthypoxic Myoclonus (Lance-Adams Syndrome)

The first cases of posthypoxic myoclonus (PHM) were described in 1963 by Lance and Adams (Jankovic, 2015c). PHM is a generalized myoclonus that occurs with recovery from the acute effects of severe brain hypoxia. The most common etiologies of the hypoxia are respiratory arrest (especially asthmatic), anesthetic and surgical accidents, cardiac disease, and drug overdose. The typical patient is in coma for several days to 2 weeks. Myoclonus and seizures may be present during the comatose phase. After recovery from coma, myoclonic jerks become apparent, especially with voluntary movements, which trigger volleys of high-amplitude jerks and intermittent pauses in the activated body part. The myoclonic movements typically flow to body parts not directly involved in the voluntary movements. The amplitude of the myoclonus is directly proportional to the delicacy of the attempted task, producing extreme disability in the performance of activities of daily living. Gait is disturbed not only by positive myoclonic jerks but also by negative myoclonus, resulting in falls. Other neurological signs are always present and include seizures, dysarthria, dysmetria, ataxia, and cognitive impairment.

CSF studies have shown low levels of 5-hydroxyindoleacetic acid (5-HIAA), the main metabolite of serotonin. A role for GABA in this disorder is suggested by the production of myoclonus by injecting GABA antagonists into the rat thalamus. Autopsies in patients with PHM show changes related to hypoxic brain damage but do not reveal any specific structural changes in brainstem raphe nuclei. Myoclonus in posthypoxic rats responds to serotonin agonists that stimulate particular subtypes of serotonin receptors (5-$HT_{1B}$, 5-$HT_{2A}/_{2B}$, and possibly 5-$HT_{1D}$). Other studies in rat models have suggested that basal serotonin levels are normal, but there is an abnormality in release of serotonin by potassium chloride and NMDA. There is some tendency for improvement in myoclonus over time, but most patients have significant disability related to the movements.

GABAergic drugs such as valproic acid and clonazepam are usually used in the treatment of PHM. Each is associated with improvement in approximately 50% of treated patients. Levetiracetam has been reported to be effective in some patients, but other GABAergic drugs such as vigabatrin and gabapentin are usually not helpful (Jankovic, 2015c). Piracetam, available in Europe and Canada but not in the United States, may also improve myoclonus by an imperfectly understood mechanism that does not involve serotonin or GABA. L-5 hydroxytryptophan (L-5HTP) administered with carbidopa may be useful, but this investigational agent is no longer available, and gastrointestinal side effects limit its tolerability.

### Startle and Hyperekplexia

Hyperekplexia is a startle syndrome characterized by muscle jerks in response to unexpected stimuli. Families with autosomal dominant and recessive inheritance have been described. Two forms of startle have been described. The major form of the illness is characterized by continuous stiffness beginning in infancy and exaggerated startle culminating in falls. Some patients have seizures and low intelligence. In the minor form, there is only excessive startle with hypnic myoclonic jerks. The hereditary form is typically caused by mutations in the gene coding for the $\alpha_1$ subunit of the inhibitory glycine receptor *(GLRA1)* on chromosome 5. The disorder is also caused by mutations in the β subunit of the inhibitory glycine receptor (GLRB), by mutations in the gephyrin gene *(GPHN)*, and by mutations in *SLC6A5*, which encodes the presynaptic glycine transporter 2. The *SLC6A5* mutations are predominately associated with recessive hyperekplexia, symptoms of which include life-threatening neonatal apnea and breath-holding spells.

Startle in patients with hyperekplexia differs from normal startle because it has a lower threshold, is more generalized, and fails to normally habituate with repeated stimuli. Electrophysiological studies in well-characterized cases suggest the origin of the pathological startle in the lower brainstem, possibly the medial bulbopontine reticular formation. The disorder is genetically heterogeneous, with most mutations occurring in patients with the major form of the illness. Symptomatic hyperekplexia has been reported to result from infarct, hemorrhage, or encephalitis. Clonazepam is the treatment of choice, although it may be only partially effective.

### Palatal Myoclonus

*Palatal myoclonus*, sometimes also referred to as *palatal tremor*, is characterized by rhythmic movements of the soft palate. Since the movement consists of repetitive rather than oscillatory contractions of agonists only, it is also classified as *segmental myoclonus* rather than tremor. There are two types of PM, depending on the presence or absence of a structural lesion of the brainstem or cerebellum. Patients without an underlying structural lesion are considered to have *essential PM*, and those with underlying structural lesions are considered to have *symptomatic PM*. Essential and symptomatic PM can be distinguished by clinical features and neuroimaging.

Essential PM is very rare. It affects men and women equally. Patients with essential PM complain of audible ear clicks. The movements usually disappear during sleep. In essential PM, the palatal movements are produced by rhythmic movement of the tensor veli palatini muscle. Symptomatic PM is more common than essential PM and affects men more often than women. Symptomatic or secondary PM is not associated with ear clicks because the levator veli palatini rather than the tensor veli palatini is involved. Simultaneous tremor of other regional structures with cranial nerve innervation may be seen. Some patients have oscillopsia from pendular nystagmus. Laryngeal involvement may interrupt speech or cause rhythmic involuntary vocalizations. Rhythmic limb tremor may be seen. In patients with symptomatic PM, hypertrophy of the superior olive is demonstrable on MRI brain scans. Symptomatic PM may be associated with slow rhythmic movement in the face and limbs, called myorhythmia, and is often associated with structural lesions found in the brainstem or cerebellum within the Guillain-Mollaret triangle, which connects the dentate nucleus with the contralateral red nucleus and inferior olive (Baizabal-Carvallo et al., 2015). Many underlying etiologies have been reported: neurodegenerative, infectious, inflammatory, demyelinating, traumatic, ischemic, and even psychogenic. Characteristic pathological changes include enlargement of olivary neurons with vacuolation of the cytoplasm. Astrocytic proliferation with aggregates of argyrophilic fibers may also be seen.

The pathophysiology of PM is incompletely understood, but it is believed that in symptomatic PM, damage to the dentato-olivary tract

**BOX 96.5 Drugs Associated with Myoclonus**

Anesthetics: etomidate, chloralose
Antibiotics, anthelmintics, antiviral drugs: penicillin, imipenem, quinolones, piperazine, acyclovir
Anticonvulsants: phenytoin, phenobarbital, primidone, valproic acid, carbamazepine, gabapentin, lamotrigine, vigabatrin
Amantadine
Antihistamines
Sodium bicarbonate (baking soda)
Benzodiazepine withdrawal
Psychotropic medications: tricyclic antidepressants, selective serotonin reuptake inhibitors, monoamine oxidase inhibitors, lithium, buspirone, neuroleptics
Antineoplastic drugs: chlorambucil, prednimustine, ifosfamide
Narcotics: morphine, meperidine, hydromorphone, fentanyl, sufentanil, diamorphine

induces synchronization of cells in the inferior olive. The firing rhythm appears to be determined by membrane properties of the olivary neurons. This rhythm is then propagated through the inferior cerebellar peduncle to the contralateral cerebellar hemisphere, where it interferes with oculomotor, cerebelloreticular, and cerebellospinal systems.

Treatment of PM is difficult. Because of the rarity of the condition, there have been no randomized controlled clinical trials of therapeutic agents. Phenytoin, carbamazepine, clonazepam, diazepam, trihexyphenidyl, and baclofen are considered first-line agents in the treatment of PM. Second-line drugs include 5-HTP and presynaptic antidopaminergic drugs such as tetrabenazine. Sumatriptan has been reported to aid a single patient. Injections of botulinum toxin into the tensor veli palatini muscle have been reported beneficial in essential PM.

### Spinal Myoclonus

Spinal myoclonus is a syndrome of involuntary rhythmic or semirhythmic myoclonic jerks in a muscle or group of muscles. The myoclonic jerks may be unilateral or bilateral. In some cases, they are stimulus sensitive. The jerks relate to spontaneous motoneuron discharge in a limited area, often a single segment of the spinal cord. Propriospinal myoclonus is a more widespread disorder in which myoclonic jerks are propagated up and down the spinal cord from a central generator. Most patients with propriospinal myoclonus have had minor spinal cord trauma with normal MRI findings, but the disorder has been reported in severe spinal cord injury, multiple sclerosis, human immunodeficiency virus, Lyme infection, syringomyelia, spinal cord tumors, and spinal cord infarction. Propriospinal myoclonus has been reported to affect particularly the transition from wake to sleep. An increasing number of cases of propriospinal myoclonus have been documented to be of psychogenic origin.

### Toxin- and Drug-Induced Myoclonus

A number of drugs and environmental agents with CNS toxicity have been shown to cause myoclonus (Box 96.5). Criteria for drug- or toxin-induced myoclonus include verified exposure, temporal association, and exclusion of genetic or other causes. The myoclonus produced by drugs and toxins is often multifocal or generalized, stimulus- and action- or stimulus-sensitive, and accompanied by other suggestive nervous system signs, particularly by encephalopathic signs. Metrizamide and diclofenac may cause segmental myoclonus. Treatment requires withdrawal of the causative drug and symptomatic treatment, if required, with clonazepam or levetiracetam.

There are many other causes of myoclonus, but autoimmune disorders, such as opsoclonus-myoclonus, NMDAR encephalitis, progressive encephalomyelitis with rigidity and myoclonus, and Hashimoto encephalopathy should be considered, particularly when the onset is subacute (Baizabal-Carvallo and Jankovic, 2018).

## TARDIVE DYSKINESIA

### Classic Tardive Stereotypy

TD is a movement disorder that develops in the context of chronic dopamine receptor blockade, usually in patients who are chronically treated with antipsychotics or antiemetics (Savitt and Jankovic, 2018). With the decline in the use of typical antipsychotics and metoclopramide and introduction of atypical antipsychotics there has been a slight decline in the incidence of TD. TD usually requires a minimum of 6 weeks or more of dopamine receptor blockade, but onset as soon as after the first dose has been reported. Reported risk factors include old age, female gender, affective disorder, edentulousness, diabetes mellitus, and prior CNS injury. Although orofacial stereotypy is the most common hyperkinetic movement disorder associated with TD, other hyperkinetic disorders such as chorea, akathisia, dystonia, tics, and myoclonus may be seen. Tardive parkinsonism has also been reported, but some patients with parkinsonism persisting years after withdrawal of the offending neuroleptic have been found to have pathological evidence of PD. The classic appearance of TD is repetitive stereotypic (e.g., chewing) movements of the mouth, tongue, and lower face (oral-buccolingual dyskinesias) (Savitt and Jankovic, 2018). In contrast to HD, the upper face tends to be spared (see Chapter 24) (Jankovic and Roos, 2014). Choreic movements may also affect the trunk and pelvis, causing pelvic thrusting movement and respiratory dyskinesia (Mehanna and Jankovic, 2010). Limb chorea and restlessness (akathisia) may also be seen.

The pathophysiology of TD is incompletely understood, but the drugs that cause this syndrome appear to exhibit potent binding to postsynaptic $D_2$ receptors (Savitt and Jankovic, 2018). Denervation supersensitivity of the postsynaptic dopamine receptor has been proposed as a possible mechanism. There are other theories, including oxidative stress and insufficiency of GABA. Evidence is accumulating that suggests that neuroleptics are toxic to the striatum, and apoptotic cell death has been described in animals chronically exposed to neuroleptics. Genetic susceptibility factors that might be involved in increased risk of TD include polymorphisms of the dopamine $D_3$ receptor gene and the 5-$HT_{2C}$ serotonin receptor gene.

The most important intervention in TD is to prevent its occurrence. In prospective studies, high-risk individuals treated with atypical rather than typical antipsychotics appear to have a reduced risk of TD compared with historical controls. Because patients may not complain about early or mild movements, the clinician must carefully examine neuroleptic-treated patients for early signs of TD. Neuroleptics should be discontinued if possible. Mild TD may improve with benzodiazepines or baclofen. Deutetrabenazine and valbenazine, dopamine-depleting drugs (VMAT2 inhibitors), have been approved by the US FDA for the treatment of TD (Bashir and Jankovic, 2020; Savitt and Jankovic, 2018).

### Tardive Dystonia

Tardive dystonia should be differentiated from transient acute dystonic reaction and from the more typical TD. In contrast to TD, which tends to affect more elderly women, young men are more likely to develop tardive dystonia. All of the typical antipsychotics, as well as antiemetics with dopamine receptor-blocking properties, have been associated with the development of tardive dystonia (Savitt and Jankovic, 2018). Symptoms begin insidiously after days to decades of neuroleptic therapy. Although rare cases have been reported after a short duration of therapy, the median duration of exposure to neuroleptics at the time of onset is 5.1 years. Tardive dystonia usually presents as focal or segmental dystonia (e.g., blepharospasm) or oromandibular or cervical dystonia, but the most typical presentation is a truncal dystonia with opisthotonic posturing in a young man associated with pronating movements of arms and extension of the elbows. There is a relationship between age at onset and distribution of the dystonic movements, with trunk and leg symptoms in younger persons and face, jaw, and neck involvement in older persons. In comparison with primary focal or segmental dystonia, there is more retrocollis and anterocollis. Dystonic symptoms may improve over a period of 5 years if the offending neuroleptic agent is withdrawn, although recovery is less common than in patients with choreic or stereotypic TD. Young patients with a shorter duration of neuroleptic exposure have the greatest likelihood of remission.

As with TD, the primary treatment of tardive dystonia is prevention, but once it has developed, every attempt should be made to rid the patient of the offending neuroleptic. Neuroleptic-dependent patients should be managed with atypical antipsychotics if possible. VMAT2 inhibitors, anticholinergics, benzodiazepines, and baclofen have all been reported to help patients with tardive dystonia. Botulinum toxin injections can be particularly helpful in patients with disabling focal or segmental dystonia such as blepharospasm or cervical and truncal dystonic movements (Jankovic, 2018b). Oral and intrathecal baclofen infusions may also be helpful.

## STEREOTYPIES

Stereotypies are involuntary or unvoluntary (in response to or induced by inner sensory stimulus or unwanted feeling), coordinated, patterned, repetitive, rhythmic, seemingly purposeless movements or utterances. Stereotypies can be seen in a variety of conditions, such as TD, but when they occur in children they are often seen in the setting of autism or intellectual impairment (Oakley et al., 2015). In this situation typical motor stereotypies include body rocking, head nodding, head banging, hand waving, fluttering of fingers in front of the face, repetitive and sequential finger movements, lip smacking, pacing, skin picking, and various self-injurious behaviors such as biting, scratching, and hitting.

Although TD is one the most common causes of adult-onset stereotypies, there are many other causes of coordinated, repetitive movements. One of the most common causes of repetitive movements is the "leg stereotypy syndrome" (Lotia et al., 2018), This is defined as a repetitive, continuous movement present almost exclusively in the legs while the patient is seated. The characteristic features of leg stereotypy disorder include continuous or intermittent flexion–extension, abduction–adduction, movement of proximal legs when seated with feet resting on the floor or flexion–extension of the knees or ankles when legs are crossed in a sitting position. When standing there is often swaying movement of the trunk and shifting of weights from one to the other. Leg stereotypy syndrome must be differentiated from other sensorymotor disorders, such as RLS. Although both conditions are familial the latter is characterized by diurnal pattern, is worse at night, and is associated with unpleasant sensations such as "crawling," "tingling," "creeping," "pulling," "electric," "itching," "burning," "prickly," and other sensory phenomenon (Patel et al., 2014). Also, in contrast to leg stereotypy syndrome, RLS often requires treatment with medications such as gabapentin, DAs, or even opiates (Wijemanne and Jankovic, 2015).

## MISCELLANEOUS MOVEMENT DISORDERS

### Hemifacial Spasm

The prevalence of HFS is 14.5 per 100,000 in women and 7.4 per 100,000 in men, but the prevalence seems to be much higher in Asian populations (Wu et al., 2010; Yaltho and Jankovic, 2011). HFS is characterized by twitching of the muscles supplied by the facial nerve. The disorder usually begins in adulthood, with an average age at onset of 45–52 years. Although there are some familial cases, most are sporadic. In typical cases, twitching first affects the periorbital muscles but spreads to other ipsilateral facial muscles over a period of months to years. The spasms are synchronous in all affected muscles. In approximately 5% of patients, the opposite side of the face becomes affected, but when bilateral, the spasms are never synchronous on the two sides. The spasms of HFS may be clonic or tonic, and often a paroxysm of clonic movements culminates in a sustained tonic contraction. Although the spasms occur spontaneously, they may be precipitated or exacerbated by facial movements or by anxiety, stress, or fatigue. The affected muscles may be weaker than their contralateral counterparts. Some patients have evidence of regional cranial neuropathy, such as altered hearing or trigeminal function. Detailed neuroradiological work-ups using routine and specialized MRI techniques may demonstrate compressing vascular structures in the facial nerve root entry zone in most patients with HFS. More advanced scanning techniques such as high-resolution T1- and T2-weighted spin echo or gradient echo imaging with gadolinium provide maximum visualization of the root entry zone. Yet, serious underlying causes are rare, and many clinicians do not routinely image patients with typical HFS unless the clinical picture is atypical or the patient is being considered for surgery.

HFS is an example of peripherallyinduced movement disorder, thought to result from compression of the facial nerve at the root exit zone, usually by vascular structures (Yaltho and Jankovic, 2011). The facial nerve root entry zone generally shows axonal demyelination or nerve degeneration. Vessels commonly implicated are the posterior inferior cerebellar artery, the anterior inferior cerebellar artery, and the vertebral artery. Tumors or other space-occupying lesions are found in approximately 5% of patients. Epidermoid tumors, neuroma, meningioma, astrocytoma, and parotid tumors are most common.

There are two main theories of pathogenesis. The first proposes that in the area of compression-induced demyelination, an *ephapse*, or false synapse, forms. Mechanical irritation or other regional changes induce ectopic activity in the region, which is then conducted antidromically within the nerve fiber. The main competing theory proposes that the aberrant signals arise from the facial nerve nucleus, which is reorganized as a result of deranged afferent information.

Traditionally, patients with HFS were treated with anticonvulsants, baclofen, anticholinergics, and clonazepam, but the introduction of botulinum toxin injections revolutionized treatment of the disorder. Botulinum toxin injected into the periorbital subcutaneous tissue produces clinically meaningful improvement in almost 100% of patients, and side effects are mild and transient. Botulinum toxin injections must be administered every 3–6 months. Follow-up of chronically treated patients shows the injections retain efficacy for at least 15 years.

A number of surgical techniques have been used in HFS. These include removal of the orbicularis oris or other affected muscles, selective destruction of parts of the facial nerve, decompression of the facial canal, and radiofrequency thermocoagulation of the nerve. Intracranial microvascular decompression of the nerve is successful in relieving spasms in up to 90% of patients, but complications such as facial nerve injury and hearing loss occur in as many as 15% of patients.

## Painful Legs–Moving Toes Syndrome

PLMTS is a very rare condition characterized by pain in the legs and spontaneous movements of the foot and toes. The pain usually precedes the onset of involuntary movements and varies in constancy and intensity. In some cases, the condition is painless. The toe and foot movements are complex, combining flexion, extension, abduction, and adduction in various sequences at frequencies of 1–2 Hz. The movements may be precipitated or aborted by moving or repositioning the foot or toes, but they cannot be simulated voluntarily. Similar movements have been described in the arms, with or without accompanying pain. In most cases, there is an underlying cause, although there is little consistency from case to case. PLMTS has been associated with injuries to the spinal cord and cauda equina, spinal nerve roots, peripheral neuropathy, and soft-tissue or bony limb trauma. EMG studies show that the movements are produced by long bursts of normal motor unit firing with normal recruitment patterns. PLMTS doubtless has a central origin. Central reorganization consequent to altered afferent information from the periphery has been proposed, but a precise location and mechanism of these changes remain unknown.

Treatment of PLMTS is very difficult. Many medications have been tried—baclofen, benzodiazepines, anticonvulsants, and antidepressants—but none has emerged as effective. Lumbar sympathetic block or epidural stimulation may give transient relief. Spontaneous resolution is very unusual.

## Stiff Person Syndrome

SPS is a rare autoimmune movement disorder, characterized by progressive rigidity of axial and proximal appendicular muscles, exaggerated lumbar lordosis, and a stiff gait (Baizabal-Carvallo and Jankovic, 2012, 2018). Intense spasms are superimposed on a background of continuous muscle contraction. Spasms and stiffness improve with sleep and are eliminated by general anesthesia and neuromuscular blocking agents. Clinical criteria for diagnosis include insidious development of limb and axial (thoracolumbar and abdominal) stiffness, clinical and electrophysiological confirmation of co-contraction of agonist and antagonist muscles, episodic spasms superimposed on chronic stiffness, and no other underlying illness that would explain the symptoms. Some authors divide SPS into three syndromes: stiff trunk syndrome, stiff limb syndrome, and rapidly progressive encephalomyelitis with rigidity. EMG examination shows continuous firing of normal motor units.

SPS is associated with autoimmune disorders such as type 1 diabetes, thyroiditis, myasthenia gravis, pernicious anemia, and vitiligo. High titers of antibodies to the 65-kD fraction of GAD and to other antigens are present. It is thought that SPS results from dysfunction of descending suprasegmental pathways possibly secondary to immune-mediated inhibition of GABA synthesis. Paraneoplastic SPS has been reported with breast and other cancers.

Untreated, SPS progresses to extreme disability. Diazepam at doses of 20–400 mg/day is the most effective symptomatic treatment. Clonazepam, baclofen, valproic acid, clonidine, vigabatrin, and tiagabine have also been reported to be effective. Intrathecal baclofen and local intramuscular injections of botulinum toxin have been helpful in some cases. Plasmapheresis, intravenous immunoglobulin (IVIG), and immunosuppression have been reported to have variable effects on the condition. In a recent placebo-controlled crossover study of IVIG, active treatment was associated with clinical improvement and decreases in anti-GAD antibody titers. Newer agents such as rituximab are currently under study for the treatment of SPS.

## Functional (Psychogenic) Movement Disorders

Functional movement disorders (FMDs), previously referred to as "psychogenic movement disorders," represent about 5% of patients in a movement disorders clinic, but the relative frequency is increasing as patients with atypical movement disorders, many of whom have FMD, are referred to specialized centers (see Chapter 113). In many cases, the symptoms are abrupt in onset and associated with a specific trigger. Clinically, distractibility is common, as are stimulus sensitivity and entrainment with voluntary activities. Other functional (psychogenic) symptoms are often present. Approximately 25% of patients have a comorbid organic movement disorder. About half have an Axis 1 psychiatric disorder, most often depression. The predominant movement disorders diagnosed as psychogenic (functional) include tremor, often manifested by irregular, distractible shaking of variable amplitude and frequency, dystonia, typically manifested by fixed abnormal posture, myoclonus, parkinsonism (Jankovic, 2011), tics (Baizabal-Carvallo and Jankovic, 2014), and a variety of other movement disorders (Stone et al., 2016; Thenganatt and Jankovic, 2019).

The pathophysiology of FMDs is poorly understood (Baizabal-Carvallo et al., 2019). Although stressful events on a background of depression and anxiety are common precipitants of FMDs, this link is not always possible to establish in all patients. While usually attributed to some psychiatric causes, several neurobiological abnormalities differentiate patients with FMD from normal controls. These include evidence of strengthened connectivity between the limbic and motor networks, increased activation of areas implicated in self-awareness, self-monitoring, and active motor inhibition such as the cingulate and insular cortex, coupled with decreased activation of the SMA and pre-SMA. Furthermore, the sense of agency defined as the feeling of controlling external events through one's own action also seems to be impaired in individuals with FMDs.

Some studies have correlated a recall of real-life events with abnormalities on functional imaging studies suggesting that the chief mechanism of functional (psychogenic) disorders involves repression of memories and conversion to somatic symptoms (Aybek et al., 2014).

Treatment of patients with functional (psychogenic movement disorders) is very challenging and requires tactful disclosure of the diagnosis, followed by insight-oriented and physical therapy, supplemented by treatment of underlying anxiety, depression, and other psychological and psychiatric issues (Thenganatt and Jankovic, 2019; see Chapter 113).

*The complete reference list is available online at https://expertconsult.inkling.com/.* 

97

# Disorders of Upper and Lower Motor Neurons

*Conor Fearon, Brian Murray, Hiroshi Mitsumoto*

## OUTLINE



It is important for the practicing clinician to make the distinction between the term *motor neuron disease* (MND) and *motor neuron diseases* (MNDs). The intention of the first term, coined by Brain in 1969, is to refer to a specific disorder of both upper and lower motor neurons, otherwise known as *amyotrophic lateral sclerosis* (ALS). The second term refers to the broader family of disorders that may affect the upper and/or lower motor neuron system as well as nonmotor systems. Within this heterogeneous family are included familial and sporadic disorders, inflammatory and immune disorders, and others of undetermined cause. Many are distinct entities, but some (e.g., primary lateral sclerosis [PLS], progressive muscular atrophy [PMA]) may be variations of a single multisystem disorder that predominantly involves motor neurons. This chapter reviews the causes, diagnosis, and treatment of the motor neuron diseases according to whether the disorder affects upper motor neurons (UMNs), lower motor neurons (LMNs), or both UMNs and LMNs.

## DISORDERS OF UPPER MOTOR NEURONS

### Neuroanatomy of Upper Motor Neurons

The UMN is a motor neuron, the cell body of which lies within the motor cortex of the cerebrum, and the axon of which forms the corticobulbar and corticospinal tracts. The LMNs, lying in the brainstem motor nuclei and the anterior horns of the spinal cord, directly innervate skeletal muscles. The UMNs are rostral to the LMNs and exert direct or indirect supranuclear control over the LMNs (Box 97.1).

#### Motor Cortex

In the cerebral cortex, UMNs are located in the primary motor cortex (Brodmann area 4) and the premotor areas (Brodmann area 6), which are subdivided into the supplementary motor area (sometimes called the *secondary motor cortex*) and the premotor cortex, respectively. Betz cells (giant pyramidal neurons) are a distinct group of large motor neurons in layer 5 of the primary motor cortex and represent only a small portion of all primary motor neurons with axons in the corticospinal tracts. Individual motor neurons in the primary motor cortex initiate and control the contraction of small groups of skeletal muscles subserving individual movements. The entire motor area of the cerebral cortex controls the highest levels of voluntary muscle movement, including motor planning and programming of muscle movement.

***Corticospinal and corticobulbar tracts.*** Axons from the motor areas form the corticospinal and corticobulbar tracts. Axons arising from neurons in the primary motor cortex constitute only one-third of all the corticospinal and corticobulbar tracts. Among these, Betz cell axons make up 3%–5% of the tract, and the remaining fibers from the primary motor cortex arise from other neurons in layer 5 of the primary motor cortex. Another one-third of the axons in these tracts derive from Brodmann area 6, which includes the supplementary motor and the lateral premotor cortex. The remaining third derives from the somatic sensory cortex (areas 1, 2, and 3) and the adjacent temporal lobe region. The corticobulbar tract projects bilaterally to the motor neurons of cranial nerves V, VII, IX, X, and XII. Most corticospinal fibers (75%–90%) decussate in the lower medulla (pyramidal decussation) and form the lateral corticospinal tract in the spinal cord (the pyramidal tracts). The remaining fibers descend in the ipsilateral ventral corticospinal tract. The lateral corticospinal tract projects to ipsilateral spinal motor neurons and their interneurons that control extremity muscle contraction, whereas the anterior corticospinal tract ends bilaterally on ventromedial motor neurons and interneurons that control the axial and postural muscles. These corticospinal axons provide direct glutamatergic excitatory input to alpha motoneurons.

***Brainstem control.*** Several brainstem nuclei exert supranuclear influence on the LMN population in the spinal cord through highly complex projections. The fibers originating in the medial and inferior vestibular nuclei in the medulla descend in the medial vestibulospinal tract and terminate both on medial cervical and thoracic motor neurons and on interneurons. They excite ipsilateral motor neurons but inhibit contralateral neurons. The lateral vestibulospinal tracts originating in the lateral vestibular nucleus (Deiters nucleus) activate the extensor motor neurons and inhibit the flexor motor neurons in all limbs.

The brainstem reticular formation also strongly influences the spinal motor neurons, exerting widespread polysynaptic inhibitory input on extensor motor neurons and excitatory input on flexor motor neurons. The reticulospinal tracts modulate various reflex actions during ongoing movements. The brainstem reticular formation receives supranuclear control from the motor cortex via the cortical reticulospinal pathway to act as a major inhibitor of spinal reflexes and activity. Therefore, a lesion of the corticoreticular pathway can disinhibit reticulospinal control of the LMNs. The tectospinal tract originates in the superior colliculus and controls eye and head movement. Variations in the balance between inhibitory input (mediated by the dorsal reticulospinal tract) and facilitatory input (mediated by the medial reticulospinal tract) alter muscle tone. To some extent, the vestibulospinal tract alters tone by input to muscle stretch receptors.

***Limbic motor control.*** The limbic system is involved in emotional experience and expression and associated with a variety of autonomic, visceral, and endocrine functions. It strongly influences the somatic motor neurons. The emotional status and experience of an individual determines overall spinal cord activity, and the limbic motor system also influences respiration, vomiting, swallowing, chewing, and licking (at least in animal studies). Furthermore, the generation of signs of pseudobulbar hyperemotionality (pseudobulbar affect, emotional incontinence) in ALS is closely related to an abnormal limbic motor control, particularly in the periaqueductal gray and nucleus retroambiguus. The latter nuclei project to the somatic motor neurons that innervate pharyngeal, soft palatal, intercostal, diaphragmatic, abdominal, and probably laryngeal muscles. Pseudobulbar hyperemotionality symptoms may appear when UMN control over these motor nuclei is impaired, and thus limbic motor control is disinhibited. There appears to be some degree of emotional regulation by the cerebellum. The "cerebellar cognitive affective syndrome" can arise when stroke, tumor, or infection interrupts connections between the cerebellum and cerebral association and paralimbic regions (Schmahmann and Sherman, 1998).

### BOX 97.1 Upper Motor Neurons and Their Descending Tracts

**The motor areas**

The primary motor neurons (Betz giant pyramidal cells and surrounding motor neurons)

**The premotor areas (the supplementary motor area and premotor cortex)**

Corticospinal and corticobulbar tracts
Lateral pyramidal tracts
Ventral (uncrossed) pyramidal tracts

**Brainstem control**

Vestibulospinal tracts
Reticulospinal tracts
Tectospinal tracts

**Limbic motor control**

## Signs and Symptoms of Upper Motor Neuron Involvement

### Loss of Dexterity

Loss of dexterity is one of the most characteristic signs of UMN impairment. Voluntary skillful movements require the integrated activation of many interneuron circuits in the spinal cord; such integration is ultimately controlled by the corticospinal tract and thus by UMNs. Loss of dexterity may express itself as stiffness, slowness, and clumsiness in performing any skillful motor actions. Asking the patient to perform rapid repetitive motions such as foot or finger tapping assesses loss of dexterity at the bedside. It is useful to assess both sides of the body, as many motor neuron disorders are asymmetrical (Box 97.2).

### Loss of Muscle Strength (Weakness)

The degree of muscle weakness resulting from UMN dysfunction is generally mild. Extensor muscles of the upper extremities and flexor muscles of lower extremities may become weaker than their antagonist muscles because the UMN lesion disinhibits brainstem control of the vestibulospinal and reticulospinal tracts.

### Spasticity

Spasticity is the hallmark of UMN disease, but its pathophysiology is complex and controversial. It seems to reflect altered firing of alpha motoneurons and interneurons within the spinal cord, together with increased activity of group II nerve fibers derived from muscle spindles. An excess level of excitatory input to gamma motoneurons exists via excess synaptic levels of excitatory neurotransmitters such as serotonin, norepinephrine, and glutamate. In addition, there is reduced inhibitory glycinergic and γ-aminobutyric acid (GABA)ergic neurotransmission. The result is a state of sustained increase in muscle tension when the muscle lengthens. Clinically, muscles exhibit a sudden resistive "catch" midway during passive movement of the limb. However, when a sustained passive stretch is continued, spastic muscles quickly release the tension and relax, an event often described

### BOX 97.2 Signs and Symptoms of Upper Motor Neuron Involvement

Loss of dexterity
Loss of muscle strength (mild weakness)
Spasticity
Pathological hyperreflexia
Pathological reflexes (Babinski, Hoffmann sign, loss of abdominal reflexes)
Increased reflexes in an atrophic limb (*probable* upper motor neuron sign)
Pseudobulbar (spastic bulbar) palsy (emotional lability, brisk jaw jerk, hyperactive gag, forced yawning, snout reflex, suck reflex, slow tongue movements, spastic dysarthria)

as the "clasp-knife phenomenon." In muscles that are severely spastic, passive movement becomes more difficult and even impossible. Sustained increases in muscle tone lead to a slowing in motor activities.

### Pathological Hyperreflexia and Pathological Reflexes

Pathological hyperreflexia is another crucial manifestation of UMN disease. The Babinski sign (extensor plantar response) is perhaps the most important sign in the clinical neurological examination and is characterized by extension of the great toe (often, but not universally, accompanied by fanning of the other toes) in response to stroking the outer edge of the ipsilateral sole upward from the heel with a blunt object. This sign may only evolve at a later stage of disease and may be absent in the setting of marked atrophy of the toe extensor muscles.

### Pseudobulbar (Spastic Bulbar) Palsy

Pseudobulbar palsy (or spastic bulbar palsy) develops when there is disease involvement of the corticobulbar tracts that exert supranuclear control over those motor nuclei that control speech, mastication, and deglutition. The prefix *pseudo* distinguishes this condition from true bulbar palsy that results from pure LMN involvement in brainstem motor nuclei. Articulation, mastication, and deglutition are impaired in both pseudobulbar and bulbar palsies, but the degree of impairment in pseudobulbar palsy is generally milder. Spontaneous or unmotivated crying and laughter uniquely characterize pseudobulbar palsy. This is also termed *emotional lability*, *hyperemotionality*, *labile affect*, or *emotional incontinence* and is often a source of great embarrassment to the patient.

## Laboratory Evidence of Upper Motor Neuron Involvement

Several promising imaging and electrophysiological techniques are under investigation as potential markers of UMN involvement in neurological disease. However, a thorough bedside examination is the easiest and most effective means to detect UMN disease.

### Neuroimaging

The use of brain magnetic resonance imaging (MRI) in ALS is largely to exclude other conditions but sometimes shows abnormal signal intensity in the corticospinal and corticobulbar tracts as they descend from the motor strip via the internal capsules to the cerebral peduncles. In ALS, signal changes, best appreciated on proton density images of the internal capsules, probably represent Wallerian degeneration; similar changes also appear on conventional T2-weighted and fluid-attenuated inversion recovery (FLAIR) sequences. However, these changes do not appear to be sufficiently sensitive, and efforts continue to evaluate other potential MRI techniques such as diffusion tensor imaging (DTI) and high-field volumetric MRI, which may serve as markers of UMN disease (Foerster et al., 2013).

### Magnetic Resonance Spectroscopy Imaging

Proton density magnetic resonance spectroscopy ($^1$H-MRS) is a noninvasive nuclear magnetic resonance technique that combines the advantages of MRI with in vivo biochemical information. A significant reduction of *N*-acetylaspartate, a neuronal marker, relative to creatine or choline (used as internal standards) exists in the sensorimotor cortices of patients with ALS who have UMN signs. Alterations in the measured levels of these metabolites using $^1$H-MRS are useful in the detection of UMN dysfunction early in the evolution of ALS and are useful for monitoring progression over time. MRS still requires further technological improvements before it comes into widespread use.

### Transcranial Magnetic Stimulation

Transcranial magnetic stimulation (TMS) is an electrophysiological technique that has detected cortical hyperexcitability/impaired inhibition as well as cortical motor neuron and long-tract degeneration in ALS. The stimulus is a brief, high-intensity electromagnetic pulse generated from a series of capacitors and discharged through wire coils applied at the scalp over the motor cortex and the evoked response measured at skeletal muscle. Several different techniques are under investigation, including single-pulse TMS, cortical silent period measurement, paired pulse TMS, and repetitive TMS (Geevasinga et al. 2019). Overall, this promising, noninvasive tool requires further evaluation as a marker of UMN dysfunction. Recent evidence suggests that it may be useful in combination with other tools such as DTI.

## Primary Lateral Sclerosis

PLS, first described by Erb in 1875, is a rare UMN disease variant that accounts for 2%–4% of all cases of ALS and is traditionally distinguished by a lack of LMN involvement. In fact, the latter feature would lead some to argue that PLS is an entity that is distinct from ALS (Kolind et al., 2013). The Pringle criteria for PLS stipulated that disease be restricted to the UMN system for at least 3 years from the time of clinical onset (Pringle et al., 1992), but a figure of 4 years is now proposed during which there is neither clinical nor neurophysiological evidence of LMN involvement. In a recent study comparing the evolution of disease in PLS versus UMN-predominant ALS and typical ALS, the median time to development of electromyographic (EMG). LMN features after onset in those with an evolving ALS was 3.17 years; in those patients, clinical signs of LMN disease occurred on average about 6 months later. Nonetheless, later development of LMN signs may occur and require reclassification as ALS in some cases, which therefore necessitates constant longitudinal review of each case (Gordon et al., 2009). Indeed, it is possible to divide PLS patients into subgroups based on clinical and molecular characteristics. A recent study identified two broad clinical groups presenting with PLS; those with bulbar/dysphagia and those with urinary urgency. Furthermore, there were PLS-like presentations due to mutations in C9Orf72 but also in PARK2, SPG7, and DCTN1 (Mitsumoto et al., 2015).

PLS typically presents in patients in their early 50s (about a decade younger than typical MND/ALS patients) as a very slowly evolving spastic paraparesis that spreads to the upper limbs and eventually causes pseudobulbar palsy. In rare instances, onset is in the bulbar system or follows a slowly ascending or descending hemiplegic pattern (Mills hemiplegic variant), but a bulbar-onset presentation should make the clinician wary of later LMN signs elsewhere. Other features include cramps and fasciculations, but such complaints are neither prominent nor universal. Bladder dysfunction is rare and, if it occurs at all, tends to be a late feature. Although muscle weakness is present, the main deficits are due to spasticity in dexterity and gait. The rate of progression can be exceedingly slow, often progressing over many years to the point where the patient manifests a robotic gait, debilitating generalized spasticity, and prominent pseudobulbar palsy. Muscle atrophy, if it occurs at all, is a very late feature. No clinically detectable sensory changes occur. Neuropsychological test batteries may define subtle cognitive deficits due to frontal cortical involvement, but dementia is not a prominent feature. A few patients may exhibit abnormal saccadic voluntary eye movements. Corticobasal syndrome can develop rarely in patients who initially present with a pure upper motor neuron syndrome (Johnson et al., 2015). Breathing is usually unimpaired in PLS, and as a consequence, forced vital capacity (FVC) is not affected (Gordon et al., 2009).

The prognosis is significantly better than for MND/ALS: one series had a median disease duration of 19 years and another series exhibited a range of survival from 72 to 491 months (Murray, 2006). The underlying pathogenesis of PLS remains undefined. Pathological changes include a striking loss of Betz cells in layer 5 of the frontal and prefrontal motor cortex (and other smaller pyramidal cells) together with laminar gliosis of layers 3 and 5 and degeneration of the corticospinal tracts. Spinal anterior horn cells are characteristically unaffected.

### Diagnosis

The diagnosis of PLS is essentially one of exclusion (Table 97.1). Rare reports of UMN-onset ALS exist where the interval between onset of UMN signs and subsequent LMN signs has been up to 27 years. As such, it is vital to reassess patients diagnosed with PLS, as late signs of LMN involvement may occur that would reclassify their disorder as UMN-onset ALS.

Appropriate testing must exclude all definable causes for generalized UMN involvement. These include structural abnormalities (Chiari malformation and intrinsic and extrinsic spinal cord lesions) and myelopathies such as multiple sclerosis (MS) spondylotic cervical myelopathy, human immunodeficiency virus (HIV) myelopathy, human T-lymphotropic virus type 1 (HTLV-1) myelopathy, Lyme disease, syphilis, or adrenomyeloneuropathy. Spondylotic cervical myelopathy and MS are probably the most common causes among these disorders. The family history must be negative to rule out hereditary spastic paraplegia (HSP)/familial spastic paraparesis, spinocerebellar ataxia (SCA), hexosaminidase-A (Hex-A) deficiency, familial ALS (FALS), or adrenomyeloneuropathy. It is now apparent that some forms of HSP, including spastin and paraplegin mutation-associated HSP, may lack a family history; it is worthwhile to carry out genetic testing for HSP in patients presenting with symptoms and signs that are restricted to the lower extremities (Brugman et al., 2009). Paraneoplastic syndromes (especially in association with breast cancer) and Sjögren syndrome may clinically resemble PLS. Thus, it is important to consider paraneoplastic diseases, particularly in an older woman presenting with a pure upper motor syndrome and other genetic mimics.

### Treatment

No specific pharmacotherapy is available, and treatment therefore focuses on symptom control and supportive care. However, antispasticity drugs such as the GABA-B agonist baclofen and the central $\alpha_2$-agonist tizanidine may be tried for symptomatic treatment. Severe spasticity sometimes requires the insertion of an intrathecal baclofen pump. Tricyclic antidepressants, selective serotonin reuptake inhibitors, or dextromethorphan/quinidine may control pseudobulbar affect lability (Brooks et al., 2005).

## Hereditary Spastic Paraplegia

HSP (or familial spastic paraparesis) is a genetically and clinically heterogeneous group of disorders rather than a single entity. The clinical feature common to all cases is progressively worsening spasticity of the lower extremities, often with variable degrees of weakness. The characteristic pathology is retrograde degeneration of the longest nerve fibers in the corticospinal tracts and posterior columns due to mutations affecting vesicular trafficking, axonal transport, lipid metabolism, mitochondrial dynamics, and myelination. Its estimated prevalence is 3–10 per 100,000, but its worldwide prevalence may actually be underestimated because of the benign nature of the disease in many families (Blackstone, 2012). It may be inherited in an autosomal dominant, autosomal recessive, or X-linked fashion, but it should be borne in mind that a number of cases will lack a family history, as stated below (Depienne et al., 2006, Lan et al., 2015).

Although most cases present in the second to fourth decades, onset is from infancy into the eighth decade. The clinical syndrome is broadly divisible into the pure form and the complicated form. In the pure form, patients develop only lower-extremity spasticity, but some of these cases eventually become complicated. However, the complicated form may also include optic neuropathy, pigmentary retinopathy, deafness, ataxia, ichthyosis, amyotrophy, peripheral neuropathy, dementia, autoimmune hemolytic anemia/thrombocytopenia (Evans syndrome), extrapyramidal dysfunction, cerebellar dysfunction, ptosis, ophthalmoparesis, intellectual disability, and bladder dysfunction (Video 97.1).

There is an ever-expanding list of genes and genetic loci in the HSP family. Over 70 genetic subtypes have been described (de Souza et al., 2017; Table 97.2). Novel techniques such as exome sequencing are valuable in discovering new genes. Inheritance of most pure HSP is autosomal dominant, whereas complicated forms are more often autosomal recessive. For example, approximately 40% of autosomal dominant pure HSP worldwide is due to mutations of the *SPAST* gene on chromosome 2p22–21, which encodes spastin, a 616-amino acid protein. Mutations of various types (missense, nonsense, frameshift, splice site) may affect this gene (McDermott, 2006). Spastin is a highly conserved member of the AAA family of proteins (adenosine triphosphatase [ATPase] associated with various cellular activities). The exact role of mutant spastin in the pathogenesis of HSP is not known, although a disturbance in maintenance of the microtubule cytoskeleton may exist, thus disrupting axonal transport. More than half of all cases do not

**TABLE 97.1 Disorders of Upper Motor Neurons and Their Key Characteristics**

| Disorders | Key Characteristics |
|---|---|
| Primary lateral sclerosis | A diagnosis of exclusion |
| Hereditary spastic paraplegia | Heredity, usually autosomal dominant, spastin gene mutation, other mutations (see text), "sporadic" |
| HTLV-1-associated myelopathy | Slowly progressive myelopathy, endemic, and positive HTLV-1 |
| HTLV-2-associated myelopathy | Amerindian, IV drug abuser, concomitant HIV |
| Adrenomyeloneuropathy | X-linked recessive inheritance, adrenal dysfunction, myelopathy, very long-chain fatty acid assay |
| Lathyrism | History of consumption of chickling peas |
| Konzo | Eastern African, cassava root consumption |

*HIV*, Human immunodeficiency virus; *HTLV*, human T-lymphotropic virus; *IV*, intravenous.

TABLE 97.2 **Hereditary Spastic Paraplegia Known Phenotype-Genotype Disorders**

| Phenotype (OMIM Reference) | Gene | Location | Proposed Mechanism | Mode of Inheritance | Key Clinical/Radiographic Features | Gene OMIM Reference |
|---|---|---|---|---|---|---|
| Spastic paraplegia 1/MASA syndrome/ CRASH syndrome (#303350) | *L1CAM* | Xq28 | Neuronal migration, myelination production | X-linked | Mental retardation, aphasia, shuffling gait, short stature, and adducted thumbs, corpus callosum hypoplasia, hydrocephalus | *308840 |
| Spastic paraplegia 2 (#312920) | *PLP1* | Xq22.2 | Myelin production | X-linked | Onset in childhood, highly variable phenotype including cerebellar signs/ optic atrophy/contractures/mental retardation | *300401 |
| Spastic paraplegia 3A (#182600) | *ATL1* | 14q22.1 | Membrane trafficking | AD | Early-onset (often before age 5–10), slowly progressive, pes cavus, sphincter disturbance. | *606439 |
| Spastic paraplegia 4 (#182601) | *SPAST* | 2p22.3 | Microtubule dynamics | AD | Variable age at onset, symptom severity and rate of symptom progression. Pes cavus, sphincter disturbance, mild dysarthria | *604277 |
| Spastic paraplegia 5A (#270800) | *CYP7B1* | 8q12.3 | Lipid metabolism | AR | Variable age at onset, mostly pure but variable cerebellar involvement, optic atrophy, reduced vibration/proprioception | *603711 |
| Spastic paraplegia 6/Familial spastic paraparesis (#600363) | *NIPA1 (SPG6)* | 15q11.2 | Membrane transport/lysosomal degradation | AD | Insidious onset in 2nd–3rd decade, variable severity, seizures, tremor | *608145 |
| Spastic paraplegia 7 (#607259) | *SPG7, (PGN CMAR, CAR)* | 16q24.3 | Mitochondrial dysfunction | AR, some heterozygous mutations | Onset in 3rd–5th decade, variable cerebellar signs/optic atrophy/eye movement abnormalities/attention deficits, cortical/cerebellar atrophy | *602783 |
| Spastic paraplegia 8 (#603563) | *KIAA0196* | 8q24.13 | Protein aggregation | AD | Onset 18–60 years, upper limb spasticity, amyotrophy, severe phenotype | *610657 |
| Spastic paraplegia 9A (#601162) | *ALDH18A1* | 10q24.1 | Amino acid metabolism | AD | Juvenile or adult, ALS-like, short stature, cataracts, pes cavus. | *138250 |
| Spastic paraplegia 10 (#604187) | *KIF5A* | 12q13.3 | Membrane transport | AD | Onset 3rd–4th decade, with or without axonal sensorimotor neuropathy. Can be associated with amyotrophy, parkinsonism, cerebellar ataxia | *602821 |
| Spastic paraplegia 11 (#604360) | *SPG11* | 15q21.1 | Unknown, presumed membrane transport | AR | Onset in adolescence, mental impairment, cerebellar ataxia, parkinsonism, amyotrophy, thin corpus callosum, "ears-of-the-lynx sign" | *610844 |
| Spastic paraplegia 12 (#604805) | *RTN2* | 19q13.32 | Tubular endoplasmic reticulum network dysfunction | AD | Onset 1st–2nd decade, pure phenotype, rapidly progressive | *603183 |
| Spastic paraplegia 13 (#605280) | *HSPD1 (SPG13, HSP60, HLD4)* | 2q33.1 | Mitochondrial protein instability | AD | Variable age at onset, pure phenotype, severe spasticity | *118190 |
| Spastic paraplegia 15/Spastic paraplegia and retinal degeneration/ Kjellin syndrome (#270700) | *ZFYVE26* | 14q24.1 | Unknown, presumed membrane transport | AR | Onset in 1st–2nd decade, variable intellectual disability/dysarthria/retinal degeneration, distal amyotrophy, parkinsonism, seizures, axonal neuropathy, thin corpus callosum, cerebral atrophy, white matter hyperintensities | *612012 |
| Spastic paraplegia 17/Silver spastic paraplegia (#270685) | *BSCL2* | 11q12.3 | Tubular endoplasmic reticulum network dysfunction | AD | Variable age at onset, distal amyotrophy | *606158 |

*Continued*

**TABLE 97.2 Hereditary Spastic Paraplegia Known Phenotype-Genotype Disorders—cont'd**

| Phenotype (OMIM Reference) | Gene | Location | Proposed Mechanism | Mode of Inheritance | Key Clinical/Radiographic Features | Gene OMIM Reference |
|---|---|---|---|---|---|---|
| Spastic paraplegia 18 (#611225) | *ERLIN2* | 8p11.23 | Endoplasmic reticulum-associated degradation pathway | AR | Onset in infancy, severe psychomotor retardation, joint contractures, global muscle weakness and atrophy, high arched palate, kyphosis/scoliosis, speech absent or limited, occasional seizures | *611605 |
| Spastic paraplegia 20/Troyer syndrome (#275900) | *SPG20* | 13q13.3 | Microtubule dynamics | AR | Onset in early childhood, distal amyotrophy and contractures, short stature, hypertelorism, maxillary overgrowth, tongue dyspraxia | *607111 |
| Spastic paraplegia 21/Mast syndrome (#248900) | *SPG21* | 15q22.31 | Dysregulation of CD4 activity | AR | Onset 2nd–3rd decade, presenile dementia, parkinsonism, cerebellar signs, thin corpus callosum and white matter abnormalities | *608181 |
| Spastic paraplegia 23 | *DSTYK* | 1q32.1 | Unknown | AR | Vitiligo, hyperpigmentation, lentigines, facial features, mental retardation, mild neuropathy | *612666 |
| Spastic paraplegia 26 (#609195) | *B4GALNT1* | 12q13.3 | Sphingolipid metabolism | AR | Onset in 1st -2nd decades of life, slowly progressive, distal amyotrophy, intellectual disability, axonal sensorimotor neuropathy, dysarthria, variable cerebellar signs, extrapyramidal signs, cortical atrophy, and white matter hyperintensities | *601873 |
| Spastic paraplegia 28 (#609340) | *DDHD1* | 14q22.1 | Lipid metabolism | AR | Onset in childhood or adolescence, slowly progressive pure phenotype | *614603 |
| Spastic paraplegia 30 (#610357) | *KIF1A* | 2q37.3 | Microtubule dynamics | AR | Onset 1st–2nd decade, variable cerebellar involvement/peripheral neuropathy | *601255 |
| Spastic paraplegia 31 (#610250) | *REEP1* | 2p11.2 | Tubular endoplasmic reticulum network dysfunction | AD | Bimodal age of onset (usually 1st–2nd decade), variable severity, mostly pure HSP, occasionally complicated (e.g., bulbar dysfunction, distal amyotrophy) | *609139 |
| Spastic paraplegia 33 (#610244) | *ZFYVE27* | 10q24.2 | Dysfunction of membrane trafficking | AD | Adult onset, pure phenotype | *610243 |
| Spastic paraplegia 35/Fatty acid hydroxylase-associated neurodegeneration (#612319) | *FA2H* | 16q23.1 | Lipid metabolism | AR | Onset in 1st decade, dysarthria, mild cognitive decline, variable dystonia/optic atrophy/seizures, leukodystrophy and occasional evidence of neurodegeneration with brain iron accumulation, atrophy of cerebellum/brainstem/corpus callosum | *611026 |
| Spastic paraplegia 39/NTE-related motor neuron disorder (#612020) | *PNPLA6* | 19p13.2 | Unknown, presumed lipid/myelination related | AR | Childhood onset, distal upper and lower extremity wasting, cerebellar signs, spinal cord atrophy | *603197 |
| Spastic paraplegia 42 (#612539) | *SLC33A1* | 3q25.31 | Glycoprotein and ganglioside metabolism in Golgi apparatus | AD | Variable age at onset, pure phenotype | *603690 |
| Spastic paraplegia 43 (#615043) | *C19orf12* | 19q12 | Mitochondrial transmembrane protein, function unknown | AR | Onset in 1st decade, decreased vibration, distal muscle atrophy, reduced reflexes, contractures | *614297 |

TABLE 97.2 **Hereditary Spastic Paraplegia Known Phenotype-Genotype Disorders—cont'd**

| Phenotype (OMIM Reference) | Gene | Location | Proposed Mechanism | Mode of Inheritance | Key Clinical/Radiographic Features | Gene OMIM Reference |
|---|---|---|---|---|---|---|
| Spastic paraplegia 44 (#613206) | *GJC2* | 1q42.13 | Disruption of oligodendrocyte homeostasis | AR | Onset of mild symptoms in 1st–2nd decade with progression in adulthood, cerebellar signs, hearing loss, seizures, hypomyelinating leukodystrophy and thin corpus callosum | *608803 |
| Spastic paraplegia 45 (#613162) | *NT5C2* | 10q24.32-q24.33 (10q24.3-q25.1) | Purine/pyrimidine nucleotides metabolism | AR | Onset before age 2, intellectual disability, contractures, optic atrophy, dysplastic corpus callosum | *600417 |
| Spastic paraplegia 46 (#614409) | *GBA2* | 9p13.3 | Sphingolipid metabolism | AR | Onset in childhood cerebellar involvement, variable cognitive impairment/cataracts/kyphoscoliosis/testicular atrophy, variable cerebral, cerebellar, and corpus callosum atrophy | *609471 |
| Spastic paraplegia 47 (#614066) | *AP4B1* | 1p13.2 | Membrane transport | AR | Onset at birth, severe mental retardation with poor or absent speech development, stereotyped laughing, spastic tongue protrusion, variable dysmorphic features | *607245 |
| Spastic paraplegia 48 (#613647) | *AP5Z1* | 7p22.1 | Membrane transport/DNA repair | AR | Adult onset, pure phenotype, mild cervical spine hyperintensities | *613653 |
| Spastic paraplegia 49 (#615031) | *TECPR2* | 14q32.31 | Interruption of intracellular autophagy pathway | AR | Onset in the first 2 years of life, moderate to severe intellectual disability, dysmorphic features, episodes of central apnea, thin corpus callosum, cerebral and cerebellar atrophy | *615000 |
| Spastic paraplegia 50 (#612936) | *AP4M1* | 7q22.1 | Membrane transport | AR | Neonatal hypotonia, severe mental retardation, dysmorphism, speech absent or limited, pseudobulbar signs, ventriculomegaly, white-matter abnormalities, and variable cerebellar atrophy | *602296 |
| Spastic paraplegia 51 (#613744) | *AP4E1* | 15q21.2 | Membrane transport | AR | Presents with neonatal hypotonia, severe intellectual disability, speech absent or limited, dysmorphic features, seizures, stereotypic laughing, contractures, ventriculomegaly, cerebral/cerebellar atrophy, and leukodystrophy | *607244 |
| Spastic paraplegia 52 (#614067) | *AP4S1* | 14q12 | Membrane transport | AR | Presents at birth with neonatal hypotonia, severe intellectual disability, speech absent or limited, talipes equinovarus, decreased shank muscle mass, short stature, dysmorphic features and microcephaly, stereotypic laughing | *607243 |
| Spastic paraplegia 53 (#614898) | *VPS37A* | 8p22 | Endosomal sorting | AR | Onset in infancy, mild-moderate cognitive impairment, dystonia, pectus carinatum, marked kyphosis | *609927 |
| Spastic paraplegia 54 (#615033) | *DDHD2* | 8p11.23 | Lipid metabolism | AR | Onset of spasticity by age 2 years, intellectual disability, short stature, foot contractures, dysarthria, dysphagia, variable optic hypoplasia, strabismus, telecanthus, thin corpus callosum and periventricular white-matter lesions, MR spectroscopy shows an abnormal lipid peak | *615003 |

*Continued*

TABLE 97.2 **Hereditary Spastic Paraplegia Known Phenotype-Genotype Disorders—cont'd**

| Phenotype (OMIM Reference) | Gene | Location | Proposed Mechanism | Mode of Inheritance | Key Clinical/Radiographic Features | Gene OMIM Reference |
|---|---|---|---|---|---|---|
| Spastic paraplegia 55 (#615035) | *C12orf65* | 12q24.31 | Mitochondrial dysfunction | AR | Onset in 1st decade, axonal peripheral neuropathy, optic atrophy, strabismus, mental retardation, arthrogryposis of small joints, thin corpus callosum | *613541 |
| Spastic paraplegia 56 (#615030) | *CYP2U1* | 4q25 | Unknown, gene may play a role in immune functions | AR | Onset birth to 8 years, upper limb involvement, dystonia, thin corpus callosum, basal ganglia calcification | *610670 |
| Spastic paraplegia 57 (#615658) | *TFG* | 3q12.2 | Endoplasmic reticulum and microtubule function | AR | Early onset, optic atrophy, wasting of hand and leg muscles and contractures, axonal demyelinating sensorimotor neuropathy | *602498 |
| Spastic paraplegia 61 (#615685) | *ARL6IP1* | 16p12.3 | Protein transport | AR | Present in first 2 years of life, sensorimotor neuropathy, severe mutilating acropathy | *607669 |
| Spastic paraplegia 62 (#615685) | *ERLIN1* | 10q24.31 | Endoplasmic reticulum function | AR | Cerebellar ataxia, distal amyotrophy | *611604 |
| Spastic paraplegia 63 (#615686) | *AMPD2* | 1p13.3 | Purine nucleotide metabolism | AR | Present in first 2 years of life, short stature, white-matter changes, thin corpus callosum | *102771 |
| Spastic paraplegia 64 (#615683) | *ENTPD1* | 10q24.1 | Purine nucleotide metabolism | AR | Onset in childhood, intellectual disability, microcephaly, delayed puberty, dysarthria | *601752 |
| Spastic paraplegia 72 (#615625) | *REEP2 (SGC32445, C5orf19)* | 5q31.2 | Shaping of endoplasmic reticulum, membrane interactions | AD or AR | Onset in early childhood, slowly progressive, postural tremor | *609347 |
| Spastic paraplegia 73 (#616282) | *CPT1C* | 19q13.33 | Altered lipid metabolism | AD | Onset in early adulthood, slowly progressive, mild amyotrophy | *608846 |
| Spastic paraplegia 74 (#616451) | *IBA57* | 1q42.13 | Mitochondrial dynamics | AR | Onset in first decade, slowly progressive, optic atrophy, distal amyotrophy | *615316 |

*AD*, Autosomal dominant; *AR*, autosomal recessive.

manifest symptoms and signs until after age 30 years. Although this is normally a pure HSP, complicated forms occur, and some cases can develop a late-onset cognitive decline. Pathologically, degeneration of the longest corticospinal tracts and, to a lesser degree, the posterior columns of the spinal cord is seen.

Mutations in the *SPG3A* gene on 14q11–q21 encoding the novel protein, atlastin, give rise to another autosomal dominant, often early-onset (<10 years of age) pure HSP, which accounts for about 10% of autosomal dominant cases. This protein shares structural homology with guanylate-binding protein 1, which is a member of the dynamin family. Dynamins are important in intracellular trafficking of various kinds of vesicles. Mutations in *KIF5A* (*SPG10*, Chr 12q), a kinesin motor domain that is critical in intracellular transport, can cause both early- and late-onset spastic paraparesis with distal amyotrophy (Blair et al., 2006). Spastic paraplegia 11 (*SPG11*) is an autosomal recessive complicated HSP (thin corpus callosum, neuropathy, cognitive impairment) due to mutations in the spatacsin gene on chromosome 15q. This protein is of unknown function and does not appear to interact with the Golgi apparatus or microtubules. The cause of autosomal dominant pure HSP, linked to 2q24–34, is a mutation in the *SPG13* gene, which encodes a mitochondrial heat shock protein. Recessively inherited complicated HSP links to chromosome 16q and is caused by a mutation in a gene encoding a mitochondrial protein known as *paraplegin*; this disorder can be either pure or complicated (cerebellar signs, pale optic discs, and peripheral neuropathy). The genes for two different X-linked complicated HSP have been identified. In the first, mutant L1 (neural) cell adhesion molecule (L1CAM) may disrupt neuronal migration or differentiation; in the second mutant proteolipid protein (PLP1) is found in association with changes in white matter (duplication mutations in this same gene can also cause Pelizaeus-Merzbacher disease). Spastic paraplegia 17 (*SPG17*) is caused by mutations in the seipin gene on chromosome 11q12–q14. Also known as *Silver syndrome*, this disorder is an autosomal dominant complicated form of HSP with distal hand and foot amyotrophy beginning in the late teens to early 30s. Mutations in this gene are also the cause of a form of distal hereditary neuropathy (Charcot-Marie-Tooth [CMT] disease type 5).

Using novel techniques such as exome sequencing, it is evident that there are multiple genes, some likely yet to be discovered, mutations of which can lead to a HSP phenotype. The terms "the HSPome" and "the HSP interactome" have been coined to highlight the ways in which known and candidate genes are connected. For example, known mutations are associated with various pathogenic mechanisms which affect cellular transport or the metabolism and development of axons and synapses (Novarino et al., 2014) (see Video 97.1 and Table 97.2).

### Diagnosis

The basis for diagnosis of HSP is evidence of a family history in the setting of progressive gait disturbance, evidence of lower-extremity spasticity, and sparing of craniobulbar function. However, difficulties arise when there is no clear family history in recessive or X-linked disease and in cases of apparently sporadic HSP. Furthermore, considerable variation in disease expression exists between and within HSP families. In the absence of a family history or a demonstration of a known mutation, it is important to consider alternative causes for the clinical presentation, including structural disease (e.g., cerebral palsy, hydrocephalus, myelopathy), degenerative/infiltrative/inflammatory disease (e.g., MS, ALS, SCA, leukodystrophy), infections (syphilis, HIV, HTLV), levodopa-responsive dystonia, metabolic/toxic damage (vitamin $B_{12}$ deficiency [subacute combined degeneration of the spinal cord (SCDC)], vitamin E deficiency, copper deficiency, lathyrism), and paraneoplastic disorders. MRI may reveal that cervical and thoracic spinal cord diameters are significantly smaller in both pure and complicated HSP than in controls (Sperfeld et al., 2005). Perhaps the most important differential diagnosis is that between apparently sporadic pure HSP and PLS, especially as the later may present with a slowly evolving spastic paraparesis for many years prior to the development of upper limb or bulbar features. The only reliable way to distinguish such disorders is through genetic testing; age at onset, urgency of micturition, and signs of dorsal column involvement (clinical or abnormal somatosensory evoked potentials [SSEPs]) are not accurate indicators of HSP versus PLS (Brugman et al., 2009).

### Treatment

At present, treatment of spastic paraplegia is limited to symptomatic interventions, supportive care to reduce spasticity, and appliances and orthotics such as canes, walkers, and wheelchairs. Antispasticity drugs such as baclofen, tizanidine, diazepam, and dantrolene are often suboptimal, and patients with very disabling spasticity may require intrathecal baclofen administered through an implanted pump.

## Human T-Lymphotropic Virus Type 1-Associated Myelopathy, or Tropical Spastic Paraparesis

HTLV-1 causes a chronic progressive myelopathy that is referred to as *tropical spastic paraparesis* (TSP) in the Caribbean or HTLV-1–associated myelopathy (HAM) in Japan. This retrovirus is endemic in the Caribbean area, southwestern Japan, equatorial Africa, South Africa, parts of Asia, Central America, and South America, where it infects between 10 and 20 million people. The true incidence and prevalence figures are likely an underestimate (Gessain and Cassar, 2012). While between 2% and 3% of those infected can develop adult-onset T-cell leukemia, an estimated 2.5%–3.8% can develop a chronic inflammatory myelopathy, with up to 20/100,000 affected in the Caribbean population and 3/100,000 in Japan. Recent evidence implicates high levels of activated HTLV-1–specific helper T cells and cytotoxic T cells in the pathogenesis of this syndrome; these immune cells appear to activate in response to interactions with retroviral env and tax proteins with greatest activity within the thoracic cord. Increased susceptibility for neurological disease appears to depend on both viral and host factors, with differences in certain HTLV-1 subgroups, proviral load, and HLA background being important. This may also explain differences in susceptibility between ethnic populations (Bassi et al., 2014; Saito, 2010). Mode of transmission is through contaminated blood, sexual activity, breastfeeding, and very rarely in utero.

HAM/TSP is a chronic, insidiously progressive myelopathy that typically begins after age 30 years (but can occur as early as the first decade). In addition to slowly progressive spastic paraparesis, patients complain of lower-extremity paresthesias, a painful sensory neuropathy, and bladder dysfunction, and some patients may also develop optic neuropathy. Examination reveals UMN signs in the legs (weakness, spasticity, pathological reflexes, hyperreflexia), although reflexes may also be brisk in the arms. Overall, evidence of LMN involvement may be scant, and objective sensory findings may be difficult to detect. MRI may reveal increased signal on T2-weighted sequences in periventricular white matter and atrophy of the thoracic cord, but these findings may not be specific to HTLV-1. The definitive diagnosis of HAM/TSP requires HTLV-1–positive serology in blood and cerebrospinal fluid (CSF). To be sensitive and specific, CSF should reveal a combination of a polymerase chain reaction (PCR) amplification of HTLV-1 deoxyribonucleic acid (DNA), together with evidence of an increased HTLV-1–specific antibody index and oligoclonal bands (Puccioni-Sohler et al., 2012). At present, no antiviral agents effectively treat HAM/TSP, but a case report showed partial benefit of plasmapheresis (Narakawa et al., 2001). As more is learned about the molecular etiology of HAM/TSP, future therapies will likely target the pathogenic effect of HTLV-1–reactive T cells.

## Human T-Lymphotropic Virus Type 2-Associated Myelopathy

Though phylogenetically similar in many respects, HTLV-1 and HTLV-2 are still antigenically distinct. Nonetheless, using enzyme-linked immunosorbent assay (ELISA) and Western blot techniques, many laboratories worldwide often report the presence of sero-indeterminate HTLV-1/2. It has long been thought that myelopathy in such sero-indeterminate cases is due to HTLV-1 rather than HTLV-2, but rare cases are now being described of a syndrome characterized by spastic paraparesis, diffuse hyperreflexia, spastic bladder, and periventricular white-matter changes on MRI in patients infected with HTLV-2 but not HTLV-1. This retrovirus is endemic in some Native American tribes and is now often encountered worldwide among intravenous (IV) drug abusers. It is worthwhile to test CSF and serum for the presence of this virus in known IV drug abusers who present with a spastic paraparesis (Silva et al., 2002). However, coinfection with HIV-1 is a confounding factor in many cases of presumed HTLV-2–associated neurological disease. It has been suggested that such coinfection, rather than infection with HTLV-2 alone, increases the likelihood of neurological manifestations (Araujo and Hall, 2004; Posada-Vergara et al., 2006).

## Adrenomyeloneuropathy

Adrenomyeloneuropathy is a variant of adrenoleukodystrophy, an X-linked recessive disorder caused by mutations in the *ABCD1* gene on chromosome Xq28 that encodes a ubiquitously expressed integral membrane peroxisomal ATPase-binding cassette transporter protein. Mutations in this gene lead to abnormal peroxisomal β-oxidation, which results in the harmful accumulation of very long-chain fatty acids (VLCFAs) in affected cells. Excessive levels of VLCFAs may interfere with the membrane components of both neurons and axons. The most common phenotype, adrenoleukodystrophy, is an inflammatory disorder of brain and spinal cord that affects young boys 4–8 years of age, who develop severe adrenal insufficiency, progressive cognitive deterioration, seizures, blindness, deafness, and spastic quadriparesis. Adrenomyeloneuropathy is a noninflammatory axonopathy of the spinal cord that involves descending corticospinal tracts in the thoracic and lumbosacral regions and the ascending posterior columns in the cervical region. The characteristic clinical picture is a slowly progressive spastic paraparesis and mild polyneuropathy in adult men (in their late 20s), with or without sensory symptoms and sphincter disturbances. Adrenal insufficiency may be present and may predate onset of neurological symptoms by several years. Adult female carriers may present with an age-related slowly progressive spastic paraparesis (Habekost et al., 2014). Approximately 20% of men with adrenomyeloneuropathy also develop cerebral changes on MRI that may accompany cognitive/language/behavioral deterioration. Rare cases may present as a spinocerebellar degeneration. Considerable phenotypic variation exists even within individual families. Female carriers may manifest more subtle symptoms such as cramps, back pain, or arthralgias. The diagnosis should be suspected in male cases with progressive sensorimotor deficits in the legs and a family history of a myelopathy (including supposed MS). Progressive sensorimotor deficits in the lower extremities with a history of memory loss or "attention deficit disorder" should also prompt testing for adrenomyeloneuropathy, as should a history of idiopathic childhood epilepsy or primary adrenal failure (Mukherjee et al., 2006). Sural nerve biopsies show loss of both myelinated and unmyelinated axons, with some degree of onion bulb formation. Ultrastructural examination may show characteristic inclusions (empty lipid clefts) in Schwann cell cytoplasm. Nerve conduction studies and needle electrode examination may reveal a predominantly axon-loss type of sensorimotor polyneuropathy with a lesser component of demyelination, and SSEPs may show reduced or absent responses. There may be signal abnormalities seen in the corticospinal tracts and parieto-occipital white matter on MRI (Teriitehau et al., 2007). The diagnostic test of choice is to demonstrate increased VLCFA levels in plasma, red blood cells, or cultured skin fibroblasts. No specific therapy exists for adult-onset adrenomyeloneuropathy.

## Plant Excitotoxins

### Lathyrism

Lathyrism is a chronic toxic nutritional neurological disease caused by long-term (or subacute) ingestion of flour made from the drought-resistant chickling pea (*Lathyrus sativus*). It is an important example of a disease in which a natural excitotoxin causes selective UMN impairment. The responsible neurotoxin is β-*N*-oxalylamino-l-alanine (BOAA), an α-amino-3-hydroxyl-5-methyl-4-isoxazolepropionic acid (AMPA) glutamate receptor agonist. Ingestion of this neurotoxin results in increased intracellular levels of reactive oxygen species and subsequent impairment of the mitochondrial oxidative phosphorylation chain. Degeneration is most prominent in those Betz cells of the motor cortex (and the longest corresponding pyramidal tracts) that subserve lower-extremity function. Lathyrism occurs in the indigenous populations of Bangladesh, China, Ethiopia, India, Romania, and Spain. It also occurred in regional concentration camps during World War II. The condition may occur in epidemic form when malnourished populations increase consumption of flour made from *L. sativus* chickling peas during times of food shortage due to droughts. An analysis of an epidemic of neurolathyrism in Ethiopia showed a higher incidence in boys aged 10–14 years. The increased risk was associated with cooking grass pea foods in traditional clay pots (Ngudi et al., 2012). The onset of clinical toxicity is either acute or chronic, manifesting as muscle spasms, cramps, and leg weakness. In addition to spastic paraparesis, sensory (including leg formications) and bladder dysfunction may occur. Occasionally there is a coarse tremor of the upper extremities. Although irreversible, the disorder is not progressive (unless there is continuing intoxication), and lifespan is not affected.

### Konzo

Konzo ("tied legs") is another toxic nutritional disorder of cortical motor neurons caused by chronic dietary ingestion of a neurotoxin derived from flour made from cassava roots that have not been soaked for a sufficient time. The disorder is endemic in protein-deficient communities in Tanzania, Zaire, and Eastern Africa and in times of famine can occur in epidemic form. The neurotoxic effect of chronic cassava root ingestion likely is derived from the liberation of cyanohydrins (cyanoglucoside linamarin) from the flour, which may be further metabolized to thiocyanate. The latter in turn may excessively stimulate the AMPA glutamate receptor subtype, causing excitotoxic neuronal injury. As with lathyrism, there appears to be a selective effect on Betz cells of the cerebral cortex and the longest corresponding corticospinal tracts. Patients typically present with spastic paraparesis (although some may exhibit only lower-extremity hyperreflexia). Occasionally one may detect weakness of the upper extremities, but not to the same degree as that of the lower extremities.

# DISORDERS OF LOWER MOTOR NEURONS

## Neuroanatomy of Lower Motor Neurons

### Interneurons

The interneurons constitute most of the anterior horn cells of the spinal cord and determine the final output of the LMNs. The interneuron system receives supranuclear excitatory and inhibitory motor control from the brainstem descending tracts, corticospinal tracts, and limbic system; this system also receives afferent information, directly and indirectly, from the afferent peripheral nerves. The interneuron system forms intricate neuronal circuits involving automatic and stereotyped spinal reflexes to coordinate and integrate the activation of synergist muscles while inhibiting antagonist muscles, contralateral muscles, and sometimes even a distant motor pool. The same interneuron network that mediates such automatic and stereotyped reflex behavior also acts as the basic functional unit involved in highly skillful voluntary movements. Ultimately, all of the interneuronal paths converge on the LMNs that innervate skeletal muscles, which Sherrington called the *final common path*.

### Lower Motor Neurons

LMNs are located in the brainstem and spinal cord and send out motor axons that directly innervate skeletal muscle fibers. Spinal cord LMNs, also known as *anterior horn cells*, cluster in nuclei forming longitudinal columns; those innervating the distal muscles of the extremities are located in the dorsal anterior horn, whereas those innervating proximal muscles of the extremities are in the ventral anterior horn. Those LMNs that innervate the axial and truncal muscles are the most medially located. The normal cervical and lumbar enlargements of the spinal cord are the result of markedly enlarged lateral anterior horns containing the LMNs for the upper and lower limb muscles.

Large spinal cord LMNs called *alpha motoneurons* are the principal motor neurons innervating muscle fibers. Medium-sized motor neurons (*beta motoneurons*) innervate both extrafusal and intrafusal (muscle spindle) fibers, and intermediate and small motor neurons (*gamma motoneurons* or *fusimotor neurons*) innervate only spindle muscle fibers. The rest of the small anterior horn cells are interneurons.

Alpha motoneurons are among the largest neurons of the nervous system. Each has a single axon that branches to its target muscles and a number of large dendrites that provide an extensive receptive field. The motor unit is the smallest unit of the motor system and consists of one alpha motoneuron, its axon, and all of its target muscle fibers.

## Clinical Features of Lower Motor Neuron Involvement

### Loss of Muscle Strength (Weakness)

The loss of an LMN results in denervation of its motor unit, whereas an impaired LMN may lead to abnormal or impaired activation of its motor unit. In either case, the number of fully functional motor units decreases, which reduces overall muscle twitch tension.

In a disease causing chronic motor unit depletion, neighboring axons belonging to healthy motor neurons may reinnervate denervated muscle fibers belonging to a diseased motor unit by collateral sprouting. In this way, existing motor units continually modify in the face of persistent losses of motor axons to maintain muscle strength.

For example, in patients who have recovered from acute poliomyelitis, depletion of more than 50% of LMNs occurs before residual muscle weakness is clinically detectable. Healthy individuals have sufficient motor units available to offset an unexpected loss of motor neurons (Box 97.3).

***Muscle atrophy and hyporeflexia.*** Muscle fiber denervation causes muscle fiber atrophy, and progressive LMN involvement results in reduced overall muscle bulk. Hyporeflexia occurs with LMN involvement because the loss of active motor units reduces the overall muscle twitch tension; thus, muscle stretch reflexes elicit less tension (diminished reflexes) or no visible twitch (absent reflexes).

***Muscle hypotonicity or flaccidity.*** *Hypotonicity*, or *flaccidity*, refers to the decrease or complete loss of normal muscle resistance to passive manipulation. In contrast to spasticity, the muscle tone is flaccid.

### Fasciculations

Fasciculations are spontaneous contractions of muscle fibers belonging to a single (or part of a) motor unit (Video 97.2). Clinically, fasciculations appear on the muscle surface as fine, rapid, flickering, and sometimes vermicular contractions that occur irregularly in time and location. The impulse for the fasciculation appears to arise from hyperexcitable motor axons anywhere in their course. Fasciculations can occur both in healthy individuals and in patients with LMN involvement, so fasciculations themselves do not indicate LMN disease.

In general, larger muscles have larger motor units and therefore larger fasciculations. In tongue muscles, fasciculations produce small vermicular movements on the tongue surface. Fasciculations usually do not cause any joint displacement but when they occur in muscles moving the fingers, joint movements can occur (mini-polymyoclonus) (see Video 97.2). Large fasciculations may occur in muscles undergoing extensive chronic reinnervation, such as chronic spinal muscular atrophy (SMA), Kennedy disease, and the postpoliomyelitis syndrome.

### Muscle Cramps

Muscle cramps are common in the general population and are a common symptom of LMN involvement and many chronic neuromuscular diseases. The pathogenesis of cramps in all these diseases, as in normal individuals, is poorly understood. Cramps and fasciculations are likely to share a common pathogenic mechanism such as hyperexcitability of the motor neurons. Muscle cramps are an abrupt, involuntary, and painful shortening of the muscle, accompanied by visible or palpable knotting, often with abnormal posture of the affected joint. Relief of cramps is by stretching or massaging.

## Laboratory Evidence of Lower Motor Neuron Involvement

### Electrodiagnostic Examination

The electrodiagnostic examination (EDX) consists of nerve conduction studies and needle electrode examination (see Chapter 36). The loss of motor units reflects in the loss of the amplitude of the maximal compound muscle action potential (CMAP). In a primarily demyelinating process, conduction velocity slows, and, in severe cases, conduction block occurs. In a primarily axon loss process, there is usually only a modest degree of conduction velocity slowing commensurate with dropout of large myelinated axons. Sensory nerve conduction studies are normal in pure LMN disorders.

The needle electrode examination EMG is crucial in obtaining electrophysiological evidence of abnormal motor units in LMN disorders. Actively denervated muscle fibers discharge spontaneously, producing fibrillation potentials and positive sharp waves. Fasciculation potentials may also be detectable, but as an isolated EDX finding, they are not sufficient evidence to diagnose an axon-loss disorder. The recruitment pattern during voluntary muscle activation is also altered in neurogenic disease, with a reduced number of motor units that have an increased firing rate; this reflects a compensatory effort on the part of surviving motor units to maintain a particular force. Because denervation of muscle fibers triggers a reinnervation process, motor units continuously remodel. Early in the reinnervating process, newly formed neuromuscular junctions are electrically unstable, and thus an individual motor unit action potential will vary in amplitude during repeated firing. Furthermore, newly regenerated axons that reinnervate denervated muscle fibers tend to have slow conduction velocities, causing a prolonged conduction time within one motor unit. All these changes alter the configuration of the motor unit potential so that it becomes irregular and polyphasic. In a chronic reinnervating process, surviving motor units may reinnervate a greater number of muscle fibers, resulting in a potential that is broader in duration and higher in amplitude. Therefore, the shape of a typical chronic neurogenic motor unit potential is polyphasic, broad, and high in amplitude.

Motor unit number estimation (MUNE) and similar techniques are specialized neurophysiological tools that can estimate the number of functioning motor units that remain in a progressive neurogenic process.

### Muscle Biopsy

Although EDX usually provides sufficient evidence of LMN involvement, muscle biopsy may also reveal early evidence of muscle fiber denervation and rule out other causes of muscle weakness. Denervated muscle fibers are small, angular, and stain darkly by oxidative enzyme and nonspecific esterase stains. As the denervation process progresses, small groups of atrophied muscle fibers (group atrophy) may appear. In normal human muscle, the different muscle fiber types that are distinguished using myosin ATPase stain appear in a random distribution, sometimes mistakenly termed a "checkerboard pattern." In chronic denervating disease, repeated denervation and reinnervation eventually results in loss of this random pattern, and in very chronic neurogenic disease (such as SMA), large areas of the biopsy consist of just one muscle fiber type, a process called *fiber-type grouping*. However, in a relatively rapid disorder of motor unit loss such as ALS, there is insufficient time to develop marked fiber-type grouping.

## Acute Poliomyelitis and Other Viral Acute Flaccid Paralyses

Poliomyelitis has long been considered the most important cause of virus-associated acute flaccid paralysis. However, due to the widespread use of polio vaccine, it is evident now that other enteroviruses and, indeed, arboviruses are more likely causes of these presentations. Poliovirus, a single-stranded ribonucleic acid (RNA) enterovirus belonging to the picornavirus family has three subtypes, with type

**BOX 97.3 Signs and Symptoms of Lower Motor Neuron Involvement**

- Loss of muscle strength (moderate to severe weakness)
- Muscle atrophy
- Hyporeflexia
- Muscle hypotonicity or flaccidity
- Fasciculations
- Muscle cramps

I being responsible for most cases of the epidemic paralytic disease. Wild-type polioviruses spread via the fecal-oral route. Before the introduction of poliovirus vaccine in the late 1950s, epidemics of acute paralytic poliomyelitis were relatively common in temperate zones and primarily affected children and young adults (infantile paralysis). In 1988, the World Health Organization resolved to eradicate poliomyelitis worldwide, but this remains unachieved as outbreaks still occur (e.g., in Nigeria, Pakistan, Afghanistan, Syria). The live oral polio vaccine can itself cause poliomyelitis and there are occasions when a parent will decline polio vaccination for their child. Thus, even in the developed world, it is still important that physicians be acquainted with this syndrome.

Acute paralytic disease caused by other viruses such as West Nile flavivirus, Japanese encephalitis flavivirus, enterovirus D68 (EV-D68), enterovirus A71 (EV-A71), and various coxsackievirus species is very similar to acute poliomyelitis. Awareness of EV-D68 as a major cause of acute flaccid paralysis increased on the back of an outbreak in 2014 in North America, Europe, and Asia. Small outbreaks continue to occur in clusters. This re-emergence has been postulated to be due to genetic evolution of the virus over time. EV-A71 was first isolated in California in the 1960s but the largest outbreaks have been in Asia in association with hand, foot, and mouth disease (HFMD) or herpangina. This is largely transmitted by the fecal-oral route but transmission can be respiratory. Severe disease occurs in up to 30% of children hospitalized and in addition to acute flaccid paralysis, patients can develop autonomic dysregulation and brainstem encephalitis.

A number of arboviruses have been implicated in similar acute paralysis presentations, including West Nile virus, Japanese encephalitis virus, and European tick-borne encephalitis virus. Of these, the most important is West Nile virus (WNV), an arthropod-borne flavivirus that causes epidemics of meningitis, encephalitis, and in some instances an acute polio-like flaccid paralysis. Approximately 80% of those who are infected are asymptomatic, and 20% develop a flu-like illness (termed *West Nile fever*). Less than 1% present with neuroinvasive disease. There is a predilection for adults rather than children, with a mean age of presentation of 56 years (Sejvar et al., 2005). Following the 1999 outbreak in New York, an epidemic spread across the North American continent and peaked in 2002/2003. Epidemics also occurred in multiple countries. WNV is now endemic in North America and is a leading cause of arboviral encephalitis in the United States. WNV is a zoonotic pathogen that has crossed over from birds to humans, the latter serving as incidental hosts. The prime bridge vector is the *Culex* mosquito, and the spread of disease appears to have followed the migration patterns of bird populations (Kilpatrick et al., 2006). Human-to-human transmission can occur via blood transfusion, organ transplant, intrauterine exposure, and breastfeeding: hence the need to screen for the virus among blood donors.

## Clinical Features

Most cases of poliomyelitis are abortive and present as a mild flu-like illness lasting up to 3 days. An aseptic meningitis can occur but this is also self-limiting in most patients. The paralytic polio (which affects less than 1% of infected patients) typically develops 2–5 days after the prodromal flu-like illness and commences with myalgias, meningism, paresthesiae, and fasciculations. Muscle weakness then develops over the following 1–2 days. Any skeletal muscle can weaken, including bulbar muscles and muscles of respiration, but the leg muscles are the most commonly affected and often this occurs in a monomelic fashion (Bitnun and Yeh, 2018). Acute flaccid paralysis in children can be particularly grave.

EV-D68 is clinically similar to poliomyelitis but spread is largely respiratory. Often the prodrome features respiratory symptoms and then improves. Within 5 days, weakness, develops along with fever, headache, and pain (in other words, a biphasic mode of presentation similar to childhood poliomyelitis). The patterns of weakness are similar to poliomyelitis.

The EV-A71 initial presentation may be with herpangina or HFMD, with paralysis beginning between 2 and 6 days later. In addition to acute flaccid paralysis, there can be elements of meningitis, encephalomyelitis, and transverse myelitis.

WNV can present dramatically with an acute asymmetrical flaccid paralysis in a febrile patient with or without meningitis, encephalitis, and cranial neuropathies (including hearing loss). Aching pains in affected limbs often accompany the paralysis, but actual sensory loss is not a feature. Respiratory failure and death may occur, and up to one-third of cases suffer bladder and bowel dysfunction. Recovery is very slow, and, from the available evidence, incomplete.

Physical examination in acute flaccid paralysis reveals severe LMN-type muscle weakness with hypoactive or absent deep tendon reflexes, decreased muscle tone, and fasciculations. With time, muscle atrophy occurs (usually beginning about 3 weeks after onset). Objective signs of sensory loss are not characteristic. In polio, the risk of paralytic disease seems to increase with patient age and with the level of virulence of the virus. Most patients with paralytic polio recover significant strength. Improvement may begin as early as the first week after the onset of paralysis, and estimates are that 80% of recovery occurs by 6 months. Further improvement may be modest, but it may continue over the ensuing 18–24 months. Up to two-thirds of patients have some degree of functional impairment. Long-term outcome in EV-D68 is still being evaluated but full recovery appears to be rare. There is significant variability in recovery from EV-A71 but in one study only 12.5% of patients had muscle weakness at 6-month follow-up, suggesting a more favorable outcome (Hu et al., 2015). In WNV, respiratory failure and death may occur, and up to one-third of cases suffer bladder and bowel dysfunction. Recovery is very slow, and, from the available evidence, incomplete.

## Laboratory Features

Motor nerve conduction studies performed 21 or more days after the onset may reveal low-amplitude maximum CMAPs. No evidence of significant demyelination-related motor conduction slowing or block exists. Sensory nerve action potentials (SNAPs) are normal. EMG examination in the acute phase shows profuse axon loss in the form of positive sharp waves and fibrillation potentials. In addition, fasciculations may be prominent. As motor axon loss progresses, evidence of neurogenic MUP changes may be detected. The CSF typically shows increased protein content with normal glucose and a pleocytosis, with polymorphonuclear cells predominating during the acute stages and lymphocytes predominating later in the disease in all of the above infections. Poliovirus-, EV-D68-, and EV-A71-specific antibodies are only rarely detected in CSF. Microbiological diagnosis is most frequently made from respiratory tract and stool samples. If EV-A71 encephalitis has occurred, detection rates in CSF are higher. Acute West Nile virus is most accurately detected in blood samples.

In light of the knowledge that most new cases of poliomyelitis are vaccine-derived, PCR is important to distinguish wild-type from vaccine–induced disease.

## Treatment

The treatment of acute flaccid paralysis consists of aggressive general supportive care. Most patients will require hospitalization in an intensive care unit to optimize close monitoring of ventilatory and cardiovascular function. After the acute illness, aggressive rehabilitation is the mainstay of continued treatment. All healthcare staff treating patients with acute paralytic poliomyelitis require prior immunization. There is no proven specific treatment for EV-D68. The WHO Guide to Clinical Management recommends use of intravenous immunoglobulin (IVIG) therapy for EV-A71 in patients who develop autonomic dysfunction or central nervous system (CNS) disease (Cardosa et al., 2011).

### Vaccination

The best treatment for polio is prevention. Two vaccines are available, the Sabin (live-attenuated) and the Salk (inactivated). The Sabin trivalent oral poliovirus vaccine, in widespread use since the early 1960s, contains all three live attenuated serotypes of poliovirus. It is almost 100% effective in preventing acute paralytic poliomyelitis. Adults who plan to travel to areas where poliomyelitis is prevalent should receive an extra dose of this vaccine. However, the oral poliovirus vaccine itself (specifically the type 2 serotype) is responsible for very rare cases of acute paralytic poliomyelitis in the developed world. For this reason, there is a move toward a bivalent vaccine containing only serotypes 1 and 3 (Bitnun and Yeh, 2018, Diop et al., 2014). A vaccine has been developed for EV-A71 and has gained use in China. There is evidence that the vaccine has prevented 600,000 cases of HFMD/herpangina and 435 deaths. Although a vaccine for WNV is available for horses and also for birds in zoos, no vaccine for humans exists. The best way to prevent this condition is to avoid mosquito bites through judicious use of appropriate clothing and insect repellants (Petersen et al., 2013). A recent trend toward parents declining to vaccinate their children remains a potential cause of future outbreaks.

## Postpolio Syndrome/Progressive Postpoliomyelitis Muscular Atrophy

In the United States alone, it is estimated that over 570,000 people have had poliomyelitis, of which between 15% and 80% may develop postpolio syndrome (PPS) (Lo and Robinson, 2018). Many years after recovery from acute poliomyelitis, these patients experience progressive functional impairment, with muscle fatigue, pain, sleep disturbances, cold intolerance, depression, dysphagia, and dysarthria. If progressive muscle weakness and wasting occurs in this setting, the term *progressive postpoliomyelitis muscular atrophy* (PPMA) is used. By definition, patients with postpolio syndrome/PPMA have recovered from acute poliomyelitis, and the disease course has been stable for at least 10 years after the recovery (Box 97.4).

**BOX 97.4 Characteristic Features of Postpolio Syndrome/Progressive Postpoliomyelitis Muscular Atrophy**

Medical history:
- Recovery from acute poliomyelitis
- A long, stable course—at least 10 years

Signs and symptoms:
- Progressive weakness, usually in previously affected muscles
- Accompanying overstressed muscle pains and arthralgia

Laboratory studies:
- EMG is helpful to identify evidence of previous polio infection
- No test is specific for PPMA

Diagnosis:
- Exclusion of other treatable diseases

Treatment:
- Symptomatic and supportive care

*EMG*, Electromyography; *PPMA*, postpoliomyelitis muscular atrophy.

### Etiology

The etiology of postpolio syndrome/PPMA is not established. Numerous studies have failed to identify chronic persistent poliovirus in PPMA, and solid evidence is lacking to implicate a persistent immune-mediated mechanism, although CSF and muscle biopsy samples show some chronic inflammation. The "peripheral disintegration model" is the most widely held theory. This theory proposes that an oversprouting of new axon terminals from surviving LMNs occur in the immediate aftermath of the acute paralytic poliomyelitis. This compensatory distal reinnervation expands the size of motor units and provides effective motor function; this stabilizes muscle strength for many years. However, this extensive nerve sprouting also increases the metabolic burden of surviving LMNs; so, after many years, an unidentified process first causes nerve terminal dysfunction, presenting as fatigue, and then nerve terminal disintegration, presenting as muscle weakness and atrophy. It is possible that normal age-related neuronal loss may be the process causing this late degeneration.

### Clinical Features

Patients who develop postpolio syndrome/PPMA previously had a stable course for many years (on average >15 years) after the acute poliomyelitis infection. These patients then experience progressive symptoms of new muscle weakness and new atrophy in previously affected muscles or sometimes in muscles apparently not affected by the original poliomyelitis; this deterioration occurs over a protracted timeframe of at least 1 year. EMG examination reveals that muscles thought to be clinically unaffected by acute poliomyelitis often have evidence of previous disease (characterized by chronic neurogenic motor unit potential (MUP) changes with or without some acute denervation). Weakness can involve limbs and/or bulbar musculature. Muscle cramps and fasciculations may accompany new weakness, but they are often present in stable muscles also. Generalized fatigue is characteristic and can be the most disabling accompaniment, often called the *polio wall*. Other common symptoms include pain, sleep disturbances, cold intolerance, depression, hypoventilation (manifesting as dyspnea), dysphagia, and dysarthria. The proposal is that these new symptoms should have persisted for a full year if one is to consider the diagnosis of postpolio syndrome. The neurological examination reveals focal and asymmetrical muscle weakness and atrophy, but it may be difficult to determine whether the weakness and atrophy is new and progressive or remote and static. Fasciculations can be unusually coarse and large in keeping with the giant motor units detectable during EMG examination.

### Laboratory Features

Because EMG provides definitive evidence of remote poliomyelitis and can help exclude diseases mimicking PPMA, it is an indispensable test when suspecting PPMA, though it cannot confirm the diagnosis. In patients with PPMA, the motor nerve conduction studies may be abnormal (low maximum CMAP amplitudes) when recorded from affected muscles. The needle electrode examination of affected weak muscles typically shows a reduced number of motor units and chronic neurogenic MUPs. Giant motor units may be present, indicative of chronic denervation and reinnervation. Modest numbers of fibrillation potentials and occasional fasciculations may occur in affected muscles, but such electrophysiological evidence of acute muscle fiber injury is not necessary to make the diagnosis. Sensory nerve conduction studies are normal. The muscle biopsy specimen usually shows acute and chronic neurogenic atrophy and often marked group muscle fiber atrophy and fiber-type grouping; however, these biopsy findings are not diagnostic of PPMA.

### Diagnosis

A history of clinical stability for at least 10 years after recovery from acute poliomyelitis is a prerequisite for considering the diagnosis of PPMA. When this requirement is satisfied, PPMA is then a diagnosis of exclusion. Exclude all potential diseases causing progressive, focal, and asymmetrical weakness. Myelopathy, radiculopathy, electrolyte abnormalities, endocrine diseases, diabetic amyotrophy, connective tissue disorders, entrapment neuropathies, inflammatory myositis, inflammatory neuropathy, and vasculitis are among the diseases to exclude by appropriate laboratory studies. The symptoms of progressive focal muscle weakness in PPMA may raise the possibility of the PMA variant of ALS. Approach this diagnosis with great caution in the setting of a history of prior paralytic polio.

### Treatment

No specific pharmacotherapy for postpolio syndrome exists. Care focuses on symptom relief (Gonzalez et al., 2010). A randomized controlled trial of IVIG (2 courses of IVIG at a dose of 90 g per course over 3 days, with a 3-month interval) reported a significant improvement in muscle strength but not quality of life in 135 patients (Gonzalez et al., 2006). Other agents have also been studied but at present there is insufficient evidence to support use of any of these (IVIG included) in postpolio syndrome (Koopman, 2015; Patwa et al., 2012).

The care plan should focus on avoiding fatiguing activities that aggravate symptoms, modifying activities to conserve energy, weight reduction for those who are overweight, and treating underlying medical disorders that reduce overall well-being. Careful screening and treatment for possible sleep apnea and depression are important. Those patients who have worsening of preexisting ventilatory muscles may require noninvasive positive-pressure ventilation (NIPPV) or noninvasive bilevel positive airway pressure (BiPAP) ventilation.

Physical therapy should focus on nonfatiguing aerobic exercise, modest isometric/isokinetic exercise, and range-of-motion stretching maneuvers. The goal should be to maintain exercise in affected muscles but not to the point of overuse, while also limiting the disuse of unaffected muscles. Low-impact exercise in warm water can be particularly helpful and also appears to help control fatigue and pain. In patients with more serious functional decline, prescribe appropriate assistive devices to maintain activities of daily living. Pulmonologists must evaluate those who develop respiratory insufficiency to rule out primary pulmonary disease and to prevent/treat chest infections. Patients whose employment or lifestyle involves significant physical exertion need to modify their work duties and other activities.

## Multifocal Motor Neuropathy

A complete description of multifocal motor neuropathy is in Chapter 106. The condition is believed to be autoimmune in nature, and most cases have evidence of focal demyelination in the peripheral nerves (multifocal motor neuropathy with conduction block [MMNCB]) similar to that in chronic inflammatory demyelinating peripheral neuropathy. The clinical presentation, however, is with pure LMN involvement. The condition enters into the differential diagnosis of benign focal amyotrophy and the PMA variant of ALS. It is important to search for this condition since it is treatable by high-dose immunoglobulin infusions or other immunotherapy.

## Benign Focal Amyotrophy

The terms *benign focal amyotrophy*, *brachial monomelic amyotrophy*, *benign calf amyotrophy*, *Hirayama disease*, or *juvenile segmental muscular atrophy* are used to describe disorders characterized by LMN disease clinically restricted to one limb. The etiology is unknown. Autopsy studies have shown the affected region of spinal cord flattened, the anterior horn markedly atrophied and gliotic, and a reduction in the numbers of both large and small motor neurons. Based upon neuroradiological studies, Hirayama, who established the disease entity, has proposed a mechanically induced limited form of ischemic cervical myelopathy, being the result of local compression of the dura and spinal cord against vertebrae during repeated neck flexion/extension, in turn due to disproportionate growth between the contents of the dural sac and the vertebral column (Hirayama, 2008; Hirayama and Tokamaru, 2000). However, surgical decompression has not altered the course of the disease, and this theory is no longer widely held. Another school of thought is that this is a segmental, perhaps genetically determined, SMA, but the actual cause is still unknown.

The disease usually begins in the late teens, but many cases can present in the fourth decade. More than 60% of patients are men. Although originally described in Indian and Japanese patients, the disorder is now recognizable around the world. The most common presentation is one of an idiopathic, slowly progressive, painless weakness and atrophy in one hand or forearm. The distribution of muscle weakness varies markedly from case to case, but a characteristic feature is that the condition remains limited to only a few myotomes in the affected limb. The most common pattern is unilateral atrophy of C7–T1 innervated muscles, with sparing of the brachioradialis (the "oblique atrophy" pattern). Muscle stretch reflexes are invariably hypoactive or absent in the muscles innervated by the involved cord segment but are normal elsewhere. UMN signs are not present, and if they are, one should consider the onset of ALS instead. Approximately 20% have hyperesthesia to pinprick and touch, usually located on the dorsum of the hand. The cranial nerves, pyramidal tracts, and the autonomic nervous system are normal. Weakness and atrophy may progress steadily for the initial 2–3 years, but most patients have stabilized within 5 years. The arm is the affected limb in approximately 75% of the patients and the leg in the remaining 25% (benign calf amyotrophy). Spread may occur to the contralateral limb in about 20% of cases (Gourie-Devi and Nalini, 2003), and rare patients later develop an ALS-like picture.

No pathognomonic laboratory or electrodiagnostic tests exist for this condition; their main purpose is to exclude alternative diagnoses. Motor nerve conduction studies are either normal or reveal only reduction in the maximum CMAPs; a modest reduction in SNAPs occurs in up to one-third of patients. The EMG examination may show some fibrillation and fasciculation potentials, and chronic neurogenic motor unit changes are prominent. The C5–T1 myotomes are most commonly involved when the arms are affected. Careful EMG examination may reveal mild neurogenic changes on the asymptomatic contralateral side. The serum creatine kinase (CK) concentration may be modestly elevated, but other routine laboratory test results are normal. Cervical MRI may reveal segmental spinal cord atrophy or occasionally an area of increased signal on T2-weighted scans of the cervical spinal cord enlargement. "Incidental" spondylosis and cervical spinal canal stenosis detected by MRI require careful evaluation before the diagnosis of benign focal amyotrophy is established.

### Differential Diagnosis

Two diseases require distinction from benign focal amyotrophy: ALS, which is almost always a relentlessly progressive terminal disease, and MMNCB, which is a treatable peripheral motor neuropathy. A small proportion of ALS presents as an LMN monomelic disease, albeit in an older patient population. It is only with follow-up examination that the more widespread anterior horn cell disorder becomes apparent and UMN signs appear. Deep tendon reflexes are almost always hyperactive early in the evolution of ALS. Furthermore, the electrodiagnostic finding of generalized widespread acute and chronic motor neuron loss distinguishes ALS from the segmental motor neuron involvement of benign focal amyotrophy. The slowly progressive focal weakness that is distinctive of benign focal amyotrophy may also be the presenting picture of MMNCB, but detailed motor nerve conduction studies and serum tests for elevated titers of anti-GM1 antibodies can differentiate these two conditions.

Cervical or lumbosacral radiculopathy may also appear in a manner somewhat akin to benign focal amyotrophy. However, radicular pains and sensory impairment are typical of radiculopathies. Neuralgic amyotrophy/Parsonage-Turner syndrome typically begins with severe pain before the onset of weakness and wasting in the distribution of predominantly motor nerves derived from the brachial plexus. It may also involve selected sensory nerves. Most cases are monophasic and do not progress over years, as does benign focal amyotrophy, although hereditary neuralgic amyotrophy can present as recurrent bouts of brachial plexopathy. Cervical syringomyelia or a benign tumor involving nerve roots or the spinal cord may also cause progressive weakness in a monomelic fashion. Careful EMG studies and neuroimaging should differentiate these diseases.

### Treatment

The term *benign* in *benign focal amyotrophy* distinguishes it from malignant motor neuron disease, as seen in ALS. This condition is not life threatening, but it nevertheless severely impairs motor function in the involved extremity (although most patients adapt very well to their disability). Supportive care consists of physical and occupational therapy and effective use of assistive devices (splinting and braces). Tendon transfers are a consideration in selected patients with focal weakness in a muscle group whose function is crucial for certain activities of daily living.

## Spinal Muscular Atrophy

SMA is a group of disorders caused by degeneration of anterior horn cells and, in some subtypes, of bulbar motor neurons. Almost all cases are genetically determined, with most being autosomal recessive due to homozygous deletions of the survival motor neuron *(SMN)* gene on chromosome 5. Traditionally, SMA is classified as one of the four types based on the age at onset: SMA type 1 (infantile SMA or Werdnig-Hoffmann syndrome), SMA type 2 (intermediate SMA), SMA type 3 (juvenile SMA or Kugelberg-Welander disease), and SMA type 4 (adult-onset SMA, pseudomyopathic SMA). A very severe prenatal form of SMA (type 0 SMA) can manifest prenatally with reduced fetal movements and respiratory distress at birth. It is also important to consider the maximum function that a child achieves in terms of sitting and walking; this is of prognostic significance. In the less severe forms of the disease, there can be periods where the child will improve or plateau, but long-term studies have demonstrated a net deterioration (Russman, 2007) (Table 97.3). The estimated incidence of infantile and juvenile recessive SMA is 1 in 6000 to 10,000 live births, with an approximate carrier frequency of 1 in 35 of the general population, making it a leading genetic cause of infant mortality, although the carrier frequency is lower in people of sub-Saharan African origin (Sangaré et al., 2014). True adult-onset disease accounts for probably less than 10% of all cases of SMA, with an estimated prevalence of 0.32 in 100,000. The mean age at onset is the mid-30s but ranges from 20 to the late 40s. Up to 95% of all childhood cases are due to deletion of the survival motor neuron (SMN1, telomeric SMN, SMNT) gene located on chromosome 5q11.2–13.3. The remaining cases are due to small SMN mutations (rather than full deletions). SMN1 is located within an inverted gene duplication, the other half of which is occupied by the almost identical SMN2 (centromeric SMN, SMNC) gene. The SMN1 protein product is functionally absent in the vast majority (95%–98%) of cases of SMN-mutated SMA, and small amounts are present in the remaining few percent. The SMN2 protein is present in all patients, but the copy number can vary considerably. Only 1%–2% of childhood-onset SMA is unrelated to the SMN locus on chromosome 5.

SMN1 protein is a 38-kDa polypeptide important in the processing of the primary transcripts of other genes. Although a ubiquitous protein, expression is great within spinal motor neurons, and this may be why the disorder manifests as a motor neuron disease. It is associated with both nuclear and cytoplasmic complexes involved in messenger RNA (mRNA) splicing and interacts with other proteins that are important in the regulation of ribosomal RNA processing and modification. Within the nucleus, SMN1 forms macromolecular complexes with other nuclear proteins important in the assembly of spliceosomal small nuclear ribonucleoproteins (snRNPs). It is thus possible that SMA develops because of disruption in mRNA transport and/or SMN-dependent snRNP biogenesis. SMN2 protein is almost identical to SMN1 protein but only has about 10% of the activity of SMN1 protein because of a C-to-T transition within exon 7 that alters splicing. The full-length SMN1 transcript has all 9 exons, whereas 90% of the transcripts from SMN2 lack exon 7. Thus, only 10% of the SMN2 output is the full-length SMN transcript, the remainder being unstable and rapidly degraded. Therefore, despite the near-identical nature of the two proteins, SMN 2 cannot compensate fully for loss of SMN1. Motor neuron health requires at least 23% full-length SMN protein. The SMN genome is rather unstable and, as a consequence, increased copy numbers of SMN2 are possible through a process of gene conversion from SMN1 to SMN2. This has major implications for

**TABLE 97.3 Childhood and Adult Spinal Muscular Atrophies**

| SMA Type | Age at Onset | Maximum Function Achieved | Survival/Prognosis | Inheritance | Defective Gene |
|---|---|---|---|---|---|
| 0. Prenatal | Prenatal | Needs respirator support at birth | Fatal at birth without respirator support | AR | *SMN* gene |
| 1. Infantile SMA (Werdnig-Hoffmann) | Birth to 6 months | Sits with support | Death by age 2 years | AR | *SMN* gene |
| 2. Intermediate SMA | Before 18 months | Sits independently | No walking, adulthood | AR | *SMN* gene |
| 3. Juvenile (Kugelberg-Welander) | After 18 months | Walks independently: approx. 25 steps | Adulthood | AR | *SMN* gene |
| 4. Adult-onset SMA (pseudomyopathic SMA) | After 5 years (most >30 years) | Walks normally | Slow progression Proximal or distal | AR, AD "Sporadic" | *SMN* gene VAPB, dynactin unknown, distal overlap with HMN-V |

*AD*, Autosomal dominant; *AR*, autosomal recessive; *HMN-V*, hereditary motor neuropathy type V; *SMA*, spinal muscular atrophy; *SMN*, survival motor neuron; *VAPB*, vesicle-associated membrane protein B.

the clinical phenotype: the infantile form is very severe because most of these children have no SMN1 and only two copies of SMN2, thus producing about 9% of full-length functional transcript, whereas multiple copies of SMN2 (3–5) are associated with mild SMA (Hirth et al., 2005; Kostova et al., 2007; Monani, 2005). A study from Japan showed that the type of SMA mutation itself is also an independent determinant of severity (Yamamoto et al., 2014).

Most (about 70%) adult-onset type 4 SMA is autosomal recessive, is allelic with SMA types 1, 2, and 3, and is due to mutations or deletions in the SMN1 gene. Gene conversion events occur in some cases with SMA type 4 whereby SMN1 is "converted" to SMN2. The remaining adult-onset SMA cases are autosomal dominant, autosomal recessive (but not linked to chromosome 5), or are apparently sporadic. One rare form of adult-onset SMA described in a large Brazilian family was caused by a missense mutation in the vesicle trafficking protein, vesicle-associated membrane protein (VAPB). This can present with typical ALS or with a late-onset SMA (Nishimura et al., 2004).

## Clinical Features

***Spinal muscular atrophy type 1, infantile form (Werdnig-Hoffmann disease).*** SMA type 1 begins within the first few months of life. By definition, children with this disease are never able to sit without support. Symptoms include severe hypotonia, a weak cry, and respiratory distress. These children are unable to lift their heads when placed prone and demonstrate severe head lag when pulled from a supine to a seated position (Fig. 97.1). The baby's posture at rest also takes a characteristic "frog-leg" position, with the thighs externally rotated and abducted and the knees flexed (a "floppy" baby). Limb weakness is severe, generalized, and worse proximally. The infant is unable to sit and raise its arms or legs from the examining table, but there may be antigravity movements of the hands and flickering movements of the feet. Muscle stretch reflexes are usually absent, and the sensory examination is normal. Observation of the fingers may reveal fine, small-amplitude involuntary movements called *minipolymyoclonus* that are due to dense fasciculations. Contractures usually do not develop in the early phases but may develop after several months of immobilization. Bulbar muscle weakness makes feeding laborious, causes a continuous gurgling, and eventually leads to aspiration pneumonia. Fasciculations of the tongue occur in about 50% of affected infants. In contrast to bulbar and extremity muscles, the facial muscles are only mildly weak, giving these children an alert expression. Extraocular movements are always normal. Intercostal muscles are severely weak, but diaphragmatic strength preserves until late in the disease. This dysequilibrium of ventilatory muscle function causes outward flaring of the lower ribcage and gives rise to a bell-shaped chest deformity. Death from respiratory failure, pneumonia, and malnutrition usually occurs before age 2 years. A rare form of atypical infantile SMA, spinal muscular atrophy with respiratory distress (SMARD) (Viguier et al., 2019), is associated with respiratory distress, cardiomyopathy, and lactic acidosis. This disorder is not due to SMN1 deletion but caused by mutations in the gene for immunoglobulin mu-binding protein 2 (IGHMBP2). It is interesting that this gene has homology to SETX, the gene responsible for ALS4, which can cause a familial form of distal amyotrophy, oculomotor apraxia–cerebellar ataxia, or juvenile ALS.

***Spinal muscular atrophy type 2, intermediate form (chronic spinal muscular atrophy).*** The signs and symptoms of SMA type 2 usually begin between the ages of 6 and 18 months. Delayed motor milestones are often the first clue to neurological impairment, with more prominent leg weakness then arm weakness. A fine hand tremor due to minipolymyoclonus suggests the diagnosis. The distribution, pattern, and progression of weakness is similar to that found in SMA type 1, but type 2 disease is quantitatively much milder, and progression is slower. Most children eventually are able to roll over and sit unsupported, but they rarely achieve independent walking. Weakness of trunk muscles produces a characteristic rounded kyphosis

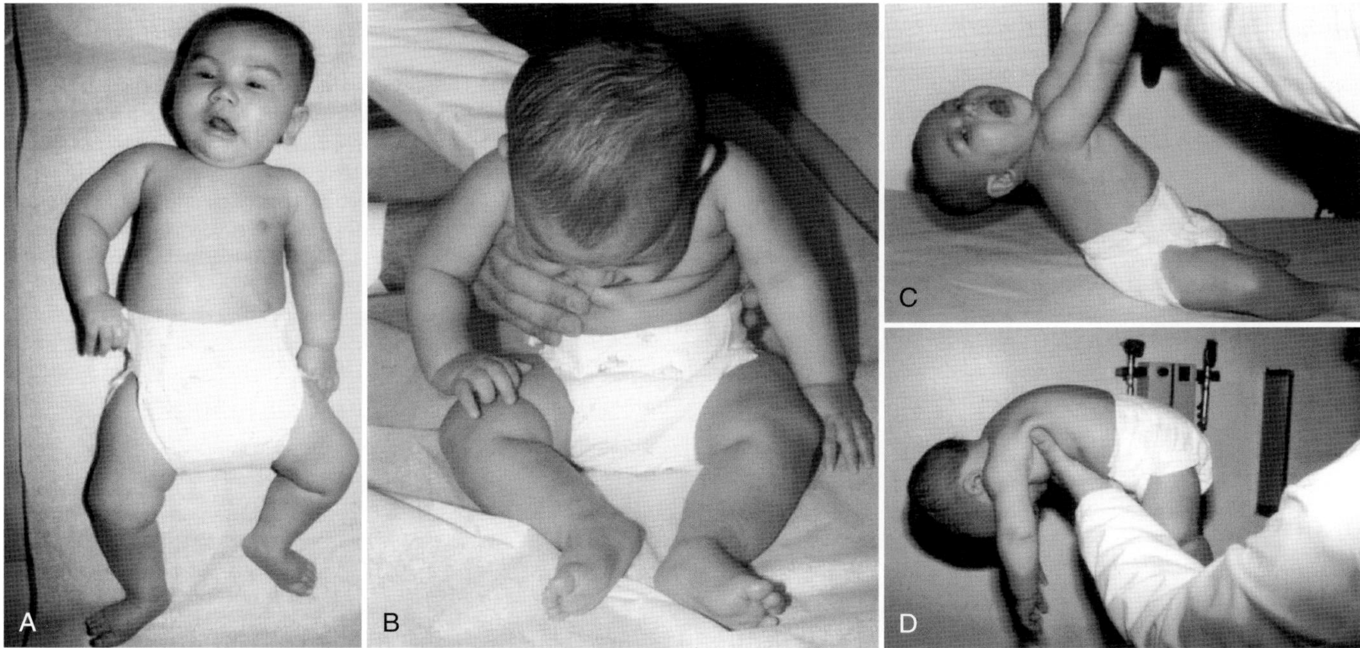

**Fig. 97.1 A 6-Month-Old Baby with Werdnig-Hoffmann Disease. A,** The baby has a typical "frog leg" posture; mouth is triangular, and facial expression suggests facial weakness. **B,** On sitting, the baby cannot sustain his head upright. **C,** When the baby is pulled by the arms, the head falls back. **D,** When the body is held supine, the head and extremities drop by force of gravity, and there is no active body motion. *(Courtesy Neil Friedman, Cleveland Clinic.)*

in the seated position, and, as the shoulders weaken, the child becomes less mobile and eventually wheelchair confined. Contractures of the hips and knees, clubfoot deformities, severe scoliosis, and dislocation of the hips may eventually develop. The long-term prognosis varies markedly; some die in childhood because of respiratory failure, but many others survive into the third or fourth decade of adulthood.

Another rare childhood-onset form of SMA that is distinct from SMA type 2 is Fazio-Londe disease. This is a form of sporadic autosomal dominant or autosomal recessive progressive facial and bulbar palsy of late childhood. Affected children are normal at birth but develop progressive bulbar palsy (PBP) and eventual respiratory failure in the second decade of life, with little or no evidence of involvement of other motor neurons and with usually normal extraocular motility. The differential diagnosis includes a structural brainstem lesion, myasthenia gravis, and the Miller Fisher variant of Guillain-Barré syndrome (GBS).

***Spinal muscular atrophy type 3, juvenile form (Kugelberg-Welander disease).*** The onset of the juvenile form of SMA is typically after 18 months of age (usually between 5 and 15 years) and presents with difficulty in walking. Patients with onset before the age of 3 years are subclassified as SMA type 3a and those after age 3 years as SMA type 3b. The disorder has an appearance not unlike a limb-girdle muscular dystrophy. As weakness in hip-girdle muscles increases, the child develops a waddling (Trendelenburg) gait, with a protuberant abdomen due to an exaggerated lumbar lordosis, and trouble climbing stairs. As weakness progresses, the Gowers maneuver is used to arise from lying supine on the floor. Pseudohypertrophy of the calf muscles sometimes occurs, but this may be an illusion resulting from relative preservation of calf muscles as compared to thigh muscles. Eventually, wasting and weakness of the neck, shoulders, and arms develop, but, as with SMA type 2, weakness in the lower extremities is nearly always more severe than in the upper extremities. Fasciculations are more prominent than in SMA types 1 and 2, and a fine action tremor is common. Tendon reflexes uniformly reduce and are lost, and the sensory examination is normal.

The clinical course of SMA type 3 is one of slowly progressive limb-girdle weakness, but there may be long periods of stability that last for years. The eventual degree of disability is difficult to predict, but if onset is after the age of 2 years, it is likely that the patient will remain ambulatory into the fifth decade of life and enjoy a normal lifespan.

***Spinal muscular atrophy type 4, adult-onset.*** Most cases of autosomal recessive, 5q-associated, adult-onset SMA appear to affect proximal muscles. The characteristic clinical presentation is that of a slowly progressive limb-girdle weakness leading to difficulty in walking, climbing stairs, and rising from a chair or the floor. Fasciculations are an important finding and occur in 75% of patients. Quadriceps muscle weakness is often a prominent feature. Muscle cramps occur but are not prominent. Bulbar signs, bony deformities such as scoliosis, and respiratory weakness are rare. Many cases have a distribution of weakness reminiscent of the limb-girdle muscular dystrophies, leading to the older term, *pseudomyopathic SMA* (Fig. 97.2).

Many cases of autosomal dominant adult-onset SMA (also known as *Finkel-type SMA*) are clinically similar to the recessive form described earlier. Finkel-type SMA usually begins in the third decade of life, is proximal in distribution, is very slowly progressive, and involves the legs before the arms. Most patients remain ambulatory for decades after clinical onset. One of the autosomal dominant missense mutations causing adult-onset Finkel-type SMA affects VAPB. It is interesting that some patients with this mutation develop the clinical features of ALS rather than SMA (Nishimura et al., 2004). DYNCH1H1 and BIC2D (both autosomal dominant) can cause a phenotype of lower extremity predominant SMA (SMALED) (Beecroft et al., 2017; Wan et al., 2019 ). TRP4V-associated disease is very variable but can include a scapuloperoneal-type presentation (Biasini et al., 2016). CHCHD10 autosomal dominant disorders are also highly variable and can be ALS-like, frontotemporal-type dementia (FTD)-like, myopathy-like, or SMA-like (Penttila et al., 2015).

A relatively new class of adult-onset SMA has recently emerged and is sometimes referred to as *SMA-5* to help distinguish a distal rather than proximal pattern of slowly PMA. The classification of these rare disorders is rather vague, and considerable overlap with distal CMT (see later discussion) exists. Several patterns of inheritance occur, including autosomal dominant, autosomal recessive, and X-linked recessive. Some lack any apparent pattern of inheritance. Distal-predominant adult-onset SMA and some of the neuronal forms of CMT disease appear to overlap both clinically and genetically: indeed, the difference may be purely semantic. Motor-predominant CMT variants such as hereditary motor neuronopathy type 5 (HMN-5), itself a heterogeneous group of conditions, present with a slowly progressive LMN-predominant disorder affecting distal limb muscles. Mutations in the glycyl-tRNA synthetase (GARS) gene, for example, were identifiable in multiple families around the world. Patients usually present with very indolent symmetrical or asymmetrical weakness, clumsiness, and wasting of intrinsic hand muscles (with a particular predilection for thenar muscles) in the absence of any proximal weakness or sensory findings. There is little functional disability (Del Bo et al., 2006; Dubourg et al., 2006). Mutations in the p150Glued subunit of the dynactin gene, a microtubule protein important in axonal transport, cause another distal-predominant atrophic disorder that also has a predilection for thenar muscles. Unlike the GARS-associated disorder, involvement of the face and vocal cords may occur (Puls et al., 2005).

## Laboratory Studies

The first-line investigation in autosomal recessive proximal SMA (types 0–4) is molecular genetic analysis to identify homozygous deletions in the *SMN* gene on chromosome 5q and, if confirmed, no further work-up is necessary. However, if a homozygous deletion of SMN1 is not detectable in a patient with a clinical picture consistent with SMA, one can assay for the combination of a deleted SMN allele on one gene and a point mutation on the other. PCR is able to distinguish the single nucleotide change in exon 7 that determines SMN2 from SMN1. It requires measurement because it has prognostic importance. Serum CK may be elevated up to 10 times normal levels in SMA type 3 but is typically normal in the infantile and intermediate types. EMG is valuable in supporting the diagnosis, although it may be technically limited in children by the need to carry out the test under conscious

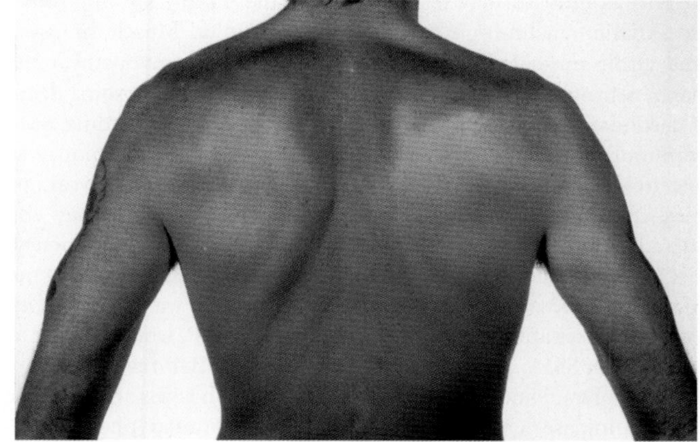

**Fig. 97.2** Patient with mild adult-onset proximal spinal muscular atrophy and marked shoulder-girdle muscle atrophy. Note subluxation at both shoulder joints and marked deltoid muscle atrophy.

sedation. CMAPs may be reduced in amplitude, but conduction velocities and sensory nerve conduction study results are normal. The needle electrode examination may reveal evidence of acute denervation (fibrillation potentials and positive sharp waves) along with fasciculation potentials and evidence of chronic motor unit remodeling due to a chronic process of denervation and reinnervation. Reduced recruitment of large polyphasic motor units is therefore characteristic, although sedation hampers full voluntary activation. Complex repetitive discharges are an electrodiagnostic feature of SMA type 3. Muscle biopsy reveals a highly characteristic pattern called *grouped fascicular atrophy* (especially in typical Werdnig-Hoffmann SMA): entire fascicles or groups of fascicles are atrophied, whereas neighboring fascicles (often made up entirely of type 1 fibers) are composed of hypertrophied fibers. It is important to remember that myopathic changes, including fiber size variability, fiber splitting, internal nuclei, and fibrosis, complicate long-standing denervating disorders such as childhood and juvenile SMA.

While serum CK and aldolase are often normal in adults with SMA type 4, they may be elevated to levels less than 10-fold the normal values. Motor nerve conduction studies reveal normal conduction velocities and reduced CMAPs in the presence of normal SNAPs. Needle electrode studies show marked chronic neurogenic motor unit changes, which are modest if any evidence of acute denervation. Myopathic changes due to secondary myopathic degenerative changes in motor units are also common. Fasciculation potentials may occur in involved muscles. When molecular genetic testing fails to help with diagnosis, it can be very useful to get a muscle biopsy, which typically shows evidence of a markedly chronic denervation similar to that described in SMA type 3 but with more frequent changes of secondary myopathy.

### Differential Diagnosis

For infantile SMA type 1, one must exclude all other causes of infantile hypotonia. This includes Pompe disease, centronuclear myopathy, nemaline myopathy, congenital muscular dystrophy, central core disease, and congenital or infantile myotonic dystrophy. For older children with suspected types 2 and 3 SMA, the differential diagnoses include myasthenia gravis, various muscular dystrophies, inflammatory myopathies, and a variety of structural, metabolic, and endocrine myopathies. Clinical, laboratory, and muscle biopsy features usually distinguish these disorders with relative ease. Limb-girdle muscular dystrophy may be difficult to distinguish from adult-onset proximal SMA; it can be autosomal recessive, is often adult-onset, and affects predominantly proximal muscles. The pattern of muscle weakness often points to the diagnosis; for instance, in adult-onset SMA, the triceps muscles may be weaker than the biceps, the opposite of the situation in limb-girdle muscular dystrophy. Muscle biopsy in limb-girdle muscular dystrophy reveals a primary myopathy rather than a neurogenic process, but one should be aware that some degree of secondary myopathic changes can occur in long-standing SMA. Immunohistochemistry and Western blotting on muscle biopsy are able to distinguish SMA from dystrophinopathies, sarcoglycanopathies, calpainopathies, and dysferlinopathies. Other myopathies considered include polymyositis and adult-onset acid maltase deficiency.

Chronic inflammatory demyelinating polyneuropathy (CIDP) may mimic SMA because of chronic proximal muscle weakness, but the tendon reflexes are usually diffusely absent in CIDP, whereas some are preserved in SMA. Electrodiagnostic studies in CIDP reveal a demyelinating polyradiculoneuropathy, and CSF protein levels are increased. Hexosaminidase-A deficiency in adults has a similar phenotype to adult-onset SMA, but several nonmotor symptoms typically arise. In the absence of a family history of SMA, it can be most difficult to distinguish adult-onset distal-predominant SMA from the PMA variant of ALS. However, adult-onset SMA progresses very slowly, whereas PMA progresses relatively rapidly (albeit slower than classic ALS). Furthermore, muscle biopsy and EDX assessment in adult-onset SMA reveals a markedly chronic disease, whereas PMA findings are consistent with more subacute denervation and thus more modest evidence of neurogenic motor unit remodeling.

### Treatment

A major breakthrough in specific treatment of SMN1 gene SMA has been made with the approval of intrathecal antisense oligonucleotide (ASO) therapy (nusinersen) in SMA types 1, 2, and 3a. Indeed, the potential for this therapy to transform Werdnig-Hoffmann disease from a universally fatal disorder to a slow chronically progressive disease must be considered a medical triumph. ASOs are complementary to "sense" strand nucleic acids to which they bind and control gene expression: nusinersen binds to the intronic splicing sequencer N1 (ISS-N1) and thus promotes exon 7 production in the final transcript (the production of full-length protein from SMN2). The treatment improves rates of survival/freedom from use of a ventilator at 24 months. In those with later-onset disease, there are demonstrable improvements in motor function (Michelson et al., 2018). Intrathecal administration can be challenging in the older age groups due to scoliosis and respiratory difficulties and a multidisciplinary approach is recommended (Wurster et al., 2019). An issue with this treatment is the expense of the ASO therapy itself; cost–benefit analyses are important when considering this form of therapy (Zuluaga-Sanchez et al., 2019). Additional treatment focuses on supportive care, including physiotherapy, respiratory care, nutritional support, orthotics, and orthopedic interventions. Typical Werdnig-Hoffmann disease is almost uniformly fatal by age 2 years. However, because some affected infants survive beyond infancy and live into childhood, aggressive management including physiotherapy and respiratory therapy is essential in all cases.

The management objectives in young children with the intermediate form are twofold: (1) maintain active mobility and independence as long as possible and (2) prevent the development of contractures and kyphoscoliosis. Any devices, even a scooter board, should be considered to maintain mobility. Because all patients invariably become wheelchair confined, the use of an electric-powered wheelchair is required. However, the timing of wheelchair use is critical because it hastens the development of contractures and scoliosis. Stretching exercises in major joints should be part of the patient's daily routine.

Patients with SMA have normal or increased intelligence. They attend school and as adults often live and work outside the home. A well-coordinated multidisciplinary approach is essential when attempting to optimize residual function, especially during periods of disease progression. Physical therapy, occupational therapy, orthopedic evaluation, and emotional support are essential.

Maintaining an upright position delays the development of scoliosis. Therefore, a specialized evaluation for a wheelchair at a comprehensive seating clinic is critical. A back brace potentially delays the development of scoliosis. However, bracing remains controversial because it does little to retard the onset or progression of scoliosis and may actually impair function in some patients by reducing spinal flexibility and respiratory vital capacity. Potential benefits from bracing include reduced back discomfort and the ability to sit for longer periods.

Progressive scoliosis eventually requires surgical correction in most patients with juvenile SMA. In general, delay surgery until growth ceases. However, in some patients who have never ambulated or who lost ambulation very early, consider surgical intervention for severe scoliosis even before growth ceases. Improved aesthetics, balance, and seating comfort are among the benefits; however, lack of body flexibility, reduced pulmonary function, and general decline in overall motor function may occur after surgery. Pros and cons for scoliosis surgery must be openly discussed with the patient, although for most, the benefits outweigh the disadvantages. Preoperative and postoperative physical and occupational therapy assessments are critical steps for the patient who contemplates spinal fusion for progressive scoliosis in SMA.

### Genetic Counseling and Prenatal Diagnosis

SMA is one of the most devastating diseases of childhood, and the parents of affected children and their relatives should receive genetic counseling, including determination of carrier status of SMN genes. The available carrier detection tests determine the SMN1 and SMN2 gene dosages and are best carried out in a family where an SMN deletion has been found previously in an affected individual or for an individual who is about to marry a known carrier. Noncarriers will have a single copy of the normal SMN1 on each chromosome, whereas carriers will have only one normal and one deleted SMN gene. Determination of the SMN2 gene dosage in the setting of an SMN deletion is of particular prognostic importance: the more copies of SMN2, the better the prognosis.

## Kennedy Disease (X-Linked Recessive Bulbospinal Neuronopathy)

In 1968, Kennedy and colleagues reported a new X-linked recessive SMA with bulbar involvement and gynecomastia. The primary pathology was thought to be in the LMNs, but sensory system involvement was later recognized, which led to the term *bulbospinal neuronopathy*. Molecular genetics research has shown Kennedy disease to be a trinucleotide repeat expansion disease. Though rare, it is more common than adult-onset SMA (Box 97.5).

### Pathogenesis

In 1991, La Spada and colleagues found the gene abnormality responsible for Kennedy disease: a cytosine-adenine-guanine (CAG) trinucleotide repeat expansion on the androgen receptor gene located on the X chromosome. In normal individuals, the repeats range from 17 to 26 in this coding region, whereas in patients with Kennedy disease, the repeats range from 40 to 65. Two independent components exist for the symptoms of Kennedy disease, one androgen dependent and the other androgen independent. The gynecomastia and testicular atrophy seen in Kennedy disease may be associated with the classic function of the androgen receptor, and thus the severity of symptoms might relate directly to the receptor's affinity for androgen. Studies of cultured scrotal skin fibroblasts found that direct high-affinity dihydrotestosterone binding decreases in some patients. The abnormal expansion of CAG repeats involves the first exon, an amino-terminal transactivating domain of the androgen receptor protein. The expansion of the CAG repeat in an androgen receptor causes a linear decrease in the transactivation function but does not completely eliminate androgen receptor activity. The residual androgen receptor activity is sufficient to ensure normal development of male primary and secondary sexual characteristics, as evidenced by the fact that affected men are phenotypically male and usually fertile.

The subtle decline of androgen receptor transactivation may eventually lead to the loss of integrity of certain tissues that require continuously high androgen levels. Androgens are crucial for normal male development of motor neurons in the rat spinal bulbocavernosus nucleus and for regenerating facial motor neurons in rats and hamsters. Therefore, continuous androgen receptor function may be crucial to maintain normal motor neuron function throughout life.

As with most other trinucleotide repeat expansion disorders such as Huntington disease and several spinocerebellar ataxias, the trinucleotide repeat expansion mutation appears to confer a toxic gain-of-function on the gene product rather than a loss of function. In fact, complete absence of the androgen receptor leads to an entirely different disorder called *androgen-insensitivity syndrome*. The mutant androgen receptor leads to an altered receptor–DNA interaction or receptor–protein interaction that interferes with neuronal function. The CAG repeat encodes an unusually long polyglutamine tract in the androgen receptor protein, which appears to alter the normal protein moiety, resulting in mutant protein aggregation. This may in turn interfere with proteasomal breakdown of other cellular proteins and/or interfere with tubulin-mediated cellular transport. Mutant protein may also interfere with mitochondrial function and transcription regulation and contribute to endoplasmic reticulum stress (Cortes and La Spada, 2018).

**BOX 97.5 Characteristic Features of Kennedy Disease**

Pathogenesis:
- X-linked recessive inheritance
- Abnormal CAG expansion in the gene encoding androgen receptor protein

Neurological manifestations:
- Slowly progressive limb-girdle muscle weakness
- Early tremor
- Slowly progressive moderate bulbar dysfunction
- Muscle cramps and prominent fasciculations
- Facial fasciculations

Systemic manifestations:
- Gynecomastia (60%–90%)
- Endocrine abnormalities (testicular atrophy, feminization, infertility)
- Diabetes mellitus

Laboratory studies:
- Markedly abnormal sensory nerve conduction studies
- Elevated serum creatine kinase
- Abnormal sex hormone levels
- Abnormal CAG repeats in the androgen receptor gene

*CAG*, Cytosine-adenine-guanine.

### Clinical Features

As is often seen in an X-linked syndrome, this is a disorder of men, who remain largely asymptomatic until after age 30 years. Hand tremor and subtle speech disturbance are early features that are followed by LMN muscle weakness, initially involving either the proximal hip extensor or shoulder girdle muscles, and associated with decreased or absent reflexes, muscle atrophy, and occasionally calf pseudohypertrophy. Kennedy disease usually causes no respiratory muscle weakness. Coarse muscle fasciculations can be prominent in the extremities and trunk and muscle cramps can be a first symptom in many (Rhodes et al., 2009). Facial and perioral fasciculations are present in more than 90% of patients (Video 97.3). The tongue shows chronic atrophy, often as a longitudinal midline furrow. However, despite weakness of facial and tongue muscles, significant bulbar symptoms are usually a relatively late feature. Neurological examination of the sensory system may reveal only modest impairment. Progression is slow, with most cases remaining independent of assist devices until late into the fifth decade of life (Atsuna et al., 2006). If bulbar dysfunction is severe, the prognosis becomes less favorable. Partial androgen insensitivity is an important element of this condition, and gynecomastia is one of the unique features of Kennedy disease that can be found in 60%–90% of patients (Fig. 97.3). Other endocrine abnormalities include testicular atrophy, infertility (40%), and diabetes mellitus (10%–20%). It is now recognized that female carriers may manifest subtle neurological deficits such as late-onset bulbar dysfunction.

This disorder often exhibits genetic anticipation—that is, the greater the number of repeats, the younger the age at onset. However, the number of repeats has no correlation with other features such as severity of weakness, serum CK level, and presence or absence of gynecomastia, impotence, or sensory neuronopathy. Furthermore, there is marked variation in phenotypical expression within and among families.

### Laboratory Studies

Molecular genetic testing is available to identify the abnormal expansion of the CAG repeat in the exon 1 of the androgen receptor gene on the X chromosome. CK levels may be elevated as high as 10 times normal. Serum androgen levels are either normal or decreased, whereas estrogen levels are elevated in some patients. The estrogen-to-androgen ratio increases in some patients, but there is no consistent finding regarding sex hormone levels, and evidence of partial androgen resistance may not develop for several years after disease onset.

Motor nerve conduction study results are generally normal, although one-third of the patients have reduced amplitudes of CMAPs. EMG examination of these patients is always abnormal and shows modest acute but prominent chronic denervation changes in motor units. EDX reveals a sensory neuronopathy in 95% of patients (Ferrante and Wilbourn, 1997). Another unique change is the presence of prominent fasciculation potentials in the face (especially in the perioral region) and limbs.

Muscle biopsy shows modest denervation, prominent reinnervation, and fiber-type grouping similar to that seen in other forms of adult-onset SMA. Sural nerve biopsy usually reveals a loss of myelinated fibers.

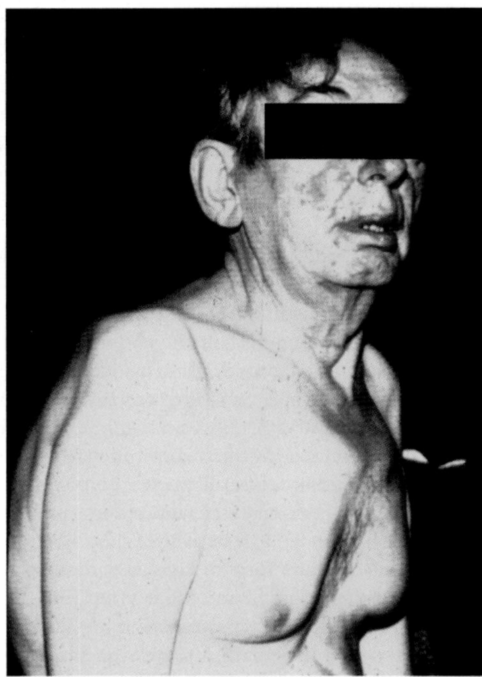

**Fig. 97.3** A man with X-linked recessive bulbospinal muscular atrophy (Kennedy disease), showing gynecomastia. *(From Perkin, G.D., Miller, D.C., Lane, R.J.M., Patel, M.C., Hochberg, F.H., 2011. Atlas of Clinical Neurology, third ed. pp. 28–56. © Saunders.)*

### Differential Diagnosis

The clinical features (e.g., progressive limb-girdle weakness, bulbar signs, muscle cramps, prominent fasciculations) resemble those of ALS, but a careful physical examination should provide sufficient clues to distinguish one from the other. The most characteristic features are gynecomastia, perioral fasciculations, calf pseudohypertrophy, and hand tremor. Generally, ALS progresses rapidly, whereas Kennedy disease is a largely indolent disorder. The EDX in Kennedy disease shows abnormal sensory nerve conduction studies, which is unusual for any motor neuron disease. Kennedy disease may also be easily mistaken for adult-onset SMA because of the slowly progressive limb-girdle weakness in both, but bulbar involvement and gynecomastia are unlikely features of SMA. Hereditary sensorimotor neuropathy, limb-girdle dystrophy, or facioscapulohumeral muscular dystrophy also may mimic Kennedy disease. Careful clinical examination, EDX studies, and muscle or nerve biopsy distinguishes these disorders. Ultimately, a molecular gene study to identify the abnormal CAG repeats in the androgen receptor gene will yield the answer.

### Manifesting Carrier

The female children and mother of an affected male patient are all obligate carriers (except in rare instances of a de novo mutation). Male children of affected individuals cannot inherit the mutant gene on the X chromosome. Female siblings of an affected patient have a 50% chance of carrying the affected gene on the X chromosome. Through a process known as *skewed X chromosome inactivation* (lyonization), female carriers can present with neuromuscular symptoms such as exertional muscle pain, cramps, and late-onset bulbar dysfunction, and the EDX may detect mild chronic denervation in both upper and lower limb muscles.

### Treatment

Supportive and symptomatic therapy is the key to treatment, as outlined in the section on adult-onset SMA. Muscle cramps may be problematic but are often relieved by baclofen, clonazepam, or vitamin E. Patients with symptomatic diabetes require appropriate medical management.

In Kennedy disease, dysarthria and dysphagia may cause marked disability. Although severe loss of bulbar function is rare, offer speech therapy and appropriate communicative devices when appropriate. Careful nutritional management is also important. Enteral feeding provided via gastrostomy is the most effective and practical means to meet nutritional and fluid requirements. Genetic counseling is important for patients, potential carriers, and male siblings. A natural history-controlled study recently showed that long-term use of leuprorelin, a gonadotrophin analogue, improves elements of functional decline and also reduces respiratory complications and death in Kennedy disease (Hashizume et al., 2017).

## Progressive Muscular Atrophy

PMA, first described by Aran in 1850, is a clinical LMN disorder during its entire clinical course and comprises approximately 5%–8% of all adult-onset motor neuron diseases. It is an overwhelmingly sporadic disease, but rare genetic diseases, such as those due to mutations in dynactin, VAPB, and A4V SOD1, may present with a pure LMN disorder, so a careful family history is important. Although PMA occurs in both sexes, men are more often affected than women. In a recent study, the average age of onset of PMA was about 3 years older than that of ALS, but other studies report a younger age at onset (Kim et al., 2009; Murray, 2006). Several studies have demonstrated that PMA progresses more slowly than ALS, so the average survival is significantly longer. The mean duration of disease was 159 months in one series of cases, and in another study, the 5-year survival was 63.7% in PMA versus 36.8% in ALS. Most of the very longest-duration cases of "ALS" have the PMA variant. Interestingly, the recent paper by Kim et al. showed that the development of UMN signs was unrelated to survival time after diagnosis (Kim et al., 2009; Murray, 2006). However, Visser et al. (2007) showed that patients with a low vital capacity baseline with an early decline in pulmonary function in the first 6 months had an especially poor prognosis.

It has been questioned whether PMA is an independent disease or represents one end of the spectrum of ALS. However, if followed over time, many patients with PMA go on to develop clinical features of upper motor neuron disease, which allows reclassification to ALS (and thus eligibility for entry into clinical trials). In a recent retrospective study of 916 cases diagnosed with ALS at a major neurological center, in 91, the original diagnosis was PMA; 20 of these developed UMN signs within 61 months of the original diagnosis. Autopsy studies have also demonstrated UMN involvement in some cases classified as PMA in life. Studies using magnetic resonance spectroscopy and/or TMS reveal evidence for upper motor neuron involvement in PMA patients. Furthermore, cognitive/behavioral changes similar to those seen in ALS are also detected in PMA (Kim et al., 2009; Maragakis et al., 2010; Rowland, 2006).

### Etiology

All hypotheses about the cause of ALS are also applicable to PMA (see Etiology, under Amyotrophic Lateral Sclerosis, later in this chapter).

### Clinical Features

By definition, the signs and symptoms of PMA are LMN in type throughout the entire clinical course. A common presentation is that of focal asymmetrical muscle weakness in the distal extremities, with gradual spread to other contiguous muscles. The weakness and muscle atrophy are purely LMN in type and eventually involve both the upper and lower extremities. A less common presentation is that of proximal rather than distal muscle weakness. Bulbar and respiratory involvement eventually develops but is not as common in the early stages as in classic "spinal" ALS.

### Laboratory Studies

The serum CK concentration may be moderately elevated, especially when patients are physically active, but never attains levels more than 10 times normal. Patients with PMA do not have high titers of anti-GM1 antibodies. The EMG examination reveals findings consistent with a widespread disorder of anterior horn cells and is useful to exclude other diagnostic possibilities such as CIDP, MMNCB, or myopathy. Muscle biopsy will show denervation atrophy, but it is usually unnecessary to perform this test unless the clinical features are unusual enough to suggest an alternative diagnosis.

### Differential Diagnosis

PMA is usually a fatal disease and has no cure. Therefore, the diagnosis of PMA requires the exclusion of all other potentially treatable or definable diseases. Indeed, PMA-like disease is the most common type of presentation in the "mimic" disorders spectrum (Cortes-Vicente et al., 2017). In a previous review, 17 of 89 patients originally diagnosed with PMA were later diagnosed with MMNCB, CIDP, inflammatory myopathy, and myasthenia gravis (Visser et al., 2002). MMNCB is the most important of the alternative conditions that may present with focal and asymmetrical weakness in the absence of UMN signs (for more detailed description, see Chapter 106). The classic form is associated with EDX evidence of multifocal demyelination conduction blocks and elevated titers of antibodies against GM1 gangliosides. Clinically, patients develop slowly progressive multifocal muscle weakness but less prominent muscle atrophy. The treatment of choice is human IVIG (Van den Berg-Vos et al., 2000). The clinical and electrodiagnostic findings of sensory involvement, high CSF protein levels, and response to immunotherapy readily separate CIDP and PMA. Important clues that should lead one to suspect inclusion body myositis (IBM) are elevated serum CK to levels more than expected in typical PMA and a selective weakness in wrist flexors, finger flexors, and quadriceps muscles, without fasciculations. EMG in IBM should show evidence of a primary myopathy with increased insertional activity but without fasciculations. In IBM, additional neurogenic changes are common, and quantitative EMG may be required to clearly identify the myopathic nature of this disorder. Muscle biopsy characteristically reveals rimmed vacuoles and nuclear inclusions. Adult-onset SMA is a far more indolent disorder than PMA, and the very chronic process of denervation and reinnervation in SMA leads to fiber-type grouping on muscle biopsy, which is not a prominent feature of the less-protracted PMA. It is important to carry out regular follow-up examinations on patients with PMA to search for signs of UMN involvement that indicate the diagnosis of ALS. The pure motor neuropathy forms of CMT (especially hereditary motor neuropathy type V) present with a slowly progressive distal pattern of weakness and wasting, with no sensory changes. A familial pattern is usual, and genetic testing may reveal mutations in different genes such as GARS or seipin. A paraneoplastic motor neuronopathy has been described with clinical features that are similar to PMA, albeit with more rapid progression and with later development of nonmotor features. Many such cases have anti-Hu antineuronal antibodies in the setting of solid cancers (especially small-cell lung cancer). A similar subacute presentation may also occur in patients with lymphoma or other lymphoproliferative disorders, although signs of corticospinal tract dysfunction may become apparent in over 50% of cases. The onset of lymphoma may or may not coincide with onset of motor features.

### Treatment

The treatment of PMA is identical to that of ALS, as summarized later in this chapter.

## Subacute Motor Neuronopathy in Lymphoproliferative Disorders

A subacute, progressive, and painless motor neuron syndrome may rarely develop in patients who have Hodgkin and non-Hodgkin lymphoma with or without a paraproteinemia (Rowland, 2006; Rudnicki and Dalmau, 2000). The lymphoma may or may not temporally coincide with the motor neuron disorder, and one or other disorder may present first. Although UMN signs may develop later in more than half of all cases, a LMN-onset syndrome is typical, with patchy, asymmetrical, lower extremity–predominant muscle weakness and wasting. Neuropathology shows a loss of anterior horn cells and ventral root nerve fibers; some have evidence of inflammation in the anterior horns of the spinal cord, and half have corticospinal tract degeneration. In some patients, the disease may be relatively benign. The rate of progression of muscle weakness and atrophy tends to slow down with time, and, in rare instances, the motor syndrome may respond to treatment of the underlying lymphoproliferative disorder. However, the prognosis appears to be less favorable in those who develop a combined UMN and LMN disorder. Twenty percent of all cases so far reported with motor neuron presentations in the setting of lymphoproliferative disease had myeloma or macroglobulinemia. The pathogenesis of this ALS-like disorder is undetermined, but an immune mechanism may be at play; small patient series and case reports reveal that some patients who develop this LMN syndrome may have various autoantibodies (such as antisulfatide antibody), paraproteinemia, increased CSF protein, and/or oligoclonal bands.

### Postirradiation Lower Motor Neuron Syndrome

Radiation directed to the retroperitoneal paraaortic area for the treatment of testicular or lymphoid cancers can cause a pure LMN syndrome in the lower extremities that first appears many years after the irradiation. Sensory abnormalities and sphincter dysfunction are rare, and the EDX findings are consistent with a disorder of the lumbosacral motor neurons or the cauda equina (the SNAPs are spared). Myokymic discharges and nonresolving conduction blocks are characteristic electrodiagnostic features. The disease usually progresses over the first few years after symptom onset but subsequently becomes stable. There is debate as to the exact mechanism. There is only anecdotal evidence that antiinflammatory therapies may be of benefit (Chamberlain et al., 2011).

## DISORDERS OF BOTH UPPER AND LOWER MOTOR NEURONS

### Amyotrophic Lateral Sclerosis

ALS is a neurodegenerative disorder of undetermined etiology that primarily affects the motor neuron cell populations in the motor cortex, brainstem, and spinal cord. It is progressive, and most patients eventually succumb to respiratory failure. The first detailed description was by Jean Martin Charcot in 1869, in which he discussed the clinical and pathological characteristics of "la sclérose latérale amyotrophique," a disorder of muscle wasting (amyotrophy) and gliotic hardening (sclerosis) of the anterior and lateral corticospinal tracts (Gordon, 2006) involving both upper and lower motor neurons. ALS is known by several other names including *Charcot disease*, *motor neuron disease*, and, in the United States, "Lou Gehrig disease" in remembrance of the famous "Iron Horse" of baseball who was diagnosed with ALS in 1939.

The World Federation of Neurology Research Group on Neuromuscular Disorders has classified ALS as a disorder of motor neurons of undetermined cause, and several variants are recognized. Included in this group are PLS and PBP. As previously mentioned, PMA is also thought to be a variant of ALS, despite its exclusion from current clinical research trial criteria. It is important to recognize that ALS is a progressive dynamic disorder. Some cases present with the classic combination of UMN and LMN signs, but others may have UMN onset, LMN onset, bulbar onset, or dyspnea at onset and only later develop signs of involvement of the other parts of the motor system (Box 97.6).

Between 5% and 10% of ALS is familial rather than sporadic, the most common inheritance pattern being autosomal dominant. Thus one comes across the terms *sporadic ALS* (SALS) and *familial ALS* (FALS). A few other conditions have a phenotypical expression similar to that of ALS, including Western Pacific ALS-parkinsonism-dementia complex (PDC) (or Guamanian ALS) and juvenile ALS.

The incidence and prevalence rates for sporadic ALS are surprisingly uniform throughout the world. The estimated incidence in North America and Europe is about 2 per 100,000, and the prevalence is about 5–7 per 100,000 (Mehta et al., 2016). In sporadic spinal ALS, the male-to-female ratio is 1.2–1.4 : 1, but a slight female predominance exists in the bulbar-onset variety. ALS may occur as early as in the second decade of life, but the peak incidence is in the 65- to 74-year-old age bracket (McGuire and Nelson, 2006). The mean disease duration from symptom onset to death is approximately 3 years, but roughly 1 in 5 patients survive to 5 years, and 1 in 10 patients survive to 10 years (Murray, 2006). The disease process may be more aggressive in patients with bulbar onset, older age at onset, and certain genotypes (Al-Chalabi and Hardiman, 2013). No specific environmental, occupational, or physical factors link with absolute

**BOX 97.6 Practical Classification of Amyotrophic Lateral Sclerosis**

Sporadic or acquired ALS:
- Classic (spinal-onset) ALS
- Mills hemiplegic variant
- Pseudoneuritic presentation
- Flail-arm presentation
- Monomelic presentation
- UMN onset
- LMN onset
- Bulbar onset
- Dyspnea onset
- Progressive muscular atrophy
- Primary lateral sclerosis
- Progressive bulbar palsy
- Western Pacific ALS

Familial ALS:
- ALS1: SOD1 missense mutations, chr 21q-22.1, adult, AD (rare AR)
- ALS2: ALSIN mutations, chr 2q330, juvenile onset, AR
- ALS3: gene unknown, chr 18q, adult, AD
- ALS4: senataxin gene, chr 9q34, juvenile onset, AD
- ALS5: linked to chr 15q15, juvenile onset, AR
- ALS6: FUS/TLS, chr 16p, adult, FTD overlap, AD (some AR)
- ALS7: gene unknown, chr 20p, adult, AD
- ALS8: VAPB, chr 20q, adult, AD
- ALS9: angiogenin, chr 14q, adult, AD
- ALS10: TDP-43, chr 1q, adult, FTD overlap, AD
- ALS11: FIG4, chr 6q, adult, AD
- ALS12: optineurin, chr 10p15, AD
- ALS13: ATXN2 12q24, association
- ALS14: VCP, Chr 9p13
- ALS15: UBQLN2, chr X
- ALS16: SIGMAR1, chr 9p13
- ALS17: CHMP2B, chr 2q, adult, AD
- ALS18: PFN1, chr 17p13
- ALS19: ERBB4, chr 2q34
- ALS20: HNRNPA1, chr 12q13
- ALS21: MATR3, chr 5q31.2
- ALS22: TUBA4A, chr 2q35
- ALS23: ANXA11, chr 10q22.3
- ALS24: NEK1, chr 4q33
- ALS25: KIF5A, chr 12q13.3
- ALS due to rare mutations (e.g., p150 dynactin subunit mutation, DAO mutation, SQSTM1 mutation, hnRNPA1 mutation, ERLIN2 mutation, UNC13A mutation, cytochrome oxidase gene mutation, NF heavy chain gene mutation, peripherin, APEX nuclease gene mutation)

FTD-ALS overlap:
- ALS-FTD, C9orf72, chr 9p21, adult, AD (can present as pure ALS also or as pure FTD)
- FTD with some ALS features; tau gene on chr 17 and progranulin gene on chr 17.

*AD*, Autosomal dominant; *ALS*, amyotrophic lateral sclerosis; *AR*, autosomal recessive; *chr*, chromosome; *FTD*, frontotemporal dementia; *LMN*, lower motor neuron; *UMN*, upper motor neuron.

certainty to an increased risk of ALS. Areas of interest include chronic exposure to electromagnetic fields, high levels of physical activity (e.g., ex-National Football League players; Lehman et al., 2012), high dietary intake of glutamate, environmental toxins, and a history of military service in the Persian Gulf War. Smoking appears to be an independent risk factor for sporadic ALS, with a higher risk for those who have smoked for many years (Armon, 2009; Gallo et al., 2009). Several environmental trace elements have been evaluated as potential causative agents for ALS, including selenium, aluminum, iron, manganese, copper, zinc, cadmium, and lead, but there is no convincing evidence that any one of these plays a major part in ALS pathogenesis.

### Pathology

The pathological hallmarks of ALS are the degeneration and loss of motor neurons, with astrocytic gliosis and microglial proliferation in the presence of intraneuronal inclusions in degenerating neurons and glial cells. UMN cell loss occurs in the motor cortex, with loss of Betz cells from Brodmann area 4 and astrocytic gliosis and axonal loss in corticospinal tracts. There is loss of LMNs in the brainstem and spinal cord, with both TAR DNA binding protein 43-positive and FUS-positive ubiquitinated inclusions in remaining neurons. Small eosinophilic cytoplasmic inclusions called *Bunina bodies* are common. Extramotor pathology may also be found in the frontotemporal cortex, hippocampus, thalamus, spinocerebellar tracts, dorsal columns, and substantia nigra.

### Etiology

The cause for sporadic ALS is unknown. A significant body of basic and clinical research lends strong support to a theory of ALS pathogenesis which proposes selective motor neuron damage from a complex chain of injurious events involving excitotoxins, oxidative stress, neurofilament dysfunction, altered calcium homeostasis, mitochondrial dysfunction, enhanced motor neuron apoptosis, and proinflammatory cytokines. Genetic factors may play a role in "sporadic" disease: several proposed ALS susceptibility genes include APOE, SMN, peripherin, apex nuclease gene, and vascular endothelial growth factor (VEGF) gene. Indeed, it has been proposed that onset of ALS is a multi-step process in which a genetic mutation represents one of several steps in the development of the disease (Al-Chalabi and Hardiman, 2013).

***Protein aggregation.*** One of the pathological hallmarks of sporadic ALS is the presence of TDP43- and FUS-positive ubiquitinated intraneuronal inclusion bodies in neurons and glial cells. TDP43 and FUS, both implicated in the pathogenesis of FALS and SALS, are normally nuclear proteins, but in ALS they are mislocalized to the cytoplasm in the form of distinct aggregates (inclusion bodies); how the mislocalization contributes to neuronal loss is still unclear. Several other pathological intracellular aggregates described in ALS can contain neurofilament proteins, chaperone proteins (14-3-3), and copper-zinc superoxide dismutase (SOD1). Furthermore, mutations in other ALS-associated genes, such as UBQLN2, C9orf72, SIGMAR1, PFN1, DAO, and ATXN2, are also associated with aggregate formation (Finsterer and Burgunder, 2014). It is still unclear whether protein aggregation is directly toxic to cells or is a defense mechanism to reduce intracellular aggregation of toxic proteins.

***Glutamate excitotoxicity and free radical injury.*** Glutamate, which is the most abundant free amino acid in the CNS, is one of the major excitatory amino acid (EAA) neurotransmitters. Glutamate produces neuronal excitation and participates in many neuronal functions, including neuronal plasticity. In excess, however, it causes neurotoxicity. The role of glutamate excitotoxicity in neurodegeneration is strengthened by the observation that exogenous glutamate receptor agonists result in clinically observable neurotoxicity, as seen in lathyrism, Guamanian ALS, and Konzo (see previous section on UMN disease). Domoic acid is another potent non-*N*-methyl-D-aspartic acid (NMDA) receptor agonist that can cause motor weakness. An outbreak of food poisoning caused by ingestion of mussels contaminated with domoic acid–producing phytoplankton diatoms led to an amnestic syndrome and, in some cases, significant muscle weakness (sometimes manifesting as an alternating hemiplegia) (Costa et al., 2010).

Impaired glutamate transport reduces clearance of glutamate from the synaptic cleft, which may leave excessive amounts of free excitatory neurotransmitter to repeatedly stimulate the glutamate receptor and thus allow calcium ions to enter the neuron. Regional differences in the levels of activity of calcium buffering systems and in glutamate receptor subtype expression may explain the selective vulnerability of certain motor neuron pools within the CNS.

***Immunological and inflammatory abnormalities.*** Several pieces of evidence implicate an inflammatory process in the pathogenesis, if not the initiation, of ALS. It is now understood that there is a complex interplay between astrocytes, microglial cells, proinflammatory cytokines, and cell adhesion molecules as part of the pathogenesis of both sporadic and familial ALS. However, immunotherapies have been ineffective to date. Whether these inflammatory responses are part of the pathogenesis or are indeed part of a protective response remains to be elucidated (Haukedal and Freude, 2019). Unfortunately, various strategies aimed at modulation of the immune system have failed to alter the course of ALS in treatment trials to date.

***Mitochondrial dysfunction.*** Disturbances in mitochondrial function and structure occur in both human ALS and in transgenic animal models of the SOD1-associated disease, which suggests a role for aberrant redox chemistry in the earlier stages of disease. In effect, mitochondrial damage may impair the cellular energy production system. Mutant SOD1 aggregates appear to clump together on mitochondrial membranes and may also interfere with chaperone-assisted mitochondrial protein folding. Furthermore, axonal transport of mitochondria along axons may be disrupted (Shi et al., 2010). Recent evidence reports that Betz cells that display TDP-43 inclusions show dysfunction at the level of the mitochondria, endoplasmic reticulum, and the nuclear membrane. Furthermore, these changes emerge early in the disease (Gautam et al., 2019). Experimental ALS models also display a role for mitochondrial dysfunction in FUS-associated disease (Cozzolino et al., 2013).

***Neurofilament and microtubule dysfunction.*** Abnormalities of axonal transport likely play a significant part in the pathogenesis of ALS. Mutations in the genes for neurofilament subunits (neurofilament heavy chain and peripherin), although rare, appear to confer increased risk for the later development of SALS (Robberecht and Philips, 2013). It has been shown that mutations in profilin 1 (PFN1), which is an important protein involved in the polymerization of actin, can cause ALS, as can mutations in VAPB and dynactin (see Familial Amyotrophic Lateral Sclerosis section). Antibodies to phosphorylated neurofilament heavy subunit or neurofilament light subunit have emerged as new diagnostic biomarkers for ALS, although their use in detecting disease progression over time appears to be limited (Mitsumoto and Saito, 2018).

***Aberrant RNA processing.*** *RNA metabolism* refers to the various steps in the life of RNA molecules from pre–mRNA splicing through RNA editing and processing, and then on to transport, reassembly into polyribosomes, and degradation. An evolving theory, and perhaps the most important one in ALS pathogenesis is that mutations in such proteins as C9orf72, TDP43, FUS/TLS, senataxin, peripherin, SMN1, SOD1, and angiogenin may result in aberrant interactions in RNA metabolism (Chew et al., 2019, Finsterer and Burgunder, 2014; Haeusler et al., 2014; Robberecht and Philips, 2013).

## Clinical Features

The typical clinical picture in ALS is that of a patient with a progressive motor deterioration manifesting with both UMN and LMN symptoms and signs. Thus, one should consider this diagnosis when a patient presents with a combination of marked weakness and wasting but with brisk reflexes, spasticity, and pathological reflexes. Of course, not all patients present with this classic pattern: muscle weakness in ALS usually begins in a focal area, first spreading to contiguous muscles in the same region before involvement of another region. The first presentation may appear very similar to a focal mononeuropathy, sometimes called the *pseudoneuritic* or *flail leg presentation* (Wijesekera et al., 2009). More commonly, however, single-limb weakness appears to occur in muscles derived from more than one peripheral nerve and/or nerve root distribution; this is a *monomelic presentation.* Onset of muscle weakness is more common in the upper than the lower extremities (classic, spinal ALS), but in approximately 25% of patients, weakness begins in bulbar-innervated muscles (bulbar-onset ALS). On rare occasions (1% or 2% of patients, more often male), the weakness starts in the respiratory muscles (dyspnea or respiratory onset). Some patients present with weakness that is restricted to one side of the body (Mills hemiplegic variant), and up to 10% of patients appear with bilateral upper-extremity wasting, which is known as the *flail arm* or *flail person in the barrel variant.* The latter is more commonly seen in males and typically presents in proximal muscles of the upper limb before spreading distally into the hands, and then much later (one study used a 12-month interval) into other regions. Reflexes may be retained or even brisk in the markedly weakened limbs (Video 97.4).

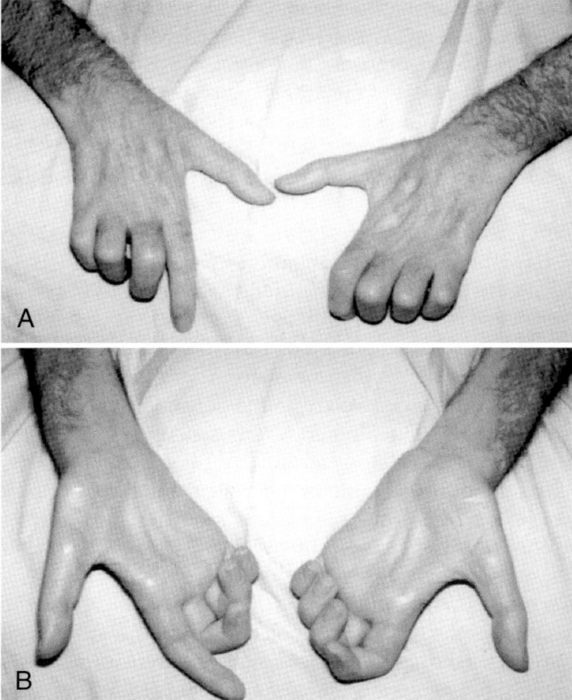


**Fig. 97.4** **A, B,** Severe intrinsic hand muscle atrophy in a patient with amyotrophic lateral sclerosis. Note the "claw hand" and atrophy of muscles innervated by both ulnar and medial nerves.

Symptoms of muscle weakness vary, depending on which motor function is impaired. For example, when weakness begins in the hand and fingers, patients report difficulty in turning a key, buttoning, opening a bottle cap, or turning a doorknob (Fig. 97.4). When weakness begins in the lower leg, foot drop may be the first symptom, or the patient may complain of instability of gait, falling, or fatigue when walking (see Video 97.3). When bulbar muscles are affected, the first symptoms may be slurred speech, hoarseness, or an inability to sing or shout, soon followed by progressive dysphagia (Fig. 97.4; see Video 97.4). Patients with bulbar-onset ALS often initially consult ear, nose, and throat (ENT) specialists and not only experience progressive impairment in bulbar function but also excessive drooling (sialorrhea) and weight loss. Pseudobulbar palsy may present with inappropriate or forced crying or laughter (see Signs and Symptoms of Upper Motor Neuron Involvement, earlier in this chapter), which is often a source of great emotional distress for patients. Excessive forced yawning may also be a manifestation of pseudobulbar palsy. In the rare patient who presents with progressive respiratory muscle weakness, the first consultation may be with a pulmonologist or even admission to the intensive care unit; the diagnosis of ALS may be established when the patient fails weaning from the ventilator. Head drop (or droop) may be a feature in ALS, caused by weakness of cervical and thoracic paraspinal muscles (Fig. 97.6). Fasciculations are not commonly the presenting

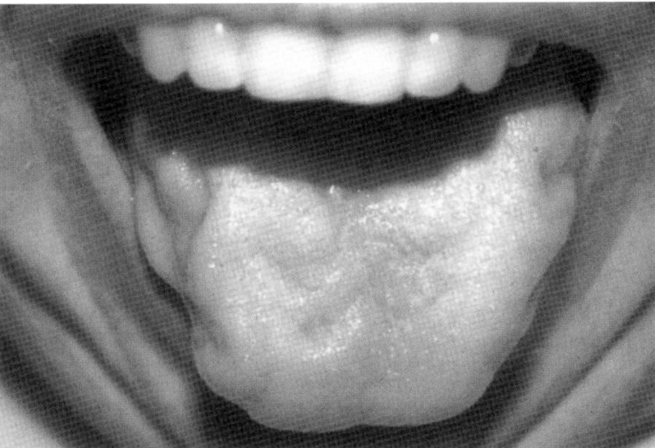

**Fig. 97.5** Atrophy of the Tongue in Amyotrophic Lateral Sclerosis.

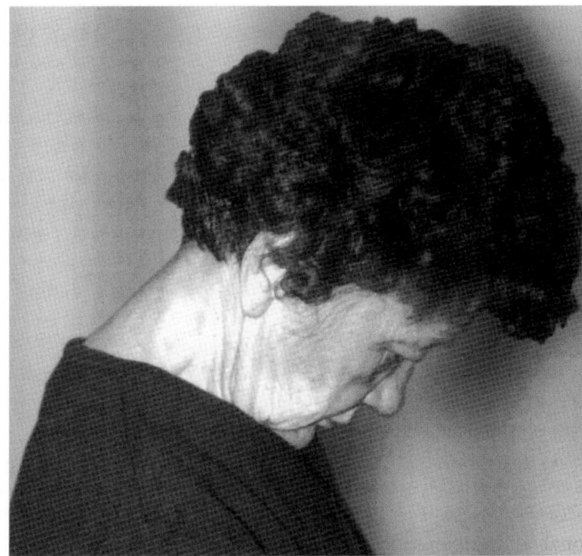

**Fig. 97.6** Patient with amyotrophic lateral sclerosis, showing head droop caused by weakness of the thoracic and cervical paraspinal muscles.

feature of ALS, but they develop in almost all patients soon after onset, and their absence should prompt one to reconsider the diagnosis. In some patients, waves of fasciculations spread across the chest or back. Muscle cramps are one of most common symptoms in patients with ALS and often precede other symptoms by many months. In ALS they can occur in unusual muscles such as in the thigh, abdomen, back, or tongue. Spasticity develops in wasted muscles, and patients may suffer painful flexor spasms in limbs.

As dysphagia worsens, reduced caloric intake worsens fatigue and accelerates muscle weakness. Aspiration of liquids, secretions, and food becomes a risk. Patients may complain that they produce copious amounts of abnormally thick oral secretions, which may drool excessively from the mouth. This sialorrhea is made worse as perioral muscles weaken and/or head drop develops. Weight loss is often rapidly progressive; this does not simply reflect poor caloric intake but represents a form of ALS cachexia. Marked loss of muscle bulk exposes joints and associated connective tissues to abnormal mechanical stresses that can lead to joint contractures, joint deformities, painful shoulder pericapsulitis, and bursitis. Sleep disturbances in the form of increased awakenings from hypopnea and hypoxia are common in ALS and contribute to daytime sleepiness, morning headaches, and fatigue. As respiratory difficulty worsens, patients may be unable to lie supine because of worsening diaphragmatic weakness and thus compensate by using multiple pillows. In more advanced stages, patients are unable to lie in bed at all. Other manifestations of ventilatory failure include dyspnea on exertion and eventually dyspnea at rest. As the disease advances, motor function is progressively impaired, and activities of daily living (e.g., self-hygiene, bathing, dressing, toileting, walking, feeding, and verbal communication) become difficult. Accordingly, a patient's quality of life progressively deteriorates. It may be difficult to distinguish daytime fatigue, broken sleep, affect lability, and sighing from depression, but it is vitally important to be aware of the latter, as both fatigue and depression may occur in ALS (McElhiney et al., 2009).

FTD and/or cognitive impairment is present in many patients with ALS, albeit on a spectrum from apparently normal to a florid FTD. These observations lend support to the notion that ALS is not a pure disorder of motor neurons, but rather a disorder that primarily affects motor neurons, with the potential to involve nonmotor systems. One needs to be cautious when assessing apparently cognitively normal patients with ALS because the deficits may be so subtle as to require specific assessments of personality, behavior, praxis, verbal fluency, visual attention, and verbal reasoning. Dysarthria may mask language disturbances (especially anomia). With appropriate testing, cognitive deficits may be found in about 50% of patients with ALS, but the full clinical (Neary) criteria for a diagnosis of FTD are met in only about 15%–20% of cases (Lomen-Hoerth, 2011). Many of the genetic causes of ALS can also present with frontotemporal dementia (e.g., C9orf72) (see section on familial ALS below, Box 97.6).

## Atypical Features

Extrapyramidal dysfunction, eye movement abnormalities, autonomic disturbances, and abnormal sphincter control are extremely rare in ALS, and their presence should always prompt one to reconsider the diagnosis. Eye movement abnormalities, however, occur in rare cases maintained on ventilators, and sphincter disturbances have appeared in a few reports. Although sparing of the sensory system is characteristic, some patients do report vague sensory symptoms such as numbness or aching, and there is electrophysiological evidence that ascending afferent pathways may be involved, despite the absence of objective sensory loss on physical examination. The motor neurons of Onufrowicz in the sacral cord are essentially not involved in ALS, and thus patients generally do not complain of significant problems with sphincter control (although some may report mild urgency of micturition). Similarly, eye movements are typically normal in ALS; it takes detailed quantitative testing to be able to identify abnormal vertical ocular saccades. Approximately 5% of patients with ALS exhibit signs of extrapyramidal tract dysfunction, usually in the form of retropulsions during attempted ambulation.

## Natural History of the Disease

Evidence exists for a preclinical phase in ALS. Patients lose motor neurons before they become aware of weakness. Wohlfart (1958) estimated that collateral reinnervation could offset the development of clinical weakness until at least 30% of anterior horn cell motor neurons had been lost. Swash and Ingram described a case of sporadic ALS who complained of muscle fatigue for 6 years before onset of weakness, wasting, and fasciculations. However, once the clinical phase is evident, a generally linear decline in motor function occurs over time. The pattern of disease spread is predictable. When onset is in one arm, spread is often first to the contralateral side, then the ipsilateral leg, the contralateral leg, and finally the bulbar region. Onset in the leg often follows a similar pattern, yet again with final involvement of the bulbar region. Bulbar-onset ALS tends to spread to the hands first, with spread to thoracic myotomes, and then the legs. Overall, the pattern suggests that rostral-caudal involvement is faster than caudal-rostral spread. During the course of the disease, transitory improvement, plateaus, or sudden worsening can occur, but spontaneous improvement, although reported, is exceedingly rare.

## Prognosis

The median duration of ALS from clinical onset ranges from 22 to 52 months and the mean duration from 23 to 43 months, with an average 5-year survival rate of 22% (roughly 1 in 5) and a 10-year survival rate of 9.4% (roughly 1 in 10) (Murray, 2006). The most robust poor prognostic factors in ALS are older age at onset and bulbar-onset pattern (Chio et al., 2009). Other important poor prognostic factors include short interval between onset and clinical diagnosis (correlating with a more aggressive presentation), rapid progression rate as assessed on return visits, low body mass index, FTD-ALS presentation, dyspnea at onset, and rapid rate of decline in pulmonary function. PLS and PMA (clinically UMN- or LMN-only presentations) usually portend a better prognosis, whereas several other clinical subtypes, including Mills hemiplegic variant, the pseudoneuritic presentation (flail leg), and the flail-arm variant, harbor a better prognosis. Those who have younger age at onset and those who are psychologically well adjusted have a better prognosis. Those who have low-amplitude CMAPs in the setting of normal sensory potentials (the generalized low motor-normal sensory pattern) as revealed by nerve conduction studies appear to have a poor prognosis. Low serum chloride levels are associated with a short-term survival without ventilatory support because they reflect accumulation of bicarbonate due to respiratory failure. There may be differences in natural history and prognoses in different parts of the world; a natural history study in China revealed that Chinese ALS is somewhat younger in onset (mean age, 49.8 years) and with less bulbar presentations and a median survival time of 71 months (Chen et al., 2015)

## Laboratory Studies

The diagnosis of clinically definite ALS can sometimes be established on the history and clinical examination alone, but owing to the seriousness of the diagnosis, ancillary investigations are necessary to exclude other possibilities. All such testing is an extension of a thorough history and physical examination and includes blood tests, the EDX, and neuroimaging.

Several blood tests are commonly performed as part of the evaluation of patients with suspected ALS. The list includes serum CK concentration, blood count, chemistry panel (including calcium, phosphate, and magnesium), Venereal Disease Research Laboratories (VDRL) test results, HIV, GM1 autoantibody titers, sedimentation rate, serum protein immunofixation or immunoelectrophoresis, angiotensin converting enzyme (ACE) and glycosylated hemoglobin ($HbA_{1c}$), thyroid function studies including thyroid-stimulating hormone, serum parathormone (if calcium is raised), and vitamin $B_{12}$ levels. The serum CK concentration may be modestly elevated, particularly early in the disease and in active males. Patients older than 50 years and smokers of any age should have a chest radiograph taken. If any chest lesion is identifiable, or if the presentation is subacute with atypical features such as sensory loss, an anti-Hu antibody level should be determined. Certain patients may have clinical features that suggest a disorder of the neuromuscular junction and should have testing for antibodies against the acetylcholine receptor or voltage-gated calcium channel. If there is biochemical evidence of adrenal insufficiency, it is prudent to obtain a VLCFA assay to investigate for possible adrenomyeloneuropathy. Young-onset ALS with atypical clinical features such as early dementia, cramps, and tremor should prompt the physician to obtain a leukocyte Hex-A assay. Young age at onset, with perioral fasciculations and gynecomastia, should prompt genetic assessment for the trinucleotide repeat expansion on the androgen receptor gene that is present in Kennedy disease. If there is a positive family history in otherwise typical ALS, it is important to counsel the patient in preparation for appropriate mutation analysis. Reserve CSF examination for cases with features suggestive of an infectious or infiltrative process such as lymphoma or basal meningitis or suspected CIDP. No specific features on muscle biopsy distinguish ALS from other neurogenic disorders; reserve biopsy for cases that are more suggestive of a myopathy.

The EDX is an invaluable tool in the investigation of ALS and its variants (see Chapter 36). It serves as an adjunct to the clinical examination and is particularly useful in determining the presence or extent of LMN disease. Again, none of the EDX findings are ALS specific, but they can strongly support the diagnosis. Furthermore, repeated investigations at intervals monitor disease progression. Sensory nerve conduction studies are characteristically normal unless the patient happens to have a coincidental mononeuropathy or polyneuropathy. Motor nerve conduction study results may be normal, although the conduction velocity and CMAP amplitude may diminish in keeping with the extent of motor axon loss. There should be no evidence of conduction slowing or block, which would suggest a primarily demyelinating disorder. Severe motor axon loss may give rise to the "generalized low motor-normal sensory" EDX pattern, which may portend a poorer prognosis.

The EMG examination characteristically reveals a combination of acute (positive sharp waves and fibrillation potentials) and chronic (reduced neurogenic firing pattern with evidence of increased amplitude and duration, polyphasic MUPS) changes in a widespread distribution that is not in keeping with any single root or peripheral nerve distribution. Fasciculation potentials are common and typically of complex morphology; their absence should prompt an investigation for another disorder. The Awaji-shima algorithm for the neurophysiological diagnosis of suspected ALS stresses the importance of fasciculation potentials: the presence of fasciculations potentials is evidence of acute denervation in the same way that one regards fibrillation potentials and positive sharp waves. Moment-to-moment amplitude variation, indicating impaired motor unit stability, is also an important sign of denervation (Carvalho and Swash, 2009). Mention should be made of a special EDX finding, the split-hand phenomenon; in some patients with ALS, EDX reveals severe changes in muscles of the lateral hand (thenar eminence) but relative sparing of the medial hand (hypothenar eminence). EDX changes should be observed in a certain topographical distribution and ideally should be carried out in at least three of the four regions of the neuraxis (bulbar, cervical, thoracic, and lumbosacral).

The most important role for neuroimaging studies in ALS is to exclude structural, inflammatory, or infiltrative disorders that may mimic this disease, and therefore all patients should undergo appropriate imaging of brain and spinal cord. On occasion, one may discern abnormal signal in the motor tracts when viewed with proton density–weighted MRI scans of brain; this signal change is due to Wallerian degeneration and if seen occurs in patients with more severe disease. FLAIR and T2-weighted fast-spin echo sequences are less specific in their ability to detect such corticospinal tract signal changes. Nonspecific atrophy of the frontal and parietal cortex may also occur. Ultrasound may have a role in detection of tongue fasciculations that may not be otherwise found by EMG (Misawa et al., 2011; O'Gorman et al., 2017). The search for ALS biomarkers has led to the investigation of other imaging techniques such as magnetization transfer ratio (MTR) imaging, magnetic resonance voxel-based morphometry, magnetic resonance spectroscopy, and DTI (Mazon et al., 2018). Functional imaging studies with blood oxygenation level–dependent (BOLD) functional MRI and magnetoencephalography may reveal abnormal activity in motor and nonmotor areas in ALS, but further studies are needed to determine their role in UMN assessment (Agosta et al., 2010; Turner et al., 2009). Similarly, additional research is necessary to clarify the role of TMS, whether used alone or in combination with DTI in the evaluation of the UMN system (Foerster et al., 2013; Mitsumoto et al., 2007; Vucic and Rutkove, 2018).

While erect forced vital capacity is the most commonly measured index of pulmonary function in ALS, supine FVC provides a more accurate assessment of diaphragmatic weakness. The maximal inspiratory pressure (MIP) and nocturnal oximetry are possibly more effective for the detection of nocturnal hypoventilation. Transdiaphragmatic sniff pressure (sniff Pdi) and the sniff nasal pressure (SNP) are also useful indicators of hypercapnia and nocturnal hypoxemia (Carratù et al., 2011; Miller et al., 2009; Niedermeyer et al., 2019).

## Diagnosis

In May 1990, at El Escorial, Spain, the World Federation of Neurology established diagnostic criteria for ALS, which were later modified at Airlie House, Virginia (1998) (http://www.wfnals.org). These criteria (Table 97.4) include clinical, electrodiagnostic, and pathological components. The clinical criteria divide candidates into those with definite, probable, laboratory-supported probable, possible, and FALS-based on a careful history and examination of four regions of the neuraxis: bulbar, cervical, thoracic, and lumbosacral. The purpose of establishing these criteria was to facilitate entry of appropriate candidates into clinical research trials, but they prove invaluable in the assessment of all patients with ALS.

A patient is referred to as having "definite ALS" if there is clinical evidence of both UMN and LMN signs in three or more regions. "Probable ALS" is UMN and LMN signs in two regions. "Possible ALS" implies that a patient either has UMN and LMN signs in one region only or has UMN signs alone in two regions. In addition, "possible ALS" may be applied to those with LMN signs in two regions as long as these are detected rostrally to the UMN signs. "Probable ALS-laboratory supported" refers to those patients who have clinical evidence of possible ALS but also have EDX evidence of more widespread

**TABLE 97.4 Diagnostic Criteria for the Clinical Diagnosis of Amyotrophic Lateral Sclerosis**

| | |
|---|---|
| Definite ALS | UMN and LMN signs in at least 3 regions (bulbar and 2 spinal regions or 3 spinal regions without bulbar) |
| Probable ALS | UMN and LMN signs in 2 regions, with some UMN signs rostral to LMN signs |
| Probable ALS, lab-supported | UMN and LMN signs in 1 region, with UMN signs alone in another region and EMG evidence of LMN involvement in at least 2 limbs |
| Possible ALS | UMN and LMN signs in 1 region; or UMN signs alone in 2 or more regions; or LMN signs are rostral to UMN signs |
| Familial ALS, lab-supported | Otherwise unexplained UMN or LMN signs in at least 1 region, with gene mutation in the proband or a positive family history of family member with a disease-causing gene mutation |

*ALS*, Amyotrophic lateral sclerosis; *EMG*, electromyographic; *LMN*, lower motor neuron; *UMN*, upper motor neuron.
*Adapted from revised World Federation of Neurology Criteria for the Diagnosis of ALS. Available at http://www.wfnals.org.*

LMN involvement. The proposal is that one should apply the Awaji neurophysiological algorithm to the revised El Escorial criteria to clarify the El Escorial electrodiagnostic criteria and improve diagnostic sensitivity. The Awaji algorithm has increased the importance of fasciculation potentials as being representative of acute denervation as long as there is evidence of chronic denervation in the same muscles. Using both sets of criteria together, Carvalho and Swash demonstrated an increased sensitivity in the diagnosis of bulbar-onset ALS from 38% with revised El Escorial alone to 87% when both sets of criteria were used. Another group achieved a specificity of over 95% when using both sets of criteria together (Carvalho and Swash, 2009; Douglass et al., 2010, Gawel et al., 2014). More recently, a combination of clinical, electrophysiological, and TMS measures can generate an entity known as the ALS diagnostic index (ALSDI), which may help distinguish suspected ALS from mimics (Geevasinga et al., 2019). Follow-up examinations may be helpful in assessing patients with ALS, as disease progression may move a patient up a category, which not only may clarify the diagnosis but also may allow entry of that patient into research trials.

### Differential Diagnosis

The differential diagnosis of ALS is rather extensive; motor symptoms and signs may be present in many other neurological and systemic disorders. Because there are no specific diagnostic markers for ALS, differentiating all other motor neuron diseases that may produce signs and symptoms of UMN, LMN, or both UMN and LMN involvement is essential for establishing the correct diagnosis. One may approach this task in an anatomical fashion and consider how ALS may appear similar to other disorders of the brain, brainstem, spinal cord, anterior horn cell, nerve root, peripheral nerve, neuromuscular junction, and muscle. Alternatively, one may approach this task in terms of the presentation: Is it UMN only, LMN only, combined UMN-LMN, bulbar only, and so on? Are there any atypical features such as prominent bladder or sensory involvement that suggest another diagnosis? For example, when UMN involvement is prominent, PLS, spastic paraparesis, or HAM should be considered, whereas pure LMN involvement suggests that one should also consider PMA, IBM, MMNCB, adult-onset SMA, Lambert-Eaton myasthenic syndrome, or Kennedy disease.

Severe cervical spondylosis may impinge upon both the cervical cord and the nerve roots and thus present with both UMN and LMN signs. Because pain, spastic bladder, and posterior column signs are not always present, EMG and neuroimaging may be required to distinguish it from ALS. Neuroimaging is also invaluable in assessing other disorders of the brainstem and spinal cord that may superficially mimic certain features of ALS such as intrinsic or extrinsic tumors, foramen magnum meningiomas, syringobulbia, and syringomyelia. MS usually presents with UMN signs, but on rare occasions, LMN signs develop when demyelinating plaques affect the ventral root exit zones. Neuroimaging and lumbar puncture studies should distinguish the two conditions. CIDP may manifest as a predominantly LMN disorder, but some patients also have demyelinating lesions in the CNS that cause additional UMN signs.

It may be difficult to differentiate PBP from bulbar myasthenia gravis, as even repetitive stimulation studies and testing for serum antibodies against acetylcholine receptor may be negative in the latter. Follow-up examinations, however, usually reveal the insidiously progressive nature of the motor neuron disorder. Bulbar symptoms in ALS may be mistaken for brainstem stroke, but the progressive nature of bulbar symptoms and negative brainstem MRI will usually clarify the picture. On rare occasions, the increased tone, dysarthria, and sialorrhea of Parkinson disease may be confused with ALS. However, the former is characteristically responsive to L-dopa, and tremor is often prominent. Multiple-system atrophy may present with a combination of UMN and LMN signs together with dysarthria and dysphagia, but cerebellar ataxia, eye-movement abnormalities, sphincter disturbance, and dysautonomia are usually prominent features. SCA types 2 and 3 (Machado-Joseph disease) are also part of the differential diagnosis. Other diseases that mimic ALS include adult Hex-A deficiency, adrenomyeloneuropathy, and certain motor paraneoplastic syndromes. Hyperthyroidism may present with hyperreflexia, weight loss, and fasciculations but also tremor, heat intolerance, and tachycardia. Hyperparathyroidism may present with a LMN or even myopathic disorder that mimics PMA. Both the benign fasciculation syndrome and cramp-fasciculation syndrome may lead to referrals for the evaluation of ALS, but these patients have no other symptoms or signs that suggest a widespread progressive disorder of motor neurons.

### Treatment

Treatment of ALS is outlined in Box 97.7 and Table 97.5.

***Presentation of the diagnosis of amyotrophic lateral sclerosis.*** The first step in the management of ALS is to present the diagnosis in a compassionate yet informative manner. Allow adequate time to present the diagnosis. Whenever possible, the patient should not be

**BOX 97.7 Comprehensive Care and Management for Patients With Amyotrophic Lateral Sclerosis**

- Presentation of the diagnosis of ALS
- Specific pharmacotherapy
- Symptomatic treatment
- Team approach at ALS clinic
- Ethical and legal issues
- Physical rehabilitation
- Speech and communication management
- Nutritional care
- Respiratory care
- Home care and hospice care

*ALS*, Amyotrophic lateral sclerosis.

**TABLE 97.5 Symptomatic Treatment in Amyotrophic Lateral Sclerosis**

| Symptoms | Pharmacotherapy | Other therapy |
|---|---|---|
| Fatigue | Pyridostigmine bromide<br>Antidepressants<br>Methylphenidate<br>Amantadine<br>Modafinil | Energy conservation<br>Work modification<br>Sleep study: BiPAP if abnormal |
| Spasticity | Baclofen<br>Tizanidine<br>Dantrolene sodium<br>Diazepam | Physical therapy<br>Range-of-motion exercises<br>Botulinum toxin injections |
| Jaw clenching | Benzodiazepines | Botulinum toxin injections into masseters |
| Cramps | Quinine sulfate<br>Baclofen<br>Vitamin E<br>Clonazepam | Massage<br>Physical therapy |
| Fasciculations | Carbamazepine | Assurance |
| Sialorrhea | Hyoscyamine sulphate<br>Diphenhydramine<br>Scopolamine patch<br>Glycopyrrolate<br>Atropine<br>TCAs | Suction machine<br>Botulinum toxin injection into salivary glands<br>Parotid gland radiation therapy<br>Steam inhalation<br>Nebulization<br>Dark grape juice |
| Pseudobulbar laughing or crying | TCAs<br>SSRIs, L-dopa/carbidopa<br>Lithium<br>Mirtazapine<br>Venlafaxine<br>Quinidine/dextromethorphan | |
| Thick phlegm | Guaifenesin<br>Nebulized *N*-acetylcysteine<br>Nebulized saline<br>Propranolol | Insufflation-exsufflation<br>High-flow chest wall oscillation therapy<br>Cool mist humidifier<br>Rehydration<br>Pineapple or papaya juice<br>Reduced intake of dairy products, caffeine, alcohol |
| Aspiration | Cisapride | Modified food consistency<br>Tracheostomy<br>Modified laryngectomy and tracheal diversion |
| Joint pains | Antiinflammatory drugs<br>Analgesics | Range-of-motion exercises<br>Heat |
| Depression | TCAs<br>SSRIs, venlafaxine, mirtazapine, bupropion | Counseling<br>Support group meetings, psychiatry |
| Insomnia | Zolpidem tartrate<br>Lorazepam<br>Opioids<br>TCAs | Pressure air pad/gel mattress<br>Noninvasive positive pressure ventilation where appropriate |
| Laryngospasm | Sublingual lorazepam | |
| Respiratory failure | Bronchodilators<br>Morphine sulfate | Hospital bed<br>Nocturnal noninvasive ventilator IPPB |
| Constipation | Increase oral liquid<br>Metamucil<br>Dulcolax suppositories<br>Lactulose and other laxative | Exercise<br>"Power pudding": prune juice, prunes, applesauce, bran |

*BiPAP,* Bilevel positive airway pressure; *IPPB,* intermittent positive-pressure breathing; *SSRIs,* selective serotonin reuptake inhibitors; *TCAs,* tricyclic antidepressants.

alone. A second appointment, a short time later, is often required because many patients and their families find it difficult to absorb the information at first. At the appropriate time, it is important to bring up issues such as advance directives and issues regarding terminal care (Mitsumoto and Rabkin, 2007; Mitsumoto and Saito, 2018) (see also Chapter 114). Providing information on progress in research, available pharmacotherapies, and the possibility of active participation in clinical trials may increase hope for patients. It is also important to convey the concept of the multidisciplinary care team. Owing to the serious nature of the diagnosis, it is important to facilitate a second opinion if so requested. ALS is almost invariably a relentlessly progressive and terminal disorder, and physicians must raise the issues of the living will and durable power of attorney for health care relatively early after diagnosis to allow the patient and family to prepare ahead. Such decisions are not final and are reversible at any time. Furthermore, some patients either do not wish to or cannot make such decisions (Miller et al., 2013).

***Specific pharmacotherapy.*** In 1996, the US Food and Drug Administration (FDA) approved riluzole (Rilutek) as the first specific drug for the treatment of ALS. It principally functions as an antiglutamate agent, but its mechanism of action is uncertain. The two studies that led to riluzole approval showed that survival was significantly longer in patients with ALS who took 50 mg of riluzole twice a day compared with those who took placebo, although this survival benefit was only modest and was disproportionately beneficial in bulbar-onset disease. A Cochrane meta-analysis of the controlled riluzole trials has shown that 100 mg daily results in a 9% increase in the probability of survival for 1 year and prolongs median survival by 2–3 months when taken for 18 months (Miller et al., 2012). Side effects are relatively uncommon and include fatigue, gastrointestinal upset, dizziness, and an increase in liver function tests. To minimize side effects, we recommend 50 mg per day in the evening, and after a week or two, the patient can increase to the regular dose of 50 mg twice a day. Not all patients with ALS receive riluzole therapy; the cost of the drug is one of the main factors in this regard, although generic versions have mitigated this cost somewhat.

Intravenous edaravone, a free radical scavenger, has been recently approved in Japan and then the results were presented to the FDA, which approved the medication without any additional trials. This agent was originally developed for acute stroke treatment in Japan and subsequently found to be useful in treatment of ALS (Abe et al., 2014). A further study was undertaken in responders only (ALS 19 Study Group, 2017). Over a 6-month trial period, it has been shown to improve the ALS Functional Rating Scale-revised (ALSFRS-R) to a modest degree. However, most patients were also taking concomitant riluzole and strict inclusion criteria suggest that it may only prove effective in a small cohort of patients.

Assessment of several agents with antiglutamate activity revealed no clinical benefit, although dextromethorphan-quinidine has benefit in the treatment of pseudobulbar emotional lability.

Many other agents have been trialed in ALS, including neurotrophic factors, antiinflammatory agents, creatine, coenzyme $Q_{10}$, lithium and minocycline and other antibiotics, but none have been found to be effective (Mitsumoto et al., 2014). The rating scale used in most ALS trials is the ALSFRS-R. It has been argued that this measure may fail to show positive outcomes in trials, in part explaining the plethora of negative ALS trials. Other functional scales such as the King's College and MiToS staging systems have been proposed to more accurately monitor progression of disease in clinical trials (Corcia et al., 2018). Perhaps one of the reasons for so many disappointing results over the years is that much promising preclinical work was based upon the mutant SOD1 mouse model, which is not representative of the pathogenesis of most ALS. It remains to be seen whether novel agents with relevance to TDP43 or FUS mislocalization might show more promise, and the search continues for new agents and techniques for the specific treatment of ALS. Research is ongoing into the potential role for stem cell therapy and gene therapy in patients with ALS (Chia et al., 2018; Gordon et al., 2013; Madigan et al., 2017; Staff et al., 2016). It is critical to improve the selection of candidate therapies, clinical trial methodology, and clinical trial practice. To this end, the Airlie House ALS clinical trial guidelines have been updated and renewed using the modified Delphi consensus method.

***Aggressive symptomatic treatment.*** Although specific pharmacotherapy is still markedly limited for the treatment of ALS, symptomatic treatment can substantially improve a patient's symptoms and discomfort. Table 97.5 summarizes specific pharmacological and nonpharmacological symptomatic treatments (Miller et al., 2009, 2012).

***Multidisciplinary team approach at amyotrophic lateral sclerosis clinic.*** The care of patients with ALS has become increasingly complex. As a consequence, many patients receive care by a multidisciplinary team in a specialized ALS center rather than by a single treating physician. The team often consists of neurologists, a nurse coordinator, physical therapists, occupational therapists, dietitians, speech pathologists, and social workers. Pulmonary specialists and other health professionals should also be available. Using this holistic approach, the aim is to maintain physical independence for as long as possible and to provide psychosocial support to patients and families. As such, specialized multidisciplinary clinic referrals should be offered to patients to optimize and improve quality of life and possibly prolong survival (Miller et al., 2009, 2012).

***Physical rehabilitation.*** The main goal of rehabilitation for patients with ALS is to improve their ability to carry out activities of daily living for as long as possible without causing undue physical or emotional strain. Physical therapy also prevents complications secondary to disuse of muscles and immobilization, such as a frozen shoulder. Employ various types of exercise that maintain or enhance strength, endurance, and range of motion. There have been concerns that exercising ALS-affected muscles to the point of fatigue may actually be harmful, but this has not been borne out in the literature. The occupational therapist is another valuable member of the ALS care team. A range of assistive and adaptive devices are available to improve mobility and comfort and help carry out activities of daily living. For example, walkers, wheelchairs, splints, and collars are useful to manage wrist drop, foot drop, head drop, and gait instability. Successful rehabilitation also includes an evaluation of the home environment; customized home equipment can easily help preserve a patient's independence and safety.

***Speech and communication management.*** Speech and communication dysfunction is one of the most serious factors reducing quality of life in the patient with ALS. Ideally, speech pathologists should assess speech and communication soon after establishing the diagnosis so the patient can maintain independent communication for as long as possible. Follow-up is thus required at regular intervals. Assessment and care should incorporate intelligibility strategies, energy-conserving techniques, nonverbal techniques (gestures and other body language), and assistive/augmentative communication devices. Numerous communication devices are available that vary in sophistication and complexity, ranging from simple and relatively inexpensive mechanical devices such as alphabet or picture boards to specialized computer devices such as a voice synthesizer.

***Nutritional care.*** Dysphagia and aspiration are distressing and dangerous complications of ALS and are particularly prominent in the bulbar-onset variety. As oral intake progressively declines, there is acceleration in weight loss and malnutrition, which not only aggravates muscle weakness but also shortens survival. Therefore, in every patient with ALS, evaluate the nutritional status at each visit. Although physicians can take such a history, evaluation by an experienced dietitian is often most helpful. Initially, patients should change the form and texture of their food and use a high-calorie food supplement, but eventually such measures become insufficient to maintain the patient's weight, and proactive enteral tube feeding becomes imperative.

Percutaneous endoscopic gastroscopy (PEG) is a standard minor surgical procedure that may improve quality of life but with unproven effect on survival (Katzberg and Benatar, 2011). PEG is also probably effective in helping patients maintain weight/body mass index (Miller et al., 2009, ProGas Study Group, 2015).

Although it is a relatively simple surgery for otherwise healthy patients who have dysphagia, patients with ALS pose particular difficulties and often have impending respiratory failure that may complicate the procedure. Guidelines advocate placement of a PEG tube in consenting patients with dysphagia whose seated predicted forced vital capacity is more than 50%, but PEG may be performed for patients with a forced vital capacity of less than 50% predicted if NIPPV is also used during the procedure (Gregory et al., 2002).

Radiologically inserted gastrostomy and percutaneous radiological gastrostomy are alternative approaches that may be preferable in such cases but are not yet in widespread use. It is important to emphasize that those who receive a PEG tube can continue to eat by mouth, and that the purpose of enteral feeding is to provide calories and fluid. Indeed, aspiration is a continued risk to the patient even after PEG tube insertion, and if recurrent aspiration of PEG contents becomes a persistent problem, one can either recommend percutaneous enteral jejunostomy (PEJ), which further reduces (but still does not eliminate) the risk, or a tracheostomy.

***Respiratory care.*** Respiratory failure is the most common cause of death in ALS. Indeed, dyspnea-onset ALS presents with obvious ventilatory difficulties, and it is for this reason that it harbors a particularly poor prognosis. It is important to make patients and family members aware that almost all forms of ALS will eventually end by ventilatory failure, although symptoms may go largely unnoticed until relatively late in the disease course. The patient must be made aware that although ventilation via a tracheostomy may indefinitely prolong life, there is no effect on the disease itself. In fact, by prolonging the natural history of the disorder, there is a strong possibility that atypical symptoms may arise, such as visual changes or even sensory loss. Nonetheless, some patients choose to have a tracheostomy and invasive ventilation; this option should be a consideration to improve the quality of life of such individuals (Niedermeyer et al., 2019). Most patients and their physicians opt for the noninvasive ventilation (NIV) approach. Evidence exists that patients should be offered NIV at the onset of dyspnea when the forced vital capacity falls to less than 50% predicted or when a rapid, progressive weakness and wasting of perioral muscles may prevent adequate use of the NIV mask. Nasal pillows can be helpful in this circumstance and are often better tolerated than the mask at all stages. Several factors should be borne in mind when offering this form of treatment. Evidence exists that NIV improves quality of life and may prolong survival in ALS (Bourke et al., 2006; Miller et al., 2009), but NIV does not prolong life indefinitely, and these patients still face the difficult decision of whether to use an invasive ventilator. Diaphragmatic pacing has been approved for use in patients with ALS, but its clinical effectiveness and long-term safety require further study (Amirjani et al., 2012). When making the decision to withdraw ventilatory support or when noninvasive means of ventilatory assistance are insufficient, it is imperative that all attempts focus on effective and compassionate palliative end-of-life care. Hospice care and judicious amounts of opioids, oxygen, and anxiolytics should be prescribed to allow patients to live their final days with dignity and in as much comfort as possible.

***Home care and hospice care.*** When the patient's condition deteriorates, home hospice care or admission to a residential hospice care facility is required (Mitsumoto et al., 2005). Close collaboration between patients, their caregivers, home-care nurses, and ideally the ALS clinic team will ensure effective and satisfying home care. When a patient has no caregiver, choose a site other than the home for extended care. Hospice care provides highly effective palliative services to patients and their families. Just as important, hospice philosophy strongly affirms life, so that patients who are in the terminal stages of their disease can maintain their independence and dignity to the greatest degree possible (Connolly et al., 2015; Mitsumoto, 2009).

## Familial Amyotrophic Lateral Sclerosis

Between 5% and 10% of all ALS is an inherited trait, in which case it is termed *familial ALS* (FALS). It is quite possible that the true frequency of FALS is higher because anything less than a detailed family history may fail to identify an affected family member, and reduced penetrance may account for some apparently sporadic disease. There are autosomal dominant, autosomal recessive, and X-linked forms, some being juvenile onset and others being adult onset (see Box 97.6). Over 30 genes have been implicated as causative, increasing the risk of developing ALS, or accelerating the disease, but many of these account for only rare cases (Oskarsson et al., 2018). The clinical presentation varies considerably, not just in terms of age and site of onset but also in terms of disease duration. FALS is currently classified from ALS1 to ALS25.

Mutations in C9orf72 (open reading frame 72 on chromosome 9) are the most common cause of familial ALS (circa 40%) and a significant percentage of apparently sporadic ALS (circa 7%) (Balendra and Isaacs, 2018). The mutation is one of a hexanucleotide expansion repeat. Presentation can be that of ALS, particularly with bulbar onset. However, it can also present as an ALS-FTD overlap or indeed a pure behavioral variant FTD (which can include psychosis). Some versions can include ataxia and parkinsonism and the repeat expansion has recently been found to cause Huntington disease phenocopies (Hensman Moss et al., 2014) (Video 97.5). Age of onset is apparently slightly younger and there is more rapid progression with shorter survival. Penetrance of the gene increases with age and in one study was shown to reach 100% above the age of 80 years (Majounie et al., 2012). The function of C9orf72 still remains to be clearly elucidated but its structure suggests that it might function as a GDP-GTP exchange factor for RAB GTPases, in turn implying a role in cell signaling and autophagy. The hexanucleotide repeats lead to the formation of pathogenic DNA-RNA "quadruplexes" which appear to generate abnormal transcripts that in turn lead to nucleolar stress (Haeusler et al., 2014). Whether the mutation leads to a loss of function, toxic gain of function, or indeed both, remains to be seen (Robberecht and Philips, 2013). Cerebral imaging may reveal symmetrical frontal and temporal atrophy (Yokoyama and Rosen, 2012).

Up until recently, *SOD1* (which encodes superoxide dismutase 1), located on chromosome 21q21, was considered the most important gene in ALS. ALS1 is a form of late-onset (usually > age 30) motor neuron disorder associated with mutations in *SOD1* that accounts for 15%–20% of all cases of FALS (and thus 1%–2% of all ALS) (Rosen et al., 1993). Inheritance in most is in an autosomal dominant pattern, but a recessive variant occurs (Andersen et al., 1996). Mutations in *SOD1* confer toxic gain of function, leading to disease through multiple possible mechanisms, including oxidative stress, protein aggregation, apoptosis, and impairment of axonal transport. There is a large degree of phenotypical variability in the expression of SOD1-associated FALS, not only between different families but also between individual members of the same family. Furthermore, penetrance is rather variable and age dependent. Generally, establishing the diagnosis of FALS is only by the fact that other family members in successive generations are, or were, affected by ALS. The clinical features of individual FALS patients overlap considerably with those of patients with SALS.

ALS2 is a rare recessively inherited disorder mapped to a gene on chromosome 2q33 that encodes a novel protein called alsin. Analysis of the original families revealed that all were due to truncated protein product from frameshift or nonsense mutations, but missense mutations occur. This juvenile ALS, originally described in consanguineous families from Tunisia, was also discovered in families from Saudi Arabia and Kuwait. The phenotype of this disorder varies according to the family of origin; in the Tunisian family, it presents as a slowly progressive ALS-like disorder with mean age of onset at age 12 years; in the

Kuwaiti family, the phenotype is similar to early-onset PLS. Sequence homology analysis of this protein supports that it is a guanine-nucleotide exchange factor for Rab 5 and is thus important in intracellular cell signaling, endosomal dynamics, mitochondrial trafficking, and cytoskeleton organization. In contrast to the toxic gain-of-function theory of pathogenesis in ALS1, it appears that loss of function of the gene product is responsible for the selective injury to, and dysfunction of, the corticospinal tract in ALS2. Alternate splicing of the *alsin* gene results in both long and short transcripts. Frameshift and nonsense mutations cause an ALS phenotype when there is homozygous loss of both the short and long forms, whereas the PLS presentation occurs with homozygous loss of the long form alone. Missense mutations may cause an unstable protein product or lead to a protein product that is directly toxic to the cell via aberrant regulation of the apoptotic pathway. Certain mutations in the *alsin* gene also give rise to an infantile ascending hereditary spastic paraparesis, which demonstrates the link between ALS and related motor neuron diseases (Eymard-Pierre et al., 2006; Panzeri et al., 2006). ALS3 describes a large European family with adult-onset autosomal dominant ALS linked to chromosome 18q21 (Hand et al., 2002). The gene for this disorder has not yet been identified. ALS4 is a juvenile-onset, slowly progressive, dominantly inherited distal amyotrophy with UMN signs but sparing bulbar features. It is caused by mutations in the senataxin gene *(SETX)* on chromosome 9q34, which has a DNA/RNA helicase domain suggesting a role in DNA repair and RNA processing. *SETX* has homology to *IGHMBP2,* the gene responsible for SMARD1, a rare form of SMA. Mutations in *SETX* also cause a recessively inherited disorder called *oculomotor apraxia and cerebellar ataxia*. However, it has recently been shown that caution should be exercised as not all missense mutations are pathogenic and functional assays are required (Arning et al., 2013). A form of slowly progressive, usually mild, recessive juvenile ALS (ALS 5) described in North African and European families is due to mutations in the spatacsin *(SPG11)* gene (and thus is also a cause of hereditary spastic paraparesis; see Table 97.2). ALS6 is an autosomal dominant ALS that can also be associated with frontotemporal dementia and hallucinations. Mutations on the *FUS/TLS* (fused in sarcoma/translocated in liposarcoma) gene on chromosome 16q12 have the pathological characteristic of FUS-immunoreactive skein-like cytoplasmic inclusion bodies. FUS is normally a nuclear protein, so this is yet another example of protein mislocalization in neurodegenerative disease. *FUS* mutations have a worldwide distribution and account for about 5% of FALS; they are also detectable in about 1% of SALS (Lai et al., 2010). Furthermore, it has recently been shown that *FUS*-immunoreactive cytoplasmic inclusions are common in both SALS and non-SOD1 FALS and are also immunoreactive to TDP43 and ubiquitin (Deng et al., 2010). ALS7 is a rare, late-onset, autosomal dominant disorder linked to chromosome 20p13. The cause for ALS8 is a mutation in a vesicle trafficking protein gene called *VAPB* (vesicle-associated membrane protein/synaptobrevin-associated membrane protein B) on chromosome 20q13.3. The clinical presentation displays quite marked heterogeneity: some patients develop a slowly progressive ALS-like picture with prominent tremor and onset between the ages of 31 and 45 years, whereas others present with a late-onset SMA or a severe, rapidly progressive ALS (Nishimura et al., 2004). ALS9 results from mutations on the angiogenin gene on chromosome 14q. This is an autosomal dominant disorder of adults (from the fourth to the eighth decade). Angiogenin may help protect motor neurons from excitotoxic- and hypoxia-induced injury, but it may also play an important role in RNA transcription as well as interact with cellular cytoskeletal proteins. ALS10, which accounts for 2%–5% of FALS, is caused by mutations in the *TDP43* gene on chromosome 1 and presents clinically as ALS with either limb or bulbar onset. Despite the association of TDP inclusions with some forms of FTD, cognitive deficits do not occur in *TDP43* mutation–associated ALS. TDP43 immunoreactive ubiquitinated inclusions are present in degenerating neurons and glial cells just as they in sporadic ALS (Kuhnlein et al., 2008; Van Deerlin et al., 2008). The *TDP43* gene product is a dual DNA/RNA binding protein mainly expressed in the nucleus and may play an important part in the regulation of RNA trafficking and translation. TDP43 can modulate human low-molecular-weight neurofilament mRNA stability, which in turn underlies neurofilament aggregates, sometimes seen in ALS (Strong et al., 2006). TDP43 inclusion bodies are in fact seen in several disorders apart from ALS, including FTD, frontotemporal lobar degeneration with motor neuron degeneration, corticobasal degeneration, Guamanian ALS–PD complex, and hippocampal sclerosis. While this might suggest that TDP43 inclusion bodies are a nonspecific marker of neuronal injury or indeed representative of a physiological cell response to injury, the frequency of *TDP43* mutations (30 to date) in both SALS and FALS suggests a pathogenic role. ALS11 is due to mutations of the *FIG4* gene on chromosome 6q21, which encodes a phosphoinositide 5-phosphatase, a regulator of a signaling lipid on the surface of endosomes. Mutations in this gene are known to cause a recessively inherited severe axonal sensorimotor form of Charcot–Marie–Tooth known as CMT4J, which is usually early onset (although one family presented with an adult disorder resembling ALS). *FIG4* mutations can cause an ALS or PLS presentation, and additional personality changes were noted in two cases. Of the nine cases with *FIG4* mutations, only three were FALS, the rest apparently being sporadic (Chow et al., 2009). Mutations in the *OPTN* gene for optineurin, a negative regulator of tumor necrosis factor alpha (TNF-α)–induced activation of nuclear factor kappa B (NF-κB) cause ALS12. OPTN may also play a role membrane trafficking, exocytosis, and maintenance of the Golgi apparatus. Mutations in this gene are known to cause primary open angle glaucoma. For patients presenting with ALS, the inheritance patterns were both autosomal recessive and autosomal dominant, with onset between the ages of 30 and 60 years and long-disease duration. One case which came to autopsy showed optineurin-positive cytoplasmic inclusion bodies in anterior horn cells; the investigators also showed that TDP43- and SOD1-positive inclusions in SALS and SOD1 FALS were co-labeled with optineurin, suggesting a broader role for this protein in the pathogenesis of ALS (Maruyama et al., 2010). It is proposed that certain individuals with *ATX2* mutations in the intermediate range may suffer an increased risk of ALS *(ALS 13)* through an interaction between the polyglutamine repeat and TDP43 resulting in mislocalization of the latter to the cytoplasm (Elden et al., 2010). Another adult onset autosomal dominant ALS which can be associated with FTD is ALS14, caused by mutations in the *VCP* gene. Pathologically, ubiquitin positive inclusions can be seen in neurons. Interestingly, *VCP* mutations can also cause an inclusion body myopathy with Paget disease and FTLD. ALS15, due to *UBQLN2* mutations, can in fact be sporadic as well as inherited and again can be a cause of both ALS and FTD. Mutations in this gene lead to disturbances in the proteasomal pathway. ALS16 is a juvenile-onset ALS which is only rarely associated with FTD. It is due to mutations in *SIGMAR1,* which normally encodes an endoplasmic reticulum chaperone protein, thus suggesting a role for altered ER (ER) and Golgi function in disease pathogenesis. Again, *SIGMAR1* mutations can cause ubiquitinated inclusions in the proximal axon. Mutations in *CHMP2B* cause ALS17, an adult-onset, progressive disorder with predominantly lower motor neuron involvement, and can also cause FTD. Mutations of the gene appear to confer injury to the motor neurons through abnormalities in protein breakdown and clearance within cells. Mutations in *PFN1* (ALS18), which encodes profilin, can cause an FTD overlap or ALS alone. Profilin is important in axonal transport. ALS19 is due to mutations in *ERBB4,* which normally encodes a receptor tyrosine kinase, and mutations of which disrupt neuregulin pathway. This presents with typical autosomal dominant ALS of late onset. ALS20 is caused by *HNRNPA1* gene mutations on chromosome 12, which may lead to inclusion body formation due to dysregulated protein polymerization. Although not formally classified as a familial ALS (it has been described as a spinal and bulbar muscular atrophy), it is apparent that mutations in the p150Glued subunit of the dynactin gene may cause ALS-like presentations. Furthermore, a family history is not always evident (Munch et al., 2004). Dynactin 1 is a vital component of the dynein-dynactin motor complex and is important in retrograde axonal transport. Puls et al. have described a particular LMN disorder caused by a mutation in the p150Glued subunit of dynactin 1. The clinical phenotype is distinctive, with early bilateral vocal cord paralysis followed by prominent involvement of intrinsic hand muscles (especially those of the thenar eminence), the legs, and the face (Puls et al., 2005).

## Amyotrophic Lateral Sclerosis–Parkinsonism-Dementia Complex (Western Pacific Amyotrophic Lateral Sclerosis)

In 1954, Mulder and colleagues described an unusually high incidence of ALS in the adult native Chamorro population on the Western Pacific island of Guam. Soon afterwards, a related disorder of high incidence characterized by dementia and parkinsonism was also found in this population, with some patients displaying overlap features between ALS, parkinsonism, and dementia. A similar disorder was subsequently described in western New Guinea and the Kii peninsula of Japan, with an ALS incidence between 50 and 150 times higher than elsewhere (Kaji et al., 2012). Clinically, about 5% of patients develop a predominantly ALS type of disorder, whereas 38% manifest principally with a combination of parkinsonism and dementia. The pathology of this unusual disorder bears similarities to that of Alzheimer disease, with prominent loss of CNS neurons and the presence of abundant tau-immunoreactive neurofibrillary tangles. However, the characteristic pathology of Guamanian ALS and PDC is by TDP43-positive inclusions in neurons and glial cells. α-Synuclein pathology also is detectable in the amygdala of affected brain tissue (Mimuro et al., 2018). Multiple members of a single family may be affected, and it has recently been shown that first-degree relatives of patients with ALS-PDC have a significantly higher risk of developing the disease than controls. Despite these observations and a genetic association study implicating the tau gene as a susceptibility gene for ALS-PDC, accumulated epidemiological evidence strongly suggests that an environmental factor rather than a genetic factor is more important in disease pathogenesis. Various environmental toxins have been implicated in the pathogenesis of ALS-PDC, chief among them being neurotoxins derived from the native cycad seed. This seed contains β-methylamino-L-alanine (BMAA), an amino acid that is toxic to cortical and spinal motor neurons and thought to be the product of cyanobacterial activity in the roots of the cycad palm. Cycad seed also contains a carcinogenic substance called *cycasin* that may act either alone or in concert with BMAA to damage motor neurons. Toxic sterol glucosides have also been isolated from washed cycad flour, and they can cause the release of glutamate (Khabazian et al., 2002). However, the role of cycad seeds in neurotoxicity is still subject to debate (Snyder et al., 2011). The cyanobacteria/BMAA hypothesis has wider implications for research in SALS worldwide. It has been recently shown that protein-bound BMAA is present in the brains of North American patients dying with ALS and Alzheimer disease and it has been hypothesized that such patients may be genetically susceptible to BMAA-induced neurodegeneration (Bradley and Mash, 2009). The cycad seed has many uses: in West Papua and Guam as a topical medicine for skin lesions and in Japan as an oral medicine (Spencer et al., 2016). Cox and Sacks (2002) proposed a process of biomagnification of cycad toxins in Guam through the Chamorro practice of eating flying foxes, which themselves feed on cycad seeds. The incidence of the Guamanian ALS variant has rapidly declined over the past several decades, a process thought to reflect the Westernization of the region. The decline in the incidence of ALS-PDC in Guam may reflect the dwindling flying fox population on Guam through a massive increase in commercial hunting using firearms introduced to the island in the decades following World War II. However, other social and dietary shifts have occurred in Guam that might be responsible for the decrease.

## Spinocerebellar Ataxia Type 3 (Machado-Joseph Disease)

Machado-Joseph disease is an autosomal dominant syndrome with onset varying from the third to seventh decade of life. Although cerebellar ataxia is the predominant clinical feature, patients often present with slowly progressive generalized spasticity, cramps, muscle wasting, and fasciculations of the face and tongue. Other characteristic findings include extrapyramidal signs such as dystonia and rigidity, protuberant eyes, and progressive external ophthalmoparesis. Affected patients have a twofold to threefold expansion of a CAG trinucleotide repeat on the ataxin-3 gene on chromosome 14q32.1. The expanded triplet repeat results in a mutant gene product containing an expanded polyglutamine tract. This appears to aggregate into intranuclear neuronal inclusion bodies and may interfere with the function of the cellular proteasome in degradation of proteins (Schmidt et al., 2002). The Machado-Joseph disease phenotype may also occur in SCA-2, with slowly progressive ataxia, eyelid retraction, and facial fasciculations. Patients often have slow saccades or ophthalmoparesis and may have reduced or absent deep tendon reflexes. The cause of SCA-2 is an expanded polyglutamine-encoding CAG triple repeat sequence on chromosome 12q.

## Adult Hexosaminidase-A Deficiency

Adult Hex-A deficiency is an autosomal recessively inherited late-onset GM2 gangliosidosis (the other subtypes being infantile and juvenile). All three subtypes are caused by an abnormal accumulation of GM2 ganglioside in neurons due to a deficiency in the activity of the lysosomal enzyme. Hex-A is encoded by a gene on chromosome 15q23–q24 and normally degrades GM2 ganglioside. Only about 10% of Hex-A activity is required for normal health, but in the severe infantile form of this disorder, also known as *Tay-Sachs disease*, mutations in the α subunit of Hex-A result in complete deficiency of enzyme activity. Juveniles and adults with Hex-A deficiency, however, are compound heterozygotes with varying degrees of residual enzymatic activity and thus have a later-onset disorder with considerable variability in the phenotype. It is more common in males and those of Ashkenazi Jewish ancestry, but females and non-Jewish persons can also develop this disorder.

The adult form has a mean of onset of about 18 years and usually presents as slowly progressive weakness of predominantly proximal muscles of the upper and lower extremities (Barritt et al., 2017; Neudorfer et al., 2005). In some patients, severe cramps may present in association with muscle weakness, mimicking SMA. In others, however, a combination of dysarthria, spasticity, and LMN signs may resemble ALS. Additional sensory, cerebellar, cognitive, psychiatric, and extrapyramidal features may later develop. The EDX may reveal prominent complex repetitive discharges and abnormal SNAPs. Generally, this constellation of symptoms and signs is not easily mistaken for ALS, but in the relatively early stages, patients with Hex-A deficiency may not manifest many features other than motor system dysfunction. Genetic counseling is important before assaying a patient's serum or leukocytes for deficiency of Hex-A activity.

## Allgrove Syndrome (Four-A Syndrome)

Four-A syndrome (Allgrove syndrome) is a very rare autosomal recessive disorder that derives its name from the combination of achalasia, alacrima, adrenocorticotropic insufficiency, and amyotrophy. The *AAAS* gene is located on chromosome 12q13 and encodes a ubiquitous protein called aladin which heavily expresses in the neuroendocrine system and may be important in regulation of the cell cycle, cell signaling, intracellular transport, and the cell cytoskeleton. The syndrome can manifest from the first decade of life with dysphagia and adrenocortical insufficiency, but a wide a range of neurological problems can arise later in life, including cognitive deterioration, optic atrophy, seizures, autonomic disturbance (dry mouth, postural hypotension, and syncope), and bulbospinal amyotrophy (amyotrophy of limbs and tongue, with tongue fasciculations and pyramidal signs) (Ikeda et al., 2013; Kimber et al., 2003).

## Adult Polyglucosan Body Disease

Polyglucosan body disease is a very rare, late-onset, slowly progressive disorder characterized by a combination of UMN and LMN signs, cognitive decline, distal sensory loss, and disturbances of bladder and bowel function. MRI of the brain may reveal diffuse white-matter signal increase on T2-weighted images. The diagnosis is clinched by the finding of characteristic pathological changes in tissue from peripheral nerve, cerebral cortex, spinal cord, or skin. Axons and neural sheath cells contain non-membrane-bound cytoplasmic periodic acid–Schiff-positive polyglucosan bodies. Ultrastructural examination shows that the inclusions consist of 6- to 8-nm branched filaments and are most abundant in myelinated nerve fibers. In Ashkenazi Jewish patients (and one reported non-Ashkenazi Jewish patient), the disorder was caused by mutations of the glycogen-branching enzyme *(GBE)* gene, with subsequent deficiency of the protein product. However, adult polyglucosan body disease (APBD) occurs in many different populations, and considerable molecular heterogeneity has been noted, with otherwise typical cases lacking *GBE* mutations despite deficiency of enzyme activity (Klein et al., 2004). The recent (albeit inadvertent) generation of muscle polyglucosan bodies in a transgenic mouse engineered to overexpress glycogen synthase in the presence of normal levels of glycogen-branching enzyme suggests that an imbalance in the activities of these two enzymes is the possible molecular mechanism underlying this unusual disorder (Raben et al., 2001). It is interesting to note that two types of polyglucosan body may be seen in ALS—Lafora bodies and corpora amylacea—although neither is considered a characteristic pathological feature.

## Paraneoplastic Motor Neuron Disease

There is evidence that motor neuron disease may rarely be a paraneoplastic phenomenon, although there is a possibility that the ALS and the neoplasm are chance associations. (Corcia et al., 2014). Patients may present with features that are rather typical of pure "spinal" ALS or manifest in a manner akin either to PMA or to PLS. Other motor neuron manifestations may represent only one part of a larger paraneoplastic syndrome, such as anti-Hu antibody associated encephalomyelitis, with atypical features such as dysautonomia or ataxia. Unfortunately, most paraneoplastic motor disorders are unresponsive to treatment of the underlying tumor. Rare motor disorders have been described in association with other paraneoplastic antibodies, including anti-Yo antibody in a patient with ovarian carcinoma and a novel antineuronal antibody in a patient with breast cancer. A subacute painless and progressive LMN-predominant disorder has been well characterized in lymphoma (both Hodgkin and non-Hodgkin types: see earlier discussion). Patients may eventually develop UMN signs, and some may improve either with treatment of the cancer or spontaneously. Elevated CSF protein levels or the presence of a paraprotein in the blood should prompt a detailed investigation for lymphoma. Although there is insufficient evidence to conclude that there is increased risk of cancer in ALS, a combination of UMN and LMN signs has been well described in patients with breast, uterine, ovarian, and non–small-cell cancer. This ALS-like disorder is quite rapidly progressive and does not appear to respond either to treatment of the underlying cancer or to immune therapies. UMN signs and symptoms that mimic PLS may rarely occur in patients with breast tumors and may in fact precede the cancer diagnosis by a few months. In general, one should investigate for a paraneoplastic disorder if there are atypical features such as ataxia, sensory loss, and dysautonomia, and it would seem to be prudent to carry out breast screening on women with a PLS presentation.

## Human Immunodeficiency Virus Type 1-Associated Motor Neuron Disorder

A retrospective review of 1700 cases of HIV-1-infected patients with neurological symptoms identified 6 cases presenting as a reversible ALS-like syndrome (Moulignier et al., 2001), representing a 27-fold increased risk of developing an ALS-like disorder in that particular HIV-1 patient population. Overall, patients were somewhat younger than the normal ALS population, all but one being younger than 40 years at the time of diagnosis. Onset was characteristically in a monomelic pattern followed by a very rapid spread to other regions over a period of weeks. There were clinical features of both UMN and LMN involvement, with fasciculations, cramps, and bulbar symptoms. Two patients also had rapidly progressive dementia, with other features suggesting an additional diagnosis of AIDS-dementia complex. Sensory and sphincter disturbances were not apparent. CSF protein levels were sometimes mildly increased, and a lymphocytic pleocytosis was evident in three patients, but all remaining laboratory results (HIV-1 seropositivity apart) were negative. EDX revealed a widespread disorder of anterior horn cells in the absence of demyelinating conduction block, and MRI in one patient showed diffuse white-matter signal increase suggestive of AIDS-dementia complex. At the pathological level, there are some features that are shared between ALS and HIV encephalitis; HIV cases also develop TDP-43 deposits (Douville and Nath, 2017).

In each case, antiretroviral therapy was beneficial either in stabilizing or (in two instances) curing the disease. No similar cases have been identified in this particular study population since the introduction of highly active antiretroviral combination chemotherapy in the management of HIV infection. Another case report found similar clinical features in a 32-year-old HIV-positive patient who also enjoyed a complete response to antiretroviral therapy. MRI of brain showed increased T2-weighted signal in the brachium pontis with some minimal contrast enhancement. The resolution of motor symptoms coincided with a lack of detectable HIV in plasma and CSF. In addition, the abnormal MRI signal almost completely resolved (MacGowan et al., 2001). Flail-arm ALS-like variants have also been described, with MRI signal changes in the anterior cervical spinal cord (Henning and Hewlett, 2008; Nalini et al., 2009). Other forms of HIV may also relate to the pathogenesis of motor neuron disease; a pure LMN syndrome occurred in a woman who was seropositive for HIV-2. Overall, there seems to be sufficient evidence to implicate HIV as a potential cause of an ALS-like disorder, but one must also consider the possibility of coincidental HIV infection in patients who have true sporadic ALS.

*The complete reference list is available online at https://expertconsult.inkling.com/.* 

98

# Channelopathies: Episodic and Electrical Disorders of the Nervous System

*Min K. Kang, Geoffrey A. Kerchner, Louis J. Ptáček*

## OUTLINE



Channelopathies are disorders caused by ion channel dysfunction. Because of the great diversity of ion channel proteins and their expression in different tissues, channelopathies comprise a wide variety of clinical diseases (Table 98.1), the discovery of which helps elucidate how ion channels function in both illness and health. The *periodic paralyses*—the first group of ion channel disorders characterized at a molecular level—defined the field of channelopathies, which now encompasses diseases not only in muscle but also in the kidney (Bartter syndrome), epithelium (cystic fibrosis), and heart (long QT syndrome), as well as neurons. Because muscles and neurons are electrical organs, it is not surprising that most channelopathies are associated with neurological disease. Despite significant heterogeneity, a pervasive feature of neurological channelopathies is a paroxysmal phenotype of various neurological presentations, encompassing myopathy, peripheral neuropathy, epilepsy, migraine headache, and episodic movement disorders. After a brief introduction to ion channels, this chapter describes disorders caused by congenital and acquired dysfunction of ion channels expressed in skeletal muscle, neurons and neuromuscular junction.

## ION CHANNELS

One needs a basic understanding of channel structure and function before addressing channelopathies and their clinical manifestations. Ion channels are transmembrane glycoprotein pores that underlie cell excitability by regulating ion flow into and out of cells across the lipid bilayers of the cell membrane. They are composed of distinct protein subunits, each encoded by a separate gene. The categorization of most channels, depending on their means of activation, is as *voltage-gated* or *ligand-gated*. Changes in membrane potentials activate and inactivate voltage-gated ion channels. They are named according to the physiological ion preferentially conducted (e.g., $Na^+$, $K^+$, $Ca^{2+}$, $Cl^-$). Ligand-gated ion channels respond instead to specific chemical neurotransmitters (e.g., acetylcholine, glutamate, γ-aminobutyric acid [GABA], glycine).

Distributed ubiquitously in excitable tissues, voltage-gated ion channels are critical for establishing a resting membrane potential and generating action potentials, especially in tissues where rapid conduction of messages is required (e.g., nerves, cardiac cells, or skeletal muscles). Most channels have a similar basic structure, consisting of one or more pore-forming subunits (generally referred to as *α-subunits*) and a variable number of accessory subunits (often denoted β, γ, etc.). An α-subunit is composed of four homologous domains (I–IV) and typically has six transmembrane segments (S1–S6). The S4 segment has positively charged residues and serves as "a sensor." The S5–S6 segments usually form the ion pore. These segments determine ion selectivity for the α-subunits, and voltage sensing is conferred by the S4 segment, while the remaining accessory subunits act as modulators.

Voltage-gated channels are "gated" with high sensitivity to changes in transmembrane potential. The conductance is tightly regulated by changes in conformations of the channel, as channels exist in one of three states: open, closed, or inactivated. Voltage-gated channels open (or activate) with threshold changes in membrane potential, then transition after a characteristic interval to either a closed or an inactivated state. From the closed state, a channel can reopen with an appropriate change in membrane potential. In the inactivated state, a change in membrane potential normally sufficient to open the channel is ineffective and the channels will not conduct current. Inactivation is both time and voltage dependent, and many channels display both fast and slow components of inactivation. Inactivation is a means of negative regulation of the channel, influencing electrical stability in excitable cells.

TABLE 98.1 **Genetic Channelopathies**

| Disease | Ion Channel | Gene | Chromosome |
|---|---|---|---|
| **Muscular Channelopathies** | | | |
| Andersen-Tawil syndrome | Kir2.1*; potassium (inward rectifier) | KCNJ2 | 17q23.1–q24.2 |
| | Kir3.4; potassium (inward rectifier) | KCNJ5 | 11q24 |
| Central core disease | Calcium (ryanodine receptor) | RYR1 | 19p13.1 |
| Congenital myasthenic syndromes | nAChR $\alpha_1$-subunit | CHRNA1 | 2q24–q32 |
| | nAChR $\beta_1$-subunit | CHRNB1 | 17p12–p11 |
| | nAChR $\delta$-subunit | CHRND | 2q33–q34 |
| | nAChR $\varepsilon$-subunit | CHRNE | 17p13–p12 |
| | (nAChR anchoring protein: rapsyn) | RAPSN | 11p11.2–p11.1 |
| Hyperkalemic periodic paralysis | Nav1.4; sodium $\alpha_4$-subunit | SCN4A | 17q23.1–q25.3 |
| Hypokalemic periodic paralysis | Cav1.1; calcium (L-type) | CACNA1S | 1q32 |
| | Nav1.4; sodium $\alpha_4$-subunit | SCN4A | 17q23.1–q25.3 |
| Malignant hyperthermia | Calcium (ryanodine receptor) | RYR1 | 19q13.1 |
| | Cav1.1; calcium (L-type) | CACNA1S | 1q32 |
| Myotonia congenita | Chloride | CLCN1 | 7q35 |
| Paramyotonia congenita | Nav1.4; sodium $\alpha_4$-subunit | SCN4A | 17q23.1–q25.3 |
| Potassium-aggravated myotonia | Nav1.4; sodium $\alpha_4$-subunit | SCN4A | 17q23.1–q25.3 |
| **Neuronal Channelopathies** | | | |
| ADNFLE | nAChR $\alpha_4$-subunit | CHRNA4 | 20q13.2–q13.3 |
| | nAChR $\beta_2$-subunit | CHRNB2 | 1q21 |
| | KCa4.1; potassium (sodium-activated) | KCNT1 | 9q34.3 |
| ADPEAF | (Potassium channel regulator) | LGI1 | 10q24 |
| Alternating hemiplegia of childhood | ($Na^+/K^+$-ATPase) | ATP1A2 | 1q21–q23 |
| BFNS | Kv7.2; potassium (M channel) | KCNQ2 | 20q13.3 |
| | Kv7.3; potassium (M channel) | KCNQ3 | 8q24 |
| BFNIS, BFIS | Nav1.2; sodium $\alpha_2$-subunit | SCN2A | 2q23–q24.3 |
| | ($Na^+/K^+$-ATPase†) | ATP1A2 | 1q21–q23 |
| Childhood absence epilepsy | $GABA_A$ receptor $\gamma_2$-subunit | GABRG2 | 5q31.1–q33.1 |
| | $GABA_A$ receptor $\beta_3$-subunit | GABRB3 | 15q11.2–q12 |
| | Cav3.2; calcium (T-type) | CACNA1H‡ | 16p13.3 |
| | Cav2.1; calcium (P/Q-type) | CACNA1A‡ | 19p13 |
| Congenital stationary night blindness | Cav1.4; calcium (L-type) | CACNA1F | Xp11.23 |
| Deafness (nonsyndromic type 2) | Kv7.4; potassium | KCNQ4 | 1p34 |
| Episodic ataxia 1 | Kv1.1; potassium | KCNA1 | 12p13 |
| Episodic ataxia 2 | Cav1.4; calcium (P/Q-type) | CACNA1A | 19p13 |
| Episodic ataxia 5 | Calcium $\beta_4$-subunit | CACNB4 | 2q22–q23 |
| Episodic ataxia 6 | (EAAT1†) | SLC1A3 | 5p13 |
| Familial hemiplegic migraine 1 | Cav1.4; calcium (P/Q-type) | CACNA1A | 19p13 |
| Familial hemiplegic migraine 2 | ($Na^+/K^+$-ATPase) | ATP1A2 | 1q21–q23 |
| Familial hemiplegic migraine 3 | Nav1.1; sodium $\alpha_1$-subunit | SCN1A | 2q24 |
| Familial temporal lobe epilepsy / febrile seizures | (Carboxypeptidase†) | CPA6 | 8q13.2 |
| GEFS+ | Nav1.1; sodium $\alpha_1$-subunit | SCN1A | 2q24 |
| | Sodium $\beta_1$-subunit | SCN1B | 19q13.1 |
| | Nav1.2; sodium $\alpha_2$-subunit | SCN2A | 2q23–q24.3 |
| | Nav1.7; sodium $\alpha_9$-subunit | SCN9A | 2q24 |
| | $GABA_A$ receptor $\gamma_2$-subunit | GABRG2 | 5q31.1–q33.1 |
| | $GABA_A$ receptor $\delta$-subunit | GABRD | 1p36.3 |
| Hereditary hyperekplexia | Glycine receptor $\alpha_1$-subunit | GLRA1 | 5q32 |
| | Glycine receptor $\beta$-subunit | GLRB | 4q31.3 |
| | (Glycine transporter†) | GLYT2 (SLC6A5) | 11p15.2–p15.1 |
| JME | $GABA_A$ receptor $\alpha_1$-subunit | GABRA1 | 5q34–q35 |
| | Calcium $\beta_4$-subunit | CACNB4‡ | 2q22–q23 |
| | (R-type calcium channel regulator†) | EFHC1‡ | 6p12–p11 |
| Mental retardation, autosomal dominant | Glutamate receptor NR2B subunit | GRIN2B | 12p13.1 |
| PED | (GLUT1†) | SLC2A1 | 1p34.2 |
| PKD | (Proline-rich transmembrane protein 2†) | PRRT2 | 16p11.2 |

*Continued*

**TABLE 98.1 Genetic Channelopathies—cont'd**

| Disease | Ion Channel | Gene | Chromosome |
|---|---|---|---|
| PNKD with epilepsy | KCa1.1; potassium (BK) | KCNMA1 | 10q22.3 |
| PNKD without epilepsy | (PNKD protein†) | PNKD | 2q35 |
| Primary erythermalgia | Nav1.7; sodium $\alpha_9$-subunit | SCN9A | 2q24 |
| Scapuloperoneal spinal muscular atrophy/ congenital distal spinal muscular atrophy/ CMT2C/HMSN2 | TRPV4 | TRPV4 | 12q24.1 |
| Spinocerebellar ataxia type 6 | Cav2.1; calcium (P/Q-type) | CACNA1A | 19p13 |
| **Nonneurological Channelopathies** | | | |
| Bartter syndrome antenatal 1 | Na-K-2Cl cotransporter | SLC12A1 | 15q15–q21.1 |
| Bartter syndrome antenatal 2 | Kir1.1; potassium (inward rectifier) | KCNJ1 | 11q24 |
| Bartter syndrome 3 | Chloride | CLCNKB | 1p36 |
| Cystic fibrosis | Chloride | CFTR | 7q31.2 |
| Dent disease | Chloride | CLCN5 | Xp11.22 |
| FPHHI | Potassium (accessory subunit) | ABCC8 | 11p15.1 |
| | Kir6.2; potassium (inward rectifier) | KCNJ11 | 11p15.1 |
| Liddle syndrome 1 | Sodium (non-voltage-gated) | SCNN1A | 12p13 |
| | Sodium (non-voltage-gated) | SCNN1B | 16p13–p12 |
| | Sodium (non-voltage-gated) | SCNN1G | 16p13–p12 |
| LQT1 | Kv7.1; potassium | KCNQ1 | 11p15.5 |
| LQT2 | Kv11.1; potassium | KCNH2 | 7q35–36 |
| LQT3 | Nav1.5; sodium $\alpha_5$-subunit | SCN5A | 3p21–24 |
| LQT4 | (anchoring protein ankyrin-B†) | ANK2 | 4q25–q27 |
| LQT5 | Potassium (accessory subunit) | KCNE1 | 21q22.1–q22.2 |
| LQT6 | Potassium (accessory subunit) | KCNE2 | 21q22.1 |

*ADNFLE*, Autosomal dominant nocturnal frontal lobe epilepsy; *ADPEAF*, autosomal dominant partial epilepsy with auditory features; *BFNS*, benign familial neonatal seizures; *BFNIS*, benign familial neonatal–infantile seizures; *BFIS*, benign familial infantile seizures; *CMT2C*, Charcot–Marie–Tooth disease type 2C; *EAAT1*, excitatory amino acid transporter 1; *FHM*, familial hemiplegic migraine; *FPHHI*, familial hyperinsulinemic hypoglycemia of infancy; *GEFS+*, generalized epilepsy with febrile seizures plus; *HMSN2*, hereditary motor and sensory neuropathy type 2; *JME*, juvenile myoclonic epilepsy; *LQT*, long-QT syndrome; *nAChR*, nicotinic acetylcholine receptor; *PED*, paroxysmal exercise-induced dyskinesia; *PKD*, paroxysmal kinesigenic dyskinesia; *PNKD*, paroxysmal nonkinesigenic dyskinesia.

*Where appropriate, ion channel names are provided according to the International Union of Basic and Clinical Pharmacology Committee on Receptor Nomenclature and Drug Classification (NC-IUPHAR).

†These associated genes/proteins may not be ion channels; they may instead contribute indirectly to ion channel function, regulate neurotransmitter kinetics, or possess other or unknown functions.

‡Unproven association.

A neuron typically has a resting potential of –75 mV, with the intracellular side being negative relative to the extracellular space. When the resting potential reaches a threshold or more positive membrane potential of –55 mV, depolarization occurs, which leads to the production of an action potential. This is achieved by opening a specific ion channel—a voltage-gated sodium channel—in which case sodium ions will rush into the cells down the concentration gradient. In order to reach the action potential, the sodium channel changes its confirmation from a closed or resting state to an open state. When the membrane potential reaches its peak, about 40 mV, the sodium channels close and become inactive. Then, repolarization occurs, due to the opening of another voltage-gated channel, such as a potassium channel. This leads to a rapid return to the resting potential via an outflux of potassium ions (down the potassium concentration gradient). Before achieving a stable resting potential, the membrane potential becomes "hyperpolarized" for a short time. Slowly, the sodium channels return to the closed state from the inactivated state. While in the inactivated state, sodium channels are not responsive to voltage changes. However, in the closed state, they become sensitive to voltage changes again.

Different tissues and cells express different ion channels; thus, dysfunction of a specific ion channel can lead to a broad spectrum of phenotypes, depending on the tissue/cell type/ion channel involved. This is particularly important in the nervous system, where there is tremendous heterogeneity of the cells with regard to ion channel expression. Each subtype is encoded by a different gene, and its expression is highly cell specific.

Depending on the location within the channel, mutations could alter voltage-dependent activation, ion selectivity, or time and voltage dependence of inactivation. Thus, two different mutations within the same gene can result in dramatically different physiological effects. For example, a mutation that prevents or slows inactivation could lead to a persistent ionic current. Conversely, a mutation elsewhere in the same gene that prevents activation will decrease ionic current. *Phenotypic heterogeneity* describes how different mutations in a single gene cause distinct phenotypes. For instance, mutations in the skeletal muscle voltage-dependent sodium channel can result in hyperkalemic periodic paralysis, hypokalemic periodic paralysis, potassium-aggravated myotonia (PAM), or paramyotonia congenita (PMC; see Table 98.1 and Fig. 98.1). In contrast, *genetic heterogeneity* occurs when a consistent clinical syndrome results from a variety of underlying mutations in distinct genes. For example, familial hypokalemic periodic paralysis can result from distinct mutations in the *SCN4A* or *CACNA1S* genes.

Ion channel mutations may lead to either "loss of function" or "gain of function" in each case. Generally speaking, loss-of-function mutations cause reduced permeability, whereas gain of function implies the gain of an abnormal function (e.g., increased permeability or altered selectivity vs. normal permeability in the wrong part of the cell). Furthermore, genetic channelopathies are not restricted to mutation of the channels, but other mutations involving regulatory, modifiers, posttranscriptional, and posttranslation changes can also result in ion channel dysfunction (Fig. 98.2)

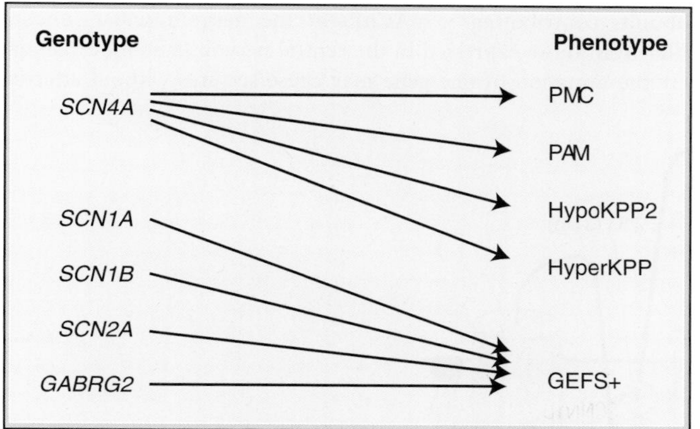


**Fig. 98.1** Illustration of the principle that various mutations within a single gene (e.g., *SCN4A*) can lead to distinct clinical syndromes; conversely, mutations in different genes may result in a single recognized clinical entity. *GEFS+*, Generalized epilepsy with febrile seizures plus; *hyperKPP*, hyperkalemic periodic paralysis; *hypoKPP2*, hypokalemic periodic paralysis type 2; *PAM*, potassium-aggravated myotonia; *PMC*, paramyotonia congenita.

## Ion Channel Classification

Voltage-gated potassium channels (VGKCs) consist of four homologous α-subunits that combine to create a functional channel. Humans possess many distinct *VGKC* genes, and the resulting channels exhibit specialized properties and display rich tissue-type and cellular-compartment specificity. Each α-subunit of voltage-gated channels contains six transmembrane segments (S1–S6) linked by extracellular and intracellular loops (Fig. 98.3). The S5–S6 loop penetrates deep into the central part of the channel and lines the pore. The S4 segment contains positively charged amino acids and acts as the voltage sensor. These channels serve many functions, most notably to establish the resting membrane potential and to repolarize cells following an action potential. A unique class of potassium channel, the inwardly rectifying potassium channel, is homologous to the S5–S6 segments of the VGKC. Because the voltage-sensing S4 domain is absent, voltage dependence results from a voltage-dependent blockade by magnesium and polyamines rather than from the movement of the positively charged S4 domain in response to membrane depolarization.

Voltage-gated sodium and calcium channels are highly homologous and share homology with VGKCs, from which they evolved. The α-subunits contain four highly homologous domains in tandem within a single transcript (DI–DIV; Fig. 98.4). Each domain resembles a VGKC α-subunit, with six transmembrane segments, as described earlier. Sodium and calcium channels differ in several regards, despite their many similarities. The amino acid sequence forming the selectivity

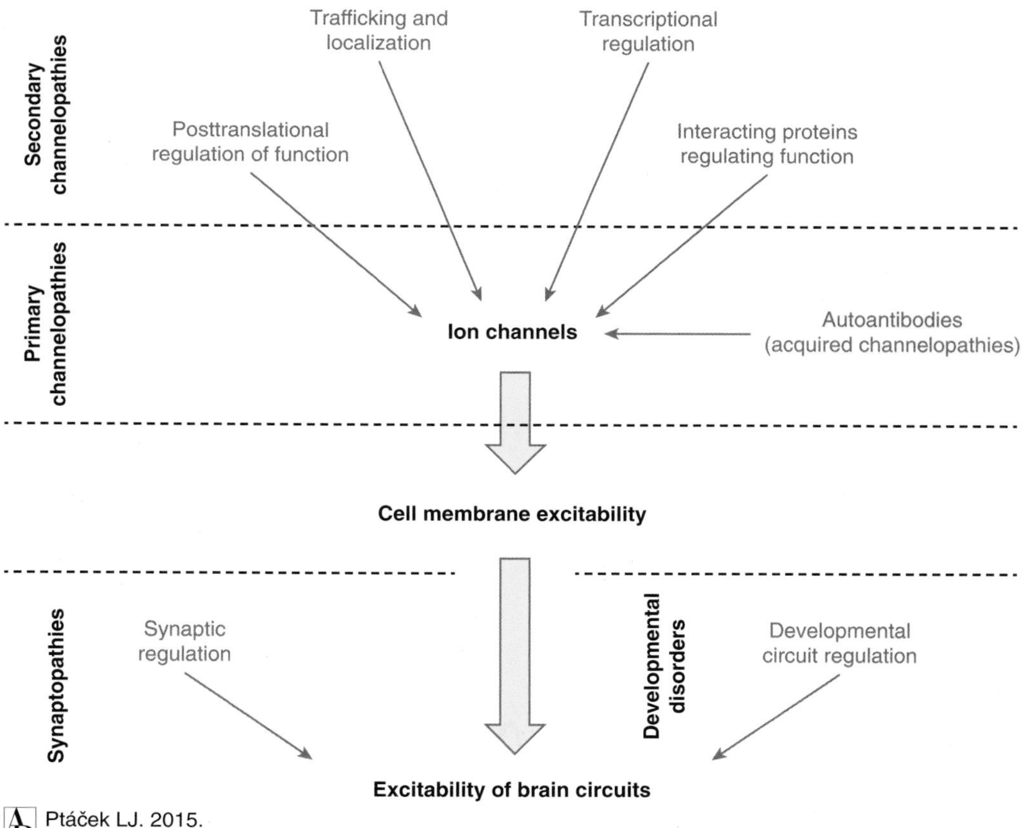


**Fig. 98.2 Proposed Classification Scheme for Electrical and Episodic Disorders.** Channelopathy is referred to as an abnormal function of ion channels themselves or secondary to disrupted orchestration of signaling from other proteins.

filter and the modulatory auxiliary subunits are different. The sodium channel is composed of an α- and a β-subunit, and the calcium channel is composed of a pore-forming $\alpha_1$-subunit, an intracellular β-subunit, a membrane-spanning γ-subunit, and a membrane-anchoring $\alpha_2\delta$-subunit. Sodium channels mediate fast depolarization and underlie the action potential, whereas voltage-gated calcium channels (VGCCs) mediate neurotransmitter release and allow the calcium influx that leads to second messenger effects.

Ligand-gated ion channels activate on binding with their respective agonists. $GABA_A$, glycine, and nicotinic acetylcholine receptors (nAChRs) are examples of ligand-gated ion channels with known disease-causing mutations. Although distinguished by their ligand binding and ion permeability, channels gated by GABA, glycine, and acetylcholine share several structural similarities. Five intrinsic membrane subunits assemble to form hetero- or homopentamers. Each subunit contains four transmembrane domains (M1–M4), the second of which lines the pore and determines ionic selectivity (Fig. 98.5). Subunits contributing to nAChRs at the neuromuscular junction differ from those expressed in the central nervous system, explaining why the mutation of one gene may cause seizures without affecting

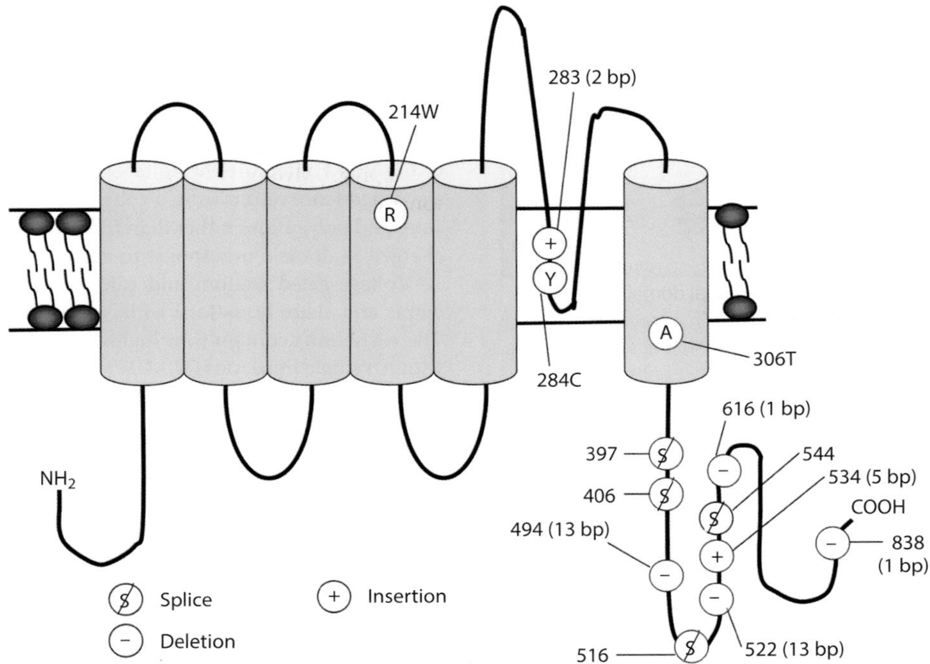


**Fig. 98.3 Proposed Structure of the Voltage-Gated Potassium Channel, Kv1.1 (KCNA1), Implicated in Episodic Ataxia Type 1.** Voltage-dependent potassium channels comprise four subunits that form a channel pore. Each subunit contains six transmembrane domains, with the S4 segment containing positively charged amino acids that act as the voltage sensor. Mutations associated with episodic ataxia type 1 are illustrated. Disease-causing mutations are indicated by the one-letter amino acid representation. Amino acids with circles are wild-type, and the corresponding mutation is indicated by a connecting line with the corresponding position and amino acid.

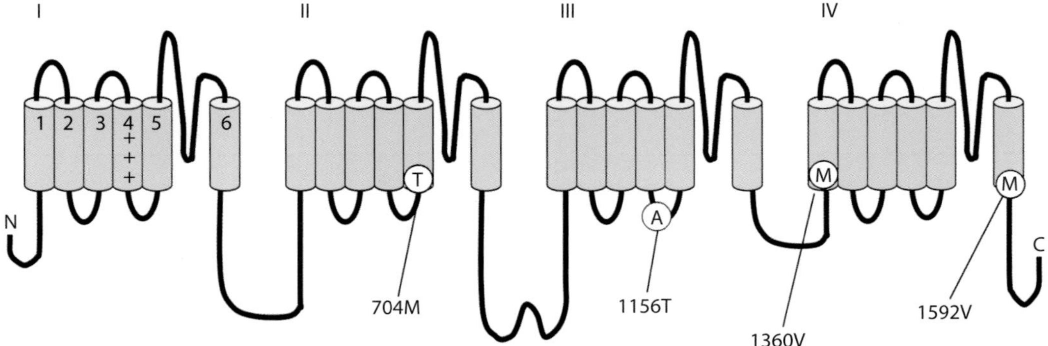


**Fig. 98.4 Diagram of the Voltage-Gated Sodium Channel and the Four Most Common Mutations Causing Hyperkalemic Periodic Paralysis.** The α-subunit consists of four highly homologous domains (I to IV), each containing six transmembrane segments (S1–S6). When inserted into the membrane, the four domains fold so as to encircle a central ion-selective pore lined by the S5–S6 loops. Analogous to the potassium channel (see Fig. 98.3), the S4 segments contain positively charged residues conferring voltage dependence on the channel. Auxiliary β-subunits are not shown.

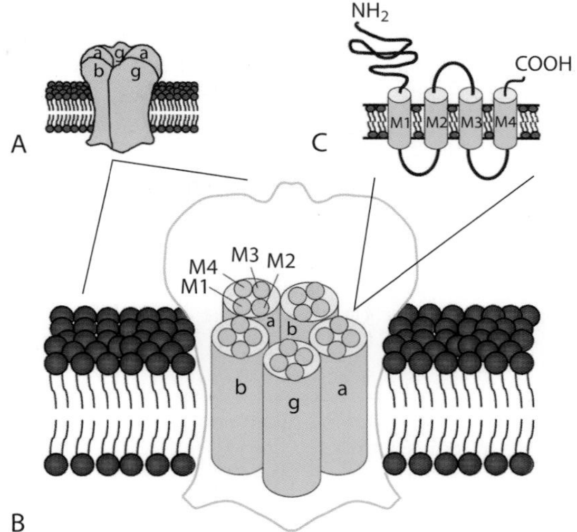


**Fig. 98.5 Molecular Structure of the Nicotinic Acetylcholine Receptor.** **A,** Three-dimensional model showing a pentameric protein forming a pore. Two molecules of acetylcholine (ACh) bind to the α-subunits to open the channel. **B,** Each subunit contains four α-helical domains, labeled M1 to M4. The M2 domain forms the channel pore. **C,** An enlarged diagram of the α-subunit showing the extracellular N and C termini and the four transmembrane domains. The amino acids at boundaries of the M2 domain are negatively charged, forming a selectivity filter for cations.

neuromuscular transmission, or vice versa. Binding of acetylcholine opens the channel, which conducts monovalent cations ($Na^+$ and $K^+$) with little or no selectivity, and some are additionally permeable to calcium. Channel activation results in membrane depolarization and excitation of the postsynaptic neuron or muscle fiber.

The $GABA_A$ and glycine receptors belong to the nAChR superfamily and similarly consist of five subunits. $GABA_A$ receptors include α-, β-, and either γ- or δ-subunits. The predominant glycine receptor is a heteropentamer of three α-subunits and two β-subunits. In either case, agonist binding opens the channel and allows the flux of chloride ($Cl^-$) into the cell, generally causing hyperpolarization and decreased excitability. Therefore, both GABA and glycine mediate inhibitory synaptic transmission.

Channelopathies encompass a variety of diseases in multiple systems, including neurological, cardiac, endocrine, and kidney disorders, as summarized in Table 98.1. In the nervous system, most channelopathies are characterized by episodic attacks. Phenotypically, it ranges from muscle disease and peripheral neuropathy to episodic movement disorders, epilepsy, and migraine headache. Patients experience recurrent "attacks" throughout life, usually with complete resolution between attacks. Although there are strikingly diverse presentations, depending on the expression pattern of the gene, this group of disorders shares many similarities. First, as mentioned earlier, they are episodic with various frequencies of attacks. Second, these disorders have triggers or precipitating factors such as stress, sleep deprivation, and certain dietary factors that often precede the onset of an attack. Third, these disorders typically have a similar natural history, with an onset in childhood to young adulthood, worsening through adolescence and young-adult life, and improvement in middle- and late-adult life.

## GENETIC DISORDERS OF MUSCULAR ION CHANNELS

Skeletal muscle channelopathies are characterized by periodic paralyses and nondystrophic myotonia. These disorders include familial hypokalemic periodic paralysis (hypoKPP), hyperkalemic periodic paralysis (hyperKPP), PMC, myotonia congenita, PAM, and Andersen-Tawil syndrome (ATS). The patients with these disorders present with episodic muscle weakness, lasting minutes to hours, typically with full recovery between episodes. With recurrent episodes, one can develop permanent and fixed weakness later in life. Inheritance is autosomal dominant, with high penetrance, though for some mutations, there can be sex-dependent penetrance. Usually, there are triggers, as mentioned earlier, including stress, alcohol, recent illness, exercise followed by rest, fasting, or glucose-rich meals. Weakness can be regional or generalized, while bulbar and respiratory involvement is rare. Carbonic anhydrase inhibitors such as acetazolamide can be used to reduce the frequency of attacks of weakness. Sodium channel blockers like mexiletine are sometimes effective in reducing myotonic symptoms and signs (see Table 98.2).

The patients may describe myotonia as muscle "stiffness" or "cramping." Myotonia can be found clinically, and subclinical myotonia can be detected using electromyography (EMG). Myotonia is enhanced muscle excitability that leads to sustained bursts of discharges. Due to hyperexcitability of the muscle, one experiences involuntary contraction in said muscle, resulting from the inability to relax after forceful voluntary contraction. This can be demonstrated in the exam room, asking the patient to make a tight fist or forceful eye closure, and it is called "action myotonia." Percussion myotonia is another supporting exam finding of muscle channelopathies. When a muscle, such as the gastrocnemius muscle, is tapped with a reflex hammer, a persistent dimpling of the muscle can be seen. Myotonia is a nonspecific sign found in several other diseases, including myotonic dystrophy 1, myotonic dystrophy 2 (proximal myotonic myopathy), myotonia congenita, PMC, and hyperKPP. The "paramyotonia" in paramyotonia congenital describes the ability to demonstrate worsening of myotonic stiffness with repeated muscle contractions and is best seen in the orbicularis oculi. This can be also be precipitated by muscle cooling (i.e., a temperature-sensitive phenotype). PMC is one disorder in this group with a distinct clinical finding of paramyotonia, commonly demonstrated with repeated forceful eye closure, leading to increasing myotonia of the orbicularis oculi.

Clinical and subclinical myotonia can be demonstrated using EMG, which shows sustained bursts of muscle after-discharges that persist following voluntary contraction or occur in response to insertion of an EMG needle. It produces a characteristic "dive-bomber" discharge, with waxing and waning discharges (20–80 Hz).

In addition to distinct myotonic discharges using EMG, nerve conduction studies (NCS), in particular the short and long exercise tests (SET and LET), can be further utilized to narrow down the differential diagnosis (Fournier et al., 2004). The compound motor action potentials (CMAPs) are recorded at a basline and every 10 seconds after 10 seconds of short isometric exercise up to 60 seconds. This 60 second set of CMAP recording is repeated twice, with a resting period of 1 minute between each set. It is noteworthy that maintaining a warm temperature is important, as cooling may change the pattern with decreased CMAP amplitude yet increased CMAP duration. The LET is performed by isometric exercise for 5 minutes. CMAPs are recorded every minute during the exercise, after exercise, and every 5 minutes after exercise, for 40–45 minutes.

The pattern of decrement and increment of CMAP amplitude over time are helpful to identify distinct subgroups of mutations causing periodic paralysis. Fournier et al. (2004) analyzed the patterns after short and long exercises and categorized muscle channelopathies into 5 groups, as summarized in Table 98.4.

TABLE 98.2 Clinical Features of the Periodic Paralyses and Nondystrophic Myotonias

| | HypoKPP | HyperKPP | PMC | MC | PAM |
|---|---|---|---|---|---|
| Age at onset | 2nd decade | 1st decade | Infancy | 1st decade | 1st–2nd decade |
| Duration of attack | Hours–days | Minutes–hours | Hours | Minutes–hours | N/A |
| Severity of attack | Moderate–severe | Mild–moderate | Mild–moderate | Mild–moderate | |
| Triggers | Postexercise, CHO load | Postexercise, fasting, K load | Cold, postexercise | Rest | K |
| Myotonia | Absent | Present | Present | Present | Present |
| Serum $K^+$ | Usually low | Normal or high | Variable | Normal | Normal |
| Progressive weakness | Some patients | Some patients | Absent | Present in Becker myotonia | Absent |
| Treatment for weakness | CAI | CAI | CAI | N/A | N/A |
| Treatment for myotonia | N/A | Mexiletine | Mexiletine | Mexiletine, phenytoin | CAI |

*CAI*, Carbonic anhydrase inhibitor; *CHO*, carbohydrate; *hyperKPP*, hyperkalemic periodic paralysis; *hypoKPP*, hypokalemic periodic paralysis; *MC*, myotonia congenita; *PAM*, potassium-aggravated myotonia; *PMC*, paramyotonia congenita; *K*, potassium.

## Hypokalemic Periodic Paralysis (hypoKPP)

### Clinical

The prevalence of hypoKPP is approximately 1 per 100,000. Episodes of limb weakness accompanied by hypokalemia usually begin during adolescence. Attacks usually occur in the morning and are often triggered either by the ingestion of a carbohydrate load and high salt intake the previous night or by rest following strenuous exercise. Generalized muscle weakness and reduced or absent tendon reflexes are characteristic. Heralding the weakness may be sensory changes, fatigue, or a feeling of heaviness or aching in the legs or back. During paralysis, level of consciousness and sensation are preserved. Paralysis either spares the facial and respiratory muscles or causes only mild weakness, making medical intervention rarely necessary. The frequency, length, and severity of attacks vary. Although attacks may occur several times a week, they more often occur at intervals of weeks or months. Attack duration varies from minutes to days, typically lasting several hours. Occasionally the attacks are sufficiently brief to cause difficulty in documenting the accompanying hypokalemia. Patients usually recover full strength, although mild weakness may persist for several days or (more rarely) be permanent. A progressive permanent myopathy with mild proximal weakness may develop later in life, although it is rare.

### Pathophysiology

There are largely two genes that are responsible for hypoKPP. HypoKPP1 is up to 70% of cases, and it is caused by mutations in the *CACNA1S* gene encoding the $\alpha_1$-subunit of the dihydropyridine-sensitive L-type voltage-gated skeletal muscle calcium channel, $Ca_v1.1$, on chromosome 1q32.1 (Venance et al., 2006).

$Ca_v1.1$ is the slow-inactivating, L-type calcium channel and can be blocked by 1,4-dihydropyridine (e.g., amlodipine and nifedipine), phenylalkamines (e.g., verapamil), and benzothiazepines (e.g., diltiazem; Fialho et al., 2018). This channel functions as the voltage sensor of the ryanodine receptor and plays an important role in excitation–contraction coupling in skeletal muscle. Four mutations in the S4 segments alter voltage sensitivity. Two mutations, involving arginine-to-histidine substitutions within the highly conserved S4 segments of DII and DIV (Arg-528-His and Arg-1239-His), account for most cases. The others involve arginine-to-glycine substitutions at the same locations.

HypoKPP2 is caused by a mutation in *SCN4A* gene on chromosome 17q23.3 encoding the pore-forming α-subunit of the skeletal muscle voltage-gated sodium channel, $Na_v1.4$. Approximately 10%–20% of families with hypoKPP have this mutation. This is the same channel implicated in hyperKPP and other disorders described later (see Fig. 98.1). Evidence suggests that this sodium channel–associated syndrome is phenotypically different from the more common CACNA1S form. A proposed separate clinical entity, hypoKPP2, may be distinguishable from hypoKPP1 associated with CACNA1S by the presence of myalgias following paralytic attacks, and the presence of tubular aggregates instead of vacuoles in the muscle biopsy. In some patients, acetazolamide worsens symptoms (Bendahhou et al., 2001; Sternberg et al., 2001). In a large retrospective series, hypoKPP2 was associated with an older age of onset and shorter duration of attacks than classical hypoKPP1 (Miller et al., 2004).

Whether involving *SCN4A* or *CACNA1S*, virtually all mutations causing hypoKPP involve an S4 voltage-sensor domain. In the case of the sodium channel, these mutations allow a leak current to pass through the "gating pore" at resting membrane potentials, bypassing the central channel pore and leading to inappropriate muscle fiber depolarization and consequent channel inactivation and action potential failure (Sokolov et al., 2007). Speculation exists that this phenomenon may also occur in mutated VGCCs.

### Diagnosis

An accurate medical history is essential for the diagnosis because observation of attacks is unusual, and patients are often normal between attacks. Characteristic features of hypoKPP that distinguish it from hyperKPP are that paralytic attacks are less frequent, longer lasting, precipitated by a carbohydrate load, and often begin during sleep (see Table 98.2). Potassium concentrations are usually low during an attack, less than 3.0 mM, although concentrations less than 2 mM should suggest a secondary form of periodic paralysis. Electrocardiogram (ECG) changes such as increased PR and QT intervals, T-wave flattening, and prominent U waves suggest an underlying hypokalemia. Provocative testing can be dangerous and is not routine. Test performance requires a hospitalized setting with continuous cardiac monitoring and should be performed only in patients without cardiac or renal disease. After giving an oral glucose load (2–5 g/kg up to a maximum of 100 g) with or without subcutaneous insulin (0.1 U/kg), one performs serial examinations of strength while monitoring serum glucose and potassium concentrations. Myotonia is not found in hypoKPP, either clinically or with EMG. EMG may reveal membrane irritability with myopathic changes but often is normal. Short and long exercise tests reveal Fournier pattern V, with decrement CMAPs following the long exercise test without significant change in the SET. Creatine kinase (CK) can be normal but may be elevated. Potassium between attacks is normal. Muscle

**TABLE 98.3 Acetazolamide**

| | |
|---|---|
| Use | Prophylactic agent for some channelopathies (see text). |
| Mechanism | Inhibits carbonic anhydrase. |
| Dosing | *Adults:* start 125 mg daily, titrating as needed up to a maximum daily dose of 1000–1500 mg, divided bid–qid. An extended release formulation is available.<br>*Children:* consult a pharmacist. |
| Side effects | Taste changes (especially for carbonated drinks), fatigue, paresthesias, metabolic acidosis, blurred vision, myelosuppression, nephrolithiasis, etc. (Increased dietary citrate might be recommended to compensate for decreased urinary citrate observed during acetazolamide therapy.) |
| Monitoring | Check electrolytes, BUN, creatinine, and CBC at baseline and periodically throughout therapy. |
| Metabolism | None; excreted unchanged by kidneys. |

*bid*, Twice daily; *BUN*, blood urea nitrogen; *CBC*, complete blood cell count; *qid*, four times daily.
Please note that this table is for brief informational purposes only. Prescribing physicians should consult a pharmacist or an appropriate reference for complete and updated information.

histology reveals nonrimmed vacuoles within muscle fibers in biopsies in hypoKPP1 or tubular aggregates in hypoKPP2. Genetic testing should render muscle biopsy and provocative testing obsolete for diagnosis.

Thyrotoxic periodic paralysis (TPP) may be clinically indistinguishable from hypoKPP, except that it is not familial and serum potassium levels are often lower than in familial hypoKPP (<2.5). TPP is more common in Asian adults and in men more than women. Some cases may be associated with a mutation in *KCNJ18*, the gene encoding a novel inwardly rectifying potassium channel (Ryan et al., 2010). All patients with hypoKPP require screening for hyperthyroidism, as the treatment—correction of the thyroid disorder—differs from that outlined for familial hypoKPP. Treatment of hypothyroidism would prevent further attacks of weakness. Beta-blockade is often effective in reducing the frequency and severity of the paralytic attacks (Amato and James, 2016). One needs to exclude other secondary forms of hypokalemic paralysis when serum potassium concentrations remain low between attacks. Renal, adrenal, and gastrointestinal causes of persistent hypokalemia are common, and thiazide diuretic use and licorice (glycyrrhizic acid) intoxication must also be considered.

### Treatment

An effective holistic approach to treatment includes lifestyle modifications and acute and chronic pharmacological intervention. Dietary modification to avoid high carbohydrate loads and refraining from excessive exertion help prevent attacks. Prophylactic use of acetazolamide (Table 98.3) decreases the frequency and severity of attacks. Dichlorphenamide is another carbonic anhydrase inhibitor that effectively prevents attacks, as demonstrated in a randomized clinical trial (Tawil et al., 2000) where the average dose was 100 mg daily. More potent than acetazolamide, dichlorphenamide may be useful when the efficacy of the former begins to fail. A clinician may keep in mind that hypoKPP2 caused by SCAN4A has less benefit from carbonic anhydrase inhibitors compared to patients with hypoKPP1 (Matthews et al., 2011). Potassium-sparing diuretics (e.g., loop diuretics) or angiotensin-converting enzyme inhibitors may be of prophylactic benefit in patients with normal renal function in whom other more conservative measures are insufficient. Many believe that reducing the frequency or severity of paralytic attacks provides protection against the development of myopathy based on anecdotal experience, although this has never been formally tested in a controlled trial. Inhibition of Na, K, Cl cotransporter (NKCLC), particularly with bumetanide (which is a NCLC blocker) is currently in clinical trial.

During an acute attack, the preferred method of treatment is oral potassium chloride given at 0.5–1.0 mEq/kg, not exceeding 200 mEq in a 24-hour period. If a patient is unable to take oral potassium (e.g., arrhythmia due to hypokalemia or airway compromise due to altered mental status), then intravenous potassium (KCl bolus 0.05–0.1 mEq/kg or 20–40 mEq/L of KCl in 5% mannitol) is indicated. Cardiac monitoring is important during the administration of potassium.

## Hyperkalemic Periodic Paralysis (hyperKPP)

### Clinical

Characteristic of this disorder is episodic weakness precipitated by hyperkalemia. Although the weakness is generally milder than in hypoKPP, it can be sufficiently severe in hyperKPP to cause flaccid quadriparesis. As in hypoKPP, respiratory and ocular muscles are unaffected and consciousness is preserved. The frequency of attacks varies from several per day to several per year. Attacks are usually brief, lasting 15–60 minutes, but may last up to days. Unlike hypoKPP, myotonia is present between attacks. Onset is usually in infancy or childhood, and characteristic attacks occur by adolescence. Triggers include rest after vigorous exercise, foods high in potassium, fasting, stress, and fatigue. Despite its name, hyperKPP is often associated with a normal serum potassium concentration during an attack (see the following Diagnosis section). Most patients experience a subacute onset, and some describe paresthesia or a sensation of muscle tension prior to attacks. In these situations, mild exercise may abort or lessen the severity of the attack. The thigh and calf muscles are often involved. Generalized weakness is uncommon, making hyperKPP distinct from hypoKPP. Mild weakness may persist afterward, and the later development of a progressive myopathy is common.

### Pathophysiology

HyperKPP is an autosomal dominant disorder, with high penetrance, and there are some sporadic cases. The disorder links to *SCN4A*, the same gene responsible for a minority of hypoKPP cases. Among several identified missense mutations, four account for about two-thirds of cases (see Fig. 98.1). Functional expression of naturally occurring mutations demonstrated a decrease in the voltage threshold of channel activation or abnormally prolonged channel opening or both (Bendahhou et al., 2002; Hayward et al., 1999), effectively increasing the depolarizing inward current. If sustained long enough, this would lead to inactivation of the sodium channels, transitory cellular inexcitability, and weakness.

### Diagnosis

Despite advances in defining the underlying genetic mutations, a thorough medical and family history and physical examination remain the best diagnostic tools. Serum potassium is normal between attacks and even during many attacks. Unlike hypoKPP, potassium administration may precipitate an attack. In the absence of provocative testing, the basis for diagnosis is the clinical presentation. Hyperkalemia itself can cause weakness; thus secondary causes of hyperkalemia should be considered, especially if the potassium levels are greater than 7 mEq/L. Myotonia is present in many patients between attacks, either spontaneously or after muscle percussion, and failure to produce myotonia discriminates hypoKPP from hyperKPP (see Table 98.2). Take care not to confuse subjective muscle stiffness with objective changes. Peaked T waves on ECG suggest hyperkalemia and are an aid to diagnosis. As in hypoKPP, serum CK concentrations are often normal but sometimes can be elevated. A potassium-loading test provokes an attack but is not usually necessary and can be dangerous.

Electrodiagnostic studies are useful for demonstrating subclinical myotonic discharges, not seen in hypoKPP. Myopathic findings such as fibrillation potentials and small polyphasic motor unit potentials occur during late stages of disease. Interictal NCS are usually normal, but the CMAPs during the attack may be reduced. The SET and LET reveal a Fournier pattern IV, (Table 98.4) where the SET shows increased amplitude after the first trial, which is further increased in subsequent trials, and the LET shows a transient increase in amplitude after exercise, followed by a gradual decrement in amplitude over 40 minutes.

### Treatment

The goal of therapy is to abort the acute attacks and prevent future attacks. Acute attacks are often sufficiently brief and mild, so as not to require acute intervention. In more severe attacks, aim treatment at lowering extracellular potassium levels. Mild exercise or eating a high sugar load (juice or a candy bar) may suffice, as insulin drives extracellular potassium into cells. Thiazide diuretics and inhaled β-adrenergic agonists are similarly helpful, and intravenous glucose, insulin, or calcium gluconate may be used for severe weakness. To prevent attacks, a diet low in potassium and high in carbohydrates may obviate the need for prophylactic drug therapy. Patients are also advised to avoid fasting, strenuous exercise, and cold. Oral dichlorphenamide (50–150 mg/day) was useful for prophylaxis in one randomized controlled trial (Tawil et al., 2000). Acetazolamide (see Table 98.3) and thiazide diuretics are useful as well. Successful prophylaxis may decrease the later onset of myopathy, although direct proof of this hypothesis is lacking. Finally, myotonic symptoms are troublesome in some patients; sodium channel blockers, such as mexiletine, can be used for symptomatic management. Obtaining ECGs is advised due to QT prolongation. (Amato et al., 2016)

## Paramyotonia Congenita

### Clinical

The characteristic features of PMC are paradoxical myotonia, cold-induced myotonia, and weakness after prolonged cold exposure. Unlike classic myotonia, which shows a warm-up phenomenon (see the later section Myotonia Congenita), patients with PMC often show exacerbation of myotonia after repeated muscle contraction. Symptoms may be recognized in infants and certainly by childhood and usually remain unchanged throughout life, although one may develop progressive permanent weakness over time. Infants may be noted to have difficulty opening their eyes after crying due to myotonia of the orbicularis oculi. Myotonia affects all skeletal muscles, although the facial muscles and muscles of the neck and hands are the most common sites of myotonia in the winter. The onset of weakness is often during the day, lasts several hours, and is exacerbated by cold, stress, and rest after exercise. Many patients are asymptomatic when warm. However, cold-induced stiffness may persist for hours even after the body warms, and percussion myotonia is present even when the patient is otherwise asymptomatic.

### Pathophysiology

The cause of PMC is point mutations in the *SCN4A* gene on chromosome 17q. Thus, PMC is allelic to hyperKPP, PAM, and less commonly, hypoKPP. Mutations of the gene, which include substitutions at T1313 on the DIII to DIV linker and at R1448 on the DIV–S4 segment, cause defects in sodium channel deactivation and fast inactivation. The resting membrane potential rises from −80 up to −40 mV when intact muscle fibers cool. Mild depolarization results in repetitive discharges (myotonia), whereas greater depolarization results in sodium channel inactivation and muscle inexcitability (weakness).

### Diagnosis

A family history of exercise- and cold-induced stiffness or difficulty of relaxation after forceful contraction strongly supports the diagnosis of PMC. When asked to close their eyes forcefully and repeatedly, affected individuals exhibit progressive difficulty with relaxation and are eventually unable to open their eyes; this is called paramyotonia, the name derived from paradoxical reaction to exercise. Furthermore, muscle cooling may elicit an increase in myotonia, a reduction in isometric force of 50% or more, and a prolongation of the relaxation time by several seconds after muscle cooling supports the diagnosis. Serum potassium concentration may be high, low, or normal during attacks, and serum CK concentrations may be elevated 5–10 times normal. Electrodiagnostic studies are useful in establishing the diagnosis. EMG reveals fibrillation-like potentials and myotonic discharges that are accentuated by muscle percussion, needle movement, and muscle cooling. Muscle cooling elicits an initial increase in myotonia, then a progressive decrease in myotonia, followed by a decrease in CMAP amplitude that correlates respectively, with muscle stiffness and weakness. The SET commonly reveals postexercise myotonic potentials (PEMPs) after a short exercise on the motor conduction studies. CMAP amplitudes show delayed decrement after second and third trials, particularly in patients with *T1313M* mutation. The SET in patients with Q270K mutation shows prominent decrement with cooling. The LET shows decrement in CMAP amplitudes during and after exercise without return to its baseline. These SET and LET patterns are categorized to Fournier pattern I, which is distinctive for PMC (Table 98.4). Muscle pathology shows only nonspecific changes, and biopsy is unnecessary.

### Treatment

Symptoms are generally mild and infrequent. Direct treatment, when required, at either myotonia or weakness or both. Sodium channel blockers such as mexiletine are effective in reducing the frequency and severity of myotonia, as shown in a randomized trial (Statland et al., 2012). Patients with weakness often respond to agents used to treat hyperKPP (e.g., thiazides, acetazolamide). A single case report suggests the possible use of pyridostigmine (Khadilkar et al., 2010). Cold avoidance reduces the frequency of attacks.

## Myotonia Congenita

### Clinical

Inheritance of myotonia congenita (MC) is either as an autosomal dominant (Thomsen disease) or recessive (Becker myotonia) trait. The main feature is myotonia or delayed muscle relaxation after contraction. Forceful movement abruptly initiated after several minutes of rest causes the most pronounced myotonic stiffness. The myotonia of MC displays a *warm-up phenomenon* in which the myotonia decreases or vanishes completely when repeating the same movement several times, in contrast to the myotonia seen in patients with PMC. Unlike PMC, cold temperature does not exacerbate the clinical or electrical myotonia or weakness (Subramony et al., 1983) The onset of Thomsen

**TABLE 98.4 Electrodiagnostic Pattern**

| Fournier Pattern | Short Exercise Test | Long Exercise Test | Clinical Phenotype |
|---|---|---|---|
| I | Postexercise amplitude decrement that worsens with each trial | Postexercise amplitude decrement that does not return to baseline over 40 minutes | Paramyotonia congenita (T1313M or R1448C sodium) |
| II | Postexercise amplitude decrement that improves with each trials | No postexercise amplitude change or small transient decrement | Myotonia congenita (chloride channel mutation) |
| III | No postexercise amplitude change | No postexercise amplitude change | Other forms of myotonia (G1306A, 1693T sodium) |
| IV | Postexercise amplitude increment that increases with each trial | Transient postexercise amplitude increment followed by late continuous decrement over 40 minutes | HyperKPP (T704M sodium) |
| V | No postexercise amplitude change | Late continuous postexercise amplitude decrement over 40 minutes | HypoKPP-1 (R528H calcium) |

disease is often within the first decade, whereas the onset of Becker myotonia is generally at 10–14 years of age. Although myotonia can affect all skeletal muscles, it is especially prominent in the legs, where it is occasionally severe enough to impede a patient's ability to walk or run. In rare cases, sudden noise causes sufficient generalized stiffness to make the patient fall to the ground and remain rigid for several seconds. The recessive and dominant forms share many similarities, but some clinical features help distinguish the two. In general, patients with recessive disease experience transitory bouts of weakness after periods of disuse and may develop progressive myopathy (Kornblum et al., 2010); in addition, muscle hypertrophy and disease severity are greater than in the dominant form. Becker myotonia is more common than Thomsen disease. In contrast to myotonic dystrophies, affected individuals have no systemic disorders such as cardiomyopathy, cataracts, endocrinopathies, ventilatory weakness, and skeletal deformities.

### Pathophysiology

Electrical instability of the sarcolemma leads to muscle stiffness by causing repetitive electric discharges of affected muscle fibers. Early in vivo studies in myotonic goats revealed greatly diminished sarcolemmal chloride conductance in affected muscle fibers. This causes a depolarization of the sarcolemmal membrane and muscle hyperexcitability. Genetic linkage analysis for both recessive and dominant forms of MC pointed to a locus on chromosome 7q, where the responsible gene, *CLCN1*, encodes the major skeletal muscle chloride channel. More than 70 mutations have been identified within *CLCN1*, and, interestingly, some of these mutations are recognized to cause both dominant and recessive forms (Zhang et al., 2000). Examination of the functional effects of several myotonia-causing *CLCN1* mutations in heterologous expression systems reveals effects on channel gating or membrane expression levels, usually resulting in a decreased chloride conductance (Desaphy et al., 2014; Zhang et al., 2000).

### Diagnosis

On clinical exam, patients may display muscle hypertrophy, often giving patients a muscular or athletic appearance. Muscle strength and reflexes are normal, although there may be mild proximal weakness. Tapping the belly of a muscle with a percussion hammer can elicit percussion myotonia that lasts for several seconds. Action myotonia can be also demonstrated by having patients make a strong grip or closing the eyes tightly and then opening them. With repetitive contractions, one may find relaxation easier, due to a warm-up phenomenon.

Electrodiagnostic testing is also helpful. NCS may find decremental CMAP amplitudes on repetitive stimulation at 10 Hz or higher. EMG also demonstrates myotonia. The SET and LET may show transient decrease in CMAP after the first trial and no significant change in amplitudes after exercise, respectively (Fournier pattern II, Table 98.4). This pattern is seen more commonly in individuals with the autosomal recessive form. Greater than 20% decrement of amplitude-and-area during SET is specific for MC (Tan et al., 2011). Biopsy is usually nonspecific, showing enlarged fibers in hypertrophied muscle, increased numbers of internalized nuclei, and decreased type 2B fibers (Table 98.4).

### Treatment

Many patients (especially with Thomsen disease) experience only mild symptoms and do not require treatment. For those with more severe myotonia (especially with Becker myotonia), sodium channel blocking agents remain the mainstay of treatment. Mexiletine is the most commonly used and was shown to be effective in treating myotonia in a preliminary randomized placebo-controlled study (Statland et al., 2012). Other sodium channel blockers such as tocainide, phenytoin, procainamide, and quinine exhibit variable degrees of efficacy.

## Potassium-Aggravated Myotonia

### Clinical

PAM is a rare autosomal dominant disorder with clinical features similar to MC, except that the myotonia fluctuates and worsens with potassium administration. Distinguishing PAM from other nondystrophic myopathies is important because PAM patients respond to carbonic anhydrase inhibitors. Episodic weakness and progressive myopathy do not occur. Symptom severity varies, with some patients experiencing only mild fluctuating stiffness and others a more protracted painful myotonia. PAM now encompasses the conditions previously known as *myotonia fluctuans*, *myotonia permanens*, and *acetazolamide-sensitive myotonia*. Exercise or rest after exercise, potassium loads, and depolarizing neuromuscular blocking agents aggravate myotonia, whereas cold exposure has no objective effect. Prominent myotonia of the orbicularis oculi and painful myotonia suggest the diagnosis.

### Pathophysiology

PAM links to chromosome 17q, where mutations in the *SCN4A* gene cause the disease. This sodium channel is the same one implicated in hyperKPP, PMC, and the sodium channel subtype of hypoKPP (see the earlier discussion and Fig. 98.1). Functional expression studies reveal that the disease-causing mutations lead to a large persistent sodium current secondary to an increased rate of recovery from inactivation and an increased frequency of late channel openings (Wu et al., 2001). The cause of myotonia is enhanced inward current, which leads to prolonged depolarization and subsequent membrane hyperexcitability.

### Diagnosis

Diagnosis can often be made clinically and screening for the mutated gene is becoming more available. Distinguishing PAM from other episodic nondystrophic myotonias may be difficult. Unlike hyperKPP and PMC, PAM patients do not experience weakness. Another distinction between PAM and PMC is the lack of response to muscle cooling, either clinically or on EMG. The SET and LET show no change or decrement (Fournier pattern III), although other patterns have been seen. (Table 98.4)

### Treatment

Carbonic anhydrase inhibitors markedly reduce the severity and frequency of attacks of myotonia. Acetazolamide is most commonly used (see Table 98.3).

## Andersen-Tawil Syndrome

### Clinical

ATS is a rare autosomal dominant disorder characterized by the tetrad of periodic paralysis, cardiac arrhythmias, dysmorphic features (including hypertelorism, micrognathia, low-set ears, high-arched or cleft palate, dental findings, short stature, and clinodactyly) and distinct neurocognitive deficits in executive function and abstract reasoning (Yoon et al., 2006a, 2006b). The periodic paralysis, often triggered by rest after exercise, prolonged rest, and stress, is often the presenting symptom and can be hypo-, normo-, or hyperkalemic. The cardiac phenotype, often discovered later, includes prolonged QT intervals, but bidirectional ventricular tachycardia is common. Despite the known association of cardiac arrhythmias in rare periodic paralysis patients, ATS was only recognized as a separate entity in 1971. In families segregating an ATS allele, the phenotypic expressivity can vary greatly. Patients can manifest one, two, three, or four features of the tetrad, and the severity of any single feature can be extremely variable. Rare individuals are asymptomatic disease-gene carriers.

### Pathophysiology

Mutations in the *KCNJ2* gene on chromosome 17q account for approximately two-thirds of ATS probands. *KCNJ2* encodes a widely expressed inwardly rectifying potassium channel (Plaster et al., 2001). Interestingly, among all identified probands, about 50% have an autosomal dominant disorder, and identification of sporadic cases with de novo mutations is common. The mechanisms of channel dysfunction are heterogeneous, including impaired phospholipid binding, pore function, or protein trafficking. Because VGKCs are tetrameric complexes, many (if not all) of the mutations are dominant negative. *KCNJ5*, encoding another inwardly rectifying potassium channel, may represent a second ATS-associated gene, as a mutation there was identified in one patient with ATS who did not harbor any *KCNJ2* mutation (Kokunai et al., 2014).

### Diagnosis

Previous studies that took into account the variable penetrance of ATS classified individuals as affected if two of three criteria were met: paroxysmal weakness, prolonged QT interval with or without ventricular dysrhythmias, or characteristic dysmorphic features (Yoon et al., 2006a). ATS should be included in the differential diagnosis of any individual with documented long-QT syndrome, even in the absence of periodic paralysis or dysmorphism. Some family members of patients with the full clinical triad show only prolonged QT intervals. Similarly, perform ECG on all patients with suspected periodic paralysis for careful measurement of the QT interval.

Often the diagnosis of ATS is established when an individual with paroxysmal weakness presents during an acute phase with ECG abnormalities. However, one often overlooks the diagnosis because the cardiac abnormalities, as with periodic muscle weakness, can be transitory and missed on routine ECG. A Holter monitor can capture episodic dysrhythmias or longer tracings for QT-interval analysis when ATS is suspected and the standard ECG is normal. Cardiac monitoring under provocative maneuvers such as tilt-table testing or graded exercise protocols may allow dysrhythmias to surface and should be utilized when the diagnosis of ATS is highly suggested but prior cardiac evaluation is unremarkable.

Creatine kinase concentrations are often normal during episodes of weakness but are occasionally elevated. Depending on the particular mutation, potassium concentrations during an attack are usually low but can be high or normal. Provocative testing in any case of periodic paralysis may be risky, and hypokalemic challenges in ATS may be particularly dangerous because of the potential to exacerbate preexisting QT prolongation and trigger life-threatening ventricular arrhythmias.

### Treatment

The goal of therapy is to control underlying cardiac arrhythmias and to decrease the frequency, severity, and duration of attacks of weakness. Unfortunately, in some families, treatments for arrhythmias can produce weakness, and treatments for weakness may exacerbate cardiac dysrhythmias. The periodic paralysis usually responds to carbonic anhydrase inhibitors. In ATS with hypokalemic weakness, oral potassium ingestion treats acute attacks. Prophylaxis with daily sustained-release potassium tablets may prevent attacks of weakness. Maintaining a high serum potassium level (>4.5 mEq/L) also has the additional advantage of narrowing the QT interval, thus reducing the likelihood of developing ventricular arrhythmias.

Treatment of the prolonged QT interval depends on the severity of the underlying arrhythmias. The use of beta-blockers is a mainstay of treatment in long QT. Clinical experience shows that patients with ATS tolerate these agents well. In the presence of syncope due to sustained ventricular tachycardia, the placement of an implantable defibrillator is useful. Some evidence suggests that flecainide may be effective in the treatment of severe ATS-associated ventricular arrhythmias (Bökenkamp et al., 2007; Pellizzón et al., 2008).

## Malignant Hyperthermia

Malignant hyperthermia is an uncommon syndrome that manifests as a hypermetabolic reaction to volatile anesthetics and depolarizing neuromuscular blocking agents. Inheritance is usually autosomal dominant, but multifactorial inheritance also occurs. Further complicating efforts to define the inheritance and the incidence is that many people with malignant hyperthermia do not develop symptoms on all exposures, and some never experience exposure to inciting agents.

Malignant hyperthermia displays genetic heterogeneity. Disease-causing mutations have been identified in *RYR1*, the gene encoding the skeletal muscle ryanodine receptor, and *CACNA1S*, the L-type VGCC implicated in hypoKPP. The ryanodine receptor is a calcium channel expressed on the endoplasmic reticulum mediating calcium release in excitation–contraction coupling. To date, more than 20 disease-causing point mutations in *RYR1* have been identified in humans, accounting for half of affected families.

Clinical manifestations of malignant hyperthermia include tachypnea, tachycardia, rigidity, acidosis, rhabdomyolysis, and hyperthermia. Unfortunately, an intraoperative diagnosis often becomes apparent when symptoms develop. In patients in whom there is a family history suggestive of the diagnosis or in those who have had an event during previous anesthesia, the *caffeine-contracture test* remains the best-available test for diagnosis. A thin strip of explanted muscle is stimulated electrically to achieve maximal contraction and then exposed to caffeine; increased contracture signifies the disease. Although this test is useful, results are highly operator dependent. Therefore, if any possibility of this condition exists, the standard of practice is the pretreatment of every patient undergoing anesthesia with dantrolene. Although malignant hyperthermia is always a consideration in patients who become weak with anesthesia, a periodic paralysis—distinguished by flaccidity rather than rigidity—may be uncovered during periods of stress.

Immediate termination of exposure to anesthesia, immediate effective core cooling, and the administration of dantrolene sodium, an inhibitor of calcium release from the sarcoplasmic reticulum, are the mainstays of treatment for this condition and have significantly reduced mortality since their introduction into clinical use.

### Congenital Myasthenic Syndromes

The congenital myasthenic syndromes are a rare, heterogeneous, nonimmune group of disorders of neuromuscular transmission. Chapter 108 covers these disorders in detail.

## GENETIC DISORDERS OF NEURONAL ION CHANNELS

The disorders considered here involve inherited ion channel defects in neurons. Like muscle channelopathies, these defects also result in episodic phenotypes. Many such mutations cause epilepsy, considered separately in a later section.

### Familial Hemiplegic Migraine

#### Clinical

Familial hemiplegic migraine (FHM) is a rare autosomal dominant subtype of migraine with motor aura, characterized by lateralized motor weakness of variable intensity—hemiparesis to hemiplegia. Other aura symptoms such as visual aura, paresthesia, ataxia, fever, or lethargy may present during the attack. Motor symptoms often start in the hand and gradually spread to other areas, over 20–30 minutes, although it may occur suddenly mimicking a stroke. The duration of the symptoms can be variable, from a few hours to weeks. The diagnostic hallmark is episodic, reversible, unilateral motor weakness, along with at least one other kind of aura.

Cortical spreading depression (CSD) is a widely accepted physiology underlying the migraine aura. CSD is a slow self-propagating wave of neuronal and glial depolarization, followed by hyperpolarization.

Four subtypes, genetically defined (see later discussion), are distinguishable by clinical characteristics. FHM type 1 (FHM1) accounts for about 50%–75% of families. FHM1 is commonly associated with cerebellar degeneration. In addition to weakness, auras always involve additional symptoms, including sensory, visual, and language disturbances (Ducros et al., 2001). Severe aura attacks may last days or weeks and may involve fever, meningismus, and impaired consciousness, ranging from confusion to coma. Recovery between attacks is typically complete, although 30%–50% of patients with FHM1 exhibit permanent progressive cerebellar signs that include nystagmus, gait or limb ataxia, or dysarthria. These manifestations of FHM1 overlap with episodic ataxia type 2 (EA2) and spinocerebellar ataxia type 6 (Fig. 98.6), which are allelic with *CACNA1A* mutations (see the following discussion). By contrast, the characteristic features of FHM2 are an absence of cerebellar signs and a tendency for lower penetrance than in FHM1. FHM2 accounts for less than 25% of cases. Ataxia does not occur in FHM3, a rarer and more recently defined entity. FHM4 is diagnosed if there is no known genetic mutation of FHM. Importantly, patients with FHM exhibit a spectrum of disease expression, and subtype classification is likely to evolve with our knowledge of underlying genetics.

#### Pathophysiology

FHM is a genetically heterogeneous condition that links to three loci on chromosomes 1q, 2q, and 19p; other loci are possible (Ducros et al., 1997). FHM1 includes the 50%–75% of families that show genetic

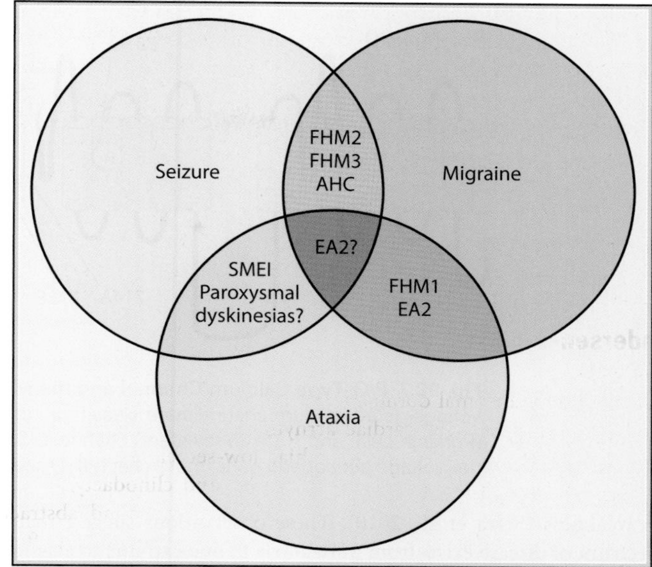


**Fig. 98.6 Venn Diagram Showing Phenotypic Overlap Among Various Channelopathies.** *AHC*, Alternating hemiplegia of childhood; *EA*, episodic ataxia; *FHM*, familial hemiplegic migraine; *SMEI*, severe myoclonic epilepsy of infancy.

linkage to chromosome 19p13, with causative missense mutations in the *CACNA1A* gene (Ophoff et al., 1996). This gene encodes the pore-forming $\alpha_{1A}$-subunit of the neuronal P/Q-type VGCC, which is distributed widely throughout the brain. It is present at motor nerve terminals and the neuromuscular junction and is the principal calcium channel expressed by cerebellar Purkinje and granular neurons. These channels play an integral role in the action potential–triggered presynaptic calcium influx at nerve terminals that triggers vesicular fusion, playing an important role in neurotransmitter release. At least 17 different missense mutations and one nonsense mutation (Jen et al., 1999) are reported in CACNA1A (Fig. 98.7). These cause a variety of altered but not lost functions: changes in channel conductance, kinetics of inactivation, and current density (Hans et al., 1999; Kraus et al., 2000). Indeed, these mutations may confer gain of function, because many appear to cause a hyperpolarizing shift in the activation voltage, meaning that channels open and permit calcium influx at abnormally low membrane potentials. In one extreme case, the S218L mutation confers both the tendency to open near the resting potential of many neurons (−60 to −50 mV) and overall slowing and reduction in channel inactivation, thus causing marked increases in overall calcium influx. In keeping with this extreme biophysical profile, S218L produces a severe clinical phenotype of aura attacks triggered by minor head trauma and leading to deep coma and prolonged cerebral edema (Tottene et al., 2005). On the other hand, some loss-of-function mutations associated with episodic ataxia type 2 (EA2) may also cause migraine symptoms (Jen et al., 2004), suggesting that a direct correlation between presynaptic VGCC-mediated calcium entry and disease severity is too simplistic. Importantly, the mechanism linking altered channel biophysics to disease expression is controversial and defies a simple model.

As mentioned earlier, other mutations in *CACNA1A* cause different dominantly inherited neurological disorders, including EA2 and spinocerebellar ataxia type 6 (SCA6). Although most patients with FHM1 also suffer persistent cerebellar deficits, a few mutations in *CACNA1A* cause only hemiplegic migraine (Ducros et al., 2001), and one mutation appears to cause classical migraine with aura but

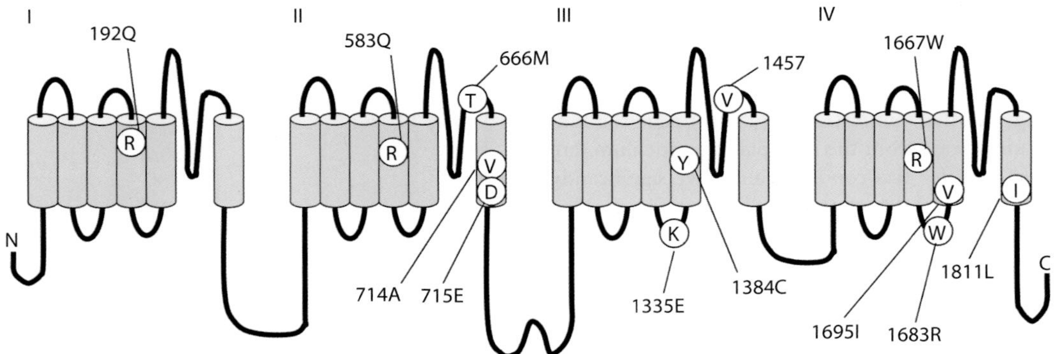


**Fig. 98.7** P/Q-Type Calcium Channel and the Mutations Causing Familial Hemiplegic Migraine Type 2. Voltage-gated calcium channels are classified into transient (T-type), long-lasting (L-type), N (neuronal), P/Q (Purkinje cell), and R (toxin-resistant) channels. Shown is the *CACNA1A*-encoded $\alpha_{1A}$-subunit, which forms the voltage sensor and pore of the channel. Disease-causing missense mutations are illustrated.

no weakness (Serra et al., 2010). These observations suggest that a spectrum of disease exists from pure ataxia at one extreme to classical migraine at the other.

Patients with FHM2, representing 10%–20% of all FHM sufferers, exhibit mutations in the *ATP1A2* gene encoding the $\alpha_2$-subunit of the $Na^+/K^+$-ATPase, a protein responsible for maintaining the membrane potential in neurons and other cells (De Fusco et al., 2003). This pump plays a critical role in establishing transmembrane ionic gradients and is in this way directly integral to the function of innumerable ion channels and other proteins. Many missense mutations have been identified, probably resulting in a loss of function but not loss of surface expression (De Fusco et al., 2003), possibly by a reduced affinity for potassium (Segall et al., 2004). Although an ionic mechanism is likely, the precise pathophysiological connection to hemiplegic aura or head pain remains obscure. Additional mutations in *ATP1A2* may also cause a form of benign familial infantile seizures (see the later section on Epilepsy; Vanmolkot et al., 2003) and alternating hemiplegia of childhood (Swoboda et al., 2004). A single mutation was found to cause hemiplegic migraine with cerebellar findings (Spadaro et al., 2004), challenging the conception that this association is specific for *CACNA1A* mutations.

FHM3 involves mutations in the *SCN1A* gene on chromosome 2q24 that encodes a neuronal voltage-gated sodium channel $\alpha_1$-subunit. To date, three missense mutations have been identified, and the two that have been characterized electrophysiologically each confer upon the channel more rapid recovery from fast inactivation and thus the potential for faster firing frequency and neuronal hyperexcitability (Castro et al., 2009; Dichgans et al., 2005). Other mutations in *SCN1A* cause some cases of severe myoclonic epilepsy of infancy and generalized epilepsy with febrile seizures plus (see the later section on Epilepsy). Interestingly, mutations causing epilepsy occur near those causing FHM3, and one mutation—L263V—causes both clinical phenotypes (Castro et al., 2009). Epilepsy has also been reported in cases of FHM1 and FHM2, pointing to the intriguing possibility of a pathogenic link between seizure and migraine.

## Diagnosis

Genetic testing is now commercially available, but the diagnosis is mostly made clinically. Family history is clearly helpful in demonstrating autosomal dominance, but it is important to note that typical migraine syndromes may also show a strong (if less regular) familial pattern. Certain clinical elements of FHM help distinguish it from classical migraine with aura. Although the aura symptoms may be similar to those in classical migraine, FHM patients are more likely to experience motor, speech, and sensory symptoms. Furthermore, the duration of the headache, as well as the duration of the visual and sensory components of the aura, are typically greater in FHM patients (Thomsen et al., 2002). Although patients with classical migraine often experience the aura in isolation from the headache, FHM patients experience an associated headache virtually all the time. Infrequently, FHM patients may experience bilateral weakness, whereas this is generally not the case in patients with classical migraine. Finally, although defined genetically, one might clinically suspect FHM based on an association with cerebellar abnormalities or seizures (see Fig. 98.6).

## Treatment

Anecdotal evidence suggests that acetazolamide reduces the frequency of migraine attacks (Battistini et al., 1999; Jen et al., 2004). As suggested by functionally enhanced calcium currents in many cases of FHM, the calcium channel blocker verapamil aborted an attack when administered intravenously (Yu and Horowitz, 2001). To date, no controlled study has tested the efficacy of these or other agents in FHM. The guidelines for treating common migraine may be applied, except that triptans and ergotamine are not used, out of concern—possibly unwarranted—for stroke (Artto et al., 2007). Nimodipine is contraindicated because of the risk of worsening symptoms (Mjåset and Russell, 2008).

# Familial Episodic Ataxias

The familial episodic ataxias (EAs) are rare, dominantly inherited diseases characterized by episodes of ataxia of early onset, often with completely normal cerebellar function between attacks (Jen et al., 2007). Of the seven syndromes now recognized (EA1–EA7), the two most common forms, EA1 and EA2, are best described.

## Clinical

Characteristic of EA1 are attacks of cerebellar incoordination with jerking limb movements, often accompanied by slurred speech, that last for seconds to minutes. The episodes can occur spontaneously, but common triggers include exertion, infection, stress, or startle. Between attacks, patients may show *myokymia*, muscle rippling resulting from motor nerve hyperexcitability, especially in the hands and around the eyes. Symptom onset is in infancy, with spontaneous resolution in the second to third decade. Frequency, duration, and intensity of attacks vary greatly. EA1 is associated with epilepsy and hearing impairment (Spillane et al., 2016).

Patients with EA2 experience episodes of truncal ataxia lasting hours to days, precipitated by exertion and stress. Age of onset varies between childhood and young adulthood but is most frequently in the second decade. Vertigo, nausea, and vomiting are present in more than half of patients, and many exhibit spontaneous nystagmus that is not seen interictally. Between episodes, the patient returns to normal but frequently displays gaze-evoked nystagmus with features typical of rebound nystagmus (Jen et al., 2007). Less commonly, positional and, later in the disease course, spontaneous downbeat nystagmus occurs. Approximately half of EA2 patients report headaches that meet criteria for migraine. Since mutations causing EA2 are in the same gene as in FHM1, this is not surprising.

### Pathophysiology

The mutation underlying EA1 is on chromosome 12. At least 15 missense mutations have been described in the responsible gene, *KCNA1*, which encodes a delayed rectifier VGKC ($K_v$1.1) that opens with a delay after membrane depolarization, allowing $K^+$ efflux and membrane repolarization (see Fig. 98.3). Co-expression of mutant and wild-type channels results in delayed outward potassium current and impaired membrane repolarization following an action potential (Zerr et al., 1998), a dominant-negative effect that could lead to increased neuronal excitability and neurotransmitter release. The delayed rectifier potassium channel is widely expressed in the nervous system, with highest levels in the cerebellum and myelinated axons of peripheral nerves. In the cerebellum, an imbalance between inhibition and excitation could result in brief episodic incoordination. Similarly, in the peripheral motor nerves, impaired repolarization could lead to repetitive neuronal activity and resultant myokymia. Suggesting that these two effects may be mechanistically distinct is a *KCNA1* missense mutation that causes an episodic ataxia more akin to EA2 without myokymia (Lee et al., 2004a) and another missense mutation resulting in myokymia without ataxia (Rea et al., 2002).

EA2 is caused by mutations in *CACNA1A*, which encodes $Ca_v$2.1, a pore-forming α1A subunit of the calcium channel (Ophoff et al., 1996). In addition to FHM1, *CACNA1A* mutations also causes SCA6, resulting in cerebellar dysfunction. While FHM and EA are paroxysmal, SCA is not paroxysmal but characterized by progressive cerebellar degeneration. Various mutations have been found; however, the common pathophysiology appears to be cortical depression from neural hyperexcitability (Vincent et al., 2007). Whereas FHM1 is associated with missense mutations in the same gene, the genetic alterations associated with EA2 seem more dramatic. Of the approximately 30 mutations described so far, most are truncating, a few are missense, one is insertional, and one is due to expansion of a triplet CAG domain. Functional expression studies of some of these mutations reveal loss of voltage sensitivity or complete loss of channel function (Guida et al., 2001), suggesting that haploinsufficiency may underlie the phenotype. Some mutations may additionally interfere with protein folding and trafficking (Wan et al., 2005).

EA5 results from mutation of the VGCC $\beta_4$-subunit gene *CACNB4*, also implicated in idiopathic generalized epilepsy (see the later section on Epilepsy); it is clinically similar to EA2, except that seizures are an additional feature (Escayg et al., 2000a). Mutations in *SLC1A3*, the gene encoding the excitatory amino acid transporter EAAT1, cause EA6, an episodic ataxia associated with hemiplegia and seizures (Jen et al., 2005). The genes for EA3 (1q42), EA4, or EA7 (19q13) have not been identified.

### Diagnosis

Diagnosis is mostly clinical. Family history is helpful in making the diagnosis, despite rare cases of de novo mutations. The probability of examining a patient during an attack is low, so careful examination for interictal signs is important. Although almost half of EA1 patients

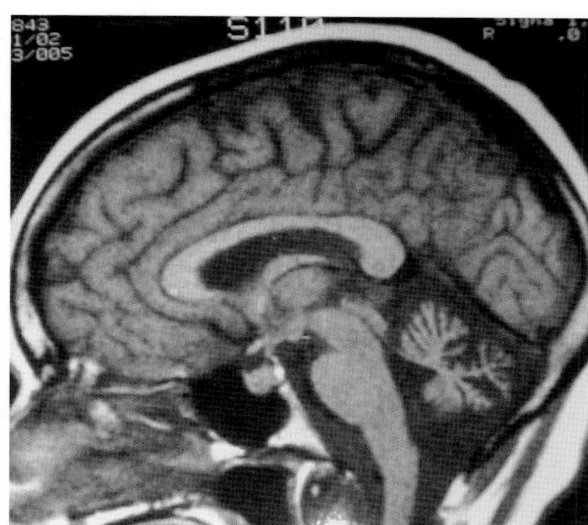

**Fig. 98.8 Sagittal Magnetic Resonance Image From a Patient with Episodic Ataxia Type 2.** Note the significant cerebellar atrophy from this relatively advanced case. Type 1 patients do not display cerebellar atrophy (not shown).

complain of diplopia, they do not have nystagmus, which helps distinguish them from EA2 patients. The brevity of attacks and the persistent interictal myokymia seen in EA1 also help distinguish this from EA2. EA2 patients may demonstrate interictal end-point tremor or impaired suppression of the vestibulo-ocular reflex. They tend to have subtle and slowly progressive interictal cerebellar signs, particularly gaze-evoked nystagmus. Although progressive ataxia often develops, it is rarely severe enough to prevent walking without assistance. Magnetic resonance imaging (MRI) may detect cerebellar atrophy, especially of the anterior vermis (Fig. 98.8), whereas EA1 patients have no cerebellar atrophy. Interestingly, there appears to be an increased incidence of epilepsy in both EA1 and EA2 patients, emphasizing the overlapping symptoms, possibly due to shared mechanisms (see Fig. 98.6). Genetic testing is available clinically and on a research basis.

### Treatment

Acetazolamide reduces the severity of attacks. Response to treatment varies among families, but generally, patients with EA2 have a greater response than those with EA1. Carbamazepine or 4-aminopyridine (Strupp et al., 2004) are beneficial in some patients. Because stress and strenuous exercise often exacerbate attacks, lifestyle modification can be quite effective.

## Hereditary Hyperekplexia

### Clinical

Human startle disease, or hereditary hyperekplexia, is a rare hereditary disease characterized by an exaggerated startle response to sensory stimuli, plus neonatal hypertonia, hyperreflexia, and myoclonic jerks. It was first described in a Swedish family with startle reflexes and violent falls due to generalized stiffness (Kirstein et al., 1958). The usual inheritance is autosomal dominant, but several recessive mutations exist. Patients have generalized stiffness immediately after birth, which resolve over time (Koning-Tijsssen et al. 2000). The normal startle response is a primitive reflex that manifests as a stereotyped sequence of blinking, grimacing, neck flexion, and arm abduction and flexion. Both pathological and normal startle responses originate from the caudal brainstem, spreading rostro-caudally, as demonstrated using EMG in different muscles (Bakker et al., 2009). Patients exhibit

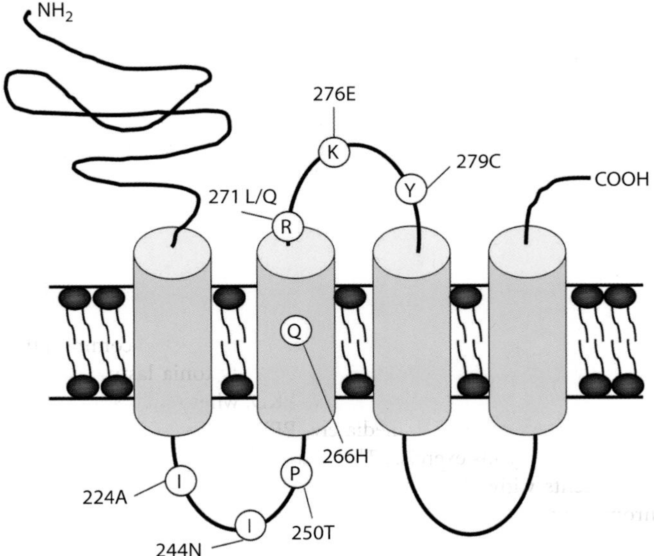


**Fig. 98.9 The α1-Subunit of the Human Glycine Receptor and Pathogenic Mutations Underlying Hyperekplexia.** The glycine receptor shares significant homology with the nicotinic acetylcholine receptor, possessing five subunits to form a channel pore.

an overreaction to unexpected visual, tactile, or particularly auditory stimuli, with sudden generalized myoclonic jerks followed by stiffness, often resulting in uncontrolled falling during standing and walking. Following a startle reflex, there is generalized stiffness for a few seconds (Suhren et al., 1966). Consequently, patients often develop a characteristic slow, wide-based, cautious gait. Consciousness is preserved during the attacks, which helps distinguish this from startle epilepsy. Attack frequency may increase during times of stress, fear, lack of sleep, or the expectation of being frightened. The onset of symptoms may be as early as the neonatal period, with rigidity or generalized hypertonia, nocturnal limb jerking, and an exaggerated startle response. Attacks vary in severity and frequency and may be so severe as to cause apneic episodes and even death. Affected children may show a slight delay in motor development. A minor form of hyperekplexia, less common than the major form, manifests as an exaggerated startle response without associated symptoms, such as neonatal stiffness.

### Pathophysiology

Since being first reported in 1958, there are many reported mutations responsible for hereditary hyperekplexia, including *GLRA1, GLRB, GPHN, GLYT2* (also named *SLC6A5*), and *ARHGEF9* (Harvey et al., 2004, Rees et al., 2002, 2003). Eighty percent of hereditary hyperekplexia is caused by a mutation in the *GLRA1* gene on chromosome 5q encoding the glycine receptor $\alpha_1$-subunit. The glycine receptor is a heteropentameric ligand-gated chloride channel composed of three ligand-binding $\alpha_1$-subunits and two β-subunits, located in postsynaptic membrane, mediating fast inhibitory neurotransmission in the brainstem and spinal cord. Several dominant, recessive, and de novo *GLRA1* missense point mutations are seen in familial hyperekplexia patients. Most mutations flank the M2 pore-forming domain (Fig. 98.9). The physiological consequence of mutations in the $\alpha_1$-subunit is decreased glycine sensitivity, impaired channel opening, and uncoupling of agonist binding from channel activation. These changes reduce glycinergic inhibition and increase neuronal excitability.

Mutations in the gene encoding the glycine receptor β-subunit *(GLRB)* also cause hyperekplexia. An example is a compound heterozygous patient with spontaneous hyperekplexia possessing a missense mutation on one allele and a splice-site mutation on the other (Rees et al., 2002). Electrophysiological studies showed reduced sensitivity of the mutant channel to agonist, suggesting impaired binding of glycine to the channel.

Finally, loss-of-function mutations in *GLYT2* (also named *SLC6A5*), the gene encoding the presynaptic glycine transporter 2 protein, have been identified in three families with hereditary hyperekplexia. Glycine transporters mediate synaptic reuptake of the neurotransmitter, and its genetic deletion reproduces hyperekplexia in mice (Eulenburg et al., 2006). Reduction of glycine transporter function is expected to prolong glycine neurotransmission; how this leads to hyperekplexia is unknown.

### Diagnosis

Physical examination may reveal diffuse hyperreflexia. The diffuse hypertonicity in infancy generally resolves with time, and adults have normal tone between attacks. An exaggerated *head-retraction reflex* is common in these patients. Tapping the forehead or root of the nose downward with a reflex hammer causes a brisk involuntary backward jerk of the head. This reflex is generally absent in unaffected individuals. Distinguish this condition from startle epilepsy, a rare seizure disorder characterized by startle-induced tonic spasm of a limb followed by a complex partial seizure; asymmetrical tonic posturing occurs during spells, and patients often have developmental delay and focal neurological signs. Neuroimaging in startle epilepsy reveals cortical dysplasia, although an interictal electroencephalogram (EEG) rarely shows a clear seizure focus. By contrast, familial hyperekplexia patients typically have normal development, display no ictal EEG findings to suggest a seizure disorder, have normal brain imaging, and maintain full consciousness during attacks. Brainstem pathology, including pontine hemorrhage or infarction, multiple sclerosis, vascular brainstem compression, and brainstem encephalitis, may cause a syndrome similar to hyperekplexia. Rarely, sporadic cases of hyperekplexia occur; therefore, do not exclude the diagnosis in patients lacking a family history.

### Treatment

Treatment with benzodiazepines helps reduce neonatal hypertonia and significantly reduces the severity and frequency of startle-induced attacks in some patients. Although clonazepam is the standard treatment, low-dose clobazam is effective in the treatment of hyperekplexia and well tolerated in infants. Benzodiazepines act by increasing GABA-mediated inhibition and have no effect on glycinergic transmission. This suggests that enhancing the GABA-mediated inhibition may compensate for glycinergic dysfunction.

## Hereditary Peripheral Nerve Disorders

### *SCN9A* Mutation

*Primary erythromelalgia (PE)*, also known as *familial erythromelalgia* or *Weir Mitchell disease*, is an autosomal dominant disorder characterized by burning pain and redness in the limbs in response to warmth or moderate exercise (Dib-Hajj et al., 2008; Yang et al., 2004). Paroxysmal extreme pain disorder (PEPD), previously known as familial rectal pain syndrome, is characterized by burning pain in the rectal, ocular, and mandibular areas accompanied by autonomic dysfunction, such as skin flushing (Hayden, 1959). Both PE and PEPD are caused by mutations in *SCN9A*, encoding a voltage-gated sodium channel selectively expressed in small-diameter dorsal root ganglion neurons (mostly nociceptors) and sympathetic ganglion neurons. The mutations responsible for PE are gain-of-function mutations that enhance current through the channels by decreasing the voltage threshold for activation, among other effects, while mutations causing PEPD impair the fast inactivation of the sodium channel. The discovery that expression of this sodium channel is narrowly restricted to a population of pain-mediating neurons, and that its enhanced function can result in pain, raises the exciting hypothesis that selective channel blockade may result in relief of chronic pain. Mexiletine and topical lidocaine are used for PE, and carbamazepine has shown benefit in PEPD. Supporting a more general role for this gene, some polymorphisms correlate with a lowered pain threshold in patients without primary erythermalgia (Reimann et al., 2010). Loss-of-function mutations in the same gene lead to an inherited insensitivity to pain (hereditary sensory and autonomic neuropathy type IID). A selective antagonist of this channel does not yet exist.

### *TRPV4* Mutation

*Scapuloperoneal spinal muscular atrophy*, *congenital distal spinal muscular atrophy*, and *Charcot-Marie-Tooth disease type 2C* (or hereditary motor sensory neuropathy type 2) are related disorders. Characteristic of all are autosomal dominant inheritance, muscle weakness and wasting, and other features that can include arthrogryposis, scoliosis, or vocal cord paralysis. These disorders result from mutations in *TRPV4*, the gene on chromosome 12q encoding the vanilloid transient receptor potential (TRP) protein, a peripheral nerve nonselective cation channel activated by many noxious stimuli such as heat, mechanical stress, osmotic pressure, and inflammatory cytokines (Auer-Grumbach et al., 2010; Deng et al., 2010; Landoure et al., 2010). Although the pathogenic mechanism remains unclear, all known mutations affect the ankyrin repeat region of the protein, where regulatory proteins, second messengers, and other TRPV4 channels normally bind. Unlike most disorders in this chapter, the phenotypes resulting from *TRPV4* mutations are not episodic.

## Paroxysmal Dyskinesia

The paroxysmal dyskinesias are rare syndromes characterized by recurrent, episodic attacks of involuntary movements, such as dystonia, chorea, athetosis, ballism, or a combination. While some cases may be sporadic, most exhibit autosomal dominant inheritance.

*Paroxysmal non-kinesigenic dyskinesia* (PNKD) involves attacks of dystonia, chorea, or athetosis, occurring spontaneously or triggered by alcohol, coffee, stress, or fatigue. An aura of paresthesia, tension, or dizziness may precede abnormal movements that typically involve the limbs. The attacks last for minutes to hours, which is longer in duration and less frequent than paroxysmal kinesigenic dyskinesia (PKD). In a family with an autosomal dominant pattern of PKND and generalized epilepsy (mostly absence attacks, as discussed later), a mutation of *KCNMA1* on chromosome 10q was identified (Du et al., 2005). This gene encodes the α-subunit of the BK channel, a potassium channel that normally activates with both membrane depolarization and a rise in intracellular calcium; the mutation heightens calcium sensitivity, enhancing channel activity. Ethanol may also activate the BK channel (Davies et al., 2003), suggesting a mechanism whereby alcohol consumption in synergy with the mutation may precipitate a dyskinetic attack (Du et al., 2005). PNKD without epilepsy is linked to mutation of the *PNKD* gene (previously called the myofibrillogenesis regulator gene, *MR1*) on chromosome 2 (Lee et al., 2004b); subsequently, the protein encoded by this gene has been shown to encode a novel synaptic protein regulating exocytosis (Shen et al., 2015). Studies in a mouse model of the human mutations recapitulated caffeine- and ethanol-sensitive attacks and abnormal dopamine signaling. Neuropharmacological experiments showed that the abnormal signaling is being mediated through the indirect pathway of the striatum (Lee et al. 2012). Treatment of PNKD involves avoidance of triggers; benzodiazepines, including clonazepam, often help.

Another related disorder is PKD. It involves attacks triggered by sudden movement, change in direction or startle, often with auras as in PNKD. Attacks commonly manifest with choreoathetosis and dystonia, typically lasting for 5–10 seconds. It may occur as frequently as daily or only a few times per year. Mutations in the proline-rich transmembrane protein 2 *(PRRT2)* gene on chromosome 16q cause PKD and benign familial infantile seizures (as discussed later; Chen et al., 2011; Lee et al., 2012). PRRT2 function is not known but thought to be involved in neurotransmitter release and synaptic vesicle fusion (Valtorta et al., 2016). Distinguishing PKD from PNKD is beneficial, as PKD usually responds dramatically to antiepileptic therapy, like carbamazepine and phenytoin (Bruno et al, 2004).

*Paroxysmal exercise-induced dyskinesia* (PED) is less common than PKD and PNKD and involves lower limb dystonia lasting up to 30 minutes, triggered by exercise. Unlike PKD, where sudden movement may precipitate attacks immediately, PED attacks occur after 15–20 minutes of vigorous exercise. The episode lasts from 5 to 30 minutes, and patients with PED usually do not experience aura. *SLC2A1* on chromosome 1p is the gene encoding the GLUT1 glucose transporter protein, and mutations cause PED (Weber et al., 2008) or idiopathic generalized absence seizures (Suls et al., 2008); some mutations in *SLC2A1* may cause more severe clinical phenotypes that include cognitive dysfunction and microcephaly. PED is usually autosomal dominantly inherited. Treatments include trigger avoidance and a ketogenic diet.

A theme emerges from these disorders, such that mutations in certain genes may give rise to phenotypic heterogeneity, involving a spectrum of paroxysmal dyskinesia and epilepsy.

## Other Inherited Neuronal Channelopathies

The rapid proliferation and lowering cost of whole-exome sequencing have led to frequent discoveries of new, rare genetic disorders. As one example, de novo mutations in *GRIN2B*, the gene encoding the *N*-methyl-D-aspartate receptor (NMDA) subunit 2B protein, associate with mental retardation (Endele et al., 2010; O'Roak et al., 2012). NMDA receptors are well known to neuroscientists as the subtype of glutamate receptor that mediates long-term potentiation, a form of synaptic plasticity thought to underlie learning and memory, and the 2B subunit in particular has special importance in the developing brain; it is not surprising that disruption of this receptor would result in impaired learning.

# EPILEPSY

Epilepsy is a disorder with recurrent seizures that affects 1%–2% of the general population. Ion channels are crucial in regulating the excitability of the neurons. Thus the dysfunction of ion channels is believed to cause excessive electrical excitability and resultant seizure activity. In some cases, channel mutations leading to lower excitability in inhibitory neurons could have led to a common final pathway of seizures. Among 977 identified epilepsy-associated genes, 60 genes are ion channel genes (Wang et al., 2016). Although most epilepsies have a complex mode of inheritance, some rare idiopathic epilepsies are monogenic, most of which are autosomal dominant. Discussed here are syndromes associated with an identified gene. As might be expected from diseases characterized by abnormal electrical activity in the brain, familial epilepsy syndromes often result from aberrant ion channel function.

## Familial Focal Epilepsies

Unlike generalized epilepsy syndromes, which exhibit a strong genetic pattern, few focal epilepsy syndromes are genetic. Of these syndromes, only two have known causative mutations.

### Autosomal Dominant Nocturnal Frontal Lobe Epilepsy

A syndrome characterized by clusters of brief partial seizures that occur during light sleep, autosomal dominant nocturnal frontal lobe epilepsy (ADNFLE) is a monogenic disorder with a penetrance of 70%–80%. The motor seizures, which manifest as hyperkinetic tonic stiffening and clonic jerking movements, may occur several times per night, usually shortly after falling asleep or just before awakening. Aura may precede seizures, manifesting as various somatosensory, sensory, and psychic phenomena. Episodes often start with a gasp, grunt, or vocalization, followed by eye opening or staring. Secondary generalization is unusual, and patients remain conscious during the seizures. Patients become symptomatic within the first or second decade of life, although later onset occurs. Seizures generally persist throughout adult life, becoming less severe beyond the fifth decade. Suggesting an important contribution of genetic background, intrafamilial variability in seizure frequency and severity is significant, with some patients experiencing several seizures nightly and others remaining seizure-free for months. Interictal EEG is normal, and ictal EEG may show bifrontal epileptiform discharges. Because of the clinical similarities, ADNFLE is often mistaken for benign nocturnal parasomnia or night terror. Therefore, nocturnal video polysomnography is very useful in distinguishing ADNFLE from these other conditions.

ADNFLE was initially shown to be caused by a point mutation in the nAChR $\alpha_4$-subunit gene *CHRNA4* on chromosome 20q (Steinlein et al., 1995). The nAChRs are acetylcholine-activated cation channels that play an important role in postsynaptic excitation and neurotransmitter release. Four mutations in *CHRNA4* were identified in several ethnic groups. Mutations have also been identified in *CHRNB2* (Phillips et al., 2001) and *CHRNA2* (Aridon et al., 2006), encoding the nAChR $\beta_2$- and $\alpha_2$-subunits. The $\beta_2$-subunit associates closely with the $\alpha_4$-subunit, and the $\alpha_4$–$\beta_2$ combination is the dominant subtype of nAChR in the brain. Mutations in *CHRNA4* and *CHRNB2* involve M2, the second transmembrane domain and the part of the protein thought to line the channel pore. Some cases of ADNFLE link to chromosome 15q24, close to a cluster of three other nAChR subunits, although the responsible mutations have not been elucidated (Philips et al., 1998). Mutations result in increased sensitivity both to activation by acetylcholine and to block by carbamazepine. This latter in vitro observation bears clinical relevance because ADNFLE patients have a good therapeutic response to carbamazepine. Given the wide distribution of nAChRs within the brain, it remains unclear why the epilepsy is focal and why the seizures arise selectively in the frontal lobes.

Missense mutations in the sodium-gated potassium channel gene *KCNT1* on chromosome 9q were found to cause a severe form of ADNFLE. As *KCNT1* is highly expressed in frontal lobes, this may explain cognitive dysfunction and psychiatric symptoms (Heron et al., 2012). The same gene is implicated in malignant migrating partial seizures of infancy (Barcia et al., 2012), in which mutations disrupt a protein kinase C phosphorylation site and lead to constitutive channel hyperactivation, the postulated pathophysiological mechanism (Barcia et al., 2012). Furthermore, a missense mutation in the corticotropin-releasing hormone (CRH) gene has been detected in one Italian family with ADNFLE. It is an interesting finding, as this seems not directly related to channelopathy (Sansoni et al. 2013). Further physiological connection is to be elucidated.

### Familial Temporal Lobe Epilepsies

Temporal lobe epilepsies exist in both sporadic and inherited forms, and the genetics of familial syndromes remain largely unknown (Andermann et al., 2005). The onset of familial lateral temporal lobe epilepsy (FLTLE), or autosomal dominant partial epilepsy with auditory features (ADPEAF), a benign syndrome distinguished from the more common mesial form by characteristic auditory auras, is in the second or third decade, and transmission is autosomal dominant with incomplete penetrance. Approximately 50% of cases involve mutations in the leucine-rich, glioma-inactivated gene 1 *(LGI1)* on chromosome 10q (Kalachikov et al., 2002; Morante-Redolat et al., 2002), whose product was shown to complex with presynaptic A-type VGKCs (Schulte et al., 2006). Normally, *LGI1* appears to reduce channel inactivation, and its dysfunction results in faster inactivation kinetics and, likely, neuronal hyperexcitability. A different gene, *CPA6* on chromosome 8q, encodes a carboxypeptidase enzyme (not an ion channel), in which partial loss of function associates with familial temporal lobe epilepsy (heterozygous mutations) or febrile seizures (homozygous; Salzmann et al., 2012).

## Idiopathic Generalized Epilepsies

The idiopathic generalized epilepsies (IGEs) are among the most common seizure disorders, occurring at an overall frequency of 15%–20% among cohorts of adults and children (Jallon and Latour, 2005). A strong genetic component to IGE transmission exists, but the pattern of inheritance varies between individual disorders. Some rare syndromes, including benign familial neonatal seizures (BFNS) and generalized epilepsy with febrile seizures plus, are monogenic autosomal dominant traits, now known to be due to mutations in ion channel genes. Other more common syndromes—juvenile myoclonic epilepsy (JME), childhood absence epilepsy (CAE), juvenile absence epilepsy (JAE), and epilepsy with grand mal seizures on awakening (EGMA)—exhibit a more complex pattern of inheritance. These disorders, which relate to each other by a continuum of clinical phenotypes and similar EEG findings (see Chapter 100), probably encompass a broad range of individual diseases. We now know that aberrant ion channels underlie at least some of these diseases.

### Benign Familial Neonatal Seizures

BFNS is a rare autosomal dominant disorder. Multifocal or generalized tonic-clonic convulsions appear after the third day of life. Myoclonic seizures are rare. Seizures are generally brief and well controlled by antiepileptic medications, although status epilepticus occurs. Age of onset may extend up to the fourth month of life, and in most cases, seizures disappear spontaneously after a few weeks or months. Although these children usually have normal neurological examination and development, the risk of recurring seizures later in life is about 15%. These later seizures, often provoked by auditory stimuli or emotional stress, are easily controllable with antiepileptic medications. Interictal EEG activity is usually normal, whereas the ictal EEG attenuates at the onset, followed by slow waves, spikes, and a burst–suppression pattern.

Two BFNS-causing genes have been identified—one on chromosome 20q and the other on chromosome 8q. The mutated genes both encode VGKCs: *KCNQ2* and *KCNQ3*, respectively (Biervert et al., 1998; Charlier et al., 1998; Singh et al., 1998). These channels activate by membrane depolarization and contribute to the repolarization of the action potential. Reports appear of missense amino acid deletion, splice-site frameshift mutations, and gene deletions; most involve the *KCNQ2* gene (Fig. 98.10). Functional expression of mutant channels results in reduced potassium current, likely leading to impaired membrane repolarization and thus increased neuronal excitation. *KCNQ2*- and *KCNQ3*-encoded products combine to form a heteromeric channel underlying the M-current (Wang et al., 1998), a potassium conductance found widely in the central nervous system that plays a crucial role in the regulation of neuronal excitability. Co-expressing the mutant gene (*KCNQ2* or *KCNQ3*) together with its wild-type allele and its wild-type partner results in mild (25%) reduction in M-current amplitude. Although it is unclear how the mutated channels either independently or in the form of the M-current lead to seizures, KCNQ2 channels are concentrated in the septum and hippocampus, areas key for control of rhythmic brain activity and neuronal synchronization, and both associated with the generation of epileptic seizures. Thus, even slight alterations in neuronal excitability through impaired KCNQ2/KCNQ3 channel-mediated repolarization could presumably lead to aberrant neuronal synchronization and seizures. In light of reports that lamotrigine and carbamazepine enhance neocortical potassium currents in vitro, they may be of particular use in BFNS patients.

## Generalized Epilepsy with Febrile Seizures Plus

Febrile seizures are the most common seizure disorder in children, affecting 2%–5% of all children younger than 6 years. Although most febrile seizures show complex inheritance, a small proportion transmits in an autosomal dominant pattern. The disorder termed *generalized epilepsy with febrile seizures plus* (GEFS+) refers to the phenotype of individuals who have febrile seizures extending beyond 6 years of age, with or without afebrile generalized tonic-clonic seizures. Although most patients experience only febrile or febrile seizures plus, approximately 30% of patients may experience other generalized epilepsy phenotypes, such as absence, myoclonic, and atonic spells, and even partial seizures with secondary generalization. More severe phenotypes include myoclonic-astatic epilepsy and severe myoclonic epilepsy of infancy. EEG may show irregular 2.5- to 4-Hz generalized spike-and-wave or polyspike-wave discharges.

A high level of genetic heterogeneity exists in GEFS+ (see Fig. 98.1). Mutations in four voltage-gated sodium channel genes (*SCN1B* on chromosome 19q and *SCN1A, SCN2A,* and *SCN9A* on chromosome 2q; Escayg et al., 2000b; Singh et al., 2009; Sugawara et al., 2001; Wallace et al., 1998) and two $GABA_A$ receptor genes (*GABRG2* and *GABRD*) encoding the $\gamma_2$- and δ-subunits (Baulac et al., 2001; Dibbens et al., 2004) cause GEFS+ (Fig. 98.11). Evidence exists for other mutated genes not yet identified. Functional analysis of several mutated sodium channels reveals slow inactivation, enhanced inward sodium current, and thus neuronal hyperexcitability (Lossin et al., 2002). Functional studies of the two *GABRG2* mutations showed reduced channel conductance in one case and abolished benzodiazepine sensitivity in the other. The *GABRD* mutations reduce current amplitude, each leading in different ways to a decrease in synaptic inhibition and thus an increase in neuronal excitability. These functional observations evoke compelling molecular explanations for clinical disease and, like ADNFLE and BFNS, illustrate how heterogeneous genetic defects may converge on a single clinical phenotype.

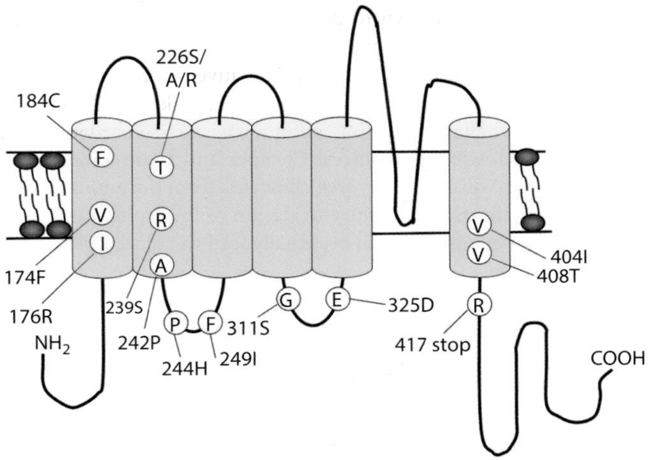


**Fig. 98.10** The neuronal potassium channel α-subunit encoded by the *KCNQ2* gene, and the proposed pathogenic mutations causing benign familial neonatal seizures. The majority of mutations have been identified in this channel, which is believed to coassemble with the *KCNQ3* gene product and underlie the M-current.

## *SCN2A* Mutation and Other Early Childhood Seizures

Other rare convulsive disorders of early childhood include benign familial infantile seizures and benign familial neonatal-infantile seizures, differentiated from BFNS by the age of onset. At least some cases involve mutations in the sodium channel $\alpha_2$-subunit gene, *SCN2A*, the same gene affected in some cases of GEFS+ (see the preceding section). Two mutations are present in families with seizures beginning at 1–3 months of age and ending at around 4 months ("neonatal-infantile"; Heron et al., 2002). Both mutations occur in cytoplasmic loops, inhibiting channel inactivation. A third mutation, also affecting a cytoplasmic loop, was identified in a family with similar seizures beginning at 4–12 months of age ("infantile"; Striano et al., 2006). Of note, *ATP1A2* mutations account for some cases of benign familial infantile seizures (see the earlier section, Familial Hemiplegic Migraine).

## Juvenile Myoclonic Epilepsy

JME accounts for 4%–10% of all epilepsy (Jallon and Latour, 2005). Featuring myoclonic jerks, generalized tonic-clonic seizures, and

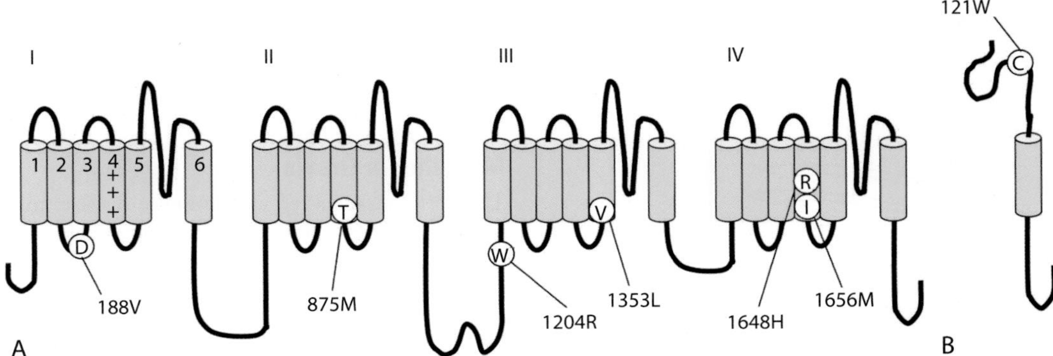


**Fig. 98.11** Mutations in the voltage-gated $Na^+$ channel causing generalized epilepsy with febrile seizures plus (GEFS+). The α-subunit is encoded by *SCN1A* **(A)**, and the $\beta_1$-subunit **(B)** is encoded by the *SCN1B* gene. Disease-causing mutations are shown. Mutations in other genes, including *SCN2A* and *GABRG2*, also cause GEFS+ (see Fig. 98.1).

absence spells, JME typically begins during adolescence (see Chapter 100). A genetic pattern is clear, but the mixed inheritance pattern suggests multiple heritable causes. One French-Canadian family suffers an autosomal dominant form of JME associated with a mutation in the $GABA_A$ receptor $\alpha_1$-subunit gene, *GABRA1* (Cossette et al., 2002), that results in loss of function and possible neuronal hyperexcitability (Krampfl et al., 2005). Less well described is the possible role of the VGCC $\beta_4$-subunit gene, *CACNB4*, in JME and episodic ataxia (see the previous discussion; Escayg et al., 2000a). GABRD variations may influence susceptibility to JME (Dibbens et al., 2004).

*EFHC1* is a gene on chromosome 6p, and five missense mutations have been identified in 6 of 44 JME families in whom it was sequenced (Suzuki et al., 2004). Although the precise function of the EFHC1 protein is unknown, it binds specifically to R-type VGCCs, alters their function, and perhaps thereby influences cell death pathways when transfected into cells in vitro. Whether or not this model turns out to be correct, it illustrates that an inherited channelopathy may result not only from mutation of a channel gene itself but also of genes whose products regulate the function of otherwise normal channels (Fig. 98.12).

Chromosome 15q has genetic loci implicated by linkage studies as possible contributors to some cases of JME. This area is known to contain, among other genes, the $\alpha_7$-subunit of the nicotinic acetylcholine receptor, CHRNA7 (Elmslie et al., 1997).

Similar to JME is familial adult myoclonic epilepsy (FAME) and autosomal dominant cortical myoclonus and epilepsy (ADCME), characterized by autosomal dominant inheritance, adult onset, varying degrees of myoclonus in the limbs, rare tonic-clonic seizures, and a benign course. These syndromes bear some similarity to JME, except for the adult onset and the highly penetrant autosomal dominant transmission. Whereas the genes are not yet known, the *FAME* gene has been mapped to chromosome 8q24 (Plaster et al., 1999) and the *ADCME* gene to chromosome 2q11.1–q12.2 (Guerrini et al., 2001).

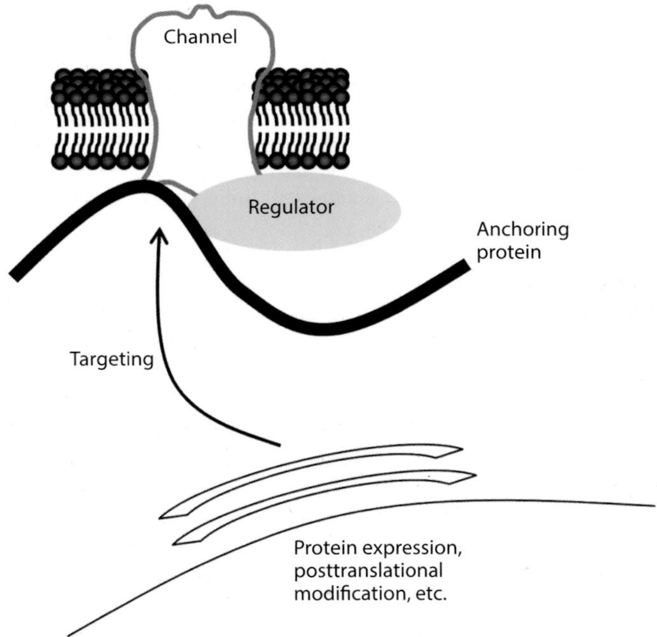


**Fig. 98.12 Normal Ion Channel Function Relies Not Only on a Normal Channel Protein.** Illustrated are examples of other processes that when defective may theoretically result in aberrant ion channel function and disease.

### Childhood Absence Epilepsy

CAE, a syndrome less common than JME and typified by brief, frequent absence spells (see Chapter 100), exhibits a multigenic pattern of inheritance. Mutations in *GABRB3*, encoding the $GABA_A$ receptor $\beta_3$-subunit, appear to cause CAE in some families (Tanaka et al., 2008; Urak et al., 2006). A mutation in the $GABA_A$ receptor $\gamma_2$-subunit gene, *GABRG2*, on chromosome 5q, conferring loss of benzodiazepine-induced enhancement of GABA-induced currents in vitro, is present in a family with CAE and an increased incidence of febrile seizures (Wallace et al., 2001). The $GABA_A$ receptor mediates phasic or tonic inhibitory transmission leading to hyperpolarization by allowing chloride anion influx through its pore (Hirose et al, 2014). Mutations in the T-type VGCC gene, *CACNA1H*, may contribute to some cases of CAE (Chen et al., 2003) and influence susceptibility to other IGEs (Heron et al., 2007). Mutations in other genes—*CACNA1A*, *GABRA1*, and a locus on chromosome 8q24—may also play a role.

### Theoretical Considerations

The phenotypic and EEG characteristics of various IGEs overlap to a considerable extent, implying that the boundaries separating some of these disorders may be blurred. Moreover, the relationships between molecular defects and clinical expression are irregular. Mutations in some genes (e.g., *SCN2A*, *GABRG2*) lead to heterogeneous clinical syndromes or genotype–phenotype divergence. Genotype-phenotype convergence is typified by ADNFLE, BFNS, and GEFS+, each of which may result from myriad underlying genetic roots (see Fig. 98.1). These considerations challenge existing definitions of disease, which will likely shift as knowledge advances. Cheaper and more widely available genetic tests will eventually free clinicians from the ambiguities of syndromic classification, and the elucidation of the molecular basis of familial epilepsy syndromes will eventually lead to tailored pharmacological treatments.

## AUTOIMMUNE CHANNELOPATHIES

Most channelopathies result from genetic mutation and are present from conception, usually with a family history of similar disorders. However, some ion channel disorders may develop in a previously normal individual. Beyond the obvious roles of drugs, toxins, and electrolyte disturbances in disrupting the function of structurally normal channels, circulating autoantibodies are the next most common known cause of acquired channelopathies. In some cases, these are autoimmune disorders, and, in some cases, they are paraneoplastic phenomena. A *paraneoplastic syndrome* is a remote nonmalignant effect of a primary tumor, thought to be caused by a cross-reactive autoimmune response against a tumor antigen. The syndrome is often apparent before the tumor itself is recognized. Therefore, paraneoplastic channelopathies are important to recognize, not only for their own sake but also because they may herald a more morbid underlying process.

### Myasthenia Gravis

The best characterized autoimmune disease, myasthenia gravis, is characterized by "fatigable weakness." This results in most cases from circulating antibodies directed against nAChRs. Polyclonal immunoglobulin G (IgG) reacts against variable extracellular nAChR epitopes at the neuromuscular junction, with the main immunogenic region located on each of two α-subunits of the heteropentameric receptor complex (Tzartos et al., 1998). Antibodies produce disease by activating complement, causing lysis of the muscle membrane, and by cross-linking AChRs, leading to accelerated protein degradation. In addition to AChR antibodies (blocking, modulating, and binding), antibodies against muscle-specific tyrosine kinase (MuSK) or LDL receptor-related protein 4 (LRP) 4 also have been found in myasthenic patients lacking the AChR antibodies. Understanding of the cause of autoantibody production is poor, but it probably results from multiple disease processes, sometimes involving thymoma or thymic hyperplasia (see Chapter 108).

## Lambert-Eaton Myasthenic Syndrome

Like myasthenia gravis, Lambert-Eaton myasthenic syndrome (LEMS) produces weakness by obstructing neuromuscular transmission. LEMS is caused by defected postsynaptic neurotransmitter transmission, typically presenting with proximal leg weakness and fatigue in middle-aged adults. Autoantibodies directed against P/Q-type VGCCs impair presynaptic calcium influx, thereby reducing action potential-triggered vesicle release. These autoantibodies are not specific to the neuromuscular junction, and patients also exhibit autonomic dysfunction. However, the antibodies probably do not cross the blood–brain barrier to a sufficient extent to cause diseases mimicking *CACNA1A* mutants—FHM1, EA2, SCA6, or seizures—although some patients may exhibit ataxia (see the later section Paraneoplastic Cerebellar Degeneration). Conversely, weakness is not a typical feature in patients with loss-of-function *CACNA1A* mutations, although EMG studies reveal expected neuromuscular abnormalities (Jen et al., 2001). Small-cell lung cancer cells express VGCCs, likely triggering immunogenesis in the large proportion of patients in whom LEMS turns out to be a paraneoplastic phenomenon. As in myasthenia gravis, polyclonal antibodies may be detectable in LEMS. The extracellular S5–S6 linker regions of the α-subunit are the proposed pathogenic epitopes (Takamori, 2004).

## Acquired Neuromyotonia (Isaacs Syndrome)

Isaacs syndrome presents with painful muscle cramps and stiffness, slow muscle relaxation after contraction, commonly affecting adolescents and young adults. Characteristic features of acquired neuromyotonia are fasciculations and myokymic and neuromyotonic discharges on EMG, reflecting motor nerve hyperactivity driven by abnormal peripheral nerve firing. Due to excessive muscle fiber activities, the patients with Issacs syndrome often present with weight loss, muscle hypertrophy, and hyperhidrosis. The syndrome may occur in association with thymoma. The autoimmune target is the VGKC found along peripheral motor axons and responsible for repolarization after action potential firing (Shillito et al., 1995). This is the same channel affected in EA1, and the mechanism of interictal myokymia is identical: reduced potassium efflux from axons and nerve terminals leads to higher membrane potentials, inappropriate action potential firing, and acetylcholine release. This same phenomenon probably also affects autonomic fibers, explaining why excessive sweating, salivation, and lacrimation are often observed. The action of these antibodies is complement-independent and appears to involve cross-linking of channels (Tomimitsu et al., 2004).

VGKC antibodies probably also cause *Morvan syndrome*, which encompasses all the clinical features of acquired neuromyotonia plus a fluctuating delirium (Barber et al., 2000; Lee et al., 1998). Supporting a role for circulating autoantibodies is the effectiveness of plasma exchange in the treatment of these patients (Liguori et al., 2001). VGKC antibodies were present in a series of patients suffering from an encephalopathy indistinguishable from limbic encephalitis, with temporal lobe-onset seizures and behavioral and cognitive disturbances, but no neuromuscular abnormality (Thieben et al., 2004). Thus, a peripheral-to-central spectrum of disease may exist, with acquired neuromyotonia on the one extreme and VGKC antibody-associated limbic encephalitis on the other.

Other antibodies have been also identified in patients with Issacs and Morvan syndrome. Patients with CASPR2 antibodies may present with neuromyotonia alone, limbic encephalitis, or Morvan syndrome. CASPR2 is not an ion channel, but this protein is important in clustering of $K_V1.1$ and $K_V1.2$, located in the juxtaparanodal regions of both peripheral and CNS axon (Amato and James, 2016). Other associated antibodies are often paraneoplastic and include nAChR, CRMP-5, amphiphysin, and antinuclear neuronal type 4.

## Paraneoplastic Cerebellar Degeneration

Paraneoplastic cerebellar degeneration (PCD), presenting as a rapidly progressive ataxic syndrome, most commonly occurs in cases of breast, ovarian, and lung malignancies. PCD probably represents a spectrum of diseases associated with distinct autoimmune targets. Among these may be the anti-P/Q-type VGCC antibodies found in small-cell cancer. Although these antibodies more typically cause peripheral disease (LEMS), they are found less commonly in the CSF of patients with PCD (Graus et al., 2002). Purkinje cell loss is the pathological hallmark of PCD; these cells express high levels of P/Q-type VGCCs, and it seems likely that antibodies directed against these channels are pathogenic. PCD associated with small-cell lung cancer may occur with or without neuromuscular dysfunction, and the factors predisposing to central versus peripheral action of the paraneoplastic antibodies are unknown. Finally, despite the fact that the same molecule may be the target of pathology in PCD and *CACNA1A*-associated diseases (FHM1, EA2, SCA6), PCD is not an episodic disorder but rather characterized by rapid deterioration, perhaps due to target cell destruction.

## Limbic Encephalitis

The term *limbic encephalitis* encompasses an array of autoimmune disorders associated with psychiatric symptoms, cognitive dysfunction, and seizures, often in the context of an underlying malignancy. Some of these disorders result from an autoantibody directed against a brain ion channel. VGKC antibody-associated limbic encephalitis, mentioned earlier, is one example. Anti–*N*-methyl-D-aspartate (NMDA) receptor limbic encephalitis is the most common antibody-mediated encephalitis (Dalmau et al., 2008). This syndrome, which occurs mainly in women, causes psychiatric symptoms, seizures, delirium, and other neurological symptoms. Like PCD, anti-NMDA receptor encephalitis strongly suggests an underlying malignancy—typically ovarian teratoma. NMDA receptors represent one of three classes of glutamate-gated ion channels in the brain; α-amino-3-hydroxy-5-methyl-4-isoxazolepropionic acid (AMPA) receptors represent another class, and antibodies against those receptors may also cause limbic encephalitis (Lai et al., 2009). Antibodies against $GABA_B$ receptors were isolated in a series of patients with limbic encephalitis and prominent seizures (Lancaster et al., 2010). While not an ion channel, this G protein-coupled GABA receptor regulates ion channels and synaptic transmission. Leucine-rich glioma inactivated-1 (LGI-1) and CASPR2 are the proteins that complex with a voltage-gated potassium channel. LGI-1 is rich in the hippocampus and neocortex. Dysfunction of LGI-1 causes secondary channel dysfunction, causing reduction of the synaptic AMPA receptor. Patients with LGI-1 antibodies often present with focal seizure, and approximately 50% of them have pathognomonic faciobrachial dystonic seizures. Seizures progress over time to an established limbic encephalitis.

As for PCD, acquired neuromyotonia, and LEMS, limbic encephalitis should be treated with intravenous immune globulin (IVIG), plasma exchange, steroids, or other immunosuppressant therapies in parallel with an aggressive search for an underlying neoplasm.

## SUMMARY

Advances in molecular biology and electrophysiology have allowed discovery and the characterization of a new group of disorders termed the *channelopathies*. Understanding the underlying pathophysiology of these diseases has not only expanded our knowledge of basic ion channel physiology but, more importantly, has also provided insight into mechanisms of common neurological disorders such as epilepsy and migraine. The channelopathies, a seemingly heterogeneous group of diseases, share striking similarities. Most have intermittent symptoms, despite the invariant presence of the mutation, with interictal return to a normal state. Exacerbating factors such as stress, exertion, and fatigue are common to many of the channelopathies. Response to treatment with carbonic anhydrase inhibitors (acetazolamide) is a common feature among these genetic disorders (see Table 98.3), leading some clinicians to use acetazolamide responsiveness as a diagnostic litmus test for the channelopathies. The mechanism by which acetazolamide prevents and ameliorates attacks is not completely understood, although recent evidence suggests the activation of potassium channels may play a role.

These similarities suggest a common underlying pathophysiological basis shared among the channelopathies. In fact, many of the channelopathies, such as EA2 and FHM, share several characteristics. This chapter has attempted to provide a clinical approach to the recognition, diagnosis, and treatment of the channelopathies. Furthermore, knowing where the genetic mutation is located does not necessarily predict the clinical phenotype. Diagnostic confusion arises from phenotypic variability within a given syndrome and phenotypic similarities among different syndromes, as well as the realization that mutations in the same gene can produce seemingly unrelated phenotypes (see Fig. 98.1). This underscores the importance of careful clinical assessment. The clinician's most useful diagnostic tool remains a detailed history and physical examination.

Genetic contributions to common seizure and headache syndromes are well known but more difficult to dissect at a molecular level. This is due to the large number of genes/proteins that almost certainly contribute to headache and epilepsy susceptibility. Further complicating this genetic heterogeneity is the complex interaction of genes and the environment. Normal variations in proteins, like those discussed earlier, occur in the general population. One exciting hypothesis is that some of these "normal" variations have functional consequences for channels (and other proteins, too). Innumerable factors contribute to net neuronal excitability, circuit dynamics, and brain function. These factors subtly increase or decrease by polymorphisms in the many ion channel proteins and in other proteins expressed by a neuron. In most families, these many polymorphisms average each other out, resulting in "normal" excitability. However, in occasional families segregating multiple hyperexcitability alleles, offspring may be more susceptible to seizure or headache than the general population and experience attacks unmasked by appropriate precipitating conditions. This model is consistent with familial clustering of such disorders, but it is inconsistent with simple Mendelian traits segregating from generation to generation. Whether clues from Mendelian episodic neurological disease ultimately bear on the complex genetics of epilepsy and migraine remains to be seen.

The example of thyrotoxic hypoKPP is quite exciting. Worldwide, thyrotoxic hypoKPP is about 10 times more common than all the familial periodic paralyses put together. However, since it is a sporadic disorder, mapping of causative genes is impossible. Clues from the familial periodic paralyses motivated the hypothesis that led to the identification of inwardly rectifying potassium channel mutations in some of these patients (Ryan et al., 2010). In this case, the mutations are segregating in families but are only "uncovered" in those (sporadic) individuals who develop thyrotoxicosis. Additional insights into many common and sporadic diseases will continue to be gained through the study of rare familial cases and better understanding of the genetics and pathophysiology.

Despite considerable progress in the understanding of channelopathies, several unanswered questions remain, such as why these syndromes are episodic, why acetazolamide is effective in such a diverse group of disorders, and how identical mutations within a gene can cause dominant or recessive behavior. Although disease-targeted pharmacological therapy is ideal, this has largely remained theoretical, and such work is still in early stages. Understanding where a certain mutation lies within a gene does not fully reveal the intricacies of the clinical phenotype, and mutational effects in vivo are likely to be considerably more complicated than those demonstrated in vitro. Thus future advances in defining the various channelopathy phenotypes and understanding the underlying molecular mechanism will greatly contribute to the understanding of these and other related disorders.

Finally, disruption of ion channel function may occur in more complex ways than simply by mutation in an ion channel gene or by an autoantibody to the channel protein itself. Our appreciation of the complex association of ion channels with other proteins that target, anchor, regulate, or otherwise influence their behavior is growing (see Fig. 98.12). Examples include EFHC1 and LGI1, discussed earlier in the chapter, which encode ion channel-regulating proteins and cause ion channel dysfunction when mutated. Mutation in ankyrin-B, an anchoring protein that co-localizes a diverse range of ion channels and other membrane proteins, causes long-QT syndrome type 4 (Mohler et al., 2003). Mutations in similar anchoring proteins are likely to be discovered in neurological disease; perhaps *Schwartz-Jampel syndrome* is an example. This rare autosomal recessive syndrome characterized by myotonia and chondrodysplasia results from mutations in *HSPG2*, the gene encoding perlecan, the heparan sulfate proteoglycan enriched in basement membranes and cartilage (Stum et al., 2006); the pathophysiological link between perlecan and myotonia has yet to be established. The spectrum of episodic and electrical disorders of the nervous system will continue to grow.

*The complete reference list is available online at https://expertconsult.inkling.com/.*

99

# Neurocutaneous Syndromes

*Monica P. Islam, E. Steve Roach*

## OUTLINE



Neurocutaneous disorders are congenital or hereditary conditions that feature lesions of both the skin and nervous system. Although each condition, or *phakomatosis*, is distinct and characterized by a unique pathophysiology, the concept of *neurocutaneous disorders* unifies those neurological disorders, whose identification depends primarily on simple visual diagnosis. These disorders may be inherited or sporadic; some of the sporadic disorders result from somatic mosaicism. Advances in clinical genetics have established the molecular basis for some of the disorders, although recognition and treatment still require an appreciation of the cutaneous and systemic symptoms. This chapter reviews the clinical features of the more common neurocutaneous syndromes.

## TUBEROUS SCLEROSIS

Tuberous sclerosis complex (TSC) is a disorder of cellular differentiation and proliferation that can affect the brain, skin, kidneys, heart, and other organs. Many clinical features of TSC result from hamartomas, but true neoplasms also occur, particularly in the kidney and brain. Abnormal neuronal migration plays a major additional role in neurological dysfunction (Roach, 2016; Roach & Sparagana, 2004).

Population-based studies suggest a prevalence of one per 6000 individuals. However, because of the striking variability of clinical expression, establishing the diagnosis of TSC can be difficult in individuals with subtle findings, and the true prevalence may be considerably higher. Cutaneous findings are usually the first clue that a patient has TSC, but other features may lead to the diagnosis. In infants, cardiac involvement and seizures frequently are presenting signs, whereas dermatological, pulmonary, or renal involvement may lead to diagnosis in older individuals. Updated guidelines have introduced genetic testing as the potential sole diagnostic criterion in addition to clinical findings (Box 99.1).

The inheritance of TSC is autosomal dominant with variable penetrance. The estimated spontaneous mutation rate for TSC varies from 66% to 86%, depending in part on the completeness of investigation of the extended family. Two genes are responsible for TSC: TSC1, coding for hamartin at chromosome 9q34.3; and TSC2, coding for tuberin adjacent to the gene for adult polycystic kidney disease at chromosome 16p13.3. The clinical features of TSC1 and TSC2 overlap, since the two gene products form a single functional unit that is an upstream modulator in the mammalian target of rapamycin (mTOR) signaling pathway. Both gene products downregulate small G-protein Ras-homolog enriched in brain (RHEB) activity in this pathway. However, genotype-phenotype studies indicate that individuals with a TSC2 mutation tend to have more severe disease, and the frequency of TSC2 mutations is greater among individuals with spontaneous mutations (Sancak et al., 2005). Multiple mutation types exist in different regions of each gene, and even individuals with identical genetic mutations can have different phenotypes. Molecular diagnostic testing—including prenatal testing—has been available since the early 2000s, and a disease-causing mutation is identified in about 85% of the individuals who meet the clinical diagnostic criteria. Some of the individuals with no mutation identified via routine gene analysis prove to have mosaicism (Roach, 2016). Large genomic deletions and rearrangements are more common in the TSC2 gene than in TSC1, and more mutations have been identified for TSC2 than for TSC1. TSC2 mutations appear more commonly than TSC1 in patients with subependymal nodules (SENs), intellectual disability, renal angiomyolipomas, and retinal phakomas. Intellectual disability and other neuropsychiatric involvement are more likely in individuals with TSC2 than in those with TSC1 mutation (Au et al., 2007).

### BOX 99.1 Updated Diagnostic Criteria for Tuberous Sclerosis Complex 2012

**A. Genetic Diagnostic Criteria**

The identification of a pathogenic mutation in either TSC1 or TSC2 is sufficient to make a definite diagnosis of TSC. A pathogenic mutation is defined as a mutation that clearly inactivates the function of the TSC1 or TSC2 proteins (e.g., out-of-frame indel or nonsense mutation), prevents protein synthesis (e.g., large genomic deletion), or is a missense mutation whose effect on protein function has been established. Other TSC1 or TSC2 variants whose effect on function is less certain do not meet these criteria and are insufficient to support a definite diagnosis of TSC. Note that 10%–25% of TSC patients have no mutation identified by conventional genetic testing, so a normal result does not exclude TSC or affect the use of clinical diagnostic criteria to diagnose TSC.

**B. Clinical Diagnostic Criteria**

***Major Features***

1. Hypomelanotic macules (≥3, at least 5-mm diameter)
2. Angiofibromas (≥3) or fibrous cephalic plaque
3. Ungual fibromas (≥2)
4. Shagreen patch
5. Multiple retinal hamartomas
6. Cortical dysplasias*
7. Subependymal nodules
8. Subependymal giant-cell astrocytoma
9. Cardiac rhabdomyoma
10. Lymphangioleiomyomatosis (LAM)†
11. Angiomyolipomas (≥2)†

***Minor Features***

1. "Confetti" skin lesions
2. Dental enamel pits (≥3)
3. Intraoral fibromas (≥2)
4. Retinal achromic patch
5. Multiple renal cysts
6. Nonrenal hamartomas

Definite diagnosis: Two major features or one major feature with ≥2 minor features

Possible diagnosis: Either one major feature or ≥2 minor features

*Includes tubers and cerebral white-matter radial migration lines.

†A combination of the two major clinical features (LAM and angiomyolipomas) without other features does not meet criteria for a definite diagnosis.

*TSC*, Tuberous sclerosis complex.

Adapted from: Northrup, H., Krueger, D.A., 2013. Tuberous sclerosis complex diagnostic criteria update: Recommendations of the 2012 International Tuberous Sclerosis Complex Consensus conference. Pediatr Neurol 49, 243–254.

### Cutaneous Features

The cutaneous lesions of TSC include hypomelanotic macules, the shagreen patch, ungual fibromas, and facial angiofibromas (Fig. 99.1). Hypomelanotic macules *(ash leaf spots)* occur in over 90% of affected individuals (Fig. 99.2). The lesions usually are present at birth but may be evident in the newborn only with an ultraviolet light (Wood's lamp). Other pigmentary abnormalities include confetti lesions (areas with stippled hypopigmentation, typically on the extremities) and poliosis (a white patch or forelock) of the scalp, hair, or eyelids. Hypomelanotic macules are common in normal individuals (Table 99.1), but three or more hypomelanotic macules greater than 5 mm is a major diagnostic criterion for TSC.

*Facial angiofibromas* (previously termed *adenoma sebaceum*) consist of vascular and connective tissue elements. Although multiple facial angiofibromas are relatively specific for TSC, they are found in only three-fourths of affected individuals and often appear several years after the diagnosis has been established by other means. The lesions typically become apparent during the preschool years as a few small red macules on the malar region; they gradually become papular, larger, and more numerous, sometimes extending down the nasolabial folds or onto the chin. Angiofibromas often become less prominent after starting an mTOR inhibitor, and topical application has been studied (Koenig et al., 2018). Forehead plaques or fibrous facial plaques resemble angiofibromas histologically, though they are not papular.

The *shagreen patch* most often is found on the back or flank area; it is an irregularly shaped, slightly raised, or textured skin lesion. About 20%–30% of patients with TSC have a shagreen patch, which may not be seen in young children.

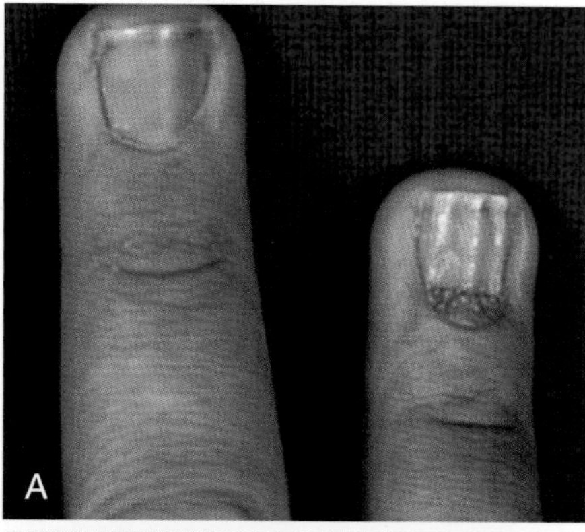


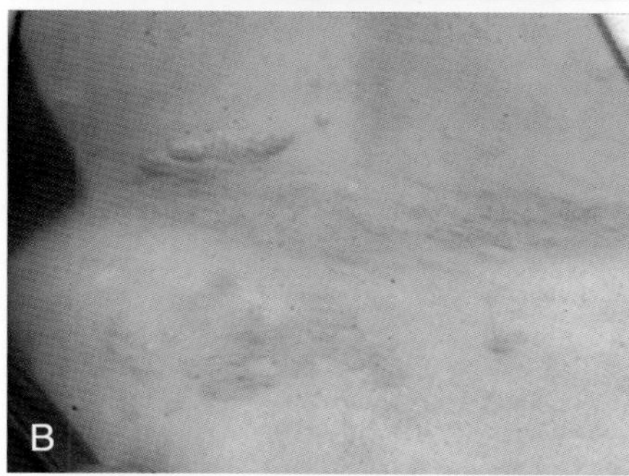


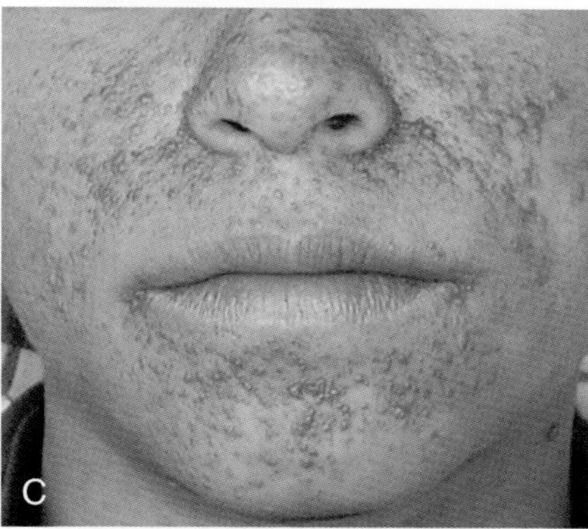


**Fig. 99.1** Classic cutaneous manifestations of tuberous sclerosis include (**A**) ungual fibromas, (**B**) shagreen patch on the lower back, and (**C**) facial angiofibromas. *(A, Reprinted with permission from Roach, E.S., Delgado, M.R., 1995. Tuberous sclerosis. Dermatol Clin 13, 151–161.)*

*Ungual fibromas* are nodular or fleshy lesions that arise adjacent to (periungual) or underneath (subungual) the nails. The presence of two or more is considered a major criterion as a single lesion can develop after trauma in individuals without TSC. Ungual fibromas are among the latest cutaneous manifestation of TSC, present in up to 80% of older adults but only 20% overall (Northrup et al., 2013).

## Neurological Features

The predominant neurological manifestations of TSC are intellectual disability, epilepsy, and behavioral abnormalities, although milder forms of the disease with little or no neurological impairment are common. Impaired cellular interaction results in disrupted neuronal migration along radial glial fibers and abnormal proliferation of glial elements. Neuropathological lesions of TSC include SENs, cortical and subcortical hamartomas (tubers), areas of focal cortical dysplasia, and heterotopic gray matter. SENs commonly arise from germinal matrix progenitors in the caudothalamic groove near the foramen of Monro. These lesions can grow over time, but usually only into adolescence, after which time they calcify. These remain asymptomatic unless they transform into subependymal giant-cell astrocytomas (SEGAs). Tubers frequently extend from the ventricle wall to the cortical surface, with a linear or wedge-shaped distribution. Similar to normal brain, tubers develop between 14 and 16 weeks, gestation, such that the tuber load is established before birth, though they may not be visible on imaging until later childhood, given myelination status. These focal malformations of cortical development most frequently involve one gyrus at a time, but more diffuse involvement such as hemimegalencephaly can occur as well. Histology of these areas demonstrates disorganized cortical lamination and underlying abnormal myelination with indistinct gray-white-matter junction architecture. Calcification frequently is present. Dysmorphic neurons are often present, and other abnormal astrocytes similar to those seen in sporadic focal cortical dysplasias are termed *balloon cells* or *giant cells* for their abundant cytoplasm (Wong, 2008).

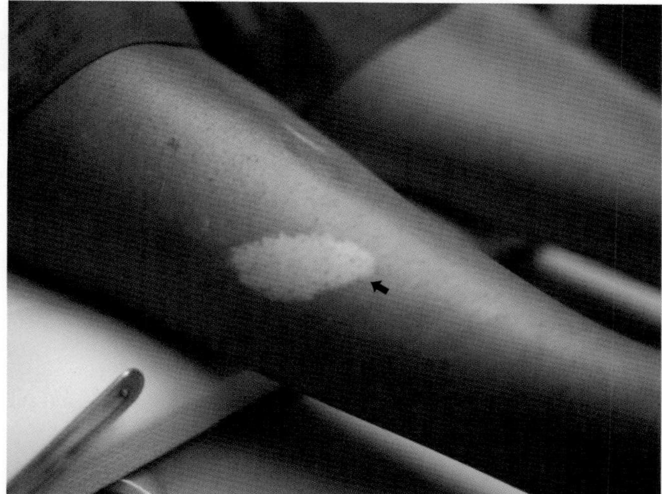

**Fig. 99.2 A Hypomelanotic Macule (Ash Leaf Spot) *(Arrow)* From the Leg of a Patient With Tuberous Sclerosis.** *(Reprinted with permission from Weiner, D.M., Ewalt, D.H., Roach, E.S., et al., 1998. The tuberous sclerosis complex: a comprehensive review. J Am Coll Surg 187, 548–561.)*

Seizures of various types occur in 80%–90% of patients. Most develop during the first year of life, which is a poor prognosticator for autism and poor cognitive development. TSC is the most common cause of infantile spasms, and one-third of children with TSC develop them. Children with infantile spasms are more likely to have a high burden of cortical lesions demonstrated by magnetic resonance imaging (MRI) and are more likely to exhibit long-term cognitive impairment. For many, vigabatrin has been a more effective treatment option than adrenocorticotropic hormone (ACTH). Resective epilepsy surgery is a consideration in individuals with seizures localizing to one or two tubers. Corpus callosotomy is an option in some children. Some individuals with prolonged seizure freedom while taking medication can successfully discontinue anti-seizure medication (Sparagana et al., 2003).

Many TSC patients have intellectual disability, but many have normal intelligence. As seen with early-onset epilepsy in general, intellectual disability in TSC often accompanies epilepsy that manifests earlier in life and that is refractory. The number of subependymal lesions does not correlate with the clinical severity of TSC, but MRI evidence of numerous cortical lesions is associated with more

TABLE 99.1 **Frequency of Lesions in Individuals With Tuberous Sclerosis Versus Other Individuals**

| Lesion | Tuberous Sclerosis Complex | Other Individuals |
|---|---|---|
| Hypomelanotic macules | Occur in over 95% of TSC patients, often with many lesions | Occur in up to 5% of the population (but usually fewer than three lesions per person) |
| Facial angiofibromas | Eventually seen in 75% but less often in children | Seen in individuals with multiple endocrine neoplasia type 1 and in a few sporadic families |
| Shagreen patch | Up to 48% | Occasional |
| Ungual fibromas | Seen in 15% but often not until adulthood | Occasionally sporadic or after nail trauma (but typically one lesion) |
| Rhabdomyomas | One or more tumors seen in 47%–65% but much more common below 2 years<br>Up to 51% of patients with rhabdomyomas have TSC | In 14%–49% of rhabdomyoma patients, there are no other signs of TSC |
| Renal AML | Often multiple AML occur in up to 80% of TSC patients by age 10 | Sporadic AML occur but are typically solitary |
| Renal cysts | Polycystic kidneys occur in 3%–5% of TSC patients<br>Smaller numbers of renal cysts are present in 15%–20% | There are both dominant and recessive polycystic kidney diseases<br>A few cysts are frequent sporadic findings in adults |
| Cortical dysplasia/tubers | 90%–95% and usually multiple lesions are present (magnetic resonance imaging yields highest detection rate) | Sporadic cortical dysplasia (typically one lesion) is common among individuals who have epilepsy not due to TSC |
| Subependymal nodules | 83%–93% | Rare, especially if calcified |
| Subependymal giant-cell tumors | Up to 15% (using radiographic criteria) | Rare in the absence of TSC |

*AML*, Angiomyolipoma; *TSC*, tuberous sclerosis.
*From Roach, E.S., Sparagana, S.P., 2010. Diagnostic criteria for tuberous sclerosis complex. In: Kwiatkowski, D.J., Whittemore, V.H., Thiele, E.A. (Eds.), Tuberous Sclerosis Complex: Genes, Clinical Features, and Therapeutics. Wiley-VCH Verlag, Weinheim, pp. 21–25. Used with permission.*

significant cognitive impairment and seizure intractability. The most abnormal regions seen on MRI tend to coincide with focal abnormalities of the electroencephalogram (EEG). The severity of intellectual disability ranges from borderline to profound intellectual disability. In addition to intellectual disability, many children with TSC have significant behavioral and psychiatric dysfunction. Autism, hyperkinesis, aggressiveness, psychosocial difficulties, and even psychosis can occur, either as isolated problems or in combination. The prevalence of autistic spectrum disorders is 25%–50% and equal between boys and girls. Behavioral problems are frequent and independent of intellectual ability. Mood disorders also are increased. De Vries and colleagues described the array of behavioral and psychiatric symptoms resulting from TSC as *tuberous sclerosis associated neuropsychiatric disorders* (TAND), and they developed a useful clinical screening tool (de Vries et al., 2015).

Computed tomography (CT) best demonstrates the calcified SENs that characterize TSC (Fig. 99.3). CT sometimes shows superficial cerebral lesions, but they are far more obvious with brain MRI (Fig. 99.4). T2-weighted sequences show evidence of abnormal neuronal migration in some patients as high-signal linear lesions running perpendicular to the cortex. SENs along the ventricular surface give the characteristic appearance of "candle guttering." More than one-fourth of patients with TSC show cerebellar anomalies.

SEGAs develop in 6%–14% of patients with TSC. Unlike the more common cortical tubers and SENs, SEGAs can enlarge (Fig. 99.5) and cause symptoms of increased intracranial pressure, particularly if extension into the lateral ventricles creates an obstructive hydrocephalus. Clinical features include new focal neurological deficits, unexplained behavior change, deterioration of seizure control, or symptoms of increased intracranial pressure. Acute or subacute onset of neurological dysfunction may result from sudden obstruction of the ventricular system by an intraventricular SEGA. Rarely, acute deterioration occurs because of hemorrhage into the tumor itself.

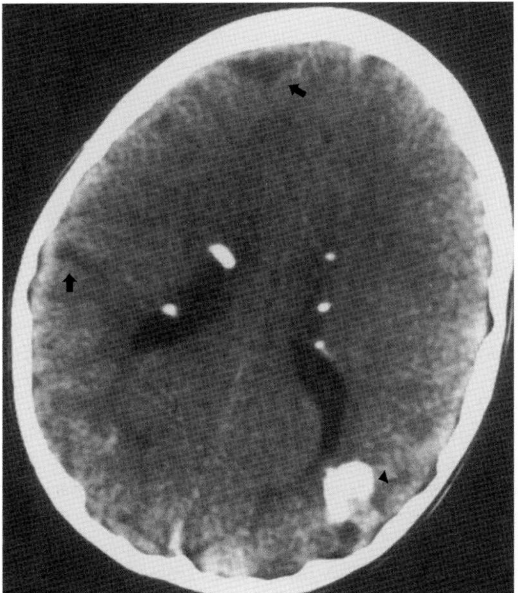

**Fig. 99.3** Computed cranial tomography scan from a child with tuberous sclerosis complex demonstrates typical calcified subependymal nodules; a large calcified parenchymal lesion *(arrowhead)* and low-density cortical lesions *(arrows)* are seen as well. *(Reprinted with permission from Roach, E.S., Kerr, J., Mendelsohn, D., et al., 1991. Diagnosis of symptomatic and asymptomatic gene carriers of tuberous sclerosis by CT and MRI. Ann N Y Acad Sci 615, 112–122.)*

SEGAs are usually benign but locally invasive, and early surgery can be curative. Identification of an enlarging SEGA before the onset of symptoms of increased intracranial pressure or appearance of new neurological deficits is ideal. Periodic screening for identifying SEGA

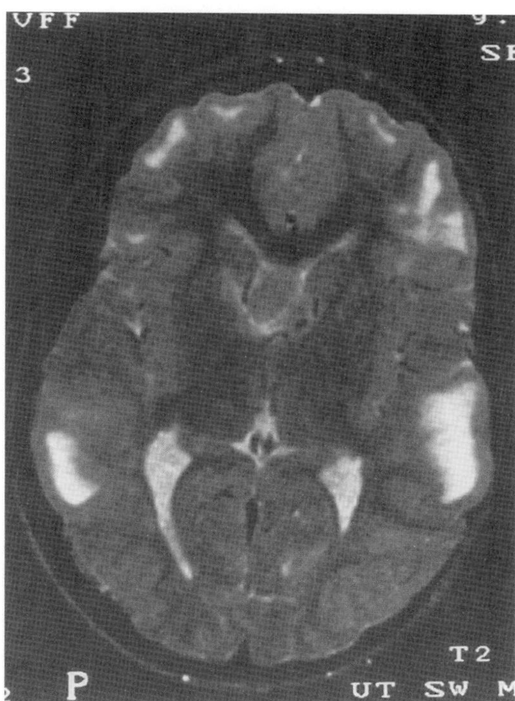


**Fig. 99.4** Noncontrast T2-weighted magnetic resonance imaging scan from a child with tuberous sclerosis demonstrates extensive high-signal cortical lesions typical of tuberous sclerosis.

may improve surgical outcome. Recent work suggests that rapamycin and the oral mTOR inhibitor everolimus inhibit the growth of SEGAs. Everolimus has approval from the US Food and Drug Administration (FDA) for the treatment of SEGAs, renal angiomyolipomas, and, most recently, seizures due to TSC (Krueger et al., 2013). There also have been reports of improvement in pulmonary lymphangioleiomyomatosis (LAM) and facial angiofibromas (Franz, 2013).

### Retinal Features

The frequency of retinal hamartomas in TSC varies from almost negligible to 87% of patients, probably reflecting the expertise and technique of the examiner. Pupillary dilatation and indirect ophthalmoscopy are important, particularly in children who may be uncooperative. Findings vary from classic mulberry lesions adjacent to the optic disc (Fig. 99.6) to plaque-like hamartoma or depigmented retinal lesions. Most retinal lesions are clinically insignificant, but some patients have visual impairment caused by large macular lesions, and very few patients have visual loss caused by retinal detachment, vitreous hemorrhage, or hamartoma enlargement. Occasionally, patients have a pigmentary defect of the iris. Funduscopic examination is valuable at the time of diagnosis, to monitor existing abnormalities or to evaluate for new symptoms.

### Cardiac Features

Approximately two-thirds of individuals with TSC have a cardiac rhabdomyoma, but few demonstrate clinical symptoms. Cardiac rhabdomyomas are hamartomas, tend to be multiple, and involute with time. These lesions sometimes are evident on prenatal ultrasound testing (Fig. 99.7), usually after 24 weeks, gestational age. Most individuals who develop cardiac dysfunction present soon after birth with heart failure. A few children later develop cardiac arrhythmias or cerebral thromboembolism from the rhabdomyomas. The cause of congestive heart failure is either by obstruction of blood flow via intraluminal tumor or by lack of sufficient normal myocardium to maintain perfusion. Some patients stabilize after medical treatment with digoxin and diuretics and eventually improve; others require surgery. Echocardiography and electrocardiography (ECG) establish the diagnosis. Arterial aneurysms can occur. Surveillance studies every 6–12 months help monitor existing rhabdomyomas until stabilization or involution occurs. The size of these lesions may increase with hormone exposure—a consideration in the neonate, pubertal individual, and child treated with ACTH for infantile spasms.

### Renal Features

Renal angiomyolipomas occur in up to three-fourths of patients with TSC, usually presenting by 10 years of age. Most of these lesions are histologically benign tumors with varying amounts of vascular tissue, fat, and smooth muscle (Fig. 99.8). Bilateral tumors and multiple tumors in a kidney are common. The prevalence and size of renal tumors increase with age, and tumors larger than 4 cm are much more likely to become symptomatic than smaller tumors. Renal cell carcinoma or other malignancies can affect TSC patients less commonly and at younger ages than the general population. Coalescing angiomyolipomas can contribute to end-stage renal disease. Endovascular embolization of the larger renal angiomyolipomas prevents hemorrhage and other complications (Ewalt et al., 2005). Rapamycin and everolimus limit the growth of these tumors, at least transiently.

Single or multiple renal cysts are also a feature of TSC; these tend to appear earlier than the renal tumors. Ultrasound or cranial CT easily identifies larger cysts, and the combination of renal cysts and angiomyolipomas is characteristic of TSC. Individual renal cysts may disappear. Surveillance imaging is recommended, at least every 2–3 years—more frequently in those with existing or symptomatic renal involvement.

### Pulmonary Features

Pulmonary disease presents after puberty in the form of LAM and is five times more common in females than in males. Pulmonary lesions, symptomatic or asymptomatic, can be demonstrated in almost half of women with TSC who undergo chest CT. Baseline pulmonary function testing, 6-minute walk test, and high-resolution CT of the chest are recommended in all symptomatic patients and asymptomatic females at age 18 years. Spontaneous and recurrent pneumothorax, dyspnea, cough, and hemoptysis are typical symptoms of pulmonary TSC. Of those who develop symptoms, 10%–12% die within 10 years of symptom onset from complications of pulmonary TSC (Cudzilo et al., 2013). Tamoxifen and progesterone may be helpful in some patients, and mTOR inhibitors have been additional treatment options.

## NEUROFIBROMATOSIS TYPE 1

Neurofibromatosis type 1 (NF1), or von Recklinghausen disease, is the most common of the neurocutaneous syndromes, occurring in approximately 1 in 3000 people. Inheritance is autosomal dominant, but approximately half of NF1 cases result from a spontaneous mutation. The clinical features are highly variable.

A mutation of the 60-exon *NF1* gene on chromosome 17q11.2 causes NF1. The NF1 gene product, neurofibromin, is a tumor-suppressor GTPase-activating protein functioning to inhibit Ras-mediated cell proliferation. Despite identification of approximately 100 mutations of *NF1* in various regions of the gene, none correlates to a specific clinical phenotype (Pasmant et al., 2012).

Several patients have developed a somatic *NF1* mutation affecting only a limited region of the body. With this mosaic NF1, one extremity may have café-au-lait lesions, subcutaneous neurofibromas, and other signs of NF1, but the rest of the body is unaffected (Garcia-

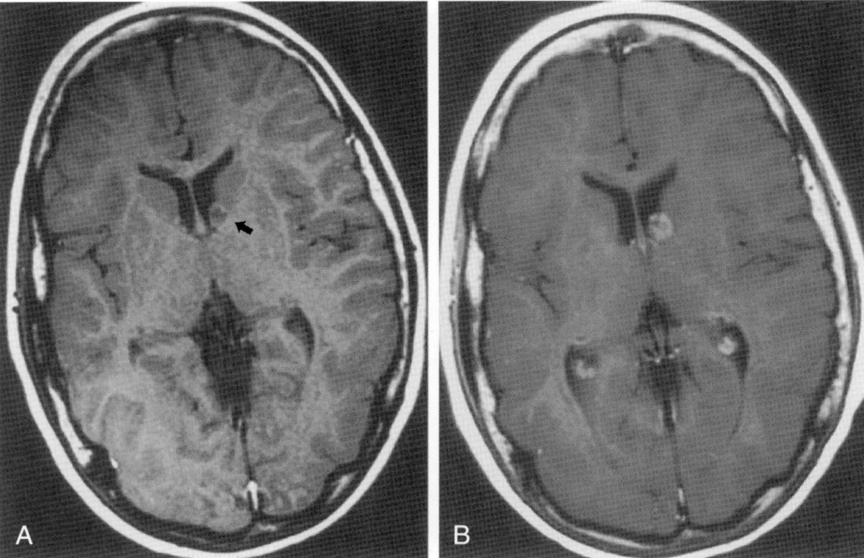


**Fig. 99.5** **A,** Noncontrast T1-weighted magnetic resonance imaging scan from a child with tuberous sclerosis shows an irregular mass *(arrow)* with a central signal void caused by calcification protruding into the left frontal horn. **B,** Another scan with gadolinium a few months later shows contrast enhancement and minimal tumor growth.

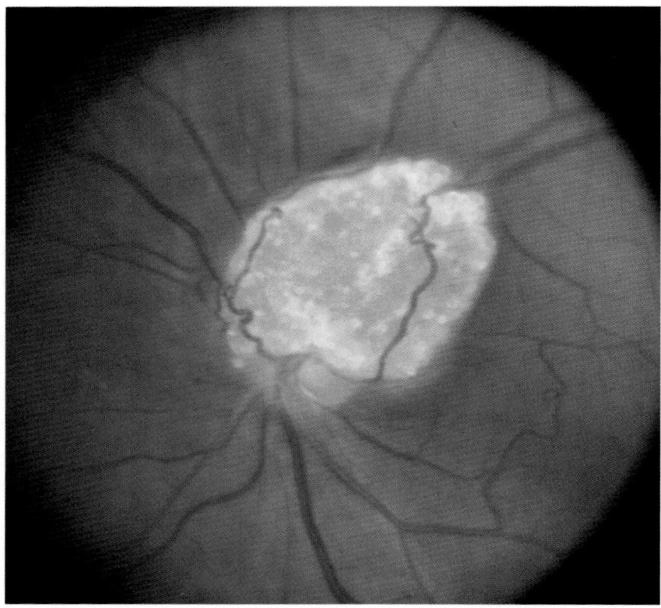

**Fig. 99.6** A retinal astrocytoma (mulberry lesion) adjacent to the optic nerve is typical of those found in tuberous sclerosis. *(Reprinted with permission from Roach, E.S., 1992. Neurocutaneous syndromes. Pediatr Clin North Am 39, 591–620.)*

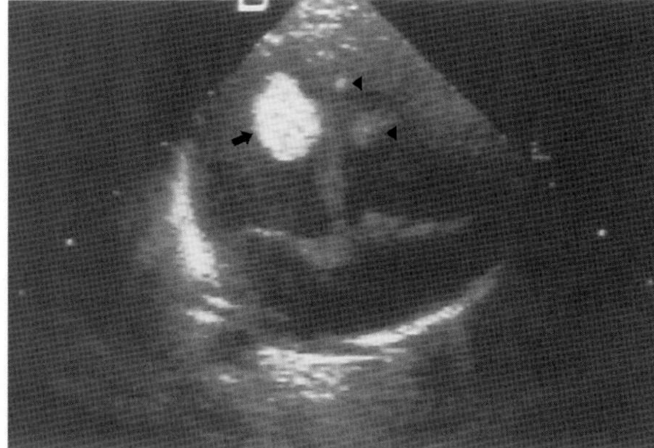

**Fig. 99.7** Prenatal ultrasound study reveals a large cardiac rhabdomyoma *(arrow)* and two smaller rhabdomyomas *(arrowheads)* in a child who subsequently proved to have tuberous sclerosis. *(Reprinted with permission from Weiner, D.M., Ewalt, D.E., Roach, E. S., et al., 1998. The tuberous sclerosis complex: a comprehensive review. J Am Coll Surg 187, 548–561.)*

Romero et al.,). Similarly, some patients with germline mosaicism have no outward manifestations of NF1 but have multiple affected offspring.

If several characteristics are present and the physician is astute, the diagnosis of NF1 is obvious, especially when another family member is affected. The diagnosis is difficult when the clinical features are atypical and the family history is negative. Very young children may have fewer apparent lesions, making definitive diagnosis difficult. Diagnostic criteria (Box 99.2) help to resolve some of these questionable cases, but specific gene testing is replacing the use of clinical criteria. Screening for the *NF1* gene is technically difficult because the gene is large and several different mutations are causative. Commercially available studies have a 30% false-negative rate.

## Cutaneous Features

Cutaneous lesions of NF1 (Fig. 99.9) include café-au-lait spots, subcutaneous neurofibromas, plexiform neurofibromas, and axillary freckling. *Café-au-lait spots* are flat, hyperpigmented areas that vary in shape and size. They typically are present at birth but increase in size and number during the first few years of life. Later in childhood, skin freckling, 1–3 mm in diameter, often occurs symmetrically in the axillae *(Crowe sign)* and other intertriginous regions. Most children with six or more café-au-lait spots as their only diagnostic criterion will go on to meet diagnostic criteria, usually by age 6 years.

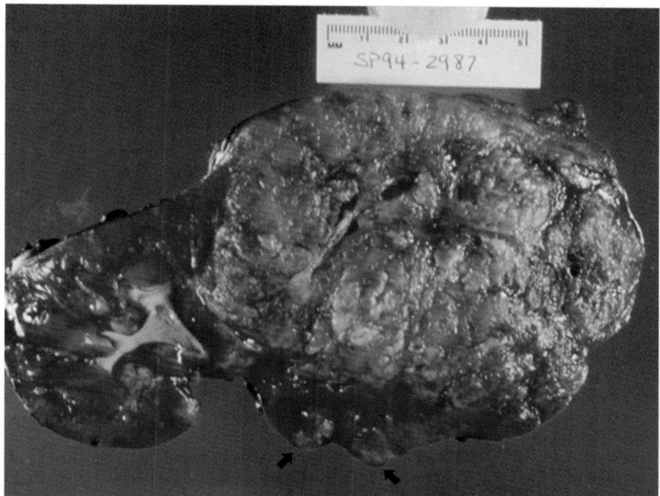


**Fig. 99.8** A large angiomyolipoma of the lower pole of a kidney removed at surgery; several smaller angiomyolipomas *(arrows)* can be seen in the same specimen. *(Reprinted with permission from Weiner, D.M., Ewalt, D.E., Roach, E.S., et al., 1998. The tuberous sclerosis complex: a comprehensive review. J Am Coll Surg 187, 548–561.)*

**BOX 99.2 Diagnostic Criteria for Neurofibromatosis**

**Neurofibromatosis Type 1 (Any Two or More)**

Six or more café-au-lait lesions more than 5 mm in diameter before puberty and more than 15 mm in diameter afterward
Freckling in the axillary or inguinal areas
Optic glioma
Two or more neurofibromas or one plexiform neurofibroma
A first-degree relative with neurofibromatosis type 1
Two or more Lisch nodules
A characteristic bony lesion (sphenoid dysplasia, thinning of the cortex of long bones, with or without pseudoarthrosis)

**Neurofibromatosis Type 2**

Bilateral eighth nerve tumor (shown by magnetic resonance imaging, computed tomography, or histological confirmation)
A first-degree relative with neurofibromatosis type 2 and a unilateral eighth nerve tumor
A first-degree relative with neurofibromatosis type 2 and any two of the following lesions: neurofibroma, meningioma, schwannoma, glioma, or juvenile posterior subcapsular lenticular opacity

*Data derived from Neurofibromatosis. Conference statement, 1988. National Institutes of Health Consensus Development Conference. Arch Neurol 45, 575–578.*

*Neurofibromas* are benign tumors arising from peripheral nerves. These tumors are composed predominantly of Schwann cells and fibroblasts but contain endothelial, pericyte, and mast cell components. Neurofibromas can develop at any time; their size and number often increase after puberty.

*Plexiform neurofibromas* often occur on the face and can cause substantial deformity. Patients with plexiform tumors of the head, face, or neck and those who presented before 10 years of age are more likely to do poorly (Needle et al., 1997). Plexiform neurofibromas have a 5%–13% lifetime risk of malignant degeneration into malignant peripheral nerve sheath tumors (MPNSTs). MPNSTs carry poor 5-year survival rates despite treatment with surgery, chemotherapy, and radiation. PNFs and MPNSTs are difficult to distinguish radiographically and sometimes even pathologically.

## Neurological Features

NF1 affects the nervous system in several ways, but the clinical features vary even within the same family. Tumors occur in the brain, spinal cord, and peripheral nerves. Compared to the general population, there is higher incidence of learning disability and attention disorders. Accompanying moyamoya syndrome predisposes to stroke.

*Optic nerve glioma* (Fig. 99.10) is the most common CNS tumor caused by NF1. Approximately 15% of patients with NF1 have unilateral or bilateral optic glioma. The growth rate of these tumors varies, but they tend to behave less aggressively in patients with NF1 than those without NF1. When symptomatic, the presenting features are optic atrophy, progressive vision loss, pain, or proptosis. Precocious puberty is a common presenting feature of chiasmatic optic nerve tumors in children with NF1. Management options include observation with serial brain MRI or treatment with radiation, chemotherapy, or small-molecule therapies that specifically target signaling pathways downstream of activated Ras. Radiation is less favored, especially given possible exacerbation of vasculopathy in this population.

Ependymomas and meningiomas of the CNS occur in patients with NF1 less often than in patients with neurofibromatosis type 2. Neurofibromas and schwannomas are common but not always symptomatic; they develop on either cranial nerves or spinal nerve roots. The symptoms from these tumors (discomfort, pain, numbness, weakness, and bowel/bladder dysfunction) reflect their size, location, and rate of growth.

Macrocephaly is seen in half of NF1 patients, typically attributable to megalencephaly related to increases in white-matter volume. Macrocephaly is independent of hydrocephalus accompanying aqueductal stenosis, which also occurs in this disorder. Approximately 60%–78% of patients with NF1 have increased signal lesions within the basal ganglia, thalamus, brainstem, and cerebellum on T2-weighted MRIs (Fig. 99.11). These areas are not routinely visible with CT. The origin and significance of these radiographic lesions are unclear, and they are referred to at times as *unidentified bright objects* (UBOs). Whether these MRI lesions correlate with the likelihood of cognitive impairment is still debatable; radiographic findings do not correlate with neurological deficits. Patients with NF1 tend to have full-scale intelligence quotient (IQ) scores within the low-normal range and to exhibit behavioral problems. Deep gray-matter radiological findings tend to decrease with time, while cortical and subcortical findings do not decrease or increase.

## Systemic Features

Lisch *nodules* are pigmented iris hamartomas (Fig. 99.12). They are pathognomonic for NF1. Lisch nodules do not cause symptoms; their significance lies in their implications for the diagnosis of NF1. Lisch nodules are often not apparent during early childhood, so their absence does not exclude the diagnosis of NF1. Rarely, children with NF1 have retinal hamartomas, but these usually remain asymptomatic.

Dysplasia of the renal or carotid arteries occurs in a small percentage of patients with NF1. Renal artery stenosis causes systemic hypertension. Another potential cause of hypertension is pheochromocytoma. Several forms of cerebral artery dysplasia occur, most commonly moyamoya syndrome, which promotes cerebral infarction in children and brain hemorrhage in adults. Arterial aneurysms occur as well.

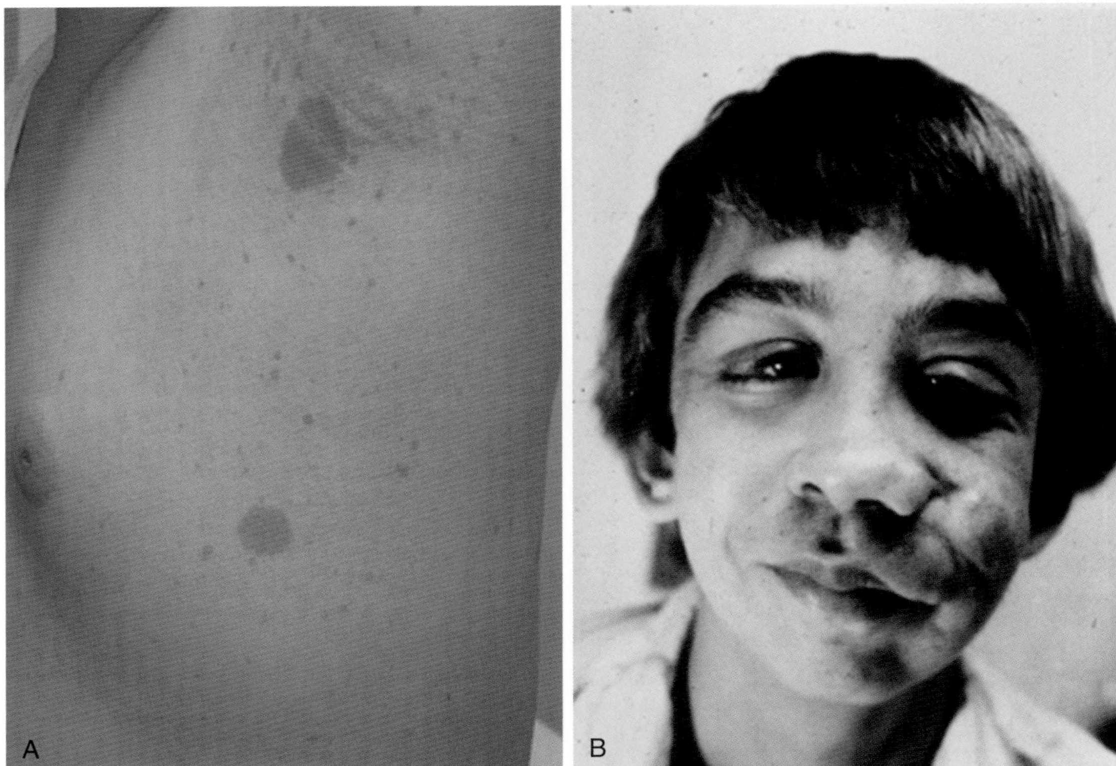


**Fig. 99.9** A, Typical café-au-lait spots and axillary freckling in an individual with neurofibromatosis type 1. B, Plexiform neurofibroma in a boy with neurofibromatosis type 1. *(B, Reprinted with permission from Roach, E.S., 1988. Diagnosis and management of neurocutaneous syndromes. Semin Neurol 8, 83–96.)*

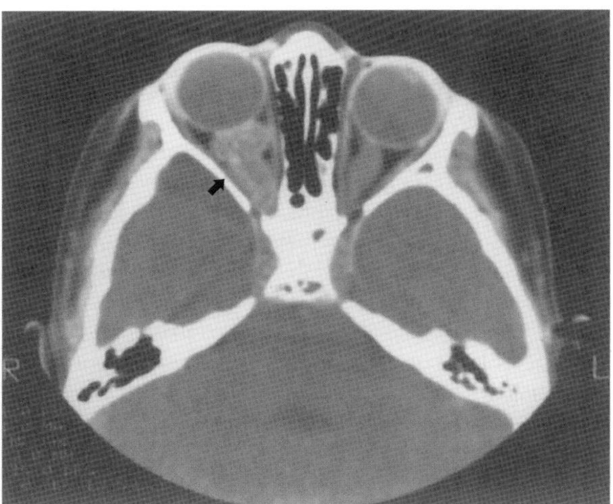

**Fig. 99.10** Computed cranial tomography scan from a child with neurofibromatosis type 1 shows bilateral optic nerve gliomas, larger in the right optic nerve *(arrow)* than the left. *(Reprinted with permission from Roach, E.S., 1992. Neurocutaneous syndromes. Pediatr Clin North Am 39, 591–620.)*

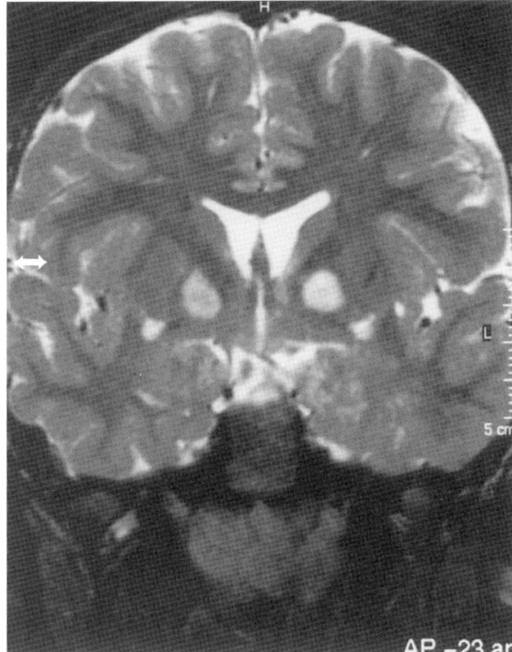

**Fig. 99.11** Coronal T2-weighted magnetic resonance imaging scan shows bilateral high-signal lesions in the basal ganglia, abnormalities typical of neurofibromatosis type 1.

The most common skeletal manifestations in NF1 consist of short stature and macrocephaly. Other skeletal abnormalities include long-bone dysplasia (resulting in pathological fractures and subsequent pseudoarthrosis), scoliosis, and bony erosion secondary to adjacent tumor. Dysplasia of the sphenoid wing is common.

A mimic of NF1 is LEOPARD syndrome (*l*entigenes, *E*CG conduction abnormalities, *o*cular hypertelorism, *p*ulmonary stenosis, *a*bnormal (male) genitalia, *r*etardation of growth, *d*eafness) is an autosomal dominant disorder whose features also include café-au-lait spots and obstructive cardiomyopathy. The café-au-lait spots and cardiac abnormalities may suggest NF1. Legius syndrome is another autosomal dominant NF-like syndrome; it is characterized by similar cutaneous features but little tumorigenesis.

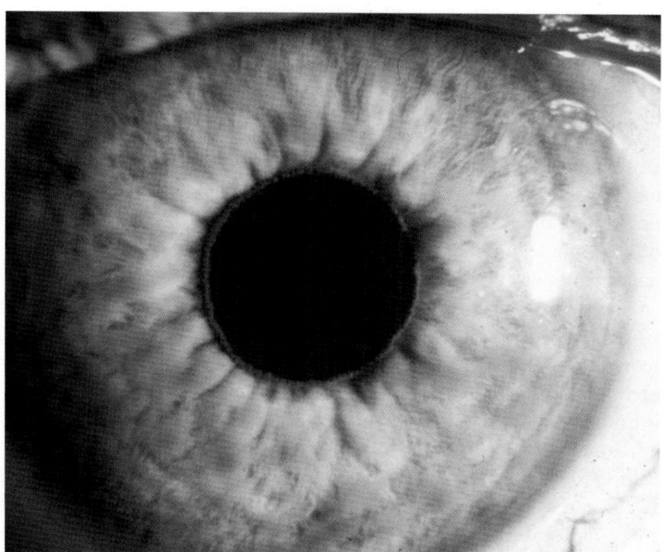

**Fig. 99.12** Lisch Nodules of the Iris in a Patient With Neurofibromatosis Type 1.

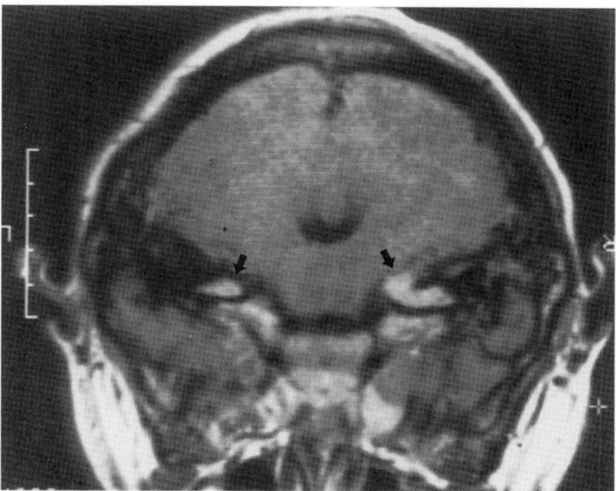

**Fig. 99.13** Cranial magnetic resonance imaging scan from a child with neurofibromatosis type 2 shows bilateral vestibular tumors *(arrows)*. As these grow larger, there is an increased likelihood of symptoms. *(Reprinted with permission from Roach, E.S., 1992 Neurocutaneous syndromes. Pediatr Clin North Am 39, 591–620.)*

## NEUROFIBROMATOSIS TYPE 2

Designated fully a separate entity from NF1 in the late 20th century, neurofibromatosis type 2 (NF2) is characterized by bilateral vestibular schwannomas and often is associated with other brain or spinal cord tumors. Similar to NF1, the inheritance is autosomal dominant. Some suggest the diagnosis of NF2 based on multiple meningiomas or nonvestibular schwannomas even without family history or classic bilateral vestibular schwannomas. NF2 occurs in only 1 in 35,000 to 50,000 people.

A mutation of the *NF2* gene on chromosome 22 causes NF2. The NF2 protein product is schwannomin or merlin, moesin-ezrin-radixin-like protein. The *NF2* gene is a tumor suppressor. Dysfunction of the *NF2* gene accounts for the occurrence of multiple central nervous system (CNS) tumors in patients with NF2. Several different mutations have been documented in the *NF2* gene. The clinical severity may be related to the nature of the *NF2* mutation; missense mutations that allow some protein function tend to produce milder clinical forms, whereas frameshift and nonsense mutations that produce stop codons preventing the production of any protein often cause severe disease (Halliday et al., 2017).

### Clinical Features

Patients with NF2 have few cutaneous lesions, and these tend to be subtle. Instead, patients often have multiple types of CNS tumors (thus, the designation of *central NF*). Café-au-lait spots and subcutaneous neurofibromas are less common than in NF1. Some patients exhibit presenile posterior subcapsular cataracts.

Most patients who meet established diagnostic criteria for NF2 (see Box 99.2) eventually develop bilateral vestibular schwannomas, previously termed acoustic neuromas (Fig. 99.13). Symptoms of NF2 typically develop in adolescence or early adulthood but can begin in childhood. Common complaints with large acoustic tumors include hearing loss, tinnitus, vertigo, facial weakness, poor balance, and headache. Unilateral hearing loss is relatively common in the early stages. Consider screening with annual auditory brainstem responses or brain MRI.

Other CNS tumors occur much less often than vestibular schwannomas. The term *MISME syndrome* (*m*ultiple *i*nherited *s*chwannomas, *m*eningiomas, and *e*pendymomas) applies to this disorder. The clinical features of these tumors depend primarily on their location within the brain and spinal cord. Schwannomas of other cranial nerves occur in some patients. Meningiomas, ependymomas, and astrocytomas also occur with increased frequency. Patients with NF2 may develop multiple simultaneous tumor types, and baseline imaging at the time of diagnosis should include the brain and spinal cord.

*Merlin* is a novel regulator of TSC/mTORC1 signaling, so mTOR inhibitors are being evaluated in the management of NF2 tumors (James et al., 2009) and also have been under study for the treatment of plexiform neurofibromas in NF1.

## STURGE-WEBER SYNDROME

The characteristic features of Sturge-Weber syndrome (SWS) are a facial cutaneous angioma (port-wine nevus) and an associated leptomeningeal and brain angioma. The findings usually are ipsilateral but can be bilateral or even contralateral. In addition to the facial nevus, other findings include intellectual disability, seizures, contralateral hemiparesis and hemiatrophy, and homonymous hemianopia (Thomas-Sohl et al., 2004). However, the clinical features are variable, and individuals with cutaneous lesions and seizures but with normal intelligence and no focal neurological deficits are common. The syndrome occurs sporadically and in all races. A somatic mutation in *GNAQ* has been identified in patients with port-wine stains with or without SWS. This activating mutation disrupts the q class of G-protein alpha subunits and contributes to reduced GTPase activity; this results in increased cell signaling activity (Shirley et al., 2013).

### Cutaneous Features

The nevus typically involves the forehead and upper eyelid but also may involve both sides of the face and extend onto the trunk and limbs (Fig. 99.14). Nevi that involve only the trunk, or facial nevi that spare the upper face, rarely are associated with an intracranial angioma. The facial angioma is usually obvious at birth; it may thicken over time and develop a nodular texture. Reactive hypertrophy of adjacent bone and connective tissue may occur. Some children have the characteristic neurological and radiographic features of SWS, yet have no skin lesions. More frequently, the typical cutaneous and ophthalmic findings are present without clinical or radiographic evidence of an intracranial lesion. Only 10%–20% of children with a port-wine nevus of the forehead have a leptomeningeal angioma. Although the leptomeningeal angioma is typically ipsilateral to a unilateral facial nevus, bilateral brain lesions occur in at least 15% of patients, including some with a unilateral cutaneous nevus.

## Ocular Features

Glaucoma is the main ophthalmological condition associated with SWS. The risk of developing glaucoma has two age peaks, the first in infancy and the second in late childhood. Amblyopia and buphthalmos (enlarged globe) are present in some newborns. In others, the glaucoma becomes symptomatic later and, if untreated, causes progressive blindness. Periodic measurement of the intraocular pressure is mandatory, particularly when the nevus is near the eye. Patients with SWS also may develop choroid angiomas or heterochromasia of the iris ipsilateral to the nevus.

## Neurological Features

Epilepsy, intellectual disability, and focal neurological deficits are the principal neurological abnormalities of SWS. Seizures often begin in conjunction with hemiparesis or other focal deficits. Seizure onset before age 2 years increases the likelihood of future intellectual disability and refractory epilepsy. Intellectual disability is likely in children with refractory seizures, whereas children who never experience seizures usually have normal intelligence. Few children who have normal cognition at age 3 years will later develop severe intellectual impairment.

Epilepsy eventually develops in 72%–80% of patients with SWS with unilateral lesions and in 93% of patients with bihemispheric involvement. Although some begin in adult life, 75% of seizures begin during the first year, 86% by age 2, and 95% before age 5. Focal motor seizures or generalized tonic-clonic seizures are the most typical seizure type initially associated with SWS. Other initial seizure types are infantile spasms, myoclonic seizures, and atonic seizures. The first few seizures are often focal, even in patients who later develop generalized tonic-clonic seizures or infantile spasms. Seizures can be refractory or may remain well controlled with medication for long intervals.

The neurological impairment caused by SWS depends in part on the site of the intracranial vascular lesion. Because the occipital region frequently is involved, visual-field deficits are common. Hemiparesis often develops acutely in conjunction with the initial flurry of seizures. Although often attributed to postictal weakness, hemiparesis may be permanent or persist longer than typical of a postictal deficit. Some children develop sudden weakness without seizures, either as repeated episodes of weakness similar to transient ischemic attacks or as a single stroke-like episode with persistent neurological deficit. Not all patients have permanent focal neurological signs.

Early developmental milestones may be normal, but mild to profound mental deficiency eventually develops in approximately half of patients. Only 8% of the patients with bilateral brain involvement are intellectually normal. Behavioral concerns are frequent, even in patients who are not intellectually disabled. The clinical condition eventually stabilizes, resulting in residual hemiparesis,

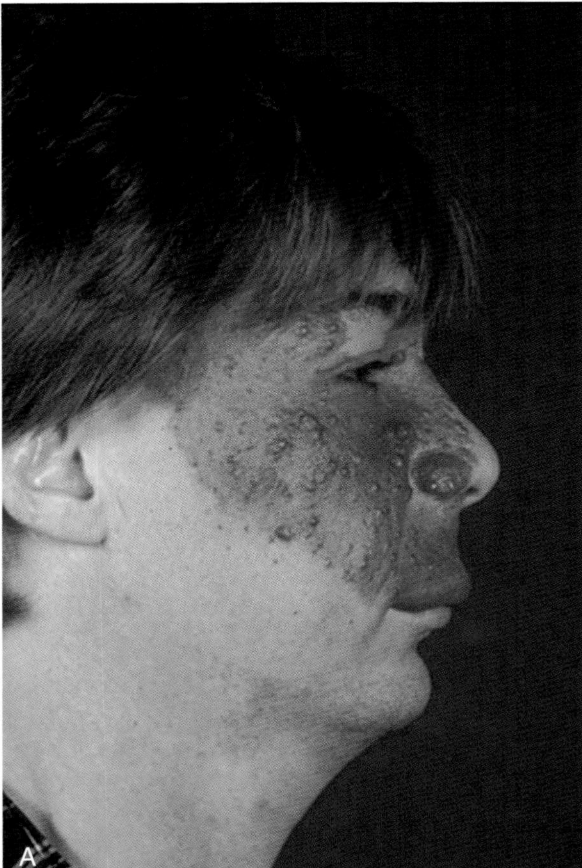

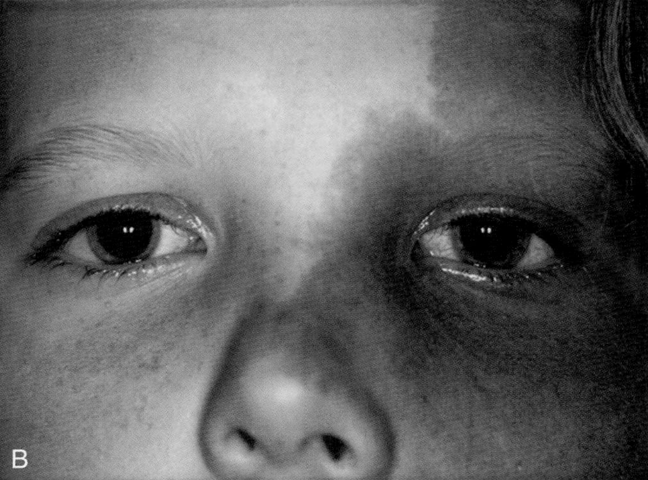

**Fig. 99.14** Two patients with the classic distribution of the port-wine nevus of Sturge-Weber syndrome on the face and eyelid. **A,** The nevus has developed a nodular texture. **B,** Episcleral or conjunctival angiomas can occur on the affected side.

hemianopia, intellectual disability, and epilepsy, but without further deterioration.

## Diagnostic Studies

Most children with a facial port-wine nevus do not have an intracranial angioma. Neuroimaging studies help distinguish children with SWS from those with isolated cutaneous lesions. Although gyral calcification is a typical feature of SWS, the tram-track appearance first described on standard radiographs is uncommon and is almost never present in neonates. CT shows intracranial calcification much earlier (Fig. 99.15) than standard skull radiographs. Extensive cerebral atrophy is apparent even with CT, but MRI more readily shows subtle atrophy.

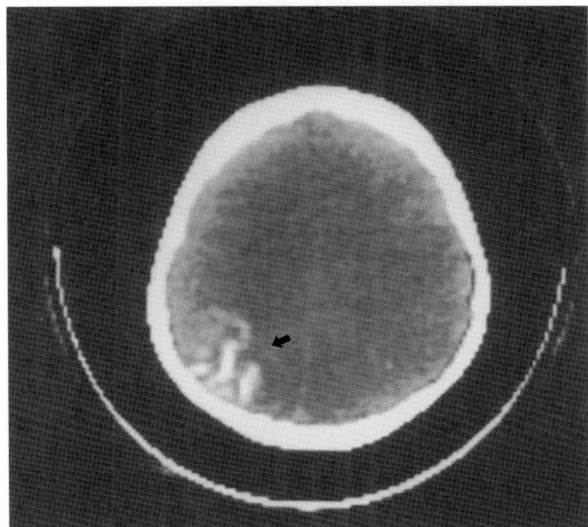

**Fig. 99.15** Computed tomographic scan from a typical patient with Sturge-Weber syndrome; the occipital gyriform calcification pattern *(arrow)* is easily seen. *(Reprinted with permission from Garcia, J.C., Roach, E.S., McClean, W.T., 1981. Recurrent thrombotic deterioration in the Sturge-Weber syndrome. Childs Brain 8, 427–433.)*

MRI with gadolinium contrast (Fig. 99.16) effectively demonstrates the abnormal intracranial vessels in most patients with SWS. Positron emission tomography (PET) demonstrates reduced metabolism of the brain adjacent to the leptomeningeal lesion. However, patients with recent-onset seizures may have increased cerebral metabolism near the lesion. Single-photon emission computed tomography (SPECT) shows reduced perfusion of the affected brain. Both PET and SPECT often reveal vascular changes extending well beyond the area of abnormality depicted by CT (Maria et al., 1998). Although functional imaging is not necessary for all patients, it may help initially to establish a diagnosis and may help characterize the extent of abnormality before surgery.

Cerebral arteriography is no longer routine in the evaluation of SWS but is sometimes useful in atypical patients or prior to surgery for epilepsy. The veins are more abnormal than the arteries, with enlarged, tortuous, subependymal, and medullary veins and sparse superficial cortical veins. Failure of the sagittal sinus to opacify after ipsilateral carotid injection may be due to obliteration of the superficial cortical veins by thrombosis; the abnormal deep venous channels probably have a similar origin as they form collateral conduits for nonfunctioning cortical veins. Microscopic hemorrhages are sometimes evident on pathology specimens, although significant intracranial hemorrhage is rare.

## Treatment

Generally, the more extensive the intracranial lesion, the more difficult it is to control seizures with medication. Resection of a localized brain vascular lesion or hemispherectomy can often improve seizure control and may promote better intellectual development (Bourgeois et al., 2007). Despite general agreement on the efficacy of surgical resection, debate remains concerning patient selection and the timing of surgery. Almost one patient in five has bilateral cerebral lesions, limiting the surgical options unless one hemisphere is clearly responsible for most of the seizures. Often the patient selected for surgery is

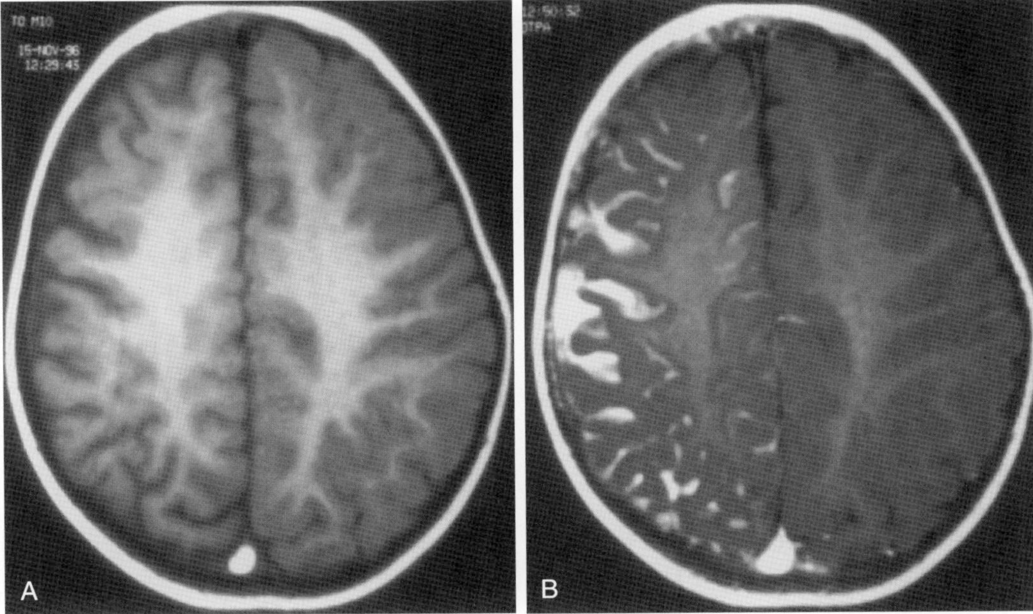


**Fig. 99.16** **A,** Magnetic resonance imaging study from a child with Sturge-Weber syndrome; this T1-weighted axial view without contrast infusion is normal. **B,** Scan on the same child with gadolinium reveals leptomeningeal and intraparenchymal angioma.

one with refractory seizures, clinical dysfunction (e.g., hemiparesis, hemianopia) of the area selected for resection, and failure to respond to an adequate trial of anticonvulsants. Patients with less extensive lesions should have a limited resection rather than a complete hemispherectomy. The limited resection preserves as much normal brain as possible, even at the risk of having to do another operation later. Corpus callosotomy is useful for patients with refractory tonic or atonic seizures and extensive disease. In effect, the surgical considerations in children with SWS are similar to those used with other patients with epilepsy. Low-dose aspirin has been offered to patients with SWS in an effort to minimize the burden of stroke-like episodes, seizures, or cognitive impairment (Lance et al., 2013). Aspirin is generally well-tolerated, but its efficacy has not been established.

## VON HIPPEL-LINDAU SYNDROME

Von Hippel-Lindau (VHL) syndrome is an autosomal dominant inherited disorder characterized by hemangioblastomas arising in the retina and CNS, as well as visceral cysts and tumors. Hemangioblastomas may occur sporadically but are usually multiple and more likely to occur in young persons. Current prevalence estimates of this disorder are approximately 1 in 40,000.

*Hemangioblastomas* are benign slow-growing vascular tumors that cause symptoms from hemorrhage or local mass effect. Histologically, hemangioblastomas are composed of endothelium-lined vascular channels surrounded by stromal cells and pericytes. Mast cells are present and may produce erythropoietin.

The initial symptoms of VHL usually arise from effects of the vascular anomalies in the CNS, but some patients may present with pheochromocytoma or renal, pancreatic, hepatic, or epididymal tumors. One classification system categorizes patients according to whether pheochromocytoma is present. The most common pattern of VHL findings includes retinal and CNS hemangioblastomas and pancreatic cysts (Lonser et al., 2003).

### Neurological Features

In the CNS, the most common site of hemangioblastomas is the cerebellum in approximately half of patients (Fig. 99.17), followed by spinal and medullary sites. Cerebral hemangioblastomas are present in less than 5% of patients with VHL. The cerebellar hemispheres are affected far more frequently than the cerebellar vermis. Cerebellar hemangioblastomas typically present in the second decade of life.

Early symptoms of cerebellar and brainstem hemangioblastomas include headache, the most common symptom, followed by ataxia, nausea and vomiting, and nystagmus. Symptoms are often intermittent or slowly progressive, but up to 20% of patients have an acute onset of symptoms following mild head trauma. Spinal hemangioblastomas typically present with focal back or neck pain and sensory loss or weakness. Because of their typical intramedullary location, spinal hemangioblastomas frequently lead to syringomyelia. The conus medullaris and the cervicomedullary junction are the most common sites. Brainstem hemangioblastomas tend to arise in the area postrema in the medulla, where they may be associated with syringobulbia. Occasionally, hemangioblastomas occur in the cerebral hemispheres or sites near the third ventricle, such as the pituitary gland or its stalk, the hypothalamus, or optic nerve. The incidence of cerebellar hemangioblastomas increases with age, and 84% of patients with VHL will develop at least one such tumor by age 60 years (Maher et al., 1990).

Hemangioblastomas are best visualized using contrast-enhanced MRI. Routine screening of the brain and spinal cord should include precontrast and postcontrast T1-weighted images with thin sections through the posterior fossa and spinal cord and surface coil

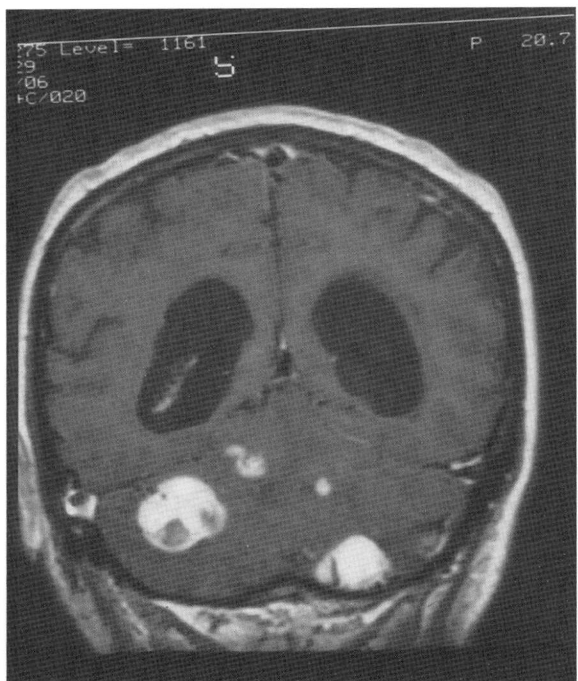

**Fig. 99.17** Magnetic resonance imaging showing multiple cerebellar hemangioblastomas in a patient with Von Hippel-Lindau syndrome.

imaging of the entire spinal cord. Arteriography is not necessary for diagnosis but is valuable in demonstrating the feeding vessels if surgical resection is planned.

Endolymphatic sac tumors occur in 10%–15% of these individuals. Sometimes they are bilateral. Presenting symptoms can be abrupt change in hearing accompanying hemorrhage or vertigo and tinnitus (Butman et al., 2008).

### Ocular Features

Childhood onset of symptoms is unusual, but retinal hemangioblastomas may occur in children as young as 1 year. Retinal hemangioblastomas may be asymptomatic, especially if they occur in the periphery of the retina. Vision loss occurs when the lesions are large and centrally located, even in the absence of hemorrhage. Arteriovenous shunting leads to fluid extravasation. Hemorrhage may lead to retinal injury and detachment, glaucoma, uveitis, macular edema, and sympathetic ophthalmitis.

### Systemic Features

Renal cysts are present in more than half of individuals with VHL, although, as with CNS and retinal hemangioblastomas, the patients may be asymptomatic. Extensive renal cysts rarely lead to renal failure. Of greater concern is renal cell carcinoma, which develops in more than 70% of patients and is the leading cause of death. These tumors are usually multiple and tend to occur at a younger age than sporadic renal cell carcinoma (Ashouri et al., 2015). Simple renal cysts arise from distal tubular epithelium, whereas renal cell carcinoma tumors arise from proximal tubular epithelium.

Pheochromocytomas occur in 7%–19% of patients and may be the only clinical manifestation of VHL, even in carefully screened individuals. Tumors may be bilateral and occur outside the adrenal glands. Symptoms of pheochromocytoma include episodic or sustained hypertension, severe headache, and flushing with profuse sweating—or even hypertensive crises, stroke, myocardial infarction, and heart failure. Diagnostic laboratory investigation demonstrates excessive catecholamine concentrations in serum and urine.

Cysts and tumors of the pancreas and epididymis are also features of VHL. Pancreatic tumors include nonsecretory islet cell tumors, simple cysts, serous microcystic adenomas, and adenocarcinomas. Pancreatic cysts are the most common of these lesions and are asymptomatic unless they obstruct the bile duct or become numerous enough to cause pancreatic insufficiency. Islet cell tumors coincide frequently with pheochromocytomas, possibly because both tumors derive from neural crest cells. Epididymal cystadenomas also may be asymptomatic but palpable and cause discomfort.

### Molecular Genetics

Confirming initial suspicions, the VHL gene is a tumor-suppressor gene located on chromosome 3p25–26. A mutation in the VHL gene also occurs in many sporadic clear-cell renal carcinomas that present later in life, as compared with those with VHL disease. This gene plays a role in the function of hypoxia-induced factor HIF2$\alpha$. This regulation contributes to increased vascularization and upregulation of proangiogenic genes and other oxygen-sensitive genes via hypoxia response elements (HREs). These genes include vascular endothelial growth factor (VEGF), platelet-derived growth factor (PDGF), transforming growth factor alpha (TGF-$\alpha$), glucose transporter-1 (GLUT1), carbonic anhydrase IX, and erythropoietin (EPO), among others. In particular, VEGF is important in angiogenesis; its level in ocular fluid of patients is significantly higher than in unaffected subjects. Recognition of these affected genes has focused trials of certain therapies (Clark & Cookson, 2008).

Hundreds of known mutations exist. Despite complex genotype-phenotype relationships, some clinical correlations are possible. Missense mutations in this gene are associated with pheochromocytoma, whereas nonsense, frameshift, and splice-site mutations as well as deletions predominate in families without pheochromocytomas. Microdeletions and microinsertions, nonsense mutations, or deletions appear in 56% of families with VHL type 1, whereas missense mutations account for 96% of those responsible for VHL type 2 (Chen et al., 1995). Specific mutations in codon 238 account for 43% of the mutations responsible for VHL type 2, and one group of patients (type 2C) appears to be at low risk for any feature of VHL except pheochromocytoma.

### Treatment

Careful screening (Box 99.3) is the most important aspect of management of VHL. Screening is mandatory for all first-degree relatives in a family with VHL or pheochromocytoma. Other indications for clinical screening include pancreatic cysts, multiple or bilateral renal cell tumors, retinal hemangiomas, and cerebellar hemangioblastomas. Availability of molecular analysis for the VHL gene reduces the number of asymptomatic relatives requiring surveillance; only relatives who have inherited the VHL mutation need annual screening.

## HEREDITARY HEMORRHAGIC TELANGIECTASIA

Hereditary hemorrhagic telangiectasia (HHT), also known as *Rendu-Osler-Weber syndrome* or *Osler-Weber-Rendu syndrome*, is a highly penetrant autosomal dominant disorder characterized by telangiectasias of the skin, mucous membranes, and various internal organs. The prevalence is 1 in 10,000. Two different genes are responsible for most cases. One gene on chromosome 9q33–34 (HHT1) encodes for endoglin (ENG), a TGF-$\beta$ binding protein. The other gene, on chromosome 12q13 (HHT2), encodes for activin A receptor type II-like 1 kinase, or ACVRL1. In some, a SMAD4 gene mutation leads to juvenile polyposis and HHT. Up to 30% of cases arise from spontaneous mutations. The clinical features and the age at presentation are highly variable. Diagnostic criteria known as the *Curacao criteria* include spontaneous recurrent epistaxis, visceral manifestation, and an affected first-degree relative; these were formulated in 2000 (Shovlin, 2000). Consensus guidelines regarding surveillance in 2009 recommend sequence analysis of ENG and ACVRL1 in index cases to guide testing at-risk family members or to assist diagnosis in individuals who do not meet the requisite three of the four clinical criteria (Faughnan et al., 2011)

Cutaneous telangiectasias most often occur on the face, lips, and hands and are less common on the trunk. Telangiectasias of the nasal mucosa often cause epistaxis well before other complications of the disease occur and can be severe enough to contribute to iron-deficiency anemia. Approximately one-third of patients have conjunctival telangiectasias, and 10% have retinal vascular malformations, although vision loss from these lesions is uncommon. Telangiectasias are not prominent during the first decade, but they tend to enlarge and multiply thereafter.

Widespread vascular dysplasia of the lungs, gastrointestinal tract, or genitourinary system, depending on which site is predominantly affected, can produce hemoptysis, hematemesis, melena, or hematuria. Other involved organs and tissues can include the thyroid, diaphragm, liver, pancreas, spleen, vertebrae, or aorta. Pulmonary arteriovenous malformations (AVMs) occur in 15%–20% of patients, and 60%–90% of all pulmonary AVMs are associated with HHT. Screening includes chest radiograph, arterial blood gas on oxygen, and bubble contrast echocardiogram to evaluate for pulmonary shunting. Repeat screening is helpful every 5 years or at times when the number and size of AVMs increase, such as during puberty or pregnancy. Other tests include chest CT and pulmonary angiography.

### Neurological Features

Neurological complications are common. Frequent complaints include headache, dizziness, and seizures. Less common complications include paradoxical embolism with stroke, intraparenchymal or subarachnoid hemorrhage, and meningitis or brain abscess.

Paradoxical embolism via a pulmonary arteriovenous fistula (AVF) leads to cerebral infarction. Rarely, a clot may form within the

**BOX 99.3 Cambridge Screening Protocol for von Hippel-Lindau Disease**

**Affected Patient**

- Annual physical examination and urine testing
- Annual direct and indirect ophthalmoscopy with fluorescein angioscopy or angiography
- Cranial magnetic resonance imaging (MRI) or computed tomography (CT) every 3 years to age 50 and every 5 years thereafter
- Annual renal ultrasound, with abdominal CT scan every 3 years (more frequently if multiple renal cysts are discovered)
- Annual 24-h urine collection for vanillylmandelic acid

**At-Risk Relative**

- Annual physical examination and urine testing
- Annual direct and indirect ophthalmoscopy from age 5 years
- Annual fluorescein angioscopy or angiography from age 10 years until age 60
- Cranial MRI or CT every 3 years from age 15 to 40 and every 5 years until age 60
- Annual renal ultrasound, with abdominal CT scan every 3 years from age 20 to 65 years
- Annual 24-h urine collection for vanillylmandelic acid

fistula itself before migrating into the arterial circulation. Intermittent symptoms with subsequent improvement result from repeated small emboli. The cause of transient ischemic attacks during hemoptysis is air embolism from a bleeding pulmonary AVF. Approximately 1% develop cerebral abscess or meningitis, probably because septic microemboli bypass the normal filtration of the pulmonary circulation via a pulmonary AVF.

Vascular anomalies may be found anywhere in the brain, spinal cord, or meninges, and more than one type of lesion may be present in the same patient—making this a diagnosis for consideration in patients with multiple cerebrovascular malformations. Approximately one-fourth of HHT patients are likely to have a cerebral vascular malformation. AVMs, high-flow pial fistulae, and telangiectasias are most common; cavernous malformations, venous angiomas, and vein of Galen malformations also occur, but less commonly.

Screening should begin with MRI and MR angiography (MRA) of the brain, although cerebral angiography is most sensitive. Angiography every 5 years with interim surveillance is recommended. MRI is the best procedure for patients with known AVMs.

### Treatment

As with most of the neurocutaneous syndromes, treatment of HHT is limited to the management of complications. Because many of the neurological complications of the disease arise secondary to a pulmonary AVF, resection or embolization of the fistula is essential. Treatment of cerebral AVMs is embolization, excision, or radiosurgery. Periodic transfusion and chronic iron administration may be necessary. To reduce risk of brain abscess in cases of undiagnosed pulmonary AVM, antibiotic prophylaxis is a recommendation prior to dental procedures (Faughnan et al., 2011).

## HYPOMELANOSIS OF ITO

Hypomelanosis of Ito (HI) is a heterogeneous and complex neurocutaneous disorder affecting the skin, brain, eye, skeleton, and other organs. Ito named the disorder *incontinentia pigmenti achromians*, but the present name is *hypomelanosis of Ito* to avoid confusion with incontinentia pigmenti. It is the third most frequent neurocutaneous disease after NF1 and the TSC. HI is usually a sporadic disorder with minimal recurrence risk.

### Cutaneous Features

The skin findings are distinctive and in fact are the only constant feature of HI. Hypopigmented whorls, streaks, and patches are present at birth and tend to follow *Blaschko lines*, pathways demarcating embryonic skin development. In HI, the hypopigmented skin lesions are usually multiple, involve several body segments, and may be unilateral or bilateral. They may be observable at birth but commonly develop in infancy, depending on the degree of skin pigmentation. Wood's lamp examination may enable detection of hypopigmented lesions. The degree or distribution of skin depigmentation does not appear to correlate with either the severity of neurological symptoms or associated organ pathology. The hypopigmented lesions follow Blaschko lines in two-thirds of patients and are patchy in others. Other skin findings in patients with HI include café-au-lait spots, cutis marmorata, aplasia cutis, nevus of Ota, trichorrhexis, focal hypertrichosis, and nail dystrophy. Electron microscopy of the hypopigmented lesions consistently shows a marked reduction of melanocytes (Cavallari et al., 1996). In the proximity of preserved melanocytes, the basal keratinocytes contain a nearly normal content of melanosomes. Depigmented areas contain an increased number of Langerhans cells.

Many different cytogenetic anomalies occur in HI. Most patients are mosaic for aneuploidy or unbalanced translocations, with two or more chromosomally distinct cell lines either within the same tissue or between tissues. Genetic alterations in HI include ring chromosome 22, mosaic trisomy 18, 18/X translocation, and others. Mosaicism for sex chromosome aneuploidy also occurs. Many individuals have normal lymphocyte karyotypes, but it is important to recognize that mosaicism may be tissue specific, so karyotype abnormalities may be demonstrable in fibroblasts but not in lymphocytes.

### Neurological Features

The frequency of neurological abnormalities in patients with typical skin lesions ranges from 50% to 80% (Nehal et al., 1996). Epilepsy and intellectual disability are the most common neurological abnormalities. Approximately half of patients with HI have seizures, usually with onset in the first year of life. Focal seizures are most common.

Macrocephaly is more common than microcephaly. Generalized cerebral or cerebellar hypoplasia is the most common abnormality on imaging. Severe cortical neuronal migration anomalies, hemimegalencephaly, and lissencephaly occur as well. Hemimegalencephaly may be ipsilateral or contralateral to the cutaneous hypopigmentation. Extensive periventricular white-matter lesions are another common finding. Small periventricular cysts and gray-matter heterotopias occur as well. About a third of patients with HI have normal cranial MRI studies.

### Systemic Features

Some 50%–70% of patients with HI have noncutaneous defects. Ocular findings include microphthalmia, heterochromia iridis, dacryostenosis, pannus, corneal opacities, cataract, optic atrophy, retinal detachment, and pigmentation anomalies of the retina. The most common musculoskeletal anomaly is hemihypertrophy, but other anomalies include short stature, pectus carinatum and excavatum, cleft palate, butterfly vertebrae, scoliosis, and clinodactyly and polysyndactyly. Dental anomalies are frequent, including conical or hypoplastic teeth, hypoplastic dental enamel, and cleft lip and palate. Cardiac defects include tetralogy of Fallot, pulmonary stenosis, and septal defects. Disorders of endocrine and renal development occur infrequently.

## INCONTINENTIA PIGMENTI

Incontinentia pigmenti (IP) is a rare X-linked dominant condition affecting the skin, eyes, and CNS. Skeletal and dental anomalies are common and variable. A transitory leukocytosis (predominantly eosinophilic) of uncertain clinical significance can occur. Skin biopsy was instrumental in making the diagnosis in the past, but now gene testing is widely available. Skin biopsy from hyperpigmented regions shows free melanin granules in the dermis.

### Cutaneous Features

The skin manifestations are characteristic. Skin abnormalities progress in stages any time from the newborn period to adulthood. The duration of each stage is variable and may overlap with other stages. The lesions typically evolve from blister (stage 1) to verrucous (stage 2) to linear and pigmented (stage 3) and finally to atrophic and hypopigmented (stage 4) (Fig. 99.18). Skin lesions develop along Blaschko lines. The blister or bullous stage often presents in the neonatal period and is often evaluated as an infectious process. Verrucous transformation is most typical during infancy, and abnormalities of the nails and teeth as they erupt become notable. The hyperpigmented stage is prominent in childhood and adulthood but begins to fade in the second or third decade. The hypopigmented or atretic stage may demonstrate loss of

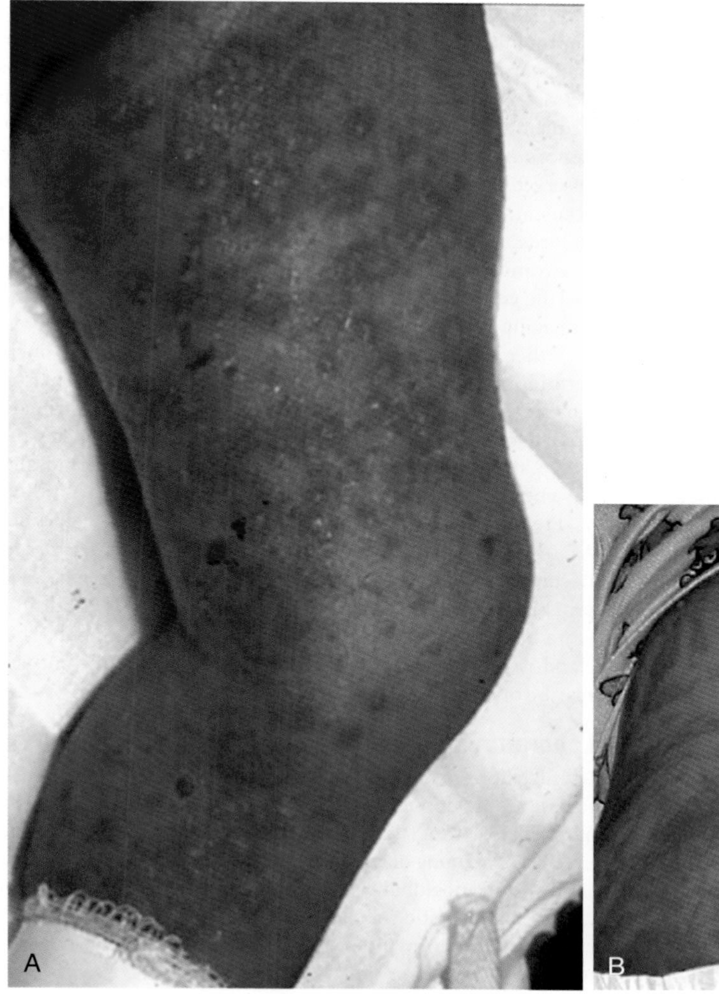


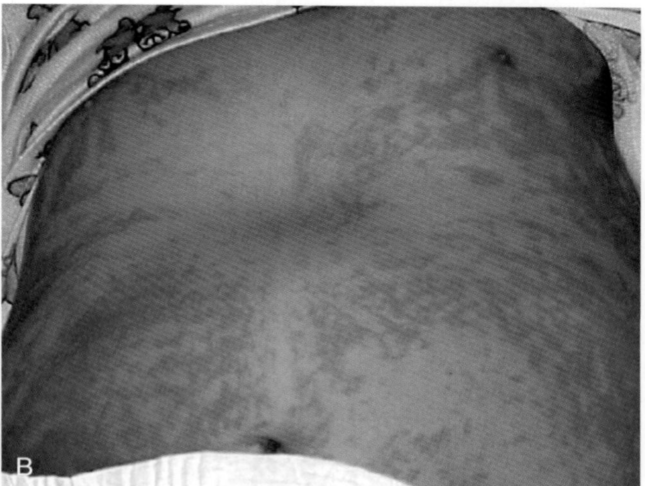


**Fig. 99.18** Features of incontinentia pigmenti change over time from blister-like and verrucous in the infant (**A**) to hyperpigmented in an older individual (**B**).

normal hair and subcutaneous structures in addition to changes in coloration. Not all stages occur in all individuals, especially the hypopigmented stage.

Abnormalities of hair include alopecia in areas that may have been previously affected or unaffected by skin pigmentation changes. Scalp hair may be thin or coarse. Abnormalities of eyebrows may be present as well. Nails may be brittle or demonstrate pits; these findings may wax and wane and raise concern for fungal infection. Tooth abnormalities may include abnormal shape or malpositioning.

IP carries an increased risk of retinal detachment. This is most likely to occur in early childhood and is rare after 6 years of age. Dilated funduscopic examination demonstrates retinal neovascularization as a precursor to detachment. Frequent surveillance ophthalmological examination is important, especially early in life, and may be helpful in making the diagnosis in at-risk family members not otherwise symptomatic.

### Neurological Features

Neurological abnormalities have been overestimated in the past, and the incidence appears less with laboratory confirmation available. Seizures occur more frequently in this population. Most affected females have normal intelligence. Affected males are more likely to have developmental delay. Neurological abnormalities are more likely to occur in individuals with ocular abnormalities. Some demonstrate cerebral or cerebellar atrophy.

### Genetics

Transmission is X-linked dominant, and nuclear factor kappa B (NF-κB) essential modulator (NEMO) is the causative gene—more recently termed *IKBKG* (Greene-Roethke, 2017). Deletion in exons 4–10 is the responsible mutation in 80%–90% of patients (Nelson, 2006). This protein is involved in prevention of apoptosis. The mutation is expected to be lethal in males; however, males with somatic mosaicism or an additional X chromosome, as in Klinefelter syndrome, have survived. These individuals demonstrate immunodeficiency and ectodermal dysplasia rather than the characteristic skin findings described.

## ATAXIA-TELANGIECTASIA

Ataxia-telangiectasia (AT) is a neurodegenerative disorder that begins in early childhood as a slowly progressive ataxia. Telangiectasias (dilated small blood vessels), immunodeficiency, and cellular sensitivity to ionizing radiation develop later. The distinctive skin lesions predominantly involve the sclerae, earlobes, and bridge of the nose, with less common involvement of the eyelids, neck, and antecubital and popliteal fossae. The combination of these telangiectasias in a child with progressive ataxia is pathognomonic for AT. The most striking non-neurological feature of AT is an increased frequency of sinopulmonary infections and a dramatically increased risk for malignancy of the lymphoreticular system, especially leukemia and lymphoma. The estimated prevalence of AT, an autosomal recessive disorder, ranges from 1 in 40,000 to 1 in 100,000. The gene frequency is as high as 1% in the general population.

### Cutaneous Features

Telangiectasias typically do not develop until age 3–6 years, well after the onset of ataxia. Two other dermatological features of AT that may be overlooked are hypertrichosis and occasional gray hairs. Hypertrichosis is noticeable particularly over the forearms. These often-overlooked features in the context of a child with slowly progressive ataxia provide clues to the correct diagnosis. Progeric changes such as poikiloderma, loss of subcutaneous fat, and sclerosis also have been associated. Abnormal radiosensitivity may underlie reports of basal cell carcinomas in young adults. Cutaneous granulomas, commonly associated with immunodeficiency states such as severe combined immunodeficiency and X-linked hypogammaglobulinemia, may appear as the initial cutaneous manifestation of AT (Chiam et al., 2011).

### Neurological Features

Ataxia, the first manifestation of AT, appears when the child learns to walk in the second year of life. Truncal ataxia predominates early in the course of the disorder, affecting sitting, balance, and gait. Muscle strength is normal, and attainment of early gross motor milestones is usually on time. The ataxia is slowly progressive, and children typically require a wheelchair by the age of 12 years. As the child matures, limb ataxia, intention tremor, and segmental myoclonus become apparent. Choreoathetosis may be difficult to distinguish from dysmetria and intention tremor, but it may dominate the clinical picture in older children. At times, the choreoathetosis may resemble segmental myoclonus of the limbs or trunk. Progressive dystonia of the fingers may appear in the second and third decades of life. Axial muscles are affected, and a stooped posture gradually develops. Progressive dysarthria is present.

Abnormal eye movements are nearly universal in children with AT. Voluntary ocular motility is impaired; nystagmus and apraxias of voluntary gaze such as disorders of smooth pursuit and limitation of upgaze are the most common abnormalities. Oculomotor apraxia may precede appearance of the telangiectasias but is often misidentified as an attention-seeking behavior. Strabismus is seen in many young children with AT, but it is often transitory and does not warrant corrective surgery.

In adult patients with AT, the neurological features include progressive distal muscular atrophy and fasciculations, with relative preservation of proximal strength. The gradual loss of vibration and position sense indicates involvement of the spinal cord dorsal columns, and neuropathological and electrophysiological studies reveal a primarily axonal peripheral polyneuropathy (Verhagen et al., 2007).

Serial brain imaging in older children and adults shows nonprogressive cerebellar atrophy. Autopsy studies confirm the radiographic impression of cerebellar degeneration, with reduced numbers of Purkinje cells, granular and basket cells of the cortex, and neurons in the nuclei of the vermis. Degenerative changes are more extensive in adults, involving the substantia nigra, brainstem nuclei, and spinal cord. Relative sparing of the cerebral cortex is associated with fewer significant neuropsychological deficits (Hoche et al., 2014).

### Immunodeficiency and Cancer Risk

Approximately 10%–15% of patients with AT develop a lymphoid malignancy by early adulthood (Taylor et al., 1996). T-cell malignancies are more common than B-cell tumors, although both are more frequent than in the general population. This increased risk of T-cell tumors may be due to the increase in chromosomal rearrangement observed in T lymphocytes from patients with AT. T-cell tumors may occur at any age, whereas B-cell lymphomas tend to arise in older children. AT is in a family of disorders (including Nijmegen breakage syndrome, Bloom syndrome, and Fanconi anemia) characterized by specific cellular defects in response to deoxyribonucleic acid (DNA)-damaging agents.

Other tumor types reported in association with AT include dysgerminoma, gastric carcinoma, liver carcinoma, retinoblastoma, and pancreatic carcinoma. In fact, nonlymphoid tumors, primarily carcinomas, represent approximately 20% of all malignancies in patients with AT. Cerebellar astrocytoma, medulloblastoma, and glioma also have been linked to AT in case reports.

Frequent sinopulmonary infections are another characteristic of AT. A third of patients have a potentially severe immune deficiency. Recurrent or chronic sinusitis, bronchitis, pneumonia, and chronic progressive bronchiectasis were frequent causes of death in previous years but now usually respond to antibiotic treatment. The thymus gland is often small or absent on chest radiography, and at autopsy may be only rudimentary.

### Laboratory Diagnosis

Useful laboratory tests in the diagnosis of AT include serum α-fetoprotein, immunoglobulins (Igs), and cellular radiosensitivity tests. Nearly all patients with AT have an elevated α-fetoprotein level, which is utilized as a screening diagnostic test. Approximately 80% have decreased serum immunoglobulin—IgA, IgE, or IgG, especially the IgG2 subclass. Characteristic cellular features are reduced life span in culture, cytoskeletal abnormalities, chromosomal instability, hypersensitivity to ionizing radiation and radiomimetic agents, defective radiation-induced checkpoints at the G1, S, and G2 phases of the cell cycle, and defects in signal transduction pathways (Rotman & Shiloh, 1997).

The gene associated with AT, ataxia telangiectasia mutated (ATM), is a large gene located at chromosome 11q22–23, and more than 100 ATM mutations occur widespread throughout the ATM gene. Although the function of the ATM gene product is not clear, it belongs to a family of large proteins involved in cell cycle progression and checkpoint response to DNA damage. One postulation is that oxidative stress specifically activates ATM by initiating signal transduction pathways responsible for protecting cells from such insults (Savitsky et al., 1995). Thus, the production of reactive oxygen species by ionizing radiation may play an important role in mutagenesis in cells with absent or abnormal ATM.

The high risk of malignancy in AT underscores the importance of early diagnosis in affected individuals and subsequent routine surveillance for leukemia and lymphoma. Treatment of the neurological deficits is symptomatic at present. Whether neuroprotective medications or medications that modulate neuronal growth factors can slow neurodegeneration in AT is unknown. Treatment options include vitamin E, α-lipoic acid, and folic acid for their theoretical role in reduction in chromosomal breaks and subsequent translocations or inversions. Genetic counseling and prenatal diagnosis are available.

## EPIDERMAL NEVUS SYNDROME

The term *epidermal nevus syndrome* (ENS) encompasses several disorders that have in common an epidermal nevus and neurological manifestations such as epilepsy or hemimegalencephaly. The syndrome name represents the predominant cell type of the nevus; for example, *nevus verrucosus* (keratinocytes), *nevus comedonicus* (hair follicles), and *nevus sebaceous* (sebaceous glands). Several subtypes of ENS exist and should be differentiated from one another: *nevus sebaceous syndrome* (Schimmelpenning-Feuerstein-Mims syndrome), *Proteus syndrome*, *CHILD* (congenital hemidysplasia with ichthyosiform nevus and limb defects) syndrome, *Becker nevus associated with extracutaneous involvement* (pigmented hairy ENS), *nevus comedonicus syndrome*, and *phakomatosis pigmentokeratotica* (Happle, 1995). Terms such as *Schimmelpenning syndrome*, *organoid nevus syndrome*, and *Jadassohn nevus phakomatosis* describe combinations of neurological findings and sebaceous nevi. It is probably best to consider ENS a heterogeneous group of disorders characterized by epidermal and adnexal hamartomas and other organ system involvement.

### Cutaneous Features

Epidermal nevi are linear or patchy slightly raised lesions that typically present at birth but may appear first in early childhood. The most common location is on the head or neck. Only 16% of congenital nevi subsequently enlarge, compared with 65% of nevi arising after birth. Nevi on the head and neck rarely enlarge, whereas more than half of lesions elsewhere extend beyond their original boundaries.

Most nevi contain more than one tissue type, complicating dermatological classification; the nevus name typically reflects the predominant tissue. Verrucous nevi are the most common type.

### Neurological Features

Neurological involvement is variable but more likely when other extracutaneous disease is present. The location of the nevus appears to correlate with the likelihood of neurological symptoms, with neurological complications of ENS most often occurring in the setting of an epidermal nevus on the face or scalp (Asch & Sugarman, 2018). Cognitive deficits are common, and seizures occur in more than half of those affected. Usually ipsilateral to the nevus, focal epileptiform discharges and focal slowing are the most common EEG abnormalities. Infantile spasms with hypsarrhythmia may occur. Other neurological symptoms include cranial nerve palsies, hemiparesis (especially in patients with hemimegalencephaly), microcephaly, and behavior problems. Spina bifida and encephaloceles rarely occur.

Cerebrovascular anomalies occur in approximately 10% of patients with ENS. Intracranial blood vessels may be dysplastic, dilated, or occluded. A few patients have had AVMs and aneurysms. Ischemia or hemorrhage from intracranial blood vessel anomalies may result in porencephaly, infarctions, and dystrophic calcification.

### Other Features

Tumors occur with moderate frequency in association with ENS. The nevus itself may undergo malignant transformation, often into a basal cell carcinoma. Extracutaneous tumors have included astrocytomas, Wilms tumors, rhabdomyosarcomas, and gastrointestinal carcinomas, among others.

Skeletal abnormalities are quite frequent but often secondary to neurological dysfunction that alters skeletal development. Certain skeletal anomalies may be a primary part of ENS, such as abnormal vertebrae. Limb anomalies include clinodactyly, limb reduction defects, syndactyly, polydactyly, bifid thumbs, and talipes equinovarus.

Half of patients with ENS have ocular abnormalities such as colobomas. Disorders of globe growth include either microphthalmia or macrophthalmia. Retinal lesions such as scarring, degeneration, and detachment may occur. Strabismus and lipodermoid lesions of the conjunctivae are more frequent but less serious findings.

Approximately 10% of patients with ENS have cardiovascular and genitourinary malformations. Single reports describe hypoplastic left-sided heart, ventricular septal defect, coarctation of the aorta, pulmonic stenosis, patent ductus arteriosus, and dilated pulmonary artery. Horseshoe kidney, cystic kidneys, duplicated collecting system, and ureteropelvic junction obstruction also occur.

### Neuroimaging

Megalencephaly ipsilateral to the epidermal nevus is the most frequent finding on neuroimaging, but bilateral involvement is common also. In some patients, megalencephaly results from asymmetrical growth of the skull, with the brain being of normal size. MRI of the skull may show a widened diploic space. Often, enlargement of the calvarium and the ipsilateral cerebral hemisphere are present together. In addition, several types of cerebral dysplasia are associated with ENS, also primarily ipsilateral to the epidermal nevus. Focal pachygyria is the most common type of cortical dysplasia in ENS. The surface of the affected hemisphere may be smooth, the cortical mantle thickened, and the adjacent white matter abnormal.

## NEUROCUTANEOUS MELANOSIS

Neurocutaneous melanosis (NCM) is a congenital disorder of melanotic cell development that involves the CNS, especially the leptomeninges (Agero et al., 2005). Congenital melanocytic nevi may occur without CNS involvement, and, conversely, melanin is found normally in the CNS in the absence of congenital nevi. NCM is apparently not hereditary and affects male and female subjects with equal frequency. The incidence of NCM is unknown, but it is very uncommon, with only 100–200 cases reported in the literature.

Although the precise pathogenesis is not well understood, a disorder involving neural crest cell differentiation and melanocyte embryogenesis is suspected. The prominent involvement of the leptomeninges and skin over the spine supports the suggestion that the primary defect is abnormal migration of nevus cell precursors, although the embryological origin of nevus cells has not been determined. Alternatively, melanin-producing cells may be produced in excessive numbers. It has also been speculated that nevi located over the spine result from an error early in nevus cell migration or differentiation, whereas nevi are restricted to the extremities if the error occurs later in development (Pavlidou et al., 2008).

### Cutaneous Features

The characteristic lesions are dark to light brown hairy nevi present at birth (Fig. 99.19). Multiple small nevi (satellite nevi) usually are present around one giant nevus that most commonly appears on the lower trunk and perineal area (swimming trunk nevus). A giant nevus is absent in 34% of patients with NCM. Approximately one-third of patients have a large nevus over the upper back (cape nevus). The giant nevi may fade over time, but satellite nevi continue to appear during the first few years of life.

Diagnostic criteria for NCM have been suggested: (1) large or multiple (three or more) congenital nevi (large is ≥20 cm in an adult, 9 cm on the scalp of an infant, or 6 cm on the body of an infant); (2) no evidence of cutaneous melanoma, except in patients in whom the examined portions of the meningeal lesions are benign; and (3) no evidence of meningeal melanoma, except in patients in whom the examined areas of the cutaneous lesions are benign (Marghoob et al., 2004). Some authors argue that a definitive diagnosis of NCM requires histological confirmation of the CNS lesions. However, in the context of the

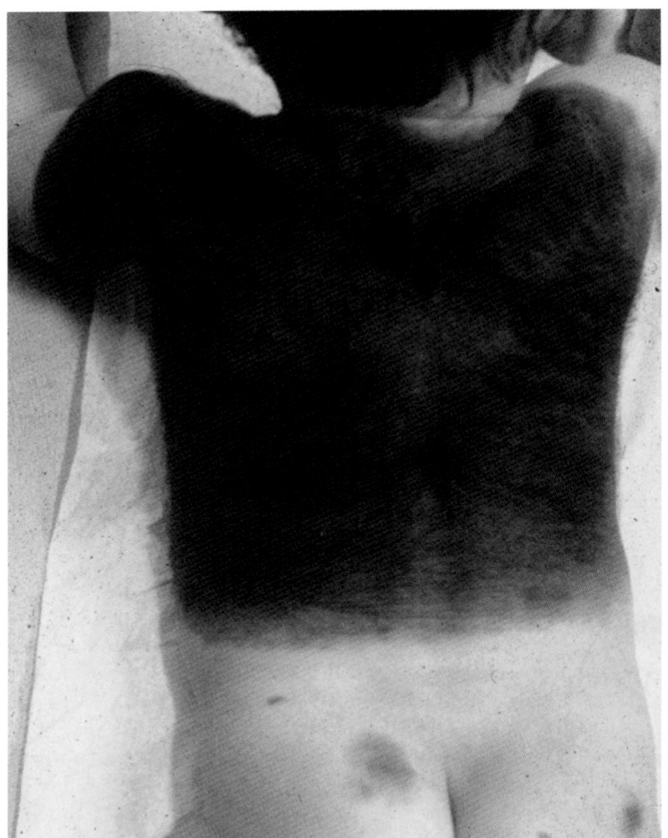

**Fig. 99.19** Large, Dark, Hairy Nevus Covering most of the back of an Infant with Neurocutaneous Melanosis.

typical melanocytic cutaneous nevi and characteristic neuroimaging findings, leptomeningeal or brain biopsy is unnecessary.

Biopsy of a congenital nevus reveals extension of the nevus cells into the deep dermis or even the subcutis between collagen bundles and around nerves, hair follicles, and blood vessels. Nevus cells tend to form cords or nests. Sheets of nevomelanocytes in the dermis may display a few mitoses and large atypical cells positive for S100 and HMB45 antibodies and formaldehyde-induced green-specific fluorescence. The occurrence of atypical mitoses in the dermis may constitute an early stage of malignant melanoma. The greatest risks in NCM are the high incidence of malignant transformation of melanotic cells and spinal and intracranial pathology.

## Neurological Features

Neurological symptoms may result from leptomeningeal melanosis, intracranial melanoma, or intracerebral or subarachnoid hemorrhage. Malformations of the vertebral column, spine, and brain also may impair neurological function. The median age of neurological complications is 2 years, but infants may be affected (DeDavid et al., 1996). Leptomeningeal melanosis is probably the most common cause of neurological symptoms, especially in children. This tends to occur at the base of the brain along the interpeduncular fossa, ventral brainstem, upper cervical cord, and ventral surface of the lumbosacral cord. Marked leptomeningeal melanosis (Fig. 99.20) is present in the vast majority of patients with NCM and associated with interruption of cerebrospinal fluid (CSF) flow. This leads to hydrocephalus and increased intracranial pressure with typical symptoms of irritability, vomiting, seizures, and

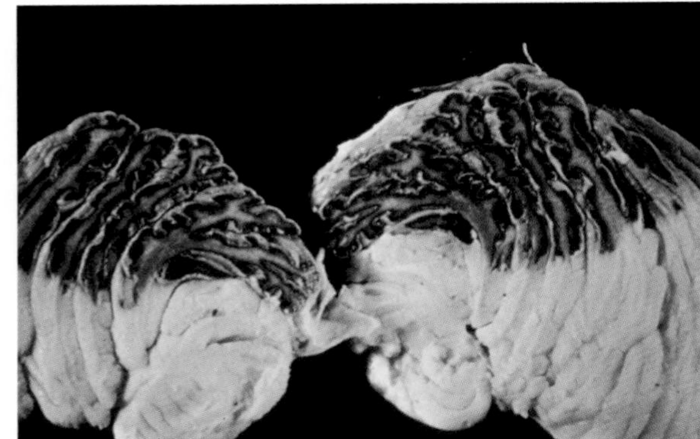

**Fig. 99.20** Leptomeningeal Melanosis at Autopsy in a Patient With Neurocutaneous Melanosis. *(Photo courtesy Dr. John Bodensteiner. Reprinted with permission from Miller V.S. 2004. Neurocutaneous melanosis, In: Roach E.S., Miller V.S. (Eds.), Neurocutaneous Disorders. Cambridge University Press, Cambridge, pp. 71–76.)*

papilledema. In infants, symptoms may include rapidly increasing head circumference or tense anterior fontanelle. Cranial nerve deficits such as limitation of upgaze and lateral gaze are common. Myelopathy occurs when leptomeningeal proliferation affects the spinal cord or spinal nerves.

The likelihood of symptomatic neurological involvement correlates with location of large nevi. Large congenital melanocytic nevi occur in a posterior and midline position in nearly 80% of affected patients (Agero et al., 2005). In one series, all 33 patients with neurological symptoms had a nevus over the back, whereas none of 26 patients with nevi restricted to the limbs had neurological abnormalities. Patients occur with leptomeningeal melanosis confirmed by biopsy and CNS involvement but without skin lesions.

## Laboratory Findings

CSF from patients with neurological symptoms may show a mild pleocytosis and elevated pressure and protein. CSF cytopathology shows numerous round cells with abundant cytoplasm and ovoid nuclei, and light brown cytoplasmic granules (presumably melanin) may be seen. The most characteristic histological feature is the presence of numerous irregular fingers projecting from the cell body, which may aid in diagnosis of NCM.

## Neuroimaging

Approximately half of neurologically asymptomatic children with NCM have abnormal cranial neuroimaging study results. Cranial MRI demonstrates lesions with T1 shortening in the cerebellum, in the anterior temporal lobe (especially the amygdala), and along the basilar meninges (Fig. 99.21). Some of these lesions also show T2 shortening. The pons, medulla, thalami, and base of the frontal lobe often are affected (Ramaswamy et al., 2012). Gadolinium-enhanced MRIs rarely may show enhancement of the pia-arachnoid. In one study, five of six children with neurological symptoms of increased intracranial pressure showed leptomeningeal thickening and enhancement. Conversely, asymptomatic children never showed leptomeningeal thickening. Inferior vermian hypoplasia and Dandy-Walker malformation have been reported. Spinal MRI study results are usually normal.

It may be difficult to distinguish radiological evidence of CNS melanoma from benign melanin deposits. Serial imaging studies are the best way to follow clinically suspect MRI lesions. Certain neuroimaging findings help distinguish benign intracranial melanosis from

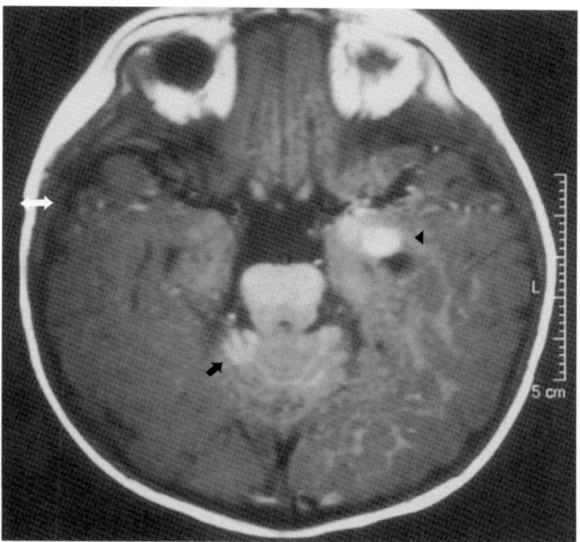


**Fig. 99.21** T1-weighted cranial magnetic resonance imaging scan showing leptomeningeal melanosis over the cerebellum *(arrow)* and focal melanosis or melanoma in the temporal lobe *(arrowhead)*.

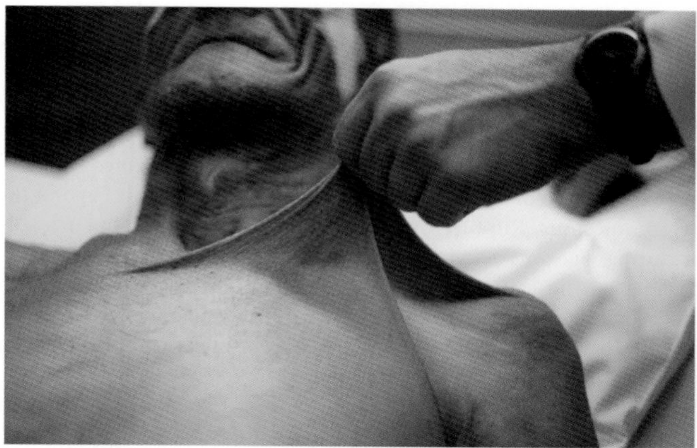

**Fig. 99.22** Cutaneous hyperelasticity of the anterior chest in a patient with Ehlers-Danlos syndrome without cerebrovascular disease.

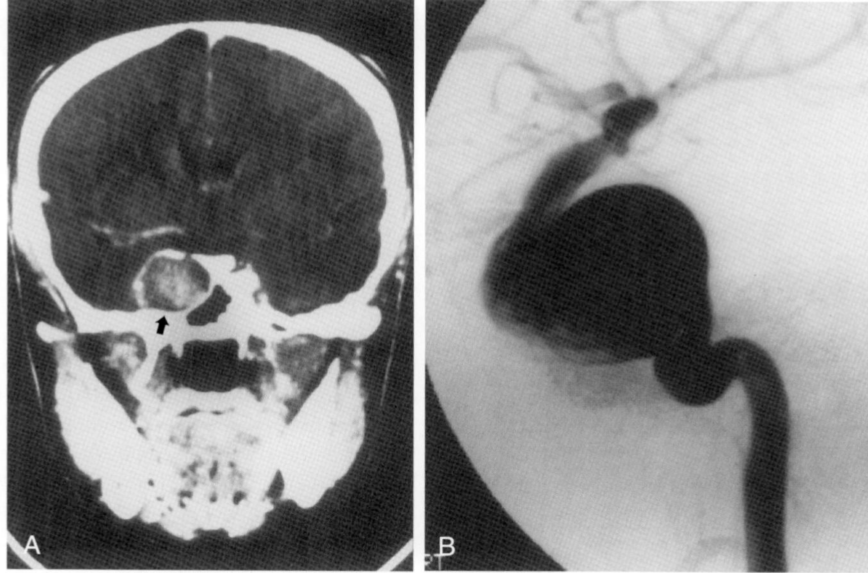


**Fig. 99.23** **A,** Computed tomographic scan with contrast from an 18-year-old patient with headache and a family history of type IV Ehlers-Danlos syndrome reveals a giant aneurysm *(arrow)* of the right intracavernous carotid artery. **B,** Right internal carotid angiogram confirms the giant aneurysm of the intracavernous carotid artery. *(Reprinted with permission from Roach, E.S., Zimmerman, C.F., 1995. Ehlers-Danlos syndrome, In: Bogousslavsky, J., Caplan, L.R. (Eds.), Stroke Syndromes. Cambridge University Press, London, pp. 491–496.)*

melanoma; necrosis, perilesional edema, contrast enhancement, and hemorrhage are features of melanoma. Unfortunately, melanoma may not exhibit any of these findings until late in its course when metastasis is likely to have already occurred.

## EHLERS-DANLOS SYNDROME

At least 10 subtypes of Ehlers-Danlos syndrome (EDS) exist, defined by the clinical features, inheritance pattern, and even specific molecular defects. Together these syndromes are characterized by fragile or hyperelastic skin (Fig. 99.22), hyperextensible joints, vascular lesions, easy bruising, poor wound healing, and excessive scarring. Some patients develop peripheral neuropathy caused by lax ligaments, and others may present with neonatal hypotonia or weakness. Neuromuscular kyphoscoliosis can develop. However, vascular lesions such as aneurysm (Fig. 99.23) and arterial dissection are the most serious threat to the nervous system. (See also Chapter 65 and 104.)

More than 80% of EDS patients have type I, II, or III, and the other subtypes are individually uncommon. Type IV most often leads to neurovascular complications, and its prevalence is 1 in 50,000 to 500,000. Often, a delay in the diagnosis of type IV EDS occurs because of a decreased incidence of hyperelastic skin or hyperextensible joints compared to other types. Transmission of all familial type IV EDS cases with a documented abnormality of type III collagen is autosomal dominant. Various defects of the COL3A1 gene (which codes for the $\alpha_1$ chain of type III collagen) on chromosome 2 have been identified (Schwarze et al., 1997). Mutations of this gene are rare in patients with aneurysm without type IV EDS (Hamano et al., 1998).

### Neurovascular Features

There is a risk of aneurysms, and the most commonly affected intracranial vessel is the internal carotid artery, typically in or just beyond the cavernous sinus. Rupture of the aneurysm can occur spontaneously or during vigorous activity. Rupture within the cavernous sinus may create a carotid-cavernous fistula. Less often, the aneurysm occurs in other intracranial arteries and presents with subarachnoid hemorrhage. Most individuals become symptomatic in early adulthood, but some begin in childhood and adolescence.

Some patients develop a fistula after minor head trauma, but most occur spontaneously and even without an aneurysm. Clinical features of carotid-cavernous fistula include proptosis, chemosis, diplopia, and pulsatile tinnitus. The vascular fragility of type IV EDS makes both standard angiography and intravascular occlusion of the fistula difficult.

Arterial dissection occurs in both intracranial and extracranial arteries, and the initial features depend primarily on which artery is affected. One patient with a vertebral dissection developed a painful pulsatile mass of the neck. Dissection of an intrathoracic artery secondarily can occlude cervical vessels, and distal embolism from a dissection can cause cerebral infarction. Surgery is difficult because the arteries are friable and difficult to suture, and handling the tissue leads to tears of the artery or separation of the arterial layers. Type IV EDS should be considered in children and young adults with arterial dissection.

## CEREBROTENDINOUS XANTHOMATOSIS

Cerebrotendinous xanthomatosis (CTX) is an autosomal recessive disorder of bile acid synthesis characterized by tendon xanthomas, cataracts, and progressive neurological deterioration (Box 99.4). The underlying defect consists of the enzyme, sterol 27-hydroxylase, whose gene (CYP27A1) is located on chromosome 2q. The enzyme deficiency leads to deposits of cholesterol and cholestanol, a metabolic derivative of cholesterol, in virtually every tissue, particularly the Achilles tendons, brain, and lungs. Bile acid production decreases markedly, which leads to reduced chenodeoxycholic acid (CDCA) concentration in bile. Excretion of bile acid precursors increases in bile and urine. Serum cholesterol levels are typically not elevated in CTX syndrome.

**BOX 99.4 Clinical Features of Cerebrotendinous Xanthomatosis**

**Neurological**
Progressive dementia
Ataxia
Nystagmus
Dysarthria
Hyperreflexia
Bulbar symptoms
Palatal and pharyngeal myoclonus
Peripheral neuropathy
Electroencephalographic abnormalities
Parkinsonism
Cerebral and cerebellar atrophy
Cataracts

**Behavioral Abnormalities**
Personality changes
Irritability
Agitation
Aggressiveness
Paranoid ideation
Auditory hallucinations
Catatonia

**Musculoskeletal**
Xanthomas
Osteoporosis and bone fractures
Large paranasal sinuses

### Neurological Features

Personality changes and decline in school performance may be the earliest neurological manifestations of this syndrome. Progressive loss of cognitive function typically begins in childhood, but some patients remain intellectually normal for many years. EEG shows nonspecific characteristics of metabolic encephalopathy such as slowing. Seizures may occur. Ataxia with gait disturbance, dysmetria, nystagmus, and dysarthria are common. Psychosis with auditory hallucinations, paranoid ideation, and catatonia occur rarely, but examination for cataracts and tendon xanthomas should be included in the evaluation of patients with new-onset psychosis. Parkinsonism may be the only neurological symptom. Cranial MRI typically shows involvement of the dentate nuclei (Gallus et al., 2006). Other findings include cerebral and cerebellar atrophy and diffusely abnormal white matter, presumably reflecting sterol infiltration with demyelination. Focal lesions of the cerebral white matter and globus pallidus are sometimes demonstrable on MRI.

Peripheral neuropathy is a prominent feature of CTX, with signs of pes cavus, areflexia, and loss of vibration perception. Sural nerve biopsy may show reduced densities of both myelinated and unmyelinated axons, and teased fibers show axonal regeneration and remyelination. Large-diameter myelinated nerve fibers particularly are affected. Schwann cells contain foamy macrophages and lipid droplets. Short-latency somatosensory evoked potentials may show prolonged central conduction times with tibial nerve stimulation, but normal conduction velocities with median nerve stimulation. Brainstem auditory evoked potentials and visual evoked potentials are abnormal in approximately half of patients studied. These electrophysiological parameters correlate with the ratio of serum cholestanol to cholesterol concentration and may improve with treatment with CDCA.

### Xanthomas

The Achilles tendon is the most common site of tendon xanthomas, but the quadriceps, triceps, and finger extensor tendons also show xanthomatous involvement. Tendon xanthomas usually appear after the age of 20 years but may occur earlier. A substantial number of patients never develop xanthomas. Compared with xanthomas found in patients with familial hypercholesterolemia or hyperlipoproteinemia, these xanthomas appear similar grossly but contain high amounts of cholestanol and little cholesterol. The presence of early-onset cataracts, progressive dementia, and tendon xanthomas is pathognomonic of CTX syndrome (Salen & Steiner, 2017). The differential diagnosis includes Marinesco-Sjögren syndrome multiple sclerosis, hereditary spastic paraparesis, olivopontocerebellar atrophy, and spinocerebellar degeneration.

### Other Clinical Features

Onset of cataracts by age 10 years and chronic diarrhea are a characteristic combination in CTX. Cataracts can be bilateral and asymptomatic.

Osteoporosis may lead to an increased risk of skeletal and vertebral fractures. Large paranasal sinuses occur in association with CTX. Renal disorders reported in patients with CTX include nephrolithiasis, nephrocalcinosis, and renal tubular acidosis.

### Treatment

Treatment of CTX focuses on lowering cholestanol levels, primarily with CDCA. Other lipid-lowering agents such as cholestyramine or β-hydroxymethylglutarate-CoA inhibitors are not as effective alone, but the latter in combination with CDCA constitutes the most effective treatment. Long-term therapy can lead to striking improvement in neurological function, resolution of peripheral and intracranial xanthomas, and improvement of EEG and peripheral nerve conduction abnormalities as well as visual and somatosensory evoked potentials. It may be that early treatment is required, which ideally would begin before onset of clinical symptoms in individuals with a family history of CTX. The possibility that early treatment may improve the neurological symptoms of CTX underscores the importance of careful screening and genetic counseling of asymptomatic relatives of patients with this disorder. Treatment with cholic acid is also an option and may produce fewer side effects (Mandia et al., 2019).

## PROGRESSIVE FACIAL HEMIATROPHY

Progressive facial hemiatrophy (Parry-Romberg syndrome) occurs sporadically. The relationship of this disorder to *en coup de sabre*, morphea, and linear scleroderma is still debated (Peterson et al., 1995). Traditionally, progressive facial hemiatrophy involves the upper cranium, whereas *en coup de sabre* tends to affect the lower face as well. Scleroderma and morphea affect other parts of the body. However, understanding of pathogenesis is poor, and they may prove to have a similar origin. An arbitrary distinction based on the anatomical distribution does have at least one practical use: as a rule, only patients whose upper face and head are affected are likely to develop cerebral complications.

### Clinical Features

Progressive facial hemiatrophy is characterized by unilateral atrophy of the skin, subcutaneous tissue, and adjacent bone (Fig. 99.24). The atrophic area is characteristically oblong or linear and sometimes begins as a raised erythematous lesion. The lesion sometimes begins after trauma to the area. The atrophy eventually stabilizes, leaving facial disfigurement.

Epilepsy is probably the most common neurological problem associated with progressive facial hemiatrophy. Some patients develop a usually mild hemiparesis. Less common neurological features include cognitive impairment, cranial neuropathy, or even brainstem signs. Cerebral calcifications and white-matter lesions are common neuroimaging findings (Fig. 99.25); abnormalities typically lie beneath the cutaneous lesion (Fry et al., 1992).

Understanding of the cause of progressive facial hemiatrophy and related disorders is poor. Proposed mechanisms (e.g., cortical dysgenesis, dysfunction of the sympathetic nervous system, chronic localized meningoencephalitis) are inadequate to explain all of the clinical features.

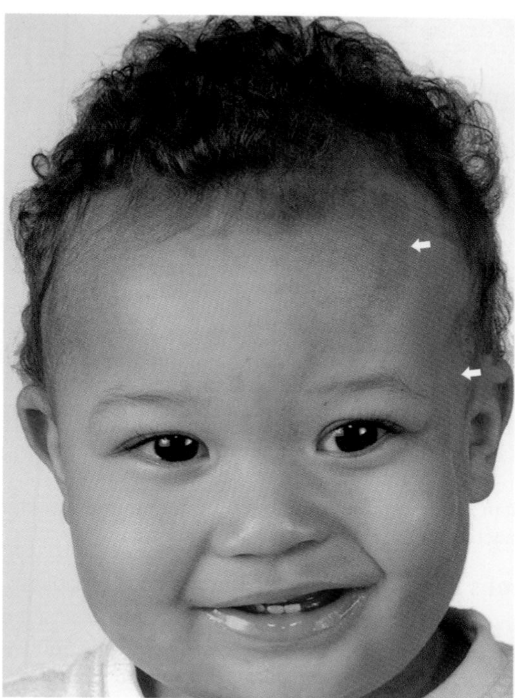

**Fig. 99.24** Unilateral atrophy of the skin and subcutaneous tissue *(arrows)* in a young boy with progressive hemifacial atrophy.

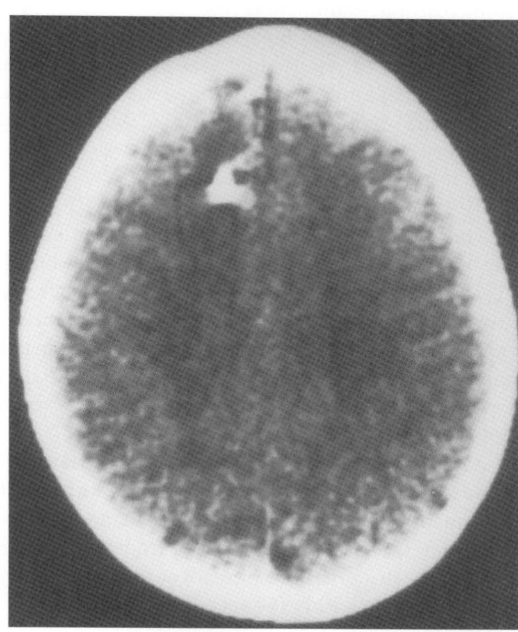

**Fig. 99.25** Computed tomographic scan revealing right frontal encephalomalacia and calcification in a patient with progressive facial hemiatrophy.

## KINKY HAIR SYNDROME (MENKES DISEASE)

Kinky hair syndrome, also known as *Menkes disease* or *trichopoliodystrophy*, is an X-linked recessive disorder of connective tissue and neuronal metabolism caused by inborn disorders of copper metabolism:namely, impaired cellular export of copper, leading to accumulation in all tissues except the liver and brain. The estimated frequency is 1 in 40,000 to 1 in 298,000 live births. In the classic form of kinky hair syndrome, the neurological symptoms begin in the first year of life, and the course is rapidly progressive, with death by the third year of life in more involved cases. Death is commonly due to infection, cerebrovascular complications, or the neurodegenerative process. Documented cases of late-onset cases and apparently asymptomatic individuals are in the literature. Clinical features in affected girls are similar to but

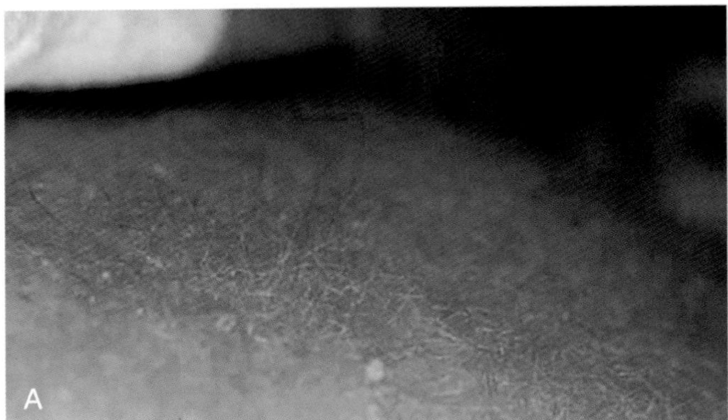


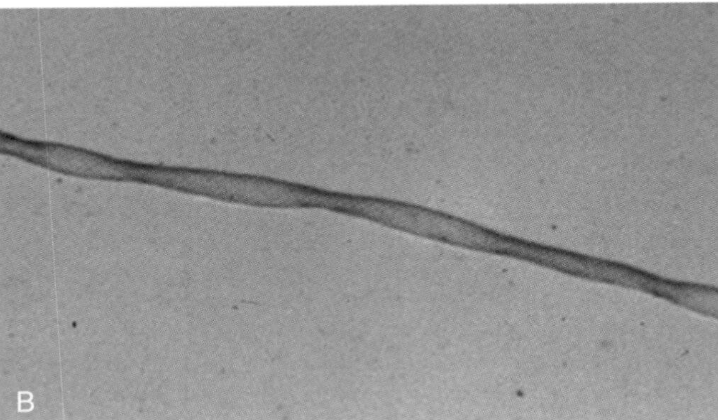


**Fig. 99.26** A, Brittle, light-colored hair seen in kinky hair syndrome. B, Hair shaft from a patient with kinky hair syndrome.

milder than those seen in typical neonatal-onset cases; genetic analysis reveals inactivation of the normal X chromosome.

## Cutaneous Features

Connective tissue abnormalities are a major feature of kinky hair syndrome and include loose skin, hyperextensible joints, bladder diverticula, and skeletal anomalies. The enzyme lysyl oxidase has copper-dependent steps that are impaired in the establishment of elastin and collagen cross-linking. Keratin cross-linking and melanin production also depend on copper, and copper deficiency leads to characteristic cutaneous features. The hair is light-colored and brittle and on microscopic examination (Fig. 99.26) appears as pili torti (twisted hair) and trichorrhexis nodosa (complete or incomplete fractures of the hair shafts at regular intervals). Trichorrhexis nodosa is not pathognomonic of kinky hair syndrome; it also occurs in biotinidase deficiency and argininosuccinic aciduria. Skin may be diffusely hypopigmented or normal.

## Other Clinical Features

Kinky hair syndrome covers a clinical continuum from nearly normal to the severe classic infantile-onset form (Box 99.5). Newborns may be more prone to cephalohematomas or spontaneous bone fractures and develop temperature instability, diarrhea, and failure to thrive in early infancy. Sympathetic adrenergic dysfunction, including hypotension, hypothermia, anorexia, and somnolence, is attributable to the impairment of dopamine β-hydroxylase that requires copper for the synthesis of norepinephrine and other neurotransmitters.

One variant of kinky hair syndrome is the occipital horn syndrome in which connective tissue symptoms predominate, and cognitive and motor involvement is variable. This disorder is named for the characteristic exostoses ("orbital horns") resulting from calcification of the trapezius and sternocleidomastoid muscles at their attachment to the occipital skull.

### BOX 99.5 Neurological and Systemic Features of Infantile-Onset Kinky Hair Syndrome

- Premature birth, low birth weight
- Neonatal jaundice
- Hypothermia
- Decreased facial expression
- Prominent forehead
- Full cheeks
- Narrow palate
- Hypopigmented skin
- Cutis laxa
- Pili torti
- Inguinal hernia
- Hepatomegaly
- Deafness
- Bladder diverticula
- Joint laxity
- Skeletal anomalies:
  - Pectus excavatum
  - Wormian skull bones
  - Metaphyseal spurring of long bones
- Ataxia
- Seizures
- Intracranial hemorrhage
- Neuroimaging findings:
  - Cerebellar and cerebral atrophy
  - White-matter abnormalities
  - Subdural fluid collections
  - Dilated and tortuous intracranial and extracranial blood vessels
  - Cerebral edema

## Neurological Features

In early-onset cases, hypotonia develops in the first few weeks to months and gradually develops into spastic quadriparesis with clenched fists, opisthotonus, and scissoring. Seizures are a prominent feature of this disorder, appearing by age 2–3 months, and may be focal or generalized. Myoclonic seizures are especially common. Developmental delay and regression appear between ages 4 and 6 months in the classic form.

Intracranial and extracranial blood vessels may be tortuous, kinked, and dilated (Kim & Suh, 1997); the cause may be defective or deficient elastin fibers in the walls of these blood vessels. Neuropathological studies show diffuse neuronal loss and gliosis that is particularly prominent in the cerebrum and cerebellum. Microscopic findings include abnormal dendritic arborization in the cerebellar cortex.

## Neuroimaging

Cranial MRI and CT studies show diffuse cerebral atrophy with secondary subdural fluid collections, which may be large enough to cause mild compression of the ventricular system. The presence of large subdural fluid collections and metaphyseal fractures in an infant can lead to the erroneous diagnosis of child abuse. In older children, MRI studies typically reveal diffuse white-matter signal abnormalities suggestive of demyelination and gliosis, whereas in infants the white matter may be only focally affected. Diffuse brain atrophy, subdural effusions or hemorrhages, infarction, or edema also may be present. MRI shows tortuous intracranial blood vessels, better seen by MRA or conventional angiography. Skull radiographs may show wormian bones.

### Genetic Studies

A gene involved in transmembrane copper transport, ATP7A (also referred to as *MNK*), has been implicated in both kinky hair syndrome and occipital horn syndrome. ATP7A maps to Xq13.3 and is highly homologous to the gene implicated in Wilson disease. ATP7A mRNA is present in several cell types and organs except liver, which explains the clinical observations that liver does not accumulate excess copper and is largely unaffected in kinky hair syndrome.

Infantile-onset kinky hair syndrome results from extensive mutations of ATP7A (e.g., large deletions, frameshift mutations), whereas occipital horn syndrome is associated with promoter and splicing efficiency mutations, possibly leading to reduced levels of an otherwise normal protein product. Mutations of the ATP7A gene in the patients with the occipital horn syndrome have been base pair substitutions affecting normal messenger ribonucleic acid (mRNA) splicing (Tumer & Horn, 1997). Copper deficiency impairs the function of multiple enzymes that require copper as a cofactor: tyrosinase, cytochrome C oxidase, dopamine β-hydroxylase, and Cu/Zn superoxide dismutase, among others.

### Diagnosis and Treatment

When suspected clinically, low serum copper and ceruloplasmin support the diagnosis. Plasma catecholamine analysis to evaluate for dopamine β-hydroxylase deficiency also may be helpful. Specialized centers can determine intracellular accumulation of copper. The large size of the ATP7A gene and the variety of mutations make detection of a specific genetic defect difficult, unless previously established for a given family. Carrier status is difficult to assess, although prenatal testing for copper content in chorionic villi or cultured amniotic-fluid cells is available.

The focus of treatment approaches is to restore copper to normal levels in brain and other tissues. Careful medical care is particularly important in extending the life span. Copper histidine administered parenterally (subcutaneously) is the most promising treatment, and substantial clinical improvement in a small number of patients has been reported. Undoubtedly, response to copper histidine treatment partly depends on the specific mutation of ATP7A involved. Such correlations are not yet well characterized.

Aggressive copper replacement beginning in early infancy may be necessary to significantly improve neurological outcome (Tang et al., 2008). Replacement therapy does not appear to help the connective tissue abnormalities in kinky hair syndrome. Preservation of some residual activity of adenosine triphosphatase (ATPase) may be required for significant clinical efficacy from copper replacement treatment, since it did not normalize neurological outcome in two children with the Q724H splicing mutation, which yields a nonfunctioning ATPase.

## XERODERMA PIGMENTOSUM

Xeroderma pigmentosum (XP) is a group of uncommon neurocutaneous disorders characterized by susceptibility to sun-induced skin disorders and variable (but typically progressive) neurological deterioration. Inheritance of XP is autosomal recessive, often in the setting of parental consanguinity, and occurs in 1 in 30,000 to 1 in 250,000 or higher. It occurs more frequently in Japan and Egypt than in the United States and Europe. Several gene mutations involving nucleotide excision repair and DNA transcription have been associated with XP and related syndromes such as Cockayne syndrome, trichothiodystrophy, and De Sanctis-Cacchione syndrome.

### Complementation Groups

Complementation analysis has been important in understanding the genetic basis of XP. If two particular cell types with different metabolic abnormalities are fused, the cell produced may function normally. These two cell types have different complementation groups and presumably have a different genetic basis. In XP, eight complementation groups have been identified (XP-A through XP-G and a variant group). Although some general genotype–phenotype correlations among these complementation groups exist, considerable clinical overlap exists between them (Copeland et al., 1997). Complementation groups XP-A, XP-C, and XP-D are the most common. Despite the few individuals with XP-B available, cloning of the responsible gene (XPBC) was successful. The XPBC gene is located on chromosome 2q21 and encodes a protein that is a component of the basal transcription factor TFIIH/BTF2. This protein helps regulate both DNA transcription initiation and nucleotide excision repair.

Mutations in the XPCC gene, located on chromosome 3p25.1, cause XP-C. Patients with XP-C generally do not have prominent neurological dysfunction. The XPCC gene codes for a protein involved in global genome repair, but full understanding of its exact role is lacking. Complementation group D is the third most common complementation group. Characteristic of the abnormalities are mild to severe neurological dysfunction. The gene associated with XP-D is at chromosome 9q13. The gene product in XP-D is a component of TFFIIH/BTF2, as is XP-B, and accordingly, XP-B and XP-D have similar clinical features. Complementation group E (XP-E) is uncommon and associated with mild neurological and cutaneous symptoms. The precise localization and function of the XP-E gene of its associated protein, XPEC, has not been determined. No neurological symptoms occur in patients from complementation groups F or G or the variant group.

### Related Syndromes

De Sanctis-Cacchione syndrome is a variant of XP in which patients have severe and progressive cognitive deficiency, dwarfism, and gonadal hypoplasia. Trichothiodystrophy and similar syndromes link to XP complementation groups B and D. Patients with trichothiodystrophy have brittle hair and nails because of sulfur-deficient matrix proteins, ichthyosis, and intellectual disability. Patients with photosensitivity (P), ichthyosis (I), brittle hair (B), impaired intelligence (I), possibly decreased fertility (D), and short stature (S) fit into the PIBI(D)S syndrome. DNA repair studies of patients with trichothiodystrophy demonstrate reduced ultraviolet-induced DNA repair synthesis, and one patient assigned to XP-D. A variant of trichothiodystrophy is Tay syndrome, in which dysplastic nails and lack of subcutaneous fatty tissue are characteristic. Low birth weight, short stature, and intellectual disability are also features of this disorder.

Cockayne syndrome combines cutaneous sunlight sensitivity, dwarfism, intellectual disability, microcephaly, dental caries, peripheral neuropathy, and sensorineural deafness. The combined features of XP and Cockayne syndrome within complementation groups XP-B, XP-D, and XP-G indicate that there is considerable clinical heterogeneity and phenotypical overlap within the subsets of these complementation groups. Trichothiodystrophy may present with congenital ichthyosis (collodion baby) but persistent ichthyosis of the scalp, trunk, palms, and soles is the main feature.

### Cutaneous and Ocular Features

Cutaneous and ocular features of XP result primarily from ultraviolet light exposure (Box 99.6). The onset of cutaneous symptoms in XP is

**BOX 99.6 Cutaneous and Ocular Features of Xeroderma Pigmentosum**

**Cutaneous Features**

Sunlight sensitivity
Freckling
Atrophy
Xerosis and scaling
Telangiectasia
Actinic keratosis
Angioma
Keratoacanthoma
Fibroma
Malignant tumors
Basal cell carcinoma
Squamous cell carcinoma
Melanoma
Fibrosarcoma

**Ocular Features**

***Eyelids***

Atrophy leading to loss of lashes, ectropion, entropion
Neoplasm

***Conjunctiva***

Conjunctivitis
Inflammatory lesions such as pinguecula
Pigmentation, telangiectases, dryness
Symblepharon, inflammatory nodules
Neoplasm

***Cornea***

Exposure keratitis leading to corneal clouding, dryness, ulceration, scarring, and vascularization
Neoplasm

***Iris***

Iritis, synechiae, atrophy

usually early; the median age of onset is 1–2 years, typically freckling or erythema and bullae formation after sun exposure. Nearly half of patients develop malignant skin lesions, with the median age of first skin neoplasm being only 8 years. The estimated incidence of non-melanoma skin cancer under the age of 20 years is 10,000-fold greater than that observed for the general US population (DiGiovanna & Kraemer, 2012). Light-skinned infants develop erythema and bullae after even brief sun exposure. Sun exposure also induces prominent macule formation (freckling or solar lentigenes), which over time enlarge and coalesce. Telangiectasias and epidermal and dermal atrophy develop in later years, and the skin becomes dry. Actinic keratosis, angiomas, keratoacanthomas, and fibromas also occur. Ocular tissues are particularly susceptible to ultraviolet damage. Keratitis and conjunctivitis with photophobia are common in patients with XP. Atrophy of the eyelids leads to loss of lashes and ectropion or entropion. Neoplasms of the eyelid, conjunctiva, and cornea include squamous cell carcinoma, epithelioma and basal cell carcinoma, and melanoma. The tip of the tongue, gingiva, and palate also are susceptible to sun exposure.

Most of what is known about the neurological features in XP comes from studies of Japanese patients with XP-A. Research indicates that the severity of neurological symptoms correlates with particular mutations within the XPAC gene, and presumably this is true in other types of XP (Maeda et al., 1995). The principal neurological symptoms in XP-A are progressive dementia, sensorineural hearing loss, tremor, choreoathetosis, and ataxia. Progressive dementia begins in patients with XP-A during the preschool years, and IQ scores after 10 years of age are invariably less than 50. Sensorineural hearing loss has a later onset, but most patients older than 10 years have hearing impairment. Cerebellar signs develop at approximately the same time as the hearing loss. Microcephaly is present in about half of patients.

EEG studies most often show nonspecific generalized slowing, but focal slow waves and focal spike discharges occasionally occur. Peripheral neuropathy is a prominent feature that may begin in the first decade of life. Deep tendon reflexes are absent in nearly all patients older than 6 years. Motor nerve conduction velocities are normal during the first 3 years of life but slow by 6 years. Similarly, all patients older than 6 years had either absent or prolonged sensory nerve conduction velocities. Electromyography shows a neuropathic pattern with large, prolonged, polyphasic motor unit potentials and incomplete recruitment of motor units. Nerve biopsy may show an age-dependent decrease of myelinated fibers, which was associated with rare acute axonal degeneration, sparse axonal regeneration, rare axonal atrophy, and few onion bulb formations, consistent with a neuropathic process.

Neural tissue lacks exposure to sun-induced DNA damage. Therefore, the cause of neurodegeneration in patients with XP remains unexplained. The high frequency of neurological symptoms in XP-B and XP-D but not in XP-C, XP-F, XP-G, and the variant group supports the notion that one cause of the neurological dysfunction in XP is dysfunction of DNA transcription rather than nucleotide excision repair. Deficits in excision repair may closely link to skin cancer susceptibility. In addition, recent work suggests that in XP, the cause of neurological injury is partly defective repair of lesions produced in nerve cells by reactive oxygen species generated as by-products of an active oxidative metabolism. Specifically, two major oxidative DNA lesions, 8-oxoguanine and thymine glycol, are excised from DNA in vitro by the same enzyme system responsible for removing pyrimidine dimers and other bulky DNA adducts.

## Treatment

Cancer surveillance and avoidance of precipitating factors is the most important aspect of health screening of individuals with XP. There is hope that gene therapy will reduce cancer risk and perhaps improve neurological outcomes. In vitro studies offer hope that, eventually, recombinant retroviruses can transfer and stably express the human DNA repair genes in XP cells to correct defective DNA repair (Zeng et al., 1997). Using the recombinant retroviral vector LXSN, successful transfer of human XP-A, XP-B, and XP-C–complementary DNAs (cDNAs) into primary and immortalized fibroblasts obtained from patients with XP-A, XP-B, and XP-C occurred. After transduction, monitoring of the complete correction of DNA repair deficiency and functional expression of the transgenes included ultraviolet survival, unscheduled DNA synthesis, and recovery of RNA synthesis. In a similar study, XP-FR2 cells expressed a high level of XP-F protein and ERCC1 protein following the cloning of XP-F cDNA into a mammalian expression vector plasmid and introduction into group F XP (XP-F) cells. The XP-FR2 cells expressed a high level of XP-F protein and ERCC1 protein. They showed ultraviolet resistance comparable to that in normal human cells and had normal levels of ultraviolet-induced unscheduled DNA synthesis and normal capability to remove DNA adducts. This demonstrates that the nucleotide excision repair defect in XP-F cells is fully corrected by overexpression of XP-F cDNA alone.

## OTHER NEUROLOGICAL CONDITIONS WITH CUTANEOUS MANIFESTATIONS

Many other conditions with cutaneous stigmata also manifest neurological symptoms primarily or secondarily. Fabry disease is an X-linked lysosomal disorder with prominent cutaneous angiokeratoma corporis diffusum, sensory neuropathy, and risk of stroke (see Chapters 68 and 106). A connective tissue disorder known as *pseudoxanthoma elasticum* demonstrates characteristic skin plaques, and vascular involvement leads to cerebrovascular compromise (see Chapter 65). Wyburn-Mason syndrome (or Bonnet-Dechaume-Blanc syndrome) is a rare sporadic neurocutaneous syndrome characterized by retinal, facial, and intracranial AVMs.

## CONCLUSIONS

Neurocutaneous syndromes long have been defined on the basis of cutaneous features and neurological involvement guiding diagnosis of a syndrome—and the awareness of clinical features accompanying these syndromes remains of utmost importance. Regardless of which sign or symptom manifests first, the pathophysiology arising from angiogenic proliferation or loss of tumor suppression function has guided prognosis across multiple body systems. Imaging technology has enabled surveillance of involvement at presymptomatic stages. Significantly, the understanding of affected genes and gene protein function has not only advanced the phenotypic breadth of clinical involvement but also has begun to expand the availability of interventions that might slow or halt progression across multiple systems and syndromes.

*The complete reference list is available online at https://expertconsult.inkling.com/.* 

100

# Epilepsies

*Bassel W. Abou-Khalil, Martin J. Gallagher, Robert L. Macdonald*

## OUTLINE



## SEIZURES AND EPILEPSY DEFINITIONS

*Seizures* are transient events that include symptoms and/or signs of abnormal excessive hypersynchronous activity in the brain (Fisher et al., 2005). The traditional definition of epilepsy required the occurrence of two unprovoked seizures. It is known that the risk of seizure recurrence after two unprovoked seizures is greater than 60% (Hauser et al., 1998), and treatment would normally be initiated with an antiseizure medication (ASM) in that setting. There are situations where the risk of seizure recurrence after a single seizure is equally high, suggesting an enduring predisposition to have recurrence. Treatment would normally be initiated in these situations, and there was a desire to include this in the definition of epilepsy. In 2014, the International League Against Epilepsy (ILAE) revised the definition of *epilepsy* as a disease of the brain with (1) at least two unprovoked (or reflex) seizures occurring greater than 24 hours apart, or (2) one unprovoked (or reflex) seizure and a probability of further seizures similar to the general recurrence risk (at least 60%) after two unprovoked seizures, occurring over the next 10 years, or (3) diagnosis of an epilepsy syndrome (Fisher et al., 2014).

A variety of seizure types exist, and epilepsy is not a single entity but rather a collection of disorders/diseases that have in common the occurrence of seizures. Hence, a need exists for classification of seizures and of epilepsies and epileptic syndromes. The classification is important for communication and diagnostic purposes, but also for evaluating drug specificity and prescribing the most appropriate therapy. The diagnosis of certain seizure types can predict response to therapy and prognosis. The newest classification has three levels, starting with classification of seizure types (Scheffer et al., 2017). The classification of seizures requires a description of signs and symptoms during a seizure.

## ICTAL PHENOMENOLOGY

### Glossary of Seizure Terminology and Other Definitions

The terms frequently used in the description of seizures follow. Whenever possible, the definition is derived from the glossary of descriptive terminology for ictal semiology, reported by the ILAE task force on classification and terminology (Blume et al., 2001). The term *ictal semiology* means the signs and symptoms associated with seizures.

*Motor manifestations* refer to involvement of the musculature, usually with an increase in muscle contraction that produces a movement. A motor manifestation can also be negative, associated with a decrease in muscle contraction. The term *positive motor* can be used to specifically indicate an increase in muscle contraction.

Several qualifiers for motor manifestation exist. *Elementary motor* refers to the contraction of a muscle or group of muscles that is usually stereotyped and does not include multiple phases. Elementary motor manifestations include *tonic*, which means a sustained increase in muscle contraction lasting up to minutes. *Tonic activity* includes epileptic spasms that are a sudden flexion and/or extension which is more sustained than a myoclonic jerk but yet very short in duration, affecting predominantly proximal or truncal muscles. *Postural manifestation* suggests tonic activity that results in a posture. This will usually involve contraction of more than one muscle. *Versive manifestation* indicates a sustained or forced deviation of the eyes or the head to one side (Fig. 100.1). This may be associated with a truncal rotation. *Dystonic posturing* is a sustained contraction that results in an abnormal posture with a rotating or twisting motion (Fig. 100.2). A *myoclonic jerk* or *myoclonus* refers to a very brief involuntary contraction usually lasting less than 100 ms. This can affect any distal or proximal body part and may also be generalized. *Negative myoclonus* refers to an interruption of tonic muscle activity for less than 500 ms without prior positive contraction. Negative myoclonus may produce a jerk-like motion in association with a transitory loss of posture of that body part. Negative myoclonus would not be visible if the affected body part were resting. *Clonic activity* refers to a regularly repetitive jerking that is prolonged. Clonic activity is further described as being *without a march* if it remains confined to the same body part from beginning to end. Clonic activity has a *Jacksonian march* if it spreads through contiguous body parts on the same side, reflecting horizontal spread of seizure activity over the motor strip. *Tonic-clonic activity* is a sequence of initial tonic posturing that evolves to a clonic phase. *Atonic activity* refers to a sudden decrease or loss of muscle tone usually lasting more than 1 second. This can affect the head, trunk, or limbs, usually bilaterally. However, focal atonic activity can also occur. *Astatic* refers to a loss of erect posture; an astatic seizure is synonymous with a drop attack.

*Automatisms* are repetitive motor activities that are more or less coordinated and resemble a voluntary movement but are not purposeful. Automatisms usually occur in association with altered sensorium, and the individual is usually amnestic to their occurrence. Automatisms may be an inappropriate continuation of previously ongoing activity. This is referred to as *perseverative automatisms*. Automatisms that start after seizure onset are called *de novo automatisms*. Automatisms may be reactive—for example, fumbling with an object that was present or newly placed in the patient's hand.

Automatisms can be described by the part of the body affected. Some of the most common are oroalimentary automatisms, which include lip smacking, chewing, swallowing, and other mouth movements (Video 100.1). Ictal spitting and ictal drinking can be considered forms of oroalimentary automatisms. Automatisms affecting the distal extremities are manual or pedal. Manual or pedal automatisms can be bilateral or unilateral. *Gestural automatisms* include extremity movements such as those used to enhance speech. More recently, introduced categories for upper extremity automatisms are manipulative and nonmanipulative (Kelemen et al., 2010). *Manipulative automatisms* involve picking and fumbling motions, typically reflecting interaction with the environment (see Video 100.1). *Nonmanipulative upper extremity automatisms* tend to be rhythmic and do not involve interaction with the environment (Video 100.2). Distal nonmanipulative upper-extremity automatisms have been described with the acronym RINCH (rhythmic ictal nonclonic hand) movements (Kuba et al., 2013; Lee et al., 2006; Zaher et al., 2020). *Hyperkinetic automatisms* imply an inappropriately rapid sequence of movements that predominantly involve axial and proximal limb muscles. The resulting motion can be thrashing, rocking, pelvic thrusting, kicking, or bicycling motions. Seizures with hyperkinetic automatisms are often referred to as *hypermotor* (Video 100.3). 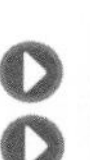 *Gelastic* refers to abrupt laughter or giggling (Video 100.4), while *dacrystic* refers to abrupt crying, both inappropriate.

Seizures may include a variety of subjective or sensory phenomena. *Sensory phenomena* are described as *elementary* if they involve a single primary sensory modality with unformed phenomena. This is applied predominantly to visual or auditory hallucination. *Elementary visual phenomena* could consist of flickering or flashing lights and other simple patterns such as spots, scotomata, or visual loss. *Elementary auditory phenomena* include buzzing, ringing, or humming sounds or single tones, but may also be negative, with loss of hearing. *Somatosensory phenomena* can include tingling and other paresthesias, shock-like sensations, numbness, pain, or a sense of movement or a desire to move a body part. Somatosensory phenomena can remain confined to the same body part or could also have a Jacksonian march, in which case the sensation moves to adjacent body parts on the same side, reflecting spread of the seizure discharge in the sensory cortex. *Olfactory hallucinations* are most often disagreeable and usually difficult to characterize. A variety of *gustatory hallucinations* can occur, particularly with a metallic taste. A *cephalic sensation* is a sensation in the head that can be described variably, including tingling, fullness, pressure, or lightheadedness.

The category of *experiential phenomena* is wide and includes affective experiences such as fear, sadness, elation; dysmnesic phenomena such as feelings of familiarity (déjà vu) or unfamiliarity (jamais vu); and complex hallucination (such as seeing people or hearing music) and illusions (alterations of perception). *Dyscognitive* describes events in which the predominant feature is alteration of cognition including perception, attention, memory, or executive function. The most recent classification of seizures reorganized experiential phenomena into cognitive category and emotional or affective category (Fisher et al, 2017).

*Autonomic phenomena* are very common in seizures. They may be subjective, including an epigastric sensation, nausea, a feeling of palpitation, or a feeling of flushing, or can be objective, including pupillary dilation, piloerection, pallor or flushing, vomiting, and even flatulence.

## CLASSIFICATION OF SEIZURES

Two classifications developed by the ILAE were used widely: the Clinical and Electroencephalographic Classification of Epileptic Seizures published in 1981 (Commission on Classification and Terminology of the International League Against Epilepsy, 1981; Box 100.1) and the Classification of Epilepsies and Epileptic Syndromes introduced in 1989 (Commission on Classification and Terminologyof the International League Against Epilepsy 1989; Box 100.2). These classifications were recently revised based on advances made in the last three decades (Fisher et al., 2017; Scheffer et al., 2017). The current chapter uses the newer terminology but offers the corresponding older established terminology.

The 1981 classification of seizures has a major dichotomy based on whether seizures start in one part of one hemisphere or in both hemispheres simultaneously. Seizures that start in one part of one hemisphere are classified as *partial* (or *partial-onset*) *seizures*, whereas those that start in both hemispheres simultaneously are classified as *generalized* (or *generalized-onset*) *seizures*. Partial-onset seizures are subclassified as *simple partial* if there is no impairment of consciousness, *complex partial* if there is impairment or loss of consciousness at any point in the seizure, and *partial seizures evolving to generalized*

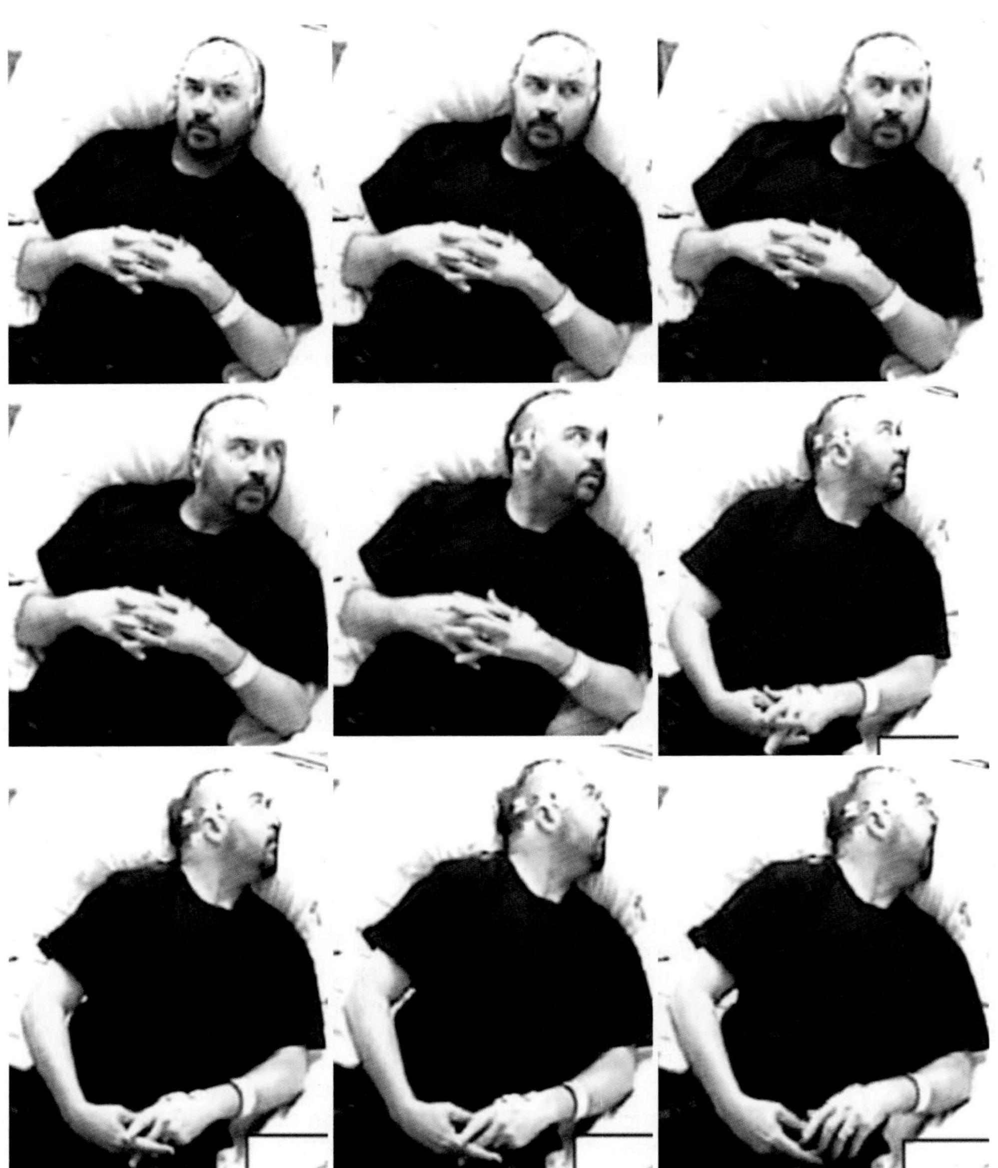

**Fig. 100.1** Versive eye and head turning in transition to bilateral tonic posturing in a subject with right frontal lobe seizures. Note the associated neck extension.

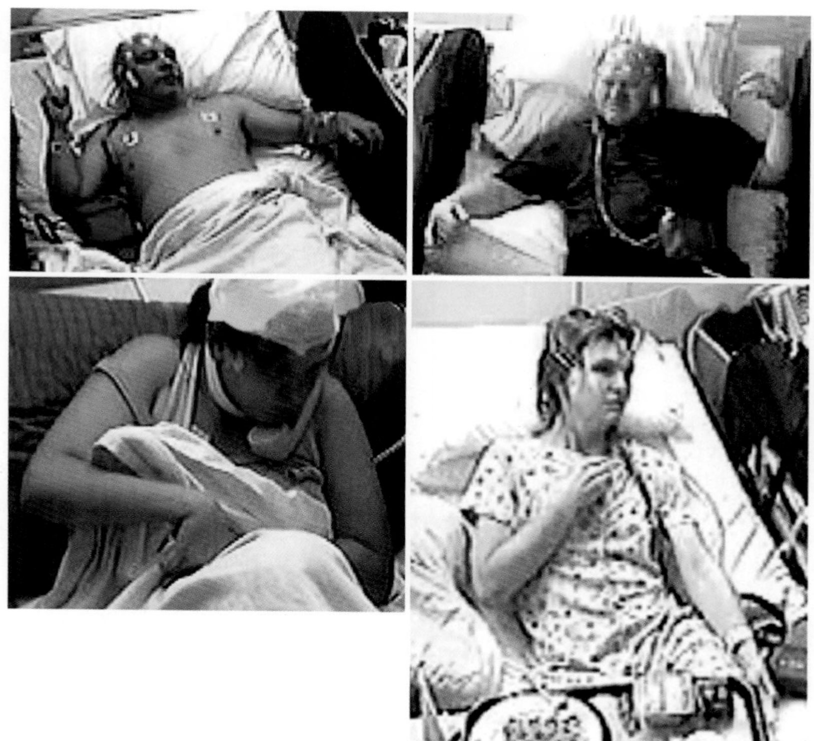

**Fig. 100.2** Dystonic posturing (DP): variable pattern demonstrated in four patients with temporal lobe epilepsy. *Left to right: top,* right arm DP, left arm DP; *bottom,* right arm DP, right arm DP.

*tonic-clonic (GTC) convulsions*. Simple partial seizures can have motor signs, somatosensory or special sensory symptoms, autonomic symptoms and signs, or psychic symptoms. Under the heading of generalized seizures were included *generalized absence* (typical or atypical), *myoclonic, clonic, tonic, tonic-clonic,* and *atonic seizures*. Acknowledging that some seizures cannot be classified into partial or generalized onset, the classification also includes a category of unclassified seizures.

One important criticism of the 1981 classification is that it requires both clinical and electroencephalographic (EEG) information, and assumptions on correlation of clinical and EEG features may be incorrect. A purely semiological classification of epileptic seizures was proposed, based solely on observed clinical features (Luders et al., 1998). The semiological seizure classification includes somatotopic modifiers to define the somatotopic distribution of the manifestations and allows demonstration of evolution of ictal manifestations using arrows to link sequential manifestations (Luders et al., 1998). Although this classification was not adopted by the ILAE, it is considered an optional seizure classification system that is useful for localization purposes in epilepsy surgery centers.

The latest ILAE revision of the seizure classification (Figure 100.3) has maintained the division of seizures based on generalized or focal onset but has recommended replacing the term *partial* with *focal* (Fisher et al., 2017). The latest revision updated the definition of *focal seizures* as "originating within networks limited to one hemisphere," with the possibility of the seizures being discretely localized or more widely distributed, and possibly originating in subcortical structures. *Generalized seizures* were defined as "originating at some point within, and rapidly engaging, bilaterally distributed networks," which do not necessarily include the entire cortex (Fisher et al., 2017). The revised concepts acknowledge that generalized seizures can be asymmetrical (Fisher et al., 2017). The category of focal-onset seizures underwent major changes. The terms "simple partial" and "complex partial" were abandoned. Level of consciousness during seizures can still be used to classify focal-onset seizures, if it is known, but it is no longer obligatory. The aspect of consciousness chosen for classification is the patient's awareness during a seizure. Focal seizures are *focal aware seizures (FAS)* if awareness is totally preserved for the whole duration of the seizure or *focal impaired awareness seizures (FIAS)* if there is any alteration of awareness during any part of the seizure. Secondarily generalized seizures were renamed *focal to bilateral tonic-clonic seizures (FBTCS)*. The term "generalized" was reserved for seizures that are generalized from onset. Another important level of classification for focal seizures is by the first clinical manifestation at onset. Thus, focal seizures can be classified as motor or nonmotor, or if possible with the specific initial sign or symptom under these headings (Fig. 100.3). As an exception, for a seizure to be classified as *behavior arrest seizure*, behavior arrest has to be the dominant clinical feature for the whole duration of the seizure. The other major change in the classification is that it allows some classification of unknown onset seizures. The new classification allows some seizure types such as tonic or myoclonic to be focal or generalized. Table 100.1 summarizes some of the key terminology changes between the old and the new classifications.

## Other Seizure Terminology

*Convulsion* is an old term typically used to denote a GTC seizure. It may also be used to indicate a seizure with prominent motor

**BOX 100.1 1981 International League Against Epilepsy Classification of Epileptic Seizures**

I. Partial (Focal, Local) Seizures
   A. Simple partial seizures (consciousness not impaired)
      1. With motor symptoms
      2. With somatosensory or special sensory symptoms
      3. With autonomic symptoms
      4. With psychic symptoms
   B. Complex partial seizures (with impairment of consciousness)
      1. With simple partial onset followed by impairment of consciousness
      2. With impairment of consciousness at onset
   C. Partial seizures evolving to secondarily generalized seizures
      1. Simple partial seizures evolving to generalized seizures
      2. Complex partial seizures evolving to generalized seizures
      3. Simple partial seizures evolving to complex partial seizures evolving to generalized seizures
II. Generalized Seizures (Convulsive or Nonconvulsive)
   A. Absence seizures
      1. Typical absence seizures
      2. Atypical absence seizures
   B. Myoclonic seizures
   C. Clonic seizures
   D. Tonic seizures
   E. Tonic-clonic seizures
   F. Atonic seizures
III. Unclassified Epileptic Seizures

*From Commission on Classification and Terminology of the International League Against Epilepsy, 1981. Proposal for revised clinical and electroencephalographic classification of epileptic seizures. Epilepsia 22, 489–501.*

**BOX 100.2 1989 International League Against Epilepsy Classification of Epilepsies and Epileptic Syndromes**

1. Localization-related (focal, local, partial) epilepsies and syndromes
   1.1. Idiopathic (with age-related onset)
   1.2. Symptomatic
   1.3. Cryptogenic
2. Generalized epilepsies and syndromes
   2.1. Idiopathic (with age-related onset, listed in order of age appearance)
   2.2. Cryptogenic or symptomatic (in order of age)
   2.3. Symptomatic
      2.3.1. Nonspecific etiology
      2.3.2. Specific syndromes
3. Epilepsies and syndromes undetermined as to whether they are focal or generalized
   3.1. With both generalized and focal seizures
   3.2. Without unequivocal generalized or focal features
4. Special syndromes
   4.1. Situation-related seizures (Gelegenheitsanfälle)
      4.1.1. Febrile convulsions
      4.1.2. Isolated seizures or isolated status epilepticus
      4.1.3. Seizures occurring only when there is an acute metabolic or toxic event

*From Commission on Classification and Terminology of the International League Against Epilepsy, 1989. Proposal for revised classification of epilepsies and epileptic syndromes. Epilepsia 30, 389–399.*

activity. *Convulsive* is an adjective indicating the presence of prominent motor activity such as tonic or clonic or both. *Nonconvulsive* refers to a seizure or status epilepticus without prominent clonic or tonic motor activity. The term is most commonly used with status epilepticus to indicate that seizure activity is predominantly affecting consciousness or behavior, with minimal or no motor activity. The term *grand mal* is also an old term that is usually synonymous with GTC seizure. The term is discouraged in scientific writing because it does not specify whether the onset is focal or generalized. Patients may use the term *grand mal* simply to indicate a big seizure, and the neurologist has to convert this term into official terminology. The term *petit mal* is an old synonym for *childhood absence epilepsy* (CAE) but is also used to describe absence seizures. Again, the term is commonly used by patients to indicate a small seizure, which may actually be a focal seizure. A *primary generalized seizure* or *primarily generalized seizure* is a synonym for *generalized-onset seizure*. *Primary generalized epilepsy* is a synonym for *idiopathic generalized epilepsy* (IGE). *Secondarily generalized seizure* is an old term for a focal seizure that evolves to bilateral tonic-clonic activity. This is to be distinguished from *secondary generalized epilepsy*, which is a synonym of *symptomatic generalized epilepsy*, an old term for generalized epilepsy of structural/metabolic etiology, where most seizures are usually of generalized onset. The term *secondary generalized epilepsy* should be discouraged because of confusion with secondarily generalized seizure.

## SEIZURE TYPES

### Focal Seizures (Partial Seizures)

#### Focal Aware Seizures (Simple Partial Seizures)

FAS are seizures in which awareness is not altered at any point in the course of the seizure. FAS of purely subjective nature are often referred to as *auras* or *isolated auras*. The manifestations of FAS depend on the brain region involved in the ictal discharge. However, it is important to recognize that the seizure activity may originate in silent areas, and the first clinical manifestations may reflect seizure spread to other brain regions. Nevertheless, FAS and auras may have important lateralizing and localizing value. For example, focal clonic or tonic activity is usually contralateral to the hemisphere involved in seizure activity. Somatosensory auras, visual auras, and auditory auras are often useful in suggesting localization and lateralization of the epileptogenic zone. However, some auras are nonspecific and may be seen with a variety of localizations.

Auras are typically short in duration, lasting seconds to minutes. Some patients may experience a *prodrome*, a difficult-to-describe feeling that a seizure may occur. Prodromes may last hours or even days and have to be distinguished from auras. On the other hand, auras may occasionally be prolonged, in which case they are called *aura continua*, which is a form of focal nonconvulsive status epilepticus without impairment of consciousness.

#### Focal Impaired Awareness Seizures (Complex Partial Seizures)

*FIAS* are characterized by altered awareness during the seizure. Impairment may be very subtle, manifesting with slight confusion, fuzziness, or slowing of responses. A patient may have some recollection of events or total amnesia for the event. FIAS may start with an aura or may start with loss of awareness. It is sometimes difficult to determine if awareness was impaired. The patient may be totally

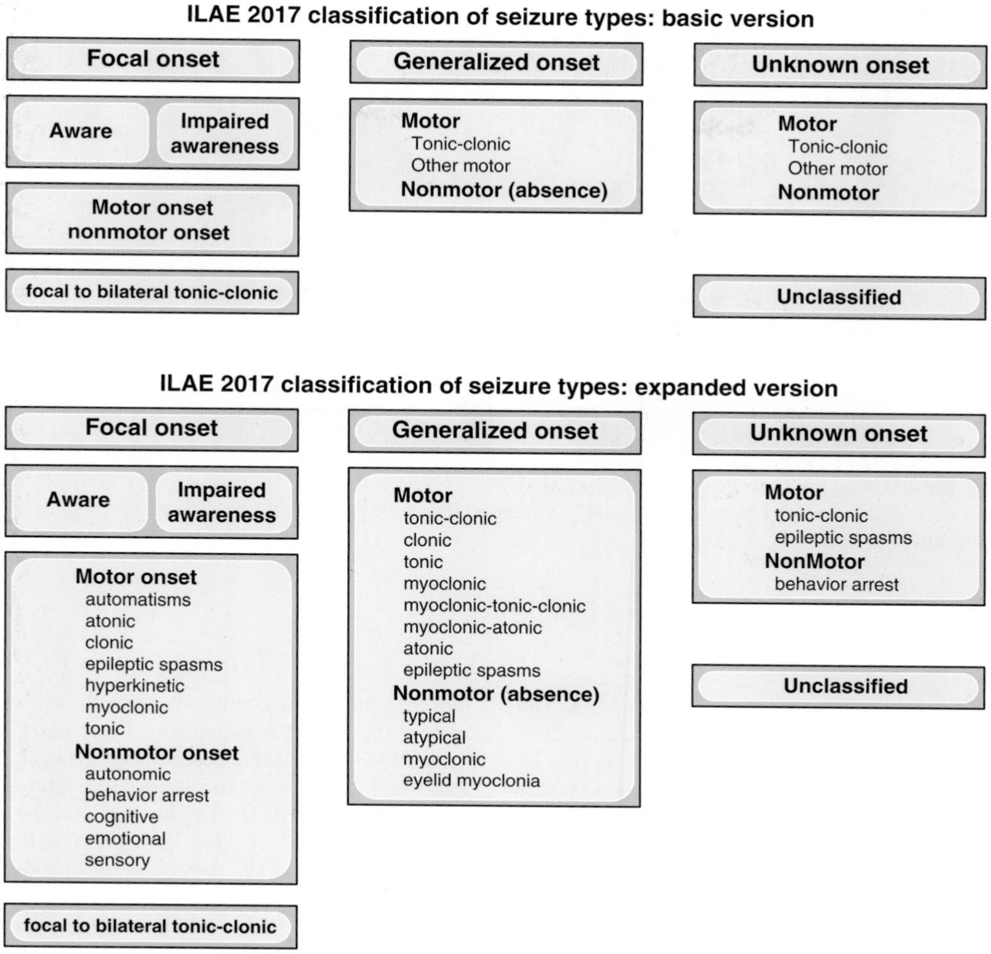

**ILAE 2017 classification of seizure types: basic version**

| Focal onset | Generalized onset | Unknown onset |
|---|---|---|
| Aware / Impaired awareness | **Motor**<br>Tonic-clonic<br>Other motor<br>**Nonmotor (absence)** | **Motor**<br>Tonic-clonic<br>Other motor<br>**Nonmotor** |
| Motor onset<br>nonmotor onset | | |
| focal to bilateral tonic-clonic | | Unclassified |

**ILAE 2017 classification of seizure types: expanded version**

| Focal onset | Generalized onset | Unknown onset |
|---|---|---|
| Aware / Impaired awareness | **Motor**<br>tonic-clonic<br>clonic<br>tonic<br>myoclonic<br>myoclonic-tonic-clonic<br>myoclonic-atonic<br>atonic<br>epileptic spasms<br>**Nonmotor (absence)**<br>typical<br>atypical<br>myoclonic<br>eyelid myoclonia | **Motor**<br>tonic-clonic<br>epileptic spasms<br>**NonMotor**<br>behavior arrest |
| **Motor onset**<br>automatisms<br>atonic<br>clonic<br>epileptic spasms<br>hyperkinetic<br>myoclonic<br>tonic<br>**Nonmotor onset**<br>autonomic<br>behavior arrest<br>cognitive<br>emotional<br>sensory | | Unclassified |
| focal to bilateral tonic-clonic | | |

**Fig. 100.3** The 2017 ILAE Operational Classification of Seizure Types.

**TABLE 100.1 Select Terminology in New Versus Old Seizure and Epilepsy Classifications**

| 1981 Terminology | 2017 Terminology |
|---|---|
| **Seizure Classification** | |
| Partial seizure | Focal seizure |
| Simple partial seizure | Focal aware seizure |
| Complex partial seizure | Focal impaired awareness seizure |
| Secondarily generalized seizure | Focal to bilateral tonic-clonic seizure |
| **Epilepsy Classification** | |
| Localization related epilepsy | Focal epilepsy |
| Idiopathic generalized epilepsy | Idiopathic generalized epilepsy or genetic generalized epilepsy (both terms are acceptable) |
| Cryptogenic epilepsies | Epilepsies of unknown cause |
| Symptomatic epilepsies | Structural/metabolic epilepsies secondary to specific structural or metabolic lesions or conditions, but which do not fit a specific electroclinical pattern. |
| Benign | Self-limited or pharmacoresponsive |
| Epilepsies undetermined as to whether focal or generalized | (1) Combined generalized and focal (if both seizure categories coexist) or (2) Unknown (if the seizure type cannot be determined) |

conscious but unable to respond verbally because of aphasia or unable to respond or react because of motor inhibition.

Impaired awareness seizures may arise from any lobe but most commonly arise from the temporal lobe; the frontal lobe is the second most common site of seizure origin. The most common type of motor activity in this seizure type is automatism, described earlier. The different seizure manifestations in seizures arising from different lobes of the brain are discussed in the next section.

### Focal to Bilateral Tonic-Clonic Seizures (Partial Seizures Evolving to Generalized Tonic-Clonic Activity)

These seizures may start as focal aware or FIAS. The transition to bilateral tonic-clonic activity usually involves versive head turning in a direction contralateral to the hemisphere of seizure onset (see Fig. 100.1), and focal or lateralized tonic or clonic motor activity. The pattern of evolution may be clonic-tonic-clonic in some instances. The bilateral tonic phase may be asymmetrical, with flexion on one side and extension on the other. This has been called *figure-of-four posturing* (Kotagal et al., 2000; Fig. 100.4). Some asymmetry and asynchrony may also occur in the clonic phase, resulting in a slight degree of side-to-side head jerking (Niaz et al., 1999). The evolution from tonic to clonic activity is gradual and not always simultaneous in all affected body parts. A phase of high-frequency tremor has been referred to as the *tremulous* or *vibratory phase* of the seizure (Theodore et al., 1994). Clonic activity typically decreases in frequency over time, with longer

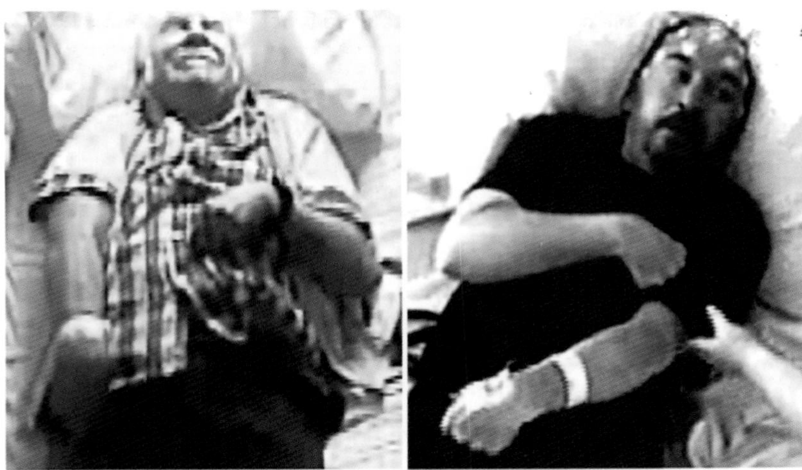

**Fig. 100.4** A, Figure-of-four posturing, usually seen in transition from focal to generalized activity. The sign lateralizes seizure activity contralaterally to the extended upper extremity (left hemisphere on the left, right hemisphere on the right).

intervals between jerks toward the termination of the seizure. The clonic activity may end on one side of the body first so that clonic activity may then appear lateralized to one side. In addition, there may be a late head turn ipsilateral to the hemisphere of seizure origin (Wyllie et al., 1986). After the motor activity stops, the individual is usually limp and has a loud snoring respiration often referred to as *stertorous respiration* (Video 100.5). During the course of recovery, there may be variable agitation. The speed of recovery is expected to be slower with longer and more severe seizures.

## Focal Seizure Semiology in Relation to Localization

***Focal seizures of temporal lobe origin.*** Temporal lobe seizures most often are of mesial temporal amygdalohippocampal origin, in association with the pathology of hippocampal sclerosis. Patients commonly have isolated auras, and FIAS tend to start with an aura. The most common aura is an epigastric sensation frequently with a rising character (French et al., 1993). Other auras occur less commonly and include fear, anxiety, and other emotions, déjà vu and jamais vu, nonspecific sensations, and autonomic changes such as palpitation and gooseflesh. Olfactory and gustatory auras are uncommon and are more likely with tumoral mesial temporal lobe epilepsy (MTLE).

FIAS may start with an aura or with altered consciousness. With nondominant temporal lobe seizures, the patient may remain responsive and verbally interactive. However, recollection of conversations is unusual. Altered consciousness is often associated with an arrest of motion and speech. *Speech arrest* is not synonymous with *aphasia* and does not distinguish dominant and nondominant temporal lobe seizures. Automatisms are one of the most prominent manifestations, and oroalimentary automatisms are the most prevalent. Extremity automatisms also occur and are most commonly manipulative, with picking or fumbling (see Video 100.1). This type of automatism is not of direct lateralizing value. However, the contralateral upper extremity is commonly involved in dystonic posturing (Kotagal et al., 1989) or milder degrees of posturing and immobility (Fakhoury and Abou-Khalil, 1995; Williamson et al., 1998). This reduces the availability of the contralateral arm for automatisms, so manipulative automatisms tend to be ipsilateral, involving the unaffected upper extremity. Nonmanipulative automatisms typically consist of rhythmic movements either distally or proximally. These tend to be contralateral, often preceding overt dystonic posturing (Kuba et al., 2013; Lee et al., 2006; Zaher et al., 2020). Head turning occurs commonly. Early head turning is not usually forceful. It typically occurs at the same time as dystonic posturing and is most often ipsilateral (Fakhoury and Abou-Khalil, 1995; Williamson et al., 1998). Late head turning most often occurs during evolution to bilateral tonic-clonic activity (see Video 100.5). This is usually contralateral to the side of seizure origin (Williamson et al., 1998). Well-formed ictal speech may occur during seizures of nondominant temporal lobe origin (Gabr et al., 1989). Verbal output may at times be tinged with a fearful tone. FIAS of temporal lobe origin usually last between 30 seconds and 3 minutes. Postictal manifestations may be helpful in lateralizing the seizure onset. Postictal aphasia is commonly seen after dominant temporal lobe seizures (Gabr et al., 1989). In one study, patients with dominant left temporal seizure origin were unable to read a test sentence correctly in the first minute after seizure termination, but patients with nondominant right temporal lobe origin were able to read the test sentence within 1 minute of seizure termination (Privitera et al., 1991).

Seizures of lateral temporal origin or neocortical temporal origin are much less common than those of mesial temporal origin. They cannot be reliably distinguished based on their semiology, but certain features suggest lateral temporal origin. Auditory auras are the most common auras referable to the lateral temporal cortex, usually implying involvement of the Heschl gyrus. Other types of auras referable to the lateral temporal cortex are vertigo and complex visual hallucinations (usually posterior temporal). Oroalimentary automatisms are less common, and the pattern of contralateral dystonic posturing and ipsilateral extremity automatisms is also less common (Dupont et al., 1999). Early contralateral or bilateral facial twitching may be seen as a result of propagation to the frontal operculum (Foldvary et al., 1997). Seizures of lateral temporal origin tend to be shorter in duration and have a greater tendency to evolve to bilateral tonic-clonic activity than seizures of mesial temporal origin. Seizures originating in the temporal lobe may have hypermotor semiology characteristic of frontal lobe origin, due to propagation to the frontal lobe (Vaugier et al., 2009; Yu et al., 2013). This is commonly seen with seizure origin in the temporal pole (Wang et al., 2008).

***Focal seizures of frontal lobe origin.*** Many different seizure types can originate in the frontal lobe, depending on site of seizure origin and propagation. FAS can be motor with focal clonic activity, can originate in the motor cortex, or can be the result of spread to the motor cortex. These seizures may or may not have a Jacksonian march. Asymmetrical tonic seizures or postural seizures are usually related to involvement of the supplementary motor area in the mesial frontal cortex anterior to the motor strip. The best-known posturing pattern is the *fencing posture* in which the contralateral arm is extended and the ipsilateral arm is flexed. Tonic posturing may involve all four extremities and is occasionally symmetrical. When these seizures originate in the supplementary motor area, consciousness is usually preserved (Morris et al., 1988). Supplementary motor seizures are an important exception to the rule that bilateral motor activity during a seizure should be associated with loss of consciousness. Supplementary motor seizures are usually short in duration and frequently arise out of sleep. They tend to occur in clusters and may be preceded by a sensory aura referable to the supplementary sensory cortex. The pattern of posturing described with supplementary motor area seizures can occur as a result of seizure spread to the supplementary motor area from other regions of the brain. In that case, consciousness is frequently impaired. Subjective FAS may also occur with frontal lobe origin, the most common being a nonspecific cephalic aura.

FIAS of frontal lobe origin tend to be very peculiar. They may be preceded by a nonspecific aura (most commonly cephalic) or they may start abruptly, often out of sleep. Their most characteristic features are hyperkinetic automatisms with frenzied behavior and agitation (Jobst et al., 2000; Williamson et al., 1985). These are often referred to as hypermotor seizures. There may be various vocalizations including expletives. The manifestations can be so bizarre as to suggest a psychiatric origin (Video 100.6). The seizure duration is short, often less than 30 seconds, and postictal manifestations are brief or nonexistent, further adding to the risk of misdiagnosis as psychogenic seizures. Frontal lobe FIAS arise predominantly from the orbitofrontal region and from the mesial frontal cingulate region. However, they can arise from other parts of the frontal lobe. It may be difficult to determine the region of origin in the frontal lobe based on the seizure manifestations. It has been suggested that the presence of tonic posturing on one side points to a mesial frontal origin, as does rotation along the body axis, which sometimes leads to turning prone during the seizure (Leung et al., 2008; Rheims et al., 2008). Ictal pouting, also known as "chapeau de gendarme," tends to arise in the anterior cingulate region (Souirti et al., 2014).

Seizures originating in the frontal operculum are associated with profuse salivation, oral facial apraxia, and sometimes facial clonic activity (Williamson and Engel, 2008). Seizures originating in the dorsolateral frontal lobe may involve tonic movements of the extremities and versive deviation of the eyes and head. The head deviation preceding evolution to bilateral tonic-clonic activity is contralateral, but earlier head turning can be in either direction (Remi et al., 2011). Seizures may begin with forced thinking. Focal seizures of frontal origin may at times resemble absence seizures (So, 1998). It is important to recognize that seizures originating in the frontal lobe can propagate to the temporal lobe and produce manifestations typical of mesial temporal lobe seizures.

***Focal seizures originating in the parietal lobe.*** The best-recognized seizure type that originates in the parietal lobe is focal seizure with somatosensory manifestations. The somatosensory experience can be described as tingling, pins and needles, numbness, burning, or pain. The presence of a sensory march is most suggestive of involvement of the primary sensory cortex. Sensory phenomena arising from the second sensory area and the supplementary sensory area are less likely to have a march. Somatosensory auras tend to be contralateral to the hemisphere of seizure origin, but they may be bilateral or ipsilateral when arising from the second or supplementary sensory regions. Other auras of parietal lobe origin are a sensation of movement in an extremity, a feeling of the body bending forward or swaying or twisting or turning, or even a feeling of an extremity being absent (Salanova et al., 1995a, 1995b). Some patients may complain of inability to move a limb. Vertigo has been reported, as well as visual illusions of objects going away or coming closer or looking larger (Siegel, 2003). Some patients may have initial auras suggesting spread to the occipital or temporal lobe. Seizures involving the dominant parietal lobe may produce aphasic manifestations. Motor manifestations tend to reflect seizure spread to the frontal lobe. These include tonic posturing of the extremities, focal motor clonic activity, and version of the head and eyes (Cascino et al., 1993; Ho et al., 1994; Williamson et al., 1992a). Negative motor manifestations may occur, with ictal paralysis (Abou-Khalil et al., 1995). Seizures may spread to the temporal lobe, producing oroalimentary or extremity automatisms (Siegel, 2003). In one study, motor manifestations were more likely with superior parietal epileptogenic foci, and oroalimentary and extremity automatisms more likely with inferior parietal epileptogenic foci (Salanova et al., 1995a). Visual manifestations seemed more likely with posterior parietal lesions.

***Focal seizures originating in the occipital lobe.*** The best-recognized occipital lobe seizure semiology is that of FAS with visual manifestations (Salanova et al., 1992). The most common are elementary visual hallucinations that are described as flashing colored lights or geometrical figures. These are usually contralateral but may move within the visual field. Complex visual hallucinations with familiar faces or people may also occur. Negative symptoms may be reported, with loss of vision in one hemifield. Ictal blindness may occur, with loss of vision in the whole visual field. Objective seizure manifestations include blinking, nystagmoid eye movements, and versive eye and head deviation contralateral to the seizure focus. This version may occur while the patient is still conscious or could be a component of impaired awareness seizures.

Seizure manifestations that are related to seizure spread to the temporal or frontal lobe are very common. Oroalimentary automatisms are typical of seizures that spread to the temporal lobe, whereas asymmetrical tonic posturing typifies spread to the frontal lobe; both types of spread can be seen in the same patient (Williamson et al., 1992b). Spread to the temporal or frontal lobe is so common with occipital lobe seizures that it is at times reported in most patients (Jobst et al., 2010b). Ictal semiology cannot distinguish seizures originating from the mesial versus lateral occipital region (Blume et al., 2005). Evolution of occipital seizures to bilateral tonic-clonic activity is commonly reported.

### Focal Seizures Originating in the Insular Cortex

Insular epilepsy is uncommon and frequently unrecognized because of the inability to record directly from the insula with scalp electrodes. Subjective symptoms that should suggest seizure origin in the insula include laryngeal discomfort, possibly preceded or followed by a sensation in the chest or abdomen, shortness of breath, and paresthesias around the mouth or also involving other contralateral body parts (Isnard et al., 2004). Objective seizure manifestations include dysarthria/dysphonia, sometimes evolving to complete muteness. With seizure progression in some patients, tonic spasm of the face and upper limb, head and eye rotation, and at times generalized dystonia occur (Isnard et al., 2004). Hypersalivation is also very common and can be impressive. Insular-onset seizures may spread to other brain regions and can be disguised as temporal lobe, parietal lobe, or frontal lobe epilepsy (Jobst et al., 2019; Ryvlin, 2006; Ryvlin et al., 2006).

## Generalized Seizures

### Generalized Absence Seizures

Typical absence seizures are characterized by a sudden blank stare with motor arrest, usually lasting less than 15 seconds (Commission on Classification and Terminology of the International League Against Epilepsy, 1981). The individual is usually unresponsive and unaware. The seizure ends as abruptly as it starts, and the patient returns immediately to a baseline level of function with no postictal confusion but may have missed conversation and seems confused as a result (Video 100.7). If the only manifestation is altered responsiveness and awareness, with no associated motor component, the absence seizure is classified as *simple absence*. Most often, generalized absence seizures include mild motor components and are classified as *complex absence*. The most common motor components are automatisms such as licking the lips or playing with an object that was held in the hand before the seizure. Other motor components include clonic, tonic, atonic, and autonomic manifestations. Clonic activity may affect the eyelids or the mouth. An atonic component may manifest with dropping an object or slight head drop or drooping of the shoulders or trunk. Tonic components may manifest with slight increase in tone.

The EEG hallmark of a typical generalized absence seizure is generalized 2.5- to 4-Hz spike-and-wave activity with a normal interictal background (Fig. 100.5). Atypical absence seizures are diagnosed primarily based on a slower (<2.5 Hz) frequency of the EEG spike-and-wave activity. Less important distinctions are that the onset and termination of an atypical absence seizure may be less abrupt and the motor components a bit more pronounced than seen with typical absence seizures. Atypical absence seizures usually occur in individuals with impaired cognitive function. Affected individuals usually have associated seizure types such as generalized tonic, generalized atonic, and GTC seizures.

Additional generalized absence seizure types recently recognized by the ILAE include *myoclonic absences*. The key manifestation of these seizures is a prominent rhythmic myoclonus predominantly affecting the limbs (Bureau and Tassinari, 2005b). Otherwise, myoclonic absences resemble typical absence seizures with respect to impairment of consciousness. Another related seizure type recently recognized is *eyelid myoclonia with absence*. The eyelid myoclonia consists of pronounced rhythmic jerking of the eyelids, usually associated with an upward deviation of the eyes and retropulsion of the head (Caraballo et al., 2009). There may or may not be associated generalized spike-and-wave activity on EEG. Absence seizures may evolve to GTC activity (Mayville et al., 2000; Video 100.8).

### Generalized Myoclonic Seizures

Myoclonic seizures are muscle contractions lasting a fraction of a second (<250 ms), in association with an ictal EEG discharge (Blume et al., 2001). The myoclonic jerk can be generalized, affecting the whole body, or could affect just the upper extremities or (rarely) the head or trunk, or even the diaphragm. The myoclonic jerks may affect one side of the body at one time, but typically the other side is affected at other times. The jerks can be single or could occur in an arrhythmic cluster ( Video 100.9). It should be noted that myoclonus is not always epileptic (Faught, 2003). Myoclonus can be generated anywhere along the central nervous system (CNS). Epileptic myoclonus is generated in the cerebral cortex and is usually associated with a single or brief serial spike-and-wave or polyspike-and-wave activity.

Negative myoclonic seizures consist of a very brief pause in muscle activity rather than a brief muscle contraction (Rubboli and Tassinari, 2006). Just as with positive myoclonus, negative myoclonus can be generalized, bilateral with limited distribution, or even focal, typically with shifting lateralization.

Generalized myoclonic seizures may be immediately followed by a loss of tone. The seizure type is called *myoclonicatonic*. Historically it was called *myoclonicastatic*. The seizures are brief (1 second or less) but may be associated with falls and injuries (Video 100.10). The EEG shows generalized spike-and-wave or polyspike-and-wave discharge. The slow wave is prolonged and associated with the electromyographic (EMG) silence characteristic of the atonic phase. Myoclonic seizures may precede a more sustained tonic contraction, and the resultant seizures may be referred to as *myoclonic-tonic seizures* (Berg et al., 2010). Generalized myoclonic seizures may cluster just before a GTC seizure occurrence (Video 100.11).

### Generalized Clonic Seizures

Unlike myoclonic seizures, which are single jerks (but may occur in arrhythmic clusters), each generalized clonic seizure consists of a series of rhythmic jerks. Generalized clonic seizures are uncommon and particularly rare in adults (Noachtar and Arnold, 2000). They are more frequently seen in certain epileptic syndromes of infancy and childhood. For example, clonic seizures are a common seizure type of severe myoclonic epilepsy of infancy (Dravet syndrome). Clonic seizures are also noted in progressive myoclonic epilepsies.

### Generalized Tonic Seizures

Generalized tonic seizures are typically brief seizures, lasting a few seconds to 1 minute (Video 100.12). Their onset may be gradual or abrupt. They may be initiated with a myoclonic jerk. They can vary in severity from subtle, with slight increase in neck tone with upward deviation of the eyes, to massive, with involvement of the axial muscles and extremities. Proximal muscles are the most affected. Most commonly there is neck and trunk flexion as well as abduction of the shoulders and flexion of the hips. However, extension may also occur. Tonic seizures may be asymmetrical, which could result in turning to one side. The pattern of muscle involvement may change over time so that there may be a change in the position of the limbs over the course of the seizure. Autonomic changes may occur, with tachycardia, pupil dilation, and flushing. Involvement of respiratory muscles could cause apnea and cyanosis. The tonic contraction may end with one or more pauses that result in a few clonic jerks. A postictal state with confusion may occur, but recovery is usually rapid. However, tonic seizures may be followed by atypical absence, resulting in what appears to be a more prolonged postictal state. This has been referred to as *tonic-absence seizure* (Shih and Hirsch, 2003). Generalized tonic seizures occur most often out of sleep and drowsiness.

### Epileptic Spasms

Epileptic spasms have similarities to generalized tonic seizures but a shorter duration that is intermediate between generalized myoclonic and generalized tonic seizures (Blume et al., 2001), with a typical duration of 0.5–2 seconds. The pattern of contraction is "diamond-shaped," with intensity of contraction maximal in the middle of the spasm and less at the beginning and end. Epileptic spasms were also called *infantile spasms* and *salaam attacks*. Because their occurrence is not restricted to infants, the preferred current term is *epileptic spasms*. The classic epileptic spasm involves neck and trunk flexion and arm abduction with a jackknife pattern, but extension may be seen. Epileptic spasms typically occur in clusters recurring every 5–40 seconds. In a cluster, the initial spasms may be subtle or mild, increase in intensity as the cluster progresses, and decrease in intensity again toward the end of the cluster (Bleasel and Lüders, 2000).

### Generalized Tonic-Clonic Seizures

GTC seizures are dramatic and the best recognized form of seizures. They are commonly referred to as *grand mal*, but this term is archaic

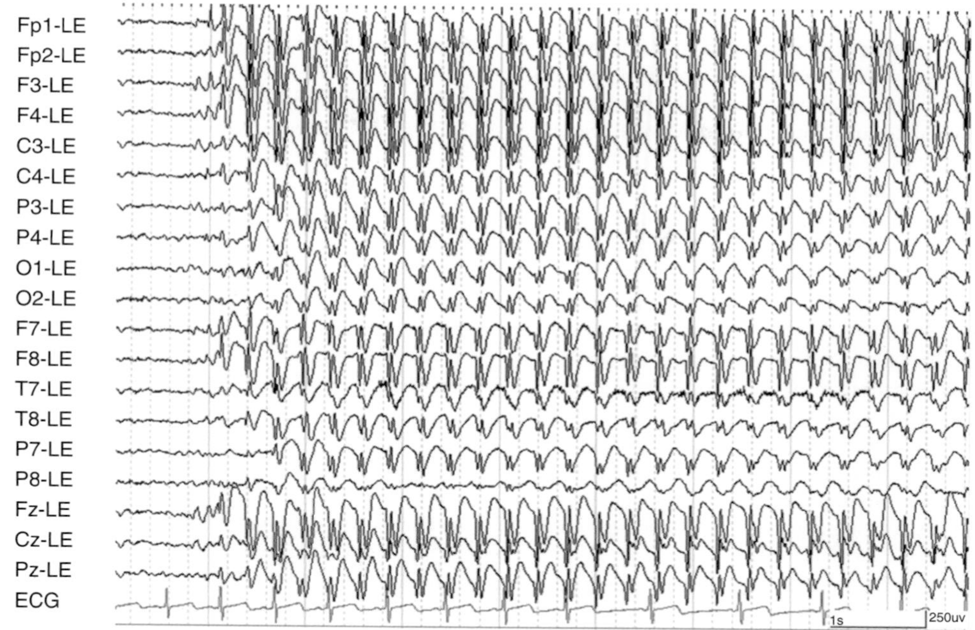


**Fig. 100.5** Generalized absence seizure displayed with referential montage using linked ear reference. Spike-and-wave discharges are bifrontally predominant.

and does not distinguish seizures of focal onset from those with a generalized onset. GTC seizures do not have an aura, but they may be preceded by a prodrome—the vague sense a seizure will occur—lasting up to hours. Seizure onset is abrupt, most often with loss of consciousness and a generalized tonic contraction, but some seizures may be initiated with a series of myoclonic jerks, leading to the term *myoclonic-tonic-clonic seizure* (see Video 100.11). The tonic phase may have asymmetrical movements, and these often change from seizure to seizure. One such commonly encountered asymmetry is versive head turning, which is not evidence of a focal onset (Chin and Miller, 2004; Niaz et al., 1999). The tonic phase includes an upward eye deviation with eyes half open and the mouth open. Involvement of the respiratory muscles usually produces a forced expiration that produces a loud guttural vocalization, often referred to as the *epileptic cry*. Cyanosis may occur during the tonic phase in association with apnea. The tonic phase gradually evolves to clonic activity. The transition can be with initially high-frequency and low-amplitude motion, often referred to as a *vibratory phase*. With seizure progression, the frequency of clonic jerks decreases, and the amplitude may initially increase but later decreases just before the seizure stops. In the immediate postictal state the individual is limp and unresponsive. Respiration is loud and snoring in character *(stertorous)*. The postictal state is often followed by sleep, although the individual may awaken briefly with postictal confusion. Tongue biting commonly occurs and most often affects the side of the tongue. Incontinence of urine is common, and incontinence of stool may also occur. After awakening, patients often have a pronounced headache and generalized muscle soreness. GTC seizures rarely last more than 2 minutes. The severity may vary. The postictal state seems to correlate with severity and duration.

### Generalized Atonic Seizures

Generalized atonic seizures are associated with very brief, sudden loss of tone and vary from extremely subtle, manifesting with only a head drop, to generalized loss of tone and falling. Atonic seizures may result in falling if the person is standing, called a *drop attack*. However, drop attacks may be the result of both generalized atonic and generalized tonic seizures. There is a very brief loss of consciousness and brief postictal confusion. Seizures are usually very brief, lasting 1 second to a few seconds. They may be preceded by a brief myoclonic jerk, in which case the seizure type is called *myoclonic-atonic* (see Video 100.10). Very brief myoclonic-atonic seizures are typical of the syndrome of myoclonic-astatic epilepsy (Doose syndrome) (Oguni et al., 2001). More prolonged atonic seizures can be seen with Lennox-Gastaut syndrome or other symptomatic generalized epilepsies. Despite their brief duration, generalized atonic seizures can result in serious injury and are an important cause of morbidity in epilepsy.

### Generalized-Onset Seizures with Focal Evolution

Generalized-onset seizures rarely may evolve to focal seizures (Deng et al., 2007; Linane et al., 2016; Williamson et al., 2009). This seems to occur with either myoclonic or absence seizures. The clinical manifestations most often are behavioral arrest and staring, with minor automatisms. However, focal motor manifestations may also occur. This type of seizure tends to be prolonged and may be associated with postictal confusion (Linane et al., 2016; Williamson et al., 2009).

## CLASSIFICATION OF EPILEPSIES AND EPILEPTIC SYNDROMES

The classification of seizures addresses single seizure events and not epilepsy as a condition. The 1989 classification of epilepsies and epileptic syndromes tried to organize epilepsies and epilepsy syndromes (commission on classification and terminology of the International League Against Epilepsy, 1989). It defined an epileptic syndrome as "an epileptic disorder characterized by a cluster of signs and symptoms customarily occurring together; these include such items as type of seizure, etiology, anatomy, precipitating factors, age of onset, severity, chronicity, diurnal and circadian cycling, and sometimes prognosis." A syndrome does not necessarily have a common etiology and prognosis. Two important divisions were used in the classification. The first separated epilepsies with generalized-onset seizures, called *generalized epilepsies*, from epilepsies with focal-onset seizures, referred to as *localization-related*, *partial*, or *focal epilepsies*. The other division separated epilepsies of known etiology (named *symptomatic epilepsies*) from those of unknown etiology. Epilepsies of unknown etiology were named *idiopathic* if they were pure epilepsy and "not preceded or occasioned by another condition." These epilepsies were considered to have no underlying cause other than a possible hereditary predisposition. Thus, they were presumed genetic. The idiopathic epilepsies were also defined by an age-related onset and clinical and EEG characteristics. Epilepsies of unknown etiology were called *cryptogenic* if they were presumed symptomatic, but with an occult etiology. Although the term *cryptogenic* was widely used in the epilepsy field, confusion existed concerning its exact meaning, which resulted in a recommendation to replace it with the term *probably symptomatic* (Engel, 2001). The 1989 classification of epilepsies and epileptic syndromes also subdivided symptomatic partial epilepsies based on lobar anatomical localization of the epileptogenic zone into temporal, frontal, parietal, and occipital lobe epilepsy. Temporal lobe epilepsy was further subdivided into amygdalohippocampal and lateral temporal, and frontal lobe epilepsy into seven subgroups: supplementary motor, cingulate, anterior frontopolar, orbitofrontal, dorsolateral, opercular, and motor cortex. The abbreviated classification is found in Box 100.2.

The 1989 classification of epilepsies and epileptic syndromes merited updating based on new knowledge. In 2010 the ILAE commission on classification suggested eliminating the division of localization-related and generalized epilepsies (Berg et al., 2010), and instead listing epilepsies by age of onset, distinctive constellations, or underlying cause (Box 100.3). The list incorporated newly identified or characterized epileptic conditions. In 2017 the ILAE published an updated classification of epilepsies (Scheffer et al., 2017). The classification had three levels: seizure types (from the classification of epileptic seizures), epilepsy types, and epilepsy syndromes (Fig. 100.6). Although achieving all three levels of classification is desirable, it is not feasible for all patients. In some instances, classification of the seizure type(s) may be the only level achieved, particularly where medical resources are limited. However, at every level of classification physicians are encouraged to consider/investigate the etiology of the epilepsy and address comorbidities. The epilepsy types maintained the two major categories of focal and generalized epilepsies, but also added a category of *combined generalized and focal* epilepsies to include patients who have both focal-onset and generalized-onset seizures. The list of etiology categories comprises structural, genetic, infectious, metabolic, immune, and unknown etiology, with the possibility that more than one category may apply for some epilepsies.

## Select Epilepsies, Epileptic Syndromes, and Related Disorders

An *epileptic syndrome* was defined as a complex of signs and symptoms that define a unique epilepsy condition with different etiologies. A syndrome must involve more than just a seizure type (Engel, 2006). One common important attribute of syndromes is a characteristic age at onset. Below are descriptions of select epileptic syndromes or constellations.

### Benign Familial Neonatal Epilepsy

Benign familial neonatal epilepsy was previously referred to as *benign familial neonatal convulsions* (Plouin and Anderson, 2005). This rare, dominantly inherited disorder is due to mutations affecting voltage-gated potassium channel genes (*KCNQ2, KCNQ3*) (Biervert and Steinlein, 1999). Affected infants are usually full term and appear normal at birth. In 80% of instances, seizures start on the second or third day of life, although some infants may develop seizures later in the first month of life. The seizures are typically clonic but often preceded by a tonic component. They are more often unilateral but can also be bilateral. The seizures remit within 2–6 months. There is a slight increase in the risk of later epilepsy (11%–15%).

### Early Myoclonic Encephalopathy and Ohtahara Syndrome

Early myoclonic encephalopathy and Ohtahara syndrome have much in common, including age at onset in the neonatal period, severe seizure manifestations, and an EEG pattern of burstsuppression, in which periods of high-voltage EEG activity are separated by periods of generalized attenuation (Aicardi and Ohtahara, 2005; Djukic et al., 2006; Ohtahara and Yamatogi, 2006).

Early myoclonic encephalopathy is characterized by focal myoclonus involving limbs or face that is very frequent, sometime continuous, shifting from one region to another. Generalized massive myoclonus may appear shortly thereafter, as will focal motor seizures. Epileptic spasms typically develop later in the course of the disorder. Neurological status is abnormal, either at birth or with the development of clinical seizures. Most infants are hypotonic. The prognosis is poor. There is increased mortality in the first few years of life, and survivors have considerable developmental delay.

Ohtahara syndrome is characterized by epileptic spasms as the predominant seizure type, but a third of affected infants also have other seizure types, including focal motor seizures, hemiconvulsions, and generalized motor seizures. The epileptic spasms are associated with generalized attenuation on EEG. The prognosis is also poor, with

**BOX 100.3 ILAE Classification of Status Epilepticus (SE) (Trinka et al., 2015)**

**(A) With Prominent Motor Symptoms**

- A.1 Convulsive SE (CSE, synonym: tonic–clonic SE)
  - A.1.a. Generalized convulsive
  - A.1.b. Focal onset evolving into bilateral convulsive SE
  - A.1.c. Unknown whether focal or generalized
- A.2 Myoclonic SE (prominent epileptic myoclonic jerks)
  - A.2.a. With coma
  - A.2.b. Without coma
- A.3 Focal motor
  - A.3.a. Repeated focal motor seizures (Jacksonian)
  - A.3.b. Epilepsia partialis continua (EPC)
  - A.3.c. Adversive status
  - A.3.d. Oculoclonic status
  - A.3.e. Ictal paresis (i.e., focal inhibitory SE)
- A.4 Tonic status
- A.5 Hyperkinetic SE

**(B) Without Prominent Motor Symptoms (i.e., Nonconvulsive SE, NCSE)**

- B.1 NCSE with coma (including so-called "subtle" SE)
- B.2 NCSE without coma
  - B.2.a. Generalized
    - B.2.a.a Typical absence status
    - B.2.a.b Atypical absence status
    - B.2.a.c Myoclonic absence status
  - B.2.b. Focal
    - B.2.b.a Without impairment of consciousness (aura continua, with autonomic, sensory, visual, olfactory, gustatory, emotional/psychic/experiential, or auditory symptoms)
    - B.2.b.b Aphasic status
    - B.2.b.c With impaired consciousness
  - B.2.c Unknown whether focal or generalized
    - B.2.c.a Autonomic SE

SE, Status epilepticus.

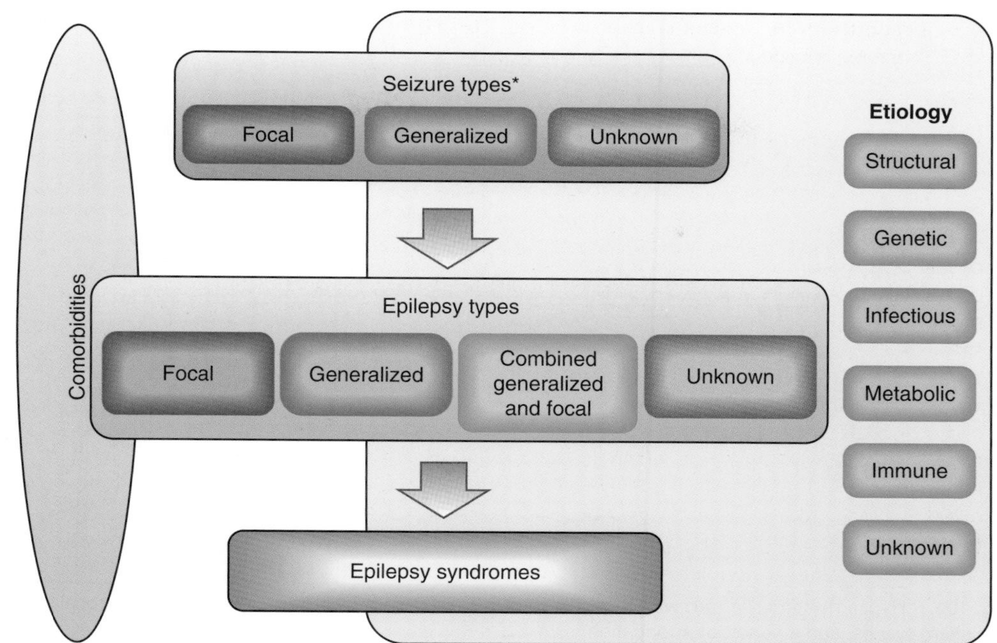


**Fig. 100.6** The International League Against Epilepsy (ILAE) 2017 Classification of the Epilepsies. *denotes onset of seizure.

very high mortality in the first few years of life, and severe mental and physical handicap in survivors. The EEG may evolve from the initial suppression-burst pattern to a hypsarrhythmia pattern, typical of West syndrome.

### West Syndrome

West syndrome has a later age at onset, with a peak onset between 3 and 7 months of age. It is characterized by a clinical triad of epileptic spasms, arrest or deterioration of psychomotor development, and a characteristic EEG pattern called *hypsarrhythmia* (Dulac and Tuxhorn, 2005). The disorder is heterogeneous in its etiology. Epileptic spasms are usually the initial manifestation. They tend to occur in clusters, sometimes multiple times a day. Approximately two-thirds of infants have brain lesions. Psychomotor development may be abnormal prior to onset, but there is a clear deterioration after onset. The spasms may have asymmetries, which are more likely when there is a focal brain lesion. The prognosis is variable, with a small proportion of patients recovering quickly without sequelae. This is more likely to happen in the absence of brain pathology. Otherwise, more than 70% develop intellectual disability and other cognitive disabilities. The treatment of infantile spasms has some important differences from treatment of other seizure types. Steroids such as corticotropin (adrenocorticotropic hormone [ACTH]) and prednisone are helpful, particularly in the absence of underlying known pathology.

Hypsarrhythmia is characterized by high-voltage disorganized EEG activity with slow waves and multifocal spikes and sharp waves punctuated by periods of generalized attenuation (Fig. 100.7). When a spasm occurs, it is usually during a period of attenuation. The attenuation may have superimposed high-frequency, low-voltage EEG activity. The periods of attenuation are typically very short in duration, lasting 1–2 seconds.

### Dravet Syndrome

Dravet syndrome, also called *severe myoclonic epilepsy of infancy*, is usually due to a de novo mutation affecting the *SCN1A* gene encoding the $\alpha_1$ sodium channel subunit (Claes et al., 2001). De novo mutations account for about 95% of cases. It may also be due to a nonsense mutation of the GABRG2 $\gamma$-aminobutyric acid A ($GABA_A$) receptor subunit (Huang et al., 2012). Dravet syndrome and related epileptic or developmental encephalopathies may be caused by a number of other genetic mutations (Steel et al., 2017). The typical clinical presentation is that a previously normally developing infant has febrile status epilepticus at around 6 months of age, and then recurrent generalized or shifting hemiclonic seizures are seen, often triggered by fever. After 1 year of age, other seizure types appear, including myoclonic seizures, absence seizures, and FIAS as well as atonic seizures at times. The seizures are drug resistant and may be exacerbated by some sodium channel blockers such as carbamazepine and lamotrigine. A delay or arrest in development may occur, and even regression may be seen, typically after episodes of prolonged seizure activity (Dravet et al., 2005; Scheffer et al., 2009). The prognosis is poor; the majority of individuals develop intellectual disability and at times ataxia and spasticity.

Borderline severe myoclonic epilepsy of infancy may include variations such as epilepsy with the absence of myoclonic seizures or even other seizure types.

It has now become recognized that Dravet syndrome accounts for a large proportion of individuals previously diagnosed with vaccine encephalopathy (Berkovic et al., 2006). The fever associated with vaccination may cause an earlier age at onset of Dravet syndrome, but it does not affect the eventual course of the condition (McIntosh et al., 2010).

### Genetic Epilepsy with Febrile Seizures Plus

Genetic epilepsy with febrile seizures plus (GEFS+) appears to be autosomal dominant in inheritance, often due to a sodium channel mutation, most often in the *SCN1A* or *SCN1B* gene (Escayg et al., 2001; Wallace et al., 2002). It can also be due to a mutation in the $\gamma_2$ subunit of the $GABA_A$ receptor (Harkin et al., 2002). No mutation has been identified in the majority of families. The condition has a heterogeneous phenotype in affected individuals, even within the same kindred (Scheffer and Berkovic, 1997; Singh et al., 1999; Fig. 100.8). Some individuals have only the typical febrile seizure phenotype, with

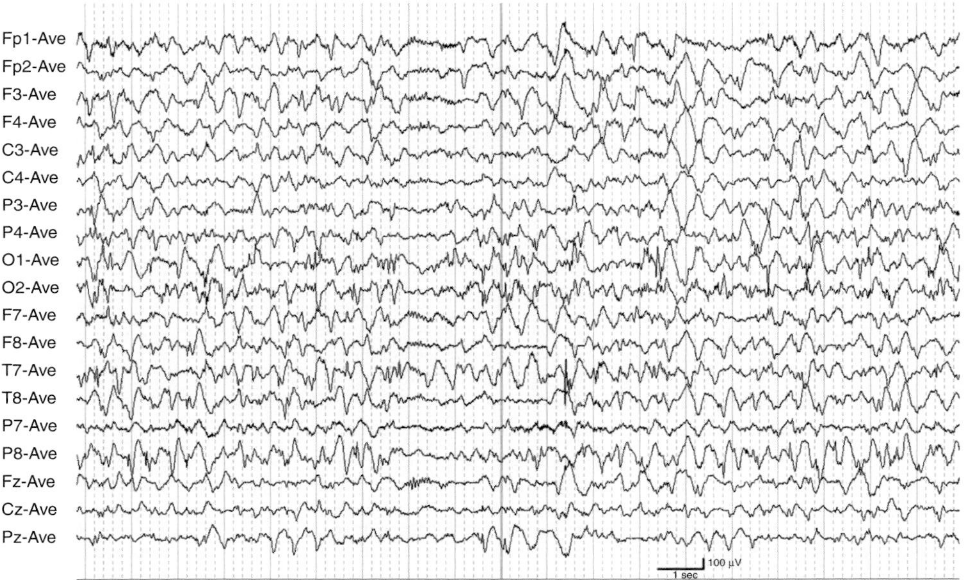


**Fig. 100.7** Hypsarrhythmia pattern with disorganized high-voltage slow background activity, multifocal spikes and sharp waves, and a period of attenuation.

febrile seizures disappearing by 6 years of age. Other individuals have *febrile seizures plus*, which refers to febrile seizures persisting beyond 6 years of age or febrile seizures intermixed with afebrile GTC seizures. Other individuals even have other seizure types such as generalized absence or myoclonic seizures. Less common seizure types are myoclonic-atonic and focal seizures typical of temporal lobe origin (Abou-Khalil et al., 2001; Scheffer et al., 2007).

### Panayiotopoulos Syndrome

The onset of seizures in Panayiotopoulos syndrome is typically between 1 and 14 years of age, with a peak at 4–5 years (Covanis et al., 2005). Seizures include autonomic manifestations, particularly ictal vomiting, altered responsiveness and arrest of activity, and deviation of the eyes to one side. Autonomic manifestations are particularly pronounced (Caraballo et al., 2007). Seizures can be very prolonged, lasting longer than 30 minutes, qualifying for focal nonconvulsive status epilepticus. Seizures predominate during sleep. The EEG shows multifocal spikes but with posterior predominance. Despite the alarming seizure manifestations, prognosis is generally good. Seizures are infrequent, with about a quarter of patients having only one seizure and half having two to five at most. Remission typically occurs within 1–3 years of onset.

### Epilepsy with Myoclonic-Atonic Seizures (Myoclonic-Astatic Epilepsy or Doose Syndrome)

This presumed genetic epilepsy is characterized by seizure onset between 18 and 60 months of age (Guerrini et al., 2005). The characteristic seizure types are myoclonic and myoclonic-atonic seizures, present in all affected children. Tonic-clonic seizures are also seen in a majority of children. Atypical absence seizures are also common and frequently associated with reduced muscle tone. Pure atonic seizures may also occur. Generalized tonic seizures are less frequently seen. GTC seizures are most often the seizure type that results in the diagnosis of epilepsy, with smaller seizures noticed thereafter. Seizures can be easily precipitated by inappropriate treatment with carbamazepine. The course of the condition is somewhat unpredictable. In more than half of affected children, the seizures go into remission. More than half of patients also have normal cognitive function, with less than half having mild to severe intellectual disability. A worse prognosis is predicted by GTC seizures in the first 2 years of life and early status epilepticus (Kelley and Kossoff, 2010).

### Self-Limited Epilepsy with Centrotemporal Spikes

Self-limited epilepsy with centrotemporal spikes, previously known as benign epilepsy with centrotemporal spikes (BECTS) is also referred to as *benign rolandic epilepsy*. This is the most common form of idiopathic focal epilepsy in children (Dalla Bernardina et al., 2005). Seizures begin between 3 and 13 years of age, with a peak between 5 and 8 years. Affected children will have had a normal development and normal cognitive function. Seizures typically start with paresthesias affecting one side of the face, particularly around the mouth, then contraction of that side of the face evolving into clonic activity of the face. Increased salivation and drooling occurs. Consciousness is preserved in the vast majority of children if the seizure does not evolve to bilateral tonic-clonic activity. Seizures are typically nocturnal and generally have a low rate of recurrence, so treatment is not always necessary. The natural history is characterized by spontaneous remission around the time of puberty. Patients with BECTS may have cognitive and behavioral problems while the condition is active, but long-term prognosis is excellent (Camfield and Camfield, 2014).

BECTS has long been thought to have a genetic basis, but the concordance in identical twins is low, suggesting that other mechanisms may play a role (Vadlamudi et al., 2004). The diagnosis of BECTS depends on the clinical presentation as well as the EEG. The typical EEG abnormality is high-voltage central-midtemporal blunt sharp waves activated in sleep (Fig. 100.9). These can become bilateral independent in deeper sleep. Atypical fields are common, particularly posterior temporal or parietal. The incidence of generalized spike-and-wave discharges in affected individuals is increased (Beydoun et al., 1992; Drury and Beydoun, 1991).

### Autosomal Dominant Nocturnal Frontal Lobe Epilepsy

Age at seizure onset in autosomal dominant nocturnal frontal lobe epilepsy is highly variable but is most often younger than age 20, with a mean between 8 and 11 years. Seizures typically arise out of sleep. In their most pronounced expression, they may be hypermotor with vigorous frenetic movements of the extremities such as thrashing, kicking,

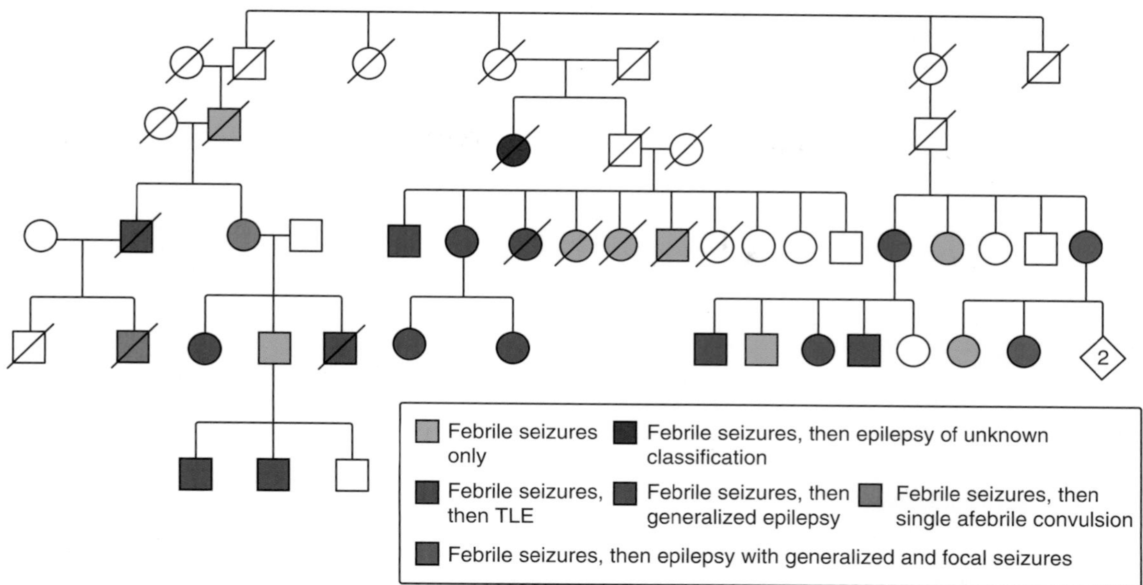


**Fig. 100.8** Pedigree of a family with autosomal dominant genetic epilepsy with febrile seizures plus, demonstrating phenotypic heterogeneity in affected individuals. *TLE,* Temporal lobe epilepsy.

or bicycling. The seizures may be asymmetrical tonic, sometimes with evolving posturing, or may have a mixture of hypermotor and tonic manifestations. The seizures are usually stereotyped. They are typically short in duration, lasting less than 30 seconds. They can be so short as to simply manifest with paroxysmal arousal (Provini et al., 1999). The condition is often misdiagnosed as a sleep disorder or psychogenic seizures (Scheffer et al., 1995).

This disorder is genetically heterogeneous (De Marco et al., 2007) but typically due to mutations in the neuronal nicotinic acetylcholine receptor (Steinlein et al., 1995). Carbamazepine appeared particularly effective in this condition. Interestingly, the mutated nicotinic receptors were found to be more sensitive to carbamazepine than to valproate (Picard et al., 1999).

## Late-Onset Childhood Occipital Epilepsy (Gastaut Type)

The age at onset of seizures in late-onset childhood occipital epilepsy ranges from 3 to 16 years, with a mean age of 8 (Covanis et al., 2005). The seizures are of occipital lobe onset and manifest with visual symptoms. The ictal phenomena include elementary visual hallucinations, complex visual hallucinations and illusions, visual loss in one field or total blindness, eye deviation, and eye blinking. There may be progression of seizure manifestations with spread beyond the occipital lobe, particularly lateralized or GTC activity. Consciousness is usually preserved if seizure activity does not spread beyond the occipital lobe. Postictal headache is a very common symptom, resulting in confusion with migraine. The interictal EEG is characterized by occipital spikes and sharp waves that can be extremely frequent, and typically activated with eye closure. The discharges can be so frequent as to raise concern for an ictal pattern.

## Epilepsy with Myoclonic Absences

Epilepsy with myoclonic absences is a syndrome with male predominance and starts between 1 and 12 years of age, with a mean of 7 years (Bureau and Tassinari, 2005a). Its most distinctive seizure type is myoclonic absences. These seizures include impairment of consciousness of variable degree and very prominent myoclonus involving primarily the upper extremities but also the legs. The duration varies from 10 to 60 seconds, and seizures typically recur several times a day. The associated EEG usually shows 3-Hz generalized rhythmic spike-and-wave activity similar to what is seen in typical absence seizures. Approximately two-thirds of patients also have other seizure types, particularly GTC seizures. Seizures tend to be resistant to monotherapy and often require dual therapy with valproate and ethosuximide or one of these agents in combination with lamotrigine.

Myoclonic absences tend to disappear over time, but GTC seizures may persist. Patients may have intellectual disability preceding the onset of the seizures, and some may show decline over time, particularly those with GTC seizures.

## Lennox-Gastaut Syndrome

Lennox-Gastaut syndrome is defined by a triad of several seizure types including generalized tonic, generalized atonic, and atypical absence seizures, a characteristic interictal EEG abnormality of generalized slow spike-and-wave discharges (<2.5 Hz) in waking and bursts of paroxysmal fast activity (≈10 Hz) in sleep (Fig. 100.10), and cognitive dysfunction (Arzimanoglou et al., 2009; Beaumanoir and Blume, 2005). Drop attacks due to either generalized atonic or generalized tonic seizures tend to be the most debilitating seizure type because of associated injuries. The age of onset is between 3 and 10 years, with a peak between 3 and 5 years. Lennox-Gastaut syndrome may start de novo or may evolve, for example from West syndrome. Seizures tend to be drug resistant. Lennox-Gastaut syndrome tends to be a chronic disorder even though epilepsy may become less active over time. Almost half of these patients may appear normal before onset of seizures, but deterioration occurs, and the cause is probably multifactorial.

## Epileptic Encephalopathy with Continuous Spike-and-Wave during Sleep and Landau-Kleffner Syndrome

The common features of the related conditions of epileptic encephalopathy with continuous spike-and-wave during sleep (CSWS) and Landau-Kleffner syndrome (LKS) are a decline in cognitive function in association with an EEG pattern of continuous spike-and-wave activity during slow-wave sleep (Fig. 100.11). In both conditions the associated seizures are often easy to control, and the predominant clinical manifestations are related to the EEG abnormality in sleep (Nickels and Wirrell, 2008; Tassinari et al., 2005).

In the case of LKS, the cognitive decline is specifically in the area of speech. The condition is often called acquired epileptic aphasia. This

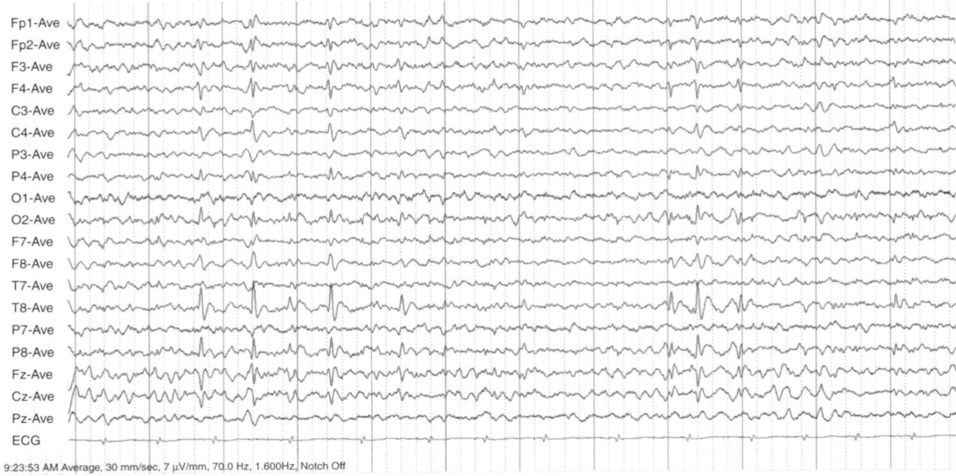


**Fig. 100.9** Characteristic sleep electroencephalographic recording in patient with benign epilepsy with centrotemporal spikes, demonstrating frequent negative right midtemporal sharp waves (at *T8*) with field extending to right posterior temporal *(P8)* and right central *(C4)* regions. Note simultaneous positivity in bifrontal regions.

disorder typically appears between 2 and 8 years of age, with a peak between 5 and 7 years. The most common initial manifestation is verbal auditory agnosia. The language disturbance will usually progress despite good control of clinical seizures. In fact, clinical seizures may not even occur in about a quarter of patients. The evolution is variable. Spontaneous remissions may occur within the first year. Classical ASMs may be ineffective. Benefits have been reported with valproate, levetiracetam, and benzodiazepines, which reduce the EEG abnormality. Steroids and immunoglobulins have been reported to be helpful. Surgical treatment with multiple subpial transections (MSTs) has been advocated (Morrell et al., 1995).

CSWS differs from LKS in that a larger proportion of individuals have pre-existing neurological abnormalities, and the cognitive regression is more likely to be global and associated with motor impairments.

### Childhood Absence Epilepsy

CAE syndrome, previously referred to as *petit mal* or *pyknolepsy*, typically starts between the ages of 4 and 10 years with a peak between 5 and 7 years (Hirsch and Panayiotopoulos, 2005). Affected children are normal in their development and neurological status. The key seizure type is generalized typical absence seizures occurring many times a day. In association with seizures, the EEG shows generalized synchronous and symmetrical spike-and-wave activity with a frequency around 3 Hz. It is not unusual for the spike-and-wave frequency to be initially faster (up to 4 Hz) and drop by approximately 0.5–1 Hz by the end of the ictal discharge. Seizure duration is brief, usually less than 15 seconds. Seizure frequency is very high, with multiple daily seizures. In 2005 the ILAE proposed strict criteria to define the syndrome, which include the absence of GTC or myoclonic seizures prior to or during the active stage of absence seizures. The criteria also exclude eyelid and perioral myoclonia, high-amplitude rhythmic jerking of the limbs, and arrhythmic jerks of the head, trunk, or limbs (Hirsch and Panayiotopoulos, 2005). With this strict definition of the syndrome, many patients with a predominance of absence seizures are excluded and cannot be classified as having CAE (Ma et al., 2011; Valentin et al., 2007), but a very favorable prognosis is expected. Only 8% of patients fulfilling the strict criteria had GTC seizures, compared to 30% of those who did not (Grosso et al., 2005), and 65% of those satisfying the stricter criteria had a complete seizure remission, compared to 23% of those who did not. Persistence or relapse of seizures tends to be predominately related to GTC seizures. In some instances, CAE evolves into juvenile myoclonic epilepsy (JME) in the second decade. This will be discussed later under that heading.

CAE is thought to be genetically determined, with high concordance for monozygotic twins (Berkovic et al., 1998). However, the exact mode of inheritance is unknown. Although some families had a single gene mutation (including $GABA_A$ receptor and calcium channel mutations), most are thought to have polygenic inheritance (Hughes, 2009; Wallace et al., 2001).

For children with pure absence seizures, ethosuximide is the treatment of choice (Glauser et al., 2010). Coexistence of other seizure types requires a broader-spectrum ASM. Absence seizures beginning before 4 years of age could be due to glucose transporter 1 (GLUT1) deficiency in 12% of patients (Arsov et al., 2012). This condition responds well to the ketogenic diet.

### Juvenile Absence Epilepsy

Juvenile absence epilepsy is very similar to CAE except that the age at onset is in the second decade, with a peak between ages 10 and 12 (Wolf and Inoue, 2005). The absence seizures are not as frequent as in CAE. In addition, the majority of patients also have GTC seizures. This condition has a greater tendency for persistence of seizures into adulthood than is the case with CAE.

### Juvenile Myoclonic Epilepsy

Juvenile myoclonic epilepsy (JME), also known as *juvenile myoclonic epilepsy of Janz* or *impulsive petit mal*, is common (Thomas et al., 2005) and accounts for up to 10% of all cases of epilepsy. The age at onset is typically between 12 and 18, but epilepsy may start in the first decade in a subgroup of patients who appear to have CAE early on. The defining seizure type is generalized myoclonic seizures, which occur in all patients by definition. Generalized myoclonic seizures typically occur after awakening, particularly with sleep deprivation. They are typically mild, predominately affecting the upper extremities. Although they are the first seizure type to appear, they are often not recognized as seizures and not brought to medical attention. Patients typically come to medical attention after a GTC seizure, which is most likely to occur after sleep deprivation or binge drinking of alcohol. The physician has to ask about myoclonus in order to make the diagnosis. Approximately one-third of patients also have generalized absence seizures. JME is clinically and genetically heterogeneous (Martinez-Juarez et al., 2006).

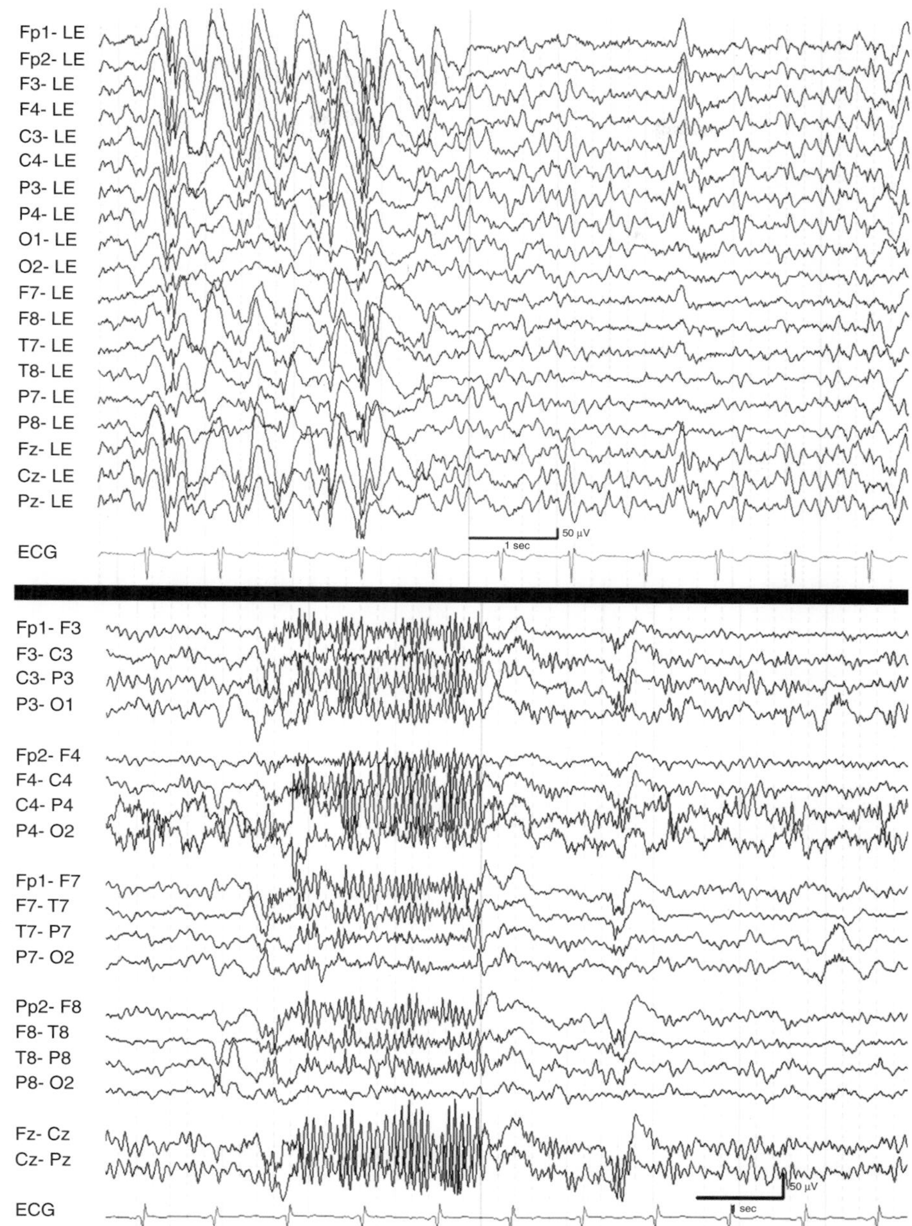


**Fig. 100.10** Typical electroencephalographic findings in Lennox-Gastaut syndrome, with slow spike-and-wave activity in waking *(top)* and paroxysmal fast activity in sleep *(bottom)*.

The most important group is classic JME, and the second largest is CAE evolving to JME. The latter tends to be more treatment resistant.

The diagnosis of JME is based on the clinical history and EEG, which shows generalized irregular 4- to 6-Hz spike-and-wave activity occurring in bursts. The EEG is most likely to record discharges after awakening (Labate et al., 2007). JME is predominantly a lifelong condition, with less than 25% of patients seizure free off medication in long-term follow-up (Camfield and Camfield, 2009; Geithner et al., 2012; Senf et al., 2013). However, the majority of patients can have seizure remission with medication therapy. The prognosis for seizure freedom is lowest in individuals with CAE leading to JME and in individuals who have all three seizure types: generalized myoclonic, GTC, and generalized absence seizures (Gelisse et al., 2001; Martinez-Juarez et al., 2006). Valproate appears to be the most effective medication for all three seizure types, but its teratogenicity and some adverse effects limit its use in women of childbearing age (Montouris and Abou-Khalil, 2009). Seizures may be aggravated by several ASMs that are specific for focal epilepsy (Gelisse et al., 2004; Genton et al., 2000).

JME is thought to have predominantly polygenic inheritance. It is genetically heterogeneous. There have also been some families with autosomal dominant inheritance and several identified mutations (Delgado-Escueta et al., 2013), including a mutation of the $GABA_A$ receptor (Cossette et al., 2002).

### Epilepsy with Generalized Tonic-Clonic Seizures Alone

Epilepsy with GTC seizures alone includes so-called epilepsy with grand mal on awakening as well as epilepsy with GTC seizures that are random in timing. Although the onset is in the second decade in the

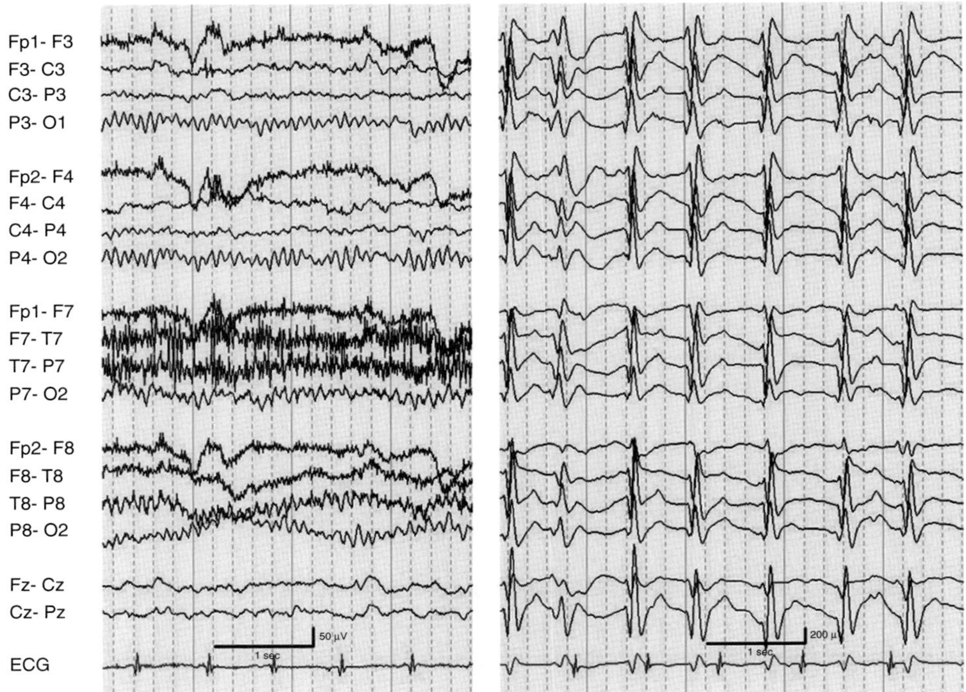


**Fig. 100.11** Electroencephalogram in patient with epileptic encephalopathy with continuous spike-and-wave during sleep with normal background in waking *(left)* and continuous spike-and-wave activity in deep sleep *(right)*.

majority of individuals, there is a very wide range. As noted with other IGE syndromes, sleep deprivation is a frequent precipitant. Seizures generally respond well to treatment, similarly to what has been noted with JME.

## Autosomal Dominant Epilepsy with Auditory Features

Autosomal dominant epilepsy with auditory features (ADEAF) is usually related to a mutation in the leucine-rich glioma-inactivated-1 (*LGI1*) gene (Ottman et al., 2004), but may also be caused by reelin mutations (Michelucci et al., 2017). Inheritance, as the name indicates, is autosomal dominant. Seizures typically begin in adolescence or adulthood, with a mean age at onset of 24. Affected subjects commonly report an elementary auditory aura such as buzzing, ringing, humming, or even loss of hearing. Seizures may start with aphasic manifestations when the onset is in the dominant lateral temporal lobe (Gu et al., 2002).

## Familial Mesial Temporal Lobe Epilepsy

Familial MTLE is a heterogeneous condition. There is a benign syndrome, first identified in twins, in which the most prominent aura is déjà vu with frequent FAS, infrequent FIAS, and rare FBTCS (Berkovic et al., 1996; Perucca et al., 2017). Prior febrile seizures are uncommon, and magnetic resonance imaging (MRI) is normal with no hippocampal sclerosis. The epilepsy is frequently not recognized when the only seizure type is subjective FAS, but when recognized is very responsive to medical therapy.

Other familial MTLE may be associated with prior febrile convulsions, hippocampal sclerosis on MRI, and less responsiveness to medical therapy, at times requiring surgical treatment (Cendes et al., 1998).

Familial MTLE is most probably polygenic in inheritance for most families, even though there are reports of autosomal dominant inheritance (Chahine et al., 2013; Crompton et al., 2010; Hedera et al., 2007). No gene mutation has yet been identified.

## Mesial Temporal Lobe Epilepsy with Hippocampal Sclerosis

MTLE with hippocampal sclerosis is one of the most common epilepsies in epilepsy referral centers. Mesial temporal or hippocampal sclerosis is the most common pathology noted in surgical specimens from patients undergoing temporal lobectomy for drug-resistant temporal lobe seizures. It is characterized by neuronal loss and gliosis predominately affecting CA1 and CA3 sectors of the hippocampus, with relative sparing of CA2. Patients with MTLE and hippocampal sclerosis frequently have a history of antecedent febrile seizures (up to 80%) (French et al., 1993). The febrile seizures are usually complex, in particular prolonged. Even though febrile status epilepticus is known to injure the hippocampus in some instances, it is not clear that this is the only factor at play (VanLandingham et al., 1998). Some studies have shown evidence of prior hippocampal malformation that may predispose to injury (Fernandez et al., 1998; Park et al., 2010a). In addition, hippocampal sclerosis has been reported in familial MTLE without prior febrile seizures (Kobayashi et al., 2003). The age at onset of habitual afebrile seizures is variable but most commonly is in late childhood or adolescence. The presence of hippocampal sclerosis predicts poor response to medical therapy (Semah et al., 1998). However, the exact percentage of individuals who are drug resistant has varied between studies. It is not unusual for seizures to be drug responsive initially, with long remissions but later evolution to drug resistance (Berg et al., 2006).

The seizure pattern has already been described. The clinical seizure characteristics cannot reliably distinguish MTLE due to hippocampal sclerosis from that due to lesions (Wieser, 2004).

The hippocampal sclerosis is usually identified on MRI showing decreased volume and increased signal in the affected hippocampus (Fig. 100.12). Positron emission tomography (PET) usually shows temporal hypometabolism that is predominant in the mesial temporal region on the affected side (Fig. 100.13).

Neuropsychological evaluation commonly demonstrates memory dysfunction which may be material specific, with greater involvement of verbal memory when the left hemisphere is involved or visual-spatial memory when the right hemisphere is involved. Memory impairment tends to be greater with longer duration of uncontrolled seizures, suggesting evidence of progression.

While drug resistance is common, the response rate for surgical therapy is excellent. After temporal lobectomy or selective amygdalohippocampectomy, 60%–80% of individuals are seizure free (Wieser, 2004).

### Rasmussen Syndrome

Rasmussen syndrome is a chronic progressive disorder of unknown etiology, and probably heterogeneous (Hart and Andermann, 2005). Seizures most commonly start between 1 and 14 years of age with focal-onset motor seizures. The seizures can remain focal aware or evolve to focal impaired awareness or FBTCS. Seizures usually start in the same hemisphere. They become progressively more frequent with episodes of status epilepticus. Progressive hemiparesis and other deficits occur, depending on the affected hemisphere. General intellectual decline occurs at the time of hemiparesis. Imaging shows progressive hemiatrophy, with lesser atrophy on the other side (Fig. 100.14). An abnormal increased T2 signal is initially most pronounced in the perisylvian region. PET reveals marked decreased metabolism in the affected hemisphere.

An autoimmune etiology is suspected. In some patients, antibodies to the GluR3 subunit of the glutamate receptor have been identified (Rogers et al., 1994). Some benefit may occur with intravenous immunoglobulin (IVIG), plasmapheresis, and corticosteroids, but hemispherectomy is generally required to achieve seizure control.

### Progressive Myoclonus Epilepsies

Progressive myoclonus epilepsies (PME) are a heterogeneous group of genetic disorders characterized by myoclonus, GTC seizures, and progressive neurological dysfunction, predominately with cerebellar ataxia and often with dementia (Genton et al., 2005). Included in the group are Unverricht-Lundborg disease, Lafora body disease, mitochondrial encephalopathy with ragged red fibers, and ceroid lipofuscinosis, among others. Unverricht-Lundborg disease was also called *Baltic myoclonus*, but it is recognized now as a worldwide condition. It is due to a mutation in the *cystatin B* gene (Genton, 2010). The onset is typically between 7 and 16 years of age, initially with action myoclonus, then later development of tonic-clonic or clonic-tonic-clonic seizures. The myoclonus worsens progressively and greatly limits motor function. Ataxia occurs and is generally mild, but it can be very aggravated by the use of phenytoin. Phenytoin can also cause mild dementia.

Lafora disease typically starts between 6 and 19 years of age. Initial seizures are GTC or myoclonic, but affected individuals may also have focal aware visual seizures. The condition progresses with increasingly severe myoclonus, ataxia, and dementia. Death typically occurs 2–10 years after onset of symptoms. The condition is caused by loss-of-function mutations in *EPM2A* or *NHLRC1*, which encode laforin and malin, resulting in accumulation of abnormal glycogen in Lafora bodies (Nitschke et al., 2018). The diagnosis can also be made by detection of Lafora bodies in skin biopsies.

Myoclonic epilepsy with ragged red fibers (MERRF) has a variable age at onset. In addition to myoclonus, GTC seizures, and ataxia, there may be signs to suggest mitochondrial disease, such as deafness, myopathy, optic atrophy, or lipomas. More than one mitochondrial mutation causes MERRF. It could be diagnosed with muscle biopsy showing typical ragged red fibers. The condition can also be diagnosed with genetic testing from skin or muscle.

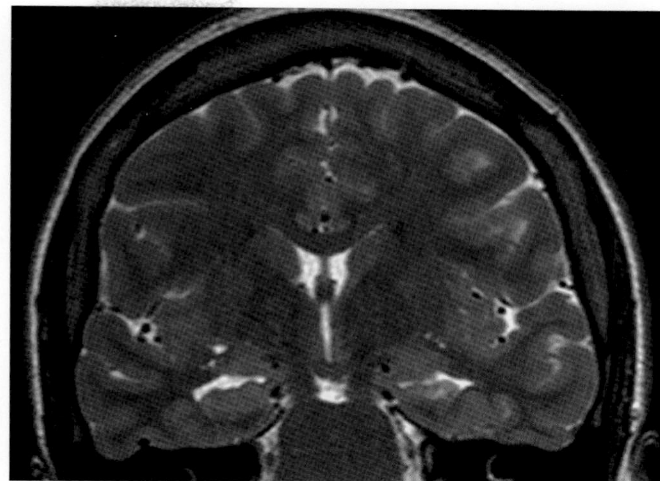

**Fig. 100.12** Left hippocampal sclerosis identified on magnetic resonance imaging T2-weighted oblique coronal image. Note hippocampal asymmetry, with relatively decreased volume and increased T2 signal in affected left hippocampus.

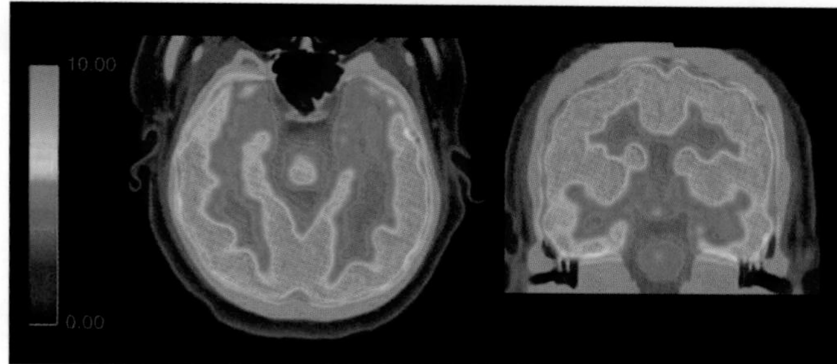


**Fig. 100.13** Fluorodeoxyglucose positron emission tomography co-registered with computed tomography, demonstrating left temporal hypometabolism predominant in mesial temporal region. Patient had left hippocampal sclerosis.

Treatment for progressive myoclonic epilepsy remains symptomatic at this time. Seizures are often resistant to medical therapy. Valproate is considered the drug of choice for most patients, but other broad-spectrum seizure medications have a role. In particular, there is anecdotal evidence of perampanel being particularly effective against myoclonus and GTC seizures in some patients (Ferlazzo et al., 2017).

### Gelastic Seizures with Hypothalamic Hamartoma

Gelastic seizures with hypothalamic hamartoma typically starts with gelastic seizures in early life, with other seizures also becoming associated later on (Berkovic et al., 2003). There may be cognitive and behavioral disturbances. Some individuals have precocious puberty and a short stature. MRI reveals a hypothalamic hamartoma that can vary in size and appearance (Fig. 100.15). Seizures originate within the hamartoma.

### Febrile Seizures

Febrile seizures are not traditionally diagnosed as a form of epilepsy per se, even though the condition is characterized by epileptic seizures (Berg et al., 2010). The condition affects 2%–5% of children, mostly between 3 months and 6 years of age. It is the most common form of seizure in children (Knudsen, 2000) and a benign disorder in the vast majority of those affected. Most febrile seizures are GTC in semiology. They are typically symmetrical, last less than 15 minutes, and usually only one seizure occurs in association with a particular illness. Febrile

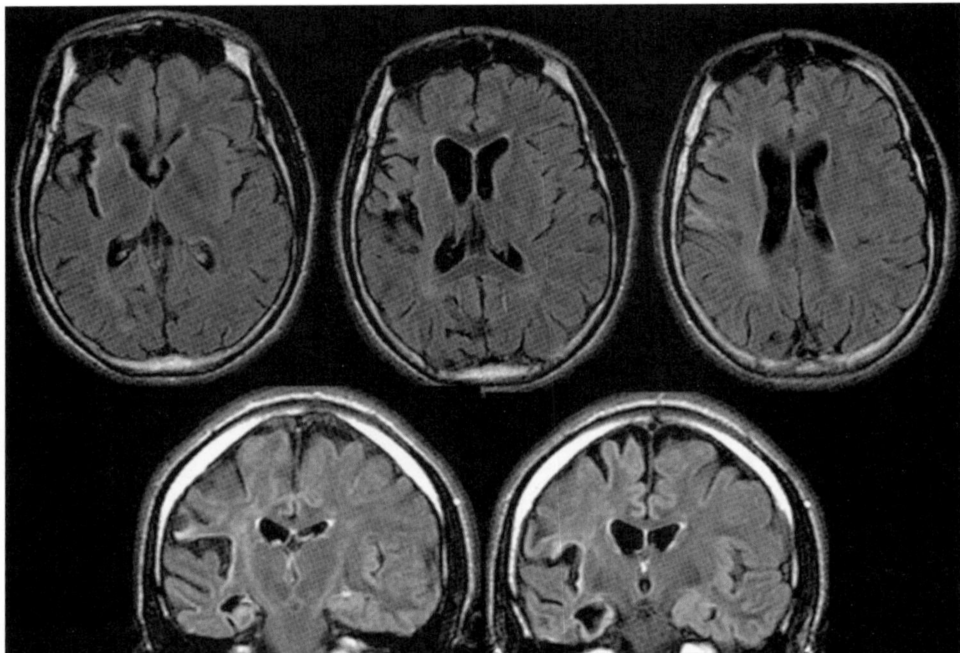

**Fig. 100.14** Rasmussen encephalitis in an 18-year-old man with left focal motor seizures since age 3 and progressive left hemiparesis. Fluid-attenuated inversion recovery magnetic resonance imaging (FLAIR MRI) shows right hemisphere atrophy with widening of sulci and ventricular enlargement. Atrophy is very pronounced in the right hippocampus. There is also increased T2 signal on the right most pronounced in the right insular region.

seizures that satisfy the above criteria are called *simple febrile seizures*. *Complex febrile seizures* are defined by one or more of the following three criteria: prolonged duration of greater than 15 minutes, focal features (either focal ictal features or lateralized postictal weakness), or the occurrence of more than one seizure in 24 hours or with the same febrile illness. Most affected children will not have a recurrence of a febrile seizure in their lifetime. Approximately 30%–40% will have at least one recurrence, but multiple recurrences are infrequent. Predictors of recurrence are early age at onset (<1 year), the presence of epilepsy or febrile seizures in first-degree relatives, and attendance at daycare, which increases the risk of febrile infectious illnesses.

Even though febrile seizures are a benign condition and the vast majority of affected children never develop afebrile seizures, they do increase the risk of later epilepsy. In one important study, the risk of later epilepsy was 7% by age 25 years (Annegers et al., 1987). In another study of children seen in the emergency room for their first febrile seizure, the risk of afebrile seizures was 6% at 2 years (Berg and Shinnar, 1996). The factors that predict later epilepsy include preexisting neurodevelopmental abnormalities, complex features (prolonged duration, focal features, and multiple occurrences per day), a family history of epilepsy, and recurrent febrile seizures. The presence of one complex feature increases the risk to 6%–8%, two complex features, 17%–22%, and all three complex features, 49% (Annegers et al., 1987). Complex features tend to predict an increased risk of focal epilepsy, while a large number of febrile seizures and a positive family history of epilepsy increase the risk of later generalized epilepsy. Febrile seizures may be prolonged to qualify for the definition of febrile status epilepticus. Febrile status epilepticus may injure the hippocampus (VanLandingham et al., 1998), with unilateral increased hippocampal T2 signal on MRI in about 11.5% of affected children (Shinnar et al., 2012). This acute MRI finding is frequently followed by development of hippocampal sclerosis on follow-up imaging (Lewis et al., 2014). Another 10.5% of children with febrile status epilepticus had a hippocampal malformation, most commonly hippocampal malrotation, suggesting that this congenital malformation may have predisposed them to febrile status epilepticus (Shinnar et al., 2012). It is not yet known if these radiological findings are associated with development of temporal lobe epilepsy.

Evidence exists that febrile seizures have a strong genetic influence. The inheritance is most probably polygenic in the majority of children, but several reports indicate clear autosomal dominant transmission in some families. Several mutations have been described, some in families with pure febrile seizures and others in families with both febrile seizures and epilepsy.

Some genetic epilepsy syndromes are known to start with febrile seizures. One of these is Dravet syndrome or severe myoclonic epilepsy of infancy (see earlier discussion). The febrile seizures in this condition tend to be prolonged and often asymmetrical. Fever appears to be a trigger for seizures, but the subsequent course of the condition is progressive, with afebrile seizures and neurological decline eventually developing. Dravet syndrome is usually due to a truncating mutation in the *SCN1A* sodium channel or *GABRG2* $GABA_A$ receptor subunit gene. GEFS+ is an autosomal dominant syndrome with heterogeneous clinical expression. Some individuals have the typical febrile convulsion syndrome with some febrile seizures that disappear by age 6 years, while others have febrile seizures persisting beyond age 6 or occurring in conjunction with other seizure types (see Fig. 100.8).

Single febrile seizures are more likely to be polygenic, whereas families with single-gene inheritance are more likely to include recurrent febrile seizures. Digenic inheritance has been described (Baulac et al., 2001); affected individuals had two mutations, and those unaffected had either one or no mutation.

Since most febrile seizures are benign, there is usually no need to treat affected patients with prophylactic daily medication. Intermittent medication may be given at the time of fever. For example, diazepam may be given orally or rectally in patients with frequent recurrent

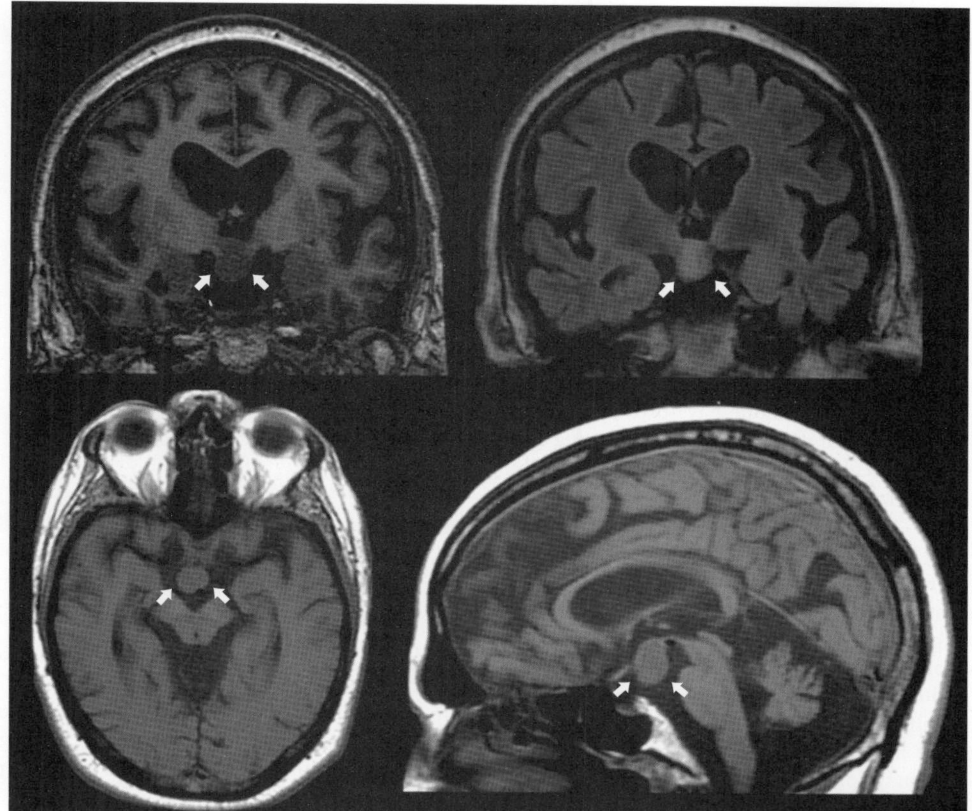

**Fig. 100.15** Hypothalamic hamartoma (see *arrows*) in a subject with gelastic seizures and short stature. *Left to right, top row,* T1-weighted coronal, fluid-attenuated inversion recovery (FLAIR) coronal; *bottom row,* T1-weighted axial, T1-weighted sagittal section. There is also cerebral atrophy with widened sulci and ex-vacuo ventricular enlargement.

febrile seizures. Rectal diazepam can be administered for prolonged febrile seizures (Knudsen, 2000).

## Causes and Risk Factors

Seizures and epilepsy can result from inherited or acquired factors or a combination of both. Several genetic epilepsy syndromes were described earlier. The following discussion will focus on acquired causes and risk factors, which vary considerably depending on age.

In children, developmental brain malformations are an important cause of epilepsy. These can be generalized, hemispheric, or focal. They are also classified as related to abnormal cell proliferation or differentiation, including tuberous sclerosis, focal cortical dysplasia, and hemimegalencephaly; as related to abnormal neuronal migration, including lissencephaly, subcortical band heterotopias, and periventricular nodular heterotopias; and as related to abnormal cortical organization, including polymicrogyria and schizencephaly. Some of these malformations are genetically determined—for example, tuberous sclerosis, lissencephaly, subcortical band heterotopia, and bilateral periventricular nodular heterotopia. Many of these malformations have other associated neurological disorders or physical findings, and most are easily diagnosed on MRI. Focal malformations associated with epilepsy are less likely to have other neurological manifestations than hemispheric or generalized malformations. The severity of epilepsy and its response to therapy can be quite variable, but it is commonly drug-resistant, prompting evaluation for surgical treatment.

Risk factors for epilepsy in early life include neonatal seizures and febrile seizures, both of which are conditions not considered forms of epilepsy. However, it is difficult to consider these risk factors as causes of later epilepsy.

Infections are an important risk factor for epilepsy. The risk of later epilepsy is higher for both meningitis and encephalitis if seizures occur during the acute illness. The relative risk of later epilepsy was increased 16-fold after encephalitis and 4-fold after bacterial meningitis (Annegers et al., 1988). The risk of later epilepsy was greatest with infection prior to age 5. Early occurrence of meningitis or encephalitis prior to age 4 predicted mesial temporal localization with hippocampal sclerosis, and better outcome with temporal lobectomy (O'Brien et al., 2002).

### Head Trauma

Head trauma is an important risk factor for epilepsy, with the greatest risk seen in association with penetrating head injury, head injury with depressed skull fracture, and severe head trauma with prolonged loss of consciousness. In a landmark study, *mild traumatic brain injury* (characterized by absence of fracture and a loss of consciousness or post-traumatic amnesia for <30 minutes) was associated with only a 1.5-fold increase in risk of epilepsy, which was not statistically significant (Annegers et al., 1998). Patients with *moderate head injury*, defined as loss of consciousness or post-traumatic amnesia for 30 minutes to 24 hours or a skull fracture, had a 2.9-fold increase in risk, while those with *severe head injury*, including brain contusion or intracranial hematoma or loss of consciousness or post-traumatic amnesia for more than 24 hours, had a 17-fold increased risk. The risk was highest in the first year after the injury but remained increased thereafter for a duration that varied with severity of the injury. For those with moderate brain injuries, the risk was markedly increased for up to 10 years only; for those with severe traumatic brain injury, the risk continued to be increased. The Vietnam Head Injury Study (VHIS), in which 92% of subjects had penetrating head injuries, found a 53% prevalence of post-traumatic epilepsy approximately 15 years after the injury. The risk was 580 times higher than that of the general age-matched population in the first year after injury, and it was still 25 times higher after 10 years (Salazar et al., 1985). A follow-up study in a subgroup of the original patients found that 12.6% of individuals who had post-traumatic epilepsy developed epilepsy more than 15 years after the injury (Raymont et al., 2010). Early seizures appeared to be a strong risk factor for late seizures, but early seizures were usually related to the severity of the head injury and intracranial lesions.

Changes in the brain reflecting the process of epileptogenesis are likely in the latent period between the head injury and onset of chronic epilepsy. Among several therapeutic measures tested for efficacy in preventing epilepsy after head injury, none have proven effective (Temkin, 2009). However, phenytoin was effective in preventing seizures in the first week (Temkin et al., 1990). Levetiracetam was equally effective in preventing early seizures (Inaba et al., 2013).

## Vascular Malformations

The two vascular malformations most commonly associated with epilepsy are arteriovenous malformations (AVMs) and cavernous malformations. Venous malformations, also called *venous anomalies*, may be accidental findings not directly related to epilepsy unless associated with a cavernous malformation. *Arteriovenous malformations* are high-pressure vascular malformations with arteriovenous shunting. They are a tangle of feeding arteries and draining veins without intervening capillary bed. They may come to attention during evaluation for seizures or after they bleed; they may also be incidental when imaging is performed for unrelated reasons. Because of the high pressure, they are susceptible to bleed at a rate of 1%–3% per year, which is the main reason they require therapy. Surgical treatment is effective, with one series reporting 94% of patients seizure free, most on no ASMs (Piepgras et al., 1993). Patients with small AVMs were more likely to present with hemorrhage, whereas those with large AVMs were more likely to present with seizures. The best seizure outcome was seen with resection of small AVMs. Endovascular treatment with embolization and radiosurgery can also improve seizure control, though to a lesser extent. Stereotactic radiosurgery rendered more than 50% of patients seizure free and was more likely to be successful when the preoperative seizure frequency was low and the AVM was small (Schauble et al., 2004).

*Cavernous malformations* consist of blood-filled epithelium-lined caverns with no discrete arteries or veins (Kraemer and Awad, 1994). On MRI they have a characteristic "popcorn" appearance with mixed signal within the lesion and a rim of decreased signal, reflecting hemosiderin (Fig. 100.16). They may be multiple in approximately a third of cases. Cavernous malformations are low-pressure lesions with a much smaller risk of bleeding than AVMs. They are strongly associated with epilepsy. If seizures are controlled with medical therapy, there is no clear indication for surgical resection. However, when epilepsy is drug resistant, resection of the cavernous malformation is associated with excellent results, provided the hemosiderin-stained brain tissue surrounding it is removed (Awad and Jabbour, 2006). Intraoperative monitoring with electrocorticography can also improve surgical outcome (Van Gompel et al., 2009). Excellent results were also reported with stereotactic laser ablation, which may be an alternative to open surgery (Willie et al., 2019).

Anterior temporal encephaloceles are emerging as an underrecognized etiology of temporal lobe epilepsy with important therapeutic implications. They are usually in the floor or anterior aspect of the middle cranial fossa, most often medially. They are easily overlooked on MRI imaging, and have to be specifically looked for in patients with presumed nonlesional temporal lobe epilepsy. Their diagnosis may be supported by identification of a defect in the floor of the anterior middle cranial fossa on three dimensional CT images. When confirmed as etiology of drug-resistant temporal lobe epilepsy, an excellent postsurgical outcome can be predicted. There is evidence that a limited inferior temporal pole resection sparing the hippocxampus may be sufficient for excellent outcome (Tse et al 2020).

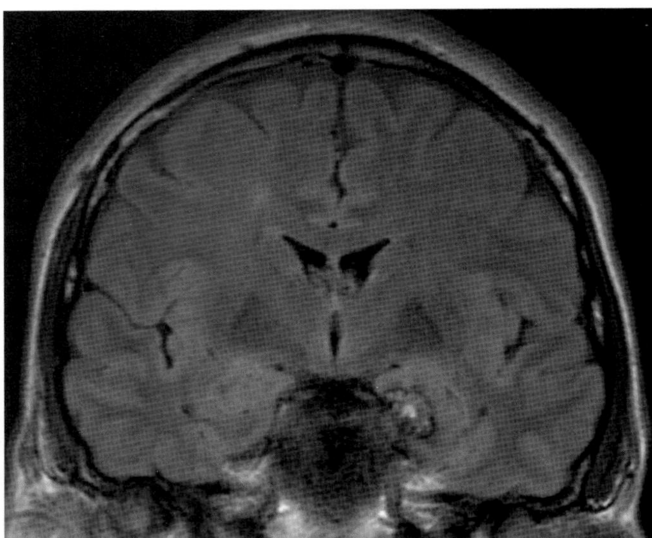

**Fig. 100.16** Left Mesial Temporal Cavernous Malformation.

## Brain Tumors

Brain tumors are a common cause of epilepsy, particularly drug-resistant epilepsy. Most drug-resistant epilepsy occurs with low-grade tumors, especially those in the temporal lobe (Rajneesh and Binder, 2009). Low-grade tumors associated with epilepsy are gangliogliomas, dysembryoplastic neuroepithelial tumors (DNETs), and low-grade gliomas. Excellent seizure control most often occurs after removal of gangliogliomas and DNETs. As expected, incomplete resection is associated with less likelihood of seizure control.

Seizures contribute to the morbidity of malignant brain tumors in approximately a quarter of patients. Grade 3 anaplastic astrocytomas are more likely to present with seizures at onset than glioblastoma multiforme (Moots et al., 1995).

## Parasitic Infections

Neurocysticercosis is thought to be the leading cause of acquired epilepsy in adulthood in the developing world, but it is an uncommon cause of epilepsy in developed countries. Seizures are thought to occur in 70%–90% of patients (Pal et al., 2000). Seizures in most patients can be controlled with ASMs. When epilepsy is drug resistant, patients with living cysticerci in the brain can benefit from albendazole, an antiparasitic treatment, in combination with dexamethasone (Garcia et al., 2004).

Other parasitic infections are also common causes of seizures and epilepsy in the developing world, particularly cerebral malaria with *Plasmodium falciparum*.

## Stroke

Stroke increases the risk of seizures and epilepsy at any age, but it is the most common cause of seizures in the elderly (Menon and

Shorvon, 2009). As in post-traumatic seizures, early seizures that occur within 2 weeks of the stroke most often do not progress to chronic epilepsy, but they do increase the risk of chronic epilepsy. As with head trauma, the risk of chronic epilepsy is highest in the first year after stroke, with a 17-fold increase in the risk compared to population in the community. Approximately 30% of individuals who have early post-stroke seizures develop later epilepsy. This is a 16-fold increase in risk compared to individuals who did not have early seizures. Seizures and even status epilepticus can be a presenting symptom of acute stroke.

As expected, strokes involving the cortex are more likely to produce epilepsy than deep white-matter strokes. The incidence of seizures is also higher in patients with intracerebral hemorrhage.

### Inflammatory and Autoimmune Disorders

Immune disorders increase the risk of epilepsy and seizures (Ong et al, 2014). In systemic lupus erythematosus, the risk of seizures is 12%–20% and is more likely with anticardiolipin and anti-Smith antibodies (Najjar et al., 2008). The risk of epilepsy is also increased in primary CNS inflammatory conditions such as multiple sclerosis. Between 2% and 6% of patients with multiple sclerosis have seizures. Those who do tend to have more extensive cortical involvement with inflammatory disease. Seizures are more likely to occur in the context of acute relapse, but some patients develop chronic epilepsy. Seizures are a more common acute manifestation of acute disseminated encephalomyelitis, noted in approximately 50% of patients. However, chronic epilepsy is much less likely, with only about 5% affected.

Hashimoto encephalopathy is a steroid-responsive encephalopathy usually presenting with behavioral-cognitive abnormalities. Seizures occur in 60% of individuals. Patients have elevated antithyroid antibodies, but it is not clear that these antibodies are responsible for the clinical manifestations (Castillo et al., 2006).

Autoimmune limbic encephalitis is an increasingly recognized cause of seizures and epilepsy. Suggested diagnostic criteria include (1) subacute onset of short-term memory loss, altered mental status, or psychiatric symptoms, (2) at least one of new focal CNS findings, seizures not explained by prior epilepsy, cerebrospinal fluid (CSF) pleocytosis, or MRI features suggestive of encephalitis, and (3) reasonable exclusion of alternative causes (Graus et al., 2016). It can be paraneo-plastic or nonparaneoplastic. The most commonly associated neoplasms are small-cell lung cancer, testicular cancer, thymoma, breast cancer, or teratoma. Perhaps the most meaningful classification of autoimmune limbic encephalitis is by the antibody target; associated antibodies may be directed against intracellular cytoplasmic/nuclear antigens or against antigens on the plasma membrane. The latter have a better prognosis with appropriate therapy, with a greater possibility of reversing the clinical manifestations. The most common antibodies directed against intracellular targets are anti-Hu, anti-Ma, anti-amphiphysin, and anti-CV2/CRMP5 (Gaspard, 2016). Anti-glutamic acid decarboxylase (Anti-GAD) antibodies may fall into this category, but it is not clear if the antibodies are pathogenic or an epiphenomenon (Spatola and Dalmau, 2017). The most common antibodies against plasma membrane antigens include anti–*N*-methyl-D-aspartate (NMDA) receptor antibodies (Dalmau et al., 2008; Titulaer et al., 2013) and anti-LGI1 antibodies previously thought to represent anti-potassium channel antibodies (LGI1 is a component of the potassium channel complex) (Lai et al., 2010). Anti-NMDA receptor antibody encephalitis most often presents with psychiatric symptoms, but most patients will have seizures in the course of the disease. Anti-LGI1 encephalitis often presents with faciobrachial dystonic seizures, with distinctive brief unilateral dystonic posturing of the arm and face, often before the appearance of the other manifestations of memory loss, MRI changes, and hyponatremia (Irani et al., 2011). These seizures respond very well to immunotherapy, but poorly to ASMs (Irani et al., 2013; Thompson et al., 2018). Other neuronal cell membrane targets include α-amino-3-hydroxy-5-methyl-4-isoxazole-propionic acid (AMPA) and $GABA_A$ and $GABA_B$ receptors (Bataller et al., 2010; Hoftberger et al., 2013; Petit-Pedrol et al., 2014).

An immune basis of epilepsy should be suspected in individuals who have other autoimmune disease, abrupt or recent onset of seizures (particularly if resistant to ASMs and progressive in frequency and severity), associated manifestations such as behavioral changes and psychosis, faciobrachial dystonic seizures, severe memory disturbances, and abnormal signal on MRI in the hippocampi. A scoring system has been suggested to identify patients with serum antibodies suggesting an autoimmune etiology (Dubey et al., 2017). The identification of immune origin is important for treatment of seizures. ASMs alone are often ineffective while immunotherapy is particularly effective, especially in patients with antibodies directed against cell membrane targets (de Bruijn et al., 2019; Malter et al., 2010).

An immune origin is suspected in several well-described epileptic syndromes. These include West syndrome, Lennox-Gastaut syndrome, LKS, and Rasmussen syndrome. All are discussed earlier in the chapter.

### Other Risk Factors

Other risk factors have been specifically investigated in older adults. Several risk factors for stroke are independently associated with increased risk of epilepsy, without evidence of any stroke. For example, hypertension is associated with a 1.57-fold increase in the risk (Ng et al., 1993). Left ventricular hypertrophy without diuretic treatment was associated with an 11-fold increased risk (Hesdorffer et al., 1996). Diuretics were protective, as left ventricular hypertrophy treated with diuretics carried no increase in risk (Hesdorffer et al., 1996).

Dementia, particularly Alzheimer disease, has been associated with epilepsy, with up to a 10-fold increase in risk compared to a reference population (Hauser et al., 1986). Patients who developed seizures had a younger age at onset of dementia, with seizures tending to be a late feature first seen an average of 6.8 years after onset (Mendez et al., 1994). Using very conservative criteria, the incidence of seizures was found to be 1.5%, but still with an eightfold increase in risk compared to an age-matched population (Scarmeas et al., 2009).

Major depression seemed to increase the risk of epilepsy sixfold in patients 55 years or older. This was the case without any prior neurological insult (Hesdorffer et al., 2000). Attempted suicide also increased the risk of epilepsy (Hesdorffer et al., 2006).

Alcohol abuse is known to be associated with acute withdrawal seizures within 48 hours of stopping alcohol. However, chronic alcohol intake was also associated with increased risk of chronic epilepsy, related to the amount of alcohol use. The increased risk was almost 20-fold for the heaviest drinkers (Ng et al., 1988).

Heroin increased the risk of unprovoked seizures threefold, while marijuana seemed to confer protection (Ng et al., 1990). Cocaine may reduce seizure threshold in individuals with epilepsy, but it is not clear that it is an important risk factor for chronic epilepsy (Koppel et al., 1996).

### Causes of Acute Symptomatic Seizures

Acute symptomatic seizures occur in close temporal relationship with an acute CNS insult—metabolic, toxic, structural, infectious, or inflammatory (Beghi et al., 2010). Many of the causes of epilepsy already discussed can also cause acute symptomatic seizures. Metabolic and toxic causes of acute symptomatic seizures do not usually cause chronic epilepsy.

Metabolic disturbances known to cause seizures include hypoglycemia, hyperglycemia, hyponatremia, hypocalcemia, hypomagnesemia, and uremia (Beghi et al., 2010). Withdrawal from chronic alcohol abuse may be associated with GTC seizures as well as other manifestations of withdrawal, typically within 48 hours of the last alcohol intake. Acute withdrawal from benzodiazepines and barbiturates can also be associated with withdrawal seizures, more commonly when short-acting agents are involved.

Several illicit drugs produce acute symptomatic seizures, particularly cocaine and other stimulants taken in excess.

Several medications can trigger acute symptomatic seizures at high doses or in susceptible individuals. These same medications, as well as metabolic derangements, can also trigger seizures in people with epilepsy, at lower thresholds than for people without epilepsy.

## SEIZURE PRECIPITANTS

Some patients with epilepsy report seizure precipitants that will not trigger seizures in unaffected individuals. More than 50% of subjects with epilepsy reported at least one precipitant (Frucht et al., 2000; Nakken et al., 2005). Emotional stress and sleep deprivation were the most commonly reported precipitants. Other precipitants were fatigue, fever or illness, flickering light, and menstruation. In some epileptic syndromes and epilepsies (e.g., BECTS, frontal lobe epilepsy), seizures occur preferentially in sleep.

Several medications can reduce the seizure threshold, including tricyclic antidepressants, bupropion, various antipsychotics, CNS stimulants, fluoroquinolone antibiotics, older antihistaminics, meperidine, and tramadol. Fever can reduce the threshold for seizures in patients with known epilepsy. Hyperventilation is well known to precipitate generalized absence seizures. It can also precipitate other seizure types to a much lesser extent (Arain et al., 2009; Guaranha et al., 2005).

One likely common reason for precipitation of seizures is missing antiepileptic medication doses. Breakthrough seizures can occur with missing any of the ASMs. However, carbamazepine and oxcarbazepine are associated with more severe seizures upon abrupt withdrawal (Azar et al., 2008b; Marciani et al., 1985).

A prominent precipitation of seizures in association with the menstrual cycle has been termed *catamenial epilepsy*. This is reported in approximately 55% of women (Herzog, 2008). The most common pattern of clustering of seizures is perimenstrual, typically in the 3 days before and 3 days after onset of the period. Less common patterns are periovulatory (occurring around ovulation) and luteal, in association with inadequate luteal phase cycles. The mechanism of catamenial epilepsy is thought to be related to the opposite effects of estradiol and progesterone on seizure threshold. Estradiol is a proconvulsant, whereas progesterone has an anticonvulsant effect. Progesterone therapy has been suggested as a treatment when catamenial epilepsy is not responsive to standard ASMs (Herzog et al., 2012).

## EPIDEMIOLOGY OF EPILEPSY AND SEIZURES

### Descriptive Epidemiology

The *incidence of epilepsy* is defined as number of new cases in a unit of time divided by the total population at risk. The overall incidence in North America, adjusted for age, varied from 16 to 51 per 100,000 persons per year (Banerjee et al., 2009). The incidence is similar in European studies, but figures were at times higher in developing countries, up to 111 per 100,000 in a study in rural Chile. Incidence is high in the first decade of life, lowest in adult years until the fifth decade of life, then higher thereafter. In US studies, the highest incidence was after age 75. The increased incidence in older age was not seen in developing countries. Incidence is slightly higher in males and higher in groups with lower socioeconomic status. The finding was not accounted for by known risk factors such as head injury and stroke.

*Prevalence of epilepsy* is defined as number of individuals with epilepsy divided by total population at a point in time. This is most often *active prevalence*, referring to active epilepsy at the time of the study, as opposed to *lifetime prevalence*, which includes anyone who developed epilepsy prior to the study. The age-adjusted prevalence tends to be lower in developed countries. In door-to-door surveys, the age-adjusted prevalence ranged from 2.7 per 1000 in Italy to 7.1 per 1000 in Mississippi. Prevalence is higher in males and also higher in groups with low socioeconomic status.

*Cumulative incidence* is the estimate of the proportion of individuals who will have developed epilepsy by a certain age. In Rochester, Minnesota, at age 80 the cumulative risk of epilepsy was 4%, and the cumulative risk for all unprovoked seizures was more than 5% (Hauser et al., 1993). The cumulative incidence of all epilepsy was 1.2% through age 24 (Hauser et al., 1993).

### Epidemiology of the First Unprovoked Seizure

Studies of recurrence after the first unprovoked seizure have predominantly focused on patients who present with a GTC seizure, with or without focal onset. Milder seizures are much less likely to present to medical attention after their first occurrence. A meta-analysis of observational studies estimated a 2-year recurrence risk of approximately 40% (Berg and Shinnar, 1991). Two large randomized trials gave slightly different estimates for recurrence in patients randomized to treatment (Berg, 2008). One predicted a recurrence risk of 51% at 2 years after the initial seizure (First Seizure Trial Group, 1993), and the other estimated the risk at 39% at 2 years, 51% at 5 years, and 52% at 8 years (Marson et al., 2005). The risk of recurrence is highest in the first 2 years. Treatment reduced the risk by 60% in one study (First Seizure Trial Group, 1993) and 30% in the second study (Marson et al., 2005).

The two factors that most influenced recurrence rate were an abnormal EEG and an abnormal neurological status. Individuals with a normal EEG and normal neurological status had a risk of recurrence of 25% at 2 years and 30% at 4 years (Kim et al., 2006).

The risk of recurrence increases remarkably after a second seizure. In one prospective study in adults the 2- and 5-year risks of recurrence after the first seizure were 27% and 33%, and after the second seizure were 61% and 73% (Hauser et al., 1998).

## MORBIDITY AND MORTALITY

### Morbidity and Comorbidity

Compared to the general population, individuals with epilepsy are at risk for increased morbidity and mortality. A large European cohort study of predominantly young patients diagnosed within the previous 5 years showed a significantly greater cumulative probability of illness than controls (49% by 12 months and 86% by 24 months in patients vs. 39% and 75% in controls) (Beghi and Cornaggia, 2002). The chance of illness tended to increase with number of seizures, and there was also a significant correlation between the number of illnesses and seizure frequency. However, most of the illnesses reported were trivial. Patients with epilepsy differed from controls predominantly in ear, nose, and throat complaints. Accidents were also considerably more common in patients than controls (17% and 27% by 12 and 24 months compared to 12% and 17% for controls). The number of wounds increased with the number of ASMs, which may reflect impairment of attention as a result of seizure medications. Nervous system disorders that were more common in patients than in controls included headache and vertigo/dizziness (van den Broek and Beghi, 2004).

Several studies support an increased incidence of psychiatric disorders in epilepsy. A cross-sectional study that included 5834 individuals with epilepsy suggested that persons with epilepsy have double the risk of psychiatric disorders and an increased risk for neurodegenerative conditions, particularly dementias and Parkinson disease, cardiovascular disorders, cerebrovascular disorders, upper-gastrointestinal hemorrhages, fractures, pneumonia, chronic lung diseases, diabetes, and brain tumors (Gaitatzis et al., 2004). A US survey also found an almost threefold greater frequency of serious mental illness and an increase in physical comorbid conditions including cancer, arthritis, heart disease, stroke, asthma, severe headaches, lower back pain, and neck pain (Strine et al., 2005). It is likely that individuals with longer duration of epilepsy and drug-resistant epilepsy contribute to the higher morbidity in the cross-sectional surveys.

A survey designed to measure a wide spectrum of neuropsychiatric and pain comorbidities found several neuropsychiatric disorders to be more than twice as prevalent in patients with self-reported epilepsy as in those without epilepsy (Ottman et al., 2011). These disorders included bipolar disorder, attention-deficit/hyperactivity disorder (ADHD), and movement disorders/tremor. The last two had not been reported in previous national surveys. A survey of frequency and severity of depressive symptoms in community-based patients with epilepsy or asthma found evidence of depression in 36.5% of epilepsy subjects compared to 27.8% of asthma subjects and 11.8% of healthy controls. Patients with epilepsy are more likely to be depressed than patients with asthma, suggesting that depression is not solely related to a chronic illness (Ettinger et al., 2004). The presence of depression was associated with worse quality-of-life scores. As a result, clinicians evaluating patients with epilepsy are advised to discuss mood and quality of life as part of the evaluation (Ettinger et al., 2004).

Psychiatric symptoms need to be detected early and treated effectively, avoiding the erroneous supposition that depression is a normal reaction to the epilepsy (Garcia-Morales et al., 2008). The presence of depression should influence the selection of ASMs, avoiding drugs that are known to be associated with depression and favoring medications such as lamotrigine with a known positive mood effect. In addition, there should be a low threshold for prescribing specific antidepressant or mood-stabilizing medications, as well as consulting a psychiatrist. Compared to controls, the risk of suicidal behavior and suicide is increased in persons with epilepsy. The relationship between depression/suicidality and epilepsy is bidirectional, with a higher risk of developing epilepsy in those with a past history of suicidality, and a higher risk of suicidality in individuals with epilepsy (Hesdorffer et al., 2006). In subjects who developed epilepsy, the incidence of depression, anxiety, and suicide attempts was increased even 3 years before epilepsy diagnosis, suggesting that some mechanisms underlying reduced seizure threshold may also increase the risk for psychiatric disorders and suicide (Hesdorffer et al., 2012a). Psychiatric comorbidity at time of epilepsy diagnosis is an unfavorable prognostic indicator for seizure freedom with pharmacological therapy (Hitiris et al., 2007; Petrovski et al., 2010). Lifetime psychiatric history was also a predictor of worse outcome after anterior temporal lobectomy for drug-resistant temporal lobe epilepsy (Kanner et al., 2009).

Other comorbidities associated with epilepsy include migraine. The rate ratio for migraine was 2.4 for individuals with epilepsy in comparison with controls (Ottman and Lipton, 1994). In addition, specific epileptic syndromes have a greater association with migraine (Kossoff and Andermann, 2010). The comorbidity of migraine may influence the choice of ASM. Some ASMs such as topiramate and valproate have proven effective in migraine prophylaxis and are approved for this indication by the US Food and Drug Administration (FDA).

Sleep disorders are also a known comorbidity of epilepsy. Epilepsy patients frequently have excessive daytime sleepiness, which is multifactorial (Manni and Tartara, 2000). Several studies have suggested that the prevalence of obstructive sleep apnea may be relatively high in individuals with epilepsy as compared with controls (Kaleyias et al., 2008; Manni and Terzaghi, 2010; Manni et al., 2003). Sleep apnea is even more prevalent in individuals with drug-resistant epilepsy (Malow et al., 2000b) and may play a role in drug resistance. Sleep apnea may worsen seizure control by fragmenting nocturnal sleep and mimicking sleep deprivation. In one study in older epilepsy patients, obstructive sleep apnea was more common in those with new-onset or newly worsened epilepsy than in individuals with stable or well-controlled epilepsy (Chihorek et al., 2007). In those patients with coexistent epilepsy and sleep apnea, there is evidence that treatment of the sleep apnea may have a beneficial effect on seizure control (Malow et al., 2008). Other sleep disorders associated with epilepsy include insomnia. In particular, sleep-maintenance insomnia was reported more frequently than in controls (Khatami et al., 2006). Polysomnography in patients with epilepsy demonstrates reduced percentage of sleep time spent in rapid eye movement (REM) sleep, increased waking after sleep onset, prolonged REM latency, and increased number of stage shifts (Touchon et al., 1991). The findings are more common with temporal lobe epilepsy. The decrease in REM is more pronounced if seizures occurred during the early part of the night (Bazil et al., 2000).

## Mortality in Epilepsy

Epilepsy carries a two to three times higher mortality rate than that of the general population (Tomson, 2000). The standardized mortality ratio in an early study was 2.3 through 29 years of follow-up (Hauser et al., 1980). The most significant increase in standardized mortality ratio was noted early after diagnosis (Neligan et al., 2011). The standardized mortality ratio does depend on the seizure type. For example, GTC seizures were associated with increased mortality, while absence seizures were not (Hauser et al., 1980). Patients who became seizure free after epilepsy surgery had the same mortality rates as the general population (Sperling et al., 1999). The highest mortality is found in epilepsy patients with intellectual disability or cerebral palsy (Forsgren et al., 2005). Premature mortality in epilepsy may be seizure-related, may be due to the underlying cause of epilepsy, or may be a result of conditions only indirectly related to epilepsy, such as cerebrovascular disease, pneumonia, and neoplastic disorders (Forsgren et al., 2005). There is also increased mortality due to suicide (Bell et al., 2009). Seizure-related deaths include death from status epilepticus, accidents and drowning, and sudden unexpected death in epilepsy (SUDEP) (Forsgren et al., 2005).

SUDEP is defined as "sudden, unexpected, witnessed or unwitnessed, nontraumatic and nondrowning death, occurring in benign circumstances, in an individual with epilepsy, with or without evidence for a seizure and excluding documented status epilepticus" (Nashef et al., 2012). Sudden unexpected death has a 27-fold higher rate than in controls and is the most common cause of epilepsy-related death (Holst et al., 2013). When SUDEP is witnessed, it is most often associated with a GTC seizure near the time of death (Tomson et al., 2005), and the vast majority of unwitnessed SUDEP is associated with tongue biting or incontinence, suggesting recent GTC seizures (Langan, 2000). The most important risk factor for SUDEP is a high frequency of bilateral tonic-clonic seizures (Hesdorffer et al., 2012b). SUDEP is most commonly sleep-related and unwitnessed, and patients are found in a prone position (Liebenthal et al., 2015), with similarity to infant death syndrome. There is strong evidence that central apnea plays an important role in SUDEP. Ictal apnea and hypoxia are common (Bateman et al., 2008; Nashef et al., 1996). Pronounced oxygen desaturation occurred even in focal seizures that did not progress to bilateral convulsions, most commonly with seizures of temporal lobe onset. The duration of the seizure and electrographic evidence of contralateral spread influenced the degree of desaturation. An EEG analysis suggested that prolonged generalized EEG suppression was more commonly seen with seizures recorded in individuals who later died of SUDEP. Beyond 80 seconds of postictal generalized EEG suppression, the odds of SUDEP were quadrupled. It is thought that the generalized EEG suppression reflects profound postictal cerebral dysfunction that may be a mechanism for central apnea (Lhatoo et al., 2010).

It is now increasingly recognized that patients deemed at high risk for SUDEP need to be informed about this potential complication. Education about SUDEP is not necessary in patients with well-controlled seizures, but it is important for noncompliant individuals who could reduce the risk of SUDEP with improved compliance, and for patients with drug-resistant epilepsy who are excellent candidates for epilepsy surgery, which reduces the risk of SUDEP when successful (So et al., 2009).

## PATHOPHYSIOLOGY AND MECHANISMS

Seizures are transient neurological events resulting from excessive and hypersynchronous brain activity that present in a multitude of forms such as brief, abrupt behavior arrest and staring (typical absence), impaired awareness and automatisms (FIAS) and tonic-clonic seizures. Seizures exhibit such diverse behavioral manifestations because each seizure type activates different brain circuits. Therefore, discussions of epilepsy pathophysiology must be done in context of the circuits that produce each seizure. The two most-extensively studied seizure circuits are the ones that produce typical absence seizures and hippocampal focal seizures. Therefore, in this section, we will describe the circuits that engaged in each of these seizure types as well as known pathophysiological mechanisms that produce the excessive and hypersynchronous activity within the circuits during a seizure.

### Typical Absence Seizures

Generalized seizures such as typical absence seizures engage widespread regions in both cerebral hemispheres extremely rapidly and thus give the appearance on clinical EEG of activating the entire cortex instantaneously. However, functional MRI (fMRI) (Carney et al., 2012; Gotman et al., 2005), magnetoencephalography (MEG) (Miao et al., 2014; Stefan et al., 2009; Tenney et al., 2014; Westmijse et al., 2009), and high-density EEG (Holmes et al., 2004) studies revealed that generalized seizures engage distinct brain networks that often involve the thalamus and frontal and parietal cortices.

In rodent models, typical absence seizures also activate discrete, interconnected cortical and thalamic regions including the somatosensory barrel cortex ($S1^{bfd}$) and the thalamic reticular (nRT) and ventroposterior medial (VPM) nuclei (for in-depth reviews, see Fogerson and Huguenard, 2016; Luttjohann and van Luijtelaar, 2015). Three key anatomical/physiological features of this cortico-thalamo-cortical (CTC) circuitry promote oscillations. First, excitatory neurons in VPM project to the inhibitory GABAergic neurons in nRT, which then provide feedback inhibition to VPM. Second, VPM neurons fire in two modes—tonic and bursting. In the bursting mode, a VPM neuron pacemaker-like current ($I_h$) activates upon hyperpolarization and the resultant depolarization activates a T-type calcium channel (T-type current) that transiently further depolarizes the neurons allowing a brief period of repetitive action potentials. The action potentials are transmitted from VPM to $S1^{bfd}$ to form EEG spikes as well as to nRT, which provides feedback inhibition to VPM. Third, VPM and nRT neurons are highly interconnected—both within and between the thalamic nuclei. The interconnectedness produces the synchrony of neurons during the oscillation

In nonepileptic individuals, VPM burst-mode firing and CTC oscillations produce sleep-related low-frequency delta activity and high-frequency sleep spindles. Absence seizure research has focused on identifying physiological conditions that cause this naturally oscillating circuit to produce pathological spike-wavedischarges (SWDs). High-resolution electrophysiological recordings in CAE animals revealed that SWD spikes originate in $S1^{bfd}$ and spread to the thalamus within 10–100 ms (Meeren et al., 2002; Polack et al., 2007). Selective modulation of $S1^{bfd}$, nRT, and VB by lesioning, pharmacological, and optogenetic methods revealed that all three circuit elements play critical roles in SWD and elucidated some of the physiological conditions that promote seizures. First, unilateral inhibition of somatosensory cortex $GABA_A$ receptors produces SWDs (Steriade and Contreras, 1998) whereas blockade of action potentials in $S1^{bfd}$, but not other cortical regions, abolish bilateral SWDs (Polack et al., 2009; Sitnikova and van Luijtelaar, 2004). These results highlight a principal role of somatosensory cortex in absence seizures. Similarly, in nRT, bilateral increased tonic or phasic $GABA_A$ inhibition (Hosford et al., 1997; Liu et al., 1991) and unilateral lesioning (Meeren et al., 2009) reduces/eliminates SWDs whereas bilateral $GABA_A$ antagonism increases them (Aker et al., 2002). Finally, tonic VB hyperpolarization increases SWDs (Cope et al., 2009; Hosford et al., 1997; Liu et al., 1991; Sorokin et al., 2017), whereas facilitation of synaptic VB $GABA_A$ signaling does not change them (Hosford et al., 1997). Conversely, reduction of VB tonic inhibition decreases SWDs (Cope et al., 2009; Sorokin et al., 2017). It should be noted that while enhanced tonic inhibition can produce SWDs, it is not necessary for their formation (Zhou et al., 2015).

Although typical absence seizures can arise in patients with acquired brain lesions (Wakamoto, 2008), they occur most often with IGE syndromes that, by definition, are not associated with gross anatomical changes. Most IGE cases arise from complex inheritance, but some IGE syndromes are monogenic (familial or sporadic [de novo]) (Macdonald et al., 2010), and the mutations often occur in synaptic protein genes such as neurotransmitter receptor and voltage-gated ion channel genes. These monogenic epilepsy mutations have specific molecular consequences for the mutant proteins they encode. This has been studied in detail for mutations in genes for subunits of the inhibitory $GABA_A$ receptors, which have been associated with multiple genetic epilepsies syndromes, including CAE, JME, GEFS+, Lennox-Gastaut syndrome, infantile spasms, Dravet syndrome, and Doose syndrome (Macdonald et al., 2010). We will discuss the human $GABA_A$ receptor subunit gene (GABR) mutations that produce CAE in *GABRA1*, *GABRB3*, and *GABRG2* to illustrate some of the effects of *GABR* mutations that produce *CAE* and *SCN1A* mutations to produce Dravet syndrome, since the results reported for *GABRs* and *SNC1A* could be generalizable to *CAE* and Dravet syndrome mutations in other synaptic protein genes.

The $GABA_A$ receptor is a ligand-gated, chloride-selective ion channel responsible for most synaptic inhibition in the CNS and is a heteropentamer whose expression and current kinetic properties are determined by the subunit combination of the receptor. While there are numerous genes that encode subunits and subunit subtypes of the $GABA_A$ receptor ($\alpha$1–6, $\beta$1–3, $\gamma$1–2, $\delta$, $\varepsilon$, $\theta$, and $\pi$), the majority of the $GABA_A$ receptors in the CNS are composed of 2 $\alpha$, 2 $\beta$, and a single $\gamma$ or $\delta$ subunit. To date, numerous *GABR* mutations have been associated with autosomal dominant monogenetic epilepsy syndromes, which are primarily in *GABRA1, GABRB1, GABRB2, GABRB3,* and *GABRG2* subunit genes. All the the GABR epilepsy mutations reported thus far have resulted in loss- or reduction- in function of the corresponding GABAAR subunit. However, the currently studied mutations produce loss of function by a variety of different mechanisms including messenger (m)RNA through nonsense-mediated decay, misfolding, and degradation of the nascent polypeptides, dominant negative reductions in wild-type $GABA_A$ receptor expression, impaired receptor oligomerization, formation of insoluble protein aggregates, and altered electrophysiological properties. Specific potential therapies for each of these molecular consequences have been proposed.

The human S326fs328X mutant α1 subunit causes CAE (Maljevic et al., 2006). The mutation impairs $GABA_A$ receptor function by causing loss-of-function due to frameshift or deletion of GABRA1 that produces degradation of the mutant mRNAs by nonsense mediated mRNA decay (NMD). Electrophysiological studies demonstrated that heterozygous loss of the α1 subunit expression reduces synaptic $GABA_A$ currents in excitatory neurons in both cortical layer VI and VB without changing VB tonic inhibition (Zhou et al., 2013, 2015).

The human P11S, S15F, and G32R mutant β3 subunits cause CAE (Tanaka et al., 2008) by decreasing $GABA_A$ receptor current. The current reduction is due to impaired function of surface $GABA_A$ receptors without altering surface expression of mutant β3 subunits (Tian and Macdonald, 2012).

The human IVS6+2T>G mutant γ2 subunit also causes CAE (Kananura et al., 2002). The decrease of $GABA_A$ receptor current is produced by a premature stop codon in the mutant gene that produces NMD, thus decreasing γ2-subunit mRNA and surface $GABA_A$ receptors.

Neurons express α1β3γ2 subunits, nRT neurons express α3β3 subunits, and VBn neurons express α1β2γ2 subunits, suggesting that locations that express ternary α1β3γ2 receptors and binary α3β3 β3 subunit-containing receptors are responsible for generating CAE. In contrast it is likely that locations that express β1 or β2, but not β3, subunits do not generate CAE.

Thus, the *GABRA1* and *GABRG2* mutations that produce typical CAE cause degradation of mutant mRNA by NMD without altering the function of successfully assembled and trafficked receptors. The resultant reduced subunit expression reduces cell-surface expression of the mutated subunit. In contrast, the *GABRB3* mutation that produces typical CAE alters the function of the ion channel without altering receptor function.

Altered inhibitory neurotransmission may also contribute to the pathology of Dravet syndrome, a genetic epilepsy syndrome that confers febrile seizures and generalized seizures including myoclonic seizures and atypical absence seizures. Approximately 85% of Dravet patients possess mutations in the *SCN1A* gene, which encodes the α subunit of the neuronal voltage-gated sodium channel type 1. The majority (78%) of Dravet syndrome *SCN1A* mutations are predicted to be particularly disruptive to protein function; these disruptive mutations include amplification, frameshift, truncation, deletion, or duplication mutations. Interestingly, both pyramidal and GABAergic neurons derived from induced pluripotent stem cells from two Dravet patients showed increased, not decreased, sodium channel currents, hyperexcitability, and spontaneous bursting (Liu et al., 2013). These findings suggested the possibility that overcompensation by a different sodium channel α subunit could also contribute to the pathophysiology of Dravet syndrome. However, different results are obtained when Dravet syndrome is modeled in mice. Both heterozygous Scn1a deletion mice (Yu et al., 2006) and mice that heterozygously contained the Dravet-associated Scn1a R1407X nonsense mutation (Ogiwara et al., 2007) experienced spontaneous seizures. The hippocampi of Scn1a deletion mice exhibited reduced sodium currents in the interneurons, but not the pyramidal neurons. The R140X mutation reduced spike amplitudes in cortical layer II/III interneurons. These findings suggested that Dravet syndrome mutations reduce interneuron function, resulting in disinhibition.

## Hippocampal Focal-Onset Seizures

The current epilepsy classification system (Fisher et al., 2017) does not group focal seizures based upon the presumed region of onset (e.g., frontal, temporal, etc.), a decision made in light of current research that revealed that focal-onset seizures, like generalized-onset seizures, engage and influence long-range brain networks. Nevertheless, unlike generalized epilepsies, focal epilepsies, especially those that initially engage the mesial temporal lobe, are very responsive to targeted surgical ablation (Hoyt and Smith, 2016; Jermakowicz et al., 2017) and thus it is practical to consider the pathophysiological processes that produce excessive and hypersynchronous discharges in these distinct structures. Therefore, we will examine the processes thought to form seizures in the hippocampus, the most extensively studied structure in mesial temporal lobe seizures.

Much of the neuronal signaling through the hippocampus is mediated through the so-called "trisynaptic circuit" consisting of (1) entorhinal cortex perforant path projections to dentate gyrus granule cells (DGCs), (2) DGC axons (mossy fibers) projections to CA3 pyramidal neurons, and (3) Schaffer collaterals from CA3 cells to CA1 pyramidal neurons. In the nonepileptic animals, DGCs are relatively nonexcitable and thus perforant path stimulation produces few action potentials ("sparse activation"), a property thought to be important for cognitive functions such as memory encoding and pattern separation (Cayco-Gajic and Silver, 2019; Hainmueller and Bartos, 2018). In addition, DGC sparse activation limits the propagation of seizures from the entorhinal cortex to the cortex (Behr et al., 1996, 1998; Dreier and Heinemann, 1991), a property referred to as "dentate gating" (Dengler and Coulter, 2016; Dudek and Sutula, 2007). Consistent with these early studies, optogenetic inhibition and excitation selectively applied to DGC have reduced and increased, respectively, the frequency and duration of electrographic seizures as well as the progression to a convulsive seizure (Bui et al., 2018; Krook-Magnuson et al., 2015; Tung et al., 2018). In addition, optogenetic excitation of dentate gyrus mossy cells decreased seizure duration and the fraction of electrographic seizures that evolved into a convulsion (Bui et al., 2018), a result consistent with the feedforward inhibition of mossy cells to DGC.

Much of the research into the pathogenesis of hippocampal focal-onset seizures has focused on uncovering mechanisms by which dentate gating is diminished. Unlike the absence seizure network, there is little evidence to suggest that genomic mutations play the predominant role in altering neural transmission through the dentate gate. Therefore, this section will discuss alterations in dentate gyrus microcircuitry, DGC excitability, and GABAergic inhibition, that modify DRG sparse activation.

Histological analysis of dentate gyri from both humans and epileptic animals demonstrate that DGC mossy fibers form collateral connections (mossy fiber sprouting) on DGC dendrites in the dentate gyrus inner molecular layer. These aberrant connections provide recurrent synaptic excitation to DGC (Scharfman et al., 2003) and thus may be the mechanism by which dentate gating is reduced. However, the epileptogenic role of mossy fiber sprouting is unclear. The recurrent excitatory signaling is weak (Scharfman et al., 2003) and, in one mouse model, administration of rapamycin, an inhibitor of the mammalian target of rapamycin (mTOR) signaling pathway reduced mossy fiber sprouting but did not change seizure frequency (Buckmaster and Lew,

2011; Heng et al., 2013), a result that suggested that although mossy fiber sprouting is a very common histological finding, it may be an epiphenomenon that does not disrupt dentate gating or promote seizures. However, because rapamycin affects many cellular processes, including the sprouting of inhibitory interneuron axons (Buckmaster and Wen, 2011), it is possible that antiepileptogenic reductions in mossy fiber sprouting could be counterbalanced by other pro-epileptogenic effects. The development of techniques to selectively reduce mossy fiber sprouting is needed to clarify its role in disrupted dentate gating.

Altered DGC electrophysiological properties may also contribute to reduced dentate gating and hippocampal seizures. Compared with controls, DGCs from epileptic rats exhibited depolarized resting potentials, increased action potential firing rates, and prolonged action potential waveforms (Althaus et al., 2015). In addition, ectopic DGC, neurons born in the dentate gyrus subgranular proliferative zone that mature after the epileptogenic insult and fail to migrate properly to the granule zone (Kron et al., 2010), possess increased firing rates compared with their normotopic counterparts (Althaus et al., 2015). Therefore, ectopic DGC also likely increase dentate gyrus excitability. The presence of increased slow-wave oscillations (SWO, 0.1–2.0 Hz) in membrane potential may increase seizures in the epileptic dentate gyrus. Although healthy DGCs rarely exhibit spontaneous SWO, status epilepticus produces strong, long-duration SWO that are in phase with neocortical oscillations (Ouedraogo et al., 2016). Depolarizing phases of the SWO will facilitate dentate transmission at the time of increased neocortical neural activity and thus promote seizures.

Finally, reduced inhibitory GABAergic signaling may also disrupt dentate gating. Animal models of hippocampal epilepsy have reduced parvalbumin-, somatostatin-, and neuropeptide Y-expressing GABAergic inhibitory interneurons in the dentate (Kobayashi and Buckmaster, 2003; Sun et al., 2007) and fewer fibers in the dentate inner molecular layer express the inhibitory neuromarker, cholecystokinin (Sun et al., 2014). Although exceptions exist (Dengler et al., 2017), DGCs in epilepsy models exhibit a lower frequency of inhibitory postsynaptic currents (IPSCs) (Kobayashi and Buckmaster, 2003; Sun et al., 2014; Zhang et al., 2007), a finding consistent with reduced presynaptic inhibitory interneurons. In addition to reduced frequency, several (Dengler et al., 2017; Kobayashi and Buckmaster, 2003; Zhang et al., 2007) (but not all [Sun et al., 2014]) studies found reduced synaptic DGC ISPC amplitudes. The finding that supplementation of glutamine, a GABA precursor, restores dentate gating in epileptic mice (Dengler et al., 2017) suggests that reduced presynaptic GABA biosynthesis is a factor that reduces DGC IPSC amplitudes.

In conclusion, seizure pathophysiology is complex and must be studied in the contexts of the neural circuits that produce each seizure. The networks that generate typical absence and hippocampal focal seizures have been most thoroughly studied. Absence seizures are associated with many different genetic mutations that alter the physiology of different components of the thalamocortical networks. In contrast, hippocampal focal seizures are associated with post transcriptional changes, some of which may alter physiology in the dentate gyrus. Studies of both these networks have revealed distinct areas that can be modulated to reduce seizures.

## DIFFERENTIAL DIAGNOSIS

Seizures and epilepsy have many imitators, some of which are age specific. In infants, the list includes apnea, either central or obstructive, which can be a seizure manifestation but can also be nonepileptic. Jitteriness associated with a variety of metabolic disturbances can imitate clonic or myoclonic seizures. Exaggerated startle can also be mistaken for tonic seizures. After the neonatal period, early childhood imitators of seizures include shuddering attacks and stereotypies or repetitive behaviors that can be mistaken for seizures. Gastroesophageal reflux may be associated with posturing (Sandifer syndrome); a greater occurrence of spells following feeding may be a clue to the diagnosis. Breath-holding spells represent a form of syncope that may be associated with tonic posturing and a few jerks (Laux and Nordli, 2005). Either cyanosis or pallor can accompany these breath-holding spells, and both are precipitated by injury or frustration, but cyanotic spells are preceded by crying.

Imitators of epilepsy that are more common in old age include transient ischemic attacks (TIAs) and transient global amnesia. Transient ischemia generally causes negative symptoms.

With loss of function such as weakness or numbness, whereas seizures involving sensory or motor cortex are more likely to produce positive symptoms such as twitching or paresthesias. However, seizures may occasionally present with only negative symptoms, and TIAs rarely present with limb shaking. Limb shaking as a feature of TIAs has been associated with high-grade stenosis or occlusion of the internal carotid artery (Persoon et al., 2010). Although TIAs tend to be longer in duration than seizures (most seizures last <2 minutes and most TIAs last >2 minutes), limb-shaking TIAs are short, usually shorter than 5 minutes and even shorter than 1 minute. One feature that could distinguish them from seizures is precipitation by rising or exercise and association with weakness of the affected limb (Persoon et al., 2010). TIAs can be misdiagnosed as seizures, but the more common scenario is to misdiagnose negative motor seizures or sensory seizures as TIAs. The presence of a sensory march should be suggestive of an epileptic nature.

*Transient global amnesia* is a condition in older individuals characterized by memory loss without impairment of other cognitive function, and affected subjects are able to engage in complex activities. Most transient global amnesia episodes last hours and are single events, although they may repeat in a minority of individuals. The nature of transient global amnesia is not totally clear.

Conditions that can imitate seizures and epilepsy through much of the life span include nonepileptic psychogenic seizures, syncope, classical migraine, and a number of sleep and movement disorders. These will be discussed in greater detail.

### Psychogenic Nonepileptic Seizures

*Psychogenic nonepileptic seizures* (PNES), also called *psychogenic nonepileptic events*, *pseudoseizures*, or *pseudoepileptic seizures*, are the most common imitators of seizures and epilepsy in referral centers. These are emotionally triggered attacks not associated with any paroxysmal epileptic activity in the brain. Most are the result of somatoform disorder, with a variety of reported traumatic antecedents, particularly sexual or physical abuse in women (Duncan and Oto, 2008). Antecedents or historical precipitants of PNES include head injury, which is also a common and important risk factor for epilepsy. In one study, 33% of patients with head injury and seizures had PNES on video-EEG monitoring (Hudak et al., 2004). PNES may also appear after surgery and can be one explanation for apparent failure of epilepsy surgery (Ney et al., 1998; Parra et al., 1998; Reuber et al., 2002). This emphasizes the need for video-EEG evaluation of patients who have had recurrence of seizures after epilepsy surgery. A diagnosis of fibromyalgia or a history of chronic pain were found to be predictors of PNES (Benbadis, 2005). The neurobiology of PNES is not known, but imaging studies have suggested altered functional connectivity of several brain regions in patients with PNES as compared to normal controls (Perez and LaFrance, 2016).

PNES are diagnosed in a considerable proportion of patients referred for drug-resistant seizures. The population-based incidence has been estimated at between 1.4 and 4.6 per 100,000 person-years of observation. In one study, the incidence was highest between 15 and 24 years of age (Sigurdardottir and Olafsson, 1998) and in another between 25 and 45 years of age (Szaflarski et al., 2000). All studies agree that there is a higher prevalence in women (70%–80%). The various patterns of clinical manifestations of PNES can be classified in three broad categories: psychogenic motor seizures with prominent motor activity, psychogenic minor motor or trembling seizures with tremor of the extremities, and attacks with motionless unresponsiveness or collapse (Groppel et al., 2000; Meierkord et al., 1991; Selwa et al., 2000). In children, prolonged staring and unresponsiveness was the most common pattern, while motor activity was more common in adolescents (Kramer et al., 1995).

The diagnosis of PNES depends on prolonged video-EEG monitoring with recording of typical attacks. The use of suggestion may facilitate the precipitation and recording of attacks. Hyperventilation and photic stimulation are usually adequate suggestion techniques; suggestion methods should not involve patient deception. In some individuals, suggestion may precipitate atypical attacks; to verify that recorded events are typical of what occurs at home, it is crucial to seek the input of family members who have witnessed attacks. PNES may coexist with epilepsy. Early studies suggested that more than 50% of patients with PNES also have epilepsy, but most studies now agree on a much smaller proportion, probably not more than 10% or 15% (Benbadis et al., 2001; Lesser et al., 1983; Martin et al., 2003).

A number of studies have tried to identify features that suggest PNES origin (Avbersek and Sisodiya, 2010). In a comparison of epileptic GTC seizures and PNES with motor activity, features that predicted PNES were out-of-phase upper and lower extremity movements, absence of vocalization or vocalization at the very onset of seizures, forward pelvic thrusting, absence of whole-body rigidity, and side-to-side head movements. No single feature was totally predictive by itself, and these features were particularly strong predictors when combined (Gates et al., 1985), but such clinical features can also be seen in frontal lobe FIAS and other hypermotor seizures (Saygi et al., 1992). Other features that may help discriminate PNES from epileptic seizures include pseudosleep at onset (Benbadis et al., 1996b); preictal behavioral changes (Moore et al., 1998); discontinuous seizure activity; prolonged seizure duration; eye closure during unresponsiveness (Chung et al., 2006; DeToledo and Ramsay, 1996); resistance to eye opening; eye fluttering; certain vocalizations such as stuttering, gagging, gasping, screaming, weeping, or moaning; emotional display during events; emotional triggers; precipitation of typical events by suggestion; and attacks occurring in the clinic waiting room or admitting office. Tongue biting and incontinence occur more commonly with epileptic seizures but are also frequently reported by patients with PNES (Peguero et al., 1995). Injuries to the tongue during epileptic seizures tend to affect the side of the tongue. Biting the tip of the tongue or the lip was suggestive of PNES (DeToledo and Ramsay, 1996). Self-injury was also reported by patients with PNES, but one study suggested that burn injuries were specific for epileptic seizures (Peguero et al., 1995). The presence of postictal stertorous respiration is very helpful to diagnose epileptic convulsive seizures (Sen et al., 2007), whereas shallow rapid respiration was more likely after PNES (Azar et al., 2008a).

The gold standard for diagnosing PNES is the recording of typical attacks with EEG-video and demonstrating typical semiology and absence of EEG changes peri-ictally with habitual attacks (Perez and LaFrance, 2016). Neurologists have to be aware that some epileptic seizures have no EEG correlate. For example, frontal lobe FIAS of orbitofrontal or cingulate origin commonly have no associated EEG changes, nor do supplementary motor seizures. For definitive diagnosis, it is often necessary to record multiple attacks and observe changes in conjunction with ASM withdrawal. Epileptic seizures may evolve to bilateral tonic-clonic activity, which provides a definitive diagnosis. In one study comparing patients with frontal lobe FIAS and patients with PNES, there was no significant difference in the history of psychiatric disease, ictal pelvic thrusting, rocking of body, side-to-side head movements, or rapid postictal recovery (Saygi et al., 1992). Of interest, turning to a prone position occurred only in frontal lobe FIAS. Nocturnal occurrence, short ictal duration, younger age at onset, stereotyped movements, and abnormal MRI or EEG favored frontal lobe FIAS. Others have also suggested that while epileptic seizures are very stereotyped, PNES tend to have a lot of variability. However, this notion has been disputed (Seneviratne et al., 2010).

Pseudo-status epilepticus is a common occurrence in PNES, reported in a greater proportion of patients than status epilepticus in patients with epilepsy (Dworetzky et al., 2006). As expected, it tends to be resistant to treatment with ASMs, until the development of stupor or coma, which may lead to intubation. Its early recognition is essential to prevent potentially harmful interventions.

## Syncope

*Syncope* is an abrupt transient loss of consciousness caused by decreased cerebral perfusion. It is an important condition in the differential diagnosis of epilepsy in the elderly as well as teenagers and young adults. Although syncope is mostly recognized by loss of posture and limp unresponsiveness, the majority of closely observed individuals will have brief transient motor manifestations early after loss of consciousness. The most common motor manifestation is myoclonus that is most often multifocal and arrhythmic (Lempert et al., 1994). Other motor manifestations may also occur, including posturing, head turning, upward eye movement, oral automatisms, and righting movements (Lempert et al., 1994). The motor manifestations, particularly myoclonus, are an important factor in the misdiagnosis of syncope as seizures. Although syncope with myoclonus has been referred to as "convulsive syncope," there is no associated EEG discharge, and the origin is thought to be in the brainstem. Syncope can have a variety of mechanisms, some benign and others serious. In younger individuals, the most common is neurally mediated syncope. This can be triggered by a variety of factors, including intense pain, emotion, and standing for prolonged periods of time in hot or crowded places. In addition, syncope can be precipitated in some individuals by micturition, defecation, or cough. Neurally mediated syncope tends to have a prodrome of lightheadedness, nausea, pallor, cold sweating, graying of vision, and hearing becoming distant, as well as other visual or auditory hallucinations (Carreño, 2008; Crompton and Berkovic, 2009; Lempert et al., 1994). Syncope may also be due to orthostatic hypotension, cardiac arrhythmias, and structural cardiopulmonary disease (Carreño, 2008; Crompton and Berkovic, 2009). Syncope due to cardiac arrhythmia is usually more abrupt with no preceding symptoms. In the differentiation of syncope from seizures, features that favor syncope include known heart disease, prior confirmed syncope, precipitation by prolonged standing or rising to an upright position, presence of dehydration, the typical neurocardiogenic syncope prodrome described earlier, description of pronounced pallor by witnesses, absence of tonic or clonic activity, description of multifocal myoclonus lasting less than 15 seconds, and recollection of loss of consciousness. Features that would favor seizures include previous seizures, known cortical brain lesion, presence of tongue biting, incontinence, cyanosis, postictal confusion, postictal headache, and lack of recollection of loss of consciousness (Crompton and Berkovic, 2009). Syncope may rarely trigger an epileptic seizure (Stephenson et al., 2004). These seizures, referred to as *anoxic-epileptic seizures*, are to be distinguished from the much more common nonepileptic "convulsive" syncope.

### Migraine

Epilepsy and migraine both present with paroxysmal manifestations as a result of cerebral cortex involvement (Kossoff and Andermann, 2010). Types of migraine that are most likely to be confused with seizures are classical migraine with visual or somatosensory aura, basilar migraine, and acute confusional migraine (Carreño, 2008; Kossoff and Andermann, 2010). Occipital lobe seizures may be followed by a migraine-like headache that makes it hard to distinguish them from a classical migraine with a visual aura. Helpful distinguishing features include duration of the aura. The aura in migraine typically lasts 5–60 minutes (Carreño, 2008), reflecting that cortical spreading depression (the main pathophysiology of migraine) results from a slow depolarization that spreads at about 3 mm/min (Crompton and Berkovic, 2009). In contrast, epileptic discharges propagate at a much higher speed; epileptic auras are usually less than 30 seconds in duration. Another helpful distinction is that the visual aura in migraine is most commonly a fortification spectrum or scintillating scotoma, whereas colored circles are the most common aura in occipital lobe seizures (Carreño, 2008; Kossoff and Andermann, 2010). Migraine without headache, also called *migraine equivalent*, can be an even more difficult diagnostic challenge. Basilar migraine starts with brainstem manifestations that include dysarthria, vertigo, changes in hearing, diplopia, and ataxia, and then involves loss of consciousness.

Migraine and epilepsy have a greater overlap than would be expected by chance. The prevalence of each is increased in the presence of the other, and some epileptic syndromes (e.g., benign epilepsy with occipital paroxysms, BECTS) have a particularly higher incidence of migraine (Kossoff and Andermann, 2010). In addition, a rare condition referred to as "migralepsy" (or *migraine-triggered epilepsy* or *migraine-triggered seizures*) is characterized by seizures that occur during or shortly after the migraine aura. Certain antiseizure medications such as valproate and topiramate are used successfully in migraine prophylaxis, but others such as oxcarbazepine or carbamazepine do not seem to be effective. However, acute abortive therapy for the two conditions is totally different.

### Sleep Disorders

*Parasomnias* are the most important imitators of seizures in the category of sleep disorders (see Chapter 101). These include sleep walking (somnambulism), sleep talking, night terrors, confusional arousals, and REM behavior disorder. They may imitate frontal lobe seizures that occur preferentially or even exclusively in sleep. Somnambulism, sleep talking, and night terrors typically start in childhood and tend to disappear in adolescence. They are most likely to arise out of slow-wave sleep in the first half of the night, usually after a latency of 90 minutes from sleep onset. Frontal lobe seizures are more likely to arise out of stage 1 or 2 sleep (Carreño, 2008). These events are more likely to be seizures if they occur in the first hour of sleep or in the transition between waking and sleep. REM behavior disorder is characterized by loss of muscle atonia during REM sleep, which results in acting out dreams. The behavior includes verbalization and vocalization, as well as motor activity that may be violent (e.g., kicking, punching) and getting out of bed. Affected individuals will be aware that they have been dreaming and may report the content of their dreams. REM behavior disorder is more likely in the second half of the night when REM sleep is most likely to occur (Carreño, 2008). REM behavior disorder rarely starts before age 50; it is most often a chronic disorder associated with a synucleinopathy, particularly Lewy body dementia (Crompton and Berkovic, 2009). The differentiation of parasomnias and frontal lobe seizures may be aided by the use of a scale (Derry et al., 2006) or a structured interview (Bisulli et al., 2012).

Some manifestations of narcolepsy can imitate seizures. These include sleep attacks, cataplexy, sleep paralysis, and hallucinations during the transition between waking and sleep. Attacks of cataplexy are brought on by emotional stimuli and are characterized by loss of muscle tone, which may result in loss of posture. Cataplexy may include some jerky motions that could imitate seizure activity. However, an important distinguishing feature is total preservation of consciousness and complete memory of the events. The association with other manifestations of narcolepsy should help establish the diagnosis.

### Paroxysmal Movement Disorders

Paroxysmal movement disorders that can be confused with epilepsy include nonepileptic myoclonus, paroxysmal dyskinesia, and hyperekplexia (Crompton and Berkovic, 2009). Myoclonus may be generated at any level of the CNS; epileptic myoclonus is generated at the level of the cortex and is usually associated with a scalp EEG discharge. In the case of focal cortical myoclonus, the distinction can be harder to establish (Crompton and Berkovic, 2009). Paroxysmal dyskinesia can be classified into two broad categories: kinesigenic and noinkinesigenic, both usually familial (Fahn and Frucht, 2008). In *paroxysmal kinesigenic dyskinesia*, the attacks are often brought on by a sudden movement or startle, usually after a period of inactivity. The movements are any combination of chorea, athetosis, ballism, and a dystonic posture (Fahn and Frucht, 2008). They can be bilateral or alternate sides, which is helpful in distinguishing them from epileptic seizures that generally produce consistently unilateral posturing. Other helpful distinguishing features are that consciousness is always preserved, and there is no postictal change. However, the condition responds very well to ASMs. The attacks in *paroxysmal nonkinesigenic dyskinesia* are longer (minutes to hours as compared to seconds), less frequent, and precipitated not by movement but rather by alcohol, caffeine, stress, excitement, or fatigue. The attacks do not usually respond to ASMs (Fahn and Frucht, 2008). *Hyperekplexia* is an inherited disorder in which there is an exaggeration of startle reflexes (Crompton and Berkovic, 2009). The exaggerated startle has to be distinguished from startle-evoked seizures, which are most often of supplementary motor origin.

## EVALUATION AND DIAGNOSIS

The clinical history is always a cornerstone in the evaluation of seizures and epilepsy. Other elements of the evaluation depend on the clinical presentation; different testing is recommended in patients presenting with new-onset seizures, patients with recently drug-resistant seizures, or patients pursuing epilepsy surgery. This section will therefore be subdivided based on the particular presentation.

### Evaluation of Recent-Onset Seizures and Epilepsy

Evaluating an individual with one or more attacks that could represent seizures always starts with an in-depth history. Tests such as EEG and brain imaging should primarily supplement the history and help classify seizures/epilepsy and identify underlying pathology. Ideally, at the end of the evaluation, the seizure diagnosis and classification are confirmed, an epilepsy syndrome has been diagnosed if that is possible, and any structural etiology has been identified. The best treatment options can then be determined, and in some cases it may be possible to predict prognosis.

#### History

The patient with possible seizures should be asked about potential seizure triggers, any symptoms preceding the event, and recollection of what happened during the event. However, in many instances the patient can only provide an incomplete or distorted account because of altered consciousness; it is therefore crucial to obtain an independent history from a witness. If possible, more than one witness should be interviewed to assess the consistency of the description, because the recollection of events by the witness may also be distorted by panic. The final account of the event should list its components in temporal order starting with prodrome, aura, objective manifestations, and then postictal signs and symptoms. The interviewer should ask about urinary incontinence, tongue biting, postictal confusion, and postictal muscle soreness. Additional questions to be asked depend on the specific differential diagnosis in each case. In instances when multiple attacks have occurred, the family may have captured events on home video. Review of such video segments can be extremely helpful.

The past medical history may identify important risk factors for epilepsy or for other disorders. This should include a history of gestation, birth, developmental milestones, and illnesses in infancy and childhood. Of particular importance are febrile seizures and CNS infections such as meningitis or encephalitis, all of which are associated with increased risk of epilepsy. Any head trauma should be investigated with questions about loss of consciousness and its duration, and history of depressed skull fracture or other intracranial pathology. Other epilepsy risk factors to investigate will depend on age at onset—for example, history of stroke becomes important when epilepsy starts in old age.

Family history of afebrile seizures and other paroxysmal disorders as well as family history of febrile seizures should be obtained. The family history can be optimized by first asking the patient or informed relative about the number of first-degree and second-degree relatives in every category. This may help with the recall of who is affected. It is often best to obtain family history from a senior female relative who is likely to be more informed about the family than younger and male members.

Review of systems should be expanded with respect to CNS abnormalities. If specific syndromes are suspected, the review of systems should include symptoms related to other organs that may be affected in these syndromes.

## Physical and Neurological Examination

The most important aspects of the examination will vary depending on age and specific circumstances. In children, careful examination of the skin is important for identification of neurocutaneous disorders that are often associated with epilepsy. Dysmorphic features may suggest certain chromosomal abnormalities. The neurological examination may reveal abnormalities of mental status or motor and reflex asymmetries that could help with lateralization of the epileptogenic zone in focal epilepsy. However, most individuals will have a normal neurological examination.

## Electroencephalography

The EEG is a graphic representation of voltage change over time. Each EEG channel records the potential difference between two electrode positions on the scalp. In referential recordings, the first input in each channel represents the active electrode, while the second input represents the reference, which should be ideally neutral but often is not. In bipolar recordings, each channel represents the difference in potential between adjacent electrodes organized in a logical montage. Digital EEG recordings that have become standard allow reformatting of EEG montages and the judicious use of filters to optimally visualize interictal EEG activity as well as the ictal onset. When the history is consistent with seizures or epilepsy, the EEG is the most helpful test to confirm the diagnosis, help classify the epilepsy as focal or generalized, and even help identify the specific syndrome in some instances.

The routine EEG is typically 20–30 minutes long. It should include standard activation procedures such as hyperventilation and photic stimulation. The waking recording should include eyes-open and eyes-closed conditions. Ideally there should also be a recording of drowsiness and sleep, but that may be difficult to obtain without sleep deprivation. Routine EEG is unlikely to record seizures, with the exception of generalized absence seizures that can be easily precipitated by hyperventilation in the untreated patient. The main contribution of a routine EEG is the recording of interictal epileptiform activity, which includes spikes, sharp waves, spike-and-wave discharges, and polyspike-and-wave discharges.

A number of criteria help identify discharges as epileptiform. They are typically of high voltage in comparison with the surrounding EEG activity. Their duration is 70–200 ms for sharp waves and less than 70 ms for spikes; when recorded from the scalp, epileptiform discharges are usually longer than 20 ms. Epileptiform discharges tend to have more than one phase, and the predominant component is negative. That negative component tends to be asymmetrical; when the epileptiform discharge is recorded from the first input in a channel, it has a shorter and lower-voltage ascending segment and a longer and higher-voltage descending segment (Gotman, 1980; Fig. 100.17). Epileptiform discharges tend to have an aftergoing slow wave, and they tend to arise from an abnormal background. The criteria mentioned above are not necessarily all satisfied. However, the more criteria satisfied, the more confident one can be about the epileptiform nature of the discharge. Many physiological potentials and normal variants are sharp in configuration and may be misdiagnosed as epileptiform. In fact, misinterpretation of the EEG is one of the most common reasons for overdiagnosis/misdiagnosis of epilepsy. Another reason is inadequate history and failure to obtain a thorough description of events from witnesses (Smith et al., 1999).

The first interictal EEG is normal in about 50% of patients with epilepsy (Salinsky et al., 1987). Additional routine EEGs can improve the yield, but there is little to be gained after four normal EEGs. With multiple recordings, more than 90% of individuals with epilepsy will have epileptiform EEG abnormalities recorded (Salinsky et al., 1987). Several studies have explored ways to improve the yield of the first EEG in epilepsy. One study found that a sleep-deprived EEG was superior to a routine EEG and to an EEG with medication-induced sleep (Leach et al., 2006). Prolonging recording time increases the yield of EEG. One study found that a 4-hour outpatient video-EEG study added considerably to the yield of a 20-minute EEG, particularly in patients with focal epilepsy (Modur and Rigdon, 2008). Even shorter extension of recording time from 30 minutes to ≥45 minutes increased detection of epileptiform discharges by about 20% and event capture by around 30% (Burkholder et al., 2016). Timing of the EEG is also important. In generalized epilepsy, a morning EEG is more likely to yield epileptiform abnormalities than an afternoon EEG (Labate et al., 2007). In patients with JME, a slightly sleep-deprived EEG obtained predominantly after a nap is the most useful, since both seizures and epileptiform discharges are more likely after arousal from sleep.

Epileptiform discharges are more likely to be focal in patients with focal seizures and more likely to be generalized in patients with generalized-onset seizures. The EEG can record generalized absence seizures, which are reliably precipitated with hyperventilation in the untreated child, and can demonstrate interictal epileptiform discharges that are characteristic of certain syndromes (see Figs. 100.5, 100.7, 100.9–100.11). For most patients with focal seizures, the localization of epileptiform discharges corresponds to the epileptogenic

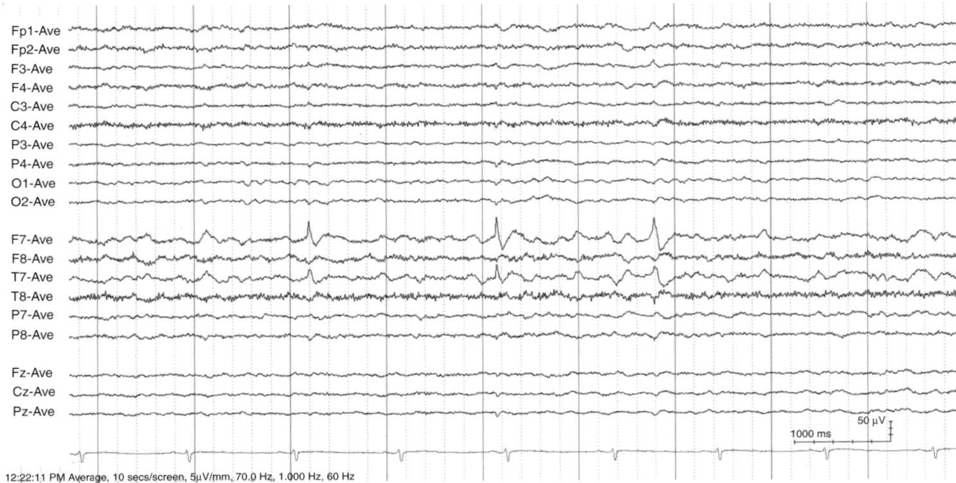


**Fig. 100.17** Left temporal epileptiform discharges emanating from an abnormal background. Note the asymmetrical waveform of sharp waves.

zone, but this is not always true. Some patients with seizures arising from one temporal lobe may have bitemporal independent epileptiform discharges. Temporal lobe epileptiform discharges may also be predominant in patients who have epilepsy of frontal, parietal, or occipital origin. Some patients with generalized-onset seizures may have focal or multifocal epileptiform discharges in addition to generalized discharges.

Besides its diagnostic role, the EEG can help determine prognosis after a first seizure. An abnormal EEG has been consistently associated with an increased risk of seizure recurrence in both children and adults, particularly if the abnormality is epileptiform. In untreated patients, the risk of seizure recurrence was increased by a factor of 1.54 if the EEG was abnormal (Kim et al., 2006).

The routine EEG has important limitations. It is an indirect assessment because it does not usually record the ictal events for which the patient is seeking evaluation. Some patients may have both epileptic and nonepileptic seizures or may have nonepileptic seizures together with epileptiform EEG abnormalities that reflect a seizure tendency in the absence of actual seizures. Some patients with focal epilepsy may have generalized EEG abnormalities that reflect an inherited generalized seizure tendency even though they do not have generalized-onset seizures. Because of all these reasons, prolonged EEG-video monitoring may be superior for definitive diagnosis of events in question. However, prolonged video-EEG monitoring is expensive and therefore reserved for patients who have had recurrent attacks with atypical manifestations and a nondiagnostic routine or sleep-deprived EEG. Video-EEG monitoring is also indicated for patients who continue to have seizures despite adequate treatment, raising the possibility of incorrect seizure diagnosis or classification.

### Neuroimaging

Neuroimaging is always indicated in adults with new-onset seizures or epilepsy to identify structural causes of epilepsy, some of which may require treatment of their own (Krumholz et al., 2007). After the first unprovoked seizure, imaging in adults has an approximately 10% yield of clinically significant findings, leading to the diagnosis of disorders such as a brain tumor or other structural lesions. Computed tomography (CT) remains the test most likely to be obtained in the emergency room after the initial seizure, but CT will often miss temporal lobe pathology because of bone streak artifact. MRI is the imaging modality of choice for identifying brain pathology in patients with new-onset seizures or epilepsy, and in that setting is preferably obtained with and without contrast. If it is possible to wait for an MRI, the emergency CT scan can be skipped.

In children with new-onset seizures, imaging may require conscious sedation or general anesthesia. An imaging study is not always required and may be omitted in children with a confident diagnosis of a genetic epilepsy syndrome such as CAE or BECTS. If there is any indication for a neuroimaging study, MRI is preferred. Published guidelines recommend elective MRI in the presence of unexplained cognitive or motor impairment or neurological exam abnormality, focal-onset seizure, an EEG not characteristic of a benign focal epilepsy of childhood or IGE, or in children younger than 1 year of age (Hirtz et al., 2000). Emergency imaging is also recommended in any child exhibiting a prolonged postictal focal deficit.

### Other Testing

Most patients presenting to the emergency room with their first seizure will have blood studies performed routinely, but the value of such testing is not established. While a small proportion of patients have metabolic abnormalities with the first seizure, most abnormalities are not clinically significant. Metabolic blood testing should be guided by specific clinical circumstances based on the history and examination. Published guidelines suggested obtaining blood glucose, blood cell counts, and electrolyte panels, particularly sodium, in specific clinical circumstances (Krumholz et al., 2007). A lumbar puncture is only indicated if there is reason to suspect an infectious or inflammatory etiology (e.g., if the patient is febrile). Toxicology screening should similarly be restricted to specific clinical circumstances.

## Evaluation of Drug-Resistant Seizures and Epilepsy

When seizures are drug resistant, it is important to reassess the diagnosis of epilepsy. Reevaluation of the history may identify features suggestive of a nonepileptic origin of attacks or incorrect classification of seizures that resulted in an incorrect therapeutic choice. The task may be facilitated by having the description of multiple events to assess precipitating factors and variability or consistency of the seizure manifestations. The patient should be questioned about potentially remediable factors such as alcohol or drug abuse, abuse of caffeine, the use of concomitant medications that can reduce the seizure threshold, sleep deprivation, or poor compliance with prescribed treatment. Most often, additional investigation is needed, particularly prolonged video-EEG recordings to capture typical events for definitive diagnosis.

### Prolonged Electroencephalographic Recordings

Prolonged EEG or video-EEG monitoring increases the probability of capturing events. Modalities include *short-term video-EEG* for 2–8 hours, *ambulatory EEG* with or without video, and *long-term video-EEG*. Short-term monitoring is ideal for individuals whose attacks are very frequent or can be provoked by certain stimuli. It is often very useful for young children who tend to have multiple daily attacks. Its advantages include that it can be an outpatient procedure, making it convenient and less expensive. Ambulatory EEG also has the advantage of being an outpatient procedure, and it allows for patients to be evaluated in their natural environment with its stressors and other seizure triggers. Although it can theoretically be performed with concomitant video, video monitoring is not usually part of this procedure, and the exact correlation between EEG and clinical changes is not possible. The absence of concomitant video makes it difficult to eliminate artifact as the source of apparent discharges. Ambulatory EEG is nevertheless useful to evaluate EEG changes with attacks that occur daily and involve loss of consciousness, since events with loss of consciousness are expected to produce EEG changes if they are epileptic in nature. Ambulatory EEG is less useful for evaluation of subjective events or other events without altered consciousness, which may be FAS. This is because FAS often have subtle or even no associated EEG change. Home video-EEG monitoring allows review of event semiology and may be appropriate if medication withdrawal is not needed to precipitate events.

Inpatient video-EEG monitoring may be the most definitive long-term video-EEG modality, as it allows observation in conjunction with ASM withdrawal. This is necessary when attacks are infrequent and partially controlled with medications. The recording can continue for several days up to weeks if needed. Withdrawal of ASMs may unmask epileptiform EEG abnormalities (true with some ASMs such as benzodiazepines, valproate, and levetiracetam) and may also allow greater seizure propagation that can confirm the diagnosis for some seizures of unclear nature. Methods that can be used to help precipitate attacks include hyperventilation, photic stimulation, sleep deprivation, and other precipitants reported by the patient. Inpatient long-term video-EEG monitoring is the best modality for localization of the epileptogenic zone in patients undergoing evaluation for epilepsy surgery.

## Evaluation of Patients for Epilepsy Surgery

Some 35% of patients with focal-onset seizures are resistant to ASM therapy (Kwan and Brodie, 2000a), making them candidates for epilepsy surgery. Unless there is a clear contraindication to such surgery, these patients typically undergo a presurgical evaluation, the goal of which is to localize the epileptogenic zone. The *epileptogenic zone* is defined as the zone whose resection is necessary and sufficient to eliminate seizures (Lüders, 2008; Rosenow and Luders, 2001). This zone cannot be directly defined by any test but can be estimated by a number of other zones.

The *ictal onset zone* (also called *seizure onset zone* or *pacemaker zone*) is the area of cortex that is generating seizures (Carreño and Lüders, 2008). This zone, if accurately defined, is contained within the epileptogenic zone but may be smaller than the epileptogenic zone. Thus it is possible that seizures start in a section of the epileptogenic zone, but other parts of that zone are able to take on the function of seizure generation once the ictal onset zone is removed. Identifying and defining the ictal onset zone can be challenging, since the earliest detected ictal activity may have already undergone considerable spread from where the seizure actually originated. Even when recording the EEG directly from the brain with implanted electrodes, the ictal onset zone may be missed unless the electrodes were placed directly over that zone.

The *irritative zone* is the zone that generates interictal epileptiform discharges. In the most straightforward situation, the irritative zone is localized within the epileptogenic zone. However, in some cases there may be multiple irritative zones, only one of which corresponds to the epileptogenic zone. One of the more common scenarios is bilateral mesial and lateral temporal irritative zones in a patient with a unilateral mesial temporal epileptogenic zone. The relationship between the irritative zone and the epileptogenic zone may be even more complex. For example, a mesial frontal epileptogenic zone may have a corresponding mesial frontal irritative zone that cannot be detected by scalp EEG, and bilateral temporal irritative zones that do not generate seizures.

The *ictal symptomatogenic zone* is the region that produces the seizure manifestations. If the epileptogenic zone is in primary sensory or motor cortex, the initial seizure manifestations may be related to the function of that cortex; in that situation, the ictal symptomatogenic zone corresponds to the ictal onset zone. However, in many instances, the ictal onset zone is located in silent cortex, and the initial clinical manifestations reflect activation of distant nonsilent areas along the path of seizure propagation. The ictal symptomatogenic zone may be more valuable for lateralization than exact localization because it is most likely that seizures will spread within the hemisphere of origin before spreading to the contralateral hemisphere. However, this is not always the case.

The *epileptogenic lesion* is a structural brain abnormality that is presumed to be the cause of the epilepsy and is usually identified on MRI. The relationship of the epileptogenic lesion to the seizure onset zone is variable. Some lesions such as cortical dysplasia or hypothalamic hamartoma are intrinsically epileptogenic, and seizures may arise from within the lesion. On the other hand, seizures usually arise from brain-surrounding cavernous malformations and benign tumors. In the case of very large lesions, seizures may arise from one aspect of the surrounding brain. It is important to keep in mind that certain lesions are incidental and not necessarily related to the epilepsy. For example, arachnoid cysts and venous malformations are often unrelated or indirectly related to the epilepsy (through association with cortical malformation) (Arroyo and Santamaria, 1997; Morioka et al., 2006; Paetau et al., 1992). Another important factor to keep in mind is that there may be multiple lesions, only one of which is responsible for seizure generation. In general, the identification of an epileptogenic lesion greatly improves the confidence of congruent electrical localization of the ictal onset and irritative zones. Failure to remove the epileptogenic lesion partially or completely is an important cause of surgical failure (Cendes et al., 1995; Clarke et al., 1996).

The *functional deficit zone*, responsible for functional deficits, can be measured in a variety of ways including neurological examination, neuropsychological testing, interictal EEG focal attenuation and slow activity, local glucose uptake by PET, or local cerebral blood flow by interictal PET with [$^{15}$O]$H_2O$ or interictal single-photon emission computed tomography (SPECT). While the functional deficit zone may include the epileptogenic zone, it is often considerably larger. For example, hypometabolism may involve the whole temporal lobe and even extend beyond the temporal lobe in patients with temporal lobe epilepsy and hippocampal sclerosis, in whom the epileptogenic zone may be limited to the hippocampus and parahippocampal gyrus (Henry and Roman, 2011).

The remainder of this section will discuss individual elements of the presurgical evaluation.

## Neurological History

Identifying specific risk factors in the history can help predict the epileptogenic lesion. For example, a history of febrile status epilepticus in infancy has a strong correlation with the pathology of hippocampal sclerosis (Cendes et al., 1993). Meningitis and encephalitis occurring prior to age 5 are also associated with temporal lobe epilepsy and hippocampal sclerosis, whereas the same risk factors occurring after age 5 appear to predict neocortical epileptogenic zones (Marks et al., 1992; O'Brien et al., 2002). Similarly, earlier head trauma may also predict hippocampal sclerosis, though hippocampal sclerosis may also be seen after head trauma at an older age (Diaz-Arrastia et al., 2000; Marks et al., 1995). The description of the seizure aura and other early seizure semiology helps with the localization of the ictal symptomatogenic zone. Certain auras such as rising epigastric sensation are characteristic of mesial temporal localization, while elementary auditory hallucinations at seizure onset favor a lateral temporal localization and elementary visual hallucinations favor an occipital localization (Henkel et al., 2002; Palmini and Gloor, 1992). The description of seizure semiology by witnesses is also helpful, particularly for lateralization. However, since the recording of clinical seizures is an important component of presurgical evaluation, analysis of video-EEG recorded seizure semiology supersedes the description provided by witnesses for the purpose of localization and lateralization.

## Neurological Examination

The neurological examination can identify focal neurological deficits that help define the functional deficit zone, but the examination is most often noncontributory.

## Electroencephalographic and Video-Electroencephalographic Recordings

EEG/video-EEG is a cornerstone of the presurgical evaluation, contributing to the localization of four zones. The interictal focal attenuation and focal slow activity contribute to the definition of the functional deficit zone; the fields of the interictal epileptiform discharges define the irritative zones; and the electrographic localization of seizure onset helps define the ictal onset zone. However, it is important to recognize that what appears to be the initial localization of the ictal discharge may represent seizure activity propagated from a distant location not directly accessible to EEG electrodes. There is evidence to suggest that for ictal EEG activity to be visible on scalp EEG, it should involve at least 10 $cm^2$ of cortex (Tao et al., 2007). Therefore, the initial ictal onset may be visible only after considerable seizure spread. The use of additional electrodes beyond the International 10–20 electrode placement can be useful. This includes additional closely spaced electrodes in the 10-10 system, or electrodes outside of the 10-10 system, such as true anterior temporal electrodes, sphenoidal electrodes, zygomatic electrodes, or cheek electrodes. The International Federation of Clinical Neurophysiology has recommended the standard addition of six inferior temporal electrodes to the 10–20 electrode placement to improve detection of epileptiform activity (Seeck et al., 2017). While clinical scalp EEG is two-dimensional, three-dimensional localization of interictal and ictal EEG signals is possible with *electrical source imaging*. This technique's precision is enhanced with higher-density EEG using at least 64 electrodes from the 10-10 system. Source imaging is used more often with MEG, discussed later in this chapter. For patients in whom the ictal onset zone cannot be properly defined by scalp EEG, it may be necessary to implant intracranial electrodes, discussed later in this section.

The analysis of seizure semiology by video-EEG provides several localizing and lateralizing signs that help define the ictal symptomatogenic zone (Loddenkemper and Kotagal, 2005). For example, early head turning in temporal lobe epilepsy tends to be ipsilateral to the seizure focus, and late head turning preceding evolution to bilateral tonic-clonic activity tends to be contralateral (Fakhoury and Abou-Khalil, 1995). Lip smacking and other oroalimentary automatisms are characteristic of temporal lobe involvement. Extremity dystonic posturing is a strong contralateral lateralizing sign (Kotagal et al., 1989). While extremity automatisms are not directly lateralizing in general, manipulative automatisms tend to be ipsilateral to the seizure onset zone when associated with contralateral dystonic posturing (Dupont et al., 1999). Nonmanipulative automatisms, particularly RINCH motions, tend to be contralateral (Kelemen et al., 2010; Kuba et al., 2013; Lee et al., 2006). Unilateral eye blinking tends to be ipsilateral to the seizure focus (Benbadis et al., 1996a). Well-formed ictal speech is usually indicative of nondominant temporal lobe involvement, whereas postictal aphasia suggests dominant temporal lobe involvement (Gabr et al., 1989). Ictal vomiting, ictal spitting, ictal drinking, and postictal urinary urgency have all been associated with right temporal lobe origin, but exceptions have been reported (Knake et al., 2005; Loddenkemper and Kotagal, 2005). Ictal pouting suggests anterior cingulate localization (Souirti et al., 2014).

## Magnetic Resonance Imaging

A high-resolution MRI is crucial for definition of the epileptogenic lesion (see Figs. 100.12 and 100.16). For optimal detection of mesial temporal sclerosis, the MRI should include oblique coronal images perpendicular to the axis of the hippocampus, including T1-weighted, T2-weighted, and fluid-attenuated inversion recovery (FLAIR) sequences. These images should ideally have a slice thickness of at most 1.5 mm. Ideally the MRI should also include a sequence with T1-weighted thin adjacent images for reformatting and surface rendering. The use of surface coils together with 3-tesla MRI can be very helpful in the definition of cortical dysplasia (Knake et al., 2005). In addition, methods of postprocessing, such as texture or morphometric analysis, can also be very helpful in identifying cortical dysplasia (Bernasconi et al., 2001; Wagner et al., 2011). Diffusion tensor imaging helps define white-matter tracts. Asymmetries may help in lateralization in temporal lobe epilepsy (Ahmadi et al., 2009). Three-dimensional reconstruction of white-matter tracts, also known as *tractography*, allows visualization of altered connectivity in association with cortical dysplasia (Colombo et al., 2009). Diffusion-weighted imaging is occasionally useful in localization and lateralization (O'Brien et al., 2007; Wehner et al., 2007).

## Positron Emission Tomography

PET imaging uses positron-emitting isotopes to image metabolism, perfusion, synthesis of neurotransmitters, and receptor density. The synthesis of positron-emitting ligands requires a cyclotron on site. As a result, PET availability has been relatively limited to major academic centers. At present, the most commonly used ligand is $^{18}$F-fluorodeoxyglucose (FDG), which allows the imaging of glucose uptake/metabolism in the brain. FDG-PET is almost always an interictal study; ictal PET is usually fortuitous and difficult to plan. FDG-PET contributes to the definition of the functional deficit zone. Approximately 80% of patients have a discrete region of hypometabolism that has a good correlation with the side of the epileptic focus in temporal lobe epilepsy (Abou-Khalil et al., 1987). The region of PET hypometabolism is usually larger than the epileptogenic zone (see Fig. 100.13). PET hypometabolism has a greater correlation with the ictal onset zone than scalp EEG-defined ictal onset (Engel et al., 1982). FDG-PET is particularly useful in patients without MRI abnormalities. The identification of temporal hypometabolism corresponding to well-localized electrographic ictal onset and interictal epileptiform activity on EEG may permit sufficient confidence to proceed with epilepsy surgery without invasive monitoring (Carne et al., 2004). FDG-PET can be misleading in some patients with extratemporal epilepsy, showing temporal hypometabolic zones (Radtke et al., 1994). As with other diagnostic techniques, FDG-PET cannot be used in isolation.

PET using flumazenil images central benzodiazepine receptor density. Zones of decreased benzodiazepine receptor density are smaller than, and encompassed in, areas of hypometabolism by FDG-PET. They have a greater specificity for the ictal onset zone (Burdette et al., 1995; Savic et al., 1993). In addition, flumazenil PET may identify heterotopic neurons not visible on MRI (Hammers et al., 2005). PET scanning using $^{11}$C-α-methyl-l-tryptophan (AMT) images serotonin synthesis and is helpful in identifying the epileptogenic tuber in patients with tuberous sclerosis and multiple tubers (Chugani et al., 1998; Fedi et al., 2003). The epileptogenic tuber usually has increased serotonin synthesis. This PET modality has also been found useful in cortical dysplasia (Chugani et al., 2011; Juhasz et al., 2003).

### Single-Photon Emission Computed Tomography

SPECT uses a gamma-emitting tracer to image regional cerebral blood flow. The technique is widely available and is less expensive than PET. Interictally, regions of reduced metabolism also tend to have reduced blood flow, but interictal SPECT is less sensitive than interictal FDG-PET and therefore is not widely used. The main benefit of SPECT is ictal imaging. When the ligand is injected intravenously (IV) at the very onset of seizures, greater uptake is noted in the ictal onset zone (Fig. 100.18). However, if the injection is late, the focal hyperperfusion may represent seizure propagation. The value of ictal SPECT is enhanced by subtraction and co-registration with MRI (SISCOM) (O'Brien et al., 1998, 2000; Van Paesschen et al., 2007). SISCOM is particularly valuable in extratemporal epilepsy and in patients who have had persistent seizures after epilepsy surgery (Wetjen et al., 2006; see Fig. 100.18).

### Magnetic Resonance Spectroscopy

Magnetic resonance spectroscopy (MRS) provides quantitative histochemical information, applied mostly to the hydrogen atom and, to a lesser extent, phosphorus. The most commonly measured substances are *N*-acetyl aspartate (NAA), which is localized in neurons and decreased with neuronal injury, and creatine and choline, which are increased with gliosis and increased membrane turnover. The NAA-to-creatine ratio is highly sensitive in detecting mesial temporal structural and functional abnormalities. The ratio is decreased in abnormal regions. When data are acquired in parallel from a large number of voxels, the voxels that are statistically abnormal can be color coded, generating a map of abnormal areas. In patients with MTLE, there are decrements in the NAA/creatine ratio that extend along the majority of the hippocampal formation and are more pronounced anteriorly (Hetherington et al., 2004). The contralateral hippocampus is involved to a lesser degree, so asymmetries are useful in lateralization of MTLE. The NAA/creatine ratio appears to have a large functional component. The ratio improves contralaterally with successful epilepsy surgery (Kuzniecky et al., 2001). MRS can also be used to measure other compounds such as lactate and GABA (Petroff et al., 2001).

### Magnetoencephalography

Electric currents which produce voltages on the scalp that serve as the basis for EEG also produce magnetic fields that can be measured with MEG. Just like EEG, MEG can track magnetic brain activity in real time. It has an advantage over EEG in that magnetic signals are not distorted by differences in conductivity between the brain, skull, and scalp. However, MEG has similar signal drop-off with distance, which is the inverse square of the distance from the source. MEG does not detect pure hippocampal spikes but can detect propagated spikes, and the dipole orientation is then helpful to distinguish mesial from lateral sources (Knowlton and Shih, 2004). MEG appears slightly more sensitive for convexity neocortical sources than EEG, detecting sources involving 3–4 cm$^2$ of cortex as opposed to 6 cm$^2$ of cortex for the EEG. The latest-generation MEG machines typically contain 300 or more sensors covering most of the head and allowing accurate estimation of the magnetic source dipole origin.

By using fiducial markers, structural MRI, and core registration, the magnetic source can be displayed on the structural MRI, which has been referred to as *magnetic source imaging* (Knowlton and Shih, 2004; Stefan et al., 2011). Magnetic source imaging can be applied to spontaneous magnetic activity as well as to event-related magnetic fields. MEG is used mostly for evaluation of interictal epileptiform activity and thus helps define the irritative zone. While EEG is best at recording epileptiform discharges with a vertical dipole (perpendicular to the gyral surface), MEG best records horizontal dipoles parallel to the surface, so MEG and EEG are complementary in this regard. Availability of MEG remains limited to major academic centers.

MEG is also very useful for localization of cortical functions prior to epilepsy surgery, through the recording and localization of event-related fields. MEG has been used effectively for localization of sensory and language functions (Abou-Khalil, 2007; Papanicolaou et al., 2004). There is evidence to also suggest that it may be able to lateralize memory functions (Ver Hoef et al., 2008).

### Functional Magnetic Resonance Imaging

Local cerebral activation produces a local increase in glucose metabolism, cerebral blood flow, and cerebral metabolic rate for oxygen. The cerebral blood flow increase tends to surpass the increase in cerebral metabolic rate for oxygen so that cerebral activation results in an increase in the capillary and venous oxygenation level and a relative reduction in deoxyhemoglobin. Deoxyhemoglobin is paramagnetic, so an increase in oxygenation produces an increase in magnetic signal. Blood oxygenation level-dependent (BOLD) contrast is the basis of fMRI; fMRI has been used predominantly for localization of cortical functions that have to be spared in epilepsy surgery. It can effectively localize motor and sensory cortex as well as language cortex (Chakraborty and McEvoy, 2008; Janecek et al., 2013). There is also increasing evidence that it can localize memory functions (Binder et al., 2010).

The use of fMRI for epilepsy localization is more experimental at this point. It usually requires concomitant EEG recording during fMRI acquisition (Gotman et al., 2006; Zijlmans et al., 2007). Interictal epileptiform discharges are associated with a hemodynamic change that usually has a latency of several seconds. The hemodynamic change can reflect activation, deactivation, or both. Defining the regions of the brain with hemodynamic changes in response to interictal epileptiform discharges helps define the irritative zone. The most significant hemodynamic response was recently found to correspond to the seizure onset zone in most patients (Khoo et al., 2017). However, only patients with frequent epileptiform discharges can be studied with EEG-fMRI.

### Neuropsychological Testing

Neuropsychological testing helps in the definition of the functional deficit zone. The battery of tests evaluates cortical functions of left and right temporal, frontal, parietal, and occipital lobes. Some tests also help identify mesial versus lateral temporal dysfunction. Localizing information helps to support other tests in the presurgical evaluation. Neuropsychological testing can also help predict postoperative

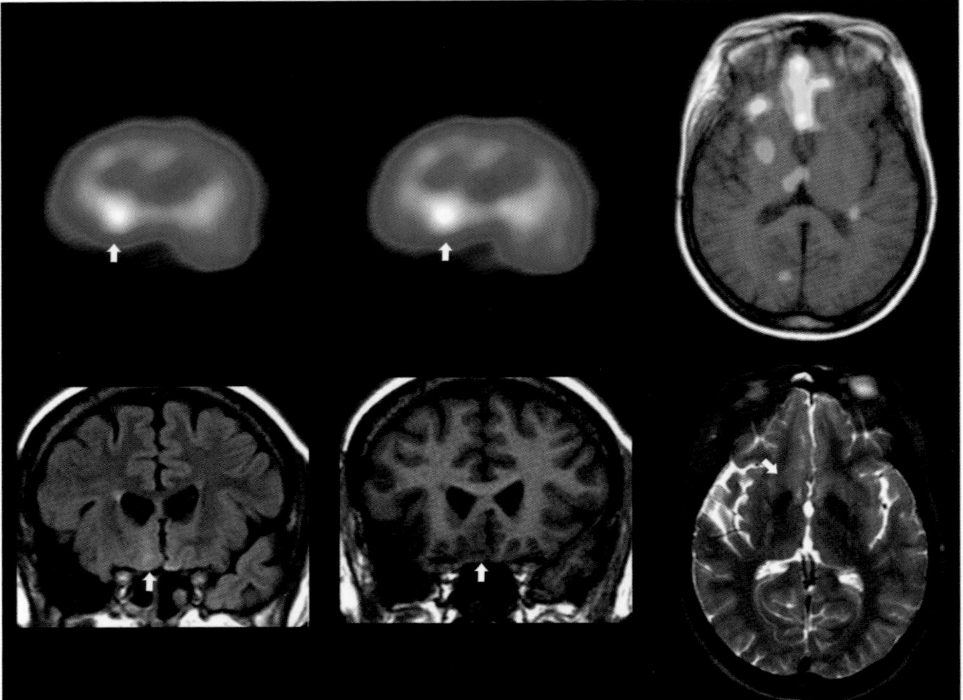

**Fig. 100.18** Ictal single-photon emission computed tomography (SPECT) *(top left and middle)*, magnetic resonance imaging (MRI) *(bottom)*, and subtracted ictal SPECT co-registered to MRI (SISCOM) *(top right)* in patient with drug-resistant seizures persisting after right temporal lobectomy. The two coronal ictal SPECT images demonstrate right orbitofrontal hyperperfusion *(arrows)* corresponding to a region of subtle increased T2 signal, thickened cortex, and blurred gray/white junction on MRI *(arrows)*. MRI images from left to right are coronal fluid-attenuated inversion recovery (FLAIR), coronal T1, and axial T2 images. Surgical pathology was cortical dysplasia with balloon cells. SISCOM demonstrates hyperperfusion corresponding to the orbitofrontal pathology.

deficits, particularly when the planned resection will remove functioning cortex.

### Wada Test

The Wada test involves intracarotid injection of anesthetic, usually amobarbital, to examine language and memory functions in the contralateral hemisphere. The Wada test was initially designed to lateralize language function, but its use was later expanded to examine memory lateralization and assess the risk of memory loss after temporal lobe surgery. It is also useful for defining the functional deficit zone in the mesial temporal region. For example, if a patient fails memory testing after injection of the left hemisphere but passes memory testing after injection of the right hemisphere, this suggests that the right mesial temporal structures are functionally inadequate to support memory. Because the Wada test is invasive, there have been many efforts to replace it (Abou-Khalil, 2007); fMRI and MEG can reliably identify the hemisphere dominant for language functions and can obviate the need for Wada test when memory testing is not necessary.

### Invasive Electroencephalographic Recordings

Surgery may proceed without invasive testing if presurgical results are congruous, if there is a structural or clear functional lesion corresponding to consistent electrical localization, and if there is no definite risk to eloquent cortex. Indications for invasive EEG include:

- An epileptogenic zone that is well lateralized but not well localized; for example, unclear whether frontal or temporal, anterior temporal or posterior temporal, or mesial or lateral temporal.
- Bitemporal ictal onsets or bitemporal frequent epileptiform activity.
- An epileptogenic zone that overlaps with functional cortex.
- Extratemporal or neocortical nonlesional epilepsy.
- Ill-defined epileptogenic zone or incongruent data. It is generally essential to have a hypothesis for the location of the epileptogenic zone in one or two regions prior to invasive recording.

Different types of electrodes can be used for different indications for invasive EEG. Subdural grid electrodes are useful for better localization of a well-lateralized epileptogenic zone and for mapping of functional cortex with electrical stimulation in order to preserve it at the time of surgery. Depth electrodes are useful for lateralization of ictal onset in a patient with apparent bilateral mesial temporal foci, or for recording from relatively inaccessible regions, such as the insula, depth of sulci, or heterotopias. Subdural or epidural strip electrodes are useful for bilateral coverage or for sampling large areas without craniotomy. Foramen ovale electrodes, inserted through the foramen ovale to record from mesial temporal cortex, are useful for lateralization of the epileptogenic zone in patients with apparent bilateral mesial temporal foci. Epidural peg electrodes are inserted into an opening in the skull, outside the dura. Their use eliminates muscle artifact. They can be used to sample electrical activity from large superficial cortical regions.

Subdural electrodes allow mapping of cortical functions with electrical stimulation if there is a possibility that surgery may put these functions at risk. Stimulation of primary motor or primary sensory cortex typically produces positive responses, whereas stimulation of association cortex produces disruption of function if the patient is engaged in a task that requires the function of that cortex. Localization of language cortex requires the patient to be involved in language activities during electrical stimulation. Depth electrodes implanted stereotactically have become the dominant method of invasive EEG recording due to greater tolerability, lower complication rate, and superior flexibility (Mullin et al., 2016; Schmidt et al., 2016).

## MEDICAL THERAPY

Medical therapy is generally the first-line treatment after the diagnosis of epilepsy has been made (Fig. 100.19). Its goal should be complete seizure freedom in the absence of medication side effects. Since the choice of therapy depends on seizure and epilepsy classification, ideally there should be enough evidence to diagnose the seizure type and the epilepsy syndrome prior to deciding on initial therapy. The treating physician must have a low threshold for reevaluating the diagnosis when therapy fails, particularly when the diagnosis of epilepsy is based on history alone without supportive EEG or imaging data.

Pharmacotherapy is not always necessary after a single unprovoked seizure, particularly when the risk of recurrence appears low, based on known predictors (e.g., with a normal EEG and MRI; see earlier discussion of epidemiology of the first unprovoked seizure) (Krumholz et al., 2015). Delay in initiation of therapy until after the second unprovoked seizure does not affect the odds of subsequent long-term remission. Rarely, some mild forms of epilepsy may not require therapy. For example, in BECTS, seizures may be infrequent, occur in sleep, and remit at puberty. In some patients with JME, seizures are clearly linked to sleep deprivation or binge alcohol consumption, and may be managed with lifestyle adjustments only, especially when myoclonic seizures are the only seizure type. In the vast majority of individuals, however, medical therapy is necessary.

### Initiating Therapy

The many ASMs available for prescription include classical ASMs that were marketed before 1980 and many new ASMs that have been marketed since 1993. Knowledge of their pharmacokinetic properties is essential for safe and effective use (Table 100.2). Choice of the first ASM depends primarily on the classification of seizure type and epilepsy syndrome (Table 100.3) but should also take into consideration factors such as age, gender, comorbid conditions, and individual circumstances. The ASM choice should consider the ASM's spectrum of efficacy, its specific pharmacological properties in relation to the patient's specific needs, its

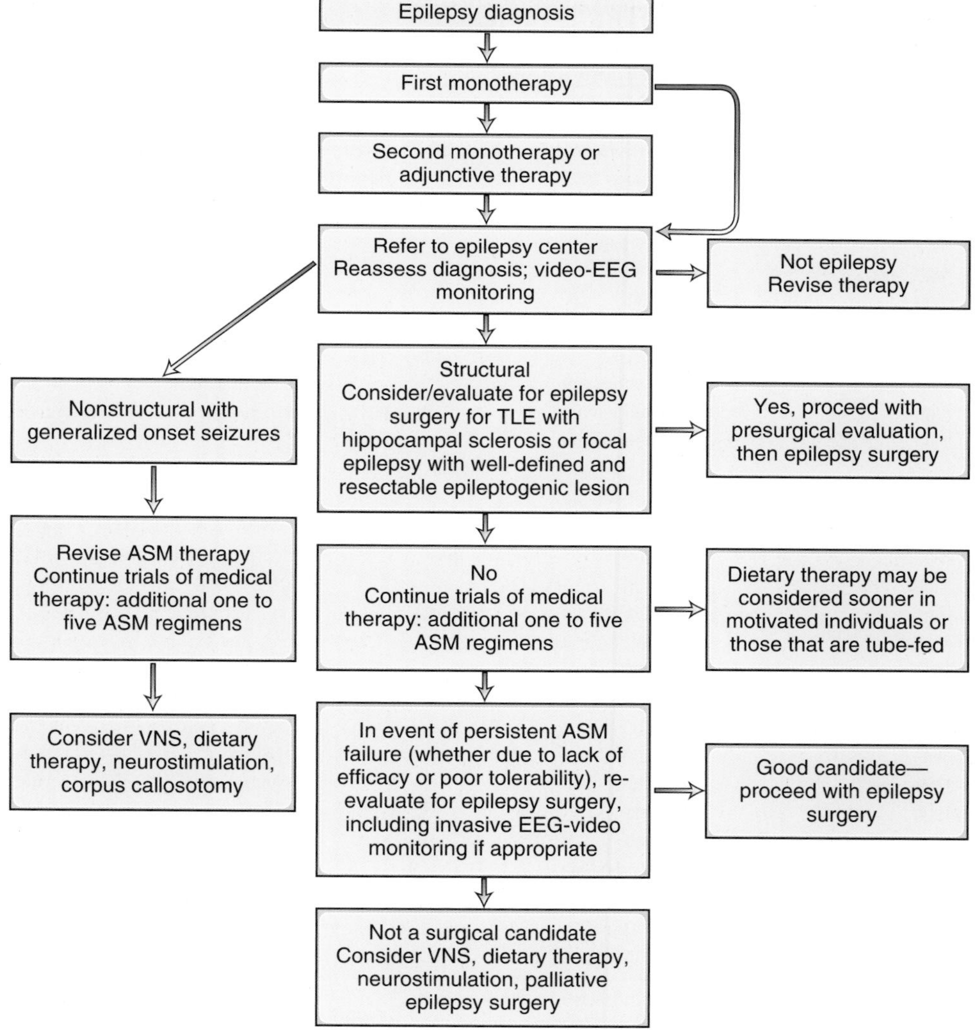


**Fig. 100.19 Treatment Algorithm for Epilepsy.** Additional steps assume that seizures are not controlled despite adequate trial of well-tolerated medication. *AED,* Antiepileptic drug; *EEG,* electroencephalographic; *TLE,* temporal lobe epilepsy; *VNS,* vagus nerve stimulation.

safety profile in the patient's age and gender group, as well as its efficacy in the patient's comorbid conditions. Whenever possible, these determinations should be based on solid evidence derived from well-designed studies. The ASMs with FDA-approved indications outside of epilepsy include clonazepam (panic attacks); carbamazepine (trigeminal neuralgia, bipolar disorder); valproate (migraine prophylaxis, acute treatment, and maintenance for mania/bipolar disorder); gabapentin (postherpetic neuralgia); lamotrigine (maintenance for bipolar disorder); topiramate (migraine prophylaxis); and pregabalin (diabetic peripheral neuropathy, postherpetic neuralgia, fibromyalgia). However, several ASMs are used off-label for a variety of nonepilepsy indications ranging from insomnia to restless legs syndrome and essential tremor, based on trial data or anecdotal evidence (Azar and Abou-Khalil, 2008).

For focal-onset seizures, carbamazepine or phenytoin may be used first, but newer drugs have clear pharmacokinetic advantages, particularly absence of enzyme induction (French et al., 2004). Oxcarbazepine and topiramate were the only ones with official FDA indications, until 2016 when the FDA allowed a drug's efficacy as adjunctive therapy in adults to be extrapolated to efficacy in monotherapy (Abou-Khalil, 2019). Lamotrigine, gabapentin, levetiracetam, zonisamide, lacosamide, and eslicarbazepine acetate have clinical trial evidence supporting their use as initial monotherapy (Kanner et al., 2018a). A large community-based study found that lamotrigine was significantly better than carbamazepine, gabapentin, and topiramate and had a nonsignificant advantage compared to oxcarbazepine with respect to time to treatment failure (Marson et al., 2007a). However, lamotrigine requires slow titration and would not be an appropriate first choice when a rapid onset of action is needed. When rapid therapeutic effect is required, oxcarbazepine and levetiracetam may be the drugs of choice because they can be started at an effective dose. Topiramate also requires slow titration. Because of its cognitive adverse effects, it is not generally the first drug of choice unless comorbidities (e.g., migraine, obesity) favor its use.

For generalized-onset seizures, the initial ASM is dependent on the seizure type(s). For pure generalized absence seizures, ethosuximide is the first drug of choice, based on a comparative trial with valproate and lamotrigine, in which it had the best balance of efficacy and tolerability (Glauser et al., 2010). Valproate was equally effective and may be the best choice if there are concomitant GTC seizures or generalized myoclonic seizures because ethosuximide efficacy is limited to generalized absence seizures. For IGE with GTC seizures, valproate was

**TABLE 100.2 Antiepileptic Drug Absorption, Elimination Half-Life, Formulations (Displayed in Order They Were Marketed in the United States)**

| Antiseizure Medication | Oral Bioavailability<br>High: ≥90%<br>Intermediate: ≥70–<90%<br>Low: <70% | Half-Life (Hours)*<br>Short: ≤10<br>Intermediate: >10–<30<br>Long: ≥30 | Intravenous Formulation | Extended-Release Oral Formulation | Requires Slow Titration |
|---|---|---|---|---|---|
| Phenobarbital | High | Long | X | | |
| Primidone | High | Intermediate | | | X |
| Phenytoin | High | Intermediate | X† | X | |
| Methsuximide‡ | High | Long | | | |
| Ethosuximide | High | Long | | | |
| Clonazepam | High | Long | | | |
| Carbamazepine | Intermediate | Intermediate | | X | X |
| Valproate | High | Intermediate | X | X | |
| Felbamate | High | Intermediate | | | |
| Gabapentin | Low§ | Short | | | |
| Lamotrigine | High | Intermediate | | X | X |
| Topiramate | Intermediate | Intermediate | | X | X |
| Tiagabine | High | Short | | | X |
| Levetiracetam | High | Short | X | X | |
| Oxcarbazepine‡ | High | Intermediate | | X | |
| Zonisamide | High | Long | | | |
| Pregabalin | High | Short | | | |
| Lacosamide | High | Intermediate | X | | |
| Rufinamide | Intermediate | Short | | | X |
| Vigabatrin | High | Short¶ | | | |
| Ezogabine/retigabine | Low | Short | | | X |
| Clobazam | High | Long | | | |
| Perampanel | High | Long | | | |
| Eslicarbazepine | High | Intermediate | | | |
| Brivaracetam | High | Short | X | | |
| Cannabidiol | Low | Long | | | + |
| Cenobamate | Intermediate | Long | | | X |

*The $t_{1/2}$ for antiseizure medication (ASM) given as monotherapy in a young adult.
†Parenteral formulation is also available as fosphenytoin, a phenytoin prodrug that can be administered intramuscularly.
‡Applies to active metabolites (*N*-desmethyl methsuximide for methsuximide, monohydroxy derivative [MHD] for oxcarbazepine).
§Gabapentin bioavailability decreases with increasing dose, ranging from ≈60% after a single 300 mg dose to ≈30% at 4800 mg/day given in three divided doses.
¶The duration of ASM effect is much longer than expected for the short $t_{1/2}$.

**TABLE 100.3 Established Efficacy of Antiseizure Medications by Seizure Type (FDA Indications and Class I–III Evidence)**

| | Fda-Approved Indications | | | | | | | | Other Noteworthy Efficacy Evidence |
|---|---|---|---|---|---|---|---|---|---|
| | Monotherapy Versus Adjunctive Therapy Indication* | | Seizure Type or Syndrome Indication | | | | | | |
| Antiseizure Medication | Monotherapy | Adjunctive | Focal | Generalized Tonic-Clonic | Absence | Myoclonic | LGS | IS | Therapy and Seizure Type |
| Phenobarbital | X | X | X | | | | | | |
| Primidone | X | X | X | | | | | | |
| Phenytoin | X | X | X | X | | | | | |
| Methsuximide | X | X | | | X | | | | Two class IV trials supporting efficacy for focal-onset seizures |
| Ethosuximide | X | X | | | X | | | | |
| Clonazepam | X | X | | | X[†] | X | | | |
| Carbamazepine | X | | X | X | | | | | |
| Valproate | X[‡] | X | X | X[‡] | X | X[‡] | | | Initial monotherapy for generalized tonic-clonic and myoclonic seizures |
| Felbamate | Conversion to monotherapy[§] | X | X | X[‖] | | | X[‖] | | |
| Gabapentin | | X | X | | | | | | Initial monotherapy for focal seizures |
| Lamotrigine | Conversion to monotherapy[§] | X | X | X | | | X[‖] | | Initial monotherapy for absence seizures |
| Topiramate | X | X | X | X | | | X[‖] | | |
| Tiagabine | | X | X | | | | | | |
| Levetiracetam | | X | X | X | | X | | | Initial monotherapy for focal seizures |
| Oxcarbazepine | X | X | X | | | | | | |
| Zonisamide | | X | X | | | | | | Initial monotherapy for focal seizures |
| Pregabalin | | X | X | | | | | | |
| Lacosamide | X | X | X | | | | | | |
| Rufinamide | | X | | | | | X[‖] | | |
| Vigabatrin | X[¶] | X | X | | | | | X[¶] | |
| Ezogabine/retigabine | | X | X | | | | | | |
| Clobazam | | X | | | | | X | | |
| Perampanel | X | X | X | X | | | | | Efficacy against myoclonic seizures |
| Eslicarbazepine | X | X | X | | | | | | |
| Brivaracetam | X | X | X | | | | | | |
| Cannabidiol | | X | | | | | X (also DS) | | |
| Cenobamate | X | X | X | | | | | | |

*DS*, Dravet syndrome; *FDA*, US Food and Drug Administration; *IS*, infantile spasms; *LGS*, Lennox-Gastaut syndrome.

*The FDA indications for older antiseizure medications (ASMs) (first 7 rows) are less specific with respect to monotherapy versus adjunctive indication, and even with respect to seizure type. Official labeling may not specify monotherapy versus adjunctive therapy for older ASMs marketed prior to 1993.

†For patients who have failed ethosuximide.

‡The official FDA indication is initial monotherapy for absence or partial seizures and adjunctive therapy "in patients with multiple seizure types that include absence seizures." Valproate is widely considered a monotherapy drug of choice in patients with idiopathic generalized epilepsy with tonic-clonic or myoclonic seizures.

§For partial-onset seizures only.

‖Adjunctive in LGS.

¶Monotherapy only for infantile spasm.

significantly better than both lamotrigine and topiramate for time to treatment failure (Marson et al., 2007b) and may be the first drug of choice for men, in the absence of prohibitive comorbidities. However, valproate is teratogenic, with dose-related increased risk of major congenital malformation, permanent cognitive impairment, and increased risk of autism in the exposed fetus. A different ASM should be used first in women with IGE, but valproate may be used at a low dose if other ASMs fail to control seizures (Montouris and Abou-Khalil, 2009). While no ASM has official FDA initial monotherapy indication for generalized myoclonic seizures, valproate is clearly effective, and levetiracetam, which has FDA approval as adjunctive therapy for generalized myoclonic seizures (Noachtar et al., 2008), may also be effective in monotherapy. Weaker evidence exists for efficacy of topiramate, zonisamide, and lamotrigine (lamotrigine may even aggravate myoclonic seizures in some individuals) (Biton and Bourgeois, 2005; Crespel et al., 2005; Genton et al., 2006; Prasad et al., 2003). The newest drugs perampanel and brivaracetam also have anecdotal evidence of efficacy.

For all epilepsy indications, treatment is initiated with an ASM monotherapy. In the absence of urgency, it is preferable to start at a low dose and titrate slowly, even for ASMs that can be started at a higher effective dose. The initial target dose is often the minimal effective dose that has been demonstrated in clinical trials, keeping in mind that the pivotal clinical trials may have underestimated or overestimated that dose in some instances. If the initial target dose is not sufficient, the ASM dose can then be titrated gradually until efficacy is established. For patients with infrequent seizures, it may take a long time to determine when an effective dose has been reached. Therefore it is wise for the initial target dose to be an average rather than a minimum effective dose. Before a medication can be considered ineffective, it usually has to be titrated to the highest tolerated dose. If a medication fails due to lack of efficacy, the neurologist may choose either replacement monotherapy or adjunctive therapy with another medication. The available evidence is that the two options do not differ significantly in either efficacy or tolerability (Beghi et al., 2003; Kwan and Brodie, 2000b). If the initial therapy has been completely ineffective, then replacement monotherapy is the best choice. If the initial therapy was partially effective, adjunctive therapy may be a consideration. If medication failure is due to lack of tolerability, then replacement monotherapy is the clearly preferable option. Replacement monotherapy usually requires initially adding the new ASM before withdrawing the old agent. However, overnight switch is possible for some ASMs such as carbamazepine and oxcarbazepine (Albani et al., 2004).

Adjunctive therapy should take into consideration any possible pharmacodynamic or pharmacokinetic interactions between the medications in question (Table 100.4). Ideally, the added medication should not have adverse pharmacokinetic or pharmacodynamic interactions (Abou-Khalil, 2017). All ASMs are appropriate for adjunctive therapy (Kanner et al., 2018b). Some ASM combinations have a suggestion of synergy. For example, the lamotrigine and valproate combination seems to have greater efficacy than what would be predicted by the efficacy of each ASM alone (Brodie and Yuen, 1997). There is also evidence favoring the combination of lamotrigine and levetiracetam (Kinirons et al., 2006).

At present, the ASM mechanism of action (Table 100.5) is not crucial for initial ASM selection (Guimaraes and Ribeiro, 2010), but there is a suggestion that combining two ASMs with different mechanisms may have a greater chance of efficacy than combining two ASMs with the same mechanism (Brodie and Sills, 2011; Margolis et al., 2014). Mechanism of action may be a predictor of adverse effects from pharmacodynamic interactions. For example, dizziness, ataxia, and diplopia are more likely when combining lacosamide with another agent that acts on the sodium channel (Novy et al., 2011; Sake et al., 2010). The neurologist will often need to reduce the dose of the initial ASM when adding a second ASM with a similar mechanism of action. A better understanding of the epilepsy pathophysiology in individual patients may improve the selection of ASMs in the future, with a greater role for mechanism of action.

There are limited examples of epilepsy genetics predicting ASM efficacy. Autosomal dominant nocturnal frontal lobe epilepsy is particularly responsive to carbamazepine and its analog, oxcarbazepine (Picard et al., 1999; Raju et al., 2007). Dravet syndrome, which is usually caused by a sodium channel mutation, may have seizure aggravation with the use of agents acting on the sodium channel, particularly lamotrigine (Guerrini et al., 1998).

## Antiseizure Medication Considerations Based on Age and Gender

Age and gender may have an influence on ASM selection (Azar and Abou-Khalil, 2008). In the pediatric age group, specific epilepsy syndromes have implications for ASM efficacy. Tolerability profiles may also be different for children and adults, which may influence the risk/benefit ratio for specific agents. Serious rashes from lamotrigine, behavioral adverse effects from levetiracetam, and oligohidrosis from topiramate and zonisamide are more likely in children, while hyponatremia from oxcarbazepine and aplastic anemia from felbamate are much less likely. Valproate-induced liver failure is more likely in children younger than 2 years of age. In women of childbearing potential, certain ASMs may reduce the efficacy of oral contraception, and valproate is to be avoided for two important reasons: higher risk of congenital malformations in the exposed fetus and increased risk of polycystic ovaries and hyperandrogenism (Lofgren et al., 2007).

In the elderly, a key consideration is interaction with other medications, which favors newer nonenzyme-inducing ASMs (Arain et al., 2009). Some ASM adverse effects are more likely in the elderly—for example, reversible parkinsonism and cognitive impairment from valproate (Armon et al., 1996) and hyponatremia from oxcarbazepine, particularly when combined with diuretics or other agents that may lower sodium (Dong et al., 2005). Several trials have examined the comparative efficacy and tolerability of ASMs in the elderly. Lamotrigine and gabapentin were better tolerated than immediate-release carbamazepine in new-onset geriatric epilepsy (Brodie et al., 1999; Rowan et al., 2005), but no difference was found between lamotrigine and extended-release carbamazepine (Saetre et al., 2007).

## Pharmacoresistance, Tolerance, and Seizure Aggravation

Persistence of seizures despite ASM therapy should always prompt reevaluation of the diagnosis; one of the most common causes of apparent drug resistance is misdiagnosis of nonepileptic psychogenic seizures. Other causes of apparent pharmacoresistance include breakthrough seizures related to noncompliance, sleep deprivation (particularly in IGE), alcohol or drug abuse, and co-medications that reduce the seizure threshold. In addition, seizures may appear resistant because of incorrect ASM selection or inadequate ASM use.

Approximately a third of individuals with epilepsy will not become seizure free at follow-up despite adequate ASM therapy (Chen et al., 2018; Kwan and Brodie, 2000a). However, the definition of the exact time point when epilepsy is considered drug resistant has not been agreed upon. An ILAE task force recommended the definition of *drug-resistant epilepsy* as "failure of adequate trials of two tolerated, appropriately chosen and used antiepileptic drug schedules (whether as monotherapies or in combination) to achieve sustained seizure freedom" (Kwan et al., 2010).

**TABLE 100.4 Hepatic Metabolism, Enzyme Induction/Inhibition, Pharmacokinetic Interactions, and Protein Binding**

| Antiseizure Medication | Hepatic Metabolism | Hepatic Enzyme Induction | Autoinduction | Hepatic Enzyme Inhibition | Affected by Enzyme Inducers | Affected by Enzyme Inhibitors | Protein Binding |
|---|---|---|---|---|---|---|---|
| | High: >90%<br>Intermediate: ≥50% to ≤90%<br>Low: <50% | +Minimal<br>++Intermediate<br>+++Pronounced<br>−Absent | | | +Affected<br>−Not Affected | | High: ≥85%<br>Low: <85% |
| Phenobarbital | Intermediate | +++ | − | − | + | + | Low |
| Primidone | Intermediate | +++ | − | − | + | + | Low |
| Phenytoin | High | +++ | − | − | + | + | High |
| Methsuximide | Low | + | − | − | + | − | Low |
| Ethosuximide | Intermediate | − | − | − | + | − | Low |
| Clonazepam | Intermediate | − | − | − | − | − | High |
| Carbamazepine | High | +++ | +++ | − | + | + | Low |
| Valproate | High | − | − | +++ | + | + | High |
| Felbamate | Intermediate | + | − | ++ | + | + | Low |
| Gabapentin | None | − | − | − | − | − | None |
| Lamotrigine | High | + | + | − | + | + | None |
| Topiramate | Low | +* | − | +* | + | − | Low |
| Tiagabine | High | − | − | − | + | − | High |
| Levetiracetam | None | − | − | − | ± | − | Low |
| Oxcarbazepine | High | ++† | − | +† | + | + | Low |
| Zonisamide | Intermediate | − | − | − | + | + | Low |
| Pregabalin | None | − | − | − | − | − | None |
| Lacosamide | Low | − | − | − | + | − | Low |
| Rufinamide | High | + | − | + | + | + | Low |
| Vigabatrin | None | + | − | − | − | − | None |
| Ezogabine/retigabine | Intermediate | − | − | − | + | − | Low |
| Clobazam | High | + | − | + | + | + | Low |
| Perampanel | High | + | − | − | + | − | High |
| Eslicarbazepine | High | + | − | + | + | − | Low |
| Brivaracetam | High | − | − | − | + | − | Low |
| Cannabidiol | High | − | − | + | + | + | High |
| Cenobamate | High | + | − | ++ | + | − | Low |

*Applies to dose ≥200 mg.
†Applies to dose ≥900 mg.

Drug resistance may be related to the underlying epilepsy pathology. Idiopathic epilepsy is less likely to be drug resistant than symptomatic epilepsy (Berg et al., 2001b). In one large study, 82% of patients with generalized idiopathic epilepsy were seizure free for the past year as compared with only 35% of symptomatic focal epilepsy, 25% of patients with cerebral dysgenesis, 11% of patients with temporal lobe epilepsy due to mesial temporal sclerosis, and 3% of patients with dual pathology (Semah et al., 1998). Initial seizure frequency was also a predictor (Berg et al., 2001a). In one study, drug resistance was seen in 51% of individuals who had more than 20 seizures before starting treatment, versus 29% of those who had fewer than 20 seizures (Kwan and Brodie, 2000a). Other predictors of drug resistance were history of acute symptomatic or neonatal status epilepticus and focal EEG slow activity. Age at onset between 5 and 9 years predicted a lower risk of resistance (Berg et al., 2001a).

Resistance to the first ASM predicts resistance to the next ASM. In the landmark study of Kwan and Brodie, 47% of patients with newly treated epilepsy became seizure free with the first ASM monotherapy, 13% with the second ASM monotherapy, and 1% with the third ASM monotherapy. Among patients who failed the first ASM, 11% became seizure free if the first ASM was ineffective, while 41%–55% became seizure free if the first ASM was not tolerated owing to side effects or idiosyncratic reaction (Kwan and Brodie, 2000a). In a follow-up report of 1795 patients, the 1-year seizure-free rate was 50.5% on the first drug regimen, 11.6% on the second regimen, and 4.4% on the third regimen (Chen et al., 2018).

Other studies have suggested that continued ASM trials have a greater chance of achieving remission than suggested by the study of Kwan and Brodie. In one study of continued ASM trials in drug-resistant epilepsy, 14% achieved a 6-month terminal seizure remission after 3 years of follow-up with medication therapy only (Callaghan et al., 2007). In a separate study, about 16% of all drug introductions resulted in seizure freedom for more than 12 months, and 28% of patients were rendered seizure free by a drug introduction over 5 years of follow-up (Luciano and Shorvon, 2007). Negative clinical predictors in these studies included history of status epilepticus, younger age at intractability, greater number of failed drug therapies, and presence of intellectual disability. Shorter-duration epilepsy and idiopathic epilepsy were favorable predictors. Failure of ASM therapy suggests the need to consider alternative therapies discussed later in this chapter.

**TABLE 100.5 Key Known Antiseizure Medication Mechanisms of Action**

| Antiseizure Medication | Sodium Channels | Potassium Channel | Enhancing GABA | Glutamate Receptor | High-Voltage Activated Calcium Channels | T-Calcium Channels | $\alpha_2\delta$-Subunit of Voltage-Activated Calcium Channels | SV2A | Comment |
|---|---|---|---|---|---|---|---|---|---|
| Phenobarbital | | | X | X | X | | | | |
| Primidone | | | X | X | | | | | |
| Phenytoin | X | | | | | | | | |
| Methsuximide | ? | | | | | X | | | |
| Ethosuximide | | | | | | X | | | |
| Clonazepam | | | X | | | | | | |
| Carbamazepine | X | | | | | | | | |
| Valproate | X | | X | | | X | | | |
| Felbamate | X | | X | X | X | | | | NMDA receptor antagonism |
| Gabapentin | | | | | | | X | | |
| Lamotrigine | X | | | | X | | | | |
| Topiramate | X | | X | X | | | | | Kainate and AMPA receptor antagonism |
| Tiagabine | | | X | | | | | | Inhibition of GABA reuptake |
| Levetiracetam | | | | | | | | X | |
| Oxcarbazepine | X | | | | | | | | |
| Zonisamide | X | | | | | X | | | |
| Pregabalin | | | | | | | X | | |
| Lacosamide | X | | | | | | | | Selective enhancing of slow inactivation of voltage-gated sodium channels |
| Rufinamide | X | | | | | | | | |
| Vigabatrin | | | X | | | | | | Irreversible inhibition of GABA transaminase |
| Ezogabine/retigabine | | X | | | | | | | Enhancing of transmembrane potassium currents |
| Clobazam | | | X | | | | | | |
| Perampanel | | | | X | | | | | Noncompetitive antagonism of AMPA glutamate receptors |
| Eslicarbazepine | X | | | | | | | | |
| Brivaracetam | | | | | | | | X | |
| Cannabidiol | | | X | | | | | | Also modulates intracellular calcium |
| Cenobamate | X | | X | | | | | | |

*AMPA*, α-Amino-3-hydroxy-5-methyl-4-isoxazole-propionic acid; *GABA*, γ-aminobutyric acid; *NMDA*, *N*-methyl-D-aspartate; *SV2A*, synaptic vesicle protein 2A.

Drug resistance does not always manifest early in the course of epilepsy. It may develop after a variable latency, may be overcome with the use of a new ASM, and may be punctuated by periods of drug responsiveness, particularly with the use of new ASMs (Schmidt and Loscher, 2005a). In the follow-up study by Brodie and colleagues of 1098 patients with newly diagnosed epilepsy, 68% were seizure free for at least 1 year at the last clinic visit. Upon reviewing the course of seizure control, 37% achieved early and sustained seizure freedom, 22% had sustained seizure freedom after a delay, 16% had a pattern of alternating seizure freedom and relapse, while 25% never attained seizure freedom (Brodie et al., 2012). In one group of patients evaluated for resective epilepsy surgery, the mean latency to failure of the second

ASM was 9.1 years (range, 0–48), and 26% of patients reported at least 1 year of seizure freedom after the second unprovoked seizure (Berg et al., 2003).

Pharmacoresistance may have more than one mechanism. One proposed mechanism is that ASMs do not reach the epileptogenic zone in sufficient concentration because of multidrug transporters that transport ASMs out of neurons. A number of findings support this hypothesis indirectly, but there is no direct evidence of causality (Schmidt and Loscher, 2009). Another key hypothesis is that the ASM target (e.g., channels, receptors) is no longer sensitive to the ASM. Disease severity may play a role and may have common neurobiological factors with pharmacoresistance (Schmidt and Loscher, 2009). Another explanation for the loss of an ASM response is tolerance, which is established with benzodiazepines but likely occurs with other ASMs as well (Loscher and Schmidt, 2006).

Seizure aggravation may occur with a number of medications (Chaves and Sander, 2005). This is most common in generalized epilepsy, where ASMs such as carbamazepine, oxcarbazepine, phenytoin, tiagabine, gabapentin, or vigabatrin may increase the number of seizures or provoke the appearance of new seizure types (myoclonic or absence seizures) at a therapeutic level. In addition, any ASM may cause a paradoxical increase in seizures in some patients. This phenomenon has been documented with levetiracetam (Nakken et al., 2003). A number of ASMs have been reported to increase seizure frequency or severity as a manifestation of toxicity, with ASM serum levels above "therapeutic" range. This is well documented for phenytoin but may also occur with other agents. Finally, seizure exacerbation may occur in the setting of ASM-induced encephalopathy or with sedation. For example, seizures may be exacerbated with valproate-induced encephalopathy, and sedative ASMs may exacerbate tonic seizures in patients with Lennox-Gastaut syndrome.

## Medication Adverse Effects

It is essential to know the most common and the most serious adverse effects of ASMs before using them. Such potential adverse effects should be discussed with the patient before prescribing any medication. The most common adverse effects are dose dependent and will predictably occur if titration continues (Toledano and Gil-Nagel, 2008). Their appearance indicates that the dose should be reduced. These adverse effects are most likely to occur at the time of greatest serum concentration following medication intake, in which case they could be alleviated without dose reduction by splitting the dose, taking the medication with food, or using an extended-release preparation. Some dose-dependent adverse effects can be predicted by the mechanism of action. For example, the most common dose-dependent adverse effects with medications acting on the sodium channel (phenytoin, carbamazepine, oxcarbazepine, lamotrigine) are dizziness, ataxia, and diplopia. Sedation is common and sometimes unavoidable with benzodiazepines and barbiturates acting on the GABA receptor. In general, dose-dependent adverse effects are reversible with dose reduction or medication discontinuation. Cognitive and behavioral adverse effects of ASMs could be considered in the category of dose-dependent adverse effects, although some individuals may be predisposed by virtue of genetic or other factors. Barbiturates and benzodiazepines are best known to affect cognition, but any ASM can cause impairment of concentration and memory. Among the new ASMs, topiramate and zonisamide are the most likely to impair cognition, while lamotrigine is the least likely. Depression may occur with any ASM, and psychosis is an uncommon adverse effect of many ASMs but seems more likely associated with topiramate, vigabatrin, and levetiracetam.

Long-term adverse effects of ASMs are often overlooked but could be more concerning because they are difficult to reverse or at times are irreversible. Common examples include weight gain seen with valproate and pregabalin, and weight loss noted with topiramate and zonisamide. Barbiturate chronic use may be associated with frozen shoulder and Dupuytren contractures. One of the more recently appreciated chronic adverse effects of ASMs is reduction in bone mineral density. This is most likely to occur with chronic use of enzyme-inducing ASMs but has also been associated with valproate and other nonenzyme-inducing agents (Ensrud et al., 2004, 2008; Farhat et al., 2002). It is unclear whether any ASM is not detrimental to bone density, and bone mineral density reduction may have different mechanisms with different drugs. It is therefore advisable to monitor bone density with chronic ASM therapy, and to supplement vitamin D and calcium. The enzyme-inducing ASMs carbamazepine and phenytoin have been associated with serological markers of vascular risk, ameliorated upon switching to lamotrigine or levetiracetam (Mintzer et al., 2009). Another long-term adverse effect of ASMs is potential for teratogenicity (Kluger and Meador, 2008) as well as reduced IQ in exposed infants. This adverse effect is most pronounced with valproate (Meador et al., 2009). Valproate in utero exposure also increases risk of autism (Christensen et al., 2013).

Idiosyncratic adverse effects are not dose dependent but rather depend on individual patient genetic predisposition. They most commonly affect organs such as the liver, skin, and blood. Examples include hepatotoxicity, which may occur with valproate and felbamate; Stevens-Johnson syndrome, which may occur with several ASMs including phenytoin, carbamazepine, and lamotrigine; and aplastic anemia, which may occur with felbamate and (more rarely) carbamazepine. There are some predictors for these serious adverse effects. For example, valproate hepatotoxicity is more likely in children younger than 2 years, particularly those with mitochondrial disease (Bjornsson, 2008). Stevens-Johnson syndrome and toxic epidermal necrolysis with carbamazepine are more likely in individuals of Asian descent who carry the *HLA-B1502* allele. Prior immune disorder and prior cytopenia are risk factors for felbamate-associated aplastic anemia (Pellock et al., 2006). In some instances, genetic testing may identify individuals at greater risk of idiosyncratic reactions, but there is a need for progress in the field of epilepsy pharmacogenomics (Kasperaviciute and Sisodiya, 2009).

## Therapeutic Drug Monitoring

Monitoring ASM levels should be used predominantly as an adjunct to clinical decision making rather than the determinant of ASM dose. An ASM is typically titrated to the lowest dose known to be effective, but titration may stop earlier if it is clear that seizure freedom has already been achieved at a lower dose. Once a clinically effective dose has been reached, a serum drug level is then obtained for future reference. Routine drug levels are not necessary, and the level does not have to be repeated after that unless a breakthrough seizure occurs. The new level can be compared to the baseline reference level to determine whether a drop in the level played a role in the seizure. A serum level can also be helpful to determine how much room there is to increase the dose if seizures have not yet come under control. ASM serum levels are valuable to help explain lack of ASM efficacy at what appears to be a relatively high dose or appearance of adverse effects at a relatively low dose. One explanation for lack of efficacy is noncompliance. If seizures have not come under control and the ASM serum level is 0, it is likely that the patient is not actually taking the medication. Another reason for a low serum level may be fast metabolism, either due to genetic factors or due to enzyme induction by a concomitant medication. Similarly, serum levels can be useful to explain toxicity at a relatively low dose. Adverse effects may be due to an elevated serum level as a result of slow metabolism (either due to genetic factors or to hepatic or renal dysfunction) or pharmacokinetic interaction.

A therapeutic range is quoted for some ASMs, particularly classical ASMs such as phenytoin, carbamazepine, and valproate. Although a useful guide, a value outside the range should never be the only basis for dosage change. This therapeutic range may be helpful for patients with infrequent seizures, for whom ascertainment of effective seizure control may take a very long time. For these patients, aiming for a level in the middle of the range may be advisable. The classical ASM for which serum levels may be the most helpful is phenytoin. Phenytoin has nonlinear kinetics, and its serum level can fluctuate widely with small changes in dose or bioavailability. When the dose is being titrated in a patient with difficult-to-control seizures, it may be difficult to predict when to stop increasing the dose, and the level may have to be checked intermittently during this process. The usually quoted therapeutic range is 10–20 μg/mL. If the level is found to be at 20 μg/mL, additional titration may result in toxicity. Nevertheless, it is ill advised to reduce the dose for a level above 20 if the patient has good seizure control and no adverse effects. A therapeutic range is less established for many of the new-generation ASMs. Lamotrigine levels have been better evaluated than other new ASMs. Toxic adverse effects are likely to occur with a level greater than 20 μg/mL, and few patients are expected to derive therapeutic benefit beyond this point (Hirsch et al., 2004).

For two medications that are highly protein bound, protein-free levels may have added value. Phenytoin and valproate are approximately 90% protein bound, and the protein-free portion is responsible for efficacy and toxicity (Levy and Schmidt, 1985). The total level is usually a good predictor of the free level. However, in instances where the proportion of protein binding may be altered, the total serum level is a poor predictor of the protein-free level. These situations include low-protein states such as malnutrition, hepatic failure, and renal failure, the combined use of phenytoin and valproate, which compete for protein binding, and pregnancy. The elderly may also have a greater protein-free portion. Valproate has saturation kinetics for protein binding such that there is a greater proportion of free valproate at higher levels. Protein-free serum levels have greater value in guiding therapy in the special situations noted.

### Discontinuation of Antiseizure Medication Therapy

Owing to the potential adverse effects of ASMs, particularly long-term adverse effects, discontinuation of ASM therapy should be considered when it is no longer necessary. Although there are several predictors of sustained remission on no medications, there is never a guarantee that seizures will not recur after ASM discontinuation. The decision to withdraw ASMs is easiest to make when the epileptic syndrome is known to remit. One example of such a syndrome is BECTS, which is known to remit at puberty. On the other hand, JME, the most common idiopathic generalized epilepsy syndrome, is known to have a very high risk of seizure recurrence; pharmacological therapy is expected to be lifelong in the majority of patients.

Most patients will not be diagnosed with a specific syndrome whose course is well known. In a study of 294 children with nonsyndromic epilepsy followed for more than 10 years, complete remission, defined as 5 years seizure free and medication free, was achieved by 58% of children (Berg et al., 2011). Good seizure outcome at 2 years and no known underlying cause of epilepsy were predictors of remission, while older age at onset was independently associated with a poorer chance of complete remission.

The decision to withdraw medications must balance the potential consequences of seizure relapse and the potential benefits of eliminating medication side effects and costs on an individual basis (Shih and Ochoa, 2009). The risk of seizure recurrence after ASM discontinuation is lower in children than in adults, and the potential psychosocial consequences of recurrent seizures are fewer in children. Hence ASM withdrawal is considered sooner in children, usually after 1 or 2 years of seizure freedom. In a meta-analysis of ASM discontinuation, the overall risk of relapse after ASM discontinuation was 25% at 1 year and 29% at 2 years. Relapse was more likely in patients with remote symptomatic seizures than in patients with idiopathic seizures, and with adolescent-onset versus childhood-onset epilepsy; an abnormal EEG was associated with a relative risk of 1.45. One study found a greater predictive value for serial EEGs obtained after initiating ASM withdrawal (Galimberti et al., 1993). Other factors associated with a greater risk of recurrence in other studies are focal seizures and longer than 5 years to attain seizure freedom. Early ASM response predicted successful ASM withdrawal in children (Shih and Ochoa, 2009). A prospective multicenter randomized study of continued ASM treatment versus slow withdrawal over 6 months reported that 41% of those in the withdrawal group relapsed at 2 years, compared to 22% of patients on continued treatment (Medical Research Council Antiepileptic Drug Withdrawal Study Group, 1991).

Additional factors predicting recurrence in adults have included longer duration of active disease, shorter number of years of seizure remission, abnormal psychiatric examination, presence of hippocampal atrophy, abnormal neurological findings, IQ below 70, increased number of seizures, focal-onset seizures, and multiple seizure types (Shih and Ochoa, 2009). Seizure relapse in adults will restrict driving privileges and may endanger employment, particularly in certain occupations. There is also a concern that seizure control may be difficult to regain (Schmidt and Loscher, 2005b). Hence, discontinuation of ASMs in seizure-free adults is usually delayed for at least 4 years and occasionally postponed indefinitely.

The optimal rate of ASM withdrawal after remission has not been established scientifically. Abrupt discontinuation of ASMs is not appropriate in this setting. Severe seizures have been reported during withdrawal of some ASMs, including benzodiazepines, carbamazepine, and oxcarbazepine. It is generally agreed that ASMs in general and medications associated with tolerance (e.g., benzodiazepines) in particular should be withdrawn gradually.

## SURGICAL THERAPY

### Timing

If seizures fail to come under control with medications, surgical therapy is considered. An ILAE task force suggested that failure of *two* tolerated, appropriately chosen, and used ASM schedules constitutes medical failure (Kwan et al., 2010). This was in part based on the finding that when two ASM monotherapies have failed, the chances that additional medical therapy will provide complete seizure control diminish considerably (Kwan and Brodie, 2000a). It is reasonable at that point to refer the patient to an epilepsy center, particularly if the underlying epilepsy is surgically remediable and surgical results are expected to be excellent. Examples include temporal lobe epilepsy with hippocampal sclerosis and focal epilepsy with underlying focal epileptogenic lesion. However, if expected surgical results are less favorable, it is reasonable to continue medical therapy using different monotherapies and various combinations (see Fig. 100.19). In a study by Selwa et al., (2003), continued changes in ASM regimen rendered about 20% of patients who were not candidates for epilepsy surgery seizure free at 4-year follow-up. It is important to keep in mind that surgical outcome and chances of seizure freedom after postoperative ASM withdrawal are better with earlier surgery, so epilepsy surgery should not be delayed for too long (Simasathien et al., 2013).

Evaluation for epilepsy surgery should probably not be pursued for patients who are noncompliant with medications—and therefore have not actually failed medical therapy. Nor should surgery be pursued for patients with only brief, subjective FAS (i.e., isolated auras) since these seizures often persist after epilepsy surgery.

## Presurgical Evaluation

An extensive presurgical evaluation is necessary before considering epilepsy surgery and has already been discussed in detail (see Evaluation and Diagnosis). Its purposes are to (1) localize the epileptogenic zone (whose resection is necessary and sufficient to eliminate seizures), (2) identify incongruent evidence that may indicate the need for additional tests including invasive EEG, and (3) determine whether planned surgical resection poses risk to cerebral functions. Essential elements of the presurgical evaluation include interictal and ictal EEG, video analysis of recorded seizures, and structural imaging with MRI to identify an epileptogenic lesion. Interictal PET scanning with FDG and neuropsychological testing are also commonly part of the presurgical evaluation. In cases where interictal EEG abnormalities are consistently focal and congruent with a focal unilateral structural epileptogenic lesion, some have advocated skipping ictal EEG recordings, particularly where resources are limited. Complex scenarios where there is incongruence in the presurgical data require additional testing that should include functional imaging with PET, ictal SPECT, MEG, or even invasive EEG with implanted intracranial electrodes. The decision to proceed with surgery should balance the predicted benefits of epilepsy surgery against the predicted risks of functional deficits that might result from surgery.

## Surgical Approaches

Epilepsy surgery can be classified as either curative or palliative. The aim of curative surgery is to eliminate seizures completely and potentially produce permanent remission without the need for ASMs. Palliative surgery is considered only if "curative" surgery is not viable.

The most common epilepsy localization is mesial temporal, specifically amygdalohippocampal. The most common surgical approach has been a *temporal lobectomy* in which lateral temporal cortex is resected first, followed by resection of the amygdala and hippocampus. The resection size is typically different for dominant and nondominant resection. The lateral resection usually measures around 6 cm from the temporal pole on the right but is less extensive on the left to reduce the chance of language deficits. The typical left dominant temporal lobectomy measures about 4 cm from the temporal pole (Wiebe et al., 2001). Dominant temporal lobectomies often spare the superior temporal gyrus in an effort to reduce risk of language disturbance, but a randomized prospective trial did not suggest that this was associated with benefit (Hermann et al., 1999). Some centers tailor the resection based on preoperative language functional mapping with electrical stimulation or fMRI. The hippocampal resection usually measures about 3 cm. One study suggested that a more complete hippocampal resection was associated with greater chance of postoperative seizure freedom (Wyler et al., 1995), but the findings were not confirmed in a second study (Schramm et al., 2011).

For individuals with clear hippocampal sclerosis, *selective amygdalohippocampectomy* (SAH) is an alternative approach with less risk to language functions and equal outcome for seizure control (Tanriverdi et al., 2008). The original approach advocated by Yasargil was trans-sylvian (Siegel et al., 1990), but the same operation could use a transcortical approach through the middle temporal gyrus, or an inferior temporal approach. No clear difference in surgical outcome was noted in a study comparing transcortical and trans-sylvian approaches, but phonemic fluency was significantly improved after transcortical but not after trans-sylvian SAH (Lutz et al., 2004). The "Spencer" approach involves resection of the anterior 3 cm of the temporal pole to expose mesial temporal structures for resection (Spencer et al., 1984). A favorable surgical outcome with respect to seizure control requires inclusion of the parahippocampal gyrus in the surgical resection (Siegel et al., 1990). Recently, laser ablation under real-time MR thermographic guidance has been proposed as an alternative to open resection in patients with hippocampal sclerosis (Gross et al., 2018). Its main advantages are decreased surgical morbidity and better cognitive outcome (Drane et al., 2015). This approach can also be used for other small deep epileptogenic lesions. Radiofrequency thermoablation has been used less frequently to lesion deep epileptogenic foci. It can be applied via depth electrodes already implanted for localization purposes, but with the disadvantage of less temperature control (Voges et al., 2018).

*Lesionectomy* is a suitable surgical approach when there is a well-defined structural lesion such as benign tumor or cavernous malformation. In the latter case, the resection must include hemosiderin-stained tissue surrounding the malformation. There is some evidence to support the use of intraoperative electrocorticography to guide the extent of resection (Van Gompel et al., 2009).

Nonlesional neocortical epilepsy usually requires a *tailored resection* after the ictal onset zone and cortical functions have been defined through intracranial recordings, most often using subdural grids.

*Hemispherectomy* is the preferred surgical approach when the epileptogenic zone is well lateralized but widespread in one hemisphere, and the hemisphere functions are impaired or expected to become impaired (Limbrick et al., 2009). Examples of conditions for which hemispherectomy is often the recommended procedure include Rasmussen syndrome, Sturge-Weber syndrome, and hemimegalencephaly. The current *functional hemispherectomy* technique removes temporal and centroparietal regions, leaving the frontal and occipital poles with their blood supply but disconnected from the remainder of the brain. Hemispherectomy provides complete seizure control in approximately three-quarters of patients and improved seizure control in the majority of the remainder (Limbrick et al., 2009). The disappearance of seizures will often improve the function of the remaining hemisphere such that cognitive function and behavior are often improved at follow-up.

If the epileptogenic zone includes eloquent cortex, resection may not be possible without unacceptable deficits, and the technique of MST is then considered (Morrell et al., 1989). MST involves disconnection of horizontal intracortical fibers while preserving the integrity of vertical connections. The procedure is based on evidence that the ictal discharge often spreads along horizontal fibers, while cortical functions tend to follow a vertical columnar organization. MST on eloquent cortex is most often performed in conjunction with resection of adjacent nonessential cortex. More recently, hippocampal transection was proposed as a memory-sparing procedure for patients with MTLE without hippocampal sclerosis, who are at risk of memory decline from hippocampal resection (Uda et al., 2013).

*Corpus callosotomy* (CC) is a palliative surgical procedure involving partial or complete disconnection of the corpus callosum. The procedure is most often used for drop attacks and is thought to disrupt rapid bilateral seizure spread responsible for sudden loss of consciousness or loss of posture without warning. CC can change seizure characteristics such that seizures may become focal or patients may have a warning, giving them time to protect themselves before further seizure progression. In seizure types where bihemispheric synchrony is required for seizure expression, CC may potentially eliminate clinical seizure manifestations. Drop attacks are the seizure type most helped by CC, with benefit in about three-quarters of patients and freedom from drop attacks in more than a third (Tanriverdi et al., 2009). GTC seizures are also helped. A two-thirds anterior callosotomy is generally performed first, with the possibility of extending the callosotomy later if there is insufficient improvement. CC is not effective for focal seizures, including FIAS of temporal lobe epilepsy. It is reserved for patients with severe epilepsy, falls, and injuries. The most appropriate candidates have symptomatic generalized epilepsy, but CC may be considered for patients with highly refractory GTC seizures in the setting of IGE (Cukiert et al., 2009; Jenssen et al., 2006b).

### Surgical Results and Predictors of Surgical Freedom

Epilepsy surgery can be a very effective treatment for patients who are found to be good candidates after a presurgical evaluation. The best surgical outcome has been reported in temporal lobe epilepsy surgery. The efficacy of temporal lobe epilepsy surgery was confirmed in a randomized controlled trial in which 80 patients with temporal lobe epilepsy were randomly assigned to immediate temporal lobectomy or additional ASM therapy for 1 year. At 1 year, the difference between the two groups was highly significant: 58% of patients in the surgical group and 8% in the medical group were free of seizures impairing awareness; 38% in the surgical group and 3% in the medical group were free of all seizures, including auras (Wiebe et al., 2001).

Many other studies have confirmed efficacy of surgery, with generally better results for MTLE than neocortical epilepsy. In a seven-center prospective observational study of resective epilepsy surgery in patients aged 12 years and older, 339 operated patients (297 mesial temporal, 42 neocortical) were followed over 2 years (Spencer et al., 2005). Of these, 66% (223) experienced 2-year remission, not significantly different between mesial temporal and neocortical resections (68% and 50%, respectively). Seizure remission was defined as 2 years completely seizure free after hospital discharge, with or without auras. Only absence of GTC seizures and presence of hippocampal atrophy were significantly and independently associated with remission, and only in the mesial temporal resection group.

Epilepsy surgery significantly improved quality-of-life score measures within 6 months after surgery; subsequent changes over time were sensitive to seizure-free and aura-free status (Spencer et al., 2007). Other factors reported in some studies as predictors of postoperative seizure freedom after temporal lobe surgery include discrete abnormalities (lesions and hippocampal sclerosis), unilateral ictal and interictal epileptiform discharges, and antecedent febrile convulsions (not consistently reported). The etiology of head trauma, normal MRI, and absence of hypometabolism on PET were unfavorable predictors in some studies. Postoperative seizures and epileptiform activity on postoperative EEG were also unfavorable predictors. In neocortical epilepsy, well-circumscribed lesions (e.g., tumor, cavernoma), complete lesion resection, and focal beta or gamma activity at ictal onset were favorable predictors, while absence of a lesion and generalized spike-and-wave EEG pattern were unfavorable predictors.

ASMs usually have to be continued for at least a period of time after successful epilepsy surgery, but the number and dose of ASMs may be reduced prior to that time. Most commonly, medications are tapered after 1–2 years of complete seizure freedom. However, there is a risk of recurrence in approximately one-fifth to one-third of patients (Kim et al., 2005; Lee et al., 2008; Park et al., 2010b; Rathore et al., 2011; Schiller et al., 2000; Schmidt et al., 2004). The risk seems lower in pediatric patients (Lachhwani et al., 2008). Factors associated with greater likelihood of recurrence included older age at surgery and longer duration of epilepsy (Al-Kaylani et al., 2007; Kim et al., 2005; Lee et al., 2008). Other factors associated with recurrence were ASM reduction before 10 months (Lee et al., 2008) and normal preoperative MRI (Schiller et al., 2000).

Late relapse is not a rare event. Relapse after a 2-year remission occurred in 25% of mesial temporal and 19% of neocortical epilepsy patients in the seven-center study. Only delay to remission predicted relapse, and only in mesial temporal epilepsy patients (Spencer et al., 2005). In a study of anterior temporal lobectomy for temporal lobe epilepsy in 325 patients followed for a mean of 9.6 years, 55.3% of patients were seizure free at 2 years, 47.7% at 5 years, and 41% at 10 years (McIntosh et al., 2004). Patients who were seizure free at 2 years postoperatively had a 74% probability of seizure freedom at 10 years after surgery. Long-term postoperative outcome was examined specifically in 171 patients with MRI-defined hippocampal sclerosis (Janszky et al., 2005a). Seizure freedom was noted in 80% at 6 months, 71% at 2 years, 66% at 3 years, and 58% at 5 years. Predictors of outcome varied at different time points: preoperative FBTCS and ictal dystonia were negative predictors at 2 years; longer epilepsy duration and ictal dystonia at 3 years; and only longer epilepsy duration at 5 years.

About a third of patients who are not seizure free immediately after surgery eventually achieve long-term seizure freedom (Janszky et al., 2005b). Normal MRI findings and FBTCS preoperatively were unfavorable predictors; rare postoperative seizures and ipsilateral temporal interictal epileptiform discharges were associated with seizure-free outcome. Newly administered levetiracetam also showed a significant positive effect on the postoperative outcome, independent of other prognostic factors (Janszky et al., 2005b).

Patients who have failed epilepsy surgery can be considered for reoperation, usually after at least 1–2 years. Reoperation is more likely to be successful if the initial surgery missed the epileptogenic zone or epileptogenic lesion, or if the initial resection was incomplete. Between one- and two-thirds of reoperations result in seizure freedom or near-seizure freedom (Germano et al., 1994; Gonzalez-Martinez et al., 2007; Holmes et al., 1999; Ramantani et al., 2013; Salanova et al., 2005; Siegel et al., 2004). If the first presurgical evaluation was extensive and the surgery was appropriate based on the findings, reoperation is unlikely to be successful.

Epilepsy surgery has potential adverse effects that may be expected in some instances, as well as unexpected complications. A contralateral upper-quadrant visual-field loss is to be expected after temporal lobectomy, but this is usually not of functional consequence to the patient (Hughes et al., 1999). Cognitive changes may occur. Dominant temporal lobe epilepsy surgery carries risks of verbal memory loss in 44% and reduced naming in 34% of patients (Sherman et al., 2011). Memory may continue to decline for up to 2 years after surgery (Alpherts et al., 2006). There is a suggestion of increased risk for memory decline in patients with larger hippocampal volumes (Baxendale et al., 2008). On the other hand, memory deficits associated with the function of the contralateral temporal lobe may improve postoperatively in some patients with unilateral hippocampal sclerosis (Baxendale et al., 2008).

## OTHER THERAPIES

Other therapies are often considered only after medical therapy fails and when surgical therapy is not possible or has also failed (Cascino, 2008). However, alternative nonpharmacological therapy should also be considered when patients may be candidates for surgery, but expectations for complete seizure freedom are low. These alternatives include dietary therapy, stimulation therapies, and radiosurgery.

## Dietary Therapy

Dietary therapy is a very old treatment of epilepsy, first proposed in 1921 to mimic the effects of fasting by producing ketosis, acidosis, and dehydration (Sinha and Kossoff, 2005). Interest in a ketogenic diet decreased with the introduction of many new ASMs in the 1990s but increased again with the realization that the newer ASMs had only a modest impact on drug-resistant epilepsy. The *ketogenic diet* is a very low-carbohydrate, high-fat, and low-to-adequate protein diet that includes some restriction of total calories (≈75% of age recommendations). The amount of protein is based on age requirement: carbohydrates are only 5–10 g/day, and the remaining calories come from fat. The ratio of fat to protein plus carbohydrate ranges from 2:1 to 4:1. The diet is typically initiated with a fast. Although the fasting is not necessary for therapeutic efficacy, it does provide a faster onset of action that may help improve compliance. Initiation with fasting requires hospital admission, which may also be helpful for monitoring unexpected adverse effects of the diet and reviewing medications for possible carbohydrate components (Sinha and Kossoff, 2005). Efficacy of the ketogenic diet in children was confirmed in a randomized controlled but unblinded trial: 38% of children who received the diet had a greater than 50% reduction versus only 6% of controls, and 7% had a greater than 90% reduction versus none of the controls (Neal et al., 2008). A blinded crossover study in children with Lennox-Gastaut syndrome did not reach significance, but this may have been due to methodological problems (Freeman et al., 2009). In a prospective study of the ketogenic diet in 150 children with drug-resistant epilepsy, 3% were seizure free at 3 months and 7% at 12 months; 27% had a greater than 90% decrease in seizure frequency at 1 year (Freeman et al., 1998). A multicenter study similarly showed that 10% of children with highly refractory epilepsy were seizure free at 1 year, and 40% had a 50% or greater decrease in seizure frequency (Vining et al., 1998).

The ketogenic diet is a little less effective in adolescents and adults than in children and is also limited by a higher rate of noncompliance in adolescents. The onset of action is very fast. In one study the median time to first improvement was 5 days, with a range of 1–65 days. The onset of improvement was faster in children who were fasted (5 vs. 14 days), but there was no difference between 1 and 2 days of fasting. Fasting had no effect on long-term efficacy. Some 75% of children improved within 14 days. Improvement was unlikely if no benefit had been seen by 2 months, although exceptions did exist (Kossoff et al., 2008b).

The mechanism of the ketogenic diet is not well understood. Its benefit may be related to acidosis, ketosis, calorie restriction and decrease in blood glucose, dehydration, or increase in certain lipids (Sinha and Kossoff, 2005). Predictors of success included concomitant use of the ketogenic diet and vagus nerve stimulation (Kossoff et al., 2007; Morrison et al., 2009). Children receiving phenobarbital in combination with a ketogenic diet were less likely to benefit. Adverse effects of the ketogenic diet include constipation and worsening of reflux, both of which can be managed with minor adjustments and stool softeners. Acidosis may occur, mostly at initiation and in association with acute illness; it can be managed with hydration. Unexplained fatigue could be helped by supplementation with carnitine. The potential adverse effect of decreased growth is most likely to occur in the youngest children. Renal calculi have been reported in 5%–6% of individuals and may be averted with improved hydration. Hyperlipidemia is of unknown long-term significance.

Indications for the ketogenic diet include refractory seizures, regardless of classification. Individuals unable to tolerate ASM therapy are particularly good candidates for the diet. The ketogenic diet is easiest to manage in tube-fed patients or infants receiving formula. A ketogenic diet is particularly beneficial and could be considered first-line therapy for children with GLUT deficiency and pyruvate dehydrogenase deficiency. Other syndromes where the ketogenic diet has been reported to be especially beneficial include myoclonic-astatic epilepsy, tuberous sclerosis, Rett syndrome, Dravet syndrome, and infantile spasms (Kossoff et al., 2009). Absolute contraindications include mitochondrial disorders, pyruvate carboxylase deficiency, and β-oxidation defects.

Patient compliance with the ketogenic diet has proven difficult, so other diets have been explored in the treatment of epilepsy. The *modified Atkins diet* was created to be more palatable and less restrictive than the ketogenic diet. It only restricts carbohydrates (10 g/day for children and 15 g/day for adults), not protein, fat, or calories. It is modified from the standard Atkins diet in that the induction phase limiting carbohydrates is indefinite, and that fat is not only allowed but also encouraged. Weight loss is not the goal of this diet, but weight loss has been associated with improvement.

The efficacy of the Atkins diet has been studied prospectively in children and adults. In one pediatric study, 65% of children had a greater than 50% reduction in seizures (Kossoff et al., 2006), and in an adult study, 47% had greater than 50% reduction at 3 months and 33% at 6 months, but 33% discontinued the diet before 3 months. The modified Atkins diet also seems to work fairly rapidly; median time to seizure reduction was 2 weeks. In the adult prospective study, a higher level of ketosis was associated with improvement early on and weight loss later on (Kossoff et al., 2008c). Another study suggested consistently strong ketosis was important for maintaining the efficacy of diet therapy (Kang et al., 2007). The Atkins diet has advantages over the ketogenic diet in that it is easier to initiate in an outpatient setting and requires only limited dietician input. It is more tolerable and has fewer adverse effects than the ketogenic diet. The presence of obesity in other family members may encourage them to try the diet as well, thus improving the chances of success for the patient. The modified Atkins diet has also been proposed as an inexpensive treatment option in developing countries (Kossoff et al., 2008a).

The suggestion that a lower glucose level played a role in dietary efficacy prompted a trial of a *low glycemic index diet* (Muzykewicz et al., 2009). This diet selectively restricts high glycemic index foods that produce a substantial postprandial increase in blood glucose and insulin. The diet allows only low glycemic index carbohydrates, with an overall carbohydrate intake of 40–60 g/day. There was a greater than 90% improvement in seizure control in about 25% at 3 months, with another 25% experiencing 50%–90% improvement. There was a correlation between efficacy and blood glucose at 1 month and 12 months of treatment.

Overall, the advantages of dietary therapy are that it is effective, has a rapid onset of action, and has different adverse effects than seen with ASMs. Disadvantages include that dietary therapy may be socially isolating, and compliance is difficult to maintain. The less-restrictive diets are easier to follow, but they also give more opportunity for cheating (Muzykewicz et al., 2009).

## Vagus Nerve Stimulation

Vagus nerve stimulation (VNS) was first approved in 1997 as the only device for the adjunctive treatment of refractory focal-onset seizures in adults and adolescents aged 12 years or older. More recently, VNS was also FDA approved as adjunctive long-term treatment for chronic or recurrent depression that has not responded to antidepressants. Animal data suggested that VNS has acute abortive effects, terminating seizures that have already started (McLachlan, 1993), and acute prophylactic effects, reducing seizure frequency and severity during intermittent stimulation (Takaya et al., 1996). Efficacy in patients with drug-resistant epilepsy was confirmed in two pivotal randomized blinded controlled studies that demonstrated 24.5%–28% short-term reduction in seizure frequency (Handforth et al., 1998; The Vagus Nerve Stimulation Study Group, 1995). The long-term continuation studies suggested increasing benefit over time, with median seizure reduction of 34% 3 months after the end of the second double-blind trial, and 45% by the end of 1 year. In one cohort followed for 12 years, mean reduction in seizure frequency was 26% after 1 year and 52% after 12 years of treatment (Uthman et al., 2004). However, seizure freedom is reported in less than 10% of patients (Ben-Menachem, 2002). Hence, individuals who are excellent candidates for epilepsy surgery should be advised of the much greater chance of seizure freedom with surgical therapy.

Even though there are no randomized trials of VNS in patients with drug-resistant generalized epilepsy, several studies have supported VNS efficacy in both idiopathic and symptomatic generalized epilepsy (Ben-Menachem, 2002; Elliott et al., 2011; Kostov et al., 2009; Ng and Devinsky, 2004); the same is true for VNS efficacy in children. Thus VNS efficacy does not seem to be specific for a particular form of epilepsy or particular age. The mechanism of action of VNS for epilepsy is not totally clear. Approximately 80% of the vagus nerve is composed of afferent myelinated fibers projecting to the nucleus of the tractus solitarius, which itself has widespread projections (Ben-Menachem, 2002). In humans with implanted VNS, imaging of blood flow with PET showed that VNS increased blood flow in some regions and decreased blood flow in others. Increased blood flow in the thalamus correlated with long-term seizure control (Henry et al., 1999). In another study using SPECT, acute reduction in amygdala perfusion and chronic reduction in hippocampal perfusion correlated with clinical efficacy (Van Laere et al., 2002).

The VNS device consists of a generator, usually implanted over the chest under the left clavicle, and electrodes that are placed around the left vagus nerve and tunneled under the skin to connect with the generator. VNS implantation is usually an outpatient surgical procedure with rare complications, the most important of which is infection. Asystole (with full recovery) has been reported during routine intraoperative lead testing, approximately once for every 1000 implantations. VNS is usually programmed to stimulate for 30 seconds, alternating with 5 minutes of rest, but the duration of stimulation time on and stimulation time off can be changed. Some patients seem to derive greater benefit from "rapid-cycle" stimulation, with 7 seconds of stimulation alternating with 12 seconds of rest. The first parameter to be titrated is current intensity, which is increased by 0.25 mA steps as needed to achieve benefit. Other output current parameters that can be programmed are frequency and pulse width. The optimal stimulation parameters have not been well defined and may vary between individuals. In addition to the recurring output current cycles, a single on-demand stimulation train can be programmed separately to abort seizures with the use of a magnet. On-demand stimulation is particularly helpful to abort or attenuate seizures in individuals who have an aura (Morris, 2003). However, the clinical efficacy of on-demand stimulation is difficult to confirm with rigorous investigation. Newer VNS models also offer responsive stimulation upon detection of sudden increase in heart rate. This is based on the observation that ictal tachycardia is an early sign observed in the majority of patients (Eggleston et al., 2014; Hirsch et al., 2015).

The most common VNS adverse effect is hoarseness, which occurs during stimulation cycles. This is to be expected in most patients, but it does improve over time. The same is true of other stimulation-related adverse effects of coughing, throat pain, dyspnea, and paresthesias (Ben-Menachem, 2002). VNS may also exacerbate obstructive sleep apnea, so it is important to diagnose and treat sleep apnea before initiating VNS therapy (Malow et al., 2000a; Marzec et al., 2003).

The main advantages of VNS are that it does not have the ASM adverse effects of sleepiness, tiredness, dizziness, or cognitive dysfunction. It may improve mood and promote alertness, and it gives patients and families a sense of control with the use of on-demand stimulation to abort seizures. In addition, compliance does not require patient effort. However, it does require surgical implantation, and the battery has to be changed every 3–10 years depending on the stimulation parameters. It is difficult to predict who will benefit from this therapy, but the best candidates are patients who are not good candidates for epilepsy surgery, have frequent seizures, and have a consistent aura or a slow seizure progression, so that on-demand stimulation could be used to abort seizures. VNS has also become frequently used in symptomatic generalized epilepsy before proceeding with CC (Nei et al., 2006; Rosenfeld and Roberts, 2009; You et al., 2008).

## Other Stimulation Therapies

*Trigeminal nerve stimulation*, which had an antiepileptic effect in a rodent model of epilepsy, can be delivered noninvasively in humans and is being investigated as an alternative stimulation modality. In a small open-label pilot study, bilateral stimulation of the ophthalmic branch produced a mean reduction in seizure frequency of 59% at 12 months (DeGiorgio et al., 2009). A larger blinded randomized controlled trial in 50 subjects with focal-onset seizures showed a reduction in seizure frequency as measured by the response ratio, but there was no significant difference between groups in the 50% responder rates (30.2% for the treatment group and 21.1% for the active control group) (DeGiorgio et al., 2013). Of note is that the active treatment group showed a significant improvement in responder rate over the treatment period, from 17.8% at 6 weeks to 40.5% at 18 weeks.

*Repetitive transcranial magnetic stimulation* (rTMS), a noninvasive cortical stimulation method, was also investigated as a treatment for drug-resistant epilepsy, with variable results:L rTMS modulates cortical excitability, with high-frequency rTMS enhancing and low-frequency rTMS decreasing cortical excitability in most individuals (Gangitano et al., 2002). Most studies used daily rTMS sessions for about 1 week, then evaluated efficacy 2–4 weeks later. A meta-analysis deduced that low-frequency rTMS is moderately beneficial, with more improvement in subjects who have cortical dysplasia or neocortical epilepsy, probably because of greater and more precise access of rTMS therapy to the more superficial seizure foci (Hsu et al., 2011).

Various brain targets have been explored for stimulation, including cortical and subcortical targets. Scheduled *open-loop stimulation* to various cortical and subcortical structures, including the thalamus, subthalamic nucleus, cerebellum, and hippocampus, demonstrated variable success (Jobst et al., 2010a). Bilateral stimulation of the anterior nucleus of the thalamus was proven effective in a multicenter double-blind randomized trial (Fisher et al., 2010). Median seizure reduction was 14.5% in the control group and 40.4% in the stimulated group during the blinded phase, and there was a 56% median reduction in seizure frequency by 2 years. However, participants in the stimulated group were more likely to report depression or memory problems as adverse events. Bilateral deep brain stimulation of the anterior nucleus of the thalamus for epilepsy was first approved in Europe in 2010, then by the US FDA in 2018 (Salanova, 2018). The FDA approval is for adjunctive therapy in individuals 18 years of age or older diagnosed with focal epilepsy "refractory to three or more anti-epileptic medications."

Responsive *closed-loop stimulation* delivers a stimulus to the presumed seizure onset zone in response to seizure detection (Jobst et al., 2010a). The concept is based on evidence that brief stimulation can terminate seizure activity if delivered early after seizure onset. The generator is implanted in the skull and connected to either depth or subdural strip electrodes to deliver stimulation directly to one or two seizure onset zones. The responsive stimulator device was found to be effective in a pivotal randomized double-blind, sham stimulation controlled trial in patients with drug-resistant focal-onset seizures. The reduction in seizure frequency over the blinded evaluation period was 37.9% in the treatment group compared to 17.3% in the sham stimulation group (Morrell, 2011). In the open-label extension, median percent reduction in seizures was 44% at 1 year and 53% at 2 years, suggesting progressive improvement with time (Heck et al., 2014). The device was approved by the FDA as an adjunctive therapy in individuals 18 years or older with focal-onset seizures who have undergone diagnostic testing that localized no more than two epileptogenic foci, are refractory to two or more antiseizure AEMs, and currently have frequent and disabling seizures. Responsive stimulation is a suitable treatment option for patients with bilateral independent seizure foci or with an epileptogenic zone in eloquent cortex not suitable for surgical resection.

In general, the advantages of stimulation include that it is reversible and adjustable, unlike resective surgery. However, the optimal stimulation parameters are not generally well defined, and, to date, stimulation therapies have been predominantly palliative. The decision to pursue stimulation therapy has to balance risks and benefits in comparison with other available therapies.

### Radiosurgery

Radiosurgery uses a stereotactic frame to immobilize the head while radiation beams are precisely directed from different angles to a target. The method delivers radiation to the target with a steep gradient so that regions within a few millimeters of the target receive a substantially reduced radiation dose (Romanelli and Anschel, 2006). Radiosurgery was initially used for treatment of brain tumors and AVMs not readily accessible to standard surgery, with beneficial effect on seizure control. It has also been used successfully for hypothalamic hamartoma. More recently, radiosurgery was explored for MTLE. A prospective study in three European centers reported 65% of patients seizure free at 2 years after radiosurgery. Five patients had transient side effects, including depression, headache, nausea, vomiting, and imbalance. No permanent neurological deficit was reported, except nine visual-field deficits. However, seizure freedom was delayed for most patients, the main improvement occurring between 12 and 18 months; some patients only became seizure free after 2 years post treatment.

A US multicenter prospective study randomized patients to high- or low-dose radiosurgery. At 36 months of follow-up, 76.9% of patients randomized to the high dose and 58.8% randomized to the low dose were free of seizures for the prior 12 months (Barbaro et al., 2009). Seizure remission correlated with appearance of vasogenic edema demonstrated on serial imaging after approximately 9–12 months (Chang et al., 2010). The degree of radiation-induced local vascular insult and neuronal loss was dose dependent and predicted long-term seizure remission (Chang et al., 2010). Neuropsychological testing showed no definite change in cognitive measures from baseline at 2 years after radiosurgery (Quigg et al., 2011). A single-blinded multicenter controlled trial randomized 58 adult subjects with drug-resistant unilateral MTLE to either stereotactic radiosurgery or standard temporal lobectomy (Barbaro et al., 2018). Seizure remission was achieved in 52% of the radiosurgery and 78% of the temporal lobectomy patients.

Radiosurgery may have a place in the treatment of drug-resistant mesial temporal epilepsy for patients who are opposed to or at greater risk for complications with standard epilepsy surgery. However, the long-term risk/benefit ratio of radiosurgery needs better definition.

## QUALITY-OF-CARE STANDARDS IN THE MANAGEMENT OF EPILEPSY

The American Academy of Neurology developed standardized quality measures for epilepsy care (Fountain et al., 2011) that have since been updated based on new evidence and performance gaps (Fountain et al., 2015; Patel et al., 2018). The latest quality measurement set includes the following:

- Counseling for women of childbearing potential, at least once a year
- Comprehensive epilepsy care center referral for discussion for patients with intractable epilepsy
- Quality-of-life assessment, at least once
- Quality-of-life outcome, at a visit at least 4 weeks after initial assessment
- Depression and anxiety screening at every office visit

The measures were primarily developed for quality improvement projects. Providers were encouraged to identify measures most meaningful for their patients and to implement these measures to drive improvement in practice (Patel et al., 2018).

## SEIZURE CLUSTERS AND STATUS EPILEPTICUS

*Seizure clusters,* also called *acute repetitive seizures* and *serial seizures,* are closely grouped seizures representing an increase in seizure frequency compared to baseline, usually occurring over the span of minutes to a couple days. Seizure clusters may include any type of seizure and may vary in severity, but by definition there is complete recovery in between seizures. Seizure clusters are more common in patients with drug-resistant epilepsy, particularly those with remote symptomatic epilepsy and extratemporal epilepsy. Patients with seizure clusters are more likely to have a history of status epilepticus. Seizure clusters themselves may or may not progress to prolonged seizures or even status epilepticus. Such progression may be predictable for individual patients, based on their seizure history. This may determine the most appropriate treatment for seizure clusters. Mild clusters can be treated with oral doses of benzodiazepines. However more severe clusters, particularly those known to progress to severe prolonged seizures or status epilepticus, may require other routes of administration. Rectal diazepam was the only FDA-approved treatment for out-of-hospital administration by nonmedical caregivers (Cereghino et al., 1998), until intranasal midazolam spray was approved in 2019 (Detyniecki et al., 2019). Buccal midazolam is in wide clinical use in Europe and various countries (Nakken and Lossius, 2011), but has not been approved in the United States. Intranasal diazepam was approved by the US FDA in 2020. The efficacy of intramuscular diazepam delivered by autoinjector was demonstrated in a blinded controlled trial (Abou-Khalil et al., 2013), but this did not lead to FDA approval or marketing. Other approaches that were evaluated include buccal diazepam and staccato midazolam.

*Status epilepticus* was previously broadly defined as seizure activity that continues for 30 minutes, or recurrent seizures without recovery between attacks. The 30-minute duration has been the subject of debate, since it may delay aggressive therapy, particularly when prolonged duration can be predicted in the absence of therapy. Experimental evidence suggests that irreversible neuronal injury may start after 20–30 minutes of generalized convulsive status epilepticus (GCSE) (Fujikawa, 1996; Meldrum and Brierley, 1973), so every effort has to be made to stop seizure activity prior to that. A large body of evidence suggests that the bilateral tonic-clonic phase if focal or generalized onset seizures does not last longer than 2 minutes (Jenssen et al., 2006a; Theodore et al., 1994) except when it evolves into status epilepticus. As a result, it has been suggested that vigorous therapy for status epilepticus be initiated after 5 minutes of bilateral tonic-clonic activity (Lowenstein et al., 1999). There is also evidence that FIAS that last longer than 10 minutes will likely evolve into status epilepticus (Jenssen et al., 2006a). Based on the above, the ILAE defined status epilepticus as a condition "resulting from the failure of the mechanisms responsible for seizure termination or from the initiation of mechanisms which lead to abnormally prolonged seizures (after time point $t_1$), and can have long-term consequences (after time point t2)" (Trinka et al., 2015). The time point t1 for status epilepticus was 5 minutes for bilateral tonic-clonic seizures, 10 minutes for focal seizures, and 10–15 minutes for absence seizures.

Any seizure type may evolve into status epilepticus. Status epilepticus may be classified based on the seizure type it evolves from. The most dangerous type of status epilepticus, GCSE, may evolve from a primary GTC seizure or more often from a FBTCS. One form of status epilepticus with a low likelihood of irreversible neuronal injury is generalized absence status epilepticus, which evolves from generalized absence seizures.

The most recent ILAE classification of status epilepticus (see Box 100.3) includes the two major categories of status epilepticus with prominent motor symptoms and status epilepticus without prominent motor symptoms, which is synonymous with nonconvulsive status epilepticus. Status epilepticus with prominent motor symptoms includes *convulsive status epilepticus*, which has been made synonymous with *tonic-clonic status epilepticus*, *myoclonic status epilepticus* (with coma or without coma), *focal motor status epilepticus*, *tonic status epilepticus*, and *hyperkinetic status epilepticus*. Convulsive status epilepticus can be generalized, focal evolving to bilateral tonic-clonic, or unknown whether focal or generalized in onset. *Nonconvulsive status epilepticus* can be with coma or without coma. Nonconvulsive status epilepticus without coma can be generalized as in absence status epilepticus, or focal, with or without impairment of consciousness. Focal nonconvulsive status epilepticus without impairment of consciousness is often referred to as *aura continua*.

Nonconvulsive status epilepticus without coma is generally considered a less serious medical emergency than convulsive status epilepticus. However, nonconvulsive status epilepticus with coma, including what was previously referred to as *subtle convulsive status epilepticus* is extremely serious, difficult to treat, and has a poor prognosis. Nonconvulsive status epilepticus with coma may evolve from convulsive status epilepticus in which treatment has been delayed or has been ineffective. It may also be seen without prior overt convulsive status epilepticus when there has been a serious brain insult such as severe traumatic brain injury, hypoxic injury, or massive strokes. In generalized absence status epilepticus, the patient usually appears awake but may be either unresponsive to verbal stimuli or may have slowed or inappropriate responses. In focal nonconvulsive status epilepticus with impaired consciousness, there is a wide spectrum of impairment of consciousness, responsiveness, or behavior. There may be considerable cyclical fluctuations in the clinical manifestations.

The definitive diagnosis of nonconvulsive status epilepticus requires confirmation with EEG. Even convulsive status epilepticus has to be differentiated from psychogenic status epilepticus or pseudostatus epilepticus, which may require video-EEG for definitive diagnosis. However, the EEG patterns of status epilepticus, particularly nonconvulsive status epilepticus, are not totally specific (Kaplan, 2007). When the EEG pattern is not specific, the definitive diagnosis also requires observation of a definite clinical response to treatment, or at least restoration of normal EEG activity that was previously absent. In convulsive status epilepticus, a sequence of EEG patterns was reported, starting with discrete recurrent seizures separated by interictal slow activity, merging seizures with waxing and waning ictal discharge, continuous ictal discharge, continuous ictal discharge punctuated by generalized attenuation, and then periodic discharges on a relatively flat background (Treiman et al., 1990). This sequence was proven in an animal model of status epilepticus, and also suspected in human status epilepticus based on EEGs of patients studied at different stages of the condition. A similar sequence may also occur in focal status epilepticus, with asymmetrical or focal EEG features. The last pattern in the sequence, periodic discharges on a relatively flat background, is somewhat problematic because periodic discharges are not specific.

The incidence of status epilepticus is likely underestimated by published studies. The highest overall incidence, 41 cases per 100,000 per year, was found in the prospective population-based study of status epilepticus in Richmond, Virginia (DeLorenzo et al., 1996). The incidence of status epilepticus is elevated early in life, decreases after that, then increases in the elderly, with up to 98.9 annual cases per 100,000 persons in that age group (Vignatelli et al., 2003).

The etiology of status epilepticus is very dependent on age. The most common cause in children is febrile status epilepticus, accounting for more than half of cases (Rosenow et al., 2007). In adults, status epilepticus is much more often due to acute cerebrovascular accidents, hypoxia, metabolic causes, and low ASM levels (Rosenow et al., 2007). It is important to recognize that the majority of patients in status epilepticus do not have a history of epilepsy.

Status epilepticus is a neurological emergency that requires prompt intervention. The goal of therapy is to stop seizure activity in the brain before neuronal injury has started. In addition, delay in initiating therapy is associated with resistance to treatment (Treiman et al., 1998), probably due to alteration in the functional properties of $GABA_A$ receptors (Goodkin et al., 2008; Jones et al., 2002; Macdonald and Kapur, 1999). Since convulsive status epilepticus is the most serious form, its treatment will be discussed first. Treatment of status epilepticus may have to start before arrival in the emergency room. Individuals known to have recurrent status epilepticus may respond to rectal diazepam administered by a parent or care partner. There is also evidence to support the use of buccal midazolam, nasal midazolam, and nasal lorazepam (Arya et al., 2011). Even when prehospital treatment was not effective and status epilepticus had persisted upon arrival in the emergency room, there was evidence that prehospital treatment with rectal diazepam was associated with a shorter duration of status after arrival to the emergency department (Chin et al., 2008). For individuals not prepared for home treatment of status epilepticus, the use of 2 mg of IV lorazepam by paramedics was associated with termination of status before arrival to the emergency room in 59.1% of individuals, compared to 21.1% treated with placebo (Alldredge et al., 2001). Intramuscular autoinjector administration of midazolam by paramedics was found at least as safe and effective as IV lorazepam for prehospital seizure cessation (Silbergleit et al., 2012). Intramuscular midazolam could be administered faster than IV lorazepam. At arrival in the emergency department, 73.4% of 448 subjects in the intramuscular midazo-lam group were free of seizure activity, as compared with 63% of 445 subjects in the IV-lorazepam group.

Upon arrival in the emergency room, treatment of convulsive status epilepticus begins with basic life support measures, specifically attention to airway, breathing, and circulation (Treiman, 2007). Blood samples should be drawn for hematological and serum chemistry values, as well as ASM levels for patients who are already taking these medications. If blood glucose is low or cannot be measured rapidly, IV glucose should be administered, in conjunction with IV thiamine if there is a concern for malnutrition. Based on the landmark Veterans Affairs Status Epilepticus Cooperative Study, lorazepam 0.1 mg/kg was the most effective agent, terminating overt convulsive status epilepticus within 20 minutes in 64.9% of patients (Treiman et al., 1998). It was much less effective in subtle convulsive status epilepticus (nonconvulsive status epilepticus with coma), terminating it within 20 minutes in only 17.9% of patients with a verified diagnosis. Lorazepam was superior to phenytoin alone, which controlled overt convulsive status within 20 minutes in only 43.6% of patients with verified diagnosis. If the first treatment failed to control status epilepticus, the chances of control with the second treatment were minimal and mortality was twice as high (Treiman et al., 1998).

A standard treatment protocol is necessary for the hospital treatment of convulsive status epilepticus. The American Epilepsy Society issued an evidence-based guideline in 2016 (Glauser et al., 2016). It recommended initiating treatment in adults with either intramuscular midazolam, IV lorazepam, IV diazepam, or IV phenobarbital for a bilateral convulsive seizure that has lasted at least 5 minutes. Lorazepam is usually the first agent used for terminating status. If lorazepam is successful in stopping seizure activity, the decision to add another agent depends on the underlying etiology. Lorazepam's duration of action is approximately 12–24 hours. If the etiology is reversible (e.g., status epilepticus due to metabolic or toxic factors), lorazepam may be the only treatment necessary. Intravenous diazepam is not recommended as the only treatment because of its rapid redistribution in adipose tissue, markedly shortening its duration of action following IV administration. Another longer-acting ASM is needed if the underlying etiology is not rapidly reversible.

If convulsive status epilepticus is not controlled after lorazepam 0.1 mg/kg, a second-line therapy should be initiated within 20 minutes of seizure onset. Choices include IV infusion of 20 mg/kg of fosphenytoin (no faster than 150 mg/min) or 40 mg/kg of valproic acid, or 60 mg/kg of levetiracetam (Kapur et al 2019). Lacosamide is a more recently introduced option, supported with retrospective studies. If convulsive status epilepticus is still not responsive after 40 minutes, endotracheal intubation is necessary at this point, followed by general anesthesia using midazo-lam, propofol, or pentobarbital. The purpose of general anesthesia is to control electrical status epilepticus in the brain. EEG monitoring is necessary at this point because electrical status epilepticus may continue after motor activity stops. If the EEG continues to show ictal activity, the anesthesia has to be deepened to a burst-suppression pattern and even to complete suppression in some cases. Patients who require general anesthesia to control status epilepticus will generally require long-term maintenance with ASMs. Serum levels of ASMs must be in a high therapeutic zone prior to discontinuation of general anesthesia. If seizure activity recurs upon withdrawal of general anesthesia, a number of agents have been used successfully. ASMs with IV formulation are used more often (Agarwal et al., 2007; Aiguabella et al., 2011; Albers et al., 2011; Alvarez et al., 2011; Chen et al., 2011; Goodwin et al., 2011; Kellinghaus et al., 2011; Koubeissi et al., 2011; Misra et al., 2006; Moddel et al., 2009), but high-dose topiramate and felbamate have also been advocated as treatment options (Wasterlain and Chen, 2008). During the treatment of refractory status epilepticus with ASMs, the cause of status has to be investigated and treated appropriately (Shorvon, 2011). Immunotherapy may be indicated if an autoimmune therapy is suspected.

The treatment of other forms of status epilepticus may be less aggressive, depending on the type of status encountered. In nonconvulsive status epilepticus with impaired consciousness, or focal motor status epilepticus, aggressive treatment should avoid depressing level of consciousness. It is still recommended to start with one of the benzodiazepines listed above, followed by second-line agent IV agents, including fosphenytoin, valproate, levetiracetam, and lacosamide. The use of general anesthesia should be avoided if at all possible, because of associated increased risk of infection and death (Sutter et al., 2014).

Generalized absence status epilepticus may respond to IV lorazepam but may require additional IV valproate for control. Generalized myoclonic status epilepticus can be treated with IV lorazepam, valproate, or IV levetiracetam. Levetiracetam is the only ASM approved by the FDA for treatment of myoclonic seizures based on class I clinical trial evidence.

Outcome of status epilepticus depends on the underlying cause, patient age, duration and severity of status epilepticus, and rapidity of therapy initiation. In the Richmond status epilepticus study, mortality was 3% for children and 26% for adults (DeLorenzo et al., 1996). Status epilepticus of less than 1-hour duration had a 2.7% mortality rate after 1 month, compared to 32% for status epilepticus persisting longer than 1 hour (Towne et al., 1994). Patient age and depth of coma at presentation were the strongest predictors of outcome (Neligan and Shorvon, 2011). However, depth of coma is related to duration of status (including delay in initiating therapy) and underlying illness.

*The complete reference list is available online at https://expertconsult.inkling.com/.* 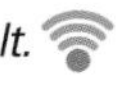

# 101

# Sleep and Its Disorders

*Alon Y. Avidan*

## OUTLINE



Since antiquity, scientists, philosophers, writers, and religious scholars from all cultures and continents have repeatedly raised two fundamental questions—(1) what is sleep? and (2) why do we sleep?—without satisfactory answers.

Some 2000 years ago, Lucretius postulated that sleep is an absence of wakefulness. Macnish, in 1830, proposed a variation of Lucretius's concept, defining *sleep* as "suspension of sensorial power in which the voluntary functions are absent but the involuntary functions, such as circulation, respiration, and other functions controlled by the autonomic nervous system, remain intact." Sleep, however, is not simply an absence of wakefulness, nor is it simply suspension of sensorial power; it results from a combination of passive withdrawal of afferent stimuli to the brain and activation of certain neurons in selective brain areas.

Three basic physiological processes of life consist of *wakefulness*, *nonrapid eye movement* (NREM) *sleep*, and *rapid eye movement* (REM) *sleep*, with independent functions and controls. The invention of the electroencephalogram (EEG) in 1929, fundamental physiological studies to understand consciousness, sleep, and wakefulness in the 1930s and 1940s, and the discovery of REM sleep by Aserinsky and Kleitman in 1953 ushered in the golden age of sleep medicine. In the second half of the last century, substantial advances were made in our scientific understanding of sleep and its disorders, and sleep medicine was established as an important clinical discipline. Scientific progress in sleep medicine has accelerated markedly in recent years, particularly in our appreciation of the glymphatic system and the adverse consequences of poor or insufficient sleep. Neurologists are in a unique position to screen for sleep disorders for three key reasons: (1) sleep disturbances occasionally precede the diagnosis of key neurological conditions (insomnia in the case of Alzheimer dementia and REM sleep behavior disorder in the case of Parkinson disease [PD]); (2) sleep disorders, when untreated/unrecognized often increase the severity of the primary neurological disease (i.e. untreated sleep apnea in the setting of epilepsy) and worsens quality of life for both patients and bedpartners/caregivers; (3) sleep disorders when identified and managed represent a unique window of opportunity in lessening the disease burden and may in the future help delay and even reverse the progression of a neurodegenerative condition. Neurologists must be aware of the importance of disorders and ask their patient at least one question about their satisfaction with, or quality of, their sleep.

This chapter is intended to provide a brief overview and definition of sleep covering the following attributes of sleep: architecture, requirements, function, ontogeny, dreams, the neurobiology of sleep and wakefulness, and review chronobiology and sleep-wake circadian rhythm. Discussion will focus on physiological changes in normal sleep and will transition to a focus on sleep deprivation, excessive sleepiness, and causes/consequences of excessive daytime sleepiness. This chapter will review the classification of sleep disorders, outline a pragmatic approach to a patient with sleep complaints, review clinical spectrum of sleep disturbances, underlying pathophysiogy, best practices for assessment,and management. For more in-depth information about sleep disorders, the reader is referred to the growing number of sleep medicine textbooks (Avidan, 2018; Chervin, 2014; Chokroverty and Billiard, 2015; Kirsch, 2013; Kryger, 2013; Kryger, Avidan, Berry, 2013; Kryger, Roth, and Dement, 2021).

This review of sleep medicine is written during these unprecedented times due to the COVID-19 pandemic and the associated sleep disorders related to anxiety, depression, and poor sleep quality related to physical and social isolation, quarantine, anxiety, stress, or financial losses. As new data are emerging, neurologists are encouraged to appreciate the patterns and emergence of sleep disturbances, insomnia, sleep disordered breathing, nightmares, fatigue, exhaustion, and complex nocturnal behaviors. Current data highlights that fatigue, central hypersomnolence, and REM sleep behavior disorder might be conferred by severe acute respiratory syndrome coronavirus 2 (**SARS-CoV- 2**) infection per se, while rising rates of insomnia ("coro/covidnosomnia") might be related mainly to confinement, anxiety, and psychosocial factors (Partinen, 2020).

## DEFINITION OF SLEEP

Sleep is defined on the basis of both behavioral and physiological criteria (Table 101.1). The behavioral criteria include lack of mobility or slight mobility, closed eyes, a characteristic species-specific sleeping posture, reduced response to external stimulation, quiescence, increased reaction time, elevated arousal threshold, impaired cognitive function, and a reversible unconscious state. Physiological criteria (see Sleep Architecture and Sleep Stages, later) are based on EEG, electro-oculography (EOG), and electromyography (EMG) findings as well as other physiological changes in ventilation and circulation.

The moment of sleep onset is characterized by gradual shift of EEG wave rhythms, cognition, and mental processing. The onset of sleep occurs even prior to entrance to stage N1 NREM sleep and is defined as subjective heaviness and ptosis of the eyelids; clouding of the sensorium; and a decrement in logical or rational perception of visual and auditory stimuli and reduced capacity to respond with appropriate logic. The term *predormitum* was originally coined by Critchley (1955) to describe this moment of sleep onset. The moment of sleep offset, or awakening, is also a gradual process similar to the moment of sleep onset, but is pathologically prolonged in the setting of sleep disturbances such as sleep apnea or sleep deprivation, leading to grogginess and significant cognitive performance decrements, an impairment defined as sleep inertia (Hilditch and McHill, 2019).

### Sleep Architecture, Sleep Hypnogram, and Sleep Stages

Sleep is divided into two independent states: NREM and REM sleep based on physiological correlates. NREM sleep is further divided into three stages, primarily on the basis of EEG criteria. NREM and REM sleep alternate, with each cycle lasting for approximately 90–100 minutes. Four to six such cycles are noted during a normal sleep period. The first two cycles are dominated by slow-wave sleep (stage N3), but in later cycles, these stages are noted only briefly and sometimes not at all. Conversely, the duration of the REM sleep cycle increases from the first to the last cycle, and toward the end of the night, the longest REM cycle may last as long as 1 hour. Thus, the first third of a normal sleep episode is dominated by slow-wave sleep, and REM sleep dominates the last third as illustrated in Fig. 101.1, *A–C*.

The hypnogram is a pictorial representation of the sleep stages of sleep from sleep onset to offset and is helpful following sleep study staging and interpretation in serving as a fingerprint of a patient's sleep patterns at baseline and prior to and following treatment.

In their 1968 criteria, Rechtschaffen and Kales (RK) divided NREM sleep into stages 1, 2, 3, and 4. In 2007, this staging was modified slightly by an American Academy of Sleep Medicine (AASM) Task Force, and NREM sleep is now divided into three stages: N1, N2, and N3 (slow-wave sleep). In the modified staging criteria adopted by the AASM (Iber et al., 2007), the traditional RK stage 1 NREM sleep was labeled N1, RK stage 2 was labeled N2, and RK stages 3 and 4 were combined into one stage, N3. Sleep scoring and staging is a procedure whereby the sleep recording is broken up into 30-second segments, "*epochs*," of a polysomnographic (PSG) tracing with a paper or monitor speed of 10 mm/sec.

*Stage Wake* (Fig. 101.2): Stage W is scored when more than 50% of the epoch consists of alpha EEG frequency. Chin EMG is relatively high tone reflecting the high-amplitude muscle contractions and movement artifacts. From stage W, patients typically proceed to stage N1, but infrequently they may enter REM sleep or stage N2 sleep directly, if the pressure to do so is high (reflecting a state of severe pathological sleep deprivation such as in observed in narcolepsy).

*NREM Sleep*: Accounts for the highest proportion (75%–80%) of sleep time in adults and is made up of stages N1, N2 (light sleep), and N3 (deep or slow-wave sleep).

*Stage N1 Sleep* (Fig. 101.3): Makes up approximately 3%–to-8% of total sleep time. It is demarcated by a significant shift of alpha rhythms (8–13 Hz), a characteristic of wakefulness, which diminishes to less than 50% of the epoch. N1 sleep is demarcated by the emergence of a mixture of slower theta rhythms (4–7 Hz) and beta waves (>13 Hz). The EMG activity drops slightly, and slow rolling eye movements may be recorded. Vertex sharp waves are noted toward the end of stage N1 sleep.

*Stage N2 sleep* (Fig. 101.4): Begins after approximately 10–12 minutes of stage N1 sleep. The characteristic EEG findings of stage N2 sleep include *sleep spindles* (12–18 Hz, most often 14 Hz) and biphasic *K complexes* intermixed with vertex sharp waves. The EEG recording contains theta activity and fewer than 20% slow waves (0.5–2 Hz). Stage N2 sleep lasts for approximately 30–60 minutes.

*Stage N3 sleep* (Fig. 101.5): N3 or slow wave sleep comprises 15%-to–25% of total sleep. The patient is less responsive to environmental stimuli. It is defined by the presence of a minimum of 20 percent delta waves ranging from 0.5–to-2 Hz and having a peak-to-peak amplitude >75 μV. It is an important sleep stage as it is the most restorative form of sleep, but also where one is most likely to observe disorders of arousal (none-REM parasomnias) such as somnambulism and sleep terrors (Previous criteria defined stage N3 with 20–50 percent delta waves and a stage N4 with greater than 50 percent delta waves. However, at present time N2 and N4 are combined as stage N3.

**TABLE 101.1 Behavioral and Physiological Criteria of Wakefulness and Sleep.**

| Attribute | Awake | Asleep: Nonrapid Eye Movement Sleep | Asleep: Rapid Eye Movement Sleep |
|---|---|---|---|
| Posture | Erect, sitting, or recumbent | Recumbent | Recumbent |
| Activity | Present | Moderately reduced, immobile; postural shifts | Absent. When present may signify REM sleep behavior disorder. |
| Response to stimulation | Normal | Mildly to moderately reduced | Moderately reduced to no response |
| Level of alertness | Alert | Unconscious but reversible | Unconscious but reversible |
| Eyelids | Open | Closed | Closed |
| Eye movements | Waking eye movements | Slow rolling eye movements | Rapid eye movements |
| EEG | Alpha waves; desynchronized | Synchronized | Theta or sawtooth; mixed frequency, desynchronized |
| PSG (PSG: EEG, EOG, EMG) | | | 1 sec |
| Neurochemistry Modulating Activity (cerebrum, c.c., thalamus, cerebellum, olfactory bulb, pituitary gland, pons, medulla) | | | |
| Acetylcholine (Ach) | ↑ | ↓ | ↑ |
| Norepinephrine (NE) | ↑ | ↓ | ↓ |
| Serotonin (5-HT) | ↑ | ↓ | ↓ |
| Histamine | ↑ | ↓ | ↓ |
| Hypocretin / Orexin | ↑ | ↓ | ↓ |
| Dopamine (Da) * | | | |
| EMG (muscle tone) | Normal (Augmented) | Mildly to moderately reduced | Severely reduced or absent (Atonic) |
| EOG | Waking eye movements | Slow rolling eye movements | Rapid eye movements |

Comparison between EEG presentation, physiology, and neurotransmitter dominance in wakefulness, NREM sleep, and REM sleep. Neuromodulator activity is primarily cholinergic during wake and REM sleep *(green arrows)*; wake is supported by activity of monoamines, histamine, and hypocretin/orexin *(green arrows)*. In sleep, monoaminergic systems, including norepinephrine and serotonin and attenuated activity *(pink arrows)*, and are silent in REM sleep *(red arrows)*. Whereas dopamine levels do not change dramatically across the sleep-wake cycle *(asterisks)*, phasic events.
*EEG*, Electroencephalogram; *EMG*, electromyogram; *EOG*, electro-oculogram. *PSG* Polysomnography.
*From PSG and Neurochemistry Source: Nir, Y., Tononi, G., 2010. Dreaming and the brain: from phenomenology to neurophysiology. Trends Cogn. Sci. 14(2), 88–100. https://doi.org/10.1016/j.tics.2009.12.001. Copyright © 2010 Published by Elsevier Inc.*

*R or REM Sleep* (Fig.101.6): The first REM sleep (R sleep) episode is noted 60–90 minutes after the onset of sleep. REM sleep accounts for 20%–25% of sleep time. Based on EEG, EMG, and EOG characteristics, REM sleep can be subdivided into two stages: tonic-REM and phasic-REM. However, this subdivision is not recognized in the recently modified staging. The EEG tracings during REM sleep are characterized by fast rhythms and theta activity, some of which may have a sawtooth appearance. A desynchronized EEG, atonia of the major muscle groups, and depression of monosynaptic and polysynaptic reflexes are characteristics of the *tonic stage. Phasic REM sleep* is characterized by REMs in all directions, as well as phasic swings in blood pressure and heart rate, irregular respiration, spontaneous middle-ear muscle activity, and tongue movements. A few periods of apnea or hypopnea may arise during REM sleep.

Under normal circumstances, one observes an orderly progression from wakefulness to sleep onset to NREM sleep proceeding to REM sleep. A relaxed wakefulness is characterized by a behavioral state of quiescence and a physiological state of alpha and beta frequencies on the EEG recording, waking eye movements, and increased muscle tone. Deviation from this progression may be seen in conditions of sleep state instability such as in narcolepsy, characterized by short sleep onset of REM sleep, or sleep fragmentation related to conditions such as sleep-disordered breathing (SDB). Certain medications (such as antidepressants) may reduce and sometimes eliminate normal appearance of slow-wave or REM sleep.

Table 101.2 summarizes EEG sleep stage frequencies and Table 101.3 highlights the proportion of each sleep stage during NREM and REM sleep states.

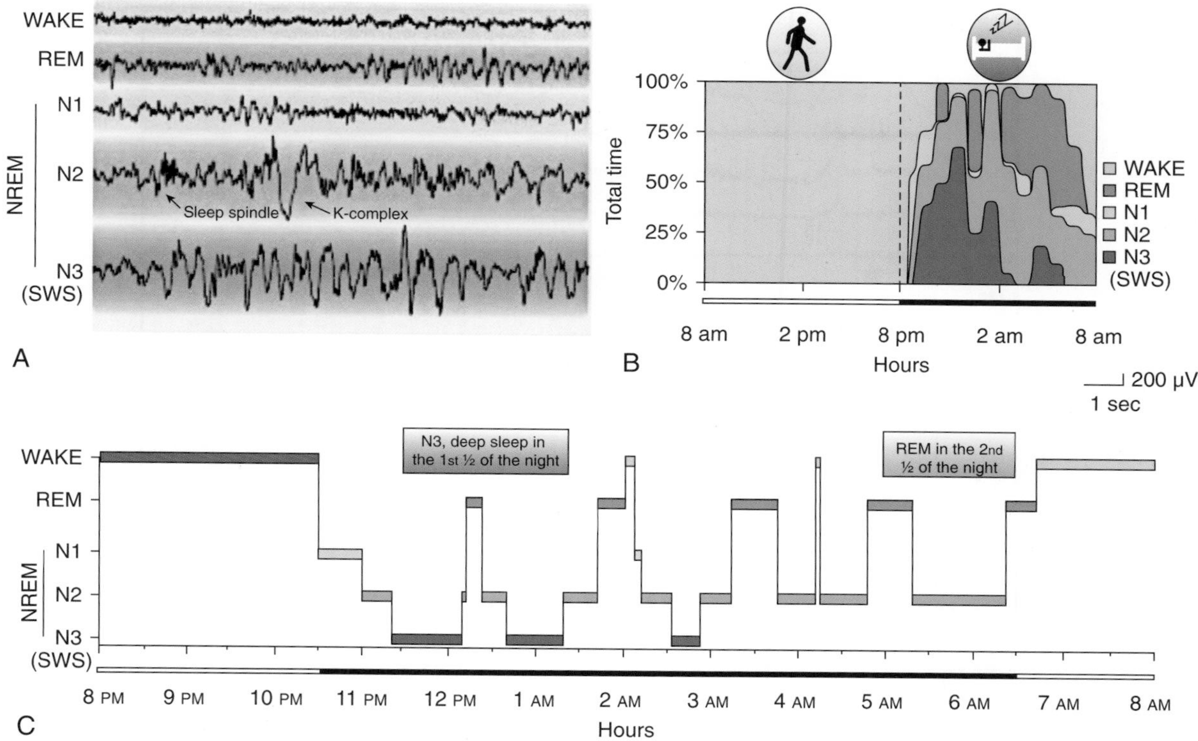


**Fig. 101.1 Sleep Hypnogram. A,** Depiction of electroencephalogram (EEG) wake-sleep patterns in humans for each vigilance state: wakefulness (*WAKE*, in *yellow*), REM sleep (*REM*, in *red*), non REM sleep (*NREM*, in *blue*). In humans NREM sleep is indicated with the 3 substages (N1, N2, and N3, in different *blue* shades); N3 represents the sleep characterized by slow waves (slow-wave sleep, *SWS*). **B,** Percentages of time spent in each vigilance state over 24 hours in humans. **C,** Sleep hypnogram provides for a dynamic biometric assessment of an individual's sleep over 12 hours. Hypnogram is illustrated horizontally by convention, with time plotted on the x-axis, against the stage of sleep on the y axis (and other physiological measures such as oxygen levels, position, apneas, and limb movements).

Fig. 101.7 illustrates the percent sleep stage distribution during the night. Sleep staging and scoring address normal adult sleep and 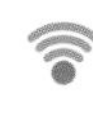 the macrostructure (eBox 101.1) and microstructure (eBox 101.2) of sleep. In patients with sleep disorders such as sleep apnea, parasomnias, or nocturnal seizures disrupting sleep, such assessments may be difficult.

## Sleep Microstructure

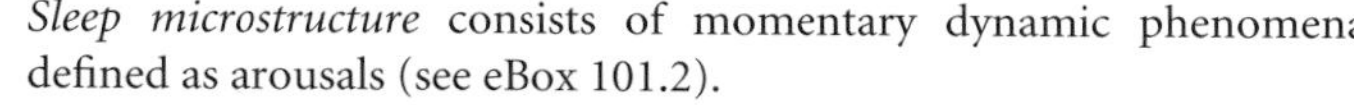

*Sleep microstructure* consists of momentary dynamic phenomena defined as arousals (see eBox 101.2).

An *arousal* is a shift in EEG frequency, and an *arousal index* is defined as the number of arousals per hour of sleep; up to 10 can be considered a normal arousal index, while a higher index signifies sleep fragmentation.

*Cyclic alternating pattern* (CAP) consist of repetitive cortical EEG pattern that is noted mainly during NREM sleep, lasts for 2–60 seconds, and implies predisposition toward sleep instability. A phase of CAP is marked by increased EEG potentials, with contributions from both synchronous high-amplitude slow and desynchronized fast rhythms in the EEG recording. A CAP cycle consists of an unstable phase (phase  A) and a relatively stable phase (phase B) (eFig. 101.8). During phase A, heart rate, respiration, blood pressure, and muscle tone increase. The rates of CAP cycles and arousals increase in both older individuals and a variety of sleep disorders such as parasomnias. A period without CAP is thought to indicate a state of sustained stability and may be used to understand normal and abnormal sleep.

## Ontogeny of Sleep Patterns with Age

The evolution of EEG and wake-sleep states from the fetus, preterm infant, term infant, preschooler, adolescent, to adult follows in an orderly manner depending on the maturation of the central nervous system (CNS). Neurological, environmental, and genetic factors, as well as comorbid medical or neurological disorders, will have significant effects on such ontogenetic changes. Sleep requirements change dramatically from infancy to old age. Newborns have a polyphasic sleep pattern with 16 hours of sleep per day. The sleep requirement decreases to approximately 10 hours per day by age 3–5 years. In preschool children, sleep assumes a biphasic pattern. Adults exhibit a monophasic sleep pattern, with an average duration of 7.5–8 hours per night.

The newborn infant spends approximately 50% of the time in REM sleep, but by age 6 years this time is decreased to the normal adult pattern of 25% (Fig. 101.9). On falling asleep, a newborn baby goes immediately into REM sleep, or active sleep, which is accompanied by restless movements of the arms, legs, and facial muscles. In premature babies, it is often difficult to differentiate REM sleep from wakefulness. By age 3 months, the NREM-REM cyclical pattern of adult sleep is established. However, the duration of the NREM-REM cycle is shorter in infants, lasting for approximately 45–50 minutes and increasing to 60–70 minutes by age 5–10 years, and to the normal adult cyclical pattern of 90–100 minutes by age 10 years. Sleep spindles begin to appear at about 3 months of age; K complexes are seen by about 6 months (Fig. 101.10).

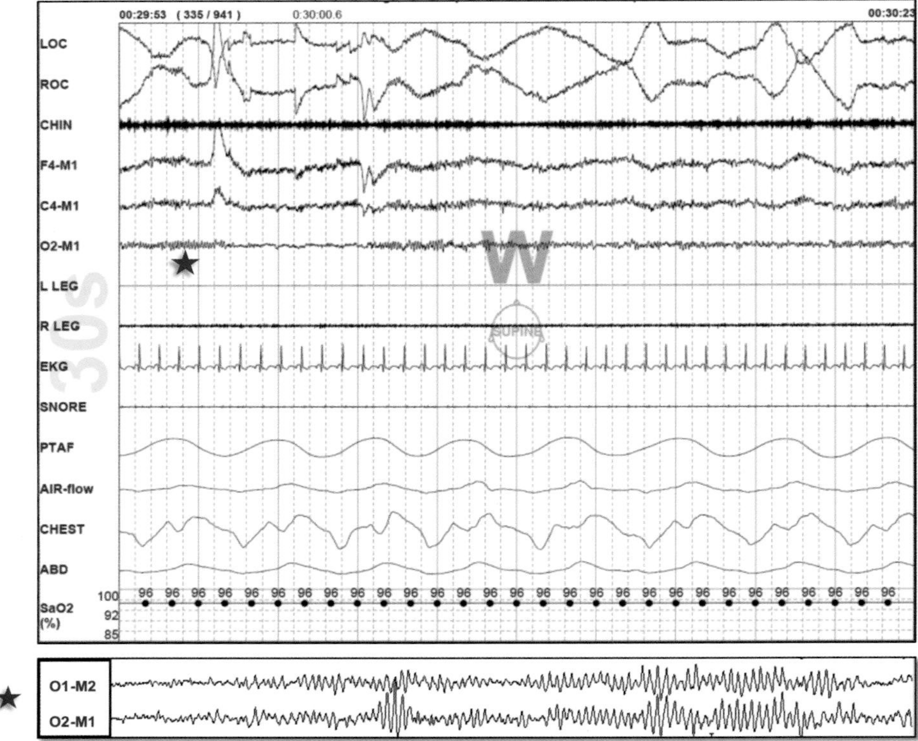


**Fig. 101.2 Polysomnographic Recording Depicting Wakefulness in an Adult.** The electroencephalograms (EEG) portion of the diagram demonstrates posterior dominant 10-Hz alpha rhythm intermixed with a small amount of low-amplitude beta rhythms (international nomenclature). Waking eye movements are seen in the electrooculogram (EOG) in the left *(LOC)* and right *(ROC)* electrodes. Stage W is defined by the presence of alpha rhythm noted in the occipital leads (★) increased chin EMG tone (*CHIN* electrode) rapid eye movements of wakefulness (LOC, ROC). Stage W is scored when more than 50% of the epoch is composed on alpha EEG frequency over the occipital region. Submental EMG depicts relatively high tone and will reflect the high-amplitude muscle contractions and occasionally, movement artifacts. The EOG channels will show eye blinks. As the patient becomes drowsy, with the eyes closed, the EEG will show predominant alpha activity, while the EMG activity will become less prominent. The EOG channels may show slow rolling eye movements. Electrooculogram (EOG): Left, LOC-A2; right, ROC-A1; LOC and ROC left and respectively right outer cantus electrooculography (EOG) electrodes. Electroencephalogram (EEG): *M1*, Left mastoid electrode location (Reference Electrode); *M2*, Right mastoid electrode location (Reference Electrode); C3 and *O1*, left central and left occipital respectively; C4 and *O2*, right central and occipital respectively; F4, Right frontal electrode location. Electromyogram (EMG): CHIN electromyogram (EMG), (Chin 1–chin 2); Limb EMG (L = left leg, R = right leg), LAT1–LAT2 (AT: Anterior Tibias Muscle); L & R ARM, L & R LEG: Left, Right, Arm and Legs EMG; Electrocardiogram (EKG). Respiratory Channels: SNORE, Snore sensor sound; ORAL/N/O AIR-flow, Nasal–oral airflow; THOR/CHEST and ABD, chest and abdominal walls motion effort; $EtCO_2$, End tidal carbon dioxide; PTAF, Pressure transducer airflow; $SaO_2$%, oxygen saturation by pulse oximetry (finger probe).

## Sleep in Older Adults

A characteristic feature of sleep in old age is marked attenuation of the amplitude of slow waves; therefore, during scoring of slow sleep, which depends not only on the rate but also on the amplitude of slow waves, the percentage of slow waves decreases, time awake increases, and light sleep (stage N1) increases (Fig. 101.11). The other characteristic feature during old age is repeated awakenings throughout the night, including early-morning awakenings. Older people spend more time awake in bed than younger people and undergo deterioration in the quality of sleep: Sleep is lighter and more fragmented with increasing age, with reductions of slow-wave sleep. Total sleep time and sleep efficiency decrease. The percentage of slow-wave sleep is reduced and is accompanied by an increase in the percentage of non-REM N1 and N2 sleep. An increase in sleep latency and time spent awake after sleep onset also occurs. While sleep need is similar to younger people, the ability to sleep is impaired. Fig. 101.12 schematically shows the evolution of sleep state distribution in newborns, infants, children, adults, and older adults as a function of time.

## Sleep Habits

Additional text available at http://expertconsult.inkling.com. 

## Sleep Requirements and Quantity of Sleep

Sleep need is determined by heredity rather than by different personality traits or other psychological factors. Social or biological factors may also play a role.

Sleep requirement is defined as the optimal amount of sleep required to remain alert and fully awake and to function adequately throughout the day. Sleep requirement for an average adult is approximately 7.5–8 hours regardless of environment or cultural differences. The 2015 Join Consensus Statement from the AASM and Sleep

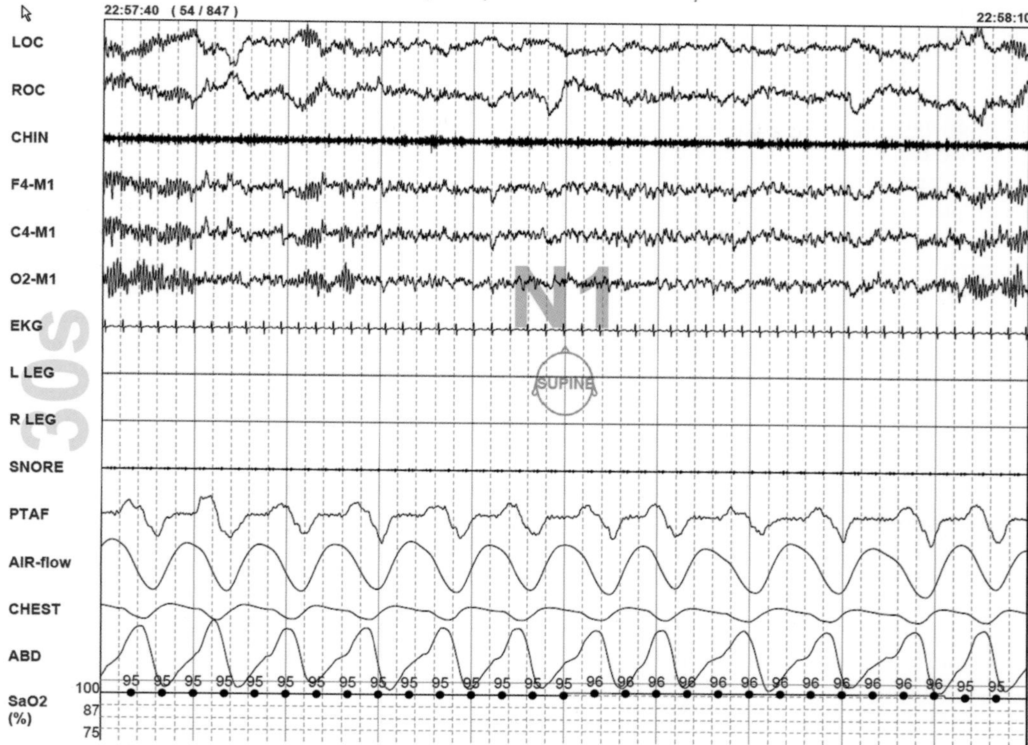


**Fig. 101.3 Polysomnographic Recording Shows Stage 1 Nonrapid Eye Movement (NREM) Sleep (N1) in an Adult.** The epoch demonstrates a decrease of alpha activity to less than 50% and low-amplitude beta and theta activities. Alpha rhythm is best visualized in the posterior regions of the head (O2-M1), appearing when closing the eyes and relaxing (at the beginning of the epoch), and disappearing when opening the eyes (at the end of the epoch). Stage N1 sleep is scored if the alpha rhythm is attenuated or replaced by low-amplitude, mixed-frequency activity (4–7 Hz) for more than half of the epoch. The EMG shows less activity than in wake, but the transition is gradual. During stage N1 sleep, breathing becomes shallow, heart rate becomes regular, blood pressure falls, and the patient exhibits little or no body movement. The monitored patient is still easily awakened and might even deny having slept.

Research Society (SRS) recommended that adults should sleep 7 or more hours per night on a regular basis to promote optimal health. The recommendations went on to highlight that sleeping *less than* 7 hours per night regularly is associated with greater predisposition to adverse health outcomes, including weight gain, insulin resistance, cardiovascular disease, stroke, impaired immune function, increased pain, impaired performance, increased errors, psychiatric conditions such as depression, and greater risk of accidents (Watson et al., 2015). Fig. 101.13 illustrates the Join Consensus Statement from the AASM and SRS sleep duration recommendations from infancy to older age.

## Chronic Sleep Deprivation

Modern society appears to be chronically sleep deprived. Data demonstrate detrimental loss of vigilance with progressive sleep loss, confirming the possibility that sleep deprivation's consequences are serious. Fig. 101.14 shows psychomotor vigilance task (PVT) performance lapses under varying doses of daily sleep, confirming the data of serious lapses when sleep is curtailed beyond 8 hours. A poll by the National Sleep Foundation (NSF) in 2000, 2001, and 2002 indicated that the average sleep duration for Americans had fallen to 6.9–7.0 hours. Across the board, over the last half of the 20th century, sleep duration has diminished by 1.5–2 hours leading to an epidemic of sleep deprivation, where most people are in bed for only 5–6 hours per night on a regular basis. A more recent Sleep in America poll from the NSF found that a majority of the public (65%) reported that getting enough sleep makes them a "more effective person," yet 41% admit to rarely taking into account how much sleep they need in planning for the next day and ranked sleep second to last when asked which of five items were most important to them personally (Knutson et al., 2017).

## Sleep and Dreams

Additional text available at http://expertconsult.inkling.com.
Additional text available at http://expertconsult.inkling.com.

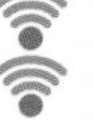

## Neurobiology and Pharmacology of Sleep and Wakefulness

The neuroanatomical substrates for wakefulness and sleep (REM and NREM) are located primarily within the diencephalon and brainstem (McCarley, 2007, 2009; Steriade and McCarley, 2005; Gent, Bassetti, and Adamantidis, 2018; Knutson et al., 2017; Luppi and Fort, 2019; Saeed et al., 2019). Fig. 101.16 summarizes the determination of sleep-wake states according to the specific site and the corresponding neurotransmitter responsible for either wakefulness or sleep. Neuronal networks for achieving wake/sleep are both interconnected and redundant.

Brain pathways regulating wakefulness use the cholinergic, noradrenergic (AKA NE=norepinephrine), dopaminergic, and histaminergic neurons Fig. 101.17, *A*. The cholinergic neurons fire at the highest rate during wakefulness and REM sleep but decrease their rates of firing at the onset of NREM sleep. Wakefulness-promoting aminergic neurons include noradrenergic neurons in the locus coeruleus, serotonergic neurons in the dorsal raphe of the brainstem, histaminergic neurons in the tuberomammillary nucleus of the hypothalamus, dopaminergic neurons in the ventral tegmental area, substantia nigra, and ventral periaqueductal area.

After a period of uncertainty regarding the role of dopamine, it has recently been confirmed that the midbrain dopaminergic system (A8–A10), particularly the dopaminergic neurons in the ventral periaqueductal gray (vPAG), play an active role in maintaining wakefulness through their widespread reciprocal connections with sleep/wake regulatory systems of neurons (Fuller and Lu, 2009). Norepinephrine-containing locus coeruleus neurons show their highest firing rates during wakefulness, their lowest during REM sleep, and intermediate rates during NREM sleep. Pharmacological studies suggest that posterior hypothalamic histaminergic neurons also help maintain wakefulness.

The excitatory amino acids, glutamate and aspartate, are intermingled within the ARAS and are present in many neurons projecting to the cerebral cortex, forebrain, and brainstem. These excitatory amino acids are maximally released during wakefulness. The discovery of hypothalamic hypocretin neurons and their widespread CNS projections has directed attention to the role of the hypocretin system in sleep/wake regulation. In 1998, deLecea and coauthors described two neuropeptides in the lateral hypothalamus and perifornical region that were termed *hypocretin 1* and *hypocretin 2*. Independently in the same year, Sakurai and colleagues (1998) described two neuropeptides in the same region, which they named *orexin A* and *orexin B* (corresponding to hypocretin 1 and hypocretin 2, respectively).

It was shown thereafter that these hypocretin systems have widespread ascending and descending projections to the locus coeruleus, dorsal raphe, ventral tegmental area, tuberomammillary nuclei of the posterior hypothalamus, laterodorsal tegmental (LDT) and pedunculopontine tegmental (PPT) nuclei, VLPO neurons in the hypothalamus, basal forebrain, limbic system (hippocampus and amygdala), cerebral cortex, thalamus (intralaminar and midline nuclei), and autonomic neurons (nucleus tractus solitarius [NTS], dorsal vagal nuclei, and intermediolateral neurons of the spinal cord). Hypocretin systems promote wakefulness mainly through excitation of tuberomammillary histaminergic, locus ceruleus noradrenergic, and midline raphe serotonergic neurons as well as dopaminergic neurons. Reduced activity of hypocretin systems may be partly responsible for inducing sleepiness. These systems also suppress REM sleep through activation of the aminergic neurons (REM-off), which in turn inhibit REM-on neurons in the LDT/PPT nuclei. Brainstem arousal centers were identified and characterized, and support was later provided for the concept of *sleep-promoting circuitry* in the anterior hypothalamus/preoptic area, where the VLPO nucleus contains sleep-active cells that contain the inhibitory neurotransmitters γ-aminobutyric acid (GABA) and galanin (Gal), which promote sleep eFig. 101.7.

Fig. 101.17 summarizes the neuroanatomical substrates of wakefulness, REM and NREM sleep highlighting the neuroanatomy, neurochemistry, and corresponding physiological activity during polysomnography.

Additional text available at http://expertconsult.inkling.com.

## MECHANISM OF MUSCLE ANTONIA DURING RAPID EYE MOVEMENT SLEEP

Muscle hypotonia or atonia during REM sleep is thought to depend on inhibitory postsynaptic potentials generated by dorsal pontine interneurons sending descending axons as depicted in Fig. 101.19. The pathway from the peri-locus coeruleus (Pre-Coeruleus, in the diagram) alpha region ventral to the locus coeruleus, to the lateral tegmental reticular tract, and then to the medial medullary region (demarcated as the magnocellular reticular formation) and the reticulospinal tract projecting to the spinal interneuron of the spinal cord controls REM sleep-induced muscle atonia. An experimental lesion (☆) in the peri-locus coeruleus alpha region and in the medial medullary region (Panel B) produced REM sleep without muscle atonia (RSWA). In addition to DEB associated with RSWA, it is thought that a structural or functional alteration of the pathway maintaining muscle atonia during REM sleep is most likely responsible.

Advances in neuroimaging studies, including positron emission tomography (PET) and single-photon emission computed tomography (SPECT) scans, have been able to visualize dramatic changes in function in cortical and subcortical neuronal networks in different sleep states and stages, advancing our understanding of the functional neuroanatomy of sleep/wakefulness (Dang-Vu et al., 2007). PET scans have shown marked activation of the amygdala and the anterior cingulate region (part of the limbic system) during REM sleep, which is, of course, generated by brainstem neurons. In contrast, in NREM sleep, neuroimaging techniques have shown declining function in the thalamocortical circuits, including the association cortex of the frontoparietal and temporal lobes. Thus, the brainstem, hypothalamic, and forebrain sleep/wake-promoting neurons modulate functions of widespread forebrain cortical areas, keeping in balance cortical and subcortical circuits to control sleep/wake.

Additional text available at http://expertconsult.inkling.com.

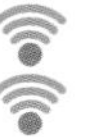

Additional text available at http://expertconsult.inkling.com.

### Circadian Rhythm and Chronobiology of Sleep

The 18th-century French astronomer de Mairan (1731) first directed our attention to the existence of circadian rhythm when he noted that in a heliotrope plant, the leaves closed at sunset and opened at sunrise even when the plant was kept in darkness (see Chokroverty, 2015a). This observation clearly pointed to a 24-hour rhythm controlled by an internal clock. The existence of such a circadian rhythm in human beings and other animals was confirmed toward the last half of the last century. The term *circadian rhythm* originates from the Latin *circa*, meaning "about," and *dies*, meaning "day." Human circadian rhythm generally has a cycle length close to 24 hours (approximately 24.2 hours) (Czeisler and Gooley, 2007). The existence of circadian rhythms independent of environmental stimuli has been clearly demonstrated by experimental isolation of humans from all environmental time cues (the German term, *Zeitgeber*, or "time giver"), as in a cave or underground bunker, to study free-running rhythms.

The paired SCN, the paired nuclei above the hypothalamus, function as the body clock to control circadian rhythm (Fig. 101.20). The recent discovery of anatomical projections from SCN to the lateral hypothalamic neurons containing hypocretin (wake-promoting) and anterior hypothalamic VLPO containing sleep-promoting neurons suggested that the SCN may also affect sleep regulation and homeostasis independent of circadian rhythm generation (Turek and Vitaterna, 2011) (Video 101.1).

The existence of environment-independent autonomous rhythms suggests that the human body also has an internal biological clock. The SCN receives photic information from the retinohypothalamic tract, which sends signals to multiple synaptic pathways in other parts of the hypothalamus, the superior cervical ganglion, and the pineal gland where melatonin is produced and released (A). Through a polysynaptic projection, the SCN inhibits the activity of the superior cervical ganglia (SCG), which supply the pineal gland with an excitatory, noradrenaline (NA)-containing input (B). This mechanism allows light to suppress the production and release of melatonin from the pineal gland and, subsequently, melatonin secretion is enhanced in the dark period (de Bodinat et al., 2010). Melatonin is a critical modulator of

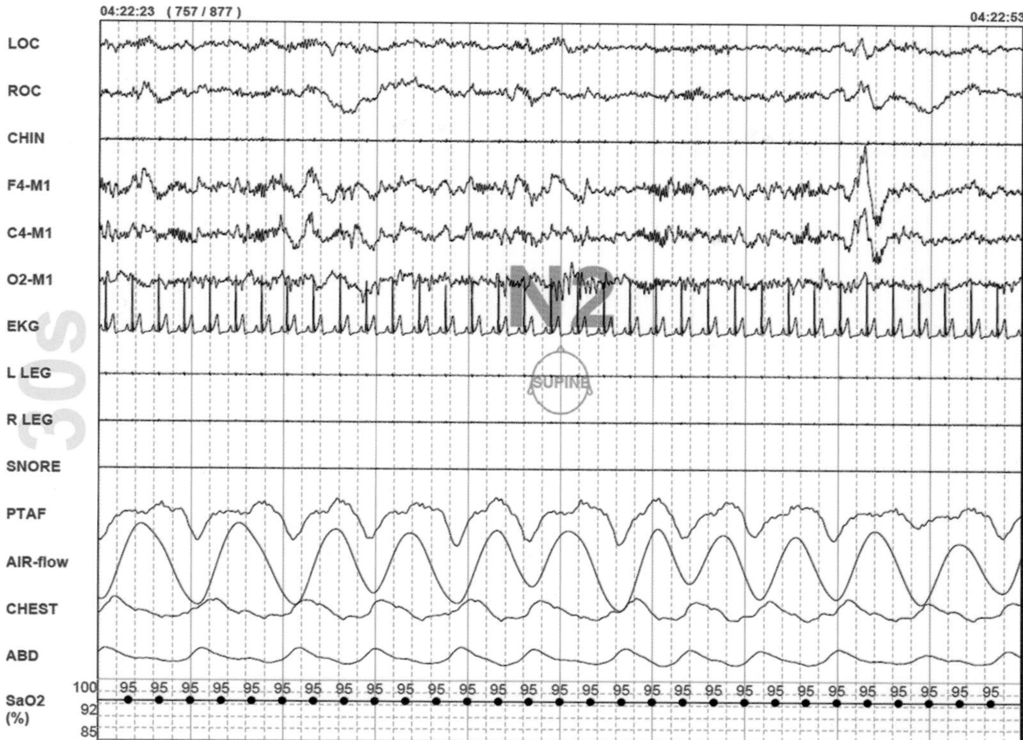


**Fig. 101.4 Stage N2 Sleep.** Unique features of stage N2 sleep include 12- to 14-Hz sleep spindles and biphasic K complexes intermixed with delta waves (0.5–2 Hz) and up to 75 μV in amplitude occupying less than 20% of the epoch. Stage N2 is an intermediate stage of sleep, but it also accounts for the bulk of a typical polysomnographic recording. It follows stage N1 sleep and initially lasts about 20 minutes. Stage N2 can begin to be scored if one or more K complexes or sleep spindles are noted during the first half of the epoch or the last half of the previous epoch. K complexes are biphasic in morphology consisting of negative (upward deflection) sharp waves followed by a slower positive (downward deflection) component with a total duration of greater than 500 ms. Sleep spindles are generated in the midline thalamic nuclei, are characterized by 12- to 14-Hz sinusoidal EEG activity in the central vertex region and must persist for at least 0.5 seconds. Stage N2 sleep is associated with a relative diminution of physiological bodily functions with attenuation of blood pressure, brain metabolism, gastrointestinal secretions, and cardiac activity.

human circadian rhythm for entrainment by the light/dark cycle. The melatonin level rises fairly abruptly in the evening and then reaches its maximum level between 3:00 AM and 5:00 AM, after which it decreases to low levels during the daytime. Melatonin reciprocally activates the SCN at two melatonin receptors (C): melatonin type 1 ($MT_1$) and melatonin type 2 ($MT_2$) receptors. Serotonergic input from the raphe nucleus modulates the SCN through actions at serotonin (also known as 5-hydroxytryptamine; 5-HT) receptor 5-$HT_{2C}$. Daily activity and behaviors likewise influence output from the SCN—the neuronal master clock for coordinating circadian rhythms—including key physiological processes such as the sleep/wake cycle, body temperature, and neuroendocrine secretion. The SCN also receives key signals vital for metabolism (Fig. 101.21) and derives "time of day" information from environmental light cues captured by specialized cells within the retina.

Sleep scientists have begun to identify the molecular basis of the mammalian circadian clock. A total of eight or nine genes (e.g., CLOCK, PER, Bmal) and their protein products have been identified within the circadian clock system; understanding of these is still evolving (Turek and Vitaterna, 2011). Remarkable progress has been made in the past few years in the key components of the circadian clock in both fruit flies *(Drosophila)* and mammals. Dysfunction of circadian rhythm results in some important human sleep disorders. The molecular mechanism of two human circadian rhythm disorders—advanced sleep phase syndrome (ASPS) and delayed sleep phase syndrome (DSPS)—has been uncovered by applying gene sequencing techniques. ASPS occur due to a mutation of the PER2 gene (a human homolog of the period 2 gene in *Drosophila*) causing advancing of the clock (i.e., alteration of the circadian timing of sleep propensity). DSPS is due to polymorphism of the PER3 gene.

## Circadian, Homeostatic, and Other Sleep Factors

Sleep and wakefulness are controlled by both homeostatic and circadian factors. The duration of prior wakefulness determines the propensity to sleepiness (homeostatic factor), whereas circadian factors determine the timing, duration, and characteristics of sleep. There are two types of sleepiness: physiological and subjective (Dinges, 1995). *Physiological sleepiness* is the body's propensity to sleepiness. There are two highly vulnerable periods of sleepiness: 2:00–6:00 AM, particularly 3:00–5:00 AM, and 2:00–6:00 PM, particularly 3:00–5:00 PM. The propensity to physiological sleepiness (e.g., midafternoon and early-morning hours) depends on circadian factors. The highest number of sleep-related accidents have been observed during these periods. *Subjective sleepiness* is the individual's perception of sleepiness; it depends on several external factors such as a stimulating environment and ingestion of coffee and other caffeinated beverages.

Physiological sleepiness depends on two processes: homeostatic factor and circadian phase. *Homeostatic factor* refers to a prior period of wakefulness and sleep debt. After a prolonged period of wakefulness, there is an increasing tendency to sleep. The recovery from sleep debt is aided by an additional amount of sleep, but this

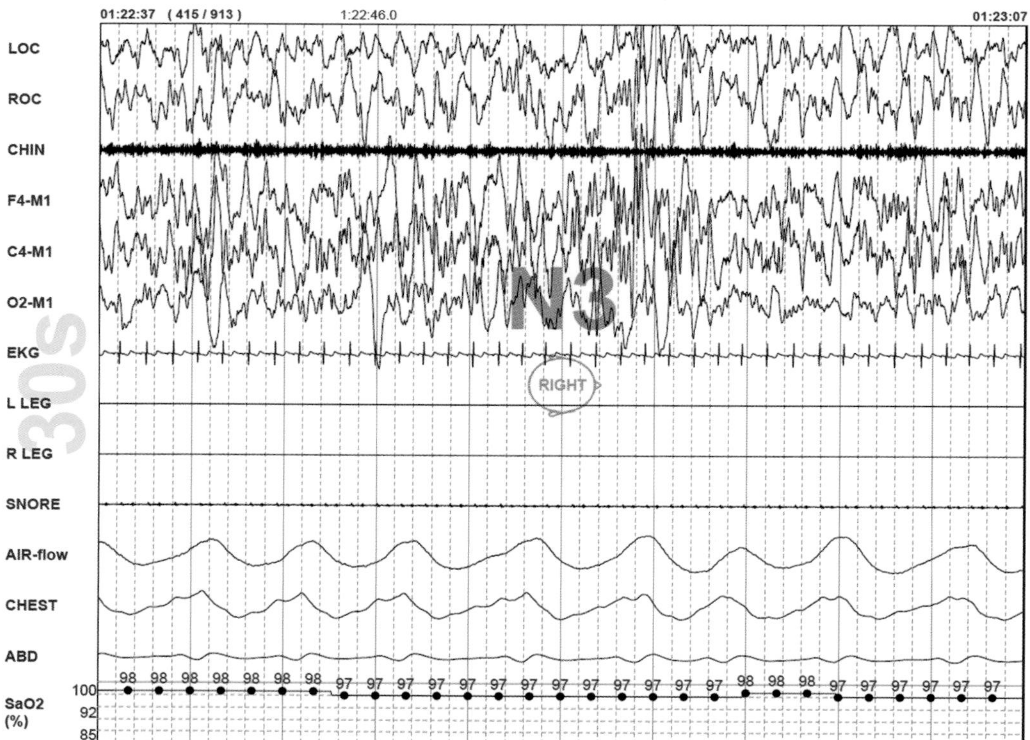


**Fig. 101.5 Stage N3 Sleep.** Polysomnographic recording of Stage N3, also termed *deep sleep, slow-wave sleep (SWS)*, or *delta sleep*. The updated American Academy of Sleep Medicine Sleep (AASM) Sleep Stage Scoring collectively refers to stage N3 as being comprised of *Rechtschaffen and Kales (R & K) sleep scoring* stage 3 and 4 together and does not make a distinction between them as such distinction probably does not appear to serve clear clinical significance. N3 sleep is marked by high-amplitude slow waves (0.5-to-2 Hz) with minimum amplitude of 75 microvolts as measured over the frontal regions. Slow-wave activity must be present for greater than or equal to 20% of the epoch to be scored stage N3 sleep. No specific criteria for EOG and EMG exist for stage N3 sleep, but in general, muscle tone is further decreased and there is no eye movement activity. This stage of sleep has the highest threshold for arousal and is associated with disorders of arousal.

recovery is not linear. Thus, an exact number of hours of sleep are not required to repay sleep debt; rather, the body needs an adequate amount of slow-wave sleep for restoration. The interaction between the circadian and the homeostatic drive producing alertness is depicted in Fig. 101.22. The *circadian factor* determines the body's propensity to maximal sleepiness between 3:00 AM and 5:00 AM. The second period of maximal sleepiness (3:00–5:00 PM) is not as strong as the first. Sleep and wakefulness and the circadian pacemaker have a reciprocal relationship: the biological clock can affect sleep and wakefulness, and sleep and wakefulness can affect the clock. There are two variables that seem to play a role in regulating the timing of sleep. First is the homeostatic sleep drive, which increases as the day progresses and the longer a person is awake. The second is timing information from the SCN. In this two-process model, the SCN promotes wakefulness by stimulating arousal networks. The activity of the circadian system appears to oppose that of the homeostatic sleep drive, and thus the alerting mediated by the SCN increases during the day. The propensity to be awake or asleep at any time is related to the homeostatic sleep drive and the opposing SCN alerting signal. At normal bedtime, both the alerting drive and the sleep drive are at their highest level. The two melatonin receptors, MT1 and MT2 receptor subtypes, are directly involved in the regulation of sleep and circadian regulation. Stimulation of MT1 receptors is believed to decrease the alerting signal from the SCN, while MT2 stimulation is thought to be involved in synchronizing the circadian system.

Various sleep factors have been identified, but their role in maintaining homeostasis has not been clearly established (Krueger et al., 2011). Several cytokines, such as interleukin-1, interferon-α, and tumor necrosis factor, promote sleep. Other sleep factors increase in concentration during prolonged wakefulness and infection. It has been shown that adenosine in the basal forebrain can fulfill the major criteria for the neural sleep factor that mediates the somnogenic effect of prolonged wakefulness by acting through adenosine A1 and A2A receptors. Several other endogenous compounds may serve as sleep factors, including delta sleep-inducing peptides, muramyl peptides, cholecystokinins, arginine vasotocin, vasoactive intestinal peptides, growth hormone-releasing factors, and somatostatins. Finally, neurologists need to be mindful of how the circadian clock regulates how the body responds to an illness, such as COVID-19. It is particularly relevant these days to appreciate the role of chronotherapy when matching immunotherpy to the body's circadian rhythm in impacting recovery from illness.

## Functions of Sleep

The function of sleep remains the greatest biological mystery of all time. There are several theories about the function of sleep (eBox 101.3), but none are satisfactory (Crick and Mitchison, 1995; Kavanau, 1997; Mahowald et al., 1997). Sleep deprivation experiments in animals have clearly shown that sleep is necessary for survival, but from a practical point of view, complete sleep deprivation for a prolonged period cannot be conducted in humans. Sleep deprivation studies in humans have shown an impairment of performance, which demonstrates the need for sleep. The performance impairment of prolonged sleep deprivation results from a decreased motivation and frequent "microsleeps." Overall, human sleep deprivation experiments have proven that sleep deprivation causes sleepiness and impairment of

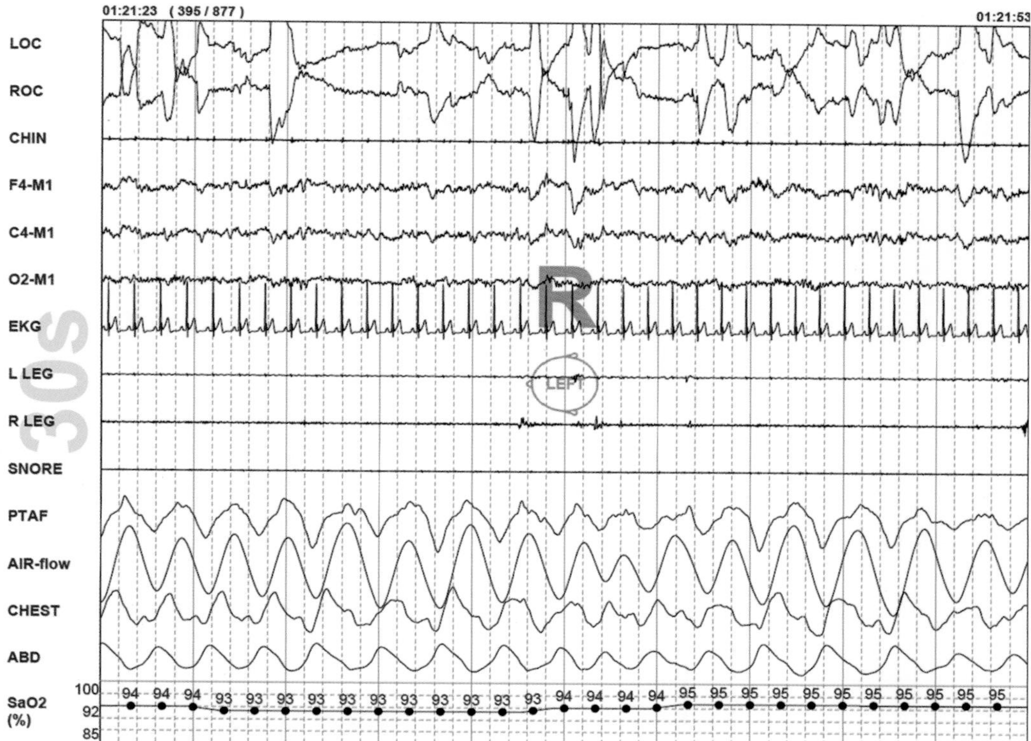


**Fig. 101.6 Stage REM (R) Sleep.** Polysomnographic recording of Stage R sleep shows rapid eye movement (REM) depicting mixed-frequency theta, low-amplitude beta, characteristic sawtooth waves. Chin electromyogram (EMG) shows marked hypotonia. Stage R sleep is also referred to as *paradoxical sleep*, or *active sleep*, typically occurs between 90 and 120 minutes after sleep onset in adults, and occupies between 20% and 25% of overnight adult sleep. Rapid eye movements are conjugate, irregular, sharply peaked eye movements. Chin EMG tone should be at the lowest level of any sleep stage. Unlike the progressive relaxation noted during the NREM sleep stages N1, N2, and N3, physiological activity during REM sleep is significantly higher. Blood pressure and pulse rate may increase dramatically or may show intermittent fluctuations. Breathing becomes irregular and brain oxygen consumption increases. If patients are awakened from stage R sleep, they may often recall dreaming. Pathologically short REM sleep latency may point to a state of acute or cumulative sleep deprivation, may be caused by abrupt discontinuation of REM sleep–suppressing agents (such as antidepressants), central nervous system hypersomnias, and may also suggest a major affective disorder.

performance, vigilance, attention, concentration, and memory. Sleep deprivation may also cause some metabolic, hormonal, and immunological effects. Sleep deprivation causes immune suppression; even partial sleep deprivation reduces cellular immune responses. Studies from Van Cauter's (Spiegel et al., 1999) group include a clearly documented elevation of cortisol level following even partial sleep loss, suggesting an alteration in hypothalamic-pituitary-adrenal axis function. This has been confirmed even in chronic sleep deprivation that causes impairment of glucose tolerance. Glucose intolerance may contribute to memory impairment as a result of decreased hippocampal function. Chronic sleep deprivation may also cause a decrement of thyrotropin concentration, increased evening cortisol level, and sympathetic hyperactivity, which may serve as risk factors for obesity, hypertension, and diabetes mellitus. Further data from the same group demonstrated that increase in ghrelin levels associated with short sleep reduced leptin. These differences in leptin and ghrelin may induce increased appetite, possibly explaining the increased body mass index (BMI) observed with short sleep duration in the study populations. The authors correctly indicate that in Western societies, where chronic sleep restriction is common and food is ubiquitous, alterations in appetite regulatory hormones with sleep curtailment may contribute to obesity.

The *restorative theory* suggests that sleep is needed to restore cerebral function after periods of waking. The findings of increased secretion of anabolic hormones (e.g., growth hormone, prolactin, testosterone, and luteinizing hormone) and decreased levels of catabolic hormones (e.g., cortisol) during sleep, as well as the subjective feeling of being refreshed after sleep, may support the theory of body and brain tissue restoration by sleep. The role of NREM sleep in restoring the body is further supported by the presence of increased slow-wave sleep after sleep deprivation. The critical role of REM sleep for CNS development in young organisms and increased protein synthesis in the brain during REM sleep may support the theory of restoration of brain function by REM sleep. Although data remain scant and controversial, studies of brain basal metabolism that suggest an enhanced synthesis of macromolecules such as nucleic acids and proteins in the brain during sleep provide an argument in favor of the restorative theory of sleep.

The *energy conservation theory* is somewhat inadequate. The fact that animals with a high metabolic rate sleep longer than those with slower metabolism has been cited in support of this theory. It should, however, be noted that during 8 hours of sleep, only 120 calories are conserved.

The *adaptation theory* suggests that sleep is an instinct that allows creatures to survive under a variety of environmental conditions.

Some recent advances have been made in understanding the molecular mechanisms of *memory consolidation* during sleep (Stickgold and Walker, 2007). Studies have revealed that new memories can be strengthened by sleep. In other words, sleep can rescue memories that are lost during wakefulness during the daytime, and consolidated memories can be reconsolidated when they are reactivated. Memory is stored in

## TABLE 101.2 Key Brain Wave Morphologies, Frequencies, and Landmarks Used in Sleep Staging

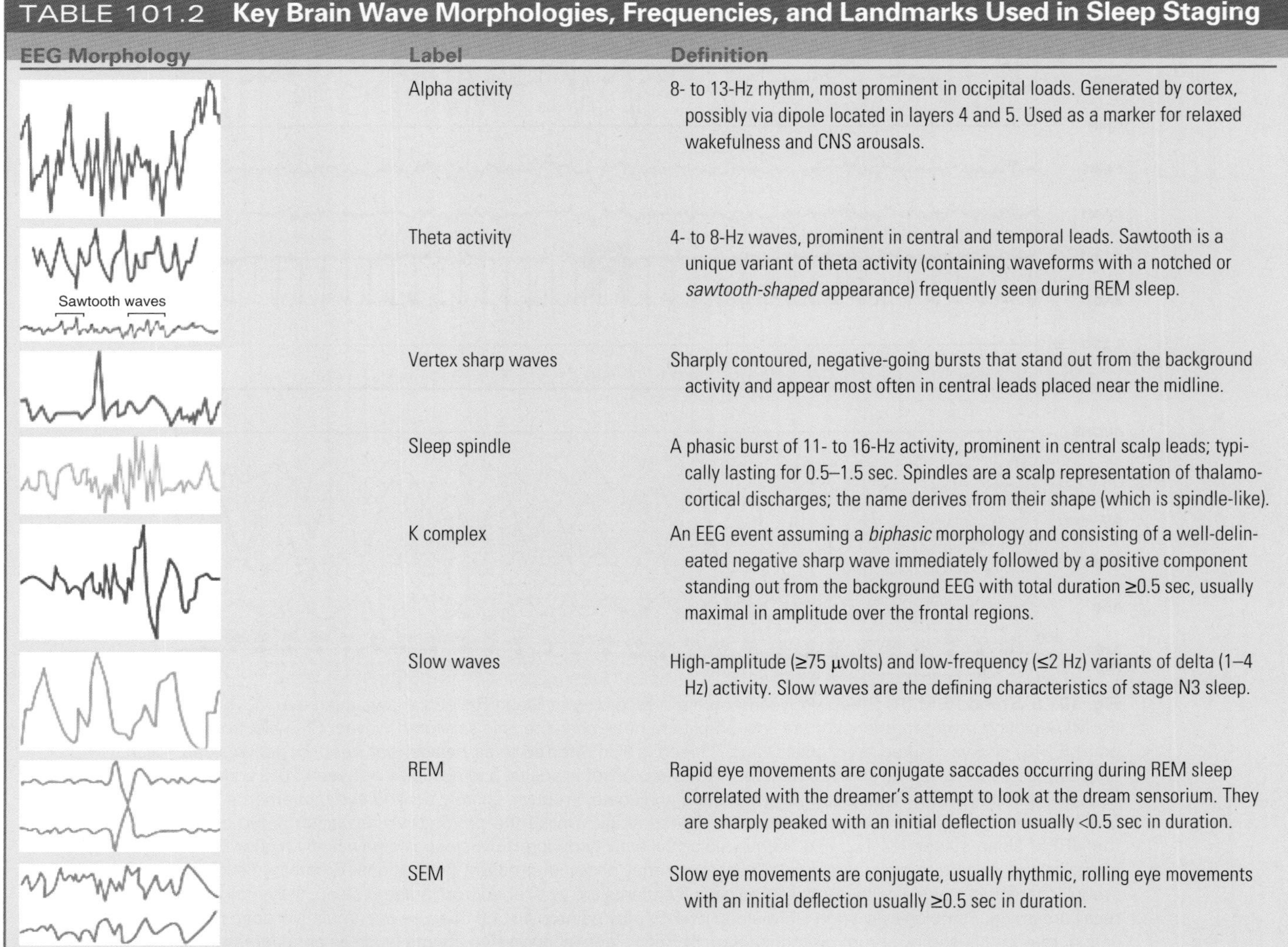

| EEG Morphology | Label | Definition |
|---|---|---|
| | Alpha activity | 8- to 13-Hz rhythm, most prominent in occipital loads. Generated by cortex, possibly via dipole located in layers 4 and 5. Used as a marker for relaxed wakefulness and CNS arousals. |
| Sawtooth waves | Theta activity | 4- to 8-Hz waves, prominent in central and temporal leads. Sawtooth is a unique variant of theta activity (containing waveforms with a notched or *sawtooth-shaped* appearance) frequently seen during REM sleep. |
| | Vertex sharp waves | Sharply contoured, negative-going bursts that stand out from the background activity and appear most often in central leads placed near the midline. |
| | Sleep spindle | A phasic burst of 11- to 16-Hz activity, prominent in central scalp leads; typically lasting for 0.5–1.5 sec. Spindles are a scalp representation of thalamocortical discharges; the name derives from their shape (which is spindle-like). |
| | K complex | An EEG event assuming a *biphasic* morphology and consisting of a well-delineated negative sharp wave immediately followed by a positive component standing out from the background EEG with total duration ≥0.5 sec, usually maximal in amplitude over the frontal regions. |
| | Slow waves | High-amplitude (≥75 μvolts) and low-frequency (≤2 Hz) variants of delta (1–4 Hz) activity. Slow waves are the defining characteristics of stage N3 sleep. |
| | REM | Rapid eye movements are conjugate saccades occurring during REM sleep correlated with the dreamer's attempt to look at the dream sensorium. They are sharply peaked with an initial deflection usually <0.5 sec in duration. |
| | SEM | Slow eye movements are conjugate, usually rhythmic, rolling eye movements with an initial deflection usually ≥0.5 sec in duration. |

*CNS*, Central nervous system; *EEG*, electroencephalogram; *REM*, rapid eye movement.
*Modified from Kryger, M.H., Avidan, A., Berry, R., 2013. Atlas of Clinical Sleep Medicine, second ed. Saunders/Elsevier, Philadelphia.*

## TABLE 101.3 Summary of Nonrapid Eye Movement and Rapid Eye Movement Sleep States

| Sleep State | % Sleep Time |
|---|---|
| NREM sleep | 75–80 |
| N1 | 3–8 |
| N2 | 45–55 |
| N3 | 13–23 |
| REM sleep (stage R) | 20–25 |
| Tonic stage | Continuous |
| Phasic stage | Intermittent |

*NREM*, Nonrapid eye movement; *REM*, rapid eye movement.

two stages: short-term memory, which is labile, and long-term memory, which is stable and consolidated, requiring synthesis of new ribonucleic acid (RNA) and proteins by the neurons. Recent studies have clearly shown a significant contribution of sleep to memory consolidation. It has been suggested that memory consolidation occurs during both slow-wave and REM sleep. There is a further suggestion that REM-NREM sleep cycling is also important for memory consolidation.

The theory of *maintenance of synaptic and neuronal network integrity* is an emerging concept that is concerned with the primary function of sleep. Intermittent stimulation of neural network synapses is necessary to preserve CNS function (Kavanau, 1997).

Gene expression (Cirelli and Tononi, 2011) studied by deoxyribonucleic acid (DNA) microarray technique identified sleep- and wakefulness-related genes (brain transcripts) subserving different functions (e.g., energy metabolism, synaptic excitation, long-term potentiation, and response to cellular stress during wakefulness and protein synthesis, memory consolidation, and synaptic downscaling during sleep). Fig. 101.23 provides a basis for the *synaptic homeostasis theory*.

The top panel of the figure illustrates schematically how a net increase in synaptic strength occurs during wakefulness when many circuits in the brain become potentiated (red lines in the brain schematic), resulting in overall cellular and systems costs, followed by synaptic renormalization during sleep. This is that time when most, if not all, circuits undergo synaptic down-selection (green lines). The bottom portion of the figure highlights how parameters are used to test SHY. The color gradient in the column labeled "synaptic strength" highlights that while objectively verifiable indicators of structural and molecular measures were more likely to reveal a state of synaptic strength, electrophysiological measures such as firing rates and evoked responses can be strongly affected by other factors that modulate intrinsic neuronal excitability, including

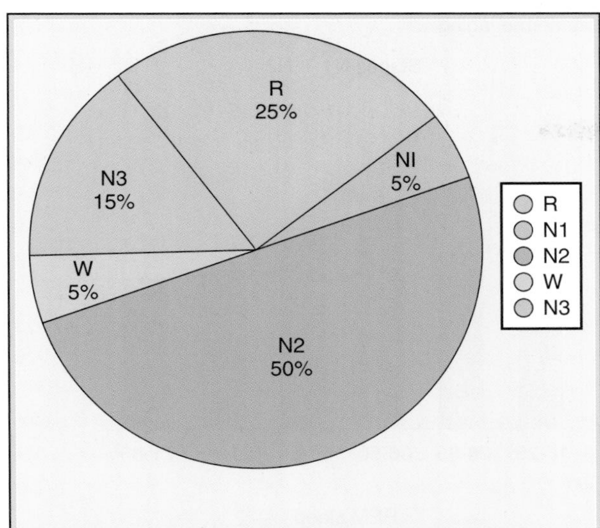


**Fig. 101.7 Pie Graph Demonstrates Proportion of Time During the Night That an Adult Spends in Various Sleep Stages.** Wakefulness *(W)* in sleep usually makes up less than 5% of the night. Stage *N1* sleep generally makes up 2% to 5% of sleep; stage *N2*, 45% to 55%; stage *N3*, 3% to 15%. Nonrapid eye movement (NREM) sleep therefore usually makes up 75% to 80% of sleep. Stage rapid eye movement *(R)* sleep typically makes up between 20% and 25% of total sleep of the night, occurring in three to six discrete episodes. *(Modified from Kryger, M.H., Avidan, A., Berry, R., 2013. Atlas of Clinical Sleep Medicine, second ed. Saunders/Elsevier, Philadelphia).*

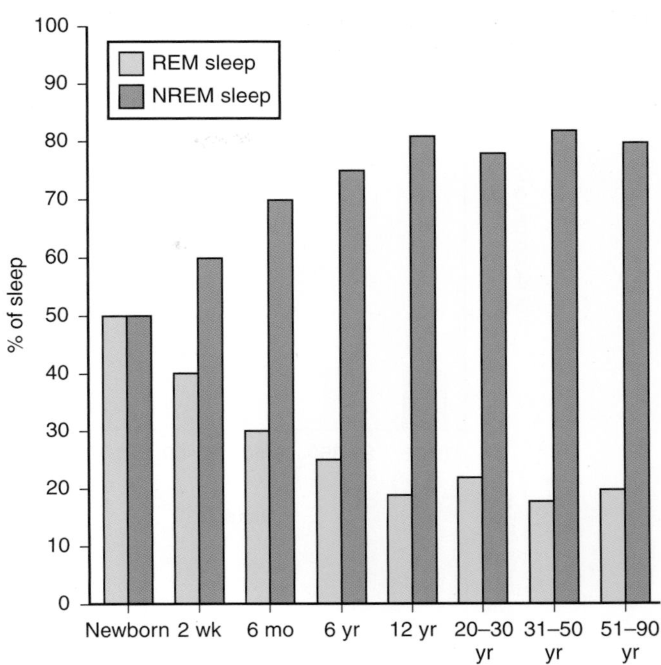


**Fig. 101.9** Schematic diagram showing percentages of rapid eye movement *(REM)* and nonrapid eye movement *(NREM)* sleep at different ages. Note the marked changes in REM sleep in the early years. *(Modified and adapted from Roffwarg, H.P., Muzzio, J.N., Dement, W.C., 1966. Ontogenic development of the human sleep-dream cycle. Science 152, 604).*

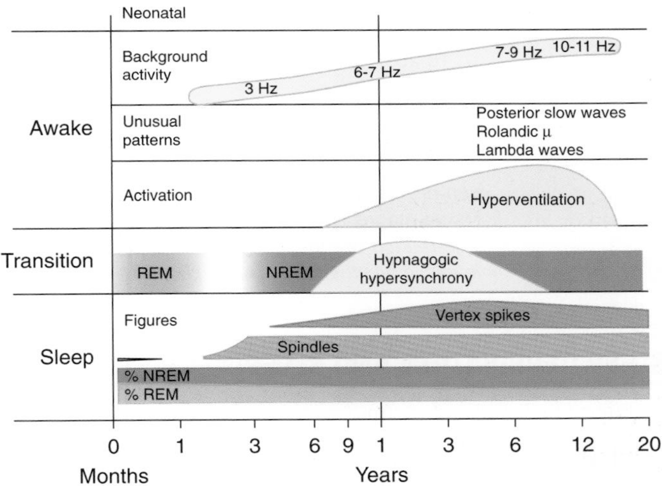


**Fig. 101.10 Maturation of the Brain Wave Patterns in Sleep.** Development, appearance, and disappearance of electroencephalographic landmarks from prematurity to 3 months post term to age 20. Sleep spindles and vertex transients generally appear around 48 weeks of conception. *NREM,* Non rapid eye movement; *REM,* rapid eye movement. *(From Hrachovy, R.A., 2000. Development of normal EEG. In: Levin, K.H., Luders, H.O. [Eds.], Comprehensive Clinical Neurophysiology. WB Saunders, Philadelphia, pp. 387–413).*

the levels of neuromodulators and the overall balance between excitation and inhibition. However, these cannot be used alone to infer synaptic strength. In the upper panels (structural and molecular), the red line indicates the axon to spine interface (ASI), and the yellow area outlines the head of the spine. Excitatory glutamatergic receptors (AMPARs) are shown as squared boxes close to the ASI. Minis = miniature excitatory synaptic currents (Cirelli, 2017; Cirelli and Tononi, 2015).

The *thermoregulatory function theory* is based on the observation that thermoregulatory homeostasis is maintained during sleep, whereas severe thermoregulatory abnormalities follow total sleep deprivation. The preoptic anterior hypothalamic neurons participate in thermoregulation and NREM sleep. These two processes are closely linked by preoptic anterior hypothalamic neurons but are clearly separate. Thermoregulation is maintained during NREM sleep but is suspended during REM sleep. Thermoregulatory responses such as shivering, piloerection, panting, and sweating are impaired during REM sleep. There is a loss of thermosensitivity in the preoptic anterior hypothalamic neurons during REM sleep.

A fascinating new theory proposes a sleep state-dependent enhanced brain flushing as depicted by enhanced CSF flow through a relatively newly discovered drainage system, the so-called glymphatic system (Iliff et al., 2012). In mice, data revealed that enhanced CSF-flow, during sleep state, increased the removal of β-amyloid metabolites. The glymphatic system allows for CSF circulation through the brain, exchanging fluid allowing for enhanced clearance waste products across the blood–brain barrier into the nearby blood vessels for further transportation, as illustrated in Fig. 101.24 (Herculano-Houzel, 2013). Emerging new data shows that the glymphatic (paravascular) system mediates liquid flux through the brain, highlights that the circadian clock probably plays a critical role in this context, and likely holds new research paradigms to further elucidate the role of sleep-state depended CSF-flow in delaying and preventing neurodegenerative disease-associated metabolites during sleeping, including alpha-synucleinopathies and tauopathies (Larson et al., 2012). The glymphatic fluid transporting system could provide an additional source of apoE and then delivers it to brain via the periarterial space. By inference, when the glymphatic fluid flow and interstitial fluid (ISF) clearance system fails in this essential physiological role, one would presume a high likelihood of apoE isoform-specific disorders chronically (Achariyar et al., 2016).

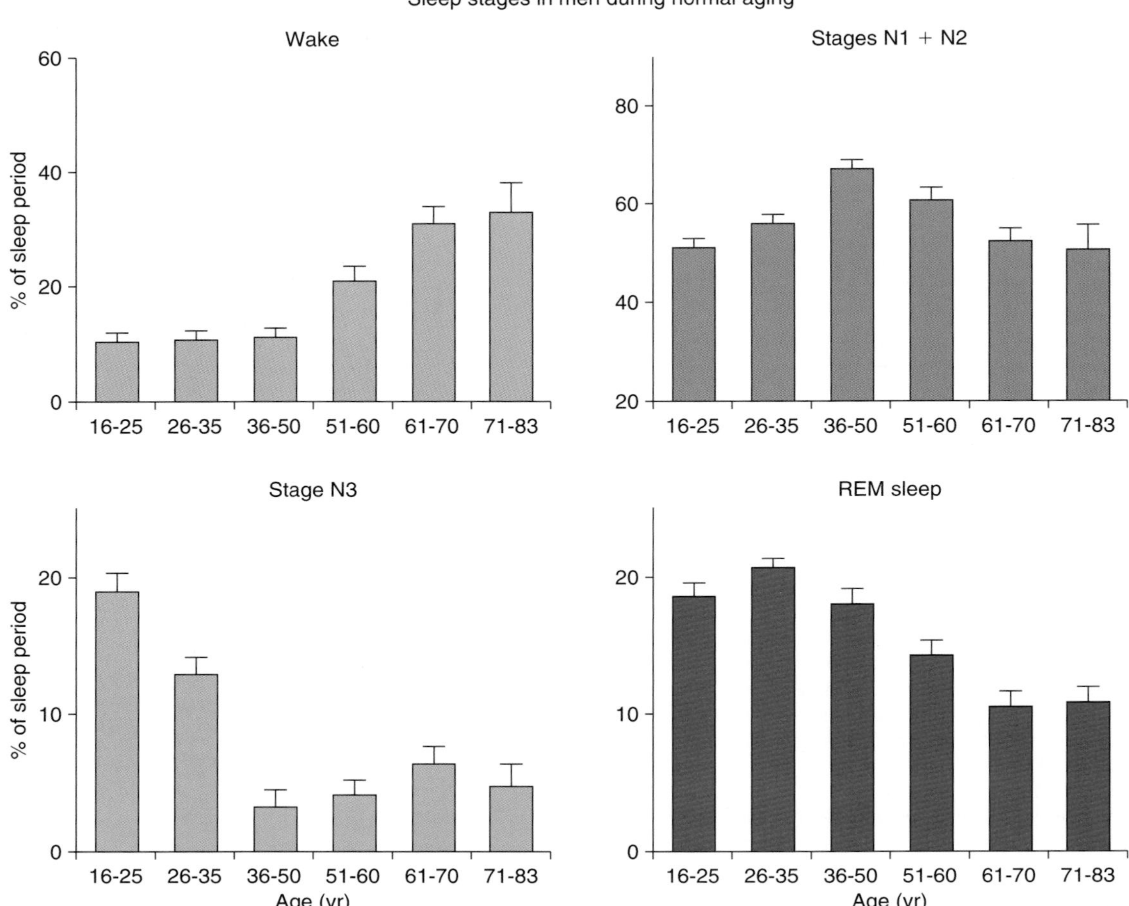


**Fig. 101.11 Sleep Changes with Age.** Age-related changes in sleep stages occur with different chronologies for slow-wave sleep (stage N3) and rapid eye movement *(REM)* sleep. From young adulthood to midlife, deep slow-wave sleep is replaced by lighter stages of sleep without significant changes in sleep fragmentation or REM sleep. From midlife to late life, sleep is more fragmented at the expense of decreases in both lighter stages of sleep (N1 + N2) and REM sleep. *(Modified from Van Cauter, E., Leproult, R., Plat, L.,2000. Age-related changes in slow-wave sleep and REM sleep and relationship with growth hormone and cortisol levels in healthy men. JAMA 284, 861–868. With permission.)*

## SLEEP DEPRIVATION AND SLEEPINESS

 Additional text available at http://expertconsult.inkling.com.

### Total Sleep Deprivation

 Additional text available at http://expertconsult.inkling.com.

### Partial and Selective Sleep Deprivation

 Additional text available at http://expertconsult.inkling.com.

### Consequences of Excessive Daytime Sleepiness

 The consequences of excessive daytime sleepiness (EDS) presented in eBox 101.4 principally affect four key domains: (1) performance and productivity at work and school, (2) higher cerebral functions, (3) quality of life and social interactions, and (4) morbidity and mortality (Roth and Roehrs, 1996).

#### Performance and Productivity at Work and School

Impaired performance and reduced productivity at work for shift workers, reduced performance in class for school and college students, and impaired job performance in patients with narcolepsy, sleep apnea, circadian rhythm disorders, and chronic insomnia are well-known adverse effects of sleep deprivation and sleepiness. Sleepiness and associated morbidity are worse in night shift workers, older workers, and female shift workers. Recent data indicates that chronic sleep deprivation is associated with poorer academic performance as assessed by grade point average (GPA) (Chen and Chen, 2019). The ramifications of chronic sleep loss may also predict the likelihood of obtaining a college degree. Students who experienced sleep deprivation from their freshman to senior years had a lower chance of graduation than students who were not sleep deprived (Chen and Chen, 2019).

#### Higher Cerebral Functions

Sleepiness interferes with higher cerebral functions, causing impairment of short-term memory, concentration, attention, cognition, and intellectual performance. Psychometric tests document increased reaction time in patients with excessive sleepiness. These individuals make increasing numbers of errors, and they need increasing time to reach the target in reaction time tests (Dinges, 1995). Sleepiness can also impair perceptual skills and new learning. Insufficient sleep and

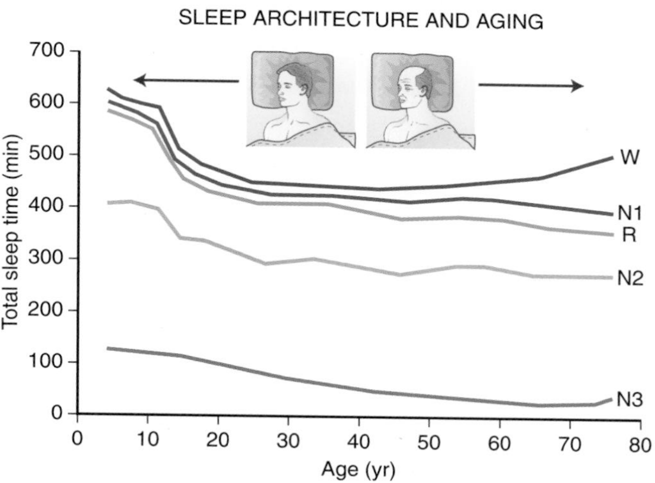


**Fig. 101.12 Ontogeny of Sleep.** Changes in sleep stage in infants, children, adults, and elder adults, demonstrating the evolution of sleep by sleep stage. *W*, wake; *R*, rapid eye movement (REM) sleep; *N1, N2, N3*, stages N1, N2, and N3 NREM sleep, respectively. Compared with early life, older adults spend more time awake in bed, less time in R and N3 sleep, and more time in lighter stages of sleep.

excessive sleepiness may cause irritability, anxiety, and depression. Learning disabilities and cognitive impairment due to impaired vigilance have also been described (Roth and Roehrs, 1996).

### Morbidity and Mortality

Persistent daytime sleepiness causes individuals to have an increased likelihood of accidents. Estimates by the US National Highway Traffic Safety Administration showed that approximately 56,000 police-reported crashes per year resulted from drivers who were "asleep at the wheel." New York state police estimate that 30% of all fatal crashes along the New York State Thruway occur because the driver fell asleep at the wheel. Approximately 1 million crashes annually (one-sixth of all crashes) are thought to be produced by driver inattention or lapses. Sleep deprivation and fatigue make such lapses more likely to occur. Truck drivers are especially susceptible to fatigue-related crashes (Lyznicki et al., 1998). Many truckers drive during the night while they are sleepiest. Truckers also may have a high prevalence of sleep apnea. The US Department of Transportation estimates that 200,000 automobile accidents each year may be related to sleepiness. Nearly one-third of all trucking accidents that are fatal to the driver are related to sleepiness and fatigue. A general population study by Hays and colleagues (1996) involving 3962 elderly individuals reported an increased mortality risk of 1.73 in those with EDS, defined by napping most of the time.

The presence of sleep disorders (see Primary Sleep Disorders Associated with Excessive Daytime Sleepiness, later) increases the risk of crashes. Individuals with untreated insomnia, sleep apnea, and narcolepsy, as well as shift workers, have more automobile crashes than other drivers (Costa de Silva et al., 1996). A 1991 Gallup Organization national survey found that individuals with chronic insomnia reported 2.5 times as many fatigue-related automobile accidents as those without insomnia. The same 1991 Gallup survey found serious morbidity associated with untreated sleep complaints, as well as impaired ability to concentrate and accomplish daily tasks, impaired memory, and interpersonal difficulties. Sleep deprivation has an adverse impact on cognition and leads to increases in number of failures to carry out intended actions, which may have severe consequences in safety-critical situations (Grundgeiger et al., 2014).

A 1994 telephone survey of drivers by the New York State Task Force estimated that approximately 25% reported that they had fallen asleep at the wheel at some time. Young male drivers are especially susceptible to crashes caused by falling asleep, as documented in a study in North Carolina in 1990, 1991, and 1992 (e.g., in 55% of the 4333 crashes, the drivers were predominantly male and age 25 or younger). In the October 1995 Gallup poll, 52% of all adults surveyed said that in the past year, they had driven a car or other vehicle while feeling drowsy; 31% of adults admitted dozing off while at the wheel of a car or other vehicle, and 4% reported having had an automobile accident because of tiredness during driving. Sleep deprivation increases morbidity and mortality due to metabolic derangements and accidents. A number of national and international catastrophes involving industrial operations, nuclear power plants, and all modes of transportation have been related to sleepiness and fatigue (Dinges, 1995). Some of the more infamous examples are the Exxon Valdez oil spill in Alaska; the nuclear disaster at Chernobyl in the former Soviet Union; the near-nuclear disaster at Three Mile Island in Pennsylvania; the gas leak disaster in Bhopal, India, resulting in 25,000 deaths; and the Challenger space shuttle disaster. In postgraduate medical training, data has repeatedly shown a dose response relationship between average hours of sleep per night and personal stress, reports of working while professionally and personally impaired. Studies comparing extended call shift with a revised schedule allowing for sleep recovery revealed the rate of diagnostic errors was 5.6 times higher in the traditional schedule than the intervention schedule as depicted in Fig. 101.26 (Lockley et al., 2004). These reports among others have catalyzed the Institute of Medicine (IOM) to proposed new work hours schedules which were accepted by the Accreditation Council for Graduate Medical Education (ACGME, 2010) and went into effect in July 2011.

## Causes of Excessive Daytime Sleepiness

Excessive sleepiness may result from both physiological and pathological causes (eBox 101.5).

### Physiological Causes of Sleepiness

It is important to first differentiate sleepiness from fatigue or tiredness. Based on the behavioral definition, fatigue can be differentiated by absence of the previously mentioned criteria for the presence of sleep. Fatigue defines a state of sustained lack of energy coupled with a lack of motivation and drive, but without the behavioral criteria of sleepiness such as heaviness or drooping of the eyelids, sagging or nodding of the head, and yawning. In addition, fatigue is often a secondary consequence of sleepiness. Sleep deprivation and sleepiness due to lifestyle and habits of going to sleep and waking up at irregular hours can be considered to result from disruption of the normal circadian and homeostatic physiology. Groups who are excessively sleepy because of lifestyle and inadequate sleep include young adults and elderly individuals, workers on irregular shifts, healthcare professionals (e.g., physicians, particularly the residents, and nurses), firefighters, police officers, train drivers, pilots and flight attendants, commercial truck drivers, and those individuals with competitive drives to move ahead in life, sacrificing hours of sleep and accumulating sleep debt. Among young adults, high school and college students are particularly at risk for sleep deprivation and sleepiness. The reasons for excessive sleepiness in adolescents and young adults include both biological and psychosocial factors. Some of the causes for later bedtimes and sleep deprivation in these groups include social interactions with peers; homework in the evening; sports, employment, or other extracurricular activities; early wake-up times to start school; and academic obligations requiring additional school or college work at night. Biological factors may play a role but are not well studied. For example, teenagers may need extra hours of sleep. Also, the circadian timing system may change with sleep phase delay in teenagers. EDS associated with shift work has been described (see Primary Sleep Disorders Associated with Excessive Daytime Sleepiness, later).

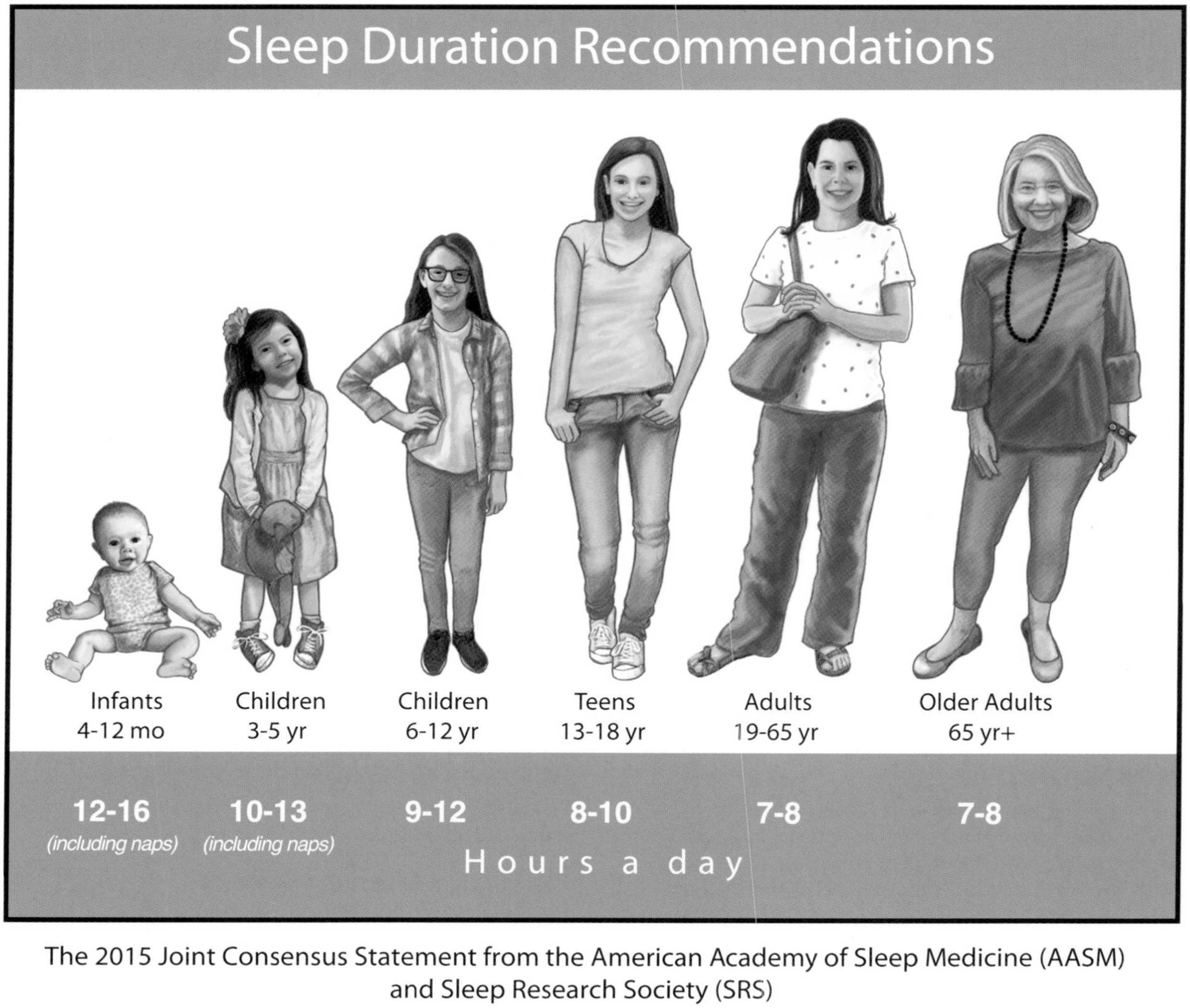

Sleep Duration Recommendations

Infants 4-12 mo | Children 3-5 yr | Children 6-12 yr | Teens 13-18 yr | Adults 19-65 yr | Older Adults 65 yr+

12-16 (including naps) | 10-13 (including naps) | 9-12 | 8-10 | 7-8 | 7-8

Hours a day

The 2015 Joint Consensus Statement from the American Academy of Sleep Medicine (AASM) and Sleep Research Society (SRS)

**Fig. 101.13 Sleep Duration Recommendations.** In 2015, the American Academy of Sleep Medicine (AASM) and Sleep Research Society (SRS) developed a consensus recommendation for the proper amount of sleep needed to promote optimal health in adults *(From Watson, N.F., Badr, M.S., Belenky, G., et al., 2015. Recommended amount of sleep for a healthy adult: a joint consensus statement of the American Academy of Sleep Medicine and Sleep Research Society. Sleep. 38 [6], 843–844. Published 2015 Jun 1. https://doi.org/10.5665/sleep.4716.)*

## Pathological Causes of Sleepiness

Neurological causes of excessive sleepiness may include CNS tumors and vascular lesions affecting the ARAS and its projections to the posterior hypothalamus and thalamus, leading to daytime sleepiness. It should be noted that lesions of this system often cause coma rather than just sleepiness. Brain tumors (e.g., astrocytomas, suprasellar cysts, metastases, lymphomas, and hamartomas affecting the posterior hypothalamus, pineal tumors, and astrocytomas of the upper brainstem) may produce excessive sleepiness. Prolonged hypersomnia may be associated with tumors in the region of the third ventricle. "Secondary" narcolepsy with or without cataplexy with hypocretin deficiency resulting from craniopharyngioma and other tumors of the hypothalamic and pituitary regions has been described. Cataplexy associated with sleepiness, sleep paralysis, and hypnagogic hallucinations has been described in patients with rostral brainstem gliomas with or without infiltration of the walls of the third ventricle. Narcolepsy-cataplexy also has been described in a human leukocyte antigen (HLA) DR2-negative patient with a pontine lesion documented by MRI.

Other neurological causes of EDS include bilateral paramedian thalamic and sometimes other cortical and subcortical infarcts (Bassetti and Valko, 2006), post-traumatic hypersomnolence, and multiple sclerosis (MS) (Kanbayashi et al., 2009). Narcolepsy-cataplexy has been described in occasional patients with MS (Nishino and Kanbayashi, 2005) and arteriovenous malformations in the diencephalon.

EDS has been described in association with encephalitis lethargica and other encephalitides, as well as with encephalopathies, including Wernicke encephalopathy. It was noted that the lesions of encephalitis lethargica described by Von Economo in the beginning of the last century, which severely affected the posterior hypothalamic region (eFig. 101.27), were associated with the clinical manifestation of extreme somnolence. These lesions apparently interrupted the ascending arousal systems projecting to the posterior hypothalamus through a variety of mechanisms including cerebrovascular accidents (Scammell et al., 2001). While encephalitis lethargica is now extinct, lesions in the diencephalon due to CNS and comorbid medial reasons may occasionally be encountered on the neurology wards. Cerebral sarcoidosis, Whipple disease, and tumors involving the hypothalamus may cause symptomatic or secondary narcolepsy, which may present with severe hypersomnolence with or without hypothalamic deficiencies.

Cerebral trypanosomiasis, or African sleeping sickness, is transmitted to humans by tsetse flies: *Trypanosoma gambiense* causes Gambian

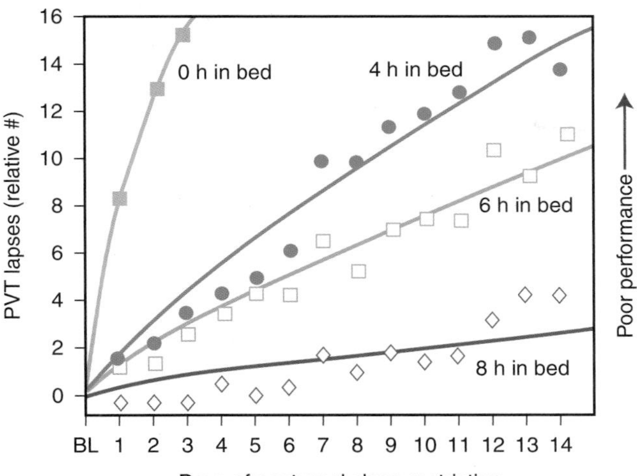


**Fig. 101.14 Sleep Deprivation and Performance.** Data depicting a "dose relationship" between poor performance and the Psychomotor Vigilance Task *(PVT)* performance lapses under varying doses of daily sleep. Displayed are group averages for subjects in the 8-hour *(diamond)*, 6-hour *(light square)*, and 4-hour *(circle)* chronic sleep period time in bed (TIV) across 2 weeks, and in the 0-hour *(dark square)* sleep condition across 3 days. Subjects were tested every 2 hours each day; data points represent the daily average (07:30–23:30) expressed relative to baseline *(BL)*. Curves through data points represent statistical nonlinear, model-based, best-fitting profiles of the response to sleep deprivation for subjects in each of the four experimental conditions. *(Adapted from Van Dongen, H.P., Maislin, G., Mullington, J.M., et al., 2003. The cumulative cost of additional wakefulness: dose-response effects on neurobehavioral functions and sleep physiology from chronic sleep restriction and total sleep deprivation. Sleep 26, 117–126.)*

or West African sleeping sickness, and *Trypanosoma rhodesiense* causes East African sleeping sickness.

Certain neurodegenerative diseases such as Alzheimer disease (AD), PD, and multisystem atrophy (MSA) also may cause EDS (Raggi and Ferri, 2010). The causes of EDS in AD include degeneration of the SCN, resulting in circadian dysrhythmia, associated sleep apnea-hypopnea, and frequent periodic limb movements in sleep (PLMS). In PD, excessive sleepiness may be due to the associated PLMS, sleep apnea, and depression. EDS in MSA associated with cerebellar-parkinsonism or parkinsonian-cerebellar syndrome and progressive autonomic deficit may be caused by the frequent association with sleep-related respiratory dysrhythmias, impaired melatonin secretion, and possible degeneration of the reticular activating arousal systems (Cao et al., 2018; Devine, Lee Khemani, and Carter, 2019; Nakamura et al., 2018; Rekik et al., 2018; Silvestri, 2018).

Sleep disorders are being increasingly recognized as a feature of PD and other parkinsonian disorders. Although some studies have attributed the excessive daytime drowsiness and irresistible sleep episodes (sleep attacks) to antiparkinsonian medications (Ondo et al., 2001), sleep disturbances are also an integral part of PD (Arnulf et al., 2002). In one study of 303 patients with PD, 21% reported falling asleep while driving (Ondo et al., 2002). Several studies also reported a relatively high incidence (10%–20%) of symptoms of restless legs syndrome (RLS) in patients with PD (Hening et al., 2009; Krishnan et al., 2003; Ondo et al., 2002). There is also increasing awareness about the relationship between parkinsonian disorders and REM sleep behavior disorder (RBD). RBD as well as its associated PSG biomarker—RSWA—may be the presenting feature of PD, MSA, and other parkinsonian disorders, long before the appearance of the motor manifestations (Boeve, 2010; Boeve et al., 2007; Iranzo et al., 2014; Postuma et al., 2010a; Raggi and Ferri, 2010; McCarter et al., 2019; Nepozitek et al., 2019).

The following question was found to have 94% sensitivity and 87% specificity in detecting RBD: "Have you ever been told, or suspected yourself, that you seem to 'act out your dreams' while asleep (for example, punching, flailing your arms in the air, making running movements, etc.)?" (Postuma et al., 2012).

These and other studies provide evidence supporting the notion that dopamine activity is normally influenced by circadian factors (Rye and Jankovic, 2002). For example, tyrosine hydroxylase levels fall several hours before waking, and their increase correlates with motor activity. The relationship between hypocretin and sleep disorders associated with PD is of considerable interest especially since recent data has linked depletion of hypothalamic hypocretin/orexin neurons as positively correlating with impaired memory in animal models of PD (Oliveira et al., 2019) Myotonic dystrophy and other neuromuscular disorders may cause EDS due to associated sleep apnea-hypopnea syndrome and hypoventilation. In addition, in myotonic dystrophy, there may be involvement of the ARAS as part of the multisystem membrane effects noted in this disease.

***Excessive daytime sleepiness associated with general medical disorders.*** Several systemic diseases such as hepatic, renal, or respiratory failure and electrolyte disturbances may cause metabolic encephalopathies that result in EDS. Patients with severe EDS drift into a coma. The other medical causes for EDS include congestive heart failure and severe anemia. Hypothyroidism and acromegaly also may cause EDS due to the associated sleep apnea syndrome. Hypoglycemic episodes in diabetes mellitus and severe hyperglycemia are additional causes of EDS.

***Primary sleep disorders associated with excessive daytime sleepiness.*** A number of primary sleep disorders cause excessive sleepiness (see eBox 101.5). The most common cause of EDS in the general population is behaviorally induced insufficient sleep syndrome which is associated with significant adverse health and social outcomes including association with 7 of the 15 leading causes of death and has been declared to be a "public health epidemic" (Chattu et al., 2018). The next most common cause is obstructive sleep apnea syndrome (OSAS) followed with narcolepsy and idiopathic hypersomnolence. Most patients with EDS referred to the sleep laboratory have OSAS. Other causes of EDS include circadian rhythm sleep disorders, periodic limb movement disorder (PLMD), RLS, and inadequate sleep hygiene and certain CNS acting agents.

Many sedatives and hypnotics cause EDS. In addition to the benzodiazepine and nonbenzodiazepine hypnotics and sedative antidepressants (e.g., tricyclic antidepressants and trazodone), nonbenzodiazepine neuroleptics, antihistamines, antipsychotics, most older generation antiepileptic drugs, and narcotic analgesics including tramadol also cause EDS. Beta-blockers for treatment of hypertension may occasionally cause excessive sleepiness.

Toxin and alcohol-related hypersomnolence can occur as well. Many industrial toxins such as heavy metals and organic toxins (e.g., mercury, lead, arsenic, and copper) may cause EDS. These may sometimes also cause insomnia. Individuals working in industrial settings using toxic chemicals routinely are at risk. These toxins also may cause systemic disturbances such as alteration of renal, liver, and hematological function. There may be an impairment of nerve conduction. Chronic use of alcohol at bedtime may produce alcohol-dependent sleep disorder. Usually this causes insomnia, but sometimes the patients may have excessive sleepiness in the daytime. Many of these patients suffer from chronic alcoholism. Acute ingestion of alcohol causes transient sleepiness.

## CLASSIFICATION OF SLEEP DISORDERS

### International Classification of Sleep Disorders

The latest edition of the *International Classification of Sleep Disorders* (ICSD-III) (AASM, 2014) listed seven broad categories of disordered sleep, along with several subcategories under each category as

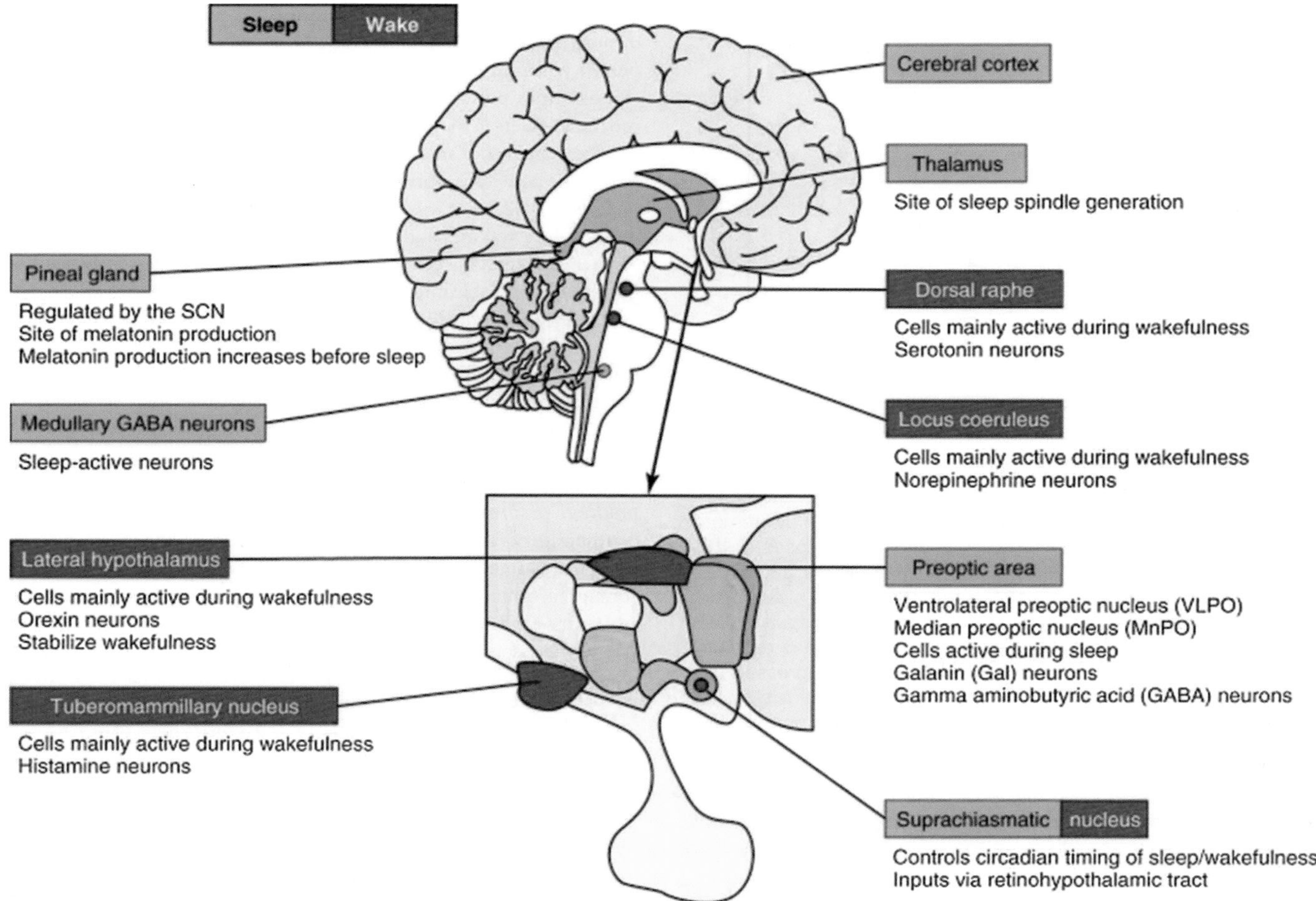


**Fig. 101.16** Neuroanatomy and Neuromodulators of Wake *(blue)* and Sleep *(red)*. The brain in the awake state illustrates important arousal and sleep centers and pathways of neurotransmission. Current models of wakefulness and sleep hold that wakefulness is maintained by the combined excitatory influence of forebrain-projecting noradrenergic (locus coeruleus), histaminergic (tuberomammillary nucleus), serotoninergic (dorsal raphe), and cholinergic (not shown) cell groups located at or near the mesopontine junction. Sleep, on the other hand, is initiated and maintained by neurons in the median preoptic *(MnPO)* and ventrolateral preoptic *(VLPO)* nuclei via inhibitory projections to the more rostrally situated wakefulness-promoting cell groups. Hypocretin (orexin) neurons located in the lateral hypothalamus reinforce activity in the brainstem arousal pathways and also stabilize both sleep and wakefulness. Disruption of the hypocretin system leads to narcolepsy. The suprachiasmatic nuclei *(SCN)* determine the timing of the sleep-wake cycle and help to "consolidate" these behavioral states. The pineal gland, located in the epithalamus, produces melatonin, a hormone thought to function as a hypnotic signal. The cerebral cortex and medullary brainstem also contain subpopulations of γ-amino butyric acid (GABA)-ergic sleep-active neurons. *(From Biology of Sleep Kryger MH, Avidan, AY, Berry, R. Atlas of clinical sleep medicine. Second edition. ed. Philadelphia, PA: Elsevier/Saunders; 2013 Chapter 3, 22-64.)*

well as Appendices A and B (see eBox 101.6). Appendix A includes sleep-related medical and neurological disorders, including sleep-related epilepsy and headache, fatal familial insomnia (FFI), as well as sleep-related laryngospasm, sleep-related gastroesophageal reflux, and sleep-related myocardial ischemia. Appendix B includes substance-induced (e.g., alcohol, opioid, cannabis, sedative, hypnotic or anxiolytic, cocaine, other stimulants, hallucinogens, nicotine, inhalants, and other psychoactive substances) sleep disorders. The seven broad categories consist of insomnia, sleep-related breathing disorders (SBDs), central disorders of hypersomnolence, circadian rhythm sleep disorders, parasomnias, sleep-related movement disorders, and other sleep disorders. The ICSD-III reflects a major change from the ICSD-II predominantly in simplification of the insomnia disorders, an expansion of the SBDs, classification of narcolepsy into type 1 and type 2, consolidating the ICSD-II idiopathic hypersomnias into single entity and recurrent hypersomnia into a singly entry with a subtype.

## Approach to a Patient with Sleep Complaints

The approach to a patient with a sleep complaint must begin with a clear understanding of sleep disorders as listed in the International Classification of Sleep Disorders (ICSD). Some common sleep complaints are trouble falling asleep and staying asleep *(insomnia)*; falling asleep during the day *(daytime hypersomnolence)*; and inability to sleep at the right time *(circadian rhythm sleep disorders)*. Other common complaints are thrashing and moving about in bed with repeated leg jerking (parasomnias and other abnormal movements, including nocturnal seizures) and RLS.

Cardinal manifestations in a patient complaining of insomnia include all or some of the following: difficulty falling asleep; frequent awakenings, including early-morning awakening; insufficient or total

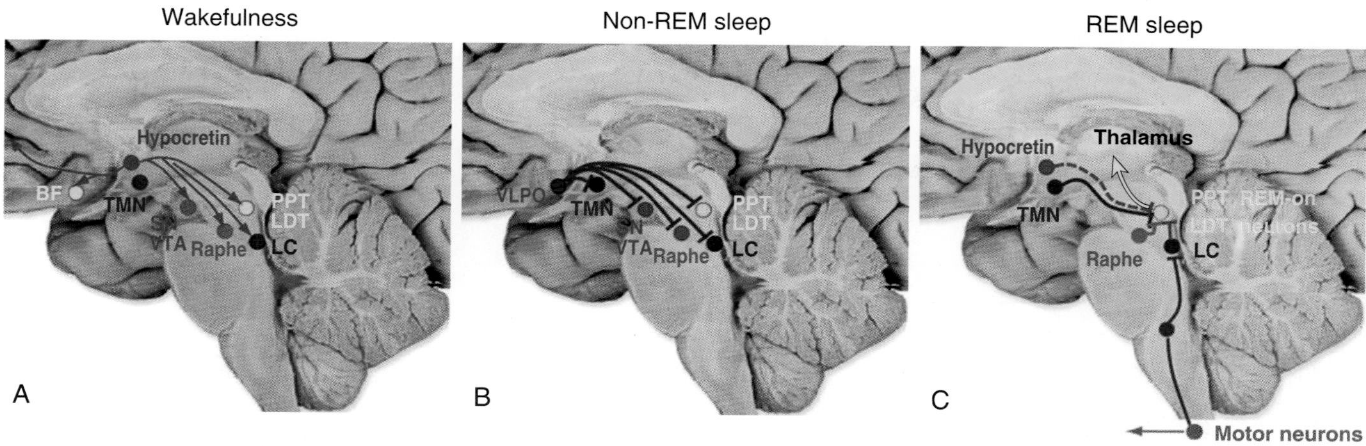


| Neurochemistry | Wakefulness<br>A | Nonrapid eye movement sleep (non-REM) sleep<br>B | Rapid eye movement (REM) sleep<br>C |
|---|---|---|---|
| BF: Acetylcholine | ++++ | + | ++++ |
| LDT: Acetylcholine | ++++ | +++ → 0 | ++++ |
| Dorsal and median raphe: Serotonin | ++++ | ++ | 0 |
| Loceus coeruleus : (NE) | ++++ | ++ | 0 |
| TMN: (Histamine) | ++++ | ++ | 0 |
| Posterior/lateral hypothalamus (Hypocretin/orexin) | ++++ | + | + |
| Ventrolateral preoptic area (GABA) | + | +++ | ++++ |

| Neurophysiology | Wakefulness | Nonrapid eye movement sleep (non-REM) sleep | Rapid eye movement (REM) sleep |
|---|---|---|---|
| Posture | Erect, sitting, or recumbent | Recumbent | Recumbent |
| Mobility | Normal | Slightly reduced or immobile; postural shifts | Moderately reduced or immobile; myoclonic jerks |
| Response to stimulation | Normal | Mildly to moderately reduced | Moderately reduced to no response |
| Level of alertness | Alert | Unconscious but reversible | Unconscious but reversible |
| Eyelids | Open | Closed | Closed |
| Eye movements | Waking eye movements | Slow rolling eye movements | Rapid eye movements |
| EEG | Alpha waves; desynchronized | Synchronized | Theta or sawtooth; desynchronized |
| EMG (muscle tone) | Normal | Mildly reduced | Moderately to severely reduced or absent |
| EOG | Waking eye movements | Slow rolling eye movements | Rapid eye movements |

**Fig. 101.17 Neuroanatomy and Neuromodulators of Wake Nonrapid Eye Movement and Rapid Eye Movement Sleep.** The brain in the awake state illustrates important arousal and sleep centers and pathways of neurotransmission. Schematic representation of wake/sleep pathways and localization of strategic arousal and sleep centers in the brain. Midsagittal view is shown with superimposed schematic representation of circuits most relevant for wakefulness (**A**), non-REM sleep (**B**), and REM sleep (**C**). **A, Mechanism of** Wakefulness (**Arousal**): Summary: hypocretin/orexin neurons project to, and excite, the other wake-promoting brainstem nuclei, as well as the basal forebrain, and widely throughout the cortex *(red arrows)*. Cholinergic input *(orange)* from the laterodorsal tegmental (LDT) and pedunculopontine (PPT) nuclei project through the thalamus and facilitate thalamocortical transmission of *arousal signals*. A second pathway projects through the hypothalamus to cortical centers and facilitates the processing of thalamocortical inputs that arise from midbrain centers, including the noradrenergic *(blue)* locus coeruleus (LC); the serotonergic *(purple)* dorsal raphe (Raphe); the histaminergic *(pink)* tuberomammillary nucleus (TMN); and the dopaminergic *(yellow)* ventral periaqueductal grey matter (VPAG). This pathway also receives input from the cholinergic *(orange)* basal forebrain (BF) and the peptidergic neurons of the lateral hypothalamus (LH) and perifornical neurons (PeF), which contain hypocretin or melanin-concentrating hormone *(light green)*. The melatonergic *(red)* neural network affects *arousal and sleep* through regulation of circadian rhythms. This internal biological clock originates in the suprachiasmatic nucleus (SCN), projects through the dorsomedial hypothalamus (DMH), and sends inhibitory signals to the γ-aminobutyric acid (GABA)-ergic *(grey)* ventrolateral preoptic nucleus (VLPO) of the hypothalamus. *During non-REM sleep*, the ventrolateral preoptic nucleus (VLPO) projects to, and inhibits, the wake-promoting nuclei *(green lines)*. *During REM sleep*, the LDT and PPT cholinergic neurons lack the wake-inhibition (from hypocretin/orexin, TMN, raphe, and LC), and excite the thalamus *(yellow)*. Medullary interneurons inhibit motor neurons, causing atonia in REM. *BF*, Basal forebrain; *LC*, locus coeruleus; *LDT*, laterodorsal tegmentum; *PPT*, pedunculopontine nucleus; *SN*, substantia nigra; *TMN*, tuberomammillary nucleus; *VLPO*, ventrolateral preoptic nucleus; *VTA*, ventral tegmental area. *(Adapted from Nishino, S., [ed.]. 2013. Basic sleep concepts, science, deprivation, and mechanisms of neurotransmitters and neuropharmacology of sleep/wake regulations. Encyclopedia of Sleep. Stanford University School of Medicine, Palo Alto, CA, pp 395–406. With permission.)*

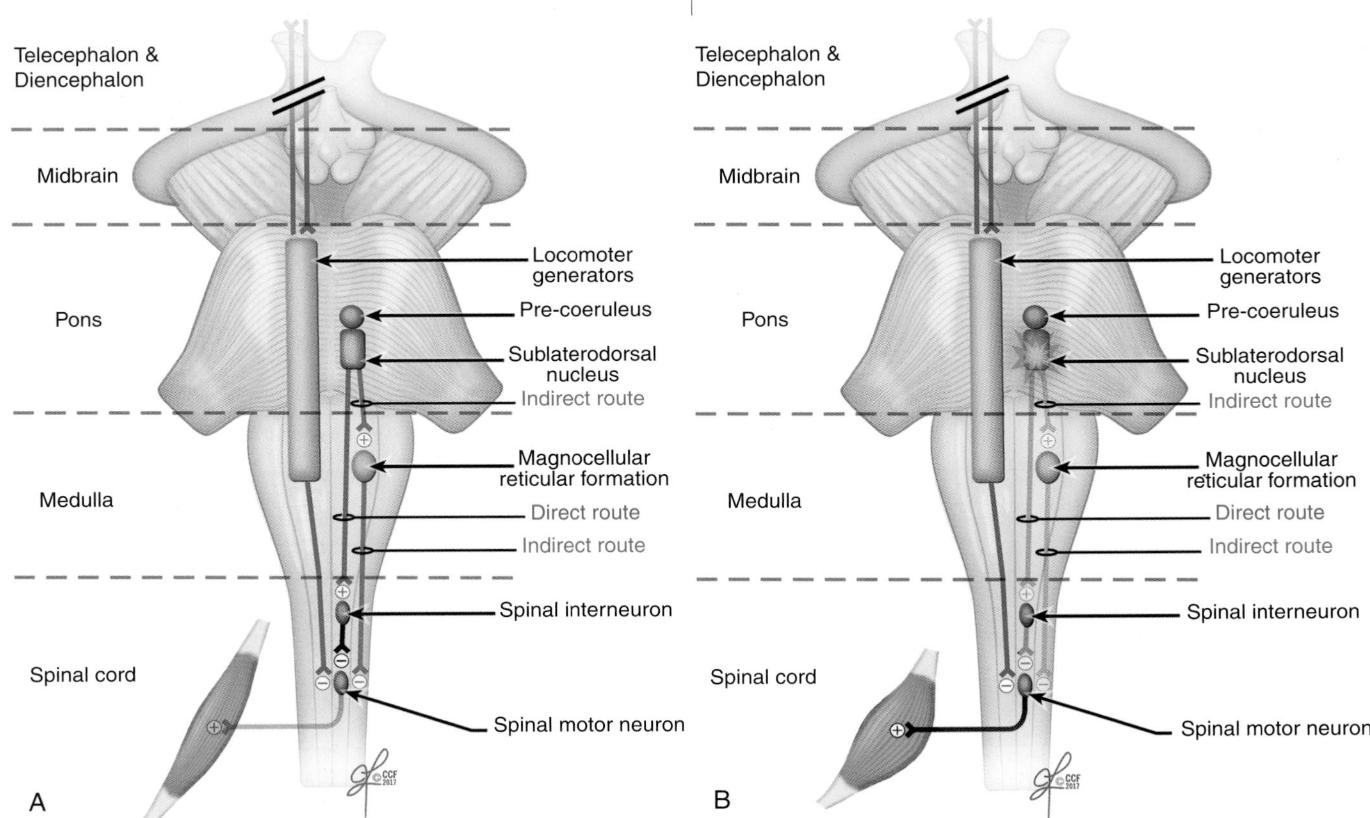


**Fig. 101.19 Neurophysiology and Neuropathology of Rapid Eye Movement (REM) Sleep Motor Control.** A, Physiology of normal rapid eye movement *(REM)* sleep muscle atonia: The "REM-on" regions consisting of the pre-coeruleus and sublaterodorsal nucleus (SLD) activate two inhibitory pathways, referred to as the direct route and indirect route. The SLD nucleus stimulates an inhibitory spinal interneuron via the direct route and this nucleus in turn inhibits or hyperpolarizes the alpha motor neuron to induce skeletal muscle atonia. The SLD nucleus activates the medullary magnocellular reticular formation (MCRF) through the indirect route causing the MCRF to inhibit the motor neuron and thus produce skeletal muscle atonia. B, Pathophysiology in the setting of REM sleep behavior disorder. Dysfunction of the SLD nucleus and/or its afferent or efferent neuropathways results in loss of the normally present inhibition of the motor neuron thus permitting skeletal muscles to become active during REM sleep culminating in augmentation of EMG tone (RSWA) and dream enactment behavior (DEB) diagnostic of RBD. Rapid eye movement sleep behavior disorder, chest. *(Adapted from Boeve, B.F., Silber, M.H., Saper, C.B., et al., 2007. Pathophysiology of REM sleep behaviour disorder and relevance to neurodegenerative disease. Brain 130 [Pt 11], 2770–2788.)*

lack of sleep; daytime fatigue, tiredness, or sleepiness; lack of concentration, irritability, anxiety, and sometimes depression and forgetfulness; and preoccupation with psychosomatic symptoms, such as aches and pains.

Cardinal manifestations of hypersomnia include EDS, falling asleep in an inappropriate place and under inappropriate circumstances, no relief of symptoms after additional sleep at night, daytime fatigue, inability to concentrate, and impairment of motor skills and cognition. Additional symptoms depend on the nature of the underlying sleep disorder (e.g., snoring and apneas during sleep witnessed by a bed partner in patients with OSAS; attacks of cataplexy, hypnagogic hallucinations, sleep paralysis, automatic behavior, and disturbed night sleep in patients with narcolepsy).

Sleeplessness and EDS are symptoms; therefore, every attempt should be made to find a cause for these complaints. Insomnia may be due to a variety of causes. The etiological differential diagnosis for EDS may include OSAS; central sleep apnea (CSA); narcolepsy; idiopathic hypersomnia; several psychiatric, neurological, and other medical illnesses; drug or alcohol abuse; and periodic hypersomnolence (Kleine-Levin syndrome [KLS]). Sometimes a patient with RLS may complain of EDS. Abnormal movements and behavior during sleep include REM and NREM sleep parasomnias and other abnormal movements (e.g., PLMS), some daytime movement disorders that persist during sleep, and nocturnal seizures.

The physician must evaluate the patient first on the basis of the history and physical examination before undertaking laboratory tests, which must be determined by the clinical diagnosis. The first step in the assessment of a sleep-wakefulness disturbance is careful evaluation of the sleep complaints. The history should include information on the patient's entire 24 hours and must include a detailed sleep history, with a sleep questionnaire as well as a sleep log or diary (Fig. 101.28). It must also include psychiatric, neurological, medical, drug-alcohol, and family and past histories. The history must be followed by a physical examination to uncover medical or neurological causes of insomnia, hypersomnia, and parasomnias (Avidan, 2018). Physical examination of patients with OSAS may uncover upper airway anatomical abnormalities.

It is advisable to interview the bed partner, caregiver, or parents of children to get an adequate history, particularly the history during

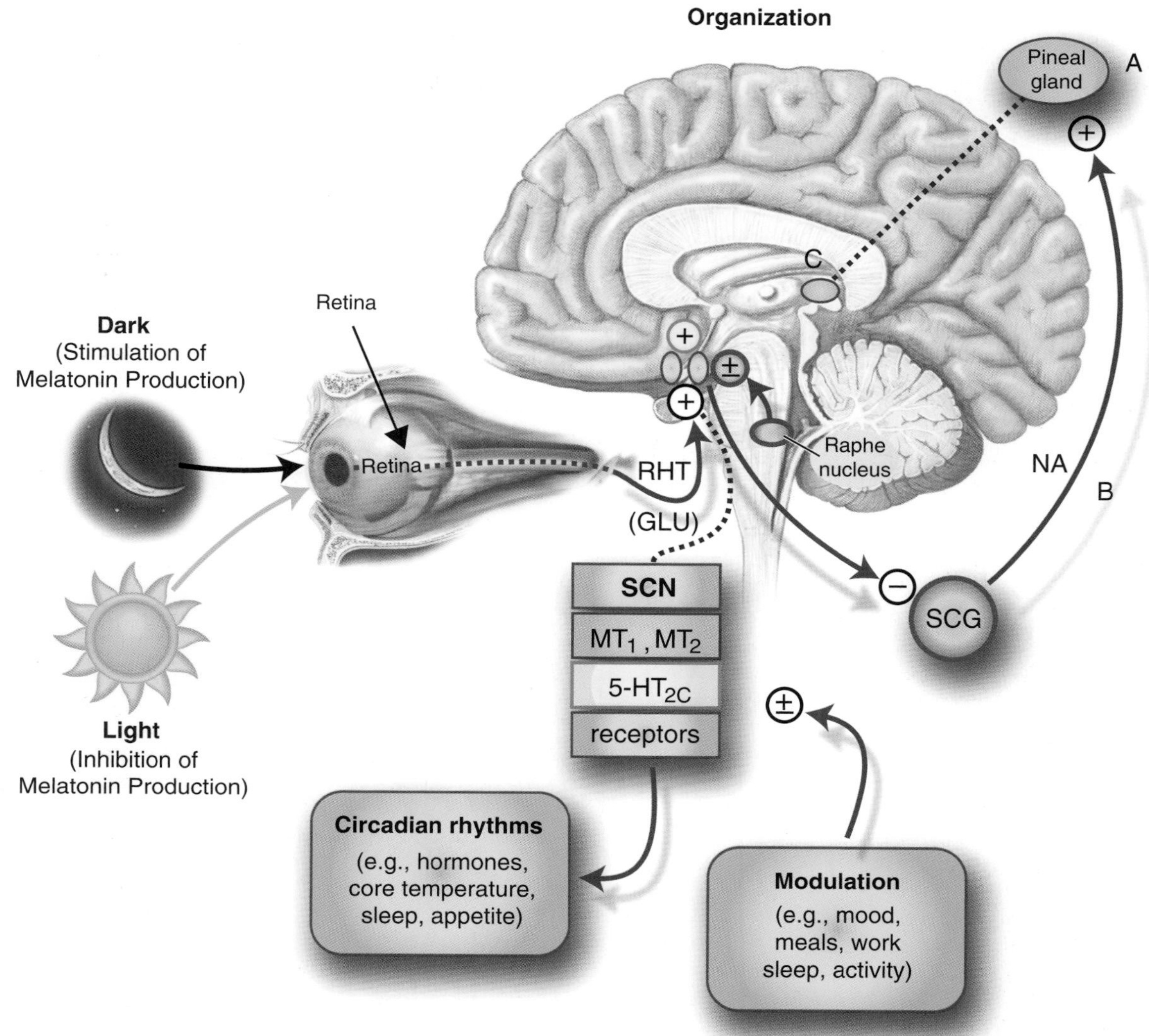


**Fig. 101.20 The Suprachiasmatic Nucleus Sends Timing Information to the Brain and Periphery.** The circadian pacemaker is located in the hypothalamic suprachiasmatic nucleus (SCN). It is responsible for generating the internal circadian rhythms in gene expression, electrophysiology, and hormone secretion. Direct projections from the retina carry information about the cycle of light and darkness to the SCN, which in turn synchronizes a phase of SCN rhythms with the external environment. *(From de Bodinat, C., Guardiola-Lemaitre, B., Mocaer, E., Renard, P., Munoz, C., Millan, M.J. 2010. Agomelatine, the first melatonergic antidepressant: discovery, characterization and development. Nat. Rev. Drug Discov. 9[8], 628–642.)*

sleep at night, which may have an effect on daytime functioning. A sleep questionnaire containing a list of pertinent questions relating to sleep complaints; sleep hygiene; sleep patterns; medical, psychiatric, and neurological disorders; and drug and alcohol use may be filled out by the patient to save time during the history taking. A sleep log kept over a 2-week period also is a valuable indicator of sleep-wake-patterns and is of fundamental importance in screening for causes of sleep deprivation. Such a log should include bedtime, rise time on weekdays and weekends, daytime naps, amount of time needed to fall sleep, number and duration of nighttime awakenings, total sleep time, and subjective feelings upon awakening.

Pertinent questions can help diagnose primary sleep disorders. For example, a history of snoring and apneas witnessed during sleep at night would suggest OSAS. Unusual movements during sleep at night may suggest PLM. A history of sleep attacks and REM-sleep intrusion phenomena such as cataplexy, hypnagogic hallucinations, sleep paralysis, and disturbed night sleep in a young adult suggests narcolepsy. Nonrefreshing sleep or no benefit from additional sleep may suggest sleep apnea syndrome and idiopathic hypersomnia. Identification of an irregular sleep-wake schedule and delayed sleep onset and awakening and inquiry into the patient's lifestyle to uncover sleep deprivation and insufficient sleep are important for the diagnosis of sleepiness. An urge to move the limbs in the early evening may suggest RLS. A family history is important in primary sleep disorders such as narcolepsy, RLS, and advanced/delayed circadian patterns

## Subjective Measures of Sleepiness

A variety of scales have been developed to assess the subjective degree of sleepiness. The most well-known is the Epworth Sleepiness Scale (ESS), which assesses the level of sleepiness (Johns,

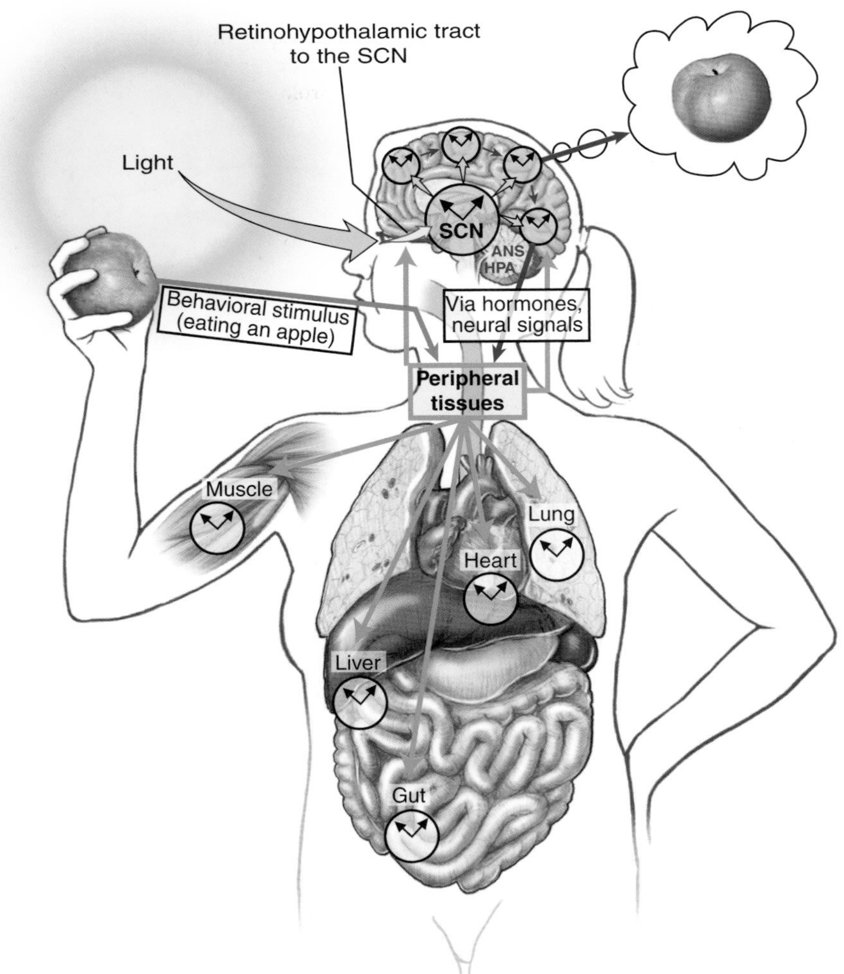


**Fig. 101.21** The suprachiasmatic nucleus *(SCN)* derives "time of day" information from environmental light cues captured by specialized cells within the retina. This information is relayed via the retinohypothalamic tract to the SCN, which conveys timing information to the brain including the paraventricular, arcuate nuclei subparaventricular zone, medial preoptic area, intergeniculate leaflet, and paraventricular nucleus of the thalamus. The SCN also provides timing cues to peripheral tissues via the autonomic nervous system and hormones, which together organize complex behaviors from the sleep/wake to the feeding/fasting rhythm "peripheral oscillators." *(From Arble, D.M., Sandoval, D.A., 2013. CNS control of glucose metabolism: response to environmental challenges. Front. Neurosci. 7, 20. https://doi.org/10.3389/fnins.2013.00020.)*

1998) in a variety of situations. The patient is rated on eight situations with a score of 0–3 (3 being the highest chance of dozing off). The maximum score is 24, and a score greater than 10 suggests the presence of excessive sleepiness (Box 101.7). This scale has been weakly correlated with multiple sleep latency test (MSLT) scores, which is the gold standard measurement at present for daytime sleepiness, and normal values do not necessarily imply the lack of clinically significant daytime sleepiness. However, it is high in vulnerable population such as people with narcolepsy, sleep apnea, and sleep-deprived residents as depicted in Fig. 101.29 (Avidan, 2013; Lipford et al., 2019; Papp et al., 2004).

The Stanford Sleepiness Scale (SSS) (eBox 101.8) is a seven-point scale that measures subjective sleepiness but may not be reliable in patients with persistent sleepiness. The scale may detect sleepiness as it waxes and wanes over the course of a day. Advantages include its brevity, its ease of administration, and its ability to be administered repeatedly, but normative data do not exist, making it difficult to use for clinical decision making or comparisons between persons.

The Karolinska Sleepiness Scale (KSS) is another subjective measure of sleepiness somewhat similar to the SSS measuring responses on a 9-point scale (1 = very alert to 9 = very sleepy), while scores of 7 or above are considered pathologic. The KSS is useful when evaluating sleepiness in drug trials, and fatigue in flight crews. Similarly to the SSS, it lacks normative data, and diurnal pattern and the impact of stress, sleep quality, sex, illness, and age (Akerstedt et al., 2017).

Another scale is the visual analog scale of alertness and well-being. In this scale, subjects are asked to indicate their feelings on an arbitrary line.

Laboratory tests should be used to confirm the clinical diagnosis and must be subservient to the clinical history and physical examination. The tests to uncover suspected sleep disorders are resource intensive and are best planned in consultation with a sleep specialist; they are described in later sections of this chapter.

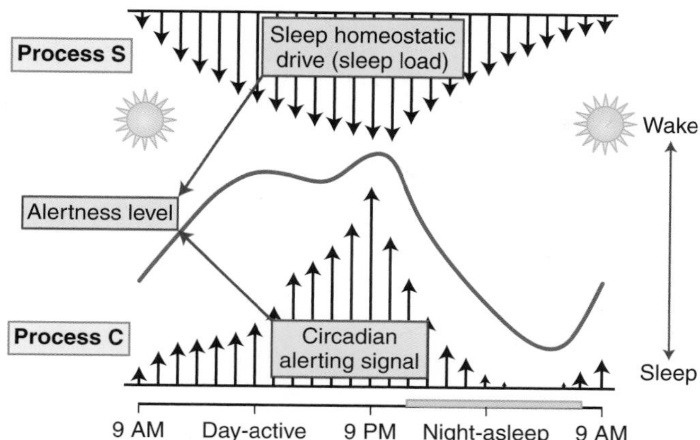


**Fig. 101.22 Circadian Mediation of Sleep and Wakefulness.** Sleep and wakefulness are regulated by two processes operating simultaneously: the homeostatic process (Process S) which primarily regulates the length and depth of sleep, and endogenous circadian rhythms (Process C: "biological time clocks"), which influence the internal organization of sleep and timing and duration of daily sleep/wake cycles.

## CLINICAL PHENOMENOLOGY

In this section, pertinent features of some common primary sleep disorders are described, along with a summary of sleep dysfunction in neurological, medical, psychiatric, and pediatric disorders.

### Insomnia

Insomnia is the most common sleep disorder affecting the population and the most common disease encountered in the practice of sleep medicine (Morin and Benca, 2011, 2015). Several population surveys of adults have determined that approximately 35% of the general public has had insomnia complaints; in 10%, this is a persistent problem (Jaussent et al., 2017; Morin, LeBlanc, et al., 2006; Ohayon, 2002; Roth and Roehrs, 2003). *Insomnia* is defined as an inability to initiate, maintain sleep, or early awakening, despite an adequate opportunity for sleep, culminating in poor sleep quality associated with a lack of feeling restored and refreshed in the morning, leading to a dissatisfaction with sleep and poor daytime functioning (AASM, 2014). The ICSD-III (AASM, 2014) classifies insomnia into three types: short-term insomnia disorder, chronic insomnia disorder, and other insomnia disorder.

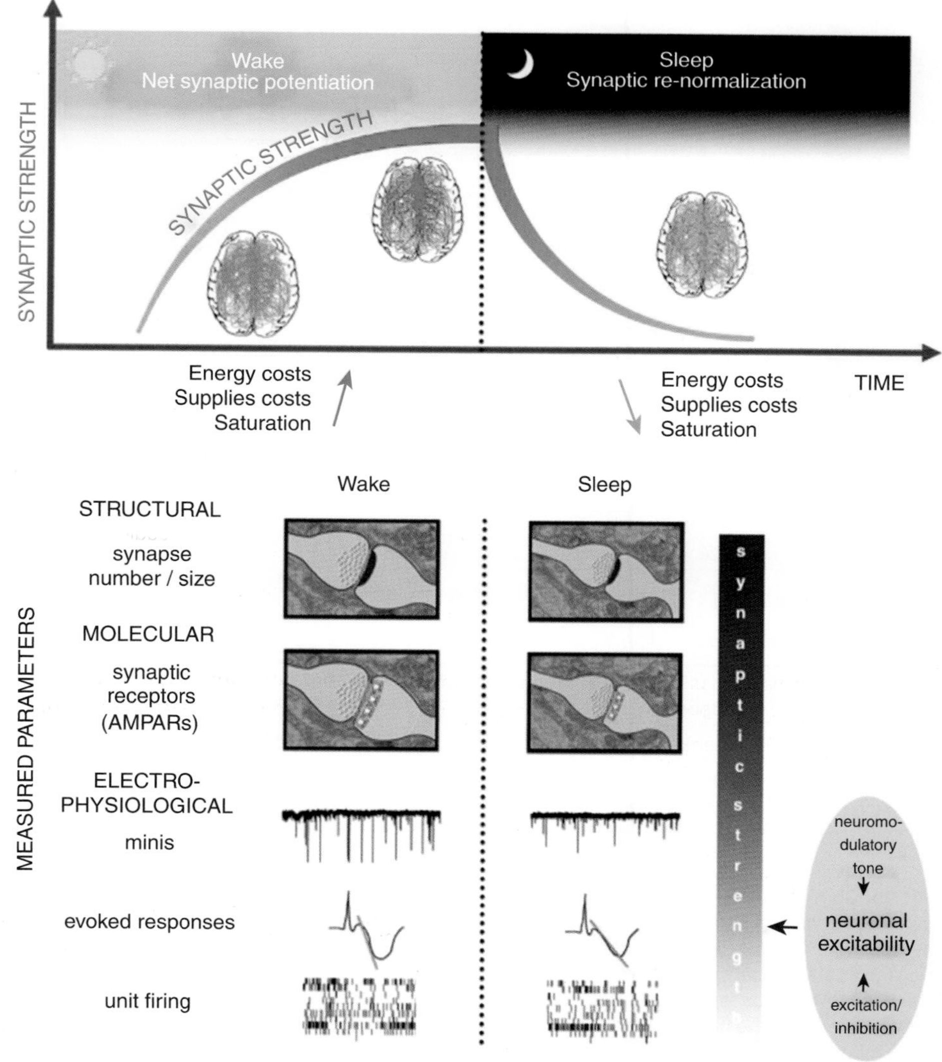


**Fig. 101.23 Sleep, Synaptic Homeostasis and Neuronal Firing Rates.** (*From Cirelli, C., 2017. Sleep, synaptic homeostasis and neuronal firing rates. Curr. Opin. Neurobiol. 44, 72–79. © 2017.*)

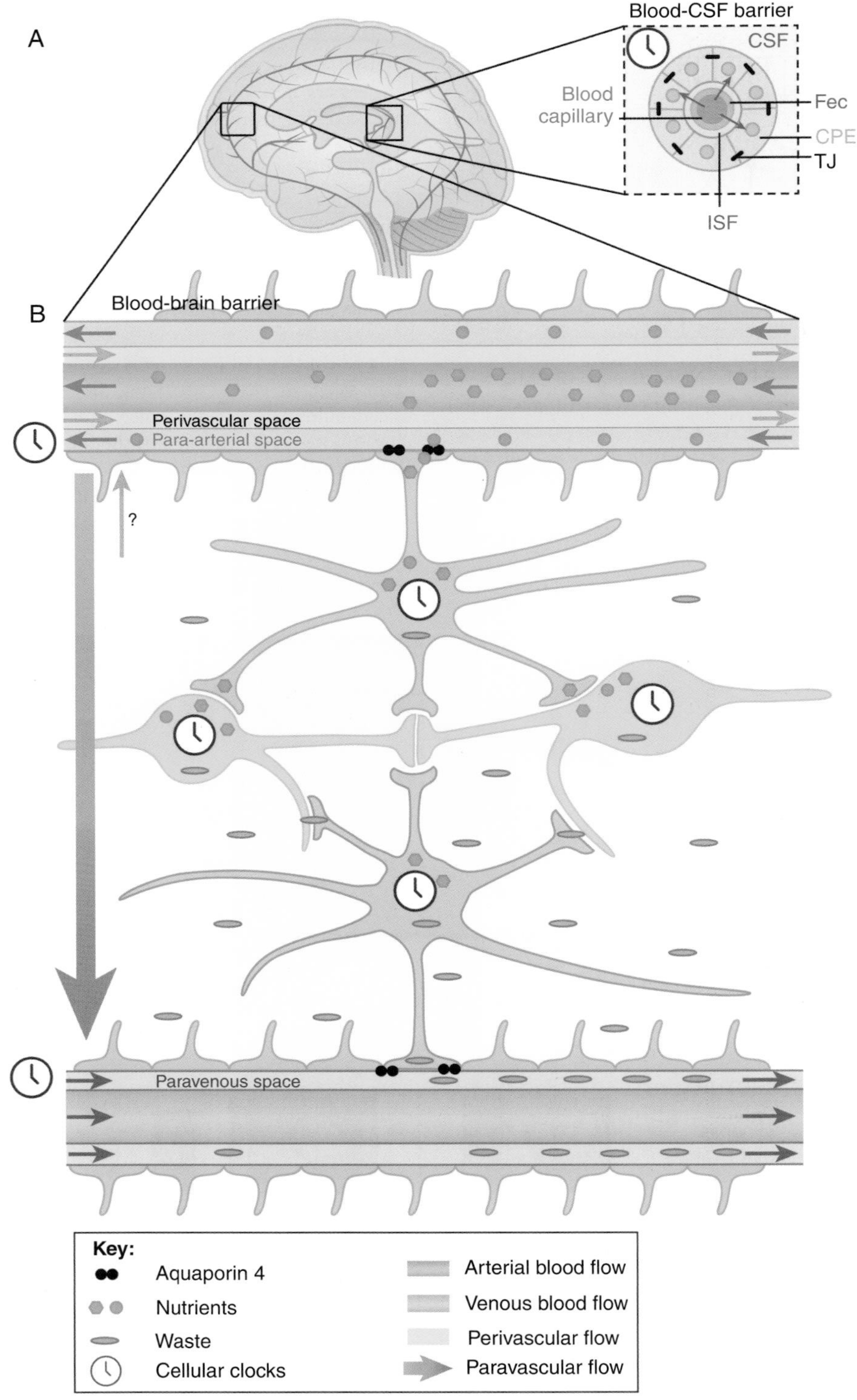


Trends in neurosciences

**Fig. 101.24 Glymphatic Waste Clearance System and Relationship to Sleep. A,** Representation of the fluid compartments and barriers of the brain. **B,** Waste clearance route through the blood–brain barrier with a paravascular flow (red–blue shaded arrow) from arteries *(red)* to veins *(purple)*. Astrocytes *(green)* take up fluid from the para-arterial space via aquaporin 4 channels and distribute it to neurons *(orange)* and the intercellular space. Waste loaded fluid is then cleared by astrocytes via aquaporin 4 into the paravenous space and transported out of the brain. A perivascular flow *(yellow arrows)* is also hypothesized. *CSF*, Cerebrospinal fluid; *CPE*, choroid plexus epithelial cell; *Fec*, fenestrated endothelial cell; *ISF*, interstitial fluid; *TJ*, tight junction. *(Adapted, with permission, from [41, 55]. Urs Albrecht, Jürgen A. Ripperger, Circadian Clocks and Sleep: Impact of Rhythmic Metabolism and Waste Clearance on the Brain, Trends in Neurosciences, Volume 41, Issue 10, 2018, Pages 677–688, ISSN 0166-2236, https://doi.org/10.1016/j.tins.2018.07.007. (http://www.sciencedirect.com/science/article/pii/S0166223618301905.)*

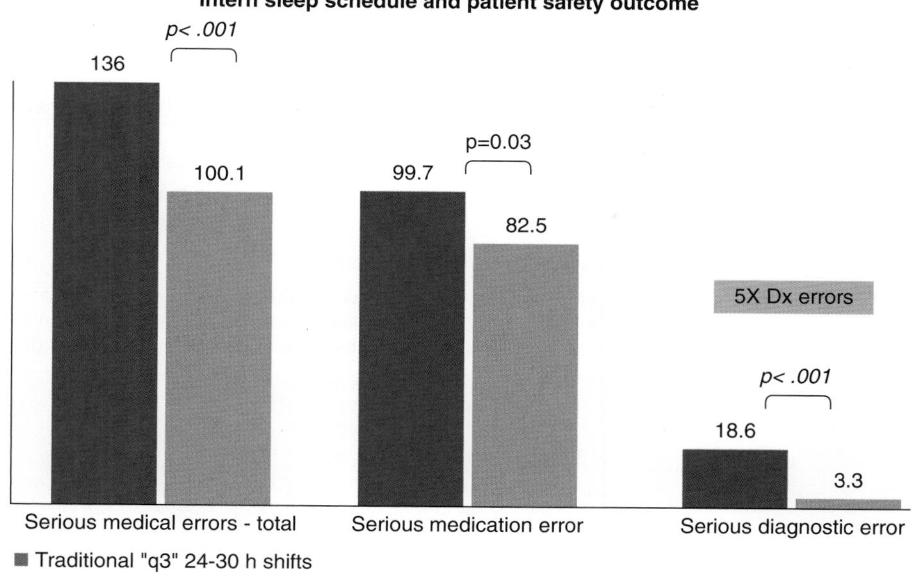


**Fig. 101.26 Intern Sleep Schedule and Patient Safety Outcome.** Twenty interns studied under two conditions: a "traditional on-call schedule" with 30-hour shifts scheduled every other shift and an "intervention schedule" in which shifts were limited to 16 hours. Sleep times were collected from sleep logs and, during ICU shifts, the logs were supplemented by continuous ambulatory polysomnographic recordings. Objectively verifiable indicators of attentional failures included periods of slow rolling eye movements intruding during wakefulness. Failures were documented in a subgroup of recordings from between 11 PM and 7 AM. The number of attentional failures during the night in the traditional condition was more than twice the number of attentional failures in the intervention condition. Medical errors were determined by direct observation of interns and chart review, voluntary repor ts, and computerized event-detection monitoring and reported as errors per 1000 pt days. Errors consisted of procedural, medication, and diagnostic errors. The study included 2203 patient days, 634 admissions, and 5888 hours of direct observation. Interns made 35.9% more serious errors during the traditional schedule than during the intervention schedule. The rate of diagnostic errors was 5.6 times higher in the traditional schedule than the intervention schedule.

The perception of insomnia does not necessarily depend on total hours of sleep obtained, because there is considerable individual variation in sleep requirement. There is an increasing association of insomnia with age, female sex, low socioeconomic status, divorce, widowhood, separation, recent stress and depression, and drug or alcohol abuse, with higher predilection among women (Martikainen et al., 2003).

### Short-Term Insomnia Disorder (Acute Insomnia)

This type of insomnia is characterized by short-term difficulty in initiating or maintaining sleep that results in general sleep dissatisfaction and is accompanied by daytime distress about the poor sleep quality or impairment in social, family, occupational, academic, or other important areas of functioning. The disorder and its associated symptoms occur despite having adequate time and circumstances to obtain necessary sufficient sleep (AASM, 2014). In many cases of short-term insomnia lasting less than 3 months, there is an identifiable cause that serves as the precipitant. In other cases, insomnia occurs episodically, often coincident to daytime stressors that account for the insomnia (AASM, 2014). Once the stressful event is removed and the patient adjusts to the event, the sleep disturbance resolves. Causes of acute insomnia are listed in Box 101.9.

### Chronic Insomnia

Most cases of insomnia are chronic and comorbid with other conditions (Morin and Benca, 2015, 2011). Common comorbidities include psychiatric, medical, primary sleep-related (i.e., OSAS), neurological disorders, pain syndrome, or drug and alcohol abuse. eBox 101.10 lists the causes of chronic insomnia. These comorbid insomnias were classified as secondary insomnia in the past, but this signifies causation; no definite evidence exists that these conditions are responsible for insomnia (National Institutes of Health, 2005). 

In addition to short-term effects of disturbed sleep and inadequate daytime functioning, people with insomnia report impaired work performance and productivity, reduced social and physical functioning, reduced overall quality of life, and a two- to fivefold increased risk for developing subsequent depression associated with significant suicidal behavior. There are also suggestions of increased mortality and morbidity from coronary artery disease, hypertension, obesity, and diabetes mellitus (Ayas et al., 2003a, 2003b; Knutson and Turek, 2006). A longitudinal sleep laboratory follow-up study for 14 years, however, found increased mortality in men with chronic insomnia with objectively measured short sleep duration that could not be explained by comorbid type 2 diabetes mellitus or hypertension (Vgontzas et al., 2010). The clinically significant consequences (both short-term and long-term) of insomnia most typically develop when sleep difficulties occur at least three times per week and persist for at least 3 months. Hence those frequency and duration criteria must be met for a diagnosis of chronic insomnia disorder (AASM, 2014).

### Two-week sleep diary

**Instructions:**

1. Write the date, day of the week, and type of day: work, school, day off, or vacation.
2. Put the letter "C" in a box when you have coffee, tea, cola, or anything else with caffeine. Put "M" in a box when you take any medicine. Put "A" in a box when you drink alcohol. Put "E" in a box when you exercise.
3. Put a downward arrow to show when you go to bed. Shade in the box when you think you fell asleep.
4. Shade in all the boxes that show when you are asleep at night or when you take a nap during the day.
5. Put an upward arrow to indicate when you got out of bed.
6. Leave boxes unshaded to show when you are awake at night and during the day.

**Sample entry below:** On a monday when I worked, I jogged on my lunch break at 1:00 pm, had a glass of wine with dinner at 6:00 pm, fell asleep watching television from 7:00-8:00 pm, went to bed at 10:30 pm, fell asleep around midnight, woke up and stayed awake between 4:00-5:00 am, went back to sleep between 5:00-7:00 am, and had coffee and breakfast and took medicine at 7:00 am.

| | Today's date | Day of the week | Type of day (work, school, vacation) | Noon | 1 PM | 2 | 3 | 4 | 5 | 6 PM | 7 | 8 | 9 | 10 | 11 | Midnight | 1 AM | 2 | 3 | 4 | 5 | 6 AM | 7 | 8 | 9 | 10 | 11 AM |
|---|---|---|---|---|---|---|---|---|---|---|---|---|---|---|---|---|---|---|---|---|---|---|---|---|---|---|---|
| | Sample | Mon. | Work | | E | | | | | A | | | | ↓ | | | | | | | | ↑ | C M | | | | |
| Week 1 | | | | | | | | | | | | ↓ | | | | | | | | | | | | | ↑ | | |
| | | | | | | | | | | | ↓ | | | | | | | | | | | | | ↑ | | | |
| | | | | | | | | | | | ↓ | | | | | | | | | | | | | | | ↑ | |
| | | | | | | | | | | | | | | | ↓ | | | | | | | | | | | ↑ | |
| | | | | | | | | | | | | ↓ | | | | | | | | | | | | | ↑ | | |
| | | | | | | | | | | | | ↓ | | | | | | | | | | | | ↑ | | | |
| | | | | | | | | | | | ↓ | | | | | | | | | | | | | ↑ | | | |
| Week 2 | | | | | | | | | | | | | | | ↓ | | | | | | | | | ↑ | | | |
| | | | | | | | | | | | | | | | | ↓ | | | | | | | | | | | ↑ |
| | | | | | | | | | | | | ↓ | | | | | | | | | | | ↑ | | | | |
| | | | | | | | | | | | | | | ↓ | | | | | | | | | | | | ↑ | |
| | | | | | | | | | | | | ↓ | | | | | | | | | | | | | | ↑ | |
| | | | | | | | | | | | | | | | | ↓ | | | | | | | | | | ↑ | |
| | | | | | | | | | | | | | | | ↓ | | | | | | | | | | | | ↑ |

**Adapted with permission from:** The American Academy of Sleep Medicine.
Form available at: http://sleepeducation.org/docs/default-document-library/sleep-diary.pdf.

**Fig. 101.28** Sample Sleep Log (Sleep Diary). A sleep log is a record of an individual's sleeping and waking times, usually tabulated over a period of several weeks. The patient is instructed to record the following data: Time required to fall asleep; time he/she thinks they fell as leep; number, time, and length of any nocturnal awakenings; time he/she woke up; time he/she got out of bed; time he/she wanted to wake up; a comment on how he/she felt during the day; start and end times of any daytime naps; potential medications used. *(Adapted with permission from The American Academy of Medicine. Available at: http://sleepeducation.org/docs/default-document-library/sleep-diary.pdf.)*

## Proposed Mechanism and Physiological Profiles of Patient with Insomnia

The proposed basis and evolution of insomnia as a disorder of hyperarousal (Fig. 101.30) and its evolution during early life to adulthood and from acute to chronic forms is summarized in Fig. 101.31, as it transforms to chronic insomnia. Patients suffering from insomnia may suffer from a general disorder of hyperarousal due to a functional alteration in the anatomical substrates for sleep/wake states conferred by hyperactivity of wake-promoting neurons or hypoactivity of sleep-generating neurons that is genetically determined. Evidence of hyperarousal is provided by the following observations in these patients (Morin and Benca, 2011, 2015) and is highlighted in Fig. 101.31:

- Increased heart rate
- Elevated sympathetic and decreased parasympathetic tone (as measured by spectral analysis to show heart rate variability)
- Increased 24-hour and evening cortisol levels and increased 24-hour corticotropin levels (indicating abnormal hypothalamic–pituitary–adrenal axis)
- Increased brain glucose metabolism
- Increased EMG activity, as noted in the frontalis muscle
- EEG spectral analysis showing increased beta activity
- Decreased nocturnal melatonin and increased diurnal melatonin levels
- Increased latencies on MSLT, despite disturbed nocturnal sleep
- Neuroimaging findings of subcortical (ARAS) hyperarousal. The data support that in people with insomnia, during transition from waking to sleep, there is a state of increased cerebral metabolism due to a lack of a reduction in activity in subcortical structures compared to people without insomnia (Nofzinger et al., 2004).

Hyperarousal dysfunction is supported by functional neuroanatomy, where PET imaging designed to measure regional brain

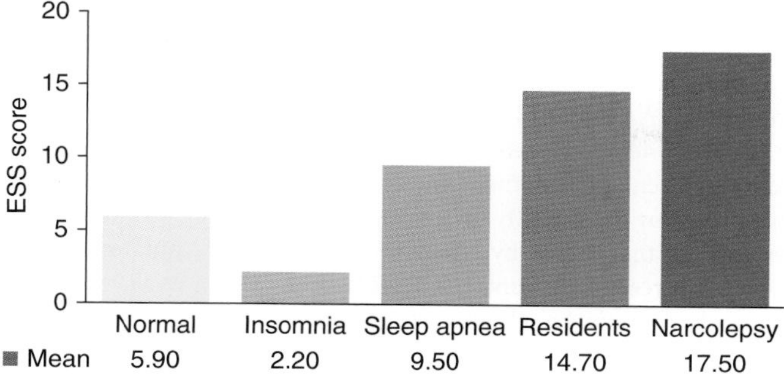


**Fig. 101.29 The Epworth Sleepiness Scale (ESS) Across Populations.** The diagram highlights ESS for normal subjects and patients with representative sleep disorders (insomnia, obstructive sleep apnea, and narcolepsy) as well as medical residents. Sleepiness in medical residents is equivalent to that found in patients with serious sleep disorders such as narcolepsy. The ESS is an 8-item self-report which asks respondents to rate their likelihood of "dozing" under several specified conditions. The individual rates each situation from 0 to 3, with 3 indicating the highest likelihood. The highest possible score is 24. The generally accepted value for the upper limit of "normal" is 11. Values between 11 and 13 are considered mild, 14 and 17 moderate, and greater than 17 severe.

**BOX 101.9 Causes of Acute Insomnia**

| | |
|---|---|
| Internal (patient-related factors) | Acute medical or surgical illnesses (including intensive care unit stays)<br>Stimulant medications (e.g., theophylline, beta-blockers, corticosteroids, thyroxine, bronchodilators, or withdrawal of central nervous system depressant medications) |
| External (environmental factors) | A change of sleeping environment (most common cause of transient insomnia, the so-called first night effect)<br>Jet lag<br>Unpleasant sleep environment (excessively hot/cold room temperature)<br>Excessive environmental noise (living close to the motor way/train track/airport)<br>Excessive environmental light exposure |

**BOX 101.10 Chronic Insomnia Phenotypes**

Idiopathic or primary insomnia
Psychophysiological insomnia
Paradoxical insomnia (sleep state misperception)
Inadequate sleep hygiene
Insomnia comorbid with psychiatric disorders
Insomnia comorbid with general medical disorder
Insomnia comorbid with neurological disorder
Insomnia due to drug or other substance abuse

metabolism demonstrates that patients with insomnia show increased activity during the transition from waking to sleep onset as compared to healthy subjects, suggesting that there is an overall cortical hyperarousal in insomnia (eFig. 101.32). Furthermore, patients with insomnia have less reduction of activation from waking to NREM sleep in the ARAS, hypothalamus, insular cortex, amygdala, hippocampus, anterior cingulate, and medial prefrontal cortices, as illustrated in the figure (Nofzinger et al., 2004; Nofzinger et al., 2006).

Additional insomnia subtypes mentioned in the ICSD-II are provided for historical reasons. This outline as well as insomnia criteria from the ICSD-III along with a listing of medical and neurological comorbidities are provided in Boxes 101.11 and 101.12 at http://expertconsult.inkling.com.

The section below covers insomnia subtypes of described in the ICSD-III (AASM, 2014).

## Idiopathic and Psychophysiological Insomnia

The onset of idiopathic insomnia occurs in early childhood, as highlighted in Fig.101.31 and contributing to a "Predisposition" to develop insomnia Fig. 101.33, as demarcated by the red column. Patients generally have lifelong difficulty with initiating or maintaining sleep, or both, resulting in poor daytime functioning. Diagnosis depends on the exclusion of concomitant comorbid medical, neurological, psychiatric, or psychological disturbances. Psychophysiological insomnia may transpire during young adulthood, and the symptoms may persist for decades. This is chronic insomnia is characterized by hypervigilance and hyperarousal and it is fueled by learned sleep-preventing associations. Patients are overconcerned on sleep problems, but they may not have generalized anxiety or any other psychiatric disorders. Sometimes a family history exists. The development of conditioned responses incompatible with sleep is the predominant feature of psychophysiological insomnia. Insomnia is an event precipitated or initiated by a stressor such as acute life events such as a new job, death of a loved one, COVID19 and surgery, but it persists even after that initial stress is gone (see Fig.101.33, demarcated by the yellow column). Factors contributing to negative conditioning in the setting of insomnia are "perpetuating" factors include excessive fear and frustration about being unable to initiate and maintain sleep, and the identification of the bedroom as an arousal sign and environmental and disadvantages life-style factors that perpetuate the insomnia Fig. 101.33, blue column including alcohol, caffeine, artificial and excessive blue light exposure from light exposure, television and electronics high temperatures and excessive environmental noise. Patients generally sleep poorly during nocturnal polysomnogram, a phenomena referred to as "the first night effect", although occasionally patients sleep better because they are removed from their usual sleep environment (reverse first-night effect). Patients with psychophysiological insomnia confine anxiety to sleep-related issues, which differentiates them from patients with generalized anxiety disorders. New data provide good evidence to support the view that primary psychophysiological insomnia is a true conflict between the sleep system and inappropriate activation of CNS (Riemann, 2010).

## Paradoxical Insomnia

Paradoxical insomnia is a sleep state misperception characterized by subjective complaints of sleeplessness without objective evidence (e.g., PSG evidence of insomnia). Patients often complain of severe sleep disturbance but lack supportive objective evidence to corroborate the degree of sleep disturbance claimed. (AASM, 2014). There is an increased propensity for these patients to underestimate the amount of sleep they are actually getting. In essence, they are thought to perceive much of the time they actually sleep as wakefulness. Actigraphy (an accelerometer which measures sleep/wake activities) or PSG recording documents normal sleep patterns in such patients.

## Inadequate Sleep Hygiene

Patients with inadequate sleep hygiene negate the good sleep measures that promote sleep. Such measures include avoidance of caffeinated beverages, alcohol, and tobacco in the evening; avoidance of intense mental activities close to bedtime (this has been seriously questioned in recent literature); avoidance of daytime naps and excessive time spent in bed awake; and adherence to a regular sleep/wake schedule.

Insomnia commonly coexists or precedes the development of a number of psychiatric illnesses. Surveys have shown that individuals with insomnia are more likely to develop new psychiatric disorders, particularly major depression, within 6–12 months. Anxiety disorders, depression, and schizophrenia are some of the major psychiatric disorders associated with insomnia.

Medical and neurological disorders comorbid with insomnia are  listed in eBoxes 101.11 and 101.12. RLS, PLMD, and circadian rhythm disorders are some of the other causes of chronic insomnia. In some patients, insomnia may coexist with sleep apnea.

### Mechanism of Insomnia in Neurological Diseases

Insomnia in neurological disorders may result from the following suggested mechanisms:

- Hypofunction (metabolic or structural) of the hypothalamic VLPO neurons or the lower brainstem hypnogenic neurons in the region of the NTS and dysfunction of thalamus may alter the balance between the waking and sleeping brain, causing sleeplessness.
- Neurological disorders may cause pain, agitation and confusion, alteration of the sensory-motor system, and abnormal movements during sleep, which may interfere with normal progression and cycling of NREM-REM sleep.
- Medications used to treat neurological illnesses (e.g., corticosteroids, antiepileptic drugs such as lamotrigine, zonisamide, and levetiracetam, dopaminergic medications, decongestants) may cause insomnia.
- Certain neurological disorders may alter circadian rhythm in the SCN causing insomnia. (This is particularly true in the case of Alzheimer dementia, but also PD and traumatic brain injury [TBI].)
- Neurological illnesses have a bidirectional relationship with psychiatric conditions, particularly depression and anxiety, which promote sleeplessness.
- Neurological disorders such as MSA, MS and neuromuscular disorders such as myotonic dystrophy type 2 have strong association with primary sleep disorders such as SDB, resulting in sleep fragmentation, excessive sleepiness impaired quality of life.

## Central Disorders of Hypersomnolence

Since the French physician Gelineau used the term *narcolepsy* in 1880 to describe irresistible sleep attacks and astasia, which includes all the features of cataplexy, there have been many reports of patients with narcolepsy-cataplexy syndrome (Nishino, 2007; Nishino and Mignot, 2011; Scammell, 2003). The prevalence of narcolepsy is estimated to be approximately 1 in 2000 individuals in the United States, 1 in 600 people in Japan, and 1 in 500,000 individuals in Israel. Reports of adequate epidemiological studies in different parts of the world are, however, lacking (Video 101.2).

### Genetics of Narcolepsy

Most cases of human narcolepsy are sporadic, but some are dominant. There is, however, a 10–40 times greater prevalence of narcolepsy in families than in the general population. For example, approximately one or two first-degree relatives of narcoleptic patients, compared with 0.02%–0.18% in the general population, manifest the illness. Twin studies show that the majority of monozygotic twins are discordant, and only 25%–31% are concordant, suggesting an influence of environmental factors in the etiology of narcolepsy. From 95% to 100% of white and Japanese patients carry the HLA. It has been established that HLA-DQB1*0602 is a marker for narcolepsy on chromosome 6 across all ethnic groups. However, cases of narcolepsy not carrying HLA-DR2 or HLA-DQ1 antigens have been reported. In addition, 12%–38% of the general population carries the same HLA alleles, but narcolepsy is present in only 0.02%–0.18% of the population. Clinically, *HLA-DQB1*0602* typing may be indicated when considering a CSF hypocretin measurement. Hypocretin levels are generally normal if the patient is HLA-negative, unless the patient has a diencephalic lesion that explains the CNS hypersomnia (narcolepsy type due to a medical condition) (AASM, 2014).

***Pathogenesis of narcolepsy-cataplexy syndrome.*** The most exciting recent development in sleep medicine is the pathogenetic role played by the recently discovered hypocretin (orexin) peptidergic systems in the lateral hypothalamus. Reports of mutation of the hypocretin receptor 2 gene (HCRTR2) in dogs (Lin et al., 1999) and pre-prohypocretin knockout mice (Chemelli et al., 1999) producing the phenotype of human narcolepsy brought narcolepsy research to the forefront of the molecular neurobiology field. Most cases of human narcolepsy and cataplexy have decreased hypocretin 1 in the cerebrospinal fluid (CSF) (Bourgin et al., 2008; Fronczek et al., 2009; Nishino, 2007). Hypocretins are noted to be depleted in narcoleptic brains at autopsy, as can be seen in Fig. 101.34 (Thannickal et al., 2000) with a proposed mechanism involving an environmental trigger which produces an autoimmune response in genetically venerable individuals (Overeem et al., 2008). In addition, mutation of the pre-prohypocretin gene has been identified in one child with severe narcolepsy (Peyron et al., 2000). Therefore, the contemporary theory for the pathogenesis of narcolepsy-cataplexy syndrome suggests that the condition results from a depletion (degeneration or autoimmune disorder) of the hypocretin neurons in the lateral and perifornical region of the hypothalamus, as can be appreciated in Fig. 101.35. Narcolepsy-cataplexy syndrome thus can be considered a hypocretin (orexin) deficiency syndrome, which is how the condition is being referred to in the updated version of the ICSD-III (AASM, 2014). The possibility of an autoimmune disorder has been raised because of the association of narcolepsy with HLA-DQB1*0602 haplotype; however, all attempts to find evidence of autoimmune disorder in narcolepsy have so far failed (Overeem et al., 2008). There is no evidence of inflammatory processes or immune abnormalities, presence of classical autoantibodies, or an increase of oligoclonal bands in the CSF in these patients. Erythrocyte sedimentation rate, serum immunoglobulin levels, C-reactive protein, complement levels, and lymphocyte subset ratio are all found to be normal in these patients, pointing against an autoimmune disorder. On the other hand, increased levels of streptococcal antibodies in narcoleptic patients in some reports and evidence of gliosis in the lateral hypothalamus by Thannickal and colleagues (2000) indicate that further exploration for possible immune-related dysfunction in narcolepsy is needed. Finally, the presence of autoantibodies (patient serum binding to rat hypocretin neurons) in one out of nine narcolepsy-cataplexy patients keeps the autoimmune theory very much in the forefront (Knudsen et al., 2007). Environmental considerations such as streptococcal infection, seasonal influenza, and more recent reports implicating the 2009 influenza pandemic A/H1N1 raise even stronger concerns for an immunological mechanism for narcolepsy. Proposed immunological mechanisms that could trigger specific destruction and subsequent elimination of hypocretin producing neurons include molecular mimicry or bystander activation and are likely a combination of genetic and environmental factors, such as upper airway infections (Mahlios et al., 2013).

In the summer of 2010 concerns were raised in Scandinavia about a possible association between narcolepsy and ASO3 adjuvanted A/H1N1 2009 pandemic vaccine following observation of a potential temporal association by clinicians in sleep centers in these countries. A follow-up study of children in England depicted a comparable association of increased risk (Miller et al., 2013). The earlier data from Finland described a 13-fold increased risk of narcolepsy following vaccination of patients aged 4–19, the majority of whom developed narcolepsy symptoms within 3 months after vaccination (Fig. 101.36) and almost

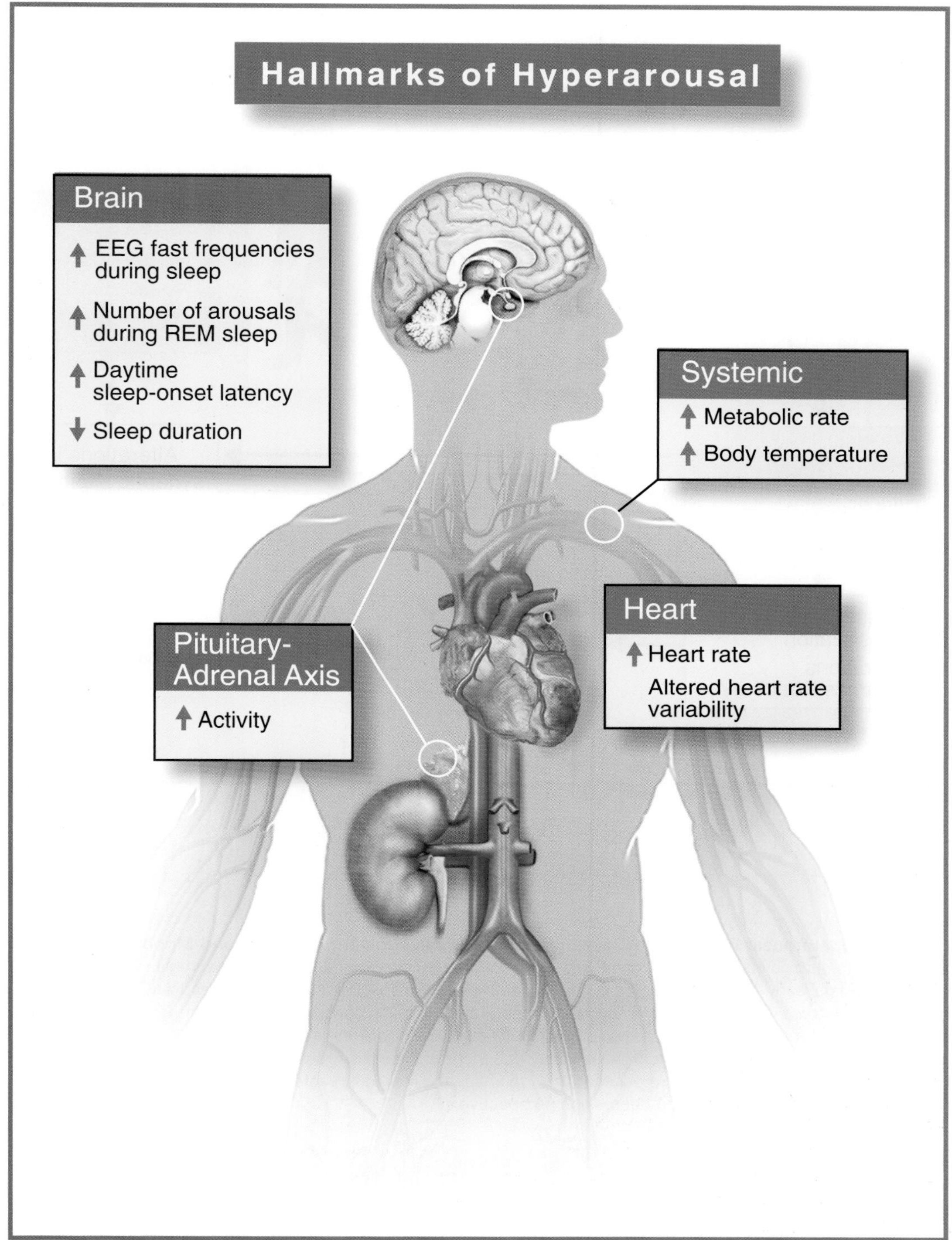


**Fig 101.30 Indicators of Hyperarousal in Insomnia.** Insomnia disorder is characterized by physiological hyperarousal consisting of increased activity of the hypothalamic–pituitary–adrenal axis. Such activity is supported by increased levels of cortisol and amplification of sympathetic autonomic nervous system activity demarcated by an increased resting heart rate, metabolic rate, and increased body temperature. Quantified sleep electroencephalography *(EEG)* and polysomnographic data demonstrate reduction in sleep duration and efficiency, arousals, and is supported by an increased sleep-onset latency during daytime investigations of sleepiness utilizing the Multiple Sleep Latency Test (MSLT). This is also consistent with the lowest ESS score observed among patients with insomnia in figure 101.29. *REM*, Rapid eye movement.

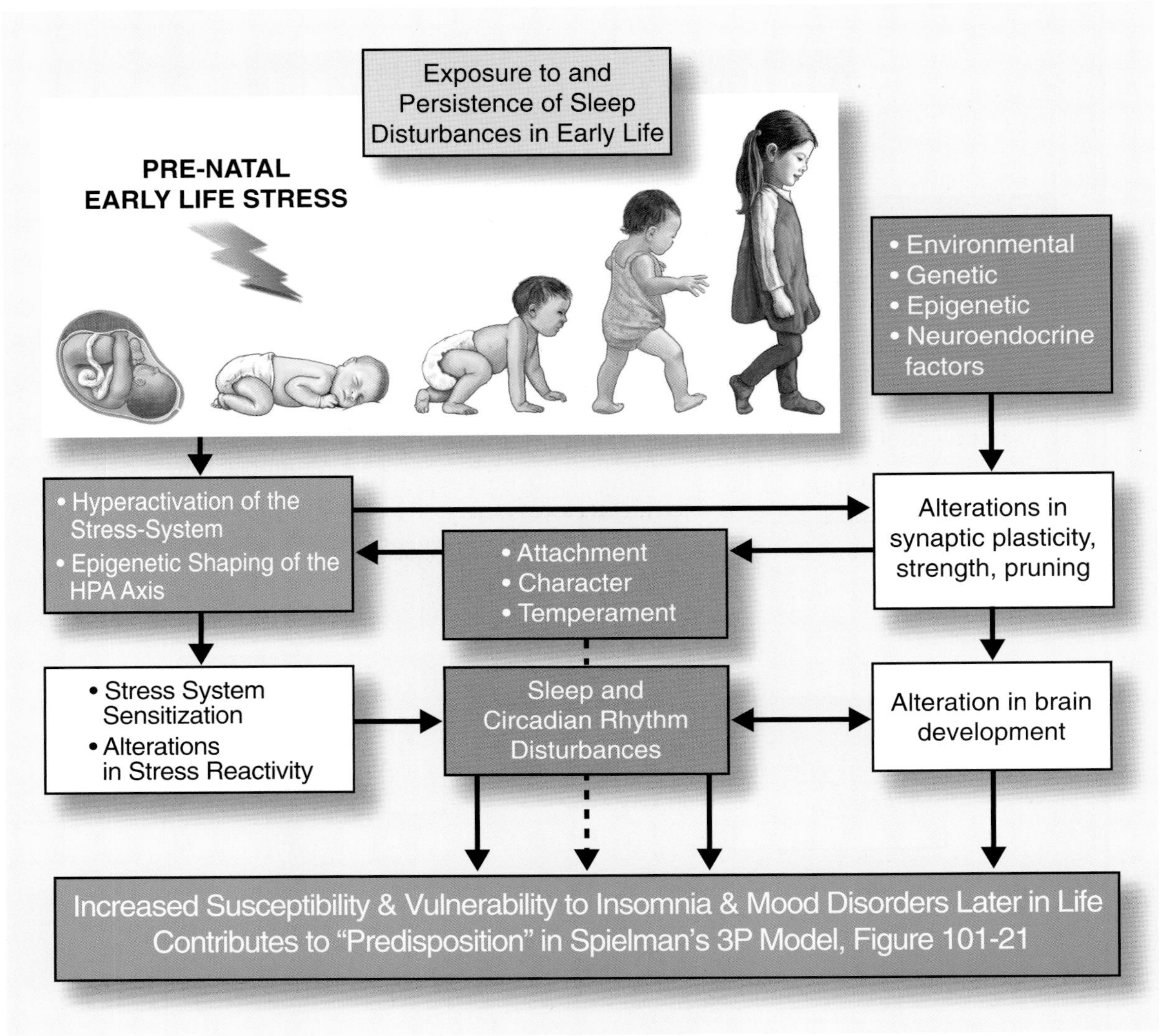

**Fig 101.31** Indicators of Hyperarousal in Insomnia Developmental Pathways toward Insomnia and Mood disorders in Adult Life. Sleep disturbances and pathways to chronic insomnia and mood disorders in adult life. The model of chronic insomnia in the setting of mental disorders emerges initially in early-prenatal/early life stress occurs within the framework of the complex-genetic –and environmental predisposition that is mediated through exposure to stress. Programming may occur in prenatal and postnatal periods, which constitute highly sensitive periods during the development of an individual and may subserve the basis of predisposition to insomnia and mental health pathologies later in life possibly through epigenetic mechanisms. Since disturbed sleep is one of the key consequences of early life stress it is hypothesized that disturbed sleep due to prenatal early life stress, possibly mediated by epigenetic processes, may re-shape the individual's stress system contributing to an increased vulnerability to stress-related disorders, particularly insomnia and depression prospectively.

all within 6 months (Nohynek et al., 2012; Wijnans et al., 2013). New data from Stanford University implicated a small epitope of pH1N1 that resembles hypocretin and is likely involved in molecular mimicry (De la Herran-Arita et al., 2013). Fig. 101.37 highlights a few pathophysiological mechanisms for narcolepsy which points toward selective venerability (conferred through HLA positivity), a trigger, and a reaction leading to destruction of the vulnerable populations of orexin neurons. It is believed that the underlying pathology of narcolepsy is related to genetic, environmental, and acute triggering factors. The implications of genetic factors (specifically HL A-DQB1*06:02 positivity) are a strong predisposition to narcolepsy. The first clinical marker of such a predisposition is a short sleep latency period before onset of REM sleep. Environmental exposures to bacterial and viral pathogens in early life might alter immune system development.

## Clinical Manifestations of Narcolepsy

The onset of the disorder in most cases is in adolescents and young adults, with a peak incidence between ages 15 and 30. However, rare cases have been described in children younger than age 5 and adults older than age 50. The ICSD-III divides narcolepsy into two types: narcolepsy type 1 (with cataplexy, or low hypocretin levels), and narcolepsy type 2 (without cataplexy, and with normal hypocretin levels) (AASM, 2014) eTable 101.6.  Secondary narcolepsy due to a known underlying CNS disorder is referred to as narcolepsy type 1 due to a medical condition (when hypocretin levels are low) or narcolepsy type 2 due to a medical condition (when hypocretin levels are normal). Diseases impacting the major clinical manifestations of narcolepsy include sleep attacks (100%), cataplexy (60%–70%), sleep paralysis (25%–50%), hypnagogic hallucinations (20%–40%), disturbed night

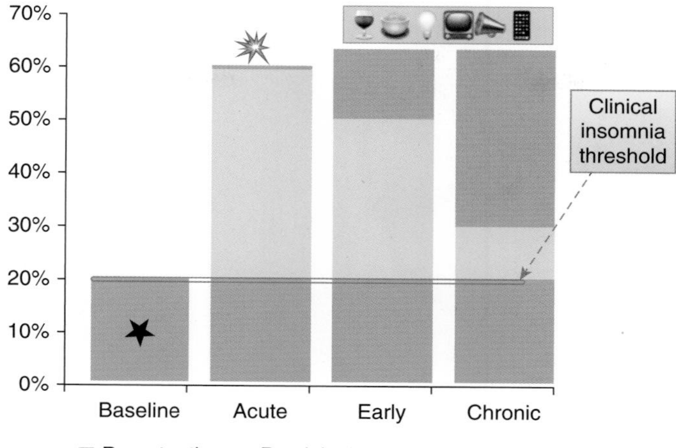


**Fig. 101.33** **3-P Model of Insomnia Etiology.** The 3-P Model of Insomnia Etiology explains that all express a certain vulnerability to express insomnia (Predisposing Factors, 1st P). Insomnia disorder occurs when a precipitating event pushes patients above the insomnia threshold (2nd P). When the precipitating factor ★ diminishes, the insomnia is kept above threshold when patients develop behavioral conditioned arousal response associated with the bedroom environment that perpetuates the insomnia. These perpetuating (3rd P) factors are shown in the figure by alcohol too close to bedtime, caffeine too late during the day, excessive light, TV, light-emitting electronic devices).

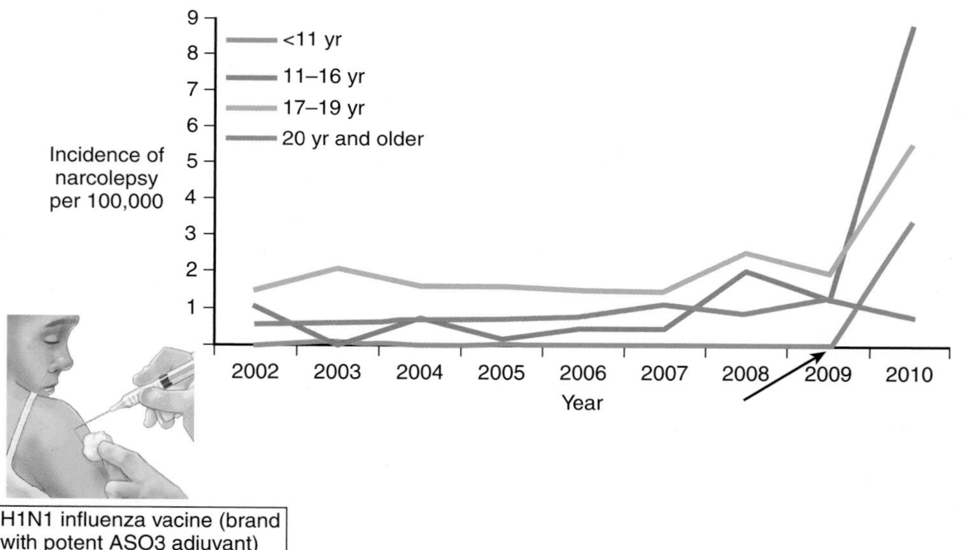


**Fig. 101.36** **Narcolepsy Incidence Following Administration of the H1N1 Vaccine.** Epidemiological data following vaccination of children in Finland and Sweden with a monovalent 2009 H1N1 influenza vaccine (brand with potent ASO3 adjuvant). The data demonstrate 8- to 12-fold increase in narcolepsy following vaccination as demarcated by the arrow. The Centers for Disease Control (CDC) in the United States did not find any association between US-licensed H1N1 or seasonal influenza vaccine and narcolepsy following review of data collected by the Vaccine Adverse Event Reporting System (VAERS). *(Data from Nohynek, H., Jokinen, J., Partinen, M., et al., 2012. As03 adjuvanted AH1N1 vaccine associated with an abrupt increase in the incidence of childhood narcolepsy in Finland. PLoS ONE 7 [3], e33536.; Wijnans, L., Lecomte, C., de Vries, C., et al., 2013. The incidence of narcolepsy in Europe: before, during, and after the influenza A(H1N1) pdm09 pandemic and vaccination campaigns. Vaccine 31 [8], 1246–1254.)*

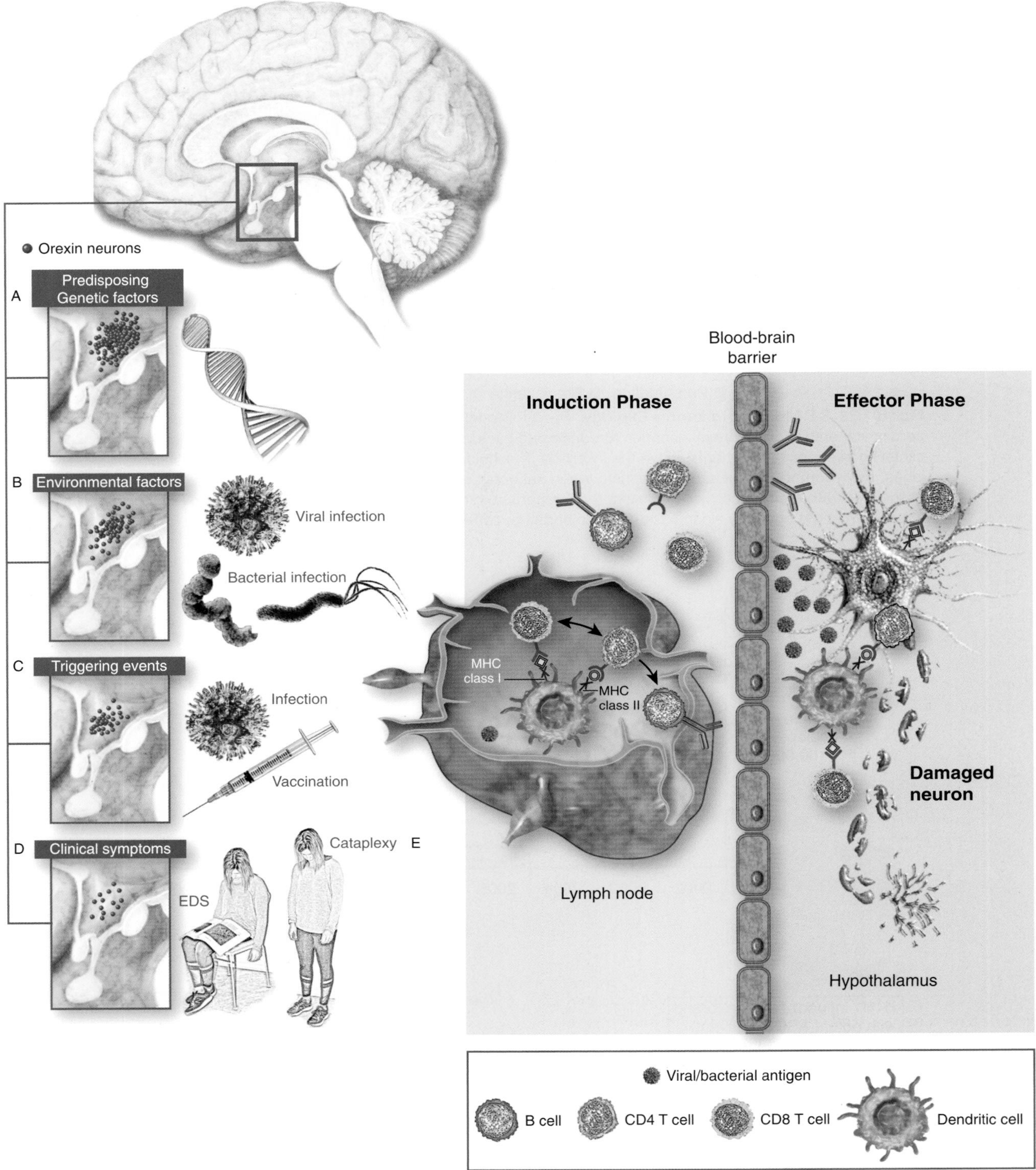


**Fig. 101.37 Plausible Disease Mechanism in Narcolepsy.** It is believed that the underlying pathology of narcolepsy is related to genetic, environmental, and acute triggering factors. The implications of genetic factors (specifically HL A-DQB1*06:02 positivity) are a strong predisposition to narcolepsy **A**. The first clinical marker of such a predisposition is a short sleep latency period before onset of rapid eye movement (REM) sleep. **B,** Environmental exposures to bacterial and viral pathogens in early life might alter immune system development in susceptible individuals and predispose these individuals to narcolepsy later in life. One hypothesis implicates these changes directly or indirectly cause the loss of some orexin neurons. An alternative explanation is that these genetic and environmental factors might only increase the vulnerability of these neurons. **C,** Triggering events could include vaccinations and infections by viruses such as influenza type A (H1N1) and bacteria such as Streptococcus spp. induce or reactivate the immune response, leading to the selective destruction of venerable orexin neurons (induction phase) resulting in the clinical manifestation of narcolepsy (D).

**Fig. 101.37, cont'd** **D,** The clinical symptoms of narcolepsy progress over days to weeks and perhaps even years, as an increasing number of orexin neurons is destroyed or silenced, causing an imbalance in brainstem sleep and wake pathways (effector phase) that leads to full-spectrum narcolepsy with cataplexy. **E,** The exact sequence of events leading to the selective and preferential destruction of orexin neurons in the hypothalamus is still under investigation, but presumed inflammatory cytokines and activated immune cells (dendritic cells, antigen-specific CD4+ T cells, and cytotoxic CD8+ T cells), which eventually cross the blood–brain barrier, are thought to be involved. Antibodies can cross a disrupted blood–brain barrier and might also contribute to neuronal destruction. *EDS*, Excessive daytime sleepiness; *MB*, mammillary body; *OT*, optic tract. *(From Bassetti, C.L.A., Adamantidis, A., Burdakov, D. et al., 2019. Narcolepsy—clinical spectrum, aetiopathophysiology, diagnosis and treatment. Nat. Rev. Neurol. 15, 519–539. https://doi.org/10.1038/s41582-019-0226-9.)*

**TABLE 101.5 Major Clinical Features of Narcolepsy**

| MAJOR MANIFESTATIONS | |
|---|---|
| Excessive sleepiness | 100% |
| Cataplexy | 70% |
| Sleep paralysis | 25%–50% |
| Hypnagogic/hypnopompic hallucinations | 20%–40% |
| Disturbed night sleep | 70%–80% |
| Automatic behavior | 20%–40% |

sleep (70%–80%), and automatic behavior (20%–40%) (Nishino, 2007; Nishino and Mignot, 2011; Overeem et al., 2001) (Table 101.5).

The classic *narcoleptic sleep attack* is an irresistible desire to fall asleep in inappropriate circumstances and at inappropriate places (e.g., while talking, driving, eating, playing, or when involved in boring or monotonous circumstances) as illustrated in Fig. 101.38. These spells last from a few minutes to as long as 20–30 minutes, and the patient generally feels refreshed on waking. There are wide variations in frequency of attacks—anywhere from daily, weekly, monthly, or every few weeks to months. Attacks generally persist throughout the patient's lifetime, although fluctuations and rare temporary remissions may occur. Patients often show a decline in performance at school and work and encounter psychosocial and socioeconomic difficulties as a result of sleep attacks and EDS.

*Cataplexy* is defined as a sudden loss of tone in all voluntary muscles with the exception of the respiratory and ocular muscles. By definition, cataplexy is universally preceded by a prodromal of emotion leading to a transient episode of muscle weakness. The typical emotions that trigger cataplexy are positive phenomena and include laughter and excitement, rage, or anger more than 95% of the time. The attacks may be complete or partial but are rarely unilateral. Most commonly, patients momentarily have head nodding, sagging of the jaw, buckling of the knees, dropping of objects from the hands, dysarthria, or loss of voice, but sometimes they may slump or fall forward to the ground for a few seconds. The duration is usually a few seconds to a minute or two, and consciousness is retained completely during the attack. During brief cataplectic spells, neurological examination reveals flaccidity of the muscles and absence or markedly reduced muscle stretch reflexes. H reflex and F responses are decreased or absent. Generally, cataplectic spells occur months to years after the onset of sleep attacks, but occasionally cataplexy is the initial manifestation. It is a lifelong condition but is generally less severe and may even disappear in old age. Rarely, status cataplecticus occurs, particularly after withdrawal of anticataplectic medications. An EEG recording shows evidence of wakefulness during brief cataplectic spells, but if the attack lasts longer than 1 to 2 minutes, the EEG shows REM sleep. A potential pathogenetic mechanism postulated for cataplexy is illustrated in Fig. 101.39 and is based on activation, during awake state, of brainstem neuronal circuitry that normally induces skeletal muscle atonia during REM sleep. During cataplexy, muscle weakness is generated by decreased excitation of noradrenergic neurons and increased inhibition of skeletal motor neurons by GABA-releasing or glycinergic neurons (Dauvilliers et al., 2014) (Bassetti et al., 2019). The medial prefrontal cortex and amygdala contain neural networks through which positive emotions conceivably trigger cataplectic attacks (Dauvilliers et al., 2014).

*Sleep paralysis* occurs in approximately 25%–50% of patients and is generally noted months to years after the onset of narcoleptic sleep attacks. The sudden apparent paralysis of one or both sides of the body or one limb occurs either during sleep onset (hypnagogic) or on awakening (hypnopompic) in the morning. The patient is unable to move or speak and is frightened, although he or she retains consciousness. The attacks last from a few minutes to 15–20 minutes.

*Hypnagogic hallucinations* are found in 20%–40% of narcoleptic patients. They occur either at sleep onset or on awakening in the morning and generally appear months to years after the onset of sleep attacks. Hallucinations are most commonly vivid and visual (and often fear-inducing) but are sometimes auditory, vestibular, or somesthetic in nature. In 30% of patients, three of the four major manifestations of the narcoleptic tetrad (sleep attacks, cataplexy, sleep paralysis, and hypnagogic hallucinations) occur together, and in about 10% of cases, all four major features occur together.

***Disturbed night sleep and automatic behavior.*** Disturbed night sleep is commonly noted in 70% to 80% of patients. In approximately 20%–40% of cases, automatic behavior characterized by repeated performance of a single function such as speaking or writing in a meaningless manner, driving on the wrong side of the road, or driving to a strange place without recalling the episode is noted. These episodes of automatic behavior may result from partial sleep episodes, frequent lapses, or microsleeps.

The clinical presentation of narcolepsy with cataplexy in children may be different from that of adults (AASM, 2014). Children may present with prolonged nocturnal sleep or paradoxically may present with hyperactive behavior, insomnia, and bizarre hallucinations. Children may present with characteristic *cataplectic facies* (facial weakness with tongue protrusion) not associated with emotion, or cataplexy may be manifested with perioral dystonic movements (Fig. 101.40) (Postiglione et al., 2018).

***Comorbid conditions.*** In addition to the major manifestations, patients with narcolepsy may also have several important comorbid conditions (see eTable 101.6): sleep apnea, PLMS, and RBD. Sleep  apnea is noted in approximately 30% of narcoleptic patients; most commonly central apnea is seen, but obstructive or mixed apnea is also reported. Associated sleep apnea may aggravate sleep attacks. It is important to diagnose obstructive sleep apnea (OSA) in these patients because treatment with continuous positive airway pressure (CPAP) will relieve apnea, with curtailment of EDS. RBD generally occurs in

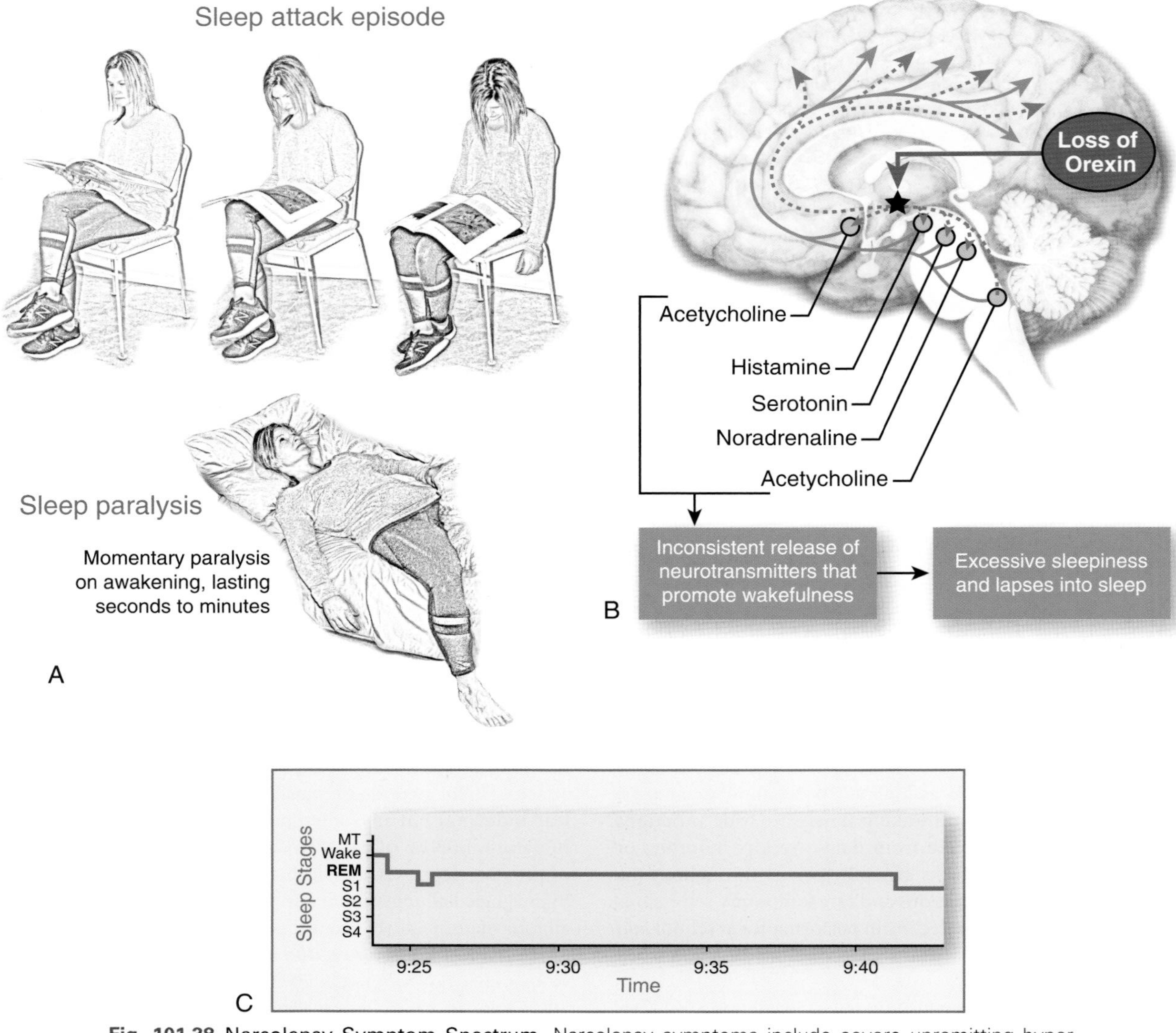


**Fig. 101.38 Narcolepsy Symptom Spectrum.** Narcolepsy symptoms include severe unremitting hypersomnolence with sleep attacks in virtually all patients, cataplexy in the majority, as well as sleep paralysis, hypnagogic hallucinations, disturbed night sleep, and automatic behavior. The underlying mechanism of excessive daytime sleepiness has recently been linked to loss of orexin neurons. This pathology reduces excitatory input to the cortex, thalamus, and wake-promoting neurotransmitter systems in multiple brain regions, resulting in persistent sleepiness throughout the day. **A,** Sleep episode/involuntary nap during quiet reading. **B,** The specific loss of orexin-producing neurons in patients with narcolepsy accompanied by cataplexy leads to erratic firing of the brainstem neurons responsible for arousal. This change results in excessive daytime sleepiness and a predisposition to lapses into sleep. **C,** A neurophysiological recording made during a multiple sleep latency test (MSLT) documents the transition from wakefulness into sleep. A shortened sleep latency period is evident, and a so-called sleep-onset rapid eye movement (REM) period (SOREMP) occurs within 15 min. In patients with narcolepsy accompanied by cataplexy, SOREMPs occur in ~50% of sleep episodes (detected by MSLT or night-time polysomnography). *(A, B, C Adapted from Bassetti, C.L.A., Adamantidis, A., Burdakov, D.* et al. *Narcolepsy — clinical spectrum, aetiopathophysiology, diagnosis and treatment.* Nat. Rev. Neurol. *15, 519–539 (2019). https://doi.org/10.1038/s41582-019-0226-9. With permission.)*

men with narcolepsy—in up to 36% of all patients with the disorder. Mostly commonly, the stimulants and tricyclic antidepressants or selective serotonin reuptake inhibitors (SSRIs) used to treat narcolepsy-cataplexy syndrome may induce or exacerbate RBD. PLMS have been noted in 10%–60% of narcoleptic patients. There is a high prevalence (exact percentage is not known in limited studies) of both eating disorder (Droogleever-Fortuyn et al., 2008) and increased BMI (Schuld et al., 2002) not related to each other in narcoleptic patients, as well as anxiety disorders, depression, and fatigue which is distinct from sleepiness.

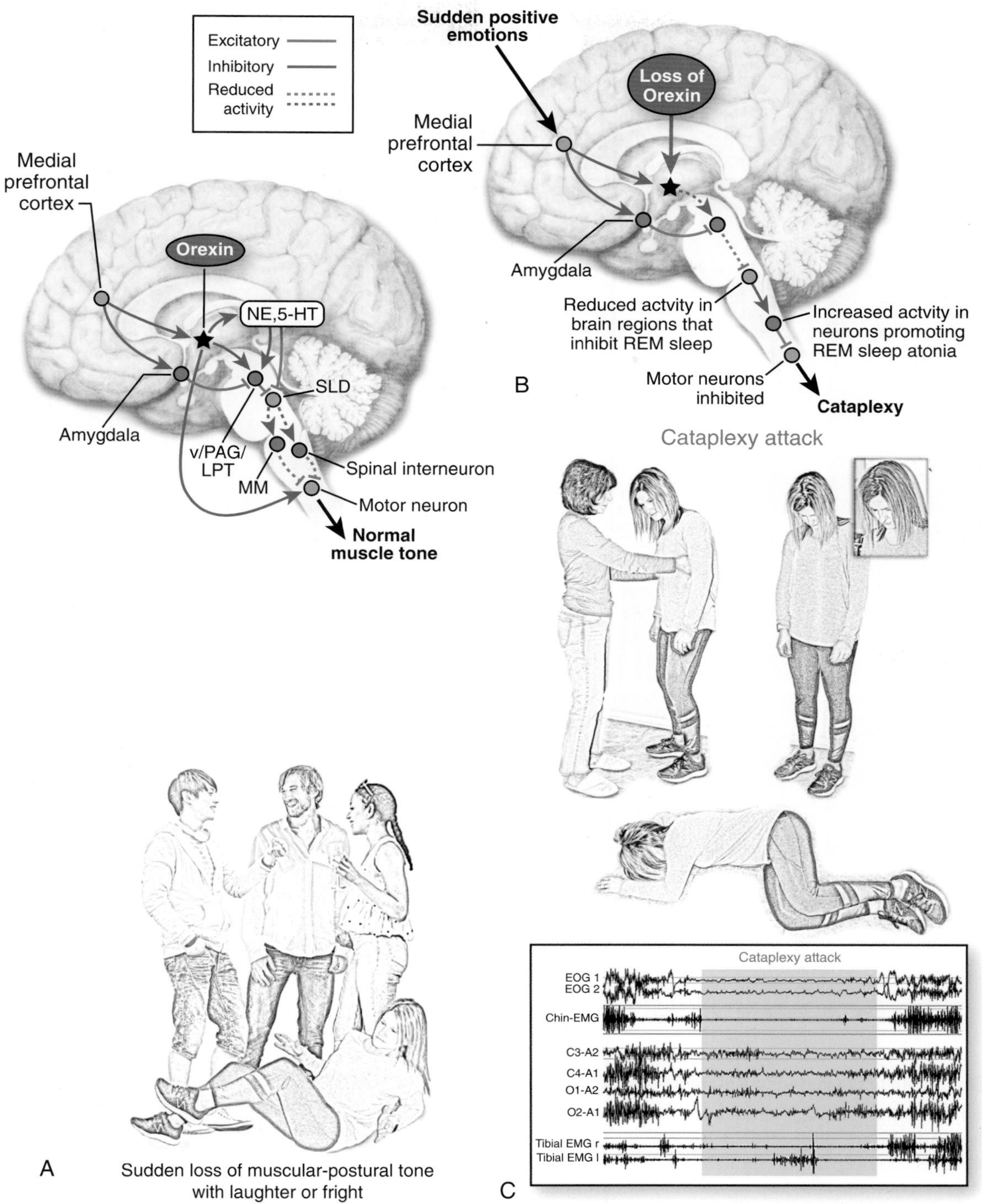


**Fig. 101.39 Cataplexy in the Setting of Narcolepsy Type 1.** The patient with cataplexy attack depicts a fairly rapidly progressive bilateral loss of skeletal muscle tone, ptosis, loss of control of facial muscles, and loss of tone of the neck and upper extremity muscles during laughter triggered by tickling. Consciousness is preserved, and mild muscle twitching or face grimacing can occur. **B,** Sudden, positive emotions activate neurons in the vicinity of the medial prefrontal cortex that excite orexin neurons in the lateral hypothalamus and the central amygdala. The absence of orexin, however, leads to reduced activity of GABAergic neurons in the periaqueductal grey area that inhibit rapid eye movement (REM) sleep and enhances the activity of glutamatergic neurons in the sublaterodorsal tegmental nucleus involved in REM atonia. The imbalance in this pathway results in the activation of descending pathways that inhibit spinal motor neurons and eventually to cataplexy. Pathways shown in blue are excitatory, while those in red are inhibitory. Open circles indicate neuron-cell bodies. Dotted lines indicate reduced activity. **C,** An electromyography (EMG) recording during a cataplexy episode *(shaded area)* documents a loss of muscle tone in multiple channels with superimposed bursts of increased muscle phasic activity (which present clinically as motor phenomena such as muscle twitching and face grimacing). *EOG,* Electro-oculography channel; *l,* left; *r,* right. *(Adapted from Bassetti, C.L.A., Adamantidis, A., Burdakov, D. et al., 2019. Narcolepsy—clinical spectrum, aetiopathophysiology, diagnosis and treatment. Nat. Rev. Neurol. 15, 519–539. https://doi.org/10.1038/s41582-019-0226-9. With permission.)*

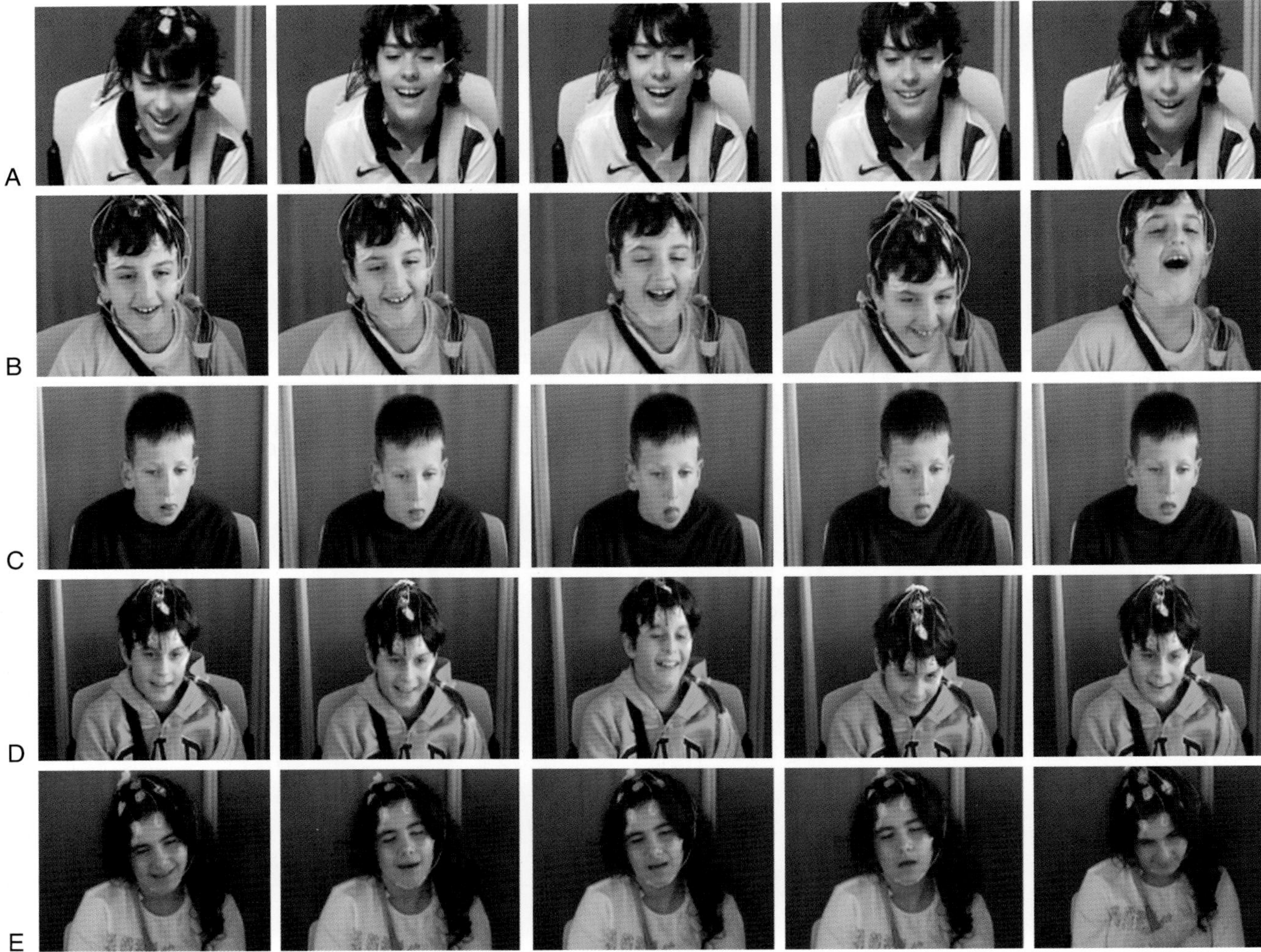

**Fig. 101.40 Cataplectic Facies Phenotype.** Unique facial aspects (cataplectic facies) and complex movements of cataplectic attacks close to disease onset. **A**, Facial weakness, ptosis with onward head and trunk flexion with active shoulder raising; (**B**) head drop and opposing neck hyperextension viewing (when looking at something); (**C**) perioral movement with mouth opening and tongue protrusion; (**D**) bilateral ptosis with active eyebrow raising and head swaying; (**E**) generalized facial hypotonia with bilateral ptosis, asymmetrical facial contraction. *(From Postiglione, E., et al., 2018. The clinical spectrum of childhood narcolepsy. Sleep Med. Rev. 38, 70e85. © 2017 Elsevier Ltd. All rights reserved.)*

### Differential Diagnosis of Narcolepsy-Related Sleep Attacks

The most common conditions that should be differentiated from narcoleptic sleep attacks are illustrated in Box 101.13 and Table 101.7. Narcolepsy-related sleep attacks should be differentiated from other causes of EDS. These include sleep deprivation and insufficient sleep syndrome, OSAS, alcohol- and drug-related hypersomnolence, idiopathic hypersomnia (Aldrich, 1996), circadian rhythm sleep disorders, and other medical, neurological, and psychiatric disorders causing hypersomnolence. OSAS (which will be reviewed later in the chapter) is the most common cause of EDS in patients referred to a sleep laboratory for evaluation. It is characterized by repeated episodes of obstructive and mixed apneas during NREM and REM sleep in overnight PSG recordings. These patients have prolonged daytime sleep episodes followed by fatigue and drowsiness on awakening, which contrasts with a fresh feeling in narcoleptic patients on awakening from brief sleep attacks. All patients with hypersomnolence can be excluded after careful history and physical examination and overnight PSG recording.

**BOX 101.13 Differential Diagnosis of Narcoleptic Sleep Attacks**

Obstructive sleep apnea syndrome
Sleep deprivation
Insufficient sleep syndrome
Alcohol/drug-related hypersomnolence
Periodic hypersomnolence
Medical, neurological, and psychiatric disorders causing hypersomnolence
Idiopathic hypersomnia
Circadian rhythm sleep disorders

Idiopathic hypersomnia (see later discussion) closely resembles narcolepsy syndrome. In contrast to narcolepsy, the sleep episodes in idiopathic hypersomnia are prolonged, and the sleep is not refreshing. PSG recordings and MSLT scores do not show sleep-onset REM sleep but do show pathological sleepiness. There is no disturbance of

REM-NREM organization on PSG recordings. Some patients with idiopathic hypersomnia may have a positive family history.

### Differential Diagnosis of Cataplexy and Other Features of Narcolepsy

Cataplectic attacks may be mistaken for partial complex seizures, absence spells, atonic seizures (as well as gelastic-atonic seizures characterized by laughing followed by loss of muscle tone), drop attacks, basilar migraines, vertebrobasilar insufficiency, syncope, and pseudocataplexy (Box 101.14). Pseudocataplexy is a functional disorder, often seen in patients with cataplexy, in which there are negative thoughts rather than laughter, the typical precipitant of true cataplexy, and characterized by spells extending over minutes to hours rather than the seconds to minute/s characteristic of *bona fide* cataplexy (Plazzi et al., 2010; Shankar et al., 2010). A partial complex seizure, however, is characterized by an altered state of consciousness, unlike cataplexy. In addition, patients with seizures may have generalized tonic-clonic movements, postictal confusion, and epileptiform discharges on EEG. Absence spells are characterized by staring with vacant expression lasting up to 30 seconds, with an altered state of alertness associated with characteristic 3-Hz spike-and-wave patterns in the EEG. Atonic seizures are accompanied by transient loss of consciousness and EEG evidence of slow spike-and-wave discharges or multiple spike-and-wave discharges.

Sleep paralysis, in the context of narcolepsy, should be differentiated from isolated physiological and familial sleep paralysis in which other manifestations of narcolepsy are absent. Automatic behavior should be differentiated from the automatisms observed in partial complex seizures and psychogenic fugue. The clinical history, pre/post event triggers/confusion, physical examination, and EEG should be helpful in differentiating these conditions. Differential diagnosis of narcolepsy and cataplexy are summarized in Table 101.7 (Postiglione et al., 2018).

"Symptomatic narcolepsy" or "secondary narcolepsy" is the previously used term to describe narcolepsy associated with underlying structural, genetic, inflammatory, or vascular abnormality impacting the hypothalamus and leading to severe CNS hypersomnolence with or without cataplexy or abnormal CSF hypocretin levels. Depending on the presence of cataplexy/reduced CSF hypocretin levels, narcolepsy type 1 and 2 may be found. Leading CNS causes include diencephalic and midbrain tumors, MS, strokes, cysts, vascular malformations, encephalitis, cerebral trauma, and paraneoplastic syndrome with anti-Ma2 antibodies and it may present with narcoleptic-like sleep attacks and other manifestations (Nishino, 2007; Nishino and Mignot, 2011; Clavelou et al., 1995). Cataplexy may develop in children affected with Niemann-Pick disease type C. Fig. 101.41 illustrates a scenario from the authors' practice of a gentleman with a history of neurosarcoid of the diencephalon and hypocretin deficiency illustrating a case of secondary/symptomatic narcolepsy (Panossian and Avidan, 2016).

### Idiopathic Hypersomnia

Idiopathic hypersomnia (IH) is characterized by a greater than 3-month duration of EDS and an irrepressible need to sleep or daytime lapses into sleep in the absence, and after correction, of sleep deprivation (AASM, 2014).

The onset of the disease is generally around the same age as narcolepsy (15–30 years). The sleep pattern, however, is different from that of narcolepsy. The patient generally sleeps for hours, and the sleep is not refreshing. Total 24-hour sleep time is 660 minutes or more (typically 12–14 hours) on 24-hour PSG monitoring or wrist actigraphy recording. The MSLT shows a mean sleep onset latency of 8 minutes or less, with less than two sleep-onset REM sleep periods. Table 101.7 lists

**BOX 101.14 Differential Diagnosis of Cataplexy**

- Partial complex seizure
- Absence spell
- Atonic seizure
- Drop attack
- Syncope
- Vertebrobasilar insufficiency
- Basilar migraines
- Pseudocataplexy

ICSD-III classification (AASM, 2014) of three major central disorders of hypersomnolence and their differentiating features. Supportive features also include profound sleep inertia, known as sleep drunkenness (elucidated as prolonged difficulty waking up accompanied by irritability and repeated returns to sleep), mental fatigability, dependence on other people for awakening them, and long (>1 hour) unrefreshing naps (AASM, 2014; Vernet et al., 2010). Because of EDS, the condition may be mistaken for sleep apnea. However, the patient does not give a history of cataplexy, snoring, or repeated awakenings throughout the night. As part of the sleep drunkenness spectrum, some patients may have automatic behavior with amnesia for the events. Physical examination uncovers no abnormal neurological findings. This disabling and lifelong condition should be differentiated from other causes of EDS (see eBox 101.5). Some recent data propose that IH may be a dysfunction of the autonomic nervous system as patients sometimes present with perception of temperature dysregulation, orthostatic disturbance, headache, and peripheral vascular complaints (Raynaud-type phenomena with cold hands and feet) (AASM, 2014; Bruck and Parkes, 1996). Sleep paralysis and hypnagogic hallucinations may also be reported, but the frequency is uncertain (4%–40% in different series). Finally, there is no clear association between idiopathic hypersomnia and HLA.

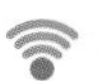

### Kleine-Levin Syndrome (aka Recurrent Hypersomnia, Periodic Hypersomnolence)

KLS is a form of recurrent hypersomnia associated with symptoms of hyperphagia and megaphagia, cognitive impairment, and hypersexuality affecting mostly adolescent patients (males > females) (Arnone and Conti, 2016; Arnulf, 2015; Miglis and Guilleminault, 2016; Sum-Ping and Guilleminault, 2016). During the episodic sleep attacks, the patient sleeps for 16–18 hours a day or more and upon awakening eats voraciously. Other behavioral disturbances during the episodes include hyperorality, memory impairment, confusion, hallucinations, and polydipsia. The ICSD-III requires that there be at least two episodes of excessive sleepiness lasting between 2 days and 5 weeks in duration, more frequent than once a year and once every 18 months, with periods of normalcy between episodes (normal alertness, cognition, and mood) (AASM, 2014). During candidate periods, KLS is likely when at least one of the following is present: disinhibited behavior (e.g., hypersexuality), cognitive impairment, altered perception, eating abnormality, so long as the hypersomnia is not better explained by another disorder, especially bipolar disorder (AASM, 2014).

Sleep studies in KLS reveal normal sleep cycling and MSLTs show pathological sleepiness without sleep-onset REM. The cause of the condition is undetermined; a limbic-hypothalamic dysfunction has been suspected but not proven. Reports of thalamic and hypothalamic hypoperfusion on SPECT study, as seen in eFig. 101.42, support this hypothesis (Hong et al., 2006; Huang et al., 2005). While no evidence-based treatments are currently available

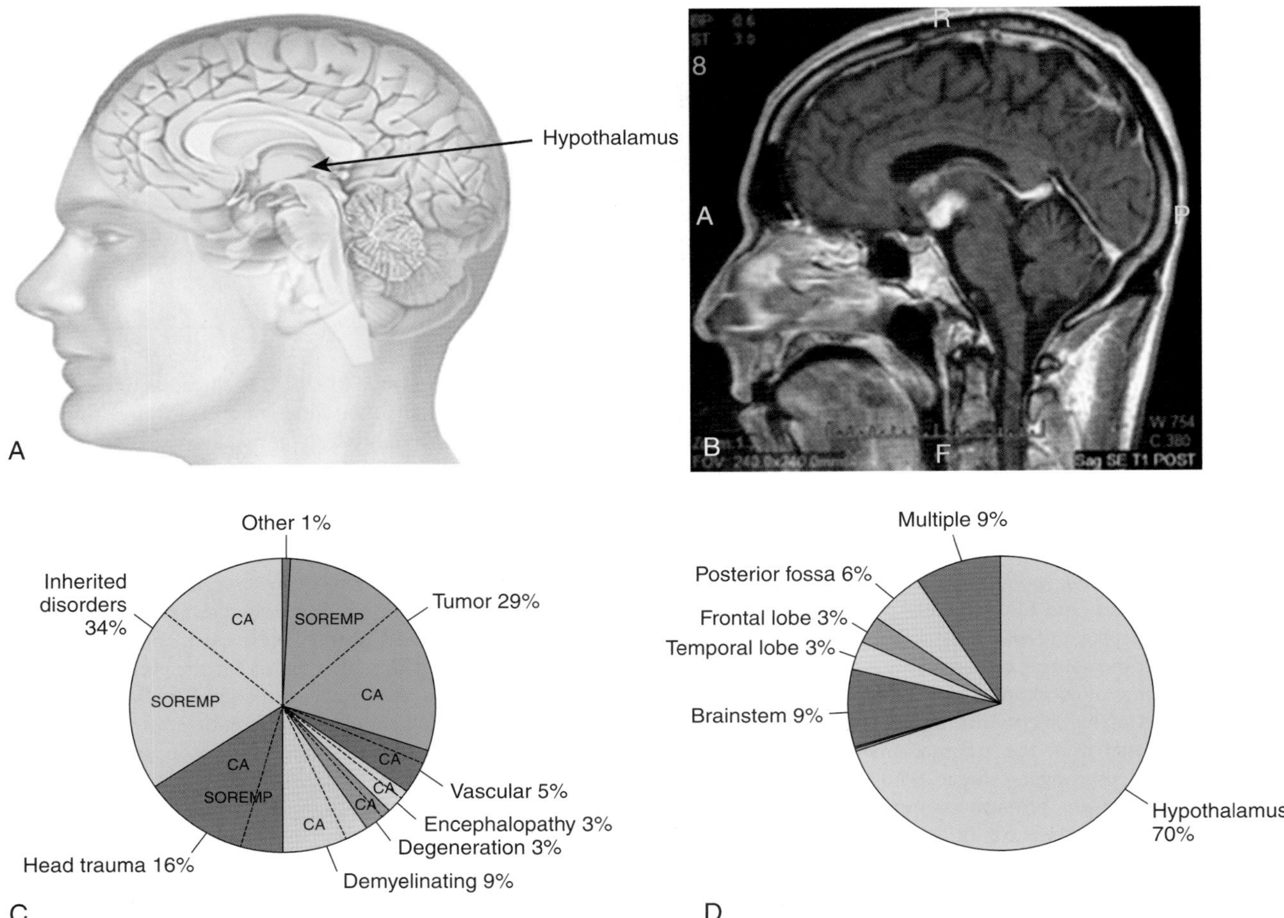


**Fig. 101.41 Secondary or "Symptomatic" Narcolepsy.** Secondary narcolepsy is caused by diencephalic injury in the setting of neurosarcoidosis. **A,** The location of the diencephalon, where the wake-stabilizing hypocretin-producing cells are localized. **B,** Brain MRI indicated sarcoid involvement of the hypothalamus, showing postcontrast hyperintensity within the anterior hypothalamus. The patient did not experience any brainstem involvement, nor were any appreciable lesions found in the locus coeruleus or raphe nuclei. **C** and **D,** Neurological diseases and location of brain lesions in 113 cases of secondary narcolepsy. **C,** Neurological diseases are shown by category reported as secondary narcolepsy. Reported here are tumors, inherited disorders, and head trauma, which are the 3 most frequent causes. The percentage of cataplexy *(CA)* or sleep-onset REM periods (SOREMP) is denoted in each category with a dashed line. **D,** Location of brain lesions in symptomatic patients with narcolepsy associated with brain tumor; the hypothalamus and adjacent structures are the most common location. Included are 113 symptomatic cases of narcolepsy. *(A, Copyright © Alon Y. Avidan, MD, MPH; B, Copyright © Alon Y. Avidan, MD, MPH; C, D, Modified from Kanbayashi, T., Sagawa, T., Takemura, F., et al., 2011. The pathophysiologic basis of secondary narcolepsy and hypersomnia. Curr. Neurol. Neurosci. Rep. 11 [2], 235–241.)*

for KLS, lithium treatment has been found to be effective (Oliveira et al., 2013, Sveinsson, 2014) and recent reports also suggest possible treatment intervention with clarithromycin and flumazenil (Kelty et al., 2014; Rezvanian and Watson, 2013; Trotti et al., 2014) (Video 101.3).

## Sleep Apnea Syndrome

Sleep apnea syndrome is broadly divided into two types: upper airway OSAS and central sleep apnea syndrome (CSAS), depending on pathophysiological mechanisms. OSAS is the most common sleep disorder referred to sleep laboratories for PSG recordings. Two groups of neurologists, Gastaut, Tassinari and Duron from France (Gastaut et al., 1965), and Jung and Kuhlo from Germany, in 1965 (Jung and Kuhlo, 1965) independently located the site of obstruction in OSAS in the upper airway. In CSAS, the problem lies in the ventilatory control mechanism in the CNS.

Upper airway OSA-hypopnea syndrome remains undiagnosed or underdiagnosed because of insufficient knowledge and awareness of serious consequences resulting from this disorder. OSAS causes significant morbidity and mortality and is often associated with a variety of comorbid conditions (Banno and Kryger, 2007; Korson and Guilleminault, 2015). Cardinal features of OSAS include habitual loud snoring, witnessed apneas during sleep, and daytime hypersomnolence as well as hyperactivity and nocturnal enuresis, particularly in children. OSAS is characterized by repetitive episodes of complete (apnea) or partial (hypopnea) upper airway obstruction during sleep, resulting in arterial oxygen desaturation and arousal from sleep.

## Sleep-Disordered Breathing Terminology

The spectrum of SDB includes a variety of breathing patterns based on analysis during overnight PSG recordings. Fig. 101.43 schematically shows some patterns of SDB. Apnea or cessation of breathing consists of three types: obstructive, central, and mixed. Cessation of airflow with no respiratory effort defines central apnea, during which both diaphragmatic and intercostal muscle activities as well as gas exchange through the nose or mouth are absent (see Fig. 101.43, *C*). In contrast, during obstructive apnea, airflow stops while the effort continues (see Fig. 101.43, *B*); in mixed apnea, there is an initial cessation of airflow with no respiratory effort (central apnea) followed by a period of upper airway OSA (see Fig. 101.43, *D*).

There are two separate rules for scoring hypopnea in the recent AASM Scoring Manual (Iber et al., 2007). The rule requires a reduction of the signal by 30% or more of the baseline for at least 10 seconds accompanied by oxygen desaturation of 3% or more, or the event is associated with an arousal within 3 seconds of the event. The "alternate" rule requires a reduction of nasal pressure or the alternative airflow sensor signal by 30% or more of the baseline amplitude for at least 10 seconds accompanied by oxygen desaturation of 4% or more from the pre-event baseline. In both these rules the amplitude reduction must be present for at least 90% of the event's duration.

To be clinically significant, the number of apneas and hypopneas per hour of sleep (Apnea-Hypopnea Index, or AHI) must be at least 5. Most clinicians, however, use this index in the context of the clinical presentation (severe sleepiness, impairment of function) as well as underlying comorbidities (such as atrial fibrillation, recent stroke, neuromuscular disorder) when deciding on clinical significance and management. An *arousal* is defined as either a transient return of alpha activities (8–13 Hz) or beta rhythms (>13 Hz) or a change from delta to theta activities in the EEG lasting from 3 to 14 seconds. *Paradoxical breathing* is characterized by movements of the thorax and abdomen in opposite directions, indicating increased upper airway resistance and upper airway obstruction (see Fig. 101.43, *B*). Repeated arousals temporally related to paradoxical breathing (Fig. 101.44) and at times crescendo snoring which result in sleep fragmentation signifies the presence of upper airway resistance which is an important factor causing EDS (Berry, 2012). Upper airway resistance syndrome (UARS) is characterized by repeated abnormal respiratory efforts during sleep without apnea, accompanied by recurrent arousals and EDS. The Respiratory Disturbance Index (RDI) includes all these abnormal breathing events, including respiratory effort-related arousal. *Cheyne-Stokes breathing* is a unique form of SDB characterized by cyclical and periodic breathing changes in breathing with a crescendo-decrescendo sequence separated by central apneas or hypopneas (Fig. 101.45) (Abraham et al., 2015) (Video 101.4).

*Dysrhythmic breathing* (Fig. 101.46, *I*) is characterized by nonrhythmical respiration of irregular rate, rhythm, and amplitude that becomes worse during sleep. This type of breathing may result from an abnormality in the automatic respiratory pattern generator in the brainstem. *Apneustic breathing* (see Fig. 101.46, *L*) is characterized by prolonged inspiration with an increase in the ratio of inspiratory to expiratory time. This type of breathing may result from a neurological lesion in the caudal pons disconnecting the apneustic center in the lower pons from the pneumotaxic center in the upper pons. *Inspiratory gasp* (see Fig. 101.46, *K*) is characterized by short inspiratory time and a relatively prolonged expiration and has been noted in association with a lesion in the medulla. *Ataxic breathing* (see Fig. 101.46, *H*) is characterized by clusters of cyclic breathing followed by recurrent periods of apnea (the apnea length is greater than the ventilatory phase). *Biot breathing* (see Fig. 101.46, *J*) is a variant of ataxic breathing characterized by two to three breaths of nearly equal volume separated by long

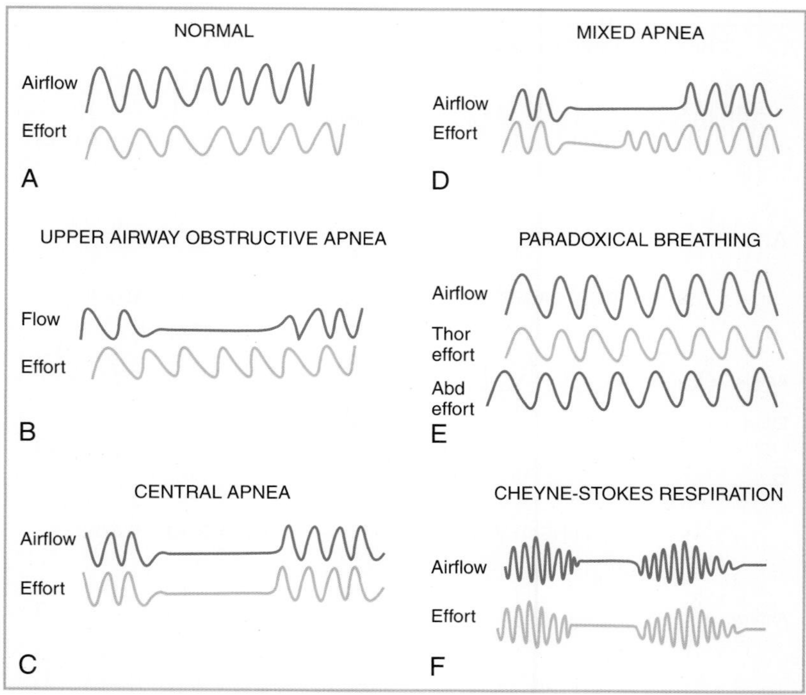


**Fig. 101.43 Schematic Diagram Showing Different Types of Breathing Patterns in Neurological Illnesses (Part 1). A,** Normal breathing pattern. **B,** Upper airway obstructive apnea. **C,** Central apnea. **D,** Mixed apnea (initial central followed by obstructive apnea). **E,** Paradoxical breathing. **F,** Cheyne-Stokes breathing. *(From Chokroverty, S., 2009. Sleep Disorders Medicine: Basic Science, Technical Considerations, and Clinical Aspects, third ed. Saunders, Philadelphia, Fig. 29.6.)*

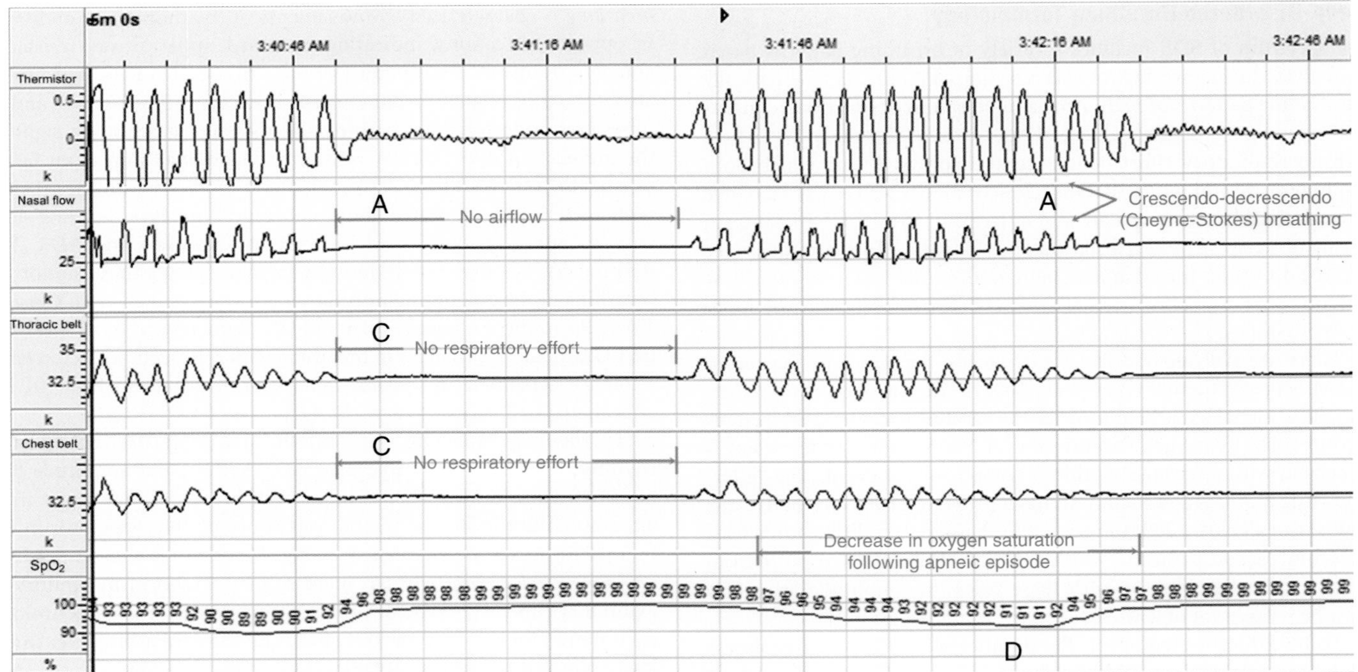


**Fig. 101.45 Cheyne-Stokes Breathing (CSB) Crescendo-Decrescendo Pattern from an Overnight Polysomnographic (PSG).** The CSA breathing morphology is uniquely characterized by cycles of deep, rapid, crescendo-decrescendo breathing pattern (**A**), punctuated by periods of slower, shallower breathing or no breathing at all (**B**) with no respiratory effort in between (**C**), with some delay due to chemoreceptor signal processing and circulatory delay (**D**), with resumption of breathing and recovery of the arterial $O_2$ saturation ($SpO_2$). "D" is pathologically protracted in patients with congestive heart failure and a prolonged circulation time. Each individual episode contributes a discrete hypoxic episode and a release of norepinephrine and continued insults accelerate the downward cycle toward heart failure. *(From Abraham, W. T., et al., 2015. Phrenic nerve stimulation for the treatment of central sleep apnea. JACC Heart Fail. 3 [5], 360–369.)*

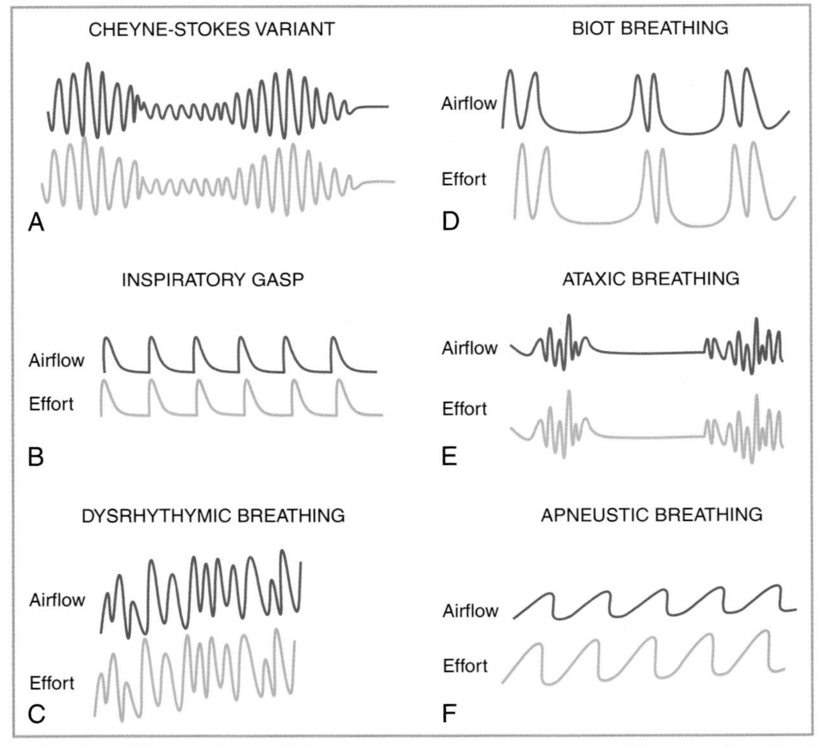


**Fig. 101.46 Schematic Diagram Showing Different Types of Breathing Patterns in Neurological Illnesses (Part II). A,** Cheyne-Stokes variant pattern. **B,** Inspiratory gasp. **C,** Dysrhythmic breathing. **D,** Biot breathing, a special type of ataxic breathing characterized by 2 to 3 breaths of nearly equal volume followed by a long period of apnea. **E,** Ataxic breathing. **F,** Apneustic breathing. *(From Chokroverty, S., 2009. Sleep Disorders Medicine: Basic Science, Technical Considerations, and Clinical Aspects, third ed. Saunders, Philadelphia, Fig. 29.6.)*

periods of apnea. Ataxic (including Biot) breathing is often noted in medullary lesions.

*Hypoventilation is illustrated in* Fig. 101.47 I, II and refers to a reduction of alveolar ventilation accompanied by hypoxemia and hypercapnia without any apnea or hypopnea; it may be noted in patients with neuromuscular disorders and kyphoscoliosis and those with underlying lung or chest-wall abnormalities that impair gas exchange during wakefulness. During sleep hypoventilation, the partial pressure of arterial carbon dioxide ($Paco_2$) rises at least 10 mm above the supine awake values (Iber et al., 2007; Pepin et al., 2016).

## Epidemiology of Obstructive Sleep Apnea Syndrome

No study has been specifically designed to determine the incidence of OSAS in a previously healthy population. Based on a definition of 15 or more apneas or hypopneas per hour of sleep accompanied by EDS, the recent Wisconsin sleep cohort study data listed prevalence figures of moderate to severe OSAS at 10% in men and 3% in women aged 30–49 years but 17% in men and 9% in women aged 50–70 years. There is a strong association between OSAS and male gender, increasing age, and obesity. The condition is common in men older than age 40, and among women the incidence of OSAS is greater after menopause. Approximately 85% of patients with OSAS are men, and obesity is present in about 70% of OSAS patients. There is an increased prevalence of OSAS in those with a thick neck and large abdomen. Men with a neck circumference measuring more than 17 inches and women with a neck measuring more than 16 inches are at risk for OSAS. Fig. 101.48 demonstrates the compromised retroglossal airspace in the setting of sleep apnea and the anatomical sites that might participate in the pathology of OSA: The normal airspace (green) is severely compromised because of restriction of the upper airway, intranasal space, and retropalatal and the retroglossal spaces.

Race may be a factor, given that a high prevalence of SDB is noted in Pacific Islanders, Mexican Americans, and African Americans. There are also family aggregates of OSAS. Other factors with a high association are alcohol, smoking, and drug use. Other risk factors include nasal allergies or congestion, endocrine diseases (e.g., hypothyroidism, acromegaly), disorders with autonomic failure or those associated with craniofacial abnormalities (e.g., Marfan, Down, and Pierre-Robin syndromes). The risk factors associated with OSAS are listed in eBox 101.15.

## Evaluation and Assessment

Detailed sleep history as well as the daytime history, and careful physical examination should be focused on specific associated and risk factors, specifically BMI, cardiopulmonary examination, and an examination

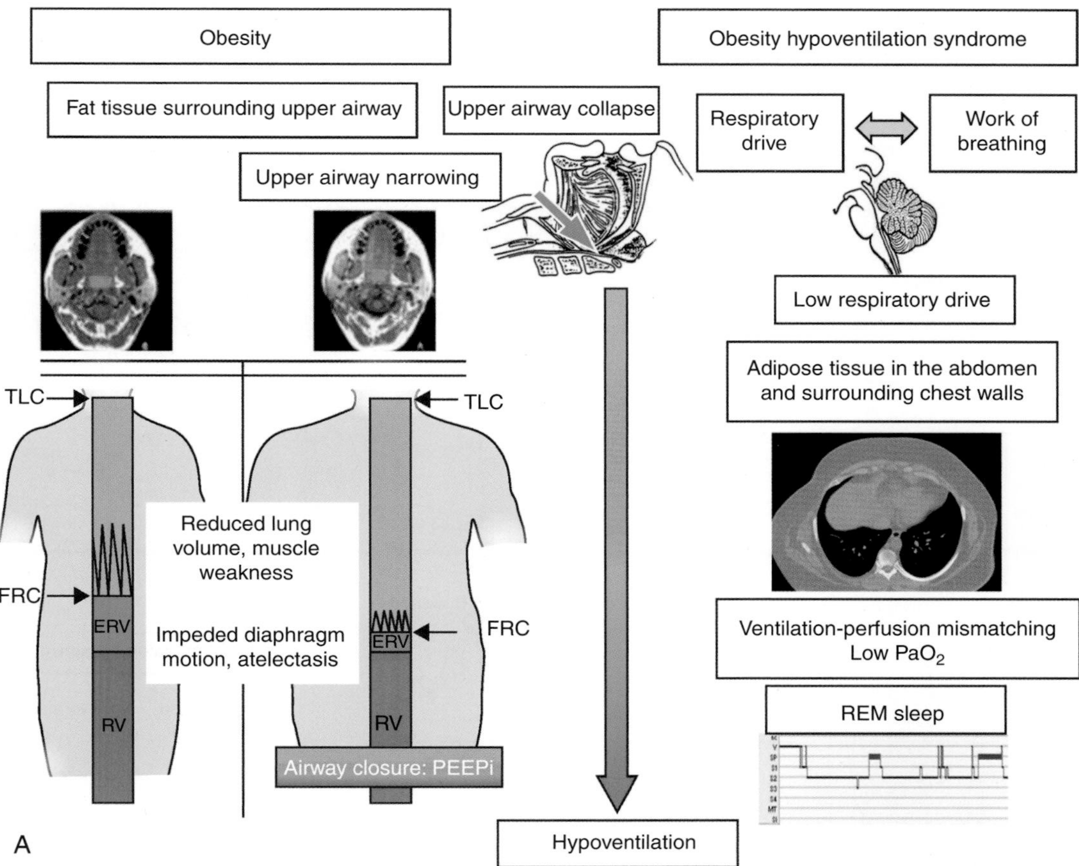


**Fig. 101.47 Hypoventilation Syndrome in the Setting of Obesity.** I: Obesity-related alterations in the respiratory system, respiratory drive, and in breathing during sleep. *ERV*, Expiratory reserve volume; *PEEPi*, intrinsic positive end-expiratory pressure; *REM*, rapid eye movements; *RV*, residual volume; *TLC*, total lung capacity;. II: (**A**) Evolution of nocturnal transcutaneous $CO_2$ in a typical patient with obesity hypoventilation syndrome. Panel A shows a hypnogram (PSG attributes vs. time) during wakefulness reference $TcPCO_2$. Panel B depicts increase in $TcPCO_2$ due to long-lasting apneas and hypopneas. Panel C highlights the increase in $PtCO_2$ corresponding to REM sleep hypoventilation (red circles).

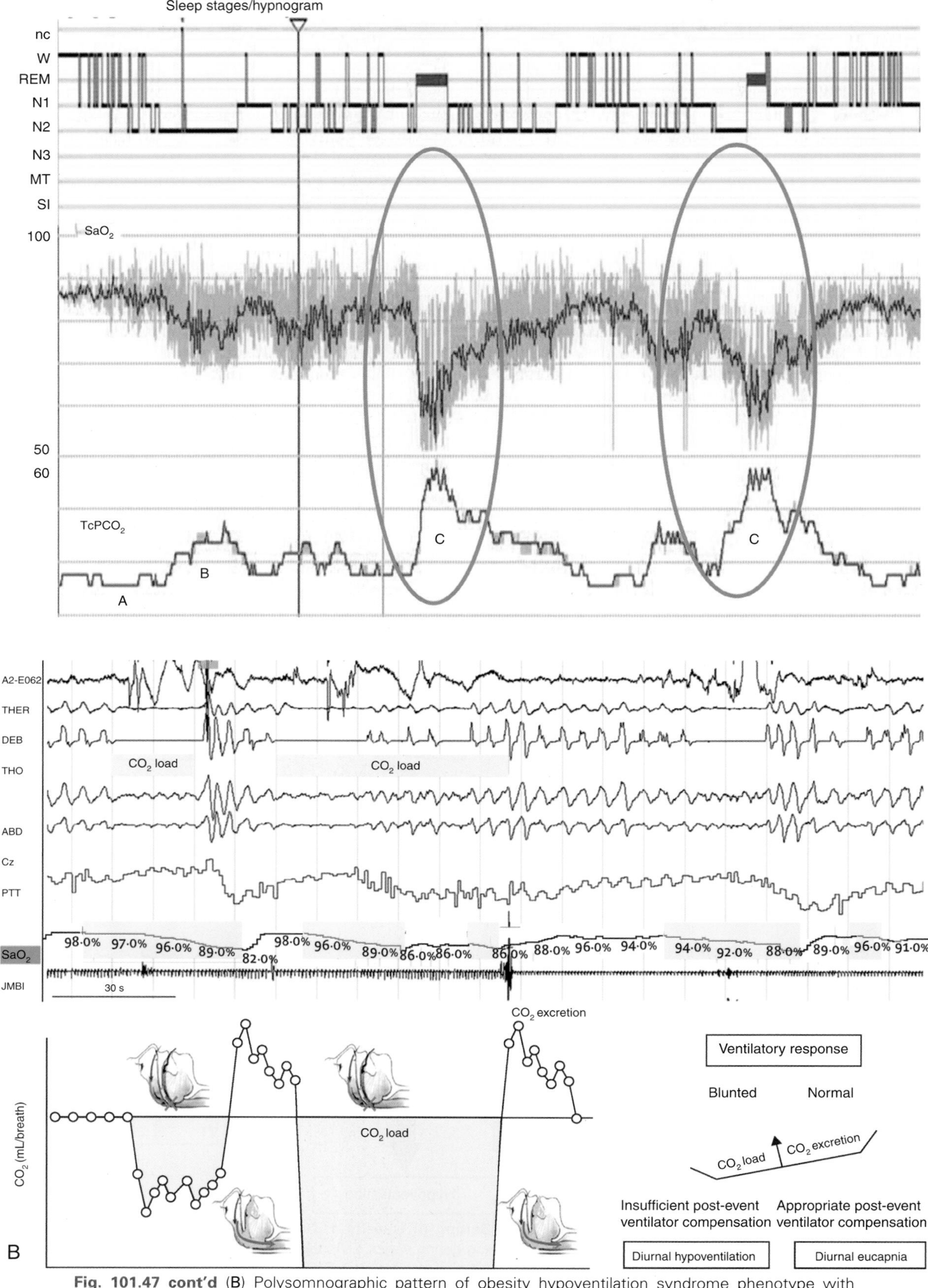


**Fig. 101.47 cont'd** (B) Polysomnographic pattern of obesity hypoventilation syndrome phenotype with long-lasting apneas as the main contributor to daytime hypercapnia. The insufficient post-event ventilatory compensation leads to a progressive hypercapnia ($CO_2$ overload) across the night contributing to the pathogenesis of diurnal hypoventilation via alteration of ventilatory drive. ABD=abdominal movements. *Cz*, Electroencephalography; *DEB*, flow; *JMB1*, leg movements; *PTT*, pulse transit time; *SaO*$_2$, oxygen blood saturation; *SAT*, $SpO_2$; *THER*, oronasal thermistor; *THO*, thoracic movements. *(From Pepin, J.L., et al., 2016. Prevention and care of respiratory failure in obese patients. Lancet Respir. Med. 4 [5], 407–418.)*

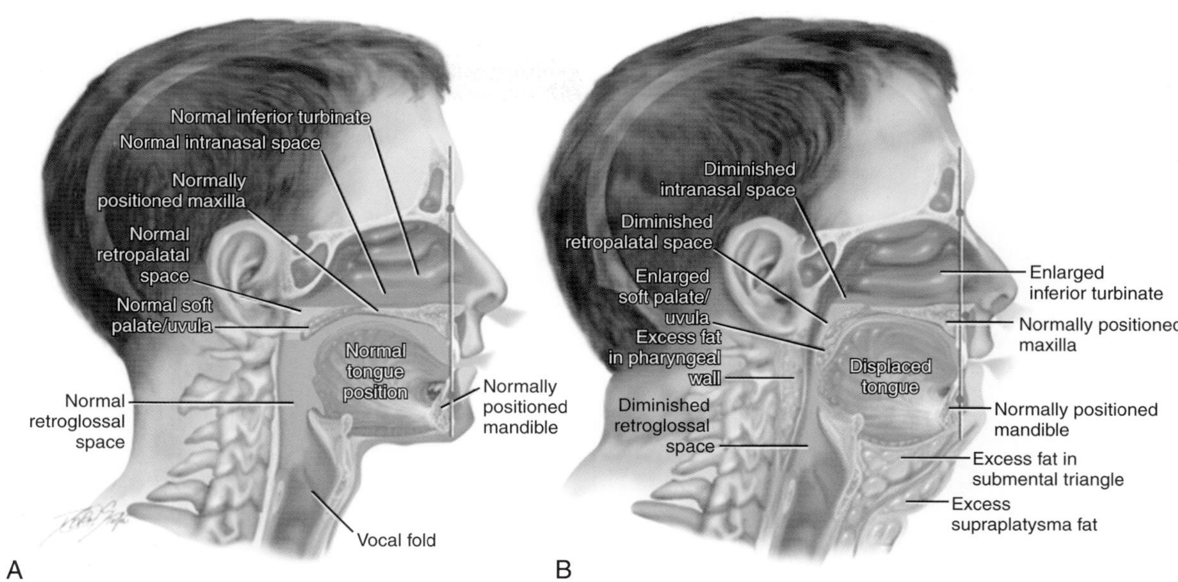


**Fig. 101.48 The Airway Anatomy in Sleep Apnea: The Perfect Storm.** Normal and abnormal airway anatomy. **A,** this illustrated midline sagittal cross-section of the head and neck depicts the normal upper airway and maxillofacial spaces and anatomy of a healthy, normal-weight 20-year-old man. The patient has a normal upper and lower facial skeleton and normal soft tissue indicators (soft palate, tongue, tonsils, and adenoids), without any compromise of the intranasal cavity. **B,** with increasing age and weight gain, the same individual three decades later has an elevated body mass index. Although the anatomy of the upper and lower facial skeleton remains fixed without any changes, fatty tissue consisting of adipose cells has expanded and infiltrated the crevices and space in the upper airway. Particularly compromised are the retropharyngeal and the lateral pharyngeal tissues, the soft palate, and the floor of the mouth, culminating in restricted airflow. At age 20 years, the patient had normal upper airway space (the intranasal, retropalatal, and the retroglossal sites were all well visualized and with appropriate space for air flow to proceed smoothly and unimpeded. At age 50 years, he has developed obstructive sleep apnea: The normal airspace (green) is severely compromised because of restriction of the upper airway, intranasal space, and retropalatal and the retroglossal spaces. A perfect storm indeed. *(From Posnick, J.C., 2014. Obstructive sleep apnea: evaluation and treatment. In: Posnick, J.C. [ed.]. Orthognathic Surgery: Principles and Practice. Elsevier, Philadelphia:, pp. 992–1058.)*

of the upper airways (neck circumference, airway size, as highlighted in Fig. 101.49) (Myers et al., 2013). The Modified Mallampati and tonsillar size classification are useful in evaluating patient airway size and gauging the possible risk for OSA (Fig. 101.40 New) (Friedman et al., 2013; Waters and Cheng, 2009) The laboratory assessment and management are described in this chapter, under Laboratory Assessment of Sleep Disorders.

Physical examination may reveal obesity in approximately 70% of the cases, with increased BMI and increased neck circumference, in addition to upper airway anatomical abnormalities causing reduction of the upper airway space (e.g., low-hanging soft palate, large edematous uvula, large tonsils and adenoids, especially in children, retrognathia, and micrognathia) as is highlighted in Fig. 101.50 (Avidan, 2018; Myers et al., 2013). In severe cases physical examination may reveal evidence of congestive heart failure, cardiac arrhythmias, hypertension, and polycythemia.

### Clinical Manifestations of Obstructive Sleep Apnea Syndrome

The symptoms of OSAS can be divided into two groups (Flemons, 2002; Korson and Guilleminault, 2015): those occurring during sleep  and those occurring during waking hours (eBox 101.16). Nocturnal symptoms include habitual loud snoring, choking during sleep, cessation of breathing, and abnormal motor activities during sleep (e.g., jerking and shaking movements, confusional arousals, or sleep walking), severe sleep disruption, gastroesophageal reflux causing heartburn, nocturnal enuresis (noted mostly in children), and profuse sweating at night. The daytime symptoms include EDS characterized by sleep episodes lasting 0.5–2 hours and occurring mostly when the patient is relaxing. The prolonged duration and the unrefreshing nature of these sleep attacks in OSAS differentiate these from narcoleptic sleep attacks. The other daytime symptoms include impairment of memory and motor skills, irritability, morning headache in some patients, automatic behavior, retrograde amnesia, and hyperactivity (in children). Erectile dysfunction in men is often associated with severe and long-standing OSAS.

OSAS is associated with increased morbidity and mortality as a result of both short-term (Strohl et al., 2013) consequences (impairment of quality of life and increasing traffic and work-related accidents) and long-term consequences resulting from associated and comorbid conditions such as hypertension, heart failure, MI, cardiac arrhythmias, stroke due to both supratentorial and infratentorial infarctions, and transient ischemic attacks as well as cognitive dysfunction, depression, and

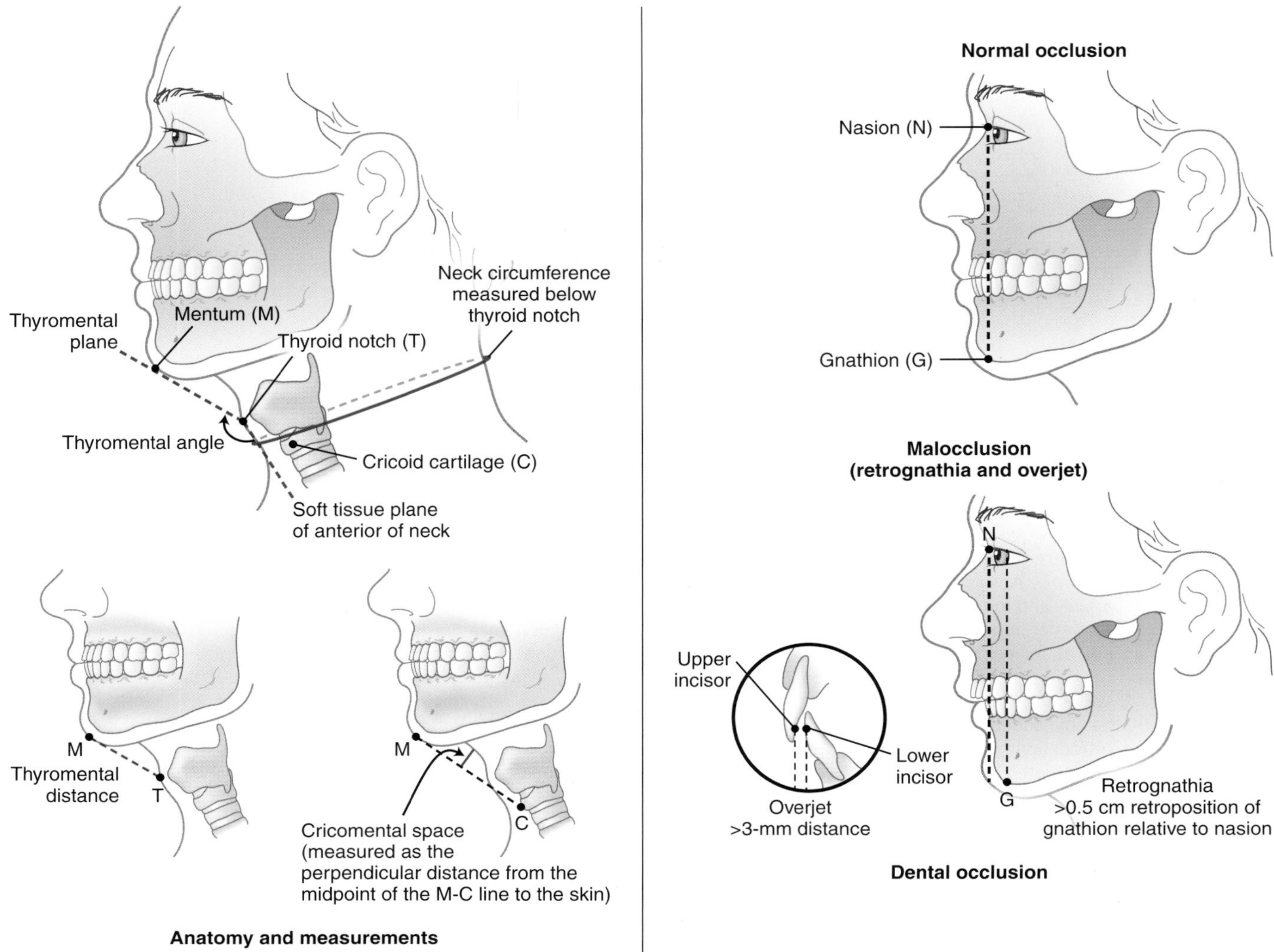


**Fig. 101.49** Anatomy and Surface Measurements in the Assessment of a Patient with Suspected Obstructive Sleep Apnea. Retrognathia, overjet, and reduced cricomental space are key craniofacial properties that are predictive of obstructive sleep apnea. (*From Myers, K.A., Mrkobrada, M., Simel, D.L., 2013. Does this patient have obstructive sleep apnea? The rational clinical examination systematic review. JAMA 310, 731–741.*)

insomnia as summarized in Fig. 101.51. (Gaspar et al., 2017; Banno and Kryger, 2007; Cordero-Guevara et al., 2011; Flemons, 2002; Kendzerska et al., 2014; Kohler et al., 2013; Korson and Guilleminault, 2015; Marin et al., 2005; Redline et al., 2010; Somers et al., 2008; Vlachantoni et al., 2013; Zamarion et al., 2013). Several prospective longitudinal studies (Nieto et al., 2000; Peppard et al., 2000; Young et al., 1997) have shown a clear association between OSAS and systemic hypertension, which may be noted in approximately 50% of patients with OSAS. The factors that cause hypertension in OSAS include repeated hypoxemias during sleep at night causing an increased sympathetic activity. OSAS is frequently noted in about 30% of cases of essential hypertension. Several studies have shown improvement of hypertension or reduction of need for antihypertensive medications after effective treatment of OSAS with CPAP titration (Banno and Kryger, 2007; Faccenda et al., 2001; Hla et al., 2002; Kendzerska et al., 2014; Kohler et al., 2013; Pepperell et al., 2002; Vlachantoni et al., 2013; Zamarion et al., 2013). Pulmonary hypertension is also noted in approximately 15%–20% of cases. Cardiac arrhythmias in the form of premature ventricular contractions, ventricular tachycardia, sinus pauses, and third-degree heart block as well as sudden cardiac death have been attributed to OSAS. Heart failure, mostly systolic heart failure but also diastolic heart failure (in which the studies are limited), is associated with both obstructive and CSAs, but more CSAs, including Cheyne-Stokes breathing, than obstructive apneas (Arias et al., 2007; Javaheri, 2006; Javaheri and Somers, 2011; Kendzerska et al., 2014; Levy et al., 2013; McNicholas et al., 2007; Randerath and Javaheri, 2015; Somers et al., 2008). The presence of central apnea, including Cheyne-Stokes breathing, increases the mortality in patients with heart failure. Cognitive dysfunction, which is noted in moderately severe to severe OSAS patients (Lim and Pack, 2014), shows improvement after satisfactory treatment with CPAP titration (Atwood and Strollo, 2015). Recently awareness about the presence of depression and insomnia in patients with OSAS has grown, but adequate studies have not been conducted to find the prevalence and impact of these conditions on OSAS (Glidewell, 2013). There has been an increased association between OSAS and impaired quality of life, metabolic syndrome, hypertension, increased risk for metabolic disease, (increased insulin resistance with type 2 diabetes, hypertriglyceridemia, and obesity), depression, cognitive decline, drowsy driving and motor vehicle accidents, and cognitive

A. Friedman Classification: Palate Positions
*(Modified Mallapati)*

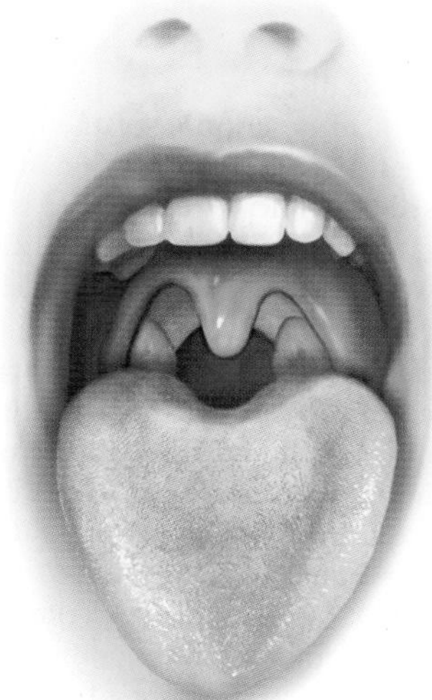

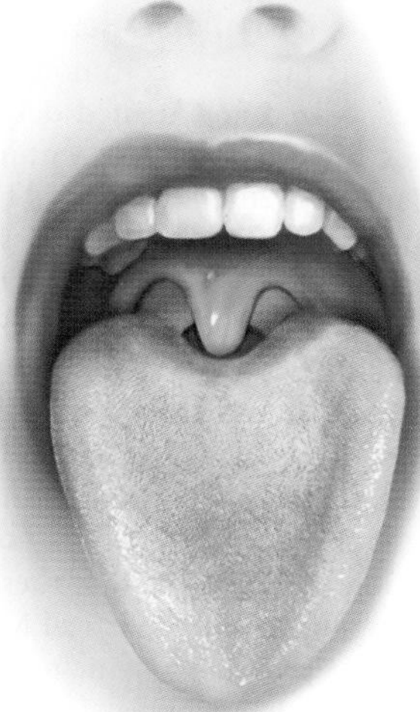

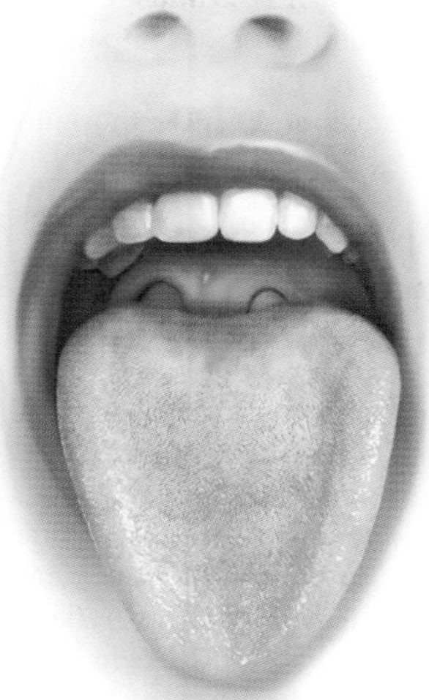

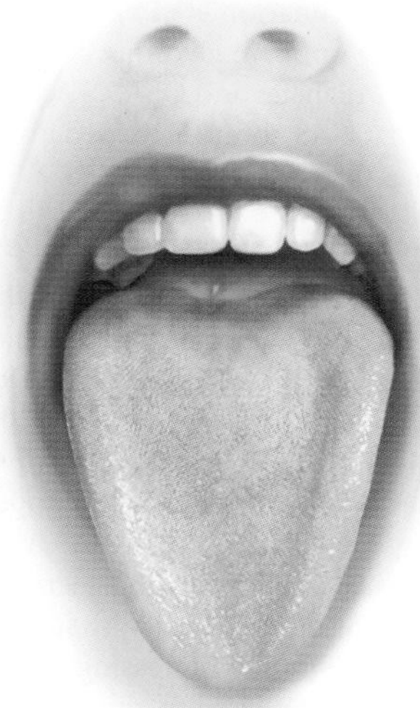

Position I
Allows visualization of the entire uvula and tonsils/pillars
Position II
Allows visualization of the uvula but not the tonsils
Position III
Allows visualization of the soft palate but not the uvula
Position IV
Allows visualization of the hard palate only

B. Tonsillar-Size Classification

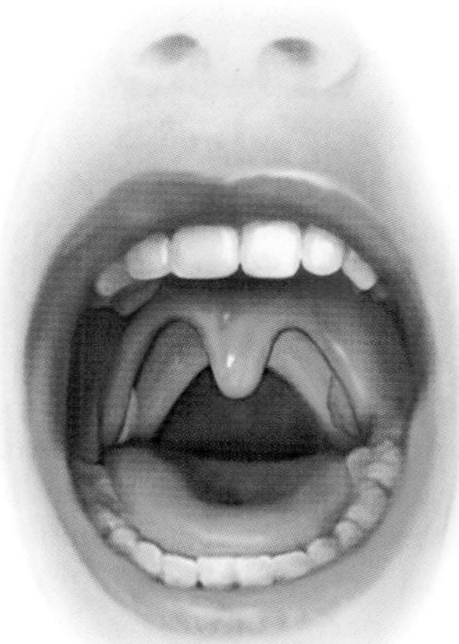

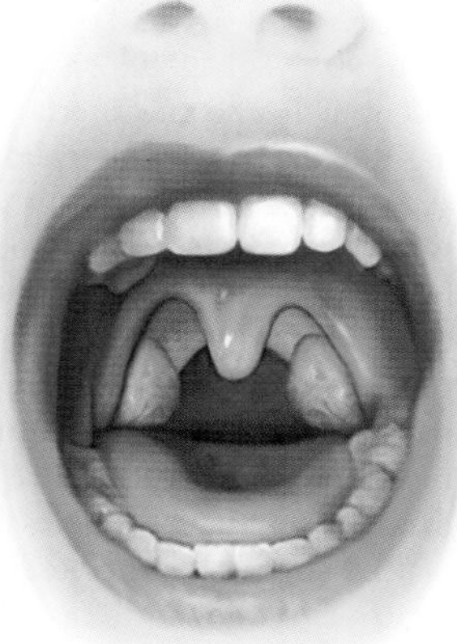

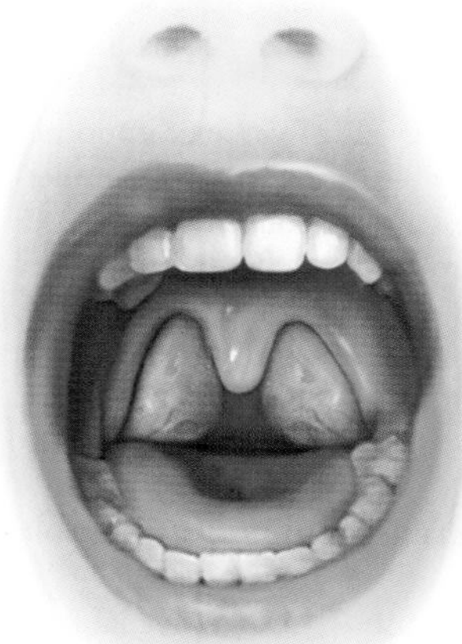

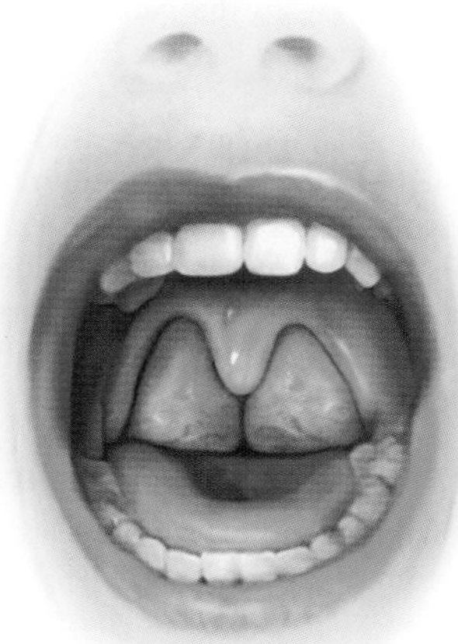

Grade 1
Within tonsillar fauces
Grade 2
Outside tonsillar fauces, up to 50% of airway to midline
Grade 3
Outside tonsillar fauces, up to 75% of the distance to the midline
Grade 4
Outside tonsillar fauces, > 75% of the lateral airway dimension

**Fig. 101.50 New Sleep Medicine Examination. A,** The Modified Mallampati classification describes tongue size relative to oropharyngeal size. The test is conducted with the patient in the sitting position, the head held in a natural position, the mouth wide open and relaxed and with the tongue inside the mouth without any protrusion or phonation. The subsequent classification is assigned based upon the pharyngeal structures that are visible. Class I = visualization of the soft palate, fauces, uvula, anterior and posterior pillars. Class II = visualization of the soft palate, fauces, and uvula. Class III = visualization of the soft palate and the base of the uvula. Class IV = soft palate is not visible at all. If the patient phonates, this falsely improves the view. If the patient arches his or her tongue, the uvula is falsely obscured. The test was initially adapted to predict ease of intubation but can be used to predict the potential severity of obstructive sleep apnea. **B,** Clinical of tonsillar size is based on the following scheme. Grade 1: within tonsillar fauces; Grade 2: outside tonsillar fauces, up to 50% of the airway to the midline; Grade 3: outside tonsillar fauces and up to 75% of the distance to the midline; and Grade 4: >75% of the lateral airway dimension. (*Modified from Mallampati, S.R., Gatt, S.P., Gugino, L.D., et al., 1985. A clinical sign to predict difficult tracheal intubation: a prospective study. Can. Anaesth. Soc. J. 32, 429–434.*)

decline. The mechanisms accounting for OSA include hypoxia, sleep fragmentation, and systemic inflammation (Dumortier and Bricout, 2019; Walia, 2019). (a combination of) (Oyama et al., 2012; Sharma et al., 2011; Zamarion et al., 2013). However, CPAP treatment did not significantly improve glycemia control or insulin resistance in patients with type 2 diabetes and OSAS. Recent studies have also shown an association of OSAS to an increased risk of cancer and cancer mortality (Martinez-Garcia et al., 2014).

### Pathogenesis of Obstructive Sleep Apnea Syndrome

The factors contributing to the pathogenesis of OSAS include local anatomical, neurological, and vascular factors as well as familial predisposition (Banno and Kryger, 2007; Dempsey et al., 2010; Joosten et al., 2014; Korson and Guilleminault, 2015). Collapse of the pharyngeal airway is the fundamental factor in OSA. During sleep, muscle tone decreases, including that of the upper airway dilator muscles, which maintain upper airway patency. As a result of this decreased tone, these muscles relax, causing increased upper airway resistance and narrowing of the upper airway space. Defective upper airway reflexes may also play a role. Increasing familial occurrence of OSAS in some patients may be related to abnormal craniofacial features. In children, adenotonsillar enlargement and craniofacial dysostosis causing narrow upper airway space are important factors. Neurological factors include reduced medullary respiratory neuronal output and ventilatory control instability which may create excessive response to respiratory muscles (high loop gain) promoting upper airway collapse and obstruction in susceptible individuals. Other neurological factors include autonomic activation during sleep-related breathing events, contributing toward development of hypertension and cardiac arrhythmias. Vascular factors contributing to the pathogenesis and long-term adverse consequences (Banno and Kryger, 2007; Javaheri and Somers, 2011) include increased endothelin 1 (a vasoconstrictor), reduced nitric oxide (a known vasodilator), and increased serum levels of vascular endothelial growth factor (glycoprotein responsible for vascular remodeling and atherosclerosis). It has been shown that after effective CPAP titration, these vascular abnormalities are reversed. Thus, a complex interaction of peripheral upper airway anatomical, central neural, vascular, and genetic factors contributes to the syndrome of upper airway OSAS.

### Upper Airway Resistance Syndrome

Additional text and eFig. 101.34 are available at http://expertconsult.inkling.com.

*Central sleep apnea syndrome.* Additional text is available at http://expertconsult.inkling.com.

### Central Sleep Apnea Syndrome

CSAS includes primary CSA, CSA with Cheyne-Stokes breathing, CSA due to high altitude periodic breathing, CSA due to a medical disorder without Cheyne-Stokes breathing, CSA due to drug or substance abuse (e.g., use of opiates) (Javaheri and Randerath, 2014), primary CSA of infancy, primary CSA of prematurity, and treatment emergent CSA (ICSD-III; AASM, 2014). Primary CSAS is rare, and the patient may present with EDS and frequent awakenings due to repeated episodes of central apnea followed by arousals. The patient may also present with insomnia. Cheyne-Stokes breathing as previously highlighted in Fig. 101.44 noted in patients with congestive heart failure (Javaheri, 2006; Javaheri and Somers, 2011; Javaheri and Dempsey, 2013) and sometimes in renal failure. The presence of Cheyne-Stokes breathing in cardiac failure increases mortality. Patients with primary CSA usually are normocapnic or hypocapnic, with $Paco_2$ of 40 mm Hg or lower. The other important point of differentiation is that the cycle length (apnea plus ventilatory duration) is more than 45 seconds in Cheyne-Stokes breathing and less than 45 seconds in primary CSA.

## Restless Legs Syndrome

### Clinical Manifestations

RLS is the most common movement disorder but is uncommonly recognized and treated despite a lucid description of the entity in the middle of the last century (Hening et al., 2009; Wijemanne and Jankovic, 2015). Diagnosis is based on clinical grounds and is based on the International Restless Legs Syndrome Study Group (IRLSSG) criteria first established in 1995 (Walters, 1995) and modified slightly in 2003 (Allen et al., 2003), and modified again in 2012 (Allen et al., 2014). These criteria include five essential diagnostic criteria (Box 101.17). In addition, there are supportive clinical features as well as specifiers for clinical significance and clinical course of RLS (Box 101.18). The IRLSSG diagnostic criteria are consensus criteria established by the international experts in RLS after careful deliberation. It is notable that these differ from the AASM (2014) and the Diagnostic and Statistical Manual (DSM-V) diagnostic criteria. The AASM criteria must include the specifier for clinical significance (see Box 101.18), whereas DSM-V (2013) criteria require a frequency of at least three times a week and a duration of at least 3 months for symptoms. This division into three different requirements amongst three groups of physicians is unfortunate but it is hoped that in future these three groups would merge the criteria into uniform and consistent diagnostic criteria to avoid confusion among physicians in different specialties (Video 101.5).

RLS is a lifelong sensory-motor neurological disorder (Earley, 2003; Patel et al., 2014) that often begins at a very young age but is mostly diagnosed in the middle or later years. Prevalence of RLS increases with age and plateaus for some unknown reason around age 85 to 90 (Allen et al., 2001; Earley, 2003; Earley et al., 2011). All five essential diagnostic criteria (see Box 101.17) are needed for establishing the diagnosis. The overall prevalence of RLS has been estimated at about 7.2% for all adult populations when severity was not considered, but at 2.7% for moderate to severe cases, particularly those in North American and European populations (Allen et al., 2005; Chokroverty, 2014). The prevalence appears to be much less in some surveys from Asia (<1%–3%), suggesting the possibility of ethnic, racial, and environmental influence in susceptibility to disease. In most surveys, the prevalence is greater in women than in men, and the disease is gradually progressing (Hening et al., 2004). Family studies of RLS suggest an increased incidence (≈40%–50%) in first-degree relatives of idiopathic cases. A high concordance (83%) in monozygotic twins and complex segregation analysis suggest an autosomal dominant mode of inheritance (Hening et al., 2009). Linkage analysis documented significant linkage to at least five different chromosomes (12q, 14q, 9p, 2q, and 20p). Recent genome-wide association and linkage analysis have documented common variations in certain genomic regions, conferring more than 50% increase in risk to RLS-PLMS (Stefansson et al., 2007; Winkelmann et al., 2007). Four allelic variations in different genes have been identified on chromosomes 2p, 6p, 15q, and 12q. Recent review of the genetics of RLS can be reviewed elsewhere (Jimenez-Jimenez et al., 2018; Khan et al., 2017; Rye, 2015; Winkelmann et al., 2017).

The sensory manifestations of RLS include intense disagreeable feelings described as creeping, crawling, tingling, burning, aching, cramping, knifelike, or itching sensations. These creeping sensations occur mostly between the knees and ankles, causing an intense urge to move the limbs to relieve these feelings. Sometimes, similar symptoms occur in the arms or other parts of the body, particularly in advanced stages of the disease or when the patient develops

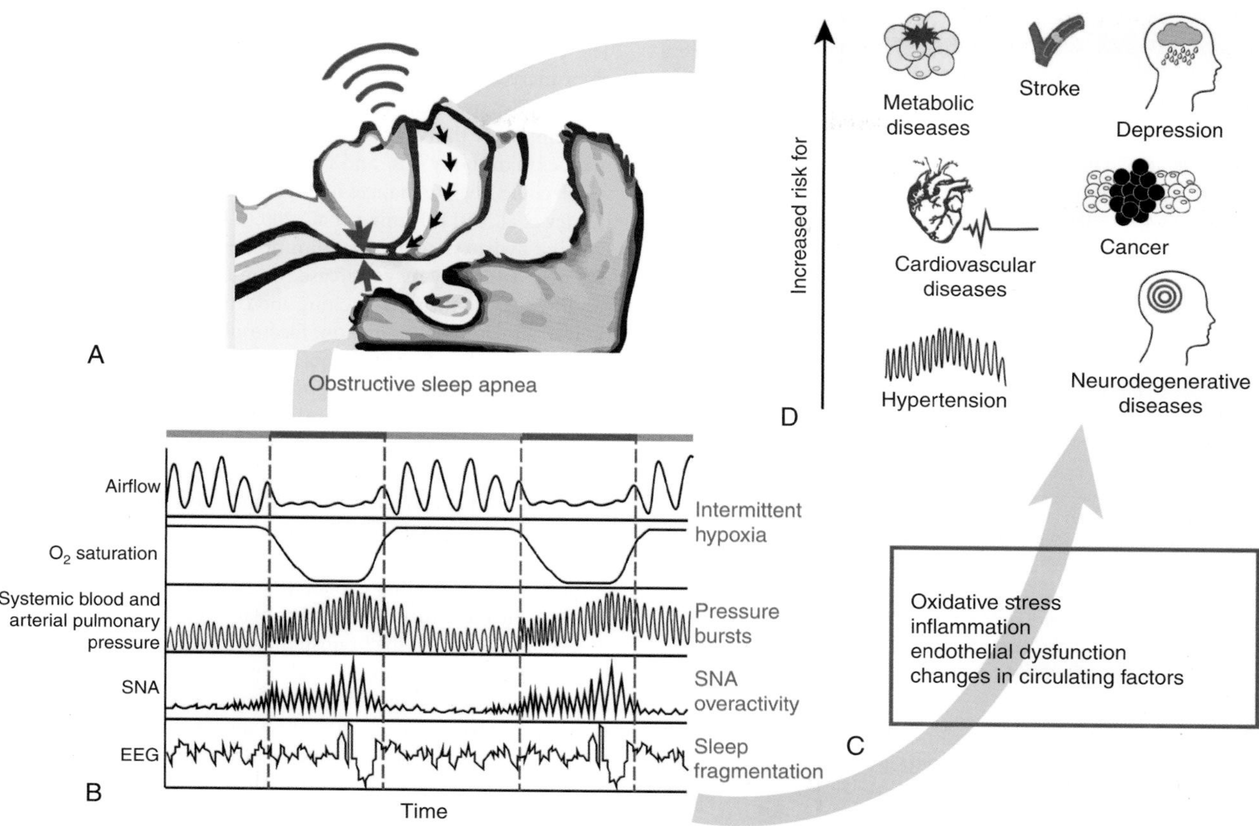


**Fig. 101.51 Consequences of Untreated Obstructive Sleep Apnea.** Pathophysiological Mechanisms and Outcomes of Obstructive Sleep Apnea (OSA). Representative scheme of the pathophysiological mechanisms of OSA and associated consequences: (**A**) OSA is characterized by recurrent episodes of complete (apnea, represented in this figure) or partial (hypopnea) obstruction of the upper airway during sleep. (**B**) Apnea episodes (between red broken lines) result in cessation of the airflow, often accompanied by reduced oxygen ($O_2$) saturation and increased systemic blood and arterial pulmonary pressure. As a result, sympathetic neural activity *(SNA)* increases and apnea episodes end with an arousal of the central nervous system to restore upper airway patency, marked by an increased electroencephalogram *(EEG)* wave frequency. Thus, repetitive obstruction episodes while sleeping culminate in cyclical deoxygenation–reoxygenation (intermittent hypoxia; IH), overactivation of SNA, bursts in systemic blood and arterial pulmonary pressures, and several arousals and microarousals that result in sleep fragmentation (SF). (**C**) As a result, OSA is associated with oxidative stress, inflammation, endothelial dysfunction, and changes in circulating factors. (**D**) Untreated OSA has been associated with an increased predisposition for several impairments and diseases, including hypertension, cardiovascular diseases, metabolic disorders, stroke, depression, cancer, and neurodegenerative diseases (*From Gaspar, L.S., Alvaro, A.R., Moita, J., Cavadas, C. 2017.Obstructive sleep apnea and Hallmarks of aging. Trends Mol. Med. 23 [8], 675–692. https://doi.org/10.1016/j.molmed.2017.06.006. Copyright © 2017 Elsevier Ltd.*)

augmentation (a hypermotor syndrome with symptoms occurring at least 2 hours earlier than the initial period, with intensification and spread to other body parts) resulting from long-standing dopaminergic medications (Allen et al., 2003, 2014; Garcia-Borreguero et al., 2007; Garcia-Borreguero and Williams, 2010). Up to 30%–50% of RLS/WED patients complain of actual pain (more of an ache rather than a sharp burning pain) and not just uncomfortable sensation (Allen et al., 2014). Most of the movements, particularly in the early stages, are noted in the evening while the patients are resting in bed. In severe cases, however, movements may be noted in the daytime while subjects are sitting or lying down. At least 80% of RLS patients have PLMS, and many also have periodic limb movements in wakefulness (Video 101.6).

The condition may have a profound impact on sleep. Patients often seek medical attention for sleep disturbance—generally a problem of initiation, although difficulty maintaining sleep owing to associated PLMS can occur. Neurological examination is generally normal in the idiopathic form. As stated earlier, RLS often begins in childhood, but diagnosis of childhood RLS may be difficult based on the National Institutes of Health (NIH) consensus conference criteria established in 2002 (Allen et al., 2003) and updated recently (Picchietti et al., 2013). To make a correct diagnosis, RLS must be differentiated from conditions mimicking RLS (Box 101.19) or those associated (comorbid) with RLS (Chokroverty, 2009b) (eBoxes 101.20 and 101.21). An important and often difficult condition to differentiate from RLS is akathisia (see eBox 101.21).

**BOX 101.17 Five Essential Diagnostic Criteria for Restless Legs Syndrome**

**Criterion 1.** An urge to move the legs, usually but not always accompanied by uncomfortable sensations in the legs.*

**Criterion 2.** The urge to move the legs with any accompanying unpleasant sensations begins or worsens during periods of inactivity or quiescence such as lying down or sitting.

**Criterion 3.** The urge to move the legs with any accompanying unpleasant sensations is partially or totally relieved by movement, such as walking or stretching, as long as the activity continues.

**Criterion 4.** The urge to move the legs with any accompanying unpleasant sensations during rest or inactivity only occurs or is worse in the evening or night than during the day.

**Criterion 5.** The above features are not accounted for by another medical or behavioral condition (e.g., myalgia, arthritis, venous stasis, leg cramps, positional discomfort, or habitual foot tapping).

*The adult and the pediatric diagnostic criteria are merged together except that the description of these symptoms in criterion 1 should be in the child's own words.

*From Allen, R.P., Picchietti, D.L., Garcia-Borreguero, D., et al., 2014. Restless legs syndrome/Willis Ekbom disease diagnostic criteria: Updated International Restless Legs Syndrome Study Group (IRLSSG) consensus criteria e history, rationale, description, and significance. Sleep Med 15, 860e73. (Marelli et al., 2015).*

**BOX 101.18 Supportive Features and Specifiers for Clinical Significance and Clinical Course of Restless Legs Syndrome**

- Following features (not essential for diagnosis) will support the diagnosis of restless legs syndrome (RLS) in case of some doubt about diagnostic certainty:
  1. Periodic limb movements in sleep (PLMS) or wakefulness (PLMW) at a frequency or intensity greater than expected for age
  2. Response to dopaminergic treatment at least initially
  3. Positive family history of RLS among first-degree relatives
  4. Lack of profound daytime sleepiness
- Specifier for clinical significance:

RLS symptoms cause significant distress in social, occupational, educational, or other important areas of functioning by impacting sleep, energy/vitality, activities of daily living, behavior, cognition, or mood.

- Specifier for clinical course (these criteria do not apply to pediatric age group pregnancy, or drug-induced RLS):
  1. Intermittent RLS: symptoms occur on average less than twice per week with at least five lifetime events.
  2. Chronic-persistent RLS symptoms occurring on average at least twice weekly for the past year.

In the differential diagnosis, it is important to look for clues including subtle signs based on history and physical findings that point to the correct diagnosis. The history should include a detailed description of the present complaint, duration and nature of the sensory-motor complaints, as well as past, family, psychiatric, and drug histories. For the diagnosis of RLS, five IRLSSG essential criteria must be met (see Box 101.17), with or without the supportive features. For the diagnosis of mimicries and conditions associated with RLS, characteristic clinical features of the particular condition should help in arriving at the correct diagnosis.

### Pathophysiology

The pathophysiology and the site of CNS dysfunction in idiopathic or primary RLS remain unclear (Allen et al., 2013; Earley et al., 2011; Trenkwalder and Paulus, 2004; Trenkwalder and Winkelman, 2003). Contemporary thinking in the pathophysiology of RLS suggests abnormalities in the body's use and storage of iron and dopamine dysfunction, which could involve changes in dopamine receptors or dopamine uptake (Earley et al., 2011; Hening et al., 2009). Iron is a necessary cofactor for tyrosine hydroxylase, the rate-limiting enzyme in dopamine synthesis, and iron deficiency may decrease the number of dopamine $D_2$ receptor binding sites, so the most exciting and current research focus is centered on iron-dopamine dysfunction. Electrophysiological (blink reflex excitability, back-averaging technique, EEG beta oscillations) and magnetic brain stimulation studies using the paired stimulation technique show increased cortical excitability and decreased subcortical inhibition, suggesting the site of the CNS dysfunction in RLS in the subcortical loci (Earley et al., 2011; Hening et al., 2009). One study suggested a possible spinal mechanism, based on a flexor reflex study showing increased flexor reflex excitability during sleep compared to waking, in contrast to decreased excitability in control subjects (Bara-Jimenez et al., 2000). A spinal mechanism may explain PLMS (Clemens et al., 2006) but does not explain the entire RLS symptomatology. Functional MRI (fMRI) points to locations in the brainstem, cerebellum, and thalamus (Bucher et al., 1997). PET and SPECT studies gave contradictory reports regarding presynaptic and postsynaptic dopaminergic dysfunction (Earley et al., 2011; Hening et al., 2009). CSF analysis, special MRI, and neuropathological studies demonstrate reduction in CNS iron or ferritin or both, as can be seen in Fig. 101.52 (Allen and Earley, 2001; Earley et al., 2011; Hening et al., 2009). In summary, currently there are multiple and inconsistent theories challenging researchers seeking to make advances in treatment, for example, the most plausible iron-dopamine connection theory in a subset of patients, an alternative neurotransmitter or neuronal pathway (e.g., the activation of thalamic glutamate or hypoxic pathway, both central and peripheral), opioid pathway, reduced thalamocortical connectivity coupled with genetic predisposition (Allen et al., 2013; Ku et al., 2014; Jimenez-Jimenez et al., 2018; Khan et al., 2017; Rye, 2015; Winkelmann et al., 2017).

### Periodic Limb Movements in Sleep

PLMS (AASM, 2014) is a PSG finding (Fig. 101.53) characterized by periodically recurring stereotyped limb movements, particularly dorsiflexion of the ankles and sometimes flexion of the knees and hips at an average interval of 20–40 seconds (range, 5–90 seconds), a duration of 0.5–10 seconds during predominantly NREM sleep, and occurring for at least four consecutive movements (Box 101.22). PLMS appears most commonly in RLS but may also occur in a large number of other medical, neurological, and sleep disorders and with ingestion of medications (e.g., SSRIs, tricyclic antidepressants) and even in normal individuals, particularly in those older than age 65. In the current ICSD-III (AASM, 2014), PLMD characterized by PSG findings of PLMS with a frequency of greater than 5/hour in children or greater than 15/hour in adults without associated RLS causing repeated awakenings and sleep fragmentations associated with impaired daytime functioning which cannot be explained by another medical, neurological, psychiatric, or other sleep disorder is listed as a separate entity. There is a growing body of evidence that PLMS may simply be a PSG observation and may have no specific clinical significance except its presence in the majority of patients with RLS (Mahowald, 2002; Montplaisir et al., 2000; Video 101.7).

**BOX 101.19 Conditions That Mimic Restless Legs Syndrome**

**Presenting with Excess Restlessness**

| | |
|---|---|
| Restless legs syndrome | Symptoms occur during wakefulness but with a specific demonstratable circadian pattern predilection to manifest during the evening time. Diagnosis made by clinical history, often based on description of an urge to move described as an uncomfortable creepy-crawling sensation brought on at time of inactivity or rest (sitting and lying). Movement of symptomatic limb leads to partial or complete relief. Symptomatic relief is persistent as long as movement continues. Demonstrates presence of circadian pattern. |
| PLMD (periodic limb movement disorder) | Polysomnographic manifestation of leg movements. Diagnosis made by sleep study. Does not include sensory symptoms such as an urge to move as in restless legs syndrome (RLS). Patients may endorse sleep disturbance and complaints of daytime fatigue and sleepiness. Must exclude other causes of PLMS, including sleep disorder breathing. |
| Nocturnal leg cramps | Painful muscular contraction in the back of the legs readily differentiates this condition from RLS, e.g., cramps or "Charlie horse cramps" are a common experience. Though symptoms may occur at night and relief may be achieved with stretching, unlike RLS, cramps are experienced as a usually painful muscular contraction. |
| Neuropathic pain | Commonly reported as numbness, burning, tingling, and pain—descriptors not as commonly seen in RLS. Although the sensory symptoms may become more noticeable at night, the symptoms are usually also present throughout the day. Unlike RLS, significant relief is not obtained with walking or during sustained movement. |
| Hypotensive akathisias | Feeling of restlessness, often localized to the legs, brought on by sitting still. Should not occur while lying down but might be relieved with movement. Occurs in individuals with orthostatic hypotension. |
| Arthritis lower limb | Discomfort centered more in joints, does not usually have prominent circadian pattern as seen in RLS. |
| Volitional movements, foot tapping, leg rocking | Occurs in individuals who fidget, especially when bored or anxious, but usually do not experience associated sensory symptoms, discomfort, or conscious urge to move. Usually lacks a circadian pattern. |
| Positional discomfort | Often comes on with prolonged sitting or lying in the same position but usually relieved by a simple change in position as opposed to ongoing movement, unlike RLS. |
| Neuroleptic induced akathisia | Usually generalized as opposed to limb-predominant. No pronounced circadian pattern, and often no relief with movement. Should have history of specific medication exposure. |
| Spasticity | An involuntary, velocity-dependent, increase in muscle tone secondary to central nervous system damage that results in resistance to movement. |

Akathisia:
- Neuroleptic induced
- Antidepressant induced
- Related to central nervous system

Degenerative disease
Disorders of abnormal muscular activity
Myokymia
Hypnic jerks
Essential myoclonus
Orthostatic tremor
Anxiety/depression
Periodic limb movement disorder
Restlessness due to orthostatic hypotension
Attention-deficit hyperactivity disorder

**Presenting with Nocturnal Leg Discomfort**

"Growing pains"
Small-fiber neuropathies
Claudication
Venous stasis/varicose veins
Myalgias
Arthritis
Radiculopathies
Delusional parasitosis

**Presenting with Unusual Motor Activity Combined with Leg Discomfort**

Painful muscle cramps including nocturnal leg cramps
Syndrome of painful legs and moving toes
Variant of painless legs and moving toes
Causalgia-dystonia syndrome
Muscular pain-fasciculation syndrome

*Reproduced with permission from Chokroverty, S., 2009. Differential diagnosis of restless legs syndrome. In: Hening, W.A., Allen, R.P., Chokroverty, S., et al. (Eds.), Restless Legs Syndrome. Saunders, Philadelphia, p. 111.*

## Circadian Rhythm Sleep Disorders

Circadian rhythm sleep disorders result from a mismatch between the body's internal clock and the geophysical environment, either as a result of malfunction of the biological clock or a shift in the environment causing this to be out of phase (ICSD-III; Abbot and Zee, 2015; Reid and Zee, 2011). The patients have difficulty sleeping as a result of desynchronization between their internal circadian rhythms and external time. The most common circadian rhythm sleep disorders are jet lag (associated with high-speed air travel across several times zones) and shift work sleep disorder (seen in patients who work nonstandard shifts). A schematic reorientation of the various circadian derangements is provided in Fig. 101. 54 (Chokroverty and Thomas, 2014).

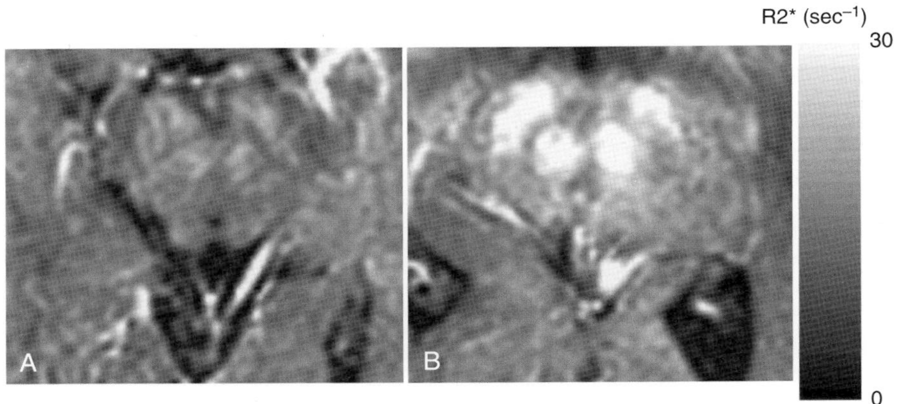


**Fig. 101.52** Reduced brain iron tissue concentrations on MRI. R2* images in a 70-year-old restless legs syndrome (RLS) patient (**A**) and a 71-year-old control (**B**). Much lower R2* relaxation rates are apparent in the RLS case in both red nucleus and substantia nigra. (*From Earley, C.J., Barker, P.B., Horská, A., et al., 2006. MRI-determined regional brain iron concentrations in early- and late-onset restless legs syndrome. Sleep Med 7, 458–461.*)

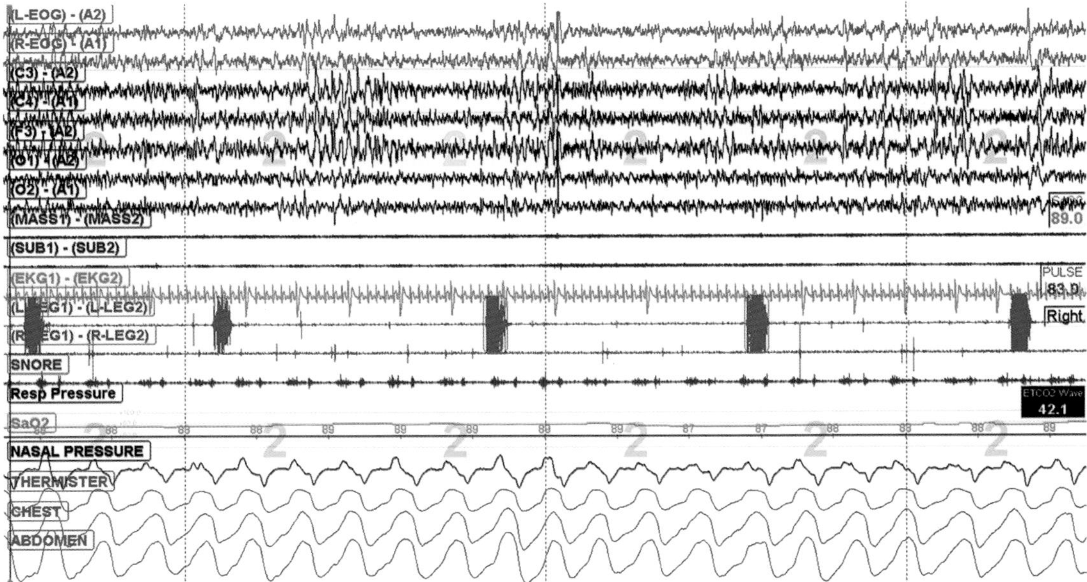


**Fig. 101.53 Periodic Leg Movements of Sleep (PLMS).** A 2-minute sleep epoch from a diagnostic polysomnogram of a patient with PLMS associated with an irresistible urge to move her legs. Her husband reports that she has frequent nighttime kicking and jerking movements that disrupt his sleep. A succession of 5 periodic limb movements are shown (circled in purple), occurring in the right and left legs (anterior tibialis muscles). According to the American Academy of Sleep Medicine, periodic leg movements are diagnosed when more than 15 leg movements per hour of sleep are captured. Four or more consecutive movements are required and the interval between movements is typically 20 to 40 seconds. The movements should appear at sequence of 4 or more separated by an interval of more than 5 and less than 90 seconds and have an amplitude of greater than or equal to 25% of toe dorsiflexion during the calibration. Reference electrodes (F4, C4, $O_2$) are referenced to mastoid electrode (M1) or average (AVG). *ABD*, Abdominal respiratory effort; *CHEST*, chest respiratory effort; *Chin*, Chin electromyogram; *EKG*, electrocardiogram; *L*, left; *LOC*, left electro-oculogram; *PTAF*, nasal pressure; *R*, right; *R LEG*, right anterior tibias surface electromyogram; *ROC*, right electro-oculogram; *SNORE*, snore sensor air flow, nasal and oral airflow; *$SpO_2$*, pulse oximetry. (*From Rama, A.N. Zachariah, R., Kushida, C.A., 2009. Sleep Med. Clin. 4 [3], 361–372.*)

### Jet Lag

The experience of *jet lag* follows eastward or westward jet travel that crosses several time zones, disrupting synchronization between the body's inner clock and external cues; north-south travel does not evoke this disorder. Jet lag symptoms include difficulty maintaining sleep, frequent arousals, and EDS, typically resolving within a few days to 2 weeks.

### Shift-Work Sleep Disorder

Shift-work sleep disorders may affect up to 5 million workers in the United States. Symptoms include sleep disruption, fatigue, gastrointestinal symptoms, increasing chances of being involved in traffic accidents, and making errors on the job. Adjustment of the work time schedule rarely improves the symptoms of shift-work sleep disorder.

**BOX 101.22 Features of Periodic Limb Movements in Sleep**

1. Repetitive, often stereotyped movements during NREM sleep
2. Usually noted in legs and consisting of extension of great toe, dorsiflexion of ankle, and flexion of knee and hip; sometimes seen in arms
3. Periodic or quasi-periodic at an average interval of 20–40 sec (range, 5–90 sec) with a duration of 0.5–10 sec and as part of at least 4 consecutive movements
4. Occurs at any age, but prevalence increases with age
5. May occur as an isolated condition or may be associated with a large number of other medical, neurological, or sleep disorders and medications
6. Seen in at least 80% of patients with restless legs syndrome
7. *Occurs predominantly during NREM*, nonrapid eye movement. Appearance of PLMS during REM raises suspicion for narcolepsy.

*NREM*, Nonrapid eye movement; *PLMS*, periodic limb movements in sleep; *REM*, rapid eye movement.

### Delayed Sleep Phase State

In DSPS the patient's major sleep episode is delayed in relation to desired clock time, causing sleep-onset insomnia or difficulty awakening at the desired time (ICSD-III). A typical schedule consists of going to sleep late between 2:00 AM and 6:00 AM, and waking up during the late morning between 10:00 AM and 2:00 PM. These patients have great difficulty functioning adequately during daytime hours if they must wake up early in the morning to go to school or work. They cannot function normally in society due to their disturbed sleep schedule; however, their sleep architecture is generally normal if these individuals are allowed to follow their own uninterrupted sleep schedule. Onset generally occurs during childhood or adolescence. Sometimes a history of DSPS in other family members exists, and some patients may complain of depression. An unusually long intrinsic period owing to an abnormality in the biological clock in the SCN is the fundamental problem.

### Advanced Sleep Phase State

Advanced sleep phase state is the converse of DSPS (ICSD-III). Patients go to sleep early in the evening and wake up early in the morning. The patient experiences sleep disruption and daytime sleepiness when not going to sleep at early hours. The condition is often seen in patients with depression and in normal elderly individuals. Familial ASPS has been ascribed to mutation in the *HPER2* gene (Jones et al., 2013).

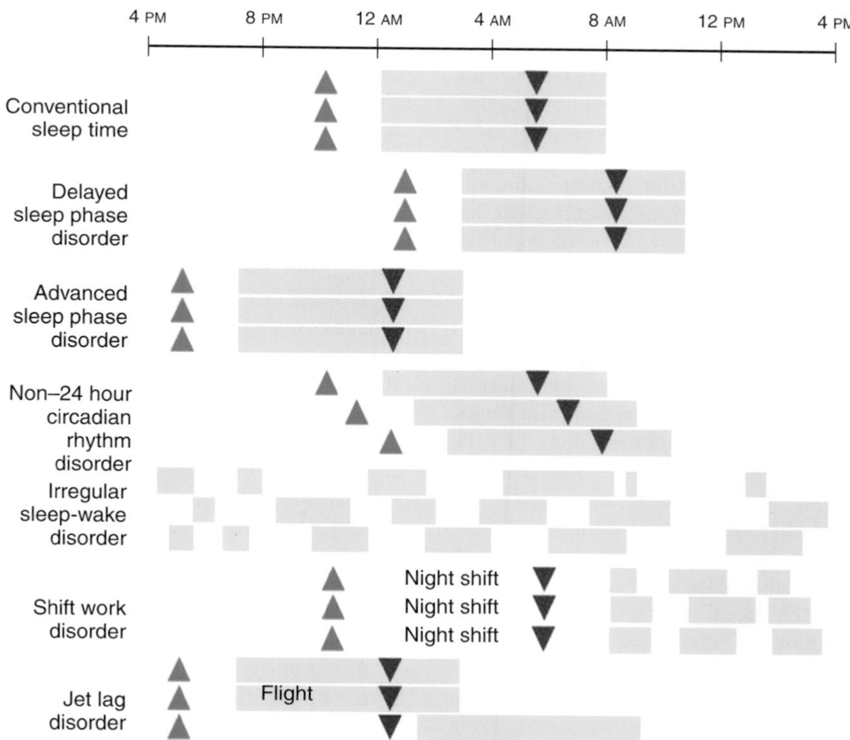


**Fig. 101.54 Schematic Representation of the Circadian Rhythm Sleep Disorders.** Circadian rhythm sleep disorders occur due to a misalignment between an individual's behavioral sleep and wake patterns and endogenous biological circadian rhythms timing system or from misalignment between circadian phase and. Disruption of circadian timing results in insomnia, excessive daytime sleepiness, and impaired performance. Symptoms may cause disruption in social, occupational, and other areas of function. *Blue rectangles* denote sleep time. *Green triangles* denote the dim-light melatonin onset, which occurs 2 hours before biological sleep-onset time. *Red triangles* denote the core body temperature nadir. (*From Malkani, R., Zee, P.C., 2014. Basic Circadian Rhythms and Circadian Sleep Disorders. Atlas of Sleep Medicine. Chokroverty & Thomas, pp. 119-126, Chapter 5.*)

### Free-Running Circadian Rhythm Disorder

Circadian rhythm sleep disorder, free-running type (nonentrained type or non-24-hour sleep-wake syndrome) is characterized by a patient's inability to maintain a regular bedtime and sleep onset that occurs at irregular hours (ICSD-III). The patient displays increasing delay of sleep onset by approximately 1 hour during each 24-hour sleep-wake cycle, causing an eventual progression of sleep onset through the daytime hours into the evening. There is no entrainment or synchronization with the usual time cues such as sunlight or social activities. This disorder is most often seen in blind people.

### Irregular Sleep/Wake Circadian Rhythm Disorder

Circadian rhythm sleep disorder, irregular sleep-wake type (irregular sleep-wake rhythm) is characterized by a lack of clearly defined circadian rhythm of sleep and wake. Patients are seen to be napping throughout the 24-hour period, but total sleep time is normal. This condition may be seen in patients with degenerative neurological disorders such as dementia and children with mental retardation. Actigraphy recordings are useful in diagnosing any of the circadian rhythm sleep disorders.

## Neurological Disorders and Sleep Disturbance

Neurological disorders may affect sleep/wake-generating neurons, causing profound sleep disturbances that may include insomnia, hypersomnia, parasomnia, circadian rhythm disorders, and abnormal movements in sleep at night. These sleep disturbances may adversely affect the natural course of the neurological illness. Neurological causes of insomnia are described elsewhere in this chapter, and neurological  disorders causing EDS or hypersomnia are listed in eBox 101.5. EDS can result from tumors and vascular lesions affecting the ARAS and its projections to the posterior hypothalamus and thalamus. Other causes of EDS include astrocytomas, suprasellar cysts, metastatic tumors, lymphomas and hamartomas affecting the posterior hypothalamus, pinealomas, and astrocytoma of the brainstem. Symptomatic narcolepsy may occasionally result from craniopharyngioma and other tumors of the hypothalamic and pituitary regions, rostral brainstem gliomas, MS, arteriovenous malformations of the diencephalon, and cerebral sarcoidosis involving the hypothalamus. Neuromuscular disorders, neurodegenerative diseases, encephalitis, and encephalopathies may also cause EDS.

### Sleep and Epilepsy

There is a reciprocal relationship between sleep and epilepsy (Gibbon, Maccormac, and Gringras, 2019). Sleep affects epilepsy and epilepsy, in turn, affects sleep. Sleep increases interictal epileptiform discharges, causing repeated arousals and sleep fragmentation resulting in EDS, which again triggers seizures and epileptiform discharges, thus repeating the cycle. Most of the time, seizures are triggered during stages N1 and N2 sleep; occasionally, however, they are triggered during slow-wave sleep. In epileptic patients, NREM sleep acts as a convulsant, causing excessive synchronization and activation of seizures in an already hyperexcitable cortex. In contrast, in REM sleep, there is desynchronization of EEG coupled with an inhibition of interhemispheric transfer of impulses, causing an attenuation of epileptiform discharges and limitation of propagation of generalized epileptic discharges to a focal area (Fig. 101.55). Sleep deprivation is another important seizure-triggering factor. Sleep deprivation increases epileptiform discharges by causing sleepiness as well as by increasing cortical excitability. Seizures may occur predominantly during sleep (nocturnal seizure), in the daytime (diurnal), or during both sleep at night and daytime (diffuse epilepsy). Approximately 10% of epileptic patients experience nocturnal seizures.

***Effect of sleep on epilepsy.*** Certain types of seizures are characteristically observed during sleep, including nocturnal frontal lobe epilepsy, tonic seizure as a component of Lennox-Gastaut syndrome, benign focal epilepsy of childhood with rolandic spikes, juvenile myoclonic epilepsy, early- or late-onset childhood occipital epilepsy, benign focal epilepsy with occipital paroxysms in EEG, generalized tonic-clonic seizures on awakening, nocturnal temporal lobe epilepsy (a subgroup of partial complex seizures), Landau-Kleffner syndrome, and continuous spike-and-wave discharges during NREM sleep (AASM, 2014).

The tonic seizures of *Lennox-Gastaut syndrome* are typically activated by sleep, are much more frequent during NREM sleep than during wakefulness, and are never seen during REM sleep. The typical EEG finding consists of trains of fast spikes intermixed with slow spike-and-wave discharges at 2–2.5 Hz.

*Benign focal epilepsy of childhood with rolandic spikes* is characterized by focal clonic facial twitchings, often preceded by perioral numbness, seen most frequently during drowsiness and sleep. The EEG shows centrotemporal or rolandic spikes or sharp waves. These discharges are present throughout the night in all stages of sleep.

*Continuous spike-and-wave* is a disease of childhood characterized by generalized continuous slow spike-and-wave discharges seen during at least 85% of NREM sleep and suppressed during REM sleep.

*Juvenile myoclonic epilepsy* is characterized by massive bilaterally synchronous myoclonic jerks which are most frequently noted on awakening. It commonly occurs in young adults aged 13–19 years. A typical EEG shows synchronous and symmetrical multiple spikes and spike-and-wave discharges.

*Sleep-related epilepsy (Formerly Nocturnal frontal lobe epilepsy)* includes nocturnal paroxysmal dystonia, paroxysmal arousals and awakenings, episodic nocturnal wanderings, and autosomal dominant nocturnal frontal lobe epilepsy (Chokroverty and Nobili, 2015; Derry et al., 2009; Derry and Duncan, 2013; Ferini-Strambi et al., 2012; Foldvary-Schaeffer and Alsheikhtaha, 2013; Nobili et al., 2007; Tinuper et al., 2005; di Corcia et al., 2005). All these disorders share common features of abnormal paroxysmal motor activities during sleep. Most cases respond favorably to antiepileptic medications, but more than a third of cases, particularly those with complex forms, are resistant to such treatment. These seizures most likely represent partial seizures arising from discharging foci in the deeper regions of the brain, particularly the frontal cortex, without any concomitant scalp evidence of epileptiform activities. The onset is anywhere from infancy to middle age. Nocturnal frontal lobe epilepsy occurs exclusively during sleep at night, but other types of frontal lobe seizures may be both diurnal and nocturnal. The episodes are characterized by sudden onset of ballismic, choreoathetoid, or dystonic movements, as well as bipedal, bimanual, and bicycling complex movements with motor and sexual automatisms occurring in NREM sleep with sudden termination (Box 101.23). The duration is mostly less than 1 minute but sometimes may be 1–2 minutes with brief postictal confusion. The spells often occur in clusters. Ictal and interictal EEGs may remain normal, but sometimes interictal EEG may show spikes; occasionally, depth recording is needed for a diagnosis.

***Effect of epilepsy on sleep.*** A variety of sleep abnormalities are noted in the PSG recording and include increased sleep-onset latency, increased number and duration of awakenings after sleep onset, reduced sleep efficiency, reduced sleep spindles and K complexes, reduced REM sleep, increased stage shifts, abnormal sleep cycling, and sleep state instability, making classification of staging difficult or impossible. Epileptic patients may present with EDS as well as insomnia. The various factors responsible for EDS in epileptics

NREM SLEEP

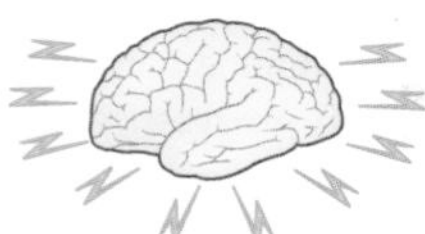

"Seizure promotor"

NREM Sleep:
Synchrony of thalamo-cortical synaptic activity
Greater tendency for propagation of epileptiform discharges

SYNCHRONIZED SLEEP
Excessive diffuse cortical synchronization
Enhancement in interhemispheric impulse traffic

REM SLEEP

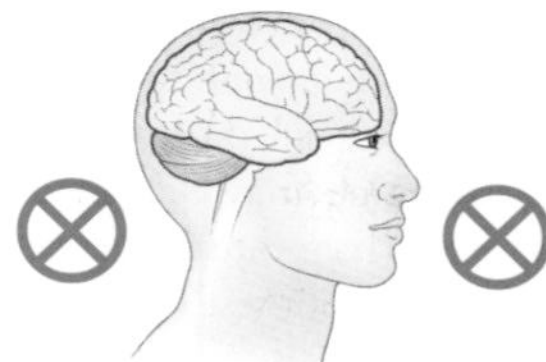

"Seizure protector"

REM Sleep:
Desynchronized neuronal discharge patterns
Relative resistance to propagation of EEG potentials
Skeletal muscle paralysis

DESYNCHRONIZED SLEEP
Inhibition of thalamocortical synchronization,
tonic reduction in interhemispheric impulse traffic

**Fig. 101.55** Sleep State and Epileptogenicity. *EEG*, Electroencephalogram; *NREM*, nonrapid eye movement; *REM*, rapid eye movement.

**BOX 101.23 Features of Sleep-Related Epilepsy**

Sporadic, occasionally familial (dominant)
Oftentimes exclusively nocturnal
Sudden onset in nonrapid eye movement sleep with sudden termination
Duration: mostly less than 1 min, sometimes 1–2 min with short postictal confusion
Often occur in clusters
Semiology: Stereotyped, tonic, clonic, bipedal, bimanual, and bicycling, ballismic and choreoathetoid movements; motor and sexual automatisms; contralateral dystonic posturing or arm abduction with or without eye deviation
Ictal EEG may be normal; interictal EEG may show spikes; sometimes depth recording is needed

*EEG*, Electroencephalogram.

include clinical seizures, particularly nocturnal seizures, frequent ictal epileptiform discharges, antiepileptic medications, associated primary sleep disorders, and depression. Insomnia in epileptics may be related to frequent arousals and sleep fragmentation resulting from nocturnal seizures and interictal epileptiform discharges, depression, anxiety, associated primary sleep disorders, and a specific effect of some antiepileptic medications (e.g., lamotrigine).

Sudden unexpected death in epilepsy (SUDEP) is defined as unexpected, sudden, non-traumatic, non-drowning death in a person with epilepsy. While the annual rates range between 0.3 and 6 cases of SUDEP per 1000 adult persons with epilepsy and 1 case of SUDEP per 4500 children, the etiology cannot be determined at autopsy. A known risk factor is recurrent generalized tonic-clonic seizures and the most effective SUDEP prevention is seizure control (Whitney and Donner, 2019). Given that SUDEP occurs at night, some have proposed disrupted sleep as a potential mechanism facilitating SUDEP and proposed exercising proper sleep hygiene; identify and treat insomnia and sleep apnea. More data are needed to determine whether patients with epilepsy are at greater risk of SUDEP when sleep-deprived, and whether primary sleep disorders such as sleep apnea, chronic insomnia, and daytime sleepiness may play a role in the pathophysiology (Somboon et al., 2019).

***Differential diagnosis.*** Sleep seizures should be differentiated from other nocturnal events such as NREM and REM parasomnias, nocturnal panic attacks, psychogenic dissociated states, PLMS, hypnic jerks, drug-induced nocturnal dyskinesias, jerking movements of sleep apnea, and other parasomnias such as bruxism, benign neonatal sleep myoclonus, and rhythmic movement disorders. There is probably an increased prevalence of sleep apnea in epilepsy, as reported by scattered case reports, but systematic study to determine the true prevalence of sleep apnea has not been undertaken (Chokroverty et al., 2006). It is, however, important to recognize the coexistence of epilepsy and sleep apnea, because treatment of sleep apnea by CPAP titration may improve seizure control (Video 101.8).

### Degenerative Dementia and Sleep Dysfunction

***Sleep and neurodegeneration: General perspectives.*** Dementia is characterized by progressive deterioration of memory and cognition followed by language dysfunction, hallucinations, other psychotic features, depression, and sleep disturbance. In advanced stages, the patient becomes bedridden, mute, and incontinent. Sleep dysfunction with or without abnormal motor activity during sleep is increasingly recognized in patients with irreversible chronic dementing illnesses (Chokroverty, 2009a; Chokroverty et al., 2015; McCurry and Ancoli-Israel, 2003; MacKenzie, 2000). AD is the most common cause of chronic dementia, accounting for at least 60% of all cases. It is estimated that by 2025 more than 10 million and by 2050 about 20 million cases of AD will be present in the United States. Other conditions include diffuse Lewy body disease (DLBD), accounting for at least 15%–20% of cases (Mackenzie, 2000); PD with dementia, frontotemporal dementia in about 10%, corticobasal ganglionic degeneration, progressive supranuclear palsy (PSP), multi-infarct or vascular dementia, Huntington disease, Creutzfeldt-Jakob disease, and FFI account for the rest of the cases. The major sleep disturbances in dementing illnesses include insomnia, hypersomnia, circadian sleep/wake rhythm disorders, excessive nocturnal motor activity, "sundowning," and respiratory dysrhythmias. Table 101.9 differentiates the key dementias based on the reported sleep disorders unique to each group (Video 101.9).

### Sleep Disorders in the Tauopathies

The *tauopathies* result from misprocessing of tau, a protein associated with microbules, and include AD, PSP, frontotemporal dementia-Pick disease, and corticobasal degeneration. Despite intensive motor activity and abnormal behavior during REM sleep, patients with RBD do not usually complain of EDS. There is a potential for injury to self and others in patients with RBD; therefore, recognition and treatment are important. Circadian sleep/wake rhythm disturbances are noted in some conditions, most prominently in AD, and may present as a cyclical agitation syndrome popularly known as the *sundowning syndrome*. Another commonly encountered excessive nocturnal motor activity that may cause sleep disturbance is PLMS, which may be noted in many of these dementing illnesses. Sleep-related respiratory dysrhythmias and loud snoring during sleep occur in some of these conditions, particularly in patients with AD, PD, and DLBD.

The following factors may be cited as causing sleep disturbances in dementing illness: accelerated normal physiological changes of aging, which include changes in sleep architecture and stages adding to the burden of sleep disturbance in dementia; status of apolipoprotein E (ApoE)-eE4 (Bliwise, 2002) genotype; and MAO-A 4-repeat allele (Craig et al., 2006) genotype. The ApoE-eE4 genotype shows an association with sleep apnea and AD, although contradictory reports have also been published. In a recent report, a quantitative sleep disturbance score was found to be slightly higher in patients with MAO-A 4-repeat allele genotypes; in the same report, however, ApoE-eE4 had no influence on the development of an altered sleep genotype. Another finding was that environment (e.g., institutionalization) aggravates sleep disturbance, especially in AD patients. Comorbid medical disturbances (e.g., congestive heart failure, COPD, pain from arthritis, nocturia, gastroesophageal reflux disease); medications used to treat AD, PD, and other dementing illnesses; comorbid primary sleep disorders (e.g., OSAS, RLS, and PLMS); inadequate sleep hygiene; circadian rhythm disruptions; and comorbid psychiatric disorders (e.g., depression) may all have adverse effects on sleep.

## Sleep in the Setting of Alzheimer Dementia

Sleep dysfunction in AD may occur even in the early stage and scientists recently showed that sleep loss may even precede AD symptoms (Ju et al., 2013), but it is more common and severe in advanced stages. In addition to sundowning, these patients often sleep early in the evening, waking up frequently and staying awake most of the night. Their sleep is fragmented and fractionated throughout a 24-hour period. Sleep apnea has been noted in more than 33% to 53% of patients with AD, more frequently in those with the ApoE-eE4 allele (Bliwise, 2002). These patients remain somnolent most of the time in the advanced stages. Sleep dysfunction in DLBD includes RBD (which often precedes the onset of illness), sleep apnea, nocturnal visual hallucinations, insomnia, and daytime hypersomnolence.

## Sleep Disruption, Inflammation and the Risk of Alzheimer Dementia

Recent evidence has linked disturbed sleep, inflammation, and risk of AD dementia precipitated by a cascade of events involving activation of systemic inflammation (as measured by mediators such as proinflammatory cytokines and C-reactive protein). This cascade results in the formation of primed and dysfunctional, microglial cell which displays an amoeboid morphology resulting in reduced and impaired clearance of amyloid from the CSF. This step results in an increase in the production of proinflammatory cytokines, and local inflammation within the CNS (Irwin, 2019; Irwin and Vitiello, 2019). This cascade of events is the final common pathway which precipitates AD dementia progression. This is illustrated in Fig. 101. 56.Additional recent data support the hypothesis that AD pathology itself can lead to sleep and circadian disruptions. Supporting this idea is an observation that certain pathophysiological processes associated with AD, such as Aβ deposition in the brain, disrupt sleep, and forever alter circadian rhythms. Given the observation that Aβ deposition in the brain and cognitive dysfunctions are detectable years prior to the clinical onset of AD, one may conclude that disruptions to the sleep-wake cycle may be a consequence rather than cause of AD pathogenesis (Cedernaes et al., 2017). Recent data from humans support the hypothesis that AD pathology itself can lead to sleep and circadian disruptions. Past research demonstrated that pathophysiological processes associated with AD, such as Aβ deposition in the brain, alter sleep, as well as disrupt circadian rhythms. Since Aβ deposition in the brain and cognitive dysfunctions are detectable years prior to the clinical onset of AD, this suggests that disruptions to the sleep-wake cycle may be a consequence rather than cause of AD pathogenesis. Alternatively, existing evidence leads us to propose that there exists a mechanistic interplay between AD pathogenesis and disruptions to sleep and interrelated circadian rhythms as summarized in Fig. 101.57.

## The Alpha Synucleinopathies

*The alpha Synucleinopathies* are a group of disorders with abnormal deposition of α-synuclein in the cytoplasm of neurons or glial cells, as well as in extracellular deposits of amyloid. The main synucleinopathies causing dementing illnesses include PD and DLBD. The parasomnia most commonly associated with some degenerative dementing illnesses is RBD. It has been suggested that in the setting of degenerative dementia or parkinsonism, RBD is a manifestation of evolving synucleinopathies but is rare in tauopathies (Boeve, 2010; Boeve et al., 2007; Iranzo et al., 2009, 2010, 2014; Postuma et al., 2009, 2009a, 2010a, 2010b, 2010c, 2013; Barone and Henchcliffe, 2018; Mahowald and Schenck, 2018; Pilotto et al., 2019).

DLBD may be mistaken for AD or PD with dementia. However, the core diagnostic features of DLBD include fluctuating cognition, recurrent visual hallucinations, and parkinsonian features (e.g., rigidity, postural instability, akinesia, bradykinesia) coupled with other features such as repeated falls, neuroleptic sensitivity, and RBD (McKeith et al., 2005; Mackenzie, 2000).

In PD, sleep dysfunction is present in 70%–90% of cases, with progressive impairment with the progression of the disease (Chokroverty, 2009a; Chokroverty and Provini, 2015). Sleep-onset and maintenance insomnia, and sleep fragmentation are common (Peeraully et al., 2012). Several nocturnal motor abnormalities are noted: RBD, PLMS, sleep-onset blinking, REM-onset blepharospasm, and intrusion of REMs into NREM sleep. Respiratory dysrhythmias are noted to be more common in PD than in age-matched controls although there are contradictory reports. Another characteristic feature in PD is daytime hypersomnolence and irresistible sleep attacks, which may be due to a combination of the intrinsic disease process and dopaminergic medications.

In PSP, sleep disturbance is present in almost all cases. Most common sleep disruptions include sleep-onset and maintenance insomnia, which is worse than in AD or PD. Sleep disturbance increases with the severity of motor abnormalities. Important PSG findings include frequent arousals, reduced REM and stage N2 NREM sleep, and RSWA (Arnulf et al., 2005; Chokroverty, 2009a; Sixel-Doring et al., 2009).

Sleep disturbance in Huntington disease is noted in approximately 20% of cases. Most commonly, sleep disruption with fragmentation is noted with increasing disease severity. Another characteristic finding is increased sleep spindle density in PSG.

Sleep dysfunction in frontotemporal dementia and corticobasal degeneration resembles that noted in AD, but adequate studies have not been conducted in these conditions to characterize sleep disruption.

Sleep apnea is more common in vascular dementia than in AD and is very common in MSA and DLBD.

*Fatal familial insomnia* is a rare and rapidly progressive autosomal dominant prion disease with a missense mutation at codon 178 of the prion protein gene (PrP) (Montagna, 2011). FFI was originally

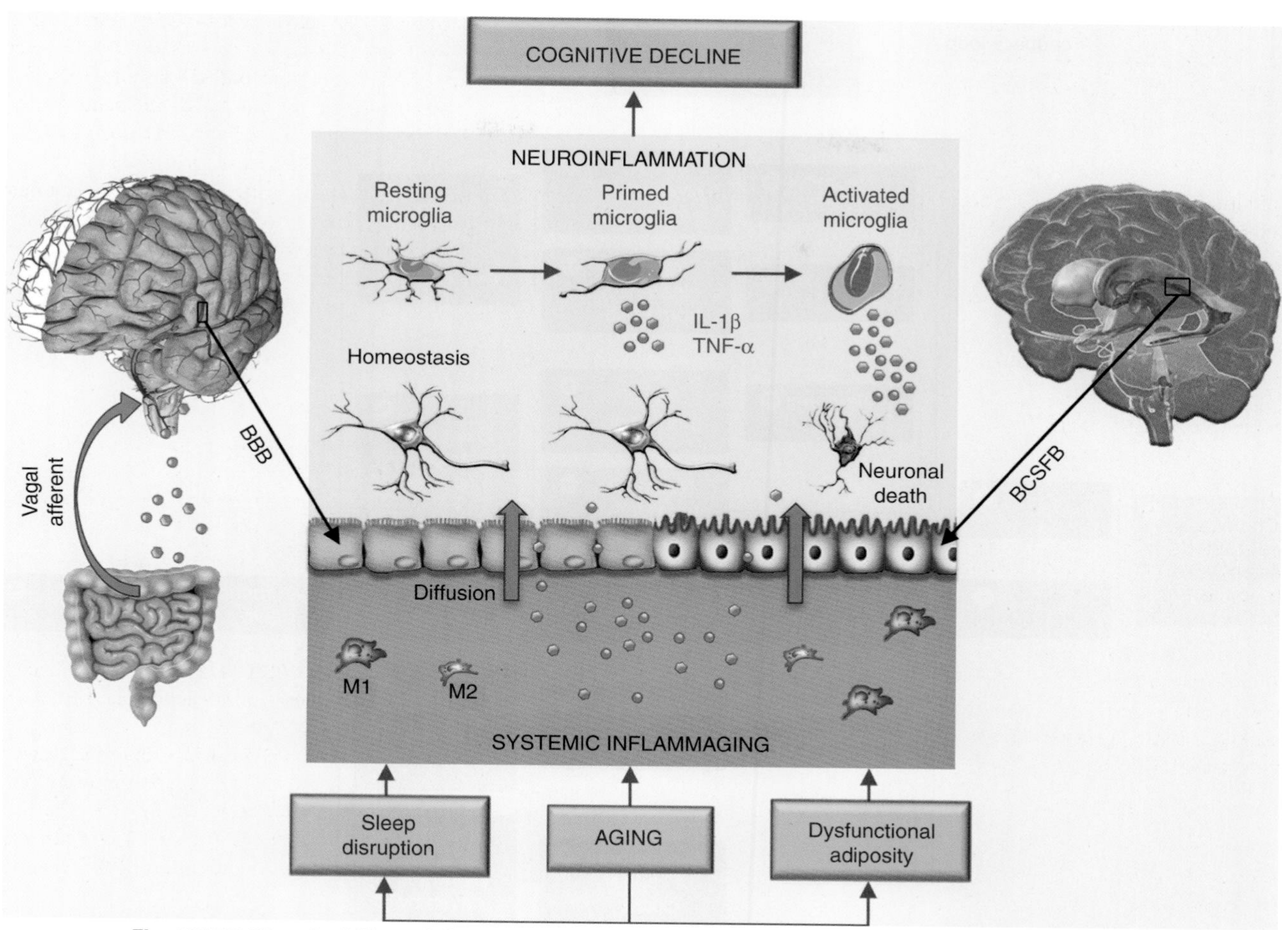


**Fig. 101.56 Disturbed Sleep, Inflammation, and Risk of Alzheimer Disease.** The impact of sleep disruption and dysfunctional aging-related cognitive decline through the common pathway of neuroinflammation. The aging process and its consequences for sleep and regional fat redistribution contribute to low-grade inflammation in the periphery. Systemic inflammation primes microglia through neural and humoral pathways (diffusion across the blood-brain barrier, BBB or blood-cerebrospinal fluid barrier, BCSFB). Primed microglia are activated to enhance synthesis of proinflammatory compounds that ultimately damage the neuron and contribute to cognitive decline. M1: classic macrophage activation; M2: alternative macrophage activation. (*From Atienza, M., Ziontz, J., Cantero, J.L., 2018. Low-grade inflammation in the relationship between sleep disruption, dysfunctional adiposity, and cognitive decline in aging. Sleep Med. Rev. 42, 171–183. ISSN 1087-0792, https://doi.org/10.1016/j.smrv.2018.08.002.*)

described in a family with a progressive neurological illness characterized by insomnia and dysautonomia that terminated in death. Clinical manifestations are impaired control of the sleep/wake cycle, including circadian rhythms; autonomic and neuroendocrine dysfunction; and somatic neurological, cognitive, and behavioral manifestations. Profound sleep disturbances and, in particular, severe insomnia are noted from the very beginning of the illness. PSG shows almost total absence of sleep pattern and only short episodes of REM sleep, lasting for a few seconds or minutes, without muscle atonia. This abnormal sleep pattern is associated with DEB in the form of complex gestures and motions and myoclonus. The terminal stage of the illness is characterized by progressive slowing on the EEG, with the patient drifting into coma. Autonomic function tests reveal evidence of sympathetic hyperactivity with preserved parasympathetic activity. Neuroendocrine functions in FFI show a dysfunction of the pituitary-adrenal axis, as manifested by striking elevation of serum cortisol but normal corticotropin, indicating abnormal feedback suppression of corticotropin. Persistently elevated serum catecholamine levels associated with abnormal secretory patterns of growth hormone, prolactin, and melatonin are noted. The nocturnal secretory peaks of growth hormone are absent. Plasma melatonin levels progressively decrease, and in the most advanced stage of the illness, there is a complete abolition of melatonin rhythm. Somatic neurological manifestations are present in all cases, particularly in the later stage of the illness and consist of dysarthria, dysphagia, ataxia, evidence of pyramidal tract dysfunction, myoclonus, tremor, and bizarre astasia-abasia (Cortelli et al., 2013). Neuropsychological studies reveal impairment of attention, vigilance, and memory. The disease progresses rapidly and ends in coma and death.

The neuropathological hallmark of FFI is severe atrophy of the thalamus, particularly the anterior ventral and dorsomedial thalamic nuclei associated with variable involvement of the inferior olive, striatum, and cerebellum. There are no spongiform changes, except in those with the longest duration of symptoms, who show mild to moderate spongiform degeneration of the cerebral cortex. Severe hypometabolism of the thalamus and mild hypometabolism of the cingulate cortex are the main findings on PET study in FFI

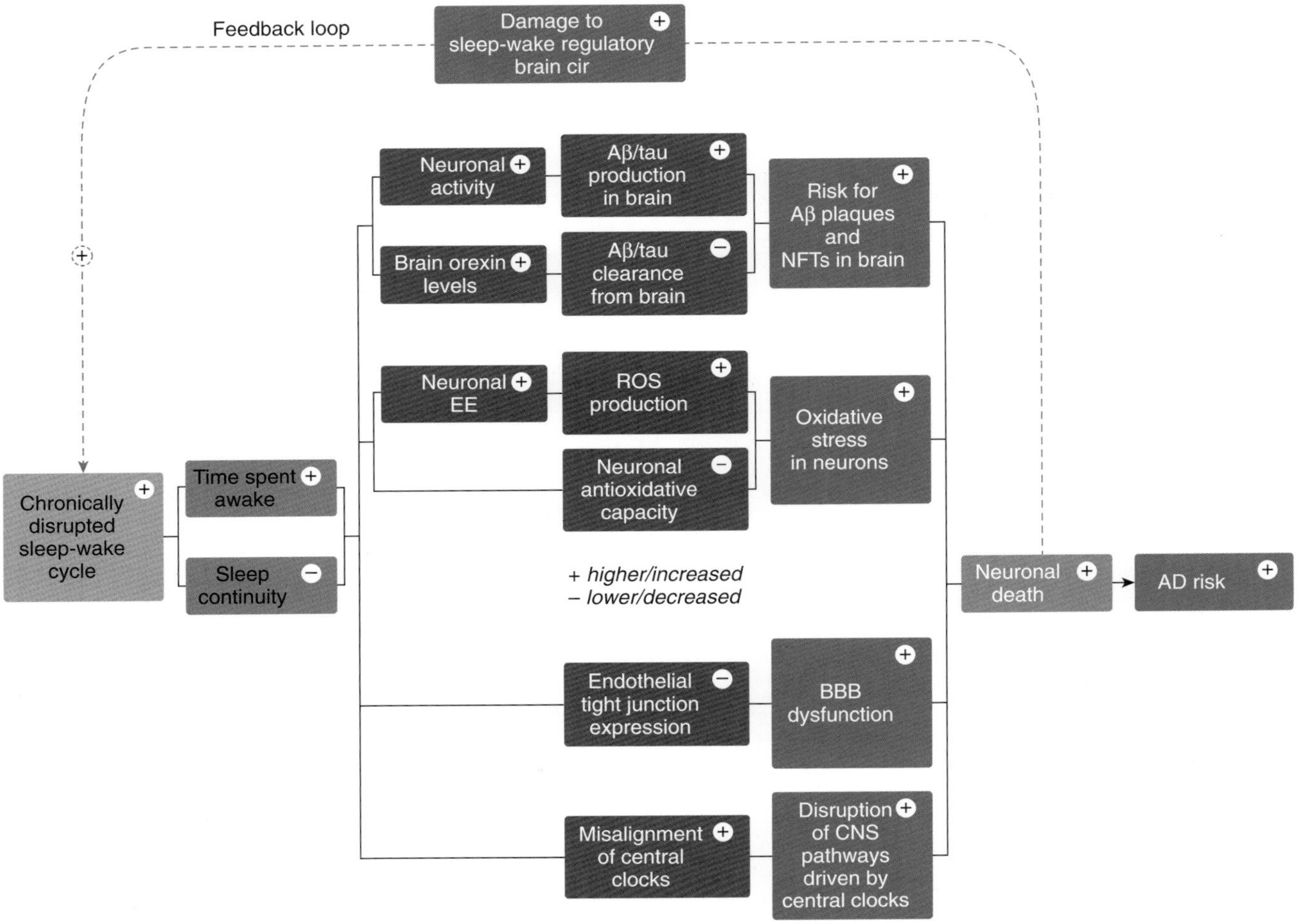

**Fig. 101.57** Overview of proposed mechanisms by which disruptions to the sleep-wake cycle may catalyze AD pathogenesis in humans. *Aβ*, amyloid beta; *AD*, Alzheimer disease; *BBB*, blood–brain barrier; *CNS*, central nervous system; *EE*, energy expenditure; *NFTs*, neurofibrillary tangles.

patients. Based on biochemical, genetic, and transmission studies, it has been concluded that FFI is a transmissible prion disease resulting from a mutation at codon 178 of PrP, associated with substitution of aspartic acid with asparagine along with the presence of a methionine codon at position 129 of the mutant allele. All human prion diseases (e.g., Creutzfeldt-Jakob disease and Gerstmann-Sträussler-Scheinker disease) should be considered in the differential diagnosis. Approximately 30 unrelated families of patients with FFI have been identified so far. FFI has been transmitted to experimental animals and is thus a transmissible prion disease, representing the third most common hereditary prion disease worldwide. Sporadic instances, however, have also been reported. The study of FFI has rekindled investigation of the role of the thalamus in sleep/wake regulation. Gemignani et al. (2012), based on a single case cross sectional EEG study in FFI, showed that the thalamus is essential for the generation of slow-wave sleep, and also suggested a role for prions in sleep regulation. FFI has clinical features in common with delirium tremens and Morvan chorea, leading to the concept of "agrypnia excitata," a clinical condition associated with disruption of a sleep-wake cycle and hyperactivity of the motor, sympathetic, and aminergic systems, and episodes of oneiric stupor related to pathological changes in the thalamolimbic circuits (Lugaresi et al., 2011). In Creutzfeldt-Jakob disease, prominent sleep disruption is noted even in the early stage and is characterized by sleep-onset and maintenance insomnia with daytime hypersomnolence. PSG shows decreased REM sleep, loss of sleep spindles and K complexes, and disruption of REM/NREM cycling similar to that noted in FFI (eFig. 101.58, *A–C*) (Baldelli and Provini, 2019). In FFI, prominent pathological findings include neuronal loss in anteroventral and dorsomedial thalamic nuclei, accounting for the sleep disturbances, but in many cases of Creutzfeldt-Jakob disease, these characteristic neuropathological findings of FFI are lacking.

## Sleep Disorders Associated with Neuromuscular Disorders

Clinicians first became aware of sleep-related respiratory dysrhythmias in patients with neuromuscular diseases by observing hypoventilation in poliomyelitis. Sleep disturbances in neuromuscular diseases are generally due to respiratory dysrhythmias associated with these diseases (Bhat et al., 2012b; Chokroverty, 2011a; Chokroverty et al., 2015). In neuromuscular disorders, sleep disturbances are due to involvement of respiratory muscles, phrenic and intercostal nerves, or neuromuscular junctions of the respiratory and oropharyngeal muscles. The most common complaint is EDS resulting from transient nocturnal hypoxemia and hypoventilation, causing repeated arousals and sleep fragmentation. In addition to the sleep-related respiratory dysrhythmias, some patients—particularly those with painful polyneuropathies, muscle pain, muscle cramps, and immobility due to muscle weakness—may complain of insomnia. Patients with neuromuscular diseases often complain of breathlessness, particularly in the supine position.

Respiratory disturbances are generally noted in the advanced stage of primary muscle disorders or myopathies, but respiratory failure may appear in an early stage. Sleep complaints and sleep-related respiratory dysrhythmias are common in Duchenne and limb–girdle muscular dystrophies as well as in myopathies associated with acid maltase deficiency (Guilleminault and Shegill, 2002). They may also occur in other congenital or acquired myopathies, mitochondrial encephalomyopathy, and polymyositis.

Many patients with myotonic dystrophy have been described with central, mixed, and upper airway OSAS, alveolar hypoventilation, daytime fatigue, and hypersomnolence (Bhat et al., 2012a; Chokroverty et al., 2015; Romigi et al., 2011). Nocturnal oxygen desaturation accompanies alveolar hypoventilation and apneas and worsens during REM sleep. EDS in myotonic dystrophy often occurs in the absence of sleep apnea. An entity called *proximal myotonic myopathy* (PROMM) has been described. PROMM, also called *DM2*, is a hereditary myotonic disorder that is differentiated from myotonic dystrophy by absence of the chromosome 19 CTG trinucleotide repeat that is associated with classic myotonic dystrophy. In PROMM there is mutation of the gene encoding for zinc finger 9 of chromosome 3q21 causing CCTG repeat. Sleep disturbances in these patients consist of difficulty initiating sleep, EDS, snoring, and frequent awakenings during sleep and alpha-NREM intrusion in overnight PSG, which suggests involvement of the REM- and NREM-generating neurons as part of a multisystem membrane disorder (Bhat et al., 2012b; Chokroverty et al., 1997; Chokroverty et al., 2015; Romigi et al., 2014). In some patients (unpublished observations), upper airway OSAs and REM-hypoventilation have also been observed (Bhat et al., 2012b; Chokroverty et al., 2015). Most of the findings are derived from case series. There is also a report of increased prevalence of RLS/WED (Lam et al., 2013a). One female patient with DM2 had RBD (Chokroverty et al., 2012).

In polyneuropathies, involvement of the nerves supplying the diaphragm and the intercostal and accessory muscles of respiration may cause breathlessness on exertion and other respiratory dysrhythmias. These may worsen during sleep, causing sleep fragmentation and daytime hypersomnolence. In painful polyneuropathies, patients may have insomnia.

Neuromuscular junctional disorders (e.g., myasthenia gravis, myasthenic syndrome, botulism, and tic paralysis) are characterized by easy fatigability of the muscles, including the bulbar and other respiratory muscles, as a result of nerve impulses of the neuromuscular junctions not being transmitted. Patients with myasthenia gravis may have central, obstructive, and mixed apneas and hypopneas accompanied by oxygen desaturation (Chokroverty, 2011a). A sensation of breathlessness on awakening in the middle of the night and early-morning hours may indicate respiratory dysfunction. Sleep-related hypoventilation and sleep apnea in neuromuscular junctional disorders may be severe enough to require assisted ventilation (Gonzalez et al., 2002). Impaired sleep quality and RLS/WED are thought to be more prevalent compared with controls in myasthenia gravis patients.

## Sleep and Spinal Cord Diseases

Sleep disturbances related to respiratory dysfunction can occur in some patients with high cervical spinal cord lesions. Patients with poliomyelitis, amyotrophic lateral sclerosis (ALS) affecting the phrenic and intercostal motor neurons in the spinal cord, spinal cord tumors, spinal trauma, spinal surgery (e.g., cervical cordotomy or anterior spinal surgery), and nonspecific or demyelinating myelitis may all have sleep disturbances. The most common symptom is hypersomnia due to sleep-related respiratory arrhythmias. Occasionally, patients with spinal cord diseases may complain of insomnia as a result of immobility, spasticity associated with flexor spasms, neck pain, and central pain syndrome.

***Sleep disturbances in poliomyelitis and postpolio syndrome.*** Respiratory disturbances worsening during sleep may occur in many patients during the acute and convalescent stages of poliomyelitis. Some are left with the sequelae of sleep-related apnea or hypoventilation, requiring ventilatory support, especially at night. Another group of patients develops symptoms decades later that constitute postpolio syndrome, in which sleep disturbances and sleep apnea or hypoventilation have also been noted (Bhat et al., 2012a; Chokroverty, 2011a; Chokroverty and Provini, 2015). Postpolio syndrome is manifested clinically by increasing weakness or wasting of the previously affected muscles and by involvement of previously unaffected regions of the body, fatigue, aches and pains, and sometimes symptoms secondary to sleep-related hypoventilation (e.g., EDS and tiredness).

***Sleep dysfunction in amyotrophic lateral sclerosis.*** ALS, a motor neuron disease, is the most common degenerative disease of the motor neurons in adults, affecting the spinal cord, brainstem, motor cortex, and corticospinal tracts. It is characterized by progressive degeneration of both upper and lower motor neurons, manifesting as a varying combination of lower motor neuron (e.g., muscle weakness, wasting, fasciculation, dysarthria, and dysphagia) and upper motor neuron (e.g., spasticity, hyperreflexia, and extensor plantar responses) signs. ALS can be associated with profound sleep disturbances, which are characterized by EDS as a result of repeated arousals and sleep fragmentation due to nocturnal hypoventilation, recurrent episodes of sleep apnea, hypopnea, hypoxemia, and hypercapnia (Bhat et al., 2012a; Chokroverty, 2011a; Chokroverty et al., 2015). Insomnia may be present in some patients, which is related to other factors such as decreased mobility, muscle cramps, anxiety, and difficulty swallowing. There is no significant relationship between bulbar involvement and severity of SDB or other types of respiratory events. Sleep-related breathing disturbances in ALS may result from weakness of the upper airway, diaphragmatic, and intercostal muscles due to involvement of the bulbar, phrenic, and intercostal motor neurons. In addition, degeneration of central respiratory neurons may occur, causing central and upper airway OSAs. Generally, respiratory failure in ALS occurs late, but occasionally this may be a presenting feature, requiring mechanical ventilation. Diaphragmatic weakness resulting from degeneration of phrenic motor neurons is noted frequently in ALS and is mainly responsible for nocturnal hypoventilation, initially during REM sleep.

## Sleep and Headache Syndromes

Sleep-related headaches are a heterogeneous group of unilateral or bilateral headaches occurring during sleep or on awakening from sleep (AASM, 2014). In day-to-day practice, headaches and sleep complaints are common. Most sleep-related headaches are daytime headaches that may also occur during sleep. The ICSD-III (AASM, 2014) includes cluster headache, chronic paroxysmal hemicrania, migraine, and hypnic headache under the heading of sleep-related primary headaches. PSG recordings in patients with cluster headaches show a strong relationship between REM sleep and attacks of headache. Migraine headaches may occur during the day and both slow-wave and REM sleep. Cluster headaches are thought to be related to REM sleep but may sometimes be triggered by NREM sleep. Chronic paroxysmal hemicrania, which is probably a variant of cluster headache, is most commonly associated with REM sleep. Significant sleep disruption in the form of decreased total and REM sleep time, accompanied by an increased number of awakenings during REM sleep, has been described in patients with chronic paroxysmal hemicrania. PSG recordings have documented sleep apnea in some patients with chronic recurring headache syndromes. The relationship between early-morning headache and upper airway OSAS has been somewhat controversial, with contradictory reports. There are occasional reports of the coexistence of OSAS and cluster headache, with improvement of headache after CPAP titration (Zallek and Chervin, 2000).

An uncommon type of headache syndrome called *hypnic headache syndrome* is described in patients older than 50. The headache awakens the patient from sleep, lasts for at least 15 minutes with a range up to 190 minutes, and with a frequency of at least 15 times per month. In many patients it occurs at a constant time each night. Hypnic headache tends to occur during REM sleep but also has been reported to occur in Stage N3. Hypnic headache syndrome is differentiated from chronic cluster headache by generalized distribution, age of onset, and lack of autonomic manifestation. This disorder often responds to lithium, indomethacin, or caffeine treatment.

Sleep-related secondary headaches include medical (e.g., hypertension), neurological, psychiatric, and primary sleep disorders (e.g., OSAS).

### Stroke and Sleep/Wake Disturbance

Sleep disturbances and sleep complaints have been described in patients with cerebral hemispheric, paramedian thalamic, and brainstem infarctions (Bassetti and Hermann, 2011; Chokroverty et al., 2015; Davis et al., 2013; Dyken et al., 2011; Johnson and Johnson, 2010; Mansukhani et al., 2011). Sleep apnea, snoring, and stroke are intimately related; sleep apnea may predispose to stroke, and stroke may predispose to sleep apnea. There is an increased frequency of sleep apnea in both infratentorial and supratentorial strokes (Bassetti and Hermann, 2011; Bassetti and Valko, 2006; Davis et al., 2013; Johnson and Johnson, 2010; Mansukhani et al., 2011). Based on findings of an AHI of 10 or greater, it has been estimated that approximately 50%–70% of all stroke patients have sleep apnea. The SBDs improve after the acute phase of stroke, but up to 60% of patients may still exhibit AHI of 10 or greater 3 months after the acute event. Many confounding variables such as hypertension, cardiac disease, age, BMI, smoking, and alcohol intake, which are common risk factors for sleep apnea and stroke, must be considered before a clear relationship can be established among these conditions. Reports by Yaggi and colleagues (2005) and Valham et al (2008) demonstrated an increased prevalence of stroke in patients with OSAS following a longitudinal follow-up study. Patients valuated for stroke risk using the Berlin questionnaire determined that up to 60% were at high risk for OSA. They also found that those with a previous diagnosis of OSA were at increased risk of death within the first month after stroke. In an earlier meta-analysis of 29 articles, Johnson and Johnson (2010) found that up to 72% of stroke patients (AHI ≥5) and up to 63% with AHI of ≥10 had SDB (primarily OSA). The meta-analysis also found that OSA was more common in those with recurrent and cryptogenic (unknown etiology) strokes, and the type and location of stroke were irrelevant factors. It is important to make a diagnosis of sleep apnea in stroke patients because of the possible adverse effects on the long-term outcome and because currently available data appear to suggest improvement of long-term survival in those who are compliant with CPAP treatment (Davis et al., 2013), although adherence (compliance) to CPAP treatment remains a problem. The Sleep SMART (Sleep for Stroke Management and Recovery Trial) represnts the first large scale trial designed to evalaute whether positive pressure therpay (PAP) for obstructive sleep apnea after stroke/transient ischemic attack improves/reduces stoke outcome by pospective evaluation for improved functional recovery, rates of recurrent vascular events or death (Brown et al., 2020).

### Traumatic Brain Injury and Sleep Disturbances

TBIs include concussion, contusion, laceration, hemorrhage, and cerebral edema. Insomnia, hypersomnia, and circadian rhythm sleep dysfunction may occur after TBI (Castriotta, 2015; Mathias et al., 2012; Mollayeva et al., 2013), but objective sleep studies documenting sleep disturbances in such patients have not been adequately performed (Rao and Rollings, 2002). After a severe TBI, brainstem function is compromised, and the patient becomes comatose. Many EEG studies have examined patients with coma after head trauma. However, no studies have adequately addressed the sleep/wake abnormalities in these patients after recovery from coma or in patients after minor brain injuries that did not result in coma. Many of these patients experience the so-called post-concussion syndrome, which is characterized by a variety of behavioral disturbances, headache, and sleep/wake abnormalities. A few reports list subjective complaints of sleep disturbance but do not include formal sleep studies. In one report of patients with closed head injury, PSG studies documented sleep-maintenance insomnia with an increased number of awakenings and decreased night sleep. The mechanism of these sleep abnormalities is unknown. Post-traumatic hypersomnia is listed under *hypersomnia due to medical condition* in the ICSD-III (AASM, 2014). TBIs may cause central and upper airway OSA (prevalence may range from 25%–35% (Mollayeva et al., 2013) by inflicting functional or structural alterations on the brainstem respiratory control system. Many of these patients may, however, have had sleep apnea syndrome before sustaining a TBI. Circadian rhythm sleep disturbances have been described in patients with TBI (Ayalon et al., 2007). There are reports of DSPS after TBIs (Quinto et al., 2000; Smits and Nagtegaal, 2000).

### Sleep and Multiple Sclerosis

Sleep-related breathing abnormalities and other sleep difficulties including insomnia, EDS, and depression have been described in patients with MS. Sleep disturbances in MS are thought to result from immobility, spasticity, urinary bladder sphincter disturbances, secondary narcolepsy, RBD, circadian rhythm disturbance, RLS-PLMS, pain, and sleep-related respiratory dysrhythmias due to affected respiratory muscles or impaired central control of breathing (Chokroverty et al., 2015). Fig. 101.59 summarizes the etiology of sleep problems in MS, based on direct and indirect causes.

### Sleep Disorders in Multisystem Atrophy

In a consensus statement by the American Autonomic Society and the American Academy of Neurology (Gilman et al., 1999, 2008), the term *multisystem atrophy* was suggested to replace the term *Shy-Drager syndrome* (see Chapters 96 and 108). MSA defines a sporadic adult-onset progressive disorder of multiple systems characterized by autonomic dysfunction, parkinsonism, and ataxia in various combinations (eBox 101.24).  *Striatonigral degeneration* is the name used when the predominant feature is parkinsonism, whereas *olivopontocerebellar atrophy* is used when the cerebellar features are the predominant manifestations. The term *Shy-Drager syndrome* is still used when the autonomic feature is predominant. Sleep dysfunction is common in MSA and consists of insomnia with sleep fragmentation, RBD, and sleep-related respiratory dysrhythmias (Chokroverty et al., 2015). RBD is common (present in 80%–95% of MSA patients) and may precede the illness, present concomitantly, or present after the onset of MSA (Boeve et al., 2007; Iranzo et al., 2006; Plazzi et al., 1997). PET and SPECT findings indicate that RBD in MSA is related to nigrostriatal dopaminergic deficit (Gilman et al., 2003). The most severe sleep disturbance in patients with MSA results from respiratory dysrhythmias associated with repeated arousals and hypoxemia. Sleep-related respiratory dysrhythmias in MSA may include obstructive, central, or mixed apneas, hypopneas, and Cheyne-Stokes breathing or a variant of Cheyne-Stokes breathing. Other breathing disorders during sleep in MSA are nocturnal inspiratory stridor, apneustic breathing, inspiratory gasping, or dysrhythmic breathing. Hypersomnia often results from nocturnal sleep disruption. Sudden nocturnal death in patients with MSA, presumably from cardiorespiratory arrest, has been reported. The current

SLEEP PROBLEMS IN MULTIPLE SCLEROSIS

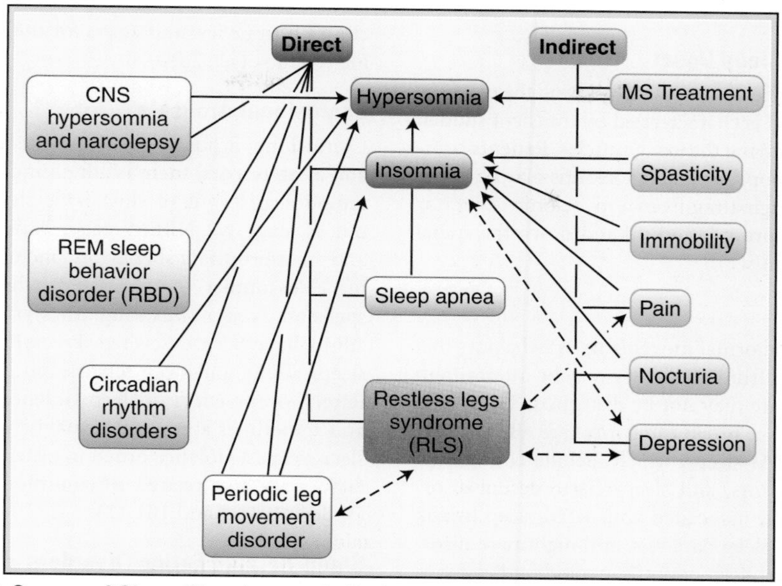

**Fig. 101.59 Direct and Indirect Causes of Sleep Disturbances in Patients with Multiple Sclerosis.** Solid-line arrows demonstrate a causative effect; double dotted-line arrows highlight bidirectional effects discussed in text. (*From Braley, T., Avidan, A., 2011. Sleep in multiple sclerosis. In: Giesser, B., [Ed.] Primer on Multiple Sclerosis. Cambridge.*)

diagnostic criteria including those derived from the second consensus statement (Gilman et al., 2008) consider dementia as a nonsupporting feature, but there is compelling emerging evidence of cognitive impairment (mainly frontal executive dysfunction) in both subtypes of MSA patients (Stankovic et al., 2014). This finding may lead to a future consensus statement to revise the diagnostic criteria.

Both direct and indirect mechanisms are responsible for the pathogenesis of sleep disruption in MSA. These may include one or more of the following: degeneration of the sleep/wake-generating neurons in the brainstem and hypothalamus; degeneration of the respiratory neurons in the brainstem or direct involvement of projections from the hypothalamus and central nucleus of the amygdala to the respiratory neurons in the NTS and nucleus ambiguus; interference with vagal inputs from the peripheral respiratory receptors to the central respiratory neurons; sympathetic denervation of the nasal mucosa, promoting upper airway obstructing apnea; and loss of cholinergic neurons in the medullary arcuate nucleus region, contributing to central alveolar hypoventilation during sleep. SPECT findings by Gilman and colleagues (2003) suggested decreased pontine cholinergic projections to the thalamus as contributing to OSA in MSA.

## Sleep-Related Movement Disorders

This category of sleep-related movement disorders in the ICSD-III (these movements consist of relatively simple stereotyped movements disturbing sleep) includes seven specific disorders: RLS, PLMS, rhythmic movement disorder, bruxism, sleep-related leg cramps, benign sleep myoclonus of infancy, and propriospinal myoclonus at sleep onset (Chokroverty et al., 2013). RLS and PMLS have been described in this chapter.

### Rhythmic Movement Disorder

Rhythmic movement disorder is noted mostly before age 18 months and is a benign condition, which disappears later in childhood. It is a sleep-wake transition disorder with three characteristic movements: head banging, head rolling, and body rocking. Rhythmic movement disorder is a benign condition, and the patient outgrows the episodes.

### Sleep-Related Leg Cramps

These are intensely painful sensations accompanied by muscle tightness that occur during sleep. The spasms usually last for a few seconds but sometimes persist for several minutes. Cramps during sleep are generally associated with awakening. Many normal individuals have nocturnal leg cramps; the cause remains unknown. Local massage or movement of the limbs usually relieves the cramps. Pharmacological therapy, however, has not been shown to provide long-term significant benefit and current practice guidelines have not been conducted.

### Bruxism

Bruxism often presents between age 10 and 20, but it may persist throughout life, often leading to secondary problems such as temporomandibular (TMJ) joint syndrome. Both diurnal and nocturnal bruxism may be associated with various movement and degenerative disorders such as oromandibular dystonia and Huntington disease (Tan et al., 2000). It is also commonly noted in children with mental retardation or cerebral palsy. Nocturnal bruxism is noted most prominently during stages N1 and N2 sleep and REM sleep. The episode is characterized by stereotypical tooth grinding and is often precipitated by anxiety, stress, and dental disease. Occasionally, familial cases have been described. Local injections of botulinum toxin into masseter muscles may be used to prevent dental and TMJ complications (Tan and Jankovic, 2000) and may improve total sleep time as well as the frequency and duration of bruxing episodes (Ondo et al., 2018; Video 101.10).

### Benign Sleep Myoclonus of Infancy

Benign sleep myoclonus of infancy occurs during the first few weeks of life and is generally seen in NREM sleep but sometimes during REM sleep. Episodes often occur in clusters involving arms, legs, and sometimes the trunk. The movements consist of jerky flexion, extension, abduction, and adduction. The condition is benign, needing no treatment.

### Propriospinal Myoclonus at Sleep Onset

Propriospinal myoclonus occurs between wakefulness and the moment of sleep onset *(predormitum)* and is characterized by transient sudden muscle jerks predominantly involving the axial muscles. Patients complain of sleep-onset insomnia. Propriospinal myoclonus may be a special type of spinal myoclonus originating from a myoclonic generator in the midthoracic region with propagation up and down the spinal cord at a very slow speed (3–16 m/sec).

## Parasomnias

*Parasomnias* can be defined as abnormal movements or behaviors that occur in sleep or during arousals from sleep; they may be intermittent or episodic, and sleep architecture may not be disturbed. The ICSD-III classifies parasomnias into three broad categories (see eBox 101.6): disorders of arousal (from NREM sleep), which include confusional arousals, sleepwalking, sleep terrors, and sleep-related eating disorder (SRED); parasomnias usually associated with REM sleep, which include RBD, recurrent isolated sleep paralysis, and nightmare disorder; other parasomnias including sleep enuresis, exploding head syndrome, sleep-related hallucinations, and parasomnia due to drugs or substances, medical conditions, or unspecified.

This classification thus lists 15 items, and some of these entities are rare. Some parasomnias, particularly somnambulism, night terror, confusional arousals, sleep enuresis, RBD, and nightmares may be mistaken for nocturnal seizures, particularly of the complex partial seizures type. The intersection of parasomnias, psychiatric diseases, and nocturnal seizures (as can be appreciated in Fig. 101.60) presents a clinical challenge and a diagnostic enigma. Characteristic clinical features combined with EEG and PSG recordings are essential to differentiate these conditions (Thorpy and Plazzi, 2010). Fig. 101.61 depicts a diagrammatic representation of the common disorders of arousals (NREM parasomnias), based on clinical semiology as a function of time (Derry et al., 2009).

### Somnambulism (Sleepwalking)

Sleepwalking is common in children between the ages of 5 and 12 (eBox 101.25). Sometimes it persists into adulthood or (rarely) begins in adults. Sleepwalking starts with the abrupt onset of motor activity arising out of slow-wave sleep during the first one-third of sleep. Episodes generally last less than 10 minutes. There is a high incidence of positive family history. Injuries and violent activity have been reported during sleepwalking episodes, but generally individuals can negotiate their way around the room. Sleep violence, associated with amnesia to the event, leading to injury and homicide have been reported, and are probably precipitated by conditions that deepen slow-wave sleep such as sleep deprivation, fatigue, concurrent illness, and sedatives (Mahowald et al., 2005; Shneerson, 2009; Siclari et al., 2010). Contrary to prior suggestions, alcohol probably does not play a role in triggering somnambulism (Pressman et al., 2013).

### Sleep Terrors (Pavor Nocturnus)

Sleep terrors also occur during slow-wave sleep (eBox 101.26 and Fig. 101.62). Peak onset is between 5 and 7 years of age. As with sleepwalking, there is a high incidence of familial cases of sleep terror. Episodes of sleep terrors are characterized by intense autonomic and motor symptoms including a loud, piercing scream. Patients appear highly confused and fearful. Many also have a history of sleepwalking episodes. Precipitating factors are similar to those described with sleepwalking. A recent study found that migraine is strongly associated with a history of sleep terrors in adolescents. Therefore, a previous clinical picture compatible with sleep terrors in early life, should prompt the clinician to review and assess for the probability of migraines later in life (Fialho et al., 2013).

### Confusional Arousals

Confusional arousals occur mostly before age 5. As in sleepwalking and sleep terrors, there is a high incidence of familial cases, and the episodes arise out of slow-wave sleep but occasionally may occur out of stage N2 NREM sleep. Patients may have some automatic and inappropriate behavior, including abnormal sexual behavior ("sexsomnia" or sleep sex) when this occurs in adults. Most spells are benign, but sometimes violent and homicidal episodes in adults have been described. Precipitating factors are the same as in sleepwalking and sleep terrors and in adults may also include SDB. Rarely, occurrences of sleep violence homicide have been reported, and sometimes abnormal sexual behavior (sexsomnia) occurs. As in sleep-related violence noted in other arousal disorders, precipitating factors are also related to conditions that deepen slow-wave sleep (Videos 101.11 and 101.12).

### Sleep-Related Eating Disorders

SRED is an important disorder of arousal common in women between the ages of 20 and 30 and consists of recurrent episodes of involuntary eating and drinking during partial arousals from sleep. Patients with SRED display strange eating behavior (e.g., consumption of inedible or toxic substances such as frozen pizza, raw bacon, and cat food). Episodes cause sleep disruption with weight gain; occasionally injury has been reported. The condition can be either idiopathic or comorbid with other sleep disorders (e.g., sleepwalking, RLS-PLMS, OSAS, irregular sleep/wake circadian rhythm disorders, and use of medications such as triazolam, zolpidem, quetiapine, and other psychotropic agents) (Nzwalo et al., 2013; Santin et al., 2014; Winkelman et al., 2011). More recent data highlight an important relationship between amnestic SRED in the setting of RLS misclassified and incorrectly treated with hypnotic agents. Hypnotics, specifically benzodiazepine modulators, could suppress memory and executive function, and therefore disinhibit amnestic SRED, suggesting that the latter could represent a nonmotor manifestation of RLS (Howell and Schenck, 2012). Clinically, it is indeed mandatory to investigate eating behavior in patients presenting with RLS symptoms as abnormal nocturnal eating could be a major risk factor for increased BMI (Antelmi et al., 2014) and poor glucose control in RLS patients with diabetes.

The most common PSG findings are multiple confusional arousals with or without eating, arising predominantly from slow-wave sleep but also from other stages of NREM sleep and occasionally from REM sleep.

### Rapid Eye Movement Sleep Behavior Disorder

RBD is a critically important REM sleep parasomnia seen in older persons (eBox 101.27). A characteristic feature of RBD is intermittent loss of REM sleep-related muscle hypotonia or atonia and the appearance of various abnormal quasi dream enactment motor activities during sleep (Fig. 101.63). The patient experiences violent DEB during REM sleep, often causing self-injury (Fig. 101.64; see Fig. 101. 63) or injury to the bed partner (Iranzo et al., 2009, 2010; Olson et al., 2000; Schenck and Mahowald, 2003; Schenck et al., 2009). Some patients have been known to construct specific restraining contraptions to prevent themselves from enacting their violent dream and sustaining injury, as is illustrated from the author's sleep clinic in Fig. 101.65 (Videos 101.13 and 101.14).

RBD may be idiopathic or secondary; however, most cases are now thought to be secondary and associated with neurodegenerative diseases. It is seen with increasing incidence in patients with PD, MSA,

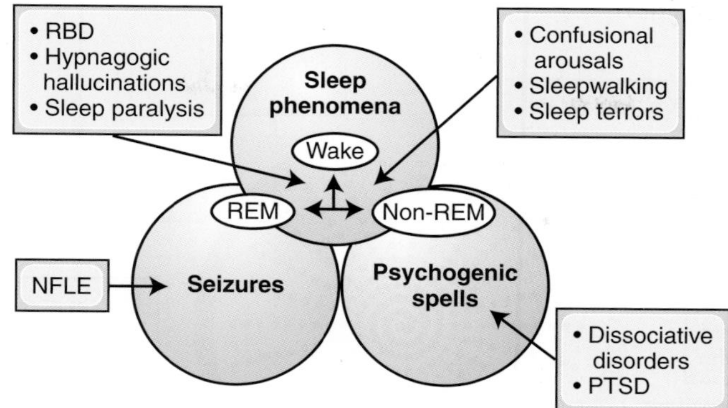


**Fig. 101.60 Overlapping States of Being as Described by Mahowald and Schenck.** Parasomnias are explainable on the basic notion that sleep and wakefulness are not mutually exclusive states but may dissociate and oscillate rapidly. The abnormal admixture of the three states of being—nonrapid eye movement *(NREM)* sleep, REM sleep, and wakefulness—may overlap, giving rise to parasomnias. REM parasomnias are due to the abnormal intrusion of wakefulness into REM sleep, and NREM parasomnias such as sleepwalking are due to abnormal intrusions of wakefulness into NREM sleep. Other nocturnal spells that may be confused with parasomnias include nocturnal frontal lobe epilepsy *(NFLE)* and psychogenic spells such as post-traumatic stress disorder *(PTSD)* and dissociative disorders. *RBD*, REM sleep behavior disorder.

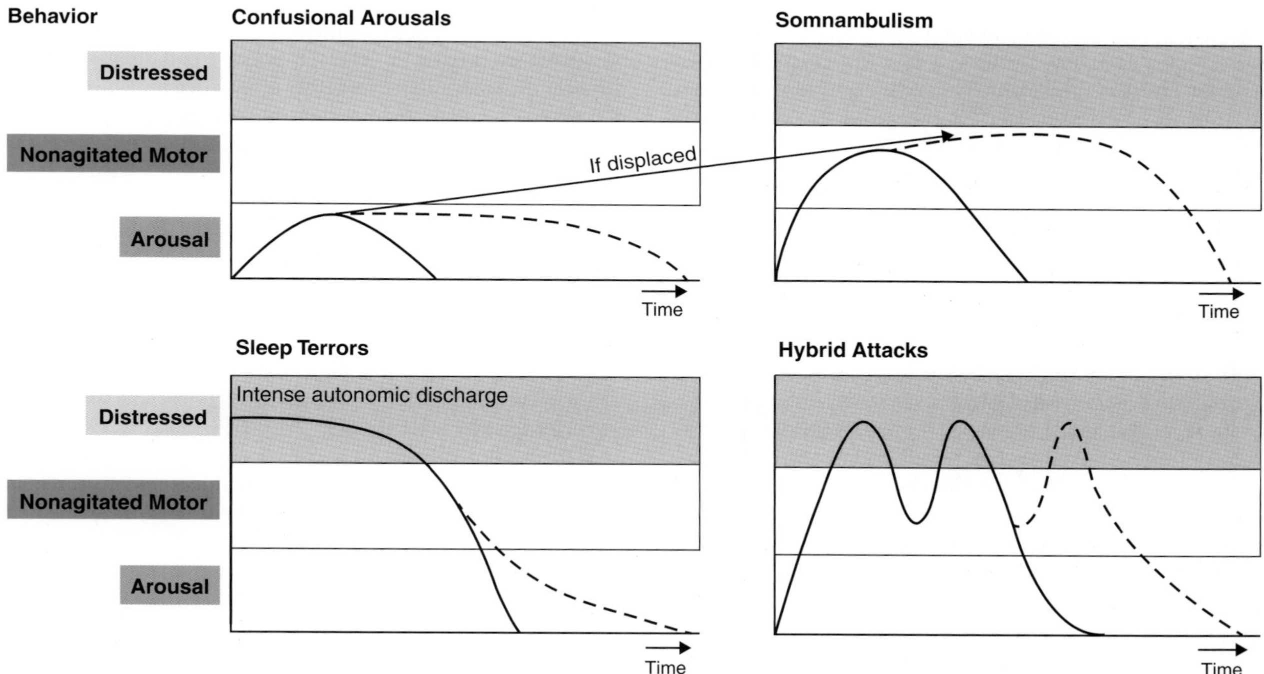


**Fig. 101.61** Diagrammatic representation of the common disorders of arousals (nonREM parasomnias), based on clinical semiology, represented as hierarchical combinations of the 3 fundamental behavior states on the *y* axis (Arousal ➔ nonagitated motor ➔ distressed state) and as a function of time (1–10 min) on the x axis. Panel 1 represents a typical confusional arousal spell. The parasomnia consists of normal arousal behaviors but of abnormal duration only. Panel 2 depicts a classic somnambulistic event comprised of normal arousal behaviors at onset, proceeding to nonagitated motor behavior. Panel 3 illustrates typical sleep terrors, beginning with a distressed, predominantly negative emotional behavior of sudden onset. Motor and normal arousal behaviors are usually also seen during these events, either at onset or offset. Panel 4 is a mixed type, an admixture of two arousal disorders, comprising waxing and waning of the multiple behavior types. All events usually start in stage N3 NREM sleep and terminate either in wakefulness or lighter NREM sleep. The episodes are typically brief (solid lines) but can sometimes be prolonged (hatched lines). (*From Derry, C.P., Harvey, A.S., Walker, M.C., Duncan, J.S., Berkovic, S.F., 2009. NREM arousal parasomnias and their distinction from nocturnal frontal lobe epilepsy: A video EEG analysis. Sleep 32 [12], 1637–1644.*)

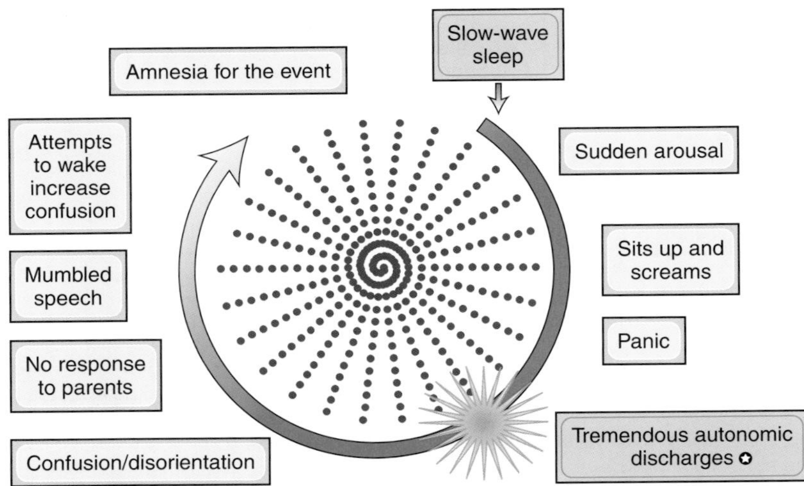


**Fig. 101.62** Sleep terrors are characterized by a sudden arousal associated with a scream, agitation, panic, and heightened autonomic activity. Inconsolability is almost universal. The child is incoherent and has altered perception of the environment, appearing confused. This behavior may potentially be dangerous and could result in injury.

corticobasal degeneration, DLBD, olivopontocerebellar atrophy, and PSP. Many patients with narcolepsy, a probable autoimmune disease causing depletion, may also present with RBD. Some authors (Boeve, 2010; Boeve et al., 2001, 2007) proposed that RBD may be an α-synucleinopathy disorder, because α-synuclein inclusions have been observed in many of the associated neurodegenerative diseases (e.g., PD, MSA, and DLBD). RBD may precede many of these degenerative diseases (Classen et al., 2010). One recent study from Spain demonstrates a "dose response" relationship between the onset of "prodromal" form of RBD to isolated RBD and later on to the development of a neurodegenerative syndrome (Fig. 101.66). The time interval between the emergence of IRBD diagnosis to neurodegenerative disorder phenoconversion was 33.1% at 5 years, 75.7% at 10 years, and 90.9% at 14 years, with a median conversion time of 7.5 years (Iranzo et al., 2014), as depicted in Fig. 101.67. Data from other cohorts reveal a similar trend, with a 5-year risk of neurodegenerative disease of 17.7%, 10-year risk of 40.6%, and a 12-year risk of 52.4% (Postuma et al., 2009). A follow-up by the group which initially discovered RBD as a sleep diagnosis recently revealed that often following a prolonged dormant interval, the majority of patients initially diagnosed with iRBD eventually developed a parkinsonian disorder or dementia, where the specificity of iRBD converting to parkinsonism/dementia is striking (Schenck et al., 2013a).

Studies have demonstrated several potential markers of neurodegenerative diseases in idiopathic RBD (Iranzo et al., 2010; Postuma et al., 2009a, 2009b, 2010a, 2010b, 2010c; Stockner et al., 2009). These markers may be present along with RBD in the "prodromal" phase of the disorder and include a heterogeneous set of biomarkers including impaired cognition, visuospatial dysfunction, impaired color vision, olfactory deficits, autonomic dysfunction (particularly orthostatic hypotension), EEG slowing, midbrain hyperechogenicity, and decreased dopamine transporter imaging. RBD may sometimes be drug induced (e.g., sedative-hypnotics, tricyclic antidepressants, anticholinergics) or associated with alcoholism and structural brainstem lesions. RBD has been linked to dopamine cell dysfunction, based on PET scan findings of reduced striatal presynaptic dopamine transporter and SPECT scan findings of reduced postsynaptic dopamine $D_2$ receptors.

Experimentally, similar behavior has been noted after bilateral perilocus coeruleus lesions in cats and a current putative neuroanatomical explanation implicated the glutamatergic pontine SLD as the key factor for RBD (Krenzer et al., 2013). A possible pathophysiological scheme to help the reader appreciate RBD is provided in Fig. 101.68.

RSWA is the most important phenotype based on PSG findings. However, when formal polysomnography is not available or cannot be obtained, one can employ a number of well validated questionnaires to help establish a probable RBD diagnosis to facilitate time-sensitive assessment, enhance the diagnostic accuracy, and allow for monitoring of disease progress of RBD (Lam et al., 2013b). At our center, we employ the Mayo Sleep Questionnaire (MSQ), which asks bed partners of patients with the suspected condition if they have ever seen the patient appear to "act out his/her dreams" while sleeping (i.e., punching or flailing arms in the air, shouting, or screaming) (Boeve et al., 2013). The MSQ yielded a sensitivity of 100% and specificity (SP) of 95% for the diagnosis of RBD.

The author points out a crucial message that RBD provides an important window with important clinical and research implications in the converging disciplines of neurology, sleep medicine, and neuroscience, highlighting the impotence of conducting future prospective research analysis evaluating putative neuroprotective agents to slow down and delay the progression to parkinsonism (Schenck et al., 2013a). The International Rapid Eye Movement Sleep Behavior Disorder Study Group (IRBD-SG) has recently published that while iRBD patients are ideal candidates for neuroprotective studies, to date there are no agents with proven evidence of either disease-modification or neuroprotective properties in PD (Schenck et al., 2013b). Nevertheless, the IRBD-SG provides an important platform for international collaboration to develop studies on RBD reviewing the role of environmental risk factors for iRBD, and candidate active treatment studies for both symptomatic and neuroprotective therapy (Schenck et al., 2013b). One recent imitative is the development of the North American Prodromal Synucleinopathy (NAPS) Consortium which facilitates collaborative efforts across geographically diverse institutions to help shed more light on characterizing RBD phenotypes with the shared purpose of planning for a clinical trials which

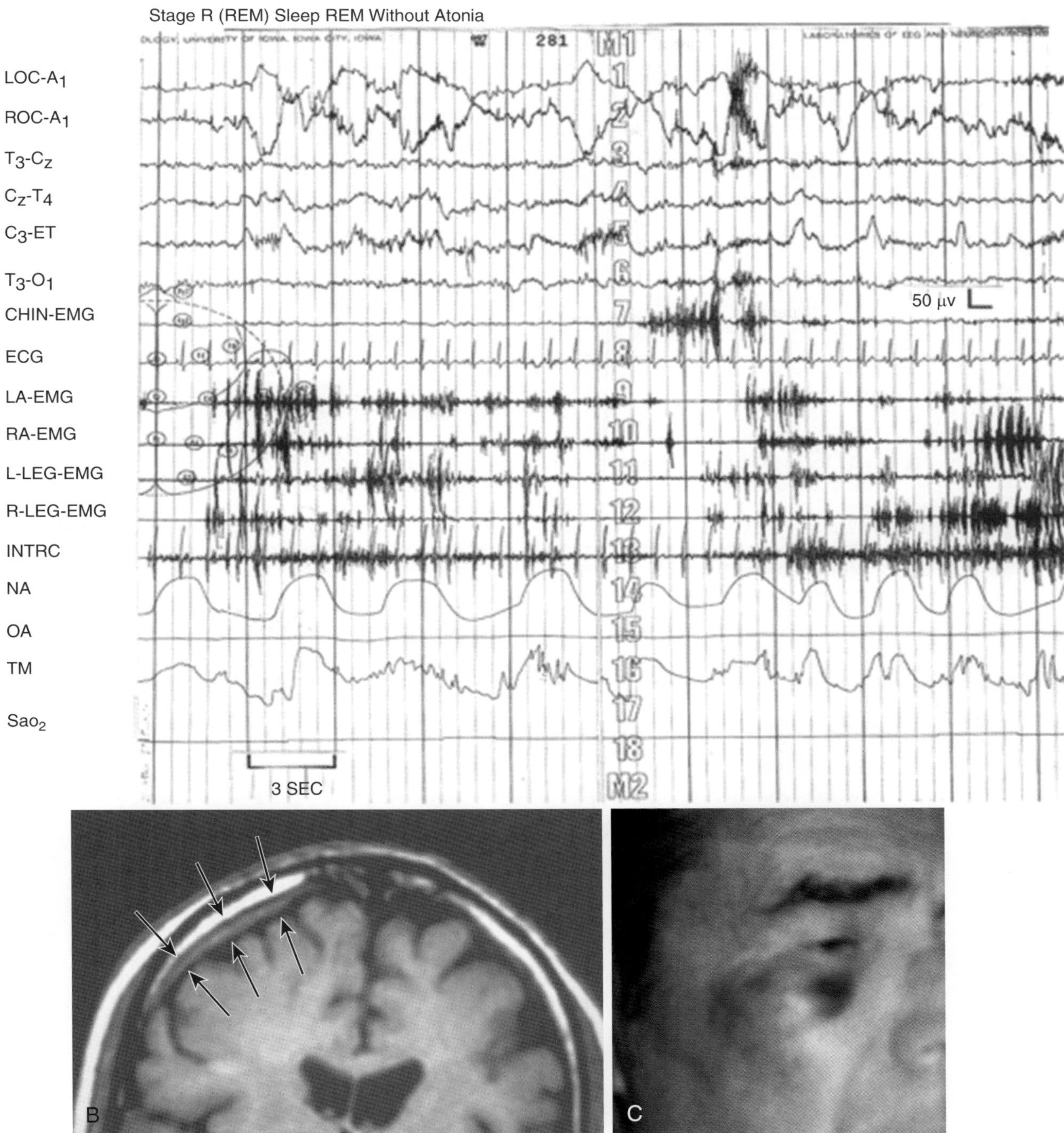


**Fig. 101.63 The Rapid Eye Movement Sleep Behavior Disorder Leading to a Subdural Hemorrhage in a 73-Year-Old Man with a Decade History of Aggressive Dream Enactment Behavior. A,** The nocturnal polysomnograph depicts an unusually high level of electromyographic (EMG) augmentation during rapid eye movement sleep consistent with REM Sleep Without Atonia (RSWA). *ET,* Ears tied; *O,* occipital; *INTRC,* intercostal EMG; *LA,* left arm; *L-LEG,* left leg; *LOC,* Left outer canthus; *NA,* nasal airflow; *OA,* oral airflow; *RA,* right arm; *R-LEG,* right leg; *ROC,* right outer canthus; *T,* temporal; *C,* central; *TM,* thoracic movement. **B,** A magnetic resonance imaging scan of the brain and brainstem showed a right subdural hematoma following an injury sustained during a dream enactment. **C,** Physical examination demonstrating skin abrasion and right infraorbital hematoma. (*A, From Dyken, M.E., Yamada, T., Lin-Dyken, D.C., 2001. Polysomnographic assessment of spells in sleep: nocturnal seizures versus parasomnias. Semin. Neurol. 21 [4], 377–390; B, C, From Dyken, M.E., Lin-Dyken, D.C., Seaba, P., et al., 1995. Violent sleep-related behavior leading to subdural hemorrhage. Arch Neurol. 52, 318–321.*)

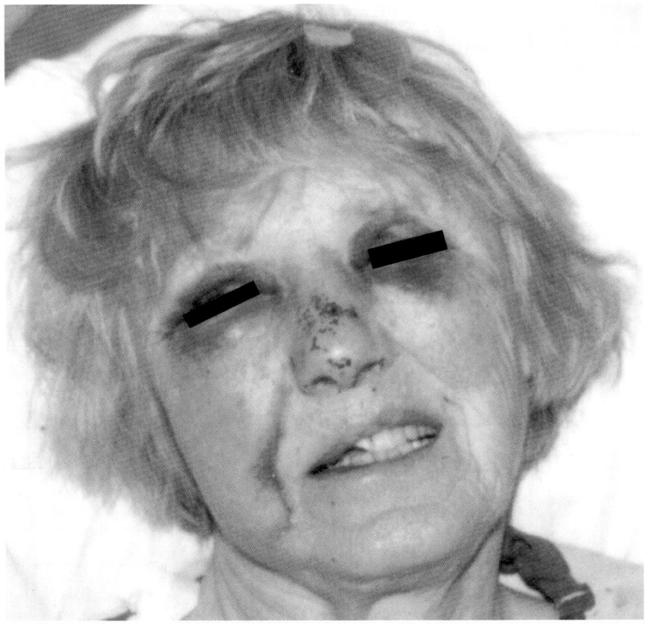

**Fig. 101.64** Photograph of a 74-year-old patient with REM sleep behavior disorder (RBD) who experienced severe facial and dental injuries following a dream enactment episode when she "dove out of her bed" and landed on the corner of a piece of furniture. This example exemplifies the need to carefully assess the bedroom environment of patients with this REM parasomnia and intervene by removing sharp objects and furniture (Level A evidence) and when appropriate intervene with pharmacological treatment using clonazepam or melatonin (Level B evidence). (*From Schenck, C.H., Lee, S.A., Bornemann, M.A., Mahowald, M.W., 2009. Potentially lethal behaviors associated with rapid eye movement sleep behavior disorder: Review of the literature and forensic implications. J. Forensic Sci. 54 [6], 1475–1484.*)

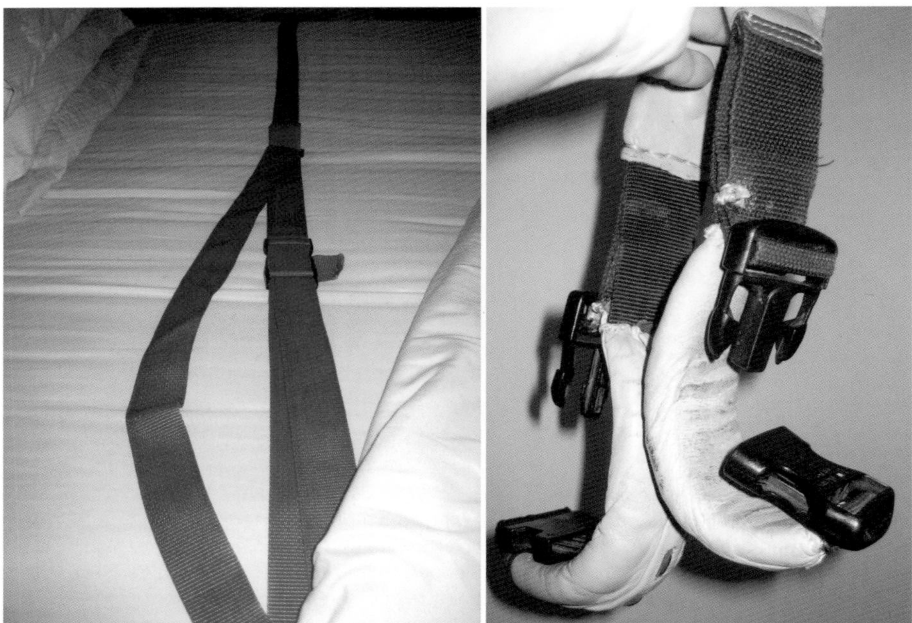

**Fig. 101.65** Set of handcuffs and mattress belt constructed by a 65-year-old man with a history of dream enactment episodes to prevent himself from moving and hurting himself and his wife. The nocturnal episodes became extremely dangerous in the last few months before presentation at a sleep disorder clinic. (*From Avidan, A.Y., 2009. Parasomnias and movement disorders of sleep. Semin. Neurol. 29, 372–392.*)

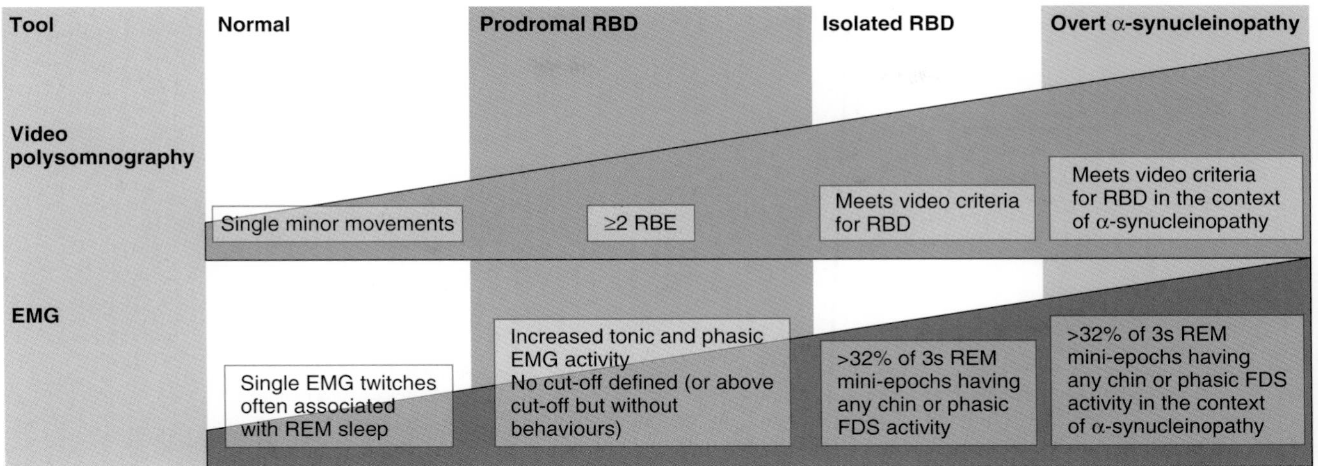


**Fig. 101.66** The New Concept of Prodromal Rapid Eye Movement Sleep Behavior Disorder. Neurophysiological and behavioral findings on polysomnography and signature EMG (electromyography) findings of augmented tone probably represent the earliest sign of an emergent α-synucleinopathy which progress along a continuum over time. From initially normal findings, patients enter a prodromal stage of rapid eye movement (REM) sleep behavior disorder (RBD) that progresses into isolated RBD, and eventually into RBD with overt α-synucleinopathy. *FDS*, Flexor digitorum superficialis; *RBEs*, REM sleep behavioral events. (*From Högl, B., Stefani, A., Videnović, A., 2018. Idiopathic REM sleep behaviour disorder and neurodegeneration—an update. Nat. Rev. Neurol. 14, 40–55.*)

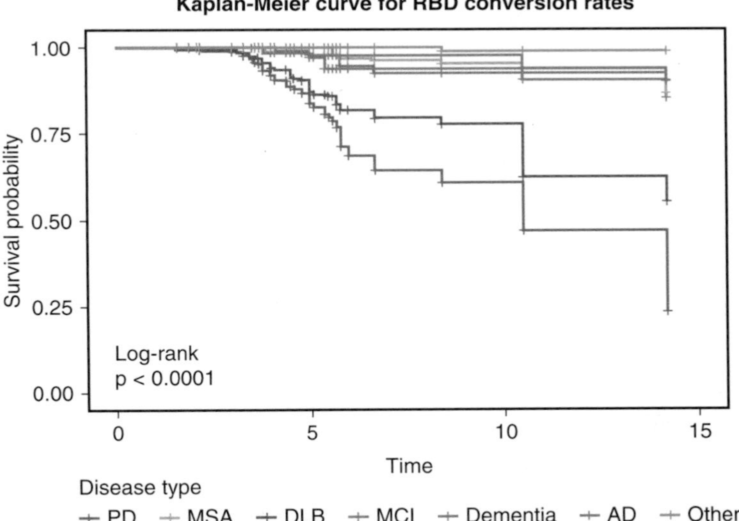


**Fig. 101.67** Rates of neurological-disease-free-survival according to the time of iRBD diagnosis in a sample of 174 patients from Spain utilizing Kaplan-Meier analysis. There is a "dose response" relationship between the years since documenting RBD episodes to phenoconversion to a neurodegenerative disease in the following relationship: 5 years -> 33%, 10 years -> 76%, 14 years -> 91%. Emerging diagnoses were dementia with Lewy bodies (DLB), Parkinson disease (PD), multiple system atrophy (MSA), and mild cognitive impairment (MCI). (*From Iranzo, A., Fernández-Arcos, A., Tolosa, E., et al., 2014. Neurodegenerative disorder risk in idiopathic REM sleep behavior disorder: study in 174 Patients. PLoS ONE 9 [2], e89741.*)

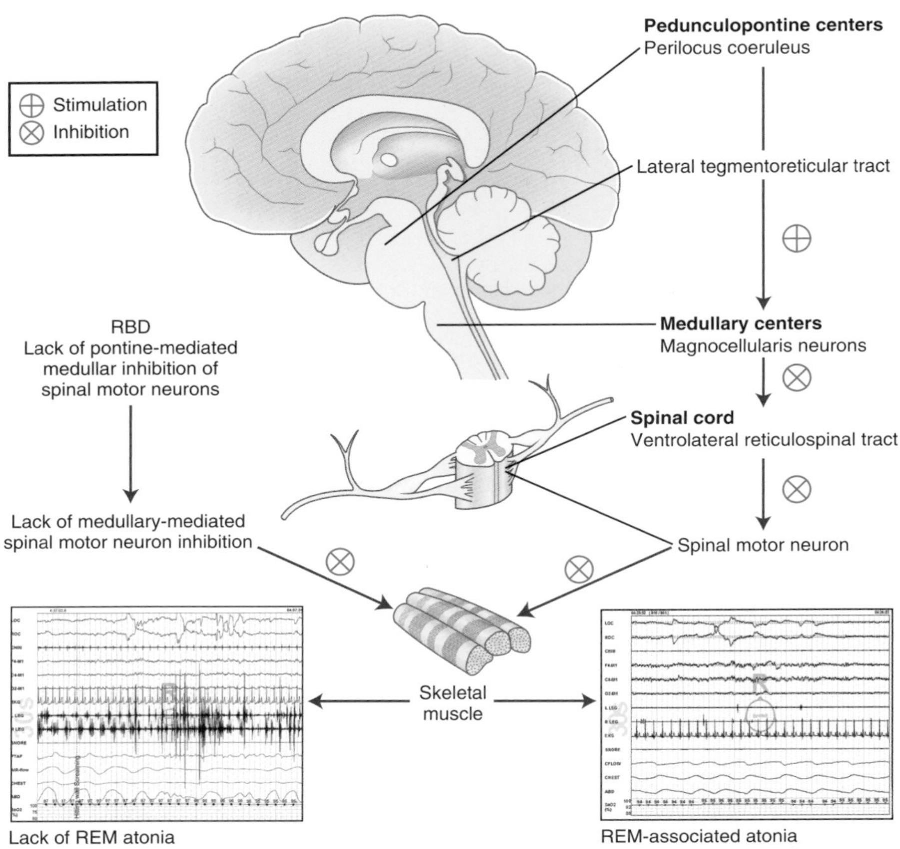


**Fig. 101.68** The normally generalized muscle atonia during rapid eye movement (REM) sleep results from pontine-mediated peri-locus coeruleus inhibition of motor activity. This pontine activity exerts an excitatory influence on medullary centers (magnocellularis neurons) via the lateral tegmentoreticular tract. These neuronal groups in turn hyperpolarize the spinal motor neuron postsynaptic membranes via the ventrolateral reticulospinal tract. In REM sleep behavior disorder (RBD), the brainstem mechanisms generating the muscle atonia normally seen in REM sleep may be disrupted. The pathophysiology of RBD in humans is based on the cat model. In the cat model, bilateral pontine lesions result in a persistent absence of REM atonia associated with prominent motor activity during REM sleep, similar to that observed in RBD in humans. The pathophysiology of the idiopathic form of RBD in humans is still not very well understood but may be related to reduction of striatal presynaptic dopamine transporters. (*Modified with permission from Avidan, A.Y., 2005. Sleep disorders in the older patient, In: Lee-Choing, T. [Guest Ed.], Primary Care: Clinics in Office Practice, vol. 32, Sleep Medicine. Elsevier, St. Louis, pp. 563–586.*)

would be ready to enroll patients for treatments trials in the hope of delaying/preventing neurodegenerative diseases before the condition is irreversible (https://www.naps-rbd.org/ https://clinicaltrials.gov/ct2/show/NCT03623672 Vvidenovic A, Ju Y-eS, Arnulf i, *et al. J Neurol Neurosurg Psychiatry* 2020;**91**:740–749.).

## Nightmares (Dream Anxiety Attacks)

Nightmares are fearful, vivid, often frightening dreams, mostly visual but sometimes auditory, and seen during REM sleep. Nightmares may accompany sleep talking and body movements. These most commonly occur during the middle to late part of sleep at night. Nightmares are mostly a normal phenomenon. Up to 50% of children, perhaps even more, have nightmares beginning at age 3–5 years. The incidence of nightmares continues to decrease as the child grows older, and elderly individuals have very few or no nightmares. Very frightening and recurring nightmares (e.g., one or more per week) are not common and may occur in a very small percentage (<1%) of individuals. Nightmares can also occur as side effects of certain medications such as antiparkinsonian drugs (pergolide, levodopa), anticholinergics, and antihypertensive drugs, particularly beta-blockers. Nightmares are common after sudden withdrawal of REM sleep-suppressant drugs (e.g., tricyclic antidepressants, SSRIs). Benzodiazepines (e.g., diazepam, clonazepam) often suppress nightmares, but withdrawal from these drugs may precipitate nightmares. Nightmares have also been reported after alcohol ingestion or sudden withdrawal from barbiturates. Nightmares may sometimes be the initial manifestation of schizophreniform psychosis, along with severe sleep disturbance. Many people with a certain personality type have nightmares throughout life. Nightmares generally do not require any treatment except reassurance. In patients with recurring and fearful nightmares, however, combined behavioral or psychotherapy and REM sleep-suppressant medications may be helpful.

### Isolated Symptoms, Apparently Normal Variants, and Unresolved Issues

This category (see eBox 101.6), listed under a separate sleep disorder in ICSD-II, has been eliminated as a separate category in ICSD-III and incorporated into the seven major categories of sleep which are most relevant to these entities. These isolated symptoms and normal variants include long sleeper, short sleeper, snoring, sleep talking, sleep starts, benign sleep myoclonus of infancy, hypnagogic foot tremor, alternating leg muscle activation during sleep, and excessive fragmentary myoclonus (EFM).

#### Sleep Talking *(Somniloquy)*

Sleep talking is apparently very common, occurring in as many as 50% of children. Sleep talking that significantly disturbs others is rare. In adults, sleep talking seems to be more common in males than in females, and it has a familial tendency. Clinically, sleep talking consists of utterances of speech or sounds that occur during the sleep episode without awareness of the event. The episodes are generally brief, infrequent, and devoid of signs of emotional stress. The course is usually self-limited and benign.

#### Catathrenia (Expiratory Groaning)

This is characterized by recurrent episodes of expiratory groaning (high-pitched, loud humming, or roaring sounds) and occurs in clusters, predominantly during REM sleep, but it may also occur during NREM sleep. PSG findings resemble central apnea with protracted expiratory bradypnea without oxygen desaturation. Simultaneous audio recordings will bring out the characteristic groaning. The clinical relevance and pathophysiology of this condition remain unknown.

#### Sleep Starts

Additional text available at http://expertconsult.inkling.com.

#### Pediatric Sleep Disorders

Despite a high incidence of sleep disturbance in children, the field of pediatric sleep disorders remains neglected. Several recent surveys found that approximately 25% of children aged 1–5 years have some kind of sleep problem. Mentally handicapped children and those with ADHD and Tourette syndrome have higher rates of sleep disorders than normal children (Hanna et al., 2013). The common sleep problems in children include a variety of parasomnias such as sleepwalking, nightmares, sleep talking, sleep enuresis, bruxism, sleep terrors, and rhythmic movement disorder; sleeplessness due to a specific childhood-onset disorder or food allergy; EDS (e.g., narcolepsy or OSA); and DSPS or ASPS. ICSD-III (AASM, 2014) does not separately list pediatric sleep disorders but these are scattered throughout other categories. Some specific examples include OSA, pediatric; congenital central alveolar hypoventilation syndrome; primary CSA of infancy; primary CSA of prematurity; irregular sleep wake rhythm disorders in childhood autism spectrum disorder, and ADHD. ADHD should be conceptualizing as a 24-hour disorder with significant relevance to sleep which requires the clinician to evaluate sleep/wake schedule patterns and sleep symptoms such as sleepiness, snoring, leg discomfort as potential opportunities for interventions in individuals with ADHD (Becker, 2020).

*Behavioral insomnia of childhood* includes difficulty falling asleep, staying asleep, or both, related to specific behavior such as inappropriate sleep-onset associations or inadequate limit setting. *Sleep-onset association* includes impairment of sleep onset because of the absence of a certain object or set of circumstances (e.g., using a bottle, sucking on a pacifier, being rocked, watching television, or listening to the radio). Sleep is normal when the particular association is present. *Limit-setting type* is characterized by child's stalling or refusing to go to sleep at an appropriate time as a result of inadequate enforcement of bedtime by the caregiver. As the child grows older, behavioral insomnia generally resolves.

***Obstructive sleep apnea in children.*** OSAS occurs in children, but there are certain differences from OSAS in adults (AASM, 2014). Children may present with EDS, but common symptoms include hyperactivity and behavioral problems during the daytime, impaired school performance, intellectual changes, increased motor activity, disturbed sleep at night, and nocturnal snoring for many months or years (eBox 101.28). Some young children may have obstructive 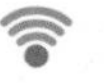 hypoventilation consisting of prolonged periods of partial upper airway obstruction associated with oxygen desaturation and hypercapnia. Obstructive hypoventilation with continuous snoring as well as paradoxical breathing are commonly present in children. Another important feature is that the upper airway obstruction is noted predominantly in REM sleep. All apneic episodes may not be followed by cortical arousals, but they do have autonomic activation following the apneic episodes. Sleep architecture in children with OSA is often normal with an adequate amount of slow-wave sleep. Some children may have UARS with a similar presentation as in adults. An important cause in children is enlargement of tonsils and adenoids. If OSAS is suspected, an overnight PSG study is indicated for documenting OSA. In contrast to adults, removal of the tonsils and adenoids in children promotes symptomatic improvement. Some occurrences of sudden infant death syndrome have been linked to sleeping in the prone position, and every attempt must be made to keep the infant in the supine position.

*Primary sleep enuresis* (listed under other parasomnia in the ICSD-III) is a condition of recurrent involuntary bedwetting after age 5 years occurring at least twice a week and present for at least 3 months in a patient who has never been consistently dry during sleep for 6 consecutive months (AASM, 2014). If the child or adult began to have bed wetting at least twice a week for at least 3 months after remaining dry for 6 consecutive months, then it is considered secondary sleep enuresis. Enuretic episodes occur during all stages of sleep, most commonly during the first one-third of the night. SBD is reported in 8%–47% of children with enuresis. Treatment includes behavioral modification and tricyclic antidepressants (e.g., imipramine) and desmopressin, either as a nasal spray or tablets.

ADHD includes symptoms of *inattention* and *hyperactivity/impulsivity*. There is an increased prevalence of RLS, PLMS, and sleep disordered breathing (DB) in children with ADHD. It is important to diagnose associated conditions such as SDB because treatment of the condition may improve the patient's symptoms of inattention and hyperactivity.

## LABORATORY ASSESSMENT OF SLEEP DISORDERS

Laboratory investigation for sleep disorders should be considered an extension of the history and physical examination. First and foremost, in the diagnosis of a sleep disorder is a detailed history, including sleep and other conditions, as outlined under Approach to a Patient with Sleep Complaints. This should be followed by a careful physical examination to uncover any underlying medical, neurological, or other causes of sleep dysfunction. Laboratory tests should include a diagnostic workup for the primary condition causing secondary sleep disturbance and a workup for the sleep disturbance itself. The two most important laboratory tests for diagnosis of sleep disturbance are PSG and the MSLT. Various other tests are also important for assessment of a patient with sleep dysfunction (Box 101.29).

#### Polysomnographic Study

An overnight PSG study is the single most important laboratory test for the diagnosis and treatment of patients with sleep disorders, particularly those associated with EDS. An all-night PSG study is

**BOX 101.29 Diagnostic Tests for Assessing Sleep Disorder**

- Diagnostic workup for the primary or comorbid condition causing sleep disturbance
- Laboratory tests for the diagnosis and monitoring of sleep disorders:
  Overnight polysomnography (PSG)
  Specialized PSG (i.e., with electroencephalography (EEG)/EMG montage to evaluate for nocturnal seizures, RBD, other parasomnias and movement disorders of sleep.
  Multiple sleep latency tests (MSLT)
  Maintenance of wakefulness test (MWT)
  Actigraphy
  Video-PSG with multiple muscle montage
- Laboratory tests for suspected seizure disorders
  Standard EEG
  Video-EEG monitoring for suspected seizure disorders
  Video-PSG with special seizure montage
- Imaging studies:
  Upper airway imaging for obstructive sleep apnea syndrome
  Neuroimaging studies (e.g., computed tomography, magnetic resonance imaging [MRI], MR-angiography, diffusion tensor MRI, and MR tractography) and cerebral angiography in cases of suspected neurological illness causing sleep disorder
  Positron emission tomography and single-photon emission computed tomography in special situations
  Positron emission tomography (PET) with Fludeoxyglucose (FDG)/amyloid imaging
  Cardiac MIBG scintigraphy and midbrain transcranial sonography in idiopathic RBD to uncover preclinical markers for neurodegeneration
  Fiberoptic endoscopy and cephalometric radiographs of the cranial base and facial bones to locate site of the upper airway collapse, and to assess posterior airway space in OSA patients
- Miscellaneous tests:
  Standard blood and urine analysis
  Pulmonary function tests including arterial blood gases (ABGs) in cases of suspected bronchopulmonary and neuromuscular disorders causing sleep-disordered breathing
  Histocompatibility leukocyte antigen for suspected narcolepsy (HLA DQB1*0602)
  Cerebrospinal fluid hypocretin-1 levels in suspected narcolepsy (1 narcolepsy had measured CSF concentrations below 110 ng/mL in this assay [mean value of <50 pg/mL]) CSF amyloid-β42 and tau protein.
  Serum iron, ferritin levels and transferrin for patients with RLS
  Electromyography and nerve conduction studies to exclude comorbid or secondary RLS
  Cardiological investigations including electrocardiogram (EKG), Holter EKG, and echocardiogram
  Endocrine tests
  Autonomic function tests in patients with suspected autonomic and sleep-related breathing disorders
- Home Sleep Apnea Tests (HSAT)
  Indications
  May be alternatives for the initial evaluation of OSA in patients with a high pretest probability for the conditions
  Contraindications to portable sleep study:
  1. Pediatric setting/patient is 18 years old or younger
  2. Moderate or severe chronic obstructive pulmonary disease (COPD)—$FEV_1/FVC$ less than or equal to 0.7 and $FEV_1$ less than 80% of predicted
  3. Moderate or severe congestive heart failure (CHF)—NYHA class III or IV
  4. Cognitive impairment (inability to follow simple instructions)
  5. Neuromuscular impairment
  6. Suspicion of a sleep disorder other than OSA (e.g., central sleep apnea, narcolepsy, restless legs syndrome, circadian rhythm disorder, parasomnias, periodic limb movement disorder)
  7. Previous technically suboptimal home sleep study (2 nights of study attempted)
  8. Previous 2-night home sleep study which did not diagnose OSA in a patient with ongoing clinical suspicion of OSA
  9. Patient is oxygen dependent for any reason
  10. History of cerebrovascular accident (CVA) within the preceding 30 days
  11. History of ventricular fibrillation or sustained ventricular tachycardia

*EMG*, Electromyography; *$FEV_1$*, forced expiratory volume in 1 second; *FVC*, forced vital capacity; *MIB*, metaiodobenzylguanidine; *NYHA*, New York Heart Association; *OSA*, obstructive sleep apnea; *RBD*, REM sleep behavior disorder; *RLS*, restless legs syndrome.

required rather than a single-day nap study. A daytime single-nap study generally misses REM sleep, and the most severe apneic episodes are noted during REM sleep. Maximum oxygen desaturation also occurs at this stage, so a daytime study cannot assess severity of symptoms. For CPAP titration, an all-night sleep study is essential. To determine the optimal level of pressure during CPAP titration, both REM and NREM sleep are required. In this section, the PSG study is described under three headings: technical considerations, indications for a PSG study, and characteristic PSG findings in various sleep disorders.

### Technical Considerations

A PSG study includes simultaneous recording of various physiological characteristics, which allows assessment of sleep stages and wakefulness, respiration, cardiocirculatory functions, and body movements. Sleep staging is based on EEG, electro-oculogram, and EMG of some skeletal muscles, especially chin muscles. Multiple EEG channels of recordings are preferable to one or two channels for documentation of focal and diffuse neurological lesions, accurate localization of epileptiform discharges in patients with seizure disorders, and more accurate determination of various sleep stages, awakenings, and transient events such as microarousal episodes. The Rechtschaffen and Kales (1968) technique of sleep scoring, despite limitations, remained the standard for sleep staging until the recent publication of the *AASM Manual for the Scoring of Sleep and Associated Events* (Iber et al., 2007). Ideally, sleep scoring should be performed manually; computerized scoring is unreliable. This manual also lists criteria for sleep and other event scoring in children older than 2 months of age. For newborn infants, the technique recommended by Anders et al. (1971) may be used. The following terms are essential for sleep staging and scoring (Iber et al., 2007):

- *Total sleep period:* time from sleep onset to final awakening.
- *Total sleep time:* total time spent between sleep onset and final awakening, excluding time spent awake during sleep time.
- *Sleep latency:* time from lights-out to sleep onset.
- *REM sleep latency:* time from sleep onset to the first REM sleep onset.
- *Sleep efficiency:* ratio of total sleep time to total time in bed, expressed as a percentage.
- *Sleep stages:* NREM sleep stages and REM sleep, expressed as a percentage of total sleep time. NREM sleep is now divided into *stage N1*, *stage N2*, and *stage N3* (slow-wave sleep); REM sleep is now labeled as *stage R.*
- *Wake after sleep onset:* time spent awake during total sleep period.

**BOX 101.30 Indications for Overnight Polysomnography**

- A polysomnography (PSG) study is routinely indicated:
  - For the diagnosis of sleep-related breathing disorders
  - For continuous positive airway pressure (CPAP) titration in patients with sleep-related breathing disorders
  - Before undergoing uvulopalatopharyngoplasty (UPPP)
  - For assessment, the efficacy of mandibular advancement devices (MAD) for treatment of obstructive sleep apnea syndrome (OSAS)
  - To evaluate for parasomnias in patients with atypical features, semiology, unusual or atypical or if the behaviors are violent or otherwise potentially injurious to the patient or others
  - To support the diagnosis of rapid eye movement sleep behavior disorder (RBD).
- An overnight PSG, preferably video-PSG with multiple channels of electroencephalography (EEG), is indicated in patients suspected of having sleep-related epilepsy
- A PSG study may be indicated for patients whose insomnia has not responded satisfactorily to a comprehensive behavioral or pharmacological treatment program for the management of insomnia. However, if a sleep-related breathing disorder or associated periodic limb movements in sleep (PLMS) is strongly suspected in a patient with insomnia, a PSG study is indicated.
- A follow-up PSG is indicated:
  - When the clinical response is inadequate or when symptoms reappear despite a good initial treatment with CPAP
  - After substantial weight loss or weight gain, which may have occurred in patients previously treated successfully with CPAP.
- Overnight PSG followed by multiple sleep latency tests (MSLT) the next day is routinely indicated in patients with suspected narcolepsy.
- An overnight PSG is required in persons with suspected PLMS or PLM disorder but is not routinely performed to diagnose restless legs syndrome (RLS).

- *Sleep cycles:* number of sleep cycles, including REM cycles, during total sleep period.
- *Stage shifts:* a change from one stage to another during NREM sleep.
- *State shifts:* a change from NREM to REM sleep or to wakefulness.
- *Arousal index*: number of arousals per hour of sleep.

The PSG study should also include airflow, respiratory effort, continuous recording of oxygen saturation by finger oximetry, an ECG and muscle activity, particularly mental or submental and bilateral EMG recordings of the tibialis anterior muscles (Chokroverty et al., 2011). It is advantageous to record snoring and body positions. Thermistors or thermocouples are generally used to qualitatively record oronasal airflow, but these are not reliable for accurate determination of hypopnea. Most laboratories now record nasal pressure using a nasal cannula-pressure transducer, which is more sensitive than a thermocouple or thermistor for detecting airflow limitation (Ayappa et al., 2000). Respiratory efforts can be recorded by use of strain gauges or inductance plethysmography. Inductance plethysmography and a piezoelectric strain gauge are the preferred methods; they can be used in a qualitative or semiquantitative fashion to monitor chest and abdominal movements. Intraesophageal balloon recording, an invasive method, accurately determines intrathoracic pressure swings and is essential for documentation of UARS. EMG recordings of the intercostal muscles using surface electrodes may also be helpful in determining respiratory effort. SDB events are recorded as an AHI or RDI score. PLMS are recorded from tibialis EMG recordings. The PLMS index is expressed as the number of PLMS per hour of sleep. The upper limit of the normal PLMS index is 5. For the diagnosis of PLMD in adults, an index of 15 or more is suggested. Details on the technical aspects of PSG recording are beyond the scope of this chapter.

### Indications for Polysomnography

Box 101.30 lists the indications for overnight PSG proposed by the AASM (Kushida et al., 2005). These include diagnosis of SBD, positive airway pressure titration in patients with SBD, follow-up treatment to assess effectiveness in OSAS patients, preoperative procedure in patients undergoing upper airway surgery for OSAS, evaluation of suspected narcolepsy, evaluation of atypical or violent parasomnias including RBD, and diagnosis of PLMD and nocturnal seizures.

### Polysomnographic Findings in Sleep Disorders

Characteristic PSG findings in OSAS include recurrent episodes of apnea and hypopnea, which are mostly obstructive or mixed, and few episodes of central apnea accompanied by oxygen desaturation and followed by arousals with resumption of breathing (Chokroverty, 2010; Chokroverty et al., 2015). An AHI score of 5 or below is considered normal. An AHI score of 5–15 may be considered evidence of mild OSAS, 16–29 as evidence of moderate OSAS, and 30 or more as evidence of severe OSAS. Similarly, 85%–89% oxygen saturation may be found in mild OSAS, whereas in moderate OSAS, 80%–84% is typical, and in severe OSAS, 79% and below is the usual finding. An arousal index of up to 10 is considered normal; 10–15 can be considered borderline. An arousal index above 15 is definitely abnormal. There are some sleep architectural changes in OSAS (reduction of slow-wave and REM sleep); most of the sleep is spent in stage N2 sleep. Other findings include short latency, increased time spent awake after sleep onset, and excessive snoring. In patients with CSA syndrome, the apneas are all central. PSG findings in patients with Cheyne-Stokes breathing consist of a characteristic crescendo-decrescendo pattern of breathing followed by apnea or hypopneas.

## Video Polysomnographic Study

A video PSG study is important for documenting abnormal movements and behavior during sleep at night in patients with parasomnias including RBD, nocturnal seizures (Fig. 101.69, *A* and *B*), and other unusual movements occurring during sleep. Parasomnias are generally diagnosed on the basis of the clinical history, but sometimes a video PSG study is required to document the condition. For suspected nocturnal epilepsy, a video PSG study using additional electrodes to include multiple-channel EEG and multiple montages covering both parasagittal and temporal regions bilaterally is required for optimal detection of epileptiform activities. Ideally, if sleep epilepsy is suspected, the video PSG recording should be interpreted using EEG analysis at the standard EEG speed of 30 mm/sec to identify epileptiform discharges. Multiple EMG channels to record from additional muscles (e.g., forearm flexor and extensor muscles, masseter and other muscles) are recommended in patients with suspected RBD.

## Multiple Sleep Latency Test

The MSLT is an important test to effectively document EDS. Narcolepsy is the single most important indication for performing MSLT. The presence of two sleep-onset REMs on four or five nap studies (a SOREMP in the preceding overnight sleep may substitute for one MSLT SOREMP) and sleep-onset latency of less than 8 minutes strongly suggest a diagnosis of narcolepsy (AASM, 2014). Abnormalities of REM sleep regulatory mechanisms (e.g., OSAS, insufficient sleep syndrome, use of REM suppressant medications) or circadian rhythm sleep disturbance may also lead to REM sleep abnormalities during MSLT.

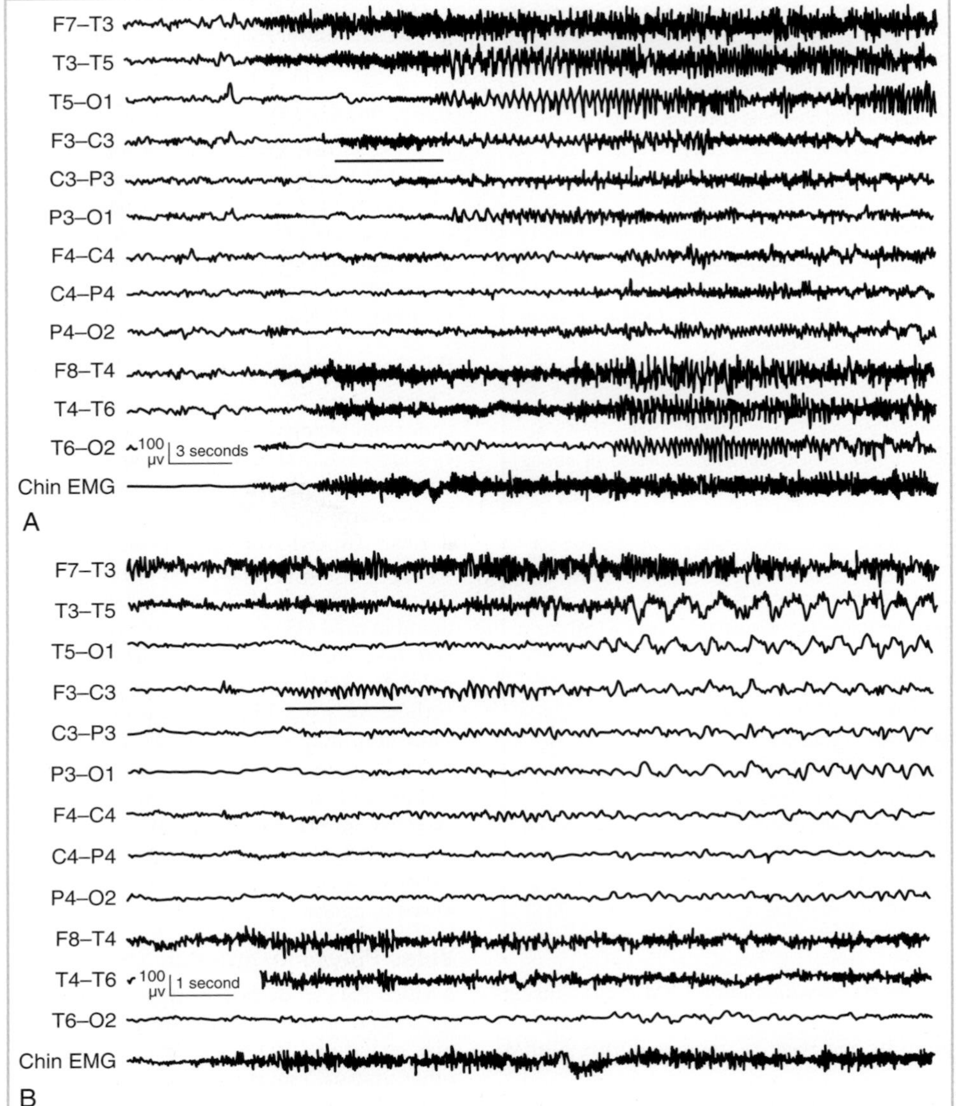


**Fig. 101.69** Portion of polysomnographic recording showing the onset of a partial seizure using (**A**) 10 mm/sec and (**B**) 30 mm/sec paper speed. Twelve channels of electroencephalogram ([EEG] International Ten-Twenty electrode placement) and chin electromyogram are shown. Underlying activity represents rhythmic ictal discharges beginning at F3-C3 (left frontocentral) and spreading rapidly to the right hemisphere, and it is accompanied by clinical seizure. The underlying activity superficially resembles muscle artifacts at 10 mm/sec paper speed (A), but it is obvious at 30 mm/sec paper speed (B) that this activity is the beginning of the rhythmic epileptiform discharges in the EEG. (*Reproduced with permission from Aldrich, M., Jahnke, B., 1991. Diagnostic value of video-EEG polysomnography. Neurol. 41, 1060.*)

## Actigraphy

Actigraphy is another laboratory test for assessing sleep disorders. It uses an actigraph (also known as an *actometer*) worn on the nondominant wrist or ankle to record acceleration or deceleration of body movements (Fig. 101.70, *A*), which indirectly indicates sleep or wakefulness. The actigraph can be worn for days or weeks, and this test complements a sleep log or diary in diagnosing circadian rhythm sleep disorders and other primary sleep disorders such as insomnia and idiopathic hypersomnia (see Fig. 101.60, *B*) or assessing a patient's treatment such is in the case of a patient with AD with irregular sleep-wake disorder (see Fig. 101.70, *C*) and those with prolonged daytime sleepiness.

## Special Electroencephalographic Studies in Nocturnal Seizure

In addition to standard EEG recording, 24-hour ambulatory EEG recording and long-term video EEG monitoring may be needed for documentation of seizures. If the results of the EEG recording, including long-term monitoring, and neuroimaging are discordant in localizing the focus, or in making a diagnosis of seizure in a patient strongly suspected to have it, the patient should be referred to a specialized epilepsy center for intracranial recordings.

## Neuroimaging Studies

Neuroimaging studies include anatomical and functional (physiological) studies. These studies are essential when a neurological illness is suspected of causing a sleep disturbance.

In addition to computed tomography (CT) and magnetic resonance imaging (MRI), which are important for detecting structural lesions of the CNS (e.g., tumors, infarction, vascular malformations), cerebral angiography—including digital subtraction arteriography and magnetic resonance angiography (MRA)—may be necessary in investigations for strokes. MRI is also helpful in patients with demyelinating and degenerative

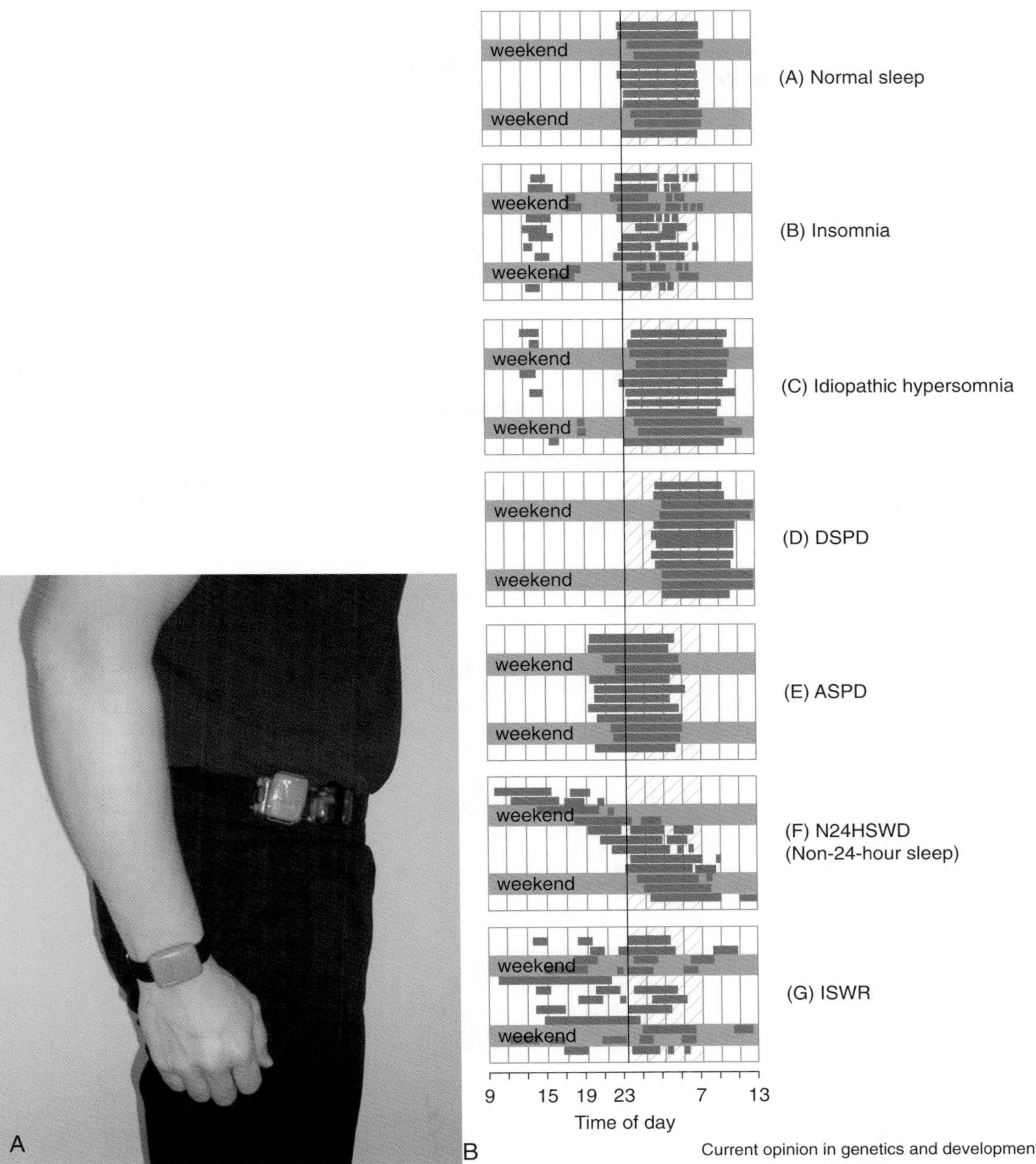


**Fig. 101.70 The Application of Actigraphy in Sleep Medicine.** (A) The Actigraph. Actigraphs are miniature computerized wristwatch-like devices that measure limb activity, based on which sleep and wake periods can be indirectly calculated. Actigraphs help to determine whether sleep is insufficient and to confirm sleepiness. (B) Actigraphy in Representative Sleep-Wake Disorders: **Normal Sleep** (A): Normal sleep in health patients with normal sleep duration (7 hrs) and sleep regularity; **Insomnia** (B): Reduced ability to imitate and maintain sleep, despite sufficient opportunity for sleep; **Idiopathic Hypersomnia** (C): uninterrupted sleep of long duration (≥11 hour/day); **DSPD** (Delayed Sleep phase disorder) (D): Stable delay of the habitual sleep period; **ASPD** (Advanced Sleep phase disorder) (E): Stable advance of the habitual sleep period; **N24HSWD** (Non-24 Hour Sleep Wake Disorder) (F): Chronic but stable delay of daily sleep and wake schedule by 1-2 hours; **ISWR** (Irregular Sleep-Wake Rhythm) (G): Absence of a clearly visible sleep-wake circadian rhythm.

*Continued*

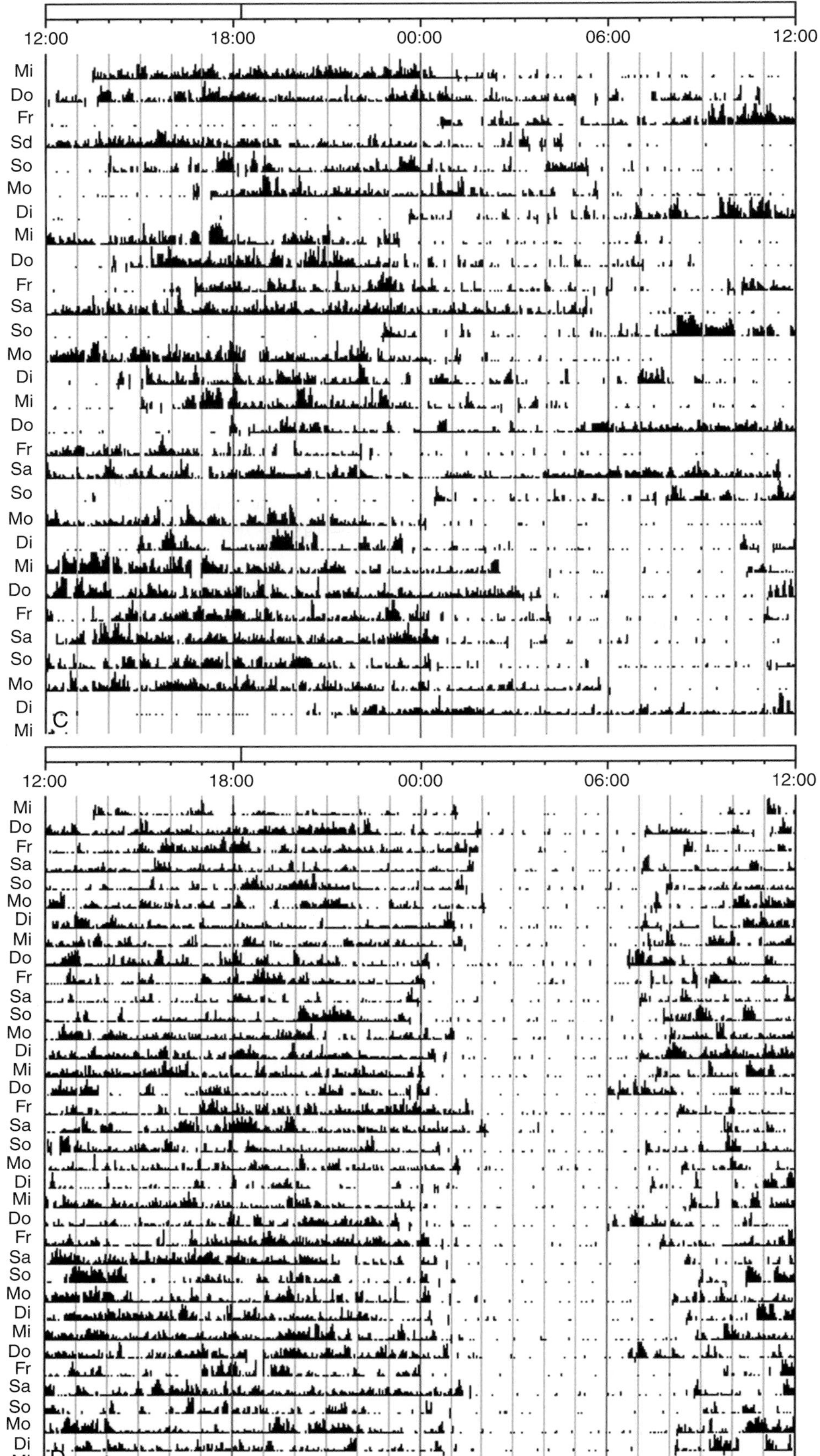


**Fig. 101.70 Cont'd** (C) Actigraphy in the setting of Irregular sleep-wake rhythm prior to light therapy (**C**), depicting an irregular sleep onset and wakeup time and establishing of a more regular rhythm following (**D**) light therapy (from the sun). The sleep period is indicated by white areas, and waking period is indicated by black bars, while physiological body shifts and movements during sleep are indicated by a few black bars in the white areas. *(**A**, From Rowlands, A.V., Stiles, V.H., 2012. Accelerometer counts and raw acceleration output in relation to mechanical loading. J. Biomechan. 45 [3], 2; 448–454; **B** From Wulff, K., et al., 2009. Sleep and circadian rhythm disturbances: multiple genes and multiple phenotypes. Curr. Opin. Gen. Dev. 19 [3], 237–246; **C, D**, From Steinig, J., Klösch, G., Sauter, C., Zeitlhofer, J., Happe, S., 2007. Sleep Med. 8 [2], 184–185, Copyright © 2006 Elsevier B.V.).*

neurological disorders that may be responsible for disturbed sleep and sleep-related breathing dysrhythmias. Other imaging studies which may be helpful include diffusion tensor MR imaging, MR tractography, and functional MRI (these are currently used mostly for research purposes).

A PET study dynamically measures cerebral blood flow, oxygen uptake, and glucose utilization and is helpful in the diagnosis of dementing, degenerative (e.g., PD and MSA), and seizure disorders. SPECT, which dynamically measures regional cerebral blood flow, may be useful for patients with cerebrovascular disease, AD, or seizure disorders. PET and SPECT can also be performed to investigate dopamine $D_2$-receptor changes in RLS-PLMS as well as narcolepsy and RBD, which may also show reduced striatal presynaptic dopamine transporter uptake. Functional MRI can be useful to study the generators and areas of activation in RLS-PLMS. Doppler ultrasonography is an important test for investigation of stroke due to extracranial vascular disease. Myelography other than CT and MRI is important for diagnosis of spinal cord diseases. Finally, meta-iodobenzylguanidine (MIBG) cardiac scintigraphy may also show reduced cardiac uptake, and midbrain transcranial sonography may show hyperechogenicity in RBD.

In selected patients, fiberoptic endoscopy may be performed to locate the site of collapse of the upper airway, and cephalometric radiographs of the cranial base and facial bones may be obtained to assess posterior airway space or maxillomandibular deficiency. These are important when surgical treatment is planned. For research investigations, cross-sectional areas of the upper airway during wakefulness may be measured by CT and MRI (Korson and Guilleminault, 2015).

### Pulmonary Function Tests

Additional text available at http://expertconsult.inkling.com.

### Other Laboratory Tests

Appropriate laboratory tests should always be performed to exclude any suspected medical disorders that may be the cause of patients' insomnia or hypersomnia. These tests may include blood analysis and urinalysis, ECG, Holter ECG, echocardiogram, chest radiography, and other investigations to rule out gastrointestinal, pulmonary, cardiovascular, endocrine, and renal disorders. In rare patients, when autonomic failure causes a sleep disturbance or SBD, autonomic function tests may be required for the diagnosis of the primary condition. In patients with narcolepsy, HLA typing may be performed because most of the patients with narcolepsy show positivity for HLA DR2DQ1 and DQB1*0602 antigens (Mignot, 1998). Another important test is measurement of CSF hypocretin 1 levels, which are found to be low (<110 pg/mL) in patients with narcolepsy type 1 who are HLA DQB1*0602 positive (Mignot et al., 2002). In patients with narcolepsy type 2 and in some other neurological conditions, CSF hypocretin may be low normal. In selected patients suspected of having a psychiatric cause of EDS, neuropsychiatric testing (e.g., the Minnesota Multiphasic Personality Inventory) may be helpful.

In patients with RLS, EMG and nerve conduction studies are important to exclude polyneuropathies or lumbosacral radiculopathies and other lower motor neuron disorders that may be associated with RLS or cause symptoms resembling idiopathic RLS. Other important laboratory tests in patients with RLS include those necessary to exclude diabetes mellitus, uremia, anemia, and other associated conditions. It is particularly important to obtain levels of serum iron (including serum ferritin and transferrin), serum folate, fasting blood glucose, blood urea, and creatinine. In a subgroup of patients with RLS, serum iron and ferritin levels are found to be low; it is important to measure these because correction of these abnormalities may improve the condition. The role of nerve biopsy remains controversial. In the vast majority of patients, a nerve biopsy is not necessary, but it may be obtained for research purposes and when there is a strong suspicion of polyneuropathy.

**BOX 101.31 Sleep Hygiene Measures**

Maintain a regular sleep-wake schedule, especially on weekends.
Avoid caffeinated beverages after lunch.
Avoid tobacco compounds, especially in the evening.
Avoid alcohol in the evening and bedtime.
Restrict time in bed awake
Adjust bedroom environment to be conducive to sleep (cooler temperature, dark, noise free)
Do not engage in any work planning the next day's activities at bedtime.
Exercise regularly for about 20–30 min in the afternoon.
Foods high in tryptophan and melatonin precursors may have a soporific effect (i.e., tart cherry juice).
Avoid exposure to blue light especially from computer, light emitting devices/tablets, TV, and other light emitting devices in the evening.
Go to bed only when sleepy.
Get out of bed if unable to fall asleep within 20 min and go to another room and either read something with low intensity light or listen to some light relaxing music. Return to bed only when sleepy. Repeat this step as many times as necessary throughout the night.
Do not watch television, read, eat, worry, or stay awake while in bed.
Remember the 3S for bedroom activities: sleep, sex, sickness.
Set an alarm clock to wake up at a fixed time each morning, including weekends.
Strategic naps during the day may consist of 15–20 minute "power naps" between 1 and 3 PM, but longer naps that are outside of this time window are ill advised.

## PRINCIPLES OF MANAGEMENT OF SLEEP DISORDERS

The principle of treatment of sleep disorders is first to find the cause for sleep disturbance and vigorously treat the primary or comorbid condition causing it. If a satisfactory treatment is not available for the primary condition or does not resolve the problem, then treatment should be directed at a specific sleep disturbance. It is beyond the scope of this chapter to discuss the management of various neurological and medical disorders causing sleep disturbance, and the reader is referred to the standard texts. Some general sleep hygiene measures (Box 101.31) should apply to all sleep disorder patients. The treatment of most commonly encountered sleep disorders is briefly discussed here.

### Treatment of Narcolepsy and Cataplexy

Treatment of narcolepsy and cataplexy includes nonpharmacological and pharmacological measures. Nonpharmacological measures include scheduled short daytime naps, sleep hygiene measures, and periodic attendance at narcolepsy support groups. For management of EDS, administration of a wake promoting agent such as armodafinil and modafinil, and a stimulant such as methylphenidate, dextroamphetamine, or methamphetamine is the treatment of choice. New treatment options include the selective histamine H3 receptor inverse agonist, Pitolisant, which was recently approved to treat excessive sleepiness in patients with NT1 and NT2. Solriamfetol, a phenylalanine derivative with dopaminergic and noradrenergic activity is also a fairly new therapeutic option to treat EDS in NT1 and NT2. Modafinil, armodafinil (the R-isomer of racemic modafinil), sodium oxybates [sodium salt of gamma-hydroxybutyrate (GHB)] and solriamfetol. (Thorpy, 2020). Methylphenidate may also be used based on data indicating a significant improvement of EDS and sleep attacks can be obtained. Treatment of cataplexy or other auxiliary symptoms of narcolepsy depends on the severity and/or frequency of the episodes. For cataplexy, treatments with tricyclic antidepressants (e.g., protriptyline, imipramine, clomipramine) and SSRIs such as fluoxetine are used with success. In some patients, viloxazine, a combined SSRI and norepinephrine reuptake inhibitor, has been useful when other drugs have failed. Pitolisant, Sodium oxybate and

**BOX 101.32 Drug Treatment of Narcolepsy—Types I and II**

**Drugs Used for Management of Excessive Sleepiness in the Setting of Narcolepsy**

Modafinil (Provigil)* 200 mg/day, up to a maximum of 400 mg/day

Armodafinil (Nuvigil): *,† start with 75 mg/day and increase if needed to 150 mg/day (maximum 250 mg/day)

**Sodium oxybate (Xyrem): 3–9 g in two divided doses, first dose at bedtime and second dose up to 2–4 h later (*)

**Calcium, magnesium, potassium, and sodium oxybates (Xywav): 3–9 g in two divided doses, first dose at bedtime and second dose up to 2–4 h later.‡

Methylphenidate (Ritalin): 5 mg in the morning and another day at noon, with a maximum dose of 50 mg/day and rarely 100 mg/day; may need to combine regular and extended release medication

Dextroamphetamine (Dexedrine): 5 mg bid, up to 50 mg/day

Methamphetamine (Methedrine): 5 mg bid, up to 50 mg/day

Solriamfetol (Sunosi): 75–150 mg/day in the morning

Pitolisant (Wakix): 9–36 mg/day in the morning

*(*) Only formal approval for treatment of pediatric patients aged 7–17 years with narcolepsy*

**Drugs Used to Treat Cataplexy and Other Auxiliary Symptoms**

Sodium oxybate (Xyrem): 3–9 g in two divided doses, first dose at bedtime and second dose up to 2–4 h later (*)

Venlafaxine (Effexor): Initiate at 37.5 mg/day bid with usual dose (75–100 mg bid)

Fluoxetine (Prozac): 20 mg/day, up to a maximum of 80 mg/day

Sertraline (Zoloft): 50 mg/day. Usual dose (50–150 mg), Maximum dose: 200 mg

Protriptyline (Vivactil): 5–10 mg/day TID/BID, Maximum dose: 30 mg/day

Clomipramine (Anafranil): 5 0 mg/day 75–125 mg/day, Maximum dose: 250 mg/day

* Half-life approximately 15 h, reduces efficacy of steroidal oral contraceptives, can cause serious rashes and allergic reactions.

† Armodafinil is the longer-acting isomer of modafinil (R-(-)-modafinil).

** Indicated in the management of cataplexy or excessive daytime sleepiness (EDS) in patients with narcolepsy ages seven and older.

‡ Adults may be initiated dosage at 4.5 g per night orally, divided into two doses at night and titrated to effect in increments of up to 1.5 g per night per week with the recommended dosage range at 6 g to 9 g per night orally. For patients 7 years and older, the recommended starting pediatric dosage, titration regimen, and maximum total nightly dosage are based on patient weight. Prescribers are encouraged to review the product information profile https://www.xywavhcp.com and https://pp.jazzpharma.com/pi/xywav.en.USPI.pdf for specific recommendations.

calcium, magnesium, potassium, and sodium oxybate, are indicated for the treatment of cataplexy as well as daytime sleepiness (Thorpy, 2020; Wakix (pitolisant) [prescribing information], 2020; Xyrem (sodium oxybate) [prescribing information], 2021.). Sodium oxybates acts as a hypnotic and consolidates REM and slow-wave sleep. Because of its short half life, sodium oxybates have to be given in two divided nightly doses at bedtime and 2.5–4 hours later. Pitolisant is a histamine 3 receptor antagonist/inverse agonist which activates histamine release in the brain and decreases excessive daytime sleepiness and cataplexy rates. Solriamfetol, is a dopamine and norepinephrine reuptake inhibitor with activity mediated through its inhibition of dopamine/norepinephrine reuptake. In refractory cases of narcolepsy-cataplexy, a combination of drugs may have to be given. Box 101.32 lists the medications for treatment of narcolepsy-cataplexy. The treatment of idiopathic hypersomnia is similar to the stimulant treatment of narcolepsy, but the therapeutic response is less satisfactory supporting that it is a different disease entity than narcolepsy.

## Treatment of Obstructive Sleep Apnea Syndrome

The treatment of upper airway OSAS consists of general measures, pharmacological therapy, mechanical devices, and surgical procedures (Box 101.33). The general measures include avoidance of alcohol, particularly in the evening, and of sedatives and hypnotics, because these agents aggravate SBD. Lifestyle modification of critical importance include measures weight loss through diet, exercise and bariatric surgery for people with high BMI, avoidance of sleep deprivation, and avoidance of supine sleeping position.

**BOX 101.33 Treatment of Upper Airway Obstructive Sleep Apnea Syndrome**

**General Measures**

Avoid alcohol and sedative-hypnotics, especially in the evening

Reduce body weight if overweight

Avoid sleep deprivation

Participate in regular exercise program

Avoid supine sleeping position

Treat nasal congestion/allergies

**Mechanical Devices**

Continuous positive airway pressure (CPAP) titration

Bilevel positive airway pressure titration

Auto-CPAP

Mandibular advancement devices (MAD, also known as oral appliances), including various mandibular advancement devices

Tongue-retaining device

**Surgical Techniques**

Weight loss surgery (bariatric surgery/gastric bypass surgery)

Uvulopalatopharyngoplasty (UPPP)

Radiofrequency UPP (somnoplasty)

Nasal surgery

Maxillomandibular advancement

Anterior hyoid advancement

Tonsillectomy and adenoidectomy (pediatric obstructive sleep apnea )

Tracheostomy (under rare circumstances)

Neurostimulators

Upper airway stimulation system

Hypoglossal nerve stimulator

### Pharmacological Treatment

Pharmacological therapy remains unsatisfactory (Morgenthaler et al., 2006); in very mild cases, partial relief has been obtained with protriptyline and medroxyprogesterone, but these drugs are generally not used today. There have been isolated reports of the use of SSRIs in mild cases and topical nasal corticosteroids for OSAS in children, with minimal benefit. In a subset of OSAS patients on adequate CPAP titration complaining of residual daytime sleepiness, armodafinil or modafinil, a novel wake-promoting agent, has been useful as an adjunct treatment.

### Positive Airway Pressure (PAP) Therapy

The devices useful for OSAS (Kushida et al., 2006a) include nasal CPAP with or without expiratory pressure relief, bilevel positive airway pressure (BPAP), and auto-CPAP and auto-BPAP titration. The treatment of choice for moderate to severe OSAS patients is CPAP titration, which is effective in more than 70% of cases. CPAP acts as a pneumatic splint, opening the upper airway passages and thereby eliminating obstructive apneas, hypoxemias, snoring, and sleep fragmentation. The optimal pressure for CPAP must be determined during an overnight PSG recording. Some patients may require BPAP titration, which delivers a higher pressure during inspiration and a lower pressure during expiration. A regular follow-up visit, particularly shortly after recommending CPAP treatment, is essential for good adherence. The unit must be used regularly during nightly sleep. The goal of treatment is to improve quality of life and prevent life-threatening complications such as cardiac arrhythmias, congestive heart failure, pulmonary and essential hypertension, strokes, and cognitive impairment. Recently, auto-CPAP machines that automatically titrate pressure according to detected abnormal breathing events have been introduced. The role of these devices remains to be determined. Despite using a 2-cm reduction in mean pressure compared to fixed-pressure CPAP, there is so far no benefit in increasing adherence with auto-CPAP. In patients with neuromuscular disorders, intermittent positive-pressure ventilation through a nasal mask may be needed to treat sleep hypoventilation or apnea.

### Alternative to PAP Therapy

Non-PAP therapy is beneficial in carefully selected patients who are not compliant with PAP or in patients with mild to moderate disease who refuse CPAP therapy. Mandibular advancement devices (dental devices) appliances (Kushida et al., 2006b) can reduce snoring and help patients control mild to moderate sleep apnea but predicting which patients will respond to a particular treatment is not always predictable. Upper airway surgery for sleep apnea (such as uvulopalatopharyngoplasty, UPPP) has been proposed and utilized for years. Unfortunately, as of 2021, uniform consensus regarding the role of surgery in people with sleep apnea is lacking. This is most likely due to the various sleep apnea phenotypes, varying degrees of severity and anatomical collapse, and the lack of consistent screening and objectively verifiable indicators to predict success (Epstein et al., 2009). In children with OSAS, tonsillectomy and adenoidectomy have been successful if not curative in most cases (Overland et al., 2021). Upper airway stimulation improves upper airway patency during sleep by stimulating the genioglossus muscle. Activation of this muscle via stimulation of the hypoglossal nerve is a creative new approach for treatment of OSA (Strollo, 2014).

Severe respiratory compromise or severe apnea associated with dangerous cardiac arrhythmias creating a life-threatening situation may require emergency tracheostomy.

### Treatment of Cheyne-Stokes Breathing and Central Sleep Apnea

CSA, including Cheyne-Stokes breathing associated with heart failure, requires aggressive treatment of heart failure (e.g., beta-blockers, digoxin, diuretics) and, if needed, heart transplant. Measures to improve ventilation include CPAP or BiPAP titration, oxygen administration, and gas modulation with inhaled carbon dioxide through the nasal mask as well as administration of theophylline and acetazolamide. Acetazolamide has been found to be useful in Cheyne-Stokes breathing associated with high altitude. CPAP titration was thought to improve the mortality in patients with heart failure, but a recent large-scale Canadian study (Bradley et al., 2005) showed no improvement in mortality, although there was improvement in ejection fraction and other measures; a later reanalysis of the data supported the usefulness of CPAP in heart failure. Another treatment that has been found to be useful in patients with Cheyne-Stokes breathing and CSA is adaptive servo ventilation (Randerath and Javaheri, 2015; Philippe et al., 2006; Randerath et al., 2009). The role of this treatment measure in terms of long-term benefit remains to be determined (Randerath, 2012).

### Treatment of Insomnia

The first step in the treatment of insomnia is an assessment of the type of insomnia (see eBoxes 101.6 and 101.10 and Box 101.9) and

**TABLE 101.8 Classification of Central Disorders of Hypersomnolence**

| ICSD-III | Alternate Names | Cataplexy | Hypocretin | Sleep Studies | HLA Titers |
|---|---|---|---|---|---|
| Narcolepsy type 1 | Hypocretin deficiency syndrome, narcolepsy-cataplexy, narcolepsy with cataplexy | Yes | Hcrt-1 ≤110 pg/mL or 1/3 of normal mean values | Mean MSLT SL ≤8 min with ≥2 SOREMPs (1 may be on prior PSG) | HLA DQB1*0602 positivity= 100% (except in narcolepsy type 1 due to medical condition) |
| Narcolepsy type 2 | Narcolepsy without cataplexy | No | Hcrt-1 >110 pg/ml or 1/3 of normal mean values<br>In the absence of cataplexy, if measured at ≤110 pg/mL or 1/3 of normal mean values, reclassify as narcolepsy type 1 | Mean MSLT SL ≤8 min with ≥2 SOREMPs (1 may be on prior PSG) | HLA DQB1*0602 positivity= 25% (except in narcolepsy type 1 due to medical condition) |
| Idiopathic hypersomnia | Idiopathic CNS hypersomnolence | No | Hcrt-1 >110 pg/mL or 1/3 of normal mean values | MSLT shows (1 of 2):<br><2 SOREMPs on MSLT or no SOREMPs on prior PSG where REM latency ≤ 15 minutes<br>AND.<br>The presence of one of the following:<br>(a) MSLT shows mean sleep latency of ≤ 8 minutes.<br>(b) Total 24-h sleep time ≥660 min on 24-h monitoring by PSG (after correction of sleep deprivation) or wrist actigraphy averaged over 7 days with unrestricted sleep | |

*CNS*, Central nervous system; *HLA*, human leukocyte antigen; *ICSD*, International Classification of Sleep Disorders; *MSLT*, multiple sleep latency test; *PSG*, polysomnographic; *SOREMP*, sleep-onset rapid eye movement (REM) period.

*Adapted from American Academy of Sleep Medicine. 2014. International Classification of Sleep Disorders, third ed. American Academy of Sleep Medicine, Darien, IL.*

**TABLE 101.8A Currently Approved Hypnotic for the Management for Insomnia (Approval as of February, 2021)**

| Class of Hypnotic and Name | Doses (mg) | Half-life (h) | Indications | Most Common Side Effects | DEA Class | Pregnancy Category |
|---|---|---|---|---|---|---|
| **Benzodiazepine Immediate Release** | | | | | | |
| Flurazepam (Dalmane) | 15, 30 | 48–120 | "Treatment of insomnia characterized by difficulty in falling asleep, frequent nocturnal awakenings, and/or early morning awakening" | Dizziness, drowsiness, lightheadedness, staggering, loss of coordination, falling | IV | X |
| Temazepam (Restoril) | 7.5, 15, 22.5, 30 | 8–20 | "Short-term treatment of insomnia" | Drowsiness, dizziness, lightheadedness, difficulty with coordination | IV | X |
| Triazolam (Halcion) | 0.125, 0.25 | 2–4 | "Short-term treatment of insomnia" | Drowsiness, headache, dizziness, lightheadedness, "pins and needles" feelings on your skin, difficulty with coordination | IV | X |
| Quazepam (Doral) | 7.5, 15 | 48–120 | "Treatment of insomnia characterized by difficulty in falling asleep, frequent nocturnal awakenings, and/or early morning awakenings" | Drowsiness, headache | IV | X |
| Estazolam (Prosom) | 1, 2 | 8–24 | "Short-term management of insomnia characterized by difficulty in falling asleep, frequent nocturnal awakenings, and/or early morning awakenings, administered at bedtime improved sleep induction and sleep maintenance" | Somnolence, hypokinesia, dizziness, abnormal coordination | IV | X |
| **Nonbenzodiazepine Immediate Release** | | | | | | |
| Zolpidem (Ambien) | 5, 10 | 1.5–2.4 | "Short-term treatment of insomnia characterized by difficulties with sleep initiation" | Drowsiness, dizziness, diarrhea, drugged feelings | IV | C |
| Zaleplon (Sonata) | 5, 10 | 1 | "Short-term treatment of insomnia, shown to decrease the time to sleep onset" | Drowsiness, lightheadedness, dizziness, "pins and needles" feeling on your skin, difficulty with coordination | IV | C |
| Eszopiclone (Lunesta) | 1, 2, 3 | 5–7 | "Treatment of insomnia… administered at bedtime decreased sleep latency and improved sleep maintenance" | Unpleasant taste in mouth, dry mouth, drowsiness, dizziness, headache, symptoms of the common cold | IV | C |
| **Nonbenzodiazepine Extended Release** | | | | | | |
| Zolpidem ER (Ambien CR) | 6.25, 12.5 | 2.8–2.9 | "Treatment of insomnia characterized by difficulties with sleep onset and/or sleep maintenance (as measured by wake time after sleep onset)" | Headache, sleepiness, dizziness | IV | C |
| **Nonbenzodiazepine Alternate Delivery** | | | | | | |
| Zolpidem Oral spray (Zolpimist) | 5, 10 | ~2.5 | "Short-term treatment of insomnia characterized by difficulties with sleep initiation" | Drowsiness, dizziness, diarrhea, drugged feelings | IV | C |
| Zolpidem Sublingual (Edluar) | 5, 10 | ~2.5 | "Short-term treatment of insomnia characterized by difficulties with sleep initiation" | Drowsiness, dizziness, diarrhea, drugged feelings | IV | C |
| Zolpidem Sublingual (Intermezzo) | 1.75, 3.5 | ~2.5 | "As needed for the treatment of insomnia when a middle-of-the-night awakening is followed by difficulty returning to sleep" | Headache, nausea, fatigue | IV | C |

**TABLE 101.8A Currently Approved Hypnotic for the Management for Insomnia (Approval as of December 2019)—cont'd**

| Class of Hypnotic and Name | Doses (mg) | Half-life (h) | Indications | Most Common Side Effects | DEA Class | Pregnancy Category |
|---|---|---|---|---|---|---|
| **Selective Melatonin Receptor Agonist** | | | | | | |
| Ramelteon (Rozerem) | 8 | 1–2.6 | "Treatment of insomnia characterized by difficulty with sleep onset" | Drowsiness, tiredness, dizziness | None | C |
| **Selective Histamine $H_1$ Receptor Antagonist** | | | | | | |
| Doxepin (Silenor) | 3, 6 | 15.3 | "Treatment of insomnia characterized by difficulties with sleep maintenance" | Somnolence/sedation, nausea, upper respiratory tract infection | None | C |
| **Hypocretin (Orexin) Receptor Antagonist** | | | | | | |
| Suvorexant (Belsomra) | 5, 10, 15, 20 | 12 | "Treatment of insomnia, characterized by difficulties with sleep onset and/or sleep maintenance" | Somnolence, depression, rare but possible risk of REM intrusion phenomena. | IV | C |
| Lemborexant | 5, 10 | 17–24 h | Treatment of insomnia, characterized by difficulties with sleep onset and/or sleep maintenance" | Somnolence, headache, and sleep paralysis | IV | C |

**TABLE 101.8B Currently Approved Hypnotic for the Management for Insomnia: (Approval as of December 2019)**

| Agent | Initiates Sleep | Maintains Sleep | Sleep with Limited Opportunity | Required inactivity (hr) | Dose (mg) |
|---|---|---|---|---|---|
| Eszopiclone | √ | √ | | 8+ | 1, 2, 3 |
| Zaleplon | √ | | √ | 4 | 5, 10 |
| Zolpidem | √ | | | 7–8 | 5, 10 |
| Extended release | √ | √ | | 7–8 | 6.25, 12.5 |
| Sublingual zolpidem (Intermezzo) | | √* | √ | 4 | 1.75, 3.5 |
| Oral spray zolpidem (Zolpimist) | √ | | | 4 | 5, 10 |
| Sublingual zolpidem for sleep initiation (Edluar) | √ | | | 4 | 5, 10 |
| Ultra-low-dose doxepin (Silenor) | | √ | | 7–8 | 3, 6 |
| Ramelteon (Rozerem) | √ | | | — | 8 |
| Suvorexant (Belsomra) | √ | √ | | 7–8 | 5, 10, 15 and 20 |
| Lemborexant | √ | √ | | 7–8 | 5, 10 |

*Provided that 4 additional hours of sleep/time in bed are available. Currently available hypnotics agents: Drug selection is based on the timing of the insomnia (i.e., sleep initiation, sleep maintenance): age, gender, history of drug abuse behavior and comorbidities. Benzodiazepine modulators, $H_1$ receptor antagonists, and melatonin agonists. The reader is advised to review US Food and Drug Administration bulletins about these agents, especially regarding dose adjustments in unique cohorts (i.e., susceptible individuals such as women and older adults) paying close attention to the development of adverse effects. Physicians' desk reference 2014.

treatment of comorbid conditions associated with it (see eBoxes 101.11 and 101.12). Treatment should be broadly divided into two classes: pharmacological and nonpharmacological.

### Pharmacological Treatment

Hypnotic medication used judiciously is the mainstay of treatment for acute, transient, or short-term insomnia. This treatment should last for a few nights to a maximum of 4 weeks. The most commonly used hypnotics are the benzodiazepine receptor agonists, which act on the $GABA_A$ receptor complex. In the past, benzodiazepines were mostly used, but because of their side effects and the availability of newer nonbenzodiazepine receptor agonists with shorter half-lives and fewer side effects, the older drugs are used infrequently now. The most frequently used newer benzodiazepine receptor agonists include zolpidem (regular and controlled-release), zaleplon, and eszopiclone. Melatonin receptor agonists (e.g., ramelteon) may also be used for sleep-onset insomnia. Patients who do not respond to these medications may be given benzodiazepines, especially intermediate-acting (e.g., temazepam). Ultra-low-dose doxepin, a histamine $H_1$ receptor antagonist, has also received FDA approval for the treatment of chronic sleep initiation and maintenance insomnia.

For chronic insomnia, nonpharmacological measures combined with judicious use of hypnotics are the best treatment. Intermittent use of hypnotics is particularly useful for patients with chronic primary

**TABLE 101.9 Neurodegenerative Conditions and their Associated Sleep Disorder**

| Amyloidopathy | Synucleinopathy | Tauopathy | TDP-43-opathy |
|---|---|---|---|
| Alzheimer disease | Parkinson disease<br>Lewy body dementia<br>Multiple system atrophy | Frontotemporal dementias<br>Progressive supranuclear palsy<br>Corticobasal degeneration | ALS<br>Frontotemporal dementia (FTLD-U) |
| Insomnia<br>Circadian rhythm changes<br>Somnolence later | Insomnia<br>Excessive somnolence<br>REM sleep behavior disorder | None characteristic (all possible, but tend to be less prominent) | ALS: SDB |

*ALS*, Amyotrophic lateral sclerosis; *REM*, rapid eye movement.

**TABLE 101.10 Cognitive and Behavioral Therapy for Insomnia**

| | | |
|---|---|---|
| Sleep Restriction | Excessive time spent in bed; fragmented sleep | Therapist instructs patient to curtail the time in bed to the actual sleep time. The time in bed is subsequently adjusted based on sleep efficiency. Time in bed can be increased by 15–20 min/wk if sleep efficiency is >85% and decreased if sleep efficiency is <80%. Daytime sleepiness is a potential side effect of this behavioral therapy, which may impact adherence |
| Stimulus Control Therapy | Excessive time spent in bed; fragmented sleep | Therapist instructs patient to curtail the time in bed to the actual sleep time. The time in bed is subsequently adjusted based on sleep efficiency. Time in bed can be increased by 15–20 min/week if sleep efficiency is >85% and decreased if sleep efficiency is <80%. Daytime sleepiness is a potential side effect of this behavioral therapy, which may impact adherence. Improve sleep continuity by limiting time spent in bed awake. |
| Relaxation Techniques | High physiologic, cognitive, or emotional hyperarousal | The goal of relaxation therapy is to reduce arousal at bedtime or on nighttime awakening by reducing somatic tension using progressive muscle relaxation or intrusive thoughts such as imagery training, meditation. |
| Sleep Hygiene | Behaviors that undermine good quality sleep target inadequate sleep hygiene (e.g., irregular bed and wake time, caffeine and alcohol before bedtime, excessive naps, watching TV in bed). Excessive time awake in bed, irregular sleep–wake schedules, hyperarousal and activities incompatible with sleep | Encourage habits that promote sleep, provide rationale for subsequent instructions. Sleep hygiene education includes guidelines about health practices (e.g., diet, exercise, substance abuse) and environmental factors (e.g., light, noise, temperature) that may promote or interfere with sleep |
| Cognitive Therapy | Unrealistic sleep expectations, misconceptions about sleep, anxiety associated with sleep anticipation, and poor cognitive coping skills | The goal of cognitive therapy is to modify dysfunctional sleep cognitions (such as changing faulty beliefs and attitudes about sleep). Reduce arousal and decrease anxiety (progressive muscular relaxation, transcendental meditation, yoga, biofeedback). Facilitate the development of more rational thoughts about sleep and the consequences of sleep loss. |

CBTi is a structured program that helps patients with insomnia identify and replace thoughts and behaviors known to cause or exacerbate insomnia with habits that promote sound sleep. The program is most effective when supervised and coached by a sleep psychologist. The table summarizes the specific technique, the abnormal insomnia behavior that the technique targets, and the overall goal.
*Adapted from Bootzin, R.R., Perlis, M.L., 1992. Nonpharmacologic treatments of insomnia. J Clin Psychiatry 53(suppl), 37–41 [Evidence Level C]; Hauri, P.J., 1998. Insomnia. Clin Chest Med 19, 157–168 [Evidence Level C].*

and psychophysiological insomnia or when the patient does not respond adequately to nonpharmacological measures. The efficacy of non-nightly use (e.g., 3–5 nights/week) has been proven in some clinical trials, but further studies are needed to confirm the usefulness of this approach (Hajak, 2006). Hypnotic medications in general should be discouraged for chronic insomnia. Hypnotic use is contraindicated in pregnancy and should also be avoided or used judiciously in patients with alcoholism or renal, hepatic, or pulmonary disease. Hypnotics should be avoided in patients with sleep apnea syndrome. Sedative antidepressants (e.g., trazodone, amitriptyline, doxepin, mirtazapine) have been used in patients with insomnia comorbid with depression, but double-blind placebo-controlled studies to understand the effectiveness of these drugs have not been undertaken. The newer antipsychotics that have hypnotic properties (e.g., olanzapine, quetiapine, risperidone) should not be used in chronic insomnia unless the insomnia is associated with psychosis. Many patients with chronic insomnia use over-the-counter medications (e.g., diphenhydramine, melatonin, valerian). These medications have some hypnotic properties, but there are many side effects and the long-term effects are not known; therefore, their use should be discouraged. Orexin/hypocretin antagonists, suvorexant, and lemborexsant are available to manage both sleep onset and maintenance insomnia and may have utility in managing insomnia in the setting of Alzheimer dementia. Table 101.8 lists the pharmacological agents used to treat insomnia.

### Nonpharmacological Treatment

Nonpharmacological measures should be the mainstay of treatment for chronic insomnia and consists of sleep hygiene measures, stimulus control, sleep restriction, relaxation, and cognitive therapies. A combination of all these measures constitutes *cognitive behavioral therapy*

## BOX 101.34 Nonpharmacological Treatment of Restless Legs Syndrome

General sleep hygiene measures (see Box 101.31)
 Avoid the following:
Caffeine and caffeinated beverages
- Smoking (tobacco compounds)
- Alcohol
- Antidepressants (e.g., tricyclic antidepressants, selective serotonin reuptake inhibitors, venlafaxine), exception is bupropion
- Antihistamines (especially over-the-counter sleep aids that may contain these compounds)
- Dopamine antagonists (e.g., most antipsychotics, antiemetics, some calcium channel blockers)
- Sleep deprivation

Encourage the following:
- Mild to moderate exercise
- Vibratory stimulation pads
- Physical activity (e.g., leg stretching) and massaging legs before bedtime
- Hot bath 2–3 h before bedtime or cold compresses (in some patients)
- Remain mentally engaged

(Table 101.10). Sleep hygiene measures are simply some commonsense steps to address both homeostatic and circadian factors (see Box 101.31). Stimulus control therapy is directed at discouraging learned associations between bedroom and wakefulness and re-establishing the bedroom as the major stimulus for sleep. These techniques have been reported to improve insomnia complaints in approximately 50% of individuals after 1 year.

Relaxation therapy includes progressive muscle relaxation; biofeedback may be added to reduce somatic arousal. Sleep restriction therapy is based on the principle that restricting total sleep time in bed may improve sleep efficiency. Total sleep time is then gradually increased to improve the level of daytime function and overall sleep quality. Some 25% of patients with insomnia benefit from such a regimen. The best nonpharmacological approach has not been established, but cognitive behavioral therapy is associated with the most sustained improvement in sleep (Morin and Benca, 2015; Morin et al., 1999). Recent data support the use of a novel forehead temperature-regulating device that promotes improvement in insomnia supported by PSG measures of the patients' ability to fall asleep by delivering frontal cerebral thermal therapy. The therapy utilizes frontal cerebral hypothermia therapy at 14–16°C, equivalent to 57–61°F) with a benign safety profile, and may

## TABLE 101.11 Pharmacological Treatment of Restless Leg Syndrome

| Generic/Brand | Dose | Risks |
|---|---|---|
| **Iron** | | |
| Ferrous sulfate | 325 mg BID/TID<br>Recommended for Ferritin < 75 µg | GI side effects: constipation. Role in treatment under current investigation |
| **Dopamine Agonists** | | |
| Pramipexole * | 0.125–0.5 mg, 1.5–2 hr before bedtime. | Augmentation, rebound, impulse control behaviors, sleepiness, nausea reported in some cases, headaches, dizziness. Hypotension, hallucinations. Application site allergic reaction (specific to rotigotine) |
| Ropinirole * | 0.25–2 mg 1.5–2 h before bedtime (+) | |
| Rotigotine patch * | 1–3 mg applied QD | |
| **Dopamine Precursor Agents** | | |
| Levodopa/Carbidopa (Sinemet) | 25/100 mg: 1/2 tab-3 tabs 30 min before bedtime | Nausea, sleepiness, augmentation of daytime symptoms, insomnia, sleepiness, gastrointestinal disturbances. Not recommended to be used chronically due to significant risks of augmentation. May be useful when used intermittently, in an "on demand" pattern |
| **Alpha-2-Delta Ligands** | | |
| Gabapentin (Neurontin) | 300–2700 mg/day initially in the evening, later divided if needed for daytime symptoms | Excessive daytime sleepiness, nausea, headache, dizziness |
| Gabapentin Enacarbil * | 300–600 mg Q5PM | |
| Pregabalin | 50–300 mg in the evening | |
| **Benzodiazepines** | | |
| Clonazepam | 0.125–0.5 mg at bedtime | Nausea, sedation, dizziness; caution in sleep apnea patients because of depressing effects on breathing and upper airway muscles |
| **Central Alpha-2 Adrenergic Agonist** | | |
| Clonidine (Catapres) | 0.1 mg BID<br>May be helpful in patients with hypertension | Dry mouth, drowsiness, constipation, sedation, weakness, depression (1%), hypotension |
| **Opioids** | | |
| Darvocet (Darvocet-N) | 300 mg/day | Nausea, vomiting, restlessness, constipation. Addiction, tolerance may be possible |
| Darvon (Propoxyphene) | 65–135 mg at bedtime | |
| Codeine, methadone; also oxycodone | 30 mg/day | |

*FDA-indicated as of February, 2021

**BOX 101.35 First-Line Medication and Treatment Consideration in Newly Diagnosed Restless Legs Syndrome**

α2δ ligands as suggested as first-line therapy given the lack of augmentation, which is problematic in the setting of dopamine agonists. Gabapentin Enacarbil may be preferred as long-term studies have not been performed with gabapentin in restless legs syndrome (RLS) and absorption is variable, thereby complicating dosing.

If dopamine agonists are used the treatment should keep dopaminergic load as low as possible with regular screening for augmentation.

The clinician should also weigh in the following factors in selecting the appropriate medication:

| Attributes to Consider | Treatment Choice |
|---|---|
| Time of day (daytime symptoms) | Select a long-acting agent, or Twice-a-day dosing of a short-acting agent |
| Sleep disturbance disproportionate to other symptoms of RLS e.g., severe insomnia | $\alpha_2\delta$ ligand |
| Comorbid insomnia | $\alpha_2\delta$ ligand |
| Pregnancy risk | Avoid both DAs and $\alpha_2\delta$ ligands<br>Consider the use of iron |
| Impaired renal function | Select a drug that is not renally excreted or reduce dose of renally excreted drugs (pramipexol, $\alpha_2\delta$ ligand) |
| Increased risk of falls | Dopamine-receptor agonist (DA) |
| Painful restless legs | $\alpha_2\delta$ ligand |
| RLS with comorbid pain syndrome | $\alpha_2\delta$ ligand |
| History of impulse control disorder | $\alpha_2\delta$ ligand |
| History of alcohol or substance abuse | DA agonist or $\alpha_2\delta$ ligand |
| Very severe symptoms of RLS | DA |
| Obesity, metabolic syndrome | DA |
| Availability or cost of drug | DA or $\alpha_2\delta$ ligand |
| Comorbid depression | CA |
| Comorbid generalized anxiety disorder | $\alpha_2\delta$ ligand |
| Higher potential for drug interactions | Select drug that is not hepatically metabolized (pramipexol, gabapentin enacarbil) |
| Symptomatic periodic limb movements in sleep | Dopamine-receptor agonist |

*Adapted from Garcia-Borreguero, D., Silber, M.H., Winkelman, J.W., Hogl, B., Bainbridge, J., Buchfuhrer, M., et al., 2016. Guidelines for the first-line treatment of restless legs syndrome/Willis-Ekbom disease, prevention and treatment of dopaminergic augmentation: a combined task force of the IRLSSG, EURLSSG, and the RLS-foundation. Sleep. Med. 21, 1–11. https://doi.org/10.1016/j.sleep.2016.01.017: Garcia-Borreguero, D., Kohnen, R., Silber, M.H., et al., 2013. The long-term treatment of restless legs syndrome/Willis-Ekbom disease: evidence-based guidelines and clinical consensus best practice guidance: a report from the international restless legs syndrome study group. Sleep Med. 14(7), 675–684; Silber, M.H., Becker, P.M., Earley, C., Foundation Medical Advisory Board of the Willis-Ekbom Disease, 2013. Willis-Ekbom disease foundation revised consensus statement on the management of restless legs syndrome. Mayo Clin. Proc. 88(9), 977–986; Silber, M.H., Krahn, L.E., Morgenthaler, T.I., 2010. Sleep Medicine Clinical Practice, second ed. Informa Healthcare, London.*

be suggested to complement existing therapies for the treatment of chronic insomnia (Roth et al., 2018).

## Treatment of Restless Legs Syndrome-Periodic Limb Movements in Sleep

Both pharmacological and nonpharmacological measures are used to treat RLS (Hening et al., 2009; Wijemanne and Jankovic, 2015). In a mild case, nonpharmacological measures (Box 101.34) may be the only treatment needed, and these should also be used in combination with medications in moderate to severe cases. Nonpharmacological treatments include sleep hygiene measures (see Box 101.31), avoidance of sleep deprivation, and avoidance of agents that trigger or aggravate RLS (e.g., caffeine, alcohol, smoking, antihistamines, neuroleptics, tricyclic antidepressants, SSRIs and other antidepressants, certain antinausea medications). A hot bath or leg massage at bedtime and mild to moderate exercise may also be helpful, particularly in mild cases.

Pharmacological treatment (Table 101.11) includes four groups of drugs (Garcia-Borreguero et al., 2013): dopaminergic agents (e.g., carbidopa-levodopa and dopamine agonists such as pramipexole, ropinirole, and rotigotine parch), benzodiazepines (e.g., clonazepam, temazepam), anticonvulsants (e.g., gabapentin, gabapentin enacarbil, pregabalin), and opiates (e.g., codeine, propoxyphene, oxycodone, hydrocodone, methadone). Rotigotine, a nonergoline dopaminergic agent delivered through a transdermal patch—ensuring continuous delivery over 24 hours, sustaining a near-constant blood level—has been FDA approved in addition to pramipexole, ropinirole, and gabapentin enacarbil for treatment of moderate to severe primary RLS. Due to the risk of augmentation, the most appropriate initial treatment in most cases is an alpha 2 delta agent or perhaps a dopamine agonist provided that dopamine load is kept low and augmentation is screened for regularly (Garcia-Borreguero et al., 2016). In mild cases, one may start with nonpharmacological measures with or without additional gabapentin or pregabalin. In patients who are intractable, a combination of two or three drugs may have to be used. The principle of treatment is to start at the lowest possible dose and then increase by one tablet every 5–7 days until maximum benefit is reached or side effects are noted. Medication is generally given 1.5–2 hours before bedtime. Depending on the timing of symptoms, the medication may have to be given in two divided doses—for example, early in the evening and later at bedtime. In some severe cases, when daytime symptoms are present, a daytime dose may be added; however, symptoms should be differentiated from augmentation, which is a drug-related exacerbation of symptoms noted mostly with carbidopa-levodopa but also seen with other dopamine agonists (Chokroverty, 2011b). In many idiopathic RLS patients, serum iron or ferritin levels may be low; appropriate treatment with ferrous sulfate combined with ascorbic acid, which promotes iron absorption, is recommended. Box 101.35 lists specific recommendations in mild or intermittent, moderate, and severe cases. In most cases RLS can be treated medically, but when the symptoms are severe and disabling despite optimal medical therapy deep brain stimulation targeting the globus pallidus may be considered as a very last resort (Ondo et al., 2012).

Nonpharmacological therapy for RLS has been reviewed and may include exercise later in the day, repetitive transcranial magnetic stimulation, compression devices, and counterstrain manipulation, which

**TABLE 101.12 Pharmacological and Nonpharmacological Treatment of Disorders of Arousal**

| Parasomnia | Treatment |
|---|---|
| Somnambulism (sleep walking) | Safeguard the sleep environment and protect the patient<br>Avoid precipitants:<br>Sleep deprivation<br>Lithium<br>Nonbenzodiazepine receptor agonists.<br>Anticipatory awakenings<br>Benzodiazepines<br>Clonazepam (0.5–1 mg)<br>Diazepam (10 mg)<br>Triazolam (0.25 mg)<br>Imipramine (50–300 mg) |
| Confusional arousal | Reassurance of benign nature<br>Avoid precipitants:<br>Sleep deprivation<br>Alcohol<br>CNS depressants<br>Escitalopram (10 mg)—*for sexsomnia* |
| Sleep terrors | Reassurance of benign nature<br>Cognitive Behavior Therapy<br>Paroxetine (20–40 mg)<br>Clonazepam (0.5–1 mg) |
| Sleep-related eating disorder | Topiramate<br>Pramipexole (when comorbid with RLS [WED]) |

*CNS*, Central nervous system; *RLS*, restless legs syndrome.

were significantly more effective for RLS severity than control conditions. However, other modes including vibration pads, yoga, cryotherapy, compression devices, and acupuncture may have some role in improving sleep-related outcomes but may be more limited in RLS per se. (Harrison et al., 2019) (Video 101.15).

## Treatment of Circadian Rhythm Sleep Disorder

The most effective treatment for DSPS is exposure to bright light (5000–10,000 lux). The patient sits in front of the light for about 30 minutes in the morning; in addition, the room light must be reduced in the evening to achieve the desired result. Melatonin at bedtime has also been used in combination with bright light therapy in these patients. Chronotherapy (intentional delay of sleep onset by 2–3 hours on successive days until the desired bedtime has been achieved) is helpful in many patients with DSPS, at least in the beginning. In ASPS, bright light therapy may be given in the evening, and light must be restricted in the morning. Melatonin has also been found to be useful in some subjects with jet lag and shift-work sleep disorders, as well as in patients with circadian rhythm disorder, free-running type (non-24-hour circadian rhythm disorder). Jet lag and shift-work sleep disorder may also be treated with zolpidem or the melatonin receptor agonist, ramelteon. Armodafinil (sustained action) or modafinil has been approved for shift-work sleep disorder to treat excessive sleepiness.

## Treatment of Parasomnias

Most parasomnias require no special treatment. Preventive measures to protect patients from injuring themselves or others should be instituted in patients with partial arousal disorders and REM behavior disorder. If attacks of sleepwalking or sleep terrors are frequent or violent, treatment with a tricyclic antidepressant or small doses of benzodiazepine (e.g., clonazepam) may be used for a short period (Table 101.12).

**TABLE 101.13 Pharmacological Treatment of REM Sleep Behavior Disorder**

| Drug* | Dose | Level of Recommendation | Special Considerations |
|---|---|---|---|
| Melatonin | 3–12 mg before bedtime (regular formulation) or 5-15 mg (sustained release) | Suggested† | Effective in patients with alpha-synucleinopathies, memory problems, and sleep-disordered breathing.<br>Side effects include headaches, sleepiness, and delusions/hallucinations. |
| Clonazepam | 0.25–2.0 mg before bedtime (usual recommended dose is 0.5–2.0 mg) | Suggested† | Use with caution in patients with dementia, gait disorders, or concomitant OSA.<br>Side effects include sedation, impotence, motor incoordination, confusion, and memory dysfunction. |
| Zopiclone | 3.5–7.5 mg before bedtime | May be considered†† | Side effects include rash and nausea. |
| Yi-Gan San | 2.5 mg tid | May be considered†† | Studied mainly on patients that could not take clonazepam. No side effects were reported when used for the treatment of RBD. |
| Sodium oxybate | Unknown | May be considered†† | |
| Donepezil | 10–15 mg | May be considered†† | |
| Rivastigmine | 4.5–6 mg bid. | May be considered†† | Studied mainly on patients with dementia of Lewy body. |
| Temazepam | 10 mg | May be considered†† | |
| Alprazolam | 1–3 mg | May be considered†† | |
| Desipramine | 50 mg qhs | May be considered†† | |
| Carbamazepine | 500–1500 mg qd | May be considered†† | |

*Not FDA approved for the treatment of RBD.
†Supported by sparse high-grade evidence data, or a substantial amount of low-grade data and/or clinical consensus.
††Supported by low-grade data.
*Adapted from Aurora, R.N., Zak, R.S., Maganti, R.K., et al.,2010. Committee Standards of Practice, and Medicine American Academy of Sleep, 2010. Best practice guide for the treatment of REM sleep behavior disorder (RBD). J Clin Sleep Med 6(1), 85–95.*

**BOX 101.36 Treatment of Sleep Disturbance in Alzheimer Disease and Related Dementias**

**General Measures**

Reduce or eliminate medications that may contribute to sleep disturbance or sleep apnea
Treat associated depression or anxiety
Eliminate alcohol or caffeine in the evening
Institute regular sleep/wake schedule and sleep hygiene
Avoid excessive daytime naps
Encourage regular exercise (e.g., walking)
Attend to environmental factors
Timed exposure to bright light in the evening and in the morning may be helpful

Most cases of RBD respond dramatically to a small dose of clonazepam (e.g., 0.5–2 mg at night). For patients who do not respond to clonazepam, melatonin or pramipexole may be tried. In resistant cases, a combination of clonazepam and melatonin may be useful. A recent practice guideline published by the AASM has provided some consensus in approaching RBD therapy, listing the data for both clonazepam and melatonin as primary agents for this disorder with level B evidence of therapy and safety measures (removal of sharp objects from the bedroom area as level A evidence) (Aurora et al., 2010) (Table 101.13).

### Treatment of Sleep Dysfunction Associated with Neurological Disorders

Treatment of neurological disorders associated with insomnia, SBD, circadian rhythm sleep disorders, and parasomnias should follow the previously outlined principles of treatment. For the treatment of patients with AD and related dementias associated with sleep disturbance, certain general measures, as outlined in Box 101.36, should be instituted. For nocturnal agitation and sundowning, the patient should be treated with antipsychotics including the newer agents (haloperidol, 0.5–1.5 mg; thioridazine, 10–100 mg; risperidone, 1–1.5 mg; olanzapine, 5–10 mg; quetiapine, 12.5–100 mg). Depression is often an important feature in patients with AD, so a sedative-antidepressant may be helpful. Frequency of urination in such patients may result from infection or enlarged prostate and may disturb sleep at night. Appropriate measures should therefore be taken in such conditions. In some patients, timed exposure to bright light in the evening may improve nighttime sleep.

Sleep has not been consistently improved in patients with PD following antiparkinsonian medications. In those patients with reactivation of parkinsonian symptoms during sleep at night, adjustment in the timing and choice of medication may be helpful. Dopamine agonists or longer-acting preparations of levodopa at bedtime may benefit sleep in some patients. Antihistamines such as diphenhydramine may promote sleep in addition to the modest antiparkinsonian effect. A small dose of carbidopa-levodopa, with a second dose later at night when the patient awakens, may sometimes help those with insomnia. Nocturnal dyskinesias related to levodopa causing insomnia may respond to a reduction in the dose of dopamine agonists or the addition of a small dose of a benzodiazepine. In patients with psychosis and severe nocturnal hallucinations, clozapine or newer drugs such as olanzapine may be used with considerable benefit. During clozapine treatment, the usual precautions of monitoring blood cell count and testing liver function should be taken. Patients with PD associated with RBD should be treated with a small dose of clonazepam or melatonin. Patients with PD with OSAS associated with oxygen desaturation and repeated arousals should be treated with CPAP titration. In some patients with insomnia, judicious short-term use of hypnotics may be recommended. Some patients with PD showing the phenotype of narcolepsy with EDS not associated with OSAS may be treated with a small dose (100 mg in the morning) of modafinil or armodafinil (150 mg in the morning). This is, however, an off-label indication.

## CONCLUSION

In conclusion, an explosive growth in sleep medicine and increasing awareness about the importance of sleep in everyday life has propelled the topic of sleep to the forefront of neuroscience. It is more important than ever for all physicians, particularly neurologists and general practitioners, to take sleep medicine seriously and gain a basic understanding and adequate knowledge of this discipline as it applies to clinical practice. This chapter has attempted to give an overview of the science of sleep to stimulate physicians to be familiar with sleep medicine. Sleep deprivation at night related to either lifestyle habits or sleep disorders is associated with increasing morbidity and mortality, and it is time for the medical profession to recognize and not neglect this silent epidemic. Many sleep disorders remain undiagnosed and underdiagnosed, but effective treatment is available to prevent short- and long-term adverse consequences. This chapter has outlined approaches to a patient with sleep complaints and methods to diagnose and treat these disorders. Sleep/wake generating neurons are located within the CNS, and patients with neurological illnesses are particularly susceptible to sleep/wake dysfunction. Because sleep may adversely affect neurological disorders, it is especially incumbent upon neurologists to have a basic understanding of sleep and its disorders, which may encroach upon almost every aspect of neurology in clinical practice.

*The complete reference list is available online at https://expertconsult.inkling.com/.* 

102

# Headache and Other Craniofacial Pain

*Ivan Garza, Carrie E. Robertson, Jonathan H. Smith, Mark A. Whealy*

## OUTLINE



## PAIN TRANSMISSION AND MODULATION AS RELATED TO HEADACHE

Headache arises from activation of pain-sensitive intracranial structures. In the 1930s, Ray and Wolff identified which intracranial components were pain sensitive and mapped the pattern of pain referral based on studies in which various intracranial structures were stimulated during intracranial surgery performed during local anesthesia. Intracranial pain-sensitive structures include the arteries of the circle of Willis and the first few centimeters of their medium-sized branches, meningeal (dural) arteries, large veins and dural venous sinuses, and portions of the dura near blood vessels. More recent data from patients during awake craniotomies also suggest that, contrary to prior belief, the pia mater and small cerebral vessels are pain-sensitive (Fontaine et al., 2018). Pain-sensitive structures external to the skull cavity include the external carotid artery and its branches, scalp and neck muscles, skin and cutaneous nerves, cervical nerves and nerve roots, mucosa of sinuses, and teeth. Cranial nerves (CN) V, VII, IX, and X, in addition to cervical spine nerve/nerve roots, carry pain from these structures.

Trauma, inflammation, traction, compression, malignant infiltration, and other disturbances of pain-sensitive structures lead to headache. Superficial structures tend to refer pain locally, whereas deeper-seated lesions may refer pain imprecisely. A purulent maxillary sinus, for example, causes pain over the involved sinus, whereas within the cranial vault, nociceptive signals reach the central nervous system (CNS) largely by way of the first division of the trigeminal nerve (CN V), so an occipital lobe tumor may refer pain to the frontal head region. Infratentorial lesions tend to refer pain posteriorly because innervation of this compartment is by the second and third cervical nerve roots, which also supply the back of the head. However, posterior lesions or cervical spine pathological conditions may also produce frontal headache, because the caudal portion of the trigeminal nucleus extends down as far as the dorsal horn at the C3 level. Impulses arriving from C2 to C3 converge on neurons within the trigeminal nucleus and may refer pain to the somatic distribution of CN V.

Afferent pain impulses into the trigeminal nucleus are modulated by descending facilitatory and inhibitory input from brainstem structures, including the periaqueductal gray matter, rostral ventromedial medulla, locus ceruleus, and dorsal raphe nuclei. Opioids diminish pain perception by activating the inhibitory systems, whereas fear, anxiety, and overuse of analgesics may activate the facilitatory systems, thereby aggravating pain.

## CLASSIFICATION

In 1988, the Headache Classification Committee of the International Headache Society introduced a detailed classification of headaches. This has been subsequently revised, most recently in 2018, into what is now the International Classification of Headache Disorders 3rd edition (ICHD-3) (*Headache Classification Committee of the International Headache Society* [IHS], 2018). Its four main parts include: (1) primary headaches, (2) secondary headaches, (3) painful cranial neuropathies, other facial pain, and other headaches, and (4) appendix (Box 102.1). Secondary headaches are those in which head pain is a symptom of an underlying disease affecting pain-sensitive structures, while in primary headache disorders head pain occurs in the absence of such disease. The purpose of the appendix in the ICHD-3 is to present research

**BOX 102.1 Classification of Headache Disorders**

**Part One: The Primary Headaches**

1. Migraine
2. Tension-type headache
3. Trigeminal autonomic cephalalgias
4. Other primary headache disorders

**Part Two: The Secondary Headaches**

5. Headache attributed to trauma or injury to the head and/or neck
6. Headache attributed to cranial and/or cervical vascular disorder
7. Headache attributed to nonvascular intracranial disorder
8. Headache attributed to a substance or its withdrawal
9. Headache attributed to infection
10. Headache attributed to disorder of homeostasis
11. Headache or facial pain attributed to disorder of the cranium, neck, eyes, ears, nose, sinuses, teeth, mouth, or other facial or cervical structure
12. Headache attributed to psychiatric disorder

**Part Three: Painful Cranial Neuropathies, Other Facial Pain, and Other Headaches**

13. Painful lesions of the cranial nerves and other facial pain
14. Other headache disorders

**Part Four: Appendix**

*From Headache Classification Committee of the International Headache Society (IHS). 2018. The International Classification of Headache Disorders, third ed. Cephalalgia 38 (1), 1–211. https://doi.org/10.1177/0333102417738202.*

criteria for multiple entities that have not been sufficiently validated. If better scientific data become available, some of these may move to the main body of the classification in future revisions (IHS, 2018). Careful definition of migraine subtypes and other primary headache disorders has helped rid research and clinical publications of the confusing and often poorly defined terminology of earlier work.

## SECONDARY HEADACHES

### Headache Attributed to Nonvascular, Noninfectious Intracranial Disorders

Intracranial lesions that occupy space, or "mass lesions," produce head pain by traction on or compression of pain-sensitive veins, venous sinuses, arteries, cranial nerves, and possibly by causing inflammation around pain-sensitive structures in the head (Obermann et al., 2011). The nature, location, and temporal profile of headache produced by an intracranial mass depend on many factors, including lesion location, rate of growth, effect on cerebrospinal fluid (CSF) pathways, and any associated cerebral edema. The intracranial mass lesion may be neoplastic, inflammatory, or cystic. Mass lesions can result in either localized or generalized head pain.

#### Tumors

The estimated prevalence of headache in patients with brain tumors (see Chapters 71 and 74) varies from 50% to 70%. The likelihood of developing headache is probably mediated by the tumor size, type, and location, and on patient age and personal history of a preceding headache disorder (Obermann et al., 2011; Valentinis et al., 2010). Infratentorial tumors and intraventricular tumors might be more likely to cause headache than supratentorial tumors. In gliomas, specifically, infratentorial and right-sided tumors are more frequently associated with headache presence at onset (Russo et al., 2018). Progressive headaches (i.e., those with increases in intensity, frequency, and duration of pain) can be due to worsening of cerebral edema, the presence of midline shift, and hydrocephalus. Factors that increase the risk of brain tumor–related headaches include a personal history of a primary headache disorder and younger age at diagnosis (Valentinis et al., 2010).

Although headache is typically not an isolated symptom at the time of brain tumor diagnosis, not uncommonly it can be the first and most severe symptom that the patient experiences (Valentinis et al., 2010). In a prospective study of 211 patients with brain tumors, headache was the most frequent initial manifestation of the tumors (22% of the patients) and headache was the sole presenting symptom in 19% (Valentinis et al., 2010). In a series of 527 adults with glioma, 12.5% indicated headache as a presenting symptom of their disease (Russo et al., 2018).

There is wide variation in the characteristics of headaches attributed to intracranial tumors. Most commonly, such headaches are considered "nonclassifiable," meaning that their phenotype does not meet the phenotypic characteristics of a primary headache disorder such as migraine or tension-type headache (Valentinis et al., 2010). A headache phenotype that is "nonclassifiable" is followed in frequency by headaches that resemble tension-type headache and then migraine (Valentinis et al., 2010). Specifically in gliomas, however, tension-type headache was the most common phenotype (47% of cases) in a recent series (Russo et al., 2018). Most brain tumor headaches are felt bilaterally and are described as causing a pressure sensation. There is substantial variability in the frequency, duration, and specific location of pain. The location of headache pain does not reliably predict the location of the underlying brain tumor (Valentinis et al., 2010).

Rapidly growing tumors are more likely to produce headache than indolent lesions, but slowly enlarging lesions can eventually produce pain by compromising the ventricular system or exerting direct pressure on a pain-sensitive structure. When the CSF circulation is partially obstructed, resulting in high intracranial pressure (ICP), headache is often worse when supine, aggravated by coughing, straining, and Valsalva, and is often associated with nausea and vomiting. When tumors interfere with CSF flow and cause periodic increases in ICP, the periods of elevated ICP may correlate with increasing headache severity, vomiting, decreased consciousness, or a change in respiration.

Tumors growing in the ventricular system are rare, but they can manifest dramatically. The classic presentation of a colloid cyst of the third ventricle is a sudden headache of great severity, rapidly accompanied by nausea and vomiting and sometimes by loss of consciousness. Intraventricular meningiomas, choroid plexus papillomas, and other intraventricular tumors can present in this manner if they suddenly obstruct the ventricular outflow pathways. A positional change may precipitate such an event; similarly, adoption of a different posture may rapidly relieve the headache and other symptoms. Colloid cysts of the third ventricle generally lead to slowly enlarging hydrocephalus that may result in a generalized and constant headache with superimposed episodes of catastrophic increases in headache intensity. Headaches that have a rapid onset and/or are associated with loss of consciousness should lead the examiner to seek a secondary cause.

Infiltrating tumors such as gliomas can reach considerable size without causing pain, because they may not deform or stretch the pain-sensitive vessels and nerves. Such lesions are more likely to present with focal neurological symptoms or with seizures rather than headache. Sudden worsening of the neurological state due to hemorrhage into the tumor may present with sudden headache. Infarction of a tumor can cause edema and swelling that result in a similar dramatic onset of head pain and neurological deficit.

Tumors that are intracranial but extraparenchymal (e.g., meningioma, acoustic neuroma, pinealoma, craniopharyngioma) and pituitary tumors can all produce headaches, but the clinician must carefully consider whether the headaches and these tumors are causally related or coincidental. When headaches are truly associated with these tumors, there are no specific headache patterns. Headaches can be near the lesion, referred to a more distant site in the cranium, or generalized when ICP increases. A family history of primary headaches and cavernous sinus invasion appear to be risk factors for headaches associated with pituitary nonfunctioning adenomas (Yu et al., 2017). Meningiomas and meningeal sarcomas can invade the skull and even cause a mass externally by direct tumor spread or by overlying hyperostosis. Such tumors are often associated with localized head pain. Meningeal carcinomatosis (carcinomatous meningitis) produces a headache in most subjects, but the associated cranial nerve involvement and other neurological symptoms are generally more striking.

The headache associated with other intracranial mass lesions such as cerebral abscess and intracranial granuloma is no more specific than that due to a cerebral neoplasm.

Features that should serve as warnings that a patient's headaches may not be of benign origin and that raise the possibility of an intracranial mass lesion are: subacute and progressive; new onset in adults; change in pattern; associated with nausea or vomiting; nocturnal or upon awakening in the morning; precipitated or worsened by changes in posture or Valsalva maneuver; associated with confusion, seizures, weakness, and/or abnormal neurological examination.

### Syndrome of Transient Headache and Neurological Deficits With Cerebrospinal Fluid Lymphocytosis

Although originally termed "migrainous syndrome with CSF pleocytosis," several later reports used various terms, including headache with neurological deficits, CSF lymphocytosis, and pseudomigraine with temporary neurological symptoms and lymphocytic pleocytosis. This self-limited syndrome consists of one to several episodes of variable neurological deficits accompanied by moderate to severe headache and sometimes fever. Each episode lasts hours, with total duration of the syndrome being from 1 to 70 days. CSF abnormalities have included a lymphocytic pleocytosis varying from 10 to more than 700 cells/mm, elevation of CSF protein, and in some patients, elevated opening pressure. MRI and CT are normal in the vast majority of reported cases. Some patients may have evidence of gray-matter swelling or hemispheric hypoperfusion (Quintas et al., 2018; Yilmaz et al., 2010). Results of microbiological studies are usually negative. The cause of the syndrome is unclear, although an immune response to a viral infection is speculated. No treatment alters the self-limited course of this disorder. In contrast to this syndrome, episodes of Mollaret meningitis (see Chapters 76 and 103) are separated by months to years and are typically not accompanied by focal neurological symptoms.

## Headaches Due To Elevated Intracranial Pressure

Lesions that prevent free egress of CSF from the ventricular system result in obstructive hydrocephalus. If this occurs before closure of the cranial sutures, enlargement of the skull occurs, usually without producing headache. Ventricular obstruction after closure of the sutures leads to raised ICP and often to headache. The pain is often worse on awakening, occipital in distribution, and associated with neck stiffness. Vomiting, blurred vision, and transitory obscuration of vision due to papilledema may follow, as well as failing vision due to optic atrophy.

Rapidly developing obstruction due to a posterior fossa mass lesion or a ball-valve tumor, such as a third ventricular colloid cyst, can lead to a rapidly increasing headache followed by vomiting, impaired consciousness, and increasing neurological deterioration. Slowly developing hydrocephalus may result in massively dilated ventricles and may be associated with little or no headache.

Congenital obstruction of the foramina of Luschka and Magendie (the Dandy-Walker syndrome) can lead to ballooning of the fourth ventricle and deformity of the cerebellum. Minor degrees of this malformation can remain asymptomatic until later in life and then manifest with obstructive hydrocephalus and headache. Similarly, the Chiari malformation can obstruct free circulation of CSF and lead to hydrocephalus and headache and can cause symptoms via direct compression of the brainstem by herniated cerebellum (Graxzzi and Andrasik, 2012). This malformation can result in an occipital-suboccipital headache worsened or even initiated by a Valsalva maneuver during lifting, straining, or coughing. Thus, the Chiari malformation is one of the causes of an exertional or Valsalva maneuver–induced headache and cough headache. Other symptoms of Chiari malformation include visual phenomena (e.g., wavy lines, flashing lights, scotoma), blurred vision, photophobia, dizziness, disequilibrium, pressure in the ears, tinnitus, decreased hearing, nystagmus, dysphagia, and dysarthria. Other symptoms might be present if there is concurrent spinal cord syrinx. The clinician must be careful to differentiate between mild cerebellar tonsillar descent, a condition that is unlikely to cause symptoms, and a true Chiari malformation, a condition that can be associated with headache.

In communicating hydrocephalus, free communication exists between the ventricular system and the subarachnoid space, but CSF circulation or absorption is impaired. Obstruction in the basal cisterns or at the arachnoid granulations may follow subarachnoid hemorrhage and meningitis. Venous sinus occlusion can impair absorption of CSF. Headache may be a prominent symptom of both obstructive and communicating hydrocephalus, except in the case of normal-pressure hydrocephalus, which is generally painless (see Chapter 86).

### Idiopathic Intracranial Hypertension

Idiopathic intracranial hypertension (IIH) is a condition of increased intracranial pressure which typically manifests with papilledema and headaches and has no identifiable cause.

***Symptoms and signs.*** In recent years, the IIH treatment trial (IIHTT) has extensively expanded the available data on this condition (Friedman et al., 2014; Smith and Friedman, 2017). Analysis of clinical profiles at baseline confirmed previous observations that IIH is almost exclusively a disease of obese young women. The mean age was 29.0 years, 97.6% were women, and the average body mass index was 39.9 kg/m$^2$ (Wall et al., 2014). Headache was the most common initial symptom reported at study entry, followed by visual loss, pulsatile tinnitus, and diplopia, in that decreasing order. Frequency of most common symptoms at study entry was: headache in 84%, transient visual obscurations in 68%, back pain in 53%, and pulse synchronous tinnitus in 52% of patients. The headaches in IIH can be constant, daily, or intermittent and may or may not be classifiable according to phenotypes of primary headaches. In the IIHTT, the most common headache phenotypes were migraine in 52% and tension-type headache in 22% of patients, with the rest not fulfilling complete criteria for other primary headaches. Visual obscurations are a direct result of raised ICP leading to papilledema, while diplopia most often results from a lateral rectus palsy. Only 32% reported visual loss in the IIHTT (Wall et al., 2014).

***Evaluation.*** Most IIH patients have papilledema, which should not be confused with pseudopapilledema (e.g., drusen). An ophthalmologist should be involved in the diagnostic evaluation to confirm this and assess threat to vision if papilledema is present. One of the most common errors in diagnosing IIH is inaccurate ophthalmoscopic examination (Fisayo et al., 2016). Brain

**TABLE 102.1 Idiopathic Intracranial Hypertension Diagnostic Criteria**

**IIH**

A. Papilledema
B. Normal neurological exam (except 6th cranial nerve palsy)
C. Neuroimaging: normal brain parenchyma, venous thrombosis excluded.
D. Normal CSF constituents
E. Elevated lumbar puncture pressure >25 cm

**IIH Without Papilledema (IIHWOP)**

- Criteria B-E for IIH plus: unilateral or bilateral 6th cranial nerve palsy.

*CSF*, Cerebrospinal fluid; *IHH*, idiopathic intracranial hypertension.
*From Mollan, S.P., Davies, B., Silver, N.C., Shaw, S., Mallucci, C.L., Wakerley, B.R., et al., 2018. Idiopathic intracranial hypertension: consensus guidelines on management. J. Neurol. Neurosurg. Psychiatry. 89 (10), 1088–1100. https://doi.org/10.1136/jnnp-2017-317440.*

neuroimaging, ideally brain magnetic resonance imaging (MRI) with contrast, is mandatory before lumbar puncture (LP) to rule out an intracranial mass as the cause for symptoms and signs. Cerebral venography (usually with magnetic resonance venography [MRV]) should also be pursued, if possible, to rule out cerebral venous sinus thrombosis (an IIH mimic) and to assess for bilateral distal transverse cerebral venous sinus stenoses, which are present in most if not all IIH patients and may aid the diagnostic evaluation. Whether these stenoses are the cause or a consequence of IIH remains a matter of debate. It has been proposed, however, that bilateral transverse sinus stenosis (or stenosis of a dominant transverse venous sinus) might lead to the following sequence of events: decreased venous outflow drainage, cerebral venous hypertension, impairment of CSF passive resorption, further incrementing CSF pressure resulting in external compression of the transverse venous sinuses, leading to worsened venous stenosis and vicious cycle perpetuation (Bidot et al., 2015). Other described brain MRI findings in IIH include: empty sella, posterior sclera flattening, optic nerve sheath distention, optic nerve vertical tortuosity, and optic nerve head enhancement (Bidot et al., 2015). None of these brain MRV and MRI findings are specific for IIH, however; they can be seen in other causes of intracranial hypertension. Normal subjects may also have bilateral cerebral venous sinus stenoses.

Following the determination that there is no intracranial mass, ventricular system obstruction, or thrombosis of a dural venous sinus, the high CSF pressure can be confirmed by LP manometry. Opening pressure via LP of at least 250 mm CSF (in adults) is required for the diagnosis of IIH (Mollan et al., 2018). Importantly, pressure should ideally be measured in lateral decubitus, which provides the most accurate readings. Opening pressures obtained while the patient is sitting are not valid. Pressures measured while prone during fluoroscopy are typically difficult to interpret because of overestimation of pressure, although some suggest a table tilt while prone may improve interpretation (Schwartz et al., 2013). CSF composition should be normal in IIH. Removal of CSF to achieve a normal closing pressure relieves the headache and temporarily prevents visual obscurations. Table 102.1 summarizes IIH diagnostic criteria. Importantly, IIH mimics or "secondary pseudotumor cerebri" causes should be ruled out prior to diagnosing IIH (Table 102.2).

***Management.*** Prevention of permanent visual field loss is the main goal of therapy. Once the diagnosis of IIH is established, treatment in the absence of immediate threat for vision loss consists of weight loss and acetazolamide. Acetazolamide is typically started at 500 mg twice daily and is gradually increased if needed and tolerated. Most

**TABLE 102.2 Secondary "Pseudotumor Cerebri"**

**Cerebral Venous Abnormalities**

- Cerebral venous sinus thrombosis
- Bilateral jugular vein thrombosis or surgical ligation
- Middle ear or mastoid infection
- Increased right heart pressure
- Superior vena cava syndrome
- Arteriovenous fistulas
- Decreased CSF absorption from previous intracranial infection or subarachnoid hemorrhage
- Hypercoagulable states

**Medications and Exposures**

- Antibiotics
  - Tetracycline, minocycline, doxycycline, nalidixic acid, sulfa drugs
- Vitamin A and retinoids
  - Hypervitaminosis A, isotretinoin, all-trans retinoic acid for promyelocytic leukemia, excessive liver ingestion
- Hormones
  - Human growth hormone, thyroxine (in children), leuprorelin acetate, levonorgestrel (Norplant system), anabolic steroids
- Withdrawal from chronic corticosteroids
- Lithium
- Chlordecone

**Medical Conditions**

- Endocrine disorders
  - Addison disease
  - Hypoparathyroidism
- Hypercapnia
  - Sleep apnea
  - Pickwickian syndrome
- Anemia
- Renal failure
- Turner syndrome
- Down syndrome

*CSF*, Cerebrospinal fluid.
*From Friedman, D.I., Liu, G.T., Digre, K.B., 2013. Revised diagnostic criteria for the pseudotumor cerebri syndrome in adults and children. Neurology 81 (13), 1159–1165. https://doi.org/10.1212/WNL.0b013e3182a55f17.*

patients in the recent IIHTT tolerated >1 g/day for 6 months (ten Hove et al., 2016). This trial has also provided support for the safe use of acetazolamide up to 4 g daily with weight loss for effective treatment of mild vision loss in IIH, with associated improvements in papilledema, increased ICP, and quality of life (Smith and Friedman, 2017). Other diuretics and topiramate are used in patients who cannot take acetazolamide, although these have not been studied in controlled fashion. The amount of weight loss required for IIH to remit is not known, but up to 15% of weight loss has been reported (Mollan et al., 2018). An ophthalmologist should follow patients together with the neurologist to properly monitor vision. Headache is usually managed according to its phenotype (e.g., migraine or tension-type), when present.

Patients who have significant visual field loss at presentation and those that have progressive visual field loss and/or progressive worsening of visual acuity despite medical management may require surgical intervention, traditionally CSF shunting or optic nerve sheath fenestration. Cerebral venous sinus stenting has been reported to improve symptoms of intracranial hypertension. The role of neurovascular stenting in IIH, however, has not yet been established. Stenting may be useful for highly selected IIH patients with venous sinus stenosis with an elevated pressure gradient in whom traditional therapies have not been effective (Mollan et al., 2018).

Of note, headaches sometimes persist even after proper management of IIH. In the IIHTT, 41% of patients reported a prior history of migraine (Wall et al., 2014). In addition, 37% of headache sufferers at baseline were overusing symptomatic headache medications (Friedman et al., 2017). Possibly, in some cases, persistent headaches may occur on the basis of other processes (e.g., migraine with or without medication overuse headache) different from intracranial hypertension.

## Headache Attributed to Low Cerebrospinal Fluid Pressure

The headache of low CSF pressure/volume from spinal CSF leaks is characteristically orthostatic, developing or worsening when a person is upright and resolving or significantly improving with recumbency. It most commonly occurs after a LP via loss of CSF volume due to the removal of CSF for diagnostic purposes, and/or continued leakage of CSF through the hole in the arachnoid and dural layers left by the LP needle. Loss of CSF can result in brain sagging and traction on pain-sensitive structures such as bridging veins and sensory nerves. Recumbency removes the effect of gravity, and the traction headache is relieved. The headache that occurs after a spinal tap usually resolves spontaneously within a few days. Spontaneous recovery is estimated to occur in 24% of patients within the first 2 days, an additional 29% of patients within 3–4 days, and an additional 19% within 5–7 days (Turnbull and Shepherd, 2003). The healing process might be hastened when the patient has relative bed rest and good hydration. When these conservative measures fail, relief can usually be obtained by the application of an epidural blood patch. An epidural blood patch consists of approximately 20 mL of the patient's own venous blood being injected into the epidural space close to the site of the original LP. The resulting compression of the thecal sac and the presumed elevation of subarachnoid pressure presumably explains the resulting headache resolution. The increased pressure resulting from the epidural blood patch presumably causes temporary cessation of the CSF leak, thereby allowing the dura and arachnoid to heal. The success rate of a single epidural blood patch is estimated between 70% and 98% (Turnbull and Shepherd, 2003).

Similar low-CSF pressure/volume headaches can occur when a spinal leak spontaneously develops, a condition still often referred to as "spontaneous intracranial hypotension" by some. Although indeed a significant number of patients with this condition have low (sometimes negative) CSF opening pressure when measured via LP, most have normal pressures (Kranz et al., 2016b). Because low CSF volume may better explain the low pressure, headache, and neuroimaging findings seen in spontaneous spinal CSF leaks, "CSF hypovolemia" has been proposed as an alternative term (Mokri, 1999). Skull-based CSF leaks, however, rarely if ever present with the classic syndrome in the setting of spontaneous spinal CSF leaks (Schievink et al., 2012). The remaining discussion pertains to "headaches secondary to spontaneous spinal CSF leaks (SSCSFL)," the authors' preferred term for this syndrome.

Spontaneous spinal CSF leaks are most commonly located in the thoracic or cervico-thoracic regions. Three main types have been identified in observational studies: the dural tear, the meningeal diverticulum, and the CSF-venous fistula (Schievink et al., 2016). Although a precipitating event for symptoms is often absent or uncertain, many patients with SSCSFL recall having a very minor injury, coughing, sneezing, or performing a Valsalva maneuver just prior to onset of symptoms. Most commonly headache is orthostatic, but not infrequently can be purely precipitated by Valsalva-like maneuvers (e.g., coughing, sneezing, laughing) or present as a combination of these two. A large series of SSCSFL specifically secondary to CSF-venous fistula reported an even greater percentage of patients experienced Valsalva-induced headache exacerbation or precipitation compared to orthostatic headache, features that should raise suspicion for occult CSF-venous fistula (Duvall et al., 2019). Occasionally, headaches secondary to SSCSFL are preceded by a single "thunderclap headache." Other common symptoms of SSCSFL include auditory muffling, tinnitus, nausea and vomiting, and neck pain. Patients who have had the condition for a prolonged time can lose the orthostatic component

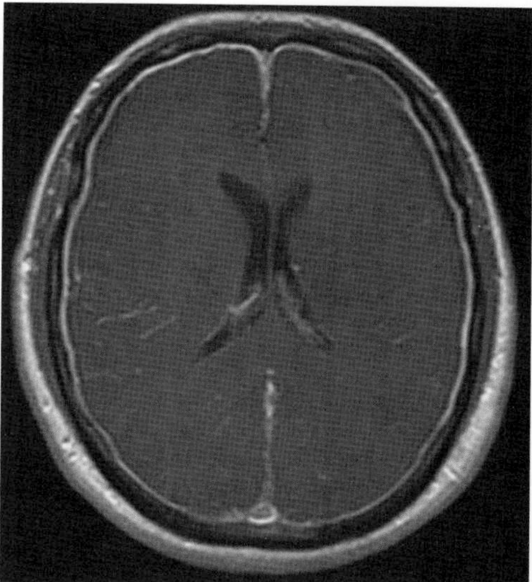

**Fig. 102.1** Axial T1-weighted magnetic resonance image with gadolinium in a patient with a spontaneous spinal cerebrospinal fluid leak and orthostatic headache demonstrates diffuse pachymeningeal thickening and enhancement.

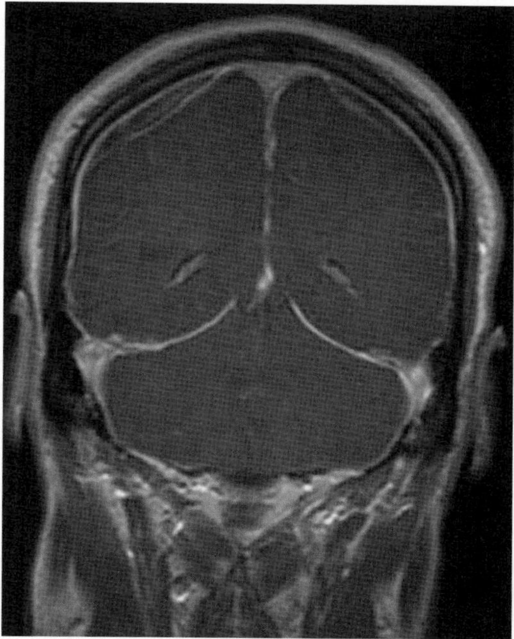

**Fig. 102.2** Coronal T1-weighted magnetic resonance image with gadolinium of a patient with orthostatic headache secondary to a SSCSFL demonstrates subdural fluid collections and pachymeningeal enhancement.

to their headache. Such patients might have constant headaches or so-called "end-of-the-day" headaches (headache starting late in the day and getting worse as the day goes on). As additional cases have been reported in the literature, the clinical picture of CSF leaks has been found to take many forms (Mokri, 2004).

When a SSCSFL is suspected, the initial diagnostic test is brain MRI with gadolinium. MRI findings supportive of a diagnosis of SSCSFL include diffuse pachymeningeal gadolinium enhancement, brain sagging (i.e., cerebral and cerebellar tonsillar descent, inferior displacement of the optic chiasm), flattening of the anterior aspect of the pons, and venous dilation (Figs. 102.1 and 102.2; eFig. 102.3). While an "acquired Chiari" from brain sagging can commonly be distinguished fairly easily from a congenital Chiari I malformation, sometimes this can be challenging. Subdural fluid collections (subdural hygromas and subdural hematomas) might occur in up to 50% of patients with SSCSFL (Schievink et al., 2005). The patient with classical symptoms of SSCSFL and classical brain MRI findings of the disorder might not need additional diagnostic tests prior to treatment with conservative measures or epidural blood patch. However, increasing symptom duration associates with decreased prevalence of abnormal dural enhancement; brain MRI can be normal in 20%–30% of cases (Kranz et al., 2016a). When the diagnosis is uncertain a complete spine MRI and/or radioisotope cisternography (RICG) may help establish the presence of a SSCSFL although they rarely localize the exact leak site. Spine MRI findings suggestive of CSF leak include dural enhancement, dilated epidural veins, epidural venous plexus engorgement, and/or epidural fluid collections. Large longitudinal epidural fluid collections often suggest the presence of a high flow or "fast" SSCSFL. On RICG, delayed radioactive tracer ascent to cerebral convexities and/or early isotope tracer appearance in the urinary bladder are findings suggestive of CSF leak. Although measurement of opening pressure via LP can aid diagnosis if low opening pressure is found, LP should be avoided when possible due to the risk of worsening symptoms following the procedure. Importantly, a normal CSF opening pressure does not rule out a spontaneous CSF leak. If RICG is pursued, however, we typically measure opening pressure during the LP part of the procedure.

In patients with the typical clinical and radiographic features of SSCSFL, treatment may be conservative with bed rest and hydration for 1–2 weeks. If this is either impractical or ineffective, treatment with an epidural blood patch is warranted. If the CSF leak site is suspected, a "targeted" patch can be attempted close to the suspected leak site, but the patch is often done "blindly" in the lumbar spine when no clear leak site is known or suspected. Although epidural blood patches are effective in a substantial number of patients, many require more than one blood patch, and some require as many as four to six blood patches (Mokri, 2004) with 1–2 months between individual attempts.

Patients with SSCSFL who fail to respond to conservative measures are best investigated with myelography, the most effective study at present to identify the precise spinal CSF leak site. Myelography can also be pursued even prior to attempting epidural blood patching in patients with SSCSFL when a more precise diagnosis and a more definitive treatment plan are desired. Conventional computed tomography (CT) myelography is often the first modality used. Dynamic CT myelography is an alternative modality, particularly helpful to localize high-flow leaks. Digital subtraction myelography may be particularly helpful in those with suspected occult CSF-venous fistula and in patients with SSCSFL with negative conventional CT myelogram. If myelography identifies the CSF leak site, targeted epidural blood patching can be attempted. However, CSF-venous fistulas appear to respond poorly to epidural blood patching (Duvall et al., 2019) and are often best managed with surgical repair in centers with expertise. For other resistant leaks that can be precisely localized, surgical repair may also be attempted.

## Headache Attributed to Trauma or Injury to the Head and/or Neck

Headaches are a common symptom following injuries to the head and neck. Direct causality between the injury and headache is typically difficult to prove, since there are no headache characteristics that are specific or sensitive for a diagnosis of posttraumatic headache. Thus, the interval between trauma and onset of headaches is relied upon for making a diagnosis of a posttraumatic headache. Although controversial, diagnostic criteria stipulate that headaches must begin within the first 7 days following trauma in order to be considered "posttraumatic" or within 7 days of regaining consciousness following a head injury or within 7 days of discontinuing medications that impair the ability to sense or report headache following head injury (IHS, 2018). In addition, the diagnosis of headaches attributed to whiplash requires that there is neck pain and/or headache at the time of whiplash. Posttraumatic headaches are considered "acute" when they have been present for less than 3 months and "persistent" when they last longer than 3 months (IHS, 2018). Posttraumatic headaches can be due to direct or indirect forces to the head and/or neck.

Headaches attributed to head injuries are typically subdivided into those associated with mild head injury and those associated with moderate to severe injury. Headache is the most common symptom following mild head injury and headaches might be more common following mild traumatic brain injury compared to moderate or severe injury (Packard, 2005). Other risk factors for the development of posttraumatic headaches might include presence of pre-injury headaches, female sex, and presence of comorbid psychiatric disorders (Stovner et al., 2009).

Most often, posttraumatic headaches phenotypically resemble migraine or tension-type headaches and less often resemble cervicogenic headache or occipital neuralgia (Lew et al., 2006). Headache may be an isolated symptom following head trauma or can be part of the post-concussion syndrome, a syndrome consisting of headache, dizziness, fatigue, cognitive dysfunction, psychomotor slowing, insomnia and personality changes (Evans, 2004; Yang et al., 2009). When considering a diagnosis of posttraumatic headache, it is essential to exclude structural traumatic injuries such as cervical spine injuries, skull fractures, intracranial hemorrhages, cerebrospinal fluid leaks, and cervical artery dissections.

Treatment of post-concussion syndrome and posttraumatic headache can be difficult, and an evidence base from which to select optimal therapies is absent. Posttraumatic headaches are thus treated according to the primary headache disorder that they most resemble (e.g., a posttraumatic headache that resembles migraine is treated with medications and other therapies typically used to treat migraine). Optimizing treatment requires that coexisting symptoms such as myofascial pain and spasm, sleep disorders, and anxiety be recognized and addressed. Nonpharmacological treatments (e.g., physical therapy, biobehavioral therapy) should be considered in addition to medication therapy.

## Headache Attributed to Infection

Inflammation of pain-sensitive structures such as the meninges and intracranial vessels produces the severe headache frequently associated with both meningitis and meningoencephalitis. Headache is the most common symptom in acute bacterial meningitis, occurring in nearly 90% of cases (van de Beek et al., 2004). Acute bacterial meningitis characteristically produces a severe holocephalic headache with neck stiffness and other signs of meningismus, including photophobia and irritability. Pain may be retro-orbital and may worsen with eye movement. The presence of the classic triad of fever, neck stiffness, and altered mental status has a low sensitivity for the diagnosis of meningitis; however, nearly all patients present with at least two of these symptoms and/or headache (van de Beek et al., 2004). Jolt accentuation of headache (i.e., worsening of headache with sudden movements) is a common feature of bacterial meningitis but its absence does not rule it out.

Chronic meningitis due to fungal or tuberculous infection may lead to headache that may be severe and unrelenting. The headache of intracranial infection is nonspecific but merits consideration, especially in immunocompromised patients. The diagnosis can be confirmed only by examination of the CSF. Further discussion of meningitis can be found in Chapters 4, 75, 76, and 77.

Sinusitis, mastoiditis, epidural or intraparenchymal abscess formation, and osteomyelitis of the skull can all cause either focal or generalized headache. The diagnosis is usually suspected in the context of other associated symptoms and signs. After craniotomy, increasing pain and swelling in the operative site may be due to osteomyelitis of the bone flap. Plain skull roentgenograms may reveal the typical mottled appearance of the infected bone, necessitating removal of the flap.

Mollaret meningitis is a rare and recurrent aseptic meningitis (see Chapters 76 and 103). The CSF cellular response includes large epithelioid cells (Mollaret cells). The pathogenesis is unknown but may relate to the herpes simplex virus. The condition may recur every few days or every few weeks for months or years. Headache, signs of meningismus, and low-grade fever accompany each attack. Treatment is mainly symptomatic.

Headache can accompany systemic infections due to viruses (e.g., influenza), bacteria (e.g., leptospirosis) and other infectious agents (e.g., *Borrelia burgdorferi*). These typically nonspecific headaches can be mild or can be a prominent symptom of the systemic infection (Gladstone and Bigal, 2010). Headaches attributable to systemic infections might be a result of the microorganisms activating pain-sensitive structures, release of inflammatory mediators, presence of fever, and/or dehydration.

## Headache Attributed to Cranial or Cervical Vascular Disorders

### Aneurysms and Arteriovenous Malformations

Intracranial aneurysms are rarely responsible for headache unless they rupture or rapidly enlarge. Large aneurysms may produce pain by exerting pressure upon cranial nerves or other pain-sensitive structures. Such pain is most commonly associated with aneurysms of the internal carotid and posterior communicating arteries. Enlargement of an aneurysm may occur shortly before rupture, and the pain is therefore an important clinical sign.

Parenchymal arteriovenous malformations (AVMs) should be considered in a patient presenting with a cranial bruit or the classic triad of migraine, seizures, and focal neurological deficits. Headache may be a presenting symptom in about 16% of patients and is often ipsilateral to the AVM. Similar to aneurysms, the pain may increase in intensity and frequency before hemorrhage. Though photophobia and phonophobia are uncommon, large AVMs can be associated with ipsilateral or bilateral throbbing cephalgia, resembling migraine. Occipital AVMs may frequently have migraine characteristics, and it is thought that the occipital location may be linked with cortical spreading depression, causing secondary migraine headaches. The visual disturbances associated with occipital AVMs may resemble migrainous aura. MR or CT angiography can usually exclude the presence of clinically significant aneurysms and AVMs.

Both aneurysms and AVMs can produce mild subarachnoid hemorrhages that result in sentinel headaches. Such headaches may be abrupt, mild, and short-lived. More catastrophic subarachnoid hemorrhages classically present as the worst headache the patient has ever had, all the more worrisome when associated with neck stiffness or pain, transient neurological symptoms (e.g., extraocular nerve palsy), or fever. Patients having any suggestion of a sentinel bleeding episode or who describe a recent thunderclap-like headache (see thunderclap headache discussion below) require emergent examination and CT to detect the presence of subarachnoid blood. If the CT is normal, perform a LP, looking for blood or xanthochromia.

### Subarachnoid Hemorrhage and Thunderclap Headache

The term *thunderclap headache* describes a severe headache occurring with instantaneous onset (within seconds) and without warning, like a clap of thunder. While multiple processes can present like this, a subarachnoid hemorrhage is the most worrisome. Rupture of an intracranial aneurysm or AVM results in a subarachnoid hemorrhage, with or without extension into the brain parenchyma. The headache of a subarachnoid hemorrhage is characteristically explosive in onset and of overwhelming intensity. Patients may relate that they thought they were hit on the head. The headache rapidly generalizes and may quickly be accompanied by neck and back pain. Loss of consciousness may also occur, but many patients remain alert enough to complain of the excruciating headache. Vomiting often accompanies the headache, which may aggravate the pain. Extension of blood into the ventricles and basal cisterns or distortion of the midline structures can each contribute to the rapid development of hydrocephalus, which frequently worsens the headache.

Suspicion of the diagnosis is easily confirmed by an unenhanced CT scan that reveals blood in the subarachnoid cisterns or within the parenchyma and often early hydrocephalus. When a CT unequivocally shows blood in the subarachnoid spaces it is not necessary or advisable to perform a LP, because the resultant reduction of CSF pressure may cause herniation of the brain or may remotely induce further bleeding from the aneurysm. Demonstration of subarachnoid hemorrhage generally indicates the need for cerebral angiography. The timing of this procedure and the subsequent mode of treatment are detailed elsewhere (see Chapter 65). The headache that occurs after a subarachnoid hemorrhage may be persistent, lasting up to 7–10 days. Rarely, a chronic daily headache (CDH) may persist for months to years.

Movement aggravates a subarachnoid hemorrhage headache, and photophobia and phonophobia are often associated. Therefore, these patients require a dark, quiet room, as well as comfort measures that minimize straining with bowel movements, vomiting, and coughing.

Other conditions which can also manifest with thunderclap headache in addition to subarachnoid hemorrhage include cerebral venous sinus thrombosis, cervicocephalic arterial dissection, pituitary apoplexy, acute hypertensive crisis, spontaneous spinal CSF leaks, meningitis, embolic cerebellar infarcts, pheochromocytoma (Angus, 2013; Heo et al., 2009), and reversible cerebral vasoconstriction syndromes (RCVS) (Calabrese et al., 2007; Schwedt, 2013). These entities can be associated with significant neurological morbidity and may not be easily seen on the initial CT image, thus underscoring the need for MRI and magnetic resonance angiography (MRA)/MRV in this group if results of the initial workup are negative. There is also a rarely seen category of thunderclap headache, referred to as primary thunderclap headache, for which there is no underlying cause established (see the section "Other Primary Headaches" later in the chapter).

### Subdural Hematoma

Bleeding into the subdural space is generally due to tearing of the bridging veins that cross the subarachnoid space to reach the venous sinuses. Chronic subdural hematomas may cause headache via enlargement of the lesion and may present without serious neurological signs for a considerable time. Midline shift was the most influential factor for headache in one study, which has led some to consider that the likely cause of headache may be stretching or twisting of the pain-sensitive meninges and meningeal arteries or veins (Yamada et al., 2018). Changes in personality, alterations in cognitive abilities, subacute dementia, and nonspecific symptoms such as dizziness and excessive sleepiness may be present for weeks or months. Focal seizures, focal weakness, sensory changes, and ultimately, decreasing levels of consciousness may occur. Symptoms of chronic subdural hematoma, including headache and focal neurological symptoms, may fluctuate and occur intermittently, thereby mimicking transient ischemic attacks (TIAs). Headache is the single most common symptom of subdural hematoma and often presents as a severe bitemporal pain. Headache due to subdural hematoma is more common in young people; the cerebral atrophy seen in many elderly patients may be protective in the setting of any space-occupying intracranial lesion. Subdural hematoma should be considered in an elderly person with recent onset of headaches, especially in the context of a traumatic injury of even mild severity. Once suspected, exclude the presence of a subdural hematoma with CT or MRI. Treatment of subdural hematomas is discussed in Chapter 60. Headaches tend to resolve after resolution of the bleed.

### Parenchymal Hemorrhage

A hemorrhage into the cerebral or cerebellar tissue is a potent source of headache of rapid onset and increasing severity. The intraparenchymal mass causes headache by deforming and shifting the pain-sensitive vascular, meningeal, and neural structures. As the hematoma enlarges, it may obstruct the normal circulation of CSF and lead to increases in ICP. Initially, the pain of a cerebral hemorrhage is often ipsilateral, but it may generalize in the presence of hydrocephalus and elevated ICP. Rupture of the hematoma into the subarachnoid space or leakage of the blood into the basal cisterns through the CSF pathways may cause the headache to intensify and may also be associated with neck stiffness and other signs of meningeal irritation. Disorders leading to cerebral and cerebellar hemorrhages are more thoroughly discussed elsewhere (see Chapter 64).

Cerebellar hemorrhages account for about 10% of all intraparenchymal bleeds and are neurological emergencies with potentially fatal outcomes. An enlarging hematoma in the cerebellum rapidly compresses vital brainstem structures and obstructs the outflow of CSF from the ventricular system. This leads to occipital headache followed rapidly by vomiting, impaired consciousness, and various combinations of brainstem, cerebellar, and cranial nerve dysfunction.

### Cerebral Ischemia

Cerebral infarctions and TIAs may be associated with transient head pain in up to 40% of patients. The headache may be either steady or throbbing and is rarely explosive or severe (Kropp et al., 2013). The location of the pain is a poor predictor of the vascular territory involved, though unilateral headaches tend to be ipsilateral to the infarct. Cerebral ischemia-related headache is more common in younger patients and patients who are female. It is also more common in patients with larger infarcts and infarcts in the posterior cerebral and vertebrobasilar arterial distributions (Kropp et al., 2013). A recent MRI voxel-based symptom lesion-mapping study suggests headache phenotypes may be related to specific ischemic lesion patterns (Seifert et al., 2018). In this study, pulsatile headache occurred with widespread cortical/subcortical strokes, noise sensitivity was associated with cerebellar lesions, nausea was associated with posterior circulation territory infarcts, and cranial-autonomic symptoms were related to parietal lobe, somatosensory cortex, and middle temporal cortical lesions (Seifert et al., 2018).

If a large cerebral or cerebellar infarct produces significant mass effect as a result of edema, the associated headache may worsen. Obstruction of the ventricular system frequently results in hydrocephalus and further aggravation of the pain. The pain may be pulsatile and may worsen with straining or the head-low position. Hemorrhagic transformation of an ischemic infarct may be associated with worsening of headache. As the infarct decreases in size and the phase of hyperemia subsides, headache generally eases, although in some, headache following stroke becomes chronic and often resembles tension-type headache (Hansen et al., 2015).

Paroxysmal visual and sensory disturbances commonly associated with migraine aura may mimic symptoms of cerebrovascular disease, occasionally making the differentiation between the two a challenge. The visual aura of migraine is typically a positive phenomenon, perceived with the eyes open or closed. Visual disturbances due to ischemic lesions of the visual pathway or retina are usually associated with negative phenomena such as vision loss or a negative scotoma; however, emboli to the retinal artery can result in showers of bright flashes, and calcarine ischemia can occasionally produce scintillating scotoma. While visual disturbances associated with stroke and TIA are usually abrupt and fixed, the migraine aura tends to march across the visual field over the course of a few minutes and is generally followed by headache after a latent interval. The headache associated with stroke and TIA typically has a more variable relationship to the visual disturbances.

### Carotid and Vertebral Artery Dissection

Dissection of the cervical portion of the carotid or vertebral arteries is associated with headache, neck pain, or face pain in approximately 80% of patients. The headache may be isolated or associated with an ipsilateral Horner syndrome or stroke symptoms. An ipsilateral Horner syndrome is more common in carotid than vertebral dissections, and the sympathetic hypofunction may be due to interference with the sympathetic fibers around the internal carotid artery as they ascend from the superior cervical ganglion to the intracranial structures. In internal carotid artery dissections, the headache is typically unilateral and ipsilateral to dissection. Facial pain is common and ipsilateral cranial nerve palsies, especially of lower cranial nerves, are not infrequent. Cerebral or retinal ischemic symptoms are the initial manifestations in a minority of patients. Vertebral artery dissections present most often with headache with or without neck pain, followed by a delay of focal CNS ischemic symptoms. In uncomplicated intracranial vertebral artery dissection, the headache usually is acute in onset with a persistent and temporal feature and in many cases the pain appears to be throbbing and severe in the ipsilateral and occipitonuchal area. Additionally, the headache often is aggravated by head flexion/ rotation and relieved by head extension and being supine (Kim et al., 2015).

Cervicocephalic arterial dissections can result from intrinsic factors that predispose the vessel to dissection, including fibromuscular dysplasia, cystic medial necrosis, and other connective tissue disorders such as Marfan syndrome or Ehlers-Danlos syndrome. Extrinsic factors such as trivial trauma may play a pathogenic role when superimposed on structurally abnormal arteries. Severe head and neck trauma may occasionally be the proximate cause of dissection. Importantly, in patients >60 years old, pain and mechanical triggers may be absent, making the diagnosis of cervical artery dissection more challenging in these older patients (Traenka et al., 2017). MRI or MRA usually confirms the diagnosis of arterial dissection. At the level of involvement, the lumen of the artery typically appears as a dark circle of flow void of smaller caliber than the original vessel, and the intramural clot appears as a hyperintense and bright crescent or circle (in both T1- and T2-weighted images) surrounding the flow void (eFig. 102.4). Catheter angiography is rarely required. The pain associated with cervicocephalic dissections is of variable duration and may require treatment with potent analgesics. Patients with evidence of distal embolization are usually treated with either antiplatelet agents or anticoagulation.

### Giant-Cell Arteritis

Giant-cell arteritis is a vasculitis of elderly persons and is one of the most ominous causes of headache in this population. When

**TABLE 102.3 Symptoms of Giant-Cell Arteritis in 166 Patients***

| Symptom | Patients with Symptom (%) | Patients in whom it was Initial Symptom (%) |
|---|---|---|
| Headache | 72 | 33 |
| Polymyalgia rheumatica | 58 | 25 |
| Malaise, fatigue | 56 | 20 |
| Jaw claudication | 40 | 4 |
| Fever | 35 | 11 |
| Cough | 17 | 8 |
| Neuropathy | 14 | 0 |
| Sore throat, dysphagia | 11 | 2 |
| Amaurosis fugax | 10 | 2 |
| Permanent vision loss | 8 | 3 |
| Claudication of limbs | 8 | 0 |
| Transient ischemic attack/stroke | 7 | 0 |
| Neuro-otological disorder | 7 | 0 |
| Scintillating scotoma | 5 | 0 |
| Tongue claudication | 4 | 0 |
| Depression | 3 | 0.6 |
| Diplopia | 2 | 0 |
| Tongue numbness | 2 | 0 |
| Myelopathy | 0.6 | 0 |

*Some patients had coincident onset of more than one symptom.
*Data from Caselli, R.J., Hunder, G.G., Whisnant, J.P., 1988. Neurologic disease in biopsy-proven giant cell (temporal) arteritis. Neurology 38, 352–359.*

unrecognized and untreated, it may lead to permanent blindness. Patients with this disorder most commonly see neurologists for new headaches of unknown cause.

***Clinical symptoms.*** The clinical manifestations of giant-cell arteritis result from inflammation of medium and large arteries. Table 102.3 summarizes clinical symptoms in 166 patients examined at the Mayo Clinic between 1981 and 1983 (Caselli et al., 1988). Headache was the most common symptom, experienced by 72% of patients at some time and the initial symptom in 33%. The headache is most often throbbing, and many patients report scalp tenderness. Headache is associated with striking focal tenderness of the affected superficial temporal or, less often, occipital artery. One-third of patients with headache may have no objective signs of superficial temporal artery inflammation.

More than half of patients with giant-cell arteritis experience *polymyalgia rheumatica*, which is the initial symptom in one-fourth. Fatigue, malaise, and a general loss of energy occur in 56% of patients and are the initial symptoms in 20%. Jaw claudication is common and the initial symptom in 4% of patients. Tongue claudication is rare.

*Amaurosis fugax* is one of the most ominous symptoms in giant-cell arteritis; 50% of affected patients subsequently become partially or totally blind if untreated. In the Mayo Clinic series, 10% of patients experienced amaurosis fugax, and 35% of those cases were bilateral. Horizontal or vertical diplopia also occurs in giant-cell arteritis.

Some 14% of patients have a neuropathy, which is a peripheral polyneuropathy in 48%, multiple mononeuropathies in 39%, and an isolated mononeuropathy in 13%. Limb claudication occurs in 8% of patients and usually involves the upper limbs. TIAs and strokes occur in 7% of patients, and the ratio of carotid to vertebral events is 2 : 1. Vertigo and unilateral hearing loss can occur. An acute myelopathy, acute confusional state, and subacute stepwise cognitive deterioration are rare manifestations.

***Physical findings.*** About 49% of patients with histologically verified giant-cell arteritis have physical signs of superficial temporal artery inflammation, including erythema, pain on palpation, arterial nodularity and/or thickening, or reduced pulsation on the affected side. Rarely, ischemic necrosis of the scalp and tongue occurs. Almost a third of patients have large-artery bruits or diminished pulses, which usually affect the carotid artery. The upper-limb arteries are more commonly affected than those in the lower limbs.

Ocular findings in giant-cell arteritis may be striking. In patients with amaurosis fugax, sludging of blood in the retinal arterioles may be observed. With infarction of the optic nerve, vision loss precedes the funduscopic signs of an anterior ischemic optic neuropathy by up to 36 hours. During the acute stage, there may be optic disc edema, optic disc pallor, and resulting visual field defects which tend to be altitudinal. Optic disc edema is commonly followed by the gradual development of optic atrophy. Restrictions in eye movements may indicate involvement of specific extraocular muscles. Oculosympathetic paresis (Horner syndrome) occasionally occurs.

Up to one-third of patients have clinically significant large-artery disease. The most common causes of vasculitis-related death are cerebral and myocardial infarction. In fatal occurrences, vertebral, ophthalmic, and posterior ciliary arteries are involved as often and as severely as the superficial temporal arteries. Rupture of the aorta is rare. In patients with peripheral neuropathic syndromes, ischemic infarction of peripheral nerves due to vasculitis is demonstrable. Intracranial vascular involvement is rare.

***Laboratory studies, and imaging.*** The laboratory abnormality most often associated with giant-cell arteritis is elevation of the erythrocyte sedimentation rate (ESR) (mean, 85 ± 32 mm in 1 hour with the Westergren method), which has a sensitivity of about 84%. C-reactive protein levels may be more sensitive than the ESR, though one study showed that both can be normal in 4% of biopsy-proven patients (Kermani et al., 2012). Patients are usually anemic (mean hemoglobin value 11.7 ± 1.6 g/dL) and show a mild thrombocytosis (mean platelet count 427 ± 116 × $10^3$/μL). As all of these laboratory tests are nonspecific, the confirmatory diagnosis rests on a temporal artery biopsy. However, the sensitivity for this procedure is low, with a high false-negative rate of 15%–40% (Chong and Robertson, 2005).

Imaging, particularly with temporal artery MRI or ultrasound, may supplement the diagnostic investigation and may be helpful in decision making about proceeding to biopsy. The superficial cranial arteries along with the mural and luminal properties can be investigated with a contrast-enhanced, high-resolution, temporal artery MRI (Bley et al., 2005). Doppler ultrasound has been advocated by some, but its practical value is difficult to assess because of the heterogeneous study findings and high operator dependence for image acquisition (Bienvenu et al., 2016). Currently, temporal artery imaging is not considered to support the diagnosis with as much certainty as temporal artery biopsy (Bienvenu et al., 2016). An angiogram of the aortic arch vessels may show long segments of smoothly tapered stenosis and occlusions of subclavian, brachial, and axillary arteries. Fluorodeoxyglucose positron emission tomography (FDG-PET)/CT may supplement the diagnostic investigation by identifying vessel inflammation. The spatial resolution of FDG-PET is best for vessels greater than 4 mm in diameter, so it is most useful when involvement of larger vessels, such as the aorta or the subclavian, vertebral, and carotid arteries, is suspected.

***Pathology.*** The histopathological features of arterial lesions include intimal proliferation with consequent luminal stenosis, disruption of the internal elastic membrane by a mononuclear cell infiltrate, invasion and necrosis of the media progressing to panarteritic involvement by mononuclear cells, giant-cell formation with granulomata within the mononuclear cell infiltrate, and (variably) intravascular thrombosis  (eFig. 102.5). Involvement of an affected artery is patchy, with long segments of the normal unaffected artery flanked by vasculitic foci known as *skip lesions*, which may begin to normalize within days after treatment. For these reasons, biopsy specimens of the superficial temporal artery should be generous (4- to 6-cm-long specimens), multiple histological sections should be taken, and bilateral biopsy considered. Employing these strategies may increase the diagnostic yield of temporal artery biopsy up to 86%.

***Immunology, etiology, and pathogenesis.*** Giant-cell arteritis is an idiopathic autoimmune disease. Although vasculitic processes are often systemic, giant-cell arteritis is usually more focal than polyarteritis nodosa and characterized by a mononuclear cell infiltrate with giant-cell formation, suggesting differences in immunopathogenesis. No distinctive antigen has been identified to explain the particular tropism of giant-cell arteritis, although the possibility that the immune reaction is directed against the internal elastic lamina (which is absent from cerebral vessels shortly after they pierce the dura) may explain the paucity of intracranial involvement. Lymphocytes sensitized to the purported antigen infiltrate the internal elastic lamina and release a host of lymphokines which attract a mononuclear cell infiltrate. Activated macrophages release lysosomal proteases and may transform into epithelioid and multinucleate giant cells. T cells themselves, by antibody-dependent cell-mediated cytotoxicity or natural killer cell actions, may also be involved. In addition, the demonstration of antibody and complement deposits at the internal elastic lamina suggests that humoral mechanisms are involved.

***Epidemiology.*** The incidence of biopsy-confirmed giant-cell arteritis ranges between 9.5 and 29.1 per 100,000 per year, significantly increases after 50 years of age, and peaks in the eighth decade (Gonzalez-Gay et al., 2009). It is the most common vasculitic process in both Europe and North America, appears to be most common among individuals of Scandinavian descent, and is significantly less common among Asians. The reported female-to-male ratio in giant-cell arteritis is as high as 4 : 1.

***Treatment and management.*** Once giant-cell arteritis is suspected, histological confirmation should be obtained, and treatment started immediately. Treatment consists of oral corticosteroids given initially in high doses and gradually tapered over months. Treatment should not be withheld pending the result of temporal artery biopsy. Prednisone may be initiated at 40–60 mg/day and continued for 1 month, after which time, start a cautious taper of less than 10% of the daily dose per week. If, at the time of presentation, ischemic complications are imminent or evolving, parenteral high-dose corticosteroids should be given until these complications stabilize. Intravenous (IV) pulse corticosteroids, typically in the form of methylprednisolone 1000 mg/day for 3 days, has been advocated for patients with transient, partial, or complete vision loss at presentation (Hoffman, 2016). Some studies have shown antiplatelet therapy with low-dose aspirin to be associated with a lower risk for developing visual loss and cerebrovascular infarcts (Nesher et al., 2004). A Cochrane review of the literature published in 2014, however, found that there is no evidence from randomized controlled trials to determine the safety and efficacy of low-dose aspirin as an adjunctive treatment in giant-cell arteritis (Mollan et al. 2014). The adjunctive use of anticoagulants for patients with ischemia may be tried, but their efficacy in this setting is unproven.

Disease activity must be monitored both clinically and by monitoring the ESR. A flare of symptoms accompanied by an increase in the ESR mandates increasing the corticosteroid dose at least to the last effective dose and often boosting it temporarily to a higher level. Relapses generally reflect too rapid a taper, and resumption of a more slowly tapering regimen is indicated after the relapse has stabilized. Some patients may require continuation of low-dose (7.5–10 mg/day) prednisone for several years, although complete withdrawal remains the eventual goal. There is some evidence that treatment with methotrexate 10 mg/wk may be an effective adjunctive treatment that allows for more rapid tapering of the prednisone dose. Recently, the US Food and Drug Administration (FDA) approved the use of tocilizumab as a steroid-sparing agent for giant-cell arteritis treatment.

The multitude of well-known adverse effects associated with exogenous corticosteroids (e.g., vertebral body compression fractures, myopathy, a confusional state, among others) may influence management by prompting a more rapid taper, thereby exposing the patient to the risks that accompany a relapse of the vasculitis.

***Course and prognosis.*** The clinical onset of giant-cell arteritis may be acute, subacute, or chronic. Although the median duration of symptoms before diagnosis is 1 month, patients may rarely present with a history of up to several years of polymyalgia rheumatica.

Within days of corticosteroid treatment, symptoms and laboratory abnormalities may begin to normalize. With tapering doses, relapses may occur and may present as a reactivation of prior symptoms or with new symptoms altogether. Neurological complications, including neuropathies and cerebrovascular events, are not always preventable by corticosteroid administration and have a median onset of 1 month after initiation of treatment. Similarly, large-artery involvement can occur up to 7 months after initiation of treatment.

Although the occurrence of amaurosis fugax often brings a patient with undiagnosed giant-cell arteritis to medical attention, permanent loss of vision rarely occurs with adequate treatment. In patients with acute and incomplete loss of vision, some visual function may return with immediate institution of corticosteroid therapy, but this is rare.

## Headache Associated With Disorders of Homeostasis

Sleep apnea may result in both an independent headache type and may also be an aggravating factor among individuals with migraine. Individuals with nocturnal or morning-predominant headaches should be asked about sleep apnea risk factors, such as snoring and observed apneic episodes. A body mass index greater than 35 kg/m$^2$, and neck circumference greater than 40 cm, further increase the likelihood of obstructive sleep apnea. The mechanism may involve hypercarbia and/or hypoxemia.

Despite common belief, mild to moderate hypertension does not directly cause headache, as demonstrated by a lack of correlation between headache diaries and 24-hour ambulatory blood pressure analysis. Conversely, hypertensive emergency is commonly associated with headache, where a diagnosis of posterior reversible encephalopathy syndrome should also be considered. In a patient with a short-duration headache associated with diaphoresis and palpitations, the possibility of pheochromocytoma should be pursued. Similarly, headache may be a sign of pre-eclampsia during pregnancy.

*Cardiac cephalalgia* occurs as a direct result of myocardial ischemia and may present in the complete absence of chest pain. The headache is characteristically brought on by exertion, improved with rest, and unlike most primary headache disorders, improved by nitroglycerin. Failure to identify this diagnostic entity may be associated with dire consequences. A cardiac evaluation should be considered in patients over the age of 50 who present with new headaches (especially if exertional) and vascular risk factors.

## Headache Caused by Disorders of the Cranium, Neck, Eyes, Ears, Nose, Sinuses, Teeth, Mouth, or Other Facial or Cranial Structures

### Ocular Causes of Headache

In the absence of injection of the conjunctiva or other obvious signs of eye disease, headache and eye pain rarely have an ophthalmic cause. The maxim is that a white eye is rarely the cause of a monosymptomatic painful eye. Acute angle-closure glaucoma is a rare but often dramatic event. The patient may present with extreme eye and frontal head pain with associated vomiting. The sclera is injected, the cornea is cloudy, the globe is stony hard, and unlike cluster headache, the pupil is fixed in mid-position.

Refractive errors, imbalance of external eye muscles, amblyopia, and "eyestrain" are not causes of headache in most instances. In children and teenagers, however, refractive errors, especially hyperopia, can produce dull frontal and orbital headaches from straining to achieve accommodation at school. Myopic children are unaffected. Trochleitis may produce a periorbital headache and be either idiopathic or secondary to an autoimmune disorder. The headache is characteristically aggravated by vertical ductions of the eye, as the tendon of the superior oblique muscle runs through this structure. Cluster headache, migraine, and other primary headaches, as well as carotid artery dissection, can cause orbital and retro-orbital pain. Each is discussed elsewhere in this chapter.

### Nasal Causes of Headache and Facial Pain

Acute purulent rhinosinusitis causes local and referred pain. The distribution of the pain depends on the sinuses involved. Maxillary sinusitis causes pain and tenderness over the cheek. Frontal sinus disease produces frontal pain; sphenoid and ethmoidal sinusitis causes pain behind and between the eyes, and the pain may refer to the vertex. Acute rhinosinusitis is commonly associated with fever, purulent nasal discharge, and other constitutional symptoms. The pain is worse when the patient bends forward and is often relieved as soon as the infected material drains from the sinus. Chronic rhinosinusitis is considered to be a risk factor for CDH, where the headache most often resembles chronic tension-type headache in features (Aaseth et al., 2010). Intracranial infections may occur as a complication of untreated sinusitis. Acute infection involving the sphenoid sinus can be especially dangerous because of its close proximity to the cavernous sinus.

Commonly, migraine headaches are erroneously diagnosed as sinus headaches, because they are associated with cranial autonomic symptoms, have prominent facial involvement, and/or are triggered (e.g., by a change in altitude/weather, an exposure to pollens, or a seasonal predilection). Most patients with a diagnosis of "sinus headaches" have migraine headaches (Cady et al., 2005).

Malignant tumors of the sinuses and nasopharynx can produce deep-seated facial and head pain before involving cranial nerves or otherwise becoming obvious. Trigeminal sensory loss is an important neurological sign which is associated with neurological involvement, often by perineural spread. MRI scanning is the optimal technique for detecting these cryptic lesions.

### Temporomandibular Joint Disorders

In 1934, Costen first drew attention to the temporomandibular joint (TMJ) as a cause of facial and head pain. Until recently, Costen syndrome was a rare diagnosis. During the past 2 decades, however, interest in disorders of the TMJ, the muscles of mastication, and the bite as they relate to headaches has been increasing. Painful temporomandibular dysfunction is most common between the ages of 35 and 45, after which spontaneous resolution is often seen. Mechanical disorders of the joint, alterations in the way the upper and lower teeth relate, and congenital and acquired deformities of the jaw and mandible can all produce head and facial pain and are very occasionally responsible for the episodic and chronic pain syndromes seen by neurologists.

The neurologist evaluating head or facial pain should be familiar with the criteria for identification and localization of TMJ disorders. Temporomandibular joint pain should relate directly to jaw movements and mastication and commonly associates with tenderness in the masticatory muscles or over the TMJ on palpation. Anesthetic blocking of tender structures should confirm presence and location of the pain source. A sudden change in occlusal relationship of the teeth, restriction of mandibular movement, and interference with mandibular movement (clicking, incoordination, and crepitus) are all symptoms and signs suggestive of TMJ dysfunction.

Bruxism, teeth clenching, and chronic gum chewing are important in the production of pain in the masseter and temporalis muscles. Arthritis and degenerative changes in the TMJ, loss of teeth, ill-fitting dentures or lack of dentures, and other dental conditions can all lead to the TMJ or myofascial pain dysfunction syndrome, which manifests as facial and masticatory muscle pain. Head pain and facial pain, even when associated with the above-discussed criteria, require full evaluation, which should include a detailed history and examination, appropriate radiographs, and laboratory studies to exclude other more serious causes. If TMJ dysfunction is thought to be the source of pain, further evaluation and treatment are in the province of the appropriate dental specialist. Even when TMJ dysfunction is believed to be responsible for facial or head pain, conservative management with analgesics, anti-inflammatory agents, application of local heat, and nonsurgical techniques to adjust the bite generally provide relief. Before using surgical modalities on the TMJ or mandibles, the diagnosis must be secure and other causes of head and facial pain excluded by appropriate investigations.

### Other Dental Causes of Craniofacial Pain

Pulpitis and root abscess generally produce dental pain that a patient can localize. The cracked tooth syndrome results from an incomplete tooth fracture, most commonly involving a lower molar. The initial pain is usually sharp and well localized, but thereafter the pain is often diffuse and hard to locate. After a fracture, the tooth is sensitive to cold. Pain may be felt in the head and face ipsilateral to the damaged tooth. With time, infection develops in the pulp, leading to extreme and well-localized pain. Confirmation of the diagnosis and treatment of the cracked tooth require the expertise of a dentist.

## Headaches and the Cervical Spine

Cervicogenic headache is often a controversial diagnosis with potential medicolegal implications. Many common cervical spine pathologies, such as degenerative spondylosis, occur just as often in individuals with or without headache. Therefore, the diagnosis rests on establishing the cervical spine as a pain generator either through clinical signs, or a diagnostic nerve block. Cervicogenic headache should be strongly suspected as a diagnosis when there is occipital headache, especially when unilateral, and associated with constant neck pain.

Migraine in particular frequently presents with pain in the occipital and nuchal regions, which are innervated by the greater occipital nerve. Furthermore, muscle hypersensitivity and tenderness, restriction of neck movements, and hyperalgesia may accompany the pain. Similarly, pain of cervical origin or cervicogenic headache is prominent in the occipital region but may also spread to trigeminal territories. The referral of pain observed in cervicogenic headache and migraine reflects the convergence of trigeminal and cervical afferents onto the same neurons in the trigeminal-cervical complex. Despite this anatomical overlap, the provocation or exacerbation of the headache by neck movement, a persistent rather than intermittent headache, and lack of photophobia, phonophobia, and nausea, are features that may be helpful in distinguishing cervicogenic headache from migraine. Diagnostic blocks performed accurately and under controlled conditions are the only currently available means by which a cervical source of pain can be established. A positive response to occipital nerve block should be interpreted with caution, however, given the fact that many primary headaches, including migraine and cluster headache, may respond to this procedure. The use of intra-articular steroids and long-acting anesthetics may provide relief that can last several months, and complete relief of headache can occasionally be achieved by radiofrequency neurotomy in patients whose headache stems from the C2 to C3 zygapophysial joint (Bogduk, 2004). Physical therapy may also be helpful in the treatment of cervicogenic headache.

## Medication Overuse Headache

Overuse of acute medications by patients with frequent headache may lead to a daily headache syndrome, now known as *medication overuse headache (MOH)*. Previously referred to as rebound or medication-induced headache, this syndrome is induced and maintained by the very medications used to relieve the pain. Diagnostic criteria according to ICHD-3 are designed to improve sensitivity, requiring only the presence of chronic daily headache (CDH) in the setting of exposure to an overused analgesic (IHS, 2018). The risk for development of medication overuse headache varies with individual substances. Opioids, butalbital-containing compounds, and some combination analgesics appear to have the highest risk; triptans carry moderate risk, and nonsteroidal antiinflammatory drugs (NSAIDs) the lowest risk. In fact, migraine prevention guidelines include recommendations for daily NSAID exposure in the preventive treatment of migraine (Silberstein et al., 2012). Further, there is longitudinal epidemiological evidence that NSAID use among individuals with <10 headache days per month is associated with a dose-dependent reduction in the development of chronic migraine (Lipton et al., 2013).

The population prevalence of CDH associated with acute medication overuse has been estimated to be 1.4% (Colas et al., 2004). The proportion of patients in the population with CDH who overuse acute medications ranges from 18% to 33%, indicating that medication overuse is not necessary for the development of CDH, nor is the overuse of acute medication synonymous with MOH. In other words, tapering and discontinuing the overused medication does not always return the patient to an episodic pattern of headache.

The most frequently overused acute medications include analgesics, opioids, butalbital-containing products, ergotamine, and triptans, alone or in combination. The delay between the frequent intake of these medications and the development of CDH appears to be shortest for triptans (1.7 years), longer for ergots (2.7 years), and longest for analgesics (4.8 years). The duration of withdrawal symptoms after discontinuation and the recidivism rate are also shortest/lowest for triptans and longest/highest for analgesics.

The pathogenesis of MOH is unclear. A leading hypothesis suggests facilitation of central trigeminal sensitization caused by a medication-induced impairment of descending inhibition of nociceptive trafficking. In rats, chronic morphine exposure increases the pain, facilitating "on" cell activation in the rostral ventromedial medulla (RVM) that may alter the balance between the descending inhibition from the nucleus reticularis dorsalis (NRD) and the facilitation from the RVM in favor of a pro-nociceptive increased descending facilitation from the RVM (Meng and Harasawa, 2007; Okada-Ogawa et al., 2009). Similar neural adaptations may contribute to opiate-induced MOH in humans by increasing the responsiveness of the nociceptive system, as well as increasing the transmission of pain signals at the medullary dorsal horn (De Felice and Porreca, 2009). Animal studies have found that sustained or repeated administration of triptans can also induce pro-nociceptive neural adaptations, enhance responses to established triggers of migraine headache, and lower cortical spreading depression threshold, the latter of which can increase the activation of the trigeminal nucleus caudalis (De Felice et al., 2010; Green et al., 2014). Some individuals may possess a genetically determined liability to medication overuse. A FDG-PET study in patients with chronic analgesic overuse in migraine sufferers demonstrated persistent hypometabolism of the orbitofrontal cortex (especially in patients overusing combination analgesics) even after withdrawal of the overused medication. Persistent orbitofrontal hypofunction is known to occur in substance abuse (Fumal et al., 2006).

Treatment of MOH is challenging and requires aggressive nonpharmacological and appropriate acute and preventive headache treatment. Rigorous controlled data are lacking, with current evidence supporting preventive therapy alone, withdrawal of overuse analgesics alone, and the combination of the two. It is generally considered that lifestyle modifications such as limiting or eliminating caffeine consumption, exercise, and establishing regular mealtimes and sleep schedules can be beneficial for some patients. Depression, anxiety, and sleep disturbances occur in more than half of patients and must be addressed. Training in relaxation techniques and biofeedback may be helpful, especially if stress or anxiety is a frequent provocative trigger. Patients should always be provided with support and close follow-up, particularly during the first 8 weeks after treatment is initiated.

Pharmacological treatment involves tapering or discontinuing the overused medication. Abrupt drug withdrawal is the treatment of choice except with barbiturates, benzodiazepines, and opioids. Typical withdrawal symptoms last 2–10 days (mean 3.5 days) but may persist for 2–4 weeks. In most patients, the withdrawal can be managed on an outpatient basis. Patients with coexistent medical or psychiatric illnesses and overuse of agents containing opioids, benzodiazepines, and barbiturates may need hospitalization or withdrawal in a controlled environment. Prednisone 60 mg daily for 5 days as a transitional and short-term treatment during the withdrawal phase to reduce withdrawal symptoms can be considered and may decrease the need for acute treatment during this time (Evers and Jensen, 2011; Rabe et al., 2013). Preventive medication aimed at the underlying primary headache disorder should be started from the outset while initiating the taper of the overused substance.

Studies have indicated a high rate of relapse following withdrawal of acute headache medications in patients with presumed MOH. One prospective study reported a relapse rate of 41% in the first year and 45% after 4 years (Katsarava et al., 2005). In another report with 4 years of follow-up, only one-third of patients initially treated for CDH and analgesic overuse were successful in refraining from chronic overuse of medication.

To avoid MOH relapse, in general, it is best to avoid the use of opioids and/or butalbital for the regular management of primary headache disorders. To prevent relapse, limit NSAIDs, aspirin, or acetaminophen use to ≤14 days/month and limit combination analgesics, triptans, ergot derivatives, or opioids to ≤9 days/month. Although data are limited, the effectiveness of headache preventive medications may be decreased by overuse of acute medications (Mathew et al., 1990).

## PRIMARY HEADACHES

### Migraine

#### Definition and Classification

The term *migraine* derives from the ancient Greek word *hemikranios*, which means "half head," underscoring the unilateral distribution of head pain that is present in about 60%–75% of people with migraine (Kelman, 2005; Wober-Bingol et al., 2004). Although not all people with migraine experience all potential phases of a migraine attack, the migraine attack can consist of up to four phases: the premonitory phase, aura, headache phase, and postdrome. In addition to head pain, the "headache phase" consists of a combination of photophobia, phonophobia, osmophobia, cutaneous allodynia, nausea, and vomiting. Although osmophobia is not part of the formal diagnostic criteria for migraine, when present, is considered to be highly specific for the disorder (Chalmer et al., 2018). Box 102.2 shows the classification of different encountered forms of migraine, including episodic migraine with aura, episodic migraine without aura, and chronic migraine (IHS, 2018).

#### Epidemiology

A survey of a sample of 20,000 households estimated 27.9 million migraine patients in the United States. More than 90% of patients report an impaired ability to function during migraine attacks, and 53% report severe disability requiring bed rest. Approximately 31% of patients with migraine missed at least 1 day from work or school in the preceding 3 months due to migraine (Lipton et al., 2001). Indirect costs of migraine related to decreased productivity and lost days of work have been calculated to be $13 billion per year; estimates are that the equivalent of 112 million bedridden days per year are due to migraine (Hu et al., 1999). The World Health Organization has declared migraine to be among the most disabling medical conditions experienced worldwide.

Migraine has a 1-year prevalence of 12% in the general population, including 18% of women and 6% of men (Lipton et al., 2007; Rasmussen, 1995). Migraine afflicts prepubescent boys and girls with a similar frequency. At puberty, the incidence of migraine increases sharply in both boys and girls, but preferentially so in girls. Peak migraine prevalence for both sexes occurs in the fourth decade of life, during which time approximately 24% of women and 7% of men have migraine (Lipton et al., 2007). Migraine tends to manifest with fluctuating frequencies of attacks throughout one's life, with a typical trend towards milder and less frequent migraines late in life. The lifetime prevalence of migraine is about 33% in women and 13% in men (Launer et al., 1999).

Due to headache and other migraine symptoms, migraine causes substantial pain and disability. During a migraine attack, the vast majority of migraineurs have at least mild disability and about half have severe disability, often requiring rest in a dark and quiet room (Lipton et al., 2007). Overall, migraineurs have lower physical, emotional, and social quality of life.

There is a genetic predisposition for developing migraine. Compared to the general population, first-degree relatives of people who have migraine without aura are about twice as likely to develop migraine without aura, while first-degree relatives of people who have migraine with aura are about four times more likely to have migraine with aura (Russell and Olesen, 1995).

#### Migraine Attack Frequency

The majority of people with migraine have attacks 1–4 times per month (Lipton et al., 2007). These migraineurs are considered to have "episodic migraine," meaning they have headaches on fewer than 15 days per month. However, 2% of the general population has "chronic migraine," meaning that they have headaches on at least 15 days per month, including at least 8 days per month on which they have symptoms of full-blown migraine attacks (Natoli et al., 2010). On average, people with chronic migraine have 22 headache days per month. An estimated 7.5% of patients with episodic migraine when followed quarterly will meet criteria for chronic migraine at least once within a 15-month period, as compared to the 2.5% transformation rate observed when patients are evaluated annually (Bigal et al., 2008b; Serrano et al., 2017).

#### Triggers of the Migraine Attack

At least three-quarters of migraineurs can identify triggers of their migraine attacks (Kelman, 2007). However, it seems that the susceptibility of the migraine brain to potential migraine attack triggers fluctuates from day to day. Thus, many migraineurs will find that exposure to a potential trigger does in fact trigger a migraine attack on some days and does not on other days. The most commonly identified migraine attack triggers include emotional stress, fluctuating female hormones, missed meals, weather factors, sleep disturbance, odors, certain visual stimuli, alcohol, muscle tension, physical exercise, and being overheated (Kelman, 2007). It has been noted that self-reported triggers are not consistently validated when formally studied experimentally. For example, photophobia, a hallmark of migraine often present during the prodrome, may be misinterpreted by a patient as light triggering their headache.

#### The Migraine Attack

***Migraine prodrome.*** Many patients with migraine report that a prodromal phase precedes the headache, typically starting 1–2 hours prior to onset of migraine headache (Kelman, 2004). The most frequent prodromal symptoms include fatigue, mild cognitive dysfunction, irritability, neck pain, light and noise sensitivity, blurred vision, excessive yawning, and excessive thirst. When premonitory symptoms are observed by the migraineur, a migraine develops within the next several days about three-quarters of the time.

***Migraine aura.*** Migraine auras occur in about one-third of migraine patients (Cutrer and Huerter, 2007). Most patients who have migraine attacks with aura also have attacks without aura, with only one-fifth of migraine-with-aura patients having aura with every migraine attack. Typical aura symptoms develop and progress gradually over several minutes and then resolve within 60 minutes. The resolution of aura symptoms often coincides with the onset of headache. Much less commonly, aura symptoms can occur during the headache phase of the migraine attack, after the headache phase, or in the absence of headache altogether ("acephalgic migraine" or "aura without headache"). Individual aura symptoms may occur in isolation during an individual migraine attack or more than one aura symptom may occur sequentially.

Visual phenomena are the most common aura symptom, reported by over 80% of patients with migraine aura (Eriksen et al., 2004; Russell and Olesen, 1996). Like all migraine aura symptoms, visual symptoms progress slowly, moving across the visual field. Visual auras consist of positive symptoms such as seeing flashing lights and wavy lines ("scintillating scotoma"), often followed by negative scotomas within the same distribution of the preceding positive visual phenomena.

Sensory aura, the second most common aura type, is, like the visual aura, characterized by positive symptoms (paresthesias) followed by negative symptoms (numbness), which slowly spread or migrate (Eriksen et al., 2004; Russell and Olesen, 1996). Sensory aura is usually unilateral and has a predilection for the hand, arm, shoulder, and face.

This may be due to the large representation of these structures in the sensory cortex or thalamus. Commonly, sensory symptoms begin in the hand and then slowly spread up the ipsilateral arm to the shoulder and face with perioral and tongue involvement. The rate of spread of a sensory aura is important to help distinguish it from a sensory seizure and the sensory disturbance of a TIA. Just as a visual aura spreads across the visual field slowly, taking as long as 20 minutes to reach maximum, the paresthesias may take 10–20 minutes to spread from the point at which they are first felt to their maximal distribution. This is slower than the spread of a sensory seizure and much slower than the spread of sensory symptoms associated with TIA. A migrainous sensory aura generally resolves over the course of 20–60 minutes, most often within 30 minutes.

After sensory aura, the next most common type is a language aura (Eriksen et al., 2004; Russell and Oleson, 1996). Expressive dysphasias, including paraphasic errors, are the most common language symptoms of migraine aura, with receptive dysphasias being less common. Language symptoms of migraine aura are typically of mild severity.

When unilateral motor weakness is present with migraine aura, the diagnosis is "hemiplegic migraine." Hemiplegic migraine can be "familial" or "sporadic." Motor weakness of hemiplegic migraine most often involves the hand and arm. Although the term "-plegia" suggests paralysis, the motor symptom of hemiplegic migraine is usually weakness as opposed to true paralysis. In addition to the hemiparesis, there must be at least one other aura symptom, including a visual, sensory, or language/speech symptom. Like with all migraine auras, the aura symptoms of hemiplegic migraine have a slow spreading onset over several minutes, with each symptom resolving within 60 minutes. However, the motor weakness of hemiplegic migraine can endure for several days. The genetics of familial hemiplegic migraine are discussed further under Migraine Genetics.

When aura consists of at least two brainstem symptoms but no motor or retinal symptoms, the diagnosis is "migraine with brainstem aura" (previously called "basilar migraine"). Migraine with brainstem aura consists of a combination of fully reversible visual, sensory, and language/speech symptoms with at least two brainstem symptoms including dysarthria, vertigo, tinnitus, hypacusis, diplopia, ataxia, and decreased level of consciousness. Each aura symptom resolves within 60 minutes.

When a migraine aura is not followed by a headache, the episode is termed *migraine aura without headache*, a *migraine equivalent*, or *acephalgic migraine*. Most commonly encountered in patients who have a past history of migraine with aura, the episodes can begin de novo, usually after 40 years of age, but they can occur at almost any age. Migraine equivalents are easily recognizable when the attacks occur on a background of migraine with aura. In the absence of such a history, the transitory disturbance may be difficult to distinguish from an episode of transient cerebral or brainstem ischemia, and thus diagnostic tests might be required.

***Headache phase.*** The headache of migraine is typically a moderate to severe unilateral throbbing pain that is exacerbated by routine physical activities. In addition to the headache, patients are hypersensitive to visual, auditory, olfactory, and somatosensory stimuli, often resulting in the migraine patient desiring rest in a dark and quiet room. Nausea, vomiting, and neck pain are frequent accompaniments.

A migraine headache can be felt anywhere throughout the head, including retro- and periorbital locations, frontal, occipital, temporal, vertex, and parietal regions. Pain is unilateral in 60%–75% of patients and bilateral in others (Kelman, 2005; Russell et al., 1996; Wober-Bingol et al., 2004). Often, pain starts unilaterally and then becomes bilateral as the migraine attack endures. Pain is most commonly described as throbbing/pulsating, but other pain qualities are also common. Headache intensity increases over approximately 90 minutes before reaching moderate to severe intensity. Pain is intensified by physical activity in the majority of patients.

During a migraine attack there is a hypersensitivity to visual, auditory, cutaneous, and olfactory stimuli. Most migraineurs have hypersensitivity to light and visual patterns, exposure to which results in generalized discomfort, visual discomfort, and worsening headache. Similarly, exposure to normal and loud volume sound results in discomfort and worsening headache intensity in most migraineurs. Increased sensitivity to odors is present in a minority of migraineurs. Scents that more commonly result in olfactory hypersensitivity include perfumes, food smells, and cigarette smoke.

The experience of nonpainful stimuli (e.g., washing the face, combing the hair) as painful on the skin is known as cutaneous allodynia, which develops in about two-thirds of migraineurs during a migraine attack (Ashkenazi et al., 2007; Bigal et al., 2008a; Lipton et al., 2008). The allodynic migraineur experiences pain or discomfort with normally nonnoxious stimulation of the skin, such as occurs with light touch of the face or scalp, wearing eyeglasses, shaving the face, and wearing a tight collar or necklace. Although allodynia symptoms are most commonly noted within the trigeminal nerve distribution, about one-fourth of migraineurs develop extracephalic allodynia, typically involving the upper extremity (Mathew et al., 2004). The identification of this feature is highly clinically relevant. The presence of allodynia during an attack tends to predict a less robust response to acute treatments (Lipton et al., 2017). Further, a history of allodynia increases ones risk of developing chronic migraine (Louter et al., 2013), but then also predicts having a more favorable response to treatment with onabotulinumtoxinA (Mathew et al., 2008b).

Nausea is present during the migraine attack in the majority of patients and vomiting occurs in about half. Besides the obvious discomfort of vomiting itself, vomiting can complicate the migraine attack by leading to dehydration and preventing the absorption of orally administered medications. Even when vomiting is absent, the absorption of orally administered migraine medications might be unpredictable due to the presence of gastric stasis (Aurora et al., 2006).

Untreated, the migraine headache phase usually lasts from 4 to 72 hours, with the majority subsiding within a day or after a night's sleep. When the migraine attack is debilitating and endures for longer than 72 hours, "status migrainosus" is diagnosed.

***Migraine postdrome.*** The majority of migraineurs continue to have migraine symptoms for up to 24 hours following resolution of the migraine headache (Kelman, 2006). The constellation of symptoms, commonly referred to by patients as the "migraine hangover," is very similar to those symptoms experienced during the premonitory phase of the migraine attack. Symptoms often include fatigue, mild cognitive dysfunction, atypical mood, generalized weakness, feeling dizzy, neck stiffness, light and sound hypersensitivity, and excessive thirst (Kelman, 2006).

## Physical Findings

Between attacks, the migraineur should have a normal neurological examination, with abnormalities on examination increasing the suspicion for a secondary headache disorder. In addition to the usual physical and neurological examinations, attention should be paid to examination of the temporal arteries, fundoscopy, cervical and cranial muscles, and temporomandibular joint. During an attack of migraine, the scalp vessels may be distended and tender. The blood pressure is likely to be elevated due to the pain. Many

**BOX 102.2 Migraine**

Migraine without aura
Migraine with aura:
- Migraine with typical aura
- Migraine with brainstem aura
- Hemiplegic migraine
- Retinal migraine

Chronic migraine
Complications of migraine:
- Status migrainosus
- Persistent aura without infarction
- Migrainous infarction
- Migraine aura-triggered seizure

Probable migraine:
- Probable migraine without aura
- Probable migraine with aura

Episodic syndromes that may be associated with migraine:
- Recurrent gastrointestinal disturbance
- Benign paroxysmal vertigo
- Benign paroxysmal torticollis

*Adapted from Headache Classification Committee of the International Headache Society (IHS). 2018. The International Classification of Headache Disorders, third ed. Cephalalgia 38 (1), 1–211. https://doi.org/10.1177/0333102417738202.*

patients are pale and clammy during the attack, especially if nauseated. The patient is likely to object to the lights of the examination room and try to avoid the glare of the ophthalmoscope during the eye examination.

## Diagnostic Testing

The majority of patients presenting with migraine do not require diagnostic testing. There are no tests that help to rule in the migraine diagnosis. Diagnostic tests may be needed to evaluate for other headache causes when a patient has atypical or worrisome features identified during the patient interview and when there are unexplained abnormalities on the neurological examination. Although such investigations must be chosen based upon the clinician's suspicions for specific causes for a secondary headache, testing may include blood tests (e.g., thyroid stimulating hormone, ESR), MRI of the brain in non-acute settings, imaging of the cervical and intracranial arteries, imaging of the intracranial venous sinuses, cervical spine imaging, LP, sleep studies, and others.

## Migraine Genetics

Although prior familial migraine studies have shown no clear Mendelian inheritance patterns, recent genetic epidemiological surveys and large national registry-based twin studies strongly support the hypothesis of a genetic contribution. Perhaps the most striking evidence of a genetic basis for migraine has come to us over the past decade from investigation of familial hemiplegic migraine.

Familial hemiplegic migraine (FHM) is a rare autosomal dominant subtype of migraine with aura in which, in the context of otherwise typical migraine attacks, patients experience hemiplegia. Thus far, three genes for FHM have been identified: *CACNA1A*, *ATP1A2*, and *SCNA1A*. A mutation in *CACNA1A*, a gene located on chromosome 19p13 that codes for the $\alpha_1$ subunit of a brain-specific voltage-gated P/Q-type calcium channel, is associated with FHM1 (Ophoff et al., 1996). The gene mutation for FHM2 is on chromosome 1q23 in the *ATP1A2* gene, a gene that encodes the $\alpha2$ isoform of the major subunit of the sodium-potassium ATPase pump (De Fusco et al., 2003). FHM3 is associated with a mutation in the gene *SCN1A* on chromosome 2q24, *SCN1A* encoding the $\alpha$ subunit of a neuronal voltage-gated sodium channel (Dichgans et al., 2005). Although FHM is a rare genetic subtype of migraine with aura, the clinical similarities (with typical migraine, with and without aura) suggest at least the possibility of a shared pathophysiology. The discovery of a genetic locus for FHM has generated considerable interest and prompted a large effort in the field of molecular genetics to find the fundamental defects in the more common forms of migraine.

Common forms of migraine (e.g., migraine without aura, migraine with aura) have complex underlying genetic profiles. It is estimated that about half of the underlying propensity toward developing migraine is due to additive gene effects, while the other half is attributable to environmental factors (Gasparini et al., 2013; Silberstein and Dodick, 2013). A meta-analysis of migraine genome-wide association studies (GWAS), including 375,000 individuals, revealed 44 genetic variants involving 38 distinct loci across the genome that are associated with either increased or decreased susceptibility to migraine (Gormley et al., 2016). Incredibly, both genes with previously known roles in nociception and ion channels were uncommon among the GWAS susceptibility loci. The identified genes were demonstrated to be enriched predominantly in smooth and vascular tissue, as well as certain brain regions. Known functions of identified genes are diverse and include cell–cell interactions, vascular biology, and synaptic regulation.

Given that susceptibility loci identified through GWAS each confer only a very small individual effect size, researchers have used polygenic risk scores to understand the cumulative impact of these common genetic variants. Interestingly, polygenic risk scores are larger in cases of familial migraine than in individual population cases, indicating that an aggregation of common variants contribute to the genetic architecture seen in families with migraine (Gormley et al., 2018). An accumulation of common variants is observed to an even greater extent among families with typical aura than without, and most prominently in cases of hemiplegic migraine. Polygenic risk scores are also being studied in migraine to understand pleiotropy—where a single genetic variant contributes to two distinct phenotypes. One example of this was a demonstration of shared genetic susceptibility between migraine and stroke, which may, in part, account for the observed clinical comorbidity (Malik et al., 2015).

## Pathophysiology

***Vascular versus neuronal.*** Whereas the migraine attack was once considered attributable to vascular dysfunction, the migraine attack is now considered to be primarily due to brain dysfunction, perhaps with secondary vascular effects. Historically, the migraine aura was thought to be due to cerebral vasoconstriction while the headache was thought to be due to cerebral vasodilation. However, there has been evidence building against the role of the intracranial vasculature in generating the migraine attack. First, there is solid evidence from functional MRI studies that a phase of focal hyperemia precedes the phase of oligemia during the migraine aura. Second, headache may begin while cortical blood flow remains reduced, thereby rendering obsolete the theory that vasodilatation is the sole mechanism of the pain. The oligemia that spreads across the cerebral cortex at a rate of 2–4 mm/min during migraine aura does not conform to discrete vascular territories, making it also unlikely that vasospasm of individual cerebral arteries, with subsequent cerebral ischemia, is the source of the aura. Furthermore, a MRA study of nitroglycerin-triggered migraine attacks showed no change in cerebral artery diameters during the migraine attack (Schoonman et al., 2008). Thus, the current prevailing theory is that the migraine attack is due to an alteration in normal brain function.

Atypical brain function during migraine likely involves widespread areas of the brain, including regions within several different functional networks that are responsible for processing pain, visual stimuli, auditory stimuli, olfactory stimuli, regulating sleep and wakefulness, and awareness (Charles, 2013). Atypical activity within these functional networks and atypical interactions between them could associate with migraine symptoms such as headache, allodynia, photosensitivity, phonosensitivity, olfactory hypersensitivity, fatigue, and decreased ability to concentrate.

***A migraine generator.*** The existence of a "migraine generator," a brain region that is responsible for triggering the migraine attack, is a matter of debate. Searches for a migraine generator typically center around pain-modulating regions of the brainstem and on the hypothalamus. In support of a brainstem region serving as a possible migraine generator, functional MRI studies performed during migraine attacks have demonstrated activation of brainstem regions (e.g., dorsal rostral pons) prior to activation of cortical regions and prior to onset of migraine symptoms (Stankewitz and May, 2011). The hypothalamus has also been considered a possible migraine generator, since many symptoms of the premonitory phase (e.g., mood changes, thirst, food cravings, excessive yawning, and drowsiness) are suggestive of hypothalamic dysfunction. A PET study of nitroglycerin-triggered migraine attacks found premonitory phase activations in posterolateral hypothalamus, several brainstem regions (e.g., midbrain tegmental area, periaqueductal gray, dorsal pons), and several cortical areas (Maniyar et al., 2014). Another study used daily functional MRI in one patient over 31 days and was able to capture three migraine attacks. This showed increased activity in the hypothalamus 24 hours prior to the onset of headache pain, as well as functional coupling of the hypothalamus with spinal trigeminal nuclei and with the dorsal rostral pons (Schulte and May, 2016).

While a single brain region might generate the migraine attack, or functional alteration within a single brain region might reduce the threshold for the migraine attack to be generated, it seems probable that there is not a single "migraine generator" shared by all people with migraine and that there is not a single "migraine generator" within individuals from attack to attack. Migraine symptoms are quite variable from attack to attack and from patient to patient. There is not a specific symptom that is reliably identified as the first symptom from migraine attack to migraine attack. In fact, during the migraine attack there is substantial co-occurrence of symptoms, meaning that multiple symptoms are present in an overlapping pattern, as opposed to there being a linear cascade of one symptom leading to the next. These clinical features of the migraine attack might suggest "parallel alteration" in the functional activity of several different brain regions and/or networks, as opposed to a "linear cascade" of dysfunction in one region leading to dysfunction in subsequent regions (Charles, 2013).

***Cortical spreading depression.*** Cortical spreading depression (CSD) is considered the electrophysiological substrate of the migraine aura. CSD tends to start in the occipital lobe and spreads forward over the cerebral hemisphere at a rate of about 2–4 mm/min. The CSD wave causes disruption in ionic gradients contributing to depolarization followed by a period of hyperpolarization. Secondary to this CSD wave, there is a corresponding initial phase of hyperemia followed by oligemia.

In humans, CSD has been studied indirectly using functional imaging. One study using blood oxygenation level–dependent (BOLD) functional MRI during visual aura was able to demonstrate waves of increased BOLD response followed by diminished BOLD signal, travelling over the occipital cortex at 3.5 mm/min, a rate similar to the CSD in animal models (Hadjikhani et al., 2001). The period of brain activation followed by the period of brain deactivation might correspond with the pattern of "positive" symptoms (e.g., visual scintillations) followed by "negative" symptoms (e.g., visual scotoma) typical of the migraine aura, a notion supported by another more recent functional imaging study (Arngrim et al., 2017). The cortical spreading depression wave is not confined within the distribution of any particular cerebral artery, but crosses the areas perfused by the middle and posterior cerebral arteries while advancing with a distinct wave front until some major change in cortical cellular architecture is reached (e.g., at the central sulcus).

It is debated whether or not cortical spreading depression can lead to activation of the trigeminocervical system and thus trigger the headache phase of the migraine attack (Burstein et al., 2012). Some data suggest that cortical spreading depression evokes a series of cortical, meningeal, and brainstem events consistent with the development of headache. In rat models, focal stimulation of the visual cortex induced CSD, and approximately 14 minutes later, triggered long-lasting activation of the meningeal nociceptors (Zhang et al., 2010). Some believe that this activation of meningeal nociceptors triggers dura mater protein extravasation and release of vasoactive neuropeptides such as calcitonin gene-related peptide (CGRP) and pituitary adenylate cyclase-activating polypeptide (PACAP), contributing to signaling along the trigeminovascular pathway (Dodick, 2018).

Interestingly, blockade of the trigeminal ganglion does not appear to disrupt the CSD-induced activation of second-order neurons in the trigeminal nucleus caudalis (Lambert et al., 2011), suggesting peripheral stimulation of this trigeminocervical system may not be the only mechanism by which the headache phase of the migraine attack is triggered. Furthermore, the majority of patients do not have migraine aura, or may experience aura without headache, or aura after the headache phase has begun. Although there is some evidence to the contrary, presumably CSD does not occur prior to onset of migraine without aura attacks. Thus, other mechanisms for trigeminocervical activation and development of migraine headache likely exist. It may be that physiological events during the premonitory phase contribute to both the aura and migraine attack in genetically susceptible individuals (Dodick, 2018).

***The trigeminocervical system and migraine headache.*** The trigeminocervical system is the basic anatomical system that underlies the migraine attack. The trigeminocervical system consists of the trigeminal and cervical sensory afferents from the pain-sensitive intracranial and extracranial structures (e.g., dura mater, cerebral and meningeal blood vessels, and posterior head/neck); the projections to the trigeminal ganglion and trigeminal nucleus caudalis (extending caudally to include input from C2 and C3 nerve roots); ascending fibers from the trigeminal nucleus caudalis to multiple brainstem, thalamic, hypothalamic, and basal ganglia nuclei; and the projections from these nuclei to higher-order cortical areas.

Activation of the trigeminocervical system results in transmission of impulses centrally toward the first synapse within laminae I and IIo of the trigeminal nucleus caudalis. From this point, nerve impulses travel rostrally to the cortex via thalamic relay centers. Activation of the trigeminocervical system leads to release of vasoactive neuropeptides from sensory afferents that innervate the major intracranial arteries, a process termed "neurogenic inflammation" (Akerman et al., 2013). Neuropeptides that are released include CGRP, substance P, vasoactive intestinal polypeptide (VIP), nitric oxide (NO), and PACAP (Gasparini et al., 2013). Release of these vasoactive neuropeptides results in vasodilation, plasma protein extravasation, inflammation, and likely contributes to causing the headache of the migraine attack.

***The hyperexcitable migraine brain.*** The migraine brain has exuberant responses to sensory stimuli, a hyperexcitability likely linked to the allodynia, photosensitivity, phonosensitivity, and olfactory hypersensitivity of migraine. Functional MRI studies consistently show the migraine brain to have greater stimulus-inducted activations of regions that facilitate the perception of stimuli compared to the nonmigraine brain (Datta et al., 2013; Moulton et al., 2011; Schwedt et al., 2015). It is not yet clear whether these exuberant activations are attributable to intrinsic cortical excitability, a lack of cortical inhibition, or a combination of both processes (Diener et al., 2012). In the migraine brain, brainstem regions that are primarily pain inhibiting have been demonstrated to hypoactivate in response to pain, further enhancing the migraine pain experience (Moulton et al., 2008). Furthermore, electrophysiological and functional imaging studies have shown that the interictal migraine brain lacks the normal habituating response to recurrent or prolonged stimuli, making the migraine patient less likely to acclimate to such stimuli (Stankewitz et al., 2013).

Recurrent and/or prolonged activation of the trigeminocervical system can lead to peripheral and central sensitization. Sensitized neurons have lower thresholds for activation, increased spontaneous activity, and receptive field expansion. Approximately three-fourths of people with migraine have evidence of central sensitization (e.g., reduced pain thresholds within trigeminal nerve and extratrigeminal nerve territories) during the migraine attack (Burstein et al., 2000). Approximately two-thirds of all people with migraine develop cutaneous allodynia during a migraine attack, a clinical manifestation of sensitization (Ashkenazi et al., 2007; Bigal et al., 2008a; Lipton et al., 2008). Existence of sensitization during a migraine attack results in increased pain and discomfort and might reduce the effectiveness of migraine abortive therapies.

### Treatment and Management

The nature of the disorder should be explained to the patient and reassurance given that although it is a painful and potentially disabling disorder, migraine has an overall favorable prognosis. Explain that migraine is now thought of as a genetic disorder of the brain that causes headache and sensitivity to the environment. Explain that a cure for migraine is lacking, but management is available. It is important that patients feel the physician understands that their headaches represent a medical problem and does not consider them to arise from psychological factors. In fact, physicians underestimate that an explanation of the condition may be a primary outcome the patient wants out of the visit. A normal head CT or MRI scan may offer considerable reassurance. Some patients are more interested in knowing that they do not have a brain tumor or other potentially lethal condition than they are in obtaining relief from the pain.

Avoidance of trigger factors, especially those that are noxious in nature (e.g., strong perfumes, gasoline) is important in the management of migraine, but simply advising a patient to avoid stress and relax more is usually meaningless. In fact, the standard advice to avoid triggers has been challenged by a clinical trial demonstrating that habituation strategies to certain triggers (e.g., bright lights) are associated with prospective reductions in headache days, as opposed to avoidance (Martin et al., 2014). The concept is highlighted by the common experience of perceiving bright lights upon exiting a dark movie theater, where avoidance of light causes a maladaptive increased sensitivity over time.

Advice to reduce excessive caffeine intake, to stop smoking, and to reduce alcohol intake is often useful. Medication use should be reviewed and modified if necessary. The use of drugs known to cause headaches (e.g., proton-pump inhibitors, reserpine, nifedipine, theophylline derivatives, caffeine, vasodilators [including long-acting nitrates], alcohol) should be discontinued, or substituted for other agents if possible. Use of estrogens and oral contraceptives should be discontinued if they are suspected of contributing to the headaches, although in some patients this may not be possible. Exercise programs to promote well-being, correction of dietary excesses, and avoidance of prolonged fasts and irregular sleeping habits can be helpful.

The topic of dietary factors in migraine is difficult. Radical alterations in the diet are rarely justified and seldom effective. A diet favoring both an increase in omega-3 and reduction in omega-6 fatty acid intake is both healthy and may be useful in longitudinal headache reduction (Ramsden et al., 2013). Avoidance of foods containing nitrites (e.g., hot dogs, preserved cold cuts) and prepared foods containing monosodium glutamate can be helpful. Avoiding monosodium glutamate can be difficult because it is a constituent of many canned and prepared foods and is widely used in restaurants, especially in the preparation of Chinese dishes. Ripened cheeses, fermented food items, red wine, chocolate, chicken liver, pork, and many other foods have been suspected of precipitating headaches. These foods mostly contain tyramine, phenylethylamine, and octopamine. An occasional patient identifies an offending foodstuff, but in our experience, dietary precipitation of migraine is uncommon. Other headache authorities disagree. In some migraineurs, strong odors, especially of the perfume or aromatic type, precipitate attacks. Avoiding the use of strong-smelling soaps, shampoos, perfumes, and other substances can be helpful for some individuals.

Persons with migraine may note that stress is a trigger for attacks but helping them deal with or avoid stress is difficult. Long-term stress management may require the help of a psychologist or other appropriately trained professional. Useful self-management techniques include biofeedback, relaxation training, hypnosis, and cognitive behavioral training.

***Pharmacotherapy.*** Medical therapy can be administered prophylactically to prevent attacks of migraine or symptomatically to relieve the pain, nausea, and vomiting of an attack. Prophylactic therapy is needed when the frequency or duration of attacks seriously interferes with the patient's lifestyle. Other indications for prophylaxis include severe or prolonged neurological symptoms or lack of response to symptomatic treatment. In general, prophylaxis should be considered if attacks occur as often as 1–2 days a week. Patients with frequent migraine headaches commonly need both symptomatic and prophylactic treatments.

### Symptomatic Treatment

An individualized strategy for migraine treatment is necessary because no single approach is effective for all patients. Symptomatic treatment should start as early in the development of an attack as possible. If an aura is recognized, patients should take medications during it rather than waiting for the pain to begin. An evidence assessment of acute migraine pharmacotherapies from the American Headache Society (AHS) has been published (Marmura et al., 2015). Limits should be explained regarding frequency of acute treatment use to guard against medication overuse headache (see Medication Overuse Headache section, previously).

For many, nonspecific medications such as simple oral analgesics (e.g., aspirin, acetaminophen, naproxen, ibuprofen), or an analgesic combination with caffeine, may be effective if pain is not very severe. Caffeine aids absorption, helps induce vasoconstriction, and may reduce the firing of serotonergic brainstem neurons. Another nonspecific combination analgesic which may be useful in the symptomatic treatment of migraine is the sympathomimetic agent isometheptene mucate. It is available in proprietary preparations combined with acetaminophen and dichloralphenazone and has the advantages of not increasing nausea and being well-tolerated, but it may fail to give relief for severe attacks. Table 102.4 lists some commonly used nonspecific acute migraine treatments. Certain aromatic oils (e.g., lavender) may provide relief. The patient may need rest in a dark, quiet room with an ice pack on the head. This provides the best situation for the analgesic to relieve the pain. If sleep occurs, the patient often awakens headache free.

Migraine-specific drugs (triptans and ergot derivatives) can be used if nonspecific analgesics do not provide adequate relief or if pain is severe from onset, these are discussed below. Migraine-specific drugs are more efficacious than nonspecific analgesics, particularly when migraine headaches are disabling. Triptans are easier to use and have fewer adverse effects than dihydroergotamine. Lasmiditan, a selective 5-$HT_{1F}$ agonist without vasoconstrictive properties has shown comparable efficacy to triptans in phase III clinical trials.

It must be recalled, that once the migraine attack is fully developed, oral preparations are almost always less effective because of decreased gastrointestinal motility and poor absorption. If severe nausea or vomiting develops, nonoral routes of administration are often necessary (suppository, intranasal, and/or injections). Antiemetics may be needed as adjunctive treatment, in addition to nonspecific and/or migraine-specific medications when nausea and vomiting are present.

Combining acute treatments with different mechanisms of action (e.g., rationale polytherapy) is more effective than a single agent. In the case of migraine, a combination of an NSAID, triptan or ergot, and an antiemetic with dopamine receptor type 2 antagonist properties (e.g., prochlorperazine, metoclopramide) targets multiple substrates of acute migraine pathophysiology. A randomized clinical trial has demonstrated superiority of stratified (medication choice based on attack severity and disability) over step (always taking NSAID first and waiting to take a triptan) care in the acute treatment of migraine (Lipton et al., 2000). Across 6 attacks, more favorable outcomes for stratified treatment were reported for headache response rates, headache disability, and direct costs of care.

Symptomatic treatment of migraine with typical aura is essentially the same as that described previously, although some data suggest subcutaneous sumatriptan may not be effective if taken during the aura phase before headache onset. This, however, remains an unsettled controversy. Modification of the aura is rarely possible or needed.

***Triptans.*** The development of sumatriptan heralded a new class of antimigraine agents that are highly selective at certain 5-HT receptors. These agents, collectively called *triptans*, together with the less-selective ergot preparations, have strong agonist activity at the 5-$HT_{1B}$ receptor, which mediates cranial vessel constriction, and at the 5-$HT_{1D}$ receptor, which leads to inhibition of the release of sensory neuropeptides from perivascular trigeminal afferents. Experiments show that activation of 5-$HT_{1B}$/5-$HT_{1D}$ receptors can attenuate the excitability of cells in the TNC, which receives input from the trigeminal nerve. Accordingly, 5-$HT_{1B}$/5-$HT_{1D}$ agonists may act at central as well as peripheral components of the trigeminal vascular system, and at least part of their clinical action may be centrally mediated.

Administration of sumatriptan can be oral, intranasal, and by subcutaneous injection (Table 102.5, eTables 102.6 and 102.7). Self-administered as a 6-mg subcutaneous injection, either using the manufacturer's auto-injector device or conventional subcutaneous injection, sumatriptan results in significant pain relief at 1- and 2-hour time points after drug administration (see eTable 102.6). For patients who had no significant pain relief after 1 hour, administration of a second dose of 6 mg provided little further benefit. Side effects of sumatriptan by injection include local reaction at the injection site, usually of mild or moderate severity, and a transient tingling or flushed sensation that may localize or generalize. A more unpleasant sense of heaviness or pressure in the neck or chest occurs in a small percentage of recipients. It rarely lasts more than a few minutes and is generally not associated with electrocardiogram (ECG) changes or other evidence of

**TABLE 102.4 Some Commonly Used Oral Nonspecific Acute Migraine Treatments**

| Agent | Single Dose |
|---|---|
| Acetaminophen | 1000 mg |
| Aspirin | 500–1000 mg |
| Ibuprofen | 200–400 mg |
| Naproxen sodium | 550 mg |
| Diclofenac potassium | 50–100 mg |
| Ketoprofen | 75–100 mg |
| Flurbiprofen | 100 mg |
| Acetaminophen/aspirin/caffeine | 500/500/130 mg |
| Acetaminophen 325 mg/isometheptene mucate 65 mg/dichloralphenazone 100 mg | 2 CAP, then 1 CAP q 1 h PRN; maximum 5 CAP/12 h |

**TABLE 102.5 Serotonin (5-HT) Agonists Used in Acute Migraine Treatment**

| Drug | Route(s) | Dose | May Repeat Doses if Headache Recurs (h) | Maximum Dose per 24 h (mg) |
|---|---|---|---|---|
| Dihydroergotamine | IV | 0.5, 1 mg | 1 | 3 |
| (DHE-45) | IM | 0.5, 1 mg | 1 | 3 |
| | SQ | 0.5, 1 mg | 1 | 3 |
| (Migranal) | Nasal spray | 2 mg (0.5 mg/spray) one spray in each nostril, repeat in 15 min | | 3 |
| Almotriptan (Axert) | Oral | 6.25, 12.5 mg | 2 | 25 |
| Eletriptan (Relpax) | Oral | 20, 40 mg | 2 | 80 |
| Frovatriptan (Frova) | Oral | 2.5 mg | 2 | 7.5 |
| Naratriptan (Amerge) | Oral | 1 mg, 2.5 mg* | 4 | 5 |
| Rizatriptan (Maxalt) | Oral | 5 mg, 10 mg* | 2 | 30 |
| Sumatriptan (Imitrex) | Oral | 25 mg, 50 mg, 100 mg | 2 | 200 |
| | SQ | 4, 6 mg | 1 | 12 |
| | Intranasal | 5 mg, 20 mg* | 2 | 40 |
| Zolmitriptan (Zomig) | Oral | 2.5 mg,* 5 mg | 2 | 10 |
| | Intranasal | 5 mg | 2 | 10 |

*IM*, Intramuscular; *IV*, intravenous; *SQ*, subcutaneous.
*These are the recommended starting dosages based on efficacy and tolerability.

myocardial ischemia. However, because sumatriptan has been shown to produce a minor reduction in coronary artery diameter, it should be used with caution in patients who have significant risk factors for coronary artery disease and should not be given to patients with any history suggestive of coronary insufficiency. It is also contraindicated in patients with untreated hypertension, ischemic or vaso-occlusive cerebrovascular disease, peripheral vascular disease, and in those using ergot preparations. It is contraindicated in women during pregnancy and in patients with hemiplegic migraine or migraine with brainstem aura (previously "basilar-type migraine"). Per the American Academy of Pediatrics, at present, sumatriptan belongs to the group of medications usually compatible with breast feeding.

Seven triptans are now available in the United States. All seem to have a beneficial effect on migraine-associated symptoms, including nausea, photophobia, and phonophobia, which also improves the patient's ability to return to normal functioning. eTable 102.7 provides a comparison of the currently available oral triptans. The potential side effects are quite similar: tingling, flushing, and a feeling of fullness in the head, neck, or chest. In general, the indications and contraindications for all 5-$HT_1$ agonists are similar. They are not safe when administered within 24 hours of ergot preparations or other members of the triptan class.

At this time, no evidence exists to allow accurate prediction of which of these agents will be most effective in a given patient. A few practical guidelines are available, based on the clinical situation and knowledge about available agents. If severe nausea or vomiting occurs early in an attack, the parenteral or intranasal routes should be used. Some patients may prefer nasal or injectable routes (sumatriptan and zolmitriptan). Zolmitriptan is available as an oral and intranasal preparation. For patients with benign but intolerable side effects from this group of medications, consider naratriptan, almotriptan, or frovatriptan, given their favorable side-effect profiles. Recurrence of headache after initial relief may necessitate a repeat dose. With future attacks, a higher dose (if available) may be used, or the triptan can be combined with an NSAID and/or an antiemetic. If one agent fails, it seems reasonable, barring major side effects, to try another agent in the class. Since there is evidence that some of these agents have a lower oral bioavailability when taken by patients with migraine, both during an attack and interictally (Aurora et al., 2006), it is logical to consider combining them with metoclopramide to improve gastric emptying.

***Ergots.*** Although increasingly less available and supplanted in many cases by newer agents, ergot preparations still have a role in the symptomatic treatment of migraine. The actions of ergotamine tartrate and other ergot preparations are complex. They are both vasoconstrictors and vasodilators, depending on the dose and the resting tone of the target vessels, and probably exert their effects on migraine via agonist activity at 5-HT receptors. Oral preparations are far less effective than those given rectally or parenterally.

If selected for use, 2 mg of ergotamine tartrate by mouth should be taken as soon as the patient recognizes the symptoms of an acute migraine attack. This dose, combined with a simple oral analgesic-caffeine combination, can be taken again in 1 hour. Possibly a better regimen, but inconvenient and unpleasant to some patients, is ergotamine tartrate by rectal suppository. The patient should be instructed to insert a 1- or 2-mg rectal suppository of ergotamine tartrate at the onset of the aura or pain and take a simple analgesic orally. The ergot preparation can be repeated in 60 minutes if needed. Experience over the course of several attacks is useful to determine the amount of ergotamine needed to obtain relief. With subsequent attacks, the entire dose can be taken at onset. If nausea is troublesome, metoclopramide in doses of 10 mg orally aids absorption of the ergotamine tartrate and may prevent vomiting. For patients who are close to vomiting or who are vomiting, an antiemetic suppository such as chlorpromazine (25–100 mg) or prochlorperazine (25 mg) can be helpful. If more than 6 mg of ergotamine is required per week, use an alternative preparation.

Ergotamine must be used cautiously by patients with hypertension and those with peripheral vascular disease. It is contraindicated in patients with coronary artery disease and in women who are pregnant. It is unwise to administer ergotamine to patients in whom the aura is particularly prolonged or characterized by a major neurological deficit. The fear of potentiating the vasospasm to the point of cerebral infarction may be unjustified but avoid the potential risk by withholding potent vasoconstrictors.

Dihydroergotamine (DHE) has been a treatment for migraine since the 1940s. Its poor oral bioavailability limits its administration to the parenteral and intranasal routes (see Table 102.5 and eTable 102.6). Patients can self-administer this drug by each of these routes. This medication should be considered when nausea and vomiting limit the use of oral medications or when other medications are ineffective. Although DHE's effects are slower than sumatriptan (see eTable 102.6), efficacy after 2 hours is similar, and the drug is associated with a lower recurrence of headache in 24 hours. Increased nausea in some patients may require combination with an antiemetic agent. When given intravenously in an acute medical care setting, use of an antiemetic is mandatory. A new inhaled formulation of DHE is currently being evaluated for US FDA approval. This new formulation may provide a means of administering DHE without IV infusion.

**Status migrainosus.** For many patients, an attack of migraine becomes a harrowing experience. After a variable period, they go to an emergency room or physician's office for further treatment. Status migrainosus is described as a debilitating migraine attack lasting for more than 72 hours (IHS, 2018). While there are no concrete guidelines currently available for status migrainosus treatment, several strategies have been used by some in the past. At our institution we have developed consensus among headache specialists for adult status migrainosus management recommendations based on available evidence, guidelines, and clinical experience (Fig. 102.6; Garza and Cutrer, n.d.). These do not replace clinical judgment but may assist the provider with decision making when encountering status migrainosus. Although, strictly defined, status migrainosus is a migraine headache lasting >72 hours, treatment often needs to start earlier if associated with significant uncontrolled vomiting and/or dehydration. In this model, if IV access is present, initial treatment consists of IV hydration, IV ketorolac 30 mg, and a neuroleptic antiemetic of choice (commonly prochlorperazine, metoclopramide, or promethazine) as needed. Specific status migrainosus treatment protocols using neuroleptic antiemetics have been published (Bell et al., 1990; Fisher, 1995; Lane et al., 1989; McEwen et al., 1987; Richman et al., 2002; Tek et al., 1990; Wang et al., 1997). To avoid extrapyramidal reactions with neuroleptic antiemetics, consideration can be given to pretreating with 1 mg oral (PO), intramuscular (IM), or IV benztropine mesylate. Benztropine is typically given to patients with a history of an extrapyramidal reaction to the chosen antiemetic, but not routinely. If IV access is not available, IM ketorolac with or without promethazine may be a good alternative. Patients with significant dehydration, complex coexisting medical problems and those requiring prolonged parenteral treatment may need to be hospitalized (Garza and Cutrer, n.d.). If initial measures fail and proper expertise is available, consideration can be given to extracranial nerve blocks directed to the area or areas of pain such as occipital, supraorbital, or auriculotemporal nerves and/or the sphenopalatine ganglion. If DHE is needed for a patient in a short-term stay setting

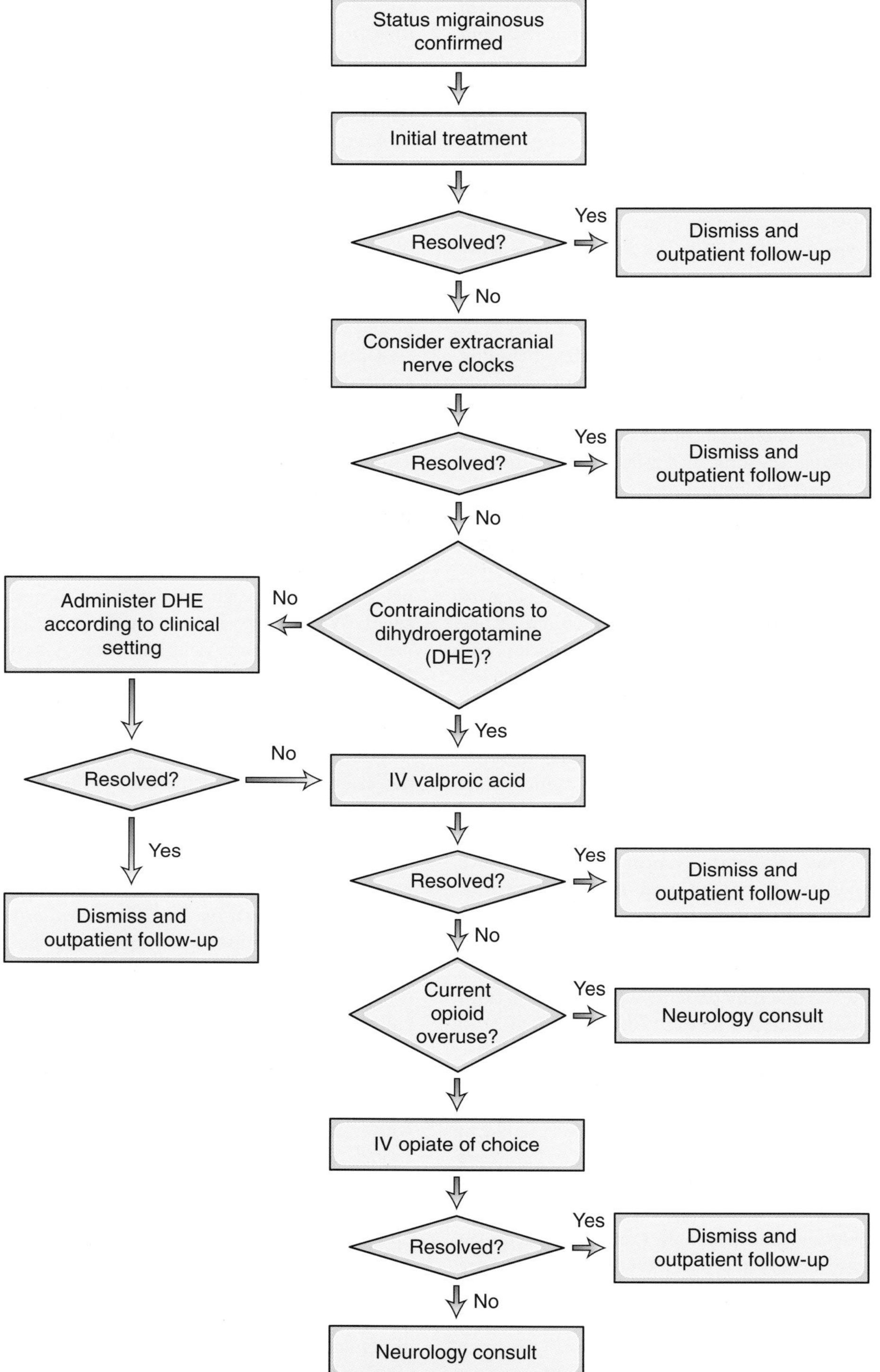


**Fig. 102.6 Status Migrainosus Management Recommendations for Adult Patients at our Institution.** *IV,* Intravenous. *(Adapted from (Garza and Cutrer, n.d.). Used with permission of Mayo Foundation for Medical Education and Research, all rights reserved.)*

such as the emergency room, it is administered as a 0.5 mg IV test dose and if tolerated may repeat DHE 0.5 mg IV 30–60 minutes later (total 1 mg). If inpatient, however, DHE is administered instead with IV 0.5–1.0 mg doses (depending on tolerance every 8 hours as needed ("Raskin protocol") (Raskin, 1990) for up to 2–5 days or via continuous IV DHE infusion ("Ford protocol") (Ford and Ford, 1997). In the latter, DHE initiates at 3 mg in 1000 mL normal saline and is administered IV at 42 mL/h but if significant nausea the rate is reduced to 21–30 mL/h (may continue up to 7 days if needed). Patients getting IV DHE are commonly pretreated with IV metoclopramide (with or without benztropine mesylate as discussed above) if no other antiemetic has been given, and the antiemetic is repeated as needed while on IV DHE treatment. When used, IV valproic acid starts with a loading dose of 15 mg/kg in D5W (5% dextrose in water) or normal saline at 20 mg/min and is followed by 5 mg/kg every 8 hours as needed (Schwartz et al., 2002). An alternative IV valproic acid protocol is 1 g in 250 mL normal saline over 1 hour (Edwards et al., 2001). A very common valproic acid IV dosing, however, is 500 mg at 20 mg/min × 1 dose (after 1000 mL normal saline) (Garza and Cutrer, n.d.). One of the main goals of this approach is to avoid opiate/opioid use as much as possible when managing status migrainosus, to minimize the risk of medication overuse headache. Dexamethasone (10 mg IV) may be given prior to dismissal to help prevent headache recurrence (Garza and Cutrer, n.d.).

### Prophylactic Treatment

A preventive program is appropriate when attacks occur weekly or several times a month, or when they occur less often but are very prolonged and debilitating. The most effective prophylactic agents available typically reduce headache frequency by at least 50% in approximately 50% of patients.

Preventive medications are generally titrated gradually to the minimum effective or maximum tolerated dosage. This target dosage is maintained for at least 3 months, and if there is a beneficial response, the medication is continued until there has been clinical stabilization for at least 6–12 months. The full benefit of a preventive medication may take up to 6 months to be realized. In a clinical trial evaluating the impact of discontinuing preventive therapy, patients taking topiramate were randomized for 6-months to either continue topiramate or switch to a placebo (Diener et al., 2007a). Remarkably, although patients continuing topiramate tended to have overall better headache outcomes, patients switching to placebo maintained improvements, compared to their pre-treatment baseline. Therefore, a discussion regarding treatment discontinuation is reasonable after 6 months if patients are doing well.

Multiple guidelines exist for the selection of preventive therapies for episodic migraine, including the American Academy of Neurology (AAN)/American Headache Society (AHS), Canadian Headache Society and the European Federation of Neurological Societies (Loder et al., 2012). The levels of recommendation made by the AAN/AHS are based on the strength of efficacy data alone, while the Canadian and European guidelines factor in a balance of potential benefits and harms. First-line therapies, including topiramate, divalproex, metoprolol, and propranolol are given first-line recommendation status by all guidelines (Loder et al., 2012). In our practice, a process of shared decision making with consideration for the strength of available clinical trial data, potential side effects, and individual patient treatment preferences and goals is employed. Table 102.8 lists some commonly used migraine preventive medications in our practice.

***β-Adrenergic blockers.*** β-Adrenergic antagonists are widely used for prophylaxis of migraine headaches (Silberstein et al., 2012). Propranolol in doses of 80–240 mg/day, if tolerated, should be given a trial of 2–3 months. Compliance increases with the use of a long-acting form of propranolol given once daily. Side effects are not usually severe. Lethargy or depression may occur and may be a reason for discontinuation of the medication. Hypotension, bradycardia, impotence, insomnia, and nightmares can all occur. As with all β-adrenergic blocking agents, propranolol should be discontinued slowly to avoid cardiac complications. It is contraindicated in persons with a history of asthma or severe depression and should be used with caution in patients using insulin or oral hypoglycemic agents, because it may mask the adrenergic symptoms of hypoglycemia. Timolol, nadolol, atenolol, and metoprolol probably have approximately the same benefit in migraine as propranolol. The mechanism of action is not known. The only pharmacological trait that separates β-adrenergic blocking agents effective in migraine from those that are not is a lack of sympathomimetic activity.

***Calcium channel blockers.*** Although the relevant mechanism by which calcium channel antagonists affect migraine is not known, their use in migraine was originally based on their ability to prevent vasoconstriction and on their other actions, including prevention of platelet aggregation and alterations in release and reuptake of serotonin. Several clinical trials have indicated some benefit for verapamil and flunarizine in preventing recurrent migraine. Little evidence exists to support the use of nimodipine. Verapamil in doses of 80–160 mg three times a day reduces the incidence of migraine with aura, but it is not as useful in migraine without aura. Experience with diltiazem is too limited to permit an assessment of its value at this time.

***Antidepressants.*** Amitriptyline and other tricyclic antidepressants can be helpful in migraine prophylaxis (Silberstein et al., 2012). The benefit seems to be independent of their antidepressant action, which typically requires doses higher than that used for migraine. Used in doses of 10–150 mg at night, amitriptyline, nortriptyline, imipramine, or desipramine may all provide some reduction in attacks of migraine, although evidence of efficacy in clinical trials is available only for amitriptyline. Protriptyline is an alternative without sedating properties, although there is no support in the literature for its use in chronic migraine. Side effects can be rather troublesome. Morning drowsiness, dryness of mouth, weight gain, tachycardia, and constipation are common. The anticholinergic side effects may decrease with time. If tolerated, give the tricyclic agents a trial of at least 3 months after reaching a therapeutic dose. The optimal dose for migraine prophylaxis is determined by titration to the effective or maximum tolerated dose within the therapeutic range (e.g. usually 50–150 mg for amitriptyline and nortriptyline).

**TABLE 102.8 Some Commonly Used Migraine Preventive Medications**

| Drug | Initial Dose (mg) | Typical Daily Dose Range | Common Adverse Effects | Serious Adverse Effects |
|---|---|---|---|---|
| Amitriptyline | 10–25 | 25–150 | Weight gain, constipation, sedation | Cardiac dysrhythmias |
| Nortriptyline | 10–25 | 25–150 | Weight gain, constipation, sedation | Cardiac dysrhythmias |
| Protriptyline | 5–10 | 10–30 | Constipation, sedation | Cardiac dysrhythmias |
| Topiramate | 15–25 | 75–200 | Paresthesias, fatigue, weight loss, cognitive impairment | Glaucoma, hyperthermia, metabolic acidosis, nephrolithiasis |
| Divalproex sodium | 250–500 | 750–1500 | Alopecia, weight gain, tremor, nausea | Pancreatitis, liver failure, thrombocytopenia |
| Gabapentin | 300 | 900–2400 | Dizziness, fatigue, edema, sedation | |
| Propranolol | 40–60 | 40–240 | Depression, fatigue | Bradyarrhythmia |
| Atenolol | 25 | 50–100 | Depression, fatigue | Bradyarrhythmia |
| Verapamil | 80–160 | 160–480 | Edema, constipation | Hypotension, dysrhythmias |

*Adapted from Garza, I., Swanson, J.W., 2006. Prophylaxis of migraine. Neuropsychiatr. Dis. Treat. 2 (3), 281–291.*

Selective serotonin reuptake inhibitors have not consistently proven to be effective for migraine prophylaxis and in some cases may elicit or aggravate headaches. Given the frequent comorbidity of generalized anxiety disorder and panic disorder, a serotonin-norepinephrine reuptake inhibitor such as venlafaxine may be considered if a single agent is desired. Venlafaxine is probably used less commonly than the tricyclic antidepressants discussed above. Nonetheless, venlafaxine was found to be effective in a placebo-controlled trial and remains an option which may prevent migraine headaches in some. Among patients with comorbid generalized anxiety disorder, venlafaxine may be an appropriate weight-neutral treatment option to facilitate dual treatment.

There are uncontrolled studies to support the use of the monoamine oxidase inhibitor (MAOI) phenelzine for migraine prophylaxis. Unfortunately, the dietary restrictions that must be carefully followed if a hypertensive crisis is to be avoided limit the widespread use of these inhibitors for prevention of migraine. Dangerous drug interactions can occur with preparations such as sympathomimetic agents, central anticholinergics, tricyclic antidepressants, and opioids, especially meperidine. Side effects of MAOIs include hypotension as well as hypertension, agitation, hallucinations, retention of urine, and inhibition of ejaculation.

***Anticonvulsants.*** Antiepileptic medications are in general a highly efficacious class of prophylactic treatment. Their mechanisms of action in migraine prophylaxis are unknown.

In the early 1990s, several blinded placebo-controlled studies showed a beneficial effect of valproate in the prophylactic treatment of migraine; 50% of patients showed a response with a 50% or better reduction in migraine incidence. Valproic acid, given in the form of divalproex sodium, is generally effective (Silberstein et al., 2012) at a range of 500–1750 mg/day, taken in divided doses. Side effects include sedation, dizziness, increased appetite, increased bleeding time, increased fragility of hair, and an asymptomatic increase in liver function test values. Valproate is contraindicated in women who are at risk for becoming pregnant, because it is associated with an increased risk for neural tube defects. While only limited evidence is available to support its use, gabapentin does appear to be effective in the reduction of migraine frequency in clinical practice. It also has beneficial effects in somatic pain and may be a good choice if a patient has neck pain, back pain, or painful peripheral neuropathy as well as migraine. It appears relatively well tolerated, although dizziness and sedation may limit its use in some patients. The usual therapeutic dose range for gabapentin is 900–2400 mg/day. Topiramate's efficacy for migraine was demonstrated in pivotal large randomized trials (Brandes et al., 2004). Topiramate has effects not only on γ-aminobutyric acid (GABA) but also on non-*N*-methyl-D-aspartate glutamate and carbonic anhydrase activity. It may have prominent sedating and cognitive side effects, making a slow gradual titration of the drug (15–25 mg/wk initially) to the therapeutic range of 75–200 mg/day the most successful strategy. Too rapid a titration schedule increases the risk of precipitating depression, especially if there is a personal or family history (Mula et al., 2009). Other side effects include paresthesia and weight loss, the latter making topiramate a particularly attractive choice for many patients. It is also associated with a mildly increased risk for calcium phosphate kidney stones. Zonisamide may be a good alternative in topiramate-intolerant patients who had previously experienced a good response (Mohammadianinejad et al., 2011).

***Other prophylactic agents.*** Cyproheptadine is a peripheral serotonin antagonist, typically used in pediatric patients. For younger patients unable to swallow pills, cyproheptadine is available in a syrup formulation. At all ages, it causes drowsiness and may cause significant weight gain. Methysergide, a peripheral serotonin antagonist and central serotonin agonist, is no longer available in the United States and Canada. Historically, it was a very useful agent despite its potential for producing serious complications.

Two small clinical trials have demonstrated efficacy of an extract of butterbur root in migraine prophylaxis, at a total daily dose of 150 mg daily (in two or three divided doses). The treatment is well tolerated, but gastrointestinal symptoms may occur. Recently, the safety of butterbur root has come into question due to potential for hepatotoxicity and carcinogenesis.

Riboflavin administered orally in a dose of 400 mg/day has been shown by Schoenen to be effective in migraine prophylaxis in a prospective randomized controlled study that enrolled a relatively small number of subjects. Its effect on the frequency of attacks was not statistically significant until the third month of the trial. There are minimal side effects associated with this agent.

Evidence is mixed regarding the efficacy of magnesium in migraine prophylaxis. Oral magnesium supplementation with 600 mg of a chelated or slow-release preparation is the recommended dosage. Magnesium-induced diarrhea and gastric irritation are the most common side effects.

Aspirin, 325 mg, taken every other day for the prevention of cardiovascular disease, may slightly reduce the frequency of migraine. NSAIDs are being increasingly recognized as having benefit in migraine prophylaxis and may be associated with reduced risk of chronic migraine development in individuals with less than 10 headache days per month based on epidemiological studies (Lipton et al., 2013).

OnabotulinumtoxinA injection in the treatment of chronic migraine is now supported by two large multicenter placebo-controlled randomized clinical trials and is currently the only FDA-approved treatment specifically for chronic migraine (Dodick et al., 2010) (see chronic migraine discussion). OnabotulinumtoxinA is established as ineffective and should not be offered for episodic migraine (Simpson et al., 2016).

Candesartan (angiotensin II receptor blocker), at a dose up to 16 mg daily, and lisinopril (angiotensin converting enzyme inhibitor), at a dose from 10 to 20 mg daily, are antihypertensives that are probably used less often than other blood-pressure medications discussed here previously. Nonetheless, both have been found to be effective as migraine preventives in randomized controlled trials and remain an option when other more commonly used preventives fail or are not tolerated.

### Neurostimulation

In March 2014, a transcutaneous supraorbital nerve stimulator was approved by the FDA for migraine prevention following a small clinical trial showing modest benefit among patients with episodic migraine (Schoenen et al., 2013b). The device is considered to be safe; however, efficacy has not been independently confirmed by other investigators.

Transcranial magnetic stimulation (TMS), a noninvasive technique utilizing a magnetic pulse hypothesized to disrupt cortical spreading depression, has now been approved by the FDA for the symptomatic treatment of migraine with aura. Single-pulse TMS (sTMS) was studied in a randomized, double-blinded, sham-controlled study, where greater pain-free responses were observed at 2 hours, with a sustained effect noted at 24 and 48 hours after treatment of migraine with aura (Lipton et al., 2010). In a prospective, open-label study of 263 patients with migraine with or without aura, scheduled twice-daily treatment with sTMS for 3 months, 46% of the patients reduced their headache frequency by half or more, and no serious adverse effects were observed (Starling et al., 2018).

A noninvasive vagal nerve stimulator was evaluated for acute treatment of migraine in a double-blind, randomized, sham-controlled trial (Tassorelli et al., 2018). When attacks were initially treated within 20 minutes, superior efficacy for pain freedom was observed at early (30- and 60-minute) time points, but not at a later (2-hour) time point. No serious adverse events were observed.

### Calcitonin Gene-Related Peptide Targeted Therapies

There has been a long-standing literature documenting a fundamental role for CGRP in the pathophysiology of migraine (Edvinsson, 2017). Along these lines, elevated levels of CGRP can be measured in the internal jugular vein during an acute attack of migraine, which then normalize with treatment with sumatriptan. Further, experimental infusion of CGRP triggers migraine in patients with migraine but not controls. The development of oral CGRP antagonists ("-gepants") have largely been hampered by hepatotoxicity in clinical trials; however, at least two agents (rimegepant and ubrogepant) have demonstrated efficacy and safety in phase III clinical trials for acute treatment of migraine.

Four different monoclonal antibodies have demonstrated safety and efficacy for preventive treatment of migraine in phase III trials. Prospective data indicate that these medications remain effective even among patients who have failed up to four prior preventive trials. Injection site discomfort is the most common side effect, with small numbers of patients also reporting constipation. Three of these monoclonal antibodies have been licensed in the United States: erenumab which targets the CGRP receptor, and fremanezumab and galcanezumab, both of which target CGRP.

The AHS has released a consensus statement offering guidance as to how to incorporate CGRP-based immunotherapies into clinical practice (American Headache Society, 2019) based on number of headache days per month and headache-related disability, as measured by the Migraine Disability Assessment Scale or the Headache Impact Test. For patients reporting 4–7 monthly headache days and at least moderate disability despite at least two 6-week trials of AAN level A or B preventive therapies, CGRP-based immunotherapy would be indicated. For patients reporting 8–14 monthly headache days, a CGRP-based immunotherapy is indicated at any disability level if at least two 6-week trials of preventive therapies have not been successful. Finally, CGRP-based immunotherapies are indicated for patients with chronic migraine if they have not responded to either two 6-week oral preventive trials or two quarterly injection cycles of onabotulinumtoxinA.

Despite general enthusiasm for the availability of a novel class of pharmacotherapy with a benign side-effect profile, significant pre-clinical concerns warrant caution pending longer term post-marketing experience. Specifically, CGRP is known to exert several protective physiological roles including vasodilation, raising concerns that worse outcomes could be observed if a patient exposed to treatment were to experience a vascular event (Deen et al., 2017). Nonetheless, open-label experience now reported out to 3 years fortunately has not documented such adverse outcomes.

### Hormones and Migraine

Migraine occurs equally in both sexes before puberty, but it becomes three times more common in women after menarche. Approximately 25% of women have migraine during their reproductive years. The changing hormonal environment throughout a woman's life cycle, including menarche, menstruation, oral contraceptive use, pregnancy, menopause, and hormone replacement therapy (HRT), can have a profound effect on the course of migraine.

***Menstrual migraine.*** Migraine attacks are generally associated with menses in one of two ways. The attacks may occur exclusively during menstruation and at no other time during the cycle. This association is referred to as *pure menstrual migraine* (PMM), and it has been proposed that PMM be defined as attacks that occur between days −2 and +3 of the menstrual cycle. The prevalence of PMM according to this definition is about 7%. More commonly, migraine attacks occur throughout the cycle but increase in frequency or intensity at the time of menstruation (menstrually related migraine). This association occurs in up to 60% of female migraineurs. Menstrual migraines have a tendency to be more severe, disabling, and treatment-refractory. Aura is uncommon. Finally, headache may be a symptom of the premenstrual syndrome, where depression, irritability, fatigue, appetite changes, bloating, backache, breast tenderness, and nausea characterize the disorder. These different relationships between migraine and the menstrual cycle can be determined by reviewing headache diaries, and their distinction is important because the pathophysiology may differ, as would the therapeutic approach.

Numerous mechanisms have been proposed to explain the pathogenesis of menstrual migraine. There is abundant clinical and experimental evidence to support the theory that estrogen withdrawal before menstruation is a trigger for migraine in some women. Estrogen withdrawal may modulate hypothalamic β-endorphin, dopamine, β-adrenergic, and serotonin receptors. This complex relationship causes significant downstream effects such as a reduction in central opioid tone, dopamine receptor hypersensitivity, increased trigeminal mechanoreceptor receptor fields, and increased cerebrovascular reactivity to serotonin. These changes, which occur during the luteal phase of the cycle, may be germane to the pathogenesis of menstrual migraine.

Several lines of investigation have implicated both prostaglandins and melatonin in the pathogenesis of menstrual migraine. Prostaglandins and melatonin are important mediators of nociception and analgesia, respectively, in the CNS. The concentrations of prostaglandin $F_2$ and nocturnal melatonin secretion increase and decrease, respectively, during menstruation in female migraineurs. These observations are the basis for the clinical use of NSAIDs and melatonin for menstrual migraine prophylaxis.

### Management of Menstrual Migraine

To establish a direct link between menstruation and headache attacks, ask the patient to keep a diary of migraine attacks and menstrual periods for at least 3 consecutive months. The nature of this relationship determines subsequent therapy. For example, for patients who have both menstrual and nonmenstrual migraine, a standard prophylactic medication might be used throughout the cycle rather than the perimenstrual use of a prophylactic agent. Clearly outline the goals of therapy in addition to the dosages, benefits, and side-effect profile of each recommended medication. Ideally, the headache diary can help identify other nonhormonal triggers. Biofeedback and relaxation therapy can be helpful in selected patients and should be used whenever possible.

***Acute menstrual migraine therapy.*** The goal of acute menstrual migraine therapy is to decrease the severity and duration of pain as well as the associated symptoms of an individual migraine attack, including nausea, vomiting, photophobia, and phonophobia. Some women may control attacks of menstrual migraine quite adequately with abortive therapy only (see Migraine/Symptomatic Treatment section, previously). The acute management of menstrual migraine does not differ from the treatment of migraine unassociated with menstruation (see Migraine/Symptomatic Treatment section, discussed previously).

***Prophylactic menstrual migraine therapy.*** Prophylaxis may either be perimenstrual (cyclic) (Box 102.3) or continuous (noncyclic, see Migraine/Prophylactic Treatment section, discussed previously). Many of the regimens suggested for perimenstrual migraine prophylaxis depend on regular menstruation and the ability to predict headache

**BOX 102.3 Cyclic (Perimenstrual) Prophylaxis for Menstrual Migraine**

Nonsteroidal anti-inflammatory drugs (days −3 through +3):
- Naproxen sodium, 550 mg bid
- Mefenamic acid, 250 mg tid
- Ketoprofen, 75 mg tid

Ergots (days −3 through +3):
- Ergotamine tartrate + caffeine (Wigraine), 1 mg qhs or bid
- Dihydroergotamine, 0.5–1 mg (subcutaneous, intramuscular, or intranasal) bid

Triptans:
- Naratriptan, 1 mg bid for 5 days
- Frovatriptan, 2.5 bid for 6 days
- Zolmitriptan, 2.5 mg bid or tid for 7 days

*bid*, Twice daily; *qhs*, every day at bedtime; *tid*, three times daily.

onset in relationship to menses. Perimenstrual prophylaxis commences a few days before the period is expected and continues until the end of menstruation. In women whose cycles are difficult to predict, continuous prophylaxis with standard migraine prophylactic agents is called for (see Migraine/Prophylactic Treatment section, discussed previously).

NSAIDs are considered first-line agents for perimenstrual prophylactic therapy in patients with either menstrual-associated migraine, or PMM, when the timing of menstruation is predictable. Different classes of NSAIDs should be tried because response may vary in a given individual. Ergot derivatives can also be effective when used as perimenstrual prophylactic drugs around the time of menstruation. Risks for rebound headaches are minimal, given the limited duration of treatment when drugs are used perimenstrually. Frovatriptan, naratriptan, and zolmitriptan have been found to be effective for perimenstrual prophylaxis and are included in the AAN and AHS guidelines on migraine prophylaxis (Silberstein et al., 2012). It is worth noting that severe menstrually related migraine may respond better to short-term or perimenstrual prophylaxis while on a chronic (continuous, noncyclic) preventive agent.

***Other treatments.*** For those with PMM, attacks are also preventable by stabilizing estrogen levels during the late luteal phase of the cycle. Estrogen levels can be stabilized by maintaining high levels with estrogen supplements. These should be directed by the patient's gynecologist.

The use of magnesium for acute and prophylactic treatment of migraine and menstrual migraine may be considered. Women with menstrual migraine have low levels of systemic magnesium, and MRS studies have demonstrated reduced levels of intracellular magnesium in the cerebral cortex of migraineurs. Low levels of intracellular magnesium may lead to neuronal hyperexcitability and spontaneous depolarization, which may be the central process initiating a migraine attack. This has led some investigators to study the effect of magnesium on menstrual migraine management.

Some physicians still advocate the use of hysterectomy and oophorectomy in women with intractable PMS and menstrual migraine whose headaches respond to medical ovariectomy. No long-term follow-up or controlled studies exist that conclusively substantiate this position. Because no study has been placebo controlled, the positive results seen in some studies may reflect the daily postoperative use of estrogen. Although two-thirds of women who have physiological menopause experience migraine relief, the opposite effect may occur with surgical menopause with bilateral oophorectomy. In a retrospective study of 1300 women, Granella and colleagues also demonstrated the unfavorable effects of surgical menopause on migraine. Therefore, until convincing evidence demonstrates otherwise, hysterectomy with or without oophorectomy is not currently a recommendation for women with menstrual migraine.

### Oral Contraception in Female Migraineurs

Migraine prevalence is highest in women during their reproductive years, the very population who use oral contraceptive therapy. Oral contraceptives have a variable effect on migraine. Migraine may begin de novo after a woman starts taking oral contraceptives, pre-existing migraine may worsen in severity or frequency, or the characteristics of the migraine attack may change (e.g., development of aura symptoms in a woman who for years had migraine without aura). Migraine attacks may also lessen after starting an oral contraceptive, particularly in women whose migraine attacks had a very close relationship to menstruation. In the majority of women, however, the pattern of migraine does not change appreciably after they start taking an oral contraceptive, particularly with the lower doses of estrogen and progestin now found in most oral contraceptives.

The concern about the use of synthetic estrogen in women with migraine pertains to the increased risk for ischemic stroke in this population, relative to age-matched women without migraine. There is now convincing evidence that female migraineurs have a small, but measurably increased risk of experiencing ischemic stroke. A 1995 case-control study found migraine to be strongly associated with the risk for ischemic stroke in young women (odds ratio [OR], 3.5), and this association was independent of other vascular risk factors. The risk for ischemic stroke was particularly increased in women with migraine who were using oral contraceptives (OR, 13.9), were heavy smokers (OR, 10.2), or who had migraine with aura (OR, 6.2). The estimated incidence of ischemic stroke in young women with migraine with aura who use oral contraceptives is 28 per 100,000 women aged 25–34, and 78 per 100,000 aged 35–44. This is in contrast to the incidence of ischemic stroke of approximately 4 and 11 per 100,000 women in the general population in the same respective age groups. Although the relative risk for ischemic stroke is increased in this group, it is important to bear in mind that the absolute risks are still small. Further, there is no convincing evidence that exposure to very low dose estrogen (<20 μg ethinyl estradiol) confers additional risk to individuals with migraine, who do not smoke and are normotensive.

The International Headache Society Task Force developed evidence-based recommendations for the use of oral contraceptives and HRT in migraineurs (Bousser et al., 2000). When prescribing combination oral contraceptives (COCs) in women with migraine, their recommendations were as follows:

- Identify and evaluate risk factors.
- Diagnose migraine type, particularly the presence of aura.
- Women with migraine should stop smoking before starting COCs.
- Treat other conditions such as hypertension and hyperlipidemia.
- Consider non–ethinyl estradiol methods in women at increased risk for ischemic stroke. Progestogen-only hormonal contraception may not increase ischemic stroke risk.
- High-dose COCs (50 μg ethinyl estradiol) are not recommended for routine use.
- Low-dose formulations (<50 μg ethinyl estradiol) containing either second- or third-generation progestogens should be used when possible.

Migraine symptoms that may necessitate further evaluation or cessation of COC include new persisting headache, new onset of migraine aura, increased headache frequency or intensity, and/or development of unusual aura symptoms, particularly prolonged aura.

With respect to contraindications for the use of HRT, the Task Force concluded that there was no evidence proving that migraine is a risk factor for ischemic stroke in women older than age 45. In addition, there are insufficient data to support an increased risk for ischemic stroke in women with any type of migraine who are using HRT. Consequently, the usual indications and contraindications for HRT should apply.

***Migraine and pregnancy.*** Pregnancy has a variable effect on migraine (see Chapter 111) Although approximately 70% of women experience improvement or remission of migraine symptoms during pregnancy, the attacks can either remain unchanged or worsen. Moreover, migraine may begin for the first time during pregnancy. Remission or improvement occurs more often in women with preexisting menstrual migraine, whereas worsening is more common in those with a history of migraine with aura. Most women who develop migraine during pregnancy have migraine with aura. Although there is a trend for improvement in the second and third trimesters, there is no significant correlation between improvement or worsening of migraine and a specific trimester.

If remission occurs during pregnancy, migraine often recurs in the postpartum period, particularly in those with a history of menstrual migraine or migraine associated with estrogen withdrawal. Postpartum migraine occurs most often 3–6 days after delivery. Migraine may be experienced for the first time in the postpartum period, but this is a very rare occurrence.

The use of medication to treat migraine during pregnancy should be limited. For most mild to moderate attacks, use nonpharmacological treatment, including biofeedback, rest, and relaxation therapy. Acetaminophen may be combined with codeine, but the indiscriminate use of codeine may present a risk to the fetus during the first or second trimester.

For patients with severe attacks or status migrainosus, the risk to the developing fetus may be greater than the judicious use of medications. The IV use of neuroleptics, supplemented with either IV opioids or corticosteroids, can be an effective strategy. Chlorpromazine or prochlorperazine (10 mg) delivered in 4 mL of crystalloid or 50 mL of normal saline as a bolus over 10–15 minutes can be effective for the headache as well as the nausea and vomiting associated with a severe attack. Methylprednisolone (50–250 mg) delivered IV can also be an effective method to terminate a severe acute migraine attack or status migrainosus during pregnancy. Intravenous magnesium sulfate (1 g) may be an effective alternative.

Cefaly, a wearable device, can likely be used safely as both a; preventive and abortive treatment during migraine. If the benefits of treatment outweigh any potential risks to the fetus then propranolol or amitriptyline could be considered for migraine prophylaxis (Pringsheim et al., 2012).

***Migraine in menopause.*** Just as with pregnancy, the effect of menopause on the course of migraine is somewhat unpredictable. In two-thirds of women with a previous history, migraine decreases with a physiological menopause, but it can either regress or worsen at menopause; in a minority of women, migraine or its functional equivalents may begin after menopause.

Women with menopausal symptoms resulting from erratic or diminished estrogen secretion may benefit from hormone replacement therapy (HRT), but consider potential risks. Few published studies have assessed the effects of HRT on migraine in perimenopausal women, but the available evidence appears to highlight the importance of both route and method of administration. With any preparation of estrogen, use the lowest effective dose. In general, parenteral or transdermal preparations provide a physiological ratio of estradiol to estrone and a steady-state concentration of estrogen. They are also more suitable delivery systems for women with migraine or for those whose headaches worsen by oral estrogen replacement therapy. Also, continuous rather than interrupted HRT may be more effective in female migraineurs whose headaches had been associated with estrogen withdrawal.

Cyclic progestins may worsen migraine. For women who require combined estrogen and progesterone therapy after hysterectomy, a transdermal progestin patch usually circumvents this problem.

## Chronic Daily Headache

*Chronic daily headache* (CDH) is a descriptive term that encompasses several different specific headache diagnoses. The designation of "chronic" in CDH refers either to the frequency of headaches or to the duration of the disease, depending on the specific headache type. For example, in chronic tension-type headache and chronic migraine, "chronic" indicates a headache frequency of at least 15 days per month. In chronic cluster headache and chronic paroxysmal hemicrania, however, "chronic" refers to a duration of at least 1 year without remission or with remissions lasting less than 3 months. In keeping with the Headache Classification Committee of the International Headache Society (IHS, 2018) and conventional clinical standards, clinicians must distinguish between primary and secondary headache disorders that present with more than 15 headache days per month. The disorders that can present with secondary CDH are numerous and include disorders of CSF dynamics (e.g., idiopathic intracranial hypertension, spontaneous spine CSF leaks), intracranial space-occupying lesions, inflammatory disorders (e.g., giant-cell arteritis), cerebrovascular disease, cervicogenic headache, TMJ disorders, trauma, infections including chronic meningitis, and medication overuse headache, among others. The development of progressively frequent and severe headaches within 3 months, neurological symptoms, focal or lateralizing neurological signs, papilledema, headaches aggravated or relieved by assuming upright or supine posture, headaches provoked by a Valsalva maneuver (cough, sneeze), systemic symptoms (e.g., weight loss, fever, myalgias), a history of sudden-onset headache, and onset after age 50 years are features that should prompt a diagnostic investigation with appropriate laboratory tests and imaging. Because these disorders are covered elsewhere in this chapter, this discussion will focus on primary CDH disorders.

If a secondary cause of headache is excluded, efforts are then focused on diagnosing the primary CDH subtype so that a treatment strategy can be established. The first decision point in making a diagnosis of a specific primary CDH disorder is to determine whether there are distinct episodes of headache with intervening headache-free periods. When discrete headache episodes are present, the usual duration of individual episodes and their frequency and timing must be determined. CDH disorders of short duration, usually defined as less than 4 hours, include cluster headache, paroxysmal hemicrania (PH), hypnic headache, SUNCT/SUNA and primary exertional and cough headache. These disorders are covered elsewhere in this chapter.

Primary CDH disorders of long duration in which individual headache episodes last longer than 4 hours include chronic migraine (CM), chronic tension-type headache, hemicrania continua, and new daily persistent headache. Indeed, patients who suffer from any of these disorders may have a continuous background daily headache with superimposed bouts of severe and disabling headache. CM and medication overuse headache (MOH) are the most common types of CDH encountered in clinical practice. Although strictly speaking, MOH is not a primary subtype of CDH, it frequently coexists with CM (see Medication Overuse Headache section, in Secondary Headaches section) and warrants simultaneous management along that of chronic migraine. Risk factors for the development of CM identified in population-based and clinic-based prospective studies include baseline high attack frequency, obesity, stressful life events, snoring, cutaneous allodynia, and overuse of certain classes of medications, particularly opioid and barbiturate combination products (Lipton, 2009; Louter et al., 2013). These risk factors may help clinicians identify those who may be at highest risk for the development of CM. It is important to recognize and address coexistent sleep and mood disorders that can lead to exacerbation of the underlying headache condition.

### Chronic Migraine

Chronic migraine, previously referred to as *transformed migraine*, is characterized by headaches (tension-type and/or migraine) on 15 or more days per month in a patient with prior migraine history, with at least 8 days per month being migraine for at least 3 months (IHS, 2018).

Patients with CM usually have a history of episodic migraine that began in their second or third decade of life. In the majority, the evolution from episodic migraine to chronic migraine is gradual, but the transition can be abrupt in about 30% of patients. Population studies estimate that patients with episodic migraine will transition to CM at the rate of approximately 2.5% per year (Lipton, 2009). For the patient with CM, on some days the headaches and associated symptoms (nausea, photo/phonophobia) may retain characteristics of migraine, whereas on other days, symptoms may be indistinguishable from a tension-type headache. These patients do not have "mixed" or "combined tension-vascular headaches," antiquated terms that are still used (Dodick, 2006).

Treatment of CM requires preventive medications and judicious use of acute medications. Only topiramate, onabotulinumtoxinA, and, more recently, erenumab, fremanezumab, galcanezumab, and eptinezumab have been studied specifically in chronic migraine via controlled studies. Two randomized double-blind placebo-controlled studies demonstrated that topiramate was effective and achieved significant reductions in migraine frequency (Diener et al, 2007b; Silberstein et al., 2007). A pooled analysis of results from two large phase-III placebo-controlled studies (PREEMPT 1 and 2) demonstrated a mean decrease from baseline in frequency of headache days, with statistically significant between-group differences favoring onabotulinumtoxinA over placebo at week 24 (−8.4 vs. −6.6; $P < .001$) (Dodick et al., 2010). While the therapeutic gain over placebo for this and many of the PREEMPT trials' outcomes appeared to be modest, onabotulinumtoxinA has been found to significantly reduce chronic migraine impact and improve quality of life (Lipton et al., 2011). Botulinum toxin blocks the release of glutamate from nociceptive terminals and therefore may reduce or inhibit the development of peripheral and central trigeminal sensitization. The mechanism of action may be referable to the observation that single trigeminal afferents may have both dural and extracranial projections (Schueler et al., 2013). The excellent tolerability of onabotulinumtoxinA makes it an extremely attractive alternative for patients who fail to tolerate oral prophylactics. The injection protocol used in the PREEMPT trials is currently the most widely accepted method of administration (Blumenfeld et al., 2010). The injections are given every 12 weeks and at least 2–3 cycles are recommended to determine response (Silberstein et al., 2015). In onabotulinumtoxinA responders, commonly a continued need and a cumulative benefit is observed over time (Aurora et al., 2014). Monoclonal antibodies targeting the CGRP receptor (erenumab) and the CGRP molecule (fremanezumab, galcanezumab, and eptinezumab) have now been developed. At the time of this publication erenumab, fremanezumab, galcanezumab, and eptinezumab have been FDA approved for the prevention of migraine. All of the CGRP monoclonal antibodies have been studied in chronic migraine and have shown favorable results.

While not rigorously studied for the treatment of CM, gabapentin, divalproex sodium, amitriptyline, and β-adrenergic blockers among other preventives used for episodic migraine prophylaxis are also frequently used in CM prevention, based on evidence for their effectiveness in patients with episodic migraine and a long clinical experience with these medications for migraine prevention (for more details, see Migraine/Prophylactic Treatment section, earlier).

Similarly to episodic migraine management (see previous discussion), preventive medications are generally titrated to the minimum effective or maximum tolerated dosage over the course of 1–2 months. This target dosage is maintained for at least 3 months, and if there is a beneficial response (>50% reduction in headache days), the medication is continued until there has been clinical stabilization for at least 6–12 months. It must be remembered that the full benefit of a preventive medication may take up to 6 months to be realized. An attempt to taper and discontinue the preventive medication is reasonable, but only after consultation with the patient and after a reasonable period of stability (>6–12 months).

Patients with chronic migraine should limit acute treatment use to prevent development of medication overuse headache (see Medication Overuse Headache section, previously).

## Cluster Headache

Among the many painful conditions that affect the head and face, cluster headache is without doubt the most painful recurrent headache, and the one that produces the most stereotyped attacks. In episodic cluster headache, attacks of pain occur in periods lasting 7 days to 1 year, separated by pain-free periods lasting 3 months or longer. In chronic cluster headache, attacks of pain occur for more than 1 year without remission or with remissions lasting less than 3 months (IHS, 2018). This chronic form of the disease may develop de novo or may evolve from episodic cluster headache. Approximately 90% of patients have episodic cluster headache, and 10% have the chronic form.

### Epidemiology

Compared with tension headache and migraine, the syndrome of cluster headaches is considerably less common. In many headache clinic populations, migraine is 10–50 times more common than cluster headache. The prevalence of cluster headache is about 1 person per 500. It occurs approximately three times more often in men than in women but is clinically identical in both genders. Although not universally observed, there is a tendency for cluster headache symptoms to remit with age (May, 2005). Unlike migraine, cluster headache has not been considered until recently to be an inherited condition. Several twin studies have demonstrated 100% concordance in monozygotic twins. Two genetic epidemiological surveys suggest that first-degree relatives may have up to an 18-times higher risk and second-degree relatives a 1- to 3-times higher risk of cluster headache than the general population. The increased familial risk of cluster headaches suggests a genetic underpinning. Inheritance is likely to be autosomal dominant with variable penetrance; nonetheless, in some families it may be autosomal recessive or multifactorial (Russell, 2004).

### Clinical Features

Onset typically begins in the third decade of life, although it has been described as early as 1 year of age and as late as the seventh decade. Periodicity is a cardinal feature of cluster headache. In most patients, the first cluster of attacks, the *cluster period*, persists on average for

6–12 weeks and is followed by a remission lasting for months or even years. The duration of the cluster period is often strikingly consistent for a given patient. A common pattern is one or two cluster periods per year. With time, however, the clusters may become seasonal and then occur more often and last longer. During a cluster, patients typically experience from 1 to 3 or more attacks in 24 hours. The attacks commonly occur at similar times throughout the 24 hours for several weeks to months. Onset during the night, or 1–2 hours after falling asleep, is common. In some patients, these may occur at the onset of rapid eye movement (REM) sleep. At times, several attacks per night can result in sleep deprivation in patients with chronic cluster headache, particularly when they avoid sleep for fear of inducing a further attack. With increasing age, the distinct clustering pattern may be less recognizable.

The attacks of pain are similar among individuals. The pain is strictly unilateral and almost always remains on the same side of the head from cluster to cluster. Rarely it may switch to the opposite side in a subsequent cluster or even (less frequently) during a single attack (Capobianco and Dodick, 2006). The pain is generally felt in the retro-orbital and temporal regions (upper syndrome) but may be maximal in the cheek or jaw (lower syndrome). It is usually described as steady or boring and of terrible intensity (so-called suicide headache). Graphic descriptions of feeling the eye being pushed out or an auger or hot poker going through the eye are common.

Onset is usually abrupt or preceded by a brief sensation of pressure in the soon-to-be-painful area. An occasional patient may describe tension and discomfort in the limbs and neck ipsilateral to the pain, either during the attack or just preceding it. Infrequently, aura symptoms (as seen in migraine) may precede cluster attacks. The pain intensifies very rapidly, peaking in 5–10 minutes and usually persisting for 45 minutes to 2 hours. Toward the end of this time, brief periods of relief may be followed by several transient peaks of pain before the attack subsides over a few minutes. Occasionally, attacks last twice as long or, less commonly, attacks may seem to merge together, producing 12 or more hours of pain. After the attack, the patient is pain free but exhausted; however, the respite may be transient because another attack may occur shortly.

During the pain, patients almost invariably avoid the recumbent position because doing so increases pain intensity. Unlike patients with migraine, they are restless and prefer to pace or sit during an attack. Some remain outdoors even in freezing weather for the duration of the attack. Interestingly, some may find relief or even abort an attack with physical exertion such as push-ups. Otherwise rational persons may strike their heads against a wall or hurt themselves in some other way as a distraction from the intense head pain. Most patients prefer to be alone during the attack. Some apply ice to the painful region, others prefer hot applications; almost all press on the scalp or the eye to try to obtain relief. During the pain, some patients consider suicide; a few attempt it.

During the pain of cluster headache, the nostril on the side of the pain is generally blocked; this blockage in turn can be followed by ipsilateral lacrimation. The conjunctiva may be injected ipsilaterally, and the superficial temporal artery may be visibly distended. Profuse sweating and facial flushing on the side of the headache have been described but are rare. Nasal drainage usually signals the end of the attack. Ptosis and miosis on the side of the pain may occur. This Horner syndrome may persist between attacks and is believed to be due to compression of the sympathetic plexus secondary to vasodilatation or other changes in the region of the carotid siphon. Migrainous symptoms such as nausea, photophobia, phonophobia, and/or osmophobia commonly accompany cluster headache (Bahra et al., 2002). Facial swelling, most often periorbital, may develop with repeated attacks. Rarely, transient localized swelling of the palate ipsilateral to the pain can be observed. Cluster headache patients tend to have coarse facial skin, deep nasolabial folds, and an increased incidence of hazel eye color. Many of the patients are heavy cigarette smokers and tend to use more alcohol than age- and sex-matched control subjects. Most patients, however, abstain from alcohol during a cluster period, since it commonly triggers attacks.

## Pathophysiology

The pathogenesis of cluster headache is not entirely understood. While the pain is likely mediated by activation of the trigeminal nerve pathways, the autonomic symptoms are due to parasympathetic outflow and sympathetic dysfunction. The periodicity suggests a defect in CNS cycling mechanisms that is likely related to hypothalamic dysfunction. The most direct evidence in support of a role of the hypothalamus in cluster headache comes from neuroimaging. PET imaging studies have shown activation in the ipsilateral ventral diencephalon during nitroglycerin-induced cluster attacks. In addition, a morphometric study of MRI scanning technology has shown an increase in volume in the diencephalon. Asymmetric facilitation of trigeminal nociceptive processing predominantly at a brainstem level has been detected in patients with cluster headache (Holle et al., 2012).

Although vasodilatation has been generally believed to be responsible for the pain, PET studies have shown that carotid artery dilation is not specific for cluster headache but is seen with other types of ophthalmic division pain; it appears to be an epiphenomenon of a primary neural process.

In 1993, Moskowitz emphasized the role of the trigeminovascular connections and substance P in the pathogenesis of vascular head pain. Further evidence suggested activation of the trigeminovascular system as manifested by increased levels of CGRP in blood sampled from the external jugular vein ipsilateral to an acute spontaneous attack of cluster headache. Vasoactive intestinal polypeptide levels were similarly elevated in the cranial venous blood during a cluster attack, demonstrating activation of the cranial parasympathetic nervous system. Parasympathetic activation is believed to be responsible for the ipsilateral conjunctival injection, lacrimation, nasal congestion, rhinorrhea, and/or eyelid edema. Trigeminal-parasympathetic overactivity may result in perivascular edema compromising the carotid canal, leading to neurapraxic injury of postganglionic sympathetic fibers and hence a Horner syndrome manifested in ptosis and miosis (May, 2005). The fact that low-frequency sphenopalatine ganglion (SPG) stimulation can provoke cluster-like headaches with autonomic features suggests efferent parasympathetic outflow from this ganglion may give rise to autonomic symptoms and activate the trigeminovascular sensory afferents which may initiate pain (Schytz et al., 2013).

## Investigations

In most patients, the diagnosis is certain on clinical grounds alone. However, imaging studies are recommended for all patients at the time of diagnosis, particularly for those presenting with an atypical episodic cluster ("cluster-like") headache or for patients with headache in the chronic phase. "Cluster-like" headaches can be associated with underlying intracranial or neck structural lesions such as neoplasms, paranasal sinus disease, vascular malformations, and cervicocephalic arterial aneurysms or dissections (Capobianco and Dodick, 2006). Therefore, as part of the evaluation, a contrast-enhanced brain MRI scan is recommended to help reassure the patient, their relatives, and physicians that the extremely painful attacks are not due to some major abnormality. Clinical judgment guides the necessity for further testing.

## Differential Diagnosis

The diagnosis of cluster headache is essentially clinical. It is helpful to have confirmation from the spouse or relatives of the periodicity, rapidity of onset and resolution, and presence of conjunctival injection, rhinorrhea, ptosis, and altered behavior during the attack. Despite the stereotyped nature of the attacks from episode to episode and from patient to patient, the diagnosis is often missed for several years. Conditions that cause episodic unilateral head and facial pain should be considered, but they are easy to exclude. Trigeminal neuralgia, sinusitis, dental disease, and glaucoma may superficially mimic the pain of cluster headache, but, in each, the temporal profile, lack of associated autonomic features, and past history allow easy differentiation. Similarly, migraine, temporal arteritis, and the headache of intracranial space-occupying lesions should not be difficult to differentiate from cluster headache. Orbital, retro-orbital, and frontal pain associated with Horner syndrome can result from ipsilateral dissection of the carotid artery; unlike the pain of cluster headache, however, it is not episodic and does not produce the restlessness so characteristic of this condition. The pain associated with Tolosa-Hunt syndrome and Raeder paratrigeminal syndrome is accompanied by oculomotor or trigeminal nerve dysfunction, a feature that should easily prevent confusion with cluster headache. Similarly, pain from compression of the third cranial nerve by an aneurysm should be easy to distinguish from cluster headache pain, especially when partial or complete third cranial nerve palsy is detected.

Cluster headache is a member of the primary headache syndromes collectively referred to as the *trigeminal-autonomic cephalalgias* (TACs); the other TACs have to be differentiated from cluster headache, since their management is usually different. These are discussed elsewhere in this chapter.

## Treatment and Management

The patient should be reassured that the syndrome, even though unbearably painful, is benign and not life threatening. Pain reduction but not cure should be promised.

The frequency, severity, and brevity of individual attacks of cluster headache and their lack of response to many symptomatic measures necessitate the use of a prophylactic treatment regimen for most patients. The treatment plan is determined by several factors, including whether the phase is episodic or chronic and whether other disease states such as hypertension and coronary or peripheral vascular insufficiency are present.

### *Pharmacological management*

**Acute (symptomatic) therapy.** Given the rapid onset and short time to peak intensity of the pain of cluster attacks, fast-acting symptomatic treatment is imperative. Oxygen, subcutaneous sumatriptan, and subcutaneous or intramuscular DHE provide the most rapid, effective, and consistent relief for cluster headache attacks.

Oxygen inhalation is one of the most effective symptomatic treatments for cluster headache. Its advantages are that it has no established adverse effects, it can be administered several times daily, it can be combined with other treatments, and it is inexpensive. Inhaled oxygen at 100% for 15–20 minutes via a nonrebreathing face mask can be dramatically effective for aborting a cluster attack. Rates of oxygen delivered at 12 L/min have been demonstrated to be effective (Cohen et al., 2009). Flow rates of 15 L/min may be effective when lower rates are not (Rozen, 2009). The best position for oxygen inhalation is sitting on the edge of a chair or bed and leaning forward with arms on knees. The mechanism of action of oxygen remains to be fully elucidated; recent data suggest that the beneficial response is mediated through its effects on the parasympathetic outflow via the facial/greater petrosal nerve, with no direct effect on trigeminal afferents (Akerman et al., 2009). Although portable regulators are available, the major drawbacks to oxygen use are the inconvenience, lack of accessibility, and need to have a regulator and canister available at all times. Unfortunately, in some cases, oxygen merely delays an attack rather than aborting it (Capobianco and Dodick, 2006).

Administration of sumatriptan by subcutaneous injection in a dose of 4–6 mg is an effective means of aborting an individual cluster attack. Sumatriptan nasal spray is less effective than the subcutaneous formulation.

DHE is available in injectable and intranasal formulations. DHE-45 administered IV provides prompt and effective relief of a cluster attack. The intramuscular and subcutaneous routes of administration provide slower relief. The potential role of intranasal DHE (2 mg) has not been validated in a controlled fashion.

Other potential symptomatic options include zolmitriptan nasal spray, octreotide, and intranasal lidocaine administered by dripping 4% viscous lidocaine into the nostril ipsilateral to the pain.

**Preventive pharmacotherapy.** Use of an effective preventive regimen cannot be overemphasized. The goals of preventive therapy are to produce a rapid suppression of attacks and maintain remission over the expected duration of the cluster period. Preventive therapy in cluster headache can be divided into transitional and maintenance prophylaxis.

**Transitional prophylaxis.** Transitional prophylaxis involves the short-term use of corticosteroids, occipital nerve blocks, ergotamine, or DHE. This typically induces a rapid suppression of attacks while one of the maintenance agents can take effect.

During the initial cluster or when the patient's past history suggests that a cluster will be of limited duration, relief can usually be obtained by administering a short course of corticosteroids. Several regimens are effective, such as 60 mg of prednisone as a single daily dose for 3–4 days, followed by a 10-mg reduction after every third or fourth day, to thereby taper the dose to zero over 18 or 24 days. Alternatively, an intramuscular injection of triamcinolone (80 mg) or methylprednisolone (80–120 mg) can be used to give a tapering corticosteroid blood level. Whichever treatment regimen is used, the patient usually obtains relief from the headaches until the lower doses or blood levels of corticosteroids are approached. The course can be repeated several times, but thereafter the risk for side effects suggests that an alternative prophylactic regimen should be used if the cluster has not run its course.

Ergotamine tartrate can be given orally or by rectal suppository on retiring to prevent nocturnal attacks of headache. This approach may only postpone the attack until morning, when it may be more troublesome if it occurs when the patient is at work. Prophylactic use of ergotamine tartrate can nevertheless be valuable, but great care must be taken to regulate the dose if chronic ergotism is to be avoided. Most patients with cluster headache can be given 2 mg of ergotamine tartrate daily for several days without adverse effects; however, caution must be used with ergotamine, triptans, and analgesics to avoid the development of MOH (Paemeleire et al., 2006). DHE is a well-tolerated ergot derivative that can be given in a dose of 0.5–1 mg every 6–8 hours in an attempt to prevent headaches, but this dose should be continued for only a few days to avoid ergotism.

In addition, an occipital nerve block ipsilateral to the cluster headache may be useful as a transitional measure in some patients when the use of other medications may be contraindicated or poorly tolerated.

Repeating this every 3 months may benefit some with chronic cluster headache (Lambru et al., 2014a).

**Maintenance prophylaxis.** *Maintenance prophylaxis* refers to the use of preventive medications throughout the anticipated duration of the cluster period. The preventive medication is initiated at the onset of the cluster period, typically in conjunction with corticosteroids, and is continued after the initial suppressive medication is discontinued.

The calcium channel blockers (Leone et al., 2009), particularly verapamil, are considered first-line preventive therapy for both episodic and chronic cluster headache. They are generally well tolerated and can be used safely in conjunction with ergotamine, sumatriptan, corticosteroids, and other preventive agents. The initial starting dose of verapamil is 80 mg three times a day after a normal ECG has been demonstrated. The authors have encountered several patients who appear to have an improved response with the nonsustained release formulation. The daily dose can be increased in 40- to 80-mg increments every 7–14 days until the attacks disappear, adverse effects occur, or the maximum daily dose of 720 mg is achieved (Leone et al., 2009). Doses as high as 960 mg daily may be required (Goadsby, 2012). These doses are considerably higher than those used for hypertension and heart disease (Rozen, 2009). If a patient requires more than 240 mg/day, an ECG is recommended before each dose increment, 2 weeks after the last adjustment, and periodically thereafter if verapamil is used long term (Cohen et al., 2007). The most common side effect of verapamil is constipation, but lightheadedness, hypotension, fatigue, peripheral edema, and bradycardia can also occur.

Methysergide can be effective for reducing or preventing cluster headache in about 60% of patients, but it is no longer available in the United States or Canada.

For patients who have chronic cluster headache with attacks that occur daily for years, relief may be obtained with lithium. Lithium carbonate, 300 mg three times a day, can be given initially and the dose adjusted at 2 weeks to obtain a serum lithium level of about 1 mEq/L. Side effects at this level include a mild tremor of the limbs, gastrointestinal distress, and increased thirst. The therapeutic range is very narrow, and blood levels of more than 1.5 mEq/L are to be avoided. Nephrotoxicity, goiter formation, and a permanent diabetes insipidus-like state have been reported after lithium treatment. In chronic cluster headache, lithium may have a beneficial effect within 1 week, but the response is typically delayed for several weeks. Although attacks may recur after some months, a renewed response to lithium may occur if the drug is withdrawn and then reintroduced after a few weeks. In patients whose headaches respond to lithium, use of the drug should be discontinued every few months to determine whether the cluster headaches have subsided. While lithium is being given, it is necessary to monitor the blood level at regular intervals to avoid the development of serious side effects. Thiazide diuretics should not be used concurrently because they can cause a rapid elevation of blood levels of lithium.

Despite the available treatments, management of patients with chronic cluster headache can be extremely difficult because many of their headaches do not respond or respond only briefly to the treatment regimens already described. In such patients, a combination of several medications may give relief. On the basis of clinical experience, the combination of verapamil and topiramate or verapamil and lithium can prove effective. For particularly resistant headaches, triple therapy may be necessary, consisting of verapamil with either topiramate or valproate plus lithium. The authors have had some success with onabotulinumtoxinA injections for chronic cluster headache, although there are no controlled studies available for its use in cluster headache. Corticosteroids can be useful in chronic cluster headache to provide brief remissions for fixed periods. Nonetheless, long-term use of corticosteroids in patients with chronic cluster headache must be resisted. Given the role that CGRP plays in cluster headache, the monoclonal antibodies targeting CGRP or its receptor could prove to be viable options in the prophylaxis of headache. Only galcanezumab has been studied in cluster headache, but as of this publication has not been FDA-approved for cluster headache.

In patients for whom conventional first-line therapy is ineffective, poorly tolerated, or contraindicated, one may consider adjunctive therapy with a number of potential agents including melatonin, baclofen, and intranasal civamide (Francis et al., 2010; May et al., 2006).

***Surgical treatment.*** Surgery is a last resort for medication-resistant chronic cluster headache, an option to be considered when all pharmacological treatment options have been thoroughly exhausted (Leone et al., 2009). Ablative procedures reported as potentially successful include radiofrequency thermocoagulation of the gasserian ganglion, trigeminal sensory rhizotomy, microvascular decompression of the trigeminal nerve, and sphenopalatine ganglion radiofrequency ablation (Leone et al., 2009; Narouze et al., 2009). Unfortunately, adverse events of these procedures can be severe and include corneal anesthesia, keratitis, and anesthesia dolorosa. Furthermore, the benefit may be less than robust and short-lived. These procedures have therefore been for the most part abandoned and are now used only rarely.

Neurostimulation procedures involving central or peripheral nervous system targets have been employed to treat refractory chronic cluster headache (Leone et al., 2009). At present, these are preferred over the previously discussed interventions but should only be considered in patients with medically intractable CH in tertiary headache centers, and the least invasive options should be considered first (Martelletti et al., 2013).

In 2003, Franzini and colleagues reported a complete response in five patients with medically refractory chronic cluster headache after stereotactic implantation of a stimulating electrode into the periventricular hypothalamus. The rationale for this procedure is based on the activation of the periventricular hypothalamus seen on PET scanning of patients during attacks of cluster headache. Sixteen patients with intractable chronic cluster headache were successfully treated by hypothalamic stimulation, with no significant adverse events in this series (Leone et al., 2005). At a mean follow-up of 23 months, 13 of the 16 patients were persistently pain free or almost pain free, while the rest were improved (Leone et al., 2006). Similar results from approximately 60 treated patients have been reported thus far. Hypothalamic deep brain stimulation may therefore be an efficacious procedure to relieve intractable chronic cluster headache. There have been, however, several intracranial hemorrhages reported with this procedure, including one death from such a hemorrhage. Less-invasive interventions are therefore favored prior to considering deep brain stimulation.

Peripheral stimulation of the occipital nerve has been employed in several open-label trials of patients with medically intractable cluster headache. One used bilateral stimulators in eight patients (Burns et al., 2007), and the other used unilateral stimulation (side ipsilateral to headaches) in eight patients (Magis et al., 2007). Substantial improvement occurred in a majority of individuals in each study, which was durable for a mean follow-up of 20 months and 15 months, respectively. The favorable outcome of 14 patients with medically intractable chronic cluster headache implanted with bilateral electrodes in the suboccipital region was published (Burns et al., 2009). Others have reported similar outcomes (Leone et al., 2017; Miller et al., 2017). This approach deserves additional study via prospective randomized controlled trials to further determine its role in cluster headache management. Factors predictive of a beneficial response to occipital nerve stimulation have failed to be elucidated; pain relief after greater occipital nerve block does not predict efficacy (Leone et al., 2009).

Schytz has shown that high-frequency stimulation of the SPG can abort cluster headaches (Schytz et al., 2013). Of very recent interest are the encouraging results from a randomized, sham-controlled study stimulating the SPG in medically refractory chronic cluster headache. Throughout a period up to 8 weeks, 19 of 28 (68%) patients had a clinically significant improvement: seven (25%) achieved pain relief in ≥50% of treated attacks, 10 (36%) a ≥50% reduction in attack frequency, and two (7%), both. Results suggest a potential dual benefit (acute pain relief and attack prevention) (Schoenen et al., 2013a). Other studies are necessary to confirm these findings.

## Other Trigeminal Autonomic Cephalalgias

Paroxysmal hemicrania (PH), short-lasting unilateral neuralgiform headache attacks (SUNCT/SUNA), and hemicrania continua (HC) are all classified along with cluster headache as trigeminal autonomic cephalalgias by the Headache Classification Committee (IHS, 2018). PH and SUNCT/SUNA are distinguished from cluster headache by having shorter attack durations and higher attack frequencies. PH and HC (the most prolonged TAC), respond completely to preventive treatment with indomethacin, which is not the circumstance in cluster headache or SUNCT/SUNA. Although rare, the occurrence of concomitant different TACs may manifest in single individuals (Totzeck et al., 2014).

### Paroxysmal Hemicrania

Paroxysmal hemicrania has a typical onset in the third decade of life. The female-to-male ratio is approximately 1:1, which contrasts with cluster headache, for which there is an overwhelming male predominance (Cittadini et al., 2008). Chronic PH and episodic PH differ in their temporal profile. In chronic PH, attacks occur for more than a year without remission or with remission periods lasting less than 3 months. Episodic PH is characterized by bouts of attacks occurring in periods lasting from 7 days to 1 year and separated by pain-free remission periods lasting at least 3 months (IHS, 2018). The headache bouts can range from 4 to 24 weeks, and remission periods can last 12–376 weeks. While active, both disorders are associated with daily attacks of severe short-lived unilateral pain, which is often maximally felt in the orbital/retro-orbital or temporal region, although extra-trigeminal pain in the occiput can occur. The mean attack frequency in one study was 11 in 24 hours, with a median of 9 attacks in 24 hours and a range from 2 to 50 attacks per day (Cittadini et al., 2008). The mean length of attacks was 17 minutes, with a median of 19 minutes and a range from 10 seconds to 4 hours. Similar to cluster headache, each paroxysm is accompanied by at least one robust ipsilateral autonomic feature, which may include lacrimation, miosis, ptosis, eyelid edema, conjunctival injection, nasal congestion, rhinorrhea, or forehead/facial sweating. Numerous cases of secondary PH have been reported and underline the importance of MRI of the brain in every case. PH typically responds completely to indomethacin. The dose required ranges from 25 to 300 mg/day. Most patients require around 150 mg/day. In a patient with suspected PH, the usual indomethacin trial includes indomethacin 25 mg 3 times a day for 3 days, then 50 mg 3 times a day for 3 days, and then finally 75 mg 3 times a day for 3 days. If at the end of this trial there is minimal or no response, discontinue indomethacin and consider an alternative diagnosis. If there is an absolute response to the indomethacin trial, however, indomethacin is continued as long as it is tolerated. The headache usually resolves within 1–2 days of initiating the effective dose. Dose adjustments are often needed to address clinical fluctuations. Skipping or delaying doses may result in recurrence of the headache. Efforts should be placed for patients to find the lowest dose possible that controls the pain. We typically place patients on gastric mucosa protective agents while they take daily indomethacin. In patients with episodic PH, the indomethacin can be continued for roughly 2 weeks beyond the typical headache bout duration, and then a trial of tapering can be undertaken. Some patients are able to discontinue indomethacin without recurrence (presumably representing a transition from chronic to episodic PH), so treatment should be tapered periodically to ensure that patients are still symptomatic. During this taper, we usually decrease the indomethacin dose by 25 mg every 3 days until either the headache recurs or the patient gets completely off indomethacin. Despite the differences in typical attack frequency and duration between cluster headache and PH, in some circumstances cluster headache and PH can be clinically indistinguishable. Thus, any patient presenting with what appears to be cluster headache but is refractory to usual cluster headache treatments should have an indomethacin trial. The therapeutic response to indomethacin is the most reliable differential diagnostic criterion for cluster headache and PH. Other treatments reported to be effective in PH include celecoxib, rofecoxib, botulinum toxin A, verapamil, nicardipine, flunarizine, ibuprofen, ketoprofen, aspirin, piroxicam, naproxen, diclofenac, phenylbutazone, acetazolamide, topiramate, prednisone, lithium, ergotamine, sumatriptan, oxygen, greater occipital nerve block, occipital nerve stimulation, and hypothalamic stimulation (Boes and Swanson, 2006; Goadsby et al., 2010).

### Short-Lasting Unilateral Neuralgiform Headache Attacks

Short-lasting unilateral neuralgiform headache attacks are attacks of moderate or severe, strictly unilateral head pain lasting seconds to minutes, occurring at least once a day and usually associated with prominent lacrimation and redness of the ipsilateral eye. This disorder has two clinical phenotypes. When the attacks are associated with both conjunctival injection and lacrimation (tearing) it is referred to as SUNCT (short-lasting unilateral neuralgiform headache with conjunctival injection and tearing). When only one or neither of conjunctival injection or lacrimation is present it is diagnosed as SUNA (short-lasting unilateral neuralgiform headache attacks with cranial autonomic symptoms) (IHS, 2018). SUNCT and SUNA are rare disorders and their treatment is entirely prophylactic, in general using the same medications.

Knowledge of SUNCT is more ample when compared to SUNA, as the latter has been described more recently. SUNCT's painful paroxysms are usually felt in or around the eye and can sometimes be triggered by cutaneous stimuli. Single stabs last on average 58 seconds, groups of stabs usually last 396 seconds, and a sawtooth attack (many stabs between which the pain does not totally resolve) typically lasts 1160 seconds (Cohen et al., 2006). Attacks may occur 2–600 times a day, with a mean of 59 attacks per day. The associated ipsilateral conjunctival injection and lacrimation are very prominent. Unlike trigeminal neuralgia, most of the pain in SUNCT is in a V1 distribution, and tears often run down the face. Only 4% of patients with trigeminal neuralgia have pain in the ophthalmic division alone (Boes and Swanson, 2006). Unlike trigeminal neuralgia, 95% of SUNCT patients have no refractory period. The brevity and high frequency of attacks in SUNCT should make the distinction from cluster headache quite clear. Numerous cases of secondary SUNCT have been reported and underline the importance of MRI of the brain in every case. Lamotrigine has been effective in several patients when given in an open fashion. Topiramate, carbamazepine, and gabapentin are all reasonable alternatives to consider. Other options with uncontrolled evidence include oxcarbazepine, verapamil, clomiphene, zonisamide, onabotulinumtoxinA, corticosteroids, and IV lidocaine. Indomethacin has no effect. The role of neurosurgical intervention directed at the trigeminal nerve in the treatment of SUNCT is unclear, and it should only be considered as a last resort. Other treatments reported to be effective in SUNCT include occipital nerve block, opioid blockade of the superior cervical ganglion, hypothalamic stimulation, and surgical removal of a pituitary microadenoma.

Both SUNCT and SUNA have been reported to respond to trigeminal nerve microvascular decompression (Williams et al., 2010). Out of 16 patients, 75% have become pain free for up to 32 months (Favoni et al., 2013). Of more recent interest in medically refractory SUNCT and SUNA is the possible role of bilateral occipital nerve stimulation (ONS). Out of nine patients in a recent study, all but one obtained substantial relief. Because ONS is not cranially invasive or neurally destructive, it might be considered the surgical treatment of choice for medically intractable SUNCT and SUNA (Lambru et al., 2014b). The precise role these two interventions may have in the management of medically refractory SUNCT/SUNA remains to be determined.

### Hemicrania Continua

As the name implies, hemicrania continua is characterized by a continuous unilateral headache of moderate intensity that may involve the entire hemicranium or simply be confined to a focal area. The female-to-male ratio is approximately 2:1, and the average age of onset is 28 years (range, 5–67 years). Although invariably continuous, this disorder may sometimes resemble a prolonged unilateral migraine attack lasting several days to weeks, with headache-free remissions. The continuous headache is typically punctuated by painful unilateral exacerbations lasting 20 minutes to several days. These periods of increasing pain intensity are accompanied by one or more autonomic features that are usually subtler than those seen in PH or cluster headache and about two-thirds report a sense of restlessness or agitation (Cittadini and Goadsby, 2010). Primary stabbing headache ("icepick headache") is often a feature of this disorder, usually on the ipsilateral side and usually during a period of exacerbation. About a third report an ipsilateral eye itch and most have migrainous features including photo- and phonophobia (unilateral in half of patients) and motion sensitivity (Cittadini and Goadsby, 2010). Because of its daily persistence, hemicrania continua may be seen in the context of medication overuse, which may alter the clinical features. Therefore, a higher index of suspicion may be required in these cases. It is reasonable to consider a trial of indomethacin in any patient with a chronic unilateral daily headache that does not respond to other conventional medications, especially if autonomic features are present. Several cases of secondary hemicrania continua have been reported, highlighting the importance of brain MRI in the evaluation of these patients. Hemicrania continua patients respond completely to prophylactic indomethacin. The indomethacin regimen is similar to that described for PH. Unfortunately, about a fourth of patients do not tolerate indomethacin, mainly from gastrointestinal side effects. Without indomethacin, treatment can be challenging. Cases of hemicrania continua have been reported that have not recurred after stopping indomethacin. It is therefore reasonable to periodically withdraw treatment (Boes and Swanson, 2006). Complete response to rofecoxib, celecoxib, aspirin, naproxen, ibuprofen, diclofenac, and piroxicam in hemicrania continua has been reported. Dihydroergotamine, methysergide, corticosteroids, acemethacin, acetaminophen with caffeine, lamotrigine, gabapentin, topiramate, melatonin, valproic acid, verapamil, onabotulinumtoxinA, and lithium have been reported to be effective in some cases. Other treatments include occipital or supraorbital nerve blocks and occipital nerve stimulation.

## Other Primary Headaches

### Tension-Type Headache

Almost everyone has a headache at some time when stressed, overworked, anxious, or subject to prolonged muscular strain. Such headaches rapidly subside with relaxation, sleep, or ingestion of simple analgesics. *Tension-type headaches* have historically been ascribed to persistent contraction of scalp, neck, and jaw musculature. However, the concept of muscle contraction causing headache has been questioned. Electromyographic (EMG) studies and other observations have led some to believe tension-type headache and migraine may be extreme ends of a spectrum.

In the past, the term "tension" had been tacitly taken to mean either emotional or muscle tension, thus implying both pathogenesis and pain mechanism. The current classification places the word "type" after "tension," and the term *tension-type headache* is now used to bring attention to the fact that actual muscle tension may not be a key factor in the pathophysiology.

The prevalence of tension-type headache ranges in the general population from 30% to 78% (IHS, 2018). In the United States, an epidemiological study showed a higher prevalence in Caucasian women and in patients aged 30–39 (Schwartz et al., 1998).

Tension-type headaches can begin at any age, are generally bilateral, and are often described as a sense of pressure or wearing a tight band around the head. The pain is of mild to moderate intensity, tends to not be aggravated by routine physical activity, and may wax and wane throughout the day or may be present and steady for days, weeks, or even years at a time. Tension headaches have no associated nausea or vomiting and are much less commonly associated with light and sound sensitivity than migraine.

The pathophysiology of tension-type headache is incompletely understood. That emotional tension leads to muscle tension and hence to headache is too simplistic. A far more complex central mechanism is likely responsible for the pain, likely involving interaction between peripheral myofascial input and sensitization of second-order nociceptive neurons in the trigeminal nucleus and spinal dorsal horn (Fumal and Schoenen, 2008). A lower-pressure pain tolerance threshold has been shown in the fingers of patients with chronic tension-type headache compared to healthy controls, suggesting the presence of allodynia and hyperalgesia in patients with this disorder.

Physical examination in acute tension-type headache is generally unrevealing. Chronic tension-type headache may be associated with craniocervical musculature tenderness. In elderly patients, the ESR should be determined to help exclude giant-cell arteritis. If the headache is new or progressively worsening, a CT or MRI of the brain can help rule out serious structural intracranial diseases mimicking tension-type headache. Cervical spine imaging may be needed to rule out secondary causes of sustained contraction of the cervical and scalp muscles. Patients with obstructive sleep apnea (OSA) have a higher likelihood of developing tension-type headache than patients without it. (Chiu et al., 2015). We routinely screen for OSA in patients with frequent or chronic tension-type headache.

For occasional mild tension-type headache, treatment with aspirin, acetaminophen, or NSAIDs may be sufficient. More severe headaches usually require a prescription analgesic, but no specific preparation has been shown to be better than another. The combination of acetaminophen with isometheptene and dichloralphenazone may be useful for moderately severe headaches. The frequent use of combination analgesics with codeine, propoxyphene, or butalbital with or without caffeine should be avoided to prevent nedication overuse headache.

The most effective prophylactic drug is possibly amitriptyline. Controlled trials have shown more than 50% improvement in over 65% of patients. The usual dose is 50–150 mg/day. The drug is better tolerated if given as a single bedtime dose. Other tricyclic antidepressants, gabapentin, mirtazapine, sodium valproate, or topiramate may be used as prophylactics if amitriptyline is not tolerated or contraindicated. Techniques to promote relaxation of the scalp and neck muscles (e.g., biofeedback, neck massage) can help in the short term, but their long-term benefit has not been established (Fumal and Schoenen, 2008).

In contradistinction to the infrequent variety, chronic tension-type headache (more than 15 headache days a month) can persist for years and can be difficult to manage.

## Primary Cough Headache

Cough headache is a headache of sudden onset that is precipitated by a brief, nonsustained Valsalva maneuver such as coughing, laughing, sneezing, or bending over. The pain is typically bilateral, explosive, and lasts seconds to minutes (Chen et al., 2009; Pascual, 2009). As a rule, the patient is free from pain between attacks. The mean age at onset of primary cough headache is around 60 years. The proportion of patients who have an underlying structural cause has varied between 11% and 59% in studies done in the MRI era. Chiari type I malformation is the most common structural abnormality found on imaging, but other entities have been described, such as headache secondary to spontaneous spine CSF leak, middle cranial or posterior fossa brain tumors, brain metastases, pituitary tumors, posterior fossa arachnoid cysts, basilar impression, sphenoid sinusitis, subdural hematoma, RCVS, and possibly unruptured intracranial aneurysm and carotid stenosis (Chen et al., 2009; Evans and Boes, 2005; Kato et al., 2018; Pascual et al., 2008). As a spontaneous spine CSF leak can present as cough headache without an orthostatic component, all patients presenting with cough headache should get an MRI with gadolinium to look for pachymeningeal enhancement (Evans and Boes, 2005). In a large series of spontaneous spinal CSF leaks secondary to CSF-venous fistulas headache occurred in isolation to Valsalva maneuvers in 12% of patients; a finding that warrants considering this entity early in the differential diagnosis of Valsalva-induced ("cough") headache (Duvall et al., 2019). Whether an unruptured intracranial aneurysm can present with cough headache is unclear but given this possibility as well as the possibility of reversible cerebral vasoconstriction, it would be reasonable to obtain an MRA of the intracranial circulation in most cases. Typically cervical vessels do not need to be imaged unless symptoms of cerebral ischemia are present.

The treatment of choice is indomethacin, administered in a regimen similar to that described for PH. The response to indomethacin does not confirm a benign etiology. Other reports suggest that primary cough headache may respond to topiramate, acetazolamide, methysergide, or LP (Chen et al., 2009; Medrano et al., 2005). Any chest disease that may be causing the cough should be identified and treated.

## Primary Exercise Headache

Primary exercise headache (previously called *primary exertional headache*) is a bilateral throbbing headache that is precipitated by prolonged physical exercise. The ICHD-3 differentiates the exercise with this type of headache as more sustained strenuous effort rather than a short burst of effort (like a Valsalva maneuver) that may trigger primary cough headache, though the two headaches may occasionally co-occur in the same patient (IHS, 2018; Sjaastad and Bakketeig, 2002). The headache is not explosive in onset but rather builds in intensity and lasts between 5 minutes and 48 hours. The headache can be prevented by avoiding excessive exertion, particularly in hot weather or at high altitude. In one prospective study, the average age at onset for primary exertional headache was 40 years, whereas the average age at onset for primary cough headache was 60 years (Pascual et al., 2008). Similar to cough headache, this disorder can be benign or symptomatic of an underlying cause. In one series, 12 of 28 patients with exertional headache were found to have underlying causes (Pascual et al., 1996). These patients, however, were older (mean age 42 vs. 24 years), developed acute severe bilateral headaches lasting 1 day to 1 month, and developed accompanying symptoms of vomiting, diplopia, or neck rigidity. Potential causes of secondary exertional headache include subarachnoid hemorrhage, cerebral metastases, intracranial hypertension, pansinusitis, and pheochromocytoma. Exercise-induced cardiac ischemic pain can refer to the head and neck and is referred to as *cardiac cephalalgia*. A patient with risk factors for coronary artery disease presenting with an exertional headache should get an exercise stress test or comparable investigation.

Preventive treatment with a beta-blocker or indomethacin on a daily basis is effective in some primary exertional headache patients. Other migraine preventives may show benefit. Ergotamine or indomethacin preemptively before exercise may be effective. A prescribed warm-up period can sometimes prevent exertional headache (Pascual, 2009).

## Primary Headache Associated With Sexual Activity

Headaches precipitated by sexual activity can occur as a dull bilateral ache which gradually increases with sexual excitement (previously called *preorgasmic headache*) or an abrupt explosive headache at orgasm (previously called *orgasmic headache*), with some patients experiencing both (IHS, 2018). The pain is usually bilateral with a median duration of 30 minutes (severe pain may last 1 minute to 24 hours). The mean age at onset ranges from the second to the fourth decade, and there is a clear male predominance (Cutrer and DeLange, 2014). Three-quarters of patients have their headaches in bouts.

Symptomatic headaches precipitated by sexual activity share a similar differential to secondary causes of exercise-induced headaches. With orgasmic headache in particular, it is mandatory to exclude such conditions as subarachnoid hemorrhage, arterial dissection, pheochromocytoma, and RCVS. In patients with risk factors for coronary artery disease, the possibility of cardiac cephalalgia should also be investigated.

Approximately 50% of patients can ease the headache by taking a more passive role during sexual activity. Indomethacin (25–50 mg) given 30–60 minutes prior to sexual activity may prevent the headache. For those intolerant of or unresponsive to indomethacin, an oral triptan can be tried 30–45 minutes before sexual activity (Frese et al., 2006). For patients with frequent attacks, daily propranolol, metoprolol, or diltiazem may be effective.

## Primary Thunderclap Headache

A "thunderclap headache" is a severe headache that reaches maximal intensity in less than 1 minute (IHS, 2018). It is the rapidity with which the headache reaches maximum intensity that differentiates a thunderclap headache from other severe headache types. As discussed previously, there are numerous potential causes of a thunderclap headache, including but not limited to subarachnoid hemorrhage, spontaneous spine CSF leak, RCVS, cervical artery dissection, cerebral venous sinus thrombosis, pheochromocytoma, and hypertensive crisis (see Subarachnoid Hemorrhage and Thunderclap Headache section). When no underlying cause for the thunderclap headache is identified following a comprehensive evaluation, a diagnosis of "primary thunderclap headache" is given. It is not clear if primary thunderclap headaches are a true entity or if they represent missed diagnoses of underlying causes for the thunderclap headache such as mild forms of the RCVS or RCVS with delayed angiographic appearance of vasoconstriction.

### Cold-Stimulus Headache

Cold-stimulus headache is a generalized headache that follows exposure to a cold stimulus that is either applied externally, ingested, or inhaled. For example, this might include exposure to cold weather, diving into cold water, or passing a solid or liquid cold material over the palate or posterior pharynx (previously known as *ice cream headache*) (IHS, 2018). A lifetime prevalence of 15% was found in a cross-sectional epidemiological survey of a 25- to 64-year-old general population (Rasmussen and Olesen, 1992). Whether this disorder is more common in migraineurs is a matter of debate. The pathophysiology is not completely understood. Clinically, after exposure to the cold stimulus, the pain begins within seconds, peaks over 20–60 seconds, and then subsides within 10 minutes after removal of the stimulus (or up to 30 minutes after removal of an external cold stimulus). The headache location is most commonly midfrontal, followed by bitemporal or occipital. In patients with migraine, the pain might be referred to the usual site of their migraine headaches. Cold-stimulus headache is best prevented by avoiding the known stimulus. Cheshire and colleague suggest divers can prevent the headaches by using a Neoprene hood when exposed to very cold waters (Cheshire and Ott, 2001).

### External-Pressure Headache

External-pressure headache refers to headache which arises from compression or traction on the scalp, without actual tissue damage. The headache should exclusively come on within an hour of stimulus exposure and remit within an hour of removal. Reported examples include headache from helmet wearing, swimming goggles, and traction from a ponytail.

### Primary Stabbing Headache

Patients with primary stabbing headache describe brief, extremely sharp jabs of pain that occur without warning and can be felt anywhere in the head, including the orbit. These recur with irregular frequency, one or many times per day. The pains are described as being like a spike driven into the skull: hence, the previous term *icepick headache*. Similar pains have been described under different terms by other investigators (e.g., *jabs and jolts, ophthalmodynia periodica*). There are no associated cranial autonomic features and no trigeminal distribution trigger points (Pascual, 2009). Stabbing pains more commonly occur in patients subject to migraine, cluster headache, or hemicrania continua. Icepick-like head pain has also been described in patients with giant-cell arteritis. Because of the brevity of the pain, the sporadic nature of attacks, and the common occurrence of spontaneous remissions, treatment is not usually required and reassurance generally suffices. However, in patients with "icepick status," in whom stabs of pain occur often, the treatment of choice is indomethacin, administered in a regimen similar to that described for PH. Cyclooxygenase-2 (COX-2) inhibitors, gabapentin, and melatonin (3–12 mg orally at night) have also been reported to be useful (Ferrante et al., 2010; Franca et al., 2004).

### Nummular Headache

Nummular headache, previously called *coin-shaped headache*, describes a focal head pain felt in one small, fixed, well-defined rounded or elliptical area of the head, typically 1–6 cm in diameter. Pain is commonly described as pressure or stabbing, and is frequently accompanied by hypesthesia, dysesthesia, paresthesia, allodynia, and/or tenderness (IHS, 2018).

A minority of patients may develop trophic changes such as hair loss or a patch of skin depression. Hair heterochromia has been described in one patient (Dabscheck and Andrews, 2010). Similar headaches have been related to structural lesions such as meningiomas, arachnoid cysts, and fibrous dysplasia of the skull. It is therefore important to perform imaging with an MRI to rule out underlying structural etiologies. Local subcutaneous anesthetic injections are generally not felt to be helpful. Small series suggest that gabapentin (300–1800 mg daily), tricyclic antidepressants, and onabotulinumtoxinA may be useful (Cuadrado et al., 2018; Guerrero et al., 2012). Twenty-five units of onabotulinumtoxinA divided among 10 injection sites in and around the circumscribed affected areas of pain has been reported to help some (Mathew et al., 2008a), the procedure is repeated approximately every 3 months if a favorable response is obtained. While one series also suggests local arterectomy may help in a select subset of patients (Guyuron et al., 2018), this is not a treatment we recommend performing routinely at present.

### Hypnic Headache

Hypnic headache is a primary headache disorder wherein the attacks of headache occur exclusively during sleep, often between 2 a.m. and 4 a.m. (Holle et al., 2013). The mean age of onset is 63 years. The pain is usually mild to moderate, but 20% of patients report severe pain. The pain is bilateral in about two-thirds of cases. The attack usually lasts from 15–180 minutes, but longer durations have been described. In contrast to cluster headache, hypnic headache usually has no autonomic features.

Caffeine before bedtime (one strong cup of regular coffee or an espresso if available) is often helpful in preventing that night's hypnic headache. Lithium, melatonin, and indomethacin can also be helpful in preventing hypnic headache. Patients responsive to gabapentin, pregabalin, verapamil, acetazolamide, onabotulinumtoxinA, topiramate, and hypnotics have also been reported (Garza and Swanson, 2007).

### New Daily Persistent Headache

New daily persistent headache (NDPH) is a daily headache that is unremitting from onset or very soon after onset (within 24 hours at most) (IHS, 2018). The vast majority of patients can pinpoint the exact date their headache started. Infection, flu-like illness, surgery, and stressful life events may precede NDPH. How these may result in NDPH is unclear and more than half of patients do not recognize a triggering or precipitating event (Rozen, 2016). Clinically, NDPH may have features suggestive of either migraine or tension-type headache. Secondary headache disorders, particularly spontaneous spine CSF leaks and cerebral venous sinus thrombosis, need to be ruled out. In general, if no secondary headache cause is found, it is recommended to classify the dominant headache phenotype, whether it is migraine or tension-type headache, and treat with preventives accordingly. Even with aggressive treatment, however, unfortunately many patients do not improve and become treatment refractory (Garza and Schwedt, 2010).

## OTHER HEADACHES AND FACIAL PAINS

### Neck-Tongue Syndrome

Neck-tongue syndrome describes paroxysmal sharp pain in the neck, occiput, or both, associated with ipsilateral sensory changes in the tongue, precipitated by neck movement. The pain lasts seconds to minutes and may be associated with sensory changes over the neck and occipital region. Though this syndrome may occur from early childhood to adulthood, the majority of reported cases in the literature have had an onset of symptoms before age 21 (Gelfand et al., 2018). The exact mechanism remains speculative. Proprioceptive fibers from the tongue travel in the lingual nerve, anastomose with the hypoglossal nerve within the tongue, then travel via the ansa cervicalis to the ventral ramus of the C2 nerve root. Evidence supports that subluxation of the atlantoaxial joint, among other conditions, may compromise the second cervical dorsal root during sudden neck rotation, resulting in numbness, paresthesia, or a sense of involuntary movement in the ipsilateral tongue (Orrell and Marsden, 1994). In general, the condition is benign. In the absence of any structural abnormality, management is conservative and may include antiinflammatory agents, temporary immobilization of the neck in a cervical collar, and possibly physical therapy exercises (Niethamer and Myers, 2016).

## Painful Trigeminal Neuropathy

Painful trigeminal neuropathy describes head and/or facial pain in the distribution of one or more branches of the trigeminal nerve and is associated with nerve damage. In contrast to the paroxysmal lancinating pain of trigeminal neuralgia, painful trigeminal neuropathy tends to be a more persistent pain of highly variable character and intensity, often associated with numbness, dysesthesia, or paresthesia. There is a broad differential for neuropathy of the trigeminal nerve, including trauma, demyelination, infection, inflammation, and neoplasm (Smith and Cutrer, 2011). Unexplained neuropathy, especially with progressive worsening, warrants further investigation with MR imaging, with special attention to the course of the trigeminal nerve. Isolated involvement of the mental nerve, with resultant chin numbness (i.e., *numb chin syndrome*), is a red flag for a potential metastatic lesion, and may require more detailed imaging of the mandible (Smith et al., 2015).

### Painful Trigeminal Neuropathy Attributed to Herpes Zoster

Painful trigeminal neuropathy may occur acutely during herpes zoster infection, and in some patients may persist for longer than 3 months (referred to as *postherpetic neuralgia*, though technically a neuropathy/neuronopathy). Pain may be burning, stabbing, itching, or aching, often with sensory abnormalities and allodynia. The diagnosis is suggested if there is a history of a vesicular rash in the distribution of pain (or pale purple scars present as sequelae of herpetic eruption). In rare cases where there is no rash present, the diagnosis can be confirmed by varicella zoster viral DNA in the CSF (IHS, 2018).

Pain during the acute phase of herpes zoster trigeminal neuropathy is severe and may require opioid analgesics. Antiviral drugs and prednisone can decrease the pain during this stage. Once developed, postherpetic neuralgia may persist indefinitely, although with time it may become less severe. Many elderly patients with this distressing pain become depressed, lose weight, and become withdrawn. Treatment of established postherpetic neuralgia is difficult and in many instances ineffective. Tricyclic antidepressants, gabapentin, pregabalin, opioids, and lidocaine patches may all be helpful in select patients (Dubinsky et al., 2004).The use of topical capsaicin is not practical in this disorder. Procedures to denervate the affected area of skin, trigeminal destructive procedures, and trigeminal tractotomy have been used for control of pain, but they are rarely used at present.

When the herpes zoster infection affects the ophthalmic division of the trigeminal nerve (i.e., herpes zoster ophthalmicus), it can affect the eye and vision, sometimes leading to a keratitis that can permanently scar the cornea. For this reason, aggressive management with systemic antivirals is recommended (Schuster et al., 2016).

### Painful Posttraumatic Trigeminal Neuropathy

Painful posttraumatic trigeminal neuropathy, previously called *anesthesia dolorosa*, consists of persistent painful anesthesia or hypesthesia in the distribution of the trigeminal nerve or one of its divisions following traumatic injury. Often related to surgical trauma of the trigeminal nerve or ganglion, it most frequently occurs as a complication of rhizotomy or thermocoagulation done to treat trigeminal neuralgia. In different series of patients treated for trigeminal neuralgia, anesthesia dolorosa has developed in anywhere from 0% to 3%, depending on the specific procedure performed (Barker et al., 1996; Maarbjerg et al., 2017). This painful numbness can be even more unbearable than the pain from trigeminal neuralgia itself, warranting careful decision making when considering surgical treatment for this condition.

## Persistent Idiopathic Facial Pain

Previously known as *atypical face pain*, persistent idiopathic facial pain (PIFP) is essentially a facial pain of unknown cause with no associated neurological deficit. The diagnosis of PIFP should be considered only when all facial pains due to disturbances of anatomy and pathophysiology have been excluded, including trigeminal neuropathy. Exhaustive radiographic and other imaging techniques may be necessary to exclude conditions such as nasopharyngeal and sinus neoplasms, bony abnormalities of the base of the skull, and dental conditions such as cryptic mandibular and maxillary abscesses. Evaluation may also require a chest roentgenogram or chest CT scan if referred pain from lung cancer is suggested by the history (smoker) or examination (digital clubbing).

Patients in whom PIFP is eventually diagnosed are usually middle-aged and predominantly female. A subset of patients may develop PIFP after insignificant trauma to the face, teeth, or gums, suggesting that PIFP and traumatic trigeminal neuropathy may represent extremes on a continuum of injury-induced neuropathic pain (Benoliel and Gaul, 2017). Pain is commonly felt in the nasolabial fold or on one side of the chin but can spread to wider areas of the face and neck. Patients complain of deep, poorly localized pain. Generally unilateral, but occasionally bilateral, the pain may be described in graphic terms such as *tearing*, *ripping*, or *crushing*, or often as *aching* and *boring*. The pain is usually present all day and every day, and gradually worsens with time. It is not influenced by factors such as alcohol consumption, heat, or cold or by factors that trigger trigeminal neuralgia. Local anesthetic blocks of the trigeminal nerve do not relieve the pain. Many patients have already undergone extensive dental, nasal, or sinus operations to no avail. Pain may be associated with other comorbid pain conditions such as chronic widespread pain and irritable bowel syndrome (IHS, 2018).

When no symptomatic etiology is identified, tricyclic antidepressants such as amitriptyline are considered first line. Medications used to treat central neuropathic pain, such as gabapentin, pregabalin, or duloxetine, may also be tried.

## Cranial and Facial Neuralgias

### Trigeminal Neuralgia

***Clinical symptoms.*** Trigeminal neuralgia describes paroxysmal pain felt within the distribution of one or more divisions of the trigeminal nerve. The pain is often triggered by a sensory stimulus to the skin, mucosa, or teeth within the area innervated by the ipsilateral trigeminal nerve. The trigger zone most commonly occurs near the nasolabial fold and may be remote from the site of pain. Chewing, teeth brushing, talking, and even cool breeze striking the face are commonly reported triggers. The pain is described as electric shock-like, shooting, or lancinating. Each attack lasts only seconds, but the pain may be repetitive at short intervals, so that the individual attacks blur into one another. After many attacks within a few hours, the patient may describe a residual lingering facial pain. Attacks of trigeminal neuralgia are most common in the second and third divisions of the nerve. Pain confined to the ophthalmic division is extremely rare. Attacks of pain during sleep are uncommon but do occur. Frequent attacks may be associated with weight loss, dehydration, or depression.

In the current ICHD-3 classification, *classical trigeminal neuralgia* refers to trigeminal neuralgia with evidence of vascular compression of the trigeminal nerve (by MRI or surgery), with associated nerve root atrophy or displacement. *Secondary trigeminal neuralgia* is due to an underlying disease such as multiple sclerosis or a space-occupying lesion, and may present as both paroxysmal pain and a concomitant continuous or near-continuous pain. If evaluation shows no underlying etiology and no clear morphological change (atrophy or displacement) in the nerve root related to blood vessel contact, the term *idiopathic trigeminal neuralgia* is preferred (IHS, 2018).

***Physical findings.*** In classical trigeminal neuralgia, there is no sensory impairment, and the motor division of the nerve is intact. The presence of physical signs such as sensory loss or masticatory muscle weakness suggests a secondary cause for trigeminal neuralgia, though a more accurate description in this case would be *trigeminal neuropathy*. This could be secondary to a lesion or mass affecting the gasserian ganglion, main sensory root, or root entry zone in the pons.

***Laboratory and radiological findings.*** Idiopathic trigeminal neuralgia has no accompanying laboratory or radiographic abnormalities. EMG and nerve stimulation (such as blink reflex studies) are normal. Imaging with MRI is done primarily to look for structural lesions such as a pontine lacunar infarct, demyelinating plaque, meningioma or schwannoma of the posterior fossa, or malignant infiltration of the skull base. High-resolution MRI and MRA may be able to identify vascular compression in select cases.

***Pathogenesis and etiology.*** Classical trigeminal neuralgia cases are felt to be related to neurovascular compression of the trigeminal nerve by neighboring vessels, including the superior cerebellar artery, anterior and posterior inferior cerebellar arteries, and superior petrosal vein. Vascular compression is believed to increase with age and contribute to focal demyelination of primary trigeminal afferents near where the trigeminal nerve enters the pons (i.e., *nerve root entry zone*). In pathology studies, vacuolated neurons, segmental demyelination, vascular changes, and other abnormalities were more common in gasserian ganglia from patients with a history of trigeminal neuralgia than in control specimens. This focal demyelination of axons in the main sensory root is hypothesized to contribute to focal hyperexcitability, leading to ectopic and repetitive neuronal discharges. In secondary trigeminal neuralgia, structural lesions may contribute to pain through a similar pathophysiological mechanism (Maarbjerg et al., 2017).

***Epidemiology.*** Trigeminal neuralgia begins after the age of 40 years in 90% of patients. It is slightly more common in women. The incidence progressively increases with increasing age (Manzoni and Torelli, 2005). Rare familial cases have been described, suggesting that genetics may play a role in some families.

***Course and prognosis.*** Trigeminal neuralgia frequently has an exacerbating and remitting course over many years. During exacerbations, the painful attacks may occur many times a day for weeks or months at a time. A spontaneous remission may occur at any time and last for months or years. The reasons for these fluctuations are unknown.

***Treatment and management.*** Treatment of trigeminal neuralgia due to a focal lesion compressing the sensory root of the trigeminal nerve is surgical exploration and decompression of the nerve. Management of classical trigeminal neuralgia can be either medical or surgical.

Sodium channel blockers, such as carbamazepine or oxcarbazepine, are considered the drugs of choice for treatment of trigeminal neuralgia, with a highly favorable response in a majority of patients. Administration of carbamazepine must be initiated with small doses of 50–100 mg and increased slowly as tolerated. Vertigo, drowsiness, and ataxia are common side effects if the preparation is introduced too quickly, especially in elderly patients. Therapeutic doses generally range from 600 to 1200 mg/day in divided dosing. The appropriate dose is the lowest dose needed to control the pain. Once the pain is controlled completely, the dose can be tapered every few weeks to determine whether a remission has developed. Oxcarbazepine may be better tolerated, but may be associated with sometimes prominent hyponatremia. When starting these medicines, regular blood counts (monitoring for agranulocytosis), liver function tests, and serum sodium should be performed for the first few months and once a year thereafter.

Second-line options for the management of trigeminal neuralgia include gabapentin, pregabalin, phenytoin, and baclofen. Other drugs that have been used include lamotrigine, valproate, clonazepam, and topiramate (Cheshire, 2007; Maarbjerg et al., 2017). Second-line drugs should be considered for trial, alone or in combination, when sodium channel blockers are either unhelpful or not tolerated. Given the beneficial effects of gabapentin in other neuropathic conditions and its benign side-effect profile, an initial trial with this drug may be an alternative option to carbamazepine/oxcarbazepine.

On occasion, one may encounter a patient in the midst of a severe attack. A useful technique in this situation is the administration of IV fosphenytoin at a dose of 15–20 mg phenytoin sodium equivalents (PE)/kg. Anesthetizing the ipsilateral conjunctival sac with the local ophthalmic anesthetic proparacaine has also proved effective in providing relief from pain for several hours to days.

A patient who is refractory to medical therapy may be a candidate for a surgical procedure. The most commonly performed surgical procedures include percutaneous procedures on the trigeminal nerve or gasserian ganglion (rhizotomy), Gamma Knife radiosurgery, and microvascular decompression. Picking the best surgical option often involves a discussion with the patient about the potential risks of the procedure based on their age and comorbidities, as well as the risk of pain recurrence.

The simplest nonmedical therapy is an alcohol block of the peripheral branch of the division of the trigeminal nerve that is painful. The mental or mandibular nerve can be blocked with 0.5–0.75 mL of absolute alcohol to control mandibular division trigeminal neuralgia. The infraorbital and supraorbital nerves can also be injected for pain involving the second and first divisions, respectively. Relief of pain occurs in a high proportion of patients so treated, but relapse is likely in most after 6–18 months. The procedure can be repeated once or twice, but thereafter it is prudent to perform a more proximal and lasting procedure because the further injection of alcohol is likely to be ineffective. The advantages of a peripheral alcohol injection include low morbidity and the temporary nature of sensory loss. Preservation of corneal sensation is also an advantage.

For many patients, especially those who are elderly or have complicating medical conditions, percutaneous radiofrequency thermocoagulation of the trigeminal nerve sensory root as it leaves the gasserian ganglion is the procedure of choice. Investigators have reported pain relief in up to 93% of patients. Recurrence rates vary with the period of follow-up. The procedure can be repeated when relapse occurs. Complications include damage to the carotid artery, adjacent cranial nerves, and the trigeminal nerve motor root. Corneal sensory loss in V1 lesions can lead to serious eye complications. Troublesome dysesthesias of the face are commonly encountered. Posttraumatic trigeminal neuropathy (previously *anesthesia dolorosa*), a distressingly painful sensation in the numb area, occurs occasionally.

Percutaneous balloon compression of the trigeminal ganglion has been shown to be an effective and technically simple treatment. The early recurrence rate, however, is higher than that reported for radiofrequency thermocoagulation, with pain recurring 2–3 years later. Stereotactic radiosurgery with the Gamma Knife has also been shown to be an effective therapy for trigeminal neuralgia and is a less invasive surgical option. However, it is also associated with a relatively high recurrence rate, and patients who have previously undergone surgical procedures may have an increased risk of facial dysesthesia following Gamma Knife radiotherapy.

In patients who are felt to be healthy enough for more invasive surgery, the preferred procedure is microvascular decompression (MVD). This involves craniotomy and posterior fossa exploration to identify the area of neurovascular compression, dissection of the offending vessel away from the trigeminal nerve, and placement of a synthetic padding to prevent future compression. In Jannetta's series of 1155 patients, 70% had excellent relief of pain continuing 10 years after the trigeminal nerve and the compressing vessel were separated. Relief of pain without the production of anesthesia is the major advantage of the procedure. Disadvantages include the need for a posterior fossa exploration, with a reported mortality rate of 1% and a risk for injury to other cranial nerves, most commonly CN IV, VII, and VIII, dependent on the experience of the surgeon. Despite the inherent risks of a retromastoid craniectomy, MVD is associated with the longest duration of pain relief, preserves facial sensation, and remains the only surgical treatment that directly addresses the presumed mechanism. When no vascular loop is found at the time of operation, the options include performing a partial or complete sensory root section or subsequently performing a radiofrequency procedure.

For a young patient unresponsive to medical treatment, posterior fossa MVD should be considered. For an elderly patient or a patient with other medical complications, however, peripheral procedures targeting the trigeminal ganglion, such as radiofrequency thermocoagulation or balloon compression, would be considered procedure of choice because of the ease of performance. Specific recommendations relating to the various interventional or surgical procedures cannot be made. Rather, the treatment must be individualized to the particular needs of the patient.

### Glossopharyngeal Neuralgia

The pain associated with neuralgia of the ninth cranial nerve is similar in quality and periodicity to that of trigeminal neuralgia. The pain is lancinating and episodic and may be severe. It is felt in the distribution of the glossopharyngeal nerve and the sensory distribution of the upper fibers of the vagus nerve. Pain in the throat, the tonsillar region, the posterior third of the tongue, the larynx, the nasopharynx, and deep in the ear is often described by patients with this rare neuralgia. The pain is usually triggered by swallowing, speaking, laughing, or coughing and is unilateral in most patients. Bilateral involvement does occur, but it is very rare. The age group involved is generally older than 40 years. Bradycardia and syncope can occur when the painful attack strikes.

Most glossopharyngeal neuralgia occurrences have been thought to be idiopathic, but vascular compression of the ninth cranial nerve has been described. Secondary glossopharyngeal neuralgia may also be due to oropharyngeal malignancies, peritonsillar infections, and other lesions at the base of the skull. Therefore, presenting patients should be evaluated with an MRI of the brain and soft tissues of the neck, with specific attention to the glossopharyngeal nerve.

Carbamazepine and phenytoin have been administered with mixed success in glossopharyngeal neuralgia. Intracranial section of the glossopharyngeal and upper rootlets of the vagus nerve almost always produces complete pain relief. A series of 47 patients treated with microvascular decompression reported 98% found immediate relief after the procedure (Sampson et al., 2004).

### Nervus Intermedius Neuralgia (Geniculate Neuralgia, Hunt Neuralgia)

This is a rare disorder characterized by brief paroxysms of pain felt deeply in the auditory canal (IHS, 2018). The intermediate nerve of Wrisberg (the nervus intermedius), a small sensory branch of the facial nerve (cranial nerve VII), and/or the geniculate ganglion are believed to be the affected structures. The accurate incidence, prevalence, and risk factors associated with this condition are unknown, since it is so rare. Middle-aged women seem to be more frequently affected. Clinically the pain is described as brief (seconds to minutes), severe, paroxysmal, and limited to the depths of the ear, associated with a trigger zone in the posterior wall of the ear canal. The pain can be sharp or burning and is not necessarily lancinating, as occurs in other cranial neuralgias. The diagnosis is made on clinical grounds. Importantly, because of the complex ear sensory innervation, other referred sources of ear pain should be considered in the differential diagnosis when evaluating a neuralgic otalgia. Nerves referring pain to the ear include branches of cranial nerves V, VII, IX, and X, and upper cervical roots (De Lange et al., 2014; Fig. 102.7).

Nervus intermedius neuralgia can develop during an episode of Ramsay-Hunt syndrome (herpes zoster virus involving the geniculate ganglion/facial nerve, causing ipsilateral facial paralysis); therefore patients with this deep stabbing ear pain should be checked for vesicles in the external auditory canal, pinna, and tonsillar fossa. Because this type of deep stabbing ear pain can be referred from the throat, imaging of the soft tissues of the neck should be included in the evaluation (DeLange et al., 2014).

For treatment, a trial with carbamazepine is appropriate. If not effective, other drugs used to treat cranial neuralgias and neuropathic pain (e.g., oxcarbazepine, gabapentin, phenytoin, lamotrigine, baclofen) can be tried. Neurosurgery is a last resort when pharmacotherapy fails, and may involve excision of the nervus intermedius and geniculate ganglion with or without exploration and/or section of CN V, IX, and X. Lovely and Jannetta (1997) reported good long-term results in up to 90% of patients in a series using microvascular decompression of CN V, IX, and X, with or without section of the nervus intermedius.

### Occipital Neuralgia

Occipital neuralgia can cause a headache in the occipital region. It is a paroxysmal jabbing pain in the greater (C2), lesser (C2–C3), and/or third (C3) occipital nerve distribution, sometimes accompanied by diminished sensation or dysesthesia in the affected area. The true incidence and prevalence of occipital neuralgia are not known, possibly because the diagnosis is frequently arbitrarily given to any pain in the occipital region (Bogduk, 2004). Injuries to the C2–C3 nerve roots through different mechanisms (entrapment, trauma, inflammation, whiplash, etc.) might contribute to occipital neuralgia.

Clinically, the pain has a sudden onset and is described as a severe stabbing, electric shock-like, or sharp shooting pain that starts at

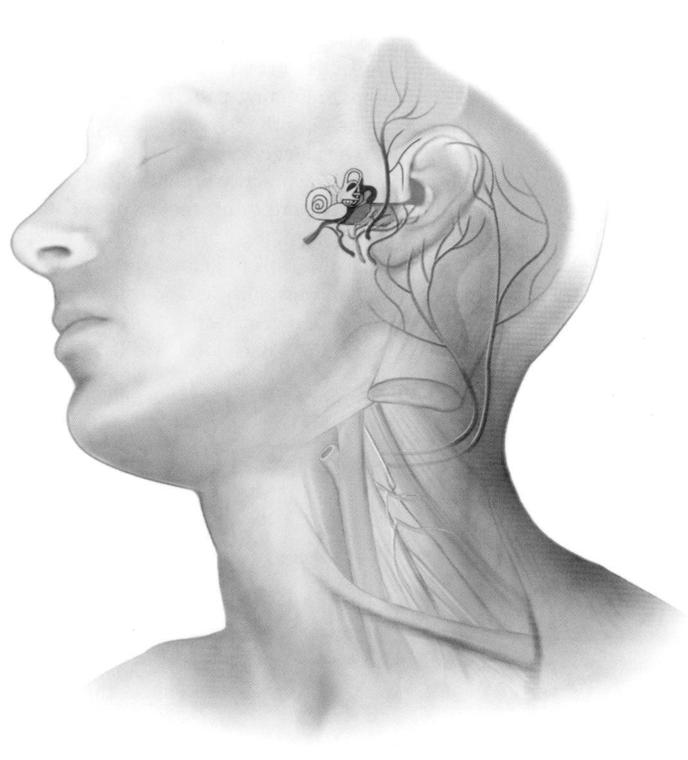


**Fig. 102.7 Sensory Innervation of the Ear and its Surrounding Structures.** Boxes with their corresponding colors illustrate each nerve's distribution. Note that sensory distributions may overlap. (*From DeLange, J.M., Garza, I., Robertson, C.E. A 50-Year-Old Woman With Deep Stabbing Ear Pain. American Academy of Neurology; 2014. Used with permission of Mayo Foundation for Medical Education and Research, all rights reserved.*)

the nuchal region and then immediately spreads toward the vertex. Paroxysms can start spontaneously or, as in other neuralgias, be provoked by specific maneuvers such as brushing the hair or moving the neck. Most often, occipital neuralgia is unilateral. Between attacks, there may be a dull occipital discomfort as a background. On examination, pressure, palpation, or percussion over the occipital nerve trunks may reveal local tenderness. These maneuvers may also trigger painful paroxysms, exacerbate the background discomfort, or elicit paresthesias following the nerve's distribution. Cervical range of motion may be restricted, and local posterior neck muscle spasms may be found. The neurological examination may find sensory deficits in the individual occipital nerve distribution but is usually otherwise unremarkable. An abnormal neurological examination should alert the clinician for potential alternative or underlying causes of the symptoms. Since structural and infiltrating lesions can cause occipital neuralgia, a cervical spine and brain MRI is commonly considered when evaluating occipital neuralgia.

In the proper clinical scenario, the diagnosis is confirmed when the pain is transiently relieved by a local occipital anesthetic block. A local anesthetic block, however, is a nonspecific intervention, so symptomatic relief does not indicate a specific etiology.

## HEADACHE IN CHILDREN AND ADOLESCENTS

Headaches are very common in children, and more so in adolescents. The prevalence of headache of any type is in the range of 37%–51% in 7 year olds, increasing to 57%–82% in 15 year olds (Lewis et al., 2002). Prepubertal boys are more often afflicted than girls, whereas, after puberty, headaches occur more often in girls (Abu-Arafeh et al., 2010; Lewis et al., 2002).

Obtaining the child's history of head pain can be challenging because most patients younger than 10 years old are unable to give clear details about the temporal profile of the headache, its frequency, and its characteristics. For this reason, the clinician must depend on parental observations of the child's behavior. Does the youngster continue to play, want to go to bed, avoid light or sound, refuse food, refuse to go to school, and then appear to recover? The neurological examination in a child should evaluate the same factors as in an older patient, including careful assessment of the optic fundus. In addition, head size should be measured, and developmental markers checked.

Laboratory and other investigations are undertaken after a thorough history and physical examination. Neuroimaging is not done routinely. Features associated with the presence of a space-occupying lesion include (1) headache onset of less than 1 month, (2) absent family history of migraine, (3) abnormal neurological findings on examination (including gait abnormalities or papilledema), (4) the presence of seizures, and (5) progressive worsening of headaches. Headache in a child younger than 3 years old is uncommon and is a red flag for a secondary etiology for headache. Therefore, it would be reasonable to perform neuroimaging for new headache in a child less than 6 years old (Gofshteyn and Stephenson, 2016). The child with a constant nonprogressive headache may need a psychological evaluation, and the family dynamics may require full evaluation. Reports from teachers are of value in assessing the child's performance.

## Migraine and Migraine Variants

Migraine is the most common cause of headaches in children referred to a neurologist, and is estimated to affect 10%–12% of children and adolescents (Abu-Arafeh et al., 2010; Slater et al., 2018). Although migraine can manifest all the features seen in older patients, migraine attacks in children are often shorter and occur less often than those in adults. The description of headache tends to evolve as age increases. In younger children, migraine pain tends to be bilateral and non-throbbing, while unilateral pain and headache pulsation tend to become more typical in adolescence (Virtanen et al., 2007). Migraine can be triggered by similar factors at all ages, including stress, fever, head trauma, and sleep and eating pattern changes. In girls, the onset of migraine may coincide with menarche.

In addition to headache, approximately 10% of migraine patients in a pediatric neurology practice present with recurrent discreet symptoms thought to be variants or precursors of migraine (Table 102.9). In the ICHD-3 classification, these are referred to as "episodic syndromes that may be associated with migraine," and include recurrent attacks of stereotyped symptoms such as abdominal pain or nausea/vomiting, episodic attacks of dizziness, unsteadiness, or torticollis (Gelfand, 2015; IHS, 2018; Lagman-Bartolome and Lay, 2015).

*The complete reference list is available online at https://expertconsult.inkling.com/.* 

**TABLE 102.9 Episodic Syndromes That May Be Associated With Migraine**

| | Typical Age of Onset | Characteristics | Associated Features |
|---|---|---|---|
| Infantile colic | Peaks at 5–6 wk; typically improves by 3–4 mo | Excessive frequent crying in an otherwise healthy, well-fed infant<br>Episodes last ≥3 h/day, ≥ 3 days/wk for ≥ 3 wk | Crying tends to be late afternoon and evening hours |
| Benign paroxysmal vertigo (BPV) | Typically 2–5 years old; may resolve around age 5–6 | Brief spontaneous attacks of vertigo lasting minutes to hours | Nystagmus, pallor, ataxia, vomiting, fearfulness<br>Normal audiometric/vestibular testing between attacks |
| Alternating hemiplegia of childhood | Starts before 18 mo | Recurrent attacks of hemiplegia alternating between sides (occasionally quadriparesis) | Should have one other paroxysmal symptom (tonic spells, dystonic posturing, choreoathetosis, oculomotor abnormalities movements, autonomic disturbance) |
| Abdominal migraine | Around 4–7 yr | Recurrent attacks of abdominal pain (dull, moderate to severe, in the midline abdomen) lasting 2–72 h | Anorexia, nausea/vomiting, pallor<br>Symptom free between attacks<br>Exclude gastrointestinal/renal disease |
| Benign paroxysmal torticollis | Starts around 5–6 mo, typically resolves by age 3–4 | Recurrent episodes of head tilt to either side, lasting minutes to days.<br>Often in regular intervals (like monthly) | Pallor, irritability, drowsiness, vomiting, ataxia<br>May evolve into BPV or migraine with aura |
| Cyclic vomiting syndrome | Around 4–7 yr | Episodic attacks of repeated vomiting (≥4/h) and severe nausea; attacks last hour to 10 days, separated by at least 1 wk | Pallor, lethargy |

# 103

# Cranial Neuropathies

*Janet C. Rucker, Meagan D. Seay*

## OUTLINE



## OLFACTORY NERVE (CRANIAL NERVE I)

See Chapter 19.

## OPTIC NERVE (CRANIAL NERVE II)

See Chapters 16 and 43.

## OCULOMOTOR NERVE (CRANIAL NERVE III)

### Anatomy

Paired oculomotor nuclei are located in the dorsal midbrain ventral to the periaqueductal gray matter at the level of the superior colliculus. Each nucleus is composed of a superior rectus subnucleus providing innervation to the contralateral superior rectus; inferior rectus, medial rectus, and inferior oblique subnuclei providing ipsilateral innervation; and an Edinger-Westphal nucleus supplying preganglionic parasympathetic output to the iris sphincter and ciliary muscles (Che Ngwa et al., 2014; eFig. 103.1). A single midline caudal central subnucleus provides innervation to both levator palpebrae superioris muscles.

A third nerve fascicle originates from the ventral surface of each nucleus and traverses the midbrain, passing through or near to the red nucleus and in close proximity to the cerebral peduncles before emerging ventrally as rootlets in the lateral interpeduncular fossa. In the interpeduncular fossa, the rootlets converge into a third nerve trunk that continues ventrally through the subarachnoid space toward the cavernous sinus, passing between the superior cerebellar artery and the posterior cerebral artery. It travels parallel to the posterior communicating artery (PCOM) and is very near to this vessel at the vessel's junction with the intracranial internal carotid artery. In the cavernous sinus, the third nerve is located within the dural sinus wall, just lateral to the pituitary gland. From the cavernous sinus, the third nerve enters the orbit via the superior orbital fissure. Just prior to entry, the nerve anatomically divides into superior and inferior divisions in the anterior cavernous sinus, although careful evaluation of brainstem lesions and their corresponding patterns of pupil and muscle involvement suggests that functional division occurs in the midbrain (Bhatti et al., 2006; Vitosevic et al., 2013). Within the orbit, the superior division innervates the superior rectus and the levator palpebrae superioris, and the inferior division innervates the inferior and medial recti, the inferior oblique, and the iris sphincter and ciliary muscles (Fig. 103.2). Prior to innervating the ciliary and sphincter muscles as the short ciliary nerves, parasympathetic third nerve fibers synapse in the ciliary ganglion within the orbit (see Fig. 103.2).

### Clinical Lesions

#### Oculomotor Nucleus

In addition to potentially causing ipsilateral weakness of the medial rectus, inferior rectus, and inferior oblique muscles, an oculomotor nuclear lesion may result in bilateral superior rectus weakness. Ipsilateral subnucleus involvement affects the contralateral superior rectus because of the completely crossed nature of superior rectus innervation (see eFig. 103.1). A unilateral oculomotor nuclear lesion may affect these unilateral originating fibers destined for decussation, as well as those fibers that originated contralaterally and are already decussated. If the single midline levator palpebrae superioris

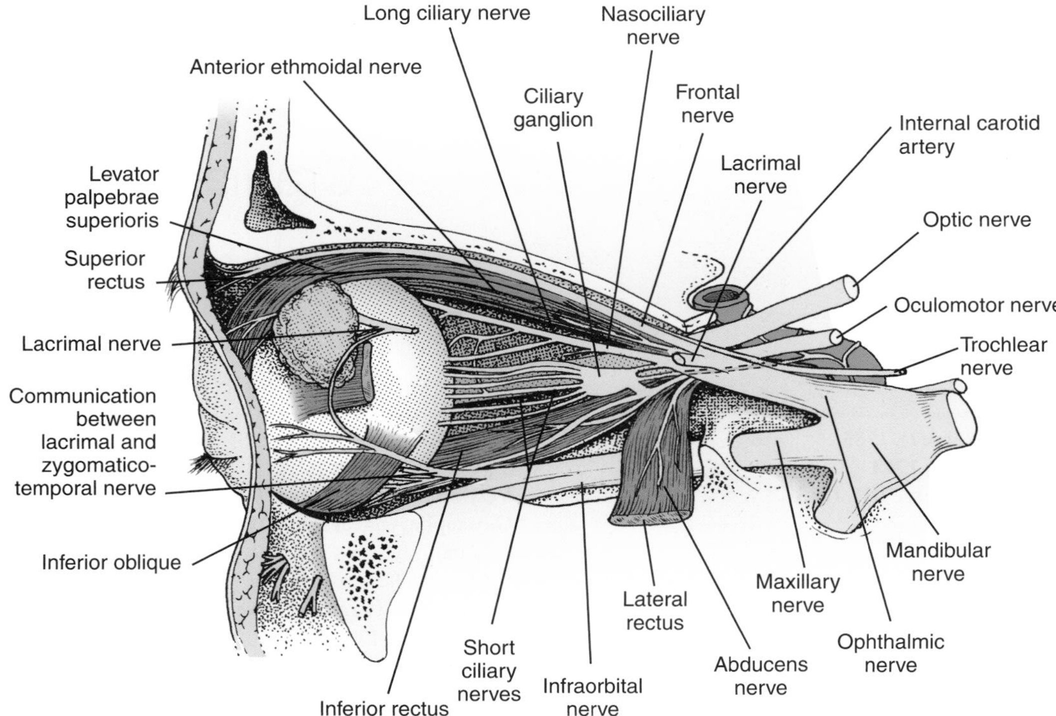


**Fig. 103.2** Oculomotor, Trochlear, Abducens, and Trigeminal Nerve Distributions in the Orbital Apex and Orbit. (*From Standring, G., 2005. Gray's Anatomy, thirty-ninth ed. Churchill Livingstone, Philadelphia.*)

subnucleus is involved in an oculomotor nuclear lesion, bilateral ptosis results. Isolated bilateral ptosis or isolated paresis of a single extraocular muscle is also possible from a small focal nuclear lesion, given the functional division of the subnuclei (Al-Sofiani and Kwen, 2015). Involvement of the rostral and dorsally located Edinger-Westphal nucleus will lead to pupil involvement. Common brainstem lesions include ischemia, hemorrhage, demyelination, infectious and noninfectious inflammation, and neoplasm.

### Oculomotor Palsy Appearance

A complete oculomotor nerve palsy has the following ipsilateral examination features: eye deviation inferiorly and laterally ("down and out"); absence of ocular elevation, depression, and adduction; and complete ptosis. A complete oculomotor palsy may be further described as complete involving the pupil with an enlarged and nonreactive pupil or as a pupil-sparing otherwise complete oculomotor palsy. A partial, or incomplete, third nerve palsy may present with any combination of deficits of third nerve innervated structures. Great emphasis is often placed on the presence of pupil involvement versus pupil sparing with regard to probable lesion etiology; however, neither this, nor the presence or absence of pain or other demographic features can fully rule out potential neurologically devastating emergent etiologies, such as a PCOM aneurysm or pituitary apoplexy (Newman and Biousse, 2017; Tamhankar et al., 2013) (see section below on Interpeduncular Fossa and Subarachnoid Space and section on Isolated Oculomotor Nerve Palsy).

### Brainstem Fascicle

*Claude syndrome* is the combination of an ipsilateral oculomotor nerve palsy and contralateral hemiataxia (Table 103.1 and Videos 103.1 and 103.2; Liu et al., 1994). Although historically the syndrome was described as involving the oculomotor fascicle and the red nucleus, the ataxia is likely due to involvement of the superior cerebellar peduncle at the caudal end of the red nucleus or the pedunculopontine nucleus, a component of the mesencephalic locomotor region (Hathout and Bhidayasiri, 2005). *Nothnagel syndrome* is the combination of ipsilateral oculomotor nerve palsy and ipsilateral hemiataxia from involvement of the oculomotor fascicle and superior cerebellar peduncle or pedunculopontine nucleus (see Table 103.1). *Weber syndrome* is the combination of an ipsilateral fascicular oculomotor nerve palsy and contralateral hemiparesis from cerebral peduncle involvement (see Table 103.1). *Benedikt syndrome* involves the oculomotor fascicle and red nucleus, causing an ipsilateral oculomotor nerve palsy and contralateral chorea or tremor (see Table 103.1). Common brainstem lesions include ischemia, hemorrhage, demyelination, infectious and noninfectious inflammation, and neoplasm (Kremer et al., 2013; Ogawa et al., 2016).

### Interpeduncular Fossa and Subarachnoid Space

The most common etiology of oculomotor dysfunction in this region is compression by a PCOM aneurysm (Fang et al., 2017). Pupillary fibers are located superomedially near the surface of the nerve and are particularly prone to compression by a PCOM aneurysm. As a result, "rules" with regard to interpretation of pupillary involvement have been defined to guide diagnostic evaluation. These will be reviewed for completion's sake, though it is now fairly well accepted that *all* oculomotor palsies warrant imaging evaluation for a PCOM aneurysm (Newman and Biousse, 2017; Tamhankar et al., 2013; Trobe, 2009). Without controversy, any pupil-involving or pupil-sparing incomplete oculomotor palsy requires immediate evaluation for a PCOM aneurysm, given the high risk of subarachnoid hemorrhage and mortality if left undiagnosed and untreated (Connolly et al., 2012; Lv et al., 2016). Some patients with an aneurysmal incomplete oculomotor nerve palsy will lack pupillary involvement at initial presentation, but the majority will progress to pupillary involvement within 1 week. Spontaneous improvement in oculomotor nerve function may occur with an aneurysm and should not

TABLE 103.1 **Named Cranial Nerve Syndromes**

| Syndrome* | Symptoms and Signs | Involved Structures |
|---|---|---|
| Claude | Ipsilateral III | III—brainstem fascicle |
| | Contralateral ataxia | Red nucleus/superior cerebellar peduncle |
| Nothnagel | Ipsilateral III | III—brainstem fascicle |
| | Ipsilateral ataxia | Superior cerebellar peduncle |
| Weber | Ipsilateral III | III—brainstem fascicle |
| | Contralateral hemiparesis | Cerebral peduncle |
| Benedikt | Ipsilateral III | III—brainstem fascicle |
| | Contralateral chorea or tremor | Red nucleus |
| Tolosa-Hunt | Ipsilateral III, IV, VI | Cavernous sinus |
| | Ipsilateral first and second branches of V | III, IV, VI, first and second branches of V |
| | Ipsilateral Horner syndrome | Sympathetic nerves |
| Wallenberg lateral medullary syndrome | Ipsilateral facial numbness and ↓ pinprick | Spinal trigeminal tract and nucleus |
| | Contralateral hemibody ↓ pain and temperature | Spinothalamic tract |
| | Dysphagia and ↓ gag reflex | Nucleus ambiguus |
| | Limb ataxia | Inferior cerebellar peduncle |
| | Horner syndrome | Sympathetic nerves |
| | Vertigo | Vestibular nuclei |
| Opalski syndrome | Wallenberg in addition to ipsilateral hemiparesis | Corticospinal fibers caudal to pyramidal decussation |
| Gradenigo | Facial and mastoid area pain | Petrous apex—temporal bone V, VI, VII |
| | Ipsilateral 1st branch of V | |
| | Ipsilateral VI and VII | |
| Foville | Ipsilateral VI and VII | VI and VII—brainstem |
| | Contralateral ataxia | Mid-cerebellar peduncle |
| | Ipsilateral Horner syndrome | Sympathetic nerves |
| | Ipsilateral deafness | Vestibulocochlear nerve/fascicle |
| | Ipsilateral ↓ taste and facial sensation | Spinal trigeminal tract/nucleus solitarius |
| Millard-Gubler | Ipsilateral VI and VII | VI and VII—brainstem |
| | Contralateral hemiparesis | Pyramidal tract |
| Raymond | Ipsilateral VI | VI—brainstem |
| | Contralateral hemiparesis | Pyramidal tract |
| Bell's palsy | VII | VII—intratemporal nerve and geniculate ganglion |
| Ramsay Hunt | VII | VII |
| | Vesicular otic or oral rash ± ↓ hearing | ±VIII |
| Melkersson-Rosenthal | VII | VII—distal branches |
| | Facial edema | |
| | Fissured tongue | |
| Eagle | IX | XI—elongated styloid process or ossified stylohyoid ligament |
| Vernet | IX, X, XI | Jugular foramen |
| Villaret | IX, X, XI | Jugular foramen |
| | XII | Hypoglossal canal |
| | Horner syndrome | Sympathetic nerves |
| Collet-Sicard | IX, X, XI | Jugular foramen |
| | XII | Hypoglossal canal |
| Avellis | X | X—brainstem or peripheral |
| | Contralateral hemiparesis | Pyramidal tract |
| Tapia | X and XII | X and XII—brainstem or peripheral |
| Dejerine medial medullary syndrome | Ipsilateral XII | XII—nuclei or fascicle |
| | Contralateral hemiparesis | Pyramidal tract |
| | Contralateral hemisensory deficit | Medial lemniscus |
| Babinski-Nageotte | Combined symptoms and signs of Wallenberg and Dejerine syndromes | Hemi-medullary: lateral and medial medulla |

*Descriptions of named syndromes vary slightly, depending on reference used.
↓, Decreased.

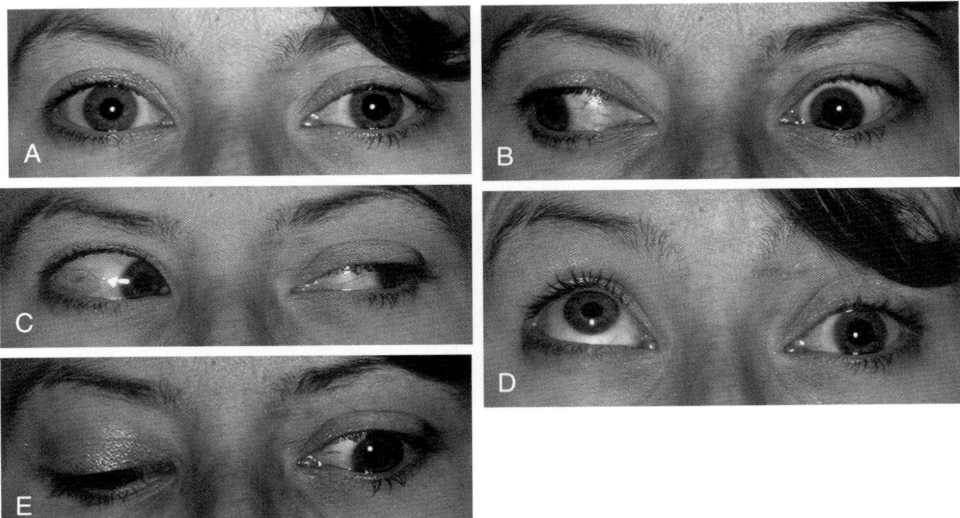

**Fig. 103.3** Traumatic left oculomotor palsy 3 months following a motor vehicle accident with closed head injury and loss of consciousness. Patient initially had complete left ptosis and complete absence of adduction, elevation, and depression. Results of magnetic resonance imaging and magnetic resonance angiography were normal. **A,** Central position with slight left ptosis, exotropia (outward deviation), and left pupillary enlargement. **B,** Impaired adduction of left eye with right gaze. Note aberrant regeneration with anomalous elevation of left lid upon adduction of left eye. **C,** Normal left gaze. **D,** Significant impaired elevation of left eye with upgaze. **E,** Impaired depression of left eye with downgaze.

preclude diagnostic testing. A pupil-sparing otherwise complete oculomotor palsy is exceedingly unlikely to result from PCOM aneurysmal compression and the urgency of imaging in this setting is controversial (Miller 2017; Newman and Biousse, 2017). However, immediate imaging is favored to avoid errors in exam interpretation that increase the risk of a missed diagnosis with high morbidity and mortality and because both basilar aneurysm and pituitary apoplexy have been reported with pupil-sparing otherwise complete oculomotor palsy (Lustbader and Miller, 1988; Tamhankar et al., 2013). Onset of oculomotor dysfunction following mild-moderate head trauma should also prompt investigation for an underlying aneurysm, though one may not always be found (Levy et al., 2005; Tajsic et al, 2017; Fig. 103.3).

Magnetic resonance angiography (MRA) and computed tomographic angiography (CTA) are the preferred diagnostic tests for aneurysm detection, but it is important to recognize that reliable interpretation of these studies requires a high level of experience, skill, and time (Chaudhary et al., 2009; Elmalem et al., 2011). The majority of PCOM aneurysms large enough to cause an oculomotor palsy are at least 4 mm in size. For aneurysms larger than 5 mm, the sensitivity of both MRA and CTA are higher than 95%; however, for aneurysms smaller than 5 mm, CTA sensitivity remains above 90% when interpreted by a neuroradiology expert, but MRA sensitivity in some studies is lower, leading some to advocate CTA as the initial diagnostic evaluation for PCOM aneurysms (Chaudhary et al., 2009). Neither MRA nor CTA is 100% sensitive, and conventional angiogram is still warranted when strong clinical suspicion for a PCOM aneurysm is present, and noninvasive studies are unrevealing.

Surgical clipping for aneurysms causing oculomotor nerve palsies results in a higher rate of oculomotor recovery compared to endovascular coiling in many (78% for surgery vs. 44% for endovascular coiling in a comparison review of retrospective studies) (Micieli et al., 2017), but not all (Zhong et al., 2019) studies. Furthermore, surgery is associated with higher periprocedural morbidity and decisions regarding treatment must take into account patient status, aneurysmal morphology, and treating physician experience (Micieli et al., 2017). Factors such as initial palsy severity and pretreatment palsy time may also play a role in recovery potential (Zhong et al., 2019).

In the subarachnoid space, the oculomotor nerve passes in close proximity to the medial temporal lobe. Herniation of the temporal lobe uncus ipsilateral to a space-occupying supratentorial lesion secondary to increased intracranial pressure may result in compression of the oculomotor nerve, manifested clinically as sudden enlargement and poor reactivity of the pupil ipsilateral to the lesion—the *Hutchison pupil* (Koehler and Wijdicks, 2015). Rarely, a unilateral enlarged and poorly reactive pupil may occur contralateral to the supratentorial lesion (Chung and Chandran, 2007). Oculomotor nerve involvement in the interpeduncular fossa and subarachnoid space may also occur secondary to inflammatory or neoplastic meningitis, in which case it may be isolated or accompanied by signs of meningeal inflammation such as meningismus or additional neurological signs. Enlargement and enhancement of the oculomotor nerve in the subarachnoid and interpeduncular locations may be seen on magnetic resonance imaging (MRI) in meningitis, with oculomotor nerve schwannomas, in association with ganglioside antibodies such as GQ1b (with persistent or transient oculomotor palsy), and in so-called ophthalmoplegic migraine, a rare condition with recurrent oculomotor paresis and pain usually seen in children (see Chapter 102; Choi et al., 2019; Qureshi et al., 2017; Shin, 2015; Wang et al., 2013; eFig. 103.4). 

### Cavernous Sinus

An oculomotor palsy in the cavernous sinus may occur in isolation or accompanied by dysfunction of other structures located in this space, including the abducens and trochlear nerves, the first and second divisions of the trigeminal nerve, and sympathetic fibers. Tolosa-Hunt syndrome is a painful of idiopathic self-limited inflammation of the cavernous sinus, typically responsive to corticosteroids (Mullen et al., 2018; see Table 103.1 and Videos 103.3 and 103.4).  Cavernous sinus infiltration by metastatic disease may be clinically and radiographically identical to Tolosa-Hunt syndrome and should be suspected, especially in older patients. Cavernous sinus lymphoma is typically steroid responsive and should be considered, especially if disease recurs with corticosteroid taper. Inflammation associated with systemic rheumatological disease or angioinvasive fungal infection, infiltration from adjacent nasopharyngeal neoplasm, carotid-cavernous fistulas, cavernous sinus thrombosis (more common in the intensive care unit than the outpatient setting), and mass effect from an intracavernous internal artery aneurysm or meningioma may also cause a cavernous sinus syndrome (Weerasinghe and Lueck, 2016). Pituitary apoplexy should be considered in the differential diagnosis for sudden-onset painful unilateral or bilateral oculomotor palsies, with or without accompanying visual loss or other ocular motor cranial nerve involvement (Hage et al., 2016).

### Orbital Apex

Oculomotor dysfunction in the orbital apex is typically accompanied by dysfunction of neighboring structures including the abducens and trochlear nerves, the first division of the trigeminal nerve, and the optic nerve. Features of orbital disease such as proptosis, chemosis, and conjunctival injection may be present. Idiopathic inflammation (orbital inflammatory pseudotumor and immunoglobulin G4 [IgG4]-related inflammation), infection (particularly aspergillosis and mucormycosis in diabetic or immunosuppressed patients), neoplastic infiltration, and inflammation or compression from adjacent sphenoid sinus infection or mucocele should be considered (Kashi, 2014; Mombaerts et al., 2017). As in cavernous sinus idiopathic inflammation (Tolosa-Hunt syndrome) versus lymphoma, idiopathic orbital inflammatory pseudotumor and lymphoma at the orbital apex are both likely to be steroid responsive, and lymphoma should be considered, especially if pain is absent and if disease recurs with corticosteroid taper. Anatomical division of the oculomotor nerve into superior and inferior branches occurs just before this location, and isolated involvement of either branch is not uncommon.

### Isolated Oculomotor Nerve Palsy

Isolated oculomotor dysfunction may occur from any lesion along the course of the nerve. Microvascular ischemia, a common cause in older patients with vascular risk factors (Fang et al., 2017; Keane, 2010), is typically pupil-sparing; however, relative pupil involvement with an average of 0.8 mm of anisocoria may be seen in up to one-third of patients with microvascular oculomotor nerve ischemia, but the pupil generally remains reactive (Jacobson, 1998). Confidence in the absence of a PCOM aneurysm may only be present when all oculomotor-innervated muscles other than the pupil are severely and completely impaired. In this era of modern noninvasive neuroimaging, it is prudent to perform emergent noninvasive vascular neuroimaging for all oculomotor palsies to avoid missing a PCOM aneurysm or other emergent etiology (see above section on Interpeduncular Fossa and Subarachnoid Space). The location of ischemia with a microvascular palsy may be anywhere along the course of the nerve but is typically peripheral and often considered to be in the cavernous sinus, although it is not visible with neuroimaging. Pain in the ipsilateral brow and eye is present in two-thirds of patients and may be severe (Wilker et al., 2009); however, the presence and characteristics of pain do not distinguish microvascular from aneurysmal oculomotor palsies (Fang et al., 2017). Spontaneous resolution over 8–12 weeks is typical for a microvascular etiology. An isolated oculomotor palsy may also arise from temporal arteritis; thus, erythrocyte sedimentation rate (ESR), C-reactive protein, and complete blood cell count (CBC) should be obtained on all elderly patients with an isolated oculomotor palsy and neuroimaging should be considered (Chou et al., 2004; Tamhankar et al., 2013; Thurtell and Longmuir, 2014). In the absence of complete spontaneous resolution with a suspected microvascular oculomotor palsy, neuroimaging is essential.

Elevation of the eyelid or constriction of the pupil upon adduction or depression of the eye is indicative of aberrant regeneration (anomalous axon innervation). When aberrant regeneration develops following an acute oculomotor palsy, a PCOM artery aneurysm or traumatic etiology is likely (see Fig. 103.3, *B*). When it develops spontaneously without a pre-existing acute palsy, a cavernous sinus meningioma or internal carotid artery aneurysm is likely, although this may also rarely occur with an unruptured PCOM aneurysm. Aberrant regeneration should not occur following a microvascular oculomotor palsy.

## TROCHLEAR NERVE (CRANIAL NERVE IV)

### Anatomy

Paired trochlear nuclei lie close to the dorsal surface of the midbrain just below the inferior colliculus. The fascicles emerge from the nuclei and course dorsally only 3–9 mm before decussating in the anterior medullary velum, and exiting the brainstem. The trochlear nerves are the only cranial nerves to emerge from the dorsal brainstem surface. After emergence, the nerves wrap around the surface of the midbrain to travel ventrally within the subarachnoid space toward the cavernous sinus. In the cavernous sinus, the trochlear nerve is located in the lateral dural wall, inferior to the oculomotor nerve. From the cavernous sinus, the nerve passes into the superior orbital fissure and ultimately innervates the superior oblique muscle contralateral to the nucleus of origin (see eFig. 103.1). The superior oblique muscle is an intorter of the eye, as well as a depressor of the adducted eye.

### Clinical Lesions

#### Trochlear Nucleus and Fascicle

It is difficult to differentiate a trochlear nuclear lesion from a tegmental (ventral and dorsolateral to the periaqueductal gray matter) fascicular lesion prior to the decussation of the fascicle. Both locations will result in paresis of the contralesional superior oblique muscle. Brainstem lesions posterior to the cerebral aqueduct in the tectal (dorsomedial to the periaqueductal gray matter) fascicle after its decussation may give rise to ipsilesional superior oblique paresis (Jeong et al., 2016). Isolated nuclear or fascicular involvement occurs rarely; it may occur in isolation or in association with other brainstem signs such as Horner syndrome, internuclear ophthalmoplegia, or cerebellar ataxia. Brainstem lesions include ischemia, hemorrhage, demyelination, infectious and noninfectious inflammation, and neoplasm (Jeong et al., 2016; Sudhakar and Bapuraj, 2010).

#### Trochlear Palsy Appearance

Trochlear nerve dysfunction results in impaired intorsion of the eye, impaired depression of the adducted eye, elevation of the affected eye (hypertropia), and vertical or oblique diplopia. The diplopia and hypertropia are worse with downgaze when the eye is in an adducted position, as this is the direction of action of the superior oblique muscle. Impaired depression of the affected eye in the adducted position may be seen but is often subtle (Fig. 103.5). A resting head tilt in the direction away from the paretic eye (e.g., right trochlear palsy, left head tilt) may be present and is considered a sign of chronicity. Because the superior oblique is an intorter of the eye, diplopia is minimized when a contralateral head tilt places the affected eye in an extorted position. The Parks-Bielschowsky three-step test (see Chapter 18 for additional information) is an examination technique utilized to assess the diplopia and hypertropia for conformation to the "pattern of a trochlear palsy" and consists of assessment of (1) which eye is hypertropic, (2) whether the hypertropia is worse in right or left gaze, and (3) whether the hypertropia is worse in right or left head tilt. The pattern of a fourth is a hypertropia on the side of the trochlear palsy, worsening in the

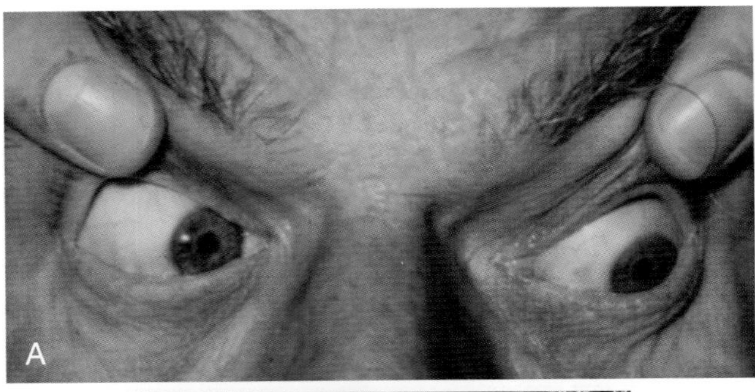


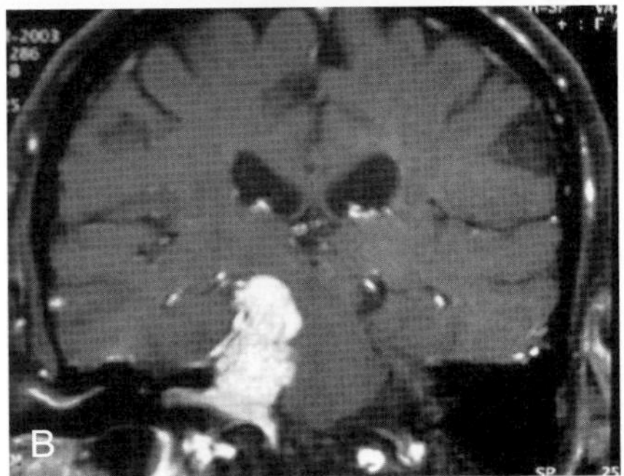


**Fig. 103.5 Right Trochlear Palsy From a Large Right Petroclival Meningioma.** Patient also had decreased hearing in right ear and cerebellar truncal ataxia. **A,** Note impaired depression of right eye in adducted position. **B,** Preoperative T1-weighted coronal magnetic resonance imaging with gadolinium reveals an extensive mass in the pontine cistern, with significant brainstem compression.

contralateral gaze direction and upon ipsilateral head tilt (Muthusamy et al., 2014). A fourth step is assessment of the hypertropia in the upright versus supine position; reduction in size of the hypertropia in the supine position suggests a skew deviation, given gravity dependence of the otolith vestibular organs (Hernowo and Eggenberger, 2014; Wong, 2010).

Evaluation for superior oblique paresis in the setting of oculomotor nerve dysfunction with impaired adduction from medial rectus paresis is best assessed with the affected eye in an abducted position, where intact intorsion during downgaze suggests intact trochlear function.

### Subarachnoid Space

Within the subarachnoid space, the nerves are near the tentorium cerebelli and are prone to unilateral or bilateral traumatic injury (Keane, 2005). Unlike traumatic oculomotor palsy, which usually occurs following severe head trauma with loss of consciousness, the trochlear nerves are injured more easily by minor degrees of head trauma (Dhaliwal et al., 2006).

Trochlear nerve involvement in isolation or accompanied by signs of meningeal inflammation, such as meningismus, or additional cranial nerve palsies, may occur secondary to inflammatory or neoplastic meningitis. Enhancement of the nerve as it travels around the midbrain may be present on MRI. An increasingly recognized cause of such enhancement in the setting of normal cerebrospinal fluid is trochlear nerve schwannoma (Elmalem et al., 2009; Torun et al., 2018; eFig. 103.6).

### Cavernous Sinus

Trochlear palsy in the cavernous sinus is generally accompanied by dysfunction of other structures including the abducens and oculomotor nerves, the first and second divisions of the trigeminal nerve, and sympathetic fibers. Idiopathic inflammation, inflammation associated with systemic rheumatological disease or angioinvasive fungal infection, infiltration from adjacent nasopharyngeal neoplasm, carotid-cavernous fistulas, and mass effect from an intracavernous internal artery aneurysm or meningioma are common causes. Pituitary apoplexy very rarely, if ever, results in isolated trochlear paresis (Hage et al., 2016).

### Orbital Apex

See Orbital Apex section above under Oculomotor Nerve, Clinical Lesions.

### Isolated Trochlear Nerve Palsy

Congenital, traumatic, and microvascular ischemic trochlear palsies are common causes of neurologically isolated trochlear paresis (Dosunmu et al., 2018; Hata et al., 2013; Tamhankar et al., 2011). Identification of a long-standing head tilt in old photographs of the patient and increased vertical fusional amplitudes (a test of the amount of image misalignment with which the individual can maintain binocular fusion—tends to be high with congenital lesions) can help confirm the diagnosis of a congenital trochlear nerve palsy. Overaction of the inferior oblique muscle, manifested by excessive elevation upon adduction of the eye ipsilateral to the trochlear weakness, and hypertropia worsening in upgaze rather than downgaze may also suggest a congenital etiology (Ivanir and Trobe, 2017; Siatkowski, 2017).

## TRIGEMINAL NERVE (CRANIAL NERVE V)

### Anatomy

The trigeminal nerve consists of afferent sensory, efferent motor, and parasympathetic fibers. The ophthalmic (V1), maxillary (V2), and mandibular (V3) trigeminal sensory nerve branches emerge from the anterior surface of the trigeminal (gasserian) ganglion in the Meckel cave (a dural cavity overlying the apex of the petrous bone) and innervate the facial skin, mucous membranes of the nose and mouth, teeth, orbital contents, and supratentorial meninges (Fig. 103.7; also see eFig. 103.1). The ophthalmic division courses in the lateral wall of the cavernous sinus inferior to the trochlear nerve and exits the skull via the superior orbital fissure. It is the anatomical substrate for the afferent limb of the corneal reflex. The maxillary division also courses in the lateral wall of the cavernous sinus, exiting the skull via the foramen rotundum to enter the sphenopalatine (also called the pterygopalatine) fossa and the inferior orbital fissure. The mandibular division exits the skull through the foramen ovale. Sensory input from these three branches travels centrally from the trigeminal ganglion via the trigeminal sensory root in the prepontine subarachnoid cistern to the trigeminal sensory nucleus, which is composed of a mesencephalic subnucleus receiving proprioceptive input from V3, a principal (main) sensory subnucleus mediating tactile sensation, and descending spinal subnuclei (oralis, interpolaris, and caudalis) that descend to the cervical spinal cord and mediate pain and temperature. Sensory information ultimately ascends to the contralateral thalamus.

The motor efferents originate in the motor trigeminal nucleus in the pons, medial to the principal sensory nucleus, emerge from the ventral pons as the motor root, travel inferior to the trigeminal ganglion and then alongside the mandibular sensory division to innervate the muscles of mastication (masseter, temporalis, pterygoids) and the mylohyoid, tensors tympani and palatini, and anterior belly of the digastric. Trigeminal nerve branches carry efferent postganglionic parasympathetic innervation from the pterygopalatine ganglia to the lacrimal gland and from the submandibular ganglia to the salivary glands. Preganglionic parasympathetic fibers travel in the facial nerve.

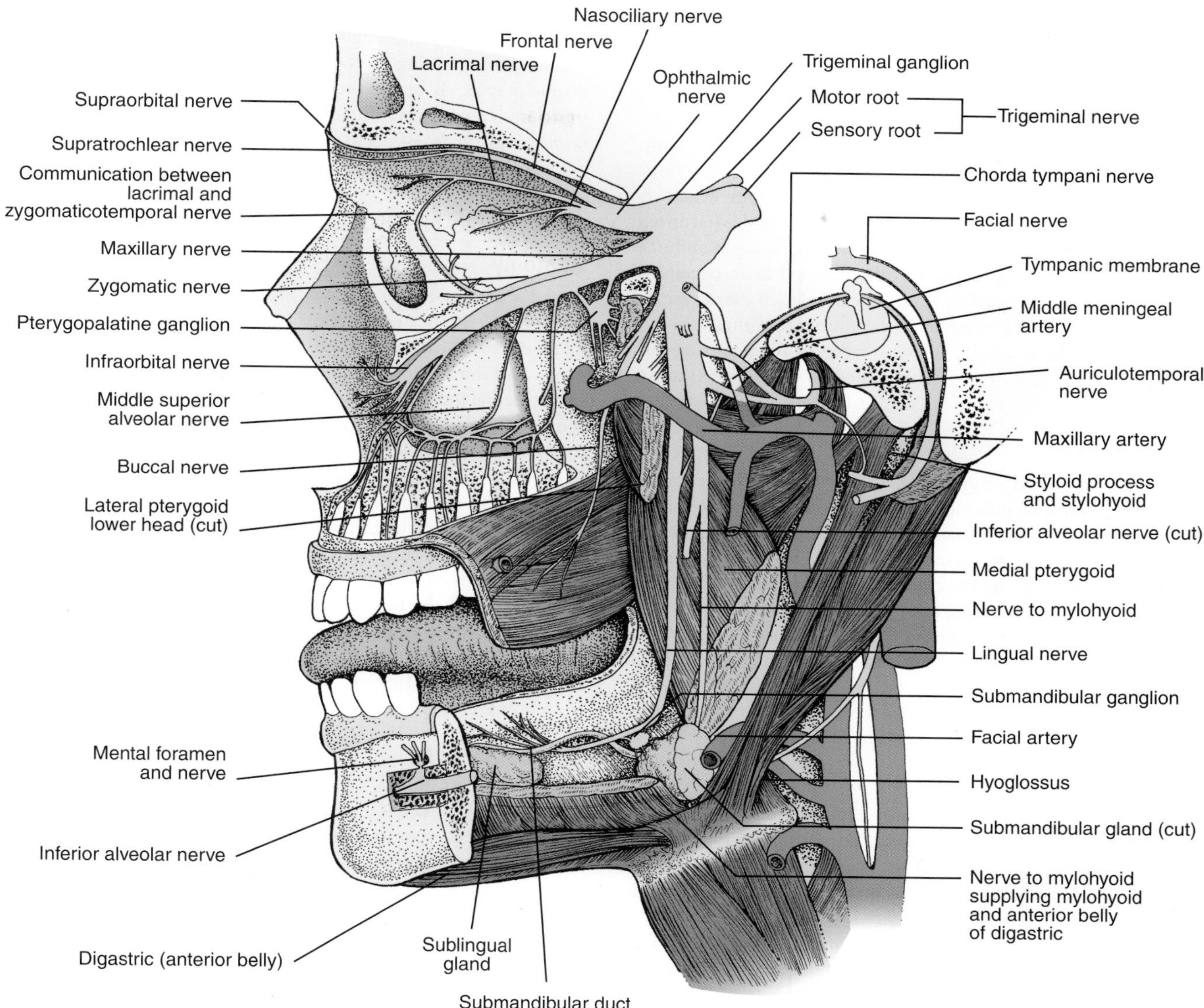


**Fig. 103.7** Trigeminal nerve ophthalmic (1), maxillary (2), and mandibular (3) branches emerging from the semilunar (trigeminal or gasserian) ganglion. (*From Standring, G., 2005. Gray's Anatomy, thirty-ninth ed. Churchill Livingstone, Philadelphia.*)

## Clinical Lesions

### Trigeminal Nucleus

The extension of the trigeminal nuclear complex throughout the entire brainstem renders it susceptible to involvement from any pathological brainstem process. Trigeminal lesions are particularly common with demyelinating disease, may involve either the nuclei or sensory root, and may be clinically silent or symptomatic (Kremer et al., 2013; Zakrzewska et al., 2018). Ischemia, hemorrhage, infectious and noninfectious inflammation, and neoplasm are other causes of trigeminal brainstem involvement (Kim et al., 2013). Additional brainstem signs are frequently present. *Wallenberg syndrome* from lateral medullary ischemia typically causes ipsilateral facial numbness and impaired pinprick sensation secondary to descending spinal tract and nucleus involvement (see Table 103.1).

### Subarachnoid Space: Nerve Roots

Classic trigeminal neuralgia is characterized by seconds-long stereotyped episodes of intensely painful electric-like shocks along one or more of the trigeminal nerve branches, though a large percentage of patients also have concomitant persistent pain (Maarbjerg et al., 2017). Pain is often elicited by sensory stimuli on the face, such as shaving or wind. There is no accompanying sensory loss or motor weakness in the affected distribution on examination. The second and third branches are most commonly affected, with less than 5% of patients experiencing involvement of the ophthalmic division. Many cases are attributable to compression of the sensory nerve root, typically at the transition between central and peripheral myelin, by a vascular structure, most often the superior cerebellar artery or anterior inferior cerebellar arteries (Haller et al., 2016). Evidence-based support for this vascular compressive etiology is provided by surgical outcome data showing that the pain is often amenable to surgical decompression, especially in cases of classic pain paroxysms (Barker et al., 1996; Sivakanthan et al., 2014). Because vascular contact with the sensory or motor nerve roots is a relatively common finding in cadavers and asymptomatic controls, vascular contact alone may be insufficient to cause trigeminal neuralgia (Yousry et al., 2004). Compression or indentation of the nerve root is likely necessary, with resultant axonal loss and demyelination (Haller et al., 2016;

Miller et al., 2009). See Chapter 102 for additional discussion of trigeminal neuralgia and other facial pain syndromes. eTable 103.2, available in the online version of this chapter at http://www.ExpertConsult.com, outlines current treatments for facial palsy and trigeminal and glossopharyngeal neuralgia.

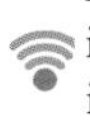

Classic trigeminal neuralgia must be differentiated from symptomatic trigeminal neuralgia secondary to an underlying neoplastic, inflammatory, paraneoplastic, or meningitic cause, from which the pain characteristics may be clinically indistinguishable (Gronseth et al., 2008; Kalanie et al., 2014; Maarbjerg et al., 2017; Wanibuchi et al., 2012). It must also be carefully differentiated from trigeminal neuropathy with differing qualitative and temporal pain characteristics and sensory deficits on examination. Cerebellopontine angle acoustic schwannomas frequently involve the sensory nerve root, causing ipsilateral facial sensory symptoms accompanied by ipsilateral tinnitus, deafness, and vertigo from vestibulocochlear nerve involvement.

### Trigeminal Ganglion

Middle cranial fossa malignant infiltration, compressive neoplastic lesions, and autoimmune inflammation are among the most common causes of trigeminal ganglion pathology. The trigeminal ganglion is a location in which the varicella-zoster virus (VZV) often lies latent, sometimes reactivating along the course of the trigeminal ophthalmic branch later in life to cause herpes zoster ophthalmicus and a pain syndrome that may occur with or without an accompanying zoster rash (Birlea et al., 2014; Vrcek et al., 2017). Identification of skin lesions along the side of the nose *(Hutchinson sign)* corresponding to the nasociliary branch of the ophthalmic division strongly predicts subsequent ocular complications (Nithyanandam et al., 2010).

### Trigeminal Nerve Branches

Dysfunction of the ophthalmic branch results in numbness or paresthesias in the anterior scalp, forehead, and supraorbital regions, and an abnormal corneal reflex. A lesion of the maxillary branch affects the cheek, lower eyelid, and upper lip. A lesion of the mandibular branch affects the lower lip, chin, and lateral face anterior to the ear. Motor involvement in a trigeminal nerve lesion is often clinically undetectable. Although it is tempting to localize a trigeminal nerve lesion based on symptom distribution, the complex branching pattern and organization of the trigeminal nuclei and ganglion prohibit such simple localization. It is common for lesions proximal to the peripheral nerve branches to evoke symptoms in a single trigeminal branch distribution.

Lesions of a single branch may result from inflammation, compression, or neoplasm (Briani et al., 2013; Perera et al., 2014). Damage to small distal branches may occur after dental procedures. The ophthalmic branch may be involved in *Gradenigo syndrome* in combination with the abducens and facial nerves from a lesion at the petrous apex, most common clinically as inflammation following otitis media in children (Vitale et al., 2017; see Table 103.1). Both the ophthalmic and maxillary branches may be affected by a cavernous sinus lesion, in which setting dysfunction of the oculomotor, trochlear, and abducens nerves is often present.

Two particularly ominous clinical scenarios are (1) insidious development of facial numbness or paresthesias in a patient with a history of facial skin malignancy, and (2) the "numb chin" or "numb cheek" syndromes. In the first situation, perineural invasion of the trigeminal branches is likely (Erkan et al., 2017; Warden et al., 2009). This is most frequently seen with head and neck adenoid cystic carcinoma, squamous cell carcinoma, and melanoma. The *numb chin syndrome* results from involvement of the mental nerve branches of the mandibular division and is most commonly due to focal metastatic nerve infiltration within the mandible, most often from breast, lung, prostate, or hematological malignancies (Assaf et al., 2014; Maeda et al., 2018; Sanchis et al., 2008), though it may also be a secondary effect of radiation or pharmacological therapies (Fortunato et al., 2018). This syndrome may rarely be the presenting manifestation of malignancy but more often represents recurrence or progression of known disease. The *numb cheek syndrome* occurs when branches of the maxillary division are involved.

## ABDUCENS NERVE (CRANIAL NERVE VI)

### Anatomy

Paired abducens nuclei are located in the dorsal pons in the floor of the fourth ventricle in close proximity to the fascicle of the facial nerve. Each nucleus contains abducens motoneurons that form the abducens nerve, and interneurons that decussate at the nuclear level and ascend in the medial longitudinal fasciculus (MLF) to the contralateral oculomotor medial rectus subnucleus to facilitate conjugate horizontal gaze in the direction ipsilateral to the abducens nuclear origin of the interneurons. The abducens fascicle exits the ventral surface of the nucleus, traverses the brainstem, emerges from the ventral pontomedullary sulcus at the caudal pontine surface, and travels in the subarachnoid space, where it ascends near the clivus. It pierces the dura and passes under the petroclinoid (Gruber) ligament into the Dorello canal, then travels through the body of the cavernous sinus lateral to the internal carotid artery (unlike the oculomotor, trochlear, and trigeminal nerves, which are housed in the lateral dural wall), and ultimately into the superior orbital fissure to innervate the ipsilateral lateral rectus muscle (see eFig. 103.1).

### Clinical Lesions

#### Abducens Nucleus

Because the abducens nucleus contains the interneurons destined to ascend in the contralateral MLF to the contralateral oculomotor medial rectus subnucleus to permit conjugate horizontal gaze, abducens nuclear lesions cause conjugate horizontal gaze palsy toward the side of the lesion. Isolated horizontal gaze palsy may occasionally occur but accompanying ipsilateral facial palsy with lower motor neuron facial weakness is typically present. Lesions involving both the abducens nucleus and ipsilateral MLF cause the *one-and-a-half syndrome*, with an ipsilateral conjugate gaze palsy and an ipsilateral internuclear ophthalmoplegia with impaired adduction of the ipsilesional eye and abducting nystagmus of the contralateral eye (see Chapter 21). Common brainstem lesions include ischemia, hemorrhage, demyelination, infectious and noninfectious inflammation, and neoplasm. Periventricular necrosis from Wernicke encephalopathy also frequently results in horizontal gaze or abducens palsy from involvement of the abducens nucleus or fascicle, respectively.

#### Abducens Palsy Appearance

Abducens nerve dysfunction results in impaired ipsilateral abduction of the eye and deviation of the eyes toward one another *(esotropia)* (Fig. 103.8 and Videos 103.5 and 103.6). Binocular horizontal diplopia and the esotropia are worse with gaze in the direction of the abduction deficit.

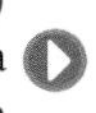

#### Brainstem Fascicle

The original *Foville syndrome* was the combination of ipsilateral abducens palsy, ipsilateral lower motor neuron facial palsy, and contralateral hemiparesis from corticospinal tract involvement (see Table 103.1). It is now more commonly applied to the combination of ipsilateral abducens and facial palsies with contralateral ataxia, ipsilateral Horner syndrome, ipsilateral deafness, and ipsilateral loss of taste and facial

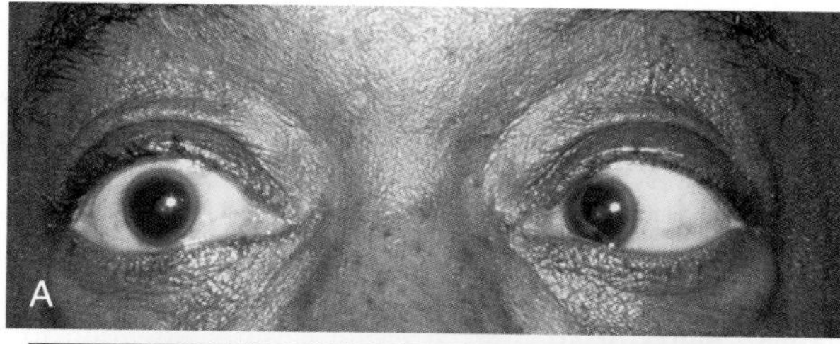


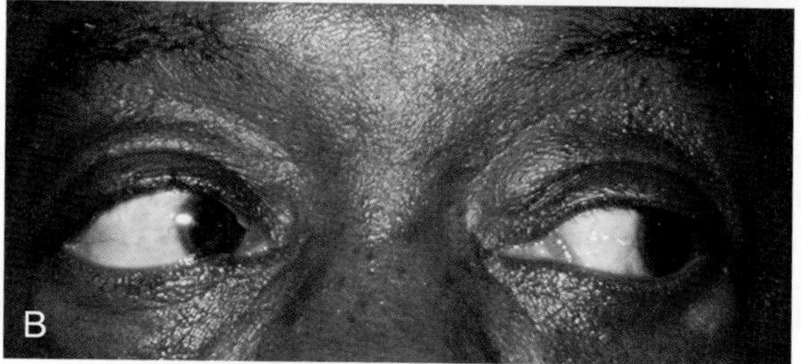


**Fig. 103.8 Right Microvascular Abducens Palsy. A,** Right gaze with impaired abduction of right eye. **B,** Normal left gaze.

sensation. *Millard-Gubler syndrome* is the combination of ipsilateral abducens and facial palsies with contralateral hemiparesis (see Table 103.1). *Raymond syndrome* is the combination of ipsilateral abducens palsy and contralateral hemiparesis (see Table 103.1). Common brainstem lesions include ischemia, hemorrhage, demyelination, infectious and noninfectious inflammation, and neoplasm. Isolated abducens palsy from fascicular involvement is rarely the presenting manifestation of cavernoma, demyelination, metastatic disease, or paraneoplastic brainstem encephalitis (Hammam et al., 2005; Mallery et al., 2012).

Quantitative assessment of the velocity of abducting saccades via eye movement recordings may help differentiate a central fascicular abducens lesion from a peripheral abducens palsy. With an acute abducens palsy (<1 month), saccadic velocities are reduced in both fascicular and peripheral lesion locations. However, after 2 months, saccadic velocities return to normal with peripheral lesions and remain impaired with fascicular lesions (Wong et al., 2006).

### Subarachnoid Space and Dorello Canal

Abducens palsy may occur in isolation or in combination with other cranial nerve palsies from infectious, inflammatory, or neoplastic meningitis, or in association with ganglioside antibodies such as GQ1b (Choi et al., 2019). The abducens nerve is in close approximation with the clivus and the basilar and vertebral arteries in its subarachnoid segment and may be affected by a neoplastic or inflammatory clivus or other skull-based process or compressed by an aneurysm, inferior petrosal sinus thrombosis, or dolichoectatic artery (Mittal et al., 2017).

The abducens nerves are particularly prone to dysfunction from alterations in intracranial pressure and from trauma. Unilateral or bilateral abducens palsies may be seen with spontaneous or post-lumbar puncture intracranial hypotension and with intracranial hypertension from any cause, the latter often accompanied by papilledema (Porta-Etessam et al., 2011). It has been suggested historically that the abducens nerve is prone to such injury because of its long intracranial course; however, it has a shorter course than the trochlear nerve, which is not prone to injury from raised intracranial pressure. Rather, it is likely tethering of the abducens nerve at the pontomedullary sulcus and Dorello canal that predispose the abducens subarachnoid portion to stretch and distortion injury with alterations in intracranial pressure and with trauma (Dhaliwal et al., 2006; Hanson et al., 2004; Tubbs et al., 2012).

### Petrous Apex

Abducens palsy is common in *Gradenigo syndrome* in combination with trigeminal ophthalmic division and facial nerve involvement from a lesion at the petrous apex (see Table 103.1). This is most commonly seen clinically as inflammation following otitis media in children (Vitale et al., 2017).

### Cavernous Sinus

An abducens palsy in the cavernous sinus may occur in isolation or accompanied by dysfunction of other structures including the oculomotor and trochlear nerves, the first and second divisions of the trigeminal nerve, and sympathetic fibers. The combination of abducens palsy and ipsilateral Horner syndrome is highly suggestive of an ipsilateral cavernous sinus lesion, because the sympathetic fibers travel along the surface of the abducens nerve briefly in the posterior cavernous sinus (Kang et al., 2011). Idiopathic inflammation, inflammation associated with systemic rheumatological disease or angioinvasive infection, infiltration from adjacent nasopharyngeal neoplasm, carotid-cavernous fistulas, and mass effect from an intracavernous internal carotid artery aneurysm or meningioma are common causes. The abducens nerves are the most frequently involved ocular motor cranial nerves in pituitary apoplexy (Hage et al., 2016), though isolated involvement is rare (Saffra et al., 2011).

### Orbital Apex

See Orbital Apex section above under Oculomotor Nerve, Clinical Lesions.

### Isolated Abducens Palsy

Isolated painful abducens palsy often represents microvascular ischemia, especially in older patients with vascular risk factors (see Fig. 103.8). Spontaneous resolution over 8–12 weeks is typical. A small percentage of patients will have an underlying structural lesion or temporal arteritis; thus, ESR, C-reactive protein, and CBC should be obtained on all elderly patients with an isolated abducens palsy and a low threshold for immediate neuroimaging is appropriate (Chou et al., 2004; Elder et al., 2016; Tamhankar et al., 2013). In the absence of complete spontaneous resolution, neuroimaging is essential. Head trauma, even if mild, is another cause of abducens palsy (Dhaliwal et al., 2006). Impaired ability to abduct the eye past midline or bilateral presentation predicts poor spontaneous recovery. The abducens nerve is the ocular motor cranial nerve most commonly affected bilaterally in isolation. This occurs most often from trauma and increased intracranial pressure (Keane, 2005).

## FACIAL NERVE (CRANIAL NERVE VII)

### Anatomy

The facial nerve comprises afferent gustatory, afferent sensory, efferent motor, and parasympathetic fibers. It innervates taste buds in the anterior two-thirds of the tongue (Fig. 104.9). Unipolar neurons with cell bodies in the geniculate ganglion within the temporal bone carry taste information from the taste buds via the chorda tympani facial nerve branch, which is joined by the lingual branch of the trigeminal nerve. The chorda tympani nerve branch joins the main trunk of the facial nerve just proximal to the stylomastoid foramen. From the geniculate ganglion, taste information travels proximally to enter the solitary tract and ultimately the rostral solitary (or gustatory) nucleus in the rostral medulla via the nervus intermedius, which passes through the internal auditory canal. Afferent sensory information from the soft palate, middle ear, tympanic membrane, and external auditory canal travel in the facial nerve.

The motor efferents originate in the motor facial nucleus in the lateral tegmentum of the caudal pons. Supranuclear innervation is bilateral to the rostral portion of the nucleus, which innervates the upper facial muscles, but unilateral to the caudal portion, which innervates the lower facial muscles. Prior to exiting the brainstem, these motor efferent fibers ascend rostrally and wrap around the abducens nucleus as the genu of the facial nerve fasciculus that protrudes into the floor of the fourth ventricle to form the facial colliculus. Fascicular fibers then traverse the brainstem to exit the lateral pons. The motor fibers travel through the cerebellopontine angle to enter the petrous temporal bone via the internal auditory canal, travel through the geniculate ganglion without synapsing, and exit the stylomastoid foramen after a tortuous course through the temporal bone and facial canal. Prior to exiting the skull via the stylomastoid foramen, a small branch is given off to the stapedius muscle (see Fig. 103.9). After exiting the stylomastoid foramen, the motor nerve enters the substance of the parotid gland before branching into temporal, zygomatic, buccal, mandibular, and cervical branches to innervate the muscles of facial expression, stylohyoid, and posterior belly of the digastric. Muscles of facial expression include the orbicularis oculi, orbicularis oris, buccinator, and platysma. Efferent motor fibers to the orbicularis oculi are the anatomical substrate for the efferent limb of the corneal reflex.

The facial nerve carries efferent preganglionic parasympathetic innervation for the lacrimal gland in the greater superficial petrosal nerve, the first branch off of the peripheral facial nerve near the geniculate ganglion (see Fig. 103.9). This is joined by the deep petrosal nerve carrying sympathetic fibers from the internal carotid artery plexus to form the nerve of the pterygoid canal (Vidian nerve) that proceeds to the pterygopalatine ganglion. Preganglionic parasympathetic innervation for the salivary glands originates in the brainstem superior salivatory nucleus and travels via the nervus intermedius and chorda tympani to the submandibular ganglion (see Fig. 103.9). Postganglionic fibers are carried in trigeminal nerve branches.

## Clinical Lesions

### Facial Palsy Appearance

Facial nerve dysfunction results in unilateral upper and lower facial weakness manifested by flattening of the nasolabial fold, an asymmetrical smile, poor eyebrow elevation, decreased forehead wrinkling, and weak eye closure (Fig. 103.10 and Video 103.7). The palpebral fissure is widened on the affected side, and deviation of the eye upward and laterally with attempted eye closure *(Bell phenomenon)* may become visible with blinks or attempts at eyelid closure. Attention to adequacy of corneal protection with provision of appropriate lubrication and protection will minimize the risk for permanent corneal damage from exposure due to incomplete eye closure. Lesions proximal to the greater superficial petrosal nerve increase the risk for corneal damage by impairing lacrimal secretion (for treatments, see eTable 103.2, available in the online version of this chapter at http://www.ExpertConsult.com).

Although it is theoretically possible to localize a facial nerve lesion to a specific nerve portion with specialized tests of tear production, stapedial muscle reflex, salivation, and taste, the primary clinical manifestation of facial nerve dysfunction is facial weakness. This must be distinguished from upper motor neuron facial weakness that causes only lower facial weakness because of bilateral supranuclear innervation to the upper facial muscles. Upper motor neuron facial weakness may also result in selective facial weakness for either volitional or emotional facial movements, whereas lower motor neuron facial weakness from facial nerve palsy affects both equally.

### Facial Nucleus and Fascicle

Although isolated lower motor neuron weakness occasionally occurs from a brainstem lesion, accompanying brainstem signs, such as horizontal gaze palsy from abducens nuclear involvement, are typically present. The original *Foville syndrome* was the

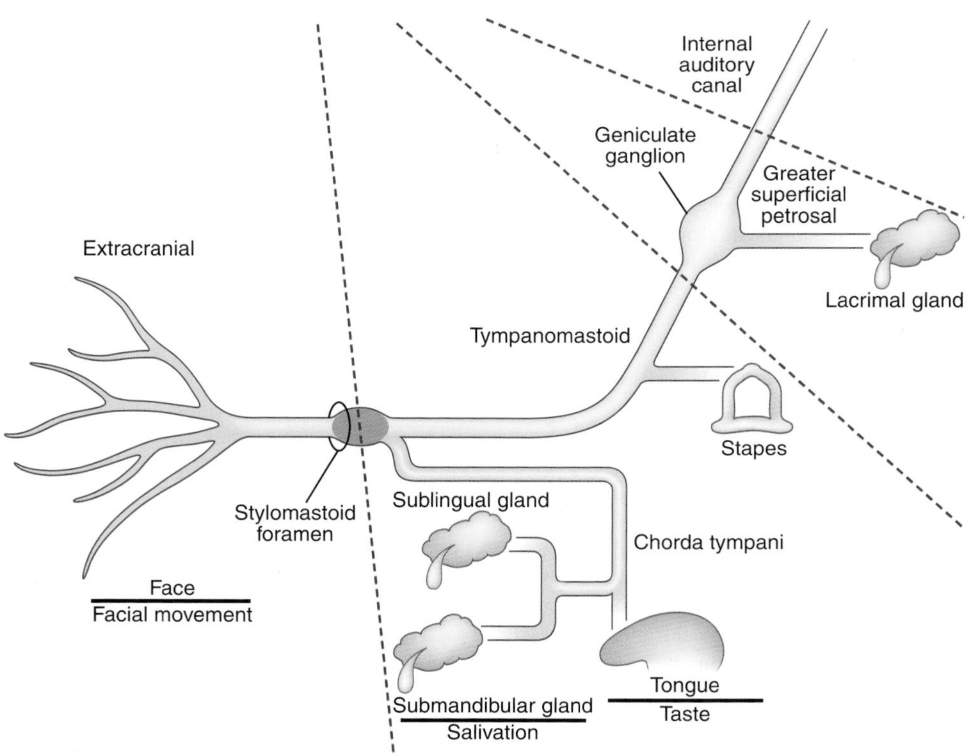


**Fig. 103.9** Facial Nerve Schematic Showing the Major Subdivisions and Their Principal Functions. *(Courtesy Patrick Sweeney, MD.)*

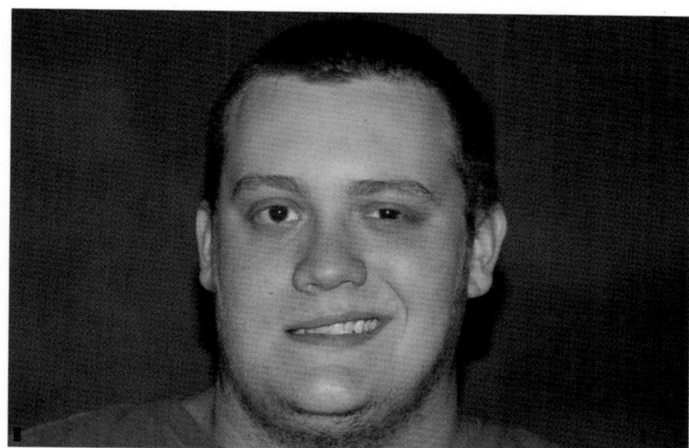

**Fig. 103.10 Right Facial Palsy.** Upon attempting to smile, there is little right facial action, the right palpebral fissure remains widened, and the right lower face fails to fully activate.

combination of ipsilateral abducens palsy, ipsilateral lower motor neuron facial palsy, and contralateral hemiparesis from corticospinal tract involvement (see Table 103.1). It is now more commonly applied to ipsilateral abducens and facial palsies with contralateral ataxia, ipsilateral Horner syndrome, ipsilateral deafness, and ipsilateral loss of taste and facial sensation. *Millard-Gubler syndrome* is the combination of ipsilateral abducens and facial palsies with contralateral hemiparesis (see Table 103.1). Common brainstem lesions include ischemia, hemorrhage, demyelination, infectious and noninfectious inflammation, and neoplasm (Agarwal et al., 2011; Kremer et al., 2013). Continuous twitching of individual facial muscles, called *facial myokymia*, is most commonly seen with demyelination and brainstem gliomas.

### Subarachnoid Space: Nerve Root

Hemifacial spasm (HFS) is characterized by involuntary episodic contractions of the muscles innervated by the facial nerve (see Videos 103.7 and 103.8; Stamey and Jankovic, 2007; Yaltho and Jankovic, 2011). It is most often unilateral and may be caused by compression and indentation of the facial motor nerve root at its brainstem exit by an aberrant vascular loop or dolichoectatic artery (Choi et al., 2013). HFS infrequently results from neoplastic compression or inflammation of the nerve root or from intrapontine lesions such as cavernoma, tumor, or demyelination (Arita et al., 2012; Collazo et al., 2018). Features suggestive of psychogenic (functional) HFS include bilateral asynchronous hemifacial involvement, isolated lower facial involvement, downward deviation of the mouth's angle, lack of the "other Babinski sign" (unilateral frontalis muscle contraction leading to eyebrow elevation simultaneous with eye closure due to orbicularis oculi contraction) (Stamey and Jankovic, 2007), ipsilateral downward movements of the eyebrow, and association with tremor or dystonia (Baizabal-Carvallo and Jankovic, 2017).

Facial weakness in isolation or in combination with other cranial nerve palsies may result from infectious, inflammatory, or neoplastic meningitis (Hiraumi et al., 2014). Cerebellopontine angle mass lesions, such as meningioma, facial schwannoma, or acoustic schwannoma, may cause facial nerve involvement (Leonetti et al., 2016). The facial nerve and vestibulocochlear nerves form a complex as they exit the brainstem, and sensorineural hearing loss is typically the primary feature of acoustic schwannomas. Acoustic schwannomas may be difficult to differentiate from facial nerve schwannomas in the cerebellopontine angle, but the latter tend to have earlier clinical facial weakness and the radiological appearance of a "labyrinthine tail," as the facial schwannoma extends into the facial canal in the temporal bone (Jacob et al., 2012; Mastronardi et al., 2018).

### Intratemporal Facial Nerve and Geniculate Ganglion

*Bell palsy*, one of the most common causes of facial nerve palsy, is a self-limited, typically monophasic facial nerve palsy of acute-subacute onset (Hohman and Hadlock, 2013; Ozkale et al., 2014; see Fig. 103.10 and Table 103.1). Pain accompanies facial weakness in 60% of patients, impaired lacrimation in 60%, taste changes in 30%–50%, and hyperacusis in 15%–30%. Ipsilateral facial sensory symptoms are not uncommon and are hypothetically explained by extension of inflammation from the facial nerve to the trigeminal nerve via the greater superficial petrosal nerve. Internal auditory canal MRI often reveals enhancement of the facial nerve, most commonly at the geniculate ganglion. Eighty-five percent of patients spontaneously recover normal facial function in 3 weeks. Bell palsy occurs with increased frequency during pregnancy, in which setting it is associated with a poorer recovery rate (Hussain et al., 2017). Residual abnormalities after acute Bell palsy occur in 12% of patients and include persistent severe facial weakness in 4% and synkinetic contraction and twitching of the upper and lower facial muscles in 17% that can worsen for up to a year after the acute Bell palsy (Beurskens et al., 2010; Fujiwara et al., 2015; Kanaya et al., 2009; see Video 103.7). Acutely, the nasolabial fold is flattened and the palpebral fissure is widened on the affected side; however, with chronicity, the affected side often becomes hypercontracted, with a deepened and prominent nasolabial fold and a narrowed palpebral fissure. Aberrant regeneration involving the lacrimal gland may result in tearing with facial muscle contraction (syndrome of "crocodile tears"), particularly during eating. Electromyographic presence of spontaneous fibrillation in facial muscles 10–14 days after onset of facial weakness is predictive of poor outcome in Bell palsy. Bell palsy may be recurrent, but alternative causes such as Lyme disease or sarcoidosis must be considered. Bilateral facial weakness is also common with acute inflammatory demyelinating polyneuropathy, Lyme disease, sarcoidosis, and Epstein-Barr virus infection (Coddington et al., 2010; Hansen et al., 2013).

Although Bell palsy is considered idiopathic, herpes simplex virus and VZV reactivation in the geniculate ganglion have been implicated in its pathogenesis. Evidence exists that Bell palsy treatment with oral corticosteroids provides benefit in preventing unsatisfactory facial recovery. Treatment with antiviral agents alone is not associated with a reduced risk of unsatisfactory recovery; however, co-administration of corticosteroids and antiviral agents may provide added benefit over corticosteroids alone (Almeida et al., 2009; Fu et al., 2018; Gronseth et al., 2012; Madhok et al., 2016; Thaera et al., 2010).

*Ramsay Hunt syndrome* consists of facial nerve palsy accompanied by a vesicular otic or oral rash due to VZV, with or without vestibulocochlear symptoms (see Table 103.1). The vesicular outbreak may occur before, after, or simultaneous with the facial weakness. Diagnosis is confirmed by a rise in serological VZV titers or positive VZV polymerase chain reaction (PCR). Serological detection or positive VZV PCR in facial palsy without a vesicular rash suggests zoster sine herpete. Facial weakness is more severe and spontaneous recovery less common in Ramsey Hunt and zoster sine herpete than in idiopathic Bell palsy (Kim et al., 2019). Early diagnosis and initiation of corticosteroid and antiviral treatment significantly improve recovery.

Intratemporal facial nerve schwannomas within the facial canal, traumatic fractures, occult skull-based neoplasms of the temporal bone, and complicated otitis media with mastoiditis may also affect the facial nerve (Leonetti et al., 2016). These entities should be considered when the onset of facial weakness is insidious and the course progressive and accompanied by hearing loss, given the proximity of the vestibulocochlear nerve. *Gradenigo syndrome* results from inflammation of the petrous apex and causes facial nerve palsy in combination with trigeminal and abducens nerve impairment (see Table 103.1). Traumatic temporal bone fractures may cause immediate or delayed facial nerve palsy (Nash et al., 2010).

### Facial Nerve Branches

Parotid neoplasms, surgical procedures, and infiltration of facial skin cancers along facial motor nerve branches may result in weakness of individual facial nerve innervated muscles (Durstenfeld et al., 2014; Hohman et al., 2014; Leonetti et al., 2016). Taste changes and hyperacusis do not typically occur with these lesions, given their distal nature, and either the upper or lower facial muscles may be affected in isolation. This may lead to diagnostic confusion with an upper motor neuron lesion when only the lower facial musculature is involved. Peripheral branches may also be affected by Lyme disease and sarcoidosis in the absence of meningeal inflammation. *Melkersson-Rosenthal syndrome* is a rare granulomatous disease with a triad of facial nerve palsy, facial edema, and tongue fissures (Elias et al., 2013; see Table 103.1). The complete triad occurs in only a quarter of patients.

## VESTIBULOCOCHLEAR NERVE (CRANIAL NERVE VIII)

See Chapters 21 and 22.

## GLOSSOPHARYNGEAL NERVE (CRANIAL NERVE IX)

### Anatomy

The glossopharyngeal nerve contains afferent gustatory, afferent sensory, efferent motor, and parasympathetic fibers and innervates taste buds in the posterior one-third of the tongue. Unipolar glossopharyngeal neurons with cell bodies in the superior and inferior (petrosal) ganglia of the glossopharyngeal nerve at the jugular foramen in the base of the temporal bone carry taste information from the taste buds to the ganglia, and then proximally into the brainstem solitary tract and rostral solitary (or gustatory) nucleus in the rostral medulla. Afferent sensory information from the uvula, tonsil, pharynx, auditory canal, middle ear, and carotid sinus and bulb travels in the glossopharyngeal nerve via the petrosal ganglion. This sensory information provides the afferent limb of the gag reflex, with the efferent limb provided by glossopharyngeal and vagus motor fibers to the pharynx. Within the brainstem, sensory information is carried to the solitary nucleus and pain information to the spinal nucleus of the trigeminal nerve. The carotid sinus and carotid body are located at the bifurcation of the internal and external carotid arteries. The carotid sinus is a baroreceptor involved in blood pressure maintenance; the carotid body is an oxygen sensor or chemoreceptor, playing an important role in respiratory reflexes. The nerve to the carotid sinus (nerve of Hering) has a connection to the dorsal vagal nucleus that creates a pathway for glossopharyngeal detection of alterations in blood pressure and oxygen saturation, and vagal-mediated corrective responses.

The motor efferents originate in the rostral nucleus ambiguus in the medulla, exit the brainstem dorsolateral to the inferior olive, and exit the skull via the jugular foramen in the temporal bone, while traversing the petrosal ganglion without synapsing. After exiting the jugular foramen, glossopharyngeal branches innervate the stylopharyngeus muscle and the superior pharyngeal constrictors.

The glossopharyngeal nerve carries efferent preganglionic fibers from the brainstem inferior salivatory nucleus via the main glossopharyngeal trunk. The tympanic nerve branch (Jacobson nerve) comes off of the main trunk at the jugular foramen and carries parasympathetic information to the otic ganglion via the lesser superficial petrosal nerve. Postganglionic fibers travel from the otic ganglion in the auriculotemporal nerve, a branch of the trigeminal nerve, to reach the parotid gland.

### Clinical Lesions

#### Glossopharyngeal Palsy Appearance

Glossopharyngeal dysfunction results in loss of the gag reflex ipsilateral to the lesion and poor pharyngeal elevation with speaking and swallowing, which appears clinically as dysarthria and dysphagia. Taste in the posterior tongue may be impaired, and patients may complain of a dry mouth from decreased salivary secretory functions.

#### Subarachnoid Space: Nerve Root

Glossopharyngeal neuralgia is characterized by paroxysmal severe episodes of unilateral stabbing pain in the tongue base, tonsilar fossa, pharynx, or middle ear. Pain is often triggered by oropharyngeal movements such as chewing, swallowing, or yawning. It may rarely be associated with syncope when simultaneous vascular compression of the glossopharyngeal and vagus nerve roots results in dysfunction of the glossopharyngeal-vagal reflex arc, with precipitation of bradycardia or asystole. Glossopharyngeal neuralgia is much less common than trigeminal neuralgia, but like trigeminal neuralgia, neurovascular compression of the nerve root is likely a common etiology, and surgical neurovascular decompression or rhizotomy may result in symptom relief (see Chapter 102) (Kandan et al., 2010; Rey-Dios and Cohen-Gadol, 2013) (for treatments, see Table 103.2).

Compressive lesions of the nerve root, such as cerebellopontine angle neoplasms or Chiari I malformations, may also cause glossopharyngeal neuralgia. Brainstem pathology, such as tumor and demyelination, is an infrequent cause. *Eagle syndrome* from compression of the glossopharyngeal nerve by an elongated styloid process or ossified stylohyoid ligament may mimic glossopharyngeal neuralgia, but the pain tends to be more persistent and dull in nature and accompanied by a foreign body sensation in the throat and dysphagia (Badhey et al., 2017; Ferreira et al., 2014; Ledesma-Montes et al., 2018; see Table 103.1).

#### Petrosal Ganglion and Jugular Foramen

Neoplasia, blunt and penetrating trauma, inflammation, infection (especially VZV), and internal carotid artery dissections may affect glossopharyngeal function at the jugular foramen. *Vernet syndrome* is a pure jugular foramen syndrome with involvement of the glossopharyngeal, vagus, and spinal accessory nerves (Ferreira et al., 2018; see Table 103.1). Since the jugular foramen is in close proximity to the hypoglossal canal that houses the hypoglossal nerve, simultaneous involvement of cranial nerves IX through XII is not uncommon. When accompanied by Horner syndrome from sympathetic involvement, the combination of cranial nerves IX through XII is called *Villaret syndrome* (posterior retropharyngeal syndrome) and is most commonly due to internal carotid artery dissection or neoplasm (Okpala et al., 2014; see Table 103.1). In the absence of Horner syndrome, the combination of cranial nerves IX through XII is called *Collet-Sicard syndrome* (see Table 103.1), which may occur with carotid dissection, jugular vein thrombosis, neoplasm, inflammation, or trauma (Handley et al., 2010; Kohli and Gandotra, 2011; Lee et al., 2017).

Glomus jugulare tumors of the jugular bulb are the most common tumors in the jugular foramen (Fayad et al., 2010). They are slow-growing, hypervascular, benign paragangliomas that present with a neck mass, pulsatile tinnitus, lower cranial nerve dysfunction, and hearing loss from extension into the middle ear (Carlson et al., 2015; Shapiro et al., 2018). Examination of the lower cranial nerves reveals the deficits to be strictly unilateral, and skull-base imaging reveals the lesion. Glomus tumors may also occur in the middle ear tympanic plexus, on the vagus nerve, and in the carotid body. Schwannomas, meningiomas, and metastases also occur in the jugular foramen. Glossopharyngeal schwannomas more often present with vestibulocochlear dysfunction than glossopharyngeal involvement (Vorasubin et al., 2009).

### Glossopharyngeal Nerve Branches

Direct pressure or stretch injury of the branches may occur from surgical intervention, particularly with suspension laryngoscopy and tonsillectomy (Ford and Cruz, 2004). Postoperative taste changes and impaired swallowing are usually transient. *Reflex otalgia*, or referred middle ear pain, occurs with oropharyngeal neoplasms owing to the anatomical neural connections between the oropharyngeal and tympanic branches. It is generally a poor prognostic sign that increases the likelihood of tumor recurrence after treatment (Thoeny et al., 2004). Syncope in a patient with a history of head and neck cancer may be an ominous harbinger of recurrent disease. *Carotid hypersensitivity syndrome* (syncope provoked by carotid massage), *glossopharyngeal neuralgia with syncope*, and *parapharyngeal space-lesion syncope syndrome* (syncope in the absence of neuralgia or carotid massage) are all occasionally seen from focal neoplastic infiltration of the glossopharyngeal nerve and the glossopharyngeal-vagal reflex arc.

## VAGUS NERVE (CRANIAL NERVE X)

### Anatomy

The vagus nerve contains afferent gustatory, afferent sensory, efferent motor, and parasympathetic fibers. The vagus nerve innervates taste buds in the epiglottis. Unipolar vagus neurons with cell bodies in the inferior (nodose) ganglion of the vagus nerve, at the jugular foramen in the base of the temporal bone, carry taste information from the taste buds to the ganglion, and then proximally into the brainstem solitary tract and rostral solitary (or gustatory) nucleus in the rostral medulla. Afferent sensory information from the larynx, trachea, bronchi, esophagus, stomach, intestines, colon, and aortic sinus and bulb travels in the vagus nerve via the inferior (nodose) ganglion. Within the brainstem, the sensory information is carried to the solitary nucleus. Afferent sensory information from the external ear and meatus travels in the vagus nerve via the superior (jugular) ganglion of the vagus nerve and proximally into the brainstem caudal spinal trigeminal nucleus.

The motor efferents originate in the nucleus ambiguus and dorsal motor nucleus in the medulla, exit the brainstem laterally, and exit the skull via the jugular foramen in the temporal bone while traversing the nodose ganglion without synapsing. After exiting the jugular foramen, branches innervate the palatal constrictors and intrinsic laryngeal muscles. Pharyngeal innervation by the vagal and glossopharyngeal nerves provides the efferent limb of the gag reflex, with the afferent limb provided by glossopharyngeal sensory fibers to the pharynx. The superior laryngeal branch exits the main vagus trunk just inferior to the nodose ganglion, and the inferior laryngeal branch (recurrent laryngeal nerve) exits the main trunk in the thorax. The course of the left and right recurrent laryngeal nerves differs, with the right nerve crossing under the right subclavian artery and ascending in the neck and the left nerve wrapping under the aorta to ascend more vertically. Both nerves enter the larynx.

The vagus nerve carries efferent preganglionic fibers from the nucleus ambiguus and dorsal motor nucleus to the cardiac, pulmonary, esophageal, gastric, mesenteric, and myenteric plexi. The parasympathetic fibers descend in the neck, with motor and sensory fibers in the main vagus trunk within the carotid sheath, which also contains the internal jugular vein and internal carotid artery.

### Clinical Lesions

#### Vagus Palsy Appearance

Vagus dysfunction results in unilateral loss of pharyngeal and laryngeal sensation, unilateral loss of sensation in the external ear, dysphagia, hoarseness of the voice, unilateral paralysis of the uvula and soft palate, and deviation of the uvula contralateral to the lesion. Otolaryngological examination reveals unilateral paralysis of the vocal cords.

#### Vagus Nucleus

Nuclear lesions may result from ischemia, hemorrhage, infectious and noninfectious inflammation, neoplasm, and demyelination (Kremer et al., 2013; Oks et al., 2018). *Wallenberg syndrome* from lateral medullary ischemia affects the nucleus ambiguus, causing dysphagia with bilateral impairment of pharyngeal and laryngeal function, possibly explained by involvement of bilateral cortical prenuclear inputs into each nucleus (Oshima et al., 2013; see Table 103.1). Swallowing impairment is accompanied by hoarseness of the voice, decreased gag reflex, ipsilateral facial sensory disturbances from trigeminal involvement, limb ataxia from cerebellar peduncle involvement, ipsilateral Horner syndrome, contralateral body impaired pain and temperature sensation from spinothalamic tract involvement, and vertigo from vestibular involvement. *Opalski syndrome* is a variant of the lateral medullary syndrome accompanied by ipsilateral hemiparesis due to extension of the lesion into the cervical spinal cord, affecting corticospinal fibers caudal to the pyramidal decussation (Kk et al., 2014). Ipsilateral palatolaryngeal paresis in combination with contralateral hemiparesis (*Avellis syndrome*) occurs most commonly from medullary pathology, although the initial description of the syndrome was secondary to extramedullary vagus nerve involvement, presumably from a large lesion causing ventral brainstem compression with hemiparesis (see Table 103.1). Nuclear involvement in multisystem atrophy and Lewy body disease may explain the cardiovagal failure and gastrointestinal symptoms in these diseases (Benarroch et al., 2006). Evidence suggests the pathological hallmark of Parkinson disease—Lewy bodies—initially develop in the enteric nervous system and propagate in a retrograde fashion to the central nervous system via the dorsal motor nucleus of the vagus nerve (Uemura et al., 2018). Motor neurons in the nucleus ambiguus are preferentially affected in amyotrophic lateral sclerosis.

#### Nodose Ganglion and Jugular Foramen

Neoplasm, blunt and penetrating trauma, inflammation, infection (especially VZV), and internal carotid artery dissection may affect vagus function at the jugular foramen. *Vernet syndrome* is a pure jugular foramen syndrome with involvement of the glossopharyngeal, vagus, and spinal accessory nerves (Ferreira et al., 2018) (see Table 103.1). Simultaneous involvement of cranial nerves IX through XII is common because of the proximity of the jugular foramen and hypoglossal canal. As noted earlier, when accompanied by Horner syndrome, the combination of cranial nerves IX through XII is called *Villaret syndrome* (posterior retropharyngeal syndrome). In the absence of Horner syndrome, the combination of cranial nerves IX through XII is called *Collet-Sicard syndrome*. The combination of vagus and hypoglossal nerve lesions is called *Tapia syndrome* (see Table 103.1), although the original description was of a patient with a brainstem lesion and contralateral hemiparesis. Airway manipulation and vertebral dissection may cause this syndrome (Al-Sihan et al., 2011; Gevorgyan and Nedzelski, 2013).

Glomus jugulare tumors of the jugular bulb were described earlier in this chapter in the section on Glossopharyngeal Nerve (Cranial Nerve IX), Petrosal Ganglion and Jugular Foramen.

### Vagus Nerve Branches

Direct pressure or stretch injury of the branches may occur from surgical intervention, particularly recurrent laryngeal nerve injury with thyroid or esophageal surgery, or vagus nerve stimulator placement for the treatment of epilepsy or refractory depression. Peripheral branches may be affected by herpes zoster, paragangliomas, thoracic lymphadenopathy, and neoplasms. Referred ear pain may occur with chest neoplasms, owing to direct infiltration or compression of nerve branches connected via the trigeminal nuclear system to sensory vagus nerve branches to the ear. Peripheral branch involvement in Parkinson disease, especially of the superior laryngeal nerve, may explain the dysphagia often experienced by these patients (Mu et al., 2013).

## SPINAL ACCESSORY NERVE (CRANIAL NERVE XI)

### Anatomy

The spinal accessory nucleus is located in the dorsolateral ventral horn of the cervical spinal cord. Motor neurons from this nucleus exit the cervical cord as distinct nerve rootlets that converge and ascend through the foramen magnum to form the main trunk of the spinal accessory nerve, which exits the cranium via the jugular foramen with the glossopharyngeal and vagus nerves (Fig. 103.11). After exiting the jugular foramen, nerve branches innervate the ipsilateral sternocleidomastoid and trapezius muscles. Contralateral epileptic head turning and sternocleidomastoid function following hemispheric strokes indicate that each cerebral hemisphere innervates the ipsilateral sternocleidomastoid muscle, seemingly after a double decussation in the brainstem.

According to classic anatomical teaching, fibers originating in the caudal nucleus ambiguus travel through a cranial accessory branch to join the spinal accessory branch as it travels through the jugular foramen. These cranial accessory fibers then join the vagus nerve to innervate palatal and laryngeal muscles. Some anatomical studies call into question the existence of this cranial branch, though a recent cadaver study demonstrated the existence of the cranial branch in the majority of humans (Tubbs et al., 2014).

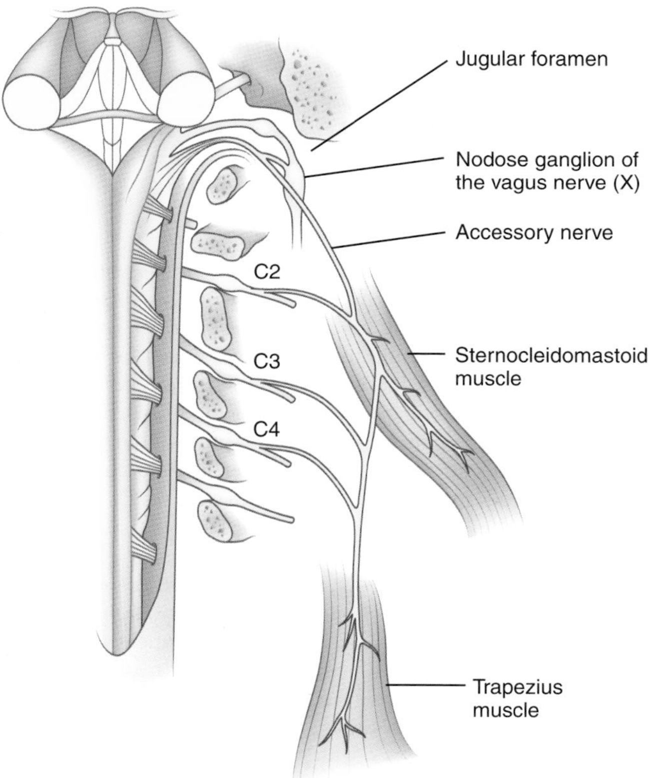


**Fig. 103.11** Spinal Accessory Nerve Course.

Afferent proprioceptive sensory information from the sternocleidomastoid and trapezius travels in the spinal accessory nerve branches via unipolar neurons with cell bodies in the cervical dorsal root ganglia.

### Clinical Lesions

#### Spinal Accessory Palsy Appearance

Spinal accessory nerve dysfunction results in weakness of contralateral head turning and ipsilateral shoulder elevation. Unilateral atrophy of the sternocleidomastoid and trapezius occurs with chronic lesions (eFig. 103.12). Scapular winging with active external shoulder rotation may be seen (Chan and Hems, 2006). Pain in the neck or shoulder is common.

#### Spinal Accessory Nucleus

Amyotrophic lateral sclerosis preferentially involves the spinal accessory and other motor neurons in the ventral horns of the spinal cord. Intrinsic spinal cord pathology such as neoplasm or syrinx may affect these motor neurons in combination with other spinal tracts.

#### Jugular Foramen

Vernet, Villaret, and Collet-Sicard syndromes are described earlier and in Table 103.1.

#### Spinal Accessory Nerve Branches

Iatrogenic injury during lymph node biopsy or dissection for head and neck cancers is the most common cause of spinal accessory nerve dysfunction (Camp and Birch, 2011). Variations in individual branch anatomy make the nerve particularly prone to difficult identification and traction or ischemic injury. Involvement of the dominant arm, scapular winging, and limited arm elevation are poor prognostic indicators. Spinal accessory branches may be intentionally injured in treatment for cervical dystonia. Trauma and isolated peripheral neoplasms occur rarely.

## HYPOGLOSSAL NERVE (CRANIAL NERVE XII)

### Anatomy

The hypoglossal nucleus is located in the medial medulla. Supranuclear inputs are generally considered to be bilateral and symmetrical, but evaluation of tongue weakness in patients with hemispheric strokes suggests asymmetry with a greater contralateral innervation. Motor neurons emerge from the ventral surface of the nucleus, forming the hypoglossal fasciculus that traverses the brainstem ventrolaterally, to exit as rootlets anterior to the inferior olive. The hypoglossal nerve exits the skull via the hypoglossal canal in the occipital condyle of the occipital bone. It then descends near the extracranial internal carotid artery, ultimately branching to innervate the styloglossus, hypoglossus, and intrinsic tongue muscles (Fig. 103.13). Fibers from cervical motor nerve roots form the ansa cervicalis, which has multiple connections with the hypoglossal nerve.

### Clinical Lesions

#### Hypoglossal Palsy Appearance

Hypoglossal nerve dysfunction results in atrophy and fasciculation of the ipsilateral tongue muscles and ipsilateral deviation of the tongue upon protrusion from the mouth (Stino et al., 2016; Yu et al., 2016; Fig. 103.14).

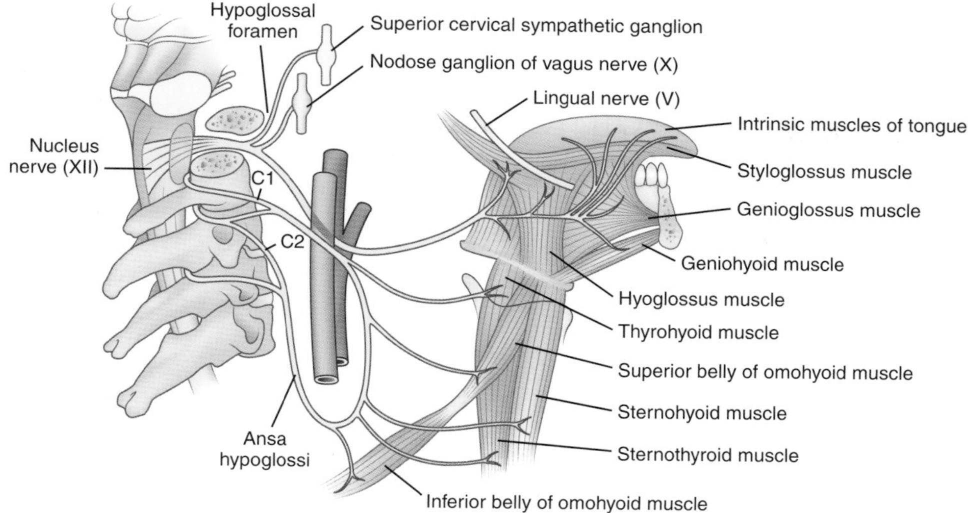


**Fig. 103.13** Hypoglossal Nerve Course.

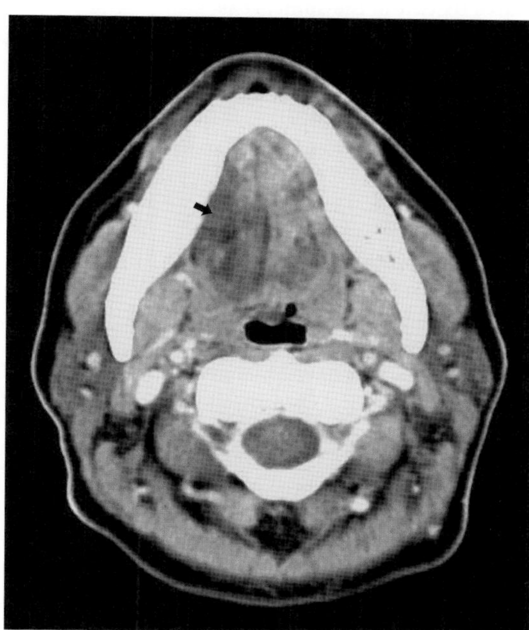

**Fig. 103.14** Axial Computed Tomography Scan Through Tongue in Patient with Right Hypoglossal Palsy. Note tongue atrophy on right side *(black arrow)*. (*Courtesy Miral Jhaveri, MD.*)

## Hypoglossal Nucleus and Fasciculus

The *medial medullary syndrome of Dejerine* consists of ipsilateral tongue weakness, contralateral hemiplegia from pyramidal tract involvement, and contralateral hemisensory loss from medial lemniscal involvement (see Table 103.1). More common than isolated medial medullary syndrome is the *hemi-medullary syndrome of Babinski-Nageotte* that combines the Dejerine and Wallenberg syndromes with deficits of swallowing impairment, hoarseness of the voice, decreased gag reflex, facial pain, limb ataxia, Horner syndrome, contralateral hemibody impaired pain and temperature sensation, and vertigo (see Table 103.1). As with the other cranial nerves, there are multiple etiologies of these brainstem syndromes. Although neurovascular compression as the hypoglossal nerve roots exit the brainstem is not classically considered a cause of hypoglossal palsy, case reports suggest this as a diagnostic possibility (Osburn et al., 2010; Straube and Linn, 2008).

## Hypoglossal Canal

Neoplasm, blunt and penetrating trauma with occipital condyle fractures, inflammation, and post-radiation injury may affect hypoglossal function at the hypoglossal canal. Since the hypoglossal canal is in close proximity to the jugular foramen, simultaneous involvement of cranial nerves IX through XII is not uncommon. Villaret, Collet-Sicard, and Tapia syndromes are described earlier and in Table 103.1.

## Hypoglossal Peripheral Branches

Mechanisms of hypoglossal branch disease are similar to those in the hypoglossal canal. Hypoglossal dysfunction is an ominous clinical finding; 50% of cases are caused by neoplasm, typically malignant. Nasopharyngeal carcinoma and skull-based metastatic disease are among the most common malignancies affecting the hypoglossal nerve. The combination of hypoglossal dysfunction with abducens palsy is highly suggestive of an aggressive clival malignancy. Retropharyngeal mass lesions other than malignancy include granulomatous inflammation and abscess. Hypoglossal palsy may be the presenting manifestation of carotid artery dissection or aneurysm and may occur iatrogenically after carotid endarterectomy (Jurkiewicz et al., 2019).

*The complete reference list is available online at https://expertconsult.inkling.com/.* 

104

# Disorders of Bones, Joints, Ligaments, and Meninges

*Christopher D. Geiger, Michael W. Devereaux, David Hart*

## OUTLINE



The bones, joints, ligaments, and meninges that support and protect the tissues of the nervous system can give rise to numerous illnesses that affect the nervous system. These disorders sometimes border on other medical disciplines unfamiliar to the neurologist and hence can be enigmatic or difficult to diagnose. They may involve cognitive functions, disrupt cerebrospinal fluid (CSF) flow dynamics, or slowly compress and distort central and peripheral neural structures. They have a mixture of genetic, developmental, traumatic, degenerative, infectious, and inflammatory mechanisms. For the clinical neurologist, awareness greatly strengthens diagnostic skill, therefore this chapter reviews many of these disorders. Chapters of overlapping interest include Chapters 27, 33, 58, 85, 89.

For an expanded version of this chapter that includes figures and boxes that are only available online, please visit http://www.expertconsult.com.

## HERITABLE DISORDERS OF CONNECTIVE TISSUE

Heritable disorders involving the major connective tissues of the body are among the most common human genetic diseases. The focus will be on those disorders that have neurological impact (Box 104.1). Many of these are being better understood at a molecular level: osteogenesis imperfecta (OI), Ehlers-Danlos syndrome (EDS), chondrodysplasias, and Marfan syndrome, to name a few.

Classifications of heritable disorders of connective tissue can rely on pattern of inheritance, clinical features, anatomical pattern, or known molecular defects. To date, genetic or molecular classification is not always helpful clinically because there are significant genotype-to-phenotype inconsistencies, testing is not widely available, and our understanding of many disorders is incomplete. Connective tissues contain

**BOX 104.1 Classification of Hereditary Disorders of Connective Tissue**

**Skeletal (Primarily Type I Collagen)**
Osteogenesis imperfecta

**Dermis, Tendons, and Ligaments (Primarily Type I Collagen)**
Hypermobile Ehlers-Danlos syndrome (type III)
Classic Ehlers-Danlos syndrome (type I)
Vascular Ehlers-Danlos syndrome

**Cartilage (Primarily Fibrils of Type II Collagen, Proteoglycans)**
Chondrodysplasias
Achondroplasia
Pseudoachondroplasia
Stickler syndrome
Craniosynostosis (syndromic)

**Skeletal, Cardiovascular, and Eye (Type I and Type III Collagen, Fibrillin, Elastin)**
Marfan syndrome
MASS phenotype (mitral valve prolapse, aortic dilation, skin, and skeletal features)
Loeys-Dietz syndrome
Beals syndrome (congenital contractual arachnodactyly)
Dermal/epidermal (keratin, laminin, type VII collagen, plectin, integrin)
Epidermolysis bullosa
Basal lamina (type IV collagen, laminin, nidogen)
Alport syndrome

a wide range of complex macromolecules assembled in the extracellular matrix. There are at least 28 different types of collagen in bone, skin cartilage, tendons, and ligaments. Other molecules including fibrillin, elastin, proteoglycans, fibronectin, hyaluronate, osteonectin, and osteocalcin contribute to tensile strength and elasticity. Forces that control the three-dimensional organization of these components remain largely unknown. In growth and development, collagen fibrils in all these supporting tissues undergo repeated synthesis, degradation, and resynthesis. Nutrition, gravitational forces, trauma, other physical stresses, endocrine factors (such as glucocorticoids), and inflammation all modify these tissues (Prockop and Czarny-Ratajczak, 2008).

## Osteogenesis Imperfecta

The various types of OI or "brittle bone disease" (incidence ≈1:20,000 births) are inherited, predominantly autosomal-dominant connective tissue disorders caused by gene mutations that affect type 1 collagen. Rare recessive inheritance has been reported (Pyott et al., 2013). This disorder is characterized by brittle osteopenic bones and recurrent fractures (Basel and Steiner, 2009). As many as nine types are known, with wide variations in severity and associated findings such as short stature, blue sclera, progressive hearing loss, poor dentition, scoliosis, and skeletal abnormalities (osteopenia, irregular ossification, multiple fractures). Laboratory studies show a molecular defect in type I procollagen in two-thirds of patients.

Potential neurological complications of OI include communicating hydrocephalus, basilar invagination, macrocephaly, kyphoscoliosis, skull fractures, subdural hematomas, and epilepsy. The basilar invagination can lead to brainstem compression (Menezes, 2008). Spinal cord compression, syringomyelia, Chiari I malformation, Dandy-Walker cysts, leptomeningeal cysts, microcephalus, or central nervous system (CNS) tumors are rarer associations. Progressive, variably conductive and sensorineural hearing loss usually begins in the second decade and affects more than half of patients by age 30 years. Joint laxity, indistinguishable from that of EDS, can result in permanent dislocations. Rarely, OI is complicated by cervical artery dissection resulting from fragility of large blood vessels (Grond-Ginsbach and Debette, 2009). Aortic regurgitation, floppy mitral valves, and mitral incompetence can lead to cerebrovascular complications. For unknown reasons, some patients develop a hypermetabolic state with elevated serum thyroxine levels, hyperthermia, and excessive sweating. Wide phenotypic variation is characteristic and appears to be related to the abundance of over 900 unique mutations in the type I procollagen *COL1A1* and *COL1A2* genes, combined with undefined chance events during embryonic and fetal development (Prockop and Czarny-Ratajczak, 2008).

Treatment is symptomatic and tailored to the severity of symptoms, though women require special attention during pregnancy and after menopause when the risk of fractures increases. More severely affected children require more comprehensive physical therapy and orthopedic management. For severe hearing loss, stapedectomy or cochlear implant may prove helpful. Neurological complications relating to potential brainstem and spinal compression require appropriate attention. Oral or intravenous bisphosphonates are commonly prescribed to individuals with OI. Although studies demonstrate increased bone mineral density as a result, it is unclear whether bisphosphonates improve clinical status (Dwan et al., 2016).

## Ehlers-Danlos Syndrome

The EDSs are a rare group of disorders with an overall frequency of 1:5000. They are a clinically and genetically heterogeneous group of inherited connective tissue disorders characterized by joint hypermobility, skin hyperextensibility and tissue fragility. The Villefranche nosology in 1998 identified 6 EDS subtypes based on clinical features, mode of inheritance, and biochemical and genetic findings (Malfait et al., 2017). In 2017 the EDS Consortium revised the classification to now include 13 subtypes. However, given the vast genetic heterogeneity and phenotypic variability of the subtypes and the clinical overlap between the subtypes, a definitive diagnosis of all EDS subtypes (except for the hypermobile subtype) relies on identification of the causative genetic variant (Malfait et al., 2017).

Of importance is that many of these subtypes can include neurological features that may lead a patient to a neurologist for evaluation before a diagnosis of EDS has been established. Neurological features include a number of neuromuscular symptoms such as weakness, hypotonia, myalgia, and paresthesia (Voermans et al., 2009). Uncommon neuromuscular disorders include axonal polyneuropathy and compression neuropathies. In addition, skeletal disorders include cranial cervical instability and scoliosis. Postural orthostatic hypotension (POTS) may occur. Any of the above symptoms/signs coupled with joint hypermobility, a feature present to a greater or lesser degree in most subtypes, and skin changes as noted above, should raise the suspicion for EDS. The Beighton joint flexibility score is a useful screening tool for the degree of joint mobility (Table 104.1)

The differential diagnosis includes Marfan syndrome and OI. If EDS is suspected, referral to a clinical geneticist is essential.

## Chondrodysplasias

Chondrodysplasias, also referred to as *skeletal dysplasias*, are heritable skeletal disorders characterized by dwarfism and abnormal body proportions. These are the most common cause of abnormally short stature. This category also includes some patients with craniosynostosis (see later discussion) who have cranial and facial malformations associated with ocular change and cleft palate but normal stature and body proportions; this is more common in the more severe

**TABLE 104.1 The Beighton Score**

| | | | |
|---|---|---|---|
| Thumb to forearm | ☐ Right | | ☐ Left |
| Bending little fingers back to 90 degrees or more | ☐ Right | | ☐ Left |
| Elbows hyperextend to 10 degrees or more (i.e., bend backwards 10 degrees or more in the wrong direction) | ☐ Right | | ☐ Left |
| Knees hyperextend to 10 degrees or more (i.e., bend backwards 10 degrees or more in the wrong direction) | ☐ Right | | ☐ Left |
| Palms flat to floor with legs straight | ☐ Able | *or* | ☐ By history |
| Total score | | | |

Score 1 point for each positive indicator of hypermobility. Maximum score is 9 points; a score of 4 or more is indicative of hypermobility. *Adapted from Beighton, P.H., Horan, F., 1969. Orthopedic aspects of the Ehlers-Danlos syndrome. J Bone Joint Surg. Br. 51, 444–453.*

**BOX 104.2 Neurological Complications of Achondroplasia**

Macrocrania, with or without hydrocephalus
Foramen magnum abnormalities with cervicomedullary compression
Respiratory disturbances, including sleep apnea and sudden infant death syndrome
Syringomyelia, diastematomyelia
Spinal stenosis with spinal cord or nerve root compression
Infantile hypotonia
Cortical atrophy
Atlantoaxial subluxation
Psychomotor delay (most have normal intelligence)

*Adapted with permission from Ruiz-Garcia, M., Tovar-Baudin, A., Del Castillo-Ruiz, V., et al., 1997. Early detection of neurological manifestations in achondroplasia. Childs Nerv. Syst. 13, 208–213.*

chondrodysplasias. Many patients develop premature degenerative joint disease. Mild chondrodysplasias in adults may be difficult to differentiate from primary generalized osteoarthritis.

They encompass over 400 disorders, which vary from mild distortions of cartilaginous structures and the eye to severe malformations that are fatal in early life (Bonafe, 2015). A number are unique and identified by eponyms based on isolated case reports. Among the features of these syndromes are high forehead, hypoplastic facies, cleft palate, short extremities (with gross distortions of the epiphyses, metaphyses, and joint surfaces), cataracts, degeneration of the vitreous, and retinal detachment. We will highlight those types most prone to neurological complications.

### Achondroplasia

Achondroplasia is an autosomal dominant disorder of endochondral bone formation. A specific mutation of a fibroblast growth factor receptor gene (*FGFR3*) is present in over 90% of patients. It is the most common skeletal dysplasia in humans. Approximately three-fourths of cases occur because of spontaneous new mutations. The syndrome is the most common cause of short-limbed dwarfism accompanied by macrocephaly and dysplasias of the metaphyses of long bones. The mutant genotype has complete penetrance. The diagnosis can be confirmed by pathognomonic radiographic changes and/or by deoxyribonucleic acid (DNA) testing. Neurological complications associated with achondroplasia are common (Box 104.2). Young achondroplastic children should be observed for complications such as hydrocephalus, compression at the foramen magnum, thoracolumbar kyphosis, and sleep apnea. Neurological complications of spinal stenosis tend to occur later in life.

### Pseudoachondroplasia

Pseudoachondroplasia, another autosomal dominant cause of short stature, is due to gene mutations for the cartilage oligomeric matrix protein (COMP), a protein that interacts with both collagens and proteoglycans in cartilage. Patients have leg deformities, short digits, vertebral anomalies, and proclivity to develop severe osteoarthritis. However, neurological complications are less common than in true achondroplasia. Nonetheless, patients are at risk for atlantoaxial (AA) dislocation. Children who carry both the achondroplasia and pseudoachondroplasia mutations have been reported, with early onset of neurological complications from lumbar or foramen magnum stenosis.

## Marfan Syndrome

Marfan syndrome is an autosomal dominant disorder of fibrous connective tissue with variable penetrance and variation of phenotypic expression; its most prominent features affect the skeleton, heart, great vessels, and eye. More than 90% of patients have a mutation in the *fibrillin-1* gene. Fibrillin-1 is an important matrix component of both elastic and nonelastic tissues. The classic patient is tall with inordinately long limbs and digits. Other skeletal changes are anterior chest deformity, scoliosis, thoracic lordosis, high arched palate with crowded teeth, and some ligamentous laxity. Ocular problems include myopia, flat corneas, and ectopia lentis. The major life-threatening problem is aortic aneurysm or dissection; aortic and mitral valves can also be affected. Case reports link Marfan syndrome to intracranial vascular abnormalities such as arterial dissections, giant aneurysms, or hemifacial spasm associated with vascular compression of the facial nerve. However, aneurysms or dissections are rare in patients with Marfan syndrome, and their highest risk of stroke is from cardiogenic emboli, especially if they have prosthetic heart valves or atrial fibrillation (Wityk et al., 2002). Patients with Marfan syndrome can have sleep apnea, possibly secondary to their skeletal deformities.

*Dural ectasia*, dilation of the caudal thecal sac, occurs in 90% of patients with Marfan syndrome and is a major diagnostic criterion. Ectasia varies in severity, increases with age, and can cause lumbar radiculopathy. Leakage from ectatic dura can cause intracranial hypotension. Case reports link Marfan syndrome to Chiari I malformation (CM-I). It is not clear whether these patients had classic CM-I or tonsillar herniation secondary to CSF hypotension. Patients can have axonal neuropathy or mild myopathy.

Many patients with Marfan-like features have neither Marfan syndrome nor any other currently identified mutations. These patients are sometimes labeled as having *MASS syndrome* (mitral valve, aorta, skeletal, and skin involvement) and vary widely in severity of manifestations (Loeys et al., 2010). A few examples of Marfan-like syndromes of neurological import are:

1. Homocystinuria, a group of autosomal recessive disorders that can cause marfanoid skeletal changes, myopia, and lens ectopia. It is important to distinguish homocystinuria from Marfan syndrome, since the former can cause mental retardation and hypercoagulability leading to strokes and because it can be treated with vitamin $B_6$, folate, and vitamin $B_{12}$.
2. Loeys-Dietz aneurysm syndrome is similar to Marfan syndrome in skeletal and aortic manifestations but does not have lens ectopia and is often associated with craniosynostosis. Neurological manifestations can include Chiari I malformation, hydrocephalus, and developmental delay. It is usually due to mutations in either *TGFB2* or the closely related *TGFB1* genes.

3. Shprintzen-Goldberg syndrome is also characterized by marfanoid features, normal lenses, and craniosynostosis. Neurological issues can include hypotonia, Chiari I malformation, developmental delay, mental retardation, and obstructive sleep apnea.
4. Beals syndrome (congenital contractural arachnodactyly [CCA]) can cause marfanoid features, joint contracture, and some features of OI. Like Marfan syndrome, it is autosomal dominant, but the mutated gene is for fibrillin-2 rather than fibrillin-1.

## CONGENITAL AND INHERITED CRANIOSPINAL MALFORMATIONS AND DEFORMITIES

Craniospinal malformations result from abnormalities of the bones of the skull and spinal column, connecting ligaments, or other soft tissues and may cause hydrocephalus, brain deformation, spinal cord compression, and syringobulbia or syringomyelia (Menezes, 1997). Many of these are congenital. Magnetic resonance imaging (MRI) and computed tomography (CT) scanning have improved the detection, understanding, and treatment of these anomalies.

### Craniosynostosis

Craniosynostosis is among the most common and relatively benign abnormalities, affecting about 1 in 2500 live births. It is caused by premature closure of one or more of the sutures of the skull bones. For babies who have abnormal skull shapes, CT scans can distinguish craniosynostosis from results of fetal head position, birth trauma, or positional plagiocephaly—flattened or misshapen areas on the head that may develop due to sleeping position. Fig. 104.1 illustrates the various types of craniosynostosis.

Craniosynostosis often occurs alone, but about 20% of cases are associated with syndromes affecting other parts of the body; the most common of these are Crouzon and Apert syndromes. However, there are over 150 syndromes associated with craniosynostosis, with considerable overlap of symptoms between them. Clinical evaluation by a geneticist may be necessary to determine the most appropriate diagnosis. Most patients with syndromic craniosynostosis appear to have a mutation in the related *FGFR2* gene. Genetic testing may be necessary to confirm the diagnosis of a specific syndrome. A family history of abnormal head shape can sometimes be found with genetic syndromes, though many syndromes are caused by de novo mutations.

### Occipitalization of the Atlas

*Occipitalization* or *assimilation of the atlas* refers to congenital partial or complete fusion of the atlas to the occiput (eFig. 104.2). The anterior arch of the atlas may fuse to the lower end of the clivus, or the posterior arch of the atlas may fuse to the occiput. The anomaly is often asymptomatic until early adult life but may become symptomatic sooner after trauma. Unilateral occipitalization of the atlas is one cause of torticollis in young children. The loss of movement between the occiput and atlas increases the stresses at the AA joint, predisposing it to gradual degeneration or traumatic dislocation. Patients with occipitalization of the atlas may have associated anomalies such as the Klippel-Feil anomaly, basilar impression, or Chiari malformation (Ghalue, 2007).

### Basilar Impression

*Basilar impression* or *invagination* refers to caudal settling of the foramen magnum onto the cervical spine, generally with encroachment of the odontoid process into the foramen magnum, often resulting in brainstem and/or upper cervical spinal cord compression. Several radiological lines (Chamberlain, McGregor, McRae, digastric) (eFig. 104.3) and measurements can be used to make the diagnosis. Congenital basilar impression may occur in isolation or may be associated with conditions such as achondroplasia, occipital dysplasia, Down syndrome, Hurler syndrome, Klippel-Feil anomaly, and cleidocranial dysplasia. Some instances of basilar impression are familial. The skeletal anomaly is often accompanied by anomalies of the neuraxis, including Chiari I or II malformation and syringomyelia (Milhorat et al., 2007). Basilar impression can cause compression of the brainstem (eFig. 104.4), the cerebellum, or (rarely) the vertebral artery, leading to vertebrobasilar ischemia. It is often asymptomatic, particularly when mild and unaccompanied by other anomalies.

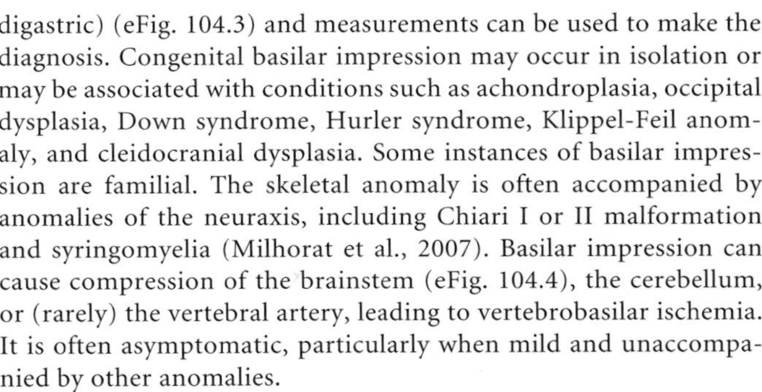

*Platybasia*, or flattening of the skull, refers to straightening of the angle between the clivus and the floor of the anterior fossa. It infrequently accompanies basilar impression and can also occur as an isolated radiographic finding without any adverse neurological consequences.

### Klippel-Feil Anomaly

Patients with the Klippel-Feil anomaly (congenital synostosis of the cervical vertebrae) (eFig. 104.5) typically have short necks, low hairlines, and limitation of cervical motion. The diagnosis is confirmed by radiographic demonstration of any two or more spontaneously fused cervical vertebrae. The condition is congenital, caused by failure of normal segmentation of the cervical vertebrae between the third and eighth weeks of fetal development. Although familial instances occur, most cases are isolated and idiopathic. The anomaly can cause direct nerve root, cervical spinal cord, and vertebral or spinal artery compression. Patients may have cervical ribs, predisposing them to thoracic outlet syndrome. Neck pain is common. Hearing loss is the most common cranial nerve symptom. Klippel-Feil syndrome is the anomaly most likely to cause *mirror movements* (synkinesia), particularly of the hands. Patients with mirror movements can have abnormal clefts or division of the spinal cord near the cervicomedullary junction, which can be detected by MRI (Royal et al., 2002). Patients with Klippel-Feil anomaly can have a wide variety of associated abnormalities of brain, spinal cord, or skeletal development, especially congenital scoliosis or Sprengel deformity with unilateral scapular elevation. Patients may develop hydrocephalus, syringomyelia, or syringobulbia. However, many patients with Klippel-Feil anomaly have no neurological symptoms or signs.

### Atlantoaxial Subluxation

Various congenital or acquired conditions can disrupt the integrity of the AA joint, leading to its dislocation (Box 104.3). In horizontal subluxation, C1 usually moves anteriorly to C2. The movement can be assessed by measuring the separation between the dens and the anterior arch of C1 on flexion, extension, and neutral radiographs; in adults, the separation should not exceed 3.5 mm. This measurement is known as the atlantodental interval (ADI). An alternative measurement is the PADI, or posterior atlantodental interval, which is measured between the posterior border of the dens and the anterior surface of the posterior arch of C1. This measurement, therefore, represents the "space available for the cord" and more accurately reflects the risk of neurological compromise than the ADI. Patients with horizontal AA joint subluxation are likely to compress their spinal cords if the diameter of the spinal canal at the level of the dens is less than 14 mm. This is unlikely to occur if the diameter is more than 17 mm. The actual relationship between the cord and the subluxing bones is best imaged with MRI, which should include flexion and extension views if plain radiographs show significant subluxation on flexion/extension imaging.

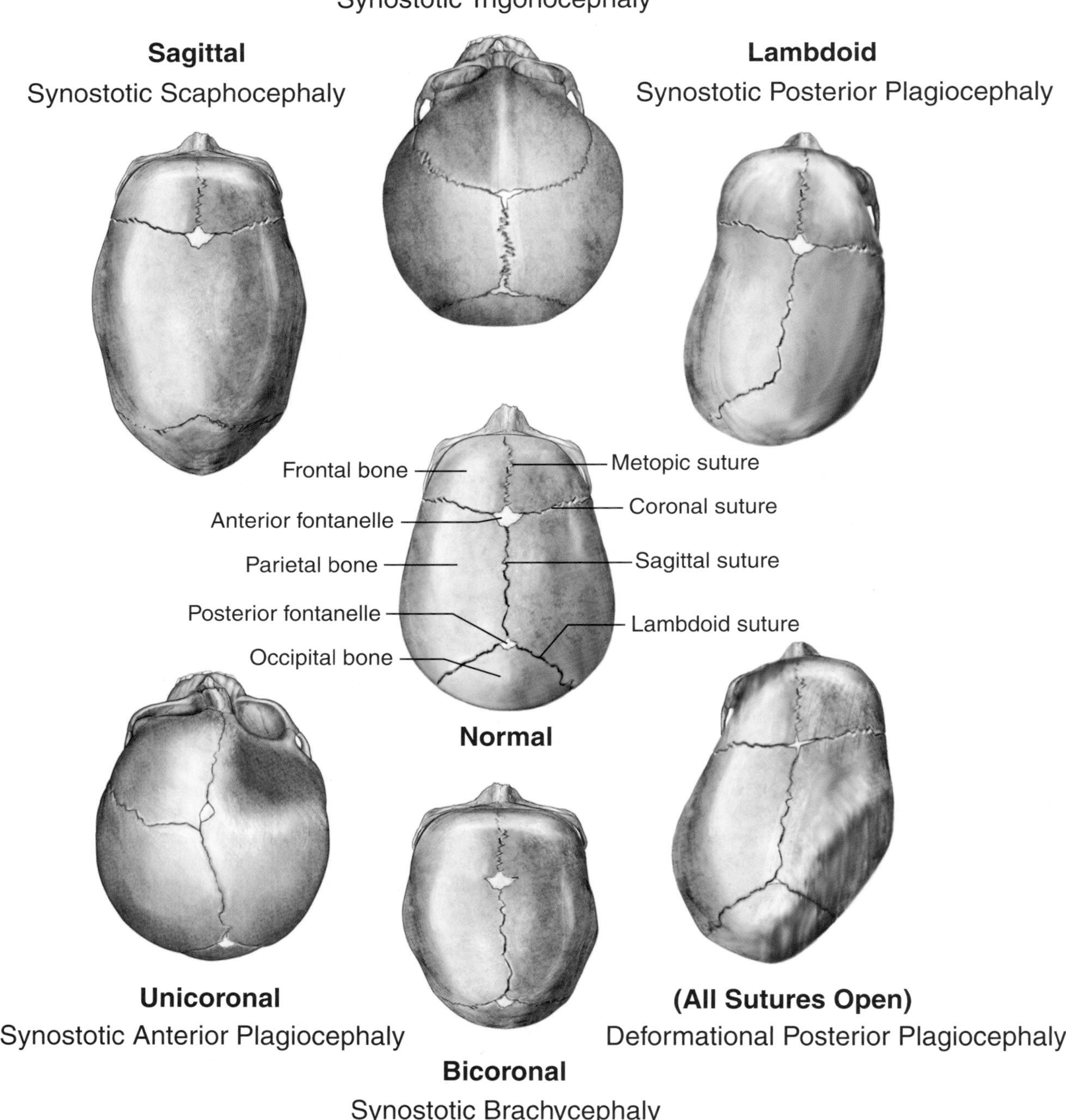


**Fig. 104.1** Craniosynostosis. *(Courtesy Han Wang, MD.)*

If MRI is contraindicated, then CT myelography is a consideration (Manczak et al., 2017). AA subluxation is very frequently encountered as part of the spectrum of cervical spine disease seen in rheumatoid arthritis (RA). The three cardinal cervical spine manifestations in RA are AA subluxation, subaxial spondylolisthesis (often multiple levels), and formation of retro-odontoid pannus. The pannus is an inflammatory mass of tissue that is often at least partially calcified, and can be very adherent to the dura, making its resection potentially very hazardous. The combination of AA subluxation and pannus formation can frequently result in significant myelopathy. Both conditions can be treated with surgical fusion of C1 and C2, which corrects the subluxation and also usually causes the pannus to resorb at least partially over several weeks to months. In patients with rapidly progressive myelopathy it might not be safe to wait for this process to alleviate the spinal

**BOX 104.3 Mechanisms of Atlantoaxial Subluxation**

I. Congenital
  A. Os odontoideum (failure of odontoid to fuse with body of axis)
    1. Isolated
    2. With connective tissue dysplasias (e.g., Down syndrome, pseudoachondroplasia, multiple epiphyseal dysplasia, spondyloepiphyseal dysplasia, Morquio disease, Klippel-Feil anomaly, Conradi syndrome)
  B. Hypoplastic dens
    1. With connective tissue dysplasia
    2. With incomplete segmentation (e.g., occipital assimilation of atlas, basilar invagination, incomplete segmentation of C2, C3, etc.)
  C. Other anomalies of C2 (e.g., bifid dens, tripartite dens with os apicale, agenesis of all or part of dens)
  D. Laxity of transverse atlantal ligament (e.g., Down syndrome)

II. Acquired
  A. Traumatic, acute or chronic un-united dens fracture
  B. Infectious
  C. Neoplastic (e.g., neurofibroma)
  D. Arthritic (e.g., rheumatoid arthritis, ankylosing spondylitis, renal amyloidosis)
  E. Bone disease (e.g., vitamin D-resistant rickets and others associated with basilar invagination)

cord compression, and direct resection of the pannus is required. This is a difficult operation, usually performed via transoral approach. (See also section below on RA.) Patients with congenital AA dislocation may have associated abnormalities such as Chiari I malformation or diastematomyelia. They can develop secondary syringomyelia. AA subluxation in patients with long-standing RA is a prime example of acquired abnormality of the AA joint and is discussed in more detail later in this chapter. Patients with AA subluxation may be asymptomatic, particularly if their spinal canal diameter is generous. However, they are vulnerable to spinal cord trauma during intubation or other neck motion under anesthesia, or as a result of a whiplash injury. Patients at risk for AA dislocation, such as those with Down syndrome or chronic RA, should have lateral flexion and extension cervical spine radiography performed before general anesthesia so the anesthesiologist can plan appropriate care during intubation.

## Chiari I Malformation

John Cleland first described a series of structural defects in the skull base and cerebellum in 1883. Hans Chiari classified the malformations into four types in 1891. Julius Arnold further expanded the definition of Chiari II malformations in 1894. In current usage, the terms Arnold-Chiari and Chiari malformations are often used interchangeably for all four types. Chiari malformations II, III, IV are discussed in the section on Spinal Dysraphism. In addition to the four classic types of Chiari malformations, several subtypes not in common use have been added: The Chiari 0 malformation and the Chiari 1.5 malformation (similar to CM-II, but without a cervical syrinx) (Schijman, 2004; Tubbs et al., 2001).

Chiari I malformation (CM-I) (Fig. 104.6), the most common type, is characterized by abnormally shaped cerebellar tonsils with resultant

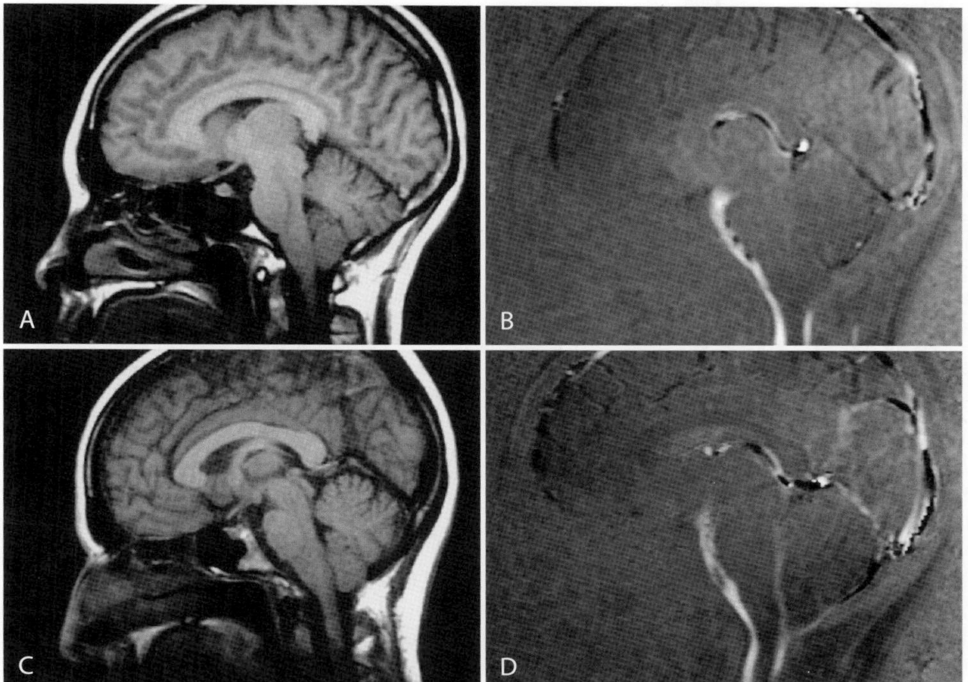


**Fig. 104.6** **A,** Sagittal magnetic resonance imaging (MRI) scan of a patient with Arnold-Chiari type I malformation. Midline T1-weighted image demonstrates low cerebellar tonsils, 8 mm below foramen magnum. **B,** MRI cerebrospinal fluid (CSF) flow study of same patient demonstrates diminished flow signal at cerebellar tonsils, indicative of CSF flow propagation abnormality. Note normal CSF flow signal below tonsils and anterior to brainstem. **C,** Sagittal MRI of a patient with low-lying cerebellar tonsils at 6 mm below foramen magnum. **D,** CSF flow study demonstrating normal flow signal at level of cerebellar tonsils, indicative of normal propagation of CSF flow through foramen magnum.

**TABLE 104.2 Summary of Posterior Cranial Fossa Morphology in Patients With Chiari Malformations**

| | Occipital Bone Size | PCFV | FM |
|---|---|---|---|
| CM-I/classic type | Small | Small | Small |
| CM-I/craniosynostosis | Small | Small | Small |
| CM-II/with myelodysplasia | Small | Small | Large |
| CM-I/tethered cord syndrome | Normal | Normal | Large |
| CM-I/cranial settling | Normal | Normal | Normal |
| CM-I/intracranial space-occupying lesions | Normal | Normal | Normal |
| CM-I/lumboperitoneal shunt | Normal | Normal | Normal |

*CM-I*, Chiari malformation type I; *CM-II*, Chiari malformation type II; *FM*, foramen magnum; *PCFV*, posterior cranial fossa volume.
*Adapted with permission from Milhorat, T.H., Nishikawa, M., Kula, R.W., et al., 2010. Mechanisms of cerebellar tonsil herniation in patients with Chiari malformations as guide to clinical management. Acta Neurochir. (Wien) 152, 1117–1127.*

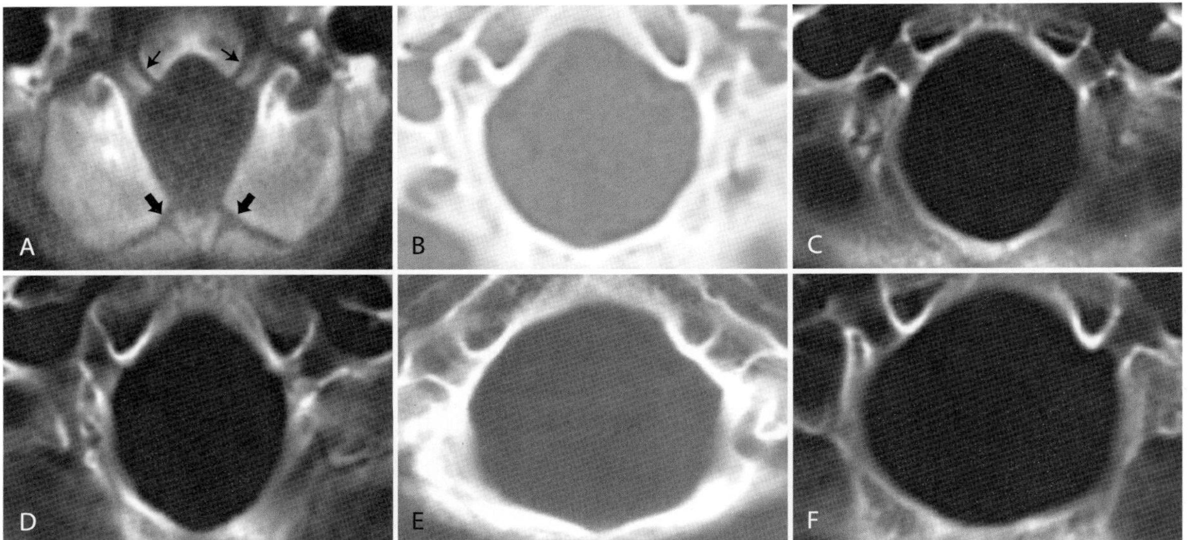


**Fig. 104.7 Morphometric Assessments of Foramen Magnum at Level of Superior Outlet Using Axial Computed Tomography Images. A,** Normal foramen magnum in 10-month-old male showing patent basi-exoccipital *(small arrows)* and exosupraoccipital synchondroses *(large arrows)*. **B,** Normal foramen magnum in 30-year-old female. **C,** Abnormally small foramen magnum in 28-year-old female with classical Chiari I malformation (CM-I). **D,** Abnormally small foramen magnum in 25-year-old female with CM-I and craniosynostosis (Crouzon syndrome). **E,** Abnormally large foramen magnum in 27-year-old female with CM-I and tethered cord syndrome. **F,** Abnormally large foramen magnum in 17-year-old male with CM-II. (*From Milhorat, T.H., Nishikawa, M., Kula, R.W., et al., 2010. Mechanisms of cerebellar tonsil herniation in patients with Chiari malformations as guide to clinical management. Acta Neurochir. [Wien] 152, 1117–1127.*)

tonsillar herniation through the foramen magnum (5 mm or more in young adults); this definition is anatomically precise, but can be confusing because there are many causes of abnormal tonsillar herniation that are not Chiari malformations. Classic CM-I is a congenital mesodermal malformation resulting in a hypoplastic posterior fossa, compressing neural tissue and forcing the cerebellar tonsils down through the foramen magnum. Distinguishing classic CM-I from other mechanisms of tonsillar herniation clarifies treatment despite overlapping clinical features (Milhorat et al., 2010). Other potential disorders causing tonsillar herniation that are unrelated to skull-base hypoplasia include hydrocephalus, intracranial mass lesions, CSF leaks, prolonged lumboperitoneal shunting, hereditary disorders of connective tissue associated with occipitoatlantoaxial joint instability and cranial settling, tethered cord syndrome, and miscellaneous conditions such as craniosynostosis, acromegaly, and Paget disease. Milhorat and colleagues have correlated measurements of the posterior cranial fossa with clinical findings in 752 patients with Chiari malformations (Milhorat et al., 2010; Table 104.2).

Patients with classic CM-I have a small posterior cranial fossa with constriction increasing below the *Twining's line*, which extends from the anterior tuberculum sellae to the internal occipital protuberance. The foramen magnum is constricted transversely and has reduced outlet area (Fig. 104.7). These findings suggest premature stenosis of the basi-exoccipital and exosupraoccipital synchondroses (see Fig. 104.7, *A*) which, if normal, would permit lateral expansion of the foramen magnum during somatic growth. Failure of the foramen magnum to expand normally during development may explain the conical shape of the posterior fossa in CM-I. Patients with achondroplasia can also have a stenosed foramen magnum and small posterior fossa, but the posterior fossa constriction is more generalized than in classic CM-I, suggesting an additional pathogenic mechanism in achondroplasia. Crouzon syndrome (see Fig. 104.7, *D*), Apert syndrome, nonsyndromic craniosynostosis,

**TABLE 104.3 Mechanisms of Cerebellar Tonsil Herniation**

| Cranial Constriction | Spinal Cord Tethering | Cranial Settling | Intracranial Hypertension | Intraspinal Hypotension |
|---|---|---|---|---|
| **"Squeeze down"** | **"Pull down"** | **"Shake down"** | **"Push down"** | **"Suck down"** |
| CM-I | Tethered cord syndrome | HDCT (e.g., EDS) | Hydrocephalus | Prolonged LPS |
| Craniosynostosis | CM-II | Posttraumatic CCI | Posterior fossa cysts, tumors | CSF leaks |
| Achondroplasia | | Osteogenesis imperfecta | Subdural hematoma | Dural ectasia |
| Acromegaly | | | Intracranial mass lesions | |
| Paget disease | | | | |

*CCI*, Craniocervical instability; *CM*, Chiari malformation; *CSF*, cerebrospinal fluid; *EDS*, Ehlers-Danlos syndrome; *HDCT*, hereditary disorders of connective tissue; *LPS*, lumbar peritoneal shunt.

*Adapted with permission from Milhorat, T.H., Nishikawa, M., Kula, R.W., et al., 2010. Mechanisms of cerebellar tonsil herniation in patients with Chiari malformations as guide to clinical management. Acta Neurochir. (Wien) 152, 1117–1127.*

**TABLE 104.4 Symptoms of Chiari I Malformation**

| Symptom | % of CM-I Patients (364) |
|---|---|
| Suboccipital headache (frequent retro-orbital component); exertional and postural accentuation | 81 |
| Ocular disturbances: floaters, blurring, photophobia, diplopia | 78 |
| Acoustic and vestibular complaints: dizziness/dysequilibrium, tinnitus | 74 |
| Dysesthesias: tenderness, numbness/tingling, burning | 59 |
| Chronic fatigue | 58 |
| Bulbar and coordinative problems: | 52 |
| • Dysphagia/dysarthria, sleep apnea | |
| • Palpitations (23 points with paroxysmal atrial tachycardia) | |
| • Tremors, clumsiness | |
| Segmental pain | 44 |
| Impaired memory or concentration | 39 |
| Cervical pain | 34 |
| Low back pain | 24 |
| Urinary incontinence | 17 |

*From Milhorat, T.M., Chou, M.W., Trinidad, E.M., et al., 1999. Chiari I malformation redefined: clinical and radiographic findings in 364 symptomatic patients. Neurosurgery 44, 1005–1017.*

achondroplasia, acromegaly, and Paget disease are other causes of a small posterior fossa. In each of these conditions, the constricting small posterior fossa is the apparent cause of cerebellar tonsillar herniation.

Some patients have a small posterior fossa with the conical configuration typical of classic CM-I, but do not have tonsillar herniation; this has been called *Chiari 0 malformation*. This designation remains controversial. It is thought that these patients can have symptoms similar to CM-I secondary to abnormalities in the flow of CSF within the skull and spinal canal (Schijman, 2004; Tubbs et al., 2001).

When patients with CM-I have other abnormalities such as hydrocephalus, basilar impression, occipitalization of the atlas, retroflexed odontoid processes, elongated styloid processes, or C1-level spina bifida occulta, the mechanism of the tonsillar herniation varies. In contrast to CM-I, patients with tonsillar herniation due to hydrocephalus, intracranial mass lesions, occipitoatlantoaxial joint instability, or prolonged lumboperitoneal shunting have normal occipital bone size, posterior cranial fossa volume, and foramen magnum size; in these conditions, mechanisms other than a small posterior fossa cause the tonsillar herniation. In patients with hydrocephalus or intracranial mass lesions, raised intracranial pressure causes compartmental shifts that push the brain caudally. In patients with occipitoatlantoaxial joint instability, cranial settling is the main cause of the herniation. In patients undergoing prolonged lumboperitoneal shunting, overdrainage of CSF apparently creates a pressure differential between the cranial and spinal compartments, drawing cerebellar tonsils downward. When the drainage is stopped, the pressure gradient can resolve, and the herniation often reverses. Low spinal fluid pressure can also cause tonsillar herniation in patients with spinal CSF leaks, dural ectasias, and myelodysplasia. Table 104.3 outlines five distinct mechanisms of cerebellar tonsil herniation; each mechanism has its own diagnostic and therapeutic implications.

Measurements of the posterior cranial fossa enhance neuroradiological diagnosis of Chiari malformations. Computer analysis of standard MR and CT images is quick and easy. Diagnosis starts by assessing the size of the posterior fossa; an abnormally small posterior fossa shows that the CM-I is likely due to cranial constriction. A normal-sized posterior fossa necessitates a search for alternative mechanisms of tonsillar herniation such as cranial settling, spinal cord tethering, raised intracranial pressure, or intraspinal hypotension. Measurement of the foramen magnum helps in the differential diagnosis of tonsillar herniation because the foramen is enlarged in tethered cord syndrome and Chiari malformation II but stenosed in classic CM-I, craniosynostosis, and miscellaneous disorders such as achondroplasia.

### Clinical Presentation

Tonsillar herniation, once considered rare, is now easily recognized on sagittal brain MRI and has a prevalence of 0.1%–0.5% (Speer et al., 2003). New genetic studies support a hereditary tendency, with a transmissibility rate approaching 12%. Women are affected three times more often than men.

Patients with CM-I may experience no symptoms or first have symptoms in adolescence or early adulthood (Meadows et al., 2000; Table 104.4). At least a quarter of patients first have symptoms following relatively minor head or neck injury. Most symptomatic patients have pressing occipital headache and neck pain. Other manifestations can include visual disturbances, neuro-otological complaints, cranial nerve dysfunction, cognitive difficulties, and sleep-related breathing disorders (Milhorat et al., 1999). Patients with CM-I often have associated syringomyelia (discussed later), but motor, sensory, sphincter, and reflex disturbances suggestive of myelopathy can occur whether or not a syrinx is present. Clinical severity correlates generally but not perfectly with the extent of tonsillar herniation and the degree of obstruction to CSF flow. In more severe cases, the medulla descends below the foramen magnum; in which case brainstem dysfunction is more likely to be among the clinical findings (Yamada et al., 2004).

**TABLE 104.5 Suggested Upper Limits of Normal for Position of Cerebellar Tonsils Below Foramen Magnum**

| Decade of Life | Distance Below Foramen Magnum (mm) |
|---|---|
| First | 6 |
| Second or third | 5 |
| Fourth to eighth | 4 |
| Ninth | 3 |

*Data used with permission from Mikulis, D.J., Diaz, O., Egglin, T.K., et al., 1992. Variance of the position of the cerebellar tonsils with age: preliminary report. Radiology 183, 725–728.*

Deciding whether common symptoms such as memory concerns, back pain, or fatigue are caused by CM-I in an individual patient is a clinical challenge. Despite speculation and public interest, there is no scientific confirmation of an association between CM-I and fibromyalgia or chronic fatigue syndrome (Garland and Robertson, 2001).

Slight extension of the tonsils below the foramen is normal in childhood, and normal values decrease with increasing age (Table 104.5). When young children have symptoms, they can have oropharyngeal dysfunction and scoliosis. Children younger than age 3 can have vomiting and gastric reflux as the sole symptoms of CM-I.

The posterior fossa or "Chiari" headache has diagnostically helpful characteristics: it is a suboccipital pressing head pain that is usually continuous, waxing and waning but not episodic, and radiating at times behind the eyes or to the vertex (Kula, 2006). The headache is almost never hemicranial and is often exaggerated by physical activity and Valsalva maneuvers including bearing down with bowel movements, with laughter, crying, coughing, and sneezing. Exacerbations can be explosive rather than throbbing or pounding. There is no aura, but visual sparkles and scotomas can punctuate the peaks of headache. Neck pain without radicular features is common. Patients may have evanescent hand paresthesias and other generalized musculoskeletal complaints.

CM-I patients with "Chiari" headaches and little else may coincidently have migraine without aura, which can result in a diagnostic dilemma. Both headaches occasionally can share some similar features such as occipital location and perimenstrual accentuation. "Chiari" headaches are not likely to respond to migraine abortive agents such as the triptans or prophylactic agents including beta-blockers and serotonin reuptake inhibitors (SRIs). However, "Chiari" headaches like migraine may respond to topiramate, presumably because it is a carbonic anhydrase inhibitor and lowers CSF pressure. Patients may have tonsillar herniation on MRI and not yet have any CM-I–related symptoms. However, these patients can have migraine. It is therefore important to first rule out migraine as a cause of headache before aggressively treating a CM-I malformation. This is even more important in those patients diagnosed with Chiari 0. Neurological examination of patients with CM-I may show subtle abnormalities but is often completely normal. The most typical finding is a vestibular-generated dysequilibrium and difficulty in tandem standing and walking. Nystagmus is difficult to appreciate even with Fresnel lens examination. Objective findings frequently elude sophisticated vestibular testing, which only occasionally reveals nystagmus of possible central or peripheral etiology. Classic downbeat nystagmus is rarely seen even with tonsillar herniation as striking as 20 mm.

The malformation is best seen on a T2-weighted sagittal MRI scan of the brain and cervical spine, which allows for assessment of the shape of the posterior fossa and may detect an accompanying syrinx as well as the extent (if any) of brainstem compression. Flow of CSF at the foramen magnum can be evaluated using phase-contrast MRI and cardiac gating to acquire images throughout the cardiac cycle (Clarke et al., 2013). Symptomatic Chiari I malformations can cause an increase in peak systolic CSF flow velocity and decreased uniformity of flow.

### Management

The severity and nature of symptoms of CM-I vary greatly, so naturally therapy should also vary from patient to patient. The minority of patients require surgery. Headache symptoms sometimes respond to carbonic anhydrase inhibitors, simple approaches to associated paracervical pain, or head elevation during sleep. Minor traumatic events can aggravate symptoms, and patients should avoid activities that risk head and neck injury.

Management of labor and delivery in patients with CM-I is somewhat controversial. Although avoiding epidural or spinal anesthesia has been recommended by some, there is a literature suggesting these techniques can be employed safely in CM-I parturients for vaginal or cesarean deliveries (Leffert et al., 2013). For women with syringomyelia, a cesarean section is advisable to avoid intrathoracic and abdominal pressure alterations associated with vaginal deliveries (Chntigian et al., 2002). Surgical decompression of the posterior fossa is appropriate treatment for the minority of patients who have significant functional impairment due to persistent headache despite medical therapy or have progressive syringomyelia. It is not indicated for symptoms limited to chronic fatigue, musculoskeletal pain, or vertigo, or for prophylaxis against worsening of headache or of syringomyelia. Kula (2006) discusses treatment in detail and provides a comprehensive management algorithm.

## SPINAL DYSRAPHISM

*Spinal dysraphism* is congenital failure of the primitive neural tube to close during fetal development and includes a number of disorders of fusion of dorsal midline structures of the spinal canal or skull (Copp et al., 2013). Neural tube defects are one of the most common congenital malformations, with 70,000–100,000 disabled individuals in the United States alone (Blencowe, 2018). The neural tube normally closes during the first 3 weeks following conception. There are genetic causes, but environmental causes are important in most cases. The most extreme form is anencephaly, characterized by absence of the entire cranium at birth; the undeveloped brain lies at the base of the skull as a small vascular mass without recognizable nervous structures.

### Spina Bifida Occulta

Spina bifida occulta is the most common and least symptomatic (usually asymptomatic) form of dysraphism. In this anomaly, the vertebral elements fail to fuse posteriorly, but the thecal and neural elements remain within the spinal canal. It is most common at posterior elements of L5–S1 and is usually noted as an incidental finding on spinal plain radiography (eFig. 104.8). Cutaneous abnormalities may be associated (Box 104.4). Orthopedic foot deformities, urinary or rectal sphincter dysfunction, or focal neurological abnormalities can indicate that the spina bifida occulta is associated with compression or malformation of neural tissues or with spinal cord tethering.

### Myelomeningocele and Encephalocele

In myelomeningocele *(spina bifida)* and meningocele *(spina bifida cystica)*, congenital defects of midline closure are accompanied by eventration of meninges and even of neural tissue. Spinal defects are often visible on examination of the back of the newborn (eFig. 104.9,

**BOX 104.4 Dorsal Midline Skin Findings Associated With Spina Bifida Occulta**

Asymmetrical gluteal fold
Dermal sinus or dimple
Hairy tuft
Hemangioma
Lipoma
Nevus
Pilonidal sinus
Rudimentary tail
Spinal aplasia cutis

Figs. 104.10 and 104.11). At times the skin and vertebral canal are open, and a sac of meninges is directly visible. The defect is most common in the lumbar region. If the sac contains nerve roots or spinal cord, it is a *myelomeningocele*; if neural elements are absent from the sac, it is a *meningocele*. These brain and spinal cord malformations may be associated with CSF leakage into adjacent structures, posing a risk of meningitis. Neurological deficits are directly related to the anatomical extent of the malformation and vary from insignificant to grave.

Either defect is often accompanied by hydrocephalus or by Chiari II malformation, in which the cerebellar vermis and caudal brainstem descend through an enlarged foramen magnum (Stevenson, 2004; Tubbs and Oakes, 2004). The extent of brainstem herniation is variable, including portions of the medulla or even of the pons. Hydrocephalus and syringomyelia are common accompanying features, and patients often have various associated anomalies such as a small posterior fossa, kink in the medulla, and polymicrogyria. These infants are at risk for later development of tethered cord syndrome, spinal dermoid, and epidermoid inclusion cysts. In Chiari III malformation, the displaced cerebellar and brainstem tissue extends into an infratentorial meningoencephalocele. An important cause is maternal folate deficiency, and most cases could be prevented if women with childbearing potential routinely took folic acid daily. Other risk factors include family history of neural closure defects and maternal treatment with some antiepileptic drugs such as valproic acid and carbamazepine. Pregnant women can be screened at 14–16 weeks for serum α-fetoprotein (AFP) levels, which are elevated about 85% of the time when the fetus has neural closure defects. The defects also can be detected by fetal ultrasonography. Ultrasound detects greater than 90% of neural tube defects at 18–20 weeks (coupled with AFP >95%).

Planning treatment for affected infants, potentially including surgery, is difficult. Initial surgical treatment in utero or in the neonatal period can provide cosmetic repair and decrease the risk for meningitis (Adzick, 2011). Also hydrocephalus can be shunted. Any existing myelopathic or radiculopathic neurological deficit is likely to persist after surgery. Some patients, especially infants with progressive brainstem dysfunction, are treated with decompression of the rostral spinal canal. Less than 30% of such patients survive beyond the first year, and long-term problems including mental retardation and paraplegia are often severe. Few patients with myelomeningocele are mentally normal, but most of those with lumbar meningocele are.

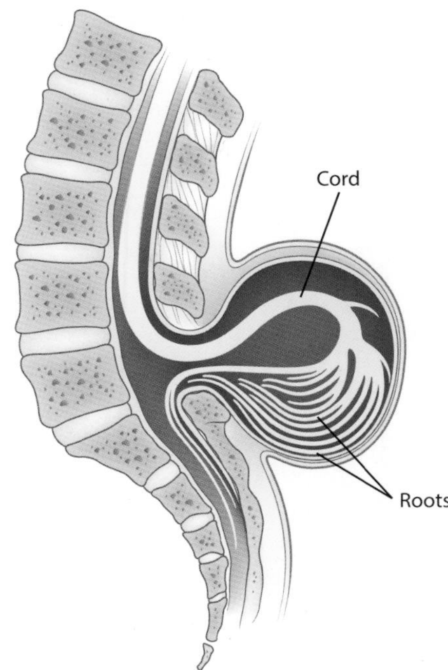


**Fig. 104.10** Diagrammatical Representation of Myelomeningocele.

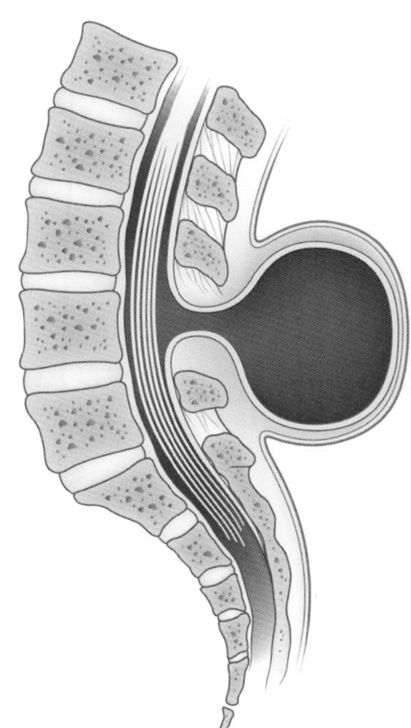

**Fig. 104.11** Diagrammatical Representation of Meningocele.

## Dandy-Walker Syndrome

Dandy-Walker syndrome results from the failure of development of the midline portion of the cerebellum. A cyst-like structure associated with a greatly dilated fourth ventricle, expanding the midline, is often seen (Fig. 104.12). The malformation typically causes the occipital bone to bulge posteriorly and displaces the tentorium and torcula upward. The cerebellar vermis is aplastic, and the corpus callosum may be deficient or absent. There is usually dilation of the aqueduct as well as the third and lateral ventricles. Chiari IV malformation is characterized by cerebellar and brainstem hypoplasia rather than displacement and is probably a variant of the Dandy-Walker malformation.

## Tethered Cord Syndromes

Congenital abnormalities of the spinal cord or cauda equina can result in spinal cord tethering, in which stretching and tension develops within the cord tissue as the spinal column elongates during early life, resulting in the conus medullaris being found at an abnormally low vertebral

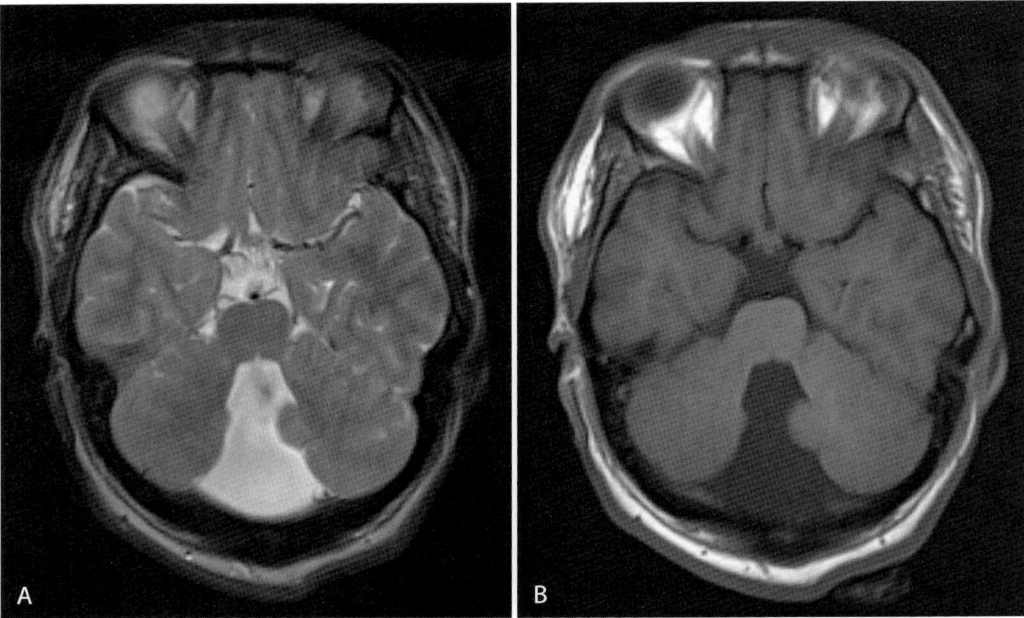


**Fig. 104.12** Dandy-Walker Malformation. A, T2-weighted magnetic resonance imaging (MRI). B, T1-weighted MRI. (*Courtesy Michael Coffee, MD.*)

**BOX 104.5 Causes of Tethered Spinal Cord**

**Primary Causes**
Dermal sinus tract
Diastematomyelia
Dural bands
Intraspinal lipoma or tumor
Meningocele, myelomeningocele, anterior sacral meningocele
Neuroenteric cyst
Sacral agenesis
Tight filum terminale

**Secondary Causes**
Arachnoiditis
Dermoid
Re-tethered spinal cord
Suture granuloma
Trauma

*Adapted with permission from McLone, D.G., La Marca, F., 1997. The tethered spinal cord: diagnosis, significance, and management. Semin. Pediatr. Neurol. 4, 192–208.*

level (Michelson and Ashwal, 2004; Box 104.5). Imaging studies, such as spinal MRI, showing the conus medullaris caudad to the lower endplate of L2, can be evidence of tethering. A child or even an adult with these abnormalities can develop progressive neurological dysfunction due to traction on the cord or nerve roots. One presentation is lower motor neuron dysfunction in one or both lower extremities, but patients can also have sensory loss, upper motor neuron signs, orthopedic foot deformities, and scoliosis. A tethered spinal cord can, in addition, cause isolated sphincter dysfunction as subtle as intermittent urinary incontinence.

The so-called occult tethered cord syndrome is an area of controversy (Drake, 2006; Selden, 2006). Uncontrolled surgical series suggest that children with neurogenic voiding dysfunction and normal spinal MRI might also have cord tethering. For some children, voiding dysfunction reportedly improved after lysis of the filum terminale, which microscopically can be abnormally thickened, fatty, and fibrous, even though the filum and conus medullaris appear normal on MRI. A few cases of cerebellar tonsillar herniation seem to be due to occult cord tethering; other features are syrinx development below the T5 level and scoliosis (Milhorat et al., 2009). In contrast to patients with classic CM-I, patients with this variation of CM-I with cord tethering have normal posterior fossa volume and an enlarged foramen magnum. Supporting the role of cord tethering as a cause of the tonsillar descent are reports of increasing herniation of the cerebellar tonsils with somatic growth, cerebellar prolapse following Chiari decompression surgery, and anatomical improvements including ascent of the conus medullaris, ascent of the cerebellar tonsils, and resolution of brainstem elongation following section of the filum terminale.

Split spinal cord malformation (SSCM), formally termed diastematomyelia, is a congenital malformation of the spinal cord characterized by sagittal division of a portion of the cord into two hemicords. In most instances, the division is located in the lower thoracic or lumbar regions. SSCM is often accompanied by skin abnormalities such as a tuft of hair at the level of the lesion. Two types of SSCM are described: type I, in which each hemicord has its own dural sheath, and type II in which both hemicords are enclosed in a single dural sheath. Neurological deficits, scoliosis, and congenital foot deformities are more common in type I. Bony and cartilaginous spurs between the hemicords are also more common with type I. Finally, surgical repair is more effective in type I and can be combined with distal untethering if a tethered cord is present as well. The spur tethers the spinal cord, leading to progressive neurological dysfunction when the vertebral column lengthens during growth. The diagnosis can often be suspected on plain radiography, which shows widening of the interpedicular distance and a posterior bony bridge at the level of the lesion. MRI or CT myelography can confirm the diagnosis (eFig. 104.13).  Surgical therapy consists of attempts to free all structures tethering the cord by removing the spurs and dura in the cleft and cutting the filum terminale if abnormally tethered.

## SYRINGOMYELIA AND SYRINGOBULBIA

*Hydromyelia* is an abnormal dilation of the central spinal canal with "excess" CSF contained within the ependymal lining. When fluid

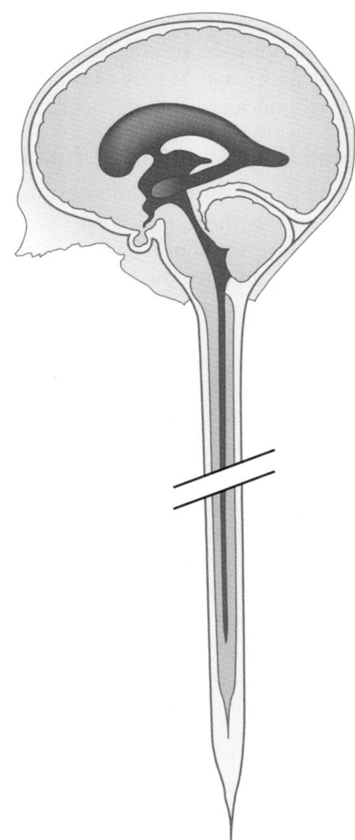

**Fig. 104.14** Diagrammatic representation of persistent central canal extending throughout length of spinal cord.

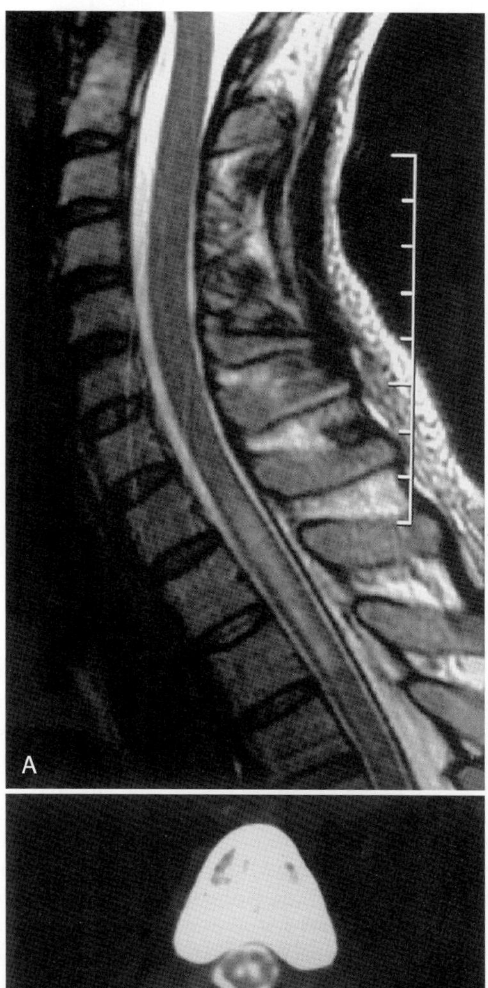


**Fig. 104.15** **A,** Sagittal T2-weighted magnetic resonance imaging demonstrates intramedullary signal abnormality posterior to T1–T3 level of spinal cord. Possible causes include edema, myelomalacia, or syringomyelia. **B,** Axial computed tomographic myelogram performed at a 3-hour delay demonstrates filling of area of signal abnormality with myelographic contrast that had been injected into lumbar subarachnoid space. Filling of cavity with contrast is consistent with syringomyelia but would not be expected in cases of cord edema or myelomalacia.

dissects into the surrounding white matter, forming a cystic cavity or syrinx, the term *syringomyelia* is applied. A *syrinx*, then, is a cavity in the spinal cord (syringomyelia) or brainstem *(syringobulbia)* (Figs. 104.14, 104.15, and 104.16). Hydromyelia and syringomyelia often coexist, and many physicians use the terms interchangeably.

The widespread use of spinal MRI has greatly increased the detection of cervical syringomyelia, which often produces nonspecific symptoms such as neck pain and at times no symptoms at all. Estimated prevalence in the United States is between 1:1300 and 1:1900.

The central canal of the spinal cord is normally wide open during embryonic life and becomes atretic after birth. It is occasionally patent in adults (see Fig. 104.14). Cervical or thoracic MRI in an adult will occasionally reveal an incidental asymptomatic hydromyelia, which is typically linear or fusiform on sagittal images; extends over several levels, sometimes discontinuously; and is round, central, and up to 4 mm in diameter on axial images (Batzdorf, 2005).

## Clinical Presentation

The prototypical presentation of a symptomatic syrinx is the presence of lower motor neuron signs at the level of the lesion, usually in the upper extremities, or in the case of syringobulbia, the lower cranial nerves. Furthermore, it can present as a myeloradiculopathy with lower motor neuron findings in the upper extremities and upper motor neuron findings in the lower extremities. In addition, there is often a dissociated, suspended sensory loss with impaired pain and temperature sensation, but preserved dorsal column sensation (i.e., light touch). However, few patients show this total picture. The clinical features vary with the size, location, and shape of the cavity; the rapidity of its evolution; and any associated neurological conditions such as a Chiari I malformation. Symptoms are more related to the pace of evolution of the syrinx than to its absolute size. Otherwise healthy patients with slit-like syrinx cavities may present with severe localized spinal and radicular pain. Other patients with syrinx cavities displacing as much as 90% of the spinal cord mass may be virtually asymptomatic.

Pain is a prominent symptom in most patients with syringomyelia. Common complaints include neck ache, headache, back pain, radicular pain, and areas of segmental dysesthesia. Painful dysesthesias are most likely to occur at or adjacent to the caudal extent of the syrinx cavity. Some patients have trophic changes corresponding to segmental loss of pain sensation. Syringomyelia can cause neuropathic monoarthritis (Charcot joint), most commonly in a shoulder or elbow.

Most syringes are in the cervical spinal cord. Those developing from hydromyelia are usually associated with Chiari I or II malformations,

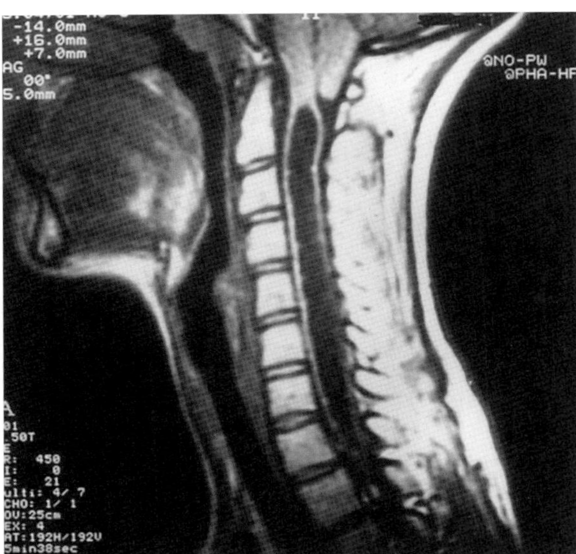


**Fig. 104.16** Magnetic resonance image demonstrates a large syringomyelic cavity in the cervical cord.

communicating hydrocephalus, or abnormalities at the craniovertebral junction. Asymptomatic hydromyelia and syringomyelia may be incidentally discovered by MRI while investigating unrelated cranial symptomatology, such as a Chiari malformation. A syrinx associated with a spinal cord tumor or trauma can occur at any level of the spinal cord. Although either CT or MRI can demonstrate a syrinx, MRI is more sensitive for complete evaluation of the cord and surrounding soft tissues. In patients in whom MRI is contraindicated, CT myelography may be useful in discerning syringomyelia, which will commonly fill with contrast on delayed images due to communication with the CSF through the central canal of the spinal cord (see Fig. 104.15).

## Communicating and Noncommunicating Syringes

The terms *communicating* and *noncommunicating syringes* indicate whether the syrinx is in communication with the CSF pathways. However, it is often difficult to determine this, even at autopsy, so these terms are mainly of use in discussions of etiology. It is better to classify syringomyelia according to its associations.

## Abnormalities of the Cervicomedullary Junction

Abnormalities of the cervicomedullary junction and posterior fossa, such as Chiari anomalies types I and II and the Dandy-Walker malformation, are the most common cause of nonidiopathic syringes. Up to 70% of nonidiopathic syringes are associated with CM-I. The mechanism of formation of these syringes is controversial (Di Lorenzo and Cacciola, 2005). Patients with cervical syringomyelia and no Chiari malformation often have a small posterior fossa or disturbed flow of CSF near the foramen magnum (Bogdanov et al., 2004). Syringes can extend beyond hydromyelia as an outpouching of the dilated central canal (see Figs. 104.15 and 104.16). One hypothesis is that the posterior fossa abnormalities interfere with the passage of CSF from the fourth ventricle through the foramina of Luschka and Magendie into the subarachnoid space. The consequence is transmission of bulk flow and the various pressure waves of the CSF (arterial, venous, respiratory) down the central canal of the spinal cord, leading to dissection of a syrinx into the substance of the spinal cord. Noncongenital abnormalities at the cervicomedullary junction that sometimes cause syringomyelia include arachnoiditis and meningiomas.

In CM-I, the large majority (80%) occur within the cervical cord. The thoracic cord can, however, be affected in isolation, and, more rarely, a lumbosacral syrinx may appear associated with spinal cord tethering secondary to a thickened and restrictive filum terminale.

## Syrinx Associated With Spinal Cord Tumors

Syringes are associated with intramedullary tumors often enough that any cystic process in the spinal cord should be considered an intramedullary tumor until proven otherwise. Syringomyelia accompanies 25%–60% of intramedullary spinal tumors; conversely, 8%–16% of syringes are caused by tumors (eFig. 104.17).  Intramedullary tumors in von Hippel-Lindau syndrome and neurofibromatosis are particularly likely to be accompanied by syringes. The syrinx extends from the tumor, more often rostrally than caudally. Ependymomas, which represent up to 10% of childhood CNS tumors and affect adults as well, are particularly likely to produce syringes because of their central location. Less than 2% of extramedullary tumors in the spinal canal (e.g., meningiomas, neuromas) are associated with syringes.

## Syrinx Associated With Spinal Cord Trauma

Syringes can develop as a late effect of serious spinal cord trauma (Carroll and Brackenridge, 2005). Estimates of the prevalence of syringes after trauma vary widely from 0.2% to 64%. However, delayed progressive intramedullary cystic lesions complicates 3%–4% of dramatic spinal cord injuries. Symptoms of ascending long-tract or segmental spinal cord dysfunction usually develop within 5 years after the acute traumatic myelopathy has stabilized, improved, or even become asymptomatic. Pain or other sensory symptoms are often prominent. Findings usually evolve gradually but occasionally worsen suddenly after events such as a cough or Valsalva maneuver. The cavities are typically eccentric and can be multiple, arising from areas of posttraumatic myelomalacia and then spreading rostrally or caudally. Severe posttraumatic spinal deformity or arachnoid scarring can also cause posttraumatic syringes.

## Syrinx Associated With Other Focal Spinal Cord Pathologies

Any illness causing arachnoiditis can lead to formation of a noncommunicating syrinx. Reported causes include meningitis, subarachnoid hemorrhage, spinal trauma, epidural infections, epidural anesthesia, and spinal surgery, but many cases of focal arachnoiditis are idiopathic. Syringes can develop as a complication of various intramedullary pathologies, including trauma and tumors (see previous discussion), spinal ischemic or hemorrhagic strokes, radiation necrosis, or transverse myelitis.

### Treatment

Indications for and approaches to surgical therapy for syringes are far from standardized. In patients with Chiari I malformations, the syrinx often improves after decompression of the malformation with various combinations of suboccipital craniectomy, upper cervical laminectomy, and/or dural grafting. The exact surgical technique is debated, and remains controversial, but it is agreed that the goal is adequate restoration of normal CSF flow and pressure across the craniocervical junction. Two recent meta-analyses have both concluded that adding a duraplasty to posterior fossa decompression results in improvement in syringomyelia, but is associated with higher rates of CSF leak and aseptic meningitis (Chai, 2018; Lin, 2018). Concerningly, another recent study has concluded that 50% of patients treated with posterior fossa decompression will require an additional surgery for persistent, progressive, and/or recurrent syringomyelia (Soleman et al., 2019). When the syrinx extends from an intramedullary tumor, resection of the tumor usually leads to regression of the syrinx, so no specific surgical drainage of the cavity is needed. When the syrinx extends from an area of localized arachnoiditis or other obstruction of the subarachnoid space, some patients benefit from resection of the arachnoiditis and restoration of CSF flow patterns with an expansile duraplasty; shunting or entering the cavity (syringotomy) is a less desirable surgical approach (Batzdorf, 2005). In patients with Chiari I malformation and syrinx, pain and other sensory symptoms are more likely to improve if the foramen magnum is decompressed within 2 years of onset of the sensory symptoms (Attal et al., 2004). Among patients undergoing surgery for syrinx in the absence of Chiari malformation, slightly more than half improved or stabilized, but over a third required more than one operation (Batzdorf, 2005).

### Clinical Correlations

A single patient often has more than one of the conditions discussed (Williams, 1991). Thus, a patient with one of the Chiari hindbrain malformations also may have some combination of bony abnormalities of the foramen magnum or cervical spine, syringomyelia, and myelomeningocele. The clinical manifestations of craniocervical deformities are protean depending on which neural structures and associated anomalies are involved. When a patient has these problems, diagnosis and treatment starts by analyzing each component. MRI and CT scans, especially with measurements of the foramen magnum and posterior fossa, have greatly eased the analytical process. Many patients are asymptomatic or first present with neurological complaints in adult life. Patients may have short necks or abnormal neck posture or movement, particularly if there is an element of skeletal deformity (e.g., Klippel-Feil anomaly, occipitalization of the atlas). Findings attributable to the brainstem or cerebellum may occur with Chiari malformations, compression of the brainstem (e.g., basilar impression, vertical displacement of the dens), or syringobulbia. Uncommonly, AA disease or basilar invagination can cause compromise of vertebrobasilar circulation, causing posterior circulation strokes or transient ischemic attacks. Specific findings suggestive of disease at the foramen magnum include downbeat nystagmus or the combination of long-tract signs with lower motor neuron dysfunction in the lower cervical spinal cord; lower motor neuron dysfunction has been attributed to impaired spinal venous drainage at the foramen magnum.

Spinal cord syndromes can be caused by syringomyelia or by extramedullary cord compression (e.g., by the dens with AA dislocation, by spinal stenosis in Klippel-Feil anomaly). Additional neurological dysfunction can occur when the anomalies form part of more widespread developmental failure (e.g., lumbar effects of myelomeningocele in Chiari II malformation, accompanying cerebral malformations in Klippel-Feil anomaly).

## SPINAL DEFORMITIES AND METABOLIC BONE DISEASE

### Osteoporosis

Osteoporotic vertebral compression fractures occur most commonly in the thoracic and thoracolumbar spine, especially in postmenopausal women (Fig. 104.18). By age 75 years, nearly a fourth of women have vertebral compression fractures. Although these fractures may lead to kyphosis ("dowager hump") and loss of body height, most are painless. The presence of a vertebral fracture in a postmenopausal woman or older man is a very strong predictor of subsequent fracture risk and an indication for pharmacological treatment of osteoporosis. In younger men and women, acute traumatic compression fractures are more likely to be painful. The pain usually is centered at the level of the compression and accompanied by loss of spinal range of motion. Pain increases with activity, decreases with bed rest, and resolves slowly, though sometimes incompletely.

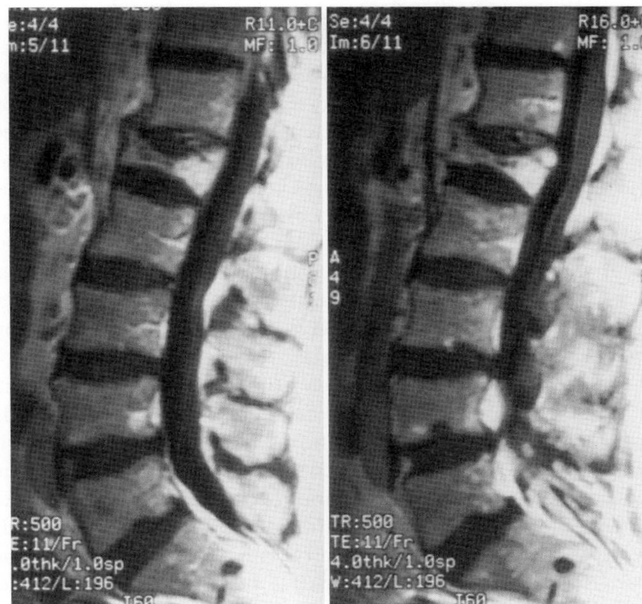


**Fig. 104.18** Spinal magnetic resonance image of a patient with vertebral compression fracture secondary to osteoporosis. T1-weighted images of lumbar spine show 70%–80% loss of height of midportion of L1 vertebral body, with relative preservation of height of posterior portion of vertebral body. Bright appearance of vertebra indicates preservation of fat within marrow compartment, which would be dark if replaced by tumor. (*Courtesy Erik Gaensler.*)

Patients with more disabling pain can be management challenges, sometimes requiring hospitalization. Initial management includes activity modification and pain control utilizing analgesics ranging from nonsteroidal antiinflammatory drugs (NSAIDs) to opioids depending on the severity of the pain. Bracing for a short period of time in the acute phase may prove helpful. For patients not responding to conservative treatments a vertebral augmentation procedure (vertebroplasty or kyphoplasty) may be considered. While controversy continues regarding the overall efficacy of these procedures for pain management and which procedure should be utilized for a given patient, there is some consensus that when administered to properly selected patients with severe pain within a 6-week period of onset there can be some reduction in the severity of pain and a shortening of the length of hospitalization (Rodriquez, 2017; Chandra, 2018). Once pain is controlled, an exercise program—including aquatic therapy, smoking reduction, and, if indicated, reduced alcohol consumption—may help reduce the risk of subsequent compression fractures.

Nonmetastatic compression fractures infrequently lead to spinal cord or nerve root compression. When a compression fracture accompanies a focal neurological compression syndrome, a metastatic vertebral lesion should be considered. MRI features that favor a malignant cause of the compression fracture include decreased T1-weighted and increased T2-weighted signal in the vertebral body, with bulging of the posterior cortical wall, pedicle involvement, and associated epidural or paravertebral mass. Use of fluorodeoxyglucose positron emission tomography (FDG-PET)/CT imaging can also be useful in this diagnosis (Cho and Chang, 2011).

### Osteomalacia and Rickets

Osteomalacia and rickets are conditions of deficient bone mineralization. In adulthood, the most common mechanism for the development of osteomalacia is vitamin D deficiency, either due to dietary restriction, malabsorption, chronic kidney disease, or lack of sunlight exposure. The most specific screening test in otherwise normal individuals is a serum 25-hydroxyvitamin D (25[OH]D) level, though additional biochemical findings may include: low serum calcium, low serum phosphate, elevated serum alkaline phosphatase, and elevated parathyroid hormone (Kennel et al., 2010). A technetium (Tc-99m) bone scan can show increased activity as a result of widespread osteoblast activation. Radiographs may reveal pseudofractures, bands of decreased bone density along the cortical surface. Long bones are typically more involved than the spine. Spinal pain, kyphosis, and compression fractures can occur in osteomalacia, but compression of spinal cord or nerve roots is rare. Basilar impression can occur in patients with osteomalacia.

Osteomalacia can result in bone pain, fractures, impaired gait, and muscle cramps. A painful proximal muscle weakness, especially in the hip girdle, can also occur. The mechanism of this myopathy is thought to be related to the aforementioned hyperparathyroidism. The physical examination reveals diminished muscle power, hypotonia, atrophy, and a "waddling" quality in the gait. When there is secondary hyperparathyroidism with hypercalcemia, tendon reflexes may be brisk. Needle electromyography (EMG) may show small-amplitude, short-duration, polyphasic motor units, without electrophysiological evidence of active denervation. Muscle biopsy may show type II atrophy. Strength can improve after adequate vitamin D replacement.

## Osteopetrosis

The osteopetroses are a group of rare inherited diseases characterized by increased bone density due to impaired bone resorption (Jenkins et al., 2013; eFig. 104.19). Varied genetic defects can cause osteopetrosis, resulting in three clinical variants: infantile severe autosomal recessive, intermediate autosomal recessive, and autosomal dominant. Osteopetrosis of the skull can cause cranial neuropathies (most often optic neuropathy), basilar impression, hydrocephalus, or syringomyelia. Osteopetrosis of the spine can contribute to spinal canal stenosis with secondary compressive myelopathy. Other complications include thrombocytopenia, anemia, osteomyelitis, and fractures. Some patients can be treated by hematopoietic stem cell transplantation. Other rare sclerosing bone disorders like progressive diaphyseal dysplasia (Camurati-Engelmann disease) or endosteal hyperostosis occasionally have neurological complications (Grond-Ginsbach and Debette, 2009).

Very rarely, infants present with both osteopetrosis and infantile neuraxonal dystrophy and follow a course of neurodegeneration and death in infancy; neuropathology of these children includes neuronal ceroid lipofuscin and eosinophilic axonal spheroids.

## Paget Disease

Paget disease of the bone (osteitis deformans) is a focal metabolic bone disease of excessive osteoclastic bony destruction coupled with reactive osteoblastic activity (Ralston et al., 2008) (Fig. 104.20). The incidence increases with age and varies among ethnic groups, with a high incidence (nearly 5%) in elderly Caucasians of Northern European descent. Men are slightly more commonly affected. Paget disease appears to be caused by a combination of genetic and environmental factors, including possible roles of calcium or vitamin D deficiency, toxins, and infections, especially with paramyxovirus. Paget disease is usually asymptomatic and discovered only because of laboratory or radiographic abnormalities. However, it may cause symptoms by bone or joint distortion, fractures, compression of neurological tissue by calcification, hemorrhage, or focal ischemia due to a vascular steal by the metabolically hyperactive bony tissue. Uncommonly, neoplasms, especially osteogenic sarcoma, can develop in pagetic bone.

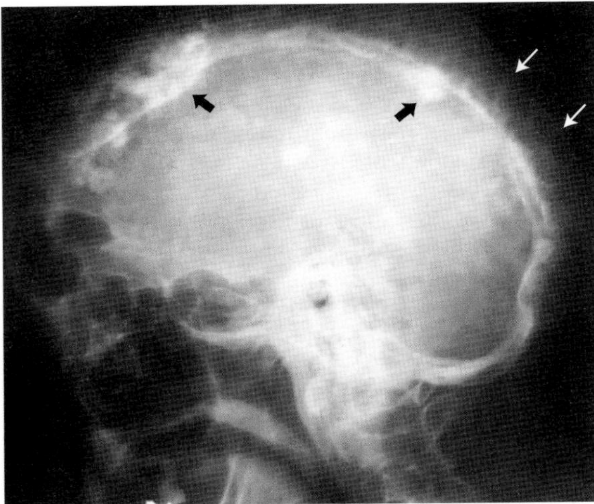

**Fig. 104.20** Radiograph of a patient with Paget disease of the skull. Note thickening of calvaria *(white arrows)* and bony sclerosis with a cotton-wool appearance *(black arrows)*. Patient has basilar invagination; note high position of dens with respect to clivus. (*Courtesy Erik Gaensler.*)

A few families have an autosomal dominant illness, which has now been characterized as valosin-containing protein (VCP) disease, and includes the triad of inclusion body myositis, frontotemporal dementia, and Paget disease of bone (Mehta et al., 2013).

### Diagnosis

Paget disease usually can be diagnosed by characteristic radiographic findings of mixed osteolytic and osteoblastic lesions (see Fig. 104.20). Osteolytic activity can cause well-demarcated round patches of low bone density in the skull *(osteogenesis circumscripta)*. Osteoblastic activity leads to thickening of cortical bone and then to a general increase in bone density, often with distortion of normal organization.

Although most patients with Paget disease have elevation of serum bone alkaline phosphatase and markers of bone resorption, focal skeletal disease with neurological complications may occur in patients without laboratory abnormalities. Alkaline phosphatase levels, when elevated, are helpful not only in making the diagnosis but also in following response to treatment. Evaluation of serum calcium and 25(OH)D levels should be completed to exclude other potential causes for the alkaline phosphatase level. Biopsy is often not required but should be considered when radiographic findings are atypical. Potential mimics include blastic lesions from metastatic disease or lytic lesions seen in multiple myeloma.

### Cranial Neurological Complications

Neurological complications with cranial involvement are common in Paget disease (Rubin and Levin, 2009). Paget disease of the skull can lead to head enlargement. Patients often complain of headache. The most common focal neurological manifestation is hearing loss. Paget disease of the cribriform plate can disrupt olfaction. Other cranial mononeuropathies (e.g., optic neuropathy, trigeminal neuralgia, hemifacial spasm) are much less frequent. Perhaps a third of patients with Paget disease of the skull have some degree of basilar invagination, but symptomatic complications such as brainstem or cerebellar compression, hydrocephalus, or syringomyelia are rare (Raubenheimer et al., 2002). Patients with Paget disease of the skull occasionally develop seizures. The pagetic skull is more vulnerable to bleeding from minor trauma, which can lead to epidural hematoma.

### Spinal Neurological Complications

Symptomatic Paget disease of the spine occurs most often in the lumbar region, where it can cause back pain, monoradiculopathies, or cauda equina syndrome. The disease may involve adjacent vertebral bodies and the intervening disk space or may cause root compression by extension from a single vertebral body. The differential diagnosis in patients with Paget disease and neurological dysfunction in a single limb includes peripheral nerve entrapment by pagetic bone.

Paget disease of the spine leading to myelopathy is more often thoracic than cervical. A variety of mechanisms are reported, including extradural extension of pagetic bone, distortion of the spinal canal by vertebral compression fractures, spinal epidural hematoma, or sarcomatous degeneration leading to epidural tumor. In a small number of patients with myelopathy, imaging shows no evident spinal cord compression, thus suggesting a vascular steal phenomenon by hypermetabolic bone in the vertebral body resulting in cord ischemia. In support of this hypothesis, drug treatment of Paget disease in these patients can improve spinal cord function, sometimes within a few days.

### Treatment

Potent nitrogen-containing bisphosphonates (e.g., zoledronic acid, pamidronate, risedronate) are the drugs of choice for treatment of Paget disease. Bone resorption decreases within days. Within 1–2 weeks of treatment, bone pain may improve. Osteoblastic bone formation and falling serum alkaline phosphatase levels occur after 1 or 2 months of therapy. Some patients experience significant neurological improvement after treatment, but improvement is often delayed 1–3 months. In cases with severe cord compression, surgical decompression is indicated, but drug treatment before surgery decreases the risk of operative bone hemorrhage. Calcitonin is an alternative treatment for patients unable to take bisphosphonates or who require more immediate surgery (Wootton et al., 1978). Patients with cranial neuropathy have less impressive responses to drug therapy. Hydrocephalus can be treated successfully with ventriculoperitoneal shunting (Roohi et al., 2005). Additional interventions such as hearing aids, analgesics, physical therapy, and orthotics are often required once the excessive bone turnover has been addressed (Siris et al., 2006).

## Juvenile Kyphosis

Juvenile kyphosis *(Scheuermann disease)* manifests as thoracic or thoracolumbar kyphosis in adolescents. This is a self-limited disorder which arises due to uneven vertebral bone growth with respect to the sagittal plane. Spinal pain is more likely to accompany lumbar than thoracic disease. Spinal radiography shows anterior vertebral wedging, increased Cobb angle, and elongated sagittal balance (horizontal distance between the center of C7 and the superior-posterior border of the S1 endplate). Neurological abnormalities are uncommon, but spinal cord compression can occur from thoracic disk herniation or direct effects of severe kyphosis.

## Scoliosis

Scoliosis can be congenital, acquired secondary to an underlying disease, or idiopathic. The most common form is idiopathic scoliosis, with or without kyphosis, that usually develops painlessly in childhood and adolescence. A few cases of acquired scoliosis are associated with tumor, spondylolisthesis, or neurological pathology such as syrinx, myelomeningocele, or Chiari I malformation. Among patients with acquired scoliosis, indications for spinal MRI include abnormal neurological examination or atypical curve features such as sudden progression, left thoracic curvature, or absent apical segment lordosis (Davids et al., 2004). Spinal cord compression is a rare complication of idiopathic scoliosis and is particularly rare if no kyphosis is present. In each patient presenting with scoliosis and myelopathy, an important consideration is whether the myelopathy caused, rather than resulted from, the scoliosis.

Patients with congenital scoliosis, unlike those with idiopathic childhood scoliosis, usually have anomalous vertebrae and may have other associated developmental problems such as Klippel-Feil anomaly or diastematomyelia. Scoliosis due to skeletal disease (e.g., achondroplasia) is more likely than idiopathic scoliosis to lead to spinal cord compromise. Myelopathy can result from spinal cord distraction during treatment of scoliosis with traction or surgery.

Scoliosis can also be caused by various neurological diseases including cerebral palsy, spinocerebellar degenerations (e.g., Friedreich ataxia), inherited neuropathies (e.g., Charcot-Marie-Tooth disease), myelopathies (e.g., syringomyelia), paralytic poliomyelitis, spinal muscular atrophy, dysautonomia (e.g., Riley-Day syndrome), and myopathies (e.g., Duchenne disease) (Vialle et al., 2013). Excessive curvature of the spine can also be due to various causes of axial extensor muscles weakness (Mika et al., 2005) or due to overactivity of abdominal flexors, as can be seen in stiff-person syndrome. Scoliosis is the most common skeletal complication of neurofibromatosis type 1. Scoliosis that develops in adulthood can often be traced to an underlying cause such as trauma, osteoporotic fracture, degenerative spondylosis, or ankylosing spondylitis; it can result in local back pain, nerve root compression, or spinal canal stenosis.

## Diffuse Idiopathic Skeletal Hyperostosis

Diffuse idiopathic skeletal hyperostosis (DISH) *(Forestier disease, ankylosing hyperostosis)* is a syndrome of excessive calcification that develops with aging, more often in men than in women. The diagnosis is made by spinal radiographs that show "flowing" calcifications along the anterior and lateral portion of at least four contiguous vertebral bodies, without loss of disk height and without typical radiographic findings of ankylosing spondylitis (eFig. 104.21). Patients are often asymptomatic but may have spinal pain or limited spinal motion. Large anterior cervical calcifications can contribute to dysphagia, hoarseness, sleep apnea, or difficulty with intubation. A rare complication is myelopathy due to spinal stenosis if the calcifications are also present within the spinal canal. Like patients with ankylosing spondylitis, patients with DISH can develop spinal fractures after relatively minor trauma. Treatment is focused on symptomatic management.

## Ossification of the Posterior Longitudinal Ligament or Ligamentum Flavum

Ossification of the posterior longitudinal ligament anterior to the spinal canal (Fig. 104.22) and ossification of the ligamentum flavum posterior to the spinal canal are uncommon syndromes of acquired calcification. The posterior longitudinal ligament extends the length of the spine, separating the posterior aspects of the disks and vertebral bodies from the thecal sac. The ligamentum flavum is in the dorsal portion of the spinal canal, attaching the laminae and extending to the capsules of the facet joints and the posterior aspects of the neural foramina. Either ligament can ossify in later life, apparently independently of the usual processes of spondylosis and degenerative arthritis. Ossification of the posterior longitudinal ligament occurs more commonly in Asians than in non-Asians and with a roughly 2:1 male:female ratio. It may be visible on lateral spinal radiography but is usually asymptomatic. It is better seen by CT scan, in which it is distinguished from osteophytes by favoring the middle of the vertebral bodies rather than concentrating at the endplates. Thickness of the calcification can range from 3 to 15 mm. Ossification of the posterior longitudinal ligament is most likely to be symptomatic in the cervical spine, where it can contribute to cord

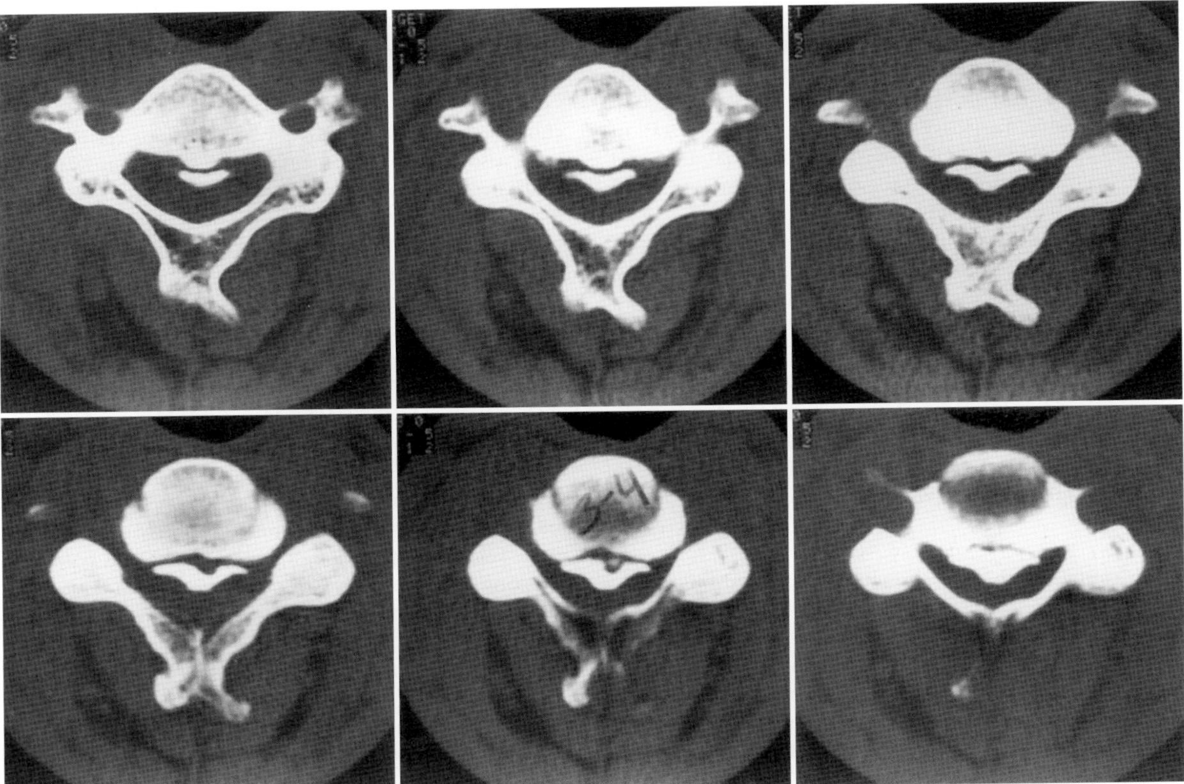

**Fig. 104.22 Computed Tomographic Scan of a Patient With Posterior Longitudinal Ligament Ossification.** Note continuous bony ridge present at every level, not just at disk space. In contrast to calcified degenerative spurs, these ligamentous calcifications are not connected to vertebral bodies. (*Courtesy Erik Gaensler.*)

compression if it is thick or if the canal is further narrowed by congenital and degenerative changes.

The ligamentum flavum can contribute by hypertrophy or ossification to spinal stenosis, most often in the lower thoracic or lumbar spine, affecting the cord or cauda equina. Risk factors for development of ossification of the ligamentum flavum include trauma, hemochromatosis, calcium pyrophosphate deposition disease, DISH spondylitis, or ossification of the posterior longitudinal ligament.

## DEGENERATIVE DISEASE OF THE SPINE

### Spinal Osteoarthritis and Spondylosis

Osteoarthritis of the spinal facet joints manifests radiographically as joint narrowing, sclerosis, and osteophyte formation. *Spondylosis* refers to degenerative disease of the intervertebral disks, visible on radiography as disk-space narrowing, vertebral endplate sclerosis, and osteophyte formation. Spinal osteoarthritis and spondylosis are inevitable consequences of aging that are visible on routine spinal radiography in more than 90% of people by the age of 60 years. They are usually asymptomatic, but cause compression of the spinal cord or nerve roots in a minority of people. Nonetheless, they are the most common cause of compressive myelopathy or radiculopathy, accounting for far more neurological disease than all the other conditions discussed in this chapter combined.

In youth, the intervertebral disks consist of a gelatinous central nucleus pulposus and a firm collagenous annulus fibrosus. Disk herniation syndromes occur when the nucleus pulposus bursts through a tear in the annulus fibrosus. This herniation can compress the nerve roots or spinal cord, depending on the spinal level involved. Rarely, disk material breaks into the thecal sac or a fragment ruptures into an epidural vein. Disk herniation is most likely to occur in young adults.

By age 40 years, most adults have some disk degeneration with dehydration and shrinkage of the nucleus pulposus, necrosis and fibrosis of the annulus fibrosus, and sclerosis and microfractures of the subchondral bone at the vertebral endplate. Compression of neurological tissue can develop from a combination of disk herniation, osteophyte formation, ligament hypertrophy, congenital stenosis of the spinal canal, low-grade synovitis, and deformity and misalignment of the spine.

### Cervical Spondylosis

Cervical osteoarthritis and spondylosis are ubiquitous with increasing age (eFig. 104.23). These disorders can rarely be attributed to specific activities or injuries. An exception is patients with dystonia and other cervical movement disorders, who seem predisposed to premature cervical spinal degeneration. Because cervical osteoarthritis and spondylosis are so commonplace, it is usually difficult to ascertain their role in contributing to the pathogenesis of chronic neck pain or headache. Cervical spine surgery in the setting of degenerative pathology is rarely if ever indicated for treatment of headache or neck pain in the absence of cervical radiculopathy or myelopathy.

### Cervical Radiculopathy

#### Clinical Presentation

The symptoms of cervical radiculopathy often appear suddenly (Carette and Fehlings, 2005). Although disk herniation or nerve root contusion can be caused by acute trauma, most cases become symptomatic without an identifiable preceding traumatic event. Disk herniation is more likely to be the cause in patients younger than 45 years; neuroforaminal stenosis by degenerative changes is more common than disk herniation and becomes more likely with increasing age. Classic cervical radicular pain originates from the neck and radiates down the arm with or without dysesthesias, paresthesias, numbness, or even weakness. Subscapular or interscapular pain is common with lower cervical radiculopathy (C7 especially, but also C6, C8, and/or T1). Radiculopathic arm pain may increase with coughing or Valsalva maneuver. Arm pain may increase with a combination of neck extension, rotation to the side of the pain, and downward axial compression of the head *(Spurling maneuver)*.

Spondylosis, osteophytes, and disk herniations at the C4–C5 level can affect the C5 root, causing pain, paresthesias, and sometimes loss of sensation over the shoulder, with weakness of the deltoid, biceps, and brachioradialis muscles. The biceps and supinator reflexes may be lost. Spread of the biceps reflex to the finger flexors, an increased triceps reflex, or a paradoxical biceps reflex (absent or reduced biceps reflex with reflex contraction of the finger flexors, or rarely the triceps) suggest the presence of myelopathy. Pathology at the C5–C6 level can affect the C6 root and cause sensory changes in the first two digits and/or lateral distal forearm, with possible weakness in the brachioradialis and wrist extensors. The biceps and brachioradialis reflexes may be diminished or inverted. Lesions at the C6–C7 level compressing the C7 root cause sensory changes in the index, middle, and/or ring fingers, and weakness in C7-innervated muscles such as the triceps, wrist flexors, and pronators. The triceps tendon reflex may be diminished.

The C5, C6, and C7 roots are the ones most commonly involved in cervical spondylosis because they are at the level of greatest mobility where disk degeneration is greatest in the cervical spine. The relative frequency of root lesions in cervical spondylosis varies in different series. Clinically evident compression of the C8 root or of roots above C5 is less common.

## Diagnostic Testing

Cervical plain-film radiography is of little value in diagnosing or excluding cervical radiculopathy. MRI scanning of the cervical spine is usually helpful in identifying nerve root compression in patients with cervical radiculopathy, as well as diagnosing causes of myelopathy, and is the imaging study of choice in most cases. Cervical myelography followed by CT scanning is sometimes more sensitive than MRI (Fig. 104.24), and is particularly helpful in patients with MRI-incompatible pacemakers, spinal cord stimulators, severe claustrophobia, and other patients who cannot undergo MRI scanning. MRI images are often degraded by the presence of hardware from prior cervical spine fusion surgeries, making CT myelography particularly useful in these patients as well. However, MRI may show nerve root compression, particularly in the neural foramina, which is invisible by CT myelography if the site of compression is lateral to the subarachnoid space, thus not filled with contrast agent. CT myelography is also better than MRI for distinguishing noncalcified disk herniation from osteophytes or calcified disk herniations. All of that said, cervical MRI or CT myelography must be interpreted with caution because degenerative abnormalities are so commonly seen in the asymptomatic spine.

Needle EMG and nerve conduction studies (NCS) can be useful in difficult diagnostic cases, both by identifying an affected motor nerve root and myotome and by helping exclude other diagnoses such as brachial plexopathy or peripheral neuropathy (Hakimi et al., 2013). NCS yield a particular pattern in cervical radiculopathy: there may be loss of amplitude in the affected compound muscle action potential (CMAP), but preservation of sensory nerve action potential (SNAP). This discrepancy occurs with intraspinal nerve root compression, which

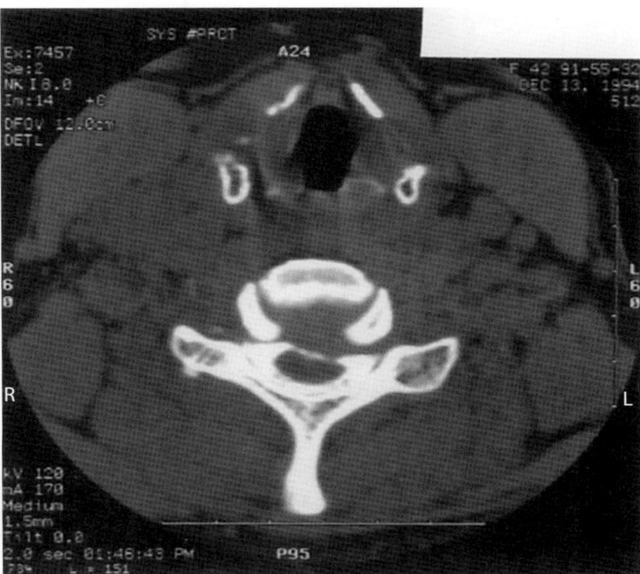


**Fig. 104.24 Computed Tomographic Scan of Cervical Spine With Intrathecal Contrast Shows a Herniated Cervical Disk.** Spinal cord *(gray)* and thecal sac *(white)* are distorted on the left by the disk. *(Reprinted with permission from Rosenbaum, R.B., Campbell, S.M., Rosenbaum, J.T., 1996. Clinical Neurology of Rheumatic Disease. Butterworth-Heinemann, Boston.)*

effectively separates motor nerve fibers from their cell body, the anterior horn cell within the spinal cord. This same lesion usually affects the root proximal to the dorsal root ganglion, allowing the sensory fibers to remain in continuity with their cell bodies. Needle EMG may reveal electrophysiological evidence of active denervation in the form of fibrillation potentials and/or positive sharp waves. Other spontaneous activity such as fasciculation potentials or complex repetitive discharges can suggest ongoing or remote motor neuron pathology, respectively. With volitional activation of the tested muscle, motor units may be large in amplitude and/or long in duration, suggesting prior denervation with subsequent reinnervation.

There are several limitations to consider when interpreting electrodiagnostic (EDX) testing for the diagnosis of radiculopathy. First, the study is of low diagnostic yield in the hyperacute period. The electrodiagnosis of radiculopathy is insensitive in detecting radiculopathy in the absence of axonal loss. Therefore, one must allow for the completion of Wallerian degeneration following an injury before the study is performed. This process typically takes 5–6 days for motor fibers and 8–9 days for sensory fibers. Needle EMG in isolation has been said to have moderate diagnostic sensitivity, with different series citing 50%–71%. Root compression resulting in intermittent ischemia or mechanical deformation may result in isolated root demyelination without secondary axonal loss. In this scenario, a patient may experience classical radicular symptoms without any objective evidence of the disease. For these reasons it is important to have concordant clinical, radiographical, and electrophysiological data when making the diagnosis. A judicious approach helps to avoid unnecessary and potentially harmful surgical procedures.

## Treatment

Most instances of cervical radiculopathy improve significantly over 4–8 weeks regardless of treatment. Various treatments such as NSAIDs, temporary/situational use of a soft cervical collar, physical therapy, or cervical traction give similar results. Other treatments such as chiropractic manipulation, acupuncture, and epidural steroid injections remain in widespread use despite contradictory, conflicting, controversial, and/or

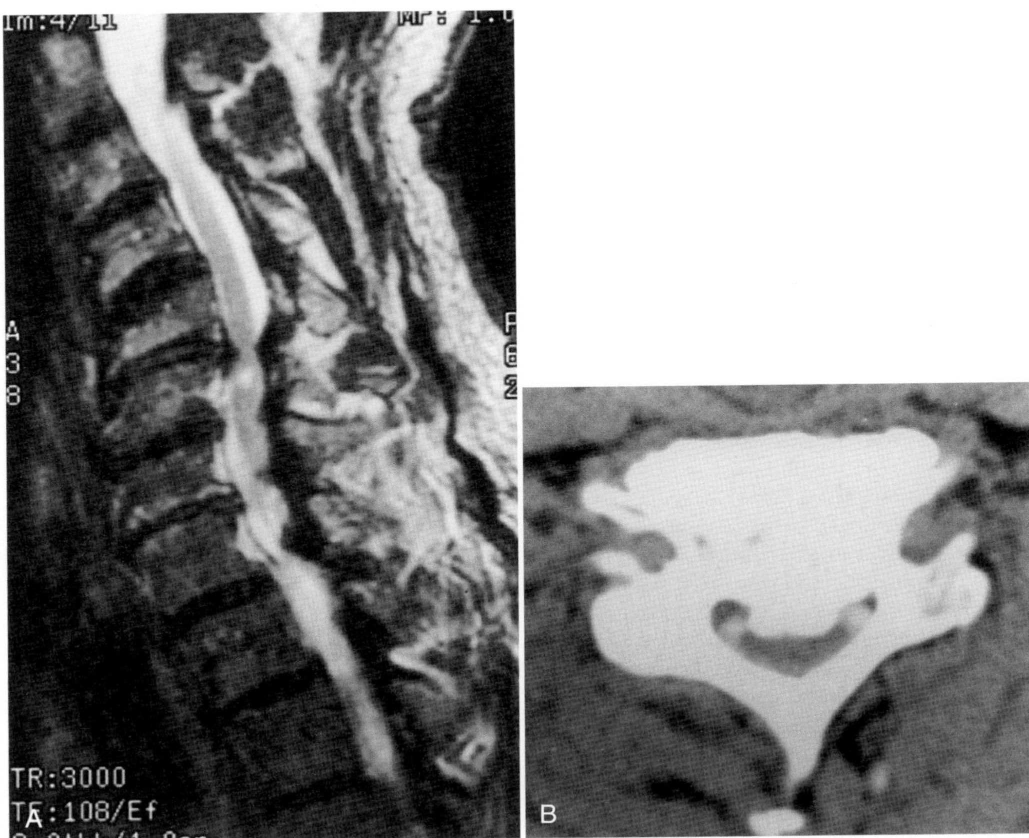


**Fig. 104.25 Cervical Spondylotic Myelopathy. A,** Sagittal T2-weighted magnetic resonance imaging scan shows maximal compression of thecal sac and spinal cord at C5–C6. **B,** Axial computed tomographic scan with intrathecal contrast at this level shows a large osteophyte arising from posterior aspect of vertebral body; spinal cord at this level is compressed, and thecal sac is so compressed that little of the white intrathecal contrast is visible. (*Reprinted with permission from Rosenbaum, R.B., Campbell, S.M., Rosenbaum, J.T., 1996. Clinical Neurology of Rheumatic Disease. Butterworth-Heinemann, Boston.*)

lacking scientific data. Patients with a typical clinical presentation and little or no neurological deficit usually can be managed with these noninvasive approaches without imaging or EDX studies. When patients with radiculopathy have marked and/or progressive weakness, intractable pain, or have not improved with nonoperative therapy, surgical nerve root decompression is usually successful; however, there is little randomized controlled comparison of nonoperative therapy and surgery (Nikolaidis et al., 2010). Anterior cervical discectomy, with either fusion or total disk arthroplasty, or posterior cervical laminoforaminotomy, have all been shown to be effective surgical techniques. Selection of one technique versus another is a complex decision and is beyond the scope of this chapter. Such a determination depends on many factors, including sagittal alignment (kyphosis vs. lordosis), site of pathology (dorsal vs. ventral vs. both), number of levels to be treated, and others.

## Cervical Spondylotic Myelopathy

Cervical myelopathy related to spondylosis and osteoarthritis usually develops insidiously, but it may be precipitated by trauma or progress in stepwise fashion. Typical clinical findings include: leg spasticity; upper-extremity weakness or clumsiness; and sensory changes in the arms, legs, or trunk. Either spinothalamic tract–mediated or posterior column–mediated sensory modalities may be impaired. Sphincter dysfunction, if it occurs, is often preceded by the motor and/or sensory deficits. Commonly, neck pain is not a prominent symptom, and neck range of motion may or may not be impaired. Some patients experience leg or trunk paresthesia induced by neck flexion *(Lhermitte sign).*

The anterior-posterior diameter of the cervical spinal cord is usually 10 mm or less. Patients rarely develop cervical spondylotic myelopathy (CSM) if the congenital diameter of their spinal canal exceeds 16 mm. In congenitally narrow canals, disk protrusion, osteophytes, hypertrophy of the ligamentum flavum, ossification of the posterior longitudinal ligament, and vertebral body subluxations can combine to compress the spinal cord. MRI, CT, or myelography provide excellent images of relation between the spinal canal and the spinal cord (Fig. 104.25). MRI is the imaging study of choice in most cases, and provides detailed information about intramedullary pathology such as secondary cord edema or gliosis. CT provides better images of calcified tissues. Even with excellent cross-sectional imaging of the spinal canal, the clinical correlation between neurological deficit and cord compression is imperfect; dynamic changes in cord compression and vascular perfusion undoubtedly contribute to the pathogenesis of CSM.

The natural history of CSM is variable. Some patients have stable neurological deficits for many years without specific therapy, whereas other patients have gradual or stepwise deterioration. Some patients improve with treatments such as bed rest, soft collars, or immobilizing collars, but these treatments have not been assessed in controlled trials. Many patients with CSM are treated by surgical decompression, with variable surgical results (Fig. 104.26). Surgical treatment tends to be highly effective at halting progressive loss of function, although recovery of lost function is less reliable, and depends on the severity and duration of symptoms prior to surgery, with better results when symptoms are milder, have been present less than 12 months, and when

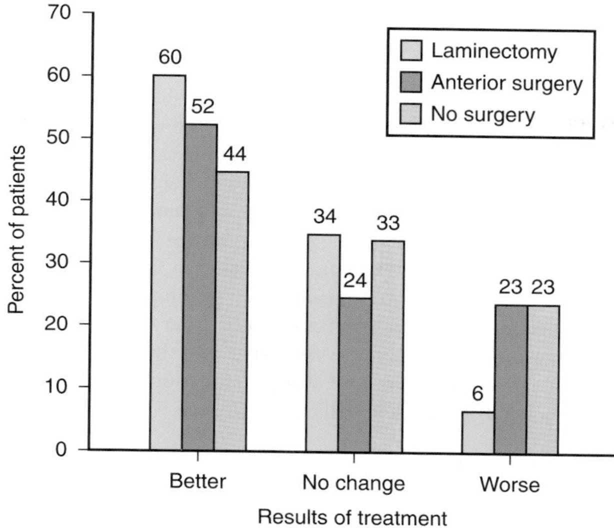


**Fig. 104.26** Results of Treatment of Cervical Spondylotic Myelopathy. *(Reprinted with permission from Rosenbaum, R.B., Campbell, S.M., Rosenbaum, J.T., 1996. Clinical Neurology of Rheumatic Disease, Butterworth-Heinemann, Boston. [Data from Rowland, L.P., 1992. Surgical treatment of cervical spondylotic myelopathy: time for a controlled trial. Neurology 42, 5.])*

the patient is younger than 70 years. Anterior cervical discectomy and fusion, anterior cervical corpectomy and fusion, posterior laminectomy, laminectomy with fusion, and laminoplasty are all potential options. As is the case with choice of surgical options for cervical radiculopathy, the choice of one technique over another is multifactorial and must be tailored to each individual patient's situation. Currently available literature remains inconclusive regarding which surgical approach is best for CSM; a recent systematic review examined the literature for anterior versus posterior treatment of CSM and concluded that both approaches are highly effective for improving CSM symptoms, that anterior approaches may have slightly higher quality of life (QOL) outcomes, and that posterior approaches have higher direct costs and slightly higher complication rates. However, the authors of this study emphasize that the studies they reviewed were all level 2 and 3 data, and that prospective randomized controlled trials will be necessary to settle this debate (Alvin et al., 2013).

## Vertebral Artery Stroke Caused by Cervical Osteoarthritis

Compression of a vertebral artery by an osteophyte is a rare cause of stroke in the vertebrobasilar distribution (Bulsara et al., 2006). The vertebral arteries pass through foramina in the transverse processes from C6 to C2. Osteophytes from the uncovertebral joint can compress the arteries. The compression may occur with something as benign as head rotation. However, the rotation often leaves the contralateral vertebral artery uncompressed, so ischemic symptoms are usually limited to those patients who have both osteophytic arterial compression on one side and a contralateral hypoplastic, absent, or occluded artery. Aggressive chiropractic neck manipulation should be discouraged since it can lead to vertebral artery dissection at the AA loop with resultant vertebrobasilar distribution embolic strokes (Devereaux, 2000).

## Thoracic Spondylosis

Degenerative changes are less common in the thoracic than in the lumbar or cervical spines given the relative lack of mobility and thus infrequency of spondylosis (Vanichkachorn and Vaccaro, 2000). Thoracic osteophytes are more likely to develop on the anterior or lateral aspects of the vertebral bodies and infrequently cause clinical radiculopathy. Thoracic disk herniations are visible on MRI in many asymptomatic individuals. Thoracic disk herniations occur most often in the lower thoracic spine. When a thoracic nerve root is impinged, the patient may note severe, sharp pain and paresthesias involving the abdominal or chest wall. There can also be associated abdominal muscle weakness resulting in a bulge or "pseudohernia" (Fig. 104.27). While pain may be significant and difficult to control in the acute phase, symptoms are often self-limited (Chaudhuri et al., 1997).

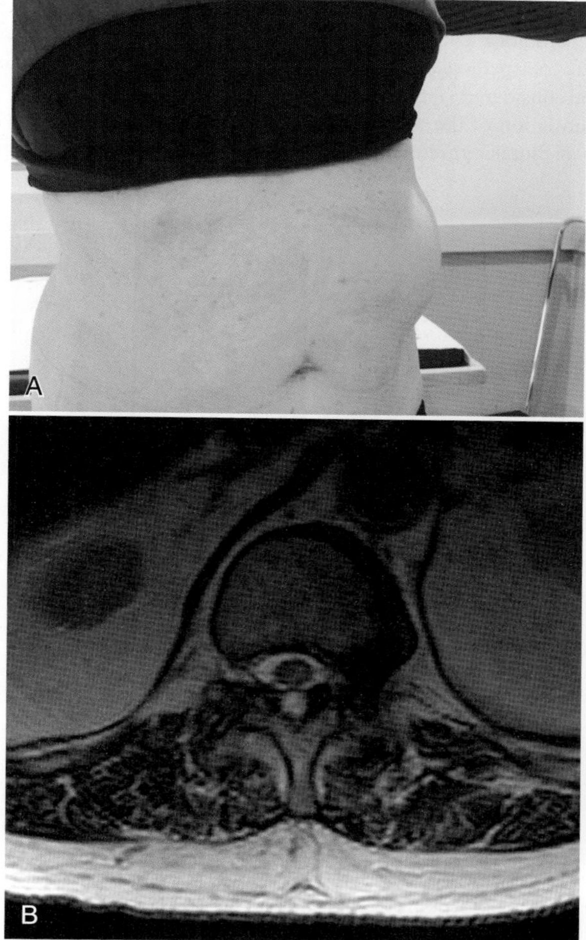


**Fig. 104.27** A, Left abdominal "pseudohernia" resulting from weakened abdominal wall musculature within a single thoracic myotome. B, Left, lateral disk bulge compressing the exiting T8 root. *(Courtesy Bashar Katirji, MD.)*

Thoracic myelopathy due to disk herniation probably has an annual incidence of approximately 1 case per 1 million. Most cases occur between ages 30 and 60 years. Symptoms often develop insidiously without identifiable preceding trauma. Back pain may or may not be present. Patients have some combination of motor and sensory findings of myelopathy; sphincter dysfunction is present in more severe cases. Thoracic MRI, CT, or myelography can confirm the diagnosis (Fig. 104.28). The treatment is surgical decompression when there is clear clinical and radiographic evidence of thoracic radiculopathy and/or myelopathy, but should be assiduously avoided when only axial back pain is present. Surgical options include transthoracic discectomy via open thoracotomy, thoracoscopy or minimally invasive thoracotomy; if the pathology is located laterally enough, a posterolateral approach such as transpedicular discectomy, open or minimally invasive, could also be considered (Fig. 104.29).

Herniation of the thoracic spinal cord into the dura is a very rare cause of thoracic myelopathy (Sasani et al., 2009). The most common presentation is a Brown-Séquard syndrome that can slowly evolve over a few years. Thoracic spine MRI shows the spinal cord ventrally deviated, often with a kink at one level between T2 and T7, and with increased dorsal subarachnoid space. CT myelography will show similar changes and confirm that there is no subarachnoid space ventrally where the spinal cord is attached to the dura. This condition can be extremely difficult to differentiate radiographically from a dorsal thoracic arachnoid cyst pushing the cord anteriorly, unless very blatant flattening of the dorsal cord surface is present, suggesting pressure from a mass lesion rather than anterior tethering alone. The adjacent vertebral body may appear scalloped. Spinal cord herniation can be idiopathic, presumably due to congenital defects in the dura, or occur after trauma or thoracic spinal surgery. Rare instances are associated with thoracic disk herniation. Some patients improve after surgical reduction of the herniation, but this is a highly technically challenging surgery.

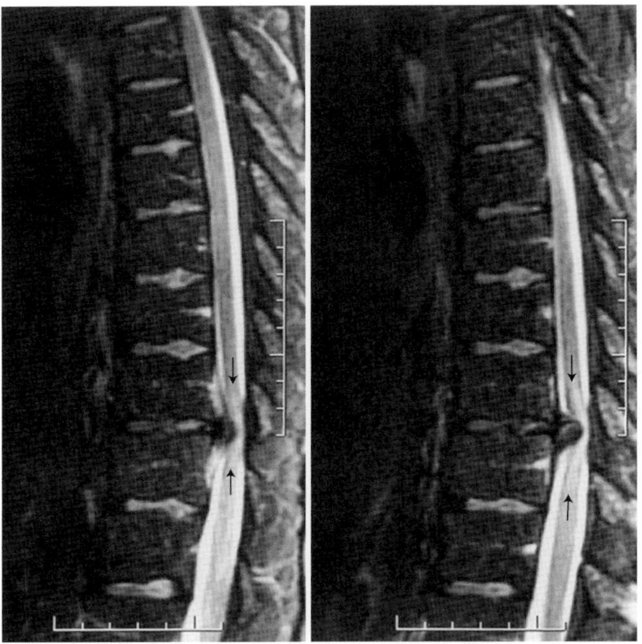

**Fig. 104.28 Thoracic Magnetic Resonance Images of a Patient With Thoracic Disk Herniation.** This large acute disk herniation at T10–T11 consists of extrusion of most of the nucleus pulposus into the spinal canal. There is secondary narrowing of the disk space and spinal cord edema *(arrows)* above and below the level of spinal cord compression. (*Courtesy Erik Gaensler.*)

## Lumbar Spondylosis

### Low Back Pain

Episodes of acute low back pain, which usually resolve within a few days, are experienced by some 80% of persons. These episodes often recur, and approximately 4% report chronic low back pain. Pain-sensitive structures in the lumbar region include the nerve roots, zygapophyseal joints, sacroiliac joints, intervertebral ligaments, muscles, fascia, annulus fibrosis and circumferential portions of the disks, and vertebral periosteum. Controlled local anesthetic injection studies suggest that in some patients, the cause of low back pain can be localized to specific zygapophyseal or sacroiliac joints. In other patients, injection of contrast media into lumbar disks reproduces pain, suggesting that the lumbar disk is the source of pain. However, this localization cannot be achieved reliably by history or physical examination, and, when attempted, localization of the source of pain is often unsuccessful. Thus, in clinical practice, "nonspecific low back pain" is a commonly made diagnosis.

The findings of osteoarthritis and lumbar spondylosis on radiography (osteophytes, endplate sclerosis, disk-space narrowing) appear gradually with increasing age and are rarely absent by age 60 years (see

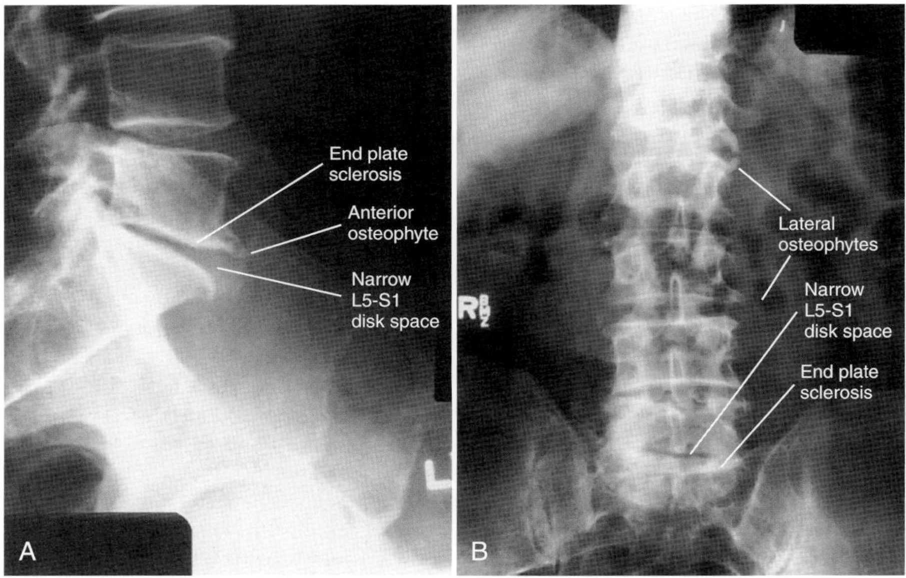


**Fig. 104.29** Lateral **(A)** and anteroposterior **(B)** radiographs of lumbar spine showing osteophytes, disk-space narrowing, and sclerosis of vertebral body articular plates. (*Reprinted with permission from Rosenbaum, R.B., Campbell, S.M., Rosenbaum, J.T., 1996. Clinical Neurology of Rheumatic Disease. Butterworth-Heinemann, Boston.*)

**BOX 104.6 Indications for Lumbar Spine Radiography in Patients With Acute Low Back Pain**

**Red Flags for Trauma**
Major trauma (e.g., motor vehicle accident, fall from height)
Minor trauma or even strenuous lifting in older or potentially osteoporotic patient
Prolonged corticosteroid use
Osteoporosis
Age >70 years

**Red Flags for Tumor or Infection**
Age >50 years or <20 years
History of cancer
Constitutional symptoms (e.g., fever, chills, weight loss)
Risk factors for spinal infection (e.g., recent bacterial infection, intravenous drug use, immunosuppression)
Pain that is worse when supine or is severe at night

*Adapted with permission from Agency for Health Care Policy and Research, 1994. Acute Low Back Problems in Adults. Assessment and Treatment: Quick Reference Guide for Clinicians. US Department of Health and Human Services, Rockville, MD.*

Fig. 104.29). The presence or absence of these findings does not correlate with symptoms and demonstrating them is of no diagnostic or therapeutic value. Therefore, radiography of the lumbar spine is indicated only when alternative diagnoses such as compression fractures, neoplasia, or infections are being seriously considered. The Agency for Health Care Policy and Research has recommended that spinal radiography be reserved for patients with "red flags," which include history of and/or signs of trauma, tumor, or infection, or any neurological deficit, but not pain alone (Box 104.6). Even limiting radiography to patients meeting these guidelines results in many needless radiographs. For example, back pain in a patient older than 50 years need not be an indication for imaging studies unless other findings suggest a condition more serious than nonspecific low back pain.

There are many causes of lumbar disk disease, including body habitus, type and amount of physical activity, acute injury, history of tobacco abuse, and genetic predisposition, which is complex and polygenic with a number of known candidate genes (Kalichman and Hunter, 2008).

### Spondylolysis and Spondylolisthesis

*Spondylolisthesis* is displacement of one lumbar vertebral body relative to an adjacent vertebral body. The most common type of spondylolisthesis is degenerative, which usually results from deterioration of the facet joints, ligaments and disk. The increased laxity allows a certain degree of anterolisthesis, but high-grade (beyond grade II) slippage is rare with this type. This occurs most commonly in the lumbar spine at L4–L5. The second-most common cause is spondylolysis, a discontinuity in the vertebral pars interarticularis, which disrupts the normal stabilizing effect of the facet joints. This is known as "isthmic" or "spondylolytic" spondylolisthesis, can result in high-grade slippage, and is most common at L5–S1. Other causes of spondylolisthesis include congenital vertebral anomalies and vertebral trauma. Spondylolysis occurs in 5%–7% of the population and is usually asymptomatic. Spondylolisthesis is often painless or may cause low back pain that sometimes radiates to the buttocks. Spondylolytic spondylolisthesis is a common cause of back pain in adolescents. Occasionally, spondylolisthesis can advance to the point of compressing nerve roots in the neural foramina or causing lumbar canal stenosis. In patients with convincing radicular symptoms, mild spondylolisthesis and no clear neuroforaminal stenosis by MRI, flexion and extension radiographs can be considered. In some cases, imaging in a neutral position may fail to demonstrate significant foraminal compromise, but flexion/extension films may reveal an unstable or "dynamic" spondylolisthesis (Even et al., 2014).

## Lumbar Radiculopathies

The back and leg neurological examination is central to decision making in patients with low back pain. Perhaps 1%–2% of patients with acute low back pain have significant lumbar nerve root compression. Three syndromes merit specific diagnostic consideration.

## Monoradiculopathy

### Clinical Presentation

Patients with an acute lower lumbar or lumbosacral monoradiculopathy due to nerve root compression typically present with unilateral leg pain *(sciatica)* radiating into the buttock, posterolateral thigh, and typically distally into the leg, foot and/or toe(s), sometimes with sensory disturbance and/or weakness. Patients often also have localized, low back pain. Pain may increase with movement, coughing, sneezing, or Valsalva maneuver and decrease with rest or recumbent positioning. Pain often increases when the straightened ipsilateral leg is raised while the patient is supine *(straight leg-raising test, Lasègue sign)* or when the leg is straightened at the knee while the patient is seated (seated straight leg-raising). The most commonly compressed nerve roots are L5, usually by L4–L5 disk herniation, or S1, usually by L5–S1 disk herniation. These localizing guidelines are variable, in part due to different sites of nerve root compression that are possible in the lumbar spine. For example, a paracentral disk herniation at L4–L5 will usually compress the traversing L5 nerve root, while a far lateral/intraforaminal disk herniation at L4–L5 will compress the exiting L4 root. For L5 radiculopathy, the findings are typically anterior leg, dorsal foot, and hallux pain, paresthesia (especially on the medial dorsal foot), and weakness in the extensor hallucis longus muscle, ankle dorsiflexors, and peroneal muscles. L5 radiculopathy can be clinically similar to peroneal mononeuropathy, but these can be differentiated by noting the presence of weakness of foot inversion with L5 radiculopathy, which is not seen with peroneal neuropathy (see Chapter 105). S1 nerve root compression can lead to plantar and lateral foot pain and paresthesia, depressed ankle jerk, and weakness of peroneal muscles and (less frequently) ankle plantar flexors. When the radiculopathy is mild, the patient may have pain without obvious objective neurological deficits.

### Diagnostic Studies

Disk herniations, osteophytes, spondylolysis, spondylolisthesis, facet joint hypertrophy, and hypertrophy or calcification of intraspinal ligaments can compress nerve roots of the cauda equina within the spinal canal or in the lateral recesses and neural foramina through which the roots exit the spinal canal. The anatomical relations between the nerve roots and the surrounding tissues are well visualized by lumbar MRI or CT myelography (Fig. 104.30, *A*, eFig 104.30, *B*). Each technique has high sensitivity for demonstrating causes of nerve root compression. On occasion, when a patient has strong clinical evidence of lumbar radiculopathy, but initial imaging studies do not show the cause of the compression, a second complementary imaging study is indicated. For example, imaging with a lumbar MRI usually is sufficient for most clinical purposes, but occasionally a patient also needs CT myelography to clarify the anatomy. Unfortunately, all spinal imaging modalities frequently show anatomical abnormalities that are not the cause of symptomatic nerve root dysfunction; all imaging results must be interpreted carefully in clinical context.

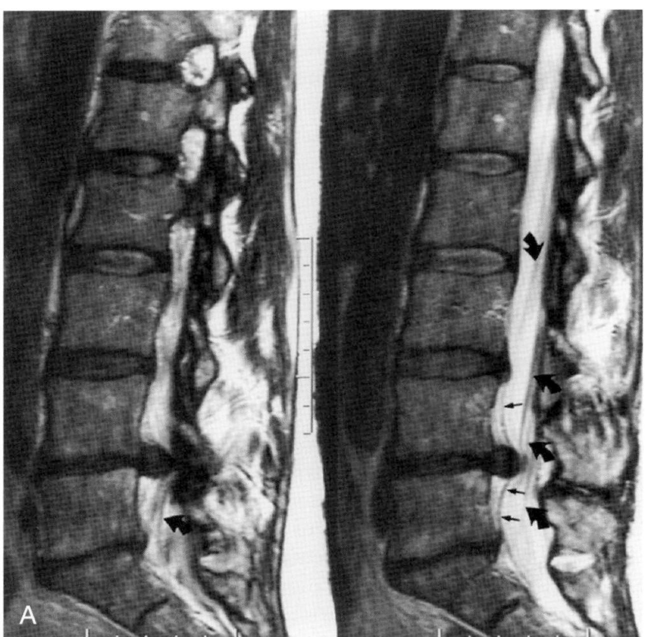


**Fig. 104.30** A, Lumbar magnetic resonance image of a patient with lumbar disk herniation at L4–L5. Ventral dura is displaced *(straight arrows)* posteriorly. Roots of cauda equina are compressed *(curved arrows)*. (A, *Courtesy Erik Gaensler.*)

As in cervical radiculopathy, EDX studies are usually performed when confirmation of the clinical diagnosis of lumbosacral radiculopathy is needed. This includes in patients whose history or examination are limited; when a more distal lesion (e.g., lumbosacral plexopathy, lower extremity mononeuropathy) needs to be excluded; or in patients in whom the clinical significance of an imaging abnormality is unclear. In addition to confirming the presence of root compression, the EDX study helps in the localization of the compression to either a single or to multiple roots; in defining the age and activity; and the severity of the lesion.

Needle EMG remains by far the most sensitive EDX tool in patients with suspected lumbosacral radiculopathy. The presence of fibrillation potentials is the most objective EMG finding. The diagnosis is confirmed by the presence of denervation in a segmental myotomal distribution with or without denervation of the paraspinal muscles along with a normal SNAP in the corresponding dermatome.

EMG sensitivity is greater with a more severe or predominantly motor radiculopathy. The needle EMG may be normal if only the dorsal root is compressed and not the ventral root (such as in patients with only pain and/or paresthesias); if the injured root lacks adequate myotomal representation (such as L1, L2, and C4 roots); or, as previously mentioned, the pathophysiology is entirely demyelinating. EMG and imaging studies are often complementary in the diagnosis of lumbosacral radiculopathy. EMG provides information about nerve root function, whereas imaging studies provide information about the anatomy of the nerve roots and surrounding structures. The agreement between imaging and EMG is higher in patients with abnormal neurological examinations.

## Treatment

Most sufferers of acute low back pain and sciatica recover within 6 weeks using simple nonoperative therapies such as brief periods of bed rest, activity limitations as required by pain, and simple nonopioid analgesics. Chronic lower back pain and sciatica are much more difficult to manage. Conservative measures can include physical therapy, judicious use of nonopioid medications, and behavioral therapies. Prolonged immobilization is detrimental, and early mobilization results in more rapid recovery. Many patients with acute low back pain and sciatica can be managed initially based on clinical examination without spinal imaging studies. Patients who have progressive weakness or sensory loss or who have severe pain that fails to improve after 6 weeks of nonoperative therapy can be considered for surgical nerve root decompression. Patients least likely to benefit from lumbar nerve root surgery are those who lack radicular pain, objective neurological signs of nerve root dysfunction, or corresponding imaging evidence of nerve root compression.

Invasive techniques such as steroids and local anesthetics injected epidurally or into facet joints are used for some patients with low back pain or radiculopathy, but we still lack consistent proof of their long-term efficacy or cost-effectiveness from randomized controlled trials (Chou et al., 2009). Lumbar epidural steroid injections may result in some improvement in radicular symptoms if pain is assessed 2–6 weeks after injections, but the injections do not have proven longer-lasting value (Armon et al., 2007).

A few patients develop a chronic low back pain syndrome or have repeated exacerbations of acute low back pain. Back-strengthening exercises and the avoidance of maneuvers that put strain on the lower back, together with the judicious use of NSAIDs, generally improve such patients' pain. Workers who are off work with low back pain for longer than 6 months have a guarded prognosis for return to work. Physicians caring for patients with low back pain lasting longer than 4 weeks need, whenever possible, to emphasize exercise, to avoid deconditioning, and to enable early return to graded work.

When surgery is performed for lumbar nerve root compression, the surgical technique depends on the clinical details such as the cause of compression and the number of nerve roots compressed. In patients with lumbar radiculopathy due to disk herniation, the most common surgical approach is microsurgical discectomy with minimal removal of the lamina. In controlled trials, this surgery provided better relief of symptoms than nonoperative therapy, based on results 2–3 months after treatment; however, the advantage of surgery decreased with longer follow-up (Chou et al., 2009). Perhaps 90% of patients report excellent relief of neuropathic pain after surgery. Many are able to return to physically strenuous work. However, a small proportion of patients postoperatively present with severe chronic pain problems *(failed back surgery syndrome)*, which particularly occurs when patients selected for surgery have neither clinical evidence of radiculopathy nor corresponding neuroimaging evidence of nerve root compression. While chronic and ongoing pain after lumbar surgery is less common after simple discectomy than it is after multilevel laminectomy, or particularly after lumbar fusion surgery, it does still occur. Recurrent disk herniation, or incomplete discectomy, are both common causes of poor postoperative condition. Less common causes include excessive epidural scarring with compression and/or tethering of nerve roots, arachnoiditis, hematoma, or postoperative spinal instability. Other problems such as misdiagnosis prior to surgery, or even possible confounding psychiatric and/or psychosocial issues, must be considered.

## Acute Cauda Equina Syndrome

Acute cauda equina syndrome presents as low back and bilateral leg pain, motor weakness of the legs, and sphincter dysfunction caused by compression of multiple lumbosacral nerve roots within the spinal canal. Particularly worrisome findings are sacral sensory loss or impaired function of the rectal and urinary sphincters. Acute cauda equina compression occurs in less than 1% of all patients who have lumbar or lumbosacral disk prolapses. The cause is usually a large midline disk herniation, most often at L4–L5 or L5–S1, but multiple other causes can be seen, including fractures, fracture/dislocation, spinal tumors, lumbar epidural abscess, or rarely, very extreme cases of degenerative canal stenosis. When acute cauda equina compression occurs, the patient needs urgent spinal imaging and decompressive surgery because the window of opportunity for restoration of neurological function is limited to 24 hours, or perhaps 48 hours in some cases, with only partial recovery being the most likely outcome in many cases.

### Lumbar Canal Stenosis

Lumbar canal stenosis results from subnormal cross-sectional area of the spinal canal due to varied anatomical changes, including congenitally small canal size, degenerative osteophytes, spondylolisthesis, facet joint hypertrophy, thickening of the ligamentum flavum, disk-space narrowing, and disk herniation (Katz and Harris, 2008). It usually develops insidiously with aging and rarely becomes symptomatic before age 40 years unless due to congenital stenosis or skeletal changes like those of achondroplasia. Men are more often affected than women.

Stenosis is often asymptomatic; however, patients can have low back pain. A particularly characteristic pattern is back and lower extremity pain that develops while standing but is absent while sitting or supine. When ambulating, patients with lumbar canal stenosis may develop *neurogenic intermittent claudication*. This manifests as progressive lower extremity pain and/or paresthesia, which abates within minutes following flexion at the waist or sitting. Some patients are more comfortable if they bend forward while they walk (the "shopping cart sign") or can bicycle without difficulty. They may develop leg symptoms with sustained erect posture or after lying with their back straight. In contrast, vasogenic intermittent claudication can be elicited by almost any lower extremity exercise, but is not elicited or relieved by any specific postures. Vascular claudication does not induce paresthesia in the lower extremities. Since both these conditions generally occur in older patients, they can occur together, which can be a diagnostic challenge. Physical examination signs of pallor, hair loss, delayed capillary refill, and lack of palpable pulses in the feet should prompt attention toward diagnostic vascular testing. A simple and inexpensive test for this is an ankle-brachial index (ABI).

Most patients with neurogenic intermittent claudication do not have objective signs of nerve root dysfunction, likely as a result of intermittent nerve root ischemia without subsequent axonal loss. Nerve stretch signs such as pain with straight leg raising are usually absent, but infrequently a patient has progressive neurological deficits from chronic cauda equina compression. Some patients develop leg weakness or other abnormal neurological signs following exercise; neurological examination before and after precipitation of the pain can be a helpful part of the evaluation of neurogenic claudication. Patients with congenital lumbar canal stenosis often have accompanying congenital stenosis of the cervical canal and should be checked for signs of a cervical myeloradiculopathy.

***Diagnostic studies.*** Spinal canal stenosis is generally evaluated by MRI and less often CT (Fig. 104.31). MRI is best at demonstrating sagittal relationships such as the role of spondylolisthesis in narrowing the canal. CT is best at studying calcified tissues and distinguishing disk from osteophyte, especially within the neural foramina. No imaging modality quantifies the extent of nerve root compression, and clinical correlations between symptoms and apparent reduction in size of the spinal canal are imperfect. In choosing which patients would benefit from decompressive surgery, one should rely more heavily on clinical findings than on the appearance of the canal in imaging studies. EMG is also a very useful tool in patient selection for decompressive surgery by helping to establish/confirm the presence of radiculopathy/cauda equina syndrome.

***Treatment.*** Patients who have neurogenic intermittent claudication may have stable symptoms for many years without developing progressive neurological deficit. Some even note regression of symptoms after months of recurrent claudication. These patients may be managed with mild analgesics. Some describe decreased discomfort if they walk with a slight stoop or using a cane. Those patients with intractable leg pain or progressive neurological deficit can be treated with wide laminectomy of the stenosed spinal canal, which usually improves the symptoms of claudication and may help back pain (Chou et al., 2009; Weinstein et al., 2008). Laminectomy, especially multilevel laminectomy, can potentially increase spinal instability, and if instability is present preoperatively or is expected to result from the decompression, the patient should be treated with both laminectomy and fusion. For many decades, debate has persisted regarding the optimal surgical treatment strategy for patients with lumbar spinal stenosis with or without associated instability, usually in the form of degenerative spondylolisthesis. Even in the presence of spondylolisthesis, many authors have advocated for treatment with laminectomy alone, while others have recommended supplemental lumbar fusion. Many studies have addressed this question over the years, with ultimately conflicting results. Two recent randomized controlled trials were published in the same issue of the *New England Journal of Medicine*. Ghogawala et al. (2016) randomized 66 patients, all with lumbar stenosis and degenerative spondylolisthesis, to treatment with either laminectomy and fusion or laminectomy alone. At 4-year follow-up, they found slightly improved clinical outcome based on Short-Form 35 (SF-36) but not Oswestry Disability Index (ODI) with laminectomy plus fusion, although this surgery was associated with higher blood loss and longer hospital stay. They also found a significantly higher reoperation rate (34% vs. 14%) for laminectomy alone. The authors concluded that laminectomy plus fusion results in slightly greater, but clinically meaningful, improvement compared to laminectomy alone. Conversely, Forsth et al. (2016) randomized 247 into four groups based on presence or absence of spondylolisthesis and laminectomy alone versus laminectomy and fusion. They found no significant clinical differences between the treatment groups at 2 years or 5 years. When they analyzed only the subgroup with spondylolisthesis, again no clinical difference in outcomes was found, even when this was applied to patients with anterolisthesis of 7.5 mm or greater. Reoperation rates were similar, as were complication rates. The authors of this study concluded that there was no benefit to adding fusion to the laminectomy, even in the presence of spondylolisthesis. They also noted an increased cost of $6800 per surgery with the addition of fusion. Neither study can be said to be definitive, and larger studies will be needed to refine our understanding of this issue.

Patients with 1- or 2-level stenosis can also be excellent candidates for minimally invasive laminectomy. A less-invasive treatment option, reserved for patients with classic neurogenic claudication relieved by sitting and forward flexion, is placement of an interspinous process blocking device. This treatment is best for patients who are elderly, as it does not stop progression of the underlying degenerative cascade, and, for that reason, may have limited longevity. It can be implanted under local anesthetic with or without light sedation, making it an appropriate alternative for those who are too frail to be put under full general anesthesia.

## INFECTIOUS DISEASES OF THE SPINE

### Pyogenic Vertebral Osteomyelitis and Epidural Abscess

Vertebral osteomyelitis and spinal epidural abscess (see Chapter 79) are uncommon conditions that present with focal spinal pain and tenderness (Curry et al., 2005; Zimmerli, 2010). Epidural abscesses in the anterior spinal canal are more likely than those in the posterior canal

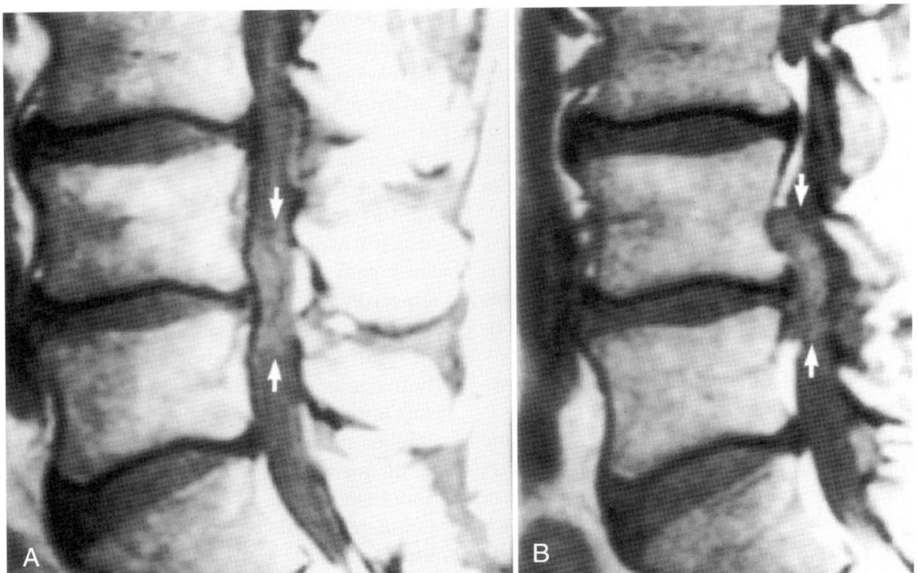


**Fig. 104.31 Magnetic Resonance Image of Patient With Lumbar Spinal Stenosis.** Midline (**A**) and parasagittal (**B**) images of lumbar spine show narrow anteroposterior dimensions of spinal canal consistent with spinal canal stenosis. (*Courtesy Erik Gaensler.*)

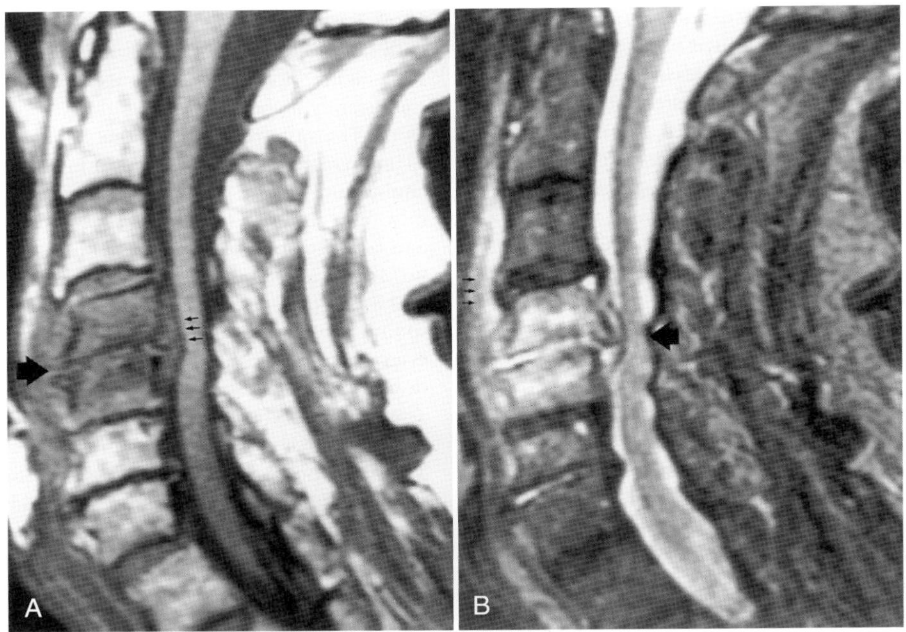


**Fig. 104.32 Magnetic Resonance Image of a Patient With Pyogenic Vertebral Osteomyelitis. A,** T1-weighted sagittal image shows replacement of normal marrow fat of C4 and C5 vertebrae with low signal intensity edema, with narrowing of disk space *(arrow)* and thickening of epidural soft tissue *(small arrows)*. **B,** T2-weighted image shows mild spinal cord compression *(arrow)* and hyperintensity of anterior longitudinal ligament, consistent with superior extension of infectious process *(small arrows)*. (*Courtesy Erik Gaensler.*)

to be associated with osteomyelitis. In either location, they can cause radiculopathic pain, compromise nerve root function, or lead to spinal cord compression. Some patients with spinal epidural abscess or vertebral osteomyelitis are afebrile at presentation, but most have an elevated erythrocyte sedimentation rate (ESR) and/or C-reactive protein (CRP). Early in the infection, routine spinal radiography may be normal. If the diagnosis is being considered, an MRI scan (Fig. 104.32) of the involved area is sensitive for detecting vertebral body abnormalities and is particularly helpful to assess for epidural or paravertebral infection. Spinal CT or radionuclide scanning are useful if MRI is unavailable or contraindicated.

Osteomyelitis may involve any vertebral body but is least common in the cervical vertebrae. Often in pyogenic, but infrequently in granulomatous osteomyelitis, the MRI shows involvement of the adjacent disk space. Osteomyelitis and spinal epidural abscess usually occur by hematogenous spread and are more likely following septicemia.

The most common causative organism is *Staphylococcus aureus*, but a wide variety of other bacteria can be responsible. Polymicrobial infection is uncommon after hematogenous infection but can occur when the source is open trauma or contiguous spread from other tissues. Diabetes, infective endocarditis, alcoholism, acquired immunodeficiency syndrome (AIDS), and other forms of immunosuppression increase the risk of its development. Other risk factors are intravenous drug use and spinal trauma. Cases may be iatrogenic following spinal surgery.

The annual incidence of hospitalization for vertebral osteomyelitis in the United States from 1998 to 2013 rose from 2.9 to 5.4 per 100,000 people. Reasons for this increase include the following (Berbari, 2015; Issa, 2018):

- Increasing rates of bacteremia due to the greater utilization of intravascular devices and various types of instrumentation
- The increasing age of the population
- The increasing number of patients receiving renal dialysis
- The increasing utilization of immunosuppressive therapies

Vertebral osteomyelitis and discitis are generally treated medically with long-term antibiotic therapy. CT-guided needle biopsy of the vertebral body and/or disk space can provide a causative organism and thus help tailor antibiotic therapy. In cases where extensive erosive and destructive changes have caused spinal instability, bracing is suggested until the infection is cleared, at which point surgical stabilization can be performed. Spinal epidural abscess, however, is almost always a surgical emergency, particularly above the level of the cauda equina (i.e., where spinal cord is present). This is because even in the absence of marked neurological compression the abscess can trigger an acute inflammatory thrombophlebitis, causing acute cord infarction and irreversible neurological compromise. This can occur rapidly even in a patient who is neurologically normal at presentation. Many patients, however, develop an epidural phlegmon ("burned-out" post-infectious inflammatory tissue that enhances) without any free pus within it (lack of rim enhancement on MRI) that is often misread as an abscess. The presence of phlegmon does not require surgical intervention unless there is mass effect on the spinal cord.

### Granulomatous Vertebral Osteomyelitis

Tuberculosis (TB) of the spine *(Pott disease)* is one of the more common forms of nonpulmonary TB and by far the most common granulomatous spinal infection. The risk is highest in regions or populations where TB is endemic. In the United States, high-risk factors are immigration from an endemic area, AIDS, homelessness, and drug or alcohol abuse. Other organisms capable of causing granulomatous osteomyelitis include brucellosis, a variety of fungi, *Nocardia*, and *Actinomyces*. Granulomatous spinal infection typically presents with insidious progression of back pain. The patient often has symptoms of systemic infection such as weight loss, fever, night sweats, or malaise.

Pott disease classically presents with destruction of vertebral bodies. Routine spine radiography results are usually abnormal by the time the diagnosis is made, and spinal deformity (gibbus deformity, a form of structural kyphosis) is a common complication. MRI is the preferred imaging study to assess for contiguous abscess in the epidural or paraspinal spaces and to evaluate possible nerve root or spinal cord compression when the spine is deformed (Fig. 104.33). Compression of spinal cord or nerve roots can occur in vertebral TB by vertebral deformity or collapse, epidural abscess, granulation tissue, or bony sequestrum. Patients may develop delayed neurological complications after apparently successful treatment of the infection. This may be due to infarction from endarteritis obliterans, delayed degenerative bony changes, or reactivation of infection. Compression of nervous structures is most common with thoracic vertebral disease: hence the eponym *Pott paraplegia*. Cauda equina compression is uncommon in TB. Treatment of vertebral TB requires long-term multiple-drug anti-tuberculous therapy. Spinal surgery may be needed, depending on the degree of spinal destruction or deformity, and is often required in cases of compression of neurological structures.

## INFLAMMATORY JOINT DISEASE

### Rheumatoid Arthritis

RA is a chronic, inflammatory, symmetrical, destructive, immune-mediated polyarthritis. In population studies, 0.2%–2% of the population is affected, women twice as often as men. Typically, patients may complain of joint pain, swelling, and "morning stiffness." Alternative systemic inflammatory conditions such as systemic lupus erythematosus, psoriasis, and rheumatic disease must be ruled out. The exact cause of RA is unknown, but genetic factors are evident in familial cases, and susceptibility is linked to certain human leukocyte antigen (HLA)-DR types (Okada, 2014). The most commonly affected regions are the small joints of the hands and feet. The diagnosis is based primarily on the patient's history of polyarthritis of greater than 6 weeks, duration and the presence of characteristic clinical findings. The presence of anti-cyclic citrullinated peptide, rheumatoid factor, and acute phase reactants (e.g., ESR, CRP) may strengthen the clinical suspicion. That said, many patients have seronegative RA, and conversely, there are numerous other causes for elevation of rheumatoid factor. Radiography, sonography, and MRI may reveal changes suggestive of synovitis; however, these modalities do not have an established role in the diagnosis of RA as outlined by the American College of Rheumatology (Aletaha, 2010).

#### Pathogenesis

The immunopathogenesis of RA is complex and includes T- and B-cell activation, angiogenesis and cellular proliferation in the synovium, inflammation in soft tissue, and eventual destruction of cartilage and bone matrix. Cytokine release, immune complex deposition, and vasculitis can all contribute to the inflammatory process. The inflamed proliferative rheumatoid synovium is called *pannus*. In the spine, pannus can disrupt stabilizing ligaments, particularly of the AA joint, and thick pannus can add to central canal stenosis with subsequent compression of nervous tissue. Rheumatoid inflammatory material can form nodules in soft tissue. On the rare occasions that these nodules form in the dura, they can contribute to rheumatoid pachymeningitis.

#### Neurological Manifestations

RA can result in complications of the CNS, peripheral nervous system, and muscle. Some of the most common neurological complications of RA are carpal tunnel syndrome and other nerve entrapments, peripheral neuropathy, and myopathy; these are discussed in Chapters 28, 105, and 106. RA can evolve to a rheumatoid vasculitis that, like other medium-sized vessel vasculitides, has the potential to cause ischemic mononeuritis, mononeuritis multiplex, or (rarely) stroke.

Headache and neckache are common in patients with RA. These are often caused by rheumatoid disease of the cervical spine. Focal neurological dysfunction is a rare and later manifestation of spinal RA. Unsurprisingly, patients develop ubiquitous changes of spinal osteoarthritis and spondylosis. In addition, early in RA, cervical radiography may show rheumatoid changes such as erosions and sclerosis at vertebral endplates and apophyseal joints. Patients may have cervical subluxations. Disk-space narrowing may occur at upper cervical disks, without associated osteophytosis.

Patients with progressive RA can develop subluxation at the AA joint. Lateral AA joint subluxation rarely causes focal neurological dysfunction but can contribute to neck ache and headache. Sagittal

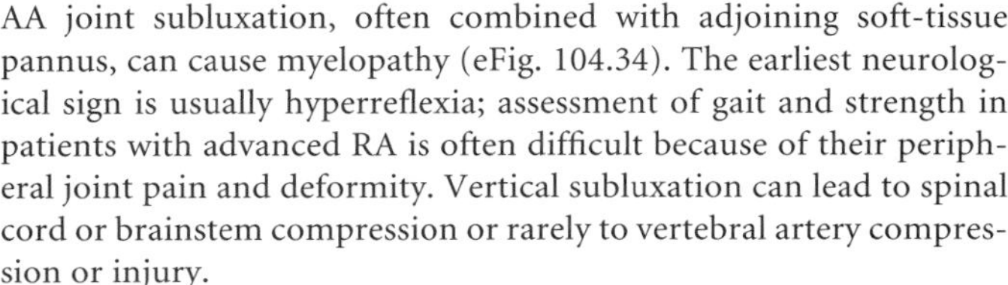

**Fig. 104.33 Magnetic Resonance Image of a Patient With Tuberculous Vertebral Osteomyelitis.** T2-weighted images show destruction of posterior inferior portion of T12 vertebra, with a soft-tissue mass projecting posteriorly into spinal canal, compressing conus medullaris *(black arrows)*. Note that T12 and L1 disks *(white arrows)* are relatively well preserved, a distinguishing feature of spinal tuberculosis. (*Courtesy Erik Gaensler.*)

AA joint subluxation, often combined with adjoining soft-tissue pannus, can cause myelopathy (eFig. 104.34). The earliest neurological sign is usually hyperreflexia; assessment of gait and strength in patients with advanced RA is often difficult because of their peripheral joint pain and deformity. Vertical subluxation can lead to spinal cord or brainstem compression or rarely to vertebral artery compression or injury.

Choosing which patients will benefit from surgical stabilization of the subluxed joint is a clinical challenge. Findings of progressive myelopathy or brainstem dysfunction are usually indications for surgery if the general health of the patient permits. Neurological dysfunction caused by AA subluxation usually occurs in patients who are already severely debilitated by their disease. Many patients do not regain neurological function after surgical stabilization of the subluxation; goals are limited to preventing deterioration. The 5-year survival of patients at this late stage of RA is perhaps 50%.

A rare late manifestation of RA is rheumatoid pachymeningitis. The dura may develop either focal rheumatoid nodules or diffuse infiltration by inflammatory cells. In rare instances, focal dural disease can lead to compression of spinal cord, cauda equina, or cranial nerves. It may also result in focal cerebral complications such as seizures. Patients may experience encephalopathy, headaches, fever, cranial nerve dysfunction, or weakness. MRI may reveal meningeal thickening or enhancement. CSF analysis is typically bland, though protein may be elevated. In these cases, a course of glucocorticoids may improve neurological symptoms (Ikeda, 2010).

Entrapment neuropathies are present in up to 45% of patients with RA (Nadeau, 2002). Pure sensory, sensorimotor, and/or autonomic neuropathies have been described in up to one-fifth of RA patients (Fleming, 1976). Muscle weakness can result from the primary affects of RA in the form of overlap myositis or as an unintended consequence of chronic steroid use. Furthermore, patients may develop generalized weakness from disuse or deconditioning on account of chronic joint pain and immobility.

## Inflammatory Spondyloarthropathies

### Clinical Presentation

The inflammatory spondyloarthropathies (SpA) include ankylosing spondylitis, reactive arthritis, psoriatic arthritis, and the arthritis of inflammatory bowel disease. This is a group of heterogeneous disorders but share the common finding of inflammation in axial joints. *Ankylosing spondylitis* is characterized by inflammatory low back pain, loss of spinal range of motion, sacroiliitis, and as it advances, radiographic evidence of sacroiliitis and spondylitis (eFig. 104.35). The clinical symptoms of inflammatory spine disease are the insidious onset of low back (and sometimes buttock) pain lasting more than 3 months, prominent morning stiffness, and improvement with activity. Nocturnal back pain may be present. Some patients with inflammatory back pain do not meet diagnostic criteria for an inflammatory SpA (Heuft-Dorenbosch et al., 2007). Most patients become symptomatic before age 40 years, and men are affected more commonly than women. Other organ systems are affected commonly in patients with inflammatory SpA; manifestations include uveitis, mucocutaneous lesions, peripheral arthritis, gastrointestinal disease, cardiac disease, and *enthesopathy* (inflammation at sites of insertion of ligament or tendon to bone). The syndesmophytes that form where spinal ligaments join vertebral bodies are one form of enthesopathy. Examples of other sites of enthesopathy are the foot (Achilles tendonitis, plantar fasciitis, heel pain), fingers or toes (dactylitis or sausage digits), and symphysis pubis, clavicle, and ribs.

*Reactive arthritis* (formerly called *Reiter syndrome*) is classically preceded by venereal or gastrointestinal tract infection. The triad of reactive arthritis is arthritis, conjunctivitis, and urethritis, but many patients do not have all three manifestations. Inflammatory low back pain is common in patients with reactive arthritis, and up to one-fourth of patients develop radiological evidence of sacroiliitis or spondylitis.

### Pathogenesis

The inflammatory SpAs are generated by a combination of genetic and environmental factors. In ankylosing spondylitis, the genetic factor is

**TABLE 104.6 Spinal Complications of Ankylosing Spondylitis Based on 105 Hospitalized Patients**

| | Anatomically Abnormal | Neurologically Abnormal |
|---|---|---|
| Spinal fracture | 13 | 7 |
| Diskovertebral destruction | 4 | 0 |
| Atlantoaxial subluxation | 1 | 0 |
| Spinal canal stenosis | 2 | 2 |

*Data from Weinstein, P., Karpman, R.R., Gall, E.P., et al., 1982. Spinal injury, spinal fracture, and spinal stenosis in ankylosing spondylitis. J. Neurosurg. 37, 609–616. Reprinted from Rosenbaum, R.B., Campbell, S.M., Rosenbaum, J.T., 1996. Clinical Neurology of Rheumatic Disease. Butterworth-Heinemann, Boston.*

clearest, with perhaps 90% of patients expressing the gene for HLA-B27, but only about 5% of people expressing this gene develop ankylosing spondylitis. In the other SpA subtypes, the prevalence of HLA-B27 positivity is lower. The exact mechanism by which HLA-B27 induces autoreactivity remains poorly understood. These diseases are largely mediated by cyclooxygenase (COX), tumor necrosis factor (TNF)-α, and interleukin (IL)-17A. All of these compounds play a role in inducing and organizing a host of pro-inflammatory mediators, resulting in autoimmunity (Veldhoen, 2017). The gut microbiome has also been implicated in stimulating a systemic immune response (Vieira-Sousa, 2015). In some patients a breakdown of the epithelial barrier in the gut allows the microbiome to infiltrate a host and set off an inflammatory cascade.

In reactive arthritis, the environmental factors are clearest, with many patients experiencing a preceding gastrointestinal or genitourinary tract infection with organisms such as *Shigella*, *Salmonella*, *Yersinia*, *Campylobacter*, or *Chlamydia*. Autoimmune T cells with tissue specificity presumably mediate the inflammatory process at sites such as joints, entheses, and eyes.

### Spinal Neurological Complications

The neurological complications of the inflammatory SpA generally do not occur until spinal disease is clinically advanced (e.g., loss of spinal range of motion, kyphosis) and radiologically evident (e.g., vertebral body squaring, syndesmophytes). Spinal complications include AA joint subluxation, spinal fractures and pseudoarthrosis, diskovertebral destruction, spinal canal stenosis, and cauda equina syndrome due to lumbar arachnoid diverticula (Table 104.6).

Subluxation of the AA joint is a late and uncommon complication of inflammatory spondyloarthropathy. Diagnosis and management issues are the same as those for patients who develop AA disease as part of RA. The fused spondylitic spine is particularly susceptible to fracture, especially in the midcervical region. The most common fracture site is C6, followed by C5 and C7. After even minor trauma, the patient with advanced spondylitis needs radiographic assessment of the cervical spine to detect fractures, if possible before myelopathic complications. Much more rarely, patients with spondylitic rigid spines develop posttraumatic myelopathy caused by epidural hematomas or cord contusions.

Destruction of a disk, particularly in the low lumbar or high thoracic region, is a late complication of spondylitis (eFig. 104.36). The adjacent vertebral bodies also may be involved. An initiating trauma is not always identified. The destruction may be asymptomatic or painful. The pain increases with movement and decreases at rest, in contrast to typical inflammatory low back pain. An epidural inflammatory response leading to cord compression can occur.

**BOX 104.7 Examples of Neurological Complications of Reactive Arthritis**

Acute transverse myelitis
Brainstem dysfunction
Encephalitis
Neuralgic amyotrophy
Personality change
Seizures
Unilateral ascending motor neuropathy

*Reprinted with permission from Rosenbaum, R.B., Campbell, S.M., Rosenbaum, J.T., 1996. Clinical Neurology of Rheumatic Disease. Butterworth-Heinemann, Boston.*

Cauda equina syndrome with insidious evolution of lower extremity pain, sensory loss, weakness, and sphincter dysfunction is a late complication of inflammatory spondyloarthropathy. Imaging studies (MRI, CT, myelography) show posterior lumbosacral arachnoid diverticula (eFig. 104.37). Although arachnoiditis may play a role in development of this syndrome, the presence of the diverticula distinguishes it from most cases of chronic adhesive arachnoiditis.

Other complications of spondyloarthropathy include lumbar radiculopathy secondary to disk herniation or osteophytes, spinal canal stenosis, and from the era when spinal radiation was used to treat spondylitis, radiation-induced cauda equina sarcoma.

### Nonspinal Neurological Complications

Rare nonspinal complications of inflammatory SpA include brachial plexopathy or entrapment neuropathies. Proximal weakness and atrophy, sometimes with mild elevations of serum creatine kinase (CK) level, often occur in advanced cases of spondylitis, suggesting an inflammatory myopathy. In patients with psoriatic arthritis, the myopathy is occasionally painful. A number of case reports detail unusual neurological illnesses in patients with reactive arthritis (Box 104.7).

### Laboratory Abnormalities

Like RA, patients may have an elevated acute phase response. High ESR and/or CRP levels are seen in approximately 50%–70% of patients with active disease (Rudwaleit, 2009). Patients with inflammatory SpA sometimes have mild elevations of CSF protein levels, with normal glucose and cell counts. They can have unexplained abnormalities of visual, auditory, and somatosensory evoked responses.

## EPIDURAL LIPOMATOSIS

Epidural lipomatosis is a non-neoplastic accumulation of unencapsulated adipose tissue within the thoracic or lumbar epidural space which can lead to spinal canal stenosis and neural compromise. This phenomenon can occur idiopathically but is more commonly a complication of chronic corticosteroid excess, obesity, or hypothyroidism (Fogel et al., 2005). This condition is very frequently underdiagnosed, and often missed on imaging studies. On axial MRI there is often encroachment on the dural sac posteriorly in a "Y"-shaped configuration. Signal characteristics follow fat on all sequences (i.e., high on T1, low on T1 fat suppression, high on T2). A typical patient has been on corticosteroids for more than 6 months and is obese and cushingoid; spinal radiography typically shows diffuse osteoporosis. Epidural lipomatosis is also a rare manifestation of the lipodystrophy that can complicate highly active antiretroviral therapy in the treatment of human immunodeficiency virus (HIV) infection. Symptomatic segmental spinal cord or nerve root compression is typically associated with epidural fat thickness of more than 7 mm in the region of compression; however, the diameter of the spinal canal and other factors affect the manifestations, so the epidural fat can be thickened asymptomatically. Patients with epidural lipomatosis usually have a body mass index of more than 27.5 kg/m$^2$ (eFig. 104.38). The compressive tissue can regress when corticosteroid doses are decreased and it responds extremely well to aggressive weight loss in morbidly obese patients. When neurological symptoms are severe, resulting in cauda equina syndrome, decompressive laminectomy may be required and usually has favorable outcomes (Bodelier et al., 2005).

## CHRONIC MENINGITIS

Most cases of chronic meningitis are due to infection (see Chapter 78), neoplasia (see Chapter 76), or sarcoidosis (see Chapter 58). A comprehensive differential diagnosis includes Behçet syndrome, isolated CNS angiitis (see Chapter 70), systemic lupus erythematosus, Sjögren syndrome, or granulomatosis with polyangiitis (formerly Wegener granulomatosis). Some other chronic or recurring meningitic syndromes merit discussion; however, a cause is not found in many cases of chronic meningitis.

### Chronic Adhesive Arachnoiditis

Focal or diffuse inflammation of the spinal theca can cause neurological symptoms caused by inflammation, adhesion, and distortion of nerve roots or spinal cord. This condition is termed *chronic spinal arachnoiditis* or *chronic adhesive arachnoiditis*. However, the process usually involves all layers of the meninges and in its chronic stages may be fibrotic rather than inflammatory. Calcification of the meninges *(arachnoiditis ossificans)* is an occasional late finding. Clinically, the condition manifests as a gradually ascending, painful cauda equina syndrome followed by a myelopathy as the arachnoiditis reaches the spinal cord. Death may result in 3–10 years from decubiti, urosepsis, and other complications of severe paraplegia.

Adhesive arachnoiditis occasionally complicates a variety of surgical or medical violations of the thecal sac (eBox 104.8). Historically, severe cases of TB or syphilis invaded the spine and caused arachnoiditis. In recent years, fungal meningitis from tainted epidural steroid injections has been a culprit. Arachnoiditis of the spinal cord is less common but can also occur after apparently successful treatment of epidural or vertebral infection and can lead to myelopathy. Involvement at the craniocervical junction can be a cause of acquired syringomyelia. Focal arachnoiditis is most common in the cauda equina following lumbar disk surgery or myelography, particularly if oil-based contrast has been used for the latter. Oil-based myelography dye has fallen out of use for many years, but some patients can still be seen who had such agents used when they were young. The symptoms of arachnoiditis can include local or radicular pain, radicular paresthesia, and less commonly more severe findings of polyradiculopathy such as motor loss or sphincter dysfunction. The diagnosis can usually be made by spinal MRI, which may show clumping of nerve roots, nodules in the subarachnoid space, loculation of spinal fluid, and local areas of enhancement. The nerve roots may clump at the periphery of the thecal sac, usually adjacent to an area of previous surgery, or in the center of the sac, usually in areas of spinal stenosis. The extent of the MRI findings correlates poorly with the severity of the clinical nerve root dysfunction. Spinal fluid may show increased CSF protein levels and mild to moderate mononuclear pleocytosis. Surgical debridement of the arachnoiditis is almost never attempted, is usually unsuccessful and may lead to increased scarring and progression of neurological deficits. Epidural or intrathecal corticosteroids are sometimes tried, but there is no proof of their efficacy, and there are reports of arachnoiditis caused by their use. Therefore, most treatment is aimed at symptomatic management. Spinal cord stimulator implantation has been shown to have some clinical efficacy for reducing pain associated with arachnoiditis. Additional interventions include multimodal analgesics, physical therapy, and psychotherapy.

### Recurrent Meningitis

Patients with recurrent attacks of acute bacterial meningitis need to be screened for dural CSF leaks or fistulas, parameningeal infections, and immunodeficiency (see Chapter 78; Tebruegge and Curtis, 2008). Recurrent meningitis can also be caused by chemical irritants leaked from tumors like dermoids, epidermoids, or craniopharyngiomas. Drug-induced meningitis, most common as an idiosyncratic reaction to NSAIDs, can recur with repeated drug exposures. Rarely, recurrent meningitis can complicate systemic inflammatory diseases such as systemic lupus erythematosus, Sjögren syndrome, Behçet disease, Lyme disease, familial Mediterranean fever, or sarcoidosis.

*Recurrent benign lymphocytic meningitis*, sometimes called *Mollaret meningitis*, can cause multiple self-limited attacks with symptoms such as headache, fever, and meningismus. Each attack generally lasts a few days (Shalabi and Whitley, 2006). Transient neurological features that may include seizures, hallucinations, diplopia, cranial nerve palsies, or altered consciousness can accompany the syndrome, implying that some cases are actually meningoencephalitis. The spinal fluid shows a mixed pleocytosis, sometimes including large macrophage-like cells (Mollaret cells). Most cases are due to herpes virus infections, especially HSV2. In other cases, echovirus, coxsackie, and Epstein-Barr have been identified. Antiviral therapies (e.g., acyclovir, valacyclovir, famciclovir) have been trialed in patients, though there is no controlled trial data to support their efficacy in preventing disease recurrence (Pearce, 2008). Some argue that the eponym *Mollaret meningitis* should be reserved for those cases without an identified causative organism: in other words, idiopathic recurrent aseptic meningitis.

The uveomeningal syndromes are a group of disorders which commonly involve the uvea, retina, and meninges. The combination of chronic or recurrent meningitis and uveitis has a specific differential diagnosis (Yeh et al., 2011; eBox 104.9). Specific entities include: granulomatosis with polyangiitis, sarcoidosis, Behcet disease and acute posterior multifocal placoid pigment epitheliopathy (Brazis et al., 2004). Often, ophthalmological characterization of the uveitis can refine the differential diagnosis. For example, the uveitis of Vogt-Koyanagi-Harada syndrome is bilateral and often causes retinal elevations and retinal pigmentary changes. Vogt-Koyanagi-Harada syndrome also causes skin and hair findings such as vitiligo, poliosis, and focal alopecia.

### Pachymeningitis

Pachymeningitis is a rare condition, visible on MRI scans as thickened gadolinium-enhancing dura (Kupersmith et al., 2004; Fig. 104.39). The differential diagnosis is extensive (eBox 104.10). Low CSF pressure from causes such as post-lumbar puncture or idiopathic intracranial hypotension can also cause apparent dural "enhancement" on MRI secondary to venous engorgement. The enhancement when the CSF pressure is low is usually diffuse and smooth, whereas pachymeningitis can cause diffuse or localized irregular areas of enhancement. *Idiopathic hypertrophic pachymeningitis* refers to those cases for which cultures, serology, and dural biopsy fail to reveal a causative infection, tumor, or systemic inflammatory disease. These patients can present with headache, cranial neuropathies, ataxia, or seizures. Pachymeningitis in the spinal canal can cause radiculopathy or myelopathy. CSF may show high protein or lymphocytic pleocytosis, but is sterile. Dural biopsy shows small mature lymphocytes, plasma

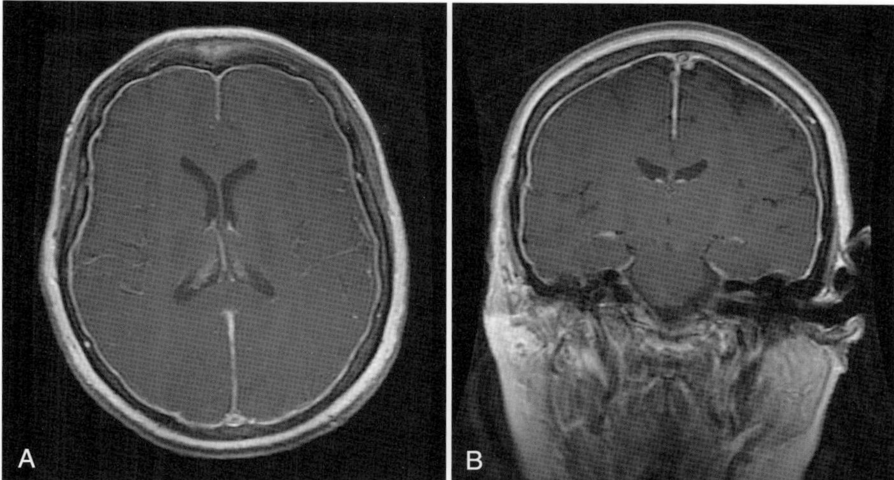


**Fig. 104.39 Dural Enhancement.** Axial (A) and coronal (B) T1-weighted images following gadolinium infusion. In this case of pachymeningitis, the enhancement pattern is thin and diffuse; other cases show more localized or irregular thickening.

cells, and epithelioid histiocytes. Immunoglobulin G4-related disease (IgG4-RD) is an increasingly recognized immune-mediated cause of hypertrophic pachymeningitis. IgG4-RD has been previously described to cause autoimmune pancreatitis, sclerosing cholangitis and other systemic disorders (Kamisawa et al., 2015). While rare, isolated CNS involvement has been described and it is an important entity to be aware of (Hayashi et al., 2018). Patients can improve after treatment with corticosteroids, sometimes supplemented with steroid-sparing immunosuppressants such as azathioprine and methotrexate.

### Superficial Hemosiderosis

Superficial hemosiderosis is a neurodegenerative disorder resulting from recurrent leakage of blood into the subpial space. Analysis of CSF often reveals xanthochromia, red blood cells, and/or elevated protein. Not all patients have an identifiable source of hemorrhage. Possible sources include brain or spine trauma, neurosurgery, cerebral or spinal aneurysms or vascular malformations, cerebral amyloid angiopathy, or spinal dural defects. Some patients with spinal dural leaks develop both superficial hemosiderosis and intracranial hypotension (Kumar et al., 2007). Common neurological clinical manifestations include gait ataxia and sensorineural deafness. These are sometimes accompanied by other upper motor neuron exam findings: limb spasticity, brisk reflexes, extensor plantar responses, bladder disturbance, or sensory signs (Kumar et al., 2006). Less common features include dementia, anosmia, or anisocoria, and, more rarely, extraocular motor palsies, neck or backache, or radicular pain. While the clinical presentation and examination are often nonspecific, the neuroradiological abnormalities are striking. MRI shows a black rim around the posterior fossa structures and spinal cord and less often the cerebral hemispheres on T2-weighted images (Fig. 104.40). These paramagnetic signal changes represent encrustation of the brain surfaces with hemosiderin. The adjacent neural tissue atrophies, with accumulation of ferritin in microglia and Bergmann cells in the cerebellum. The pattern of hemosiderin deposition can sometimes be a clue to the underlying etiology. Focal involvement is more likely the result of trauma or an underlying vascular anomaly. Whereas disseminated superficial siderosis appears to be more specific for cerebral amyloid angiopathy (Charidimou et al., 2013). Another clinically important phenomenon related to cerebral amyloid angiopathy and secondary hemosiderosis is transient neurological symptoms. Patients can experience recurrent, brief, stereotyped episodes of weakness, sensory disturbance, or other focal deficits which spread over contiguous body parts (Charidimou et al., 2012) It is this gradual spread of symptoms which differentiate these spells from transient ischemic attacks. The underlying mechanism is thought to be focal seizure activity or spreading cortical depression in response to small underlying hemorrhages. This theory has been supported by anecdotal evidence that anticonvulsant medications are efficacious in alleviating these spells (Greenberg et al., 1993). In addition to supportive measures, treatment is focused on arresting the source of bleeding once identified. In the case of cerebral amyloid angiopathy there should be an attempt to medically optimize underlying vascular risk factors (e.g., hypertension, hyperglycemia, dyslipidemia). Finally, given the elevated hemorrhage risk, caution should be exercised when placing this population on anticoagulants or antiplatelet agents.

## FIBROMYALGIA

Fibromyalgia, a syndrome defined by chronic, diffuse musculoskeletal or soft-tissue pain and multiple tender points, is part of the differential diagnosis of many patients with spinal pain. Patients may have numerous other complaints across multiple organ systems, though their physical examinations are typically normal. The sheer volume of seemingly unconnected symptoms and the lack of objective data to support those grievances are often a source of great frustration to healthcare providers. Similarly, patients may feel as though their ailment is not taken seriously or that there is some occult disease which has yet to be recognized. This frustration on both sides is compounded by the general lack of understanding regarding the disease itself. Although many mechanisms have been proposed, no consensus has been reached as to the underlying pathogenesis of the condition. That said, some believe the entity to be within the continuum of central sensitization syndromes, arising from dysfunction of central pain processing pathways (Clauw et al., 2011).

The American College of Rheumatology has proposed diagnostic criteria for fibromyalgia and for the monitoring of symptom severity (SS). They suggest that a patient must have "widespread" pain and multiple somatic symptoms. The pain must persist for greater than 3 months and must not otherwise be explained by a separate disorder. A widespread pain index (WPI) is defined as the number of painful areas out of 19 predetermined locations. Patients are also given an SS score which describes the degree to which their condition impedes

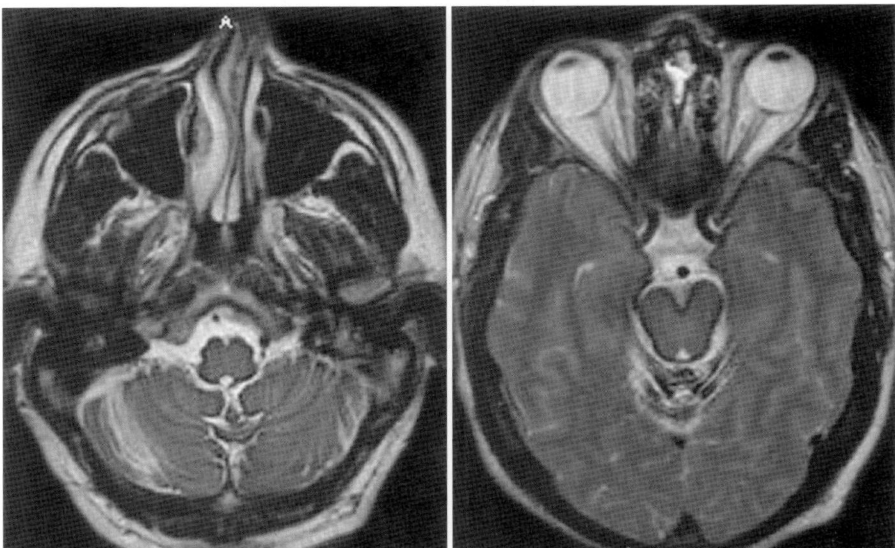

**Fig. 104.40** Axial T2-weighted magnetic resonance images demonstrate a thin ring of hypointensity surrounding the medulla and midbrain, indicating hemosiderin deposition along the leptomeninges. *(Courtesy Jim Anderson, Oregon Health Sciences University, Portland, OR.)*

their daily functioning. A score between 0 (no problems) and 3 (severe, pervasive problems) are assigned for three symptoms: fatigue, waking unrefreshed, and cognitive symptoms. The number of somatic symptoms (e.g., headache, dizziness, cramps, paresthesias, chest pain, etc.) are tallied from a review of systems. Somatic symptoms are also given a score between 0 (no symptoms) and 3 (a great deal of symptoms). The SS is calculated by combining the four values, with a maximum score of 12. A patient satisfies the diagnostic criteria for fibromyalgia when the WPI is ≥7 and SS is ≥5 or when the WPI is ≥3 and the SS is ≥9 (Wolfe et al., 2011).

Chronic pain syndromes, such as fibromyalgia, result in significant psychosocial impairment, lost wages, and higher (often unnecessary) healthcare utilization. A number of pharmacological and nonpharmacological treatments have been explored. Current evidence suggests that small doses of tricyclic antidepressants, cardiovascular exercise, cognitive behavioral therapy, and patient education have utility, but often provide incomplete or unsatisfactory results (Talotta, 2017). The cause of most cases of fibromyalgia is unknown. Behavioral and biological factors both contribute to the clinical presentation of the syndrome. Neuroscientific research on the pathogenesis of fibromyalgia has examined muscle, sleep, neuroendocrine function, and central pain processing, including studies using functional brain imaging (Nebel and Gracely, 2009). Symptoms and signs of fibromyalgia can occur in association with autoimmune diseases such as systemic lupus erythematosus or other systemic illness such as hypothyroidism. Focal trauma can cause localized self-limited soft-tissue myofascial pain. The pathogenic role of trauma, on-the-job injury, or workplace stress is controversial. Treatment includes a supportive doctor–patient relationship, aerobic exercise, and avoiding inactivity. Pregabalin, duloxetine, and milnacipran are now approved by the US Food and Drug Administration (FDA) for treatment of fibromyalgic pain. Other drugs for chronic pain (e.g., tricyclic antidepressants) are sometimes tried off-label. Small short-term controlled studies have suggested that some patients benefit from acupuncture.

*The complete reference list is available online at https://expertconsult.inkling.com/.* 

105

# Disorders of Nerve Roots and Plexuses

David A. Chad, Michael P. Bowley

## OUTLINE



## DISORDERS OF NERVE ROOTS

The spinal nerve roots serve as the transition from the peripheral nervous system to the central nervous system (CNS). Each spinal nerve is derived from anterior (ventral) and posterior (dorsal) nerve roots; the anterior roots carrying efferent motor information from anterior horn cells of the spinal cord, and the posterior nerve roots carrying afferent sensory information as the central axons of the pseudo-unipolar dorsal root ganglia cells. Both anterior and posterior nerve roots are susceptible to diseases specific to their location and to many of the disorders that affect peripheral nerves in general. Although surrounded by a rigid bony canal, they are delicate structures subject to compression and stretching. Bathed by cerebrospinal fluid (CSF), they may be exposed to infectious, inflammatory, and neoplastic processes that involve the leptomeninges. Separated from the blood by an incomplete blood–nerve barrier, the dorsal root ganglion (DRG) neurons may be injured by circulating neurotoxins.

In the clinical sphere, it is usually not difficult to recognize symptoms or signs attributable to lesions of a single nerve root. Radicular pain and paresthesias are accompanied by sensory loss in the *dermatome* (the area of skin innervated by a nerve root), weakness in the *myotome* (defined as muscles innervated by a spinal cord segment and its nerve root), and diminished deep tendon reflex activity subserved by the nerve root in question. However, when multiple roots are involved by a disease process *(polyradiculopathy)* the clinical picture may resemble a disorder of the peripheral nerves, as in a polyneuropathy, or of the anterior horn cells, as in the progressive muscular atrophy form of amyotrophic lateral sclerosis (ALS). In these complicated clinical settings, clinicians may often turn to serological, radiological, and electrodiagnostic studies to aid in diagnosis.

A disorder of the nerve roots is favored by abnormalities of the CSF (raised protein concentration and pleocytosis), paraspinal muscle needle electromyographic (EMG) examination (presence of positive sharp waves and fibrillation potentials), and spinal cord magnetic resonance imaging (MRI) (compromise or contrast enhancement of the nerve roots per se).

The sections that follow cover some anatomical features relevant to an understanding of the pathological conditions that affect the nerve roots, as well as specific nerve root disorders.

### Anatomical Features

Each nerve root is attached to the spinal cord by four to eight rootlets that are splayed out in a longitudinal direction (Rankine, 2004). The dorsal rootlets are attached to the spinal cord at a well-defined posterolateral sulcus, whereas the ventral rootlets are more widely separated and emerge over a greater area of the anterior surface of the spinal cord. For each spinal cord segment, a pair of dorsal and ventral roots unite just beyond the DRG to form a short mixed spinal nerve that divides into a thin dorsal ramus and a thicker ventral ramus (Fig. 105.1). The dorsal ramus innervates the deep posterior muscles of the neck and trunk (the paraspinal muscles) and the skin overlying these areas. The ventral ramus, depending on its spinal segment, contributes to an intercostal nerve, or to the cervical, brachial, or lumbosacral plexi and thereby supplies the trunk or limb muscles.

Directly adjacent to the spinal cord, the nerve roots lie freely in the subarachnoid space, covered by a thin root sheath, composed of a layer of flattened cells, that is continuous with the pial and arachnoidal coverings of the spinal cord. Compared with spinal nerves, the roots have fewer connective tissue cells in the endoneurium and considerably less collagen. Moreover, they lack an epineurium, as this dense connective

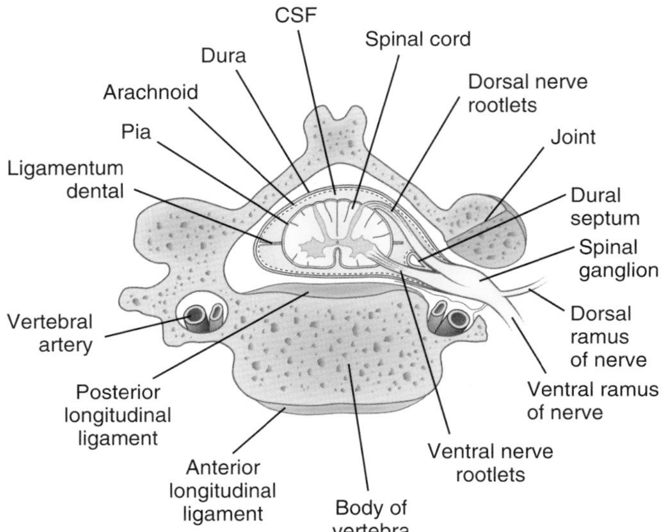


**Fig. 105.1 Relations of Dura to Bone and Roots of Nerve Shown in an Oblique Transverse Section.** On the right, the relations between the emergent nerve and the synovial joint are seen, but the joint between the vertebral bodies is not in the plane of the section. Dorsal and ventral roots meet at the dorsal root ganglion in the intervertebral foramen to form the mixed spinal nerve. The small dorsal ramus is the most proximal branch of the mixed spinal nerve and serves the cervical paraspinal muscles (not shown). The dura becomes continuous with the epineurium of the mixed spinal nerve at the intervertebral foramen. The posterior longitudinal ligament helps contain the intervertebral disk (not shown), preventing protrusion into the spinal canal. *CSF*, Cerebrospinal fluid. *(Reprinted with permission from Wilkinson, M., 1971. Cervical Spondylosis: Its Early Diagnosis and Treatment. Saunders, Philadelphia.)*

tissue layer is contiguous with the dura mater. A capillary network derived from the radicular arteries provides the blood supply to the spinal nerve roots (Becske and Nelson, 2009).

Where the nerve roots form the mixed spinal nerve, the pial covering of the root becomes continuous with spinal nerve perineurium, and the nerve takes the dural nerve root sheath through the intervertebral foramen to become continuous with the epineurium of the mixed nerve. At the intervertebral foramen, the root–DRG–spinal nerve complex is securely attached by a fibrous sheath to the transverse process of the vertebral body. At cervical and thoracic levels, the DRG is located in a protected position within the intervertebral foramina, but at the lumbar and sacral levels, the DRG may reside proximal to the neural foramina in an intraspinal location (Levin, 2002) and therefore may be vulnerable to direct compression as a result of disk herniation or from bony changes induced by osteoarthritis and lumbosacral spondylosis.

Nerve fibers, together with their meningeal coverings, occupy 35%–50% of the cross-sectional area of an intervertebral foramen. The remaining space is occupied by loose areolar connective tissue, adipose tissue (fat), and blood vessels. On computed tomographic (CT) and MRI scans, the fat acts as an excellent natural contrast agent that defines the thecal sac and nerve roots, allowing the detection of nerve root compression.

The dorsal roots contain sensory fibers that are central processes of the DRG. On reaching the spinal cord, these fibers either synapse with other neurons in the posterior horn or pass directly into the posterior columns. In the ventral root, most fibers are essentially direct extensions of anterior horn motor neurons or of neurons in the intermediolateral horn (preganglionic sympathetic neurons found in lower cervical and thoracic segments). In addition, ventral roots contain a population of unmyelinated and thinly myelinated axons that come from sensory and sympathetic ganglia (Hildebrand et al., 1997).

There are 31 pairs of spinal nerves that run through the intervertebral foramina of the vertebral column: 8 cervical, 12 thoracic, 5 lumbar, 5 sacral, and 1 coccygeal (Fig. 105.2). Each cervical nerve root exits above its corresponding vertebral segment, with the sole exception being the C8 nerve root, which exits below C7 and above T1. At thoracic, lumbar, and sacral levels, each root exits below its corresponding vertebral level. An additional feature of clinical relevance is the pattern formed by the lumbar and sacral roots as they leave the spinal cord and make their way to their respective DRG to form spinal nerves. In the adult, the spinal cord is shorter than the spinal column, ending usually between L1 and L2. Therefore, the lumbar and sacral roots descend caudally from the spinal cord to reach the individual intervertebral foramina, forming the cauda equina. The concentration of so many nerve roots in a confined area makes this structure vulnerable to a range of pathological processes.

## Traumatic Radiculopathies

### Nerve Root Avulsion

As noted earlier, each spinal root is composed of lesser amounts of collagen and is not supported by a dense epineural sheath compared to the mixed spinal nerves they form. This lack of reinforcement results in the spinal roots having approximately one-tenth the tensile strength of their corresponding peripheral nerves. Thus, the nerve root is the weakest link in the nerve root–spinal nerve–plexus complex, leading to root avulsion in the setting of traumatic traction injuries. Ventral roots are more vulnerable to avulsion than dorsal roots, a consequence of the dorsal roots having the interposed DRG and a thicker dural sheath. In most cases, root avulsion occurs in the cervical region. Lumbosacral nerve root avulsions are rare, and when they occur are generally associated with fractures of the sacroiliac joint with diastasis of the symphysis pubis or fractures of the pubic rami (Chin and Chew, 1997).

Avulsion at the level of the cervical roots can be total or may result in two clinical syndromes of partial avulsion. One is *Erb-Duchenne palsy*, in which the arm hangs at the side, internally rotated, and extended at the elbow because of paralysis of C5- and C6-innervated muscles (the supraspinatus, infraspinatus, deltoid, and biceps). The second is *Dejerine-Klumpke palsy*, in which there is weakness and wasting of the intrinsic hand muscles, with a characteristic claw-hand deformity due to paralysis of C8- and T1-innervated muscles. Injuries responsible for Erb-Duchenne palsy are those that cause a sudden and severe increase in the angle between the neck and shoulder, generating stresses that are readily transmitted in the direct line along the upper portion of the brachial plexus to the C5 and C6 roots. Today, motorcycle accidents are the most common cause of this injury, but the classic paradigm is C5 and C6 root avulsions occurring in newborns during obstetrical procedures. Brachial plexus injuries in the newborn are discussed in Chapter 112. Dejerine-Klumpke palsy occurs when the limb is elevated beyond 90 degrees and tension falls directly on the lower trunk of the plexus, C8, and T1 roots. Such an injury may occur in a fall from a height in which the outstretched arm grasps an object to arrest the fall, or during obstetrical traction on the extended arm when a newborn is delivered arm first.

***Clinical features and diagnosis.*** At the onset of root avulsion, flaccid paralysis and complete anesthesia develop in the myotomes and dermatomes served by the affected ventral and dorsal roots, respectively. Clinical features supplemented by electrophysiological and radiological studies help determine whether the cause of severe weakness and sensory loss is root avulsion or an extraspinal lesion of plexus or nerve.

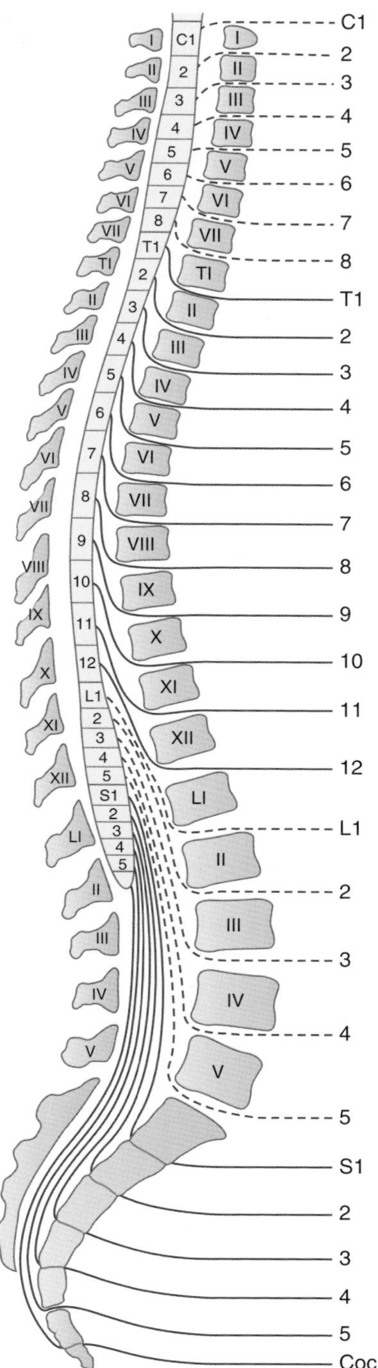


**Fig. 105.2 Relationship of Spinal Segments and Nerve Roots to Vertebral Bodies and Spinous Processes in the Adult.** Cervical roots C1–C7 (i.e., all except C8) exit through foramina above the vertebral body of the same number. The C8 root passes through the C7–T1 neural foramen, and all thoracic, lumbar, and sacral roots leave the spinal canal below the body of the vertebrae of the same number. The spinal cord is shorter than the spinal column, ending between vertebral bodies L1 and L2. Lumbar and sacral roots form the cauda equina and descend caudally, beside and below the spinal cord, to exit at the intervertebral foramina. *(Reprinted with permission from Haymaker, W., Woodhall, B., 1953. Peripheral Nerve Injuries, second ed. Saunders, Philadelphia.)*

For example: in the setting of a suspected C5 nerve root avulsion, one would predict marked weakness of the rhomboids and spinati muscles (innervated primarily by C5) and a lesser degree of weakness of those muscles of the upper trunk of the brachial plexus (deltoid, biceps, brachioradialis) which receive additional innervation from C6.

A clinical sign of T1 root avulsion is an ipsilateral Horner syndrome caused by damage to preganglionic sympathetic fibers as they traverse the ventral root to their destination in the superior cervical ganglion.

Electrophysiological tests that are valuable in differentiating a root avulsion from traumatic plexus or nerve injury include the measurement of a sensory nerve action potential (SNAP) and needle EMG examination of the cervical paraspinal muscles. In the setting of a dorsal root avulsion, the patient may experience complete anesthesia in the dermatome, yet the SNAP is preserved as the DRG cell bodies and the peripheral portions of their axons remain intact. Needle EMG of the cervical paraspinal muscles permits separation of damage of the plexus and of ventral root fibers because the posterior primary ramus, which arises just beyond the DRG and proximal to the plexus as the first branch of the spinal nerve, innervates these muscles (see Fig. 105.1). Thus, cervical paraspinal fibrillation potentials support the diagnosis of root avulsion.

In most cases, these tests are helpful in ascertaining whether root avulsion has occurred, but clinical assessment may be challenging, and testing results may be ambiguous. The physical examination may be limited because of severe pain. An absent SNAP indicates sensory axon loss distal to the DRG but does not exclude coexisting root avulsion. Even when this test of sensory function points to avulsion of the dorsal component of the root, the status of the ventral root may remain uncertain if paraspinal fibrillation potentials are not found. Paraspinal fibrillation potentials may be absent for two reasons. First, they do not appear for 7–10 days after the onset of axonotmesis; and second, even if the timing of the needle EMG is right, they may not be seen because of the innervation of paraspinal muscles from multiple segmental levels.

Paraspinal muscles have also been evaluated radiologically in the setting of root avulsion. Contrast-enhanced MRI studies of the cervical paraspinal muscles showing severe atrophy were accurate in indicating root avulsion injuries, and abnormal enhancement in the multifidus muscle was the most accurate among paraspinal muscle findings (Hayashi et al., 2002). Intraspinal neuroimaging using postmyelographic CT or MRI usually demonstrates an outpouching of the dura filled with contrast or CSF at the level of the avulsed root (Rankine, 2004). This posttraumatic meningocele results from tears in the dura and arachnoid sustained during root avulsion.

***Treatment.*** Root avulsion produces a severe neurological deficit that was once considered untreatable. In recent decades, microsurgical techniques and intraoperative electrophysiological studies have improved prospects for recovery for many patients with severe injury to peripheral nerves. The procedures of *neurolysis* (freeing intact nerve from scar tissue), *nerve grafting* (bridging ruptured nerves), and *neurotization*, or nerve transfer (attaching a donor nerve to a ruptured distal stump), have all been employed in the management of root avulsion injuries (Rankine, 2004). After C5 and C6 root avulsion injuries, for example, the plegic elbow flexors may be restored by several procedures that provide for neurotization of the musculocutaneous nerve, including reinnervating the biceps with nerve fascicles from an unaffected donor nerve (Rankine, 2004; Samil et al., 2003; Sulaiman et al., 2009; Teboul et al., 2004). Carlstedt and colleagues (1995) pioneered another approach—nerve root repair and reimplantation. They reported on a patient who had an avulsion injury involving C6–T1 in whom they were able to successfully implant two ventral roots (C6 directly and C7 via sural nerve grafts) into the spinal cord through slits in the pia mater. The successful reimplantation of avulsed ventral roots is time dependent, with better outcomes in motor strength seen if repair is attempted within 4 weeks of injury (Carlstedt, 2009). The surgical treatment of patients with avulsion injuries is an area of active ongoing investigation with the promise that if continuity between spinal cord and nerve roots can be restored, subsequent recovery of function may be possible. For example, measurement of power in upper extremity muscles years after cervical root reimplantation is associated with a proximal to distal gradient of successful recovery with shoulder girdle muscles (serratus anterior, pectoralis major and minor, and supraspinatus) potentially achieving Medical Research Council (MRC) grade 4 or 5 strength, proximal upper extremity muscles (deltoid, biceps) achieving grade 3 or 4 strength and forearm and hand muscles demonstrating little meaningful recovery (Carlstedt, 2009). While functional motor recovery varies, the oft intractable pain of cervical root avulsion injuries is more responsive to surgical intervention in most patients (Kato et al., 2006).

## Disk Herniation

Beginning in the third or fourth decade of life, cervical and lumbar intervertebral disks are liable to herniate into the spinal canal or intervertebral foramina and impinge on the spinal cord (in the case of cervical disk herniations), nerve roots (in both cervical and lumbosacral regions), or both (at the cervical level where on occasion large central and paracentral disk herniations may produce a myeloradiculopathy) (see Chapter 104).

Two factors contribute to this alteration in the intervertebral disks: degenerative change and trauma. An intervertebral disk is composed of a central, gelatinous, nucleus pulposus, and, surrounding, fibrocartilaginous, annulus fibrosus. With age, the fibers of the annulus fibrosus lengthen, weaken, and fray, thereby allowing the disk to bulge posteriorly. In the setting of such changes, relatively minor trauma leads to further tearing of annular fibers and ultimately to herniation of the nucleus pulposus. This “soft-disk” herniation occurs mainly during the third and fourth decades of life when the nucleus is still gelatinous. In fact, although disk herniations may be preceded by unaccustomed strain or direct injury, in many instances there is no history of clinically significant trauma preceding the onset of radiculopathy.

Reinforcing the annulus fibrosus posteriorly is the posterior longitudinal ligament, which in the lumbar region is dense and strong centrally, and less well developed in its lateral portion. Because of this anatomical feature, the direction of lumbar disk herniations tends to be posterolateral, compressing the nerve roots in the lateral recess of the spinal canal. Less commonly, more lateral (foraminal) herniations compress the nerve root against the vertebral pedicle in the intervertebral foramen (Fig. 105.3). On occasion, the degenerative process may be particularly severe. This leads to large rents in the annulus and posterior longitudinal ligament, thereby permitting disk material to herniate into the spinal canal as a free fragment with the potentially damaging capacity to migrate superiorly or inferiorly and compress two or more nerve roots. Most cervical disk herniations are posterolateral or foraminal.

In the cervical and lumbar regions, alteration in the integrity of the disk space is a component of a degenerative condition termed *spondylosis*, characterized by osteoarthritic changes in the joints of the spine, the disk per se (desiccation and shrinkage of the normally semisolid, gelatinous nucleus pulposus), and the facet joints. Because it spawns osteophyte formation, spondylosis leads to compromise of the spinal cord in the spinal canal and the nerve roots in the intervertebral foramina. Restriction in the dimensions of these bony canals may be exacerbated by thickening and hypertrophy of the ligamentum flavum, which is especially detrimental in patients with congenital cervical or lumbar canal stenosis.

In the cervical region, nerve root compression in patients older than 50 years is often due to disk herniation superimposed on chronic spondylotic changes. Isolated “soft” cervical disk herniation tends to occur in younger people in the setting of neck trauma. In the lumbosacral region, isolated acute disk herniation is a common cause of radiculopathy in the younger patient (<40 years), whereas bony root entrapment with or without superimposed disk herniation is the more typical cause of lumbosacral radiculopathy in the patient older than 50.

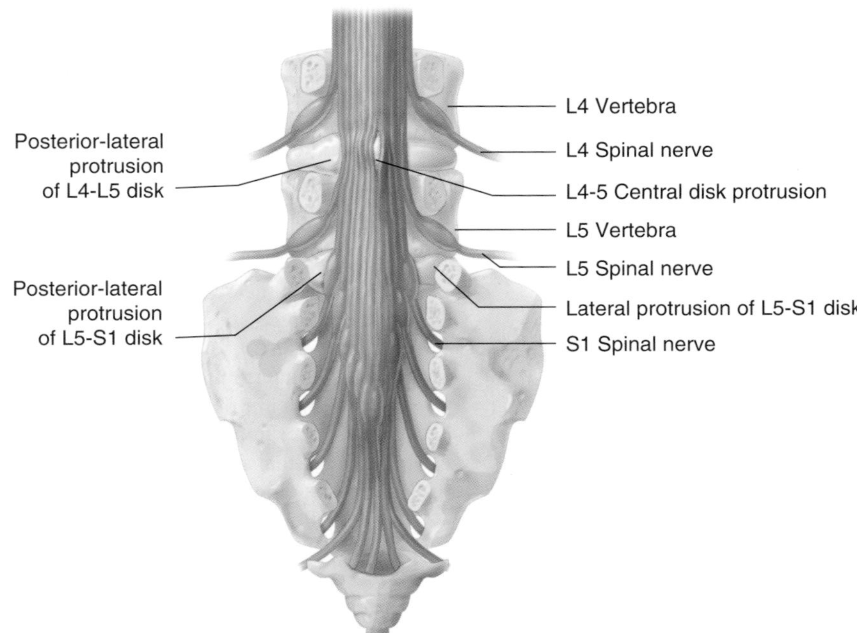


**Fig. 105.3** Dorsal View of Lower Lumbar Spine and Sacrum, Showing the Different Types of Herniations and How Different Roots and the Cauda Equina Can Be Compressed.

***Clinical features.*** Root compression from disk herniation gives rise to a distinctive clinical syndrome comprising radicular pain, dermatomal sensory loss, weakness in the myotome, and reduction or loss of the deep tendon reflex subserved by the affected root (Carette and Fehlings, 2005). Nerve root pain is variably described as knife-like or aching and is widely distributed, projecting to the *sclerotome* (defined as deep structures such as muscles and bones innervated by the root). Typically, root pain is aggravated by coughing, sneezing, and straining at stool (actions that require a Valsalva maneuver and raise intraspinal pressure). Accompanying the pain are paresthesias referred to the specific dermatome, especially to the distal regions of the dermatomes; indeed, these sensations strongly suggest that the pain has its origins in compressed nerve roots rather than spondylotic facet joints. Sensory loss caused by the compromise of a single root may be difficult to ascertain because of the overlapping territories of adjacent roots, although loss of pain is usually more easily demonstrated than loss of light touch sensation (Fig. 105.4).

Most radiculopathies occur in the lumbosacral region; compressive root lesions in this area account for 62%–90% of all radiculopathies. Cervical radiculopathies are less common, comprising 5%–36% of all radiculopathies encountered.

In the lumbosacral region, 95% of disk herniations occur at the L4–L5 or L5–S1 levels; L3–L4 and higher lumbar disk herniations are uncommon (Deyo and Weinstein, 2001). In perhaps only 10% of cases of the disk herniating far laterally into the foramen is there compression of the exiting nerve root. More commonly, the posterolateral disk herniation compresses the nerve root passing through the foramen below that disk, so L4–L5 and L5–S1 herniations usually produce L5 and S1 radiculopathies, respectively (see Fig. 105.3).

In an S1 radiculopathy, pain radiates to the buttock and down the back of the leg (classic *sciatica*), often extending below the knee; paresthesias are generally felt in the lateral ankle and foot. The ankle jerk is generally diminished or lost, and weakness may be detected in the plantar flexors, knee flexors, and hip extensors.

In an L5 radiculopathy, the distribution of pain is similar, but paresthesias are felt on the dorsum of the foot and the outer portion of the calf. The ankle reflex is typically normal, but there may be reduction of the medial hamstring reflex. Weakness may be found in L5-innervated muscles served by the peroneal nerve (including the extensor hallucis longus, tibialis anterior and peronei), tibial nerve (tibialis posterior), and the superior gluteal nerve (including gluteus medius). Weakness may be restricted to the extensor hallucis longus, or be more extensive and involve the tibialis anterior, resulting in foot drop.

A positive straight leg–raising test result is a sensitive indicator of L5 or S1 nerve root irritation. The test is deemed positive when the patient complains of pain radiating from the back into the buttock and thigh with leg elevation to less than 60 degrees. The test result is positive in up to 83% of patients with a proven disk herniation at surgery. A less sensitive but highly specific test is the crossed straight leg–raising test when the patient complains of radiating pain on the affected side with elevation of the contralateral leg.

The less common L4 radiculopathy is characterized by pain and paresthesias along the medial aspect of the knee and lower leg. The patellar reflex is diminished, and weakness may be noted in the quadriceps and hip adductors (innervated by the femoral and obturator nerves, respectively). When large herniations occur in the midline at either the L4–L5 or the L5–S1 level, many of the nerve roots running past that level to exit through intervertebral foramina below that level may be compressed, producing the *cauda equina syndrome* of bilateral

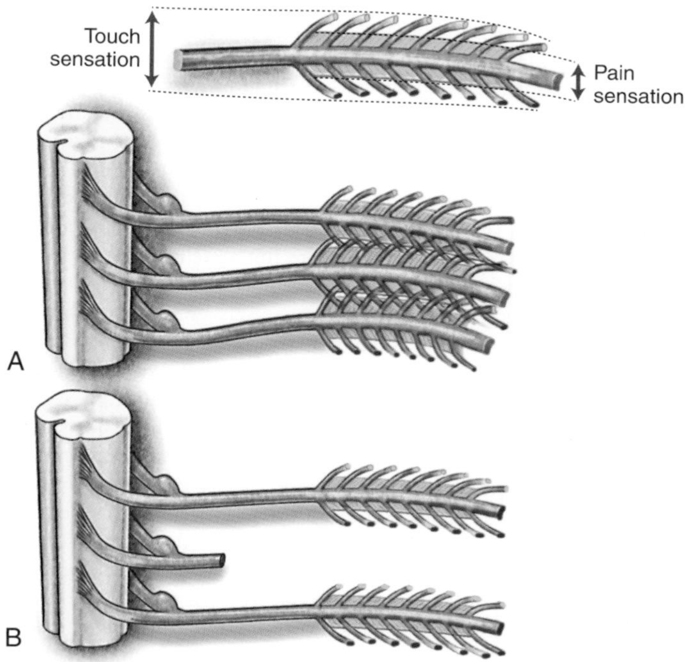


**Fig. 105.4 The Zones of Radicular Touch and Pain Sensation.** The area for touch sensation *(dark orange)* supplied by one single root is wider than the area of pain sensation *(light orange)*. Areas of pain sensation do not overlap or at most overlap incompletely, whereas areas of touch sensation of a single root are completely overlapped by those of the adjacent roots (**A**). Accordingly, monoradicular lesions (**B**) produce a hypalgesic or analgesic zone, while touch sensation remains intact or only minimally impaired. Only after two roots are involved is an anesthetic zone present.

radicular pain, paresthesias, weakness, attenuated reflexes below the disk level, and urinary retention. This is a surgical emergency requiring urgent decompression.

In the cervical region, it is likely that the greater mobility at levels C5–C6 and C6–C7 promotes the development of cervical disk degeneration with annulus fraying and subsequent disk protrusion. As previously noted, cervical nerve roots emerge above the vertebra that share their same numerical designation. Therefore, C7 exits between C6 and C7, and spondylotic changes with or without additional acute disk herniation would be expected to compress the C7 nerve root. Similarly, disk protrusion at C5–C6 and C7–T1 would compress the C6 and C8 roots, respectively. In the classic study of Yoss and associates (1957), clinical and radiological evidence of radiculopathy was found to occur most often at C7 (70%), less frequently at C6 (19%–25%), and uncommonly at C8 (4%–10%) and C5 (2%). Radiculopathy involving the T1 root is a clinical rarity (Levin, 1999).

Involvement of C6 is associated with pain at the tip of the shoulder radiating into the upper part of the arm, lateral side of the forearm, and thumb. Paresthesias are felt in the thumb and index finger. The brachioradialis and biceps reflexes are attenuated or lost. Weakness may occur in the muscles of the C6 myotome supplied by several different nerves, including the biceps (musculocutaneous nerve), deltoid (axillary nerve), and pronator teres (median nerve). The clinical features of C5 radiculopathies are similar, except that the rhomboids and spinati muscles are more likely to be weak.

When the C7 root is compressed, pain radiates in a wide distribution to include the shoulder, chest, forearm, and hand. Paresthesias involve the dorsal surface of the middle finger. The triceps reflex is usually reduced or absent. A varying degree of weakness usually involves one or more muscles of the C7 myotome, especially the triceps the flexor carpi radialis and the pronator teres.

Less common C8 root involvement presents a similar clinical picture with regard to pain. Paresthesias, however, are experienced in the fourth and fifth digits, and weakness may affect the intrinsic muscles of the hand, including finger abductor and adductor muscles (ulnar nerve), thumb abductor and opponens muscles (median nerve), finger extensor muscles (posterior interosseous branch of the radial nerve), and flexor pollicis longus (anterior interosseous branch of the median nerve).

Variations in cervical root innervation to the brachial plexus can complicate the interpretation of symptoms and signs of suspected cervical radiculopathy. A well-appreciated anatomical variant is the "pre-fixed" brachial plexus, whereby cervical root innervation is caudally displaced by one spinal segment, such that the C4 nerve root offers a greater contribution to the brachial plexus, and the T1 nerve root has less representation. A pre-fixed variant is believed to be present in 22%–40% of dissected plexi and should be considered when there is poor correlation between clinical signs and radiographic findings. For example, in one retrospective study of 31 patients with clinical and electrophysiological evidence supporting a C8 radiculopathy, 16% were attributable to compression of the C7 nerve root at the C6–C7 spinal level (Hehir et al., 2012).

***Diagnosis.*** Diagnosis is aided by a variety of imaging techniques (e.g., plain radiography, CT myelography, MRI) and EMG testing (Carette and Fehlings, 2005) (see Chapter 104). Both diagnostic modalities—the imaging approach that reveals anatomical details and the EMG techniques that disclose neurophysiological function—agree in the majority of patients (60%) with a clinical history compatible with cervical or lumbosacral radiculopathy, although only the results of one study will be positive in a significant minority of patients (40%) (Nardin et al., 1999). Although plain radiography is unhelpful in the identification of a herniated disk per se, in both the cervical and the lumbar area, it reveals spondylotic changes when present. It also may be useful for identifying less common disorders that produce radicular symptoms and signs: bony metastases, infection, fracture, and spondylolisthesis, for example.

In the cervical region, the best methods for assessing the relationship between neural structures (spinal cord and nerve root) and their fibro-osseous surroundings (disk, spinal canal, and foramen) are post-myelography CT (unenhanced CT reveals little more than the presence of bony changes) and MRI. MRI is equivalent in diagnostic capacity to post-myelography CT and therefore is preferred. In the lumbosacral region, CT is an effective method for evaluating disk disease, but when available, MRI is considered the superior imaging study. Its excellent resolution, multiplanar imaging, the ability to see the entire lumbar spine including the conus, and the absence of ionizing radiation make it highly sensitive in detecting structural radicular disorders (Ashkan et al., 2002).

A variety of neurophysiological tests are used to assess patients with disk herniation: motor and sensory nerve conduction studies, late responses, somatosensory evoked potentials, nerve root stimulation, and needle electrode examination. Sensory conduction studies are useful in the evaluation of a patient suspected of radiculopathy because SNAPs are typically normal (because the lesion is proximal to the DRG in the intervertebral foramina) even in the face of clinical sensory loss, in contrast to the situation in plexopathy and peripheral nerve trunk lesions, where SNAPs are attenuated or absent. However, in the specific instance of L5 radiculopathy, because the L5 DRG may reside proximal to the neural foramen, if intraspinal pathology is severe enough, compression of the L5 DRG may lead to attenuation or loss of the superficial peroneal nerve SNAP (Levin, 1998).

Needle EMG is the most useful electrodiagnostic procedure in the diagnosis of suspected radiculopathy (Wilbourn and Aminoff, 1998). A study is considered positive if abnormalities—especially acute changes of denervation including fibrillation potentials and positive sharp waves—are present in two or more muscles that receive innervation from the same root, preferably via different peripheral nerves. No abnormalities should be detected in muscles innervated by the affected root's rostral and caudal neighbors. Reduced *motor unit potential* (MUP) recruitment (manifested by decreased numbers of MUPs firing at an increased rate) and MUP abnormalities of reinnervation (high-amplitude, increased duration, polyphasic MUPs) are also sought by the needle electrode but are not as reliable as fibrillation potentials in establishing a definitive diagnosis of radiculopathy. However, the absence of fibrillation potentials does not exclude the diagnosis of radiculopathy. Two main reasons for this exist. First, examination in the first 1–3 weeks after onset of nerve root compromise may be negative because it takes approximately 2 weeks for these potentials to appear. At the early stages in the process of nerve root compression, the only needle electrode examination manifestation of radiculopathy might be reduced MUP recruitment resulting from axon loss, focal demyelination with conduction block, or both. Second, fibrillation potentials disappear as denervated fibers are reinnervated by axons of the same or an adjacent myotome beginning 2–3 months after nerve root compression (Fig. 105.5). Thus, in the later phases of nerve root compression, the only needle EMG changes indicative of radiculopathy might be chronic neurogenic changes of reduced recruitment and MUP remodeling. The distribution of fibrillation potentials is relatively stereotyped for C5, C7, and C8 radiculopathies, whereas C6 radiculopathy has the most variable presentation. In about half of patients, the findings are similar to C5 radiculopathy, whereas in the other half, findings are identical to C7 radiculopathy (Levin et al., 1996).

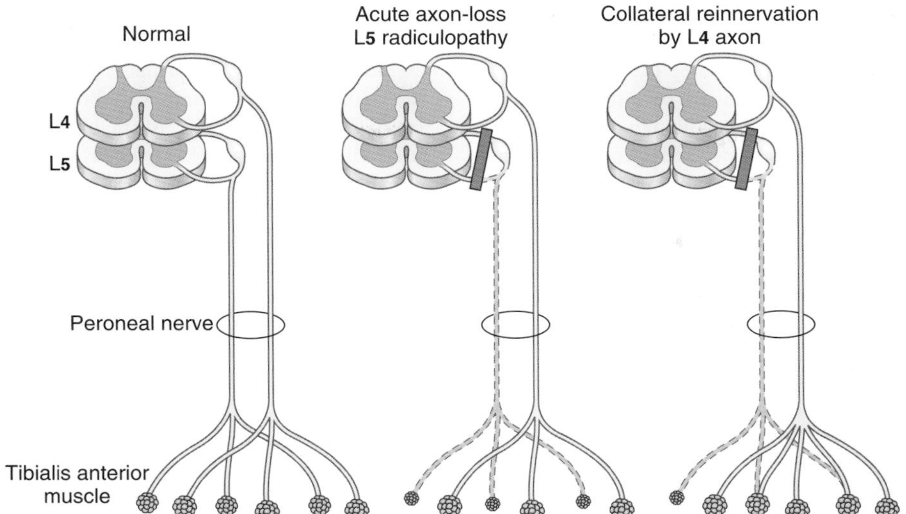


**Fig. 105.5 Diagram Illustrating How Muscle Fibers Denervated by a Radiculopathy are Reinnervated by Collateral Sprouting Despite Persisting Root Compression.** *(Reprinted with permission from Wilbourn, A.J., Aminoff, M.J., 1988. AAEE minimonograph #32: the electrophysiologic examination in patients with radiculopathies. Muscle Nerve 11, 1099–1114.)*

***Treatment.*** For cervical disk protrusion and spondylotic radiculopathy, the mainstay of treatment is conservative management—a combination of a period of reduced physical activity with use of a soft cervical collar, physiotherapy, and antiinflammatory and analgesic agents. Most patients improve, even those with mild to moderate motor deficits. Indeed, in some cases, herniated cervical disks have been observed to regress on MRI images, a circumstance that appears more likely to occur if disk material has extruded and becomes exposed to the epidural space (Mochida et al., 1998). Although there appears to be a short-term benefit to surgical decompression of an affected nerve root with regard to pain, weakness, or sensory loss, at 1 year there is no significant difference between the outcomes of surgical or conservative management (physical therapy or hard cervical collar immobilization) (Endquist et al., 2013). However, a surgical approach may be warranted in selected cases: (1) if there is unremitting pain despite an adequate trial of conservative management; (2) if there is progressive weakness in the territory of the compromised nerve root; or (3) if there are clinical and radiological signs of an accompanying new onset of myelopathy, although in a group of patients with mild or moderate myelopathy, those managed surgically had the same outcome (degree of functional disability) as those allocated to conservative treatment (Nikolaidis et al., 2010).

In the lumbosacral region, disk herniation and spondylotic changes respond to conservative management in more than 90% of patients. Bed rest had been recommended as the centerpiece of patient care, but controlled trials have demonstrated that back-strengthening exercises under the direction of a physical therapist, performed within the limits of the patient's pain, result in more rapid resolution of pain and return to normal function (Dahm et al., 2010). Follow-up MRI studies in conservatively managed patients indicate reduction in size or disappearance of herniated nucleus pulposus corresponding to improvement in clinical findings (Komori et al., 1996). Epidural corticosteroid injection may help relieve pain but does not improve neurological function or reduce the need for surgery (Carette et al., 1997). Relief of radicular pain due to paracentric lumbosacral disk herniations may best be predicted by the severity of root compression on MRI (Ghahremann and Bogduk, 2011). In a study of 71 patients receiving epidural steroid injections, those with low-grade herniations, characterized as either root effacement without displacement or root displacement with preservation of the periradicular CSF demonstrated a significantly higher incidence of subjective pain relief (74%) as compared to patients with more severe root displacement with obliteration of the periradicular CSF or morphological distortion of the nerve root (26%) (Ghahremann and Bogduk, 2011). Lumbosacral level, duration of pain, and the presence of sensory changes, motor weakness, or lost reflexes did not predict a response to epidural steroid injections. A single intravenous (IV) bolus of methylprednisolone (500 mg) given to patients with acute discogenic sciatica of less than 6 weeks' duration provided short-term improvement in leg pain, but the effect was relatively small, with no effect on functional disability, and was quite transitory (3 days) (Finckh et al., 2006). When a patient population with sciatica due to a herniated lumbar disk is followed at regular intervals for more than 10 years, surgically treated patients report more complete relief of leg pain and improved function and satisfaction compared with the nonsurgically treated group. However, improvement in the patient's predominant symptom and work or disability outcomes were similar in the two groups (Atlas et al., 2005). Three situations occur in which surgical referral is indicated: (1) in patients presenting with cauda equina syndrome for whom surgery may be required urgently, (2) if the neurological deficit is severe or progressing, or (3) if severe radicular pain continues after 4–6 weeks of conservative management.

## Diabetic Polyradiculoneuropathy

Diabetic neuropathies can be classified anatomically into two major groups: symmetrical polyneuropathies and asymmetrical focal or multifocal disorders. Examples of the latter include the cranial mononeuropathies and the conditions covered in this section: cervical, thoracoabdominal, and lumbosacral polyradiculoneuropathies. Though treated separately in the following paragraphs, they often coexist in an individual patient.

Diabetic polyradiculoneuropathy tends to affect patients in the sixth or seventh decade of life who have noninsulin-dependent diabetes of several years' duration. The syndrome of painful polyradiculoneuropathy, whether referable to cervical, thoracic or lumbosacral roots, may be the presenting manifestation of diabetes. In 30%–50%

of patients, the disorder is preceded by substantial weight loss of 30–40 pounds.

When there is predominant involvement of the thoracic roots, the presenting symptoms are generally pain and paresthesias of rapid onset in the abdominal and chest wall. The trunk pain may be severe, described variably as burning, sharp, aching, and throbbing. It may mimic the pain of acute cardiac or intraabdominal medical emergencies and may simulate disk disease, but the rarity of thoracic disk protrusions and the usual development of a myelopathy help exclude this diagnosis. Findings of diabetic thoracoabdominal polyradiculoneuropathy include heightened sensitivity to light touch over affected regions; patches of sensory loss on the anterior, lateral, or posterior aspects of the trunk; and unilateral abdominal swelling due to localized weakness of the abdominal wall muscles (Longstreth, 2005).

Diabetic lumbosacral polyradiculoneuropathy involves the legs, especially the anterior thighs, with pain, dysesthesia, and weakness, reflecting the major involvement of upper lumbar roots. A variety of names have been used to describe it, including *diabetic amyotrophy, proximal diabetic neuropathy, diabetic lumbosacral plexopathy, diabetic femoral neuropathy*, and *Bruns–Garland syndrome*. Because it is likely that the brunt of nerve pathology falls on the nerve roots, it can be designated as *diabetic polyradiculoneuropathy*. Motor, sensory, and autonomic fibers are all affected by the disease process (Dyck et al., 1999).

In most patients, onset is fairly abrupt, with symptoms developing over days to a couple of weeks. Early in the course of the condition, the clinical findings are usually unilateral and include weakness of muscles supplied by L2–L4 roots (iliopsoas, quadriceps, and hip adductors), reduced or absent patellar reflex, and mild impairment of sensation over the anterior thigh. As time passes, there may be *territorial spread*, a term used by Bastron and Thomas (1981) to describe proximal, distal, or contralateral involvement as the polyradiculoneuropathy evolves. Worsening may occur in a steady or a stepwise fashion, and it may take several weeks to progress from onset to peak of the disease. At its peak, weakness varies in severity and extent from a mildly affected patient with slight unilateral thigh weakness to a profound degree of bilateral leg weakness in the territory of the L2–S2 nerve roots. Rarely, the process of territorial spread is so extensive that it involves a multiplicity of nerve roots along the entire spinal cord and leads to profound generalized weakness, a condition designated *diabetic cachexia*.

Diabetic cervical polyradiculoneuropathy has also been described (Massie et al., 2012), and may occur independently or in temporal association with lumbosacral polyradiculoneuropathy. Similar to the lumbosacral form, it is characterized as an acute or subacute onset of unilateral limb pain, followed by focal hand and forearm weakness that may then progress to involve multiple myotomes or focal nerve territories in the affected limb. Though less common than the polyradiculoneuropathy of lumbosacral onset, progression to the contralateral upper extremity is seen in up to 35% of patients, and involvement of cranial, thoracic, and lumbosacral regions may also occur.

Laboratory studies disclose elevated fasting blood glucose in the vast majority of patients; when values are normal, they are found in treated diabetics. The erythrocyte sedimentation rate is usually normal. The typical electrodiagnostic findings comprise features of a sensorimotor axon-loss polyneuropathy (diminished sensory and motor action potentials, normal or slightly prolonged distal latencies, and normal or mildly slowed conduction velocities) with additional needle electrode examination findings of active and chronic denervation changes in paraspinal, pelvic girdle, and limb muscles. Taken together, the findings reflect multifocal axonal damage to the nerve roots and brachial or lumbosacral plexus (Amato and Barohn, 2001). Although clinical findings may point to unilateral involvement, the electrodiagnostic examination generally discloses bilateral signs. Imaging studies are almost always necessary to exclude a structural abnormality of the nerve roots that may simulate diabetic polyradiculopathy. Both CT and myelography studies are typically normal. MRI of the brachial plexus in diabetic cervical polyradiculoneuropathy is typically abnormal with an increase in T2 signaling at the root, trunk, cord, or individual nerve level being the most common finding, often in a more extensive distribution than the clinical presentation would suggest (Massie et al., 2012). Nerve hypertrophy and increased T2 signal in muscle (suggestive of edema) were also observed. The CSF protein level is usually increased to an average of 120 mg/dL, but in some patients, values exceed 350 mg/dL; pleocytosis is not a feature of this condition. Biopsy of proximal nerve sensory branches reveals axon loss and demyelination; in more severely affected patients, inflammatory cell infiltration and vasculitis is found (Said et al., 1997). Further studies of nerve biopsy specimens indicate that a microscopic vasculitis (involvement of small arterioles, venules, and capillaries) leads to ischemic injury, which in turn causes axonal degeneration and secondary segmental demyelination (Dyck et al., 1999). The presence of a small-vessel vasculitis with distinctive pathological features including transmural polymorphonuclear leukocyte infiltration of postcapillary venules and endothelial deposits of immunoglobulin (Ig)M and activated complement supports an immune-mediated inflammatory pathogenesis for this disorder (Kelkar et al., 2000).

The natural history of diabetic polyradiculoneuropathy is for improvement to occur in most patients, although the recovery phase is lengthy, ranging between 1 and 18 months with a mean of 6 months. Pain and dysesthesias improve or disappear entirely in 85% of patients; numbness improves or recovers in 50%; and strength is partially or completely restored in 70%. In some patients, episodes recur.

Therapy is usually directed toward ameliorating the severe pain of this condition. The tricyclic antidepressants (e.g., amitriptyline and nortriptyline), selective serotonin reuptake inhibitors (e.g., sertraline, nefazodone hydrochloride), selective serotonin and norepinephrine reuptake inhibitors (e.g., duloxetine, venlafaxine), anticonvulsants (e.g., gabapentin, pregabalin, carbamazepine), and topical capsaicin may have a role separately or in combination. Histopathological findings indicative of an immune-mediated pathogenesis has led to treatment of selected patients with intravenous immunoglobulin (IVIG) or other immunosuppressive treatments. A comprehensive and critical review of the literature on the role of immunotherapy of diabetic polyradiculopathy concludes that treatment remains controversial because the natural history is for spontaneous improvement, the side effects of immunotherapy may be significant, and information on efficacy is lacking from controlled clinical trials (Amato and Barohn, 2001). Prospective studies have suggested a role for immunotherapy in the treatment plan of diabetic polyradiculoneuropathy where electrophysiological findings are those of chronic inflammatory demyelinating polyneuropathy (CIDP) (Ayyar and Sharma, 2004), although the degree of improvement has been shown not to be as robust as in the immunotherapy of idiopathic CIDP (Gorson et al., 2000).

The major differential diagnostic considerations are polyradiculoneuropathies related to degenerative disk disease, infection, inflammatory or autoimmune mediated disease, and neoplastic processes. These can usually be excluded by history, examination, and routine laboratory investigations including CSF analysis. However, in our experience, the clinical presentation provoking the most anxiety is the frail elderly patient not known to be diabetic who has weight loss and abrupt onset of lower-extremity pain and weakness that progresses over months. In such a patient, the specter of neoplasia looms large, and thorough imaging studies of the nerve roots and plexuses are mandatory.

## Neoplastic Polyradiculoneuropathy (Neoplastic Meningitis)

A wide variety of neoplasms are known to spread to the leptomeninges. These include solid tumors (carcinoma of the breast and lung, gastrointestinal tract, and melanoma), non-Hodgkin lymphomas, leukemias, and intravascular lymphomatosis (Clarke, 2012). Although neoplastic polyradiculoneuropathy usually occurs in patients known to have an underlying neoplasm, meningeal symptoms may be the first manifestation of malignancy. Neoplastic meningitis occurs in approximately 5% of all patients with cancer (Chamberlain, 2006). The clinical features of neoplastic polyradiculoneuropathy include radicular pain, dermatomal sensory loss, areflexia, weakness of a lower motor neuron type, and bowel/bladder dysfunction (Mammoser and Groves, 2010). Often the distribution of the sensory and motor deficits is widespread and simulates a severe sensorimotor polyneuropathy. Associated clinical manifestations (e.g., nuchal rigidity, confusion, cranial polyneuropathies) result from infiltration of the meninges.

At postmortem examination, the cauda equina shows discrete nodules or focal granularity (Fig. 105.6). Microscopy discloses spinal roots encased by tumor cells, which appear to infiltrate the root. Malignant cells have the capacity to penetrate the pial membrane and invade the spinal nerves (Mammoser and Groves, 2010). It is presumed that disturbed nerve root function results from several mechanisms including nerve fiber compression and ischemia.

The most revealing diagnostic procedure is lumbar puncture, which is usually abnormal, disclosing one or more or the following: mononuclear pleocytosis, reduced CSF glucose, elevated protein, and neoplastic cells (Clark, 2012). By contrast, spinal fluid cytological analysis may be initially negative in more than one-third of patients who have compelling evidence of leptomeningeal carcinomatosis. Sensitivity of CSF cytology can be improved with repeated sampling, analysis of larger CSF volumes (>10 cc), and when spinal fluid is sampled near the main focus of metastatic involvement (Taillibert et al., 2005). A sensitive, albeit nonspecific, electrophysiological indicator of nerve root involvement is an abnormal F wave. In the symptomatic patient with cancer, prolonged F-wave latencies or absent F responses should raise suspicion of leptomeningeal metastases. Post-myelography CT adds strong evidence in support of the diagnosis if it demonstrates multiple nodular defects on the nerve roots, but spinal MRI, especially with gadolinium enhancement, is the initial test of choice in the cancer patient in whom leptomeningeal involvement of the spine is suspected (Gleissner and Chamberlain, 2006). Approximately 50% of patients with neoplastic meningitis and spinal symptoms have abnormalities on these studies. Gadolinium-enhanced MRI of the brain discloses abnormalities, including contrast enhancement of the basilar cisterns or cortical convexities and hydrocephalus.

Standard therapy for neoplastic meningitis is essentially palliative; it does, however, afford stabilization and protection from further neurological deterioration (Chamberlain, 2006). A multidisciplinary approach is recommended, with input from medical oncology, neuro-oncology, radiation oncology, and neurosurgery (Mammoser and Groves, 2010). With treatment that includes radiotherapy to sites of symptomatic disease, intrathecal or intraventricular chemotherapy (methotrexate, thiotepa, and cytosine arabinoside), and optimal management of the underlying malignancy, median survivals of 2–5 months may be achieved (Clarke, 2012; Chamberlain, 2006). On occasion, longer-term survival is observed in patients with neoplastic meningitis accompanying breast cancer (13% survival rate at 1 year and 6% at 2 years), melanoma, and lymphoma (Jaeckle, 2006).

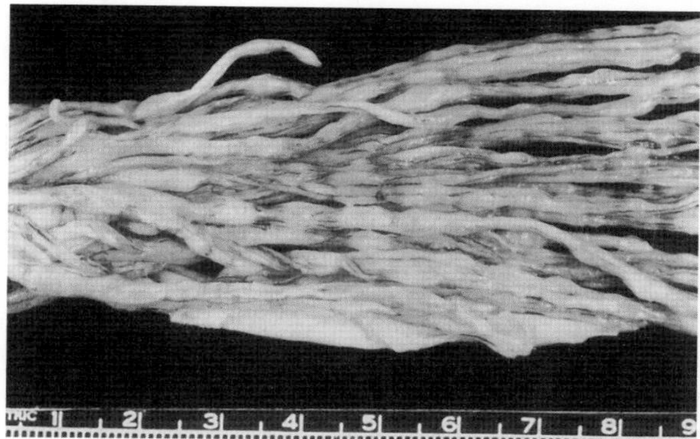


**Fig. 105.6 Cauda Equina in Leptomeningeal Carcinomatosis.** Seeding of multiple nerve roots by adenocarcinoma produces a nodular appearance. *(Courtesy Dr. T.W. Smith, Department of Pathology [Neuropathology], University of Massachusetts Medical Center, Worcester, MA.)*

## Polyradiculopathy Associated with Sarcoidosis

Sarcoidosis is a systemic, multiorgan, inflammatory granulomatous disease. Neurological involvement of any kind is rare, observed in approximately 5% of patients, and characterized by granulomatous infiltration of CNS parenchyma, meninges, peripheral nerves and their roots. Predominant involvement of motor and sensory roots has been described (Koffman et al., 1999), manifesting in the lower extremities with subacute onset of proximal more than distal weakness, sensory loss, and pain in the back or legs. Deep tendon reflexes are often attenuated in keeping with a pure radiculopathy, although concomitant intraparenchymal involvement may occur, leading to upper motor neurons signs with hyperreflexia and extensor plantar responses. More acute onset presentations mimicking the Guillain-Barré syndrome (GBS) also have been described (Fahoum et al., 2009).

Sarcoidosis characteristically presents in late adolescence through middle age, with a higher incidence in African Americans in North America. Establishing the diagnosis of neurosarcoidosis may be challenging. The gold standard of diagnosis is pathological evidence of noncaseating granulomas in involved nervous tissue. When this level of certainty cannot be achieved, clinicians turn to serum, CSF, and radiological testing to help support the diagnosis. Serum angiotensin-converting enzyme (ACE) levels are of limited utility, and do not correlate well with CSF ACE levels (Pawate et al., 2009). Elevated serum ACE levels should spur further diagnostic investigation, whereas a negative test result should not dissuade the clinician from a potential diagnosis of neurosarcoidosis. CSF analysis typically discloses elevated total protein, hypoglycorrhachia, and a lymphocytic pleocytosis, although not all patients will have all three abnormalities. The most common CSF abnormality is a high protein concentration. MRI may be most helpful in demonstrating increased T2 signal or post-gadolinium enhancement of involved nerve roots, meninges, or brain and spinal cord parenchyma. When neurosarcoidosis is suspected as the initial manifesting symptom of sarcoidosis, a diagnostic work-up to assess for systemic disease should also be pursued. This should include a plain chest x-ray or high-resolution CT to look for hilar lymph node or pulmonary involvement. Consideration should also be given to fluorodeoxyglucose positron emission tomography (FDG-PET) evaluating for pulmonary or extrapulmonary involvement that would subsequently allow for targeted biopsy of a more accessible involved organ (Glaudemans et al., 2013).

Formal evaluation of drug therapy in neurosarcoidosis is nonexistent, though convention favors initial treatment with oral or IV corticosteroids. Many patients improve with corticosteroid therapy, though long-term immunosuppression with corticosteroid-sparing agents such as azathioprine, mycophenolate mofetil, and methotrexate may be required. In the spinal column, where granulomatous infiltration may be associated with significant mass effect, decompressive laminectomy may be required.

## Infectious Radiculopathy

### Tabes Dorsalis

Tabes dorsalis, the most common form of late neurosyphilis, begins as a spirochetal *(Treponema pallidum)* meningitis (see Chapter 78). After 10–20 years of persistent infection, damage to the dorsal roots is severe and extensive, producing a set of characteristic symptoms and signs. Symptoms are lightning pains, ataxia, and bladder disturbance; signs include Argyll Robertson pupils, areflexia, loss of proprioceptive sense, Charcot joints, and trophic ulcers. Lancinating or lightning pains are brief, sharp, or stabbing in quality and are more apt to occur in the legs than elsewhere. Sensory disturbances such as coldness, numbness, and tingling also occur and are associated with impairment of light touch, pain, and thermal sensation. Episodes of visceral crisis, characterized by the abrupt onset of epigastric pain that spreads around the body or up over the chest, occur in some 20% of patients.

Most of the features of tabes dorsalis can be explained by lesions of the dorsal roots, dorsal root ganglia, and posterior columns (Gilad et al., 2007). Ataxia is due to the destruction of proprioceptive fibers, insensitivity to pain follows partial loss of small myelinated and unmyelinated fibers, and bladder hypotonia with overflow incontinence, constipation, and impotence is the result of sacral root damage. Pathological studies disclose thinning and grayness of the posterior roots, especially in the lumbosacral region, and the spinal cord shows degeneration of the posterior columns. A mild reduction of neurons in the DRG occurs, and there is little change in the peripheral nerves. Inflammation may occur all along the posterior root.

The CSF may be normal in tabes dorsalis or may show a mild lymphocytic pleocytosis (10–50 cells/μL) and elevated protein concentration (45–75 mg/dL). While up to 25% of patients are found to have nonreactive CSF-Venereal Disease Research Laboratory (VDRL), the serum treponemal tests fluorescent treponemal antibody absorption (FTA-ABS), Treponema pallidum particle agglutination assay (TPPA), and syphilis enzyme immunoassay (EIA)), remain reactive for life in virtually all patients regardless of previous treatment (Marra, 2014). The preferred treatment is aqueous penicillin G, 2–4 million units IV every 4 hours for 10–14 days, with careful CSF follow-up. CSF examination 6 months after treatment should demonstrate a normal cell count and decreasing protein content. If not, a second course of therapy is indicated. The CSF examination should be repeated every 6 months for 2 years or until the fluid is normal.

### Polyradiculoneuropathy in Human Immunodeficiency Virus-Infected Patients

Cytomegalovirus (CMV) polyradiculoneuropathy is a rapidly progressive opportunistic infection that usually occurs late in the course of human immunodeficiency virus (HIV) infection when the CD4 count is very low (<50 cells/mL) and acquired immunodeficiency syndrome (AIDS)-defining infections are present. Uncommonly, it is the initial manifestation of AIDS (Anders and Goebel, 1998). Patients often have evidence of systemic CMV infection (retinitis, gastroenteritis). The presentation is marked by rapid onset of pain and paresthesias in the legs and perineal region, associated with urinary retention and progressive ascending weakness of the lower extremities (Robinson-Papp and Simpson, 2009). Examination discloses a severe cauda equina syndrome, the combination of flaccid paraparesis, absent lower-limb deep tendon reflexes, reduced or absent sphincter tone, and variable loss of light touch, vibration, and joint position sense. The upper extremities and cranial nerves may be involved in advanced cases (Robinson-Papp and Simpson, 2009).

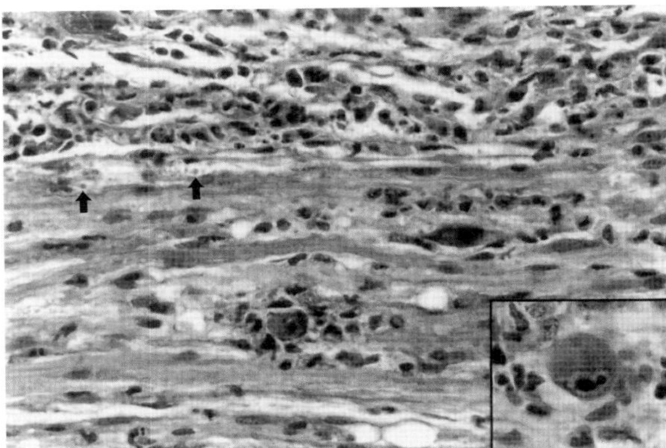

**Fig. 105.7 Cytomegalovirus Polyradiculoneuropathy.** Numerous mononuclear inflammatory cells are apparent, and the presence of myelin ovoids *(arrows)* reflects axon loss (hematoxylin and eosin stain, ×100). *Inset,* Cytomegalic cell with intranuclear inclusion (hematoxylin and eosin stain, ×150). *(Courtesy Dr. T.W. Smith, Department of Pathology [Neuropathology], University of Massachusetts Medical Center, Worcester, MA.)*

A gadolinium-enhanced MRI of the lumbosacral spine is necessary to exclude a compressive lesion of the cauda equina and is generally the first study performed (Robinson-Papp and Simpson, 2009). The MRI in CMV polyradiculoneuropathy is usually normal, but adhesive arachnoiditis has been described. The CSF has an elevated protein level, depressed glucose level, polymorphonuclear pleocytosis, and a positive CMV polymerase chain reaction (PCR) (Anders and Goebel, 1998). CMV may be isolated from CSF cultures. The needle EMG discloses widespread fibrillation potentials in lower-extremity muscles, and sensory conduction studies may reveal an associated distal sensory neuropathy that is common in the late stages of HIV infection. The pathological features are marked inflammation and extensive necrosis of dorsal and ventral roots. Cytomegalic inclusions may be found in the nucleus and cytoplasm of endothelial and Schwann cells (Fig. 105.7).

Untreated CMV polyradiculoneuropathy is rapidly fatal within approximately 6 weeks of onset. The antiviral nucleoside analog ganciclovir may benefit some patients if treatment is instituted early; improvement occurs over weeks to months. Viral resistance to ganciclovir is suggested by persistent pleocytosis and depressed CSF glucose (Cohen et al., 1993) and should prompt consideration of alternate, or combination therapy with an antiviral agent such as foscarnet, which, unlike ganciclovir, does not require intracellular phosphorylation for its effect.

Other causes of rapidly progressive lumbosacral polyradiculoneuropathy in the HIV-infected patient are meningeal lymphomatosis, *Mycobacterium tuberculosis*, and axonal polyradiculoneuritis associated with HIV infection per se (Corral et al., 1997). Additionally, one must consider acute inflammatory demyelinating polyradiculoneuropathy, syphilitic polyradiculoneuropathy (which often has an accelerated course in the patient with AIDS), herpes simplex virus type 2 and varicella-zoster virus infections. *Toxoplasma gondii* may also cause myelitis, presenting as a subacute conus medullaris syndrome that simulates the clinical features produced by CMV polyradiculoneuropathy. In the case of *T. gondii*, MRI may reveal abscess formation.

### Lyme Radiculoneuropathy

Lyme disease is caused by the spirochete *Borrelia burgdorferi*, transmitted by the deer tick *Ixodes dammini*, and is most prevalent in the

American northeast and upper Midwest, where risk of infection is greatest during the spring and summer months. A European form, caused by the spirochetes *B. afzelii* and *B. garinii*, is also well recognized in temperate climates of central Europe and Asia. Lyme is a multisystem disease affecting the skin, peripheral nervous system, CNS (referred to as *neuroborreliosis*), musculoskeletal system, and heart. To help bring order to the understanding of this illness, it may be divided into three clinical stages (Bratton et al., 2008). Stage 1 follows within 1 month of the tick bite and is marked by a characteristic rash in 60%–80% of patients, designated *erythema chronica migrans* (oval or annular shape with a clear center in the area of the bite), and influenza-like symptoms of fatigue, fever, headache, stiff neck, myalgias, and arthralgias. Stage 2, the *stage of dissemination* of the spirochete from the initial lesion, may occur within weeks of the rash, and may result in peripheral nerve, joint, and cardiac abnormalities. Stage 3, caused by late or persistent infection, may occur up to 2 years after the tick bite and is characterized by chronic neurological syndromes, among them neuropathy, myelopathy, psychiatric disturbances, and migratory oligoarthritis.

Nerve root and peripheral nerve abnormalities that characterize stage 2 develop in about 4%–5% of untreated patients (Halperin, 2010). Possible manifestations occurring within weeks after the onset of erythema chronica migrans most commonly include headache with lymphocytic (aseptic) meningitis, cranial neuropathy (especially facial mononeuropathies, bilateral in 25% of cases), and a multifocal radiculoneuropathy or mononeuritis multiplex. With nerve root involvement there may be an associated myelitis at adjacent spinal cord levels, with accompanying long tract signs on examination (Halperin, 2010). The clinical features of nerve root involvement include burning radicular pain with sensory loss, weakness, and hyporeflexia in the territory of the involved roots. Nerve conduction studies provide evidence for an associated primarily axon-loss polyneuropathy. The rare patient with *chronic neuroborreliosis*, seen in stage 3, may develop a stocking-glove patterned axon-loss polyneuropathy, that may in fact represent confluence of multiple mononeuropathies (Bratton et al., 2008; Halperin, 2008). In a non-human primate model of neuroborreliosis, the spread of *B. burgdorferi* within the nervous system—leptomeninges, motor and sensory roots, DRG, but not the brain parenchyma—has been demonstrated. In peripheral nerves from such animals, spirochetes were seen in the perineurium (Steere, 2001).

The diagnosis of Lyme disease can be made on the grounds of history and clinical presentation alone especially when there is evidence of erythema migrans. Serological testing for antibodies against *B. burgdorferi* (and confirmatory Western blot in those with borderline or positive results) can be beneficial, though neurological manifestations can be seen prior to the appearance of IgM antibodies in the blood as part of the early humeral response. Thus, antibody testing in a patient with suspected exposure within 3–6 weeks of presentation may be negative (Halperin, 2013). CSF analysis may be reserved for those with suspected CNS involvement, and will typically be abnormal with a lymphocytic pleocytosis, elevated protein, and normal glucose.

Treatment of Lyme radiculoneuropathy with IV ceftriaxone (cefotaxime and penicillin G are acceptable alternates) for 2–4 weeks is associated with resolution of symptoms and signs in most patients. Oral doxycycline (100 mg twice daily), has been shown to be equally efficacious in the treatment of European forms of neuroborreliosis, including radiculopathy (Ljøstad et al., 2008), while studies comparing IV versus oral antibiotics for the treatment of North American Lyme disease are lacking. After successful treatment, serum antibodies will often remain positive and their presence or absence offers no clinical utility in determining efficacy of treatment.

### Herpes Zoster

Herpes zoster, also known as *shingles*, is a common painful vesicular eruption occurring in a segmental or radicular (dermatomal) distribution and due to reactivation of latent varicella-zoster virus in DRG (see Chapter 77). Primary infection presents as varicella (chickenpox) earlier in life (Cohen, 2013), usually in epidemics among susceptible children. Involvement may occur at any level of the neuraxis but is most commonly seen in the thoracic dermatomes, followed by the face. Zoster, when involving the ophthalmic division of the trigeminal nerve (herpes zoster ophthalmicus), may be accompanied by keratitis, a potential cause of blindness requiring immediate treatment. When isolated to the seventh nerve, it is associated with a facial palsy and ipsilateral external ear or hard palate vesicles known as *Ramsay Hunt syndrome* (Cohen, 2013). Rarely, the viral episode can present as dermatomal pain without a rash, known as *herpes sine herpete*.

Zoster occurs during the lifetime of 10%–20% of all people, with an incidence in the general population of approximately 3–5 per 1000 per year. The incidence is low in young people and increases with age—among persons older than 75 years it exceeds 10 cases per 1000 person-years—and when immunocompetence is compromised. For example, the incidence among HIV-positive individuals was reported as 15-fold greater than that of a control group (Gnann and Whitley, 2002).

During primary infection, the virus colonizes the DRG and remains latent for many decades until it is reactivated, either spontaneously or when virus-specific cell-mediated immunity declines secondary to specific conditions (e.g., lymphoproliferative disorders, treatment with immunosuppressive drugs, organ transplant recipients, seropositivity for HIV) or normal aging, and travels down sensory nerves. Pathological changes, which are characterized by lymphocytic infiltration and variable hemorrhage, are found in the skin, DRG, and spinal roots. Involvement of the ventral roots and, on occasion, the spinal cord, explains the development of motor signs in some patients (see later discussion).

Herpes zoster is characterized by sharp or burning radicular pain associated with itching, numbness, *dysesthesias* (altered sensation), and/or *allodynia* (a painful response to normally non-noxious stimulation) typically in a single dermatome (Cohen, 2013). The cutaneous eruption, unilateral and respecting the midline, begins as an erythematous maculopapular rash and progresses to grouped clear vesicles that continue to form for 3–5 days (Cohen, 2013). These become pustules by 3–4 days and form crusts by 10 days. In the normal immunocompetent host, lesions resolve in 2–4 weeks, often leaving a region of reduced sensation, scarring, and pigmentation. Pain usually disappears as vesicles fade, but 10%–50% of patients experience persistent severe pain, that when present for more than 30 days after rash onset or following cutaneous healing is termed *postherpetic neuralgia* (PHN; Cohen, 2013). This complication is more likely to develop in the elderly, occurring in 50% of patients over 60 years of age. In half of patients affected with PHN, the pain resolves within 2 months, and 70%–80% of patients are pain free by 1 year. Rarely, pain persists for years.

In the immunologically normal host, dissemination of the virus is rare, occurring in fewer than 2% of patients. In the immunocompromised patient, however, dissemination occurs in 13%–50% of patients. Most often, spread is to distant cutaneous sites, but involvement of the viscera (lung, gastrointestinal tract, and heart) and CNS may occur. A serious complication of herpes zoster ophthalmicus is delayed contralateral hemiparesis caused by cerebral angiitis. The syndrome usually develops 1 week to 6 months after the onset of zoster and occurs in patients of all ages, 50% of whom are immunologically impaired. The mortality rate from cerebrovascular complications is 25%, and only approximately 30% of survivors recover fully.

A complication of cutaneous herpes zoster is segmental motor weakness, which occurs in up to 30% of patients with zoster reactivation (Bahadir et al., 2008). Segmental zoster paresis is about equally divided between the arms and legs, with predominantly proximal muscle weakness reflecting weakness in cervical and lumbar—C5, C6, and C7 or L2, L3, and L4—myotomes, respectively. The diaphragm and abdominal muscles may be affected, and bladder and bowel dysfunction may occur in the setting of lumbosacral zoster (Gilden et al., 2013). The interval between skin eruption and paralysis is approximately 2 weeks, with a range of 1 day to 5 weeks and a rare instance reported of delayed (4.5 months) onset of diaphragmatic paralysis. Weakness peaks within hours or days and generally follows the dermatomal distribution of zoster eruptions (Yaszay et al., 2000); spread to muscles served by unaffected segments is very uncommon (<3% of cases). The prognosis for recovery is good, with nearly complete return of function in two-thirds of patients over the course of 1–2 years, 55% showing full recovery, and another 30% showing significant improvement. One in five patients is left with severe and permanent residua.

Prognosis for recovery in patients with diaphragmatic paralysis is not as good as it is with segmental paresis involving the limb muscles, probably owing to the challenge of axonal regeneration along the long course of the phrenic nerve (Bahadir et al., 2008). The histopathological correlate of herpes zoster is inflammation and neuronal loss in the DRG that correspond to the affected segmental levels. In the case of segmental zoster paresis, there is lymphocytic inflammation and vasculitis involving adjacent motor roots and the spinal cord gray matter, with resulting motor fiber degeneration (Gilden et al., 2013). A low-grade viral ganglionitis may contribute to PHN (Quan et al., 2005).

The major goals of treatment are to relieve local discomfort, prevent dissemination, and reduce the severity of PHN (Sandy, 2005). Acyclovir, valacyclovir, and famciclovir are indicated for the immunocompetent patient older than 50 years with herpes zoster and should be started within 48 hours of the viral episode to receive the most benefit from therapy. These drugs reduce the duration of viral shedding, limit the duration of new lesion formation, and accelerate healing and pain resolution. They are all safe and well tolerated, but because of superior pharmacokinetic profiles and simpler dosing regimen, the latter two are preferred to acyclovir (Cohen, 2013). IV acyclovir is the treatment of choice in immunocompromised patients, having been shown to halt disease progression, prevent dissemination, and speed recovery in immunocompromised patients (Robinson-Papp and Simpson, 2009). In 2017, the US Food and Drug Administration (FDA) approved a non-live recombinant glycoprotein E vaccine for use in the United States to reduce the risk for herpes zoster in older adults (≥60 years). The vaccine requires two intramuscular injections, separated by 2–6 months, and is effective in preventing herpes zoster and reducing risk of post-herpetic neuralgia (Lal et al., 2015).

The pain of PHN—described variably as continuous deep aching, burning, sharp, stabbing, and shooting, and triggered by light touch over the affected dermatomes—is often debilitating and difficult to treat (Johnson and Rice, 2014). Singly or in combination, tricyclic antidepressants, selective serotonin reuptake inhibitors (sertraline or nefazodone hydrochloride), anticonvulsants (carbamazepine and gabapentin), oral opioids (oxycodone), and topical capsaicin cream or lidocaine patches are helpful for about 50% of patients. IV acyclovir followed by oral valacyclovir was found to reduce the pain of PHN in more than 50% of treated patients (Quan et al., 2005).

## Acquired Demyelinating Polyradiculoneuropathy

Acquired demyelinating polyradiculoneuropathy has two major clinical forms. One develops acutely and is known as *Guillain-Barré syndrome* (GBS); the other is chronic, progressive, or relapsing and remitting and is designated CIDP. These disorders are described in detail in Chapter 106 but are mentioned here briefly because pathological changes may be pronounced in the spinal nerve roots, especially the ventral roots. There is a dense mononuclear inflammatory infiltrate of lymphocytes, monocytes, and plasma cells (Fig. 105.8), and segmental demyelination with relative sparing of axons. Neuroimaging with MRI discloses contrast enhancement of lumbosacral roots in both GBS and CIDP (Bertorini et al., 1995; Koller et al., 2005). The predilection for nerve root involvement in these conditions helps explain certain features, including CSF and some neurophysiological findings, as well as disturbances in autonomic function that may be especially problematic in patients with GBS.

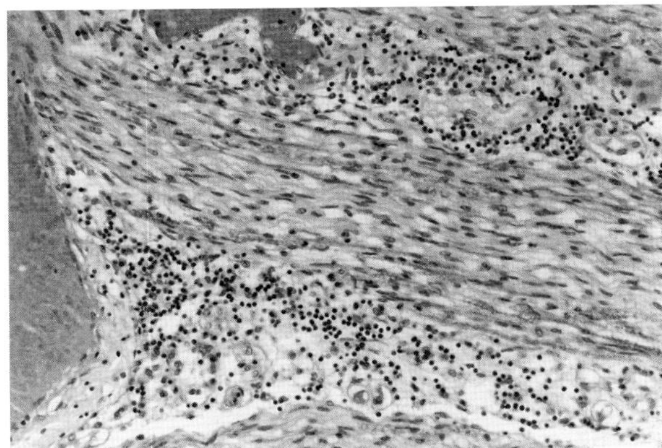

**Fig. 105.8 Cauda Equina in Guillain–Barré Syndrome.** A dense mononuclear infiltrate in the connective tissue surrounding the nerve roots is shown (hematoxylin and eosin stain). *(Courtesy Dr. T.W. Smith, Department of Pathology [Neuropathology], University of Massachusetts Medical Center, Worcester, MA.)*

A CSF profile of albuminocytological dissociation is characteristic of this syndrome and is seen in 50%–66% of patients in the first week of symptoms and in more than 75% of patients 2 weeks after symptom onset. A high lumbar CSF protein concentration in the face of a normal cisternal protein level supports the hypothesis that increased CSF protein derives largely from capillaries of the spinal roots. Nerve conduction studies usually disclose slowed motor conduction velocities, dispersed motor responses, and partial conduction block, but additional abnormalities include delayed or unobtainable F-wave responses or H-reflexes, reflecting demyelination in nerve roots (Koller et al., 2005). Indeed, abnormalities of these late responses may be the sole finding in 10%–20% of patients with GBS in the first few weeks of the illness. The autonomic disturbances that occur in GBS may be due to involvement of preganglionic sympathetic fibers, which travel in the ventral roots en route to the paravertebral sympathetic ganglia.

There is increasing recognition of rare variants of CIDP with a clear predilection for the dorsal or ventral spinal roots, with apparent sparing of more peripheral structures: termed chronic inflammatory sensory (CISP), sensorimotor (CISMP) or motor (CIMP) polyradiculopathy, based on the preferential involvement of sensory and/or motor roots (Khaldikar et al., 2017; O'Ferrall et al., 2013; Sinnreich et al., 2004). CISP is a chronic, progressive syndrome of ataxia, numbness, and paresthesias involving the limbs and/or trunk. Neurological examination reveals normal strength, marked large fiber sensory abnormalities with absent vibratory and joint position sense, less severe decrements in small fiber sensory modalities, and hypo- or areflexia. Distal nerve conduction studies are normal with abnormal late responses (prolonged or absent F-waves or H-reflexes) or absent somatosensory evoked potentials. MRI of the brain and spinal cord parenchyma is normal with thickened and/or enhanced lumbar spinal nerve roots. CSF analysis demonstrates albuminocytological dissociation without oligoclonal bands. Pathological analysis of lumbar dorsal rootlets reveals thickened rootlets, endoneurial edema with prominent staining for macrophages, and onion-bulb formations. There is a normal density of myelinated nerve fibers though with an abnormal size distribution of myelinated fibers, with a preferential decrease in the number of large-diameter myelinated nerve fibers. Peripheral sensory nerve biopsies are normal. Treatment of this inflammatory sensory or sensorimotor polyradiculopathy with oral or IV methylprednisolone, or immunoglobulin, is associated with favorable outcomes.

CISMP presents similar to CISP, though with concurrent weakness of proximal and distal muscles, predominantly in the lower limbs (Khaldikar et al., 2017). Nerve conduction studies, MRI findings, and CSF abnormalities are the same, and treatment with glucocorticoids was met with clear functional improvement in both patients, which was sustained with transitions to steroid-sparing immunomodulators.

A single case report of a pure motor variant, CIMP, has also been reported (O'Ferrall et al., 2013), characterized by insidious onset of progressive, symmetric weakness of the bilateral distal lower extremities, and attenuated reflexes, with sparing of sensation as well as bowel and bladder function. Nerve conductions show attenuated lower extremity compound motor action potentials (CMAPs) and normal SNAPs, and needle EMG shows denervation and partial reinnervation changes in muscles of multiple myotomes. MRI again shows hypertrophied lumbar spinal roots. Pathological analysis showed onion-bulb formations and a decreased number of large-diameter myelinated nerve fibers on root biopsy. This patient had a poor response to IVIG and Solu-Medrol (methylprednisolone) but had functional improvement in lower-extremity strength with plasma exchange.

## Acquired Disorders of the Dorsal Root Ganglia

The dorsal root ganglia may be selectively vulnerable to a variety of malignant and nonmalignant conditions. The resulting neurological disorder is a sensory neuronopathy syndrome whose clinical features are explained by the loss of large- and small-diameter DRG neurons. Large-cell dropout leads to kinesthetic sensory impairment, poor coordination, loss of manual dexterity, ataxia, and areflexia, whereas small-cell depletion contributes to a hyperalgesic state marked by burning pains and painful paresthesias. The sensory neuronopathies are characterized by asymmetric, non-length-dependent abnormalities of SNAPs, a global decrease in SNAP amplitudes, and hyperintensities on T2-weighted MR images of the dorsal spinal cord (Kuntzer et al., 2004; Lin and Chiu, 2008). Clinical and electrophysiological criteria have been proposed to help separate patients with sensory neuronopathy from those with predominantly sensory polyneuropathy (Camdessanche et al., 2009). Favoring the diagnosis of *neuronopathy* are the following findings: the presence of limb ataxia early in the disease, asymmetrical sensory loss at onset, upper-limb sensory loss, lost or attenuated upper-limb sensory action potentials, and relatively normal motor conduction studies.

Perhaps the best known of these uncommon conditions is *paraneoplastic sensory neuronopathy* (PSN), a disorder developing over weeks to months and characterized by ataxia and hyperalgesia while muscle strength is well preserved (Graus and Dalmau, 2013). Some patients have clinical signs of brainstem and cerebral dysfunction, reflecting a more widespread encephalomyelitis. The neuronopathy may antedate the diagnosis of cancer, usually small-cell lung carcinoma, by months to years. The CSF profile discloses elevated protein concentration and a mild mononuclear cell pleocytosis. Nerve conduction studies reveal widespread loss of sensory potentials. Neuropathological features include inflammation and phagocytosis of the sensory neurons in the DRG. PSN is associated with the presence of specific antineuronal (anti-Hu) antibodies that are complement-fixing polyclonal IgG antibodies that react with the nuclei of the neurons of the CNS and sensory ganglia but not with non-neuronal nuclei; most (80%–85%) but not all patients with PSN are found to have anti-Hu antibodies and therefore CT imaging of the chest is recommended when patients present with an acute to subacute onset of a sensory neuronopathy (Gozzard and Maddison, 2010). The antigens recognized by the anti-Hu antibodies have been characterized as proteins with molecular weights of 35–40 kD. The presence of identical protein antigens in small-cell lung cancer cells and neuronal nuclei supports the view that the pathogenesis of paraneoplastic subacute sensory neuropathy is immunologically mediated, with tumor antigens triggering the production of cross-reactive antibodies. Morphological studies provide evidence for both cytotoxic T-cell-mediated attack and humoral mechanisms in the pathogenesis of this condition. Response to immunotherapy is disappointing; however, early diagnosis of cancer gives the best chance of helping the neurological disorder before it becomes devastating (Kuntzer et al., 2004).

Other causes of DRG neuronopathy include hereditary, toxic, and autoimmune disorders (Kuntzer et al., 2004). Hereditary sensory neuropathies are usually marked by their chronicity, acrodystrophic ulcerations, fractures, bouts of osteomyelitis, and lack of paresthesias. Pyridoxine (vitamin E) abuse and cisplatin neurotoxicity are generally easily recognized. Sjögren syndrome, an autoimmune disease involving lymphocytic infiltration of exocrine glands (notably the lacrimal and salivary glands) resulting in marked dry eyes and dry mouth, may be accompanied by ataxia and kinesthetic sensory loss very similar to subacute sensory neuropathy. Diagnosis of primary Sjögren syndrome is made independent from any associated neurological manifestations. Following American and European consensus criteria (Vitali et al., 2002), diagnosis is based on four of six criteria, including subjective ocular or oral symptoms by patient history, objective measures of ocular or oral symptoms, histopathological evidence on minor salivary gland biopsy, and autoantibodies to extractable nuclear antigens Ro (SSA) or La (SSB), with one of the latter two criteria being required. In some cases of Sjögren sensory neuronopathy, cervical MRI shows cervical cord atrophy with increased T2 signal intensity at the dorsal columns, which probably stems from Wallerian degeneration of neurons in the dorsal root ganglia (Lin and Chiu, 2008). Improvement from courses of IVIG may occur in some patients when treated early in the course of the illness.

## Radiculopathies Simulating Motor Neuron Disease

Disorders of the motor roots may lead to clinical features that resemble those encountered in motor neuron disease. Detailed study of such motor neuron syndromes is important because it might provide clues to the pathogenesis of the most common form of motor neuron disease, ALS. Clinicians should consider the possibility of an ALS-mimic syndrome when a patient with clinical features of lower motor neuron involvement is found to have a monoclonal gammopathy (Chad and Harris, 1999). In this instance, investigations must vigorously pursue the possibility that physical findings stem from ventral root involvement rather than anterior horn cell degeneration. An elevated CSF protein level, the presence of a monoclonal gammopathy, along with a demyelinating process identified by nerve conduction studies, suggest a potentially treatable lymphoproliferative disease manifesting as motor polyradiculoneuropathy. In some instances of IgM monoclonal gammopathy, there is antibody specificity for the gangliosides GM1, asialo-GM1, and GD1b, among others. In rare instances, immunotherapy that reduces the serum concentrations of IgM gangliosides is associated with improvement in the lower motor neuron syndrome, thereby suggesting a possible pathogenic role of antiganglioside antibodies.

The association between lower motor neuron findings and lymphoma has been known for many years and is designated *subacute motor neuronopathy*, but the site of major pathology is not certain and could be at the root and/or neuronal level. It is characterized by subacute, progressive, painless, often patchy and asymmetric weakness of the lower motor neuron type, with greater involvement of the arms than the legs. The illness often progresses independently of the activity of the underlying lymphoma and tends to follow a relatively benign course, with some patients demonstrating spontaneous improvement.

A post-radiation lower motor neuron syndrome affecting the lumbosacral region, probably a polyradiculopathy, has been described occurring 4 months to 25 years after radiation therapy to the lower spine and cauda equina for treatment of testicular cancer, vertebral metastases, and lymphoma (Hsia et al., 2003). In some patients, MRI shows gadolinium enhancement of the conus medullaris and cauda equina that may mimic a leptomeningeal tumor (Hsia et al., 2003). Neuropathological study in a case of testicular cancer disclosed radiation-induced vasculopathy of proximal spinal roots with preserved motor neurons (Bowen et al., 1996). The course of the disorder is typically one of progression for 1–2 years followed by eventual stabilization.

## DISORDERS OF THE BRACHIAL PLEXUS

### Anatomical Features

The brachial plexus is formed by five spinal nerve ventral rami (C5–T1), each of which carries motor, sensory, and postganglionic sympathetic fibers to the upper limb. It is a large and complex peripheral nervous system structure that contains more than 100,000 individual nerve fibers (Ferrante, 2012). The five rami unite above the level of the clavicle to form the three trunks of the brachial plexus (Fig. 105.9): C5 and C6 join to form the upper trunk; T1 and C8 unite to form the lower trunk; and C7, the largest of the five rami, continues as the middle trunk. Beneath the clavicle, each trunk divides into an anterior and posterior branch leading to six divisions, which become the three cords of the brachial plexus: the lateral, medial, and posterior. The cords, which lie behind the pectoralis minor, take their names from their relationship to the subclavian artery. The lateral and medial cords carry motor fibers to the ventral muscles of the limb. The lateral cord is formed from anterior divisions of the upper and middle trunks, the medial cord from the anterior division of the lower trunk. The posterior cord carries motor fibers to the dorsal muscles of the limb; it is formed from posterior divisions of the upper, middle, and lower trunks.

The major named nerves of the upper limb are derived from the cords. After contributing a branch to the formation of the median nerve, the lateral cord continues as the musculocutaneous nerve. Similarly, after making its contribution to the median nerve, the medial cord continues as the ulnar nerve. The posterior cord divides into a smaller axillary nerve (which leaves the axilla via the quadrangular space to supply the deltoid and teres minor) and the larger radial nerve. Also, from the level of the cords, branches are distributed to the pectoralis major and minor muscles (from the lateral and medial cords, respectively) and to the subscapularis, latissimus dorsi, and teres major muscles (from the posterior cord). Cutaneous sensory branches also originate at the cord level, with the posterior cutaneous nerve of the arm arising from the posterior cord, and the medial cutaneous nerve of the arm and medial cutaneous nerve of the forearm emerging from the medial cord.

Nerve branches to the serratus anterior, levator scapulae, rhomboids, supraspinatus, and infraspinatus muscles derive from more proximal levels of the plexus. The first three muscles are supplied by branches of the anterior primary rami: the serratus anterior from C5, C6, and C7 (the long thoracic nerve) and the levator scapulae and rhomboids from branches of C5 (the dorsal scapular nerve). The supraspinatus and infraspinatus muscles are supplied by the suprascapular nerve, a branch of the upper trunk of the plexus.

### Clinical Features and Diagnosis

Not surprisingly, disorders of the brachial plexus are determined in large part by its anatomical relationships (Ferrante, 2012). Because of its location between two highly mobile structures, the neck and the shoulder, it is vulnerable to trauma. In addition, with its spatial proximity to neighboring tissues such as lymph nodes, blood vessels, and the lung parenchyma (which may themselves be targets of a variety of disease processes), the brachial plexus may be secondarily affected.

### Neurological Examination

Patients with a brachial plexopathy present with a variety of patterns of weakness, reflex changes, and sensory loss, depending on whether the whole or a portion of the plexus is disturbed. Most commonly encountered are three patterns resulting from involvement of the entire plexus, the upper trunk, or the lower trunk; less commonly seen are partial plexopathies caused by selective cord lesions.

In a panplexopathy, paralysis of muscles supplied by segments C5 through T1 occurs. The arm hangs lifelessly by the side, except that an intact trapezius allows shrugging of the shoulder. The limb is flaccid and areflexic, with complete sensory loss below a line extending from the shoulder diagonally downward and medially to the middle of the upper arm.

Lesions of the upper trunk produce weakness and sensory loss in a C5–C6 distribution. Affected muscles include the supraspinatus and infraspinatus, deltoid, biceps, brachialis, and brachioradialis, so the patient is unable to abduct the arm at the shoulder or flex at the elbow. If a lesion is so proximal that it involves the C5 ramus, the rhomboids and levator scapulae are also affected. The arm hangs at the side internally rotated at the shoulder, with the elbow extended and the forearm pronated in a "waiter's tip" posture. The biceps and brachioradialis reflexes are diminished or absent, and sensory loss is found over the lateral aspect of the arm, forearm, and thumb.

Lesions of the lower trunk produce weakness, sensory loss, and reflex changes in a C8–T1 distribution. Weakness is present in both median- and ulnar-supplied intrinsic hand muscles and in the medial finger and wrist flexors. The finger flexion reflex is diminished or absent, and there is sensory loss over the medial two fingers, the medial aspect of the hand, and the forearm.

Cord lesions are usually found in the setting of trauma. A posterior cord lesion produces weakness in the territory of muscles innervated by both radial and axillary nerves. Sensory loss occurs in the distributions of the posterior cutaneous nerve of the forearm and the radial and axillary nerves. This results in sensory loss over the posterior aspect of the arm, the dorsal surface of the lateral aspect of the hand, and a patch of skin over the lateral aspect of the arm. Lateral cord injuries produce weakness in muscles supplied by the musculocutaneous nerve, as well as weakness in the muscles of the median nerve supplied by the C6 and C7 roots (the pronator teres and flexor carpi radialis muscles). The median and ulnar nerve fibers originating from C8 and T1 segments are spared, and thus there is no intrinsic hand muscle weakness. In medial cord lesions, there is weakness in all ulnar nerve–supplied muscles and in the C8 and T1 median nerve–supplied muscles.

### Electrodiagnostic Studies

Nerve conduction studies and needle EMG provide helpful information for confirming the clinical diagnosis of brachial plexopathy, determining the character of the lesion—predominantly axon loss,

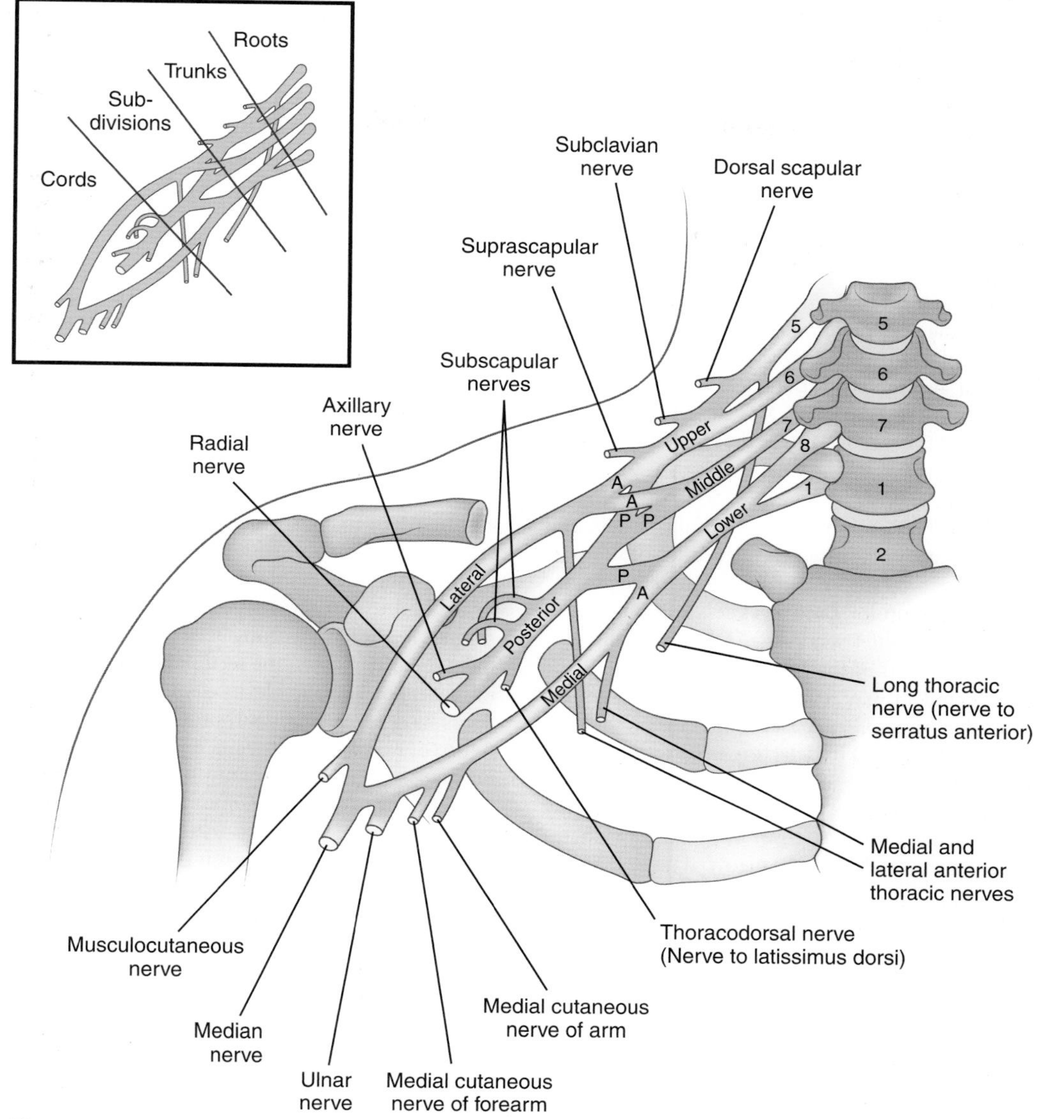


**Fig. 105.9 Brachial Plexus.** Components of the plexus have been separated and drawn out of scale. The five ventral rami (C5–T1) unite to form the upper, middle, and lower trunks of the plexus above the clavicle. Beneath the clavicle, each trunk divides into anterior *(A)* and posterior *(P)* divisions. Three cords (lateral, posterior, and medial) lie below the pectoralis minor muscle (not shown). Major upper limb nerves originate from the cords. (*Reprinted with permission from Haymaker, W., Woodhall, B., 1953. Peripheral Nerve Injuries, second ed. Saunders, Philadelphia.*)

demyelinating, or both—and arriving at a judgment with respect to prognosis for recovery of function. In axon-loss brachial plexopathies, SNAPs and CMAPs are attenuated or lost depending on the severity of the disease process as the amplitude of these responses correlates directly with the number of conducting fibers. In preganglionic lesions (at a root level) sensory responses are expected to be spared, and only motor responses will be affected. As long as at least some fast-conducting fibers are spared, the conduction velocities and distal latencies are unaffected. Conversely, in the case of demyelinating lesions, nerve conduction velocities are typically slowed, motor evoked responses dispersed, and distal latencies prolonged. Most brachial plexus lesions are axon loss in nature (Ferrante, 2012). The needle examination is very sensitive for detecting even mild motor fiber loss because fibrillation potentials develop in affected muscles by 3 weeks after the onset of a disease process.

Axon-loss brachial plexus neuropathies fall along a spectrum of severity that may be determined by the results of the electrodiagnostic study. In the context of a minimal lesion affecting both sensory and motor fibers, SNAPs and CMAPs will typically be unaffected, but needle examination will disclose fibrillation potentials because the loss of one motor axon will result in denervation of hundreds of muscle fibers. With an increase in lesion severity, SNAPs become attenuated while CMAPs are still spared. The most severe lesions compromise sensory and motor responses. Ferrante and Wilbourn (2002) also observed that it is the CMAPs that are most useful for quantifying the amount of loss suffered by a nerve. In contrast, SNAPs may be attenuated, even absent, with only partial lesions; and needle electrode examination, as we have seen, may reveal prominent fibrillation potentials with only mild motor axon loss. The needle examination is helpful in evaluating recovery from axon-loss lesions as features of MUP remodeling (increased duration and complexity of MUPs) indicate an ongoing process of collateral reinnervation, distal-to-proximal reinnervation, or both.

In a postganglionic plexopathy, numbness and sensory loss are associated with reduced or absent SNAPs because the lesion is located distal to the DRG. By contrast, in a pure radiculopathy, sensory loss is found in the face of a normal SNAP because the lesion is proximal to the DRG. In certain conditions, preganglionic and postganglionic lesions coexist, so electrodiagnostic studies disclose paraspinal muscle fibrillation and absent SNAPs. This situation is encountered most commonly in patients with trauma that damages both the plexus and avulses nerve roots. It is also found in some peripheral radiculoplexus neuropathies such as diabetes and in malignant plexopathies in which tumor not only injures the plexus but also infiltrates the nerve roots by tracking through the intervertebral foramina. Specific EMG changes are covered under individual disorders of the plexus, later in the chapter.

## Radiological Studies

Plain films of the neck and chest are often very helpful in evaluating arm weakness that is thought to be caused by a disorder of the brachial plexus. The presence of a cervical rib or long transverse process of C7 may provide an explanation for hand weakness and numbness, as seen in neurogenic thoracic outlet syndrome. A lesion in the pulmonary apex, erosion of the head of the first and second rib, or the transverse processes of C7 and T1 may reveal the cause of a lower brachial plexopathy, as found in cases of Pancoast tumor. High-resolution CT and MRI scanning are also useful in detecting mass lesions of the plexus and may allow early diagnosis and specific therapy (Amrami and Port, 2005). Magnetic resonance neurography, incorporating diffusion-weighted imaging and diffusion tensor imaging, is an emerging imaging modality offering both morphometric data and information regarding pathophysiology in plexus lesions (Noguerol et al., 2017). CT-guided biopsy can be used to obtain cytological or histological material for precise diagnosis.

## Traumatic Plexopathy

Three general categories of traumatic brachial plexus injury exist: (1) direct trauma; (2) secondary injury from damage to structures around the shoulder and neck, such as fractures of the clavicle and first rib; and (3) iatrogenic injury, most commonly seen as a complication of the administration of nerve blocks. The most pronounced of the lesions affecting the brachial plexus are preganglionic, characterized by a nerve root avulsion when rootlets are torn from the spinal cord. Lesions affecting the postganglionic portion of the plexus may be severe because of nerve rupture or of lesser severity if caused by nerve stretch (Giuffre et al., 2010). Direct injury may be either open (gunshot wounds and lacerations) or closed (stretch or traction). The main causes of traumatic brachial plexus palsies are traction and heavy impact. Injuries are usually secondary to motorcycle and snowmobile accidents, but sporting accidents in football, bicycling, skiing, and equestrian events are also important. Supraclavicular injuries are more common and more severe and have a worse prognosis than infraclavicular injuries (Ferrante, 2012). Another form of brachial plexus traction is seen in rucksack paralysis. The straps of a rucksack or backpack pressed to the shoulders may exert heavy pressure in the region of the upper trunk of the brachial plexus and thus lead to weakness in the muscles supplied by the suprascapular and axillary nerves, with sensory loss in the C5–C6 distributions.

### Early Management

The consequences of brachial plexus injury are weakness and sensory loss referable to a part or the whole of the plexus. The ultimate objective in management is to restore as much neurological function as possible with the hope of returning the limb to its pre-injury status, but one must first ensure that the cardiovascular and respiratory systems are stable. In open injuries, there may be damage to great vessels in the neck and injury to the lung, in which case immediate operative intervention is necessary. At the time of this early acute intervention, it is important to assess to what degree the various elements of the plexus have been injured. As far as possible, disrupted elements should be tagged for later repair. It may be difficult to suture damaged fascicles, and the formation of scar may prevent successful nerve regeneration. Most researchers agree that nerve resection, grafting, and anastomosis are all very difficult in the acute situation because nerve continuity may be difficult to assess. However, if portions of a plexus have been sharply transected, then primary repair should be carried out.

### Long-Term Management

Once the patient's general condition has stabilized, a careful assessment of motor and sensory function should be made. At this stage, an important issue is whether there has been root avulsion. This is a critical determination with implications for management because the outlook for return of motor and sensory function in territories supplied by avulsed roots is currently not good, although promising results of surgical repair have recently been noted. Root avulsion and its management are discussed in the section on Disorders of Nerve Roots, earlier in this chapter. If the plexus elements are in continuity and the nerve fibers have received a neuropraxic injury with minimal axonotmesis, return of normal strength and sensation is expected. In the face of axonotmesis, the main factor limiting return of function is the distance the regenerating axon sprouts must traverse before contacting end organs. Unless the muscles and sensory receptors are reinnervated within about 1 year, a good functional result is unlikely. Thus, recovery of proximal muscle strength from upper portions of the plexus is more likely than recovery of hand function when lower elements have been damaged.

Often, surgery must be performed to provide an exact intraoperative definition of the lesion's extent (see Chapter 63). Intraoperative motor evoked potentials are helpful in assessing the functional state of anterior motor roots and motor fibers. Depending on the findings, innovative microsurgical techniques are available to provide an array of options: direct nerve repair, nerve grafting, replantation, nerve transfers, and free-functioning muscle transfers (Giuffre et al., 2010). Primary nerve reconstruction combined with joint fusion and tendon transfers provides a worthwhile return of function to many patients. The joint and tendon surgeries are best performed as secondary operations after a period of physiotherapy. Intensive physiotherapy and use of orthoses are often necessary to help restore maximum function. In general, the outcome after nerve grafting is relatively good for the recovery of elbow flexors and extensors and for those of the shoulder girdle, but it is very poor for forearm and hand intrinsic muscles. Quality-of-life surveys after brachial plexus surgery indicate that 83% of patients report satisfaction with the surgical outcome (Kretschmer et al., 2009). In a large series of more than 1000 patients treated over a 30-year period (Kim et al., 2003), the results of repair by suture and grafts were best for injuries located at the C5, C6, and C7 levels, the upper and middle trunk, the lateral cord to the musculocutaneous nerve, and the median and posterior cords to the axillary and radial nerves. Results were poor for injuries at the C8 and T1 levels and for lower trunk and medial cord lesions, and the chance of recovery was reduced with delays of more than 6 months in undertaking repair.

## Neurogenic Thoracic Outlet Syndrome

True neurogenic thoracic outlet syndrome is a rare entity, seen only a few times a year in our EMG laboratory. Most patients are women. The mean age at onset is 32 years, but patients as young as 13 and as old as 73 have been reported. The clinical and electrophysiological findings point to a lesion of the lower trunk of the brachial plexus. Pain is usually the first symptom, with either aching noted on the inner side of the arm or soreness felt diffusely throughout the limb. Tingling sensations accompany pain and are felt along the inner side of the forearm and in the hand. Most patients note slowly progressive wasting and weakness of the hand muscles. The physical examination discloses hand muscle weakness and atrophy, most marked in the lateral part of the thenar eminence. In a smaller number of patients, there is mild atrophy and weakness in the forearm muscles. Sensory loss is present along the inner side of the forearm. Except for the occasional Raynaud-type episode, vascular symptoms and signs are uncommon. Electrodiagnostic studies on the affected side disclose a reduced median motor response with normal median sensory amplitudes, along with a mildly reduced ulnar motor response and reduced ulnar sensory amplitude. The needle electrode examination typically discloses features of chronic axon loss with mild fibrillation potential activity in C8- and T1-innervated muscles.

In many cases, cervical spine roentgenograms disclose small bilateral cervical ribs or enlarged down-curving C7 transverse processes. When not visualized in anteroposterior radiographs of the cervical spine, they can be seen on oblique views. MRI of the thoracic outlet is a useful diagnostic method, revealing deviation or distortion of nerves or blood vessels and suggesting the presence of vascular or nervous compressions (Aralasmak et al., 2012). Levin and colleagues (1998) have refined our understanding of the precise lesion localization of the neurogenic thoracic syndrome. They compared electrophysiological results between a group of patients with true neurogenic thoracic outlet syndrome and a group with "brachial plexopathy" stemming from median sternotomy. In the former group, the findings pointed to severe axon loss in the medial antebrachial cutaneous nerve and the abductor pollicis brevis, both sharing T1 root innervation. In the latter, an iatrogenic disorder resulting from rib retraction, the findings indicated axon loss in the ulnar sensory and motor nerves, conforming most to involvement predominantly of C8. These findings suggest that thoracic outlet syndrome and median sternotomy brachial plexopathy are due to damage to the mixed spinal nerve fibers at the level of the anterior primary rami distal to the C8 or T1 nerve roots but proximal to the lower trunk of the brachial plexus (Levin, 2002).

In most patients, a fibrous band extending from the tip of a rudimentary cervical rib to the scalene tubercle of the first rib causes angulation of either the C8 and T1 roots or the lower trunk of the brachial plexus (Fig. 105.10). Surgical division of the fibrous band can be expected to relieve pain and paresthesias and arrest muscle wasting and weakness in the majority of patients; however, return of muscle bulk and strength is unlikely.

## Metastatic and Radiation-Induced Brachial Plexopathy in Patients with Cancer

### Metastatic Plexopathy

Damage to the brachial plexus in patients with cancer is usually secondary to either metastatic plexopathy or radiation-induced injury (Jaeckle, 2010). Lung and breast carcinoma are the tumors that most commonly metastasize to the brachial plexus; lymphoma, sarcoma, melanoma, and a variety of other types are less common. Tumor metastases spread via lymphatics, and the area most commonly involved, the C8 and T1 nerve roots along with the lower trunk of the plexus, is adjacent to the lateral group of axillary lymph nodes.

The hallmark of metastatic plexopathy is pain, which is often severe. It is generally located in the shoulder girdle and radiates to the elbow, medial portion of the forearm, and fourth and fifth digits of the hand. In many patients, the neurological examination discloses signs referable to the lower plexus and its divisions; more than half of patients have Horner syndrome, whereas few have lymphedema of the affected limb. Some patients have signs indicating involvement of the entire plexus. However, in most of these patients, cervical CT myelography or MRI discloses epidural deposits that involve the C5 and C6 nerve roots, thereby explaining the upper plexus signs on examination.

An important syndrome first described by Pancoast in 1932 is a superior pulmonary sulcus tumor, the vast majority of which are non–small- cell bronchogenic carcinomas. The tumor arises near the pleural surface of the apex of the lung and grows into the paravertebral space and posterior chest wall, invading the C8 and T1 extraspinal nerves, the sympathetic chain and stellate ganglion, the necks of the first three ribs, and the transverse processes and borders of the vertebral bodies of C7 through T3. The tumor may eventually invade the spinal canal and compress the spinal cord. Presenting signs and symptoms include: severe shoulder pain radiating to the head and neck, axilla, chest, and arm; pain and paresthesias of the medial aspect of the arm and the

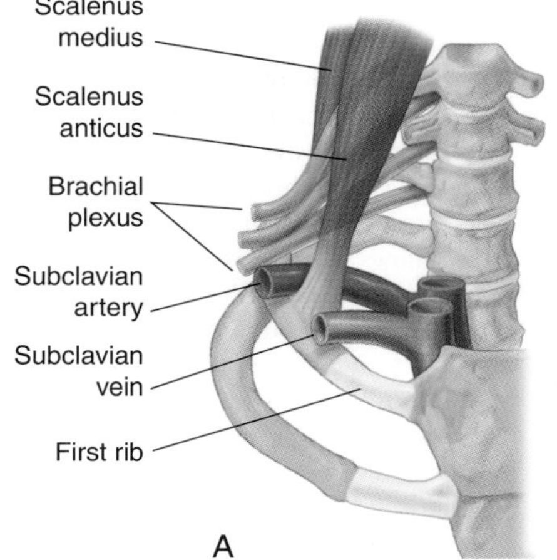


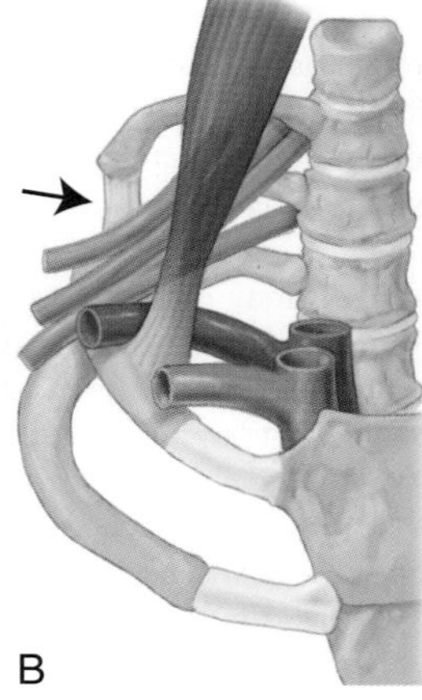


**Fig. 105.10** **A,** Normal relationships of subclavian artery and brachial plexus as they course over the first rib between the scalenus medius and anterior muscles. **B,** From the end of a short cervical rib arises a fibrous band *(arrow)*, which attaches to the upper surface of the normal first rib. This stretches and angulates chiefly the lower trunk of the brachial plexus, causing neurogenic thoracic outlet syndrome.

fourth and fifth digits; and weakness with atrophy of intrinsic hand muscles.

On occasion, metastatic brachial plexopathy may be difficult to distinguish from radiation plexopathy (see the following section on Radiation-Induced Plexopathy). Imaging studies are usually informative. In patients with metastatic disease, MRI may identify a mass adjacent to the brachial plexus and reveal whether the tumor has encroached on the epidural space. Magnetic resonance neurography is a noninvasive means of helping to exclude radiation-induced tumor in patients presenting with brachial plexopathy who have undergone prior radiation therapy to the brachial plexus (Du et al., 2010).

Results of the treatment of metastatic plexopathy are disappointing. Radiotherapy to the involved field and chemotherapy of the underlying tumor are the mainstays of treatment. Radiotherapy may relieve pain in 50% of patients but has little effect on return of muscle strength. A variety of procedures have been implemented to ameliorate the severe pain of this condition, including opioid analgesics and nonopioid adjuvant analgesics such as antidepressants and antiepileptic drugs, transcutaneous stimulation, paravertebral sympathetic blockade, and dorsal rhizotomies.

In the patient with Pancoast tumor, trimodal treatment with preoperative chemotherapy and radiotherapy followed by extended surgical resection is the most common treatment, with an overall 5-year survival rate of 41%–53% (Nikolaos et al., 2014).

### Radiation-Induced Plexopathy

Delayed injury to the structures of the brachial plexus following radiation exposure is thought to involve two factors: (1) radiation-induced endoneural and perineural fibrosis with obliteration of blood vessels, triggered by small-vessel or microvascular endothelial injury, and (2) direct radiation-induced damage to myelin sheaths and axons. Dropcho (2010) points out that breast carcinoma is the tumor most often associated with radiation plexopathy, accounting for 40%–75% of patients, followed by lung carcinoma then lymphoma.

Radiation-induced plexopathy is unlikely to occur if the dose is less than 6000 cGy. If more than 6000 cGy is given, the interval between the end of radiation therapy and the onset of symptoms and signs of radiation plexopathy ranges from 3 months to 26 years, with a mean interval of approximately 6 years. Improvements in irradiation techniques over the past several decades have allowed the use of lower radiation doses, and as such the incidence of delayed post-radiation brachial plexopathy has declined precipitously (66% in the 1950s, compared to <1%–2% today; Delanian et al., 2012). In addition to fraction size, concomitant cytotoxic therapy adds additional risk in developing a delayed radiation-induced plexopathy.

Limb paresthesias and swelling are common complaints. Although the pain of radiation plexopathy is usually less intense than that of metastatic plexopathy, it may nonetheless be problematic (severe and persistent), requiring opioids and chemical sympathectomy (Fathers et al., 2002). Weakness is usually most prominent in muscles innervated by branches of the upper trunk, but involvement of the entire limb from damage to the upper and lower portions of the plexus has also been described. Indeed, in a group of women with radiation plexopathy following treatment for carcinoma of the breast, progressive weakness resulted in loss of hand function in 90% of patients (Fathers et al., 2002). The relative resistance of the lower trunk of the brachial plexus to radiation injury is perhaps explained by the protective effect of the clavicle and the relatively shorter course of the lower trunk and its divisions through the radiation field.

The natural history of radiation-induced plexopathy is that of steadily increasing deterioration, although at times a plateau may be reached after 4–9 years of progression. Unfortunately, treatment options are not very satisfactory. Surgical treatment using neurolysis has been reported to relieve pain in some patients, but there is little information on the long-term outcome, and surgery may cause significant deterioration in motor and sensory function (Dropcho, 2010). Combination therapy with a phosphodiesterase inhibitor, pentoxifylline, tocopherol (vitamin E), and a bisphosphonate, clodronate, have been reported to improve motor strength in patients with radiation-induced radiculopathy, presumably by reducing radiation-induced fibrosis and myelin destruction (Delanian et al., 2008).

A diagnostic dilemma arises when symptoms and signs of brachial plexopathy develop in a patient who is known to have had cancer and radiation in the region of the brachial plexus, raising concern for tumor recurrence, a radiation-induced tumor, or radiation-induced plexopathy. A painful lower-trunk lesion with Horner syndrome strongly suggests metastatic plexopathy, whereas a relatively painless upper-trunk lesion with lymphedema favors radiation-induced plexopathy. MRI does not always discriminate between metastatic tumor infiltration and radiation-induced nerve fibrosis, as each may be associated with high signal intensity of nerves on T2-weighted images and contrast enhancement on T1-weighted images (Wouter van Es et al., 1997). Features which favor radiation fibrosis include thickening and diffuse enlargement of the brachial plexus without a focal mass (Wittenberg and Adkins, 2000). Magnetic resonance neurography may be useful to exclude intrinsic nerve tumor (Du et al., 2010) and FDG-PET scanning may be useful for identifying metastatic breast cancer in or near the brachial plexus, not clearly imaged by CT or MRI (Dropcho, 2010). In the early and middle stages of radiation plexopathy, nerve conduction studies disclose features of demyelinating conduction block, but as time passes, there is conversion to axon loss (Ferrante and Wilbourn, 2002). Needle EMG is helpful in separating radiation-induced plexopathy from neoplastic plexopathy by the presence of myokymic discharges in the former. These are spontaneously occurring grouped action potentials (triplets or multiplets) followed by a period of silence, with subsequent repetition of a grouped discharge of identical potentials in a semi-rhythmic manner. They appear to result from spontaneous activity in single axons induced by local membrane abnormalities. They have not been reported in cases of tumor plexopathy.

## Idiopathic Brachial Plexopathy

The terms idiopathic brachial plexopathy, brachial plexus neuritis, neuralgic amyotrophy, and Parsonage–Turner syndrome all refer to the clinical syndrome of severe pain followed by rapid paresis and atrophy of muscles in an upper extremity. It occurs in all age groups, particularly between the third and seventh decades of life. Men are affected two to three times more often than women. Although half the cases seem unrelated to any precipitating event, in others the plexopathy follows an upper respiratory tract infection, a flu-like illness, vigorous exercise (weight lifting, gymnastics, wrestling), strenuous activity (yard work), an immunization, surgery, psychological stress, or in the postpartum period (van Alfen and van Engelen, 2006).

Beyond the two cardinal manifestations of pain and weakness, the clinical phenotype of idiopathic brachial plexopathy is quite heterogeneous (Van Alfen, 2011). Patients often describe abrupt onset of a sharp, stabbing, throbbing, or aching pain involving the shoulder, scapular area, trapezius ridge, or upper arm, forearm, or hand. Within hours, this pain will have escalated to a peak severity that is often beyond anything the patient will have previously experienced, and then will persist for up to 4 weeks on average before gradually resolving (though rapid resolution of pain within 24 hours and intractable pain lasting months may be seen in 5% and 10% of cases, respectively). During this period, the patient may hold their arm in a characteristic posture, flexed at the elbow and adducted against the body, in an effort to minimize traction on the plexus, which may exacerbate pain symptoms.

Weakness of the upper extremity likely evolves during this period of intense pain, but may not be immediately appreciated by the patient, who is reluctant to move the limb and further exacerbate their pain. This often results in the classic description of weakness that is coincident with a lessening or resolution of the patient's pain. The pattern of weakness seen is highly variable, with the majority of patients having weakness referable to the upper brachial plexus, a third with weakness involving both upper and lower parts of the plexus, and approximately 15% with evidence of lower plexus involvement alone.

Patchy weakness is common, with sparing of one or more muscles in the same root, trunk, or cord distribution. Similarly, there is increasing recognition that this illness need not always be associated with circumscribed lesions of trunks or cords but may present as discrete lesions of individual peripheral nerves, including the suprascapular, axillary, musculocutaneous, long thoracic, median, and anterior interosseous or posterior interosseous nerves. A minority of patients may have involvement of nerves outside the brachial plexus proper, including the phrenic nerves, cranial nerves VII and X, and the lumbosacral plexus (van Alfen, 2011). In a small number of patients, unilateral or bilateral diaphragmatic paralysis occurs with no abnormalities on clinical or electrodiagnostic examinations of the limbs (Tsao et al., 2006). In such cases, the combination of acute shoulder pain with respiratory symptoms should suggest the diagnosis.

Sensory loss, found in two-thirds of patients and most commonly over the outer surface of the upper arm and the radial surface of the forearm, is usually less marked than the motor deficit, although the spectrum of brachial plexus neuropathy includes patients with isolated clinical and electrophysiological sensory deficits (Seror, 2004). One-third of cases are bilateral, but few are symmetrical. Rarely, symptoms may recur episodically for a year or more (van Alfen and van Engelen, 2006).

A familial form of brachial plexus neuropathy, so-called hereditary neuralgic amyotrophy, is an autosomal dominant disorder causing repeated episodes of intense pain, paralysis, and sensory disturbances in an affected limb (Chance, 2006). Like the idiopathic disorder, there may be similar antecedent triggering events. Onset is at birth or early childhood, with a good prognosis for recovery after each attack. Three-point mutations have been found in the gene *SEPT9* encoding the septin-9 protein, in 49 pedigrees with hereditary neuralgic amyotrophy linked to chromosome 17q25 (Hannibal et al., 2009; Kuhlenbaumer et al., 2005). In some individuals, associated findings include relative hypertelorism, occasional cleft palate, and skin folds or creases on the neck or forearm (Hannibal et al., 2009).

## Diagnosis

The major differential diagnostic consideration in a patient with acute arm pain and weakness is radiculopathy related to cervical spine disease. However, in this condition pain is usually persistent, neck stiffness is invariable, and it is unusual for radicular pain to subside as weakness increases. Nonetheless, an upper trunk brachial plexopathy can simulate a C5 or C6 radiculopathy. The cervical paraspinal needle EMG done several weeks after the onset of pain should be normal in brachial plexus neuropathy but show increased insertional activity and fibrillation potentials in cervical radiculopathy. Another differential diagnostic consideration is neoplastic plexopathy, discussed earlier in this chapter. This entity is usually unremittingly painful, and neurological findings are most often referable to lower plexus elements. A third consideration might be a focal presentation of motor neuron disease, but, in such cases, pain is not a feature, and sensation is always spared.

Electrodiagnostic testing is helpful in confirming the diagnosis and ruling out other conditions. Findings suggest axonal lesions of peripheral nerves occurring singly (mononeuritis) or in various combinations (mononeuritis multiplex) (van Alfen and van Engelen, 2006). Sensory studies are abnormal in up to one-third of patients; the most common abnormality is reduced amplitude of one or more sensory action potentials of the median, ulnar, and radial nerves and the lateral and medial antebrachial cutaneous nerves. Van Alfen and colleagues (2009b) found sensory abnormalities in less than 20% of nerves studied, even when the nerve was clinically affected, suggesting that the pathology may be in the nerve roots. Needle EMG is helpful because it shows an absence of fibrillation potentials in the cervical paraspinal muscles, thereby pointing to a pathological process distal to the DRG. Needle EMG is also helpful in sorting out the problems of localization, identifying lesions localized to the brachial plexus, individual peripheral nerves, or peripheral nerve branches. Finally, in a small number of patients, needle EMG is abnormal on the asymptomatic side as well as the symptomatic side, indicating that brachial plexus neuropathy can sometimes be subclinical. MRI of the brachial plexus is important in excluding structural lesions that might simulate this disorder and should be performed where there is failure to recover function (van Alfen and van Engelen, 2006). The MRI appearance in idiopathic brachial plexopathy reveals findings of diffuse high T2 signal intensity abnormalities and fatty atrophy of involved muscles (Gaskin and Helms, 2006). There are additional laboratory findings of interest (van Alfen and van Engelen, 2006). Among the group of patients with severe bilateral brachial plexus neuropathy with phrenic nerve involvement, elevated liver enzymes are found, possibly reflecting an antecedent subclinical hepatitis. In 25% of patients, antiganglioside antibodies are found, and CSF protein elevations with oligoclonal bands are also noted in some patients, reflecting the likelihood of an immune pathogenesis for this condition.

## Pathophysiology and Etiology

The pathophysiology and pathogenesis of the disorder are unclear, though genetic factors, immune-mediated mechanisms, and biomechanical factors have each been implicated (van Alfen, 2011). A likely genetic predisposition for some patients with idiopathic brachial plexopathy is based on the discovery of the *SEPT9* gene in the hereditary form of the disorder. The *SEPT9* gene gives rise to six isoforms of septin-9, a cytoskeletal protein involved in cell division and cell polarity. How exactly mutations in this gene confer susceptibility to brachial plexus injury remains unclear. Nerve biopsy studies of patients with autosomal dominant attacks of brachial plexus neuropathy during symptomatic phases disclosed prominent perivascular inflammatory infiltrates with vessel wall disruption, suggesting that the hereditary disorder has an immune pathogenesis possibly caused by genetic abnormalities of immune regulation (Klein et al., 2002). Complement-dependent antibody-mediated demyelination may have participated in the peripheral nerve damage and nerve biopsy findings in four cases of brachial plexus neuropathy revealed florid multifocal mononuclear infiltrates, suggesting a cell-mediated component as well (Suarez et al., 1996). Antecedent illness or vigorous exercise raises the possibility for a mechanistic role of both autoimmune disease and biomechanical injury in the pathogenesis of idiopathic brachial plexopathy as well. As an example, an increased incidence of brachial plexopathy in northeast Czechoslovakia occurred following contamination of the water supply with Coxsackie virus type A2 (indicating a possible post-viral immune-mediated pathophysiology), yet was particularly prevalent in knitting factory workers in this region that were required to bend and stretch their arms repeatedly throughout the day (suggesting an additional biomechanical component to injury) (van Alfen, 2011). Clinical features of the illness have also suggested other pathophysiological mechanisms. An abrupt onset might suggest an ischemic mechanism. In some cases, rapid recovery bespeaks demyelination and remyelination; in others, a long recovery period is more in keeping with axonal degeneration followed by axonal regeneration. Indeed, a biopsy of a cutaneous radial branch in a severe case of plexopathy showed profound axonal degeneration. In most patients, electrophysiological abnormalities are restricted to the affected limb, while in a small number of cases there is evidence of a more generalized polyneuropathy.

### Treatment and Prognosis

In the acute stage of the disorder, long-acting nonsteroidal antiinflammatory drugs (NSAIDs) and opioid analgesics are required to control pain (van Alfen, 2007). Evidence from one open-label retrospective series suggests that oral prednisone given in the first month after the onset can shorten the duration of the initial pain and leads to earlier recovery in some patients (van Alfen et al., 2009b). Arm and neck movements often aggravate pain, so immobilization of the arm in a sling is helpful. With the onset of paralysis, range-of-motion exercises help prevent contractures. Following the phase of acute pain, van Alfen (2007) reported two additional categories of pain. The first, experienced by nearly 80% of patients, is a shooting or radiating neuropathic pain, believed to originate from the heightened mechanical sensitivity of damaged nerves of the plexus and lasting for weeks to months. This pain may respond to gabapentin and tricyclic medications. A second type of pain that develops in many is a musculoskeletal-type pain localized to the origin or insertion of the paretic or compensating muscles, especially in the periscapular, cervical, and occipital regions. This pain requires physical therapy modalities. Up to 30% of patients who have experienced neuralgic amyotrophy will have long-standing pain for an average follow-up of 6 years (van Alfen, 2007). Accordingly, pain management becomes the mainstay of therapy for these individuals and requires a multidisciplinary approach that blends pharmacotherapy with physical and occupational modalities.

The natural history of brachial plexus neuropathy is benign; improvement occurs in the vast majority of patients, even in those with considerable muscle atrophy. Thirty-six percent have recovered by the end of 1 year, 75% by the end of 2 years, and 89% by the end of 3 years. Although some patients think they have made a full functional recovery, careful examination may disclose mild neurological abnormalities such as isolated winging of the scapula, slight proximal or distal weakness, mild sensory loss, or reduced reflex activity. In two-thirds of patients, onset of improvement is noted in the first month after symptoms begin. Those who continue to be bothered by pain and lack any signs of improvement within the first 3 months of the illness take a longer time to recover.

## DISORDERS OF THE LUMBOSACRAL PLEXUS

### Anatomical Features

The lumbar plexus is formed within the psoas major muscle by the anterior primary rami of lumbar spinal nerves L1, L2, L3, and L4. Branches of the lumbar plexus include the iliohypogastric and ilioinguinal nerves arising from L1 (with a contribution from T12), the lateral femoral cutaneous nerve of the thigh originating from the posterior divisions of L2 and L3, and the genitofemoral nerve arising from the anterior division of L1 and L2. Other branches are the femoral nerve, formed from the posterior divisions of L2, L3, and L4 within the substance of the psoas muscle, and the obturator nerve, formed by the anterior divisions of L2, L3, and L4.

The lumbar plexus communicates with the sacral plexus via the anterior division of L4 (Fig. 105.11, *A*), which joins with L5 to form the lumbosacral trunk at the medial border of the psoas at the

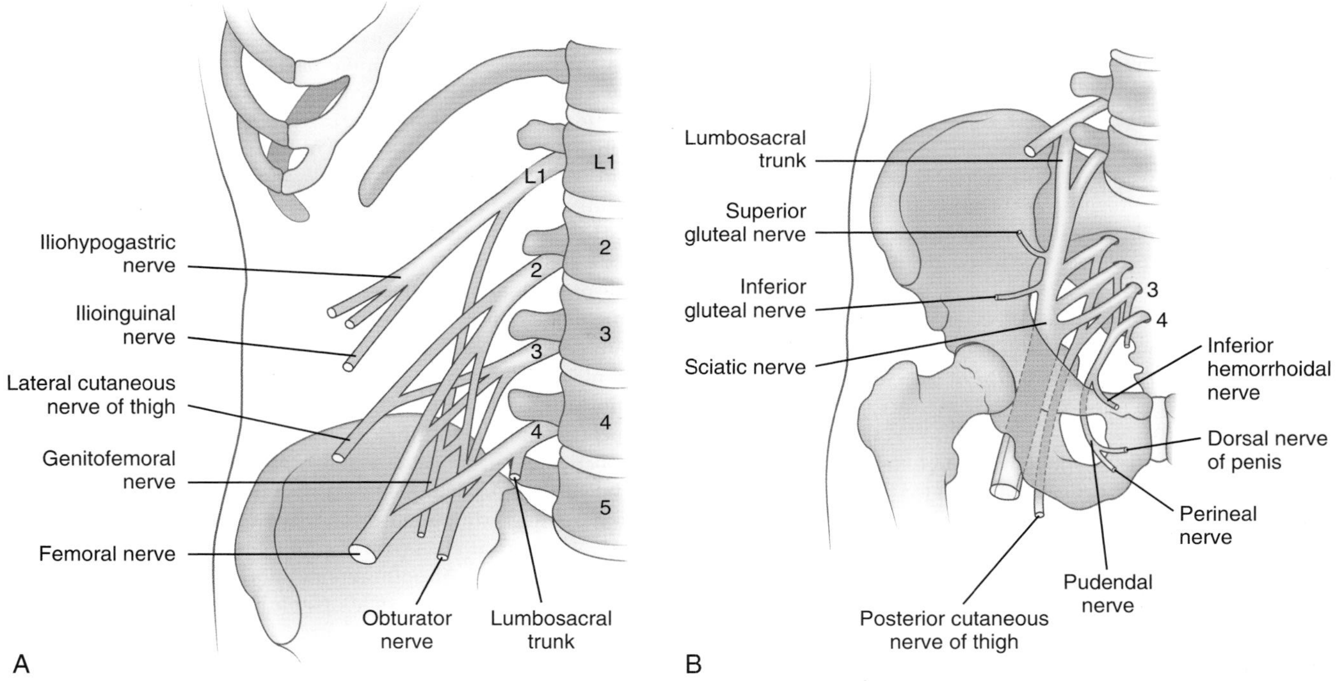


**Fig. 105.11 A,** Lumbar plexus is formed by anterior primary rami of lumbar spinal nerves L1, L2, L3, and L4 (note branches that arise from plexus). **B,** Sacral plexus is connected to lumbar plexus by the lumbosacral trunk (note branches that arise from plexus in pelvis). (*Reprinted with permission from Haymaker, W., Woodhall, B., 1953. Peripheral Nerve Injuries, second ed. Saunders, Philadelphia.*)

ala of the sacrum. The trunk enters the pelvis and joins the sacral plexus in the piriformis fossa. The sacral plexus, derived from the anterior rami of spinal nerves L4, L5, S1, S2, and S3, forms in front of the sacroiliac joint (see Fig. 105.11, *B*). Like the lumbar plexus, the sacral plexus has anterior and posterior divisions. The anterior division contributes to the tibial portion, and the posterior division contributes to the peroneal portion of the sciatic nerve, which leaves the pelvis through the greater sciatic notch. A number of important branches come from the sacral plexus in the pelvis; the superior and inferior gluteal nerves arise from posterior divisions of the sacral plexus and supply the gluteus medius and minimus muscles and the gluteus maximus, respectively. The posterior cutaneous nerve of the thigh is formed by the anterior divisions of S1, S2, and S3. It passes through the greater sciatic foramen into the buttock. The pudendal nerve originates from the undivided anterior primary rami of spinal nerves S2, S3, and S4 and extends into the gluteal region via the greater sciatic foramen.

## Clinical Features

### Neurological Examination

Lumbar plexopathy produces weakness, sensory loss, and reflex changes in segments L2 through L4, whereas sacral plexopathy leads to similar abnormalities in segments L5 through S3. Characteristic findings in lumbar plexopathy include weakness and sensory loss in both obturator- and femoral-innervated territories. Weakness of hip flexion, knee extension, and hip adduction, with sensory loss over the anteromedial aspect of the thigh occurs; the knee jerk is absent or depressed. This combination of hip flexor and adductor weakness marks the disorder as either a plexopathy or radiculopathy. More precise localization depends on laboratory studies, including needle EMG, CT, and MRI.

Findings in sacral plexopathy include weakness and sensory loss in the territories of the gluteal (motor only), peroneal, and tibial nerves. Leg weakness is typically extensive and involves the hip extensors and abductors, knee flexors, and ankle plantar flexors and dorsiflexors. Sensory loss is found over the posterior aspect of the thigh, the anterolateral and posterior aspects of the leg below the knee, and the dorsolateral and plantar surfaces of the foot. Vasomotor and trophic changes also may be found in these areas. The ankle jerk is reduced or absent. Weakness of the gluteal muscles points to involvement of sacral plexus fibers proximal to the piriformis muscle in the true pelvis or to a more proximal sacral root level. As in lumbar plexopathy, accurate diagnosis often depends on electrodiagnostic studies and neuroimaging procedures.

### Electrodiagnostic Studies

Electrodiagnostic studies are performed for several reasons. First, the EMG is helpful in identifying a motor-sensory syndrome as a plexopathy and not a radiculopathy. The diagnosis of plexopathy is confirmed if the EMG discloses denervation (fibrillation potentials and positive sharp waves) and reduced recruitment (reduced numbers of motor units, firing rapidly) in muscles innervated by at least two lumbosacral segmental levels and involving at least two different peripheral nerves. An isolated plexopathy should not be associated with EMG abnormalities in paraspinal muscles. However, as will be seen, a number of pathological processes including diabetes, radiation-induced changes, inflammation, vasculitis, and neoplasia may all involve the roots in addition to the plexus and produce a radiculoplexopathy. Second, EMG findings help determine whether a lumbosacral plexopathy is associated with a polyneuropathy. In the presence of the latter, signs of denervation and reinnervation are found bilaterally, especially in the distal muscles. Third, EMG findings may strongly suggest a particular type of plexopathy; for example, myokymic discharges point to the diagnosis of radiation plexopathy.

Routine nerve conduction studies may help establish the diagnosis of plexopathy. Reduced SNAP amplitude (sural and superficial peroneal) indicates loss of axons distal to the DRG of S1 and L5, respectively. Prolongation in F-wave latency with normal motor nerve conduction studies distally suggests a proximal lesion, either at a root or a plexus level.

### Neuroimaging Studies

Bone destruction found in plain radiographs of lumbar and sacral vertebrae and the pelvis provides evidence for a structural plexopathy. CT scanning of the abdomen and pelvis from a rostral point at the level of L1–L2 to a caudal point below the level of the symphysis pubis allows the regional anatomy of the entire lumbosacral plexus to be scrutinized (see Chapter 40).

The resolution of modern CT and MRI scanners allows identification of individual plexus components. The administration of contrast is usually required to demonstrate the extent of structural abnormalities of the lumbosacral plexus, but it may not differentiate benign and malignant neoplasms, inflammatory masses, and hematoma. A normal MRI makes a structural plexopathy very unlikely. Clues to the nature of a plexopathy are given in Box 105.1. An approach to evaluation of a plexopathy is summarized in Fig. 105.12.

## Differential Diagnosis

The differential diagnosis of lumbosacral plexopathy includes spinal root disorders (e.g., lumbosacral radiculopathy, polyradiculoneuropathy, cauda equina syndrome, anterior horn cell disorders) and myopathic conditions. Radiculopathies are usually painful, and the pain follows a predictable radicular distribution. Weakness is usually found in several muscles supplied by the same root, and the EMG usually demonstrates paraspinal muscle involvement. It is sometimes difficult to separate plexopathy from radiculopathy on clinical grounds alone, especially if several roots are involved.

Anterior horn cell disorders give rise to painless progressive weakness with atrophy and fasciculation in the absence of sensory loss. When fully developed, such disorders should not be confused with lumbosacral plexopathy. However, in rare cases, a restricted anterior horn cell disorder (focal spinal muscular atrophy involving one leg) is seen. Absence of pain and sensory loss, normal imaging studies, and absence of diabetes and vasculitis all help point away from a disturbance of the lumbosacral plexus.

Myopathies are rarely confused with lumbosacral plexopathy. Myopathies with a focal lower-extremity onset can be distinguished from lumbosacral plexopathy by elevation of muscle enzymes, myopathic features on EMG, and muscle biopsy.

## Structural Lumbosacral Plexopathy

### Hematoma

Patients with hemophilia and those receiving anticoagulants can develop hemorrhage in the iliopsoas muscle complex. It is important to recall that major components of the lumbar plexus, the femoral and obturator nerves, course from their origins in the lumbar paravertebral regions to their destinations in the thigh under cover of a tight layer of fascia. Over the iliac muscle, it is referred to as the *fascia iliaca*, and it becomes progressively thicker as it passes down behind the inguinal ligament; at this site, it forms a dense and nondistensible funnel enclosing the lower portions of the iliacus and psoas.

**BOX 105.1 Clues to the Nature of a Plexopathy**

Structural disorders:
- History or presence of malignancy
- Hemophilia or treatment with an anticoagulant
- Pelvic trauma
- Known atherosclerotic vascular disease and hypertension (aortic, hypogastric, common iliac aneurysm)
- Pregnancy, labor, delivery
- Abdominal (pelvic) surgery

Nonstructural disorders:
- Diabetes mellitus*
- Vasculitis
- Previous pelvic radiation

* Diabetics may develop a polyradiculoneuropathy that simulates a lumbosacral plexopathy.

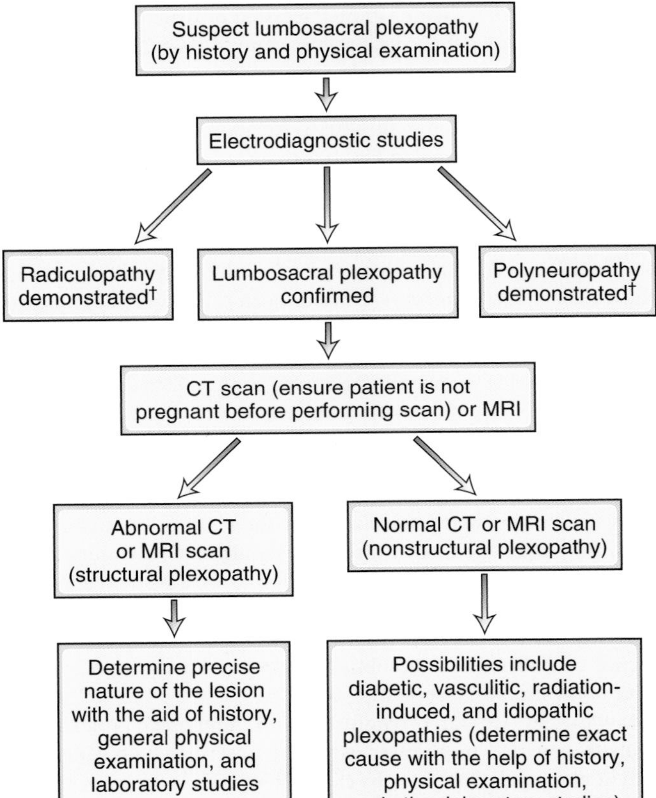


**Fig. 105.12 Approach to Evaluation of Lumbosacral Plexopathy.** Electrophysiological identification of radiculopathy may require spinal computed tomographic *(CT)* myelography or magnetic resonance imaging *(MRI)* for confirmation and precise diagnosis. *Radiculopathy is associated with plexopathy in diabetes, vasculitis, radiation, and malignancy. †Polyneuropathy may accompany plexopathies due to diabetes, vasculitis, and certain malignancies (paraneoplastic neuropathies).

Two major anatomical syndromes are associated with iliopsoas hematoma. In the first, the femoral nerve is the sole affected portion of the lumbar plexus. The hematoma arises in the iliacus and causes distention of the dense overlying fascia above the inguinal ligament. In the second syndrome, hemorrhage arises in the psoas muscle or begins

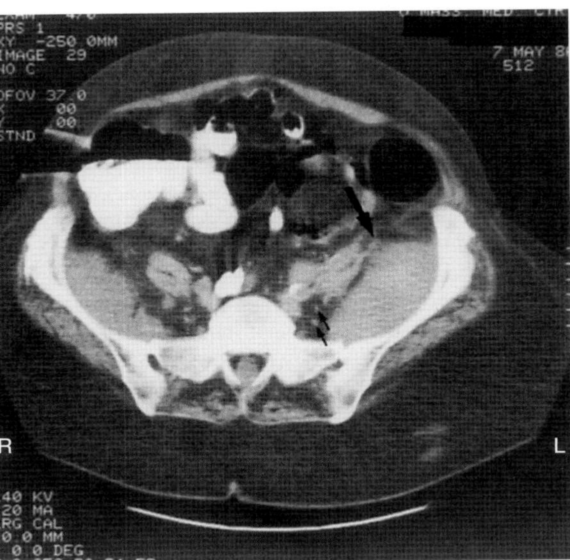


**Fig. 105.13 Hemorrhagic Lumbosacral Plexopathy.** Computed tomographic scan at L5–S1 level shows enlargement of iliacus muscles, especially on left side, owing to iliacus hematoma *(large arrow). Small arrows* indicate plexal elements. This large hematoma compresses the femoral and obturator nerves and the lumbosacral trunk.

in the iliacus muscle and extends into the psoas. In this case, other components of the plexus, the obturator and lateral femoral cutaneous nerves, are involved.

Pain, often severe, is usually the first manifestation of a retroperitoneal hematoma. The pain is present in the groin and radiates to the anterior thigh and lumbar region. It is associated with gradually increasing paresthesias and weakness. When the femoral nerve is involved, weakness and sensory loss occur in its territory; when other components of the plexus are involved, changes are more extensive and conform to the territories supplied by the involved branches of the plexus. If the hemorrhage is large, a mass may develop in the lower abdominal quadrant and be associated with systemic signs like tachycardia, hypotension, and a falling hematocrit (Parmer et al., 2006). It typically arises from the lateral wall of the pelvis and can be seen in a CT scan to obscure the normal concavity of the inner aspect of the wing of the ilium (Fig. 105.13). Because of iliacus muscle spasm, the patient usually lies in a characteristic posture with the hip flexed and laterally rotated because hip extension aggravates the pain. Several days after the onset of the hematoma, a bruise may appear in the inguinal area or anterior thigh. In some patients, especially those with relatively small hematomas and mild neurological deficits, recovery may be satisfactory with conservative measures including reversing anticoagulation, although 10%–15% of patients show no improvement. Accordingly, some centers explore the abdomen through a limited retroperitoneal incision after reversing the coagulopathy; a complete iliacus fasciotomy is performed and the hematoma is evacuated, thus relieving compression on the femoral nerve and enhancing the prospects for full recovery (Parmer et al., 2006). Clear indications for surgical exploration would include hemodynamic instability or worsening neurological dysfunction.

## Abscess

Psoas abscess was more common when tuberculosis was prevalent, but neurological complications, such as lumbar plexopathy and femoral neuropathy, were rare. This phenomenon was explained by the slow distention of the psoas sheath and by the fact that the abscess ruptured through the psoas fascia before the femoral nerve could be damaged by raised intrapsoas compartment pressure. Similarly, an acute nontuberculous psoas abscess rarely produces nerve compression, presumably because the psoas fascia is distensible. However, femoral neuropathy does occur with iliacus muscle abscess because the fascia iliaca is relatively nondistensible. Rarely, lumbar plexopathy is a complication of pelvic hydatidosis caused by the tapeworm *Echinococcus granulosus* (Serradilla et al., 2002).

## Aneurysm

Back and abdominal pains are often early manifestations of abdominal aortic aneurysms. Knowledge of abdominal and pelvic regional anatomy helps explain the radiating characteristics of these pains. An expanding abdominal aortic aneurysm may compress the iliohypogastric or ilioinguinal nerve, leading to pain radiating into the lower abdomen and inguinal areas. Pressure on the genitofemoral nerve produces pain in the inguinal area, testicle, and anterior thigh. Compression of nerve trunks L5 through S2, which lie directly posterior to the hypogastric artery, may give rise to sciatica (Shields et al., 1997); 13% of patients with aneurysms of the iliac artery will present with features of sciatica (Delgado-Garcia et al., 1999).

Hemorrhage from an abdominal aortic aneurysm may produce prominent neurological problems because of the retroperitoneal location of the hemorrhage or false aneurysm formation. In the case of an abdominal aortic aneurysm, a large retroperitoneal hematoma may injure the femoral and obturator nerves and even branches of the sacral plexus. Rupture of a hypogastric or common iliac artery aneurysm extends into the pelvis, compressing the L5 through S2 nerve trunk.

Early recognition of an aneurysm is important because the mortality rate for operation on unruptured aneurysms is 5%–7%, whereas that for ruptured aneurysms is 35%–40%. Unexplained back pain, leg pain, or pain radiating in the distribution of cutaneous nerves coming from the lumbar plexus should raise the suspicion of an aneurysm of the aorta or its major branches. A pulsatile mass felt while palpating the abdomen or, rarely, on rectal examination strongly suggests the presence of an aneurysm. Lumbosacral radiographs show a curvilinear calcific density, and abdominal sonography or CT scanning can confirm an aneurysm.

## Trauma

Because of the relatively protected position of the lumbosacral plexus, traumatic lesions are uncommon. However, fracture of the pelvis, acetabulum, or femur, or surgery on the proximal femur and hip joint may injure the lumbosacral plexus. Sacral fractures or sacroiliac joint separation accounts for most cases of traumatic lumbosacral plexopathy (68%), while acetabular and femoral fractures are much less frequently implicated (14% and 9%, respectively) (Kutsy et al., 2000). However, the latter are more likely to cause injury to proximal nerves originating from the plexus. The mechanism of posttraumatic paresis in lumbosacral plexopathies may involve a number of factors, including nerve crush caused by fractured bone fragments; retroperitoneal hemorrhage; and traction as a result of hyperextension, hyperflexion, or rotation around the hip joint. Conservative measures appear to be the most appropriate way to manage posttraumatic injuries. More than two-thirds of patients show good or moderate recovery of paresis after 18 months of follow-up after injury.

## Pregnancy

The lumbosacral trunk may be compressed by the fetal head during the second stage of labor. This tends to occur in prolonged labor with mid-forceps rotation in a small primigravida mother carrying a relatively large baby. A day or so after delivery when the patient gets out of bed, she notes difficulty walking because of foot dorsiflexor weakness. Examination discloses weakness in dorsiflexion and inversion, with reduced sensation over the lateral aspect of the leg and dorsal surface of the foot. Nerve conduction studies disclose attenuation or absence of the superficial peroneal SNAP on the affected side, and needle EMG reveals denervation in muscles innervated by L5 below the knee (Katirji et al., 2002). The primary pathology is predominantly demyelination, and the prognosis for complete recovery within 5 months is very good. In subsequent pregnancies, a trial of labor can be allowed so long as there is no evidence of disproportion or malpresentation. If labor proceeds, forceps should be used with great caution. Mid-forceps use in a woman with a previous obstetrical lumbosacral trunk palsy invites danger. It is prudent to perform cesarean section if the trial of labor is unsuccessful or if the infant is large.

Femoral neuropathy may occur in a thin patient during cesarean section in cases managed with self-retaining retractors (Alsever, 1996). In the thin abdominal wall, a deep lateral insertion of retractor blades exerts pressure on the psoas and may injure the femoral nerve. After surgery, the patient notes weakness and numbness in the territory of the femoral nerve. Recovery is usually rapid and full. The obturator nerve may be compressed by the fetal head or forceps near the pelvic brim. Patients note pain in the groin and anterior thigh as well as weakness and sensory loss in the territory of this nerve.

## Neoplasia

The lumbosacral plexus may be damaged by tumors that invade the plexus either by direct extension from intraabdominal neoplasm or by metastases. Most tumors involve the plexus by direct extension (73%), whereas metastases account for only one-quarter of cases. The primary tumors most frequently encountered are colorectal, cervical, and breast, as well as sarcoma and lymphoma (Jaeckle, 2010). Three clinical syndromes occur: upper plexopathy with findings referable to the L1–L4 segments (31%); lower plexopathy with changes in the L4–S1 segments (51%); and panplexopathy with abnormalities in the L1–S3 distribution (18%). Neoplastic plexopathy typically has an insidious onset over weeks to months. Severe and unrelenting pain is a prominent early manifestation and is aching or cramping in quality; it typically radiates from the low back to the lower extremities. Weeks to months after pain begins, numbness, paresthesias, weakness, and leg edema develop. Incontinence or impotence occurs in fewer than 10% of patients. The most commonly encountered tumors are colorectal in upper plexopathy, sarcomas in lower plexopathy, and genitourinary in panplexopathies. The majority of neoplastic plexopathies are unilateral, although bilateral plexopathies, caused usually by breast cancer, occur in approximately 25% of patients. The prognosis in lumbosacral plexopathy due to neoplasm is poor, with a median survival of 5.5 months.

Three special syndromes do not fit easily into upper, lower, or panplexopathy categories. In the first, there are paresthesias or pain in the lower abdominal quadrant or groin, with little or no motor abnormality. These patients are found to have a tumor next to L1, leading to involvement of the ilioinguinal, iliohypogastric, or genitofemoral nerves. A second group has numbness over the dorsomedial portion of the foot and sole, with weakness of knee flexion, ankle dorsiflexion, and inversion. These patients have a lesion at the level of the sacral ala, with involvement of the lumbosacral trunk. A third group present with perineal sensory loss and sphincter weakness and have neoplastic involvement of the coccygeal plexus, caused usually by rectal tumors.

Neuroimaging with CT or MRI usually establishes the diagnosis of neoplastic plexopathy, but MRI is probably more sensitive (Taylor et al., 1997). Because pelvic neoplasms may extend into the epidural space, most often below the conus medullaris, MRI of the lumbosacral spine is indicated in most patients. On occasion, a plexus neoplasm is difficult to discern by the best neuroimaging procedures. Two main explanations for this phenomenon exist. First, patients who have received previous radiotherapy may have developed tissue fibrosis that cannot be distinguished from recurrent tumor. Second, some tumors track along the plexus roots and do not produce an identifiable mass. In these instances, ancillary imaging tests (high-resolution MRI, bone scan, plain films, intravenous pyelography [VP]), a biopsy of the plexus, or both may be required to determine the etiology. Prostate cancer may cause a lumbosacral radiculoplexopathy when tumor advances into the lumbosacral plexus by perineural spread, a process that may evolve for up to 8 years, is associated with prominent urinary dysfunction, and leads to an MRI appearance of asymmetrical nerve enlargement but otherwise normal pelvic and abdominal imaging (Ladha et al., 2006).

## Nonstructural Lumbosacral Plexopathy

### Radiation Plexopathy

Radiation plexopathy usually produces slowly progressive painless weakness (Jaeckle, 2010). Dropcho (2010) points out that the radiation injury to the plexus most commonly occurs after treatment of pelvic tumors, testicular tumors, or tumors involving para-aortic lymph nodes. Pain develops in approximately half of patients with radiation plexopathy but is usually not early or severe (Dropcho, 2010). Most patients with radiation plexopathy eventually develop bilateral weakness, which is often asymmetrical and affects any muscles innervated by L2 through S1 but typically has an L5–S1 predominance (Dropcho, 2010). In most patients, leg reflexes are absent, and superficial sensation is impaired. Symptoms referable to bowel or urinary tract are usually the result of proctitis or bladder fibrosis. The latent interval between radiation and the onset of neurological manifestations is between 1 and 31 years (median 5 years), although very short latencies of less than 6 months have also been reported. An acute presentation of lumbosacral plexopathy 10 weeks following completion of radiation therapy for cervical cancer has also been observed (Abu-Rustum et al., 1999). No consistent relationship is evident between the duration of the symptom-free interval and the amount of radiation.

In most patients, radiation plexopathy is gradually progressive and results in significant or severe disability. CT and MRI of the abdomen and pelvis are typically normal though may be useful in ruling out metastatic disease involving the lumbosacral plexus (Dropcho, 2010). EMG discloses paraspinal fibrillation potentials in 50% of patients, suggesting that radiation damages the nerve roots in addition to the plexus; hence, a more appropriate designation is *radiation radiculoplexopathy*. In almost 60% of patients, the EMG discloses myokymic discharges, a feature that is only rarely seen in neoplastic plexopathy.

### Vasculitis

Vasculitic neuropathy has generally been associated with the pattern of multiple mononeuropathy, but other neuropathic syndromes have also been described, including painful lumbosacral plexopathy. The portions of the peripheral nervous system most susceptible to vasculitis-induced ischemia are the segments of peripheral nerve located at the midhumerus and midfemur levels, regions of nerve that appear to be watershed zones between vascular territories of the vasa nervorum. Proximal nerve trunks and nerve roots may also be vulnerable to the vasculitic process.

When a lumbosacral plexopathy syndrome occurs in a patient known to have a vasculitis, such as polyarteritis nodosa or rheumatoid arthritis, vasculitic plexopathy is an obvious diagnosis. The clinical diagnosis is more difficult in the setting of a seemingly idiopathic polyneuropathy or plexopathy because the process may be monosystemic and restricted to the peripheral nervous system. In such a case, a nerve biopsy may be required to establish the correct diagnosis.

## Idiopathic Lumbosacral Plexopathy

Because lumbosacral plexopathy may occur in the absence of a recognizable underlying disorder, it can be considered a counterpart of idiopathic brachial plexus neuropathy (van Alfen and van Engelen, 2006). It may begin suddenly with pain, followed by weakness, which progresses for days or sometimes many weeks. In many patients, the condition stabilizes, but in some, the course is chronic progressive or relapsing/remitting. Weakness is found in the distribution of the upper and lower portions of the lumbosacral plexus in 50% of cases; major involvement occurs in the territory of the upper portion in 40% and in the lower portion in only 10% of patients. Most patients recover over a period of months to 2 years, although recovery is often incomplete. The EMG discloses a patchy pattern of denervation in the distribution of part or all of the lumbosacral plexus, but the paraspinal muscles are spared, indicating that the process does not affect the lumbosacral roots. Dyck and colleagues (2001) designated idiopathic lumbosacral plexopathy as *nondiabetic lumbosacral radiculoplexus neuropathy* and found that it resembles diabetic polyradiculoplexopathy in terms of its clinical presentation (subacute, asymmetrical, and painful with delayed and incomplete recovery) and pathological findings (ischemic injury and microvasculitis) and suggested that it probably has an immune pathogenesis. MRI has been reported to show gadolinium enhancement in the lumbar plexus that disappeared in association with resolution of symptoms and signs of plexopathy following IV gamma globulin treatment (Ishii et al., 2004). Immune-modulating therapy may be beneficial for a subgroup of patients with idiopathic lumbosacral plexopathy (Dyck and Windebank, 2002).

*The complete reference list is available online at https://expertconsult.inkling.com.* 

106

# Disorders of Peripheral Nerves

Bashar Katirji

## OUTLINE

## CLINICAL APPROACH TO DISORDERS OF PERIPHERAL NERVES

Peripheral nerve disorders are common neurological problems caused by dysfunction of peripheral motor, sensory, or autonomic nerves. The causes of neuropathies are disparate and their clinical presentations highly variable. The main causes of neuropathy are entrapments, systemic diseases, inflammatory and autoimmune disorders, inherited disorders, ischemic settings, paraneoplastic conditions, deficiency states, infections, and toxins.

### Structure of Peripheral Nerves

The peripheral nerve is a cable-like structure containing bundles of both unmyelinated and myelinated fibers and their supporting elements. The unmyelinated axons are surrounded only by the plasma membrane of a Schwann cell. The myelinated axons are engulfed by a Schwann cell that wraps around the axons multiple times, thereby insulating the axon with multiple layers of lipid-rich cell membrane. The myelinated axon is surrounded completely by myelin and Schwann cells except at regular gaps called the *nodes of Ranvier*, which measure approximately 1 μm in adults (see Fig. 64.2 in Chapter 64, Peripheral Nerve Trauma). The propagation of action potentials from one node of Ranvier to the next *(saltatory conduction)* is maintained by a thick myelin sheath with low capacitance and high resistance to electric current and by a high concentration of voltage-gated sodium channels at the nodes of Ranvier.

### Pathological Processes Involving Peripheral Nerves

Despite the large number of causes for neuropathy, the pathological reactions of peripheral nerves to various insults remain limited. In general, these pathological processes are divided into four main categories: (1) wallerian degeneration, which is the response to axonal interruption, (2) axonal degeneration or axonopathy, (3) primary neuronal (perikaryal) degeneration or neuronopathy, and (4) segmental demyelination or myelinopathy. The patient's symptoms, the type and pattern of distribution of signs, and the characteristics of nerve conduction study abnormalities provide information about the underlying pathological changes.

Compression, traction, laceration, thermal, chemical, or ischemic nerve injury that causes interruption of axons leads to *wallerian degeneration*—that is, distal degeneration of axons and their myelin sheaths. Immediately following injury, motor weakness and sensory loss occur in the distribution of the damaged nerve. On needle electromyography (EMG), there is complete loss of voluntary activity (with a complete lesion) or a decrease in motor unit action potential (MUAP) recruitment (with a partial lesion). However, the axons remain excitable distally since distal conduction failure is not completed until 10–11 days later as the distal nerve trunk becomes progressively unexcitable. On nerve conduction studies, the amplitude of the compound muscle action potential (CMAP), evoked by stimulation distal to the lesion site, begins to decline by the second day after injury and reaches its nadir by the fifth to sixth. For sensory axons, the loss of sensory nerve action potential (SNAP) is delayed by another 2–3 days; distal SNAP remains normal for 5–6 days and then decreases rapidly to reach its nadir by 10–11 days after injury (see Fig. 36.9 in Chapter 36). The temporal sequence of wallerian degeneration is length dependent, occurring earlier in shorter than in longer distal nerve stumps. Denervation potentials (fibrillation potentials) are typically seen on needle EMG in some affected muscles (mostly proximal ones) 10–14 days after injury and become full after 3 weeks from acute nerve injury. Axonal interruption initiates secondary morphological changes of the nerve cell body, termed *chromatolysis*, and the proximal axonal caliber becomes smaller. Regeneration from the proximal stump begins as early as 24 hours following transection but proceeds slowly at a maximal rate of 2–3 mm/day and is often incomplete. Sprouting of intact axons also starts locally in partial lesions, becoming noticeable on needle EMG after 1 month of axonal injury. The quality of recovery depends on the degree of preservation of the Schwann cell/basal lamina tube and the nerve sheath and surrounding tissue, the distance of the site of injury from the cell body, and the patient's age.

*Axonal degeneration* (or axonopathy), the most common pathological reaction of peripheral nerve, signifies distal axonal breakdown and is presumably caused by metabolic derangement within neurons or vascular compromise leading to ischemia. Systemic metabolic disorders, toxin exposure, vasculitis, and some inherited neuropathies are the usual causes of axonal degeneration. The myelin sheath breaks down concomitantly with the axon in a process that starts at the most distal part of the nerve fiber and progresses toward the nerve cell body: hence the term *dying-back* or *length-dependent polyneuropathy* (Fig. 106.1). A similar sequence of events may occur simultaneously in centrally directed sensory axons, resulting in distal degeneration of rostral dorsal column fibers. The selective length-dependent vulnerability of distal axons could result from failure of the perikaryon to synthesize enzymes or structural proteins, from alterations in axonal transport, or from regional disturbances of energy metabolism. In some axonopathies, alterations in axon caliber, either axonal atrophy or axonal swelling, may precede distal axonal degeneration. Clinically, dying-back polyneuropathy presents with symmetrical distal loss of sensory and motor function in the lower extremities that extends proximally in a graded manner. The result is sensory loss in a stocking-like pattern, distal muscle weakness and atrophy, and loss of distal limb myotatic reflexes. As the polyneuropathy ascends, it affects the hands and distal upper extremities, giving a glove-like sensory loss (hence the term *stocking and glove sensory loss*), and hand weakness and atrophy. Axonopathies result in low-amplitude SNAPs and CMAPs, but they affect distal latencies and conduction velocities only slightly. Needle EMG of distal muscles shows acute and/or chronic denervation changes (see Chapter 36). Because axonal regeneration proceeds at a maximal rate of 2–3 mm/day, recovery may be delayed and is often incomplete.

*Neuronopathy* designates loss of nerve cell bodies with resultant degeneration of their entire peripheral and central axons. Either anterior horn or dorsal root ganglion cells may be affected. Focal weakness without sensory loss occurs when anterior horn cells are affected, as in anterior poliomyelitis or motor neuron disease. *Sensory neuronopathy*, or *dorsal polyganglionopathy*, means damage to dorsal root ganglion neurons that results in sensory ataxia, sensory loss, and diffuse areflexia (Fig. 106.2). A number of toxins, such as organic mercury compounds, doxorubicin, and high-dose pyridoxine, or deficiency states, such vitamin E deficiency, produce primary sensory neuronal degeneration. Immune-mediated inflammatory damage of dorsal root ganglion neurons occurs in paraneoplastic sensory neuronopathy (anti-HU syndrome) and Sjögren syndrome (Hlubocky and Smith, 2014). It is often difficult to distinguish between neuronopathies and axonopathies on clinical grounds alone. Once the pathological processes are no longer

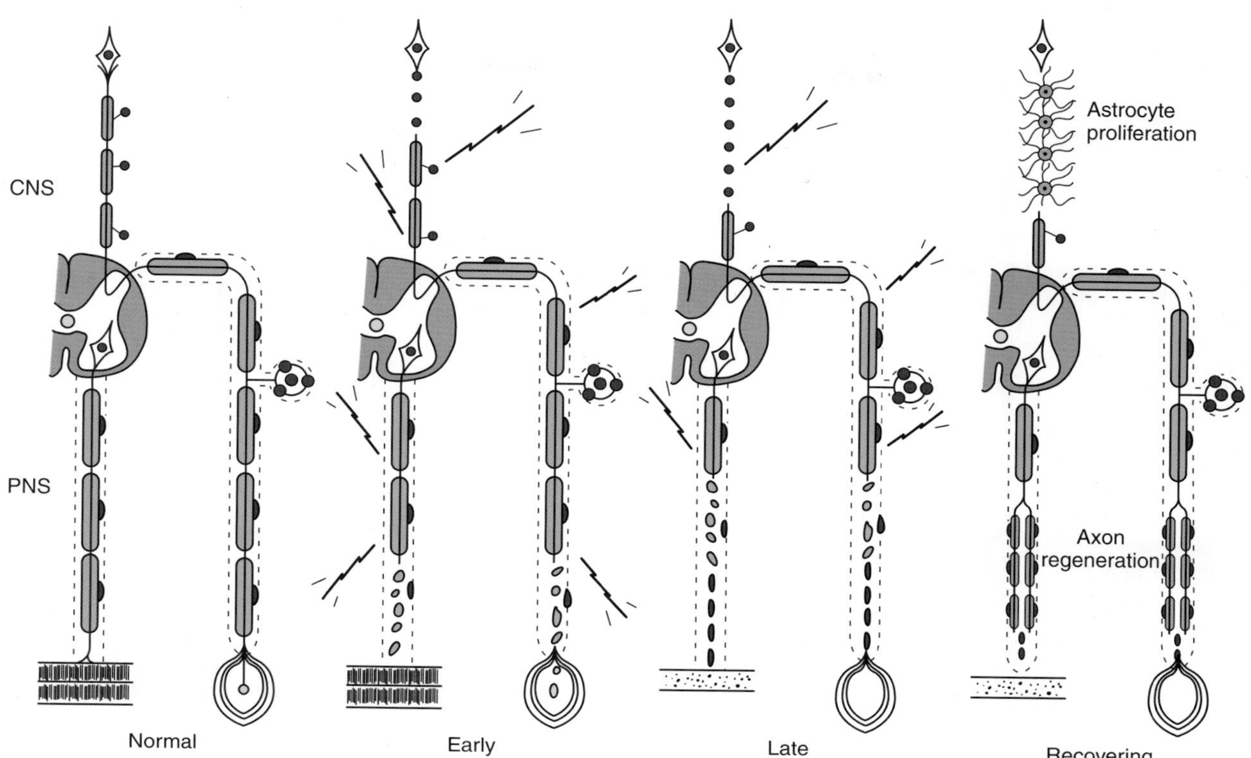


**Fig. 106.1 Diagram of the Main Pathological Events of Distal Axonal Degeneration or Axonopathy.** *Jagged lines* indicate that either a toxin or a metabolic insult acts at multiple sites along motor and sensory axons in the peripheral nervous system *(PNS)* and central nervous system *(CNS)*. Axonal degeneration begins at the most distal part of the nerve fiber and progresses proximally by the late stage. Recovery occurs by axonal regeneration but is impeded by astroglial proliferation in the CNS. *(Adapted from Herskovitz, S., Scelsa, S., Schaumburg, H.H., 2008. Disorders of Peripheral Nerves, Oxford University Press, New York.)*

active, sensory deficits become fixed, and little or no recovery takes place.

The term *segmental demyelination* (or *myelinopathy*) implies injury of either myelin sheaths or Schwann cells, resulting in breakdown of myelin with sparing of axons (Fig. 106.3). This occurs mechanically by acute nerve compression or chronic nerve entrapment and in immune-mediated demyelinating neuropathies and hereditary disorders of Schwann cell/myelin metabolism. Primary myelin damage may be produced experimentally by myelinotoxic agents such as diphtheria toxin or by acute nerve compression. Remyelination of demyelinated segments usually occurs within weeks. The newly formed remyelinated segments have thinner-than-normal myelin sheaths and internodes of shortened length. Repeated episodes of demyelination and remyelination produce proliferation of multiple layers of Schwann cells around the axon, termed an *onion bulb*. The physiological consequence of acquired demyelination, such as in inflammatory or compressive demyelination but not hereditary myelinopathies, is conduction block, which results in loss of the ability of the nerve action potential to reach the muscle, thereby producing weakness. Because the axon remains intact, there is little muscle atrophy. Relative sparing of temperature and pinprick sensation in many demyelinating polyneuropathies reflects preserved function of unmyelinated and small-diameter myelinated fibers. Early generalized loss of reflexes, disproportionately mild muscle atrophy in the presence of proximal and distal weakness, neuropathic tremor, and palpably enlarged nerves are all clinical clues that suggest demyelinating polyneuropathy. Nerve conduction studies or analysis of single teased nerve fiber preparations stained with osmium can confirm demyelination. Demyelination is present if motor and sensory nerve conduction velocities (NCVs) are reduced to less than 70% of the lower limits of normal, with relative preservation of CMAP and SNAP amplitudes. The presence of partial motor conduction block, temporal dispersion of CMAPs, and marked prolongation of distal motor and F-wave latencies are all features consistent with acquired demyelination (see Chapter 36). Recovery depends on the extent of remyelination, and therefore clinical improvement may occur within weeks. In many demyelinating neuropathies, axonal degeneration may also coexist, as evidenced by some distal limb atrophy and active denervation and reinnervation changes on needle EMG.

## Classification of Peripheral Nerve Disorders

There are several patterns of peripheral nerve disease (Box 106.1). Brachial, lumbar, and sacral plexopathy are discussed in Chapter 105, and radiculopathies are discussed in Chapter 97.

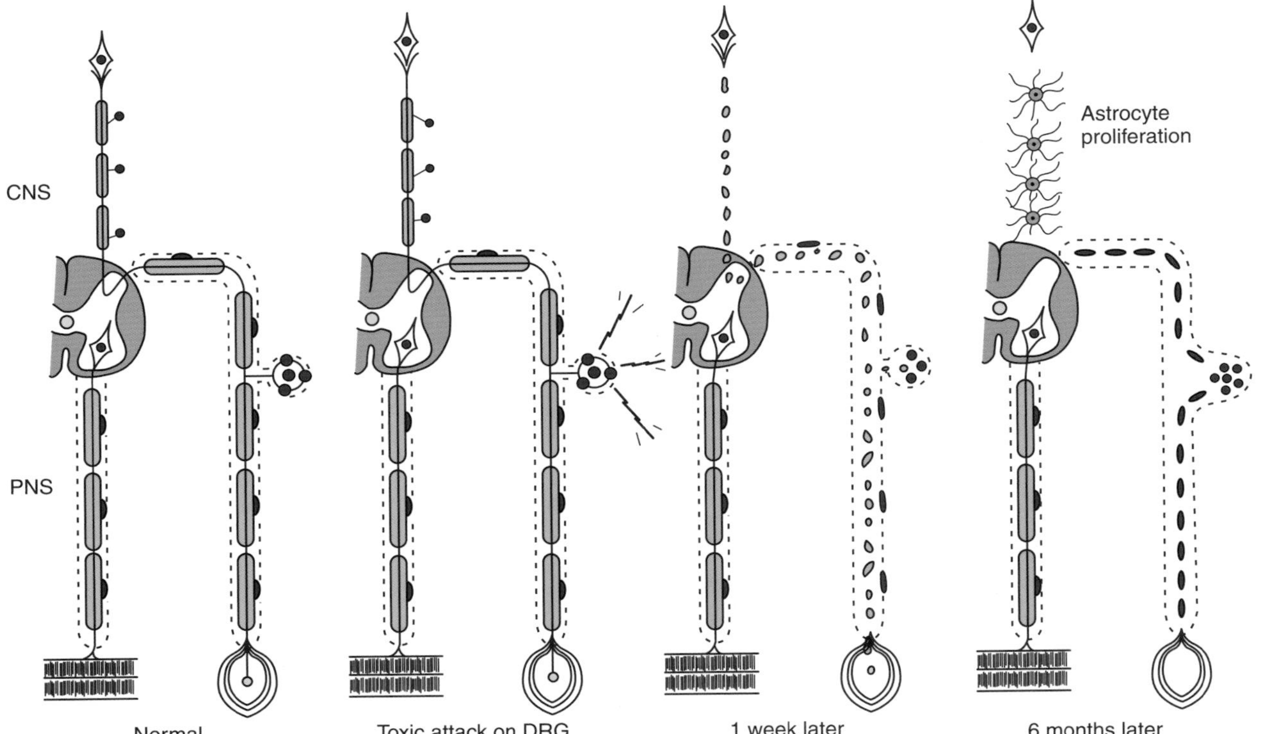


**Fig. 106.2 Diagram of the Main Pathological Events of a Sensory Neuropathy or Gangliopathy.** A toxin *(jagged lines)* produces destruction of dorsal root ganglion *(DRG)* neurons, which results in degeneration of the peripheral-central axonal processes. Recovery is poor, as no axonal regeneration can take place. *CNS*, Central nervous system; *PNS*, peripheral nervous system. *(Adapted from Herskovitz, S., Scelsa, S., Schaumburg, H.H., 2008. Disorders of Peripheral Nerves. Oxford University Press, New York.)*

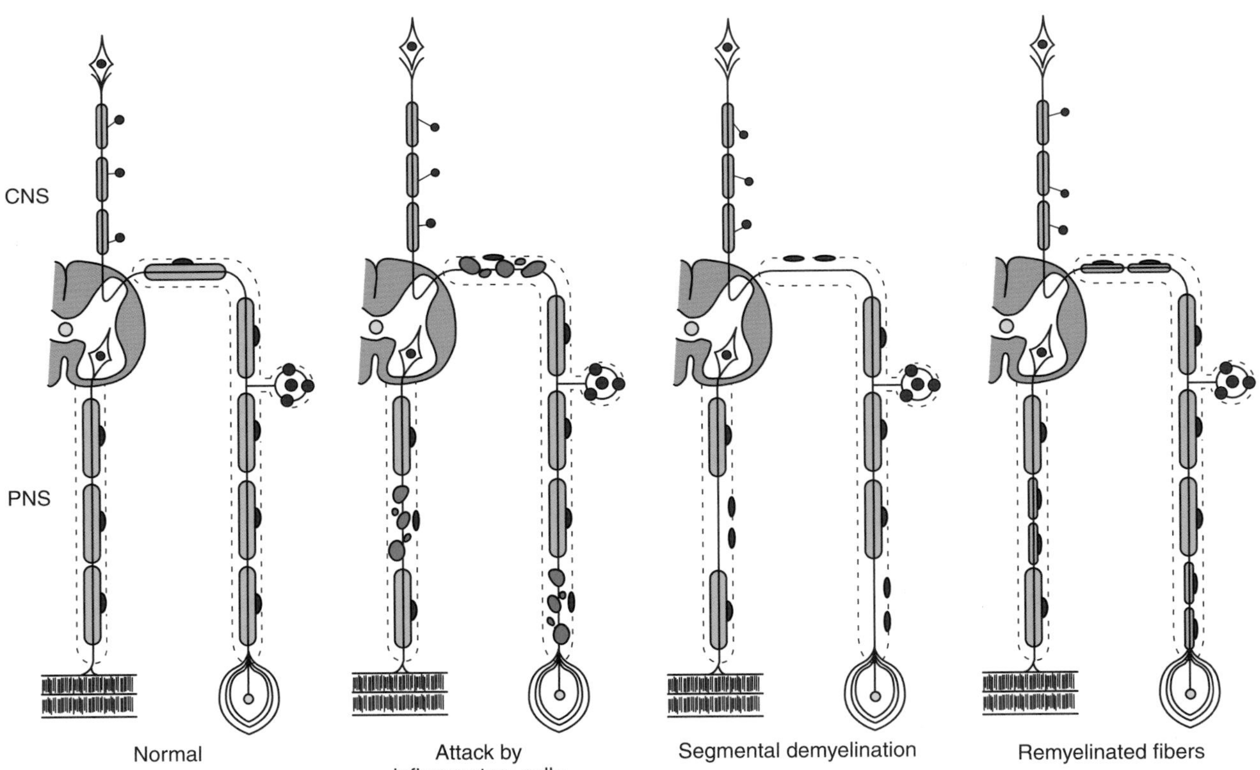


**Fig. 106.3 Diagram of the Main Pathological Events of Primary Segmental Demyelination in Immune-mediated Inflammatory Polyradiculoneuropathies.** Attack by inflammatory cells causes patchy multifocal demyelination along nerve fibers but spares their axons. Recovery occurs by remyelination. Demyelinated segments become invested by several Schwann cells, resulting in a decrease in internodal length of those areas. *CNS*, Central nervous system; *PNS*, peripheral nervous system. *(Adapted from Herskovitz, S., Scelsa, S., Schaumburg, H.H., 2008. Disorders of Peripheral Nerves. Oxford University Press, New York.)*

**BOX 106.1 Classification of Peripheral Nerve Disease**

Mononeuropathy
Plexopathy:
- Brachial plexopathy
- Lumbar plexopathy
- Sacral plexopathy

Radiculopathy:
- Cervical radiculopathy
- Thoracic radiculopathy
- Lumbosacral radiculopathy

Multiple mononeuropathy (mononeuropathy multiplex)
Polyneuropathy:
- Symmetrical polyneuropathy
- Asymmetrical polyneuropathy

Polyradiculoneuropathy

A *mononeuropathy* means focal involvement of a single nerve and implies a local process. Direct trauma, compression, entrapment, vascular lesions, and neoplastic compression or infiltration are the most common causes. Electrophysiological studies provide a more precise localization of the lesion than may be possible by clinical examination, distinguish axonal loss from focal segmental demyelination, and sometimes may reveal a more widespread change indicating an underlying generalized polyneuropathy that has made the nerve susceptible to entrapment, as occurs in diabetes mellitus (DM), hypothyroidism, acromegaly, alcoholism, hereditary amyloidosis, and hereditary neuropathy with liability to pressure palsy (HNPP).

*Multiple mononeuropathies*, or *mononeuropathy multiplex*, signify simultaneous or sequential damage to multiple noncontiguous nerves. Confluent multiple mononeuropathies may give rise to motor weakness with sensory loss that can simulate a length-dependent peripheral polyneuropathy.

*Polyneuropathy* is most commonly characterized by symmetrical distal motor and/or sensory deficits that typically have a graded increase in severity distally and distal attenuation of reflexes. The sensory and motor deficits generally follow a length-dependent stocking-glove pattern. Most polyneuropathies are fairly symmetrical, but some are asymmetrical and sometimes the result of a confluent mononeuropathy multiplex. A small number of polyneuropathies (e.g., that associated with acute intermittent porphyria [AIP]) may be predominantly proximal. It is helpful to determine the relative extent of sensory, motor, and autonomic neuron involvement, although most polyneuropathies produce mixed sensorimotor deficits and some degree of autonomic dysfunction.

## Diagnosis of Peripheral Nerve Disorders

The "shotgun" approach of ordering several panels of diagnostic tests without an adequate understanding of their significance and usefulness should be avoided. A logical systematic diagnostic approach to peripheral neuropathies consists of a detailed history, comprehensive physical and neurological examinations, a limited set of laboratory studies, and detailed electrodiagnostic (EDX) studies. Additional ancillary testing, such as autonomic testing, skin biopsy, or nerve biopsy, may be considered in special clinical situations. This approach confirms the presence of a peripheral nerve disorder; characterizes the fiber type, pattern, time course, and type of deficit of the peripheral nerve disease; shortens the list of diagnostic and etiological possibilities; and prevents misdiagnoses. Further laboratory or pathological studies to determine a specific diagnosis are sometimes performed based on the findings of the initial evaluation.

### Diagnostic Clues from the History

The symptoms of peripheral nerve disorders are due to motor, sensory, or autonomic disturbances. The inquiry should seek both negative and positive symptoms. *Negative motor symptoms* are weakness, atrophy, and walking difficulties. Muscle cramps, fasciculations, myokymia, and tremor are *positive motor manifestations*. In polyneuropathies, negative motor symptoms include early distal toe and ankle extensor weakness, resulting in tripping on rugs or uneven ground. However, a complaint of difficulty walking in itself does not distinguish muscle weakness from sensory, pyramidal, extrapyramidal, or cerebellar disturbance. If the fingers are weak, patients may complain of difficulty opening jars or turning a key in a lock.

*Positive sensory symptoms* include prickling, searing, burning, and tight band-like sensations. *Paresthesias* are unpleasant sensations arising spontaneously without apparent stimulus. The presence of spontaneously reported paresthesias is helpful in distinguishing acquired (>60% of patients) from inherited (<20% of patients) polyneuropathies. *Allodynia* refers to the perception of nonpainful stimuli as painful, and *hyperalgesia* is painful hypersensitivity to noxious stimuli. Neuropathic pain, the extreme example of a positive symptom, is a cardinal feature of many neuropathies. Neuropathic pain often has a deep, burning, or drawing character that may be associated with jabbing or shooting pains that typically increase at night or during periods of rest.

*Negative sensory manifestations* include loss or reduction of pain, temperature, or touch sensation. Imbalance and gait disturbance are common negative sensory symptoms of polyneuropathy, implying loss of proprioception. However, the negative sensory symptoms may be caused by a central myelopathic disorder, including dorsal column dysfunction as occurs with vitamin $B_{12}$ deficiency.

*Symptoms of autonomic dysfunction* are helpful in directing attention toward specific neuropathies that have prominent autonomic symptoms. It is important to ask about orthostatic intolerance (lightheadedness, presyncopal symptoms, or syncope), reduced or excessive sweating, heat intolerance, and bladder, bowel, and sexual dysfunctions. Anorexia, early satiety, nausea, and vomiting are symptoms suggestive of gastroparesis. The degree of autonomic involvement can be documented by noninvasive autonomic function studies (see Chapter 107).

Historical information regarding onset, duration, and evolution of symptoms provides important clues to diagnosis. Knowledge about the time course of disease (acute, subacute, or chronic) and the course (monophasic, progressive, or relapsing) narrows diagnostic possibilities. Guillain-Barré syndrome (GBS), acute porphyria, vasculitis, neuralgic amyotrophy, and some forms of toxic neuropathies have acute presentations. A relapsing course is found in chronic inflammatory demyelinating polyradiculoneuropathy (CIDP), acute porphyria, Refsum disease, HNPPs, hereditary neuralgic amyotrophy, and repeated episodes of toxin exposure.

In patients with a chronic indolent course over many years, inquiries about similar symptoms and bony deformities (such as pes cavus) in immediate relatives often point to a familial polyneuropathy. Inherited polyneuropathies are a major cause of undiagnosed polyneuropathies, accounting for about 30% of patients referred to tertiary centers for diagnosis. Molecular genetic testing or the clinical and electrophysiological evaluation of relatives of patients with undiagnosed neuropathy may corroborate that the disorder is familial. The presence of constitutional symptoms such as weight loss, malaise, and anorexia suggests

**BOX 106.2 Causes of Mononeuropathy Multiplex**

**Axonal Mononeuropathy Multiplex**
Vasculitis (systemic, nonsystemic)
Diabetes mellitus
Sarcoidosis
Leprosy (Hansen disease)
Human immunodeficiency virus 1 infection

**Demyelinating Mononeuropathy Multiplex**
Multifocal motor neuropathy
Multifocal acquired demyelinating sensory and motor neuropathy (MADSAM, Lewis-Sumner syndrome)
Multiple compressive neuropathies (hypothyroidism, diabetes)
Hereditary neuropathy with liability to pressure palsies (HNPPs)

**BOX 106.3 Polyneuropathies with Predominantly Motor Manifestations**

Guillain-Barré syndrome
Acute motor axonal neuropathy*
Chronic inflammatory demyelinating polyradiculoneuropathy
Multifocal motor neuropathy*
Neuropathy with osteosclerotic myeloma
Diabetic lumbar radiculoplexopathy
Charcot-Marie-Tooth disease (hereditary motor sensory neuropathies)
Lead intoxication

* Pure motor syndromes with normal sensory nerve action potentials.

an underlying systemic disorder as a cause of the polyneuropathy. Inquiry should be made about preceding or concurrent associated medical conditions (DM, hypothyroidism, chronic renal failure, liver disease, intestinal malabsorption, malignancy, connective tissue diseases, and human immunodeficiency virus [HIV] seropositivity); drug use, including over-the-counter vitamin preparations (vitamin $B_6$); alcohol and dietary habits; and exposure to solvents, pesticides, or heavy metals.

## Diagnostic Clues from the Examination

The first step in the examination of patients with neuropathy is to determine the anatomical pattern and localization of the disease process and whether motor, sensory, or autonomic nerves are involved.

In mononeuropathy, the neurological deficit follows the distribution of a single nerve. For example, in a patient with foot drop due to a common fibular (peroneal) nerve lesion, the neurological examination reveals weakness of ankle and toe dorsiflexion and ankle eversion, but ankle inversion, toe flexion, and plantar flexion are normal, since muscles controlling these functions are innervated by the tibial nerve. Similarly, sensory loss is restricted to the lower two-thirds of the lateral leg and dorsum of the foot, but sensation on the sole of the foot is normal.

In multiple mononeuropathies (mononeuropathy multiplex), the neurological findings should point to simultaneous or sequential damage to two or more noncontiguous peripheral nerves. Confluent multiple mononeuropathies, such as with involvement of the fibular and tibial nerves or median and ulnar nerves, may give rise to motor weakness with sensory loss that can simulate a length-dependent peripheral polyneuropathy. EDX studies ascertain whether the primary pathological process is axonal degeneration or segmental demyelination (Box 106.2). Approximately two-thirds of patients with multiple mononeuropathies display a picture of axonal damage. Ischemia caused by

**BOX 106.4 Neuropathies with Facial Nerve Involvement**

Guillain-Barré syndrome
Lyme disease
Sarcoidosis
Chronic inflammatory demyelinating polyradiculoneuropathy (rare)
Human immunodeficiency virus 1 infection
Gelsolin familial amyloid neuropathy (Finnish)
Tangier disease

**BOX 106.5 Polyneuropathies with Predominantly Upper-Limb Motor Involvement**

Multifocal motor neuropathy
Multifocal acquired demyelinating sensory and motor neuropathy (MADSAM, Lewis-Sumner syndrome)
Lead neuropathy*
Porphyria
Tangier disease
Familial amyloid neuropathy type 2
Hereditary motor neuropathy (uncommon forms)

* Frequently presents with wrist drop.

systemic or nonsystemic vasculitis or microangiopathy in DM should be considered. Other less common causes are disorders affecting interstitial structures of nerve—namely, infectious, granulomatous, leukemic, or neoplastic infiltration—including leprosy and sarcoidosis. In the event focal demyelination or motor conduction blocks lead to multiple mononeuropathies, multifocal acquired demyelinating sensory and motor neuropathy (MADSAM, Lewis-Sumner syndrome), multifocal motor neuropathy (MMN), or HNPP should be considered.

In polyneuropathy, the sensory deficits generally follow a length-dependent stocking-glove pattern. By the time sensory disturbances of the longest nerves in the body (lower limbs) have reached the level of the knees, paresthesias are usually noted in the distribution of the second-longest nerves (i.e., those in the upper limbs) at the tips of the fingers. When sensory impairment reaches the midthigh, involvement of the third-longest nerves, the anterior intercostal and lumbar segmental nerves, gives rise to a tent-shaped area of hypoesthesia on the anterior chest and abdomen. Involvement of the recurrent laryngeal nerves may occur at this stage, with hoarseness. Motor weakness follows a dying-back pattern and usually is greater in extensor foot muscles than in corresponding flexors. Hence, heel walking is affected earlier than toe walking in most polyneuropathies. It is helpful to determine the relative extent of sensory, motor, and autonomic fiber involvement, although most polyneuropathies produce mixed sensorimotor deficits and some degree of autonomic dysfunction.

Motor deficits tend to dominate the clinical picture in acute and chronic inflammatory demyelinating polyneuropathies, hereditary motor and sensory neuropathies (Charcot-Marie-Tooth disease), and in neuropathies associated with osteosclerotic myeloma, porphyria, lead toxicity, organophosphate intoxication, and hypoglycemia (Box 106.3). The distribution of weakness provides important information. Asymmetrical weakness without sensory loss suggests a motor neuronopathy such as motor neuron disease or MMN. The facial nerve can be affected in several peripheral nerve disorders (Box 106.4). In most polyneuropathies, the legs are more severely affected than the arms, with several notable exceptions (Box 106.5). Polyradiculoneuropathies cause both proximal and distal muscle weakness. For example, proximal and distal weakness is encountered in acute and chronic inflammatory demyelinating polyradiculoneuropathies, osteosclerotic myeloma, porphyria, and diabetic lumbar radiculoplexopathy (amyotrophy). Nerve root involvement is confirmed by denervation in paraspinal muscles on needle EMG or enhancing roots on gadolinium magnetic resonance imaging (MRI).

Autonomic dysfunction of clinical importance is seen in association with specific acute (e.g., GBS) or chronic (e.g., amyloidosis and diabetes) sensorimotor polyneuropathies. Rarely, an autonomic neuropathy may be the exclusive manifestation of a peripheral nerve disorder, without somatic nerve involvement (Box 106.6).

Predominant sensory involvement may be a feature of polyneuropathies caused by diabetes, carcinoma, Sjögren syndrome, dysproteinemia, acquired immunodeficiency syndrome (AIDS), vitamin $B_{12}$ deficiency, celiac disease (CD), inherited and idiopathic sensory neuropathies, and intoxications with cisplatin, thalidomide, or pyridoxine. Loss of sensation in peripheral neuropathies often involves all sensory modalities. However, the impairment may be restricted to selective sensory modalities in many situations, which makes it possible to correlate the type of sensory loss with the diameter size of affected afferent fibers (Fig. 106.4). Pain and temperature sensation are mediated by unmyelinated and small myelinated Aδ fibers, whereas vibratory sense, proprioception, and the afferent limb of the tendon reflex are subserved by large myelinated Aα and Aβ fibers. Light touch is mediated by both large and small myelinated fibers. In polyneuropathies preferentially affecting small fibers, diminished pain and temperature sensation predominate, along with spontaneous burning pain, painful dysesthesias, and autonomic dysfunction. There is preservation of tendon reflexes, balance, and motor strength, and hence few abnormal objective neurological signs are found on examination. A pattern of sensory loss that is very characteristic is distal loss of pinprick sensation, above which is a band of *hyperalgesia* (exaggerated pain from noxious stimuli), with normal sensation above this level. Relatively few disorders cause selective small-fiber neuropathies (Mendell and Sahenk, 2003; Box 106.7). Selective large-fiber sensory loss is characterized by areflexia, sensory ataxia, and loss of joint position and vibration sense. Loss of joint position may also manifest as *pseudoathetosis* (involuntary sinuous movements of fingers and hands when the arms are outstretched and the eyes are closed) and/or a *Romberg sign* (disproportionate loss of balance with eyes closed compared with eyes open). Striking sensory ataxia, together with pseudoathetosis or asymmetrical truncal or facial sensory loss, directs attention to a primary disorder of sensory neurons or polyganglionopathies. The differential diagnosis of ataxic sensory neuropathies is limited (Box 106.8).

### BOX 106.6 Neuropathies with Autonomic Nervous System Involvement

**Acute**

Acute pandysautonomic neuropathy (autoimmune, paraneoplastic)
Guillain-Barré syndrome
Porphyria
Toxic: vincristine, Vacor (rodenticide)

**Chronic**

Diabetes mellitus
Amyloid neuropathy (familial and primary)
Paraneoplastic sensory neuronopathy (malignant inflammatory sensory polyganglionopathy)
Human immunodeficiency virus-related autonomic neuropathy
Hereditary sensory and autonomic neuropathy

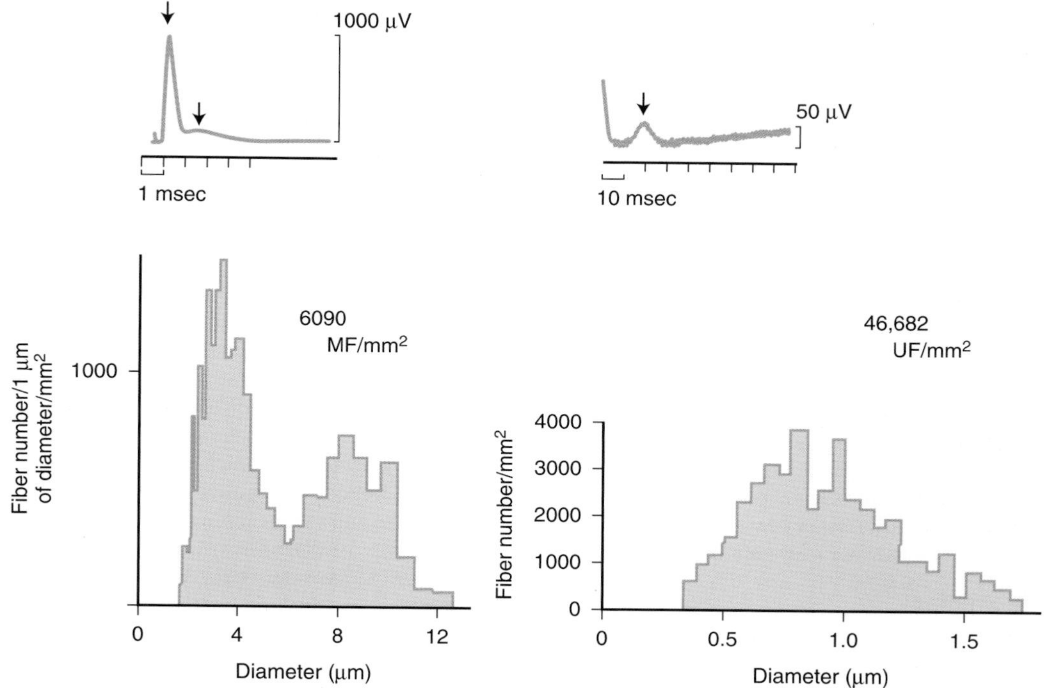


**Fig. 106.4** Myelinated fiber *(MF)* and unmyelinated fiber *(UF)* size-frequency histograms of a normal sural nerve. Fiber size distribution is bimodal for MF but unimodal for UF. MF density in normal sural nerve ranges from 6000 to 10,000 fibers/mm² of fascicular area. Number of UFs is normally about four times that of MFs. Corresponding compound nerve action potential recorded from the sural nerve in vitro is shown at top. Three distinct peaks indicated by *arrows* are, from left to right, Aa, Aa, and C-potentials, which correspond to large MF, small MF, and UF peaks, respectively.

**BOX 106.7 Small-Fiber Neuropathies**

Diabetes mellitus and impaired glucose tolerance
Sjögren (sicca) syndrome
Celiac disease
Amyloid neuropathy (early familial and primary)
Human immunodeficiency virus-associated sensory neuropathy
Hereditary sensory and autonomic neuropathies
Fabry disease
Tangier disease
Cryptogenic small-fiber neuropathy

**BOX 106.8 Sensory Ataxic Neuropathies**

Sensory neuronopathies (polyganglionopathies):
- Paraneoplastic sensory neuronopathy (malignant inflammatory sensory polyganglionopathy):
- Sjögren syndrome
- Idiopathic
- Toxic (cisplatin and analogs, vitamin $B_6$ excess)

Chronic immune sensory polyradiculopathy
Demyelinating polyradiculoneuropathies:
- Guillain-Barré syndrome (Miller-Fisher variant)
- Immunoglobulin M monoclonal gammopathy MAG** antibody

CANOMAD:*
Tabes dorsalis

* Chronic ataxic neuropathy with ophthalmoplegia, IgM paraprotein, cold agglutinins, and anti-GD1b disialosyl antibodies.
** Myelin-Associated Glycoprotein.

Palpation of peripheral nerves is an important though unreliable part of the examination. Hypertrophy of a single nerve trunk suggests either a neoplastic process (e.g., neurofibroma, schwannoma, malignant nerve sheath tumor) or localized perineurial hypertrophic neuropathy. Generalized or multifocal nerve hypertrophy is found in a limited number of peripheral nerve disorders, including leprosy, neurofibromatosis, Charcot-Marie-Tooth (CMT) disease types 1 and 3, acromegaly, Refsum disease, and rarely CIDP.

Certain telltale signs of the skin and its appendages may direct the experienced examiner to a specific diagnosis (Table 106.1): alopecia is seen in thallium poisoning; tightly curled hair in giant axonal neuropathy (GAN); white transverse nail bands, termed *Mees lines*, in arsenic or thallium intoxications; purpuric skin eruptions of the legs in cryoglobulinemia and some vasculitides; skin hyperpigmentation or hypertrichosis in POEMS syndrome (polyneuropathy, organomegaly, endocrinopathy, monoclonal gammopathy, and skin changes); telangiectasias over the abdomen and buttocks in Fabry disease; enlarged yellow-orange tonsils in Tangier disease; pes cavus and hammer toes in CMT disease; and overriding toes and ichthyosis in Refsum disease.

## Electrodiagnostic Studies

It is helpful to follow a decision-making pathway based initially on the overall pattern of distribution of deficits, followed by the electrophysiological findings, and finally the clinical course (Fig. 106.5). EDX studies, carefully performed and directed to the particular clinical situation, play a key role in the evaluation by (1) confirming the presence of neuropathy, (2) precisely locating focal nerve lesions, and (3) giving information as to the nature of the underlying nerve pathology (Gooch and Weimer, 2007; Shapiro et al., 2014; Wilbourn, 2002; see Chapter 36).

**TABLE 106.1 Neuropathies with Skin, Nail, or Hair Manifestations**

| Disease | Skin, Nail, or Hair Manifestations |
|---|---|
| Vasculitis | Purpura, livedo reticularis |
| Cryoglobulinemia | Purpura |
| Fabry disease | Angiokeratomas |
| Leprosy | Skin hypopigmentation |
| Osteosclerotic myeloma (POEMS syndrome) | Skin hyperpigmentation |
| Variegate porphyria | Bullous lesions |
| Refsum disease | Ichthyosis |
| Arsenic or thallium intoxication | Mees lines |
| Thallium poisoning | Alopecia |
| Giant axonal neuropathy | Curled hair |

*POEMS*, Polyneuropathy, organomegaly, endocrinopathy, monoclonal gammopathy, and skin changes.

Because routine sensory nerve conduction studies assess only large myelinated fibers, such studies may be entirely normal in selective small-fiber neuropathies. Quantitative sensory testing assessing cold and heat pain thresholds, tests of sudomotor function, and skin biopsy with analysis of intraepidermal nerve fiber density (IENFD) may be helpful in confirming the unmyelinated nerve fiber abnormalities (Devigili et al., 2008). Since sweating mediated by unmyelinated sympathetic cholinergic fibers is often impaired, the quantitative sudomotor axon reflex (QSART) that evaluates sweating is a highly specific and sensitive method (sensitivity of 80%) to confirm small nerve fiber damage. Quantitative sensory testing assessing both vibratory and thermal detection thresholds has become a useful addition to the bedside sensory examination in controlled clinical trials. Its use in routine clinical practice remains limited because the test is still subjective in that it requires patient cooperation and is time consuming.

## Imaging

High-resolution neuromuscular ultrasound, which is readily available and painless, is increasingly used in the diagnosis of neuromuscular disorders (Hommel et al., 2017). This technique is an extremely helpful tool in the diagnosis of mononeuropathies, including entrapment neuropathies and traumatic nerve injuries. Focal nerve enlargement, measured as cross-sectional area (CSA), is the most common indicator of nerve entrapment, including carpal tunnel syndrome (CTS) and ulnar neuropathy at the elbow (Beekman et al., 2011; Cartwright et al., 2012). More recent studies have also shown important values of neuromuscular ultrasound in the diagnosis of CIDP and in distinguishing acquired demyelinating polyneuropathies from axonal polyneuropathies. Multifocal enlargement of peripheral nerves at non-entrapment sites and of elements of brachial plexus, measured by CSA, is highly diagnostic. In addition, muscle ultrasound visualizes fasciculations in limb muscles and tongue more readily than needle EMG and increases the sensitivity of diagnosis in patients with suspected advanced life support (ALS) (Misawa et al., 2011). Muscle ultrasound is also useful in myopathies including inflammatory myopathies and muscular dystrophies by showing increased echogenicity of muscles, and delineating the distribution of muscle involvement, thus helping in diagnosis and selection of muscle biopsy sites (Noto at al., 2014; Pillen et al., 2008). It also distinguishes neurogenic from myopathic disorders such as Duchenne muscular dystrophy with severe, homogeneous increase of muscle echo intensity from spinal muscular atrophy with an inhomogeneous increase of echo intensity with severe muscle atrophy (Aydinli et al., 2003).

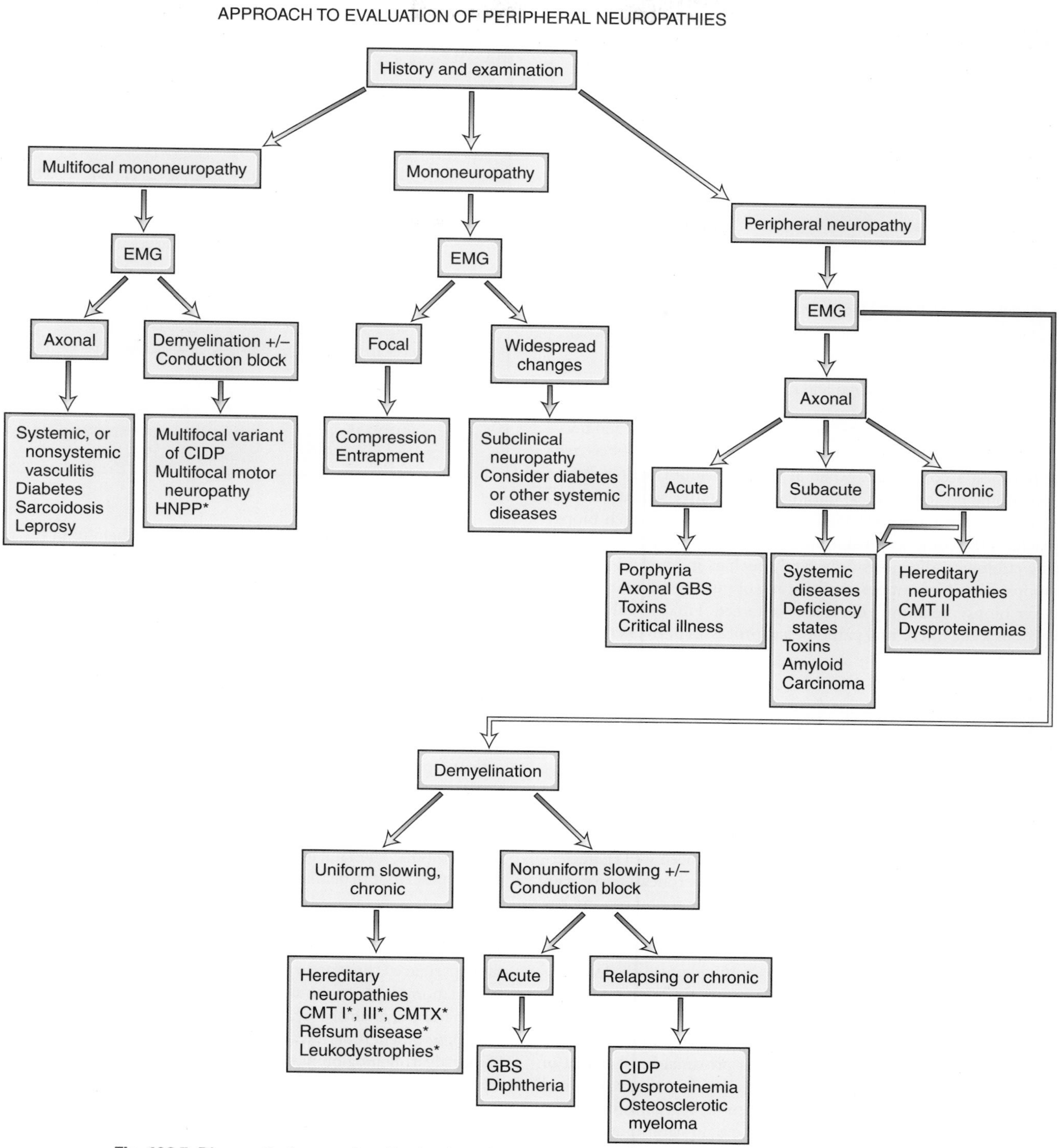

APPROACH TO EVALUATION OF PERIPHERAL NEUROPATHIES

History and examination
Multifocal mononeuropathy
Mononeuropathy
Peripheral neuropathy
EMG
EMG
EMG
Axonal
Demyelination +/– Conduction block
Focal
Widespread changes
Axonal
Systemic, or nonsystemic vasculitis
Diabetes
Sarcoidosis
Leprosy
Multifocal variant of CIDP
Multifocal motor neuropathy
HNPP*
Compression
Entrapment
Subclinical neuropathy
Consider diabetes or other systemic diseases
Acute
Subacute
Chronic
Porphyria
Axonal GBS
Toxins
Critical illness
Systemic diseases
Deficiency states
Toxins
Amyloid
Carcinoma
Hereditary neuropathies
CMT II
Dysproteinemias
Demyelination
Uniform slowing, chronic
Nonuniform slowing +/– Conduction block
Hereditary neuropathies
CMT I*, III*, CMTX*
Refsum disease*
Leukodystrophies*
Acute
Relapsing or chronic
GBS
Diphtheria
CIDP
Dysproteinemia
Osteosclerotic myeloma

**Fig. 106.5 Diagnostic Approach to Evaluation of a Patient with Peripheral Neuropathy.** Electromyography *(EMG)* denotes electrodiagnostic studies including nerve conduction studies and needle EMG. DNA diagnostic testing or specific biochemical tests are available for conditions marked with asterisks. *CIDP*, Chronic inflammatory demyelinating polyradiculoneuropathy; *CMT*, Charcot-Marie-Tooth disease; *CMTX*, Charcot-Marie-Tooth disease X-linked; *GBS*, Guillain-Barré syndrome; *HNPP*, hereditary liability to pressure palsies.

## Skin Biopsy

Skin punch or blister biopsies that demonstrate loss of intraepidermal nerve fibers are alternative methods for documenting small-fiber neuropathy (Panoutsopoulou et al., 2009). Only unmyelinated intraepidermal networks of nerve fibers can be demonstrated by immunostaining with the panaxonal marker protein gene product 9.5, studied best with the use of confocal microscopy. Age, gender, and site of skin biopsy have a profound effect on epidermal nerve fiber density. The density of intraepidermal nerve fibers is reduced in skin biopsies obtained from patients with sensory and sensorimotor polyneuropathies including idiopathic, HIV-associated, diabetic polyneuropathies (Kennedy, 2004). Skin punch biopsy is most

**BOX 106.9 Indications for Nerve Biopsy**

**Nerve Biopsy Is Diagnostic and Essential for Diagnosis**

Vasculitis*
Amyloidosis*
Sarcoidosis*
Hansen disease (leprosy)
Giant axonal neuropathy
Tumor infiltration
Polyglucosan body disease

**Nerve Biopsy Is Suggestive and Only Supportive of Diagnosis**

Charcot-Marie-Tooth disease types 1 and 3
Chronic inflammatory demyelinating polyradiculoneuropathy
Paraproteinemic neuropathy (immunoglobulin M monoclonal gammopathy with anti-myelin-associated glycoprotein antibody)

* Consider combined distal nerve and muscle biopsies.

**TABLE 106.2 Neuropathies Associated with Serum Autoantibodies**

| Autoantibody | Disease (% Positive) |
|---|---|
| **Antibodies Against Gangliosides** | |
| GM1 (polyclonal IgM) | Multifocal motor neuropathy (70%) |
| GM1, GD1a (polyclonal IgG) | Guillain-Barré syndrome (30%) |
| GQ1b (polyclonal IgG) | Miller-Fisher variant of Guillain-Barré syndrome (>90%) |
| GD1b (monoclonal IgM) | Chronic ataxic neuropathy with ophthalmoplegia, IgM paraprotein, cold agglutinins and anti-GD1b disialosyl antibodies, CANOMAD |
| **Antibodies Against Glycoproteins** | |
| Myelin-associated glycoprotein (MAG; monoclonal IgM) | Distal acquired demyelinating sensory (DADS) neuropathy or IgM neuropathy (50%–70%) |
| **Antibodies Against RNA-Binding Proteins** | |
| Anti-Hu, antineuronal nuclear antibody 1 (ANNA1) | Malignant inflammatory polyganglionopathy: that is, paraneoplastic sensory neuronopathy (>95%) |

*Ig*, Immunoglobulin.

useful in patients with suspected small-fiber neuropathy, when nerve conduction studies are normal. The diagnosis of small-fiber neuropathy is best accomplished when at least two abnormal results are met, including positive clinical findings, quantitative sensory testing, QSART, and skin biopsy (Devigili et al., 2008). Skin punch biopsy only detects the presence of skin nerve abnormalities and leads to a specific etiological diagnosis only rarely such as in amyloidosis. The skin biopsy also does not permit the study of myelinated fibers unless a thicker biopsy, including dermis, is obtained. Finally, unlike sural nerve biopsy, the interstitial pathological processes of the nerves cannot be studied.

## Nerve Biopsy

Nerve biopsy (other than for the diagnosis of vasculitis and neoplasia) should be performed only in centers with established experience with the surgical procedure, handling of nerve specimens, and pathological technique; otherwise little useful information is likely to be obtained. The sural nerve is selected most commonly for biopsy, because the resultant sensory deficit is restricted to a small area over the heel and dorsolateral aspect of the foot, and because its morphology has been well characterized in health and disease. The superficial fibular (peroneal) nerve is an alternative lower-extremity cutaneous nerve suitable for biopsy and has the advantage of allowing simultaneous biopsy of the peroneus brevis muscle through the same incision. This combined distal nerve and muscle biopsy procedure increases the yield of identifying suspected vasculitis (Collins et al., 2000; Vital et al., 2006). In contrast, adding a proximal muscle (e.g., quadriceps) to a cutaneous nerve biopsy (e.g., sural) does not significantly increase the diagnostic yield compared to nerve biopsy alone (Bennett et al., 2008). In patients with proximal involvement of the lower limbs, the intermediate cutaneous nerve of the thigh combined with a muscle biopsy can be performed. When the risk of complication is increased from a biopsy of the lower limbs (e.g., in significant distal leg ischemia, edema) or the neuropathy is preferentially more pronounced in the upper limbs, a cutaneous nerve biopsy of superficial radial or one of the antebrachial sensory nerves may be performed. When the imaging studies indicate a plexus or nerve root pathological process (e.g., inflammatory, infiltrative), a fascicular biopsy of the affected nerve by an expert surgeon may provide invaluable information. Nerve biopsy has proved to be particularly informative when techniques such as single teased fiber preparations, semi-thin sections, ultrastructural studies, and morphometry are applied to quantitate the nerve fiber pathology. Nowadays, relatively few disorders remain in which a nerve biopsy is essential for diagnosis (Pleasure, 2007; Said, 2002; Box 106.9). In general, nerve biopsy is most frequently diagnostic in suspected peripheral nerve vasculitis, amyloid neuropathy, and leprosy. It is helpful in the recognition of CIDP, hereditary demyelinating polyneuropathies, and some rare axonal polyneuropathies in which distinctive axonal changes occur, such as in giant axonal neuropathy and polyglucosan body disease. The availability of molecular genetic tests for several CMT neuropathies, HNPP, and familial transthyretin amyloidosis has decreased the necessity for nerve biopsy in these conditions.

Nerve biopsy is an invasive procedure and is associated with as high as 15% complication rate—particularly minor wound infections, wound dehiscence, and stump neuromas. Approximately one-third of patients (particularly those without much sensory loss initially) report unpleasant sensory symptoms at the sural nerve biopsy site that are still present 1 year after the biopsy (Gabriel et al., 2000). The area of the original sensory deficit declines by 90% after 18 months because of collateral reinnervation (Theriault et al., 1998). The complications may be greater if substantial foot ischemia is present or if the patient smokes cigarettes.

## Other Laboratory Tests

The clinical neuropathic patterns and the results of EDX studies guide the experienced clinician to select the most appropriate laboratory tests. A few laboratory tests should be obtained routinely in all patients with peripheral polyneuropathy. These include complete blood cell count (CBC), sedimentation rate, C-reactive protein, renal functions, fasting blood sugar, hemoglobin $A_{1C}$, thyroid studies, vitamin $B_{12}$ level, and serum protein electrophoresis with immunofixation electrophoresis. It is important to screen for monoclonal proteins in all patients with chronic undiagnosed polyneuropathy, particularly those older than 60 years, because 10% of such patients have a monoclonal gammopathy. Cerebrospinal fluid (CSF) examination is helpful in the evaluation of suspected demyelinating neuropathies and polyradiculopathies related to meningeal carcinomatosis or lymphomatosis.

Several serum autoantibodies with reactivity to various components of peripheral nerve have been associated with peripheral neuropathy syndromes, and reference laboratories offer panels of nerve antibodies for sensory, sensorimotor, and motor neuropathies. It must be emphasized that the clinical relevance of most autoantibodies has not been established for patient treatment, and their use is not cost-effective (Vernino and Wolfe, 2007). Those of greatest clinical utility are listed in Table 106.2 (Kissel, 1998). An ever-increasing number of molecular genetic tests for inherited neuropathies are available at reference laboratories (see Hereditary Neuropathies, later).

In patients with initially undiagnosed peripheral neuropathy referred to specialized centers, a definite diagnosis can be made in more than 75% of cases. Inherited neuropathies, CIDP, and neuropathies associated with other systemic diseases accounted for most diagnoses. The improved diagnostic rate resulted in large measure from detailed clinical, EDX, and laboratory evaluations and study of relatives of patients with undiagnosed neuropathy.

## MONONEUROPATHIES

### Definition and Classification of Mononeuropathies

*Mononeuropathy* is defined as a disorder of a single peripheral nerve. This may result from compression, traction, laceration, thermal, or chemical injury. The damage may involve one or more structural components of the peripheral nerve, while the pathophysiological responses to peripheral nerve lesions include axon loss, demyelination, or a combination of both.

Peripheral nerve injuries are classified based on functional status of the nerve and histological findings. Seddon divided peripheral nerve injury into three classes: neurapraxia, axonotmesis, and neurotmesis. This classification remains popular, particularly among surgeons, because of its correlation to outcome (Seddon, 1975). Later, Sunderland (1991) revised the classification into five degrees that have better prognostic implications.

#### Neurapraxia

***First-degree nerve injury.*** Neurapraxia, or first-degree nerve injury, usually results from brief or mild compression on the nerve that distorts the myelin, resulting in segmental demyelination but leaving the axons intact. The nerve conducts normally distal to but not across the lesion, resulting in conduction block, which is the electrophysiological correlate of neurapraxia. With this type of injury, recovery is usually complete following remyelination that occurs within 1–3 months if the offending cause (such as a compression) is removed.

#### Axonotmesis

Axonotmesis injury is characterized by axonal damage that results in wallerian degeneration; distal to the injury, the axons and their investing myelin sheath degenerate (wallerian degeneration) and the end organs (muscle fibers and sensory receptors) become denervated. Sunderland divided this type of nerve lesion into three further subtypes based on the disruptions of the supporting structures (endoneurium, perineurium, and epineurium).

***Second-degree nerve injury.*** The axonal loss is associated with intact endoneurial tubes as well as intact perineurium and epineurium. These lesions have fairly good prognosis, since nerve regeneration between the site of nerve injury and the target organs is well guided by the intact endoneurial tubes.

***Third-degree nerve injury.*** The axons and endoneurium are damaged while leaving the perineurium and epineurium intact. These lesions have fair prognosis and may require surgical intervention, mostly because of axonal misdirection and formation of neuromas.

***Fourth-degree nerve injury.*** The axons, endoneurium, and perineurium are disrupted, but the epineurium is intact. These lesions have poor prognosis and often require surgical repair.

#### Neurotmesis

***Fifth-degree nerve injury.*** Neurotmesis, or fifth-degree nerve injury, is the most severe type of nerve injury. It involves complete disruption of the nerve and all supporting structures. The nerve is transected, with loss of continuity between its proximal and distal stumps.

*Entrapment neuropathy* is defined as a mononeuropathy caused by focal compression or mechanical distortion of a nerve within a fibrous or fibro-osseous tunnel or less commonly by other structures such as bone, ligament, other connective tissues, blood vessels, or mass lesions. Compression, constriction, angulation, and stretching are important mechanisms that produce nerve injury at certain vulnerable anatomical sites (see Tables 106.3 and 106.5). The term *entrapment* is a useful one in that it implies that compression occurs at particular sites where surgical intervention is often required to release the entrapped nerve, such as in the case of the median nerve at the wrist in moderate to severe CTS. Overuse has been implicated as the cause of entrapment neuropathies in certain occupations, including playing of musical instruments by professional musicians.

In chronic entrapment, mechanical distortion of the nerve fibers leads to focal demyelination or, in severe cases, to wallerian degeneration. Morphological studies show a combination of active demyelination, remyelination, wallerian degeneration, and axonal regeneration at the site of entrapment. Endoneurial swelling, collagen proliferation, and thickening of perineurial sheaths accompany the nerve fiber changes. Ischemia is not a significant contributing factor to nerve fiber damage in chronic compression. In contrast, ischemia plays a more significant role in nerve injury associated with acute compression secondary to space-occupying lesions such as hematoma or compartment syndromes.

The characteristic electrophysiological feature of entrapment neuropathy is either short-segment conduction delay (i.e., focal slowing) or conduction block across the site of entrapment (see Chapter 36). In severe cases, wallerian degeneration gives rise to denervation and reinnervation in affected muscles. Nerve conduction studies together with needle EMG are essential for diagnosis and reliable documentation of the site and severity of nerve entrapment. Neuromuscular ultrasound has had an increasing role in the diagnosis of entrapment neuropathies, particularly when EDX studies are more difficult (such as in young children) or show only signs of nonlocalizing axonal loss such as with severe ulnar neuropathies (Alrajeh and Preston, 2018). In contrast, plain radiography, computed tomography (CT), and MRI may be of occasional value in identifying rare structural abnormalities, but these imaging procedures are often not necessary for routine diagnosis.

### Mononeuropathies of the Upper Extremities

Entrapment neuropathies of the upper extremities are shown in Table 106.3.

#### Median Nerve

***Applied anatomy.*** The median nerve, formed from contributions of the lateral cord (C6 and C7 fibers) and medial cord (C8 and T1 fibers) of the brachial plexus, runs into the forearm between the two heads of the pronator teres. It then gives off branches to the pronator teres, flexor carpi radialis, flexor digitorum sublimis, and the palmaris longus muscles, as well as the anterior interosseous nerve. The anterior interosseous nerve is the largest branch of the median nerve and is a pure motor nerve. It arises from the median nerve distal to these motor branches in the upper forearm and innervates the flexor pollicis longus, pronator quadratus, and median part of the flexor digitorum profundus muscles of the index and middle fingers. The median nerve then enters the wrist through the carpal tunnel, formed by the carpal bones and the transverse carpal ligament, the latter forming its roof. Before reaching the wrist, the median nerve gives off the palmar cutaneous sensory branch, which runs subcutaneously (not through the carpal tunnel) to innervate the skin over the thenar eminence. Distal to the carpal tunnel, the median nerve divides into motor and sensory divisions. The motor division innervates the first and second

TABLE 106.3 Entrapment/Compressive Neuropathies of Upper Limbs

| Nerve | Site of Compression | Predisposing Factors | Major Clinical Features |
|---|---|---|---|
| Median | Wrist (carpal tunnel syndrome) | Tenosynovitis, arthritis, repetitive wrist motions | Nocturnal paresthesia, pain, hypesthesia lateral 3 fingers, thenar atrophy |
| | Anterior interosseous | Strenuous exercise, trauma, neuralgic amyotrophy | Abnormal pinch sign, normal sensation |
| | Elbow (pronator teres syndrome) | Repetitive elbow motions | Tenderness of pronator teres, no weakness, sensory loss |
| Ulnar | Elbow (ulnar groove or cubital tunnel syndrome) | Elbow leaning, remote trauma (tardy ulnar), trauma, entrapment | Clawing, Froment sign, sensory loss of fourth and fifth fingers |
| | Guyon canal | Mechanics, cyclists, ganglion cyst | Interosseous atrophy, normal sensation of dorsum of fourth and little fingers |
| Radial | Axilla | Crutches | Wrist drop, triceps involved, sensory loss extending into forearm and sometimes arm |
| | Spiral groove | Abnormal sleep postures | Wrist drop, triceps spared, sensory loss of dorsum of hand only |
| | Posterior interosseous | Elbow synovitis, neuralgic amyotrophy | Paresis of finger extensors, radial wrist deviation |
| | Superficial sensory branch (cheiralgia paresthetica) | Wrist bands, hand cuffs | Paresthesias in dorsum of hand |
| Suprascapular | Suprascapular notch | Blunt trauma, neuralgic amyotrophy | Atrophy of supraspinatus and infraspinatus muscles |
| Axillary | Axilla | Shoulder dislocation or surgery | Weakness of arm abduction |
| Long thoracic | Shoulder | Neuralgic amyotrophy, stretch | Posterior scapular winging |
| Lower trunk of the brachial plexus or T1 roots | Thoracic outlet | Cervical rib, cervical band with enlarged C7 transverse process | Atrophy of intrinsic hand muscles (mostly thenar), paresthesias of medial hand and forearm |

lumbricals and most muscles of the thenar eminence including the opponens pollicis, abductor pollicis brevis, and superficial head of the flexor pollicis brevis. The sensory fibers of the median nerve innervate the skin of the thumb, index, middle, and lateral half of the ring fingers.

***Median nerve entrapment at the wrist (carpal tunnel syndrome).*** CTS is by far the most common entrapment neuropathy seen in clinical practice. CTS prevalence in a primary care population is about 36 per 10,000 people, with an annual incidence of 19 per 10,000 for men and 36 per 10,000 for women (Burton et al., 2018). Both the incidence and prevalence of CTS seem to be increasing.

This entrapment occurs in the tunnel through which the median nerve and long finger flexor tendons pass. Because the transverse carpal ligament is an unyielding fibrous structure forming the roof of the tunnel, tenosynovitis or arthritis in this area often produces pressure on the median nerve. The syndrome is frequently bilateral and usually of greater intensity in the dominant hand.

Symptoms consist of nocturnal pain and paresthesias, most often confined to the thumb, index, and middle fingers, but may be reported to involve the entire hand. Patients complain of tingling numbness, and burning sensations, which often awaken them from sleep. Referred pain may radiate to the forearm and even as high as the shoulder (Stevens et al., 1999). Symptoms are often provoked after excessive use of the hand or wrist or during ordinary activities such as driving or holding a phone, book, or newspaper, in which the wrist is assumed in either a flexed or extended posture. Objective sensory changes may be found in the distribution of the median nerve, most often impaired two-point discrimination, pinprick and light touch sensation, or occasionally hyperesthesia, in the thumb, index, and middle fingers, most evident in finger tips, with sparing of the skin over the thenar eminence. Thenar (abductor pollicis brevis muscle) weakness and atrophy may be present in advanced cases of CTS (Fig. 106.6). *Phalen maneuver* (flexing the patient's hand at the wrist for 1 minute) or *reversed Phalen maneuver* (hyperextension of the wrist for 1 minute) often reproduces

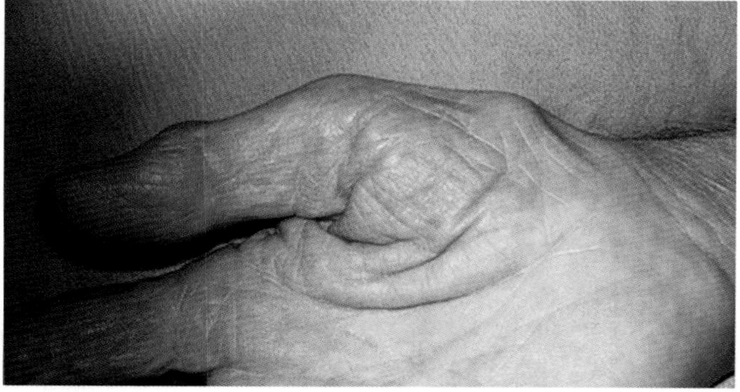

**Fig. 106.6** Thenar Atrophy in Chronic Bilateral Carpal Tunnel Syndrome.

the symptoms; it is present in about 80% of patients, and is rarely false positive (Padua et al., 2016). A positive *Tinel sign*, in which percussion of the nerve at the carpal tunnel causes paresthesias in the distribution of the distal distribution of the median nerve, is present in approximately 60% of affected patients but is not as specific for CTS and may be false positive.

Work-related wrist and hand symptoms (repetitive motion injury) from cumulative trauma in the workplace have received increasing attention by the general public in recent years (Thomsen et al., 2002). Although a proportion of these cases have bona fide CTS, longitudinal natural history data suggest that the majority of industrial workers do not develop symptoms of CTS (Nathan et al., 1998). Symptoms consistent with hand and wrist arthritis in a variety of occupational settings are now recognized as being much more common than CTS (Dillon et al., 2002). CTS appears to occur in work settings that include repetitive forceful grasping or pinching, awkward positions of the hand and wrist, direct pressure over the carpal tunnel, and the use of

**TABLE 106.4 Internal Comparison of Nerve Conduction Studies in the Evaluation of Carpal Tunnel Syndrome**

| Study | Median-Ulnar Palmar Mixed Study | Median-Ulnar Sensory Study to Ring Finger | Median-Ulnar Motor Study to Second Lumbrical Interossei | Median-Radial Sensory Study to Thumb |
|---|---|---|---|---|
| Technique | Palm stimulation of median and ulnar nerves, recording at the wrist | Median and ulnar nerves stimulation at the wrist, recording ring fingers | Median and ulnar nerves stimulation at the wrist, recording second lumbrical and second interossei, respectively (second interosseous space) | Median and radial nerves stimulation at the wrist, recording thumb |
| Abnormal values | Median-ulnar peak latency difference ≥ 0.4 ms | Median-ulnar peak latency difference ≥ 0.4 ms | Median-ulnar onset latency difference ≥ 0.5 ms | Median-radial peak latency difference ≥ 0.4 ms |

handheld vibrating tools. Increased risk for the syndrome has been found in meat packers, garment workers, butchers, grocery checkers, electronic assembly workers, musicians, dental hygienists, and housekeepers. The highest reported incidence of work-related CTS, based on the number of carpal tunnel surgeries performed, was 15% among a group of meat packers. Though using the computer keyboard may aggravate symptoms of CTS, keyboard use does not increase the risk of developing CTS (Mediouni et al., 2014; Shiri and Falah-Hassani, 2015; Stevens et al., 2001).

Diseases and conditions that have been found to predispose to the development of CTS include pregnancy, diabetes, obesity, age, rheumatoid arthritis, hypothyroidism, amyloidosis, gout, acromegaly, certain mucopolysaccharidoses, arteriovenous shunts for hemodialysis, old fractures at the wrist, and inflammatory diseases involving tendons or connective tissues at the wrist level (Becker et al., 2002). On rare occasions, CTS may be familial, and some patients with CTS have carpal tunnels that are significantly narrower than average.

The most commonly performed EDX tests for CTS are the median nerve sensory and motor conduction studies, which exhibit delayed sensory or motor latencies across the wrist in about 70% of patients. However, these studies are not sensitive enough in the diagnosis of CTS and fail to detect up to a third of patients with CTS, particularly those with mild and early symptoms. Recording the median latency at short distances over the course of the median nerve from palm to wrist and/or comparing this latency with the latency for the ulnar or radial nerve at the same distance (internal comparison nerve conduction studies) increase the sensitivity of these nerve conduction studies (Basiri and Katirji, 2015; Stevens, 1997; Table 106.4).

Mild CTS must be distinguished from proximal median neuropathies, upper brachial plexopathy, C6 or C7 radiculopathies, and polyneuropathy involving the hands. Occasionally, a transient ischemic attack may mimic the symptoms of CTS.

Ultrasound is increasingly used in the diagnosis of CTS. Thickening of the median nerve, best expressed as an increase in the CSA of the median nerve at the carpal tunnel inlet (more than 13 mm; normal <10–13 mm), or flattening of the nerve at the level of the hamate are the best diagnostic criteria (Fig. 106.7) (Cartwright et al., 2012; Tai et al., 2012). The majority of studies have found that the diagnostic utility of ultrasound and EDX studies are equal (Mondelli et al., 2008; Viser et al., 2008). MRI is most useful when a space-occupying lesion, such as ganglion, hemangioma, or bony deformity, is suspected in patients with CTS.

In cases with only mild sensory symptoms, treatment with splints in neutral position, nonsteroidal antiinflammatory drugs (NSAIDs), and local corticosteroid injection often suffice (Padua et al., 2016). Local corticosteroid injection is slightly better than splinting (Chesterton

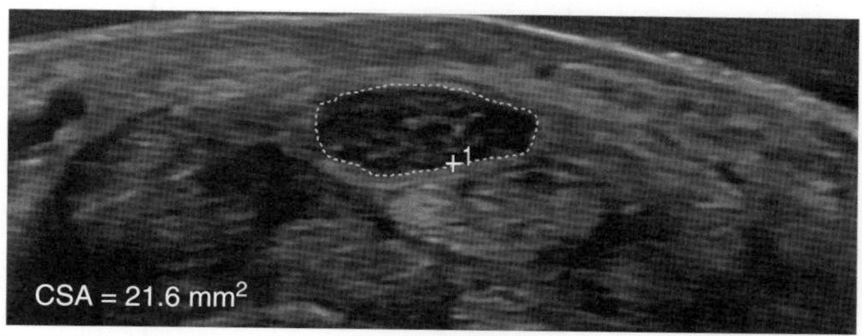


**Fig. 106.7** Ultrasound of the median nerve at the wrist showing a hypoechoic and enlarged median nerve at the carpal tunnel inlet with a cross-sectional area *(CSA)* measuring 21.6 mm$^2$ (normal < 10–13 mm)

et al., 2018). Withdrawal of provoking factors is also important. Although nonoperative treatments have been advocated (Osterman et al., 2002), a comparison of splinting versus surgery suggested that the latter may have a better long-term outcome than the former (Gerritsen et al., 2002). Use of a range of devices and appliances to protect the hand against CTS, including gel-padded gloves, has shown little if any improvement in objective measures of nerve function. There is conflicting evidence that NSAIDs, diuretics, laser, and ultrasound are effective. Exercise therapy is not useful (Piazzini et al., 2007). Methylprednisolone injections for CTS significantly relieve symptoms for a few months and reduce the need for surgery, but a significant number of patients will ultimately need surgical treatment (Atroshi et al., 2013). Oral steroids are also effective but are associated with side effects. Severe sensory loss, thenar atrophy, and active denervation on needle EMG of thenar muscles suggest the need for surgical carpal tunnel release. Open surgical sectioning of the volar carpal ligament or fiberoptic techniques are often successful, with more than 90% of patients having prompt resolution of pain and paresthesias (Louie et al., 2013; Mirza and King, 1996). Improvement in distal latencies may lag behind the relief of symptoms. Comparing with preoperative values, nerve conduction studies demonstrate improvement in those with moderate abnormalities preoperatively, whereas patients with severe or no abnormalities on baseline nerve conduction studies have poorer results (Bland, 2001). A correlation between patients seeking workers' compensation who hire attorneys and poorer operative outcomes has also been reported (Katz et al., 2001a). Older individuals may not improve as much as younger patients (Porter et al., 2002), and factors such as poor mental health, significant alcohol consumption, longer disease duration, and male gender also portend a poorer outcome. Rarely, symptoms persist after operation. Poor surgical results usually are associated with incomplete sectioning of the transverse ligament, surgical damage of the palmar cutaneous branch of the median nerve by an improperly placed skin incision, scarring within the carpal tunnel, or an incorrect preoperative diagnosis. Surgical re-exploration may be required in certain cases with poor response to the initial operation (Steyers, 2002).

***Median nerve compressions at the elbow***

**Anterior interosseous nerve syndrome.** Isolated acute involvement of the anterior interosseous nerve is often a presentation of neuralgic amyotrophy (idiopathic brachial plexus neuropathy, Parsonage-Turner syndrome) (England and Sumner, 1987; Katirji, 1986). The majority of these lesions are fascicular lesions of the median nerve in the arm involving the anterior interosseous nerve fascicle selectively (Pham et al., 2014). Fascicular torsion of the anterior interosseous fascicle in the lower arm has also been advocated to be due to the high mobility of the anterior interosseous nerve fascicles during elbow flexion leading to torsion injury or inflammation/edema followed by intraneural adhesions (Noda et al., 2017). In chronic and indolent lesions, a restricted form of MMN with conduction block should be considered and a careful and detailed electrophysiological study may reveal involvement of other nerves. The anterior interosseous nerve may be externally compressed following anterior elbow dislocations or complex elbow fractures, or rarely by fibrous bands attached to the flexor digitorum superficialis muscle, an anomalous Gantzer muscle which is an accessory portion of the flexor pollicis longus or the flexor digitorum profundus (Caetano et al., 2018).

Patients often complain of an acute or subacute onset of pain in the forearm or elbow. The patient is unable to flex the distal phalanges of the thumb and index finger, making it impossible to form a circle with those fingers *(pinch or O sign)*. Sensory and motor nerve conduction studies of the median nerve are usually normal. Needle EMG reveals denervation in muscles innervated by the anterior interosseous nerve, including the flexor pollicis longus, pronator quadratus, and flexor digitorum profundus muscles of the index and middle fingers. Spontaneous recovery usually occurs within 3–12 months, and therefore surgery may not be necessary unless penetrating injury, fracture, or progressive deterioration and weakness are detected. Patients with torsion injury showed good recovery after interfascicular neurolysis.

**Pronator teres syndrome.** In the pronator teres syndrome, the median nerve is compressed in the proximal forearm between the two heads of the pronator teres muscle, a fibrous arcade of the flexor digitorum superficialis muscle, or the lacertus fibrosus (a thick fascial band extending from the biceps tendon to the forearm fascia). This extremely rare and controversial entrapment may develop in individuals engaged in repetitive pronating movements of the forearm. Patients usually experience a vague aching pain in the volar aspect of the elbow and forearm, beginning or worsening during activities involving grasping or pronation or both. There is also an insidious onset of paresthesias and numbness of the palm of the hand, mimicking CTS but without the nocturnal symptoms. Resistance to pronation produces pain in the proximal forearm. The pronator teres may be firm and tender on palpation, and the Tinel sign may be elicited over the median nerve in the region of the elbow. Weakness of median-innervated muscles such as the flexor pollicis longus, pronator quadratus, and abductor pollicis brevis (but not of pronator teres) is rarely demonstrated, in contrast to traumatic cases such as following elbow dislocation, forearm fracture, or intracompartmental hemorrhage. Nerve conduction studies in the median nerve are usually normal and do not show the distal median motor and sensory latencies at the wrist that accompany CTS. Needle EMG is also usually normal, with no definite signs of denervation. Injection of corticosteroids into the pronator teres muscle, NSAIDs, and immobilization of the arm with the elbow flexed to 90 degrees and in mild pronation often provide relief of symptoms. Surgery is controversial but may be occasionally necessary, though patients may gain only partial relief.

**Median nerve entrapment at the ligament of Struthers.** An often bilateral supracondylar spur of the humerus is present in approximately 1% of normal individuals. This beadlike bony or cartilaginous projection arises from the anteromedial surface of the humerus, located about 5 cm above the medial epicondyle. A fibrous band, the ligament of Struthers, extends from this spur to the medial epicondyle and may rarely compromise the median nerve and the brachial artery above the elbow. Clinical symptoms resemble the pronator teres syndrome, but sometimes the radial pulse diminishes when the forearm is fully extended in supination because of the concomitant entrapment of the brachial artery. Elbow extension causes aggravation of the pain. On needle EMG, there is sometimes denervation in the abductor pollicis brevis, flexor pollicis longus, pronator quadratus, and pronator teres. Involvement of the pronator teres muscle theoretically allows differentiation of the ligament of Struthers syndrome from the pronator teres syndrome. Treatment consists of surgical excision of the spur and ligament.

## Ulnar Nerve

***Applied anatomy.*** The ulnar nerve derives its fibers from the C8 and T1 roots via the lower trunk and originates from the medial cord of the brachial plexus, along with the medial brachial and antebrachial cutaneous sensory nerves. The ulnar nerve gives no branches in the arm. At the elbow, the nerve becomes superficial and enters the ulnar groove formed between the medial epicondyle and the olecranon process. Normally, the ulnar nerve remains in the groove, but in some individuals or when there is an unusual degree of physiological cubitus valgus, the nerve may be unduly mobile, tending to slip forward (sublux) over the medial epicondyle when the elbow is flexed. In a small number of individuals, a dense fibrotendinous band and/or an accessory epitrochleoanconeus muscle may be present between the medial epicondyle and the olecranon process. Slightly distal to the groove in the proximal forearm, the ulnar nerve travels under the tendinous arch of the two heads of the flexor carpi ulnaris muscle, known as the *humeral-ulnar aponeurosis*, which forms the entrance of the cubital tunnel. Muscular branches originate to the flexor carpi ulnaris and the flexor digitorum profundus (ulnar part to the little and ring fingers). The ulnar nerve continues under the flexor carpi ulnaris and then exits in the distal forearm between the deep fascia separating the flexor carpi ulnaris and flexor digitorum profundus. Some 5–8 cm proximal to the wrist, the dorsal ulnar cutaneous sensory branch exits to innervate skin on the dorsal medial hand and the dorsal little and ring fingers. The palmar cutaneous sensory branch originates at the level of the ulnar styloid to supply sensation to the proximal medial palm. The ulnar nerve then enters the wrist through the Guyon canal, which is formed between the pisiform bone and the hook of the hamate and is covered by the volar carpal ligament and the palmaris brevis muscle. Within the Guyon canal, the ulnar nerve divides into its terminal deep palmar and superficial ulnar branches. Because the palmar cutaneous sensory and dorsal cutaneous sensory branches do not pass through the Guyon canal, the deep palmar branch is purely motor and supplies muscular innervation to the hypothenar muscles, the palmar and dorsal interossei, the third and fourth lumbricals, and two muscles in the thenar eminence, the adductor pollicis, and the deep head of the flexor pollicis brevis.

***Ulnar nerve entrapment at the elbow.*** Ulnar mononeuropathy is the second most common entrapment or compression mononeuropathy, although it is considerably less common than CTS. Compression of the ulnar nerve by a thickened, fibrotic flexor carpi ulnaris aponeurosis (humeral-ulnar aponeurosis) at the entrance of the elbow's cubital tunnel is a common cause of ulnar neuropathy *(cubital tunnel syndrome)*. Patients with a subluxed ulnar nerve are at high risk for compression at the elbow. Also, prolonged and frequent resting of the flexed elbow on a hard surface such as a desk or armchair may result in external pressure to the nerve *(ulnar groove syndrome)*. Occupations involving repeated flexion of the elbow may on occasion cause symptoms of ulnar neuropathy. A flexed elbow position increases both the intraneural and extraneural pressure on the nerve. The nerve at the site of repeated compression is associated with fibrous thickening, when a spindle-shaped swelling may be felt. Other possible sources of injury of the ulnar nerve at the elbow include direct compression when the patient uses the arms to raise up in bed following surgical operations (Stewart and Shantz, 2003) or after periods of prolonged unconsciousness. The ulnar nerve at the elbow may be acutely injured as a result of fracture or dislocation involving the lower end of the humerus and the elbow joint. Occasionally, however, the nerve becomes chronically compressed years after such an injury, which often has led to cubitus valgus deformity *("tardy ulnar palsy")*. The nerve may be damaged by osteophyte outgrowths resulting from arthritis of the elbow joint, by a ganglion or lipoma, by a Charcot elbow, and by the epitrochleoanconeus muscle and/or its dense fibrotendinous band. The ulnar nerve may also be involved in conditions that are known to increase the susceptibility of nerves to compression, such as DM or HNPP. Ulnar neuropathy at the elbow segment may also occur without any apparent cause.

Ulnar nerve lesions at the elbow result in numbness and tingling of the little and ring fingers, with variable degrees of hand weakness. Less commonly, patients present with weakness and wasting with no clear sensory symptoms. There is also variable weakness of the flexor carpi ulnaris and the flexor digitorum profundus of the ring and little fingers (ulnar part). Grip strength is reduced secondary to weakness of the adductor pollicis, flexor pollicis brevis, and palmar and dorsal interosseous muscles. To compensate for adductor pollicis weakness during an attempt to pinch a piece of paper between the thumb and index fingers, the flexor pollicis longus, a median nerve-innervated muscle, becomes involuntarily active and flexes the distal phalanx of the thumb *(Froment sign)*. Weakness of the interossei muscles results in an inability to forcefully extend the interphalangeal joints, as is necessary in finger-flicking movements. Prominent atrophy of hand muscles ensues and is most noticeable at the first dorsal interosseous muscle. Lumbrical weakness leads to clawing of the fourth and fifth fingers and flexion of the proximal and distal interphalangeal joints, with secondary hyperextension of the metacarpophalangeal joints *(benediction posture or ulnar clawing)*. Weakness of the third palmar interosseous muscle results in abduction of the little finger, which may get caught when the patient tries to put the hand in a pocket *(Wartenberg sign)*. In chronic ulnar neuropathies, the weakness and atrophy of small muscles of the hand is always more severe than the weakness and atrophy of the forearm muscles. Sensory loss or hypoesthesia involves the fifth finger, part of the fourth finger, and the hypothenar eminence and includes the dorsum of the hand but does not extend above the wrist level. Pain around the elbow and tenderness of the ulnar nerve with deep palpation is common, but distal hand or finger pain is rare. A Tinel sign at the elbow may be elicited, but this sign as well as provocative tests (flexion compression test, palpating for local ulnar nerve tenderness and nerve thickening) have poor diagnostic values (Beekman et al., 2009).

Ulnar nerve lesions at the elbow should be distinguished from ulnar nerve lesions at the wrist, lower brachial plexus lesions (lower trunk or medial cord), and C8 radiculopathy. Confirmed sensory loss that extends more than 3 cm above the wrist into the medial forearm and arm, the territories of the medial brachial and antebrachial cutaneous nerves, is inconsistent with an ulnar neuropathy at the elbow and suggests a more proximal lesion of the lower plexus or C8 or T1 roots. Similarly, weakness of median and radial innervated C8 muscles such as the flexor pollicis longus or the long finger extensors points to a plexopathy or radiculopathy.

Compared to evaluating other entrapment neuropathies such as CTS, the EDX studies used to confirm and localize ulnar nerve entrapment at the elbow are more challenging. Localizing ulnar neuropathy at the elbow relies upon the demonstration of focal demyelination across the elbow, namely slowed motor conduction velocity (>10–15 m/sec) or conduction block (localized reduction in CMAP amplitude and area of >20%–30%) or both. Focal slowing or conduction block may be found in the elbow segment in more than 75% of cases (Azrieli et al., 2003). Performing an additional ulnar motor conduction study, recording the first dorsal interosseous muscle in addition to recording the abductor digiti minimi muscle, increases the yield of finding focal slowing or conduction block. In the remaining patients, localization becomes less precise because of predominant axonal loss. To provide the extra nerve length needed during elbow flexion, the ulnar nerve is anatomically redundant in the ulnar groove when the elbow is extended, and this can cause measurement errors. A flexed position of the elbow (70–90 degrees) is preferred to the extended position when doing ulnar motor conduction studies to localize an ulnar lesion at the elbow.

Reference values to determine absolute across-elbow ulnar motor conduction velocity slowing or relative slowing in across-elbow versus forearm conduction velocities have varied depending on study design and population studied. In addition, the optimal distance for measuring ulnar motor NCV around the flexed elbow continues to be debated between 6 and 10 cm (Logigian et al., 2014). To improve diagnostic accuracy and reduce false-positive and false-negative results, different diagnostic criteria are advocated for patients with different pretest probability of ulnar neuropathy across the elbow (Logigian et al., 2014). Patients with high pre-test probability of ulnar neuropathy across the elbow (i.e., with typical clinical symptoms and signs) should have less stringent diagnostic criteria (for example >14 m/sec velocity difference or <47 m/sec velocity), while those with low pre-test probability of ulnar neuropathy across the elbow (i.e., with atypical or inconsistent clinical symptoms and signs) should have more strict diagnostic criteria (such as >23 m/sec velocity difference and <38 m/sec velocity). Short-segment incremental studies ("inching") by stimulating the ulnar nerve in successive 1- or 2-cm increments across the elbow, looking for either an abrupt drop in amplitude or increase in latency, are useful techniques that help to precisely localize the ulnar nerve lesion (Omejec and Podnar, 2015; Visser et al., 2005). Electrophysiological tests are helpful in differentiating between an ulnar neuropathy and a C8 nerve root or brachial plexus lesion. Ulnar sensory nerve conduction sparing points to C8 radiculopathy and normal needle EMG of C8 muscles innervated by the median nerve (e.g., abductor pollicis brevis, flexor pollicis longus) and radial nerve (e.g., extensor indicis proprius) help exclude a C8 root lesion or a lower brachial plexopathy.

High-resolution ultrasonography at the elbow is also useful by accurately detecting enlargement of the ulnar nerve at the elbow (Beekman et al., 2004). MRI of the elbow may reveal a space-occupying lesion or anomalous structures impinging on the nerve or demonstrate nerve enlargement and increased signal intensity, even in the absence of localizing electrophysiological abnormalities (Vucic et al., 2006).

Conservative treatment should be attempted in patients with mild or intermittent sensory symptoms or in those with symptoms brought on by occupational causes. Avoidance of repetitive elbow flexion and extension or direct pressure on the elbow may alleviate the symptoms. Elbow protectors are helpful in patients with a history of excessive elbow leaning. Conservative treatment should be continued for at least 3 months before surgery is considered. Several surgical approaches to an ulnar nerve lesion at the elbow are possible, each with its proponents and critics. Techniques include simple release of the flexor carpi ulnaris aponeurosis, anterior transposition of the nerve trunk, and resection of the medial epicondyle. The choice of procedure should be tailored to the specific lesion found at surgery and may be assisted by short-segment incremental electrophysiological studies ("inching"). Transposition of the nerve trunk carries a higher rate of complications than ulnar neurolysis (Biggs and Curtis, 2006). Depending on the type of surgery and the severity and duration of neuropathy, response to these procedures will vary. Only about 60% of patients, especially those with symptoms of less than 1 year's duration, benefit from surgery; some experience worsening of symptoms. It appears that those with more thickening of the nerve at the time of diagnosis (as determined by sonography) have a more unfavorable outcome, and those with electrophysiological signs of demyelination across the elbow, specifically significantly greater than 50% conduction block, have a more favorable course (Beekman et al., 2004; Dunselman and Visser et al., 2008).

***Ulnar nerve entrapment at the wrist.*** Distal entrapment of the ulnar nerve at the wrist (Guyon canal) or hand is a relatively uncommon condition. Ulnar nerve entrapment in the Guyon canal occurs much less frequently than at the elbow. Aside from direct trauma and laceration, the most common cause is a ganglion cyst. Other usual causes are chronic or repeated external pressure by hand tools, bicycle handlebars, the handles of canes, or excessive push-ups. Compression also may be caused by degenerative wrist joint changes, rheumatoid arthritis, or distal vascular anomalies.

Ulnar nerve entrapment at the wrist may present with a confusing array of sensory and motor symptoms or both, depending on which branches of the nerve are involved. Most cases of ulnar nerve entrapment at the Guyon canal, however, involve solely motor fibers and present with painless unilateral hypothenar and interossei weakness or atrophy. Because the palmar cutaneous and dorsal cutaneous branches leave the ulnar nerve in the distal forearm and do not enter the Guyon canal, sensation in the proximal hypothenar region and the dorsum of the little and ring fingers is not impaired in all cases of ulnar nerve lesions at the wrist or hand. The sensory loss, if present, is confined to the palmar surface of the ulnar-innervated fingers (the little finger and usually the ulnar half of the ring finger) and the distal hypothenar region. Compression at the distal portion of the Guyon canal (also referred to as the *pisohamate hiatus*) results in selective involvement of the deep motor branch, with interossei weakness and atrophy and complete or relative sparing of the hypothenar muscles as well as sensation (Katirji and Dokko, 1996).

The diagnosis is confirmed by EDX studies, often by demonstrating low amplitude (with or without prolonged distal motor latencies) to the first dorsal interosseous or abductor digiti minimi muscles or both, along with denervation of the ulnar-innervated hand muscles that parallels the clinical manifestations. Ulnar SNAP may or may not be abnormal. These EDX studies are also important in excluding an ulnar neuropathy at the elbow. Several features on the EDX examination are inconsistent with an ulnar neuropathy at the wrist: low amplitude or absent dorsal ulnar SNAP, focal slowing or conduction block across the elbow, or denervation of the flexor carpi ulnaris or the flexor digitorum profundus (ulnar portion).

Plain radiograph of the wrist may reveal a fracture of the pisiform or hook of the hamate bone. Neuromuscular ultrasound or MRI is extremely helpful and may demonstrate a structural lesion such as a ganglion cyst. Sources of occupational or recreational trauma should be eliminated. In patients with fractures, ganglia, or mass lesions, surgical intervention is necessary. The prognosis is usually good after surgical decompression with effective reinnervation.

## Radial Nerve

***Applied anatomy.*** The radial nerve is the largest nerve in the upper extremity. In the arm, lying medial to the humerus, the radial nerve innervates all three heads of the triceps muscle and the anconeus muscle. The nerve passes obliquely behind the humerus and then through the spiral groove, a shallow groove formed deep to the lateral head of the triceps muscle. Before entering the spiral groove in the midarm, it gives three sensory branches: the posterior cutaneous nerve of the arm (which innervates a strip of skin overlying the triceps muscle), the lower lateral cutaneous nerve of the arm (which innervates the lateral half of the arm), and the posterior cutaneous nerve of the forearm (which innervates the skin of the extensor surface of the forearm). In the anterior compartment of the arm, the radial nerve, lying lateral to the humerus, innervates the brachioradialis and the extensor carpi radialis longus. The nerve then passes anterior to the lateral epicondyle and innervates the extensor carpi radialis brevis and supinator. The "radial tunnel" is a space (not an anatomical tunnel) where the radial nerve travels in the upper forearm from the humeroradial joint past the supinator muscle. Within that space, the radial nerve divides into its terminal branches, the superficial radial and posterior interosseous nerves (PINs). The PIN, a terminal pure motor branch, passes under the proximal edge of the supinator muscle *(arcade of Frohse)* and travels in the forearm and innervates all the remaining wrist and finger extensors. The superficial radial nerve is a terminal pure sensory nerve and innervates the skin of the proximal two-thirds of the extensor surfaces of the thumb, index, and middle fingers, and half of the ring finger, along with the corresponding dorsum of the hand.

***Radial nerve compression in the arm.*** Radial nerve compression in the arm often occurs at the spiral groove of the humerus during drunken sleep wherein the arm is draped over a chair *(Saturday-night palsy)* (Spinner et al., 2002). The radial nerve may also be injured following fractures of the humerus. Radial nerve lesions at the axilla are much less common; they may result from misuse of crutches or from the weight of a sleeping partner's head *(honeymoon palsy)* or follow shoulder joint replacement. The radial nerve is also often involved in isolation or in combination with other single nerves in MMN with conduction block.

In radial nerve lesions in the spiral groove or midarm, there is weakness of the brachioradialis, wrist, and finger extensors, while the triceps is spared. Sensory abnormalities may occur over the dorsum of the hand, thumb, index finger, and middle finger. In lesions at the axilla, there is additional weakness of the triceps, and the sensory loss may extend into the extensor surface of the forearm and lateral half of the arm and over to the triceps owing to involvement of the posterior cutaneous nerve of the forearm and the lower lateral cutaneous and posterior cutaneous nerve of the arm.

The EDX studies are essential in confirming the site and extent of the lesion, excluding other causes of wrist drop, and estimating severity and prognosis. Low-amplitude or absent radial SNAP is common except when the pathology at the spiral groove is purely demyelinating. Conduction block across the spiral groove is seen in segmental demyelinating lesions, or the radial motor responses are low in amplitude in axon-loss lesions. Mixed lesions are also common. Needle EMG reveals denervation of all finger and wrist extensors, as well as the extensor carpi radialis and the brachioradialis. The triceps and anconeus are spared in midarm lesions and denervated in axillary lesions. Ultrasonography is a useful additional tool to electrodiagnosis for diagnosing radial neuropathy across the spiral groove. Enlarged radial nerve as determined by CSA above at 5.75 $mm^2$ is a highly specific finding (Song et al., 2018).

As with other peripheral nerve lesions, the prognosis depends on the primary pathology. Radial nerve lesions due to demyelinative conduction block, such as in most cases of Saturday-night palsy, usually improve in 6–8 weeks. Axon-loss lesions such as those often associated with humeral fracture, however, have a less favorable prognosis, with a protracted course and often incomplete recovery.

***Posterior interosseous neuropathy.*** Lesions of the PIN are uncommon and usually occur in association with trauma, fracture, soft-tissue masses (e.g., lipomas, gangliomas), or exuberant synovium motor neuropathy (i.e., rheumatoid arthritis). Occasionally, a PIN lesion, in isolation or in combination with other single nerves is a manifestation of neuralgic amyotrophy, with acute arm pain followed within a few days by weakness (Van Eijk et al., 2015). The clinical manifestations of a PIN lesion are dropped fingers and inability to extend them at the metacarpophalangeal joints. Radial deviation of the wrist on wrist extension is often pathognomonic and is due to weakness of the extensor carpi ulnaris muscle with sparing of the extensor carpi radialis muscle, the latter innervated by the main trunk of the radial nerve. EMG study confirms the diagnosis by demonstrating normal radial SNAP and denervation of the muscles supplied by the PIN, with sparing of more proximal radial-innervated muscles including the brachioradialis, extensor carpi radialis, and triceps muscles.

In rheumatoid arthritis, local injection of corticosteroids may be helpful. If the syndrome is progressive, surgical exploration, including synovectomy or decompression of the PIN, may become necessary (Shergill et al., 2001).

***Radial tunnel syndrome.*** Patients with persistent tennis elbow (lateral epicondylitis) are sometimes given a diagnosis of radial tunnel syndrome, an extremely rare and highly controversial entrapment of the radial nerve or its posterior interosseous branch within the radial tunnel (Rosenbaum, 1999). The nerve appears most vulnerable to entrapment at the level of the supinator muscle. These patients present with forearm pain and tenderness at the lateral epicondyle and slightly distally into the forearm, with no associated muscle weakness or sensory loss in the radial or PIN distribution. Pain is induced by extension of the middle finger or supination with the elbow extended. The EMG study, including radial nerve conduction studies recording the extensor digitorum communis and extensor indicis proprius, is almost always normal. Local steroid injection may temporarily relieve symptoms. In patients with persistent pain, surgical division of the supinator muscle has been advocated, with variable results.

***Superficial radial sensory neuropathy (cheiralgia paresthetica).*** *Cheiralgia paresthetica* is a mononeuropathy of the superficial dorsal sensory branch of the radial nerve. It occurs as a result of trauma from tight wristbands or handcuffs, or may result from intravenous cannulation, fracture of the wrist, or wrist surgery (e.g., plating of forearm bones after fracture). The use of one-way (only tighten) ratcheting mechanism of handcuffs increases the risk of cheiralgia paresthetica (Grant and Cook, 2000). In up to 50% of nontraumatic cases, it is also associated with *de Quervain tenosynovitis*, an inflammatory condition of thumb extensor muscles, predominantly extensor pollicis brevis (Lanzetta and Foucher, 1995). In de Quervain tenosynovitis, there is tenderness of the anatomical snuffbox and thumb extensor tendons with forced ulnar deviation while holding the thumb wrapped in the palm (Finkelstien sign). Paresthesias and pain in the distribution of the superficial sensory branch of the radial nerve characterize this benign self-limiting condition. A small area of hypoesthesia in the dorsoradial aspect of the hand is frequently identified. Nerve conduction study often shows a low-amplitude or absent dorsal radial SNAP with normal needle EMG including all radial innervated muscles.

### Musculocutaneous Nerve

The musculocutaneous nerve arises from the lateral cord of the brachial plexus, with fibers originating from the C5 and C6 roots via the upper trunk. The nerve innervates and penetrates the coracobrachialis muscle and courses down the anterior aspect of the upper arm between the two muscles it innervates—the biceps brachii and brachialis. It then terminates as a sensory nerve, the lateral antebrachial cutaneous nerve, which innervates the lateral forearm to the base of thumb. This nerve may be damaged with shoulder dislocations, following general anesthesia, or with vigorous exercise such as weight lifting or repetitive movements such as occur in carpet carriers, where the nerve is repeatedly compressed by carrying carpets on the shoulder while held in place by the arm (Sander et al., 1997). The musculocutaneous nerve may also be involved in neuralgic amyotrophy (Parsonage-Turner syndrome; Van Eijk et al., 2015). The differential diagnosis includes C5 or C6 radiculopathy, upper trunk or lateral cord brachial plexopathy, and rupture of the biceps tendon.

Clinically, patients with musculocutaneous mononeuropathy present with weakness and atrophy of the biceps brachii and brachialis muscles, diminished biceps brachii reflex, and sensory loss over the lateral aspect of the forearm anteriorly. Nerve conduction studies show reduced musculocutaneous CMAP amplitude recording the biceps muscle and a low-amplitude or absent lateral antebrachial cutaneous sensory response. Needle EMG demonstrates denervation limited to the biceps brachii and brachialis muscles, often sparing the coracobrachialis muscle.

Spontaneous recovery is the rule. Local corticosteroid injection may provide some relief of pain. Surgical decompression is contemplated if no improvement occurs.

### Suprascapular Nerve

The suprascapular nerve is a pure motor branch of the upper trunk of the brachial plexus with innervation from the C5 and C6 roots. It then passes through the suprascapular notch, covered by the transverse scapular ligament, to innervate the supraspinatus muscle. It wraps around the spinoglenoid notch of the scapular spine and innervates the infraspinatus muscle. Entrapment at the suprascapular notch occurs after repetitive forward traction of the shoulders—a condition seen in certain athletes, especially volleyball players. This nerve also may be involved in a restricted form of neuralgic amyotrophy (Parsonage-Turner syndrome, Van Eijk et al., 2015). Diffuse aching pain in the posterior aspect of the shoulder exacerbated by overhead activities is a cardinal symptom. The pain has an articular characteristic because the acromioclavicular joint and surrounding structures are innervated by the suprascapular nerve. Atrophy and weakness are confined to the infraspinatus and supraspinatus muscles. Slow and steady abduction of the arm starting from a vertical position alongside the chest is not possible with a severe lesion of the suprascapular nerve. Tendon ruptures of the rotator cuff have to be considered in the differential diagnosis. EMG shows denervation restricted to the supraspinatus and infraspinatus muscles. Local corticosteroid injection may give temporary relief of pain, although surgery is sometimes required (Antoniou et al., 2001). In entrapment at the spinoglenoid notch, pain is usually absent, and there is atrophy, weakness, and denervation of the infraspinatus muscle only.

### Intercostobrachial Nerve

The intercostobrachial nerve is a cutaneous sensory nerve derived from the second and third thoracic nerve roots. It supplies the skin on the medial surface of the upper arm and axilla, as well as the adjacent chest wall. It may be injured in a modified radical mastectomy and other surgical procedures involving the axilla and lateral pectoral region (Wallace et al., 1996).

### Double Crush Syndrome

When a sizable cohort of patients with EDX evidence of distal upper-limb entrapment neuropathies was found to have either electrophysiological or radiological and clinical evidence of cervical radiculopathy, Upton and McComas proposed that focal compression of single nerve fibers proximally might so alter axoplasmic transport as to render the distal nerve more susceptible to symptomatic entrapment neuropathy (Upton and McComas, 1973). They termed this the *double crush syndrome*. Although the concept of double crush syndrome has since been invoked in a wide variety of entrapment neuropathies, often as an explanation for failure or dissatisfaction with decompressive surgeries of the neck or limb or as a rationale to decompress a nerve in multiple proximal-to-distal sites along its course, this phenomenon is of uncertain validity (Kane et al., 2015; Wilbourn and Gilliatt, 1997).

## Mononeuropathies of the Lower Extremities

Entrapment neuropathies of lower limbs are shown in Table 106.5.

### Sciatic Nerve

***Applied anatomy.*** The sciatic nerve is formed from nerve roots L4 through S3 and is composed of two distinct nerves, the common peroneal (renamed the *fibular nerve* by the Federative Committee on Anatomical Terminology [FCAT], owing to confusion between the terms *peroneal* and *perineal*) and tibial nerves, which share a common sheath from the pelvis to the popliteal fossa. Usually the sciatic nerve emerges from the pelvis by passing beneath the piriformis muscle, but sometimes the fibular division only passes through or above the piriformis muscle. The sciatic nerve innervates all the hamstring muscles via the tibial nerve except the short head of the biceps femoris, which is innervated by the common fibular nerve. The common fibular and tibial nerves separate completely in the upper popliteal fossa or slightly above.

***Sciatic neuropathy at the sciatic notch.*** The sciatic nerve is occasionally vulnerable to entrapment as it crosses over the sciatic notch leaving the pelvis. Most sciatic nerve lesions are complications of hip replacement surgery (Cherian and Li, 2019; Plewnia et al., 1999). Traumatic lesions include bullet and stab wounds, fractures, dislocations, hematomas in the posterior thigh compartment, and misplaced intramuscular injections. Recurrent sciatic mononeuropathy may be caused by endometriosis involving the nerve at the sciatic notch. Direct compression of the sciatic nerve is rare but occasionally occurs during coma, anesthesia, or prolonged sitting on a hard surface (*"toilet seat palsy"*). Either or both divisions of the nerve may be compressed by a Baker cyst in the popliteal fossa.

A complete sciatic nerve lesion results in weakness of knee flexors and all muscles below the knee, as well as sensory loss of the entire foot and leg below the knee except for a region supplied by the saphenous nerve over the medial leg. The fibular division is more commonly involved than the tibial in proximal lesions of the sciatic nerve. Partial sciatic nerve lesions often affect the fibular nerve more than the tibial nerve and may mimic a more distal common fibular neuropathy. This is explained by the fewer fascicles with limited supportive tissue within the fibular nerve, which is also taut and secured at the sciatic notch and fibular neck. In such patients, evidence of denervation in the short head of the biceps femoris and tibialis posterior muscles and abnormal sural or medial plantar SNAPs help localize partial proximal sciatic nerve lesions (Yuen and So, 1999). Occasionally, the common fibular nerve gets injured selectively (Katirji and Wilbourn, 1994). Young age, lack of severe initial weakness, and recordable distal motor or sensory responses are predictors of favorable outcome (Cherian and Li, 2019; Yuen and So, 1999).

***Piriformis syndrome.*** On rare occasions, the piriformis muscle may entrap the sciatic nerve trunk as it passes through or over the piriformis muscle. Since the term was coined in 1947 by Robinson, the *piriformis syndrome* has been subject to controversy (Fishman and Schaeffer, 2003; Stewart, 2003). The syndrome fell out of fashion with the advancement of radiological techniques (myelography, CT, MRI) that often demonstrate that most patients with sciatica have nerve root compression and occasionally lesions of the sacral plexus or sciatic nerve at other locations.

The typical patient with piriformis syndrome has a history of buttock trauma and experiences maximal buttock pain during prolonged sitting (e.g., driving, biking), bending at the waist, or activity that requires hip adduction and internal rotation (e.g., cross-country skiing) (Kirschner et al., 2009). The neurological and EDX examinations are usually normal. A bedside test maneuver in which the hip is placed passively in adduction, internal rotation, and flexion of the hip (*AIF maneuver*) may reproduce the pain and is considered diagnostic. Imaging is usually normal but occasionally shows hypertrophy of the piriformis muscle or abnormal vessels or bands in the region of the

**TABLE 106.5 Entrapment/Compressive Neuropathies of Lower Limbs**

| Nerve | Site of Compression | Predisposing Factors | Major Clinical Features |
|---|---|---|---|
| Sciatic | Sciatic notch | Endometriosis, intramuscular injections | Pain down thigh, flail foot, absent ankle jerk |
| | Hip | Fracture, dislocations | Pain down thigh, flail foot, absent ankle jerk |
| | Piriformis muscle | Remote fall on buttock | Pain on sitting only, no weakness |
| | Popliteal fossa | Popliteal Baker cyst | Normal hamstrings |
| Fibular (Peroneal) | Fibular neck | Weight loss, leg crossing, squatting, intraoperative compression, intraneural ganglion | Foot drop, weak ankle eversion, sensory loss in dorsum of foot |
| | Anterior compartment | Muscle edema | Severe pain. foot drop |
| Tibial | Medial malleolus (tarsal tunnel syndrome) | Ankle fracture, tenosynovitis, high heel shoes | Sensory loss over sole of foot, Tinel sign at flexor retinaculum |
| Femoral | Inguinal ligament | Lithotomy position | Weak knee extension, absent knee jerk |
| | Pelvis | Intraoperative compression (retractor) | Weak hip flexion and knee extension, absent knee jerk |
| Lateral femoral cutaneous | Inguinal ligament (meralgia paresthetica) | Weight gain, diabetes, pregnancy, tight clothing, utility belts | Sensory loss in lateral thigh |
| Ilioinguinal | Abdominal wall | Trauma, surgical incision | Direct hernia, sensory loss in the iliac crest, crural area |
| Obturator | Obturator canal | Tumor, surgery, pelvic fracture | Sensory loss in medial thigh, weak hip adduction |

piriformis muscle. MR neurography may show sciatic nerve hyperintensity at the sciatic notch, a more specific sign of nerve entrapment (Filler et al., 2005). Treatment consists of exercises that include prolonged stretching of the piriformis muscle by flexion, adduction, and internal rotation of the hip. CT- or MRI-guided corticosteroid injection into the piriformis muscle may alleviate the symptoms; a positive response is used as a confirmatory test. Surgical sectioning of the piriformis muscle is indicated in cases resistant to conservative therapy. Although good outcome is expected in carefully selected patients (Filler et al., 2005), severe postoperative sciatic nerve injury was recently reported as a serious complication (Justice et al., 2012).

### Common Fibular (Peroneal) Nerve

***Applied anatomy.*** As noted earlier, the confusing similarity between *peroneal* and *perineal* led FCAT to rename the peroneal nerve the *fibular nerve.* Soon after the sciatic nerve divides close to the popliteal fossa, the common fibular nerve gives off the lateral cutaneous nerve of the calf, which innervates the skin over the upper third of the lateral aspect of the leg, and the fibular communicating nerve which joins the sural nerve. The common fibular nerve then winds around the fibular neck and passes through the origin of the peroneus longus muscle ("fibular tunnel"). Near that point, the common fibular nerve divides into its terminal branches, the deep and superficial fibular nerves. The deep fibular nerve traverses the lateral and then anterior leg compartments and innervates the tibialis anterior, extensor hallucis longus, peroneus tertius, and extensor digitorum longus. It then divides close to the ankle joint to innervate the extensor digitorum brevis and the skin of the web space between the first and second toes. The superficial fibular nerve innervates the peroneus longus and brevis and the skin of the lower two-thirds of the lateral aspect of the leg and the dorsum of the foot (except for the first web space). An accessory deep fibular nerve, seen in up to 28% of individuals, arises from the superficial fibular nerve, passes behind the lateral malleolus, and innervates the lateral part of the extensor digitorum brevis.

***Common fibular (peroneal) neuropathy at the fibular neck.*** Compression of the common fibular nerve is the most frequent compressive neuropathy in the lower extremity. This nerve is particularly vulnerable to direct pressure in the region of the fibular neck as it passes through the origin of the peroneus longus muscle. Intraoperative compression due to improper positioning or padding during anesthesia is the leading cause of acute common fibular neuropathy at the fibular neck (Katirji and Wilbourn, 1988). Weight loss, habitual leg crossing, or unrecognized pressure on the nerve in hospitalized critically ill, debilitated, or unconscious patients may also be responsible for this nerve injury (Aprile et al., 2005; Katirji, 1999). Devices that may compress the fibular nerve include casts, orthoses, pneumatic compression, antithrombotic stockings, bandages, and straps. Fibular nerve stretch injury may result from an acute forceful foot inversion or prolonged squatting (strawberry pickers palsy). Blunt trauma (e.g., post fibular fracture, knee dislocation) and open injury (e.g., lacerations) account for a significant number of cases. Postpartum peroneal neuropathy may be due to stirrups compression, prolonged squatting, or direct hand compression. Fibular nerve injury is also a known complication of knee surgery, including arthroscopic surgery and lateral meniscus repair. Up to half of patients without a clear cause of fibular mononeuropathy across the fibular head have intraneural ganglia (Young et al., 2009). These are formed when disruption of the capsule of the superior tibiofibular joint results in dissection of synovial fluid along the articular branch of the fibular nerve into the tibialis anterior motor branch (Hebert-Blouin et al., 2010). Other mass lesions such as osteochondromas or schwannomas are much less common.

A common fibular nerve lesion leads to weakness of foot and toe extension and foot eversion, with a foot drop and steppage gait. Sensory impairment is found over the lateral aspect of the lower two-thirds of the leg and the dorsum of the foot. Foot eversion and sensory loss may be spared (except for the first web space of the foot) when the lesion is selective, involving the deep fibular nerve. Pain is rare except with intraneural ganglia.

Fibular mononeuropathy is most often confused with other causes of unilateral foot drop, including L5 radiculopathy, sciatic nerve lesions (especially when predominantly affecting the common fibular nerve), and lumbosacral plexopathy (particularly when involving the lumbosacral trunk). A fibular nerve lesion must be differentiated from *anterior tibial compartment syndrome*, in which the deep fibular nerve is compressed by muscle swelling within the anterior compartment secondary to injury, heavy exercise, trauma, or ischemia. This results in an acute syndrome of severe lower leg pain, swelling, and weakness of foot and toe extensors. The anterior tibial compartment must be decompressed rapidly by fasciotomy to prevent irreversible nerve and muscle damage.

EDX studies are useful for localizing lesions and may provide clues to the underlying cause and a guide to prognosis. Although it is often possible by nerve conduction studies to demonstrate focal conduction block across the fibular head, contrary to common belief, the most frequent pathophysiological process is axonal loss, regardless of the cause (Katirji and Wilbourn, 1988). Axon-loss lesions reveal diffusely low or absent fibular motor and sensory amplitudes. In contrast to ulnar lesions across the elbow and CTS, localized slowing in the region of the fibular head is not common. Needle EMG demonstrates denervation in common fibular-innervated muscles but not in the short head of the biceps femoris (innervated by the common fibular division of the sciatic nerve in the thigh), in the L5 nerve root-innervated muscles, such as the tibialis posterior, flexor digitorum longus, tensor fascia lata and gluteus medius, or the low lumbar paraspinal muscles.

Ultrasound and MRI are effective in visualizing intraneural ganglia and other soft-tissue masses or tumors. Ultrasound is slightly more accurate than MRI in compressive fibular neuropathies (Bignotti et al., 2017). It shows thickened fibular nerve (cross-sectional area >8 $mm^2$) in about 70% of patients (Visser et al., 2013), and establishes involvement of the anterior fascicles (corresponding to fibers for the deep fibular nerve) in the majority of compressive fibular neuropathies (Bignotti et al., 2016).

The prognosis is uniformly good in cases of acute demyelinating lesions, whereas recovery is delayed in those with axonal lesions and stretch injuries. The distal fibular motor amplitude recording tibialis anterior serves as an accurate estimate of the extent of axonal loss and a good prognostic indicator of foot drop. Hence, fibular nerve studies should be performed bilaterally and compared. Bracing with a custom-made plastic ankle-foot orthosis is necessary to improve the gait in the presence of severe foot drop. The few patients who do not improve spontaneously after 3 months, or those who have pain or a slowly progressive fibular nerve lesion, may require MRI studies and surgical exploration (Kim and Kline, 1996).

### Tibial Nerve

***Applied anatomy.*** The tibial nerve innervates all the hamstring muscles except the short head of the biceps femoris. It then separates from the common fibular nerve, usually in the upper popliteal fossa, and gives off the sural sensory nerve, which is often joined by a branch from the common fibular nerve, the sural communicating nerve, to innervate the skin over the lateral aspect of the lower leg and foot, including the little toe. In the upper calf, the tibial nerve passes underneath the soleus muscle and innervates the gastrocnemius, soleus, tibialis posterior, flexor digitorum profundus, and flexor hallucis longus. At the ankle, the tibial nerve passes under the laciniate ligament, which covers the tarsal tunnel through which the nerve passes together with the tendons of the tibialis posterior, flexor digitorum longus, and flexor hallucis longus muscles and the tibial artery and veins.

***Tarsal tunnel syndrome.*** Entrapment of the tibial nerve occurs behind and immediately below the medial malleolus. Burning pain is experienced in the toes and the sole of the foot. If the calcaneal sensory branches are involved, pain and numbness also involve the heel. Examination usually reveals plantar sensory impairment and wasting of the intrinsic foot muscles. Percussion at the site of nerve compression or eversion of the foot often elicit pain and paresthesias. EDX study results should confirm entrapment of the tibial nerve at the tarsal tunnel by demonstrating slowing of motor fibers to the abductor hallucis and/or abductor digiti minimi muscles, as well as involvement of the medial and/or lateral plantar mixed potentials fibers, with sparing of the sural nerve sensory action potential. Unfortunately, medial and/or lateral plantar mixed (or sensory) potentials are technically very difficult and may be unelicitable in normal subjects with plantar calluses, foot edema, previous surgical procedures in the foot, or in adults over the age of 45. Needle EMG shows denervation of the abductor hallucis and/or abductor digiti minimi muscles and normal S1-innervated and proximal muscles such as the gastrocnemius, soleus, biceps femoris, and gluteus maximus muscles. The majority of suspected cases of tarsal tunnel syndrome, particularly when symptoms are bilateral, turn out to have generalized peripheral neuropathy, S1 radiculopathy, or non-neurological foot pain such as plantar fasciitis, stress fracture, arthritis, or bursitis. Ultrasound plays an important role in identifying the cause (Samarawickrama et al., 2016). This is particularly useful in elderly or patients with foot edema, calluses, or previous surgery as EDX studies may be difficult to perform or interpret.

Local injection with corticosteroids underneath the laciniate ligament may temporarily relieve symptoms. Surgical decompression is needed for permanent results in those rare cases in which objective evidence of this syndrome exists.

### Sural Nerve

Although the vast majority of sural nerve lesions are iatrogenic as the result of diagnostic sural nerve biopsy or sural nerve harvesting for nerve grafts, mononeuropathy of the sural nerve has been reported with a number of other conditions including lower-limb vein-stripping surgery, ankle liposuction, Baker cyst or ankle joint surgery, local trauma such as with tightly laced high-topped footwear such as ski boots or ice skates, and rarely as the initial presentation of vasculitic mononeuritis multiplex (Li and Lederman, 2014; Stickler et al., 2006; Thammongkolchai and Katirji, 2017).

### Femoral Nerve

***Applied anatomy.*** The femoral nerve is formed in the pelvis from the posterior divisions of the ventral rami of L2, L3, and L4 spinal roots, where it innervates the psoas muscle. It then passes within the iliacus compartment and innervates the iliacus muscle via a motor branch that originates 4–5 cm before the nerve crosses underneath the inguinal ligament. In the anterior thigh, the femoral nerve innervates the quadriceps and sartorius muscles and the skin of the anterior thigh and gives off the saphenous sensory nerve, which innervates the skin of the medial surface of the knee and medial leg.

***Femoral nerve lesions.*** The majority of femoral nerve lesions are iatrogenic (Al-Hakim and Katirji, 1993). Pelvic lesions follow a variety of gastrointestinal, vascular, urological, or gynecological operations such as abdominal hysterectomy, radical prostatectomy, renal transplantation, and abdominal aortic repair. During these procedures, the femoral nerve becomes compressed between the lateral blade of the retractor and the pelvic wall. Risk factors include the use of self-retaining retractors, a thin body habitus, and transverse abdominal incision (Chan and Manetta, 2002). Acute retroperitoneal hematoma is often iatrogenic following anticoagulant therapy, pelvic operations, or femoral vessel catheterization such as for cardiac catheterization. At the inguinal ligament, the femoral nerve may become kinked during lithotomy positioning, particularly when the leg is held in extreme hip flexion and external rotation, used during vaginal delivery, vaginal hysterectomy, prostatectomy, and laparoscopy. Total hip replacement, particularly surgical revisions and complicated reconstructions, may result in femoral nerve injury.

Femoral nerve injury due to spontaneous retroperitoneal hematoma may occur in hemophiliacs, patients with blood dyscrasias, or following a ruptured abdominal aortic aneurysm. Pelvic lymphadenopathy, primary malignancy of the colon or rectum, and neurofibromas or schwannomas are rare causes of femoral neuropathies. Hip hyperextension, such as in dancers or during Yoga exercise, may also cause a femoral stretch injury.

Femoral nerve lesions manifest with acute thigh weakness and anterior thigh and medial leg numbness. Thigh weakness often leads to falls. Pain is usually absent except in cases due to retroperitoneal hematomas. On examination, there is weakness of knee extension, with absent or depressed knee jerk. Thigh adduction is normal. Hip flexion is usually weak when the lesion is within the pelvis, although it may be difficult to assess hip flexion in the setting of severe quadriceps weakness.

Needle EMG reveals denervation of the quadriceps muscle. The iliacus muscle is often normal in inguinal lesions but shows denervation in femoral nerve lesions in the pelvis. Needle EMG of the thigh adductor muscles, innervated by the L2, L3, L4 roots via the obturator nerve, helps distinguish femoral nerve lesions from upper lumbar radiculopathy or plexopathy. Nerve conduction studies have prognostic value, since the amplitude and area of the femoral CMAP is a very good quantitative measure of motor axonal loss (Kuntzer et al., 1997). CT or MRI of the pelvis are urgently indicated in patients with suspected retroperitoneal hematoma or pelvic mass lesion.

Apart from patients with confirmed retroperitoneal hematoma who may require emergent drainage, most other femoral nerve lesions are treated conservatively. A knee or knee-ankle-foot orthosis is helpful for patients with unilateral severe weakness of the quadriceps and will assist in walking and prevent falls. Prevention of femoral nerve injury is of paramount importance. The surgeon should limit hip flexion, abduction, and external rotation during lithotomy positioning, particularly when "candy cane" stirrups are used. The incidence of femoral nerve lesions after pelvic and gynecological operations is significantly reduced when self-retractors are avoided; the retracting blades should also cradle the rectus muscle without compressing the psoas muscle (Chan and Manetta, 2002).

### Saphenous Nerve

Saphenous nerve lesions may follow stripping of a long saphenous varicose vein, harvesting the vein for a coronary artery bypass, or surgical and arthroscopic operations on the knee. Entrapment of the saphenous nerve is rare and may occur as it exits the subsartorial (adductor or Hunter) canal or by pes anserine bursitis. Patients with saphenous mononeuropathy have sensory loss or hyperesthesia of the medial leg that may extend into the medial arch of the foot.

Saphenous nerve lesions should be differentiated from L4 radiculopathy, lumbar plexopathy, and femoral mononeuropathy. In addition to the clinical examination, EDX studies can confirm that the quadriceps, iliacus, and thigh adductors are normal in patients with saphenous nerve lesions. Saphenous SNAP is often unilaterally absent or low in amplitude, but this response is difficult to elicit, particularly in elderly or obese patients. Saphenous nerve lesions improve spontaneously with time; decompression underneath the subsartorial canal is occasionally performed.

### Other Lower-Extremity Mononeuropathies

***Lateral femoral cutaneous nerve entrapment (meralgia paresthetica).*** The lateral femoral cutaneous nerve, which is a pure sensory nerve, passes medial to the anterior superior iliac spine under the inguinal ligament to enter the thigh under the fascia lata that it penetrates to supply the skin of the anterolateral part of the thigh. The site of entrapment is usually at the level of the inguinal ligament. Rarely, the nerve may be affected in its proximal segment by retroperitoneal tumors or be injured during appendectomy. The disorder occurs in about 4 per 10,000 individuals. It is most often seen in association with obesity, diabetes, and advancing age (Parisi et al., 2011). It is a common entrapment neuropathy during pregnancy, particularly the third trimester, and usually recovers after delivery. It may occur with ascites, or in other conditions that increase intraabdominal pressure. Direct compression by a belt, corset, beeper, or cellular phone; fracture of the anterior portion of the ilium; or pelvic tilt causing undue stresses on the abdominal musculature are other causes.

Patients develop numbness, painful burning, and itching over the anterolateral thigh. Pressure at the inguinal ligament medial to the anterior superior iliac spine may elicit referred pain and dysesthesias. Some patients report relief of pain when assuming a supine position.

Lateral femoral cutaneous nerve SNAP is technically difficult to measure and may be absent in healthy subjects, particularly women and obese individuals. Asymmetrical low-amplitude or absent potential on the symptomatic side is a confirmatory finding. Electrophysiological studies of the femoral nerve and quadriceps femoris and iliacus muscles are normal, which helps exclude lumbar radiculopathy and plexopathy. A local anesthetic nerve block may have diagnostic value (Haim et al., 2006). Treatment consists of symptomatic measures such as rest, analgesics, and weight loss. Postural abnormalities should be corrected. Neurolysis is rarely beneficial.

***Ilioinguinal neuropathy.*** The ilioinguinal nerve is analogous to an intercostal nerve. Muscle branches innervate the lower portion of the transverse abdominal and internal oblique muscles. The cutaneous sensory nerve supplies the skin over the inguinal ligament and the base of the scrotum or labia. As the nerve takes a zigzag course, passing through the transverse abdominal and internal oblique muscles, it is subject to mechanical compression such as with a direct inguinal hernia. Trauma, surgical procedures, scar tissue, and increased abdominal muscle tone caused by abnormal posture are frequently responsible. Pain is referred to the groin, and weakness of the lower abdominal wall may result in the formation of an asymmetrical bulging of the lower abdominal wall.

Conservative treatment includes rest and NSAIDs. Neurolysis may be required in refractory cases when a mechanical lesion is suspected.

***Obturator neuropathy.*** The obturator nerve is vulnerable to entrapment as it passes through the obturator canal (e.g., by an obturator hernia or osteitis pubis). An obturator neuropathy is most often associated with pelvic malignancies (prostate, cervical, or uterine cancers). It can also be seen with trauma and synovial cyst of the hip or as a surgical complication, especially with extensive retroperitoneal surgeries or laparoscopic pelvic lymphadenectomies and during total hip replacement.

Entrapment produces radiating pain from the groin down the inner aspect of the thigh, often difficult to distinguish from the pain of a recent procedure or trauma. There is weakness of hip adduction and sensory impairment in the upper medial thigh. Many patients appear to have hip-flexor weakness as a false localizing sign. Although this phenomenon may be explained by pain, it is more likely due to mechanical disadvantage of the hip flexors in the presence of weak thigh adductors. CT or MRI scanning of the pelvis is helpful in finding primary or metastatic pelvic tumors. EMG testing is essential for diagnosis by detecting selective denervation of the thigh adductor muscles, with normal quadriceps and iliacus muscles, thus excluding other causes of hip weakness including femoral nerve lesions, upper lumbar (L2, L3, or L4) radiculopathy or plexopathy, and diabetic amyotrophy (diabetic proximal neuropathy or radiculoplexopathy) (Sorenson et al., 2002).

This entrapment neuropathy is treated conservatively, which often provides good results, especially in those with acute onset of symptoms. If such treatment fails or if symptoms progress to involve other nerves in the region, a careful search for occult pelvic or retroperitoneal malignancy must be pursued.

### Migrant Sensory Neuritis of Wartenberg

In this rarely reported but not uncommon condition, a pure and relapsing-remitting sensory mononeuritis multiplex is associated with loss of sensation and pain in the distribution of the affected nerves. The onset is usually sudden, and pain is precipitated by movements and (especially) stretching of the affected limbs. Many different cutaneous nerves may be involved. Commonly involved nerves include the superficial and deep peroneal sensory nerves, the median and ulnar digital nerves, the femoral and saphenous nerves, and the radial sensory nerve (Nicolle et al., 2001). Motor nerve fibers are not affected. Laboratory tests fail to detect any underlying cause, but on occasion a sural nerve biopsy demonstrates inflammatory changes or a vasculitis, with patchy loss of nerve fibers and evidence of axonal degeneration suggestive of an ischemic process. Rarely, immunoglobulin (Ig) G deposits are also observed around blood vessels. The pain and areas of sensory loss often recover over weeks to months, but the improvement may be partial. Symptoms may recur at the same or other sites. The discrete areas of sensory deficit and nerve irritation in several cutaneous nerves should indicate the proper diagnosis. The differential diagnosis should always include conditions like DM, leprosy, vasculitis, sarcoidosis, sensory perineuritis, and rarely HNPP (Nicolle et al., 2001; Zifko and Hahn, 1997).

### Localized Perineurial Hypertrophic Mononeuropathy

A slowly progressive painless mononeuropathy that cannot be localized to entrapment sites and is caused by a focal fusiform enlargement of the affected nerve, termed *localized hypertrophic neuropathy* or *perineurioma*, is an uncommon condition affecting young adults (Simmons et al., 1999). Although any nerve may be involved, it often occurs in the radial, posterior interosseous, tibial, and sciatic nerves. The fusiform enlargement is mainly composed of "onion bulblike whorls" formed by layers of perineurial cells. The lamellae of the whorls stain for epithelial membrane antigen. The cause of the perineurial cell proliferation is unknown. It typically results in painless, slowly progressive weakness and atrophy in the distribution of the affected nerve. Sensory symptoms are minor, although sensory nerve fibers are obviously involved. EDX study shows an axonal mononeuropathy and help in the precise localization of the focal nerve lesion. MRI shows a focal enlargement of the affected nerve, increased signal on T2-weighted images, and enhancement with gadolinium.

Surgical exploration and a fascicular biopsy by a surgeon experienced in peripheral nerve microsurgery may confirm the diagnosis and exclude malignant peripheral nerve sheath tumors, which are difficult to exclude without biopsy. Surgical resection of the involved nerve segment with graft repair has been proposed, but because of the benign nature of the "tumor" and its very slow progression, the involved nerve should be preserved if it has even partial function.

## HEREDITARY NEUROPATHIES

The hereditary neuropathies constitute a complex heterogeneous group of diseases that usually share the clinical features of insidious onset and indolent course over years to decades. The number of hereditary disorders for which a metabolic or molecular defect is known is rapidly increasing, allowing a more accurate classification. For those inherited neuropathies for which the underlying genetic abnormality has yet to be identified, the classification still depends on the clinical phenotype, mode of inheritance, and class of neurons predominantly affected. Major advances in understanding the molecular basis of inherited neuropathies have come from identifying chromosomal loci or causative genes for a given disease phenotype, leading to identification of an ever-increasing number of genes coding for a specific gene product essential to myelin or axonal function (Bassam, 2014; Berger et al., 2002; Fridman and Reilly, 2015; Kamholz et al., 2000; Scherer, 2006).

Hereditary neuropathies are common disorders, accounting for nearly 40% of chronic polyneuropathies, and as many as 50% of previously unidentified peripheral polyneuropathies. Their inherited nature may go unrecognized in a surprisingly large percentage of patients (Klein, 2007). Eliciting historical evidence of long-standing neuromuscular symptoms; obtaining detailed family histories; looking for skeletal abnormalities such as hammer toes, high arches, or scoliosis; performing neurological and electrophysiological evaluations in relatives of patients; and, more importantly, testing for confirmed genes are essential in identifying a previously unsuspected inherited neuropathy. Because of the paucity of positive symptoms, patients may not volunteer information about their own or relatives' conditions. For example, paresthesias are spontaneously reported three times more commonly in acquired than in inherited neuropathies. Even in the face of a truly negative family history, the possibility of an inherited neuropathy cannot be dismissed. Such a situation may arise in cases of early death of one or both parents, few blood relatives, or autosomal recessive (AR) disease. Also, available diagnostic deoxyribonucleic acid (DNA) testing has shown that about a third of isolated cases of inherited neuropathies may arise from de novo gene mutations (Boerkoel et al., 2002). It is advisable to consider the possibility of an inherited neuropathy in any patient with a chronic polyneuropathy that remains cryptogenic or refractory to treatment.

### Charcot-Marie-Tooth Disease (Hereditary Motor and Sensory Neuropathy)

The syndrome of peroneal muscular atrophy, or CMT disease, was first described in 1886 by Charcot and Marie in Paris and Tooth in London (Charcot and Marie, 1886; Tooth, 1886). CMT disease is the most common inherited neuropathy, with an estimated prevalence of 1 per 2500 individuals (Martyn and Hughes, 1997).

Major advances have been made in recent years in the molecular genetics of CMT disease (Bennett and Chance, 2001; Berger et al., 2002; Kamholz et al., 2000). Mutations in more than 80 genes cause CMT (Inherited Neuropathy Variant Browser: http://hihg.med.miami.edu/neuropathybrowser). These mutations in CMT affect proteins involved in Schwann cell membrane structure (PMP22, MPZ, Cx32) mitochondrial movement (MFN2), signal transduction (GDAP1), cell cycle (MTMR2), cytoskeleton (NEFL, INF2, gigaxonin), transcription factors (EGR2), and protein degradation (LITAF/SIMPLE).

CMT may be classified by mode of inheritance (autosomal dominant [AD], X-linked [XL], and AR), electrophysiological studies, chromosomal locus, or causative genes (Table 106.6). CMT1 and the vast majority of subtypes of CMT2 display AD inheritance. A minority of cases occur sporadically or in siblings only and have therefore been attributed to AR inheritance or to de novo gene mutations. Because a great variability in clinical expression exists among affected kin in the dominant disorders, a recessive inheritance can only be accepted if the clinical and electrophysiological examinations of both parents have proved to be normal. Even when the cause is nonparental, most of these patients phenotypically resemble CMT1.

The majority of CMT neuropathies are demyelinating, although up to one-third are primary axonal disorders. Clinical studies combined with electrophysiological studies of a large number of families allowed a simple separation of CMT into two main groups: (1) *the demyelinating form, or CMT1* (sometimes known as hereditary motor and sensory neuropathy [HMSN-I]), in which there are marked reductions in motor NCVs and nerve biopsy findings of demyelination and onion bulb formation; and (2) *the axonal form, or CMT2* (HMSN-II), in which motor NCVs are normal or near normal, and nerve biopsy reveals axonal loss without prominent demyelination (Harding, 1995). A more severe phenotype of severe demyelinating polyneuropathy with onset occurring in early childhood and very slow conduction velocities (<10 m/sec in forearm) is referred to as *Dejerine-Sottas disease* (DSD). DSD, formerly CMT3, may no longer be a useful designation because it is genetically heterogeneous, caused by different structural myelin protein and transcription factor gene mutations. A CMT phenotype without sensory involvement on either clinical or electrophysiological examination has been classified as *hereditary motor neuropathy* or *hereditary distal spinal muscular atrophy*.

More recent discoveries and phenotype-genotype correlations have identified patients with CMT and intermediate conduction velocities with X-linked inheritance (CMTX), thus revising the electrophysiological classification of patients with suspected CMT. These are now divided into at least four groups based on *forearm (ulnar or median) motor conduction velocities*: *Group 1* are patients with velocities ranging from *15 to 35 m/sec*, with the majority diagnosed as CMT1 (mostly CMT1A); *Group 2* are patients with normal or near-normal velocities *(>45 m/sec)*, with most patients diagnosed as CMT2; *Group 3* are patients with intermediate velocities *(35–45 m/sec)*, diagnosed as CMTX, but also sometimes CMT1; and *Group 4* are patients with extremely slow velocities *(<15 m/sec)*, many presenting in early childhood as DSD phenotype and others presenting in adolescence or early adulthood as CMT1 phenotype.

The classification of CMT remains fluid and continues to change as experts alter and revise these designations based on new molecular findings. The classification of CMT subtypes based on alphabet has become unwieldy as the number of genes and mutations have increased steadily; most neurologists, including specialists in neuromuscular medicine and neurogenetics, do not memorize this nomenclature. In addition, recent studies have confirmed that the same gene defect may manifest as different phenotypes. For example, mutations in MPZ causes AD demyelinating CMT1B as well AD axonal varieties (CMT2I/J). A recent proposal is to abandon the cumbersome numerical designation of CMT subtypes and precisely identify the disorder by using the mode of inheritance (AD, AR, X), electrophysiological hallmark (De, Ax, In), and name of the gene (Magy et al., 2018; Mathis et al., 2015). For example CMT1A would be named as AD-CMTDe-PMP22dup (i.e., AD CMT, demyelinating due to PMP22 duplication). Similarly, CMT2A would be AD-CMTAx-MFN2 (AD CMT, axonal due to MFN2 mutation) and CMTX would be XL-CMTIn-GJB1 (X-linked CMT, intermediate due to GJB1 mutation).

#### Charcot-Marie-Tooth Disease Type 1

In CMT1, symptoms often begin during the first or second decade of life. It is characterized by slowly progressive weakness, muscular wasting, and sensory impairment predominantly involving the distal legs. Foot deformities and difficulties in running or walking resulting from

**TABLE 106.6 Molecular Genetic Classification of Charcot-Marie-Tooth Disease and Related Disorders.**

| Disorder | Locus | Gene | Mechanism | Testing Available |
|---|---|---|---|---|
| **CMT1** | | | | |
| CMT1A | 17p11.2 | PMP22 | Duplication > pm | Yes |
| CMT1B | 1q22-q23 | MPZ | Pm | Yes |
| CMT1C | 16p13.1 | LITAF | Pm | Yes |
| CMT1D | 10q21 | EGR2 | Pm | Yes |
| CMT1E | 17p11.2 | PMP22 | Pm | Yes |
| CMT1F | 8p21 | NEFL | Pm | Yes |
| **CMTX** | | | | |
| CMTX1 | Xq13.1 | GJB1 (Cx32) | Pm | Yes |
| CMTX4 | Xq24 | AIFM1 | Pm | Yes |
| CMTX5 | Xq22.3 | PRPS1 | Pm | Yes |
| CMTX6 | Xq22.11 | PDK3 | Pm | Yes |
| **CMT2** | | | | |
| CMT2A2 | 1p36.22 | MFN2 | Pm | Yes |
| CMT2A1 | 1p36.22 | KIFBβ | Pm | — |
| CMT2B | 3q21.3 | RAB7 | Pm | Yes |
| CMT2B1 | 1q22 | LMNA | Pm | Yes |
| CMT2B2 | 19q13.33 | MED25 | Pm | Yes |
| CMT2C | 12q24 | TRPV4 | Pm | Yes |
| CMT2D | 7p15 | GARS | Pm | Yes |
| CMT2E | 8p21 | NEFL | Pm | Yes |
| CMT2F | 7q11-21 | HSPB1 | Pm | Yes |
| CMT2I | 1q23.3 | MPZ | Pm | Yes |
| CMT2J | 1q23.3 | MPZ | Pm | Yes |
| CMT2K | 8q21.11 | GDAP1 | Pm | Yes |
| **HNPP** | | | | |
| HNPP | 17p11.2 | PMP22 | Deletion > pm | Yes |
| **DSD Phenotype** | | | | |
| DSD-A | 17p11.2 | PMP22 | Pm | Yes |
| DSD-B | 1q22-q23 | MPZ | Pm | Yes |
| DSD-C | 10q21-q22 | EGR2 | Pm | Yes |
| **AR CMT (CMT4)** | | | | |
| CMT4A | 8q21 | GDAP1 | Pm | Yes |
| CMT4B1 | 11q22 | MTMR2 | Pm | — |
| CMT4B2 | 11p15.4 | SBF2 | Pm | Yes |
| CMT4C | 5q23-q33 | SH3TC2 | Pm | Yes |
| CMT4D | 8q24 | NDRG1 | Pm | Yes |
| CMT4E | 10q21-q22 | EGR2 | Pm | Yes |
| CMT4F | 19q13 | Periaxin | Pm | Yes |
| CMT4G | 10q23 | HK1 | Pm | — |
| CMT4H | 12q11.1-q13.11 | FGD4 | Pm | — |
| CMT4J | 6q21 | FIGURE4 | Pm | Yes |

*AIFM1*, Apoptosis-inducing factor, mitochondria-associated, 1; *AR*, autosomal recessive; *CMT*, Charcot-Marie-Tooth disease; *CMTX*, X-linked CMT; *Cx32*, connexin-32; *DSD*, Dejerine-Sottas disease; *EGR2*, early growth response 2 gene; *FGD4*, FYVE, RhoGEF, and PH domain-containing protein 4; *FIGURE4*, factor-induced gene 4 protein (polyphosphoinositide phosphatase); *GARS*, glycyl tRNA synthetase; *GDAP1*, ganglioside-induced differentiation-associated protein 1; *HK1*, hexokinase 1; *HNPP*, hereditary neuropathy with liability to pressure palsies; *HSPB1*, *HSPB8*, heat shock proteins; *KIF1Bβ*, microtube motor KIF1Bβ; *LITAF*, lipopolysaccharide-induced tumor necrosis factor-α factor; *LMNA*, Lamin A/C; *Med25*, Mediator complex subunit 25; *MFN2*, Mitofusin 2; *MPZ*, myelin protein zero gene; *MTMR2*, myotubularin-related protein 2; *NDRG1*, N-myc downstream regulated gene 1; *NEFL*, neurofilament light chain gene; *PDK3*, pyruvate dehydrogenase kinase, isoenzyme 3; *pm*, point mutations; *PMP22*, peripheral myelin protein-22; *PRPS1*, phosphoribosylpyrophosphate synthetase 1; *RAB7*, RAS associated protein 7; *SH3TC2*, SH3 domain and tetratricopeptide repeats-containing protein 2.

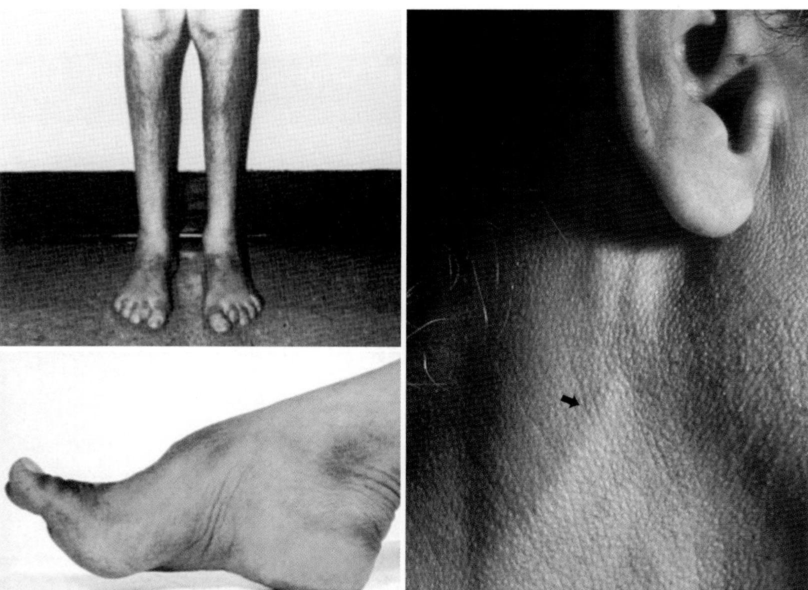

**Fig. 106.8** Leg atrophy, pes cavus, and enlarged great auricular nerve *(arrow)* are evident in a patient with Charcot-Marie-Tooth type 1 disease.

symmetrical weakness and wasting in the intrinsic foot, peroneal, and anterior tibial muscles are often present. In two-thirds of patients, the upper limbs are involved later in life. Inspection reveals pes cavus and hammer toes in nearly 75% of adult patients, mild kyphosis in approximately 10%, and palpably enlarged hypertrophic peripheral nerves in 25% of patients (Fig. 106.8). The foot deformities occur because of long-term muscular weakness and imbalance between the intrinsic extensor and long extensor muscles of the feet and toes (a similar process causes clawing of the fingers in more advanced cases). Absent ankle reflexes are universal and frequently associated with absent or reduced knee and upper limb reflexes. Some degree of distal sensory impairment (diminished vibration sense and light touch in the feet and hands) is usually discovered by examination but rarely gives rise to positive sensory symptoms. Occasionally, patients have an essential or postural upper-limb tremor. Such cases have been referred to as *Roussy-Lévy syndrome*, but current evidence suggests that this is not a separate clinical or genetic entity.

Severity of neuropathy in affected family members varies considerably. Approximately 10% of patients with slowed NCVs may remain asymptomatic. In women with CMT1, the disease may exacerbate during pregnancy. Such worsening is temporary in about a third of patients but becomes progressive in the remainder. Slow deterioration in strength and decline in axonal function continues throughout adulthood, although much of this deterioration likely represents the effects of aging superimposed on decreased reserves (Verhamme et al., 2009).

SNAPs are usually absent with surface recordings. Motor nerve conduction studies show uniform slowing to less than 75% of the lower limits of normal in all nerves. Motor conduction velocities of upper-limb nerves prove more useful than studies of lower-extremity nerves because distal denervation in the feet is often severe and sometimes complete. A motor conduction velocity below 35 m/sec in the forearm segment of the median or ulnar nerves is a proposed cutoff value to distinguish CMT1 from CMT2 and CMTX. Although this cutoff is useful, it can be misleading if applied too rigidly. The conduction slowing evolves over the first 5 years of age and does not change appreciably afterward. Neurological deficits correlate with reductions in CMAP and SNAP amplitudes rather than conduction velocity, indicating that clinical weakness results from loss of axons.

Uniform conduction slowing is often used to differentiate CMT1 from acquired demyelinating neuropathies. Uniform slowing along the entire length of nerves and among neighboring nerves suggests an inherited myelinopathy affecting conduction in all nerves and nerve segments in the upper extremities or lower extremities to the same degree. In contrast, acquired demyelinating neuropathies result in multifocal or nonuniform conduction slowing together with excessive temporal dispersions and conduction blocks. Uniform conduction slowing is found in CMT1A with PMP22 duplication or point mutations; CMT1B with MPZ point mutations; DSD phenotype, including PMP22, MPZ, and EGR2 gene mutations; as well as metachromatic leukodystrophy (MLD); Cockayne disease; and globoid cell (Krabbe) leukodystrophy (Lewis et al., 2000).

Neuromuscular ultrasound in adults and children with CMT1 displays significantly larger nerve CSA compared with control (Zaidman et al., 2013). Nerve enlargement is commonly diffuse and more pronounced than in acquired demyelinating polyneuropathies (such as CIDP and MMN), where the enlargement is often regional. In children with CMT1A, the CSA correlates with neurological disability and the expected increase in nerve CSA with age is disproportionately greater in CMT1A, suggesting ongoing nerve hypertrophy throughout childhood (Yiu et al., 2015).

Routine hematological and biochemical studies are normal. CSF is also normal, which helps differentiate the condition from chronic inflammatory demyelinating polyneuropathy (CIDP), in which the CSF protein is usually elevated. Sural nerve biopsy typically shows the changes of a hypertrophic neuropathy, characterized by onion bulb formation, increased frequency of fibers with demyelinated and remyelinated segments, an increase in endoneurial area, and loss of large myelinated fibers (Fig. 106.9). Gene mutations, predominantly affecting genes for myelin and Schwann cell proteins, have been recognized that account for more than three-quarters of families with CMT1 (Fig. 106.10). CMT1A is the most common CMT subtype, accounting for 70%–80% of CMT1 cases and more than 50% of all CMT cases. The disease is caused by duplication of a 01.5-Mb fragment in the short arm of chromosome 17p11.2-12 harboring peripheral myelin protein 22 (PMP22). Rarely, the disease is caused by PMP22 point mutation. PMP22 is a membrane glycoprotein found in the compact portion of the peripheral myelin sheath. The precise function of PMP22 in normal nerve remains unknown. Deletion of the same 1.5-megabase region on chromosome 17p11.2 results in a

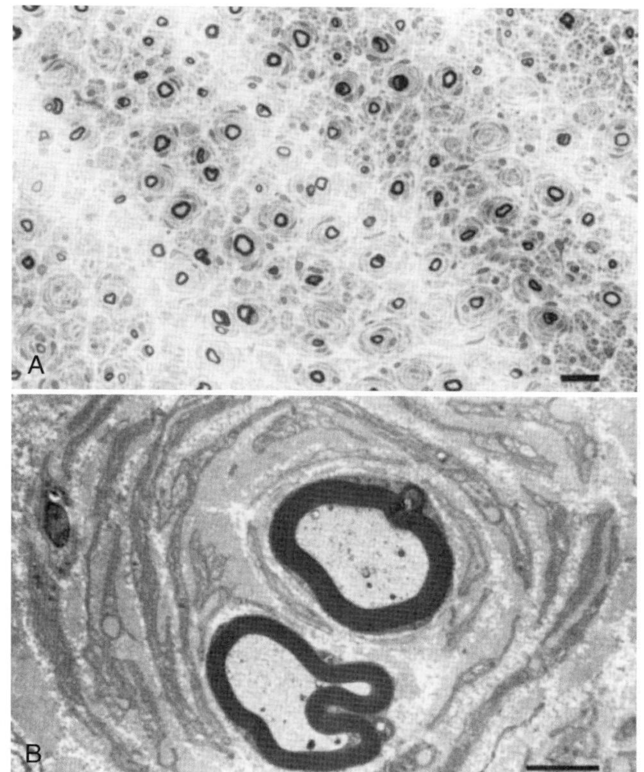

Fig. 106.9 Charcot-Marie-Tooth Type 1 Disease. A, Semi-thin transverse section of sural nerve showing numerous onion bulbs. (Toluidine blue; bar = 20 μm.) B, Electron micrograph of an onion bulb formation; two small myelinated fibers are surrounded by multiple layers of Schwann cell processes. (Bar = 0.5 μm.)

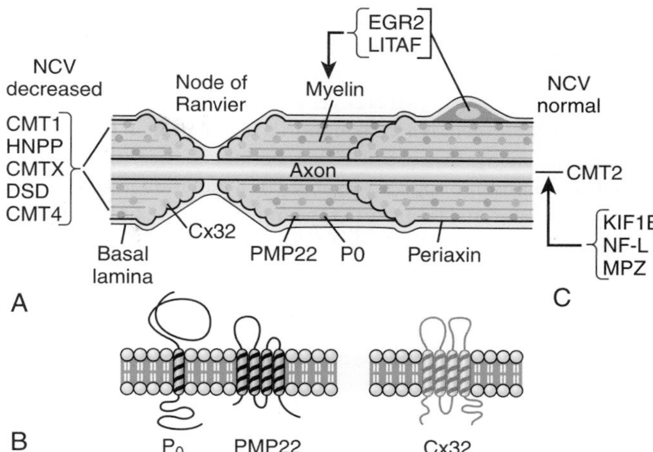


Fig. 106.10 A, Charcot-Marie-Tooth disease *(CMT)* and related disorders: CMT1, CMT with X-linked inheritance *(CMTX)*, hereditary neuropathy with liability to pressure palsies *(HNPP)*, Dejerine-Sottas disease *(DSD)*, and most of CMT4 are inherited disorders of myelin. CMT2 is a primary axonal disorder. Alterations in dosage of peripheral myelin protein 22 (PMP22) gene account for the majority of patients with CMT1A and HNPP. B, Point mutations of these genes (connexin-32 [Cx32], myelin protein zero [MPZ, P0], PMP22, EGR2, periaxin) result in CMTX, CMT1B, CMT1A, DSD, and CMT4. Mutations of the LITAF gene result in CMT1C. C, Point mutations of the KIF1B and NF-L genes and specific MPZ missense mutations result in CMT2. *NCV*, Nerve conduction velocity. *(Adapted with permission from Lupski, J.R., 1998. Molecular genetics of peripheral neuropathies. In: Martin, J.D. (Ed.), Molecular Neurology. Scientific American, New York. All rights reserved.)*

single copy of the normal PMP22 gene, a finding observed in 85% of patients with HNPP. The CMT1A duplication or HNPP deletion is caused by reciprocal recombination events that occur in male germ cell meiosis. The PMP22 duplication or deletion can be detected in blood samples using pulse-field electrophoresis followed by hybridization with specific CMT1A duplication junction fragments or cytogenetic testing with a PMP22 probe by fluorescence in situ hybridization.

CMT1B is clinically indistinguishable from CMT1A but it only accounts for 4% to 5% of CMT1 cases. It is caused by mutations in the *myelin protein zero* (P0; gene symbol, MPZ) gene, mapped to chromosome 1q22-23. MPZ is the major peripheral myelin glycoprotein and is thought to function as an adhesion molecule in the formation and compaction of peripheral myelin. It is a member of the immunoglobulin superfamily, with distinct extracellular transmembrane and intracellular domains. Mutations in the gene encoding for MPZ have also been associated with DSD, and congenital hypomyelination neuropathy. Different MPZ mutations result in divergent morphological effects on myelin sheaths, consisting of uncompacting of myelin or focal myelin foldings (Gabreëls-Festen et al., 1996). Motor conduction block was reported rarely in CMT1B patients with specific MPZ mutations (Street et al., 2002). Specific MPZ missense mutations have also been reported with a CMT2 phenotype, showing only mild slowing of NCVs (Marrosu et al., 1998). The Thr124 Met mutations in the MPZ gene have been detected in several families with a distinct CMT2 phenotype (CMT2J) characterized by late onset, marked sensory loss, and sometimes deafness, chronic cough, and pupillary abnormalities (De Jonghe et al., 1999).

CMT1C is caused by a mutation in lipopolysaccharide-induced tumor necrosis factor-alpha (LITAF/SIMPLE) gene, mapped to chromosome 16p13-12 expressed on Schwann cells. This gene encodes a lysosomal protein that may play a role in protein degradation pathways (Street et al., 2003). Affected individuals in these families manifest characteristic CMT1 symptoms.

CMT1D is mapped to chromosome 10q21-q22 and is due to mutation of the early growth response 2 gene (EGR2) which encodes a zinc-finger transcription factor expressed in myelinating Schwann cells that regulates the expression of myelin proteins including PMP22, P0, Cx32, and periaxin (Kamholz et al., 2000). EGR2 gene missense mutations have also been reported in patients with DSD, or congenital hypomyelination neuropathy (Timmerman et al., 1999; Warner et al., 1998). Respiratory compromise and cranial nerve dysfunction are commonly associated with EGR2 mutations (Szigeti et al., 2007). Other rare CMT1 subtypes include CMT1E and CMT1F.

### Charcot-Marie-Tooth Disease Type 2

CMT2 constitutes about one-third of all AD CMT disease. It is associated with mutations in genes affecting intracellular processes such as axonal transport, membrane trafficking, and translation (see Chapter 48). Clinical symptoms begin later than in CMT1, most commonly in the second decade, but may be delayed until middle age or beyond. Foot and spinal deformities tend to be less prominent than in CMT1. The clinical features closely resemble those of CMT1 but differ in that peripheral nerves are not enlarged, and upper limb involvement, tremor, and diffuse areflexia occur less frequently. However, in individual cases, it is often impossible to determine the type of CMT disease on the basis of clinical manifestation alone. Approximately 20% of affected individuals are asymptomatic.

CMT2A is the most common CMT2 subtype and accounts for 30% of CMT2 cases (see Table 106.6). CMT2A2, which is responsible for most CMT2 families, shares clinical features of weakness and atrophy with other CMT variants, but has an earlier onset and is more severe, often resulting in earlier disability and wheelchair dependence. It may also be associated with optic atrophy. It is caused by mutations in the mitofusin 2 (MFN2) gene, with a locus on chromosome 1p36.22. MFN2 protein is a mitochondrial fusion protein ubiquitously expressed in many tissues including peripheral nerves. CMT2A1, linked to chromosome 1p36.22, is caused by a mutation in kinesin protein involved in axonal transport of synaptic vesicles (Saito et al., 1997; Zhao et al., 2001). In CMT2B, which is linked to chromosome 3q13-22, there is prominent sensory loss with foot ulcerations (De Jonghe et al., 1997). A mutation in the RAB7 gene, which encodes a small guanosine triphosphatase (GTPase) late endosomal protein, has been found to be causative (Verhoeven et al., 2003). This form of CMT is clinically very similar to hereditary sensory neuropathy type 1 (HSN1) but lacks spontaneous lancinating pain. CMT2B1 and CMT2B2 are AR disorders, caused by mutation in the lamin A/C gene on chromosome 1q22, and mediator of RNA polymerase II transcription, subunit 25 gene (MED25) on chromosome 19q13.33, respectively. Another distinct subgroup of severely affected patients, designated CMT2C (mapped to chromosome 12q24), develop vocal cord, intercostal, and diaphragmatic muscle weakness (Klein et al., 2003). Because of respiratory failure, the life expectancy of these patients is shortened. CMT2D, mapped to chromosome 7p14, is characterized by weakness and atrophy that is more severe in the hands than in the feet (Ionasescu et al., 1996b). In CMT2E, some patients within the same kindred and with an otherwise typical CMT2 phenotype may exhibit slowed motor nerve conduction that is much below the forearm cutoff value of 38 m/sec and a more severe clinical phenotype. This form of CMT is caused by mutations in genes that encode neurofilament light (NEFL) subunit, and patients may have axonal swelling (giant axons) and significant secondary demyelination on sural nerve biopsies (Fabrizi et al., 2006; Jordanova et al., 2003). CMT2F, caused by mutations in small heat shock protein 27 (Hsp27), is characterized by later onset (35–60 years), mild sensory impairment, and moderate to severely slowed NCVs of lower limbs but normal or mildly reduced velocities in the upper limbs. Mutation in Hsp27 may impair formation of the stable neurofilament network that is essential for the maintenance of peripheral nerves. CMT2G has the same gene locus as CMT4H (see later discussion on type 4 disease) on chromosome 12q12-q13.3, with the age onset from 9 to 76 years. CMT2I and CMT2J are designated as CMT2 with MPZ (myelin protein zero) gene mutations. CMT2J is associated with pupillary abnormalities (Adie pupil) and hearing loss.

Motor NCV may be normal or mildly reduced. SNAPs are either absent or reduced in amplitude. Sural nerve biopsy specimens show preferential loss of large myelinated fibers, without significant demyelination; there may be clusters of regenerating myelinated fibers, a hallmark of axonal regeneration.

### X-Linked Charcot-Marie-Tooth Disease

X-linked Charcot-Marie-Tooth disease (CMTX) is phenotypically similar to CMT1. CMTX1 is caused by many mutations in gap junction protein B1 (GJB1), the gene that encodes connexin 32 (Cx32), on chromosome Xq13.1. Affected male subjects tend to be more severely affected, and females with the gene mutation are asymptomatic or may have a mild neuropathy. CMTX1 should be considered in any patient whose family history does not exhibit a male-to-male transmission. CMTX1 accounts for 7%–16% of all forms of CMT, making it the second most common form of CMT (following CMT1A).

The connexins are a family of highly related genes encoding a group of channel-forming proteins. Cx32 is a gap junction protein found in noncompacted paranodal loops and Schmidt-Lanterman incisures of Schwann cell cytoplasm, which is encoded by a four-exon gene located on chromosome Xq. As a gap junction protein, Cx32 forms small channels that facilitate transfer of ions and small molecules between Schwann cells and axons. More than 200 different mutations in Cx32 have been identified in CMTX1 families. Genotype-phenotype correlations among patients with Cx32 mutations suggest that most missense mutations result in a mild clinical phenotype, whereas nonsense and frameshift mutations produce more severe phenotypes (Ionasescu et al., 1996a).

Cx32 is expressed in Schwann cells and oligodendrocytes, regions of noncompact myelin (incisures and paranodes), as well as other non-neural cells. Some mutations of Cx32 have been reported to be associated with central nervous system (CNS) involvement with white-matter MRI and MR spectroscopy abnormalities, abnormal brainstem auditory evoked potentials, and deafness (Murru et al., 2006). An interesting phenomenon of transient and acute ataxia, dysarthria, and weakness occurring after visiting high altitudes and associated with CNS white-matter MRI abnormalities has been described in patients with two mutations: R142W and C168Y (Paulson et al., 2002). This suggests that CMTX1 patients should be cautioned about travel to high-altitude locations. It has been proposed that Cx32 mutations may cause these abnormalities by reducing the number of functional gap junctions between oligodendrocytes and astrocytes, making them more susceptible to changes in intercellular ions and small-molecule exchange that occur in situations of metabolic stress (e.g., high altitude or physical activity).

Men with CMTX1 show significant slowing in NCV, and brainstem auditory evoked responses are often abnormal. A picture of both axonal loss and demyelination is revealed on nerve biopsy. There is debate as to whether CMTX1 should be classified as a primary axonal or demyelinating disorder (Birouk et al., 1998). However, careful studies of individual patients suggest nonuniform conduction slowing consistent with demyelination (Gutierrez et al., 2000; Lewis, 2000). NCVs in males with CMTX1 with Cx32 mutations are often slow, usually in the intermediate, slowing between 35 and 45 m/sec. Conduction slowing in heterozygous women may be subtle and frequently is in the range found in patients with axonal polyneuropathies leading to a suspected diagnosis of CMT2. The absence of male-to-male transmission on family history, the presence of mild to intermediate conduction velocities (>42 m/sec) in female carriers, and delayed brainstem auditory evoked response latencies in affected men is highly suggestive of CMTX1 and Cx32 mutations (Nicholson et al., 1998). Much less common X-linked CMT subtypes have been described (see Table 106.6)

### Dejerine-Sottas Disease (Charcot-Marie-Tooth Disease with Dejerine-Sottas Phenotype)

DSD, previously designated as CMT3, is an uncommon progressive hypertrophic neuropathy with onset in childhood. Although originally the disorder was thought to be AR, most cases are sporadic and in some instances have been shown to result from a de novo dominant mutation. The majority of patients have mutations that are common in other types of CMT, including PMP22 duplication or point mutation, MPZ mutation, or EGR2 mutation.

Motor development is delayed; proximal weakness, global areflexia, enlarged peripheral nerves, and severe disability are the rule. Motor conduction velocities are markedly slowed, often to less than 10–15 m/sec in the forearms. Temporal dispersion and amplitude reduction on proximal stimulation may be found in such cases, owing to high electrical stimulation thresholds in hypertrophic nerves. CSF protein is frequently increased. Pathologically, pronounced onion bulb changes are associated with hypomyelination and loss of myelinated fibers. Defective myelination is confirmed by an increased axon-to-fiber diameter ratio. Cases of congenital hypomyelination neuropathy probably represent a variant of DSD at the far end of a spectrum of defective myelination. DSD is genetically heterogeneous and is caused by different structural myelin protein and transcription factor gene mutations (see Chapter 48).

TABLE 106.7 **Selected Charcot-Marie-Tooth Phenotypes and Molecular Diagnostic Testing**

| Test | CMT1 | HNPP | CMTX | CMT2 | DSD/CHN |
|---|---|---|---|---|---|
| PMP22 dup/del FISH | X, duplication | X, deletion | — | — | X, duplication |
| DNA sequencing: | | | | | |
| Cx32 | X | | | | X |
| PMP22 | X | | | | X |
| MPZ | X | | | | X |
| EGR2 | X | | | | |
| Periaxin | | | | X | |
| NEFL | | | | X | |

*CMT1*, Charcot-Marie-Tooth disease type 1; *CMTX*, X-linked CMT; *Cx32*, connexin-32, *DSD/CHN*, Dejerine-Sottas syndrome/congenital hypomyelination neuropathy; *EGR2*, early growth response 2 gene; *FISH*, fluorescence in situ hybridization; *HNPP*, hereditary neuropathy with liability to pressure palsies; *MPZ*, myelin protein zero; *NEFL*, neurofilament light chain gene; *PMP22 dup/del*, peripheral myelin protein 22 duplication or deletion is detected by pulse field gel electrophoresis or cytogenetic testing with FISH.

### Charcot-Marie-Tooth Disease Type 4

The majority of Charcot-Marie-Tooth disease type 4 (CMT4) patients have AR inheritance. They are less common, accounting for less than 10% of all CMT cases. They are characterized by onset in early childhood and progressive weakness leading to inability to walk in adolescence. Both demyelinating and axonal types have been identified (Dubourg et al., 2006). Common to all the demyelinating subgroups is a disturbance in normal myelination of the axons; clinical and electrophysiological features are similar in several of these subtypes with severe forms of CMT1 or DSD. Conduction velocities are slowed (20–30 m/sec). CSF protein is normal. Nerve biopsy shows loss of myelinated fibers, hypomyelination, and onion bulbs.

CMT4 consists of several subgroups (see Table 106.6). Each subgroup is rare and tends to be more common in certain inbred populations. CMT4A is the most common and accounts for 25%–30% of all AR cases. The disease has been mapped to chromosome 8q13 because of ganglioside-induced differentiation-associated protein 1 (GDAP1) mutations, the most common cause of CMT4, and may result in demyelinating as well as axonal phenotypes (Nelis et al., 2002). CMT4B1 is mapped to chromosome 11q21 caused by myotubularin-related protein 2 (MTMR2) mutations, with findings of redundant loops of focally folded myelin (Houlden et al., 2001b), while CMT4B2 is mapped to chromosome 11p15.4 caused by set-binding factor-2 gene (SBF2) mutations. In both, irregular folding and redundancy of loops of myelin are evident on nerve biopsies. Children affected with CMT4B2 also exhibit congenital glaucoma, leading to loss of vision. CMT4C, characterized by frequent and severe scoliosis, is linked to chromosome 5q31-q33 and is caused by SH3TC2 gene mutation (Azzedine et al., 2006). CMT4D has onset in childhood but may progress into the fifth decade of life. It is associated with dysmorphic features and hearing loss. CMT4E is a form of congenital hypomyelinating neuropathy, often diagnosed as DSD, associated with mutations in PMP22 and ERG2 (early growth response) genes. The phenotypic presentation of CMT4F is also severe, similar to that for DSD phenotype, but the mutations occur in the periaxin gene, which produces a membrane-associated protein solely expressed in myelinating Schwann cells. Periaxin is a cytoskeleton-associated protein that links the cytoskeleton of the Schwann cell with the basal lamina, a necessary function to stabilize the mature myelin sheath (Takashima et al., 2002). CMT4H is similar to CMT2G in terms of genetic locus but is more severe clinically, with an onset in early childhood and prominent nerve hypomyelination.

### Complex Forms of Charcot-Marie-Tooth Disease

Some dominant forms of CMT have displayed features intermediate between CMT1 and CMT2, with conduction velocities between 35 and 45 m/sec. These forms have been classified separately as dominant intermediate CMT (DI-CMT) and include types A, B, C, and D. DI-CMTA maps to chromosome 10q24-25, but its gene defect has not been discovered. DI-CMTB is caused by mutations in the dynamin 2 (DNM2) gene and maps to chromosome 19p12-13. This typically presents as a classic mild to moderately severe CMT phenotype. Some families with this variety have developed neutropenia and early cataracts (Claeys et al., 2009). A mutation in tyrosyl-tRNA (transfer ribonucleic acid) synthetase has been found to be the cause of DI-CMTC, which maps to chromosome 1p34-35 and typically displays a mild, very slowly progressive course (Jordanova et al., 2006). DI-CMTD maps to chromosome 1q22 MPZ gene mutations.

A number of families with CMT exhibit additional features such as optic atrophy, pigmentary retinal degeneration, deafness, and spastic paraparesis. Cardiac involvement is encountered in occasional patients, but prospective family studies find no association between cardiomyopathy and CMT disease. A syndrome of CIDP responding to prednisone and immunosuppression has been reported in patients with inherited CMT disease due to MPZ mutation (Watanabe et al., 2002), providing evidence that nongenetic factors may play a role in clinical expression of the mutant gene. It has been suggested that any patient with a hereditary neuropathy who suffers a recent rapid deterioration should be considered as having a secondary CIDP and be treated with immunosuppressants such as corticosteroids or high-dose intravenous immunoglobulin (IVIG).

### Practical Molecular Diagnostic Testing for Patients with Charcot-Marie-Tooth Disease and Related Disorders

Molecular diagnostic testing should be considered in CMT and related peripheral neuropathies. Commercial reference laboratories can detect point mutations or PMP22 duplication/deletion by DNA sequencing of PMP22, Cx32, MPZ, EGR2, periaxin, GDAP1, and NEFL, among others, in samples of peripheral blood (Table 106.7). It is, however, advisable to use the clinical and EDX findings supplemented by a detailed family history and plan a logical approach to obtaining DNA studies. An all-inclusive "battery" of available genetic tests of CMT disease is tempting but interpretation of results may be more difficult because of frequent detection of genes with variants of unknown significance. Population studies confirmed that CMT1A (PMP22 duplication or PMP22 deletion), CMT1X (Cx32 mutation), CMT1B (MPZ mutation), and CMT2A (MFN2 mutation) account for about 65%–70% of all CMT cases (Bassam, 2014; Boerkoel et al., 2002).

- In families with at least two generations with the disease, known male-to-male transmission, and uniform conduction slowing (<35 m/sec if forearm), CMT1A should be considered first and the PMP22 duplication test should be obtained.

- If normal, PMP22 sequencing should be done.
- If normal, CMT1B should be excluded by obtaining MPZ DNA sequencing.
- Patients who have neither the PMP22 duplication nor male-to-male transmission should be screened for CMTX1 by looking for Cx32 mutations.
- For patients displaying an axonal pattern, the MFN2 mutation should be investigated first, as this is the most common type of CMT2 (England et al., 2009a).
- Given the high spontaneous mutation rate, the diagnosis of CMT1A should be considered even in the absence of a positive family history.
- The PMP22 duplication test followed by DNA sequencing of PMP22, MPZ, EGR2, and periaxin should be considered in childhood cases with severe demyelinating neuropathy suggestive of DSD or congenital hypomyelination neuropathy.
- Because of the severe reactions to vincristine and other chemotherapeutic neurotoxic drugs in CMT patients, before initiating cancer chemotherapy it is best to rule out CMT1A in any patient with either unexplained chronic neuropathy or a family history of neuropathy (Graf et al., 1996).

### Treatment and Management

The rates of progression of CMT1 and CMT2 are slow, disability occurs relatively late, and lifespan may be normal. Management is mainly symptomatic. Patients should be instructed in proper foot care and advised to wear broad, well-fitting shoes. Insoles may be used to distribute body weight more evenly in patients with a foot deformity. Ankle-foot braces or orthopedic procedures are indicated to correct severe foot drop. Patients should be warned to avoid neurotoxic drugs because of greater susceptibility to agents such as vincristine. Issues like genetic counseling, family planning, prenatal diagnosis, and psychological concerns must be carefully approached, preferably by a multidisciplinary team including a genetic counselor. Recent studies suggest that CMT is associated with higher risk for complication during delivery (Hoff et al., 2005). Also, during pregnancy the symptoms of CMT may worsen.

Despite astonishing advances in the molecular genetics of CMT, there is still no effective treatment available for any form of the disease. Rats overexpressing PMP22 worsen with progesterone administration. This has led to proposed use of progesterone antagonists for CMT1A, though potentially unacceptable side effects have prevented such trials. The same animal model showed a convincing clinical and pathological improvement following administration of ascorbic acid (vitamin C), a known promoter of myelination. Though pharmacological treatment trials in CMT are rare, this discovery prompted a multicenter double-blind placebo-controlled study on the use of ascorbic acid at 1 or 3 g/day in CMT1A. Ascorbic acid was found to be well tolerated, but no significant benefit was demonstrated in the CMT neuropathy score at 12 months, concluding vitamin C does not improve the course of CMT1A in adults or children (Gess et al., 2015; Micallef et al., 2009). The possibly beneficial role of neurotrophins, particularly neurotrophin 3 (NT3), in CMT1A and nerve regeneration has recently been demonstrated in a small pilot study (Sahenk et al., 2005). Treating cells with curcumin, derived from the curry spice turmeric, releases the MPZ mutants from the endoplasmic reticulum into the cytoplasm, thus reducing the number of apoptotic cells and becoming a potential treatment for CMT1B (Khajavi et al., 2005). Some CMT2 patients with MPZ mutations may respond to corticosteroids (Donaghy et al., 2000).

## Hereditary Neuropathy with Liability to Pressure Palsies

HNPP is an AD disorder of peripheral nerves leading to increased susceptibility to mechanical traction or compression. It occurs with an estimated prevalence of 16 per 100,000 population. Patients have recurrent episodes of isolated mononeuropathies, typically affecting, in order of decreasing frequency, the fibular nerve, ulnar nerve, brachial plexus, radial nerve, and median nerves. Painless brachial plexopathy is seen in up to a third of patients. Most HNPP patients experience the initial episode in the second or third decade of life. Attacks usually are provoked by minor compression, slight traction, or other trivial trauma. Most episodes are of sudden onset, painless, and usually followed by complete recovery within days or weeks. Less-common presentations include transient positionally induced sensory symptoms, progressive mononeuropathy, chronic sensory polyneuropathy, mild CMT phenotype with pes cavus, and a diffuse chronic sensorimotor neuropathy resembling CIDP (Mouton et al., 1999). About 15% of mutation carriers remain asymptomatic.

Nerve conduction studies in patients with HNPP associated with PMP22 deletion typically demonstrate a characteristic pattern of prolonged distal motor latencies with only mild slowing in forearm segments of median and ulnar nerves, focal slowing and conduction blocks of median, ulnar, and fibular nerves at compression sites, and diffuse reduction of SNAP amplitudes (Dubourg et al., 2000; Mouton et al., 1999). The median forearm motor NCV is typically above 38 m/sec, but sensory studies demonstrate velocities in the demyelinating range and reduced or absent SNAPs. The sural SNAP is absent or abnormal in more than 90% of patients, while the tibial motor nerve is slowed in about 60% of the patients. The most common focal entrapment neuropathy at compressive sites are the ulnar nerve at the elbow and median nerve at the wrist, each occurring in more than three-fourths of patients, followed by the fibular nerve at the fibular head, seen in one-third of the patients (Takahashi et al., 2017). Prolonged median distal motor latencies and abnormal sensory conduction studies are frequently found in asymptomatic carriers (Infante et al., 2001).

Sural nerve biopsy specimens demonstrate focal sausage-like thickenings of myelin, termed *tomacula* (Fig. 106.11), segmental demyelination, and axonal loss. Linkage studies show a 1.5-megabase deletion of chromosome 17p11.2-12 that includes the PMP22 gene and corresponds to the duplicated region in CMT1A in 85% of affected patients with HNPP. The remaining patients have a variety of mutations in PMP22 that lead to frameshift or nonsense mutations causing functional changes in the protein (Lenssen et al., 1998; van de Wetering et al., 2002). Exactly how the deletion of PMP22 causes HNPP remains unclear, though loss of function of the PMP22 protein is the likely explanation for HNPP, and a toxic gain of function in CMT1A (Katona et al., 2009; Li et al., 2004). Molecular diagnosis of the 17p11.2 deletion has replaced nerve biopsy for the diagnosis of HNPP. Testing should be considered regardless of family history in any patient presenting with painless multiple mononeuropathies, brachial plexopathy, or recurrent demyelinating neuropathy (Tyson et al., 1996). The primary treatment strategy in HNPP is to prevent nerve injury by avoiding pressure damage.

## Hereditary Neuralgic Amyotrophy

Recurrent brachial plexopathy, often preceded by severe ipsilateral limb pain, is the hallmark of hereditary neuralgic amyotrophy, an AD disorder. Most patients recover over weeks to a few months, with accumulating evidence of residual neurological deficit over time. Patients also have dysmorphic features, including hypotelorism, epicanthal folds, microstomia, and dysmorphic ears. The disorder maps to chromosome 17q25 and is associated with mutations in the SEPT9 gene (Kuhlenbäumer et al., 2005).

Other hereditary neuropathies, including GAN, hereditary sensory and autonomic neuropathy (HSAN), neuropathy associated with spinocerebellar, primary erythromelalgia, familial amyloid polyneuropathy (FAP), porphyric neuropathy, Fabry disease, leukodystrophies with neuropathy, Refsum disease, Tangier disease, Bassen-Kornzweig syndrome, and mitochondrial cytopathies and polyneuropathy are discussed in the online version of this chapter, available at http://www.experconsult.com. 

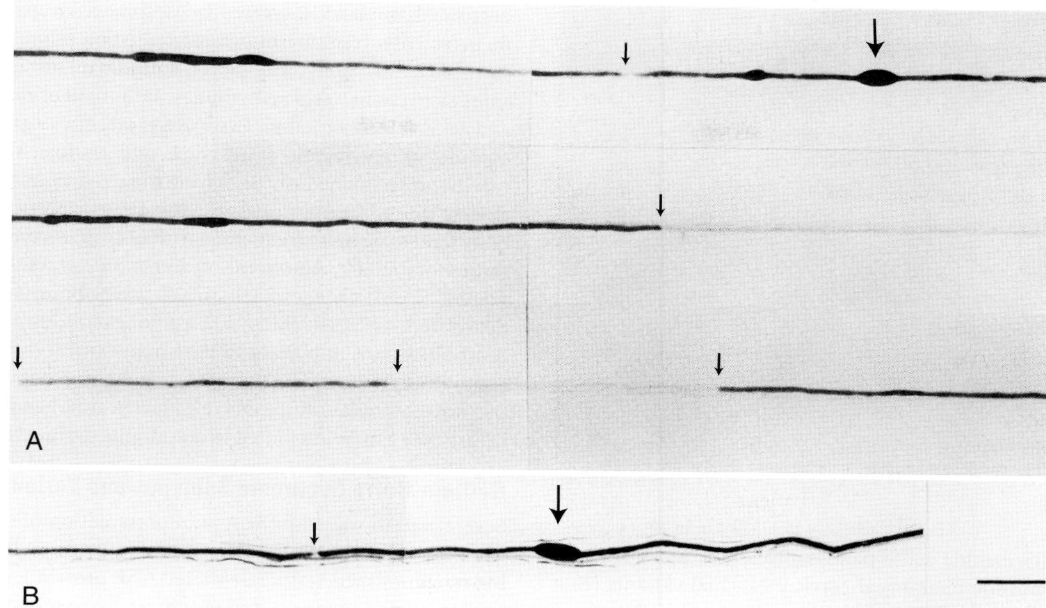


**Fig. 106.11** Single teased nerve fibers from a patient with hereditary liability to pressure palsies, showing examples of focal sausage-shaped enlargements of the myelin sheath *(large arrows)* in two fibers (**A, B**). Fiber A shows thinly remyelinated internodes. Successive nodes of Ranvier *(thin arrows)* can be followed from left to right. (Bar = 100 μm.) *(Reprinted with permission from Bosch, E.P., Chui, H.C., Martin, M.A., et al., 1980. Brachial plexus involvement in familial pressure-sensitive neuropathy: electrophysiological and morphological findings. Ann Neurol 8, 620–624.)*

## INFLAMMATORY DEMYELINATING POLYRADICULONEUROPATHIES

Inflammatory demyelinating polyradiculoneuropathies are acquired immunologically mediated polyneuropathies classified on the basis of their clinical course into two major groups: (1) GBS, and (2) CIDP. In GBS, the maximal deficits develop over days or weeks (maximum 4 weeks), followed by a plateau phase and gradual recovery. Chronic forms pursue either a slowly progressive (2 months or more) or a relapsing-remitting course.

### Guillain-Barré Syndrome

In 1916, Guillain, Barré, and Strohl emphasized the main clinical features of GBS: motor weakness, areflexia, paresthesias with minor sensory loss, and increased protein in CSF without pleocytosis *(albuminocytological dissociation)*. Our current understanding of the pathology was greatly enhanced when multifocal inflammatory demyelination of spinal roots and peripheral nerves was described. The frequent finding of motor conduction blocks and reduced conduction velocities provided further electrophysiological confirmation of the widespread demyelination. Improvement in modern critical care has dramatically changed outcomes in GBS, including a reduction in the mortality rate from 33% before the introduction of positive-pressure ventilation to the current rate of approximately 1%–5% (Alshekhlee et al., 2008a).

The diagnosis of GBS depends on clinical criteria supported by electrophysiological studies and CSF findings (Box 106.10). These diagnostic criteria define acute inflammatory demyelinating polyneuropathy (AIDP), which is the most common form of GBS in Europe and North America. However, in recent years, it has been recognized that GBS is a heterogeneous syndrome, and not all GBS cases are due to acute demyelination and resemble experimental allergic neuritis. An axonal immune-mediated injury may also produce a similar clinical presentation. This axonal subtype of GBS is called *acute motor-sensory axonal neuropathy* (AMSAN) because of involvement of both motor and sensory fibers and is known for its severity and poor recovery. A second, pure motor axonal subtype called *acute motor axonal neuropathy* (AMAN) was first described in northern China, where it occurs in summer epidemics in children and young adults (Yuki and Hartung, 2012). The *Miller-Fisher syndrome* (MFS) variant accounts for 6% of total GBS cases in Western countries, whereas in Taiwan the proportion is as high as 18%, suggesting a geographical difference. Other

**BOX 106.10 Diagnostic Criteria for Guillain-Barré Syndrome**

**Features Required for Diagnosis**
Progressive weakness of both legs and arms
Areflexia or hyporeflexia

**Clinical Features Supportive of Diagnosis**
Progression over days to 4 weeks
Relative symmetry of symptoms and signs
Mild sensory symptoms or signs
Bifacial palsies
Autonomic dysfunction
Absence of fever at onset
Recovery beginning 2–4 weeks after progression ceases

**Laboratory Features Supportive of Diagnosis**
Elevated cerebrospinal fluid protein with <10 cells/μL
Electrodiagnostic features of nerve conduction slowing or block

*Adapted from Ashbury, A.K., Cornblath, D.R., 1990. Assessment of current diagnostic criteria for Guillain-Barré syndrome. Ann Neurol 27(Suppl), S21–S24.*

**BOX 106.11 Classification of Guillain–Barré Syndrome Subtypes and Variants**

**Common Subtypes**

Acute inflammatory demyelinating polyradiculoneuropathy (AIDP)
Acute motor axonal neuropathy (AMAN)
Acute motor-sensory axonal neuropathy (AMSAN)

**Rare Variants**

Miller-Fisher syndrome
Ataxic variant (acute ataxic neuropathy)
Pharyngeal-cervical-brachial variant
Multiple cranial neuropathy variant
Facial diplegia with paresthesias
Paraparetic variant
Acute pandysautonomia

rare variants of GBS include acute pandysautonomia, facial diplegia with paresthesias, and the pharyngeal-cervical-brachial variants (Box 106.11). The classification of GBS subtypes and variants is based on the clinical picture and electrophysiological and pathological findings (Griffin et al., 1996).

## Clinical Features

The classic form of GBS is a nonseasonal illness that affects persons of all ages, but males are more often affected than females (1.5:1). With the virtual eradication of acute poliomyelitis, GBS has become the leading cause of acute paralytic disease in Western countries. The mean annual incidence is 1.8 per 100,000 population and has remained stable over the past three decades (Flachenecker, 2006). Incidence rates increase with age from 0.8 in those younger than 18 years to 3.2 for those 60 years and older.

Patients with classic GBS initially present with weakness with or without paresthetic sensory symptoms, often worse in the hands and fingers. The fairly symmetrical weakness of the lower limbs ascends proximally over hours to several days and may subsequently involve arms, facial, and oropharyngeal muscles, and in severe cases, respiratory muscles. Less often, weakness may be descending and begin in the upper limbs or cranial innervated muscles. Its severity varies from mild, in which patients are still capable of walking unassisted, to a nearly total quadriplegia. Hyporeflexia or areflexia are the invariable features of GBS but may be absent early in the course of the disease.

Cranial nerve involvement occurs in 45%–75% of cases in different series. Facial paresis, usually bilateral, is found in at least half of patients. Involvement of extraocular muscles and lower cranial nerves is seen less often. Occasional patients may develop facial myokymia. Pseudotumor cerebri with papilledema occurs as a rare complication and is almost always due to chronically elevated intracranial pressure. The proportion of patients developing respiratory failure and requiring assisted ventilation seems to increase with age and ranges from 9% to 30% in hospital-based series (Alshekhlee et al., 2008a).

Sensory loss is not a prominent feature and is frequently limited to distal impairment of vibration sense. Moderate to severe pain in the extremities, interscapular area, or back occurs in about 70% of patients during the acute phase of illness, and this may persist for a year in a third of those affected (Ruts et al., 2010b). Dysesthetic pain, described as burning or tingling of the limbs, or joint stiffness is less common (Moulin et al., 1997).

Autonomic dysfunction of various degrees has been reported in 65% of patients admitted to the hospital. Most of the clinically significant autonomic dysfunction occurs within the first 2–4 weeks of the illness, the peak period of paralysis. Its varied and complex manifestations may be related to either increased or decreased sympathetic-parasympathetic activity, resulting in orthostatic hypotension, urinary retention, gastrointestinal atony, iridoplegia, episodic or sustained hypertension, sinus tachycardia, tachyarrhythmias, anhidrosis or episodic diaphoresis, and acral vasoconstriction. Excessive vagal activity accounts for sudden episodes of bradycardia, heart block, and asystole. These "vagal spells" may occur spontaneously or may be triggered by tracheal suctioning or similar stimuli. Serious cardiac arrhythmias with hemodynamic instability tend to be more frequent in patients with severe quadriparesis and respiratory failure. Autonomic dysfunction can result in electrocardiographic (ECG) changes, including T-wave abnormalities, ST-segment depression, QRS widening, QT prolongation, and various forms of heart block. It is important to note that some of the common medical complications, including pulmonary embolism, hypoxia, and pneumonia, lead to similar symptoms (e.g., tachycardia) and must be excluded before they can be attributed to autonomic dysfunction.

## Guillain-Barré Syndrome Subtypes and Variants

Several variations from the typical presentation of GBS exist (see Box 106.11). Their link to GBS is supported by preceding infectious episodes, diminished reflexes, elevated CSF protein levels, and, in many of them, an acknowledged immune-mediated origin.

A GBS subtype, AMAN was first reported in epidemic proportions among children and young adults in northern China during summer months; AMAN is now considered the most common GBS subtype in Asia. Sporadic cases of AMAN presenting with acute flaccid paralysis without clinical or electrophysiological involvement of sensory nerves are reported from Europe and North America, often scattered within large series of patients with GBS. AMAN differs from GBS in electrophysiological studies that demonstrate normal SNAPs and reduced CMAP amplitudes with no signs of demyelination as supported by normal motor distal latencies and conduction velocities. Autopsy studies of some cases have shown noninflammatory wallerian-like degeneration of ventral roots and motor axons in mixed nerves. However, nerve biopsy studies in others have shown intrusion of macrophages between the axon and the surrounding myelin sheath, with relatively little axonal degeneration. Most patients with AMAN improve as rapidly as patients with AIDP (Ho et al., 1997). The rapid clinical improvement rates and the paucity of pathological findings in some fatal cases could be explained either by conduction failure of motor axons at nodes of Ranvier because of macrophage intrusion or by axonal degeneration of motor nerve terminals as confirmed by motor point biopsy. Antecedent *Campylobacter jejuni* infection is detected by using serological tests in 76% of AMAN patients from northern China. AMAN represents a very good example of molecular mimicry in which the immune system, in its efforts to eradicate *C. jejuni*, elaborates antibodies against neural antigens who share ganglioside-like epitopes with the lipopolysaccharides of the organism. These antibodies, mainly anti-GM1 or anti-GD1a antibodies, bind to the axolemma at the node of Ranvier, leading to membrane-attack complex formation and conduction failure.

A fulminant and less common subtype of GBS, AMSAN, carries a poor prognosis for recovery. All patients develop an acute and rapidly progressive course leading to a maximum deficit in less than 7 days, often profound quadriparesis with severe muscle wasting and requiring prolonged ventilatory support. EDX studies show markedly reduced or absent CMAPs, without significant conduction slowing, and absent SNAPs. The subsequent appearance of abundant fibrillation potentials on needle EMG, together with persistently inexcitable motor nerves and poor recovery are compatible with a primary axonopathy as the underlying disease process. Extensive wallerian axonal degeneration without significant inflammation or demyelination has been described in ventral and dorsal roots and in peripheral nerves at autopsy (Griffin et al., 1996).

*MFS,* which accounts for about 5% of cases, is characterized by the triad of ophthalmoplegia, ataxia, and areflexia. Patients present with diplopia followed by gait and limb ataxia. Ocular signs range from complete ophthalmoplegia, including dilated and unreactive pupils, to external ophthalmoparesis with or without ptosis. Cranial nerves other than ocular motor nerves may be affected. The ataxia is attributed to a peripheral mismatch between proprioceptive input from the muscle spindles and the kinesthetic information from joint receptors. Motor strength is characteristically preserved, although overlap with typical GBS seems to occur when some patients progress to develop quadriparesis. EDX studies demonstrate an axonal process affecting predominantly sensory nerve fibers, with no or only mild motor nerve conduction abnormalities. SNAP amplitudes are normal in half of the patients and reduced or absent with a sural sparing pattern in one-third of patients (Lyu et al., 2013). Motor conduction studies, F-wave latencies, and needle EMG are usually normal. Most patients have increased CSF protein without pleocytosis 1 week after the onset. Brain MRI is usually normal, though rarely the MRI may show brainstem lesions or gadolinium enhancement of ocular motor nerves. About 20% of patients with MFS have followed *C. jejuni* infection and 8% followed *Haemophilus influenzae* infection. Serum IgG antibodies to the ganglioside GQ1b are detected in acute-phase sera of 98% of patients with MFS and in many patients with GBS with ophthalmoplegia and ataxia, especially in those with a preceding *C. jejuni* infection, suggesting that the antibodies are disease specific and related to the pathogenesis (Yuki and Koga, 2006). GQ1b is abundantly present in paranodal regions of ocular nerves, explaining the association between high titers of this antibody and ophthalmoplegia. Other antiganglioside antibodies such as anti-GT1a, anti-GD3, and anti-GD1b have also been associated with MFS but with a lesser frequency. MFS has a favorable prognosis, with recovery after a mean of 10 weeks and a corresponding reduction in the antibody titers.

*Acute pandysautonomia,* considered to be another variant of GBS, is rare and characterized by the rapid onset of combined sympathetic and parasympathetic failure without somatic sensory and motor involvement. The deep tendon reflexes are usually lost during the course of the illness. These patients develop severe orthostatic hypotension, heat intolerance, anhidrosis, dry eyes and mouth, fixed pupils, fixed heart rate, and disturbances of bowel and bladder function. About half of patients have autoantibodies to ganglionic acetylcholine receptors, which may play a pathogenetic role by blocking cholinergic transmission in autonomic ganglia (Vernino et al., 2000). Ganglionic receptor-blocking antibodies serve as serological markers of autoimmune autonomic neuropathies and are elevated in both acute pandysautonomia and paraneoplastic autonomic neuropathy.

GBS may be strictly regional, as in the *pharyngeal-cervical-brachial variant.* Patients present with rapid onset of symmetrical multiple cranial nerve palsies (polyneuritis cranialis), most notably bilateral facial palsy. Isolated *facial diplegia with distal paresthesias* may be a forme fruste of this variant of GBS (Susuki et al., 2009).

The existence of a *sensory ataxic variant* of GBS affecting mainly sensory nerve fibers has long been suspected but rarely confirmed. Such patients present with acute ataxia, sensory loss, areflexia, high levels of CSF protein, and nerve conduction features of demyelination (Oh et al., 2001). SNAPs are intact in 60% and reduced or absent in the rest. Clinically, this variant is similar to the MFS, except for the lack of ophthalmoplegia and reduced occurrence of elevated GQ1b antibodies (65% vs. 98% in MFS). An *acute and painful small-fiber neuropathy* that is claimed to be another variant of GBS is reported to be responsive to corticosteroids, unlike the other variants (Dabby et al., 2006). It has been suggested that GBS following cytomegalovirus (CMV) infection is more likely to have prominent or predominant sensory involvement.

## Diagnostic Studies

CSF examination and serial EDX studies are important ancillary studies for confirming the diagnosis of GBS. Other laboratory studies are of limited value. Mild transient elevations in liver enzymes without obvious cause are found in about a third of patients. Hyponatremia is seen most frequently in ventilated patients because of inappropriate secretion of antidiuretic hormone. Deposition of immune complexes may rarely lead to glomerulonephritis and result in microscopic hematuria and proteinuria.

In the first week of neurological symptoms, the CSF protein may be normal in up to 50% of patients but then becomes elevated on subsequent examinations. In approximately 10% of cases, the CSF protein remains normal throughout the illness. Transient oligoclonal IgG bands and elevated myelin basic protein levels may be detected in the CSF of some patients. The increase in CSF protein and immunoglobulins is not usually associated with a cellular response *(albuminocytological dissociation).* In about 10% of patients, there is a slight lymphocytic pleocytosis greater than 10 cells/mm. However, moderate CSF pleocytosis (usually >50 cells) is a distinctive feature of GBS associated with HIV or Lyme infections.

The prompt diagnosis of GBS is warranted by the need to initiate early treatment. Hence, EDX studies are increasingly requested early on when the diagnosis of GBS is considered. The EDX consultant is often asked not only to exclude other diagnoses (e.g., botulism, myasthenia gravis) but also to confirm the diagnosis of GBS. Frustration is frequently encountered within the first few weeks of illness, since nerve conduction studies may not be diagnostic early in the course of the disease. The EDX studies in patients with GBS assist in detecting the presence of multifocal demyelination, the hallmark of acquired demyelinating polyneuropathy; however, these EDX abnormalities represent an evolving picture in GBS.

Abnormalities of EDX studies are found in approximately 90% of established GBS cases, sometimes during the course of illness. EDX studies performed in patients enrolled in the North American GBS study found abnormalities of distal motor latencies and F-wave latencies in about half of patients studied within 30 days of onset (Cornblath et al., 1988). Partial motor conduction block (30%), slowing of motor conduction velocity (24%), and reduced distal CMAP amplitudes (20%) were less frequent. However, some of these abnormalities are often nonspecific and do not distinguish acquired demyelination from axonal degeneration, which is characterized by reduced CMAP and SNAP amplitudes.

The most common EDX abnormalities seen in the first 2 weeks of illness are absent H reflexes and absent, delayed, or impersistent F waves, findings that are common in polyneuropathies but not specific for the demyelinating types. Abnormal F waves in the presence of normal conduction velocities and distal latencies are more specific findings since they suggest proximal demyelination. Multiple or complex A (axon) waves, recorded from several nerves and sometimes replacing F waves, are also commonly associated with AIDP. Reduced amplitude or absent SNAPs in the upper extremity combined with normal sural SNAPs *(sural sparing pattern)* are changes highly specific for the diagnosis of AIDP and occur in about 50% of patients during the first 2 weeks of the illness (Albers and Kelly, 1989; Gordon and Wilbourn, 2001). Sural sparing combined with abnormal F waves is highly specific (96% specific) for the diagnosis of AIDP, is present in about half of the patients with AIDP and in about two-thirds of patients younger than 60 years during the first 2 weeks of illness (Gordon and Wilbourn, 2001). A sensory ratio (sural + radial SNAPs/median + ulnar SNAPs) is a good substitute for sural sparing pattern, particularly in elderly patients who have absent sural SNAP or those with preexisting CTS. A high ratio (>1) is fairly specific and distinguishes GBS from other axonal polyneuropathies such as diabetic neuropathies. Conduction block of motor axons, the electrophysiological correlate of clinical weakness, is recognized by a decrease of greater than 50% in CMAP amplitude from distal to proximal stimulation in the absence of temporal dispersion. Conduction block at non-entrapment sites is highly specific for demyelination, but it occurs only in 15%–30% of early GBS, depending on the number of nerves and nerve segments studied. Patients with weakness that is related primarily to conduction block tend to have a faster and more complete recovery than those with diffusely low motor amplitudes. Prolonged distal motor latencies, reduction in distal CMAP amplitudes, significant CMAP dispersion, and slowing of motor conduction velocities are less common and tend to occur later in the course of the disease (Cleland et al., 2006; Cros and Triggs, 1996; Gordon and Wilbourn, 2001). Needle EMG is mostly complementary in GBS, initially showing decreased motor unit recruitment. Subsequently, if any amount of axonal degeneration occurs, fibrillation potentials appear 2–4 weeks after onset.

In general, the EDX studies become more specific for multifocal demyelination during the third and fourth weeks of illness (Albers and Kelly, 1989). In fact, about half of the patients have normal NCSs during the first 4 days of illness (except for absent H reflexes), while only about 10% of them have normal studies by the first week of illness (Gordon and Wilbourn, 2001). Additionally, several EDX criteria have been advocated over the years, with sensitivities ranging from 20% to 70% (Alam et al., 1998). In general, about two-thirds of patients fulfill the criteria for highly suggestive or definite AIDP in the first 2 weeks of illness, with high specificity (95%–100%). EDX parameters are the most reliable indicators of prognosis. Mean distal CMAP amplitude of less than 20% of the lower limit of normal (LLN) was associated with poor outcome in the North American GBS study (Cornblath et al., 1988). However, low distal CMAPs may be due to distal demyelination with distal conduction block and often mimics axonal loss. Rapid recovery of low distal CMAPs and SNAPs on sequential studies is a necessary confirmatory sign of distal demyelination. Inability to distinguish demyelinating conduction block from reversible conduction failure and axon-discontinuity conduction block has caused erroneous classification in up to one-third of GBS patients where the initial classification changed after serial recordings (Rajabally et al., 2015).

The value of specific serological tests in the diagnosis of GBS is limited except in MFS and AMAN (Yuki and Hartung, 2012). There is no specific ganglioside antibody that appears to be associated with AIDP. Hence, these ganglioside antibodies are not clinically useful. However, elevated anti-GQ1b ganglioside antibodies are consistently found in about 95%–98% of patients with MFS. Preceding *C. jejuni* infection has been linked to AMAN variant and high titers of anti-GM1, anti-GD1b, anti-GD1a, and anti-GalNAc-GD1a ganglioside antibodies of the IgG class (Jacobs et al., 1996). Serological tests for *C. jejuni* infection are difficult both to perform and interpret. Other studies confirmed the presence of IgG antiglycolipid antibodies in 10%–40% of patients with GBS but failed to show a correlation with *C. jejuni* infection (Ho et al., 1995). Elevated serum antibodies to *Mycoplasma*, CMV, or *C. jejuni* can pinpoint the preceding infection. Antigalactocerebroside antibodies have been detected in patients with precedent *Mycoplasma* infection. Complement-fixing antibodies to peripheral nerve myelin are present in most patients during the acute phase of GBS.

Imaging studies, more specifically MRI of the brain and spine, are most useful to exclude brainstem or spinal cord disease as a cause of the weakness. MRI of the lumbar spine with gadolinium, however, may be abnormal in GBS and may show nerve root enhancement of the cauda equina, particularly in children with GBS (Yikilmaz et al., 2010).

### Differential Diagnosis

Care should be taken to distinguish GBS from other conditions leading to subacute motor weakness (Box 106.12). Among the polyneuropathies with acute onset, acute porphyria, diphtheria, and occasional

**BOX 106.12 Differential Diagnostic Considerations in Guillain-Barré Syndrome**

**Muscle Disorders**
- Polymyositis
- Dermatomyositis
- Necrotizing autoimmune myopathy
- Rhabdomyolysis (drugs, toxins, exercise, trauma, metabolic myopathies, etc.)
- Critical illness myopathy

**Muscle Membrane Disorders**
- Familial periodic paralysis
- Secondary hypokalemic paralysis (thyrotoxicosis, malabsorption, barium salt poisoning, or abuse of diuretics, laxatives, or licorice)

**Neuromuscular Junction Disorders**
- Myasthenia gravis (myasthenic crisis)
- Botulism
- Drug-induced neuromuscular blockade
- Toxic:
  - Organophosphate
  - Nerve gas
  - Tick
  - Black widow spider
  - Snake venoms
- Metabolic:
  - Hypermagnesemia (toxemia of pregnancy treated with parenteral magnesium, magnesium-containing antacids, or cathartics)
  - Hypophosphatemia (parenteral hyperalimentation, phosphate-bindings antacids, acute alcohol intoxication, and severe respiratory alkalosis)

**Peripheral Nerve and/Root Disorders**
- Guillain-Barré syndrome
- Acute intermittent porphyria
- Diphtheritic polyneuropathy
- Critical illness polyneuropathy
- Vasculitic neuropathy
- Heavy metal acute poisoning (thallium, arsenic)
- Diffuse polyradiculopathy:
  - Infectious (Lyme, cytomegalovirus [CMV])
  - Inflammatory (sarcoidosis)
  - Neoplastic (solid tumors, lymphomas)

**Anterior Horn Cell Disorders**
- Acute poliomyelitis (wild-type polio viruses, West Nile virus, enteroviruses)

**Spinal Cord Disorders**
- Transverse myelitis
- Cord compression (disc herniation, fracture/dislocation, epidural malignancy)
- Cord infarction (anterior spinal artery syndrome)

**Brainstem Disorders**
- Central pontine myelinolysis
- Pontine infarct (basilar artery thrombosis)

toxic neuropathies (arsenic, thallium, buckthorn, acrylamide, organophosphate compounds, and n-hexane) must be considered. Flaccid general weakness and failure to wean from the ventilator are common features of *critical illness polyneuropathy* that develops in patients confined to the intensive care unit (ICU) with sepsis and multiorgan failure. EDX features of an axonal neuropathy and normal CSF findings distinguish critical illness neuropathy from the classic form of GBS. A related syndrome, *critical illness myopathy*, follows the use of non-depolarizing neuromuscular blocking agents or IV corticosteroids or both. Metabolic disturbances (severe hypophosphatemia, hypokalemia, or hypermagnesemia), rhabdomyolysis, and inflammatory myopathies may result in rapidly progressive generalized weakness. Elevated creatine kinase (CK), abnormal serum electrolytes, and needle EMG help distinguish these disorders from GBS. Disorders of neuromuscular transmission including myasthenic crisis, botulism, and tick paralysis should also be considered. *Myasthenic crisis* is often associated with CMAP decrement on slow-frequency repetitive nerve stimulation. *Botulism* develops after the consumption of contaminated foods, with ophthalmoparesis and facial and bulbar weakness. Nerve conduction studies reveal low-amplitude CMAPs, and high-frequency repetitive nerve stimulation or maximal voluntary contraction leads to an incremental response that is typical of presynaptic neuromuscular transmission defect. Acute brainstem infarct, spinal cord compression, epidural abscess, and transverse myelitis may present diagnostic difficulties before upper motor neuron signs develop and before results of EDX and CSF studies become available. Among other signs, early urinary retention and a sharply demarcated sensory level on the trunk suggest spinal cord disease and call for urgent spinal MRI. CSF pleocytosis (>50 cells per μL) casts doubt on the diagnosis of uncomplicated GBS and suggests inflammatory or neoplastic meningoradiculopathies such as secondary to Lyme disease, HIV infection, or CMV in AIDS. Poliomyelitis caused by the wild-type polio viruses may produce a rapidly evolving asymmetrical weakness accompanied by fever and CSF pleocytosis. Poliomyelitis due to West Nile virus may lead to flaccid paralysis in up to 27% of patients with neurological complications.

## Pathology

Classic pathological studies of AIDP have demonstrated endoneurial perivascular mononuclear cell infiltration together with multifocal demyelination. The peripheral nerves may be affected at all levels from the roots to distal intramuscular motor nerve endings, although most lesions usually occur on the ventral roots, proximal spinal nerves, and lower cranial nerves. Intense inflammation may lead to axonal degeneration as a consequence of a toxic bystander effect. Ultrastructural studies have shown that macrophages play a major role in demyelination by stripping off myelin lamellae from the axon. The inflammatory infiltrates consist mainly of class II-positive monocytes and macrophages, and T lymphocytes. The expression of class II antigen is increased in Schwann cells, raising the possibility that Schwann cells may present the antigen to autoreactive T cells and activate the destruction of myelin. Pathological studies in patients with AMAN using electron microscopy have demonstrated the presence of macrophages in the periaxonal space of myelinated internodes. Extensive primary wallerian-like degeneration of motor and sensory roots and nerves without significant inflammation or demyelination is found in cases of AMSAN.

## Pathogenesis

The bulk of experimental and clinical evidence suggests that GBS is an organ-specific, immune-mediated disorder caused by a synergistic interaction of cell-mediated and humoral immune responses against peripheral nerve antigens that are still incompletely characterized (Kieseier et al., 2006a).

Approximately two-thirds of patients report a preceding event, most frequently an upper respiratory or gastrointestinal infection, surgery, or immunization 1–4 weeks before the onset of neurological symptoms (Govoni and Granieri, 2001; Table 106.11). The agent responsible for the prodromal illness often remains unidentified. Specific infectious agents linked to GBS include CMV, Epstein-Barr virus, varicella-zoster virus (VZV), hepatitis A and B, HIV, *Mycoplasma pneumoniae*, and *H. influenzae*. Recent evidence from Colombia, French Polynesia, and Puerto Rico have shown that infection with Zika virus, a mosquito-borne RNA *Flavivirus*, plays an important role in the development of GBS (Parra et al., 2016).

The most common identifiable bacterial organism linked to GBS and particularly its axonal forms is *C. jejuni*, a curved gram-negative rod that is a common cause of bacterial enteritis worldwide. Evidence of *C. jejuni* infection from stool cultures or serological tests was found in 26% of patients with GBS admitted to hospitals in the United Kingdom, compared with 2% of case controls (Rees et al., 1995). Retrospective studies from the United States, Holland, Germany, and Australia report serological evidence of recent *C. jejuni* infection ranging from 17% to 39% of patients with GBS. It should be noted that in the United States alone, an estimated 2.4 million cases of enteric infection with *C. jejuni* are reported per year, yet only about 2500 individuals develop GBS. This suggests that host-related factors or certain polymorphisms of *C. jejuni* determine the development of GBS. *C. jejuni* infection may play an even greater role in northern China, where the infection rates are 76% in patients with AMAN and 42% in patients with AIDP (Ho et al., 1995). Molecular mimicry between GM1 ganglioside and *C. jejuni* lipo-oligosaccharide is established as the pathogenic link for this association.

Epidemiological data suggested a slight increase in cases of GBS following the 1976 A/New Jersey influenza vaccine, although no excess risk of developing GBS was seen with subsequent influenza vaccines. The most recent studies suggest an even further decline of reported cases of GBS after influenza vaccination from the low levels reported a decade earlier, indicating that the risk of GBS after influenza vaccination now stands at only one additional case per 2.5 million persons vaccinated (Haber et al., 2004). A UK study also provides reassurance that the great majority of sporadically occurring GBS is not associated with immunization (Hughes et al., 2006b). For these reasons, prior GBS should not preclude administration of influenza vaccines in high-risk individuals.

Other vaccines (notably tetanus and diphtheria toxoids, rabies, oral polio, and meningococcal conjugate vaccines); drugs including

**TABLE 106.11 Antecedent Events of Guillain-Barré Syndrome**

| Antecedent Event | Percentage |
|---|---|
| Respiratory illness | 58 |
| Gastrointestinal illness | 22 |
| Respiratory and gastrointestinal illness | 10 |
| Surgery | 5 |
| Vaccination | 3 |
| Other | 2 |
| **Serological Evidence of Specific Infectious Agents** | |
| *Campylobacter jejuni* | |
| Cytomegalovirus | |
| Human immunodeficiency virus | |
| Epstein-Barr virus | |
| *Mycoplasma* pneumonia | |
| Hepatitis A and B | |
| Zika virus | |

streptokinase, suramin, gangliosides, and heroin; and Hymenoptera stings have been associated in a few cases. Several cases have occurred in immunocompromised hosts with Hodgkin lymphoma or in pharmacologically immunosuppressed patients after solid organ or bone marrow transplantation.

A preceding infection may trigger an autoimmune response through "molecular mimicry," in which the host generates an immune response against an infectious organism that shares epitopes with the host's peripheral nerves. At the onset of disease, activated T cells play a major role in opening the blood–nerve barrier to allow circulating antibodies to gain access to peripheral nerve antigens. T-cell activation markers (interleukin [IL]-6, IL-2, soluble IL-2 receptor, and interferon γ [IFN-γ]) and tumor necrosis factor α (TNF-α), a proinflammatory cytokine released by T cells and macrophages, particularly IL-23 (Hu et al., 2006), are increased in patient serum. In addition, adhesion molecules and matrix metalloproteinases are critically involved in facilitating recruitment and transmigration of activated T cells and monocytes through the blood–nerve barrier. Soluble E-selectin, an adhesion molecule produced by endothelial cells, and metalloproteinases are increased in patients with GBS during the early stages of disease. A cell-mediated immune reaction against myelin components is supported by experimental allergic neuritis, the accepted animal model for AIDP. Experimental allergic neuritis can be produced by active immunization with whole peripheral nerve homogenate, myelin, or PNS-specific myelin basic protein P2, P0, or galactocerebroside.

Several observations indicate that humoral factors also participate in the autoimmune attack on peripheral nerve myelin, axons, and nerve terminals: (1) immunoglobulins and complement can be demonstrated on myelinated fibers of affected patients by immunostaining; (2) MFS and AMAN are strongly associated with specific antiganglioside antibodies; (3) serum from MFS and AMAN patients contains IgG antibodies that block peripheral nerve transmission in a mouse nerve-muscle preparation; (4) complement C1-fixing antiperipheral nerve myelin antibody can be detected in the serum of patients during the acute phase of GBS; (5) intraneural injection of GBS serum into rat sciatic nerve results in secondary T-cell infiltration of the injection site at the time of the appearance of the hind limb weakness; and (6) plasmapheresis or immunoglobulin infusions result in clinical improvement.

Understanding of the immune mechanisms of GBS, including AIDP and its axonal subtypes, was enhanced by the detailed immunohistochemical and ultrastructural studies of clinically well-defined autopsied cases from northern China. The earliest changes seen in AIDP within days of onset consisted of deposition of complement activation products and membrane attack complex on the outermost Schwann cell surface, followed by vesicular myelin changes at the outermost myelin lamellae, with subsequent recruitment of macrophages and progressive demyelination (Hafer-Macko et al., 1996). Previously, the role of complement had been suggested by the finding of increased levels of complement activation products in CSF and soluble terminal complement complexes in serum of patients with AIDP. The immune attack in AIDP appears to begin with binding of autoantibodies to specific epitopes on the outermost Schwann cell membrane, with consequent activation of complement (Fig. 106.17). The nature of the epitope in AIDP, although still uncertain, is likely to be a glycolipid. Pathological studies of early cases of AMAN found deposition of activated complement components and immunoglobulins at the nodal axolemma. This was followed by disruption of the paranodal space, allowing the entry of complement and immunoglobulins along the axolemma, with subsequent recruitment of macrophages to affected nodes. Finally, macrophages were shown to invade the periaxonal space, leading to wallerian-like degeneration of motor fibers

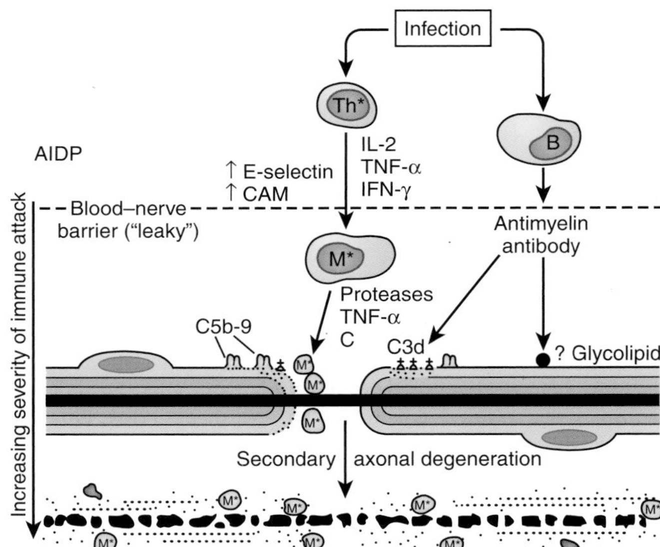


**Fig. 106.17 Immune Injury to Nerve Fibers in Acute Inflammatory Demyelinating Polyradiculoneuropathy** *(AIDP)*. Preceding infection may trigger formation of antimyelin autoantibodies and activated T-helper cells *(Th*)*. Proinflammatory cytokines (tumor necrosis factor alpha *[TNF-α]*, interferon gamma *[INF-γ]*), and upregulation of adhesion molecules (E-selectin, intercellular adhesion molecule *[ICAM]*) facilitate breakdown of blood–nerve barrier to activated T cells, macrophages, and antimyelin antibodies. Antimyelin antibodies react with epitopes on the abaxonal Schwann cell membrane, with consequent activation of complement. Deposition of complement activation products *(C3d)* and membrane attack complex *(C5b-9)* on the outermost Schwann cell membrane leads to vesicular myelin changes, followed by recruitment of macrophages *(M*)* and progressive demyelination. Intense inflammation may lead to secondary axonal degeneration. *B*, B cell; *IL-2*, interleukin 2. *(Adapted from Bosch, E.P., 1998. Guillain-Barré syndrome: an update of acute immune-mediated polyradiculoneuropathies. Neurologist 4, 211–226.)*

(Hafer-Macko et al., 1996; Fig. 106.18). These findings suggest that AMAN is caused by an antibody- and complement-mediated attack on axolemmal epitopes of motor fibers. The most attractive candidate targets are GM1- and asialo-GM1-like gangliosides, which are present in nodal and internodal membranes of motor fibers. Certain *C. jejuni* strains associated with axonal GBS and MFS variants contain GM1-like epitopes in their polysaccharide coats. Anti-GM1 and GQ1b antibodies that cross-react to these lipopolysaccharide epitopes are found in a high proportion of patients with AMAN and MFS, respectively, as well as in some patients with AIDP. These observations have led to the concept of molecular mimicry in which epitopes of the infectious agent elicit antibodies that cross-react with shared epitopes on axons. The nerve fibers thereby become the inadvertent targets of an immune response directed against an infectious organism. The antiganglioside antibodies obtained from AMAN and MFS patients block neuromuscular transmission in an in vitro nerve-muscle preparation. The blocking activity of these IgG antibodies can be neutralized by IVIG (Buchwald et al., 2002). Furthermore, rabbits immunized with GM1 develop AMAN, thereby fulfilling the postulates for confirming an autoimmune pathogenesis (Sheikh and Griffin, 2001). AMSAN may be caused by a more severe immune injury triggered by axonal epitopes because similar pathological changes affecting motor and sensory fibers have been observed in cases of AMSAN. In addition to *C. jejuni* and gangliosides, molecular mimicry for GBS is also shown with for *Mycoplasma* pneumonia and galactocerebroside, and CMV infection and moesin (Sawai et al., 2014).

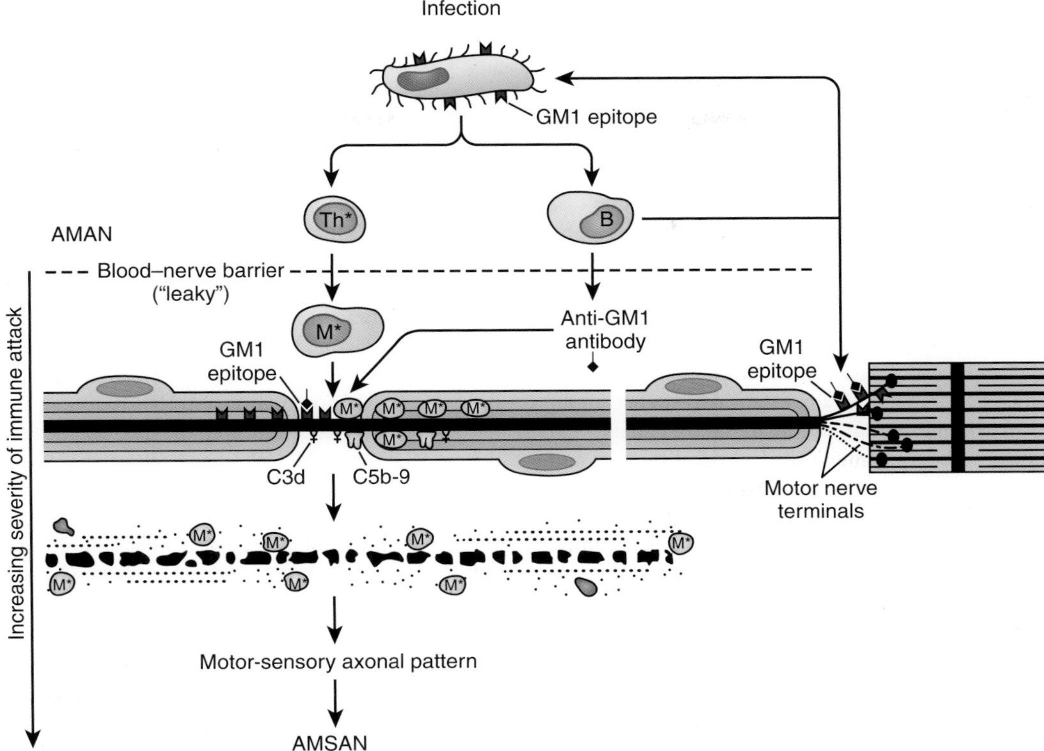


**Fig. 106.18 Immune Injury to Nerve Fibers in Acute Motor Axonal Neuropathy *(AMAN)*.** Molecular mimicry of GM1-like epitopes common to both lipopolysaccharide coats of certain *Campylobacter jejuni* strains and axonal membranes may cause an autoimmune response. Activated complement components *(C3d, C5b-9)* and immunoglobulins are found at nodes of Ranvier and along axolemma of motor fibers. Macrophages *(M*)* are recruited to targeted nodes and invade periaxonal space, leading to wallerian degeneration. Lack of blood–nerve barrier at motor nerve terminals may make these distal axons vulnerable to circulating GM1 antibodies. *AMSAN*, Acute motor sensory axonal neuropathy; *B*, B cell; *Th**, activated T-helper cells. *(Adapted from Bosch, E.P., 1998. Guillain-Barré syndrome: an update of acute immune-mediated polyradiculoneuropathies. Neurologist 4, 211–226.)*

## Treatment

General supportive management is the mainstay of treatment. Patients with rapidly worsening acute GBS should be observed in the hospital until the maximum extent of progression has been established. The reduction in mortality to less than 5% reflects improvements in modern critical care. The prevention of complications, of which respiratory failure and autonomic dysfunction are the most important, provides the best chance for a favorable outcome (Bosch, 1998). Respiratory and bulbar function, ability to handle secretions, heart rate, and blood pressure should be closely monitored during the progressive phase. Respiratory failure requiring mechanical ventilation develops in up to 30% of patients with GBS. Predictors of future need for mechanical ventilation include rapid disease progression (onset to admission in <7 days), severity of limb weakness, presence of facial weakness, and bulbar weakness (Walgaard et al., 2010). Hence, patients with one or more of these predictors, evidence of dysautonomia, or signs of respiratory insufficiency should be admitted to the ICU for closer observation. Signs of impending respiratory failure include deterioration in forced vital capacity (FVC), declining maximal respiratory pressures, and hypoxemia caused by atelectasis. Initially it may be necessary to monitor FVC and negative inspiratory pressure every 4–6 hours while the patient is awake. Patients should be monitored by pulse oximetry, especially at night, for the early detection of oxygen desaturation. Serial measures of decline in respiratory function that could predict future respiratory failure include vital capacity of less than 20 mL/kg or a decline by 30% from baseline, maximal inspiratory pressure less than 30 cm $H_2O$, and maximal expiratory respiratory pressure of less than 40 cm $H_2O$ (Lawn et al., 2001). This so-called *20-30-40 rule* allows patients at risk to be identified and transferred to an ICU for even closer monitoring. In a series of 200 patients, short disease duration, inability to lift the head from the bed, and a vital capacity of less than 60% predicted the need for mechanical ventilation in 85% of patients with all three risk factors (Sharshar et al., 2003). Elective intubation for ventilatory assistance should be performed when FVC falls below 12–15 mL/kg or below 18 mL/kg in patients with severe oropharyngeal weakness, or when arterial $PO_2$ values fall below 70 mm Hg with inspired room air. When respiratory assistance is needed for longer than 2 weeks, a tracheostomy should be performed.

In the event of cardiac arrhythmias or marked fluctuations of blood pressure, continuous ECG and blood pressure monitoring allow early detection of life-threatening situations that require prompt treatment. Antihypertensive and vasoactive drugs must be used with extreme caution in the presence of autonomic instability. Tracheal suctioning may trigger sudden episodes of hypotension or bradyarrhythmia. Back and radicular pain often respond to NSAIDs. At times, oral or parenteral opioids are required for adequate pain control. Increased metabolic requirements together with negative caloric intake caused by impaired swallowing may lead to a state of relative starvation in severely affected patients. Nutritional requirements should be met by providing a high-caloric protein diet or by beginning enteral feedings as early as possible.

Subcutaneous heparin or low-molecular-weight heparin together with calf compression devices should be ordered routinely in immobilized patients to lower the risks of venous thrombosis and pulmonary embolism. Infections of the lung and urinary tract develop in almost half of patients with GBS in the ICU. Prevention and prompt treatment of nosocomial infections are important aspects of care. Chest physical therapy and frequent oral suctioning aid in preventing atelectasis in patients with impaired cough and sigh. Skilled nursing care with regular turning and attention to skin, eyes, mouth, bowel, and bladder are essential. Exposure keratitis is avoided in cases of facial diplegia by using artificial tears and by taping the eyelids closed at night. Pressure-induced ulnar or fibular nerve palsies are prevented by proper positioning and padding. Physical therapy is started early because it helps prevent contractures, joint immobilization, and venous stasis. Psychological support and constant reassurance about the potential for recovery are important for the morale of patients and family members. In the recovery phase, skilled physical therapy and rehabilitation hasten recovery.

Among specific therapeutic interventions aimed at mitigating the harmful effects of the autoimmune reaction and autoantibodies, plasma exchange and high-dose IVIG infusions have been shown to be equally effective. Six large randomized controlled trials involving more than 600 patients have established the benefit of centrifugal plasma exchange in acute GBS by shortening the recovery time (Lehmann et al., 2006). Therapeutic plasma exchange is recommended for patients with moderate to severe weakness (defined as the ability to walk only with support or worse). Benefits are clearest when plasma exchange is begun within 2 weeks of onset. The effect of plasma exchange in mildly affected patients and the optimal number of exchanges were investigated by the French Cooperative Group on Plasma Exchange (1997). Even mildly affected patients benefited from two exchanges. Four exchanges were optimal for moderate and severe cases, and six exchanges did not have additional benefit. The recommended plasmapheresis schedule entails a series of four to five exchanges (40–50 mL/kg) with a continuous flow machine on alternate days, using saline and albumin as replacement fluid. A Cochrane review confirmed the value of plasma exchange over supportive therapy in hastening the recovery from GBS when started within 30 days after disease onset (Raphael et al., 2002). Plasmapheresis should be performed only in centers with experience in exchange techniques in critically ill patients. Most serious complications are linked to venous access problems, including hematoma formation at puncture sites, pneumothorax after insertion of central lines, and catheter-related septicemia. Septicemia, active bleeding, and severe cardiovascular instability are contraindications for plasmapheresis. Filtration-based plasma exchange techniques, which use porous membranes for filtration, has similar safety and efficiency when compared to centrifugal plasma exchange. A single study comparing these two modalities in patients with GBS demonstrated a shorter time to onset of effect and greater change in disability with centrifugal plasma exchange. However, mortality and outcome after 6 months were not different between the two therapeutic modalities (Lyu et al., 2002).

Three randomized trials comparing IVIG with plasma exchange demonstrated the benefit of five daily infusions of immunoglobulin (0.4 g/kg/day) given in the first 2 weeks of the disease (Plasma Exchange/Sandoglobulin Guillain-Barré Syndrome Trial Group, 1997). Both treatment modalities were equally effective. There was no advantage of using both together. These findings were confirmed by another Cochrane systematic review (Hughes et al., 2001b). In pediatric patients with GBS, IVIG seems to be of similar efficacy as in adults (Korinthenberg et al., 2005).

Anti-idiotypical antibodies supplied by IVIG that have the potential to bind and neutralize pathogenetic antibodies are the proposed mode of action. Minor side effects such as headaches, myalgias and arthralgias, flulike symptoms, fever, and vasomotor reactions are observed when infusion flow rates are excessive. More serious complications such as anaphylaxis in IgA-deficient individuals (1 per 1000 population, who develop anti-IgA antibodies after the first course of IgA-containing IVIG infusions), aseptic meningitis, congestive heart failure, thrombotic complications (venous thrombosis and cerebral and myocardial infarctions), and transient renal failure, have been reported (Brannagan, 2002). The rate of vascular complications, particularly cerebral and myocardial infarctions, is higher in patients with vascular risk factors treated with a more rapid infusion rate. To prevent headache and possibly aseptic meningitis, patients should be pretreated with oral acetaminophen, 500–1000 g, or ibuprofen, 800 mg, a few hours before each infusion; the dose can be repeated 6 hours later if headache develops. IVIG has become the preferred treatment for acute GBS in US hospitals, probably because of ease of administration (Alshekhlee et al., 2008b; Fig. 106.19). For patients with hyperviscosity, congestive heart failure, chronic renal failure (especially that due to diabetes), or congenital IgA deficiency, IVIG is contraindicated and plasma exchange is preferred.

The optimal effective dose of IVIG has not been well established. The IVIG dose used in the clinical trials and in practice was set arbitrarily at a total of 2 g/kg divided in 5 days (0.4 g/kg/day) empirically based on clinical experience in patients with idiopathic thrombocytopenic purpura. Six daily infusions of 0.4 g/kg were reported to be superior to three daily infusions in patients who could not receive plasma exchange (Raphael et al., 2001). GBS patients receiving the standard dose of IVIG (0.4 g/kg/day × 5 days) have a large variation of IgG levels measured 2 weeks after infusion, and those with a smaller increase in IgG level do worse, independent of other prognostic factors (Kuitwaard et al., 2009). It is not yet known whether the infusion of additional IVIG to patients who show a small increase in IgG levels is beneficial.

With both plasma exchange and IVIG, one or more episodes of deterioration following the initial improvement or stabilization after treatment, described as "treatment-related fluctuations," may be encountered in 10%–20% of patients. This may pose practical problems both in terms of treatment and in differentiating these patients from those who are developing a rapid-onset CIDP (Ruts et al., 2005). Additional rescue treatment with IVIG or plasma exchange in patients with poorly responsive or relapsing GBS may be useful (Alboudi et al., 2019); however, prospective randomized studies to either a second-line treatment or supportive management are needed for patients who do not respond or relapse after first-line treatment.

Corticosteroids are not recommended because two randomized controlled trials, one using conventional doses of prednisolone and the other using high-dose IV methylprednisolone, have found no benefit. The combination of IVIG with methylprednisolone failed to find significant long-term advantage over IVIG alone in one trial. A recent Cochrane review confirms that corticosteroids do not produce significant benefit or harm (Hughes et al., 2006c).

## Course and Prognosis

Approximately 15% of GBS patients have a mild condition, remain ambulatory, and recover after a few weeks. Conversely, 5%–20% of patients have a fulminant course and develop flaccid quadriplegia, ventilator dependence, and axonal degeneration, often within 2 days from the onset of symptoms. The recovery is delayed and virtually always incomplete and most have substantial residual motor deficits at 1-year follow-up. Patients with AMAN and electrophysiological evidence of

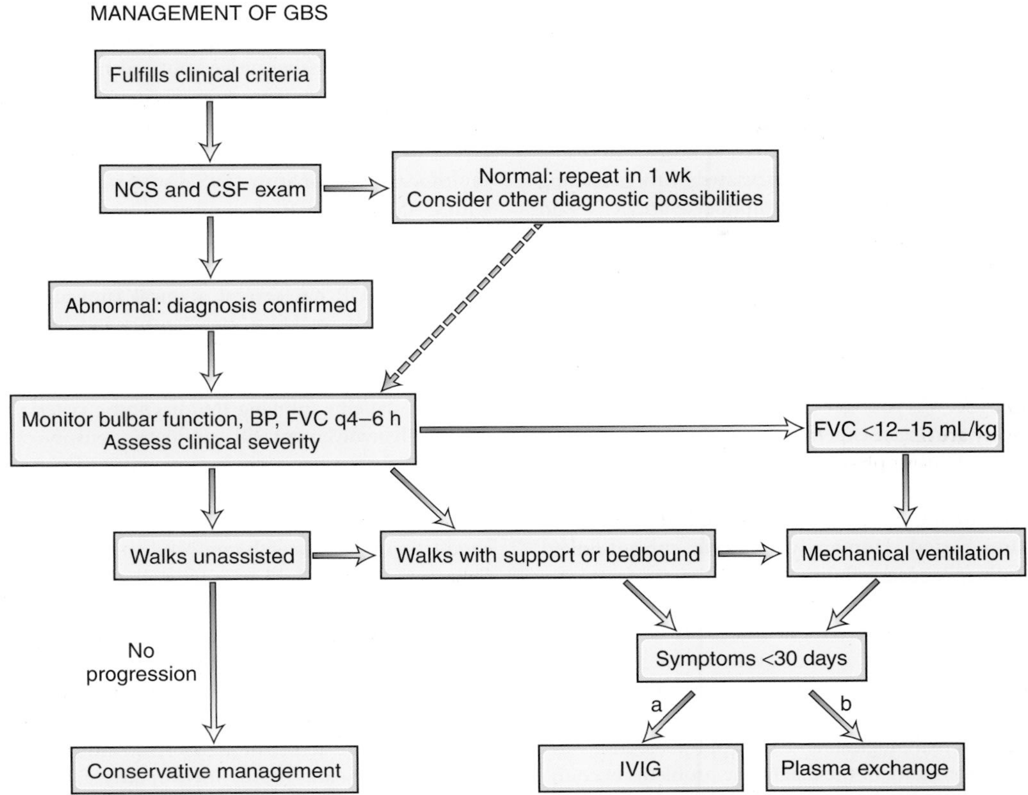


**Fig. 106.19 Decision-Making Pathway in Management of Guillain–Barré Syndrome.** Both treatment options, intravenous immunoglobulin *(IVIG) (a)* and plasma exchange *(b)*, are equally efficacious. IVIG is preferred because of its ease of administration. *BP,* Blood pressure; *CSF,* cerebrospinal fluid; *GBS,* Guillain–Barré syndrome; *FVC,* forced vital capacity; *NCS,* nerve conduction studies. *(Adapted from Bosch, E.P., 1998. Guillain-Barré syndrome: an update of acute immune-mediated polyradiculoneuropathies. Neurologist 4, 211–226.)*

axonal failure have a prognosis which is comparable to patients' AIDP. This is explained by reversible conduction failure caused by transitory dysfunction at the node of Ranvier without secondary axonal degeneration.

Because progressive axonal degeneration of nerve roots results in the disintegration of axonal membrane and release of axoskeletal proteins such as neurofilaments and tau proteins into the CSF, it has been suggested that higher levels of CSF neurofilaments and tau serve as predictors of worse motor and functional outcome (Jin et al., 2006; Petzold et al., 2006).

Up to 30% of patients with GBS develop respiratory insufficiency requiring assisted ventilation, and between 2% and 5% die of complications (Alshekhlee et al., 2008a). After progression stops, patients enter a plateau phase lasting 2–4 weeks or longer before recovery begins. Although most patients recover functionally, 20% still have residual motor weakness 1 year later. Approximately 70% of patients complete their recovery in 12 months and 82% in 24 months. Up to 5% of patients may have a recurrence following recovery. Predictors for poor recovery (<20% probability of walking independently at 6 months) include older age (>60 years), history of preceding diarrheal illness, recent CMV infection, ventilatory support, rapid progression reaching maximum deficit in less than 7 days, hyponatremia, and low distal CMAP amplitudes (20% of LLN or less) or inexcitable nerves. The overall prognosis of GBS is also influenced by the patient's age, the severity of illness at its peak, and whether immunomodulating therapies are initiated early. Complications such as acute hypoxic-ischemic encephalopathy and infectious episodes also probably worsen the prognosis.

Patients with GBS should reach their maximum deficit within 4 weeks of onset; if the disease progresses over a longer period of time, CIDP should be considered. About 5% of patients initially diagnosed with GBS develop a more protracted course similar to CIDP: hence the term *acute-onset CIDP* (Odaka et al., 2003). Acute-onset CIDP should be considered if GBS patients have one or more of these findings: (1) deteriorate after 8 weeks; (2) have more than two treatment-related fluctuations, particularly when they occur beyond 1 month of the illness; (3) have prominent sensory symptoms or signs; (4) have multifocal enlargement of peripheral nerves on ultrasound; or (5) develop new prominent demyelinating features on follow-up EDX studies many months after the initial presentation (Anadani and Katirji, 2015; Kerasnoudis et al., 2015; Ruts et al., 2010a). Recent studies have also suggested that nerve excitability techniques may be useful in distinguishing acute-onset CIDP from AIDP at the initial stage of disease (Sung et al., 2014).

## Chronic Inflammatory Demyelinating Polyradiculoneuropathy

CIDP is a heterogeneous group of immune-mediated neuropathies characterized by a relapsing-remitting or a chronically progressive clinical course, typically exceeding 8 weeks, and demyelinating features on EDX testing. Many similarities exist between CIDP and AIDP, the most common acute form of GBS. Both disorders have similar clinical features, involve the spinal roots and peripheral nerves, and share the CSF albuminocytological dissociation and the pathological abnormalities of multifocal inflammatory demyelination, with nerve conduction features reflecting demyelination. An autoimmune basis is suspected for both disorders, although the supporting evidence remains incomplete (Hughes et al., 2006a; Nobile-Orazio et al., 2014). The major differences between the two conditions are in the time course, prognosis, and their response to corticosteroids. CIDP has a more protracted clinical course, is rarely associated with preceding infections, has an association with human lymphocyte antigens, and responds to corticosteroid therapy.

Two patterns of temporal evolution of CIDP can be seen. More than 60% of patients show a continuous or stepwise progressive course over months to years, and one-third have a relapsing course with partial or complete recovery between recurrences, whereas acute-onset CIDP is rare. The age of onset may influence the course of the disease. In one large series, the age of onset was younger (mean 29 years) in those who had a relapsing course than in those experiencing a chronic progressive course (mean 51 years). A history of preceding infection is found in less than 10%. In contrast, pregnancy is associated with a significant number of relapses, occurring mainly in the third trimester and the immediate postpartum period. Human lymphocyte antigen-linked genetic factors may influence susceptibility to CIDP.

The prevalence of CIDP ranges from 1 to 9 per 100,000 of the population depending on diagnostic criteria (Rajabally et al., 2009). Although precise prevalence figures are not available for the United States, CIDP represents 13%–20% of all initially undiagnosed neuropathies referred to specialized neuromuscular centers.

The substantial clinical, pathological, and electrophysiological variability of CIDP accounts for many of the diagnostic problems encountered in clinical practice, including the commonly observed under- or overdiagnosis of this condition. Inaccurate diagnosis may result in months if not years of expensive, ineffective, and potentially harmful treatments. Misdiagnosis of CIDP is increasingly occurring due to both clinical and EDX flaws. Erroneous diagnosis of CIDP is often due to inclusion of extremely atypical forms, many patients with sensory symptoms only and reliance on wrong electrophysiological interpretation of acquired demyelination such as absence of conduction block at non-entrapment sites, presence of mild amplitude-dependent slowing in axonal polyneuropathies and diabetics, and slowing of conduction velocity at compression sites only (Allen and Lewis 2015; Allen et al., 2018). Other sources of inaccuracies include subjective perception of treatment benefit and presence of only mild or moderate elevation of CSF protein.

### Clinical Features

CIDP is a lifelong disease that invariably causes some degree of disability even with the most effective immunomodulating therapies (Lewis, 2007). It is seen at all ages, with the peak incidence in the fifth and sixth decades. The manifestations at onset are extremely variable. Most patients have symmetrical motor and sensory involvement, although occasional cases with predominantly motor involvement may be seen (Mathey et al., 2015). To fulfill diagnostic criteria for CIDP, weakness must be present for at least 2 months. Proximal limb weakness is almost as severe as distal limb weakness, indicating a non-length-dependent neuropathy. Muscle wasting is rarely pronounced. These signs provide helpful clinical clues to separate CIDP patients from those with axonal neuropathies. Both upper and lower limbs are affected, although the legs are often more severely involved. Generalized hyporeflexia or areflexia is the rule. Sensory symptoms in a stocking-glove distribution (numbness or tingling) implicating large-fiber involvement occur frequently, whereas pain occurs less frequently. Children differ from adults by having a more precipitous onset and more prominent gait abnormalities. Additional findings, listed in decreasing order of frequency, are postural tremor of the hands, enlargement of peripheral nerves, papilledema, and facial or bulbar weakness. Rarely, respiratory failure requiring mechanical ventilation or autonomic dysfunction may be seen. Massive nerve root enlargement, causing myelopathy or symptomatic lumbar stenosis, or vision loss due to progressive pseudotumor cerebri are other unusual clinical features (Midroni and Dyck, 1996). Occasionally, CIDP may be associated with a relapsing multifocal demyelinating CNS disorder resembling multiple sclerosis, with CNS demyelination confirmed by abnormal visual and somatosensory evoked potentials and brain MRI (Falcone et al., 2006).

***Chronic inflammatory demyelinating polyradiculoneuropathy variants.*** CIDP has several atypical clinical variants with different distribution of weakness and sensory deficits. These atypical CIDP variants constitute about 18%–20% of all CIDP patients (Donuddu et al., 2019).

Some patients fulfilling the diagnostic criteria for CIDP have only distal limb involvement with symmetric, sensory, or sensorimotor symptoms and signs, often with sensory ataxia *(distal acquired demyelinating symmetric neuropathy, or DADS variant)*. Electrophysiological studies showed symmetrical and uniform slowing of distal latencies more than conduction velocities with rare conduction blocks. Nearly two-thirds of these patients have IgM monoclonal gammopathies, and though they have been reported to respond poorly to therapy, some patients respond favorably to IVIG or rituximab (Dalakas et al., 2009; Katz et al., 2000).

Multifocal distribution of weakness and sensory deficits are seen in some patients. This multifocal form of CIDP, initially identified by Lewis and Sumner (hence the term *Lewis-Sumner variant*), is also described by the acronym *MADSAM* (multifocal asymmetric demyelinating sensory and motor) neuropathy. Electrophysiological studies demonstrating focal conduction block or severe slowing of nerve conduction distinguish this multifocal demyelinating neuropathy from the vasculitic axon-loss multiple mononeuropathies. Unlike MMN, patients with this multifocal variant of CIDP have clinical and electrophysiological involvement of both motor and sensory nerves, increased CSF protein, and a good response to corticosteroids.

Pure sensory and pure motor variants of CIDP are relatively common. In both variants, motor conduction studies are abnormal despite the absence of motor symptoms and signs in the sensory types.

Selective involvement of sensory nerve roots, termed *chronic immune sensory polyradiculopathy* (CISP), is likely another variant of CIDP. Such patients present with a sensory ataxic syndrome with normal motor and sensory conduction studies. Sensory nerve root involvement is suggested by abnormal somatosensory evoked responses, enlarged lumbar roots on MRI, and elevated CSF protein. In selected cases, nerve root biopsy confirms segmental demyelination, onion bulbs, and endoneurial inflammation (Sinnreich et al., 2004). These patients have a positive response to IVIG.

Selective involvement of sensory and motor nerve roots, termed *chronic immune sensorimotor polyradiculopathy* (CISMP), is increasingly recognized (Thammongkolchai et al., 2019). This is considered a variant of CIDP and is responsive to IVIG. These patients have both weakness and sensory symptoms with chronically progressive, stepwise, or recurrent symptoms. EDX studies show normal SNAPs and normal motor conduction studies (except for some reduction of CMAP amplitudes) without slowing or conduction blocks. The majority have abnormal F-waves and H-reflexes. Needle EMG is consistent with polyradiculopathy pattern with fibrillation potentials and large MUAPs with reduced recruitment involving multiple myotomes with or without involvement of the paraspinal muscles. CSF protein is elevated and MRI often shows enhancing caudal and lumbosacral roots in the majority of patients, confirming the inflammatory root pathology (Thammongkolchai et al., 2019). When regional and limited to the lower extremities, this is sometimes referred to as chronic inflammatory lumbosacral polyradiculopathy (Caporale et al., 2011).

A syndrome characterized by *chronic ataxic neuropathy and ophthalmoplegia is associated with disialosyl-ganglioside IgM antibodies and cold agglutinins* (known under the acronym *CANOMAD*) and is considered a CIDP variant. The IgM protein has autoantibodies directed against gangliosides, specifically to GD1b and GQ1b (Arbogast et al., 2007; Eurelings et al., 2001; Willison et al., 2001). Autopsies have shown dorsal root ganglionopathy with significant loss of dorsal root ganglion cells and dorsal column atrophy as well as clonal IgM anti-disialyl gangliosides secreting B lymphocytes within cranial and peripheral nerves (McKelvie et al., 2013). Optimal treatment for CANOMAD is not yet established. Plasma exchange followed by rituximab or cyclophosphamide and IVIG may halt or improve symptoms. Surgical correction of strabismus usually improves ocular motility and visual symptoms.

It is important to remember that CIDP is a syndrome with many underlying causes. Acquired demyelinating polyradiculoneuropathies meeting the diagnostic criteria for CIDP may be associated with HIV-1 infection, systemic lupus erythematosus (SLE), monoclonal gammopathy of undetermined significance (MGUS), chronic active hepatitis, and inflammatory bowel disease. Compared with idiopathic CIDP, the patients with a *monoclonal gammopathy* tend to be older, have a more protracted course but less severe functional impairment at presentation, and respond less favorably to immunomodulatory therapy (Dalakas et al., 2009).

Excluding patients with MGUS, CIDP has been reported in association with *hematological malignancies* (including Waldenström macroglobulinemia [WM], multiple myeloma, POEMS syndrome, and Castleman disease) and *lymphomas*. Onset of CIDP frequently preceded that of lymphoma. Occasional patients with *malignant melanoma* or after therapy by vaccination with melanoma lysates develop CIDP. The association between melanoma and CIDP might be explained by molecular mimicry because both melanoma and Schwann cells are derived from neural crest tissue and share common glycolipid antigens (Weiss et al., 1998).

CIDP may occasionally be *drug induced*. A demyelinating neuropathy mimicking CIDP may follow treatment with tacrolimus, a macrolide antibiotic with strong immunosuppressive properties. Similarly, CIDP may be triggered by TNF-α antagonists, including etanercept, infliximab, and adalimumab (Alshekhlee et al., 2010). The neuropathic manifestations in these patients may start as early as 2 weeks after initiation of therapy or as late as 16 months. Interferon-alpha treatment has been reported to induce CIDP and Lewis-Sumner variant as well as AIDP, neuralgic amyotrophy, and cranial neuropathies (Supakornnumporn and Katirji, 2018). Immune checkpoint–blocking antibodies are new immunotherapy tools that have shown remarkable benefit in the treatment of a range of cancer types, including melanoma, lung cancer, and urological malignancies. The majority of these agents, including ipilimumab (anti-CTL-4, cytotoxic T-lymphocyte antigen 4), nivolumab and pembrolizumab (anti-PD-1, programmed cell death 1), and atezolizumab, avelumab, and durvalumab (anti-PD-L1, programmed cell death ligand 1) have been reported to induce or worsen autoimmune diseases including myasthenia gravis and myositis (Kolb et al., 2018). CIDP and AIDP have also been reported following the use of immune checkpoint–blocking antibodies (Supakornnumporn and Katirji, 2017, 2018).

CIDP is claimed to be more than 10 times more frequent in patients with both insulin-dependent diabetes mellitus (IDDM) and noninsulin-dependent diabetes mellitus (NIDDM), and these patients respond to IVIG therapy (Sharma et al., 2002a). Appropriate laboratory studies are necessary to separate these polyradiculoneuropathies from idiopathic CIDP without concurrent disease.

### BOX 106.13 Diagnostic Criteria for Chronic Inflammatory Demyelinating Polyradiculoneuropathy

**Mandatory Clinical Criteria**

Progressive or relapsing muscle weakness for 2 months or longer
Symmetrical proximal and distal weakness in upper or lower extremities
Hyporeflexia or areflexia

**Mandatory Laboratory Criteria**

Nerve conduction studies with features of demyelination (motor nerve conduction <70% of lower limit of normal [LLN])
Cerebrospinal fluid protein level >45 mg/dL, cell count <10/μL
Sural nerve biopsy with features of demyelination and remyelination including myelinated fiber loss and perivascular inflammation

**Mandatory Exclusion Criteria**

Evidence of relevant systemic disease or toxic exposure
Family history of neuropathy
Nerve biopsy findings incompatible with diagnosis

**Diagnostic Categories**

Definite: mandatory inclusion and exclusion criteria and all laboratory criteria
Probable: mandatory inclusion and exclusion criteria and two of three laboratory criteria
Possible: mandatory inclusion and exclusion criteria and one of three laboratory criteria

*Adapted from Cornblath, D.R., Asbury, A.K., Albers, J.W., et al., 1991. Research criteria for diagnosis of chronic inflammatory demyelinating polyneuropathy (CIDP). Neurology 41, 617–618.*

### Laboratory Studies

The diagnosis of CIDP is supported by a laboratory profile including EDX, CSF, and nerve biopsy findings (Box 106.13). A pattern of nerve conduction changes strongly supports acquired multifocal and nonuniform demyelination. This includes (1) reduction in motor conduction velocities in at least two motor nerves (<80% of LLN if CMAP amplitude >80% of LLN, and <70% of LLN if CMAP amplitude <80% of LLN); (2) partial conduction block (proximal CMAP amplitude and area <50% of distal in long nerve segments, or proximal CMAP amplitude and area <20%–50% of distal in short nerve segments) or abnormal temporal dispersion in at least one motor nerve at non-entrapment sites; (3) prolonged distal latencies in at least two motor nerves (>125% of upper limit of normal [ULN] if CMAP amplitude >80% of LLN, and >150% of ULN if CMAP amplitude <80% of LLN); and (4) absent F waves or prolonged F-wave latencies in at least two motor nerves (>125% of ULN if CMAP amplitude >80% of LLN, and >150% of ULN if CMAP amplitude <80% of LLN). At least three criteria are necessary to fulfill the diagnosis of CIDP.

Neuromuscular ultrasound of peripheral nerves in patients with CIDP often shows multiple sites of nerve enlargement at non-entrapment sites, and increased intra- and inter-nerve size variabilities and increased nerve vascularization (Goedee et al., 2017; Padua et al., 2014). Enlargements of proximal median nerve segments in the arms and any trunk of the brachial plexus is highly specific and sensitive findings in confirming CIDP and its variants, and reliably distinguish them from axonal neuropathies and motor neuron disease (Goedee et al., 2017).

CSF protein values in excess of 45 mg/dL are found in 95% of cases, and levels above 100 mg/dL are common. CSF pleocytosis is rare except in HIV-associated CIDP. MRI scanning may demonstrate gadolinium

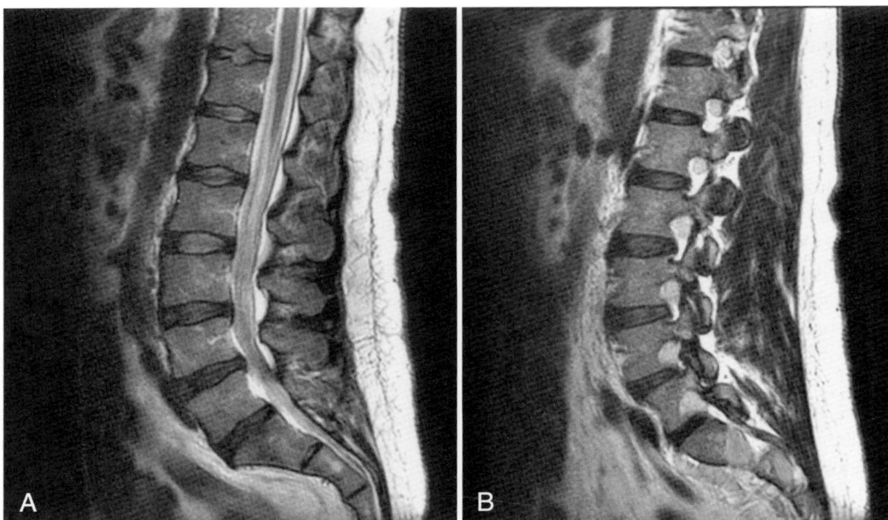


**Fig. 106.20** A, T2-weighted postgadolinium sagittal lumbar magnetic resonance image showing diffuse enlargement of cauda equina, with abnormal enhancement, in patient with chronic inflammatory demyelinating polyradiculoneuropathy. B, Hypertrophic nerve roots are best appreciated in parasagittal image.

enhancement of lumbar roots, providing radiological evidence of an abnormal blood-nerve barrier (Bertorini et al., 1995; Fig. 106.20). Blood cell counts, sedimentation rate, and biochemical screening tests are important to exclude systemic disorders. Serum and urine immunoelectrophoresis with immunofixation, a skeletal bone survey, or both are required to look for the cause of an associated monoclonal gammopathy or underlying myeloma. Antimyelin antibodies directed against MPZ (P0) have been found in a small proportion of patients (Yan et al., 2001).

About 10% of patients with CIDP have antibodies against proteins of the node of Ranvier. Antibodies of the IgG4 isotype target the paranodal proteins contactin-1 (CNTN1) and neurofascin-155 (NF155). This parallels the emerging evidence of nodo-paranodopathy as a possible key pathophysiology in CIDP and immune-mediated neuropathies. These patients tend to have more severe, mostly motor, polyneuropathy, with axonal loss and poor response to IVIG (Mathey et al., 2017; Querol and Illa, 2015).

The changes in sural nerve biopsy specimens do not fully represent the pathological process taking place in motor roots or more proximal nerve segments. In one large series of biopsies, demyelinating features were seen in only 48%; 21% had predominantly axonal changes, 13% had mixed demyelinating and axonal changes, and 18% were normal. The value of nerve biopsy as a routine diagnostic tool for CIDP has been questioned. A study conducted in 64 patients with CIDP used multivariate logistic regression analysis of sural nerve biopsy findings and other clinical and laboratory criteria to assess the value of nerve biopsy. Only high CSF protein (>100 mg/dL) and nerve conduction studies consistent with demyelination were strong predictors of CIDP, and an independent predictive value of the sural nerve biopsy could not be demonstrated (Molenaar et al., 1998). Nevertheless, sural nerve biopsy, when properly processed for semi-thin sections and teased nerve fiber preparations, is helpful in supporting the diagnosis and excluding other causes of neuropathy. Typically, moderate reduction in myelinated fibers, endoneurial and subperineurial edema, and segmental demyelination and remyelination are observed. Onion bulb formations, a sign of repeated episodes of segmental demyelination and remyelination, may be absent or abundant depending on the chronicity of the condition at the time of biopsy. Endoneurial and epineurial mononuclear inflammatory cells are a helpful diagnostic sign when present. The presence of inflammatory infiltrates can be highlighted using immunocytochemical markers. One study demonstrated epineurial T cells in perivascular clusters and endoneurial infiltration of macrophages and T cells. Rarely is the biopsy entirely normal.

### Treatment

Corticosteroids, plasmapheresis, and immunoglobulin infusion are all effective in CIDP and are the mainstays of treatment. About 50%–70% of patients respond to each of these treatments. Also, almost 50% of patients not responding to the first treatment respond to the second therapy. The efficacy of these therapies was confirmed in recent Cochrane Reviews and in consensus statements published by several neurological associations (Donofrio et al., 2009; Eftimov et al., 2009; Joint Task Force of the EFNS and the PNS, 2010; Mehndiratta and Hughes, 2002; Mehndiratta et al., 2004; Patwa et al., 2012).

Daily single-dose oral prednisone is started at 60–80 mg (1–1.5 mg/kg for children). Improvement can be anticipated to start within 2 months but may not be evident till 3–5 months (Van Schaik et al., 2010). Following improvement, the dose may be converted to an alternate-day, single-dose schedule. The initial daily dose is tapered to alternate-day prednisone by reducing the even-day dose by 10 mg/week; high-dose alternate-day prednisone is maintained until a remission or plateau phase is achieved. More than 50% of patients reach this point by 6 months. After attaining maximum benefit, a slow taper of prednisone (e.g., 10 mg/month followed by 5-mg decrements at doses below 50 mg on alternate days) can then begin. The individual patient's clinical improvement and side-effect profile serve as guides to the rapidity of the taper. Some patients are exquisitely sensitive to reduction in corticosteroid dosage, in which case this must be reduced slowly to avoid producing a severe relapse. Patients may need alternate-day prednisone (10–30 mg) for years to suppress disease activity. Side effects from prolonged oral prednisone use are significant. Osteoporosis causing vertebral compression fractures, obesity, diabetes, hypertension, and cataracts are the most common long-term complications. Patients should be followed for the development of cataracts, increased intraocular pressure, hypertension, truncal obesity, hyperglycemia, aseptic necrosis of bone, peptic ulcer disease, and susceptibility to infection. Precautions taken to diminish complications include a low-sodium (2 g/day) and low-carbohydrate diet and proton pump inhibitors for all patients. Calcium and vitamin D supplements should be initiated within a few months in an effort to limit osteoporosis, and bone density should be monitored. In patients with coexisting osteopenia or osteoporosis, bisphosphonates or nasal calcitonin may be beneficial.

Pulse corticosteroid treatment is a viable alternative treatment since it may produce fewer side effects than long-term oral prednisone. High-dose intermittent IV or oral methylprednisolone has beneficial effects for initial and long-term therapy that are equal to those of oral prednisone and IVIG, and the side-effect profile and cost of treatment are less (Lopate et al., 2005; Muley et al., 2008). Pulse oral dexamethasone (40 mg/day × 4 days every 4 weeks) resulted in a similar remission rate and side effects as oral prednisone, but the patients improved twice as fast (Van Schaik et al., 2010).

Three controlled studies have confirmed the benefit of therapeutic plasma exchange for CIDP of both chronic progressive and relapsing course. Ten plasma exchanges performed over 4 weeks resulted in substantial but transient improvement in 80% of patients (Hahn et al., 1996a). Improvement began within days of starting therapy, yet 70% of responders relapsed within 14 days after plasma exchange was stopped. The optimal schedule for plasma exchanges has not been established and probably varies from patient to patient. A common approach employs three exchanges (50 mL/kg) weekly for the first 2 weeks, followed by one or two exchanges per week from the third through the sixth week. Then the treatment frequency is adjusted according to clinical response. Plasma exchange can only be performed in medical centers with special expertise in apheresis and requires secure vascular access. Venous access problems may be overcome by placement of central venous catheters, although this approach carries the risk of pneumothorax, hematoma, brachial plexus injury, and serious infection. Plasmapheresis may be difficult to maintain for months or years, and the majority of patients needing prolonged plasmapheresis require the addition of prednisone for lasting benefit and stabilization.

The benefit of IVIG as the initial treatment of CIDP were suggested by several small studies (Fee and Fleming, 2003; Hahn et al., 1996b; Mendell et al., 2001). Improvement was seen as early as the first week of treatment, whereas maximal benefit was reached after several infusions at 2–3 months (Latov et al., 2010). Those patients who respond to the initial series of infusions may need maintenance infusions every 3–8 weeks. A randomized double-blind, placebo-controlled, crossover international trial (ICE study) used an initial IVIG dose of 2 g/kg followed by a maintenance dose of 1 g/kg every 3 weeks. The study included a 24-week placebo-controlled phase, a response-conditional crossover phase for patients who failed to improve, and a 24-week extension phase. The study showed that a statistically significant number of patients improved with IVIG compared to placebo, and the time to and probability of relapse was much lower for IVIG versus placebo (Hughes et al., 2008). This study resulted in the 2008 US Food and Drug Administration (FDA) approval of IVIG therapy (Gamunex 10%) for treatment of CIDP, the first neurological disease to be approved for such a therapy. Treatment with at least two courses of IVIG administered 3 weeks apart may be required for initial improvement, and continued maintenance therapy is necessary to achieve a maximal therapeutic response (Latov et al., 2010). The high level of effectiveness combined with low incidence of adverse events makes IVIG a good, although costly, first treatment choice.

IVIG is generally safe even in patients above the age of 60 years, including when administered in patients' homes (Lozeron et al., 2016; Souayah et al., 2018). Adverse reactions to IVIG therapy are usually minor and occur in less than 10% of patients (Brannagan, 2002; Souayah et al., 2018; Wittstock and Zettl, 2006). Headache is the most common infusion-related reaction and is usually mild to moderate and could be treated with simple analgesics. Myalgias are also common and often last 1–2 days after infusion. Severe headache, typical migraine attacks, chills, and nausea are less common. These can be controlled by reducing the rate of infusion (<200 mL/h) or by pretreatment with acetaminophen and ibuprofen (see previous discussion). Diphenhydramine or intravenous corticosteroids or both may be used as premedications for allergic manifestations like hives, seen in about 6% of patients. Aseptic meningitis is rare but could be severe. Thrombotic events including stroke, myocardial infarction, retinal vein occlusion, and deep vein thrombosis may occasionally occur in patients with cardiovascular risk factors and increased serum viscosity, particularly with infusion rates of greater than 0.4 g/kg/day. Patients with preexisting renal disease, especially the elderly, and those with DM and hypovolemia are at risk of developing worsening renal failure (Lozeron et al., 2016). This complication is often associated with IVIG products containing high concentrations of sucrose. Close monitoring of renal function, correction of hypovolemia, discontinuation of concomitant nephrotoxic drugs, and the use of products without sucrose are measures to prevent renal tubular necrosis in patients with preexisting kidney disease. The serum IgA level may be determined before the first infusion because those with very low IgA levels may have allergic or anaphylactic reactions during later infusions; however, current guidelines question the necessity of this precaution.

Comparison studies showed that the beneficial effect of IVIG is equivalent to plasmapheresis. Both treatments were equally efficacious but short lived, and most patients required continued intermittent treatment for sustained improvement. One trial compared IVIG (2 g/kg given over 1 or 2 days) with oral prednisolone (60 mg for 2 weeks followed by a taper over 4 weeks) in a crossover design. Both treatments resulted in improvement after 2 and 6 weeks, although IVIG tended to be slightly superior to oral prednisolone (Hughes et al., 2001a). A randomized controlled trial comparing the 6-month efficacy of IVIG to intravenous methylprednisolone showed that IVIG was more frequently effective and better tolerated than steroids during the first 6 months of treatment. However, when effective, steroids were more likely to induce remission and less frequently associated with deterioration after therapy discontinuation than IVIG (Nobile-Orazio et al., 2012). Subcutaneous immunoglobulin (SCIG) provides more even physiological IgG levels with less "drop off" period before next dose and less of a sharp peak in IgG levels after dose. It also has decreased severity and frequency of adverse headaches and nausea. Although SCIG may be more convenient for patients to administer at home, it requires self-injection and has potential injection site reactions. A recent randomized, double-blinded, placebo-controlled trial confirmed that SCIG administered subcutaneously via infusion pump at a weekly dose of 0.4 g/kg or 0.2 g/kg is effective as an alternative maintenance therapy for patients who were responsive to IVIG treatment (van Schaik et al., 2018).

In clinical practice, treatment with IVIG, SCIG, plasma exchange, or corticosteroids should be limited to patients with neuropathic deficits of sufficient magnitude to justify the risks and expense of treatment (Fig. 106.21). The increasing trend is to use IVIG as first-line treatment. The best IVIG dosage schedule in patients with CIDP has not been established, and much needs to be learned about the optimal dosage schedule, since each trial used different dosage and infusion regimens. The interval of repeat infusions is determined by the expected duration of the clinical benefit and should be tailored to the individual patient. Most patients receive an initial course of IVIG of 2 g/kg over 2–5 days. The standard schedule of 0.4 g/kg daily for 5 days should be used for elderly patients and patients who have impaired renal or cardiovascular function or who have high serum viscosity. A second dose within 3–4 weeks should be given, since the positive effect may require 6–8 weeks and two to three courses (Latov et al., 2010). An essential aspect of the management of CIDP is the assessment of patients at baseline and at follow-up visits after treatment, using objective and validated means

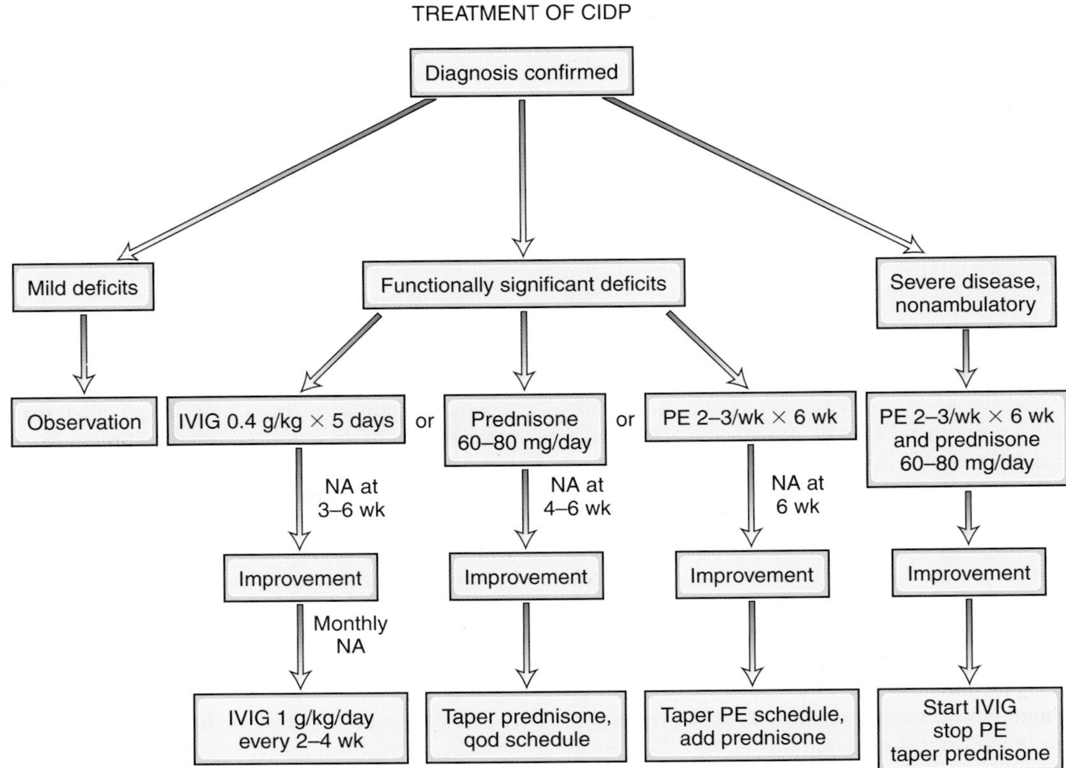


**Fig. 106.21** **Decision-Making Pathway in the Management of Chronic Inflammatory Demyelinating Polyradiculoneuropathy *(CIDP)*.** *IVIG,* Intravenous immunoglobulin; *NA,* neurological assessment; *PE,* plasma exchange; *qod,* every other day.

of determining the severity of the neuropathic deficits. Following the initial two treatment courses, responders are monitored at monthly intervals. When secondary deterioration occurs, patients are re-treated with single IVIG infusions (1–2 g/kg depending on the severity of the relapse), and the subsequent repeat infusions are set at every 3–8 weeks. For patients with residual deficits, small to moderate doses of prednisone or intermittent IV methylprednisolone may provide additional benefit. Patients who fail to respond to IVIG are treated either with plasma exchange or corticosteroids. Plasma exchange is combined with prednisone for severely affected nonambulatory patients because of the slightly higher response rates to these treatments.

Alternative forms of immunosuppressive treatment should be considered for patients with CIDP who are refractory to corticosteroids, plasma exchange, and IVIG. None of the alternative agents, however, have been tested in randomized and controlled trials (Mahdi-Rogers et al., 2017). Azathioprine, methotrexate, or mycophenolate mofetil may be used as corticosteroid-sparing adjunctive agents in long-term management (Bedi et al., 2010; Cocito et al., 2011). Use should be limited to patients with inadequate response to corticosteroids or those who require high corticosteroid maintenance doses with unacceptable side effects. Other immune interventions (Kieseier et al., 2006b) include cyclosporine A, monthly infusions of cyclophosphamide, and interferon α 29 (Gorson et al., 1998). Rituximab (375 mg/m$^2$ IV each week for 4 weeks) failed to reduce the IVIG dose in a pilot study (Gorson et al., 2007); however, rituximab may be effective in the subgroup of patients with CIDP and elevated antibodies to paranodal proteins such as CNTN1 and NF155 (Querol et al., 2015).

The absence of any therapeutic response from these immune-modulating therapies should lead to a reappraisal of the diagnosis. The most common causes of treatment failure are incorrect diagnosis, inadequate dose and duration of treatment, and the negative effects of concomitant and underlying illness.

### Prognosis

In contrast to the good prognosis in the monophasic GBS, CIDP tends to be associated with prolonged neurological disability and is less likely to have spontaneous remissions. About 50% of patients are severely disabled at some stage by their illness and 10% of patients remain disabled in spite of treatment. Although 95% of patients with CIDP show initial improvement following immunosuppressive therapy, the relapse rate is high and the degree of improvement modest. Despite the initial responsiveness, only 40% of patients remained in partial or complete remission without receiving any medication. The presence and degree of axonal loss have been considered responsible for incomplete recovery. Confirmation of this view was provided by a systematic study comparing clinical outcome and biopsy findings: Six years after onset of illness, 56% had good outcome, 24% deteriorated and failed to respond to all treatments, and 11% died of complications of the disease. Axonal loss on the nerve biopsy correlated with poorer outcome (Bouchard et al., 1999).

## Multifocal Motor Neuropathy

MMN, with a prevalence of 1–2 per 100,000, is a treatable but incurable immune-mediated motor neuropathy that bears a superficial clinical resemblance to motor neuron disease of the lower motor neuron type. Whether MMN is a distinct nosological entity or simply variably related motor neuron disease or a multifocal motor variant of CIDP is not established.

### Clinical Features

MMN is more common in men and mainly affects young adults; two-thirds of affected individuals are age 45 years or younger. It rarely occurs

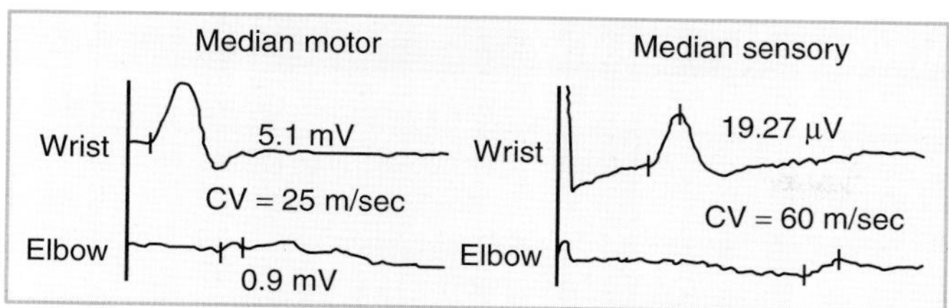


**Fig. 106.22 Partial Motor Conduction Block of Median Nerve.** Compound muscle action potential (CMAP) was recorded from abductor pollicis brevis muscle. Supramaximal stimulation at elbow produced an 80% drop in amplitude of median CMAP compared with stimulation at wrist. Sensory conduction along the same nerve segment was preserved. *CV*, Conduction velocity. (*Courtesy Dr. J.C. Stevens.*)

in childhood (Moroni et al., 2006). MMN almost always present with progressive, usually distal, asymmetric upper extremity motor weakness in the distribution of a single peripheral nerve. This may remain confined to a single nerve for several years, although MMN usually steadily progresses to affect other nerves. Several diagnostic criteria for this neuropathy have been proposed (Joint Task Force of the EFNS and the PNS, 2006; Olney et al., 2003). These criteria share the following features: progressive, asymmetrical, predominantly distal limb weakness in the distribution of two or more peripheral nerves, developing over months to years, with a striking predilection for the upper extremities and particularly hands, without upper motor signs. Wrist drop, grip weakness, or foot-drop are the most common presenting features. Despite profound weakness, muscle bulk is initially well preserved. Muscle cramps and fasciculations, particularly after exercise, are common. Profound weakness in muscles with normal bulk, or focal weakness in the distribution of individual nerves rather than in a spinal segmental pattern, are clues that should alert the clinician to suspect this disorder. Cranial nerve involvement is unusual, but rare involvements of ocular, facial, hypoglossal, and phrenic nerves—the latter resulting in respiratory failure—have been reported. Tendon reflexes are depressed or absent but may be normal. Autonomic dysfunction has not been reported. Minor transient paresthesias are commonly reported by patients, but objective sensory deficits are usually absent or may involve small patchy areas in the distal limbs. The course is slowly or less often stepwise progressive over months to years (Nobile-Orazio et al., 2005) without progression to generalized immobility.

MMN may follow immunotherapy with TNF-α inhibitor for Crohn disease, rheumatoid arthritis, and psoriasis. Most patients required IVIG and the majority improved or recovered over months to years.

## Laboratory Studies

The diagnosis depends on careful EDX studies demonstrating persistent focal motor conduction block, defined as more than 50% reduction in amplitude and area of proximally stimulated muscle evoked response compared to distally stimulated response in one or more motor nerves at sites not prone to compression (see Chapter 36). What makes MMN unique is that the conduction block is confined to motor axons. SNAPs and sensory conduction are preserved, including along the same nerve segments (Fig. 106.22). The selective vulnerability of motor fibers has not been satisfactorily explained. Other features of demyelination such as motor conduction slowing, temporal dispersion, and prolonged F-wave and distal motor latencies may be present in nerves without conduction block. When such abnormalities are prominent or if there are abnormal SNAPs, the possibility of CIDP or Lewis-Sumner syndrome (MADSAM) should be strongly considered. Transient abnormal amplitude reduction with proximal stimulation (conduction block) may occasionally be seen in vasculitic neuropathy during the early stage of wallerian degeneration. Needle EMG of the clinically weak muscles invariably shows signs of denervation, especially in advanced disease, reflecting the occurrence of as yet poorly explained axonal loss. Fasciculations are common, and myokymia may be seen.

The extent of reduction of the CMAP amplitude or area and the degree of acceptable temporal dispersion necessary for diagnosis of conduction block continue to be controversial (Chaudhry and Swash, 2006). Despite the general acceptance of conduction block as a diagnostic criterion for MMN, some investigators report patients with similar phenotypic presentation who lack conduction blocks but respond equally well to the treatment (Delmont et al., 2006). Keep in mind, however, that conduction block in some nerves may vary significantly within patients and over time. The extent of CB may decrease or even disappear after several years because of a progressive reduction of distal CMAP amplitude, which may reflect either secondary axonal degeneration or the appearance of unrecognized very distal CB. The skill of the electromyographer and the patient's cooperation are essential for the demonstration of difficult-to-detect conduction blocks and for avoiding misdiagnosis of other conditions.

The spinal fluid protein is frequently normal, although moderately increased protein levels (<100 mg/dL) may be found in a third of patients. MRI of the brachial or lumbosacral plexus (Van Es et al., 1997) or ultrasonography (Beekman et al., 2005) may be helpful by demonstrating focal enlargement and increased signal intensities of affected nerve trunks.

In 1993, Kaji and colleagues reported a patient with pure motor weakness of the arm and proximal conduction block who underwent biopsy of a motor nerve branch adjacent to the site of focal conduction block (Kaji et al., 1993). This revealed scattered demyelinated axons and small onion bulbs without inflammatory changes. Another study using fascicular biopsies of nerves at the site of conduction block of mixed upper-arm nerves found minimal evidence of inflammation but multifocal fiber loss without demyelination, remyelination, or hypertrophic changes (Taylor et al., 2004). The sural nerve frequently shows subtle pathological changes of demyelination and remyelination, quite similar to those in CIDP but of lesser degree. These morphological abnormalities indicate that sensory nerves are involved in this disorder despite the lack of clinical or electrophysiological findings. However, routine nerve biopsies are not required but can be useful in detecting an alternative cause.

Controversies remain about the possible relationship between antiganglioside antibodies and acquired lower motor neuron syndromes and multifocal motor neuropathies. Among the gangliosides, GM1 is abundantly found on the outer surface of neuronal membranes where potential binding sites could serve as antigenic targets. High titers of IgM anti-GM1 antibodies can be found in 50%–60% of patients with MMN and conduction block. High titers are occasionally seen (<15%) in amyotrophic lateral sclerosis and GBS variants including AMAN and the axonal form of GBS associated with *C. jejuni* infection, but rarely seen (<5%) in other peripheral neuropathies and non-neurological autoimmune disorders. These observations, along with conflicting results obtained from experimental studies on the pathogenic role of anti-GM1 antibodies, suggest that these antibodies are neither specific nor required for the diagnosis of MMN but can be considered a marker for the disease. Whether these antibodies are an epiphenomenon secondary to nerve damage or have a direct immunopathogenic role for nerve damage will require further studies. Similarly, the role of *C. jejuni* infection in multifocal neuropathy, despite anecdotal reports of such an association, remains unproven (Terenghi et al., 2002).

TABLE 106.12 **Differential Diagnosis of Multifocal Motor Neuropathy**

| Features | Multifocal motor neuropathy | CIDP | Amyotrophic lateral sclerosis |
|---|---|---|---|
| Lower motor neuron weakness | Distal or proximal, asymmetrical, follows peripheral nerve distribution | Proximal and distal, usually symmetrical | Distal > proximal, follows myotomal (root) distribution |
| Upper motor neuron signs | Absent | Absent | Often present |
| Sensory loss | Absent | Present | Absent |
| Motor conduction block | Prominent | Frequent | Absent |
| Sensory conduction | Normal SNAPs | Low to absent SNAPs | Normal SNAPs |
| Cerebrospinal fluid protein | Normal (70%) | Elevated | Normal |
| Anti-GM1 antibodies | 50%–60% | Absent | <15% |

*CIDP*, Chronic inflammatory demyelinating polyradiculoneuropathy; *SNAP*, sensory nerve action potential.

The differential diagnosis of progressive limb weakness and atrophy without sensory symptoms is mainly restricted to motor neuron disease, including amyotrophic lateral sclerosis and its lower motor neuron form, progressive muscular atrophy, bibrachial motor neuron disease, benign monomelic amyotrophy, CIDP, Lewis-Sumner syndrome and MMN, and HNPP (Table 107.12). Other conditions to be considered include postpoliomyelitis syndrome, lead- or dapsone-induced motor neuropathies, and hexosaminidase-A deficiency.

### Treatment

Identifying patients with MMN is important because many such patients respond to treatment. Treatment with IVIG is the preferred treatment as shown previously by several uncontrolled studies. Other treatment options are few and, unlike with CIDP, prednisone or plasma exchange have little or no benefit and may even worsen the disease in some patients.

IVIG was shown to benefit 70% of patients in open uncontrolled trials and four randomized double-blind controlled trials involving a total of 45 patients (van Schaik et al., 2005). Improvement may be quite impressive and is often rapid (within a few days to 3 weeks of treatment) but lasts for only weeks to months. Younger age at onset, a smaller number of affected limb regions, elevated GM1 antibody titers, definite conduction blocks, and higher distal CMAP amplitudes (suggestive of minimal axon loss) are associated with a favorable response (Van den Berg-Vos et al., 2000). The majority of patients require repeated IVIG infusions, though few patients experience prolonged remissions of longer than 12 months. Most patients require maintenance infusions for years, and with the passage of time, the intervals between infusions may become progressively shorter. In a double-blinded study of 44 patients, mean maximal grip strength declined 31% during placebo and increased 3.75% during IVIG, while 35% of patients had worsened during placebo and not during IVIG (Hahn et al., 2013). Based on this study, IVIG treatment was approved by the FDA for patients with MMN. Based on such observations, it is appropriate to initiate treatment with IVIG and continue maintenance infusions (0.4 g/kg once every 1–8 weeks) in patients who have a functionally meaningful response. Dose and frequency of repeated IVIG administration must be individualized for each patient, giving another dose just before the anticipated time of relapse. The decline in IVIG's effectiveness over time is attributed to the progressive and poorly understood axonal degeneration or development of new conduction blocks (Van Asseldonk et al., 2006). Equivalent doses of SCIG may be as effective (Harbo et al., 2010). The value of higher doses of maintenance IVIG (2 g/kg monthly) is not established. Treatment may reduce the number of conduction blocks, promote reinnervation, and prevent axonal degeneration (Terenghi et al., 2004). The presence of motor axon loss, as determined by low distal CMAP amplitudes, and longer disease duration without IVIG treatment denote poor longer-term prognosis (Cats et al., 2010).

Some uncontrolled studies suggest oral cyclophosphamide or interferon beta may reduce the frequency and dosage of infusions. For non-responders to IVIG, IV cyclophosphamide is indicated depending on the degree of disability and the patient's understanding of the seriousness of potential side effects such as bone marrow depression, gonadal damage, hemorrhagic cystitis, and a long-term increased risk of cancer. Pestronk and coworkers (1994) suggested that monthly IV cyclophosphamide (1 g/m$^2$) for 6–8 months, preceded on each occasion by two plasma exchanges, may be an effective treatment. However, owing to concerns over long-term side effects, cyclophosphamide was not recommended by a group of experts. As an alternative to cyclophosphamide, rituximab, a monoclonal antibody directed against the B-cell surface marker, CD20, has shown conflicting results (Gorson et al., 2007; Pestronk et al., 2003; Rojas-Garcia et al., 2003; Ruegg et al., 2004). A recent open-label study showed that rituximab was unable to reduce the amount of IVIG required for patients with MMN (Chaudhry and Cornblath, 2010). There are insufficient data to support the use of other agents such as azathioprine, mycophenolate mofetil, cyclosporine, or interferons. Mycophenolate as an adjunct therapy did not change the course of the disease (Piepers et al., 2007). New therapeutic strategies are required to develop more long-term-effective, less expensive, and possibly curative treatment of MMN. Eculizumab, a mAb that binds complement component 5 and may inhibit terminal complement activation, is a promising treatment for MMN. A single study failed to allow reduction in IVIG dosing, though some subjective motor improvements were reported. Further study is necessary to evaluate this agent efficacy.

## PERIPHERAL NEUROPATHIES ASSOCIATED WITH MONOCLONAL PROTEINS

### Monoclonal Gammopathy of Undetermined Significance

Patients undergoing evaluation for chronic peripheral neuropathy should be screened for the presence of a monoclonal protein (M protein) (England et al., 2009a). A monoclonal protein is produced by a single clone of plasma cells and is usually composed of four polypeptides: two identical heavy chains and two light chains. The M protein is named according to the class of heavy chain (IgG, IgM, IgA, IgD, and IgE) and type of light chain, κ (kappa) or λ (lambda). In two-thirds of patients with a monoclonal protein, no detectable underlying disease is found, and they are described as having MGUS (monoclonal gammopathy of unknown significance) (Rajkumar et al., 2006). MGUS is present in 1%–3% of the population, mostly elderly. MGUS has replaced the term benign monoclonal gammopathy because up to one-fourth of patients go on to develop malignant plasma cell dyscrasias in long-term follow-up. The risk of progression of MGUS to a malignant plasma cell proliferative disorder is about 1% per year (Kyle et al., 2002). This is not affected by age or

**TABLE 106.13 Relative Risk of Progression in Patients with MGUS Versus General Population**

| Condition | Relative Risk |
|---|---|
| Multiple myeloma | 25 |
| Plasmacytoma (including osteosclerotic myeloma) | 8.5 |
| Amyloidosis | 8.4 |
| Waldenström macroglobulinemia | 46 |
| Lymphoma | 2.4 |
| Chronic lymphocytic leukemia | 0.9 |

*MGUS*, Monoclonal gammopathy of undetermined significance.
*Adapted from Kyle, R.A., Therneau, T.M., Rajkumar, S.V., et al., 2002. A long-term study of prognosis in monoclonal gammopathy of undetermined significance. N Engl J Med 346, 564–569.*

**TABLE 106.14 Characteristic Findings in Monoclonal Gammopathy of Undetermined Significance**

| | |
|---|---|
| Common monoclonal type | IgM, IgG, IgA |
| Common light chain | κ |
| Quantity | <3 g/dL |
| Urine light chains | Rare |
| Marrow plasma cells | <5% |
| Skeletal lesions | Absent |
| Complete blood cell count | Normal |
| Organomegaly, lymphadenopathy | Absent |

*Ig*, Immunoglobulin.

the duration of MGUS, although the cumulative risk of progression during one's lifetime is, of course, highest in younger patients (Table 107.13). A strong predictor of progression is a rise in serum monoclonal protein concentration (Eurelings et al., 2005; Kyle et al., 2002). The characteristic features distinguishing MGUS from other plasma cell dyscrasias are listed in Table 106.14.

Routine serum protein electrophoresis frequently lacks the sensitivity required to detect small M proteins. Immunoelectrophoresis or immunofixation is required to detect small amounts of M proteins, confirm the monoclonal nature, and characterize the heavy- and light-chain types. Urine studies detect excretion of light chains (Bence Jones protein) that often accompany multiple myeloma or primary amyloidosis. All patients with neuropathy and associated M protein, as well as patients whose profiles suggest amyloidosis or myeloma, should have a 24-hour urine collection for detection of Bence Jones protein. Following discovery of an M protein, a CBC with differential, calcium, and renal profile are necessary, immunoglobulins should be quantitated, and a radiological skeletal bone survey obtained to detect lytic or sclerotic bone lesions of myeloma. If the monoclonal spike exceeds 1.5 g/dL, a bone marrow aspirate and biopsy should be obtained to differentiate a malignant plasma cell dyscrasia from MGUS. Rectal, fat, or cutaneous nerve biopsies may be required to confirm a possible diagnosis of amyloidosis (Kissel and Mendell, 1995).

Approximately 10% of patients with idiopathic peripheral neuropathy have an associated monoclonal gammopathy, which represents a sixfold increase over the general population of the same age. In contrast, about 5% of patients with MGUS have an associated polyneuropathy. The pathophysiological relationship between the M protein and the neuropathy is often obscure, but some M proteins have antibody-like properties directed against components of myelin or axolemma. When the higher frequency of MGUS in older patients is considered, the causal relationship between MGUS and this type of neuropathy becomes less clear (Notermans et al., 1996a). Finding an M protein among patients with neuropathy may lead to the discovery of underlying disorders such as primary amyloidosis, multiple or osteosclerotic myeloma, plasma cell dyscrasia, macroglobulinemia, cryoglobulinemia, Castleman disease, lymphoma, or malignant lymphoproliferative disease. The frequency of monoclonal IgM is overrepresented in patients with neuropathy (60% IgM, 30% IgG, and 10% IgA). The light-chain class is usually κ, in contrast to patients with osteosclerotic myeloma or amyloidosis (Ropper and Gorson, 1998).

### Clinical Features

The clinical presentations of the neuropathies associated with different heavy-chain classes are generally indistinguishable. Symptoms begin in later life (median age of onset in the sixth decade), appear insidiously, and progress slowly over months to years. There is a male predominance. The most common presentation is a symmetrical sensorimotor polyneuropathy which may be one of three more common subtypes: CIDP phenotype, distal acquired demyelinating symmetric (DADS) neuropathy, or an axonal sensorimotor peripheral polyneuropathy. A predominantly sensory neuropathy may be seen in up to 20% of patients. Cranial nerves and autonomic functions are preserved. Sensory impairment can be prominent, with variable involvement of light touch, pinprick, vibration, and position sense. Muscle stretch reflexes are universally diminished or absent. The lower limbs are involved earlier and to a greater extent than the upper.

Elevation of CSF protein is common, sometimes in excess of 100 mg/dL. The EDX studies show evidence of acquired demyelination or, more often, both demyelination and axonal degeneration. A small number of patients, usually with IgG MGUS, have electrophysiological features of a pure axonal polyneuropathy. SNAPs are reduced in amplitude or unobtainable. Needle EMG shows chronic and active denervation. Sural nerve biopsy findings of patients with M proteins of all three immunoglobulin classes show nerve fiber loss, segmental demyelination, and axonal atrophy and degeneration.

Though the clinical and EDX studies of peripheral polyneuropathies associated with MGUS are heterogeneous, several distinct peripheral neuropathy subgroups exist:

1. In about half of patients, a polyradiculoneuropathy occurs that shares clinical and laboratory features with CIDP. Patients with CIDP and MGUS tend to be older and have a more indolent course, with more sensory than motor findings but poorer long-term functional outcome than CIDP without M protein (Simmons et al., 1995). The M protein in these patients is often the IgG type.
2. IgM MGUS neuropathy and DADS neuropathy represents a distinct and often homogeneous group characterized by slowly progressive sensory gait ataxia. Upper-limb postural tremor can be prominent. EDX studies show slow motor conduction velocities in the demyelinating range, with a predilection for distal demyelination. SNAPs are reduced in amplitude or unobtainable. In at least 50% of patients with IgM MGUS neuropathy, the IgM monoclonal protein demonstrates reactivity against myelin-associated glycoprotein (MAG) (Steck et al., 2006): hence the term anti-MAG neuropathy. MAG is a glycoprotein that makes up only 1% of peripheral nerve myelin. It is concentrated in periaxonal Schwann cell membranes, paranodal loops of myelin, and areas of noncompacted myelin, where it serves as a cytoskeletal-associated protein playing a role as an adhesion molecule for interactions between Schwann cells and axons. Knockout mice expressing no MAG activity have significantly smaller axons than normal mice, suggesting the important role played by MAG in the proper maintenance of structure

and function of axons. Anti-MAG antibodies cross-react with other components of peripheral nerve, including several complex glycosphingolipids, PMP22, and the P0 protein of myelin. Which of these reactivities relates to the neuropathy is unclear. Antibody activity to MAG can be detected by Western blot and enzyme-linked immunosorbent assay or by immunocytochemical staining of nerves. Immunofluorescence studies show that IgM with anti-MAG activity binds to the periphery and periaxonal regions of myelinated fibers that correspond to the distribution of MAG. Ultrastructurally, the myelin lamellae show a widened periodicity (myelin splitting), which is considered the pathological hallmark of anti-MAG antibodies (Fig. 106.23). In those with IgM MGUS, predictors for progression of the neuropathy to moderate disability (Rankin Scale score of 3 or greater) include higher age at onset and demyelination. Anti-MAG antibodies, on the other hand, portend a better prognosis with respect to neuropathy-related disability (Niermeijer et al., 2010). No consistent binding of monoclonal proteins to myelinated fibers is seen in nerve biopsy specimens from patients with IgG and IgA MGUS.

The underlying mechanism of nerve fiber damage in MGUS neuropathy remains unknown, although an immune-mediated origin is suspected. The case for pathogenic activity of IgM antibodies directed against MAG and other glycosphingolipids is better established than that for other antigens or for IgG and IgA antibodies. On the other hand, the lack of correlation between the deposition of anti-MAG antibody and the degree of pathological nerve damage, as well as the poor correlation between the amount of M protein in serum and the severity of neuropathy, raise questions about the causal linkage.

3. Approximately 15% of patients with IgM MGUS neuropathy have autoantibodies directed against gangliosides, and those with IgM antibodies to GD1b and GQ1b have been associated with sensory ataxic neuropathies (Eurelings et al., 2001). Patients who have disialosyl-ganglioside IgM antibodies and cold agglutinins present with a chronic sensory ataxic neuropathy, areflexia, and fixed or relapsing-remitting ophthalmoplegia. This rare clinical syndrome has been described under the acronym CANOMAD: *chronic ataxic neuropathy, ophthalmoplegia, IgM monoclonal protein, cold agglutinins, and disialosyl antibodies* (Arbogast et al., 2007; Willison et al., 2001). Pathologically, there is significant loss of dorsal root ganglion cells, resulting in dorsal column and root atrophy as well as infiltration of cranial and peripheral nerves with clonal IgM anti-disialyl gangliosides secreting B lymphocytes (McKelvie et al., 2013).

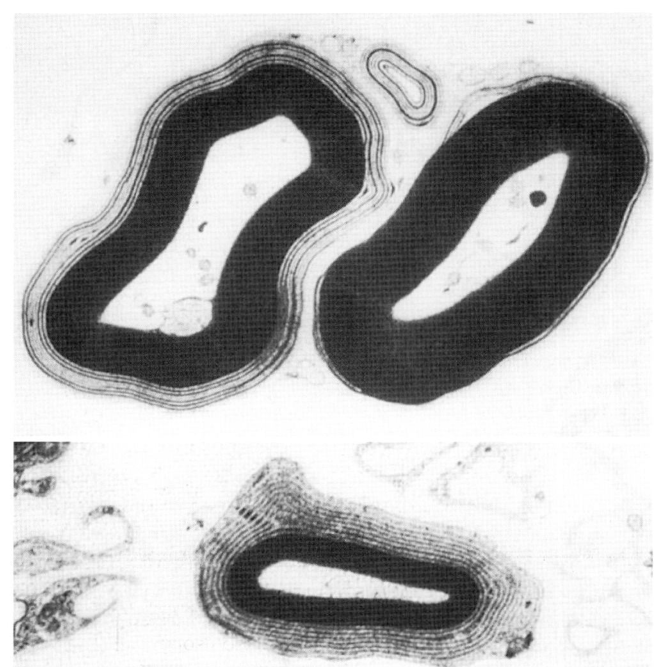

**Fig. 106.23 Electron Micrographs Showing Fibers with Myelin Splitting.** *Upper panel,* Myelinating fiber on left shows splitting of myelin lamellae at intraperiod line, whereas nerve fiber on right has normal compact myelin (×15,000). *Lower panel,* Similar myelin splitting (×20,000). Findings are characteristic of antimyelin-associated glycoprotein antibody deposits in myelin sheath. *(Reprinted with permission from Mendell, J.R., Barohn, R.J., Bosch, E.P., et al., 1994. Continuum-peripheral neuropathy. Am Acad Neurol 1, 42.)*

## Treatment

The optimal treatment of MGUS neuropathy has not been established, and few controlled trials have been conducted. Treatment decisions depend on the severity of the neuropathy and the age of the patient. Patients with minor deficits and indolent course are best followed without treatment. This view is supported by the long-term outcome of patients with IgM MGUS neuropathy. In one study, not only was the neurological impairment similar in treated and untreated patients after an average follow-up of 8 years but also the immunomodulatory treatments resulted in serious adverse events in half of the treated patients (Nobile-Orazio et al., 2000). However, in general, the more closely the neuropathy fulfills the criteria for CIDP, the more likely the patient will respond to immunomodulatory therapies. About half of the patients treated with plasmapheresis, IVIG, and prednisone, often in combination with other immunosuppressants, experienced temporary benefit. A systematic review of treatments for IgG or IgA paraproteinemic peripheral neuropathy identified one relevant randomized controlled trial with 18 participants. Results showed plasma exchange had modest improvement over sham plasma exchange over a short-term follow-up. This short-term benefit of plasmapheresis did not occur in the IgM subgroup. Patients with a CIDP-like picture and IgG gammopathy should be treated like patients with CIDP without gammopathy. When a prominent axonal neuropathy is associated with IgG paraprotein, especially in the elderly, the role of these therapies becomes less clear.

IVIG (2 g/kg given over 1–5 days) may produce only a short-term and partial benefit in 50% of patients with IgM MGUS with or without anti-MAG neuropathy (Comi et al., 2002). Patients with progressive disabling neuropathy caused by IgM MGUS, with or without anti-MAG reactivity, may respond to aggressive immune interventions aimed at lowering the IgM level. This may be achieved by intermittent courses of oral cyclophosphamide and prednisone given at 4-week intervals for 6 months; plasma exchanges followed by IV cyclophosphamide; or fludarabine, a fluorinated purine analog, used in cancer treatment (Niermeijer et al., 2006; Notermans et al., 1996b). Another purine analog, cladribine, resulted in prolonged remission in one patient with IgM neuropathy (Ghosh et al., 2002). Chlorambucil with and without corticosteroids may be effective in one-third to two-thirds of patients. The long-term effects of these therapies have not been established, since the neuropathy has a slow progression and the follow-up of the reported patients has been generally short. The long-term side effects of these agents, however, may be substantial. The initially reported benefit of interferon alfa could not be confirmed in a randomized controlled trial. Rituximab, a mouse/human chimeric monoclonal CD20 antibody directed against B cells, is reported to be effective in some cases of anti-MAG neuropathy in anecdotal reports. However, two double-blind placebo-controlled studies

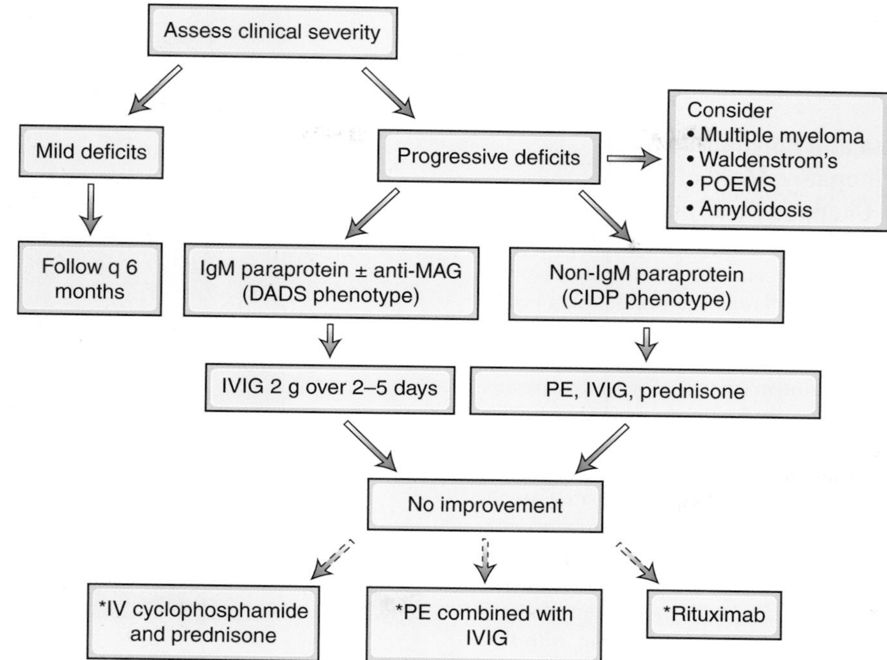


**Fig. 106.24** Decision-making pathway in the diagnosis and management of peripheral neuropathy with monoclonal gammopathy of undetermined significance *(MGUS)*. *There are anecdotes of improvement with these drugs, but controlled studies are not available to support their use. *CIDP*, Chronic demyelinating polyradiculoneuropathy; *DADS*, Distal acquired demyelinating sensory neuropathy; *IgM*, immunoglobulin M; *IV*, intravenous; *IVIG*, intravenous immunoglobulin; *MAG*, myelin-associated glycoprotein; *NP*, neuropathy; *PE*, plasma exchange; *POEMS*, Polyneuropathy, organomegaly, endocrinopathy, monoclonal gammopathy, and skin changes.

showed conflicting results (Dalakas et al., 2009; Léger et al., 2013). The reported improvement is usually associated with the reduction of serum anti-MAG antibodies. Patients may require repeated cycles of therapy to maintain improvement. An algorithm for the treatment of MGUS neuropathy is proposed in Fig. 106.24. Patients with rapid clinical deterioration of neuropathy despite treatment should be re-evaluated for the development of underlying malignant lymphoproliferative disorders or amyloidosis.

## Waldenström Macroglobulinemia

WM is characterized by proliferation of malignant lymphoplasmacytic cells in bone marrow and lymph nodes that secrete an IgM monoclonal spike of more than 3 g/dL. WM typically affects elderly men and manifests with fatigue, anemia, bleeding, and hyperviscosity syndrome. Peripheral neuropathy occurs in about a third of patients with WM and is a chronic, symmetrical, predominantly sensory polyneuropathy similar to that associated with nonmalignant IgM monoclonal proteins. Other presentations include pure painful sensory or pure motor neuropathies, multiple mononeuropathies associated with cryoglobulins, and typical amyloid neuropathy. Anti-MAG reactivity is found in approximately 50% of WM patients with neuropathy. Patients with positive anti-MAG antibodies have slowed motor NCVs and prolonged distal latencies consistent with demyelination. Nerve biopsy findings are indistinguishable from those seen in IgM MGUS neuropathy. Patients with demyelinating polyneuropathy may respond to rituximab, chemotherapy including fludarabine or cladribine, or plasmapheresis, singly or in combination, but the response appears to be less consistent than in IgM MGUS-related neuropathy. Treatment with autologous stem cell transplantation may induce positive responses even in patients resistant to other therapies (Dimopoulos et al., 2009).

## Multiple Myeloma

Polyneuropathy occurs in approximately 5% of patients with multiple myeloma. One-third of patients demonstrate abnormalities on careful EDX studies. The most common neurological complications of multiple myeloma are related to spinal cord and nerve root compression from lytic vertebral lesions. Diffuse bone or radicular pain resulting from vertebral body involvement, anemia, renal insufficiency, and hypercalcemia may provide clues to the underlying disorder. The clinical manifestations of myeloma neuropathy are heterogeneous, but most patients present with mild distal sensorimotor polyneuropathy and less frequently with a pure sensory neuropathy. Furthermore, AL (amyloid light chain) amyloidosis complicates multiple myeloma in 30%–40% of cases. These patients have a high likelihood of death within 2 years after the diagnosis and generally have a more severe sensorimotor neuropathy. Painful dysesthesias, preferential involvement of small-fiber sensory nerves, autonomic dysfunction, and CTS are suggestive of amyloid neuropathy. Rectal, abdominal fat, or sural nerve biopsy specimens in patients with progressive myeloma neuropathy may lead to confirmation of an amyloidosis diagnosis.

Nerve conduction and sural nerve biopsy studies are consistent with an axonal polyneuropathy causing loss of myelinated fibers. Treatment of the underlying myeloma may sometimes improve the neuropathy. Thalidomide, an effective agent in the treatment of multiple myeloma, may in itself cause a dose- and duration-dependent neuropathy

(Mileshkin et al., 2006). Bortezomib, a cytotoxic agent used for the treatment of refractory myeloma, also causes peripheral neuropathy (Argyriou et al., 2008).

### Osteosclerotic Myeloma and Polyneuropathy, Organomegaly, Endocrinopathy, Monoclonal Gammopathy, and Skin Changes Syndrome

Osteosclerotic myeloma occurs in less than 3% of all patients with myeloma, but 85% of these patients present with an associated peripheral neuropathy. In this disorder, the plasma cell proliferation occurs as single or multiple plasmacytomas that manifest as sclerotic bone lesions. The majority of these patients have *Crow-Fukase syndrome* or *POEMS syndrome*. POEMS is an acronym for polyneuropathy, organomegaly, endocrinopathy, M protein, and skin changes (Dispenzieri et al., 2015).

The initial symptoms in the majority of patients are related to a polyradiculoneuropathy (Li et al., 2017). The polyneuropathy usually begins with sensory changes in the lower limbs followed by sensory ataxia and motor weakness. The clinical course is often slowly progressive but is sometimes more rapidly worsening. The polyneuropathy of POEMS is different from that associated with multiple myeloma in several aspects: It occurs at an earlier age, is demyelinating, with slow motor NCVs and elevated CSF protein levels, usually in excess of 100 mg/dL. The monoclonal protein in POEMS is usually less than 2 g/dL and may not be detectable using immunofixation in up to 10% of cases. It is virtually always composed of λ light chains associated with IgG and IgA heavy chains. Vascular endothelial growth factor (VEGF) serum level is significantly elevated in POEMS but not in other demyelinating neuropathies; VEGF level above 200 pg/mL has a sensitivity of 95% and specificity of 68% in the diagnosis of POEMS (D'souza et al., 2011).

The diagnosis of POEMS syndrome requires a high index of suspicion. The diagnosis is confirmed by having *three major criteria* of the disease: (1) polyneuropathy (usually demyelinating), (2) monoclonal plasma cell disorder, and (3) elevated VEGF; along with *two minor criteria* including sclerotic bone lesions, organomegaly (hepatomegaly, splenomegaly, or lymphadenopathy), skin change, edema, endocrinopathy (hypogonadism, hyperestrogenemia, or hypoparathyroidism), polycythemia, or thrombocytosis. These criteria have 100% sensitivity and 100% specificity (Suichi et al., 2019).

The neuropathy of POEMS bears a striking resemblance to CIDP, with symmetrical proximal and distal weakness with variable sensory loss. Cranial nerves are spared except for occasional cases of papilledema. POEMS should be considered in patients carrying a diagnosis of CIDP but without good response to standard CIDP therapy, such as IVIG, plasma exchange, or corticosteroids. The clinical and electrophysiological similarities between this condition and CIDP emphasize the need to screen for an occult M protein and sclerotic bone lesions in all adult patients presenting with an acquired demyelinating polyneuropathy or possible POEMS by obtaining serum and urine immunofixation, free light chain, VEGF level, and skeletal survey.

The bony lesions may be single or multiple and tend to involve the axial skeleton; the majority of lesions occur in the spine, pelvis, and ribs. Their radiographical appearance varies from dense ivory to mixed sclerotic and lytic lesions with a sclerotic rim (Fig. 106.25). Radioisotope positron emission tomography (PET)-CT scans also identify bone lesions and assist in identifying the site for bone marrow biopsy which is usually necessary to confirm the presence of an isolated plasmacytoma (see Fig. 106.25).

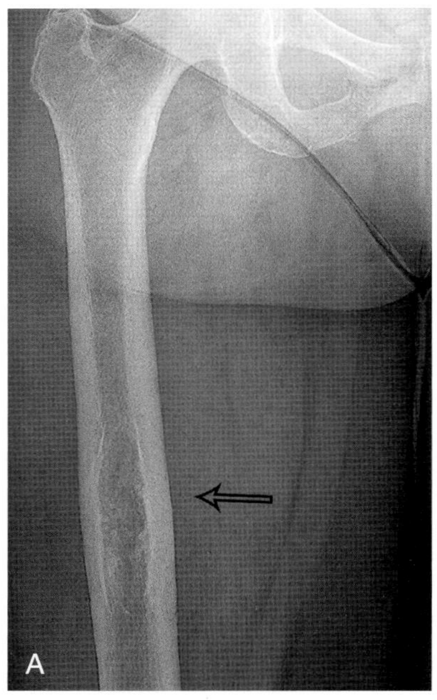


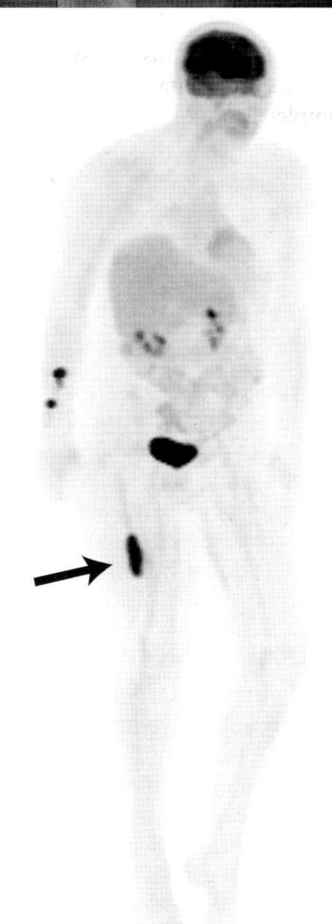


**Fig. 106.25** A 55-year-old woman with polyneuropathy, organomegaly, endocrinopathy, monoclonal gammopathy, and skin changes, initially diagnosed with chronic inflammatory demyelinating polyradiculoneuropathy and failed treatments with prednisone, intravenous immunoglobulin, and plasma exchange. She had IgG λ paraprotein (0.1 g/dL) and elevated serum vascular endothelial growth factor (VEGF) at 981 pg/mL. X- Rays showed an expansile lytic lesion of the femur with cortical scalloping (**A**) while positron emission tomography scan showed marked hyperintense metabolic activity corresponding to right femoral lesion (**B**). Biopsy of the lesion showed focal lambda restricted plasmacytoma.

Most patients develop one or more of the multisystem manifestations of the POEMS syndrome (Dispenzieri et al., 2015). Hepatosplenomegaly is often encountered. Gynecomastia and impotence in men, secondary amenorrhea in women, DM, and hypothyroidism are the most common endocrinopathies. Hyperpigmentation, hypertrichosis, diffuse skin thickening, hemangiomas, and white nail beds are dermatological features. Pitting edema of the lower limbs, ascites, pleural effusions, and clubbing of the fingers are other signs. Approximately one-fourth of patients with POEMS syndrome have no associated bone lesions. Some of these patients have Castleman syndrome (a nonmalignant form of angiofollicular lymphadenopathy), and others have a plasma cell dyscrasia restricted to the lymphoreticular system.

The pathogenesis of this multiorgan disorder is poorly understood. The associated plasma cell dyscrasia seems to play a crucial role, as clinical improvement follows the disappearance of the monoclonal proteins. Elevated levels of proinflammatory cytokines such as TNF-α, interleukins, and VEGF have been implicated in the multisystem manifestations. The alteration of endoneurial vessel permeability following an abnormal activation of endothelial cells by VEGF may explain the polyneuropathy. Increased permeability allows serum components such as complement and thrombin to diffuse into the endoneurial space and induce nerve damage.

The importance of recognizing this rare syndrome lies in its potential for treatment. Patients with solitary lesions are treated with tumoricidal irradiation, complete surgical extirpation, or both. Patients with multiple bone lesions receive radiation combined with prednisone and melphalan. High-dose chemotherapy with autologous blood stem cell support is another option for patients with multifocal bone lesions or diffuse bone marrow plasmacytic infiltration (Karam et al., 2015; Kuwabara et al., 2008). Substantial improvement of both neurological and systemic features is seen in some patients, but the response may take many months. The high serum VEGF level is usually decreased dramatically following successful treatment, implying a major role played by VEGF in the development of the syndrome and neuropathy (Kuwabara et al., 2006).

## Cryoglobulinemia

Cryoglobulinemia is a condition characterized by the presence of serum immunoglobulins that reversibly precipitate in the cold. According to their molecular composition, cryoglobulins are classified into three groups: type 1 are isolated monoclonal immunoglobulins associated with myeloma, macroglobulinemia, and other lymphoproliferative disorders; type 2 consists of a mixture of a monoclonal protein, usually IgM-κ with antirheumatoid factor activity, and polyclonal IgG; and type 3 are polyclonal IgM and IgG immunoglobulins. Types 2 and 3 are usually referred to as *mixed cryoglobulins*. Mixed cryoglobulinemia may occur as a primary condition without any apparent underlying process, termed *essential mixed cryoglobulinemia*, or may be secondary to autoimmune diseases or chronic hepatitis C virus (HCV) infections. The detection of anti-HCV antibodies and HCV RNA in serum and cryoprecipitate of most patients with essential cryoglobulinemia firmly establishes a causal role for HCV in the formation of cryoglobulins (Apartis et al., 1996). Mixed cryoglobulinemia is a systemic disease characterized by recurrent purpura of the legs and cutaneous vasculitis, often precipitated by cold temperatures, arthralgias, renal impairment, and peripheral neuropathy. The reported prevalence of peripheral neuropathy varies from 37% to 57%, using electrophysiological criteria for confirmation. The most common presentation is a painful sensory or sensorimotor polyneuropathy or, less often, mononeuropathy multiplex (Tembl et al., 1999).

EDX studies show axonal changes with denervation, particularly in distal leg muscles. In most cases, the sural nerve biopsy confirms necrotizing vasculitis or perivascular inflammation affecting small-sized epineurial vessels, together with multifocal or global myelinated fiber loss and acute axonal degeneration. Low serum complement levels and the deposition of immunoglobulin in the walls of affected vessels suggest cryoprecipitable immune complexes are responsible for the disease manifestations.

Treatment of cryoglobulinemic neuropathy rests on expert opinion and uncontrolled trials. Patients with biopsy-proven vasculitis and progressive neurological deficits initially require immunosuppression with corticosteroids and either oral or IV cyclophosphamide. Plasmapheresis has been recommended for the rapid removal of cryoglobulins during acute exacerbations of neurological deficits or glomerulonephritis. Once clinical remission is achieved, immunosuppressive therapy is tapered off, and then specific treatment directed against the underlying HCV infection is offered. The recommended treatment regimen consists of interferon alfa-2a in combination with ribavirin for 6–12 months. Rituximab, given over a period of 3 months, also proved beneficial in both clinical and electrophysiological evaluations of neuropathy in a small open prospective study for HCV-associated type 2 cryoglobulinemic neuropathy (Cavallo et al., 2009).

## Primary Systemic Amyloidosis

Systemic amyloidoses are multisystem disorders caused by extracellular deposition of insoluble fibrillar proteins arranged in a β-pleated sheet conformation in various organs and tissues throughout the body (Kwan, 2007). The β-pleated sheet configuration consisting of strands of polypeptides in zigzag formation seems to be responsible for the typical staining properties with Congo red stain, appearing red under normal light microscopy but apple-green in polarized light. Several unrelated proteins can form amyloid fibrils and cause specific acquired as well as inherited forms of amyloidosis. In both primary systemic amyloidosis and amyloidosis complicating multiple myeloma or WM, amyloid is composed of fragments of immunoglobulin light chains from the amino-terminal variable regions, or less commonly the complete immunoglobulin light chain, and is designated AL amyloidosis (Falk et al., 1997). In primary AL amyloidosis, clonal populations of nonproliferative plasma cells synthesize light-chain polypeptides that are deposited in tissues as amyloid. Between 1200 and 3200 new cases are diagnosed yearly in the United States. AL amyloidosis in association with multiple myeloma and WM is distinguished from primary amyloidosis by the number and morphology of plasma cells in the bone marrow and the amount of M protein in the serum. Amyloid fibrils from patients with familial amyloid neuropathies are composed of one of three mutant proteins: transthyretin, apolipoprotein A1, and gelsolin (see FAP, earlier). Mutations in the genes encoding fibrinogen A, apolipoprotein A2, lysozyme, and cystatin C are associated with a non-neuropathic form of familial amyloidosis. Immunohistochemical techniques using specific antibodies can distinguish the different types of amyloidogenic proteins in biopsy material.

### Clinical Features

Primary amyloidosis usually occurs after age 40, with a median age of onset of 65 years. Men are twice as likely to be affected. The initial symptoms are frequently fatigue and weight loss followed by symptoms and signs related to specific organ involvement. The organs most commonly affected, either individually or together, are the kidney, heart, liver, and the autonomic nervous system and PNS. CNS involvement is absent. Peripheral neuropathy occurs in 15%–35% of patients and is the presenting manifestation in 10% (Matsuda et al., 2011). The majority have renal or cardiac presentation, with peripheral neuropathy as a later manifestation. The neuropathy begins with painful dysesthesias in the legs and follows a chronic progressive course. Pain and temperature sensation are lost before light touch or vibratory sensation. Distal symmetrical weakness and a pansensory loss evolve later in the course of disease. Most patients develop features of autonomic dysfunction that include postural hypotension, impotence, gastrointestinal disturbances, impaired sweating, and loss of bladder control. Nearly 25% of patients develop a superimposed CTS caused by amyloid infiltration of the flexor retinaculum at the wrist. Infiltration of amyloid deposits in joints and cartilages also occurs. The constellation of painful dysesthesias, autonomic dysfunction, and a history of CTS should alert the clinician to the possibility of amyloidosis. Typical findings on examination are hepatomegaly, pitting edema related to hypoalbuminemia, spontaneous periorbital purpura caused by vascular infiltration ("raccoon eyes sign"), and macroglossia, a sign occurring in 20% of patients. Amyloid deposition between muscle fibers may cause pseudohypertrophy of muscles. Renal amyloidosis usually manifests as proteinuria and renal failure. Rapidly progressive congestive heart failure caused by cardiac amyloid infiltration is seen in a third of patients.

EDX studies show changes of axonal polyneuropathy, with low-amplitude or absent SNAPs and low-amplitude CMAPs but preserved motor conduction velocities (Matsuda et al., 2011). Distal median motor latencies are prolonged in patients with CTS. Needle EMG frequently provides evidence of active denervation. A monoclonal protein or light chains are detected in 90% of patients by means of immunofixation of serum or urine. Monoclonal λ light chains are more common than κ light chains (ratio of λ to κ, 3:1). A quantitative light-chain assay is the most sensitive method for detecting low-level monoclonal proteins. Bone marrow examination reveals slightly increased plasma cells and clonal dominance of a light-chain isotope by immunohistochemical staining.

The diagnosis is established by the histological demonstration of amyloid deposition in tissues. Abdominal fat aspiration, bone marrow aspirate, and rectal biopsy are convenient procedures that provide about an 80% yield of positive results. In patients with suspected amyloid neuropathy, combined muscle and sural nerve biopsy is the most sensitive technique to provide confirmation in more than 90% of cases. One-tenth of patients with AL amyloidosis lack monoclonal proteins in serum or urine by immunofixation, and these patients are difficult to distinguish from those with familial or secondary amyloidosis. In most of these patients, a clonal dominance of plasma cells can be identified by immunocytochemical staining of a bone marrow specimen, or positive identification of AL amyloid can be achieved in tissue samples by immunohistochemical staining using labeled antibodies specific for human light chains. If confirmation of a plasma cell clone cannot be obtained, familial amyloidosis should be considered even in the absence of a positive family history. In such patients, molecular genetic testing to identify TTR mutations is indicated (see Familial Amyloid Neuropathy, earlier page 28-e4). Amyloidogenic mutations, most often in the genes encoding for fibrinogen A and TTR, were found in 10% of 350 patients who had initially been misdiagnosed with presumed AL amyloidosis (Lachmann et al., 2002). Results of sural nerve biopsy show amyloid deposition around blood vessels and within the endoneurial space (Fig. 106.26), severe loss of myelinated and unmyelinated fibers, and active axonal degeneration. The pathogenetic mechanism of nerve fiber damage remains uncertain.

The prognosis in primary amyloidosis is poor, with a median survival of less than 18 months. Death is commonly due to progressive congestive heart failure or renal insufficiency. Patients with amyloid

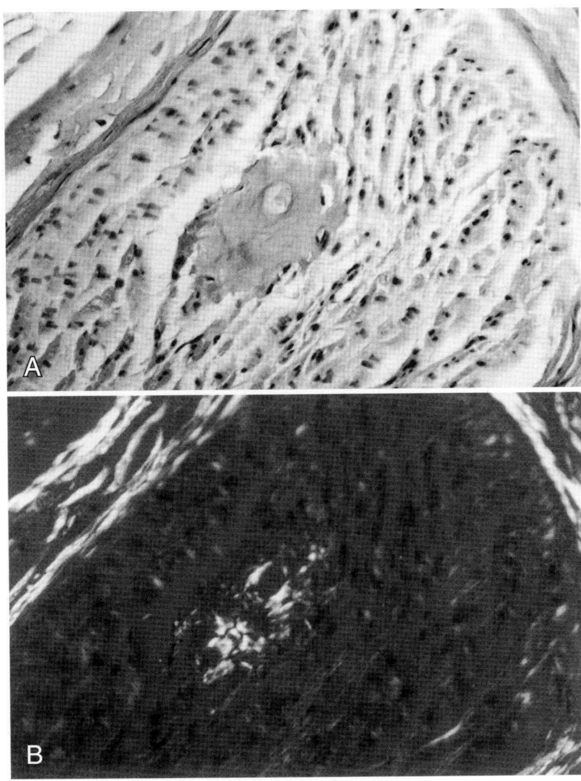


**Fig. 106.26 Amyloid Neuropathy.** **A**, Sural nerve biopsy shows deposition of amyloid in endoneurial vessel wall and loss of myelinated fibers. **B**, Under polarized light, Congo red-positive area shows apple-green birefringent deposits typical of amyloid. (Congo red, ×250.)

neuropathy without cardiac or renal involvement have a more favorable prognosis, with a median survival of 40 months. The treatment of AL amyloidosis remains unsatisfactory, but some aspects of disease may respond to chemotherapy that suppresses the underlying clonal plasma cell disorder. Intermittent oral melphalan and prednisone are reported to slow progression of renal and cardiac amyloidosis, but the treatment has no effect on the neuropathy. High-dose melphalan with autologous blood stem cell transplantation has shown promising results, with improvement of neurological deficits in selected patients. Because of high treatment-related mortality, stem cell transplantation is currently applicable to patients without significant cardiac involvement (Sanchorawala, 2006). Bortezomib and dexamethasone have also been shown to provide a benefit in survival in patients with AL amyloidosis (Lamm et al., 2010).

## NEUROPATHIES ASSOCIATED WITH SYSTEMIC DISORDERS

### Diabetic Neuropathies

DM is estimated to affect 23.6 million people in the United States, and this number is growing by an alarming rate of 5% per year (National Diabetes Information Clearinghouse, 2007). This trend is also becoming increasingly evident in other developed and developing countries, largely attributed to the increased prevalence of overweight and obesity. In addition to vasculopathies, the complications specific to diabetes include retinopathy, nephropathy, and neuropathy. Patients with IDDM or NIDDM of sufficient duration are vulnerable to these complications.

*Diabetic neuropathy* is a generic term defined as the presence of symptoms and signs of peripheral nerve dysfunction in individuals with diabetes after the exclusion of other causes. The mere association of neuropathic symptoms with DM is insufficient for the diagnosis of diabetic neuropathy, so the importance of excluding other causes that might be treated differently or have a different prognosis cannot be overemphasized (Harati, 2007). In addition, diabetic neuropathies, being common disorders, may coincide with other conditions that cause similar manifestations including CIDP, vitamin $B_{12}$ deficiency, alcoholic neuropathy, and endocrine neuropathies. Additional causes of polyneuropathy may be present in 10%–50% of patients with DM (Dyck et al., 1993; Gorson and Ropper, 2006).

Diabetes remains the leading cause of peripheral polyneuropathy in developed countries. There are different estimates on the prevalence of diabetic neuropathy, but taking the current prevalence of diabetes, it is estimated that as many as 7.7 million people in the United States have some degree of diabetic peripheral neuropathy. The varied estimates of the reported prevalence of diabetic neuropathy have been due in part to biases of patient selection and different criteria used for the definition of diabetic neuropathy. To some clinicians, the neuropathy is present only when clinical symptoms or signs appear, but others may diagnose diabetic neuropathy based solely on EDX, quantitative sensory testing, or autonomic abnormalities.

In general, the diagnosis of a definite diabetic neuropathy should be based on clinical symptoms, objective neurological signs, and EDX confirmation. Quality-of-life measurements provide an additional vantage point from which to judge the effect of neuropathy on everyday life (Padua et al., 2001). The risk of developing symptomatic neuropathy in patients without neuropathic symptoms or signs at the time of initial diagnosis of diabetes is estimated to be 4%–10% by 5 years and up to 50% by 25 years. In a population cohort of diabetic patients, two-thirds of diabetics had objective evidence of some type of neuropathy, but only about 15% had symptomatic degrees of polyneuropathy. Among 894 women older than age 65 in Maryland, both age and diabetes were found to correlate with increased vibratory detection threshold values (Resnick et al., 2001). Longer duration of diabetes and male gender may predispose to the development of neuropathy in younger patients with IDDM. Those with NIDDM have an increased risk for neuropathy over time; a Finnish study showed that 8.3% of such individuals have neuropathy at baseline, increasing to 41.9% after 10 years, with an even higher percentage in those with low serum insulin concentrations (Partanen et al., 1995). In a cohort of 775 US veterans with diabetes, 50% were found to have decreased foot sensation at baseline using monofilament sensory testing, and an additional 20% developed hypoesthesia over an average follow-up period of 2.6 years. Factors associated with decreased foot sensation included poor glycemic control, height, and age. Electrophysiological studies demonstrate subclinical conduction abnormalities in most patients with IDDM after 5–10 years of diabetes. The prevalence of neuropathy is significantly higher among diabetics who consume excessive amounts of alcohol. Tobacco use may also predispose to earlier development and more severe symptoms of neuropathy, presumably by inducing vasoconstriction and nerve ischemia (Tesfaye et al., 2005). Diabetics with lower-limb ischemia due to peripheral vascular disease also have a more severe neuropathy than diabetics without limb ischemia.

Several recent studies have shown that patients presenting with a chronic "idiopathic" axonal polyneuropathy have nearly a twofold higher frequency of undiagnosed DM and impaired fasting blood glucose than age-matched controls. These studies (Hoffman-Snyder et al., 2006) suggest that an axonal neuropathy may be the presenting or the earliest manifestation in diabetes. It is noted, however, that only 20%–30% of patients with impaired fasting blood glucose levels or glucose intolerance will progress to frank diabetes within 3 years, and many will revert to normal through weight loss, diet, and exercise. The probability that neuropathy in such patients may also improve following these interventions seems likely, but solid evidence for this is lacking.

Several peripheral nerve manifestations are associated with diabetes and are grouped into distinct clinical syndromes, each having a characteristic presentation and course. A useful classification divides the diabetic neuropathies into symmetrical polyneuropathies versus focal or multifocal neuropathies (Box 106.14). However, there is significant overlap between these syndromes.

#### Clinical Features

***Distal symmetrical polyneuropathy.*** Distal symmetrical polyneuropathy is the most common form of diabetic neuropathies.

**BOX 106.14 Classification of Diabetic Neuropathies**

**Generalized Symmetrical Polyneuropathies**
Distal sensory or sensorimotor polyneuropathy
Small-fiber neuropathy
Autonomic neuropathy
Large-fiber sensory neuropathy

**Focal and Asymmetrical Neuropathies**
Cranial neuropathy (single or multiple)
Truncal neuropathy (thoracic radiculopathy)
Limb mononeuropathy (single or multiple)
Lumbosacral radiculoplexopathy (amyotrophy, proximal neuropathy)

**Combinations**
Polyradiculoneuropathy
Diabetic neuropathic cachexia

Many physicians incorrectly assume that the term *diabetic neuropathy* is synonymous with *distal symmetrical polyneuropathy*, because the latter constitutes perhaps three-fourths of all diabetic neuropathies. In distal symmetrical polyneuropathy, however, sensory deficits predominate, and autonomic symptoms usually correlate with the severity of the neuropathy. Most patients will develop only a minor motor involvement affecting the distal muscles of the lower extremities. Sensory disturbances have a stocking-glove distribution following a length-dependent pattern. Early sensory manifestations begin in the toes, gradually spreading proximally; when these reach above knee level, the fingers and hands become affected. In more advanced cases, sensation becomes impaired over the anterior chest and abdomen, producing a truncal wedge-shaped area of sensory loss.

The distal symmetrical polyneuropathy may be subclassified further into two major subgroups, depending on the nerve fiber type most involved: large-fiber and small-fiber variants. Although diabetic sensory neuropathy frequently forms a continuous spectrum ranging between these two polar types, selective sensory nerve fiber involvement does occur, giving rise to relatively pure large- or small-fiber-type presentations.

The large-fiber neuropathy variant presents with painless paresthesias beginning at the toes and feet, impairment of vibration and joint position sense, and diminished muscle stretch reflexes. Early large-fiber involvement is often asymptomatic, but sensory deficit may be detected by careful examination. In advanced cases, significant ataxia may develop secondary to sensory deafferentation. The term *diabetic pseudotabes* is applied to patients having severe lancinating pains, loss of joint sensation, and diabetic pupillary abnormalities (pseudo-Argyll Robertson pupils).

A relatively common variant of diffuse diabetic polyneuropathy is *diabetic polyradiculoneuropathy*. Often beginning as a distal symmetrical polyneuropathy, this disorder comes to involve proximal segments of the PNS, including multiple lumbosacral roots, thoracic posterior primary rami, and (less commonly) cervical myotomes. More commonly, on needle EMG, patients with ordinary distal symmetrical diabetic polyneuropathy sometimes have low-grade active denervation changes in multiple levels of thoracic paraspinal muscles, which may herald the development of a more widespread and proximal neuropathy. The trigeminal blink reflex is often spared in advanced diabetic neuropathy and polyradiculoneuropathy, providing an important method to distinguish between this and immune-related polyradiculoneuropathies such as chronic inflammatory polyradiculoneuropathies. Much less commonly encountered is *diabetic polyradiculopathy*, in which peripheral sensory nerve conduction studies are normal. Both clinically and electrodiagnostically, the focus of the disease appears to be at the nerve root level. Occasional patients with either IDDM- or NIDDM-associated neuropathy meet the EDX criteria for CIDP (Sharma et al., 2002a). Some of these patients respond to high-dose IVIG therapy, although a controlled clinical trial has not yet been completed (Sharma et al., 2002b).

In contrast to the large-fiber neuropathy, the small-fiber neuropathy frequently presents with pain of a deep, burning, stinging, aching character, often associated with spontaneous shooting pains and allodynia to light touch. Pain and temperature modalities are impaired, with relative preservation of vibration and joint position sensation and muscle stretch reflexes. On examination, there is often touch and pin hypoesthesia, tactile hyperesthesia or allodynia, or both. These two findings when combined have excellent sensitivity (83%) and specificity (90%) for the diagnosis of neuropathic pain and diabetic small-fiber neuropathy (Spallone et al., 2012). The small-fiber variant is often accompanied by autonomic neuropathy (Santiago et al., 1999). At times, a painful small-fiber neuropathy develops soon after the onset of IDDM.

It is now clear that peripheral neuropathy can occur before the onset of clinically definite DM; this is known as *impaired glucose tolerance (IGT) neuropathy* (Hoffman-Snyder et al., 2006). Individuals with IGT, as determined by oral glucose tolerance testing (OGTT), have been demonstrated to have symptoms, EDX abnormalities, and IENFD reduction consistent with a predominantly small-fiber neuropathy, although with changes less pronounced than in their diabetic counterparts (Sumner et al., 2003). The implication for clinical practice is that patients with undiagnosed painful peripheral neuropathy should undergo OGTT (Singleton et al., 2001); early diagnosis followed by improved lifestyle may result in reversal of IGT and neuropathy.

An acute painful neuropathy may be precipitated following initiation of treatment of a diabetic patient with insulin *(treatment-induced neuropathy)*. Burning pain and paresthesias develop in the distal lower extremities shortly after the establishment of glucose control. Pain persists for weeks or up to several months, with spontaneous resolution to follow. Pathological studies demonstrate active axonal regeneration, which may act as generators of spontaneous nerve impulses. This phenomenon is said to be more common in the rare form of DM associated with a mitochondrial tRNA mutation at position 3243 (Suzuki et al., 1997).

Patients with newly diagnosed diabetes may experience transient pain and paresthesias in the distal lower extremities *(hyperglycemic neuropathy)*. The symptoms will usually resolve when the hyperglycemia is brought under control.

*Diabetic neuropathic cachexia* refers to an acute and severe painful diabetic neuropathy associated with precipitous severe weight loss, depression, insomnia, and impotence in men. Although it is rare, it imparts major challenges in diagnosis and treatment. The syndrome is more common in men with poor glucose control. Improved glucose control and weight gain often result in recovery and improvement of EDX abnormalities (Yuen et al., 2001). The reason for profound weight loss, severe pain, and spontaneous recovery remains obscure.

Sensory loss makes patients with diabetes susceptible to repetitive, often unnoticed injuries that set the stage for foot ulcers and distal joint destruction *(acrodystrophic neuropathy)*. Chronic foot ulceration is one of the more severe complications of DM, occurring in 4%–10% of patients, and is due to a combination of unnoticed traumatic tissue damage, vascular insufficiency, and secondary infection (Laing, 1998). Prevention is better than treatment. Daily inspection and proper foot care can prevent or lessen the severity of this complication (Birke et al., 2002).

*Neuropathic arthropathy*, or a *Charcot joint formation*, is a complication seen in patients with diabetes who often have foot ulcers and autonomic impairment. Unlike the Charcot joint seen in syphilis, diabetic arthropathy tends to involve the small joints in the feet. The role of pronounced inflammatory reactions and cytokines following the initial joint insult resulting in increased osteoclastogenesis has recently been emphasized (Jeffcoate et al., 2005). The abundance of osteoclasts causes progressive bone loss, leading to further fractures and potentiation of inflammation and osteoclast formation.

EDX studies are helpful in confirming the diagnosis of distal symmetrical polyneuropathy. Absent or decreased amplitudes of the sural nerve potentials and low amplitude or absent tibial H-reflexes are found in almost all patients. Active denervation in intrinsic foot muscles or decreased amplitudes of CMAPs, together with mild slowing of conduction velocities in the motor nerves, are found in more than two-thirds of patients. Abnormal sensory nerve conduction studies are found in more than half. Even in the small-fiber variant, nerve conduction studies and needle EMG examination are often abnormal.

***Autonomic neuropathy.*** Autonomic neuropathy usually correlates with the severity of somatic neuropathy. The spectrum of autonomic involvement ranges from subclinical functional impairment of cardiovascular reflexes and sudomotor function to severe cardiovascular, gastrointestinal, or genitourinary autonomic dysfunction (Low, 2002).

Orthostatic hypotension, resting tachycardia, or diminished heart-rate response to respiration are the hallmarks of diabetic cardiac autonomic neuropathy. Orthostatic hypotension occurs mainly because of failure of the sympathetic nervous system to increase systemic vascular resistance in the erect posture and impairment of compensatory cardiac acceleration. It is crucial to exclude confounding effects of medications or coexisting hypovolemia when diagnosing neurogenic postural hypotension. Vagal denervation of the heart results in a high resting pulse rate and loss of sinus arrhythmia. An increased incidence of painless or silent myocardial infarction is reported in diabetic patients with autonomic neuropathy. It is important to investigate the cardiac autonomic neuropathy of diabetes by appropriate noninvasive autonomic function tests because the presence of such autonomic dysfunction predicts cardiovascular morbidity and mortality (Astrup et al., 2006).

Gastrointestinal motility abnormalities involving the esophagus, stomach, gallbladder, and bowel, as well as fecal incontinence may occur. Delayed gastric emptying, usually of solids, leads to nausea, early satiety, and postprandial bloating. Diabetic diarrhea due to small-intestinal involvement typically occurs at night and is explosive and paroxysmal. However, constipation due to colonic hypomotility is more common than diarrhea. Associated weight loss or malabsorption is rare. Bacterial overgrowth may occur and can often be successfully treated with small doses of tetracycline (250–500 mg/day in a single dose given at the onset of a diarrheal attack) in adult patients.

Impaired bladder sensation is usually the first symptom of urinary autonomic dysfunction. Bladder atony leads to prolonged intervals between voiding, gradually increasing urinary retention, and finally overflow incontinence. The symptoms of urinary autonomic dysfunction develop insidiously and progress slowly. Patients with diabetes who have neurogenic bladder should be encouraged to void routinely every few hours to prevent urinary retention. Impotence is often the first manifestation of autonomic neuropathy in men with diabetes, occurring in more than 60% and causing serious emotional distress. Autonomic dysfunction involves both erectile failure and retrograde ejaculation. Most diabetic men with impotence have some evidence of associated distal symmetrical polyneuropathy. Autonomic neuropathy is not the only cause of impotence in diabetic males, and other factors such as vasculopathies, hormonal alterations, and psychological issues are equally important.

Sudomotor abnormalities result in distal anhidrosis, compensatory facial and truncal sweating, and heat intolerance. A peculiar hyperhidrosis called *gustatory sweating* is characterized by profuse sweating in the face and forehead immediately following food intake. This often becomes difficult to treat and socially embarrassing. Oral or topical glycopyrrolate may prove partially effective in some patients. Pupillary abnormalities include constricted pupils with sluggish light reaction, which occurs in 20% of unselected diabetic patients. This results from early involvement of sympathetic nerves that dilate the iris and an imbalance between parasympathetic and sympathetic function. A blunted autonomic response to hypoglycemia produces an inadequate sympathetic and adrenal response and hence an unawareness of hypoglycemia that may seriously complicate intensive insulin treatment (Cryer, 2006).

***Lumbosacral radiculoplexopathy (amyotrophy, proximal neuropathy).*** Since Garland coined the term *diabetic amyotrophy* to describe this special type of diabetic neuropathy, its clinical definition and limits have been the subject of debate, largely because the term itself is ambiguous. Some experts have suggested that this term be abandoned and replaced with *diabetic proximal neuropathy*, emphasizing the proximal motor weakness as a distinguishing clinical feature. Diabetic amyotrophy, thoracolumbar radiculopathy, and proximal or diffuse lower extremity weakness should probably be grouped under the single term, *diabetic lumbosacral radiculoplexopathy*, since these disorders seem to be different presentations of the same basic involvement of multiple nerve roots or proximal nerve segments. The eponymic designation *Bruns-Garland syndrome* avoids anatomical inconsistencies. As the name implies, the disorder is almost always restricted to the lower limbs. In a significant number of patients, at least one additional body region is also affected, mostly the thoracic but occasionally the cervical region. Isolated cases of diabetic cervical radiculoplexopathy were recently reported (Massie et al., 2012). Clinically, asymmetrical weakness and wasting of pelvifemoral muscles may occur either abruptly or in a stepwise progression in individuals with diabetes who are older than 50 years. The disorder is rare in young adults or children (Fernandes Filho et al., 2005). The onset is unrelated to the duration of diabetes, and the condition may develop in patients with long-standing NIDDM during periods of poor metabolic control and weight loss, but it can also occur in mild and well-controlled diabetics or be the presenting feature of diabetes. Typically, unilateral severe pain in the lower back, hip, and anterior thigh heralds the onset of neuropathy. Within days to weeks weakness ensues, affecting proximal and, to a lesser extent, distal lower-extremity muscles (iliopsoas, gluteus, thigh adductor, quadriceps, hamstring, and anterior tibialis). In some cases, the opposite leg becomes affected after a latency of days to months. Reduction or absence of knee and ankle jerks is the rule. Numbness or paresthesias are minor complaints. Weight loss occurs in more than half of patients and is more pronounced than in individuals with nondiabetic lumbosacral radiculoplexopathy (Dyck et al., 2001). The progression may be steady or stepwise and may continue for many months. The result is often a debilitating, painful, asymmetrical motor neuropathy with profound atrophy of proximal leg muscles. Pain usually recedes spontaneously long before motor strength begins to improve. Recovery takes up to 24 months because of the slow rate of axonal regeneration. In many cases, mild to moderate weakness persists indefinitely. Overlap with distal symmetrical polyneuropathy is noted in up to 60% of patients. Those with polyneuropathy more commonly have gradual onset of symptoms, bilateral findings, significant weight loss, and diffuse paraspinal muscle denervation. Typical EMG findings include low-amplitude femoral nerve motor responses, prominent fibrillation potentials in thoracic and lumbar paraspinal muscles, and active denervation in affected muscles. Neuroimaging studies of the lumbar spine, lumbosacral plexus, or both should be considered when lumbar root, cauda equina lesions, or structural lumbosacral plexopathy are suspected. Sural nerve biopsy specimens in these individuals show multifocal nerve fiber loss, suggesting ischemic injury and perivascular infiltrates in small vessels, which implies an immune mechanism (Dyck et al., 2000b; Fig. 106.27). A vascular pathogenesis of this proximal neuropathy was documented by autopsy, showing infarcts of the proximal nerve trunks and lumbosacral plexus. Although a beneficial effect of immunomodulating therapies has been proposed, controlled studies have shown no positive effect for corticosteroids in enhancing the recovery of the motor deficit.

***Truncal neuropathy.*** Diabetic truncal neuropathy or thoracic radiculopathy involving the T4 through T12 spinal nerve roots causes pain or dysesthesias in areas of the chest or abdomen, thereby producing diagnostic confusion. Bulging of the abdominal wall as a result of weakness of abdominal muscles may also occur, mimicking a hernia (Fig. 106.28).

This unique truncal pain is seen in older patients with NIDDM and may occur either in isolation or together with the typical lumbosacral

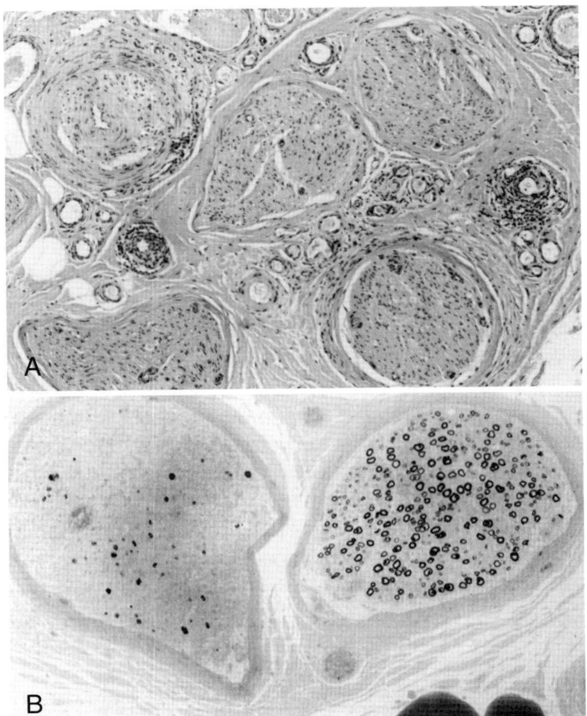


**Fig. 106.27** A, Sural nerve biopsy from patient with diabetic lumbar radiculoplexopathy. Perivascular lymphocytic inflammation involves two epineurial arterioles. (Hematoxylin and eosin, ×25.) B, In the same patient, semi-thin transverse section illustrates selective involvement of one fascicle, with marked loss of myelinated fibers, a pattern highly suggestive of nerve ischemia. (Paraphenylenediamine-stained semi-thin epoxy section, 80.) *(Courtesy Dr. P.J. Dyck, Mayo Clinic, Rochester, MN.)*

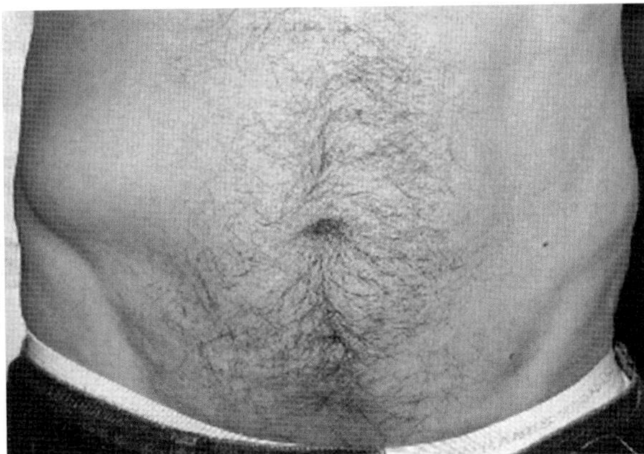

**Fig. 106.28** Bulging of right lower thoracic abdominal wall at level of umbilicus, associated with diabetic truncal monoradiculopathy.

radiculoplexopathy. The regions of sensory loss or dysesthesia involve the trunk in a highly variable pattern, affecting either the entire dermatomal distribution of adjacent spinal nerves or, more often, restricted areas limited to the distribution of the dorsal or ventral rami of spinal nerves. Patients describe burning, stabbing, boring, beltlike pain. Contact with clothing can be very unpleasant. The onset may be either abrupt or gradual and in some patients preceded or accompanied by a profound weight loss. The clinical picture may mimic intraabdominal, intrathoracic, or intraspinal disease, or even herpes zoster, requiring careful differential diagnostic consideration. Neurological findings are limited to hypoesthesia or hyperpathia over the thorax or abdomen. The symptoms may persist for several months before gradual and spontaneous resolution within 4–6 months.

EDX studies help by demonstrating active denervation in paraspinal and abdominal muscles, although these features are not specific for truncal mononeuropathy. Focal anhidrosis on the trunk correlating with the area of pain is detected with the help of the thermoregulatory sweat test (TST).

***Limb mononeuropathy.*** Single mononeuropathies, often seen in diabetic patients, are thought to be caused by two basic mechanisms: nerve infarction or entrapment. Limb mononeuropathies secondary to nerve infarction is rare and much less common than cranial mononeuropathies. They have a stereotyped presentation, with abrupt onset of pain followed by variable weakness and atrophy. Because the primary pathological lesion results in acute axonal degeneration, recovery tends to be slow. The median, ulnar, and fibular nerves are most commonly affected. Mononeuropathies due to nerve entrapment are more common than nerve infarctions. These two conditions can usually be distinguished by clinical and electrophysiological features. EDX studies demonstrate axonal loss in nerve infarction in contrast to focal conduction block or focal slowing often mixed with axonal loss in entrapment.

DM is a risk factor for single or multiple entrapment neuropathies. Diabetes is found in 8%–12% of patients presenting with CTS. Electrophysiological abnormalities consistent with CTS without symptoms are found in one-fourth of diabetic patients, whereas population-based studies have shown symptomatic CTS in 8% of diabetics. The risk for CTS is more than twofold for patients with diabetes than in the general population. The reason diabetes predisposes to nerve entrapment is unknown, but aggravation of ischemia in nerves already stressed by chronic endoneurial hypoxia may be one factor. The possibility of occult diabetes should always be kept in mind in every case of entrapment neuropathy.

***Multiple mononeuropathies.*** *Multiple mononeuropathies* refers to the involvement of two or more nerves. As in mononeuropathy, the onset is abrupt in one nerve, and then other nerves are involved sequentially at irregular intervals. Multiple mononeuropathies involving the proximal nerves are considered the cause of diabetic amyotrophy. Nerve infarction results from occlusion of the vasa nervorum. Because multiple mononeuropathies occur most frequently in systemic vasculitis, this possibility should always be considered in the differential diagnosis of diabetic multiple mononeuropathies.

***Cranial mononeuropathies.*** A detailed description of cranial mononeuropathies is given in Chapter 103. A third-nerve palsy is the most commonly encountered diabetic cranial mononeuropathy. Pupillary sparing, the hallmark of diabetic third-nerve palsy, results from ischemic infarction of the centrifascicular oculomotor axons due to diabetic vasculopathy of the vasa nervorum. The peripherally located pupillary motor fibers are spared as a result of collateral circulation from the circumferential arteries. With decreasing frequency, the fourth, sixth, and seventh nerves are also affected. Patients with Bell palsy have a significantly higher frequency of diabetes than an age-matched population. Most make a full recovery in 3–5 months.

Two serious infectious syndromes occur occasionally in patients with DM and characteristically affect one or more cranial nerves by local inflammation. *Rhinocerebral mucormycosis* and *"malignant" external otitis* were often fatal before the advent of early diagnosis and effective treatment strategies (Smith, 1998).

## Laboratory Findings and Diagnostic Studies

The revised 2003 American Diabetes Association criteria for diagnosis of diabetes (Genuth et al., 2003) define a normal fasting plasma glucose as being equal or less than 100 mg/dL (5.55 mmol/L). Impaired fasting glucose (IFG) occurs when the glucose level is above 100 mg/dL but below 126 mg/dL (6.99 mmol/L). An IGT is defined as a 2-hour plasma glucose level between 140 mg/dL (7.77 mmol/L) and 199 mg/dL (11.04 mmol/L) following ingestion of 75 g of oral glucose. Diabetes is defined as fasting blood glucose above 126 mg/dL or the 2 hours level of greater than 200 mg/dL (11.1 mmol/L) in the OGTT.

The diagnosis of IGT (prediabetes) remains challenging and often under dispute by both physicians and patients. Glycosylated hemoglobin ($HbA_{1c}$) is a useful indicator of the long-term control of hyperglycemia but is not generally used to diagnose IGT, or IFG. The diagnostic sensitivity of $HbA_{1c}$ for prediabetes is unclear, although the specificity is very high. In at-risk patients with prediabetes and normal $HbA_{1c}$, an OGTT is recommended. The American Diabetes Association recommends that two tests (fasting glucose, $HbA_{1c}$ measurement, 2-hour plasma glucose level after OGTT) obtained at two separate visits should be abnormal for confirmation of the diagnosis of diabetes (American Diabetes Association, 2018). More recently, elevated levels of fasting glucose and $HbA_{1c}$ from a single baseline blood sample was shown to have moderate sensitivity (55%) but high specificity to identify patients who will develop frank diabetes in the next 5 years of follow-up (98%), with specificity increasing to 99.6% at 15 years (Selvin et al., 2018).

The EDX features of diabetic sensorimotor peripheral polyneuropathy are characteristic of a primarily axon loss polyneuropathy. Abnormalities occur more commonly in sensory than in motor fibers, in the legs more than in the arms, and in distal more than proximal nerve segments. Sensory nerve and CMAP amplitudes are often reduced in patients with diabetic polyneuropathy. Conduction velocities are typically slower in this group than in healthy subjects, although strict criteria for demyelinating neuropathy are not often met (Herrmann and Griffin, 2002; Sharma et al., 2002a). In severe diabetic polyneuropathy, there is often complete absence of all routine sensory and motor conduction studies in the legs and absent sensory responses in the hands with very low amplitude median and ulnar motor responses in the upper limbs. Needle EMG shows long-duration, high-amplitude, and rapidly recruited MUAPs with fibrillation potentials in distal muscles. This is usually symmetrical and worse in the leg muscles distally with a distal to proximal gradient.

Autonomic testing is indicated in patients with diabetic autonomic neuropathy and provides a useful assessment in patients with distal symmetric polyneuropathy. Cardiac response to deep breathing evaluates cardiovagal functions by assessing heart rate variability to deep breathing, a very sensitive method for detecting early cardiovagal denervation. Cardiac response to Valsalva maneuvers also tests parasympathetic innervation to the heart. A tilt-table test evaluates adrenergic vasomotor function and cardiac sympathetic function and is essential when orthostatic hypotension is suspected. QSART to evaluate the postganglionic segment of the thermoregulatory pathway and TST provides a widespread "geographic" screen of the sudomotor loss. These studies are recommended (Level B) by the American Academy of Neurology (England et al., 2009b). Gastrointestinal autonomic dysfunction and atony is best assessed by demonstrating the abnormally slow passage of barium through the gut. Neurogenic urinary bladder and sphincter dysfunction is assessed by quantitating the postvoiding residual urine, cystoscopy, and urodynamic studies. Male sexual dysfunction, including erectile impotence, could be evaluated during rapid eye movement (REM) sleep by penial tumescence studies.

Skin biopsy with quantification of the IENFD is particularly useful in confirming small-fiber neuropathy (Lauria et al., 2010). Small-fiber neuropathy is closely linked to the metabolic syndrome, which consists of diabetes/prediabetes, hypertension, dyslipidemia, and central obesity (Zhou et al., 2011). Corneal confocal microscopy assesses corneal nerve fiber and nerve branch density and significantly correlates with IENFD in patients with small-fiber neuropathy (Jiang et al., 2016). In diabetics, reduced corneal sensation and corneal nerve fiber and nerve branch density correlates with disease duration and with IENFD (Cruzat et al., 2017; Jiang et al., 2016). Cutaneous nerve biopsy is rarely indicated and is kept when the diagnoses of amyloidosis or vasculitis are being considered.

## Pathology

The underlying pathological processes differ in the various types of diabetic neuropathy. Cranial and limb mononeuropathy and multiple mononeuropathies are thought to be caused by small-vessel occlusive disease. The precise location of the primary pathological process in diabetic asymmetrical proximal neuropathy remains unsettled. Postmortem examination of the obturator nerve in a single case of proximal neuropathy showed multiple infarcts due to occlusion of the vasa nervorum. However, lumbar nerve roots were not examined. Studies of peripheral sensory nerves in patients with diabetic lumbosacral radiculoplexopathy reveal microangiopathy and evidence of ischemia (Dyck et al., 2001). Whether ischemic or inflammatory lesions in multiple lumbar roots, plexus, or proximal nerve segments are responsible for this particular diabetic complication still remains to be decided.

The pathological lesions of symmetrical distal polyneuropathy have been extensively investigated (Engelstad et al., 1997). The sural nerve shows loss of myelinated fibers, acute axonal degeneration, some degree of demyelination, and, almost invariably, evidence of a small endoneurial blood vessel vasculopathy. This last condition is characterized by narrowing or closure of the endoneurial capillary lumen by hyperplastic endothelial cells, thickening of the capillary wall, and marked redundancy of basement membranes. Dying-back centripetal axonal degeneration is evident. Painless distal polyneuropathy affects predominantly the large-nerve fiber populations, whereas painful distal diabetic polyneuropathy often shows marked depletion of small myelinated and unmyelinated fibers. In the latter condition, active axonal regeneration gives rise to abnormal nerve impulses and neuropathic pain.

The demyelinating process in diabetes has been interpreted as either the result of primary progressive axonal atrophy or direct damage to Schwann cells secondary to ischemia or metabolic disturbances. Nerve fiber loss in diabetic neuropathy is distributed multifocally within individual and different fascicles (differential fascicular involvement), a pattern similar to that seen experimentally from injection of microspheres into the peripheral nerve vasculature to cause occlusion of multiple endoneurial blood vessels. Fiber depletion increases from proximal to distal in the nerves. This finding correlates with electrophysiological studies demonstrating a diffuse abnormality of NCVs with proximodistal gradients.

## Pathogenesis of Diabetic Neuropathy

Although the causes of diabetic neuropathies remain unknown, currently accepted hypotheses focus on the possibilities of metabolic and ischemic factors and their interactions in causing nerve injury. Hyperglycemia has been implicated in many different pathogenic mechanisms in diabetic neuropathy (Simmons and Feldman, 2002), but there is also a role for insulin deficiency and its effect on neurotrophic factors in the pathogenesis of neuropathy. Hyperglycemia generates rheological changes that increase endoneurial vascular resistance and reduce nerve blood flow. Hyperglycemia also causes depletion of nerve myoinositol through a competitive uptake mechanism and activates protein kinase C (Das Evcimen and King, 2007). In addition, persistently elevated blood glucose levels activate the polyol pathway in nerve tissue through the enzyme aldose reductase, which leads to the accumulation of sorbitol and fructose in nerve and enhancement of nonenzymatic glycosylation of structural nerve proteins (Thornalley, 2002). Another adverse effect of hyperglycemia is auto-oxidation of glucose, which results in the generation of toxic reactive oxygen intermediates (Sheetz and King, 2002). Overly exuberant activation of protein kinase C has been linked to vascular damage in diabetic neuropathy (Eichberg, 2002). These metabolic changes are likely to cause abnormal neuronal/axonal and Schwann cell metabolism and impaired axonal transport. Direct measurements of sugar alcohols in sural nerves from patients with diabetes confirm the correlation between increased levels of glucose, sorbitol, and fructose and the severity of the neuropathy.

Endoneurial hypoxia is produced by decreased blood flow to the nerve and increased endoneurial vascular resistance from endothelial cell hyperplasia. Once hypoxia is established, a vicious cycle of further capillary damage escalates hypoxia. Endoneurial hypoxia is thought to impair axonal transport and reduces nerve sodium-potassium-ATPase activity. The impairment of these functions causes axonal atrophy, leading to reduced NCVs. Although the precise mechanisms leading to capillary abnormalities that initiate hypoxia are unknown, the hypoxic hypothesis provides a framework for further research into the pathogenesis of diabetic neuropathy. Autoimmune mechanisms and amino acid, electrolyte, and lipid biochemical abnormalities also play a role in the neuropathies of DM.

### Treatment

The cornerstone in the treatment of diabetes and its complications remains optimal glucose control. Considerable evidence supports the idea that good diabetic control is associated with less frequent and less severe peripheral nerve complications. Although the data are less compelling for NIDDM, poor glycemic control has been associated with neuropathic deficits (Adler et al., 1997). A larger, more recent prospective study with a 6-year follow-up, however, compared intensive glucose control versus standard glucose control in a population with long-standing poorly controlled NIDDM (average $HbA_{1c}$ of 9.4%) and showed no benefit with respect to new cases of neuropathy, despite achieving the goal of a reduction of $HbA_{1c}$ by 1.5% (Duckworth et al., 2009). The Action to Control Cardiovascular Risk in Diabetes (ACCORD) trial, an even larger study of over 10,000 patients with poorly controlled NIDDM ($HbA_{1c}$ of 8.1%), specifically assessed the effect of intensive treatment of hyperglycemia on microvascular complications including neuropathy. The study, which aimed for a $HbA_{1c}$ of less than 6% in the intensive treatment group, was limited by the fact that a 22% relative risk of death from all causes was discovered at an average of 3.7 years into the 5-year planned follow-up in the group being treated with intensive therapy. Those patients in the intensive treatment group were then transitioned to standard treatment. At the end of the study, new cases of neuropathy were significantly reduced in the intensive treatment group, but no significant difference was found at the time of transition to standard therapy (Ismail-Baig et al., 2010). A third trial of over 11,000 patients with NIDDM (average $HbA_{1c}$ of 7.5%), the ADVANCE trial, also assessed vascular outcomes in patients with intensive versus standard glycemic control. New or worsening neuropathy, a secondary outcome, was not found to be significantly affected by intensive glucose control after a median follow-up of 5 years (The ADVANCE Collaborative Group, 2008). The Diabetes Control and Complication Trial (DCCT; 1995) showed that intensive glucose management by insulin pump or by multiple daily insulin injections in patients with IDDM reduces the development of neuropathy by 64% at 5 years compared to conventional therapy. Recent follow-up studies of the DCCT study cohort indicate that the beneficial effect of intensive glucose management persisted for at least 8 years after the completion of DCCT, underscoring the importance of continuous good diabetes control. Successful pancreatic transplantation is beneficial in preventing the progression of diabetic neuropathy, and the effect may be sustained in long-term follow-up (Navarro et al., 1997). Unfortunately, once the diabetic neuropathy is established, the existing damage is largely irreversible (Coppini et al., 2006). Attempts to treat diabetic neuropathy by manipulating nerve metabolism have been disappointing. Clinical trials of myoinositol supplementation have shown conflicting results, and those of aldose reductase inhibitors have so far failed to produce convincing clinical improvement or proved toxic, though there were modest changes in nerve conduction and nerve pathology.

Despite promising preliminary evidence, neurotrophin treatments for diabetic neuropathy, such as NGF, have been disappointing (Apfel, 2002). Based on experimental data suggesting that oxidative stress mediated by free-radical species may be involved in diabetic neuropathy, two large multicenter randomized controlled clinical trials of α-lipoic acid, either oral or IV, showed benefit in reducing neuropathic symptoms and deficits (Ametov et al., 2003; Ziegler et al., 2006). Despite two multicenter controlled clinical trials of α-linoleic acid in diabetic neuropathy which showed lessening of neuropathic deficits and improvement in measures of nerve conduction (Horrobin, 1997), because of licensing problems, no further trials with this substance are planned. VEGF gene transfer into small mammals has been shown to improve NCVs, increase blood vessel density, and enhance nerve blood flow (Schratzberger et al., 2001), giving impetus to pursuing this approach to treat human diabetic neuropathy. Because human C-peptide prevents neuropathy in diabetic rats in a dose-dependent fashion (Zhang et al., 2001), clinical interest has developed for this compound as well.

Symptomatic treatment for pain, autonomic manifestations, and the complications of sensory loss can be offered to mitigate the impact of neuropathic symptoms. It should be remembered that about 20% of patients with chronic painful diabetic neuropathy of over 6 months' duration demonstrate a complete remission of symptoms over time (Daousi et al., 2006). Intravenous methylprednisolone therapy for patients with diabetic lumbosacral radiculoplexopathy showed no beneficial effect in the weakness and atrophy but some lessening of pain and positive neuropathic symptoms. IVIG reversed the weakness rapidly in a teenager with diabetic lumbosacral radiculoplexopathy (Fernandes Filho et al., 2005). Use of high-dose IVIG or methylprednisolone has been reported to benefit patients with progressive deficits and biopsy evidence of inflammation in uncontrolled studies (Dyck and Windebank, 2002). The long-term use of corticosteroids in diabetic patients is, however, problematic.

Several therapeutic interventions may reduce the symptoms of autonomic dysfunction. Patients with symptomatic orthostatic hypotension are advised to sleep with the head of the bed elevated 6–10 inches. The head-up tilt prevents salt and water losses during the night and will combat supine hypertension. Practical suggestions include drinking two cups of strong coffee or tea with meals, eating more frequent small meals rather than a few large ones, and increasing the daily fluid intake (>20 oz/day) and salt ingestion (10–20 g/day). Elastic body stockings may be beneficial by reducing the venous capacitance in bed but are poorly tolerated by many patients. Plasma volume expansion can be achieved by fludrocortisone (0.1–0.6 mg/day). NSAIDs inhibit prostaglandin synthesis; ibuprofen, 400 mg four times a day, is better tolerated than indomethacin. Midodrine, an $\alpha_1$-adrenergic agonist that causes vasoconstriction, and droxidopa, a synthetic amino acid analog that is directly metabolized to norepinephrine by dopa decarboxylase, are effective in neurogenic orthostatic hypotension (Kaufmann et al., 2014; Wright et al., 1998). Both may cause supine hypertension and should not be taken late in the evening. Subcutaneous recombinant human erythropoietin has proved effective in some patients with orthostatic hypotension and anemia.

Delayed gastric emptying is often relieved with metoclopramide, a dopamine antagonist, which may induce extrapyramidal symptoms at higher doses. Diabetic diarrhea may be treated with short courses of tetracycline or erythromycin if appropriate. In some cases, clonidine has been reported to reduce the troublesome diarrhea. Genitourinary complications of diabetic autonomic neuropathy require close collaboration with a urologist. Patients with a neurogenic bladder should be encouraged to adhere to a frequent voiding schedule during the day, which helps diminish the amount of residual urine. For more severe involvement, manual abdominal compression or intermittent self-catheterization may be needed. Treatment of erectile impotence should be directed by a urologist, who can counsel the patient regarding the options of either oral treatment with sildenafil or similar drugs, direct injections into the corpora cavernosa, or penile implants. Proper skin care in diabetics with cutaneous sensory loss, impaired sweating, and vascular disease is extremely important to prevent foot ulcers.

## Peripheral Neuropathy in Malignancies

Advances in the diagnosis and management of malignancies have accelerated in recent years, leading to novel chemotherapeutic strategies and prolonged survival rates for many cancer patients. With these welcome improvements comes an increasing awareness of peripheral nerve complications in patients with various forms of neoplasm and chemotherapy. The frequency with which neuropathy occurs in cancer depends on the type of neoplasm and the method of detection. If clinical criteria alone are used, 2%–16% of cancer patients are estimated to have peripheral neuropathy. When quantitative sensory testing or electrophysiological studies are carried out, approximately 30%–40% of patients have abnormalities suggestive of peripheral nerve involvement (Amato and Collins, 1998).

Peripheral nerve complications may result from one or more mechanisms related to cancer or its treatment. These include (1) compression or invasion of nerve roots or nerve plexus by direct extension of primary or metastatic tumor; (2) meningeal metastases with involvement of multiple nerve roots; (3) remote effects of cancer affecting neuronal cell bodies, nerve axons, Schwann cells or myelin, terminal axons, neuromuscular junction, and muscle; (4) entrapment neuropathies in individuals with profound cachexia; and (5) neurotoxic effects of chemotherapy or radiation.

### Compression/Invasion of Nerves

Apart from head and neck tumors invading cranial and cervical peripheral nerves, focal neuropathies from primary neoplasms are uncommon. Salivary gland cancers are known to affect the facial and other cranial nerves, often growing insidiously by perineurial spread, thereby eluding early detection even by sophisticated imaging procedures. Nasopharyngeal carcinomas, meningiomas, and skull base tumors may interrupt cranial nerve fibers directly. Primary or recurrent neoplasms of the breast or lung apex in particular may invade the brachial plexus. Similarly, primary or recurrent pelvic or retroperitoneal cancers may involve the lumbosacral plexus.

### Metastases

Discrete single metastatic lesions may rarely cause cranial or somatic mononeuropathy. The *numb chin syndrome* results from invasion of the inferior alveolar nerve by metastases to the mandible. Patients complain of numbness of the chin and lower lip. Leukemias, lymphomas, and breast cancer are the most common neoplasms responsible for numb chin syndrome. More commonly, widespread metastases arise in the leptomeninges from carcinoma or lymphoma, leading to leptomeningeal carcinomatosis or lymphomatosis, respectively.

### Entrapment

Individuals who lose substantial weight or are bedridden are subject to fibular and ulnar compression neuropathies (Rubin et al., 1998).

### Iatrogenic Neuropathies

Chemotherapeutic agents that cause primarily peripheral neurotoxicity, including vinca alkaloids, platinum compounds, and taxanes, are discussed in the section on Toxic Neuropathies. The neurological complications of radiation plexopathy are discussed in Chapters 86, 97, and 105. Surgical resection of bulky cancers may result in trauma to peripheral nerves, though this may be unavoidable because of inextricable adherence or transit of nerve fibers through the tumor mass.

### Paraneoplastic Neuropathies

**Definition.** *Paraneoplastic neurological disorders* are remote effects of cancer that involve either the CNS or PNS alone or both. They are not caused by invasion of the tumor or its metastases or by infection, ischemia, metabolic and nutritional derangements, surgery, or other forms of tumor treatment (deBeukelaar and Sillevis Smith, 2006) (see Chapter 80). Classical syndromes including limbic encephalitis, subacute cerebellar degeneration, opsoclonus-myoclonus, subacute sensory neuronopathy, Lambert-Eaton myasthenic syndrome, or dermatomyositis. Patients are considered to have a *definite paraneoplastic neurological syndrome* if they have (Graus et al., 2004):

- A classical PNS syndrome and cancer that develops within 5 years of the diagnosis of the neurological disorder, regardless of the presence of paraneoplastic antibodies.
- A non-classical PNS syndrome that objectively improves or resolves after cancer treatment (provided that the syndrome is not susceptible to spontaneous remission).
- A non-classical syndrome with paraneoplastic antibodies and cancer that develops within 5 years of the diagnosis of the neurological disorder.
- A neurological syndrome (classical or not) with well-characterized paraneoplastic antibodies.

Small-cell carcinoma of the lung (SCLC) is the most common malignancy associated with paraneoplastic neurological syndromes, but carcinoma of breast, ovaries, kidney, prostate, thymoma, and Hodgkin and non-Hodgkin lymphoma may also trigger these syndromes. The neurological symptoms may precede the detection of the underlying cancer by 4–12 months. The clinical course is often rapidly progressive, leaving patients severely disabled in only a few weeks or months.

Paraneoplastic neurological syndromes are considered autoimmune disorders because of the presence of autoantibodies in serum and CSF that are reactive with protein antigens in the neoplastic tissue and neurons *(onconeural antibodies)*. Paraneoplastic neuropathies have been associated with an ever-increasing number of autoantibodies (Chan et al., 2001; Table 106.15). A positive antibody test mandates a thorough search for an underlying malignancy. The majority of these antibodies are directed against intracellular antigens in the nucleus or cytoplasm of neurons while others are directed at surface channels. Antibodies against surface antigens are sensitive and specific for neurological syndrome, are not highly predictive of malignancy (autoimmune variants), cause reversible loss of synaptic function rather than neuronal damage, and have better potential for recovery. In contrast, antibodies against intracellular antigens are quite specific for presence of cancer, are surrogate markers of specific immune responses and triggers cytotoxic cell-mediated immunity with inflammatory infiltrate which results in neuronal destruction of irreversible nature.

Antibodies directed against *neuronal nuclear antigens* include the type 1 antineuronal nuclear antibody (ANNA-I or anti-Hu, named

TABLE 106.15 **Autoantibodies in Neurological Paraneoplastic Syndromes**

| Antibody | Neurological Manifestations | Types of Tumors |
|---|---|---|
| ANNA-I (anti-Hu) | Sensory ataxia (MISP), GI dysmotility, autonomic N, PEM | SCLC |
| ANNA-II (anti-Ri) | Opsoclonus/myoclonus, jaw dystonia, ataxia, SMN | SCLC, breast |
| ANNA-III | Sensory N, SMN, ataxia, PEM | SCLC, adenocarcinoma of lung, esophagus |
| CRMP-5 (anti-CV-2) | Dementia, SMN, vision loss, chorea | SCLC, thymoma |
| PCA-1 (anti-Yo) | Cerebellar ataxia, SMN | Ovary, breast |
| PCA-2 | PEM, ataxia, autonomic and motor N | SCLC |
| Amphiphysin | Stiff person syndrome, sensory N | SCLC, breast |
| P/Q-type calcium channel | LEMS | SCLC |
| N-type calcium channel | LEMS, SMN | SCLC, breast, ovary |
| Ganglionic AChR | Autonomic N, GI dysmotility, PN hyperexcitability | SCLC, thymus |
| Voltage-gated potassium channel | PN hyperexcitability, Isaacs syndrome, Morvan syndrome | Thymus, lung |

*AChR*, Acetylcholine receptor; *ANNA*, antineuronal nuclear antibody; *CRMP-5*, collapsin response-mediator protein-5; *LEMS*, Lambert-Eaton myasthenic syndrome; *MISP*, malignant inflammatory sensory polyganglionopathy; *N*, neuropathy; *PCA-1*, type 1 Purkinje cell cytoplasmic antibody; *PCA-2*, type 2 Purkinje cell cytoplasmic antibody; *PEM*, paraneoplastic encephalomyelitis; *PN hyperexcitability*, peripheral nerve hyperexcitability; *SCLC*, small-cell lung carcinoma; *SMN*, sensorimotor neuropathy.

after the first two letters of the name of the patient in whom Hu antibody was first discovered). This is associated with subacute sensory neuronopathy, autonomic neuropathy, and limbic encephalomyelitis. SCLC is found in more than 80% of ANNA-I seropositive patients (Lucchinetti et al., 1998). These polyclonal IgG autoantibodies are directed against 35- to 40-kDa proteins that belong to the Hu-family of RNA-binding proteins expressed in nuclei of neurons and malignant cells. The type 2 antineuronal nuclear antibody (ANNA-II, or anti-Ri) was originally described in women with opsoclonus/myoclonus associated with breast cancer, but it may also be seen in men with peripheral neuropathy in association with lung cancer. ANNA-III is highly associated with SCLC or adenocarcinoma of the lung in patients with sensorimotor neuropathies, cerebellar ataxia, and encephalomyelitis.

Three IgG autoantibodies related to lung cancer are directed against *neuronal cytoplasmic antigens*. These are amphiphysin antibody, type 2 Purkinje cell cytoplasmic antibody (PAC-2), and the collapsin response-mediator protein-5 (CRMP-5) antibody. CRMP-5 IgG (or anti-CV-2) antibodies are associated with SCLC and (rarely) thymoma and occur in patients with multifocal neurological signs that include sensory or sensorimotor neuropathies, chorea, optic neuropathy, and disturbance of smell and taste (Yu et al., 2001). Amphiphysin antibody is associated with breast carcinoma and stiff person syndrome.

Autoantibodies directed against *neuronal surface ion-channel antibodies* include P/Q and N-type calcium channel antibodies, ganglionic acetylcholine receptor, and voltage-gated potassium channel antibodies. P/Q-type calcium channel antibodies are present in more than 90% of patients with Lambert-Eaton syndrome (LES). N-type calcium channel antibodies are markers for lung, breast, or ovarian cancers and are found in patients with various neurological manifestations, including LES and peripheral neuropathy. Ganglionic acetylcholine receptor antibodies are found in patients with both idiopathic and paraneoplastic types of autonomic neuropathy (Vernino et al., 2000). Voltage-gated potassium channel antibodies are detected in patients with autoimmune disorders of peripheral nerve hyperexcitability. These include Isaacs syndrome, Morvan syndrome, and cramp-fasciculation syndrome (Sawlani and Katirji, 2017). These rare disorders can be seen in association with thymoma, lung cancer, and Hodgkin lymphoma (Hart et al., 2002).

When a paraneoplastic neuropathy is suspected in relation to cancers, including lung cancer, screening for an entire panel of autoantibodies that includes ANNA-I, CRMP-5, amphiphysin, PCA-2, ANNA-type 2, and ANNA-type 3, and calcium channel antibodies provides an even greater diagnostic yield. However, paraneoplastic autoantibody testing may result in a large proportion of false positives, particularly in patients with clinical presentations that are not considered paraneoplastic in origin (Ebright et al., 2018). Panels that are targeted to specific clinical presentations are likely more useful.

In *paraneoplastic neuromuscular disorders*, sensory or autonomic ganglia, peripheral nerves, nerve terminals, neuromuscular junctions, and muscle may be affected, causing diverse clinical syndromes. Peripheral neuropathies associated with carcinoma may be classified according to the distribution of involvement into the following clinical types: (1) paraneoplastic sensory neuronopathy, (2) autonomic neuropathy, (3) sensorimotor polyneuropathy (either axonal or demyelinating types), and (4) mononeuritis multiplex. Any neuropathy, especially a sensory or autonomic neuropathy of subacute onset occurring in at-risk individuals such as smokers, should raise suspicion of a paraneoplastic disorder.

***Paraneoplastic sensory neuronopathy (malignant inflammatory sensory polyganglionopathy).*** The terms subacute sensory neuronopathy, carcinomatous sensory neuropathy, paraneoplastic sensory neuropathy, paraneoplastic sensory ganglionopathy, and malignant inflammatory sensory polyganglioneuropathy are synonyms to describe the distinct progressive, severe sensory neuropathy associated with cancer. Although the sensory ganglion cell is the primary site of injury, other neurons including autonomic ganglia and CNS nerve cells are often involved as well (Hlubocky and Smith, 2014). The presence of an autoantibody directed against a nuclear protein that is shared by neuronal nuclei and tumors, and the intense inflammatory response found in the affected dorsal root ganglia, support an immune-mediated mechanism.

**Clinical features.** Patients are middle-aged or older, and many are heavy smokers. Women are affected twice as often as men in the United States, in contrast to a European study and to the overall male predominance of SCLC (Graus et al., 2001). The most common underlying neoplasm is SCLC (≈90%), followed in decreasing order of frequency by breast carcinoma, ovarian cancer, and lymphoma. In 9 of 10 cases, neurological symptoms are the presenting features and precede the discovery of the tumor by several months. The median interval from onset of neuropathic symptoms to diagnosis of the underlying neoplasm is 5 months. Symptoms may develop within days in a fulminant fashion or progress more gradually over months. Numbness, painful paresthesia, and lancinating pain often begin in one limb and progress to involve all four limbs. Upper limbs are usually involved first or almost invariably involved with the progression of the disease. Occasionally the trunk, face, and scalp are affected in somatotopic regions highly suggestive of neuronopathies. There is global loss of all sensory modalities, with a striking loss of proprioception and inability to localize the limb in space, resulting in sensory ataxia and pseudoathetosis of the upper extremities. Tendon reflexes are globally reduced or absent. Although muscle strength is preserved or only mildly decreased, patients are often severely disabled and unable to walk because of their sensory deficits.

About half of affected patients have symptoms and signs reflecting more widespread involvement of the central and PNS including paraneoplastic encephalomyelitis, cerebellar degeneration, and autonomic neuronopathy, as evidenced by involvement of the myenteric plexus neurons, autonomic ganglia, spinal cord, brainstem, cerebellum, and limbic cortex. These patients display varying degrees of gastrointestinal dysmotility, autonomic dysfunction, myelopathy, cerebellar signs, brainstem findings, and subacute dementia.

**Laboratory and diagnostic studies.** The hallmark of paraneoplastic sensory neuronopathy is the absence of, or marked reduction in, SNAPs. Motor conduction studies are normal with relatively preserved amplitudes of CMAPs, though the motor conduction velocities may be mildly reduced. Needle EMG may demonstrate minor neurogenic changes. The CSF is frequently abnormal with a mild pleocytosis, elevated protein, and occasionally oligoclonal bands. The sural nerve frequently shows a combined loss of myelinated and unmyelinated fibers, axonal degeneration, and minimal axonal regeneration, sometimes with mononuclear inflammatory cells around epineurial vessels. The principal neuropathological features include degeneration of dorsal root ganglion cells with intense mononuclear cell inflammation, subsequent loss of sensory axons, and degeneration of the posterior roots, peripheral sensory nerves, and the posterior columns of the spinal cord. Many patients have pathological evidence of a more generalized encephalomyelitis characterized by inflammatory infiltrates and neuronal loss in hippocampus, brainstem, and spinal cord.

About 90% of patients with sensory neuronopathy associated with SCLC have significantly elevated titers of ANNA-I (Hu) antibodies by immunohistochemistry or Western blot analysis. Although low titers have been found in 20%–40% of patients with SCLC without neurological disease, only about 0.1% of patients with SCLC have anti-Hu paraneoplastic syndrome. Other associated tumors include breast cancer, ovarian cancer, sarcoma, and Hodgkin lymphoma. Anti-Hu antibody discovery has a specificity of 99% and sensitivity of 82% for the detection of cancer (Molinuevo et al., 1998). Hence, a positive antibody implies the presence of cancer while negative anti-Hu antibody does not exclude an underlying cancer. Seropositive patients should have chest CT because the tumor may go undetected by chest x-rays. If negative, abdominal and pelvic CT or MRI are indicated. When cancer is not found by conventional radiological procedures, PET has been shown to reveal findings suggestive of cancer in 28% of patients and leads to a diagnosis of cancer in 12% (McKeon et al., 2010).

**Differential diagnosis.** The diagnostic possibilities of acquired sensory neuronopathies include malignant inflammatory sensory polyganglioneuropathy, the ataxic sensory neuronopathy associated with Sjögren syndrome or HIV infection, and idiopathic sensory neuronopathies. These conditions share similar pathological characteristics of an inflammatory ganglionopathy. The toxic sensory neuronopathies caused by high-dose pyridoxine (generally >500 mg/day) or following chemotherapy with cisplatinum should be excluded by history. Although it may be difficult to distinguish patients with malignant inflammatory sensory polyganglioneuropathy from those with other causes of sensory neuronopathy, serological testing for ANNA-I (Hu) antibodies is extremely valuable in the differential diagnosis of ataxic sensory neuronopathies because of its high specificity (99%) and sensitivity (82%) for the detection of cancer (Molinuevo et al., 1998).

In addition, the discovery of prominent dysautonomia or presence of neurological signs suggesting disease outside the dorsal root ganglion (particularly CNS deficits) should prompt a careful search for malignancy, especially SCLC.

**Treatment and prognosis.** The outlook for patients with paraneoplastic sensory neuronopathy is poor (Vedeler et al., 2006). Early diagnosis and prompt treatment of the underlying neoplasm provide the best chance to stabilize the condition. More often the neuronopathy pursues a relentless independent course despite treatment of the underlying tumor. In the absence of a detectable tumor, antitumor treatment may be considered in patients with anti-Hu antibodies, age greater than 50 years, and with a history of smoking. Treatment with plasmapheresis, IVIG, and immunosuppressive agents has had disappointing results. Nevertheless, minor modifications of the clinical course have been observed in a few patients receiving immunomodulatory therapy (Graus et al., 2001). Symptomatic treatment is directed at neuropathic pain and accompanying dysautonomic symptoms such as orthostatic hypotension.

***Paraneoplastic autonomic neuropathy.*** Subacute panautonomic failure may be associated with malignancies, most commonly SCLC. Most patients have focal or generalized gastrointestinal dysmotility presenting with abdominal pain, nausea, vomiting, and severe constipation, with subtle or no sensory deficits. High titers of ganglionic acetylcholine receptor or ANNA-I (Hu) antibodies may be found in some patients with cancer. Although high serum titers of ganglionic acetylcholine receptor antibody may be seen in 14%–30% of patients with cancer, this antibody is found in patients with autoimmune and paraneoplastic autonomic neuropathy and is generally not a marker of malignancy (Li et al., 2015; McKeon et al., 2009; Vernino et al., 2000).

***Sensorimotor polyneuropathy.*** It is far more common for cancer patients to have distal symmetrical sensorimotor polyneuropathy than sensory neuronopathy. Clinically, these length-dependent neuropathies are often of slow onset, progress gradually, and are indistinguishable from distal axonal neuropathies in individuals without malignancy. The neoplasms reported in association with this nondescript polyneuropathy, in decreasing order of frequency, originate in lung, stomach, breast, colon, pancreas, and testis. Whether these neuropathies are truly paraneoplastic remains to be proven.

Anti-CRMP5/CV2 (collapsin response mediator protein) antibodies also occur with paraneoplastic peripheral neuropathies (Antoine et al., 2001). These patients usually have more motor involvement, less frequent upper limb involvement, and frequent cerebellar ataxia. Anti-CRMP5/CV2 antibodies are usually associated with SCLC, neuroendocrine tumors, and thymoma.

Acute and chronic inflammatory demyelinating polyradiculoneuropathies have occasionally been linked to underlying malignancies. GBS has been rarely reported in patients with Hodgkin lymphoma. CIDP may occur in association with hematological malignancies, particularly non-Hodgkin lymphoma and melanoma (Rajabally and Attarian, 2018). Molecular mimicry of common antigens shared by both melanoma and Schwann cells may explain the increased association of CIDP with melanoma. CIDP is often diagnosed before the malignancy. Atypical clinical features such as ataxia, cranial/respiratory/autonomic involvement, abdominal pain, diarrhea, constipation, poor appetite, or weight loss should raise the suspicion of an underlying malignancy. It is important to recognize these acquired acute or chronic immune-mediated polyradiculoneuropathies in the clinical setting of malignancies since both respond to immunomodulatory therapies.

***Mononeuritis multiplex.*** Paraneoplastic vasculitis is recognized to occur as a remote effect of cancer and frequently presents as cutaneous vasculitis in hairy cell leukemia and lymphoma. Peripheral nerve vasculitis is a rare complication of Hodgkin and non-Hodgkin lymphoma; SCLC; adenocarcinoma of the lung, prostate, endometrium; and renal cell cancer. Patients present with multiple mononeuropathy or painful asymmetrical sensorimotor neuropathy that precedes the discovery of tumor in most. The association of vasculitis with SCLC and seropositive ANNA-I autoantibodies supports a paraneoplastic origin. Two-thirds of patients have responded to either chemotherapy of the underlying malignancy or cyclophosphamide with or without corticosteroids (Oh, 1997).

### Lymphoma, Neurolymphomatosis, Leukemia, and Polycythemia Vera

Neurological complications of lymphoma result from (1) direct involvement of the leptomeninges, spinal cord, or brain; (2) compression of the spinal cord or nerve roots by epidural masses; (3) bacterial, fungal, and viral infections; (4) complications of treatment (e.g., chemotherapy, radiation, bone marrow transplantation); and (5) remote effects. Spinal cord compression is the most frequent complication, followed by VZV infection and toxic neuropathies related to chemotherapy (Kelly and Karcher, 2005). Peripheral neuropathy unrelated to chemotherapy is found in approximately 5% of patients with lymphoma.

*Neurolymphomatosis* is a rare condition with diffuse infiltration of peripheral and cranial nerves, plexus, or nerve roots by neurotropic neoplastic cells in a patient with a hematological malignancy. Approximately 90% of patients have non-Hodgkin lymphoma, while the remainder of patients carry a diagnosis of acute leukemia. Patients present in several ways, depending on the site of PNS involvement, as ascending paralysis mimicking GBS, progressive polyradiculoneuropathy, cauda equina syndrome, distal sensorimotor polyneuropathy, or multiple mononeuropathy. Peripheral nerves are affected most commonly (60%), followed by spinal nerve roots in 48%, cranial nerves in 46%, and plexus in 40%. Over half of patients have involvement of more than one of these regions of the PNS (Grisariu et al., 2010). The diagnosis is confirmed by positive CSF cytology or lymphomatous infiltration of nerves as seen by nerve biopsy or autopsy. Neurolymphomatosis responds poorly to systemic chemotherapy, because the nerve–blood barrier limits the access of cytotoxic drugs (Odabasi et al., 2001). Median survival is 10 months (Grisariu et al., 2010).

*Intravascular lymphomatosis*, or *angiotropic large-cell lymphoma*, is characterized by the proliferation of malignant lymphocytic cells within small blood vessels of the brain, spinal cord, peripheral nerves, and skin. Neurological manifestations include multifocal strokes, myelopathy with or without cauda equina lesions, and polyradiculoneuropathies. Intravascular lymphoma may be confirmed by biopsy of involved tissues such as skin, muscle, or peripheral nerves. A significantly raised serum lactate dehydrogenase (LDH) and sedimentation rate is seen in over two-thirds of patients (Wong et al., 2006). If untreated, the disease is rapidly fatal. Survival has been reported after chemotherapy (Oei et al., 2002).

Acute and chronic inflammatory demyelinating polyradiculopathies have been described in association with Hodgkin and non-Hodgkin lymphoma. About 8% of patients with monoclonal gammopathy have a low-grade lymphoma or lymphocytic leukemia and may develop a distal demyelinating neuropathy in association with IgM paraproteinemia.

Lymphoproliferative disorders are claimed to be overrepresented in patients with motor neuron disease. This association was initially restricted to lower motor neuron syndromes and named *subacute motor neuronopathy*, occurring as a remote effect of lymphoma. Only a few patients with pure lower motor neuron syndromes have improved following treatment of the concurrent lymphoproliferative disorder.

Neurological complications of chronic lymphocytic leukemia develop in the advanced stages of the disease. These include herpes zoster infection, followed by opportunistic infections and treatment-related complications. Peripheral nerve involvement is rare (<1%) and consists of leukemic nerve infiltrations and immune-mediated neuropathies.

Neurological complications of acute leukemias stem from hemorrhage into the brain or nerve trunks; leukemic infiltration of the brain, leptomeninges, cranial nerves, spinal roots, and peripheral nerves; CNS infections; or chemotherapy-related neurotoxicity.

Mild distal sensory neuropathy is a rare complication of polycythemia vera. Positive sensory complaints such as pruritus, paresthesias, and burning feet are common. Polycythemia vera-associated pruritus, typically precipitated by contact with water, may be an agonizing aspect of the disease. Selective serotonin reuptake inhibitors such as paroxetine or fluoxetine have been beneficial in alleviating pruritus.

### Neuropathies Related to Bone Marrow Transplantation

Peripheral neuropathy is an uncommon complication of bone marrow transplantation. In a prospective study of 115 patients with leukemia undergoing allogeneic bone marrow transplantation, 4% developed neuropathy in the first 3 months after transplantation. A number of potential neuropathic complications may occur in the post-transplant period, including neurotoxicity of drugs used in the conditioning regimen and critical illness neuropathy. Immune-mediated polyradiculoneuropathies have all been described in association with chronic graft-versus-host disease (Openshaw, 1997). The observed predominantly motor polyradiculoneuropathy meets clinical and laboratory criteria for CIDP. Patients improve after immunomodulatory therapy consisting of IVIG, plasma exchange, or immunosuppressant therapy. Acute inflammatory demyelinating polyradiculoneuropathy or GBS has also been reported in patients after allogeneic and autologous bone marrow transplantation (Wen et al., 1997). IVIG and plasmapheresis are considered effective treatments. Skin sclerosis and nodular thickening associated with chronic graft-versus-host disease may also lead to single or multiple sensory mononeuropathies such as the saphenous or antebrachial nerves (Al-Shekhlee and Katirji, 2001).

## Peripheral Nerve Vasculitis

The vasculitides represent a clinicopathological spectrum of disorders characterized by inflammation and destruction of the walls of blood vessels of different calibers, leading to luminal occlusion and ischemia or hemorrhage in the affected organ systems (Burns et al., 2007). Vasculitis can be observed in two clinical settings: primary vasculitis without known underlying cause, or secondary vasculitis occurring in the setting of infectious, malignant, or metabolic diseases or resulting from drug exposure (Collins, 2012). PNS involvement is a common complication of systemic vasculitis (50%–80%), especially in polyarteritis nodosa and small-vessel vasculitides because the small- and medium-sized vessels affected in these types of vasculitides correspond to the size of the vasa nervorum (Langford, 2003). The types of vasculitides that may affect the PNS are listed in Box 106.15. Systemic necrotizing vasculitis occurs in a diverse group of diseases affecting multiple organ systems, including the PNS and CNS. On the other hand, peripheral neuropathy may be the only manifestation of a more indolent condition—nonsystemic vasculitic neuropathy.

*Polyarteritis nodosa*, by far the most common vasculitis in this group, is characterized by necrotizing inflammation of medium-sized or small arteries affecting the kidneys, skeletal muscle, gastrointestinal

**BOX 106.15 Classification of Vasculitides Affecting the Peripheral Nervous System**

Primary systemic vasculitis:
- Predominantly large-vessel vasculitis
  - Giant cell arteritis
- Predominantly medium-vessel vasculitis
  - Polyarteritis nodosa
- Predominantly small-vessel vasculitis
  - Microscopic polyangiitis
  - Eosinophilic granulomatosis with polyangiitis (Churg-Strauss syndrome)
  - Granulomatosis with polyangiitis (formerly Wegener granulomatosis)
  - Essential mixed cryoglobulinaemia (non-hepatitis C virus [HCV])
  - Immunoglobulin A (IgA) vasculitis (Henoch-Schönlein purpura)

Vasculitis associated with systemic disease:
- Connective tissue diseases
  - Rheumatoid vasculitis
  - Systemic lupus erythematosus
  - Sjögren syndrome
  - Systemic sclerosis
  - Mixed connective tissue disease
- Infections (hepatitis B, hepatitis C, HIV, cytomegalovirus, human T cell-lymphotropic virus I)
- Malignancy

Nonsystemic vasculitis neuropathy

tract, skin, PNS, and occasionally CNS. Peripheral nerve involvement occurs in 50%–75% of patients. Hepatitis B surface antigen is found in one-third of cases. *Churg-Strauss syndrome* typically presents with asthma, sinusitis, eosinophilia, and systemic vasculitis of small and medium-sized vessels. The frequency of peripheral nerve involvement is similar to that seen in polyarteritis nodosa (Hattori et al., 1999). *Granulomatosis with polyangiitis (formerly Wegener granulomatosis)* affects the upper and lower respiratory tract and is accompanied by glomerulonephritis and necrotizing vasculitis. The PNS is involved in 10%–20% of cases. Cranial nerve involvement and external ophthalmoplegia occur in 11% of patients as a result of granulomatous infiltration of the orbit or cavernous sinus.

When vasculitis develops in association with a well-defined connective tissue disorder, the clinical and pathological features resemble polyarteritis nodosa. Among the connective tissue disorders, *rheumatoid vasculitis* is by far the most common cause of vasculitic neuropathy. Approximately 15%–30% of patients cannot be categorized and are classified as having *microscopic polyangiitis*. In the hypersensitivity vasculitides, cutaneous manifestations dominate the clinical picture, although peripheral nerves may be involved. Peripheral nerve lesions complicate giant-cell arteritis in 14% of cases. More than 10% of patients with vasculitic neuropathy present in the setting of malignancies, most commonly myeloproliferative or lymphoproliferative disorders, and infections including HIV and hepatitis B and C virus.

Hepatitis B and hepatitis C are the most common viruses associated with systemic vasculitis, usually in the context of polyarteritis nodosa and mixed cryoglobulinemia, respectively. Polyarteritis nodosa predominantly affects medium-size vessels and mixed cryoglobulinemia is more selective toward small vessels. Multiorgan involvement is common in both disorders, with gastrointestinal, renal, and cutaneous involvement being almost always present in hepatitis B- associated vasculitis/polyarteritis nodosa while cutaneous manifestations, renal failure, and hypertension are most prominent in hepatitis-C associated vasculitis/mixed cryoglobulinemia syndrome (Collins, 2012; Ferri et al., 2004; Stübgen, 2011).

## Nonsystemic Vasculitic Neuropathy

A restricted necrotizing vasculitis affecting only peripheral nerves and skeletal muscle is the most common cause of vasculitic neuropathy in patients presenting to a neurologist. One-third of patients with biopsy-proven vasculitic neuropathy lack evidence of systemic disease or a definable connective tissue disease. Multiple mononeuropathies are the most common clinical presentation with stepwise sensory-motor deficits following peripheral nerve territories. This is followed by progressive asymmetrical neuropathy or symmetrical distal polyneuropathy (Collins and Hadden, 2017; Davies et al., 1996). Generally the patients have no constitutional symptoms or serological abnormalities because joints, visceral organs, and skin are unaffected. The severity of symptoms and deficits varies considerably. The disease course may be indolent and protracted over years without ever becoming life threatening. The diagnosis depends exclusively on results of nerve and muscle biopsy, though the sedimentation rate and C-reactive protein levels may be increased. The pathological features are identical to those seen in classic polyarteritis nodosa, affecting small and medium-sized arteries in muscle and nerve.

## Pathogenesis

The precise immunological events leading to vessel injury in vasculitis are not well understood. Immune complex deposition within vessel walls and T-cell-dependent, cell-mediated cytotoxic reactions are the two basic immunopathogenic mechanisms causing destruction of vessel walls. Vascular endothelial cells may serve as antigen-presenting cells and have important functions initiating the cell-mediated immune process. Although drugs and certain infectious agents, including HIV-1 and hepatitis B and C viruses, have been implicated as triggers of the immune responses, in most instances a causal agent cannot be identified. Small-vessel vasculitis and pathological features of ischemic nerve injury have been described in peripheral sensory nerves of patients with diabetic and nondiabetic lumbosacral radiculoplexopathies (Dyck et al., 2001).

The final common pathway of vasculitic neuropathy is extensive occlusion of vasa nervorum at the level of epineurial arterioles of 50–300 μm in diameter, leading to nerve ischemia. Nerve ischemia results in axonal degeneration. Because of the random focal nature of vasculitis, axonal degeneration typically shows a pattern of asymmetrical patchy involvement both between and within nerve fascicles *(differential fascicular involvement)*. The ischemia is most pronounced in proximal nerves such as the fibular division of the sciatic nerve at the midthigh or the ulnar nerve at the mid–upper arm in watershed areas between the distributions of major nutrient arteries. The extensive branching and intermixing of nerve fibers may result in a more homogeneous nerve fiber loss in distal sensory nerves. Large myelinated fibers appear to be more susceptible to ischemia than unmyelinated fibers.

## Clinical Features

In systemic vasculitis, multisystem signs are evident together with fever, malaise, weight loss, and hypertension. The majority of patients with PNS involvement present with peripheral neuropathy as the initial manifestation of disease. Initially, acute onset of deep-seated proximal pain in the affected limb is common. Burning pain, sensory loss, and weakness in the distribution of affected nerves develop over several days. However, a more chronic and indolent course with progressive deficits is common. Irrespective of the underlying vasculitic syndrome, the clinical features of vasculitic peripheral neuropathy are similar and depend on the extent, distribution, and temporal progression of ischemia. Three types of peripheral nerve involvement can be distinguished, although considerable overlap occurs between types (Fig. 106.29):

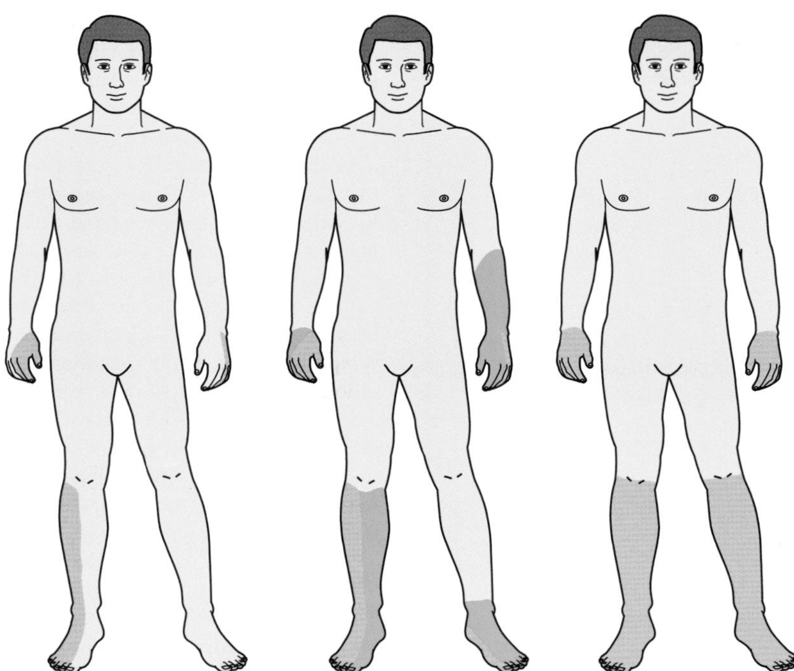

**Fig. 106.29** Clinical Patterns of Neuropathic Involvement in Vasculitic Neuropathy. *Left figure* illustrates multiple mononeuropathies or mononeuritis multiplex. *Middle figure* illustrates asymmetrical sensorimotor polyneuropathy due to overlapping multiple mononeuropathies obscuring individual nerve involvement. *Right figure* illustrates symmetrical sensorimotor polyneuropathy resulting from extensive proximal ischemic nerve lesions. *(Adapted from Mendell, J.R., Barohn, R.J., Bosch, E.P., et al., 1994. Continuum-peripheral neuropathy. Am Acad Neurol 1, 31.)*

1. Multiple mononeuropathies with motor and sensory deficits restricted to the distribution of individual nerves (10%–15%). The most common mononeuropathies affected are the fibular nerve in the lower extremity and the ulnar nerve in the upper extremity (Collins and Periquet-Collins, 2009).
2. Overlapping or confluent multiple mononeuropathies (60%–70%), in which anatomically contiguous nerves will eventually be affected, obscuring individual nerve involvement. This often results in asymmetrical flaccid weakness and pansensory loss in one or more extremities.
3. Subacute symmetrical, distal sensorimotor neuropathy caused by extensive widespread vasculitis (≈30%). This presentation of vasculitic neuropathy can be difficult to distinguish from other types of distal axonopathies and requires a high index of clinical suspicion. A detailed history may indicate that the neuropathy began focally, then followed a course of stepwise progression of deficits before becoming generalized.

## Laboratory Features

The laboratory evaluation of patients with suspected vasculitis should be directed toward identifying an underlying disorder or documenting serological abnormalities that may point to a specific vasculitic syndrome, as well as investigating involvement of other organs. These studies should include sedimentation rate, C-reactive proteins, CBC with total eosinophil count, renal function, urinalysis, hepatic enzymes, serum protein electrophoresis, angiotensin-converting enzyme, rheumatoid factor, antinuclear antibody, extractable nuclear antigens, serum complements, C-reactive proteins, antineutrophilic cytoplasmic antibodies, cryoglobulins, hepatitis B antigen and antibody, and hepatitis C antibody.

Antineutrophilic cytoplasmic antibody (ANCA) is helpful in the diagnosis of Wegener granulomatosis, Churg-Strauss syndrome, and microscopic polyangiitis. Two types of ANCA may be detected with indirect immunofluorescence by using alcohol-fixed neutrophils as substrate, producing two major staining patterns, cytoplasmic (c)-ANCA and perinuclear (p)-ANCA; c-ANCA directed against the neutrophil proteinase 3 (PR3 ANCA) is strongly (75%–90%) associated with Wegener granulomatosis; p-ANCA directed against the neutrophil enzyme myeloperoxidase (MPO-ANCA) is found with variable frequency (5%–50%) in microscopic polyangiitis, Churg-Strauss syndrome, and Wegener granulomatosis.

EDX studies are helpful in establishing the pattern of involvement and documenting axonal nerve damage. Careful study may reveal that what clinically appeared to be a symmetrical polyneuropathy may in fact be an asymmetrical neuropathy resulting from overlapping mononeuropathies. Nerve conduction studies reveal low-amplitude SNAPs and CMAPs in a multifocal distribution with normal or minimally reduced conduction velocities. Partial motor conduction block may be seen transiently with acute nerve infarcts before the completion of wallerian degeneration (Jamieson et al., 1991; Mohamed et al., 1998). EMG demonstrates more widespread denervation than anticipated clinically.

A definite diagnosis of vasculitis depends on confirmation of vascular lesions in nerve or muscle biopsies. Combined muscle and nerve biopsies may also increase the diagnostic yield (Vital et al., 2006). Of the cutaneous nerves suitable for biopsy, the sural nerve or superficial fibular nerve are preferred. A simultaneous peroneus brevis muscle biopsy can be obtained through the same incision when sampling superficial fibular nerve or, alternatively, the gastrocnemius muscle could be sampled through a second incision. However, it is not useful to obtain a vastus lateralis muscle biopsy in patients undergoing sural nerve biopsy at the ankle for the purpose of identifying vasculitis (Bennett et al., 2008). This proximal muscle biopsy may be too distant from the

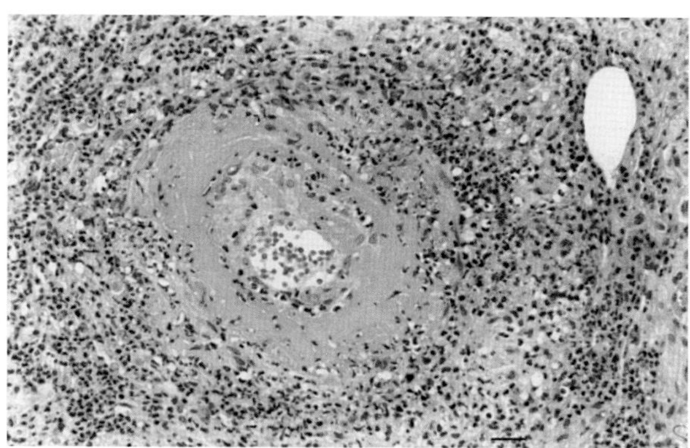

**Fig. 106.30 Sural Nerve Biopsy from Patient with Systemic Vasculitis.** A medium-sized epineurial blood vessel with fibrinoid necrosis of its wall and perivascular and transmural mononuclear cell infiltration is shown. (Hematoxylin and eosin, ×75; bar = 25 μm.)

usually distal pathological process in vasculitic neuropathy. In a cohort of patients with clinically suspected vasculitis, the estimated sensitivity of a definitely positive combined superficial fibular nerve/peroneus brevis muscle biopsy was 60% and increased to 86% if pathological features suggestive of vasculitis were included (Collins et al., 2000).

A definite *pathological diagnosis* of vasculitis requires the presence of vascular wall inflammation accompanied by vascular wall damage necrosis (Fig. 106.30). Cellular infiltrates are composed predominantly of T cells and macrophages. Additional common and supportive findings in vasculitic neuropathies include: (1) vascular deposits of immunoglobulins and complement, including membrane attack complex demonstrated by immunostaining in more than 80% of cases; (2) inflammation of microvessels without vascular damage (termed microvasculitis); and (3) differential fascicular involvement with asymmetric nerve fiber loss or multifocal subfascicular or central fascicular loss of fibers with acute axonal degeneration on cutaneous nerve biopsy. These findings are much less specific when seen in isolation (without vascular wall inflammation and damage) since they may occur in other immune nonvasculitic neuropathies.

### Treatment

In systemic necrotizing vasculitis, disease activity must be suppressed rapidly to limit ongoing organ and nerve damage. Induction therapy is often initiated rapidly with a combination of prednisone and a cytostatic agent (usually cyclophosphamide). Combination therapy was significantly more effective than corticosteroid monotherapy in inducing sustained improvement at 6 months and reducing disability. Combination immunosuppressive therapy results in an 80%–90% remission rate in Wegener granulomatosis and systemic necrotizing vasculitis. Treatment is started with daily prednisone (1 mg/kg/day) together with monthly IV cyclophosphamide at 0.75 g/m$^2$ body surface area per month for 6 months, adjusted monthly upward to 1 g/m$^2$ or downward to 0.5 g/m$^2$ on the basis of the patient's leukocyte count 2 weeks after the infusion. The dose of cyclophosphamide should be adjusted to lower the total lymphocyte count to about 750/μL, while maintaining the total leukocyte count above 3000/μL and the total neutrophil count above 1500/μL. Oral cyclophosphamide at 2 mg/kg of body weight per day may be a substitute of the intravenous form, but carries more side effects. In fulminant cases, corticosteroids may also be initiated by giving IV methylprednisolone (500–1000 mg) daily for 3–5 days followed by oral prednisone. Rituximab, at a dose of 375 mg/m$^2$ body surface area/week for 4 weeks, may be used instead of cyclophosphamide for induction therapy and is shown to be as effective for induction of remission in the ANCA-associated vasculitides (Jones et al., 2010; Stone et al., 2010). The role of plasmapheresis in the management of severe vasculitis remains controversial but may provide additional benefit in patients with life-threatening disease (Allen and Bressler, 1997). In patients with nonlife-threatening mild systemic vasculitis, prednisone given together with methotrexate (20–25 mg/week) is effective. High-dose prednisone is often adequate in patients with nonsystemic vasculitic neuropathy. The role of drugs such as mycophenolate mofetil or leflunomide in the treatment of vasculitis remains less known. Similarly, the beneficial effects of IVIG have not been proven by randomized control trials.

Cyclophosphamide is associated with substantial toxicity including bone marrow suppression, life-threatening infections, hemorrhagic cystitis, infertility, myeloproliferative disease, and bladder cancer. This is more common when using the oral form. From the onset of treatment, CBCs should be monitored frequently. Liberal fluid intake and frequent voiding may lessen the risk of hemorrhagic cystitis. Urine should be monitored for the presence of microscopic hematuria.

Once clinical remission is achieved, prednisone can be tapered over a period of 4–6 weeks to a dosage of 1 mg/kg every other day. Patients are kept on both drugs until significant improvement occurs, at which time prednisone is gradually tapered further. Cyclophosphamide, azathioprine, or methotrexate are useful in maintaining remission and should be maintained for 1 year after the disappearance of all traces of disease activity. Physical and occupational therapy is indicated to optimize activities of daily living.

Meaningful recovery has been reported in 60% of patients at 6 months and 86% at 1 year. Long-term treatment results may be complicated by chronic sequelae from organ damage, disease relapses, and medication side effects.

Other neuropathies associated with system disorders, including neuropathy in connective tissue diseases, rheumatoid arthritis, SLE, systemic sclerosis, Sjögren syndrome, trigeminal sensory neuropathy in connective tissue disorders, and neuropathy in sarcoidosis are discussed in the online version of this chapter, available at http://www.experconsult.com. 

## Alcoholic Neuropathy and Nutritional Deficiencies

### Alcoholic Neuropathy

Alcoholic neuropathy (also see Chapter 84) is one of the most common peripheral neuropathies seen in general practice. Depending on the diagnostic criteria used, its frequency varies from 12.5% to 48.6% in chronic alcoholism. Covert alcoholism may only be uncovered by a focused history provided by family members. A close association between alcoholic neuropathy and nutritional deficiency is well established. The neuropathic picture of chronic alcoholism is essentially indistinguishable from thiamine deficiency.

***Clinical features.*** The symptoms of alcoholic neuropathy begin insidiously and progress slowly. Muscle weakness begins distally and spreads to more proximal muscles. Gait difficulty, weakness, and muscle cramps are common. Sensory loss and burning paresthesias are frequent. Hyperpathia and dysesthesias are troublesome in many patients. The legs are always more affected than the arms. Distal muscle wasting, loss of tendon reflexes, and sensory loss of all modalities in a stocking-glove distribution are common. In advanced cases, sensory ataxia caused by loss of joint position sense may coexist with alcoholic cerebellar ataxia. Autonomic dysfunction due to vagal nerve or sympathetic nerve involvement may be present and is associated with higher mortality rates.

EDX studies show an axonal sensorimotor polyneuropathy. Low-amplitude or absent CMAPs or SNAPs are common, particularly in the legs. Needle EMG shows active denervation with chronic reinnervation in distal muscles. Sural nerve biopsy specimens demonstrate loss of nerve fibers of all sizes. Acute axonal degeneration is particularly common in patients after binge drinking, whereas axonal regeneration is frequently seen in chronic alcoholism.

***Etiology.*** Deficiency of thiamine and other B vitamins, caused by inadequate dietary intake, impaired absorption, and greater demand for thiamine to catalyze the metabolism of the alcohol, is considered the major cause of polyneuropathy in alcoholic patients. It is likely that in at least a subgroup of patients, the direct toxic effect of alcohol is responsible for the neuropathy (Koike and Sobue, 2006).

***Treatment.*** Abstinence from alcohol, addiction counseling, and a nutritionally balanced diet constitute the principal therapy. In one study, a good prognosis for mild to moderate polyneuropathy after 3–5 years of abstinence is reported. Supplementation with thiamine and other B vitamins is important. In patients with significant gastrointestinal symptoms, parenteral vitamin treatment is initially required. Improvement in the polyneuropathy may be very slow because it requires axonal regeneration. For the management of painful alcoholic neuropathy, see Management of Neuropathic Pain, later.

### Niacin Deficiency (Pellagra Neuropathy)

Niacin (nicotinic acid, vitamin $B_3$), an end-product of tryptophan metabolism, is incorporated into the coenzymes nicotinamide adenine dinucleotide (NAD) and NADPH, and their reduced forms. These coenzymes play important roles in carbohydrate metabolism.

Dietary deficiency of niacin is rare in developed countries but is seen in populations dependent on corn (maize) as the main source of carbohydrate because corn contains little niacin or tryptophan. Nonendemic pellagra rarely occurs in patients with alcoholism or malabsorption. Excessive conversion of tryptophan to serotonin in carcinoid syndrome also results in niacin deficiency and pellagra. Deficiency of vitamin $B_6$ and diets rich in neutral amino acids that interfere with tryptophan metabolism may also cause niacin deficiency. In Hartnup disease, in which tryptophan transport is impaired and requirement for dietary niacin is increased, a pellagra-like illness can also develop. Oral nicotinic acid (50–250 mg/day) is sufficient to treat most symptomatic patients. However, the response to treatment may be incomplete.

Deficiency of niacin leads to pellagra, which affects the gastrointestinal tract, skin, and nervous system, resulting in the triad of dermatitis, diarrhea, and dementia (the *3Ds*). A distal sensorimotor polyneuropathy develops in 40%–56% of patients with pellagra; if diarrhea and skin changes are absent, it is clinically indistinguishable from thiamine-deficiency neuropathy.

### Pyridoxine (Vitamin $B_6$) Deficiency

Vitamin $B_6$ is required for cellular functions and growth. Niacin, folate, and carnitine require vitamin $B_6$ for their metabolism. Humans and other mammals cannot synthesize vitamin $B_6$, thus requiring it from exogenous sources. The regular diet of most adults is adequate for the daily requirement of 1.5–2 mg of vitamin $B_6$. Isolated pyridoxine deficiency, however, may occur during treatment with isoniazid (INH), hydralazine, or (rarely) penicillamine. These drugs structurally resemble vitamin $B_6$ and interfere with pyridoxine coenzyme activity. Pregnant and lactating women and elderly individuals are at a greater risk of developing vitamin $B_6$ deficiency. It may also occur in chronic alcoholism, celiac disease (CD), and renal insufficiency with dialysis. The deficiency of vitamin $B_6$ can be detected by direct assay. Vitamin $B_6$-deficient peripheral polyneuropathy is characterized by distal sensory and motor deficits of insidious onset. Up to 50% of slow inactivators of INH may develop neuropathy that causes axonal degeneration of both myelinated and unmyelinated fibers. When using INH, supplementary pyridoxine (100 mg/day) is recommended. Paradoxically, high-dose (≥500 mg/day) pyridoxine may cause a predominantly sensory polyneuropathy (see Toxic Neuropathies, later).

### Folate Deficiency

Folate functions as a coenzyme or co-substrate and is involved in the metabolism of nucleic and amino acids. Its deficiency rarely exists in the pure state and is usually associated with other deficiencies. Folate deficiency is seen in alcoholism (especially with hard liquor), small-bowel diseases, "blind-loop" syndrome, partial gastrectomy, atrophic gastritis, antacid therapy, and gastric acid neutralization. Increased folate requirements are also seen in pregnant and lactating women and in hemolytic anemia. Drugs such as methotrexate that inhibit dihydrofolate reductase act as folate antagonists. Folate deficiency may cause an axonal sensory polyneuropathy characterized clinically by loss of joint position and vibratory sense and absent tendon reflexes. In addition, there may be evidence of spinal cord involvement, with spasticity of the legs and extensor plantar responses. The neuropathy of folate deficiency is, in general, similar to that of cobalamin deficiency but of a milder degree. In severe cases, encephalopathic symptoms may predominate. Macrocytic anemia is an important clue to either folate or vitamin $B_{12}$ deficiency. Patients with clinically significant folate deficiency may also have elevated plasma homocysteine levels. Coexisting vitamin $B_{12}$ deficiency must be excluded because, in such cases, folate therapy without cobalamin replacement may exacerbate neurological manifestations. Patients have been reported with neurological disease, indistinguishable from subacute combined degeneration, who rapidly responded to folate replacement.

### Vitamin $B_{12}$ Deficiency: Subacute Combined Degeneration

Cobalamin (vitamin $B_{12}$) and folate are essential vitamins necessary for effective DNA synthesis. Impaired DNA synthesis could interfere with oligodendrocyte growth and myelin formation. Animal products (meat, poultry, fish, and dairy products) are the primary dietary source of cobalamin. The average Western diet provides an excess of the vitamin (daily requirement 3–9 μg), which is stored in the liver. Excessive intake of vitamin $B_{12}$ has not been associated with any adverse effect. Within the acid environment of the stomach, cobalamin is released from dietary proteins. Free cobalamin initially binds to glycoproteins known as *R-binders*, which are secreted by salivary glands and gastric mucosa. In the duodenum, the cobalamin-R-binder complex is degraded by pancreatic enzymes, and the released cobalamin then binds avidly to intrinsic factor, a 60-kD glycoprotein produced by gastric parietal cells. The vitamin $B_{12}$–intrinsic factor complex is absorbed by means of binding to intrinsic factor receptors in the terminal ileum. A small portion of ingested cobalamin is also absorbed by passive diffusion.

Cobalamin deficiency is common, including in the elderly, and mainly produces pernicious anemia (Stabler, 2013). This results from lack of intrinsic factor caused by progressive autoimmune destruction of parietal cells in the gastric mucosa. Acquired malabsorption of vitamin $B_{12}$ may occur also following gastric and terminal ileal resection and in the setting of a wide range of gastrointestinal disorders. Large stores of cobalamin in the body may delay development of deficiency symptoms for several years after bariatric surgeries. Unusual causes include dietary insufficiency in strict vegetarians (vegans) and intestinal infection with fish tapeworms. The prevalence of cobalamin deficiency is increased in AIDS patients with neurological involvement. A low level of cobalamin may be seen in pregnancy, oral contraceptive and anticonvulsant use, and in multiple myeloma. Intraoperative use or recreational abuse of nitrous oxide, which inactivates cobalamin-dependent enzymes, may cause acute or subacute vitamin $B_{12}$-dependent neurological disease, particularly in patients with marginal cobalamin stores. Prophylactic $B_{12}$ injections given weeks before anesthesia will prevent the neurological deterioration. In a number of elderly patients with cobalamin deficiency, no specific cause is found. Intracellularly, cobalamin is converted into two coenzymes required for the formation of methionine and succinyl-CoA synthesis. Reduced methionine synthesis may be responsible for the neurological manifestations of cobalamin deficiency. Serum cobalamin level may be falsely elevated in renal failure, hepatic insufficiency, and myeloproliferative disorders.

Population surveys estimate that 2% of persons age 60 years and older have undiagnosed pernicious anemia. The disease is especially common in those of Northern European heritage and Blacks. The full-blown clinical picture of vitamin $B_{12}$ deficiency consists of macrocytic anemia, atrophic glossitis, and peripheral and central neurological complications (Toh et al., 1997). These last conditions include peripheral polyneuropathy and optic atrophy, as well as lesions in the posterior and lateral columns of the spinal cord (subacute combined degeneration of the spinal cord) and in the brain. The neurological dysfunction may be the earliest and often the only manifestation of vitamin $B_{12}$ deficiency. The peripheral polyneuropathy manifests with paresthesias and large-fiber modality sensory loss (vibration and proprioception), which may begin or be prominent in the hands. The spinal cord manifestations consist of posterior column damage, particularly of thoracic and cervical cord, which may include a truncal sensory level, and upper motor neuron signs of limb weakness, spasticity, and extensor plantar responses. Cerebral involvement ranges from subtle behavioral changes and forgetfulness to dementia or stupor. Vitamin $B_{12}$ deficiency may also cause autonomic dysfunction and orthostatic hypotension (Beitzke et al., 2002; Skrabal, 2004). An unsteady gait, positive Romberg sign reflecting a sensory ataxia, diffuse hyperreflexia, and absent ankle jerks should raise the suspicion of cobalamin deficiency.

Nerve conduction studies show low-amplitude or absent SNAPs. Conduction velocities are normal. The dorsal columns of the spinal cord may show a decreased signal on T1- and increased signal on T2-weighted MRI images, and temporary contrast enhancement involving the dorsal and lateral column may be present (Locatelli et al., 1999). CNS involvement is also suggested by abnormal visual and somatosensory evoked potentials. Evidence of axonal degeneration is found in sural nerve biopsy specimens. The diagnosis is confirmed by low serum vitamin $B_{12}$ levels (<170 pg/mL) and normal serum folate concentration. Some 30%–40% of patients with neurological symptoms due to vitamin $B_{12}$ deficiency have borderline-low levels (150–200 pg/mL). A megaloblastic anemia with elevated red cell mean corpuscular volume (>94 fL) may be absent in about 30% of patients. Elevated serum methylmalonic acid and homocysteine levels, which are the substrates for cobalamin-dependent enzymes, are helpful when there is diagnostic uncertainty or when the vitamin $B_{12}$ level is below 350 pg/mL. However, in folate and pyridoxine deficiency, hypothyroidism, psoriasis, alcohol abuse, INH use, and leukemia, as well as increased age, the homocysteine level may be elevated. Serum methylmalonic acid level may be raised in hypovolemia, renal insufficiency, or methylmalonyl-coenzyme A mutase deficiency. The two-part Schilling test confirms that vitamin $B_{12}$ deficiency is the result of intestinal malabsorption and is caused by intrinsic factor deficiency, but the test is now rarely performed owing to concerns of radiation exposure and cost. Antibodies to intrinsic factor are found in 70% of patients with pernicious anemia; antiparietal cell antibodies are more sensitive (90%) but lack specificity. A combined antiparietal cell antibody test and serum gastrin level, a marker for hypochlorhydria, may increase the accuracy of diagnosis.

Initial treatment consists of daily intramuscular injections of 1 mg of cyanocobalamin or hydroxycobalamin for the first week, followed by weekly injections of 1 mg until 12 doses have been given. The serum levels of methylmalonic acid and homocysteine will return to normal no later than 2–3 weeks after completion of the course. Maintenance schedules of monthly injections of 100 μg or 1 mg every 3 months have been found satisfactory in preventing relapses (Savage and Lindenbaum, 1995). This treatment corrects the anemia and may reverse the neurological complications completely if given soon after their onset. Major neurological improvement can be expected to occur during the first 3–6 months of therapy. If maintenance therapy is interrupted, neurological symptoms may not occur immediately because of the large stores of vitamin $B_{12}$ in the liver but may reappear as early as 6 months later (Stabler, 2013). Megaloblastic anemia may take several years before it appears. For maintenance therapy, oral administration of large quantities of vitamin $B_{12}$ (1 mg) in compliant patients is also feasible, because 1% of vitamin $B_{12}$ is absorbed without intrinsic factor mediation (Kuzminski et al., 1998). The efficacy of nasal or sublingual cobalamin delivery as well as oral preparations of intrinsic factor remains unproven. The initial severity of neurological deficits, duration of symptoms, and hemoglobin level before treatment correlate with neurological outcome. The inverse correlation between degree of anemia and neurological damage is not understood. If symptoms progress despite adequate therapy and normalization of vitamin $B_{12}$ levels, other conditions such as copper deficiency neuromyelopathy (see Copper Deficiency Myelopathy and Myeloneuropathy, later) should be investigated.

### Vitamin E Deficiency

Significant vitamin E (α-tocopherol) deficiency develops in children and young adults with chronic severe intestinal fat malabsorption, as occurs in cholestatic liver disease, cystic fibrosis, CD, following extensive intestinal resections, and in the inherited disorder of abetalipoproteinemia (see Hereditary Neuropathies, earlier). Rarely, vitamin E deficiency develops in the absence of fat malabsorption (Jackson et al., 1996). Isolated familial vitamin E deficiency is an AR disorder in which mutations in the α-tocopherol transfer protein gene cause failure to incorporate α-tocopherol into very-low-density lipoprotein in the liver. About 25%–50% of affected individuals are compound heterozygotes, which may help explain the clinical variability.

Prolonged vitamin E deficiency of any cause may lead after years to a spinocerebellar syndrome with a large-fiber sensory neuropathy, ataxia, proprioceptive loss, areflexia, ophthalmoplegia, and pigmentary retinopathy that may be indistinguishable from Friedreich ataxia. Myopathy and peripheral nerve disease may predominate in some cases. In adults with chronic cholestasis, it may take 2 years to deplete vitamin E stores and an additional 5–10 years to develop neurological complications.

Vitamin E is an antioxidant and free-radical scavenger, and its deficiency results in a central and peripheral distal axonopathy of large-caliber sensory axons affecting peripheral nerves and the posterior columns of the spinal cord. Lipofuscin-like accumulations are found in the Schmidt-Lanterman clefts of large-diameter myelin sheaths in sural nerve biopsy specimens. Impaired antioxidant protection may account for neurological and retinal lesions in long-standing deficiency. EDX study results show normal motor conduction studies and low-amplitude or absent SNAPs. Evoked potential studies may be abnormal. Vitamin E deficiency is established by low fasting plasma levels of vitamin E (<5 μg/mL). However, in the presence of hyperlipidemia, the vitamin E level may be normal even in the presence of clinical symptoms. Laboratory studies used to confirm fat malabsorption include 72-hour fecal fat determination, vitamin A and D levels, amylase levels, liver function tests, peripheral blood smear to search for acanthocytes (present in Bassen-Kornzweig syndrome), and apolipoprotein B level.

Vitamin E is abundant in many foods including vegetable oils, nuts, fruits, leafy vegetables, and cereals. Its bioavailability is dependent on the fat content of the food. Vitamin E supplementation is indicated regardless of cause in all patients with low serum vitamin E levels. An initial oral supplementation with vitamin E in large doses (1500 IU–6000 IU/day) may result in cessation of further deterioration, neurological improvement, and attainment of a normal ratio of α-tocopherol to total lipids in the serum. In isolated vitamin E deficiency, 400–1200 IU/day is sufficient. If no absorption can be documented after large oral doses of standard vitamin E, a water-soluble form of α-tocopherol is recommended.

### Neuropathy Associated with Malabsorption Syndromes

Malabsorption may occur as a result of a primary gastrointestinal disease or after extensive resection of gastrointestinal tract. Intestinal malabsorption may lead to myopathy or peripheral polyneuropathy. A careful search for occult malabsorption or CD should be part of the routine investigation of all patients with neuromuscular disease of obscure cause, particularly in patients with ataxia and peripheral neuropathy. Gluten-sensitive enteropathy or CD is the prototype of gluten-sensitive disorders and is characterized by malabsorption due to relapsing inflammatory injury to the mucosa of the small intestine after ingestion of wheat gluten in genetically predisposed individuals. The typical symptoms include diarrhea, weight loss, and dermatitis herpetiformis. More than 90% of patients with CD express the human lymphocyte antigen HLA-DQw2 or DQ8. It is a T-cell-mediated disorder and may be associated with other autoimmune conditions such as DM, dermatitis herpetiformis, Sjögren syndrome, rheumatoid arthritis, primary biliary cirrhosis, and thyroid diseases. Patients develop antibodies against gliadin, tissue transaminases, and other intestinal antigens. It is claimed that patients with or without gastrointestinal symptoms may rarely (5%–8%) develop varied neurological complications including a predominantly sensory and mostly mild axonal neuropathy, multiple mononeuropathies, autonomic neuropathy, cerebellar ataxia, myopathy, epilepsy, and encephalopathy (Grossman, 2008; Hadjivassiliou et al., 2006). The issue, however, remains contentious, since antigliadin antibodies are also raised in more than 10% of normal adults or patients with other disorders (e.g., hereditary ataxias), and a gluten-free diet may not result in a satisfactory neurological improvement or a fall in antigliadin antibodies (Gibbons and Freeman, 2005; Rosenberg and Vermeulen, 2005; Serratrice et al., 2004; Wills and Unsworth, 2002).

The cause of PNS involvement is poorly understood. Earlier studies have implicated vitamin deficiencies ($B_{12}$, E, D, folic acid, or pyridoxine). However, vitamin replacement rarely improves neurological deficits. Immunological factors have been proposed in patients without vitamin deficiencies and are supported by the common association of CD with other autoimmune disorders. The diagnosis is facilitated by the determination of more specific serological markers such as antiendomysial and tissue transglutaminase IgA antibodies. Unlike antigliadin antibodies, these antibodies are highly predictive of CD (>90%). Rapid assays for tissue transglutaminase antibodies have been developed (Nemec et al., 2006), and other tests involving antibodies to synthetic gliadin peptide are being developed. The diagnosis is established by small-bowel biopsy or HLA typing. A strict gluten-free diet, which is difficult to maintain, may stabilize the neurological disease but improvement is rare.

Severe sensorimotor or predominantly sensory polyneuropathies with ataxia or burning feet may occur in starvation. Multiple micronutrient deficiencies including thiamine, folate, cobalamin, and sulfur amino acids, in the absence of an apparent malnutrition but with high sugar intake, were thought to be responsible for the outbreak of polyneuropathy, optic neuropathy, hearing loss, and combined system degeneration that occurred in Cuba in 1992 and 1993 as a result of the US embargo.

### Neuropathy Associated with Bariatric Surgery

Bariatric surgery for morbid obesity is becoming increasingly common. Multiple surgical techniques have been employed. Of these, the Roux-en-Y gastric bypass, biliopancreatic diversion, and biliopancreatic diversion with duodenal switch are particularly known to cause deficiencies of vitamins and other micronutrients (Bloomberg et al., 2005). Vomiting, which is a common complication of obesity surgery, places these patients at a greater risk for such deficiencies. If unrecognized, these deficiencies lead to a number of metabolic and neurological complications that include neuropathy, myelopathy, optic neuropathy, and encephalopathy (Juhasz-Pocsine et al., 2007; Koffman et al., 2006). The neuropathy, which takes several forms (sensory-predominant polyneuropathy, mononeuropathy multiplex, and radiculoplexoneuropathy), is seen in about 16% of patients. Rate and absolute amount of weight loss, prolonged gastrointestinal symptoms, low serum albumin and transferrin, postoperative surgical complications, and, most importantly, poor nutritional compliance are considered the main risk factors for the development of neuropathy (Thaisetthawatkul et al., 2004). Except for vitamin $B_{12}$ and copper deficiencies in patients with myelopathy, no specific nutritional deficiency correlates with the neurological complications (Juhasz-Pocsine et al., 2007). If discovered early, the neuropathic symptoms may be reversed by adequate supplementation or reversal of the surgical bypass (Thaisetthawatkul et al., 2010).

### Copper Deficiency Myelopathy and Myeloneuropathy

Many foods are rich in copper, and therefore dietary copper deficiency is rare. After absorption in the stomach and proximal small intestine and passage through liver, about 95% of copper becomes bound to ceruloplasmin. The absorption and bioavailability of copper may be impaired by a number of factors, including excessive zinc ingestion, iron deficiency, and ascorbic acid and antacid intake. Zinc and copper compete in using a common transporter in the intestinal wall, and excessive zinc intake results in the displacement of copper. The most frequent causes of copper deficiency are malabsorption syndromes (e.g., protein-losing gastroenteropathy, CD, and Menkes syndrome), gastrointestinal surgeries (especially bariatric surgery), prolonged parenteral nutrition, and use of copper chelating agents. Ingestion of excess zinc in the form of zinc supplements, denture cream, and coins has also been associated with copper deficiency (Gabreyes et al., 2013; Nations et al., 2008; Rowin and Lewis, 2005). In some patients, no obvious cause can be identified.

Deficiency of copper impairs the function of several important oxidases. Acquired copper deficiency with hypocupremic myelopathy with or without a peripheral polyneuropathy (myeloneuropathy) may mimic combined system degeneration caused by cobalamin deficiency and follows a progressive course (Kumar, 2007). A number of hematological abnormalities may be present: macro-, micro-, and normocytic anemia; sideroblastic anemia; neutropenia; iron-containing plasma cells; vacuolated erythroid cells; megaloblastic changes; myelodysplastic syndrome; and, rarely, thrombocytopenia. These hematological features are present in more than 80% of patients. The neurological manifestations of copper deficiency may precede the hematological abnormalities and are present in 75% of patients (Gabreyes et al., 2013). The neurological, EDX, and imaging characteristics of hypocupremic myeloneuropathy are similar to those of cobalamin deficiency (combined system degeneration) with spastic paraparesis, with or without sensory polyneuropathy as the most common findings. The optic nerves or CNS may occasionally be involved (Prodan et al., 2002). The peripheral polyneuropathy is axonal and is often overshadowed by a severe myelopathy.

Patients suspected of having hypocupremic myeloneuropathy often have cytopenia. They should have their serum copper, zinc, and ceruloplasmin measured. Serum zinc may be elevated even in the absence of excessive zinc ingestion (Gabreyes et al., 2013). In copper deficiency, both serum copper and ceruloplasmin levels fall. In conditions where the level of ceruloplasmin is raised, the copper level will also increase, therefore masking a true copper deficiency. Elevation of serum ceruloplasmin, an acute-phase reactant, occurs in a large number of conditions including infections, inflammatory diseases, oral contraceptive use, pregnancy, renal and hepatic diseases, malignancies, diabetes, and in cigarette smokers. It has been suggested that the red blood cell level of zinc-copper superoxide dismutase is independent of the serum copper level and may serve as the measure of body copper stores.

Treatment consists of elimination of the cause of deficiency and copper supplementation. Identifying sources of excess zinc and its discontinuation is often sufficient to improve the condition. Oral supplementation with copper gluconate, 2 mg/day, is usually sufficient to correct the deficiency, but an equivalent IV dose may be used for 1 week before initiating the continued oral supplementation. Although hematological improvement is usually rapid and complete in more than 90% of patients, only one-fourth of patients showed improvement in their neurological function, while more than two-thirds remained unchanged (Gabreyes et al., 2013).

## Uremic Neuropathy

Peripheral neuropathy develops in 60% of patients with end-stage renal failure who require chronic dialysis. *Uremic polyneuropathy* is inexplicably more common in men than in women. The clinical features are those of a slowly progressive, predominantly sensory polyneuropathy. Severe pain is unusual, but cramps, unpleasant dysesthesias, and restless legs are common symptoms. Neurological signs include distal sensory loss, especially of vibratory sensation, absent reflexes, and symmetrical toe-extensor weakness. On occasion, a rapidly progressive, predominantly motor polyneuropathy mimicking GBS may develop during the initial weeks of dialysis. Some patients have improved by switching from conventional to high-flux hemodialysis, possibly as a result of the enhanced removal of advanced glycosylation products (Bolton et al., 1997).

Chronic renal failure and the commonly associated malnutrition render peripheral nerves (e.g., ulnar nerve at the elbow, fibular nerve at the knee) susceptible to compression neuropathies. *CTS* may develop in more than 20% of patients on hemodialysis. Nerve compression from local edema secondary to the forearm arteriovenous shunts or ischemia from a fistula-induced vascular steal syndrome are likely mechanisms in the early course of dialysis. Patients on long-term hemodialysis may develop CTS because of the deposition of $\beta_2$-microglobulin amyloid deposited in the carpal ligament. *Ischemic monomelic neuropathy* is an acute complication of the placement of a more proximal shunt between the cephalic vein and brachial artery; it usually occurs in diabetic or hypertensive patients with concomitant peripheral vascular disease (Tsao et al., 2014). This neuropathy is characterized by abrupt, painful sensory loss of the affected hand and weakness of the distal median, ulnar, and radial innervated distal muscles. The weakness and sensory loss follow a distal-to-proximal gradient starting at the level of the fistula in the affected upper limb only. The EDX studies reveal an axonal disorder with absent or low-amplitude SNAPs and CMAPs in the affected hand only. Needle EMG shows active denervation and loss of MUAPs in the affected limb in a distal-to-proximal fashion. Prompt surgical closure of the fistula is recommended to avoid permanent neurological deficits.

The diagnosis of uremic polyneuropathy should only be made in the context of chronic end-stage renal failure (creatinine clearance <10 mL/min) of at least several months' duration. Drug toxicity or other systemic diseases such as DM, vasculitis, or amyloidosis that may affect both kidneys and peripheral nerves must first be excluded. CSF protein is often elevated, but rarely beyond 100 mg/dL. Low-amplitude CMAPs and SNAPs with mild generalized slowing of motor and sensory velocities are common, and distal latencies are prolonged. Late responses (H-reflex and F-wave latencies) become abnormally prolonged early in the course of chronic renal failure at a time when motor conduction velocities are still normal. Needle EMG examination shows evidence of active denervation in distal foot muscles. Regular hemodialysis rarely improves impaired conduction velocities in patients, despite clinical improvement. Sural nerve biopsy shows axonal loss of large myelinated fibers and segmental demyelination. Morphometric investigations led to the conclusion that the segmental demyelination is secondary to primary axonal atrophy.

Occasionally, exacerbation of the polyneuropathy occurs in patients with chronic renal failure at the onset of hemodialysis. Acute fluxes of water and solutes may be the cause, and reduction in the intensity of dialysis is usually recommended.

The precise cause of uremic polyneuropathy remains unknown, although a number of potential neurotoxins accumulate in end-stage renal disease (Gallassi et al., 1998). Ethylene oxide used to sterilize dialysis tubing has been proposed as a contributing neurotoxin in patients on hemodialysis.

Severe uremic polyneuropathy has become less common as a result of earlier treatment with dialysis and renal transplantation. This is also related to the earlier initiation of dialysis in uremic patients and improved techniques using more biocompatible dialyzer membranes and high-flux dialyzers. Attention should be given to avoiding drugs such as colchicine or nitrofurantoin, which are potentially neurotoxic and may accumulate in renal insufficiency. Numerous investigations have been conducted to assess the long-term effects of hemodialysis on peripheral nerve function. A consensus has emerged that chronic hemodialysis will stabilize an existing uremic polyneuropathy in most patients. Manipulating the frequency or duration of dialysis may not alter its course. Chronic peritoneal dialysis provides no advantage over hemodialysis. Successful renal transplantation results in significant clinical, EDX, and morphological recovery over a period of 3–12 months. However, renal transplantation may have little effect on the course of the polyneuropathy in diabetic patients with end-stage renal disease.

## Peripheral Neuropathy in Liver Disease

Various peripheral neuropathies may develop as a direct consequence of acute and chronic liver disease. Although many reported series of patients with neuropathy and hepatic cirrhosis have included alcoholics, a neuropathy also occurs among nonalcoholic individuals with hepatic disease. The neuropathic syndromes associated with liver diseases include (1) cryoglobulinemic neuropathy linked to HCV infection, (2) vitamin E deficiency in chronic cholestatic liver disease, and (3) neuropathies associated with end-stage liver disease and primary biliary cirrhosis. Viral hepatitis types A, B, and C have been reported as antecedent infections in the GBS. Isolated cases of CIDP have been described in chronic hepatitis B and as a complication after orthotopic liver transplantation. Hepatitis B antigenemia is found in a third of patients with polyarteritis nodosa and vasculitis.

Although a clinically overt polyneuropathy is uncommon in patients with chronic liver disease, EDX studies are frequently abnormal. The highest frequency of neuropathy by clinical criteria (75%) and confirmed by electrophysiological studies in an even greater percentage (87%) was reported in a cohort of patients who were candidates for liver transplantation for end-stage liver disease (Iani et al., 1999). The polyneuropathy is not disabling and often remains clinically unapparent. Paresthesias in the feet, distal loss of vibratory sensation, and loss of ankle reflexes are the most common findings. EDX abnormalities consist of reduced SNAPs and mild slowing of motor conduction velocities. Histological studies of the sural nerve show evidence of demyelination and remyelination. A high incidence of autonomic dysfunction has been reported in patients with end-stage liver disease by means of formal autonomic testing. The presence of autonomic neuropathy in such patients has been associated with a fivefold increase in mortality over that seen in individuals with normal autonomic function. Early liver transplantation should be considered for patients with autonomic neuropathy.

Patients with primary biliary cirrhosis may develop a sensory polyneuropathy or sensory ganglionopathy. In a few patients with strikingly elevated serum lipid levels and cutaneous xanthomas, xanthomatous infiltration of nerves is found on nerve biopsy. The prevalence of associated autoimmune diseases, most notably Sjögren syndrome, is high in primary biliary cirrhosis, which in turn is linked to predominantly sensory neuropathies. Large-fiber sensory polyneuropathies develop in children and young adults with chronic cholestatic liver disease and secondary vitamin E deficiency.

## Endocrine Disorders Associated with Peripheral Neuropathy

### Hypothyroid Neuropathy

CTS is the most common peripheral nerve complication of hypothyroidism. One-third of patients with hypothyroidism may have clinical evidence of a general polyneuropathy, which is predominantly sensory with pain and paresthesias, muscle pain, distal sensory loss, and incoordination. This may coexist with hypothyroid myopathy and elevated serum CK level. Nerve conduction studies show absent or decreased SNAPs and slow motor conduction velocities. Sural nerve biopsy demonstrates demyelination, remyelination, and increased glycogen and lysosomes in axons and Schwann cell cytoplasm. Thyroid hormone replacement usually improves the polyneuropathy, but the improvement may be partial. Thyroid function studies should be considered in patients presenting with a sensory polyneuropathy.

### Acromegaly

CTS is a well-recognized complication of acromegaly, but a generalized polyneuropathy also may develop independent of concomitant DM. About half of affected patients have distal paresthesias, sensory loss in a stocking-glove distribution, diminished muscle stretch reflexes, and distal muscle weakness. SNAPs are reduced in amplitude, and motor NCVs are slightly reduced. Nerve biopsy shows a reduced number of myelinated and unmyelinated fibers and enlargement of nerve fascicles caused by an increase in endoneurial and subperineurial tissue.

### Hypoglycemic Neuropathy

Primary hypoglycemia due to an insulinoma may cause slowly progressive motor-sensory polyneuropathy with predominant motor features of distal muscle atrophy and weakness, especially of the upper limbs. Painful paresthesias are common, but there are usually no objective signs of sensory loss. The muscle atrophy and weakness (amyotrophy) may precede the onset of clinically apparent hypoglycemic episodes by a few years. EDX studies show evidence of acute denervation and reinnervation. Hypoglycemic neuropathy may assume a greater role among diabetic patients receiving intensive insulin therapy. In fact, an average patient with IDDM has a low plasma glucose level about 10% of the time. Experimental studies suggest that hypoglycemia preferentially causes large-nerve fiber damage (Jamali and Mohseni, 2006).

## Ischemic Monomelic Neuropathy

Ischemia due to acute thromboembolic occlusion of major limb arteries or proximal arteriovenous shunt placement infrequently causes multiple axonal mononeuropathies that develop distally in the ischemic limb (ischemic monomelic neuropathy). Abrupt lightning or burning pains affect the involved extremity. Sensory examination shows a graded impairment of all modalities, particularly those mediated by large-diameter fibers (Tsao et al., 2014). Muscle strength is usually maintained, although distal weakness may often develop in severe cases. Tendon reflexes may be preserved.

EDX studies provide evidence of multiple axonal mononeuropathies in the involved ischemic limb, with a distal-to-proximal pattern. SNAPs and CMAPs are either absent or markedly reduced in amplitude, and motor conduction velocities are slowed. Acute denervation is limited to very distal extremity muscles. Both large and small fibers appear to be affected equally. Surgical endarterectomy or bypass surgery may result in recovery of neurological deficits in a period of several months, even in long-standing ischemic neuropathy. Ischemic monomelic mononeuropathy following shunt placement demands immediate surgical closure of the arteriovenous fistula.

Severe aortoiliac occlusive disease or prolonged use of an intra-aortic balloon pump may occasionally lead to lesions of the proximal sciatic and femoral nerve or the lumbosacral plexus.

## Peripheral Neuropathy in Chronic Obstructive Lung Disease

Approximately 20% of patients with chronic obstructive lung disease may develop a mild distal sensorimotor polyneuropathy that appears to be correlated with severe hypoxemia.

## Critical Illness Polyneuropathy

Acquired weakness in ICU patients is common, tends to be underappreciated, and may be due to a myopathy or polyneuropathy; however, both critical illness neuropathy and myopathy may occur concurrently (Latronico and Bolton, 2011). *Critical illness polyneuropathy* is characterized by acute limb and respiratory weakness after prolonged residence in the ICU (Visser, 2006). Excluding cardiac and pulmonary etiologies, it is a major cause of difficulty in weaning patients from the respirator. It occurs in all ages but is rare in children. Males are affected more than females. Clinical evaluation of muscular weakness acquired in the ICU is difficult because patients are often encephalopathic or sedated, and the examination may be hindered by multiple lines required for intensive support. Most patients have generalized flaccid weakness with distal prominence and depressed tendon reflexes. Muscle wasting is absent in a third of patients. It is rare to see facial weakness or other cranial nerve involvement. Pain or paresthesias are not features of critical illness neuropathy. When prospectively investigated, at least 50% of critically ill patients with sepsis and multiple organ failure who were resident in ICUs for at least 2 weeks have EDX features indicative of an axonal polyneuropathy.

EDX studies are necessary to establish the diagnosis. Nerve conduction studies reveal a distal axonal polyneuropathy with reduced CMAP and, to a lesser extent, SNAP amplitudes in conjunction with fibrillation potentials and decreased MUAPs on needle EMG. CSF is almost always normal. Primary axonal degeneration, more severe distally than proximally, is seen at autopsy.

The polyneuropathy is thought to be a complication of the systemic inflammatory response syndrome that is triggered by sepsis, severe trauma, or burns. The pathophysiology of this syndrome is currently under intense investigation. Severe infections or trauma of any type appear to initiate a series of events that ultimately lead to impaired microcirculation and multiple organ dysfunction. In burn neuropathy, which affects 11% of severe burn patients, it is postulated that occlusion of vasa nervorum or dissemination of neurotoxins (or both) are responsible for the more severe form of critical illness neuropathy (Koualske et al., 2001).

*Critical illness myopathy* is another cause of acquired weakness in residents of ICUs and is difficult to distinguish clinically from its neuropathic counterpart. This complication usually occurs in patients with acute respiratory distress syndrome or severe asthma who have been treated with IV corticosteroids, nondepolarizing neuromuscular blocking agents, or most commonly, both. Plasma CK levels are transiently and marginally elevated. Muscle biopsy may show a necrotizing myopathy with many fibers with loss of thick myosin filaments (Lacomis et al., 1996). The presence of normal sensory conduction studies in the setting of small, short-duration, polyphasic MUAPs on needle EMG helps support a diagnosis of critical illness myopathy. In critical illness myopathy, the muscles become unresponsive to direct electrical stimulation, whereas in critical illness polyneuropathy, this response is largely preserved. The difficulty in differentiating a critical illness myopathy from polyneuropathy was demonstrated in one study in which severe weakness was found in 25% of consecutively admitted ICU patients requiring mechanical ventilation, all of whom demonstrated an axonal neuropathy on EDX testing, as well as myopathic changes unrelated to denervation on muscle biopsy (De Jonghe et al., 2002). Repetitive nerve stimulation studies should be performed to exclude a defect of neuromuscular transmission caused by defective clearance of neuromuscular blocking agents. It is of utmost importance to exclude a preexisting known or unrecognized neuromuscular condition leading to ICU admission before contemplating the diagnoses of critical illness neuropathy and myopathy.

It has been suggested that intensive insulin therapy to maintain a blood glucose level of 80–110 mg/dL in ICU patients reduces the possibility of critical illness neuropathy or myopathy (from 52% to 29%). The role of insulin in reducing inflammation and in decreasing the level of nitric oxide, which leads to the protection of endothelium, has been proposed as the mechanism of insulin effect (Langouche et al., 2005). Adequate aggressive and early treatment of sepsis and septic shock may also reduce the incidence of critical illness neuropathy and myopathy.

The prognosis of critical illness myopathy and neuropathy is directly dependent on the prognosis of the underlying illness. However, those who survive the underlying conditions improve slowly, with the myopathy having a relatively better and more favorable prognosis. Patients recover spontaneously in 3–6 months following discharge from the ICU, but many patients will require intensive rehabilitation, and some degree of persistent functional disability is common.

## TOXIC AND DRUG-INDUCED NEUROPATHIES

Peripheral neuropathy is one of the most common reactions of the nervous system to toxic chemicals. Industrial, environmental, and biological agents as well as heavy metals and pharmaceutical agents are known to cause toxic neuropathies (see Chapter 86). Medications, most notably anticancer drugs, are the leading offenders in clinical practice today. Neurotoxic agents may produce distal axonal degeneration *(axonopathy)*, nerve cell body degeneration *(neuronopathy)*, or primary demyelination *(myelinopathy)* (see Pathological Processes Involving Peripheral Nerves, earlier). For most toxic neuropathies, the biochemical mechanisms underlying the pathogenesis of nerve damage remain poorly understood.

Most toxins produce symmetrical axonal degeneration in a dying-back (length-dependent) pattern beginning in the distal segments of long, large-caliber nerve fibers, eventually spreading proximally with continued exposure. A number of *toxic axonopathies* also affect the CNS, showing evidence of concurrent degeneration of dorsal column projections of sensory neurons and optic nerve axons. Electrophysiological investigations typically disclose an axonal pattern. Central axonal involvement has been linked to incomplete clinical recovery. Agents such as n-hexane and organophosphates cause simultaneous degeneration of peripheral nerve, dorsal column axons, and corticospinal pathways, often resulting in spasticity that may become apparent following recovery from the peripheral axonopathy.

The second type of toxin-induced injury targets nerve cell bodies *(toxic neuronopathy)* such as the dorsal root ganglion cell. Cisplatin, methyl-mercury compounds, high-dose pyridoxine, and doxorubicin are examples of toxins that produce neuronal degeneration. When the neuronal insult leads to apoptosis and cell death, the resulting sensory neuropathy is often severe and irreversible with limited functional recovery.

Primary *toxic demyelinating neuropathy* is a less common neuropathy but occurs with diphtheria, buckthorn toxin, and exposure to perhexiline, amiodarone, or suramin. Slowed NCVs can also be seen in certain forms of hexacarbon neuropathy, as in habitual glue sniffers, as a result of axonal swelling from neurofilament accumulation causing secondary demyelination. In buckthorn intoxication, the neuropathy may closely resemble GBS. Ingestion of the fruit of the buckthorn shrub *(Karwinskia humboldtiana)*, which grows in Mexico, Central America, the southern United States, and Caribbean countries, results in a progressive and ascending flaccid paralysis of the limbs in 3–4 weeks. Both electrophysiological and pathological studies of the peripheral nerves show extensive demyelination. However, the CSF studies are usually normal. Recovery will occur if the amount of ingestion is limited but is usually slow and may take 6–12 months. The responsible toxins are anthracenone compound (T-514) or peroxisomicine A1, T-544, T-496, and T-516, but the exact pathophysiological mechanism responsible for Schwann cell injury remains obscure (Salazar-Leal et al., 2006). Other toxins causing demyelinating neuropathies are discussed later.

To establish a causal link between a putative neurotoxin and neuropathy, two clinical criteria should be met:

1. Exposure can be verified and temporally related to the onset of clinical symptoms. Neuropathic symptoms usually occur concurrently with the exposure or following a variable latency of up to several months. There must be neurological signs and abnormal EDX studies. Because many toxic neuropathies are subclinical, subjective symptoms may or may not occur.
2. Removal from the exposure results in cessation of progression of symptoms and deficits. This is variably followed by improvement, although in certain axonopathies, cessation of exposure may be attended by a worsening of symptoms for up to 2 months (so-called coasting) before worsening ceases.

In addition, the clinician must recognize that certain factors may increase susceptibility to toxic neuropathy. These include preexisting neuropathy (e.g., CMT), simultaneous use of multiple neurotoxic drugs or compounds, and systemic disorders that cause impaired drug metabolism (Chaudhry et al., 2003). Any of these may increase the risk and severity of toxic neuropathy.

A focused history probing for a background of occupational, environmental, or drug exposure is important. Most toxic neuropathies present clinically with length-dependent sensorimotor or purely sensory deficits. Autonomic dysfunction is rarely a prominent feature, though exceptions include acrylamide, cisplatin, and vinca alkaloids. Predominantly motor toxic neuropathy is rare, being limited to dapsone, lead, and organophosphate-induced delayed polyneuropathy. Rarely do typical pathological features such as neurofilamentous axonal swellings in hexacarbon neuropathy, axonal vacuolation in thallium, or lamellar Schwann cell inclusions in amiodarone and perhexiline intoxication allow specific identification of the cause by nerve biopsy. Attention should be paid to the systemic symptoms and a thorough general examination because many toxins cause systemic toxicity as well. The most important steps in treatment involve recognition of the offending agent and elimination of exposure. Industrial and environmental agents that cause toxic neuropathies are discussed in Chapter 86 (see also London and Albers, 2007).

Many medications can cause a peripheral neuropathy that is generally reversible when the offending drug is discontinued. If a clear causal relationship between a potentially neurotoxic drug and neuropathy is established, additional investigations to search for alternative causes may be unnecessary. Premedication with such compounds as neurotrophins may in the future allow clinicians to blunt or prevent the dose-limiting neurotoxic effects of anticancer drugs.

A careful drug history including over-the-counter nutritional supplements and vitamin preparations should be obtained for every patient with polyneuropathy. Some of the drugs reported to produce peripheral neuropathy are listed in Table 106.16. Many anecdotal reports of neuropathy possibly induced by other drugs may represent coincidental occurrences and remain to be substantiated.

## Amiodarone

Amiodarone is a class III antiarrhythmic drug used in the management of refractory ventricular arrhythmias. Nearly all patients on chronic therapy develop one or more adverse effects, including thyroid abnormalities, photosensitivity dermatitis, corneal microdeposits, hepatic dysfunction, pulmonary fibrosis, myopathy, action tremor, basal ganglia dysfunction, encephalopathy, pseudotumor cerebri, optic neuropathy, and a dose-dependent polyneuropathy. A more recent retrospective study, however, found that neurological complications are far less frequently encountered in the modern era than in the 1980s when amiodarone was introduced, owing to differences in maintenance dosages. In this study, neurological adverse events of any kind were seen in only 2.8% of patients, and peripheral neuropathy was noted in less than 1% (Orr and Ahlskog, 2008). Sensorimotor polyneuropathy, either subacute or chronic, may develop in patients receiving long-term amiodarone (400 mg/day) therapy. Length of therapy is a greater risk factor for neuropathy than dose. Moderate sensory impairment and distal and sometimes proximal muscle weaknesses occur. Electrophysiological studies show mild slowing of NCVs, as well as distal denervation. The clinical and electrophysiological features may resemble CIDP, and when motor symptoms predominate and the course is rapid, GBS. Nerve biopsy demonstrates variable findings of loss of myelinated and unmyelinated fibers, axonal degeneration, and segmental demyelination. A distinctive feature is the presence of lysosomal lamellar inclusions in Schwann cells, fibroblasts, and endothelial cells resulting from inactivation of the lysosomal enzyme sphingomyelinase. There is up to 80 times greater concentration of amiodarone and desethylamiodarone in the peripheral nerve than in the serum. Because of the prolonged half-life (up to 100 days) of amiodarone, recovery following the cessation of drug can be very slow. The long half-life also heightens the importance of correctly attributing the neuropathy to amiodarone and not to other causes. Few equivalent antiarrhythmics exist for many patients, and a lengthy observation period is required to assess whether or not the progression has halted.

## Bortezomib

Bortezomib (Velcade), used in the treatment of multiple myeloma, is a proteasome inhibitor that frequently causes a predominantly sensory reversible axonal neuropathy in a dose-dependent manner, which may rarely also affect the autonomic nervous system. The neuropathy of bortezomib is more pronounced in patients with a preexisting neuropathy or other risk factors for neuropathy such as diabetes. As the scope of bortezomib has widened to include treatment of solid tumors, early observations have suggested that neuropathy may be significantly less common. The well-documented reversibility of neuropathic symptoms after stopping or reducing the dose, however, strongly suggests a primary causative role for bortezomib. Rates of neuropathy are also high in retreatment (Argyriou et al., 2008).

**TABLE 106.16 Neuropathies Caused by Pharmaceutical Drugs**

| Drugs | Clinical and Pathological Features | Comments |
|---|---|---|
| **Antineoplastic** | | |
| Cisplatin | S, DA, N | Binds to DNA; disrupts axonal transport? |
| Suramin | SM, DA, SD | DA: inhibits binding of growth factors; SD: immunomodulating effects? |
| Taxanes (paclitaxel, docetaxel) | S, DA | Promote microtubule assembly; disrupt axonal transport |
| Vincristine | S>M, M, DA | Interferes with microtubule assembly; disrupts axonal transport |
| **Antimicrobial** | | |
| Chloroquine | SM, DA | Myopathy |
| Dapsone | M, DA | Optic atrophy |
| Isoniazid | SM, DA | Pyridoxine antagonist |
| Metronidazole | S, DA | |
| Nitrofurantoin | SM, DA | |
| **Antiviral (NRTIS)** | | |
| Didanosine (ddI) | SM, DA | Reversible neuropathy |
| Fialuridine (FIAU) | S, DA | Irreversible neuropathy; also myopathy |
| Lamivudine (3TC) | S, DA | Least common NRTI neuropathy |
| Stavudine (d4T) | SM, DA | More associated with lipodystrophy syndrome |
| Zalcitabine (ddC) | SM, DA | Single most neurotoxic NRTI |
| Zidovudine (AZT) | — | Myopathy only |
| **Cardiovascular** | | |
| Amiodarone | SM, SD | Lysosomal lamellar inclusions; myopathy |
| Hydralazine | SM, DA | Pyridoxine antagonist |
| Perhexiline | SM, SD | Lipid inclusions |
| **Other** | | |
| Colchicine | SM, DA | Neuromyopathy, raised creatine kinase levels |
| Disulfiram | SM, DA | |
| Gold | SM, DA | Myokymia |
| Lipid-lowering agents (statins) | SM, DA | May also cause rhabdomyolysis |
| Nitrous oxide | S, DA | Inhibits vitamin $B_{12}$-dependent methionine synthase; myelopathy |
| Phenytoin | SM, DA | Asymptomatic in most |
| Pyridoxine | S, N, DA | Doses > 250 mg/day |
| Thalidomide | S, N | |
| L-Tryptophan (tainted) | SM, DA | Eosinophilia-myalgia syndrome |

*DA*, Distal axonopathy; *M*, motor; *N*, neuronopathy; *NRTI*, nucleoside analog reverse transcriptase inhibitor; *S*, sensory; *SD*, segmental demyelination; *SM*, sensorimotor neuropathy.

## Chloramphenicol

Chloramphenicol can produce an often reversible peripheral and optic neuropathy following prolonged high-dose therapy. The mechanism of neurotoxicity is unclear.

## Chloroquine and hydrochloroquine

Chloroquine and hydrochloroquine are antimalarial drugs that are also used in the treatment of connective tissue disorders. Typically, a painful vacuolar myopathy with increased serum muscle enzymes develops after prolonged therapy. Both also produce only mild neuropathy. Often there is evidence of both myopathy and neuropathy. Cardiac myotoxicity may also be present. Concomitant renal dysfunction is a predisposing factor for neuromyotoxicity. Muscle and sural nerve biopsies show lamellar inclusions in muscle fibers and Schwann cells. Other antimalarial agents in the same chemical class may cause a similar neuropathy. The mechanism of toxicity is thought to be lysosomal enzyme inhibition similar to amiodarone.

## Cisplatin

Several platinum compounds are used in cancer chemotherapy. The prototype of these is cisplatin, which is used widely in the treatment of ovarian, bladder, and testicular malignancies, as well as squamous cell carcinomas. Cisplatin exerts its chemotherapeutic effects by cross-linking DNA, thereby disrupting cell division. The effect of cisplatin on tumor vasculature has also been implicated in its antineoplastic effect. Sensory polyganglionopathy is the dose-limiting side effect. Cisplatin causes a dose-dependent, predominantly sensory neuronopathy affecting large cells of long-fiber nerves, causing loss of large long myelinated fibers (Krarup-Hansen et al., 2007). Ototoxicity is common, manifested by tinnitus and high-frequency hearing loss. Paresthesias, Lhermitte sign, loss of tendon reflexes, prominent proprioceptive loss, and sensory ataxia usually occur when cumulative doses exceed 400 mg/m$^2$. At the onset of symptoms, it may be difficult to distinguish this neuropathy from a paraneoplastic neuronopathy.

Autonomic symptoms, especially gastroparesis and vomiting, are common and may reflect enteric ganglion cell loss. The neuropathy may develop as late as 4 months after the drug has been stopped (coasting). Nerve conduction studies show reduced or absent SNAPs. Nerve biopsy reveals loss of large myelinated fibers and acute axonal degeneration. Most patients receiving cumulative doses below 500 mg/m$^2$ improve following cessation of therapy, but the neuropathy may persist long after the cessation of medication (Strumberg et al., 2002). Neurotrophins to prevent or ameliorate the neurotoxicity of cisplatin and experimental gene transfer therapy with VEGF are currently being investigated. Vitamin E supplementation ($\alpha$-tocopherol 400 mg/day) has been shown to reduce the severity of neuropathy when administered along with and after cessation of cisplatin (Pace et al., 2010).

The second-generation platinum compound carboplatin is less neurotoxic. There are other available and emerging platinum compounds including oxaliplatin, nedaplatin, and lobaplatin. Up to 90% of patients receiving a cumulative dose of 540 mg/m$^2$ or greater of oxaliplatin develop a predominantly sensory neuropathy (Cersosimo, 2005; Krishnan et al., 2005). Some patients also develop Lhermitte sign. During or shortly after the infusion of oxaliplatin, many patients experience transient sensory symptoms in the limbs, perioral region, and in the throat, possibly due to a temporary dysfunction of nodal voltage-gated sodium channels of peripheral nerve.

## Colchicine

Colchicine is used primarily for the treatment of gout. Subacute proximal weakness and an associated mild distal axonal neuropathy may occur in patients with mild renal insufficiency receiving conventional doses of colchicine, or in patients receiving long-term colchicine for suppression of gout. Markedly elevated serum CK levels and EDX findings of a neuromyopathic process occur. This often is misdiagnosed as uremic myopathy and neuropathy. Grip and percussion myotonia is sometimes evident while myotonic discharges on EMG are frequently observed. Although the sural nerve biopsy shows only nonspecific changes, muscle biopsy reveals autophagic vacuoles and lysosomal accumulation. The weakness and CK elevations typically remit after the drug is discontinued. Colchicine probably causes neuropathy by interfering with axoplasmic transport and impairment of axonal microtubular assembly.

## Dapsone

Dapsone is used in the management of leprosy and other skin disorders. High doses may cause a predominantly motor neuropathy characterized by weakness and atrophy of distal muscles, particularly intrinsic hand muscles. Severe optic neuropathy may also occur. Reduction of motor NCV is slight, even in the presence of severe denervation, suggesting an axonal neuropathy. Recovery after the discontinuation of drug is slow.

## Dideoxynucleosides

Zalcitabine (dideoxycytidine [ddC]), didanosine (dideoxyinosine [ddI]), and stavudine (didehydrodeoxythymidine [d4T]) are nucleoside analogs that inhibit reverse transcriptase and are used to treat HIV-1 infection. These agents cause a dose-limiting dysesthetic sensory neuropathy (Dalakas, 2001). Combined use of these drugs increases the risk of neuropathy substantially. High doses of ddC produce an acute painful sensory neuropathy that may progress for 3 weeks, or even months, after treatment is stopped (coasting). Lower doses cause a less painful sensory neuropathy in 10%–30% of patients. Preexisting neuropathy, DM, heavy alcohol consumption, and low serum cobalamin levels are risk factors that predispose to nucleoside neuropathy. Partial reversal of symptoms following withdrawal of drug allows the ddC neuropathy to be distinguished from the clinically similar HIV-1-associated distal sensory polyneuropathy. Substantial evidence is now being accumulated on the role of mitochondrial dysfunction in the pathogenesis of nucleoside analog neuropathy. Mitochondrial alterations with mitochondrial DNA depletion in the axons and Schwann cells of sensory nerves of patients treated with ddC have been reported.

## Disopyramide

A few cases of reversible sensorimotor peripheral neuropathy have been associated with the cardiac antidysrhythmic agent disopyramide (Briani et al., 2002).

## Disulfiram

Disulfiram is used in the treatment of alcoholism. The incidence of neuropathy is dose related; most patients receiving daily doses of 500 mg or more develop nerve damage after 6 months. The clinical manifestations are initially distal sensory impairment and later progressive weakness. Nerve conduction studies and EMG indicate an axonal neuropathy. Encephalopathy or basal ganglia dysfunction may also be observed in patients receiving high doses of the drug. Acute axonal degeneration and loss of myelinated fibers, as well as accumulation of neurofilaments in the swollen axons, are seen in sural nerve biopsy specimens. After the drug is stopped, improvement takes place over a period of months. The mechanism of neurotoxicity is unknown, but toxicity caused by carbon disulfide, a metabolite of disulfiram, and mitochondrial injury have been proposed.

## Ethambutol

Ethambutol is an antituberculous drug that causes peripheral sensory and optic neuropathy after prolonged administration at doses above 20 mg/kg/day.

## Etoposide

Etoposide is a semisynthetic derivative of podophyllotoxin with established antineoplastic activity in SCLC and lymphoma. Distal sensory axonal neuropathy develops in approximately 10% of patients after high-dose therapy with this agent.

## Gold

Organic gold salts are sometimes used in the treatment of rheumatoid arthritis. Toxic allergic reactions involving skin, kidneys, and blood are well known, whereas neurotoxic complications are uncommon. A dose-related distal axonal polyneuropathy may develop in patients receiving gold therapy. Many patients have the distinctive features of profound myokymia, muscle aches, insomnia, and autonomic dysfunction such as sweating and labile hypertension. After the drug is discontinued, improvement is the rule. Isolated case reports suggest that gold therapy may precipitate a Guillain-Barré-like syndrome with rapidly ascending limb weakness, sensory paresthesia, and elevated CSF protein. In these cases, nerve conduction studies show evidence of demyelinating neuropathy.

## Heroin

Both nontraumatic brachial and lumbosacral plexopathies have been reported in heroin addicts. On resumption of heroin use after a period of abstinence, the symptoms recur in one-third of patients. Intense pain is a common clinical presentation, whereas weakness and sensory impairment are less prominent. Spontaneous recovery occurs slowly over weeks or months. The mechanism of these plexopathies is unclear. A variety of mononeuropathies, usually compression-induced, also occurs among heroin addicts.

## Hydralazine

Hydralazine is an antihypertensive drug that can produce a lupus-like syndrome and rarely produces a predominantly sensory polyneuropathy. Distal "tingling asleep numbness" in the extremities, without overt clinical signs, may develop in 15% of patients on hydralazine. The neuropathy may be caused by pyridoxine deficiency by a mechanism similar to that associated with INH. Symptoms improve after withdrawal of the drug or with low-dose vitamin $B_6$ supplementation (50–100 mg/day).

## Immune Checkpoint Inhibitors

The cytotoxic T-lymphocyte–associated antigen 4 (CTLA-4), programmed death 1 (PD-1), and programmed cell death ligand 1 (PD-L1) immune checkpoints play important roles as negative regulators of T-cell activation, prevent autoimmunity, and help tumor cells escape from recognition by the host immune system. Immune checkpoint inhibitors inhibit the immune checkpoint pathways and enhance T-cell immunity. Ipilimumab inhibits CTLA-4, nivolumab and pembrolizumab inhibit PD-1, while atezolizumab, avelumab, and durvalumab inhibit PD-L1. They are increasingly used for patients with various cancers including melanoma, non–small-cell lung cancer, and urothelial carcinoma and have shown increased overall survival (Darvin et al., 2018).

Immune-related adverse events (irAEs) due to immune checkpoint inhibitors are increasingly recognized affecting most commonly skin and gastrointestinal tract. Most of these irAEs are reversible, but some result in permanent damage and, rarely, deaths (Postow et al., 2018). Neurological irAEs of treatment with immune checkpoint inhibitors included autoimmune encephalitis, transverse myelitis, myositis, myasthenia gravis, and immune polyneuropathies (Supakornnumporn and Katirji, 2018). Most immune polyneuropathies were demyelinating and consistent with the clinical diagnoses of GBS including AIDP, MFS, and acute motor and sensory axonal neuropathy (Kolb et al., 2018; Supakornnumporn and Katirji, 2017). The onset was time locked to the use of checkpoint inhibitors, occurring 2–22 weeks from the first treatment. Slightly more than half of the patients had, in addition to elevated CSF protein, CSF pleocytosis with lymphocytic predominance. Most are treated with corticosteroids (1–2 mg/kg/day of prednisone) in addition to plasma exchange or IVIG. The prognosis of GBS as an irAE is variable with several reported lethal cases (Kolb et al., 2018). In contrast to GBS, CIDP is less commonly reported and most presently acutely fulfilling the diagnosis of acute onset CIDP (Kolb et al., 2018; Supakornnumporn and Katirji, 2018).

## Isoniazid

INH is an effective antituberculous drug that interferes with vitamin $B_6$-dependent coenzymes and thus leads to pyridoxine deficiency. INH is acetylated in the liver by the enzyme acetyltransferase. Individuals unable to acetylate at a normal rate (slow acetylators) maintain high blood levels of free INH longer than rapid acetylators and are therefore more susceptible to toxic neuropathy. The slow acetylation is inherited as an AR trait. INH polyneuropathy occurs in approximately 2% of patients receiving conventional doses (3–5 mg/kg/day), its incidence increasing with higher doses. Typically, 6 months of treatment is needed before neuropathic symptoms of paresthesias, impaired distal lower extremity sensation, and weakness begin. The primary pathological process is axonal degeneration affecting both myelinated and unmyelinated fibers, often with prominent axonal regeneration. Unless recognition of this complication is delayed, recovery is rapid. Co-administration of vitamin $B_6$ (50–100 mg/day) prevents the neuropathy.

## Leflunomide

Leflunomide is an antiinflammatory disease-modifying drug used in rheumatoid arthritis. A sensory, and sometimes motor, axonal neuropathy may develop a few months after initiation of therapy (Bonnel and Graham, 2004; Martin et al., 2005). Patients who stop the drug within 30 days of symptom onset are more likely to have improvement of symptoms or complete recovery than patients who continue to use the drug for a longer time.

## Linezolid

Linezolid is an oxazolidinone used against methicillin- and vancomycin-resistant gram-positive microorganisms. Its long-term use (>28 days) may result in a predominantly sensory and poorly reversible neuropathy with both large- and small-nerve fiber involvement. The mechanism of nerve toxicity is unknown but may be related to inhibition of nerve protein synthesis or mitochondrial dysfunction (Bressler et al., 2004; Zivkovic and Lacomis, 2005). With prolonged use, an optic neuropathy may also develop.

## Lipid-Lowering Agents

The 3-hydroxymethylglutaryl-(HMG)-CoA-reductase inhibitors, or statins, have been claimed in various case reports and a small number of case-controlled and cohort studies to cause an axonal and reversible sensorimotor polyneuropathy (Gaist et al., 2002). However, substantial controversy and doubt accompanies the true existence of such an association, its severity and extent, pathophysiology, and the benefits versus the risks of statins (Bays, 2006; Guyton, 2006; Leis et al., 2005). Even if statins do cause peripheral polyneuropathy, the attributable risk is small and should be considered in the light of the benefit of these drugs in preventing and reducing cardiovascular and cerebrovascular events (McKenney et al., 2006). The incidence of neuropathy is estimated at 12 per 100,000 person-years or a prevalence of 60 per 100,000 persons. The direct role of the underlying metabolic syndrome, hyperlipidemia, or an unrecognized IGT (Hoffman-Snyder et al., 2006) on the development of neuropathy in patients receiving statins cannot be entirely excluded.

### Metronidazole and Misonidazole

Metronidazole is commonly used for the treatment of protozoal and anaerobic bacterial infections, as well as inflammatory bowel disease, peptic ulcers caused by *Helicobacter pylori*, and genitourinary tract infections. It may produce a painful, predominantly sensory polyneuropathy or sensory neuronopathy following the chronic use of cumulative doses of drug exceeding 30 g. Patients taking large doses in a short period for acute infections may also develop such neuropathies. Axonal degeneration of both myelinated and unmyelinated fibers can occur, with slow improvement after the agent is stopped. Misonidazole, a related compound used as an experimental radiation-sensitizing agent, causes a similar sensory neuropathy. The mechanism may involve DNA binding.

### Nitrofurantoin

Nitrofurantoin is a broad-spectrum antibiotic used to treat urinary tract infections. A sensorimotor polyneuropathy of the distal axonal type may develop weeks to months after beginning therapy. Distal numbness, paresthesias, and weakness are common. At times, the neuropathy progresses rapidly. Renal insufficiency, particularly in the elderly and females, predisposes patients to the development of neuropathy because of excessive tissue concentrations of nitrofurantoin, which is normally excreted by the kidneys. Patients with preexisting diabetes are also at greater risk of developing neuropathy. Electrophysiological studies show the typical changes of distal axonopathy. Nerve biopsy shows axonal degeneration. The mechanism of toxicity is unclear but is thought to be inhibition of synthesis of acetyl-CoA by furan derivatives or accumulation of metabolites such as semicarbazide, known to cause neuropathy in experimental animals. Improvement occurs after the medication is discontinued, but it may be incomplete, especially if weakness is present.

### Nitrous Oxide

A predominantly sensory neuropathy and associated myelopathy develop in individuals repeatedly abusing or exposed to nitrous oxide ($N_2O$), an inhalation anesthetic agent that is also used in the food industry as whipping cream propellant. Neurological symptoms occur following intentional abuse or, rarely, through contamination in operating rooms or pediatric dental offices with faulty $N_2O$ scrubbers. Sharp radicular pains are common symptoms, along with numbness and distal sensory loss. A Lhermitte or reverse Lhermitte sign (neck flexion induces an electrical shock sensation traveling from the feet upward), increased reflexes, and extensor plantar signs may be present. Nerve conduction studies show decreased SNAP amplitudes. $N_2O$ inhibits the vitamin $B_{12}$-dependent enzyme methionine synthase, producing a clinical syndrome indistinguishable from vitamin $B_{12}$ deficiency. $N_2O$ anesthesia may even precipitate subacute combined degeneration in patients with unrecognized cobalamin deficiency. Serum methylmalonic acid and homocysteine can be significantly elevated. Prognosis following cessation of exposure is good unless the myelopathy is severe. Vitamin $B_{12}$ supplementation appears to be of no benefit in treating $N_2O$ myeloneuropathy.

### Perhexiline

Perhexiline maleate, now used infrequently in a few countries (but not the United States) for treatment of angina pectoris, causes a reversible demyelinating neuropathy mimicking an inflammatory demyelinating polyneuropathy.

### Phenytoin

Phenytoin, a widely used antiepileptic drug, may cause mild and largely reversible or asymptomatic polyneuropathy after many years of exposure. Typical manifestations are confined to lower-extremity areflexia, distal sensory loss, and mildly reduced motor conduction velocities. The degree of abnormality is generally proportional to the duration of phenytoin treatment. Folate deficiency, which may develop during phenytoin therapy, is unrelated to the onset of neuropathy.

### Pyridoxine

High-dose pyridoxine (vitamin $B_6$, 250–3000 mg/day) may cause a severe and remarkably uniform sensory polyganglionopathy. Painful paresthesias, sensory ataxia, perioral numbness, and Lhermitte sign are common features. Nerve conduction studies show low-amplitude or absent SNAPs. Severe depletion of myelinated fibers and acute axonal degeneration are found in sural nerve biopsy specimens. Pyridoxine use should be queried in all patients with sensory neuropathy. Although its use as a prescribed agent is now limited, it is still self-administered by patients without proof of efficacy in CTS, premenstrual syndrome, hyperemesis gravidarum, and in body building. In experimental studies, high-dose pyridoxine (300 mg/kg) produced widespread dorsal root ganglion degeneration. The vulnerability of dorsal root ganglia to circulating pyridoxine is thought to be due to weak blood–brain barrier in this region. It appears that the toxic effect is exerted by pyridoxine itself and not through its metabolites. The fact that most clinical cases gradually recover suggests that dysfunctional dorsal root ganglion neurons may regain their functional capacity despite severe sensory deficits early in the course of disease.

### Suramin

Originally introduced as an antiparasitic agent, suramin is used currently as an antineoplastic drug for refractory malignancies. It acts by inhibiting DNA polymerase activity and displacing several growth factors—insulin-like growth factor (IGF-1), epidermal growth factor (EGF), transforming growth factor (TGF), and NGF—from their respective receptors. Suramin neurotoxicity is the dose-limiting side effect leading to two distinct patterns of neuropathy: one a length-dependent axonal polyneuropathy and the other a subacute demyelinating polyradiculoneuropathy (Chaudhry et al., 1996). The distal sensorimotor neuropathy that occurs in 30%–55% of patients manifests with paresthesias and mild distal leg weakness. About 15% of patients develop a subacutely evolving, demyelinating polyradiculoneuropathy. Severe generalized flaccid weakness with bulbar and respiratory involvement, nerve conduction studies consistent with demyelination, increased CSF protein levels, and perivascular inflammation and increased macrophage numbers on sural nerve biopsy are typical features, making this neuropathy virtually indistinguishable from GBS or CIDP. The severe neuropathy occurs predominantly at peak plasma suramin concentrations above 350 μg/mL. Suramin may induce inflammatory demyelination by its many immunomodulatory effects. Patients improve after drug discontinuation and with plasmapheresis.

### Tacrolimus

Tacrolimus, a macrolide antibiotic, has a potent immunosuppressive effect and is used in organ transplantation. In about 30% of patients, adverse effects including seizures, leukoencephalopathy, occipital headaches, tremor, and akinetic mutism may develop. Rarely, it may also cause one of the two types of peripheral neuropathy: a reversible but severe axonal neuropathy that occurs days after treatment; and a demyelinating neuropathy similar to CIDP, 2–10 weeks after treatment. Electrophysiological and nerve biopsy, as well as CSF findings, are those usually observed in demyelinating neuropathies. The cause of the axonal degeneration is unknown, but the demyelinating variety may be caused by an immune-mediated process, since some patients improve following plasmapheresis or IVIG administration.

## Taxanes

Two taxanes, paclitaxel (Taxol) and docetaxel (Taxotere), have played a significant role in the treatment of a variety of malignancies. They, as well as the newer antitumor agents, epothilones, bind to β-tubulin of microtubules, thereby interfering with the dynamic assembly and disassembly of the microtubules of the mitotic spindle and leading to aborted cell division and cell death. Axonal microtubules also contain β-tubulin, and binding of these drugs to microtubules results in disruption of axonal transport. Paclitaxel may also cause axonal mitochondrial damage, further contributing to the neuropathy (Flatters and Bennet, 2006). A dose-related sensory ganglionopathy results with doses above 250 $mg/m^2$ body surface area. Cumulative dosages of greater than 1000 $mg/m^2$ invariably result in a sensory and motor neuropathy. Burning paresthesias, sensory loss affecting all sensory modalities, and areflexia are followed by sensory ataxia and mild distal weakness. Disabling weakness is rare except in the presence of additional risk factors such as preexisting diabetic neuropathy, hereditary neuropathy, or combination therapy with other neurotoxic chemotherapeutic agents such as cisplatin. Rarely, cranial neuropathies or autonomic dysfunction are also observed. The neuropathy generally improves when the dose of the drug is reduced or following the completion of therapy. This may take several months. For painful symptoms, the usual symptomatic treatment is offered. Several neuroprotective agents, including leukemia inhibitory factor, amifostine (a free-radical scavenger), glutamine, and vitamin E, have been tested experimentally and in trials. Of these, only the latter two provided a mild protective effect from neuropathy (Lee and Swain, 2006).

Docetaxel, used in metastatic breast and ovarian cancer, causes a dose-dependent sensory neuropathy similar to its parent compound. Motor symptoms are present only in the most severely affected patients (New et al., 1996).

## Thalidomide and Lenalidomide

Thalidomide was introduced as a sedative-hypnotic agent in the 1950s, but it was taken off the market when its disastrous teratogenic properties became evident. The drug has, however, been found useful in treating erythema nodosum leprosum and other rare skin conditions, graft-versus-host disease, a number of complications of HIV infection, and multiple myeloma, as well as other malignancies. This compound owes its therapeutic effects to its inhibition of TNF-α production and antiangiogenic properties. Thalidomide causes dorsal root ganglion degeneration with selective involvement of large-diameter sensory neurons or a length-dependent painful sensory axonal neuropathy. Painful distal paresthesias and numbness occur, with palmar erythema and brittle nails as prominent signs. In most patients, the neuropathy is dose related, occurring after high doses or chronic administration for more than 6 months (Bastuji-Garin et al., 2002; Tosi et al., 2005). In general, cumulative dosages greater than 100 g result in significant neuropathy, and the neuropathy is rare at cumulative doses less than 20 g. After discontinuation of the drug, symptoms and signs improve slowly, though coasting is often seen. Because thalidomide produces neurotoxicity in a dose-dependent manner, monitoring for peripheral neuropathy with clinical examination and sensory conduction studies allows for early detection of neuropathy, preventing severe disability (Cavaletti et al., 2004; Plasmati et al., 2007).

Lenalidomide, an analog of thalidomide, is a more potent immunomodulator and causes neuropathy less frequently or severely. Glutethimide, a structurally related old hypnotic compound, may produce a similar sensory polyganglionopathy in patients taking high doses for many months.

## L-Tryptophan

An unusual syndrome called *eosinophilia-myalgia syndrome* was recognized in 1989 in individuals taking preparations containing a contaminated L-tryptophan. A severe axonal sensorimotor polyneuropathy, at times associated with inflammation and vasculopathy, was a prominent feature in some patients. The syndrome was to a large extent similar to Spanish "toxic oil syndrome." Recovery from the neuropathy was slow and sometimes incomplete. Since the elimination of contaminated tryptophan, the syndrome is no longer seen.

## Tumor Necrosis Factor-α Blockers

Adalimumab (Humira), etanercept (Enbrel), and infliximab (Remicade) are immunosuppressive medications used to treat rheumatoid arthritis, inflammatory bowel disease, and other rheumatological conditions by blocking TNF-α. They have been shown to trigger a demyelinating disease in the CNS similar to multiple sclerosis. Additionally, demyelinating peripheral neuropathies, which can resemble MMN with conduction block or CIDP or its variants, may follow the use of antagonists to TNF-α (Alshekhlee et al., 2010; Stübgen, 2008). Clinically, the neuropathy is typically sensorimotor but may be purely sensory or purely motor. CSF protein may be normal to moderately elevated. Nerve conduction studies show findings typical of a sensorimotor or purely motor demyelinating polyneuropathy, with relative preservation of amplitudes distally accompanied by focal slowing and conduction blocks at non-entrapment sites. IVIG and plasma exchange typically are effective in treating the neuropathy, similar to other forms of demyelinating neuropathies. The decision of whether or not to stop the offending agent should be made on a case-by-case basis (Lozeron et al., 2009). Withdrawing the offending agent does not always reverse the immune process, and chronic immunomodulating therapy (e.g., IVIG, steroids, immunosuppressive agents) may be necessary to control the inflammatory process and improve clinical outcome (Alshekhlee et al., 2010).

## Vinca Alkaloids

Vincristine, the vinca alkaloid most used in chemotherapeutic regimens, causes a length-dependent sensorimotor polyneuropathy as its dose-limiting side effect. Vinblastine and two semisynthetic derivatives, vindesine and vinorelbine, are less neurotoxic. Vinca alkaloids function as mitotic spindle inhibitors. Like taxanes, their neurotoxicity is related to tubulin binding, which interferes with axonal microtubule assembly, thereby impairing axonal transport.

Vincristine produces a dose-dependent neuropathy with sensory symptoms beginning at 5 mg and motor symptoms at cumulative doses of 30–50 mg. There are several reports of vincristine-induced severe paralysis at conventional doses in patients with preexisting hereditary neuropathies. Paresthesias and pain, often starting in the fingers before the feet, and loss of ankle jerks are common initial findings. Distal muscle weakness and sensory impairment follow. Autonomic dysfunction—particularly gastroparesis, constipation, occasionally paralytic ileus, urinary retention, impotence, and orthostatic hypotension—may occur and is an early manifestation. Weakness, often accompanied by muscle pains, may evolve rapidly to severe motor impairment. Occasionally, isolated mononeuropathies have been reported. Cranial nerve involvement occurs infrequently and includes trigeminal sensory loss, ocular motility disorders, facial weakness, and recurrent laryngeal nerve palsies.

EDX studies reflect the degeneration of distal axons. SNAPs are reduced in amplitude, whereas NCVs are preserved. EMG shows denervation in distal muscles. The predominant pathological features are axonal degeneration and myopathic changes, with spheromembranous inclusions in the muscle fibers evident on electron microscopy. Reduction in dose or withdrawal from therapy at an early stage usually leads to eventual, though delayed, recovery. In up to 60% of patients, residual sensory symptoms and absent tendon reflexes may persist, and electrophysiological abnormalities continue. Co-administration of glutamic acid or ORG 2766, an adrenocorticotropic hormone-derived synthetic peptide, has shown promising results in reducing the severity of vincristine neuropathy in preclinical trials, but there was no benefit in a clinical trial. Neurotrophins have neuroprotective effects in experimental studies as well, although there is reticence to use these compounds in patients with established neoplasms because of the fear that growth factors may stimulate tumor growth.

## NEUROPATHIES ASSOCIATED WITH INFECTIONS

Neuropathies associated with infection, including viral, bacterial, and parasitic infections, are discussed in the online version of this chapter, available at http://www.expertconsult.com.

## CHRONIC IDIOPATHIC AXONAL POLYNEUROPATHY

Despite all efforts, a group of acquired polyneuropathies remains idiopathic. Acquired chronic sensorimotor and sensory polyneuropathies are common in individuals older than 50 years of age, with an estimated prevalence of more than 3%, and a male/female ratio of 3/2. A chronic idiopathic axonal polyneuropathy with either mixed sensorimotor features or pure or predominant small sensory manifestations afflicts patients starting the sixth decade of life and may accounts for up to 30% of all polyneuropathies (Zis et al., 2016). Patients with sensorimotor peripheral polyneuropathy complain of tingling, prickling, numbness or burning of the feet, and often stiffness of the toes. There is stocking loss of pinprick and temperature sensation in the feet, together with mild loss of vibratory sensation, absent ankle reflexes, and sometimes mild toe-extensor weakness. EDX and nerve biopsy studies in patients with cryptogenic polyneuropathy are compatible with a length-dependent axonal polyneuropathy. These abnormal signs must be distinguished from normal manifestations of aging in the PNS. Loss of vibratory sense that is restricted to the toes or absent ankle reflexes may be a normal finding in healthy elderly controls (present in about a third of individuals >65). Absent lower extremity SNAPs may also be seen in healthy elderly subjects. However, absent sural SNAPs combined with fibrillation potentials in the anterior tibialis muscle support the diagnosis of polyneuropathy, since such combined abnormalities are rarely found in healthy older individuals (Vrancken et al., 2002).

*Idiopathic small-fiber neuropathy* presents with painful burning feet, with or without numbness. The condition also occurs in older patients without associated systemic diseases or exposure to identifiable toxins (Lauria et al., 2014). Epidemiological studies have shown that this disorder is not rare, with an incidence of 12 cases per 100,000 inhabitants per year and a prevalence of 53 cases per 100,000 in the Netherlands (Terkelsen et al., 2017). Most patients have elevated thermal thresholds on quantitative sensory examination and impaired distal sweating, measured by the QSART or thermoregulatory sweat testing. Sural SNAPs are preserved if small fibers are involved exclusively, but they are frequently reduced or absent in sensory polyneuropathies affecting both large and small fibers. Reduced IENFD on punch skin biopsy provides objective evidence of involvement of distal small nerve fibers in these patients (Terkelsen et al., 2017; Zhou, 2014), without identifying the specific cause. IGT may be associated with chronic axonal sensory polyneuropathies of presumed unknown cause (Hoffman-Snyder et al., 2006; Smith et al., 2001). Among 73 patients referred for distal idiopathic sensory neuropathy and screened with glucose tolerance testing, 56% had abnormal results, either IGT (36%) or frank diabetes (Sumner et al., 2003).

Both idiopathic sensorimotor and sensory polyneuropathies pursue a very slowly progressive course or reach a stable plateau. Even after a course of more than 10 years, severe disability rarely occurs. Independent ambulation is almost always maintained.

Management of these common neuropathies centers on treating neuropathic pain, providing ankle braces in some cases, and patient education about the favorable long-term outcome (Wolfe and Barohn, 1998). Periodic re-evaluation of patients in search of a possible underlying cause cannot be overemphasized.

## PAIN IN PERIPHERAL NEUROPATHY

Pain is one of the cardinal symptoms of peripheral nerve disorders. Estimates of the population prevalence of chronic pain with neuropathic components range between 6% and 10%. The liability for pain appears to vary from person to person, from nerve to nerve, between male and female, and even with age. Neuropathic pain may occur spontaneously without provocation (i.e., is stimulus independent) or be provoked by noxious or non-noxious stimuli. *Hyperalgesia* is an increased pain response to noxious stimuli. *Allodynia* is the sensation of pain elicited by non-noxious stimuli (e.g., from contact with clothing, bed sheets, or air flow).

The sensation of pain in peripheral neuropathies is generated by nerve impulses triggered when free nerve endings (nociceptors) in sensitive tissues, particularly the skin, respond to noxious stimuli. A number of neurophysiological studies have determined that both small myelinated Aδ fibers and unmyelinated nociceptive C fibers mediate the afferent impulse of pain stimuli (Campbell and Meyer, 2006). Intraneural microstimulation of human sensory nerves has shown that stimulating Aδ nociceptors evokes an acute sensation of sharp and well-localized pain. In contrast, the stimulation of polymodal C nociceptors evokes a sensation of delayed, more diffuse burning pain. Peripheral nerve injury results in the upregulation of sodium channels in nociceptive terminals and unmyelinated axons that leads to ectopic activity in sensitized C fibers and spontaneous firing in nociceptive primary sensory neurons. The increase in peripheral activity generates a cascade of secondary changes in the dorsal horn, with the end result of central sensitization in second- and third-order neurons. The peripheral and central sensitization involves a number of recently recognized neurobiological events involving altered expression of sodium channels, increased glutamate activity at *N*-methyl-D-aspartate (NMDA) receptors, and downregulation of γ-aminobutyric acid (GABA) receptors and opioid receptors. Reorganizational changes can occur at the level of the dorsal horn and dorsal root ganglion. These include the sprouting of sympathetic axons into the dorsal root ganglion, forming baskets around nociceptive neurons, and the sprouting of non-nociceptive Aβ central axon terminals into the superficial dorsal horn (Woolf and Mannion, 1999). For a more detailed discussion of neuropathic pain mechanisms, see Chapter 52.

**BOX 106.16 Peripheral Neuropathies Frequently Associated with Pain**

Diabetic neuropathies:
- Painful symmetrical polyneuropathy
- Asymmetrical polyradiculoplexopathy
- Truncal mononeuropathy

Brachial and lumbosacral plexopathy
Vasculitic neuropathy
Toxic neuropathies:
- Arsenic, thallium
- Alcohol
- Vincristine, cisplatin
- Dideoxynucleosides

Amyloid neuropathies: primary and familial
Paraneoplastic sensory neuropathy
Neuropathy associated with Sjögren syndrome
Human immunodeficiency virus–related distal symmetrical polyneuropathy
Uremic polyneuropathy
Neuropathy associated with Fabry disease
Hereditary sensory autonomic neuropathy
Cryptogenic small-fiber neuropathy

Neuropathic pain can be a prominent presenting symptom in a great number of peripheral neuropathies (Mendell and Sahenk, 2003; Box 106.16). Pain is characteristic of neuropathies with predominant small-fiber involvement, but even in large-fiber neuropathies, a sufficient number of small fibers may be damaged to cause pain. The poor clinical correlation between morphological changes seen in nerve biopsy specimens and pain is not surprising if one considers that ectopic impulses may arise from regenerating axonal sprouts or dysfunctional fibers at more proximal or distal sites than the nerve segment examined at biopsy. Neuropathic pain is of two main types. The first, termed *dysesthetic pain*, usually affects distal skin and subcutaneous structures, may be constant or intermittent (stabbing, electrical jolts), may often have a temporal pattern of worsening at periods of rest or bedtime, and is described as searing, burning, or icy-cold. Sensory examination should use techniques to elicit abnormal positive sensory phenomena. Allodynia can be elicited by light touch or nonpainful cold stimuli. When testing for hyperpathia, single and repeated pinpricks are used. Patients with hyperpathia may often complain of *summation* (pain perception increases with repeated stimulation) and *after-sensations* (pain continues after stimulation has ceased). *Nerve trunk pain*, a second type of neuropathic pain, is a deep-seated, sharp, knifelike proximal pain along nerve roots or trunks that improves with rest or optimal position but is aggravated by movement. Nerve trunk pain seems to be mediated by spontaneous impulses arising from nervi nervorum innervating nerve sheaths of affected nerve roots or trunks. Muscle pain and tenderness may develop with acutely evolving denervation of muscle, as occurs in GBS or acute poliomyelitis.

## Management of Neuropathic Pain

The management of neuropathic pain is similar for all painful neuropathies, although results vary substantially. Symptomatic treatment of neuropathic pain is effective but seldom provides complete relief, with best therapies achieving a 30%–50% reduction in pain. Simple analgesics (aspirin, acetaminophen, NSAIDs) are rarely beneficial. Most patients require additional pharmacotherapy. Drugs from several different pharmacological classes have been shown to be safe and effective in alleviating neuropathic pain. These include antidepressants, anticonvulsants, sodium channel blockers, opioids and non-narcotic analgesics, and topical agents (Attal et al., 2006). In general, once an agent is selected for treatment, the medication is started at the lowest possible dosage and slowly titrated by increasing the dose every 3–7 days until significant pain relief or intolerable side effects occur. Many treatment failures can be attributed to insufficient dosing or intolerance caused by rapid dose escalations. The use of the following drugs is supported by the results of randomized controlled studies, most of which have been conducted in postherpetic neuralgia and painful diabetic neuropathy. It is not clear that the results of these studies can be fully extended to other neuropathies, but in practice this is often done. Guidelines on pharmacological treatment of neuropathic pain have recently been published (Attal et al., 2006).

TCAs have been established to reduce pain independent of their effect on mood. These drugs block reuptake of norepinephrine and serotonin, two neurotransmitters implicated in nociceptive modulation, and also inhibit sodium channels. TCAs are effective for both constant and lancinating paroxysmal pain, particularly in patients with painful diabetic neuropathy (Saarto and Wiffen, 2005; Sindrup et al., 2005). Treatment should be initiated with low-dose (10–25 mg) amitriptyline, desipramine, or nortriptyline given at bedtime and increased by similar increments no more than once a week. Most studies have shown that doses of tricyclics of 75–150 mg (less for elderly patients) are required for pain suppression. At such high-dose levels, sedation, confusion, anticholinergic effects (constipation, dry mouth, urinary retention), and orthostatic hypotension are common side effects, particularly in elderly patients. Desipramine and nortriptyline cause less sedation and less orthostatic hypotension and have fewer anticholinergic effects than amitriptyline. TCAs should be started with caution in elderly patients and in patients with ischemic heart disease, narrow angle glaucoma, or prostatism.

Other antidepressants are also used for neuropathic pain. Selective serotonin reuptake inhibitors are less effective than TCAs in relieving neuropathic pain. Venlafaxine (150–225 mg/day) is a potent inhibitor of norepinephrine and serotonin reuptake and has fewer side effects than TCAs, but it is likely less efficacious (Sindrup et al., 2003). Duloxetine, a dual reuptake inhibitor of 5-HT and norepinephrine, at a dose of 60–120 mg/day has a moderate effect on neuropathic pain (Wernicke et al., 2006). Bupropion (300 mg/day), a specific inhibitor of norepinephrine reuptake, reduced neuropathic pain by 30% in a small group of patients.

Anticonvulsants (gabapentin, pregabalin, carbamazepine, oxcarbazepine, topiramate, and lamotrigine) are frequently given to suppress shooting or stabbing pains. Gabapentin is an anticonvulsant with an unknown mechanism of action. Its effect may be mediated by binding to voltage-dependent calcium channels expressed in the substantia gelatinosa of the dorsal horn. Controlled studies demonstrated benefit in patients with postherpetic neuralgia and painful diabetic neuropathy. When compared head to head with amitriptyline, gabapentin had equal efficacy but fewer side effects. Treatment is initiated at 300 mg at bedtime, though smaller doses should be considered for elderly patients and those with renal insufficiency. The dose is escalated by 300-mg increments every 5–7 days until adequate pain relief is achieved. The median effective dose ranges from 900 to 1600 mg, although some patients require doses of 3600 mg/day. Pregabalin, which is structurally similar to gabapentin, has been shown to be effective at 150–600 mg/day in several trials. It should be initiated at 50–75 mg twice a day and increased every 5–7 days. Carbamazepine reduces neuronal membrane excitability by blocking sodium channels. In painful diabetic neuropathy, carbamazepine (1000–1600 mg/day) was significantly better than placebo, equivalent to that of TCAs. In practice, intolerance to side effects limits its use. It is important to initiate treatment with carbamazepine at a low dose

(100 mg twice daily) and increase slowly to avoid initial symptoms of nausea, disequilibrium, and memory impairment. Oxcarbazepine, a ketoacid analog, is better tolerated, with the effective daily dose exceeding 1200 mg (Grosskopf et al., 2006). Topiramate failed to relieve diabetic neuropathic pain in three large controlled studies and had a marginal effect in one. Lamotrigine acts by blocking sodium channels and by inhibiting the presynaptic release of glutamine. Lamotrigine (200–400 mg/day) resulted in moderate pain relief in controlled studies of painful diabetic and HIV-associated neuropathies (Eisenberg et al., 2001).

Mexiletine, the oral analog of lidocaine, is the prototype of a sodium channel blocker, but there have been inconsistent results in the use of mexiletine to control pain. Two of the studies showed a beneficial effect in patients with diabetic neuropathy, but four other studies failed to demonstrate benefit. Tramadol, a centrally acting analgesic, has proved effective in painful neuropathies related to diabetes and other causes in two clinical trials in doses ranging from 200 to 400 mg/day (Harati et al., 1998). Low-affinity binding to μ-opioid receptors and inhibition of norepinephrine and serotonin uptake contribute to its analgesic action. The drug is generally well tolerated, but transient nausea and constipation occur in about 20% of patients. High-dose dextromethorphan, a low-affinity NMDA glutamate antagonist, provided partial relief in painful diabetic neuropathy but was associated with significant sedation and ataxia.

Narcotic analgesics should be limited to patients who have failed adequate treatment trials of other agents. Randomized controlled studies of oxycodone and levorphanol have demonstrated efficacy of opioids in postherpetic neuralgia and painful diabetic neuropathies (Rowbotham et al., 2003). Specific guidelines for chronic opioid therapy in neuropathic pain have been published and should be followed.

Cannabis-based medicine (herbal cannabis, plant-derived or synthetic tetrahydrocannabinol [THC], THC/cannabidiol [CBD] oromucosal spray) is a potential treatment for neuropathic pain but its value requires further controlled studies (Mücke et al., 2018).

Topical agents that act through local skin absorption have the advantage of minimal or no systemic side effects and may be useful in patients with painful, burning feet. Capsaicin, an extract of chili peppers, presumably produces relief of pain through the depletion of substance P in unmyelinated nociceptive fibers. Capsaicin cream (0.075%) is applied to the affected area of skin three to four times a day. Its use should be continued for at least 4 weeks before rejecting its effectiveness. An initial intense burning frequently occurs during the first 1–2 weeks of application. This may be minimized by applying a local anesthetic cream (such as lidocaine 5% cream) prior to the application of capsaicin cream for the initial 2 weeks of therapy. However, even after 4 weeks, the beneficial effects of capsaicin remain marginal. Patches containing 5% lidocaine have been shown to reduce pain in postherpetic neuralgia. Some patients may receive relief from burning feet and allodynia by topical application of such patches on areas of excessive pain.

It may be necessary to use drugs in combination to achieve optimal pain relief. For example, if pain is still poorly controlled on a maximum tolerated dose of gabapentin, tramadol, an opioid, or a TCA may be added (Gilron et al., 2005). Combined gabapentin and nortriptyline is more effective than either drug given alone in treating diabetic neuropathic pain and postherpetic neuralgia (Gilron et al., 2009).

Nonpharmacological treatments, including low-intensity transcutaneous electrical nerve stimulation, spinal cord stimulation, acupuncture, medical hypnosis, and meditation, may reduce the perception of pain and suffering. A comprehensive multidisciplinary pain management program should be considered for patients with chronic refractory neuropathic pain.

*The complete reference list is available online at https://expertconsult.inkling.com/.*

107

# Disorders of the Autonomic Nervous System

*Thomas Chelimsky, Gisela Chelimsky*

## OUTLINE



The term *autonomic nervous system*, meaning "self-driven," refers to an intellectually convenient but physiologically artificial division of the neuraxis. Autonomic functions are "self-driven" only to the extent that they may not involve conscious control. However, they are highly integrated with other neural circuits, and the boundaries delineating autonomic circuits from nonautonomic circuits do not hold up to careful scrutiny. It is nonetheless convenient to describe a set of pathways traditionally called *autonomic pathways*, whose primary function constitutes the unconscious control of all nonmotor end organs in the body. The innervation of each end organ is highly tailored to a balance between the primary needs of the organ itself and the importance of some degree of control in daily function. For example, while continuous liver perfusion is crucial for survival, skin perfusion is determined more by the body's thermoregulatory needs than by skin oxygenation demands. This great difference in perfusion control requirements is reflected in divergent autonomic innervation based entirely on internal demands for some and external demands for others. The innervation of still other organs may be based on internal demands in one setting and external demands in another. For example, muscle perfusion at rest is primarily an externally controlled function, with blood diverted to or from the muscle depending on systemic blood volume and pressure requirements. However, perfusion to exercising muscle is entirely internally driven because rising lactate levels turn off the ability of sympathetic fibers to control vascular tone.

At the higher control levels in the brain, autonomic integrators and signals are integrated and expressed subconsciously through the central autonomic network (Benarroch, 1997). This overlies a strong circadian rhythm of autonomic function. The autonomic nervous system consists of two large divisions—the *sympathetic* (thoracolumbar) outflow and the *parasympathetic* (craniosacral) outflow. The two divisions are defined by their anatomical origin rather than by their physiological characteristics. The circadian rhythm of autonomic function originates in the suprachiasmatic nucleus and is conveyed to the hypothalamus and brainstem. Light falling on retinal ganglion cell dendrites (not rods or cones) in the eye and transmitted via the retinohypothalamic tract entrains this rhythm. Other key inputs to autonomic outflow originate in the insular cortex and the amygdala. The principal integration of autonomic outflow to the cardiovascular system lies in the medulla. Stretch-sensitive baroreflex mechanoreceptors in the blood vessels of the thorax and neck relay information about blood pressure and blood volume through the glossopharyngeal (from carotid arteries) and vagus (from aorta) nerves to the nucleus tractus solitarius (NTS) in the posterior medulla. Excitatory neurons from the NTS innervate the dorsal motor nucleus of the vagus, which regulates parasympathetic outflow. Inhibitory neurons project to areas in the ventrolateral medulla, from which sympathetic outflow is regulated. The most important such site is the rostral ventrolateral medulla.

The autonomic nervous system exerts widespread control over homeostasis (Goldstein, 2001). Almost every organ system receives regulatory information from the central nervous system (CNS) through the autonomic efferents (Fig. 107.1), and increasingly we recognize that afferent input into the central autonomic network regulates not only the output of the autonomic system but also much CNS function not generally considered to be autonomic in nature. The emerging concept is pervasive integration of autonomic activities with the brain and body.

Baroreceptors in each carotid sinus send information about the distention of the vessel wall to the brainstem via the glossopharyngeal nerve (cranial nerve IX). Other baroreceptors in the aortic arch and the great vessels of the thorax transmit similar information via the vagus nerve (cranial nerve X) to the same brainstem nuclei. In addition, low-pressure receptors linked by the vagus nerve to the brainstem sense the blood volume in the thorax. The brainstem structure receiving this information is the NTS, which lies in the dorsal medulla at the level of the fourth ventricle. Neurotransmitters such as glutamate and nitric oxide released in the NTS lead to cardiovascular effects. The caudal ventrolateral medulla and the rostral ventrolateral medulla are crucial brainstem structures involved in the modulation of sympathetic outflow. Afferent nerve traffic from the thorax and abdomen also provides input to central cardiovascular centers after traveling with sympathetic nerves back to the spinal cord, and then to medullary cardiovascular control centers.

## CLASSIFICATION OF AUTONOMIC DISORDERS

From a neurological perspective, autonomic disorders are best understood by using the same conceptual framework employed to classify gastrointestinal disorders. At first pass, a disorder is either structural or functional. *Structural disorders* (also referred to as *autonomic failure*) are defined as having demonstrable pathological abnormalities that directly interfere with autonomic neural pathways in the peripheral or CNS, such as multiple system atrophy (MSA), Parkinson disease (PD), or diabetic autonomic neuropathy. In contrast, *functional disorders* currently have no consistently demonstrable pathological basis, are primarily defined by symptomology, and often constitute a syndrome such as postural tachycardia syndrome (POTS), complex regional pain syndrome, and irritable bowel syndrome (IBS). Clearly, disorders will move from functional to structural as etiologies are uncovered and knowledge evolves. As one editor of this book, Dr. Robert Daroff, pointed out at Grand Rounds in Neurology at Case Western Reserve University (October 1, 2010), "When I was a resident, we sent all the patients with Crohn's disease to the psychiatrist."

Since by definition structural disorders have a known pathological substrate, they can be divided into two camps—those that involve the peripheral nervous system and those that involve central pathways. Such a division would be more challenging in functional disorders, where a specific etiopathology is generally not defined, with certain rare exceptions (see later discussion and Fig. 107.1). Peripheral disorders can be further subdivided by whether the dominant pathological process involves afferent or efferent fibers. As can be discerned from Fig. 107.1, most peripheral disorders involve efferent nerves. It should be kept in mind that few if any of the structural disorders are "pure" either in their central versus peripheral localization or in afferent versus efferent functional classification. For example, diabetes has been shown to involve central pathways, and PD involves peripheral ganglia, symbolized by the dashed line in the figure connecting that box to the efferent peripheral category.

These two basic classes of dysautonomias, structural and functional, contrast with one another in other ways as well. Patients with structural disorders, despite their extensive pathological changes in the nervous system, tend to harbor proportionally few symptoms; for example, the majority of patients do not realize when their systolic blood pressure drops by nearly 90 mm Hg (Arbogast et al., 2009). In contrast, patients with functional disorders harbor enormous numbers of complaints, just as disproportionate with the demonstrable pathological involvement of the autonomic nervous system but in the opposite sense (Chelimsky et al., 2019; Ojha et al., 2011). These disorders are now being considered as multisystem rather than involving a single end organ. A new classification is being proposed, with disorders involving hollow organs, such as IBS, interstitial cystitis, functional abdominal pain, and functional dyspepsia, classified as primarily vagally mediated disorders, and disorders involving vascular dysfunction, such as migraine headache, myofascial pelvic pain, dysmenorrhea, and complex regional pain syndrome, classified as primarily sympathetically mediated disorders (Chelimsky et al., 2019). Another difference relates to prognosis. Structural disorders in general carry a very poor prognosis. For example, diabetics with autonomic neuropathy have a 5-year mortality between 25% and 50% (Ewing et al., 1976). Patients with MSA survive only 7–9 years from onset (Schrag et al., 2008). In contrast, while functional disorders can be extremely disabling (Benrud-Larson et al., 2002; O'Leary and Sant, 1997; Spiegel et al., 2008), their prognosis for longevity is generally good.

## CLINICAL FEATURES OF AUTONOMIC IMPAIRMENT

### Vision

Visual function is generally preserved in autonomic failure. With upright posture and impaired perfusion of the CNS, dimming or tunneling of vision commonly occurs as a transitory phenomenon, usually interpreted as a sign that the patient needs to sit down to avoid passing out. Reduced blood flow in brain areas subserving vision was assumed, but a simpler mechanism may also be partly at work here.

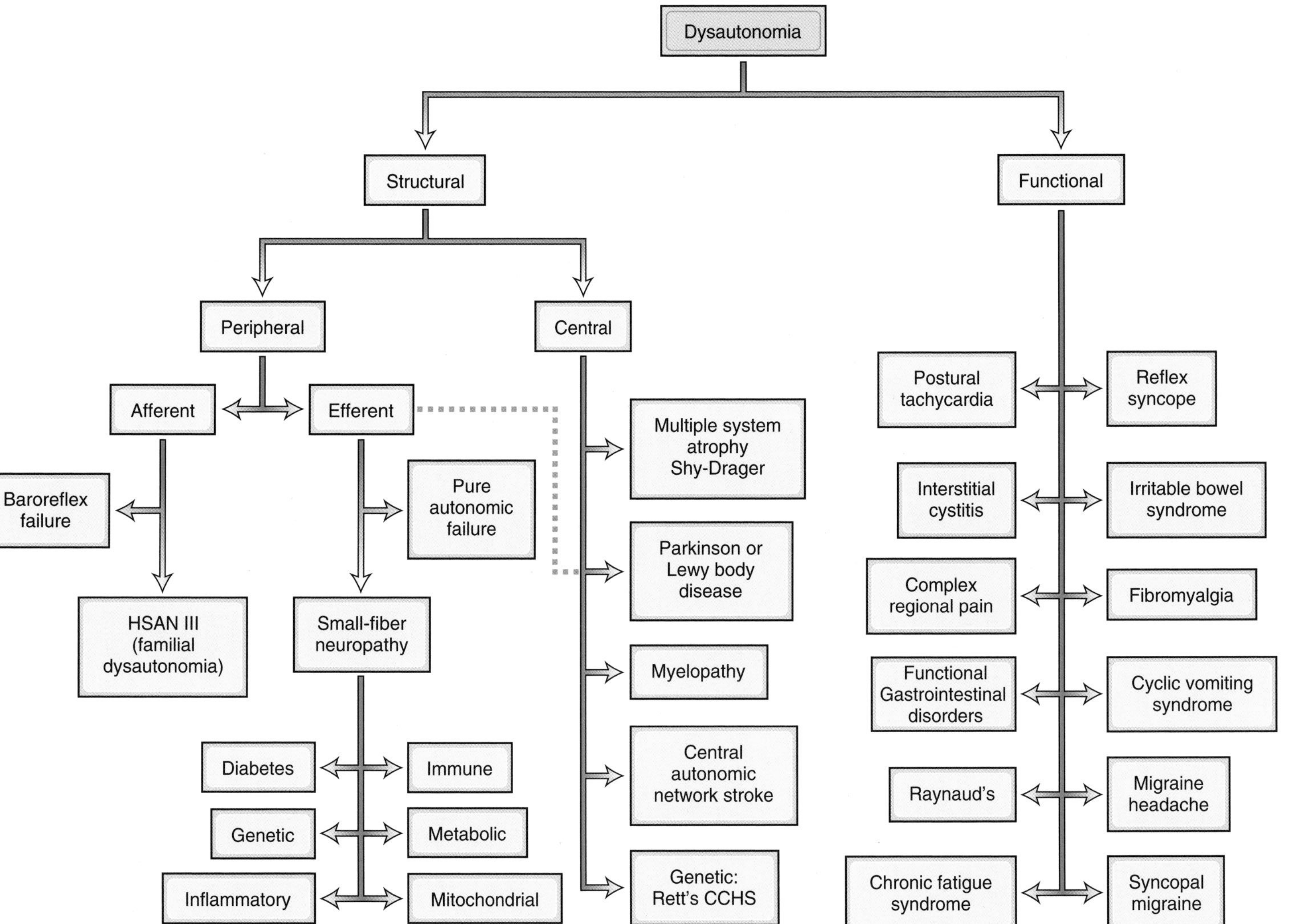


**Fig. 107.1 Classification of Autonomic Disorders or Dysautonomias.** The first conceptual division is between a structural and functional disorder. The word "functional" is being utilized in its true meaning of a disturbance in autonomic function, without clear evidence of structural damage to the autonomic nervous system, akin to the use of the word "functional" in functional gastrointestinal *(GI)* disorders, and without implication of a psychiatric etiology. In the absence of any evidence of consistent structural abnormalities, functional disorders clearly cannot be localized in the nervous system. In contrast, structural disorders can be further divided into those localized in the central and peripheral nervous systems, with the division point usually taken at the sympathetic ganglion. Finally, peripheral nervous system disorders can be further classified based on whether they primarily involve afferent or efferent nerves. It should be emphasized that there is overlap between these groups; for example, diabetes will often involve afferent nerve fibers, but this classification emphasizes the predominant fiber involvement. A *dotted line* links Parkinson disease to the peripheral efferent group since Lewy bodies are present in both the parasympathetic and sympathetic ganglia, impairing peripheral autonomic function. See below for a discussion of specific disorders. *CCHS*, Congenital central hypoventilation syndrome; *HSAN*, hereditary sensory and autonomic neuropathy.

Funduscopic examination at the moment of visual change may show a striking diminution in the caliber of vessels in the eyegrounds. It is possible that blood-flow changes in the retinal vasculature contribute to the tunneling of vision in these patients. Intraocular pressure changes greatly in patients with dysautonomias, tracking low with upright posture and hypotension and high with supine posture and hypertension. Pupillary function itself is under autonomic control and therefore often dysfunctional in dysautonomias, but night blindness from inadequate dilation of the pupil in a dark environment is quite rare. Patients not infrequently voice slowness in their ability to adapt to rapidly changing light.

## Cardiovascular

Normally when one stands, systolic blood pressure falls about 10 mm Hg, and diastolic pressure increases 5 mm Hg. Heart rate rises 5–20 beats per minute (bpm). This is due to blood redistribution with gravity, with 300–800 mL of blood pooling in the lower extremities and splanchnic venous system. Therefore, the venous return to the heart decreases. This triggers a sympathetic cardiac and blood pressure response with increase in vascular tone, increase in heart rate and cardiac contractility, and a decrease in vagal activity (Freeman et al., 2011). The muscles in the legs also play a critical role in combination with the respiratory-abdominal muscles in enhancing venous return (Miller et al., 2005).

Several abnormal responses can happen when this system fails, either by defective cardiac output or decreased vasoconstriction. In the first 10–20 seconds after being upright, some subjects experience a blood pressure drop that can exceed 30% of the baseline pressure, termed "initial orthostatic hypotension." A reflex tachycardia follows and blood pressure usually recovers within 30–60 seconds. Subjects may complain of lightheadedness while initially upright and even lose consciousness (Stewart, 2013). A fall in blood pressure of 20/10 mm Hg or more in the first 3 minutes of standing defines *orthostatic hypotension* (OH; Freeman et al., 2011). Subjects with OH may or may not have symptoms (Arbogast et al., 2009). In subjects with supine hypertension, a drop in the systolic blood pressure of >30 mmHg may be a better criterion for diagnosis (Freeman et al., 2011).

In the absence of a fall in blood pressure of 20/10 on standing, if the patient is symptomatic and experiencing tachycardia, this is usually termed "orthostatic intolerance," qualifying as POTS if the heart rate rise is greater than 30 bpm in the first 10 minutes in the upright position and, in subjects less than 19 years, an increase of >40 bpm (Freeman et al., 2011; Schondorf and Low, 1993; Stewart et al., 2018). The most common symptoms of OH are dizziness, dimming of vision, and discomfort in the neck and head. OH is greatest, and hence most easily detected, in the hour after ingesting a large breakfast. Carbohydrate acts as a depressor more than protein or fat. It is important to note that a majority of patients with OH will not have the usual expected symptoms and may present with falls only (Arbogast et al., 2009), so it is vital not to solely rely on symptom reports in the elderly population. In the new Consensus Statement (Freeman et al., 2011), the term late OH describes a drop in blood pressure occurring after the first 3 minutes upright. The significance is still unclear and may represent an early form or milder form of sympathetic adrenergic failure (Gibbons and Freeman, 2006, 2015).

In the emergency room, the most common causes of acute hypotension may be bleeding, infection, and dehydration. However, even in this context, unless the loss of volume is so severe that the patient is going into shock, the diastolic pressure rise upon standing will exceed normal, resulting in a very narrowed pulse pressure and a marked tachycardia. This clearly contrasts with the drop in diastolic pressure seen with true OH due to autonomic failure. Chronic OH is rarely due to one of the causes of acute hypotension and is easily recognizable by (1) the clear drop in diastolic pressure that accompanies the systolic drop and (2) relative paucity of related symptoms. Chronic OH often reflects a serious underlying structural autonomic disorder with poor prognosis.

Among 100 consecutive patients seen for chronic OH at one center, about two-thirds had an identifiable structural dysautonomia. Causes included MSA (Shy-Drager syndrome), autonomic neuropathy, pure autonomic failure (PAF; Bradbury-Eggleston syndrome), several genetic disorders, amyloidosis, diabetes mellitus, or malignancy (especially bronchogenic carcinoma). Causes of hypotension in the face of normal autonomic function include antidepressant therapy, diuretic abuse, mast cell activation disorder, dumping syndrome, and deconditioning. It is noteworthy that congestive heart failure improves rather than impairs orthostatic tolerance. It is important to note that OH (but not POTS) generally carries with it a poor long-term prognosis. Another center recently reviewed the 10-year survival in their patients with both OH and delayed OH. In contrast to subjects without OH or with nonprogressive delayed OH with the expected mortality rate of <10%, those with OH had a 64% mortality, and those with delayed OH that progressed to true OH had a 50% mortality—the vast majority from synucleinopathies or diabetes (Gibbons and Freeman, 2015).

## Pulmonary

Lung function is generally preserved in autonomic failure. Patients with MSA frequently experience sleep apnea, and in consequence of these apneic spells, major perturbations in blood pressure may arise acutely. This is in part dependent on the role of carbon dioxide in determining blood pressure levels in autonomic failure. Hypoventilation increases blood pressure in autonomic failure, whereas hyperventilation may lower blood pressure significantly. Patients occasionally note improved orthostatic tolerance while breathing through a dead space, although this has never been a recommendation in practice. Because of impaired swallowing in patients with MSA (Seppi et al., 2005), aspiration pneumonia occurs frequently and can be missed because the patient may not manifest the expected fever. With early diagnosis and treatment of aspiration pneumonia, patients often do well, returning to their prior state of health. Orthostatic shortness of breath has been reported as a symptom in OH (Gibbons and Freeman, 2015) and is frequently voiced in clinic by patients with POTS, presumably due to inadequate filling of the lung apex with blood in standing posture.

## Gastrointestinal

Constipation occurs in many patients with autonomic failure, but patients with diabetic dysautonomia may also have frequent and often severe diarrhea as well as significant gastroparesis. The diarrhea itself can prevent adequate blood pressure control because of the associated volatility of blood volume. Special problems sometimes occur in specific dysautonomias. For example, patients with Sjögren syndrome commonly have gastroesophageal reflux and may therefore have an increased risk of esophageal carcinoma. Patients with Chagas disease may have achalasia and enlargement of the esophagus, resulting in vomiting. Achalasia is also present in the 4 "A" syndrome (Allgrove disease) characterized by alacrima, achalasia, adrenocorticotropic hormone (ACTH) insensitivity, and autonomic neuropathy. This syndrome has been mapped to chromosome 12q13 and is produced by mutations in the *AAAS* gene (Handschug et al., 2001). Patients with some forms of genetic autonomic failure may have strikingly severe gastrointestinal fluid loss and bowel movements 10 or more times every day, which sometimes responds to low doses of clonidine. Postprandial angina may occur with food ingestion, usually without associated ST–T wave changes. Most patients with postprandial angina in practice probably have some degree of dysautonomia, and the depressor effect of food is most prominent in the setting of impaired autonomic reflexes. Postprandial angina tends to occur with upright posture following food intake (especially carbohydrates). Water intake, in association with eating, will usually help prevent this symptom.

The gastrointestinal dysfunction in two disorders with significant autonomic involvement, namely PD and diabetes, has been better evaluated and understood. For example, the role of diabetes in gastrointestinal dysmotility has been extensively studied. Diabetes can affect any part of the gastrointestinal tract. Though usually present, esophageal dysmotility produces no symptoms. In the early stages of diabetes, subjects may develop rapid gastric emptying that then progresses to gastroparesis (Yarandi and Srinivasan, 2014). A common disorder in diabetic autonomic neuropathy, gastroparesis needs to be differentiated from the gastroparesis secondary to hyperglycemia (Fraser et al., 1990). Gastroparesis may appear suddenly in patients who develop an acute diabetic autonomic neuropathy, in a syndrome that may respond to immunomodulation (see the section on diabetes specifically). Subjects with diabetic neuropathy can also have poor gastric accommodation (fundus), which may account for bloating and early satiety (Samsom et al., 1998). Diabetes widely affects the gastrointestinal tract, termed diabetic gastroenteropathy. The cause is multifactorial. In diabetes, the microvascular complications affect the neuronal environment. This neuronal microenvironment is affected by chronic hyperglycemia, oxidative stress, changes in the microbiome, increased levels of fatty acids, and decreased levels of neurotransmitters. There is also smooth muscle myopathy, which also contributes to the gastrointestinal symptoms. Other changes in the function of the enteric nervous system in diabetes may result from apoptosis of enteric neurons, where oxidative stress may play a role. An imbalance also exists in inhibitory and excitatory neuropeptides. The sum total of these changes results in cellular damage, described as glucose neurotoxicity (Meldgaard et al., 2019). These factors then result in altered gut mucosa (Chandrasekharan and Srinivasan, 2007). PD is also associated with gastrointestinal problems, affecting swallowing processes that may lead to aspiration. Salivation is not increased or may even be decreased in these patients. From early on, individuals with PD may develop delayed gastric emptying, which later in the disease may affect jejunal absorption of L-dopa. Gastric emptying of liquids is usually not delayed (Goetze et al., 2006) in PD, so alternatives when giving L-dopa are a liquid solution or administering it directly into the jejunum (Jost, 2010). Constipation is also very common in this disorder and represents the most common "autonomic" manifestation of PD, affecting 70% to 80% of patients. Often, severe constipation develops before the more typical symptoms of PD are noticed (Jost, 2010; Korczyn, 1990); the cause is multifactorial. Many of the medications prescribed to treat PD, mainly anticholinergics and (perhaps more controversial) L-dopa, may worsen constipation, but they are not the cause, since constipation is usually present before the diagnosis of PD is made and therefore before the onset of medications. Constipation is thought to be due to the degeneration of central and peripheral parasympathetic nuclei (Jost, 2010). Lewy bodies are frequently present in the bowel plexuses (Braak et al., 2006).

Other less well-characterized dysautonomias also have gastrointestinal symptoms. Individuals with POTS complain of bloating, early satiety, nausea, abdominal pain, and alternating diarrhea and constipation (Sandroni et al., 1999). In fact, more than half of the children and adults with POTS have gastrointestinal complaints, often epigastric or lower-abdominal discomfort (Chelimsky and Chelimsky, 2018; Ojha et al., 2011). Children with POTS seem to suffer nausea and vomiting more often than adults, but these findings were present in both groups (Chelimsky et al., 2015; Ojha et al., 2011; Wang et al., 2015). Interestingly, coming from the other direction, many with functional gastrointestinal problems also have cardiovascular autonomic dysfunction—primarily sympathetic. In adults, three-eighths also had parasympathetic involvement, which was not present in the pediatric group. Neuropathy is common in both groups (Camilleri and Fealey, 1990; Chelimsky and Chelimsky, 2001). Importantly, when both a functional gastrointestinal disorder and POTS are present, the gastrointestinal symptoms may resolve with treatment of the orthostatic intolerance (Fortunato et al., 2014; Sullivan et al., 2005). The cause of the gastrointestinal symptoms in POTS in unclear and may be related to blood pooling in either the lower extremities or abdomen. Electrical activity of the stomach in POTS changes from supine to the upright position (Safder et al., 2009), suggesting either lack of accommodation or gastroparesis while upright (Buchwald et al., 1987). Cyclic vomiting syndrome (CVS) has also been associated with autonomic dysfunction, and both pediatric and adult sufferers usually have POTS associated with autonomic neuropathy (Chelimsky and Chelimsky, 2007; Venkatesan et al., 2010). IBS has been associated with reduced cardiovagal modulation (Mazurak et al., 2012), which improves with cognitive behavior therapy (Jang et al., 2017), suggesting its classification in the vagally mediated functional autonomic disorders.

## Urinary Tract

In structural disorders, a reversal of the usual pattern of urine output occurs. Nocturia is brought on by recumbency and the attendant increase in blood pressure (Mathias and Bannister, 2002). The weight loss during the night is often 2–4 pounds, and the reduction in blood volume that results partially accounts for the reduction in orthostatic tolerance seen on arising each morning. The bladder is often directly involved in dysautonomias. This autonomic involvement presents as urgency, retention, incontinence, and frequency. Urological evaluation often suggests prostatic hypertrophy in men, and surgery may be a consideration. Such surgery rarely helps patients with autonomic dysfunction and should only be considered after careful consultation between the urologist and neurologist to ascertain whether a physical obstruction is truly playing a major role. Unfortunately, the $\alpha_1$-antagonist class of drugs commonly used to treat prostatic hypertrophy can worsen OH; conversely, the $\alpha_1$-agonist midodrine, used to increase blood pressure, may occasionally increase bladder symptoms. With urine retention, urinary tract infections (UTIs) occur commonly. With autonomic failure, plasma renin levels are often quite low, probably because sympathetic regulation of the kidney is impaired. However, renal function is usually well preserved in most forms of autonomic failure, except in dopamine β-hydroxylase deficiency, in which significant renal failure occurs in adulthood.

Urinary symptoms in functional disorders manifest urgency and frequency more often than incontinence and retention. For example, although interstitial cystitis requires a minimum voiding frequency of 10–12 times per day (Petrikovets et al., 2019), some severely affected patients may void up to 60 times daily and are sometimes "bathroom bound." They complain of urgency, frequency, and bladder pain that worsens as the bladder fills. This likely reflects a functional rather than a structural autonomic change, since a study comparing autonomic testing in healthy females with age- and body mass index (BMI)-matched females with interstitial cystitis did not find any difference between the groups, except a higher heart rate at baseline without any significant difference in sudomotor, cardiac sympathetic, or parasympathetic response, suggesting either no difference between groups or a functional difference (Chelimsky et al., 2014). On the other hand, cardiovascular vagal outflow was reduced in patients with interstitial cystitis, suggesting the classification of this disorder with vagally mediated disorders such as IBS and the like (Chelimsky et al., 2019a, 2019b). In addition, interstitial cystitis differs from myofascial pelvic pain in the presence of a sympathetic autonomic neuropathy in the latter disorder (Chelimsky et al., 2016), suggesting its classification with the sympathetically mediated functional disorders (Chelimsky et al., 2019).

## Sexual Function

Erectile dysfunction is often the first sign of dysautonomia in men. Most commonly, this is predominantly parasympathetic in origin and proves very difficult to treat with medication. Sildenafil (Viagra), even when cautiously employed, may induce significant hypotension. Yohimbine may help the mildly affected patient. When a disorder involves sympathetic pathways only, such as dopamine β-hydroxylase deficiency, erectile function may be normal but retrograde ejaculation occurs. In these patients, therapy with droxidopa, which restores norepinephrine, may permit antegrade ejaculation. Little information exists concerning the effects of the autonomic system on female sexual function. However, menstrual function is usually normal, and in patients of childbearing age, conception and childbirth are frequent.

## Blood

With severe autonomic failure, mild anemia, often with hematocrit in the range of 33–38, is common. This is due to inadequate levels of erythropoietin and responds to treatment with this hormone. Adolescents with POTS were found to also have lower ferritin levels, lower iron storage, and mild anemia when compared to the general population. It is still unclear whether this association leads to POTS (Jarjour, 2013).

## Sweating Abnormalities

Increases or decreases in sweating occur with disturbances of autonomic thermoregulatory function (Fealey, 2008; Low, 1997). *Hyperhidrosis* refers to conditions in which sweating is excessive for a given stimulus. It can be generalized or focal. Hyperhidrosis can be primary (episodic hypothermia with hyperhidrosis, or Shapiro syndrome) or secondary to other disorders. Typically, hyperhidrosis is episodic. Dramatic hyperhidrosis may occur in pheochromocytoma. Tumors may produce cytokines, which provoke fever and subsequently sweating when the fever breaks. Hyperhidrosis also occurs in powerful sympathetic excitation, such as delirium tremens or in the pressor surges of baroreflex failure.

Referral for localized hyperhidrosis (Table 107.1) is often to the neurologist. Evidence exists of enhanced sweat gland innervation coupled with increased activity of sympathetic fibers passing through T2–T4. This is especially prominent in young people. Perhaps 25% of such individuals have a positive family history of hyperhidrosis. Axillary or palmar hyperhidrosis may be so severe as to become disabling for normal activities (inability to grip objects due to constant pouring wetness) and social interactions (embarrassment in shaking hands, wet shirts, etc.). Several therapeutic modalities may help (Table 107.2). A major limitation in therapy of hyperhidrosis is achieving sufficient muscarinic antagonism on sweat glands without incurring unacceptable levels of muscarinic blockade elsewhere—for example, in the heart. Local application of botulinum toxin to affected skin may also be quite effective but requires repeat injections at 3- to 12-month intervals (Saadia et al., 2001). In addition, blockade of the sympathetic ganglia using pharmacological injections, radiofrequency ablations, or endoscopic gangliotomy can be very effective (Atkinson and Fealey, 2003).

Idiopathic hyperhidrosis must be distinguished from compensatory hyperhidrosis due to lower body hypohidrosis, common in dysautonomias (Klein et al., 2003), which may paradoxically be described by patients as excessive sweating in the upper body. Patients who lose their ability to perspire over most of their body may preserve it in the neck and facial area and perspire disproportionately in these areas, which captures attention more than the loss of sweating elsewhere. In this setting, hyperhidrosis actually mandates an evaluation for the cause of the anhidrosis—usually a structural dysautonomia of some type. Loss of sweating does not require specific medical therapy, but rather practical advice such as staying well hydrated, avoiding alcohol, and avoiding hot conditions. One of the most effective home remedies is a "wet shirt"—a T-shirt soaked in warm water and wrung out thoroughly before putting on provides some artificial perspiration that lasts 30–90 minutes in a hot environment. The associated surface cooling is striking and greatly increases the functional capacity of patients who must be in a hot environment.

**TABLE 107.1 Pathological Hyperhidrosis Differential Diagnosis and Some Causes of Localized Hyperhidrosis**

| Condition | Pathophysiological Mechanism of Sweating |
|---|---|
| Essential hyperhidrosis | Excessive physiological and emotional sweating affecting hands, feet, and axillae:<br>• Type 1: rest of body sweats normally<br>• Type 2: coexists with large areas of anhidrosis; probable contribution from adrenergic-mediated sweating as well as cholinergic; symmetrical distribution |
| Perilesional and compensatory hyperhidrosis | Central and/or peripheral denervation of large numbers of sweat glands produces increased sweat secretion in those remaining innervated; often asymmetrical distribution |
| Gustatory sweating | Resprouting of secretomotor axons to supply denervated sweat glands |
| Post cerebral infarct | Loss of contralateral inhibition with cortical and upper brainstem infarction |
| Autonomic dysreflexia | Uninhibited segmental somatosympathetic reflex; recent drug prescription; includes nifedipine and sublingual captopril |
| Complex regional pain syndrome | Localized sympathetic sudomotor hyperactivity; probably axon reflex vs. direct irritation/infiltration of sympathetic preganglionic or postganglionic fibers |
| Paroxysmal localized hyperhidrosis | Myopathic: transiently decreased hypothalamic setpoint temperature; responsive to clonidine, a centrally acting, $\alpha_2$-adrenergic agonist |

# ASSESSMENT OF AUTONOMIC FUNCTION

More tests of autonomic function exist than for any other neurological system. Many of these tests are readily applied at the bedside, and though easy to perform, they may be difficult to interpret in an individual patient. Measures of any function are only as valuable as the solidity of the underlying normative data—an endeavor that requires significant time and resources. Therefore, most physicians who routinely follow patients with autonomic disorders develop a small armamentarium of well-validated tests that answer questions relating to the focus of their specialty. The neurologist assessing autonomic function requires tests that localize the lesion within the neuraxis and provide information about the types of fibers involved. Therefore, tests of peripheral and central sudomotor function and tests that differentiate sympathetic from parasympathetic cardiovascular function are

**TABLE 107.2 Treatment Measures for Primary Hyperhidrosis**

| | | |
|---|---|---|
| Topical Rx | 1. 20% Aluminum chloride hexahydrate in anhydrous ethyl alcohol (Drysol). Apply half-strength to dry skin daily or every other day, mornings, and wash off.<br>2. Glycopyrronium tosylate: 3.75% topical solution (Glaser et al., 2019) | 1. Irritation of skin; less effective on palms and soles, which may require occlusive (plastic wrap) technique<br>2. Dry mouth, blurred vision, local pain, pupillary dilation |
| Tanning Rx, iontophoresis | Glutaraldehyde (2%–10%) solution; apply 2–4 times/week as needed. | Stains skin brown; for soles of feet only |
| | For palms/soles; 15–30 mA current, 20 min. at start. Drionic battery-run unit or galvanic generator needed; 3–6 treatments/week for a total of 10–15 treatments initially; 1–2 treatments/week maintenance. | Shocks, tingling may occur. Difficult to use in axilla Drionic unit; not effective when batteries low |
| Anticholinergic | Glycopyrrolate (Robinul/Robinul Forte) at 1–2 mg PO tid as needed; for intermittent/adjunctive treatment. | Dry mouth, blurred vision, Contraindicated: glaucoma, GI tract obstruction, GU tract obstruction |
| Clonidine | Useful for paroxysmal localized (e.g., hemibody) hyperhidrosis; 0.1–0.3 mg PO tid or as TTS patch (0.1–0.3 mg/day) weekly. | Somnolence, hypotension, constipation, nausea, rash, impotence, agitation |
| Excision | Second and third thoracic ganglionic sympathectomy (palmar hyperhidrosis), sweat glands (axillary liposuction); recent preference is for T2 sympathectomy to limit compensatory hyperhidrosis. | Homer syndrome, dry skin, transient dysesthetic pain. Postoperative scar or infection. Compensatory hyperhidrosis of trunk, pelvis, legs, and feet |
| Botox | 50–100 mU of botulinum toxin A into each axilla or body area treated; high doses (200 mU) prolong effect; can be repeated. | Injection discomfort, variable. Duration of effect 3–12 months Expensive. Mild grip weakness when palm is treated. Contraindicated in pregnancy, NMJ disease |

*GI*, Gastrointestinal; *GU*, genitourinary; *mU*, mouse units; *NMJ*, neuromuscular junction; *PO*, orally; *Rx*, prescription; *tid*, three times daily.
*Adapted from Fealey, R.D., 2004. Disorders of sweating. In Robertson, D., Biaggioni, I., Burnstock, G., et al. (Eds.), Primer on the Autonomic Nervous System. 2nd edn. Elsevier, New York, pp. 354–357.*

essential. The cardiologist requires tests of blood pressure and heart rate that evaluate the mechanism of any cardiovascular dysregulation. The endocrinologist measures circulating catecholamines, corticoids, sex hormones, and renin. These tests are centered on appreciating the hormonal impact and consequences of autonomic dysfunction (Raj et al., 2005). The ophthalmologist tests pupillary function, and the pharmacologist uses drug tests that assess normal or hypersensitive autonomic function response (Robertson et al., 2004). Despite such dramatically divergent diagnostic approaches, it is remarkable how much consensus is often achieved in terms of the actual diagnosis and therapy of an individual patient. Indeed, an interdisciplinary approach that involves multiple specialists from different disciplines may provide both a broader perspective on organ-system involvement and more accurate diagnosis, and may be the reason more centers are taking this direction clinically.

Regardless of the clinical evaluation setting, a careful history is obviously the critical diagnostic resource. A brief listing of important items in questioning patients is shown in Box 107.1. More detailed discussions of some of these may be found elsewhere. Key autonomic features in the physical examination are shown in Box 107.2. In this section, attention is given to highly informative autonomic tests. Table 107.3 displays a listing of widely employed tests of baroreflex function.

## Orthostatic Test

Orthostatic symptoms are usually the most debilitating aspect of autonomic dysfunction readily amenable to therapy. For this reason, the blood pressure and heart rate responses to upright posture are the starting point of any autonomic laboratory evaluation. In healthy human subjects, the cardiovascular effect of upright posture has been well defined (Low, 1997). Upon active assumption of the upright posture by standing, the vigorous contraction of large muscles leads to a transitory muscle vasodilation and a minor fall in arterial pressure for which the reflexes do not immediately compensate. However, this short-lived depressor phase is not usually seen with passive (tilt-table) upright posture if not using beat-to-beat blood pressure monitoring. This is called *initial orthostatic hypotension*, which gets restored within 30–60 seconds (Stewart, 2013). Immediately after 70- or 90-degree head-up tilt, approximately 500 mL of blood move into the veins of the legs and approximately 250 mL into the buttocks and pelvic area. A rapid increase in heart rate occurs through vagal inhibition of the sinus node, followed by a sympathetically mediated further increase. As right ventricular stroke volume declines, a depletion of blood from the pulmonary reservoir occurs and central blood volume falls. Stroke volume falls, and cardiac output decreases by about 20%. With this decline in cardiac output, blood pressure is maintained by vasoconstriction that reduces splanchnic, renal, and skeletal muscle blood flow especially, but other circulations as well.

The orthostatic test may reveal two main classes of findings. An abnormally high increase in heart rate without a drop in blood pressure defines the functional disorder of POTS, while a drop in blood pressure, with or without an increase in heart rate, defines the structural disorder of OH. These two disorders may be viewed as separate and distinct disorders that generally do not constitute part of the same pathophysiological process. However, in a progressive autonomic neuropathy, one may find a spectrum of autonomic impairment. Early, mild autonomic impairment may manifest as tachycardia, with relatively little change in blood pressure. In the presence of a still-functioning baroreflex, the increased heart rate can compensate for mild peripheral denervation, thus preventing a significant decrement in blood pressure. With moderate autonomic neuropathy, the tachycardia may still be present but may be unable to compensate completely, and mild OH may occur. As the neuropathy becomes more severe, the orthostatic fall in blood pressure becomes progressively greater, and the ability of the efferent autonomic system to manifest a tachycardia is progressively attenuated. In severe autonomic failure, the fall in blood pressure may be greater than 100 mm Hg, yet the heart rate rises little or not at all. Orthostatic tolerance is challenged by a number of factors. Important among them are food ingestion, high environmental temperature, hyperventilation, endogenous vasodilators, and many

**BOX 107.1 Key Features in the Autonomic History**

**Orthostatic Intolerance or Hypotension**
Dizziness or lightheadedness
Visual changes
Neck and shoulder discomfort
Weakness
Confusion
Slurred speech
Presyncope or syncope
Postprandial angina pectoris
Nausea
Palpitations
Tremulousness
Flushing sensation
Nocturia

**Worsened by the Following**
Bed rest
Food ingestion
Alcohol
Fever
Hot weather/environment
Hot bath
Exercise
Hyperventilation

**Hypohidrosis**
Dry skin
Dry socks and feet
Reduced skin wrinkling
Excessive sweating in intact regions

**Genitourinary Dysautonomia**
Impotence
Nocturia
Urine retention
Urinary incontinence
Recurrent urinary tract infection

**Gastrointestinal Dysautonomia**
Constipation
Postprandial fullness
Anorexia
Diarrhea
Fecal urgency and incontinence
Weight loss

**Poorly Characterized Dysautonomia Features**
Early transient autonomic hyperfunction
Anemia
Ptosis
Supine nasal stuffiness
Supine hypertension and diuresis
Fatigue

**Nonautonomic Features in Multiple System Atrophy**
Problems with balance/movement
Loud respirations/snoring
Episodic gasping respirations
Sleep apnea
Brief crying spells
Emotional lability
Leg pain
Altered libido
Hypnagogic leg jerking
Hallucinations
Difficulty swallowing
Aspiration pneumonia
Drooling
Other cerebellar and extrapyramidal symptoms

pharmacological agents. If no abnormality in orthostatic blood pressure or heart rate is detected in the hour after ingestion of a large meal, autonomic neuropathy of sufficient severity to cause cardiovascular instability is effectively excluded.

An important aspect of evaluating responses to orthostasis is the rapid reduction in total blood volume that occurs physiologically. It is not unusual for a 12% fall in plasma volume to occur within 10 minutes of the assumption of the upright posture as fluid moves from the vascular compartment into the extravascular space (Jacob et al., 2005). This accounts for the delay in the appearance of symptoms in patients with mild autonomic impairment for some minutes after the actual assumption of upright posture. Therefore, the long-stand (30 minutes) test, or Schellong test, is a much more severe orthostatic stress than the short-stand (5 minutes) test commonly employed.

**BOX 107.2 Key Features in the Autonomic Physical Examination**

**Skin**
Dry skin
Dry socks and feet
Reduced hand wrinkling
Absent pilomotor reaction
Pallor

**Eyes**
Impaired pupillary motor function
Dryness of eyes (redness and itching)
Ptosis

**Cardiovascular**
Low standing blood pressure ± tachycardia
Unchanging pulse rate on standing
Increased supine blood pressure
Loss of respiratory arrhythmia

**Gastrointestinal**
Reduced salivation
Stomach fullness
Reduced transit time
Impaired anal tone

**Genitourinary**
Impaired morning erection
Retrograde ejaculation
Urinary urgency
Sphincter weakness
Atonic bladder

**Other**
Abnormal temperature regulation
Extrapyramidal signs (rigidity > tremor)
Cerebellar signs
Impaired ocular movements
Slurred speech
Laryngeal paralysis
Muscle wasting

**TABLE 107.3 Tests of Baroreflex Function**

| Test | Afferent | Integration | Efferent | Response |
|---|---|---|---|---|
| Orthostasis | IX, X, CNS | Medulla | Autonomic | ↑HR |
| Deep breathing | X | Medulla | X | ↑HR (inspiration) |
| Valsalva maneuver | IX, X, CNS | Medulla | Autonomic | ↑HR, then ↓HR |
| Cuff occlusion | IX, X | Medulla | Autonomic | ↓BP, ↑HR |
| Saline infusion | IX, X | Medulla | Autonomic | ↑BP, ↓HR |
| Barocuff (suction) | IX | Medulla | X | ↓HR |
| Barocuff (pressure) | IX | Medulla | X | ↑HR |
| LBNP | IX, X | Medulla | Autonomic | ↑HR |
| Carotid massage | IX | Medulla | Autonomic | ↓HR, ↓BP |
| Phenylephrine | IX, X | Medulla | Autonomic | ↓HR |
| Nitroprusside | IX, X | Medulla | Autonomic | ↑HR |

*BP*, Blood pressure; *CNS*, central nervous system; *HR*, heart rate; *IX*, glossopharyngeal nerve; *LBNP*, lower-body negative pressure; *X*, vagus nerve.

### Tilt-Table Testing

Many investigators prefer the use of upright tilt to the orthostatic test to evaluate these variables. In general, analogous but not identical results are obtained. The use of upright tilt is widely used in syncope evaluation. Although no proof exists that upright tilt offers any diagnostic advantage over carefully obtained standing blood pressure and heart rate data, many investigators use tilt because of its convenience, its capacity to calibrate the gravity stimulus, its embrace by third-party payers, and its safety to the patient. In addition, the tilt test may add sensitivity if done at 70 degrees or less, by reducing the activity of the calf and thigh muscle pump and by preventing any CNS stimulus to vasoconstriction that would occur with active standing.

### Sweat Testing

Although hypohidrosis rarely dominates a patient's dysautonomia, assessment of sudomotor function is often helpful in testing for autonomic impairment (Low, 2004). Widely used tests include the thermoregulatory sweat test (TST), quantitative sudomotor axon reflex test (QSART), and sympathetic skin response (SSR).

#### Thermoregulatory Sweat Test

The TST is a sensitive semiquantitative test of sweating (Fealey et al., 1989). After a color indicator (quinizarin powder or povidone-iodine) is applied to the skin, the environmental temperature is increased until an adequate core temperature rise is attained (usually a 2°C rise in core temperature or a core temperature of 38.5°C, whichever is less) and the presence of sweating causes a change in the indicator. Thermal stimulation using infrared radiant heat lamps to directly heat the skin is also employed to provide more effective sweat stimulus. Estimating the percent of anterior surface anhidrosis quantitates the results, and the sweat rates may be measured as well. This test has also been helpful in assessing the status of dysautonomias over time. Some characteristic patterns of anhidrosis include (1) the peripheral pattern of distal anhidrosis, seen in distal small-fiber neuropathy and length-dependent axonal neuropathy; (2) the central patterns of distal sparing or segmental involvement, generally seen in MSA or PD; and (3) a sudotomal pattern suggesting involvement at the root or ganglion level, seen in disorders involving nerve roots or specific ganglia, such as diabetes, Sjögren disease, and PAF. The TST pattern is therefore helpful in distinguishing between postganglionic, preganglionic, and central lesions.

#### Quantitative Sudomotor Axon Reflex Test

The physiological basis of the QSART is elicitation of an axon reflex mediated by the postganglionic sympathetic sudomotor axon (Low, 2004). Acetylcholine (ACh) activates the axon terminal. The impulse travels antidromically, reaches a branch point, then travels orthodromically to release ACh from the nerve terminal. ACh traverses the neuroglandular junction and binds to $M_3$ muscarinic receptors on eccrine sweat glands to evoke the sweat response. The QSART specifically evaluates the functional status of postganglionic sympathetic axons.

Current is applied to one compartment of a multicompartmental sweat cell, and the sweat response is recorded from a second compartment with a sudorometer. The multicompartmental sweat cells are attached to sites on the upper and lower limbs. This distribution permits the detection of dysfunction localizable to one specific peripheral nerve territory or of a length-dependent autonomic neuropathy. An absent response indicates a lesion of the postganglionic axon. Milder axonal damage may be associated with persistent sweating or with a "hung-up" response. Many length-dependent neuropathies manifest a maximal reduction in sweat volumes distally. In most preganglionic or central disorders, the QSART is spared, although with increasing duration of the preganglionic lesion, the response may become abnormal.

#### Sympathetic Skin Response

The SSR requires the integrity of hypothalamic, brainstem, and spinal circuits, as well as postganglionic sympathetic neurons. It is performed by applying a strong electrical stimulus to the median nerve, while a long-time course (≈2 seconds) recording of skin potential is made in the contralateral palm and sole. The potential change linked to the median nerve stimulus is generated in the skin by the activation of sweat glands. Following a latency period, the typical response includes a negative (upward) deflection followed by a positive (downward) correction over several hundred milliseconds. It fatigues easily and is not always reproducible in any given individual. The SSR is usually recorded as present or absent in the hand and in the foot.

### Pharmacological Tests

Information about prevailing sympathetic and parasympathetic activation as well as denervation hypersensitivity can be achieved by the use of muscarinic and adrenergic agonists and antagonists (Robertson et al., 2004). Tables 107.4 and 107.5 provide instructive examples of how biochemical and physiological tests may be combined to make novel diagnostic discoveries.

## FUNCTIONAL AUTONOMIC DISORDERS

Functional autonomic disorders are a heterogeneous group of disorders where autonomic nervous system involvement exists, but the role of autonomic dysregulation in the pathogenesis of symptoms is unclear. Included in this group are functional gastrointestinal disorders (FGIDs), interstitial cystitis, migraine, CVS, fibromyalgia, and chronic fatigue syndrome. Many of these disorders tend to coexist in the same person. For example, about 40% of individuals with migraines have symptoms of IBS and chronic aches and pains that could represent fibromyalgia (Chelimsky et al., 2009). In our experience, children with functional gastrointestinal problems have severe fatigue, headaches, and sleep problems (Ojha et al., 2011). Whitehead et al. (2002) found a high association of FGID with fibromyalgia, chronic fatigue syndrome, temporomandibular joint disorder, and chronic pelvic pain. These disorders are now classified as chronic overlapping pain conditions (COPCs). These disorders are very common, and the prevalence from these individual COPCs ranges from 4 to 44 million based on the evaluation of cross-sectional studies (Maixner et al., 2016). A new classification of these COPCs was recently proposed, with some disorders vagally mediated and others sympathetically medicated (Chelimsky et al., 2019), as discussed in the introduction. Often POTS is a common denominator. By report, about 50% of persons with CVS and 40% with migraine report symptoms of orthostatic intolerance (Sullivan et al., 2005). Chelimsky et al. (2009) reported 24 pediatric subjects with functional gastrointestinal syndrome and either POTS or syncope, or both. Chronic fatigue has also been described in association with POTS (Hoad et al., 2008). Patients and practitioners may find it convenient to attribute all the COPCs with the POTS label. This concept is erroneous since POTS as a syndrome only includes those symptoms that develop in the upright position and resolve or greatly improve in the supine position. This concept can also lead to frustration in management.

### Reflex Syncope

Although reflex syncope is probably the most common cause of loss of consciousness, it is useful to consider the more global group of disorders that fall under "transient loss of consciousness." This

TABLE 107.4 **Tests of Neurotransmitter Receptor Responsiveness**

| Name | Administration | Receptor | Response |
|---|---|---|---|
| **Agonists** | | | |
| Phenylephrine | IV, eye | $\alpha 1$ | Pressor; pupillary dilation |
| Clonidine | Oral | $\alpha_2$, I | Depressor (central); MSNA |
| Isoproterenol | IV | $\beta_1$ | Increased HR |
| Isoproterenol | IV local | $\beta_2$ | Depressor; vascular resistance |
| Acetylcholine | IV local | Muscarinic | Decreased vascular resistance |
| Methacholine | Eye | Muscarinic | Pupillary constriction |
| Nicotine | IV | Nicotinic | Increased HR |
| **Antagonists** | | | |
| Phentolamine | IV | $\alpha_1$, $\alpha_2$ | Depressor |
| Yohimbine | IV | $\alpha_2$ | Increased BP, plasma NE |
| Propranolol | IV | $\beta_1$ | Reduced HR |
| Propranolol | IV local | $\beta_2$ | Increased vascular resistance |
| Atropine | IV | Muscarinic | Increased HR |
| Trimethaphan | IV | Nicotinic | Depressor; MSNA |
| **Neurotransmitter-Releasing Agents** | | | |
| Tyramine | IV | $\alpha$, $\beta$ | Increased BP, plasma NE |
| Hydroxyamphetamine | Eye | $\alpha_1$ | Pupillary dilation |
| **Pheochromocytoma-Provoking Agents** | | | |
| Histamine | IV | $\alpha_1$, $\beta$ | Increased BP, plasma NE |
| Glucagon | IV | $\alpha_1$, $\beta$ | Increased BP, plasma NE |

*BP*, Blood pressure; *HR*, heart rate; *I*, imidazoline; *IV*, intravenous; *MSNA*, muscle sympathetic nerve activity; *NE*, norepinephrine.

TABLE 107.5 **Other Autonomic Tests**

| Test | Afferent | Integration | Efferent | Response |
|---|---|---|---|---|
| Cold pressor | Pain fibers | CNS | Sympathoadrenal | ↑BP |
| Handgrip | Muscle afferents | CNS | Autonomic | ↑BP, ↑HR |
| Mental arithmetic | CNS | CNS | Sympathoadrenal | ↑BP |
| Startle | Auditory | CNS | Sympathoadrenal | ↑BP, ↑HR |
| Face immersion | V | Medulla | Autonomic | ↓HR |
| Pupil cycle time | Optic nerve | Edinger-Westphal | III | Dilate/constrict |
| Venous response venoconstriction (inspiratory gasp) | Spinal nerve | Cord | Sympathetic | |
| Venoarterial reflex vasoconstriction | Noradrenergic axon | Neuron | Noradrenergic axon | |
| Reflex heating | Spinothalamic | Hypothalamus | Sympathetic | Vasodilation |
| Thermoregulatory | Temperature receptors | Hypothalamus | Sympathetic | Sweating |
| QSART | Sympathetic cholinergic axon | Neuron | Sympathetic cholinergic axon | Sweating |

*BP*, Blood pressure; *CNS*, central nervous system; *HR*, heart rate; *III*, oculomotor nerve; *QSART*, quantitative sudomotor axon reflex test; *V*, trigeminal nerve.

differential diagnosis can be narrowed through three key decision points. First, the clinician must understand whether true loss of consciousness occurred, with consequent loss of memory for a short time period. If this is not the case, considerations include a fall, a vertiginous spell, an episode of near loss of consciousness, and a pseudoseizure, but not true syncope. However, if consciousness was lost, the second consideration is whether the cause was loss of brain perfusion. If this is not the case, syncope is again excluded, and possible etiologies include a true epileptic seizure (often marked by motor manifestations, lateral tongue biting, eyes open during the episode, and a prolonged postictal period), syncopal migraine (usually followed by a throbbing headache accompanied by photophobia, phonophobia, and nausea; Curfman et al., 2012), or a disorder of cerebrospinal fluid (CSF) flow (e.g., colloid cyst of the third ventricle).

When loss of perfusion is the cause of loss of consciousness, the broad diagnosis is syncope, and the third issue is determining the cause, such as cardiac arrhythmia, pulmonary embolus, or cardiovascular structural cause, or true reflex vasodilation. Only the last entity is termed *reflex syncope*. Reflex syncope (transient loss of consciousness due to loss of brain perfusion as a protective reflex) occurs at least once in 50% of healthy young adults, usually as an emotional faint with a well-recognized precipitating stimulus. Such syncope requires no medical evaluation. Syncope in the absence of a precipitating stimulus is a relatively common medical problem encountered in the office and emergency department.

Syncope is defined as a transient loss of consciousness secondary to a transient global cerebral hypoperfusion, which is of rapid onset, short duration, and spontaneous complete recovery (Moya, 2009). The guideline for the diagnosis and management of syncope emphasizes two aspects in the definition: (1) loss of consciousness and (2) being transient. The loss of consciousness is also short, usually less than 20 seconds, and recovery is very fast. When a syncopal episode is transient and nontraumatic, the causes include syncope, epilepsy, psychogenic syncope, and miscellaneous factors. The guidelines divide syncope into four groups: (1) vasovagal, produced by either orthostatic stress or emotionally mediated (fear, blood phobia, etc.); (2) situational, which can be triggered by exercise, defecation, postprandial, visceral pain cough, and so forth; (3) carotid sinus syncope; and (4) atypical without an apparent trigger or with an atypical presentation (Moya, 2009). Fainting is also classified based on the efferent branch of the autonomic nervous system most involved, sympathetic or parasympathetic. When the symptom that predominates is hypotension, syncope is usually labeled as "vasodepressor syncope" and is thought to be triggered by a lack of vasoconstriction when upright. When the symptom that predominates is bradycardia with or without a cardiac pause, syncope is usually classified as "cardioinhibitory reflex." If both efferent branches are involved, syncope is usually classified as mixed (Moya, 2009). However, at least one report suggests that both (parasympathetic and sympathetic) signals occur in every single episode (Téllez et al., 2009). Fainting is very common. In a study of medical students and their family members, 32% of the students had at least one episode of fainting in their lives. Females faint more often than males (40% vs.3 25%), and the fainting usually started during adolescence, with a mean age of 14 years. Fainting starts to increase around the age of 7 years, then increases drastically in adolescence and early adulthood, but only about 6% had their first episode of fainting after the age of 40 years. If the mother faints, the offspring of any gender is at higher risk of fainting, but if the father faints, only the sons have increased risk of fainting (Serletis et al., 2006). Clonic jerks and convulsions can happen with syncope, but there is no seizure activity associated with the abnormal movements (Stewart, 2013).

Syncope accounts for more than 1% of hospital admissions. The causes of syncope range from benign to life threatening. The common underlying mechanism of syncope is the transitory decrease in cerebral perfusion. Reflex syncope (fainting) is the most common type of syncope, especially in patients without evidence of structural heart disease (Benditt et al., 2006; Strickberger et al., 2006). Reflex syncope most commonly occurs while the patient is standing but also occurs while seated and occasionally even while lying during sleep (Jardine et al., 2006).

Unlike most conditions discussed in this chapter, reflex syncope is episodic. Between episodes, most patients appear to have normal cardiovascular function. The precise cause of reflex syncope is not understood. A clinical diagnosis can be made with a history and physical examination alone in most cases. Usually the focus is on excluding more malignant causes of syncope, especially by defining circumstances surrounding the episode of syncope, assessing symptoms before and after the event, and obtaining any collateral history from witnesses. The history may sometimes implicate structural heart disease or coexisting medical conditions that point away from reflex syncope. Worrisome features include absence of a warning, occurrence during exercise (as opposed to the cool-down period), prolonged period of loss of consciousness, and any focal neurological sign or symptom. Medications may provoke syncope, and a family history of sudden death may point to an arrhythmic cause. Historical features suggesting reflex syncope include female gender, younger age, associated warmth and diaphoresis, nausea or palpitation, and postsyncopal fatigue. A long interval between spells (from the first lifetime spell) also suggests reflex syncope.

The physical examination should focus on ruling out structural heart disease and focal neurological lesions. One widely used maneuver is carotid sinus massage. The current technique involves performing up to 10 seconds of massage to the carotid sinus in both the supine and upright posture, with a positive result requiring a drop in blood pressure or heart rate with an associated reproduction of presenting symptoms. This procedure is associated with a low rate of neurological complications, but can result in stroke if an active plaque or critical stenosis is present in the carotid being compressed.

Tilt-table testing has been widely used in evaluating syncope since the late 1980s. These tests subject patients to head-up tilt at angles of 60–80 degrees and aim to induce either syncope or intense presyncope, with reproduction of presenting symptoms. Passive tilt tests simply use upright tilt for up to 45 minutes to induce vasovagal syncope (sensitivity ≈ 40%, specificity ≈ 90%). Provocative tilt tests use a combination of orthostatic stress and drugs such as isoproterenol, nitroglycerin, or adenosine to provoke syncope with a slightly higher sensitivity but reduced specificity. Little agreement exists about the best protocol, and protocols are used increasingly less. Many physicians are more comfortable treating patients if a diagnosis is suggested by a tilt-table test. Recent studies with implantable loop recorders have called the value of tilt testing into question. The International Study on Syncope of Uncertain Etiology (ISSUE) investigators have recently reported that in the absence of significant structural heart disease, patients with tilt-positive syncope and tilt-negative syncope have similar patterns of recurrence (34% in each group over a follow-up of 3–15 months), with electrocardiographic (ECG) recording during episodes consistent with reflex syncope. Despite these recent data, tilt-table testing is still frequently used to evaluate recurrent reflex syncope. Tilt tests are relatively contraindicated in patients with severe aortic or mitral stenosis or critical coronary or cerebral artery stenosis.

Some people with reflex syncope faint only once or twice and rarely seek medical attention. Medical attention is usually sought for syncope when it becomes a recurring and troublesome disorder. Most patients do very well after assessment, with only a 25%–30% likelihood of syncope recurrence after tilt testing in patients who receive neither drugs nor a device. The cause for this apparently great reduction in syncope frequency may be spontaneous remission, reassurance, or advice about the pathophysiology of syncope and postural maneuvers to prevent it. However, patients with a greater frequency of historical syncopal spells are more likely to faint in follow-up. The time to the first recurrence of syncope after tilt testing is a simple and individualized measure of eventual syncope frequency, because those patients who faint early after a tilt test tend to continue to faint more frequently.

Many patients can simply be reassured about the usual benign course of reflex syncope and instructed to avoid those situations that precipitate fainting. The use of support stockings or increased salt intake may help. In young nonhypertensive patients, the most frequently affected, we utilize 2 g of salt in the morning and 2 g in the early afternoon. Most salt is excreted by a normal kidney within 3–4 hours. Patients should be taught to recognize an impending faint and urged to lie down (or sit down if that is not possible) quickly. This will not be enough for some patients, and other treatment options such as physical countermaneuvers (Wieling et al., 2004) and tilt training (Ector et al., 1998) may be necessary. These are covered in detail in the treatment section of the chapter, as are pharmacological and other interventions.

## Syncopal Migraine

A subgroup of patients with syncope respond poorly to the usual management of salt supplementation and tilt training. On further questioning, these patients may consistently experience a headache with migrainous features immediately prior to or after the syncopal spell. A recent review suggests that this entity, sometimes also termed *basilar migraine*, may be far more common than previously suspected, accounting for about one-third of patients with syncope referred to an autonomic specialist (presumably a more complex group of patients based on the referral bias; Curfman et al., 2012). The importance of identifying this diagnosis is its prompt response to antimigrainous medications such as verapamil and topiramate, in our experience. Further identifying features include an increased duration of loss of consciousness (up to 15 minutes in this series) and longer time to full recovery, as might be expected in a migrainous mechanism.

## Carotid Sinus Hypersensitivity

*Carotid sinus hypersensitivity* is defined as an asystole of 3 seconds, a fall in systolic pressure of 50 mm Hg, or both in response to carotid artery massage in a patient with otherwise unexplained dizziness or syncope (Fenton et al., 2000; Mathias et al., 2001). Estimates are that 35–100 patients per million per year present with this condition. Although the condition has been ensconced in the medical literature since the era of Soma Weiss (1898–1942), its definition remains controversial, in part because diagnosis is by manual massage of the carotid sinus, with its inherent variability. The test should be performed with the patient supine during continuous ECG and blood pressure monitoring and recording. Longitudinal massage should be performed for 5 seconds over the site of maximal pulsation of the right carotid sinus, located between the superior border of the thyroid cartilage and the angle of the mandible. If no response is elicited, the massage is sometimes repeated on the left side supine and ultimately also on the right and then left sides with upright tilt. Unfortunately, improved practical methods for diagnosis have not emerged. Clinically, a history may exist of syncopal symptoms associated with neck pressure, a tight collar, turning the head, shaving, or swallowing; syncope may also occur spontaneously. Hypotension, bradycardia, or both may dominate the clinical picture. The form in which bradycardia predominates may be improved by demand pacing. Some patients with carotid sinus syncope ultimately require surgical denervation. Occasionally, additional symptoms of headache, dizziness, vertigo, paresthesias, homonymous hemianopsia, and hemiplegia occur in the absence of measured blood pressure or heart rate change, but this may reflect another mechanism, such as a migrainous or ischemic process; the older literature terms this phenomenon *Weiss-Baker syndrome*.

Keep in mind that carotid sinus massage is not without risk. In our practice, we encounter a patient every 2 or 3 years who suffers a large stroke immediately after massage on the appropriate side. This presumably reflects an undetected active atherosclerotic plaque with some clot accumulation. We therefore recommend ultrasound of the carotid prior to performing carotid sinus massage on anyone older than age 40.

## Gravity-Induced Loss of Consciousness

Gravity-induced loss of consciousness (G-LOC; acceleration stress) during aerial maneuvers is a special kind of syncope seen occasionally in aircraft pilots when the aircraft pulls up quickly after descent, during which gravitational forces may be greatly increased. G-LOC occurs in at least 25% of pilots flying high-performance aircraft. Incapacitation of 30 seconds or longer may cause fatal accidents during aerial combat maneuvers. Because pilots are in an upright seated position, the vertical distance between the head and the heart is approximately 14 inches (35 cm). At about 4G, without an antigravity suit or use of the antigravity straining maneuver, blood flow to the brain will cease, and the individual loses consciousness and may then experience jerking movements of the arms or legs. With resolution of acceleration stress, consciousness recovers over the succeeding 10–60 seconds, but confusion may persist for 1–2 minutes, and impaired pilot performance may persist considerably longer.

## Postural Tachycardia Syndrome

POTS is defined as an increase of at least 30 bpm on standing (>40 bpm in subjects <19 years of age; Singer et al., 2012), associated with symptoms of sympathetic activation (Freeman et al., 2002; Jacob et al., 2000; Low, 1997). Orthostatic symptoms include light-headedness, palpitations, tremulousness, visual changes, discomfort or throbbing of the head, poor concentration, tiredness, weakness, and occasionally fainting. Usually, little or no fall in blood pressure occurs on standing (Shibao et al., 2005), and this characteristic should probably be incorporated into the definition. Patients may also have an elevated plasma norepinephrine concentration of 600 pg/mL or more on standing. Standing plasma norepinephrine levels greater than 2000 pg/mL occur, and such patients require careful study to exclude pheochromocytoma. Many POTS patients also have a bluish-red discoloration of skin in the lower extremities on standing. A reduced plasma volume of about 500 mL is often present.

POTS is estimated to affect 250,000–500,000 Americans and causes a wide range of disabilities (Benrud-Larson et al., 2002). A 4:1 female preponderance exists, typically in the 15- to 45-year age group. Symptom severity is sometimes catamenial. Possible reasons for these cyclical changes include an estrogen-dependent change in plasma volume or a direct estrogen receptor-mediated modulation of vascular reactivity. Other than essential hypertension, POTS is the most common chronic disorder of cardiovascular homeostasis. It is commonly encountered and accounts for frequent referrals to centers specializing in autonomic disorders.

The etiology of POTS is unknown; indeed, the condition has many different names (Box 107.3) and probably many causes. For many years, such patients were considered deconditioned and encouraged to pursue a vigorous exercise regimen. Although such regimens can be quite effective (Fu et al., 2010), it is nonetheless clear that the disorder did not arise from mere deconditioning. The onset of POTS may be abrupt, suddenly disabling a prior marathon runner or Olympic athlete, and often occurs in the wake of a viral infection, pregnancy, or

**BOX 107.3 Postural Tachycardia Syndrome: Alternative Names**

- Hyperadrenergic orthostatic hypotension
- Orthostatic tachycardia syndrome
- Orthostatic intolerance
- Postural orthostatic tachycardia syndrome
- Hyperadrenergic postural hypotension
- Hyperdynamic β-adrenergic state
- Idiopathic hypovolemia
- Orthostatic tachycardia plus
- Sympathicotonic orthostatic hypotension
- Mitral valve prolapse syndrome
- Soldier's heart
- Vasoregulatory asthenia
- Neurocirculatory asthenia
- Irritable heart
- Orthostatic anemia

major surgical procedure, encouraging consideration of an autoimmune etiology.

It is important to view POTS not as a disease but as a syndrome—a final common pathway by which many pathophysiological processes may present. The fundamental deficit appears to be anything that reduces the effectiveness of venous return to the heart. Some of these are simple mechanical problems that do not involve the autonomic nervous system at all, such as the congenital absence of venous valves or hypermobility disorders (e.g., Ehlers-Danlos syndrome; Gazit et al., 2003; Rowe et al., 1999), where presumably an inadequate recoil of venous elastic tissue exists to propel adequate volume back to the great veins. Other observations in patients with POTS have included the presence of autonomic neuropathy, termed *neuropathic postural tachycardia syndrome* (Al-Shekhlee et al., 2005), and the presence of very high adrenergic responsiveness, termed *hyperadrenergic postural tachycardia syndrome*, as shown in Fig. 107.2. It is not clear if these two processes are mutually exclusive. Other investigators have divided POTS into low, normal, and high blood-flow rates (Fouad et al., 1986; Stewart et al., 2007) and have found different levels of venous compliance in the three types.

Other potential pathophysiological causes include excessive venous pooling, a gravity-dependent fluid shift, diminished plasma volume or red cell mass, and dysfunction of the norepinephrine transporter. In rare specific cases, a genetic disorder has been identified. The clearest example is the illustrative but quite rare form of POTS due to norepinephrine transporter deficiency. This derives from a unique A453P mutation yielding loss of gene function. The norepinephrine transporter clears norepinephrine from the synaptic cleft. Its absence leads to a rise in synaptic and plasma norepinephrine levels with sympathetic hyperactivity (Shannon et al., 2000).

Mastocytosis may underlie POTS in some individuals (Shibao et al., 2005). The cause may be an increased number or an increased

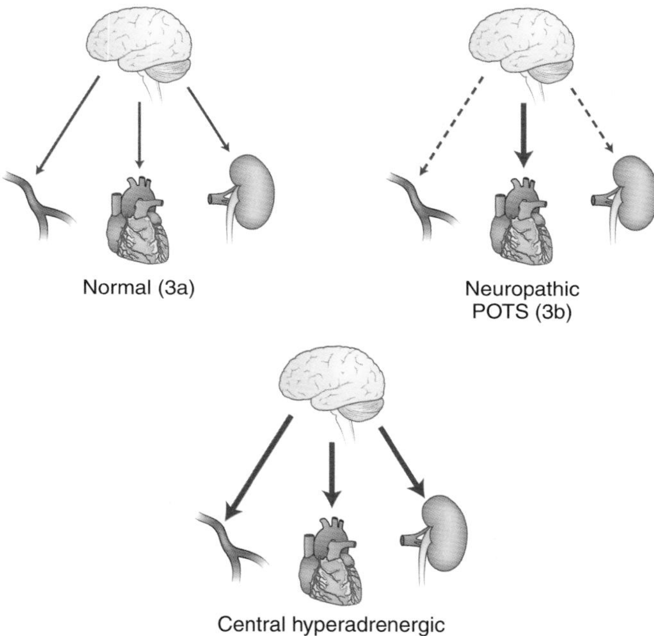


**Fig. 107.2** Pathophysiological schema in postural tachycardia syndrome (*POTS:* two of the most clearly established etiologies. Compared to normal brain control over vasculature, heart, and kidney, in neuropathic POTS, there is partial denervation that leads to relative sparing of heart-rate effects of central stimulation. In hyperadrenergic POTS, there is increased central sympathetic outflow to multiple structures, without peripheral denervation.

responsiveness of mast cells. Release of histamine and prostaglandin $D_2$ into the circulation dominate the clinical picture. Characteristic chronic skin changes (erythematous acneiform papular lesions) occur in a minority of patients, but red flushing and urticaria are common during attacks. Palpitations, with or without chest pain, headaches, nausea, vomiting, diarrhea, and dyspnea, may occur. Perhaps 25% of cases are familial (autosomal dominant). Many patients respond well to treatment with $H_1$ and $H_2$ antagonists, but some have severe attacks with hypotension, requiring treatment by epinephrine infusion. Increases in blood pressure also occur. During severe attacks, disturbances in mental status may seem out of proportion to the hypotension. Patients may also seem to be unconscious for 5–20 minutes after syncope, but they may indicate after recovery that they heard what was said to them in the minutes after syncope but were unable to speak or reply to questions. Along with histamine and prostaglandin $D_2$, substantial quantities of heparin are present in mast cells; during attacks, sometimes enough heparin is released to increase the partial thromboplastin time.

Many patients with POTS have a relatively mild disorder that may improve over succeeding weeks and months. However, in some, the symptoms are more severe, the duration of the illness may be longer, and the expected recovery may not occur. Overall, the majority of patients with POTS improve sufficiently to require no therapy after 5 years.

POTS is not a stand-alone disorder. Although specific data are still forthcoming, POTS has several comorbidities in both children and adults, such as chronic fatigue syndrome (Freeman and Komaroff, 1997; Schondorf and Freeman, 1999) and migraine. Most patients with POTS have multisystem involvement including sleep problems, upper and lower gastrointestinal complaints, headaches with migrainous features, chronic pain in various locations, Raynaud-like symptoms, and severe fatigue (Ojha et al., 2011). POTS highlights the striking contrast between structural and functional autonomic disorders. Patients with this disorder generally voice many complaints involving several systems, whereas those with severe OH (mean fall of 90 mm Hg in systolic blood pressure) frequently have minimal or no symptoms at all (Arbogast et al., 2009).

The interactions of deconditioning, sleep disturbance, chronic fatigue, and POTS itself are difficult to assess. Perhaps more challenging is the fact that many patients with POTS respond to their illness by reducing physical activity, and upon presentation to physicians, they therefore have POTS *and* are deconditioned. In individual patients, several therapies may prove helpful (Shannon et al., 2002), including propranolol 10–20 mg three times daily; increased dietary salt; fludrocortisone 0.1 mg orally daily; clonidine 0.05 mg once or twice daily; and midodrine 5 mg orally twice daily. Finally, all patients benefit from an exercise program. This should be approached cautiously, beginning in the most severe patients with no more than "orthostatic exercise," standing against a wall for incrementally increased periods each day. Therapy is discussed in more detail in the treatment section.

## Functional Gastrointestinal Disorders

Despite highly varied presenting symptom complexes, current understanding suggests a biopsychosocial model as the underlying process for most FGIDs. This model contains three main components: a genetic/environmental predisposition, pathophysiological changes, and a psychological contribution (Drossman et al., 2006). It is important to understand that the psychological contribution is not considered to be the cause of these disorders but, rather, a comorbid process either primary or secondary to the functional pain disorder. Twin and other genetic studies have demonstrated both a genetic and an environmental predisposition to the development of these disorders (Kalantar et al., 2003; Locke 3rd et al., 2000). Genetic factors have included the genotype for reduced interleukin (IL)-10 (anti-inflammatory cytokine) production, certain SERT polymorphisms (Yeo et al., 2004), increased messenger ribonucleic acid (mRNA) expression of p11 (a protein critical to 5-$HT_{1B}$ receptor function) in the sigmoid biopsies of IBS-C (Camilleri et al., 2007), and alpha-2-adrenoceptor polymorphism that affects motility (Kim et al., 2004). Environment plays a role through learned behavior from parents who seek more frequent medical attention. For example, children of patients with IBS utilize more healthcare resources than children of healthy control parents (Levy et al., 2000).

Psychological elements are often present, but these factors do not define and are not required for the diagnosis of FGID. They are modulators of the patient's experience and perhaps of treatment response. These psychological factors will also influence healthcare seeking. It is important to also consider that these individuals are frequently diagnosed as "having a psychological problem" and may not have received an appropriate diagnosis, treatment, or plan. This lack of diagnostic clarity itself in the context of a prolonged illness may contribute to psychological dysfunction.

Altered motility in the context of stress may play a role in IBS, though these mild abnormalities do not usually explain the disorder. We have also found that gastric electrical activity becomes abnormal in the upright position in children with POTS (a disorder with overlapping symptoms with FGID; Safder et al., 2010). This may explain the frequent symptom of nausea. Hyperalgesia is very common, from increased rectal sensation to distention of anal balloons to increased sensitivity and discomfort with normal physiological functions (Munakata et al., 1997; Naliboff et al., 1997). The role of either increased intestinal bacterial in the foregut (small-bowel bacterial overgrowth) or altered bacteria is well documented. Some IBS sufferers have small-bowel bacterial overgrowth; others do not fulfill the classic definition for this disease but have greater numbers of bacteria than healthy controls. Furthermore, the use of nonabsorbable antibiotics like rifaximin often improves gastrointestinal symptoms (Pimentel et al., 2000; Posserud et al., 2007). The role of bacteria in the pathogenesis of IBS is further supported by (1) the fact that a third of patients with IBS or dyspepsia describe their symptoms as having begun after an acute enteric infection (Mearin et al., 2005), and (2) the fact that about a quarter of patients who suffer an acute gastrointestinal illness will then develop an FGID (Gwee et al., 1999). More recently, these disorders that were originally defined by the absence of anatomical or inflammatory markers are now found to have increased inflammatory cells (Chadwick et al., 2002). POTS occurs frequently in these subjects, occurring in about a third of patients with FGID, as one more in a long list of comorbid disorders. There is now increasing interest in looking at the heart rate variability (HRV) in pain disorders. High-frequency (HF) heart rate peak generally reflects vagal tone, while low frequency (LF) is a marker of the baroreflex response and a general marker of autonomic tone (vagal and sympathetic) (Circulation, 1996). Reduced HF occurs in many chronic pain disorders, such as fibromyalgia (Chalaye et al., 2012), chronic neck and shoulder pain (Shiro et al., 2012), and chronic back pain (Gockel et al., 2008). According to a recent meta-analysis (Liu et al., 2013). IBS is usually associated with lower HF and a higher LF/HF ratio. However, there was no difference in the LF band between IBS subjects and healthy controls. Further studies are needed to know whether the changes in HRV are a state or trait related to the disease. It is not the goal of this chapter to enumerate every functional disorder, but to list those most commonly encountered in a general neurologist's practice. IBS is defined as 3 months of abdominal discomfort relieved by a bowel movement or associated with a change in bowel movement frequency or consistency and occurs in 10% to 20% of the general population. Chronic idiopathic nausea also occurs with some frequency. Finally, CVS is characterized by episodes of vomiting alternating with normal baseline health. Though less frequent than other disorders, it sometimes falls in the province of the neurologist because it is highly responsive to antimigrainous strategies, in particular triptans, dihydroergotamine infusion, and prevention using verapamil or tricyclic agents. A clinical clue to the diagnosis is a "switch-like" phenomenon—the patient goes from feeling and looking ill to suddenly feeling well enough to eat a large meal in the span of a few moments. This disorder has been associated with a mitochondrial polymorphism, and coenzyme $Q_{10}$ ($CoQ_{10}$) and L-carnitine supplementation may be highly beneficial in some patients (Boles et al., 2003; Ropper, 1994).

## AUTONOMIC DISORDERS CHARACTERIZED BY EXCESSIVE AUTONOMIC OUTFLOW

### Autonomic Storm and Takotsubo Cardiomyopathy

Emotional stress can cause cardiac injury and sometimes death. Until recently, neurologists have emphasized this connection more than cardiologists. Dr. Martin Samuels has been an especially forceful advocate for the study of this phenomenon (Samuels, 2007). Autonomic storms following cerebral catastrophe may have dramatic physical findings and sometimes ECG abnormalities. Indeed, some of the most dramatic T-wave inversions in the intensive care unit are observed in such patients (Rabinstein and Wijdicks, 2004). The terminology for these autonomic storms is somewhat chaotic because of lack of systematic study and a profusion of names for the condition. These hypersympathetic states have been termed *paroxysmal sympathetic storms*, *autonomic storms*, *diencephalic seizures*, *diencephalic epilepsy*, *autonomic dysreflexia*, or simply *dysautonomia*. In their extreme form, such autonomic storms result in acute alterations in body temperature, blood pressure, heart rate, respiratory rate, sweating, and muscle tone. They occur with severe head trauma, in postresuscitation encephalopathy, in intracerebral hemorrhage, with brain tumors, and sometimes in hydrocephalus. Immediately after such a catastrophe, a massive catecholamine surge occurs that can induce seizures, neurogenic pulmonary edema, and myocardial injury. Excessive sympathetic outflow declines or goes away within a few days in most patients, but some patients develop recurrent paroxysms of sympathetic overactivity for weeks or months (Rabinstein and Wijdicks, 2004).

The pathophysiology of these autonomic storms remains uncertain, but heightened activity of diencephalic or brainstem sympathoexcitatory pathways appears to be the major substrate of these episodes. Autonomic storms are probably far more common than suggested by the surprisingly sparse reports in the literature. Clinical features of autonomic storms include tachycardia, hypertension (often with widening of the pulse pressure), fever, tachypnea, sweating, flushing, and pupillary dilation. Intracranial pressure increases during the episodes, with the autonomic dysfunction usually preceding the rise in intracranial pressure. The basis for the diagnosis of autonomic storm is the characteristic dysautonomic spells in a patient with acute intracranial disease. It must be distinguished from other conditions such as neuroleptic malignant syndrome, serotonergic syndrome, malignant hyperthermia, and lethal catatonia. Additional disorders that may manifest sudden unexplained autonomic hyperactivity include Guillain-Barré syndrome (Ropper, 1994) and myelopathy. Severe hypertension, but bradycardia rather than tachycardia, are characteristic of the Cushing reflex syndrome, which occurs in patients with compression of the brainstem.

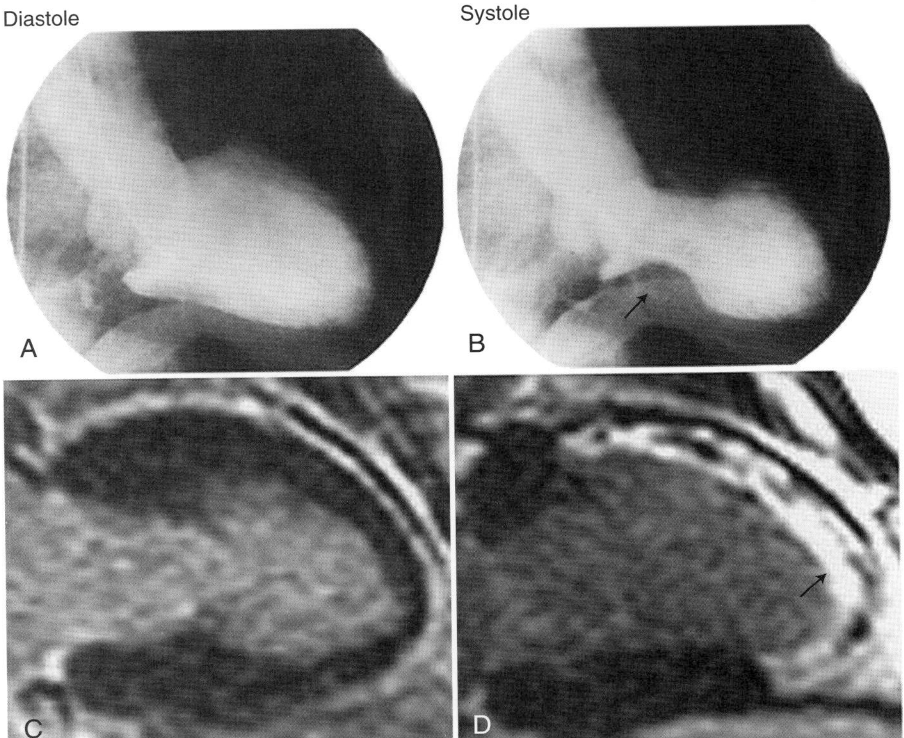


**Fig. 107.3** Ventriculography (**A** and **B**) and magnetic resonance imaging (**C** and **D**) of the heart in a patient with stress cardiomyopathy (takotsubo syndrome). In **B** the poorly contracting ventricle gives the appearance of an octopus trap, (*arrow*), hence the name. The black arrow shows the neck of the trap, where the ventricle is still contracting. *(Modified from Wittstein, I.S., Thiemann, D.R., Lima, J.A., Baughman, K.L., Schulman S.P., Gerstenblith, G., et al., 2005. Neurohumoral features of myocardial stunning due to sudden emotional stress. N. Engl. J. Med. 352, 539–548.)*

### Takotsubo "Broken Heart" Syndrome

A less dramatic but analogous condition has been recognized in postmenopausal women (Gold et al., 2005; Kurisu et al., 2002; Wittstein et al., 2005). It mimics myocardial infarction and is characterized by chest pain and shortness of breath. It was described initially in Japan as *tako tsubo* (octopus trap) *syndrome* and in the United States as *apical ballooning syndrome* or *broken heart syndrome* (Wittstein et al., 2005). The first two names describe the appearance of the left ventricle on imaging; it seems to stretch, balloon out, and weaken (Fig. 107.3). The third name derives from the severe emotional stress, such as loss of a family member, that may trigger the condition. In approximately 20% of patients, the inciting factor seems to be severe physical stress, such as trauma, surgery, or severe pain. Other names for takotsubo cardiomyopathy are *neurogenic myocardial stunning, catecholaminergic myocardial stunning*, and *stress-induced cardiomyopathy*.

Patients with takotsubo cardiomyopathy do not have coronary artery occlusion or coronary artery spasm during their presentation, but two-thirds have abnormal myocardial blood flow, apparently due to dysfunction in the microvasculature of the heart. Diagnosis is from nonspecific ST–T abnormalities, ST elevation, or QT prolongation with large negative T waves, often occurring over days in succession (Fig. 107.4). Common markers of myocardial infarction (troponin, creatine kinase) are only slightly raised, confirming that there is more stunning of the heart than permanent heart muscle damage. Plasma and urinary catecholamines are typically elevated (Wittstein et al., 2005). The reason this syndrome occurs in some individuals but not others seeming to suffer comparable levels of stress remains unknown. Treatment is supportive, and while 95% of patients experience complete recovery, approximately 10% will have recurrence over a 4-year period.

The pathophysiology of myocardial stunning probably derives from exaggerated calcium influx into the myocardial cells due to excessive norepinephrine release into the myocardium. Norepinephrine activates release of cyclic adenosine monophosphate (c-AMP), which in turn activates a calcium channel allowing calcium influx and potassium outflow. The potassium outflow may account for the frequently encountered peaked T waves seen on ECG. Pathological examination of the heart muscle reveals coagulative myocytolysis (also known as *myofibrillar degeneration* or *contraction band necrosis*) characterized by cell death in a hypercontracted state and abnormal cross-band formations. Similar lesions can be induced in animal models through stimulation of the lateral hypothalamus, limbic cortex, mesencephalic reticular formation, and stellate ganglia (Samuels, 2007).

## PREDOMINANTLY PERIPHERAL AFFERENT STRUCTURAL AUTONOMIC DISORDERS CHARACTERIZED BY IMPAIRED AUTONOMIC OUTFLOW

### Familial Dysautonomia

Familial dysautonomia (FD, also referred to as *Riley-Day syndrome* in the older literature) occurs predominantly in individuals of Ashkenazi Jewish extraction carrying mutations in the IB kinase-associated protein gene *(IKBKAP)*. The mutations cause impaired expression of the normal protein product IB kinase-associated protein (IKAP). IKAP deficiency may impair normal expression of neurotransmitters (Axelrod et al., 2006; Axelrod and Hilz, 2003). FD is part of a group of disorders termed *hereditary sensory and autonomic neuropathies* (HSANs) and is classified as HSAN III in this scheme. HSAN I and V

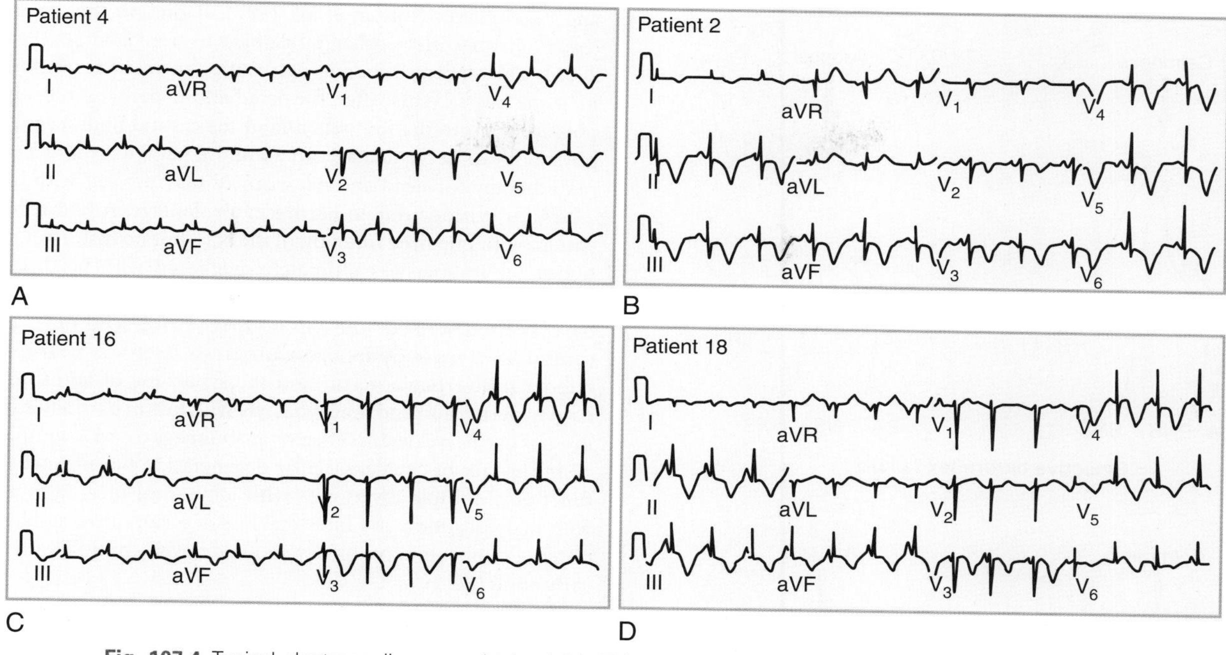


**Fig. 107.4** Typical electrocardiograms obtained 24–48 hours after presentation in four patients with stress cardiomyopathy. The abnormalities include non-specific ST changes (patient 16), ST elevation (patient 18), T wave inversion (patients 2 16 and 18), QT prolongation (patient 18). *(Modified from Wittstein, I.S., Thiemann, D.R, Lima, J.A., Baughman, K.L., Schulman S.P., Gerstenblith. G., et al., 2005. Neurohumoral features of myocardial stunning due to sudden emotional stress. N. Engl. J. Med. 352, 539–548.)*

are the other members of the group, with predominant involvement of small sensory and autonomic fibers, where loss of pain sensation is a major clinical issue. Other HSANs involve larger and generally non-autonomic fibers.

FD patients have inadequate development and limited survival of sensory and autonomic neurons. Although the literature has generally emphasized efferent sympathetic involvement, more recent studies suggest that the predominant pathophysiology originates from loss of afferent nerve function, particularly baroreceptor information (Norcliffe-Kaufmann et al., 2010), but also likely including visceral and chemoceptor information (Bernardi et al., 2003). Peripheral nerves demonstrate a reduction in the unmyelinated and small myelinated neuronal populations. In addition, there is evidence of impaired CNS myelination, especially in the optic radiation and middle cerebellar peduncle, which probably accounts for patients' frequent visual complaints and ataxia (Axelrod et al., 2010).

The diagnosis of FD is suspected clinically based on a fairly classical presentation of decreased pain and temperature perception, with relative preservation of large-fiber sensory function such as proprioception and touch sensation, labile autonomic responses, hyporeflexia, alacrima, poor oropharyngeal coordination, and absence of lingual fungiform papillae serving the taste modality of sweet. Histamine injection produces no widespread flare response but a very circumscribed response, usually measuring less than 2–3 cm in diameter, because of the absence of C-fibers that mediate the neuroinflammatory response.

Autonomic disturbances are very prominent and impose great impediments to function, especially in the neonatal period. Feeding difficulties result from poor oral coordination. Recurrent misdirection, especially of liquids, and frequent gastroesophageal reflux put the patient at risk for aspiration and chronic lung disease. Emotional or physical stress or even arousal from sleep can trigger episodes of nausea and vomiting. These episodes (dysautonomic crises) are usually associated with agitation, tachycardia, and hypertension. Vasomotor and cardiovascular perturbations, manifesting as erythematous skin blotching and hyperhidrosis, occur with excitation or eating.

Patients with FD can have either extreme hypertension or profound postural hypotension without compensatory tachycardia. Supersensitivity to cholinergic and adrenergic agents is present. Relative insensitivity to hypoxemia limits the ability to cope with pneumonia or travel to high altitudes. Ensuing hypoxemia may lead to hypotension, bradyarrhythmia, and syncope. Delayed development is common, but intelligence is usually within normal ranges.

Identification of the gene defect has not yet led to curative therapy (Tutaj et al., 2006). Preventive and supportive strategies include measures for maintaining eye moisture, fundoplication with gastrostomy to provide nutrition and avoid risk of aspiration, use of central agents such as benzodiazepines, clonidine, or carbidopa (Norcliffe-Kaufmann and Kaufmann, 2014) to control vomiting and the dysautonomic crisis, and fludrocortisone and midodrine to combat cardiovascular lability (Freeman, 2003). The result of these improved supportive measures is that approximately half of FD patients now reach adulthood.

## Baroreflex Failure

*Acute baroreflex failure*, perhaps the most dramatic neurological disorder of blood pressure regulation, may display stress-induced systolic blood pressure surges of more than 300 mm Hg. It provides evidence of the great capability of the human CNS to generate unbuffered cardiovascular excitation (Ketch et al., 2002; Timmers et al., 2003; Fig. 107.5). The clinical syndrome resembles pheochromocytoma more than a typical dysautonomia. Human baroreflexes defend against excessive peaks or dips in blood pressure. Baroreflex failure occurs when afferent baroreceptive input via the vagus or glossopharyngeal nerves or their central connections becomes impaired. Wide excursions of blood pressure and heart rate result. Such excursions may derive from endogenous factors such as anger or drowsiness, which result in high and low pressures, respectively. They may also derive from exogenous factors such as environmental stressors like excessive cold or bright light.

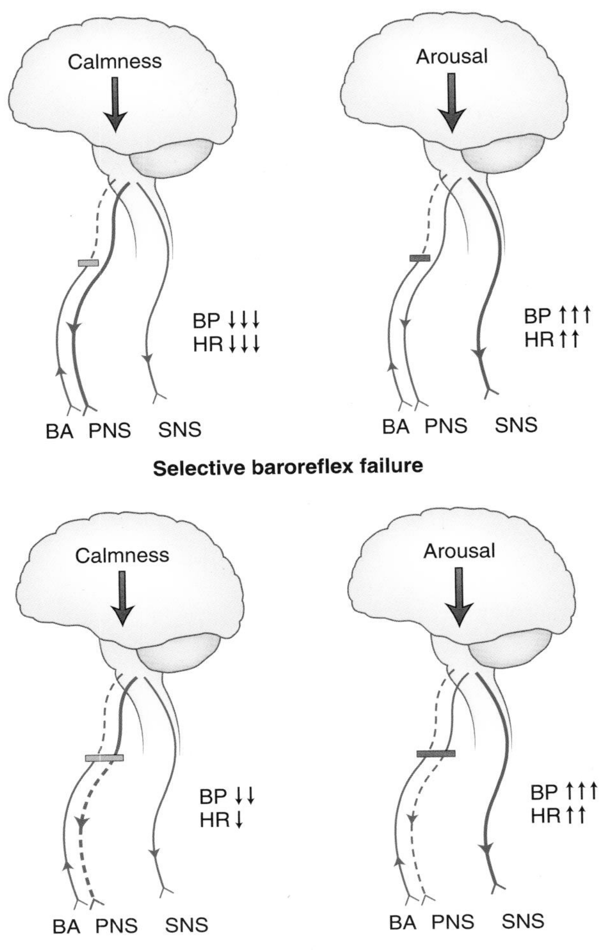


**Fig. 107.5** Selective baroreflex failure *(top)* contrasted with nonselective baroreflex failure *(bottom)*. Baroreflex afferents *(BA)* are damaged in patients with selective and nonselective baroreflex failure. Efferent sympathetic *(SNS)* and parasympathetic nerves *(PNS)* are intact in selective baroreflex failure. In nonselective baroreflex failure, efferent parasympathetic nerves are at least in part damaged. *BP*, Blood pressure; *HR*, heart rate. *(Modified from Jordan, J., Shannon, J.R., Black, B.K., Costa, F., Ertl, A.C., Furlan, R., et al., 1997. Malignant vagotonia due to selective baroreflex failure. Hypertension 30, 1072–1077.)*

Acute baroreflex impairment may produce hypertensive crisis. Over succeeding days to weeks, or in the absence of an acute event, volatile hypertension with periods of hypotension occurs; some individuals, after months to years, ultimately develop orthostatic hypotension. Usually bilateral destruction of baroreflex afferent function results in concomitant destruction of much efferent vagal function. Loss of vagal parasympathetic tone to the heart prevents bradycardia during stimuli that would ordinarily elicit parasympathetic activation (e.g., sedation, sleep). However, if the baroreflex failure occurs with relative sparing of the parasympathetic efferent vagal fibers, sleep or sedation may lead to malignant vagotonia with severe bradycardia and hypotension and episodes of sinus arrest.

Abnormalities in the vascular baroreceptors, the glossopharyngeal or vagal nerves, or their brainstem connections can all potentially lead to *chronic baroreflex failure*. Trauma from injury, tumor, radiation, surgical intervention, or brainstem stroke may also cause baroreflex failure. It occurs in familial paraganglioma syndrome owing to bilateral local tumor growth invading structures at or near the glossopharyngeal and vagal nerves (Jordan et al., 1997). Radiation therapy for throat carcinoma may incur collateral damage to cranial nerves (Seppi et al., 2005). This damage tends to occur after an interval of months and, in some cases, years after the irradiation, perhaps reflecting local fibrosis or postradiation ischemia of the carotid bodies as the pathophysiology of nerve damage. In addition, patients who have received radiotherapy for head and neck cancer may present with lightheadedness or syncope due to baroreceptor damage. A baroreflex failure patient with impaired function of the NTS but no history of radiation, tumor, or trauma was ultimately diagnosed with Leigh syndrome. Two genetic disorders that appear to entail baroreflex dysfunction have been described: the Groll-Hirschowitz syndrome, in which carotid sinus nerve dysfunction, progressive sensory neuropathy, and duodenal diverticula occur; and the syndrome of autosomal dominant hypertension and brachydactyly with loss of baroreflex buffering. Progressive nerve deafness begins at about age 6 and is complete at age 12 in the face of cochleosaccular degeneration but normal vestibular function. Multiple diverticula with jejunoileal ulceration associated with malabsorption and intestinal loss of serum protein may be associated. Peripheral nerve biopsy shows demyelination. Death occurs in early adult life.

Because of the protean manifestations of chronic baroreflex failure, the differential diagnosis can be extensive. The most important consideration is usually pheochromocytoma. The diagnosis of baroreflex failure often emerges after a negative work-up for pheochromocytoma. Other entities to be distinguished include panic attack, generalized anxiety disorder, migraine, PAF, hyperthyroidism, alcohol withdrawal, and drug use (e.g., amphetamine, cocaine). Renovascular hypertension frequently presents with volatility and brittleness and may sometimes mimic baroreflex failure. Many entities can produce orthostatic intolerance, and an equally long list can present with bradycardia and syncope.

However, despite the large differential diagnosis, key features in the evaluation of baroreflex failure make definitive diagnosis possible. The best test is to document normal or excess excursions of heart rate during normal daily activities (confirming autonomic control of heart rate) and then document an absence of bradycardic response of heart rate to the pressor effect of phenylephrine or the tachycardic heart rate response to a depressor agent. Alternatively, the observation of wide heart rate and blood pressure swings in the same direction at the same time (i.e., blood pressure rising when heart rate rises and vice versa) suggests that the baroreflex is not working and supports the diagnosis. In practice, the history of prior trauma exposure is one of the most important considerations in suspecting the diagnosis of baroreflex failure.

The typical pattern in volatile hypertension is baseline pressures in the high normal or hypertensive range (Fig. 107.6), but with pressor surges accompanied by tachycardia lasting minutes to hours. These pressor surges are elicited by mental or physical stress, during which sympathetic outflow is increased, and are characterized by palpitations and often severe headaches. Profuse sweating occurs during many attacks. Tremulousness, anxiety, and irritability are typical of these episodes, sometimes acting as the triggering event for the surge. Mild and transitory elevations in plasma glucose occasionally occur, as well as a positive correlation between blood pressure and intraocular pressure. During such pressor surges, plasma norepinephrine levels reach values not much less than those seen in pheochromocytoma.

Norepinephrine levels of 1000 pg/mL in the supine posture during a pressor surge would be typical, and values above 2000 pg/mL occur. These pressor surges can also be punctuated by hypotensive valleys, especially during periods of quiet, sedation, or sleep, when sympathetic outflow is diminished.

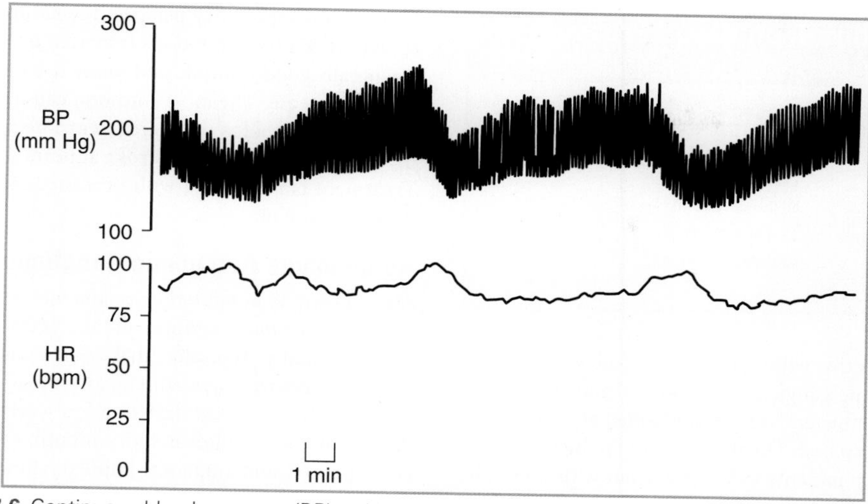


**Fig. 107.6** Continuous blood pressure *(BP)* and heart rate *(HR)* recordings at rest in a patient with baroreflex failure. Large spontaneous oscillations of HR and BP parallel each other; decreases in BP are very brisk. *(Modified from Jordan, J., Shannon, J.R., Black, B.K., Costa, F., Ertl, A.C., Furlan, R., et al., 1997. Malignant vagotonia due to selective baroreflex failure. Hypertension 30, 1072–1077.)*

Malignant vagotonia from selective baroreflex failure (Jordan syndrome; see Fig. 107.5) presents as severe bradycardia and asystole due to surges in parasympathetic tone. Along with the hypertensive episodes encountered in the other forms of baroreflex failure, patients with this form may have episodes of hypotension with a systolic pressure below 50 mm Hg. Accompanying symptoms include fatigue and dizziness with possible progression to frank syncope. The most severe episodes tend to occur during early-morning sleep, and periods of asystole longer than 20 seconds may occur. Episodes have also occurred after the administration of intravenous nitroprusside and sublingual nitroglycerin.

The treatment of baroreflex failure aims to reduce the frequency and magnitude of life-threatening surges in blood pressure and heart rate (Ketch et al., 2002). A secondary goal of therapy is to attenuate symptomatic hypotensive episodes. The pharmacological treatment of choice for blood pressure surges is clonidine (see Box 107.5). This is a physiological approach to treatment, because this agent acts centrally and peripherally to attenuate sympathetic activation and limit the extent to which pressor surges can occur. The α-adrenoreceptor blocker phenoxybenzamine has been relatively unsuccessful in reducing the frequency of pressor surges, although the magnitude of surges (but not tachycardia) is controlled. The sedative effects of $\alpha_2$-adrenoreceptor agonists such as clonidine may assist patients in preventing hypertensive episodes. In the case of clonidine, the inconvenience of frequent oral dosing can be avoided by using a transdermal preparation. Most patients with baroreflex failure will require large doses, whether oral or transdermal. To reduce the possibility of loss of a patch with consequent provocation of clonidine withdrawal, we sometimes use two #1 patches, one placed on Sunday and a second placed on Wednesday of each week, staggered this way to lessen the likelihood of inadvertent complete discontinuation of clonidine.

However, in some patients, the prevention of hypotension is also required. This is quite difficult because the hypotensive episodes are usually short-lived, and most agents have a longer half-life than spell duration. Despite its difficulties, fludrocortisone may still be the best way to treat this problem. Because some patients with baroreflex failure have reduced plasma volume as well, the fludrocortisone along with high salt intake might have beneficial effects on this variable. Generally, low doses (0.05 mg daily) are all that is required. Noteworthy, though, is that fludrocortisone requires 1 or 2 weeks for its full effect to be realized. Finally, if severe bradycardia (<40 bpm) occurs or if the patient has concomitant evidence of significant heart block, the placement of a pacemaker may be necessary.

**BOX 107.4 Differential Diagnosis of Orthostatic Hypotension**

**Autonomic Disorders**
- Pure autonomic failure
- Multiple system atrophy
- Familial dysautonomia
- Dopamine β-hydroxylase deficiency
- Baroreflex failure
- Secondary autonomic neuropathies

**Hypovolemia Disorders**
- Hemorrhage or plasma loss
- Overdiuresis
- Overdialysis
- Idiopathic hypovolemia

**Endocrinological Disorders**
- Addison disease
- Hypoaldosteronism
- Pheochromocytoma
- Renovascular hypertension

**Vascular Insufficiency**
- Varicose veins
- Absent venous valves
- Arteriovenous malformations

**Vasodilator Excess**
- Mastocytosis (histamine, prostaglandin $D_2$)
- Hyperbradykininism (bradykinin)
- Carcinoid (bradykinin)
- Hypermagnesemia

**Paroxysmal Autonomic Syncope**
- Glossopharyngeal syncope
- Micturition syncope
- Carotid sinus syncope
- Swallow syncope
- Cough syncope
- Bezold-Jarisch reflex activation

**Miscellaneous**
- Drugs and toxins
- Stokes-Adams attacks
- Gastrectomy
- Hypokinesia, weightlessness, bed rest

## PREDOMINANTLY PERIPHERAL EFFERENT STRUCTURAL AUTONOMIC DISORDERS CHARACTERIZED BY IMPAIRED AUTONOMIC OUTFLOW

### Pure Autonomic Failure

The term *pure autonomic failure* (PAF) once encompassed many causes of autonomic failure and OH (Box 107.4). This term is now

**TABLE 107.6 Stimuli on Blood Pressure in Autonomic Failure**

| Depressor | Pressor |
|---|---|
| Standing | Lying |
| Food | Water |
| Hyperventilation | Hypoventilation |
| Exercise | Water immersion |
| Straining | Abdominal binding |
| Fever, environmental heat | |

restricted to a synucleinopathy with synuclein found within Lewy bodies confined to autonomic ganglia, presenting in mid- to late life (Low, 1997; Mathias and Bannister, 2002; Robertson et al., 2004). The adrenal medulla is relatively spared. The initial feature in men is impotence, but OH usually brings patients to the physician with unsteadiness or faintness on standing. It is worst in the morning and improves as the day progresses. Supine hypertension may occur during the night while supine. Meals, exercise, fever, or environmental heat worsen OH. Other complaints include orthostatic pain in the neck, shoulders, or occiput, relieved by lying down. Although a decline in systolic blood pressure of 20 mm Hg and diastolic blood pressure of 10 mm Hg after at least 1 minute of standing defines OH, most PAF patients suffer from profound OH with a decrease in systolic blood pressure of 50 mm Hg and sometimes more than 100 mm Hg. Convulsive near-syncope may occur. Because of the variability of blood pressure, a single upright measurement may mislead the clinician regarding severity and several upright measurements are required. About 5% of PAF patients have what appears to be angina pectoris, usually in the absence of significant angiographically demonstrable coronary atherosclerosis. PAF patients tolerate high altitude very poorly, perhaps because they hyperventilate in this situation. Even with severe supine hypertension, cardiac function can be preserved and contractility may even rise (Mathias and Bannister, 2002; Robertson et al., 2004).

A reduced basal metabolic rate is typical. Hypohidrosis or at least an asymmetrical distribution of sweating is usually present. Nocturia is an invariable accompaniment of PAF and may cause the patient to get up as many as five times a night to pass substantial amounts of urine. This is due to nocturnal vascular redistribution in the microgravitational environment, as is typical of any patient with severe orthostatic hypotension. Urinary hesitancy, urgency, dribbling, and occasional incontinence may also occur related to specific bladder dysfunction. Some patients develop urine retention and may have repeated UTIs in consequence. It is noteworthy that patients with PAF do not usually experience as high a fever as healthy persons, but any fever will significantly lower their blood pressure and consequently decrease their functional capacity. A sudden decline in functional mobility in a patient with PAF is suggestive of an occult infection, often of the urinary tract.

PAF patients have greatly reduced catecholamine levels. Plasma (and urinary) norepinephrine levels are usually markedly reduced, sometimes to 10% of normal, being always less than 200 pg/mL and often under 100 pg/mL. Reduction in plasma epinephrine levels is less pronounced. Dopamine levels in urine are usually about 50% of normal values. Marked hypersensitivity to all pressor and depressor stimuli occurs (Table 107.6).

Lewy bodies characterize the pathology of PAF, along with a loss of cells in the intermediolateral column of the spinal cord and a loss of catecholamine uptake and catecholamine fluorescence in sympathetic postganglionic neurons. PAF is less disabling than MSA and PD because of the absence of cerebellar, striatal, pyramidal, or extrapyramidal dysfunction. Patients should understand the relatively benign (from a life-expectancy perspective) nature of PAF but need to learn to live within the limitations imparted by their symptoms. They have a generally good outlook, and many live for 20 years or more after the onset of disease. The most common cause of death in these patients is pulmonary embolus or intercurrent infection. The incidence of both myocardial infarction and stroke appears significantly reduced in PAF. Treatment is improving with new medications available as discussed under treatment.

## Autoimmune Autonomic Ganglionopathy

Also known as *autoimmune autonomic neuropathy* (AAN) and *acute pandysautonomia* (Vernino et al., 2000), autoimmune autonomic ganglionopathy typically strikes a previously healthy individual. Severe generalized sympathetic and parasympathetic autonomic failure unfolds over a few days to a few weeks. Orthostatic hypotension, fixed heart rate, anhidrosis, dry mouth, dry eyes, sexual dysfunction, constipation, and impaired pupillary function are present (Vernino et al., 2000). Anorexia, early satiety, postprandial abdominal pain and vomiting, constipation, or diarrhea may also be present. The spectrum and severity of dysautonomia is quite variable, however. Motor and sensory nerve abnormalities are typically absent. The most convincing evidence of an autoimmune pathogenesis is the demonstration of ganglionic nicotinic acetylcholine receptor (AChR) antibodies in high titers in a large proportion of these patients, the correlation of antibody level with dysautonomia severity, and the response of this disorder to intravenous globulin and plasma exchange (Vernino, 2005). Animal studies have demonstrated passive transfer of the disorder with infusion of patient serum. Antibody-mediated impairment of synaptic transmission occurs in autonomic ganglia (Vernino et al., 2000).

Like other autoimmune disorders, autoimmune autonomic ganglionopathy may occur in a postinfectious or postsurgical setting, in the context of other autoimmune disorders such as autoimmune thyroiditis, with pernicious anemia or type 1 diabetes, as a result of a monoclonal antibody, or as a paraneoplastic disorder. Typical malignancies include small-cell carcinoma of the lung, breast cancer, lymphoma, and a scattering of other cancers. An elevated level of serum ganglionic AChR antibody is specific for the diagnosis, but its absence does not rule it out, since not all antibodies are detectable by current methodology. Particularly suggestive of this disorder are the spectrum of neurogenic bladder, impaired pupillary function, gastroparesis, dry eyes, and dry mouth.

Treatment includes plasma exchange or intravenous immunoglobulin (Schroeder et al., 2005). Partial but incomplete improvement over time is typical. Only a third of patients experience major functional improvement of autonomic deficits. Some patients with a more insidious and progressive form (rather than the typical subacute monophasic presentation) may be clinically indistinguishable from PAF. It is likely other antibodies play a role in the production of autonomic disorders, such as antibodies to muscarinic cholinergic receptors, α-adrenergic receptors, and β-adrenergic receptors. This would typically involve dysfunction of a very selective type, involving either pure adrenergic or pure cholinergic failure, or isolated gastrointestinal dysmotility.

## Autonomic Neuropathy

Autonomic neuropathy may occur in isolation, or, more frequently as a part of a small-fiber neuropathy involving both autonomic and small unmyelinated or thinly myelinated sensory nerves. In this case, the typical presentation will include distal burning pain and changes in color of the distal limb reflecting poor vasomotor control. These symptoms may be quite disabling in their own right and particularly bothersome at night, interfering with sleep. Autonomic nerve involvement will typically affect erectile function first, may then affect bowel or bladder function with constipation or urgency, followed by parasympathetic glandular function resulting in dry eyes or mouth, and ultimately lead to OH.

Causes of autonomic and small-fiber neuropathy include diabetes or metabolic syndrome in about half of cases. Although traditional teaching might suggest that diabetic autonomic neuropathy would only occur in patients with long-standing diabetes, this is clearly no longer the case. The involvement of autonomic nerves and autonomic Schwann cells is probably an immune-mediated process that occurs at the time diabetes develops or may antedate glucose intolerance by several months or years. In one study (Hoffman-Snyder et al., 2006), more than half of patients presenting with a small-fiber neuropathy of unknown cause had occult glucose intolerance, with over a quarter being diagnosed with frank diabetes for the first time as a result of their neuropathic presentation. Neuropathy associated with diabetes treatment is increasingly recognized as well (Freeman et al., 2010) and may result from too rapid a drop in sugar levels. The triad of rapid-onset neuropathic symptoms, unexplained weight loss (probably due to diabetic gastroparesis), and new treatment initiation for diabetes should prompt strong consideration for this diagnosis, which may respond to steroid treatment early in its course (Said et al., 2003).

Sjögren syndrome (keratoconjunctivitis sicca) is probably the second most frequent cause of small-fiber neuropathy after diabetes and may present with dryness of the eyes, ears, nose, mouth, and vagina, with associated renal tubular acidosis, mononeuritis multiplex, achlorhydria, and often associated collagen disorders. Dysautonomia is relatively common from ganglionitis or cumulative mononeuritis multiplex lesions involving autonomic areas. Both primary and secondary Sjögren syndrome patients (60%) may have autoantibodies against the $M_3$ muscarinic receptor and impaired parasympathetic stimulation of bladder (Wang et al., 2004).

Other causes include multiple immunological disorders such as monoclonal protein–related neuropathy (with or without a plasma cell cancer), paraneoplastic autonomic neuropathy, postinfectious causes, and autonomic neuropathy related to various collagen vascular disorders such as lupus or rheumatoid arthritis. Infectious causes include herpes zoster, Lyme disease, and syphilis. Finally, a host of rarer metabolic and infiltrative disorders such as α-galactosidase deficiency (Fabry disease), porphyria, heavy metal poisoning, and other drugs and toxins discussed later can be responsible.

## Drug-Induced Dysautonomia

Approximately 10% of drugs used in clinical practice derive their usefulness from their effect on the autonomic nervous system (Benowitz, 2004; Low, 2004). Moreover, at least 25% of drugs may, with overdose or toxicity, exert unwanted effects on the autonomic nervous system. These observations account for the importance physicians must attach to the recognition of drug-induced autonomic impairment.

The mechanisms by which drugs cause OH include blood volume depletion; sympathoplegic effects causing impairment in the maintenance of vascular resistance, venous tone, or cardiac output; and direct vasodilatation, which lowers vascular resistance or venous tone. Vasodilators may act directly on the vasculature or indirectly by blocking the renin–angiotensin or vasopressin systems. When drugs induce OH by depleting the blood volume or by vasodilation alone, there is compensatory baroreflex-mediated sympathetic activation—that is, tachycardia, palpations, sweating, and increased circulating catecholamines. This presentation has been termed *hyperadrenergic orthostatic hypotension*. When drugs that impair central sympathetic outflow cause orthostatic hypotension, the expected sympathetic reflex response blunts or is absent (*hypoadrenergic orthostatic hypotension*).

Some drugs may cause reflex syncope (vasovagal syncope), especially those that produce hyperadrenergic OH by vasodilation. Typically such patients have an initial period of reflex tachycardia after assuming an upright posture, followed by sudden bradycardia and hypotension with signs and symptoms of cerebral hypoperfusion and parasympathetic activation. Activation of afferent ventricular mechanoreceptors, owing to the intense myocardial contractile state, may contribute to the mechanism of syncope, increasing parasympathetic and inhibiting sympathetic responses, resulting in bradycardia and vasodilation with little or no increase in plasma norepinephrine (although plasma epinephrine may increase greatly). This effect occurs in the clinical laboratory after administering isoproterenol as a stressor to patients during upright tilt testing.

Elderly patients are especially at risk for drug-induced OH, which is an important cause of syncope and falls in this population. Typically, drug-induced OH in the elderly occurs in the presence of risk factors such as reduced cardiovascular health, impaired baroreceptor function, subclinical autonomic dysfunction, and the presence of larger numbers of prescription drugs. Responsible agents include sedatives, hypnotics, antidepressants, diuretics, antihypertensive drugs, or nitrates. Tricyclic antidepressants and other norepinephrine blocking agents are the most common unsuspected cause. The effect of tricyclic antidepressants on blood pressure may come on slowly and may require more than a week after discontinuation to go away completely. Other drugs commonly involved are trimethaphan, guanadrel, clonidine, and α-adrenoreceptor blockers. In the young, chronic frequent marijuana use and excessive phenylpropanolamine use may rarely lead to hypotension.

Usually, autonomic effects of drugs are readily reversible on discontinuation, but several drugs may produce permanent injury to autonomic nerves. Wernicke encephalopathy occurs with chronic alcohol abuse, is commonly associated with OH that occurs without an adequate compensatory tachycardia, and is associated with an impaired cold pressor response together with hypersensitivity to infused catecholamines. Oncological agents such as vincristine and cisplatin can cause autonomic dysfunction and OH, from which recovery may occur over several months. Cisplatin causes both autonomic neuropathy and salt wasting, thus giving rise to OH by two different mechanisms. Paclitaxel and other chemotherapeutic agents in this class are particularly toxic to the autonomic nervous system. Most patients will get some degree of dysautonomia, which remains asymptomatic. In a minority, the autonomic neuropathy is so profound that blood pressure cannot be maintained and the drug has to be discontinued. Metronidazole has also been associated with an autonomic neuropathy in doses that usually exceed 3 g (Hobson-Webb et al., 2006). In our experience, metronidazole toxicity usually occurs in the context of another risk factor, such as diabetes or an already-present mild autonomic neuropathy that becomes markedly exacerbated by the drug. The medication should be immediately discontinued as soon as an autonomic neuropathy is uncovered. In addition, it should be avoided in patients with an extant autonomic neuropathy.

Oligohidrosis has been reported in a small number of patients receiving zonisamide, and in a proportion of these patients, hyperthermia has occurred (Low, 2004). Production of ciguatera toxin is by dinoflagellates consumed by reef fish. The presenting features of intoxication (most commonly after ingestion of barracuda, red snapper, or grouper) include vomiting, abdominal pain, myalgias, weakness, pruritus, and paresthesias of the mouth, face, and extremities. A peculiar "hot-and-cold reversal" occurs in which cold objects feel hot and vice versa. Cardiovascular features include bradycardia, hypotension, and in some cases, severe orthostatic hypotension. Increased vagal tone characterizes the nature of the autonomic disturbance. Bradycardia and, in part, OH reverse with atropine. OH is reversible in most cases, resolving within 4–6 weeks. Vacor produces severe autonomic neuropathy.

### Dopamine β-Hydroxylase Deficiency

Dopamine β-hydroxylase (DBH) deficiency is due to selective absence of norepinephrine and all its metabolites (Robertson and Garland, 2005). It is described in only a few patients but has a disproportionate importance because it illuminates human noradrenergic function. Affected patients have absent sympathetic noradrenergic function but normal parasympathetic and sympathetic cholinergic function. DBH-deficient patients exhibit profound orthostatic hypotension. Although present from birth, the disorder is often unrecognized until adulthood. Symptoms in the perinatal period include vomiting, dehydration, hypotension, hypothermia, and profound hypoglycemia requiring repeated hospitalization. Exercise capacity is poor. By early adulthood, individuals have profound orthostatic hypotension, greatly reduced exercise tolerance, ptosis of the eyelids, and supine nasal stuffiness. Presyncopal symptoms include dizziness, blurred vision, dyspnea, nuchal discomfort, and chest pain. Neuropsychiatric symptoms are surprisingly mild. CNS abnormalities are not a consideration before diagnosis driven by OH. During adult life, some DBH-deficient patients develop renal function abnormalities, including raised blood urea nitrogen and creatinine levels. Life expectancy is uncertain but appears near normal.

The diagnosis is clinical, based on the findings of OH, intact sweating, ptosis of the eyelids, and arched palate. Biochemical features include minimal or undetectable plasma, CSF, and urinary norepinephrine and epinephrine and a fivefold to tenfold elevation of plasma dopamine, a finding pathognomonic of DBH deficiency. Patients lack urinary normetanephrine, metanephrine, and vanillylmandelic acid. The molecular basis of DBH deficiency has been elucidated (Kim et al., 2002).

### Menkes Kinky Hair Syndrome (Trichopolydystrophy, X-Linked Copper Deficiency)

DBH is a copper-containing enzyme, and congenital disorders of impaired copper metabolism may present with certain features similar to DBH deficiency. Male infants with Menkes kinky hair syndrome (see Chapter 100) present with stubby, tangled, sparse hair (often white or gray in color), pudgy cheeks, spasticity, seizures, hypothermia, retarded growth, and decreased visual function. Subdural hematoma, jaundice, and osteoporosis also occur. The abnormality in copper handling leads to defective DBH functional efficiency. The incidence is between 1 in 50,000 and 1 in 100,000.

DBH deficiency is the first neurotransmitter defect with a uniquely efficacious replacement strategy. Administration of droxidopa (L-threo-3,4-dihydroxyphenylserine), or LDOPS (Freeman et al., 1999; Kaufmann et al., 2003), alleviates OH and other symptoms. Individuals do not respond well to standard therapeutic approaches for autonomic failure. Surgery can correct ptosis. Renal function should be assessed every 3 years or more often if function decreases.

## PREDOMINANTLY CENTRAL STRUCTURAL AUTONOMIC DISORDERS CHARACTERIZED BY IMPAIRED AUTONOMIC OUTFLOW

### Multiple System Atrophy

MSA, also known as *Shy-Drager syndrome*, is a progressive neurodegenerative disorder encompassing autonomic, extrapyramidal, cerebellar, and pyramidal features (Parikh et al., 2002; Seppi et al., 2005; Wenning et al., 2004). Extrapyramidal involvement (termed *MSA-P*, for *parkinsonian*) is about threefold more common than cerebellar involvement (termed *MSA-C* for *cerebellar*). Occasional patients feature both types. The pathological hallmark of MSA is neuronal loss and gliosis within multiple sites in the brain, intermediolateral columns, and the Onuf nucleus, with characteristic glial cytoplasmic inclusions (GCIs) containing α-synuclein and ubiquitin. These inclusions are quite distinct from Lewy bodies, which also contain ubiquitin, in several respects:

1. Shape: GCIs tend to be irregular in outline, in contrast to the target-shaped concentric circular Lewy bodies of PD.
2. Cellular location: GCIs are in glia, whereas Lewy bodies are in neurons.
3. Neuraxis location: GCIs dominate in the basal ganglia and pons, whereas Lewy bodies occur in the midbrain, cortex, and autonomic ganglia.

The average age of onset is 53 years; no confirmed cases exist under age 30, and onset beyond age 70 is rare. No gender predilection exists. MSA has a prevalence of 0.4 per 100,000 individuals. In some patients, the disease presents as OH or urinary tract symptoms, but in other cases, extrapyramidal or cerebellar symptoms predominate in the early stages. When OH antedates other neurological involvement, differentiation from autonomic neuropathy, PD, diffuse Lewy body disease, or PAF may be difficult (Geser et al., 2005; Kaufmann et al., 2004; Seppi et al., 2005). Even when there is full-blown parkinsonism and severe dysautonomia, MSA and PD are difficult to separate and cannot be separated on the basis of autonomic testing alone (Riley and Chelimsky, 2003). Other clinical features are better predictors of a diagnosis of MSA, such as poor response to dopamine agonists or L-dopa, absence of significant dementia, absence of tremor, and falls early in the disease course.

The clinical picture is usually dominated by three major issues: a dysautonomia manifested by severe OH and severe (most often lower motor neuron) urinary dysfunction, and a motor system disturbance that results in a wheelchair requirement early in the course of the disorder. Patients may have multiple other related complaints, including impotence, slurred speech, sleep apnea, vivid nightmares, orthostatic headache, neck pain, dimming of vision, and leg discomfort. Several specific clinical features may help in the diagnosis of MSA. Patients frequently note emotional lability, with short (sometimes only 1 or 2 minutes) episodes of crying due to happiness or sadness in response to a relatively minor environmental stimulus, such as a song or an event in a television program or movie. This is usually self-limited but may be a harbinger of depression which may respond to a selective serotonin reuptake inhibitor. Patients sometimes have periodic gasping respirations punctuating the medical interview. They only last a few seconds and are not generally deep but seem labored. Finally, many patients discontinue the use of nicotine-containing products at the onset of their disease. It sometimes appears that they no longer enjoy the nicotine. Ultimately, nicotine may provoke or worsen tremor. Some patients with MSA-C may have intermittent diplopia.

OH is usually severe, and treatment is frequently complicated by supine hypertension. Supine plasma norepinephrine levels are often near normal in patients with MSA but do not rise appropriately on standing, as expected in a disorder involving central pathways. This contrasts with the low plasma norepinephrine found in the ganglionic disorder PAF. The reduction in the lying-to-standing norepinephrine level change in MSA results from both lower-than-normal secretion with standing and higher-than-normal secretion when supine. This accounts for the sometimes severe supine hypertension seen in MSA (Shannon et al., 2000). Thus MSA does not reflect only a reduction of required autonomic outflow but an inversion of central autonomic regulation.

Involvement of the bladder occurs in most patients. The pathophysiology is complex, resulting from pathological changes in bladder-control elements at several levels in the neuraxis. Early complaints of urgency, frequency, and nocturia reflect dysfunction in upper motor neuron circuits, including loss of neuromelatonin-containing neurons in the striatum and loss of neurons in the cerebellum, raphe nuclei, and frontal cortex. The later picture is dominated by overflow incontinence, more consistent with a "lower motor neuron bladder," most likely reflecting the destruction of cells in the Onuf parasympathetic nucleus of the sacral spinal cord. Post-void residuals steadily increase from year 1 to year 5 of the disease (Ito et al., 2006). In fact, a large post-void residual in a patient with a Parkinson-like disorder suggests MSA rather than PD (Hahn and Ebersbach, 2005). Failure of bladder emptying is further compromised by loss of intermediolateral horn preganglionic sympathetic innervation to the bladder, which results in loss of control of both the sphincter and collapse of the bladder neck (Kirby et al., 1986), which remains open in 53% of patients (Sakakibara et al., 2001). Detailed reviews of the subject have been published (Fowler et al., 2008, 2010).

Prognosis in MSA is poor; 10-year survival is rare. The autonomic abnormalities are seldom the direct cause of death. Some patients develop laryngeal stridor and difficulty swallowing, which can lead to aspiration pneumonia. Some MSA patients have sleep apnea, and in some cases, this may lead to a critical loss of respiratory drive—the so-called Ondine curse. The most common causes of death in patients with MSA are pulmonary embolus, apnea, and intercurrent infection.

The pathophysiology of MSA is unknown, and no cure exists, so management continues to be symptomatic (Freeman et al., 1999; Hussain et al., 2001; Jordan and Biaggioni, 2002; Wenning et al., 2005). This includes treatment of the depression, tremor, gait disturbances, orthostatic hypotension, and possible self-catheterization when urine retention is severe. Although in the last 5 years several promising developments have occurred, mainly at the animal model, they have so far not translated into the clinical arena. A transgenic mouse model that closely mimics the disorder was developed by splicing the α-synuclein gene in front of a myelin basic protein promoter. Neurodegeneration in a transgenic mouse model of multiple system atrophy is associated with altered expression of oligodendroglial-derived neurotrophic factors (Ubhi et al, 2010). Further, rifampicin was shown to inhibit aggregation of α-synuclein in vitro and in this mouse model, leading to a National Institutes of Health–sponsored trial of rifampicin in MSA that sadly did not show that the drug halts the progression of MSA (Low et al., 2014) and may, in fact, have slightly worsened the disorder. A pilot open-label treatment with intravenous globulin showed guarded promise, showing some improvement in daily living function, but no improvement in brain imaging. A double-blind placebo control is needed to further evaluate this improvement (Novak et al., 2012). Finally, an international trial of the antiparkinsonian drug rasagiline, an inhibitor of monoamine oxidase type B, has shown no improvement (data only by abstract, not published). Several currently open trials include stem cell implantation, verdiperstat (myeloperoxidase inhibitor), intranasal insulin, sirolimus, and $CoQ_{10}$. Other drugs and approaches are also being tried in animal models.

## Parkinson Disease

From a clinical perspective, the autonomic manifestations of PD are virtually indistinguishable from those of MSA. Although some authors report a difference between the results of autonomic testing in MSA and PD (Chelimsky, 2008; Lipp et al., 2009), these studies compared patients with nonequivalent burdens of autonomic dysfunction, being much worse in MSA than in PD. Clearly, more severe abnormalities occur in patients with more severe clinical dysautonomia, causing patients with MSA to appear more severe in their test results than patients with PD. When patients in the PD group are matched with those of the MSA group for severity of autonomic involvement, autonomic testing cannot distinguish MSA from PD (Riley and Chelimsky, 2003). The autonomic dysfunction of PD can be astoundingly severe. Although autonomic dysfunction is clearly more prevalent in MSA than in PD, when a patient presents to the office with severe OH and a PD-like syndrome, PD is more likely, simply because PD is so much more common than MSA (1000 per 100,000 vs. 0.4 per 100,000; Bonuccelli et al., 2003).

The pathophysiology of autonomic dysfunction in PD is different than in MSA. Whereas MSA exclusively involves central networks and nuclei, the Lewy bodies of PD directly involve ganglia, and hence postganglionic neurons, with degeneration of peripheral autonomic fibers. One may therefore see a reduction in axon reflex sweating more frequently in PD than in MSA, though this is not always reliable. In addition, increased response to sympathetic agonists such as midodrine due to denervation supersensitivity may occur, but again this is inconsistent. Finally, this peripheral predilection in PD is the basis for the denervation seen on metaiodobenzylguanidine (MIBG) scanning of the heart, which has been touted as a diagnostic test to distinguish PD from MSA (Goldstein et al., 2009), though others do not find the same results (Geser et al., 2011). The rationale is that uptake of this compound, a congener of norepinephrine, into noradrenergic-rich tissues such as the heart will be impaired in conditions such as PAF and PD, but is comparatively normal in MSA. Finally, some authors have advocated sphincter EMG as a method of distinction, since the lower motor neuron is involved in MSA, resulting in polyphasic and bizarre motor units in this disorder but normal motor units in PD (Fowler, 2001).

Clinical classification may provide the best method at this point in time. In the recent epidemiological trial of MSA with classification based on clinical criteria, more than 100 patients were classified correctly when the classification was compared to autopsy findings.

## Myelopathy

Because sympathetic outflow (T1–L2/3) and sacral parasympathetic outflow descend in the spinal cord, cord lesions commonly result in substantial autonomic impairment. This may occur in both spinal cord injury and other disorders such as multiple sclerosis (Fowler et al., 2010), neuromyelitis optica, or spinal cord lesions of any other cause. In cervical and high thoracic levels, most sympathetic and sacral parasympathetic outflow is lost (Mathias, 2004; Mathias and Bannister, 2002). Following spinal cord injury, the initial response is hypoexcitability (spinal shock) with flaccid paralysis, impaired tendon reflexes, and spinal autonomic dysfunction presenting as atonic bladder and bowel, vasodilation, and absent spinal autonomic reflexes. This stage lasts days to weeks, and then activity below the transected cord returns. Chronically, a quite distinct autonomic dysfunction emerges (Critchley et al., 2003).

Whereas blood pressure is low following acute high thoracic cord injury, in the chronic stage blood pressure relates to the level of the spinal lesion. It is lower in high cord lesions and rises to near normal as the lesion descends. Severe hypertension may occur during autonomic dysreflexia (Head-Riddoch syndrome) after noxious stimulation below the level of the lesion—for example, related to pressure sores, abdominal visceral processes, bladder contraction or irritation from a urethral catheter, or even from skeletal muscle contraction such as muscle spasm. Any of these may elicit dramatic blood pressure elevation. These changes occur from activation below the cord lesion, whereas sweating and cutaneous dilation occur above the lesion. During autonomic dysreflexia, sympathetic nerve activity is increased. Impaired baroreflex function no doubt contributes to these effects, including the hypersensitivity to pressor and depressor agents.

Considerable morbidity occurs in autonomic dysreflexia, with severe sweating and headache, or even intracranial hemorrhage. Management consists of preventing initiation of the increased sympathetic discharge. High cord lesions are associated with warm (vasodilated) skin below the lesion. The nasal stuffiness from vasodilation in the nasal mucosa is *Guttmann sign*. There is susceptibility to hypothermia because, in addition to being unable to constrict the cutaneous circulation, shivering diminishes. However, in certain circumstances, the reverse occurs, causing hyperthermia because of the inability to sweat and vasodilate in the periphery, which would normally induce heat loss.

Environmental temperature thus needs to be carefully controlled. Hyperthermia responds to sponge bathing, the efficacy of which is enhanced by fanning. In severe cases, ice-cooled saline by intravenous infusion or urinary bladder irrigation is occasionally required. The sympathetic skin response can be useful in assessing spinal cord injury (Cariga et al., 2002). Activation of supraspinal centers and descending sudomotor neural pathways in the spinal cord are necessary for the SSR. It is absent in the feet in low spinal injuries and absent in the hand region in high spinal injuries. The presence or absence of the SSR, in addition to motor and sensory evaluation, can be a marker of spinal cord autonomic involvement and may improve classification of the extent of spinal functional deficits. The SSR can also test spinal cord sudomotor centers isolated from the brainstem that are capable of generating an SSR.

In early cord injury, vagal hyperactivity may cause excessive gastric acid secretion, with ulceration and hemorrhage (Mathias and Bannister, 2002). $H_2$ antagonists or proton pump inhibitors may be useful in such patients. In high lesions, paralytic ileus may occur, especially after the ingestion of solid food. Colon dysfunction occurs commonly but may be amenable to bowel training, modification of diet, mild laxatives, and stool softeners. Urine retention, distention, and overflow occur early after cord injury. Intermittent catheterization should be used in the early stages. Persistent infection in various sites may cause secondary amyloidosis with renal infiltration and damage.

In men, both erectile and ejaculatory failure occur in early cord injury. Conversely, in the chronic phase, priapism may occur during autonomic dysreflexia. Ejaculation is often retrograde. Various approaches that include electrical stimulation and collection of seminal fluid have been used for artificial insemination. Sildenafil (Viagra) is effective for erection in spinal injuries and autonomic failure (Hussain et al., 2001). In women, menstrual cycle disruption occurs in early cord injury. Recovery is usually within a year, and successful pregnancy has occurred in both tetraplegic and paraplegic women. In high cord lesions, uterine contractions may evoke severe autonomic dysreflexia. Such patients are particularly prone to seizures and sometimes to cerebral hemorrhage in response to very severe hypertension. These individuals require antihypertensive therapy as well as medication for seizure control.

## NONAUTONOMIC DISORDERS CAUSING HYPOTENSION OR SYNCOPE TO CONSIDER IN THE DIFFERENTIAL DIAGNOSIS

The physician must be vigilant for unexpected disorders that may be confused with autonomic dysfunction or hypotension. Some of these include the following diverse conditions.

### Aortic Stenosis

With bicuspid aortic valves, patients may develop aortic stenosis late in life. This may lead to syncopal episodes, especially with exertion. Intracardiac pressure may be high even when the cuff blood pressure is low, as when syncope occurs. Echocardiography provides a definitive diagnosis.

### Hypertrophic Cardiomyopathy

Hypertrophic cardiomyopathy is an asymmetrical hypertrophy of the ventricles. Inheritance may be autosomal dominant, but at least half of cases are sporadic. It is the most common genetic cardiac disease. Systolic function is preserved, but left ventricular outflow obstruction at rest occurs in 20% of patients and may lead to syncope, palpitations, shortness of breath, and sudden death. The echocardiogram is diagnostic.

### Subclavian Steal Syndrome (Millikan-Siekert Syndrome)

Basilar artery insufficiency results from subclavian steal; exercise of the left arm precipitates neurological symptoms including syncope, facial paresthesia, headache, and transitory loss of vision. It is due to reversal of blood flow from the vertebrobasilar system into the subclavian system.

### Innominate Artery Syndrome

Innominate artery syndrome may present with apparently low blood pressure in the right arm but be otherwise asymptomatic. It is detected by disparities of blood pressure in the two arms. However, occasionally subclavian steal occurs with proximal subclavian artery stenosis and retrograde perfusion of the vertebral artery to the distal subclavian artery.

### Sick Sinus Syndrome (Short Syndrome)

Sick sinus syndrome presents with alternating bradycardia and tachycardia. A sick sinus node is abnormally susceptible to the suppressive influence of ectopic atrial activity. It usually occurs in women after age 60, more than half of whom may experience syncope.

### Glossopharyngeal Neuralgia (Weissenberg Syndrome)

Glossopharyngeal neuralgia presents as a unilateral episodic hypotension and bradycardia in association with severe paroxysmal pain beginning in the tonsillar region, lateral pharynx, or base of the tongue and radiating deeply into the ear. Eating or talking elicits the neuralgia. This disorder sometimes occurs in the wake of injury or tumor in the neck. It may respond to treatment with yohimbine or channel blockers like mexilitene, gabapentin, or topiramate, but some patients seem very resistant to therapy. If all else fails, the division of the nerve at the area of emergence from the cranium may be required.

### Inferior Vena Cava Syndrome (Supine Hypotensive Syndrome)

Inferior vena cava syndrome occurs in the last month of pregnancy in as many as 10% of women. Assumption of the supine position causes a sudden fall in systolic blood pressure, nausea, and vomiting. Tachycardia is associated. The probable cause is decreased venous return, and hence cardiac output, from compression of the inferior vena cava by the gravid uterus.

### Pancreatic Cholera (Verner-Morrison Syndrome)

Verner-Morrison syndrome is marked by a watery diarrhea associated with an islet cell tumor and electrolyte abnormalities. It may occur with bronchogenic carcinoma or multiple endocrine neoplasia type 1. Secretion of vasoactive intestinal polypeptide is the usual cause of symptoms. In 84% of cases, the origin is the pancreas. A metabolic acidosis is usually present.

### Villous Adenoma (McKittrick-Wheelock Syndrome)

McKittrick-Wheelock syndrome arises from the severe dehydration and electrolyte depletion that occurs as a complication of colonic villous adenoma. These adenomas exude large quantities of electrolyte-rich fluid. Severe OH may occur. A key diagnostic feature is greatly elevated blood urea nitrogen with proportionately lesser elevation of serum creatinine. These findings may resolve almost completely with fluid replacement.

### Cortisol Deficiency (Addison Disease)

Hypotension and postural hypotension occur in the late stages of cortisol deficiency, as both aldosterone and cortisol itself play important roles in the maintenance of blood pressure. Aldosterone increases available intravascular volume through renal retention of sodium, while cortisol directly influences both the endothelium and vascular smooth muscle. In endothelium, cortisol inhibits the generation of vasodilators such as nitric oxide and prostacyclin, while it enables pharmacomechanical coupling of agonists such as norepinephrine in vascular smooth muscle. When cortisol is absent, hypotension and vascular collapse due to unresponsiveness of the smooth muscle to any pharmacological agonists ensue, including those given exogenously for resuscitation. In this setting, the administration of intravenous glucocorticoids is the only strategy and constitutes a medical emergency (Yang and Zhang, 2004).

## THERAPY OF DYSAUTONOMIAS

Patients with autonomic disorders have both autonomic and nonautonomic features to their illness. Some features, such as extrapyramidal and cerebellar complications in MSA and PD, are discussed elsewhere in this book (see Chapter 95). This chapter addresses treatment of the specifically autonomic aspects of these diseases, such as OH and bladder and bowel issues. For most disorders, at the time of this writing, treatment is still primarily symptomatic, even where a metabolic or genetic defect has been identified.

At the outset, however, it is important to recognize the fundamental difference between treating *hypertension* in clinical practice and treating *hypotension* in patients with autonomic disorders. When physicians treat patients with hypertension, they are not trying to improve the patient's functional capacity or symptoms, but rather an effort is being made to prevent complications of hypertension far in the future (e.g., stroke, myocardial infarction). In contrast, when we treat OH, our entire focus is on immediately improving the patient's symptoms. In rare disorders, such as most dysautonomias, evidence-based medicine drawn from studies in hundreds or thousands of people is unavailable to guide the management of hypertension. Indeed, no agent used to treat OH has been proven to attenuate long-term complications or improve patient survival. These limitations are important to keep in mind but should not prevent physicians from doing their best to keep patients as symptom free as possible.

### Nonpharmacological Interventions for Orthostatic Hypotension

Treatment of orthostasis is primarily nonpharmacological. Many measures can be used for POTS, syncope, and OH and should be implemented before moving to drugs, with approaches that are slightly different for the three disorders. When autonomic reflexes fail, certain physical maneuvers, life habits, and drugs have a much greater effect on blood pressure than they have in normal subjects. This can be used to advantage in patient management. Maintenance of physical conditioning is a fundamental principle of management. This may only be achieved with water aerobics or water jogging in shoulder-deep water if orthostasis is advanced. The water reduces the gravitational pull on blood volume to nearly a quarter of its normal value, with cerebral perfusion remaining largely intact. Great care should be exercised when coming out of the water, with return of full gravitational pull combined with a vasodilated muscular system and possibly cutaneous dilation as well, depending on water temperature. For this reason, cooler temperatures are preferred. Recumbent bicycling may also be useful.

A range of simple physical maneuvers have been identified that can improve the patient's ability to stand upright (Krediet et al., 2005; van Dijk et al., 2006); implementation is accomplished with a little education (Fig. 107.7). Physical countermaneuvers possess the additional

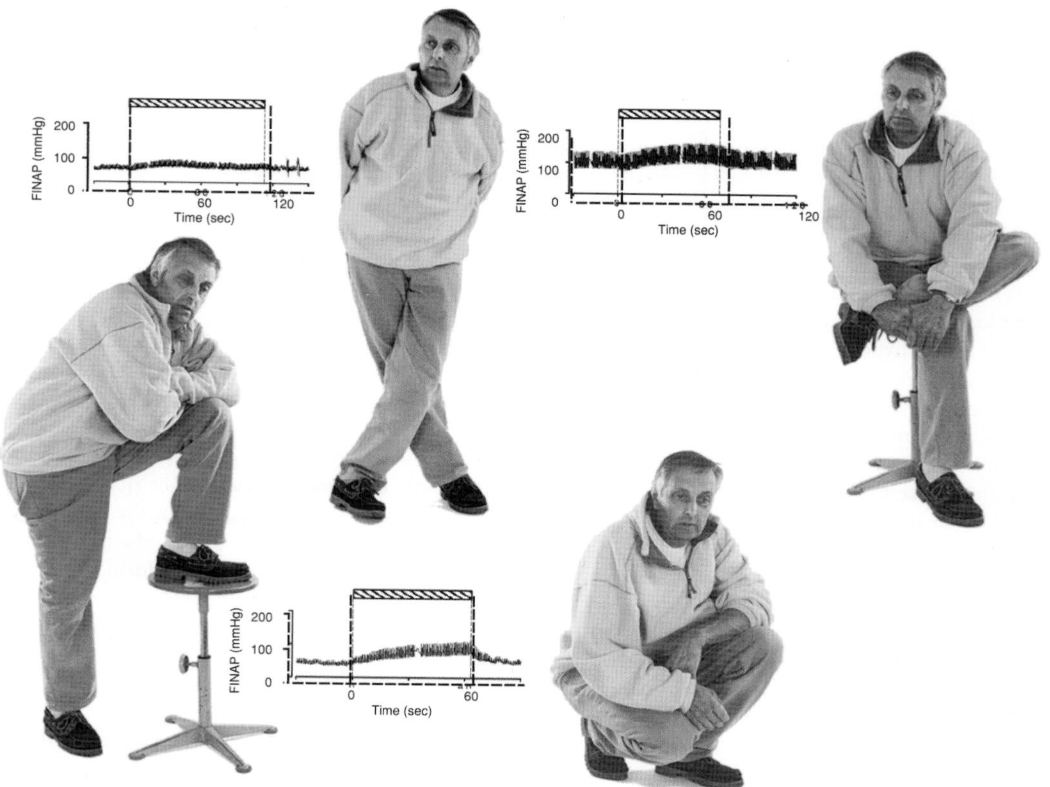


**Fig 107.7 Physical Countermaneuvers Using Isometric Contractions of Lower Limbs and Abdominal Compression.** Effects of leg crossing in standing and sitting position, placing a foot on a chair, and squatting on finger arterial blood pressure *(FINAP)* in a 54-year-old male patient with pure autonomic failure and invalidating orthostatic hypotension. The patient was standing (sitting) quietly before the maneuvers. Bars indicate the duration of maneuvers. Note blood pressure and pulse pressure increase during maneuvers. *(Courtesy M.P.M. Harms and W. Wieling, Amsterdam Medical Center, Amsterdam, The Netherlands.)*

advantage of being entirely under the patient's control, with all the convenience and self-reliance that derive from this. Such maneuvers use muscle pump action or gravity to improve circulation to the brain and forestall a faint when the person is standing; they include leg crossing, performed by crossing the legs in a scissors pattern. The patient actively stands on both legs. It is likely that this maneuver squeezes venous vessels in the legs and abdomen so that less blood pools there. Leaning forward slightly enhances the benefit of this maneuver. Crossing the legs in the seated posture may have a similar physiological basis and is quite effective, especially for individuals with the most severe orthostatic hypotension, when even the seated posture represents a challenge. One limitation of leg crossing in the upright posture is that the patient may have reduced postural stability and be more likely to fall. In particular, few patients with MSA, for example, can benefit from upright leg crossing because of their balance problems independent of their blood pressure. However, in individuals without extrapyramidal or cerebellar abnormalities, this maneuver is so strikingly useful that many patients will have discovered its value on their own and may have been using it for a number of years before they are even diagnosed with OH (Wieling et al., 2004).

Squatting is another powerful pressor maneuver. Squatting increases pressure by reducing the capacity of veins in the legs and splanchnic vasculature while also creating a mechanical impediment to arterial circulation to the legs. The usefulness of squatting to forestall a "hypotensive" emergency is very great for many patients with OH. It is noteworthy, however, that rising from the squatting position sometimes presents difficulties of its own.

Orthostatic (standing) training has been suggested as effective nonpharmacological therapy for patients with recurrent reflex syncope. This treatment involves leaning patients upright with the upper back against a wall and the feet away from the wall about 1 foot (mimicking a 70-degree angle) for 10–20 minutes once or twice a day. The maneuver should be performed on a carpeted floor with no sharp angular furniture nearby, in case of a faint. The initial results from this therapy are quite promising, and it has been subjected to an open-label trial with good results (Fowler et al., 2010). Although not proven to work in POTS or OH, orthostatic training merits being tried for both of these disorders.

Support garments over the lower part of the body benefit patients by acutely increasing blood pressure. Support garments can be used in patients with severe orthostatic hypotension, especially those who live in a relatively cool climate. A disadvantage is that the patients must be willing to take off the garments every time they lie down to preserve their effectiveness in the upright posture. This is a major inconvenience. Many patients also find the garments uncomfortable and "hot." Some individuals will save the garment for special occasions when they must stand up to speak or to carry out an important but time-limited activity in the upright posture.

## Dietary Measures

### Sodium

Dietary sodium is also an important measure in improving OH. It may seem paradoxical that salt water does not raise the pressure as much as pure water, and yet dietary sodium is salutary; salt's chronic (but not acute) effects are beneficial. Salt may be very helpful if there are no contraindications to the increase of sodium in the diet. Chronically increasing dietary salt, aiming to raise urinary sodium to 185 mmol in a 24-hour urinary collection (Wieling et al., 2004), will raise blood pressure, especially if given in concert with the mineralocorticoid fludrocortisone. The content of sodium determines the extracellular fluid volume. Patients with OH need between 6 and 10 g of sodium and 2 to 3 L of water (Shibao et al., 2012). To be assured that patients are taking enough salt, the daily 24-hour urinary excretion of sodium needs to be monitored and salt added or decreased as needed (Wieling et al., 2004). The amount of supplement will vary from patient to patient and diagnosis to diagnosis. Patients with POTS will usually require 2 g at 8:00 a.m. and 2 g at 2:00 p.m. The duration of action is 4–5 hours, so it is only needed at these two times when the patient will be upright. Salt is available in pill form by various manufacturers.

### Water Drinking

In recent years, water has been recognized as a powerful pressor agent in autonomic disorders (Jordan et al., 1999). Increases in blood pressures of 30–40 mm Hg after ingestion of 500 mL (≈16 ounces) of tap water are quite common; occasional patients may have increases in pressure of 80 mm Hg or more. The effect of water is greatest in the hour after ingestion and is almost gone 90 minutes afterward. The effect starts 5 minutes after drinking water and peaks at about 40 minutes (May and Jordan, 2011). Some patients will have discovered the benefit of water on their own, but for many others, it is important to educate them about this very useful approach to raising blood pressure (Jordan et al., 2004; Shannon et al., 2002). Once the possible effect of water is raised with patients, it usually takes only one trial for them to recognize its value. Hypotonic water works best because the sugar or salt content of other beverages attenuate pressor action. The ideal use of water is to drink it immediately upon awakening at the time medications are taken, to cover the hour window before medications begin to take effect. Interestingly, this blood pressure effect from water is only present in subjects with abnormal baroreflex regulation, either from aging or due to neurodegenerative disorders. Water drinking increases sympathetic activity through a spinal reflex, producing an increase in resting metabolic state and a vasopressor response that increases blood pressure. The response occurs after the water has exited the stomach and activates the parasympathetic system through the baroreflex, reflected in a bradycardia with increased high-frequency heart rate variability. The response may require an osmotic change in the portal tract and the liver, although the mechanism has not yet been completely elucidated. Water can be used to increase blood pressure (1) before getting up from bed; (2) before meals if the subjects have postprandial hypotension; and (3) in subjects with neurally medicated syncope, when donating blood to decrease risk of fainting or in postexercise syncope (May and Jordan, 2011). In POTS patients, water and clear soup (hyperosmolar) produced an increase in orthostatic tolerance, with less heart rate increase while upright with both liquids, more with water but not statistically significant (Z'Graggen et al., 2010).

### Food Ingestion

Ingestion of a meal, particularly one rich in carbohydrate, significantly lowers blood pressure, often about the same degree as water raises it. Desserts and other sweet foods are the most immediate and powerful depressors. Patients can use this information by adjusting their activities around meals. For example, it would be far wiser to go shopping first and eat a meal afterward, rather than the reverse.

## Drugs

### Fludrocortisone

For 50 years, fludrocortisone has been the mainstay of therapy for OH (Freeman, 2003). However, the limited success of therapy has led to many alternative agents that are sometimes helpful (Box 107.5). Fludrocortisone has two main effects: a well-known high-dose volume effect and a less well-recognized low-dose pressor effect. As a mineralocorticoid like aldosterone, fludrocortisone initially increases blood volume secondary to sodium retention. This effect requires several days to weeks to reach its peak. Although the plasma volume may

**BOX 107.5 Drug Treatment of Autonomic Failure and Nonpharmacological Measures**

Fludrocortisone (9α-fluorohydrocortisone)
Sympathomimetic amines:
- Midodrine
- Phenylpropanolamine
- Droxidopa (LDOPS)

Cyclooxygenase inhibitors:
- Indomethacin
- Ibuprofen

Ergot alkaloids:
- Ergotamine
- Dihydroergotamine mesylate

Somatostatin analogs:
- Somatostatin
- Octreotide acetate

Antihistamines:
- Diphenhydramine
- Ranitidine

Other drugs:
- Dopamine antagonists: metoclopramide, domperidone
- $\alpha_2$-Agonists and antagonists: clonidine, methyldopa, yohimbine
- β-Antagonists
- Serotonin antagonists: cyproheptadine
- Vasopressin analogs
- Vasodilators: hydralazine, minoxidil
- Erythropoietin

Nonpharmacological measures:
- Physical maneuvers
- Water
- Elevated head of bed
- Antigravity suit

return to baseline subsequently, in many patients, a residual beneficial pressor effect continues, in part due to increased peripheral vascular resistance, enhanced pressor response to norepinephrine, and extravascular fluid accumulation (edema) in the legs (van Lieshout et al., 2000), which limits blood pooling. This lesser-known effect, sensitization of α-adrenergic receptors (Davies et al., 1978), allows extremely low doses to have an impact on orthostatic homeostasis in children and young adults with POTS or syncope. We often start with a half tablet (0.05 mg) every other day, with benefit beginning at about 10 days after treatment onset. Fludrocortisone is rapidly absorbed after oral ingestion and has a plasma half-life of 2–3 hours, yet its biological half-life is much longer (several days) because of nuclear changes in sodium handling. An additional effect of fludrocortisone is that it increases sympathetic tone and pressor response (Chobanian et al., 1979; Distler et al., 1985).

Several issues must be taken into account concerning the optimal use of fludrocortisone. First, because the full pressor action of fludrocortisone is delayed for 1–2 weeks, dose alterations need not occur more frequently than at weekly intervals. The initial dose should be 0.05–0.1 mg daily or even every other day, with weekly or biweekly titration by 0.05-mg increments, aiming for a weight gain of 4–8 pounds and mild ankle swelling if using the higher dose-volume effect. The patient should be educated about the expected time course of the effect. It will be rare to find an additional benefit beyond a dosage of 0.2 mg orally daily, but doses as high as 2 mg/day are accepted. Little if any glucocorticoid effect occurs at doses in the range of 0.1–0.2 mg daily, but reduced cortisol levels due to corticotropin suppression occur after a single dose of 2 mg.

Weight is a good guide to the required dose, and the weight gain due to fluid retention should be limited to 5–8 pounds. Because much of the blood pressure effect relates to this fluid retention, the patient should be educated to accept some edema. Do not use fludrocortisone in patients who cannot tolerate fluid retention; this is rarely an issue, because such patients will rarely have significant orthostatic hypotension. If symptoms of pulmonary congestion or even pulmonary edema do develop in an autonomic failure patient after a fludrocortisone-induced increase in plasma volume, these symptoms will respond very rapidly to assumption of the seated or upright posture.

Fludrocortisone has some unusual side effects. Occasional patients may develop hypokalemia at higher doses (> 0.1mg/day). It responds to oral supplementation with potassium, which is a chronically used medication in such patients. A smaller group, perhaps 5%, will develop concomitant hypomagnesemia, and although correction of the hypokalemia will often lead to secondary correction of the hypomagnesemia, if this is not complete, small doses of magnesium sulfate (or oyster shell calcium) can be added. Fludrocortisone commonly produces mild headache in young patients but rarely in severe autonomic failure. Another common problem is the development of supine hypertension, which can be lowered acutely by elevating the head of the bed, having the patient sit or stand, or giving a carbohydrate snack. If it persists, a reduction in dosage or discontinuation of fludrocortisone may be necessary. Occasional patients on warfarin will need increased doses while on fludrocortisone. Recent improvements in our understanding of the health consequences of aldosterone antagonists in heart failure have alerted physicians to theoretical concerns about long-term mineralocorticoid receptor stimulation.

Adrenergic agonists (sympathomimetics) have increasingly supplanted fludrocortisone in therapy of autonomic failure in recent years. This is driven by the relative ease of targeting drug treatment to the times during the day when the pressor effect is most needed, whereas administration of fludrocortisone elicits a 24-hour effect, even if only one dose a day is given. Because many patients with autonomic dysfunction have supine hypertension, this is a significant disadvantage of fludrocortisone because nocturnal hypertension may worsen.

### Midodrine

The most commonly used sympathomimetic agent (Low et al., 1997), midodrine is a prodrug that is hydrolyzed in the liver to its active form, desglymidodrine, a peripherally active $\alpha_1$-adrenoceptor agonist. The peak effect of oral midodrine occurs 1 hour after administration, and its duration of action is usually 4–6 hours. Side effects are generally mild and dose related and include piloerection (goose flesh) and urinary retention (due to the α-agonist effect on the urinary sphincter). Because midodrine does not cross the blood–brain barrier, some central side effects such as those that might be seen with ephedrine, pseudoephedrine, or other sympathomimetic amines do not occur. The symptoms of goose flesh are transitory and not very problematic in most individuals, but occasional patients will find this a significant problem, especially in the scalp, and may even need to withdraw from the drug because of the side effect. Usually, however, the most severely affected patients with OH will recognize the goose-flesh sensation as a welcome signal that the blood pressure-raising effect of midodrine is present and that they will now have increased capacity to be up and around. Most patients receive 2.5–10 mg every 3–4 hours, up to a maximum of 60 mg/day. When first administering this agent to a patient who has never received it, particularly one in whom plasma norepinephrine levels are quite low, it may be worthwhile to give a 1.25-mg test dose. Midodrine should not be given after 6:00 p.m. or if the subject will be supine, owing to the risk of supine hypertension.

For older patients who nap after lunch, midodrine can be prescribed as a twice-daily drug to be taken in the morning and then after the nap around 3:00 or 4:00 p.m. A recent meta-analysis erroneously reported little to no benefit of midodrine in OH (Parsaik et al., 2013), focusing on the change in blood pressure from lying to standing, an endpoint that this drug would not affect, and which has never been used as an endpoint in any clinical trial. At this point, the weight of evidence still strongly supports the use of midodrine in OH. Midodrine may be helpful in subjects with POTS, although not all subjects with POTS seems to respond. In pediatrics, the response may depend on the change in blood pressures from supine to upright and the diastolic blood pressure while upright (Deng et al., 2014). It would make logical sense if subjects with neuropathic POTS responded better than those with hyperadrenergic POTS responded (Ross et al., 2014).

### Droxidopa

Droxidopa was approved by the US Food and Drug Administration (FDA) in 2014 for neurogenic orthostatic hypotension. Its use has generally been rising for the treatment of OH (Freeman et al., 1999; Kaufmann et al., 2003). This agent is also a kind of prodrug. It has little effect on its own but is converted in the body directly to norepinephrine by L-aromatic amino acid decarboxylase within the nerve terminal, thus allowing greater release of synaptic norepinephrine at the synapse. Droxidopa is particularly beneficial in patients with DBH deficiency because the drug directly overcomes the enzymatic defect in this genetic disorder. One DBH-deficient patient recently completed a competitive 26-mile marathon (Garland et al., 2005). However, droxidopa is also finding wider use in the treatment of other autonomic disorders, including PAF and MSA. The maximum effect of the drug occurs 5 hours after ingestion. The ultimate role of LDOPS vis-à-vis direct-acting agents such as midodrine will depend on future studies comparing these two approaches. In PD, droxidopa did not show a significant increase in blood pressure, but the subjects with PD had a significant decrease in falls with less dizziness and lightheadedness (Hauser et al., 2014). A meta-analysis of the efficacy of droxidopa in neurogenic OH showed that droxidopa is better than placebo, but after the first 2 weeks of treatment, that difference decreased and disappeared at 8 weeks. On a positive side, there were no significant side effects when compared with placebo (Elgebaly et al., 2016). A phase IV trial for long-term outcomes is under way.

### Pyridostigmine

The anticholinesterase inhibitor pyridostigmine commonly used in myasthenia gravis to increase neuromuscular junction neural traffic at the nicotinic receptor on the muscle, has been advocated for use in OH (Singer et al., 2003). It increases signal strength at the other major nicotinic receptor type, located at the autonomic ganglia, resulting in greater autonomic outflow when the system is activated. As a result, the increase in blood pressure is greater in the standing position than in the lying position, and exacerbation of supine hypertension is less of an issue than it is with drugs that work independently of central autonomic drive. Treatment usually begins with 30 mg (half a 60-mg tablet) three times daily, and the dose is gradually increased until blood pressure standing becomes acceptable, to a maximum of 90 mg three times daily.

### Erythropoietin

A mild degree of anemia is common in autonomic failure. When comparing levels of hematocrit and hemoglobin to erythropoietin in such individuals, it appears that the erythropoietin level is lower than expected for the level of anemia encountered. For this reason, erythropoietin is an indicated therapy to improve functional capacity in patients with OH and anemia. This mode of therapy is quite expensive, and third-party payers often find it difficult to understand its use for a neurological condition. The testimonials of patients about erythropoietin are quite dramatic, but long-term controlled trials are lacking. It is possible that with resolution of anemia and normalization of hematocrit, patients may look healthier to family and colleagues and may receive positive reinforcement about their condition based on this. Caution must be used in applying this mode of therapy because, in other contexts (e.g., chronic renal failure), normalization of hematocrit with erythropoietin seems to increase the mortality rate (Lau et al., 2010).

### Octreotide

Octreotide is a somatostatin analog that has significant effects on the gastrointestinal tract. At low doses in patients with autonomic impairment, it often elicits an increase in blood pressure, sometimes with minimal side effects. In our practice, we usually begin with 12.5 μg. Unfortunately, octreotide must be administered subcutaneously. Its effect appears within a few minutes and lasts a few hours. Almost all patients experience some increase in blood pressure if they have baseline autonomic impairment, but occasionally patients experience increases in blood pressure of 40 mm Hg or more and find the drug useful enough to justify subcutaneous injection. We have not had to go beyond 25 μg in managing blood pressures in our patients. However, excessively high doses may cause nausea or altered gastrointestinal motility. Long-term use (years) may increase the risk of gallstones (Veysey et al., 1999), but we have not yet encountered that complication at this low dose.

## Pacemaker Placement

Permanent dual-chamber pacemakers may sometimes be required for treatment—if, for example, severe bradycardias occur as part of the dysautonomia—but their value in reflex syncope remains controversial. They are currently not recommended, as several trials failed to show a significant benefit (Connolly et al., 1999; Mosqueda-Garcia et al., 2000). When a patient has a pacemaker already implanted, we empirically set the baseline rate slightly higher than usual (around 85 bpm or so) to maximize pump function in the context of an orthostatic disorder.

## Treatment of Supine Hypertension

Supine hypertension may sometimes be a serious problem. The physiology is now better understood. Ganglionic blockade significantly reduces supine pressure, implying that it is actually in part due to inappropriate sympathetic outflow to the vasculature in the supine position (Shannon et al., 2000)—problems of the arterial baroreflex circuits and in the renin–angiotensin–aldosterone pathways. There seems to be no involvement of the nitric oxide–induced vasodilation (Fanciulli et al., 2018). A recent consensus document from the American Autonomic Society, the European Federation of Autonomic Societies, and the European Society of Hypertension recommends, based on expert opinion, to avoid lying down during the daytime, decrease the fluid intake close to bedtime, avoid the use of fludrocortisone but rather use short-acting pressor medications, elevate the head of the bed about 30 degrees or tilt the entire bed 10 degrees, and to consume a snack that is rich in carbohydrates at bedtime (Jordan et al., 2019). Supine hypertension often requires specific treatment with short-acting antihypertensives at bedtime, such as nifedipine, losartan, or propranolol. Nifedipine should be used with caution, since it induces worse orthostatic symptoms in the morning, probably due to increased renal excretion of sodium. Furthermore, nifedipine is not recommended in the management of hypertension in the elderly (Jordan et al., 2019). Some medications affecting the nitric oxide system are useful, such as sildenafil (phosphodiesterase inhibitor), patches of nitroglycerin applied at bedtime, and nebivolol (Jordan et al., 2019). The selection of pharmacological treatment should consider the underlying cause of neurogenic supine hypertension. Clonidine works better in patients with MSA and central autonomic failure because more peripheral sympathetic nerves are preserved, which are the cause of orthostatic hypertension. Clonidine would block this effect. In contrast, in cases of disorders in which the peripheral sympathetic fibers are affected, as in PAF, clonidine would not be a good choice. Furthermore, in this group of patients, clonidine would increase the blood pressure even further (Jordan et al., 2019). In our practice, we usually treat pressures over 170/95 mm Hg or so, though no data are available as to when to treat this problem. Patients with autonomic failure do not appear to have the usually associated higher risk of stroke because high pressure is episodic rather than continuous, and the main reason to treat this is to reduce the risk associated with very high pressures (e.g., cerebral bleed).

## Bladder Issues

Early in most dysautonomias, an upper motor neuron spastic bladder dominates the clinical picture, while later a lower motor neuron flaccid process often supervenes. Urodynamics are very helpful in determining the stage of bladder dysfunction. Treatment is usually symptomatic in the early (spastic) phase, and various anticholinergic medications are available to prevent urgency and frequency. If CNS issues such as memory loss are not a problem, older agents such as oxybutynin (Ditropan) or tolterodine (Detrol) are usually adequate. Newer agents have more specific muscarinic receptor specificity and do not cross the blood–brain barrier, making them more appropriate when CNS effects should be avoided. When anticholinergics are entirely contraindicated, the β-3-adrenergic receptor antagonist mirabegron produces relaxation of the detrusor muscle. Although α-adrenergic antagonists may be helpful in patients with urgency by reducing sphincter pressure, they are relatively contraindicated in patients with OH, since they will reduce standing arterial pressure and are exact pharmacological opposites of drugs like midodrine.

Treatment of a later-stage low-pressure, flaccid detrusor employs different methods and pharmacology. The primary concern here is ureteral reflux that may lead to irreversible kidney damage. Thus, in contrast to the spastic bladder where management is primarily aimed at patient comfort, the flaccid bladder requires management from the outset to avert ureteral reflux and recurrent UTIs. Management begins by measuring a post-void residual. If over 100 mL, the risk of UTI is high, and emptying measures must be taken. This may include procholinergic medications, such as bethanechol, or acetylcholinesterase inhibitors, such as pyridostigmine, which improve detrusor contractility. If residual is still significantly over 100 mL, clean self-catheterization should be considered. Depending on the residual volume, this may be performed just once in the morning to ensure complete bladder emptying once daily; or upon awakening and before retiring; or, if needed, four times daily. The long-term prognosis for maintaining some level of detrusor function is clearly better if one allows the detrusor to work during some of the voids to maintain whatever function is still present as long as possible.

## Bowel Issues

Dysmotility associated with dysautonomias leads to upper bowel problems, such as gastroparesis and bacterial overgrowth, leading to bloating, distention, diarrhea, and lower bowel dysfunction, manifesting primarily as constipation or diarrhea, which may paradoxically be a result of obstipation with overflow stooling. All these issues demand careful thought and evaluation as the basis for appropriate management. For example, if diarrhea were due to constipation and simply treated as such with an antimuscarinic agent, the problem would become worse, not better. PD patients need a laxative approach, and polyethylene glycol (PEG) is at this time the first choice for slow transit or as a first-line treatment in other causes of constipation. It is important to work with a gastroenterologist with expertise in dysmotility. If one is not available, then a general gastroenterologist should be consulted to exclude superimposed structural disorders.

Upper-bowel dysfunction usually manifests as early satiety. It occurs commonly in diabetes and probably accounts for the profound weight loss associated with acute diabetic autonomic syndromes that may be treatment associated. Two aspects of gastric function may come as a surprise: (1) both sympathetic and parasympathetic nervous systems play key roles in gastric emptying, and pure loss of sympathetic function may lead to severe gastroparesis (Chelimsky et al., 2004); and (2) early satiety may *not* represent poor gastric emptying but rather loss of gastric accommodation (ability of the stomach to expand rapidly in compliance with a meal). To distinguish between these two possibilities, one may use a water-load test (How much water can the patient drink in 5 minutes? normal > 300 mL; Sood et al., 2002) and a gastric-emptying test with a solid and liquid diet. Upper-bowel dysmotility may benefit from promotility agents such as metoclopramide, 10 mg two or three times daily. However, metoclopramide is contraindicated in PD, owing to brain barrier passage and central effect. It should also be used with extreme caution because of the risk of tardive dyskinesia. Other motility agents are also available, including erythromycin at an adult dose of 250 mg two to three times daily. Erythromycin is a motilin agonist that improves gastric emptying and foregut motility. Octreotide is also useful in improving foregut motility, although it may produce delayed gastric emptying. It has some effect in increasing blood pressure and has been used in postprandial hypotension.

Lower-bowel dysfunction may present as constipation or diarrhea. Constipation usually requires a nonstimulating laxative such as PEG or lactulose given in generous doses until bowel function normalizes, when doses can be reduced to routine maintenance levels. A sitz marker study swallowing a capsule with many nonabsorbable rings followed by an x-ray a few days later (several protocols are available) can help determine if the constipation is due to a generalized motility disorder. When severe constipation with obstipation supervenes and is unresponsive to the standard regimen, a "home cleanout" regimen may be prescribed, consisting of bisacodyl 10 mg (2 × 5 mg tablets), followed by 1 capful of PEG in 8 ounces of liquid every 30 minutes for a total of 8–10 doses, followed by another dose of bisacodyl 4 hours later. Lubiprostone produced marked clinical improvement in a randomized double-blind placebo-controlled trial in subjects with PD, increasing daily stools in 64% of the subjects (Ondo et al., 2012). Lower-bowel dysmotility may also present with diarrhea, with a broader possible set of causes. Diarrhea may actually be a manifestation of obstipation, with liquid stool overflowing around the hard stool in the distal colon. A flat-plate abdominal radiograph is diagnostic. Other causes include small-bowel bacterial overgrowth, which may be determined by a hydrogen breath test and responds to antibiotics, in particular rifaximin, which is the current standard of care. Metronidazole should be avoided, since it may cause or worsen an autonomic neuropathy. Finally, primary lower-bowel hypermotility sometimes responds to low-dose clonidine (0.1–0.2 mg) once or twice daily.

In conclusion, autonomic disorders constitute a continuously growing field over the last decade, both in terms of pathophysiological understanding and in terms of management strategies. The discipline seems poised for an explosion of new understanding, particularly in the area of functional autonomic disorders, where new fundamental links between brain, behavior, and end-organ control may emerge.

## ACKNOWLEDGMENTS

We thank Ian Worcester for preparing the manuscript and acknowledge our friend and teacher David Robertson, whose authorship of this chapter in the fifth edition we built upon. Supported by Advancing a Healthier Wisconsin Endowment, Grant 5520298, and NIH-NIDDK R01DK083538.

*The complete reference list is available online at https://expertconsult.inkling.com/.* 

108

# Disorders of Neuromuscular Transmission

Jeffrey T. Guptill, Donald B. Sanders

## OUTLINE



Normal muscle contraction and force production require the efficient transmission of an electrical impulse from a motor axon to the muscle fibers it innervates. The neuromuscular junction (NMJ), a specialized synapse with a complex structural and functional organization, is the site of electrochemical conversion of nerve impulses into muscle fiber action potentials. The NMJ is particularly vulnerable to autoimmune disorders caused by circulating immune factors (myasthenia gravis and Lambert-Eaton myasthenia) since it has no blood–nerve barrier. Genetic abnormalities and certain toxins disrupt neuromuscular transmission (NMT) as well. Disorders of NMT produce several characteristic clinical syndromes, described in this chapter. Treatment options for autoimmune NMJ disorders remained relatively unchanged for many years, but a greater understanding of the pathophysiology of these disorders and an increasing number of targeted monoclonal antibodies and small molecules are expanding the number of treatment options.

## MYASTHENIA GRAVIS

Acquired myasthenia gravis (MG) is the most common primary disorder of NMT. In MG, the binding of autoantibodies to proteins, most commonly the acetylcholine receptor (AChR), disrupts normal NMT. This results in muscle weakness that typically predominates in certain muscle groups and fluctuates in response to effort and rest. The diagnosis depends on recognition of a distinctive pattern of weakness on history and examination, and confirmation by diagnostic tests. A number of effective therapeutic options are available, and treatment can result in minimal long-term morbidity in most patients.

### Epidemiology of Myasthenia Gravis

MG may begin at any age from infancy to very old age. Epidemiological studies report considerable variability in incidence and prevalence around the world (Deenen et al., 2015). While methodological differences may explain some of this variability, biological and genetic factors may also play a role. Estimates indicate that the US prevalence is approximately 20/100,000, or 60,000 patients total (Phillips, 2004). Epidemiological studies have shown an increasing prevalence over the past 50 years, related to an increase in the frequency of diagnosis in elderly patients, but also likely due to improved ascertainment, reduced mortality rates, and an increased longevity of the population (Carr et al., 2010). Gender and age influence the incidence of MG, women being affected nearly three times more often than are men before age 40, while the incidence is higher in males after age 50 and roughly equal during puberty. As the population ages, the average age at onset has increased correspondingly. More men are now affected than are women, and the majority of MG patients in the United States are over age 50. Detailed population-based data on clinical and serological subtypes of MG are largely lacking.

### Clinical Presentation of Myasthenia Gravis

Patients with MG seek medical attention for specific muscle weakness or dysfunction that typically worsens with activity and improves with rest. Although they may also have generalized fatigue or malaise, it is not usually the major or presenting complaint. Drooping eyelids or double vision is the initial symptom in approximately two-thirds of patients; nearly all will develop both within 2 years. Difficulty chewing, swallowing, or talking is the initial symptom in one-sixth of patients, and limb weakness in 10%. Rarely, the initial weakness is limited to

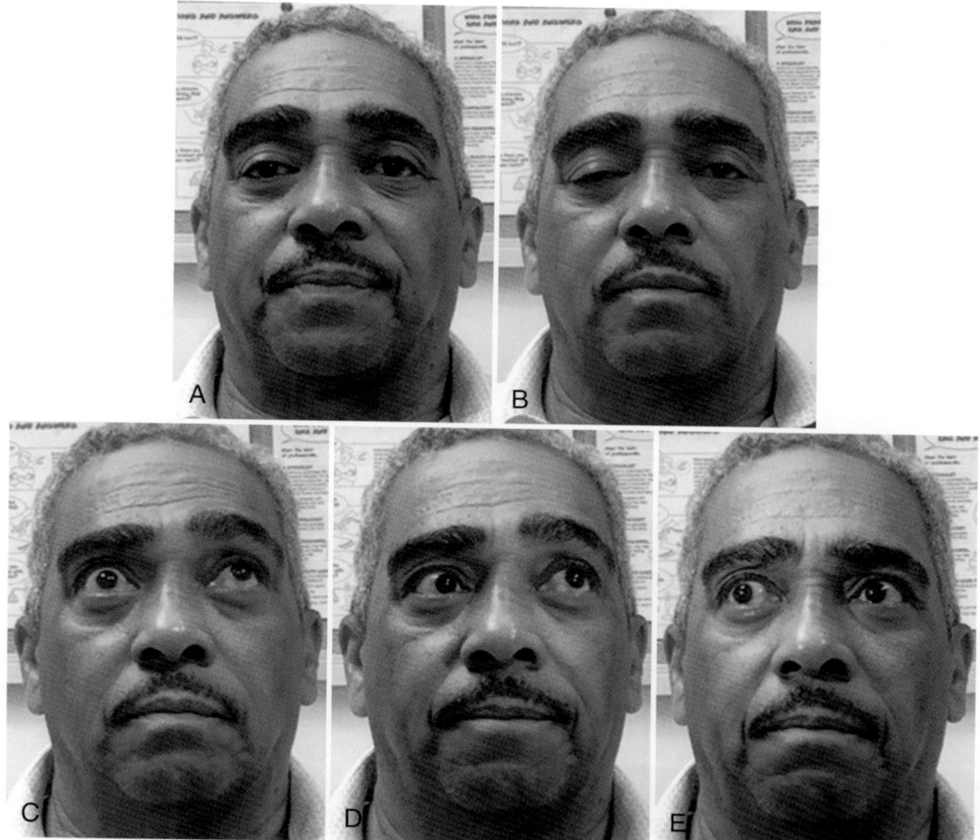

**Fig. 108.1 Ocular Motility Abnormalities In Myasthenia Gravis Due To Weakness Of Multiple Periocular Muscles In Both Eyes. A, B,** Progressive right lid ptosis during sustained forward gaze from fatigable weakness of the right levator palpebrae. **C,** Attempted upward gaze. There is incomplete superior movement of both eyes, worse in the right eye. Note the asymmetric furrowing of the forehead and elevation of the eyebrows. **D,** On left left lateral gaze, there is skew deviation with incomplete medial movement of the right eye and incomplete abduction of the left eye. **E,** On right right lateral gaze, there is incomplete movement of both eyes from weakness of right lateral rectus and left medial rectus muscles.

single muscle groups, such as neck, elbow or finger extensors, hip flexors, or ankle dorsiflexors.

Myasthenic weakness typically fluctuates during the day, usually being least in the morning and worse as the day progresses, especially after prolonged use of affected muscles. Ocular symptoms may be intermittent in the early stages, typically becoming worse in the evening or while reading, watching television, or driving, especially in bright sunlight. Many patients find that dark glasses reduce diplopia and hide drooping eyelids. Jaw muscle weakness typically becomes worse during prolonged chewing, especially of tough, fibrous, or chewy foods.

Careful questioning often reveals evidence of earlier, unrecognized myasthenic manifestations, such as frequent purchases of new eyeglasses to correct blurred vision, avoidance of foods that became difficult to chew or swallow, or cessation of activities that require prolonged use of specific muscles, such as singing. Friends may have noted a sleepy or sad facial appearance caused by ptosis or facial weakness.

The course of disease is variable but usually progressive. Weakness remains restricted to the ocular muscles in approximately 10%–15% of cases (See Ocular Myasthenia Gravis section, later in this chapter) although up to 58% has been reported in Asian populations, mainly in children (Zhang et al., 2007). In the rest, weakness progresses to involve nonocular muscles during the first 3 years and ultimately involves facial, oropharyngeal, and/or limb muscles *(generalized MG)*. Maximum weakness occurs during the first year in two-thirds of patients. Before the introduction of immunosuppression for treatment, approximately one-third of patients improved spontaneously, one-third became worse, and one-third died of the disease. Improvement, even *remission*, may occur early on but is rarely permanent (i.e., there is a subsequent *relapse*). Symptoms typically fluctuate over a relatively short period and then become more severe *(active stage)*. Left untreated, an inactive stage follows the active stage, in which fluctuations in strength still occur but are attributable to fatigue, intercurrent illness, or other identifiable factors. Although rare today, untreated weakness becomes fixed after many years, and the most severely involved muscles are frequently atrophic *(burnt-out stage)*. Factors that worsen myasthenic symptoms are emotional upset, systemic illness (especially viral respiratory infections), hypothyroidism or hyperthyroidism, pregnancy, the menstrual cycle, surgeries, drugs affecting NMT (see Treatment of Associated Diseases and Medications to Avoid section, later in this chapter), and fever.

## Physical Findings in Myasthenia Gravis

Perform the examination so as to detect variable weakness in specific muscle groups. Assess strength repetitively during maximum effort and again after rest. Performance on such tests may also fluctuate in diseases other than MG, especially if effort varies or testing causes pain. The symptoms of MG do not always vary, particularly in long-standing disease, which can make the diagnosis difficult.

### Ocular Muscles

Most MG patients have weakness of ocular muscles (Fig. 108.1; Box 108.1). Asymmetrical weakness of several muscles in both

**BOX 108.1 Ocular Findings in Myasthenia Gravis**

Weakness usually involves one or more ocular muscles without overt pupillary abnormality (Video 108.1—Ocular examination in MG).
Weakness is typically variable, fluctuating, and fatigable.
Ptosis that shifts from one eye to the other is virtually pathognomonic of MG.
With limited ocular excursion, saccades are superfast, producing ocular "quiver."
After downgaze, upgaze produces lid overshoot ("lid twitch")
Pseudo-internuclear ophthalmoplegia—limited adduction, with nystagmoid jerks in abducting eye (Video 108.2—pseudo-INO in MG).
In asymmetric ptosis, covering the ptotic eye may relieve contraction of the opposite frontalis.
Passively lifting a ptotic lid may cause the opposite lid to fall: "enhanced ptosis" or "curtain sign" (Video 108.3—"curtain sign").
Edrophonium may improve only some of several weak ocular muscles; others may actually become weaker.
Edrophonium may relieve asymmetric ptosis and produce retraction of the opposite lid from frontalis contraction.
The opposite lid may droop further as the more involved lid improves after edrophonium.
Cold applied to the eye may improve lid ptosis: "Ice-pack test" (see Fig. 108.7)

*MG*, Myasthenia gravis.

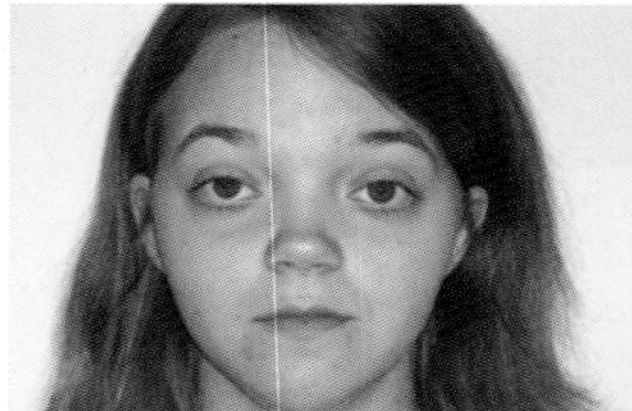
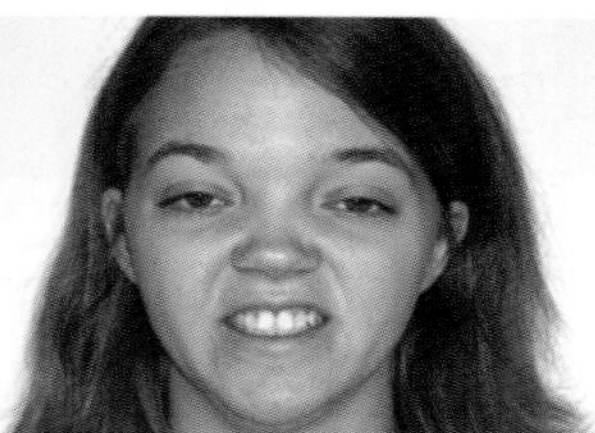

**Fig. 108.2 Typical Myasthenic Facies.** At rest *(left)*, there is slight bilateral lid ptosis, which is partially compensated by asymmetric contraction of the frontalis muscle, raising the right eyebrow. During attempted smile *(right)*, there is contraction of the medial portion of the upper lip and horizontal contraction of the corners of the mouth without the natural upward curling, producing a "sneer."

eyes is typical, the medial rectus being more frequently and usually more severely involved. The pattern of weakness cannot be localized to lesions of one or more nerves, and the pupillary responses are normal. Ptosis is usually asymmetrical (Fig. 108.2) and varies during sustained activity. To compensate for ptosis, chronic contraction of the frontalis muscle produces a worried or surprised look. Patients may also tilt their head back in compensation, which may hide subtle ptosis. Unilateral frontalis contraction is a clue that the lid elevators are weak on that side (see Fig. 108.1). When mild, ocular weakness may not be obvious on routine examination and appear only upon provocative testing, such as sustained upward gaze or red lens testing. Eyelid closure is usually weak, even when strength is normal in all other facial muscles, and may be the only residual weakness in otherwise complete remission. This is usually asymptomatic unless it is severe enough to allow soap or water in the eyes during bathing or to produce dry eyes when sleeping. With moderate weakness of these muscles, the eyelashes are not "buried" during forced eye closure (Fig. 108.3). Fatigue in these muscles may result in slight involuntary opening of the eyes as the patient tries to keep the eyes closed, the so-called *peek sign* (see Fig. 108.3).

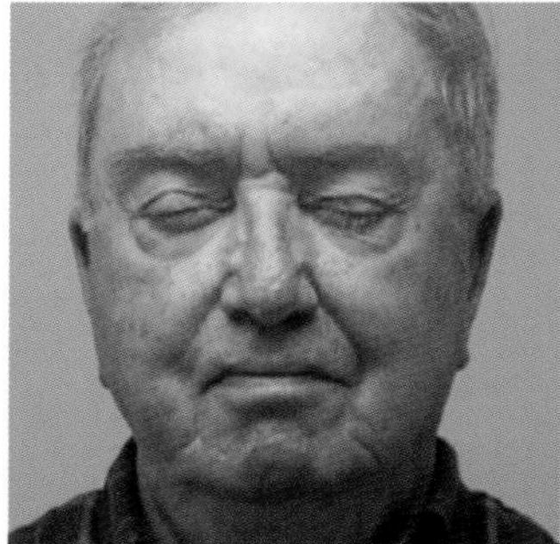
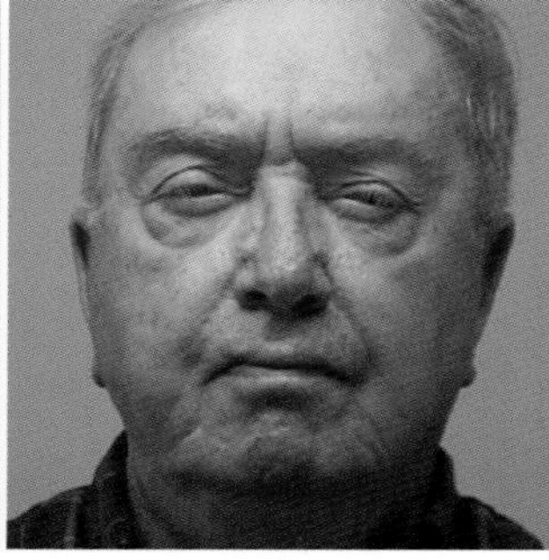

**Fig. 108.3 "Peek" Sign In Myasthenia Gravis.** During sustained forced eyelid closure the man is unable to bury his eyelashes *(left)* and, after 30 seconds, the man is unable to keep the lids fully closed *(right)*. *(Reproduced from Sanders, D.B., Massey, J.M., 2008. In Engel AG et al., Handbook of Clinical Neurology, Elsevier, figure 5, with permission.)*

### Oropharyngeal Muscles

Oropharyngeal muscle weakness causes changes in the voice, difficulty chewing and swallowing, and inadequate maintenance of the upper airway. The voice may be nasal, especially after prolonged talking, and liquids may escape through the nose when swallowing because of palatal muscle weakness. Weakness of laryngeal muscles causes hoarseness. A history of frequent choking or throat clearing or coughing after eating indicates difficulty in swallowing. Respiratory dysfunction and isolated dysphagia (without dysarthria) are rarely the initial symptoms of MG.

Myasthenic patients may have a characteristic facial appearance. At rest, the corners of the mouth often droop downward, giving a depressed appearance. Attempts to smile often produce contraction of the medial portion of the upper lip and a horizontal contraction of the corners of the mouth without the natural upward curling, which gives the appearance of a sneer (see Fig. 108.2).

Manually opening the jaw against resistance shows jaw weakness; this is not possible when strength is normal. The patient may support a weak jaw (and neck) with the thumb under the chin, the middle finger curled under the nose or lower lip, and the index finger extended up the cheek, producing a studious or attentive appearance.

### Limb Muscles

Weakness begins in limb or axial muscles in about 20% of MG patients (Kuks et al., 2004). Any trunk or limb muscle may be weak, but some are more often affected than are others. Neck flexors are usually weaker than neck extensors, and the deltoids, triceps, and extensors of the wrist and fingers and ankle dorsiflexors are frequently weaker than other limb muscles. Rarely, MG presents initially with focal weakness in single muscle groups, such as a "dropped head syndrome" due to severe neck extensor weakness, or isolated triceps weakness. In untreated patients with long-standing disease, weakness may be fixed, and severely involved muscles may be atrophic, giving the appearance of a chronic myopathy; atrophy is particularly likely in muscle specific tyrosine kinase (MuSK)-ab positive MG (See *Anti-MuSK-Antibody Positive MG*, later in this chapter).

## Immunopathology of Myasthenia Gravis

In about 80%–85% of MG patients, weakness results from the effects of circulating anti-AChR antibodies (Table 108.1). These antibodies bind to AChR on the terminal expansions of the junctional folds (Fig. 108.4) and cause complement-mediated destruction of the folds, accelerated internalization and degradation of AChR, and in some cases, they block ACh-AChR binding. Destruction of the junctional folds results in distortion and simplification of the postsynaptic region (Fig. 108.5) and

**TABLE 108.1 Myasthenia Gravis Clinical Subtypes**

| MG subtype | Age at onset | Thymic histology | Autoantibodies | Comments |
|---|---|---|---|---|
| **Ocular** | Adult in United States and Europe; childhood in Asia | Unknown | AChR (50%) | * |
| **Early Onset** | < 50 years | Hyperplasia | AChR | M:F = 1:3 |
| **Late Onset** | > 50 years | Normal | AChR<br>Titin<br>Ryanodine | M>F<br>Anti-titin, ryanodine antibodies associated with severe disease |
| **Thymoma** | >40 years (usually) | Neoplasia | AChR<br>Titin, ryanodine | May be associated with other paraneoplastic disorders |
| **MuSK** | < 40 years | Normal | MuSK | Marked female predominance; selective oropharyngeal, facial, respiratory weakness in some; IgG4 antibodies |
| **LRP4** | 30-50 years | Unknown | LRP4 | Response to therapy similar to AChR MG; IgG1 antibodies |
| **Seronegative (generalized)** | Variable | Hyperplasia in some | Abs against clustered AChR, agrin, or cortactin in some cases | *; presumed unidentified Abs in those without low-affinity AChR Abs; agrin antibodies. See text. |

*Low-affinity AChR Abs have been reported in some patients.
Abs, antibodies; *AChR*, acetylcholine receptor; *IgG*, immunoglobulin G; *LRP4*, lipoprotein receptor-related protein 4; *MG*, myasthenia gravis; *MuSK*. muscle-specific tyrosine kinase.

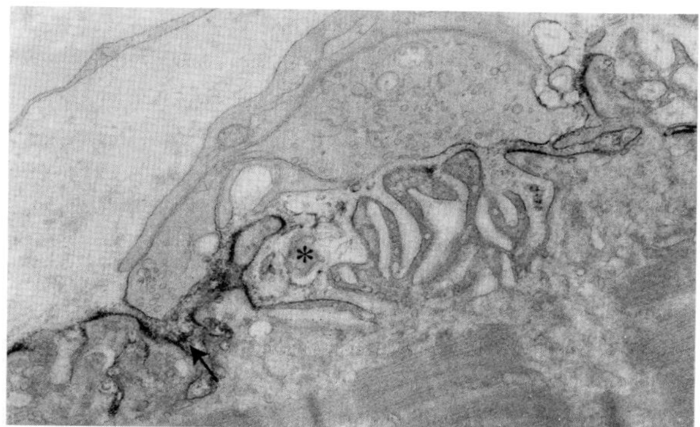

**Fig. 108.4** Localization of immunoglobulin G (IgG) at an endplate in acquired myasthenia gravis. IgG deposits have a patchy distribution, occurring on some junctional folds but not on others and on debris in the synaptic space *(arrow)*. In one region there is degeneration of junctional folds (*). *(From Engel, A.G., Lambert, E.H., Howard, F.M., 1977a. Immune complexes (IgG and C3) at the motor endplate in myasthenia gravis: ultrastructural and light microscopic localization and electrophysiologic correlation. Mayo Clinic Proc. 52, 267–280, figure 6, by permission.)*

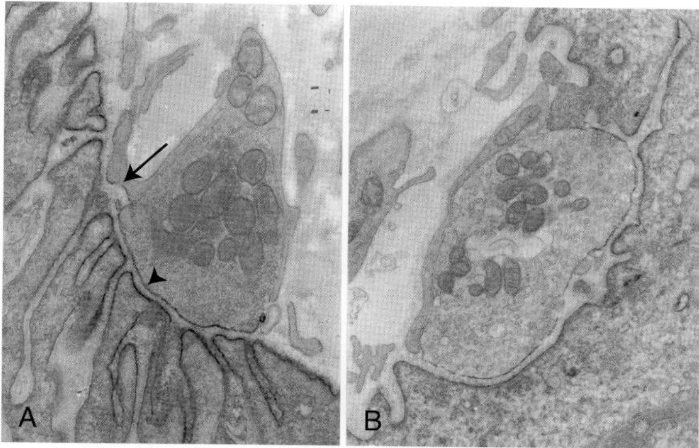


**Fig. 108.5** Ultrastructural localization of acetylcholine receptor (AChR) at the muscle endplate in a control subject (**A**) and in a patient with generalized myasthenia gravis (**B**). The AChR staining seen in A *(arrowheads)* is virtually absent in B, in which only short segments of simplified postsynaptic membrane react. *(From Engel, A.G., Lindstrom, J.M., Lambert, E.H., Lennon, V.A., 1977b. Ultrastructural localization of the acetylcholine receptor in myasthenia gravis and its experimental autoimmune model. Neurology 27, 307–315, figure 3A/B, by permission.)*

loss of functional AChR. This leads to NMT failure and muscle weakness. MG is a paradigm for an antibody-mediated disease: the physiological abnormality is passively transferrable by injection of MG immunoglobulin G (IgG) into mice, and clinical improvement follows removal of circulating antibodies by plasma exchange (PLEX; see Treatment of Myasthenia Gravis section later in this chapter).

Approximately 10% of MG patients (up to 50% of anti-AChR negative, generalized myasthenia gravis [GMG] patients) have circulating antibodies to MuSK, a surface membrane component essential in the development of the NMJ (see Table 108.1). These anti-MuSK antibodies, which are predominantly IgG4 and do not fix complement, adversely affect the maintenance of AChR clustering at the muscle endplate, leading to reduced numbers of functional AChRs (McConville et al., 2004; Niks et al., 2008a). The precise pathophysiology of the weakness and prominent muscle atrophy in MuSK-antibody myasthenia gravis (MuSK MG) is unknown. Muscle biopsy studies have shown little AChR loss, but no detailed studies of NMT in the most affected muscles are available. The events leading to autosensitization to MuSK are unknown contradicts a statement on next page.

Patients with no identifiable antibodies by these conventional assays have been termed "double-seronegative" patients. These patients may improve with conventional immunosuppressive (IS) treatments, PLEX, or even thymectomy. Recent discoveries have begun to clarify the immunopathology of these previously double-seronegative MG patients as additional autoantibodies targeting NMJ proteins have been identified. Low-affinity IgG antibodies have been found in about two-thirds of MG patients who were seronegative using conventional anti-AChR and anti-MuSK antibody assays (Leite et al., 2008). These antibodies bind to AChRs that have been clustered into high-density arrays, suggesting that they have relatively low affinity and cannot bind strongly to AChR in solution but do bind to immobilized AChRs in a native conformation. Antibodies against the proteoglycan agrin, which is released from motor neurons and binds to low-density lipoprotein receptor-related protein 4 (LRP4), have been detected in some MG patients though the clinical significance is unclear (Zhang et al.,

2014). In addition, some MuSK MG patients and 3%–54% of double-seronegative patients have IgG1 LRP4 antibodies that appear to be pathogenic (Higuchi et al., 2011; Pevzner et al., 2011; Shen et al., 2013). Additional antibodies against titin (Cordts et al., 2017; Nagappa et al., 2019), cortactin (Cortes-Vicente et al., 2016; Gallardo et al., 2014), ryanodine receptor (Nagappa et al., 2019), and agrin (Yan et al., 2018) have been reported in variable percentages of patients, but more work is needed to clarify the role of these autoantibodies in nonthymomatous MG, particularly those against intracellular proteins that are less likely to be directly related to disease pathogenesis.

T lymphocytes play a pivotal role in the initiation and maintenance of the autoimmune response against the AChR and MuSK proteins. However, the precise mechanism by which this response initiates and is maintained is incompletely understood. Activation of T cells through the T-cell receptor by major histocompatibility complex (MHC) class molecules bound with antigenic peptide ultimately leads to B-cell activation, class switching, clonal expansion, and production of autoantibodies by plasma cells. Potentially autoreactive T cells are normally controlled by a variety of immune regulatory mechanisms, including regulatory T cells, which are likely deficient or dysfunctional in MG. Accumulating research highlights the extensive dysfunction in T- and B-cell activity that contributes to MG pathogenesis (Mantegazza R, 2018; Yi et al., 2017).

### The Thymus in Myasthenia Gravis

The thymus is abnormal in most MG patients—70% have lymphoid follicular hyperplasia and more than 10% have a thymoma. Hyperplastic thymus glands from MG patients contain all the components necessary for the development of an immune response to the AChR: T cells, B cells, and plasma cells, as well as muscle-like myoid cells that express AChR. It is unlikely that the cellular alterations in the thymus are secondary to an ongoing peripheral immune response because they are absent in experimental autoimmune MG (Hohlfeld et al., 2008). In addition, thymocytes in culture spontaneously generate anti-AChR antibodies. These findings support the concept of an intrathymic pathogenesis and argue that the hyperplastic thymus is involved in the initiation of the anti-AChR immune response in patients with thymic hyperplasia. Thymic-derived AChR subunits may serve as an antigen for the autosensitization against the AChR. Expression of MuSK on human thymic myoid cells has also been reported, suggesting that the thymus may also play a role in development of MuSK MG (Mesnard-Rouiller et al., 2004).

Neoplastic epithelial cells in thymomas express numerous self-like antigens, including AChR, titin- and ryanodine receptor-like epitopes. MG-associated thymomas are also rich in autoreactive T cells. The regulation of potentially autoreactive T cells may be impaired in thymoma due to a deficiency in the expression of the autoimmune regulator gene (*AIRE*), and selective loss of T regulatory cells in human thymomas (Aricha et al., 2011; Scarpino et al., 2007; Strobel et al., 2004).

## Myasthenia Gravis Subtypes

A number of MG subtypes (see Table 108.1) can be identified based on clinical manifestations, age at onset, autoantibody profile, and thymic pathology (Gilhus et al., 2015). These subtypes appear to have unique genetic associations, strengthening the concept of distinct clinical entities and disease mechanisms.

### Ocular Myasthenia Gravis

Ptosis and/or diplopia are the initial symptoms of MG in up to 85% of patients (Grob et al., 2008), and almost all patients have both symptoms within 2 years of disease onset. Myasthenic weakness that remains limited to the ocular muscles is termed ocular myasthenia gravis (OMG), and comprises approximately 10%–15% of all MG in Caucasian populations. If weakness remains limited to the ocular muscles after 2 years, there is a 90% likelihood that the disease will not generalize. OMG is more common in Asian populations (up to 58% of all MG patients; Zhang et al., 2007).

Confirmation of the diagnosis of OMG may be a challenge as RNS studies and anti-AChR antibodies are often negative, and single-fiber electromyography (SFEMG) testing may be required.

### Generalized Myasthenia Gravis

Patients with GMG may be either early-onset (EOMG) or late-onset disease (LOMG), with the cutoff age usually defined as age 50 (see Table 108.1). EOMG patients are more often female, and typically have anti-AChR antibodies and enlarged hyperplastic thymus glands. LOMG patients are more often male and may have antibodies to striated muscle proteins such as titin and the ryanodine receptor in addition to anti-AChR antibodies. The presence of these anti-muscle antibodies, particularly anti-ryanodine receptor antibodies, has been associated with more severe, generalized, or predominantly oropharyngeal weakness, and frequent myasthenic crises (Romi et al., 2005a). LOMG patients without thymoma usually have a normal or atrophic thymus, but relatively few histological studies are available in this age group, as thymectomy has not traditionally been performed after age 50.

### Thymomatous Myasthenia Gravis

About 10%–15% of MG patients have a thymic epithelial tumor, or thymoma. Thymoma-associated MG is equally frequent in males and females and may occur at any age, with peak onset at age 50. Patients with thymomatous MG are more likely to have detectable striated muscle (e.g., titin, ryanodine receptor) antibodies.

### MuSK-Antibody Myasthenia Gravis

Antibodies to MuSK have been reported in up to 50% of patients with GMG who lack acetylcholine receptor antibodies (AChR-abs) (Guptill et al., 2010a) and have been rarely reported in OMG as well (Bau et al., 2006; Caress et al., 2005). The reported incidence of MuSK MG varies among geographic regions, the highest being closer to the equator and the lowest closer to the poles (Vincent et al., 2006). Genetic or environmental factors, or both, presumably play a role in these differences. MuSK MG predominantly affects females and may begin from childhood through middle age. In some patients, the clinical findings are indistinguishable from MuSK-negative MG, with fluctuating ocular, bulbar and limb weakness. However, many MuSK MG patients have predominant weakness in cranial and bulbar muscles, frequently with marked atrophy of these muscles (Fig. 108.6). Others have prominent neck, shoulder, and respiratory weakness, with little or no involvement of ocular or bulbar muscles. Electrodiagnostic abnormalities may not be as widespread as in other forms of MG and it may be necessary to examine different muscles to demonstrate abnormal NMT (Stickler et al., 2005). It is not uncommon for MuSK MG patients with proximal limb weakness and atrophy to be initially diagnosed with a myopathy, in part due to the distribution of weakness, but also as a result of needle EMG findings that are interpreted as myopathic. The more restricted distribution of physiological abnormalities also may limit the interpretation of microphysiological and histological studies in MuSK MG, inasmuch as the muscles usually biopsied for these studies may be normal.

Many MuSK MG patients do not improve with cholinesterase inhibitors (ChEIs)—some actually become worse, and many have profuse fasciculations with these medications (Hatanaka et al., 2005; Punga et al., 2006, 2008; Sanders et al., 2016). Disease severity tends to be

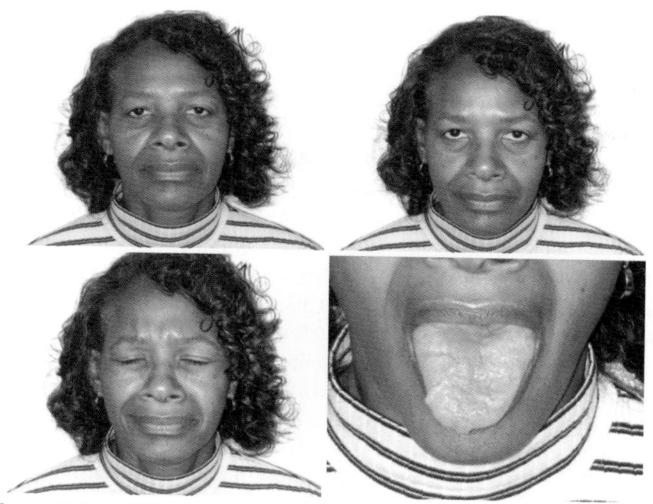

**Fig. 108.6** MuSK antibody-positive myasthenia gravis with marked upper facial muscle weakness and atrophy. At rest *(upper left)*, there is slight bilateral lid ptosis. There is no visible (or palpable) contraction of the frontalis muscle on attempted elevation of the eyebrows *(upper right)* and she does not bury the eyelashes during forced eyelid closure *(lower left)*. The tongue is markedly wasted *(lower right.)* (*From Sanders, D.B., Massey, J.M. 2008. In Engel AG et al., Handbook of Clinical Neurology, Elsevier, figure 16, by permission.*)

worse, but most improve dramatically with therapeutic PLEX or corticosteroids (Sanders et al., 2003). More immunosuppression is typically necessary, though long-term outcome is generally good (Guptill et al., 2010a). Thymic changes are absent or minimal (Lauriola et al., 2005; Vincent et al., 2005) and the role of thymectomy in MuSK MG is not yet clear (Guptill et al., 2010a; Sanders et al., 2003, 2016). Retrospective studies overwhelmingly support the benefit of rituximab (RTX) in MuSK MG (Hehir et al., 2017; Illa et al., 2008; Sanders et al., 2016). The diagnosis of MuSK MG may be elusive when the clinical features, electrodiagnostic findings, and response to ChEIs differ from typical MG.

### Seronegative Myasthenia Gravis

MG patients who lack both anti-AChR and anti-MuSK antibodies ("double-seronegative MG") are clinically heterogeneous. The true frequency of "seronegative MG" may be quite low as patients may have antibodies against novel muscle antigens or low-affinity anti-AChR antibodies that can only be detected using specialized assays (See Immunopathology of Myasthenia Gravis, above). The possibility of a rare adult onset congenital myasthenic syndrome must be considered, especially if there is no benefit from immunomodulatory therapy. Autoimmune seronegative MG patients are typically managed similarly to MG patients with AChR antibodies.

## Genetics of Myasthenia Gravis

The transmission of MG is not by classic Mendelian inheritance, but family members of patients are approximately 100 times more likely to develop the disease than is the general population (Pirskanen, 1977). In addition, 33%–45% of asymptomatic first-degree family members show jitter on SFEMG testing and anti-AChR antibodies are slightly elevated in up to 50%. These observations suggest that there is a genetically determined predisposition to develop MG.

Several correlations exist between MG and the human leukocyte antigen (HLA) genes. Certain HLA types (-DR2, -DR3, -B8, -DR1) predispose to MG (see Table 108.1), whereas others may offer resistance to disease. HLA-B8-DR2 and -DR3 types occur more commonly in patients with EOMG, HLA-B7 and -DR2 in LOMG, and HLA-DR1 in OMG (see Table 108.1). MuSK MG is associated with HLA-DR14-DQ5 (Niks et al., 2006). Different HLA associations have been reported in Asian MG patients, including an association of OMG with HLA-BW46DR9 in Chinese patients (Chen et al., 1993). Non-HLA genes (*PTPN22, FCGR2, CHRNA 1, CTLA4, TNFRSF11A*) have also been found to be associated with MG—some are also associated with other autoimmune diseases, and thus may represent a nonspecific susceptibility to autoimmunity (Avidan et al., 2014; Klein et al., 2013; Renton et al., 2015). An exception to this is the *CHRNA1* gene, which encodes the alpha subunit of the AChR and may provide pathogenetic clues specific for MG (Giraud et al., 2008) A genome-wide association study (GWAS) in European EOMG patients also found an association between *PTPN22* and TNFAIP3-interacting protein 1 (TNIP1) (Gregersen et al., 2012).

## Diagnostic Procedures in Myasthenia Gravis

The diagnosis of acquired MG is determined by demonstrating muscle weakness and one or more of the following:

- Elevated AChR or MuSK antibodies
- An unequivocal response to ChEIs
- Abnormal repetitive nerve stimulation (RNS) test or increased jitter (without nerve or muscle disease sufficient to produce a decrement or increased jitter)

In patients with childhood onset, congenital myasthenic syndromes (CMS) must be excluded (See Childhood Myasthenia Gravis section, below)

### Edrophonium Chloride Test

Edrophonium and other ChEIs impede the enzymatic breakdown of ACh by inhibiting the action of acetylcholinesterase (AChE), thus allowing ACh to diffuse more widely throughout the synaptic cleft and to have a more prolonged interaction with AChR on the postsynaptic muscle membrane. Weakness from abnormal NMT characteristically improves after administration of ChEIs; this is the basis of the diagnostic edrophonium test, which may be helpful in seronegative patients and when electrodiagnostic studies are unrevealing or unavailable. The edrophonium test is reported to be positive in 60%–95% of patients with OMG and in 72%–95% with GMG (Pascuzzi, 2003) (Video 108.4). The edrophonium test has lost favor as a diagnostic tool due to the widespread availability of autoantibody testing and it is increasingly difficult to obtain edrophonium worldwide. Details of the performance of the edrophonium test can be found in the article by Pascuzzi (2003).

### Autoantibodies in Myasthenia Gravis

***Acetylcholine receptor antibodies.*** Assays measuring antibodies that react with AChR proteins are generally regarded as specific serological markers for MG. The most widely used test for MG is the AChR-ab binding assay, which tests serum for binding to purified AChR from human skeletal muscle labeled with radioiodinated α-bungarotoxin. The reported sensitivity of this assay is approximately 85% for GMG and 50% for OMG (Stålberg et al., 2010). Nearly all thymomatous MG patients have elevated AChR-abs.

Finding elevated AChR-abs in a patient with compatible clinical features essentially confirms the diagnosis of MG, but absence of these antibodies does not exclude the disease. Assays for AChR-abs may be normal at symptom onset and become abnormal later in the disease; thus, repeat testing is appropriate when values obtained within 6–12 months of symptom onset were normal.

AChR-ab levels tend to be lower in patients with ocular or mild generalized MG but these values vary widely among patients with similar degrees of weakness, and do not predict the severity of disease in individual patients. The AChR-ab level is not a consistent marker of overall response to therapy, and may actually rise in some patients as their symptoms improve. Although antibody levels fall in most patients after

IS treatment, they also fall in patients who do not improve (Sanders et al., 2014). However, if the AChR-ab level does not fall after immunotherapy, this may indicate inadequate therapy.

False-positive AChR-ab tests are rare, but have been reported in autoimmune liver disease, systemic lupus, inflammatory neuropathies, amyotrophic lateral sclerosis, penicillamine-treated patients with rheumatoid arthritis, patients with thymoma but without MG, and in first-degree relatives of patients with acquired autoimmune MG.

Another assay for AChR-abs measures inhibition of binding of radiolabeled α-bungarotoxin to the AChR. This technique measures antibody directed against the ACh binding site on the α-subunit of the AChR. In most patients, relatively few of the circulating antibodies recognize this site, resulting in a lower sensitivity for this assay. These blocking antibodies occur in less than 1% of MG patients who do not have measurable binding antibodies and thus have limited diagnostic value.

AChR-abs cross link the AChR in the membrane and increase their rate of degradation. The AChR modulating antibody assay measures the rate of loss of labeled AChR from cultured human myotubes. About 10% of MG patients who do not have elevated binding antibodies have AChR modulating antibodies. Many patients with thymomatous MG have high levels of AChR modulating antibodies (Vernino et al., 2004).

***Antistriational muscle antibodies.*** Antistriational muscle antibodies (StrAbs), which react with contractile elements of skeletal muscle, were the first autoantibodies discovered in MG. These antibodies recognize muscle cytoplasmic proteins (titin, myosin, actin, and ryanodine receptors), and are found in 75%–85% of patients with thymomatous MG.

StrAbs are not pathogenic and are also found in one-third of patients with thymoma who do not have MG and in one-third of MG patients without thymoma. They are more frequent in older MG patients and in those with more severe disease, suggesting that disease severity is related to a more vigorous humoral response against multiple muscle antigens (Romi et al., 2005b).

StrAbs are only rarely elevated in MG in the absence of AChR antibodies and are therefore of limited use in confirming the diagnosis. The main clinical value of StrAbs is in predicting thymoma: 60% of patients with EOMG who have elevated StrAbs have thymoma and the combination of elevated AChR binding-abs and StrAbs has a 50% positive predictive value for thymoma in EOMG (DeCroos et al., 2013). Titin and other StrAbs are detectable in up to 50% of elderly patients with non-thymomatous MG, so these antibodies are less helpful as predictors of thymoma in patients over 60. StrAbs are also found in autoimmune liver disease, infrequently in Lambert-Eaton myasthenia (LEM), and in primary lung cancer.

***Anti-MuSK antibodies.*** Antibodies to MuSK are present in up to 50% of GMG patients who are seronegative for AChR-abs and in some patients with OMG (See MuSK-Antibody Myasthenia Gravis section, above).

***Anti-LRP4 antibodies.*** LRP4 antibodies are found in up to 5% of MG patients overall, and it up to one-third of those without AChR and MuSK antibodies (Gilhus et al., 2016). Patients with anti-LRP4 antibodies are predominantly women, usually have early-onset disease, and typically have mild ocular or generalized disease at symptom onset (Zisimopoulou et al., 2014). An exception appears to be the rare double-positive AChR/LRP4-MG and MuSK/LRP4-MG patients, who often have more severe symptoms than single-antibody-positive MG patients. About a third of LRP4 antibody MG patients have thymic hyperplasia, but not thymoma. LRP4 antibodies are predominantly of the complement-activating IgG1 and IgG2 subtypes. The clinical response of LRP4-MG patients to typical MG treatments is similar to patients with AChR MG. LRP4 antibodies are not specific for MG, but are also found in patients with other autoimmune disorders (Zhang et al., 2012) and in up to 23% of patients with ALS (Tzartos et al., 2014).

## Electrodiagnostic Testing in Myasthenia Gravis

RNS is the most commonly used electrophysiological test of NMT. Although a seemingly simple test, careful attention to proper technique is important to avoid technical errors. At low rates of stimulation (2–5 Hz) RNS depletes the store of readily releasable ACh at diseased motor endplates, causing failure of NMT. Characteristically in MG, there is a decrementing response of at least 10% to trains of 2–3 Hz stimulation (see Chapter 36). This may be present at baseline or after a period of exercise (post-activation exhaustion). RNS is reportedly abnormal in 53%–89% of patients with generalized MG and in 48%–67% of those with OMG (Bou Ali et al., 2016). RNS is more likely to be abnormal in a proximal or facial muscle and in clinically weak muscles. For maximal diagnostic yield, test several muscles, particularly those that are weak. If RNS is normal and there is a high suspicion for a NMJ disorder, jitter testing of at least one symptomatic muscle is recommended.

Jitter measurement (see Chapter 36) is the most sensitive clinical test of NMT and shows increased jitter in some muscles in almost all MG patients (Sanders et al., 2019; Stålberg et al., 2010). Jitter is greatest in weak muscles but is usually abnormal even in muscles with normal strength. Sixty percent of patients with OMG show increased jitter in a limb muscle, but this does not predict the subsequent development of generalized myasthenia.

In the rare patient who has weakness restricted to a few limb muscles, jitter may be abnormal only in weak muscles. This is particularly true in some patients with MuSK MG (Stickler et al., 2005) (see MuSK-Antibody Myasthenia Gravis section, above).

Increased jitter is a nonspecific sign of abnormal NMT and can be seen in other motor unit diseases. Therefore, when jitter is increased, perform other electrodiagnostic tests to exclude neuronopathy, neuropathy, and myopathy. Normal jitter in a weak muscle excludes abnormal NMT as the cause of weakness.

Jitter is now measured with concentric needle electrodes (CNEs) in most institutions because of restrictions on the re-use of sterilized material, such as SFEMG electrodes (Stålberg et al., 2009). When jitter is measured with CNE, use electrodes with the smallest recording surface, take care to minimize signal artifacts, and use reference values specific for these electrodes (Sanders, 2013; Stålberg et al., 2016, 2017).

## Ocular Cooling

Myasthenic weakness typically improves with muscle cooling. This is the basis of the "ice-pack" test, in which cooling of a ptotic lid improves lid elevation (Fig. 108.7). Assess improvement in ptosis after placing an ice pack over the ptotic eyelid, usually for 2 minutes. A meta-analysis of six studies showed this test to have high sensitivity and specificity in MG, suggesting that it may be useful in patients with lid ptosis (Larner, 2004). The test may also be positive in other NMJ disorders (Alaraj et al., 2013), but a negative ice-pack test in a ptotic lid makes MG unlikely (Fakiri et al., 2013).

## Comparison of Diagnostic Techniques in Myasthenia Gravis

Plan diagnostic testing based on the clinical presentation and distribution of weakness. The presence of AChR or anti-MuSK antibodies virtually ensures the diagnosis of MG, but their absence does not exclude it. RNS confirms impaired NMT but is frequently normal in mild or purely ocular disease. Almost all patients with MG have increased jitter, and normal jitter in a weak muscle excludes MG as the cause of

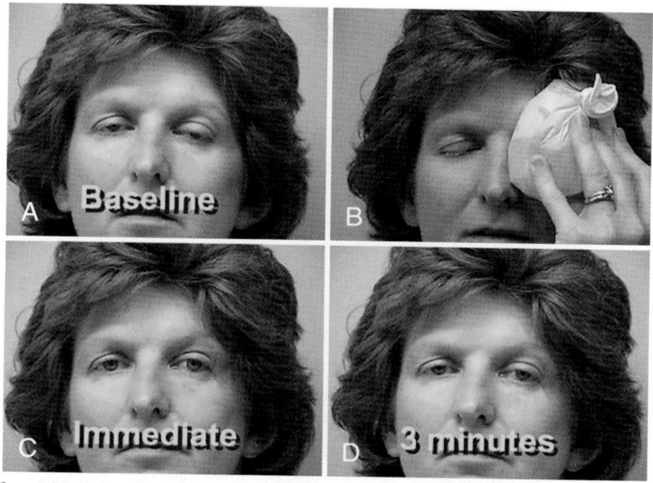


**Fig. 108.7** Ice-Pack Test In Myasthenia Gravis. Before testing (**A**) there is ptosis of both upper lids, more marked on the left. An ice pack is placed over the ptotic eye for 2 minutes (**B**). Upon removal of the ice pack, the ptosis is improved (**C**) and gradually returns (**D**).

the weakness. Neither electrodiagnostic test is specific for MG because increased jitter, even abnormal RNS, occurs in other motor unit disorders that impair NMT.

### Other Diagnostic Procedures in Myasthenia Gravis

Patients diagnosed with MG should have thyroid function tests and a chest imaging study (computed tomography [CT] or magnetic resonance imaging [MRI]) to assess for a possible thymoma. Thymoma is exceptionally rare in seronegative MG, but has been reported (Maggi et al., 2014; Rigamonti et al., 2014). Tuberculosis testing, either a TB skin test or QuantiFERON®-TB Gold Test, and testing for chronic viral infections (e.g., hepatitis C) should be considered if the use of immunosuppression is contemplated.

## Treatment of Myasthenia Gravis

The outlook for patients with MG has improved dramatically in the past 50 years, largely due to advances in intensive care medicine and the use of immunomodulating agents. In 2016, a Task Force of the MG Foundation of America published guidance statements for treating autoimmune MG based on consensus of expert opinion of an international panel of physicians experienced in the treatment of MG (Sanders et al., 2016). In addition to presenting guidance for the use of treatments for specific clinical situations, the Task Force defined the following goal of MG treatment: the patient has no symptoms or functional limitations from MG, with no more than mild side effects that require no intervention.

A number of therapeutic options are available (Table 108.2), but treatment must be individualized according to the extent (ocular vs. generalized) and severity (mild to severe) of disease, and the presence or absence of concomitant disease (including, but not limited to, other autoimmune diseases and thymoma). Treatment decisions for individual patients are determined by the predicted course of disease and the predicted response to specific treatments. Successful treatment of MG requires close medical supervision and long-term follow-up. Consider the return of weakness after a period of improvement as a herald of further progression, requiring reassessment of current treatment and evaluation for underlying systemic disease or thymoma.

### Symptom Management: Cholinesterase Inhibitors

Pyridostigmine bromide is the most commonly used ChEI and should be part of the initial treatment in most patients with MG. The initial oral dose in adults is 30–60 mg every 4–8 hours (see Table 108.2). In infants and children, the initial oral dose of pyridostigmine is 1 mg/kg. Pyridostigmine is available as syrup (60 mg/5 mL) for children or for nasogastric tube administration in patients with impaired swallowing. A timed-release tablet of pyridostigmine (180 mg) is useful as a bedtime dose for patients who are too weak to swallow in the morning. Its absorption is erratic, however, leading to possible over dosage and underdosage.

No fixed dosage schedule suits all patients and the dose should be adjusted to produce an optimal response in muscles causing the greatest disability. Patients with oropharyngeal weakness may require doses timed to provide optimal strength during meals. To avoid overdosage, aim for a dose that provides definite improvement in the most important muscle groups within 30–45 minutes and which wears off to some degree before the next dose.

The ability to reduce or discontinue pyridostigmine can be an indicator that the patient has met treatment goals, and may guide the tapering of other therapies.

Adverse effects of ChEIs result from ACh accumulation at muscarinic receptors on smooth muscle and autonomic glands and at the nicotinic receptors of skeletal muscle. Central nervous system side effects are rare with the doses used to treat MG. Common gastrointestinal complaints are queasiness, nausea, vomiting, abdominal cramps, loose stools, and diarrhea. Increased bronchial and oral secretions may be a serious problem in patients with swallowing or respiratory insufficiency. These muscarinic symptoms of overdosage may indicate that nicotinic overdose (weakness) is also occurring. Drugs that can be used to suppress the gastrointestinal side effects include glycopyrrolate, hyoscyamine sulfate, propantheline bromide, diphenoxylate hydrochloride with atropine, and loperamide hydrochloride (see Table 108.2). Be aware that some of these drugs themselves produce weakness at high dosages.

Patients with MuSK MG may become worse with ChEIs (see MuSK-Antibody Myasthenia Gravis section, above).

In two small studies, amifampridine produced improvement in some patients with acquired MG (Lundh et al., 1985; Sanders et al., 1993). Preliminary studies suggest that amifampridine may be effective symptomatic treatment in patients with MuSK MG (Bonanno et al., 2018), and more definitive clinical trials are in progress.

### Short-Term (Rapid-Onset) Immune Therapies

***Plasma exchange.*** PLEX temporarily reduces the levels of circulating antibodies, and produces improvement in a matter of days in most patients with acquired MG. It is generally used for short-term treatment of severe MG, myasthenic crisis, in preparation for surgery (e.g., thymectomy), or to prevent corticosteroid-induced exacerbations. A typical course of PLEX consists of 5–6 exchanges administered every other day; 2–3 liters of plasma are removed with each exchange. The total number of exchanges depends upon the clinical response and tolerability, but more than 6 exchanges may be required in some patients.

Benefit from a course of PLEX typically begins to wear off after 4 weeks but may persist for as long as 3 months. Longer-lasting immune therapy maintains control of symptoms thereafter. Most patients who respond to the initial course respond again to subsequent courses. Repeated exchanges do not have a cumulative benefit and we do not use PLEX as chronic maintenance therapy unless other treatments fail or are contraindicated.

Side effects during PLEX include paresthesias from citrate-induced hypocalcemia, hypotension, transitory cardiac arrhythmias, nausea, lightheadedness, chills, and pedal edema. The most serious complications relate to the use of large-bore venous access. The risks

TABLE 108.2 **Therapeutic Agents Used in Myasthenia Gravis**

| Agent | Initial Dose | Maintenance Dose | Onset of Action | Major Adverse Events | Monitoring | Comments |
|---|---|---|---|---|---|---|
| Pyridostigmine | 30–60 mg tid | 60–120 mg tid to 5x/ day, adjusted based on symptoms, typically not to exceed 480 mg/day | 15–30 minutes | Stomach cramps, nausea, vomiting, diarrhea, muscle twitching and cramps, sweating, salivation, blurred vision | Use the minimal amount that produces clinical improvement; this is best achieved by using a dose that produces observable improvement after most administrations | Can counter muscarinic adverse events with anticholinergic agents (i.e. glycopyrrolate, hyoscyamine sulfate, propantheline, diphenoxylate HCl with atropine, or loperamide |
| Prednisone | Option 1: 10–20 mg/ day, increasing daily dose by 5 mg daily equivalent every week until treatment goal achieved<br>Option 2: Start at 50–80 mg/day; this approach may require inpatient hospitalization (see text for details) | Slow alternate day taper after treatment goal achieved for several days (see text for details). Taper more slowly once ≤10 mg/ day dose equivalent. Continuing a low dose long-term can help to maintain the treatment goal | 2–4 weeks | Hypertension, diabetes, weight gain, bone loss, cataracts, GI ulcers, glaucoma, neuropsychiatric symptoms, growth retardation in children, hypothalamic–pituitary axis suppression | $HbA_{1c}$ every few months, blood pressure checks, bone density monitoring, eye exam for glaucoma and cataracts | Administer in single morning dose; temporary worsening is seen in up to 50% of patients, starting on high doses and in some patients on lower doses; IVIg or PLEX may prevent steroid-induced worsening |
| Azathioprine | 50 mg/day | Increase by 50 mg increments every 1–2 weeks to target of 2.5–3 mg/ kg/day | 2–10 months for initial response. Up to 24 months for maximum benefit | Fever, abdominal pain, nausea, vomiting, anorexia, leukopenia, hepatotoxicity, skin rash | CBC, LFTs 1–4 times in first month, then monthly to every third month.<br>Regular dermatological examinations if taken chronically | 10% of patients cannot tolerate because of flu-like reaction; major drug interaction with allopurinol; TPMT enzyme testing can be performed, if available, prior to starting treatment to identify patients at high risk of bone marrow suppression |
| Cyclosporine | 100 mg bid | Increase slowly as needed to 3–6 mg/kg/ day on bid schedule. | 1–3 months | Hirsuitism, tremor, gum hyperplasia, hypertension, hepatotoxicity, nephrotoxicity, PRES | CBC, LFTs, BUN/Cr monthly x3, then every 3 months; monitor trough drug levels | Bioequivalence differs between preparations, so avoid brand switching when possible; grapefruit juice may increase blood level; high potential for drug–drug interactions |
| Mycophenolate mofetil | 500 mg bid | 1000 to 1500 mg bid | 2–12 months | Diarrhea, vomiting, leukopenia, teratogenicity (black box warning) | CBC weekly for 4 weeks, every 2 weeks for 4 weeks, then monthly to every 3rd month; REMS program when used in women of childbearing age | Diarrhea may resolve by change to tid dosing |
| Cyclophosphamide | (1) Oral: 50 mg/day<br>(2) IV: 500 mg/m$^2$ monthly | Oral: increase by 50 mg/ week to maintenance dose of 2–3 mg/kg/day | 2–6 months | Alopecia, leukopenia, nausea and vomiting, skin discoloration, anorexia hemorrhagic cystitis, malignancy | CBC, BUN/Cr, electrolytes, LFTs, urinalysis every 2–4 weeks | IV pulse therapy may be less toxic because cumulative dose is lower |

**TABLE 108.2 Therapeutic Agents Used in Myasthenia Gravis—cont'd**

| Agent | Initial Dose | Maintenance Dose | Onset of Action | Major Adverse Events | Monitoring | Comments |
|---|---|---|---|---|---|---|
| Tacrolimus | 3–5 mg/day or 0.1 mg/kg/day | Increase dosing as needed for response following trough levels (see last column) | 1–3 months | Hyperglycemia, hypertension, headache, hyperkalemia, nephrotoxicity, diarrhea, nausea, vomiting, PRES | BUN/Cr, glucose, K+; trough drug levels every few weeks initially, then less frequently | Insulin-dependent diabetes mellitus developed in 20% of postrenal transplant patients; trough levels of 8–9 ng/ml may be effective |
| Methotrexate | 5–15 mg weekly for 2 weeks | Increase by 5 mg every 2 weeks to a maximum dose of 15–25 mg weekly | 2–6 months | Leukopenia, mouth ulceration, nausea, diarrhea, headaches, hair loss, hepatotoxicity, pulmonary fibrosis, rare nephrotoxicity, teratogenicity | CBC, LFTs monthly initially, then at least every 3 months. Monitor periodically for interstitial lung disease, a rare occurrence with doses used for immunotherapy | Consider folic acid 5 mg/day to reduce toxicity. Absolutely contraindicated in pregnancy |
| Intravenous immunoglobulin (IVIg) | 2 g/kg over 2-5 days | 0.4–1 g/kg every 4 weeks; can attempt to decrease frequency over time | 1–2 weeks | Headache, aseptic meningitis, nephrotoxicity, ischemic events, fluid overload, leukopenia, thrombocytopenia | BUN/Cr every month, decreasing to every 3rd month over time | IgA level prior to starting treatment may be useful to identify congenital IgA deficiency, a contraindication to IVIg use; avoid in patients with recent thrombotic/ischemic event. Use sucrose-free formulation for patients at risk of renal toxicity |

*From Sanders DB, Wolfe GI, Benatar M, Evoli A, Gilhus NE, Illa I, et al. International consensus guidance for the management of myasthenia gravis: Executive summary. Neurology. 2016;87:419–25.*

of subclavian lines, arteriovenous shunts or grafts for access include thromboses, thrombophlebitis, subacute bacterial endocarditis, as well as pneumothorax. These complications are minimized by using peripheral venous access (Guptill et al., 2013).

More selective removal of circulating immunoglobulins, including anti-AChR antibodies, may be accomplished using high-affinity immunoadsorption columns (Schneider-Gold et al., 2016). These columns selectively remove immunoglobulins from separated plasma, and, unlike PLEX, patients may not need replacement fresh frozen plasma or albumin. Use of immunoadsorption to treat MG is generally limited to selected regions of the world.

***Intravenous immunoglobulin.*** Intravenous immunoglobulin (IVIg) induces rapid improvement in patients with severe disease or crisis and reduces perioperative morbidity prior to surgery. Improvement is seen in 50%–100% of MG patients after infusion of a typical course of 2 g/kg, administered over 2–5 days (see Table 108.2); improvement usually begins within 1 week and lasts for several weeks or months. Class I evidence supports the use of IVIg to treat patients with refractory exacerbations of MG (Donofrio et al., 2009). In a randomized controlled trial (RCT) of MG patients with worsening weakness, IVIg induced rapid improvement in strength; this effect was more pronounced and likely more clinically significant in patients with moderate to severe disease (Zinman et al., 2007). IVIg is also used chronically in selected refractory patients, but there is little information on the optimal dosing and duration of chronic therapy.

IVIg may be particularly useful as an alternative to PLEX in children with limited vascular access. Although IVIg has demonstrated similar efficacy to PLEX in the treatment of MG exacerbations, it is unclear if it is as effective in MG crisis since the published comparison studies did not enroll enough patients in crisis and did not directly compare onset of improvement (Barth et al., 2011).

Common side effects of IVIg include headaches, chills, and fever, which usually improve when using slow infusion rates. Serious side effects are rare, but include renal toxicity, stroke, leukopenia, and aseptic meningitis. Lyophilized forms of IVIg may be associated with more frequent adverse events (Nadeau et al., 2010).

Subcutaneous administration of concentrated immunoglobulin formulations, which reduces the overall infused volume compared with IVIg, appear to be well-tolerated and may be particularly useful for patients who live in areas where home or infusion center infusions are not practical (Beecher et al., 2017; Bourque et al., 2016; Sala et al., 2018).

### Long-Term Immune Therapies

A number of IS medications are used in MG. While often quite beneficial, these medications require careful attention and should be tapered to the minimum effective dose in order to reduce the risk of long-term toxicity. Currently, there are no disease-related biomarkers to guide selection of specific IS agents; treatment is typically selected based on individual patient factors such as medical comorbidities and the desired timing of the clinical response.

***Corticosteroids.*** Corticosteroids (or other IS therapy, see below) should be used in all MG patients who have not met treatment goals after an adequate trial of pyridostigmine (Sanders et al., 2016). Prednisone produces marked improvement or complete relief of symptoms in more than 75% of MG patients and some improvement in most of the rest. Patients with recent onset of symptoms have the best responses, but those with chronic disease also may respond. The severity of disease does not predict the ultimate improvement. Patients with thymoma usually respond well to prednisone, before or after removal of the tumor.

In MG patients with generalized disease prednisone is given either as an initial high dose or an incrementing dose regimen (see Table 108.2). In the former, the initial dose is 50–80 mg/day and this is continued until sustained improvement occurs, which is usually within 2–4 weeks. Then, change to alternate day administration and taper the dose over many months to the smallest amount necessary to maintain improvement, which is ideally less than 15 mg every other day. Strength typically increases, even to remission, while the dose is being tapered. The rate of dose decrease is individualized—patients who have a rapid initial response may reduce the dose on alternate days by 20 mg each month to 60 mg every other day. If the initial response is less marked, it may be preferable to change to an alternate day dose of 100–120 mg and taper this by 20 mg each month to 60 mg every other day, then taper the dose more slowly to a target dose of 10–15 mg every other day as long as improvement persists. If weakness returns during the taper, the dose should be increased, another IS agent should be added, or both, to prevent further worsening. Discontinuing prednisone altogether almost invariably leads to return of weakness, but a very low dose (5–15 mg every other day) may be sufficient to maintain good improvement in many patients (Abuzinadah et al., 2018).

Transitory worsening occurs in approximately one-third to one-half of patients treated with high-dose daily prednisone (Pascuzzi et al., 1984). This usually begins within the first 7–10 days and lasts for several days. In mild cases, ChEIs usually manage this worsening. We recommend that patients with significant oropharyngeal or respiratory symptoms be hospitalized or receive PLEX or IVIg to minimize the steroid-induced worsening.

The incrementing dose regimen favored by some begins with prednisone 20 mg/day, increasing by 10 mg every 1–2 weeks until improvement begins. The ultimate dose is maintained until improvement is maximum, and then tapered as above. Exacerbations still may occur with this regimen, but the onset of such worsening and the therapeutic response are less predictable. A similar incrementing dose regimen is commonly used in OMG (see *Ocular Myasthenia*, in this chapter).

Prednisone is inexpensive, has a rapid onset of response, and has an established track record in MG; its use is limited by numerous and frequent side effects (Table 108.3), the severity and frequency of which increase when high doses are given for more than 1 month. Most side effects improve with dose reduction and become minimal when the dose is less than 20 mg every other day. A low-fat, low-sodium diet and exercise will minimize weight gain. Use supplemental calcium and vitamin D with bisphosphonate to counter osteopenia, particularly in postmenopausal women. Treat patients with peptic ulcer disease or symptoms of gastritis accordingly. Prednisone is contraindicated in patients with untreated tuberculosis.

Prednisone given with azathioprine (AZA), cyclosporine or mycophenolate mofetil (MMF) produces more benefit than either drug alone (see next section, Immunosuppressant drugs).

***Immunosuppressant drugs.*** A nonsteroidal IS agent should be used alone when steroids are contraindicated or refused (Sanders et al., 2016). AZA is a purine antimetabolite that interferes with T- and B-cell proliferation; expert consensus and some evidence from RCTs support its use as a first-line IS agent in MG (Palace et al., 1998). AZA improves weakness in most MG patients, but benefit may not be apparent for at least 6–12 months. The initial dose is 50 mg/day, which is increased by 50 mg/day every 7 days to a total of 150–200 mg/day (2–3 mg/kg/day). After maximum benefit has been achieved and maintained for many months, reduce the dose by 50 mg/day no more often than every 3 months to the minimal effective dose, which may be as low as 50 mg/day. Patients may respond better and more rapidly if prednisone is given concurrently. AZA allows steroid sparing during long-term therapy, which is especially beneficial in older patients (Evoli et al., 2000; Hart et al., 2007; Slesak et al., 1998).

**TABLE 108.3 Common Side Effects of Corticosteroids**

| Side Effect | Treatment/Prevention |
|---|---|
| Weight gain/fluid retention | Low-calorie, low-fat, sodium-restricted diet; exercise |
| Glucose intolerance | Monitor blood glucose/treat |
| Osteopenia/osteoporosis/avascular necrosis | Calcium and vitamin D supplementation, bisphosphonates |
| Hypertension | Monitor/treat |
| Cataracts/glaucoma | At least yearly ophthalmological evaluation |
| Steroid myopathy | Exercise/high protein diet |
| Peptic ulcer disease | Proton pump inhibitors, $H_2$ blockers |

An idiosyncratic reaction, with "flu-like" symptoms, occurs within 10–14 days after starting AZA in 15%–20% of patients—this reaction requires discontinuing the drug. The use of divided doses after meals or dose reduction minimizes gastrointestinal irritation. Leukopenia and even pancytopenia can occur at any time during treatment but are not common. Liver toxicity may also occur and is heralded by elevated serum transaminase. Monitor complete blood counts and liver enzymes every week during the first month, every 1–3 months for a year, and every 3–6 months thereafter. Reduce the dose if the peripheral white blood cell (WBC) count falls below 3500 cells/mm$^3$, then gradually increase the dose after the WBC count rises. Discontinue the drug immediately if the count falls below 1000 WBC/mm$^3$. Also discontinue treatment if the serum transaminase level exceeds twice the upper limit of normal, and restart at lower doses after values normalize. There are rare reports of AZA-induced pancreatitis, but the cost-effectiveness of monitoring serum amylase concentrations is not established. About 80% of patients treated with AZA have an increase in erythrocyte mean corpuscular volume (MCV), which is seen more often and is greater in responders than in nonresponders. Thus, a normal MCV in a patient with an incomplete AZA response suggests a higher dose may be needed.

There does not appear to be an increased risk of cancer when AZA is given for less than 10 years (Confavreux et al., 1996). Lymphoma, myelodysplastic syndromes, and serious opportunistic infections have rarely been observed in MG patients receiving AZA (Herrlinger et al., 2000; Hohlfeld et al., 1988). Data from the nephrology field indicate an increased incidence of cutaneous hyperkeratosis and skin cancer in patients taking AZA, which is attributed to the increased ultraviolet photosensitivity. Regular dermatological examinations and protection of sun-exposed areas are therefore recommended for MG patients receiving AZA chronically.

Myasthenic symptoms recur if AZA is withdrawn abruptly, even up to myasthenic crisis (Hohlfeld et al., 1985; Michels et al., 1988). In 10%–20% of MG patients, satisfactory improvement is not achieved with AZA in combination with corticosteroids, requiring the use of other IS agents.

MMF selectively blocks purine synthesis, thereby suppressing both T- and B-cell proliferation. Pilot studies and retrospective reports indicate efficacy in MG (Hehir et al., 2010; Meriggioli et al., 2003). However, data from an RCT failed to show additional benefit of MMF over 20 mg daily prednisone as initial immunotherapy of MG (Muscle Study Group, 2008) and another RCT did not show a significant steroid-sparing effect (Sanders et al., 2008a). Despite the lack of RCT evidence supporting its use in MG, MMF is widely used as monotherapy or as a steroid-sparing agent, and is recommended in several national MG treatment guidelines (Murai, 2015; Sussman et al., 2015) and in the Consensus Guidance statement for MG treatment (Sanders et al., 2016).

The usual MMF dose is 1000 mg twice daily, but doses up to 3000 mg a day have been used. In general, side effects are relatively mild and most commonly consist of diarrhea, nausea, and abdominal pain. MMF is contraindicated during pregnancy because of a high rate of malformations and spontaneous abortions (US Food and Drug Administration, 2007) and should be discontinued at least 4 months before planned pregnancies. In nonscheduled pregnancies, MMF must be discontinued immediately and sonographic examination with expert consultation initiated. Progressive multifocal leukoencephalopathy has been observed in rare heavily immunosuppressed patients receiving MMF, and isolated cases of primary CNS lymphoma and a T-cell proliferative disorder have been reported in MG patients treated with MMF (Dubal et al., 2009; Vernino et al., 2005).

Cyclosporine (CYA) is a potent IS agent that binds to the cytosolic protein cyclophilin of immunocompetent lymphocytes, especially T lymphocytes. This complex of CYA and cyclophilin inhibits calcineurin, which activates transcription of interleukin-2 (IL-2). It also inhibits lymphokine production and interleukin release and leads to reduced function of effector T cells. Evidence from RCTs (Tindall et al., 1993) and retrospective reviews (Ciafaloni et al., 2000) support the use of CYA in MG, but potential serious side effects and drug interactions limit its use. We use this agent in MG only when other IS agents are contraindicated or ineffective.

Tacrolimus is a calcineurin inhibitor similar to CYA that selectively inhibits the transcription of proinflammatory cytokines and IL-2 in T lymphocytes. Several RCTs suggest benefit of tacrolimus in MG (Cruz et al., 2015); it is approved for the treatment of MG in Japan and recommended in several national MG treatment guidelines (Fuhr et al., 2012; Murai, 2015; Sussman et al., 2015).

Tacrolimus appears to be less nephrotoxic than CYA at doses used in published MG reports, but hyperglycemia due to inhibition of insulin is relatively common in transplant patients receiving tacrolimus. Increased potassium levels often occur and there are interactions with other drugs and food, particularly grapefruit juice. Pending further study, tacrolimus should be considered as adjunctive therapy in refractory MG, as a steroid-sparing agent in patients intolerant or unresponsive to AZA and MMF, or as an alternative to prednisone in patients with contraindications when a relatively rapid clinical response is desired.

Cyclophosphamide (CP) is an alkylating cytotoxic agent that has been used after failure of standard therapy in severe, refractory GMG (de Feo et al., 2002; Drachman et al., 2003). In an RCT, patients with refractory MG had improved muscle strength and required lower steroid doses after pulsed doses of intravenous CP (500 mg/m$^2$). There are also reports of improvement in refractory MG after a one-time, high-dose (50 mg/kg) course of CP for 4 days followed by rescue therapy. Side effects of CP are common and potentially serious, including myelosuppression, hemorrhagic cystitis, and an increased risk of infection and malignancy. For this reason, CP should be reserved for patients with truly refractory, severe disease, and its use should be limited to experienced centers. The cumulative dose and duration of therapy should be monitored because of the increasing risk of infertility in both sexes after age 30 and late effects, including malignancies (about 1%, increasing in frequency with increasing dose and duration of therapy).

A single-blind prospective study provided class III evidence that methotrexate (MTX) is an effective steroid-sparing agent in generalized MG (Heckmann et al., 2011), but a subsequent RCT found no steroid-sparing effect over 12 months of treatment (Pasnoor et al., 2016). Despite the absence of high-quality data to support its use in MG, MTX has been used as a reserve treatment in the way it is used in rheumatoid arthritis—a dose of 5–15 mg oral/IV is administered once a week (Hilton-Jones, 2007). MTX is known to be teratogenic and cannot be used by males or females planning reproduction (Hilton-Jones, 2007).

RTX is a chimeric monoclonal antibody directed against the B-cell surface marker CD20. Recent studies indicate that RTX should be considered as a second-line treatment in MuSK MG patients who do not improve adequately on prednisone (Cortés-Vicente et al., 2018; Diaz-Manera et al., 2012; Guptill et al., 2010a; Iorio et al., 2015; Keung et al., 2013; Meriggioli et al., 2009)(Sanders et al., 2016). RTX may also be effective in “refractory” MG (Iorio et al., 2015; Sanders et al., 2016), but a recent RCT did not demonstrate a steroid-sparing effect of RTX in AChR MG (clinicaltrials.gov: NCT02110706). Relapses are common and may improve with repeated treatment cycles. The treatment protocol is empirical, but most patients reported receiving 4 courses of 375 mg/m$^2$.

Eculizumab is a monoclonal antibody that inhibits the cleavage of C5 into C5a and C5b, which results in blockade of terminal complement activation. Complement deposition at the NMJ is thought to play a prominent role in MG pathogenesis (Engel et al., 1987), and it is presumed that eculizumab reduces complement-mediated damage to the postsynaptic muscle membrane. In the United States, eculizumab is approved for the treatment of generalized AChR MG, and in Europe and Japan the therapy is approved only for refractory generalized AChR MG. The approval of eculizumab is based on a phase III RCT of patients with refractory AChR GMG (Howard et al., 2017). Eculizumab is not appropriate for patients with MuSK MG because complement is not thought to play a major role in the pathogenesis of MuSK MG. Eculizumab requires biweekly infusions following an induction phase. All patients must receive vaccination against Neisseria meningitis prior to treatment.

## Summary

In a review of 1000 MG patients who received IS agents for at least 1 year, all forms of MG benefited from immunosuppression: the rate of remission or minimal manifestations ranged from 85% in OMG to 47% in thymoma-associated disease (Sanders et al., 2010). Prednisone was used in the great majority of these patients and AZA was the first-choice nonsteroidal immunosuppressant; MMF and CYA were used as second-choice agents. Treatment was ultimately discontinued in nearly 20% of AChR-ab positive EOMG patients, but in only 7% of patients with thymoma. The risk of complications was related to drug dosage, treatment duration, and patient characteristics, the highest rate of serious side effects (20%) occurring in LOMG and the lowest (4%) in early-onset disease.

The goal of minimal manifestations or better is often obtained, but few patients maintain improvement unless IS therapy is continued at effective doses indefinitely. The long-term risk of malignancy is not established, so use the minimal maintenance dose of IS agents necessary to keep the MG in control. Reduce medication dosage slowly after several years of stable improvement. Avoid abrupt withdrawal of immunosuppression, as this may lead to recurrent symptoms, even myasthenic crisis (Hohlfeld et al., 1985; Witte et al., 1984). Anecdotal evidence suggests that some patients may not achieve previous levels of improvement after withdrawal and exacerbation. Opportunistic infections, lymphomas, and other serious treatment-related morbidities may occur with increasing duration of immunosuppression. Monitoring and adjustment of therapy is best done in a specialized clinic.

### Thymectomy

In an international single-blinded RCT of thymectomy in non-thymomatous generalized AChR MG, at the end of 3 years patients who underwent extended thymectomy while taking prednisone had lower Quantitative Myasthenia Gravis (QMG) scores and required less prednisone than those who took prednisone alone (Wolfe et al., 2016). A follow-up extension study showed that these benefits from thymectomy persisted at the end of 5 years (Wolfe et al., 2019).

The response to thymectomy is gradual and often continues for months or years after surgery. Clinical experience suggests that the best responses are likely in young people, especially women, early in the disease, but improvement can occur even after many years of symptoms.

In non-thymomatous MG, thymectomy is performed to potentially reduce exposure to IS agents, or if immunotherapy has been ineffective or produced intolerable side effects (Sanders et al., 2016). Thymectomy is always an elective procedure and should be performed when the patient is stable and deemed safe to undergo the procedure.

Thymectomy is generally not recommended for ocular MG, but may be an option if drug therapy is inadequate (Liu et al., 2011; Mineo et al., 2013; Roberts et al., 2001; Sanders et al., 2016; Schumm et al., 1985).

The preferred surgical approach has traditionally been a transthoracic, sternal-splitting procedure that allows wide exploration of the anterior mediastinum. Transcervical and endoscopic approaches have less postoperative morbidity and shorter recovery times, and large case series of video-assisted thoracoscopic thymectomy (VAT-T) report therapeutic results similar to the transsternal procedure (Masaoka et al., 1981; Meyer et al., 2009). Robotic video-assisted thoracoscopic thymectomy (VATS) combines the advantages of minimally invasive techniques with added maneuverability and enhanced visualization, which reportedly permits an extended thymectomy similar to that using a transsternal approach. Without a prospective study comparing different techniques, the value of different surgical approaches remains unclear. The transsternal approach is often performed in thymoma to assure complete tumor removal.

Thymectomy has usually been limited to AChR MG patients, although some reports suggest that MG patients without AChR antibodies may benefit as well (Guptill et al., 2010b; Lavrnic et al., 2005; Yuan et al., 2007); one study reported a 21% complete remission rate in both AChR-antibody negative and AChR MG patients after thymectomy (Guillermo et al., 2004).

In non-thymomatous MG, we recommend thymectomy in virtually all early-onset AChR MG patients, and as an option in AChR MG patients with onset between ages 50 and 60; others also recommend thymectomy for older patients.

We do not base the decision to recommend thymectomy on the presence of AChR antibodies alone. The role of thymectomy in MuSK MG has not yet been determined, but the majority of evidence to date suggests it is not beneficial in most patients (Sanders et al., 2016). However, we, and others, have noted stable drug-free remission in some MuSK MG patients after thymectomy (Lavrnic et al., 2005; Ponseti et al., 2009; Witoonpanich et al., 2013). Further studies are needed to assess the value of thymectomy in other groups besides AChR MG.

We consider repeat thymectomy when relapse follows a good response to the initial surgery or when there is concern that thymic tissue removal had been incomplete. MRI with appropriate cardiac gating may be useful in identifying residual thymus tissue, although many authors believe that the clinical suspicion should be the basis upon which repeat surgery is considered (Jaretzki, 2003).

Virtually all patients with thymoma should have surgical resection regardless of age and any residual normal thymus tissue should also be resected. Elderly and multimorbid patients with small tumors may be followed with periodic imaging; palliative radiation therapy may be adequate when there is little tumor spread and slow tumor progression. Stage II and WHO type B2 and B3 and all III and IV stage tumors should have radiation therapy and be treated with an interdisciplinary approach.

### Evolving Treatments

Autologous stem-cell transplantation has been performed in refractory MG patients (Pringle et al., 2005), but the role of this procedure for MG and other autoimmune disorders is unclear at this time. Other therapies in clinical development for MG include anti-neonatal Fc receptor monoclonal antibodies targeting IgG recycling (clinicaltrials.gov: NCT03052751, NCT03772587, NCT02965573), additional complement inhibitors (clinicaltrials.gov: NCT03920293, NCT03315130), a vaccine for AChR MG (clinicaltrials.gov: NCT02609022), and amifampridine for treatment of MuSK MG (clinicaltrials.gov: NCT03304054).

## Treatment Plan for Myasthenia Gravis

Individualize the treatment of MG according to the clinical presentation/subtype; this requires a comprehensive assessment of the patient's functional impairment and its effect on daily life. ChEIs may be sufficient in some patients with OMG or mild generalized disease (before or after thymectomy), but most will ultimately require immunotherapy. The therapeutic goal is to return the patient to normal function as rapidly as possible while minimizing side effects of therapy. In the long-term management of patients treated with immunotherapies, the lowest effective dose should always be used. As noted, long-term risks of infections and malignancy, while not clearly defined, have been associated with the immunosuppressants commonly used in MG.

## Association of Myasthenia Gravis With Other Diseases

MG is often associated with other immune-mediated diseases, especially hyperthyroidism and rheumatoid arthritis (Nakata et al., 2013; Ramanujam et al., 2011). Population-based studies have also shown associations with Guillain-Barré syndrome, pemphigus, and dermatomyositis (Eaton et al., 2007). Seizures occur with increased frequency in children with MG. One-fifth of our MG patients have another disease: 7% had diabetes mellitus before corticosteroid treatment, 6% have thyroid disease, 3% have an extrathymic neoplasm and fewer than 2% have rheumatoid arthritis. Extrathymic malignancies have been reported to be common in MG patients, especially in the older age group, possibly due to a common background of immune dysregulation (Levin et al., 2005).

### Treatment of Associated Diseases and Medications to Avoid

It is important to recognize the effect of concomitant diseases and their treatments on myasthenic symptoms. Thyroid disease requires vigorous treatment—both hypo- and hyperthyroidism adversely affect myasthenic weakness. Intercurrent infections require immediate attention because they exacerbate MG and can be life-threatening in immunosuppressed patients.

## BOX 108.2 Drugs to Avoid or Use with Caution in Myasthenia Gravis*

Many drugs are associated with worsening of MG. However, reported associations do not necessarily mean these medications should never be prescribed in MG. Reports are often rare or represent a coincidental association. Clinical judgment and the risk-to-benefit ratio of the drug should be considered when it is deemed important for a patient's treatment. Listed below are medications that have the strongest evidence for worsening MG.

- Telithromycin: antibiotic for community-acquired pneumonia. Not available in the US, but may be available in other countries. Should not be used in MG.
- Fluoroquinolones (e.g., ciprofloxacin, moxifloxacin, and levofloxacin): commonly prescribed broad-spectrum antibiotics that are associated with worsening MG. The US FDA has designated a "black box" warning for these agents in MG. Use cautiously, if at all. Botulinum toxin: avoid.
- D-penicillamine: used for Wilson disease and rarely for rheumatoid arthritis. Strongly associated with causing MG. Avoid.
- Quinine: occasionally used for leg cramps. Use prohibited except in malaria in the United States.
- Magnesium: potentially dangerous if given intravenously, i.e., for eclampsia during late pregnancy or for hypomagnesemia. Use only if absolutely necessary and observe for worsening.
- Macrolide antibiotics (e.g., erythromycin, azithromycin, clarithromycin): commonly prescribed antibiotics for gram-positive bacterial infections. May worsen MG. Use cautiously, if at all.
- Aminoglycoside antibiotics (e.g., gentamycin, neomycin, tobramycin): used for gram-negative bacterial infections. May worsen MG. Use cautiously if no alternative treatment available.
- Corticosteroids: A standard treatment for MG but may cause transient worsening within the first 2 weeks. Monitor carefully for this possibility (see Table 108.3).
- Procainamide: used for irregular heart rhythm. May worsen MG. Use with caution.
- Desferrioxamine: Chelating agent used for hemochromatosis. May worsen MG.
- Beta-blockers: commonly prescribed for hypertension, heart disease, and migraine but potentially dangerous in MG. May worsen MG. Use cautiously.
- Statins (e.g., atorvastatin, pravastatin, rosuvastatin, simvastatin): used to reduce serum cholesterol. May worsen or precipitate MG. Use cautiously if indicated and at lowest dose needed.
- Iodinated radiological contrast agents: older reports document increased MG weakness, but modern contrast agents appear safer. Use cautiously and observe for worsening.
- Chloroquine (Aralen): used for malaria and amoeba infections. May worsen or precipitate MG. Use with caution.
- Hydroxychloroquine (Plaquenil): used for malaria, rheumatoid arthritis, and lupus. May worsen or precipitate MG. Use with caution.
- Immune checkpoint inhibitors (ICIs): used as immunotherapy for many types of cancer. May cause MG or worsen myasthenic weakness in previously existing MG. Patients with MG and cancer who are considering ICI therapy should discuss this possible side effect with their oncologist and neurologist. Doctors evaluating new-onset weakness in cancer patients should consider MG. MG patients who have worsening weakness following ICI treatment should contact their neurologist and oncologist immediately. Examples of ICIs:

Pembrolizumab (Keytruda)
Nivolumab (Opdivo)
Atezolizumab (Tecentriq)
Avelumab ((Bavencio)
Durvalumab (Imfinzi)
Ipilimumab (Yervoy)

* See also http://myasthenia.org/What-is-MG/MG-Management/Cautionary-Drugs
*FDA*, Food and Drug Administration; *MG*, myasthenia gravis.

Use drugs that adversely affect NMT (Box 108.2) with caution. Many antibiotics fall into this category, particularly aminoglycosides, fluoroquinolones, and macrolides. Ophthalmic preparations of β-blockers and aminoglycoside antibiotics may cause worsening of ocular symptoms. When using corticosteroids to treat concomitant illness, anticipate and explain the potential adverse and beneficial effects to the patient.

MG may develop in patients during interferon α-2b treatment for malignancy and chronic active hepatitis C. In some, MG has presented with myasthenic crisis. The mechanism is unknown, but the expression of interferon-γ at motor endplates of transgenic mice results in weakness and abnormal NMJ function that improve with ChEIs. This suggests an autoimmune humoral response, similar to that in human MG.

The administration of botulinum toxin injections to patients with neuromuscular disease such as MG risks systemic side effects, including dysphagia and respiratory compromise. Administer only with great caution.

We recommend annual vaccination against influenza (including H1N1) for most patients with MG and the recombinant shingles vaccine in older patients. Vaccination against pneumococcus is a recommendation for at-risk patients before starting prednisone or other IS drugs. Never give live attenuated vaccines to immunosuppressed patients due to the risk of viral reactivation. The Centers for Disease Control and Prevention report that those taking less than 2 mg/kg per day of prednisone or every-other-day prednisone are not at risk. Patients with prior thymectomy should not receive the yellow fever vaccine.

### Checkpoint Inhibitor-Induced Myasthenia Gravis

Immune checkpoint inhibitor (ICI) drugs have revolutionized the treatment of advanced cancers. These drugs promote immune system activation to attack cancer cells by targeting CTLA-4 and PD-1 or PD-1 ligands. Neurological complications from ICIs, including MG, occur rarely and result from a loss of immune regulatory mechanisms (Pardoll, 2012). Patients may present with isolated ocular symptoms or severe MG with dysphagia and respiratory crisis (Alnahhas et al., 2016; Gonzalez et al., 2017; Kao et al., 2017). MG will often overlap with myositis and it may be difficult to distinguish between muscle and NMJ involvement on clinical grounds alone (Kimura et al., 2016; Konoeda et al., 2017). It is therefore important to perform a comprehensive evaluation, including electrodiagnostic testing and MG and myositis laboratory testing, to determine whether myositis and MG are coexisting. Biopsy of an affected muscle may also be warranted. Evidence-based treatment recommendations are lacking but we use standard MG treatments, including pyridostigmine for mild ocular symptoms, and steroids and PLEX or IVIg for severe disease. After the development of MG, if other treatment options are available or the MG disease severity was severe, avoid reinstituting an ICI. However, since many patients are receiving ICIs for advanced stage cancer with a limited life expectancy otherwise, treatment options may be limited, and restarting ICI therapy may be considered. The best candidates for restarting this class of drug may be patients with mild disease that can be controlled without aggressive interventions. Coordination with the oncology team is important at all stages of managing checkpoint inhibitor induced MG.

## Special Situations

### Myasthenic Crisis

Myasthenic crisis is respiratory failure from myasthenic weakness. An identifiable precipitating event, such as infection, aspiration, surgery, or medication change, precedes most episodes of crisis. Cholinergic crisis is respiratory failure from overdose of ChEIs and was more common before the introduction of IS therapy, when using very large dosages of ChEIs.

In MG patients with progressive respiratory symptoms, no single factor determines the need for ventilatory support. The safest approach is to admit the patient to an intensive care unit and observe closely for impending respiratory insufficiency. Serial measurements of negative inspiratory force (NIF) provide the best measure of deteriorating respiratory function in MG. Noninvasive mechanical ventilation using bilevel positive pressure ventilation (BiPAP) may avoid the need for intubation in patients in crisis without hypercapnia (Rabinstein et al., 2002).

Retrospective studies suggest that PLEX and IVIg are equally effective in stabilizing patients in crisis (Murthy et al., 2005). Others suggest that PLEX is superior, producing more rapid respiratory improvement (Qureshi et al., 1999). We use PLEX in the treatment of crisis except when there is hemodynamic instability, sepsis, coagulopathy, or during the first trimester of pregnancy.

Once ventilated, discontinuing ChEIs is safe and recommended to eliminate the possibility of cholinergic overdose and permit determination of disease severity. After addressing the precipitating factors causing crisis, add ChEIs in low doses and titrate to the optimal dose. Consider extubation when the patient has a NIF greater than −20 cm $H_2O$ and an expiratory pressure greater than 35–40 cm $H_2O$. If the patient complains of fatigue or shortness of breath, defer extubation even if these values and blood gas measurements are normal.

Prevention and aggressive treatment of medical complications offer the best opportunity to improve the outcome of myasthenic crisis.

Morning

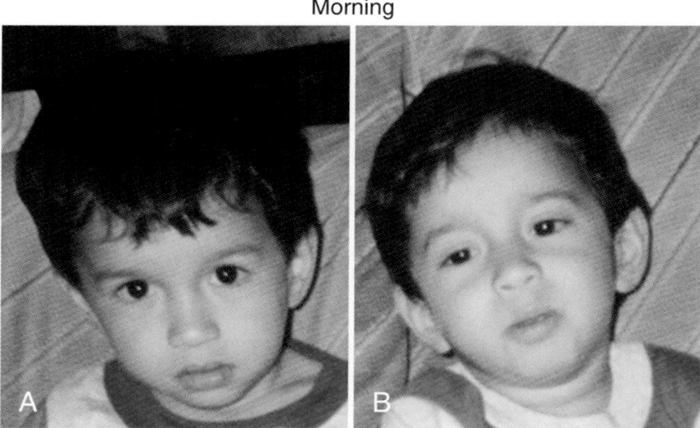


Evening

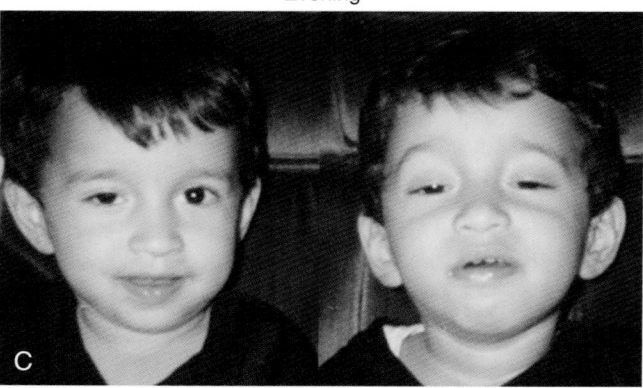


**Fig. 108.8** Twins, Age 2, Both With Acetylcholine Receptor Myasthenia Gravis (A, B). In the morning, one (B) has mild bilateral lid ptosis, slightly worse on the right; ptosis is worse or has become apparent in the evening in both boys (C).

### Anesthetic Management in Myasthenia Gravis

The stress of surgery and some drugs used perioperatively may worsen myasthenic weakness. As a rule, local or spinal anesthesia is preferred over inhalation anesthesia. Avoid the use of neuromuscular blocking agents or use them sparingly; inhalation anesthetic agents alone usually provide adequate muscle relaxation. The required dose of depolarizing blocking agents may be greater than that needed in non-myasthenic patients, whereas low doses of nondepolarizing agents cause pronounced and long-lasting blockade that may require extended postoperative assisted respiration.

### Ocular Myasthenia

While ChEIs may control symptoms adequately in some OMG patients, the benefit is usually partial and not protracted, while prednisone is often quite effective. The decision to initiate steroid therapy will depend upon the risk-benefit assessment, which is different in patients considering treatment for purely cosmetic reasons versus those in whom ocular symptoms have a profound effect on their livelihood (pilots, surgeons, etc.). Prednisone treatment may delay or reduce the frequency of progression of OMG to generalized disease (Kupersmith et al., 2003). Start prednisone at an initial dose of 10–20 mg/day with gradual increases every 3–5 days until achieving a clinical response (see Table 108.2). Alternatively, begin prednisone at a dose of 20-60mg–60 mg; the risk of steroid-induced exacerbation is less in OMG. Aim to use a maintenance dosage of prednisone that causes few major systemic adverse effects. Consider a steroid-sparing IS agent if this cannot be achieved. In general, OMG is not an indication for thymectomy, though this may be effective in some patients. (See Thymectomy section, above.)

### Childhood Myasthenia Gravis

The onset of immune-mediated MG before age 18 is referred to as *juvenile MG (JMG)* (Andrews et al., 2002; Barraud et al., 2018; Castro et al., 2013; Finnis et al., 2011; Jastrzębska et al., 2019) (Fig. 108.8). Twenty percent of JMG and almost 50% of those with onset before puberty are seronegative, which makes the distinction from CMS challenging (see Congenital Myasthenic Syndromes section, later in this chapter). Electrodiagnostic studies demonstrate abnormal NMT but features that distinguish CMS from autoimmune MG are present in only a few forms of CMS. Improvement after PLEX or IVIg may help to establish an autoimmune etiology, but failure to improve does not exclude an autoimmune etiology. Many children who are initially seronegative later develop AChR-abs. Thymomas are rare in this age group.

Treatment decisions in children with autoimmune MG should recognize that the rate of spontaneous remission is high in these patients. We recommend ChEIs alone in prepubertal children not disabled by weakness. For patients who remain symptomatic despite optimal dosing of ChEIs, prednisone is efficacious and cost-effective although the chronic side effects potentially have a long-term impact in children (growth stunting, weight gain, mood alteration, hyperglycemia, hypertension, etc.). A suggested starting dose is 0.5 mg/kg/day, with a maximum starting dose in older children of 30 mg/day. Use steroid-sparing IS drugs in more severe or refractory cases as in adult MG. PLEX and IVIg are effective short-term therapies in JMG.

Favorable results have been reported for thymectomy in JMG, even in patients less than 5 years of age, although the high rates of spontaneous remission make the assessment of benefit difficult. There are no reported adverse effects on the immune system from removing the thymus after 1 year of age (Ashraf et al., 2006; Hermes et al., 2011; Herrmann et al., 1998; Sauce et al., 2009; Tracy et al., 2009).

The value of thymectomy in the treatment of prepubertal patients with MG is unclear, but the international consensus guidance for MG management recommends thymectomy in children with generalized AChR MG if the response to pyridostigmine and IS therapy is unsatisfactory, or to avoid potential complications of IS therapy (Sanders et al., 2016).

### Pregnancy

Myasthenia may improve, worsen, or remain unchanged during pregnancy. It is common for the first symptoms of MG to begin during pregnancy or postpartum. First-trimester worsening is more common in first pregnancies, whereas third-trimester worsening and postpartum exacerbations are more common in subsequent pregnancies. Complete remission may occur late in pregnancy. The clinical status at onset of pregnancy does not reliably predict the course during pregnancy. Pregnancy is more difficult to manage at the beginning of MG and women with MG should delay pregnancy until after the disease is stable.

Therapeutic abortion is rarely, if ever, needed because of MG, and the frequency of spontaneous abortion is not increased. Oral ChEIs are the first-line treatment during pregnancy. Intravenous ChEIs may produce uterine contractions and are contraindicated. Prednisone is the IS agent of choice. Whenever possible we do not use other IS drugs during pregnancy because of theoretical potential mutagenic effects, although others feel that AZA and even CYA can be used safely during pregnancy (Ferrero et al., 2005). Increased risk of fetal malformation has been reported when men used AZA prior to conception (Norgard et al., 2004). MMF can cause birth defects and is contraindicated during pregnancy. PLEX or IVIg are useful when an immediate, albeit temporary, improvement is required during pregnancy, but avoid PLEX during the first trimester. Thymectomy should be postponed until after delivery as benefit is unlikely to occur during pregnancy.

Magnesium sulfate has neuromuscular blocking effects and is not recommended to manage pre-eclampsia; barbiturates usually provide adequate treatment. Labor and delivery are usually normal. Cesarean section is recommended only for obstetrical indications. Regional anesthesia is preferred for delivery or cesarean section. MG does not affect uterine smooth muscle and therefore does not compromise the first stage of labor. In the second stage, voluntary muscles are at risk for easy fatigue and outlet forceps or vacuum extraction may be necessary. In our experience, breast-feeding is not a problem for myasthenic mothers, despite the theoretical risk of passing maternal AChR-abs in breast milk to the newborn.

### Transient Neonatal Myasthenia Gravis

A temporary form of MG affects 10%–20% of newborns whose mothers have immune-mediated MG. The severity of symptoms in the newborn does not correlate with the severity of symptoms in the mother. Transient neonatal myasthenia gravis (TNMG) also occurs in MuSK MG (Niks et al., 2008b) and rarely in infants of seronegative mothers. Weakness may manifest in utero, particularly when maternal antibodies are directed against the fetal AChR, and may lead to arthrogryposis multiplex congenita (Barnes et al., 1995). Consider decreased fetal movement as a possible indication for PLEX or IVIg. Birth of a child with arthrogryposis should also prompt a search for MG in the mother. An affected mother who delivers an infant with TNMG is likely to have similarly affected, subsequent infants. Consider prophylactic treatment with PLEX and/or steroids in a woman with a previously affected child, as the risk of recurrent TNMG is high.

Affected newborns are typically hypotonic and feed poorly during the first 3 days. In some newborns, symptoms may be delayed for 1–2 days. Symptoms usually last less than 2 weeks but may persist for as long as 12 weeks, which correlates with the half-life of neonatal antibodies. It is not clear why some newborns develop weakness and others, with equally high antibody levels, do not. Some mothers with antibodies directed specifically against fetal AChR might themselves be asymptomatic, which makes diagnosing TNMG more difficult.

Examine all infants born of myasthenic mothers carefully at birth for evidence of myasthenic weakness. Detection of AChR or MuSK antibodies in the child provides strong evidence for the diagnosis, although seronegative mothers have delivered affected seronegative infants. Improvement following injection of 0.1 mg/kg edrophonium supports the diagnosis of TNMG, but it may be difficult to assess the response in an intubated and ventilated neonate. Improvement after edrophonium does not distinguish TNMG from some CMS. A decrementing response to RNS confirms abnormal NMT, but also does not distinguish TNMG from most CMS. Affected newborns require symptomatic treatment with ChEIs if swallowing or breathing is impaired. Consider exchange transfusion if respiratory weakness is severe.

## CONGENITAL MYASTHENIC SYNDROMES

The CMS are a group of NMJ diseases caused by genetic defects of muscle endplate molecules involved in NMT (Engel, 2008; Finlayson et al., 2013; Finsterer, 2019). Mutations in 32 genes involved in presynaptic (8), postsynaptic (15), synaptic (4), and glycosylation (5) proteins have been identified, and most have autosomal recessive inheritance (Finsterer, 2019). Symptoms are present at birth in most forms, but may go unrecognized until adolescence or adulthood, particularly when progression is gradual and clinical manifestations are mild. The most common and clinically important CMS are discussed below.

Overall, there is a 2:1 male predominance. Ophthalmoparesis and ptosis are present in most cases during infancy; mild facial paresis may be present as well. Ophthalmoplegia is often incomplete at onset but progresses to complete paralysis during infancy or childhood. Some children develop generalized fatigue and weakness, but limb weakness is usually mild compared to ophthalmoplegia. Skeletal deformities such as high-arched palate, facial dysmorphism, arthrogryposis and scoliosis are common. Muscles may be small and underdeveloped. Episodic respiratory crises may occur with any form of congenital myasthenia but are particularly common in choline acetylcholinesterase (ChAT) deficiency (see below).

The diagnosis of CMS is suggested by the clinical features and the response to ChEIs, or findings on standard electrodiagnostic studies. Determination of the specific genetic or physiological defect requires genetic studies or specialized morphological and electrophysiological studies on muscle tissue. The specific diagnosis is important since many CMS patients respond to drugs that increase the availability of ACh at the muscle endplate or alter the kinetics of the AChR. ChEIs, sometimes in very high doses, improve limb muscle weakness in some forms but worsen it in others. The weakness in some forms responds to amifampridine (Harper et al., 2000). Thymectomy and immunosuppression are not effective.

### Acetylcholine Receptor Deficiency

This is a genetically heterogeneous group with patients having various AChR subunit or rapsyn mutations. Most commonly, an ε-subunit mutation results in continued expression of the fetal γ-subunit. The age of symptom onset ranges from infancy to adulthood. Clinical manifestations include hypotonia, respiratory insufficiency, weakness of ocular and bulbar muscles, and skeletal deformities. Electrodiagnostic findings are variable and depend on the severity and distribution of weakness. RNS studies usually demonstrate a decrement but the decrement may be absent or restricted to facial muscles in mild cases. Jitter is increased in all reported cases.

These disorders respond variably to symptomatic therapy with pyridostigmine or amifampridine. Ephedrine produces benefit in some cases. Immunotherapy has no effect.

### Choline Acetyl Transferase Deficiency

This condition, previously called *congenital myasthenic syndrome with episodic apnea* or *familial infantile myasthenia,* is caused by mutations in the *CHAT* gene, which codes for endplate ChAT, the rate-limiting enzyme in the resynthesis of acetylcholine within the nerve terminal. Generalized hypotonia, ptosis, and feeding difficulties are present at birth, and the early course of the disease is punctuated by sudden episodes of severe bulbar and generalized weakness with life-threatening apnea triggered by infections or stress. Arthrogryposis may be present. Within weeks after birth, the child becomes stronger and ultimately breathes unassisted. However, episodes of life-threatening apnea occur repeatedly throughout infancy and childhood, even into adult life, and there may be a history of sudden infant death syndrome in siblings.

A decrementing response to RNS is usually present in weak muscles but may only be seen after prolonged exercise or continuous repetitive stimulation (Stålberg et al., 2010). Jitter and blocking also become progressively greater during continuous nerve stimulation (Stålberg et al., 2010), ChEIs improve strength in most children with ChAT deficiency. Symptoms tend to lessen in adolescence and adulthood when the disease resembles mild autoimmune MG or a congenital myopathy.

### Congenital Acetylcholinesterase Deficiency

Endplate AChE deficiency results from a recessive mutation of *COLQ,* the gene coding for the collagenous tail of the heteromeric AChE molecule at the muscle endplate (Ohno et al., 1999). Presentation is usually in infancy or early childhood. The symptoms are usually severe, consisting of generalized weakness, ptosis, ophthalmoparesis, bulbar and limb weakness, underdevelopment of muscles and slowed pupillary responses to light. Skeletal deformities include lordosis or scoliosis that worsens with prolonged standing. Single-nerve stimuli characteristically produce repetitive discharges and ChEIs typically make symptoms worse. Pyridostigmine is ineffective or even detrimental. Some patients respond to ephedrine (Yeung et al., 2010) or salbutamol (Padmanabha et al., 2017).

### Slow-Channel Congenital Myasthenic Syndrome

Variable expression results in a wide spectrum of clinical manifestations and severity in slow-channel congenital myasthenic syndrome (SCCMS), which has autosomal dominant inheritance. Mutations in an AChR subunit (*CHRNE, CHRNA, CHRNB* or *CHRND* genes) results in prolonged open time of the ACh channel. Severe cases present in infancy or early childhood, but mild cases may present in adulthood, as late as the seventh decade. In SCCMS neck and distal upper limb muscles; the intrinsic hand muscles and digit extensors are particularly weak and atrophic. Ptosis, ophthalmoparesis, dysarthria, dysphagia, proximal limb weakness, and respiratory insufficiency also occur in some cases. RNS shows a decrementing response. Single-nerve stimuli produce repetitive muscle discharges similar to those seen in ChEI toxicity or congenital deficiency of endplate AChE (see above). ChEIs worsen the weakness. Quinidine sulfate and fluoxetine, which reduce AChR channel open time, may improve strength (Harper et al., 2003).

### Fast-Channel Syndrome

Fast-channel syndrome is a very severe form of CMS. It results from AChR subunit mutations (*CHRNE, CHRNA,* or *CHRND* genes) that cause abnormally brief opening of the AChR ion channel. Symptoms are usually present at birth and there is severe ptosis and ophthalmoplegia. Patients have a weak cry and poor feeding, severe acral weakness, and frequent respiratory crises. Treatment is primarily supportive with ventilator support, often from birth, and gastrostomy for feeding. Patients respond to ChEIs and amifampridine but the improvement from ChEIs may wane over time.

### Rapsyn Mutations

Rapsyn is a postsynaptic protein involved in clustering AChR at the muscle endplate. Rapsyn mutations produce a CMS in which respiratory distress, hypotonia, and poor feeding are usually present at birth. There is generalized weakness and ptosis but ophthalmoplegia is uncommon. Patients have a high-arched palate and may have arthrogryposis. Respiratory crises are common until about 7 years of age in the setting of stress, such as infections, and then become less frequent. The response to ChEIs and amifampridine is good and the overall prognosis is relatively favorable, many patients being able to discontinue treatment as adults. A milder form of the disease can occur that may not be noticed during childhood and should be considered in suspected autoimmune MG that is refractory to treatment.

### *DOK-7* Mutations

DOK-7 is a muscle protein that activates MuSK and is critical in endplate development and AChR aggregation. The clinical manifestations and electrodiagnostic findings of CMS associated with *DOK-7* mutations may be indistinguishable from those of AChR deficiency (Selcen et al., 2008), including reduced fetal movements in utero and static and fatigable weakness of cranial, respiratory and limb muscles. A presentation with nonfluctuating limb girdle distribution weakness may mistakenly lead to a diagnosis of a muscular dystrophy. Ephedrine, salbutamol, or albuterol is the first choice of treatment; amifampridine may provide additional benefit. ChEIs should be avoided (Witting et al., 2014).

### *GFPT1* and *DPAGT1* Mutations

These mutations affect enzymes in glycosylation pathways and produce slowly progressive limb girdle weakness beginning in childhood or early teens (Belaya et al., 2012; Guergueltcheva et al., 2012). Some patients with the *GFPT1* mutation were initially called "familial limb-girdle myasthenia" (McQuillen, 1966). Ocular muscles are not involved and bulbar muscles are only minimally affected. EMG shows myopathic features, as well as abnormal NMT. Muscle biopsy may show tubular aggregates. ChEIs and amifampridine benefit most patients. Albuterol and ephedrine may also help.

## LAMBERT-EATON MYASTHENIA

LEM results from an immune-mediated attack against the P/Q type voltage-gated calcium channels (VGCCs) on presynaptic cholinergic nerve terminals at the NMJ and in autonomic ganglia, thereby inhibiting release of ACh (Fig. 108.9). First described in patients with lung cancer (CA-LEM), LEM also occurs as an organ-specific autoimmune disorder in the absence of cancer (NCA-LEM).

LEM is usually clinically quite distinct from MG. Most patients report gradual onset of lower extremity weakness, sometimes with muscle tenderness. Dry mouth is a common symptom of autonomic dysfunction; others are erectile dysfunction, postural hypotension, constipation, and dry eyes. Ocular and bulbar symptoms are generally not prominent

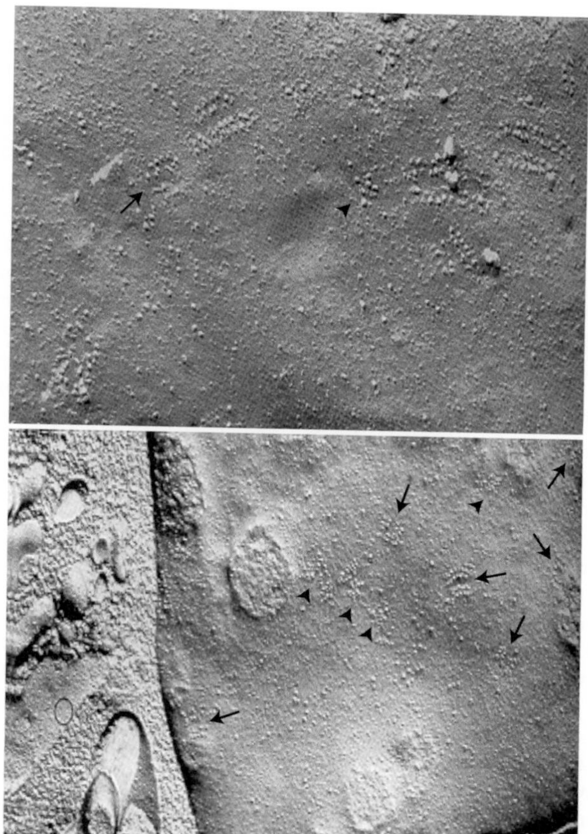

**Fig. 108.9 Freeze-Fracture Electron Micrographs Of Presynaptic Membrane P-Faces.** *Top*: control muscle. Active zones tend to be aligned along an arc *(arrow)*. Some zones display fewer than four rows of particles *(arrowhead)*. x98,000. *Bottom*: LEM muscle. Membrane leaflet shows active zones *(arrows)* and clusters of large intramembrane particles *(arrowheads)*. x59,800. *(From Fukunaga, H., Engel, A.G., Osame, M., Lambert, E.H., 1982. Paucity and disorganization of presynaptic membrane active zones in the Lambert-Eaton myasthenic syndrome. Muscle Nerve 5, 686–697, figures 2A and 4, by permission.)*

(O'Neill et al., 1988; Tim et al., 2000; Wirtz et al., 2002), but are reported in some patients, in a pattern suggesting MG (Burns et al., 2003; Titulaer et al., 2008). Prolonged apnea and ventilator dependence may follow use of neuromuscular blocking agents for surgery (Anderson et al., 1953) but respiratory failure is otherwise uncommon in the absence of primary pulmonary disease (Barr et al., 1993; Smith et al., 1996).

Symptoms usually begin after age 40, but LEM can occur in children. Males and females are equally affected. Approximately one-half the patients have an underlying malignancy—in 80% this is small-cell lung cancer (SCLC)—which may be discovered years before or years after the onset of LEM symptoms.

Examination usually demonstrates less weakness than the symptoms suggest. Tendon reflexes are almost always absent or diminished. Strength (and tendon reflexes) may facilitate briefly after exercise and then weaken with sustained activity, but this is not a universal finding. The response to edrophonium is not as robust or consistent as in MG. The weakness in LEM is not usually life-threatening and more closely resembles cachexia, polymyositis, or a paraneoplastic neuromuscular disease.

## Diagnostic Procedures in Lambert-Eaton Myasthenia

The following characteristic electrodiagnostic findings confirm the diagnosis (see Chapter 36): compound muscle action potentials (CMAPs) with low amplitude, which increases during 20–50 Hz nerve stimulation and after brief maximum voluntary muscle activation. Low-frequency RNS produces a decrementing response in a hand or foot muscle in almost all patients and almost all have small CMAPs in some distal muscle (Tim et al., 2000). The characteristic increase in CMAP size after activation is more prominent in distal muscles but it may be necessary to examine several muscles to demonstrate this important finding.

Immunoprecipitation assay demonstrates VGCC antibodies in almost all patients with CA-LEM and in more than 90% with NCA-LEM (Harper., 2002). Low titers of VGCC antibodies have also been reported in systemic lupus erythematosus and rheumatoid arthritis (Lang et al., 1993). These antibodies may not be detectable early in the disease, in which case repeat antibody testing may be useful.

Antibodies to SOX1, a transcription factor involved in neural development, were found in 64% of CA-LEM patients with SCLC and in none with NCA-LEM (Sabater et al., 2008); thus SOX1 antibodies are a marker for underlying cancer in LEM patients.

## Immunopathology of Lambert-Eaton Myasthenia

P/Q VGCCs are the target of disease-causing antibodies in LEM. The number of active zone particles in the motor nerve terminal, which represent the VGCC, is reduced (see Fig. 108.9). Similar changes occur in mice injected with IgG from LEM patients. The mechanism is probably from cross-linking of the VGCC by antibodies that downregulate VGCC expression by antigenic modulation.

SCLC cells are of neuroectodermal origin and contain high concentrations of VGCC. In CA-LEM, these antigens induce production of VGCC antibodies. In NCA-LEM, as in other primary autoimmune disorders, altered self-tolerance presumably induces production of VGCC antibodies as part of a more general immune-mediated state. VGCC antibody titers do not correlate with disease severity but the antibody levels may fall as the disease improves in patients receiving immunosuppression.

## Treatment of Lambert-Eaton Myasthenia

Once the diagnosis of LEM is established, an extensive search for underlying malignancy, especially SCLC, is mandatory. Chronic smokers should undergo bronchoscopy and/or positron emission tomography (PET) scan if chest-imaging studies are normal. The target of initial treatment is any underlying malignancy. Weakness may improve after effective cancer therapy and some patients require no further treatment. Repeat the search for occult malignancy periodically, especially during the first 2 years after symptom onset. Determine the frequency of re-evaluation by the patient's cancer risk factors.

Tailor therapy to the individual, based on the severity of weakness, underlying disease, life expectancy, and response to previous treatment. RCTs have shown that amifampridine and IVIg improve muscle strength scores and CMAP amplitudes in patients with LEM (Bain et al., 1996; Keogh et al., 2011; Maddison et al., 2005; McEvoy et al., 1989; Oh et al., 2009; Oh et al., 2016; Wirtz et al., 2009; Sanders et al., 2000; Sanders et al., 2018b). Other treatments, such as PLEX (Newsom-Davis et al., 1984), corticosteroids, and IS agents, including RTX (Maddison et al., 2011), may be of benefit in some patients but have not been tested in controlled trials. A quick clinical test that is particularly helpful to monitor therapeutic responses in LEM is the triple-timed up-and-go test (Video 108.5) (Raja et al., 2019; Sanders et al., 2018a). This validated test is sensitive to changes in clinical status and assesses the proximal lower extremity weakness and gait difficulty characteristic of LEM.

The following treatment plan for LEM is a general guide that should be modified to suit specific situations.

ChEIs improve strength in occasional LEM patients. Try pyridostigmine, 30–60 mg every 6 hours, for several days. In some patients, the major benefit is relief of dry mouth.

Amifampridine facilitates release of ACh from motor nerve terminals and produces clinically significant improvement of strength and autonomic symptoms in most LEM patients. Therapeutic responses occur with doses of 5–25 mg three to four times a day; seizures may occur at doses higher than 100 mg/day. Concomitant use of pyridostigmine, 30–60 mg, three or four times a day often enhances the response. Side effects usually are negligible: transitory perioral and digital paresthesias occur with doses greater than 10–15 mg. Cramps and diarrhea may occur when amifampridine is given with pyridostigmine and can be minimized by reducing the dose of pyridostigmine. Amifampridine has been approved for treatment of LEM at doses up to 80 mg/day.

Both PLEX and IVIg provide short-term improvement in some patients with LEM (Keogh et al., 2011). If these treatments are not effective, determine if weakness is sufficiently severe to warrant immunotherapy with prednisone, AZA, CYA, or RTX. In patients with severe weakness, use PLEX or IVIg first and add prednisone and AZA after improvement begins. It may be necessary to administer repeated courses of treatment in order to maintain improvement.

In LEM patients with cancer, the response to cancer therapy determines the prognosis. In patients without cancer who are not well treated with amifampridine, immunosuppression produces improvement in many patients, but most require substantial and continuing doses of IS medications (Abenroth et al., 2017; Maddison et al., 2001).

### Myasthenia Gravis/Lambert-Eaton Myasthenia Overlap Syndrome

The clinical presentations of MG and LEM are usually quite distinct but in some patients the clinical and electrodiagnostic findings may be similar and the correct diagnosis may not obvious. Features that favor MG include prominent ocular muscle weakness, limb weakness that predominates in the arms, and normal muscle stretch reflexes (Wirtz et al., 2002). Features that favor LEM include weakness that predominates in the hip girdle muscles, hypoactive or absent reflexes, and autonomic symptoms, especially dry mouth.

Numerous reports of patients with various overlapping features of MG and LEM have been published. These include patients with (1) clinical features of MG but facilitation on manual muscle testing or EMG, typical of LEM; and (2) clinical and EMG patterns typical of one condition initially that change to the other later; or EMG patterns typical of MG in one muscle and of LEM in another. A few reported patients appear to have a true MG/LEM overlap syndrome, with antibodies to both the AChR and VGCC (Kanzato et al., 1999; Katz et al., 1998; Newsom-Davis et al., 1991; Oh et al., 2005); we have seen one such case among 1300 patients with acquired MG and 115 with LEM. The ultimate diagnosis in patients with mixed features of MG and LEM may be moot because most treatments are the same for both conditions. Exceptions are that we do not search for cancer other than thymoma in MG, and thymectomy is not a treatment for LEM.

## BOTULISM

Botulism is caused by a toxin produced by the anaerobic bacterium *Clostridium botulinum*, which blocks the release of ACh from the motor nerve terminal (Cherington, 2007) and produces a long-lasting, severe muscle paralysis. Botulism usually follows ingestion of inadequately sterilized contaminated foods. Of eight types of botulinum toxins (A, B, $C_\alpha$, $C_\beta$, D, E, F and G), types A and B cause most cases of botulism in the United States. All toxin types block ACh release from the presynaptic motor nerve terminal and the parasympathetic and sympathetic nerve ganglia. Neuromuscular symptoms usually begin 12–36 hours after ingestion of contaminated food and are preceded by nausea and vomiting. Not all people who ingest the contaminated food become symptomatic.

### Clinical Features of Botulism

The major initial symptoms of botulism are blurred vision, dysphagia, and dysarthria. Pupillary responses to light are impaired and tendon reflexes are variably reduced. Weakness progresses for several days and then reaches a plateau. Severe respiratory paralysis may occur rapidly. Blocking of ACh release in the autonomic system produces blurring of vision from ophthalmoparesis, pupillary abnormalities, dry mouth, postural hypotension, and urinary retention. Electrophysiological findings aid the diagnosis (see below). Bioassay of the toxin by injecting serum or stool from an affected patient into mice is positive if paralysis and death of the animals follows. Polymerase chain reaction (PCR) assays are available to rapidly detect the bacteria.

Infantile botulism results from the growth of *C. botulinum* in the immature gastrointestinal tract and the elaboration of small quantities of toxin over a prolonged period (Jones, 2002). Honey is commonly incriminated as a vehicle carrying the *C. botulinum* spores that produce infantile botulism. Symptoms of constipation, lethargy, poor suck, and weak cry usually begin at approximately 4 months of age. Examination reveals weakness of the limb and oropharyngeal muscles, poorly reactive pupils, and hypoactive tendon reflexes. Most patients require ventilatory support. Demonstrating botulinum toxin in the stool or isolation of *C. botulinum* from stool culture confirms the diagnosis.

Wound botulism occurs predominantly in drug abusers after subcutaneous injection of heroin: *Clostridium* bacteria colonize the injection site and release toxin that produces local and patchy systemic weakness.

### Electromyographic Findings in Botulism

Electrophysiological abnormalities in botulism tend to evolve with time and may not be present early in the disease (Padua et al., 1999). The EMG findings in botulism include:

- Reduced CMAP amplitude in at least two muscles
- At least 20% facilitation of CMAP amplitude during tetanic stimulation
- Facilitation that persists for at least 2 minutes after activation. No post-activation exhaustion
- Short duration motor unit potentials resembling myopathy in affected muscles.

Not all patients with botulism have all these electrophysiological findings. The diagnosis is unlikely if none of these features are present.

SFEMG demonstrates markedly increased jitter and blocking in virtually every case (Padua et al., 1999). Jitter and blocking may decrease as the firing rate increases but this is not a consistent finding.

Botulinum toxin injections used in the treatment of focal dystonia and other conditions may produce focal or regional weakness, including diplopia, dysphagia, urinary incontinence, and brachial plexopathy, and may unmask or exacerbate other neuromuscular diseases, such as MG, LEM, and motor neuron disease. Jitter may be increased in muscles remote from the site of injection, and may persist for many months (Sanders et al., 1986).

### Treatment of Botulism

Treatment consists of administration of bivalent (type A and B) or trivalent (A, B, and E) antitoxin. Antibiotic therapy is not effective since the cause of symptoms (in all but infantile and wound botulism) is the ingestion of toxin rather than organisms. In infantile botulism, IV human botulism immune globulin (BIG-IV) neutralizes the toxin for several days after illness onset, shortens the length and cost of the hospital stay, and reduces the severity of illness (Arnon et al., 2006). Otherwise, treatment is supportive. ChEIs are usually not beneficial. With improvements in intensive care, the mortality rate has declined to about 20%. Depending on initial severity, recovery may be quite prolonged; many patients still have symptoms a year or more after the onset of illness.

## OTHER CAUSES OF ABNORMAL NEUROMUSCULAR TRANSMISSION

Envenomation by animal toxins is the most common cause of NMJ toxicity worldwide. Muscles of eye movement or the eyelids are most often involved, along with muscles of neck flexion and the pectoral and pelvic girdles. In more severe envenomation, bulbar and respiratory muscles are also involved. Cognition and sensation are intact and muscle stretch reflexes are often preserved or only minimally diminished, particularly early in the illness. Arthropod venoms that affect the NMJ include those of the funnel web and black widow spiders, which produce marked acute neurotransmitter release by depolarizing the presynaptic nerve terminal and increasing calcium influx into the nerve terminal. Tick paralysis results from a neurotoxin that blocks AChR function postsynaptically.

Envenomation by snakebite occurs primarily from the *Elapidae* and *Hydrophiodae* species. Snake NMJ toxins act either presynaptically or postsynaptically. Presynaptic β-neurotoxins (β-bungarotoxin, notexin, and taipoxin) impair ACh release—often there is an initial augmentation of ACh release, followed by depletion of neurotransmitter. Presynaptic toxins tend to be more potent than those that act postsynaptically. Postsynaptic α-neurotoxins produce a curare-like, nondepolarizing neuromuscular block that is variably reversible. Most venoms contain both pre- and postsynaptic neurotoxins, although one type may predominate.

Marine neurotoxins affecting the NMJ are rare and come primarily from poisonous fish (stonustoxin), a few mollusks (conotoxins), and dinoflagellates. Most marine intoxications result from ingestion. With some marine toxins, there is an increase in the concentration of toxin through successive predatory transvection up the food chain.

Heavy-metal intoxication is a rare cause of neuromuscular toxicity. Ingestion of bread made from grain contaminated with methylmercury fungicide produces weakness with characteristic decrementing responses to RNS and partial reversal by ChEIs.

Organophosphates impair NMT by irreversibly inhibiting AChE, producing a depolarizing neuromuscular block.

Abnormal NMT may be a cause of weakness in critically ill patients, and is often due to administration of drugs such as antibiotics, antiarrhythmics, and nondepolarizing neuromuscular blocking agents (Gorson, 2005). Prolonged use of these agents may result in weakness due to persistent neuromuscular blockade even hours or days after discontinuation.

NMT may also be impaired in motor unit diseases that do not primarily affect the NMJ. For example, patients with ALS may have fluctuating weakness that responds to ChEIs, a decrementing response to RNS, and increased jitter and blocking. Jitter is increased in most patients with mitochondrial disease that predominantly affects the extraocular muscles (progressive external ophthalmoplegia, PEO) (Krendel et al., 1987; Ukachoke et al., 2015), which also has clinical findings similar to MG. Features attributable to abnormal NMT have also been reported in syringomyelia, poliomyelitis, peripheral neuropathy, and inflammatory myopathy.

*The complete reference list is available online at https://expertconsult.inkling.com/.* 

109

# Disorders of Skeletal Muscle

Christopher T. Doughty, Anthony A. Amato

## OUTLINE



Disorders of skeletal muscle encompass a variety of illnesses that cause weakness, pain, and fatigue in any combination. They vary from the protean symptoms of muscle pain and fatigue that often defy any explanation to the muscular dystrophies, which one recognizes instantly on clinical grounds. Motor neuron disease (e.g., spinal muscular atrophies), neuromuscular junction disorders (myasthenia gravis, Lambert-Eaton syndrome, and congenital myasthenia), and certain polyneuropathies (e.g., chronic inflammatory demyelinating polyneuropathy) can cause similar symptoms and may be difficult to differentiate from muscle disorders on clinical grounds. Some definitions are worth reviewing. *Myopathy* simply refers to an abnormality of the muscle and has no other connotation. *Muscular dystrophies* are genetic myopathies usually caused by a disturbance of a structural protein or enzyme, resulting in necrosis of muscle fibers and replacement by adipose and connective tissue. *Congenital myopathies* are a group of illnesses that usually present in young children; many are relatively nonprogressive. However, rare "congenital myopathies" may manifest initially in adults (e.g., central nuclear myopathy, nemaline myopathy) and can be progressive. With the advent of molecular genetics, we recognize that many are allelic to what others have reported as dystrophies, further blurring their distinction as a separate category from muscular dystrophy. *Myositis* implies an autoimmune or infectious disorder in which the muscle histology shows an inflammatory response. The *myotonias* are diseases in which the occurrence of involuntary persistent muscle activity accompanied by abnormal repetitive electrical discharges distorts the normal contractile process. This occurs after percussion or voluntary contraction. *Metabolic myopathies* refer mainly to disorders of glycogen or lipid metabolism leading to impaired synthesis of adenosine triphosphate (ATP) or cause abnormal accumulation of material in the cell. The term *endocrine myopathy* refers to myopathies associated with disorders of the thyroid and parathyroid glands and to myopathies associated with corticosteroids.

Within muscle fibers chemical energy is converted into mechanical energy. The component processes include (1) excitation and contraction occurring in the muscle membranes, (2) the contractile mechanism itself, (3) various structural supporting elements that allow the muscle to withstand the mechanical stresses, and (4) the energy system that supports the activity and integrity of the other three systems. The logical categorization of myopathies is according to the part of the system involved. Abnormalities in the membrane ion channels *(channelopathies)* involved in muscle excitation cause various forms of myotonia and periodic paralysis (see Chapter 98). The complex of proteins that include dystrophin, the sarcoglycans, and α-laminin constitute a vital structural mechanism linking the contractile proteins with the extracellular supporting structures. Defects in these proteins are the basis of many forms of muscular dystrophy. Although knowledge remains incomplete, it seems reasonable to modify the classic description of the myopathies to incorporate the new information. For this reason, in the sections that follow, disease descriptions are under the heading of their known molecular defect where possible; the classic appellation appears parenthetically. Before describing the illnesses themselves, we first review the techniques used in the clinical evaluation of patients.

## MUSCLE HISTOLOGY

The technique of *muscle biopsy* is not difficult. Under local anesthesia, a small incision made over the muscle allows, with careful dissection, removal of a small strip of muscle. Needle biopsies are useful in some situations. Histochemical studies of frozen sections are essential for proper interpretation. A transverse section of normal muscle shows fibers that are roughly of equal size and average approximately 60 mm in transverse diameter (Fig. 109.1). The muscle fibers of infants and young children are proportionately smaller. Each fiber consists of hundreds of myofibrils separated by an intermyofibrillar network containing aqueous sarcoplasm, mitochondria, and the sarcoplasmic reticulum with the associated transverse tubular system. Surrounding each muscle fiber is a thin layer of connective tissue (the endomysium).

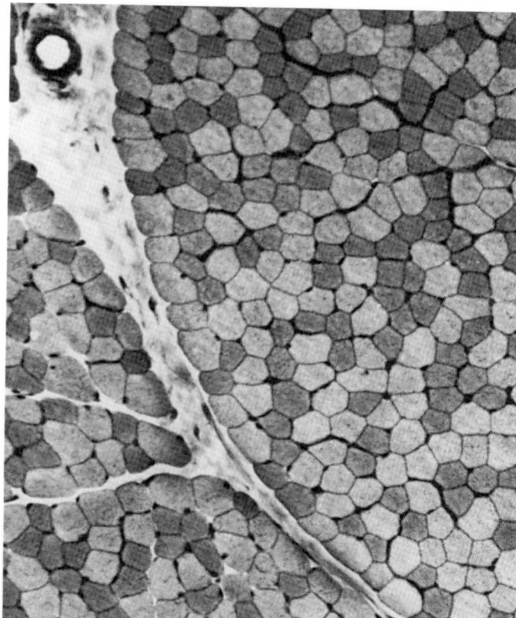

**Fig. 109.1 Normal Muscle Biopsy.** The fibers are roughly equal in size, the nuclei are peripherally situated, and the fibers are tightly apposed to each other with no fibrous tissue separating them (Verhoeff-van Gieson stain).

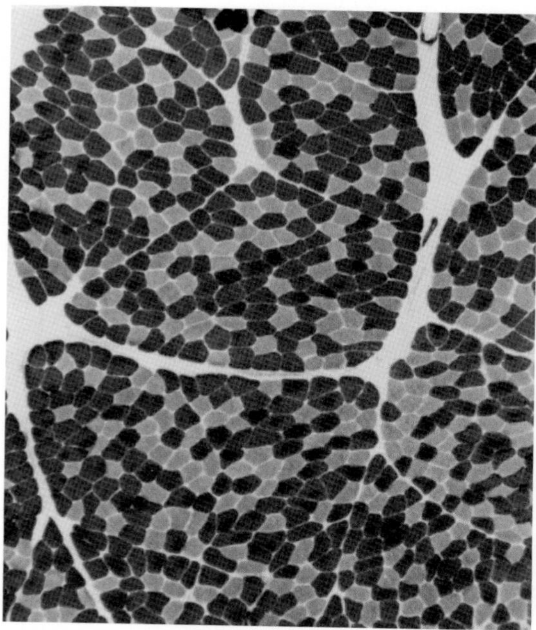

**Fig. 109.2 Normal Muscle Biopsy.** Myosin adenosine triphosphatase stain at pH 9.4 demonstrates relative proportions in size of type 1 *(light)* and type 2 *(dark)* fibers. Muscle fibers belonging to one motor unit innervated by the same anterior horn cell are uniform in type, implying there are fast and slow anterior horn cells. Subsets of fiber types are types 2A, 2B, and 2C. Metabolism of type 2A fibers is more oxidative than that of type 2B. The type 2C fiber is present in fetal muscle.

Strands of connective tissue group muscle fibers into a fascicle, separated from each other by the perimysium. Groups of fascicles are collected into muscle bellies surrounded by epimysium.

Situated at the periphery within muscle fibers are the sarcolemmal nuclei. The fibers are of different types. The simplest division is into type 1 and type 2 fibers, best demonstrated with the histochemical reaction for myosin adenosine triphosphatase (ATPase; Fig. 109.2). The type 1 and type 2 fibers are roughly synonymous with slow and fast fibers or with oxidative and glycolytic fibers in human muscle. Type 2 fibers can be further subdivided based on both staining properties and resistance to fatigue. The best demonstration of the intermyofibrillar network pattern is with the histochemical reactions for oxidative enzymes, such as reduced nicotinamide adenine dinucleotide dehydrogenase (NADH). A regular network extends across the whole fiber. In addition to the routine stains with hematoxylin and eosin, modified Gomori trichrome, myosin ATPase, and NADH, the use of other special stains demonstrates fat (Sudan black or oil red O), complex carbohydrates (periodic acid–Schiff), amyloid (Congo red), or specific enzymes (e.g., phosphorylase, succinic dehydrogenase, cytochrome oxidase [COX]). Immunocytochemical techniques demonstrate the location and integrity of structural proteins such as dystrophin. They also characterize cell types in biopsy samples with inflammatory changes.

## Changes of Denervation

When muscle loses its nerve supply, muscle fibers atrophy, often resulting in fiber squeezing into the spaces between normal fibers and assuming an angulated appearance (Fig. 109.3). Scattered angulated fibers appear early in denervation. Sometimes, picturesque changes in the intermyofibrillar network occur, as in the "target fiber," which characterizes denervation and reinnervation. This is a three-zone fiber on which the intermediate zone stains more darkly, and the central "bull's eye" stains much lighter than normal tissue (Fig. 109.4). Often a neighboring nerve twig reinnervates a denervated fiber. This results in the same anterior horn cell supplying two or more contiguous fibers. If that nerve twig then undergoes degeneration, instead of only one small angulated fiber being produced, a small group of atrophic fibers develops. Group atrophy suggests denervation (Fig. 109.5). As the process continues, large groups of geographical atrophy occur in which entire fascicles are atrophic. In addition to the change in size, a redistribution of the fiber types occurs as well. Normally a random distribution of type 1 and 2 muscle fiber types exists, sometimes incorrectly called a *checkerboard* or *mosaic pattern*. The same process of denervation and reinnervation results in larger and larger groups of contiguous fibers supplied by the same nerve twig. Because all fibers supplied by the same nerve twig are of the same fiber type, groups of type 1 fibers next to groups of type 2 fibers replace the normal random pattern. This fiber type grouping is pathognomonic of reinnervation (Fig. 109.6). When long-standing denervation is present, the atrophic muscle fibers almost disappear, leaving small clumps of pyknotic nuclei in their place.

## Myopathic Changes

Myopathies are typically associated with greater variation in pathological changes than those that occur with denervation. The type of change depends on the type of muscle disease. The normal peripherally placed nuclei may migrate toward the center of the fiber. Internalized nuclei may be seen in normal muscle (up to 2% of fibers), but when they are numerous, they usually indicate a myopathic process. Numerous internal nuclei are a feature of the myotonic dystrophies and the limb–girdle muscular dystrophies (LGMDs). Occasionally, internal nuclei are seen in certain chronic denervating conditions (e.g., juvenile spinal muscular atrophy). Necrosis of muscle fibers, in which the fiber appears liquefied and later presents as a focus of phagocytosis, occurs in many of the myopathies. These changes usually represent an active degenerative process. They often are a feature of myoglobinuria, toxic myopathies, inflammatory myopathies, and metabolic myopathies,

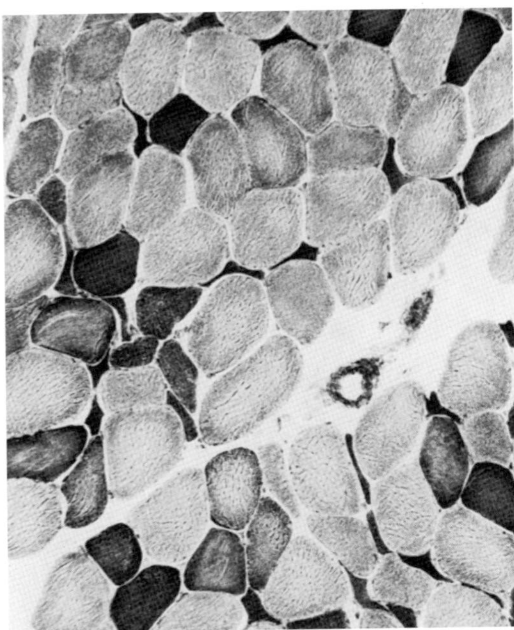

**Fig. 109.3 Denervation.** Notice the small, dark, angulated fibers demonstrated with this oxidative enzyme reaction (nicotinamide adenine dinucleotide dehydrogenase stain).

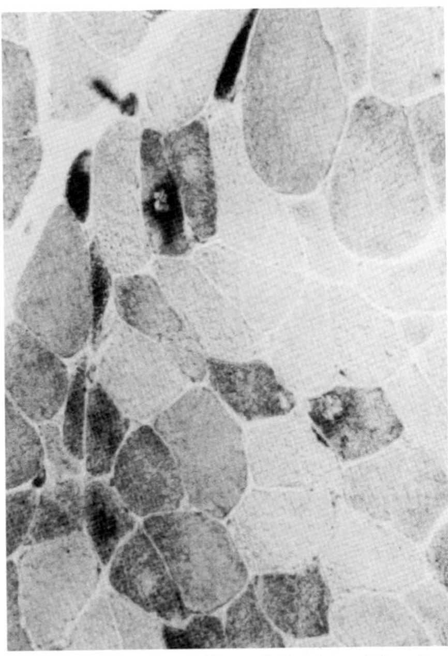

**Fig. 109.4 Denervation.** Target fibers (nicotinamide adenine dinucleotide dehydrogenase stain).

but can also be seen in dystrophies. Fiber-size variation may occur in primary diseases of muscle, with large fibers and small fibers intermingling in a random pattern. This is sometimes the only indication of a pathological process. Fiber splitting often accompanies muscle fiber hypertrophy. In transverse section, recognition of split fibers is by a thin fibrous septum, often associated with a nucleus that crosses partway but not all the way across the fiber. A detailed study of serial transverse sections may reveal more split fibers than in a single section. Fiber splitting is particularly visible in dystrophic conditions such as LGMD.

Degeneration and regeneration of fibers characterize many illnesses. When this occurs, the regenerating fibers often become basophilic, and myonuclei enlarge because of the accumulation of ribonucleic acid (RNA) needed for protein synthesis. Fiber basophilia is a sign of an active myopathy. Cellular responses include frank inflammatory reactions around blood vessels, which characterize the collagen vascular diseases and dermatomyositis (DM). Endomysial inflammation with invasion of non-necrotic muscle fibers occurs in inclusion body myositis (IBM) and polymyositis (PM). Importantly, pronounced inflammatory cellular responses may occur in dystrophies, particularly facioscapulohumeral dystrophy (FSHD) and dysferlinopathies. Even the so-called congenital inflammatory myopathies actually represent forms of congenital muscular dystrophy.

Fibrosis is another reactive change in muscle. Normally a very thin layer of connective tissue separates the muscle fibers. In dystrophic conditions, this layer thickens, and muscle fibrosis may be quite pronounced. In the inflammatory myopathies, there may be a loose edematous separation of fibers, but fibrosis is not usually characteristic in early phases of the disease except when associated with systemic sclerosis or in IBM.

Changes in the intermyofibrillar network pattern are common in myopathic disorders. There is often a moth-eaten, whorled change to the intermyofibrillar network in LGMD and FSHD (Fig. 109.7); the intermyofibrillar network loses its orderly arrangement and swirls, resembling the current in an eddying stream. These changes may be seen in several diseases but tend to be much more common in the myopathies.

## Other Changes

Selective changes in fiber types can occur. Type 2 fiber atrophy is one of the most common abnormalities seen in muscle (Fig. 109.8). Type 2 atrophy, particularly if limited to type 2B fibers, is nonspecific and indicates muscle disuse. If a limb is casted and the muscle examined some weeks later, selective atrophy of type 2 fibers is noted. Any chronic systemic illness tends to produce type 2 atrophy. It occurs in rheumatoid arthritis, nonspecific collagen vascular diseases, cancer (hence the name *cachectic atrophy*), intellectual disability in children, and pyramidal tract disease. Type 2B fiber atrophy can also result from chronic corticosteroid administration. Therefore type 2 fiber atrophy should probably be regarded as a nonspecific result of anything less than robust good health.

Type 1 fiber atrophy is more specific. It occurs in some of the congenital myopathies and dystrophies, congenital myasthenia, and is characteristic of myotonic dystrophy type 1 (Video 109.1). Changes in the proportion of fiber types are quite separate from changes in the fiber size. The name *fiber type predominance* refers to a change in the relative numbers of a particular fiber type. Type 1 fiber predominance is a normal finding in the gastrocnemius and deltoid muscles. When widespread, it is also the hallmark of congenital myopathies and many of the early dystrophies. Type 2 fiber predominance is seen in the lateral head of the quadriceps muscle. Type 2 predominance occurs occasionally in juvenile spinal muscular atrophy and motor neuron disease but is not firmly associated with any particular disease condition.

Some changes in muscle biopsy results are pathognomonic of a particular disease. *Perifascicular atrophy*, in which the atrophic fibers are more numerous around the edge of muscle fascicles, is the hallmark of DM. The presence of lipid vacuoles or abnormal pockets of glycogen characterizes the metabolic myopathies. Enzyme defects including myophosphorylase deficiency and phosphofructokinase (PFK) deficiency are detectable with appropriate histochemical stains. Interpretation of a muscle biopsy usually includes the description of a constellation of changes and the subsequent association of these

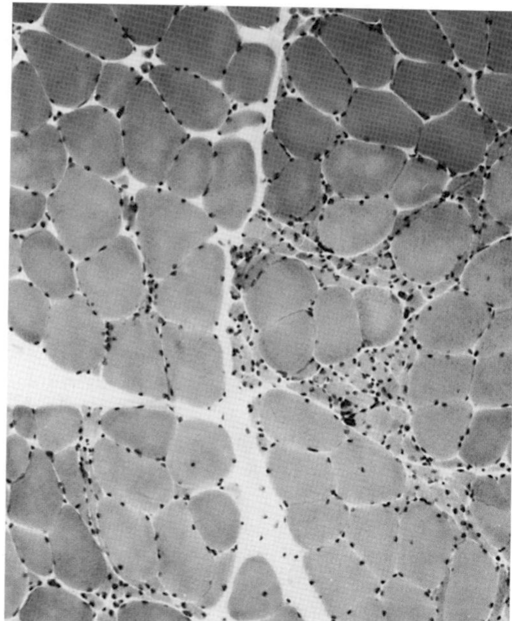

**Fig. 109.5 Denervation.** Small groups of atrophic fibers are scattered throughout the biopsy (modified Gomori trichrome stain).

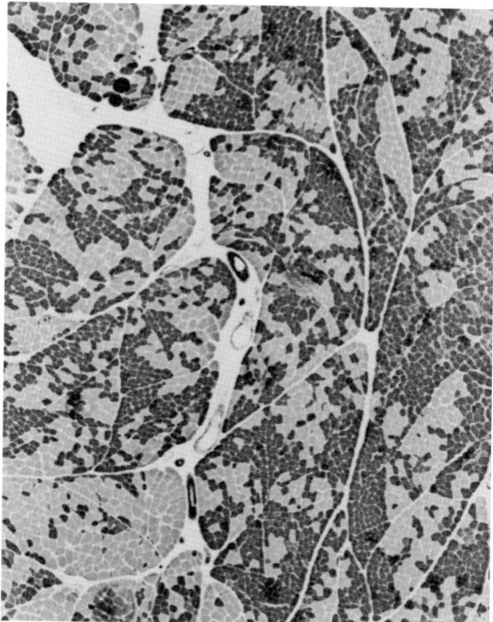

**Fig. 109.6 Chronic Denervation and Reinnervation.** Instead of the usual mosaic pattern of the two fiber types, fibers clump together, groups of one type appearing next to groups of the other type (myosin adenosine triphosphatase stain, pH 9.4).

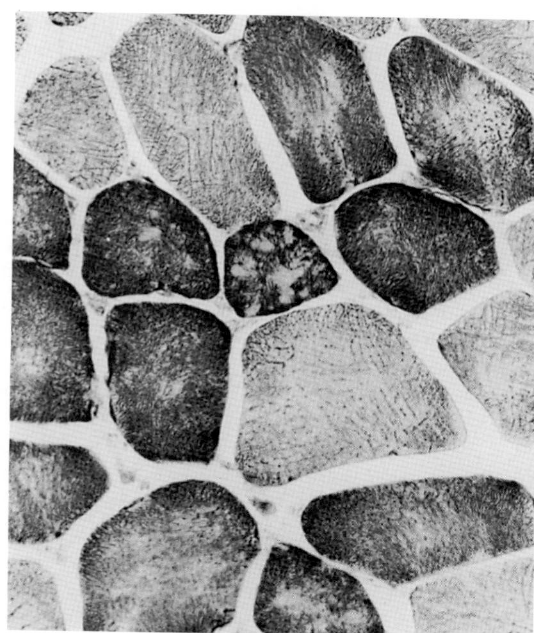

**Fig. 109.7 Myopathy.** Moth-eaten whorled fibers. Intermyofibrillar network pattern is distorted, and some areas lack proper stain (nicotinamide adenine dinucleotide dehydrogenase stain).

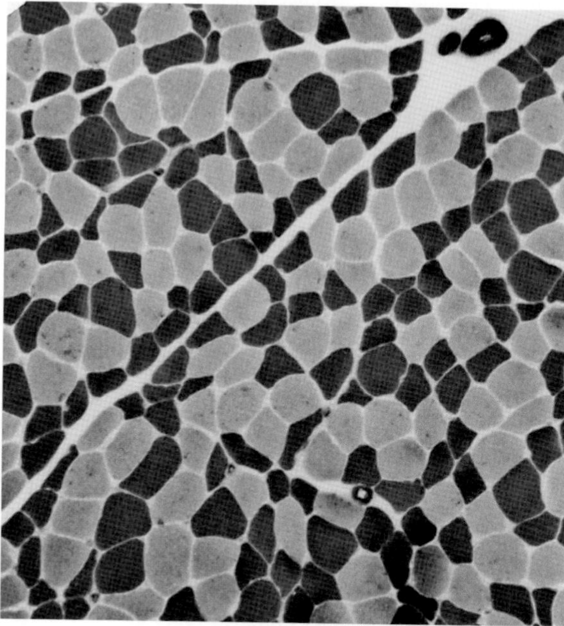

**Fig. 109.8** Type 2 fiber atrophy is a common change of disuse atrophy or steroid myopathy (myosin adenosine triphosphatase stain).

changes with a particular diagnosis when possible. Illnesses that have characteristic biopsies include infantile spinal muscular atrophy, DM, IBM, the congenital myopathies, lipid storage myopathies, and glycogen storage diseases (e.g., Pompe disease, myophosphorylase deficiency). Immunocytochemical staining can also distinguish many forms of muscular dystrophy from each other. Although not disease specific, characteristic biopsy changes differentiate chronic denervation from acute simple denervation.

## Immunohistochemistry and Immunoblot

The use of biopsy material to identify missing proteins is increasing with the greater availability of commercial antibodies to the proteins of interest. Although genetic testing is becoming easier, cheaper, and more commonly utilized, immunohistochemical testing remains useful. Identification of an absent muscle protein may allow for diagnosis when genetic testing is either unremarkable or reveals a variant of uncertain significance in a gene of interest. Immunohistochemical findings may also allow narrowing of the panel of genetic tests to be sent. For example, if a patient with suspected Duchenne muscular dystrophy (DMD) undergoes genetic testing but no pathogenic mutation is discovered, confirmation of the diagnosis may rest on demonstrating absent or abnormal dystrophin in the muscle tissue. All the sarcoglycans are demonstrated using similar techniques. Deficiency of any of the sarcoglycans causes a muscular dystrophy, and because they comprise a complex, when one is missing, all or some of the others may be absent in the biopsy. The α-sarcoglycan is particularly prone to be missing, which makes it a suitable and economical screening tool. Absence or reduction of laminin-$\alpha_2$ chain (merosin) or α-dystroglycan occurs in some forms of congenital muscular dystrophy. The lack of nuclear membrane staining with anti-emerin antibodies occurs in X-linked Emery-Dreifuss muscular dystrophy (EDMD).

Immunohistochemical techniques may give information about the type of inflammatory cell present via affinity for various markers such as CD68 (macrophages and dendritic cells), CD20 (B cells), CD3 (activated T cells), CD8 (cytotoxic T cells), and CD4 (T-helper and dendritic cells). These identify cells involved in cytotoxic, humoral, and innate immune mechanisms. Antibodies to the major histocompatibility antigen 1 (MHC1) are used to demonstrate overexpression on muscle fibers in inflammatory myopathy, while membrane attack complex (MAC) deposits may be found on the capillary endothelium in DM. Immunohistochemistry can be used to demonstrate inclusions (e.g., p62, TDP43) within muscle fibers to assist in diagnosis of IBM.

Immunoblot or Western blot of muscle biopsy is more sensitive than immunohistochemistry, particularly when dealing with an enzyme deficiency or nonstructural protein in evaluation of dystrophies. Patients with Becker muscular dystrophy may have normal-appearing immunostaining for dystrophin, because the commercial antibodies may react to that part of the dystrophin protein that is normally made. However, immunoblot reveals abnormal size or amount of dystrophin in such cases. Immunoblotting is valuable in assessing for calpainopathy (LGMD2A), dysferlinopathy (LGMD2B), and in the secondary α-dystroglycanopathies. Reductions of proteins in these disorders may be secondary, so a primary deficiency must be confirmed by genetic testing.

## SPECIFIC DISORDERS

### Muscular Dystrophies

The muscular dystrophies are a group of hereditary muscle disorders that occur at all ages and with varying degrees of severity. The traditional classification is on clinical grounds. Increasing information about the molecular basis of these disorders provides both reassurance and puzzlement to clinicians (Table 109.1). Different dystrophies are due to distinct molecular abnormalities; however, patients with similar molecular defects may show a wide variability in phenotype not always easily explained. Disorders traditionally classified as congenital myopathies on clinical grounds have been found to result from mutations in myofiber structural proteins, similar to those affected in muscular dystrophies.

For the most part, the underlying molecular abnormalities in the dystrophies involve structural proteins. Therefore it is useful to review these proteins as they occur in normal muscle. The contractile proteins, actin and myosin, are arrayed with other proteins such as troponin to form the familiar thick and thin filaments of the sarcomere. The reaction between actin and myosin results in realignment between the two molecules. In the sliding filament model, the thick and thin filaments form an array that slides back and forth.

The contractile proteins connect to the "outside" of the cell by means of a complex of proteins that ultimately links up with the basal lamina of the extracellular matrix. The first step in this connection is the protein dystrophin, located on the cytoplasmic face of the muscle membrane. This large protein (427 kD) is coded by a gene on the short arm of the X chromosome. Dystrophin consists of two ends separated by a long, flexible rod-like region. The amino terminus binds to actin, and the carboxyl terminus links dystrophin to a complex of glycoproteins in the sarcolemma. Two of these, the dystroglycans, form a direct link between dystrophin and laminin, a protein within the basal lamina. α-Dystroglycan is located extracellularly and connects to laminin. The $\alpha_2$ chain of laminin (also called merosin) provides the anchor into the extracellular matrix because it provides the attachment for α-dystroglycan. β-Dystroglycan spans the sarcolemmal membrane, linking dystrophin and α-dystroglycan. Merosin also binds to $\alpha_7\beta_1$D integrin, a protein complex located on the sarcolemma membrane. The sarcoglycan complex, composed of α-, β-, γ-, and δ-sarcoglycans, also spans the sarcolemmal membrane and link to the dystrophin-dystroglycan complex. Dystrophin, the sarcoglycans, the dystroglycans, and merosin appear to function as a unit in stabilizing the muscle membrane. Together these proteins make up the dystrophin-glycoprotein complex.

Other sarcolemmal proteins not directly linked to the dystrophin-glycoprotein complex are affected in other forms of muscular dystrophies (e.g., dysferlin, caveolin-3). Sarcomeric proteins (e.g., myosin, actin, tropomyosin, myotilin, Z-band alternatively spliced PDZ motif-containing protein [ZASP], filamin-c, desmin, titin, and telethonin, etc.), important in stabilizing the contractile apparatus, are mutated in certain dystrophies and congenital myopathies, highlighting the pathophysiological overlap of these historically clinically defined classifications. Mutations of the muscle-specific calcium-dependent protease, calpain-3 gene, are responsible for the majority of nondystrophin-related LGMDs in patients of Italian and Spanish ancestry. In addition, secretory enzymes (e.g., *O*-mannose-β-1,2-*N*-acetylglucosaminyl transferase, fukutin, and fukutin-related protein [FKRP]), which probably play a role in glucosylation of α-dystroglycan and other import proteins, are responsible for some forms of congenital muscular dystrophy, but may be associated with milder LGMD. Furthermore, mutations encoding for the nuclear envelope proteins, emerin, lamin A/C, and nesprin 1 and 2 cause EDMD.

#### Dystrophin Deficiency (Duchenne Muscular Dystrophy, Becker Muscular Dystrophy, and Atypical Forms)

An absence or deficiency of dystrophin is responsible for two disorders that cause progressive destruction of muscle. Absence of dystrophin impairs the integrity of the sarcolemmal membrane, rendering the membrane susceptible to mechanical damage. Molecules such as calcium can gain access to the fiber, initiating a chain of destructive processes ultimately leading to necrosis of the muscle fiber. Eventually, this process leads to severe loss of muscle and replacement of the muscle fibers with fibrous tissue.

The responsible gene is located on the short arm of the X chromosome at locus Xp21. The gene is extremely large, comprising more than 2.5 million base pairs and 79 exons or coding regions. Approximately 65%–75% of cases are associated with a deletion or duplication of one or more exons in the gene. Genetic testing assays designed to detect deletions and duplications should be used first, such as multiplex ligation-dependent probe amplification (MLPA) and microarray-based comparative genomic hybridization (CGH) (Hegde MR et al., 2008; Sansovic et al., 2013). "Hot spots" for these gene deletions exist, notably between exons 43 and 52 and particularly 44 and 49 (Nobile et al., 1997). The remaining 25%–35% of cases are due to point mutations (many of which introduce a premature stop codon), smaller deletions, or small insertions or duplications, which are best detected using next-generation sequencing. Whether a deletion is in frame or out of frame (see Chapter 48) determines whether dystrophin is absent

**TABLE 109.1 Molecular Defects of Muscular Dystrophies**

| Disease | Inheritance | Chromosome | Affected Protein |
|---|---|---|---|
| **X-Linked Dystrophies** | | | |
| Duchenne/Becker | XR | Xp21 | Dystrophin |
| Emery-Dreifuss | XR | Xq28 | Emerin |
| Scapuloperoneal/reducing body myopathy | XR | Xq26.3 | Four-and-a-half LIM domain 1 (FHL1) protein |
| **Limb-Girdle Muscular Dystrophies (LGMD) (Classical Classification/Proposed New Classification Where Appropriate)** | | | |
| LGMD1A/myofibrillar myopathy | AD | 5q22.3-31.3 | Myotilin |
| LGMD1B/EDMD | AD | 1q11-21 | Lamin A and C |
| LGMD1C/rippling muscle disease | AD | 3p25 | Caveolin-3 |
| LGMD1D/LGMD D1 | AD | 6q23 | DNAJB6 |
| LGMD1E/myofibrillar myopathy | AD | 2q35 | Desmin |
| LGMD1F/LGMD D2 | AD | 7q32 | Transportin 3 |
| LGMD1G/LGMD D3 | AD | | HNRNPDL |
| LGMD1I/LGMD D4 | AD | 15q15.1-21.1 | 15q15.1-21.1 |
| | | Calpain-3 | Calpain-3 |
| LGMD2A/LGMD R1 | AR | 15q15.1-21.1 | Calpain-3 |
| LGMD2B/LGMD R2* | AR | 2p13 | Dysferlin |
| LGMD2C/LGMD R5 | AR | 13q12 | γ-Sarcoglycan |
| LGMD2D/LGMD R3 | AR | 17q12-21.3 | α-Sarcoglycan |
| LGMD2E/LGMD R4 | AR | 4q12 | β-Sarcoglycan |
| LGMD2F/LGMD R6 | AR | 5q33-34 | δ-Sarcoglycan |
| LGMD2G/LGMD R7 | AR | 17q11-12 | Telethonin |
| LGMD2H/LGMD R8 | AR | 9q31-33 | E3-ubiquitin-ligase (TRIM 32) |
| LGMD2I/LGMD R9 | AR | 19q13 | Fukutin-related protein (FKRP) |
| LGMD2J/LGMD R10 | AR | 2q31 | Titin |
| LGMD2K/LGMD R11 | AR | 9q31 | POMT1 |
| LGMD2L/LGMD R12 | AR | 11p14.3 | Anoctamin 5 |
| LGMD2M/LGMD R13 | AR | 9q31-33 | Fukutin |
| LGMD2N/LGMD R14 | AR | 14q24 | POMT2 |
| LGMD2O/LGMD R15 | AR | 1p32 | POMGnT1 |
| LGMD2P/LGMD R16 | AR | 3p21 | α-Dystroglycan |
| LGMD2Q/LGMD R17 | AR | 8q24 | Plectin 1 |
| LGMD2R/myofibrillar myopathy | AR | 2q35 | Desmin |
| LGMD2S/LGMD R18 | AR | 4q35.1 | TRAPPC11 |
| LGMD2T/LGMD R19 | AR | 3p11 | GDP-mannose pyrophosphorylase B |
| LGMD2U/LGMD R20 | AR | 7p21 | Isoprenoid synthase domain containing protein |
| LGMD2V | AR | 17q25.31 | α-1,4-Glucosidase |
| LGMD2W | AR | 2p14 | LIM and senescent cell antigen like domains 2 |
| LGMD2X | AR | 6q21 | Popeye domain-containing protein 1 |
| LGMD2Y | AR | 1q25.1 | Torsin-A interacting protein 1 or lamin-associated protein 1 |
| LGMD2Z/LGMD R21 | AR | 3q13.33 | Protein O-glucosyltransferase 1 |
| LGMD R23 | AR | 6q22-23 | Laminin-$\alpha_2$ |
| LGMD R24 | AR | 3p22.1 | POMGNT2 |
| **Congenital Muscular Dystrophies (MDC)** | | | |
| Bethlem myopathy/LGMD R22 | AR | 21q22.3 and 2q37 | Collagens 6A1, 6A2, and 6A3 |
| Bethlem myopathy/LGMD D5 | AD | 21q22.3 and 2q37 | Collagens 6A1, 6A2, and 6A3 |
| MDC1A | AR | 6q22-23 | Laminin-$\alpha_2$ |
| $\alpha_7$-Integrin-related MDC | AR | 12q13 | $\alpha_7$-Integrin |
| MDC1C | AR | 19q13 | Fukutin-related protein (FKRP) |
| Fukuyama | AR | 9q31-33 | Fukutin |
| WWS | AR | 9q31 | POMT1 |
| MEB disease | AR | 1p32 | POMGnT1 |
| Rigid spine syndrome | AR | 1p35-36 | Selenoprotein N1 |
| Ullrich | AR | 21q22.3 and 2q37 | Collagens 6A1, 6A2, and 6A3 |

Continued

**TABLE 109.1 Molecular Defects of Muscular Dystrophies—cont'd**

| Disease | Inheritance | Chromosome | Affected Protein |
|---|---|---|---|
| **Distal Dystrophies/Myopathies** | | | |
| Welander | AD | 2p13 | TIA1 |
| Udd | AD | 2q31 | Titin |
| Markesbery-Griggs | AD | 10q22.3-23.2 | ZASP |
| Nonaka or hIBM/GNE myopathy | AR | 9p1-q1 | GNE |
| Miyoshi 1* | AR | 2p13 | Dysferlin |
| Miyoshi 2 | AR | 11p14.3 | Anoctamin 5 |
| Laing (MPD1) | AD | 14q11 | MyHC 7 |
| Williams | AD | 7q32 | Filamin C |
| Distal myopathy with vocal cord and pharyngeal weakness (VCPDM or MPD2) | AD | 5q31 | Matrin 3 |
| **Other Dystrophies** | | | |
| Facioscapulohumeral type 1 | AD | 4q35 | Deletion in D4Z4 region with secondary increase in DUX4 |
| Facioscapulohumeral type 2 | AD | 18p11.32 | SMCHD1 with secondary increase in DUX4 |
| Facioscapulohumeral type 3 | AD | 20q11.21 | DNMT3B (DNA methyltransferase 3B) |
| Scapuloperoneal dystrophy | AD | 2q35 | Desmin |
| | AD | 14q11 | MyHC 7 |
| | XR | Xq26.3 | Four-and-a-half LIM domain 1 (FHL1) protein |
| Emery-Dreifuss type 3 | AD | 6q24 | Nesprin-1 |
| Emery-Dreifuss type 4 | AD | 14q23 | Nesprin-2 |
| Emery-Dreifuss type 5 | AD | 3p25.1 | TMEM43 |
| Oculopharyngeal | AD | 14q11.2-13 | PABP2 |
| Myotonic dystrophy 1 | AD | 19q13.3 | DMPK |
| Myotonic dystrophy 2 | AD | 3q21 | ZNF9 |
| Myofibrillar myopathy | AD | 5q22.3-31.3 | Myotilin |
| | AD | 10q22.3-23.2 | ZASP |
| | AD | 7q32.1 | Filamin-c |
| | AD | 11q21-23 | αB-crystallin |
| | AD/AR | 2q35 | Desmin |
| | AR | 1p36 | Selenoprotein N1 |
| | AD | 10q25-26 | BAG-3 |
| | AD | 2q31 | Titin |
| **Hereditary Inclusion Body Myopathies** | | | |
| AR hIBM | AR | | GNE |
| hIBM with FTD and Paget disease | AD | | VCP |
| hIBM 3 | AD | | MyHC IIa |

*FRG1*, FSHD region gene 1; *FTD*, frontotemporal dementia; *GNE*, UDP-*N*-acetylglucosamine 2-epimerase/*N*-acetylmannosamine kinase; *hIBM*, hereditary inclusion body myopathy; *MEB*, muscle-eye-brain; *MyHC*, myosin heavy chain; *POMGnT1*, *O*-mannose-β-1,2-*N*-acetylglucosaminyl transferase; *POMT1*, *O*-mannosyltransferase gene; *VCP*, valosin-containing protein; *WSS*, Walker-Warburg syndrome; *ZASP*, Z-band alternatively spliced PDZ motif-containing protein.

*LGMD 2B and Miyoshi distal dystrophy are the same condition.

*Modified with permission from Amato, A.A., Russell, J., 2016. Neuromuscular Disease, second edition. McGraw-Hill, New York.*

from the muscle or present in a reduced altered form. This has clinical significance because the former is usually associated with the severe DMD, whereas the latter may cause the milder Becker variant (BMD). In BMD, the abnormal dystrophin preserves enough function to slow down the progress of the illness. Reading of the DNA code is triplet by triplet. Maintenance of this reading frame throughout the length of the gene is required for dystrophin production. If a deletion removes a multiple of three base pairs, the reading frame may be intact upstream and downstream and may make limited sense, as if the sentence "You cannot eat the cat" were changed to "You not eat the cat," and some modified dystrophin may be formed. This is often the situation in the mild form of dystrophin deficiency (BMD). In the severe form, the reading frame is destroyed, as if a deletion resulted in the sentence "Yoc ann ote att hec at." Exceptions to this rule exist, as frameshift deletions have been associated with the milder form of the disease, particularly at the 5′ end of the gene in exons 3–7. The prevalence of DMD in the general population is approximately 3 per 100,000, and the incidence among live-born males is 1 per 3500. BMD is approximately one-tenth

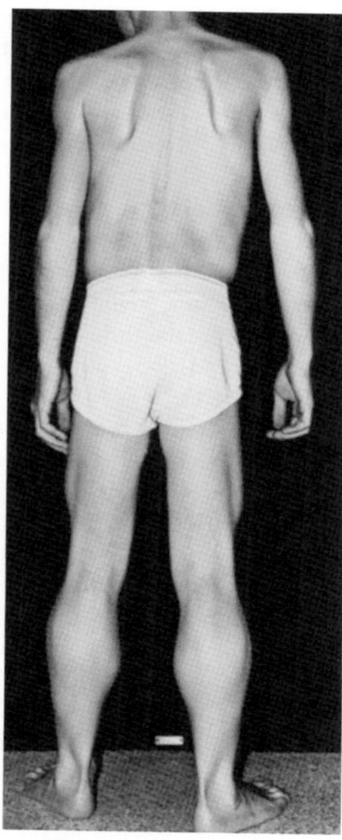

**Fig. 109.9 Duchenne Muscular Dystrophy.** Calf and thigh hypertrophy in an ambulatory 8-year-old patient.

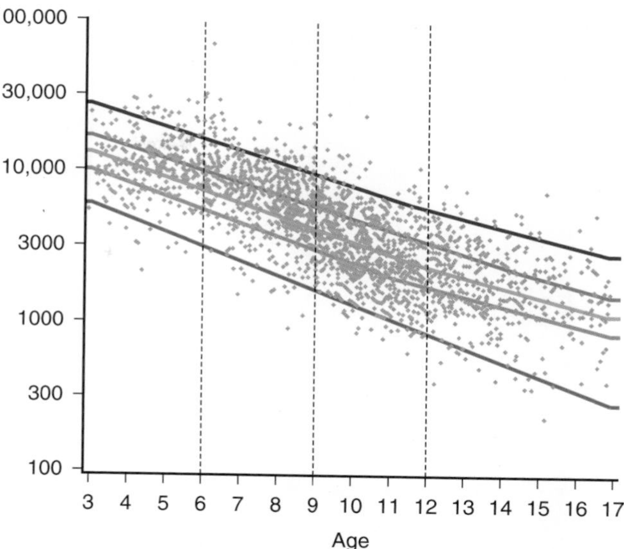


**Fig. 109.10** Duchenne muscular dystrophy: change in serum creatine kinase (CK) level with age. This is a scattergram of serum CK levels in individual patients. Lines represent the 5th, 25th, 50th, 75th, and 95th percentiles.

as common. Although the inheritance is clearly X-linked recessive, almost a third of cases are sporadic. Presumably this is due to a spontaneous mutation occurring either in the child or in the mother's ova.

***Duchenne muscular dystrophy.*** Affected children are typically normal at birth. After affected boys begin walking, however, the clumsiness seen in all toddlers persists. Progressive leg weakness, proximal greater than distal, develops through early childhood. Affected boys must place one hand on the knee to assume an upright position when rising from the floor *(Gower maneuver)*. Parents notice that the child runs improperly and is unable to jump clear of the floor with both feet. Toe-walking and a waddling gait are common. Often at this stage, the calf muscles are rather firm and rubbery *(pseudohypertrophy)* (Fig. 109.9). In the absence of therapy, tightness across several joints in the legs develops. The iliotibial bands and the heel cords are usually the first to tighten. This is particularly noticeable in boys who habitually walk on their toes. Apparent improvement may occur between ages 2 and 6 as the child gains motor skills. This is illusory because it simply represents the child's natural development, which muscle weakness has not yet outpaced.

By 5 or 6 years of age, climbing upstairs becomes difficult, requiring the use of the railing. By the age of 6 or 7, the boys often complain of sudden spontaneous falls. At first, these falls occur when the child is in a hurry or knocked off balance by playmates. The fall is quite spectacular to the onlooker; the knees collapse abruptly, and the child drops like a stone to the ground. At approximately 8–10 years of age, affected children cease to be able to climb stairs or stand up from the floor, and upper limb weakness becomes more apparent. This is typically when they begin using a wheelchair for locomotion. Earlier studies suggested that the ability to walk was lost at about age 9, but with appropriate bracing, reconstructive surgery, and physiotherapy, confinement to a wheelchair is about 12 years of age. With the increasing use of corticosteroids, many affected boys maintain ambulation even beyond 12 (Kohler et al., 2009).

Contractures of the hips, knees, and ankles become severe when the relatively untreated child spends much of the day in a wheelchair. The hips and knees lock at 90 degrees, and the feet turn downward and inward in an exaggerated position of equinovarus. It is very difficult to get normal shoes to fit them, and it is impossible for them to sleep, except in one position: usually with the knees propped up with pillows and slightly turned on one side. Handling the children at this stage becomes very difficult, and back pain and limb pain almost inevitably accompany this severe stage of muscular dystrophy. Development of a severe scoliosis compromises respiratory function.

Cardiac muscle is also affected, and clinically evident cardiomyopathy develops in one-third of patients by age 14 and virtually all patients over age 18. Screening with an electrocardiogram (ECG) and either echocardiogram or cardiac Magnetic Resonance Imaging (MRI) should be performed at diagnosis, then annually while patients are asymptomatic. Co-management with a cardiologist is essential to aid in surveillance and initiation of heart failure therapies. Progressive ventilatory muscle weakness is also uniform. Respiratory screening with once-yearly measurement of forced vital capacity (FVC) should be performed annually while boys are still ambulatory. Affected boys usually die of either cardiac or respiratory complications.

The serum concentration of creatine kinase (CK) is typically markedly elevated; levels greater than 10,000 mU/mL are common (Fig. 109.10). Electromyography (EMG) shows myopathic changes (see Chapter 36). Genetic testing has largely replaced muscle biopsy to diagnose DMD as it is less invasive and has become more widely available, but a biopsy is essential if genetic testing is unrevealing. A diagnosis may be made when immunohistochemistry reveals reduction of dystrophin on the sarcolemma or when Western blot demonstrates absent or marked reduced quantity and size of dystrophin. Three antibodies are available against the ends (Dys-2 for the carboxyl terminus and Dys-3 for the amino terminus) and the rod region (Dys-1) of the molecule. In DMD, immunostaining is absent or the stain is irregular and fragmented. Absence of the amino terminus, the end that binds with actin, appears to be associated with more severe symptoms. Variation in myofiber size, fibrosis, groups of basophilic fibers,

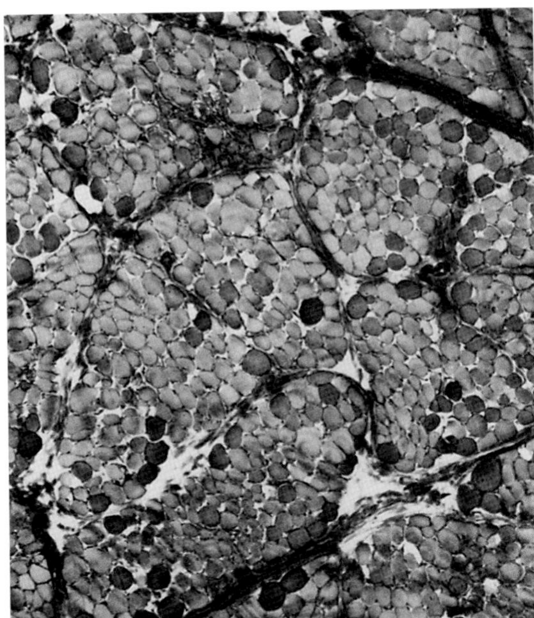

**Fig. 109.11 Duchenne Muscular Dystrophy: Muscle Biopsy.** Fibers are of variable size and separated by connective tissue. Large heavily stained opaque fibers are noted (Verhoeff-Van Gieson stain).

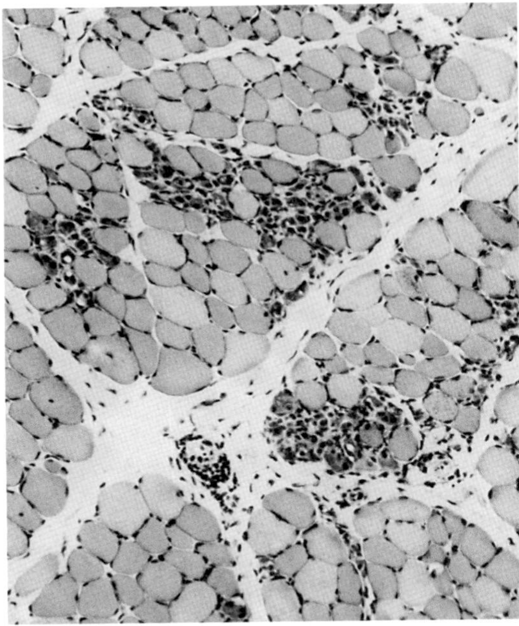

**Fig. 109.12 Duchenne Muscular Dystrophy.** Groups of small basophilic (darkly staining) fibers are scattered in the biopsy (hematoxylin and eosin stain).

and opaque or hypercontracted fibers (hyaline fibers) are typically seen (Figs. 109.11 and 109.12).

### Treatment of Duchenne muscular dystrophy

***Physical therapy.*** The primary aim of physical therapy is to keep the joints as loose as possible, avoiding contractures. Early on, the iliotibial bands and the heel cords give the greatest problems. Late in the course, elbow, wrist, and finger contractures add to functional disability. Physical therapy generally commences at 3–4 years of age, when parents learn to stretch the child's heel cords, hip flexors, and iliotibial bands daily. Passive stretching of joints is directed not at increasing the range of motion but rather at preventing any further development of contractures. This requires careful explanation to parents because they can be disheartened to see no improvement in the tightness even after many months of therapy. Night splints molded around the lower part of the legs to maintain the feet at right angles to the legs should be used starting at an early age. Ankle contractures rarely occur in patients who use these splints conscientiously. Unfortunately, some patients, particularly those 6 or 7 years or older, cannot tolerate the splints. Parents often ask about an active exercise program; such a program is largely unnecessary in a young child who runs around to the best of his ability anyway. By the time a child is having difficulty walking or is in a wheelchair, muscle weakness is severe, and exercise does not increase muscle strength.

***Bracing.*** The appropriate use of bracing may delay the child's progression to a wheelchair by approximately 2 years. A major factor responsible for inability to stand or walk is weakness of the quadriceps. Such weakness causes the knee to collapse when even slightly flexed; the only stable position is in hyperextension. The addition of a long-leg brace (knee-foot orthosis) can help solve this problem. Such a device stabilizes the knee and prevents the knee from flexing. The children walk stiff legged but do not have the same problem with falling they had previously. Generally, children are ready for bracing when they have ceased to climb stairs, are having great difficulty arising from the floor, and are having frequent daily falls. On examination, inability to straighten the knee against gravity is also an indication for bracing. Because the brace functions as a pendulum, slight elevation of the hip is sufficient to bring the leg forward so the weight of the brace is rarely a problem. There may be some advantage to a lightweight plastic knee-foot orthosis, but it may be more difficult to keep the leg straight with such a device.

***Surgery.*** Reconstructive surgery of the leg often accompanies bracing. The purpose of leg surgery is to keep the leg extended and prevent contractures of the iliotibial bands and hip flexors. Contractures of the iliotibial bands are associated with a stance in which the boy's legs are widely abducted. As noted before, the long-leg brace acts like a pendulum. If the leg is widely abducted, the child cannot swing the leg forward. Lifting the hip causes the leg to try to swing inward toward the midline, but resistance from the iliotibial band contractures renders this impossible. A simple way to maintain function in the leg is to perform percutaneous tenotomies of the iliotibial bands, knee flexors, hip flexors, and Achilles tendons. This procedure often allows a child who is becoming increasingly dependent on a wheelchair to resume walking with the aid of bracing.

Spinal stabilization is also an important option for DMD patients. Because of the extreme discomfort of severe scoliosis and the respiratory problems associated with it, spinal surgery is an acceptable procedure for managing the late stages of the disease. It is considered in patients with 35 degrees or more of scoliosis and significant discomfort. To reduce the risks associated with surgery, FVC ideally should be greater than 35% of predicted.

***Pharmacological treatment.*** Accumulating evidence suggests that corticosteroids not only improve muscle strength and pulmonary function but also delay time to disease progression milestones such as loss of ambulation (Gloss et al., Neurology 2016; Koeks et al., 2017). There is a possible but less proven beneficial effect for the associated scoliosis and cardiomyopathy, as well. Prednisone 0.75 mg/kg/daily CTD is typically initiated by the age of 5—after motor function plateaus and before substantial decline has begun; 10 mg/kg/weekend CTD is an alternative for those with side effects. The synthetic steroid deflazacort has a similar therapeutic effect and may be associated with less weight gain (Griggs et al., 2016). The usual dosing is 0.9 mg/kg/daily CTD.

Improved cardiorespiratory intervention has extended median survival dramatically from the late teens into the late 20s and early 30s (Ishikawa et al., 2011). Consensus recommendations suggest initiating an angiotensin-converting enzyme inhibitor or angiotensin receptor blocker by the age of 10. Additional treatments such as beta-blockers are used for symptomatic heart failure. Assisted ventilatory support is typically required by the age of 18.

Therapies currently in development aim to circumvent deficient dystrophin protein production. Eteplirsen is a phosphorodiamidate morpholino oligomer that binds to dystrophin gene pre-mRNA and induces exon 51 skipping (Mendell et al., 2016). Skipping this exon restores the open reading frame that is disrupted by certain dystrophin mutations. Although this actually increases the size of the deletion, it preserves translatable mRNA after the deletion, leading to production of a dystrophin protein more similar to what is seen in BMD mutations rather than DMD mutations. Thus the treatment is not curative but instead aims to convert DMD into a BMD phenotype. Approximately 13% of DMD boys are amenable to exon 51 skipping, based on which specific mutation they harbor. Eteplirsen was granted accelerated approval by the US Food and Drug Administration (FDA) in 2016 based primarily on small trials demonstrating increased dystrophin protein production in the muscle on biopsy specimens. The FDA mandated an additional clinical trial to ensure the efficacy of the drug, which is ongoing. Eteplirsen is not yet approved in Europe. Additional exon skipping therapies are in development. Ataluren, by contrast, was recently approved by the European Commission but is not yet available in the United States. Despite promising early trials, a phase III placebo-controlled trial showed no benefit for its primary endpoint, change in the 6-minute walk test (McDonald et al., 2017). It targets the estimated 11% of boys with a nonsense mutation, promoting ribosomal read-through of the stop codon.

***Becker muscular dystrophy.*** BMD shares the clinical characteristics of DMD but has a milder course (Narayanaswami et al., 2014). The disease usually begins in the first decade, although parents may notice the first signs of weakness later because of the milder symptoms. Occasionally, symptom onset is delayed until the fourth decade or later. The muscular hypertrophy, contractures, and pattern of weakness are similar to those seen in DMD. These boys, however, continue to walk independently past the age of 15 years and may not use a wheelchair until they are in their 20s or even later (Bushby et al., 1993). Teenagers with BMD often complain of leg cramps and muscle pain, often associated with exercise and often more severe than in DMD. A significant proportion of these patients have a cardiomyopathy that can be more disabling than the weakness. Cardiac transplantation has been successful in some patients with this form of the illness.

As with DMD, serum CK levels are elevated but typically not as high. EMG demonstrates myopathic features. Diagnosis requires demonstration of a mutation in the dystrophin gene or reduced quantity or size of dystrophin on muscle biopsy. In BMD, staining may be reduced but can be normal appearing. Therefore immunoblotting is required to show a decreased amount of dystrophin.

Because boys do not have much trouble in the first few years, there is a reduced need for aggressive physiotherapy, surgical reconstruction, and night splints. Patients with BMD are less prone to develop kyphoscoliosis, perhaps because they lack wheelchair confinement until after the spine has become fully mature. We have used corticosteroids only occasionally in patients with BMD. The stabilizing effect of steroids is less noticeable when the disease is already slowly progressive. In every other respect, including bracing and genetic counseling, disease treatment is the same as that for the severe form.

***Other phenotypes associated with dystrophinopathy.*** With the development of genetic testing and dystrophin analysis, it is becoming clear that dystrophin deficiency is not always associated with the BMD or DMD phenotype. Some patients have only symptoms of exercise intolerance, muscle pain, and myoglobinuria (Narayanaswami et al., 2014). Others manifest only a cardiomyopathy or are asymptomatic despite elevated serum concentrations of CK. Most female carriers of dystrophin gene mutations are asymptomatic, but approximately 8% manifest weakness and have a clinical phenotype similar to BMD or LGMD. Manifesting carriers will usually have an elevated serum CK level and myopathic EMG. Muscle biopsy will usually demonstrate a mosaic pattern or patchy staining of dystrophin on the sarcolemma.

It is impractical to perform genetic testing on all patients with neuromuscular complaints. However, the presence of muscle pain, mild weakness, an elevated serum CK, and muscle hypertrophy warrants consideration of analyzing dystrophin. Attempts to correlate the genetic abnormality with the clinical picture are inexact, but abnormalities in the amino terminus and at the carboxyl terminal domains of dystrophin are associated with the more severe form of disease. Alterations in the rod domain are more variable and may be associated with a mild phenotype. In-frame deletions and insertions are associated with a much milder phenotype than out-of-frame alterations.

***Genetic counseling.*** Because DMD and BMD are X-linked recessive disorders, we recommend testing the carrier state of all women related to an affected person by maternal linkage. Routine laboratory testing (i.e., CK elevation) and muscle biopsy are insensitive, so genetic testing is required. Up to 30% of cases may be sporadic and due to new mutations or deletions. In the experience of many clinicians, an even higher percentage of new patients arriving in the clinic are sporadic cases, perhaps because genetic counseling is widely available and the women who carry the abnormal gene decide not to have children.

Genetic analysis of all potential carriers is advisable. In a family in which the disease is associated with a deletion, there is little problem in determining whether the woman is carrying the affected X chromosome, using techniques that are presently available. Genetics laboratories can identify the presence of a mutant gene over the background contributed by the normal allele through analysis of the gene "dosage." Two normal alleles that have a double dose are compared against a deleted allele and a normal allele that have a single dose (Voskova-Goldman et al., 1997). Unfortunately, situations exist in which a mutation is identified in a boy with "sporadic" DMD but not in the mother, and yet the mother is still a carrier. This occurrence is secondary to germline mosaicism in which the mutation in the mother lies only in a percentage of her oocytes. The estimated recurrence rate of DMD is as high as 14% even in such cases. If desired, prenatal diagnosis using amniotic cells or chorionic villus biopsies can identify whether or not the fetus is affected.

### Limb–Girdle Muscular Dystrophies

There is a broad diversity in the clinical presentations of patients with forms of LGMD (Narayanaswami et al., 2014). The traditional diagnosis and classification of LGMDs was accordingly challenging. Many patients present predominantly with proximal weakness, but in others the pattern of weakness is more disparate. In some, hip weakness is greater than shoulder weakness, others the reverse. Some cases are dominantly inherited, others recessively. Onset may be late in life with mild symptoms, but in others severe and early in life.

Beginning with the discovery that a defect in one of the sarcoglycans caused a severe form of LGMD occurring in North Africa, the delineation of several other entities characterized by defects in structural proteins or enzymes followed. These include the sarcoglycans, the α2-chain of laminin (merosin), calcium-activated protease, calpain-3, and others. Those forms with *autosomal dominant* inheritance have been designated *type 1*, and those with *autosomal recessive* inheritance *type 2*. Subclassification with an alphabetical letter has traditionally characterized distinct genetic forms of LGMD1 and LGMD2 (see Table 109.1; Bushby, 1995). As more and more novel disease genes have been identified, however, this classification scheme has run out of letters for LGMD2. An updated classification schema was recently proposed which replaces 1 and 2 with A and R and the alphabetical letter with a number designating order of gene discovery as well as the gene itself. As an example, LGMD2A would be reclassified as LGMD R1 calpain-3–related (Straub et al., 2018). In this text, we will refer to both the traditional and newly proposed nomenclature.

Certain forms of LGMD have been shown to be associated with respiratory muscle weakness and/or cardiomyopathy, so identification of a specific gene can be very helpful in guiding management and informing prognosis. For some culprit genes, certain mutations have been shown to result in a LGMD phenotype while others result in other phenotypes historically classified as distinct from LGMD, such as forms of distal myopathy or congenital muscular dystrophy, autosomal dominant EDMD, exercise intolerance, or even asymptomatic hyperCKemia. Adding to the confusion, a limb–girdle pattern of weakness can also be seen in disorders not strictly classified as a form of LGMD. The following sections outline the known genetic abnormalities and then comment on the more amorphous forms of LGMD. The prevalence of these diseases as a group ranges from 1 to 2.27/100,000 (Norwood et al., 2009; van der Kooi et al., 1996). The autosomal recessive LGMDs are more common than the autosomal dominant LGMDs. Although there is heterogeneity between patients and specific disorders, as a general rule the autosomal recessive LGMDs are also more severe.

#### Autosomal dominant limb–girdle muscular dystrophies

**LGMD1A or myofibrillar myopathy (myotilin deficiency).** Patients with LGMD1A can present with proximal arm and leg weakness in their teens to late adult life or with distal leg weakness (e.g., foot drop) later in life. Some patients have early pharyngeal weakness as well (Narayanaswami et al., 2014). Serum CK concentrations can be normal or moderately elevated. Muscle biopsies may demonstrate rimmed vacuoles within muscle fibers and features of myofibrillar myopathy (MFM).

LGMD1A is allelic to one subtype of MFM and is caused by mutations in the myotilin gene located on chromosome 5q22.3-31.3 (Selcen and Engel, 2004). Myotilin is a sarcomeric protein that is present at the Z-disk. The protein is likely important in myofibrillogenesis and stabilization of the Z-disk and sarcomere.

**LGMD1B or Emery-Dreifuss muscular dystrophy (lamin A/C deficiency).** This myopathy is as also known as autosomal dominant EDMD (Bonne et al., 2000; Narayanaswami et al., 2014; van der Kooi et al., 1996). Some patients manifest with a limb–girdle pattern of weakness, while others present with a humeral-peroneal weakness. Cardiomyopathy with severe conduction defects and arrhythmias may also occur, with or without skeletal muscle involvement. Sudden death secondary to fatal arrhythmias is common, so early diagnosis is desirable and pacemaker insertion and/or implantable cardiac defibrillator (ICD) is often necessary (Kayvanpour et al., 2017). Early elbow and ankle contractures as well as spine rigidity are features seen in some patients, but not universal. Serum CK levels may be normal or elevated up to 25-fold. Muscle biopsies demonstrate dystrophic features with the rare occurrence of rimmed vacuoles.

LGMD1B is localized to mutations in the lamin A/C gene located on chromosome 1q11-21 (Bonne et al., 1999; van der Kooi et al., 1997). Alternative splicing of the lamin A/C messenger (m)RNA transcript produces lamins A and C. Lamin A/C is an intermediate-size filament located on the nucleoplasmic surface of the inner nuclear membrane, where it interacts with various lamin-associated proteins including emerin, the abnormal protein associated with X-linked EDMD. Lamin A/C may also bind to heterochromatin. Immunostaining of the nuclear membrane with anti-emerin antibodies is normal, helping distinguish this myopathy from X-linked EDMD. Electron microscopy reveals alterations in myonuclei, including the loss of peripheral heterochromatin, altered interchromatin texture, and fewer than normal nuclear pores (Sabatelli et al., 2001).

**LGMD1C or rippling muscle disease (caveolin-3 deficiency).** This rare myopathy usually presents in childhood with proximal leg weakness greater than arm weakness and exertional myalgias (Carbone et al., 2000; Minetti et al., 1998; Narayanaswami et al., 2014). Progression of weakness is variable. The clinical phenotype associated with caveolin-3 mutations is quite heterogeneous. Some patients manifest with mainly distal weakness, involving thenar, hypothenar, and intrinsic hand muscles predominantly. Others have familial hypertrophic cardiomyopathy or autosomal dominant rippling muscle disease (Aboumousa et al., 2008; Betz et al., 2001). Serum CK levels are increased 3–25 times normal. In fact, some patients manifest with asymptomatic hyperCKemia.

LGMD1C is caused by mutations in the gene encoding for caveolin-3 on chromosome 3p25 (Carbone et al., 2000; Minetti et al., 1998). Caveolins are scaffolding proteins that interact with lipids and other proteins in *caveoli*, which are flask-shaped invaginations of the sarcolemmal membrane. Immunostaining of muscle biopsies demonstrates a reduction of caveolin-3 along the sarcolemma. Electron microscopy EM reveals a decreased density of caveoli on the muscle membrane as well.

**LGMD1D or LGMD D1 DNAJB6-related.** This recently described myopathy presents in the second to sixth decade with proximal muscle or distal weakness greater in the lower extremities (Hackman et al., 2011; Harms et al., 2012; Narayanaswami et al., 2014; Sarparanta et al., 2012). Cardiorespiratory involvement was notably absent. Serum CK levels are typically slightly elevated. Muscle biopsy reveal rimmed vacuoles and features suggestive of a MFM.

**LGMD1E or myofibrillar myopathy (desmin deficiency).** This is described in the section on MFM (Greenberg et al., 2012).

**LGMD1F or LGMD D2 TNP03-related.** This recently described myopathy presents in the first to sixth decade with proximal greater than distal weakness, legs more than arms (Melià et al., 2013). Anticipation may be seen, with increasing severity in subsequent generations. CK level is normal to moderately elevated. Muscle biopsy can show rimmed vacuoles and features of MFM. It is caused by mutation in the transportin 3 (*TNP03*) gene, which encodes a nuclear import receptor for precursor-mRNA splicing factors.

**LGMD1G or LGMD D3 HNRPDL-related.** This myopathy was initially described in two kindreds, one Brazilian and one Uruguayan (Viera et al., 2014). Onset of weakness is in the second to sixth decade, with proximal lower limb weakness usually preceding upper limb weakness. Finger flexion and toe flexion weakness are typical, and early-onset cataracts may occur. It is caused by mutations in the *HNRPDL* gene, which encodes a ribonucleoprotein important in mRNA biogenesis and metabolism, mediating alternative splicing.

**Bethlem myopathy or LGMD D5 collagen 6–related.** Bethlem myopathy is allelic to the more severe Ullrich congenital muscular dystrophy (UCMD, see below) (Camacho-Vanegas et al., 2001; Bertini and Pepe 2002). Both are due to mutations encoding collagen VI (COL6A1, COL6A2, COL6A3). Onset is typically by early childhood. Joint laxity, especially distally, is common early in this disorder (Fig. 109.13). Contractures are also very common, especially at the elbows and ankles, and can lead to confusion with EDMD. Contractures can involve the wrists and fingers over time. Restrictive ventilatory deficits can be seen, presumably from a combination of weakness and

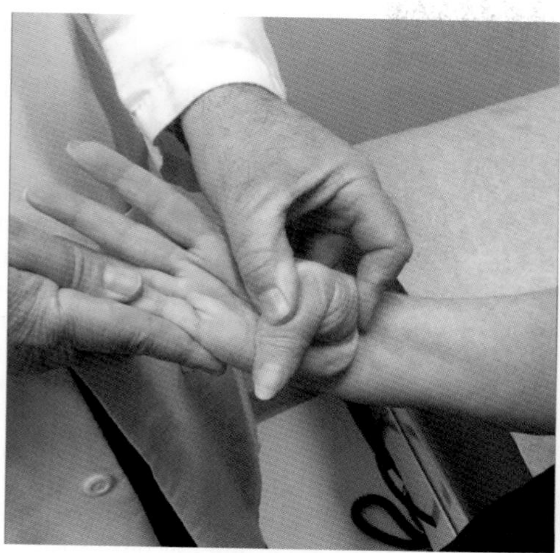
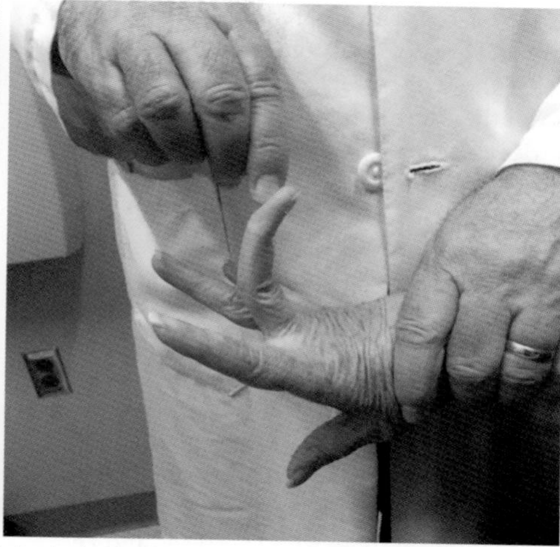

**Fig. 109.13** Bethlem Myopathy. Joint laxity in the thumb and finger.

contractures. Some patients, however, have a limb–girdle pattern of weakness without any contractures.

**LGMD2A or LGMD R1 calpain-3–related or LGMD D4 calpain-3–related.** LGMD2A was first reported in an inbred population on Reunion Island in the Indian Ocean (Fardeau et al., 1996). It is caused by mutations in the gene for muscle-specific calcium-activated neutral protease (*CANP-3* or calpain-3) (Spencer et al., 1997). Since the initial description, the disorder has shown a worldwide distribution and is the most common LGMD (Lostal et al., 2018; Vissing et al., 2016). The underlying pathophysiology of the illness is uncertain. CANP-3 is not a structural protein but an enzyme. It has been suggested that the enzyme has a regulatory role in the modulation and control of transcription factors and thus of gene expression. CANP-3 also binds to titin and can cleave filamin-C; thus it may have a role in stabilizing the sarcomere. Although most commonly autosomal recessive inheritance is seen, autosomal dominant inheritance has recently been reported in a series of 37 patients with a single 21-base-pair, in-frame deletion. These patients had a similar phenotype to traditional LGMD2A, but with milder weakness (Vissing et al., 2016).

The disease is progressive and typically begins in early adolescence but can begin in early or middle adulthood for some. Most cases have been mild to moderately progressive, with loss of ambulation in adult life. Severe forms occur. Weakness occurs in the hips first and then in the shoulders. Facial strength is preserved, and the neck flexors and extensors are strong. Scapular winging occurs, different from that seen in FSHD, with the whole of the medial scapular border jutting backward. Posterior thigh muscles and adductors are more severely affected than the knee extensors. The rectus abdominis muscles are affected early which can lead to abdominal hernias. Early contractures may develop. Mild to moderate respiratory muscle weakness can develop, commensurate with the severity of skeletal muscle weakness, but cardiac muscle is spared. The serum concentration of CK is markedly elevated early in the course and then decreases to normal concentrations later in the illness. Muscle biopsies may demonstrate endomysial inflammatory cell infiltrate with prominent eosinophils that may lead to misdiagnosis as eosinophilic myositis (Brown and Amato, 2006; Krahn et al., 2006).

**LGMD2B or LGMD R2 dysferlin-related (dysferlin deficiency).** Mutations in the gene encoding for dysferlin, located on chromosome 2p13, lead to clinically heterogeneous myopathies. Some patients show a limb–girdle pattern of weakness (LGMD2B), while others present with weakness and atrophy of the calf muscles (Miyoshi myopathy) (Harris et al., 2016). In both cases, early preferential involvement of the gastrocnemius and thigh adductors is common (Paradas et al., 2010). Dysferlinopathies account for only about 1% of LGMDs but about 60% of distal myopathies (Fanin et al., 2001). Looking at this another way, 80% of patients with dysferlinopathy manifest a distal myopathy, 8% have an LGMD pattern of weakness, and 6% have asymptomatic elevation of serum CK. Less common presentations include progressive foot drop, axial muscle weakness with bent spine syndrome/camptocormia, and rigid spine syndrome (Illa et al., 2001; Nagashima et al., 2004; Seror et al., 2008; Vilchez et al., 2005). The dysferlinopathies typically present in adolescence or early adult life. Progression is usually slow, but some patients lose ambulation in their 20s while others can walk late in life. Interestingly, intrafamilial variability exists in the pattern of weakness and disease progression.

Serum CK concentrations are markedly elevated, usually 35–200 times normal. Muscle biopsies demonstrate dystrophic features in severely affected muscles but nonspecific myopathic features in less affected muscles. Occasionally a striking endomysial or perivascular inflammatory process is appreciated, leading to an incorrect diagnosis of PM. However, unlike PM, the inflammatory cells usually do not invade non-necrotic muscle fibers. Amyloid deposition may also be evident in some cases (Spuler et al., 2008). Immunostaining and immunoblot confirm the diagnosis. Dysferlin localizes to the sarcolemmal membrane but does not directly interact with dystrophin or the sarcoglycans. Dysferlin is thought important in membrane repair (Bansal et al., 2003; Cenacchi et al., 2005; Glover and Brown, 2007).

**LGMD2C, 2D, 2E, and 2F (sarcoglycan deficiencies).** Four known sarcoglycans expressed in muscle are associated with different forms of autosomal recessive LGMD2. The genetic abnormality underlying LGMD2C, 2D, 2E, and 2F are mutations in the genes for γ-sarcoglycan, α-sarcoglycan, β-sarcoglycan, and δ-sarcoglycan, respectively. The sarcoglycans are a tightly knit family, and when one is absent, the others may also be missing. This is particularly true of α-sarcoglycan, making it both a useful screening tool and a misleading one on occasion. An absence of α-sarcoglycan is an indication to search for the abnormal gene, be it an α-, β-, γ-, or δ-sarcoglycanopathy.

Sarcoglycanopathies may account for more than 10% of patients with a limb–girdle pattern and normal dystrophin (Duggan et al., 1997; Marsolier et al., 2017). Of these, α-sarcoglycanopathies (LGMD2D) are most common, accounting for approximately 6% of cases. The most common type varies considerably between geographic areas. Sarcoglycanopathies may account for up to 50% of patients with muscular dystrophy in North Africa.

The four sarcoglycanopathies are very similar clinically and may be confused with DMD; the lack of cognitive impairment can help distinguish. Childhood-onset is common, with trunk and proximal leg weakness and a serum CK concentration of 1000 units and higher (Narayanaswami et al., 2014). Facial weakness is absent, but scapular winging and calf hypertrophy occur. Weakness is progressive and many patients require a wheelchair. Many patients experience respiratory muscle weakness and assisted ventilation may be required (Fayssoil et al., 2016). Cardiac dysfunction occurs in a minority of affected patients, more commonly in those with LGMD2C and 2E.

**LGMD2G or LGMD R7 telethonin-related.** Patients with this dystrophy may have either proximal or distal weakness (Moreira et al., 1997; Narayanaswami et al., 2014). Mean age of onset is approximately 12.5 years. Legs are affected more than arms; the quadriceps and anterior tibial muscles are affected early. Some may have a cardiomyopathy. Serum CK levels are 3–17 times normal. Muscle pathology shows dystrophic features in addition to the frequent occurrence of rimmed vacuoles within muscle fibers.

LGMD2G links to mutations in the gene that encodes for telethonin on chromosome 17q11-12 (Moreira et al., 2000). Telethonin is one of the most abundant muscle proteins, where it localizes to the sarcomere. Telethonin may interact with the large sarcomeric proteins, titin and myosin. Abnormal telethonin may disrupt normal myofibrillogenesis.

**LGMD2H or LGMD R8 TRIM 32-related.** This LGMD was initially reported in families of Manitoba Hutterite origin (Weiler et al., 1998) and is allelic with sarcotubular myopathy. Most affected individuals have a mild limb–girdle pattern of weakness, with onset from birth to the seventh decade (Narayanaswami et al., 2014). Patients may note exertional myalgias; scapular winging and facial weakness may be variably noted. Serum CKs range from 250 to over 3000 IU/L, and EMGs reveal myopathic features. Muscle biopsy features demonstrate small vacuoles that represent focal dilations of the sarcoplasmic reticulum. This myopathy is caused by mutation in the gene that encodes for E3-ubiquitin ligase (also known as *TRIM 32*) (Frosk et al., 2002). This ligase may be important for ubiquinating proteins targeted for destruction by the proteasomes (Kramerova et al., 2007). *TRIM32* mutations may lead to dysregulation of myofibrillar protein turnover.

**LGMD2I or LGMD R9 FKRP-related.** This dystrophy was initially reported in a large consanguineous Tunisian family (Driss et al., 2000). Subsequently the dystrophy has shown a worldwide distribution and is the most common type of LGMD in patients of northern European ancestry (Narayanaswami et al., 2014). The clinical phenotype is variable, with age of onset from the first to the sixth decade. The course resembles a dystrophinopathy in some, including calf hypertrophy (Mercuri et al., 2003). Difficulty running, difficulty climbing stairs, and cramps/myalgias are all common presenting symptoms. A severe cardiomyopathy can develop, and respiratory muscle weakness occurs as the disease progresses. Serum CKs are elevated 10–30 times normal in some affected younger patients but are normal in some older individuals (Brockington et al., 2001, 2002; Mercuri et al., 2003; Willis et al., 2014).

LGMD2I is caused by mutations in the gene that encodes for FKRP, a glycosyltransferase, and its deficiency is associated with abnormal glycosylation of α-dystroglycan (Brockington et al., 2002). It is unique among secondary α-dystroglycanopathies in that it more commonly causes an adult-onset LGMD rather than a form of congenital muscular dystrophy, but mutations in FKRP do also cause congenital muscular dystrophy with normal merosin (MDC1C).

**LGMD2J or LGMD R10 titin-related.** *TTN* is an enormous gene, producing the largest protein in humans. Titin is a protein that spans the entire sarcomere and serves as a ligand for calpain-3. Numerous clinical phenotypes have been described in relation to mutations throughout the gene, with varying forms of skeletal muscle involvement and/or cardiomyopathy. Autosomal dominant disorders include hereditary myopathy with early respiratory failure (HMERF), Udd distal myopathy (discussed in the Distal Myopathies section), and isolated dilated cardiomyopathy; autosomal recessive disorders include LGMD2J, adult-onset distal myopathy, proximal adult-onset rimmed vacuolar myopathy, and a congenital titinopathy (discussed in the Congenital Myopathies section) (Narayanaswami et al., 2014; Oates et al., 2018; Savarese et al., 2018). Because of its massive size, it is common to uncover novel or rare variants of uncertain significance (VUS) in the *TTN* gene when genetic testing is pursued; many of these will not be related to the patient's condition. By converse, pathogenic mutations can also be missed due to the gene's large size and complex structure.

LGMD2J is characterized by childhood-onset weakness that is more severe in the proximal muscles of the arms and legs, with distal weakness often present but mild (Udd et al., 2005). Some patients develop a cardiomyopathy. CKs are usually mildly elevated. Muscle biopsies reveal dystrophic features, and rimmed vacuoles are usually absent or rare. As the name implies, proximal adult-onset rimmed vacuolar myopathy includes rimmed vacuoles on biopsy, with a unique pattern of weakness affecting the quadriceps and soleus but sparing the tibialis anterior.

HMERF resembles Udd distal myopathy; it is autosomal dominant and associated with progressive foot drop (Narayanaswami et al., 2014; Ohlsson et al., 2012; Pénisson-Besnier et al., 2010; Pfeffer et al., 2012). However, it tends to affect patients earlier in adulthood, may also affect the proximal muscles (legs greater than arms), and is associated with early respiratory failure. Muscle biopsies reveal rimmed vacuoles and features of MFM.

**LGMD2L or LGMD R12 anoctamin 5-related.** This disorder was initially described in 14 French Canadian patients from eight different families, but has since been shown to be among the most common LGMDs in Northern Europe (Jarry et al., 2007). Subsequently, patients have been reported with a Miyoshi myopathy-like phenotype with involvement of the calves in the second decade of life, exertional myalgias, hyperCKemia, or calf hypertrophy (Bolduc et al., 2010; Mahjneh et al., 2010; Narayanaswami et al., 2014; Schessl et al., 2012). Females are more likely than males to have mild phenotypes without weakness (Penttila et al., 2012). Symptoms may begin from age 20 to 70. Those with the LGMD phenotype usually have associated quadriceps atrophy and myalgias, and weakness may be asymmetric. There is usually no cardiac or respiratory muscle involvement. Serum CK concentrations can be markedly increased. Muscle biopsies demonstrate nonspecific dystrophic features with increased endomysial connective tissue associated with basal lamina duplication and collagen disorganization infiltration. The disorder is caused by mutations in the *ANO5* gene that encodes for anoctamin 5, a transmembrane protein that may be a calcium-activated chloride channel.

**LGMD2K, LGMD2M, LGMD2N, LGMD2O, LGMD2T, and LGMD2U.** These are all secondary *α-dystroglycanopathies*, which usually present in infancy or early childhood as congenital muscular dystrophies (discussed in detail in the Congenital Muscular Dystrophy section) (Iannaccone and Castro, 2013). Rarely they present later in childhood or early adult life with a limb–girdle pattern of weakness with or without CNS involvement (Narayanaswami et al., 2014).

LGMD2K, or LGMD R11 POMT1-related, is caused by mutations in protein *O*-mannosyltransferase 1 (POMT1). This is usually associated with Walker-Warburg syndrome, but can also cause childhood onset of a milder LGMD phenotype associated with severe cognitive impairment (Godfrey et al., 2007).

LGMD2M, or LGMD R13 fukutin-related, is caused by mutations in the gene that encodes for fukutin, which usually causes Fukuyama congenital muscular dystrophy (FCMD). However, mutations in the fukutin gene have also been associated with a milder adult-onset myopathy (LGMD2M), particularly outside of Japan (Puckett et al., 2009; Vuillaumier-Barrot et al., 2009). Affected individuals can have normal intelligence and brain structure, have a mild limb–girdle weakness, present with only a cardiomyopathy, or have asymptomatic elevation of serum CK concentrations. Some patients have remarkable steroid responsiveness (Godfrey et al., 2006).

LGMD2N, or LGMD R13 POMT2-related, is caused by mutations in the gene encoding protein *O*-mannosyltransferase 2 (POMT2). Mutations in this gene can also cause Walker-Warburg syndrome and rarely are associated with a milder limb–girdle syndrome affecting hamstrings, gluteal, and paraspinal muscles with universal cognitive impairment (Østergaard et al., 2018).

LGMD2O, or LGMD R15 POMGnT1-related, is caused by mutations in *POMGnT1*, which encodes protein *O*-mannose-β-1,2-*N*-acetylglucosaminyl transferase. Mutations in this enzyme also cause muscle-eye-brain (MEB) disease. Mutations in *POMGnT1* can be associated with milder allelic variants of muscular dystrophy and normal intelligence (LGMD2N) (Clement et al., 2008; Godfrey et al., 2007).

LGMD2T, or LGMD R19 GMPPB-related, is caused by mutations in *GMPPB*, encoding guanosine diphosphate mannose pyrophosphorylase B. Those with a LGMD phenotype present from very early childhood to the fourth decade; cognitive impairment, seizures, and cataracts are common with early-onset cases (Carss et al., 2013; Cabrera-Serrano et al., 2015).

LGMD2U, or LGMD R20 ISPD-related, is caused by mutations in a gene encoding isoprenoid synthetase domain-containing protein (*ISPD*), more commonly associated with Walker-Warburg syndrome. A childhood-onset LGMD phenotype with normal intelligence has been recently reported (Cirak et al., 2013).

**LGMD2P or LGMD R16 α-dystroglycan-related.** This is a newly reported rare dystrophy that has presented with onset in the first decade, severe cognitive impairment, and with reduced α-dystroglycan expression on muscle biopsy (Dinçer et al., 2003; Hara et al., 2011; Narayanaswami et al., 2014). This dystrophy caused by a mutation in the gene encoding for α-dystroglycan.

**LGMD2Q or LGMD R17 plectin-related.** LGMD2Q has also been considered a form of congenital myasthenia and is associated with epidermolysis bullosa, in which patients develop blistering of the skin and mucous membranes, typically in infancy or early childhood (Narayanaswami et al., 2014). Affected individuals may present with congenital hypotonia or slowly progressive, proximal weakness in late childhood or adulthood. Ptosis and ophthalmoplegia may be evident. CK levels are usually elevated.

**LGMD2R or myofibrillar myopathy (desmin deficiency).** Unlike most cases of primary desminopathy, this recently reported LGMD is inherited in an autosomal recessive as opposed to autosomal dominant fashion (Cetin et al., 2013; Henderson et al., 2013). It may present in early childhood or adulthood with slowly progressive, predominantly proximal muscle fatigue and weakness and ventilatory failure. CK levels are mildly elevated. Unlike the more common autosomal dominant primary desminopathies (e.g., LGMD1E), biopsies in the reported cases did not reveal features of MFM.

**LGMD2S or LGMD R18 TRAPPC11-related.** This is another recently reported LGMD in Syrians and Hutterites (Bögershausen et al., 2013) that is characterized by an infantile onset of choreiform, athetoid or dystonic movements, seizures, truncal ataxia, and mental intellectual disability. Proximal weakness is apparent in childhood along with scoliosis and hip dysplasia; CK is mild to moderately elevated. It is caused by mutations in the transport (trafficking) protein particle complex, subunit 11 (*TRAPPC11*), which is important in trafficking proteins between endoplasmic reticulum and the Golgi complex.

**Recently described limb–girdle muscular dystrophies.** LGMD2W, attributed to a mutation in *LIMS2* (also called PINCH2), was recently reported in two Northern European siblings, both of whom developed proximal weakness, calf hypertrophy, and an enlarged triangular tongue in early childhood and later developed cardiomyopathy (Chardon et al., 2015). LGMD2X, attributed to a mutation in *BVES*, was reported in three members of an Albanian family. Those affected had second-degree heart block and an elevated CK, with the grandfather developing proximal muscle weakness in his 40s (Schindler et al., 2016). LGMD2Y, attributed to a mutation in *TOR1AIP1*, was recently reported in three patients from a consanguineous Turkish family. Weakness began in the first or second decade, along with joint contractures and rigid spine (Kayman-Kurecki et al., 2014). LGMD2Z, or LGMD R21, is attributed to mutation in *POGLUT1* and was recently reported in four patients from a consanguineous Spanish family. Proximal leg weakness began in the third decade, progressing to include upper limb weakness and loss of ambulation (Servan-Morilla et al., 2016).

***Myofibrillar myopathy.*** MFM likely results from disruption of the Z-disc. The characteristic pathological finding in MFM is myofibrillary disruption on EM and excessive sarcoplasmic accumulation of desmin and other proteins on immunostains (Amato et al., 1998; Dalakas et al., 2000; De Bleecker et al., 1996; Nakano et al., 1996, 1997; Narayanaswami et al., 2014). Desmin is a cytoskeletal protein linking the Z-disc to the sarcolemma and nucleus. This myopathy has been reported as desmin storage myopathy, desmin myopathy, familial desminopathy, spheroid body myopathy, cytoplasmic body myopathy, Mallory body myopathy, reducing body myopathy, familial cardiomyopathy with subsarcolemmal vermiform deposits, myopathy with intrasarcoplasmic accumulation of dense granulofilamentous material, Markesbery-Griggs myopathy, and hereditary inclusion body myopathy (hIBM) with early respiratory failure (Amato et al., 1998). The original classification of many such disorders was as forms of congenital myopathy, but it is now clear that MFM is a muscular dystrophy and many are allelic with forms of LGMD and distal muscular dystrophy/myopathy (Narayanaswami et al., 2014).

There is a spectrum of clinical phenotypes associated with MFM (Amato et al., 1998; Narayanaswami et al., 2014). Most patients develop weakness between 25 and 45 years of age, but onset can occur from infancy to late adulthood. Either cardiac or skeletal muscles can be involved and dominate the clinical picture. Limb weakness can be predominantly distal and affect either the arms or the legs, but in others, proximal muscles are involved more than distal muscles. Facial and pharyngeal muscles are also affected. Some patients have a facioscapulohumeral or scapuloperoneal distribution of weakness.

The cardiomyopathy may manifest as arrhythmias or conduction defects as well as congestive heart failure. Pacemaker insertion or cardiac transplantation may be required. Severe respiratory muscle weakness can also complicate MFM. In addition, there are rare reports of smooth muscle involvement leading to intestinal pseudo-obstruction.

Muscle histology demonstrates variability in fiber size, increased central nuclei, and occasionally type 1 fiber predominance (Amato et al., 1998; De Bleecker et al., 1996; Nakano et al., 1996, 1997; Narayanaswami et al., 2014). Muscle fibers with rimmed vacuoles may also be evident. Two major types of lesions are evident on light and electron microscopy: hyaline structures and nonhyaline lesions. The hyaline structures are cytoplasmic granular inclusions that are typically eosinophilic on hematoxylin and eosin, and dark blue-green or occasionally red on modified Gomori trichrome stains. They appear as cytoplasmic bodies, spheroid bodies, or Mallory bodies on EM. The nonhyaline lesions appear as dark green areas of amorphous material on Gomori trichrome stains. On EM, these nonhyaline lesions correspond to foci of myofibrillar destruction and consist of disrupted myofilaments, Z-disk–derived bodies, dappled dense structures of Z-disk origin, and streaming of the Z-disk. Immunohistochemistry reveals that both the hyaline and nonhyaline lesions contain desmin, myotilin, and numerous other proteins (Amato et al., 1998; De Bleecker et al., 1996; Nakano et al., 1996, 1997). Interestingly, abnormal muscle fibers also abnormally express several cyclin-dependent kinases in the cytoplasm, including CDC2, CDK2, CDK4, and CDK7 (Amato et al., 1998).

The pathogenesis of MFM is multifactorial (Narayanaswami et al., 2014; Selcen et al., 2004). As alluded to previously, MFM can be caused by mutations in the desmin gene, allelic with LGMD1E, and mutations in the myotilin gene, allelic with LGMD1A; the recently proposed updated classification schema of LGMDs, in fact, characterizes both disorders simply as myofibrillar myopathies and not LGMDs at all (Straub et al., 2018). Markesbery-Griggs distal myopathy, caused by mutations in the *ZASP* gene, also demonstrates MFM on pathology (Selcen and Engel, 2005). Less common mutations have been identified in the *FLNC, CRYAB, BAG3, FHL1, TTN, PLEC, ACTA1, HSPB8,* and *DNAJB6* genes, many of which encode proteins important in the formation and stabilization of the Z-disk (Kley et al., 2016). Autosomal dominant inheritance is most common, but autosomal recessive and X-linked inheritance have been reported.

### Congenital Muscular Dystrophies

The congenital muscular dystrophies, abbreviated MDC by convention, are a group of diseases typically evident at birth or soon thereafter with hypotonia and severe trunk and limb weakness (Iannaccone and Castro, 2013). All are typically autosomal recessive in their inheritance and are distinguished in part by greater or lesser central nervous system (CNS) and eye involvement (Kang, 2015). Contractures of the joints are prominent, particularly at the ankles, knees, and hips. Intellectual disability may be present, and MRI of the head shows strikingly increased white matter signal in many patients.

Several distinct forms of MDC are recognizable by clinical and genetic feature, and can be stratified based on the defective protein responsible. MDCs related to genes encoding structural proteins of the basal lamina and sarcolemma include MDC type 1 and UCMD. MDCs related to impaired glycosylation of α-dystroglycan are referred to as dystroglycanopathies (DG). Finally, mutations in selenoprotein N1 produce a unique phenotype of rigid spine syndrome.

***MDC type 1.*** MDC type 1 is the most common type of MDC in the Western Hemisphere. It is genetically heterogeneous, with approximately 50% of cases associated with primary merosin or $\alpha_2$-laminin deficiency (MDC1A). Laminin-$\alpha_2$, also known as merosin, is one of a large family of glycosylated proteins found in the basement membrane and attaches to the dystroglycan complex. The hallmark of merosinopathy includes severe weakness of the trunk and limbs and hypotonia at birth, sparing the extraocular muscles and face (Iannaccone and Castro, 2013). Prominent contractures of the feet and hips are present. Although intelligence is often normal, the incidence of epilepsy is 12% to 20%. MRI and computed tomography (CT) of the brain often reveal white-matter abnormalities. For the most part, these children are severely disabled, and many remain dependent on their caregivers for their whole lives. In milder forms of the disease, caused by partial merosin deficiency, delayed onset of symptoms and mild weakness occur (Tan et al., 1997). This situation is similar to dystrophin deficiency.

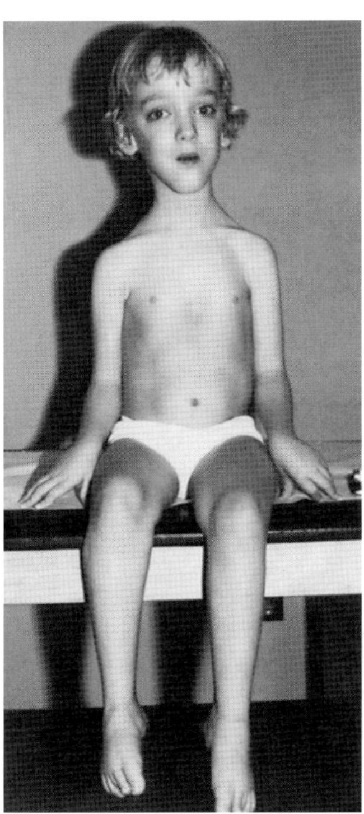

**Fig. 109.14 Congenital Muscular Dystrophy (Classic Type).** This boy also had weakness and contractures of the limbs. His illness was relatively static.

CK concentrations are elevated. EMG, in addition to demonstrating abnormalities in the muscle, shows slowed nerve conduction velocities; laminin-$\alpha_2$ is also expressed in nerve tissue. Diagnosis is established by identifying a mutation in the laminin-$\alpha_2$ gene. Demonstration of altered merosin in muscle can be helpful to guide this testing (Sewry et al., 1997). As in dystrophin deficiency, it may be advantageous to use at least two different antibodies. Skin biopsy may also reveal merosin deficiency.

There are patients with identical symptoms who do not have a mutation in the laminin-$\alpha_2$ gene (Fig. 109.14). MDC1B, for example, is caused by mutations in the gene encoding for the $\alpha_7$ subunit of $\alpha_7\beta_1$D integrin, a sarcolemmal protein that binds to merosin (Hayashi et al., 1998). Frequently the muscle symptoms are milder and progress more slowly; children may gain function as they grow older and may walk independently. Despite a shortened life span, many survive to adulthood. Certain α-dystroglycanopathies produce an identical clinical phenotype, most importantly MDC1C, which results from mutations in FKRP (Brockington et al., 2002).

***Ullrich congenital muscular dystrophy/Bethlem myopathy.*** UCMD, also known as *atonic-sclerotic dystrophy* and recently reclassified as LGMD R22 collagen 6-related, is associated with neonatal weakness, multiple contractures, and distal hyperlaxity (Bertini E, 2002). Affected children often have marked protrusion of the calcanei in their feet. The clinical course is static or slowly progressive. Serum CKs are normal or only slightly elevated. Mutations in subunits of collagen type VI cause

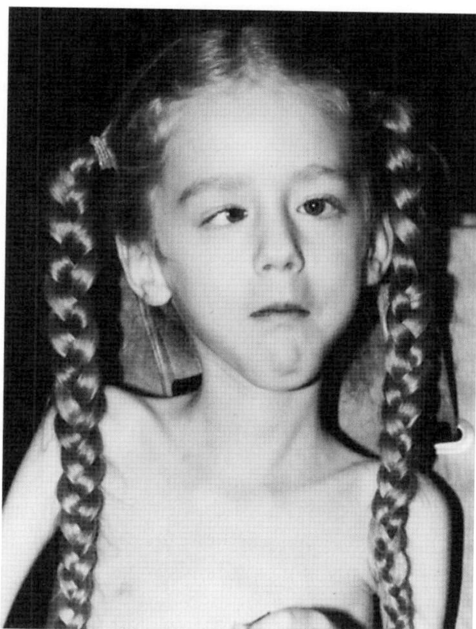

**Fig. 109.15 Congenital Muscular Dystrophy (Fukuyama Type).** This severely intellectually disabled girl had many seizures and marked contractures of the limbs. She was too weak to support her own weight. The disease was nonprogressive. Her two brothers had the same illness.

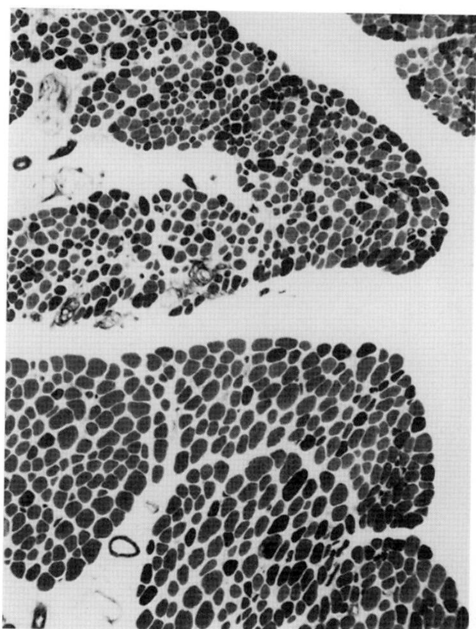

**Fig. 109.16** Biopsy from Fukuyama-type congenital muscular dystrophy. In addition to variability in fiber size and type 1 fiber predominance with fibrosis, note nonrandom distribution of atrophy. Fascicle in lower part of picture contains fibers larger than those in upper part (myosin adenosine triphosphatase stain, pH 9.4).

the disorder. UCMD is allelic to the more benign Bethlem myopathy, or LGMD D5 (see above) (Camacho-Vanegas et al., 2001). Skeletal muscle MRI scans may reveal early involvement of the thigh muscles that preferentially involve the periphery of each muscle and relatively spare the central regions along with a peculiar involvement of the rectus femoris with a central area of abnormal signal within the muscle (Mercuri et al., 2005; ten Dam et al., 2012).

***α-Dystroglycanopathies.*** At least 18 distinct genes have now been associated with forms of DG with autosomal recessive inheritance, and the resulting spectrum of disease is broad (Liewluck et al., 2018). As already described, an adult-onset LGMD2 phenotype can result in many of these patients. Most, however, result in varying severities of congenital muscular dystrophies, many of which include CNS and eye involvement. Described syndromes include MDC1C, Fukuyama congenial muscular dystrophy, Walker-Warburg syndrome, and MEB disease. A phenomenon of profound, transient weakness occurring in the setting of febrile illness has been described in patients with DG association with mutations in *FKRP, FKTN, POMT1, POMT2,* and *POMGNT1*. This typically occurs in children younger than 7, and often precedes the diagnosis of a muscular dystrophy (Carlson et al., 2017).

**Fukuyama-type muscular dystrophy** is caused by mutations in the fukutin gene (Kobayashi et al., 1998). This disease is more common in Japanese and Korean populations due to founder mutations (Kang, 2015). The glycoprotein-dystrophin complex is also expressed in the CNS, which probably accounts for the severe CNS manifestations associated with Fukuyama-type muscular dystrophy. Affected children are usually normal at birth, but some are floppy. Joint contractures are present in 70% by the age of 3 months, with the hip, knee, and ankle commonly involved. Children are often severely intellectually disabled, sometimes to the extent that speech is never developed, and either major motor or absence seizures are common (Fig. 109.15). Another curious finding is asymmetry of the skull. Weakness is diffuse, including the face and neck, and often disabling so that the child never learns to walk. The muscle disease is moderately or slowly progressive, and survival into early adult life is common. These children are completely dependent on their parents, however.

The Fukuyama variant does not resemble DMD, and the only real difficulty is in differentiating it from other forms of congenital dystrophy. Serum CK concentration is usually markedly elevated. A muscle biopsy can easily distinguish this disorder from congenital nonprogressive myopathies, as dystrophic changes with variability in fiber size and fibrosis are common. Internal nuclei are also common. The changes in fiber size may not be random, and some fascicles contain much smaller fibers than others. This nonrandom change differs from denervation atrophy, in which there is a wide random variability in fiber size within individual fascicles (Fig. 109.16).

MRI and CT scans of the brain show a variety of abnormalities, but the most striking is the presence of lucencies, particularly in the frontal area (Fig. 109.17). These changes seldom extend to the genu of the corpus callosum and spare the medial subependymal regions along the trigones and occipital horns. As the children grow older, these lucencies disappear in sequence from the occipital to the frontal region in a fashion resembling the progression of normal myelination. Occasionally, marked pallor of the myelin in the centrum semiovale, together with mild gliosis or edema, is noted. Postmortem examination reveals numerous brain malformations including agyria, pachygyria, and microgyria. The cortex may have a cobblestone appearance, absence of gray-matter lamination, and other abnormal cytoarchitectural features. Heterotopias are present in the brainstem and basal meninges, as is micropolygyria of the cerebellum. Ventricular dilatation, enlarged sulci, and aqueductal stenosis are other associated features. In short, there are marked abnormalities in the architecture of the brain.

The combination of muscular dystrophy, lissencephaly, cerebellar malformations, and severe retinal and eye malformations characterizes **Walker-Warburg syndrome** and the related **muscle-eye-brain disease** (Haltia et al., 1997). Both are associated with more severe eye abnormalities than Fukuyama-type muscular dystrophy. Walker-Warburg syndrome is the more catastrophic disease, with death often

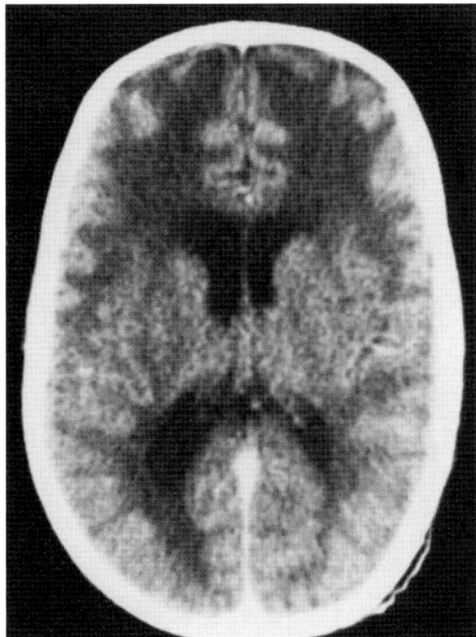

**Fig. 109.17** Computed tomographic scan of head of patient with Fukuyama congenital muscular dystrophy demonstrates lucencies in white matter, particularly toward frontal poles.

occurring within the first 2 years; eye changes include microphthalmia, colobomas, congenital cataracts and glaucoma, corneal opacities, retinal dysplasia and nonattachment, hypoplastic vitreous, and optic atrophy. MEB disease is milder and characterized by high myopia and possibly a preretinal membrane or gliosis, but severe structural abnormalities of the eye are not present.

The CNS findings are also different. MRI may be a useful technique to separate the entities (van der Knaap et al., 1997). The changes in Walker-Warburg syndrome are more severe, with various combinations of hydrocephalus, aqueductal stenosis, cerebellar and pontine hypoplasia with a small posterior vermis, Dandy-Walker malformations, and an agyric or pachygyric cobblestone cortex. T1-weighted images show diffuse decreased white-matter signal; T2-weighted images show an increased signal compatible with a defect in myelination. In MEB disease, white-matter changes are focal and the cortical changes milder.

In Walker-Warburg syndrome, mutations in *POMT1* account for 20% of cases; *POMT2*, *fukutin*, and *FKRP* are also frequent but still account for only a minority of cases (Beltran-Valero de Bernabe et al., 2002; Cormand et al., 2001; Diesen et al., 2004; van Reeuwijk et al., 2005). Some cases of muscle-eye-brain disease are caused by mutations in the gene that encodes for *O*-mannose β-1,2-*N*-acetylglucosaminyl transferase (*POMGnT1*) located on chromosome 1p3 (Yoshida et al., 2001).

***Congenital muscular dystrophies with rigid spine syndrome.*** This disorder presents in infancy with hypotonia, weakness, and delayed motor milestones. Reduced mobility of the spine is marked, and many children also develop scoliosis and contractures at the knees and elbows. Serum CK concentrations are normal to moderately elevated. Muscle biopsies may reveal type 1 predominance, increased internal nuclei, and other nonspecific myopathic features. In some kinships, the myopathy links to mutations in the selenoprotein *N1* gene located on chromosome 1p3 (Moghadaszadeh et al., 2001). Other myopathic disorders (e.g., EDMD), however, can also be associated with rigid spine syndrome.

### Other Regional Forms of Muscular Dystrophies

***Emery-Dreifuss dystrophy (emerin deficiency).*** EDMD is characterized by the triad of scapuloperoneal weakness, early contractures, and cardiac involvement. Wasting and weakness of the upper arms, shoulders, and anterior compartment muscles in the legs are typical (Narayanaswami et al., 2014). This weakness is associated with early contractures, particularly in the elbows, posterior neck, paraspinal muscles, and Achilles tendon. Elbow contractures are characteristic and are severe. As the arm extends, sudden resistance is met, which feels more like bone than the pressure of a tight tendon. EDMD can produce a rigid spine syndrome. Contractures typically develop by the teenage years. The disorder is slowly progressive and often spreads to involve other muscle groups such as those of the hip. Cardiac complications are frequent. Conduction block may explain the sometimes sudden unexpected death of these patients. Atrial paralysis occurs in which the atria are electrically inexcitable, and the heart responds only to ventricular pacing. Other cardiac problems include ventricular myocardial disease with ventricular failure. Female carriers may develop the cardiac abnormalities at a later age, and sudden death occurs. The severity of the cardiopathy in both men and women increases with age.

The most common form of EDMD exhibits X-linked inheritance and is caused by mutations in the gene *(STA)* that encodes for emerin. Emerin localizes to the inner nuclear membrane, from which it projects into the nucleoplasm (Manilal et al., 1996). Emerin belongs to a family of lamina-associated structural proteins and is important in nuclear membrane organization and its attachment to heterochromatin. EDMD-X2 is also an X-linked myopathy that can have either an "EDMD" pattern of weakness or a scapuloperoneal pattern and is caused by mutations in the *FHL1* gene that encodes for four-and-one-half LIM1 protein.

Autosomal dominant EDMD can be caused by mutations in lamin A/C, as discussed in the section on LGMD1B (Narayanaswami et al., 2014). Rare causes of autosomal dominant EDMD link to mutations in the *SYNE1* and *SYNE2* genes that encode for the nuclear proteins, nesprin-1 and nesprin-2, as well as in transmembrane protein 43 (TMEM43) or LUMA. The clinical phenotype is essentially identical to that seen with emerin and lamin A/C mutations.

Genetic testing is done to confirm the diagnosis. Because emerin is present in many tissues, skin biopsy showing that the protein is absent from nuclei in the skin confirms the diagnosis. Muscle biopsy and EMG reveal nonspecific myopathic features. The CK level is usually only slightly elevated. Every patient with the syndrome should have an ECG repeated at regular intervals, and regular ECG in other family members is recommended as isolated cardiac involvement occurs (Narayanaswami et al., 2014).

Analysis and treatment of the cardiac problems are the most pertinent parts of therapy. Most patients with EDMD need a cardiac pacemaker or intracardiac defibrillator (Narayanaswami et al., 2014) because fatal arrhythmias can be sudden, unpredictable, and fatal; it is wise to implant a pacemaker or even a defibrillator when the diagnosis is first established. It is important to realize that cardiac devices do not retard development of a cardiomyopathy and only protect the patient against the complications of conduction block. Female carriers should be screened with ECG after age 35.

***Facioscapulohumeral dystrophy.*** FSHD is an autosomal dominant disorder; however, approximately 30% of cases arise as a result of an apparently sporadic mutation (Tawil, 2015). The estimated prevalence is 1/15,000–20,000, making it the third most common muscular dystrophy. The genetic underpinnings of the disorder are complex. The disease is thought to arise from expression of a normally silenced gene, *DUX4* (double homeobox 4), which resides on chromosome 4q35. The gene is typically epigenetically repressed via methylation of a large, repetitive 3.3 kilobase sequence of DNA near the gene known as D4Z4. Normal copies of the region contain greater than 10 D4Z4 repeats. Greater than 95% of FSHD cases are caused by a deletion in the D4Z4 sequence, leading to only 1–10 repeats; this is termed FSHD1 (Tawil and Van Der Maarel, 2006). The resulting contracted D4Z4 region is hypomethylated, creating an open reading frame permissive of transcription into mRNA (de Greef et al., 2009). The situation is more complex, however, in that two allelic variants distal to the repeats (A and B) exist; only the A allele contains the polyadenylation sequence required to result in stable messenger RNA once transcribed. Both contraction of the D4Z4 repeats *and* a permissive A allele are required for the disease state. The other 5% of patients with FSHD do not have a deletion of this region, but the D4Z4 region is hypomethylated nonetheless. About 85% of these patients have mutations in the structural maintenance of chromosome's flexible hinge domain containing 1 (*SMCHD1*) gene that encodes a chromatin modifier of D4Z4, known as FSHD2 (Lemmers et al., 2012; Saconi et al., 2013). FSHD2 also requires at least one copy of *DUX4* to contain the permissive A allele. Finally, heterozygous mutations in DNA methyltransferase 3B (DNMT3B) have recently been described as an alternative cause of D4Z4 hypomethylation and FSHD (van den Boogard, 2016).

FSHD can often be reasonably suspected clinically due to the specific pattern of weakness typical in the disorder—facial, periscapular, and humeral muscles are weak early, with sparing of the deltoid. Asymmetry of the weakness is almost the rule, often leading the clinician to doubt the diagnosis of muscular dystrophy and seek a superimposed peripheral nerve lesion where none exists. Age of onset is commonly in the second decade, but can vary from infancy to well into adulthood. Facial weakness expresses itself as difficulty blowing up balloons or drinking through a straw. The child sleeps with the sclera of the eyes showing through partially opened lids. Facial expression is relatively preserved, but the smile is often flattened and transverse as opposed to the upward curve of the usual smile. When the patient attempts to whistle, the lips move awkwardly and have a peculiar pucker (Fig. 109.18). The mouth also may have a pouting quality called *bouche de tapir*.

Weakness of the shoulder muscles particularly affects fixation of the scapula. Scapular winging is expected; with the arms outstretched in front, the scapulae jut backward, with the inferomedial corner pointing backward. The deltoid muscle, by contrast, is usually bulky and its strength preserved late in the illness. The axillary folds may become horizontal and exaggerated owing to pectoral weakness and atrophy. The biceps and triceps muscles are often weak but the forearm muscles less involved, leading to the characteristic "Popeye arm" appearance. A discrepancy between the stronger wrist flexors and weaker wrist extensors as the disease progresses often supports the diagnosis.

Abdominal and paraspinal muscle weakness is very common. Exaggerated lumbar lordosis or camptocormia may occur and the abdomen may be protuberant. Preferential involvement of the lower (or less commonly the upper) abdominal muscles leads to the Beevor sign—asking the patient to lie supine and lift the head off the bed leads to displacement of the umbilicus upward or downward, away from the weaker abdominal muscles.

Despite the name, leg weakness is also common. Often the ankle dorsiflexors are involved very early in the illness and foot drop may even be the presenting complaint, creating overlap with the scapuloperineal syndromes. Hip flexor and quadriceps weakness are common, but ankle plantarflexion strength is often preserved. Rare patients present with symmetrical proximal leg weakness greater than arm weakness with sparing of facial muscles, such that they resemble an LGMD. Even in severe cases, ptosis, dysphagia, cardiomyopathy, and prominent contractures are not seen and thus should suggest an alternative diagnosis.

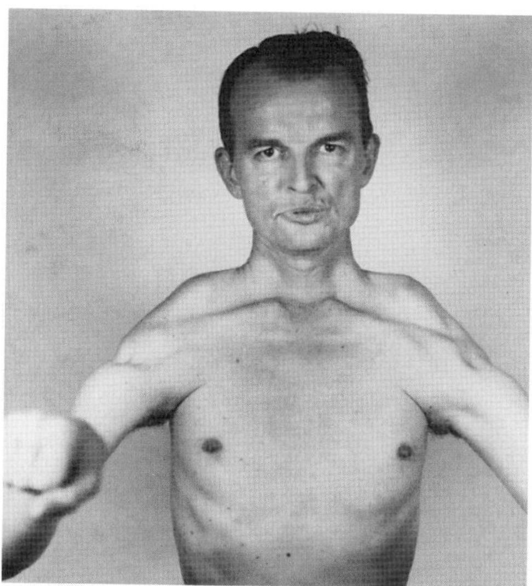

**Fig. 109.18 Facioscapulohumeral Dystrophy.** Note characteristic appearance of shoulders, downward-sloping clavicles, and bulge in trapezius muscle region due to scapula being displaced upward on attempted elevation of arms. Patient also is attempting to purse his lips.

With FSHD1, the severity of the illness bears a relationship to the size of the deletion: the smallest fragments (1–3 repeats) tend to be associated with severe illness. Another phenomenon exhibited by these families is anticipation of the illness, where cases occur with more severity and at a younger age with successive generations (Tawil and Van Der Maarel, 2006). This suggests the mutation is a dynamic one that may become increasingly severe with each generation, as is the case with myotonic dystrophy. That said, FSHD varies in severity even within the same family. Some patients may have mild facial weakness that can go unnoticed throughout life. The most severe form of FSHD, however, begins in infancy. Affected infants may have no movement at all in the face, which remains passive and expressionless. Weakness of the limbs, although it conforms to the general pattern of FSHD, is so severe that such children may lose the ability to walk by 9 or 10 years of age.

Genetic testing is available to confirm the diagnosis of FSHD1 or FSHD2, but may be unnecessary in cases with prototypical weakness and a consistent family history. The serum CK concentration usually is elevated several-fold above normal. Muscle biopsy may show general dystrophic features or tiny fibers scattered throughout the biopsy sample that suggest neuropathic change, or scattered inflammatory cellular foci associated with muscle fibers and in the interstitial tissue in patients with more severe disease (Fig. 109.19). EMG shows myopathic potentials.

Management of FSHD is supportive and includes screening for complications of the disease. The American Academy of Neurology (AAN) produced an evidence-based guideline summary in 2015 to aid clinicians in proper care (Tawil, 2015). Respiratory insufficiency occurs in an estimated 1.25% to 13% of patients, especially in those with spinal deformity or those who are wheelchair bound. Affected patients may not complain of dyspnea, as commonly respiratory insufficiency begins only during sleep—excessive daytime somnolence may be the only clue. Baseline pulmonary function testing is thus recommended at diagnosis and then annually in those with proximal leg weakness.

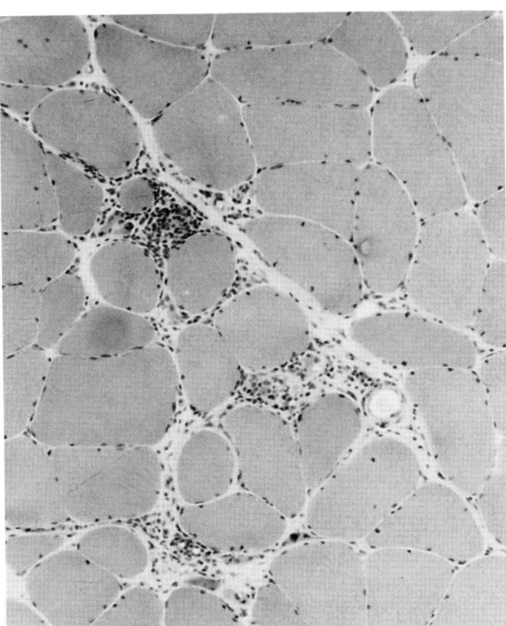

**Fig. 109.19 Facioscapulohumeral Dystrophy.** Cellular responses occur in biopsy samples from many patients with this illness. These are more often associated with necrotic fibers than with blood vessels (hematoxylin and eosin stain).

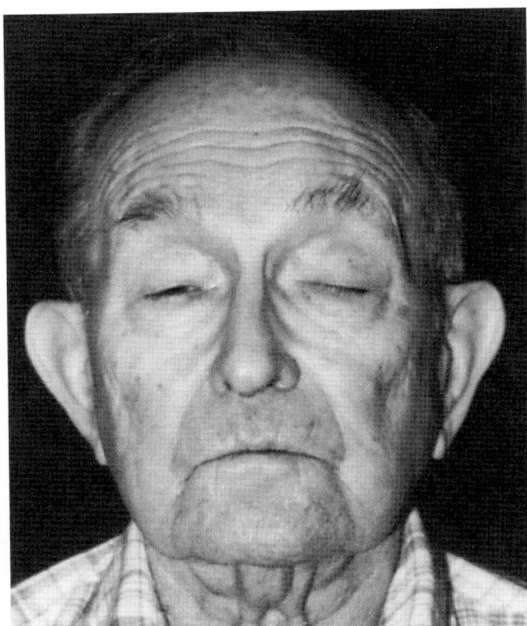

**Fig. 109.20 Oculopharyngeal Dystrophy.** Facial appearance of patient who has ptosis and no eye movements.

In severe cases, there is an association with Coats disease, an oxidative vascular degeneration of the retina. While this affects less than 1% of patients, 25% will have asymptomatic retinal abnormalities evident on examination. A baseline retinal examination is recommended; those with a low repeat number should also be followed longitudinally. Finally, sensorineural hearing loss occurs in severe cases, so affected children should be screened for hearing loss.

Management also includes offering interventions to reduce morbidity and improve functional status. Stretching and range of motion exercises are important. Physical and occupational therapy should be involved early to assist with these, as well as to assess for the need for assist devices. An ankle-foot orthosis may be beneficial for patients with foot drop. If patients have severe weakness of the anterior tibial group, overactivity of the posterior tibial muscle may be seen in an attempt to dorsiflex the foot and allow the toes to clear the ground. This results in marked inversion of the foot while walking and may lead to an equinovarus contracture. It also may make the use of an ankle-foot orthosis impossible. If lack of scapular fixation renders the patient unable to raise the arms above the head, surgical stabilization of the scapula may improve shoulder abduction and forward flexion (Twyman et al., 1996). This is particularly true in the majority of patients with preserved deltoid function. Manual fixation of the scapula at the bedside can be used to assess the potential for benefit prior to surgery. FSHD does not typically affect the life span, but 20% of those above age 50 will be wheelchair dependent.

***Scapuloperoneal syndromes.*** Weakness of the muscles of the shoulder and the anterior compartment of the lower leg is the early symptom of scapuloperoneal syndromes. Some forms of scapuloperoneal dystrophy may relate to FSHD, but most cases show no linkage to the FSH site on 4q35 (Tawil and Van Der Maarel, 2006). EDMD produces a scapuloperoneal pattern of weakness, as well. Mutations in the desmin gene on chromosome 2q35 and *FHL1* on Xq26.3 have been demonstrated to cause some cases of scapuloperoneal dystrophy; these are also categorized as myofibrillar myopathies (Narayanaswami et al., 2014). In FSHD, a discrepancy exists between the strength of the ankle dorsiflexors, which are weak, and the plantar flexors, which are strong. The same is true of the scapuloperoneal syndrome, but facial muscles are spared. Often the patient presents with a foot drop, and examination reveals the shoulder weakness. Biopsy, EMG, and other laboratory tests reveal nonspecific myopathic features. Because other hereditary scapuloperoneal syndromes due to neuropathy and anterior horn cell disease exist, it is important to confirm the diagnosis with appropriate tests in any patient with a scapuloperoneal syndrome. Preservation or even hypertrophy of the extensor digitorum brevis (used to compensate for tibialis anterior weakness) is a clinical clue toward a myopathic etiology, as this would be unlikely in a neurogenic foot drop. Ankle-foot orthoses are the only useful treatment and may improve function by correcting foot drop.

***Oculopharyngeal muscular dystrophy.*** Oculopharyngeal muscular dystrophy (OPMD) is an inherited autosomal dominant disorder with almost complete penetrance. It has an uneven geographical distribution, with foci of cases in Quebec, Germany, Uruguay (Montevideo), and the Spanish-American populations of Colorado, New Mexico, and Arizona. Isolated families also appear throughout the rest of the world. The disease is caused by an expansion of GCG repeats in the gene that encodes for polyadenylate-binding protein nuclear 1 (*PABPN1*, formerly *PABP2*) located on chromosome 14q11.2-13 (Brais et al., 1995; Stajich et al., 1996). This nuclear protein is involved in mRNA polyadenylation, but the mechanisms by which mutations cause OPMD are not yet clear.

OPMD usually begins in the fifth or sixth decade of life, but onset can be in the fourth decade. Longer *PABPN1* expansions are correlated with an earlier age of onset (Richard, 2017). Patients present with extraocular muscle weakness and mild ptosis. Initially the ptosis may be quite asymmetrical, but as the muscles weaken, both lids eventually become severely ptotic, and eye movements diminish in all directions (Fig. 109.20). Considerable variation in the severity of the extraocular palsies exists, but ptosis is constant. Concomitant with or shortly after the development of ocular symptoms, patients notice difficulty swallowing. Saliva pools in the pharynx, and at the extreme stages of the illness, dysphagia may be complete. Facial weakness occurs in a number of patients, and hip and shoulder weakness are common in the late stages. Death may occur from emaciation and starvation. The

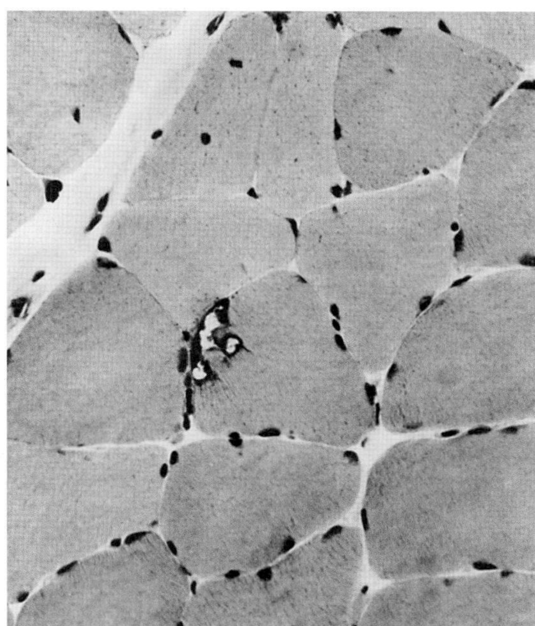

**Fig. 109.21 Oculopharyngeal Dystrophy.** Rimmed vacuoles are common in this illness (hematoxylin and eosin stain).

terminal event is often pneumonia initiated by aspiration of secretions. Although the symptoms associated with this disease may be severe, patients' life spans may be unaffected, making management of their nutritional status all the more important.

Muscle biopsy can usually be avoided, since genetic testing reveals the diagnosis. However, biopsy of weak muscles may show dystrophic findings, random variation in fiber size, necrotic fibers, some fibrosis, and occasional internal nuclei. In addition, fibers may contain autophagic vacuoles (rimmed vacuoles) (Fig. 109.21), a feature common to this illness as well as to IBM and various hereditary distal myopathies/dystrophies.

A hallmark of the illness is the presence of small 8- to 10-nm intranuclear tubulofilaments (Blumen, 1999). These occur as palisading filamentous inclusions. The filaments are unbranched and may be stacked side by side or may occur in tangles. In addition, there is often evidence of abnormal mitochondria as well as nemaline rods, particularly in pharyngeal muscles. PABPN1 is an integral part of the muscle OPMD inclusions. The inclusions also contain components of the ubiquitin-proteasome pathway, transcription factors, and mRNA-binding proteins.

Treatment of OPMD is supportive. The swallowing difficulties should be treated first by a soft diet; pureed foods represent the next step in treatment. Feeding with a nasogastric tube may be a temporary solution, but eventually gastrostomy is essential. Surgery to correct ptosis may be very successful, as opposed to results seen in other causes of ptosis such as myasthenia gravis or Kearns-Sayre syndrome (KSS).

## Distal Muscular Dystrophies/Distal Myopathies

Several muscle diseases show a predominantly distal pattern of weakness (Narayanaswami et al., 2014; Udd, 2009). Initial diagnosis of the distal myopathies is often a hereditary or acquired neuropathy or motor neuron disease, because distal dysfunction is more characteristic of neuropathic disorders. Mild elevations in serum CK occur in neuropathic disorders, but CK concentrations over 500 IU/L should raise suspicion of a myopathic process. Serum CK concentrations can be normal in some distal myopathies; therefore CK alone does not exclude a myopathy. EMG distinguishes a distal myopathy from a neuropathic disorder. Furthermore, myasthenia gravis can rarely present with predominantly distal weakness, so repetitive nerve stimulation can also be helpful. Treatment of distal myopathy is largely symptomatic. In a patient with a severe wrist drop, a cock-up splint may be helpful to preserve hand function. Similarly, an ankle-foot orthosis may treat the foot drop.

Several classically described distal myopathy syndromes are described below. Although not described in detail below, mutations in Kelch-like homologue-9 (*KLHL9*) and adenylosuccinate synthetase-like 1 (*ADSSL1*) have also been shown to lead to distal myopathy beginning in childhood. With the discovery of the genetic underpinning of these disorders, many have been found to be allelic with forms of LGMD and other disorders. Likewise, mutations in genes most commonly associated with limb–girdle phenotypes—*DNAJB6*, *MYOT*, *DES*, and *CAV3*, for example, discussed previously—have also been shown to occasionally cause a distally predominant pattern of weakness. Other myopathies associated with distal weakness include myotonic dystrophy type 1, IBM, sarcoid myopathy, focal myositis, and certain late-onset forms of congenital myopathy (e.g., centronuclear and nemaline myopathies, especially in association with *NEB*, *ACTA1*, and *RYR1* mutations). Age of onset, inheritance pattern, histopathology, and pattern of weakness are most useful in distinguishing the distal myopathies from one another. As genetic testing technology has improved and become more affordable, next-generation sequencing panels encompassing many genes have improved diagnostic yield over targeted single-gene testing (Amandine et al., 2016). Clinical and histopathological findings may still be useful when interpreting VUS or if no pathogenic mutation is found.

***Miyoshi myopathy.*** Inherited as an autosomal recessive disease, Miyoshi myopathy begins early, often in adolescence (Bejaoui et al., 1995). Mutations in the dysferlin gene that also cause LGMD2B were initially found to be responsible for Miyoshi myopathy, but subsequently mutations in the *ANO5* gene that also cause LGMD2L have been found to cause a Miyoshi phenotype (Narayanaswami et al., 2014). The weakness is characteristically in the foot plantar flexors, with severe gastrocnemius atrophy. This causes a thin, tapering leg. Patients are unable to stand on their toes, and they walk up stairs in a clumsy, jerky fashion. The illness is progressive, although it remains confined to the legs. Ultimately, hip weakness develops, and ambulation may become difficult in midlife. The serum CK concentration is extremely elevated and reaches levels of several thousand international units even before the patient becomes symptomatic. Families exist in which some members exhibit a distal myopathy and others the more traditional proximal variety. The muscle biopsy shows dystrophic changes but no autophagic vacuoles.

***Welander myopathy.*** This autosomal dominant myopathy has only been reported in Scandinavians, where it remains relatively common. Welander myopathy begins in the hands (finger and wrist drop) around age 40–60 and later involves the legs and feet (foot drop) (Narayanaswami et al., 2014). The disease is not entirely restricted to muscle. Careful evaluation may show mild distal hypesthesia and temperature loss associated with some loss of small myelinated fibers. Electrodiagnostic testing, however, shows little evidence of denervation and ample evidence of myopathy. Muscle biopsy shows myopathic findings, superimposed on which are the rimmed vacuoles characteristic of several other distal myopathies. Serum CK concentration is normal or slightly elevated. Welander myopathy is caused by mutations in T-cell-restricted intracellular antigen (*TIA1*) which is in the RNA-binding protein (Hackman et al., 2012). A particular variant in *TIA1* has been shown to cause a similar phenotype only in the presence of a second mutation in the *SQSTM1* gene. *SQSTM1* links to Paget disease of bone, as well (Niu, 2018).

***Udd myopathy.*** Udd myopathy is due to mutations in titin as discussed previously, and thus allelic with LGMD2J and HMERF. It is an autosomal dominant, adult-onset (fifth or seventh decade) dystrophy with predilection for anterior tibial muscles. Patients present with progressive foot drop typically beginning after age 35 (Hackman et al., 2002; Narayanaswami et al., 2014). Unlike other titinopathies, cardiomyopathy is rare. Serum CK concentration is normal or only slightly elevated. Muscle biopsies in Udd myopathy often demonstrate rimmed vacuoles.

***Markesbery-Griggs myopathy.*** Markesbery-Griggs myopathy is caused by mutations in *ZASP* as mentioned in the MFM section and presents with progressive foot drop, usually after age 35, and its inheritance is autosomal dominant. Over time, proximal leg and distal arm weakness (wrist and finger extensors) develops (Griggs et al., 2007; Narayanaswami et al., 2014). Cardiomyopathy is common.

Serum CK concentration is normal or usually only slightly increased. The ECG may demonstrate conduction defects or arrhythmia. An echocardiogram may reveal a dilated or hypertrophic cardiomyopathy. EMG demonstrates markedly increased insertional and spontaneous activity with fibrillation potentials, positive sharp waves, and myotonic discharges. Motor units are myopathic in morphology and recruit early. Muscle biopsies demonstrate fibers with rimmed vacuoles and other features seen in the myofibrillar myopathies (Selcen and Carpén, 2008). Therefore Markesbery-Griggs myopathy can be classified as one of the myofibrillar myopathies (Narayanaswami et al., 2014), discussed in greater detail previously.

***GNE myopathy (Nonaka myopathy/autosomal recessive hereditary inclusion body myopathy).*** Nonaka and colleagues initially described this early adult-onset distal myopathy in Japan. Other groups reported similar patients with so-called autosomal recessive hIBM (Udd, 2009). The clinical phenotype is similar to that of Markesbery-Griggs and Udd myopathies, with weakness initially involving the anterior tibial muscles in the legs and extensor forearm muscles (Narayanaswami et al., 2014). However, inheritance is in an autosomal recessive fashion and onset occurs at less than 30 years of age. The muscle biopsy results are also quite similar to those of Markesbery-Griggs, Udd, and Welander myopathies in that rimmed vacuoles are observed. Further EM reveals 15- to 18-nm tubular filaments typical of IBM. However, unlike IBM, no significant inflammatory process occurs in this hIBM.

Nonaka myopathy/autosomal recessive inclusion body myopathy is caused by mutations in the gene encoding for UDP-*N*-acetylglucosamine-2-epimerase/*N*-acetylmannosamine kinase, or *GNE,* on chromosome 9p1-q1 (Eisenberg et al., 2001). The recommended term for this disorder is now GNE myopathy. The mechanisms by which mutations in this gene lead to the myopathy are unknown but may relate to a secondary reduction in sialic acid production.

***Laing myopathy.*** This autosomal dominant distal myopathy is characterized by weakness of the anterior tibial muscle groups and the neck flexors (Laing et al., 1995; Narayanaswami et al., 2014). Onset is in childhood or early adult life. Serum CK concentrations are normal or only slightly elevated, and EMG is myopathic. Cardiomyopathy is sometimes the initial symptom. Unlike Markesbery-Griggs myopathy, Udd myopathy, and Nonaka myopathy/hIBM, rimmed vacuoles are not a feature of the muscle specimen in Laing distal myopathy. Mutations in the slow/beta cardiac myosin heavy chain 1 (*MyHC1*) gene or *MYH7* located on chromosome 14q11 are causative (Lamont et al., 2006). *MyHC* is the major myosin isoform expressed in type 1 muscle fibers. Of note, *MYH7* mutations have also been identified in hyaline body myopathy (discussed later in Congenital Myopathies) (Tajsharghi et al., 2003).

***Williams myopathy.*** This myopathy is associated with onset in the teens to fifth decade of life of predominantly lower extremity weakness that can affect proximal or distal muscles either in the arms or legs initially (Duff et al., 2011; Guergueltcheva et al., 2011; Luan et al., 2010; Narayanaswami et al., 2014; Williams et al., 2005). Some patients develop a cardiomyopathy. Serum CK is usually mildly elevated and EMG is myopathic. Muscle biopsies may reveal features of MFM.

***Vocal cord pharyngeal distal myopathy.*** This autosomal dominant myopathy typically presents in the third to fourth decade of life with preferential weakness of ankle dorsiflexion and wrist/finger extension (Feit et al., 1998; Muller et al., 2014). Weakness of the pharyngeal and vocal cord muscles is also characteristic, but not universal. As the disease progresses, respiratory muscle weakness is common. Serum CK can be normal or moderately elevated and myopathic features are commonly noted on EMG. Muscle biopsy typically reveals rimmed vacuoles; electron microscopy can show nuclei with abnormal invaginations. Mutations in the *MATR3* gene encoding matrin-3 protein have been found to be responsible (Senderek et al., 2009). Matrin-3 is a nuclear matrix protein; *MATR3* mutations have also been reported to cause amyotrophic lateral sclerosis.

### Multisystem Proteinopathy

Multisystem proteinopathy is an autosomal dominant inherited degenerative disorder that can affect multiple body systems including muscle, bone, and the CNS (Taylor, 2015). This spectrum of disease was first described with the name hIBM with Paget disease of bone and frontotemporal dementia (IBMPFD), in association with mutations in valosin-containing protein (VCP). This is a ubiquitously expressed ATPase; pathogenic mutations lead to accumulation of proteinaceous material in various body tissues, explaining the wide range of clinical phenotypes. The name multisystem proteinopathy was suggested to replace IBMPFD, as the spectrum of consequences has been shown to include type 2 CMT, parkinsonism, and motor neuron disease. An identical spectrum of disease has since been shown in association with mutations in *HNRNPA1, HNRNPA2B1,* and *SQSTM1* (Bucelli et al., 2015; Kim et al., 2013).

The myopathy that can occur in association with multisystem proteinopathy is heterogeneous, including limb–girdle and scapuloperoneal patterns of weakness. The distal form tends to preferentially ankle dorsiflexion and may be asymmetric. The onset of weakness is adultonset, typically in the 40s. Serum CK levels are normal to slightly elevated. Those with Paget disease of bone may have an elevated alkaline phosphatase. Muscle biopsy reveals rimmed vacuoles as well as inclusions that stain for ubiquitin and TDP-43. Neurogenic features such as type grouping can also be seen, perhaps due to the ability of these mutations to cause motor neuron disease.

### Myotonic Dystrophies

***Myotonic dystrophy type 1.*** Myotonic dystrophy type 1 (dystrophic myotonia type 1 or DM1) is a trinucleotide repeat disorder that affects both muscle and numerous other body systems. In addition to muscle wasting and weakness, myotonia—impaired relaxation of muscle—is characteristic of the disease. Myotonia can also be seen in some nondystrophic ion channelopathies (see below). DM1 is inherited in an autosomal dominant fashion and has an incidence of approximately 1/3000–8000 live births (Ashizawa et al., 2018). The myopathy is caused by mutations in the gene that encodes for myotonic dystrophy protein kinase (*DMPK*), located on chromosome 19q13.3. The mutation occurs in an untranslated region of the gene. This region normally contains 5–30 repeating sequences of three nucleotides (CTG

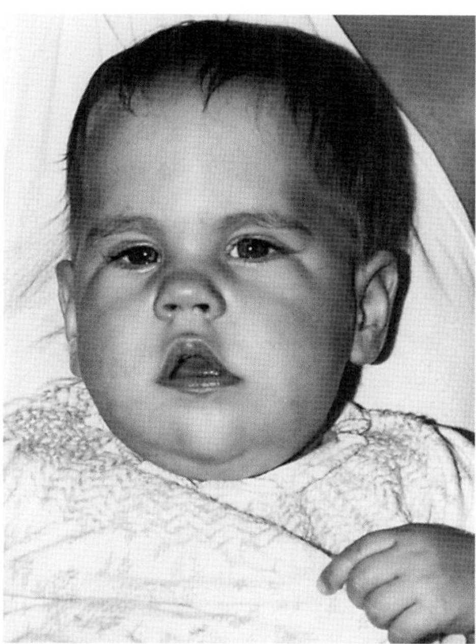

**Fig. 109.22 Infantile Myotonic Dystrophy.** This child is severely intellectually disabled and has a marked inverted-V mouth.

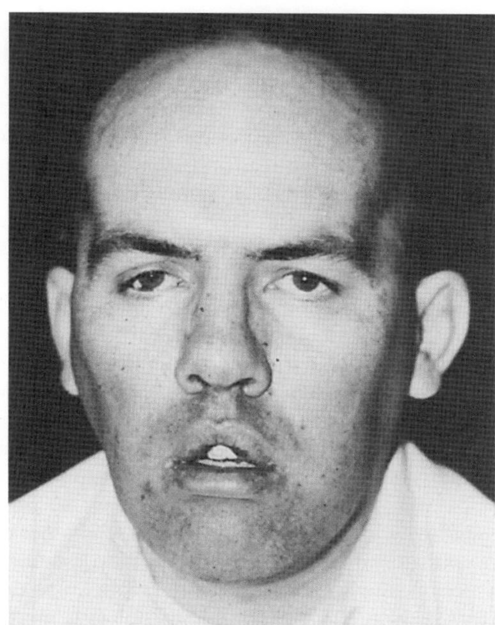

**Fig. 109.23 Myotonic Dystrophy Type 1.** Facial appearance includes ptosis, hollowing of the masseter and temples, and facial weakness.

trinucleotide repeats). In DM1, these CTG repeats expand into the hundreds or thousands.

In general, the size of the expansion reflects the severity of the illness. Children with severe congenital myotonic dystrophy may have very large expansions (>750 repeats). Mothers with more than 100 repeats are more at risk for having a child with this severe infantile form. Cardinal features are hypotonia, facial paralysis, failure to thrive, and feeding difficulties. Affected infants are prone to frequent respiratory infections, which may develop into pneumonia. The upper lip forms an inverted V or "shark mouth" (Fig. 109.22). Clubfeet are common, and the children are severely intellectually disabled. The tendency of the expansion to grow with each meiosis explains the phenomenon of anticipation, in which succeeding generations experience the illness earlier and more severely. The reverse is true of some rare patients with paternally inherited myotonic dystrophy, in which the expansion reduces in size and the clinical state may return to normal or near normal. Further complicating the issue of relating the severity of the phenotype to the genetic defect is the fact that the degree of the gene's expansion may vary among the different tissues in the body.

The mutation is not in the coding region of the gene, and other experiments with knockout mice or mice that overexpress the protein show no marked abnormality in the muscle or other systems. Studies have demonstrated that the transcribed mRNA is directly toxic, in part by sequestering RNA-binding proteins such as muscle-blind protein, thereby leading to abnormal splicing of various mRNA transcripts, including those of the muscle chloride ion channel (Mankodi et al., 2002; Mulders et al., 2009; Osborne et al., 2009; Wheeler and Thornton, 2007).

Few diseases are as easy to recognize as DM1 once the diagnosis is considered. Conversely, misdiagnosis occurs when the presenting complaint may be unrelated to the basic problem. Patients may present to many different specialists—cardiologists for heart block, gastroenterologists for gastric dysmotility, and developmental pediatricians for intellectual disability. The severity of DM1 ranges from mild weakness in some adults to profound intellectual disability and severe weakness in children.

The typical picture is of an illness beginning in early teenage life, starting with noticeable weakness of the hands and often foot drop. DM1 is one of the rare forms of dystrophy that seems to affect the distal muscles more severely. A predilection for neck muscle involvement exists, and the sternocleidomastoid muscles are often atrophic and poorly defined. A rather long face with a mournful expression is accentuated by hollowing of the temples associated with masseter and temporalis atrophy. In the fully developed disease, the eyes are hooded and the mouth slack and often tented (Fig. 109.23). The muscular weakness is not limited to the distal muscles; shoulder, hip, and leg weakness may be quite prominent.

In middle age, repeated falls are common. With time, the weakness of individual muscles becomes severe, and the myotonia may be lost. Patients with advanced disease may have no myotonia of the small muscles of the hand, although pronounced myotonia of the deltoids or forearm muscles exists. The voice alters; it may be hollow and echoing, suggesting palatal weakness. Facial weakness makes it difficult to pronounce consonants. Difficulty in swallowing is common but usually a minor complaint. Recurrent dislocation of the jaw occurs, particularly when the patient attempts to open the mouth wide, as in biting an apple.

The demonstration of myotonia is either by sharp percussion of the muscle with a reflex hammer or after firm voluntary contraction. Either maneuver elicits a sustained involuntary contraction of the muscle, which fades slowly over a matter of seconds. Percussion of the thenar eminence, a popular way of eliciting myotonia, produces a sharp abduction of the thumb and a firm contraction of the thenar eminence, which gradually relaxes and allows the thumb to return to the resting position. It is often easier to demonstrate percussion myotonia by percussion of the posterior muscles of the forearm. The normal response to percussion of the forearm is also a brisk contraction of the finger extensors or the wrist extensors, but the wrist or fingers then fall into the resting position without delay. In the myotonic patient, the fingers extend sharply, with a subsequent drift downward toward the normal position or even wrist extension that maintains for some seconds. Patients seldom complain spontaneously about myotonia, but when questioned, they may confess to finding it difficult to release a key after firmly grasping it or to let go of a hammer or vacuum cleaner, particularly in cold weather.

Cardiac disease is a common complication of DM1. Conduction disturbances and tachyarrhythmias occur commonly in addition to cardiomyopathy. The cardiomyopathy correlates in severity with the neuromuscular disease and the extent of the molecular defect in some but not all studies; the rate of progression differs widely among individuals. Sudden death is not infrequent in these patients, and may be caused by ventricular arrhythmias or complete heart block. This can even occur at an early stage of disease. Some studies show a familial tendency toward cardiac complications. The histopathology is of fibrosis (primarily in the conducting system and sinoatrial node), myocyte hypertrophy, and fatty infiltration (Phillips and Harper, 1997). EM shows prominent I-bands and myofibrillar degeneration.

Excessive daytime somnolence is a common problem in DM1 (Damian et al., 2001; Giubilei et al., 1999). The uncontrollable urge to sleep may be mistaken for narcolepsy. It is accompanied by a disturbance of the nighttime sleep pattern. Patients have an abnormal central ventilatory response, without the usual hyperpnea produced by an increasing carbon dioxide concentration. This is associated with an abnormal sensitivity to barbiturates, morphine, and other drugs that depress the ventilatory drive. General anesthetic carries some risks, and the occurrence of complications, usually respiratory, was almost 10% in one series (Mathieu et al., 1997). Anesthesiologists must be aware of the possibility of complications with these drugs. Likewise, women with DM1 are at increased risk of complications during pregnancy and delivery (Ashizawa et al., 2018). In addition to complications from analgesics and sedating medications, respiratory insufficiency and failed labor can occur. A high-risk obstetrician-gynecologist (OB-GYN) obstetrics/gynecology provider should be involved in these women's care.

Several other organs are commonly involved in the disease. Cognitive impairment is common, including executive dysfunction and visuospatial processing, and is progressive through adulthood (Gallais et al., 2017). Neurobehavioral abnormalities are also common. Cataracts are almost universal. Detection may only be by slit-lamp examination. Commonly, multihued specks appear in the anterior and posterior subcapsular zones. Endocrine abnormalities include disturbances of the thyroid, pancreas, hypothalamus, and gonads. Testicular atrophy, with disappearance of the seminiferous tubules, leads to male infertility. In the female, habitual abortion and menstrual irregularities are common. Although diabetes mellitus is no more common in the myotonic population than in the general population, a glucose tolerance test is often associated with abnormally high glucose levels, particularly late in the test. An associated overproduction of insulin seems to be due to abnormal resistance of the insulin receptor. Smooth muscle involvement accounts for several problems. Cholecystitis and symptoms referable to gallbladder function are frequent. Mild dysphagia and decreased peristalsis in the hypopharynx and proximal esophagus are present. Patients often complain of constipation and urinary tract symptoms.

DNA analysis is the definitive diagnostic test for myotonic dystrophy. Patients with clinical evidence of disease and individuals at risk require testing. Prenatal diagnosis is reliable and uses chorionic villus biopsies or cultured amniotic cells. Once a diagnosis of myotonic dystrophy has been established in one family member, other family members require genetic screening.

When clinical suspicion is not high enough to proceed straight to genetic testing, EMG is the most helpful laboratory study. In addition to the presence of myopathic features, the characteristic myotonic discharges are seen (see Chapter 36). On insertion of the needle, bursts of repetitive potentials are noted. These potentials wax and wane in both amplitude and frequency; when played over a loudspeaker, they resemble the sound of a diving propeller airplane and are called *dive bomber* or *motorcycle potentials*. Muscle biopsy in the fully developed illness is markedly abnormal (Figs. 109.24 and 109.25), demonstrating random variability in the size of fibers and fibrosis. In addition, multiple nuclei pepper the interior of the fibers. Ring fibers are numerous, in which small bundles of myofibrils are oriented at 90 degrees to the majority, rather like a thread wrapped around a stick. Other laboratory studies are less helpful. Serum CK is often abnormal. Some patients demonstrate low levels of immunoglobulin G. Abnormalities seen on

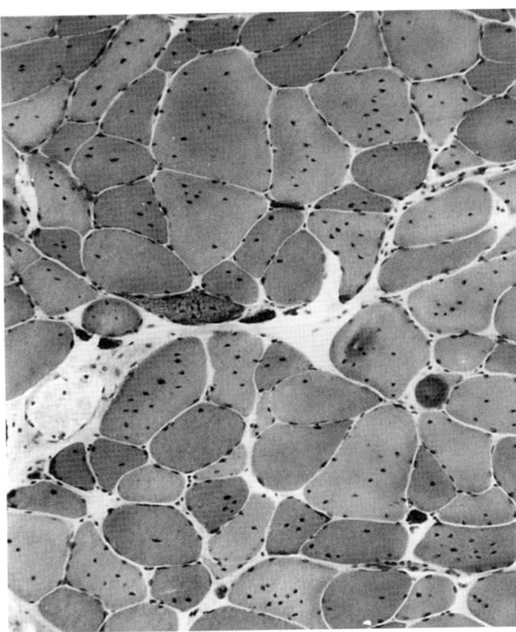

**Fig. 109.24** Myotonic Dystrophy Type 1. There are numerous internal nuclei, some scattered pyknotic nuclear clumps, and marked variability in fiber size. One ring fiber can be identified by its circular dark-staining appearance (hematoxylin and eosin stain).

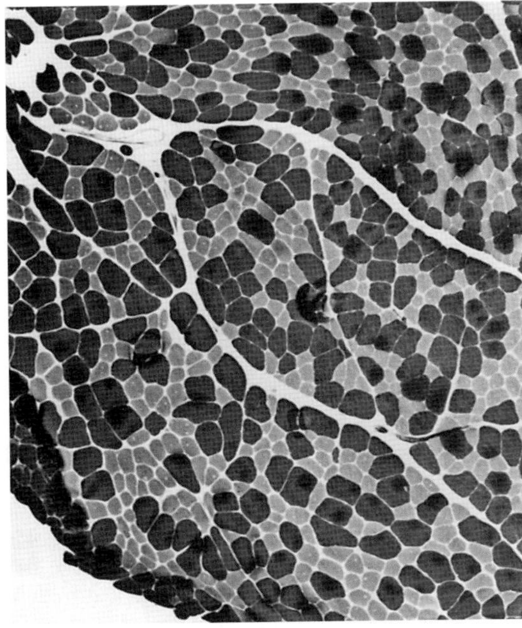

**Fig. 109.25** Myotonic Dystrophy Type 1. Myosin adenosine triphosphatase stain at pH 9.4 demonstrates that the majority of type 1 fibers are small. Type 1 fiber atrophy is noted in early cases and is obscured as the disease becomes more severe.

head MRI include cerebral atrophy, increased white-matter signals on T2-weighted images, and thickening of the cranial vault (Miaux et al., 1997). These abnormalities have little significance.

The Myotonic Dystrophy Foundation recently supported the release of expert consensus based guidelines for the supportive management of DM1 (Ashizawa et al., 2018). Because of the potential for sudden death or other serious cardiac complications even in asymptomatic patients, cardiac surveillance and management is of utmost importance. Suggestions for clinical management include a careful cardiac history and a 12-lead ECG at least every year, with a low threshold for use of 24-hour Holter monitoring. Referral to cardiology for co-management is recommended once patients develop symptoms, ECG abnormalities, or reach the age of 40. Patients may require antiarrhythmics, a pacemaker, or ICD placement. Perhaps because of vigilance regarding the cardiac manifestations of the disease, pulmonary complications are now the leading cause of death in DM1 patients. Regular monitoring of pulmonary function testing is recommended. A sleep study should be obtained in those with symptoms suggestive of sleep apnea; nocturnal ventilatory support may be required. Annual eye examinations are advised to monitor for cataracts.

Ankle-foot orthoses can be used to treat foot drop. Wrist splints are less useful. Moderate intensity exercise may be helpful. The sodium-channel blocker mexiletine was shown in a double-blind randomized placebo-controlled trial to be effective at reducing grip myotonia as measured by relaxation time (Logigian et al., 2010). Other drugs that can be used include quinine, phenytoin, procainamide, and acetazolamide. These are typically avoided in those with cardiac involvement. Patients are typically bothered more by weakness than myotonia, so their clinical utility may be modest. Modafinil, 200–400 mg/day, CTD improves hypersomnolence in DM1 patients (Damian et al., 2001).

***Myotonic dystrophy type 2 or proximal myotonic myopathy.*** Whereas DM1 has a predilection for distal muscles, patients with proximal myotonic myopathy (PROMM) experience proximal stiffness, pain, and weakness (Moxley, 1996; Udd et al., 1997). Like DM1, PROMM is an autosomal dominant trait, and cataracts are characteristic. Gonadal atrophy and cardiac abnormalities occur, but less frequently than in DM1.

Initial complaints usually arise in adult life and are a combination of muscle stiffness and unusual muscle pain, which commonly affects the thighs and may be asymmetrical. Grip myotonia is noted, and the relaxation phase is jerky. The severity of the myotonia may vary from day to day, and a "warm-up" phenomenon occurs in which the stiffness disappears after repeated contraction and relaxation. The pain is a sense of discomfort and varies from sharp to a deep visceral ache.

Prognosis is relatively good. Individuals with PROMM do not show the slow decline in ability and early cardiorespiratory death so often noted in myotonic dystrophy, but cardiac involvement can occur in a minority. Cataracts, frontal balding, and diabetes are all common associated features. EMG shows myotonic discharges only after a careful search in several muscles. Muscle biopsy shows features similar to DM1. Serum CK concentration may be elevated.

The genetic defect has been localized to mutations in the gene that encodes for zinc finger 9 (*ZNF9*) on chromosome 3q21 (Liquori et al., 2001). The mutations are expanded CCTG repeats in intron 1. As with DM1, this expanded repeat leads to expression of a toxic pre-mRNA, which as in DM1, sequesters RNA-binding proteins, leading to aberrant splicing of other mRNA species including those of ion channels (Mulders et al., 2009; Osborne et al., 2009; Wheeler and Thornton, 2007).

## Ion Channelopathies

A group of illnesses that range from myotonic syndromes to the periodic paralyses results from abnormalities in ion channels (Cannon, 2010; Matthews et al., 2010). The molecular basis for these illnesses reorients classification. The ion channels are fundamentally important in controlling the passage of ions across the cell membrane and in the shift of ions from one cell compartment to another. These proteins are associated with the cell membrane and are responsible for such phenomena as the muscle action potential. Electrical potential across the cell membrane (voltage-gated) or by ligands such as glutamate influence the proteins. Segments of these proteins have amino acid sequences that are remarkably similar across a wide range of species (conserved segments). It is logical that any change in the conserved segment of a protein might produce trouble for the organism. Some of these mutations are presumably lethal, affecting as they do such an important functional component of the cell. Other mutations may produce intermittent symptoms (e.g., the periodic paralyses).

In skeletal muscle, sarcolemmal voltage-gated calcium channels are responsible for excitation-contraction coupling. These are called L-type because of their long-lasting effect and are sensitive to dihydropyridines such as nifedipine. The calcium channel in muscle is made of five subunits: $\alpha_1$, which is the most important and forms the ion pore across the membrane; $\alpha_2$, $\beta$, $\gamma$, and $\delta$. The type of $\alpha_1$ subunit determines the sensitivity of the calcium channel. The subunit is formed from four similar transmembrane regions (domains D1–D4), each made of six membrane-spanning proteins, S1–S6, all linked in series by "loops" that extend into the cytoplasm or extracellularly; S4 is highly charged by virtue of the richness of positively charged amino acids. It may confer voltage sensitivity to the channel. Neurological conditions linked to abnormalities in the L-type calcium channel include hypokalemic periodic paralysis (Cannon, 2010; Matthews et al., 2010).

The ryanodine receptor controls the flux of calcium from the sarcoplasmic reticulum into the cytoplasm, thus playing an important part in activating the contractile mechanism of muscle. The subtype in skeletal muscle is RYR1. The ryanodine receptor is associated with the L-type calcium channel, such that when the calcium channel opens, the ryanodine receptor opens, as well. Ryanodine receptors are made of four identical subunits, each of which is approximately 550 kD. Mutations in the ryanodine receptor are associated with central core myopathy, malignant hyperthermia, and late-onset axial myopathy (e.g., bent spine syndrome).

The sodium channel is structurally very similar to the calcium channel. The $\alpha$ subunit, a 260-kD protein, confers the sodium channel activity with four domains made of six membrane-spanning proteins connected in similar fashion. Again, the S4 segment is highly charged, which might make it suitable for responding to voltage changes. Mutations in a gene for the sodium channel are the most common cause of hyperkalemic periodic paralysis and paramyotonia congenita. Some families with hypokalemic periodic paralysis (hypoKPP type 2) have mutations in the sodium channel (Bulman et al., 1999).

Defects in the chloride channel occur in some patients with either autosomal dominant or recessive myotonia congenita. The chloride channel has a different structure, being a homotetramer in which each unit contains approximately 1000 amino acids.

Finally, the potassium channels are the most ubiquitous and diverse group of ion channels. They are composed of monotetramers or heterotetramers of four $\alpha$ subunits. Mutations in various $K^+$ channel genes have been associated with hypokalemic periodic paralysis and Andersen-Tawil syndrome.

### Calcium Channel Abnormalities (Familial Hypokalemic Periodic Paralysis Type 1)

The inheritance of familial hypokalemic periodic paralysis is autosomal dominant. Most affected patients (hypoKPP1) have mutations in the *CACL1A3* gene, which encodes for the $\alpha_1$ subunit of the dihydropyridine-sensitive calcium channel located on chromosome 1q31-32.

In hypoKPP2, mutations are found in the *SCNA4A* sodium channel gene, which is more commonly associated with hyperKPP, paramyotonia congenita, and the potassium-aggravated myotonias. Most mutations in hypoKPP1 and hypoKPP2 involve the voltage-sensitive S4 segment of domains 2 and 4, resulting in a substitution of histidine for arginine. The mechanisms for the episodic weakness in hypoKPP are not completely understood, but these substitutions may result in aberrant depolarization via the proton gating pore during attacks (Cannon, 2010).

The onset of familial hypoKPP is most common in the second decade. The attacks of weakness begin with a sensation of heaviness or aching in the legs or back. This sensation gradually increases and is associated with weakness of the proximal muscles. Distal weakness may occur as the attack develops. The paralysis may be severe enough that the patient cannot get up from bed or raise the head from the pillow. Severe compromise of respiratory muscles is unusual, although a mild decrease in respiratory function may occur. At the height of the weakness, the muscle is electrically and mechanically inexcitable, and reflexes are lost. The muscles feel swollen and may be firm to palpation. Usually an attack lasts for several hours, even up to a day, and the patient's strength returns as suddenly as it left. Often a mild residual weakness clears more slowly, and permanent weakness may ensue. The attacks vary in both severity and frequency and may occur as often as several times a week but usually are isolated and separated by weeks to months. Because the disorder probably is associated with a shift in potassium, provocative factors include heavy exercise followed by a period of sleep or rest, a heavy carbohydrate load, or any other cause of increased insulin secretion. The attack often has a morning onset after waking, probably because a movement of ions such as potassium across the muscle membrane occurs during sleep. Epinephrine, norepinephrine, and corticosteroids may have a provocative effect. Attacks are most common in the third and fourth decades of life. Spontaneous improvement may occur with age.

During an attack, the serum potassium concentration falls. The weakness may commence at serum potassium concentrations at the low end of normal and become quite profound by the time the serum potassium concentration reaches 2–2.5 mEq/L. Bradycardia and ECG changes may occur. Prolongation of the PR and QT intervals and T-wave flattening are associated with prominent U waves. In patients with complete paralysis, motor nerve conduction studies may show reduced amplitudes or absent compound muscle action potentials (CMAPs). The paralyzed muscle shows no electrical activity on EMG. Between attacks, exercise testing can be helpful. Baseline ulnar CMAPs are recorded, then the patient is first instructed to exercise the muscle for 5 minutes. In half of patients, CMAPs recorded at 1-minute intervals during the exercise period demonstrate an increment of the CMAP amplitudes. Thereafter, continued periodic recording of CMAPs reveals significant decrement 10–20 minutes following exercise (Fournier et al., 2004, 2006). The test is not specific for subtype of channelopathy; however, genetic testing is available to confirm the specific diagnosis.

Muscle histology may be normal but usually shows myopathic changes. A common feature of familial hypokalemic periodic paralysis is the presence of vacuoles within the fibers, particularly in association with permanent weakness. Tubular aggregates are a feature of hypokalemic periodic paralysis caused by sodium channel mutations.

Attacks of paralysis should be treated with oral potassium. Renal function must be normal before administering potassium to a patient with paralysis. Preventive treatment has traditionally relied on acetazolamide. This drug, a carbonic anhydrase inhibitor, may produce a mild metabolic acidosis, which perhaps influences the potassium shifts that occur in the disease. Side effects of acetazolamide include tingling in the digits and a tendency for the formation of kidney stones. Hypersensitivity reactions also occur. The FDA recently approved dichlorphenamide, also a carbonic anhydrase inhibitor, specifically for treatment of both hypoKPP and hyperKPP based on a randomized, double-blind, placebo-controlled trial demonstrating significant reduction in attack frequency in patients with hypoKPP (Sansone et al., 2016). Triamterene or spironolactone is useful as an adjunctive treatment along with a low-sodium or low-carbohydrate diet for maximum effect.

### Secondary Hypokalemic Paralysis

Thyrotoxic periodic paralysis is more common in Asians and affects men more frequently than women. Inheritance is autosomal dominant and has been associated with mutations in two genes that encode for two different potassium channel proteins (Ryan et al., 2010; Wang et al., 2014).

Kidney failure or adrenal failure may be associated with changes in potassium. Renal tubular acidosis secondary to genetic defects in the kidney or the abuse of inhalants (e.g., toluene) can cause hypokalemia and paralysis as well. A more common form of potassium-induced weakness is in patients receiving potassium-depleting diuretics. Other compounds, such as licorice, are associated with potassium loss.

### Sodium Channel Abnormalities

***Potassium-sensitive periodic paralysis.*** The potassium-sensitive periodic paralyses and myotonias are associated with mutations in the *SCNA4A* gene that encodes the α subunit of the sodium channel; the gene is located on chromosome 17q (Matthews et al., 2010; Statland et al., 2012; Tan et al., 2011; Trivedi et al., 2013). Even in early descriptions of these disorders, the association of decreased electrical activity, paralysis, and signs of hyperactivity (paramyotonia) were recognized. The proper activity of the sodium channel depends on a complicated series of activation and deactivation processes that open the pore to allow the passage of sodium but also protect the cell against inadvertent excess sodium flux. The channel may exist in a number of different states: closed, open, and inactivated. Physiological studies have suggested that the domain IV S3 segment has a dominant role in the recovery of inactivated channels, whereas the S4 segment is concerned with deactivation and inactivation of the open channel (Ji et al., 1996). Among the several known mutations of the sodium channel, some impair fast inactivation of the sodium channel or shift the impulse to hyperpolarization. Evidence exists that two common mutations in hyperkalemic periodic paralysis in domain II (S5) and domain IV (S6) cause defective slow inactivation, accentuating the weakness (Hayward et al., 1997). Mutations within the domain III–IV linker, which cause myotonia with or without weakness, do not impair slow inactivation.

Studies of muscle during a paralytic attack show that it is slightly depolarized. Intracellular potassium levels decrease and sodium, water, and chloride content are increased. Studies of intercostal muscle biopsies in vitro show a high level of spontaneous muscle activity, even in normal physiological saline. Increasing the external concentration of potassium gradually depolarizes the cells and is associated with an increase in sodium conductance. Tetrodotoxin increases sodium conductance, implying that this part of the sodium channel function is unaffected. Examination of sodium currents of cultured myotubes from the muscles of patients using increased potassium concentrations in the medium resulted in an increased open time or slowed inactivation of the sodium channel associated with sustained depolarization.

In patients with paramyotonia congenita, cooling of intact muscle fibers obtained from intercostal biopsy samples reduced the resting membrane potential from approximately −80 to −40 mV, at which point the fibers were inexcitable. As the muscle cools, it passes through a phase of hyperexcitability. Tetrodotoxin prevents inexcitability by blocking sodium channels. The clinical features reflect the physiological findings.

The predominant symptom in patients with hyperkalemic periodic paralysis is weakness provoked by potassium exposure. Myotonia may be present, and some patients complain of the symptom, but the predominant difficulty is recurrent bouts of paralysis. The allelic disease paramyotonia congenita causes muscle stiffness, and bouts of weakness are mild, often provoked by exposure to cold. In some families, the distinction seems clear, but there are others with a somewhat mixed picture. The clinical features of the two conditions follow.

***Hyperkalemic periodic paralysis.*** Inheritance of potassium-sensitive periodic paralysis (hyperKPP) is autosomal dominant, with strong penetrance and involvement of both sexes (Matthews et al., 2010). Onset of symptoms is during infancy or early childhood. The infant's cry may become suddenly altered or unusual, or the child may be found lying quietly in the crib. Some parents notice an unusual stare as these babies develop, particularly on exposure to cold. The first attack commonly occurs in the first few weeks of school because of the enforced sitting. By adolescence, the attacks are characteristic. Often, rest after exercise provokes an attack, and the weakness develops quite rapidly, often within a matter of minutes. The weakness is milder than in the hypokalemic variety, and the attacks last for a shorter period. Patients may be able to walk off the symptoms if they undertake exercise early in the attack. Many prefer not to do so because an attack itself is mild and followed by a period of relative freedom from symptoms. In addition to rest after exercise, other provocative factors include exposure to cold, anesthesia, and sleep. Patients often avoid fruit juices with high potassium content, having noticed their deleterious effect. Many patients have two kinds of attacks, light and heavy. During a light attack, there is a feeling of fatigue and mild weakness that usually disappears in less than an hour. A heavy attack, however, may be associated with more severe paralysis, even to the point where the patient is unable to arise from the chair or bed. The frequency varies from two or three mild attacks a day to episodes months apart. Residual weakness may occur in middle age and beyond.

***Paramyotonia congenita.*** Mutations in the *SCNA4A* gene also lead to paramyotonia congenita. This condition may or may not be associated with episodic weakness (Matthews et al., 2010; Statland et al., 2012; Tan et al., 2011; Trivedi et al., 2013). Unlike the myotonia in myotonic dystrophy, in paramyotonia, repeated exercise accentuates myotonia, a feature most easily appreciated in the eyelids. Patients may complain of this as aching or stiffness. A clinical test is to have the patient forcibly close his or her eyes in a repetitive manner. After each repetition, the difficulty with relaxation may be accentuated until eventually the patient cannot open the eyes at all. Exposure to cold not only worsens the myotonia but may also provoke muscle weakness, symptoms patients may notice when swallowing ice cream or going out into winter weather to shovel snow. A useful test for paramyotonia is to soak a small towel in ice water and lay it over the patient's eyes for 2 minutes. Eyelid myotonia is demonstrable by having the patient sustain an upward gaze for a few seconds and then look down. The eyelids remain up, baring the sclera above the iris. When muscle is sufficiently chilled, the paramyotonia disappears, and the muscle is flaccid and paralyzed. The weakness may far outlast the exposure to cold, and it is common for the muscle not to regain its full use for hours after returning to room temperature. Strong voluntary contraction also may be associated with a long-lasting decrease in strength, which is not clearly due to an increase in myotonia. Immersing the forearm in ice water may also produce obvious weakness, which may have been lacking on the initial examination.

The diagnosis of potassium-sensitive conditions relies on demonstration of the genetic defects. However, the diagnosis should be suspected when high serum potassium levels coincide with bouts of weakness. In patients with paramyotonia, EMG of the resting muscles at room temperature shows myotonic discharges that are present on percussion or with movement of the needle. The most remarkable findings are demonstration of decrementing CMAP amplitudes on the repeated short exercise test, which is worse when performed with the extremity cooled (Fournier et al., 2004, 2006; Tan et al., 2011; Trivedi et al., 2013). Additionally, there are often after-discharges evident following brief activity on CMAP studies.

The ECG may show the changes of hyperkalemia, and the serum CK concentration may be elevated during or after an attack. Provocative testing, if considered, requires care because the administration of potassium may be dangerous. The presence of any cardiac abnormality contraindicates provocative testing. Oral potassium may be administered using approximately 1 mEq/kg. The maximum rise in potassium occurs 90–180 minutes after administration. If this dose of potassium does not provoke an attack and the index of suspicion is high, administer 2 mEq/kg orally on a subsequent occasion.

Muscle biopsies show tubular aggregates in patients with paralysis, particularly in patients with fixed weakness. Myopathic changes include internal nuclei, vacuoles, and fibrosis. The muscle biopsy may be abnormal in paramyotonia congenita, showing variability in the size of fibers, with internal nuclei and occasional vacuoles.

Acute attacks usually do not require treatment because they are mild and brief. Often patients learn to eat a candy bar or drink a sweet drink as a way of warding off an attack. Intravenous calcium gluconate treats greater weakness. Intravenous sodium chloride sometimes may abort an attack. Maintenance therapy with dichlorphenamide or acetazolamide can be helpful. The combination of hydrochlorothiazide with potassium may be effective, although the reason is unclear. Mexiletine 200 mg orally three times a day CTD may provide relief to patients with myotonia (Statland et al., 2012).

***Potassium-aggravated myotonias.*** This group of disorders includes myotonia fluctuans, myotonia permanens, and acetazolamide-responsive myotonia. Mutations in the *SCNA4A* gene are causative. Myotonia made worse by exercise or potassium ingestion, usually beginning in adolescence, is characteristic. Affected individuals do not suffer attacks of weakness. Myotonia is only sometimes evident in myotonia fluctuans but more consistently evident in myotonia permanens. The myotonia may improve with mexiletine (Statland et al., 2012). Acetazolamide-responsive myotonia resembles myotonia congenita clinically, but affected patients also often have significant muscle pain; the myotonia and pain are relieved by acetazolamide.

***Secondary hyperkalemic periodic paralysis.*** Weakness due to high levels of potassium occurs in situations other than familial hyperkalemic periodic paralysis. The difference between secondary hyperkalemic periodic paralysis and the familial condition is that extremely high levels of potassium are required in secondary hyperkalemic periodic paralysis before weakness occurs. Causes for secondary hyperkalemic periodic paralysis include renal failure or potassium administration associated with potassium-retaining diuretics.

***Hypokalemic periodic paralysis type 2.*** Although the majority of patients with hypokalemic periodic paralysis (type 1) have mutations in the calcium channel, approximately 9% of cases are due to mutation in the *SCNA4A* muscle sodium channel gene (hypoKPP2) (Bulman et al., 1999; Cannon, 2010; Sternberg et al., 2001). The clinical and laboratory features are similar to the more common type of hypokalemic periodic paralysis, but there are some differences that may help distinguish the subtypes. Patients with hypoKPP2 may be more likely to have severe myalgias following the paralytic attacks, tubular aggregates on muscle biopsy rather than vacuoles, and worsening of symptoms on acetazolamide.

### Potassium Channelopathy

***Andersen-Tawil syndrome.*** *Andersen-Tawil syndrome* (ATS) is characterized by the constellation of periodic paralysis, cardiac dysrhythmias, and dysmorphic features (Sansone et al., 1997). The disorder is a genetically heterogeneous syndrome inherited in an autosomal dominant fashion. Some cases are caused by mutations in the potassium channel gene (*KCNJ2*) located on chromosome 17q23. The attacks of paralysis may occur in early childhood or be delayed until later. Attack frequency is low and occurs with both high and low potassium. It therefore differs from the more usual hypokalemic variety, in which low potassium levels are expected. Affected members of the family often show dysmorphic features including wide-spaced eyes, low-set ears, a small chin, clinodactyly of the fifth finger, and syndactyly of the toes. Permanent muscle weakness occurs in some patients.

The importance of recognizing the syndrome lies in the frequent occurrence of cardiac involvement. This varies from a prolongation of the QT interval through ventricular tachycardia to fatal cardiac arrest. The risk of cardiac complications is sufficiently high that provocative hypokalemic or hyperkalemic testing is contraindicated. Several members of affected families have been described in whom only fragments of the syndrome exist (e.g., clinodactyly, an abnormal QT interval), so a full evaluation of the pedigree is necessary.

### Chloride Channelopathy

***Myotonia congenita.*** Two major forms of myotonia congenita exist: autosomal dominant and autosomal recessive (Matthews et al., 2010; Statland et al., 2012; Tan et al., 2011; Trivedi et al., 2013). Both are associated with abnormalities in the chloride channel, the gene for which (*CLCN1*) resides on chromosome 7q35. Introducing the mutant chloride channel into a cell system abolishes the chloride current and deranges the normal function of the chloride channel (Fahlke et al., 1997). The patient's muscles show reduced chloride conductance and greater than normal membrane resistance. The action potential in a normal muscle cell is associated with an outflow of potassium, which may accumulate in the transverse tubules simply because the physical structure of the tubule does not favor easy diffusion. Ordinarily, this does not present a problem because the chloride conductance is so large that the relatively free passage of chloride ions negates the effect of any small change in potassium. With impeded chloride conductance, the increase in potassium concentration in the transverse tubules may lead to enough depolarization to activate the sodium channels again and hence lead to repetitive electrical discharge of the membrane, producing electrical and clinical myotonia.

The original description of the dominant disease was by Thomsen among members of his family. It is usually milder than the recessive form described by Becker, in which myotonia may be associated with some weakness. It is sometimes difficult when faced with a sporadic case to decide on the pattern of inheritance. This is true because members of affected families who carry the abnormal mutation may be asymptomatic or only mildly involved. This necessitates a thorough evaluation of the family, with appropriate genetic testing.

On initial examination, especially if the patient has been sitting in the waiting room for some time, apparent weakness may be present because a severely myotonic muscle lacks full voluntary power. With repetitive activity, the muscle loosens up, and strength usually returns to normal. This is particularly true of proximal limb muscles. Symptom descriptions are stereotyped. After resting, the muscles are stiff and difficult to move. This is obvious when the patient arises from a chair. They move en bloc, with a stiff wooden appearance. As they continue, they then can walk freely and finally can run with ease. All the muscles of the body share this abnormality, and while it is most noticeable in the limbs, the face and tongue are also involved. In addition, particularly in the recessive form of the illness, muscular hypertrophy may be pronounced.

In myotonia congenita, EMG shows well-marked myotonia with none of the associated dystrophic features. In contrast with paramyotonia congenita, the short-exercise nerve conduction test demonstrates less profound decrement of CMAP amplitude that lessens with successive trials (Fournier et al., 2004, 2006; Tan et al., 2011; Trivedi et al., 2013). Muscle biopsy may demonstrate an absence of type 2B fibers, an unexplained finding, and also may reveal some increase in the size of fibers and internal nuclei as well as other mild nonspecific changes.

Unlike most patients with myotonic dystrophy, in myotonia congenita, the myotonia may be disabling. Treatment with mexiletine is often beneficial (Statland et al., 2012). Older options include quinine, procainamide, and phenytoin.

## Metabolic Myopathies

Any disturbance in the biochemical pathways that support ATP levels in the muscle inevitably results in exercise intolerance. One common symptom is muscle fatigue, a sense that the muscle will no longer perform in a normal fashion. This is true fatigue and not simply a feeling of tiredness or weariness. It may be difficult for the patient to describe the fatigue in terms the physician can understand, because it has nothing to do with the sensations experienced by a healthy person after strenuous exercise. It has an unpleasant quality, and patients describe it in terms of a barrier through which they cannot break. Other symptoms include muscle pain and sometimes muscle cramps. The normal fatigue of strenuous exercise is painless. Muscle pain after strenuous exercise (e.g., the next day) is almost universal in the untrained individual, but pain during exercise is more the hallmark of disturbed muscle function. Normally functioning muscle appears to have a series of safety mechanisms that prevent humans from exercising it to the point of destruction.

In the metabolic muscle diseases, maintenance of ATP levels is impaired, and the protective mechanism that functions in the normal person is absent. Forced exercise in patients with a metabolic myopathy causes muscle pain followed by muscle contracture, in which state the muscle is hard, swollen, and tender. This reflects actual muscle destruction. It may be associated with the release of myoglobin into the blood and urine, sometimes noticed as a change in the color of the urine, which may resemble weak tea or cola. Fatigue, muscle pain, contractures, and myoglobinuria are increasingly severe effects of the biochemical defect. In treating these illnesses, preventing the development of myoglobinuria is essential because it carries the potential for renal tubular necrosis.

This group of diseases is divisible into three major categories: disorders of carbohydrate metabolism, disorders of lipid metabolism, and disorders of mitochondrial function. Finally, there are some conditions that in theory should disturb pathways for ATP maintenance but do not seem to cause any exercise intolerance. A tissue with depleted ATP stores is probably dead tissue. Even in the metabolic myopathies, the muscle seldom reaches this critical state. What does happen, however, is that overworked support pathways produce unwelcome by-products, which probably cause the symptoms of disease.

### Disorders of Carbohydrate Metabolism

***Myophosphorylase deficiency.*** Intramuscular carbohydrate stores play an important part in the early stage of exercise, before the compensatory mechanisms of an increased supply of bloodborne metabolites and increased lipid metabolism supply the added demand. The first of the biochemical disorders to be recognized was a disorder of carbohydrate metabolism called *myophosphorylase deficiency* (McArdle disease). In 1952, McArdle noted that a young man who presented with exercise intolerance experienced pain and tightness of his muscle on forced exercise. Ischemic forearm exercise caused a painful contracture of the muscle within a minute or so. Insertion of an EMG needle showed that there was no electrical activity, thereby differentiating this contracture from a muscle cramp. McArdle commented that the phenomenon resembled the reaction of a fish muscle poisoned by iodoacetate, a compound that blocks glycolysis. Subsequent studies showed the defect to be an absence of myophosphorylase activity, encoded by a gene on chromosome 11q13. There are two forms of phosphorylase: phosphorylase a, which is the active tetramer, and phosphorylase b, an inactive dimer. Conversion of the inactive form to the active form is catalyzed by phosphorylase b kinase, which itself is activated by a protein kinase under the control of cyclic adenosine monophosphate (cAMP). Any abnormality of this cascade of reactions will result in the absence of phosphorylase activity. Both phosphorylase a and phosphorylase b kinase deficiencies are known to cause exercise intolerance. Inheritance of either illness appears inherited as an autosomal recessive trait.

Onset of symptoms is during the first 10 years of life, but only in retrospect. As children, patients may complain of being tired and unable to keep up with their playmates. The classic symptoms appear in teenage years. Fatigue and pain begin within the first few minutes of exercise, particularly if it is strenuous. There is a sensation of hitting a barrier, which causes the patient to slow down. If exercise is continued, pain develops within the muscle, which at first is deep and aching but gives way to the rapid development of a painful tightening of the muscle. The muscle is hard and contracted, and any attempt to straighten it results in great pain. The muscle contracture may last for several hours and can be differentiated from a muscle cramp on two counts: the EMG is electrically silent, and the duration of the contracture is far longer than that of a physiological cramp, which disappears after a few minutes at most.

Another aspect of McArdle disease is the development of the *second-wind phenomenon*. If, with the onset of fatigue, the patient slows down but does not stop, the abnormal sensation may disappear, and thereafter the muscle may function more normally. By gradually increasing the level of exercise, the patient may be able to break through the barrier and then may be able to exercise at an adequate level for longer periods. This second-wind phenomenon, which is related to the phenomenon normally experienced by distance runners, may be marked in patients with phosphorylase deficiency. It probably is associated with a change in the blood supply in the muscle and with an intrinsic change in the muscle's metabolism. The second-wind phenomenon usually is associated with a rise in fatty acid use and blocked by nicotinic acid.

Other unusual forms of phosphorylase deficiency exist. One such patient was an infant girl who died of respiratory failure. Phosphorylase deficiency also occurs in an occasional patient with proximal weakness and neither cramps nor fatigue. On examination, these patients are superficially normal with neither wasting nor weakness, although they may be reluctant to exert full force during muscle strength testing because of the possibility of exacerbating muscle pain.

A simple diagnostic clinical test is the *exercise forearm test*. A butterfly needle is inserted in the antecubital fossa, and baseline lactic acid and ammonia levels are obtained. The patient then opens and closes the hand repeatedly as fast as possible for 1 minute. Importantly, ischemia of the arm is unnecessary (i.e., ischemic forearm test). In fact, ischemic exercise may lead to myoglobinuria. Serum lactic acid and ammonia concentrations should be measured at 1, 2, 3, and 5 minutes after the exercise. The normal response is a three- to fourfold rise in lactic acid and ammonia. In patients with phosphorylase, phosphorylase b kinase, phosphoglycerate mutase, phosphoglycerate kinase, lactate dehydrogenase (LDH), and enolase deficiencies, the lactic acid concentration does not increase, but the ammonia concentration does. Measuring the ammonia concentrations serves as a control to ensure the patient was sufficiently exercising. A rise in lactic acid without a rise in ammonia occurs in myoadenylate deaminase deficiency.

Light microscopic examination of muscle histology may show an increase in glycogen and the presence of subsarcolemmal blebs. Muscle necrosis also may be noted. Routine stains are usually normal. However, the histochemical reaction for myophosphorylase shows reduced or no activity, and biochemical assay of muscle enzyme activity shows reduced concentrations.

***Phosphofructokinase deficiency.*** PFK is the enzyme that converts fructose 6-phosphate to fructose 1,6-diphosphate and is a step in the glycolytic chain downstream from that activated by phosphorylase. The reaction is rate limiting for glycolysis. Inheritance of PFK deficiency is as an autosomal recessive trait, the gene is on chromosome 1, and heterozygotes have decreased but not absent levels of enzyme activity.

PFK deficiency is an autosomal recessive disorder that is almost identical clinically to phosphorylase deficiency, although the second-wind phenomenon is uncommon. Most attacks are associated with nausea, vomiting, and muscle pain. There may also be mild hemolytic anemia with increased levels of bilirubin, and increased reticulocyte counts due to deficiency of red blood cell PFK. Like phosphorylase, PFK is a tetramer of different subunits, M and R. Muscle PFK is composed of identical M subunits, whereas the enzyme in the red blood cell comprises both M and R types. In PFK deficiency, the M subunit is missing but the R subunit is preserved, resulting in absence of muscle PFK and impairment of PFK in the red blood cell.

***Phosphoglycerate kinase deficiency.*** Phosphoglycerate kinase is involved in another step in the glycolytic pathway. Its absence from muscle produces a predictable picture very similar to that of phosphorylase deficiency. Venous lactate concentrations do not rise after exercise, as would be expected. The muscle biopsy histology is normal, with a normal glycogen concentration. Phosphoglycerate kinase is a single polypeptide. The gene for this disorder is on chromosome Xq13. Several different point mutations occur that produce abnormalities in the red blood cell, with hemolytic anemia, intellectual disability, and seizures.

***Phosphoglycerate mutase deficiency.*** Phosphoglycerate mutase exists as a dimer with M and B subunits. The predominant form in normal muscle is MM. A small amount of residual activity may be present in muscle because of the existence of the BB form. Patients with an absence of the enzyme have attacks of muscle pain and myoglobinuria and, in one case, typical attacks of gouty arthritis. The high uric acid level may be associated with an overactivity of the adenylate kinase/adenylate deaminase reaction. This occurs in many metabolic disorders and produces uric acid as its end product. Exercise testing shows some elevation of lactate, but not to the levels usually seen. The responsible gene is located at chromosome 7p12-13.

***Lactate dehydrogenase deficiency.*** Exercise intolerance, fatigue, and myoglobinuria are symptoms of LDH deficiency. Some differences exist in the laboratory studies between this entity and the others discussed here. In most muscle diseases, muscle LDH and serum CK concentrations fluctuate together. In this illness, not surprisingly, a marked discrepancy existed between the high levels of CK and the low levels of LDH. Furthermore, because the action of LDH in exercise is to convert pyruvate to lactate, pyruvate rises after ischemic forearm exercise, but lactate does not. The responsible gene is at chromosome 11p15.4.

***β-Enolase deficiency.*** Three patients have been reported with exercise intolerance, myalgias, and episodic hyperCKemia caused by mutations in the gene encoding β-enolase.

***α-Glucosidase deficiency (acid maltase deficiency).*** Acid maltase deficiency, or *Pompe disease*, is an autosomal recessive disorder caused by a deficiency of lysosomal α-glucosidase. Pompe disease may present in three major forms: a severe infantile form, a juvenile-onset type, or as a milder adult-onset variant (American Association of Neuromuscular and Electrodiagnostic Medicine, 2009; Katzin and Amato, 2008). Infantile Pompe disease, the classic form, is characterized by generalized weakness and hypotonia, cardiomegaly, and mild to moderate hepatomegaly with onset in the first several months of life. Infants often have an enlarged tongue (i.e., macroglossia). The weakness and cardiomyopathy are progressive, and the disease is invariably fatal by 2 years of age, secondary to cardiorespiratory failure. Juvenile-onset Pompe disease usually manifests in the first decade of life with slowly progressive proximal weakness such that it resembles Duchenne or some other form of LGMD. Ventilatory muscles may be preferentially affected, and many die in the second or third decade of life. Adult-onset Pompe disease usually manifests in the third or fourth decade (range 18–65 years, mean 36.5 years). Patients develop generalized proximal greater than distal muscle weakness resembling PM or an adult-onset type of LGMD. As in the infantile and juvenile forms of the disease, a predilection exists for involvement of respiratory muscles.

Serum CK levels are moderately elevated in Pompe disease, but adults may have normal CK levels. EMG reveals increased insertional and spontaneous activity in the form of fibrillation potentials, positive sharp waves, complex repetitive discharges, and even myotonic discharges. In mild forms of the disease, these irritative discharges may be evident only in the paraspinal muscles. ECG may demonstrate nonspecific abnormalities including Wolff-Parkinson-White syndrome. Echocardiograms can show hypertrophic cardiomyopathy. Pulmonary function tests reveal decreased FVC along with reduced maximal inspiratory and expiratory pressures that worsen in the supine position, suggestive of diaphragm involvement. Glycogen-filled vacuoles that intensely stain for acid phosphatase within muscle fibers are characteristic histopathological findings. However, in late-onset Pompe disease, muscle biopsies may reveal only nonspecific abnormalities.

Assay of α-glucosidase activity in muscle fibers, fibroblasts, leukocytes, lymphocytes, and in the urine establishes the diagnosis (American Association of Neuromuscular and Electrodiagnostic Medicine, 2009; Katzin and Amato, 2008). A good screening test is the dried blood spot, which measures enzyme activity. Diagnosis can be confirmed by genetic testing.

Diagnosis is important, particularly in the classic infantile-onset cases, as treatment is now available for this disorder. Intravenous recombinant α-glucosidase enzyme appears to be safe and beneficial for infants with Pompe disease (Kishnani et al., 2007) but has a more modest effect in late-onset Pompe disease (Kuperus et al., 2017; van der Ploeg et al., 2010).

***Treatment of the glycolytic disorders.*** Except for Pompe disease, effective medications for the glycolytic disorders are unavailable. Patients should be counseled to avoid situations that might precipitate myoglobinuria. Attempts to bypass the metabolic block by using glucose or fructose prior to any significant physical activity may help to some extent, but, while feasible, routine use would lead to weight gain. Administration of branched-chain amino acids and a protein-enriched diet also has been suggested, but there is no evidence that these regimens are any more effective than a well-balanced diet. One maneuver for patients with McArdle disease is to develop the patient's awareness of the second-wind phenomenon. Graded exercise on a treadmill can train the patient to recognize how to slow down with the first onset of symptoms and then resume exercise in small increments. This type of training requires an exercise physiology laboratory.

## Disorders of Lipid Metabolism

***Carnitine palmitoyl transferase deficiency.*** The synthesis of ATP that results from the oxidation of fatty acids requires a system as complex as that seen in glycolysis. Fatty acids, not used at the beginning of exercise, become increasingly important after 20–30 minutes of endurance exercise. After an hour, they represent the major energy supply. Consequently, defects in lipid metabolism give rise to symptoms after sustained activity. Carnitine palmitoyl transferase (CPT) is the enzyme that links carnitine to long-chain fatty acids, a linkage necessary to transport the fatty acid across the mitochondrial membrane from outside to inside (CPT-I). It is also responsible for unhooking carnitine when the complex reaches the inside (CPT-II). CPT-II deficiency is one of the more common biochemical abnormalities in muscle. Inheritance of the disorder is as an autosomal recessive trait.

Typically, CPT deficiency manifests with myoglobinuria after strenuous exercise (e.g., mountain climbing, playing four sets of tennis) sometime during the first three decades of life. Affected individuals are particularly predisposed to these attacks if exercise occurs in the fasting state or when they have an infection. This is not surprising because with fasting and infection the body is more dependent on fatty acid metabolism. Attacks of myoglobinuria in CPT deficiency are often more severe and have a greater tendency to cause renal damage than those occurring in glycolytic disorders. The cause may be that the symptoms come on so rapidly in the glycolytic disorders that cessation of exercise immediately returns the muscle to its resting condition. In disorders of lipid metabolism, the patient is often far away from home and out of necessity must use muscles that have already been damaged. Even when the muscle stops working, it still depends on fatty acid metabolism. Patients with CPT deficiency often notice that their stamina depends on their diet. Some carry a candy bar to eat during exercise. Others know that exercise in a fasting state is far more difficult for them. Despite these limitations, some patients with CPT deficiency are quite athletic and may be weightlifters or sprinters rather than marathon runners. Both activities draw on carbohydrate energy supplies and use glycolytic fibers, not the oxidative fibers. There is no abnormality on examination. Indeed, these patients are uniformly muscular, perhaps because their favorite exercise is weightlifting.

Genetic testing is available to test for mutations in the *CPT-II* gene. The CK concentration may be normal unless the patient has had a recent attack of muscle damage. The muscle biopsy in CPT deficiency is normal unless necrosis is associated with a recent bout of muscle damage. Biochemical analysis of the muscle biopsy reveals the deficiency of CPT, but the fact that one must suspect the diagnosis to ask for the assay makes it helpful only as a confirmatory test. One useful screening test is a respiratory exchange ratio (RER). The ratio of carbon dioxide produced to oxygen consumed gives an indication of the type of fuel used by the patient. In a normal individual at rest, the RER is approximately 0.8 because fatty acids are the predominant source of fuel at rest. In CPT deficiency, the RER is seldom much below 1.0, even with the patient at complete rest. It may be worthwhile to obtain incremental bicycle ergometry results because, in addition to the RER, the $Vo_2$max (maximal oxygen consumption) and work max also can be determined. Usually both are decreased. The maximum heart rate is normal, indicating full effort. Forearm exercise testing is of little value in CPT deficiency because the test stresses glycolytic pathways, and hence the results of the test are normal.

Patients with CPT deficiency should be cautioned to avoid any situation that provokes muscle pain and puts them at risk for myoglobinuria. The physiological effect of fasting should be explained and the patient warned to not attempt exercise under such conditions and not to fast when they have an infection. The use of glucose tablets or candy bars during exercise may raise exercise tolerance slightly. If myoglobinuria is noted, the patient should be admitted to the hospital and renal function monitored. Forced alkaline diuresis may be helpful in some cases. All exercise should be discontinued and the patient confined to bed rest until CK levels return to normal and renal function is uncompromised.

***Carnitine deficiency myopathy.*** Carnitine is an important compound in intermediary metabolism. It influences the balance between free coenzyme A (CoA) and acylated CoA in the mitochondria and transfers long-chain fatty acids across the mitochondrial membrane under the action of the enzyme CPT. Sources of carnitine are dietary, as well as liver and kidney synthesis. Carnitine is transported to muscle, which actively takes it up. Many metabolic processes produce acyl-CoA for use in metabolic pathways; it is then degraded by the liver or excreted by the kidneys. The formation of acylcarnitine is often a step in these processes, enabling the transport of fatty and organic acids across membranes such as the mitochondrial membrane. A surplus of acyl-CoA may cause a variety of damage. It inhibits reactions as diverse as the oxidation of pyruvate, steps in the tricarboxylic acid cycle, and gluconeogenesis. Thus an adequate amount of carnitine is necessary for normal function. One judges the adequacy of the carnitine supply from its absolute value and the percentage of free (nonacylated) carnitine. If free carnitine is absent, carnitine deficiency exists, no matter how much total carnitine is present. Because 98% of the body carnitine is in muscle, it is not surprising that carnitine deficiency is associated with neuromuscular disease. In most patients with carnitine deficiency, the loss of free carnitine is due to a defect in some other enzyme system that results in an overproduction of organic acids or a defect in acyl-CoA disposal.

Primary carnitine deficiency is caused by mutations in the sodium-dependent carnitine transporter gene, *OCTN2* (also called the *SLC22A5 gene*), located on chromosome 5q33.1 (Nezu et al., 1999). Causes of secondary carnitine deficiency include multiple acyl-CoA dehydrogenase deficiencies, resulting in an overabundance of organic acids, which then bind the available carnitine; propionyl-CoA carboxylase deficiency; methylmalonyl-CoA mutase deficiency; and a number of mitochondrial disorders. Hemodialysis, cirrhosis, pregnancy, Reye syndrome, valproate therapy, and renal Fanconi syndrome also deplete carnitine stores. In muscle carnitine deficiency, serum levels of carnitine are often normal, but muscle contains reduced total and free carnitine concentrations. Systemic carnitine deficiency includes carnitine deficiency in muscle, liver, and serum.

The most common clinical picture in muscle carnitine deficiency is a slowly progressive weakness with sudden exacerbations or a fluctuating course. Fatigue and exercise-related pains occur but usually do not constitute major complaints; myoglobinuria is usually absent. The weakness is usually proximal, and the symptoms begin during childhood or early teenage life. In addition to the limb and some trunk weakness, facial and bulbar weakness occurs.

Systemic carnitine deficiency also begins in infancy and childhood, but the muscular weakness occurs in association with an encephalopathy resembling Reye syndrome. Protracted vomiting is the initial symptom of the encephalopathy. Changing levels of consciousness, culminating in coma, follow. Hypoglycemia occurs in most patients, and there may be evidence of liver damage, with an enlarged tender liver or increased serum levels of hepatic enzymes. Hypothrombinemia, hyperammonemia, and excess lipid in the liver are also common. Fasting, because it throws the body into a dependence on fatty acids, may exacerbate the symptoms of carnitine deficiency.

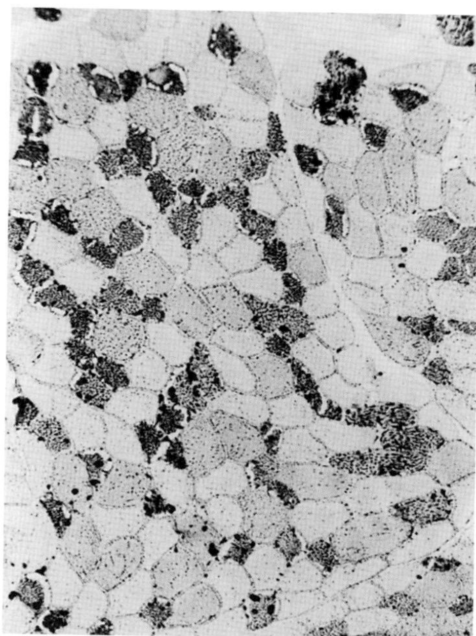

**Fig. 109.26 Carnitine Deficiency.** This lipid stain demonstrates deposition of fat in muscle fibers.

The EMG frequently appears myopathic, but no specific findings lead to the diagnosis of carnitine deficiency. The disorder may be suspected on muscle biopsy because of the accumulation of lipid droplets in muscle fibers (Fig. 109.26), but the biochemical measurement of carnitine, both free and total, is necessary to establish the diagnosis. If abnormal, it will initiate the search for the underlying defect.

The treatment of carnitine deficiency by replacing carnitine is not uniformly successful. Adults receive approximately 2–4 g/day of L-carnitine in divided doses, with the equivalent of 100 mg/kg in infants and children. No serious side effects occur, although patients may find L-carnitine unpleasant because of accompanying nausea and the fishy odor of the sweat. The results of such treatment vary. Some patients show dramatic improvement, whereas others feel no change at all. The effectiveness of other forms of treatment is equally variable. One patient responded to riboflavin in high doses and others to prednisone. Dietary manipulations such as reducing the amount of long-chain fatty acids in the diet and supplying a medium-chain triglyceride diet also are successful in some patients.

***Other disorders of lipid metabolism.*** Other less common disorders of lipid metabolism include multiple acyl-coenzyme A dehydrogenation deficiency (MADD), neutral lipid storage disease with myopathy (NLDSM), and neutral lipid storage disease with ichthyosis (NLDSI) (Ohkuma et al., 2009). These disorders can present in early childhood or adult life with weakness. MADD is an autosomal recessive disorder caused by mutations affecting electron transfer flavoprotein (ETF) or ETF dehydrogenase (ETFDH). MADD should be suspected in patients whose muscle specimens show increased lipid deposition and whose serum and urine have increased concentrations of organic acids of multiple carbon lengths. Neutral lipid storage disease is characterized by systemic accumulation of triglycerides in the cytoplasm and includes two distinct diseases: NLSDM and NLSDI (also called *Chanarin-Dorfman syndrome*). NLSDM may present as a distal myopathy with progressive foot drop and is caused by mutations in a gene that encodes adipose triglyceride lipase (ATGL). This enzyme catalyzes the initial step in triglyceride hydrolysis. A helpful laboratory feature is the presence of *Jordan bodies*, which are lipid inclusions in white blood cells seen on a blood smear. As the name implies, individuals affected with NLSDI have associated skin lesions. This disorder is caused by the mutations in the gene that encodes the coactivator of ATGL.

### Disorder of Abnormal Nucleotide Metabolism

***Myoadenylate deaminase deficiency.*** Approximately 1% to 2% of the population has a deficiency of the enzyme, myoadenylate deaminase (AMP deaminase, or AMPDA). Inheritance of the disorder is autosomal recessive. The enzyme plays a role in supporting ATP levels by acting in conjunction with adenylate kinase. Adenylate kinase converts two molecules of adenosine diphosphate to one each of ATP and AMP. Adenylate deaminase then converts AMP to inosine monophosphate, with production of ammonia. Muscle stress activates the reaction.

Early studies suggested that patients with AMPDA deficiency had myalgia or exercise intolerance. However, many people with AMPDA deficiency are asymptomatic and perfectly normal. Reports of enzyme deficiency vary from congenital hypotonia to amyotrophic lateral sclerosis. This poor correlation between the enzyme defect and the clinical symptoms makes it difficult to know how to interpret the entity.

No abnormalities on muscle biopsy under light microscopy exist, although the histochemical reaction for AMPDA is absent. The forearm exercise test is a useful screening test. Patients with AMPDA deficiency produce normal amounts of lactate but little or no ammonia and hypoxanthine, both of which are by-products of the AMPDA reaction.

## Mitochondrial Myopathies

Mitochondria are responsible for producing energy for cells by generating ATP from the by-products of carbohydrates, fatty acids, and amino acids. The clinical spectrum of mitochondrial disorders is broad and often multisystemic. Due to the high resting energy requirement of the brain, the CNS is often affected by mitochondrial disorders. The energy requirement of skeletal muscle is by contrast quite low at rest, but in exercise becomes much higher. In a group of diseases known as the *mitochondrial myopathies*, exercise intolerance results. Mitochondrial myopathies can lead to fixed weakness, as well.

Acetyl-CoA is the final product of both fatty acid metabolism and glycolysis and feeds into the tricarboxylic acid (Krebs) cycle. The final oxidative pathway, in which electrons are transferred to ATP, involves the respiratory chain in mitochondria. Under normal conditions, the rate of mitochondrial oxidation couples to the need for ATP. If ATP turnover is rapid, mitochondrial oxidation turns on, with the resulting consumption of oxygen and other metabolites. When ATP turnover is minimal, mitochondrial oxidation is relatively quiescent. The body's response to the increased demands of exercise (and increased mitochondrial oxidation) is predictable. The higher oxygen consumption necessitates augmented delivery of oxygen to the muscle, evidenced by vasodilation, tachycardia, increased cardiac output, and respiration. The heat generation that accompanies this process results in sweating. These are the normal accompaniments of vigorous exercise. When mitochondrial function is impaired, maintaining the required ATP levels even at rest may require fully activated mitochondrial oxidation. In this situation, the patient at rest may experience all the symptoms that normally accompany vigorous exercise. In addition, because the oxidative mechanisms are insufficient to cope with ATP demands, anaerobic mechanisms come into play and produce high blood lactate concentrations.

The original description of a mitochondrial disorder was by Luft and colleagues in 1962 (Luft, 1962), although the muscle symptoms were minor. Both patients were women who experienced sustained fever, profuse sweating, and heat intolerance. One preferred to spend her time in a room cooled to 4°C. Other symptoms were excessive thirst and appetite, and polyuria. General physical examination demonstrated a rapid heartbeat and respiration, profuse sweating, and warm flushed skin. Blotchy erythematous changes of the skin over the legs occurred. Although some degree of muscle weakness occurred, it was mild and not localized.

Many well-described syndromes associated with mitochondrial disorders include prominent muscle complaints. Onset of symptoms is often in childhood, with exercise bringing a heavy feeling in the limbs and muscle aches. After exercise, patients may become tired, nauseated, and breathless. Symptoms may progress over the years until patients are capable of only a limited amount of exercise. Triggers for acute attacks include unaccustomed activity, fasting, or small quantities of alcohol. Acute attacks are also often accompanied by elevated blood lactate levels.

In their most severe forms, mitochondrial diseases are detectable at rest. After excluding hyperthyroidism or intoxication with unusual compounds (e.g., dinitrophenol) that uncouple mitochondrial oxidation, few explanations exist for patients who have high pulse and respiratory rates at rest, with a serum lactate level of more than 8 mEq/L. In patients who are less severely affected, incremental bicycle ergometry is the most useful test. Increasing the workload even to low levels results in an excessive rise in pulse rate and oxygen consumption, with a low work max. This discrepancy between normal $Vo_2$max, normal heart rate, and a very low work max is characteristic of the illness. If bicycle ergometry is not available, incremental forearm exercise may demonstrate excessive lactate production for the levels of work used and unusually high venous oxygen saturation.

Muscle biopsy can demonstrate findings consistent with a mitochondrial myopathy, but rarely allows for a specific underlying genetic diagnosis. Routine light microscopy of muscle may show ragged-red fibers or may be relatively normal; EM sometimes shows abnormal mitochondria. Ragged-red fibers are not specific and are part of normal aging, although not in such quantities. The biopsy may reveal scattered fibers that lack COX—complex IV in the respiratory chain. These same fibers are frequently strongly succinate dehydrogenase (SDH) CoQ reductase positive—complex II in the respiratory chain. SDH is encoded entirely by nuclear genes. whereas COX is encoded by a mix of nuclear and mitochondrial DNA, which may explain this discrepancy. EM examination shows bizarre distortions of the mitochondria. Even though the typical clinical picture associated with ragged-red fibers in the biopsy makes the diagnosis apparent in many patients, there are some with few pathological changes and even normal biochemistry. Assay of mitochondrial enzyme activity and mutational analysis of the mitochondrial DNA (mtDNA) confirms the diagnosis.

Biochemical evaluation of the respiratory chain can help localize the defect, but, similar to history, the findings may still be nonspecific. As an example, biochemical analysis frequently shows COX deficiency; this does not guarantee a mutation in COX itself, as many upstream problems manifest as a secondary deficiency in this testing. Analysis of mitochondrial oxidation requires relatively large amounts of muscle. The introduction of noninvasive techniques to monitor muscle metabolism has had a major impact on the analysis of mitochondrial disorders, although it is perhaps less useful in the diagnosis of these conditions. Magnetic resonance spectroscopy of $^{31}$P compounds permits the analysis of ATP, creatine phosphate, inorganic phosphate, and pH in muscle. In mitochondrial disorders, a rapid fall in levels of creatine phosphate and an abnormal accumulation of inorganic phosphates exists. Equally important is a delay in the recovery of phosphocreatine levels to normal after exercise.

Genetic testing in mitochondrial disorders is complicated because mitochondrial proteins are encoded both by mitochondrial DNA and nuclear DNA—disorders can result from mutations in either. As a result, many patterns of inheritance can be seen. All the mitochondria in an embryo are derived from the mother. With hundreds of mitochondria in a single cell, typically not every mitochondria passed on carries the relevant pathogenic mutation. Mutated and normal mitochondrial DNA is thus randomly distributed among body cells in varying quantities. The number of abnormal mitochondria in a given cell must reach a certain threshold to impact energy production before any disease effects are expressed. This leads to variable phenotypic expression across body tissues. Genotype-phenotype correlation is poor, even for nuclear-encoded genes; mutations in a single gene can result in multiple different mitochondrial syndromes and a single mitochondrial syndrome can result from mutations in several distinct genes.

There is no proven therapy for mitochondrial disorders. Treatment with a "cocktail" of compounds including riboflavin, ubiquinone, vitamin C, menadione, and niacin has been popular but of unproven efficacy.

The following is a discussion of some of the more common mitochondrial disorders associated with myopathy.

### Myoclonic Epilepsy with Ragged-Red Fibers

The complete spectrum of Myoclonic epilepsy with ragged-red fibers MERRF includes myoclonus, generalized seizures (myoclonic and tonic-clonic), ataxia, dementia, sensorineural hearing loss, and optic atrophy, as well as muscular weakness and atrophy. Weakness and atrophy are usually more prominent in proximal muscles. In addition, some patients have a generalized sensorimotor polyneuropathy along with high-arched feet (pes cavus). The disorder can begin in childhood or adult life. While the course and severity are often progressive, they can be variable even within families. Cardiac muscle is also affected, and patients can develop arrhythmias or heart failure. Patients with MERRF can develop life-threatening hypoventilation in relation to surgery, sedation, or intercurrent infection.

Serum CK can be normal or mildly elevated. Serum lactate also is often elevated. Electroencephalography (EEG) may demonstrate generalized slowing of the background activity as well as bursts of spikes and slow waves. MRI or CT scan of the brain reveals cerebral and cerebellar atrophy.

Inheritance of MERRF is nonmendelian (inherited only through females). Approximately 80% of affected patients have a point mutation at nucleotide position 8344 of the mitochondrial genome resulting in an A-to-G transition in the transfer RNA for lysine ($tRNA^{Lys}$) gene. Other mutations in this gene (positions 8356 and 8366), in the transfer RNA for leucine ($tRNA^{Leu}$) gene (the gene most commonly mutated in MELAS—see next section), and several other genes also have been reported in patients with MERRF. The mitochondrial tRNA gene mutations impair the translation of mtDNA-encoded respiratory chain proteins, with resultant decreased enzymatic activity. Mutation analysis of mtDNA in leukocytes or muscle shows mutations, but the frequency of abnormal mtDNA is greater in muscle.

### Mitochondrial Encephalopathy, Lactic Acidosis, and Stroke-Like Episodes

Biochemical and morphological evidence of mitochondrial abnormalities, high lactate levels in the serum or CSF, and stroke-like episodes characterize Mitochondrial Encephalopathy, Lactic Acidosis, and Stroke-like Episodes MELAS. The onset is usually in childhood, but rare cases have onset as late as the eighth decade of life. Most patients present with recurrent migraine headaches, hemiparesis, hemianopsia, or cortical blindness. Exercise or intercurrent infection provokes attacks. Some patients develop progressive dementia after repeated attacks. Proximal muscle weakness is present in most patients, along with exercise intolerance. Many patients are short. Some patients also develop myoclonus, seizures, or ataxia.

Serum CK may be normal or elevated. Lactate levels are elevated in the serum and CSF in the majority of patients. Cortical atrophy and focal low-signal abnormalities are evident on CT and MRI scans of the brain. Muscle biopsy results are indistinguishable from those of other mitochondrial myopathies, as described earlier. Defects in the activity of complex I, III, IV, and V activities appear in muscle specimens.

Inheritance of MELAS is maternal in a nonmendelian pattern. Most cases are caused by an mtDNA mutation, an A-to-G substitution, in the gene encoding for $tRNA^{Leu}$ at nucleotide position 3243. Mutations also occur at other positions in the $tRNA^{Leu}$ gene, as well as in the genes for $tRNA^{Val}$, $tRNA^{Cys}$, and ND5 of complex 1, and in cytochrome *b* of complex III.

### Mitochondrial Myopathies Associated with Recurrent Myoglobinuria

Mitochondrial myopathy may present as exercise intolerance and recurrent myoglobinuria beginning in infancy or early adulthood. Laboratory and histopathological features are indistinguishable from other mitochondrial myopathies but serve to exclude the more common causes of myoglobinuria such as CPT2 deficiency, a glycogen storage disease, or a mild form of muscular dystrophy. This is a genetically heterogeneous group of disorders. Autosomal recessive inheritance associated with multiple mtDNA deletions, point mutations in $tRNA^{Phe}$, microdeletions within the gene encoding for cytochrome *c* oxidase III mutations in NADH dehydrogenase (ND4), and in cytochrome *b* have all been reported.

### Mitochondrial Myopathy, Lactic Acidosis, and Sideroblastic Anemia

This rare disorder typically presents in early infancy or childhood with the eponymous triad. Both exercise intolerance and fixed weakness occur. Hypertrophic cardiomyopathy and respiratory muscle insufficiency occur in nearly half. Mutations in *YARS2* and *PUS1* have been implicated (Riley et al., 2010; Somerville et al., 2017).

### Kearns-Sayre Syndrome

KSS is characterized by the clinical triad of progressive external ophthalmoplegia (PEO), retinitis pigmentosa, and heart block, with onset usually before the age of 20 years. Mild weakness of the proximal arms and legs may be apparent. KSS is also associated with short stature, sensorineural hearing loss, dementia, ataxia, depressed ventilatory drive, and multiple endocrinopathies.

Normal serum CK concentrations are typical, but lactate and pyruvate concentrations may be elevated. CSF protein is usually increased. ECG reveals conduction defects. Muscle biopsies demonstrate ragged-red fibers on Gomori trichrome stain (Fig. 109.27). The number of ragged-red fibers and COX-negative fibers correlate with the percentage of mitochondria with large deletions.

Most patients with KSS have single large mtDNA deletions of varying sizes (ranging from 1.3 to 8.8 kb). Mitochondrial DNA deletions may be present in leukocytes and other tissues, but the sensitivity is much lower than that demonstrated in muscle. The large deletions usually involve several tRNA genes, thus impairing the adequate translation of mtDNA-encoded proteins.

### Progressive External Ophthalmoplegia

Ptosis and ophthalmoparesis, with or without limb weakness, are the presenting features of PEO. Unlike in KSS, pigmentary retinopathy, cardiac conduction defects, or other systemic manifestations (e.g., endocrinopathies) are not typical. Patients with PEO can develop

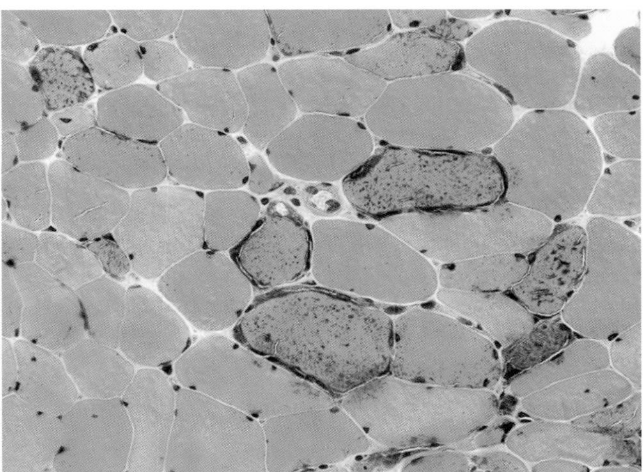

**Fig. 109.27 Kearns-Sayre Syndrome.** Typical appearance of ragged-red fibers seen in biopsy (modified Gomori trichrome stain).

hypoventilation in response to sedatives and anesthetic agents. Patients with mtDNA deletions often have dysphagia in addition to the extraocular weakness, related to cricopharyngeal achalasia.

Serum CK, serum lactate, and CSF lactate can be normal or elevated. CSF protein may be increased. In contrast to classic KSS, the ECG does not demonstrate cardiac conduction defects. Muscle pathology is indistinguishable from KSS.

This is genetically a very heterogeneous disorder (Hirano and DiMauro, 2001). Autosomal dominant and maternally inherited forms of PEO are genetically distinguishable from the sporadic subtype. Some sporadic patients with PEO have single large mtDNA deletions indistinguishable from those seen in KSS. These patients could represent partial expressions of KSS. Importantly, these deletions are sporadic in occurrence. Point mutations have been demonstrated within various mitochondrial tRNA (Leu, Ile, Asn, Trp) genes in several kinships with maternal inheritance of PEO. In addition, reports are available of multiple mtDNA deletions in a few kinships with autosomal dominant inheritance.

The molecular defects lie in nuclear genes involved in regulating the mitochondrial genome. Autosomal dominant PEO appears to be genetically heterogeneous because the disorder has been localized to mutations in the genes encoding for adenine nucleotide translocator 1 (ANT1) on chromosome 4q34-q35, Twinkle on chromosome 10q23.3-q24.3, and polymerase gamma (POLG) on 15q22-q26. ANT1 is responsible for transporting ATP across the inner mitochondrial membrane, while Twinkle and POLG1 are involved in mtDNA replication.

### Mitochondrial DNA Depletion Syndrome

The severity of muscle weakness in mitochondrial DNA depletion syndrome can vary. Fatal infantile myopathy is a severe early-onset form characterized by generalized hypotonia and weakness at birth. Weakness is progressive, leading to feeding difficulties, respiratory failure, and death usually within the first year of life. Some infants develop ptosis and ophthalmoplegia. A subclinical neuropathy is often evident on examination. Diminished or absent deep tendon reflexes are present.

A benign infantile myopathy exists that resembles the fatal form of myopathy. Generalized hypotonia, weakness, and respiratory and feeding difficulties begin in infancy or early childhood. Although ventilatory assistance may be required, muscle strength often improves during the first year of life. Motor milestones may be delayed but are usually attained. Affected individuals can have a normal life expectancy, but some die in the first two decades of life.

Serum CK can be normal or elevated, as can the serum lactate level. The associated renal tubular defect results in glycosuria, proteinuria, and aminoaciduria. MRI of the brain may reveal cerebral atrophy and patchy areas of hypomyelination of subcortical white matter. Muscle biopsies demonstrate ragged-red fibers, foci of intense NADH and SDH staining, and many COX-negative fibers.

Inheritance of this disorder is autosomal recessive and is associated with a quantitative defect in mtDNA. Several different mutations of nuclear genes (e.g., thymidine kinase gene) important in regulating the mitochondrial genome are felt to be responsible for mtDNA depletion (Saad et al., 2001). The severity of the depletion correlates with the clinical severity of the disorder. As much as a 99% reduction in mtDNA is present in the fatal infantile myopathy form of the disease, while the more benign myopathy has a smaller depletion (36%–88%) of mtDNA.

## Congenital Myopathies

Occasionally, children exhibit a lack of tone at birth or shortly thereafter. In some, obvious weakness of the limbs accompanies hypotonia, and the baby lies immobile in the crib. These children may have spinal muscular atrophy, a congenital myopathy or muscular dystrophy, a metabolic disorder (e.g., a mitochondrial myopathy), or rarely, a toxic cause (e.g., botulism). Other babies move the limbs, if not normally, at least through their full range of movement, and do so spontaneously. Determining muscle strength in a baby is difficult; however, when no obvious weakness is discernible, the category of *congenital hypotonia* is used. One of the most common causes of congenital hypotonia is damage to the CNS. Cerebral hypotonia is not due to any primary abnormality in the muscle but presumably accompanies a disturbance of reflex tone. Selective atrophy of type 2 muscle fibers occurs, and lesions occur secondary to the neurological lesion. Babies with benign congenital hypotonia do not show any neurological abnormality other than hypotonia. Tendon reflexes are preserved or slightly diminished. Muscle biopsy and EMGs are normal, and serum CK levels are appropriate to the child's age. As time progresses, the children can develop muscle tone, and normal motor development may ensue. In teenage life, these children may not gain the ranks of star high school athletes, but neuromuscular function is normal.

The only treatment necessary in all these conditions is to encourage the child to participate in play therapy, with the aim of increasing motor activity. Referrals to physical and occupational therapists are important. The subsequent sections and recent reviews discuss the more common forms of congenital myopathy (May and Joseph, 2016; North et al., 2014).

### Central Core Myopathy and Multiminicore Myopathy

Central core myopathy is inherited in an autosomal dominant fashion and is caused by a mutation in the ryanodine receptor gene (*RYR1*) (May and Joseph, 2016; North et al., 2014). It is allelic to one form of hereditary malignant hyperthermia and, not surprisingly, malignant hyperthermia and central core can occur together.

Patient with central core disease may be floppy shortly after birth, and as in so many of these myopathies, congenital hip dislocation is common. As the child grows older, delay in achieving motor milestones is the rule. At an age when the child should be running easily, he or she is often ungainly and clumsy. The family recognizes before long that the impairment is not getting any worse. Strength, although below normal, usually is not impaired enough to be severely disabling. As in some of the other illnesses, patients may be slender and short of stature. On examination, one observes diffuse weakness of the arms and legs. Mild facial and neck weakness also occur. Diminished deep tendon reflexes are the rule. Common skeletal abnormalities such as high-arched feet, a long face, and a high-arched palate are common. Some patients can have ventilatory muscle weakness. Recently, there have been reports of a late-onset axial myopathy in which patients present with truncal weakness (e.g., bent spine syndrome, neck extensor myopathy) who have *RYR1* gene mutations (Jungbluth et al., 2009; Løseth et al., 2013). EMG shows nonspecific myopathic changes in central core disease. Serum CK concentrations are usually normal, although mild elevation may occur. The muscle biopsy is diagnostic; muscle shows a combination of type 1 fiber predominance and hypotrophy with central cores, an area in the muscle fiber where the central myofibrils are in disarray. On cross-section of the muscle, many of the oxidative histochemical reactions and the periodic acid–Schiff stain demonstrate an unstained central core running through the center of the fibers (Fig. 109.28).

No specific treatment for central core disease is available. A brace may correct a deformity such as a foot drop. Advise patients about the possibility of malignant hyperthermia, a potentially fatal complication.

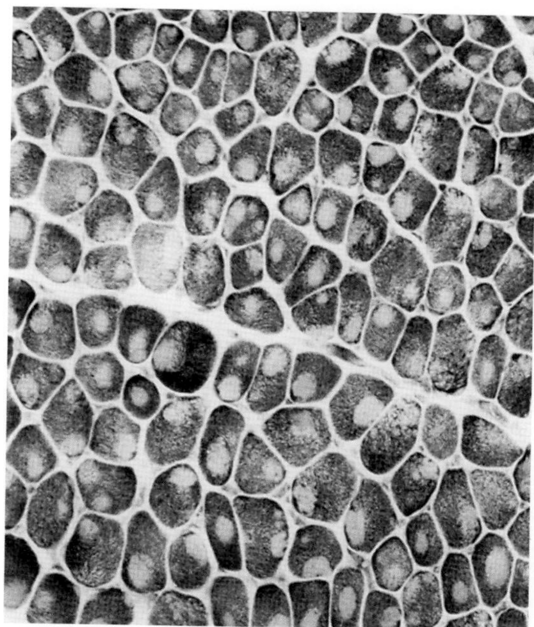

**Fig. 109.28 Central Core Disease.** Unstained area in most fibers is characteristic of this illness (nicotinamide adenine dinucleotide dehydrogenase-tetrazolium reductase stain).

## Nemaline Myopathy

The presence of small rod-like particles in muscle fibers is the basis for diagnosis of nemaline myopathy. The modified trichrome stain best displays these rods (Fig. 109.29), but EM characterizes them best. They originate in the Z-disk and exhibit structural continuity with the thin filament. They have a regular structure, presenting as a tetragonal filamentous array when cut transversely and exhibiting periodic lines both perpendicular and parallel to the long axis. Major constituents of the rods include α-actinin, desmin, and nebulin, proteins normally present in the Z-line.

The myopathy is genetically heterogenetic, with mutations having been identified in the genes that encode for α-tropomyosin (*TPM3*), β-tropomyosin (*TPN2*), nebulin (*NEB*), troponin T (*TnT1*), α-actinin (*ACTA1*), and cofilin-2 (*CFL2*) (Iannaccone and Castro, 2013; North et al., 2014; Wallgren-Pettersson and Laing, 2006). Autosomal dominant nemaline myopathy links to mutations in α-tropomyosin on chromosome 1q21-q23 (Laing et al., 1995). β-Tropomyosin is on chromosome 9p13, and cofilin-2 in chromosome 14q12 (Donner et al., 2002). Autosomal recessive nemaline myopathy has been associated with mutations in the genes that code for nebulin on chromosome 2q21.2-q22 (Pelin et al., 2002), and troponin T on chromosome 19q13 (Jin et al., 2003). Both autosomal dominant and autosomal recessive cases occur with mutations in α-actinin on chromosome 1q42.1 (Nowak et al., 1999).

The clinical picture of nemaline myopathy is heterogeneous (Iannaccone and Castro, 2013; North et al., 2014; Ryan et al., 2001; Wallgren-Pettersson, 2005). Most common is early hypotonia succeeded by diffuse weakness of the arms and legs, mild weakness of the face and other bulbar muscles, and a dysmorphic appearance. The face is long and narrow, with abnormalities of the jaw that may be either prognathous or abnormally short. The feet are often high-arched, and kyphoscoliosis is common as the children grow older. The disorder is slowly progressive. In some patients, respiratory failure out of proportion to the general weakness may ensue. Cardiomyopathy also occurs. A severe infantile variety is fatal. These children have profound hypotonia and respiratory failure. Another form may have its onset in early adulthood and present with a mild proximal or predominantly distal weakness (Wallgren-Pettersson et al., 2007). No specific treatment for nemaline myopathy is available. Bracing and surgery have a role in treatment.

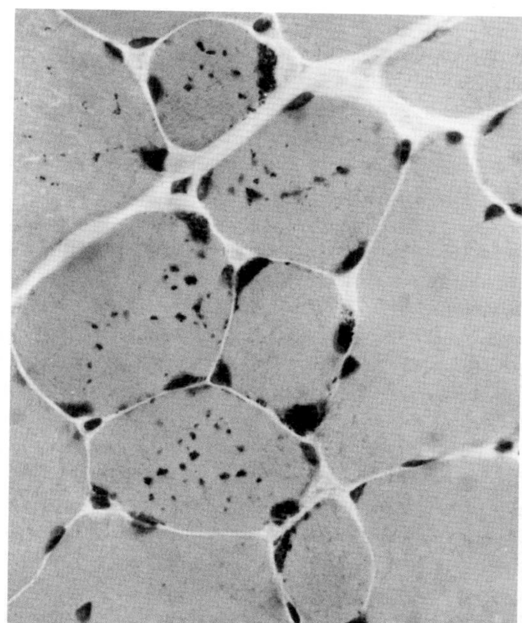

**Fig. 109.29 Nemaline Myopathy.** Although better demonstrated with the electron microscope, nemaline rods are also noted with histochemical reactions. Granular appearance of these fibers is due to the presence of many rods (modified Gomori trichrome stain).

In nemaline myopathy, EMG demonstrates the nonspecific myopathic changes. Serum CK levels may be normal or elevated. The muscle biopsy, in addition to demonstrating nemaline rods, often shows type 1 fiber predominance, selective atrophy of the type 1 fibers, and deficiency of type 2B fibers (Fig. 109.30). EM examination shows the characteristic rods. These are most often in the cytoplasm, but intranuclear rods also occur and equate with the severe infantile form (Goebel and Warlo, 1997).

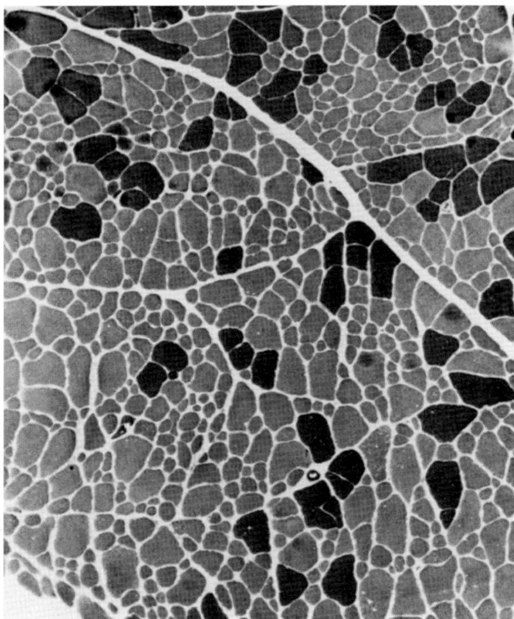

**Fig. 109.30 Nemaline Myopathy.** As in central core disease, nemaline myopathy shows predominance and atrophy of type 1 fibers. Note that the very smallest fibers in this biopsy are all type 1 (myosin adenosine triphosphatase stain, pH 9.4).

## Centronuclear Myopathy

The term *centronuclear myopathy* applies to a group of diseases in which the pathological finding is the presence of fibers with internal nuclei (Iannaccone and Castro, 2013; North et al., 2014). The most common form is an X-linked and infantile presentation of severe extraocular, facial, and limb weakness that is often fatal due to respiratory failure (Wallgren-Pettersson, 2005). This disorder is also known as *myotubular myopathy*, as muscle biopsies show atrophic fibers with central nuclei resembling myotubes. Severe hypotonia and respiratory distress are the presenting features. The disorder is usually fatal during the first few months due to respiratory failure. The weakness is severe and includes weakness of the facial and neck muscles as well as the extraocular muscles. Ptosis and ophthalmoparesis occur. The ribs are thin, and there are contractures at the hips and less often at the knees and ankles. X-linked myotubular myopathy results from mutations in the *MTM1* gene encoding for myotubularin-1 (Laporte et al., 1997). Occasional female carriers manifest less severe disease.

An autosomal dominant form of centronuclear myopathy also exists. The disorder is milder, occurs later in life, and is less common than the severe X-linked form. Ptosis, extraocular weakness, and facial weakness may be present, and moderate limb weakness gives rise to some disability. Equinovarus deformity of the feet occurs. The autosomal recessive variety, which is also less common, seems to be intermediate in severity between the other varieties. Some autosomal dominant cases of centronuclear myopathy are associated with early involvement of distal muscles and caused by mutations in the *DNM2* gene on chromosome 19p13.2 that encodes for dynamin-2 (Bitoun et al., 2005; Fischer et al., 2006). Of note, mutations in this gene cause CMT2B (Zuchner et al., 2005), explaining some of the overlapping features (distal weakness, mild sensory abnormalities).

Laboratory studies show normal or slightly elevated serum CK concentrations. EMG demonstrates marked muscle membrane instability in the form of fibrillation potentials, positive sharp waves, complex repetitive discharges, and occasionally even myotonic discharges. Muscle biopsy demonstrates characteristic features. With the routine hematoxylin and eosin or trichrome stains, marked variability in the size of fibers occurs, most of which are small. In the center of many of these fibers is a large, plump nucleus resembling the myotube stage of muscle development. With the oxidative enzyme reaction, many of the fibers have a darkly staining central spot. Almost all the fibers have a pale staining area, with an ATPase reaction that runs through the middle of the fiber. Although this looks superficially like a core, most central cores are not visible with an ATPase stain. When viewed in longitudinal section, the fiber has a long central area containing nuclei spaced at intervals. The biopsy shares features of the other congenital disorders, with type 1 fiber predominance and often type 1 fiber atrophy or hypotrophy. The biopsy findings in the X-linked recessive illness appear similar. Although the muscle fibers superficially resemble myotubes, they are in fact quite different: hence the preferred term, *centronuclear myopathy*. The differentiation into well-marked histochemical fiber types and the cytoarchitecture of the fiber more resemble the adult fiber. Two fetal cytoskeletal proteins (vimentin and desmin), which are found in fetal myotubes, have been demonstrated in fibers from patients with myotubular myopathy by immunocytochemical studies. On occasion, the EEG shows a paroxysmal disturbance.

Treatment includes respiratory and general supportive measures. Treatment of the severe infantile form requires balancing intervention against the very poor prognosis. The decision whether or not to provide life support for these children is a difficult one. Most die within the first 2 years.

## Congenital Fiber-Type Disproportion

Children affected by congenital fiber-type disproportion are floppy at birth, with varying degrees of weakness. The weakness is diffuse and frequently involves the face and neck. Sometimes in early childhood, strength improves, but whether this represents an improvement in the disease or the child's normal growth is uncertain. Contractures, particularly of the Achilles tendons, and congenital hip dislocation are common. Respiratory complications are common during the first 2 years of life, when the disease can be quite severe. As the children grow older, they remain weak and are short, with low weight. Accompanying the illness are various deformities of the feet, high-arched palate, and kyphoscoliosis.

EMG shows myopathic potentials but no evidence of muscle membrane instability (i.e., no fibrillation potentials or positive sharp waves). The serum CK concentration may be normal to slightly elevated. Muscle biopsy is diagnostic; the characteristic feature is a marked disproportion between the size of type 2 and type 1 fibers. Muscle biopsy shows the features of type 1 fiber atrophy and predominance. The original suggestion that a 15% smaller mean diameter of type 1 fibers compared to type 2 fibers was diagnostic was incorrect. The diagnosis should only be made when the discrepancy between the type 1 and type 2 fibers is greater than 45% and when more than 75% of the fibers are type 1 (Fig. 109.31). The reason for this discrepancy in fiber size is unknown.

Inheritance is autosomal dominant in approximately 40% of reported cases. This illness may represent nemaline myopathy without apparent rods, as some cases have been found with mutations in *ACTA1* and *TPN3* genes. Some patients have had mutations in the gene that encodes for selenoprotein N, which are also associated with multiminicore myopathy, congenital muscular dystrophy with rigid spine, and some cases of MFM.

## Inflammatory Myopathies

Inflammatory cell infiltrates may be seen on muscle biopsy in a wide range of myopathies and dystrophies. In many cases, this is presumably a secondary response of the immune system to the muscle fiber damage

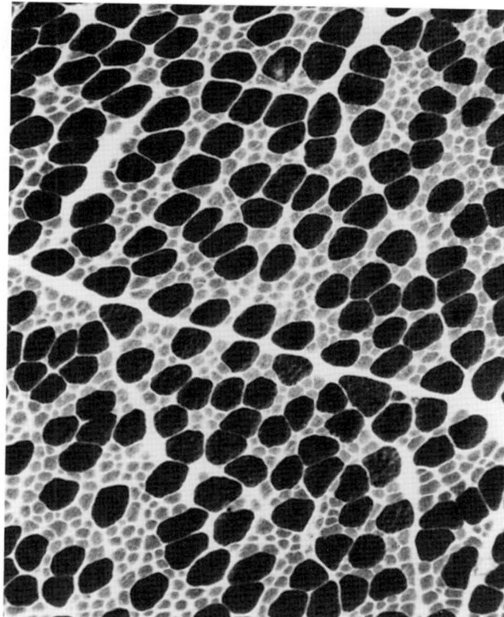

**Fig. 109.31 Congenital Fiber-Type Disproportion.** The diagnosis requires a clear discrepancy between hypertrophic type 2 fibers and atrophic type 1 fibers, as demonstrated in this picture (myosin adenosine triphosphatase stain, pH 9.4).

induced by the underlying disorder. In the inflammatory myopathies, however, the disease process is a primary result of an abnormality of the immune system itself. DM, myositis associated with antisynthetase syndrome (ASS), PM, immune-mediated necrotizing myopathy (IMNM), and IBM are the most common inflammatory myopathies (Amato and Barohn, 2009a, 2009b). The underlying pathogenesis of these inflammatory myopathies is diverse. Inflammatory myositis can occur in isolation, as a paraneoplastic manifestation of malignancy, or in association with connective tissue disorders (overlap syndromes). When myositis occurs as part of another autoimmune disease (e.g., rheumatoid arthritis), the primary condition often overshadows the myopathy. Finally, viral, bacterial, and parasitic infections can directly affect muscle; much of the muscle damage in these cases arises from the resulting immune response.

The classification of inflammatory myositis was initially based on criteria established by Bohan and Peter in 1975. Because IBM and IMNM were not yet understood to be distinct entities and because these criteria did not require muscle biopsy, the incidence of PM was overestimated and the disease likely overdiagnosed. Over time, distinct clinical and histopathological features have been described between these various disorders. Recent consensus classification schemas recognize these advances and allow for distinction between DM, PM, IBM, IMNM, and ASS (Allenbach et al., 2018; De Bleeker JL, Neuromuscul Disord, 2015; Hoogendijk, 2004). Equally important, however, an expanding array of pathological autoantibodies have been discovered in association with various myositis syndromes. Both myositis-specific antibodies (MSA)—seen only in the presence of an inflammatory myositis—and myositis-associated antibodies (MAA)—seen in myositis overlap syndromes with other autoimmune diseases—have been described. In many cases, a specific antibody can predict the underlying histopathology with high specificity and also predict clinical characteristics of the disease. In addition to securing a diagnosis, the identification of a specific autoantibody can offer the clinician important information about common associated manifestations of disease (e.g., interstitial lung disease [ILD] in ASS), risk of associated malignancy, prognosis, and expected response to various treatments. Contemporary classification schemes have incorporated these discoveries to an increasing degree. As there is not yet a perfect correlation between clinical, histopathological, and serological findings, there remains some controversy regarding appropriate categorization into strict categories of disease.

## Dermatomyositis

DM is an illness in which weakness is associated with a characteristic skin rash. It is the most common form of myositis and can present at any age from childhood through late adult life (Bendewald et al., 2010). The rash typically occurs prior to or with the onset of muscle weakness, although occasionally it will begin later. A "heliotrope rash" is characteristic—purplish discoloration of the skin over the cheeks and eyelids. An erythematous, macular rash may develop on the face, in a V-shaped distribution below the neck, the shoulders and upper back (shawl sign), or extensor surfaces of the elbows, knees, and knuckles (Gottron sign). The knuckles can also develop a papular rash (Gottron papules). The rash may spread widely over the body and be associated with edema of the skin, which frequently becomes scaly and weeping. Because the hallmark of the disease is the capillary abnormality, it may be helpful to use a hand lens to examine the skin around the nail beds. There, small hemorrhages and looped, dilated, and sometimes thrombosed capillaries may combine with avascular areas. The cuticle is discolored. In chronic long-standing DM of childhood, the skin changes may be more disabling than the muscle weakness. In the terminal stage, the skin may be a shiny, fragile, shell-like covering that cracks at the slightest movement. Soft-tissue calcification occurs in some patients as the disease progresses; it is usually late in the illness and is not necessarily an indication of active disease.

Weakness is symmetrical and affects the proximal more than distal muscles of the arms and legs. Dysphagia affects up to 30%. Muscle pain may be noted but should not be the predominant feature of the disorder. The illness often follows a relapsing-remitting course, although occasionally the illness is clearly monophasic even to the point of recovering spontaneously without treatment.

Muscle is not the only tissue involved in DM. There may be evidence of vascular abnormalities such as the Raynaud phenomenon. Cardiac involvement ranges from conduction defects to congestive cardiac failure secondary to cardiomyopathy. Interstitial pneumonitis and fibrosis may cause a nonproductive cough and respiratory distress. Chest radiographs show changes in the majority of patients, with patchy consolidation, particularly subpleural, and peribronchovascular thickening. The changes are reversible with treatment (Mino et al., 1997). Delayed gastric and esophageal emptying occurs in the illness, indicating an abnormality in the smooth muscle of the upper gastrointestinal tract. There is an increased risk for cancer in adults with DM. Approximately 10% to 15% of adults will develop a cancer within 2–3 years of presentation of the myositis (Olazagasti et al., 2015). Accordingly, all patients should undergo comprehensive screening. Breast, pelvic, testicular, and prostate examinations should be performed. We send complete blood count, electrolytes and renal function, urinalysis, and serum protein electrophoresis. We also obtain a CT scan of the chest, abdomen, and pelvis, a colonoscopy in all those over 50 or with gastrointestinal complaints, and mammography and pelvic ultrasound in women.

The serum CK concentrations are often elevated in DM but can be normal in a third of cases, particularly in patients with a very indolent course. Serum CK levels do not necessarily reflect activity of the disease, so one might see a clinical exacerbation unaccompanied by marked changes in enzyme levels of patients whose illness appears quiescent and who have moderately elevated levels of CK. The CK levels may rise

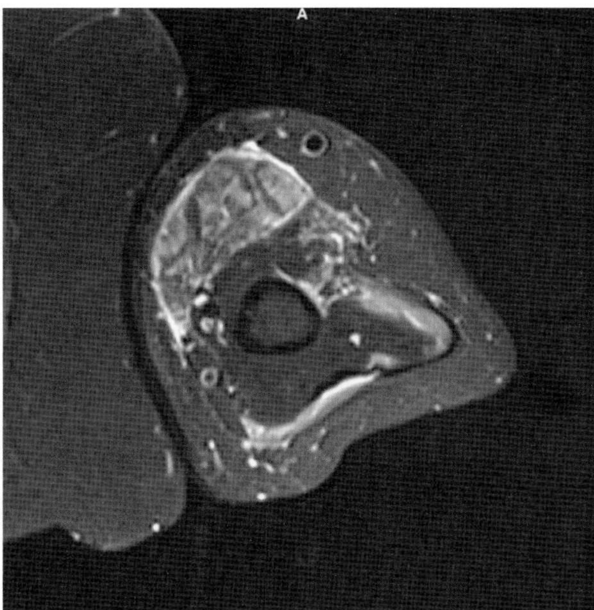


**Fig. 109.32 Dermatomyositis.** Short tau inversion recovery sequence on magnetic resonance imaging of the arm demonstrates hyperintensity consistent with muscle edema in affected muscles.

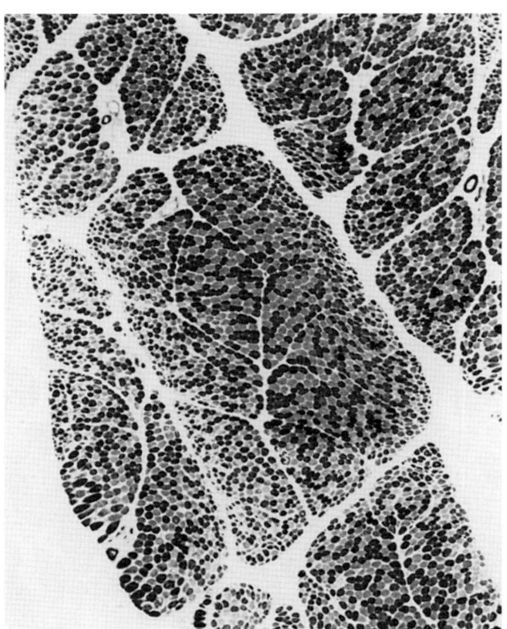

**Fig. 109.33 Dermatomyositis.** Perifascicular atrophy (myosin adenosine triphosphatase stain, pH 9.4).

several weeks before a clinical relapse occurs. In approximately 10% of patients with a normal CK, the serum aldolase may be elevated. EMG demonstrates early recruitment of small polyphasic motor unit action potentials (MUAPs), often associated with increased insertional activity, fibrillation potentials, positive sharp waves, and complex repetitive discharges. When obtained, muscle MRI may show evidence of edema in affected muscles, best seen on short tau inversion recovery (STIR) sequences (Fig. 109.32). This is not specific for inflammatory myositis, but it may be helpful in selecting which muscle to biopsy.

MSA are found in 60%–70% of patients with DM and include antibodies against Mi-2, melanoma differentiation protein 5 (MDA5), transcriptional intermediary factor 1-ϒ (TIF1-ϒ), and nuclear matrix protein 2 (NXP-2). Anti-Mi-2 occurs in 7%–30% (Pinal-Fernandez et al., 2015). Compared to other patients with DM, patients with anti-Mi-2 antibodies have a reduced risk of malignancy and more favorable response to treatment. By contrast, anti-TIF1-ϒ antibodies are seen in 14%–31% and are highly predictive of associated malignancy.

The characteristic histological feature on muscle biopsy is *perifascicular atrophy* (a crust of small fibers surrounding a core of more normal-sized fibers deeper in the fascicle) (Fig. 109.33). Perifascicular atrophy is a rather specific abnormality and is typically seen only in DM and in some overlap syndromes (see later discussion). Importantly, perifascicular atrophy is not always appreciated (occurring in <50% of biopsies in the authors' experience), particularly in adults and in patients undergoing biopsy early in the course of their illness. Prior to perifascicular atrophy, deposition of MAC may be seen on capillaries and small blood vessels.

Gene expression studies in muscle biopsies and peripheral blood in patients with DM demonstrate increased expression of type 1 interferons (IFNs) and the proteins they regulate (Walsh et al., 2007). Overexpression of IFN may be directly toxic to small capillaries and muscle fibers. There is increased expression of type 1 IFN-inducible proteins on small blood vessels and muscle fibers, with an early predilection for perifascicular muscle fibers (Greenberg et al., 2005b; Salajegheh et al., 2010). Expression of type 1 IFN-inducible proteins on perifascicular fibers is more sensitive than perifascicular atrophy for the

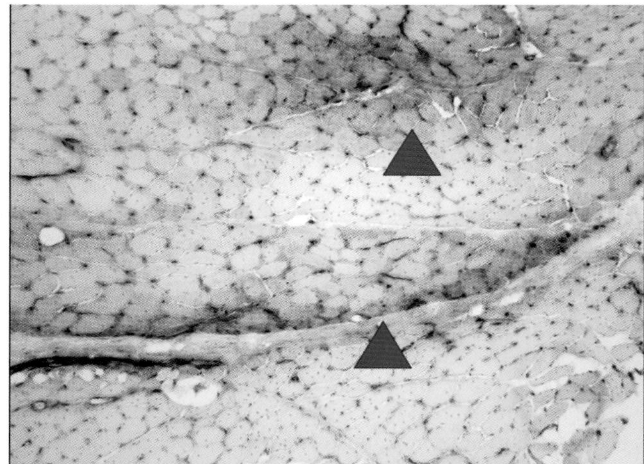

**Fig. 109.34 Dermatomyositis.** Expression of myxoma virus resistance protein on perifascicular fibers is a sensitive and specific marker of dermatomyositis.

diagnosis of DM. Expression of one such protein, myxoma virus resistance protein (MxA), has been shown to have a sensitivity of 71% and specificity of 98% for diagnosis of DM and to be more sensitive than either perifascicular atrophy or MAC deposition (Fig. 109.34) (Uruha et al., 2017). Interestingly, one role of MxA is that it may serve to form tubuloreticular inclusions surrounding RNA viruses, thereby preventing their replication. These tubuloreticular inclusions formed by MxA are similar in appearance to the inclusions seen in endothelial cells on EM of DM patients. Expression of retinoic acid inducible-gene 1 (*RIG-1*) has also been shown to be more sensitive than perifascicular atrophy (Suarez-Calvet et al., 2017).

Inflammatory infiltrate can be scant. When present, the inflammatory cells are located around blood vessels (perivascular inflammation) and in the perimysial connective tissue as opposed to the endomysium (Fig. 109.35). Further evidence for humoral rather than cytotoxic

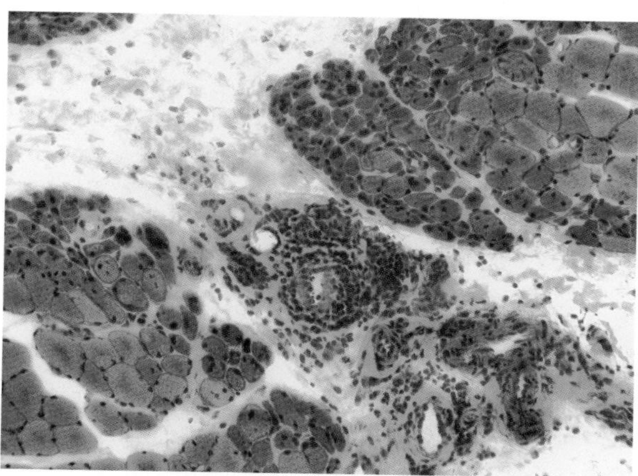

**Fig. 109.35 Dermatomyositis.** Inflammatory cells, when present, are located around blood vessels (i.e., perivascular) and are located primarily in perimysial connective tissue as opposed to endomysium, as seen in polymyositis and inclusion body myositis.

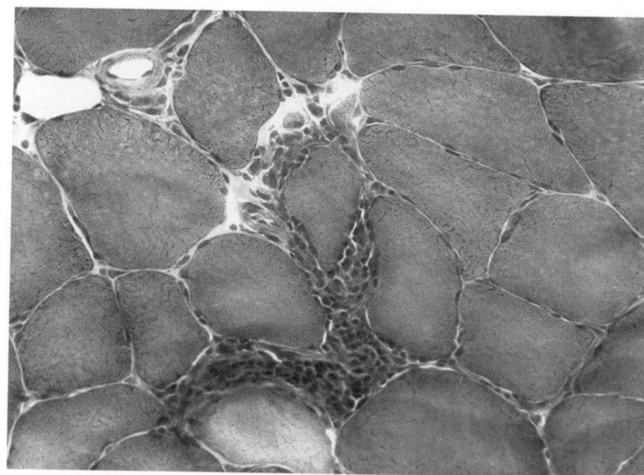

**Fig. 109.36 Polymyositis.** Mononuclear inflammatory cells composed of cytotoxic T cells and macrophages surround and invade non-necrotic muscle in endomysium.

factors is found in the relative preponderance of B and CD4 cells compared to CD8 (cytotoxic) cells in the inflammatory reaction associated with the blood vessels. Studies have demonstrated that the majority of these $CD4^{+}$ cells, once thought to be T-helper cells, are actually plasmacytoid dendritic cells (PDCs) (Greenberg et al., 2005b). PDCs are part of the innate immune system and function both as antigen-presenting cells and as secretors of type 1 IFNs. With advancing disease, destruction of capillaries may result in muscle infarction. Unlike polymyositis and IBM, endomysial inflammation with invasion of non-necrotic muscle fibers is not a feature of DM.

## Polymyositis

Polymyositis usually presents in adults in an acute or insidious fashion. The disorder is more frequent in women than in men, as are other autoimmune diseases. Weakness is symmetrical and affects the proximal more than distal muscles of the limbs. The pattern of weakness can help distinguish polymyositis from IBM (Amato et al., 1996). The weakness may be similar in distribution to that seen in many of the LGMDs. Usually when patients have severe proximal weakness (e.g., Medical Research Council grade 4 or less), examination reveals distal weakness as well. If a patient has severe proximal weakness in the absence of any distal weakness, LGMD should be suspected. Extraocular features usually are not involved. Dysphagia associated with altered pharyngeal and esophageal motility occurs, particularly in the overlap syndromes, where polymyositis is associated with other rheumatological diseases such as scleroderma.

One would expect an inflammatory disorder of the muscle to cause severe pain, but such is not the case with polymyositis. Although half of patients describe an aching, tender quality to the muscles, the more severe the pain, the less likely the diagnosis of polymyositis. Systemic symptoms are common at onset, such as malaise, fever, and anorexia. A viral prodrome sometimes precedes the illness, but such events are sufficiently common enough that the association may be coincidental.

The diagnostic studies in polymyositis are similar to those in DM and include serum CK concentrations, serum autoantibodies, EMG, and muscle biopsy. Serum CK concentration should always be elevated in polymyositis, unlike DM or IBM, in which the CK concentration may be normal.

What was traditionally considered polymyositis is likely a heterogeneous group of disorders. Revised contemporary classification criteria create a more narrow definition of PM and allow for exclusion of IBM and LGMDs, which can share histopathological features of PM (Hoogendijk JE, 2004). For example, calpainopathy (LGMD 2A), dysferlinopathy (LGMD 2B), and FSHD all commonly have inflammation evident on muscle biopsy. Polymyositis is a cell-mediated disorder in which the immune attack is directed against some unknown antigen(s) on the muscle fibers. Definitive diagnosis requires demonstration of $CD8^{+}$ T cells invading *non-necrotic* myofibers expressing MHC-I (Fig. 109.36) and the absence of rimmed vacuoles. When this finding is absent, widespread MHC-1 expression on non-necrotic myofibers can support diagnosis of PM. Perifascicular atrophy does not occur, and neither immunoglobulin nor complement deposition occurs on small blood vessels. Many cases that would traditionally be considered PM may better be conceptualized as an overlap syndrome (see below).

***Myositis associated with antisynthetase syndrome.*** The discovery of several anti-aminoacyl-tRNA synthetase (ARS) antibodies has allowed for distinct categorization of the ASS. The most common of these antibodies is anti-Jo-1, but several others have since been described. In general, these patients manifest with some combination of constitutional symptoms such as fever and weight loss, myositis, ILD, nonerosive arthritis, Raynaud phenomenon, and an erythematous skin rash. "Mechanic's hands" is most characteristic—hyperkeratotic lesions on the lateral and palmar aspects of the fingers. The propensity to develop each of these findings varies with each specific ARS. As an example, among patients with anti-Jo-1 antibodies, 90% develop myositis, 66% develop ILD, 40% develop Raynaud phenomenon, 31% develop mechanic's hands, and 27% fever. By contrast, less than 50% patients with PL-7 or PL-12 antibodies develop myositis and instead are more likely to present with ILD. Regardless of the specific antibody, patients with ASS with ILD at diagnosis should be actively screened for its later development.

As the ARS antibodies were first described, they were identified among patients traditionally thought to have both DM and PM. Findings on muscle biopsy are often similar to what is seen in DM. Recent data, however, suggest that ASS may be associated with its own distinct histopathological features, further supporting the argument that perhaps it is best to consider ASS its own distinct clinical entity. Perifascicular atrophy can be seen but compared to DM there may be more prominent myofiber necrosis, MHC-1 and MHC-2 expression, and MAC deposition in the perifascicular region. HLA-DR expression in particular may distinguish ASS from DM, as it has been reported in over 80% of patients with ASS versus 24% of patients with DM, and perifascicular expression was only observed in ASS. Fragmentation of the perimysial connective tissue with alkaline phosphatase staining has been reported. Finally, myonuclear actin filaments and rod formation has been reported, as well (Aouizerate et al., 2014; Mescam-Mancini L, Brain 2015; Mozaffar and Pestronk, 200; Stenzel et al., 2015).

### Myositis Associated with Other Collagen Vascular Diseases (Overlap Syndromes)

Systemic lupus erythematosus, mixed connective tissue disease, systemic sclerosis, rheumatoid arthritis, and Sjögren syndrome all may have weakness as a facet of the disease complex. The overlap syndromes are those in which features of these illnesses coexist with an inflammatory myopathy. The clinical features are otherwise typical of DM or polymyositis. Histopathologically, many cases resemble DM on muscle biopsy, but necrotizing myopathy or nonspecific inflammatory features may be seen. MAAs are associated with overlap syndromes and sometimes predate clinical features of a connective tissue disease in patients with myositis (Troyanov et al., 2005). These include anti-PM-Scl (associated with scleroderma myositis), anti-U1-ribonucleoprotein (RNP) (associated with mixed connective tissue disease), anti-Ku, anti-Ro, and anti-La.

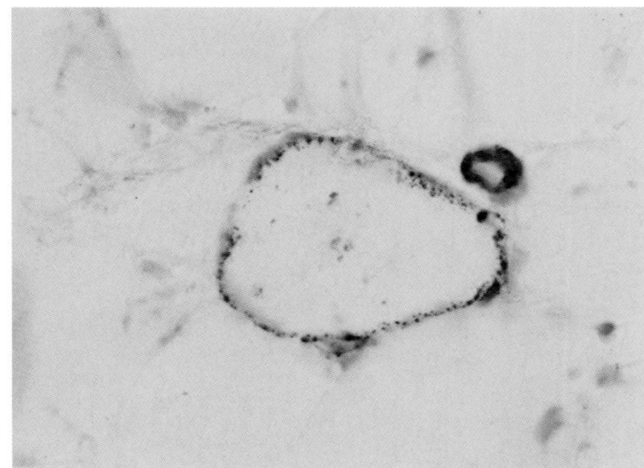

**Fig. 109.37 Immune-Mediated Necrotizing Myopathy.** Immunohistochemical staining demonstrates deposition of complement C5b-C9, the membrane attack complex, on a muscle fiber and capillary.

### Immune-Mediated Necrotizing Myopathy

IMNM clinically resembles polymyositis, with proximal upper and lower extremity weakness. Facial weakness, scapular winging, asymmetry, and prominent distal weakness are all unusual for this disorder. The onset of weakness can be quite acute but is subacute in others. IMNM has been associated with autoantibodies against 3-hydoxy-3-methylglutaryl-coenzyme A reductase (HMGCR) and against the signal recognition particle (SRP). Some patients are seronegative for both, suggesting other antibodies have yet to be discovered.

Anti-HMGCR antibodies were first discovered in statin-exposed patients who develop weakness that does not resolve after stopping the medication (Grable-Esposito et al., 2010; Mammen et al., 2011). Unlike the more common (but still rare) toxic myopathy from statins, patients with anti-HMGCR IMNM require immunomodulatory treatment for improvement in their weakness. This antibody has thus become a critical tool for making this important distinction between the toxic and autoimmune forms earlier. Anti-HMGCR antibodies can also be found in nonstatin-exposed patients with IMNM—typically younger adults and children. This disease can be subacute in children, mimicking LGMD, so it is important to consider testing for anti-HMGCR antibodies in such children without a genetic mutation found. Anti-SRP antibodies are associated with more rapid disease course and more severe weakness (Pinal-Fernandez et al., 2017). Affected patients quickly develop fibrosis and fatty replacement of muscle, so early treatment is critically important to allow for return to normal function. Neck weakness (e.g., head drop), dysphagia, and cardiac complications are also more common.

IMNM can occur in the setting of connective tissue disease as an overlap syndrome and can also occur as a paraneoplastic syndrome. Cancer screening, as described in the DM section, is recommended for all these patients. The risk of an associated cancer appears to be higher in nonstatin-exposed anti-HMGCR patients compared to anti-SRP (Allenbach et al., 2016).

Serum CK is nearly always elevated in IMNM, and the EMG should demonstrate fibrillation potentials, positive sharp waves, and myopathic motor unit potentials. On muscle biopsy, histological analysis reveals necrotic muscle fibers with minimal inflammatory cell infiltration. Deposition of MAC on non-necrotic muscle fibers and upregulation of MHC-1 are expected (Fig. 109.37; Watanabe 2016).

### Treatment of Dermatomyositis, Polymyositis, and Immune-Mediated Necrotizing Myopathy

Few randomized double-blinded trials of patients with myositis exist. Nevertheless, general agreement exists to treat these disorders with corticosteroids, some other form of immunosuppression, or a combination of these (Allenbach et al., 2018; Mammen et al., 2016). Corticosteroids are generally considered first line. We start patients with myositis on high-dose, daily prednisone (0.7–1 mg/kg/day, up to 60 mg daily). In patients with severe disease a 3–5 day pulse of intravenous methylprednisolone (1 g/daily) can be used first. This high dose should typically be maintained until strength improves and the CK normalizes; typically this requires 2–4 months. Thereafter, a slow taper of 10 mg every month is reasonable until prednisone 20 mg/day is reached. We taper more slowly thereafter.

Most patients require treatment with a second agent beyond corticosteroids. We add a second-line therapy if there has been poor response to corticosteroids after 2–4 months or if the patient relapses during taper. The development of significant side effects with corticosteroids may also necessitate a second agent. Blood glucose, serum potassium, and blood sugar should be monitored while on prednisone. We also recommend annual eye examinations. We prescribe calcium (500 mg–600 mg twice or three times daily) and vitamin D (1000 IU/daily) to all patients given the deleterious effect on bone.

Based on accumulating observational data, the subtype of myositis and specific autoantibody found in a given patient may be useful to individualize treatment. For example, among patients with DM, those with anti-Mi-2 antibodies are less likely to require a second agent (Love et al., 1991). Patient with anti-Jo-1 ASS, by contrast, frequently fail corticosteroid monotherapy (Koenig et al., 2007). Of particular importance, patients with IMNM rarely respond adequately to corticosteroid monotherapy; 90% of patients in one cohort required addition of a second-line agent within 6 months (Kassardjian et al., 2015). This observation has led some experts to recommend that patients with IMNM should be started on a second-line agent either immediately together with prednisone or within 1 month if there is no evidence of response (Allenbach et al., 2018). Moreover, it is our experience and that of others that intravenous immunoglobulin (IVIG; 2 g/kg/day over 2–5 days) may be effective as monotherapy, without corticosteroids, in patients with anti-HMGCR IMNM (Mammen et al., 2015). This is especially important in patients with contraindications to corticosteroids or severe side effects. Common complications include vasomotor symptoms, headache, rash, leukopenia, and fever. Thrombotic events occur in some patients. A controlled double-blind trial of IVIG as second-line therapy in patients with DM also showed improvement in functional ability and strength.

Methotrexate, azathioprine, and mycophenolate mofetil are commonly preferred second-line agents for myositis. We prefer methotrexate, as it appears to work much faster (e.g., within 2–3 months) compared to the other options. Methotrexate is usually administered orally at a starting dose of 7.5 mg/wk and gradually increased as necessary up to 15-25 mg/wk. If higher doses are required, we administer the drug subcutaneously or intravenously. Folate is given simultaneously. Methotrexate can cause interstitial pulmonary fibrosis. For this reason, we tend to avoid methotrexate in patients with ILD. Methotrexate is also associated with hepatotoxicity and bone marrow suppression. It is important to monitor complete blood counts (CBCs) and liver function tests in patients receiving methotrexate.

Many neurologists instead use azathioprine as their second-line agent of choice, but it can take 9 months or longer to see an effect. Most patients tolerate an oral dose of 1.5–2 mg/kg/day CTD. Before beginning treatment, a baseline CBC, platelet count, and liver function studies should be obtained. Therapy should be initiated with a low dose (e.g., 50 mg/day in an adult CTD), then the dose gradually increased while monitoring blood studies. A decrease in platelets below 150,000/mL or a total neutrophil count of less than 1000/mL are indications for drug reduction or stopping the drug temporarily. Blood studies should be monitored weekly at first and then monthly. An idiosyncratic response to azathioprine occurs in some patients. This consists of severe gastrointestinal distress with nausea and vomiting, associated with fever and some elevation of liver function tests. The response disappears when the drug is withdrawn.

Mycophenolate mofetil is another option as a second-line agent. We usually start at 1 g twice daily and go up to 1.5 g twice daily as needed CTD. Unlike azathioprine or methotrexate, this drug is not associated with liver toxicity, but as with other immunosuppressive agents, there is increased risk for malignancies in the future. Although mycophenolate mofetil appears to be beneficial, it carries an increased risk for infection (Rowin et al., 2006).

We have found rituximab to be useful in refractory patients with myositis. A double-blind, placebo-controlled trial of rituximab was negative (Oddis et al., 2013) but there were many issues with the study design. There is some evidence that rituximab may be particularly helpful in patients with anti-SRP IMNM (Allenbach et al., 2018). There is a low risk of progressive multifocal leukoencephalopathy that needs to be discussed with patients prior to use.

Observational studies suggest that 20%–40% of patients with PM and DM achieve long-term remission off pharmacological therapy, but for most the course will be either chronic or relapsing-remitting. Remission off therapy is even less common with IMNM. There is a mortality risk associated with myositis, particularly among those with ILD and/or associated malignancy.

### Inclusion Body Myositis

IBM is the most common myopathy in patients older than 50 years of age (Amato and Barohn, 2009b; Amato et al., 1996). Only rarely does it occur in people younger than age 50. Unlike DM, polymyositis, and other autoimmune disorders, IBM is much more common in men than in women. The disease characteristically affects the distal muscles of the arms and legs. The deep finger flexors, including the flexor pollicis longus, and wrist flexors are involved early and usually more than the wrist and finger extensors (Amato et al., 1996; Benveniste et al., 2011; Cox et al., 2011; Lloyd et al., 2014; Rose et al., 2013). In the legs, early involvement of the quadriceps and anterior tibial muscles occurs. Profound atrophy is appreciable in the flexor forearms and quadriceps. Muscle atrophy and weakness are often asymmetrical and may lead to an erroneous diagnosis of motor neuron disease (Dabby et al., 2001). However, unlike amyotrophic lateral sclerosis, no significant atrophy of the hand intrinsics occurs, fasciculations are absent, and deep tendon reflexes are normal or reduced. The progression is gradual but relentless, and disability may be severe. Facial weakness and dysphagia occur in one-third of patients. Myalgia is absent. Sometimes the sporadic form occurs in a familial setting (Amato and Shebert, 1998). It is important not to confuse these rare cases of familial inclusion body *myositis* with hereditary inclusion body *myopathies*.

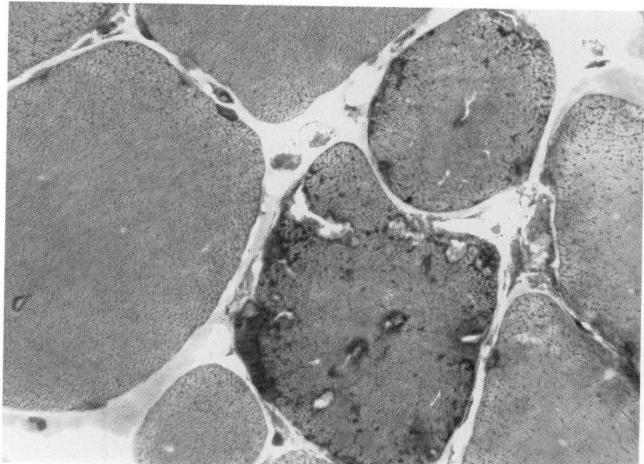

**Fig. 109.38 Inclusion Body Myositis.** Scattered muscle fibers contain one or more rimmed vacuoles (modified Gomori trichrome stain).

The clinical history and examination are the basis for suspecting the diagnosis of IBM. Recent studies have demonstrated that up to 70% of patients have autoantibodies in the serum directed against cytosolic 5′-nucleotidase 1A (cN-1A or NT5c1A) (Larman et al., 2013; Pluk et al., 2013). Specificity is reported to be greater than 90%, so these can be helpful for distinguishing IBM from other myopathies. Muscle biopsy is confirmatory. The CK concentration is typically normal or only mildly elevated (<10 times the upper limit of normal). The EMG demonstrates fibrillation potentials and positive sharp waves. A mixture of both small and large polyphasic motor unit potentials can be seen, creating diagnostic confusion and sometimes leading to an erroneous diagnosis of motor neuron disease. These large motor units were taken for some time to represent a neurogenic process; however, they represent remodeling of the motor unit that is possible with any chronic myopathy.

The muscle biopsy demonstrates endomysial inflammation and invasion of non-necrotic muscle fibers similar to polymyositis (Amato and Barohn, 2009b; Rose et al., 2013). In addition, characteristic "rimmed" vacuoles may be evident. On light microscopy, the structures have a sharply demarcated vacuole surrounded by a rim of altered tissue that stains red with the trichrome stain and bluish purple on hematoxylin and eosin (Fig. 109.38). Eosinophilic inclusions, amyloid, and other deposits are usually present in the vacuolated muscle fibers (Fig. 109.39; Rose et al., 2013; Salajegheh et al., 2009a, 2009b). Immunohistochemistry can aid in diagnosis, as these inclusions may stain for Tar DNA-binding protein-43 (TDP-43)—very specific for IBM—or for p62—very sensitive for IBM (Fig. 109.40; Hiniker et al., 2013). EM demonstrates the presence of cytoplasmic tubulofilamentous structures that are 15–21 nm in diameter, with an inner diameter of 3–6 nm. The numbers of deletions of mtDNA are increased in IBM when compared with normal age-matched controls. This probably reflects the increased number of COX-negative fibers and ragged-red fibers noted on muscle biopsy. The findings do not cast any light on the etiology of the illness, which shares no clinical features with the mitochondrial disorders (Moslemi et al., 1997).

Unfortunately, because of sampling error, the biopsy is not definitively diagnostic 20% to 30% of the time, showing only inflammatory cellular reaction without rimmed vacuoles. (Amato et al., 1996; Griggs et al., 1995; Lloyd et al., 2014). The absence of rimmed vacuole inclusions can lead to the misdiagnosis of polymyositis if the clinician

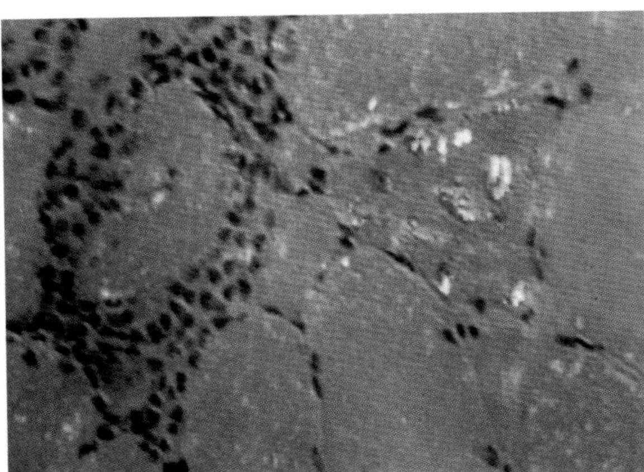

**Fig. 109.39 Inclusion Body Myositis.** Congo red stain under polarized light shows amyloid deposition within muscle fibers.

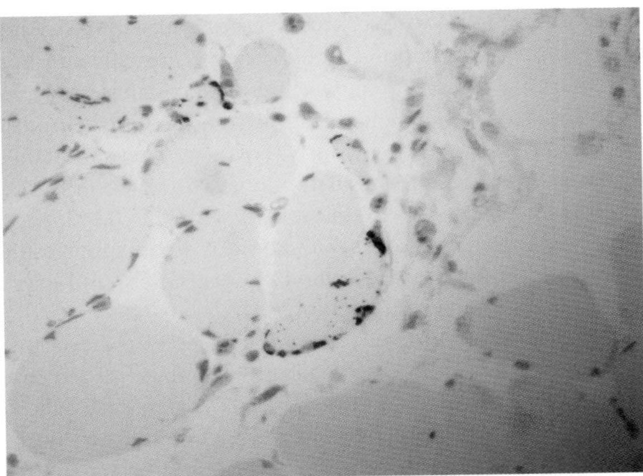

**Fig. 109.40 Inclusion Body Myositis.** p62 staining of myofiber inclusions is a sensitive finding for inclusion body myositis.

is unaware of the distinct differences in the clinical pattern of muscle weakness seen in IBM and polymyositis.

The invasion of muscle fibers by $CD8^+$ cytotoxic cells on muscle biopsy suggests that IBM results from cell-mediated cytotoxicity with an immune basis. This is reinforced by the presence of MHC class I antigens on the invaded muscle fibers. The disease, however, generally has a chronic progressive course and is considered unresponsive to prednisone and other immunosuppressive (e.g., methotrexate) and immunomodulating (e.g., IVIG) therapies (Benveniste et al., 2011; Cox et al., 2011; Griggs et al., 1995; Rose et al., 2013). Indeed, this is one criterion for suspecting the diagnosis. It is tempting to embark on a therapeutic trial when the inflammatory reaction is marked, but the side effects of corticosteroids and other immunosuppressive/immunomodulating therapies in the elderly are severe, particularly in the absence of any objective improvement with these agents in several double-blind placebo-controlled trials. Recent work has demonstrated that nearly 60% of patients with IBM have aberrant clonal populations of large granular T lymphocytes meeting criteria for T-cell large granular lymphocytic leukemia (Greenberg et al., 2016). These granular lymphocytes are seen invading muscle on biopsy of patients with IBM. This has led to the idea that autoimmune T-cell expansion in IBM might evolve into a neoplastic-like disorder, which could explain the refractoriness of this disorder to standard immune therapies.

## Other Inflammatory Conditions

Muscle frequently shows subclinical involvement in chronic granulomatous diseases such as sarcoidosis and tuberculosis. Bacterial infection (pyomyositis) is rare outside of tropical countries but does occur, particularly with the spread of human immunodeficiency virus (HIV) infection. The organism involved is often *Staphylococcus aureus* and sometimes *Streptococcus*. Usually the large muscle groups such as those of the thigh are the site of infection. The muscle is hot, painful, and swollen, and any movement exacerbates pain. Parasitic infections of muscles include those due to trichinosis, cysticercosis, and toxoplasmosis. In trichinosis, general symptoms of malaise and fever are associated with myalgia and stiffness. There may be periorbital edema, and the jaw muscles commonly are involved. Laboratory studies include muscle biopsy, which may show evidence of hypersensitivity (e.g., eosinophilia, hypergammaglobulinemia). Treatment is with thiabendazole. In-depth discussion of viral-associated myopathies can be found in Chapters 76 and 77.

## Polymyalgia Rheumatica

Severe muscle pain characterizes polymyalgia rheumatica. This diagnosis should not be given without full investigation because of two major implications: the high frequency of temporal arteritis and the effectiveness of corticosteroid therapy. The diagnosis should be limited to those with the typical picture, including increased erythrocyte sedimentation rate, and not used as an explanation for various aches, cramps, and pains. Women are affected more commonly than men, and the disorder is rare in individuals younger than age 55. The patient develops muscle stiffness, pain, and a feeling that the muscles have set. The arms are involved more commonly than the legs. Manipulation of the limb exacerbates the pain. The symptoms are particularly prominent in the morning when the patient arises and improve as the patient loosens up. These symptoms may be associated with chronic malaise, pyrexia, night sweats, and weight loss. On examination, the only specific muscle complaint is soreness. Tenderness over the temples, suggesting temporal arteritis, is an associated condition in 20% to 30% of affected individuals.

The erythrocyte sedimentation rate is elevated (often >70 mm/h), and this should be considered an essential part of the diagnosis of polymyalgia rheumatica. A mild hypochromic anemia may be associated. Otherwise, laboratory studies are generally normal. The serum CK concentration is not elevated, EMG may be normal, and muscle biopsy may show type 2 fiber atrophy, a nonspecific finding unhelpful in the diagnosis.

Polymyalgia rheumatica may be self-limiting but may take years to fade. For this reason, the recommended treatment is with prednisone and nonsteroidal antiinflammatory drugs (NSAIDs). The response to prednisone may be quite dramatic, with resolution of symptoms in hours to days. For the most part, the doses can be lower than used in other inflammatory autoimmune disorders. Maintenance on a low level of corticosteroids is often necessary for 2 years, and even then, only 24% of patients were able to stop treatment in one prospective study.

## Toxic Myopathies

Several commonly used drugs cause myopathy. Classification of the toxic myopathies is according to their presumed pathogenic mechanisms. Destruction of muscle fibers may be the result of the drug directly disrupting the sarcolemma, nuclear function, mitochondrial function, that of other organelles, or by triggering an immune attack.

### Necrotizing Myopathies

A necrotizing myopathy complicates the use of several drugs. The cholesterol-lowering agents are the most common. Most patients have only myalgias or cramps, or simply asymptomatic elevations of serum CK levels. Rarely, a toxic myopathy leading to weakness or even rhabdomyolysis develops. The myopathic signs and symptoms usually resolve after discontinuing the offending agent, but this may take weeks or sometimes months.

***Cholesterol-lowering drugs.*** Statins inhibit HMGCR, leading to lower cholesterol. Up to 20% of patients on statins complain of myalgias and/or cramps, but in many these are unrelated to the statin. Asymptomatic hyperCKemia affects 5% of statin-users. More severe myopathy, resulting in severe pain and symmetric proximal weakness, occurs in less than 0.1% of patients. Symptomatic rhabdomyolysis is rarer still, with an incidence of approximately 2–3/100,000 patient/years (Aronis et al., 2016). Statin myotoxicity most commonly occurs 1–6 months after initiation of statin. Risk is dose-dependent; male sex, age over 65 years, renal or hepatic failure, and hypothyroidism are additional risk factors (Chan et al., 2005). Concurrent use of other cholesterol-lowering agents and medications that inhibit the cytochrome P450 (CYP)3A4 enzyme also increase the risk of toxic myopathy and rhabdomyolysis. The combination of a statin and either cyclosporine or gemfibrozil is particularly problematic.

EMG of weak muscles reveals fibrillation potentials, positive sharp waves, and myotonic discharges with early recruitment of small-duration MUAPs. EMG in patients with asymptomatic serum CK elevations is often normal. Muscle histology demonstrates necrotic muscle fibers. Lipid-filled vacuoles within myofibers and COX-negative myofibers may be appreciated, but these are not a consistent finding (Phillips et al., 2002). Stopping the statin will lead to resolution of symptoms and normalization of CK in weeks to months.

As mentioned earlier, less commonly, an IMNM may be triggered by statin medications (Grable-Esposito et al., 2010; Mammen et al., 2011). This appears clinically similar to the toxic form, with proximal muscle weakness and CK elevation of 5000–10,000 U/L. However, symptoms and CK do not improve with cessation of the statin and instead patients require treatment with immunomodulatory therapy. Most patients with statin-associated IMNM develop antibodies against HMGCR; these antibodies are almost never seen in either statin-exposed healthy control patients or those with self-limited toxic myopathy (Mammen et al, 2012).

Fibric acid derivatives, niacin, and ezetimibe have also been associated with a similar spectrum of myotoxicity. With niacin and ezetimibe, this is usually with the concurrent use of a statin (Greenberg and Amato, 2006; Hodel, 2002).

## Inflammatory Myopathy

### Immune Checkpoint Inhibitors

Immune checkpoint inhibitors (ICPis) are increasingly being used for the treatment for many different cancers and often have benefit even in advanced/metastatic cases. These drugs work by targeting mechanisms used by cancer to evade surveillance and destruction by the immune system. Cytotoxic T cells, when activated via the T-cell receptor through presentation of a "non-self" antigen by an antigen presenting cell, typically require a second signal to permit action. This response is determined by a balance of this co-stimulatory signal and competing inhibitory signals. Inhibitors of two inhibitor receptors on cytotoxic T cells have been developed: cytotoxic T-lymphocyte-associated antigen-4 (CTLA-4; e.g., ipilimumab) and programmed cell death-1 receptor (PD-1; e.g., pembrolizumab and nivolumab). Inhibitors of the ligand of PD-1 (PD-L1; e.g., durvalumab) on antigen presenting cells have also been developed.

Upregulation of the immune system allows for increased antitumor activity, but also frequently leads to off-target immune-related adverse events (irAEs). These may affect any body system—hypophysitis, thyroiditis, pancreatitis, and hepatitis are common. Neurological irAEs of all varieties—peripheral neuropathy, encephalopathy, and meningitis, for example—are increasingly being recognized, affecting 2.9% of patients treated with a PD-1 inhibitor in one cohort (Kao et al., 2018).

Myositis is less frequent than other neurological irAEs but has been reported with treatment with CTLA-4, PD-1, and PD-L1 inhibitors. Weakness and myalgia typically begin after just 1 or 2 cycles of the medication. The distribution of weakness may mimic other inflammatory myopathies including axial and proximal muscle weakness, but oculomotor and bulbar weakness are also very common (Touat et al., 2018). This may lead to suspicion of myasthenia gravis, which can also occur as an irAE (Suzuki et al., 2017). In fact, overlap of myositis and MG appears common. In cases of myositis, CK values are almost always elevated; fibrillation potentials, positive sharp waves, and myopathic MUAPs are seen on EMG in most patients, as well. MSA are usually negative. In those with MG, a decremental response to slow repetitive nerve stimulation is seen instead. Acetylcholine receptor antibody positivity has also been reported. In case of both myositis and MG, concurrent myocarditis appears common, so cardiac screening should be performed. Muscle biopsies have demonstrated endomysial histiocytic and lymphocytic inflammation, with upregulation of PD-L1 and PD-1.

Development of symptomatic myositis should prompt stopping the ICPi. In mild cases, this alone may lead to resolution of symptoms. Most patients, however, will require treatment with corticosteroids (Brahmer et al., 2018). Patients improve over a period of weeks; prednisone can typically be tapered over this period, as the myositis seems to be monophasic frequently.

### Amphiphilic Drug Myopathy (Drug-Induced Autophagic Lysosomal Myopathy)

Amphiphilic drugs contain separate hydrophobic and hydrophilic regions. This results in the drug's ability to interact with the anionic phospholipids of cell membranes and organelles. Pathological autophagic vacuoles, which form through disruption of lysozymes, are characteristic. These agents can also cause a toxic neuropathy that is often more severe than the myopathy.

***Chloroquine.*** Chloroquine is used to treat malaria, sarcoidosis, systemic lupus erythematosus, and other connective tissue diseases. A rare adverse side effect is the development of slowly progressive, painless, proximal weakness and atrophy, worse in the legs than the arms. Cardiomyopathy may also occur. Reduced sensation distally and loss of deep tendon reflexes are often appreciated secondary to a concomitant toxic neuropathy. This "neuromyopathy" usually does not occur unless patients take 500 mg/day for a year or more but has been reported with dosages as low as 200 mg/day CTD. The neuromyopathy improves after chloroquine discontinuation.

Serum CK levels are usually elevated. Motor and sensory nerve conduction studies reveal mild to moderate reduction in amplitudes, with slightly slow velocities in patients with a superimposed neuropathy. Increased insertional activity and myopathic MUAPs are seen in weak proximal limb muscles. Neurogenic-appearing units and reduced recruitment may be seen in distal muscles more affected by the toxic neuropathy. Muscle and nerve biopsies demonstrate autophagic vacuoles. On EM, the vacuoles are noted to contain concentric lamellar myeloid debris and curvilinear structures.

***Amiodarone.*** Amiodarone is an antiarrhythmic medication that causes a neuromyopathy characterized by severe proximal and distal weakness along with distal sensory loss and reduced reflexes. Patients with renal insufficiency are predisposed to developing the toxic neuromyopathy. Muscle strength gradually improves following discontinuation of amiodarone. Autophagic vacuoles are seen on muscle biopsies. Myeloid inclusions may be appreciated on nerve biopsies. These lipid membrane inclusions may be evident in muscle and nerve biopsies as long as 2 years following discontinuation of amiodarone.

### Antimicrotubular Myopathy

***Colchicine.*** Colchicine is associated with a generalized toxic neuromyopathy due to its binding with tubulin and prevention of tubulin's polymerization into microtubular structures. Typically the neuromyopathy has a slow, gradual onset in the setting of chronic administration, but it can also develop secondary to acute intoxication. Risk factors are chronic renal failure and age over 50 years. Patients manifest progressive proximal muscle weakness that resolves within 4–6 months after discontinuing the colchicine.

Serum CK is usually elevated. Nerve conduction studies reveal reduced amplitudes, slightly prolonged latencies, and mildly slow conduction velocities of motor and sensory nerves in the arms and legs. Needle EMG demonstrates irritability and myopathic MUAPs.

Autophagic vacuoles containing membranous debris may be seen on muscle biopsies. The neuromyopathy appears to be the result of abnormal assembly of microtubules that disrupts intracellular movement or localization of lysosomes.

### Mitochondrial myopathy

Zidovudine (AZT), a nucleoside-analog reverse transcriptase inhibitor used to treat HIV, led to a myopathy in 17% of patients treated with AZT as monotherapy for longer than 9 months (Peters et al., 1993). Nucleoside analogs compete with natural nucleoside substrates of HIV reverse transcriptase and, accordingly, can also inhibit human mitochondrial γ-DNA polymerase. As AZT has been supplanted by other newer antiretrovirals or instead used at lower doses as part of a multidrug regimen, the incidence of myopathy is now much lower. Serum CK levels are mildly elevated and EMG typically reveals an irritable myopathy in affected patients. HIV itself may be associated with myositis, so a muscle biopsy may be required to differentiate the cause. AZT myopathy manifests with pathological signs of mitochondrial dysfunction—ragged-red fibers on modified Gomori trichrome stain and COX-negative fibers.

Myotoxicity can also complicate telbivudine, lamivudine, and entecavir—nucleoside analogs used to treat hepatitis B—though asymptomatic CK elevation is the most common manifestation. The highest incidence of symptomatic myopathy has been reported in patients with renal failure treated with telbivudine after liver transplant. Rhabdomyolysis can occur with didanosine, lamivudine, raltegravir, ritonavir, and indinavir. The mitochondrial etiology is less clearly established for these agents than with AZT.

### Myopathies of Other Mechanisms

***Corticosteroid myopathy.*** The development of proximal muscle weakness and atrophy affecting the legs more than the arms in association with a cushingoid appearance is a complication of chronic corticosteroid administration. Serum CK is normal, as are the results of needle EMG. Muscle biopsies reveal atrophy of type 2 fibers, especially the fast-twitch, glycolytic type 2B fibers. It is not known why corticosteroids cause a myopathy, but it may be due to diminished protein synthesis, increased protein degradation, alterations in carbohydrate metabolism, mitochondrial alterations, and reduced sarcolemmal excitability.

Sometimes it may be difficult clinically to distinguish corticosteroid myopathy from exacerbation of an underlying immune-mediated neuromuscular disorder (e.g., inflammatory myopathy, myasthenia gravis, chronic inflammatory demyelinating polyneuropathy) in a patient being treated with corticosteroids. If the weakness recurs as the corticosteroid agent is being tapered, then a relapse of the underlying disease process is more likely. An increasing serum CK and/or an EMG showing a prominent increase in insertional and spontaneous activity would support a flare of an underlying inflammatory myopathy. If, on the other hand, the weakness reappeared while the patient was on a chronic high dose of corticosteroids, corticosteroid myopathy is a consideration.

***Critical illness myopathy.*** Patients in the intensive care unit (ICU) may develop generalized weakness due to critical illness myopathy (CIM) or critical illness polyneuropathy (CIP). CIM has also been termed *acute quadriplegic myopathy* (AQM), *acute illness myopathy*, and *myopathy associated with thick filament* (myosin) *loss* (Lacomis et al., 1996, 1998). In a large series involving 88 patients who developed weakness while in an ICU, CIM was three times as common as CIP (42% vs. 13%) (Lacomis et al., 1998). CIP rarely occurs without concurrent CIM.

CIM typically leads to proximally predominant weakness, which can be severe and may include respiratory muscle weakness. The myopathy is often initially recognized by the inability to wean the patient from the ventilator. When present, CIP produces distally predominant weakness and sensory loss. Reflexes can be reduced or absent in either form. Patients who are critically ill due to sepsis or have multiorgan system failure are at an especially high risk for CIM/CIP, and hyperglycemia is an additional risk factor. Although it is traditionally taught that corticosteroids and neuromuscular blocking agents (NMBAs) confer an elevated risk, data are actually mixed. Critically ill patients frequently require one or both medications. A systematic review of 665 reported patients found no association between glucocorticoids or neuromuscular blocking agents (NMBAs) and development of CIM or CIP (Stevens et al., 2007).

Serum CK levels are normal or moderately elevated. Nerve conduction studies reveal marked reduced amplitudes of CMAPs, with normal distal latencies and conduction velocities (Rich et al., 1996, 1997). Sensory nerve action potential (SNAP) amplitudes should be normal or mildly reduced (>80% of the lower limit of normal). Markedly reduced-amplitude SNAPs suggest CIP, unless there is an unrelated baseline neuropathy. EMG usually demonstrates prominent fibrillation potentials and positive sharp waves and early recruitment of myopathic MUAPs. Patients with severe weakness may be unable to volitionally recruit any MUAPs, which can make it difficult to distinguish CIM from CIP in patients who may have coincidental abnormal sensory conduction studies. Muscle biopsies reveal a wide spectrum of histological abnormalities, including type 2 muscle fiber atrophy with or without type 1 fiber atrophy, scattered necrotic muscle fibers, and, importantly, focal or diffuse loss of reactivity for myosin ATPase activity. EM reveals loss of thick filaments (myosin).

## Endocrine Myopathies

Myopathy can result from endogenous steroid hormone excess (i.e., Cushing syndrome) just the same as with exogenous corticosteroid administration. Additionally, myopathy can be seen in relation with thyroid and parathyroid diseases.

### Hypothyroidism

Patients with hypothyroidism develop proximal muscle weakness about one-third of the time (Duyuff et al., 2000). Cramps and myalgia are also common. Muscle symptoms are rarely the presenting complaint, with other systemic symptoms such as fatigue, cold intolerance, and weight gain typically also present. A distal, symmetric polyneuropathy can occur as a result of hypothyroidism, and carpal tunnel syndrome is common. Rhabdomyolysis has also been reported. Patients with muscle involvement may have delayed relaxation of the muscle stretch reflexes. Direct percussion of muscle with a reflex hammer can produce painless local mounding (myoedema) in about one-third of patients; other patients have muscle hypertrophy (Salick and Perason, 1967).

The serum CK is often elevated, but may be normal. Most cases occur with primary thyroid dysfunction, so thyroid stimulation hormone (TSH) should be elevated and thyroxine (T4) and triiodothyronine (T3) levels low. Needle EMG is frequently normal, though some patients may have myopathic motor unit potentials evident in severely weak muscles—especially when the CK is elevated. Muscle biopsy is rarely required, but when performed shows nonspecific findings including type 2 muscle fiber atrophy, type 1 muscle fiber hypertrophy, rare necrotic fibers, increased internalized nuclei, and vacuoles (Laylock and Pascuzzi, 1991). With correction of the hypothyroid state, muscle strength improves in the majority of patients.

### Hyperthyroidism

Thyrotoxic myopathy also produces proximal muscle weakness, typically more rapid in onset than with hypothyroidism (Kung, 2007). Muscle atrophy, particularly of the shoulder girdle, and scapular winging can occur. In severe cases, rhabdomyolysis has been reported. Myalgias and fatigue are common, like with hypothyroidism. Occasionally patients will develop bulbar or respiratory muscle weakness. Thyroid ophthalmopathy can occur in patients with Graves disease, leading to weakness of extraocular muscles and proptosis. Myasthenia gravis has been reported in association with Graves disease, leading to some diagnostic confusion. Eye closure weakness—present with myasthenia gravis and typically absent with Graves disease—as well as fluctuating symptoms can help distinguish.

On examination, muscle strength reflexes may be brisk in contrast to hypothyroidism. Fasciculations and myokymia may also be noted. Serum CK values are commonly normal, as are NCS and EMG. With correction of hyperthyroidism, patients typically improve over months (Duyuff et al., 2000).

## Rhabdomyolysis

Rhabdomyolysis is a condition of acute and severe muscle fiber breakdown that leads to release of sarcoplasmic contents into the bloodstream, including myoglobin and potassium. Plasma myoglobin is filtered by the renal glomeruli but may precipitate in the renal tubules, producing acute renal failure. Potassium release into the bloodstream may cause cardiac arrest. The degree of muscle breakdown can cause profound muscle weakness and pain. Causes of rhabdomyolysis include crush injuries to limbs with vascular occlusion, metabolic myopathies such as CPT deficiency, and toxic myopathies such as those due to statin drugs (Nance and Mammen, 2015). However, in most cases of rhabdomyolysis, no underlying cause can be identified. Many of these patients have recurrent episodes of the condition.

*The complete reference list is available online at https://expertconsult.inkling.com/.* 

110

# Neurological Problems in the Newborn

*Jarred Garfinkle, Steven P. Miller*

## OUTLINE



Neurological problems in the newborn infant can arise from innate processes such as genetic abnormalities or disorders of nervous system development or can be the result of acquired brain injury from external insults. Both innate and acquired brain injury in the newborn have lifelong important impact on the developing person and his or her family (Moster et al., 2008). The increasing incidence of preterm delivery worldwide, currently estimated at 11%, and the improved survival of the sickest newborns require the neurologist to be aware of the neurological burden of perinatal and neonatal illness (Harrison and Goldenberg, 2016). More than half of very preterm newborns will have developmental problems ranging from attention-deficit/hyperactive disorder to cerebral palsy (Pascal et al., 2018). Almost half of neonates with hypoxic-ischemic encephalopathy (HIE) have neurodevelopmental sequelae as well (Jacobs et al., 2013). These developmental outcomes challenge the child, the family, and the community (Moster et al., 2008).

The newborn, whether term or preterm, has a limited means of manifesting injury to the central nervous system (CNS). The adult brain manifests change in many domains with regional specificity, including cognition, behavior, speech, vision, and movement. In contrast, the neonatal brain is in a state of rapid development and most commonly reveals underlying brain dysfunction in two nonspecific ways: encephalopathy and seizures. In the preterm newborn, the neurological signs of significant injury can be even more subtle or not manifest at all.

Advances in neurodiagnostic testing, and neuroimaging in particular, have enhanced our understanding of the pathophysiology of brain injury in the newborn. Digital electroencephalography (EEG) with bedside trending, such as amplitude-integrated EEG (aEEG), and remote access availability grant the clinical team a real-time window into brain function (Fig. 110.1). Neonatal neurology is a growing medical subspecialty with increasing numbers of dedicated multidisciplinary programs at academic institutions (Smyser et al., 2016). In addition to specific neuroprotective therapies, the increasing focus on the developing brain in the neonatal intensive care unit (NICU) may lead to improved outcomes via earlier recognition and treatment of neurological conditions (Bonifacio et al., 2011). A cooperative team effort often is the most effective approach to neurological problems in newborns. Many units also address fetal brain injury (Kirkham et al., 2018).

This chapter reviews the practical aspects of diagnosis and management of neonatal neurological problems commonly encountered by practicing neurologists.

## NEONATAL SEIZURES

A *seizure* is defined clinically as a paroxysmal alteration in any neurological function accompanied by seizure activity identifiable on an EEG. Unlike the child and adult, in whom unprovoked seizures

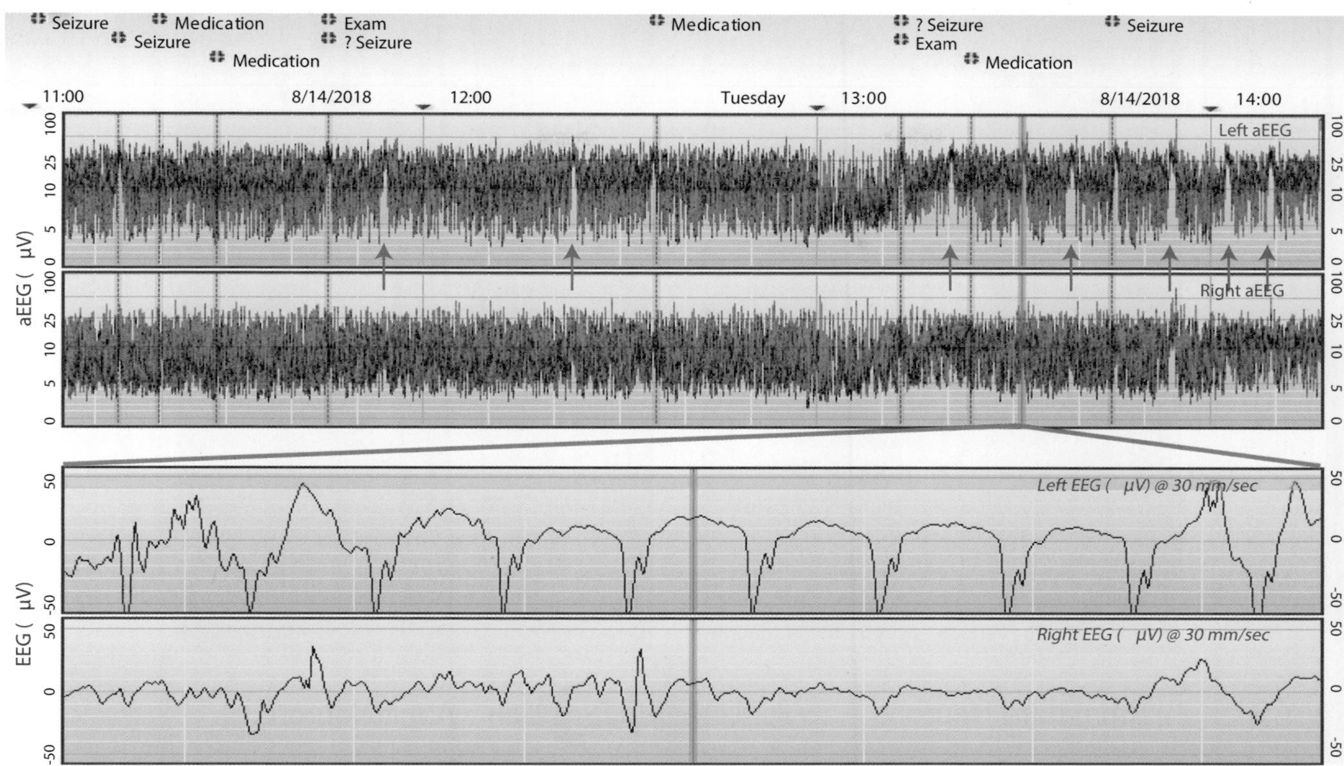


**Fig. 110.1 Amplitude-Integrated Electroencephalography *(aEEG)* of a Neonate Demonstrating Seizures.** The repetitive sudden rise in the lower margin of the aEEG trace (upper panel; marked in real-time with *green bars*) corresponds to seizures on the raw electroencephalography *(EEG)* trace in the lower panel of the image (corresponding to the *red bar*). Additional events which appear to be seizures on the aEEG, but which were not marked in real time, are indicated by *green arrows*. In this example, the seizures appear to be emanating from the left hemisphere. Notations at the top of the image were made in real time by the treating team to indicate what was transpiring at the bedside.

predominate, seizures in newborns are almost always acute symptomatic (Glass et al., 2016). They are more common in the first 28 days of life than in any other time of life and represent one of the most common manifestations of neonatal brain injury (Abend et al., 2018). The timing of onset of the seizures informs the etiology (Fig. 110.2).

## Pathophysiology

Several developmental factors leading to excess excitation and reduced inhibition influence the high rate of acute-symptomatic seizures in the neonatal period. In adult neurons, γ-aminobutyric acid A ($GABA_A$) receptor activation leads to chloride influx to produce membrane hyperpolarization and inhibition. In immature neurons, there is a net chloride *efflux* with $GABA_A$ receptor activation, which leads to membrane depolarization and excitability (Ben-Ari, 2014). The developmental fluctuations in neuronal chloride gradients are mediated largely by membrane ion transporters: NKCC1 leads to a high intracellular chloride concentration, whereas KCC2 acts as an active chloride extrusion pathway (Fig. 110.3). With increasing age, the expression of the KCC2 becomes dominant. These developmental changes in chloride influx/efflux may contribute to the often-disappointing response of neonatal seizures to GABA-agonist anticonvulsant medications such as phenobarbital.

An understanding of the adverse consequences of neonatal seizures on the developing brain is emerging and informs the need to treat subclinical and refractory seizures (Fig. 110.4). Prolonged seizures may cause neuronal injury principally via disturbances in cerebral energy metabolism, with eventual diminution of energy supplies,

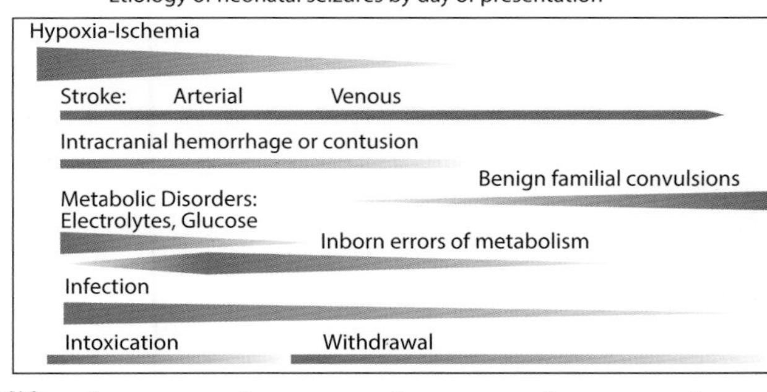


**Fig. 110.2 Common Etiologies of Neonatal Seizures.** The most common etiologies of neonatal seizures are plotted by their most common day(s) of presentation. (*Adapted from Miller, S.P., Ferriero, D.M., 2007. Neonatal brain injuries. In: Gilman, S. [Ed.], Neurobiology of Disease, first ed. Elsevier Academic Press, Burlington, p. 605.*)

and excitotoxicity (Holmes, 2009). Recurrent, shorter seizures in animal models have not demonstrated neuronal injury but have been shown to mediate long-term morphological and physiological deficits, including suppression of neuronal stem cells (Holmes, 2009). There is also growing evidence that seizures in human newborns are associated with adverse neurobehavioral outcomes. Neonatal seizures, especially if frequent, intractable, or prolonged, are independently associated with further hypoxic-ischemic brain injury as measured by magnetic resonance (MR) spectroscopy and with later neurodevelopmental impairment (Glass et al., 2009; Miller et al., 2002).

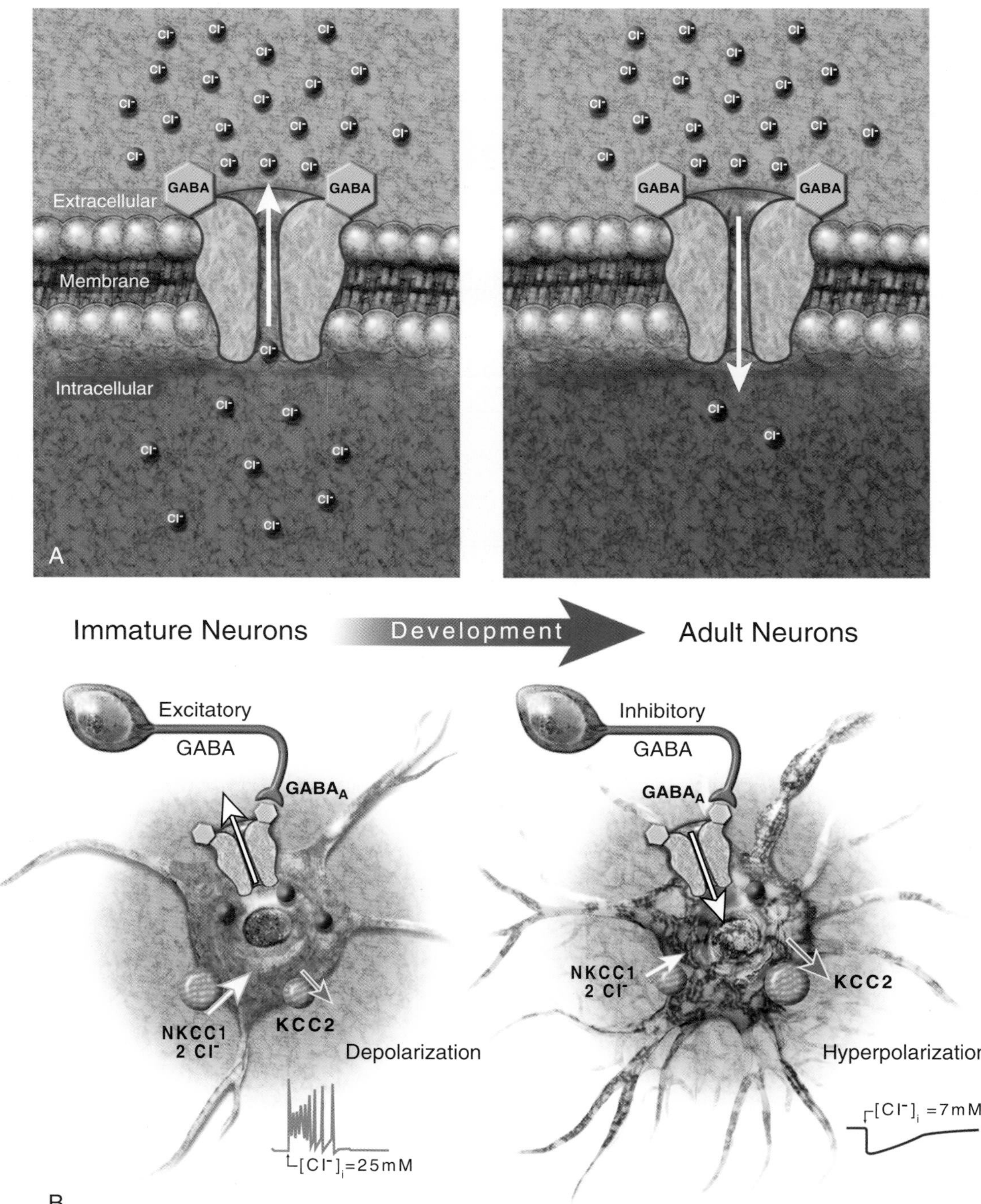


**Fig. 110.3 Schematic Diagram of the Developmental Alterations of Chloride Levels, The γ-Aminobutyric Acid *(Gaba)* Channel, and Chloride Cotransporters. (A)** The intracellular chloride ($Cl^-$) levels are higher in immature than adult neurons. **(B)** GABA depolarizes and excites immature neurons and inhibits adult ones. (*Adapted from Ben-Ari, Y., 2014. The GABA excitatory/inhibitory developmental sequence: a personal journey. Neuroscience 279, 196.*)

## Etiology

Most neonatal seizures are acute symptomatic and can follow a multitude of causes (see Fig. 110.2). The remainder relate to developmental brain abnormalities and neonatal epilepsy syndromes that are often of genetic origin. Determining the etiology, or etiologies, is important because it informs management and prognosis. HIE accounts for almost half of neonatal seizures in term newborns (Glass et al., 2016). In preterm newborns, HIE and intracranial hemorrhage each account for approximately one-third of the seizures, although the clinician should be alert for multiple concurrent etiologies (Glass et al., 2017).

Congenital CNS abnormalities account for 5%–10% of neonatal seizures and require neuroimaging for diagnosis. Hypoxic-ischemic brain injury in the second and third trimesters of gestation can result

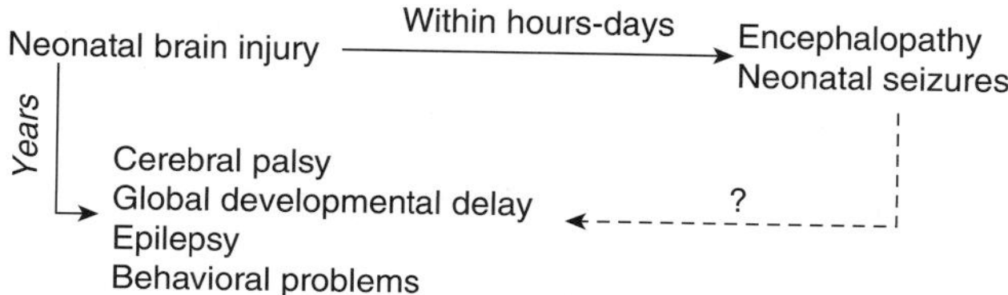


**Fig. 110.4** Schematic of the Associations Between Neonatal Brain Injury, Neonatal Seizures, and Later Neurodevelopment. (*Adapted from Garfinkle, J., Shevell, M.I., 2016. Neurodevelopmental outcomes of neonates with seizures. In: Nagarajan, L. [Ed.], Neonatal Seizures: Current Management and Future Challenges, first ed. Mac Keith Press, London, p. 164.*)

in malformation of brain development (Inder et al., 1999). Seizures in the context of cerebral dysplasia are particularly refractory and usually progress towards epilepsy.

## Neonatal Epilepsy Syndromes

Neonatal epilepsy syndromes encompass genetic channelopathies and specific metabolic deficiencies that are increasingly recognized with next-generation genetic sequencing. Channelopathies can range from benign, with resolution of seizures and normal neurodevelopment, to severe early-onset epileptic encephalopathies.

Benign familial neonatal epilepsy is an inherited autosomal dominant condition. When familial seizures are not identified, then the condition is termed benign neonatal seizures. Several gene loci which encode for voltage-gated channels, including *KCNQ2*, *KCNQ3*, and *SCN2A*, have been identified (Axeen and Olson, 2018). Seizure onset is usually in the first week of life, and seizures classically remit within the first year of life.

In early infantile epileptic encephalopathy, seizures are often initially refractory. Some families retrospectively report rhythmic movements in utero. Some of the newborns are classified as having Ohtahara syndrome, a severe epileptic encephalopathy characterized clinically by intractable tonic seizures and burst suppression on EEG and caused by an increasing number of genetic abnormalities. Early myoclonic encephalopathy is another phenotype of early infantile epileptic encephalopathy featuring erratic focal myoclonus that shifts around the body in an asynchronous pattern, often with burst suppression pattern on EEG. Patients with early infantile epileptic encephalopathies may evolve into West or Lennox-Gastaut syndromes with age (Sanders et al., 2018). Sodium channel blockers, such as phenytoin and carbamazepine, are particularly effective in managing the channelopathies (Sanders et al., 2018; Sands et al., 2016).

In the context of seizures of unknown etiology, treatable metabolic epileptic encephalopathies should be considered and appropriate therapy instituted pending diagnosis. These disorders include pyridoxine-responsive seizures and folinic acid–responsive seizures, which are both allelic to antiquitin (ALDH7A1) deficiency; pyridox(am)ine-5′-phosphate oxidase deficiency secondary to homozygous mutations of PNPO; and 3-phosphoglycerate dehydrogenase deficiency responsive to serine supplementation (Saudubray and Garcia-Cazorla, 2018). Classically, the diagnosis of pyridoxine-responsive seizures was based on a response to a single large dose (e.g., 100 mg) of intravenous pyridoxine with concurrent EEG recording. However, the pyridoxine challenge is not sensitive and can induce apnea. As such, one strategy for suspected vitamin-responsive early-onset epileptic encephalopathies is to initiate broad treatment with folinic acid and pyridoxal phosphate for 3 days and to continue the therapy if there is a clinical improvement pending genetic test results (Fig. 110.5). Elevations of urinary α-aminoadipic semialdehyde (AASA) and serum or cerebrospinal fluid (CSF) pipecolic acid are nonspecific biomarkers for pyridoxine-dependent seizures (Ficicioglu and Bearden, 2011).

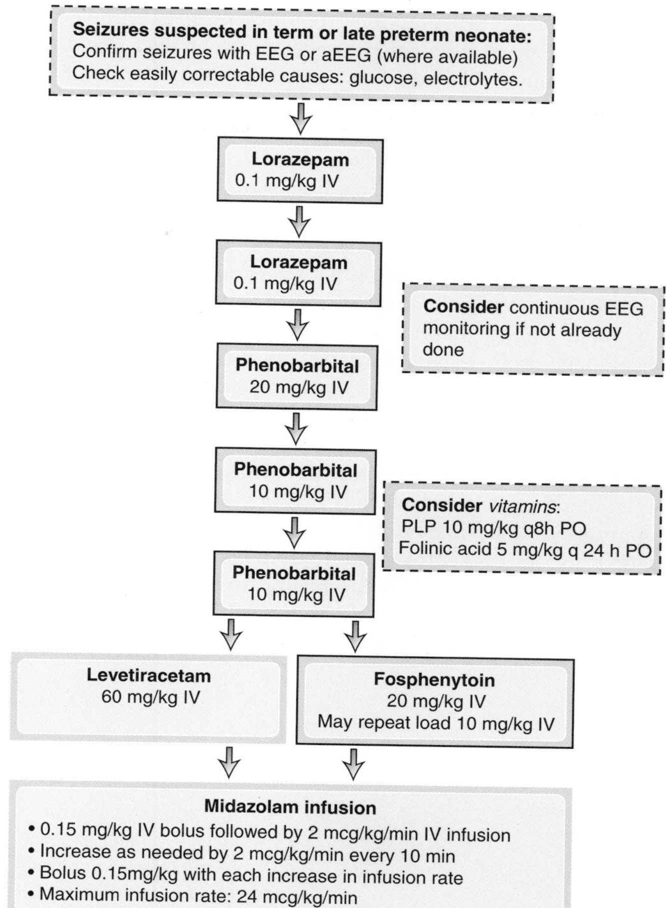


**Fig. 110.5** An Example Neonatal Seizure Management Algorithm Adapted From the Hospital for Sick Children (Toronto, Ontario, Canada). *aEEG*, Amplitude-integrated electroencephalography; *IV*, intravenous PLP, pyridoxal phosphate; PO, per os.

Many other inherited disorders can without specific treatments present with refractory neonatal seizures, such as nonketotic hyperglycinemia, peroxisomal biogenesis defects, respiratory chain disorders, sulfite oxidase deficiency, Menkes disease, and congenital disorders of glycosylation.

## Diagnosis, Semiology, and Differential Diagnosis (see Chapter 91)

Accurate diagnosis of neonatal seizures requires electrographic corroboration due to the difficulty in accurately identifying clinical seizures. Seizure manifestations in newborns differ from those in older individuals in that newborns generally do not have well-organized, generalized tonic-clonic seizures due to the immaturity of their synaptic connections. In addition, seizures in the newborn are often clinically silent and detected only on EEG; these seizures are referred to as subclinical seizures (Fig. 110.6; see later). In one study, only one-third of neonatal EEG seizures displayed clinical signs on simultaneous video recordings; only one-third of these clinical manifestations were recognized by experienced neonatal staff; and only one-quarter of clinically suspected seizures documented by staff had corresponding electrographic evidence of seizure activity (Murray et al., 2008). As such, EEG monitoring to identify seizures is an essential tool to avoid missing and undertreating seizures and to avoid overdiagnosing and overtreating seizures (Shellhaas et al., 2011). If continuous EEG is not available, then continuous aEEG can be used. aEEG is a simplified trend monitor that displays one or two channels of time-compressed, processed EEG signal on a semi-logarithmic scale (see Fig. 110.1). Compared with EEG, it is less sensitive but readily interpreted by trained bedside practitioners. The use of these brain-monitoring tools is a cornerstone of modern neonatal neurocritical care (Bonifacio et al., 2011).

Clinical seizure semiologies have been classified by Volpe, and they are summarized in Table 110.1 (Abend et al., 2018). Seizure types are not specific for etiology, but some are seen more often with certain underlying conditions. For instance, focal clonic seizures in the term "newborn" are most commonly associated with focal cerebral infarction. Subtle and generalized tonic seizures do not consistently show concomitant electrographic discharges. In these cases the abnormal movements may represent nonepileptic brainstem release phenomena or seizure discharges in deep cerebral structures which are not transmitted to surface EEG.

Nonepileptic movements must be distinguished from seizures. Physiological myoclonus, which occurs in healthy newborns, differs from myoclonic seizures, which often have a dismal outcome: the seizures are not evoked by stimuli, are nonsuppressible by touch, and occur with concomitant encephalopathy. Jitteriness, which is an exaggerated startle response, is often confused with clonic seizures, especially because both jitteriness and clonic seizures occur in similar underlying conditions, such as HIE, hypoglycemia, and drug withdrawal. The absence of associated ocular movements and autonomic changes (e.g., tachycardia, hypertension, and apnea) and the presence of stimulus sensitivity distinguish jitteriness from seizures. The predominant movement in jitteriness is tremor, in which the alternating movements are rhythmic and of equal rate and amplitude (Abend et al., 2018). In contrast, movements in clonic seizures have a fast and slow component. In addition, jitteriness stops when passively flexing the affected limb. Hyperekplexia is another abnormal movement that is nonepileptic. It is characterized by an exaggerated startle response and sustained tonic spasms in response to unexpected auditory, visual, and somesthetic stimuli and is caused by genetic mutations in genes involved in glycine neurotransmission (Shahar and Raviv, 2004).

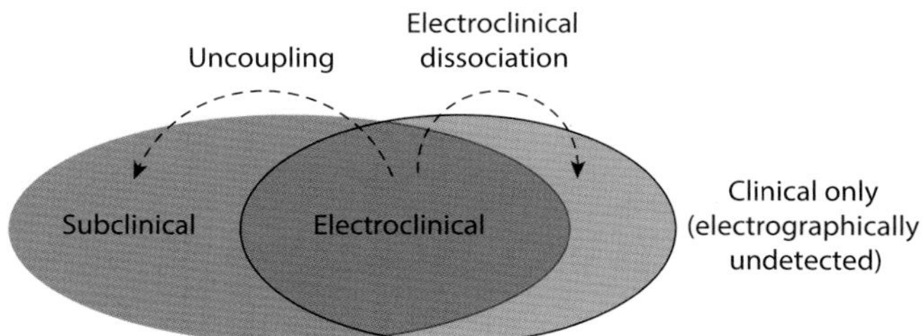


**Fig. 110.6** Venn Diagram of Neonatal Seizures Classified According to Clinical And Electrographic Manifestations.

**TABLE 110.1 Clinical Seizure Classification from Volpe**

| Clinical Seizure | Manifestations and Key Points |
|---|---|
| Subtle | Eye deviation, blinking, fixed stare<br>Repetitive mouth and tongue movements<br>Apnea, other autonomic phenomena<br>Bicycling, other rhythmic limb movements |
| Clonic: focal or multifocal | Rhythmic movements of muscle groups<br>Often represents a focal pathology |
| Tonic: focal or generalized | Sustained flexion or extension of muscle groups |
| Myoclonic focal, multifocal, or generalized | Synchronous flexion jerks<br>Must be distinguished from nonepileptic myoclonus |

*From Abend, N.S., Jensen, F.E., Inder, T.E., Volpe, J.J., 2018. Neonatal seizures. In: Inder, T.E., Volpe, J.J., Darras, B., de Vries, L., du Plessis, A., Neil, J., Perlman, J. (Eds.), Volpe's Neurology of the Newborn. Elsevier.*

## Electroencephalography

EEG and aEEG are necessary tools for the diagnosis of neonatal seizures. Continuous conventional EEG is currently recommended as the "gold standard" for diagnosis of neonatal seizures by the American Clinical Neurophysiology Society (Shellhaas et al., 2011). In most neonatal seizures, electrographic onset is focal or multifocal. Spread of the seizure within one hemisphere and secondary generalization to the contralateral hemisphere are uncommon, presumably due to the immature synapses in the newborn brain (Abend et al., 2018).

Neonatal EEG seizures have (1) a sudden electrographic change; (2) repetitive waveforms that evolve in morphology, frequency, and/or location; (3) an amplitude of at least 2 μV; and (4) a duration of at least 10 seconds (Tsuchida et al., 2013). Fig. 110.6 illustrates the terminology used to describe clinical, electrographic, and subclinical seizures. Uncoupling refers to the phenomenon by which the clinical manifestations terminate while electrographic seizures persist, and commonly occurs in neonates after the administration of anticonvulsant medications (Scher et al., 2003). Electroclinical dissociation refers to the phenomenon by which the clinical expression of a seizure occurs without an electrical correlate (Weiner et al., 1991). Although electroclinical dissociation exists (e.g., seizures emanating from the mesial temporal lobe), it is not common.

Sharp transients are normal in premature newborns and should not be confused with seizure activity. Similarly, the trace-alternant pattern of quiet sleep in normal=term infants, in which normal low-amplitude activity is preserved between bursts, must be distinguished from the abnormal burst-suppression pattern, in which long periods of voltage suppression or absence of activity are recorded between bursts of high-voltage spikes and slow waves (Andre et al., 2010). Interictal EEG has prognostic value: severe suppression of the background activity, whether interrupted by high-amplitude bursts or not, is associated with an abnormal outcome. Importantly, the severity of background disturbance is a more important predictor of seizure risk than are interictal epileptiform abnormalities in the neonate with brain injury (Glass et al., 2014).

## Management

Suspected neonatal seizures require urgent investigation for acute-symptomatic etiologies and management because prolonged and recurrent seizures are likely independently associated with brain injury and abnormal brain development, as discussed earlier. Glucose and electrolyte levels should be measured and any abnormality corrected. A full sepsis evaluation, including cultures of blood and CSF, should also be undertaken if feasible and empiric antibiotics started. Neuroimaging studies should proceed according to institutional availability; ultrasound of the head is usually readily available and can give diagnostic clues (Weeke et al., 2015).

Genetic epilepsy syndromes are diagnosed with appropriate gene panels or whole exome sequencing.

There is little in the way of evidence-based guidelines for the pharmacological management of neonatal seizures; nonetheless, treatment with anticonvulsant medications should be initiated once seizures are confirmed electrographically or if the clinical suspicion for seizures is sufficiently high. The World Health Organization (WHO) recommends phenobarbital as a first-line agent but other agents, such as phenytoin (or fosphenytoin) and benzodiazepines are acceptable alternatives and are all available intravenously (World Health Organization, 2011; Painter et al., 1999). Approximately half of seizures are controlled with a 20 mg/kg load of phenobarbital or phenytoin (Painter et al., 1999). Benzodiazepines such as lorazepam or midazolam have the advantage of a short half-life and can be particularly useful when seizures are suspected based on clinical observation alone but unconfirmed by EEG or aEEG. The use of these medications as a first-line agent may obviate the need for further therapy in neonates in whom seizures do not recur or, are later shown, via neuromonitoring, not to have any epileptic correlate. Levetiracetam is increasingly being used as well despite limited safety and efficacy data (Ahmad et al., 2017). A recent randomized controlled trial showed that levetiracetam was less effective than phenobarbital for the treatment of neonatal seizures (Sharpe et al., 2020). If seizures are not controlled after repeated loading doses of standard medications, titration of a midazolam infusion may be indicated. An example of an abridged seizure management algorithm is provided in Fig. 110.5, but individual institutions should develop their own.

### Prognosis and Progression Toward Epilepsy

The major determinant of prognosis following neonatal seizures is the underlying etiology (see Fig. 110.4). Of newborns with seizures who survive their acute injury, 25%–70% will go on to have subsequent neurodevelopmental impairments (Uria-Avellanal et al., 2013). The frequency of epilepsy following neonatal seizures is between 10% and 30% (Pisani et al., 2015). A relatively high frequency of infantile spasms has been observed among survivors of neonatal seizures (Garfinkle and Shevell, 2011).

The decision regarding maintenance antiepileptic medications after NICU discharge relates mostly to the likelihood of developing postneonatal epilepsy balanced with the potential long-term toxicity of the therapy. In most acute symptomatic seizures, the seizures remit within a few days of life. Currently, it is unknown if continuing antiepileptic treatment for up to several months is helpful or harmful. The rationale for using antiepileptic drugs at discharge is to decrease the likelihood of seizure recurrence. In the presence of risk factors for later epilepsy, antiepileptic medication may be warranted. These risk factors include status epilepticus, severe hypoxic-ischemic brain injury, and the use of more than a single antiepileptic medication to adequately control the neonatal seizures (Garfinkle and Shevell, 2011; Pisani et al., 2015). Importantly, there are theoretical concerns that some treatment strategies for neonatal seizures could be toxic to the developing brain, and, as such, it may be judicious to withhold maintenance antiepileptic medication in the absence of these risk factors for later epilepsy (Jansen, 2018).

## BRAIN INJURY IN THE PRETERM NEWBORN

The brain of the preterm newborn is in a state of rapid development and is susceptible to four overarching and overlapping forms of preterm brain injury: intraventricular hemorrhage (IVH), white matter injury (WMI), gray matter injury, and cerebellar hemorrhage.

The neurodevelopmental impact of preterm brain injury is substantial and lifelong. Among contemporary cohorts of children born very preterm, (i.e., at <32 weeks' gestation) 5%–10% have major motor deficits, including cerebral palsy, and more than half have significant cognitive, behavioral, and/or sensory deficits (Pascal et al., 2018). The principal major motor deficit is spastic diplegia, because the periventricular lesions traverse descending fibers from the motor cortex subserving lower extremity function. Although most very preterm-born children have normal intelligence and no cerebral palsy, careful assessment at school age reveals an important burden of motor dyspraxia, processing deficits in attention and executive functions, anxiety, and visually based challenges with information processing and language (Johnson and Marlow, 2017). These less overt neurodevelopmental challenges are likely linked to impairments in cerebral growth and disturbances in cerebral maturation rather than injuries that are appreciable on diagnostic brain imaging (Back and Miller, 2014).

### Intraventricular Hemorrhage

IVH is a common injury in the preterm brain, and its incidence is inversely proportional to gestational age. The bleeding originates in the subependymal germinal matrix, from which cortical neuronal and glial cell precursors develop during the late second and early third trimesters. The highly vascularized germinal matrix involutes with advancing gestation (Inder et al., 2018b).

#### Pathogenesis

The predisposition of the preterm infant to germinal matrix hemorrhage is due to several factors: arterioles lack autoregulation and exist in a pressure-passive state; blood vessels lack a supporting basement membrane; and extravascular tissue pressure is low in the first few days of extrauterine life. Thus IVH may occur in the setting of elevated venous pressure or fluctuations in cerebral blood flow triggered by factors that include respiratory distress, pneumothorax, asphyxia, left ventricular dysfunction, patent ductus arteriosus, hypotension, hypothermia, and hyperosmolarity (Ballabh, 2014). In addition, individual NICU characteristics are critical determinants of severe intraventricular hemorrhage (Synnes et al., 2006).

#### Timing, Presentation, and Grading

The risk period for IVH is highest in the first 3 or 4 days of life, with 50% of hemorrhages detectable by 24 hours and its clinical presentation is *usually clinically silent.* If large enough, it may manifest as sudden deterioration with neurological signs such as stupor, seizures, decerebrate posturing, or apnea. A tense fontanelle, together with a sudden anemia, hyperglycemia, hyperkalemia, or bradycardia, may herald an IVH; hyponatremia from inappropriate secretion of antidiuretic hormone may occur as well.

Cranial ultrasound examinations are typically performed in the first week of life to detect IVH, and the images are used to classify IVH according to the algorithm adapted from (Papile et al., 1978) (Fig. 110.7). Grade I IVH is limited to the subependymal region; grade II IVH has blood in the ventricles without ventricular distension; and grade III IVH shows enlargement of the ventricles secondary to distention. The classic grade IV IVH arises from venous infarction of the periventricular white matter rather than from a direct extension of the IVH into the parenchyma.

A larger IVH may produce an inflammatory reaction that obliterates the subarachnoid space or cerebral aqueduct with subsequent ventricular dilatation and hydrocephalus (Inder et al., 2018b). Symptoms of progressive hydrocephalus, such as increasing head circumference, a full anterior fontanelle, separation of cranial sutures, or autonomic symptoms of high intracranial pressure, such as apneas, bradycardia, or hypertension, are not sensitive or timely markers of hydrocephalus because they often appear days or weeks after the onset of ventricular dilatation.

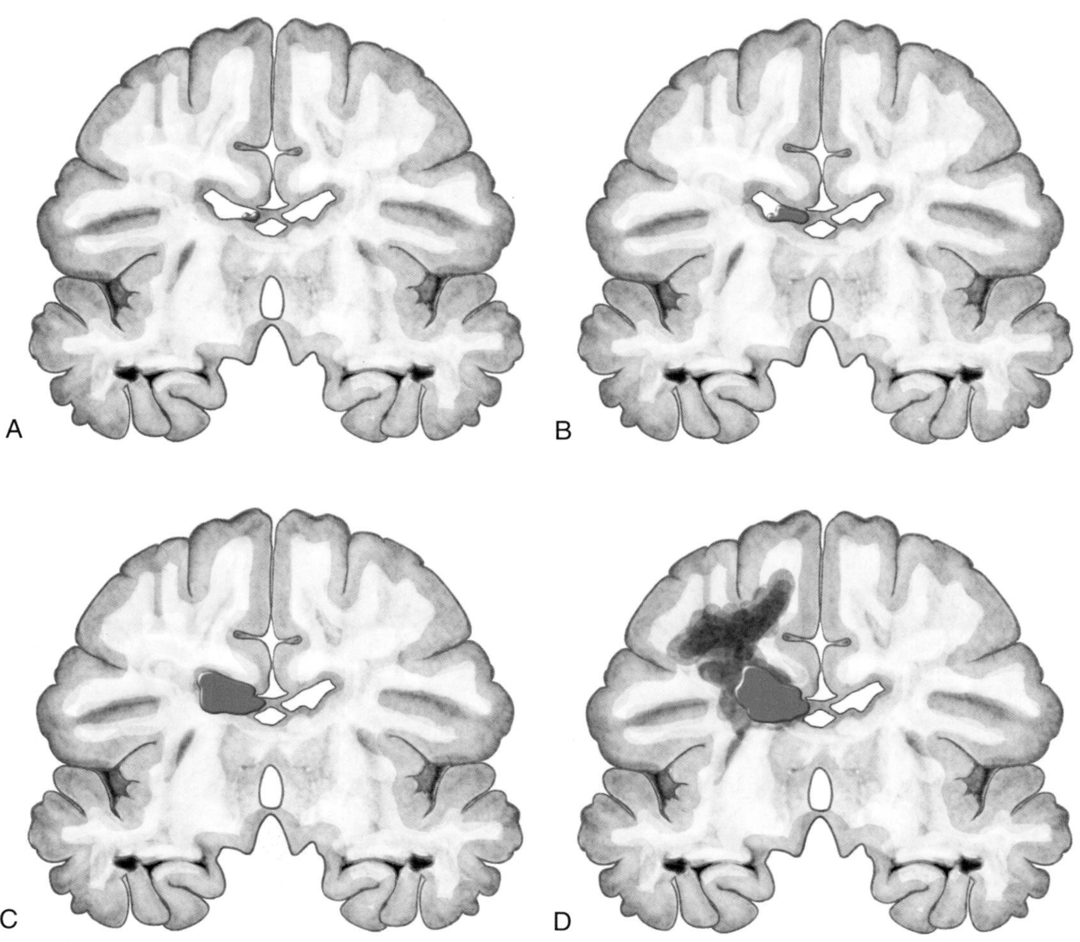


**Fig. 110.7** The Progressive Grades of Intraventricular Hemorrhage From Mildest to Most Severe. **(A)** Grade I hemorrhage involves less than 10% of the ventricular volume of the lateral ventricles. **(B)** Grade II involves 10%–50% of the ventricular volume. **(C)** Grade III involves more than 50% of the ventricular volume and is frequently associated with ventricular dilatation. **(D)** Hemorrhage is associated with periventricular hemorrhagic infarction.

### Prevention

Prenatal administration of steroids and maternal transfer to a tertiary-level hospital are the best means of preventing IVH. Practice bundles that limit fluctuations in cerebral blood flow via maintenance of partial pressure of carbon dioxide ($Pco_2$) and metabolic status within a normal range, avoidance of excessive suctioning and handling, and avoidance of rapid volume infusions and infusions of sodium bicarbonate are increasingly used (Lea et al., 2017).

### Management

Serial head ultrasound examinations are necessary in the setting of significant IVH to detect progressive ventricular dilatation. Clinical guidelines for the management of posthemorrhagic hydrocephalus are locale specific and accumulating evidence suggests that *early* removal of CSF in the setting of posthemorrhagic ventricular dilatation may reduce the need for ventriculoperitoneal shunt placement and attenuate neurodevelopmental impairment (Leijser et al., 2018). The commonest methods of CSF removal are serial lumbar punctures and insertion of a ventricular access device with a reservoir (e.g., Ommaya reservoir). Placement of a ventriculoperitoneal shunt or endoscopic third ventriculostomy are options for long-term CSF diversion for persistent hydrocephalus (Mazzola et al., 2014).

### Prognosis

Grade I and II IVH are associated with a statistically higher likelihood of later moderate or severe impairment, but most neonates with mild IVH do not have such impairments (Mukerji et al., 2015). Neonates with grade III IVH, and especially those with associated periventricular hemorrhagic infarction or posthemorrhagic ventricular dilatation, are at higher risk for poor neurodevelopmental outcome.

## White Matter Injury

WMI is the commonest form of brain injury in preterm neonates and is linked in experimental models and clinical studies to hypoxia-ischemia, infection, and inflammation (Back and Miller, 2014). The susceptibility to WMI is critically related to the timing of the insult, as, over the third trimester, distinct cell types are selectively more vulnerable to injury. Moreover, a wide variety of additional factors may synergistically sensitize the brain to injury. Such factors include nutritional status, systemic illnesses, painful procedures and exposure to glucocorticoids, sedatives, and prenatal exposure to drugs of abuse (Podrebarac et al., 2017).

WMI encompasses two major groups of pathology: focal necrosis, which itself ranges from cystic to microscopic, and diffuse nonnecrotic lesions (Back, 2017; Guo et al., 2017) (Fig. 110.8). Focal cystic necrosis, of which periventricular leukomalacia (PVL) is the most severe, occurs in the white matter adjacent to the ventricles and pathologically involves degenerative axons and phagocytic macrophages. The large necrotic lesions of PVL have become uncommon in contemporary cohorts of preterm neonates. Punctate and diffuse WMIs are currently the predominant lesions in most preterm neonates imaged with magnetic resonance imaging (MRI). Punctate WMI appears as areas of abnormal signal intensity with a characteristic topology, with most lesions occurring in the periventricular regions (Guo et al., 2017). Pathologically, diffuse WMI features selective degeneration and regeneration of preoligodendrocytes, a mitotically active progenitor cell line that peaks as a cell line between 23 and 32 weeks' gestation. In preterm diffuse WMI, the preoligodendrocytes that degenerate then fail to mature to myelin-forming oligodendrocytes; however, axons are spared (Buser et al., 2012). Over the past two decades, the prevalence of WMI seems to be decreasing in some centers (Gano et al., 2015).

Although WMI is the most commonly observed abnormality in preterm neonates on diagnostic MRI, it does not fully account for the burden of neurodevelopmental disability in this population (Chau et al., 2013). Impaired *development* of the white matter contributes more to neurodevelopmental disability following preterm birth. In other words, white matter dysmaturation, secondary to developmental arrest of preoligodendrocytes rather than injury, is the primary brain abnormality in contemporary cohorts of preterm neonates (Back and Miller, 2014).

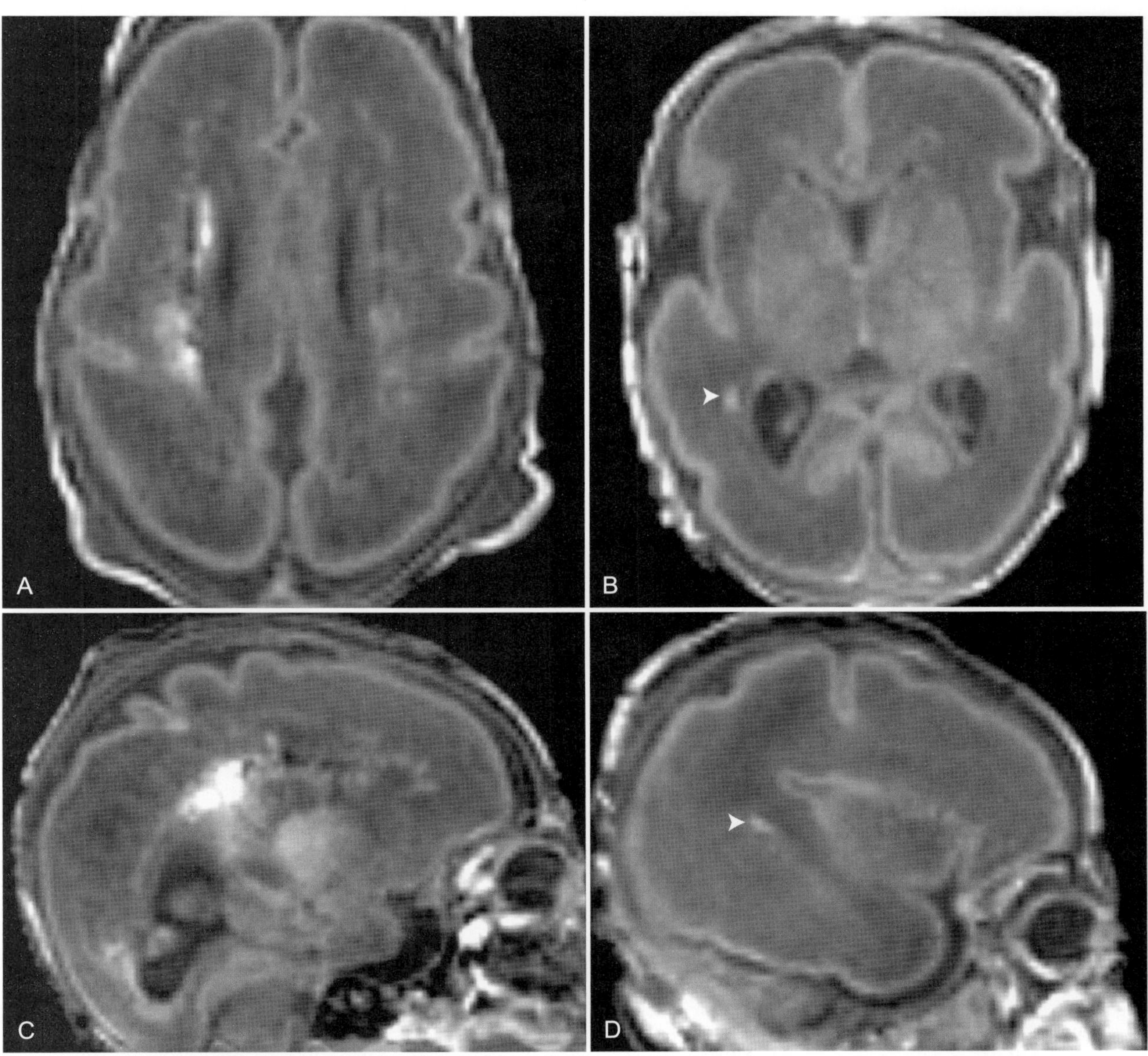


**Fig. 110.8 Different Severities of White Matter Injury in the Preterm Neonate. (A and C)** Appearance of cystic necrotic white matter injury on magnetic resonance imaging (MRI). Small areas of cavitation are appreciated as hypointensity on the sagittal T1-weighted image. **(B and D)** Punctate white matter injury on MRI has the appearance of signal hyperintensities on T1 *(arrowheads)*.

### Gray Matter Injury

Importantly, WMI is the "tip of the iceberg" following hypoxia-ischemia in the third trimester of gestation because it is most readily identified on MRI. Experimental models of preterm hypoxia-ischemia demonstrate concurrent impairments of neuronal development in the cerebral cortex and basal ganglia, as well as in transient cell populations such as the subplate (Dean et al., 2013; McClendon et al., 2017). Neuronal degeneration may occur either as a primary process or via retrograde degeneration secondary to axonal injury in foci of white matter necrosis. In contemporary cohorts studied with MRI, overt evidence of neuronal necrosis is uncommon. Rather, reduced cortical and subcortical growth is accompanied by a reduction in the complexity of the dendritic arborization (Dean et al., 2013). This process is likely reflected in reduced volumetric growth of gray matter structures on MRI (Karolis et al., 2017).

### Cerebellar Hemorrhage

Cerebellar hemorrhage is an increasingly recognized complication of preterm birth and ranges in severity from mild punctate lesions to larger hemispheric and vermian hemorrhages (Tam, 2018). Neuronal proliferation in the cerebellum occurs in either of the two major germinal zones, the ventricular epithelium or the secondary epithelium, and continues into postnatal life (Patel and Barkovich, 2002). These richly vascularized structures, like the subependymal germinal matrices adjacent to the lateral ventricles, are more vulnerable to rupture. Larger cerebellar hemorrhages can be diagnosed on ultrasound through the mastoid foramen. Punctate hemorrhages, which are typically classified as those less than 4 mm, can only be diagnosed on MRI. Although usually clinically silent, if large enough, signs of brainstem compression (e.g., apnea or bradycardia) and of obstruction to CSF flow can occur. Fortunately, these catastrophic cerebellar hemorrhages are currently rare.

Large cerebellar hemorrhages are associated with mortality and severe neurodevelopmental impairment, which may be mediated by interruption of transsynaptic trophic interactions between the cerebellum and cerebrum (Hortensius et al., 2018). However, smaller cerebellar hemorrhages are linked to reduced preschool motor and visuomotor function and more externalizing behavior in a size- and location-dependent manner (Garfinkle et al., 2020).

## HYPOXIC-ISCHEMIC INJURY IN THE TERM NEWBORN

HIE in the term neonate may be defined as a neonatal encephalopathy (NE) with a constellation of clinical features and a characteristic topography of lesions on MRI similar to that described in animal models and neuropathological studies of hypoxic-ischemic injury (Volpe, 2012). The nomenclature of HIE is inconsistent but carries significant weight medicolegally. HIE results from reduced blood flow and oxygen delivery to the brain and from the excessive accumulation of metabolites; it is often mediated by impaired prenatal and perinatal placental gas exchange (American College of Obstetrics and Gynecology, 2014).

### Etiology and Pathophysiology

The etiology of HIE includes multiple factors that interact over time but typically results from a serious hypoxic-ischemic event, be it acute or prolonged, that occurs before labor, during labor, and/or at delivery (American College of Obstetrics and Gynecology, 2014). When oxygenated blood supply is limited, the fetus adapts by binding a greater concentration of oxygen to hemoglobin, preferentially shunting oxygenated blood to tissues at greatest risk of injury and limiting oxygen consumption. Regions of the brain with the greatest metabolic demands—the Rolandic cortex, thalamus, and basal ganglia—are most vulnerable to acute hypoxic-ischemic injury (Volpe, 2018). After the initial injury and upon reperfusion of cerebral tissues, there is a transient return of cellular metabolic function. This period is followed by a *secondary* decrease in aerobic metabolism and deficiency in high-energy phosphates that results in a profound injury from excitotoxicity, apoptosis, reactive oxygen species, and inflammation (Wassink et al., 2014).

### Diagnosis

NE is defined as a condition occurring in babies born more than 35 weeks' gestational age in which there is disturbed neurological function and particularly in the degree or quality of consciousness. Other features, such as seizures and abnormal tone, movements, and reflexes, may co-occur but are not necessary for the diagnosis (American College of Obstetrics and Gynecology, 2014). Importantly, there are many causes of NE, of which hypoxia-ischemic injury is but one (Volpe, 2012). Other causes include infection, stroke, and metabolic syndromes. The diagnosis of HIE is based on suggestive signs during the pregnancy and labor/delivery and a characteristic lesion topography on imaging studies (Martinello et al., 2017). Table 110.2 lists features of the pregnancy and labor/delivery that suggest HIE.

Once diagnosed, the severity of HIE should be clinically staged. The first staging system was established by Sarnat and Sarnat in 1976 and has since been adapted by multiple groups (Table 110.3). Several others have been created and are in wide clinical use; these include the Thompson Encephalopathy Score, the National Institute of Child Health and Human Development neurological examination, and the University of California, San Francisco Encephalopathy Score (Miller et al., 2004; Shankaran et al., 2005; Thompson et al., 1997). Neonates presenting with mild encephalopathy, or Sarnat stage 1, appear hyperalert with wide-open eyes and are often jittery or agitated. Neonates with moderate encephalopathy, or Sarnat stage 2, present with lethargy, low tone, decreased primitive reflexes, and seizures. Neonates with severe encephalopathy, or Sarnat stage 3, present with stupor or coma, flaccid tone, intermittent decerebrate posturing, absent primitive reflexes, and seizures (Sarnat and Sarnat, 1976). The seizures typically present during the secondary phase of injury and before 24 hours of life.

**TABLE 110.2 Features of Pregnancy and Labor/Delivery That Are Commonly Seen in Hypoxic-Ischemic Encephalopathy**

| |
|---|
| **Pregnancy** |
| Gestational diabetes mellitus |
| Intrauterine growth restriction |
| Preeclampsia |
| Pregnancy-induced hypertension |
| **Labor and Delivery** |
| Reduced fetal movements |
| Non-reassuring fetal heart rate tracing |
| Placental abruption |
| Cord accident |
| Low cord pH |
| Low Apgar scores |
| Need for neonatal resuscitation |

## Neuroimaging

Two predominant patterns of brain injury can typically be discerned in neonatal HIE (Barkovich et al., 1995; Miller et al., 2005) (Fig. 110.9). The basal ganglia–thalamus pattern, which predominantly involves the central gray nuclei (ventrolateral thalami and posterior putamina) and perirolandic cortex, is most often seen following an acute perinatal sentinel event such as cord prolapse (Okereafor et al., 2008). The watershed predominant pattern of injury is typically seen following "prolonged partial asphyxia" without a known sentinel event. The vascular watershed zones encompassing the anterior–middle cerebral artery and posterior–middle cerebral artery territories, including white matter and the overlying cortex, are primarily affected (de Vries and Groenendaal, 2010). Less commonly, MRI reveals a periventricular pattern of injury classically associated with preterm brain injury (Li et al., 2009).

MRI abnormalities evolve with a typical time course. Diffusion restriction on diffusion-weighted imaging (DWI) usually begins soon after the injury, peaks within a few days, and "normalizes" within the first week of life. The temporal evolution of changes is also dependent on the severity of the insult, with more rapid diffusion changes seen in more severe injuries. Changes on T1- and T2-weighted imaging, including absence of a normal high-signal intensity of the posterior limb of the internal capsule on T1, may begin only around the third or fourth day of life (Barkovich et al., 2006; Rutherford et al., 1998). MR spectroscopy examines the cerebral metabolic derangements associated with HIE in the deep gray nuclei and metabolite ratios, in particular lactate:*N*-acetyl aspartate ratio, have prognostic value (Thayyil et al., 2010). Ideally, MRI is performed as soon as hypothermia treatment finishes (i.e., day 3 or 4 of life) when diffusion abnormalities are readily apparent and the diagnosis of HIE can be confirmed to inform treatment pathways.

**TABLE 110.3 Severity of encephalopathy "Sarnat stages"**

| Category | Mild encephalopathy | Moderate encephalopathy | Severe encephalopathy |
|---|---|---|---|
| **Level of consciousness** | ↑ | ↓ | ↓↓ |
| **Spontaneous motor activity** | Normal | ↓ | ↓↓ |
| **Tone** | Mild distal flexion | ↓ | ↓↓ |
| **Reflexes** | | | |
| **Muscle stretch reflexes** | ↑ | ↓ | ↓↓ |
| **Suck** | ↓ | ↓ | ↓↓ |
| **Moro** | ↑ | ↓ | ↓↓ |
| **Autonomic system** | Sympathetic | Parasympathetic | ↓↓ |
| **Clinical seizures** | None | ++ | + |
| **EEG background** | Normal | ↓ | ↓↓ |

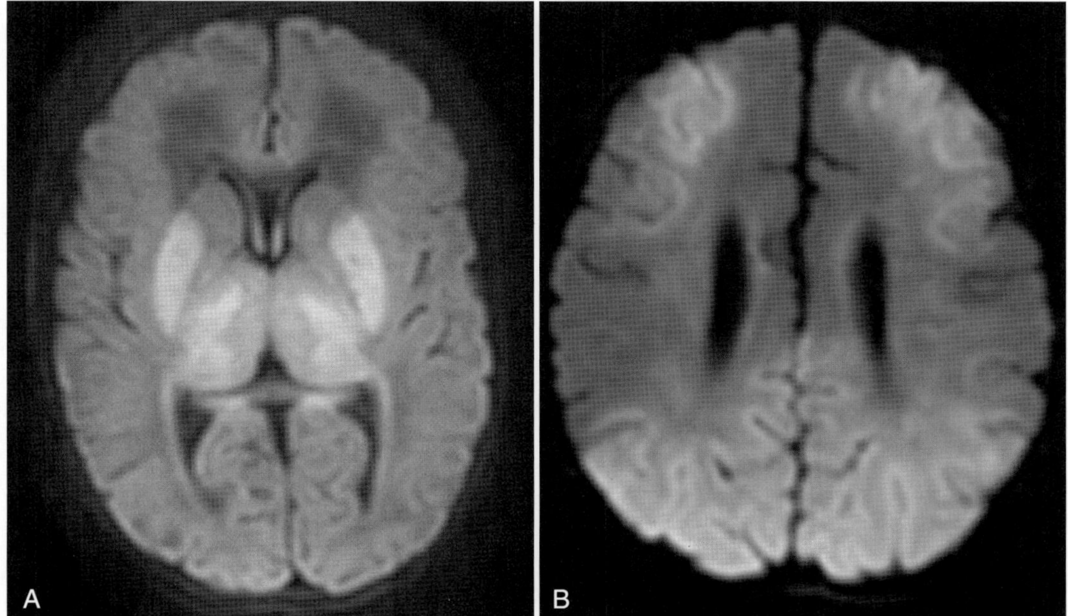


**Fig. 110.9 Predominant Patterns of Brain Injury in Term Hypoxic-Ischemic Encephalography. (A)** Basal ganglia-predominant pattern of injury is demonstrated on diffusion-weighted imaging as areas of restricted diffusion (hyperintense) in the thalami and putamina. **(B)** Watershed-predominant pattern of injury is demonstrated as areas of restricted diffusion (hyperintense) in the cortical and subcortical watershed regions.

## Management

Initial steps in management focus on appropriate resuscitation and correction of metabolic derangements. Therapeutic hypothermia, during which the neonate is cooled to 33.5°C for 72 hours or the head is placed in a cooling pack, is an effective intervention when started within 6 hours of life in the setting of moderate or severe HIE, with a number needed to treat to prevent one death or moderate or severe impairment of seven (Jacobs et al., 2013; Shankaran et al., 2005). Furthermore, an estimated 5% of cerebral palsy in term-born children following NE may be theoretically prevented with hypothermia (Garfinkle et al., 2015). Aggressive seizure management with continuous EEG monitoring may also attenuate injury (see earlier). Adjunct interventions, such as erythropoietin, are being studied and may be incorporated into the standard of care in the future (Hassell et al., 2015; Juul et al., 2018).

## Prognosis

Despite the standard provision of therapeutic hypothermia, the rate of mortality and neurodevelopmental morbidity in moderate-severe HIE remains at almost 50% (Jacobs et al., 2013). Neonates with mild HIE usually have no significant neurodevelopmental sequelae, whereas those with severe HIE often die or are severely impaired with spastic quadriparesis, intellectual disability, cortical visual impairment, and seizure disorders. The outcomes of neonates with moderate HIE are less predictable. In the original description of HIE in 1976, Sarnat and Sarnat reported that resolution of moderate encephalopathy by day of life 5 was associated with appropriate short-term neurodevelopmental outcome; persistence of encephalopathy beyond 7 days was associated with death or neurological sequelae (Sarnat and Sarnat, 1976). The relationship between the severity of NE in the first days of life with neurodevelopmental outcome holds true in contemporary cohorts treated with hypothermia as well (Gunn et al., 2008).

Electrographically, a persistently discontinuous EEG (or aEEG), burst suppression pattern, and refractory seizures all suggest significant underlying brain injury. On MRI, scoring systems have been developed to evaluate the burden of injury and prognosticate even in the hypothermia era (Rutherford et al., 2010). Clinical variables such as the Apgar score do not reliably predict the severity of HIE and prognosis.

# PERINATAL STROKE

Perinatal stroke has been defined as, "a group of heterogeneous conditions in which there is a focal disruption of cerebral blood flow secondary to arterial or cerebral venous thrombosis or embolization, between 20 weeks of fetal life through 28th postnatal day confirmed by neuroimaging or neuropathologic studies" (Raju et al., 2007). Neonates with stroke most commonly present with focal clonic seizures, and some present in the context of NE (Ramaswamy et al., 2004). However, some babies with stroke appear normal during the neonatal period and present only in later infancy or childhood, with early handedness or developmental delay. The enhanced susceptibility to stroke in the perinatal period is multifactorial: the hypercoagulable state of the mother, the mechanical stress during delivery, the transient right-to-left intracardiac shunt, and the high hematocrit and blood viscosity are all implicated (van der Aa et al., 2014).

Neonatal stroke can be divided into perinatal arterial ischemic stroke (PAIS), cerebral sinovenous thrombosis (CSVT), and neonatal hemorrhagic stroke. All three conditions share similar risk factors and clinical presentations. These clinical risk factors are not dissimilar from those associated with HIE and include intrauterine growth restriction, chorioamnionitis, meconium-stained amniotic fluid, emergency instrumented or caesarean deliveries, low Apgar scores, and need for neonatal resuscitation (see Table 110.2). Neonatal hemorrhagic strokes are often explained by hemorrhagic transformation of PAIS or CSVT or by primary conditions such as bleeding disorders and vascular malformations; however, many elude an overt explanation (Cole et al., 2017).

## Perinatal Arterial Ischemic Stroke

The pathogenesis of PAIS is not fully understood but involves passage of thrombi derived from the placenta or venous circulation through the patent foramen ovale or ductus arteriosus, resulting in occlusion of a cerebral artery. Placental pathology and clinical observations suggest that mild hypoxia-ischemia in the fetus dilates the ductus venosus, creating a direct pathway for placental debris or clots to the arterial circulation via one of the aforementioned shunts (Michoulas et al., 2011). Furthermore, the majority of PAIS is in the left middle cerebral artery (MCA) territory, perhaps because the clot has a direct route from the aorta or the ductus arteriosus to the left middle cerebral artery (MCA) via the left common carotid artery (Harteman et al., 2012).

The clinical hallmark of PAIS is focal seizures that present after 12 hours of life (Rafay et al., 2009). In preterm neonates, the presentation is most often subclinical and the strokes are detected on screening brain ultrasounds (Golomb et al., 2008).

MRI is the imaging modality of choice for neonates with suspected PAIS (Fig. 110.10). MR angiography rarely adds any value but can be done to assess for vascular anomalies. Unlike the ischemia/reperfusion injury seen in HIE, in which cytotoxic edema may manifest on DWI only after a few days, in neonatal stroke vascular occlusion leads to cytotoxic edema and DWI restriction within hours (Debillon et al., 2017; van der Aa et al., 2014).

The value of testing prothrombotic factors in the neonatal period is questionable because there is minimal association between perinatal stroke and thrombophilia, and abnormal thrombophilia testing is not associated with recurrent stroke (Curtis et al., 2017; Debillon et al., 2017; Miller et al., 2016; van der Aa et al., 2014). Some authorities also recommend an echocardiogram to detect occult cardioembolic causes or structural heart disease with a right-to-left shunt (van der Aa et al., 2014). However, cohort studies have not demonstrated value in performing an echocardiogram in this population (Lehman et al., 2017).

Acute management of PAIS is supportive and includes hydration, glucose homeostasis, and seizure management. There is no established role for thrombolytic therapy. According to the American Heart Association, long-term anticoagulation should be *considered* only for neonates with PAIS who have a severe thrombophilic disorder or multiple cerebral or systemic emboli (Roach et al., 2008). Absent these two indications, the risk of stroke recurrence is extremely low. The long-term neurological sequelae of PAIS include hemiparetic cerebral palsy, which is typically mild, epilepsy, and cognitive/behavioral challenges. Hemiparesis is more common when the cortex, posterior limb of the internal capsule, and basal ganglia are all involved (Kirton et al., 2007; Wagenaar et al., 2018).

## Cerebral Sinus Venous Thrombosis

Perinatal CSVT is increasingly recognized but still less common than PAIS. Multiple sinuses are usually involved, and the most often thrombosed sinuses are the superior sagittal sinus, the transverse sinuses, and the deep sinuses (Berfelo et al., 2010). Most clinically symptomatic CSVTs are associated with infarction, with is often hemorrhagic (see Fig. 110.10). IVH is often present and associated with infarction involving the thalamus and internal capsule; IVH in the term neonate should prompt venous vascular imaging (Wu et al., 2003). In contrast to PAIS, CSVT often presents with seizures with preceding or accompanying encephalopathy (Jordan et al., 2010).

Head ultrasound with color Doppler studies, CT with venography (CTV), MRI with venography (MRV), and conventional angiography are all suitable tests for suspected CSVT. There is no consensus on whether anticoagulation therapy is indicated for neonatal CSVT, although it is associated with reduced propagation of the thrombus without an increased risk of extension of the hemorrhage in nonrandomized studies (Rossor et al., 2018). The range of outcomes in CSVT is similar to that of PAIS and depends on the extent of infarct and hemorrhage (Kersbergen et al., 2011).

## METABOLIC BRAIN INJURY

NE can result from lack of energy substrate, as in hypoglycemia, or from toxicity, as in hyperammonemia and hyperbilirubinemia. The topography of injury on neuroimaging or neuropathology can give clues as to the underlying etiology. Long-term consequences depend on the rapidity with which the insult is recognized and addressed.

### Hypoglycemic Brain Injury

In addition to oxygen, glucose is the brain's essential energy substrate. Hypoglycemia is common in newborns, especially preterm ones, and can be caused by several different mechanisms that are beyond the scope of this chapter. When blood glucose drops to less than a certain, poorly defined threshold, cerebral blood flow increases to maintain substrate delivery and the brain attempts to maintain aerobic metabolism by using alternative fuels, such as lactate and ketone bodies (Vannucci and Duffy, 1976). Below a certain threshold, and particularly if prolonged, hypoglycemia may cause neuronal and glial injury. In addition, hypoglycemia often accompanies hypoxemic and ischemic injuries to the brain, such as HIE or stroke, and compounds these injuries by exacerbating the cerebral metabolic derangement (Wong et al. 2013). Seizures, which increase the rate of glucose utilization, exacerbate the energy deficit already present in the context of hypoglycemia. Treating hypoglycemia in neonates with HIE, stroke, and/or seizures is thus paramount.

Early on, hypoglycemia commonly produces jitteriness and lethargy, which may manifest as poor feeding and exacerbate the hypoglycemia (Thornton et al., 2015). Seizures ensue when the hypoglycemia is severe and/or prolonged or accompanied by another neuropathological process such as ischemia. Hypoglycemic injury has a characteristic predilection for the parieto-occipital cortex and subcortical white matter. The involved areas exhibit restricted diffusion on DWI (Wong et al., 2013). Visual evoked potentials may show poor or absent cortical responses (Tam et al., 2008).

Any neonate at risk for hypoglycemia, including those born preterm, small for gestational age, or to mothers with diabetes mellitus, should be screened for hypoglycemia after birth. Management guidelines vary, but treatment of hypoglycemia is universally indicated in the symptomatic neonate and a typical threshold for treatment of asymptomatic hypoglycemia is a plasma glucose of less than 50 mg/dL (<2.8 mmol/L) (Thornton et al., 2015). Treatment options include supplemental formula, dextrose buccal gel, and intravenous dextrose bolus followed by a dextrose infusion, depending on the clinical situation. The prognosis of brain injury associated with hypoglycemia depends on the topography and extent of injury. In contrast with HIE, not all early MRI changes associated with hypoglycemia progress to necrosis. Cortical visual impairment, which can range from mild impairment to blindness, is common. Epilepsy and cognitive sequelae are also common (Burns et al., 2008). More subtle deficits in executive function and visual motor function are detectable at school age in neonates who have hypoglycemia without brain injury (McKinlay et al., 2017).

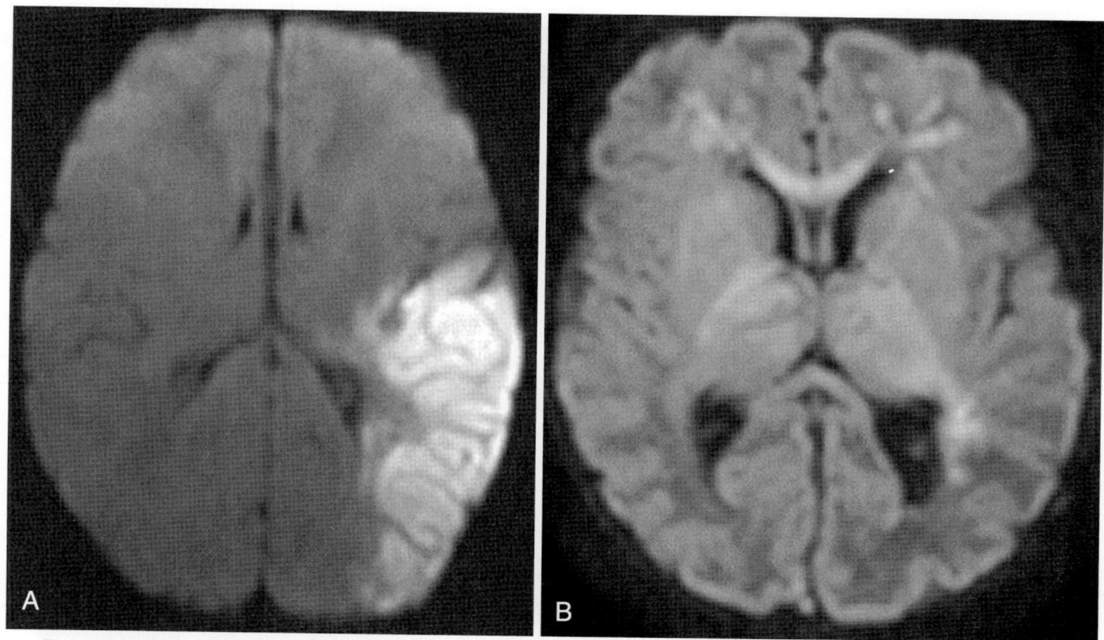


**Fig. 110.10 Acute Symptomatic Perinatal Arterial Ischemic Stroke and Perinatal Cerebral Sinus Venous Thrombosis (CSVT). (A)** Main branch left middle cerebral artery infarct in a term neonate on diffusion-weighted imaging (DWI) as area of restricted diffusion (hyperintense). **(B)** Punctate and confluent areas of restricted diffusion on DWI involving the frontal and parietal white matter and the thalami secondary to diffuse CSVT. Restricted diffusion in the internal capsules and corpus callosum may represent pre-wallerian degeneration. In addition, there is layering of blood in the occipital horn of the left lateral ventricle.

## Inborn Errors of Metabolism

Many inborn errors of metabolism lead to irreversible brain injury, and early recognition and institution of appropriate care are thus important (Saudubray and Garcia-Cazorla 2018; see chapter 91). Most inborn errors of metabolism that present in the newborn period are referred to as "small molecule" disorders and include organic acidurias, amino acidurias, urea cycle defects, and galactosemia. Another important group of inborn errors of metabolism with NE comprise the congenital lactic acidemias, which are due to severe mitochondrial defects. Inborn errors of metabolism can present at any time in life with variable acuity, but we will focus on several more common ones that present acutely in the neonatal period (Perlman and Volpe, 2018a).

The accumulation of metabolic toxins in the bloodstream can lead to NE with seizures and vomiting after an initial asymptomatic period, usually due to food intake and catabolism. Small-molecule intoxication disorders do not interfere with the embryofetal development, owing to the ability of the placenta to remove toxic metabolites. An exception to this rule is nonketotic hyperglycinemia, which presents as encephalopathy, hypotonia, and myoclonic seizures and rapidly progresses to coma as glycine accumulates (Nissenkorn et al., 2001). In utero, nonketotic hyperglycinemia manifests as dysplasia of the corpus callosum and cortex.

There are several key clinical features of small-molecule disorders, including an unusual odor of the neonate's body or urine. Initial biochemical testing may reveal ketosis, acidosis, hypoglycemia, lactic acidemia, hyperammonemia, bone marrow suppression, and characteristic changes on amino and organic acid chromatography. An elevated ammonia level can induce respiratory alkalosis. Newborn screening varies across jurisdictions but is too slow and unreliable to exclude inborn errors of metabolism in neonates with an acute or evolving encephalopathy. MRI with DWI and spectroscopy can be a valuable resource in establishing the diagnosis and the extent of brain injury, and some patterns are reviewed here (Poretti et al., 2013).

Urea cycle disorders are characterized by an enzymatic deficiency in converting ammonia to urea and biochemically are characterized by hyperammonemia and initial respiratory alkalosis. They usually present within hours to days of life, and the pattern of restricted diffusion includes a crenulated ribbon in the subcortical white matter and depths of the sulci (Poretti et al., 2013). The important exception is arginase deficiency, which will present later in life with a slowly progressive spastic diplegia.

Maple syrup urine disease is a disorder of catabolism of branched-chain amino acids caused by deficiency of the branched-chain keto acid dehydrogenase enzyme. It usually presents towards the end of the first week of life and features a sweet-smelling urine. On MRI, it is characterized by intramyelinic ("myelin splitting") edema, which is thought to be caused by energy failure resulting in a decreased $Na^+/K^+$ ATPase activity (Fig. 110.11) (Poretti et al., 2013).

Disorders involving primary energy metabolism from mitochondrial defects may have findings of cerebral dysplasia on prenatal imaging. Two such examples are pyruvate dehydrogenase complex (PDHc) deficiency, which is caused by mutations in the multienzyme PDHc that catalyzes the conversion of pyruvate to acetyl CoA, and pyruvate carboxylase deficiency, which also leads to a buildup of pyruvate. Both conditions present with NE, lactic acidosis, and seizures that may not feature a symptom-free prelude. Imaging may reveal corpus callosum dysgenesis, cortical dysplasias, and periventricular pseudocysts of germinolysis, likely due to prenatal energy failure (Soares et al., 2016). MR spectroscopy demonstrates a lactate peak.

## Hyperbilirubinemia

Neurologists should be alert to the possibility of hyperbilirubinemia because the incidence of chronic bilirubin encephalopathy is increasing (Sgro et al., 2012). Unconjugated bilirubin can cause direct injury to neurons and astrocytes via energy depletion, excitotoxicity, and free radical attack (Ostrow et al., 2004). Hyperbilirubinemia is common in the newborn period and not usually associated with brain injury; however, when the unbound portion of unconjugated bilirubin

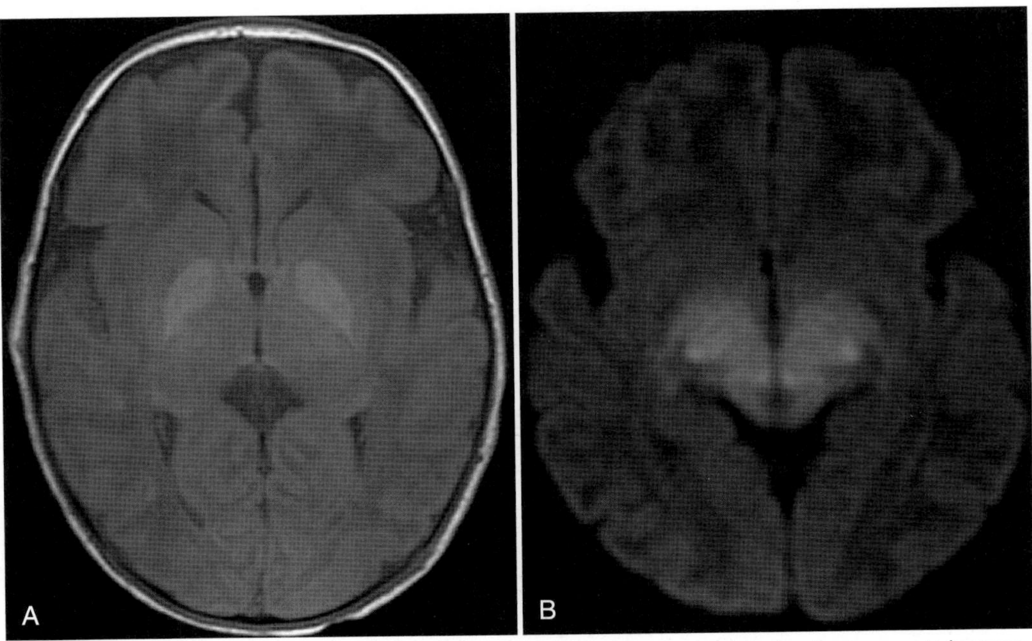


**Fig. 110.11 Metabolic Brain Injury.** (A) Kernicterus from bilirubin neurotoxicity in a term neonate is appreciated as symmetric T1 hyperintensity of the globi pallidi on magnetic resonance imaging *(arrowheads)*. (B) Myelin-splitting edema of the myelinated white matter tracts in the brainstem secondary to maple syrup urine disease, manifested as restricted diffusion on diffusion-weighted imaging.

is sufficiently high, it can enter the brain and cause neurotoxicity. Prematurity, hypoxic-ischemic injury, acidosis, and other physiological disturbances can predispose the neonate to bilirubin neurotoxicity. The classic neuropathology of acute bilirubin encephalopathy features bilirubin staining of specific nuclear groups (i.e., kernicterus) and neuronal necrosis. The classic topography of kernicterus and subsequent neuronal injury involves the basal ganglia (particularly the globus pallidus and subthalamic nucleus), hippocampus, substantia nigra, various cranial nerve nuclei (particularly the auditory, oculomotor, vestibular, and facial nerve nuclei), cerebellar nuclei, and anterior horn cells (Connolly and Volpe, 1990).

Neonates with bilirubin neurotoxicity commonly exhibit clinical symptoms encompassed by acute bilirubin encephalopathy. In contrast to NE due to hypoxic-ischemic injury or hypoglycemia, acute bilirubin encephalopathy features prominent abnormalities of brainstem function, especially with disturbed feeding and high-pitched crying (Johnson et al., 2002). In addition, as the syndrome evolves over days, there is tendency for tone to increase, likely due to extrapyramidal injury. In the advanced phase, the neonate may show retrocollis-opisthotonos and a shrill cry (Perlman and Volpe, 2018b). Seizures are uncommon but possible. Neurological manifestations of bilirubin neurotoxicity are often missed in the preterm neonate or attributed to other pathologies, such as apnea of prematurity or sepsis.

Chronic bilirubin encephalopathy always follows the acute form and has a distinct temporal evolution. Over the first year of life, the characteristic features are hypotonia (evolving from the neonatal hypertonia), active deep tendon reflexes, and delayed acquisition of motor skills. After the first 6–12 months, the classic constellation of findings becomes apparent. These include extrapyramidal movement abnormalities (athetotic and dystonic cerebral palsy), gaze disturbances (particularly upgaze), and auditory deficits with relatively preserved intellect. Dental dysplasia is also common (Johnson et al., 2002). Concomitant brain injury from prematurity may alter these manifestations.

Brainstem evoked response audiometry may detect bilirubin neurotoxicity early on, showing a central more than a peripheral sensorineural abnormality. On MRI, the most common finding is symmetric T1 hyperintensity of the globi pallidi (see Fig. 110.11). However, T1 hyperintensity may be short lasting and is often followed by a chronic T2 hyperintensity in the affected areas. Importantly, MRI may be completely normal (Wisnowski et al., 2014). Prevention and control of hyperbilirubinemia through surveillance, phototherapy, and attenuation of hemolysis are the central tenets of management (Maisels et al., 2009).

## INFECTIONS IN THE CENTRAL NERVOUS SYSTEM

A variety of infectious processes, both bacterial and viral, can disrupt and damage the neonatal brain. Infections may occur in fetal life, around the time of delivery, or in the neonatal period.

### Bacterial Meningitis

Neonatal meningitis is the most common bacterial infection of the CNS and is classified as early or late disease (Nizet and Klein, 2016). Early-onset meningitis, manifesting in the first few days of life, is likely acquired from the birth canal and is usually accompanied by multisystem disease. In contrast, late-onset disease usually presents with isolated meningitis and impressive neurological signs such as stupor, seizures, cranial neuropathies, and bulging anterior fontanelle. Late-onset meningitis can sometimes present insidiously over weeks as obstructive hydrocephalus. The most common bacterial causes of early-onset meningitis are group B streptococcus and *Escherichia coli;* bacteria involved in late-onset disease are more heterogenous. *Listeria monocytogenes* is a worrisome but uncommon pathogen.

Brain injury in meningitis follows inflammation and ischemia. The acute changes of bacterial meningitis are striking and include arachnoiditis, ventriculitis, vasculitis, cerebral edema, and infarction (Berman and Banker 1966). Presumably, hematogenously borne bacteria invade the choroid plexus with subsequent entrance of bacteria into the ventricular system and later movement to the arachnoid through normal CSF flow. Vasculitis of both arteries and veins is often complicated by arterial narrowing and, more importantly, complete occlusion of the veins with thrombosis (Friede, 1973). The increased permeability of blood vessels from vasculitis leads to vasogenic edema and can be accompanied by cytotoxic edema when parenchymal injury occurs. This edema can contribute to reduced cerebral blood flow. Herniation of supratentorial structures through the tentorial notch or of the cerebellar tonsils into the foramen magnum are rare given the separable sutures of the neonatal cranium. Neuronal injury and WMI may also ensue secondary to the inflammation from the bacterial toxins and ischemia from impaired cerebral autoregulation (Gordon et al., 2017; Shah et al., 2005). In preterm neonates with meningitis, oxidative injury may predispose toward severe WMI (Inder et al., 2002). Tissue necrosis with abscess formation complicates meningitis from certain gram-negative species, such as *Enterobacter* and *Serratia.* Hydrocephalus may develop due to obstruction of CSF flow, especially at the aqueduct (Berman and Banker, 1966).

CSF evaluation is the most important diagnostic test, and the hallmark of meningitis is an elevated white blood cell (WBC) count, predominantly comprising polymorphonuclear leukocytes, an elevated protein concentration, and a depressed glucose concentration. Normal values for CSF WBCs have not been definitively established for term or preterm neonates, owing to wide ranges of CSF parameters and the overlap in values between infected and uninfected neonates (Srinivasan et al., 2012). The administration of antibiotics prior to CSF procurement may lead to diagnostic uncertainty. In such cases, broad-based bacterial polymerase chain reaction (PCR) techniques directed against the 16S ribosomal RNA subunit have been used to identify pathogens (Gordon et al., 2017). Head ultrasounds and MRI are helpful in defining the complications of meningitis, such as empyema, infarction, and hydrocephalus (Oliveira et al., 2014).

Appropriate antimicrobial therapy is the mainstay of treatment, and there is currently no role for empiric corticosteroids in neonatal meningitis. Chemoprophylaxis of women colonized with group B streptococcus at the time of delivery is recommended by the Center for Disease Control and Prevention and is particularly effective for early-onset disease (Verani et al., 2010). Neurointensive care of the neonate with meningitis includes seizure control and monitoring for hyponatremia secondary to inappropriate antidiuretic hormone secretion. Prognosis depends on the presence and extent of brain injury, but neurodevelopment and hearing are often compromised (Ouchenir et al., 2017).

### Viral Infections

Viral and protozoan infections can complicate both the intrauterine and neonatal periods. The acronym TORCH is used as a reminder for the major nonbacterial neonatal infections: toxoplasmosis, others (such as syphilis and human immunodeficiency virus [HIV]), rubella, cytomegalovirus (CMV), and herpes simplex virus (HSV). All of the TORCH infections occur during pregnancy by transplacental inoculation, except for HSV and HIV, which usually are contracted by passage of the fetus through an infected birth canal. Although most newborns with TORCH syndromes have clinical features of disease during the first month of life, symptoms can be delayed until later infancy and childhood. In addition to the TORCH infections, enterovirus, parechovirus, parvovirus B19, rotavirus, varicella, lymphocytic choriomeningitis, and mosquito-borne alphaviruses (West Nile, chikungunya) and flaviviruses (dengue virus and Zika virus) may cause fetal or neonatal illnesses with significant brain injury. Two overarching types of pathologies can be distinguished, albeit with significant overlap: (1) inflammatory, destructive lesions and (2) malformations secondary to disturbed neuronal proliferation or migration.

### Cytomegalovirus

Occurring in approximately 1% of live newborns, CMV infection is the most common congenital viral infection and results either from primary maternal infection or from reactivation of virus in the mother. Most newborns with congenital CMV infection are asymptomatic and neurological sequelae can only occur in fetuses who acquire the infection in the first trimester (Faure-Bardon et al. 2018). Affected infants can present with microcephaly, meningoencephalitis, chorioretinitis, sensorineural hearing loss, growth restriction, hepatosplenomegaly, jaundice, and thrombocytopenia and anemia. Congenital CMV is the most common acquired cause of sensorineural hearing loss, which often develops later in infancy (Fowler and Boppana, 2018). The meningoencephalitis comprises (1) inflammatory cells in the meninges; (2) perivascular infiltrates with inflammatory cells; and (3) periventricular necrosis with calcifications that may mimic PVL on MRI (Perlman and Argyle, 1992). In addition, CMV has tropism for neural progenitor cells, resulting in cerebellar hypoplasia and neuronal migration abnormalities, such as polymicrogyria, lissencephaly, pachygyria, and schizencephaly, which are also distinctive features (Teissier et al., 2014).

CMV can be cultured or detected by PCR of saliva, urine, or blood (Fowler and Boppana, 2018). Congenital CMV cannot be diagnosed in infants after the first week of life because it can be acquired postnatally through breast milk or passage through an infected birth canal. Peripartum and postnatal acquisition of CMV does not cause neurological disease but can be associated with injury to other systems. Prevention consists of good personal hygiene, especially hand washing after contact with diapers or oral secretions of young children. Women who develop a mononucleosis-like illness during pregnancy should be evaluated for CMV infection. There is some evidence that therapy with intravenous ganciclovir or oral valganciclovir may provide clinical benefit for symptomatic newborns (Kimberlin et al., 2015). However, risks of side effects must be balanced against benefit because much of the brain injury occurs in utero.

Most asymptomatic newborns with congenital CMV infection develop normally but are at risk for later sensorineural hearing loss (Bartlett et al., 2017). Survivors of symptomatic congenital CMV may have severe neurological sequelae.

### Toxoplasmosis

Toxoplasmosis is an inflammatory and destructive parasitic infection that is acquired transplacentally and affects principally the CNS and the eye in the fetus and newborn. Pregnant women may become infected by ingesting raw or undercooked meat containing tissue cysts excreted in the feces of infected cats. Transmission is highest in the third trimester, but severity is highest when acquired early in the pregnancy (Dunn et al., 1999). The classic triad of congenital toxoplasmosis includes (1) chorioretinitis, (2) diffuse intracranial calcification, and (3) hydrocephalus (Roizen et al., 1995). Neuropathological changes include extensive necrosis and calcification of the cerebral cortex and periventricular tissue. Cerebral injury in the periaqueductal region obstructs CSF flow and causes hydrocephalus. Neurological signs in the neonate are usually absent but can be severe with bulging fontanelle, nystagmus, seizures, and abnormal tone (Desmonts and Couvreur, 1974). Other organs that may be involved are the liver, bone marrow, lungs, muscles, and myocardium.

Several tests are helpful in diagnosing congenital toxoplasmosis, including neonatal antibody screening and PCR of the amniotic fluid or placenta. Examination of the CSF may show lymphocytosis, high protein content, and trophozoites (Naessens et al., 1999). Diffuse intracerebral calcifications may be seen on skull radiography, CT, and ultrasound. Primary prevention involves avoidance of exposure to cat feces or raw meat. Secondary prevention involves detection and treatment of infected women during pregnancy before the fetus is infected. Spiramycin, pyrimethamine, clindamycin, and sulfadiazine with folinic acid are used to treat the infected mothers and infants during the first year (Peyron et al., 2016). Most survivors have significant neurological sequelae. In contrast, asymptomatic newborns have a good prognosis (Berrebi et al., 2010).

### Rubella

Although the incidence of congenital rubella infection is extremely low in North America since the widespread uptake of the rubella vaccination, it remains a significant problem in many parts of the world and should be distinguished from congenital Zika virus infection (Murhekar et al., 2018). The congenital rubella syndrome occurs when the fetus is infected before 20 weeks' gestation and frequently results in miscarriage (Ueda et al., 1979). The classic triad for congenital rubella syndrome includes (1) sensorineural hearing loss, (2) eye abnormalities (chorioretinopathy, cataracts, or microphthalmia), and (3) congenital heart disease, especially pulmonary artery stenosis and patent ductus arteriosus. Other clinical features in the newborn include fetal growth restriction, jaundice, hepatosplenomegaly, petechial rash, bone lesions, and thrombocytopenia. Neurologically, it is characterized by inflammation and tissue destruction (i.e., meningoencephalitis) and impaired neuronal proliferation, which results in microcephaly and impaired myelination (Waxham and Wolinsky, 1984). Calcifications are less common.

Diagnosis is confirmed by culture of the virus (throat swab, urine, or CSF) and demonstration of rubella-specific immunoglobulin M (IgM) in neonatal plasma. CSF often demonstrates a pleocytosis with elevated protein. Universal immunization prevents this disease.

### Herpes Simplex

Neonatal herpes simplex infection is acquired soon before or during passage through an infected birth canal in the vast majority of cases and, less commonly, postnatally. Neonatal HSV infection acquired during the peripartum or postpartum periods can present as (1) localized oral, cutaneous, or ophthalmic disease; (2) localized disease of the CNS; or (3) disseminated disease with hepatosplenomegaly, severe disseminated intravascular coagulation, and renal failure, with or without meningoencephalitis (James and Kimberlin, 2015). The risk for infection is highest when the mother has a primary infection, even if asymptomatic, and considerably lower with reactivated maternal infection. Brain disease if characterized by extensive, often hemorrhagic, meningoencephalitis. Neurological manifestations include stupor and seizures typically presenting later than other brain injuries. Presentation of disseminated herpes occurs on mean day of life 11–12, whereas presentation of localized CNS disease presents on mean day of life 15–20 (Kimberlin et al., 2001b). Indeed, the neonate with herpes localized to the CNS or disseminated disease is usually discharged from the hospital before the illness begins. Less commonly, congenital herpes infection can be acquired in utero via transplacental spread and presents with the triad of skin vesicles or scarring, eye damage, and severe manifestations of microcephaly or hydranencephaly secondary to fetal encephalitis (Hutto et al., 1987).

Intranuclear inclusions may be detected in vesicular fluid, CSF, or conjunctival scrapings. Studies of the CSF usually are consistent with viral meningoencephalitis and often show red blood cells. Diagnosis is most readily established using serum and CSF PCR. MRI, especially DWI, is useful for delineating the extent and severity of brain injury (Fig. 110.12) (Bajaj et al., 2014). Electroencephalogram characteristically shows multifocal paroxysmal or periodic discharges comprising repetitive sharp slow-wave complexes (Mikati et al., 1990). In term newborns, a 21-day course of acyclovir should be started empirically and has been shown to improve mortality and neurodevelopmental outcomes (Kimberlin et al., 2001a).

### Human Immunodeficiency Virus

Antiretroviral use during pregnancy, labor, and breastfeeding and for infant prophylaxis have drastically reduced mother-to-child transmission of HIV (Connor et al., 1994). Before the era of antiretroviral treatment and prophylaxis, the onset of neurological disease in vertically transmitted HIV was after 2 months of age (Epstein et al., 1988). Due to its rarity and postneonatal onset, we refer the reader elsewhere for a discussion of the neurological complications of HIV in children (Donald et al., 2014).

### Enterovirus and Parechovirus

Enteroviral and parechoviral meningoencephalitis are clinically and pathologically indistinct. They are typically acquired intrapartum by exposure to maternal blood or genital secretions or postnatally via the fecal-oral and respiratory routes (Harik and DeBiasi, 2018). The encephalitis mostly affects the white matter and may look like diffuse WMI on MRI (see Fig. 110.12) (Verboon-Maciolek et al., 2008). Activation of the innate immune response and microglia may lead to disturbance of the premyelinating oligodendrocytes and axons, but neuropathological studies are scant (Volpe, 2008).

The clinical features of enteroviral or parechoviral meningoencephalitis are largely indistinguishable from bacterial or herpes meningoencephalitis but more commonly feature rash, diarrhea, and myocarditis. Isolation of the virus in CSF via PCR is the most important diagnostic test as routine CSF studies are usually normal. Despite the extensive white matter abnormalities on DWI, the outcome is highly variable and not universally poor (Verboon-Maciolek et al., 2006). In addition to supportive care, investigational antivirals such as pleconaril have been increasingly used (Harik and DeBiasi, 2018).

### Zika Virus

Zika is a mosquito-borne virus that resulted in an outbreak of congenital microcephaly in Brazil and other countries in 2014 (Rasmussen et al., 2016). Zika virus infection in early pregnancy has been associated with severe brain injury, likely due to the virus's targeting of neural progenitor cells and their subsequent depletion (Tang et al., 2016). Clinically, the hallmark is profound congenital microcephaly with overlapping sutures and redundant scalp tissue, and it is often accompanied by arthrogryposis. The macula and optic nerve are visibly affected on fundoscopy. MRI reveals malformations of cortical development, ventriculomegaly, cerebellar and brainstem hypoplasia, and band-like multifocal calcifications in the cortical-subcortical junction, along with associated cortical atrophy (Ribeiro et al., 2017). Serological testing on CSF, when available, reveals IgM antibodies. Children from the original outbreak with congenital Zika are currently presenting with severe neurodevelopmental delay and epilepsy (Alves et al., 2018).

## TRAUMA TO EXTRACRANIAL, CENTRAL, AND PERIPHERAL NERVOUS SYSTEM STRUCTURES

The frequency of traumatic injuries at birth has reduced alongside improvements in obstetrical care. This section discusses the diagnosis and management of traumatic injuries according to anatomical location.

### Intracranial Hemorrhage

Intracranial hemorrhage can be classified as epidural, subdural, subarachnoid, cerebellar, intraventricular, and other forms of

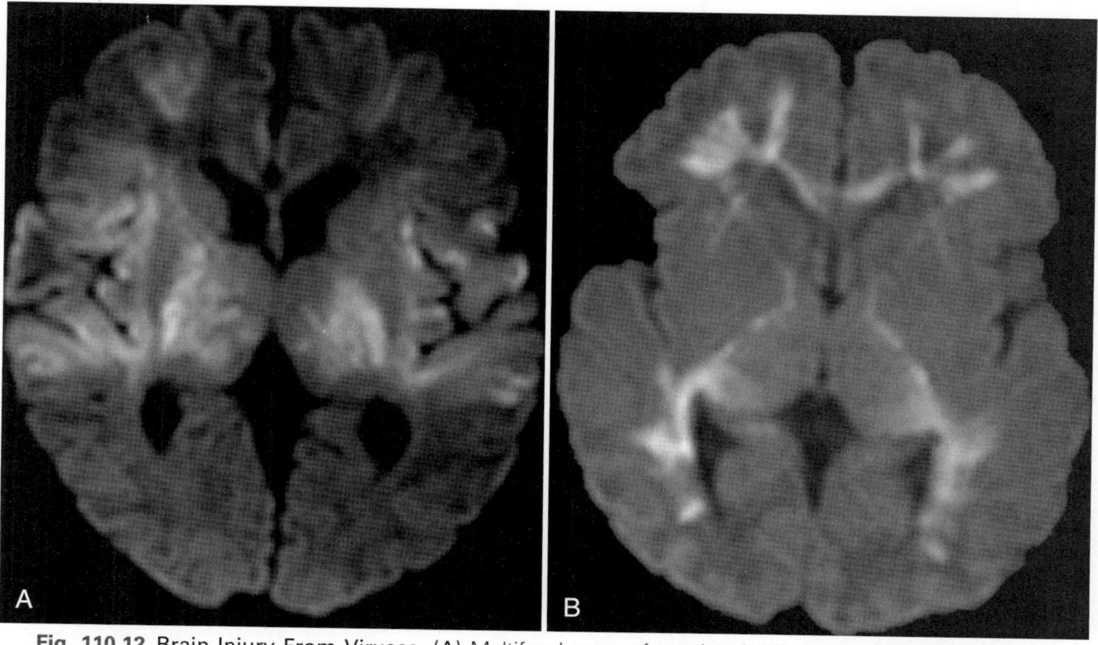


**Fig. 110.12 Brain Injury From Viruses.** **(A)** Multifocal areas of restricted diffusion on diffusion-weighted imaging without a clear pattern from herpes encephalitis. **(B)** Confluent restricted diffusion of the white matter secondary to enterovirus encephalitis.

intraparenchymal. Epidural hemorrhage is often accompanied by a linear skull fracture from traumatic labor or delivery and can present with seizures and signs of increased intracranial pressure (Takagi et al., 1978). Subdural hemorrhage results from laceration of major veins and sinuses. It is often related to excessive molding of the head from vaginal delivery and is almost always asymptomatic. When sufficiently large, symptoms can include seizures and asymmetric tone. At its most severe, rupture of a major vein or sinus secondary to tentorial laceration can result in major infratentorial bleeding and severe brainstem signs (Inder et al., 2018a). Another severe form of subdural hemorrhage, occipital diastasis, occurs with traumatic separation of the squamous and lateral parts of the occipital bones. It is usually associated with breech delivery and cerebellar laceration with infratentorial hemorrhage.

Primary subarachnoid hemorrhage is usually self-limited, originating from small vessels in the leptomeningeal plexus or bridging veins within the subarachnoid space. Infants may be asymptomatic or present with seizures in an otherwise well newborn. Hydrocephalus from obstruction of CSF flow is a rare sequela. Diagnosis may be suspected based on uniformly blood-stained or xanthochromic CSF and confirmed by CT or MRI (Tan et al., 2018).

## Extracranial Hemorrhage

Of the three extracranial hemorrhage types, only subgaleal hematomas are typically dangerous, although any hemorrhage can be a source of hyperbilirubinemia. Extracranial hemorrhages are classified according to the tissue planes involved. Caput succedaneum represents superficial hemorrhagic edema between the skin and the epicranial aponeurosis and is commonly observed after vaginal delivery. Subgaleal hemorrhage, which is often associated with delivery by vacuum extraction, is located between the aponeurosis and the periosteum of the skull and can be associated with hemorrhagic shock due to the ability of the blood to spread beneath the entire scalp. As such, rapid identification and volume resuscitation are important. Cephalohematoma occurs in the deepest plane between the periosteum and cranial bones and presents as a circumscribed boggy region confined by cranial sutures. It is usually a consequence of vacuum or forcep delivery. Cephalohematomas do not typically present with neurological symptoms and resolve in a few weeks to months (Reichard, 2008).

## Skull Fractures

Skull fractures may be linear or depressed, and in recognizing them, the clinician should become aware of the possibility of a more serious intracranial disorder. Linear skull fractures, often associated with direct compressive traumas, are usually parietal in location. Bony continuity is lost on imaging, but the clinical examination is normal and no therapy is indicated. A leptomeningeal cyst may develop at the site of a skull fracture but will usually regress over time. This unusual complication may be identified by transillumination of the region or radiographic evidence of a widening bony defect (a "growing fracture") (Johnson and Helman, 1995).

Depressed skull fractures are called *ping-pong fractures* because the bone buckles inward without loss of continuity like a depression in a ping-pong ball. Depressed skull fractures may be suspected clinically by palpation of the skull. CT or MRI should be performed to detect any intracranial hemorrhage or adjacent cerebral contusion. In the absence of intracranial lesions, treatment is required only when a depressed fracture impinges on the brain. Spontaneous elevation of the bone may occur with skull molding, or the fracture can be elevated with the use of a vacuum extractor or breast pump (Hung et al., 2005).

## Spinal Cord Injury

Spinal cord injury in the neonate is uncommon and is caused by excessive torsion or traction. Injuries associated with breech delivery (excessive traction) involve principally the lower cervical and upper thoracic regions, whereas injuries after vertex delivery (excessive torsion) more commonly involve the upper cervical and midcervical cord (Rossitch and Oakes, 1992). Injuries of the lower thoracic and lumbar spinal cord are even less common and are usually related to vascular occlusion due to umbilical artery catheterization or air embolus from peripheral intravenous injection.

The neurological features reflect the segmental level of the lesion. Newborns with high cervical lesions are often stillborn or die quickly from respiratory failure in the absence of rapid ventilatory support. Lower cervical and upper thoracic lesions cause urinary retention, hypotonia, weakness, and areflexia of all limbs, evolving subsequently to spastic paraplegia or quadriplegia. Cord injuries are distinguished from neuromuscular disorders and brain injuries by preserved facial and eye movement, a distinct sensory level of response to pinprick, urinary retention, and reduced anal tone.

## Facial Paralysis

Unilateral facial paralysis can occur in utero by compression of the facial nerve against the bony sacral promontory or by the pressure of forceps blades during delivery (Shapiro et al., 1996). The clinical features are a unilateral widened palpebral fissure and flattened nasolabial fold with the infant at rest and an inability to close the eye completely or grimace when crying. Unilateral facial paralysis must be distinguished from asymmetrical crying facies resulting from congenital aplasia of the depressor angularis oris muscle, a condition that is associated with cardiac anomalies. Neonatal facial palsy is managed by the use of artificial tears and taping the affected eye closed at night to prevent corneal injury. Most cases resolve within weeks or months without sequelae (Duval and Daniel, 2009). Surgical exploration may be indicated in the absence of clinical or electromyographic recovery (Renault, 2001).

## Brachial Plexus Injury

Brachial plexus injury occurs in large newborns with shoulder dystocia who are difficult to deliver. When the upper roots of the brachial plexus (C5 and C6) are involved, as is most common, the injury is termed Erb palsy. Klumpke palsy involves the lower cervical nerve roots down to the first thoracic root. Rare cases of brachial plexus injury have been associated with diaphragmatic paralysis caused by injury to the third to fifth cervical roots. Brachial plexus injury also may be associated with Horner syndrome, a fractured clavicle or humerus, cervical cord injury, and facial palsy.

Involvement of the upper cervical roots results in loss of wrist and finger extension. The biceps reflex on the affected side may be absent and the Moro reflex asymmetric. With involvement of the lower roots, paralysis extends to intrinsic hand muscles and includes an absent grasp reflex. The diagnosis is based on careful neurological examination. Electrodiagnostic tests, which are technically challenging in neonates, and imaging tests, which can identify evidence of nerve root avulsion injuries, are not commonly used in most decision algorithms but may be predictive of recovery (Wilson et al., 2018).

Prognosis of brachial plexus injury relates largely to the rate of initial improvement, with evidence of improved arm function within 2–4 weeks portending a full recovery. Given the absence of an effective baseline investigation, serial examinations are required to determine severity and recovery potential. Deficits persist in approximately 25% of patients (Smith et al., 2018). For all injury severities, assessment and occupational and physical therapy should be provided at specialized multidisciplinary centers by 1 month of age. Early initiation of range of motion activities is important for recovery. Children with incomplete recovery experience lifelong functional impairment; as such, surgical reconstruction of the plexus should be considered in infants with no evidence of spontaneous recovery at 3 months (Coroneos et al., 2017).

## NEONATAL ABSTINENCE SYNDROME AND ANTIDEPRESSANT EXPOSURE

Fetal exposure to certain drugs can result in transient neonatal signs consistent with withdrawal or acute toxicity and can cause lasting effects on the developing brain.

### Neonatal Abstinence Syndrome

Over the past decade, there has been a dramatic increase in the prevalence of neonatal abstinence syndrome (NAS), which manifests pursuant to passive addiction of the fetus to opioids (McQueen and Murphy-Oikonen 2016). The clinical manifestations of NAS primarily involve the central and autonomic nervous systems and the gastrointestinal system. They range from tremors and irritability to hyperpyrexia and seizures (Table 110.4). Symptom onset is within the first few days of life and varies depending on the half-life of the opioid. Identification of newborns at risk for NAS is important to ensure early intervention. In addition to self-report, procurement of biological specimens from the neonate can help to identify at-risk newborns. Scoring tools for at-risk newborns are essential and permit objective assessment (Hudak and Tan, 2012).

Ideally, initial care for the newborn with NAS should be nonpharmacological, which involves reducing exposure to noise and lights, minimizing handling, swaddling and holding the infant, and providing opportunities for nonnutritive sucking (McQueen and Murphy-Oikonen, 2016). Neonates should stay in the room with their mothers and be breastfed, if possible. Unfortunately, in most cases, nonpharmacological treatment is insufficient and treatment with oral morphine solution or methadone becomes necessary. There is emerging evidence for the use of sublingual buprenorphine as a first-line agent and for clonidine as a second-line agent. Children with NAS are more likely to have neuropsychiatric challenges, even after accounting for the numerous environmental and social factors associated with substance use (Uebel et al., 2015). As such, newborns with NAS merit close medical follow-up care and social services after discharge.

**TABLE 110.4 Typical Clinical Features of Neonatal Abstinence Syndrome**

| Typical Clinical Features |
|---|
| **Central Nervous System Manifestations** |
| Excessive sucking |
| High-pitched crying |
| Increased muscle tone |
| Irritability |
| Myoclonic jerks |
| Seizures |
| Sleep disturbances |
| Tremors |
| **Metabolic, Vasomotor, and Respiratory Manifestations** |
| Fever |
| Frequent yawning |
| Nasal stuffiness |
| Sneezing |
| Sweating |
| Tachypnea |
| **Gastrointestinal Manifestations** |
| Loose or watery stools |
| Vomiting |
| Weight loss and poor feeding |

### Antidepressant Exposure

Selective serotonin reuptake inhibitors (SSRIs) exert their effect by binding to the serotonin transporter to prevent the reuptake of serotonin by the presynaptic neuron. Neonates exposed to SSRIs during fetal life are at risk for neurobehavioral disturbances, which together have been referred to as *poor neonatal adaptation syndrome* (Grigoriadis et al., 2013). These neurobehavioral symptoms may occur because of drug withdrawal and/or serotonin toxicity (Hudak and Tan, 2012). Symptoms include agitation, irritability, tremors, spasms, hypertonia, hypotonia, poor feeding, respiratory problems, and sleep disturbance, and symptomatology can sometimes be indistinguishable from NAS. Recovery from SSRI exposure usually occurs spontaneously over days, and treatment can involve nonpharmacological support, as described earlier, and, if necessary, sedatives (Koren et al., 2009). Studies of long-term outcomes following SSRI exposure have been encumbered by the difficulty in differentiating direct drug effects from maternal mental health effects (Mezzacappa et al., 2017).

*The complete reference list is available online at https://expertconsult.inkling.com/.* 

111

# Cerebral Palsy

*Elizabeth Barkoudah, Siddarth Srivastava, Claudio Melo de Gusmao, David Coulter*

## OUTLINE



## HISTORY

What we now recognize as cerebral palsy has been known throughout history from ancient Egyptian, Greek, and Roman times to the present (Panteliadis et al., 2013). However, early writers did not always recognize the cerebral origin of the disorder. Cerebral palsy was often confused with poliomyelitis because both caused debilitating conditions. Osler's 1889 monograph clearly distinguished the upper motor neuron (UMN) origin of cerebral palsy from the spinal or lower motor neuron origin of polio (Osler, 1889). Freud reviewed the available literature in 1897 and concluded that the term "infantile cerebral paralysis" was only a clinical description and not clearly related to etiology or pathology (Freud, 1968). Little's paper in 1862 correlated the spastic diplegia pattern of cerebral palsy with birth injuries (Little, 1862) and led to the use of the term "Little's Disease" for this condition. Little, Gowers, Osler, and others believed that the etiology of cerebral palsy was related to injuries early in life, either at birth or shortly afterward, due to anoxic, infectious, or vascular causes (Panteliadis et al., 2013). Freud's careful pathological examination of cases identified congenital brain abnormalities and hereditary factors as well. He thus proposed an etiological classification of cerebral palsy into congenital causes, birth injuries, and injuries acquired after birth (Freud, 1968).

Early 20th century writers generally agreed that cerebral palsy was a "useful administrative term which covers individuals who are handicapped by motor disorders which are due to nonprogressive abnormalities of the brain" (Crothers and Paine, 1959). Much of the interest was on developing orthopedic and physical therapies. Crothers and Paine's classic monograph, "The Natural History of Cerebral Palsy," presented the results of their study of 1821 cases including 467 children whom they had followed personally at Boston Children's Hospital from 1930 to 1950 (Crothers and Paine, 1959). The founding of the American Academy for Cerebral Palsy in 1947, the United Cerebral Palsy Association in 1949 in the United States, the Spastics Society (now SCOPE) in Britain in 1952, and other related groups focused attention on research and treatment of cerebral palsy.

## DEFINITION

Morris reviewed the history of the definition and classification of cerebral palsy (Morris, 2007). An international consensus panel in 2004 developed the current definition:

*Cerebral palsy is defined as a group of permanent disorders of the development of movement and posture, causing activity limitation, that are attributed to non-progressive disturbances that occurred in the developing fetal or infant brain* (Rosenbaum et al., 2007).

Thus, to make a diagnosis of cerebral palsy, the patient must have:

1. A disorder of movement and posture (such as weakness, spasticity, dystonia, ataxia, or choreoathetosis) with onset prior to age 1–2 years.
2. Reliable evidence that the disorder is due to a disturbance in the fetal or infant brain.
3. No evidence to suggest progression or worsening over time.
4. Significant functional limitation in the performance of desired activities.
5. Reasonable expectation that the disorder will persist throughout life.

Despite having a nonprogressive nature (dubbed "static encephalopathy" by some older textbooks), the clinical expression of brain injury changes over time. Therefore cerebral palsy should be viewed as a dynamic disorder that evolves with growth and aging, contrary to what the terms "static" or "palsy" imply. A diagnosis of cerebral palsy would not be appropriate if the disorder is very mild and causes minimal activity limitation, if it may disappear as the child grows up, if the disorder begins after infancy, if the disorder is progressive, or if the disorder is due to a spinal or neuromuscular etiology.

The type of motor impairment largely depends on the location of the brain injury or malformation resulting in a variety of tone abnormalities (including but not limited to spasticity, dystonia, chorea, athetosis, and hypotonia), compromised motor planning, decreased strength, and fatigability. When present in combination, chorea and dystonia may be referred collectively as "dyskinesia." Spasticity is a motor disorder characterized by a velocity-dependent increase in tonic stretch reflexes (muscle tone) with exaggerated tendon jerks,

**TABLE 111.1 Clinical Features of the Upper Motor Neuron Syndrome**

| Positive Features | Negative Features |
|---|---|
| Increased tendon reflexes with radiation | Muscle weakness |
| Clonus | Loss of dexterity |
| Positive Babinski sign | Fatigability |
| Involuntarily activation of remote muscle | Loss of selective control of muscle and limb segments |
| Spasticity | Nonmotor changes: cognition, communication, behavioral, sleep disturbance |
| Extensor and flexor spasms | |

Positive features are an important diagnostic finding, more amenable to active intervention and may be of less relevance to one's overall disability. In contrast, negative features, which are characterized by a reduction in motor activity, are more causative to disability, have been focused on less, and have reduced responsiveness to intervention strategies.

resulting from hyperexcitability of the stretch reflex, as one component of the UMN syndrome (Feldman et al., 1980). Spasticity commonly is confused with a variety of tone and movement abnormalities, such as rigidity, clonus, and dystonia. Many features of the UMN syndrome are actually more responsible for disability than the more narrowly defined spasticity itself. The clinical features of the UMN syndrome can be divided into two broad groups—negative phenomena and positive phenomena (Purves et al., 2001) (Table 111.1).

### Classification

There are several classification systems to describe cerebral palsy, a reflection of the complexity underlying the heterogeneity of cause, distribution, type of motor involvement, and severity. For the most part, categorical labels have focused on the clinical features, rather than etiology. Notwithstanding the inherent heterogeneity in large-boundary categories, classification aids in providing common parlance to coordinating care, understanding cause, monitoring of comorbidities, treatment, prognosis, and determining estimates of long-term outcomes.

One such classification system starts by the determination of type of motor involvement: spastic or extrapyramidal. Spastic cerebral palsy can then be further truncated topographically into unilateral or bilateral (Fig. 111.1). In extrapyramidal cerebral palsy, the name implies that underlying brain damage has spared the pyramidal tracts. Therefore spasticity is absent, but different impairments in movement, coordination, and balance are seen. Clinically, these patients exhibit dystonia and/or choreoathetosis (collectively referred to as "dyskinetic") or ataxia associated with lesions in the cerebellum or its connections. Spastic cerebral palsy accounts for 80% of cases, while extrapyramidal make up 20% of cases (15% dyskinetic and 5% ataxic) (Gulati and Sondhi, 2018). Another classification system divides cerebral palsy by severity. Mild, moderate, and severe groups exist without specified criteria for each and are primarily used for diagnostic purposes. The Gross Motor Function Classification System (GMFCS) was born from a desire to categorize based on abilities and limitations in motor functioning (Fig. 111.2). Goals included improved communication for treatment decisions, research into treatment outcomes, and improved understanding and communication of the development of a child with cerebral palsy and anticipated future motor needs (Palisano et al., 1997). Importance is on usual rather than best motor performance in a variety of settings: home, school, and community.

## CLINICAL APPROACH

### Epidemiology

Cerebral palsy is the most common neuromotor disorder in childhood, with an overall incidence of approximately 2 cases per 1000 live births (Oskoui et al., 2013). Prevalence is related to gestational age and is higher in very premature infants, up to 40–60 per 1000 cases compared with 1–2 per 1000 cases for those born at term. Life expectancy is related to the severity of the disability. The primary factors limiting life expectancy are mobility and feeding. Life expectancy for 15-year-old individuals with cerebral palsy who are immobile and tube fed is 13 years, whereas life expectancy for 15-year-old individuals with cerebral palsy who are ambulatory and self-feeders is 55 years (Strauss et al., 2008). Death is related to infections (especially aspiration, pulmonary infections, urinary tract infections, and sepsis), seizures, fractures, and disorders of aging (heart attacks, strokes, etc.) (Himmelmann et al., 2015). Factors associated with higher mortality include being of female sex, cognitive impairment, and epilepsy. Among subtypes, dyskinetic cerebral palsy is associated with higher mortality when compared with diplegic, ataxic, and hemiplegic subtypes. Despite having a higher mortality rate when compared with the general population, cerebral palsy should be considered a lifelong disorder.

### Etiology

The cerebral disruption associated with cerebral palsy can occur prenatally, perinatally, or postnatally in the first 2 years of life (Koman et al., 2004), given that brain development is ongoing during this critical period (Stiles and Jernigan, 2010). Congenital cerebral palsy (due to cerebral injury/maldevelopment before or during birth) accounts for 85%–90% of total cases, while acquired cerebral palsy (due to cerebral injury after 1 month of life) is responsible for the remaining percentage of cases (Centers for Disease Control and Prevention [CDC], 2018b). There are several well-known causes of acquired cerebral palsy. The most common cause in this category is perinatal stroke, which can be ischemic, hemorrhagic, or thromboembolic in nature. The second most common cause of acquired cerebral palsy is meningitis or encephalitis during infancy (Smithers-Sheedy et al., 2016). Head trauma, for example due to abusive head trauma or motor vehicle accidents, can also result in acquired cerebral palsy (Arens and Molteno, 1989).

There are multiple risk factors which can lead to the development of congenital cerebral palsy. Prematurity confers a strong risk (Sukhov et al., 2012), and it increases with degree of prematurity: in one study, conducted in Finland, the incidence of cerebral palsy in very preterm infants (<32 weeks' gestation) was 8.7%, while the incidence in late preterm infants (34 to <37 weeks' gestation) was 0.6% (Hirvonen et al., 2014). Very low birth weight (<1500 g) is an important determinant predictor of cerebral palsy and other neurodevelopmental disorders (Linsell et al., 2016). Periventricular/intraventricular hemorrhage (frequently associated with prematurity) can also serve as a risk factor, especially when severe (Bolisetty et al., 2014; Mukerji et al., 2015 ). In a multicenter study conducted in Europe, the risk of cerebral palsy was increased in multiple births compared with single births, although this risk was largely mediated by prematurity, which is often seen in multiple births (Topp et al., 2004).

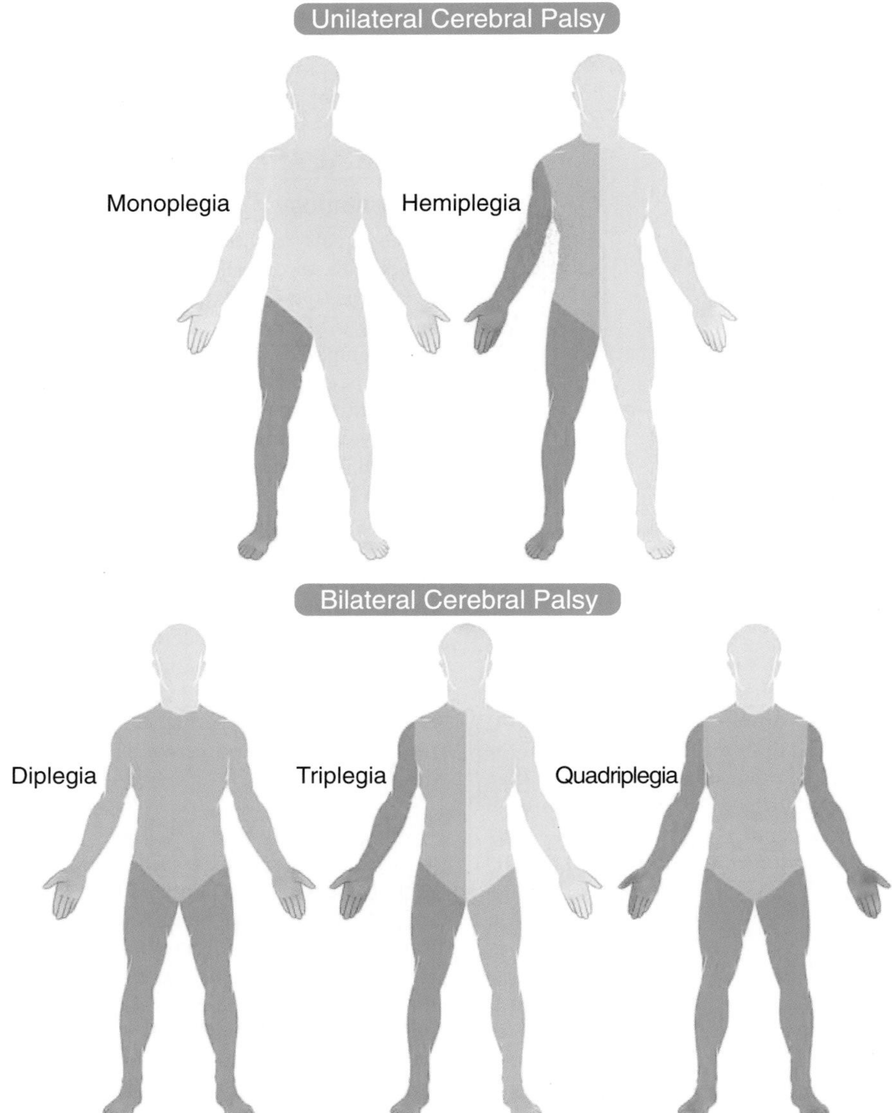


**Fig. 111.1 Topographical Description in Spastic Cerebral Palsy.** Spastic cerebral palsy accounts for 70%–80% of cases and is due to an injury of the pyramidal tracts affecting voluntary movement (Gulati and Sondhi, 2018). The neurophysiology of spasticity is due to a chronic reduction in presynaptic inhibition and hyperexcitability of motor neurons through alterations in motor neuron membrane and synaptic input. Monoplegia and hemiplegia affect one side of the body; in monoplegia one limb is affected, whereas in hemiplegia both arm and leg on one side are affected. Hemiplegia can be asymmetrical, affecting the arm or leg greater than the other extremity. Diplegia, triplegia, and quadriplegia affect both sides of the body. In diplegia, the predominant picture is involvement of the lower extremities. However, the arms can be affected, though not to the same degree. In triplegia, both lower extremities and one arm are affected. A common picture is diplegia from periventricular leukomalacia and a hemiplegia from an interventricular hemorrhage. This results in one lower extremity being more severely affected due to a dual mechanism of injury. In quadriplegia, all extremities are involved. *(From H. Kerr Graham, Jean-Pierre Lin, Peter Rosenbaum, Nigel Paneth, Bernard Dan, Diane L. Damiano , Allan Colver, Jules G. Becher, Deborah Gaebler-Spira, Dinah S. Reddihough , Kylie E. Crompton and Richard L. Lieber. Cerebral palsy. Nat. Rev. Dis. Prim. 2, 1–24.)*

Prior thinking was that perinatal asphyxia (such as from placental abruption or uterine rupture) was the driving factor behind the development of cerebral palsy, but this is not true: perinatal asphyxia is responsible for only approximately less than 12% of cases (Pappas and Korzeniewski, 2016). Maternal and fetal infections, such as chorioamnionitis and congenital cytomegalovirus, may also play a role in the pathogenesis of cerebral palsy (Ahlin et al., 2013; Bear and Wu, 2016; Smithers-Sheedy et al., 2017).

Causative factors for dyskinetic cerebral palsy include perinatal hypoxia-ischemia (in term or near-term infants), kernicterus, intracranial hemorrhage, stroke, infections, or brain maldevelopment (Himmelmann et al., 2009). In addition, several genetic and/or metabolic conditions can cause a clinical picture suggestive of dyskinetic cerebral palsy. There is an increasing trend to classify these disorders based on the genetic etiology as the primary diagnostic category, rather than lumping them into the nonspecific "cerebral palsy" header. For

## GMFCS expanded and revised between 6th and 12th birthday: descriptors and illustrations

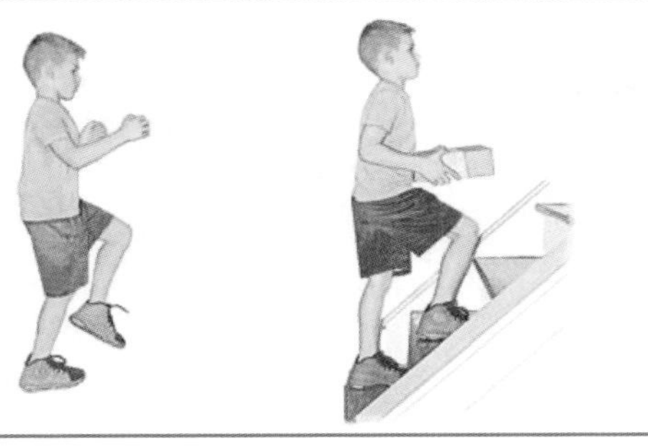

### GMFCS Level I

- Walk at home, school, outdoors and in the community
- Can climb stairs without use of railing
- Perform gross motor skills such as running and jumping, but speed, balance and coordination are limited

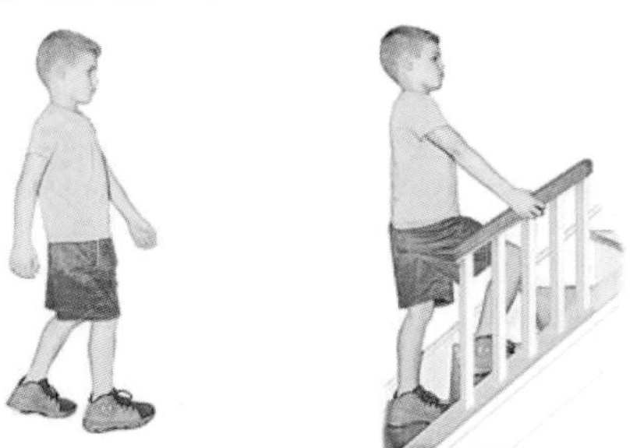

### GMFCS Level II

- Walk in most settings
- Climb stairs holding onto a railing
- May experience difficulty walking long distances and balancing on uneven terrain, inclines, in crowded areas or confined spaces
- May walk with physical assistance, a hand-held mobility device or use wheeled mobility over long distances
- Have only minimal ability to perform gross motor skills such as running and jumping

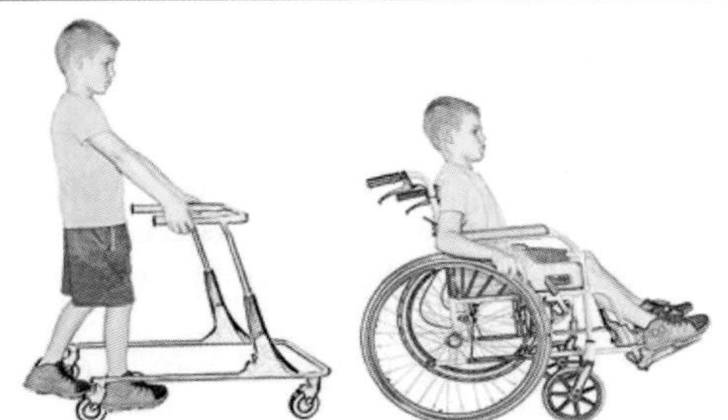

### GMFCS Level III

- Walk using a hand-held mobility device in most indoor settings
- May climb stairs holding onto a railing with supervision or assistance
- Use wheeled mobility when traveling long distances and may self-propel for shorter distances

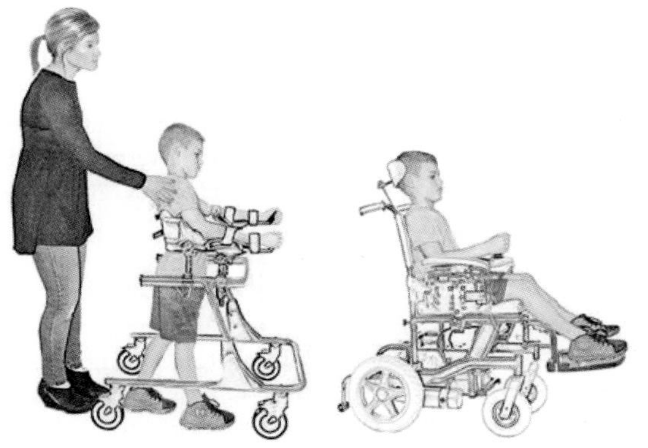

### GMFCS Level IV

- Use methods of mobility that require physical assistance or powered mobility in most settings
- May walk for short distances at home with physical assistance or use powered mobility or a body support walker when positioned
- Transported in a manual wheelchair or use powered mobility when at school, outdoors or in the community

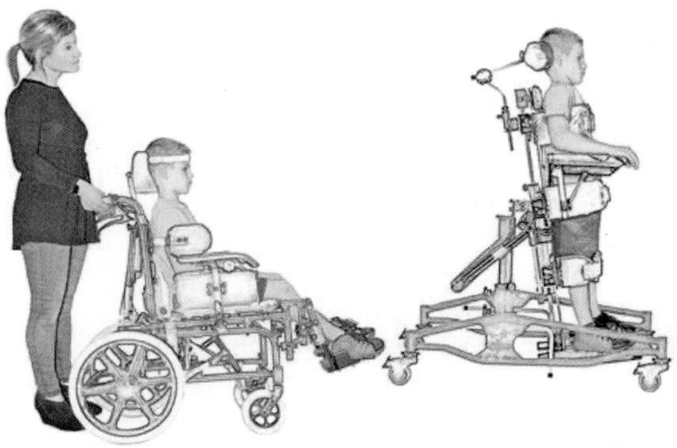

### GMFCS Level V

- Transported in a manual wheelchair in all settings
- Limited in their ability to maintain anti gravity head and trunk postures and control leg and arm movements

**Fig. 111.2** **Gross Motor Function Classification System *(GMFCS)* Expanded and Revised (E&R) for Children with Cerebral Palsy, 6–12 Years of Age.** The GMFCS uses a five-level rating system that corresponds to ability and impairment of daily motor functioning based on self-initiated movement with emphasis on sitting, walking, and wheeled mobility. GMFCS is shown here for ages 6–12, with an additional age band for youth 12–18 years of age, reflective of environmental and personal factors on mobility methods at those ages. The GMFCS E&R descriptors were devised by Palisano et al. (*Palisano, R.J., Rosenbaum, P., Bartlett, D., Livingston, M.H., 2008. Content validity of the expanded and revised Gross Motor Function Classification System. Dev. Med. Child Neurol. 50(10), 744–750. From Graham, H.K., Rosenbaum, P., Paneth, N., et al., 2016. Cerebral palsy. Nat. Rev. Dis. Prim. 2, 1–24. Images are courtesy of B. Reid, A. Harvery, and H. Kerr Graham., The Royal Children's Hospital, Melbourne, VIC, Australia. From Graham, H.K., Rosenbaum, P., Paneth, N., et al., 2016. Cerebral palsy. Nat. Rev. Dis. Prim. 2, 1–24.*)

some authors, cerebral palsy is synonymous with long-term neurological sequelae of perinatal or infantile brain injury or brain malformations. In the absence of documented risk factors or compatible neuroimaging, these conditions are considered "CP mimics" and have an underlying monogenic etiology (Pearson et al., 2019).

In fact, there is increased recognition that a growing fraction of cases may be due to an underlying genetic cause. One study found that 10% of children with cerebral palsy had a clinically relevant pathogenic chromosomal copy number variant (Oskoui et al., 2015). Another study performed whole exome sequencing, discovering that 14% of the cohort had a single gene disorder (McMichael et al., 2015). Inborn errors of metabolism can sometimes go undetected under the guise of a cerebral palsy diagnosis, some potentially treatable (Leach et al., 2014). Disorders of cortical formation may underlie some cases of cerebral palsy (Tsutsui et al., 1999), and these disorders themselves may have genetic causes (Barkovich et al., 2012).

## Diagnosis

Cerebral palsy is a clinical diagnosis that takes into account key elements from the history, physical examination, and review of neuroimaging data.

The history should focus on whether there was perinatal or postnatal injury to the brain and, if so, what factors led to this injury. Accordingly, details about the pregnancy that are important to document include, but are not limited to, the following: the gravidity and parity of the mother; illnesses or medical conditions diagnosed during gestation and their treatments; exposure to alcohol, cigarettes, illicit substances, or prescription medications; history of decreased fetal movements (acute or long-standing); and any other major complications. Prematurity is a strong risk factor for the development of cerebral palsy: so it is important to know the gestational age of the infant and the birth weight. A close review of labor and delivery is essential, especially if there were perinatal events that may have contributed to hypoxic-ischemic injury, such as placental abruption that necessitated emergency cesarean section (Morgan et al., 2018). Especially in the presence of prematurity, the neonatal course may be complicated by various issues such as intracranial hemorrhage, seizures, respiratory failure, necrotizing enterocolitis, hyperbilirubinemia, sepsis, or meningitis, each of which may serve as risk factors. The last key element is the developmental trajectory: it is important to quantify rates of development in motor, language, and visual-motor/problem-solving domains and whether the trajectory has been of continued acquisition of skills, plateauing, or regression.

There are multiple components to the physical examination that are necessary to characterize abnormalities of tone, reflexes, movements, posture, and balance that may be consistent with the diagnosis of cerebral palsy. The physical examination should focus on the following features: presence of any limb deformities, curvature of the spine, range of motion of joints, muscle tone, muscle strength, reflexes, presence of any movement disorders, and gait (Koman et al., 2004). In infants, primitive reflexes that have not yet integrated by the normative period may be an early diagnostic clue (Krigger, 2006). Individuals with cerebral palsy may adopt certain postures affecting their arms (e.g., flexion of the elbows, wrists, and fingers, with internal rotation of the shoulders and pronation of the forearms) and legs (e.g., flexion of the hips, knees, and toes, with adduction of the hips). Examples of gait abnormalities include toe walking, adduction of the hips, crouched gait, and jump gait (Koman et al., 2004). Individuals with dyskinetic cerebral palsy may exhibit predominant dystonia, chorea, or a combination of these features (Videos 111.1 and 111.2).

Once a diagnosis of cerebral palsy is suspected, the clinical classification may follow based on the predominant movement abnormality: spastic, dyskinetic, or hypotonic-ataxic. For those who have spastic cerebral palsy, cases can be further divided topographically: spastic diplegia (involvement of the legs greater than the arms); spastic hemiplegia (involvement of one side of the body, usually the arm more so than the leg); and spastic quadriplegia (involvement of all limbs in addition to the trunk and face) (CDC, 2018a). Sometimes a combination of movement disorders is encountered ("mixed" cerebral palsy).

### Neuroimaging

Neuroimaging is essential to evaluating the type, severity, and etiology of injury to, or maldevelopment of, the brain (Morgan et al., 2018). Although modalities such as head ultrasound have their use, ultimately magnetic resonance imaging (MRI) of the brain is almost always preferable. Imaging generally correlates with the findings on clinical examination and/or etiology, with involvement of the pyramidal tract in spastic cerebral palsy and of the basal ganglia or cerebellum in dyskinetic or ataxic subtypes. For example, patients with kernicterus have preferential involvement of the globus pallidus (Yilmaz et al., 2001). It is estimated that up to 70% of patients with dyskinetic cerebral palsy have imaging evidence of involvement of the thalamus and basal ganglia, with lenticular nucleus most commonly affected (Aravamuthan et al., 2016; Monbaliu et al., 2017). In patients with injury secondary to hypoxic-ischemic events, involvement of these areas is explained by their high metabolic rate, preferentially affected in the term and near-term infant. More severe presentations, when dyskinesia is combined with spasticity, can be seen with involvement of central cortico-subcortical areas and the hippocampus (Monbaliu et al., 2017; Krägeloh-Mann et al., 2007) (Fig. 111.3).

Imaging can be normal in some patients. In a case series, up to 13% of patients with dyskinetic cerebral palsy had unremarkable imaging. (Graham et al., 2016) Nevertheless, the absence of visible structural injury to the central nervous system (CNS) (especially if the history is not associated with risk factors) should raise concern for an underlying genetic condition. Recognizing such syndromes may play a major role in management as there can be specific treatments based on the diagnostic category. Examples include dopa-responsive dystonias, neurotransmitter diseases, some leukodystrophies, and several other neurometabolic conditions.

### Distinguishing Genetic Causes of Cerebral Palsy From Acquired Causes

Several different approaches exist for distinguishing genetic causes of cerebral palsy from acquired causes. One such approach, building from principles outlined in Lee et al. (2014), is as follows. There are three steps that the clinician can consider undertaking after an individual has received a diagnosis of cerebral palsy.

The first step (Step 1) is asking if the history, examination, and brain MRI are consistent with mechanisms of brain injury. The following questions are important to ask:

- Does the presumed cause of cerebral palsy match with the child's motor and cognitive presentation? (e.g., a child with spastic diplegia who has a history of prematurity and periventricular leukomalacia [PVL] on MRI).
- Is the clinical course nonprogressive?
- Is the MRI abnormal in a way that explains the child's presentation? (e.g., a child with hemiplegia with evidence of perinatal stroke on MRI)

If the answer to all of these questions is *Yes*, then no further work-up may be necessary. However, if the answer to any of these questions is *No*, then the clinician should move to the second step.

The second step (Step 2) is asking if there are any red flags that raise suspicion for an underlying genetic disorder. These include elements

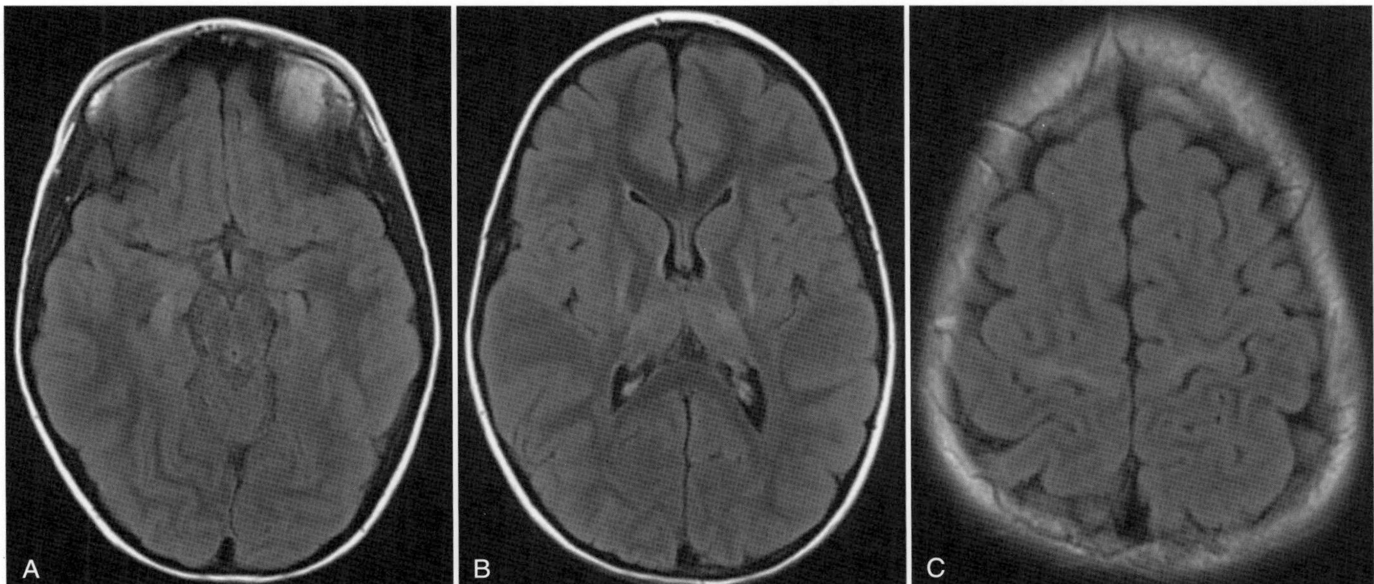


**Fig. 111.3 Magnetic Resonance Imaging of a Brain with Cerebral Palsy (CP) Secondary to Hypoxic-Ischemic Injury.** Clinically, the 5-year-old patient has mixed CP, with dyskinetic and spastic components (fluid-attenuated inversion recovery [FLAIR] sequences). **A,** Increased signal in the hippocampi. **B,** Loss of volume and increased signal change visible on the posterior putamina and thalami. **C,** Volume loss and increased signal change in the perirolandic cortices bilaterally.

from the history (severe symptoms in the absence of history of perinatal injury, developmental regression, progressively worsening symptoms); elements from the family history (multiple family members affected with cerebral palsy, especially if there is a pattern that suggests a particular mode of inheritance, history of consanguinity between the parents); elements from the physical exam (isolated hypotonia, prominent extrapyramidal symptoms such as rigidity without an adequate explanation like basal ganglia involvement due to hypoxic ischemic encephalopathy); and elements from the brain MRI (normal MRI, imaging abnormalities isolated to the globus pallidus). If the answer is *No* (meaning there are no red flags), further work-up may not be necessary. However, if the answer is *Yes*, then the individual's presentation of cerebral palsy raises concern for an underlying neurogenetic cause, and further evaluation/diagnostic testing may be warranted (Step 3).

The third step (Step 3) involves defining the predominant type of movement abnormalities to determine what genetic testing needs to be done. The type of cerebral palsy—spastic, dyskinetic (including dystonia, chorea, athetosis, hemiballismus), or ataxic-hypotonic—can pinpoint specific genetic conditions. See Table 111.2. At this stage, evaluation by a specialist in neurogenetics may be required.

## Life Span Issues

Adults with cerebral palsy outnumber children by a ratio of 3:1 in some countries (Australian Cerebral Palsy Register Group, 2013; Himmelmann et al., 2015). Guidelines have been developed to assist clinicians to improve transition to adult care (Brown et al., 2016; Cooley et al., 2011). Unfortunately, cerebral palsy is still perceived as a pediatric disorder and appropriate care centers for adults with cerebral palsy are lacking. Clinical issues in childhood relate to tone management (discussed later), orthopedic surveillance for hip and joint disorders and scoliosis, and neurological management of seizures and developmental support. Orthopedic interventions become less important in adulthood once the skeleton is mature, but the need for effective tone management continues. The need for seizure management is lifelong, but often seizures become less severe in adulthood. Developmental support in childhood and adolescence is focused on the educational system, where neurological input can be very helpful to ensure the most appropriate interventions. Guardianship, when it is appropriate, and financial planning become key issues as the patient enters adulthood. Adult neurologists need to be familiar with the service systems for adults with cerebral palsy, including state agencies for developmental disabilities, federal and private insurance agencies, and group home providers and agencies providing daytime supports. Family involvement and support are critical at all ages. Long-term planning for healthcare interventions and care directives should be proactive as the adult with cerebral palsy ages, just as it should be for everyone else.

Gait and self-care worsen in a substantial proportion of adults with cerebral palsy. A decline in balance is frequently reported (Morgan et al., 2018; Opheim et al., 2009; Turk et al., 2009). The mechanisms are likely to be multifactorial. Long-standing hypertonia and weakness can lead to anatomical changes in musculoskeletal structures, leading to joint malalignment and instability. Over time, this process is believed to cause increased effort, muscle overuse, and decreased endurance. These factors, as well as decreased access to rehabilitation, probably contribute to pain and fatigue being frequent complaints in adults with cerebral palsy (Opheim et al., 2009; Turk et al., 2009).

Dyskinetic cerebral palsy can also be complicated by degenerative changes of the cervical spine (Kim et al., 2014). Sustained involuntary movements and malalignment due to imbalanced hypertonia can predispose to spine instability; compression of neural elements may ensue with cervical myelopathy. Onset is usually in the fourth decade, and the diagnosis is often delayed (Jameson et al., 2010; Kim et al., 2014).

Furthermore, adults with cerebral palsy experience disadvantages in social life and employment (Colver et al., 2014). The prevalence of depression can be as high as double that of the general population, with higher scores correlating with higher levels of functional disability (van der Slot et al., 2012).

TABLE 111.2 **Examples of Genetic Conditions Associated With Different Types of Cerebral Palsy**

| Type of Cerebral Palsy | Categories of Associated Genetic Conditions | Specific Examples |
|---|---|---|
| **Spastic Cerebral Palsy** | | |
| | Hereditary spastic paraplegias | • Arginase deficiency (*ARG1* defect) |
| | Leukodystrophies | • Pelizaeus-Merzbacher disease<br>• Krabbe disease<br>• Metachromatic leukodystrophy<br>• Hypomyelination with atrophy of the basal ganglia and cerebellum (H-ABC) |
| | Neuronal migration disorders | • Lissencephaly<br>• Polymicrogyria<br>• Primary microcephaly |
| | Forebrain cleavage disorders | • Holoprosencephaly |
| **Dyskinetic Cerebral Palsy** | | |
| | Neurotransmitter disorders | • Disorders of tetrahydrobiopterin metabolism<br>• Disorders of catecholamines and serotonin metabolism<br>• Disorders of serine and glycine metabolism<br>• Disorders of glutamate and $\gamma$-Aminobutyric acid metabolism<br>• Disorders of folate metabolism<br>• Disorder of vitamin $B_6$ metabolism |
| | Transporter disorders | • Glucose transporter type I deficiency (*SLC2A1* defect)<br>• Monocarboxylate transporter 8 deficiency (*SLC16A2* defect) |
| | Organic acidemias | • Glutaric aciduria type 1Methylmalonic acidemia |
| | Disorders of energy metabolism | • Mitochondrial disorders<br>• Pyruvate dehydrogenase deficiency |
| | Other | • Neuronal brain iron accumulation syndromes (NBIAs)<br>• Creatine deficiency<br>• Fucosidosis<br>• H-ABC |
| **Ataxic Cerebral Palsy** | | |
| | Cerebellar malformation disorders | • Joubert syndrome |
| | Angelman syndrome | |
| | Mitochondrial disorders | • Coenzyme $Q_{10}$ deficiency |
| | Congenital disorders of glycosylation | |
| | Spinocerebellar ataxias | |
| | Leukodystrophies | • H-ABC |

Many of these categories and even specific examples can have multiple genetic causes.
*Adapted from Lee, R.W., Poretti, A., Cohen, J.S., Levey, E., Gwynn, H., Johnston, M.V., et al., 2014. A diagnostic approach for cerebral palsy in the genomic era. Neuromol. Med. 16, 821–844.*

## TREATMENT

The overarching goal of therapies for patients with cerebral palsy is to maximize functioning by improved biomechanics from tone, musculoskeletal deformities, and muscle weakness. The treatment strategy for cerebral palsy is best developed in a multidisciplinary setting, where medical interventions are embedded in a rehabilitation context considering the patient's individual goals. Besides having a patient-centered approach, communication with healthcare staff, including physiatry, orthopedic care, and primary care, as well as physical therapy, occupational therapy, and speech therapy, maximizes the chances of success. Therapeutic approaches can be divided into categories such as pharmacological, rehabilitative, and surgical. In most cases, integration of these therapies provides the most benefit rather than a sequential approach. Rehabilitative strategies include orthotics, casting, and physiotherapy, although occupational and speech therapy may be equally important. The other treatment options are discussed separately as follows.

### Spastic Cerebral Palsy

Enteral medications are commonly used as first-line agents for hypertonia, given their ease of use and known side-effect profiles. They provide benefit for more widespread spasticity. Although baclofen is routinely favored, other antispasmodic medications such as tizandine, dantrolene, and benzodiazepines are also acceptable (Chung et al., 2011; Delgado et al., 2010; Verrotti et al., 2006). Second-line medications such as clonidine or gabapentin (Lapeyre et al., 2010) may provide dual benefit for both tone management and other neurological associations, including sleep disruption, dysautonomia, pain, and neuroirritability. In contrast, for management of focal or segmental spasticity, chemodenervation agents are ideal, given their ability to target these specific locations. Examples include botulinum toxin A (BoNT-A), phenol, and ethyl alcohol (Chung et al., 2011). Targeted injections combined with rehabilitative therapies can allow for improved motor functioning and delay/avoidance of orthopedic surgery (Jr et al., 2018). These injections require repeat administration with timing, dose, and location dependent on needs. Typically, repeat injections are performed every 4–6 months, primarily to avoid the development of resistance, although as soon as 3 months may be necessary (Jr et al., 2018).

### Intrathecal Baclofen

Intrathecal baclofen (ITB) can be considered in patients whose spasticity is not adequately treated with enteral baclofen or who are experiencing side effects such as sedation, weakness, or gastointestinal symptoms (Hasnat et al., 2004; Medical Advisory Secretariat, 2005). Only a small portion of enteral baclofen crosses the blood-brain barrier to act on the γ-aminobutyric acid (GABA) receptor. By infusing baclofen directly into the cerebrospinal fluid (CSF), ITB can be administered at a fraction of the concentration directly to the site of drug action, thus avoiding many of the side effects seen with enteral baclofen. Unlike the selective dorsal rhizotomy (SDR) or orthopedic surgeries, ITB treatment is reversible.

Candidacy for placement of an intrathecal pump needs to be considered cautiously in populations including anticoagulation therapy, local or systemic infection, or anatomical spine abnormalities. Before implantation, a baclofen test dose is performed to ensure a positive response to intrathecal administration and guidance on initial starting doses. A pump, used for storage and delivery of baclofen, is surgically placed in the abdomen on one side under the skin. The pump is attached to a catheter which administers the baclofen intrathecally. Baclofen is refilled on average every 2–6 months depending on dose and concentration via silicon port by needle insertion. The pump delivers baclofen constantly throughout the day, although it can be programmed to deliver boluses at different times of the day depending on patient needs. Currently all pumps will require surgical replacement in 5–7 years due to battery life length.

Complication rates are higher in children compared with adults, with the most common being catheter related; disconnection of the catheter from the pump occurring in 9% of pumps implanted; and catheter dislodgement from the intrathecal space occurring in 8% of pumps implanted (Gooch et al., 2003). Catheter-related complications occur more frequently in pumps with catheter access ports. Other complications include 9.3% infection, 4.9% CSF leak, and 1% pump-related problem (Gooch et al., 2003).

Benefits of ITB include ease of daily activities, ease of caregiving, and comfort as reported by caregivers and patients via the Rehabilitation Institute of Chicago Care and Comfort Caregiver Questionnaire (RIC CareQ) (Baker et al., 2014). Spasticity benefit was noted in all extremities while studied over a 10-year period without diminishment of that benefit (Albright et al., 2003). Although most studies focus on ITB for the management of spasticity, there is also evidence in ITB having a beneficial role in the treatment of dyskinesias, particularly dystonia (Eek et al., 2018; Motta et al., 2008). Benefits reported are similar to those in which ITB was used for spasticity management: reduced dystonia, improved posture, and ease of caregiving. ITB for the management of dyskinetic cerebral palsy has not always been advantageous, because it has been reported that ITB can worsen dystonia or provide no benefit (Silbert & Stewart-Wynne, 1992; Walker et al., 2002).

### Selective Dorsal Rhizotomy

The origins of SDR herald from the late 1880s as a means to treat unremitting limb pain. In patients whose pain was resultant from spasticity, it was noted that both pain and tone improved following surgery. Without postsurgical rehabilitation support and unacceptable side effects (sensory abnormalities, proprioceptive loss, and ulcer formation), the rhizotomy for treatment of "congenital spastic paraplegia" was abandoned. The practice of using rhizotomy for spasticity management took a 50-year hiatus before being resurrected in the 1960s. Over time the rhizotomy was refined both clinically and technically to the now-known SDR.

Because SDR is an irreversible treatment for spasticity, optimal selection of ideal candidates from a multidisciplinary approach is necessary to avoid short- and long-term complications (Wang et al., 2018). The main goal of SDR is to improve gait or functioning. Selection criteria focus on history, examination, imaging, and gait analysis. Ideal candidates are children aged 4–10 years for whom relearning gait patterns is easier and secondary orthopedic deformities from spasticity can be avoided. These candidates function as GMFCS I–III with good selective motor control and minimal weakness. The underlying neurological etiology is PVL in the setting of prematurity with sparing of the basal ganglia and thalamus. Because the benefits from the SDR rely on the postsurgical rehabilitation, cognition and behavior of the child are essential for their participation in this therapy.

SDR's spasticity benefits are due to a partial sensory deafferentation of the spinal cord. This is achieved by resection of dorsal nerve rootlets based on abnormal motor responses to electrical stimulation. The total number of nerve rootlets resected ranges from 25% to 40%, although in some institutions it exceeds 40% (Wang et al., 2018). Complications from SDR are rare when dorsal rootlet resectioning was not excessive (<50%) and often transient. These included sensory loss, weakness, and bowel/bladder dysfunction (Munger et al., 2017; Wang et al., 2018). Poorer outcomes not as a result of surgical technique are often related to less-ideal SDR candidate selection or need for surgical orthopedic intervention. Because the primary outcome of SDR is to lessen spasticity, the need for enteral pharmacological tone management and/or BoNT should be eliminated or reduced. In patients GMFCS I–III, SDR has allowed for ongoing functional ambulation gains in childhood and protects from decline in adolescents seen on natural history studies (Hanna et al., 2009; Munger et al., 2017).

More recently SDR is being looked at for management of tone, minimizing pain, and ease of caregiving in patients functioning on a GMFCS IV–V level. SDR manages lower extremity tone equally as the ITB pump; may provide more upper extremity tone control compared with the ITB pump; and improves bladder function (D'Aquino et al., 2018). In patients GMFCS IV–V who underwent SDR after ITB pump removal, 90% of caregivers felt functional results were superior and more efficacious (Ingale et al., 2016). Compared with ITB, SDR is cheaper and has lower dependence by avoiding the need for ongoing management (refills, replacements, etc.). Outcomes of SDR use in patients GMFCS IV–V will need to be tracked longer over time to ensure these reported benefits persist.

## Dyskinetic Cerebral Palsy

The treatment approach should be also chosen according to the movement phenomenology. In general, dystonia tends to have a stronger impact in several functional domains, activity, participation, and quality of life when compared with choreoathetosis (Monbaliu et al., 2017). Most treatment modalities addressing dystonia in cerebral palsy have not been studied in a controlled fashion, and treatment is still largely determined by expert opinion. Good resources exist to review available evidence (American Academy for Cerebral Palsy and Developmental Medicine Care Pathways, 2018; Fehlings, et al., 2018). Medications used to treat dystonia include oral baclofen, benzodiazepines, trihexyphenidyl, clonidine, and gabapentin, but practice varies widely. BoNT can be injected intramuscularly for targeted chemodenervation. Surgical treatment modalities include ITB and deep brain stimulation (Eek et al., 2018; Vidailhet et al., 2009).

ITB may result in dystonia reduction, with evidence for benefit with higher catheter placement (Eel et al., 2018; Fehlings et al., 2018). The effect may be gauged after a trial administration after lumbar puncture and can be considered over deep brain stimulation if there is severe hypertonia with combined spasticity and dystonia. Deep brain stimulation is a neurosurgical procedure that evolved from the recognition that pallidotomies and thalamotomies could help patients with medically refractory dystonia. It involves the introduction of stimulating electrodes in areas of the brain such as the globus pallidus or the subthalamic nucleus, which are connected to an extracranial pulse generator that is implanted in the subcutaneous space in the thoracic or abdominal area. After the surgical procedure, the beneficial effects are not immediately visible, often taking several months. The procedure is associated with perioperative risks as well as infection and hardware complications. Therefore patient selection and consideration of the appropriate target for deep brain stimulation is key, but it remains a challenge. Most authors agree that the presence of spasticity, contractures/deformities, and myelopathy are poor predictors of response and that neurosurgical expertise, anatomical factors, and severity/time of dystonic symptoms may influence response (Koy et al., 2013; Romito et al., 2015; Vidailhet et al., 2009).

### Orthopedic Interventions

Musculoskeletal pathology in patients with cerebral palsy include fixed muscle contractures, torsion of long bones, hip displacement, and spine deformities (Kerr et al., 2016). Several surgical methods exist for lengthening the muscle-tendon units for contraction management, although these are rarely necessary before 6 years of age. Prior to this, prevention of contracture development is key and often is a combination of tone management, bracing, and stretching exercises. Femoral and tibial torsion occur respectively due to failure of remodeling fetal anteversion (Kerr et al, 2003) and mostly as a response to abnormal biomechanical forces during walking (Selber et al., 2004). Derotational osteotomies are ideally performed between 6 and 12 years of age (Kerr et al., 2016). With increasing GMFCS level comes increased risk of developing hip displacement and neuromuscular scoliosis (Persson-Bunke et al., 2012; Soo et al., 2006). Monitoring and prevention strategies are paramount because both hip displacement and scoliosis may progress with age. Conservative treatment and surgical approaches can be challenging when balancing the complexity of these surgical interventions and outcome goals defined presurgically.

## SUMMARY

Cerebral palsy is a neurological disorder that affects body movement and muscle tone, posture, or coordination caused by a nonprogressive disturbance that occurred in the developing fetal or infant brain. Although the underlying cause is nonprogressive, how the body is affected can evolve over time given maturation of the nervous system. The diagnosis of cerebral palsy remains clinically supported by additional laboratory and diagnostic studies and is one of the most commonly diagnosed physical disabilities in children. In the past, children with cerebral palsy were not expected to achieve normal life expectancies. With advances in medical management, children with cerebral palsy are surviving well into adulthood. Adults with cerebral palsy benefit from a multidisciplinary approach to manage the physical and medical comorbidities related to their disease as well as the same age-related health aspects as any adult.

*The complete reference list is available online at https://expertconsult.inkling.com/.* 

112

# Neurological Problems of Pregnancy

D. Malcolm Shaner

## OUTLINE



Diseases of the nervous system develop and continue despite pregnancy. The good neurologist maintains a broad perspective, balancing the needs of the woman, her fetus, and her loved ones. Insofar as this audience creates an atmosphere for performance, the clinician may feel like a stage character prompted by cues from scattered, incomplete, and occasionally contradictory findings reported in the literature. Still, neurologists who enjoy drama find gratification in caring for the pregnant woman with neurological disease.

## NEUROLOGICAL COMPLICATIONS OF CONTRACEPTION

The neurologist can help a woman with pre-existing neurological disease to plan a pregnancy. The expected burden of her neurological disease must be balanced against her perceived need for procreation. Asking her to consider the effect of a child on her life and how her illness might affect the child can be beneficial. For instance, a patient who is wheelchair enabled with spinal muscular atrophy (SMA) or muscular dystrophy may have difficulty with breathing during the later stages of pregnancy, may need a cesarean section to deliver the baby, and may have great difficulty lifting the baby as it grows. The neurologist might discuss prenatal genetic testing with women affected by inherited neurological disease. To address controversy concerning the best use of amniocentesis, chorionic villus sampling, or preimplantation genetic diagnosis, a geneticist's help can be enlisted. One retrospective study suggested an increased relapse rate in women with multiple sclerosis (MS) undergoing an abortion, a procedure potentially preventable with the effective use of contraception (Landi et al., 2018). Many women welcome the neurologist's calming opinion.

While sterilization, such as with tubal ligation, is a consideration, sterilization often is irreversible and performed usually for indications other than neurological disease. Approximately 4% of women with epilepsy of reproductive age report having had a tubal ligation. Sterilization is not discussed in this section.

Oral contraceptives containing more than 80 μg of estrogen are linked to increased incidence of stroke. Physicians have considered that risks of hormonal contraception (HC) nevertheless are lower than the risks associated with pregnancy. Parsimonious use of estrogen in modern preparations as low as 20 μg have demonstrably increased safety. Exclusively progestogen agents do not increase stroke risk. No progestogen preparation is safer than another. Progestogens also have been used successfully in the treatment of migraine, according to a meta-analysis (Warhurst et al., 2018) and possibly have been associated with improved seizure control. Hormonal oral contraceptives, either progestogens or combined oral estrogen and progestogen contraceptives (COCs), do not cause increased seizures in a cohort study (Beier et al., 2018), although a retrospective registry study concluded that COCs increase risk (Herzog et al., 2016). Earlier studies on the use of COCs containing less than 50 μg of estrogen in nondiabetic, nonhypertensive patients indicate that these agents pose no additional risk or at most a true relative risk of ischemic stroke of no more than 2.5 (Petitti et al., 1996). In recent studies, this increased relative risk may be as low as 1.3 (95% confidence interval [CI] 1.1–1.6) (Champaloux et al., 2017). Given the very low annual incidence of ischemic stroke (≈11.3 per 100,000 in the normal population of women 15–44 years of age), this small or nonexistent added risk can be considered safe. When women taking this dose smoke cigarettes, the risk for hemorrhagic stroke increases the odds ratio (OR) to 3.64, with a 95% CI of 0.95–13.87. Discussion of stroke in pregnancy and the puerperium occurs later in the chapter.

## Contraception, Migraine, and Stroke Risk

### Effect on Stroke Risk

The effect of COCs on stroke incidence in patients with migraine remains incompletely clear. Retrospective data from a US Nationwide Healthcare Claims Database published in 2017 add to previous case-control and cohort studies (Chang et al., 1999; Kurth et al., 2006; MacClellan et al., 2007; Tzourio et al., 1995) to show that migraine with and without aura are both associated with increased stroke risk that further is exacerbated by COCs (Champaloux et al., 2017). Patients aged 15–50 suffering an ischemic stroke are nearly twice as likely to have had a history of migraine than those without ischemic stroke (Abanoz, 2017) (Table 112.1).

Expected incidence of ischemic stroke in women aged 15–44 (strokes per 100,000 women per year) has been measured in large studies and ranges from 10/100,000 to 11/100,000. This figure is age dependent, as illustrated in Fig. 112.1.

**TABLE 112.1 Absolute Risk of Ischemic Stroke in Women Aged 20–44 Years in Relation to the Use of Hormonal Contraception and Migraine Status**

| | No Migraine | Migraine With Aura | Migraine Without Aura |
|---|---|---|---|
| Without hormonal contraception | 2.5/100,000 | 5.9/100,000 | 4.0/100,000 |
| With hormonal contraception | 6.3/100,000 | 14.5/100,000 | 10.0/100,000 |

*From Sacco, S., Merki-Feld, G.S., Ægidius, K.L., Bitzer, J., Canonico, M., Kurth, T., et al. 2018. Correction to: Hormonal contraceptives and risk of ischemic stroke in women with migraine: A consensus statement from the European Headache Federation (EHF) and the European Society of Contraception and Reproductive Health (ESC). J. Headache Pain. 19(1), 81.*

While current studies suggest that estrogen increases the disproportionate stroke risk for women with migraine, consensus recommendations and authority opinions differ. American College of Obstetrics and Gynecology (ACOG) guidelines issued in 2010 reinforce a notion that continuous or extended-cycle COCs, transdermal estrogen patch, and depot-medroxyprogesterone acetate "may afford relief of headaches for some women" based on uncontrolled studies and theoretical support (ACOG, 2010). ACOG simultaneously offered that due to the devastating consequences of a stroke, physicians "should consider" alternative means of contraception to COCs for women with migraine and "focal neurological signs," women who smoke, or women over the age of 35 (ACOG 2010, Bulletin 110). Echoing this approach in 2017, reviewers suggested that more studies are needed. However, "any form of hormonal therapy should be avoided" in patients with aura lasting longer than 60 minutes, aura with multiple neurological symptoms, including migraine with brainstem aura and hemiplegic migraine; such therapy should be discontinued for any patient without the latter symptoms but who develop aura for the first time or have worsening migraine. These patients should be monitored for worsening cardiovascular risk factors. For patients with simple aura, an individualized approach is suggested (Broner et al., 2017).

In 2017, European medical societies issued a more restrictive consensus statement recommending that physicians avoid the prescription of COCs when used for contraception in women with migraine. The European Headache Federation and the European Society of Contraception and Reproductive Health advised that they are placing foremost values of caution and safety. Additional qualifications include the application of an estimated relative risk of COCs of 2.52, higher than the observed risk of low-dose COCs in some studies (Weill et al., 2016), the elimination of age as a variable, but qualified that the evidence on which the recommendations are based is of low to medium quality. The societies issued 13 recommendations—4 strong and 9 weak (Sacco et al., 2017). Perhaps most important is that the recommendations emphasize that the amount of estrogen in each of the preparations varies and should be taken into account. A proscription against the use of any COC for any patient experiencing migraine with aura is stated. Instead, authors suggest initially using or switching to the use of condoms, intrauterine devices (IUDs), permanent methods, or

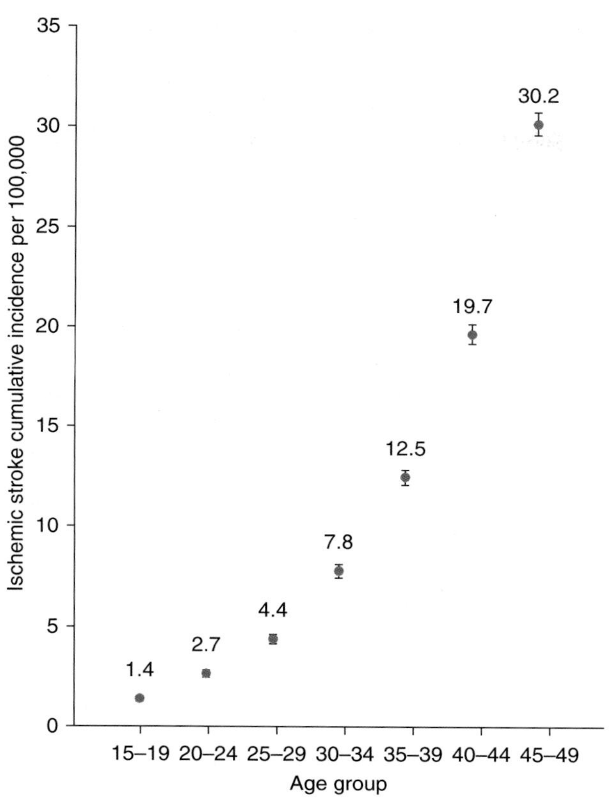


**Fig. 112.1 Average Yearly Cumulative Incidence of Ischemic Stroke, 2006–12.** Graph of ischemic stroke incidence among women of reproductive age by 5-year age group. (*From Champaloux, S.W., Tepper, N.K., Monsour, M., Curtis, K.M., Whiteman, M.K., Marchbanks, P.A., et al. 2017. Use of combined hormonal contraceptives among women with migraines and risk of ischemic stroke. Am. J. Obstet. Gynecol. 216(5), 489.e1–489.e7.*)

progestogen-only contraception, with a goal to lower the risk of ischemic stroke while balancing the woman's need to limit procreation with reasonably effective methods.

For women suffering migraine without aura associated with additional risk factors (smoking, hypertension, obesity, history of cardiovascular disease, previous history of venous thrombosis or thromboembolism) progestogen-only or non-hormonal contraception is suggested. For those women with migraine without aura and without additional risk factors, COCs containing less than or equal to 35 μg DMS of ethinylestradiol are recommended as a "possible" contraceptive option with monitoring of migraine frequency and characteristics. The consensus statement suggests that physicians planning to use COCs or progestogens to treat polycystic ovary syndrome or endometriosis should continue as clinically indicated, regardless of migraine type. When used for contraception, the statement suggests that COCs be discontinued with the development of migraine with or without aura and alternative contraceptive methods employed.

Investigators have reported migrainous infarction associated with the use of postcoital contraception when regimens containing estrogen are used within 24 hours in patients who have a history of migraine with aura (Caballero, 2009). For women with either type of migraine seeking emergency contraception, authors of the consensus statement recommended the use of levonorgestrel DMS 1.5 mg orally, ulipristal acetate 30 mg orally DMS, or the copper-bearing IUD rather than estrogen-containing products. For any woman with non-migrainous headache seeking hormonal contraception, low-dose hormonal contraception was advised.

Researchers bemoan conflicting messages from physicians received by women with migraine seeking contraceptive advice. The problem lies partially in the incompleteness of the information on actual risk and considerations with regard to how much risk is reasonable given the availability of nonestrogen contraceptive methods as alternatives.

**TABLE 112.2 Bi-Directional Drug Interactions Between Hormonal Contraceptives and Antiepileptic Drugs**

| | AED May Be Reduced by COC | Ethinyl Estradiol May Be Reduced by AED | Progestin May Be Reduced by AED |
|---|---|---|---|
| Carbamazepine | n.a. | Yes | Yes |
| Eslicarbazepine | n.a. | Yes | Yes |
| Felbamate | n.a. | Yes | Yes |
| Gabapentin | n.a. | No | No |
| Lacosamide | No | No | No |
| Lamotrigine | Yes | No | Yes |
| Levetiracetam | No | No | No |
| Oxcarbazepine | n.a. | Yes | Yes |
| Peram panel | n.a. | No | Yes* |
| Phenobarbital | n.a. | Yes | Yes |
| Phenytoin | n.a. | Yes | Yes |
| Pregabalin | n.a. | n.a. | n.a. |
| Retigabine/ezogabine | No | No | No |
| Rufinamide | No | Yes | Yes |
| Stiripentol | n.a. | n.a. | n.a. |
| Topiramate | n.a. | Yes* | No |
| Valproate | Yes | No | No |
| Zonisamide | No | No | No |

*Dose dependent.

*AED*, Antiepileptic drug; *COC*, combined oral contraceptive; *n.a.*, no data available.

*From Reimers, A., Brodtkorb, E., Sabers, A., 2015. Interactions between hormonal contraception and antiepileptic drugs: Clinical and mechanistic considerations. Seizure 28, 66–70.*

### Effect on Migraine

The effect of COCs on migraine frequency and severity is variable and difficult to investigate, worsening in 18%–50%, improving in 3%–35%, and without change in 39%–65%, in a review article (Massiou and MacGregor, 2000). Those women suffering migraine with aura were more negatively affected than those without aura. Attacks occur most frequently during the pill-free week. Continuing the administration of a hormonally active pill reduces migraine severity and frequency (Sulak et al., 2007). A history of purely perimenstrual migraine makes sensitivity to COCs more likely, although this effect may be minor (Lieba-Samal et al., 2011) and may be helped by shortening the pill-free drug regimen from 7 to 4 days (De Leo, et al., 2011).

## Contraception and Epilepsy

The risk of teratogenic effects of antiepileptic drugs (AEDs) or neurocognitive deficits in gestationally exposed children often prompt neurologists to advise safe contraceptive methods for women taking these medications. Nevertheless, contraceptive failure occurs more frequently in women with epilepsy About half of women with epilepsy discontinue oral contraception and about a quarter discontinue an IUD (Mandle et al. 2017). Reports of increasing safety of IUDs for both nulliparous and multiparous women suggest that IUDs are an obvious and superior alternative to pharmaceutical contraception in appropriately selected women taking anticonvulsants. Still, the prescription of AEDs and hormonal contraception is common. When AEDs and hormonal contraceptives are taken together, some drug interactions cause physicians to worry over risks of uncontrolled epilepsy and unplanned pregnancy. Physicians prescribing AEDs to women taking hormonal contraceptives need both general and theoretical approaches, given the introduction of newer AEDs, newer hormonal agents with lower amounts of ethinyl estradiol (20–35 μg DMS), and the use of AEDs for indications other than epilepsy, such as the treatment of neuropathic pain, migraine, anxiety, and bipolar disorder (see Table 112.2).

### Effect of Antiepileptic Drugs on Contraception

Further prospective studies are needed to confirm and refine registry data that found a more than doubled risk of spontaneous fetal loss when women with epilepsy experience unintended pregnancy. This information is coupled with findings that 65% of women with epilepsy have pregnancies that are unplanned, compared to about 45%–51% in the general US population. About one-third of women with unintended pregnancy and epilepsy engage in contraceptive methods that are known to be relatively ineffective (barrier, withdrawal, or combination), about one-third use no contraception, and about 20% use systemic hormonal contraception in combination with enzyme-inducing AEDs, which may double pregnancy risk (Herzog et al., 2018).

Anticonvulsants do not affect the efficacy of medroxyprogesterone. Although an IUD may be superior overall, medroxyprogesterone may be the contraceptive pharmaceutical of choice in women with seizure disorders. Based on theoretical considerations, some investigators recommend administering medroxyprogesterone injections every 10 weeks rather than every 12 weeks for women taking anticonvulsants that induce hepatic microsomal enzymes.

Unwanted pregnancies with levonorgestrel have occurred in women taking phenytoin and in women taking carbamazepine. Some researchers advise against the use of levonorgestrel in patients taking liver enzyme–inducing drugs of any kind, including enzyme-inducing anticonvulsants (carbamazepine, eslicarbazepine, felbamate, oxcarbazepine, phenobarbital, phenytoin, rufinamide, topiramate, perampanel). Usual-dose COCs, progestogen-only pills, medroxyprogesterone injections, and levonorgestrel implants have no known interactions and can be used in patients receiving valproic acid, vigabatrin, lamotrigine, gabapentin, tiagabine, levetiracetam, zonisamide, ethosuximide, and benzodiazepines. Failure of COCs with oxcarbazepine is reported in incomplete studies. A World Health Organization Working Group recommended against use of COCs, transdermal patch, vaginal ring, and progesterone-only pills for women taking phenytoin, carbamazepine, barbiturates, primidone, topiramate, or oxcarbazepine due to reduced contraceptive effect (Gaffield et al., 2011). Enzyme-inducing AEDs affect emergency contraception for unintended pregnancy. Doubling the first dose of levonorgestrel to 1.5 mg DMS has been recommended. However, we lack studies on efficacy of this regimen and also on the use of ulipristal (Johnson, 2018).

### Effect of Contraception on Antiepileptic Drugs

In a small prospective study, researchers find no substantial effect on AED levels for women with epilepsy using a progestogen IUD (Davis et al., 2016). The study included the use of lamotrigine, levetiracetam, oxcarbazepine, carbamazepine, lacosamide, valproate, and clobazam.

Some neurologists advise female epileptic patients taking microsomal enzyme-inducing anticonvulsants to increase the dose of estrogen in their contraceptives to at least 50 μg (O'Brien and Guillebaud, 2006). Although this adjustment may increase contraceptive effectiveness, the efficacy of the regimen is untested. The result is that barrier, spermicidal, or other contraceptive measures often are recommended for use simultaneously or exclusively.

In a careful study of small numbers of women, COCs lowered levels of lamotrigine by about 33%. This same study demonstrated that the lamotrigine levels of women in mid-luteal menstrual phase and not taking COCs dropped by about 31% (Herzog et al., 2009). Other studies report that when women take COCs, lamotrigine levels may decrease by half and some patients may suffer an increase in seizures. This effect is not seen when additional anticonvulsants are used with lamotrigine. Manufacturers of lamotrigine recommend that physicians increase that medication when patients taking lamotrigine monotherapy are placed on COCs. Adjustment of lamotrigine dose is unnecessary with progestogens.

Valproic acid (VPA) levels were lowered up to 23% with use of COCs in one small study. For patients taking VPA, an AED known to have teratogenic and neurocognitive effects on the fetus, contraception may be particularly important. An IUD may be the contraceptive of choice, and dual use of barrier methods may be advised for patients taking VPA.

### Miscellaneous Conditions

Estrogen-containing oral contraceptive agents may worsen chronic inflammatory demyelinating polyneuropathy (CIDP) and moyamoya disease, unmask systemic lupus erythematosus (SLE), worsen migraine, and produce chorea in patients with antiphospholipid antibody syndrome (APS). For young women taking COCs, the low risk for stroke in this age group approximately doubles. Some physicians advise that an individually tailored contraceptive approach may include the recommendation of COCs in antiphospholipid antibody–negative patients with inactive or moderately active stable SLE (Bermas, 2005). The heightened risk for cerebral venous thrombosis (CVT) in women taking oral contraceptive agents increases with prothrombin or factor V gene mutations. Routine screening for prothrombin gene mutation before initiating hormonal contraception probably is not useful (Bushnell et al., 2014). Some neurologists recommend against the use of hormonal contraceptives in women with activated protein C resistance.

### Summary Recommendations

For patients with migraine and epilepsy an IUD may be the contraceptive method most broadly acceptable due to its rate of efficacy, low discontinuation rate, minimal effect on the disease process, and safety associated with usual therapeutics. Medroxyprogesterone injection may be the pharmaceutical of choice for these patient groups or, in selected patients, an oral progestogen.

Due to risk of contraceptive failure, women taking liver enzyme–inducing AEDs in general should avoid COCs, etonogestrel, or levonorgestrel implants. Levonorgestrel-containing IUDs are safe and effective.

When COCs are used for patients with epilepsy, careful attention to levels of lamotrigine and valproic acid may be needed.

The use of COCs in patients with migraine increases stroke risk. Caution should be exercised with mixed recommendations from medical societies.

In general, COCs should not be used for patients with migraine when alternatives are easily available and acceptable. If they are employed, low-dose estrogen COCs are preferred for women with migraine without aura, and avoided for women with migraine with aura.

## ETHICAL CONSIDERATIONS

Partially settled and unresolved ethical difficulties complicate care of the gravid woman with neurological disease. In nearly every instance, physicians juggle competing responsibilities to, and differing goals of therapy for, the mother and fetus. In complex situations, multiple interested parties may demand a determining say, including the husband, the father (if not the husband), the family, the state, legal representatives, and political and religious groups.

When a diagnosis of maternal death by neurological criteria is confirmed for a woman carrying a fetus considered to be nonviable, judicial review in the state of Texas, a state whose laws favor fetal preservation, confirms that medical interventions need not be continued (Gostin, 2014). No consensus exists as to the conditions under which such medical interventions must be offered by physicians when the fetus is considered viable or marginally viable. Researchers reviewed 30 retrospective cases reported over 28 years of pregnant women diagnosed as dead by neurological criteria (Esmaeilzadeh et al., 2010). In this retrospective study, detailing a select fraction of those seen in medical practice, 12 infants were delivered. Medical documentation from six of these at 24 months did not include a notation of medical problems. Maternal organ procurement could be confirmed as having taken place in 10 of these patients with an "excellent" graft survival at 1 year.

Confronted with this situation, physicians who decide to offer continued medical interventions turn to the ethically appropriate surrogate(s) or legally recognized healthcare decision maker, sometimes one for the mother and one for the fetus, to discuss foreseeable possible futures in a process of shared decision making. Advice from a Committee on Bioethics or an ethics consultant is recommended in current literature (Esmaeilzadeh et al., 2010). In some states, the physician helps select surrogates. In others, a statute-driven "hierarchy" exists. Some states prohibit an appropriate surrogate from permitting the termination of pregnancy for an incapacitated patient but not when the patient is dead. Advising pregnant women to execute advance directives for medical care seems an unlikely and incomplete solution, particularly given that half the states in the United States contain some restrictions on a pregnant woman's documented preference for end-of-life care and healthcare decisions (Ecker, 2014).

## IMAGING

Computed tomography (CT) scanning employs ionizing radiation with known risks of teratogenesis, mutagenesis, and carcinogenesis. In general, physicians avoid ionizing radiation during pregnancy, particularly between 8 and 15 weeks, the gestational period most sensitive to ionizing radiation. However, the risk is not as high as perceived by some medical professionals, and several authors urge an approach balanced to the diagnostic needs of the woman and fetus. Researchers estimate the average woman receives background radiation less than 0.1 rad over 9 months. Risks of fetal malformation demonstrably increase with radiation doses above 15 rad. Induced miscarriages and major congenital malformations occur at negligibly increased risk with doses to the fetus under 5 rad. Estimated radiation dosage from a typical CT scan of the brain is less than 0.050 rad when employing precautionary lead shielding. Lumbar spine CT delivers some 3.5 rad. Acting on anxiety attributed by some to physician advice, women have opted for pregnancy termination after receiving low-dose diagnostic radiation during early gestation (Ratnapalan et al., 2008). Iodinated contrast media used for radiological procedures has the potential to depress fetal thyroid production. Most states mandate routine newborn thyroid screening; this is especially important in infants receiving iodinated contrast agents in utero.

In general, when circumstances require urgent neuroimaging, CT remains the most appropriate tool during pregnancy (Chansakul and Young, 2017) and, when contrast is required, iodinated CT contrast agents are likely safer than gadolinium-based contrast agents (ACR Committee on Drugs and Contrast Media, 2018). That said, some authors provide recommendations during pregnancy for imaging specific conditions, such as the use of noncontrasted magnetic resonance venography when CVT is suspected, MRI with or without contrast to demonstrate the pachymeningeal pathology associated with intracranial hypotension syndrome, and the relative help from both MRI and CT techniques in characterizing pituitary apoplexy (Haber and Nunez, 2018).

Magnetic resonance imaging (MRI) without contrast can be used selectively to scan the brain and the venous and arterial circulations and is useful during pregnancy. No study or clinical observation has detailed harmful effects to mother or child, but detailed longitudinal studies on children exposed in utero to MRI are lacking. Limited information involves the use of 1.5-T MRI while data detailing the safety of 3.0-T magnets are unavailable. Despite the observations by the American College of Obstetricians and Gynecologists and the American College of Radiology (ACOG, 2004; ACR Committee on Drugs and Contrast Media, 2004; Kanal et al., 2007) that there is no known adverse effect of MRI on the fetus, only two human studies on this point existed at that time, neither of which was of a design adequate to detect adverse effects that may be significant (International Commission on Non-Ionizing Radiation Protection, 2004). A more recent retrospective study of a Canadian provincial database (Ray et al., 2016) also may have been underpowered to detect rare events. The authors found that in their series, MRI during the first trimester of pregnancy was not associated with increased risk of harm to the fetus or easily detectable in early childhood. Although current safety information is optimistic, restriction of maternal brain MRI, balancing the importance of diagnostic yield to the rare but uncertain fetal risk of MRI, especially during the first trimester, continues to be prudent.

Fortunately, most MRI studies relevant to neurological disease do not require the use of gadolinium. However, definitive studies detailing the safety of gadolinium-based magnetic resonance contrast agents during pregnancy and lactation are lacking. Gadolinium crosses the placenta, finds its way into amniotic fluid, and is swallowed by the fetus. Fetal developmental delay occurs in animals receiving high doses of gadolinium. No reports of mutagenic or teratogenic effects in humans appear in reviews of available literature (ACR Committee on Drugs and Contrast Media, 2018). A small prospective study of 26 women who received gadolinium inadvertently during the periconceptional period and first trimester yielded a single child with a minor congenital anomaly (De Santis, 2007). A larger retrospective study (Ray et al., 2016) found that gadolinium-enhanced MRI at any time in pregnancy was associated with an increased fetal risk of rheumatological, inflammatory, or infiltrative skin conditions and stillbirth or neonatal death. While a theoretical risk of nephrogenic systemic fibrosis exists, no known cases have yet been reported (ACR Committee on Drugs and Contrast Media, 2018).

### Breastfeeding

A small percentage of iodinated contrast medium is excreted into breast milk and absorbed by the infant gut. The amount is calculated to be so small as to make it reasonable to declare maternal iodinated contrast material injection to be safe without a need to interrupt breastfeeding (ACR Committee on Drugs and Contrast Media, 2018). Optional interruption of breastfeeding may be suggested to last a period of 12–24 hours, but without value stopping for longer than 24 hours. Preparatory storage of milk before the contrast and discarding of milk pumped within 24 hours following contrast has been advised.

Some authorities recommend that a woman abstain from breastfeeding for 24 hours after receiving iodinated contrast agents, including gadolinium (Tang et al., 2004). Others, citing the tiny amount of contrast entering breast milk and the minute amount absorbed from the baby's gut, suggest that the potential risks are insufficient to warrant a recommendation to interrupt breastfeeding (Chen et al., 2008; Webb et al., 2005). Reasoning that only a small percentage of gadolinium-based contrast medium is excreted into milk and absorbed by the infant gut, no interruption of breastfeeding is recommended by the American College of Radiology (ACR Committee on Drugs and Contrast Media, 2018) which provides recommendations for those women wishing to further reduce risk identical to those above for CT contrast imaging while breastfeeding.

## HEADACHE

### Tension Headache

Headache during pregnancy is common. Usually a patient visits the neurologist to receive reassurance that no serious medical problem is apparent. Of the headaches that occur during pregnancy, benign tension headaches are seen most often (see Chapter 102). No known association exists with hormones and, specifically, no association with the hormonal changes of pregnancy. Treatment for mild headaches often includes cognitive behavioral therapy, adequate rest, moist heat, massage, exercise (pregnant and postpartum women should accrue 150 minutes weekly of moderately intense aerobic activity, Piercy et al., 2018), avoidance of triggering factors, and use of acetaminophen. Attempts to link in utero exposure to acetaminophen to attention-deficit/hyperactivity disorder (ADHD) and asthma have been inconclusive according to the US Food and Drug Administration (FDA), and it can be considered safe in usual doses (Liew, 2014; Wells, 2016). For severe headaches, the use of a tricyclic antidepressant such as amitriptyline or nortriptyline may be helpful. No evidence of embryopathy occurs with amitriptyline, and preschool children exposed in utero to tricyclic antidepressants have normal global IQs, language, and behavioral development. Fluoxetine may cause uncommon but serious fetal risks (Chambers et al., 2006; Diav-Citrin et al., 2008; Mills, 2006).

### Migraine Headache

More than 80% of women with migraine clearly show improvement during pregnancy, but 15% continue to have headaches, and in 5% headaches worsen. The prognosis for women with migraine without aura is better than that for women with migraine with aura. Headaches were more likely to persist with diagnosed menstrual migraine, hyperemesis, or a "pathological pregnancy course" in a prospective study. For women anticipating pregnancy, the physician may discontinue or reduce the dose of all migraine medications to lower the risk of possible fetal damage and offer vigorous treatment with behavioral therapy, moist heat, and the judicious use of acetaminophen or opioid preparations. Migraine usually lessens during the second and third trimesters. The diagnosis of complicated migraine or de novo migraine with aura during pregnancy requires a thorough consideration of other diagnoses. Migraine may increase the risk for preeclampsia, especially for patients with prepregnancy obesity (Adeney et al., 2005) and may increase the risk for peripartum stroke (James et al., 2005). While small increased incidences of low birth weight, preterm birth, and cesarean section were noted in an Asian population (odds ratios 1.16, 1.24, and 1.16, respectively), the single large study did not control for the use of medications in this population, where the authors noted equivocal clarity in the database diagnosis of migraine (Chen et al., 2010). Other studies and retrospective reviews suggest that women with migraine can expect an increased risk of gestational hypertension, preeclampsia, preterm birth, dyslipidemia, ischemic heart disease, and thromboembolic disease. While these findings lead some to suggest that pregnancy in a patient with migraine should be considered "high risk" with increased monitoring and physician visits (Wabnitz and Bushnell, 2015), the absence of prospective carefully designed studies to clearly define and confirm these risks may account for the lack of policy endorsing such an approach.

#### Before Pregnancy

Pregnancy and the anticipation of pregnancy complicate usual migraine therapy. Valproic acid causes fetal malformations. FDA labeling contraindicates the use of valproic acid for fertile women with migraine unless no substitute can be found. This contraindication may make sense in the context of an unplanned pregnancy rate in the United States that approximates 50%. For fertile women taking prophylactic valproic acid whose migraine has been unresponsive to other therapy, folic acid supplementation is advised (see the section Epilepsy and Its Treatments). Discussion of reliable contraceptive measures and the risks for fetal malformation is essential. During pregnancy, physicians advise avoidance of valproic acid to treat headache. Topiramate is fetally toxic in animals, and the magnitude of teratogenic risk of topiramate is incompletely determined in humans. When prescribing topiramate, unintended fetal exposure during the early first trimester may occur with unplanned pregnancy. Canadian labeling advises that physicians restrict therapeutic topiramate for migraine to those fertile women using reliable contraception.

The calcitonin gene–related peptide (CGRP) monoclonal antibodies used to treat migraine have long half-lives. They cross the placenta in increasing amounts throughout pregnancy in animal models. CGRPs play a theoretical role in regulating uteroplacental blood flow, myometrial uterine relaxation, and the maintenance of gestational blood pressure. Blockade of CGRP conceivably may increase the potential for gestational hypertension, preeclampsia, and eclampsia. Adverse events in animal reproduction studies were not observed with fremanezumab, galcanezumab, and erenumab. Given the absence of human pregnancy safety data, some advocate for the use of registries to help to confirm safety, to avoid the use of CGRP monoclonal antibodies in women who are planning pregnancy, and to advise contraception for women taking these medications simultaneous with their prescription (Dodick, 2019). Whether these antibodies enter breast milk is unknown.

### During Pregnancy

***Acute treatments.*** Authorities suggest that opioids and antiemetics, specifically prochlorperazine (oral or suppository) and meperidine, are the drugs of choice for migraine during pregnancy (Goadsby et al., 2008). Some physicians simultaneously treat with diphenhydramine to reduce the potential for dystonic reaction with prochlorperazine. Metoclopramide and acetaminophen are unassociated with fetal risk and are of benefit. Emergency physicians in New York commonly order a combination of acetaminophen and metoclopramide as initial treatment (Hamilton and Robbins, 2019). Although sometimes employed, the addition of diphenhydramine to metoclopramide to treat headache has been shown to be ineffective for migraine (Friedman et al., 2016).

Opioids used chronically for pain are associated with birth defects, poor fetal growth, stillbirth, and preterm delivery. However, these risks are not known to occur with occasional acute treatment of migraine, and, while of uncertain risk, opioids may provide significant benefit when initial treatment is ineffective.

The use of occasional, single-dose naproxen sodium orally or ketorolac intravenously is relatively safe throughout pregnancy, although safest when used during the first two trimesters. In the past, researchers reported possibly increased risk of miscarriage for women using nonsteroidal antiinflammatory drugs (NSAIDs) longer than 1 week during pregnancy. Larger, more recent studies were unable to support this claim. Manufacturers recommend avoiding NSAIDs altogether after 30 weeks' gestation, and cautious use during breastfeeding, primarily due to fetal cardiovascular risks.

Physicians commonly employ the use of intravenous fluids, such as normal saline over 1–2 hours, to treat acute migraine, a treatment safe during pregnancy. Data to support its use are wanting (Balbin et al., 2016).

For triptans, data are incomplete and their general use is inadvisable. Limited information suggests a low or no teratogenic potential (Kurth and Hernandez-Diaz, 2010). This reassuring but qualified news has led some to suggest that prescription of a triptan may be acceptable in pregnant women who suffer physiologically and psychologically disabling migraine, whose headaches respond to a triptan, and in whom safer medications have failed (Von Wald and Walling 2002). A prospective, cohort study suggests relative safety of sumatriptan without endorsing the use of other triptans (Spielmann et al., 2018).

During pregnancy, ergotamine and dihydroergotamine cause high rates of fetal malformation and are contraindicated. Canadian Headache Society guidelines (Orr et al., 2015) recommend against the use of dexamethasone, magnesium sulfate, tramadol, and acetaminophen for any adult presenting with acute migraine. American Headache Society guidelines (Marmura et al., 2015) find level A evidence for the use of acetaminophen and level B evidence for the use of magnesium sulfate in general migraine pharmacotherapy in adults. During pregnancy, intravenous magnesium sulfate used daily for 5 days is known to result in serious bony fetal abnormalities. The occasional use for migraine likely is safe and some physicians continue to employ magnesium when other therapies have failed. Butalbital was found to lack evidence for efficacy in the treatment of adults with migraine in American Headache Society guidelines. The safety of butalbital during pregnancy has been investigated incompletely. One study hints at a possible increased risk of serious cardiac defects (Browne et al., 2014).

***Migraine prophylaxis.*** Rare case reports describe fetal toxicity associated with propranolol, atenolol, and other beta-blockers. Although often safe during pregnancy, these drugs usually are discontinued or usage is reduced to the lowest effective dose. Prolonged use of atenolol to treat hypertension during pregnancy is associated with an increased risk of intrauterine growth restriction (IUGR) and current guidelines describe atenolol as contraindicated during pregnancy (Bushnell et al., 2014). When physician and patient are convinced that prophylactic therapy is required, the benefit of metoprolol or verapamil may outweigh risks. Incomplete data are available for lithium usage in humans. In animals, lithium is teratogenic. Physicians commonly advise that patients avoid lithium to treat headache during pregnancy.

In Australian studies, it has been shown that pregnant women commonly (20%–48%) seek alternative therapies (Frawley et al., 2013; Peng et al., 2013). A variety of products are available without prescription. One systematic review concluded that DMS riboflavin 400 mg daily taken prophylactically is well tolerated, inexpensive, and has demonstrated efficacy in reducing the frequency of migraine in adults (Thompson and Saluja, 2017). The daily allowance of riboflavin recommended by the Institute of Medicine Food and Nutrition Board during pregnancy and lactation is DMS 1.4 and DMS 1.6 mg, respectively (National Institutes of Health, 2018). The safety and efficacy of riboflavin to treat migraine during pregnancy remains unexplored.

Magnesium oxide 400–600 mg DMS daily has been found to be effective migraine prophylaxis in nonpregnant subjects, although the effect is modest. Daily allowance recommended by the Institute of Medicine in pregnant women aged 19–30 and 31–50 is 310 DMS and 360 mg DMS, respectively; and 310 and 320 mg daily DMS while breastfeeding.

Lack of safety data and known potential risks during pregnancy has led some authors to advise against the use of Petasites (butterbur) during pregnancy (D'Andrea et al., 2014). Evidence-based guidelines published by the American Academy of Neurology (AAN) in 2012 including the use of nutraceuticals in nonpregnant adults were retired over Petasites safety concerns (Holland, 2012; personal communication).

### Postpartum

Breastfeeding reduces migraine recurrence (Sances et al., 2003), but postpartum falls in estrogen are thought to trigger migraine. In general, the breastfeeding woman with migraine should avoid ergotamine and lithium. NSAIDs are safe for mothers breastfeeding healthy infants. Cautious use of triptans and some antidepressants is accepted. Sumatriptan by injection may be an ideal way to deal with disabling migraine in this period (Goadsby et al., 2008). When beta-blockers are called for during lactation, some authors favor the use of propranolol (MacGregor, 2012).

For some drugs, in the absence of empiric safety data, the American Academy of Pediatrics offers recommendations for breastfeeding based on the milk-to-plasma ratio of the drug, considering that when this relative infant dose ratio is less than 10%, some drugs can be considered to be safe, and possibly unsafe when over 25% (Hutchinson et al., 2013). Approaches sometimes include pumping and discarding breast milk associated with the use of a medication. Guidelines from manufacturers of CGRP antagonist monoclonal antibodies advise that a decision to breastfeed during therapy should consider the risk of infant exposure, the benefits of breastfeeding to the infant, and benefits of treatment to the mother.

When a woman presents with severe puerperal headache, physicians may derive some comfort that 34% of women with a history of migraine will develop headache during the first postpartum week, commonly between 4 and 6 days and usually benign. However, the puerperium also is the time serious illness may present with sudden severe or "thunderclap" headache (see Chapter 102). The differential diagnosis includes migraine, cerebrospinal fluid (CSF) hypovolemia including postdural puncture headache, CVT, preeclampsia/eclampsia, subarachnoid hemorrhage, stroke syndromes, posterior leukoencephalopathy syndrome, postpartum cerebral angiopathy, pituitary apoplexy, Sheehan syndrome, and lymphocytic hypophysitis (Gladstone et al., 2005). A careful history detailing whether and how the current headache differs in character from a woman's previous migraine may be helpful toward accurate diagnosis.

## LEG MUSCLE CRAMPS

Between 5% and 30% of pregnant women experience painful leg cramps, which do not adversely affect the fetus but bother the patient. The condition resolves rapidly postpartum. Typically, cramps occur in the morning or evening during the last trimester of pregnancy. Changes in the ionic concentrations of potassium, magnesium, sodium, and calcium may be important in the pathogenesis. Magnesium lactate or magnesium citrate tablets (122 mg DMS in the morning and 244 mg DMS in the evening) relieve or considerably lessen symptoms in approximately 80% of patients. Placebo is similarly effective in 40%. A randomized, double-blind, placebo-controlled prospective trial in Thailand using magnesium bisglycinate chelate 100 mg three times daily DMS led to a 50% reduction of cramp frequency in about 86% of those on the medication and 61% of those on placebo. The study also found those in the magnesium group noted a similar reduction in cramp severity without additional side effects (Supakatisant and Phupong, 2015). Some physicians report successful therapy with oral calcium carbonate or gluconate, 500 mg DMS three or four times daily. A randomized small study of calcium supplementation found a reduction in the frequency but not the severity of muscle cramps in an Iranian patient population (Khoramroudi et al., 2011). Passive stretch and massage are helpful for the acute cramp, while daily preventive stretching before sleep has been helpful in nonpregnant adults.

## MYASTHENIA GRAVIS

### Before Pregnancy

Fertility is unaffected by myasthenia gravis, and oral contraceptive agents do not weaken these patients. No single study offers certainty with regard to the cumulative risk pregnancy causes in the patient with known myasthenia gravis (Hoffman et al., 2007). Conditions may remain stable, improve, worsen, or both improve and worsen at different stages of pregnancy. Approximately two-thirds of patients report some worsening at some time during pregnancy or the puerperium. The puerperium and first trimester are times of greatest risk. The course of myasthenia gravis for a future pregnancy is not predictable by the course of previous pregnancies. A consensus group advises that physicians should reassure the majority of their patients with stable disease that their myasthenia gravis likely will remain stable through pregnancy (Sanders et al., 2016).

The effect of thymectomy on myasthenia gravis usually is delayed. The potential mother can be advised that the procedure may be helpful for a pregnancy beginning approximately 1 year after surgery. Generally in women with myasthenia who may become pregnant, the physician should use drugs other than azathioprine and cyclosporine. Mycophenolate is associated with an increased risk of congenital malformations and spontaneous abortion, prompting the manufacturers to recommend a negative pregnancy test within 1 week before beginning therapy and use of two reliable forms of contraception 4 weeks before and 6 weeks after therapy. Mycophenolate may affect the effectiveness of hormonal contraception. Rituximab crosses the placenta and higher levels in infants have been recorded than in the pregnant mothers. Hematological abnormalities, infections, and premature births are reported in infants born to inadvertently exposed mothers. Use is not recommended during pregnancy to treat nonlife-threatening myasthenia and the manufacturer recommends effective contraception during use of rituximab and for 12 months following its use. Myasthenia gravis does not influence the contractile strength of the smooth muscle of the uterus, the incidence of postpartum hemorrhage, or the occurrence of toxemia.

### During Pregnancy

The medical therapy of myasthenia gravis changes little with pregnancy. Anticholinesterase agents including edrophonium (Tensilon) and plasmapheresis are relatively safe. An international consensus panel advises against the use of anticholinesterase agents intravenously to avoid the risk of uterine contractions associated with their use and to consider postponing CT scans of the chest looking for thymoma in newly diagnosed myasthenia gravis until after pregnancy (Sanders et al., 2016). Rapid drug metabolism during pregnancy may require increasing the rate or dose of anticholinesterase drugs. Corticosteroids remain the immunosuppressant drugs of choice during pregnancy, although they may increase the risk for gestational diabetes and preeclampsia. Abortion does not lessen the manifestations of myasthenia gravis. Fetal ultrasound helps to detect limb deformities known as arthrogryposis fetalis, thought to be due to the reduced fetal movement associated with circulating maternal antibodies. Although the use of intravenous human immunoglobulin (IVIG) appears safe during pregnancy, the number of myasthenic patients studied is small. In animals, azathioprine is teratogenic, and low levels cross the placenta. Physicians generally advise patients with myasthenia to discontinue azathioprine in preparation for pregnancy. A few women with myasthenia gravis receiving azathioprine during pregnancy have given birth to healthy children. Some researchers point to the uncommon reports of human teratogenicity and intimate that azathioprine might be safer than animal data suggest. Proponents declare azathioprine to be safe during pregnancy and breastfeeding with slim supportive empiric information (Norwood et al., 2014). Mycophenolate is contraindicated and rituximab relatively contraindicated during pregnancy.

Regional anesthesia is preferred for cesarean section. When the patient is taking anticholinesterase agents, metabolism of procaine is slowed and poorly predictable; in these patients, lidocaine is favored for local anesthesia. Neuromuscular blocking agents such as curariform drugs must be avoided because they may have a greatly prolonged effect in patients with myasthenia gravis. The use of magnesium sulfate as a tocolytic agent or a treatment for preeclampsia may precipitate a myasthenic crisis and is contraindicated.

Theoretical risks based on neurophysiology studies and rare case reports have led some authors to suggest that physicians should avoid phenytoin and barbiturates in the myasthenic developing toxemia of pregnancy (Waters et al., 2019). This recommendation stands in contrast to common practice and the recommendations of an international consensus panel that phenytoin and barbiturates are acceptable and may be drugs of choice (Hamel and Ciafaloni, 2018; Sanders et al., 2016). We lack studies specifically on the use of levetiracetam in this clinical scenario, with case reports noting efficacy.

### Postpartum

Breastfeeding poses no significant difficulty, despite evidence that the antiacetylcholine receptor antibodies do pass to the baby in breast milk. Cyclosporine and azathioprine are secreted in breast milk; in general they should be avoided because of their risk for immunosuppression and tumorigenic potential. When medically necessary, the small but uncertain tumorigenic potential of azathioprine must be weighed against the known benefits of breast milk.

Corticosteroids also are secreted into breast milk but in small amounts. Large doses of anticholinesterase drugs taken by the mother may lead to gastrointestinal upset in the breastfed newborn.

### Pregnancy Outcome

A retrospective Norwegian study reported an increased risk for premature rupture of amniotic membranes and double the rate of cesarean section among myasthenic women. A smaller retrospective Taiwanese study found statistically insignificant increased risk of cesarean section, infants small for gestational age, low birth weight, and no difference for preterm delivery (Wen et al., 2009). Premature labor may be more common in women with myasthenia gravis but this varies considerably among multiple studies.

Perinatal mortality increases to 6%–8% for infants of women with myasthenia gravis, which is approximately five times that of the normal population. Approximately 2% of these are stillborn. Transient neonatal myasthenia affects 10%–20% of infants born to women with myasthenia gravis. Most infants who develop transient myasthenia gravis do so within the first day, but weakness may begin up to 4 days after delivery and usually resolves within 3–6 weeks. Neonates require careful observation for at least 4 days. An imperfect correlation exists between maternal levels of antiacetylcholine receptor antibodies and the likelihood that the neonate will develop transient myasthenia gravis. Intrauterine exposure to receptor antibodies rarely may result in arthrogryposis, which has a high likelihood of recurrence in future pregnancy. The role of intragestational plasmapheresis and immunosuppression to prevent this condition in subsequent pregnancies is unknown (Polizzi et al., 2000).

## MUSCULAR AND NEUROMUSCULAR DISORDERS

### Myotonic Dystrophy

Pregnancy is uncommon in women who have advanced myotonic dystrophy type 1, probably caused by progressive ovarian failure. Before the development of advanced disease, there is no significant reduction in fertility. For women who are able to conceive, pregnancy can be hazardous for both mother and fetus. Myotonic weakness often worsens during the second half of pregnancy. Congestive heart failure is reported. Ineffective uterine contractions, premature labor, and breech presentation often complicate labor. Tocolysis may result in aggravation of myotonia. Oxytocin can stimulate the myotonic uterus to produce increased contractions. Myotonic dystrophy complicates obstetric anesthesia, and regional anesthesia is preferred. Patients with myotonic dystrophy are unduly sensitive to respiratory suppression with pentobarbital. After delivery, hypotonic uterine dysfunction results in an increased risk for retained placenta and postpartum hemorrhage.

Half of children born to women with myotonic dystrophy inherit the disorder. Anticipation due to an increased number of triplet repeats (see Chapter 48) is responsible for the syndrome of congenital myotonic dystrophy in the neonate (see Chapter 109). Many neonates are hypotonic, and reported rates of morbidity are high (Awater et al., 2012). Fetal myotonic dystrophy may affect fetal swallowing, causing polyhydramnios, resulting in a mortality rate of 10%–20% in several small case series. Prenatal diagnostic testing with amniocentesis or chorionic villus biopsy is available.

Available data suggest that myotonic dystrophy type 2 (see Chapter 109) is more benign than type 1 and may not result in problems with general anesthesia or increase problems of delivery for the pregnant woman. Type 2 may not increase the risk for polyhydramnios or stillbirth or result in congenital myotonic dystrophy (Day et al., 2003). Another study noted that about 21% in their series of type 2 first presented with myotonic weakness during pregnancy, which worsened during subsequent pregnancies (Rudnik-Schöneborn et al., 2006). Some 17% of patients miscarried, half experienced preterm labor, and 27% delivered preterm.

For patients whose diagnosis of myotonic dystrophy is known before pregnancy who are unwilling to consider pregnancy termination if diagnostics indicate an affected fetus, prenatal genetic diagnosis (PGD) with in vitro fertilization may offer an alternative strategy. Patients should have resources to accept the cost of PGD, risk of misdiagnosis, and modest rate of successful outcome (Fernandez et al., 2017).

### Facioscapulohumeral Dystrophy

Information gathered in a study with self-selected and possible recall bias provides insight that the second stage of labor may be adversely affected by skeletal muscle weakness for many, and associated with worsened irreversible weakness in 12%–24% of patients with this dominantly inherited disorder. In order of frequency, complaints included worsening of generalized weakness, frequent falling, difficulty carrying the infant owing to worsening of shoulder weakness, worsening or new-onset pain, and difficulty carrying the infant caused by leg weakness. Despite the worsening, 90% of women report they would choose pregnancy again. Outcomes of pregnancy are good, with a statistically higher frequency of low birth weight (16.4%), and more than double the incidence of operative (23.8%) and forceps delivery (15.4%–19%) (Awater et al., 2012; Ciafaloni et al., 2006).

### Limb–Girdle Muscular Dystrophy

Limited information suggests that LGMD worsens in half of patients, prompting termination of pregnancy in 8.8% of total pregnancies. Abnormal fetal presentations occur in a quarter, and neonatal outcome is favorable. In Germany, cesarean section increased to 27% (Awater et al., 2012). Maternal hypercapnea and hypoxemia are blamed for the 2-month postpartum death of one woman after her second pregnancy. Some authors recommend that patients with neuromuscular disease and a vital capacity of under 1 liter be advised against pregnancy (Awater et al., 2012). Obstetric management can be challenging (von Guinneau, 2018). Therapeutic considerations include management of an accompanying cardiomyopathy and declining respiratory function requiring early cesarean section. Exaggerated lumbar lordosis exacerbated by pregnancy may complicate placement of epidural analgesia. Increased sensitivity to nondepolarizing muscle relaxants, sedatives, and analgesics and increased risk of malignant hyperthermia with succinylcholine and inhalation anesthetics call for skilled and flexible anesthesiology management.

### Inflammatory Myopathy

The diagnosis of inflammatory myopathy commonly is made in women past reproductive years. Few pregnancies have been studied. Current information suggests that pregnancy does not precipitate or exacerbate polymyositis or dermatomyositis. Retrospective interviews in Spain found that 7 of 14 pregnancies in 8 patients were associated with clinical improvement (Iago et al., 2014), with excellent pregnancy outcome. Other studies, such as information from a Chinese treatment center (Zhong et al., 2017), point out that when inflammatory disease is active, very high rates of spontaneous abortion and preterm birth can be expected. Decreased activity of myositis correlates with a more favorable outcome for the fetus (Váncsa et al., 2007). Corticosteroids and intravenous IVIG are the mainstays of therapy (Linardaki et al., 2011).

### Metabolic Myopathies

Metabolic myopathies are rare (see Chapter 109). Management during pregnancy is based on anecdotal experience and theoretical consideration. Authors describe successful management of McArdle disease (myophosphorylase deficiency) with intravenous dextrose during labor (Giles and

Maher., 2011). For those pregnant women with Pompe disease, cessation of enzyme-replacement therapy during the first trimester has been associated with clinical worsening but is the current practice until more safety data accumulate (Klos, 2017). Mitochondrial disorders such as MELAS are noted to worsen during pregnancy. A case report described a patient with MELAS and multiple complications receiving successful administration of intrathecal bupivacaine for delivery (Bell et al., 2017).

### Spinal Muscular Atrophy

Researchers conducting retrospective polls of patients with autosomal recessive SMA and pregnancy decry that only 11 of 19 patients (57%) received genetic counseling and that 74% had disease worsening, persisting after delivery in 42% (Elsheikh et al., 2017). Despite this untoward effect, patients report good pregnancy outcomes and elect additional pregnancies.

Another study of 25 patients reported a higher rate of vaginal operations and cesarean section (42.4%), preterm delivery (29.4%), and a worsening of their underlying condition in one-third of patients (Awater et al., 2012).

## NEUROPATHY

### Bell Palsy

Facial nerve palsy occurs two to four times more commonly during late pregnancy and the puerperium, usually about 35 weeks' gestation. Large studies estimate that facial palsy complicates 0.17% of pregnancies (Baugh et al., 2013). A retrospective chart review found the prognosis for recovery of facial nerve function to be worse when facial palsy occurs during pregnancy but not usually when the severity of the facial palsy is mild. Researchers find increased frequency of toxemia and hypertension in patients with gestational facial palsy and recommend careful and continued monitoring of the affected woman for these conditions (Shmorgun et al., 2002). Pharmacological therapy of Bell palsy during pregnancy remains controversial. When begun within 3 days of onset of facial weakness, prednisone 1 mg/kg for 5 days, tapering rapidly over a total 10-day course DMS, may be effective in improving the prognosis in nongravid adults and is considered safest when not used during the first trimester (Vrabec et al., 2007). The routine use of antiviral drugs simultaneously has not been proven unequivocally effective in nongravid adults in the absence of a varicella-zoster syndrome (Ramsay Hunt syndrome or zoster sine herpete), including a meta-analysis (Baugh et al., 2013; Browning, 2010; Quant et al., 2009). This combination of drugs has not been tested adequately during pregnancy. Individually, the drugs pose low risk. Documenting worsened facial function scores at least 1 year after gestational Bell palsy and the limited efficacy of steroids, researchers have suggested that a prudent approach may be to avoid steroids during the first trimester and to discuss steroids and antiviral therapy during later pregnancy (Phillips et al., 2017). Patching of the eye and lubricating eye drops may help prevent corneal irritation (see Chapter 103). No independent association with cesarean section, Apgar score, birth weight, or perinatal mortality has been demonstrated (Katz et al., 2011).

### Carpal Tunnel Syndrome

Approximately one in three pregnant women reports nocturnal hand paresthesias, primarily during the last trimester, often associated with peripheral edema. Excessive weight gain and fluid retention increase the occurrence of these complaints. Symptoms usually resolve spontaneously within weeks after parturition A large study found that of patients complaining of gestational tingling, 15% continued to report discomfort 12 months postpartum. Complaints were associated with higher scores of depression and onset in early pregnancy (Meems et al., 2017). During pregnancy, conservative therapy is indicated. Splinting of the wrist in the neutral position is helpful. Additionally, some physicians inject corticosteroids into the carpal tunnel. When hand muscles supplied by the median nerve weaken, the treatment of choice is surgical decompression using fiberoptic techniques.

### Low Back Pain

Low back pain is ubiquitous in the nongravid female population and increases during pregnancy. In retrospective questionnaires, researchers find more than half the pregnant population recall pain during their pregnancy and half of those women remembered radiation of the back pain to the extremities. As many as three-quarters of pregnant women report low back pain at some time in their pregnancy in prospective studies (Pennick and Young, 2008). A careful prospective study estimated the prevalence of "true" sciatica, radiation of the pain in a dermatomal distribution, to be less than 1% (Ostgaard et al., 1991). Investigators blame this torment and its propensity to increase after the fifth month of pregnancy on increasing lumbar lordosis, direct pressure from the enlarging uterus, postural stress, and hormonally induced ligamentous laxity. In one study, nearly all women experiencing back pain during pregnancy, serious enough to provoke loss of work, suffered recurrence of back pain in a subsequent pregnancy and low back pain recurred commonly in the nongravid state. MRI and electromyography (EMG) can be helpful rarely. Risks of EMG are negligible. Authorities advise avoiding muscles that bring the EMG needle too close to the developing fetus. Risks of MRI are discussed above. An extensive review of the literature concluded that interventions for the treatment of the low back pain of pregnancy are biased enough that unequivocal therapeutic direction cannot be indicated. The efficacy and risk of techniques to prevent low back pain are unknown. Studies of specifically tailored strengthening exercise, sitting pelvic tilt exercise programs, and water gymnastics all reported beneficial effects. The effect of physiotherapy is small but may be of some benefit, as may acupuncture. Studies on acupuncture claim better results than for physiotherapy (Pennick and Young, 2008). Distinguishing pelvic girdle pain from low back pain remains problematic although some authors describe benefit to a comprehensive and detailed approach (Vermani et al., 2010).

When minor neurological deficits accompany a syndrome suggesting compressive disk disease, authorities recommend a conservative approach based on limited case series (LaBan et al., 1995). Surgical management for compressive disk disease has been successfully employed and is suggested during pregnancy to treat severe or progressive neurological deficits and in the presence of a cauda equina syndrome (Brown and Levi, 2001; LaBan et al., 1995).

We lack studies or consensus agreement on the preferred mode of delivery for patients with herniated and symptomatic lumbosacral disk disease. LaBan et al. (1995) describe patients who underwent cesarean section successfully to avoid the theoretical increases of epidural venous pressure during the Valsalva maneuver associated with parturition. They suggest that a reflex response of skeletal muscle to pain during pregnancy may be responsible for elevated venous pressure, and that regional block anesthesia may be as effective with vaginal delivery.

### Meralgia Paresthetica

The expanding abdominal wall and the increased lordosis of pregnancy stretch the lateral femoral cutaneous nerve to the thigh as it penetrates the tensor fascia lata or at the inguinal ligament. This unilateral or bilateral affliction of late pregnancy resolves within 3 months postpartum. The condition may be exacerbated during the hip flexion and increased intraabdominal pressure of delivery and when retractors are applied for cesarean section.

### Acute Polyradiculoneuropathy (Guillain-Barré Syndrome)

Pregnancy does not affect the incidence or course of acute polyradiculoneuropathy (Guillain-Barré syndrome [GBS]), but some investigators believe the pregnant patient may be more vulnerable to complications (Chan et al., 2004) especially in the last trimester and puerperium (Sharma et al., 2015). Usually, infants of a mother without complications are born healthy. Diagnostic screening for viral causes of GBS that may affect the fetus such as cytomegalovirus (CMV), human immunodeficiency virus (HIV), and Zika virus have added implications during pregnancy. Only one case of neonatal acute polyradiculopathy resulting from maternal disease is reported. Some investigators recommend fluid loading before plasmapheresis to prevent hypotension. Others suggest avoidance of tocolytics in the presence of autonomic instability. IVIG has been used safely during pregnancy, but the number of patients who received this therapy and were studied remains small. Uterine contractions are unaffected by the disease. Cesarean section is only for obstetric indications. Severe hyperkalemia caused presumably by succinylcholine anesthesia resulting in reversible cardiac arrest has been described in a pregnant woman 3 weeks after complete recovery from acute polyradiculopathy. This case and additional related reports have prompted some authors to suggest that the combination of pregnancy and acute polyradiculopathy should lead to the cautious use or avoidance of depolarizing neuromuscular blocking agents.

### Chronic Inflammatory Demyelinating Polyneuropathy

CIDP is three times more likely to relapse during the last trimester and puerperium than in the absence of pregnancy. Infants are unaffected. Corticosteroids, plasmapheresis, and IVIG treat exacerbations during pregnancy. Oral contraceptives can worsen CIDP.

### Charcot-Marie-Tooth Disease Type 1

Small studies indicate that Charcot-Marie-Tooth disease type 1 worsens in approximately one-third to half of affected women during pregnancy. The magnitude of the effect of pregnancy on this disease remains unclear. Risk is less when weakness begins in adult life. After delivery, this deterioration improves in a third of patients and becomes persistently progressive in one-fifth to two-thirds of patients, although studies vary in their observations (Awater et al., 2012; Byrne et al., 2018; Swan et al., 2007). A retrospective Norwegian study found that affected women were twice as likely as the general population to have fetal-presentation anomalies, experience postpartum hemorrhage, and undergo cesarean section—commonly on an emergency basis. Forceps delivery occurred three times as often (Hoff et al., 2005). Epidural anesthesia for labor is safe. Preimplantation genetic diagnosis associated with in vitro fertilization and subsequent confirmation through amniocentesis and chorionic villus sampling has been applied successfully for a handful of couples. Proponents suggest potential usefulness in couples opposed to abortion, leading to improved rate of progeny unaffected by CMT1 (Kuliev, 2013).

### Gestational Polyneuropathy

Distal symmetrical neuropathy affects malnourished women. Presumably, thiamine and possibly other nutrients are deficient. The acute presentation of symmetrical neuropathy and Wernicke encephalopathy (see later discussion) in the third and fourth months may be due to the thiamine deficiency associated with hyperemesis gravidarum.

### Maternal Brachial Plexus Neuropathy

Hereditary brachial plexus neuropathy is an autosomal dominant disorder characterized by periodic attacks of asymmetrical pain, weakness, atrophy, and sensory alteration of the shoulder girdle and upper limbs attributed to involvement of proximal upper-limb nerves or the brachial plexus. Symptoms are indistinguishable from those of Parsonage-Turner syndrome (see Chapter 32). Attacks may begin as early as 3 hours postpartum despite cesarean section, may recur for weeks following parturition, and may follow subsequent pregnancies. Intravenous methylprednisolone may reduce the pain but seems not to influence the course of the disease.

### Maternal Obstetric Palsy

Peripheral nerves are occasionally compressed by the fetal head, the application of forceps, and improperly positioned leg holders. Craniopelvic disproportion, dystocia, prolonged labor, and primigravida status contribute to these injuries. Unilateral lumbosacral (L4, L5, and rarely S1) plexus injury is most common. The fetal brow strikes the nerves as they cross the posterior brim of the true pelvis (Fig. 112.2). The associated sensory deficit usually involves more widespread sensory loss than that due to peroneal neuropathy. Peroneal nerve injuries often are caused when the nerve is compressed between a leg holder and the fibular head. Less common obstetric palsies include those of the femoral and obturator nerves.

Most maternal obstetric palsies are neurapraxic and resolve within 6 weeks. In future pregnancies, women with recurrent craniopelvic disproportion, dystocia, or axonal degeneration with their initial neuropathy are candidates for cesarean delivery. Otherwise, a cautious trial of labor may be prudent.

## MOVEMENT DISORDERS

### Restless Legs

Unpleasant paresthesias (described as creeping, crawling, aching, or fidgetiness) localized deep within both legs affect 14%–30% of pregnant women (Chen et al., 2018) compared with 2%–15% of the general population. Usually they begin 30 minutes after the patient lies down. A meta-analysis described an almost threefold average prevalence increase between the first and last trimester, from 8% to 22%. Ethnic differences influence the rate at which symptoms are reported. An irresistible desire to move the legs accompanies the discomfort. Symptoms resolve sharply during the first month postpartum, after which time about 5% of women remain affected. A genetic predisposition is

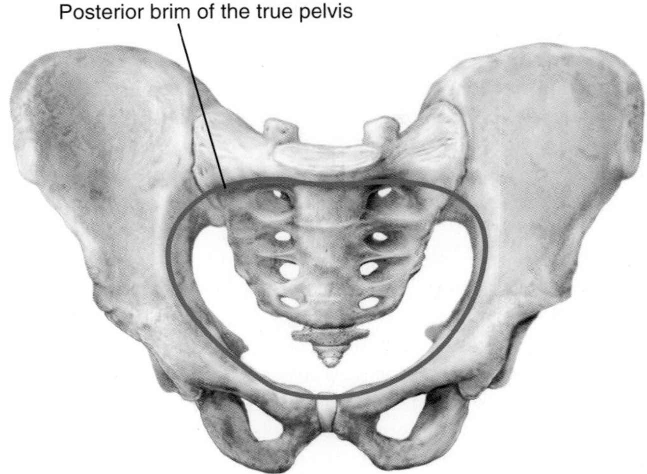


**Fig. 112.2** The fetal brow may strike nerves within the lumbosacral plexus as they cross the posterior brim of the true pelvis. *(Redrawn from Gray, H., Lewis, W.H., 2000. Anatomy of the Human Body, 20th ed. Lea & Febiger, Philadelphia, 198; Bartleby, New York)*

suggested as a possible etiology for the persistence of discomfort. A study found lower average hemoglobin and mean corpuscular volume than in healthy subjects (Manconi et al., 2004) but this association has not been confirmed (Hubner et al., 2013). A study in Thailand found that a hemoglobin of less than 11 and a history of restless legs syndrome (RLS) predicted the occurrence of RLS during pregnancy, 71% of cases diagnosed in the third trimester (Panvatanich and Lolekha, 2019). Gestational worsening may occur in about 60% of patients reporting RLS before pregnancy, but investigators also report improvement in some 12% of preexisting RLS. Approximately 80% of patients complaining of restless legs experience periodic movements in sleep (see Chapter 101). These stereotyped flexion movements of the legs during nonrapid eye movement (REM) sleep may awaken the patient, leading to sleep loss and excessive daytime somnolence. Caffeine ingestion, uremia, alcohol use, iron deficiency, hypothyroidism, vitamin deficiency, rheumatoid arthritis, peripheral neuropathy, and medications are important, if only occasional, associated factors. The importance of iron and folic acid supplementation remains unclear. Folic acid may be of benefit in treating restless legs during pregnancy. Anecdotal reports suggest a benefit from vitamin E, vitamin C, and magnesium supplements. Electric vibrators, stretching, walking, decreased activity, and massage also may be helpful. The use of dopaminergic agonists and L-dopa to treat periodic limb movements of sleep during pregnancy has not undergone systematic study. Anecdotal reports indicate success and safety with L-dopa. When a physician decides to offer either of these therapies, careful disclosure of the potential for known and also unforeseen risks to the fetus may allow the patient to make an informed decision.

## Chorea Gravidarum

Chorea of any cause beginning in pregnancy is termed *chorea gravidarum*. Historically, rheumatic heart disease (often fatal) was associated with most cases, but rheumatic heart disease has virtually disappeared. Today, the disease linked most strongly with this condition is the APS, with or without SLE. Additional etiologies include tardive dyskinesia due to neuroleptics, hyperthyroidism, Wilson disease, Huntington disease (HD), neuroacanthocytosis, vascular disease, other hypercoagulable states, and a variety of intoxications.

Chorea commonly presents during the second to fifth months of pregnancy and uncommonly may begin postpartum. Subtle, sometimes severe, cognitive change may accompany the chorea. Usually this condition resolves spontaneously within weeks to months, often shortly after delivery. Choice of therapy for this often benign condition depends on the severity of the disorder and other accompanying clinical manifestations. Expectant observation, cautious use of haloperidol, and use of corticosteroids have been successful. Oral contraceptives also have been associated with the appearance of chorea. The mechanism by which pregnancy and oral contraceptives cause chorea is unknown. Chorea may recur in subsequent pregnancies.

## Dystonia and Dystonia Gravidarum

Pregnancy does not affect dystonic symptoms in women diagnosed with dystonia before pregnancy (Gwinn-Hardy et al., 2000). Dystonia has no documented deleterious effect on the course of pregnancy, labor, or outcome. Prenatal genetic counseling is advised for those dystonias known to be autosomally dominant or when a genetic predisposition is suspect. Botulinum toxins do not cross the placenta and are not expected in circulation after intramuscular injection. Although more data are needed, the risk of botulinum toxin to the embryo or fetus appears low or nonexistent (Briggs Drugs in Pregnancy and Lactation, 2018). L-dopa treatment for dopa-responsive dystonia when continued in pregnancy crosses the placental barrier and is metabolized by the fetus. While L-dopa does not appear to present a major risk to the fetus, long-term studies of neurodevelopment are lacking.

When dystonia arises de novo during pregnancy, medications are commonly implicated, including the antiemetics metoclopramide, prochlorperazine, and promethazine. Women in distress during the hours that this condition continues often accept the low or no fetal risk of antihistamines such as diphenhydramine administered intravenously, orally, or both (Etwel et al., 2017).

Researchers describe dystonia arising and continuing during pregnancy without identifiable cause as *dystonia gravidarum*. One Chinese and two Italian cases of cervical dystonia beginning within weeks of conception and resolving by either the third trimester or postpartum were described (Buccoliero, 2007, Fasano, 2007, Lim, 2006a). Two cases were treated with clonazepam with known fetal risks. Botulinum toxin has not been employed. When needed, botulinum toxin A, used with caution, seems preferable to baclofen (Kranick et al., 2010). Sudden onset of adductor spasmodic dysphonia in pregnancy has been described in five patients (Ankola et al., 2013). Researchers suggest that the occurrence of these gestational dystonias are related to the high estrogenic state of pregnancy and combined contributing risk factors.

## Huntington Disease

We lack studies that demonstrate an effect of HD on the course of pregnancy or an effect of pregnancy on the course of HD. Physicians advise women known to have HD that the risk of transmitting the illness to a child is 50%. Most patients with HD die within 15–20 years after a symptomatic diagnosis, their later years commonly characterized by severe emotional, intellectual, and motor decline. Patients with HD have more children than the normal population. Based on this information, authorities are divided on how physicians should counsel patients. Some suggest advising fertile women with HD to consider measures to avoid pregnancy—not for the sake of the mother but to avoid the risk of propagation of HD into future generations and to avoid the predictable effect of the mother's death and disability on the child. For those women interested in planned pregnancy, genetic testing through amniocentesis or chorionic villus sampling allows women to consider pregnancy termination in the case of an affected fetus. Preimplantation genetic diagnosis associated with in vitro fertilization can be helpful but does not eliminate the need for amniocentesis and chorionic villus sampling to confirm the accuracy of a preimplantation genetic diagnosis. Physicians debate the ethics of genetic testing when patients at risk for HD are unwilling to discover their own personal risk through presymptomatic testing yet request testing of the embryo/fetus.

## Friedreich Ataxia

Little information about pregnancy and Friedreich ataxia is available. One retrospective study found no adverse outcomes in 17 women but recommended cardiac examination and monitoring during labor. Studies point to medications such as magnesium sulfate, muscle blockers, and barbiturates as possibly problematic in isolated case reports, with cautious use of these medications recommended (Kranick et al., 2010).

## Parkinson Disease

Rarely, patients suffering from Parkinson disease become pregnant. No reliable studies on the effect of pregnancy on the course of Parkinson disease or the effect of the disease on pregnancy are available. Information available from case reports is contradictory but indicates a possible adverse effect of pregnancy on the symptoms. No difficulty with pregnancy outcomes is known. Available limited data best support the cautious use of L-dopa/carbidopa and the possible avoidance of amantadine during pregnancy (Kranick et al., 2010). Limited human data suggest that L-dopa/carbidopa is compatible with breastfeeding.

### Tourette Syndrome

A study of 11 pregnancies in a mixed retrospective and prospective analysis found no unequivocal effect of pregnancy on the severity of tics in Tourette syndrome. The authors acknowledge the severe limitations of the study on a topic about which little information is otherwise available. The study also indicates the importance of this information for physicians treating patients whose tics worsen during pregnancy and for whom neurological consultation is requested (Stern et al., 2009). Management suggestions include cautious continuation of some medications. A lower-risk alternative includes trial off medication and appropriately targeted use of habit reversal training (HRT) or Comprehensive Behavioral Intervention for Tics (CBIT) (Chang et al., 2018b).

### Wilson Disease

Small case series provide limited information on which to base treatment decisions during pregnancy for women with Wilson disease. Pregnancy is contraindicated only in the presence of severe liver disease (Brewer et al., 2000). Pregnancy does not appear to have an adverse effect on the course of Wilson disease, but lack of treatment of the condition can have such an effect. Anecdotal but numerous reports of women who stop therapy during pregnancy document disease progression and maternal death. A retrospective study from Germany and the largest case series on pregnancy outcomes reported 282 pregnancies in 136 patients. Liver functions worsened in 6%, and resolved postpartum. Neurological symptoms worsened in 1% and persisted after delivery. Spontaneous abortions occurred in about one quarter. Patients who received therapy had fewer spontaneous abortions than those not taking medications. Birth defects were seen in 3% of live births. The authors concluded that although teratogenic potential is a concern, chelation therapy in pregnancy is safe and should be continued throughout pregnancy. The patient should be monitored for hepatic and neurological illness (Pfeiffenberger et al., 2018). This study underlines similar findings from India where most adverse outcomes occurred in patients untreated with chelation therapy (Sinha et al., 2004). Debate over the most effective and safest medication continues. Penicillamine and trientine are teratogenic in animals; zinc acetate is not. One review suggests an advantage of zinc acetate (Kranick et al., 2010), as do advocates of zinc therapy (Brewer et al., 2000). In a series in which zinc acetate was given during 26 pregnancies, one case of microcephaly and one cardiac defect were noted. The authors mention four miscarriages they chose not to include in the study analysis (Brewer et al., 2000) (Table 112.3).

## WERNICKE ENCEPHALOPATHY AND HYPEREMESIS GRAVIDARUM

More than three-fourths of women experience nausea and vomiting during pregnancy, most commonly between 6 and 16 weeks' gestation. When vomiting becomes severe enough to result in weight loss (5% of prepregnancy weight), metabolic derangement, or dehydration (high urine specific gravity), the condition is termed *hyperemesis gravidarum*. There is no international consensus on a definition, making studies on this entity difficult to conduct and interpret (Koot et al., 2018). Commonly, hyperemesis is isolated and idiopathic, affecting less than 1% of pregnancies. Molar pregnancy, hyperthyroidism, and hepatitis are differential diagnostic considerations. Hypokalemia associated with hyperemesis gravidarum is blamed for rare cardiac arrest, respiratory arrest, and fetal loss (Walch et al., 2018). Studies on treatment with vitamin $B_6$ (pyridoxine), 10–25 mg three times daily for 5 days DMS, showed little benefit, but enthusiasts continue to recommend this treatment, sometimes with ginger. However, a meta-analysis found that affected women taking vitamin B6 spend more days in hospital (Boelig et al., 2018). Antihistamines, metoclopramide, and steroids have been recommended in an approach proportionate to the severity of the medical condition (Niebyl, 2010). A literature review found no difference in efficacy among the use of metoclopramide, ondansetron, and promethazine, recommending that a choice may be determined based on cost and side effects of these medications (Boelig et al., 2018). Other authors suggest further investigation into the use of mirtazapine (Abramowitz et al., 2017). National guidelines describing a treatment approach have been updated (Committee on Obstetric Practice, 2018). Although US national guidelines recommend against gestational marijuana use (Committee on Obstetric Practice, Committee opinion, 2017), the practice is common in states where consumption is legal. In Northern California researchers find that use of marijuana for severe, mild, and no nausea and vomiting were 11.3%, 8.4%, and 4.5% respectively, despite lack of demonstrated efficacy or safety (Young-Wolff et al., 2018).

In the context of hyperemesis gravidarum, apathy, drowsiness, memory loss, catatonia, ophthalmoplegia, nystagmus, ataxia, and optic neuropathy, with or without optic disc edema, may result individually or together, typically between 14 and 20 weeks' gestation. These clinical features are emblematic of *Wernicke encephalopathy* (see Chapter 85). A subtle presentation can delay prompt diagnosis. This condition is sometimes associated with gestational polyneuropathy and central pontine myelinolysis. Exacerbating factors include persistence of the

**TABLE 112.3 Number of Pregnancies and Abortion Rates With Respect to WD Medical Therapy During Pregnancy**

| Therapy | Pregnancies | Live Births | Abortion Rate | Relative Risk (95% CI) | *P* Value* |
|---|---|---|---|---|---|
| WD undiagnosed | 86 | 51 (59%) | 35 (41%) | Reference | Reference |
| DPA | 118 | 98 (83%) | 20 (17%) | 0.416 (0.259–0.669) | ,001 |
| Trientine | 36 | 26 (72%) | 10 (28%) | 0.683 (0.380–1.225) | n.s. |
| Zinc | 20 | 18 (90%) | 2 (10%) | 0.246 (0.064–0.938) | ,035 |
| Combination | 8 | 7 (87%) | 1 (13%) | 0.307 (0.048–1.955) | n.s. |
| Pause | 14 | 9 (64%) | 5 (36%) | 0.878 (415–1.853) | n.s. |

**P* value adjusted according Bonferroni.
Relative risks for abortion for each therapy are shown in comparison to pregnancies in undiagnosed patients.
WD, Wilson Disease *CI*, Confidence interval; DPA, D-penicillamine *n.s.*, nonsignificant; *WD*, Wilson disease.
*From Pfeiffenberger, J., Beinhardt, S., Gotthardt, D.N., Haag, N., Freissmuth, C., Reuner, U., et al. 2018. Pregnancy in Wilson's disease: Management and outcome. Hepatology 67(4), 1261–1269.*

hyperemesis over at least 2 weeks and the administration of intravenous glucose without other nutrients.

Death or severe morbidity results when this condition is not treated. In a small study, only half of women with this condition delivered normal children. The amount and duration of parenteral thiamine supplementation required is unknown and must be titrated to the clinical state. The Royal College of Physicians endorses a protocol employing intravenous Thiamine 500 mg three times daily for 2-3 days followed by 250 mg daily for 3-5 days, then oral thiamine 100 mg three times daily. Treatment with multiple vitamins IV, correcting hypomagesemia, and potentially fatal hypokalemia remain elements essential to maternal and fetal recovery (Thomson, A, 2012). Despite therapy, some women continue to have ataxia and visual difficulties months to years afterward. Several researchers suggest treating any patient with prolonged nausea and vomiting with oral thiamine, 100 mg daily, and those admitted to the hospital with 150 mg daily DMS (Jarvis and Nelson-Piercy, 2011) (Fig. 112.3).

## MULTIPLE SCLEROSIS

### Effect of Multiple Sclerosis on Pregnancy

Studies yield conflicting results on the nature and extent of the effect of MS on pregnancy course, labor, and outcome. There is reliable support to suggest that infants of MS mothers are born with lower birth weight and there is an increased rate of cesarean section. That said, authors reviewing the literature conclude that the majority of women with MS can safely choose to become pregnant, give birth, and breastfeed children (Bove et al., 2014).

A retrospective study based on insurance claims in the United States found that the adjusted proportion of women with MS and pregnancy linearly increased between the years 2006 and 2014 from 7.91% to 9.47%. This trend stands in contrast to a simultaneous linear decrease in patients without MS from 8.83% to 7.75% (Houtchens et al., 2018a). These researchers suggest that the decreasing prevalence of pregnancy for women without MS mirrors national data. The increasing prevalence for women with MS is explained as possibly the result of MS patients having developed a more positive outlook, and reference more robust counseling by medical professionals, further characterized as improved. This study also found increased insurance claims for peripartum complications in patients with MS, including premature labor, infections, cardiovascular disease, anemia/acquired coagulation disorders, neurological complications, sexually transmitted diseases, acquired fetal damage, and congenital malformations. MS patients were slightly older. Further data in a subsequent publication revealed that a small, but possibly significant proportion of these patients were prescribed disease-modifying drugs during pregnancy and shortly before (Houtchens et al., 2018b).

In contrast, a retrospective California study from 2001 to 2009 found no significant increases in adverse pregnancy outcomes (Fong et al., 2018). This latter finding jibes with previous studies asserting that uncomplicated MS has no apparent effect on fertility, pregnancy, labor, delivery, the rate of spontaneous abortions, congenital malformations, or stillbirths. One study of a large US national database noted marginally increased risk of fetal intrauterine growth restriction (IUGR; weight <10th percentile for gestational age) and rate of cesarean section. Calculated at 2.7%, the low rate of IUGR was 1.9 times more likely than the normal population. Physicians performed cesarean section at a higher rate: 42% for women with MS compared to 32.8% for controls. The study found no increase in other adverse obstetric outcomes. The authors acknowledge significant methodological concerns. Pregnancy outcome data were unavailable (Kelly et al., 2009).

### Effect of Pregnancy on Multiple Sclerosis

Oral contraceptive agents do not affect the incidence of MS. In a small study, researchers cautiously predict an increased relapse rate in patients with MS undergoing in vitro fertilization. This effect was noted for 3 months after the procedure, possibly associated with failure of IVF and the use of gonadotropin releasing hormone agonists (Michel et al., 2012).

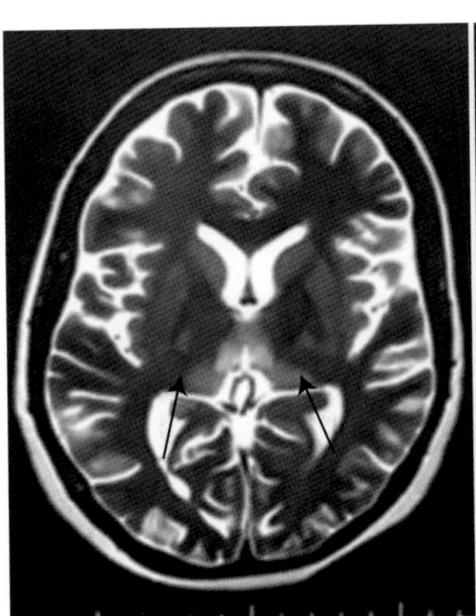
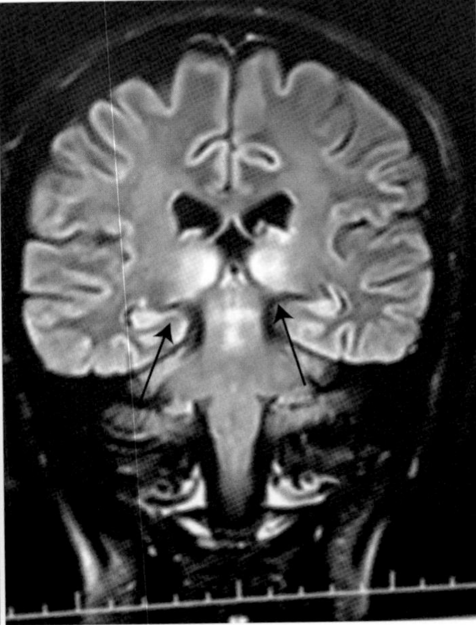
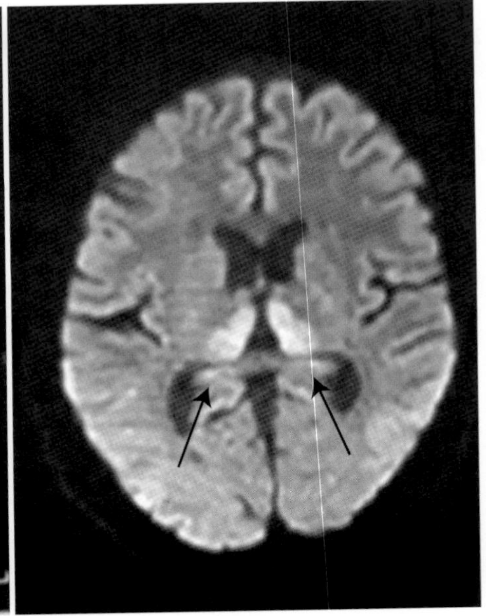

**Fig. 112.3** Magnetic resonance imaging of the brain showing hyperintense and diffusion-restricted areas in the peritectal region and bilateral medial thalami in a patient with clinical Wernicke encephalopathy associated with hyperemesis gravidarum. Left: T2 weighted image. Arrows indicate increased thalamic intensity. Middle: Diffusion weighted image. Arrows indicate thalamic involvement. Peri-tectal involvement is seen in the midline. Right: Diffusion weighted image. Arrows indicate thalamic involvement. (*From Talib, V., Sultana, S., Hamad, A. Yaqoob, U., 2018. Wernicke encephalopathy due to hyperemesis gravidarum in pregnancy: A case report. Cureus 10[7], e2991.*)

Predicting the effect of pregnancy on the course of MS for an individual patient remains challenging. Prospective analysis clarifies that for research populations, MS does not worsen overall as a result of pregnancy and suggests that for the average fertile patient with MS, the overall rate of progression of disability from MS compared to the rate of progression 1 year before pregnancy does not change for some 21 months postpartum. The exacerbation rate of MS decreases during the last trimester and increases during the 3–6 months after parturition. Postpartum relapse correlates with, but is predicted poorly by, an increased relapse rate in the prepregnancy year, an increased relapse rate during pregnancy, and a higher level of disability at pregnancy onset (Vukusic et al., 2004). In one study finding that women with increasing parity were less likely to encounter a first demyelinating event, the author claims a cumulative protective effect of pregnancy on MS (Ponsonby, 2012).

Management strategies for MS must be adapted to the individual patient. Anecdotal reports detail the success of plasmapheresis in a pregnant woman with rapidly progressive MS and in another woman with Devic syndrome. Clinical improvement has also been associated with the use of IVIG in a few case studies. Short-term courses of corticosteroids during pregnancy seem safe, but baclofen and tizanidine are not well studied.

Postpartum exclusive breastfeeding may be the best approach to suppression of relapses in MS. For patients whose disease worsens and want to continue to breastfeed, glatiramer acetate and interferon beta are most likely to be safe (Coyle, 2014). Breastfeeding women who start immunomodulating agents immediately postpartum have more relapses than those who remain untreated and breastfeed (Langer-Gould et al., 2009). In a study of the use of IVIG postpartum, more women remained relapse free if they breastfed for more than 3 months (90% vs. 71%) (Haas and Hommes, 2007). Some researchers recommend that women breastfeed for at least 2 months postpartum before considering immunomodulating therapy (Langer-Gould et al., 2009), but others maintain that current data do not exclude a possibility that some MS patients may benefit from immunomodulating therapy (Airas et al., 2010). Currently the American Academy of Pediatrics recommends breastfeeding exclusive of other oral nutrition "for about 6 months, followed by continued breastfeeding as complementary foods are introduced, with continuation of breastfeeding for 1 year or longer as mutually desired by mother and infant".

A succinct summary and description of most points of interest to patients can be obtained through the National MS Society (Giesser, 2018).

Investigators recommend discontinuing glatiramer acetate, interferon beta-1a, interferon beta-1b, natalizumab, fingolimod, teriflunomide, dimethyl fumarate, alemtuzumab, daclizumab, ocrelizumab, rituximab, cladribine, mitoxantrone, before an anticipated pregnancy, during gestation, and while breastfeeding for most patients. Contraception for fertile women taking these agents is recommended.

Discontinuation of some of these medications is complicated in the presence of safety warnings and the need for "washout" periods. A safety alert was issued for fingolimod in November 2018, advising that when fingolimod is stopped, MS can become much worse than before fingolimod was begun or being taken, and can result in permanent, severe disability more severe than usual patient relapses and unrelated to the patient's prior disease state, usually between 2 and 24 weeks after stopping fingolimod. A cohort study demonstrated clinical or imaging worsening in 35% of patients stopping fingolimod (Cerda et al., 2018). An immune reconstitution inflammatory syndrome has been described after discontinuing natalizumab associated with progressive multifocal leukoencephalopathy (PML), usually within days or weeks when plasmapheresis is employed to speed natalizumab elimination. Planning is essential for safe management. The considerate neurologist may inquire routinely whether a patient plans, foresees, or admits to the possibility of pregnancy to promote active engagement in a discussion of alternatives in the context of a possible need for abrupt discontinuation of therapies.

Depending on the half-life of the therapy and concerns regarding adverse pregnancy outcomes, manufacturers recommend a period of time without medication to avoid fetal exposure during the sensitive first trimester of organogenesis. Washout periods vary. Although glatiramer acetate is of uncertain deleterious effect during pregnancy, manufacturers advise a washout period of 1 month. In contrast, teriflunomide metabolism may take 8 months to 2 years for levels considered safe. As a result, an 11-day course of cholestyramine and charcoal to speed elimination is recommended, accompanied by confirmatory serum levels. Mitoxantrone should be discontinued at least 2–3 months before pregnancy, with a pregnancy test administered for fertile women before every dose. To obtain the latest information regarding a washout period, checking updated literature concerning a specific therapy is recommended.

Human studies of interferons suggest the possibility of increased spontaneous abortion, fetal loss, and low birth weight, supplementing the reported abortifacient data for interferons in primates (Boskovic et al., 2005; Sandberg-Wollheim et al., 2005). This information is at odds with postmarket surveillance studies that report a rate of spontaneous abortion and other adverse fetal events no different than expected in a normal population (Coyle et al., 2003). In one small study, the rate of spontaneous abortion with the use of interferon beta-1b was higher than the normal population (28%) and higher than that of interferon beta-1a (Weber-Schoendorfer et al., 2009). A larger study suggests that early first trimester interferon beta-1b exposure results in no increased risk of spontaneous abortion. Lower birth weight and length in exposed children did not result in significant fetal complications, malformation, or developmental abnormalities after a median follow-up of approximately 2 years (Amato et al., 2010).

Glatiramer acetate seems safer than interferons in animal studies, but these studies are incompletely generalizable to humans. We lack reliable information on pregnancy outcomes for significant numbers of women who take glatiramer acetate throughout pregnancy. One small study warns against the use of glatiramer acetate while describing the spontaneous abortion rate associated as "encouraging" (Wolfgang et al., 2008), and another that glatiramer acetate does not pose a major risk for developmental toxicity, stopping short of recommending its use during pregnancy (Weber-Schoendorfer and Schaefer, 2009). An analysis of studies reporting pregnancy outcomes for women taking interferon beta, glatiramer acetate, and natalizumab concludes that no excellent studies have been performed and that additional study is needed (Lu et al., 2012). Of the MS therapies commonly used, glatiramer acetate is considered least risky during pregnancy. An expert panel concluded that glatiramer acetate should be discontinued when trying to conceive, throughout gestation, and while breastfeeding. However, in pregnant women with severe or highly active MS, benefit may outweigh fetal risk (Bove et al., 2014). In 2018, its use during pregnancy was described as controversial (Houtchens et al., 2018b).

The oral agents teriflunomide, fingolimod, and dimethyl fumarate cause reproductive toxicity in animals and are contraindicated during pregnancy. Current recommendations for a woman taking teriflunomide are to employ strict contraception. When 10 women taking teriflunomide unintentionally became pregnant, there resulted three spontaneous abortions and six induced abortions. One woman treated for 31 days of the pregnancy delivered a healthy baby without health concerns noted for 2 years. Men taking teriflunomide are advised to use reliable contraception and use an accelerated elimination procedure when stopping teriflunomide to avoid fetal exposure (O'Connor, 2006, 2011). Whether teriflunomide enters breast milk is unknown.

Given current theoretical benefits of breastfeeding to both the patient with MS and to the infant, breastfeeding without teriflunomide may be the better choice.

Elimination of fingolimod takes about 2 months. Fertile women are advised to use effective contraception while taking fingolimod and to avoid pregnancy for 2 months after stopping the medication. Nevertheless, unplanned pregnancies are common and occurred in a prospective study despite strict directions to adhere to a program of double contraceptive measures. A study of 66 infants thus exposed to fingolimod during the first trimester yielded increased risk of spontaneous abortion, five children with abnormal fetal development, and two with major malformations including one with acrania (Karlsson et al., 2014). Fingolimod is secreted into the breast milk of rodents. Breastfeeding is not recommended while taking fingolimod and for 2 months after drug cessation. Whether dimethyl fumarate enters breast milk is unknown as are the risks to the breastfeeding infant.

The effects of breastfeeding on the neonate while taking immunomodulating agents are known incompletely. Until more information is available with regard to safety, some authorities advise discontinuation of these medications, explaining to patients that while not certain, breastfeeding may suppress MS disease severity.

Mitoxantrone causes fetal damage in animals and should not be used during pregnancy, and only with reliable contraception in fertile women. Methotrexate causes major malformations during pregnancy, should be avoided during lactation, and should also be used only with contraceptives. In animals, high-dose natalizumab causes abortions and crosses the placenta, but we lack reliable studies on humans. Most researchers recommend against natalizumab use during pregnancy.

## NEUROMYELITIS OPTICA SPECTRUM DISORDER—DEVIC SYNDROME

Neuromyelitis optica (NMO) may be diagnosed reliably when a patient presents with optic neuritis, myelitis, and supported by findings that include a spinal cord lesion demonstrated on MRI of three or more segments in length, NMO-IgG seropositivity, and brain MRI nondiagnostic of MS (Wingerchuk et al., 2006). Few studies are available on the effect of pregnancy on this uncommon demyelinating disease or the effect of the disease on pregnancy. Retrospective information from 20 women affected by NMO and experiencing 25 pregnancies finds a halving of the relapse rate during the first and second trimesters, a mild worsening in the third trimester, and for 3 months postpartum—a doubling. An additional retrospective study of 40 patients and 54 pregnancies found the relapse rate throughout gestation unchanged, but increased some four- to fivefold during the subsequent 6 months postpartum (Kim et al., 2012). An international study of 31 women and 46 pregnancies using a questionnaire and chart review noted an overall worsening both during pregnancy and particularly the postpartum 3 months when rate of relapse for about 10% of their patients reached three times the annualized rate (Klawiter et al., 2017). A retrospective international study of cohorts of women with aquaporin-4 antibody–positive neuromyelitis optica spectrum disorder (NMOSD) found an increased risk of miscarriage, preeclampsia, and relapse rate. Further study is needed to confirm these findings and the magnitude of the effect (Nour et al., 2016). Investigators found no negative effect of epidural anesthesia (Chang et al., 2018a) or breastfeeding. Monitoring during pregnancy and postpartum is recommended. An individualized approach to treatment during pregnancy and breastfeeding based on disease severity and known fetal risk of immunomodulating drugs has been suggested, coupled with a continuing need to investigate treatment and disease outcomes during pregnancy.

## TUMORS

### Primary Brain Neoplasms

A meta-analysis observes reduced glioma risk with hormone replacement therapy and oral contraceptive use and increased meningioma risk with hormone replacement therapy (Cowppli-Bony et al., 2011). Brain tumors of all types occur during pregnancy, but only at 38% of the rate expected in nonpregnant women of fertile age. Diminished fertility in women with these tumors may explain this reduction, because pregnancy probably does not protect against the development of neoplasms. Studies show increased numbers of abortions before the symptoms of tumor appear. The effect of pregnancy on morbidity and mortality in women with brain tumors is not known, but certain tumors grow more rapidly during pregnancy (Pallud et al., 2009). Meningiomas have estrogen receptors, which may explain the enlargement usually seen during pregnancy. The rupture rate of spinal hemangiomas increases with the duration of gestation. Pregnancy increased type II glioma growth rate, seizure frequency 40%, and further oncological treatment postpartum in a study of 12 pregnancies (Pallud et al., 2010). Postpartum remission of symptoms of meningioma, vascular tumors, and acoustic neuromas may be due to tumor shrinkage.

Gestational brain tumors tend to present at different stages dependent on tumor type: gliomas usually present problems during the first trimester, meningiomas during and after the second trimester, and vascular tumors in the third trimester.

Malignant tumors or tumors threatening compression of vital brain structures usually require surgery during pregnancy. During pregnancy, most neurosurgical procedures appear well tolerated (Cohen-Gadol et al., 2009). Surgery for some benign tumors can wait several weeks postpartum to observe for spontaneous symptomatic improvements. Most women with brain tumors deliver by cesarean section. Vaginal delivery is reserved for patients whose tumor would not pose a threat of herniation with the shifts of intracranial pressure associated with labor. Pregnancy interruption is considered when increased intracranial pressure, vision loss, or uncontrolled seizures develop as a result of the tumor. A report of neurosurgery performed on 34 patients describes that procedures are generally safe enough during pregnancy to argue for earlier operative intervention rather than delaying until postpartum (Nossek et al., 2011). A Chinese study documented relative maternal and fetal safety of surgical procedures to treat hemangioblastoma in 8 patients in a series of 24 patients (Ma et al., 2018).

Administration of corticosteroids commonly lessens symptoms of brain tumors (see Chapter 73, but fetal hypoadrenalism may result from their use. Physicians usually defer potentially teratogenic chemotherapy until after delivery. Cranial radiation therapy during pregnancy may be helpful to the mother, but no dose of radiation is completely safe for the fetus. The fetus usually is seriously affected when it receives doses greater than 0.1 Gy (10 rad), which may cause growth retardation, microcephaly, and eye malformations. The fetus may also be affected by lower amounts of radiation, particularly early in gestation. Researchers estimate that in utero exposure to 0.01–0.02 Gy of radiation increases the incidence of leukemia by one case per 6000 exposed children. Estimates of the fetal dose during radiation for brain tumors range from 0.03 to 0.06 Gy. One study suggests that alternative positioning of the patient may reduce fetal exposure to as little as 0.003 Gy when a dose of 30 Gy is delivered to the brain (Magne et al., 2001).

### Pituitary Tumors

Women with untreated hyperprolactinemia often are anovulatory and infertile. Treatment with dopamine agonists restores ovulation in 90% of patients. During pregnancy, medical therapy focuses on preventing complications of tumor growth.

Bromocriptine reduces prolactinoma size, usually within 6 weeks to 6 months. Although this drug has no demonstrated teratogenic potential, some investigators recommend discontinuation of the medication unless clearly needed during pregnancy. Bromocriptine suppresses lactation, and anecdotal reports of puerperal maternal hypertension, seizures, stroke, and cerebral angiopathy are in the literature. Data on other dopamine agonists during pregnancy are limited.

The normal pituitary gland and most pituitary tumors grow during pregnancy. The woman with a pituitary microadenoma (<10 mm) may be reassured that fewer than 5% of these tumors grow enough to become symptomatic. The risk for a macroadenoma becoming symptomatic ranges from 16% to 36% but is considerably less for patients who receive radiation or surgical therapy before pregnancy. Commonly, physicians advise women with macroadenomas to have transsphenoidal surgery before attempting pregnancy or to receive bromocriptine therapy during pregnancy. Checking visual fields every 3 months or more often based on clinical concern may reduce the need for MRI in patients with known macroadenomas (Pivonello et al., 2014). Monitoring of prolactin levels is not helpful. MRI is indicated after delivery and should be performed if symptoms are increasing. For women with a symptomatic macroprolactinoma diagnosed during pregnancy, therapeutic options include bromocriptine therapy, pregnancy termination, or surgery.

Usually, women with pituitary tumors deliver vaginally. Studies have not demonstrated tumor growth associated with breastfeeding. Pituitary apoplexy may present within days, weeks, or occasionally years after delivery. Uncommonly, a pituitary mass presenting in late pregnancy or up to 1 year postpartum may be lymphocytic hypophysitis. Some researchers find MRI to be helpful in establishing the diagnosis and possibly reducing the need for neurosurgery (Gutenberg et al., 2009). The outcome of pregnancy is good for the majority of women with macroprolactinomas and nonfunctioning pituitary adenomas (Lambert et al., 2017).

### Choriocarcinoma

Cerebral metastases are a common manifestation of this rare tumor of trophoblastic origin. The tumor metastasizes first to the lung and then from lung to brain. This often happens months after a molar pregnancy or abortion. Approximately 15% of tumors follow normal pregnancies, but most are discovered after pregnancies characterized by spontaneous abortion or by vaginal bleeding, premature labor, and an enlarged uterus due to a molar pregnancy. Women with such cerebral metastases present with seizures, hemorrhage, infarction, or gradually progressive deficits. The tumor may invade the sacral plexus, cauda equina, or spinal canal. A ratio of serum to CSF chorionic gonadotropin of less than 60 suggests the presence of choriocarcinoma brain metastasis. Chemotherapy, radiation, and surgery have yielded successful results following early diagnosis.

## IDIOPATHIC INTRACRANIAL HYPERTENSION (PSEUDOTUMOR CEREBRI)

Idiopathic intracranial hypertension (IIH) (see Chapters 16 and 88) usually worsens with pregnancy. Some researchers advise a delay in pregnancy until all signs and symptoms of pre-existing IIH abate. Termination of pregnancy is of unknown value and is not indicated. Healthy babies usually result regardless of whether IIH begins before or during pregnancy. A small study suggests that about 90% of subsequent pregnancies are unaffected by previous IIH (Golan et al., 2013). Visual loss is estimated to occur in 10%–20%.

Commonly, IIH develops during the 14th gestational week and disappears after 1–3 months, but it sometimes persists until the early puerperium and rarely presents postpartum. Typically these women are obese and gain weight rapidly with pregnancy. Brain imaging is normal. In patients with clinical features consistent with IIH, guidelines from 2011 recommend imaging the cerebral venous system to exclude CVT (Saposnik et al., 2011). Protein concentration may be slightly low in otherwise normal spinal fluid.

Frequent checks of optic fundi, visual acuity, and visual fields are recommended to monitor the condition and the results of treatment. Initial CSF pressures that exceed 350 mm $H_2O$ usually indicate more severe disease. Careful studies of the effectiveness of treatment are unavailable. Most physicians advise moderation in diet to reduce weight gain while avoiding ketosis. Two-week courses of corticosteroids, most commonly dexamethasone or prednisone, are added for vision loss. Four to six serial lumbar punctures should be performed before considering optic nerve sheath fenestration or lumboperitoneal shunting.

The use of acetazolamide remains controversial; human studies are inadequate to determine its efficacy or teratogenic potential. Nevertheless, acetazolamide has been used to treat IIH during many pregnancies productive of healthy infants. Some physicians recommend restricting its use until after 20 weeks' gestation. A retrospective study of 12 patients taking acetazolamide 500 mg twice a day DMS resulted in normal children (Lee et al., 2005) and a larger study of 158 pregnancies recommends that the medication remain a treatment option when clinically indicated (Falardeau et al., 2013). No fetal injury resulted when acetazolamide was taken during the first trimester in a small cohort of 17 pregnant patients with IIH (Huang et al., 2017). A consensus panel, citing the limited safety data felt they could not offer a "safe" recommendation to support the use of acetazolamide during pregnancy. Instead, those patients threatened with visual loss during pregnancy were recommended to receive serial lumbar punctures with consideration for a CSF diversionary procedure (Mollan, 2018).

Acetaminophen with or without codeine may improve headache. More aggressive therapy usually is reserved for vision loss. Adequate pain control during labor may decrease expected rises in intracranial pressure. Usually these patients can undergo vaginal delivery with epidural analgesia. Recurrence of IIH in a subsequent pregnancy is unusual.

## EPILEPSY AND ITS TREATMENTS

### Maternal Considerations

Women with epilepsy have approximately 15% fewer children than expected. Reasons offered for this decrease in fertility include social effects of epilepsy, menstrual irregularity, the effect of some antiepileptic medications on the ovaries, and an effect of seizures on reproductive hormones. In an Indian registry-based study, 38.4% of women with epilepsy were infertile. Researchers identified age, lower education, and polytherapy with antiepileptic medications as risk factors (Sukumaran et al., 2010). However, when women with epilepsy in the US plan pregnancy, birth rates are comparable to the general population (Pennell et al., 2018).

Maternal mortality for pregnant women with epilepsy is increased over the general population. In the United States during the hospitalization for delivery, risk of death is about 10 times that of women without epilepsy (MacDonald et al., 2015). In Denmark, mortality is five times higher (Christensen et al., 2018).

Convulsive seizures during pregnancy can result in blunt trauma to the mother. Trauma is the leading nonobstetric cause of maternal death in women with epilepsy, but the incidence is very low. The effect of pregnancy on seizure occurrence can be predicted from the control of epilepsy during the 9 months preceding gestation. The fewer seizures there are in the 9 months before conception, the lower the risk for worsening during the pregnancy. Women who have at least one seizure in a month can be expected to have more seizures during pregnancy. Women who have less than one seizure in 9 months usually do not experience an increase in seizure rate during pregnancy.

Many studies suggest that approximately one-fourth of women experience an increase in seizure rate during gestation and that somewhat less than that experience fewer seizures. Women with focal epilepsy have higher rates of seizure worsening during pregnancy compared to women with generalized epilepsy, and women with frontal lobe epilepsy have especially elevated rates of seizure worsening during pregnancy and postpartum (Voinescu et al., 2018a). Researchers postulate that for some women, increased seizure frequency may result from lowered levels of circulating unbound AEDs. Pregnancy alters protein binding of many AEDs and increases the volume of distribution and metabolism of many drugs. However, even when blood levels of drugs are maintained adequately, approximately 10% of women experience worsened seizure control during pregnancy. During labor, approximately 1%–2% of epileptic women have a convulsive seizure, and another 1%–2% have a seizure within 24 hours of delivery. Other factors that may theoretically contribute to a possible increase in seizure rate include hormonal changes, sleep deprivation, mild chronic respiratory alkalosis, the use of folic acid supplements, and emotional factors.

A prospective Finnish study is more optimistic, suggesting that the frequency of seizures during gestation does not change or may even decrease (Viinikainen et al., 2006). The International Registry of Antiepileptic Drugs and Pregnancy (EURAP) reports that nearly 60% of women with epilepsy and careful monitoring do not have seizures during pregnancy (EURAP Study Group, 2006). A consensus statement and review of the evidence available concluded that there is insufficient evidence to determine whether gestation is associated with any predictable change in the frequency of seizures or status epilepticus reported in populations of women with epilepsy (Harden et al., 2009b).

While early studies suggested that epilepsy does not affect the course of pregnancy to a clinically significant degree, a large US study found that a diagnosis of epilepsy brings with it heightened risk for preeclampsia (adjusted OR, 1.59 [95% CI, 1.54–1.63]), preterm labor (adjusted OR, 1.54 [95% CI, 1.50–1.57]), and stillbirth (adjusted OR, 1.27 [95% CI, 1.17–1.38]), and women had increased healthcare utilization, including an increased risk of cesarean delivery (adjusted OR, 1.40 [95% CI, 1.38–1.42]) and prolonged length of hospital stay (>6 days) among both women with cesarean deliveries (adjusted OR, 2.13 [95% CI, 2.03–2.23]) and women with vaginal deliveries (adjusted OR, 2.60 [95% CI, 2.41–2.80]) (MacDonald et al., 2015).

When women with epilepsy take AEDs, researchers in Norway find the risk of severe preeclampsia, early pregnancy bleeding, pregnancy induction, and cesarean section to be increased, approximately 5-, 6.4-, 2.3-, and 2.5-fold, respectively. In this same study, forceps delivery and preterm birth were increased for those women not taking AEDs (Borthen et al., 2011). More recently, investigators in Norway found that the risk of cesarean section, breech presentation, and low birth weight was doubled for their population of women with epilepsy and taking AEDs, findings unaffected by seizure frequency and without increased risk of preeclampsia (Farmen et al., 2019).

## Fetal Considerations

Nearly 90% of epileptic women deliver healthy, normal babies. However, risks for miscarriage, stillbirth, prematurity, developmental delay, smallness for gestational age, and major malformations are increased in the offspring of epileptic mothers. Available literature suggests that there is no increase in perinatal mortality. Maternal seizures, AEDs, and socioeconomic, genetic, and psychological aspects of epilepsy affect outcome. Although AEDs may cause significant problems for the fetus, the consensus among neurologists has been that maternal seizures probably are more dangerous. Convulsive seizures cause fetal hypoxia and acidosis and are associated with the potential for blunt trauma to the fetus and placenta (Holmes et al., 2001). Fetal heart rate slows during and for up to 20 minutes after a maternal convulsion, which suggests the presence of fetal asphyxia. The child of an epileptic mother experiencing convulsions during gestation is twice as likely to develop epilepsy as the child of a woman with epilepsy who does not have a convulsive seizure during gestation. A retrospective study identified five or more generalized convulsive seizures during gestation as an independent risk factor for lowered verbal IQ scores in children (Adab et al., 2004). Pregnant women may be reassured that current data do not indicate an increased risk for malformation to their fetus from an uncomplicated single seizure during the first trimester.

A prospective study in which clinicians physically examined children of epileptic mothers and controls (Holmes et al., 2001) reported the frequency of major malformations (structural abnormalities of surgical, medical, or cosmetic importance not including microcephaly, growth retardation, or hypoplasia) to be 1.8% in their normal control population. With one AED (phenytoin, carbamazepine, or phenobarbital) this rate rose to 3.4%–5.2%, and with two or more to 8.6%. Some women with a history of seizures did not take anticonvulsants during pregnancy and had a rate of major malformation statistically the same as the control population at 0%. Women who suffered seizures during the first trimester and were taking their anticonvulsant drugs had a rate of major malformation of 7.4%–7.8%. This carefully gathered information lays blame for teratogenesis primarily on the use of AEDs (Fig. 112.4).

Studies of various design suggest that valproic acid causes a higher rate of teratogenicity than other commonly used AEDs. Increased risk may be related to increasing dose of valproic acid and was 9.1% for higher valproic acid doses in one study and 10.3% in another (Morrow et al., 2006; Tomson et al., 2018). In addition, maternal use of valproic acid was associated with lower scores on sixth grade Danish language

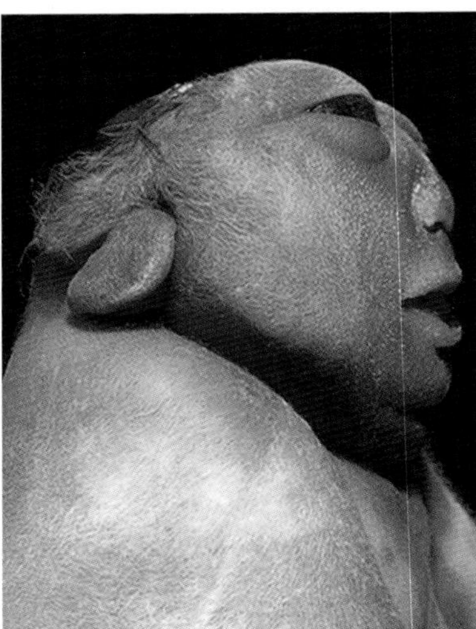

**Fig. 112.4** Anencephaly results from the lack of closure of the neural tube during the first trimester and has been associated with the use of antiepileptic drugs. *(From The University of Utah Eccles Health Sciences Library, Copyright © 1994–2015 WebPath by Edward C. Klatt, MD, Savannah, Georgia, USA. All rights reserved. http://library.med.utah.edu/WebPath/PEDHTML/PED031.html).*

and mathematics performance tests (Elkjær et al., 2018). Higher-dose lamotrigine (>200 mg/day) DMS also possibly increases teratogenicity up to 5.4% (Brodie, 2006), while lamotrigine generally had no effect on Danish performance tests. Based on these trends, some researchers have suggested caution in the use of AEDs, particularly valproic acid, in treating fertile women with epilepsy and avoidance of this medication during the first trimester if possible.

A European Registry study of 7355 pregnancies during which one of eight AEDs was taken between 1999 and 2016 (Tomson et al., 2018) offers two major conclusions. The first is that higher doses of valproic acid, carbamazepine, lamotrigine, and phenobarbital increase fetal risk for major malformations. Additionally, risks of major congenital malformation associated with lamotrigine, levetiracetam, and oxcarbazepine are within the range reported in the literature for offspring unexposed to AEDs. Scanty data for topiramate and phenytoin restrict interpretation (Table 112.4).

AEDs with known teratogenic effect exert their most serious effects during the first 2.5 months of gestation. Change medication before or during the first trimester to be maximally useful. The neural tube closes between 3 and 4 weeks. Cleft lip and palate occur with exposure before 5 and 10 weeks, respectively, whereas congenital heart disease due to anticonvulsant exposure occurs before 6 weeks' gestation.

A syndrome described initially as *fetal hydantoin syndrome*—including midfacial hypoplasia, long upper lip, low birth weight, cleft lip and palate, digital hypoplasia, and nail dysplasia—occurs with carbamazepine, primidone, and valproic acid and is more accurately called *fetal anticonvulsant syndrome*. Some minor anomalies usually disappear during the first years of life. Investigators speculate that midfacial hypoplasia associated with hypoplasia of the facial bones could be a marker for cognitive dysfunction. Trimethadione has such a high teratogenic potential that its use during pregnancy is contraindicated and should be avoided in women who might become pregnant.

Adequate human studies of newer anticonvulsant drugs during pregnancy are lacking. The teratogenic potential of gabapentin, vigabatrin, tiagabine, zonisamide, topiramate, clobazam, lacosamide, and perampanel, is incompletely understood. At this time, the physician may consider reevaluating the need for these anticonvulsants in a patient planning pregnancy or substituting an effective agent with known potential risks.

Several studies focused on cognitive effects of AEDs employed during pregnancy. One study described normal behavior in children of women with epilepsy on no AEDs during gestation, compared to matched controls. Vinten et al. (2005) found that children exposed to valproic acid in utero have significantly lower verbal IQ scores and memory function than children exposed to carbamazepine or phenytoin. While contradictions exist in published literature, the effects of carbamazepine and phenytoin may have little effect on cognition, but methodological problems hinder these analyses. A small United Kingdom pregnancy registry study compared use of valproic acid (mean dose 800 mg) DMS and levetiracetam (mean dose 1700 mg) DMS taken throughout pregnancy to a control group. Assessing development in children less than 2 years of age, 8% who were exposed to levetiracetam fell within the below average range, while the corresponding statistic was 40% for valproic acid, and 12% born to control mothers (Shallcross et al., 2011). Larger-scale prospective studies are needed to adequately quantify the cognitive effect of in utero AED exposure.

## Breastfeeding

The newborn ingests anticonvulsant drugs secreted in breast milk and may become sedated and hyperirritable. Infants may show withdrawal reactions from phenobarbital after lactational exposure. Known health benefits of breast milk probably outweigh potential subtle and theoretical effects of older AEDs on the nervous system. Little information is available on newer anticonvulsants concerning their secretion into breast milk and effects on the infant. The use of these drugs while nursing must be individualized based on the known benefits over alternatives. A published abstract describes data from a prospective, multi-institutional study of 181 children exposed in utero to AEDs. At age 6, the IQs of those children who were breastfed the milk of mothers taking AEDs versus the IQ of infants not breastfed were about 4 points higher. AEDs included monotherapy with carbamazepine, lamotrigine, phenytoin, or valproate. When interviewed, the study author suggested that when it comes to making a decision it may be better to accept the "known benefit [of breastfeeding rather] than the theoretical risk [of exposure to AEDs]" (Meador et al., 2013). Some authorities suggest measuring infant AED levels when there are parental or professional concerns (Van Ness, 2013). Despite general recommendations to breastfeed with AEDs, women with epilepsy breastfeed less (about 70%) than women without epilepsy (about 85%) (Johnson et al., 2018).

**TABLE 112.4 Prevalence of Major Congenital Malformations in Offspring Exposed Prenatally to One of Eight Different Antiepileptic Monotherapies**

| | Dose Range (mg/day) | Number of Pregnancies Exposed | Number of Major Congenital Malformation Events | Prevalence of Major Congenital Malformation Events (95% CI) |
|---|---|---|---|---|
| Lamotrigine | 25–1300 DMS | 2514 | 74 | 2·9% (2·3–3·7) |
| Carbamazepine | 50–2400 DMS | 1957 | 107 | 5·5% (4·5–6·6) |
| Valproate | 100–3000 DMS | 1381 | 142 | 10·3% (8·8–12·0) |
| Levetiracetam | 250–4000 DMS | 599 | 17 | 2·8% (1·7–4·5) |
| Oxcarbazepine | 75–4500 DMS | 333 | 10 | 3·0% (1·4–5·4) |
| Phenobarbital | 15–300 DMS | 294 | 19 | 6·5% (4·2–9·9) |
| Topiramate | 25–500 DMS | 152 | 6 | 3·9% (1·5–8·4) |
| Phenytoin | 30–730 DMS | 125 | 8 | 6·4% (2·8–12·2) |

*CI*, Confidence interval.

*From Tomson, T., Battino, D., Bonizzoni, E., Craig, J., Lindhout, D., Perucca, E., et al. 2018. Comparative risk of major congenital malformations with eight different antiepileptic drugs: A prospective cohort study of the EURAP registry. Lancet Neurol. 17, 530–538.* 

## Status Epilepticus

No special considerations exist during pregnancy when potentially fatal generalized convulsive status epilepticus is treated. Physicians agree that prompt application of a specific treatment regimen with which the physician is familiar generally assures the best chance of success. Monotherapy with phenobarbital or lorazepam/midazolam and combined therapies with phenytoin are effective. An Indian retrospective study identified the most common etiologies as eclampsia, posterior reversible encephalopathy syndrome, cortical venous thrombosis (CVT), subarachnoid hemorrhage and *N*-methyl-D-aspartate (NMDA) receptor antibody-mediated encephalitis. Six out of 10 women with refractory status epilepticus (60%) and five out of 10 fetuses (50%) had a good outcome (Rajiv et al., 2018).

## Common Advice and Management Strategy

For patients planning pregnancy, the need for AED therapy should be reevaluated before conception and valproic acid avoided if possible, particularly when employed as polytherapy. A consensus statement published by the AAN recommends that for a fertile woman taking valproic acid as monotherapy for epilepsy, avoidance of valproic acid may be considered during the first trimester (Harden et al., 2009c). Carbamazepine should be weaned in women with a family history of neural tube defects, particularly if there is a suitable substitute. The need for carbamazepine, phenytoin, and phenobarbital in particular may deserve reconsideration. Lamotrigine, levetiracetam, and oxcarbazepine are drugs least associated with major congenital malformation. When an AED is needed, monotherapy at the lowest effective dose is preferred. Serum levels while on that dose may be helpful when drawn before conception as part of a plan to monitor levels during gestation.

Once pregnancy has begun, discontinuing medications becomes problematic. A supplement to a practice parameter from the AAN states: "Although many of the recommendations in this parameter suggest minimizing AED exposure during pregnancy, for most women with epilepsy, discontinuing AEDs is not a reasonable or safe option" (Harden et al., 2009c).

Warning the patient about the effects of sleep deprivation and noncompliance with the drug regimen may be helpful when paired with a thorough description of the potential consequences of seizures and benefits of AEDs.

Physicians often monitor and adjust serum AED concentrations with increased frequency during gestation and the postpartum period. Some reviewers observe that lamotrigine levels drop more commonly during pregnancy and suggest that if there is a benefit to increased attention to AED levels, lamotrigine therapy might be most deserving of scrutiny. While individually variable, significant increased lamotrigine clearance can be seen as early as 5 weeks' gestation (Karanam et al., 2018). A review of available literature associated with a practice parameter (Harden et al., 2009a) provides a recommendation that monitoring of lamotrigine, carbamazepine, and phenytoin levels is reasonable. A small, preliminary study of 44 women taking levetiracetam, oxcarbazepine, topiramate, phenytoin and valproic acid found that levetiracetam, oxcarbazepeine, and topiramate levels also drop during pregnancy. This effect is notable for levetiracetam during the first trimester, and by the second trimester for oxcarbazepine and topiramate. Suggestions include defining a target dose for these medications before pregnancy with a goal of obtaining at least 65% of that target dose when blood levels are sampled during pregnancy (Voinescu et al., 2018b; Reisingeret al., 2013). When physicians target monitoring of lamotrigine and levetiracetam levels associated with prescription changes, doses increase. Investigators found that for lamotrigine, an increase of average dosing of 200 mg DMS can be expected from weeks 20–23 to weeks 24–27 and another 200 mg DMS increase during the following 4 weeks (28–31). For levetiracetam, average doses increased by approximately 500 mg DMS from weeks 16–19 to 20–23, and another 500 mg DMS change between weeks 23 and 31 (Makelky et al., 2018).

Women with epilepsy taking AEDs during gestation should be managed on an individual basis. During pregnancy, including after the period of organogenesis has passed, alteration of specific AED medication is likely to cause more harm than good. However, adjustment of medications to 65% at least of prepregnancy lowest effective levels may be helpful.

Women who take folic acid supplements before and during pregnancy lower their risk for delivering a child with major malformations. In addition, folic acid supplementation 4 weeks before gestation and throughout the first trimester for women taking AEDs is protective against childhood language delay (Husebye et al., 2018). The use of folic acid has become routine, but recommendations vary. The Department of Health in the United Kingdom and the Centers for Disease Control and Prevention in the United States have recommended, respectively, 5 and 4 mg of folic acid daily DMS for women who have had a child with a neural tube defect and 0.4 mg for all other women planning pregnancy. Anticonvulsants inhibit the absorption of folic acid. Occasionally, folic acid lowers anticonvulsant concentrations. Some investigators suggest that 5 mg of folic acid be given daily DMS to women treated with valproic acid or carbamazepine. Others recommend 2–4 mg DMS daily for all women with epilepsy who are taking anticonvulsants, beginning as long as 3 months before conception until 12 weeks' gestation. Folic acid supplementation may be particularly helpful for language development for children of women taking lamotrigine (Husebye et al., 2018).

In one study, women taking AEDs and a multiple vitamin supplement containing folic acid had no reduction in the risk to their infants for developing cardiovascular defects, oral clefts, or urinary tract defects compared with women who took no supplements (Hernandez-Diaz et al., 2000). One detailed review found "insufficient published information to address the dosing of folic acid and whether higher doses offer greater protective benefit" (Harden et al., 2009a). These reviewers concluded that offering women with epilepsy supplements of at least 0.4 mg of folic acid before pregnancy DMS "may be considered." A review of similar data recommended folic acid 0.4–0.8 mg DMS for all women capable of or planning pregnancy (U.S. Preventive Services Task Force, 2009). Compelling data demonstrate the beneficial effect of folic acid supplementation to reduce the incidence of neural tube defects (Fig. 112.5).

For patients taking AEDs during pregnancy, a second-trimester high-resolution ultrasound evaluation helps exclude spina bifida aperta, cardiac anomalies, and limb defects. When results of the ultrasound scan are inconclusive, consider amniocentesis and obtain α-fetoprotein and acetylcholinesterase concentrations.

A deficiency of vitamin K–dependent clotting factors occurs in some neonates born to women who take phenobarbital, primidone, carbamazepine, ethosuximide, or phenytoin. Although rarely reported, neonatal intracerebral hemorrhage may be attributable to a vitamin K deficiency. In an attempt to lower this risk, some physicians prescribe oral vitamin $K_1$ 10–20 mg daily beginning 2–4 weeks before expected delivery DMS and until birth. The American Academy of Pediatrics has recommended that physicians inject every newborn with 1 mg of vitamin $K_1$ intramuscularly DMS. When hemorrhage occurs, fresh frozen plasma corrects the hemorrhagic state acutely. Studies do not support the hypothesis that maternal enzyme–inducing AEDs increase the risk for bleeding in offspring. A literature review finds inadequate evidence to determine whether the newborns of women with epilepsy taking AEDs have an increased risk of hemorrhagic complications (Harden et al., 2009a). An accompanying practice parameter noted insufficient evidence to support or refute

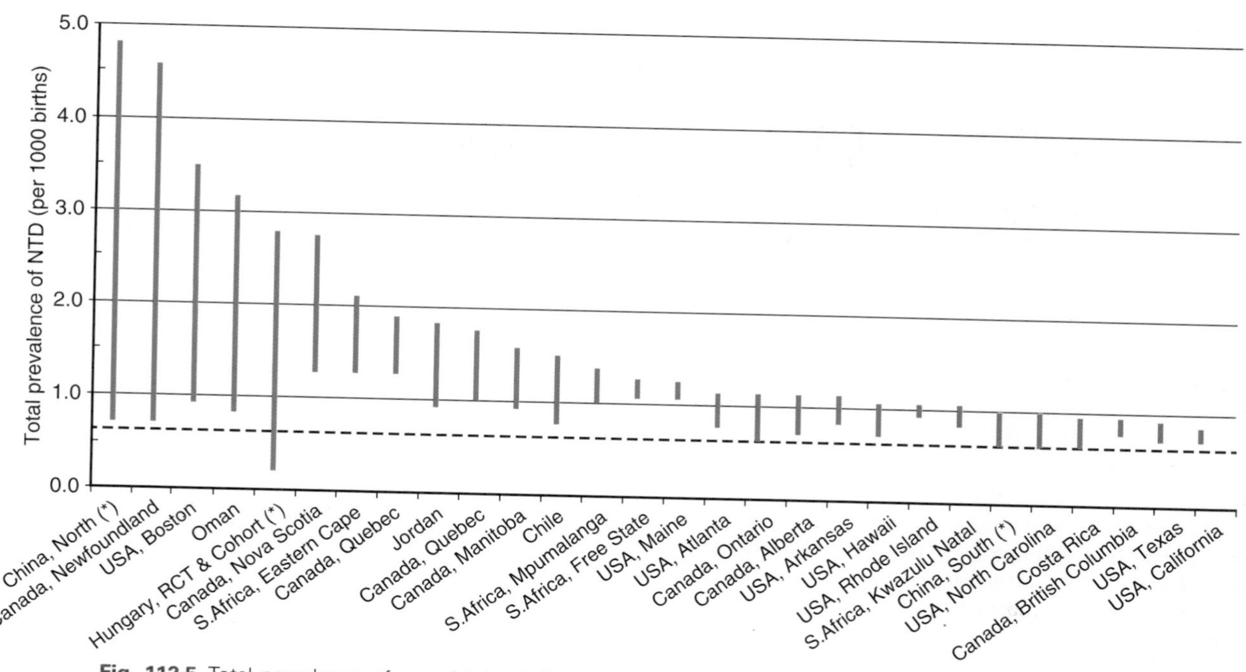


**Fig. 112.5** Total prevalence of neural tube defects (NTD) before and after the individual supplementation with folic acid or before and after the mandatory fortification in the country/region. Black lines: upper limit = total prevalence before the intervention, bottom limit = total prevalence after the intervention; *(*)* individual intervention trials, all the others: population interventions through mandatory folic acid fortification. (*From Mastroiacovo, P., Leoncini, E., 2011. More folic acid, the five questions: Why, who, when, how much, and how. Biofactors 37[4], 272–279.*)

a benefit of prenatal vitamin K supplementation (Harden et al., 2009b). A cohort study of 11,572 women found that use of liver enzyme-inducing AEDs in late pregnancy does not meaningfully increase the risks of bleeding complications, including postpartum and neonatal bleeding complications in clinical settings, where neonatal intramuscular vitamin K administration is standard of care (Panchaud et al., 2018).

Occasionally, seizures occur for the first time during pregnancy. Pregnancy has little effect on the use of diagnostic examinations and treatment considerations. The most common causes of seizures during childbearing years include idiopathic epilepsy, trauma, congenital defects, neoplasms, meningitis, intracerebral hemorrhage, and drug or alcohol toxicity. In addition, pregnancy predisposes women to certain epileptogenic conditions such as eclampsia, water intoxication, thrombotic thrombocytopenic purpura, sinus or CVT, and amniotic fluid embolus. Common iatrogenic causes of epilepsy include hyponatremia due to intravenous fluid infusion during the intrapartum period, and the use of epidural or parenteral anesthetics.

A single first-onset seizure resolving within minutes usually can be managed acutely without anticonvulsants. Once the physician determines the cause for the seizure and whether further seizures are likely, the need for anticonvulsant medication can be reviewed.

In general, breastfeeding is advised. Reviewing the latest manufacturer-provided information on breastfeeding with regard to a particular AED may be helpful in counseling parents with regard to the benefits of breastfeeding and the risks of a particular AED.

## CEREBROVASCULAR DISEASE

### Arteriovenous Malformations

The risk for repeat hemorrhage from a previously ruptured arteriovenous malformation (AVM) generally outweighs the risk from surgical excision or an obliterative procedure. Surgery can usually be performed shortly after the diagnosis is made and before pregnancy is considered. When performing proton-beam irradiation, some authorities advise women to wait 2 years before conception. The decision concerning management (excision, embolization, or irradiation) remains controversial. No specific therapeutic recommendation is available for patients planning pregnancy.

The risk for hemorrhage from an AVM (whether unruptured or previously ruptured) rises from a low point during childhood and teenage years to a higher risk during childbearing years. Whether pregnancy poses an additional risk remains uncertain. The best retrospective review suggests that risk for hemorrhage during pregnancy resulting from an unruptured AVM may be as low as 2.65%. This is probably no different from the risk to nonpregnant women with unruptured AVMs (Liu et al., 2014). Multiple pregnancies do not increase the rate of hemorrhage. A carefully constructed retrospective study using a different methodology suggests that the risk of hemorrhage from an unruptured AVM is increased during pregnancy to about 8.1% (Gross and Du, 2012) and may be as low as 1.1% annually outside pregnancy. Methodological difficulties continue to frustrate confident understanding. In the past, physicians routinely advised women with an AVM, previously ruptured or not, to avoid pregnancy. This conclusion from early retrospective studies indicated that 87% of AVMs rupture during pregnancy and that 25%–30% of initial ruptures are fatal. Subsequent analysis contradicted these dismal estimates. Still, we have no prospective studies. The clinician must exercise caution in interpreting this information.

Women whose AVM is repaired surgically can undergo vaginal delivery. Physicians usually perform cesarean section for incompletely repaired or partially treated previously ruptured AVMs. Epidural anesthesia is preferred.

### Intracranial Hemorrhage

Women presenting with pregnancy-associated stroke are as likely to have an infarct as an intracerebral hemorrhage. Compared with the nonpregnant state, intracerebral hemorrhage occurs 2.5 times more often during pregnancy and almost 30 times more often during the 6 weeks postpartum. Up to 44% of these hemorrhages are associated with eclampsia and preeclampsia. In France, nearly half of women with intracerebral hemorrhage associated with eclampsia die. Additional diagnostic considerations include vascular malformations (AVMs, aneurysms, and moyamoya disease), bleeding diatheses, cocaine toxicity, bacterial endocarditis, sickle cell disease, and metastatic choriocarcinoma. In approximately one-third of patients who have intracerebral hemorrhage, no specific cause is uncovered. The frequency of intracranial hemorrhage and its contributing causes is different in different populations (Jeng et al., 2004).

Subarachnoid hemorrhage is a common cause of nonobstetric maternal death. Hemorrhage from aneurysms and vascular malformations accounts for 25%–35% of intracranial hemorrhages. Management strategies are generally the same as those applied outside of pregnancy. Definitive therapy for AVMs may be postponed until after delivery while a more aggressive strategy may be considered for some patients, particularly when the AVM ruptures (Gross and Du, 2012). Surgery or obliterative therapy for an aneurysm usually is urgent. The effects of some treatment agents for subarachnoid hemorrhage (e.g., nimodipine) on the human fetus are not well studied. However, the potentially fatal consequences of vasospasm associated with subarachnoid hemorrhage make their use reasonable during pregnancy.

Anticonvulsants, specifically phenytoin, are unnecessary and ineffective in nongravid patients who have had an intracranial hemorrhage but have not had a seizure. Data during pregnancy are unavailable. Prophylactic anticonvulsants probably are best reserved for those women whose hemorrhage has caused a mass effect sufficient to increase the risk of cerebral herniation associated with sudden increase in intracranial pressure that sometimes occurs with a seizure. Anticonvulsant use is reasonable after a first convulsion.

Although many physicians recommend cesarean section for patients with gestational intracranial hemorrhage, mode of delivery did not affect outcome in the studies available. Vaginal delivery with epidural anesthesia is acceptable.

## Ischemic Stroke

Most women who have a stroke before gestation complete uneventful pregnancies with excellent outcomes (Coppage et al., 2004). A Chinese study found no difference in fetal outcomes when strokes occurred during pregnancy (Kang and Lin, 2010). Women with emboligenic cardiac disease, SLE, APS, or other coagulopathies have the added risk for stroke during pregnancy associated with those conditions. Stroke during one pregnancy by itself is not a risk factor for stroke in subsequent pregnancies. A review of a US national database found a stroke risk per 100,000 deliveries of 34.2 (9.2 for ischemic stroke, 8.5 for cerebral hemorrhage, 0.6 for CVT, and 15.9 for the category of "pregnancy-related cerebrovascular event") excluding subarachnoid hemorrhage. This same study suggests that the risk for gestational and peripartum stroke increases among women diagnosed with migraine, thrombophilia, SLE, heart disease, sickle cell disease, hypertension, thrombocytopenia, age over 35, being African American, and patients receiving blood transfusions (James et al., 2005). A Taiwanese study found increased stroke risk up to a year postpartum and a small increased risk with parity (Cheng et al., 2017). Cesarean delivery and gestational hypertension place women at increased risk for stroke.

Transitory neurological symptoms and preeclampsia are common during the pregnancies and puerperia of women with cerebral autosomal dominant arteriopathy with subcortical infarcts and leukoencephalopathy (CADASIL). For these women, there is no difference in the miscarriage rate, mode of delivery, neonatal birth weight, or Apgar score (Roine et al., 2005). Two-dimensional echocardiography may be the test of greatest importance when evaluating a woman with gestational stroke. CT and selective angiography are associated with a small risk to the fetus and require adequate shielding and hydration. Avoiding risks of x-irradiation may make magnetic resonance angiography preferable to selective angiography in the diagnosis of aneurysm, AVM, arteritis, venous thrombosis, or vasospasm (see Imaging section, earlier).

Eclampsia and preeclampsia are associated with approximately one-fourth of pregnancy-related infarcts in the United States and approximately half of such infarcts in France. In 25%–35% of patients suffering ischemic stroke, the cause remains unclear. In the remainder, the stroke is symptomatic of a systemic illness such as premature atherosclerosis, hypertension, cardiac disease, hyperlipidemia, diabetes, arterial dissection, Takayasu disease, vasculitis, APS, SLE, sickle cell disease, thrombotic thrombocytopenic purpura, CVT, coagulopathies, and tobacco use, cocaine use, and other drug use. Etiologies of stroke unique to pregnancy include choriocarcinoma, postpartum cerebral angiopathy, and postpartum cardiomyopathy. Stroke during labor or shortly after vaginal delivery may result from an amniotic fluid embolus. Air embolus to the heart, with subsequent generalized and focal cerebral ischemia, occurs with vaginal air insufflation during abortions performed outside medical standards, obstetric procedures including cesarean section, and orogenital sex.

A meta-analysis of stroke risk of women undergoing assisted reproductive technology (ART) found a trend toward increased risk of stroke with a pooled hazard ratio of 1.25 (Dayan et al., 2017). In a cohort study of women unable to conceive after ART, researchers noted a 21% annual relative increased risk of cardiovascular events independent of the number of treatment cycles (Udell et al., 2017). Both studies acknowledge methodological uncertainty and a need for further and confirmatory investigation. Theoretical pathophysiology for this effect includes the effect of drugs used in ART that result in ovarian hyperstimulation, subsequent imbalance in renin–angiotensin, and blood pressure dysregulation.

### Ischemic Stroke Prophylaxis

The use of aspirin at a low dose (60–150 mg/day) DMS throughout pregnancy is demonstrably safe in the second and third trimesters. No longitudinal studies have confirmed the efficacy of aspirin in preventing stroke during pregnancy. The safety and efficacy of clopidogrel and ticlopidine are unknown during pregnancy, and their use is not advisable.

The American Heart Association and American Stroke Association issued a consensus guideline (Bushnell et al., 2014) based in part on a meta-analysis of aspirin use in pregnancy in 2007, recommending that "women with chronic primary or secondary hypertension or previous pregnancy-related hypertension should take low-dose aspirin DMS from the twelfth week of gestation until delivery." These same groups also recommend calcium supplementation to reduce risk for preeclampsia based on a literature review that found calcium supplementation to approximately halve the risk of preeclampsia, stating that "calcium supplementation (of ≥1 g/day, orally DMS) should be considered for women with low dietary intake of calcium (<600 mg/day) to prevent preeclampsia." The International Society for the Study of Hypertension in Pregnancy expanded and specified these suggestions, recommending that those women with strong clinical risks for preeclampsia (prior preeclampsia, chronic hypertension, pregestational diabetes mellitus, maternal body mass index >30 kg/m$^2$, antiphospholipid syndrome, and receipt of ART) receive low-dose aspirin (75–162 mg/day) DMS, ideally before 16 weeks but definitely before 20 weeks, to prevent preterm (before 37 weeks' gestation) preeclampsia, supplemented with calcium (1.2–2.5 g/day) DMS when dietary intake of calcium is less than 600 mg/day (Brown et al., 2018). In part, these recommendations are based on a placebo-controlled study demonstrating effectiveness of aspirin at a dose of 150 mg daily until 36 weeks' gestation DMS in reducing the occurrence of preterm preeclampsia from 4.3% to 1.6%. No difference between neonatal adverse outcomes or other adverse events were noted between the groups. The authors justify their use of the dose of 150 mg, in part noting that the commonly used dose of 81 mg of aspirin per day has no appreciable effect on platelet function in up to one-third of pregnant women. Aspirin administration was recommended at night, rather than during the day (Rolhick et al., 2017).

### Acute Stroke Treatment

Selim and Molina (2013) clarify that the pregnant state is different from the nonpregnant state in that several conditions in pregnancy commonly cause stroke symptoms that are less likely or unlikely to respond to acute stroke therapy, including preeclampsia/eclampsia amniotic fluid embolism, and, additionally, the reversible cerebral vasoconstriction syndrome. Prenatal exposure to radiation and contrast agents associated with endovascular thrombolysis may damage the fetus.

Data to justify thrombolytic therapy for stroke during pregnancy are unimpressive. While very limited quantities cross the placenta due to its large molecular weight, intravenous tissue plasminogen activator (tPA) carries theoretically significant but unexplored potential risks for the fetus (Murugappan et al., 2006). Pregnant women were excluded from randomized trials on thrombolytics. The basis for thrombolytic use in this group lies in case reports, generalization from data obtained in the nonpregnant state, and the use of tPA during pregnancy for illnesses other than stroke. Current information does not justify a claim that tPA benefits the pregnant woman, the fetus, or can be considered indicated during pregnancy. Missing is a trial that demonstrates that pregnant women receiving tPA by protocol, particularly in later months, do better clinically than those not receiving tPA, and that the fetal outcomes of pregnancy are either equivalent or, if negative, are outweighed by maternal benefit. As a result, the use of tPA during pregnancy continues to be controversial.

A registry study found that physicians employ tPA uncommonly in both the pregnant and postpartum state, despite the 2015 removal of both tPA and obstetric delivery from package labeling as warnings concerning its use (Leffert et al., 2016). In this context, the American Heart Association/American Stroke Association indicated that "IV alteplase administration may be considered in pregnancy when the anticipated benefits of treating moderate or severe stroke outweigh the anticipated increased risks of uterine bleeding" with the support for this statement described as "weak" (Powers et al., 2018). Authors suggest that women at particularly high risk of hemorrhage (e.g., with placenta previa or a previous obstetric hemorrhage) may be better served by prompt catheter-based reperfusion therapy (e.g., thrombectomy) if eligible, rather than treatment with intravenous tPA (Leffert et al., 2016).

Guidelines from the American Heart Association/American Stroke Association do not recommend a specific time interval after cesarean section or vaginal delivery before considering the use of thrombolytics to be safe. Relevant advice within this guideline details that tPA is relatively contraindicated within 14 days of a surgical procedure and within 21 days after bleeding from urinary or gastrointestinal hemorrhage (poorly compressible sites) (Powers et al., 2018). Emergency cesarean section for a pregnant woman shortly following tPA may be problematic.

## Antiphospholipid Antibody Syndrome

Women with circulating antiphospholipid antibodies (APAs) and without a history of pregnancy loss do not require treatment to prevent stroke during pregnancy. Successful pregnancies without treatment are common. Routine screening of asymptomatic patients for APAs is not recommended. Women with very high antibody titers, habitual first-trimester abortion, a single miscarriage in the later trimesters, or a symptomatic APS, particularly with previous stroke, usually receive treatment. Various studies have examined the use of monotherapy or polytherapy in widely ranging doses and combinations of aspirin, prednisone, subcutaneous unfractionated heparin (UFH), IVIG, hydroxychloroquine, and occasionally placebo. Studies on low-molecular-weight heparin (LMWH) are optimistic but incomplete. Stroke in women with symptomatic antiphospholipid antibody syndrome (APS) may occur at doses of heparin sufficient to produce a usually therapeutic serological anticoagulation effect. Some researchers advise women seriously ill with APS to avoid pregnancy. Others more specifically advise that APS patients should delay pregnancy if they have experienced a thrombotic event within 6 months, and should avoid pregnancy in the presence of uncontrolled hypertension or severe pulmonary hypertension (Taylor et al., 2017). When APS becomes catastrophic during pregnancy, some researchers suggest that triple therapy may be reasonable (Hoayek et al., 2016) (Table 112.5).

**TABLE 112.5 Revised Classification Criteria for Antiphospholipid Syndrome***

| Criteria | |
|---|---|
| ***Clinical*** | |
| Pregnancy morbidity | One or more unexplained deaths of a fetus at or beyond the 10th week of gestation with normal fetal morphology documented by ultrasound or direct examination, or<br>One or more premature births of a morphologically normal neonate before 34 weeks' gestation secondary to preeclampsia with severe features, eclampsia, or placental insufficiency (IUGR, abnormal or nonreassuring fetal surveillance tests, oligohydramnios), or<br>Three or more unexplained, consecutive spontaneous abortions before the 10th week of gestation with maternal anatomical and hormonal abnormalities excluded |
| Vascular thrombosis | One or more clinical episodes of arterial, venous, or small-vessel thrombosis in any tissue or organ without significant evidence of inflammation in the vessel wall on histopathological diagnosis |
| ***Laboratory*** | |
| Lupus anticoagulant | Present on 2 or more occasions at least 12 weeks apart |
| Anticardiolipin antibody | IgM and/or IgG in serum or plasma on 2 or more occasions, at least 12 weeks apart, measured by standardized ELISA. Must be in titer >99th percentile |
| Anti-beta2-glycoprotein-I antibody | IgM anchor IgG in serum or plasma present on 2 or more occasions, at least 12 weeks apart, measured by standardized ELISA. Must be in titer >99th percentile |

*Must have 1 clinical criterion and 1 laboratory criterion to make the diagnosis.

*ELISA*, Enzyme-linked immunosorbent assay; *IgG*, immunoglobulin G; *IgM*, immunoglobulin M; *IUGR*, intrauterine growth restriction.

*From Taylor, D., Fuchs, A. Ashmead, G., 2017. Antiphospholipid syndrome in pregnancy. Top. Obstetrics and Gynecology. 37(15), 1–5; based on criteria from an international consensus agreement in 2006 (Miyakis, S., Lockshin, M.D., Atsumi, T., Branch, D.W., Brey, R.L., Cervera, R., et al. 2006. International consensus statement on an update of the classification criteria for definite antiphospholipid syndrome (APS). Journal of Thrombosis and Haemostasis 4[2], 295–306).*

## Peripartum Stroke

Debate continues over classification of syndromes described as postpartum cerebral angiopathy, delayed peripartum vasculopathy, posterior reversible leukoencephalopathy syndrome (PRES), reversible cerebral vasoconstriction syndrome, or postpartum stroke. These patients present with peripartum or puerperal focal neurological signs and symptoms, often with headache, and have hypertension without edema or proteinuria. Brain MRI scanning depicts ischemia primarily in the parieto-occipital region, and angiography commonly demonstrates vasospasm. The course often is benign, but permanent deficits may occur. When these occurrences include headache, altered sensorium, seizures, or visual loss without hemorrhage, consider the possibility of a reversible posterior leukoencephalopathy syndrome (RPLS). Other authors might suggest the diagnostic consideration of a reversible segmental cerebral vasoconstriction (RSCV) syndrome (see Chapter 65), particularly when vasospasm demonstrated by arteriography involves large blood vessels within the circle of Willis (Singhal et al., 2009). Patients have been treated with calcium channel antagonists, corticosteroids, and antihypertensive medication. Although the condition also resolves spontaneously, 5%–12% of patients may have a fulminant course. Some researchers believe peripartum stroke is a form of eclampsia/preeclampsia and suggest relaxation of requirements for diagnosis of eclampsia/preeclampsia. Researchers in Mexico found that half of patients with eclampsia showed signs of PRES on imaging studies (Camara-Lemarroy et al., 2017). Given such a hypothesis, it follows that these authors treat patients with RSCV who have suffered seizures with magnesium sulfate, and in their analysis, note a trend toward poorer outcomes in those patients treated with glucocorticoids.

Primary angiitis of the central nervous system presenting with stroke is less commonly associated with pregnancy than the cerebral vasoconstriction syndromes noted. It is associated with milder headache or none at all, but with abnormal CSF in 80%–90% of patients with pleocytosis and elevated protein. Confirmation is through biopsy and less commonly through diagnostic arteriography, which may have difficulty visualizing the disease of the small blood vessels that characterizes this condition. Prompt treatment with cyclophosphamide and prednisone is recommended (Birnbaum and Hellmann, 2009).

In one case series, Witlin et al. (2000) characterized postpartum stroke as an uncommon and unpreventable complication of pregnancy. After excluding trauma, neoplasm, infection, or eclampsia, they described women suffering ischemic or hemorrhagic stroke without specific warning; hemorrhage may follow initial ischemia with injury to blood vessel walls. In general, these events were most common around the eighth day after delivery (range 3–35 days) and were associated with cesarean delivery. Seizures in half of these patients, an increase in mean arterial pressure to 1.5 times above baseline, and headache heralded the onset. Two of 20 patients died of severe intracerebral hemorrhage. Included in this series were patients with CVT and a ruptured AVM. The investigators postulated that the hypercoagulable or thrombophilic state of pregnancy may emerge as a major risk factor, perhaps interacting with underlying coagulopathies.

## Cerebral Venous Thrombosis

Aseptic thrombosis of the cerebral venous system, in its most obvious clinical state, presents with puerperal headache that worsens over several days, a change in behavior or personality, convulsive seizures, and neurological deficits. The patient may be emotionally regressed, anxious, or lethargic, with mild to obvious neurological signs and (occasionally) papilledema. Initial symptoms generally begin 1 day to 4 weeks postpartum and peak in occurrence at 7–14 days postpartum.

CVT has been associated with hypercoagulable states, infection, sickle cell disease, dehydration, and ulcerative colitis, in addition to gestation. Women diagnosed with peripartum CVT have no known increased risk for CVT in subsequent pregnancies. Differential diagnoses include eclampsia, meningitis, and cerebral mass. A large Swedish cohort study indicated that CVT was the most common cerebrovascular disorder of women in the period between 2 days before and 1 day after delivery. The standardized incidence rate ratio increased about 115-fold for CVT, 95-fold for intracerebral hemorrhage, 47-fold for subarachnoid hemorrhage, and 34-fold for cerebral infarction. Rates between 2 days post delivery and 6 weeks postpartum continued elevated: 15-fold for CVT, 12-fold for intracerebral hemorrhage, 8.3-fold for cerebral infarction, and 1.8-fold for subarachnoid hemorrhage (Salonen Ros et al., 2001).

Brain MRI scanning with magnetic resonance venography is the initial imaging procedure of choice. Although it detects occlusion of major sinuses with high sensitivity, when smaller veins are involved, detection may be more difficult. The MRI may show multiple small infarcts involving the gray and white matter, sometimes with minor hemorrhage. More sensitive CT venography may be considered in some patients when potential benefits outweigh the risks of radiation and intravenous contrast. Digital subtraction and selective angiography/venography remain additional options.

Geographic location influences the frequency of CVT. India reports a high rate of puerperal CVT, estimated at 400–500 per 100,000 births. This high rate is primarily attributable to dehydration and has a predilection for women delivering at home. Incidence in the United States is comparatively low, approximately 9 per 100,000 deliveries. CVT associated with pregnancy is relatively more benign than that occurring without pregnancy. Researchers in Mexico describe a mortality rate of approximately 10% for gestational CVT and 33% for CVT not associated with pregnancy. In the United States, estimates of the mortality rate of CVT from all causes suggest that approximately one of ten patients dies. However, death did not occur in a national survey of 4454 patients with peripartum CVT in the United States. Cesarean section and age older than 25 are risk factors for CVT, while preeclampsia and eclampsia are not (Cantu-Brito et al., 2010).

Researchers find APAs and diminished activity of protein S in women with gestational and puerperal CVT. Occasionally, multiple defects in coagulation occur in the same woman. Current theory suggests that levels of proteins such as C4b-binding protein increase during pregnancy and the puerperium, creating a hypercoagulable state. Some women have conditions that predispose them to hypercoagulation during pregnancy, such as activated protein C resistance (factor V Leiden mutation), protein S deficiency, or antithrombin III antibodies. Homocystinuria (hyperhomocysteinemia) may increase risk. Serological testing that may be beneficial includes protein C, protein S, antithrombin deficiency, antiphospholipid syndrome, prothrombin G20210A mutation, and factor V Leiden. Generally, testing for protein C, protein S, and antithrombin deficiency is indicated 2–4 weeks after completion of anticoagulation therapy.

While pregnancy and the puerperal state may carry a more benign prognosis for CVT, current guidelines describe an aggressive approach as reasonable for all patients. During both pregnancy and the puerperium, anticoagulation with low-molecular-weight heparin (LMWH) in full anticoagulant doses is recommended regardless of the presence of intracerebral hemorrhage, which may occur in nearly half the patients (Einhäupl et al., 2010; Saposnik et al., 2011). LMWH is not associated with teratogenesis, in contrast to UFH. Full anticoagulation with LMWH should be initiated and continued throughout pregnancy, holding for labor and delivery, commonly for 24 hours before resuming LMWH or beginning warfarin for at least 6 weeks, corresponding to a total treatment duration of 3–6 months in some recommendations (Bousser and Crassard, 2012) and 6 months in others (Saposnik et al., 2011). When an underlying disorder such as APS is diagnosed, the therapeutic approach would be modified appropriately. Endovascular thrombolysis may be considered if deterioration occurs despite intensive anticoagulation treatment. Short-term anticonvulsants are recommended after a first seizure, but not before then. Steroids are not recommended unless used to treat another underlying disease. Future use of contraceptives containing estrogen for these patients is contraindicated. The patient can be reassured that recurrence of CVT in future pregnancies is low (Mehraein et al., 2003) and additional venous thrombotic events are rare (Aguiar de Sousa et al., 2017). Outcomes of future pregnancies are overwhelmingly good. A lukewarm recommendation for LMWH in future pregnancies can be considered (Saposnik et al., 2011).

## ECLAMPTIC ENCEPHALOPATHY

Preeclampsia develops in approximately 4%–8% of pregnancies in prospective studies. Increasing longitudinal incidence has been attributed to an increase in maternal age, obesity, assisted reproductive techniques, and illness such as diabetes, hypertension, and renal disease that predispose to preeclampsia. Migraine (Wabnitz and Bushnell, 2015) and snoring (Kordi et al., 2018) may be additional risk factors. Eclampsia accounts for nearly half of intracranial hemorrhages and nearly half of cerebral infarcts in pregnancy and puerperium in French hospitals. In the United States, the figures are lower (14% and 24%, respectively). Methodological problems plague these studies, and accurate estimates are difficult to obtain. Neurological symptoms are more likely when the onset of eclampsia is postpartum. Maternal morbidity and mortality increase when eclampsia occurs at 32 weeks' gestation. Preeclampsia increases the risk for stroke occurring over 42 days, postpartum by about 60% (Brown et al., 2006). In Mexico, preeclampsia and eclampsia are not risk factors for developing CVT (Cantu-Brito et al., 2010), but toxemia and CVT are described together in case reports.

### Nomenclature and Classification

Preeclampsia (toxemia gravidarum) and eclampsia remain the principal causes of maternal perinatal morbidity and death. Attempts to subsume these disorders as a vascular disorder in pregnancy or hypertensive disorder of pregnancy are frustrated by incomplete understanding of the disease pathogenesis. Definitions of preeclampsia continue to evolve. Edema, proteinuria, and hypertension after 20 weeks' gestation characterize the classic syndrome of preeclampsia. Epileptic seizures and this preeclamptic triad constitute the syndrome of eclampsia. Defining the terms *preeclampsia* and *eclampsia* in this way simplifies a complex disorder. Important and common manifestations such as hepatic hemorrhage, disseminated intravascular coagulation, abruptio placentae, pulmonary edema, papilledema, oliguria, headache, hyperreflexia, hallucinations, and blindness seem relatively neglected in this definition. Occasionally, eclamptic seizures may precede the clinical triad of preeclampsia. Reasoning that pedal edema is ubiquitous and nonspecific during pregnancy, a consensus group recommended that physicians exclude edema as a criterion for the diagnosis of preeclampsia and concluded that the dyad of hypertension and proteinuria is sufficient, more sensitive, and no less specific (National High Blood Pressure Education Program Working Group, 2000). Continuing along this parsimonious path, the ACOG eliminated the requirement for proteinuria in 2013 and indicated: "In recognition of the syndromic nature of preeclampsia, the task force has eliminated the dependence of the diagnosis on proteinuria. In the absence of proteinuria, preeclampsia is diagnosed as hypertension in association with thrombocytopenia (platelet count less than 100,000/μL), impaired liver function (elevated blood levels of liver transaminases to twice the normal concentration), the new development of renal insufficiency (elevated serum creatinine greater than 1.1 mg/dL or a doubling of serum creatinine in the absence of other renal disease), pulmonary edema, or new-onset cerebral or visual disturbances. . . . *Gestational hypertension* is blood pressure elevation greater than or equal to 140 mm Hg systolic or greater than or equal to 90 mm Hg diastolic on two occasions at least 4 hours apart after 20 weeks' gestation in the absence of proteinuria or the aforementioned systemic findings, while *chronic hypertension* is hypertension that predates pregnancy, and *superimposed preeclampsia* is chronic hypertension in association with preeclampsia" (ACOG, 2013).

ACOG and other groups also abandon previous definitions of "severe" preeclampsia, given that the syndrome can worsen abruptly, without predictive value in labeling it as "not severe." Instead, preeclampsia is described with or without severe features (Table 112.6).

### Pathogenesis

A specific laboratory test for this disorder is lacking, and understanding of the pathogenesis remains incomplete. Conditions considered to place women at added risk for preeclampsia include multifetal gestations, previous preeclampsia, diabetes mellitus, hypercoagulable states, advanced age, dyslipidemia, microalbuminuria, APS, obesity, and chronic hypertension. While some studies indicate increased risk of fetal growth restriction, spontaneous abortion, ectopic pregnancy, placenta previa, and fetal death in women who smoke during pregnancy,

**TABLE 112.6 Clinical Characteristics for the Diagnosis of Preeclampsia**

| Features | Definition |
|---|---|
| Hypertension | • Systolic ≥140 mm Hg; or diastolic ≥90 mm Hg after 20 weeks' gestation |
| Accompanied by one or more of the following: | |
| Proteinuria | • ≥300 mg of protein in 24 h urine collection or spot urine protein/creatinine ratio ≥30 mg/mmol or "2+" on dipstick testing (equivalent to ≥1 g/L) |
| Other maternal organ dysfunction | • Renal insufficiency (creatinine ≥90 μmol/L; 1.02 mg/dL)<br>• Liver involvement (elevated transaminases—at least twice upper limit of normal ± upper right quadrant or epigastric abdominal pain)<br>• Neurological complications (examples include eclampsia, altered mental status, blindness, stroke, hyperreflexia accompanied by clonus, severe headaches accompanied by hyperreflexia, persistent visual scotomata)<br>• Hematological complications (thrombocytopenia—platelet count below 150,000/dL, disseminated intravascular coagulation, hemolysis) |
| Uteroplacental dysfunction | • Fetal growth restriction (failure to achieve full growth potential in utero)<br>• Abnormal Doppler ultrasound findings |

*Adapted from the International Society for the Study of Hypertension in Pregnancy Statement: From Yong, H.E., Murthi, P., Brennecke, S.P., Moses, E.K., 2018. Genetic approaches in preeclampsia. In: Preeclampsia. Humana Press, Edts. Murthi, P., Vaillancourt, C. New York, NY, pp. 53–72.*

several studies paradoxically suggest that smoking reduces the risks of eclampsia and gestational hypertension (Yang et al., 2006).

Geneticists associate preeclampsia with a molecular variant of the angiotensinogen gene and suggest a possible genetic predisposition. Candidate genes include the *STOX1* and *ACVR2A*. A relationship to metabolic syndrome has been suggested (Yong, 2018). Some researchers postulate that damage to the fetal-placental vascular unit (e.g., defective placentation) may release products toxic to the endothelium, causing diffuse vasospasm and organ injury. Researchers point to soluble FMS-like tyrosine kinase 1 (sFlt1), a substance produced in toxic amounts by the placenta and implicated in reducing levels of angiogenic trophic factors such as vascular endothelial growth factor and placental growth factor. Lack of these trophic factors may result in the clinical and pathological syndrome of preeclampsia. Additional research efforts point to altered regulation of immune-cell populations such as decidual natural killer cells as potential therapeutic targets (Zhang et al., 2018). Short intervals between pregnancies reduce the risk for preeclampsia. No theory satisfactorily explains the tendency for preeclampsia or eclampsia to affect primarily young primigravid women.

At autopsy of patients who died of eclampsia, pathologists find cerebral edema; hypertensive encephalopathy; subarachnoid, subcortical, and petechial hemorrhages; and infarction of multiple areas of the brain and brainstem. The occipital lobes, parietal lobes, and watershed areas are most vulnerable. Although any of these lesions may cause seizures, the patient may not have a seizure. This observation has led to criticism that the definition of eclampsia solely based on a seizure is too restrictive.

Two theories compete to explain the genesis of the cerebral lesions. Elevated blood pressure may overcome protection usually provided by the precapillary arteriolar sphincter. Loss of autoregulation then leads to rupture of fragile capillaries, resulting in ring hemorrhages and thrombosis. Alternatively, diffuse cerebral endothelial dysfunction may precipitate generalized cerebral vasospasm, producing the same pathological changes.

One review observed that many women diagnosed with preeclampsia or eclampsia had, in retrospect, clinical features most consistent with other diseases. These included cerebral arterial infarction, hypertensive encephalopathy, and CVT. Eagerness to diagnose toxemia, possibly because of the rate at which the condition naturally presents, may overestimate its incidence in epidemiological studies. The neurologist must consider alternative diagnoses carefully.

Gestational hypertension (blood pressure elevation without additional elements of organ injury) complicates 6% of pregnancies. Within this group are women suffering from unrecognized chronic hypertension and transient hypertension of pregnancy. One-quarter of them will develop preeclampsia/eclampsia. Mild transitory hypertension does not affect mother or fetus. When the physician discovers end-organ damage associated with gestational hypertension, the patient is treated according to the recommendations for preeclampsia. When proteinuria (>300 mg per 24 hours) accompanies gestational hypertension, physicians may diagnose preeclampsia; although this definition has not been substantiated by research, it is commonly used.

Approximately 4%–14% of women with preeclampsia develop a syndrome called *HELLP*, an acronym for hemolysis, elevated liver enzyme levels, and low platelets. All three components must be present. Hemolysis is detectable by an abnormal peripheral blood smear, a bilirubin level of 1.2 mg/dL, or a lactate dehydrogenase level of 600 IU/L. Liver enzyme levels are elevated when aspartate aminotransferase is two times normal. A platelet count of less than $100 \times 10^3/\mu L$ is low. HELLP syndrome results from severe injury to vascular endothelium and is associated with a high rate of maternal and fetal injury. Patients complain of malaise, nausea, right upper quadrant pain, and vomiting. Occasionally, HELLP syndrome presents without preeclampsia. Debate continues whether to consider HELLP to be separable from or, as it is commonly seen, another expression of preeclampsia.

## Management

Preeclampsia can be prevented. The International Society for the Study of Hypertension in Pregnancy expanded and specified suggestions from the American Heart Association and American Stroke Association consensus guideline (Bushnell et al., 2014), recommending that those women with strong clinical risks for preeclampsia (prior preeclampsia, chronic hypertension, pregestational diabetes mellitus, maternal body mass index >30 kg/m$^2$, antiphospholipid syndrome, and receipt of ART) receive low-dose aspirin (75–162 mg/day) DMS, ideally before 16 weeks but definitely before 20 weeks to prevent preterm (before 37 weeks' gestation) preeclampsia; and supplementation with calcium (1.2–2.5 g/day) DMS when dietary intake of calcium is less than 600 mg/day (Brown et al., 2018). In part, these recommendations are based on a placebo-controlled study demonstrating effectiveness of aspirin at a dose of 150 mg daily DMS until 36 weeks' gestation in reducing the occurrence of preterm preeclampsia from 4.3 to 1.6%. No difference between neonatal adverse outcomes or other adverse events were noted between the groups. The authors justify their use of the dose of 150 mg DMS, in part noting that the commonly used dose of 81 mg of aspirin per day DMS has no appreciable effect on platelet function in up to one-third of pregnant women, and that the aspirin dose was recommended to be taken at night, rather than during the day (Rolnick et al., 2017). Folic acid supplementation 4 mg daily DMS after the first trimester is ineffective in reducing preeclampsia in at-risk populations (Wen et al., 2018) and vitamin D supplementation also is without benefit (Purswani et al., 2017).

Women diagnosed with preeclampsia require careful fetal monitoring (ACOG, 2002). When hypertension is severe (systolic pressure of 160 mm Hg or diastolic pressure of 105–110 mm Hg), consensus groups recommend methyldopa, labetalol, and nifedipine as safe and effective, and recommend that these medications be considered when blood pressure elevation is moderate (Bushnell et al., 2014). Atenolol, angiotensin receptor blockers, and direct renin inhibitors are described as contraindicated. A Cochrane Review found that treating mild to moderate hypertension reduces the risk of severe hypertension during pregnancy by half. Unfortunately, that treatment did not translate into positive outcomes such as reduced incidence of preeclampsia or fetal/maternal mortality rates. When treatment for mild to moderate hypertension is desired, calcium channel blockers and beta-blockers seem best (Abalos et al., 2018).

Eclampsia, preeclampsia with severe accompanying features, or HELLP syndrome require definitive therapy. Commonly, delivery is performed within 24–48 hours of presentation, and all gestational products are removed from the uterus by vaginal or cesarean delivery. Experts offer plans of expectant management for women able to tolerate additional time to allow fetal lung maturation and stabilization before delivery (Haddad and Sibai, 2005; O'Brien and Barton, 2005).

Parenteral magnesium sulfate is used extensively to treat symptoms of preeclampsia with severe features and eclampsia while the woman awaits delivery. In a large clinical trial, women presenting for delivery with hypertension were given either phenytoin or magnesium sulfate. Among the women receiving magnesium sulfate, fewer developed seizures. In a separate analysis of women with eclampsia, magnesium sulfate therapy reduced recurrent seizures better than regimens using either diazepam or phenytoin. The mechanism of action remains unclear. The most coherent theory suggests that magnesium sulfate affects the pathogenesis of cerebral disease, resulting in a secondary effect on the seizures. Alternatively, the anticonvulsant action may be mediated through magnesium sulfate's role as an NMDA antagonist. Usually, drug therapy continues for a day after delivery. About 10% of patients with an eclamptic seizure will have additional seizures, prompting the use of additional medication. AEDs commonly used to prevent and control eclamptic seizures include barbiturates, phenytoin, and benzodiazepines.

For some women, thrombocytopenic purpura and hemolytic-uremic syndrome may be seen with, or may complicate, toxemia and HELLP syndrome. Death and severe neurological disease are common. Survival may improve with the use of plasma transfusion and plasmapheresis.

## Future Risks Associated With Preeclampsia

Researchers found that offspring of preeclamptic women born in Helsinki, Finland, between 1934 and 1944 experienced an almost doubled risk for stroke during adulthood (Kajantie et al., 2009). A United States study estimated a hazards ratio of 1.3 (Miller et al., 2018). In Denmark, offspring of preeclamptic women have an increased risk of epilepsy—particularly when the infant is born post-term rather than preterm—varying with the severity of toxemia, from an incidence rate ratio of 1.16–5 times that expected (Wu et al., 2008).

In Denmark, vascular dementia was 3.46 times more common in women with a history of preeclampsia (Basit et al., 2018). In the United States, minor impairments in performance on tests of long-term cognitive function of women with preeclampsia were driven by metabolic and psychosocial factors rather than an independent effect of preeclampsia (Dayan et al., 2018).

These predictive studies enforce a redoubling of efforts towards improving the control of already known risk factors for stroke in these women and their offspring and emphasize the importance of preventing and treating preeclampsia. A cohort study of teachers found a potential beneficial effect of aspirin but not statins in reducing future stroke risk in women with hypertensive disorders during pregnancy and under the age of 60. Despite the size of the study, methodological limitations led authors to call for a randomized, controlled trial to establish the efficacy of prophylactic aspirin in this group of women (Miller et al., 2018) and an accompanying editorial describes the results as too preliminary to guide clinical decision making (Feske and Bushnell, 2019).

*The complete reference list is available online at https://expertconsult.inkling.com/.* 

113

# Functional and Dissociative Neurological Symptoms and Disorders

*Jon Stone, Alan Carson*

## OUTLINE



This chapter brings together an integrated clinical approach for the patient who presents with a functional or dissociative (psychogenic) neurological disorder that is with symptoms that are inconsistent or incongruent with recognized neurological disease. We focus on the most common symptoms presenting to neurologists: blackouts, weakness, sensory disturbance, and movement disorders. We discuss scientific advances in understanding the etiology and mechanisms of these symptoms and how these lead naturally to new approaches to treatment. However, our primary aim is to give practical clinical advice to the neurologist struggling with an often challenging clinical situation.

## TERMINOLOGY

Terminology in this area is problematic and reflects many different ways of conceptualizing and approaching the problem. There is no perfect solution here. The term to use will depend not only on how the cause of these symptoms is seen but also may depend on how the individual neurologist wishes to communicate the diagnosis to the patient (discussed later).

### Psychiatric Terminology

- *Conversion disorder (functional neurological symptom disorder)* is the term used in in the Diagnostic and Statistical Manual of Mental Disorders, 5th Edition (DSM-5), the American Psychiatric Association's classification system for mental disorders. The name still retains the Freudian idea that intolerable psychological conflict leads to the conversion of distress into physical symptoms, but the new criteria are simpler and require only (a) the presence of a motor or sensory symptom, (b) positive evidence of inconsistency or incongruity with disease (such as the Hoover sign), (c) the disorder to not be better explained by a neurological disease (although one may be present), and (d) distress or impairment. Psychological factors are no longer required to be judged as being "associated with the symptom onset" in recognition of the fact that in many patients no identifiable recent stressor is present. The conversion hypothesis is currently just one of many competing hypotheses trying to explain these symptoms and is often an unsatisfactory model in clinical practice (Stone et al., 2011). (For the full DSM-5 diagnostic criteria for conversion disorder, see Box 113.1.)
- *Dissociative seizure/motor disorder* (conversion disorder) (International Classification of Diseases, 10th Revision [ICD-10] F44.4–9 and ICD-11 6B60) suggests dissociation as an important mechanism in symptom production. Dissociation encompasses a variety of symptoms in which there is a lack of integration or connection of normal conscious functions. The difficulty is that not all patients with functional symptoms describe dissociative symptoms (see General Advice in History Taking, later).
- *Somatization disorder* (DSM-IV 300.81) was a term applied to a patient with a history of symptoms unexplained by disease, starting before the age of 30. The definition in DSM-IV required at least one neurological symptom, four pain symptoms, two gastrointestinal symptoms, and one sexual symptom. Somatization disorder has essentially been eliminated from DSM-5, although the concept of someone with a lifelong vulnerability to functional disorders remains clinically useful.
- *Somatic symptom disorder* replaced somatization disorder in the DSM-5, with the major distinction that it was irrelevant whether the somatic symptom had a basis in pathophysiological disease. The emphasis instead being on "Excessive thoughts, feelings, and/or behaviors related to these somatic symptoms or associated health concerns." However, early signs are that this phrase will quickly

become synonymous with somatization, despite the intentions of the authors.

- *Illness anxiety disorder* describes excessive and intrusive health anxiety about the possibility of serious disease, which the patient has trouble controlling. Typically, the patient seeks repeated medical reassurance, which only has a short-lived effect. Health anxiety (previously called hypochondriasis) is often present to varying degrees in patients with psychogenic/functional symptoms but may be completely absent.
- *Factitious disorder* (DSM-5) describes symptoms that are consciously fabricated for the purpose of medical care or other non-financial gain, in distinction to functional disorders which are genuine..
- *Munchausen syndrome* describes someone with factitious disorder who wanders between hospitals, typically changing their name and story. There is a strong association with severe personality disorder.
- *Malingering* is not a psychiatric diagnosis but describes the deliberate fabrication of symptoms for material gain.

**BOX 113.1 DSM-5 Diagnostic Criteria: Conversion Disorder and ICD-10-CM codes (Functional Neurological Symptom Disorder)**

**DSM-5 Diagnostic Criteria**

A. One or more symptoms of altered voluntary motor or sensory function.
B. Clinical findings provide evidence of incompatibility between the symptom and recognized neurological or medical conditions.
C. The symptom or deficit is not better explained by another medical or mental disorder.
D. The symptom or deficit causes clinically significant distress or impairment in social, occupational, or other important areas of functioning or warrants medical evaluation.

*Specify* if:
Acute episode: Symptoms present for <6 months.
Persistent: Symptoms occurring for 6 months or more.
*Specify* if:
With psychological stressor (specify stressor)
Without psychological stressor

**ICD Coding**

**Coding note:** The ICD-9-CM code for conversion disorder is 300.11, which is assigned regardless of the symptom type. The ICD-10-CM code depends on the symptom type (see below).

*Specify* symptom type:
(F44.4) With weakness or paralysis
(F44.4) With abnormal movement (e.g., tremor, dystonic movement, myoclonus, gait disorder)
(F44.4) With swallowing symptoms
(F44.4) With speech symptom (e.g., dysphonia, slurred speech)
(F44.5) With attacks or seizures
(F44.6) With anesthesia or sensory loss
(F44.6) With special sensory symptom (e.g., visual, olfactory, or hearing disturbance)
(F44.7) With mixed symptoms

*DSM-5,* Diagnostic and Statistical Manual of Mental Disorders, 5th Edition; *ICD-9-CM,* International Classification of Diseases, 9th Revision, Clinical Modification; *ICD-10-CM,* International Classification of Diseases, 10th Revision, Clinical Modification.

*Reprinted with permission from the Diagnostic and Statistical Manual of Mental Disorders (DSM), Fifth Edition, (Copyright 2013). American Psychiatric Association. ICD=International Classification of Diseases*

### Other Terminology

Our preferred terms for motor/sensory symptoms and blackouts unexplained by disease are *functional* and *dissociative* because (a) they describe a mechanism and not an etiology and (b) they sidestep an illogical debate about whether symptoms are in the mind or the brain (Carson et al., 2016; Edwards et al., 2014). The term *functional* is used in this chapter and is increasingly the term of choice for those in the field (Hallett et al., 2016).

- *Functional* describes in the broadest possible sense a problem due to a change in function (of the nervous system) rather than structure. It can be criticized for being too broad a term.
- *Psychogenic, psychosomatic,* and *somatization* all describe an exclusively psychological etiology.
- *Nonorganic, nonepileptic* describes what the problem is *not*, rather than what it is.
- *No diagnosis* refers to the fact that many neurologists, even when faced with clear evidence of a functional/psychogenic neurological problem, are in the habit of making no diagnosis at all and simply conclude that there is no evidence of neurological disease (Friedman and LaFrance, 2010).
- *Medically unexplained* superficially appears to be a neutral term but is often interpreted by patients and doctors as not knowing what the diagnosis is, rather than not knowing why they have the problem. Furthermore, many neurological diseases have uncertain etiology.
- *Hysteria*, an ancient term originating from the idea of the "wandering womb" causing physical symptoms, is generally viewed as pejorative.

## EPIDEMIOLOGY IN NEUROLOGY AND OTHER MEDICAL SPECIALTIES

A number of studies of neurological practice have found that approximately one-third of neurological outpatients present with symptoms the neurologist does not think relate to neurological disease. In half of these (approximately one-sixth) the neurologist makes a primary "functional" or "psychogenic" diagnosis. The rest have some neurological disease but symptoms out of proportion to that disease (Stone et al., 2010a). These figures mirror those in other medical specialties where functional symptoms comprise approximately a third to a half of patients seeing a cardiologist, gastroenterologist, rheumatologist, and other specialty practices. Table 113.1 lists functional symptoms and syndromes according to specialty. Patients with functional neurological symptoms have much higher rates of these other "non-neurological" functional symptoms (Crimlisk et al., 1998).

**TABLE 113.1 Functional Symptoms and Syndromes According to Medical Specialty**

| Specialty | Symptoms |
|---|---|
| Gastroenterology | Irritable bowel syndrome |
| Respiratory | Chronic cough, brittle asthma (some) |
| Rheumatology | Fibromyalgia, chronic back pain (some) |
| Gynecology | Chronic pelvic pain, dysmenorrhea (some) |
| Allergy | Multiple chemical sensitivity syndrome |
| Cardiology | Atypical/noncardiac chest pain, palpitations (some) |
| Infectious diseases | (Postviral) chronic fatigue syndrome, chronic Lyme disease (where physician disagrees that there is ongoing infection) |
| Ear, nose, and throat | Globus sensation, functional dysphonia |
| Neurology | Dissociative (nonepileptic) attacks, functional weakness and sensory symptoms |
| Psychiatry | Depression, anxiety |

Studies of patients with functional neurological symptoms have shown that they report just as much physical disability and have higher rates of anxiety and depression than patients with neurological disease. Most studies show that a minority of patients do not have psychiatric comorbidity. Patients with these symptoms are more likely than the general population to be out of work because of ill health (Carson et al., 2011). Findings are similar in other specialties.

## CLINICAL ASSESSMENT OF FUNCTIONAL NEUROLOGICAL DISORDERS

### General Advice in History Taking

Clinical assessment of the patient with a functional disorder requires a somewhat different approach to the standard neurological assessment, especially when there are time constraints. We suggest the following to improve the efficiency of assessment:

1. *Start by making a list of all physical symptoms.* Patients with functional disorders typically have multiple physical symptoms. Making a list at the beginning avoids symptoms cropping up later, helps to build rapport, and allows an early appreciation of the main difficulties. Always ask about fatigue, pain, sleep disturbance, memory and concentration symptoms, and dizziness. It may seem counterintuitive to be seeking more symptoms in someone who is already polysymptomatic, but sometimes these symptoms, especially fatigue, are reluctantly volunteered even though they often cause the most limitation.
2. *Dissociative* symptoms. Dizziness, if present, may turn out to be dissociative in nature (e.g., feeling "spaced out," "there, but not there," or "unreal"). Patients often have trouble describing dissociation, partly because it is hard to describe but also because they fear the symptoms indicate "craziness." *Depersonalization* describes feeling disconnected from your own body; *derealization* is a feeling of being disconnected from your surroundings (Video 113.1).
3. *Onset.* The onset in patients with weakness and movement disorders is sudden in approximately half of patients. Physical injury, pain, or acute symptoms of dissociation or panic are common in this situation. More gradual-onset symptoms are often associated with fatigue.
4. *What can the patient do?* Patients with functional symptoms have a tendency to report what they can no longer do rather than what they *can* do. Although it is helpful to hear about previous function, ask what they are able to do—do they enjoy it?
5. *Look for other functional symptoms and syndromes* (see Table 113.1). The more they have, the more likely it is that the presenting neurological complaint is functional. Some patients rotate between different specialists, with none appreciating their vulnerability to functional symptoms in general.
6. *Ask the patients what they think is wrong and what should be done.* If they or their family have been concerned or wondering about a specific neurological disease such as multiple sclerosis, Lyme disease, or "trapped nerves," this information is important to tailoring an explanation for the diagnosis later on. Do they have health anxiety? Do they think they are irreversibly damaged? Efforts at rehabilitation may be futile unless beliefs about damage can be altered. In one prospective study of outpatients, beliefs about irreversibility predicted outcome more than age, physical disability, and distress (Sharpe et al., 2010). What happened with previous doctors and why has the patient come to see you? Some patients seek diagnosis and treatment; others are simply looking for a label for a problem they do not expect to resolve.
7. *Avoid blunt questions about depression and anxiety.* It is not necessary for the purposes of neurological diagnosis to make an accurate assessment of a patient's psychological state on the first visit. The diagnosis of a functional disorder should be made on the basis of the physical examination, not the presence or absence of psychological comorbidity. It often may be wise to leave questions about emotions for later; only a minority of patients with functional symptoms believe that stress or psychological factors have anything to do with their symptoms, in contrast to patients with disease who commonly attribute their symptoms to stress (Stone et al., 2010b). Patients with functional disorders do have high rates of depression and anxiety but are often wary of questions about their emotions. They often feel that the doctor is angling to blame their physical symptoms on them personally. Blunt questions like "Are you depressed or anxious?" may not therefore yield accurate answers. Instead try the following:
   - For depression, ask about activities they can do and whether they get enjoyment from them; if not, they may have *anhedonia.* If hospitalized, do they look forward to visits from friends and family? Look at the patient—is he or she miserable or avoiding eye contact? Or try framing questions around the physical symptoms: "Does your leg weakness get you down?" Depression is likely when there is persistent anhedonia or low mood most of the time, with four or more of the following: fatigue, sleep disturbance, suicidal ideation, poor memory or concentration, psychomotor retardation/agitation, or feelings of worthlessness/guilt.
   - For anxiety, look for three out of the following six symptoms: restlessness/on edge, insomnia, fatigue, irritability, poor concentration, and/or tense muscles combined with a history of worry that is persistent and hard to control. Worry will often be primarily focused on health.
   - For panic attacks, look for four of the following: palpitations, sweating, trembling/shaking, shortness of breath, choking sensation, chest pain/pressure, nausea/feeling of imminent diarrhea, dizziness, derealization/depersonalization, afraid of going crazy/losing control, afraid of dying, tingling, or flushes/chills. Panic is a very common problem in patients with functional symptoms, especially nonepileptic attacks. Typically, they are not reported as panic attacks at all, but rather attacks where the patient unexpectedly had multiple symptoms all at once. The emotional component of the panic attack is experienced but erroneously attributed by the patient as being an understandable fear about the physical "attack" that is occurring.
8. *Do not always expect psychological comorbidity or life events.* Depression and anxiety are common, but approximately one-third of patients will have neither. Likewise, although some patients have a history of a recent life event or stress, this is only a risk factor in some patients and in others it is not present (Ludwig et al., 2018). Sometimes the panic attack or physical injury that triggered the symptom is the most stressful life event, and the presence of the symptom then serves to perpetuate the anxiety. Avoiding a diagnosis of functional symptoms in someone because they are psychologically "normal" is as great an error as making the diagnosis simply because the patient has a lot of obvious psychological comorbidity.

### Advice in Specific Physical Diagnosis

The diagnosis of functional symptoms should always be made on the basis of either:

- Clinical features typical of a functional neurological disorder (e.g., a typical thrashing dissociative [nonepileptic] attack with side-to-side head movements and eyes closed for 5 minutes); or
- Physical signs demonstrating internal inconsistency (e.g., Hoover sign for functional weakness, entrainment in functional tremor—see later discussion).

Mistakes are more likely when (1) too much weight is placed on the presence of a psychiatric history; (2) the diagnosis is made just because the problem is bizarre or unfamiliar; (3) there is failure to consider the possibility of a comorbid neurological disease (e.g., dissociative attacks and epilepsy in the same patient); or (4) when the assessing clinician is unfamiliar with a wide range of unusual neurological disorders (Stone et al., 2013).

*La belle indifference* (smiling indifference to disability) has no diagnostic value because it is just as commonly present in neurological disease (Stone et al., 2006). When it is present, it often reflects a conscious desire on the patient's behalf to appear happy in a situation where he or she is concerned that someone will make a psychiatric diagnosis, or alternatively may indicate factitious disorder.

## Blackouts/Dissociative (Nonepileptic) Attacks

Dissociative (nonepileptic) attacks, also commonly called psychogenic nonepileptic seizures, are the most common type of symptom unexplained by disease seen in neurological practice (Schacter and LaFrance, 2018). Studies have estimated that up to one in seven patients in a "first fit" clinic, 50% of patients brought in by ambulance in apparent status epilepticus, and approximately 20%–50% of patients admitted for videotelemetry have this diagnosis. Mean age of onset is in the mid-20s, but peak is late teens; females predominate 3:1. Later-onset patients in their 40s and 50s have a 1:1 gender ratio and typically have health anxiety and a history of recent "organic" health problems (Duncan et al., 2006).

Dissociative attacks most frequently involve shaking movements of the limbs with impaired awareness for the attack. The movement seen is usually a tremor rather than a jerk. Approximately 20% of attacks resemble syncope more than epilepsy and consist of the patient falling down and lying still with their eyes shut for more than 2 minutes (Tannemaat et al., 2013); very few other conditions lead to this clinical scenario. Occasionally, attacks similar to complex partial seizures may be seen. Drop attack semiology without loss of awareness can also be seen in patients who are recovering from or subsequently develop dissociative attacks, suggesting a continuity of these phenotypes in some patients.

The diagnosis is usually made on the basis of the observable features of an attack, preferably recorded using video electroencephalography (EEG) (Table 113.2; Lafrance et al., 2013). No one feature should be used on its own to make a diagnosis, but some are more reliable than others (Avbersek and Sisodiya, 2010). Data on the reliability of these signs have largely been taken from studies of videotelemetry; these signs are less reliable when based on witness descriptions.

Attention has shifted in recent years to diagnosis using subjective experience of the attack. Patients with dissociative attacks typically do not volunteer a prodrome. Indeed, studies analyzing dialogue between neurologists and patients have shown that the lack of any attempt to describe a prodrome may be of diagnostic value in itself because patients with epilepsy usually do attempt to describe their prodrome when present, compared with patients with dissociative attacks who describe the disability associated with the attack (Reuber et al., 2009). However, if questioned, many patients with nonepileptic attacks will admit to a brief prodrome with features of panic (Hendrickson et al., 2014; Fig. 113.1). If obtained, this is useful information that gives the clinician windows into understanding both the nature of the attacks (a mechanism related to panic attacks in which the patient dissociates) and possible treatment (teaching the patient distraction techniques to use during this warning phase to avert the attack and following treatment principles for panic disorder). As some patients recover, they may experience awareness during the attack itself.

Video EEG may be supplemented by an open suggestion protocol to help record an attack (McGonigal et al., 2002). Deceptive placebo induction with saline or a tuning fork is more controversial. Postictal prolactin measurement (to detect high prolactin after a generalized seizure) has fallen out of favor owing to problems with the reliability and timing of the test. Common diagnostic pitfalls include coexistent epilepsy (present in 5%–20% of patients), frontal lobe seizures, sleep-related movement disorders, and paroxysmal movement disorders.

**TABLE 113.2 Differentiating Dissociative (Nonepileptic) Attacks From Generalized Tonic-Clonic Epileptic Seizures**

| | Dissociative Attacks | Epileptic Seizures |
|---|---|---|
| **Helpful** | | |
| Duration over 2 min* | Common | Rare |
| Fluctuating course* | Common | Rare |
| Eyes and mouth closed* | Common | Rare |
| Resisting eye opening | Common | Very rare |
| Side-to-side head or body movement* | Common | Rare |
| Opisthotonus, arc de cercle | Occasional | Very rare |
| Visible large bite mark on side of tongue/cheek/lip | Very rare | Occasional |
| Dislocated shoulder | Very rare | Occasional |
| Fast respiration during attack | Common | Ceases |
| Grunting/guttural ictal cry sound | Rare | Common |
| Weeping/upset after a seizure* | Occasional | Very rare‡ |
| Recall for period of unresponsiveness* | Common | Very rare |
| Thrashing, violent movements | Common | Rare |
| Postictal stertorous breathing* | Rare | Common |
| Pelvic thrusting*,† | Occasional | Rare§ |
| Asynchronous movements*,† | Common | Rare |
| Attacks in medical situations | Common | Rare |
| **Not So Helpful** | | |
| Stereotyped attacks | Common | Common |
| Attack arising from sleep | Occasional | Common |
| Aura | Common | Common |
| Incontinence of urine or feces* | Occasional | Common |
| Injury* | Common¶ | Common |
| Report of tongue biting* | Common | Common |

*Endorsed by a systematic review (Avbersek and Sisodiya, 2010).
†These signs unhelpful in distinguishing nonepileptic attacks from frontal lobe seizures.
‡Normally sleepy.
§Frontal lobe epilepsy. Dissociative attacks do sometimes appear to arise from sleep, but video electroencephalogram (EEG) usually shows this not to be true sleep. Attacks arising from EEG-documented sleep are suggestive of epilepsy.
¶Especially carpet burns and bruising.

## Weakness/Paralysis

Weakness as a functional symptom is more common in females and typically presents in the mid-30s but like all functional symptoms can occur in children and the elderly. Estimates of incidence are approximately 5/100,000, comparable with multiple sclerosis. Comorbidity with other functional symptoms, especially fatigue and pain, is almost invariable. The most common presentation is unilateral weakness, followed by monoparesis and paraparesis. There is no good evidence for left-sided or nondominant preponderance. Complete paralysis is less common clinically than weakness (Stone et al., 2010b).

The onset is sudden in approximately 50% of patients. In the acute presentation, there are often symptoms of a panic attack, dissociative seizure, or an immediate trigger such as a physical injury, acute pain,

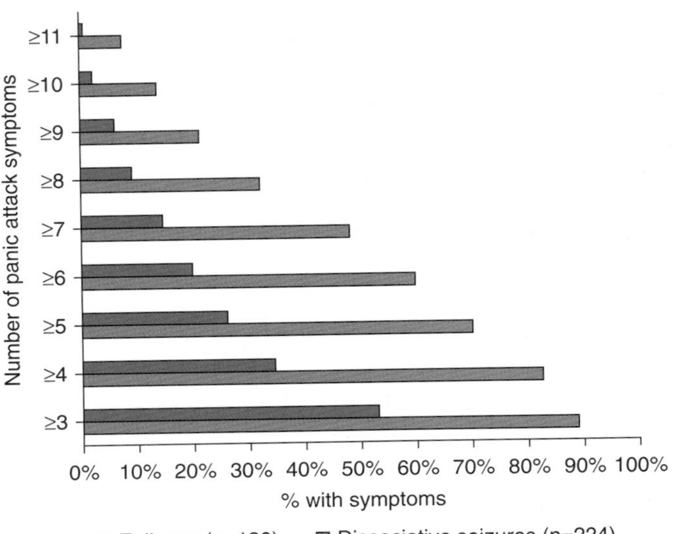


**Fig. 113.1** Prodromal symptoms of panic are much more common in dissociative (nonepileptic) attacks than epilepsy. Although they may not initially be disclosed, they provide an opportunity for treatment. *(Redrawn from Hendrickson, R., Popescu, A., Dixit, R., Ghearing, G., Bagic, A., 2014. Panic attack symptoms differentiate patients with epilepsy from those with psychogenic nonepileptic spells (PNES). Epilepsy Behav 37, 210–214.)*

migraine, a general anesthetic, or an episode of sleep paralysis (Stone et al., 2012). When the onset is more gradual, there is typically a history of fatigue, pain, or immobility on which the weakness becomes superimposed gradually over time. The weakness seen in *complex regional pain syndrome type 1* (CRPS-1) (Popkirov et al., 2019) has the same clinical features as *functional weakness.*

Subjectively, patients with functional weakness often report that the affected limb "doesn't feel as if it belongs" to them or, in extreme situations, as if it is "not there" or is "someone else's" limb (Video 113.2). They commonly report that the leg gives away or that they keep dropping things unexpectedly. The diagnosis depends on demonstrating internal inconsistency and incongruence with disease:

- *Pattern of weakness.* In functional weakness, the limb is usually globally weak or often demonstrates the inverse of pyramidal weakness, with the flexors weaker in the arms and the extensors weaker in the legs.
- *Inconsistency during examination.* This may be obvious—for example, a patient who can walk to the examination table but cannot raise the leg against gravity on examination. More commonly there is weakness of ankle movements, but the patient can stand on tiptoes or on their heels. Arm weakness may be incompatible with performance, such as removing shoes or carrying a bag.
- *Hoover sign.* Hip extension must be weak for this test to work. The presence of hip extension weakness itself in an ambulant patient is a positive sign of functional weakness. If hip extension returns to normal during contralateral hip flexion against resistance, this demonstrates structural integrity of the motor pathways (Fig. 113.2; Video 113.3). The test is easiest to do with the patient in the sitting position. We find it useful to demonstrate this sign to the patient and relatives to indicate that the diagnosis is being made on the basis of positive criteria. This test may be false positive when there is cortical neglect.
- *Hip abductor sign.* A similar test involves demonstrating weakness of hip abduction, which returns to normal with contralateral hip abduction against resistance.
- *Dragging gait.* If there is moderate or severe unilateral leg weakness, the patient may walk with a dragging gait in which the foot does not leave the ground. Often the hip is externally or internally rotated (Fig. 113.3).
- *"Give-way" weakness.* This is a pattern of weakness in which the patient transiently has normal power but then the limb gives way, sometimes just before it is touched. If the arm is very weak, it may hover for a second before collapsing. Normal power can be produced by saying to the patient, "At the count of 3, push—1 … 2 … 3 … *push.*" This is a less reliable sign and occurs more commonly in painful limbs or occasionally in myasthenia gravis.
- *Drift without pronator sign.* Sometimes patients with functional arm weakness will demonstrate a downward drift of the arm without the pronation seen in conditions such as stroke (Daum and Aybek, 2013).
- *Facial spasm (looking like weakness)* (Video 113.4). It is not uncommon to see patients who apparently have weakness of their face, usually ipsilateral to a functional hemiparesis (Fasano et al., 2012). In fact, the appearance is nearly always due to unilateral overactivity of the platysma muscle which pulls the side of the lip downwards. There may be jaw deviation and sometimes an upward deviation of the mouth instead. Contraction of the orbicularis oculi muscle can lead to an appearance with a depressed eyebrow (Fig. 113.4), which may be interpreted incorrectly as ptosis, although true functional ptosis does occur more rarely. These features can sometimes be enhanced on examination by sustained voluntary contraction of facial or periocular muscles.
- *"Altered" reflexes.* Occasionally, patients with functional weakness may have what appears to be ankle clonus, which on closer inspection has features of functional tremor. There may also appear to be reflex asymmetry if the patient is co-contracting agonist and antagonist muscles on one side of their body. Finally, in our experience it is not that unusual for the plantar response to be relatively mute on the affected side if there is marked sensory disturbance.

## Movement Disorders

Functional movement disorders have been increasingly recognized by movement disorder specialists, especially over the past decade (Baizabal-Carvalloet al., 2019). In specialist clinics, these symptoms account for up to 10% of new referrals (Hallett et al., 2011). Like weakness, the onset of functional movement disorders is often sudden or may be accompanied by pain (Pareés et al., 2014). The course may be unusual, with sudden remissions or relapses in different limbs. General clues to a functional movement disorder include improvement with distraction (many so-called organic movement disorders get worse during distraction) and worsening with attention. Many organic movement disorders, especially gait disorders, can look bizarre, but if a clinician is careful to make the diagnosis only on positive grounds, it should not be as intimidating a diagnosis as it first appears. Gupta and Lang proposed a revised classification in which *clinically definite* cases included cases *documented* through resolution with placebo or psychotherapy and cases *clinically established* with clear positive evidence on examination and *laboratory supported* with electrophysiology (Gasca-Salas and Lang, 2016). Caution is warranted insofar as organic movement disorders can also improve temporarily with placebo and because functional and organic movement disorders commonly exist together.

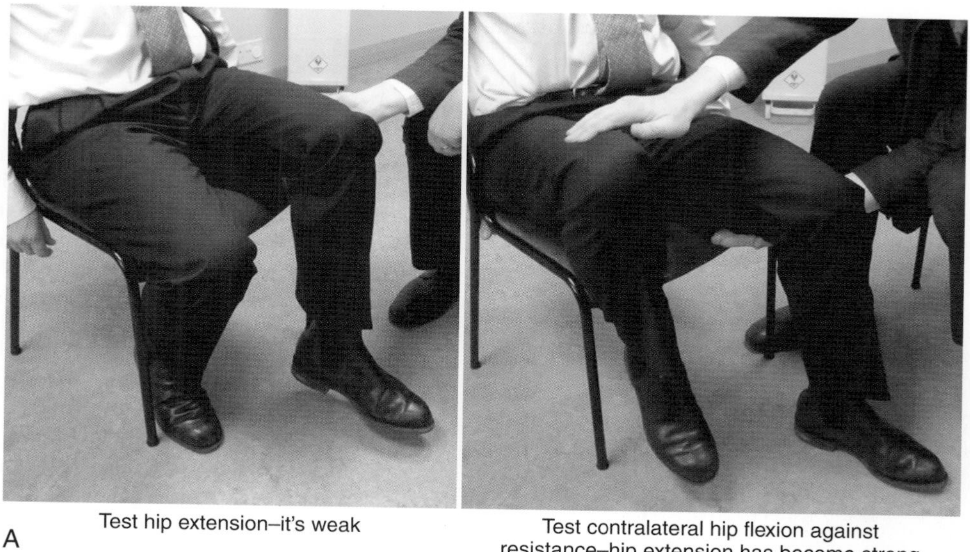
A
Test hip extension–it's weak
Test contralateral hip flexion against resistance–hip extension has become strong

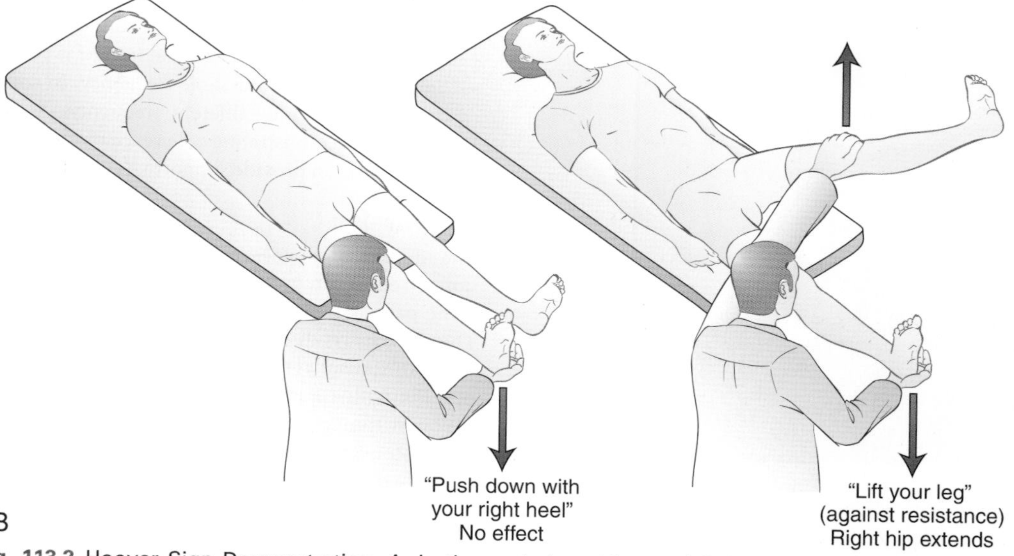
"Push down with your right heel" No effect
"Lift your leg" (against resistance) Right hip extends
B

**Fig. 113.2** Hoover Sign Demonstration. A. In the seated position and B. in the supine position *(From Stone, J., 2009. The bare essentials: functional symptoms in neurology. Pract Neurol 9, 179–189, by permission of BMJ publications.)*

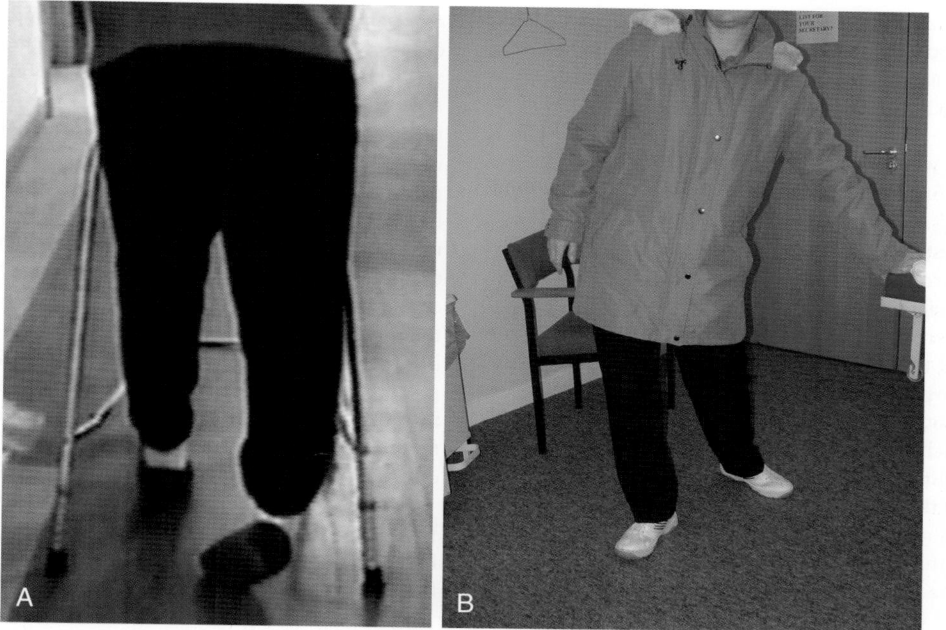
A
B

**Fig. 113.3** A dragging gait with external (B) or internal (A) hip rotation is characteristic of functional leg weakness.

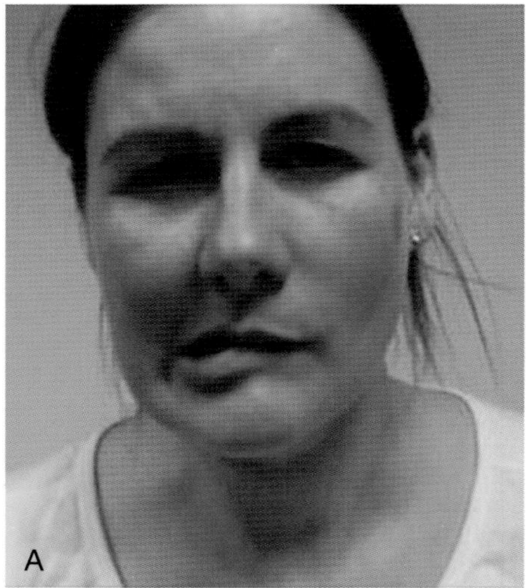


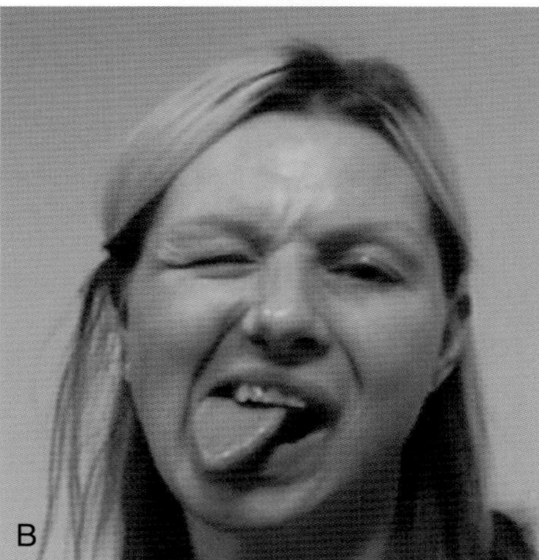


**Fig. 113.4** Functional facial spasm, leading to (**A**) deviation of the chin and downward movement of the corner of the mouth from platysma contraction and (**B**) upward contraction of the mouth and orbicularis.

## Tremor

Tremor is the most commonly encountered functional/psychogenic movement disorder (Schwingenschuh et al., 2016; Thenganatt and Jankovic, 2014). There are a number of positive clinical features, none of which are 100% reliable, that should enable a positive diagnosis to be made:

- Variable frequency, which may include starting and stopping of the tremor, is more useful than variable amplitude, which can be found in organic tremor.
- The entrainment test is carried out by asking the patient, with the unaffected limb, to copy a rhythmical tapping movement provided by the examiner, preferably using thumb and forefinger. The movement should be altered in frequency while the patient is trying to copy it, to bring out the features described as follows. If the tremor is in the legs, ask the patient to copy foot tapping movements. If it is in the trunk, then tongue or neck movements may be used. Mental distraction tasks such as mental arithmetic tend to be less effective distractors in functional tremor. In functional tremor, one of three things happens: (1) the patient is unable to copy the simple tapping movement and cannot explain why; (2) the tremor in the affected limb stops; or (3) the tremor in the affected hand entrains to the same rhythm as the examiner. False positives in this test appear to be rare, although, as with any positive functional sign, they do not exclude the possibility of an additional underlying "organic" movement disorder. In contrast, false negatives are more common, particularly if the tremor is long-standing or if the tremor relies on mechanics. For example, a heel-tapping leg tremor in someone sitting with their foot plantar-flexed on the ground is characteristic of a functional tremor (Edwards and Bhatia, 2012). Tremor recording, if available, can be helpful in recording the response to this test.
- *Ballistic movements.* Ask the patient to make sudden ballistic movements with the good hand by touching the rapidly moving finger of the examiner. Functional tremor will often stop briefly during the movement.
- *Attempted immobilization.* Attempting to immobilize the affected limb often makes a functional tremor worse. Likewise, loading the limb with weights tends to make the tremor worse, whereas organic tremor tends to improve with this maneuver.
- *Coactivation sign.* Most functional tremor is similar to voluntary tremor. Sometimes the mechanism of the tremor is different and relates to coactivation of agonist and antagonist muscles (like shivering).
- *Coherence analysis.* If functional tremor is present in more than one limb, it usually has the same frequency. In contrast, organic tremor usually has slightly different frequencies in different body parts. Therefore demonstrating coherence of the tremor between different body parts can provide supportive evidence of a functional tremor.

## Parkinsonism

The addition of slowness and postural instability to a patient with functional tremor can give the appearance of Parkinson disease, especially if the patient is also depressed and has diminished facial expression. The slowness is distractible and without the normal decrement seen in parkinsonism (Thenganatt and Jankovic, 2016). There may be stiffness but with a quality of active resistance to it. Fluorodopa positron emission tomography (PET) scanning or dopamine transporter single-photon emission computed tomography (SPECT) scanning should be normal in functional movement disorder patients.

## Myoclonus

Brief jerky movements may appear to be myoclonus. More commonly, patients have more complex hyperkinetic movements that are hard to accurately classify. Functional myoclonus may be stimulus sensitive, especially during deep tendon reflex testing, where myoclonus may occur even before the reflex hammer has made contact (Dreissen et al., 2016). Functional/psychogenic myoclonus is often associated with a Bereitschaftspotential (BP) prior to the movement. This requires recording multiple events using EEG and back-averaging according to an electromyogram (EMG) (van der Salm et al., 2012). The presence of a BP does not provide evidence of conscious intention to move but does indicate that the voluntary motor system is being used for the movement. In recent years it has become recognized that a large proportion of patients with axial myoclonic syndromes, commonly described as propriospinal myoclonus, have a BP prior to their jerks and other features in keeping with a functional movement disorder (van der Salm et al., 2014). In addition, tics as a functional/psychogenic movement disorder also rarely occur. Clinical features include a late age of onset, lack of premonitory symptoms, inability to suppress tics, and comorbidity with other functional movement disorders (Baizabal-Carvallo and Jankovic, 2014).

## Dystonia

Dystonia has a troubled past relationship with so-called hysteria. In the heyday of psychoanalysis, cervical dystonia was incorrectly interpreted as a "turning away of responsibility" and writers' cramp as evidence of sexual conflict. Nonetheless, there is currently a consensus that dystonic movements, especially fixed dystonia where the posture does not fluctuate, do occur as a functional/psychogenic phenomenon. The most common presentation is with a clenched fist, sometimes with wrist/elbow flexion or an inverted foot (Schrag et al., 2004; Fig. 113.5; Videos 113.2 and 113.5). It is most frequently seen in association with limb pain in a situation where the diagnosis of CRPS-1 may be made. As with functional weakness, there is no difference clinically between the abnormal movements seen in CRPS and those diagnosed as functional in the absence of pain (Popkirov et al., 2019). Fixed dystonia does occur without pain, commonly in a limb with functional weakness. Persistent fixed dystonia may be associated with contractures, which are best assessed under anesthetic.

Three neurophysiological studies have found it impossible to distinguish functional dystonia and organic dystonia on the basis of neurophysiological measures such as short and long intracortical inhibition, cortical silent period, and reciprocal inhibition in the forearm. One of these studies found that a measure of plasticity was increased in organic dystonia but was normal in functional dystonia (Schmerler and Espay, 2016). It is perhaps with this symptom that traditional boundaries between psychogenic/organic and functional/structural are at their most blurred.

### Gait Disorders

In studies of misdiagnosis, gait disorders figure disproportionately in cases where the initial diagnosis of a "nonorganic" problem turned out to be wrong. Clues to a functional gait disorder include a gait that varies dramatically when walking backward, jogging, or distracted by another task such as having to guess numbers written on their back or using a cell phone. Care must be taken, as some conditions (e.g., dyskinetic gaits in treated Parkinson disease and vestibular disorders) may share some of these features (Růžička et al., 2011). Common types of functional gait disorder include the following (Lempert et al., 1991):

- *Dragging gait* (as described in functional weakness).
- *Tightrope walker's gait* with short slow steps, hips and knees flexed, and sometimes with arms outstretched as if walking a tightrope; commonly associated with fear of falling; when extreme may be associated with crouching.
- *Truncal ataxia.* Tending to fall in all directions with upper body swaying and correcting leg movements.
- *Astasia-abasia*, which refers to normal limb power and sensation on the bed but inability to stand and walk. This can occur in organic truncal ataxia, sensory ataxia, and hydrocephalus.
- *Knee-buckling gait*, usually seen when the patient has unilateral functional weakness.

## Sensory Disturbances

Functional sensory symptoms are common in patients with functional weakness and in patients with chronic limb pain (Stone and Vermeulen, 2016). They do occur on their own, although even here the patient often has some signs of functional weakness on examination even in the absence of symptoms of weakness. Common patterns are the following:

- *Hemisensory disturbance.* Just as functional weakness is most commonly unilateral, the most common functional sensory symptom is the *hemisensory syndrome* in which the patient complains that one side of their body feels different from the other side (Fig. 113.6). They may complain that they feel "split down the middle" and also describe ipsilateral blurred vision or hearing problems. Functional sensory signs often occur in patients with chronic pain and complex regional pain (Rommel et al., 1999).

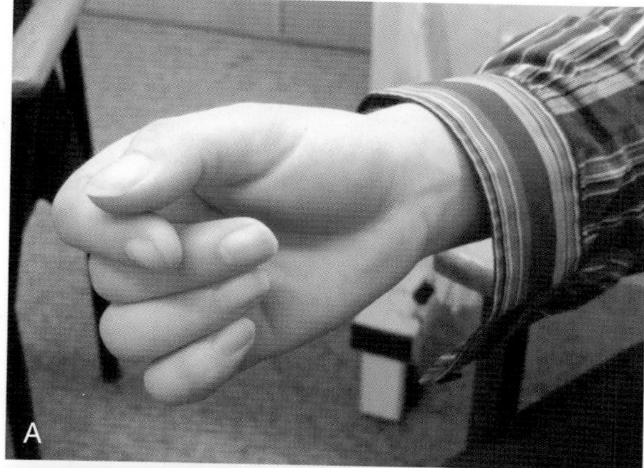


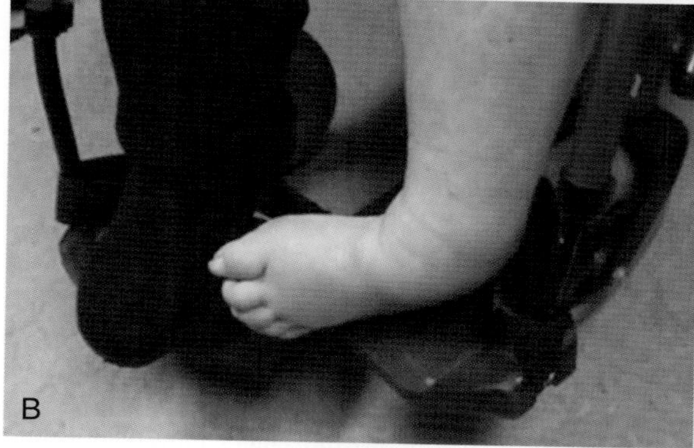


**Fig. 113.5** Functional/psychogenic dystonia typically presents with (**A**) a clenched fist or (**B**) an inverted plantar-flexed ankle. *(From Stone, J., 2009. The bare essentials: functional symptoms in neurology. Pract Neurol 9, 179–189, by permission of BMJ publications.)*

- *Sensation cutoff at the groin or shoulder.* This is usually associated with the patient's dissociative report that the limb "feels as if it's not there."
- Examination findings in functional sensory disturbance are much less reliable than motor signs, so it is best to rely on evidence of mild functional weakness if present. The following signs are sensitive but not specific:
    - Alteration of vibration sense across the forehead or sternum.
    - *Tests for complete sensory loss.* Complete anesthesia is rare, so tests such as "Say yes when you feel it and no when you don't" and "Close your eyes and touch your nose when I touch your hand" are rarely useful. The *Bowlus maneuver* involves having patients interlock their fingers behind their back and asking them to state whether the right or left fingers are being touched.
    - Other sensory tests, such as finding exact splitting of sensation at the midline or nondermatomal sensory loss, are common but even less specific for functional sensory symptoms.

## Visual Symptoms

Functional visual symptoms and methods of detection include the following:

- Intermittent blurred vision, often ipsilateral to functional weakness, and hemisensory disturbance, described elegantly as *asthenopia* in older texts. Patients may describe transiently screwing up their eyes to make it go away, which is suggestive of convergence spasm.
- *Double vision.* Binocular diplopia is usually due to convergence spasm, asymmetrical overactivity of the normal convergence response (Fekete et al., 2012). This can be demonstrated by testing convergence movements but holding the finger at a close distance

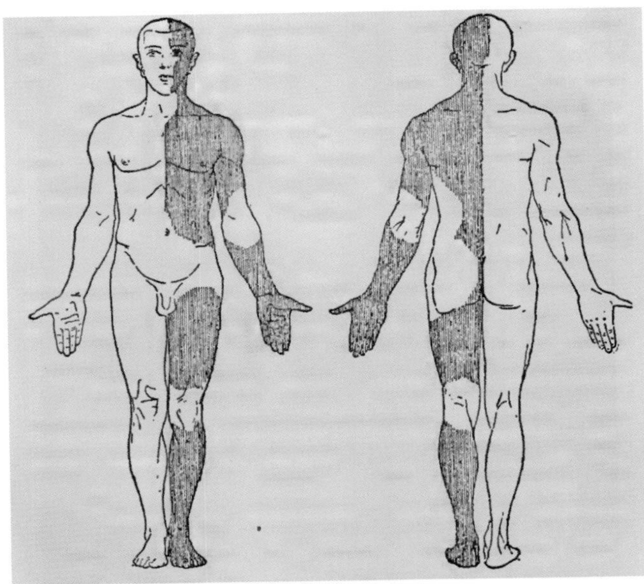

**Fig. 113.6 A Case of Hemisensory Disturbance Depicted by Jean-Martin Charcot.** *(From Charcot, J.M., 1889. Clinical Lectures on Diseases of the Nervous System. New Sydenham Society, London.)*

for longer than usual. When persistent, convergence spasm can resemble a sixth nerve palsy. Monocular diplopia is usually functional but can be due to ocular pathology. Triplopia is surprisingly usually related to an organic eye movement abnormality but can be functional (Keane, 2006).

- *Total visual loss.* Complete functional visual loss is normally relatively easy to diagnose at the bedside. Ask the patient to put his or her fingers together or sign his or her name (not a problem if organically blind). Extend a hand as if expecting a handshake, and watch him or her navigate around the room. Normal findings include pupillary response, menace reflex (sudden movements of the hand toward the eye), and optokinetic nystagmus with a rotating striped drum. There may be a convergence response to a mirror placed close in front of the face. Always consider the possibility of organic cortical blindness.
- *Monocular/partial visual loss.* At the bedside, many patients with functional monocular symptoms have a tubular field defect (Fig. 113.7, *A*). Normally the visual field is conical, such that the visual field at 2 m is twice as large as at 1 m. Another common finding is spiral, star-shaped, or pinpoint visual fields on Goldmann perimetry (see Fig. 113.7, *B*). As the test proceeds, the patient tires and reports progressively constricted fields. A large variety of other tests exist to give an objective measure of acuity (Chen et al., 2007). For example, in monocular visual problems, the "fogging test" involves deliberately and gradually worsening acuity in the good eye until the point when any acuity better than 6/60 must be coming from the affected eye. The stereoscopic test gives an estimate of acuity based on the perception of varying stereoscopic images.
- *Hemifield loss.* When this is functional, the patient will report binocular hemianopic fields, but on testing there is monocular hemianopia on the side of the hemifield loss and normal monocular vision in the other eye (Keane, 1979).
- *Nystagmus.* This can sometimes be seen as a voluntary/functional phenomenon or in patients who spend a lot of time in the dark or wearing dark glasses.
- *Gaze restriction.* This may sometimes occur as a functional phenomenon, often as a finding on examination only, or commonly in the context of functional parkinsonism.

## Speech and Swallowing Symptoms

Functional speech and swallowing symptoms commonly encountered in neurological practice include the following:

- *Articulation. Functional dysarthria* usually takes the form of intermittent slurred speech or stuttering speech with difficulty starting words (Duffy, 2016). Speech may be slow with hesitations noticeably occurring in the middle of sentences when it is harder to interrupt. In this context, speech may become telegrammatic, missing the prepositions and conjunctions of normal speech. Just as functional weakness is at its worst when directly tested, functional speech problems are worst when having to repeat words or phrases to command and, like developmental stuttering, may resolve when the patient is singing or speaking about something that makes them feel emotional or angry. Complete mutism still occurs; we have seen a man who used a computer to speak for 4 years before making a good recovery. Foreign accent syndrome can occur after stroke or other brain lesions due to a breakdown of prosody, the melody of speech, which as a by-product leads to a new accent. In functional foreign accent syndrome, there are internal inconsistencies and periods of normality (McWhirter et al., 2019).
- *Dysphonia. Functional dysphonia* is a common presenting symptom to otolaryngologists but may be seen by neurologists in combination with other functional symptoms. Speech is usually whispering in nature and may follow a genuine or perceived episode of laryngitis. At least six randomized controlled trials in this area have suggested benefit of voice therapy (Ruotsalainen et al., 2008).
- *Globus pharyngis.* This describes the symptom of "something sticking" in the throat, even when the patient is not swallowing anything. There is controversy regarding how often this symptom can be explained by gastroesophageal reflux disease, and investigation by gastroenterology or otolaryngology is usually appropriate (Selleslagh et al., 2014). More recent scholarship has cast doubt on this assumption.

### Dizziness

Approximately 20% of patients in specialist dizziness clinics have chronic dizziness that clinically appears to relate to a functional disorder. Previous terms including phobic postural vertigo, visual vertigo, and chronic subjective dizziness have now been replaced with the term persistent postural perceptual dizziness (PPPD or "triple PD") (Popkirov et al., 2018). They key defining features in the Bárány Society definition are dizziness, unsteadiness, or nonspinning vertigo on most days for 3 months, lasting for hour-long periods; exacerbation by upright posture, active or passive motion without regard to direction or position, and exposure to moving visual stimuli or complex visual patterns; and triggering by an event that causes vertigo, unsteadiness, dizziness, including vestibular, neurological, and psychiatric disorders. As with other functional neurological disorders, psychiatric comorbidity may not be present. There have been advances in understanding the pathophysiology of the condition and its treatment with vestibular habituation and/or specific psychological therapy.

## Memory and Cognitive Symptoms

Functional cognitive symptoms are a common primary presentation and comorbid complaint among patients with other functional neurological symptoms (Ball et al., 2020; McWhirter et al., 2020; Teodoro et al., 2018).

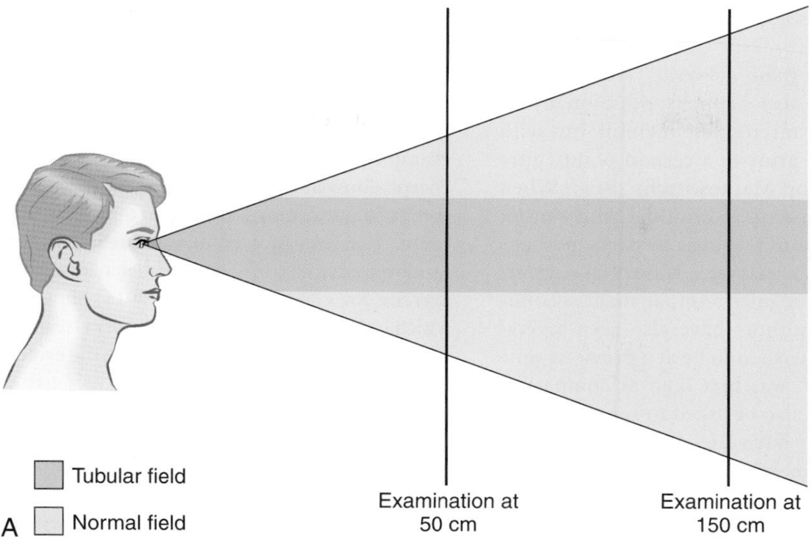


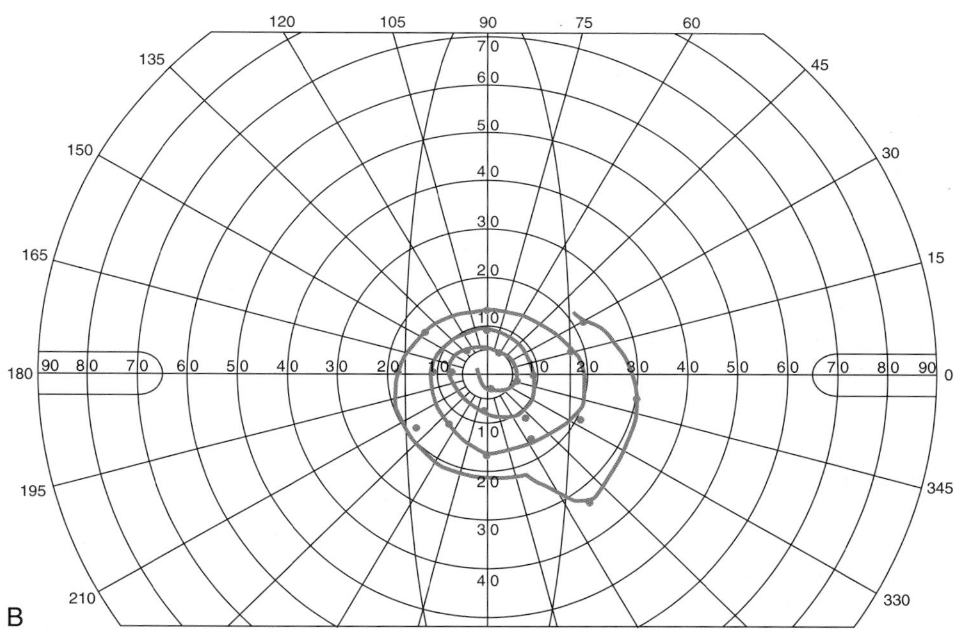


**Fig. 113.7** Functional visual symptoms can be associated with (**A**) tubular visual fields at the bedside or (**B**) spiral fields on Goldmann perimetry. *(From Stone, J., 2009. The bare essentials: functional symptoms in neurology. Pract Neurol 9, 179–189, by permission of BMJ publications.)*

They may be attributable (by both doctor and patient) to associated fatigue, anxiety, or low mood or become a presenting symptom in their own right. Presentations include the following:

- *"Normal" absent-mindedness and functional memory symptoms.* In someone who is usually not absent-minded, forgetting why they went upstairs, losing their keys, or losing track of conversation may be interpreted as abnormal. Anxiety about the cause and attention paid to the symptom can amplify the problem and lead to neurological referral. A subgroup of patients in any memory clinic presents without obvious anxiety, depression, or stress apart from anxiety about their memory symptoms. In addition to escalating absent-mindedness as described, patients with functional memory symptoms usually reports variability in their memory problems and episodes when they forgot familiar information such as their own address and then remembered it again.
- Word-finding difficulty is a common symptom among patients with other functional neurological symptoms. They may also report mixing words up with spoonerisms or neologisms, but true dysphasia is rare.
- *Poor concentration as part of a psychological disorder.* Attention and concentration may be noticeably impaired in anxiety and depression. In severe depression, the presentation may be that of a pseudodementia. Routine neuropsychological tests may give spuriously low values. Attempting to control for this with the use

of self-reported anxiety and depression scales is unreliable in the authors' experience.

- *Pure retrograde functional/psychogenic amnesia.* This memory syndrome, common to fiction, also happens occasionally in real life. It presents with normal anterograde memory but with a large chunk of absent memory prior to a certain point (pure retrograde amnesia) (Staniloiu and Markowitsch, 2014). When not associated with obvious gain (e.g., a criminal who cannot remember the crime), it can occur in response to stress, perhaps as a self-deceptive phenomenon. It may be a feature in patients who have apparent catastrophic cognitive impairment secondary to minor head injury. The authors have also seen several patients with this syndrome who wished to be at a previous time in their life, and their "amnesia" was best seen as compatible with that wish. Neurologists may also be asked to see patients in fugue states who characteristically have moved from where they normally live and then cannot remember who they are or where they live.

In the assessment of patients with functional cognitive symptoms, approximate answers to questions (e.g., "How many legs has a horse got?" Answer: "3") are classically described. This has been called *Ganser syndrome* after the 19th-century German psychiatrist who first reported it. In our experience, this is rare and is a marker of factitious symptoms. More common is the early loss of relatively "protected" knowledge such as the names of spouses or children, discrepancies between real-life function and test results, or discrepancies between results on cognitive tests that localize to the same anatomical region (e.g., memory). The individual may do better in more complex tasks in the same domain than simple ones. In such situations, cognitive "effort tests" may be useful. These are very simple tests that even patients with severe dementia or head injury should be able to perform well. For example, the coin-in-the-hand test involves 10 trials of showing patients which hand a coin is held in, asking them to close their eyes for 10 seconds, and then asking them to choose the hand with the coin (Kapur, 1994). A score at chance indicates poor effort. A score below chance is sometimes used as evidence of factitious disorder/malingering, although in reality it cannot distinguish between conscious or unconscious deception.

### Overlap With Pain and Fatigue

#### Pain

We have discussed the similarity of functional motor and sensory symptoms seen in CRPS-1 to those seen in patients without limb pain. The neurologist may also have to assess back pain in someone with functional symptoms. Certain signs, including some described by Gordon Waddell, do provide useful information (Waddell, 2004):

- *Straight leg raising while lying and sitting.* If a patient can sit comfortably on an examination table with their legs stretched out at 90 degrees to their body, any pain induced by straight leg raising in the supine position cannot be due to true sciatic nerve pain.
- *Simulated rotation.* Ask the patient to stand with his or her feet flat on the floor and rotate the trunk with the arms stabilized at the sides. This movement occurs at the knees and not the back and should not cause significant back pain.
- *Localized tenderness.* Some patients with back pain are exquisitely tender to superficial palpation.
- *Axial loading.* Pressure on the head should not cause significant back pain.

These signs are not, as is commonly assumed, proof of malingering or even exaggeration, but they do suggest that reports of back pain are heightened when the patient and doctor are paying attention to it.

#### Fatigue

Fatigue is often, for all of the patient's more obvious symptoms, to be his or her most limiting symptom, as it is in many neurological diseases (Gelauff et al., 2018). Chronic persistent fatigue in the absence of a disease cause has been labeled, defined, and conceived of in many ways—for example, chronic fatigue syndrome (CFS), neurasthenia, and myalgic encephalomyelitis (ME). One of the simpler definitions of CFS is persistent fatigue lasting longer than 6 months which is not due to another cause. The relevance of this discussion is that there have been large randomized trials of cognitive-behavioral therapy (CBT) and graded exercise for CFS (White et al., 2011) showing modest benefit overall, which have potentially helped to inform treatment for patients with functional neurological symptoms (where the evidence is more limited).

## FEIGNING AND MALINGERING

The issue of feigning remains topical in this area, firstly because these are symptoms without verifiable disease, and secondly—unlike, for example, irritable bowel syndrome—they are symptoms that relate to the voluntary nervous system (Kanaan et al., 2009). Distinguishing symptoms that are under conscious intentional voluntary control from those that are not is difficult because: (1) the positive signs used to make a diagnosis of functional symptoms would be the same if someone was feigning and (2) doctors are not trained to detect deception.

Clues to feigning include a documented history of lying or use of multiple different names, major inconsistencies in the history given to different clinicians, and avoidance of investigations. The only definitive ways to be confident that feigning is an explanation for functional neurological symptoms are if the patient is covertly observed doing something highly discrepant with what he or she has claimed to be able to do (e.g., playing tennis when he or she claims to be in a wheelchair) or if he or she confesses to feigning. Feigning of other symptoms such as posttraumatic stress disorder, pain states, or depression appears to be at least as common as feigning of neurological symptoms in medicolegal scenarios.

If apparent exaggeration is present (e.g., "My pain score is 11 out of 10"), this is often exaggeration to convince the doctor there is a problem rather than exaggeration to deceive. This exaggeration may paradoxically get worse when they feel disbelieved by the doctor. In addition, some discrepancies between reported and observed function occur because of the attentional nature of the condition. For example, in one study, 10 patients with functional tremor who explicitly knew that a "tremor watch" would record how much of the time they were shaking grossly overestimated the result (84% diary estimate vs. 4% recorded tremor). Similar to looking inside the fridge to see if the light is on, some patients with functional disorders may feel as if their symptoms are always there because they are whenever they think about them (Parees et al., 2012).

Although clinicians estimate feigning to account for approximately 5% of patients with functional symptoms, it is impossible for anyone to truly know. Most neurologists will come across patients in their career who have "hoodwinked" them, or they may boast about those they caught. It may be tempting to start believing that most patients are feigning. Several arguments stand in the way of this hypothesis: (1) the homogeneity of patient experiences as described in clinic, both of their symptoms and of their general bewilderment; (2) follow-up studies showing symptom persistence over decades; (3) the high frequency of nonepileptic attacks during video EEG even when patients have been told this is the suspected diagnosis; (4) the persistence of positive signs such as the Hoover sign even when the patient has been shown how it operates; (5) evidence of shoe wear in patients with functional gait disorders and contractures in patients with fixed dystonia; (6) similar prevalence figures between industrialized nations with welfare benefit systems and nonindustrialized countries without (Simon et al., 1996); (7) historical consistency in clinical presentation over centuries (Stone et al., 2008); and (8) differential improvement in randomized controlled trials with similar intensity of therapy (Nielsen et al., 2017).

## MISDIAGNOSIS

Although neurologists tend to worry about feigning, doctors other than neurologists, especially psychiatrists, tend to be preoccupied by the opposite concern of misdiagnosis. Studies in the 1950s and 1960s suggested high rates of the misdiagnosis of hysteria of up to 60%. A systematic review of 27 studies included 1466 patients with a mean follow-up of 5 years and found a frequency of misdiagnosis of approximately 4% since 1970, before the advent of computed tomography (CT) scans and videotelemetry (Stone et al., 2005; Fig. 113.8). This is a frequency of misdiagnosis comparable to other neurological and psychiatric disorders. A study of 1144 patients in Scotland found an even lower misdiagnosis rate at 18 months of only four patients (Stone et al., 2009). However, this is not a reason for complacency, and we would recommend that neurologists continue to be responsible for these diagnoses. For neurologists, relying on obvious psychiatric comorbidity, forgetting about neurological disease comorbidity, and making a diagnosis using gait disorder are common pitfalls (Stone et al., 2013).

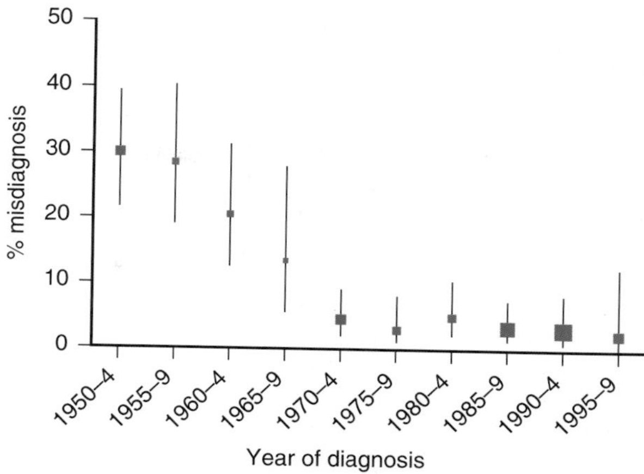


**Fig. 113.8** Frequency of misdiagnosis of conversion symptoms and hysteria (mean %, 95% confidence intervals) in 27 studies ($n$ = 1466), mean follow-up 5 years, plotted at midpoint of 5-year intervals according to when patients were diagnosed. *(From Stone, J., 2009. The bare essentials: functional symptoms in neurology. Pract Neurol 9, 179–189, by permission of BMJ publications.)*

## PROGNOSIS

Long-term follow-up studies have suggested that functional motor symptoms persist in the majority and improve in a third (Gelauff and Stone, 2016). As expected, sensory symptoms have a better prognosis than weakness, which in turn has a better outcome than fixed dystonia (Ibrahim et al., 2009). Dissociative (nonepileptic) seizures probably have a better overall outcome than motor disorders (Gelauff and Stone, 2016).

Good prognostic factors for functional neurological symptoms are a willingness to accept the potential reversibility of the symptoms, a good interaction with the doctor, short duration of symptoms, and a lack of other physical symptoms. The presence of anxiety and depression and change in marital status have been found to predict positive outcome in some studies but not others.

Poor prognostic factors include strong beliefs in lack of reversibility of symptoms/damage, anger at the diagnosis of a nonorganic disorder, delayed diagnosis, multiple other physical symptoms/somatization disorder, concurrent organic disease, personality disorder, older age, sexual abuse, receipt of financial benefits, and litigation. However, in most studies, these prognostic factors explained only a limited amount of the variance. In practice, some patients with many poor prognostic factors respond well to treatment, and some with many good prognostic features do badly.

## ETIOLOGY AND MECHANISM

Patients often ask, "Why has this happened?" It is useful to rephrase this question into two separate questions as we do for other neurological disorders such as multiple sclerosis: "Why has it happened?" (etiology) and "How has it happened?" (mechanism).

The etiology of functional symptoms is multifactorial and varies hugely between patients. Although one can individually formulate an etiology for patients based on the factors shown in Table 113.3, this model is likely to be incomplete. If there is one rule here, it is avoid generalizing. There are many useful psychological models of functional neurological disorder (Carson et al., 2016), but the notion that all patients with functional symptoms have been abused or suffered some sort of trauma is not supported by the evidence (Ludwig et al., 2018). Stress, including recent or remote events, is undoubtedly relevant for many patients (Keynejad et al., 2019). Just as relevant to understanding mechanism as "stress" is the presence of a physiological trigger such as minor injury, infection, or drug side effect, as discussed earlier (Pareés et al., 2014; Stone et al., 2012). Having a neurological disease is also an important and powerful risk factor for functional symptoms. Understanding prior vulnerabilities may help to fill in general understanding about the problem, but it is really the perpetuating factors in Table 113.3 that are the most important targets for treatment.

The neural mechanisms of functional neurological symptoms are not yet well understood, but functional imaging studies of functional motor symptoms combined with other neurophysiological techniques are adding to our understanding (Baizabal-Carvallo et al., 2019). A functional imaging study of unilateral weakness and sensory disturbance in four patients whose symptoms subsequently improved showed "dose-responsive" hypoactivation in contralateral thalamic and basal ganglia areas (Vuilleumier et al., 2001; see Fig. 113.7). Other studies are beginning to converge on a hypothesis that preemptor areas are overactive and not properly integrating with feedforward areas in the brain, such as the parietal lobe, that may be responsible for the sense of agency of movement. This might help to explain the apparent voluntariness of functional motor symptoms in the absence of a sense of intention on the part of the patient (Voon et al., 2010). Other studies have emphasized strengthened connectivity between limbic and motor networks. Another study found neural differences in patients feigning weakness compared with patients with actual functional weakness (Cojan et al., 2009). Somatosensory evoked potentials may be altered in functional disorders compared with feigning (Blakemore et al., 2013). In patients with dissociative (nonepileptic) seizures, some intriguing preliminary findings in interictal EEG are also emerging (Knyazeva et al., 2011). Neuroimaging and advances in neuroscience do hold out a promise of understanding symptoms in parallel neurological and psychiatric ways, with the hope of potentially being able to abandon the artificial distinction between the two.

**TABLE 113.3 Potential Etiological Factors in Patients With Functional Neurological Disorders**

| Factors | Biological | Psychological | Social |
|---|---|---|---|
| Factors acting at all stages | Recognized structural/metabolic disease | Emotional disorder | Socioeconomic deprivation |
| Predisposing | History of previous functional symptoms<br>Genetic factors affecting personality<br>Biological vulnerabilities in nervous system? | Personality disorder<br>Perception of childhood experience as adverse<br>Personality traits<br>Poor attachment/coping style | Life events and difficulties<br>Childhood neglect/abuse<br>Poor family functioning<br>Symptom modeling (via media or personal contact) |
| Precipitating | Abnormal physiological event or state (e.g., hyperventilation, drug side effect, sleep paralysis)<br>Physical injury/pain | Perception of life event as negative, unexpected<br>Acute dissociative episode/panic attack | |
| Perpetuating | Plasticity in central nervous system motor and sensory (including pain) pathways<br>Deconditioning<br>Neuroendocrine and immunological abnormalities similar to those seen in depression and anxiety | Illness beliefs (patient and family)<br>Perception of symptoms as being due to disease/damage/outside the scope of self-help<br>Not feeling believed<br>Avoidance of symptom provocation | Presence of a social welfare system<br>Social benefits of being ill<br>Availability of legal compensation<br>Stigma of "mental illness" in society and from medical profession<br>Ongoing medical investigations and uncertainty |

## INVESTIGATIONS

Investigations will usually be necessary, partly because the presence of a functional disorder does not exclude a comorbid underlying neurological disease, but it is worth considering how to perform them in the patient's best interest if results are likely to be normal. If there is any delay in tests, patients can benefit from being told the likely diagnosis and that clinical investigations will probably be normal or show only incidental or age-related findings (Petrie et al., 2007). It is especially worth anticipating the 15% risk of nondiagnostic high-signal lesions on magnetic resonance imaging (MRI) and other "incidentalomas" (Morris et al., 2009) and the presence of age-related degenerative change on spinal MRI which correlates poorly with symptoms (Brinjikji et al., 2015). An analogy with gray hair may be useful—everyone gets it, but it does not necessarily mean anything. Try to do all the necessary tests at the same time and not sequentially, which tends to prolong the agony of "diagnostic limbo". If there is a clear clinical diagnosis of functional neurological disorder, abnormalities on a scan should be seen as comorbid rather than refuting the diagnosis.

## TREATMENT

Fig. 113.9 shows a treatment algorithm for functional neurological symptoms described in more detail later.

### Explanation

The diagnosis of a functional disorder is made on the basis of positive neurological features on assessment, combined with a knowledge of the range of presentations of neurological disease, and not on the basis of psychiatric symptomatology—even though the latter may be relevant to etiology and treatment. Neurologists are therefore in a good position to explain the diagnosis of functional disorders (Stone et al., 2016). A really successful explanation can alter outcome dramatically, even with long-standing symptoms. Most authors agree that a good explanation is a prerequisite to successful treatment with physiotherapy or psychological therapy, and there is some evidence that it does affect outcome (Carton et al., 2003; Jankovic et al., 2006). How the diagnosis is explained to the patient will depend on the clinician's own views of why and how the symptoms are present; no method is suitable for all patients. Table 113.4 lists a series of components of explanation that we believe provide a constructive basis for further treatment. A successful explanation leaves patients feeling they have finally "got to the bottom" of what the problem is, with confidence that they do have something genuine, but potentially reversible with rehabilitation and determination. Even in those who do not improve, there is value in the peace of mind brought by a clear diagnosis. In our own practice, showing patients their positive signs, such as the Hoover sign or the tremor entrainment test, is the most transparent and effective way of explaining that this is not a diagnosis of exclusion, but one in which the physical signs indicate the potentially reversible nature of the problem (Stone and Edwards, 2012).

The issue of whether one tells the patient he or she has psychogenic symptoms, conversion disorder, functional symptoms, or dissociative symptoms—terminology discussed at the beginning of this chapter—is only one of these components and is not as important as the totality of the explanation. A psychological explanation has the advantage of being clear-cut, compatible with psychiatric referral, and consistent with psychiatric terminology. Unfortunately, words such as *psychogenic* are commonly interpreted by a patient as meaning "crazy" or "making symptoms up." Studies in primary care attempting to help patients reattribute their functional symptoms psychologically have not been successful (Gask et al., 2011). *Functional* is a more acceptable term (Edwards et al., 2014), which, along with *dissociative*, describes a mechanism and leaves the etiology more open. These terms have the advantage of allowing a more integrated description involving biological, psychological, and social factors as stressors on neural function and facilitating treatment aimed at restoring nervous system function. The common criticism is that they are too broad and open to confusion (Fahn and Olanow, 2014). One option is to use a functional explanation by default and introduce discussion of psychological factors later if relevant or necessary. Even an unspoken suspicion that most patients with functional symptoms are feigning will likely be picked up on, regardless of what is said out loud.

There are many barriers to a successful explanation other than the words used. Patients with functional disorder have often gone through a phase themselves of wondering "Is it me?" because of the variability of the symptoms but, in contrast, also experience feelings of being out

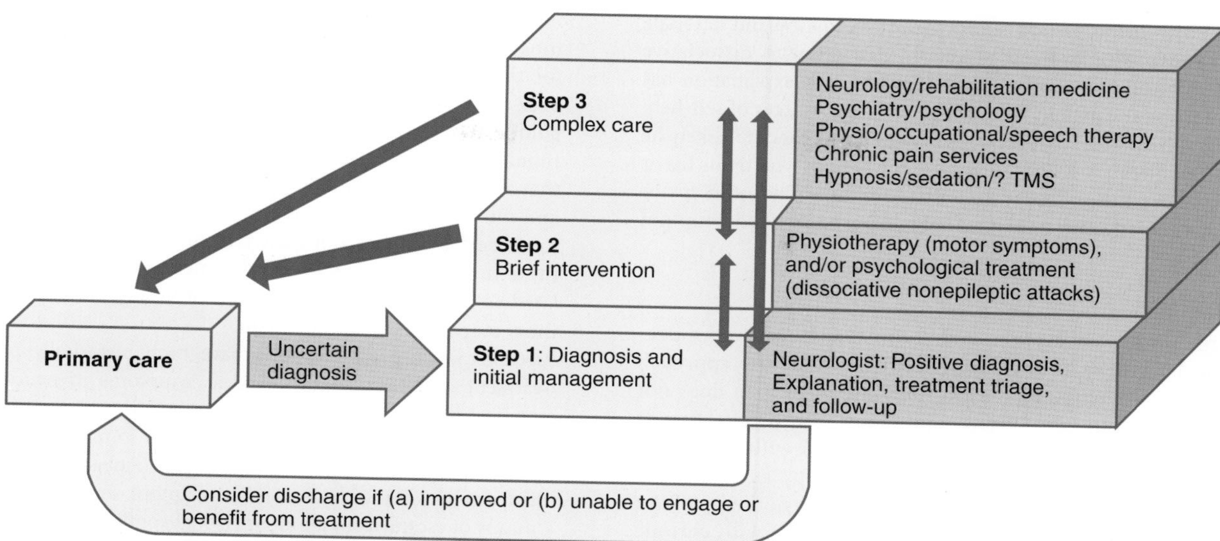


**Fig. 113.9 A Treatment Algorithm for Functional Neurological Symptoms.** Note that the neurologist has a role not just in diagnosis but in initial explanation and triaging further treatment. Patients who cannot engage with the diagnosis often do not benefit from attempts at further treatment. *TMS,* Transcranial magnetic stimulation. *(Adapted with permission from Health Improvement Scotland [2012]). (2012).)*

**TABLE 113.4 Ingredients of a Successful Explanation for Functional Symptoms/Disorders**

| Ingredient | Example |
|---|---|
| Explain what they *do* have. | "You have a functional movement disorder."<br>"You have dissociative attacks." |
| Emphasize the mechanism of the symptoms rather than the cause. | Weakness: "Your nervous system is not damaged, but it is not functioning properly."<br>Attacks: "You are going into a trancelike state, a bit like someone being hypnotized." |
| Explain how you made the diagnosis. | Show the patient their Hoover sign, tremor entrainment, or dissociative attack video, explaining why it is typical of the diagnosis you are making. |
| Indicate that you believe them. | "I do not think you are imagining/making up your symptoms/going crazy." |
| Emphasize that it is common. | "I see lots of patients with similar problems." |
| Emphasize reversibility. | "The physical signs are showing us that you have the potential to get better." |
| Emphasize that self-help is a key part of getting better. | "This is not your fault, but there are things you can do to help it get better." |
| Metaphors may be useful. | "The hardware is alright, but there's a software problem."<br>"It's like a car/piano that's out of tune." |
| Explain what they *don't* have and why. | "You do not have multiple sclerosis (epilepsy, etc.)." |
| Introduce the role of depression/anxiety. | "If you have been feeling low/worried, that will tend to make the symptoms even worse" (often easier to achieve on a second visit). |
| Use written information. | Send the patient their clinic letter; give them a website address (e.g., http://www.neurosymptoms.org, http://www.nonepilepticattacks.info). |
| Stop the antiepileptic drug in dissociative seizures. | If you have diagnosed dissociative attacks and not epilepsy, stop the anticonvulsant; leaving the patient on the drug will hamper recovery. |
| Make the psychiatric referral when appropriate. | "Dr. X has a lot of experience and interest in helping people like you to manage and overcome these kinds of symptoms." |
| Involve the family/friends. | Explain it all to them as well. |

of control. They can therefore be particularly sensitive to a diagnosis that suggests that they are doing it on purpose or in control. Even when they are comfortable with the diagnosis of a functional disorder, this is a hard thing to explain to friends, family, and employers. Neurologists for their part are often unsure what to think about this area of their practice and may prefer to dodge the whole issue by only explaining that there is no neurological disease (Friedman and LaFrance, 2010). Patient frustration is the inevitable upshot; they want to know what is wrong with them, and not just what is not.

## Further Neurological Treatment

Traditionally, many neurologists have ceased their involvement after the diagnosis, handing care back to the family doctor or referring on to a psychiatrist. However, neurologists can play an important role, with a second or further visit to reinforce the explanation and rationale for the diagnosis, stop anticonvulsants in patients with dissociative attacks, and consider onward referral. If a thorough explanation has been offered, and the patient has been given some sources of self-help yet returns with no idea what his or her diagnosis is, then it is likely he or she will be difficult to help. Conversely, the patient who trusts his or her clinician's expertise will start to understand how physiotherapy or psychological therapy may be helpful in breaking established symptom patterns.

## Physiotherapy

For a patient with a symptom such as weakness, gait, or movement disorder, there is increasing evidence that an approach which focuses on changing physical function and which does not necessarily have to involve a "talking therapy" can be effective. It is currently our practice to refer eligible patients with functional weakness or movement disorder for physiotherapy as a first-line treatment. Two randomized controlled trial of physiotherapy have shown benefit sustained for 6–12 months in patients with chronic functional motor symptoms; (Jordbru et al., 2014; Nielsen et al., 2017). Physiotherapy for patients with functional disorders does have specific features compared with those used in other neurological disorders. For example, if someone has limb weakness, rather than paying a lot of attention to the weak limb, as after a stroke, it may be helpful to use distraction techniques during movement to allow better movement. In someone with a functional tremor, asking the patient to make a voluntary large amplitude movement on top of their tremor and then to reduce the amplitude may allow them to gain control of an involuntary tremor. Principles of graded exercise as used in CFS are also likely to be helpful. As with back pain, the patient should be told to expect relapses as they increase activity. Mental imagery techniques and mirror therapy as used in CRPS may also be useful (Nielsen et al., 2013). Consensus open access recommendations for physiotherapy for functional motor disorders are currently available (Nielsen et al., 2015).

## Psychological Treatment

Because up to one-third of all neurology outpatients have functional symptoms to some degree, it is unlikely they could all have specialist psychological treatment, nor do they all need it. Patients with mild symptoms may just need to be steered in the right direction, given sensible information, and they will do the rest themselves. Patients who are struggling with disabling symptoms are likely to benefit from further treatment. Randomized controlled trials have shown benefit of CBT in dissociative (nonepileptic) attacks (Goldstein et al., 2010; LaFrance et al., 2014), a wider range of functional symptoms (Sharpe et al., 2011), and in somatization disorder (Allen and Woolfolk, 2010). Other uncontrolled studies have shown similar treatment effects for more broad-based psychotherapy in a range of functional neurological symptoms (Reuber et al., 2007). But what does (and can) a psychiatrist/psychologist actually do with patients with functional symptoms?

- *Further explanation.* A psychiatrist or psychologist must be familiar with the area and able to give the same kind of explanation the patient has received from the neurologist. This in itself may take some time.
- Detection and treatment of comorbid psychiatric problems such as anxiety, depression, posttraumatic stress disorder, or obsessive-compulsive disorder.
- *CBT.* This involves developing the patient's diagnosis to change how they think about their symptoms and behave as a consequence of them (Table 113.5). It is an approach based in learning theory and aims to provide a detailed examination of the interactions between physical symptoms, thoughts, behavior, and mood. It applies a model that patients will gain immediate reward for their actions that influence future behavior; a patient with back pain may rest at the first signs of exacerbation, removing the pain in the short term but leading to long-term poorer function. Illness and other beliefs will also feature; the patient may believe that acute exacerbation of their back pain is a sign of new damage and thus strive to avoid this and become fearful of it. This can in turn result in increased muscle tension and poor posture, making the actual occurrence more likely. Such vicious circles are postulated as contributing to the genesis of functional symptoms, and the therapy aims to unpick them.
- Psychodynamic psychotherapies have been historically popular in treatment of functional neurological symptoms in neurology, but empirical support is lacking. However, there is evidence of benefit of short psychodynamic psychotherapy in other somatic symptoms such as irritable bowel syndrome and chronic pain (Abbass et al., 2009). Such therapy is based on the premise that symptom development occurs as a means of escape from an interpersonal conflict. These conflicts are seen in the context of abnormally learned patterns of interpersonal relationships during childhood, which then go on to distort social interactions in adulthood. For example, a patient who has suffered an abusive upbringing may be prone to emotional instability, anger, or passivity which determine their interpretation and response to physical sensations as well as their interactions with health professionals when seeking help for those symptoms. Therapy based on these principles includes learning to recognize these subconscious maladaptive patterns, allowing for a more socially skilled approach to interpersonal conflict resolution, and discarding a presumed psychic need to develop physical symptoms.

### Multidisciplinary Treatment

The importance of multidisciplinary treatment for functional neurological disorders is increasingly recognized, including occupational therapy (Gardiner et al., 2018) and speech and language therapy (Barnett et al., 2018) when appropriate. Studies of specialized inpatient units have shown promising results (Demartini et al., 2014; Jacob et al., 2018; McCormack et al., 2014).

## Specific Advice for Dissociative (Nonepileptic) Attacks

In addition to the approaches described, some additional helpful measures include:

- *Stop anticonvulsant drugs.* Studies have shown this is safe to do (Oto et al., 2005). Not stopping them sends a very mixed message to the patient about how confident the physician is about the diagnosis.
- *Look carefully for warning symptoms and teach distraction techniques.* As described earlier, symptoms of panic are common, although often not initially reported, in patients with dissociative (nonepileptic) attacks. Patients need help recognizing and sometimes remembering these warning symptoms and with distraction techniques to avert an attack. When they have averted just one attack or developed more awareness of shaking, this will reinforce their confidence in the diagnosis.
- *Recognize triggers for attacks.* Patients commonly report recognizing no pattern at all to their attacks. However, they may be helped to see that attacks are more likely in situations where the consequences are especially embarrassing or inconvenient, like in shops or on stairs (because they have been worrying that the attack would happen), and conversely when they are sitting quietly undistracted (when trance like symptoms are more likely to take hold). When they are highly distracted or focused on a task, they may be less likely to occur.

**TABLE 113.5 Examples of Changes in Thoughts and Behavior That Can Help Patients With Functional Neurological Disorders**

| | Dissociative Attacks | Functional Weakness | Chronic Back Pain |
|---|---|---|---|
| Old thought | "Oh no, what's happening to me? Am I going to die during one of these attacks?" | "I've got Multiple Sclerosis, I'm going to end up in a wheelchair. No one believes me." | "My spine is damaged. I must avoid moving too much in case it makes it worse." |
| New thought | "I'm having something a bit like a panic attack where I'm losing control." | "Hmm...this is odd, but it looks as if I can get better. That doctor is right. When I'm not thinking about the leg, it does seem to move better." | "My bones are fine, it's my muscles that are stiff and out of condition." |
| Old behavior | Avoid going out. Worry constantly about attacks. | Seeing lots of specialists. Not doing very much in case it makes it worse. | Avoiding exercise/back movement. |
| New behavior | Try out distraction techniques during warning symptoms. | Gradually exercise, trying not to focus on limb weakness. Learn to expect relapses. | Gradually exercise, expecting exacerbations of pain. |

### Specific Advice for Functional Motor Symptoms

In addition to the approaches described, some additional issues include:

- *Physical aids and appliances/sickness benefits.* Patients with disability from functional symptoms may ask whether they should have a wheelchair or go on to health-related financial benefits. The advice here is not really different from any other patient with a disability that may improve. Wheelchairs and sickness benefits definitely improve independence and morale in some patients but can also create a further obstacle to rehabilitation by discouraging day-to-day movement and an early return to work (Gardiner et al., 2018).
- *Hypnosis.* This treatment has a long association with functional neurological symptoms, especially suited to functional motor symptoms. Two randomized controlled trials found it to be of benefit in patients with motor symptoms (Moene et al., 2003). Patients may be able to learn self-hypnosis and other relaxation techniques.
- *Sedation.* Patients with prolonged paralysis or fixed dystonia may benefit from examination under sedation. Rather than quiz the patient (abreaction), we suggest that the patient is held just at the point of anesthesia, to demonstrate (with video) better function under sedation than during wakefulness and to "kick start" some improvement (Video 113.6; Stone et al., 2014). A secondary function of the procedure is to look for evidence of contractures in patients with fixed dystonia. We find that it is important for the patient to be given physiotherapy immediately afterwards if they have made some improvement during the procedure.
- *Transcranial magnetic stimulation* (TMS). Promising results using TMS in acute functional motor disorders (where improvement may have occurred anyway) (Chastan and Parain, 2010) and chronic patients (Garcin et al., 2013) have been placed in context by a study that showed similar benefit from spinal TMS (Garcin et al., 2017) and negative outcome studies (McWhirter et al., 2016). Most authors agree that treatment effects in existing studies are unlikely to relate to direct alteration of neural pathways. Instead TMS provides a way for a patient to see the potential reversibility of symptoms, as well as the desire of the physician to help the patient. Peripheral nerve stimulation is also associated with good anecdotal outcomes. Electrical stimulation for patients with these disorders is nothing new and has been a feature of medicine since the early 1800s (Adrian and Yealland, 1917).

### Drug Treatment

There is no good evidence to guide the use of antidepressant drugs for patients with dissociative (nonepileptic) attacks or motor and sensory symptoms. However, there is some evidence supporting the use of antidepressant drugs across a range of other functional symptoms, with the balance of evidence favoring the use of tricyclic antidepressants (Kroenke, 2007). Outcomes do not appear to be affected by the presence or absence of depressed mood. Where comorbid anxiety, depression, or panic is present, drug treatment can be discussed on its own merits. Similarly, there is a good evidence base for the use of tricyclic antidepressants in pain or insomnia in the absence of mood disorder. Patients with functional symptoms do seem to be unusually sensitive to drug side effects, possibly via nocebo mechanisms. We advise any drugs be started at a low dose and increased slowly. It can be helpful to caution patients that they may experience side effects over the first few weeks, but if they stick with it, these will often settle down.

### When Nothing Helps

Just because a patient has a functional disorder does not mean he or she should automatically get better (see the earlier section Prognosis). Neurologists should bear in mind that only one in three patients—or much less than that for symptoms such as fixed dystonia—will improve spontaneously. It is important to maintain reasonable expectations of one's therapeutic abilities in a situation where multiple powerful perpetuating factors may exist. If despite all best efforts, a patient does not really agree with or is unable to understand the diagnosis, the neurologist has perhaps done everything possible in the circumstances. Alternatively, a patient may be fully accepting of the diagnosis, but it may be too difficult for anyone to help. Patients can be told that they have done their best for the time being and that their symptoms may improve in the future, but for now the management is to learn to manage the symptoms as much as possible. The patient's primary physician has an important role in recognizing vulnerability to symptoms, treating intercurrent mood and anxiety problems, and protecting patients from unnecessary investigations and treatments in secondary care where possible.

## SUMMARY

Functional and dissociative disorders in neurology are common, disabling, and distressing. The diagnosis should be made on the basis of positive physical signs or observation of attacks, combined with a sound knowledge of neurological disease—not on psychological grounds. Neurologists are in a good position to alter the illness trajectories of many patients with a careful and rational explanation of the diagnosis and onward appropriate referral.

Sources of free self-help for patients, created by researchers, can be found online at:

- http://www.neurosymptoms.org. Self-help material for all of the symptoms described in this chapter.
- http://www.nonepilepticattacks.info. Free self-help material specifically about nonepileptic attacks.

*The complete reference list is available online at https://expertconsult.inkling.com/.*

# INDEX

Note: Page numbers followed by "*f*" indicate figures, "*t*" indicate tables, and "*b*" indicate boxes.

## B

## D

## J

## M

## P

## S

## W

## X